The 5-Minute Clinical Consult 2013

21ST EDITION

Editor-in-Chief

Frank J. Domino, MD
Professor
Pre-doctoral Education Director
Department of Family Medicine and Community Health
The University of Massachusetts Medical School
Worcester, Massachusetts

Associate Editors

Robert A. Baldor, MD
Professor
Department of Family Medicine and Community Health
The University of Massachusetts Medical School;
Vice-Chairman
Department of Family Medicine and Community Health
UMass Memorial Health Care
Worcester, Massachusetts

Jeremy Golding, MD
Professor of Family Medicine and of Obstetrics and Gynecology
The University of Massachusetts Medical School
Quality Officer—Department of Family Medicine and Community Health
UMass Memorial Health Care—Hahnemann Family Health Center
Worcester, Massachusetts

Jill A. Grimes, MD
Clinical Instructor
Department of Family Medicine
University of Massachusetts Medical School
Worcester, Massachusetts;
Private Practice
West Lake Family Practice
Austin, Texas

Julie Scott Taylor, MD, MSc
Associate Professor of Family Medicine
Director of Clinical Curriculum
Alpert Medical School of Brown University
Providence, Rhode Island

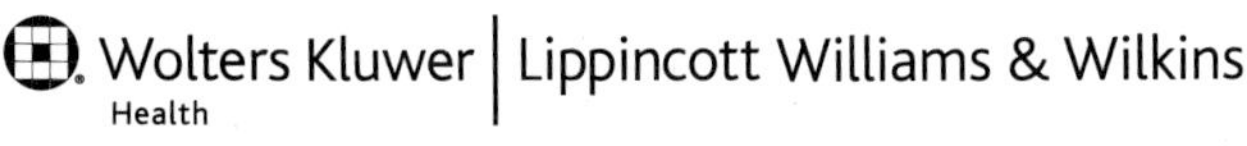

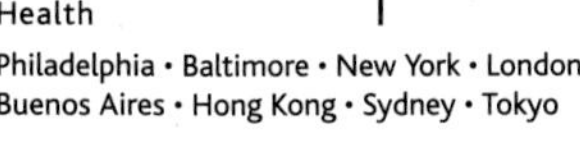

Senior Acquisitions Editor: Sonya Seigafuse
Senior Product Manager: Kerry Barrett
Vendor Manager: Bridgett Dougherty
Senior Manufacturing Manager: Benjamin Rivera
Senior Marketing Manager: Kim Schonberger
Design Coordinator: Terry Mallon
Production Service: Aptara, Inc.

Two Commerce Square
2001 Market Street
Philadelphia, PA 19103 USA
LWW.com

Printed in China

Library of Congress Cataloging-in-Publication Data

ISBN-13: 978-1-4511-3735-4
ISBN-10: 1-4511-3735-4

Care has been taken to confirm the accuracy of the information presented and to describe generally accepted practices. However, the authors, editors, and publisher are not responsible for errors or omissions or for any consequences from application of the information in this book and make no warranty, expressed or implied, with respect to the currency, completeness, or accuracy of the contents of the publication. Application of the information in a particular situation remains the professional responsibility of the practitioner.

The authors, editors, and publisher have exerted every effort to ensure that drug selection and dosage set forth in this text are in accordance with current recommendations and practice at the time of publication. However, in view of ongoing research, changes in government regulations, and the constant flow of information relating to drug therapy and drug reactions, the reader is urged to check the package insert for each drug for any change in indications and dosage and for added warnings and precautions. This is particularly important when the recommended agent is a new or infrequently employed drug.

Some drugs and medical devices presented in the publication have Food and Drug Administration (FDA) clearance for limited use in restricted research settings. It is the responsibility of the health care provider to ascertain the FDA status of each drug or device planned for use in their clinical practice.

To purchase additional copies of this book, call our customer service department at (800) 638-3030 or fax orders to (301) 223-2320. International customers should call (301) 223-2300.

Visit Lippincott Williams & Wilkins on the Internet: at LWW.com. Lippincott Williams & Wilkins customer service representatives are available from 8:30 am to 6 pm, EST.

10 9 8 7 6 5 4 3 2 1

CCS0412

In keeping with the 5-minute Clinical Consult theme, I am devoting one minute each to five different groups that deserve recognition here. In alphabetical order, just like the text.

1. To my author colleagues: *An editor's work is directly related to the quality and skill of an author. In the 5MCC enterprise, we are very fortunate to work with some of the very best authors, from a wide variety of specialties and clinical backgrounds. I have had the frequent experience of editing chapters where many of the key citations were also written by the author(s). A special thank you to senior authors who have mentored more junior authors in the chapter and algorithm writing process for helping to develop the next generation of medical writers.*

2. To my editor colleagues: *Dr. Frank Domino is a fearless leader and one of my true heroes in the field of academic family medicine. I feel very fortunate to work on one of his many successful teams. My co-editors Drs. Bob Baldor, Jeremy Golding, and Jill Grimes are a constant source of wisdom, creativity, and support, both electronically and in person. I am a better academic for being a part of this group.*

3. To my family: *My parents, my husband, and my four children think it is neat to see my name on the cover of a textbook (and I must agree). I have actually overheard Cassandra, Harrison, Amelia, and Simon Taylor debating with each other whether their mama is famous or not. And now they are famous too, since their names are in print with mine. Many thanks to my beloved extended family for their steadfast support of my late nights of editing and regular work travel. So glad you get to come on some of the trips with me.*

4. To my patients: *It is a profound honor to be a physician and to serve as your health care provider. The main reason that I am an Associate Editor is to stay up to date on the best and most current medicine. This work helps me to take the best care of you possible. I am very confident and proud this product helps other health care providers to do the same for their own patients.*

5. To my students: *The medical students at Brown University are unbelievably intelligent, talented, and service oriented. Please know you are a daily inspiration to me and the rest of your faculty. You are future leaders in clinical medicine, medical education, research, and advocacy. I look forward to working with you as colleagues in this diverse and evolving profession that is 21st-century medicine.*

–Julie Scott Taylor, MD, MSc

The 5-Minute Clinical Consult 2013

21ST EDITION

ADVISORY BOARD

PREFACE

To laugh often and much;
To win the respect of intelligent people and
The affection of children;
To earn the appreciation of honest critics and
Endure the betrayal of false friends;
To appreciate beauty,
To find the best in others;
To leave the world a bit better,
Whether by a healthy child,
A garden patch, or
A redeemed social condition;
To know even one life has breathed easier because you have lived.
This is to have succeeded.

–R. W. EMERSON

You have succeeded. Some days, should you feel the challenges of disease have won, remember, many have breathed easier because you have lived. Every single day, your presence, compassion, and care allows others to live with less worry and pain, and greater hope. We will never cure all disease, but we succeed at making every life better.

This resource provides the knowledge, but it is just one instrument in your toolbox of service. Adding to it your skill, insight, and intuition makes you a master of your craft.

I am honored to welcome you to the *2013 5-Minute Clinical Consult.* Our editorial team has again collaborated with hundreds of authors to bring you this comprehensive and current resource whose goal is to assist you and your patients.

Based on your feedback, we present this highly organized content with newly added features in print and online (5minuteconsult.com). The Standard Edition provides you with 30 day FREE access. 5minuteconsult.com provides:

- Fast, intuitive search functionality providing you with answers in <30 seconds
- Current evidence-based designations highlighted in each topic's text
- A revised and updated Health Maintenance section
- More than 900 topics
- FREE POINT of CARE CME: 1/2 hour CME Credit for every digital search
- 200+ diagnostic and treatment algorithms
- Full-color Images and Videos for procedures and treatment
- Drug database from A to Z Drugs
- More than 1,3000 patient handouts in English and Spanish

Evidence-based health care is the integration of the best medical information *with* the values of the patient and your skill as a clinician. We have updated our EBM content and its visibility, so you can focus on how to best apply.

The Health Maintenance one-page summaries have been updated through December 2011, and are based on the US Preventive Services Task Force.

The algorithm section includes both diagnostic and treatment algorithms. This easy-to-use graphic method helps you evaluate an abnormal finding and prioritize treatment.

Please view the online and mobile versions at *www.5minuteconsult.com.* Your 30 day access is **free** with book purchase, allowing you to quickly reference the 5-Minute wherever needed. Included are over 900 topics on an easy-to-use interface allowing smooth maneuverability between topics, algorithms, images, video procedures, and more as well as extra topics not in the book.

Welcome to the *2013 5-Minute Clinical Consult.* Our editorial team values your observations, so please drop me an e-mail and share your thoughts, suggestions, and constructive criticism at: 5MinConsultFeedback@lww.com.

FRANK J. DOMINO, MD
Professor
Pre-doctoral Education Director
Department of Family Medicine and Community Health
The University of Massachusetts Medical School
Worcester, Massachusetts
January 27, 2012

EVIDENCE-BASED MEDICINE

WHAT IS EVIDENCE-BASED MEDICINE AND WHY IS THIS NEW?

Remember when we used to treat every otitis media with antibiotics? These recommendations came about because we applied logical reasoning to observational studies. If bacteria cause an acute otitis media, then antibiotics should help it resolve sooner, with less morbidity. Yet, when rigorously studied (via a systematic review), we found little benefit to this intervention.

The underlying premise of evidence-based medicine (EBM) is the evaluation of medical interventions, and the literature that supports those interventions, in a systematic fashion. EBM hopes to encourage treatments proven to be effective and safe. And when insufficient data exists, it hopes to inform you, on how to safely proceed.

EBM uses as endpoints of real patient outcomes; morbidity, mortality and risk. It focuses less on intermediate outcomes (bone density), and more on patient conditions (hip fractures).

Implementing EBM *requires* 3 components: The best medical evidence, the skill and experience of the provider, and the values of the patients. Should this patient be screened for prostate cancer? It depends on what is known about the test, on what you know of its benefits and harms, your ability to communicate that information, and that patient's informed choice.

"All this in 15 minutes," you ask? This is not an easy task. My goal is to provide you with the tools to assist in this process.

This book hopes to address the first EBM component, providing you access the best information in a quick format. While not every test or treatment has this level of detail, many of the included interventions here use systematic review literature support.

The language of medical statistics is useful to interpreting the concepts of EBM. Below is a list of these terms, with examples to help take the confusion and mystery out of their use.

POPULATION INFORMATION

These terms are designed to help you and epidemiologists look at the "community" as a whole, and determine how frequently disease occurs:

Prevalence: *Proportion of people* in a population who have a disease

In the US, 0.3% (3 in 1,000) people over the age 50 have colon cancer.

Incidence: How many *new cases of a disease* occur in a population during an interval of time; for example, "the estimated incidence of colon cancer in the US is 104,000 in 2005."

TESTING INFORMATION

We often hear the words *sensitivity* and *specificity* and cringe. They are, at a minimum, very confusing. These terms are characteristics of a test, but they tell us little about the lab result we are holding in our hands. Rather, it is the *predicative value* that helps us interpret test results.

ML is a 53-year-old woman who you saw for a Health Maintenance visit; you ordered a *screening* mammogram and the report demonstrates an irregular area of microcalcifications. She is waiting in your office to receive her test results; what can you tell her?

Sensitivity (Sn): Percent of people with disease who test positive; for mammography, the sensitivity is 71–96%.

Specificity (Sp): Percent of people without disease who test negative; for mammography, the specificity is 94–97%.

Does this help in your discussion with ML? No, because these tests refer to characteristics of people who are known to have disease (sensitivity) or those that are known not to have (specificity) disease. What you have is an abnormal test result. To better explain this result to ML, you need to know the positive predictive value.

Positive predictive value (PPV): Percent of *positive* test results that are truly positive; the PPV for a woman 50–59 ~22%. Only 22% of abnormal screening mammograms in this group truly identified cancer. The other 78% are false positives.

Negative predictive value (NPV): Percent of negative test results that are truly negative.

You can tell ML only 1 out of 5 abnormal mammograms correctly identify cancer; the 4 are false positives, but the only way to know which mammogram is correct is to do further testing.

You may both find some comfort knowing the chance she has cancer is so low.

The PPV and NPV tests are population dependent, while the Sensitivity and Specificity are characteristics of the test, and have little to do with the patient in front of you. So when you receive an abnormal lab result, especially a screening test like mammography or PSA value, understand their limits based on their PPV and NPV.

TREATMENT INFORMATION

In discerning the statistics of randomized, controlled trials of interventions, first consider an example. The Scandinavian Simvastatin Survival Study (4S) (*Lancet.* 1994;344[8934]:1383–9) found using simvastatin in patients at high risk for heart disease for 5 years resulted in deaths in 8% of patients vs. 12% of those on placebo; this results in a relative risk of 0.70, a relative risk reduction (RRR) of 33%, and a number needed to treat of 25.

There are two ways of considering the benefits of an intervention with respect to a given outcome. The absolute risk reduction (ARR) is the difference in the percent of people with the condition before and after the intervention. Thus, if the incidence of MI was 12% for the placebo group and 8% for the simvastatin group, the ARR is 4% (12% − 8% = 4%).

The RRR reflects the improvement in the outcome as a percentage of the original rate and is commonly used to exaggerate the benefit of an intervention. Thus, if the risk of MI were reduced by simvastatin from 12% to 8%, then the RRR would be 33%

(4%/12% = 33%). 33% may appear better than 4%, the 4% that reflects the true outcome.

ARR is usually a better measure of *clinical* significance of an intervention. For instance, in one study, the treatment of mild hypertension was been shown to have a RRR of 40% over 5 years (40% fewer strokes in the treated group). However, the ARR was only 1.3%. Because mild hypertension is not strongly associated with strokes, aggressive treatment of mild hypertension yields only a small clinical benefit. Don't confuse Relative Risk Reduction with Relative Risk.

Absolute (or attributable) risk (AR): The percent of people in the placebo or intervention group who reach an end point; in the simvastatin study, the absolute risk of death was 8%.

Relative risk (RR): The risk of disease of those treated or exposed to some intervention (i.e., simvastatin) divided by those in the placebo group or who were untreated.

–If RR < 1.0, it reduces risk–the smaller the number, the greater the risk reduction.

–If RR > 1.0, it increases the risk–the greater the number, the greater the risk increase.

Relative risk reduction (RRR): The relative decrease in risk of an end point compared to the percent of that endpoint in the placebo group.

If you are still confused, just remember the RRR is an overestimation of the actual effect.

Number needed to treat (NNT): This is the number of people who need to be treated by an intervention to prevent one adverse outcome. A "good" NNT can be a large number (>100) if risk of serious outcome is great. If the risk of an outcome is not that dangerous, then lower (<25) NNTs are preferred.

The NNT should be compared to a similar statistic, the Number Needed to Harm (NNH). This is the number of people who have to be given treatment before one excess side effect or harm occurs. When the NNT is compared to the NNH, you and the patient can judge whether the benefit of the intervention is great enough to outweigh the risk of harm.

REFERENCES

To help you interpret diagnostic and treatment recommendations within the *5-Minute Clinical Consult*, we have graded the best information within the text, and highlighted this content.

An "A" grade means the reference is from the highest-quality resource, like a systematic review. A *systematic review* is a summary of the medical literature on a given topic that uses strict, explicit methods to perform a thorough search of the literature and then provides a critical appraisal of individual studies, concluding in a recommendation. The most prestigious collection of systematic reviews is from the Cochrane Collaboration (www.cochrane.org).

A "B" grade means the data referenced comes from high-quality randomized controlled trials performed to minimize bias in their outcome. Bias is anything that interferes with the truth; in the medical literature, it is often unintentional, but it is much more common than we appreciate. In short, always assume some degree of bias exists in any research endeavor.

A "C" grade implies the reference used does not meet the A or B requirements; they are often treatments recommended by consensus groups (like the American Cancer Society). In some cases, they may be the standards of care. But implicit in a group's recommendation is the bias of the author or the group that supports the reference. For example, the American Urological Society's recommendation around screening for prostate cancer may be motivated by their need for funding rather than patient outcomes. Compare this to the highly valid recommendations of the US Preventive Services Task Force (www.ahrq.gov), the organization that determines which health maintenance interventions are reasonable, and does so with the least bias.

BIAS

Bias is anything interferes with the truth. There are many types of bias that should be considered by the publishers of medical information. Below describes a number of bias types that often affect our care without us knowing it is present:

Publication bias occurs when research is not published; this is often when a study finds data that does *not* support an intervention. The motivation to publish information that "didn't work" is low. It is estimated that up to 40% of all medical research never gets published. So when you read of an intervention that "works," wonder if other studies were done that didn't show benefit and went unpublished.

Comparator bias occurs when research compares an intervention to placebo, when placebo isn't the standard of care. Knowing a new antibiotic is more effective than placebo for treating acute otitis media is not helpful if you typically use amoxicillin.

Why not release research comparing the new drug to the standard of care? Often, the research has been done, and the new drug proved no better. If this study does not get published, you have an example of publication bias.

Selection bias involves either using a tool that doesn't discriminate between populations selected or just reporting a just subset of study participants from a study. Either will result in the data being skewed because it can only be applied to small subset of people.

Attrition bias and the concept of intention to treat. Attrition bias is when researchers do not fully acknowledge and address how a study deals with participants who do not adhere to the research protocol or drop out completely. Intention to treat analysis hopes to diminish attrition bias by statistically considering the nonadhering or dropped out patients as unsuccessfully benefiting from the intervention.

Commercial (funder) bias involves who paid for the research being done, and do they have a vested interest in the outcome. Despite its size and scope, the recent *Jupiter* trial on treating low-risk adults with a statin has been called into question, as the company who funded the study makes the brand name drug used in the study and the lead author is part owner of the unique test employed in the trial. The data may be accurate, but until this is studied by less vested interests, some feel its outcome cannot be clinically applied.

When I was in medical school, they didn't teach us about systematic reviews, meta-analysis or forest plots. These new terms are appearing more than ever in the medical press, and they are a huge benefit to making the world of the medical literature pertinent to our practice.

Have you been annoyed how one week you learn of a randomized controlled trial that supports a treatment, to be followed the next week with a contradictory article? Statisticians have figured out how to resolve this using something called a systematic review.

Systematic reviews take all the literature on a topic, say using antibiotics to treat otitis media, and combines the data to determine if the sum of all the trials tells a different story than any single trial. The large number of participants in this type of research results in a much more statistically (and clinically) significant conclusion than any single paper. Want more? Check this out: http://musculoskeletal.cochrane.org/what-systematic-review.

A **meta-analysis** is a quantitative systematic review, and demonstrates it outcomes in the form of a forest plot. The bottom line with interpretation of a forest plot is look for the diamond on the bottom. If it is to LEFT of the vertical line, it means risk of an outcome was reduced by the intervention. If it is fully to the RIGHT, then risk of that outcome was increased. And if the diamond touches the vertical line, it means there was no statistical influence of the intervention on the outcome. To understand these concepts better, here is a great resource: http://www.cochrane-net.org/openlearning/html/mod3-2.htm.

Lastly, on the www.5minutemedicine.com Web site, we will soon be adding **comparative effectiveness reviews.** There are wonderful provider- and patient-derived tools to help you choose what treatment to select when you have a multiple options. The US Agency for Health Care Research and Quality have done us this favor; to learn more, check out: http://effectivehealthcare.ahrq.gov/index.cfm/what-is-comparative-effectiveness-research1/.

I hope this brief introduction to EBM has been informative, clear, and helpful. If any of the information above seems unclear, or if you have a question, please drop me an e-mail at 5MinConsultFeedback@lww.com

ACKNOWLEDGMENTS

This is the 21st edition of the *5-Minute Clinical Consult*, a comprehensive point of care tool to assist in the care of patients. From beginning to end, one cannot find a more current and easy to use collection of clinically useful content.

Developing and maintaining a book and Web site of this magnitude requires an equally broad effort from its supporting team. I wish to thank the dedication and tireless efforts of the team: Point-of-Care Editor, Sonya Seigafuse; Senior Product Manager, Kerry Barrett; Kim Schonberger, Senior Marketing Manager; and Lisa McAllister, Director, Electronic Product Strategy. And for their years of support, vision and friendship, thanks to Ave McCracken and Michelle LaPlante. They have given of themselves far beyond their call of duty, and I am deeply indebted to their effort. For the vision of making the 5-Minute the leading resource in health care around the world, my sincerest thanks to Diane Harnish.

This 2013 edition is the direct result of the dedication and insights of our Associate Editors. I wish to thank Drs. Robert Baldor, Jeremy Golding, Jill Grimes, and Julie Scott Taylor for their insights, hard work, and overwhelming commitment to the *5-Minute Clinical Consult*. And our Editorial Team wishes well to Dr. Taylor, who leaves our ranks as Associate Editor. Your insights and perspective will be sorely missed.

I wish to especially thank my wife, Sylvia, and my daughter, Molly, who have given greatly for this book.

The challenge of completing a book covering this broad a spectrum of medicine requires insights and skills far beyond my own.

Many thanks to my mentors Bob Baldor and Mark Quirk who are an enormous support—always there to encourage, reassure, and impart wisdom.

Many in the academic and health care worlds are due thanks for support, insight, and friendship: Daniel Lasser, Alan Chuman, Michele Pugnaire, Karen Rayla, Isabel Feliciano, Phil Fournier, Erik Garcia, Jeff Stovall, Jim Comes, Len Levin, Judy Norberg, J. Herb Stevenson, Mick Godkin, Susanna Guzman, Michael Kidd, Zainab Nawab, Sanjiv Chopra, Susan Gauquier, Vasilios (Bill) Chrisostomidis, James (Jay) Broadhurst, Danuta Antkowiak, Atreyi Chakrabarti, Kerry Morse, Mark Powicki, Steve Messineo, and the faculty and students of the University of Massachusetts Medical School.

Medicine is a challenge I have fortunately not had to meet alone. Thanks to my parents, Frank and Angela (Jean); my brother John and his family, Marylou, Cate, and Jane; Frank, Mary Anne, Diane, and David Christian; the Diana and Hymie Lipschitz family; and the Bob and Ruth Pabreza family; they are responsible for who I am and my success in life.

I am blessed with the best of friends; without them, I would not be a physician. Thanks to Bob Bacic, Ron Jautz, Richard Onorato, John Horcher, Auguste Turnier, Bob Smith, Paul Saivetz, Antoinette and (Gary) Francis, Bob and Nancy Gallinaro, Drew and Jill Grimes, Louay Toma, Laurie, Alan, Daniel, Jenny and Matt Bugos, Alan Ehrlich, Teri and Andy Jennings, Bill Demianiuk, Mark Steenbergen, John and Kathleen Polanowicz, Phil and Carol Pettine, Mark Shelton, Steve Bennett, Vicki Triolo, Michael Bernatchez, and yes, still Milo.

—Frank J. Domino, MD

CONTRIBUTING AUTHORS

Dawn Abbott, MD
Assistant Professor of Medicine
Brown Medical School
Division of Cardiology
Rhode Island Hospital
Providence, Rhode Island

Lindsay Abcunas, MD
Resident
Obstetrics and Gynecology
University of Massachusetts Medical School
Worcester, Massachusetts

CPT Alain Michael P. Abellada, MD
PGY-1, Family Medicine Residency
Carl R. Darnall Army Medical Center
Fort Hood, Texas

Humaira Abid, MD
Resident
Department of Family and Community Medicine
University of Texas Health Science Center
San Antonio, Texas

George M. Abraham, MD, MPH
Associate Professor
Department of Medicine
University of Massachusetts Medical School
Associate Program Director
Department of Internal Medicine
Saint Vincent Hospital
Worcester, Massachusetts

Luis K. Abrishamian, MD
Department of Emergency Medicine
Los Angeles County and University of Southern California Hospital
Los Angeles, California

Ali R. Abtahi, DO
The Lake Erie College of Osteopathic Medicine
Erie, Pennsylvania

Abdulrazak Abyad, MD, PhD, MBA, MPH, AGSF, AFCHSE
Director, Abyad Medical Center and Middle East Longevity Institute
Dean, Multi Media Medical University
Chairman, Middle-East Academy for Medicine of Aging
President, Middle-East Association on Age and Alzheimer's
Coordinator, Middle-East Primary Care Research Network and Middle-East Network on Aging
Editor, Middle-East Journals of Family Medicine, Age & Aging, Psychiatry and Alzheimer's, and Nursing
Associate Editor, Middle-East Journal of Internal Medicine
Tripoli, Lebanon

William B. Adams, MD
Associate Professor of Medicine (Dermatology)
University of Louisville School of Medicine
Louisville, Kentucky

Nitin Aggarwal, MD
Warren Alpert Medical School of Brown University
Providence, Rhode Island

Maria I. Aguilar, MD
Assistant Professor of Neurology
Department of Neurology, Vascular Neurology
Mayo Clinic College of Medicine
Consultant, Department of Neurology
Mayo Clinic Hospital
Phoenix, Arizona

Francisco Aguirre, MD
Department of Obstetrics/Gynecology
Johns Hopkins Hospital
Baltimore, Maryland

Yasir Ahmed, MD
Department of Ophthalmology
Alpert Medical School of Brown University
Providence, Rhode Island

Eyad Akrad, MD
Medical Resident
Department of Internal Medicine
St. Elizabeth Health Center
Youngstown, Ohio

Mushreq Alani, MD
Trauma and Critical Care Fellow
Trauma Surgery Section
Hamad General Hospital
Doha, Qatar

Mazen Albeldawi, MD
Fellow
Department of Gastroenterology and Hepatology
Cleveland Clinic
Cleveland, Ohio

Kelly J. Alberda, MD
Assistant Clinical Professor
Department of Family Medicine
University of Texas Southwestern Austin Family Medicine Residency
Blackstock Family Health Center
Austin, Texas

Howard Alfred, MD
Clinical Associate Professor of Medicine
Department of Internal Medicine
Division of Nephrology
University of Massachusetts Medical School
University of Massachusetts Memorial Health Care
Worcester, Massachusetts

Fozia A. Ali, MD
Assistant Clinical Professor
Department of Family and Community Medicine
University of Texas Health Science Center, San Antonio
University Hospital
San Antonio, Texas

Sridevi Alla, MD
University of Mississippi Medical Center
Department of Family Medicine
Jackson, Mississippi

Satya B. Allaparthi, MRCS, MD
Fellow, Robotic Laparoscopic Urology
University of Massachusetts Medical School
St. Vincent's Hospital
Worcester, Massachusetts

Andrew Allegretti, MD
Department of Internal Medicine
Harvard Medical School
Massachusetts General Hospital
Boston, Massachusetts

Richard W. Allinson, MD
Associate Professor
Department of Ophthalmology
The Texas A&M University System, Health Sciences Center
College Station, Texas
Senior Staff Physician
Department of Ophthalmology
Scott & White Clinic
Waco, Texas

Ziad Alnabki, MD
Resident Physician
Internal Medicine
University of Louisville
Louisville, Kentucky

Brian Alverson, MD
Assistant Professor
Department of Pediatrics
Warren Alpert School of Medicine
Brown University
Head of Pediatric Hospitalist Section
Department of Pediatrics
Rhode Island Hospital
Providence, Rhode Island

Kinjal Amin, PharmD
Adjunct Assistant Professor
Massachusetts College of Pharmacy and Health Sciences
Post-doctoral Global Patient Safety and Risk Management Fellow
Genzyme
Worcester, Massachusetts

Jeffrey Scott Anderson, MD
Inpatient and Consultation Psychiatrist
Department of Psychiatry
Veteran Affairs Medical Center—Nashville Campus
Nashville, Tennessee

Julia K. Anderson, MD
Department of Dermatology
University of Connecticut
Farmington, Connecticut

David Anthony, MD, MSc
Assistant Professor of Family Medicine
Warren Alpert Medical School of Brown University
Pawtucket, Rhode Island

Armin Arasheben, MD
Department of Family Medicine
State University of New York Upstate Medical Center
Department of Medical Education
St. Joseph's Hospital
Syracuse, New York

Ivan Augusto Arenas, MD, PhD
Department of Internal Medicine
Framingham Union Hospital
MetroWest Medical Center
Framingham, Massachusetts

Paul Arguin, MD
Medical Epidemiologist
Centers for Disease Control and Prevention
Atlanta, Georgia

James J. Arnold, DO
Family Medicine Faculty Physician
Assistant Program Director
Department of Family Medicine
David Grant (USAF) Medical Center
Travis Air Force Base, California

Patricia K. Aronson, MD
Assistant Professor
Generalist Division
Department of Obstetrics and Gynecology
University of Massachusetts Memorial Medical Center
Worcester, Massachusetts

James Arrighi, MD
Associate Professor of Medicine and Diagnostic Imaging
Program Director, Cardiology Fellowship
Warren Alpert Medical School of Brown University
Director, Nuclear Cardiology
Rhode Island Hospital
Providence, Rhode Island

Asma Ashraf, MBBS, BSC
Family Medicine Resident
Department of Family Medicine
Parkland Health and Hospital System
Dallas, Texas

Atena Asiaii, MD, MPH
Harvard School of Public Health
Boston, Massachusetts
Alpert Medical School of Brown University
Providence, Rhode Island

Cheryl Atherley-Todd, MD
Assistant Professor
Family Medicine
Nova Southeastern University College of Osteopathic Medicine
Fort Lauderdale-Davie, Florida

Gerard P. Aurigemma, MD
Professor
Department of Cardiology
University of Massachusetts Medical School
Director, Noninvasive Cardiology
Department of Cardiology
University of Massachusetts Medical Center
Worcester, Massachusetts

Swati B. Avashia, MD
Clinical Assistant Professor
Internal Medicine and Pediatrics
Department of Family Medicine
University of Texas Southwestern
Austin, Texas

Nelson Aweh, MD, MBBS, EdM
MetroWest Medical Center
Cambridge, Massachusetts

Jennifer L. Ayres, PhD
Clinical Psychologist
University of Texas Southwestern Medical Center Austin
Austin, Texas

Stephen J. Bacak, DO, MPH
Resident Physician
Department of Obstetrics and Gynecology
Akron General Medical Center
Akron, Ohio

Elisabeth L. Backer, MD
Clinical Associate Professor
Department of Family Medicine
University of Nebraska Medical Center
Omaha, Nebraska

Yolanda Backus, MD
Family Practice
Rockville, Maryland

Melissa Badowski, PharmD, BCPS, AAHIVE
Clinical Assistant Professor, HIV/ID
Section of Infectious Diseases
University of Illinois at Chicago
Chicago, Illinois

Drew C. Baird, MD
Associate Faculty
Uniformed Services University of Health Sciences
Bethesda, Maryland
Faculty
Family Medicine Residency Program
Carl R. Darnall Army Medical Center
Fort Hood, Texas

Sangeetha Balasubramanian, MD
Fellow
Department of Rheumatology
University of Massachusetts Medical School
Worcester, Massachusetts

Robert A. Baldor, MD
Professor
Family Medicine and Community Health
University of Massachusetts Medical School
Vice-Chairman
Family Medicine and Community Health
University of Massachusetts Memorial Health Care
Worcester, Massachusetts

Jerry Balikian, MD
Professor
Departments of Medicine and Radiology
University of Massachusetts Medical School
Worcester, Massachusetts

Vincenzo A. Barbato, DO
Department of Internal Medicine
Palmetto General Hospital
Hialeah, Florida

Brent J. Barber, MD
Assistant Professor of Clinical Pediatrics (Cardiology)
Director, UMC Pediatric Cardiac Services
University of Arizona College of Medicine
Tucson, Arizona

Katharine Barnard, MD
Assistant Professor
Department of Family Medicine
University of Massachusetts Medical School
Medical Director
Plumley Village Health Services
University of Massachusetts Memorial Medical Center
Worcester, Massachusetts

Timothy J. Barreiro, DO, FCCP, FACOI
Associate Professor of Pulmonary and Critical Care Medicine
Department of Medicine
Ohio University Heritage College of Medicine
Northeast Ohio Medical University
Director, Pulmonary Health and Research Center
St. Elizabeth Hospital
Youngstown, Ohio

Michael C. Barros, PharmD, BCPS
Clinical Assistant Professor of Pharmacy Practice
Temple University School of Pharmacy
Clinical Pharmacist, Heart Failure/Heart Transplant
Temple University Hospital
Philadelphia, Pennsylvania

Adam Barta, MD
Assistant Professor
Department of Family Medicine
University of Texas Southwestern, Austin
Austin, Texas

Ashutosh Barve, MD, PhD
Assistant Professor of Medicine
Division of Gastroenterology, Hepatology and Nutrition
Department of Medicine
University of Louisville
Louisville, Kentucky

Kay A. Bauman, MD, MPH
Professor
Department of Family and Community Medicine
University of New Mexico School of Medicine
Albuquerque, New Mexico

Dennis J. Baumgardner, MD
Professor of Family Medicine
University of Wisconsin School of Medicine and Public Health
Director of Campus Research,
Aurora UW Medical Group
Associate Director for Health Services Initiatives,
Center for Urban Population Health
Madison, Wisconsin

Chad Beattie, MD
Fellow
Primary Care Sports Medicine
University of Massachusetts Memorial Medical School
Worcester, Massachusetts

Francesca L. Beaudoin, MS, MD
Assistant Professor
Department of Emergency Medicine
Warren Alpert Medical School of Brown University
Attending Physician
Department of Emergency Medicine
Rhode Island Hospital
Providence, Rhode Island

Armando Bedoya, MD
Department of Internal Medicine
Duke University
Durham, North Carolina

Charlene Beer, RN, BSN
Department of Orthopaedics
University of Texas Southwestern
Dallas, Texas

Paul Belliveau, PharmD, RPh
Associate Professor of Pharmacy Practice
Massachusetts College of Pharmacy and Health Sciences
Worcester, Massachusetts
Clinical Pharmacist
Pharmacy
Concord Hospital
Concord, New Hampshire

Kara Keating Bench, MD, MPH
University of Massachusetts Medical School
Worcester, Massachusetts

Paul Beninger, MD
VP Global Patient Safety
Division of Infectious Disease
Genzyme—A Sanofi Company
Cambridge, Massachusetts

Kelly Bennett, MD
Assistant Professor
Department of Family and Community Medicine
Texas Tech University Health Science Center
Lubbock, Texas

Terrell Benold, MD
Clinical Assistant Professor
Department of Family Medicine
University of Texas Southwestern Medical School, Austin Programs
Austin, Texas

Andrew Bentley, MS
Clinical Herbalist
Private Practice
Center for Wellness Therapies
Lexington, Kentucky

Lionel Bercovitch, MD
Clinical Professor of Dermatology
Warren Alpert Medical School of Brown University
Department of Pediatric Dermatology
Hasbro Children's Hospital
Warren Alpert Medical School of Brown University
Providence, Rhode Island

Jamie Berkes, MD
Medical Director of Liver Transplant
Transplant Hepatology Fellowship
Program Director
Hepatology
University of Illinois at Chicago Medical Center
Chicago, Illinois

Bryan G. Beutel, MD
Physician
Department of Orthopaedic Surgery
NYU Hospital for Joint Diseases
New York, New York

Neela Bhajandas, PharmD
Clinical Assistant Professor of Pharmacy
Department of Pulmonary and Critical Care
Temple University School of Pharmacy
Philadelphia, Pennsylvania

Grace Bhak, MD
Warren Alpert Medical School of Brown University
Providence, Rhode Island

David Bick, MD
Department of Otolaryngology
Tufts Medical Center
Boston, Massachusetts

Kenneth M. Bielak, MD
Associate Professor
Department of Family and Sports Medicine
University of Tennessee Graduate School of Medicine
Knoxville, Tennessee

Cheryl Bilinski, MD, MPH
Department of Medicine
University of Connecticut School of Medicine
Farmington, Connecticut

Melissa Phillips Black, MD
Assistant Professor
Internal Medicine, Geriatrics Division
Emory University School of Medicine
Atlanta, Georgia

Robert M. Black, MD
Clinical Professor of Medicine
Department of Renal Medicine
UMass Medical School
Chief, Division of Renal Medicine
St. Vincent Hospital and Fallon Clinic
Worcester, Massachusetts

Timothy L. Black, MD
Pediatric Surgeon
Department of Pediatric Surgery
Cook Children's Medical Center
Fort Worth, Texas

Joceyln F. Blackwell, MD, MAJ, MC
Core Faculty
Family Medicine Residency Program
Carl R. Darnall Army Medical Center
Fort Hood, Texas

Lewis S. Blevins, Jr, MD
Medical Director
Neuroendocrinology
California Center for Pituitary Disorders at UCSF
Professor of Neurological Surgery and Medicine
University of California, San Francisco
San Francisco, California

Rebecca Blumhofer, MD, MPH
Department of Family Medicine
University of Massachusetts
Barre Family Health Center
Worcester, Massachusetts

Kimberly Bombaci, MD
University of Massachusetts Medical School
Worcester, Massachusetts

Bryan C. Bordeaux, DO, MPH
Department of Population Medicine
Harvard Medical School
Department of Internal Medicine
Harvard Vanguard Medical Associates
Boston, Massachusetts

Marie L. Borum, MD, EdD, MPH
Director, Division of Gastroenterology and Liver Diseases
The George Washington University Medical Center
Director of the Gastroenterology Fellowship
Associate Professor of Public Health
The George Washington University School of Public Health and Health Services
Washington, District of Columbia

Naomi F. Botkin, MD
Assistant Professor
Division of Cardiovascular Medicine
University of Massachusetts Medical School and Memorial Center
Worcester, Massachusetts

Caleb Bowers, MD
Family Practitioner
Wichita, Kansas

Captain Michael R. Brackman, DO
Department of Family Medicine
Carl R. Darnall Army Medical Center
Fort Hood, Texas

Marri K. Brackman, DO
Family Practice
Temple, Texas

Erica Braverman, MSIV
Warren Alpert Medical School of Brown University
Providence, Rhode Island

Doreen Brettler, MD
Department of Hematology/Oncology
University of Massachusetts Medical School
Worcester, Massachusetts

Renata Brindise, DO
Family Practice
Garden City, Michigan

Amy Brodsky, MD
Department of Dermatology
University of Chicago
Brodsky Dermatology
Glenview, Illinois

Benjamin P. Brown, MD
Warren Alpert Medical School of Brown University
Providence, Rhode Island

Theodore R. Brown, DO, MPH
Departments of Family, Preventive, and Occupational and Environmental Medicine
Command and General Staff College
Ft. Leavenworth, Kansas

Karen R. Browning, BSc
Warren Alpert Medical School of Brown University
Providence, Rhode Island

Brenna Brucker, MSIV
Warren Alpert Medical School of Brown University
Providence, Rhode Island

William J. Brucker, MD
Warren Alpert Medical School of Brown University
Providence, Rhode Island

Andrew M. Brunner, MD
Clinical Fellow
Department of Medicine
Harvard Medical School
Boston, Massachusetts
Department of Internal Medicine
Massachusetts General Hospital
Boston, Massachusetts

Patricio Bruno, DO
Assistant Professor
Director of Inpatient Services
Department of Family Medicine
University of Connecticut School of Medicine
Saint Francis Hospital and Medical Center
Hartford, Connecticut

Karen Bryant, MD
Hospitalist Program
Concord Hospital
Concord, New Hampshire

Karen Buch, MD
Medical Resident
Department of Internal Medicine
St. Vincent's Hospital
Worcester, Massachusetts

Stephanie Burger, DO
Lake Erie College of Osteopathic Medicine
Erie, Pennsylvania

K. John Burhan, MD
Faculty
Department of Family Medicine
Creighton University School of Medicine
Omaha, Nebraska

John R. Burk, MD
Adjunct Professor
Integrative Physiology
University of North Texas Health Science Center
Owner/Partner
Texas Pulmonary and Critical Care Consultants, PA
Fort Worth, Texas

Kristin Burke, MD
University of Massachusetts Medical School
Worcester, Massachusetts

Susanne Burkett, MD
Resident Faculty
Department of Family Medicine
Good Samaritan Family Medicine Center
Phoenix, Arizona

Leah A. Burnett, MD
Department of General Surgery
University of Pittsburgh Medical Center/Mercy Hospital
Pittsburgh, Pennsylvania

Harold J. Bursztajn, MD
Associate Clinical Professor
Department of Psychiatry
Harvard Medical School
Associate Clinical Professor
Department of Psychiatry
Beth Israel Deaconess Medical Center
Boston, Massachusetts

David E. Burtner, MD
Vice Chairman and Professor
Department of Family and Community Medicine
Mercer University School of Medicine
Macon, Georgia

Nancy Byatt, DO, MBA
Assistant Professor
Department of Psychiatry
University of Massachusetts Medical School
Attending Psychiatrist
Psychosomatic Medicine and Emergency Mental Health
Department of Psychiatry
University of Massachusetts Medical Center
Worcester, Massachusetts

Michael Bybel, Jr, DO
Resident Physician
Department of Family Medicine
Carl R. Darnall Army Medical Center
Fort Hood, Texas

Patricio Cabral, MD
Framingham, Massachusetts

Marie Ellen Caggiano, MD, MPH
Assistant Professor
Department of Family Medicine and Community Health
University of Massachusetts Medical School
Physician
Hahnemann Family Health Center
Worcester, Massachusetts

Mitchell A. Cahan, MD
Assistant Professor
Department of Surgery
University of Massachusetts Medical School
Director of Acute Care Surgery
Department of Surgery
UMass Memorial Medical Center
Worcester, Massachusetts

Kimberly Caldwell, MD
Department of Family Medicine
David Grant Medical Center
Travis Air Force Base, California

Larissa Calka, DO
Department of Family Medicine
University of Massachusetts Medical School
Worcester, Massachusetts

Katherine M. Callaghan, MD
Department of Obstetrics and Gynecology
University of Massachusetts Medical School
Worcester, Massachusetts

Angela Camacho-Duran, MD
Assistant Professor of Psychiatry
University of Massachusetts Medical School
Worcester, Massachusetts

Maya Campara, PharmD, BCPS
Clinical Assistant Professor
Department of Pharmacy Practice
University of Illinois Medical Center at Chicago
Clinical Pharmacist
Division of Solid Organ Transplant
University of Illinois at Chicago Medical Center
Chicago, Illinois

David Candelario, DO
Family Medicine Resident
Department of Family and Community Medicine
UT Southwestern Medical Center
Dallas, Texas

Jennifer A. Caragol, MD
Assistant Professor
Department of Family and Community Medicine
University of Kentucky
Lexington, Kentucky

Stephanie Carinci, MD
Central Florida Neurologic Consultants
Deland, Florida

David M. Carne, MD
Department of General Surgery
Northeast Ohio University College of Medicine
Rootstown, Ohio
Department of General Surgery
Akron General Medical Center
Akron, Ohio

Noel John M. Carrasco, MD, FAAP
Professor of Pediatrics, Integrative Medicine
Course Director
NIM Instructor for Nutrition
A.T. Still University—School of Osteopathic Medicine in Arizona
Mesa, Arizona

Stephanie Carreiro, MD
Department of Emergency Medicine
Brown University
Rhode Island Hospital
Providence, Rhode Island

Laurie A. Carrier, MD
Clinical Instructor
Department of Family and Community Medicine
Northwestern University Feinberg School of Medicine
Family Physician and Psychiatrist
Heartland International Health Center
Chicago, Illinois

Ana Isabel Casanegra, MD
Assistant Professor of Medicine
Department of Vascular Medicine
Cardiovascular Section
Vascular Medicine Program
University of Oklahoma Health Sciences Center
Oklahoma City, Oklahoma

Mary Cataletto, MD
Professor of Clinical Pediatrics
Department of Pediatrics
SUNY Stony Brook
Stony Brook, New York
Associate Director
Pediatric Pulmonology
Winthrop University Hospital
Mineola, New York

Oguz Cataltepe, MD
Associate Professor
Department of Surgery and Pediatrics
Division of Neurosurgery
University of Massachusetts Medical School
Director, Pediatric Neurosurgery
UMass Memorial Medical Center
Worcester, Massachusetts

Jan Cerny, MD, PhD
Assistant Professor of Medicine
Department of Medicine
Division of Hematology and Oncology
University of Massachusetts Medical School
UMass Memorial Medical Center
Worcester, Massachusetts

Olga M. Ceron, MD
Retina/Vitreous Specialist
Staff Physician
Massachusetts Eye Research and Surgery Institution (MERSI)
Cambridge, Massachusetts

Shaylin Cersosimo, MD, MPH
Resident, Family Medicine
University of Massachusetts Memorial Medical Center
Worcester, Massachusetts

Teresa V. Chan, MD
Assistant Professor
Department of Otolaryngology—Head and Neck Surgery
University of Texas—Southwestern Medical Center
Dallas, Texas

Allen Chang, MD
University of Massachusetts Medical School
Worcester, Massachusetts

Felix B. Chang, MD
Assistant Professor
Department of Family Medicine and Community Health
University of Massachusetts School of Medicine
Medical Director
UMass Fitchburg Family Medicine Residency Program
UMass Memorial Health Alliance Hospital
Associate Medical Director
Leominster Community Health Connections
Leominster, Massachusetts

Phillip Chang, MBBS
Visiting Medical Officer
Department of Otolaryngology
St. Vincent's Hospital
Sydney, Australia

Jason Chao, MD, MS
Professor
Department of Family Medicine
Case Western Reserve University School of Medicine
Department of Family Medicine
University Hospitals Case Medical Center
Cleveland, Ohio

Arka Chatterjee, MD
Department of Internal Medicine
University of Louisville School of Medicine
Louisville, Kentucky

Shaila V. Chauhan, MD
Assistant Professor of Obstetrics and Gynecology
Division of Reproductive Endocrinology
University of Massachusetts Medical School
Worcester, Massachusetts

Stephanie Yu-hsuan Chen, MD
Department of Psychiatry
University of Massachusetts Medical School
Worcester, Massachusetts
Tufts Medical Center
Boston, Massachusetts

Rebecca Cherner, DO
Assistant Professor of Family Medicine
Nova Southeastern University College of Osteopathic Medicine
Broward General Medical Center
Dane, Florida

Manjula Cherukuri, MD
Assistant Professor, Family Medicine
Department of Family and Community Medicine
UT Southwestern Medical Center at Dallas
Dallas, Texas

Josue Chery, MD
University of Massachusetts School of Medicine
Worcester, Massachusetts

Edward Cheung, MD
Department of Medicine
The Warren Alpert Medical School of Brown University
Providence, Rhode Island

Sanjiv Chopra, MBBS, MACP
Professor of Medicine
Faculty Dean for Continuing Education
Harvard Medical School
Senior Consultant in Hepatology
Beth Israel Deaconess Medical Center
Boston, Massachusetts

Viola Chu, MD, MS
University of Hawaii—John A Burns School of Medicine
Honolulu, Hawaii

Arlene S. Chung, MD
Resident Physician
Department of Emergency Medicine
Warren Alpert Medical School of Brown University, Emergency Medicine Residency
Providence, Rhode Island

Young-Me Chung, MD
60th Medical Squadron, MDOS/SGOF
Family Medicine Clinic
David Grant Medical Center
Travis AFB, California

Tara Chute, MD
University of Massachusetts Medical School
Worcester, Massachusetts

Brian M. Clark, MD
Associate Professor
Department of Obstetrics and Gynecology
University of Massachusetts Memorial Medical Center
Chief, Division of Reproductive Endocrinology and Infertility
University of Massachusetts Medical School
Worcester, Massachusetts

S. Lindsey Clarke, MD, FAAFP
MUSC AHEC Associate Professor
Department of Family Medicine
Self Regional Healthcare Family Medicine Residency Program
Director of Predoctoral Education
Montgomery Center for Family Medicine
Self Regional Healthcare
Greenwood, South Carolina

Lisa Clemons, MD
Clinical Assistant Professor
Department of Family Medicine
University of Texas Southwestern—Austin
Brackenridge Hospital
Austin, Texas

Jerry Michael Cline, MD
Las Vegas, Nevada

Kara M. Coassolo, MD
Attending Physician, Maternal Fetal Medicine
Department of Obstetrics and Gynecology
Lehigh Valley Health Network
Allentown, Pennsylvania

Cameron J. Codd, DO
Department of Obstetrics and Gynecology
Akron General Medical Center
Akron, Ohio

Jaye Cole, MD
Assistant Professor
Department of Family Medicine
Texas Tech University Health Sciences Center School of Medicine
Lubbock, Texas

Naida Cole, MD, MM
Alpert Medical School of Brown University
Providence, Rhode Island

Irene C. Coletsos, MD
Clinical Associate
Tufts University School of Medicine
Psychiatry Resident PGY III
St. Elizabeth's Medical Center
Boston, Massachusetts

Dana M. Collaguazo, MD
Assistant Professor, Clinical
Department of Emergency Medicine
The University of Iowa Hospitals and Clinics
Iowa City, Iowa

Nathan T. Connell, MD
Assistant Instructor in Medicine
Department of Internal Medicine
Alpert Medical School of Brown University
Rhode Island and The Miriam Hospitals
Providence, Rhode Island

Caitlin M. Connolly, MD
Department of Internal Medicine
University of Massachusetts Medical School
Worcester, Massachusetts

Kyle V. Contini, MD
Department of Family Medicine
Creighton University School of Medicine
Omaha, Nebraska

Stephanie L. Conway, PharmD
Assistant Professor, Pharmacy Practice
Massachusetts College of Pharmacy and Health Sciences
Worcester, Massachusetts
Clinical Pharmacist
University of Massachusetts- Hahnemann Family Health Center
Worcester, Massachusetts

Maryann R. Cooper, PharmD
Assistant Professor of Pharmacy Practice
Hematology/Oncology
Massachusetts College of Pharmacy and Health Sciences
Manchester, New Hampshire
Worcester, Massachusetts

Marco Cornelio, MD
Department of Family Medicine
University of Massachusetts Department of Family Medicine and Community Health
Worcester, Massachusetts

Macario C. Corpuz, Jr., MD, FAAFP
Assistant Professor
Department of Family Medicine and Community Health
University of Massachusetts Medical School
Medical Staff
Department of Family Medicine
University of Massachusetts Memorial Hospital
Worcester, Massachusetts

Bodie Correll, MD
Department of Family Medicine
Scott & White Hospital
Temple, Texas

Ryan F. Coughlin, MD
University of Massachusetts Medical School
Worcester, Massachusetts

Alissa Craft, DO, MBA
Vice Chair and Associate Professor, Pediatrics
Western University of Health Sciences College of Osteopathic Medicine of the Pacific
Lebanon, Oregon

Neil Crittenden, MD
Department of Internal Medicine
University of Louisville
Louisville, Kentucky

Jennifer Crombie, MD
Department of Medicine
University of Massachusetts Medical School
Worcester, Massachusetts

Alan J. Cropp, MD
Professor of Medicine
Department of Internal Medicine
Northeastern Ohio Universities College of Medicine and Pharmacy
Rootstown, Ohio
Medical Staff
Department of Internal Medicine
St. Elizabeth Hospital Health Center
Youngstown, Ohio

Katie Crowder, MD
Faculty Physician
Travis Family Medicine Residency
Department of Family Medicine
David Grant Medical Center
Travis Air Force Base, California

Wanda Cruz-Knight, MD
Assistant Professor
Predoctoral Director
Department of Family Medicine
Case Western Reserve School of Medicine
Cleveland, Ohio

Sandra Cuellar, PharmD, BCOP
Clinical Assistant Professor
Department of Pharmacy Practice
University of Illinois at Chicago College of Pharmacy
Clinical Oncology Pharmacist
Department of Pharmacy Practice
University of Illinois at Chicago Medical Center
Chicago, Illinois

Hongyi Cui, MD, PhD
Assistant Professor of Surgery
Department of General and Laparoscopic Surgery
University of Massachusetts Medical School
Associate Director, Acute Care Surgery
Department of Surgery
University of Massachusetts Memorial Medical Center
Worcester, Massachusetts

Paul T. Cullen, MD
Clinical Associate Professor
Department of Family Medicine
University of Pittsburgh
Pittsburgh, Pennsylvania
Residency Program Director
Department of Family Medicine
Washington Hospital
Washington, Pennsylvania

James F. Cunagin, MD
Senior Clinical Instructor and Director of Behavioral Science, Department of Family Medicine
Senior Clinical Instructor, Department of Psychiatry
University Hospitals Case Medical Center
Case Western Reserve University School of Medicine
Cleveland, Ohio

Michael P. Curry, MD
Medical Director, Liver Transplantation
Beth Israel Deaconess Medical Center
Assistant Professor of Medicine
Harvard Medical School
Cambridge, Massachusetts

Carol Curtin, MSW, LICSW
Research Assistant Professor
Department of Family Medicine and Community Health
E.K. Shriver Center
University of Massachusetts Medical School
Waltham, Massachusetts

Tyler Cymet, DO
Associate Vice President for Medical Education
American Association of Colleges of Osteopathic Medicine
Chevy Chase, Maryland

Zarna J. Dahya, MD
Department of Internal Medicine
University of Louisville
Louisville, Kentucky

Jennifer S. Daly, MD
Professor
Department of Medicine, Microbiology and Physiological Systems
University of Massachusetts Medical School
Clinical Chief
Division of Infectious Diseases and Immunology
University of Massachusetts Memorial Health Center
Worcester, Massachusetts

Akhil Das, MD, FACS
Assistant Professor of Urology
Department of Urology
Thomas Jefferson University
Attending Physician
Department of Urology
Thomas Jefferson University Hospital
Philadelphia, Pennsylvania

Janice E. Daugherty, MD, FAAFP, ABIHM
Associate Professor
Department of Family Medicine
The Brody School of Medicine at East Carolina University
Greenville, North Carolina
Patient Care Privileges
PIH County Memorial Hospital
Greenville, North Carolina

Raul Davaro, MD
Associate Professor
Department of Medicine
University of Massachusetts
Worcester, Massachusetts

Alexander E. Davidovich, DO, MS
New York College of Osteopathic Medicine of NYIT
Old Westbury, New York

AuTumn Davidson, MD
Department of Obstetrics and Gynecology
University of Massachusetts Medical School
Worcester, Massachusetts

Marin Dawson-Caswell, DO
Assistant Professor
Department of Family Medicine
Louisiana State University Health Sciences Center
New Orleans, Louisiana

Lauren Michal de Leon, MD
Warren Alpert Medical School at Brown University
Providence, Rhode Island

Garreth C. Debiegun, MD
Clinical Instructor, Emergency Medicine
Maine Medical Center and Tufts University School of Medicine
Portland, Maine

Peerawut Deeprasertkul, MD
Cardiology Fellow
Michigan State University
Lansing, Michigan

Gina M. DeFranco, DO
Assistant Professor
Department of Family Medicine
Lincoln Memorial University—DeBusk College of Osteopathic Medicine
Harrogate, Tennessee

Sophia L. Delano, MPP, MD
Pediatric Intern
Massachusetts General Hospital
Boston, Massachusetts

Konstantinos E. Deligiannidis, MD, MPH
Assistant Clinical Professor
Department of Family Medicine and Community Health
University of Massachusetts Medical School
UMass Memorial Health Care
Worcester, Massachusetts

Deborah DeMarco, MD
Senior Associate Dean for Clinical Affairs
Associate Dean, GME
Professor of Medicine
Division of Rheumatology
University of Massachusetts Medical School
Worcester, Massachusetts

Shannon Demas, MD
University of Massachusetts Medical School
Worcester, Massachusetts

Penelope H. Dennehy, MD
Professor of Pediatrics
The Alpert Medical School of Brown University
Chief, Pediatric Infectious Diseases
Hasbro Children's Hospital
Providence, Rhode Island

Amar Deshpande, MD
Assistant Professor
Division of Gastroenterology
University of Miami Miller School of Medicine
Miami, Florida

Alicia R. Desilets, PharmD
Assistant Professor of Pharmacy Practice
Department of Pharmacy Practice
Massachusetts College of Pharmacy and Health Sciences
Manchester, New Hampshire

Richard F. DeSouza, MD
Attending Physician
Department of Internal Medicine
Yale—New Haven Hospital
New Haven, Connecticut

Mathew J. Devine, DO
Assistant Professor
Department of Family Medicine
University of Rochester
Associate Medical Director
Department of Family Medicine
Highland Family Medicine
Rochester, New York

Jessica Devitt, MD
House Officer
Department of Family Medicine
University of Colorado School of Medicine
Denver, Colorado

Gretchen M. Dickson, MD, MBA
Assistant Professor
Department of Family and Community Medicine
University of Kansas—School of Medicine, Wichita
Wichita, Kansas

Dennis M. Dimitri, MD
Vice Chair and Clinical Associate Professor
Department of Family Medicine and Community Health
University of Massachusetts Medical School
Worcester, Massachusetts
Vice Chair for Clinical Services
Department of Family Medicine and Community Health
University of Massachusetts Medical Center
Worcester, Massachusetts

Frank J. Domino, MD
Professor
Pre-doctoral Education Director
Department of Family Medicine and Community Health
The University of Massachusetts Medical School
Worcester, Massachusetts

David J. Donahue, MD
Medical Director
Department of Pediatric Neurosurgery
Cook Children's Medical Center
Surgical Director
Pediatric Epilepsy Program
Cook Children's Medical Center
Fort Worth, Texas

Anna Doubeni, MD
Assistant Professor
Family Medicine and Community Health
University of Massachusetts Medical School
Worcester, Massachusetts

Cary D. Douglass, MD
President, West Lake Family Practice
West Lake Hills, Texas

Kathleen A. Downey, MD
Associate Professor
Department of Family and Community Medicine
University of Cincinnati
Cincinnati, Ohio

Raymond G. Dufresne, Jr., MD
Professor of Dermatology
Division of Dermatologic Surgery
The Warren Alpert Medical School of Brown University
Providence, Rhode Island

Kaelen C. Dunican, PharmD
Associate Professor
Department of Pharmacy Practice
Division of Community Pharmacy Practice
Massachusetts College of Pharmacy and Health Sciences
Worcester, Massachusetts

Nedim Durakovic, MD
Department of Otolaryngology
The Warren Alpert Medical School of Brown University
Providence, Rhode Island

Cheryl Durand, PharmD, RPh
Assistant Professor of Pharmacy Practice
Massachusetts College of Pharmacy and Health Sciences
Manchester, New Hampshire

William J. Durbin, MD
Professor, Residency Director
Department of Pediatric Infectious Disease
University of Massachusetts Medical School
Chair, Department of Pediatric Infectious Disease
UMass Memorial Healthcare
Worcester, Massachusetts

Geolani Dy, MD
Warren Alpert Medical School of Brown University
Providence, Rhode Island

Kylee Eagles, DO
Department of Family Medicine
Chief Family Medicine
University of Massachusetts Medical School
Worcester, Massachusetts

Alan M. Ehrlich, MD
Assistant Clinical Professor
Department of Family Practice
University of Massachusetts Medical School
Worcester, Massachusetts

Alison Ehrlich, MD
Clinical Professor of Dermatology
George Washington University
Washington, DC

William G. Elder, Jr., PhD
Associate Professor
Department of Family and Community Medicine
University of Kentucky College of Medicine
University of Kentucky Chandler Medical Center
Lexington, Kentucky

Amy Ellingson-Itzin, MD
Department of Obstetrics and Gynecology
University of Massachusetts Medical School
UMass Memorial Medical Center
Worcester, Massachusetts

Nancy Elliot, MD, FACS
Director of Montclair Breast Center
Montclair, New Jersey

Carrie Lynn Ellis, DVM, MS
Associate Veterinarian
Department of Veterinary Medicine
The Animal Hospital in Mt. Lookout Square
Cincinnati, Ohio

Robert Ellis, MD
Assistant Professor
Department of Family Medicine
University of Cincinnati College of Medicine
Cincinnati, Ohio

Pamela I. Ellsworth, MD
Associate Professor of Urology/Surgery
Department of Surgery
The Warren Alpert School of Medicine at Brown University
Pediatric Urologist
Department of Surgery
Hasbro Children's Hospital
Providence, Rhode Island

Kevin Engelhardt, MD
Department of Pediatrics
University of Arizona College of Medicine
Tucson, Arizona

Joseph K. Erbe, DO
Faculty
Department of Family Medicine
David Grant Medical Center
Travis Air Force Base
Fairfield, California

Rasai L. Ernst, MD
Senior Instructor
Department of Family Medicine
University Hospitals Case Medical Center
Cleveland, Ohio

Martin A. Espinosa Ginic, MD
Cardiology Fellow
University of Louisville
University of Louisville Hospital
Louisville, Kentucky

Janelle M. Evans, MD
Department of Obstetrics and Gynecology
University of Massachusetts Medical School
Worcester, Massachusetts

Kristyn Fagerberg, MD
West Lake Family Practice
Austin, Texas

Ashley Falk, MD
Family Practice
Offutt Air Force Base, Nebraska

Nathan P. Falk, MD
Chief, Primary Care Sports Medicine
Offutt Air Force Base/University of Nebraska Medical Center
Omaha, Nebraska

Pang-Yen Fan, MD
Associate Professor of Medicine
Department of Nephrology
University of Massachusetts Medical School
Worcester, Massachusetts

Rhonda A. Faulkner, PhD
Director, Behavioral Medicine
Department of Family Medicine
Family Medicine Residency Program
University of Illinois College of Medicine at Saint Joseph Hospital
Chicago, Illinois

Peter Fay, MD
Clinical Assistant Professor of Surgery
Department of Ophthalmology
Alpert Medical School of Brown University
Providence, Rhode Island

Neil J. Feldman, DPM
Central Massachusetts Podiatry, PC
Worcester, Massachusetts

Rebecca Feldman, MD
University of Massachusetts Medical School
Worcester, Massachusetts

Edward Feller, MD
Clinical Professor of Medicine
Adjust Professor of Community Health
Department of Gastroenterology, Public Health
Warren Alpert Medical School of Brown University
Providence, Rhode Island

Warren J. Ferguson, MD
Associate Professor
Department of Family Medicine and Community Health
University of Massachusetts Medical School
Vice Chair
Department of Family Medicine and Community Health
UMass Memorial Medical Center
Worcester, Massachusetts

Lauren Ferrara, MD
New York Medical College
Valhalla, New York

Kathleen Ferrer, MD
Assistant Professor
Department of Pediatrics
Children's National Medical Center
George Washington University School of Medicine and Health Sciences
Washington, District of Columbia

Scott A. Fields, MD
Professor and Vice Chair
Department of Family Medicine
Oregon Health and Science University
Portland, Oregon

Stanley Fineman, MD
Associate Clinical Professor
Department of Pediatrics
Emory University School of Medicine
Atlanta, Georgia
Atlanta Allergy and Asthma Clinic
Marietta, Georgia

Judy Fingergut, MD
Clinical Assistant Professor
Department of Family Medicine
Stony Brook University Hospital
Stony Brook, New York

Jonathon M. Firnhaber, MD
Clinical Assistant Professor
Department of Family Medicine
Brody School of Medicine
East Carolina University
Greenville, North Carolina

Timothy P. Fitzgibbons, MD
Fellow
Department of Cardiology
University of Massachusetts Medical School
Worcester, Massachusetts

Jonathan M. Flacker, MD
Associate Professor
Department of Medicine
Division of Geriatric Medicine and Gerontology
Emory University School of Medicine
Medical Director, Emory Clinic at Wesley Woods
Geriatrics
Wesley Woods Health Center
Atlanta, Georgia

Joseph A. Florence, MD
Professor/Director, Division of Programs
Department of Family Medicine
East Tennessee State University Quillen College
Johnson City, Tennessee

Terence R. Flotte, MD
Dean and Provost Executive Deputy Chancellor of the Medical School
Professor
Department of Pediatrics
Celia and Isak Distinguished Professorship
Department of Pediatric Pulmonary
University of Massachusetts Medical School
Professor
Department of Pediatrics
University of Massachusetts Memorial Health Center
Worcester, Massachusetts

Mary K. Flynn, MD
Department of Family Medicine and Community Health
University of Massachusetts Medical School
Worcester, Massachusetts

Harry W. Flynn, Jr., MD
J. Donald M. Gass Distinguished Chair
Professor of Ophthalmology
Department of Ophthalmology
Bascom Palmer Eye Institute
University of Miami
Miami, Florida

Jay Gar-Yee Fong, MD
Assistant Professor
Department of Pediatric Gastroenterology
University of Massachusetts School of Medicine and Medical Center
Worcester, Massachusetts

James Foody, MD
Professor of Medicine
Divisions of General Internal Medicine and Geriatrics
Vice Chair Department of Medicine for Clinical Affairs
Northwestern University
Feinberg School of Medicine
Chicago, Illinois

Nicole Foras, MD
Department of Family Medicine
St. Luke's Medical Center
Milwaukee, Wisconsin

Phillip Fournier, MD
Clinical Associate Professor
Family Medicine and Community Health
Director of Student Health
University of Massachusetts Medical School
Worcester, Massachusetts

Stanley L. Fox, MD
Dermatology
Cleveland, Ohio

Robert L. Frachtman, MD
Austin Gastroenterology, PA
Austin, Texas

Jennifer E. Frank, MD
ThedaCare Physicians—Neenah West
Neenah, Wisconsin

Samuel Frank, MD
Assistant Professor of Neurology
Boston University School of Medicine
Boston, Massachusetts

Jenny Frazier, MD
Family Practice
Austin, Texas

Nancy J. Freeman, MD
Clinical Associate Professor of Medicine
Warren Alpert School of Medicine at Brown University
Chief, Hematology/Oncology
Providence VA Medical Center
Providence, Rhode Island

Brian B. Freniere, MD
University of Massachusetts Medical School
Worcester, Massachusetts

Jerry Friemoth, MD
Associate Professor of Clinical Family Medicine
University of Cincinnati College of Medicine
Cincinnati, Ohio

Rebecca A. Frye, DO
Faculty Physician
Department of Family Medicine
David Grant Medical Center
Travis Air Force Base, California

Scott Frye, MD
Resident Physician
Department of Internal Medicine
David Grant Medical Center
Travis Air Force Base, California

Michael S. Furman, MD
Department of Internal Medicine
Alpert Medical School of Brown University
Providence, Rhode Island

Richard Gacek, MD
Director, Otology/Neurotology
UMass Memorial Medical Center
Professor of Otolaryngology
University of Massachusetts Medical School
Worcester, Massachusetts

Heidi L. Gaddey, MD
Department of Family Medicine
David Grant Medical Center
Travis Air Force Base, California

J. Scott Gaertner, MD
West Lake Family Practice
Austin, Texas

Stephanie Galica, MD
University of Massachusetts Medical School
Worcester, Massachusetts

Jessica Weston Galvin, DO
PGY-1, Traditional Rotating Intern
University Hospitals Richmond Medical Center
Richmond Heights, Ohio

Sumanth Gandra, MD, MPH
Infectious Disease Fellow
University of Massachusetts Medical School
Worcester, Massachusetts

Jennifer Gao, MD
Department of Internal Medicine
Alpert Medical School, Brown University
Providence, Rhode Island

Andrew Gara, MD
University of Massachusetts Medical School
Worcester, Massachusetts

Erik J. Garcia, MD
Assistant Professor
Department of Family and Community Medicine
UMass Memorial Medical Center
Worcester, Massachusetts

Luis T. Garcia, MD
Clinical Assistant Professor
Department of Family Medicine
University of Illinois—Chicago
Chairman and Residency Program Director
Department of Family Medicine
Saint Joseph Hospital
Chicago, Illinois

Riabianca Garcia, MD
Warren Alpert Medical School of Brown University
Providence, Rhode Island

Amit Garg, MD
Director, Residency Program
Department of Dermatology
Boston University School of Medicine
Assistant Professor
Department of Dermatology
Boston Medical Center
Boston, Massachusetts

Christopher Garofalo, MD
Active Staff
Department of Family Medicine
Family Medicine Associates of South Attleboro PC
Attleboro, Massachusetts

William T. Garrison, PhD
Professor
Department of Pediatrics
Division of Child and Adolescent Psychology
University of Massachusetts Medical School
Chief
Developmental and Behavioral Pediatrics
UMass Memorial Healthcare
Worcester, Massachusetts

Renata Gazzi, MD
Clinical Faculty
Department of Family Medicine
University of Illinois at Chicago
Clinical Faculty/Attending Physician
Department of Family Medicine
Saint Joseph Hospital
Chicago, Illinois

Gerald Gehr, MD
Assistant Professor of Medicine
Dartmouth Medical School
Hanover, New Hampshire
Hematology/Oncology Program
Dartmouth-Hitchcock Manchester
Norris Cotton Cancer Center Manchester
Manchester, New Hampshire

Bethany Gentilesco, MD
Assistant Professor of Medicine
Brown Alpert Medical School
Providence, Rhode Island
Hospitalist
The Miriam Hospital
Providence, Rhode Island

Major Dena George, MD
Assistant Professor
Department of Family Medicine
Uniformed Services University of the Health Sciences
Carl R. Darnall Army Medical Center
Fort Hood, Texas

Paul George, MD
Assistant Professor of Family Medicine
Warren Alpert Medical School of Brown University
Providence, Rhode Island

Thomas Germano, MD
Assistant Clinical Professor
Department of Emergency Medicine
Warren Alpert Medical School at Brown University
Attending Physician
Rhode Island Hospital
Providence, Rhode Island

Jeff Ray Gibson, Jr., MD
Assistant Professor
Department of Anesthesiology
The Texas A&M University Health Sciences Center College of Medicine
Senior Staff Anesthesiologist
Department of Anesthesiology
Scott & White Memorial Hospital
Temple, Texas

Timothy Gibson, MD
Assistant Professor
Department of Pediatrics
University of Massachusetts Medical School
Chief
Hanshaw Hospitalist Service
Department of Pediatrics
UMass Memorial Children's Medical Center
Worcester, Massachusetts

David B. Gilchrist, MD
Assistant Professor
Department of Family Medicine
University of Massachusetts Medical School
University of Massachusetts Memorial Hospital
Worcester, Massachusetts

Neil A. Gilchrist, PharmD
Adjunct Assistant Professor
Department of Pharmacy Practice
Massachusetts College of Pharmacy and Health Sciences
Clinical Pharmacy Specialist
Department of Pharmacy
UMass Memorial Medical Center
Worcester, Massachusetts

Cheryl L. Gilmartin, PharmD
Clinical Assistant Professor
Department of Pharmacy Practice
College of Pharmacy
University of Illinois
Clinical Pharmacist
Section of Nephrology
University of Illinois
Chicago, Illinois

Alfred Chege Gitu, MD
Faculty Physician
Department of Family Medicine
Greenwood Family Medicine Residency Program
Self Regional Healthcare
Greenwood, South Carolina

Gerald Gleich, MD
Assistant Professor of Family Medicine and Community Health
Department of Family Medicine/Geriatrics
University of Massachusetts Medical School
Worcester, Massachusetts

JL Godwin, MD
The Warren Alpert Medical School of Brown University
Providence, Rhode Island

Andrew D. Goldberg, MD
Fellow
Department of Critical Care Medicine
Mayo Clinic
Rochester, Minnesota

Dori Goldberg, MD
Assistant Professor of Medicine
Department of Dermatology
University of Massachusetts Medical School
Worcester, Massachusetts

Dan Golding, MD
Assistant Professor of Diagnostic Imaging (Clinical)
Diagnostic Imaging
Brown Alpert Medical School
Providence, Rhode Island

Jeremy Golding, MD
Professor of Family Medicine and of Obstetrics and Gynecology
The University of Massachusetts Medical School
Quality Officer
Department of Family Medicine and Community Health
UMass Memorial Health Care—Hahnemann Family Health Center
Worcester, Massachusetts

Michael Golding, MD
Senior Attending
New Hanover Hospital
Medical Director, Psych Support Inc.
Raleigh, North Carolina

Walter K. Goljan, MD
Department of Internal Medicine
Webster Square Medical Center
Worcester, Massachusetts

Leonard G. Gomella, MD, FACS
The Bernard W. Godwin Professor of Prostate Cancer Chairman
Associate Director of Clinical Affairs
Department of Urology
Jefferson Medical College
Philadelphia, Pennsylvania

Christian D. Gonzalez, MD
Clinical Director, Pain Medicine
Miami Neurological Institute
Aventura, Florida

Gerardo Gonzalez, MD
Associate Professor of Psychiatry
Director of Addiction Psychopharmacology Research Unit
Director of Addiction and Comorbidity Treatment Service (ACTS)
Director of the Addiction Psychiatry Fellowship program
University of Massachusetts Medical School
UMass Memorial Medical Center
Worcester, Massachusetts

Herbert P. Goodheart, MD
Associate Clinical Professor
Department of Dermatology
Mount Sinai College of Medicine
New York, New York
Director of Dermatology Services
Department of Dermatology
Elmhurst Hospital Center
Elmhurst, New York

Jeffrey L. Goodie, PhD
Assistant Professor
Department of Family Medicine
Uniformed Services University of the Health Sciences
Bethesda, Maryland

Mark D. Goodman, MD
Associate Professor and Interim Chairman
Department of Family Medicine
Creighton University School of Medicine
Omaha, Nebraska

Geetha Gopalakrishnan, MD
Associate Professor of Medicine
Department of Endocrinology
Alpert Medical School of Brown University
Providence, Rhode Island

Ilya Gorbachinsky, MD
Wake Forest University Baptist Medical Center
Winston-Salem, North Carolina

Joseph Gordon, MD
Department of Medicine
George Washington University
Washington, DC

Paul R. Gordon, MD, MPH
Associate Professor
Department of Family and Community Medicine
University of Arizona - College of Medicine
Tucson, Arizona

Shilpa Gowda, MD
Warren Alpert Medical School of Brown University
Providence, Rhode Island

Parag Goyal, MD
Department of Internal Medicine
New York Presbyterian Hospital-Weill Cornell Medical Center
New York, New York

Heath A. Grames, PhD
Assistant Professor and Program Director for the Marriage and Family Therapy Program
Department of Child and Family Studies
The University of Southern Mississippi
Hattiesburg, Mississippi

Anne Granfield, MD
University of Massachusetts Medical School
UMass Memorial Medical Center
Worcester, Massachusetts

Jane M. Grant-Kels, MD
Professor and Founding Chair
Department of Dermatology
Director of Dermatopathology
Director of Cutaneous Oncology and Melanoma Program
Dermatology Residency Director
Assistant Dean of Clinical Affairs
University of CT Health Center
Farmington, Connecticut

Chris Graves, MD
House Staff, Orthopaedics
University of Iowa Carver College of Medicine
Iowa City, Iowa

Michael J. Gray, MD
Department of Emergency Medicine
University of Massachusetts Medical School
Worcester, Massachusetts

Ellen Greenblatt, MD, FRCSC
Associate Professor
Department of Obstetrics and Gynecology
University of Toronto
Medical Director
Centre for Fertility and Reproductive Health
Mount Sinai Hospital
Toronto, Ontario
Canada

Jennifer J. Greene Welch, MD
Assistant Professor
Department of Pediatrics
Alpert Medical School Brown University
Attending Physician
Division of Pediatric Hematology/Oncology
Department of Pediatrics
Hasbro Children's Hospital
Providence, Rhode Island

Pamela L. Grimaldi, DO, FAAFP
Assistant Professor
Department of Family Medicine and Community Health
University of Massachusetts Medical School
Staff, Physician
Department of Family Medicine
University of Massachusetts Memorial Hospital
Worcester, Massachusetts

Drew Grimes, MD
Capital Anesthesiology Associates
Austin, Texas

Jill A. Grimes, MD
Clinical Instructor
Department of Family Medicine
University of Massachusetts Medical School
Worcester, Massachusetts
Private Practice
West Lake Family Practice
Austin, Texas

Anastasia Grivoyannis, MD
Department of Medicine
Division of Emergency Medicine
University of Washington, Harborview Medical Center
Seattle, Washington

Shanin Gross, DO
Assistant Professor, Attending Physician
Department of Family and Community Medicine
Penn State College of Medicine
Hershey Medical Center
Hershey, Pennsylvania

Marc M. Grossman, MD, FACEP, CPHM
Clinical Assistant Professor of Medicine
FIU Wertheim College of Medicine
Vol. Assistant Professor of Medicine (Emergency Medicine) and Neurology
University of Miami College of Medicine
Assistant Medical Director
Miami-Dade Fire Rescue
Miami, Florida

Neil Grossman, MD
Department of Pediatrics
University of Massachusetts Medical School
Worcester, Massachusetts

Angela L. Gucwa, MD
General Surgery Resident
Georgia Health Sciences University
Augusta, Georgia

John A. Guisto, MD
Professor, Emergency Medicine
University of Arizona College of Medicine
Tucson, Arizona

Adarsh K. Gupta, DO, MS
Assistant Professor
Department of Family Medicine
Director, Center for Information Mastery
University of Medicine and Dentistry New Jersey-School of Osteopathic Medicine
Attending Physician
Department of Family Medicine
Kennedy Memorial Hospital
Stratford, New Jersey

Neena Gupta, MD
Assistant Professor of Pediatrics
University of Massachusetts Medical School
Department of Pediatric Nephrology
University of Massachusetts Memorial Children's Medical Center
Worcester, Massachusetts

Neha Gupta, MD
Family Medicine
MSU/Kalamazoo Center for Medical Studies
Kalamazoo, Michigan

Gregory D. Gutke, MD, MPH
Department of Occupational Medicine
United States Air Force
Robins Air Force Base, Georgia

Michael S. Guy, MD
Teaching Faculty
Northeastern Ohio Medical University
Department of Obstetrics and Gynecology
Akron General Medical Center
Akron, Ohio

Andrea Haas, MSIV
University of Massachusetts Medical School
Worcester, Massachusetts

M. Tye Haeberle, MD
Intern, Internal Medicine
University of Louisville
Louisville, Kentucky

Laura Hagopian, MD
University of Massachusetts Medical School
Worcester, Massachusetts

Jessica E. Haley, MD
Department of Pediatrics
University of Arizona
University Medical Center
Tucson, Arizona

Patricia Halligan, MD
Private Practice
Rochester, New York

Ihab Hamzeh, MD
Assistant Professor of Medicine
Department of Cardiology
University of Louisville
Department of Cardiology
Robley Rex VA Medical Center
University of Louisville
Louisville, Kentucky

Kelly B. Han, MD
House Staff
Department of Internal Medicine and Pediatrics
Duke University Medical Center
Durham, North Carolina

Samson H. Hanka, MD
Department of Internal Medicine
Metro West Medical Center
Framingham, Massachusetts

Thomas J. Hansen, MD
Associate Dean for Medical Education
Associate Professor
Department of Family Medicine
Creighton University
Omaha, Nebraska

Allison Hargreaves, MD
University of Massachusetts Medical School
Worcester, Massachusetts

Amena Hashmi, MD
Department of Family and Community Medicine
The University of Texas Southwestern Medical Center
Dallas, Texas

Robert Hasty, DO, FACOI
Program Director
Palmetto General Hospital Internal Medicine Residency
Assistant Professor of Internal Medicine
Nova Southeastern University College of Osteopathic Medicine
Fellow of the American College of Osteopathic Internists
Fort Lauderdale, Florida

Fern R. Hauck, MD, MS
Associate Professor
Departments of Family Medicine and Public Health Sciences
University of Virginia School of Medicine
Charlottesville, Virginia

Kevin Heaton, DO
Primary Care Sports Medicine, Family Practice
Access Sports Medicine and Orthopaedics
Exeter, New Hampshire

Daithi S. Heffernan, MD
Department of Surgery
Division of Trauma and Surgical Critical Care
Alpert Medical School of Brown University
Rhode Island Hospital
Providence, Rhode Island

Janet O. Helminski, PT, PhD
Associate Professor, Physical Therapy
Midwestern University
Downers Grove, Illinois

Scott T. Henderson, MD
Director of Medical Services
Department of Family Medicine
Student Health Center
University of Missouri
Columbia, Missouri

Stephen Hendriksen, MD
Department of Emergency Medicine
Warren Alpert Medical School of Brown University
Providence, Rhode Island
Rhode Island Hospital
Providence, Rhode Island

Jaroslaw T. Hepel, MD
Asistant Professor
Department of Radiation Oncology
Brown University
Department of Radiation Oncology
Rhode Island Hospital
Providence, Rhode Island

Jennifer P. Herbert, MD
Assistant Professor
Associate Director for Medical Student Education
Department of Family Medicine
Georgia Health Sciences University
Augusta, Georgia

Fernando A. Hernandez, MD
Physician
Department of Family Medicine
United States Air Force

Reagan J. Herrington, MD
Resident
Department of Emergency Medicine
Rhode Island Hospital
The Warren Alpert Medical School of Brown University
Providence, Rhode Island

Kerri-Ann Hew, DO
Family Practice
Broward Health Physician Group
Fort Lauderdale, Florida

Luisa A. Hiendlmayr, MD
Resident
UMass Family Medicine
University of Massachusetts
Fitchburg, Massachusetts

Angela Y. Higgins, MD
University of Massachusetts Medical School
Worcester, Massachusetts

Benjamin Hilliker, MD
University of Massachusetts Medical School
Worcester, Massachusetts

Nadine T. Himelfarb, MD
Department of Emergency Medicine
The Warren Alpert Medical School of Brown University
Rhode Island Hospital
Providence, Rhode Island

Mia Souheil Hindi, MD
Fellow
Department of Gastroenterology
University of Miami, Miller School of Medicine
Miami, Florida

Richard Hinds, MD
Department of Medicine
Warren Alpert Medical School of Brown University
Providence, Rhode Island

W. Jeff Hinton, PhD
Associate Professor, Interim Chair
Department of Child and Family Studies
Division of Marriage and Family Therapy/Mental Health
The University of Southern Mississippi
Hattiesburg, Mississippi

Crystal L. Hnatko, DO
Affiliate Faculty
Sutter Family Residency Program
Department of Family and Sports Medicine
Vacaville, California

R. Jeffrey Hofmann, MD
Clinical Associate Professor
Department of Ophthalmology
Division of Surgery
Alpert School of Medicine, Brown University
Providence, Rhode Island

N. Wilson Holland, MD, FACP
Assistant Professor
Department of Medicine
Emory University School of Medicine
Fellowship Program Director
Division of Geriatric Medicine
Staff Physician, Geriatrics and Extended Care
VA Medical Center
Atlanta, Georgia

Michael B. Holliday, MD
Assistant Professor, University of Cincinnati
Department of Family and Community Medicine
Director, Clinical Operations
Medical Director, UC Health Primary Care at Forest Park
Cincinnati, Ohio

David M. Holmes, MD
Clinical Associate Professor
Department of Family Medicine
State University of New York at Buffalo
Buffalo, New York

Michael P. Hopkins, MD, MEd
Director Aultman Health Foundation
Professor and Chair
Department of Obstetrics and Gynecology
Northeastern Ohio University College of Medicine
Director
Department of Obstetrics and Gynecology
Aultman Health Foundation
Canton, Ohio

James Horowitz, MD
Chief Resident Internal Medicine/Attending
Department of Cardiology
New York Presbyterian Hospital
New York, New York

Evan R. Horton, PharmD
Assistant Professor of Pharmacy Practice
Massachusetts College of Pharmacy and Health Sciences
Worcester, Massachusetts
Clinical Specialist
Department of Pharmacy (Pediatrics)
Baystate Medical Center
Springfield, Massachusetts

Kim House, MD
Medical Director
Atlanta Eagle's Nest—A Community Living Center
Decatur, Georgia

Elizabeth E. Houser, MD
Staff Urologist
Department of Urology
Seton Family of Hospitals
St. David's Family of Hospitals
Westlake Hospital
Austin, Texas

Jay U. Howington, MD
Assistant Professor
Department of Surgery and Radiology
Mercer University School of Medicine
Department of Neurological Surgery
Neurological Institute of Savannah
Savannah, Georgia

Dennis E. Hughes, DO
Department of Emergency Medicine
Veterans Health Care System
Fayetteville, Arkansas

Karen A. Hulbert, MD
Associate Professor
Department of Family and Community Medicine
Medical College of Wisconsin
Milwaukee, Wisconsin

John C. Huscher, MD
Assistant Professor
Department of Family Medicine
University of Nebraska Medical Center
Omaha, Nebraska
Staff Physician
Hospitalist
Faith Regional Health Services
Norfolk, Nebraska

Lawrence M. Hwang, MD
Assistant Clinical Professor
Department of Family Medicine
University of California Los Angeles
Los Angeles, California
University of California Los Angeles Santa Monica and Orthopedic Hospital
Santa Monica, California

Robert J. Hyde, MD
Assistant Professor
Department of Emergency Medicine
University of Pittsburgh School of Medicine
Pittsburgh, Pennsylvania

Amanda Iantosca, DO
Family Medicine Residency
Department of Family Medicine
University of Massachusetts Fitchburg
Fitchburg, Massachusetts

Deborah Ikhena, MD
Resident Physician
University of Massachusetts Medical School
Worcester, Massachusetts

Sabrina A. Indyk, MD
Department of Family Medicine
Resurrection Medical Center
Chicago, Illinois

Pablo I. Hernandez Itriago, MD
Assistant Professor
Department of Family Medicine
Boston University School of Medicine
V.P. Medical Services/Medical Director
South End Community Health Center (SECHC)
Boston, Massachusetts

Christine K. Jacobs, MD
Associate Professor
Department of Family and Community Medicine
St. Louis University School of Medicine
Residency Program Director
St. Louis University Family Medicine
St. Louis University School of Medicine
St. Louis, Missouri

Deepa Jagadeesh, MD, MPH
Hematology/Oncology Fellow
Department of Medicine—Hematology/Oncology
University of Massachusetts Medical School
Worcester, Massachusetts

Neha Jakhete, MD
George Washington University School of Medicine and Health Sciences
Washington, District of Columbia

Catherine James, MD
Assistant Professor
Attending Physician
Department of Pediatrics, Division of Pediatric Emergency Medicine
University of Massachusetts School of Medicine
University of Massachusetts Memorial Medical Center
Worcester, Massachusetts

Carrie R. Janiski, DO, ATC, NASM-PES
Resident Physician
Department of Family Medicine
Michigan State University - Kalamazoo Center for Medical Studies
Kalamazoo, Michigan

Courtney I. Jarvis, PharmD
Associate Professor
Department of Pharmacy Practice
Massachusetts College of Pharmacy and Health Sciences
Worcester, Massachusetts
Clinical Pharmacy Pharmacist
Department of Family Medicine
UMass Memorial Medical Center
Barre, Massachusetts

Joselyn Jedick, DO
Department of Family Medicine
Division of Sports Medicine
Banner Good Samaritan Hospital
Phoenix, Arizona

Eric L. Jenison, MD
Professor
Department of Obstetrics and Gynecology
Northeastern Ohio Universities College of Medicine and Pharmacy
Rootstown, Ohio
Chairman and Program Director
Department of Obstetrics and Gynecology
Akron General Medical Center
Akron, Ohio

John Jenkins, MD

Pim Jetanalin, MD
Department of Rheumatology
University of California, San Diego
La Jolla, California

Samuel Joffe, MD
Cardiology Fellow
University of Massachusetts Medical School
UMass Memorial Medical Center
Division of Cardiovascular Medicine
Worcester, Massachusetts

Amanda Johnson, MD
University of Massachusetts Medical School
Worcester, Massachusetts

Kendall Johnson, MD
University of Massachusetts Medical School
Worcester, Massachusetts

Mirjana Jojic, MD
Department of Psychiatry
University of Massachusetts
Worcester, Massachusetts

Chiedza Jokonya, MD, MRCPCH
Director of Pediatric Program
Department of Family Practice/Pediatrics
Maine Dartmouth Family Medicine Residency
Augusta, Maine

Lisa O. Jolly, MD
Department of Family Medicine
University of Texas Southwestern
Dallas, Texas

Rinat Jonas, MD
Assistant Professor
Department of Pediatric Neurology
Boston University
Pediatric Clinical Neurology
Boston Medical Center
Boston, Massachusetts

Brandon Q. Jones, MD
Department of Family Medicine
David Grant Medical Center
Travis Air Force Base, California

Stacy Jones, MD
Capitol Anesthesiology Association
Austin, Texas

Maurice F. Joyce, III, MD
Department of General Surgery
Lahey Clinic
Burlington, Massachusetts

David M. Joyner, MD
Former Clinical Associate Professor
Division of Orthopedic Surgery
Acting Director of Intercollegiate Athletics
The Pennsylvania State University
University Park, Pennsylvania

Patrick W. Joyner, MD, MS
Department of Orthopaedic Surgery
Duke University Medical Center
Durham, North Carolina

Manjula Julka, MD, FAAFP
Associate Program Director, Family Practice
Assistant Professor, Predoctoral Site Director
University of Texas Southwestern Medical Center
University of Texas Southwestern Family Medicine Residency Program
Dallas, Texas

Jacqueline M. Kaari, DO, FACOP, FAAP
Assistant Professor
Department of Pediatrics
University of Medicine and Dentistry of New Jersey
Stratford, New Jersey
Acting Chairperson
Chief of Pediatrics
Kennedy Health System
Sewell, New Jersey

Jenna M. Kahn, MD
Warren Alpert Medical School at Brown University
Providence, Rhode Island

Marc Jeffrey Kahn, MD, MBA
Peterman-Professor of Medicine
Sr. Associate Dean
Department of Medicine
Division of Hematology/Medical Oncology
Tulane University School of Medicine
New Orleans, Louisiana

Monica Kaitz, MD
Warren Alpert Medical School of Brown University
Providence, Rhode Island

Abir O. Kanaan, PharmD
Associate Professor of Pharmacy Practice
Massachusetts College of Pharmacy and Health Sciences
Worcester, Massachusetts

Margo L. Kaplan Gill, MD
Assistant Professor
Department of Family Medicine
UMass Medical School
University of Massachusetts
Worcester, Massachusetts

Rahul Kapur, MD, BCSM
Director, Primary Care Sports Medicine Fellowship
Assistant Professor, Family Medicine and Sports Medicine
Department of Family Medicine and Community Health and University of Pennsylvania Sports Medicine Center
University of Pennsylvania Health System
Philadelphia, Pennsylvania

Ioannis Karakis, MD
Department of Neurology
Boston University Medical Center
Boston, Massachusetts

Atil Kargi, MD
Assistant Professor of Medicine
Department of Endocrinology
University of Miami Miller School of Medicine
Miami, Florida

Anand Karsan, MD
Clinical Instructor
Department of Emergency Medicine
University of Illinois Chicago
Chicago, Illinois

Darpreet Kaur, MBBS, DGO
Foreign Medical Graduate
Department of Obstetrics and Gynecology
Volunteer
PsychSupport Inc.
Raleigh, North Carolina

Tracy Kedian, MD
Assistant Professor
University of Massachusetts Medical School
Worcester, Massachusetts

Kristy Kedian Brown, DO
Associate Professor
Family Medicine
University of Massachusetts Medical School
Faculty
Family of Medicine
University of Massachusetts Memorial Hospital
Worcester, Massachusetts

Rick Kellerman, MD
Professor and Chair
Department of Family and Community Medicine
University of Kansas School of Medicine—Wichita
Wichita, Kansas

Brandi Kelly, PharmD
Adjunct Clinical Assistant Professor
University of Kansas School of Pharmacy
Lawrence, Kansas
University of Missouri—Kansas City School of Pharmacy
Kansas City Missouri
MedTrak Services
Overland Park, Kansas

John J. Kelly, MD
Associate Professor
Department of Surgery
University of Massachusetts Medical School
Chief
Department of Surgery
University of Massachusetts Memorial Medical Center
Worcester, Massachusetts

Susan C. Kent, PharmD, CGP
Clinical Assistant Professor
Department of Geriatric Medicine
Temple University School of Pharmacy
Philadelphia, Pennsylvania

Robert M. Kershner, MD, MS, FACS
Professor and Chairman
Department of Ophthalmic Medical Technology
Medical Director
Ophthalmic Medical Technology A.S. Degree Program
Eye Physician and Surgeon
Consultant Specialist
Pharmaceutical, Biomedical and Ophthalmic Medical Devices
Palm Beach, Florida

Benjamin M. Keyser, DO
General Surgery Residency Program
Georgia Health Sciences University
Medical College of Georgia
Augusta, Georgia

Omar A. Khan, MD, MHS, FAAFP
Clinical Assistant Professor
Department of Family Medicine
University of Pennsylvania
Jefferson Medical College
Philadelphia, Pennsylvania
Clinical Assistant Professor
University of Vermont
Burlington, Vermont
Attending Physician
Christiana Care Health System and A.I. DuPont Hospital for Children
University of Vermont
Burlington, Vermont

Salwa Khan, MD, MHS, FAAP
Pediatric Hospitalist
Department of Pediatrics
Children's Hospital of Philadelphia
Philadelphia, Pennsylvania

Birgit Khandalavala, MD
Associate Professor, Family Medicine
Creighton University
Omaha, Nebraska

Pooja Khandelwal, MD
Department of Pediatrics
University of Arizona
Tucson, Arizona

Morteza Khodaee, MD, MPH
Assistant Professor
Department of Family Medicine, Primary Care Sports Medicine CAQ
University of Colorado Denver School of Medicine
Denver, Colorado

Marie Kieras, MD
Department of Combined Internal Medicine and Pediatrics
University of Massachusetts
Worcester, Massachusetts

Daniel Y. Kim, MD
Chief, Head and Neck Surgery
Associate Professor, Otolaryngology—Head and Neck Surgery and Radiation Oncology
Department of Otolaryngology—Head and Neck Surgery
University of Massachusetts Medical School
University of Massachusetts Memorial Medical Center
Worcester, Massachusetts

Juhee Kim, MD
Resident Physician
Department of Family Medicine
David Grant Medical Center
Travis Air Force Base, California

Sam Seung Yeol Kim, MBBS, Mmed
Associate Clinical Lecturer
Department of Medicine
University of Sydney
Surgical Resident
Department of Surgery
Westmead Hospital
Westmead, Sydney, Australia

Walter M. Kim, MD, PhD
University of Massachusetts Medical School
Worcester, Massachusetts

Mitchell S. King, MD
Associate Professor of Family Medicine
Department of Family and Community Medicine—Rockford
University of Illinois College of Medicine
Rockford, Illinois

Jeffery T. Kirchner, DO, FAAFP, AAHIVS
Clinical Associate Professor
Department of Family and Community Medicine
Temple University School of Medicine
Philadelphia, Pennsylvania
Associate Director, Family Medicine Residency Program
Department of Family and Community Medicine
Lancaster General Hospital
Lancaster, Pennsylvania

Jason M. Kittler, MD, PhD, JD
Assistant Clinical Professor
Department of Internal Medicine
University of Massachusetts Medical School
Worcester, Massachusetts
Berkshire Medical Group
Pittsfield, Massachusetts

Jacob Kleinman, MD
University of Massachusetts Medical School
Worcester, Massachusetts

Michael S. Kleinman, DO
Fellow
Department of Neurology
Beth Israel Deaconess Medical Center
Boston, Massachusetts

Dagmar Klinger, MD
Assistant Professor
Department of Medicine
University of Massachusetts Medical School
Nephrologist
Department of Medicine
UMass Medical Center
Worcester, Massachusetts

Adam Klipfel, MD
Staff Surgeon
Department of Colorectal Surgery
Rhode Island Colorectal Clinic
Providence, Rhode Island

Teresa L. Knight, MD
Volunteer Clinical Faculty
Washington University School of Medicine
Volunteer Clinical Faculty
St. Louis University, Doisy College of Allied Heath
CEO, Women's Health Specialists of St. Louis
St. Louis, Missouri

Ajar Kochar, MD
The Warren Alpert Medical School at Brown University
Providence, Rhode Island

Kristen Koenig, MD, CPT, MC
Department of Family Medicine
Carl R. Darnall Army Medical Center
Fort Hood, Texas

Anjali Koka, MD
Department of Anesthesia, Critical Care and Pain Management
Massachusetts General Hospital
Boston, Massachusetts

Scott Kopec, MD
Department of Pulmonary Medicine
University of Massachusetts Medical Center
Worcester, Massachusetts

Michael Koster, MD
Assistant Clinical Professor of Pediatrics
Department of Pediatric Infectious Diseases
Alpert Medical School of Brown University
Hasbro Children's Hospital
Providence, Rhode Island

Daniel J. Kowal, MD
Division Director of Computed Tomography
Department of Radiology
St. Vincent's Hospital
Worcester, Massachusetts

Michael S. Krathen, MD
Department of Dermatology
Boston University School of Medicine
Department of Dermatology
Boston Medical Center
Boston, Massachusetts

Ronald M. Kreinbrink, MD, Capt USAF AMC 60 MDOS/SGOF
Department of Family Medicine
David Grant Medical Center
Travis Air Force Base, California

Allison Kreiner, MD
Resident
Department of Obstetrics and Gynecology
Akron General Medical Center
Akron, Ohio

Anita Krishnarao, MD MPH
Alpert Medical School of Brown University
Providence, Rhode Island

David W. Kruse, MD
Assistant Clinical Professor
Department of Orthopaedic Surgery and Family Medicine
University of California, Irvine
Irvine, California

E. James Kruse, DO, FACS
Assistant Professor of Surgery
Surgical Oncology Section
Assistant Professor of Surgery
Gynecology Oncology Section
Georgia Health Sciences University
Augusta, Georgia

Rebecca Kruse-Jarres, MD, MPH
Assistant Professor
Department of Medicine
Tulane University
New Orleans, Louisiana

Nancy Kubiak, MD
Associate Professor
Internal Medicine
University of Louisville
Louisville, Kentucky

Eric J. Kujawski, DO
Sports Medicine Fellow
Department of Family Medicine
University of Tennessee
Knoxville, Tennessee

Veena Kulchaiyawat, DO
Department of Family Medicine
University of California, Irvine
Orange, California

Alphonsus W. Kung, MD
Department of Family Medicine and Community Health
University of Massachusetts Medical School
Worcester, Massachusetts

Sindhu Kurian, MD
Clinical Instructor- Resident
Department of Family Medicine
Michigan State University/Kalamazoo Center for Medical Studies
Kalamazoo, Michigan

Jason M. Kurland, MD
Fellow, Department of Nephrology
Rhode Island Hospital/Brown University
Providence, Rhode Island

Daniel B. Kurtz, PhD
Assistant Professor
Department of Biology
Utica College
Utica, New York

Dylan C. Kwait, MD
Department of Diagnostic Imaging
Division of Diagnostic Radiology
Maimonides Medical Center
Brooklyn, New York

Mildred LaFontaine, MD
Department of Neurology
Concord Hospital
Concord, New Hampshire

Amara Lai, MD
Department of Family Medicine
Banner Good Samaritan Family Medicine
Phoenix, Arizona

Enrico C. Lallana, MD
Department of Neuro-Oncology
Kaiser-Permanente Sacramento Medical Center
Sacramento, California

Joann Lamb, MD
Family Practice Associates of Western PA, P.C.

Rahele Lameh, MD
Assistant Professor
Department of Family and Community Medicine
University of Texas Southwestern Medical Center

Stephen K. Lane, MD, FAAFP
Clinical Instructor
University of Massachusetts Medical School
Worcester, Massachusetts
Clinical Instructor
Boston University Medical School
Boston, Massachusetts

Eduardo Lara-Torre, MD
Associate Professor
Department of Obstetrics and Gynecology
Virginia Tech-Carilion School of Medicine
Associate Residency Program Director
Department of Obstetrics and Gynecology
Carilion Clinic
Roanoke, Virginia

Lars C. Larsen, MD
Professor
Department of Family Medicine
The Brody School of Medicine at East Carolina University
Greenville, North Carolina

Austin Larson, MD
Department of Pediatrics
The Children's Hospital
University of Colorado
Aurora, Colorado

Richard A. Larson, MD
Professor
Department of Medicine, Section of Hematology/Oncology
The University of Chicago
Chicago, Illinois

Lisa Laskiewicz, MD
Department of Medicine
University of Massachusetts Medical School
Worcester, Massachusetts

Tui A. Lauilefue, MD
John A. Burns School of Medicine
University of Hawaii
Honolulu, Hawaii

Margo Lauterbach, MD
Staff Psychiatrist
Neuropsychiatry Program
Sheppard Pratt Health System
Baltimore, Maryland

Justin P. Lavin, Jr., MD
Professor
Department of Obstetrics and Gynecology
Northeastern Ohio College of Medicine
Rootstown, Ohio
Vice Chairman, Chief of Maternal Fetal Medicine
Department of Obstetrics and Gynecology
Akron General Medical Center
Akron, Ohio

Matthew R. Lawler, MD
University of Massachusetts Medical School
Worcester, Massachusetts

Alexis Lawrence, MD
University of Massachusetts Medical School
Worcester, Massachusetts

Tinh Le, DO, MBA
Fort Worth, Texas

James J. Ledwith, Jr., MD
Program Director
UMass Fitchburg Family Medicine Residency
Fitchburg, Massachusetts

Damon F. Lee, MD
Assistant Professor of Family Medicine
John A. Burns School of Medicine, University of Hawaii
Honolulu, Hawaii

Daniel J. Lee, MD
Assistant Professor
Department of Otology and Laryngology
Harvard Medical School
Division of Otology and Neurotology
Department of Otolaryngology
Massachusetts Eye and Ear Infirmary
Boston, Massachusetts

Daniel T. Lee, MD
Associate Clinical Professor
Department of Family Medicine
David Geffen School of Medicine at UCLA
Los Angeles, California
Staff Attending
Department of Family Practice
UCLA Medical Center and Orthopaedic Hospital
Santa Monica, California

Juyong Lee, MD, PhD
Medical Associate
Cardiovascular Disease
St. Elizabeth's Medical Center
Boston, Massachusetts

Sarah Lee, MD
Department of Medicine
The Warren Alpert Medical School of Brown University
Providence, Rhode Island

Frederick Stuart Leeds, MD, MS
Assistant Professor
Department of Family Medicine
University of Cincinnati School of Medicine
Cincinnati, Ohio

Matthew R. Leibowitz, MD
Assistant Clinical Professor
Department of Medicine
David Geffen School of Medicine at UCLA
Attending Physician
Department of Infectious Diseases
UCLA Medical Center
Los Angeles, California

Meg Lekander, MD
Assistant Instructor in Family Medicine
Warren Alpert School of Medicine of Brown University
Providence, Rhode Island

Sergio A. Leon, MD
Rheumatology Fellow
Division of Rheumatology
University of Massachusetts Medical School
Worcester, Massachusetts

Andrew Leone, MD
Department of Urology
Brown Alpert Medical School
Rhode Island Hospital
Providence, Rhode Island

Deborah W. Leong, MD
Instructor
Harvard Medical School
Boston, Massachusetts
Department of Internal Medicine
Harvard Vanguard Medical Associates
Boston, Massachusetts

Maya Leventer-Roberts, MD, MPH
Department of Pediatrics
Mount Sinai School of Medicine
Mount Sinai Kravis Children's Hospital
New York, New York

Ruth Levesque, MD
Department of Obstetrics and Gynecology
University of Massachusetts Memorial Hospital
Worcester, Massachusetts

Jay H. Levin, MD
The Warren Alpert Medical School of Brown University
Providence, Rhode Island

Nikki A. Levin, MD, PhD
Associate Professor of Medicine
Division of Dermatology
University of Massachusetts Medical School
UMass Memorial Medical Center
Worcester, Massachusetts

Gary I. Levine, MD
Associate Professor
Residency Director
Department of Family Medicine
Brody School of Medicine
East Carolina University
Greenville, North Carolina

James H. Lewis, MD, FACP, FACG, AGAF
Professor of Medicine
Division of Gastroenterology
Georgetown University Medical Center
Washington, District of Columbia

Amy Li, DMD
General Dentist
Department of General Dentistry
Boston University
Boston, Massachusetts
University of Massachusetts
Worcester, Massachusetts

Jonathan T. Lin, MD
The Warren Alpert Medical School at Brown University
Providence, Rhode Island

Brian K. Linn, MD
Medical Staff
Department of Family Medicine/Sports Medicine
North Arkansas Regional Medical Center
Harrison, Arkansas

Jonathan Liu, MD
Warren Alpert Medical School of Brown University
Providence, Rhode Island

Kimberly E. Liu, MD, FRCSC, MSI
Assistant Professor
Department of Obstetrics and Gynecology
University of Toronto
Staff Physician
Mount Sinai Hospital
Toronto, Ontario, Canada

Nancy Y. Liu, MD
Associate Professor of Clinical Medicine
Department of Medicine
University of Massachusetts Medical School
Worcester, Massachusetts

John Paul Lock, MD
Assistant Professor
Department of Medicine
University of Massachusetts School of Medicine
Worcester, Massachusetts

Madaiah Lokeshwari, MD
Hospitalist
Department of Medicine
Heywood Hospital
Gardner, Massachusetts

David Longstroth, MD
Department of Family Medicine
Contra Costa Regional Medical Center
University of California
Martinez, California

Claudia M. Lora, MD
Instructor
Department of Medicine, Section of Nephrology
University of Illinois at Chicago
Faculty
Department of Medicine
University of Illinois Medical Center
Chicago, Illinois

Phyllis Losikoff, MD
Assistant Professor of Pediatrics
Alpert Medical School of Brown University
Providence, Rhode Island

Bency K. Louidor-Paulynice, MD
University of Massachusetts Medical School
Worcester, Massachusetts

Jane K. Louie, MD
Clinical Instructor
Department of Neurology, Division of Neurophysiology
Tufts University School of Medicine
Neurological Services, PC
Framingham, Massachusetts

Zhen (Richard) Lu, MD
Department of Family Medicine, Urgent Care
Orange Coast Memorial
Huntington Beach, California

Craig Lubin, MD
Austin Gastroenterology
Austin, Texas

Daniel Lubin, MD
Warren Alpert Medical School of Brown University
Providence, Rhode Island

Ann M. Lynch, PharmD, RPh, AE-C
Assistant Professor
Department of Pharmacy Practice
University of Massachusetts College of Pharmacy Health Science
Worcester, Massachusetts

Jonathan MacClements, MD
Professor and Chair/Program Director of the Family Medicine Department
University of Texas Health Center at Tyler
Tyler, Texas

David C. Mackenzie, MD
Assistant Instructor
Department of Emergency Medicine
The Warren Alpert Medical School of Brown University
Rhode Island Hospital
Providence, Rhode Island

Marina MacNamara, MSIV, MPH
Warren Alpert Medical School of Brown University
Providence, Rhode Island

Douglas W. MacPherson, MD, MSc(CTM), FRCPC
Associate Professor
Departments of Internal Medicine, Clinical Tropical Medicine, and Medical Microbiology
Faculty of Health Sciences, McMaster University
Hamilton, Ontario, Canada

Michelle Magid, MD
Clinical Assistant Professor
Texas A&M Health Science Center
Assistant Professor
University of Texas Medical Branch
Clinical Assistant Professor
University of Texas Southwestern, Seton Family of Hospitals in Austin
Austin, Texas
Psychiatry Director of ECT
Seton Mind Institute, Seton Family of Hospitals
Austin, Texas

Anne M. Mahoney, MD
Rush University Medical Center
Chicago, Illinois

Thomas W. Mahoney, MD
Family Medicine Resident
David Grant Medical Center Family Medicine Residency
Travis Air Force Base, California

Patrick Mailloux, DO
Assistant Professor of Medicine
Tufts University School of Medicine
Associate Program Director
Critical Care Medicine Fellowship
Baystate Medical Center
Springfield, Massachusetts

Barbara A. Majeroni, MD
Professor of Family and Community Medicine
Penn State Hershey Medical School
Hershey, Pennsylvania

M. Keenan Mak, MD
Department of Family Medicine
Creighton University Medical Centre
Omaha, Nebraska

Serena Mak, MD
Department of Diagnostic Imaging
Division of Diagnostic Radiology
Maimonides Medical Center
Brooklyn, New York

Maricarmen Malagon-Rogers, MD
Associate Professor
Department of Family Medicine
University of Tennessee Graduate School of Medicine
Director, Pediatric Nephrology
Department of Pediatrics
University of Tennessee Medical Center, Knoxville
Knoxville, Tennessee

George Malcolmson, MD
University of Massachusetts Medical School
Worcester, Massachusetts

Melanie J.S. Malec, MD
Fellow
Department of Family Medicine
Case Western Reserve University
University Hospitals Case Medical Center
Cleveland, Ohio
Family Medicine
Lake Health Physician Group
Chardon, Ohio

Shazia Malik, MD
Department of Family Medicine
Michigan State University - Kalamazoo Center for Medical Studies
Kalamazoo, Michigan

Samir Malkani, MD
Associate Clinical Professor of Medicine
Division of Endocrinology and Diabetes
University of Massachusetts Medical School
Worcester, Massachusetts

Michael A. Malone, MD
Assistant Professor
Associate Medical Director
Department of Family Medicine
Pennsylvania State Hershey College of Medicine
Staff
Department of Family Medicine
Pennsylvania State Milton S. Hershey Medical Center
Hershey, Pennsylvania

Joshua M.V. Mammen, MD, PhD
Assistant Professor
Department of Surgery
University of Kansas
Kansas City, Kansas

Lee A. Mancini, MD, CSCS, CSN
Assistant Professor
Department of Family Medicine and Community Health
University of Massachusetts Medical School
Sports Medicine Physician
Department of Family Medicine and Community Health
University of Massachusetts Medical Center
Worcester, Massachusetts

Daniel Mandell, MD
University of Massachusetts Medical School
Worcester, Massachusetts

Mark J. Manning, DO, MsMEL
Assistant Professor
Department of Obstetrics and Gynecology
University of Massachusetts Medical School
UMass Memorial Medical Center
Worcester, Massachusetts

Mariann Manno, MD
Associate Professor
Departments of Pediatrics and Emergency Medicine
University of Massachusetts Memorial Medical Center
Division Director
Department of Pediatrics
University of Massachusetts Memorial Children's Medical Center
Worcester, Massachusetts

Aaron S. Mansfield, MD
Clinician-Investigator/Fellow
Department of Medicine/Division of Hematology
Department of Oncology
Mayo Clinic
Rochester, Minnesota

Eric J. Mao, MD
Warren Alpert Medical School at Brown University
Providence, Rhode Island

Erin Marchand, MD
Travis AFB, California

Nathaniel Marchetti, MD
Associate Professor of Medicine
Department of Pulmonary and Critical Care Medicine
Temple University School of Medicine
Philadelphia, Pennsylvania

Murat Mardirossian, MD
Department of Family Medicine
University of California, Irvine
UC Irvine Douglas Hospital
Orange, California

Alina Markova, MD
The Warren Alpert Medical School of Brown University
Providence, Rhode Island

Robert A. Marlow, MD, MA
Professor of Clinical Family Medicine
Department of Family and Community Medicine
University of Arizona College of Medicine
Tucson and Phoenix, Arizona
Associate Director/Director of Research
Family Medicine Residency Program
Scottsdale Healthcare
Scottsdale, Arizona

William L. Marshall, MD
Associate Professor
Department of Medicine
University of Massachusetts Medical School
Attending Physician
Department of Medicine
University of Massachusetts/Memorial Medical Center
Worcester, Massachusetts

Michelle T. Martin, PharmD
Clinical Assistant Professor
Department of Pharmacy Practice
University of Illinois at Chicago
Clinical Pharmacist
Ambulatory Care Pharmacy
University of Illinois Medical Center at Chicago
Chicago, Illinois

Stephen A. Martin, MD, EdM
Instructor
Department of Family Medicine and Community Health
University of Massachusetts Medical School
Worcester, Massachusetts

Christina Master, MD
Associate Professor of Clinical Pediatrics
Department of Pediatrics
Perelman School of Medicine at the University of Pennsylvania
Associate Program Director, Primary Care Sports Medicine Fellowship
Department of Sports Medicine
The Children's Hospital of Philadelphia
Philadelphia, Pennsylvania

A. Raquel Mateo-Bibeau, MD
Infectious Disease Specialist
Department of Medicine
John F. Kennedy Medicine Center
St. Mary's Medical Center
Atlantis, Florida

Donnah Mathews, MD
Assistant Professor
Department of Medicine
Alpert School of Brown University
Attending Physician
Department of General Internal Medicine
Rhode Island Hospital
Providence, Rhode Island

Brent Matsuda, MD
University of Hawaii John A. Burn School of Medicine
Honolulu, Hawaii

Michele L. Matthews, PharmD, CPE, RPh
Associate Professor of Pharmacy Practice
Department of Pain Management
Massachusetts College of Pharmacy and Health Sciences
Clinical Pharmacy Specialist
Pain Management Center
Brigham and Women's Hospital
Boston, Massachusetts

Jason Matuszak, MD
Clinical Assistant Professor
Department of Family Medicine
University of Buffalo
Chief of Sports Medicine
Department of Sports Medicine
Excelsior Orthopaedics
Amherst, New York

Brandon Maughan, MD, MHS
Resident Physician
Department of Emergency Medicine
Alpert Medical School of Brown University
Rhode Island Hospital
Providence, Rhode Island

Karen L. Maughan, MD
Associate Professor
Attending Faculty
Department of Family Medicine
University of Virginia
Charlottesville, Virginia

George Maxted, MD
Faculty
Department of Family Medicine
Tufts University Family Medicine Residency at Cambridge Health Alliance
Tufts University
Cambridge, Massachusetts

Beth Mazyck, MD
Clinical Associate Professor
Department of Family Medicine and Community Health
University of Massachusetts Medical School
Worcester, Massachusetts
Vice President of Medical Services
Community Health Connections, Inc.
Family Health Center
Fitchburg, Massachusetts

Christiane Mbianda, MD
Internal Medicine Resident
Medical College of Wisconsin and Affiliated Hospitals
Milwaukee, Wisconsin

Margaret McCormick, MS, RN
Clinical Assistant Professor
Department of Nursing
Towson University
Towson, Maryland

Matthew McGuiness, MD
Clinical Fellow
Department of Cardiovascular Medicine
University of Massachusetts Medical School
Worcester, Massachusetts

Elizabeth Colman McKeen, MD
Department of Pediatrics
Harvard University
Massachusetts General Hospital for Children
Boston, Massachusetts

Patricia McQuilkin, MD
Assistant Professor
Department of Pediatrics
University of Massachusetts Medical School
Worcester, Massachusetts

Gary Mark McWilliams, MD
Executive VP Chief Ambulatory Services Officer
Ambulatory Operations
University Health System
San Antonio, Texas

Cody Mead, DO, CPT, MC, USA
Chief Resident
Family Medicine Residency
Carl R. Darnall Army Medical Center
Fort Hood, Texas

Eva Medvedova, MD
Assistant Professor
Department of Internal Medicine
University of Massachusetts Medical School
Worcester, Massachusetts

Michelle L. Mellion, MD
Assistant Professor of Neurology
Department of Neurology/Clinical Neurophysiology
Rhode Island Hospital
The Warren Alpert Medical School of Brown University
Providence, Rhode Island

Erika Mello, MD
University of Massachusetts Medical School
Worcester, Massachusetts

Priscilla Merriam, MD
Hematology/Oncology Fellow
Brown University Medical School
Providence, Rhode Island

Theo E. Meyer, MD, DPhil
Professor
Department of Cardiovascular Medicine
University of Massachusetts Medical School
Director
Cardiac Cath Lab
Department of Cardiology
University of Massachusetts Medical School
Worcester, Massachusetts

Sabrina Mia, MD
Department of Family Medicine
Summa Barberton Hospital (NEOUCOM)
Barberton, Ohio

Gregory D. Middleton, MD
Associate Professor
Department of Rheumatology
University of California, San Diego
San Diego, California

Tracy O. Middleton, DO
Chief, Family Medicine
Clinical Associate Professor
Midwestern University
Arizona College of Osteopathic Medicine
Glendale, Arizona

James P. Miller, MD
Medical Director, Pediatric Surgery
Cook Children's Medical Center
Fort Worth, Texas

Sandra Miller, MD
Assistant Director
Family Medicine Residency
Banner Good Samaritan Medical Center
Phoenix, Arizona

Jonathan Min, MD
University of Massachusetts Medical School
Worcester, Massachusetts

Jeffrey F. Minteer, MD
Clinical Associate Professor
Department of Family Medicine, Geriatrics, Palliative Medicine
University of Pittsburgh
Pittsburgh, Pennsylvania
Cinical Associate Professor
Penn State University
University Park, Pennsylvania
Department of Family Medicine
Program Director, Family Medicine Residency
Washington Hospital
Washington, Pennsylvania

Mark H. Mirabelli, MD
Assistant Professor
Department of Orthopaedics and Family Medicine
University of Rochester
Rochester, New York

Anna Mirk, MD
Instructor
Department of Medicine, Division of Geriatrics and Gerontology
Emory University School of Medicine
Atlanta VA Medical Center
Decatur, Georgia

Ann Mitchell, MD
Associate Professor of Clinical Neurology
Department of Neurology
University of Massachusetts Memorial Medical Center
Worcester, Massachusetts

Vinod P. Mitta, MD
University of Southern California Keck School of Medicine
Los Angeles, California

Payal Modi, MD, MScPH
Emergency Medicine Resident
Brown University
Rhode Island Hospital
Providence, Rhode Island

Bryan K. Moffett, MD
Assistant Professor
Department of Internal Medicine
University of Louisville School of Medicine
Hospitalist, Internal Medicine
University of Louisville
Louisville, Kentucky

Sean Monaghan, MD
Surgery Resident
Department of Surgery
Rhode Island Hospital
Alpert Brown Medical School of Brown University
Providence, Rhode Island

Jahan Montague, MD
Assistant Professor of Medicine
Department of Nephrology
University of Massachusetts Medical School
Worcester, Massachusetts

Tiffany A. Moore Simas, MD, MPH, MEd
Assistant Professor
Department of Obstetrics/Gynecology and Pediatrics
Director of Obstetrics and Gynecology Research Division
University of Massachusetts Medical School
Full-Time Generalist Obstetrician-Gynecologist
Department of Obstetrics and Gynecology
University of Massachusetts Medical Center—Memorial Campus
Worcester, Massachusetts

William J. Moran, DO
Affiliate Clinical Instructor
Department of Family Medicine
Chicago College of Osteopathic Medicine
Elmhurst, Illinois

Wynne Morgan, MD
Resident in Psychiatry
University of Massachusetts Medical School
Worcester, Massachusetts

Richard A. Moriarty, MD
Professor of Clinical Pediatrics
Department of Pediatrics
UMass Medical School
Pediatric Infectious Disease Consultant
Department of Pediatrics
UMass Memorial Health Care
Worcester, Massachusetts

Anna K. Morin, PharmD, RPh
Associate Dean
School of Pharmacy
Massachusetts College of Pharmacy and Health Sciences
Worcester, Massachusetts
Associate Professor
Pharmacy Practice
Manchester, Massachusetts
Clinical Pharmacist
Department of Pharmacy Services
Worcester State Hospital
Worcester, Massachusetts

Richard P. Moser, MD, FACS
Professor of Surgery
Director, Massachusetts Center for Translational Research in Neurosurgical Oncology
University of Massachusetts Medical School
Worcester, Massachusetts

Mohammad Ansar Mughal, MD
Family Practice
Community Medicine Associates
San Antonio, Texas

Christian Müller, PhD
Assistant Professor
Department of Pediatrics
University of Massachusetts Medical School
Worcester, Massachusetts

Herbert L. Muncie, Jr., MD
Professor
Director of Student Education
Department of Family Medicine
Louisiana State University School of Medicine
New Orleans, Louisiana

Amanda Murchison, MD
Assistant Professor
Department of Obstetrics and Gynecology
Virginia Tech—Carilion School of Medicine
Assistant Residency Program Director
Department of Obstetrics and Gynecology
Carilion Clinic
Roanoke, Virginia

Gregory Murphy, MD
University of Massachusetts Medical School
Worcester, Massachusetts

Eleftherios Mylonakis, MD
Associate Professor of Medicine
Division of Infectious Diseases
Harvard Medical School
Massachusetts General Hospital
Boston, Massachusetts

Shashidhara Nanjundaswamy, MD, MBBS, MRCP, DM
Assistant Professor
Department of Neurology
University of Massachusetts Medical School
Neurologist
Department of Neurology
University of Massachusetts Memorial Health Care
Worcester, Massachusetts

Johra Nasreen, MD
Department of Family Medicine
University Hospital
University of Texas Health Science Center
San Antonio, Texas

Beverly L. Nazarian, MD
Clinical Associate Professor of Pediatrics
Department of Pediatrics
University of Massachusetts Medical School
Pediatrician
Pediatric Primary Care
University of Massachusetts Medical Center
Worcester, Massachusetts

Donald A.F. Nelson, MD
Director of Medical Informatics
Cedar Rapids Medical Education Foundation
Active Medical Staff
Department of Family Medicine
St. Luke's Hospital
Cedar Rapids, Iowa

Elizabeth Ann Nelson, MD
Senior Associate Dean, Medicine-General Medicine
Baylor College of Medicine
Houston, Texas

Carla M. Nester, MD
Assistant Professor
Department of Medicine and Pediatrics
Division of Adult and Pediatric Nephrology
The University of Iowa Hospitals and Clinics
Iowa City, Iowa

Jessica Nguyen, DO
Department of Family Medicine
UT Southwestern
Dallas, Texas

Kim-Lien Nguyen, MD
Cardiovascular Imaging Fellow
Department of Cardiology
National Heart, Lung, and Blood Institute
Bethesda, Maryland

Maria de La Luz Nieto, MD
Obstetrics and Gynecology
University of Massachusetts Medical School
Worcester, Massachusetts

Prachaya Nitchaikulvatana, MD
Fellow, Department of Rheumatology
University of Massachusetts Medical School
Worcester, Massachusetts
New England Neurological Associates
Lawrence, Massachusetts

Thomas Noh, MD
University of Hawaii John A. Burn School of Medicine
Honolulu, Hawaii

Keith Nokes, MD, MPH
Assistant Professor
Department of Family Medicine and Community Health
University of Massachusetts Medical School
Worcester, Massachusetts
Clinical Instructor
Department of Family Medicine
Tufts University School of Medicine
Boston, Massachusetts

Rocio Nordfeldt, MD
Family Medicine Residency Program
UMass Medical School
Worcester, Massachusetts

David R. Norris, MD
Assistant Professor
Office of Student Programs
Dept. of Family Medicine
University of Mississippi Medical Center
Jackson, Mississippi

Laura L. Novak, MD
Associate Director
Barberton Family Practice Residency
Summa Barberton Hospital
Barberton, Ohio

Jennifer O'Brien, MD
Department of Internal Medicine
Alpert Medical School of Brown University
Providence, Rhode Island

Kelly O'Callahan, MD
Instructor
Department of Medicine
University of Massachusetts Medical School
Physician
Department of Gastroenterology
New England Gastroenterology Associates
Worcester, Massachusetts

Ira S. Ockene, MD
David and Barbara Milliken Professor of Preventive Cardiology
Director, Preventive Cardiology Program
University of Massachusetts Medical School
Worcester, Massachusetts

J. Michael O'Connell, Jr., MD
Associate Professor of Medicine
Department of Internal Medicine
Brown University
Providence VAMC
Providence, Rhode Island

John B. O'Donnell, MD
Associate Professor
Department of Medicine, Division of Hematology
College of Human Medicine
Michigan State University
Grand Rapids, Michigan

Jacqueline L. Olin, MS, PharmD, BCPS, CPP, CDE
Associate Professor of Pharmacy
Wingate University School of Pharmacy
Wingate, North Carolina

Jill SM Omori, MD
Associate Professor of Family Medicine and Community Health
University of Hawaii John A. Burn School of Medicine
Honolulu, Hawaii

Angeline Opina, MD
Department of Internal Medicine/Pediatrics
University of Oklahoma Health Science Center
Oklahoma City, Oklahoma

Amimi S. Osayande, MD
Assistant Professor
Department of Family and Community Medicine
UT Southwestern Medical School
Dallas, Texas

Hussam Osman, MD

Deepak K. Ozhathil, MD
University of Massachusetts Medical School
Worcester, Massachusetts

Kelly Pagidas, MD
Assistant Professor of Obstetrics and Gynecology
Obstetrics and Gynecology
Alpert Medical School of Brown University
Providence, Rhode Island

Nathan Tuaefu Palmer, MD
Capt, USAF, MC
Physician
Department of Family Medicine
David Grant Medical Center
Travis Air Force Base
Fairfield, California

Balakumar Pandian, MD
Assistant Professor
Internal Medicine and Pediatrics
University of Texas Southwestern
Hospitalist
Department of Internal Medicine
Brackenridge Hospital
Austin, Texas

Linda Paniagua, MD
Department of Internal Medicine
Alpert Medical School of Brown University
Providence, Rhode Island

Jon S. Parham, DO, MPH
Associate Professor
Department of Family Medicine
University of Tennessee, Graduate School of Medicine
Active Staff
Department of Family Medicine
University of Tennessee Medical Center
Knoxville, Tennessee

Douglas S. Parks, MD
Associate Professor
Family Medicine Residency
University of Wyoming
Chief
Division of Family Medicine
Cheyenne Regional Medical Center
Cheyenne, Wyoming

Birju B. Patel, MD, FACP
Assistant Professor of Medicine
Emory University School of Medicine
Division of Geriatrics and Gerontology
Department of Medicine
Atlanta VA Medical Center
Decatur, Georgia

Chintan K. Patel, MD
Department of Urology
Brown Alpert Medical School
Providence, Rhode Island

Deepak Patel, MD
Assistant Professor
Department of Family Medicine
Rush Medical College
Chicago, Illinois
Director of Sports Medicine
Rush-Copley Family Medicine Residency
Aurora, Illinois

Krunal Patel, MD
University of Massachusetts Medical School
Worcester, Massachusetts

Mahesh C. Patel, MD
Assistant Professor of Medicine
Division of Infectious Diseases
Department of Internal Medicine
University of Illinois
Chicago, Illinois

Mayha K. Patel, OMSIV
Department of Osteopathic Medicine
Western University of Health Sciences
Pomona, California

Neepa Patel, MD
Department of Neurology
Boston Medical Center
Boston, Massachusetts

Nihal Patel, MD
University of Massachusetts Medical School
Worcester, Massachusetts

Nilay Patel, MD
Department of Internal Medicine
Warren Alpert Medical School of Brown University
Providence, Rhode Island

Payal S. Patel, DO
Pediatric Hospitalist
Department of Pediatrics
Edward Hospital
Naperville, Illinois

Sagar C. Patel, MD
Warren Alpert Medical School of Brown University
Providence, Rhode Island

Danielle Patterson, MD, MSc
Assistant Professor, Obstetrics and Gynecology
Department of Urogynecology
University of Massachusetts Medical School
Worcester, Massachusetts

Elizabeth W. Patton, MD, MPhil
Department of Obstetrics and Gynecology
Northwestern University
Prentice Women's Hospital
Chicago, Illinois

Laura Paulin, MD, MHS
Montefiore Medical Center of the Albert Einstein College of Medicine
Bronx, New York

Liberto Pechet, MD, FACP
Professor Emeritus
Pathology and Medicine
University of Massachusetts Medical School
Director, Hematology Labs
Hospital Laboratories
University of Massachusetts Memorial Medical Center
Worcester, Massachusetts

Ernest Pedapati, MD
Cincinnati Children's Hospital
Cincinnati, Ohio

Rade N. Pejic, MD
Assistant Professor of Family Medicine
Tulane University
Lead Physician of Multi-Specialty Clinic
Department of Family Medicine
Tulane Medical Center
New Orleans, Louisiana

Elizabeth B. Pelkofski, MD
Department of Obstetrics and Gynecology
University of Massachusetts
Worcester, Massachusetts

Amy Pelletier, DO
Department of Pediatrics
Baystate Medical Center
Springfield, Massachusetts

Lisa Pelunis-Messier, PharmD
Adjunct Faculty Member
Department of Pharmacy
Clinical Pharmacy Research Services
Massachusetts College of Pharmacy
Worcester, Massachusetts

E. Anderson Penno, MD, MS
Department of Ophthalmology
Western Laser Eye Associates
Calgary, Alberta, Canada

Douglas A. Pepple, MD
Fellow
Department of Sports Medicine
University of Illinois at Chicago
University of Illinois at Chicago Medical Center
Chicago, Illinois

Ruben Peralta, MD, FACS
Director of Trauma and Critical Care Fellowship Program
Department of Surgery
Hamad Medical Corporation
Department of Medical Education
Senior Consultant, Surgery, Trauma and Care
Department of Surgery
Hamad General Hospital
Doha, Qatar, United Arab Emirates

Christine S. Persaud, MD
Clinical Assistant Instructor
Department of Family Medicine
Stony Brook University Medical Center
Stony Brook, New York

Adam B. Pesaturo, PharmD, BCPS
Critical Care Pharmacist
Department of Pharmacy Services
Baystate Medical Center
Springfield, Massachusetts

Kimberly A. Pesaturo, PharmD
Assistant Professor
Department of Pharmacy Practice
Massachusetts College of Pharmacy and Health Sciences
Clinical Specialist—Pediatrics
Department of Pharmacy
University of Massachusetts Memorial Medical Center
Worcester, Massachusetts

Bobby X. Peters, MD
Assistant Professor
Department of Emergency Medicine
University of Iowa
Iowa City, Iowa

Bruce B. Peters, DO
Associate Professor of Family Medicine
Department of Humanities, Health, and Society
The Herbert Wertheim College of Medicine
Department of Pediatrics/Internal Medicine and Addiction Medicine
Green Family Neighborhood HELP
Miami, Florida

Nicole D. Pilevsky, MD
Obstetrics and Gynecology
Capital Women's Care
Maple Lawn, Maryland

M. Halit Pinar, MD
Professor of Pathology and Laboratory Medicine
Alpert Medical School of Brown University
Providence, Rhode Island

Matthew C. Plosker, MD
Department of Family Medicine
University of Massachusetts Memorial Medical Center
Fitchburg, Massachusetts

Barbara R. Pober, MD
Geneticist
Children's Hospital Boston
Boston, Massachusetts

Edward Pokorny, MSIV
LMU-DCOM
Harrogate, Tennessee

Phyllis Pollack, MD
Associate Clinical Professor
Department of Pediatrics
University of Massachusetts Medical School
Consultant
Department of Pediatrics
University of Massachusetts Medical Center
Worcester, Massachusetts

Anna Porter, MD
Instructor of Medicine
Department of Medicine
Section of Nephrology
University of Illinois at Chicago College of Medicine
Chicago, Illinois

Michael Poshkus, MD
Assistant Professor of Medicine
The Warren Alpert Medical School of Brown University
Division of Infectious Diseases
Rhode Island Hospital
Providence, Rhode Island

Stacy E. Potts, MD, MEd
Assistant Clinical Professor
Department of Family Medicine and Community Health
University of Massachusetts
Family Physician
Department of Family Medicine and Community Health
University of Massachusetts Memorial Health Care
Worcester, Massachusetts

James Powers, DO, FACEP
Associate Dean for Clinical Affairs
Assistant Professor
Department of Emergency Medicine
Edward Via College of Osteopathic Medicine
Blacksburg, Virginia

Pia Prakash, MD
Department of Internal Medicine
The George Washington University Medical Center
Washington, DC

Abdullah Hasan Pratt, MD
Pritzker School of Medicine
University of Chicago
Chicago, Illinois

Thomas Price, MD
Assistant Professor
Division of Geriatric Medicine and Gerontology
Emory University
Chief, Department of Medicine
Wesley Woods Geriatric Hospital
Atlanta, Georgia

William A. Primack, MD
Clinical Professor of Medicine and Pediatrics
University of North Carolina Kidney Center
University of North Carolina School of Medicine
Chapel Hill, North Carolina

Kimberly Pringle, MD
Department of Emergency Medicine
Brown University/Rhode Island Hospital
Providence, Rhode Island

Colleen M. Prinzivalli, PharmD, BCPS
Clinical Medicine Pharmacist
Boston Medical Center
Boston, Massachusetts

Barbara Provo, MSN, APNP, CWOCN, FNP-BC
Coordinator, Wound, Ostomy and Continence Program
Froedtert Hospital
Nurse Practitioner
Division of Vascular Surgery and Wound Care
Wound and Ostomy Program
Froedtert Health
Milwaukee, Wisconsin

George Gunter A. Pujalte, MD
Clinical Lecturer
Department of Family Medicine
University of Michigan
University of Michigan Medical Center
Ann Arbor, Michigan

Elise H. Pyun, MD
Clinical Associate Professor
Department of Rheumatology
University of Massachusetts Medical School
Rheumatology Attending
Department of Medicine
University of Massachusetts Medical Center
Worcester, Massachusetts

Juan Qiu, MD, PhD
Associate Professor
Department of Family and Community Medicine
Pennsylvania State University College of Medicine
Attending Physician
Department of Family Medicine
Penn State Hershey Medical Group
State College, Pennsylvania

Jonna M. Quinn, DO
Aultman Hospital
Canton, Ohio

Diane Radford, MD, FACS, FRCSEd
Surgical Oncologist
Department of Surgical Oncology and Breast Surgery
St. Louis Cancer and Breast Institute
St. Louis, Missouri

Naureen B. Rafiq, MBBS, MD
Instructor, Family Medicine
Creighton University Medical Center
Omaha, Nebraska

Mhd Basheer Rahmoun, MD
Assistant Professor, Adjunct
Department of Pharmacy Practice
Massachusetts College of Pharmacy and Health Sciences
Clinical Research Fellow
Clinical Pharmacology Study Group
Worcester, Massachusetts

Amendeep Rai, MD
Department of Family Medicine
MSU/KCMS Family Medicine
Kalamazoo, Michigan

Jyoti Ramakrishna, MD
Assistant Professor
Department of Pediatrics
University of Massachusetts Medical School
University of Massachusetts Memorial Healthcare
Worcester, Massachusetts

Muthalagu Ramanathan, MD
Assistant Professor
Department of Internal Medicine
Division of Hematology/Oncology/BMT
University of Massachusetts Medical School
University of Massachusetts Medical Center
Worcester, Massachusetts

Neha P. Raukar, MD, MS
Assistant Professor of Emergency Medicine
Director, Division of Sports Medicine
Department of Emergency Medicine
Brown Alpert Medical School at Brown University
Providence, Rhode Island

Mohammed A. Razvi, BA
George Washington University School of Medicine and Health Sciences
Washington, District of Columbia

Tejesh S. Reddy, MBBS
Department of Family Medicine
Creighton University
Omaha, Nebraska

Jennifer Reidy, MD
Assistant Professor
Department of Family Medicine
University of Massachusetts Medical School
Worcester, Massachusetts

Marc Restuccia, MD
Clinical Associate Professor of Emergency Medicine
EMS Division Director
University of Massachusetts Medical School
Worcester, Massachusetts

Harlan Rich, MD
Associate Professor of Medicine
Alpert Medical School, Brown University
Director of Endoscopy
Rhode Island Hospital
Providence, Rhode Island

Derek M. Richardson, Capt USAF AMC 60 MDOS/SGOF
Department of Family Practice
David Grant Medical Center
Travis Air Force Base, California

Janet Ricks, DO
Assistant Professor
Department of Family Medicine
University of Mississippi Medical Center
Jackson, Mississippi

Katherine M. Riggert, DO
Sports Medicine Fellow
Department of Family Medicine
University of Massachusetts Medical School
Fitchburg, Massachusetts
Sports Medicine Fellow
Department of Family Medicine and Community Health
University of Massachusetts Memorial Hospital
Worcester, Massachusetts

Sheldon Riklon, MD
Assistant Professor
Third-year Clerkship Director
University of Hawaii John A. Burns School of Medicine
Honolulu, Hawaii

Daphne Robakis, MD
Resident
Department of Neurology
Boston Medical Center
Boston, Massachusetts

Teresa M. Robb, MD
Clinical Instructor
Department of Obstetrics and Gynecology
Jefferson Medical College of Thomas Jefferson University
Attending Physician
Department of Obstetrics and Gynecology
Albert Einstein Medical Center
Philadelphia, Pennsylvania

Michele Roberts, MD, PhD
Diplomate American Board of Pathology (AP/CP)
Diplomate American Board of Medical Genetics
Paxton, Massachusetts

Leslie Robinson-Bostom, MD
Associate Professor of Dermatology
Warren Alpert Medical School of Brown University
Providence, Rhode Island
Director
Division of Dermatopathology
Department of Dermatopathology
Rhode Island Hospital
Providence, Rhode Island

Ann M. Rodden, DO, MS
Assistant Professor
Department of Family Medicine
Medical University of South Carolina
Charleston, South Carolina

Jennifer L. Rogers, MD
Aultman Hospital
Canton, Ohio

Noah M. Rosenberg, MD
University of Massachusetts Medical School
Worcester, Massachusetts

Montiel T. Rosenthal, MD
Associate Clinical Professor
Department of Family and Community Medicine
University of Cincinnati
Director of Prenatal Clinic
Department of Family Medicine
The Christ Hospital
Cincinnati, Ohio

Steven E. Roskos, MD
Associate Professor
Department of Family Medicine
Michigan State University
College of Human Medicine
East Lansing, Michigan

N. Paul Rosman, MD
Professor of Pediatrics and Neurology
Boston University School of Medicine
Pediatric Neurology
Boston Medical Center
Boston, Massachusetts

Julie L. Roth, MD
Assistant Professor
Department of Neurology
The Warren Alpert Medical School of Brown University
Providence, Rhode Island

Leslie Roth, MD
Assistant Professor of Surgery
Department of Surgery
The Warren Alpert Medical School of Brown University
University Surgical Associates
Providence, Rhode Island

Jason Rothschild, MD
Warren Alpert Medical School of Brown University
Providence, Rhode Island

Michael Rousse, MD, MPH
Hospitalist Director
Department of Medicine
Northeastern Vermont Regional Hospital
St. Johnsbury, Vermont

Vibin Roy, MD
Department of Family Medicine
UT Southwestern
Dallas, Texas

Anna Rudnicki, MD
Assistant Professor
Department of Medicine
Division of Pulmonary and Critical Care Medicine
University of Massachusetts Medical School
Worcester, Massachusetts

Stephanie Ruest, MD
University of Massachusetts Medical School
Worcester, Massachusetts

Christine Runyan, PhD
Associate Clinical Professor
Department of Family Medicine and Community Health
University of Massachusetts Medical School
Department of Clinical Health Psychology in Primary Care
Hahnemann Family Health Center
Worcester, Massachusetts

Anup K. Sabharwal, MD, FACE
Clinical Assistant Professor
Department of Medicine
Herbert Wertheim College of Medicine
Florida International University
Miami, Florida

Rachel Sagor, MD
Department of Medicine
University of Massachusetts Medical School
Worcester, Massachusetts

Stanley Sagov, MD
Assistant Professor
Department of Family Medicine
University of Massachusetts
Worcester, Massachusetts
Chief of Family Medicine
Department of Medicine
Mount Auburn Hospital
Cambridge, Massachusetts

Wayra Salazar-Moreno, MD
Infectious Diseases Fellow
Department of Infectious Diseases
University of Massachusetts
Worcester, Massachusetts

Rahma Salim, MD
Trauma and Critical Care Fellow
Trauma Surgery Section
Hamad General Hospital
Doha, Qatar

Tracey Samko, MD
University of Massachusetts Medical Center
Worcester, Massachusetts

Ricardo A. Samson, MD
Professor
Department of Pediatrics
The University of Arizona
Chief
Section of Pediatric Cardiology
University Medical Center
Tucson, Arizona

Arthur B. Sanders, MD, MHA
Professor
Department of Emergency Medicine
University of Arizona College of Medicine
Tucson, Arizona

Mark A. Sanders, DO, JD, MPH, LLM, FACOFP
Chair and Associate Professor
Department of Family Medicine
Chicago College of Osteopathic Medicine
Midwestern University
Downers Grove, Illinois

David Sapienza, MD
University of Massachusetts Medical School
Worcester, Massachusetts

Dillon Savard, MD
Faculty
Family Medicine Residency
David Grant Medical Center
Fairfield, California

Shailendra K. Saxena, MD, PhD
Assistant Professor, Family Medicine
Creighton University School of Medicine
Omaha, Nebraska

Dalia Sbat, PharmD
Adjunct Faculty
Department of Pharmaceutical Science
Massachusetts College of Pharmacy and Health Sciences
Worcester, Massachusetts
Pharmacist
Walgreens Pharmacy
Shrewsbury, Massachusetts

Andres Schanzer, MD, FACS
Associate Professor of Surgery and Quantitative Health Sciences
Program Director
Vascular Fellowship and Residency
University of Massachusetts Medical School
Worcester, Massachusetts

Fred Schiffman, MD
Vice Chairman, Department of Medicine
Sigal Family Professor of Humanistic Medicine
Clinical Director, Comprehensive Cancer Center
Professor of Medicine
Alpert Medical School of Brown University
The Miriam Hospital
Providence, Rhode Island

Karl M. Schmitt, MD
Assistant Director
Residency in Family Medicine
St. Elizabeth Medical Center
Associate Professor
University of Cincinnati College of Medicine
Family Medicine
Edgewood, Kentucky
Chairman
Department of Medicine
St. Elizabeth Medical Center
Edgewood, Kentucky

Justine M. Schober, MD, FAAP
Director of Academic Research
UPMC Hamot Medical Center
Erie, Pennsylvania

Lisa M. Schroeder, MD
Assistant Director
Family Practice Residency Program
Summa Barberton Hospital
Assistant Professor of Family Medicine, NEOUCOM
Barberton, Ohio

Alexandra A. Schultes, MD
Associate Professor
Department of Family Practice
University of Massachusetts
Worcester, Massachusetts

Jennifer Schwartz, MD
Primary Care Sports Medicine Fellow
Department of Sports Medicine
University of Massachusetts
Fitchburg, Massachusetts

Christopher J. Scola, MD
Clinical Assistant Professor of Medicine
University of Connecticut School of Medicine
Rheumatology Consultant
Hartford Hospital
Hartford, Connecticut

Ingrid U. Scott, MD
Professor of Ophthalmology and Public Health Sciences
Penn State College of Medicine
Hershey, Pennsylvania

Stephen M. Scott, MD, MPH
Associate Professor
Department of Family Medicine
Weill Cornell Medical College in Qatar
New York, New York

Gail Scully, MD, MPH
Assistant Professor
Department of Internal Medicine
Division of Infectious Disease and Immunology
University of Massachusetts Medical School
Worcester, Massachusetts

David P. Sealy, MD
Clinical Professor
Department of Family Medicine
Director, Primary Care Sports Medicine Fellowship
Department of Sports Medicine
Self Regional Healthcare
Medical University South Carolina
Greenwood, South Carolina

Amber Seba, MD
Fellow
Hematology and Oncology
University of Illinois College of Medicine
Chicago, Illinois

Sheila M. Seed, PharmD, MPH
Associate Professor
Department of Pharmacy Practice
Massachusetts College of Pharmacy and Health Sciences
Worcester, Massachusetts

Harry W. Sell, Jr., MD, FACS
Chairman
Department of Surgery
UPMC Mercy
Pittsburgh, Pennsylvania

Morgan Sendzischew, MD
University of Miami Miller School of Medicine
Miami, Florida

Sudha Seshadri, MD
Professor of Neurology
Boston University School of Medicine
Boston, Massachusetts

Patricia Seymour, MD
Assistant Professor
Department of Family Medicine and Community Health
University of Massachusetts Medical School
Worcester, Massachusetts

Amy Shah, MD
Chief Resident
Department of Psychiatry
University of Cincinnati
The University Hospital
Cincinnati, Ohio

Meera Shah, MD
George Washington University School of Medicine and Health Sciences
Washington, District of Columbia

Samir A. Shah, MD
Clinical Associate Professor of Medicine
Department of Gastroenterology
Chief of Gastroenterology
The Miriam Hospital Gastroenterology Associates
Providence, Rhode Island

Daniel J. Shaheen, PharmD
Adjunct Assistant Professor
Department of Pharmacy Practice
Massachusetts College of Pharmacy and Health Sciences
Worcester, Massachusetts

Mohammad Shahsahebi, MD
Department of Community and Family Medicine
Duke University Medical Center
Durham, North Carolina

Irina Shakhnovich, MD, MS
Vascular Surgery Fellow
Medical College of Wisconsin
Milwaukee, Wisconsin

Kevin C. Shannon, MD, MPH, FAAFP
Assistant Professor
Department of Community and Family Medicine
Dartmouth Medical School
Department of Family Medicine
Dartmouth-Hitchcock Clinic
Lebanon, New Hampshire

Archit Sharma, MD
Department of Family Medicine
Creighton University Medical Center
Omaha, Nebraska

Puja Sharma, MD
PGY-3, Summa Barberton Family Practice Residency Program
Barberton, Ohio

Sanjeev K. Sharma, MD
Associate Professor
Department of Family Medicine
Creighton University School of Medicine
Omaha, Nebraska

Saurabh Sharma, MD
Assistant Professor
Department of Family Medicine
University of Massachusetts Medical School
Academic Hospitalist
University of Massachusetts Medical Center
Worcester, Massachusetts

Douglas Shemin, MD
Associate Professor
Department of Medicine
Brown University School of Medicine
Interim Director
Division of Kidney Diseases
Rhode Island Hospital
Providence, Rhode Island

Anna Shifrin, MD
Department of Internal Medicine
St. Vincent Hospital
Worcester, Massachusetts

Lisa Shives, MD
Northshore Sleep Medicine
The Linden Center for Sleep and Metabolic Disorders
Medical Director
Evanston, Illinois

Natasha Shur, MD
Assistant Professor
Department of Genetics
Alpert Medical School of Brown University
Providence, Rhode Island

Aamir Siddiqi, MD
Director
Department of Clinical Services
Norris Health Center
University of Wisconsin
Milwaukee, Wisconsin

Najmul H. Siddiqui, MBBS, MD
Department of Family Practice
Creighton University Medical Center
Omaha, Nebraska

Mark Sigman, MD
Chairman of Urology
The Miriam and Rhode Island Hospitals
The Warren Alpert School of Medicine of Brown University
Providence, Rhode Island

Hugh J. Silk, MD, MPH
Assistant Professor
Department of Family Medicine and Community Health
University of Massachusetts Medical School
Staff
Department of Family Medicine and Community Health
University of Massachusetts Memorial Medical Center
Worcester, Massachusetts

Rebecca Sills, MD
University of Massachusetts Medical School
Worcester, Massachusetts

Matthew A. Silva, PharmD, RPh, BCPS
Associate Professor of Pharmacy Practice
Department of Pharmacy Practice, Family Medicine
Massachusetts College of Pharmacy and Health Sciences
Clinical Pharmacist
Department of Family Medicine/Pharmacy
Family Health Center of Worcester
Worcester, Massachusetts

B. Brent Simmons, MD
Assistant Professor
Department of Family Medicine
Drexel University—College of Medicine
Philadelphia, Pennsylvania

Tracey G. Simon, MD
Warren Alpert Medical School of Brown University
Providence, Rhode Island

Linda Sinclair, MD
University of Massachusetts Medical School
Worcester, Massachusetts

Jaspreet Singh, DO
Assistant Professor
Department of Urology
Thomas Jefferson University Hospital
Philadelphia, Pennsylvania

Ravinder Singh, MD
Assistant Professor
Department of Family Medicine
SUNY at Buffalo
Olean, New York

Marcia Sirota, MD, FRCP(C)
Department of Psychiatry
Ruthless Compassion Institute
Toronto, Ontario, Canada

D. Ryan Skinner, DO
Department of Dermatology
O'Bleness Memorial Hospital
Athens, Ohio

Glenn Skow, MD, MPH
Clinical Assistant Instructor
Department of Family Medicine
Stony Brook University Medical Center
Stony Brook, New York

Patrick Smallwood, MD
Assistant Professor of Psychiatry
Department of Psychiatry
University of Massachusetts Medical School
Attending Psychiatrist/Medical Director of Psychosomatic Medicine and Emergency Mental Health
UMass Medical Center
Worcester, Massachusetts

Michael Smit, OD, OMS IV
Pacific Northwest University College of Osteopathic Medicine
Yakima, Washington

Gregory D. Smith, DO, FACOFP
Associate Vice President of External Affairs, Health Sciences
Senior Associate Dean, DeBusk College of Osteopathic Medicine
Lincoln Memorial University
Harrogate, Tennessee

Stanley G. Smith, MA, MB, CCFP, FCFP
Professor Emeritus
Department of Family Medicine
University of Western Ontario
Department of Family Medicine
London East Medical Centre
London, Ontario, Canada

John C. Smulian, MD, MPH
Vice Chair and Chief of Maternal Fetal Medicine
Department of Obstetrics and Gynecology
Lehigh Valley Health Network
Allentown, Pennsylvania

Rachel A. Sneed, MD
Assistant Professor
University of Cincinnati College of Medicine
Cincinnati, Ohio
Assistant Professor
Clinton Memorial Hospital Family Medicine Residency Program
Wilmington, Ohio

Kimberly Snyder, MD
Department of Emergency Medicine
Capitol Emergency Associates
Austin, Texas

Michael Snyder, MD
Professor
Department of Medicine - Hematology/Oncology, Pathology
University of Massachusetts Medical School
Worcester, Massachusetts

Albert Sohn, MD
College of Medicine, University of Illinois at Chicago
Chicago, Illinois

Augustine J. Sohn, MD, MPH
Assistant Professor
Department of Clinical Family Medicine
Department of Family Medicine
University of Illinois at Chicago
Attending Physician
Department of Family Medicine
University of Illinois Hospital
Chicago, Illinois

Patricia Solga, MD
Pediatric Orthopaedic Surgeon
Warren Alpert School of Medicine at Brown University
Providence, Rhode Island

Weily Soong, MD
Clinical Associate Professor
Department of Pediatric Allergy and Immunology
University of Alabama School of Medicine
Managing Partner
Alabama Allergy and Asthma Center
Birmingham, Alabama

Mia D. Sorcinelli, MD
Attending Physician
Department of Family Medicine
Lawrence General Hospital
Lawrence, Massachusetts

Adam J. Sorscher, MD
Assistant Professor
Department of Psychiatry
Dartmouth Medical School
Physician
Department of Family Medicine and Sleep Medicine
Dartmouth-Hitchcock Medical Center
Lebanon, New Hampshire

Leslie Soyka, MD
Associate Professor
Department of Pediatrics
Division of Pediatric Endocrinology
University of Massachusetts Medical School
Worcester, Massachusetts

Mikayla Spangler, PharmD, BCPS
Assistant Professor
Creighton University School of Pharmacy and Health Professions
Clinical Pharmacist, Creighton Family Healthcare
Omaha, Nebraska

John Spittler, MD, MS
Department of Family Medicine
University of Colorado
Aurora, Colorado

Joshua J. Spooner, PharmD, MS
Director of Clinical and Outcomes Services
Advanced Concepts Institute
University of the Sciences in Philadelphia
Philadelphia, Pennsylvania

Kellie A. Sprague, MD
Assistant Professor
Division of Hematology-Oncology
Tufts University School of Medicine
Assistant Director
Bone Marrow Transplant Program
Division of Hematology-Oncology
Tufts Medical Center
Boston, Massachusetts

Dana Sprute, MD, MPH
Assistant Professor
Department of Family and Community Medicine
University of Texas Southwestern Medical Center
Assistant Clinical Professor
University of Texas Medical Branch
Austin, Texas

Michelle St. Fleur, MD
University of Massachusetts Medical School
Worcester, Massachusetts

Joan M. Stachnik, PharmD, BCPS
Clinical Assistant Professor
Drug Information Group
Department of Pharmacy Practice
College of Pharmacy
University of Illinois Medical Center at Chicago
Chicago, Illinois

Michael S. Stalvey, MD
Assistant Professor, Pediatric Endocrinology
Department of Pediatrics
University of Alabama School of Medicine
Birmingham, Alabama

Oscar Starobin, MD
Department of Cardiology
University of Massachusetts Medical Center
Worcester, Massachusetts

Daniel Stein, BA
Boston University School of Medicine
Boston, Massachusetts

Gillian S. Stephens, MD, MSc
Assistant Professor
Department of Family and Community Medicine
St. Louis University
St. Louis, Missouri

Debora B. Sternaman, PharmD
Regional Medical Scientist
Department of Medical Affairs
Boehringer Ingelheim
Georgetown, Texas

Edward C. Sternaman II, MD
Hospitalist
Department of Internal Medicine
Seton Williamson
Round Rock, Texas

J. Herbert Stevenson, MD
Director, Sports Medicine Fellowship
Department of Family and Community Medicine
University of Massachusetts Medical School
Director, Sports Medicine
Department of Family and Community Medicine
University of Massachusetts Memorial Medical Center
Worcester, Massachusetts

Lara Stewart, DO, MPH
Family Medicine
Westchester, California

Sheila O. Stille, DMD, MAGD
Assistant Professor
Department of Family Medicine and Community Health
University of Massachusetts Medical School
Program Director, General Practice Residency in Dentistry
Department of Family Medicine and Community Health
University of Massachusetts Memorial
Worcester, Massachusetts

Christy Stine, MD, PhD
Assistant Professor
Department of Pediatrics, Division of Pediatric Neurology
University of Massachusetts Memorial Children's Medical Center
Worcester, Massachusetts

Jeffrey G. Stovall, MD
Associate Professor
Department of Psychiatry
Vanderbilt University School of Medicine
Residency Training Director, Adult Psychiatry
Vanderbilt Psychiatric Hospital
Nashville, Tennessee

Ryung Suh, MD, MPP, MBA, MPH
Assistant Professor
Health Systems Administration
Georgetown University
Washington, District of Columbia
Command Surgeon and Occupational Health Division Chief
Defense Threat Reduction Agency
Fort Belvoir, Virginia

Karyn M. Sullivan, PharmD, MPH, RPh
Associate Professor
Department of Pharmacy Practice
Massachusetts College of Pharmacy and Health Sciences
Clinical Pharmacist
Department of Pharmacy
St. Vincent Hospital
Worcester, Massachusetts

Heather Summe, MD
University of Massachusetts Medical School
Worcester, Massachusetts

Sana Syed, MD
Department of Neurology
Boston Medical Center
Boston, Massachusetts

Vassiliki P. Syriopoulou, MD
Emeritus Professor of Pediatrics
First Department of Pediatrics
Athens University
Chief of Infectious Diseases
First Department of Pediatrics
Aghia Sophia Children's Hospital
Athens, Greece

Alfonso J. Tafur, MD, RPVI
Assistant Professor of Medicine
Department of Vascular Medicine
Oklahoma University Health and Sciences Center
Oklahoma City, Oklahoma

Denisse Tafur Chang, MD
Universidad de Especialidades Espiritu Santo
Guayaquil, Ecuador

Komal Talati, MD
The Warren Alpert Medical School of Brown University
Providence, Rhode Island

Christine Tam, MD
University of Massachusetts Medical School
Worcester, Massachusetts

Emmanouil Tampakakis, MD
Chemical Biology
Massachusetts General Hospital
Boston, Massachusetts

Irene J. Tan, MD
Assistant Clinical Professor of Medicine
Columbia Presbyterian College of Physicians and Surgeons
Department of Rheumatology
Stamford Arthritis Care, LLC
Stamford, Connecticut

Weizhen Tan, MD
Pediatric Resident
Yale-New Haven Hospital
New Haven, Connecticut
University of Massachusetts Medical School
Worcester, Massachusetts

Chris Tang, MD
Occupational Medicine
Care On Site
Long Beach, California

Dawn S. Tasillo, MD
Associate Clerkship Director
Department of Obstetrics and Gynecology
University of Massachusetts Medical School
Assistant Professor
UMass Memorial Medical Center
Worcester, Massachusetts

Joao Tavares, MD
Clinical Assistant Professor of Medicine
Department of Internal Medicine
Warren Alpert Medical School of Brown University
Providence, Rhode Island

Eugene M. Tay, MD, MS
Assistant Professor
Department of Family Medicine
College of Human Medicine
Michigan State University
Grand Rapids, Michigan

Cole Taylor, MD
Family Practice Clinic Director
Misawa Air Base Hospital
Aomori Prefecture, Japan

Julie Scott Taylor, MD, MSc
Associate Professor of Family Medicine
Alpert Medical School of Brown University
Providence, Rhode Island

Trevor Tejada-Berges, MD
Assistant Professor
Department of Gynecologic Oncology
Warren Alpert School of Medicine of Brown University
Women and Infants' Hospital
Providence, Rhode Island

Stacy Temple, DMD
General Dentist
Edward M. Kennedy Community Health Center
Clinton, Massachusetts

Richard Terek, MD
Associate Professor
Department of Orthopaedic Oncology
Warren Alpert Medical School of Brown University
Providence, Rhode Island

Melicien Tettambel, DO
Professor and Chair
Department of Osteopathic Principles and Procedures
Pacific Northwest University of Health Sciences—College of Osteopathic Medicine
Yakima, Washington

Alissa A. Thomas, MD
Department of Neurology
Dartmouth Hitchcock Medical Center
Lebanon, New Hampshire

Richard J. Thomas, MD, MPH
Associate Professor
Department of Preventive Medicine and Biometrics
Uniformed Services University of the Health Sciences
Acting Department Head
Department of Occupational Medicine
National Naval Medical Center
Bethesda, Maryland

Katherine Thompson, MD
Warren Alpert Medical School at Brown University
Providence, Rhode Island

Margaret E. Thompson, MD
Associate Professor
Department of Family Practice
Michigan State University College of Human Medicine
Grand Rapids, Michigan

Michelle A. Tinitigan, MD
Assistant Clinical Professor
Department of Family and Community Medicine
University of California, San Francisco
San Francisco, California

Adam J. Tinklepaugh, MD
George Washington University School of Medicine and Health Sciences
Washington, District of Columbia

Kinga K. Tomczak, MD, PhD
Pediatric Neurology Resident, PGY-4
Boston Medical Center
Boston University Medical School
Boston, Massachusetts

Sebastian T.C. Tong, MD, MPH
Boston University School of Medicine
Health Care Management and Policy
Harvard School of Public Health
Boston, Massachusetts

Moshe S. Torem, MD, DLFAPA
Professor of Psychiatry
Department of Psychiatry
Northeastern Ohio Universities College of Medicine
Rootstown, Ohio
Chief of Integrative Medicine
Department of Medicine
Akron General Medical Center and Center for Mind-Body Medicine
Akron, Ohio

William A. Tosches, MD
Associate Clinical Professor of Neurology and Medicine
Department of Neurology
University of Massachusetts Medical School
Worcester, Massachusetts
Chief of Neurology Service
Milford Regional Medical Center
Milford, Massachusetts

Khasha Touloei, DO
Western College of Health Sciences
Pomona, California

Alyssa H. Tran, DO
Department of Family and Community Medicine
University of Texas Health Science Center
University Hospital
San Antonio, Texas

Natasha A. Travis, MD
Assistant Professor of Medicine
Department of General Internal Medicine
Medical College of Wisconsin
Froedtert Hospital
Milwaukee, Wisconsin

Samir K. Trehan, MD
Department of Orthopedic Surgery
The Warren Alpert Medical School of Brown University
Providence, Rhode Island

Zoltan Trizna, MD, PhD
Private Practice, Dermatology
Austin, Texas

Katherine Tromp, PharmD
Assistant Professor
Department of Pharmacy Practice
Lake Erie College of Osteopathic Medicine
LECOM—Bradenton School of Pharmacy
Bradenton, Florida

Richard E. Trowbridge, MD
Department of Family Medicine
David Grant Medical Center
Travis Air Force Base, California

Caroline Tschibelu, MD
Department of Emergency Medicine
Alpert Medical School at Brown University
Providence, Rhode Island

Kristin A. Tuiskula, PharmD, RPh
Assistant Professor
Pharmacy Practice
Massachusetts College of Pharmacy and Health Sciences
Worcester, Massachusetts

Deepali Tukaye, MD, PhD
Department of Internal Medicine
University of Louisville
Louisville, Kentucky

Katharine Tumilty, MD
University of Massachusetts Medical School
Worcester, Massachusetts

Auguste Turnier, MD
Internist/Gastroenterologist, Private Practice
Haddonfield, New Jersey

Lawrence E. Udom, MD, MPH
Department of Psychiatry/Family Medicine, Sports Medicine
Max Sports Medicine Program
Riverside Methodist Hospital
Columbus, Ohio

Meredith Ulmer, DO
Department of Family Medicine
Resurrection Medical Center
Chicago, Illinois

Katherine Upchurch, MD
Clinical Professor
Department of Medicine
University of Massachusetts Medical School
Clinical Chief
Division of Rheumatology
UMass Memorial Medical Center
Worcester, Massachusetts

Richard P. Usatine, MD
Professor
Department of Family and Community Medicine
University of Texas Health Science Center at San Antonio
San Antonio, Texas

Santiago O. Valdes, MD
Assistant Professor
Department of Pediatrics
University of Arizona
Tucson, Arizona

Anthony Valdini, MD, MS, FACP, FAAFP
Director of Research
Director of the Faculty Development Fellowship
Director of Faculty Development
Greater Lawrence Family Health Center
Lawrence, Massachusetts

Kelly Valla, PharmD
Department of Hematology/Oncology
University of Illinois at Chicago
Chicago, Illinois

Bonnie Vallie, MD
Department of Internal Medicine
Cleveland Clinic
Cleveland, Ohio

Ron Van Ness-Otunnu, MD
House Staff Officer
Department of Emergency Medicine
Warren Alpert Medical School of Brown University
Rhode Island Hospital
Providence, Rhode Island

Virginia VanDuyne, MD
Chief Resident
Department of Family Medicine
University of Massachusetts Family Medicine Residency Program
Worcester, Massachusetts

Elizabeth Varadian, DO, MS
Natividad Medical Center
Salinas, California

Adam P. Vasconcellos, MD
Department of Internal Medicine
Harvard Medical School
Brigham and Women's Hospital
Boston, Massachusetts

Timothy Veal, MD
Department of Psychiatry—Transitional
Naval Medical Center
San Diego, California

Jake D. Veigel, MD
University of Massachusetts Primary Care Sports Medicine Fellowship
University of Massachusetts Medical School
Fitchburg, Massachusetts

Martina Vendrame, MD, PhD
Assistant Professor in Neurology
Department of Neurology
Boston University
Boston, Massachusetts

Michael P. Vezeridis, MD
Professor of Surgery
Department of Surgery
Warren Alpert Medical School of Brown University
Providence, Rhode Island

Tiffany Victor, DO
Department of Internal Medicine
Ohio University Heritage College of Osteopathic Medicine—St. Joseph Health Center
Warren, Ohio

Siva Vithiananthan, MD
University Surgical Associates Inc.
Providence, Rhode Island

Stacey Vitiello, MD
Montclair Breast Center
Montclair, New Jersey

Emily Von Bargen, MD
Department of Obstetrics and Gynecology
University of Massachusetts Medical School
Worcester, Massachusetts

Kenton I. Voorhees, MD
Associate Professor and Vice Chair, Education
Department of Family Medicine
University of Colorado Denver School of Medicine
Aurora, Colorado

Yongkasem Vorasettakarnkij, MD, MSc
Instructor, Department of Medicine
Faculty of Medicine
Chulalongkorn University
Bangkok, Thailand
Research Fellow, Program in Cardiovascular MR
Martinos Center for Biomedical Imaging
Massachusetts General Hospital
Charlestown, Massachusetts

Kunal K. Vyas, DO
Western University of Health Sciences College of Osteopathic Medicine
Pomona, California

Jaime Wagner, MD
Department of Emergency Medicine
The Warren Alpert Medical School of Brown University
Department of Emergency Medicine
Rhode Island Hospital
Providence, Rhode Island

John B. Waits, MD
Associate Professor/Program Director-Tuscaloosa Family Medicine Residency
Department of Family Medicine/Obstetrics and Gynecology
University of Alabama School of Medicine
Physician
Department of Family Medicine/Obstetrics
DCH Regional Medical Center
Tuscaloosa, Alabama

L. Marie Walsh, MD
Family Medicine
Loveland Community Health Center
Loveland, Colorado

William V. Walsh, MD
Assistant Professor of Medicine
Division of Hematology Oncology
University of Massachusetts Medical School
UMass Memorial Medical Center
Worcester, Massachusetts

Annie R. Wang, MD
Warren Alpert Medical School of Brown University
Providence, Rhode Island

Terri Warren, MEd, BSN, MSN
Department of Sexually Transmitted Infections
Westover Heights Clinic
Portland, Oregon

Donald E. Watenpaugh, PhD
Adjunct Professor
Department of Integrative Physiology
University of North Texas Health Science Center
Fort Worth, Texas
Adjunct Professor
Department of Biomedical Engineering
University of Texas at Arlington
Arlington, Texas

Kathryn Watts, MD
George Washington University School of Medicine and Health Sciences
Washington, District of Columbia

Ramothea L. Webster, MD, PhD
Department of Family Medicine
United States Air Force Medical Corp.
Langley Air Force Base
Hampton, Virginia

Patrice Weiss, MD
Professor
Department of Obstetrics and Gynecology
Virginia Tech—Carilion School of Medicine
Residency Program Director and Vice-Chair
Department of Obstetrics and Gynecology
Carilion Clinic
Roanoke, Virginia

Frederick C. Weitendorf, RPH, RN
Assistant Clinical Professor of Pharmacy
Sullivan University College of Pharmacy
Critical Care Pharmacist
VA Medical Center
Louisville, Kentucky

Nathan Weldon, MD
Department of Family Medicine
Southern California Permanente Medical Group
Riverside, California

Lawren D. Wellisch, MD
The Alpert Medical School of Brown University
Providence, Rhode Island

Amanda Westlake, MD
Alpert Medical School of Brown University
Providence, Rhode Island

Andrew J. Westwood, MD
Department of Neurology
Boston Medical Center
Boston, Massachusetts

Vernon Wheeler, Jr., MD, FAAFP
Assistant Professor
Department of Family and Community Medicine
Uniformed Services University School of Medicine
Chief
Family Medicine Obstetrics
Carl R. Darnall Army Medical Center
Fort Hood, Texas

Chris Wheelock, MD
Faculty Southwest Washington Family Medicine
Clinical Instructor of Family Medicine University of Washington
Vancouver, Washington

Diane L. Whitaker-Worth, MD
Associate Professor of Dermatology
University of Connecticut
Farmington, Connecticut

Brett White, MD
Associate Professor
Associate Residency Director
Medical Director
Department of Family Medicine
Oregon Health and Science University
Portland, Oregon

Christopher C. White, MD, JD, FCLM
Assistant Professor
Department of Psychiatry and Family Medicine
University of Cincinnati College of Medicine
Medical Director, Psychiatric Consultation
Department of Psychiatry and Behavioral Neuroscience
University Hospital
Cincinnati, Ohio

Kelsey A. White, PharmD
Adjunct Assistant Professor
Massachusetts College of Pharmacy and Health Sciences
Worcester, Massachusetts

Michelle Whitehurst-Cook, MD
Associate Professor of Family Medicine
Associate Dean for Admissions
VCU School of Medicine
Richmond, Virginia

Janice F. Wiesman, MD
Assistant Professor
Department of Neurology
Boston University School of Medicine
Boston Medical Center
Boston, Massachusetts

Elaina C. Wild, MD
Department of Family Medicine
David Grant Medical Center
Fairfield, California

April Wilhelm, MD
Warren Alpert Medical School of Brown University
Providence, Rhode Island

Joanne E. Wilkinson, MD, MSc
Assistant Professor
Department of Family Medicine
Assistant Professor
Department of Community Health Sciences
Boston University Schools of Medicine and Public Health
Boston, Massachusetts

Alan L. Williams, MD
Adjunct Professor of Family Medicine
Department of Family Medicine
Uniformed Services University of the Health Sciences
Bethesda, Maryland

Pamela M. Williams, MD, Lt Col, USAF, MC
Assistant Professor of Family Medicine
Uniformed Services
University of Health Sciences
Program Director
David Grant Family Medicine Residency
David Grant Medical Center
Travis Air Force Base, California

Alan Williamson, MD
Department of Family Medicine/Sports Medicine
David Grant USAF Medical Center
Travis Air Force Base, California

Jessica Lenore Wilson, MD
University of Illinois at Chicago College of Medicine
Chicago, Illinois

Kathryn Wilson, MD
Resident
Department of Family Practice
University of Massachusetts Medical School
Worcester, Massachusetts

Leah Wilson, MD
Resident Physician
Department of Obstetrics and Gynecology
University of Massachusetts Medical School
Worcester, Massachusetts

Amy B. Wilson-LaMothe, PharmD
Massachusetts College of Pharmacy - Worcester
Worcester, Massachusetts

Robyn D. Wing, MD
Department of Pediatrics
University of Massachusetts Medical School
Worcester, Massachusetts

James Winger, MD
Assistant Professor
Department of Family Medicine
Loyola Stritch School of Medicine
Maywood, Illinois

Fawn Winkelman, DO
Resident Physician
Department of Family Medicine
Broward General Medical Center
Fort Lauderdale, Florida

Victoria Winn, MD
University of Massachusetts Medical School
Worcester, Massachusetts

Christopher M. Wise, MD
W. Robert Irby Professor of Medicine
Department of Internal Medicine
Division of Rheumatology
Virginia Commonwealth University Medical College of Virginia
Richmond, Virginia

Jeffrey D. Wolfrey, MD
Clinical Professor
Department of Family and Community Medicine
University of Arizona College of Medicine
Tucson, Arizona
Residency Director
Department of Family Medicine
Banner Good Samaritan Medical Center
Phoenix, Arizona

Zerlina Wong, MD
The Warren Alpert Medical School of Brown University
Providence, Rhode Island

Kyle D. Wood, MD
Department of Urology
Wake Forest University Baptist Medical Center
Winston-Salem, North Carolina

Fae G. Wooding, PharmD
Assistant Professor of Pharmacy Practice
Massachusetts College of Pharmacy and Health Sciences
Worcester, Massachusetts

Patrick J. Worth, MD
Department of Surgery
Oregon Health and Science University
Portland, Oregon

Frances Y. Wu, MD
Clinical Assistant Professor
Department of Family Medicine
UMDNJ—New Jersey Medical School
Newark, New Jersey
Assistant Director
Department of Family Practice
Somerset Medical Center
Somerville, New Jersey

Wesley Wu, MD
Warren Alpert Medical School of Brown University
Providence, Rhode Island

Hong Xiao, MD
Associate Professor
Department of Family Practice
University of Texas Southwestern Medical Center
St. Paul University Hospital
Parkland Memorial Hospital
Dallas, Texas

Joseph F. Yammine, MD
Clinical Assistant Professor of Medicine
Department of Cardiovascular Medicine
Warren Alpert Medical School of Brown University
Memorial Hospital of Rhode Island
Pawtucket, Rhode Island

Julie Yeh, MD, MPH
Assistant Professor
Department of Family, Community, and Preventive Medicine
Drexel University College of Medicine
Medical Staff
Department of Family, Community, and Preventive Medicine
Hahnemann University Hospital
Philadelphia, Pennsylvania

Gary Yen, MD
Assistant Professor
Department of Family Medicine
University of Michigan
Ann Arbor, Michigan

Robert A. Yood, MD
Clinical Professor of Medicine
Department of Medicine
University of Massachusetts Medical School
Chief
Division of Rheumatology
Fallon Clinic
Worcester, Massachusetts

Edward L. Yourtee, MD
Clinical Instructor
Department of Internal Medicine, Infectious Diseases
University of Vermont College of Medicine
Adjunct Assistant Professor of Medicine
Department of Internal Medicine, Infectious Diseases
Dartmouth Medical School
Southern New Hampshire Internal Medicine Associates
Derry, New Hampshire

Eleanor G. Yu, PharmD
Adjunct Assistant Professor
Massachusetts College of Pharmacy and Health Sciences
Worcester, Massachusetts

Leanne Zakrzewski, MD
Department of Family Medicine
University of California, Los Angeles, David Geffen School of Medicine
Los Angeles, California

Brian W. Zator, DO
Resident
Department of Family Medicine
Resurrection Medical Center
Chicago, Illinois

John K. Zawacki, MD
Professor of Medicine
Department of Medicine
Division of Gastroenterology
University of Massachusetts Medical School
UMass Memorial Health Care
Worcester, Massachusetts

Katrina Darlene Zedan, MSPAS, PA-C
Department of Acute Care/Family Medicine
University of Texas Health Science Center
First Assistant in Orthopaedic Surgery
Department of Surgery
Baptist and Methodist Health Systems
San Antonio, Texas

Di Zhao, MD, PhD
Fellow
Department of Nephrology
University of Massachusetts Medical School
Worcester, Massachusetts

Amy Zhou, MD
University of Massachusetts Medical School
Worcester, Massachusetts

D. Matthew Ziegler, MD
Resident Physician
Department of Family Medicine
North Colorado Family Medicine
Greeley, Colorado

Peter J. Ziemkowski, MD
Associate Professor
Department of Family Medicine
College of Human Medicine
Michigan State University
Clerkship Director
Family Medicine Residency Program
MSU/Kalamazoo Center for Medical Studies
Kalamazoo, Michigan

Susan Ziglar, MD
Assistant Professor
School of Pharmacy
Wingate University
Wingate, North Carolina

Richard Kent Zimmerman, MD, MPH
Professor
Department of Family Medicine
University of Pittsburgh
Pittsburgh, Pennsylvania

Thomas G. Zimmerman, DO, FACOFP
Director of Osteopathic Medical Education
Program Director
Osteopathic Family Medicine Residency
South Nassau Communities Hospital
Oceanside, New York
Clinical Assistant Professor of Family Medicine
New York College of Osteopathic Medicine
Old Westbury, New York

Gennine M. Zinner, RNCS, ANP
Clinical Instructor
Department of Nursing
MGH Institute of Health Professions
Adult Primary Care
Boston Health Care for the Homeless Program
Boston, Massachusetts

Trisna Zoltan, MD, PhD

Olivia Zurek, MD
University of Massachusetts Medical School
Worcester, Massachusetts

Susan L. Zweizig, MD
Associate Professor
Division of Gynecologic Oncology
Department of Obstetrics and Gynecology
University of Massachusetts Medical Center
Worcester, Massachusetts

CONTENTS

Topics

US Preventive Services Task Force Recommendations

This section is designed to be a quick reference to the best screening and prevention recommendations from the least biased sources. They are the US Preventive Services Task Force (USPSTF), the US Centers for Disease Control (CDC), the American Academy of Pediatrics, and the American Academy of Family Physicians.

The recommendations below should be tailored to patients' preferences. For example, **"The USPSTF recommends biennial screening mammography for women aged 50 to 74 years"** recommendation is just that, a recommendation; screening every year, or starting earlier, is a decision to be made between you and the patient. *An Informed Consent* discussion for screening empowers the patient and the clinician to use these recommendations in a patient-centered manner.

Absent in these recommendations "vested interests." Many disease-specific groups (American Cancer Society, the American Heart Association, National Osteoporosis Foundation, etc.) suggest interventions that serve *their* goals, but do not always have a strong evidence base. The USPSTF provides the most unbiased, evidence-based recommendations.

—Frank J. Domino, MD
Editor-in-Chief

Each intervention receives an evidence-based grading set by the USPSTF. They are:

2005 TASK FORCE RATINGS

Strength of Recommendations

The USPSTF grades its recommendations according to 1 of 5 classifications (A, B, C, D, I) reflecting the strength of evidence and magnitude of *net benefit* (benefits minus harms).

- **A.** The USPSTF strongly recommends clinicians provide [the service] to eligible patients. The USPSTF found good evidence that [the service] improves important health outcomes and concludes that benefits substantially outweigh harms.
- **B.** The USPSTF recommends clinicians provide [this service] to eligible patients. The USPSTF found at least fair evidence that [the service] improves important health outcomes and concludes that benefits outweigh harms.
- **C.** The USPSTF makes no recommendation for or against routine provision of [the service]. The USPSTF found at least fair evidence [the service] can improve health outcomes but concludes the balance of benefits and harms is too close to justify a general recommendation.
- **D.** The USPSTF recommends against routinely providing [the service] to asymptomatic patients. The USPSTF found at least fair evidence that [the service] is ineffective or that harms outweigh benefits.
- **I.** The USPSTF concludes the evidence is insufficient to recommend for or against routinely providing [the service]. Evidence the [service] is effective is lacking, of poor quality, or conflicting and the net benefit cannot be determined.

In 2008, the USPSTF updated their rating system for *all new recommendations*; they are:

GRADE DEFINITIONS AFTER MAY 2007

What the Grades Mean and Suggestions for Practice

The USPSTF has updated its definitions of the grades it assigns to recommendations and now includes "suggestions for practice" associated with each grade. The USPSTF has also defined levels of certainty regarding net benefit. These definitions apply to USPSTF recommendations voted on after May 2007.

Grade	Definition	Suggestions for Practice
A	The USPSTF recommends the service. There is high certainty that the net benefit is substantial.	Offer or provide this service.
B	The USPSTF recommends the service. There is high certainty that the net benefit is moderate or there is moderate certainty that the net benefit is moderate to substantial.	Offer or provide this service.
C	The USPSTF recommends against routinely providing the service. There may be considerations that support providing the service in an individual patient. There is at least moderate certainty that the net benefit is small.	Offer or provide this service only if other considerations support the offering or providing the service in an individual patient.
D	The USPSTF recommends against the service. There is moderate or high certainty that the service has no net benefit or that the harms outweigh the benefits.	Discourage the use of this service.
I Statement	The USPSTF concludes that the current evidence is insufficient to assess the balance of benefits and harms of the service. Evidence is lacking, of poor quality, or conflicting, and the balance of benefits and harms cannot be determined.	Read the clinical considerations section of USPSTF Recommendation Statement. If the service is offered, patients should understand the uncertainty about the balance of benefits and harms.

Levels of Certainty Regarding Net Benefit

Level of Certainty*	Description
High	The available evidence usually includes consistent results from well-designed, well-conducted studies in representative primary care populations. These studies assess the effects of the preventive service on health outcomes. This conclusion is therefore unlikely to be strongly affected by the results of future studies.
Moderate	The available evidence is sufficient to determine the effects of the preventive service on health outcomes, but confidence in the estimate is constrained by such factors as: • The number, size, or quality of individual studies. • Inconsistency of findings across individual studies. • Limited generalizability of findings to routine primary care practice. • Lack of coherence in the chain of evidence. As more information becomes available, the magnitude or direction of the observed effect could change, and this change may be large enough to alter the conclusion.
Low	The available evidence is insufficient to assess effects on health outcomes. Evidence is insufficient because of: • The limited number or size of studies. • Important flaws in study design or methods. • Inconsistency of findings across individual studies. • Gaps in the chain of evidence. • Findings not generalizable to routine primary care practice. • Lack of information on important health outcomes. More information may allow estimation of effects on health outcomes.

*The USPSTF defines certainty as "likelihood that the USPSTF assessment of the net benefit of a preventive service is correct." The net benefit is defined as benefit minus harm of the preventive service as implemented in a general, primary care population. The USPSTF assigns a certainty level based on the nature of the overall evidence available to assess the net benefit of a preventive service. *Current as of May 2008.*

HEALTH MAINTENANCE: BIRTH TO 10 YEARS

(www.ahrq.gov/clinic/cps3dix.htm)

Leading causes of death:

- Perinatal infections
- Congenital anomalies
- Sudden infant death syndrome (SIDS)
- Accidents (drowning, abuse)
- Motor vehicle accidents

Recommended counseling, testing, or interventions

Height, weight, growth chart	
Immunizations (*www.cdc.gov/nip* or *www.immunizationed.org*)	(DPaT, IPV, Hib, hepatitis A, hepatitis B, MMR, pneumococcal, rotavirus, varicella, influenza 6 months–18 years)
Counseling:	Injury prevention: –Car seats –Seat belts –Bicycle helmets –Smoke and carbon monoxide detector –Window/stair guards –Firearm storage
Breast-fed infants	400 IU vitamin D started before 2 months
Congenital hypothyroidism	At birth
Dental caries in preschool children	Oral fluoride supplementation for children older than 6 months whose primary water source is deficient in fluoride: –6 months–3 years 0.25 mg, –3–6 years 0.5 mg, –6–16 years 1 mg/d
Diet	Low-saturated-fat diet and physical exercise
Hearing screening	At birth
Lead screening	High risk: Minority, urban residency, low SES, house built before 1950, recent immigration
Obesity	Screen children ≥6 years for obesity and offer/refer to comprehensive, intensive behavioral interventions to promote improvement in weight status
Substance abuse prevention	Tobacco, alcohol counseling
Tuberculosis screening	High risk: Urban residency, low SES, recent immigration or exposure to recent immigrant
Vision screening: Strabismus, amblyopia, visual acuity	To be completed between ages 3 and 5 years
Gonococcal ophthalmia neonatorum	Prophylactic ocular topical medication for all newborns

Insufficient to recommend for or against

Dysplasia of the hip	By physical examination

HEALTH MAINTENANCE: 11–24 YEARS

(www.ahrq.gov/clinic/uspstf/uspstopics.htm)

Leading causes of death:

- Motor vehicle accidents
- Unintentional injuries
- Homicide
- Suicide
- Malignant neoplasms

Immunizations *(www.cdc.gov/vaccines* or *www.immunizationed.org)*

Tetanus-diphtheria-pertussis (Tdap), meningococcal (MCV4), human papilloma virus (females), varicella (2 total for those without immunity), influenza

Disease	Recommended intervention (A or B grade)
General	Height, weight, BMI, BP, injury prevention (seat belts, firearms), low-saturated-fat diet, physical exercise
Alcohol and substance abuse screening	*
Breast and ovarian cancer by BRCA mutation	If high risk: Ashkenazi, or 2 first-degree relatives with breast or ovarian cancer at <50 years of age
Cervical cancer screening	3 years after first intercourse or age 21
Chlamydia, gonorrhea and syphilis screening	If high risk: Sexually active, pregnancy, IV drug use
Depression	In clinical practices that have systems in place to assure accurate diagnosis, effective treatment, and follow-up
Diabetes mellitus (non–fasting glucose)	If BP >135/80
Domestic/family violence	If sexually active
HIV screening	If high risk: Sexually active, pregnancy, IV drug use
Hepatitis B	If high risk: Sexually active, pregnancy, IV drug use
Lipid disorders	One fasting lipid panel to identify familial hypercholesterolemia during adolescence
Tuberculosis screening	If high risk: Travel, immigrant, alcohol abuse, IV drug use
Obesity (counseling for obese patients)	Screen children ≥6 years for obesity and offer/refer to comprehensive, intensive behavioral interventions to promote improvement in weight status.
Folic acid for women	all women planning or capable of pregnancy take a daily supplement of 0.4–0.8 mg (400–800 μg) of folic acid
Tobacco cessation	Ask all adults about tobacco use and provide tobacco cessation interventions for those who use tobacco
Suicide screening	Depression*

***Additional screening**

Alcohol abuse	"Risky"/"hazardous" alcohol use: >7 drinks per week or >3 drinks on any one occasion for women, and >14 drinks per week or >4 drinks on any one occasion for men. OR Screen: "On any occasion during the last 3 months, have had >5 alcohol drinks" or CAGE: Tried to CUT down, been ANGERED by questions about your drinking, felt GUILTY about your drinking, had an EYE OPENER (drink in the morning)
Domestic violence	Screen all at-risk patients (all women, especially when pregnant) "Do you feel safe in your present relationship?" "Have you been hit, kicked, punched, or otherwise hurt in the last year?"
Substance abuse	Question about drug use and related problems should be considered in all adolescent and adult.
Suicide	Risk factors include history of mood or other mental disorder, substance abuse, and history of "deliberate self-harm."

Against (D grade)

Coronary heart disease via ECG, ETT, etc.
Hemochromatosis
Scoliosis screening
Testicular cancer

HEALTH MAINTENANCE: 25–45 YEARS

(www.ahrq.gov/clinic/cps3dix.htm)

Leading causes of death:

- Accidental overdose (narcotics, etc.)
- Motor vehicle accidents
- Cardiovascular disease
- Malignant neoplasm
- HIV

Immunizations (*www.cdc.gov/nip* or *www.immunizationed.org*)

Tetanus	Tdap every 10 years or just at age 50 (if completed primary series)
Influenza	All adults

Disease	Recommended intervention (A or B grade)
General	Height, weight, BMI, BP, injury prevention (seat belts, firearms), low-saturated-fat diet, physical exercise
Alcohol and substance abuse	*
Breast and ovarian cancer by genetic testing	Refer for genetic counseling if: Ashkenazi heritage, or 2 first-degree relatives with breast or ovarian cancer at <50 years of age
Breast cancer screening by mammography	Mammography starting at age ≥40; repeat every 1–2 years
Cervical cancer screening	Begin 3 years after first intercourse
Coronary heart disease	Evidence is insufficient to recommend using nontraditional risk factors (high-sensitivity C-reactive protein [hs-CRP], ankle-brachial index [ABI], leukocyte count, fasting blood glucose level, periodontal disease, carotid intima-media thickness [carotid IMT], coronary artery calcification [CAC] score on electron-beam computed tomography [EBCT], homocysteine level, and lipoprotein[a] level) to screen asymptomatic men and women with no history of CHD to prevent CHD events
Depression	In clinical practices that have systems in place to assure accurate diagnosis, effective treatment, and follow-up
Diabetes mellitus, type II (if BP >135/80)	Random serum glucose if sustained BP (either treated or untreated) >135/80 mm Hg
Domestic/family violence	If sexually active
Diet/obesity	Intensive behavioral dietary counseling for patients with known risk factors for cardiovascular and diet-related chronic disease
Chlamydia, gonorrhea, syphilis testing	All adults who are at increased risk (sexually active, IV drug use, etc.)
HIV screening	All adults who are at increased risk (sexually active, IV drug use, etc.)
Hepatitis B	All pregnant women and those with multiple sexual partners, IV drug use, etc.
Lipid disorders	Men: 35 and older for lipid disorders Women: 45 and older for lipid disorders
Suicide screening	If depressed*
Tobacco abuse	Ask all adults about tobacco use and provide tobacco cessation interventions for those who use tobacco
Tuberculosis screening	If high risk: Travel, immigrant, alcohol abuse, IV drug use

*Additional screening

Alcohol abuse	"Risky"/"hazardous" alcohol use: >7 drinks per week or >3 drinks on any one occasion for women, and >14 drinks per week or more than 4 drinks on any one occasion for men. OR Screen: "On any occasion during the last 3 months, have had more than 5 alcohol drinks" or CAGE: Tried to CUT down, been ANGERED by questions about your drinking, felt GUILTY about your drinking, had an EYE OPENER (drink in the morning)
Domestic violence	Screen all at-risk patients (all women, especially when pregnant) "Do you feel safe in your present relationship?" "Have you been hit, kicked, punched, or otherwise hurt in the last year?"
Substance abuse	Questioning about drug use and related problems should be considered in all adolescent and adult.
Suicide	Risk factors include history of mood or other mental disorder, substance abuse, and history of "deliberate self-harm."

Recommends against

Aspirin	The USPSTF recommends against the use of aspirin for stroke prevention in women younger than 55 years and for myocardial infarction prevention in men younger than 45 years.
Testicular cancer	The USPSTF recommends against testicular exam to screen for testicular cancer.

HEALTH MAINTENANCE: 45–65 YEARS

(www.ahrq.gov/clinic/cps3dix.htm)

Leading causes of death:

- Cardiovascular disease
- Malignant neoplasm
- Accidents
- Cirrhosis

Immunizations *(www.cdc.gov/nip* or *www.immunizationed.org)*

Tetanus	Tdap every 10 years or just at age 50 (if completed primary series)
Influenza	All adults

Disease	Recommended intervention (A or B grade)
General	Height, weight, BMI, BP, injury prevention (seat belts, firearms), low-saturated-fat diet, physical exercise
Alcohol and substance abuse	*Insufficient for population; screen at risk
Aspirin	Recommends use of aspirin for men age 45–79 and women age 55–79 years when potential benefit due to a reduction in myocardial infarctions outweighs the potential harm due to an increase in GI hemorrhage
Breast and ovarian cancer by genetic testing	Refer for genetic counseling if: Ashkenazi heritage, or 2 first-degree relatives with breast or ovarian cancer at <50 years of age
Breast cancer screening by mammography	Mammography starting at age ≥50; repeat every 1–2 years
Cervical cancer screening	Begin 3 years after first intercourse
Chlamydia, gonorrhea, syphilis testing	All adults who are at increased risk (sexually active, IV drug use, etc.)
Colon cancer	Start at age 50–75 by fecal occult blood testing, sigmoidoscopy, or colonoscopy
Coronary heart disease	Evidence is insufficient to recommend using nontraditional risk factors (high-sensitivity C-reactive protein [hs-CRP], ankle-brachial index [ABI], leukocyte count, fasting blood glucose level, periodontal disease, carotid intima-media thickness [carotid IMT], coronary artery calcification [CAC] score on electron-beam computed tomography [EBCT], homocysteine level, and lipoprotein[a] level) to screen asymptomatic men and women with no history of CHD to prevent CHD events
Depression	In clinical practices that have systems in place to assure accurate diagnosis, effective treatment, and follow-up
Diabetes mellitus, type II if BP >135/80	Random serum glucose if sustained BP (either treated or untreated) >135/80 mm Hg
Domestic/family violence	*If sexually active
Diet/obesity	Intensive behavioral dietary counseling for patients with known risk factors for cardiovascular and diet-related chronic disease
HIV screening	All adults who are at increased risk (sexually active, IV drug use, etc.)
Hepatitis B	All pregnant women and those with multiple sexual partners, IV drug use, etc.
Lipid disorders	All adults over 45 should be screened
Suicide screening	If depressed*
Osteoporosis	Only screen in women younger than 65 years if their fracture risk is equivalent to that of a 65-year-old
Tobacco abuse	Ask all adults about tobacco use and provide tobacco cessation interventions for those who use tobacco
Tuberculosis screening	If high risk: Travel, immigrant, alcohol abuse, IV drug use

*Additional screening

Alcohol abuse	"Risky"/"hazardous" alcohol use: >7 drinks per week or >3 drinks on any one occasion for women, and >14 drinks per week or >4 drinks on any one occasion for men. OR Screen: "On any occasion during the last 3 months, have had more than 5 alcohol drinks" or CAGE: Tried to CUT down, been ANGERED by questions about your drinking, felt GUILTY about your drinking, had an EYE OPENER (drink in the morning)
Domestic violence	Screen all at-risk patients (all women, especially when pregnant) "Do you feel safe in your present relationship?" "Have you been hit, kicked, punched, or otherwise hurt in the last year?"
Substance abuse	Questioning about drug use and related problems should be considered in all adolescent and adult.
Suicide	Risk factors include history of mood or other mental disorder, substance abuse, and history of "deliberate self-harm."

HEALTH MAINTENANCE: 65 YEARS AND ABOVE

(www.ahrq.gov/clinic/cps3dix.htm)

Leading causes of death:

- Cardiovascular disease
- Malignant neoplasm
- Stoke
- COPD
- Dementia

Immunizations *(www.cdc.gov/nip* or *www.immunizationed.org)*

Tetanus	Tdap every 10 years or just at age 50 (if completed primary series)
Influenza	All adults

Disease	Recommended Intervention (A or B Grade)
General	Height, weight, BMI, BP, injury prevention (seat belts, firearms), low-saturated-fat diet, physical exercise
Alcohol and substance abuse	*Insufficient for population; screen at risk
Aspirin	Recommends use of aspirin for men age 45–79 and women age 55–79 years when potential benefit due to a reduction in myocardial infarctions outweighs the potential harm due to an increase in GI hemorrhage
Breast and ovarian cancer by genetic testing	Refer for genetic counseling if: Ashkenazi heritage, or 2 first-degree relatives with breast or ovarian cancer at <50 years of age
Breast cancer screening by mammography	Mammography through age 75; repeat every 1–2 years; after age 75, at discretion
Cervical cancer screening	May cease to screen if had adequate recent screening and are not at high risk
Chlamydia, gonorrhea, syphilis testing	All adults who are at increased risk (sexually active, IV drug use, etc.)
Colon cancer	Start at age 50–75 by fecal occult blood testing, sigmoidoscopy, or colonoscopy
Coronary Heart Disease	Evidence is insufficient to recommend using nontraditional risk factors (high-sensitivity C-reactive protein [hs-CRP], ankle-brachial index [ABI], leukocyte count, fasting blood glucose level, periodontal disease, carotid intima-media thickness [carotid IMT], coronary artery calcification [CAC] score on electron-beam computed tomography [EBCT], homocysteine level, and lipoprotein[a] level) to screen asymptomatic men and women with no history of CHD to prevent CHD events
Depression	In clinical practices that have systems in place to assure accurate diagnosis, effective treatment, and follow-up
Diabetes mellitus, type II if BP >135/80	Random serum glucose if sustained BP (either treated or untreated) >135/80 mm Hg
Domestic/family violence	*If sexually active
Diet/obesity	Intensive behavioral dietary counseling for patients with known risk factors for cardiovascular and diet-related chronic disease
HIV screening	All adults who are at increased risk (sexually active, IV drug use, etc.)
Hepatitis B	All pregnant women and those with multiple sexual partners, IV drug use, etc.
Lipid disorders	All adults over 45 should be screened
Osteoporosis	All women at 65; insufficient evidence to support screening men
Suicide screening	If depressed*
Tobacco abuse	Ask all adults about tobacco use and provide tobacco cessation interventions for those who use tobacco
Tuberculosis screening	If high risk: Travel, immigrant, alcohol abuse, IV drug use

*Additional screening

Alcohol abuse	"Risky"/"hazardous" alcohol use: >7 drinks per week or >3 drinks on any one occasion for women, and >14 drinks per week or >4 drinks on any one occasion for men. OR Screen: "On any occasion during the last 3 months, have had more than 5 alcohol drinks" or CAGE: Tried to CUT down, been ANGERED by questions about your drinking, felt GUILTY about your drinking, had an EYE OPENER (drink in the morning)
Domestic violence	Screen all at-risk patients (all women, especially when pregnant) "Do you feel safe in your present relationship?" "Have you been hit, kicked, punched, or otherwise hurt in the last year?"
Substance abuse	Questioning about drug use and related problems should be considered in all adolescent and adult.
Suicide	Risk factors include history of mood or other mental disorder, substance abuse, and history of "deliberate self-harm."

Diagnosis and Treatment: An Algorithmic Approach

This section contains flowcharts (or algorithms) to help the reader in the diagnosis of clinical signs and symptoms, and treatment of a variety of clinical problems. They are organized by the presenting sign, symptom, or diagnosis.

These algorithms were designed to be used as a quick reference and adjunct to the reader's clinical knowledge and impression. They are not an exhaustive review of the management of a problem, nor are they meant to be a complete list of diseases.

ABDOMINAL PAIN, CHRONIC

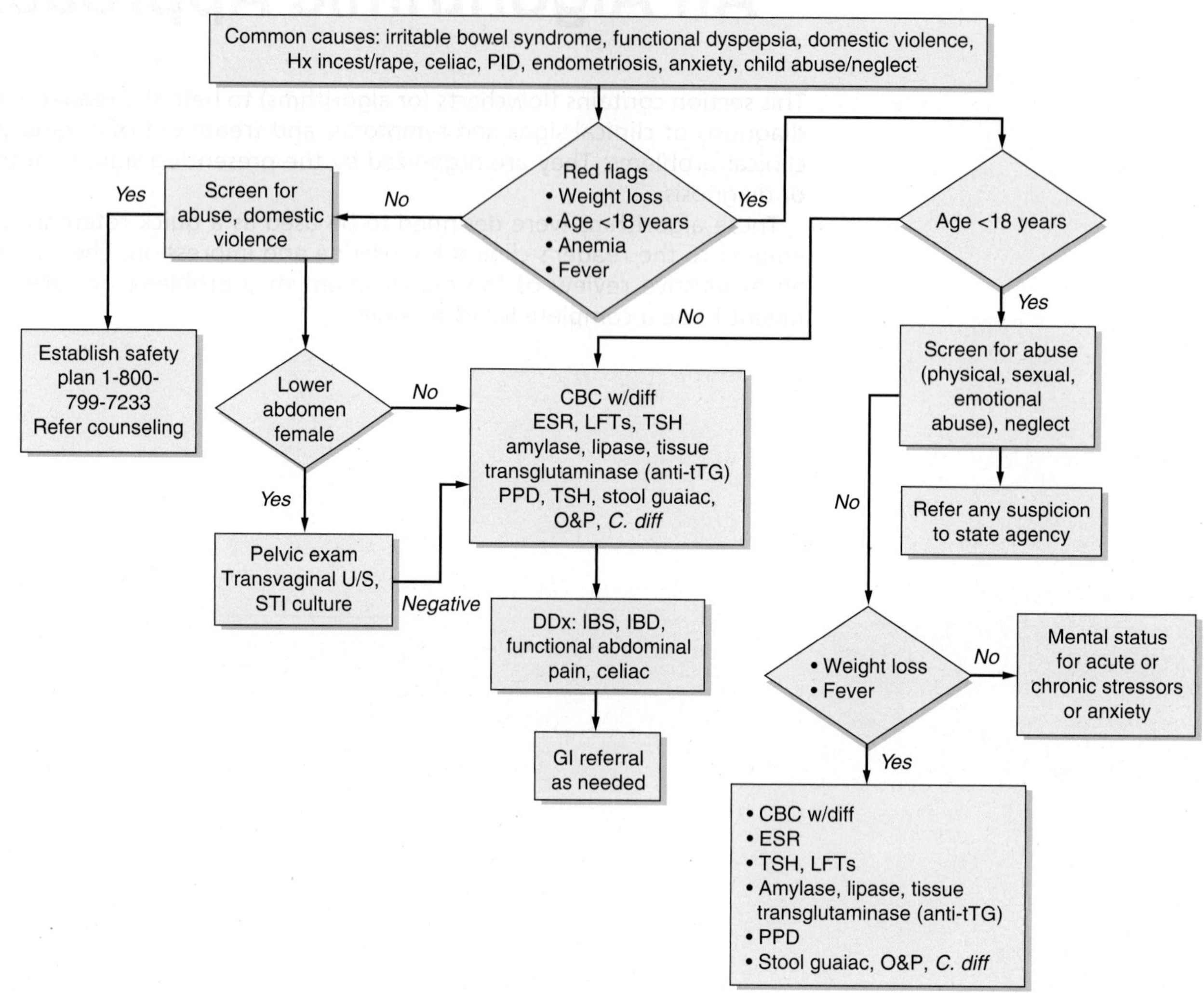
Common causes: irritable bowel syndrome, functional dyspepsia, domestic violence, Hx incest/rape, celiac, PID, endometriosis, anxiety, child abuse/neglect
Red flags
• Weight loss
• Age <18 years
• Anemia
• Fever
No
Yes
Screen for abuse, domestic violence
Yes
Establish safety plan 1-800-799-7233
Refer counseling
Lower abdomen female
No
Yes
Pelvic exam
Transvaginal U/S,
STI culture
Negative
CBC w/diff
ESR, LFTs, TSH
amylase, lipase, tissue transglutaminase (anti-tTG)
PPD, TSH, stool guaiac, O&P, C. diff
DDx: IBS, IBD, functional abdominal pain, celiac
GI referral as needed
Age <18 years
No
Yes
Screen for abuse (physical, sexual, emotional abuse), neglect
Refer any suspicion to state agency
No
• Weight loss
• Fever
No
Mental status for acute or chronic stressors or anxiety
Yes
• CBC w/diff
• ESR
• TSH, LFTs
• Amylase, lipase, tissue transglutaminase (anti-tTG)
• PPD
• Stool guaiac, O&P, C. diff

Josue Chery, MD

Neurogastroenterol Motil. 2006;18(7):499–506.

ABDOMINAL PAIN, LOWER

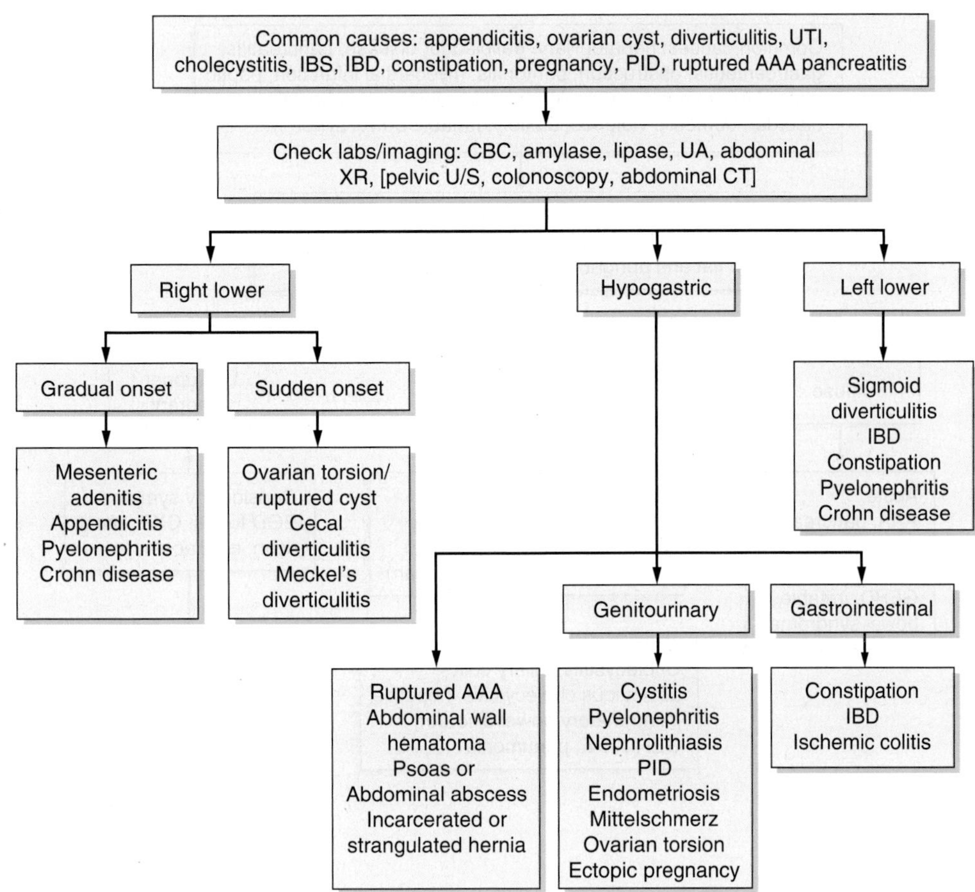

Nilay Patel, MD and Siva Vithananthan, MD

Scand J Gastroenterol. 1999;231(Suppl):3–8.

ABDOMINAL PAIN, UPPER

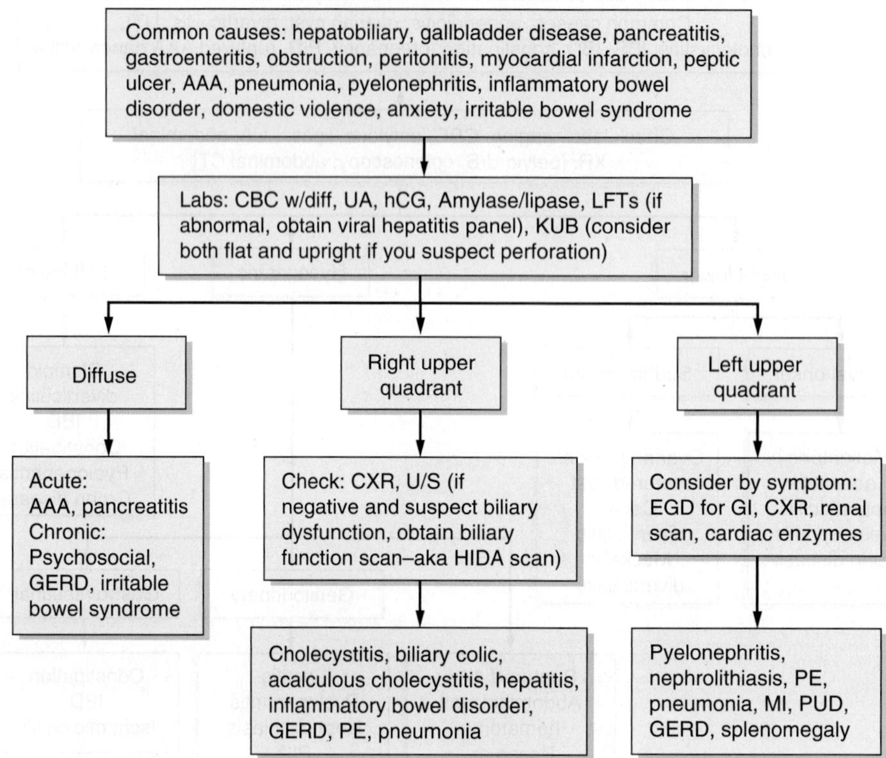

Nilay Patel, MD and Siva Vithananthan, MD

Scand J Gastroenterol. 1999;231(Suppl):3–8.

ABDOMINAL RIGIDITY

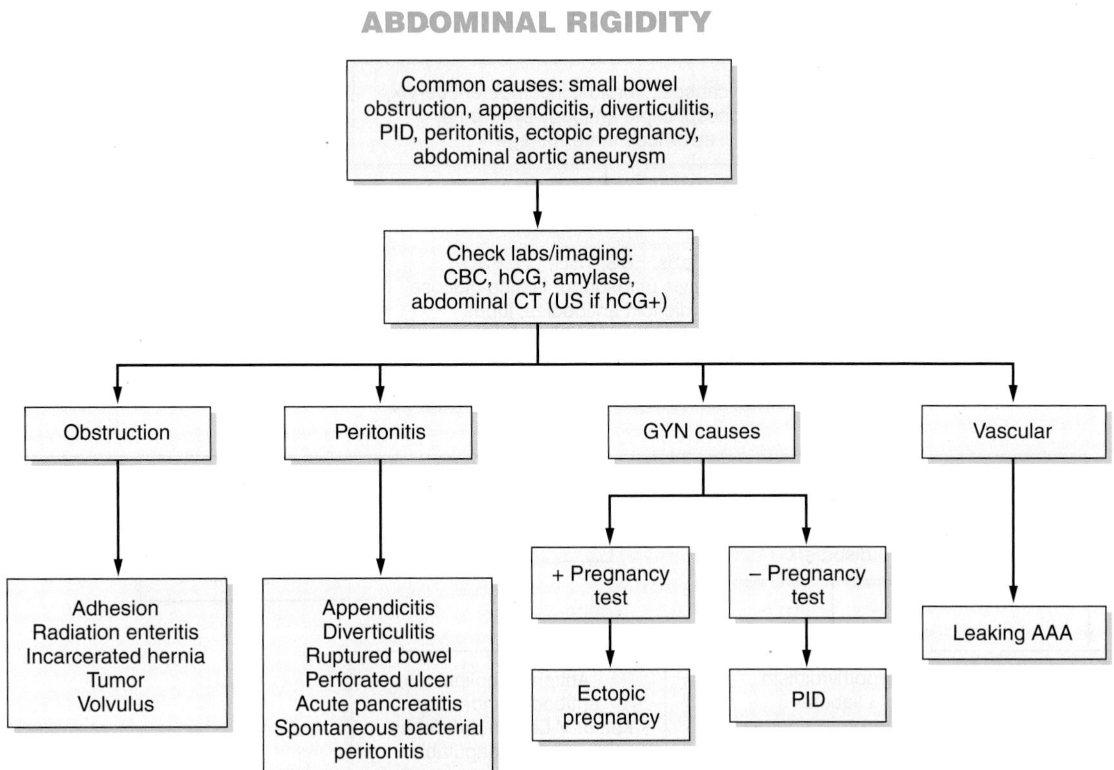

Robert A. Baldor, MD and Alan M. Ehrlich, MD

Med Clin North Am. 2008;92(3):599–625, viii–ix.

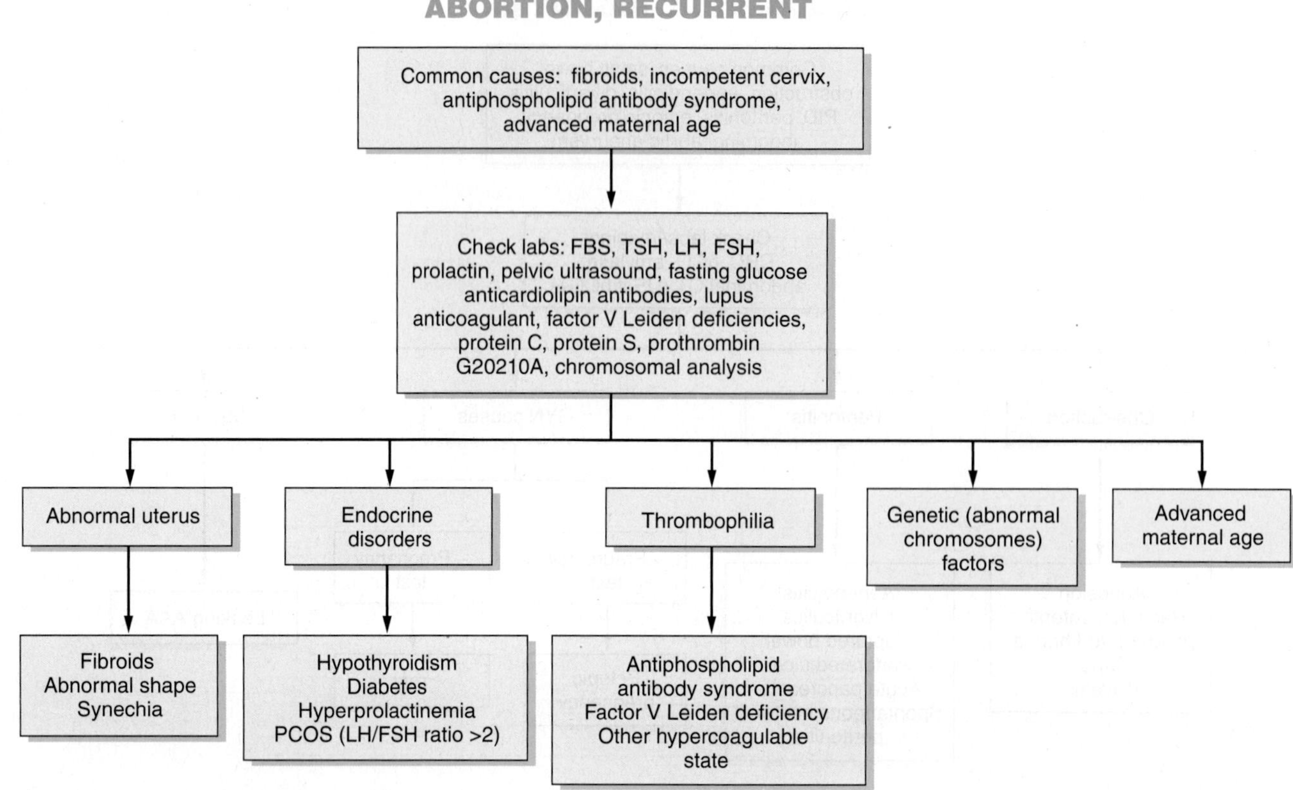

Robert A. Baldor, MD and Alan M. Ehrlich, MD

J Obstet Gynaecol Res. 2009;35(4):609–22.

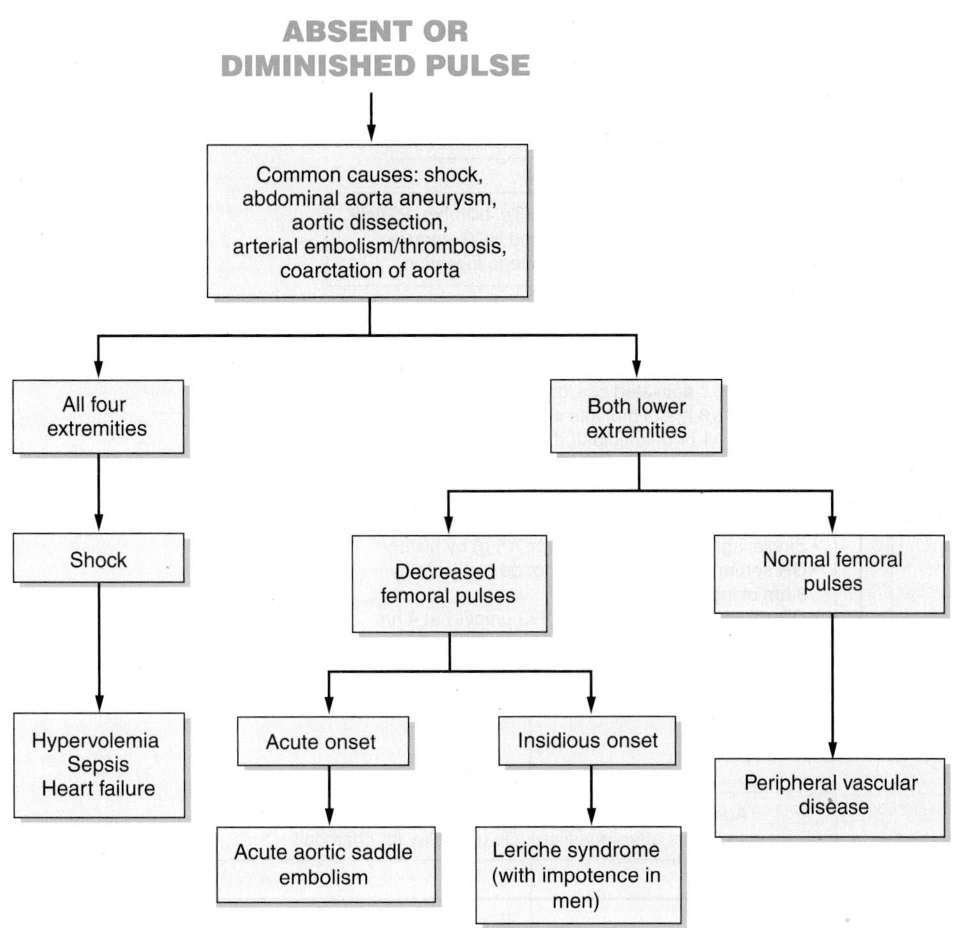

Robert A. Baldor, MD and Alan M. Ehrlich, MD

Semin Vasc Surg. 2009;22(1):10–6.

ACETAMINOPHEN POISONING, TREATMENT

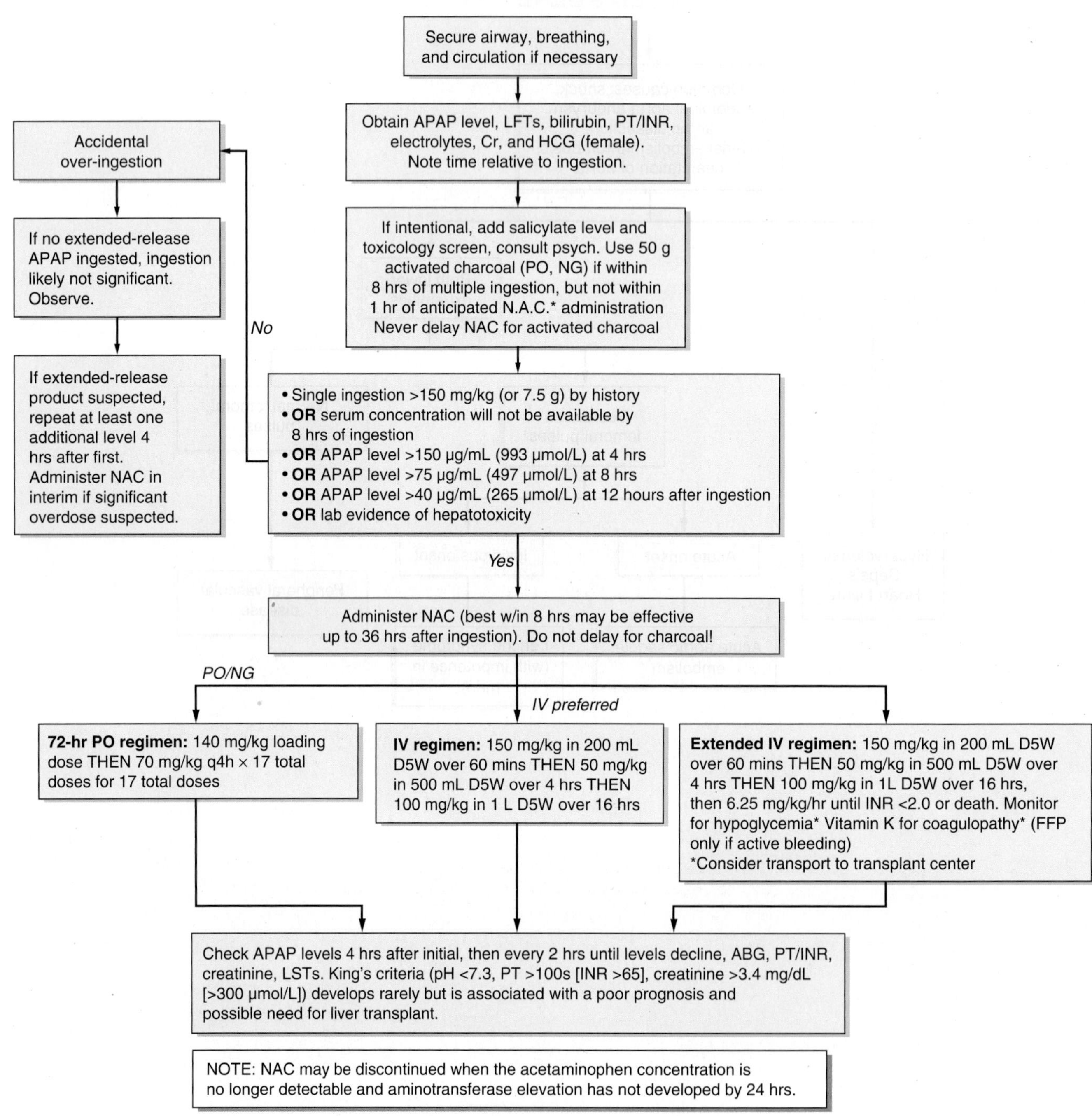

Secure airway, breathing, and circulation if necessary
Obtain APAP level, LFTs, bilirubin, PT/INR, electrolytes, Cr, and HCG (female). Note time relative to ingestion.
If intentional, add salicylate level and toxicology screen, consult psych. Use 50 g activated charcoal (PO, NG) if within 8 hrs of multiple ingestion, but not within 1 hr of anticipated N.A.C.* administration Never delay NAC for activated charcoal
• Single ingestion >150 mg/kg (or 7.5 g) by history
• OR serum concentration will not be available by 8 hrs of ingestion
• OR APAP level >150 μg/mL (993 μmol/L) at 4 hrs
• OR APAP level >75 μg/mL (497 μmol/L) at 8 hrs
• OR APAP level >40 μg/mL (265 μmol/L) at 12 hours after ingestion
• OR lab evidence of hepatotoxicity
No
Accidental over-ingestion
If no extended-release APAP ingested, ingestion likely not significant. Observe.
If extended-release product suspected, repeat at least one additional level 4 hrs after first. Administer NAC in interim if significant overdose suspected.
Yes
Administer NAC (best w/in 8 hrs may be effective up to 36 hrs after ingestion). Do not delay for charcoal!
PO/NG
IV preferred
72-hr PO regimen: 140 mg/kg loading dose THEN 70 mg/kg q4h × 17 total doses for 17 total doses
IV regimen: 150 mg/kg in 200 mL D5W over 60 mins THEN 50 mg/kg in 500 mL D5W over 4 hrs THEN 100 mg/kg in 1 L D5W over 16 hrs
Extended IV regimen: 150 mg/kg in 200 mL D5W over 60 mins THEN 50 mg/kg in 500 mL D5W over 4 hrs THEN 100 mg/kg in 1L D5W over 16 hrs, then 6.25 mg/kg/hr until INR <2.0 or death. Monitor for hypoglycemia* Vitamin K for coagulopathy* (FFP only if active bleeding)
*Consider transport to transplant center
Check APAP levels 4 hrs after initial, then every 2 hrs until levels decline, ABG, PT/INR, creatinine, LSTs. King's criteria (pH <7.3, PT >100s [INR >65], creatinine >3.4 mg/dL [>300 μmol/L]) develops rarely but is associated with a poor prognosis and possible need for liver transplant.
NOTE: NAC may be discontinued when the acetaminophen concentration is no longer detectable and aminotransferase elevation has not developed by 24 hrs.

*APAP = Acetaminophen NAC = N-acetylcysteine

John Jenkins, MD

Med J Aust. 2008;188(5):296–301.

ACID PHOSPHATASE ELEVATION

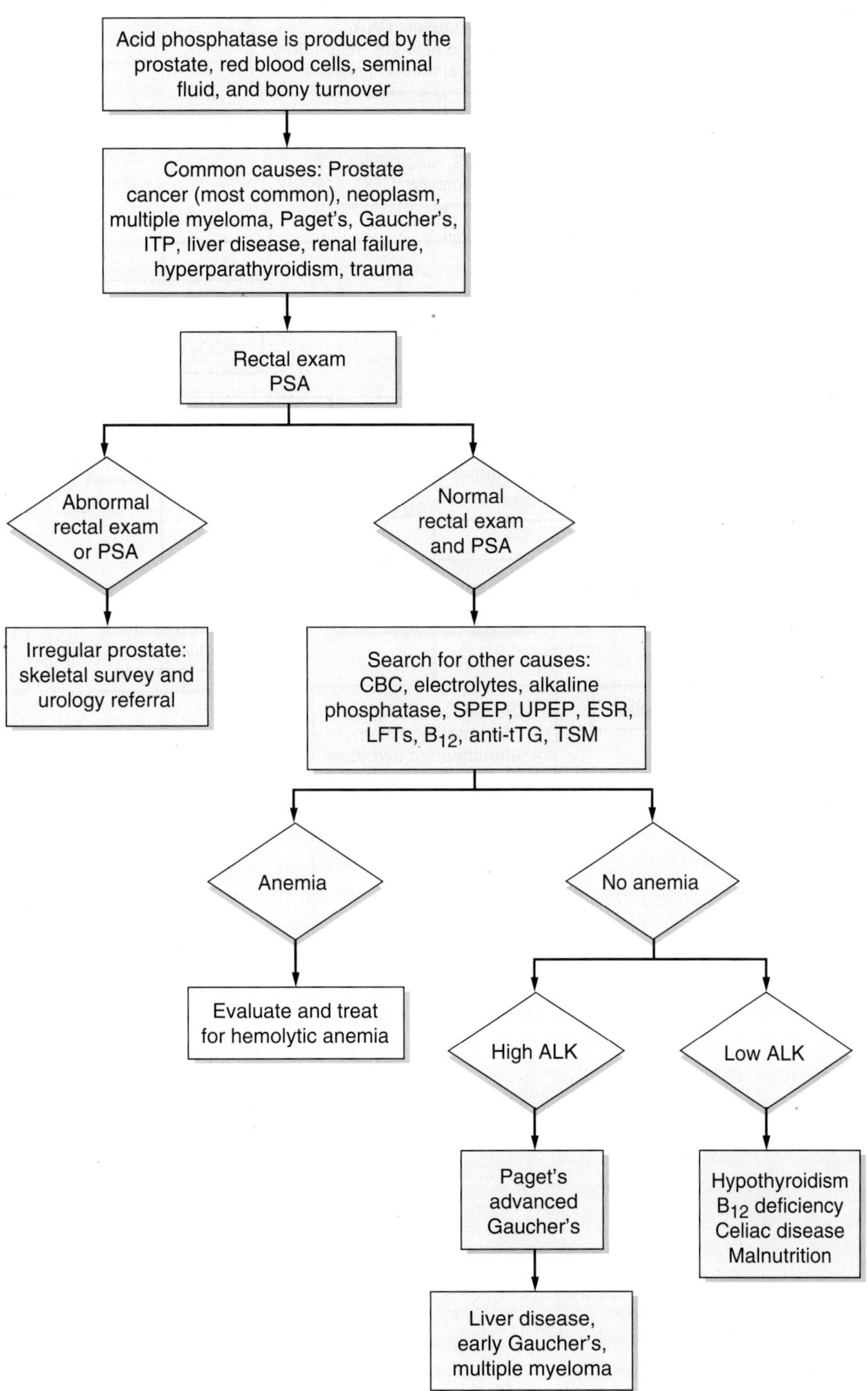

Laura Hagopian, MD and Michael Snyder, MD

Scand J Clin Lab Invest. 1991;51(6):517–24.

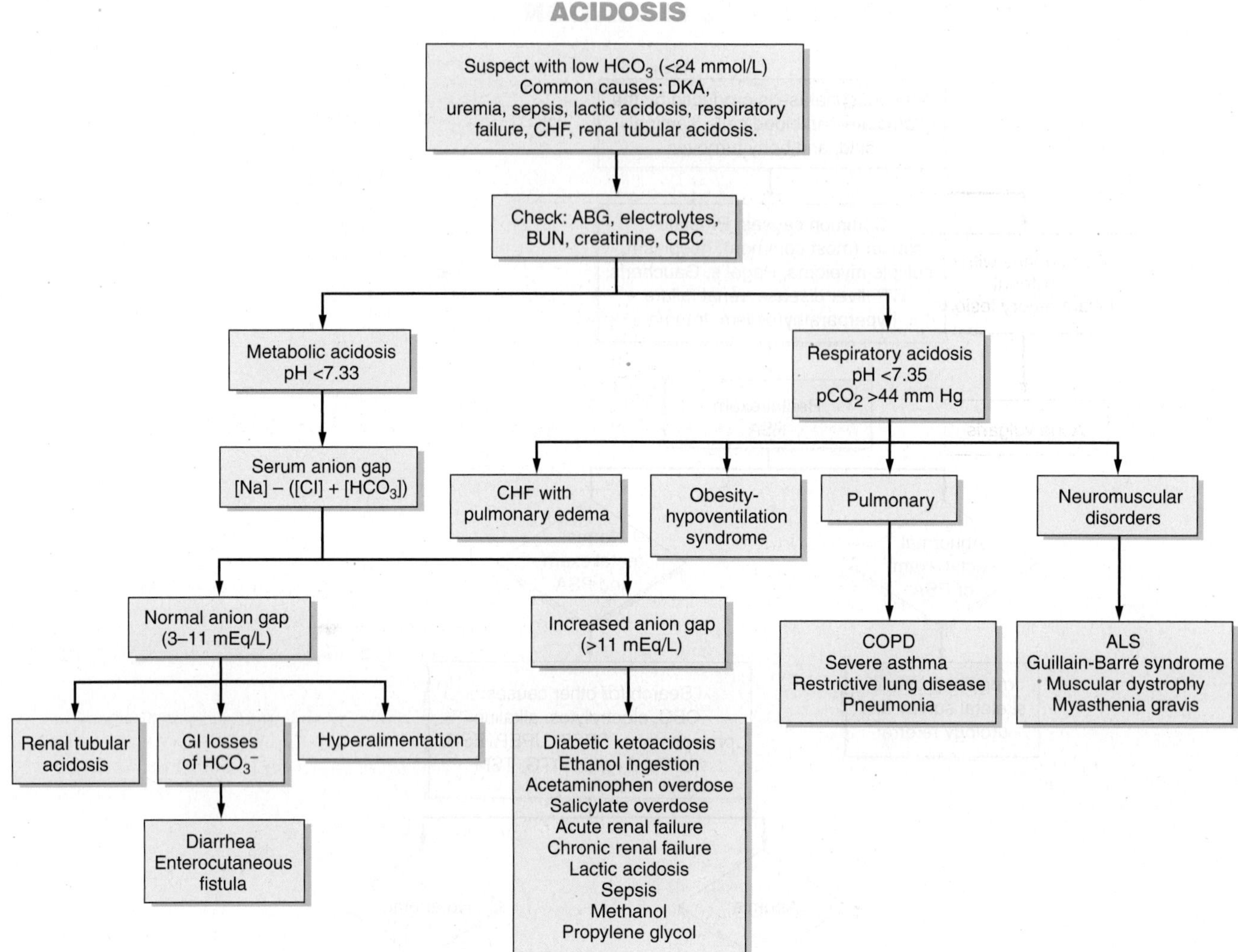

Robert A. Baldor, MD and Alan M. Ehrlich, MD

Diabetes Care. 2009;32(7):1335–43.

ACNE

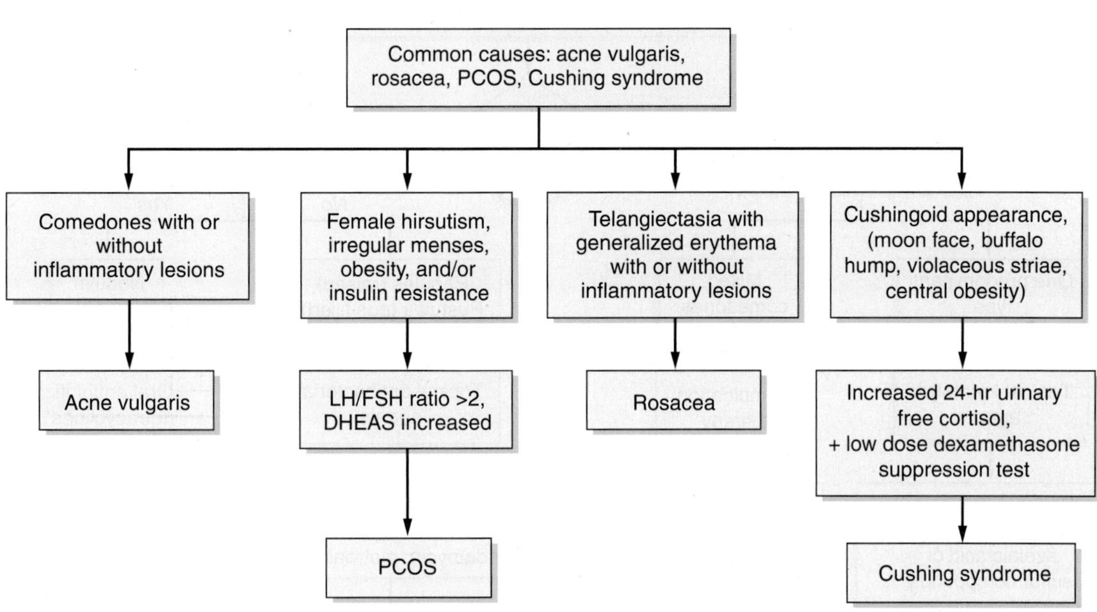

Robert A. Baldor, MD and Alan M. Ehrlich, MD

Dermatol Clin. 2009;27(4):459–71, vi.

ACNE VULGARIS, TREATMENT

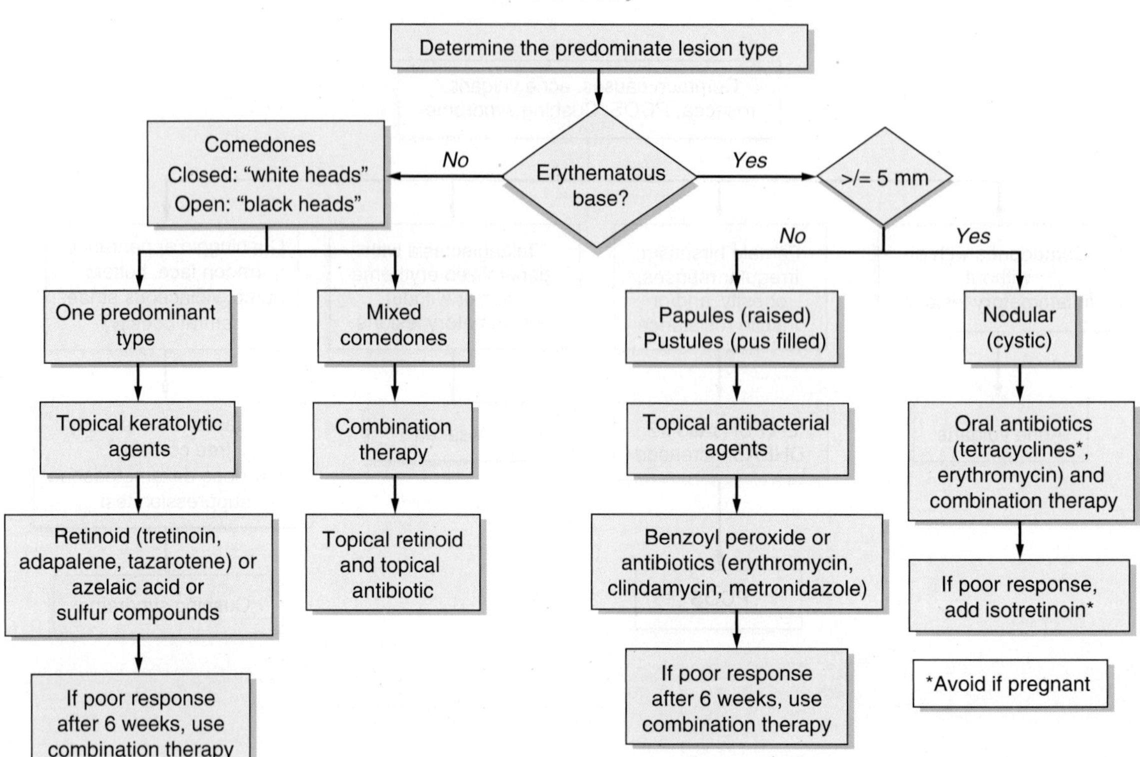

Robert A. Baldor, MD

Treat Guidel Med Lett. 2008;6(75):75–82.

ADRENOCORTICAL INSUFFICIENCY

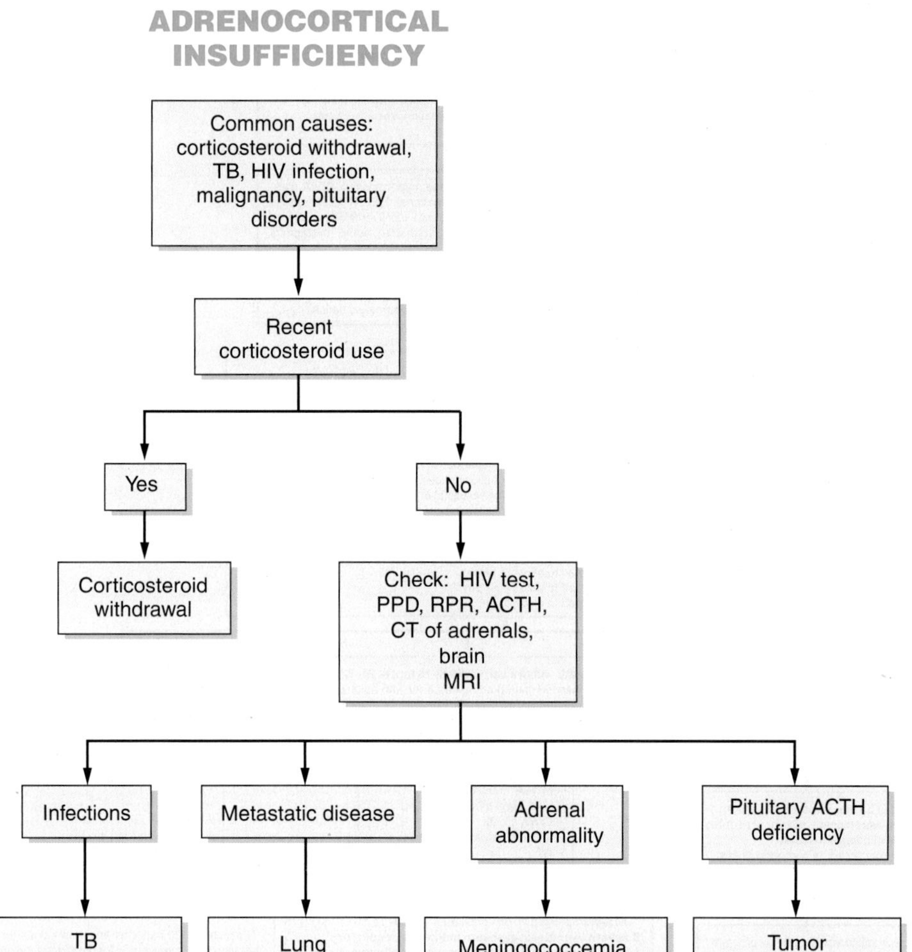

Robert A. Baldor, MD and Alan M. Ehrlich, MD

Ann Intern Med. 2003;139(3):194–204.

ALCOHOL WITHDRAWAL, TREATMENT

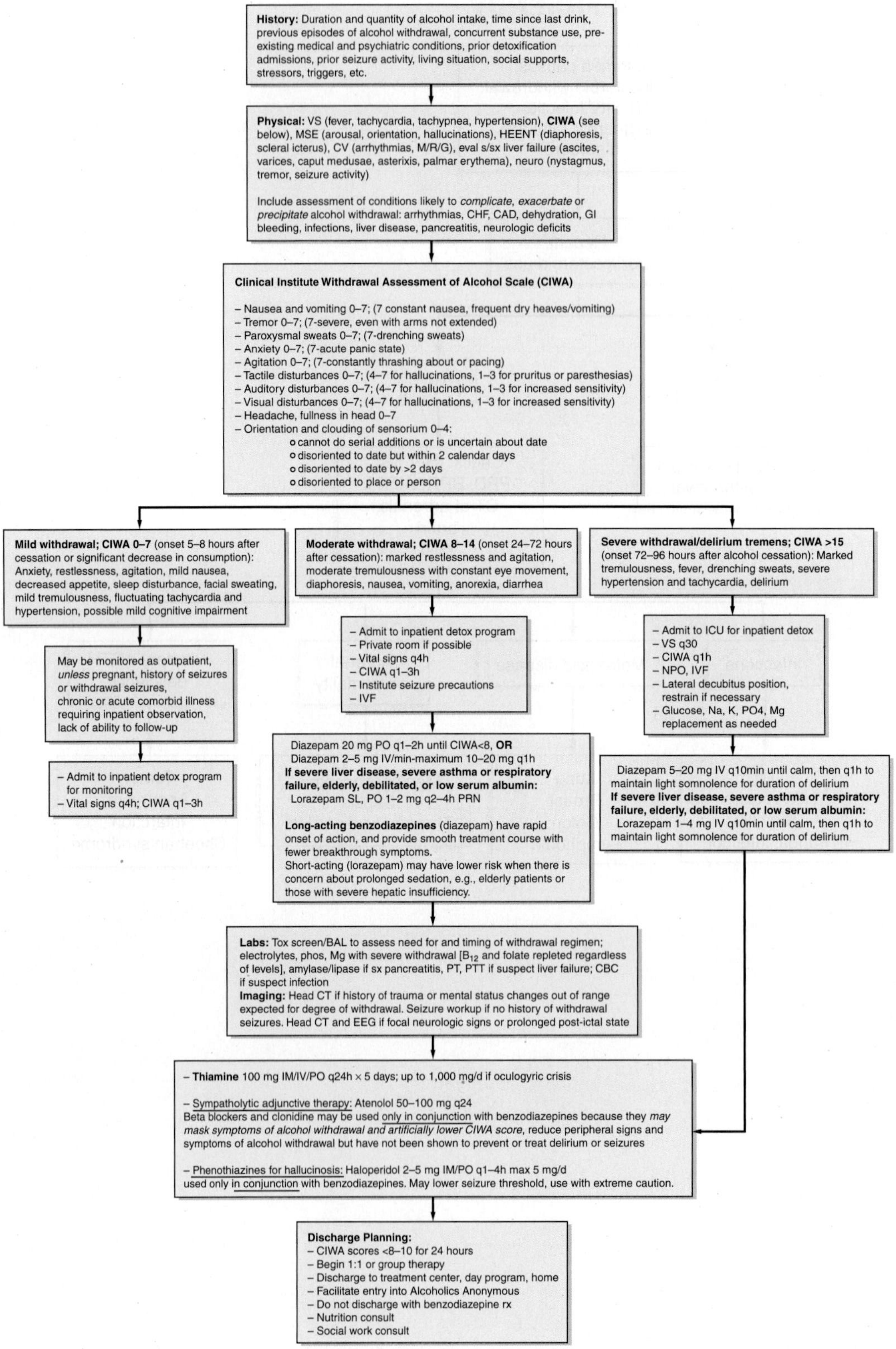

History: Duration and quantity of alcohol intake, time since last drink, previous episodes of alcohol withdrawal, concurrent substance use, pre-existing medical and psychiatric conditions, prior detoxification admissions, prior seizure activity, living situation, social supports, stressors, triggers, etc.

↓

Physical: VS (fever, tachycardia, tachypnea, hypertension), **CIWA** (see below), MSE (arousal, orientation, hallucinations), HEENT (diaphoresis, scleral icterus), CV (arrhythmias, M/R/G), eval s/sx liver failure (ascites, varices, caput medusae, asterixis, palmar erythema), neuro (nystagmus, tremor, seizure activity)

Include assessment of conditions likely to *complicate, exacerbate* or *precipitate* alcohol withdrawal: arrhythmias, CHF, CAD, dehydration, GI bleeding, infections, liver disease, pancreatitis, neurologic deficits

↓

Clinical Institute Withdrawal Assessment of Alcohol Scale (CIWA)

- Nausea and vomiting 0–7; (7 constant nausea, frequent dry heaves/vomiting)
- Tremor 0–7; (7-severe, even with arms not extended)
- Paroxysmal sweats 0–7; (7-drenching sweats)
- Anxiety 0–7; (7-acute panic state)
- Agitation 0–7; (7-constantly thrashing about or pacing)
- Tactile disturbances 0–7; (4–7 for hallucinations, 1–3 for pruritus or paresthesias)
- Auditory disturbances 0–7; (4–7 for hallucinations, 1–3 for increased sensitivity)
- Visual disturbances 0–7; (4–7 for hallucinations, 1–3 for increased sensitivity)
- Headache, fullness in head 0–7
- Orientation and clouding of sensorium 0–4:
  - cannot do serial additions or is uncertain about date
  - disoriented to date but within 2 calendar days
  - disoriented to date by >2 days
  - disoriented to place or person

↓

Mild withdrawal

Mild withdrawal; CIWA 0–7 (onset 5–8 hours after cessation or significant decrease in consumption): Anxiety, restlessness, agitation, mild nausea, decreased appetite, sleep disturbance, facial sweating, mild tremulousness, fluctuating tachycardia and hypertension, possible mild cognitive impairment

↓

May be monitored as outpatient, *unless* pregnant, history of seizures or withdrawal seizures, chronic or acute comorbid illness requiring inpatient observation, lack of ability to follow-up

↓

- Admit to inpatient detox program for monitoring
- Vital signs q4h; CIWA q1–3h

Moderate withdrawal

Moderate withdrawal; CIWA 8–14 (onset 24–72 hours after cessation): marked restlessness and agitation, moderate tremulousness with constant eye movement, diaphoresis, nausea, vomiting, anorexia, diarrhea

↓

- Admit to inpatient detox program
- Private room if possible
- Vital signs q4h
- CIWA q1–3h
- Institute seizure precautions
- IVF

↓

Diazepam 20 mg PO q1–2h until CIWA<8, **OR**
Diazepam 2–5 mg IV/min-maximum 10–20 mg q1h
If severe liver disease, severe asthma or respiratory failure, elderly, debilitated, or low serum albumin:
Lorazepam SL, PO 1–2 mg q2–4h PRN

Long-acting benzodiazepines (diazepam) have rapid onset of action, and provide smooth treatment course with fewer breakthrough symptoms.
Short-acting (lorazepam) may have lower risk when there is concern about prolonged sedation, e.g., elderly patients or those with severe hepatic insufficiency.

↓

Labs: Tox screen/BAL to assess need for and timing of withdrawal regimen; electrolytes, phos, Mg with severe withdrawal [B_{12} and folate repleted regardless of levels], amylase/lipase if sx pancreatitis, PT, PTT if suspect liver failure; CBC if suspect infection
Imaging: Head CT if history of trauma or mental status changes out of range expected for degree of withdrawal. Seizure workup if no history of withdrawal seizures. Head CT and EEG if focal neurologic signs or prolonged post-ictal state

↓

Severe withdrawal

Severe withdrawal/delirium tremens; CIWA >15 (onset 72–96 hours after alcohol cessation): Marked tremulousness, fever, drenching sweats, severe hypertension and tachycardia, delirium

↓

- Admit to ICU for inpatient detox
- VS q30
- CIWA q1h
- NPO, IVF
- Lateral decubitus position, restrain if necessary
- Glucose, Na, K, PO4, Mg replacement as needed

↓

Diazepam 5–20 mg IV q10min until calm, then q1h to maintain light somnolence for duration of delirium
If severe liver disease, severe asthma or respiratory failure, elderly, debilitated, or low serum albumin:
Lorazepam 1–4 mg IV q10min until calm, then q1h to maintain light somnolence for duration of delirium

↓ (to Thiamine box)

Management

- **Thiamine** 100 mg IM/IV/PO q24h × 5 days; up to 1,000 mg/d if oculogyric crisis

- Sympatholytic adjunctive therapy: Atenolol 50–100 mg q24
Beta blockers and clonidine may be used only in conjunction with benzodiazepines because they *may mask symptoms of alcohol withdrawal and artificially lower CIWA score,* reduce peripheral signs and symptoms of alcohol withdrawal but have not been shown to prevent or treat delirium or seizures

- Phenothiazines for hallucinosis: Haloperidol 2–5 mg IM/PO q1–4h max 5 mg/d
used only in conjunction with benzodiazepines. May lower seizure threshold, use with extreme caution.

↓

Discharge Planning:
- CIWA scores <8–10 for 24 hours
- Begin 1:1 or group therapy
- Discharge to treatment center, day program, home
- Facilitate entry into Alcoholics Anonymous
- Do not discharge with benzodiazepine rx
- Nutrition consult
- Social work consult

Alexis Lawrence, MD and Warren J. Ferguson, MD

N Engl J Med. 2003;348:1786.

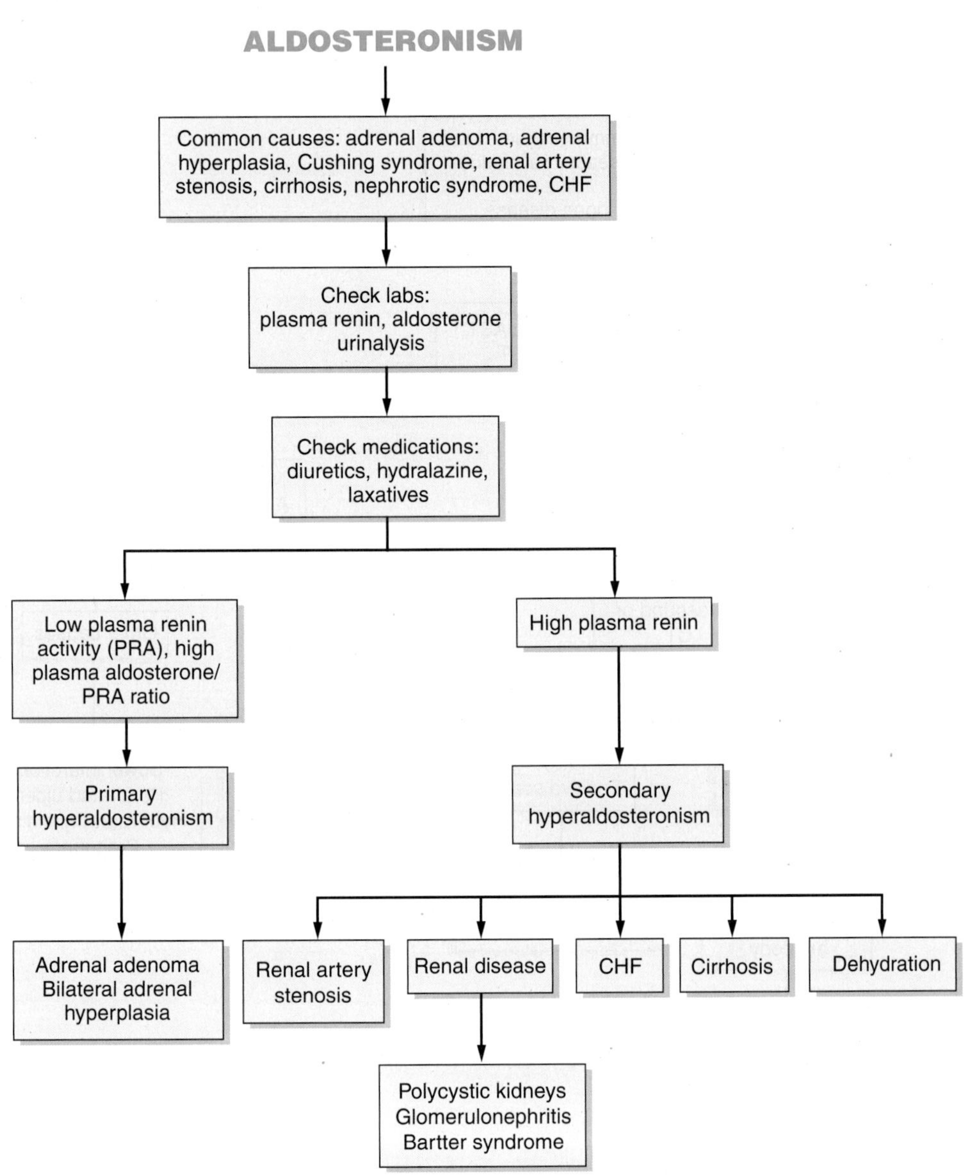

Robert A. Baldor, MD and Alan M. Ehrlich, MD

Cardiology. 1985;72(Suppl 1):57–63.

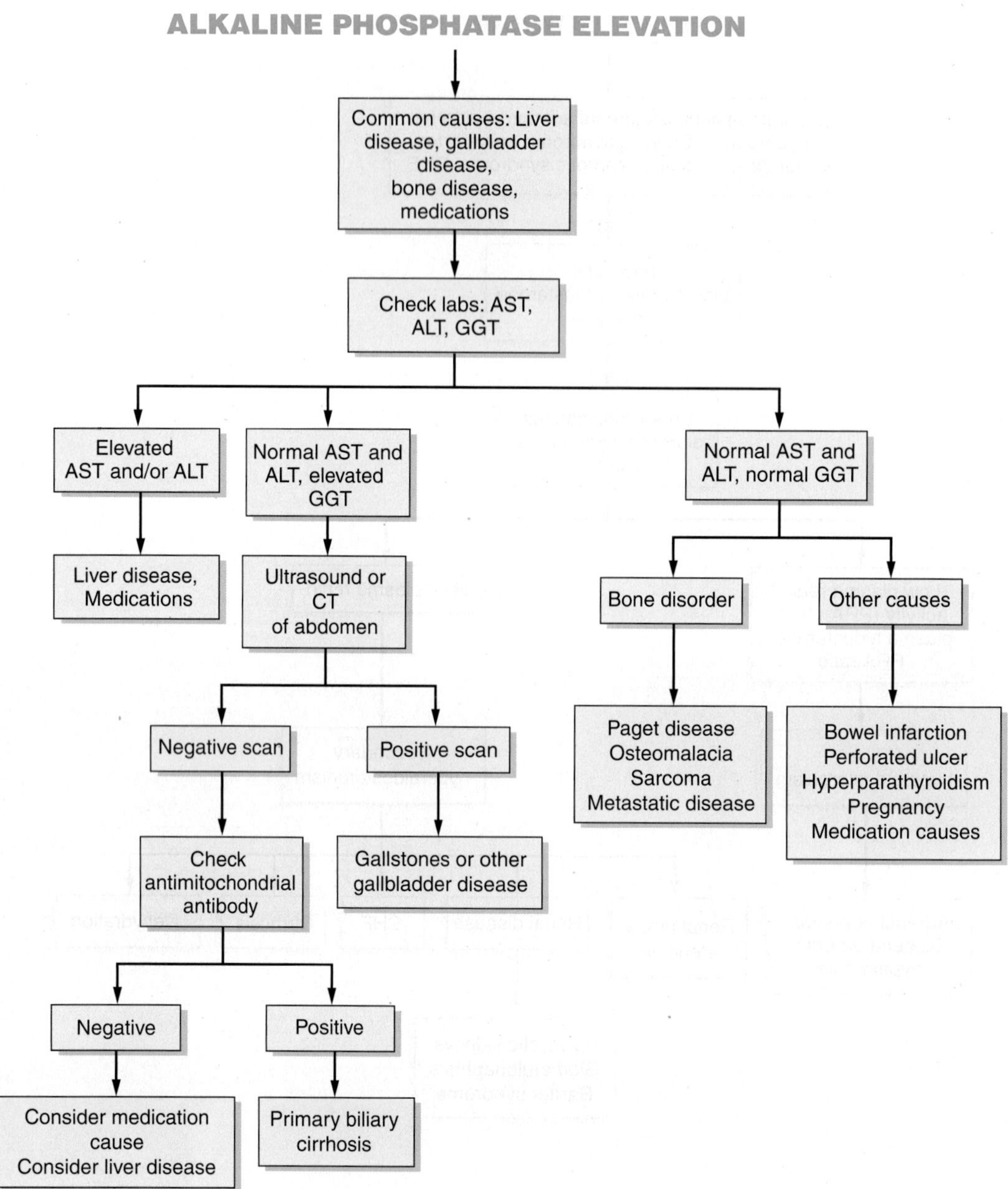

Robert A. Baldor, MD and Alan M. Ehrlich, MD

J Fam Pract. 2001;50(6):496–7.

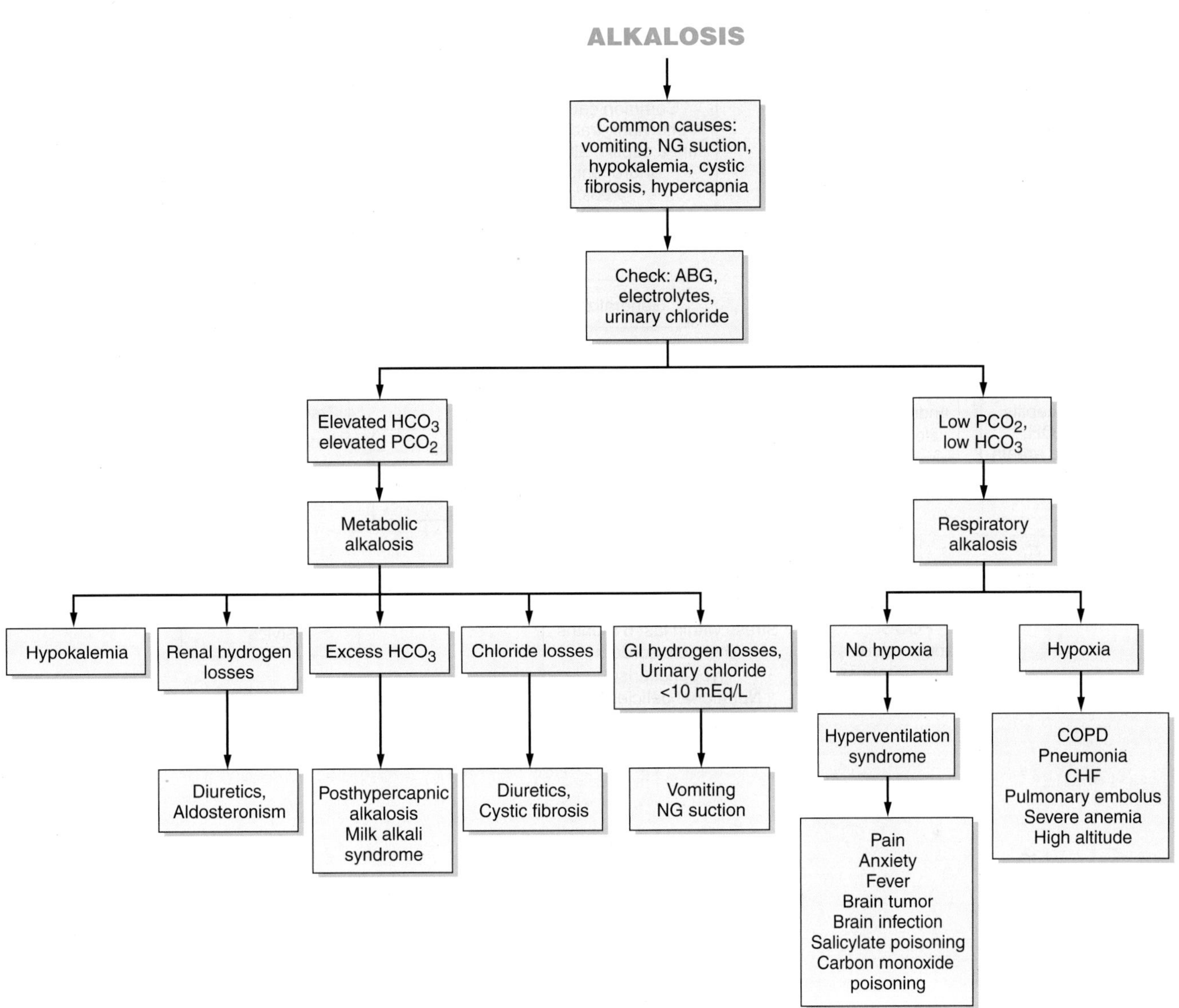

Robert A. Baldor, MD and Alan M. Ehrlich, MD

Nutr Clin Pract. 2008;23(2):122–7.

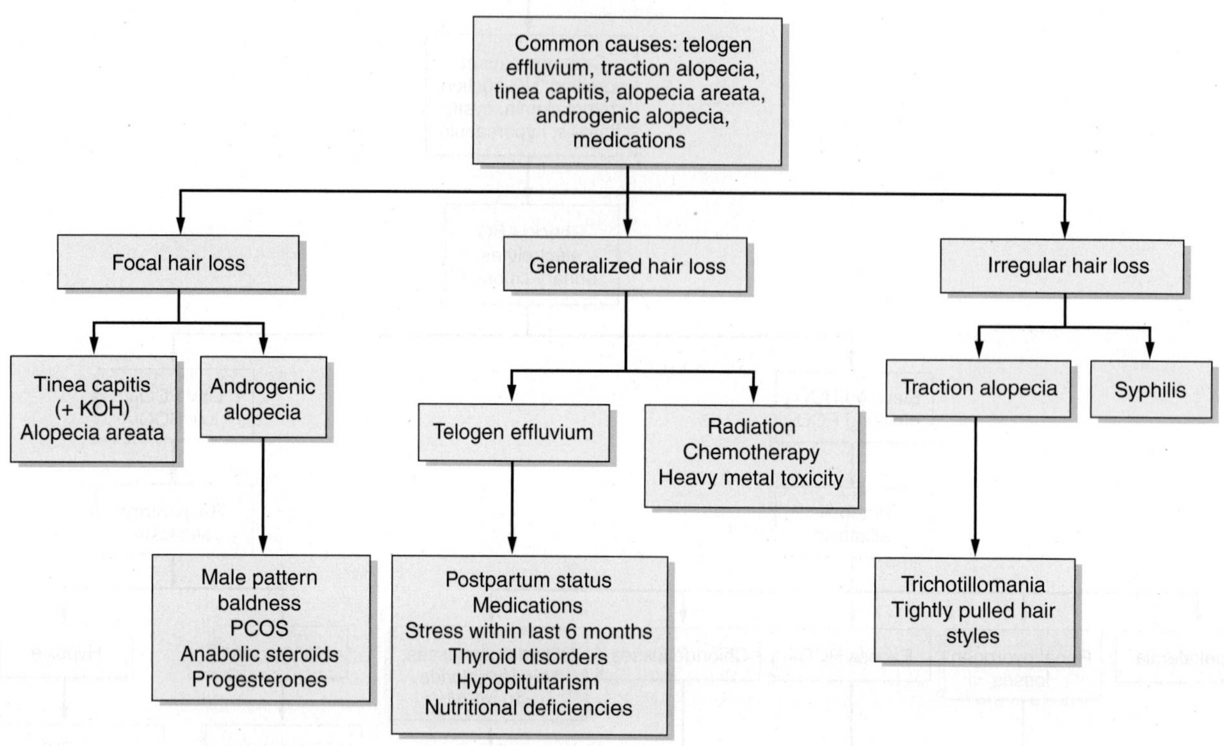

Robert A. Baldor, MD and Alan M. Ehrlich, MD

Am Fam Physician. 2009;80(4):356–62.

AMENORRHEA, PRIMARY (ABSENCE OF MENARCHE BY AGE 16)

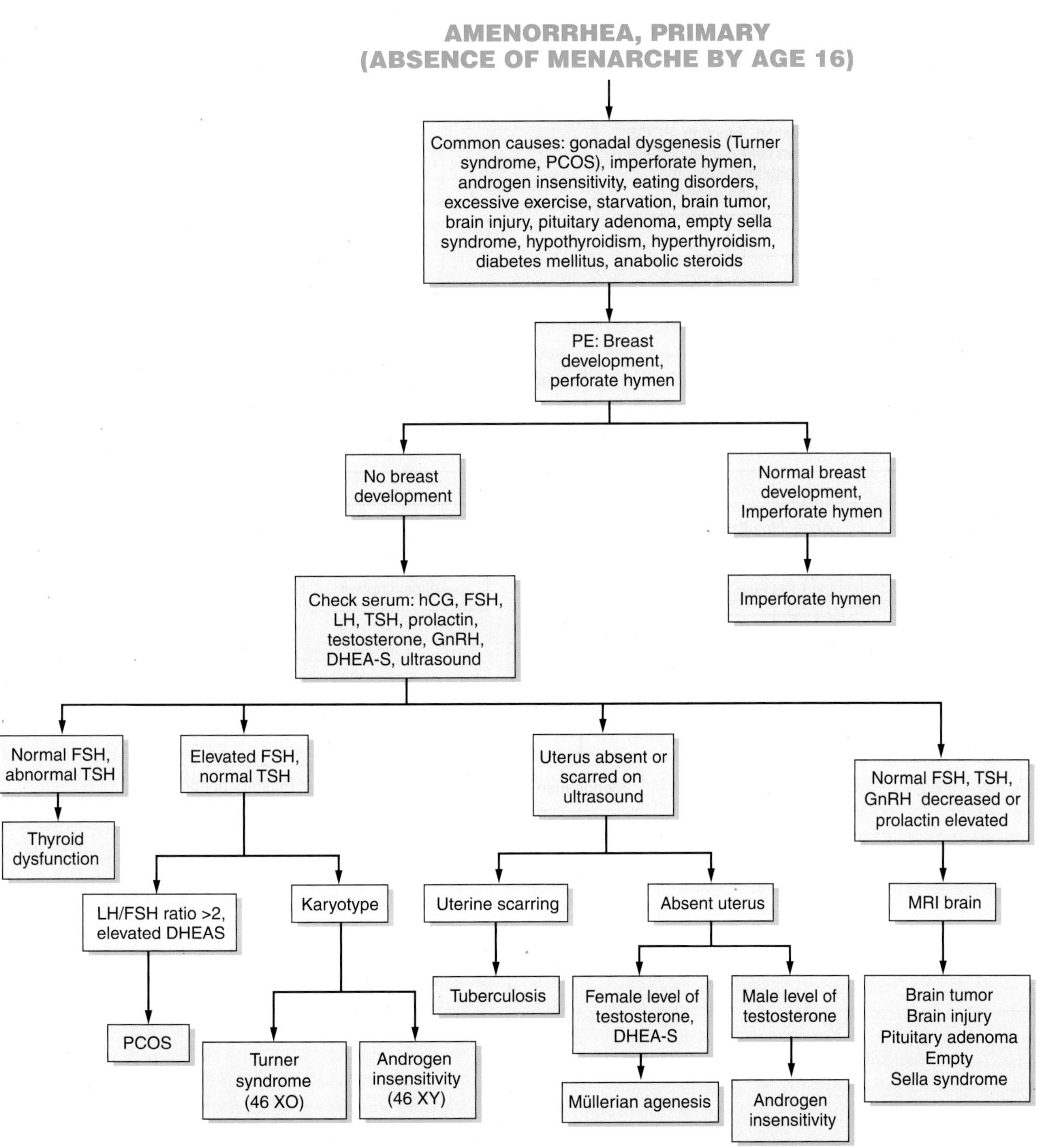

Robert A. Baldor, MD and Alan M. Ehrlich, MD

Am Fam Physician. 2006;73:1374–82.

AMENORRHEA, SECONDARY

Common causes: pregnancy, ectopic pregnancy, anorexia/ starvation, infection, PCOS, ovarian failure (menopause), pituitary adenoma hypothyroidism

↓

Urine hCG

- ⊕ → Intrauterine pregnancy; Ectopic pregnancy
- ⊖ → Vaginal/bimanual exam; FSH, LH, TSH
  - → Stress; Weight loss; Extreme exercise
  - → Acne, hirsutism, BMI >30, Deepening of voice, LH/FSH ratio >2 → Check labs: DHEA-S, testosterone (increased) → PCOS
  - → ↑ FSH; ↑ LH → Hot flashes; Sleep difficulty; Decreased libido → Menopause
  - → Medications: Oral contraceptives; Metoclopramide; Antipsychotics
  - → Galactorrhea → Increased serum prolactin → Pituitary adenoma
  - → Elevated TSH → Hypothyroidism

Robert A. Baldor, MD and Alan M. Ehrlich, MD

Am Fam Physician. 2006;73:1374–82.

AMNESIA

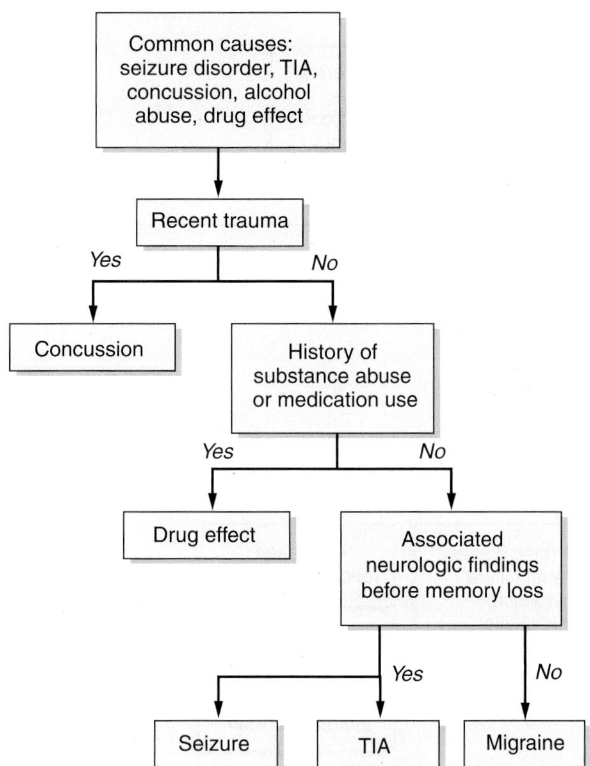

Robert A. Baldor, MD and Alan M. Ehrlich, MD

Ann Intern Med. 2007;146(6):397–405.

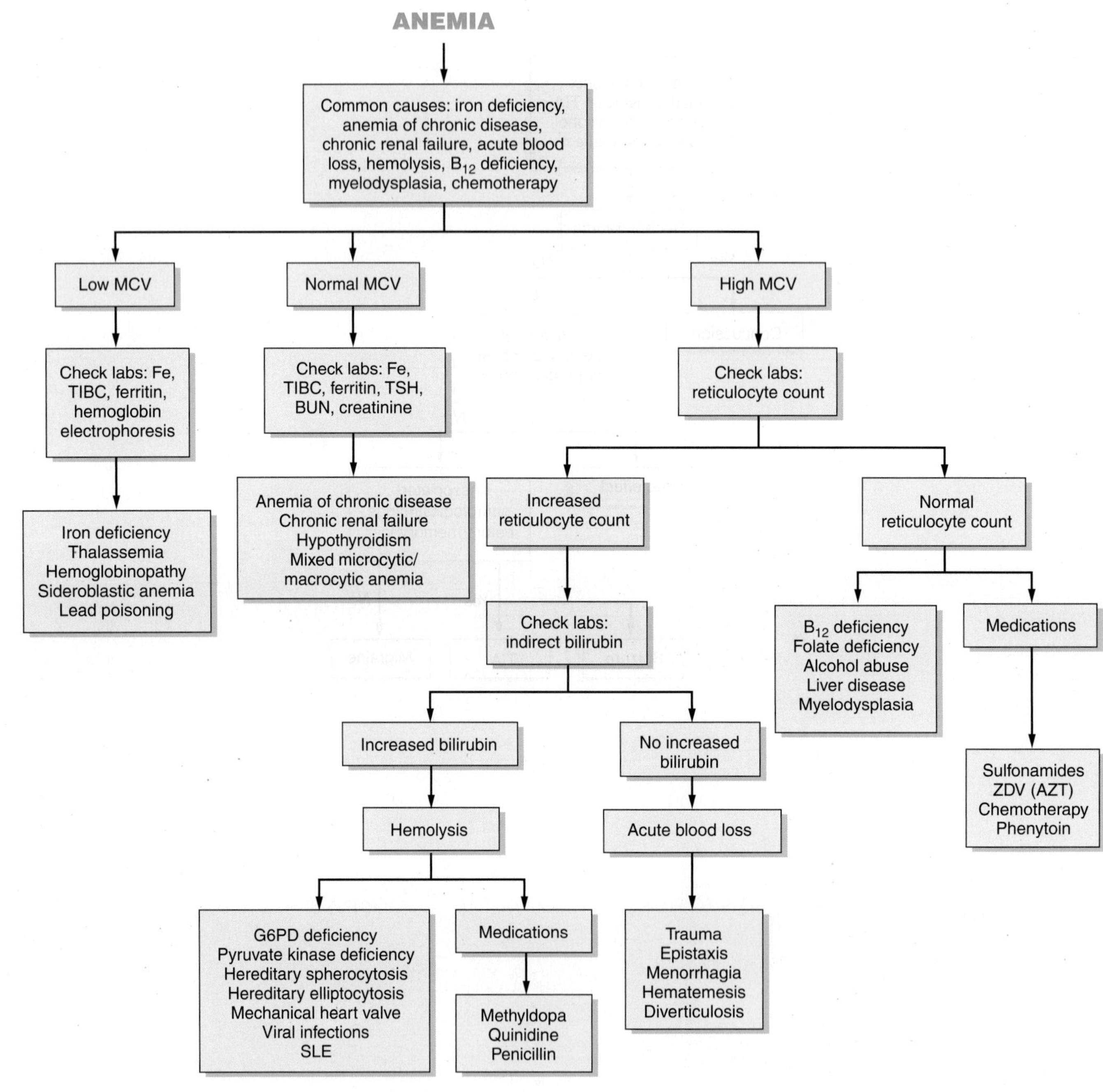
ANEMIA
Common causes: iron deficiency, anemia of chronic disease, chronic renal failure, acute blood loss, hemolysis, B12 deficiency, myelodysplasia, chemotherapy
Low MCV
Normal MCV
High MCV
Check labs: Fe, TIBC, ferritin, hemoglobin electrophoresis
Check labs: Fe, TIBC, ferritin, TSH, BUN, creatinine
Check labs: reticulocyte count
Iron deficiency
Thalassemia
Hemoglobinopathy
Sideroblastic anemia
Lead poisoning
Anemia of chronic disease
Chronic renal failure
Hypothyroidism
Mixed microcytic/macrocytic anemia
Increased reticulocyte count
Normal reticulocyte count
Check labs: indirect bilirubin
B12 deficiency
Folate deficiency
Alcohol abuse
Liver disease
Myelodysplasia
Medications
Increased bilirubin
No increased bilirubin
Sulfonamides
ZDV (AZT)
Chemotherapy
Phenytoin
Hemolysis
Acute blood loss
G6PD deficiency
Pyruvate kinase deficiency
Hereditary spherocytosis
Hereditary elliptocytosis
Mechanical heart valve
Viral infections
SLE
Medications
Methyldopa
Quinidine
Penicillin
Trauma
Epistaxis
Menorrhagia
Hematemesis
Diverticulosis

Robert A. Baldor, MD and Alan M. Ehrlich, MD

Am Fam Physician. 2000;62:1565–72.

ANOREXIA

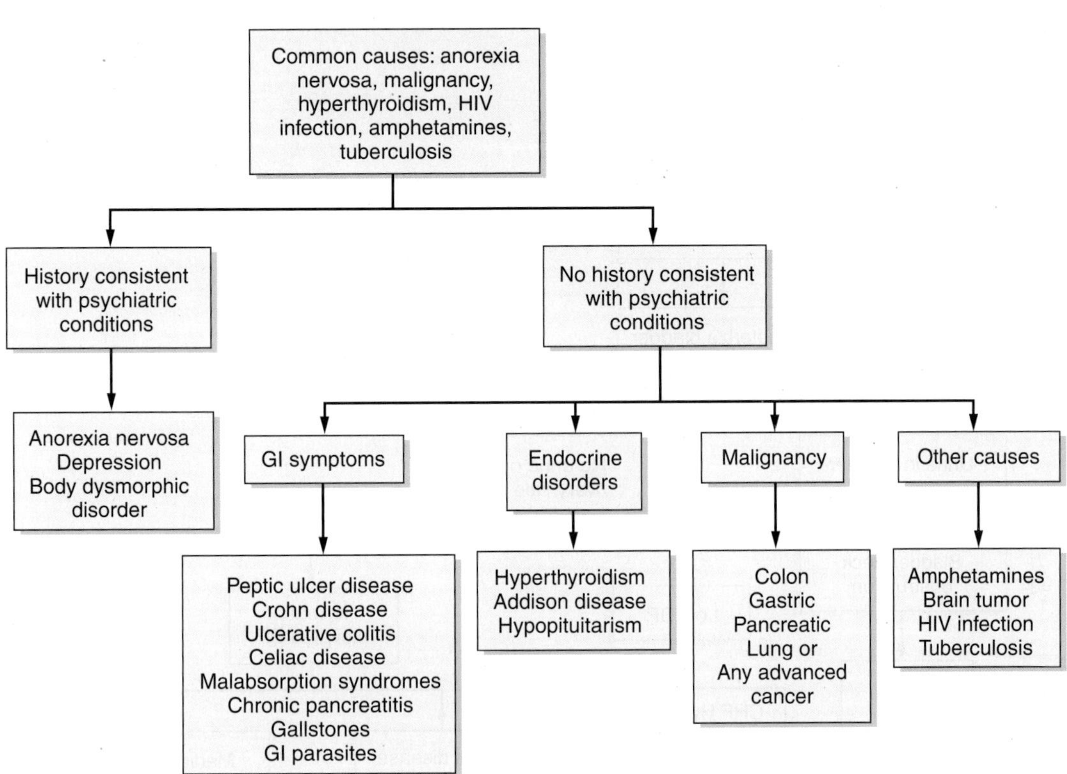

Robert A. Baldor, MD and Alan M. Ehrlich, MD

Am Fam Physician. 2003;67:297–304, 311–2.

ANURIA OR OLIGURIA

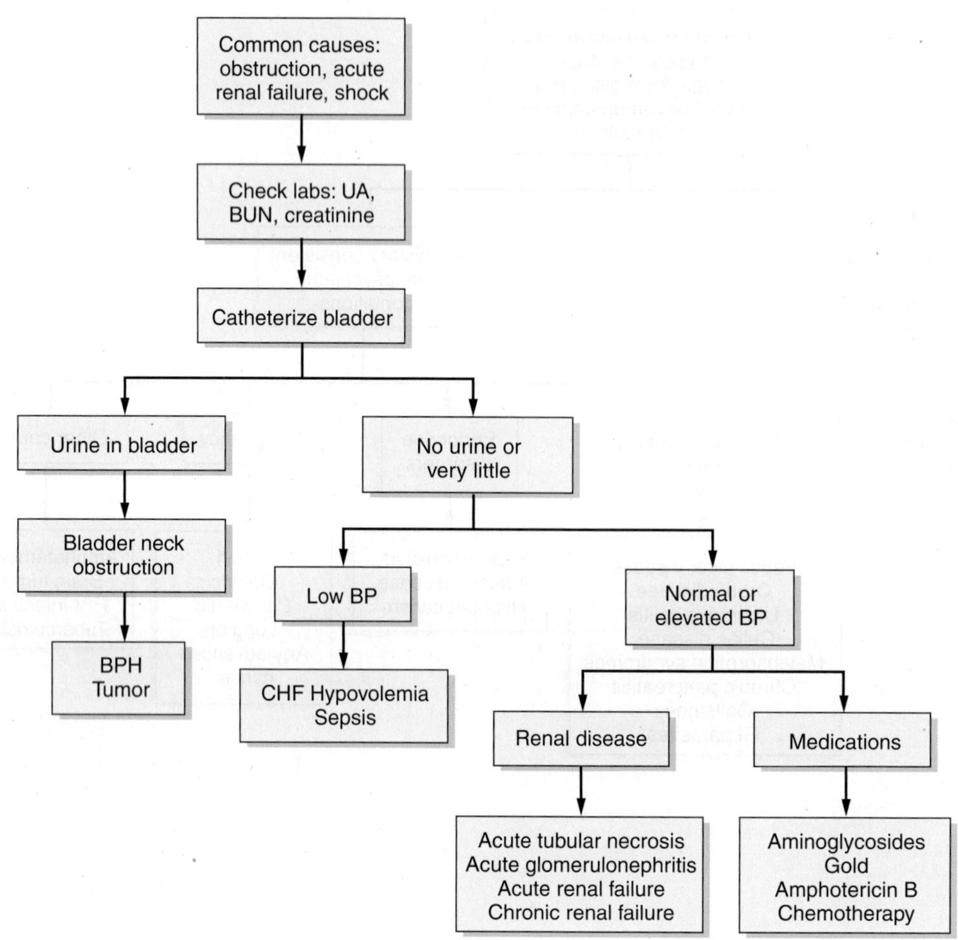

Robert A. Baldor, MD and Alan M. Ehrlich, MD

Am Fam Physician. 2000;61:2077–88.

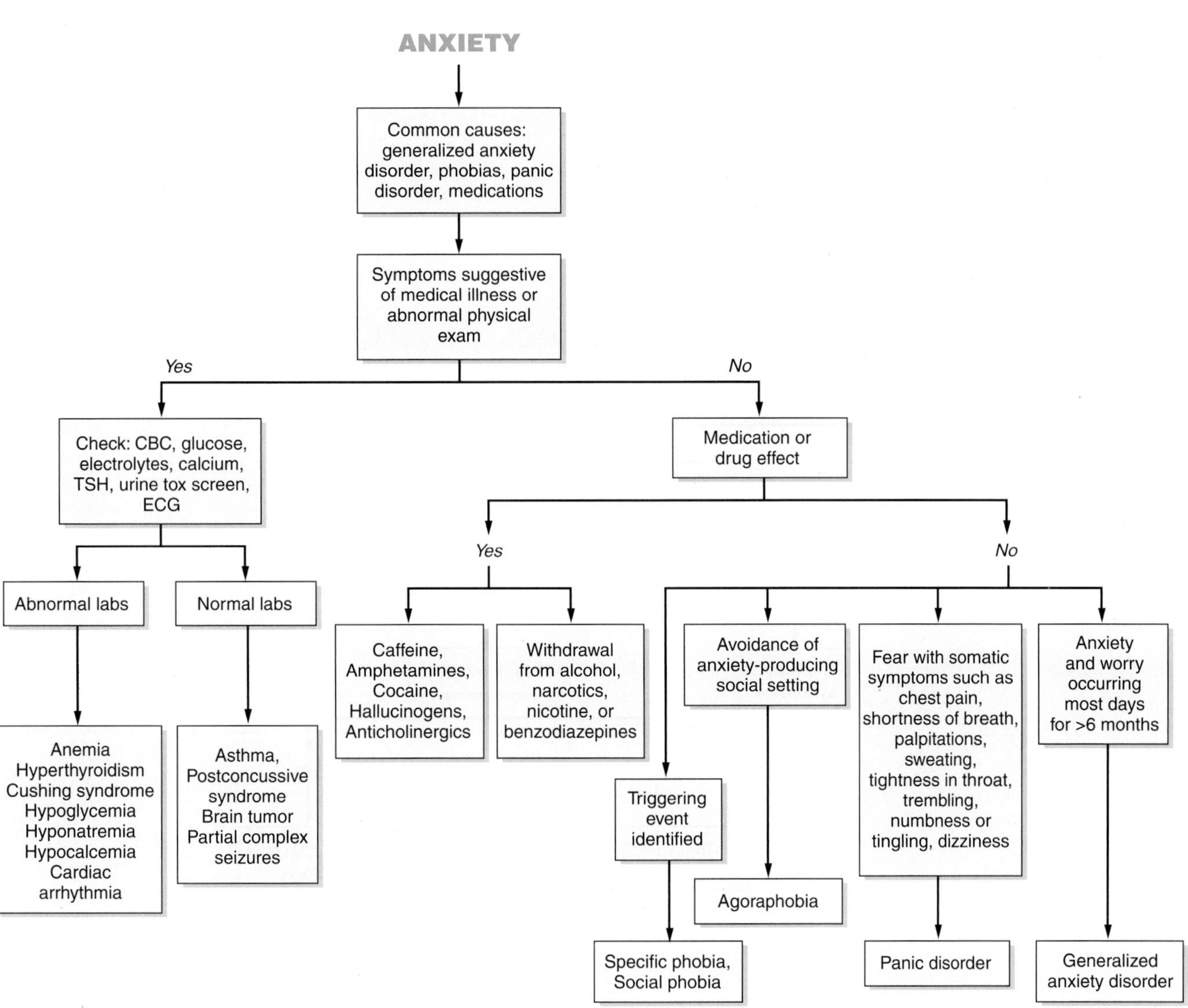

Robert A. Baldor, MD and Alan M. Ehrlich, MD

Am J Psychiatry. 1999;156:1677–85.

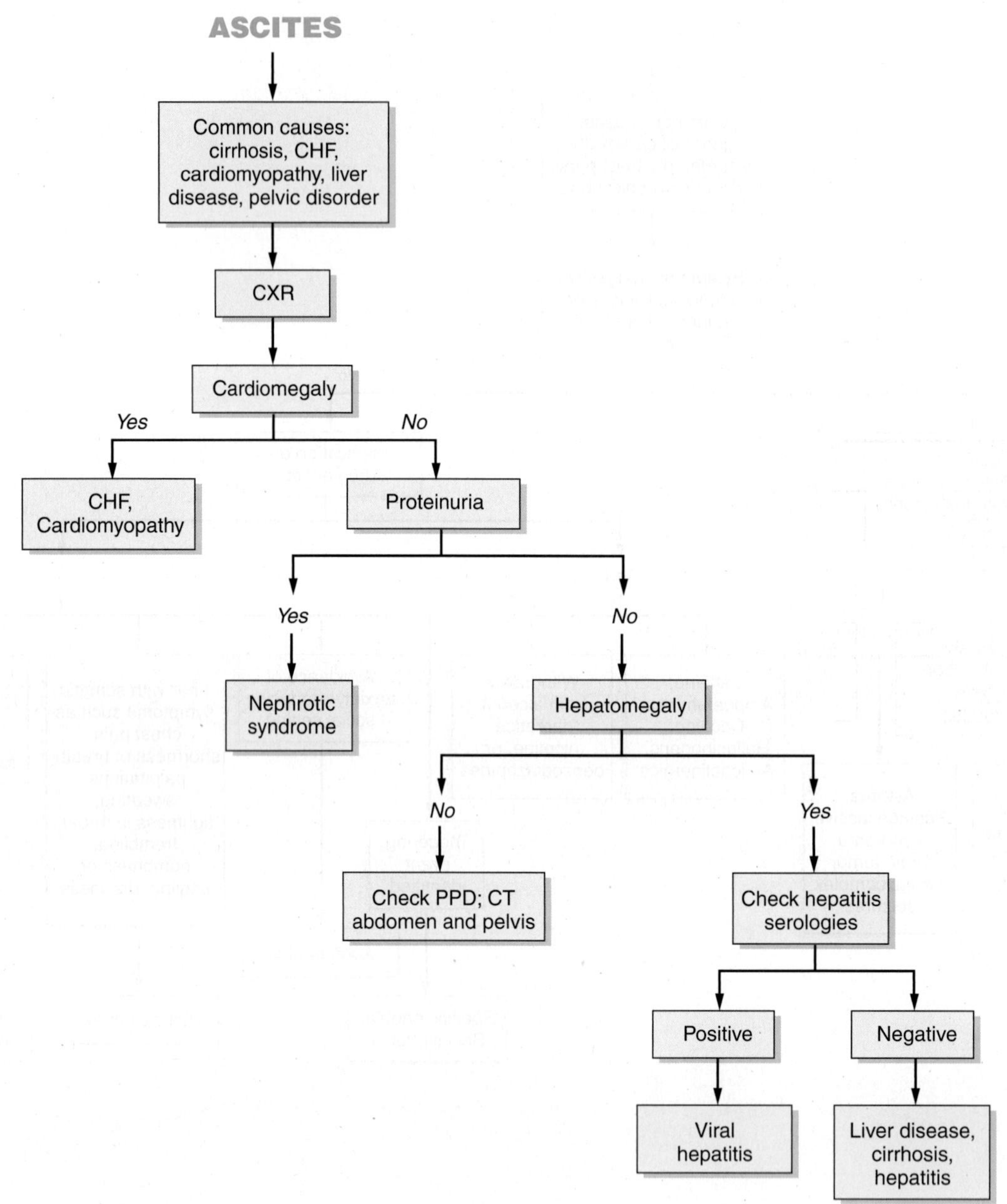

Robert A. Baldor, MD and Alan M. Ehrlich, MD

Am Fam Physician. 2006;74:767–76.

AST ELEVATION

Common causes: hemolysis, liver disease, myocardial infarction, CHF, acute renal failure, biliary obstruction, pancreatitis, muscle disorders, medications

↓

Check: LFTs, consider CBC, BUN, creatinine, hepatitis serologies, CPK, amylase, CXR, ultrasound/CT of abdomen

↓

- Jaundice → Liver disease, Biliary obstruction, Hemolysis, Viral hepatitis
- Chest pain or dyspnea → Myocardial infarction, CHF
- Abdominal pain, Elevated amylase → Pancreatitis
- Edema → CHF, Acute renal failure
- Muscle disorder or injury
- Liver toxicity → Alcohol, Medications

Robert A. Baldor, MD and Alan M. Ehrlich, MD

Am Fam Physician. 2005;71:1105–10.

ASTHMA EXACERBATION, PEDIATRIC ACUTE

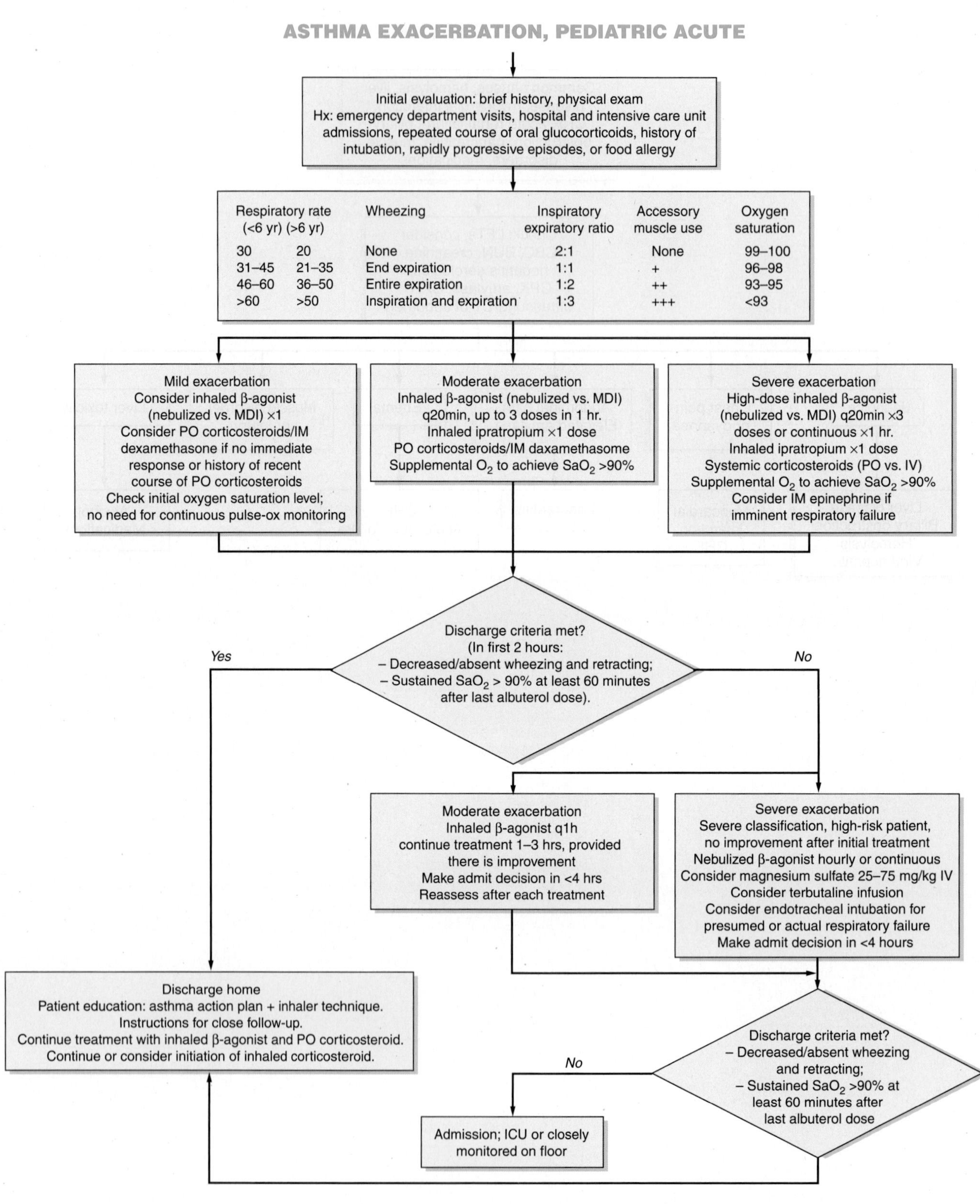

Initial evaluation: brief history, physical exam
Hx: emergency department visits, hospital and intensive care unit admissions, repeated course of oral glucocorticoids, history of intubation, rapidly progressive episodes, or food allergy
Respiratory rate (<6 yr) (>6 yr)
Wheezing
Inspiratory expiratory ratio
Accessory muscle use
Oxygen saturation
30 20 None 2:1 None 99–100
31–45 21–35 End expiration 1:1 + 96–98
46–60 36–50 Entire expiration 1:2 ++ 93–95
>60 >50 Inspiration and expiration 1:3 +++ <93
Mild exacerbation
Consider inhaled β-agonist (nebulized vs. MDI) ×1
Consider PO corticosteroids/IM dexamethasone if no immediate response or history of recent course of PO corticosteroids
Check initial oxygen saturation level; no need for continuous pulse-ox monitoring
Moderate exacerbation
Inhaled β-agonist (nebulized vs. MDI) q20min, up to 3 doses in 1 hr.
Inhaled ipratropium ×1 dose
PO corticosteroids/IM daxamethasome
Supplemental O2 to achieve SaO2 >90%
Severe exacerbation
High-dose inhaled β-agonist (nebulized vs. MDI) q20min ×3 doses or continuous ×1 hr.
Inhaled ipratropium ×1 dose
Systemic corticosteroids (PO vs. IV)
Supplemental O2 to achieve SaO2 >90%
Consider IM epinephrine if imminent respiratory failure
Discharge criteria met? (In first 2 hours:
– Decreased/absent wheezing and retracting;
– Sustained SaO2 > 90% at least 60 minutes after last albuterol dose).
Yes
No
Moderate exacerbation
Inhaled β-agonist q1h
continue treatment 1–3 hrs, provided there is improvement
Make admit decision in <4 hrs
Reassess after each treatment
Severe exacerbation
Severe classification, high-risk patient, no improvement after initial treatment
Nebulized β-agonist hourly or continuous
Consider magnesium sulfate 25–75 mg/kg IV
Consider terbutaline infusion
Consider endotracheal intubation for presumed or actual respiratory failure
Make admit decision in <4 hours
Discharge home
Patient education: asthma action plan + inhaler technique.
Instructions for close follow-up.
Continue treatment with inhaled β-agonist and PO corticosteroid.
Continue or consider initiation of inhaled corticosteroid.
Discharge criteria met?
– Decreased/absent wheezing and retracting;
– Sustained SaO2 >90% at least 60 minutes after last albuterol dose
No
Admission; ICU or closely monitored on floor

Catherine James, MD

Am Fam Physician. 2005;71:1959–68.

ATAXIA

Common causes: labyrinthitis, multiple sclerosis, stroke, BPPV normal pressure hydrocephalus alcoholism, spinal cord disorders, multisensory loss

- Acute onset
  - TIA; Stroke; Acute alcohol intoxication; Encephalitis; Head trauma; Postviral status; HIV infection; Any infection or acute metabolic disturbance in the elderly; Muscle weakness
  - Medications
    - Phenytoin; Carbamazepine; Phenobarbital; Anticholinergic drugs; Aminoglutethimide; Aminoglycosides
  - Tinnitus, vertigo, and/or hearing loss
    - Labyrinthitis; Ménière disease; Acoustic neuroma
- Gradual onset
  - Toxic exposure
    - Mercury; Lead; Thallium; Carbon tetrachloride; Toluene
  - No toxic exposures
    - Family history of ataxias
      - Friedreich ataxia; Ataxia telangiectasia
    - No family history
      - Sensory loss in extremities
        - Peripheral neuropathy; Syphilis; Spinal cord tumor or injury; Vitamin B_{12} deficiency; Multiple sclerosis; HIV infection; Multi-sensory loss
      - No sensory loss
        - Posterior fossa lesions; Multiple sclerosis; Hypothyroidism; Syphilis; Normal pressure hydrocephalus

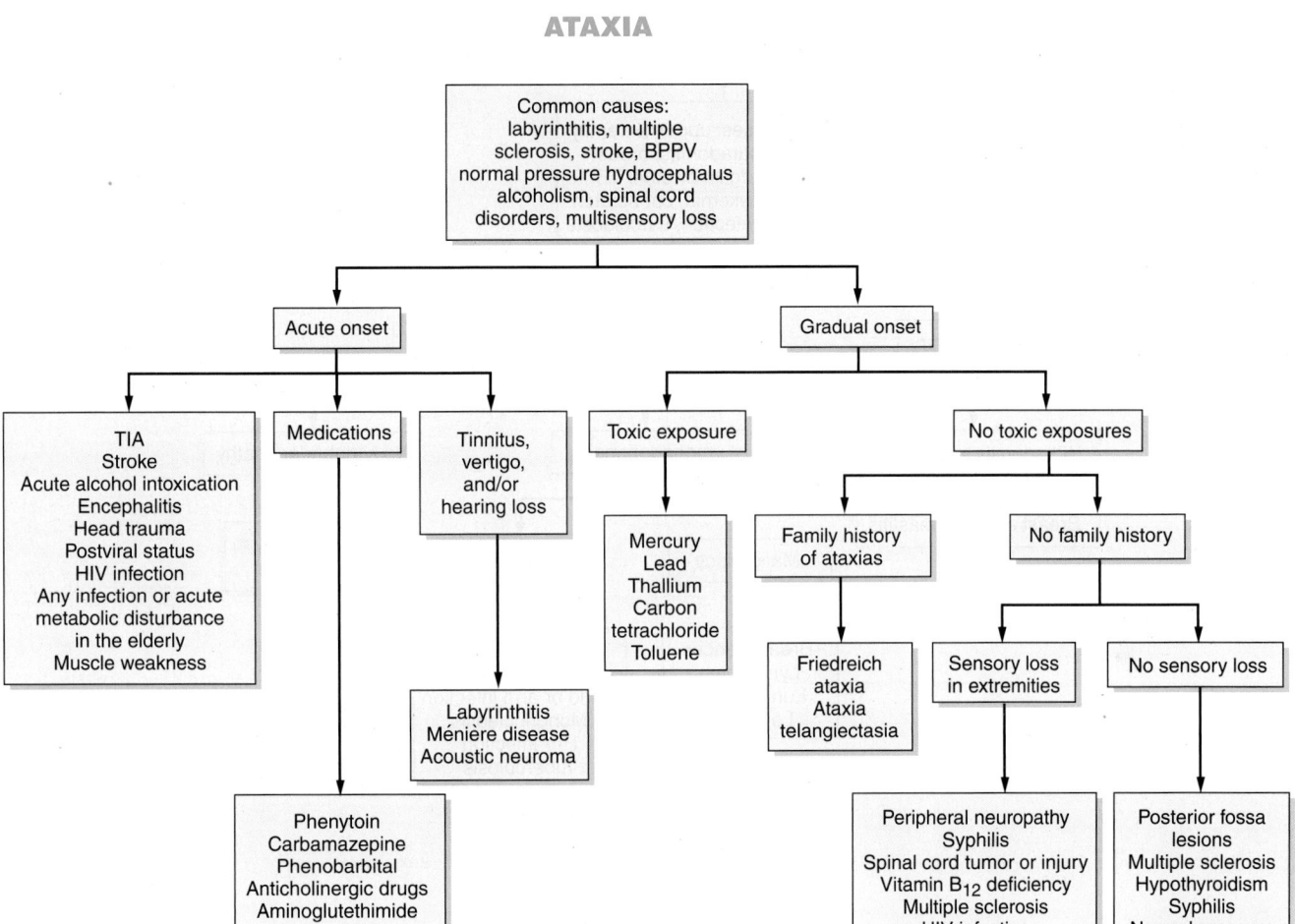

Robert A. Baldor, MD and Alan M. Ehrlich, MD

Arch Neurol. 2008;65(10):1296–303.

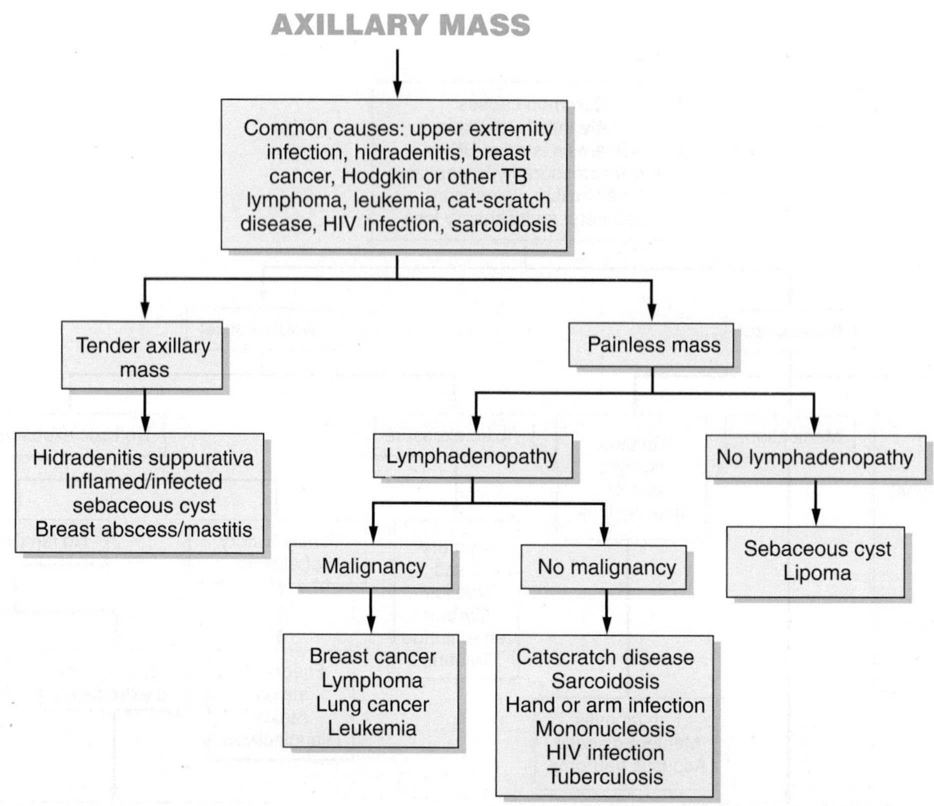

Robert A. Baldor, MD and Alan M. Ehrlich, MD

Ann Surg Oncol. 2000;7:411–5.

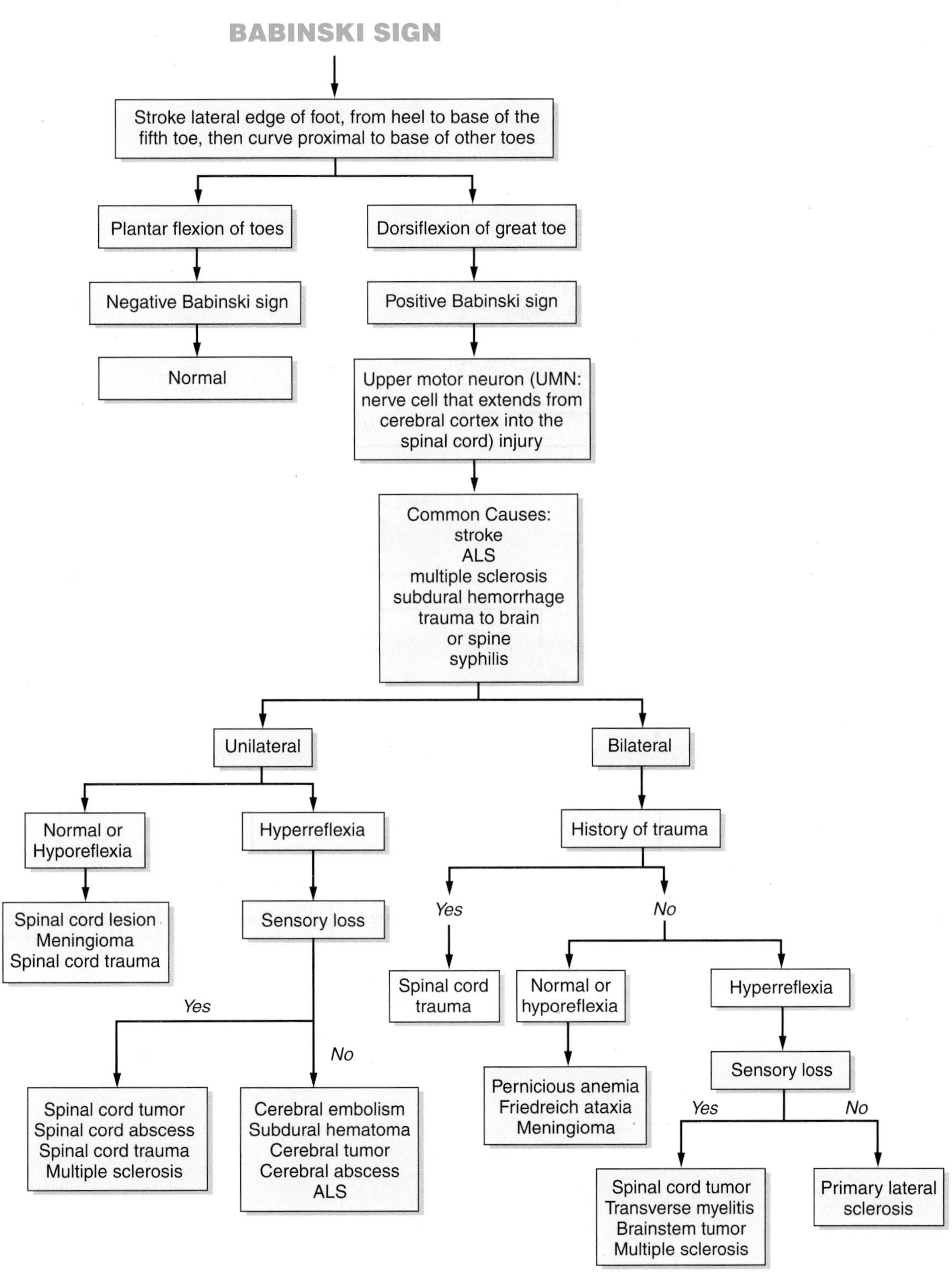

Robert A. Baldor, MD and Alan M. Ehrlich, MD

J Neurol Neurosurg Psychiatry. 2002;73(4):360–2.

BACK PAIN, ACUTE

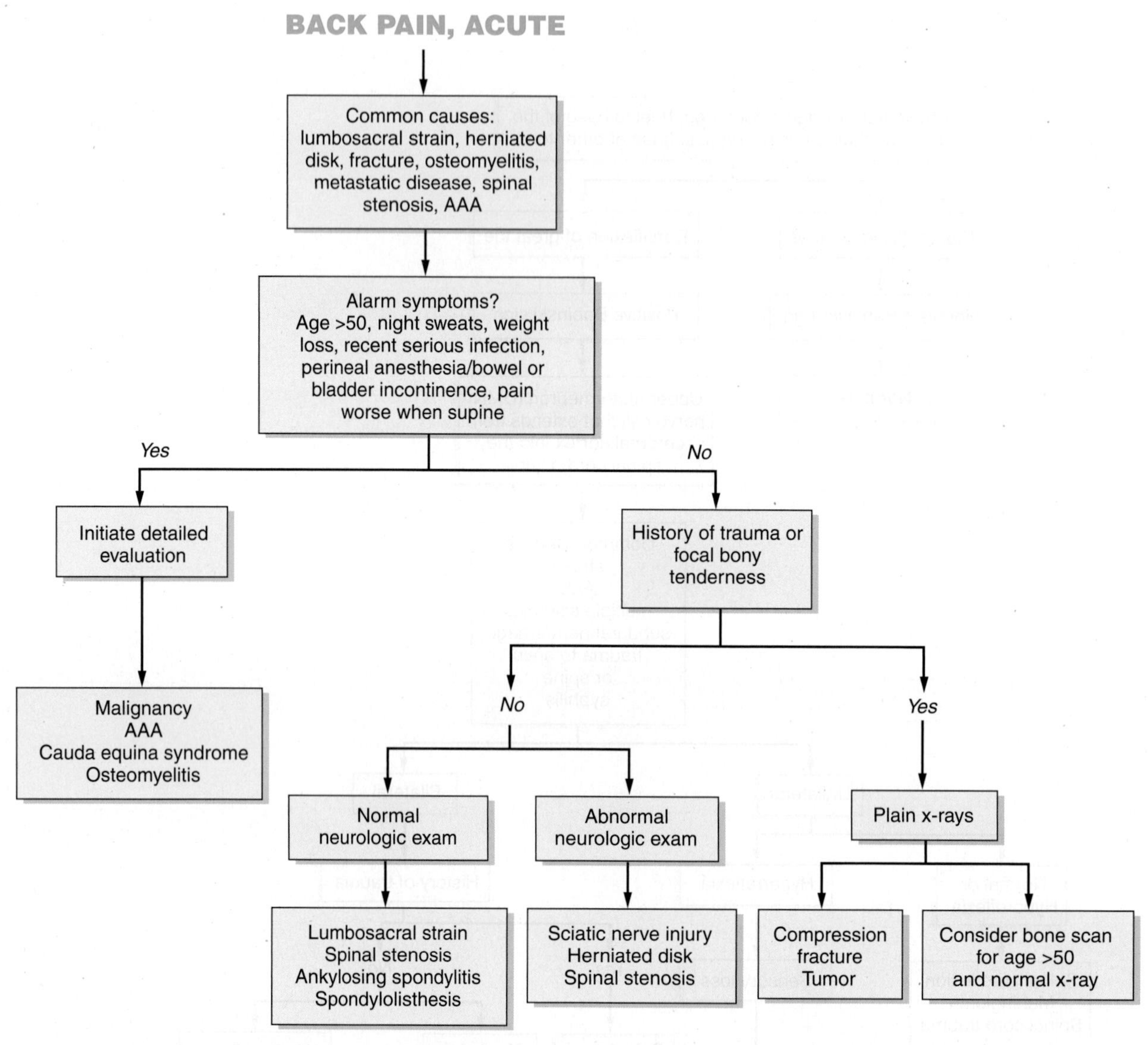

Robert A. Baldor, MD and Alan M. Ehrlich, MD

Am Fam Physician. 2007;75:1181–8.

BLEEDING GUMS

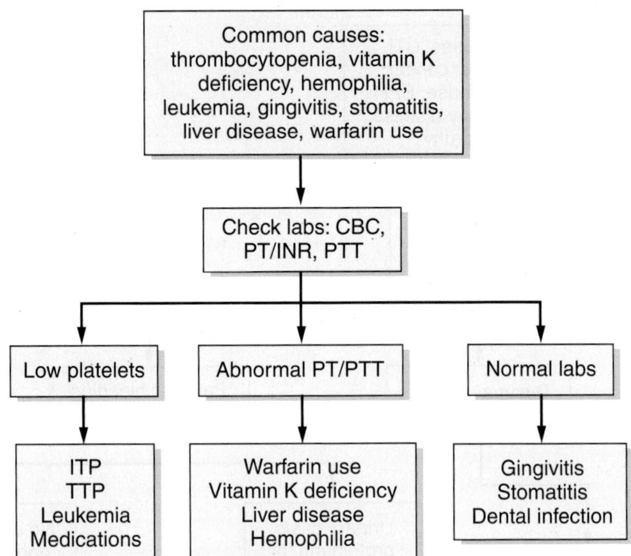

Robert A. Baldor, MD and Alan M. Ehrlich, MD

Compend Contin Educ Dent. 1999;20(10):936–40.

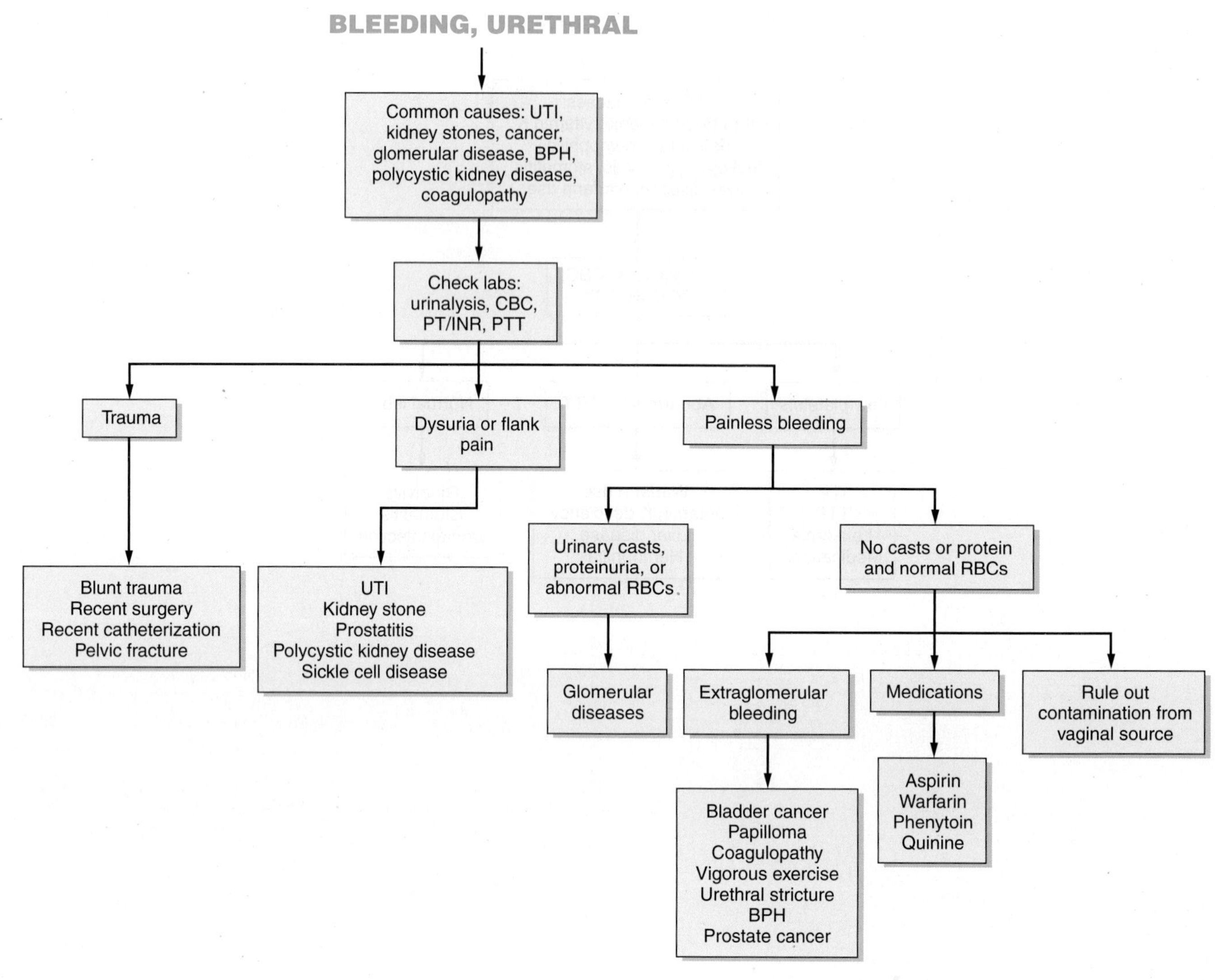

Robert A. Baldor, MD and Alan M. Ehrlich, MD

Am Fam Physician. 2001;63:1145–54.

BREAST DISCHARGE

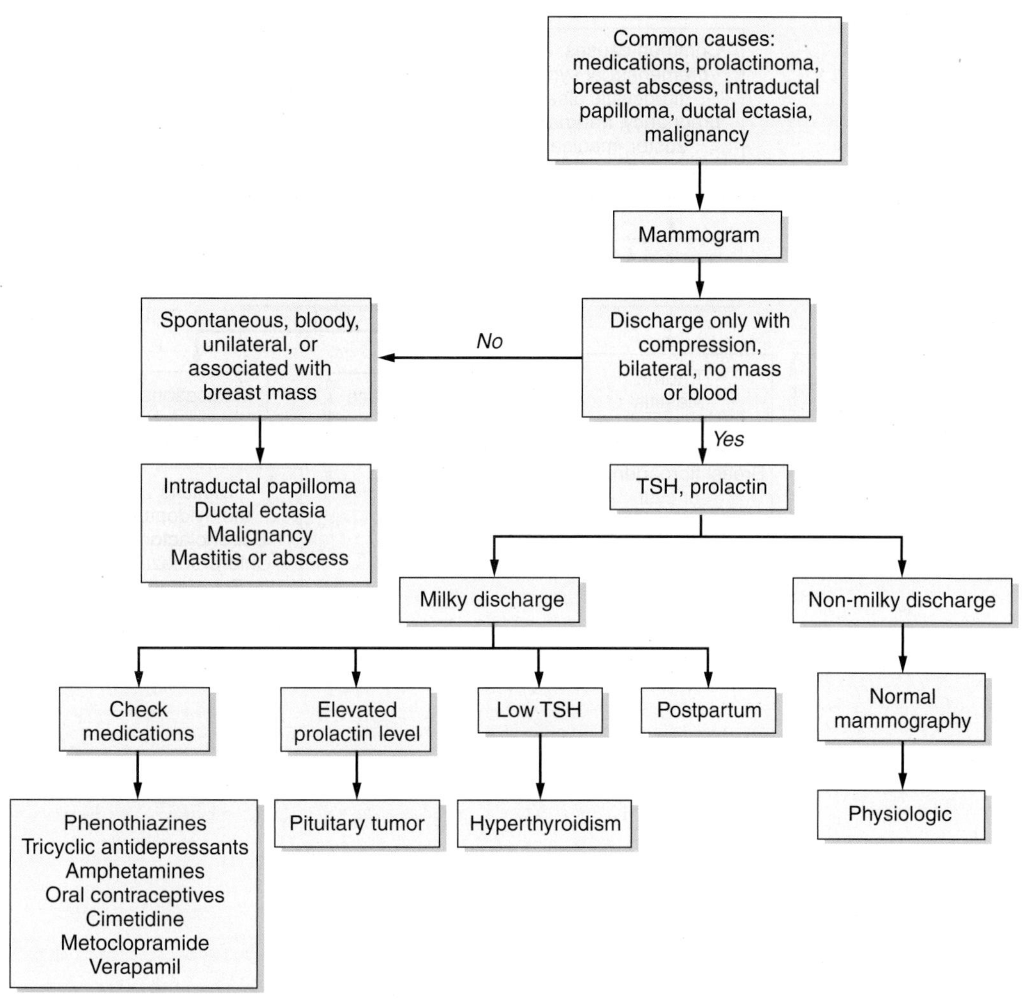

Robert A. Baldor, MD and Alan M. Ehrlich, MD

Breast J. 2009;15(3):230–5.

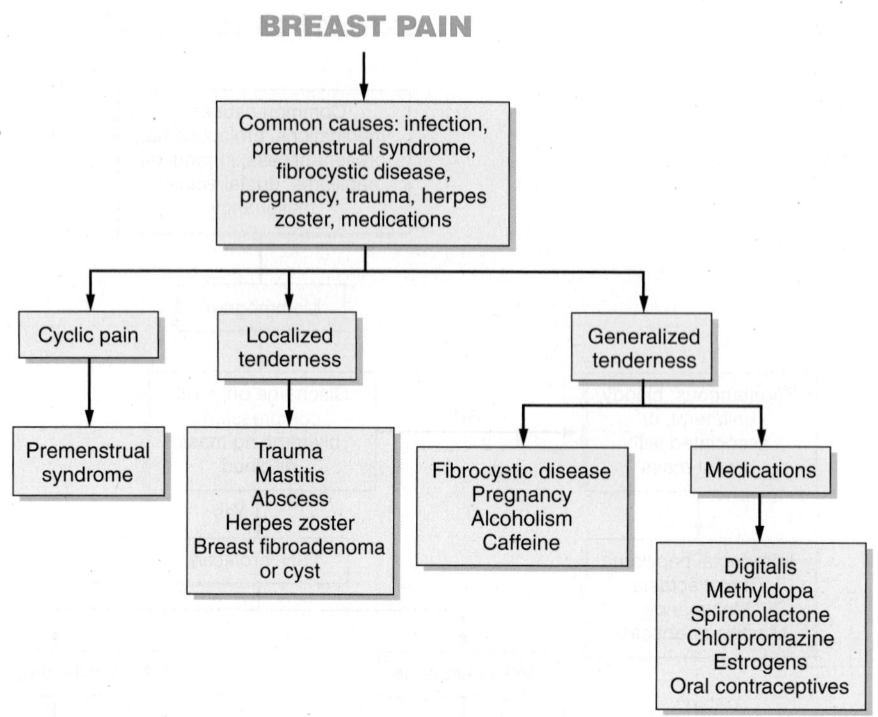

Robert A. Baldor, MD and Alan M. Ehrlich, MD

Obstet Gynecol Clin North Am. 2008;35(2):285–303.

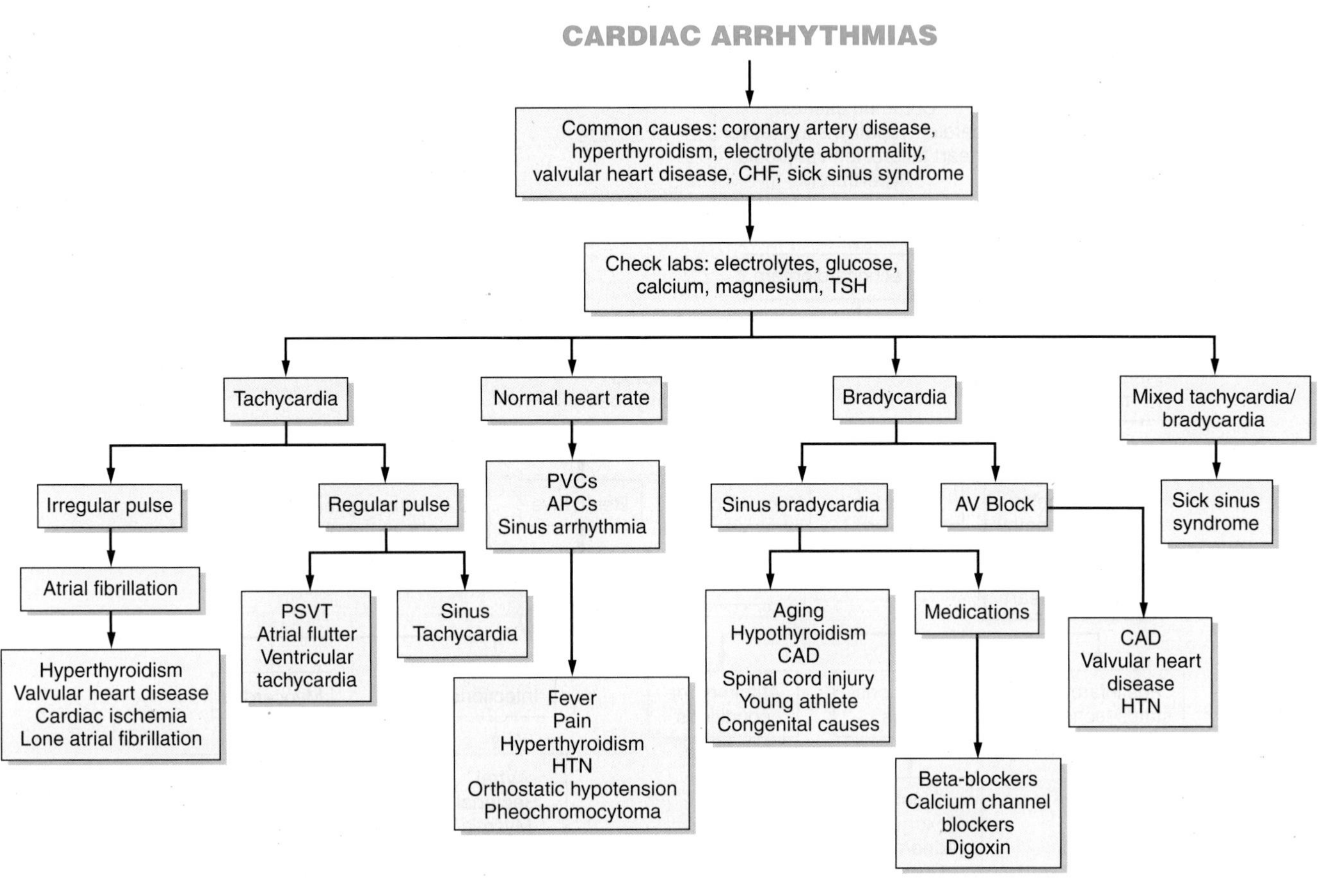

Robert A. Baldor, MD and Alan M. Ehrlich, MD

Am Fam Physician. 2005;743–50, 755–9.

CARDIOMEGALY

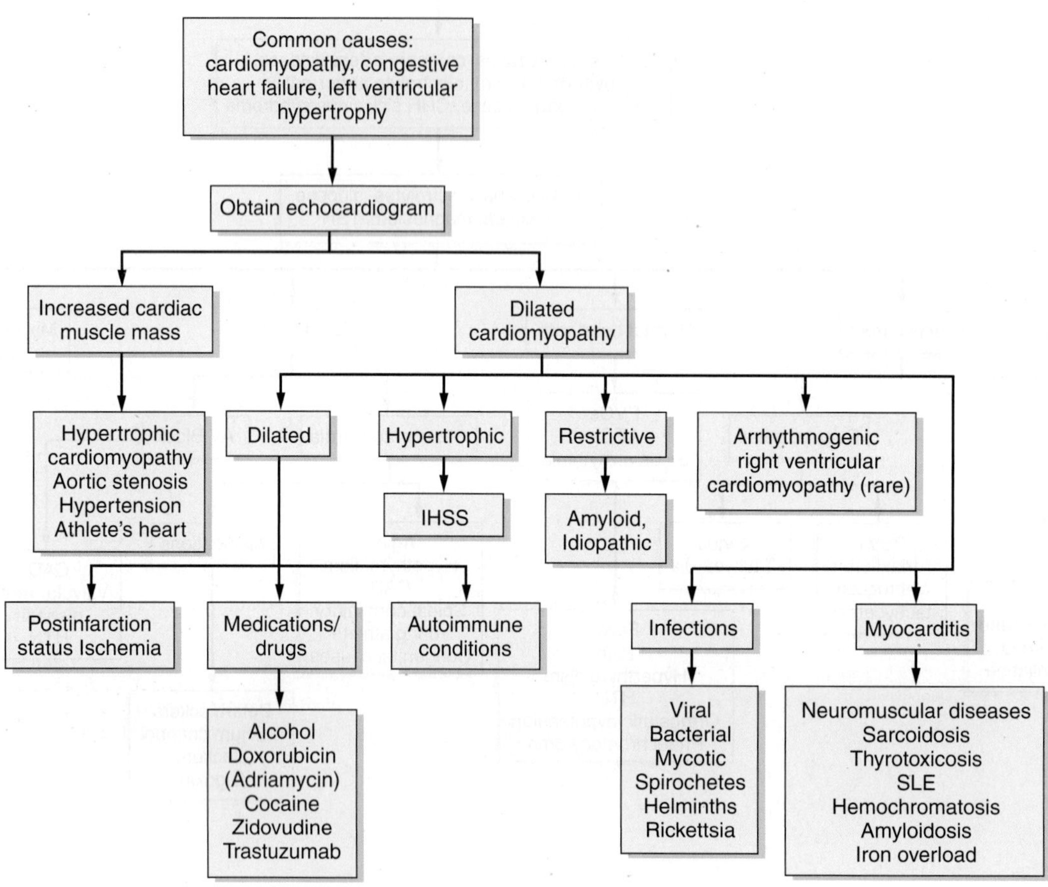

Robert A. Baldor, MD and Alan M. Ehrlich, MD

Eur J Echocardiogr. 2009;10(8):iii15–21.

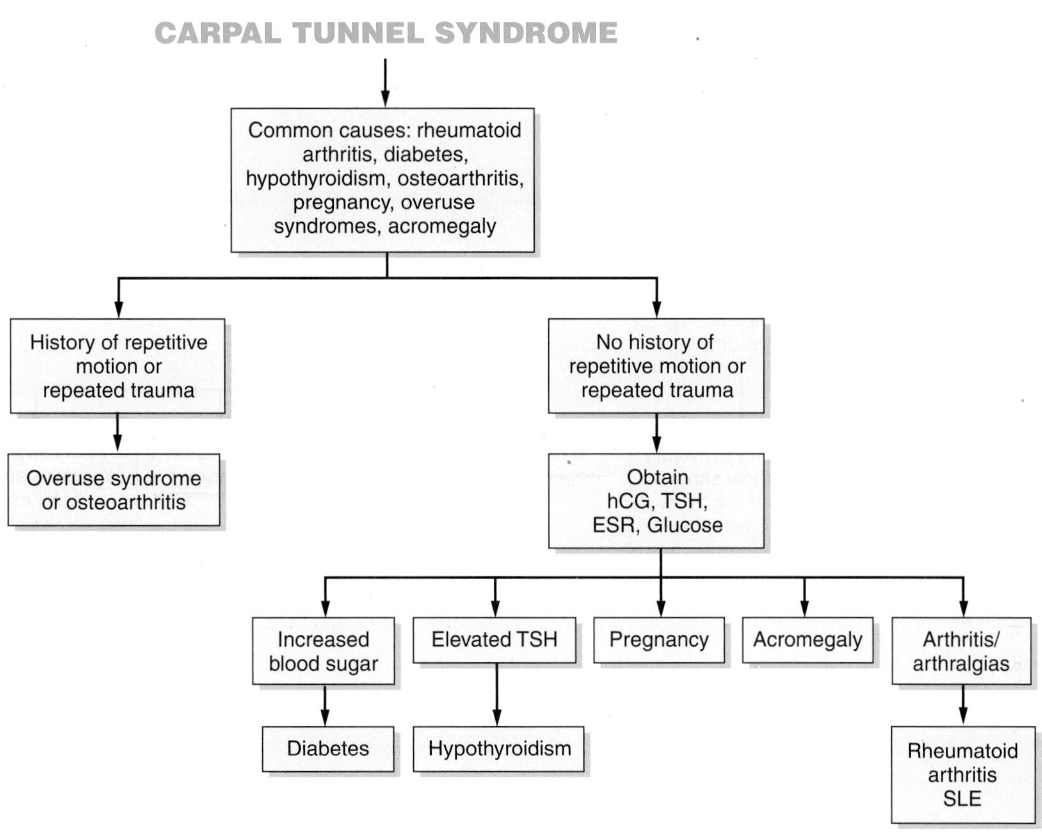

Robert A. Baldor, MD and Alan M. Ehrlich, MD

BMJ. 2007;335(7615):343–6.

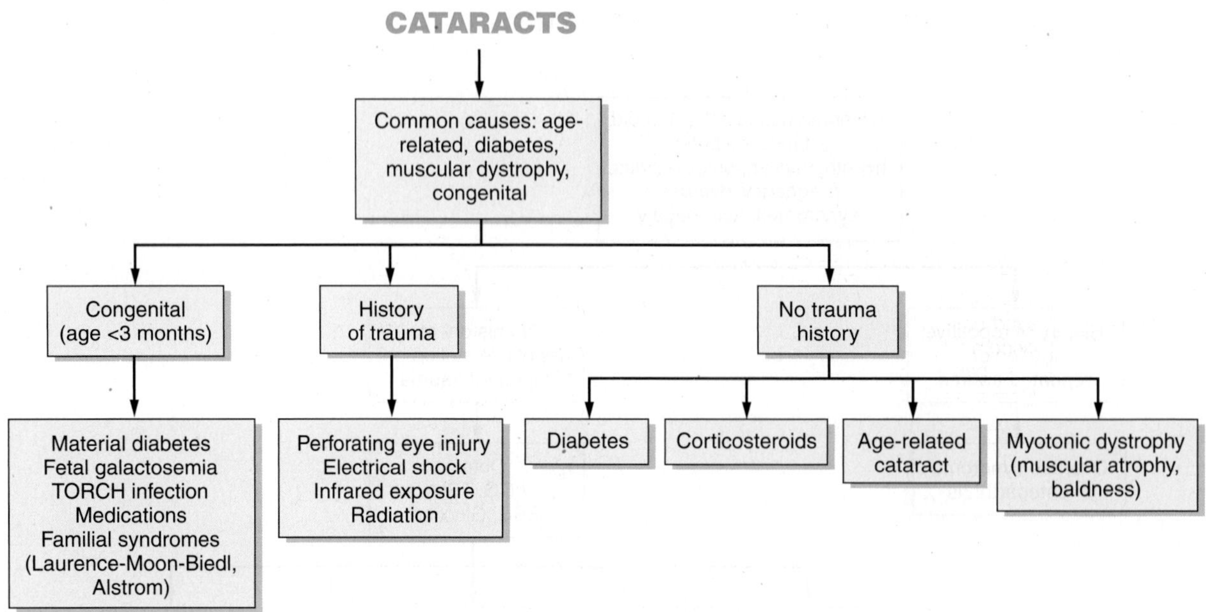

Robert A. Baldor, MD and Alan M. Ehrlich, MD

Ophthalmology. 2010;117(8):1471–8.

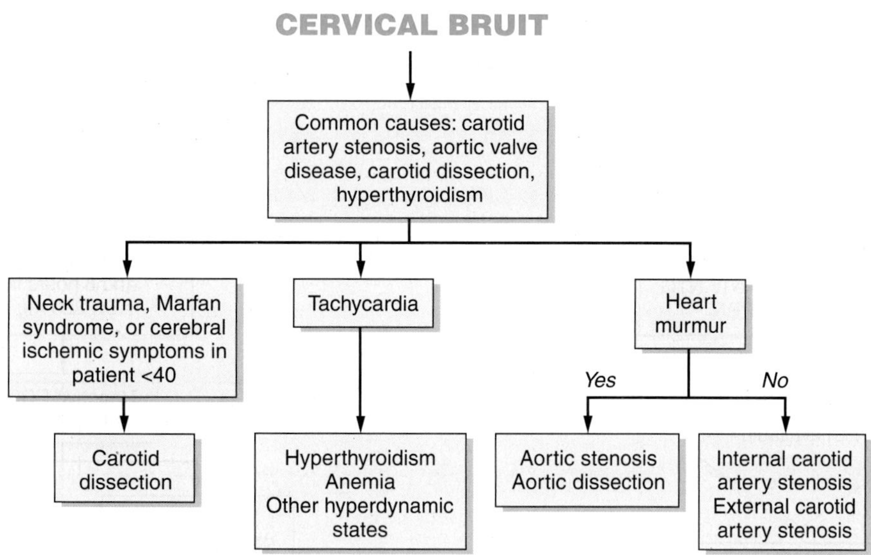

Robert A. Baldor, MD and Alan M. Ehrlich, MD

http://www.ncbi.nlm.nih.gov/bookshelf/br.fcgi?book=cm&part=A593

CHEST PAIN/ACUTE CORONARY SYNDROME

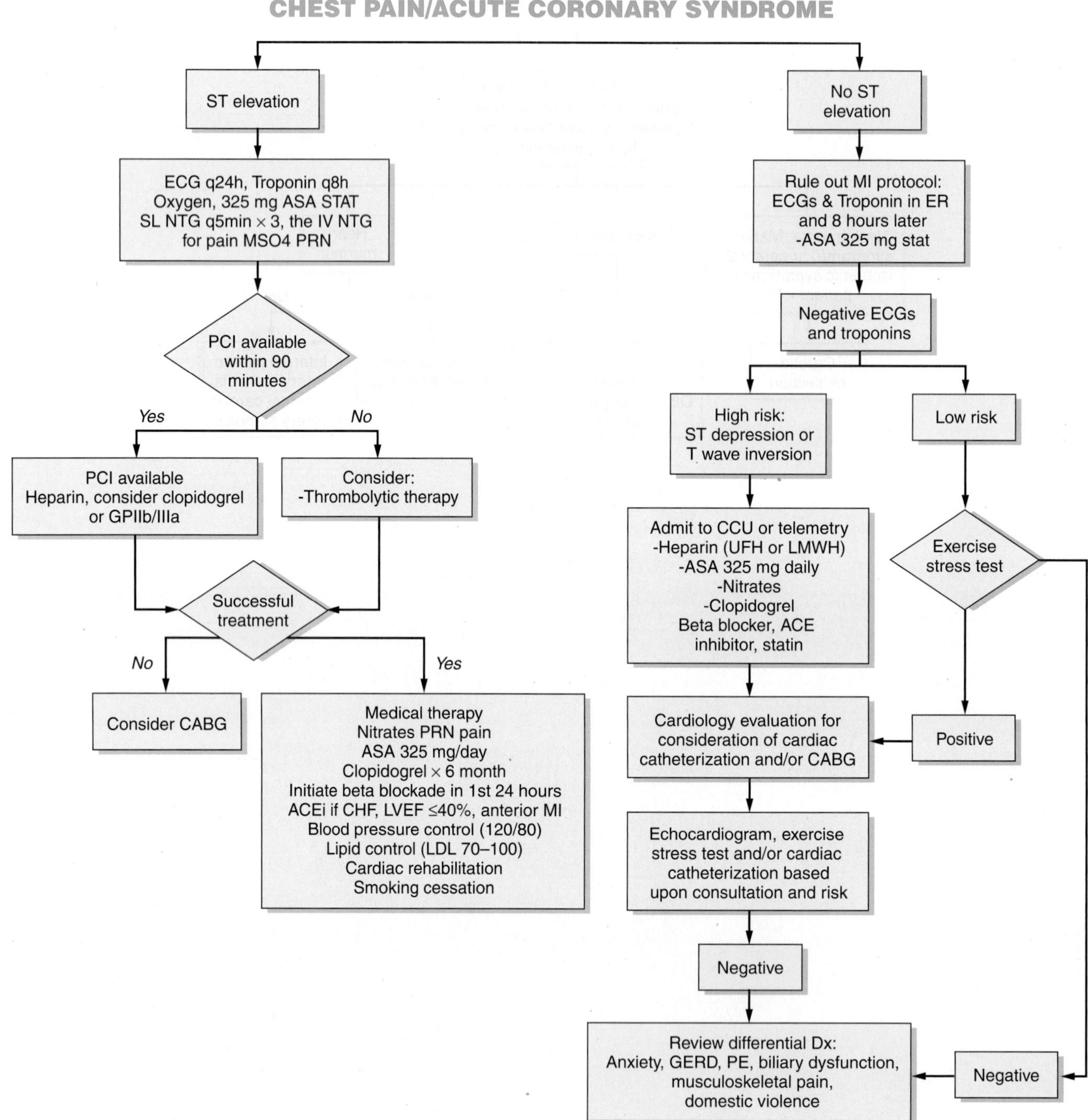

Allen Chang, MD and Naomi F. Botkin, MD

Circulation. 2005;112(22 Suppl):III55–72.

CHRONIC OBSTRUCTIVE PULMONARY DISEASE (COPD), DIAGNOSIS AND TREATMENT

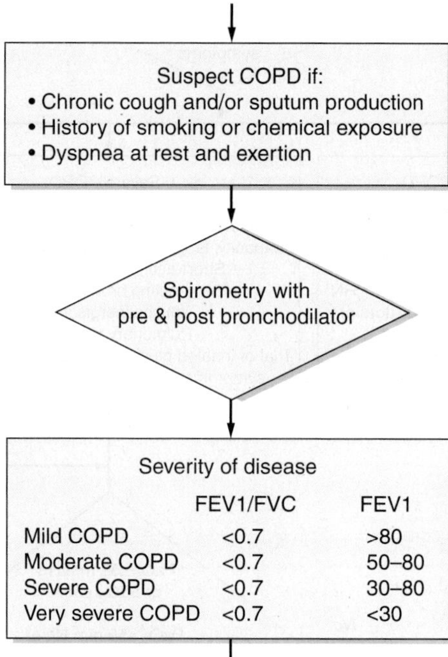

Suspect COPD if:
- Chronic cough and/or sputum production
- History of smoking or chemical exposure
- Dyspnea at rest and exertion

↓

Spirometry with pre & post bronchodilator

↓

Severity of disease

	FEV1/FVC	FEV1
Mild COPD	<0.7	>80
Moderate COPD	<0.7	50–80
Severe COPD	<0.7	30–80
Very severe COPD	<0.7	<30

↓

Functional dyspnea scale

0 Not troubled with breathlessness except with strenuous exercise.
1 Troubled by shortness of breath when hurrying or walking up a slight hill.
2 Walks slower than people of same age due to breathlessness or has to stop for breath when walking at own pace on the level.
3 Stops for breath after walking ~100 m or after a few minutes on the level.
4 Too breathless to leave the house or breathless when dressing or undressing.

↓

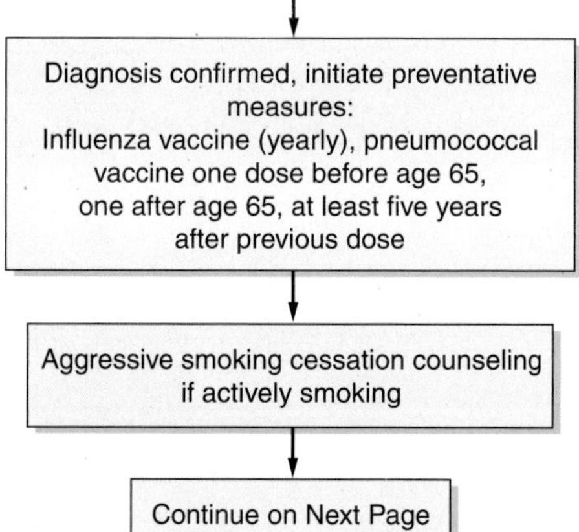

Diagnosis confirmed, initiate preventative measures:
Influenza vaccine (yearly), pneumococcal vaccine one dose before age 65, one after age 65, at least five years after previous dose

↓

Aggressive smoking cessation counseling if actively smoking

↓

Continue on Next Page

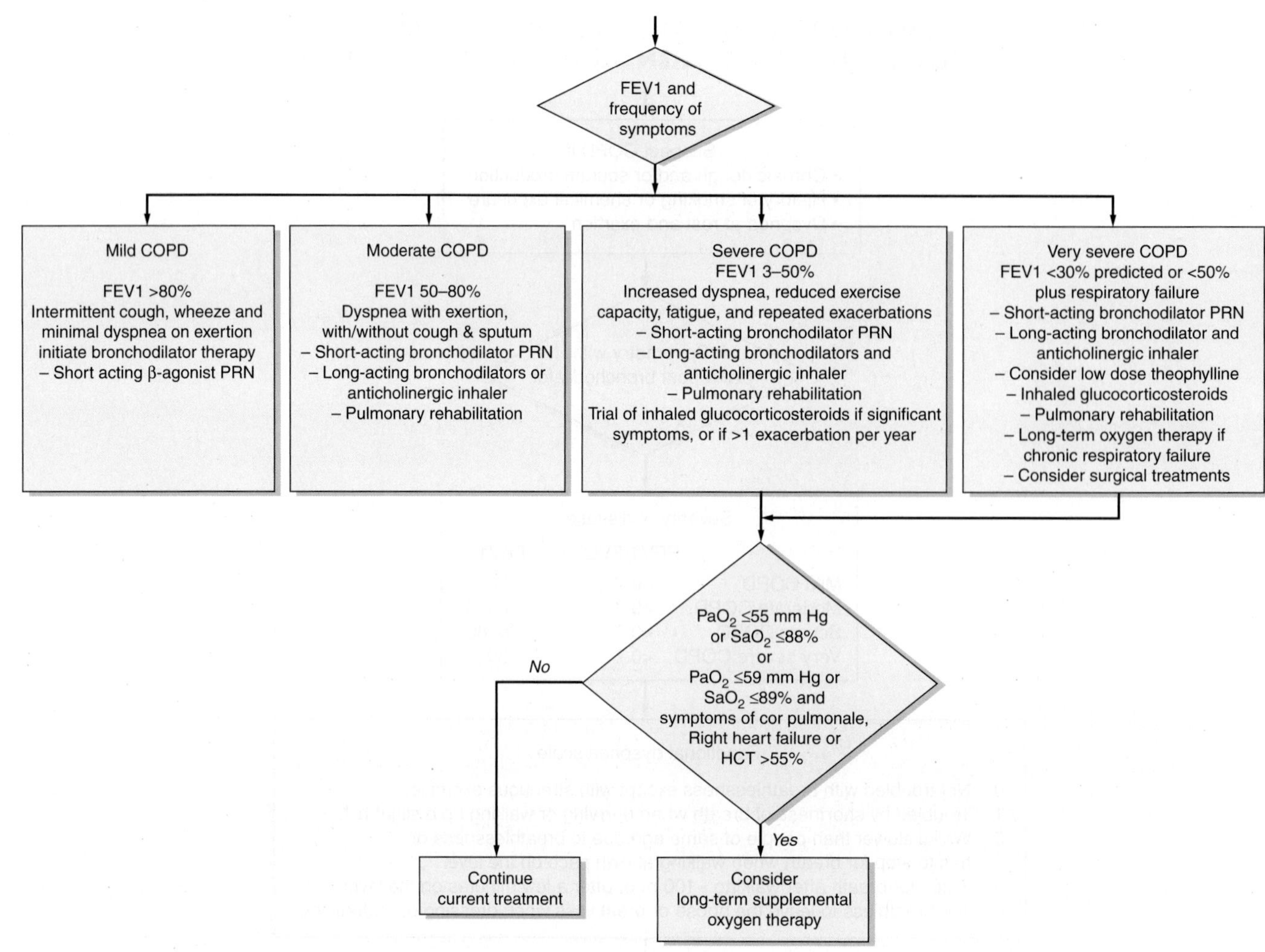

Laura Paulin, MD, MHS and Scott Kopec, MD

National Guidelines Clearinghouse. Global Initiative for Chronic Obstructive Lung Disease (GOLD); 2008.

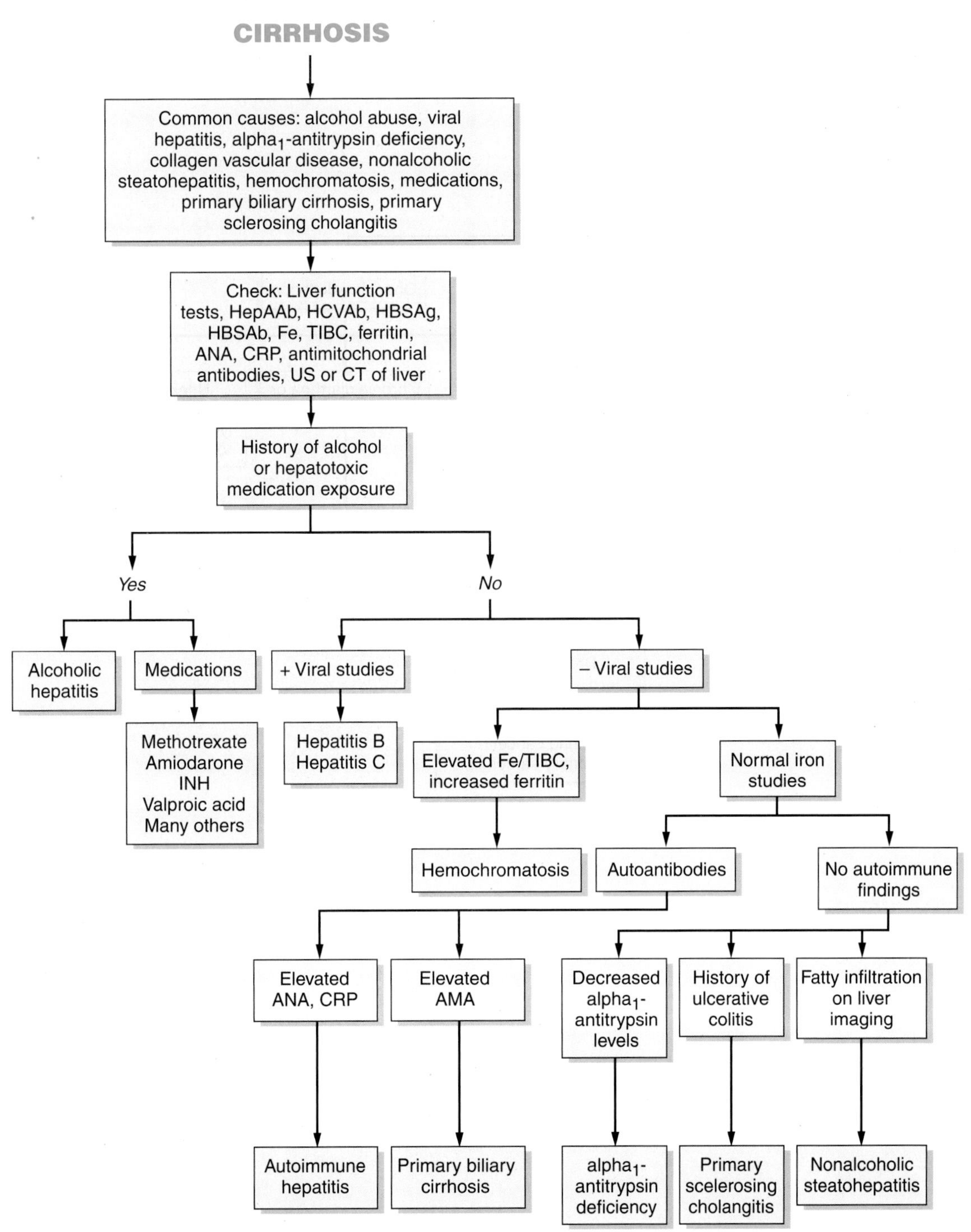
CIRRHOSIS
Common causes: alcohol abuse, viral hepatitis, alpha$_1$-antitrypsin deficiency, collagen vascular disease, nonalcoholic steatohepatitis, hemochromatosis, medications, primary biliary cirrhosis, primary sclerosing cholangitis
Check: Liver function tests, HepAAb, HCVAb, HBSAg, HBSAb, Fe, TIBC, ferritin, ANA, CRP, antimitochondrial antibodies, US or CT of liver
History of alcohol or hepatotoxic medication exposure
Yes
No
Alcoholic hepatitis
Medications
+ Viral studies
– Viral studies
Methotrexate
Amiodarone
INH
Valproic acid
Many others
Hepatitis B
Hepatitis C
Elevated Fe/TIBC, increased ferritin
Normal iron studies
Hemochromatosis
Autoantibodies
No autoimmune findings
Elevated ANA, CRP
Elevated AMA
Decreased alpha$_1$-antitrypsin levels
History of ulcerative colitis
Fatty infiltration on liver imaging
Autoimmune hepatitis
Primary biliary cirrhosis
alpha$_1$-antitrypsin deficiency
Primary sclerosing cholangitis
Nonalcoholic steatohepatitis

Robert A. Baldor, MD and Alan M. Ehrlich, MD

Med Clin North Am. 2009;93(4).

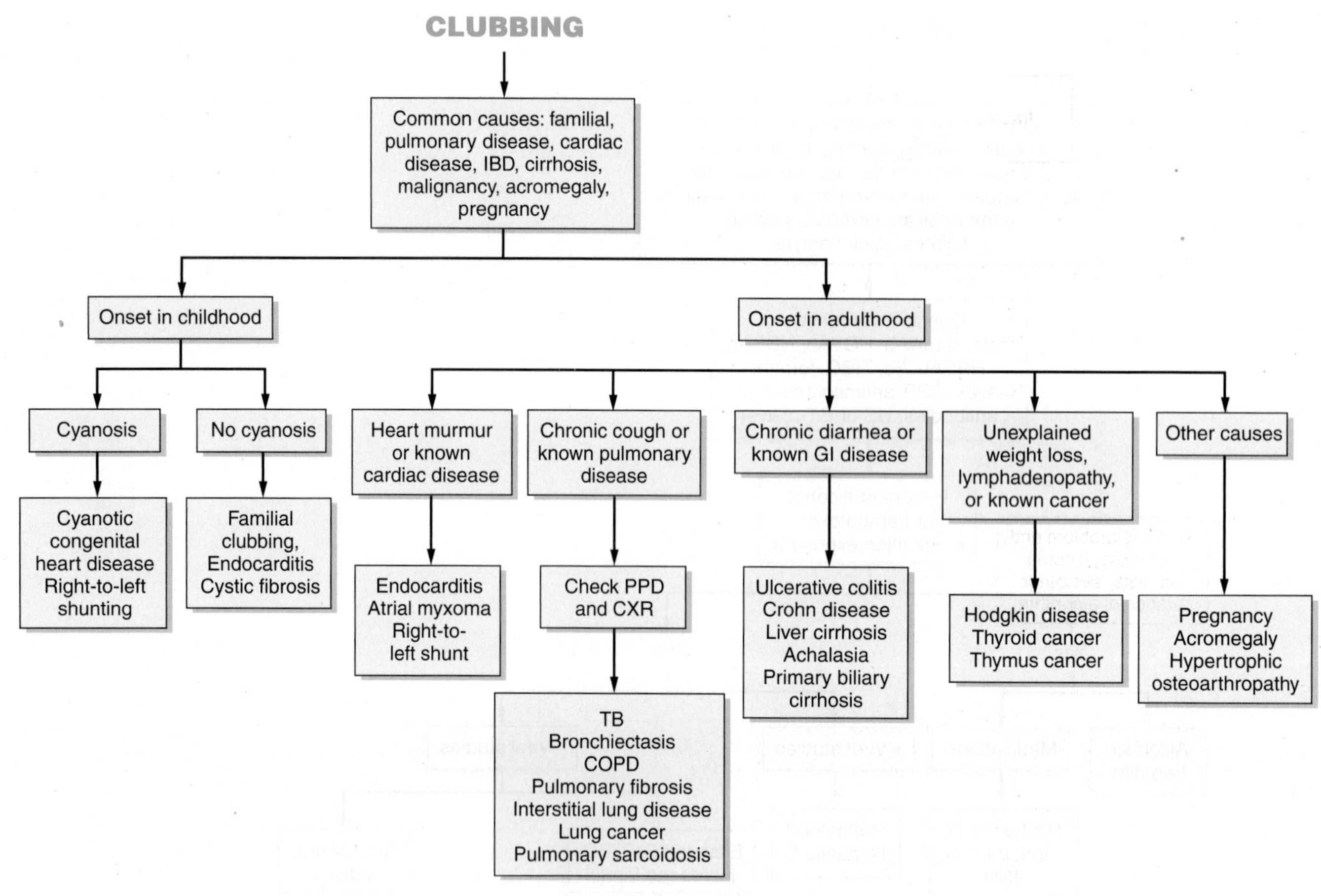
CLUBBING
Common causes: familial, pulmonary disease, cardiac disease, IBD, cirrhosis, malignancy, acromegaly, pregnancy
Onset in childhood
Onset in adulthood
Cyanosis
No cyanosis
Heart murmur or known cardiac disease
Chronic cough or known pulmonary disease
Chronic diarrhea or known GI disease
Unexplained weight loss, lymphadenopathy, or known cancer
Other causes
Cyanotic congenital heart disease Right-to-left shunting
Familial clubbing, Endocarditis Cystic fibrosis
Endocarditis Atrial myxoma Right-to-left shunt
Check PPD and CXR
Ulcerative colitis Crohn disease Liver cirrhosis Achalasia Primary biliary cirrhosis
Hodgkin disease Thyroid cancer Thymus cancer
Pregnancy Acromegaly Hypertrophic osteoarthropathy
TB Bronchiectasis COPD Pulmonary fibrosis Interstitial lung disease Lung cancer Pulmonary sarcoidosis

Robert A. Baldor, MD and Alan M. Ehrlich, MD

Clin Dermatol. 2008;26(3):296–305.

COMA

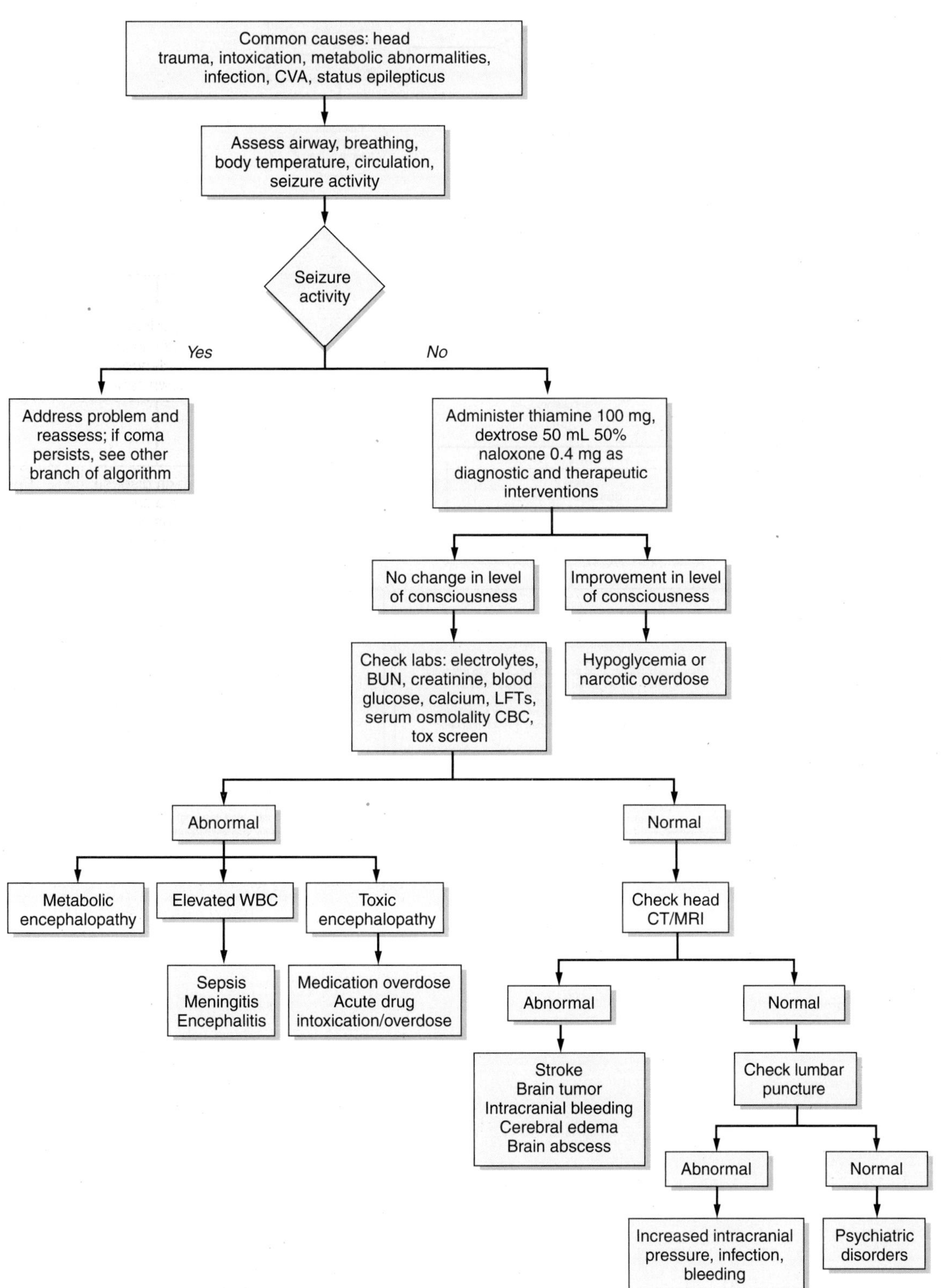

Robert A. Baldor, MD and Alan M. Ehrlich, MD

Neurol Clin. 2008;26(2).

CONCUSSION, SIMPLE EVALUATION AND MANAGEMENT (SPORTS)

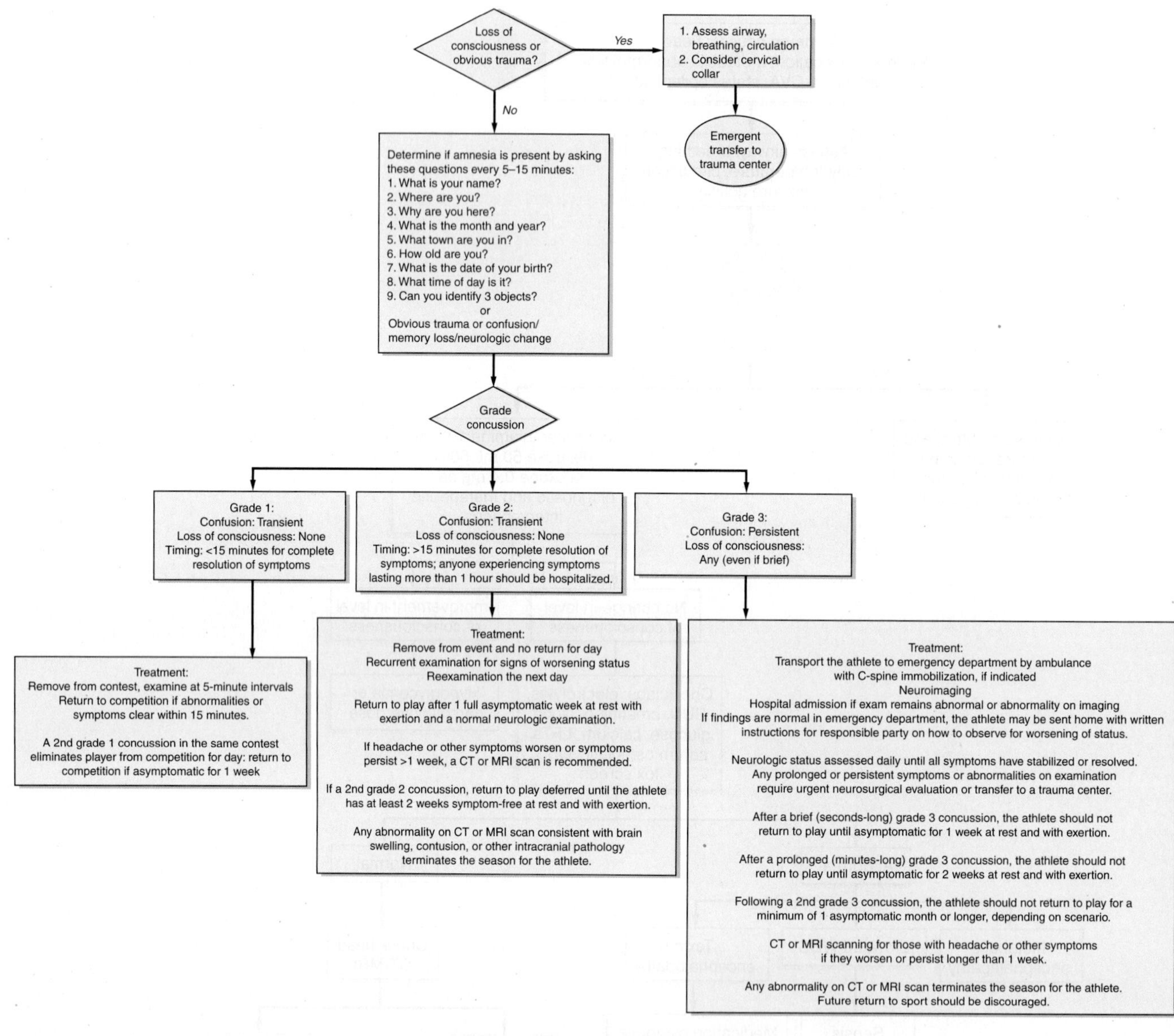

Loss of consciousness or obvious trauma?
Yes
1. Assess airway, breathing, circulation
2. Consider cervical collar
Emergent transfer to trauma center
No
Determine if amnesia is present by asking these questions every 5–15 minutes:
1. What is your name?
2. Where are you?
3. Why are you here?
4. What is the month and year?
5. What town are you in?
6. How old are you?
7. What is the date of your birth?
8. What time of day is it?
9. Can you identify 3 objects?
or
Obvious trauma or confusion/ memory loss/neurologic change
Grade concussion
Grade 1: Confusion: Transient Loss of consciousness: None Timing: <15 minutes for complete resolution of symptoms
Grade 2: Confusion: Transient Loss of consciousness: None Timing: >15 minutes for complete resolution of symptoms; anyone experiencing symptoms lasting more than 1 hour should be hospitalized.
Grade 3: Confusion: Persistent Loss of consciousness: Any (even if brief)
Treatment: Remove from contest, examine at 5-minute intervals Return to competition if abnormalities or symptoms clear within 15 minutes.
A 2nd grade 1 concussion in the same contest eliminates player from competition for day: return to competition if asymptomatic for 1 week
Treatment: Remove from event and no return for day Recurrent examination for signs of worsening status Reexamination the next day
Return to play after 1 full asymptomatic week at rest with exertion and a normal neurologic examination.
If headache or other symptoms worsen or symptoms persist >1 week, a CT or MRI scan is recommended.
If a 2nd grade 2 concussion, return to play deferred until the athlete has at least 2 weeks symptom-free at rest and with exertion.
Any abnormality on CT or MRI scan consistent with brain swelling, contusion, or other intracranial pathology terminates the season for the athlete.
Treatment: Transport the athlete to emergency department by ambulance with C-spine immobilization, if indicated
Neuroimaging
Hospital admission if exam remains abnormal or abnormality on imaging
If findings are normal in emergency department, the athlete may be sent home with written instructions for responsible party on how to observe for worsening of status.
Neurologic status assessed daily until all symptoms have stabilized or resolved. Any prolonged or persistent symptoms or abnormalities on examination require urgent neurosurgical evaluation or transfer to a trauma center.
After a brief (seconds-long) grade 3 concussion, the athlete should not return to play until asymptomatic for 1 week at rest and with exertion.
After a prolonged (minutes-long) grade 3 concussion, the athlete should not return to play until asymptomatic for 2 weeks at rest and with exertion.
Following a 2nd grade 3 concussion, the athlete should not return to play for a minimum of 1 asymptomatic month or longer, depending on scenario.
CT or MRI scanning for those with headache or other symptoms if they worsen or persist longer than 1 week.
Any abnormality on CT or MRI scan terminates the season for the athlete. Future return to sport should be discouraged.

Armin Arasheben, MD and Jason Matuszak, MD

Br J Sports Med. 2005;39:691.

CONGESTIVE HEART FAILURE: DIFFERENTIAL DIAGNOSIS

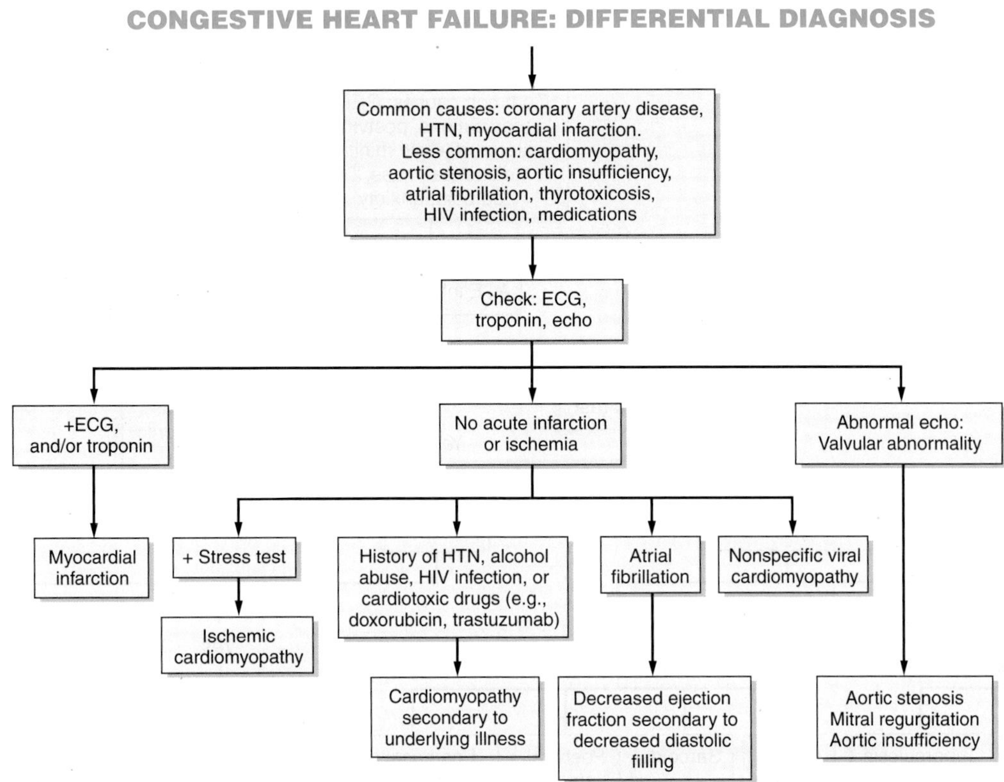

Robert A. Baldor, MD and Alan M. Ehrlich, MD

Joint ACC/AHA Guideline for Diagnosis and Management of Chronic Heart Failure in the Adult at guidelines.gov.

COUGH, CHRONIC

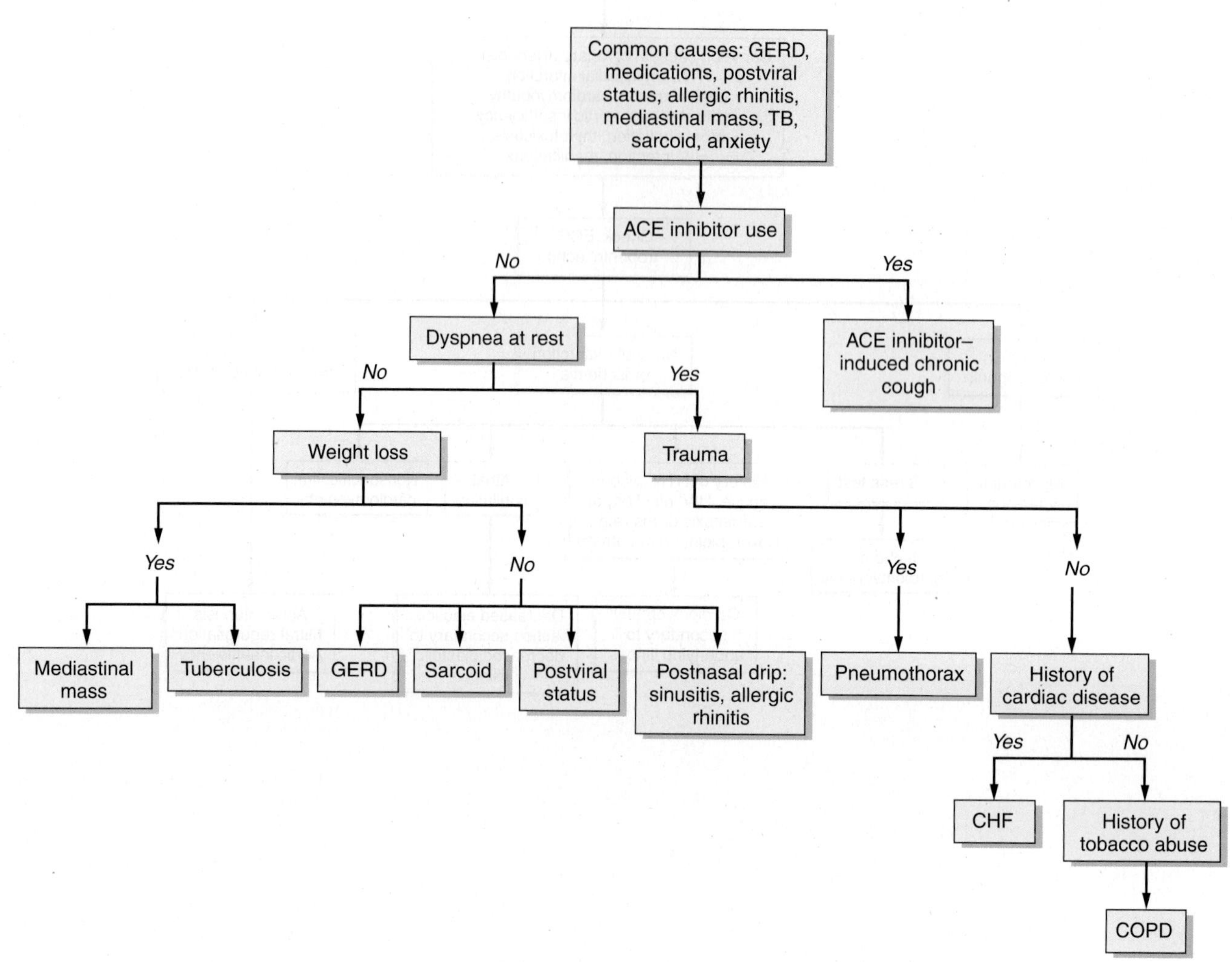

Robert A. Baldor, MD and Alan M. Ehrlich, MD

ACCP Guideline Chronic Cough Chest. 2006;129(1 Suppl):220S–1S.

CRYPTORCHIDISM (Undescended Testes)

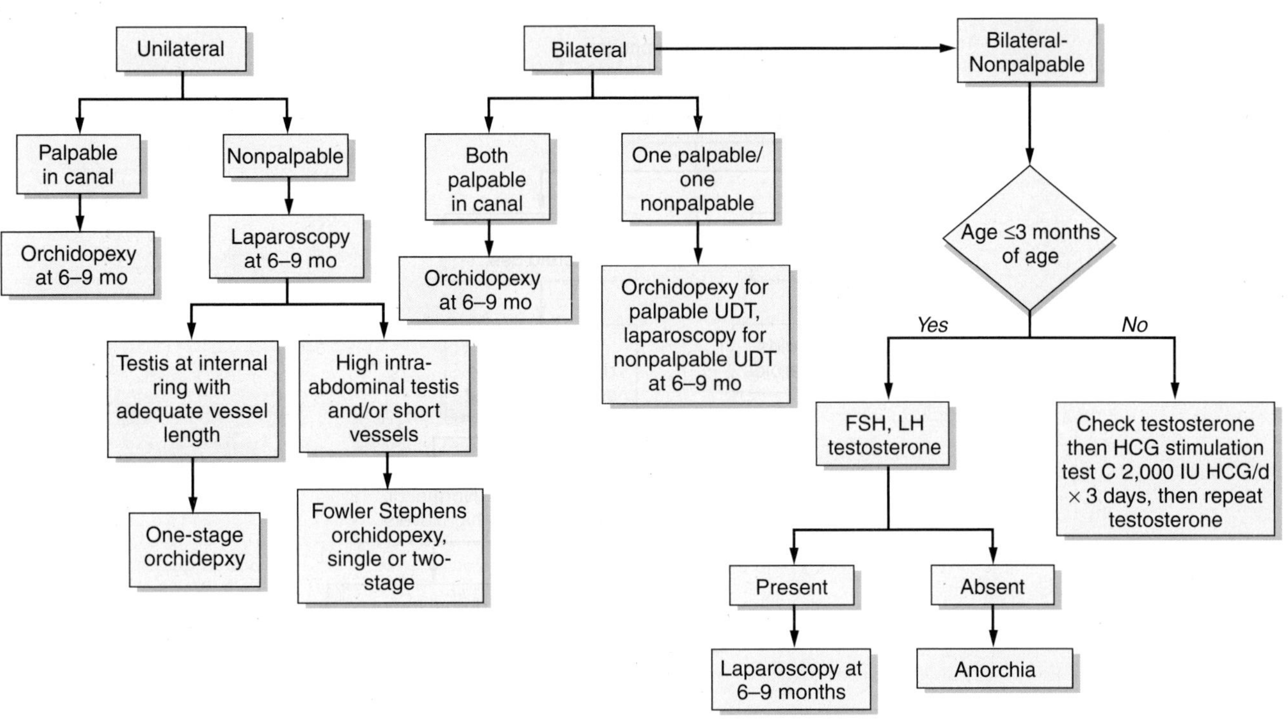

Robert A. Baldor, MD and Alan M. Ehrlich, MD

Am Fam Physician. 2000;62:2037–44, 2047–8.

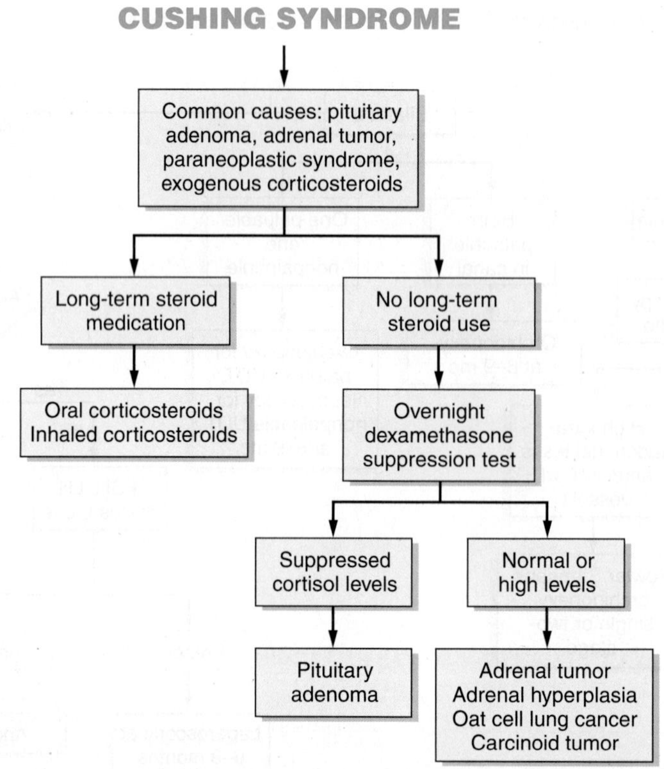

Robert A. Baldor, MD and Alan M. Ehrlich, MD

J Clin Endocrinol Metabol. 2009;94(9).

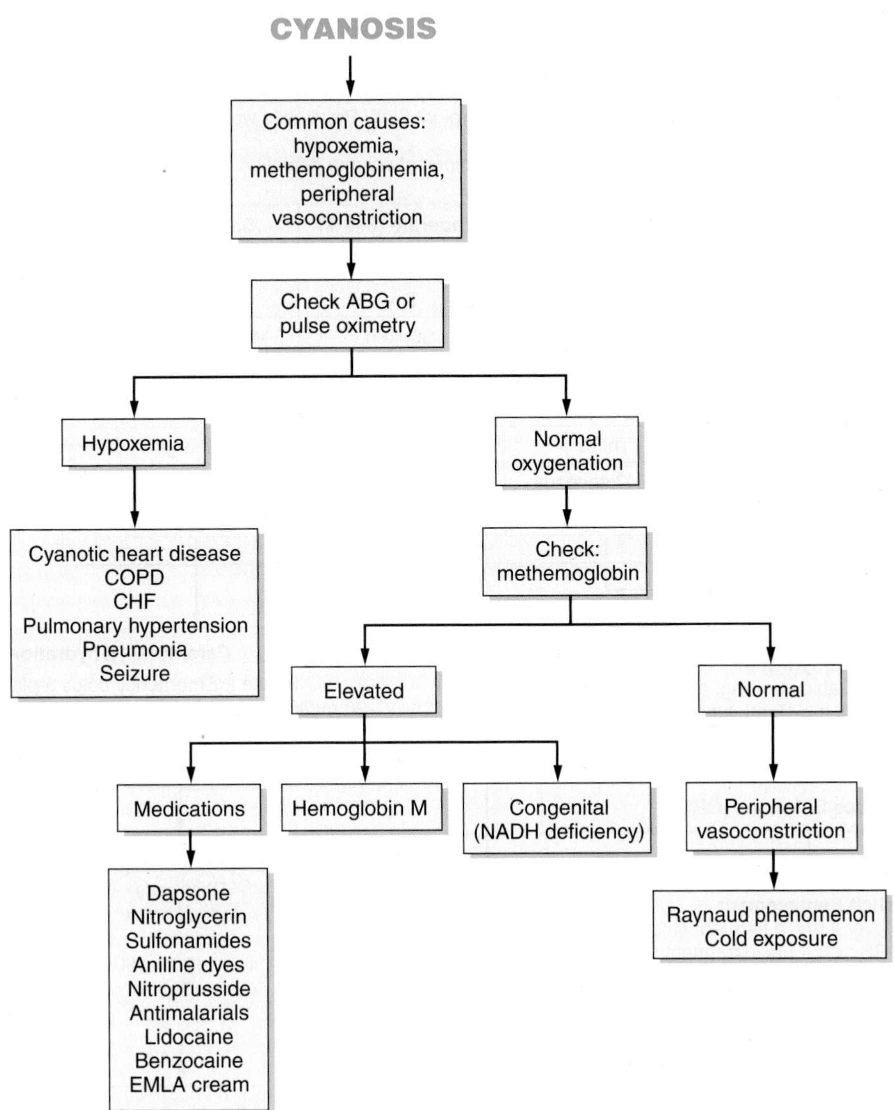

Robert A. Baldor, MD and Alan M. Ehrlich, MD

Am J Roent. 2005;189:241–7.

DEHYDRATION, PEDIATRIC

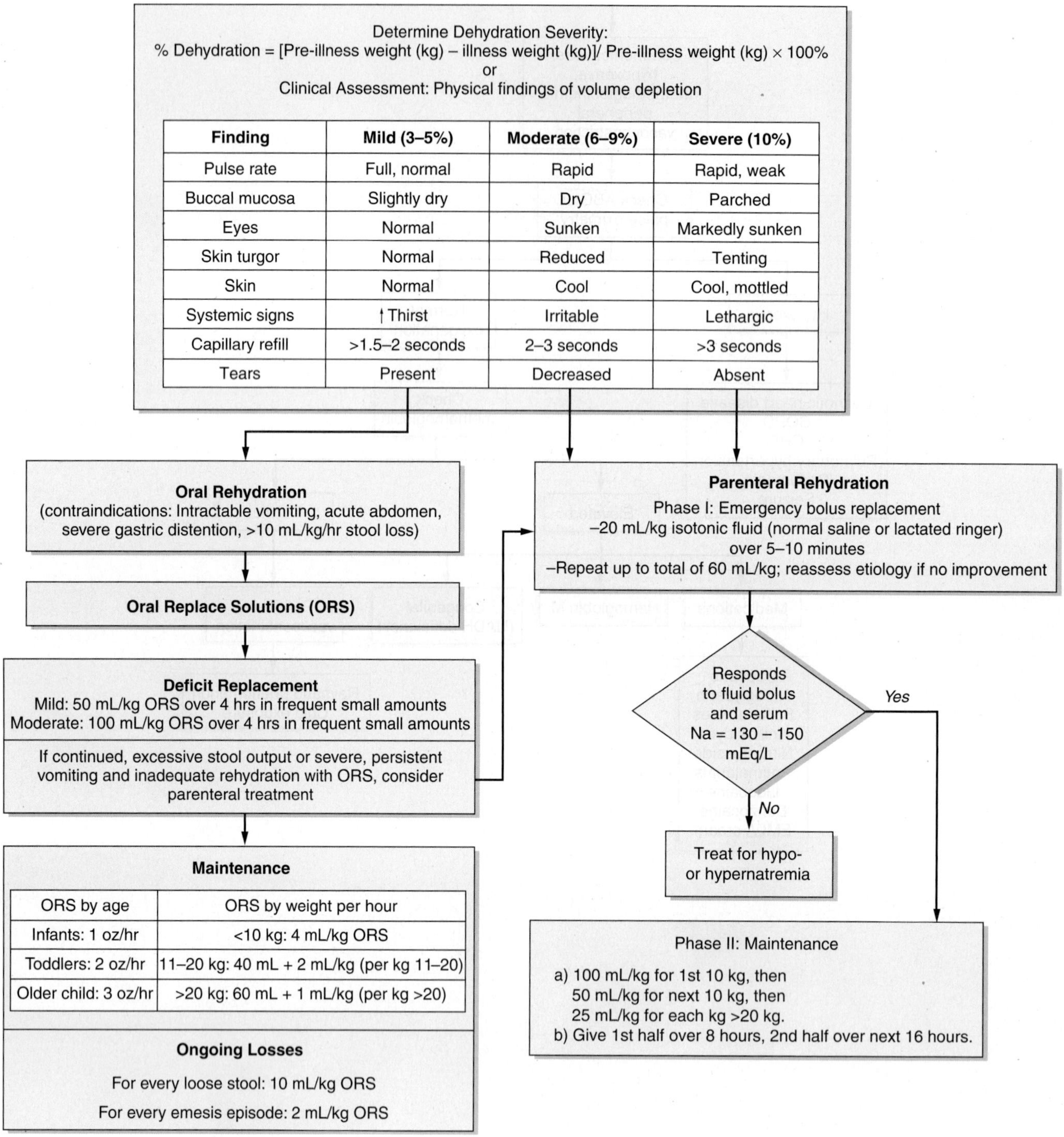

Determine Dehydration Severity:
% Dehydration = [Pre-illness weight (kg) – illness weight (kg)]/ Pre-illness weight (kg) × 100%
or
Clinical Assessment: Physical findings of volume depletion

Finding	Mild (3–5%)	Moderate (6–9%)	Severe (10%)
Pulse rate	Full, normal	Rapid	Rapid, weak
Buccal mucosa	Slightly dry	Dry	Parched
Eyes	Normal	Sunken	Markedly sunken
Skin turgor	Normal	Reduced	Tenting
Skin	Normal	Cool	Cool, mottled
Systemic signs	↑ Thirst	Irritable	Lethargic
Capillary refill	>1.5–2 seconds	2–3 seconds	>3 seconds
Tears	Present	Decreased	Absent

Mild → Oral Rehydration; Moderate, Severe → Parenteral Rehydration

Oral Rehydration
(contraindications: Intractable vomiting, acute abdomen, severe gastric distention, >10 mL/kg/hr stool loss)

↓

Oral Replace Solutions (ORS)

↓

Deficit Replacement
Mild: 50 mL/kg ORS over 4 hrs in frequent small amounts
Moderate: 100 mL/kg ORS over 4 hrs in frequent small amounts

If continued, excessive stool output or severe, persistent vomiting and inadequate rehydration with ORS, consider parenteral treatment (→ Parenteral Rehydration)

↓

Maintenance

ORS by age	ORS by weight per hour
Infants: 1 oz/hr	<10 kg: 4 mL/kg ORS
Toddlers: 2 oz/hr	11–20 kg: 40 mL + 2 mL/kg (per kg 11–20)
Older child: 3 oz/hr	>20 kg: 60 mL + 1 mL/kg (per kg >20)

Ongoing Losses

For every loose stool: 10 mL/kg ORS

For every emesis episode: 2 mL/kg ORS

Parenteral Rehydration
Phase I: Emergency bolus replacement
–20 mL/kg isotonic fluid (normal saline or lactated ringer) over 5–10 minutes
–Repeat up to total of 60 mL/kg; reassess etiology if no improvement

↓

Responds to fluid bolus and serum Na = 130 – 150 mEq/L?

- *No* → Treat for hypo- or hypernatremia
- *Yes* → Phase II: Maintenance

Phase II: Maintenance

a) 100 mL/kg for 1st 10 kg, then
50 mL/kg for next 10 kg, then
25 mL/kg for each kg >20 kg.
b) Give 1st half over 8 hours, 2nd half over next 16 hours.

Stephanie Galica, MD

Am Fam Physician. 2009;80(7):692–6.

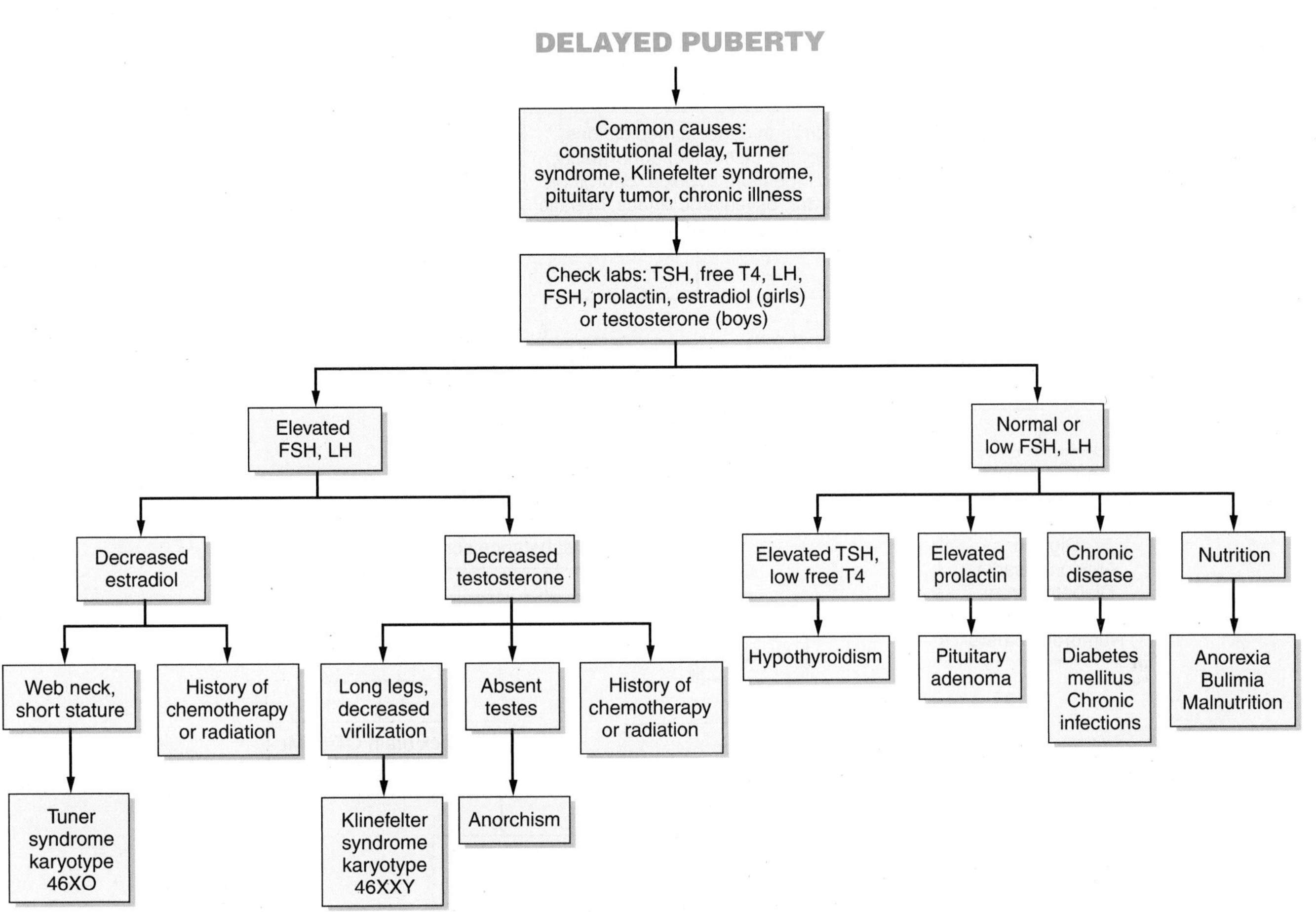

Robert A. Baldor, MD and Alan M. Ehrlich, MD

Am Fam Physician. 1999;60:209–24.

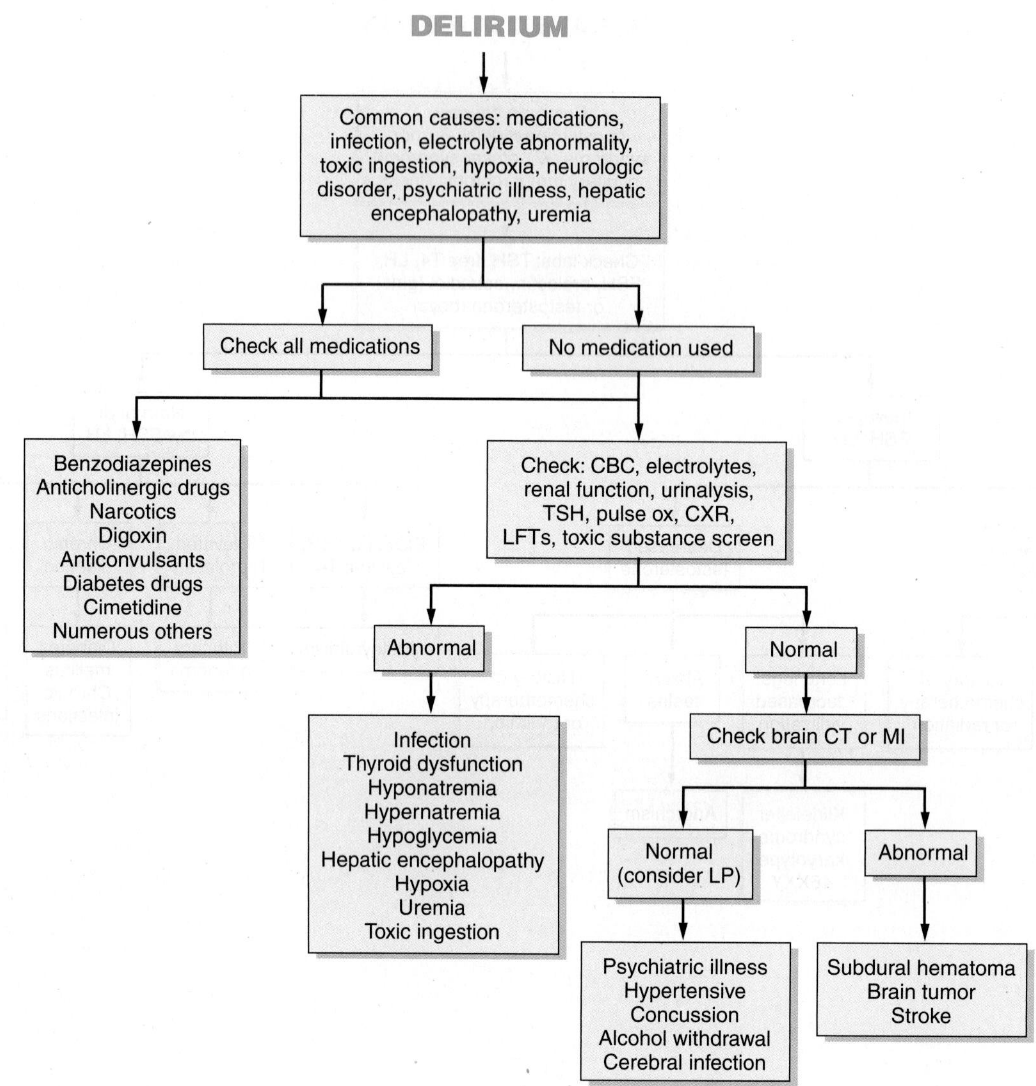
DELIRIUM
Common causes: medications, infection, electrolyte abnormality, toxic ingestion, hypoxia, neurologic disorder, psychiatric illness, hepatic encephalopathy, uremia
Check all medications
No medication used
Benzodiazepines
Anticholinergic drugs
Narcotics
Digoxin
Anticonvulsants
Diabetes drugs
Cimetidine
Numerous others
Check: CBC, electrolytes, renal function, urinalysis, TSH, pulse ox, CXR, LFTs, toxic substance screen
Abnormal
Normal
Infection
Thyroid dysfunction
Hyponatremia
Hypernatremia
Hypoglycemia
Hepatic encephalopathy
Hypoxia
Uremia
Toxic ingestion
Check brain CT or MI
Normal (consider LP)
Abnormal
Psychiatric illness
Hypertensive
Concussion
Alcohol withdrawal
Cerebral infection
Subdural hematoma
Brain tumor
Stroke

Robert A. Baldor, MD and Alan M. Ehrlich, MD

Am Fam Physician. 2003;67:1027–34.

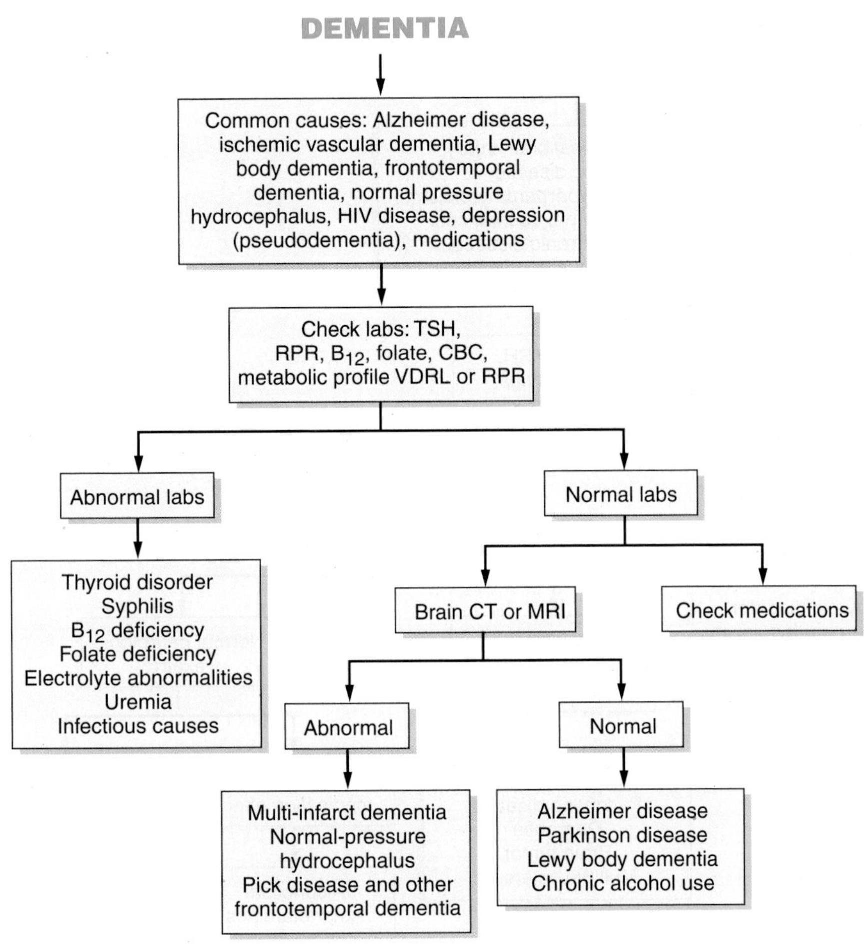
DEMENTIA
Common causes: Alzheimer disease, ischemic vascular dementia, Lewy body dementia, frontotemporal dementia, normal pressure hydrocephalus, HIV disease, depression (pseudodementia), medications
Check labs: TSH, RPR, B_{12}, folate, CBC, metabolic profile VDRL or RPR
Abnormal labs
Normal labs
Thyroid disorder
Syphilis
B_{12} deficiency
Folate deficiency
Electrolyte abnormalities
Uremia
Infectious causes
Brain CT or MRI
Check medications
Abnormal
Normal
Multi-infarct dementia
Normal-pressure hydrocephalus
Pick disease and other frontotemporal dementia
Alzheimer disease
Parkinson disease
Lewy body dementia
Chronic alcohol use

Robert A. Baldor, MD and Alan M. Ehrlich, MD

Neurology. 2001;56(9):1143–53.

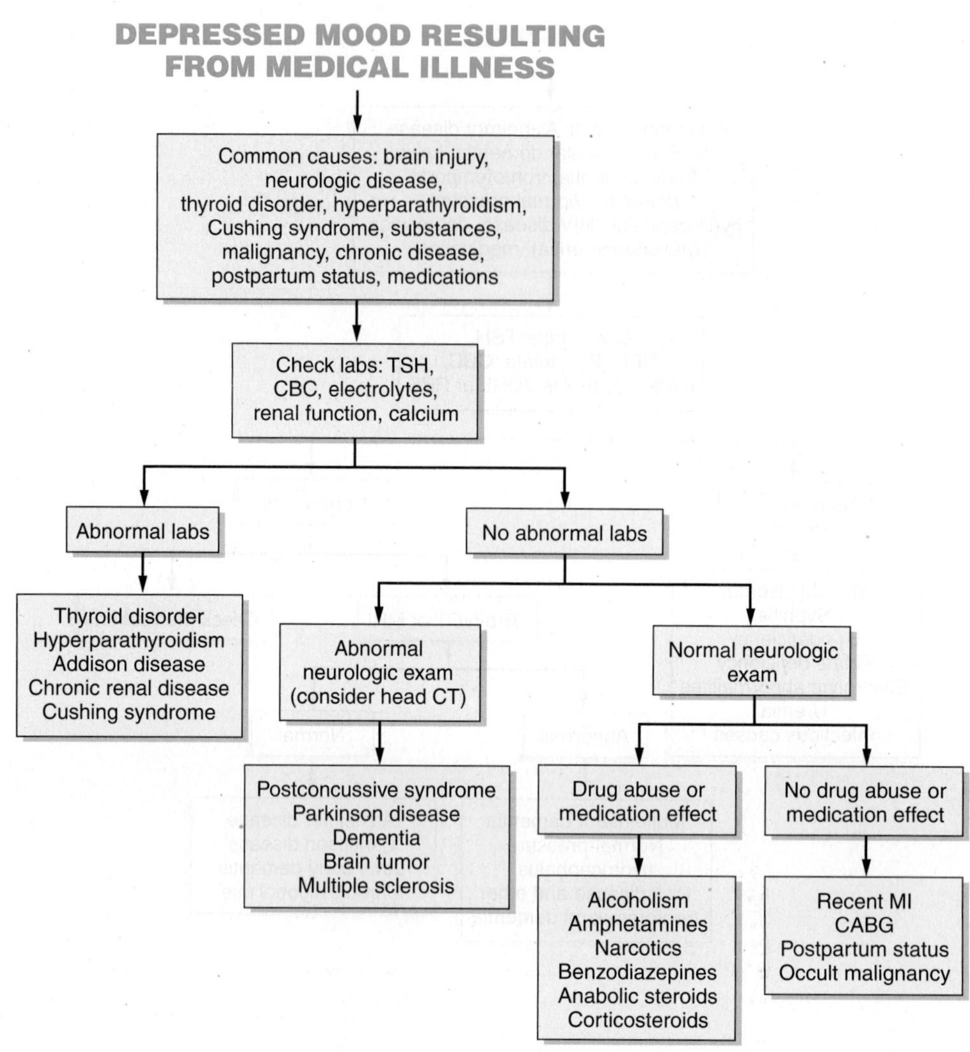

Robert A. Baldor, MD and Alan M. Ehrlich, MD

Phys Sportsmed. 2009;37(2):141–5.

DEPRESSIVE EPISODE, MAJOR

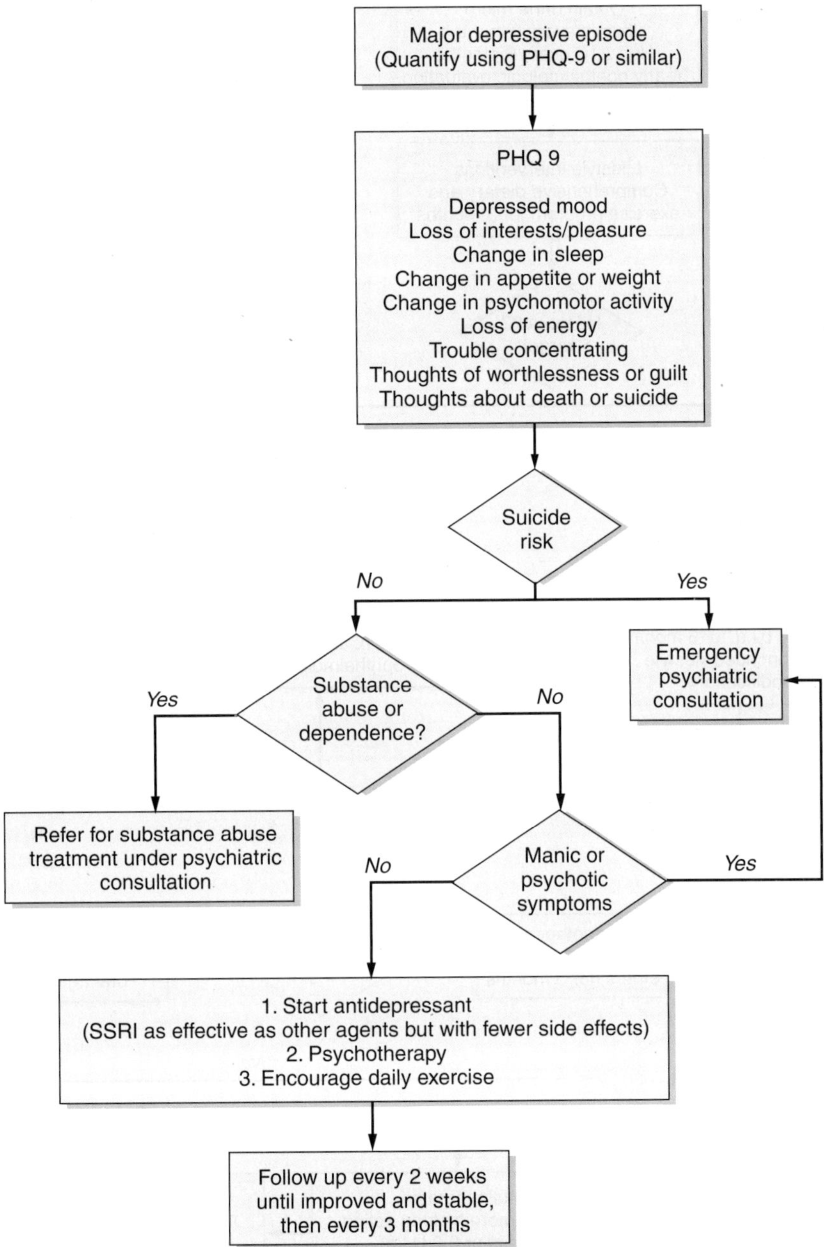

James F. Cunagin, MD

Depression. University of Michigan Health System; 2005 Oct. 20 at National Guidelines Clearinghouse.

DIABETES MELLITUS, TYPE 2

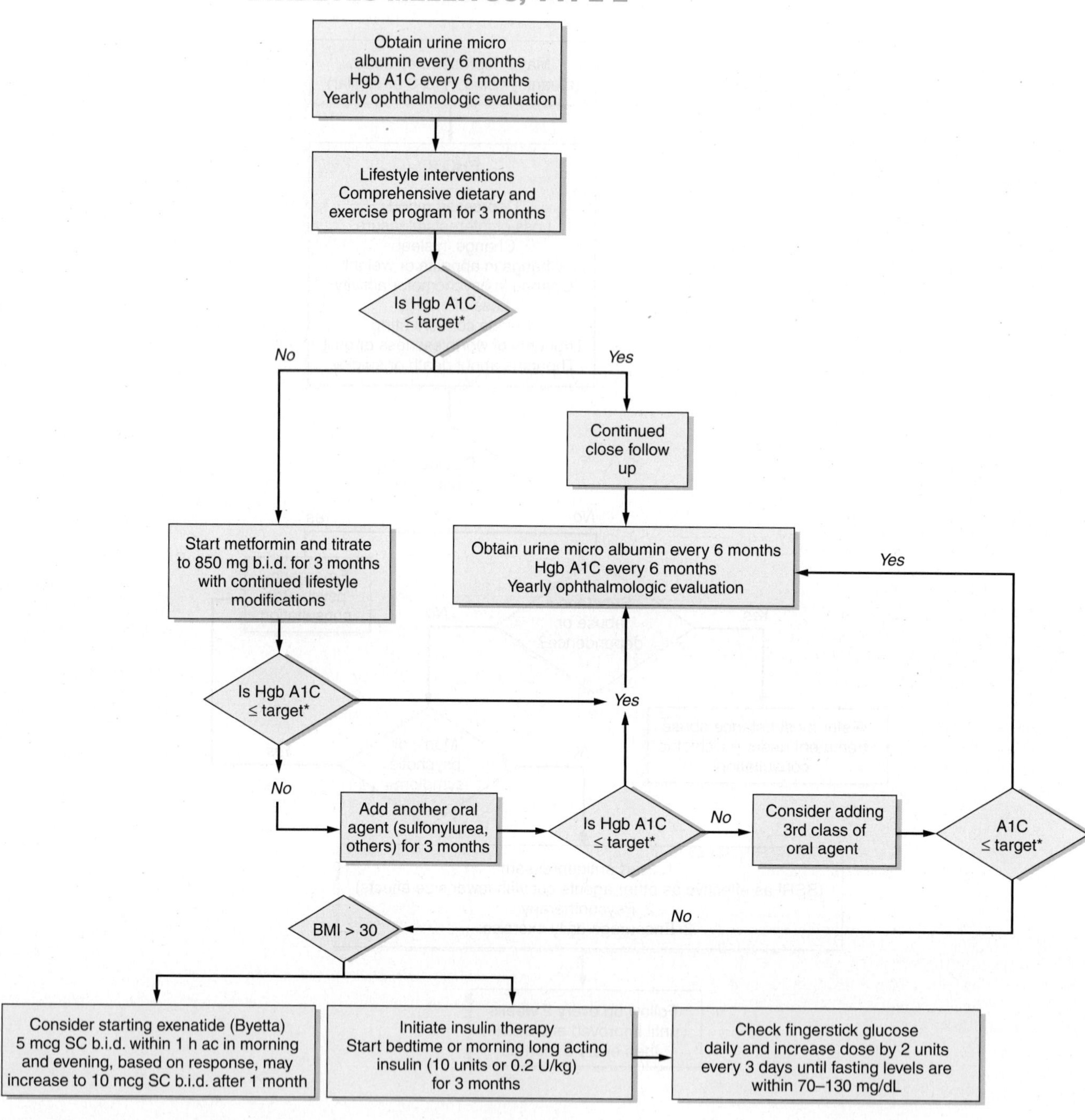

*Target uncertain. Newly diagnosed diabetics without major comorbidities, target likely <7%. Older patients and those with major comorbidities or established diabetic end-organ disease, target <8%

Frank J. Domino, MD

Am Fam Physician. 2009;79(1):29–36.

DIABETIC KETOACIDOSIS (DKA), TREATMENT

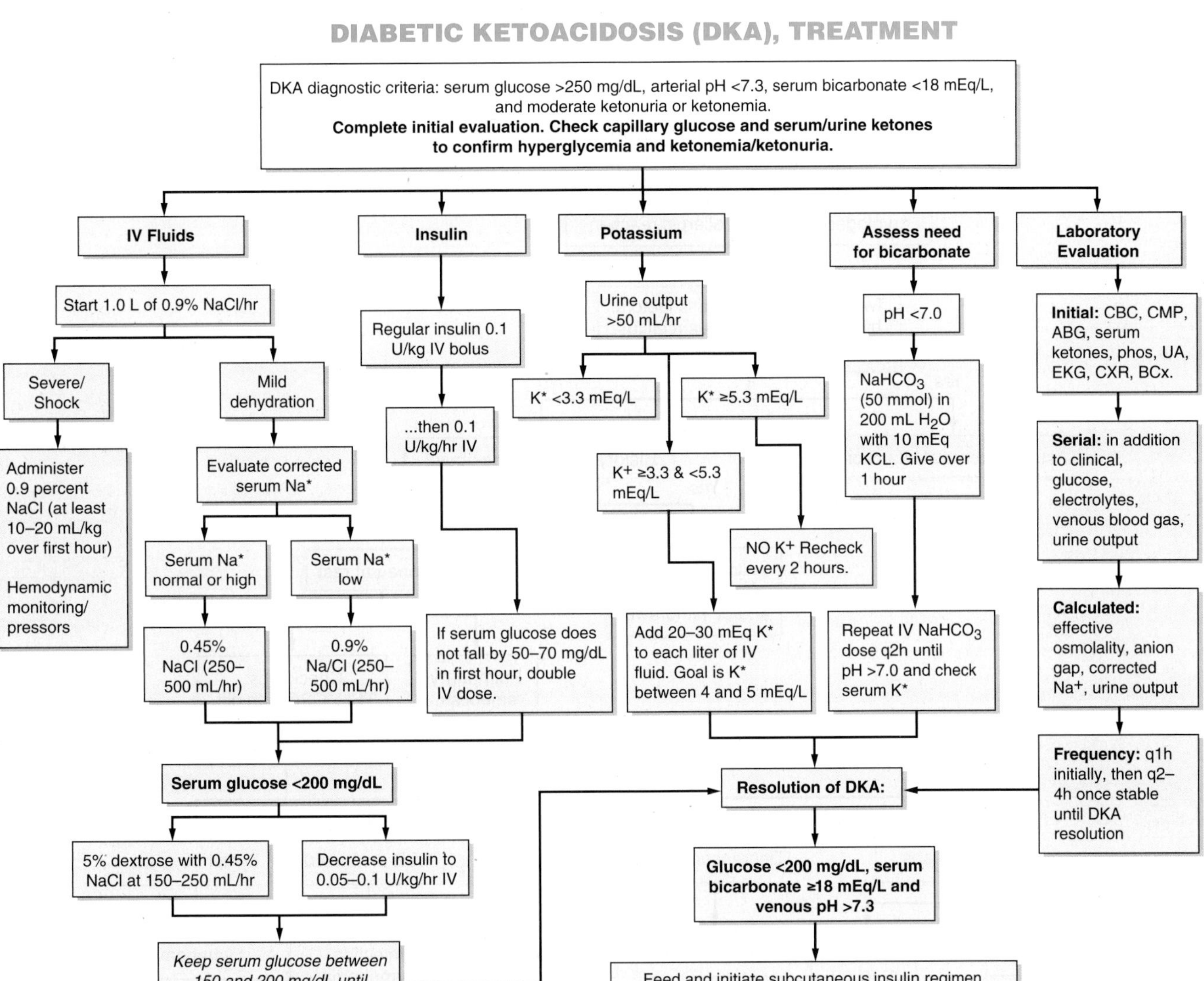
DKA diagnostic criteria: serum glucose >250 mg/dL, arterial pH <7.3, serum bicarbonate <18 mEq/L, and moderate ketonuria or ketonemia.
Complete initial evaluation. Check capillary glucose and serum/urine ketones to confirm hyperglycemia and ketonemia/ketonuria.
IV Fluids
Start 1.0 L of 0.9% NaCl/hr
Severe/ Shock
Administer 0.9 percent NaCl (at least 10–20 mL/kg over first hour)
Hemodynamic monitoring/ pressors
Mild dehydration
Evaluate corrected serum Na*
Serum Na* normal or high
0.45% NaCl (250–500 mL/hr)
Serum Na* low
0.9% Na/Cl (250–500 mL/hr)
Insulin
Regular insulin 0.1 U/kg IV bolus
...then 0.1 U/kg/hr IV
If serum glucose does not fall by 50–70 mg/dL in first hour, double IV dose.
Potassium
Urine output >50 mL/hr
K* <3.3 mEq/L
K* ≥5.3 mEq/L
K+ ≥3.3 & <5.3 mEq/L
NO K+ Recheck every 2 hours.
Add 20–30 mEq K* to each liter of IV fluid. Goal is K* between 4 and 5 mEq/L
Assess need for bicarbonate
pH <7.0
NaHCO3 (50 mmol) in 200 mL H2O with 10 mEq KCL. Give over 1 hour
Repeat IV NaHCO3 dose q2h until pH >7.0 and check serum K*
Laboratory Evaluation
Initial: CBC, CMP, ABG, serum ketones, phos, UA, EKG, CXR, BCx.
Serial: in addition to clinical, glucose, electrolytes, venous blood gas, urine output
Calculated: effective osmolality, anion gap, corrected Na+, urine output
Frequency: q1h initially, then q2–4h once stable until DKA resolution
Serum glucose <200 mg/dL
5% dextrose with 0.45% NaCl at 150–250 mL/hr
Decrease insulin to 0.05–0.1 U/kg/hr IV
Keep serum glucose between 150 and 200 mg/dL until resolution of DKA
Resolution of DKA:
Glucose <200 mg/dL, serum bicarbonate ≥18 mEq/L and venous pH >7.3
Feed and initiate subcutaneous insulin regimen (0.5–0.8 U/kg/d), keeping IV insulin going 1–2 hours after SC doses. Look for precipitating cause(s).

Kitabchi AE, Wall BM. Management of diabetic ketoacidosis. *Am Fam Physician.* 1999;60(2):455–64.
Kitabchi AE, Umpierrez GE, Miles JM, et al. Hyperglycemic crises in adult patients with diabetes. *Diabetes Care.* 2009;32(7):1335–43.
Trachetenbarg DE. Diabetic ketoacidosis. *Am Fam Physician.* 2005;71(9):1705–14.

John B. Waits, MD

LMAJ. 2003;168(7):859–6.

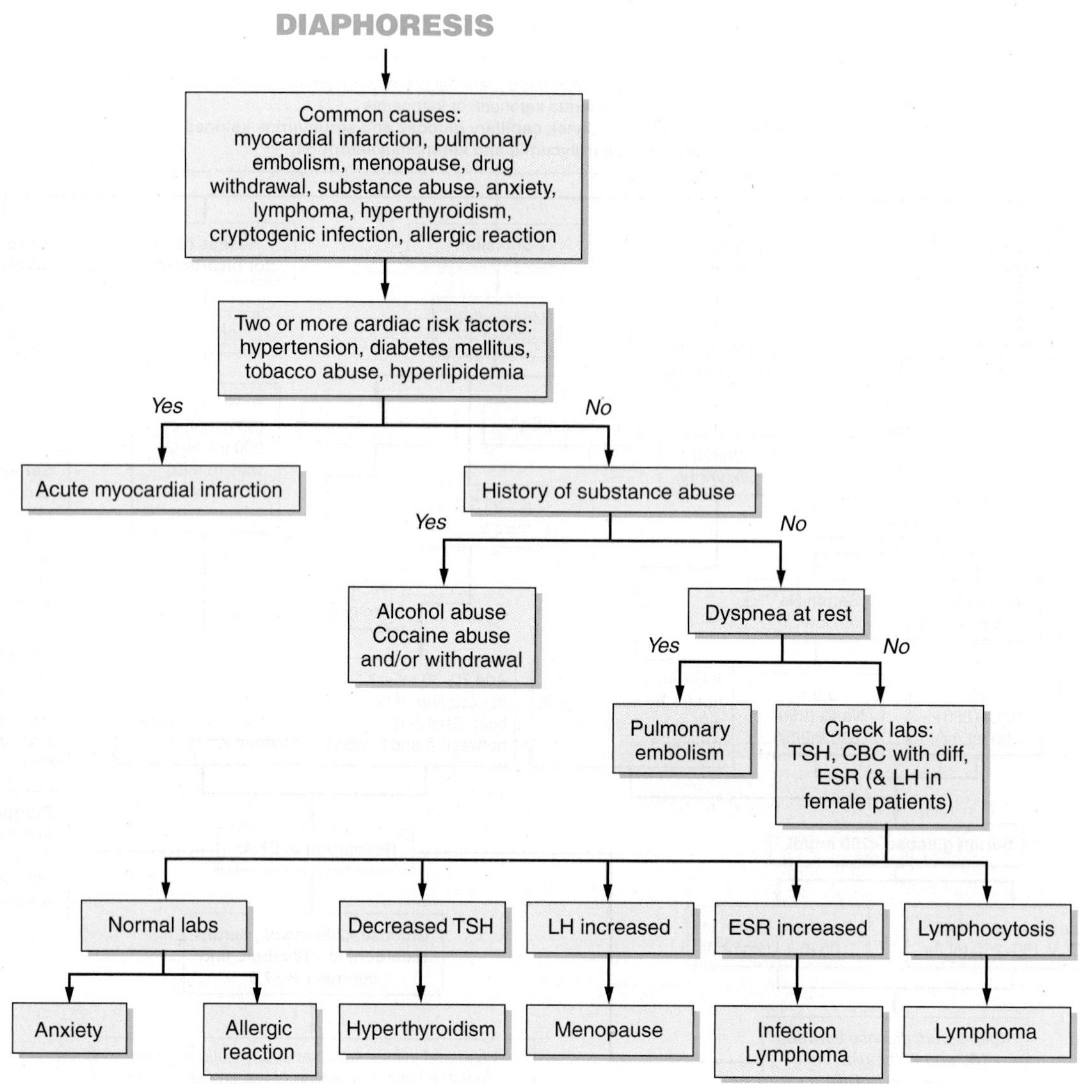

Robert A. Baldor, MD and Alan M. Ehrlich, MD

Depression University of Michigan Health System; 2005 Oct. 20 at National Guidelines Clearinghouse.

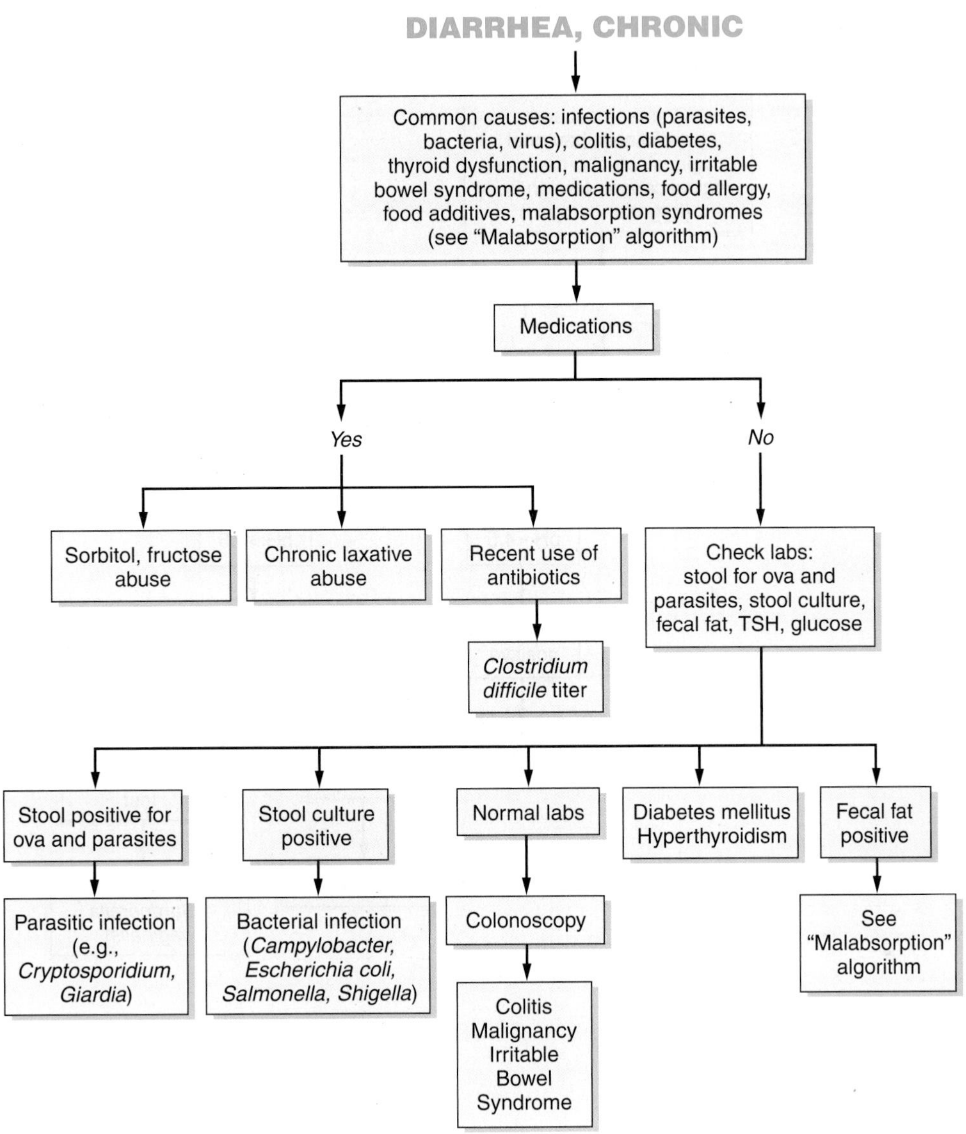

Robert A. Baldor, MD and Alan M. Ehrlich, MD

Institute for Clinical Systems Improvement (ICSI); 2009 May. 114 p. at National Guidelines Clearinghouse.

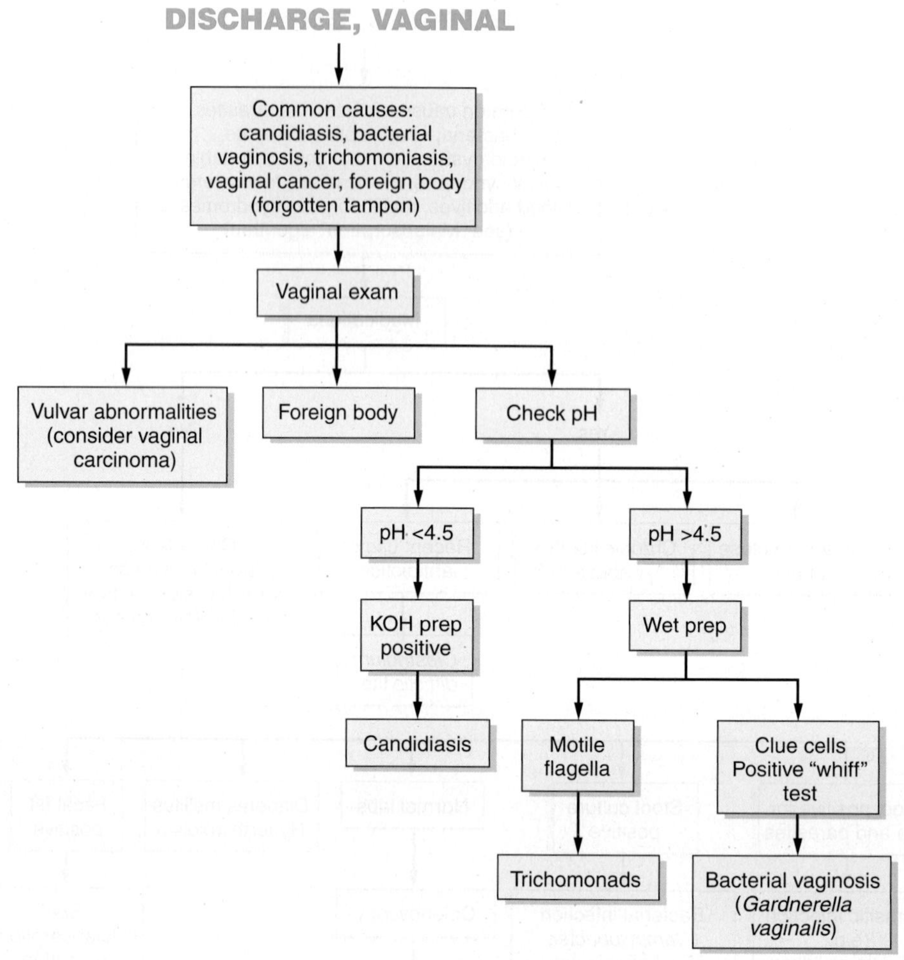

Robert A. Baldor, MD and Alan M. Ehrlich, MD

Primary Care Clin Office Pract. 2009;36(1).

DIZZINESS

- Vertigo (room spin)
- Pre-syncope (sense about to pass out)
- Dysequilibrium (instability with walking)
- True Dizziness (non-organic)

Dysequalibrium

Check patellar reflexes

- Decreased reflexes
  - Diabetic neuropathy
  - B12 deficiency
  - Hypothyroid
  - Amyloidosis
  - Syphilis (Tabes dorsalis)
- Variable
  - Cerebellar disease
  - Intoxication (EtOH, mercury, lithium, gas, solvents, glue)
- Increased
  - Cervical spondylosis
  - Spinal cord tumor
  - Multiple myeloma

Pre-syncope

Have patient hyperventilate to induce symptoms

1. Orthostatic
   - drug induced (C.V. drugs, opioids, etc.)
   - dehydration
2. Arrythmia
3. Anemia/GI bleed
4. Hypoglycemia
5. Aging autonomic nervous system
6. Anxiety

Vertigo

- Lasts for days
  - Vestibular neuritis
  - Cerebellar or brain stem stroke
- Lasts for minutes-hours
  - T.I.A.
  - Meniere's
  - Partial seizure
  - Multiple sclerosis
  - Migraine
  - Perilymphatic fistula
- Lasts seconds to minutes
  - Benign paroxysmal positional vertigo → Perform Dix-Hallpike maneuver → Rotatory nystagmus with last component toward affected ear → Treat with Epley maneuver

True dizziness

- Somatoform disorder
- Bipolar disorder
- Panic disorder

James J. Foody, MD

Am Fam Physician. 2010;82(4):361–68.

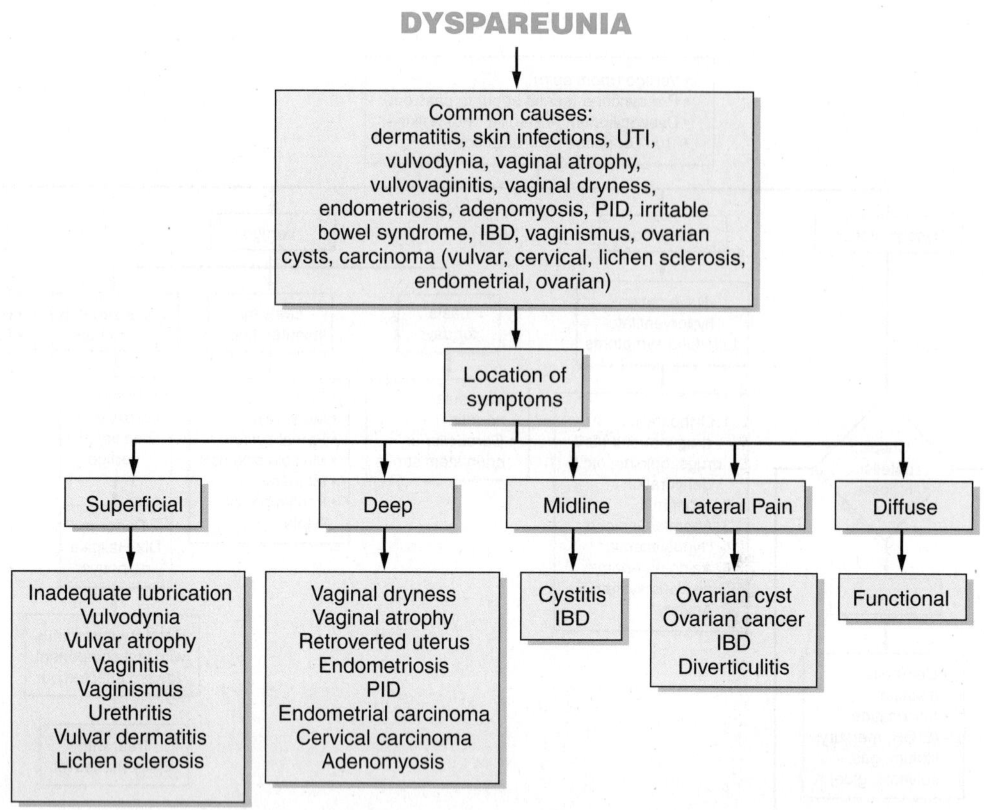
DYSPAREUNIA
Common causes: dermatitis, skin infections, UTI, vulvodynia, vaginal atrophy, vulvovaginitis, vaginal dryness, endometriosis, adenomyosis, PID, irritable bowel syndrome, IBD, vaginismus, ovarian cysts, carcinoma (vulvar, cervical, lichen sclerosis, endometrial, ovarian)
Location of symptoms
Superficial
Deep
Midline
Lateral Pain
Diffuse
Inadequate lubrication Vulvodynia Vulvar atrophy Vaginitis Vaginismus Urethritis Vulvar dermatitis Lichen sclerosis
Vaginal dryness Vaginal atrophy Retroverted uterus Endometriosis PID Endometrial carcinoma Cervical carcinoma Adenomyosis
Cystitis IBD
Ovarian cyst Ovarian cancer IBD Diverticulitis
Functional

Robert A. Baldor, MD and Alan M. Ehrlich, MD

Obstet Gynecol Clin. 2006;33(4).

DYSPEPSIA

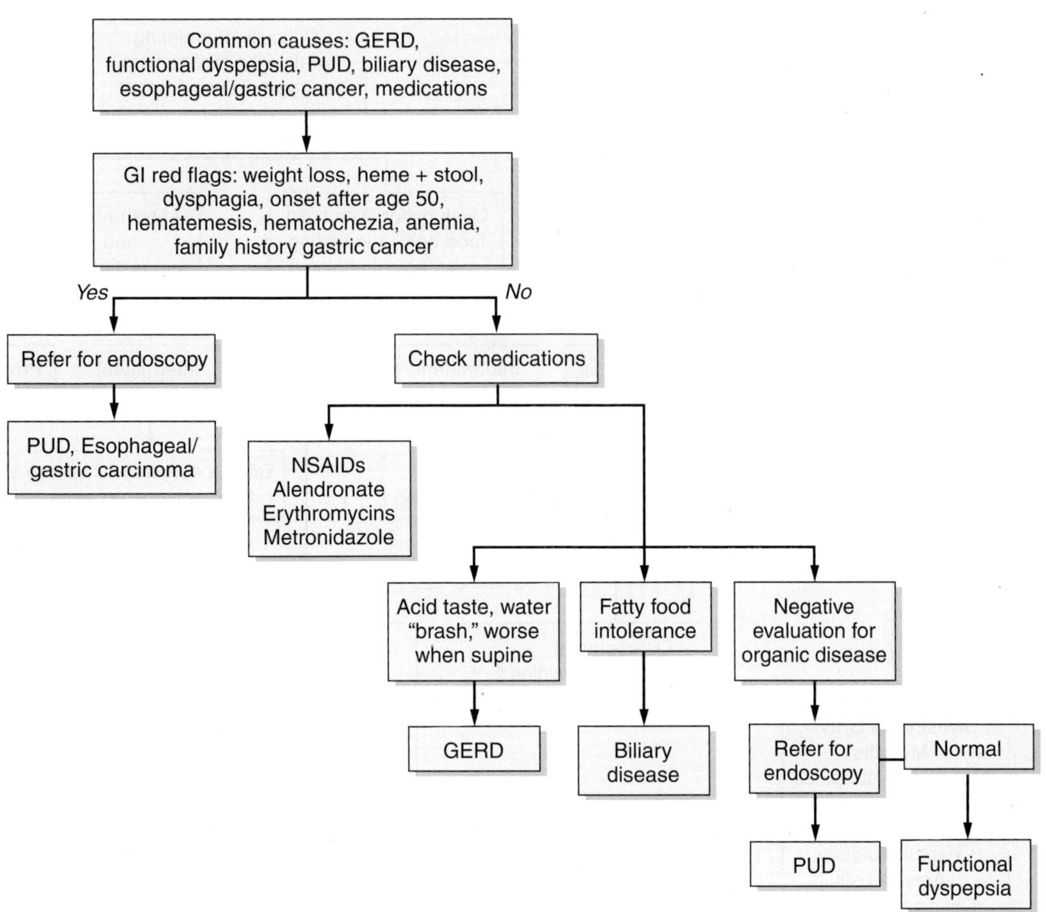

Robert A. Baldor, MD and Alan M. Ehrlich, MD

J Fam Pract. 2009;58(7 Suppl Short):S1–1.

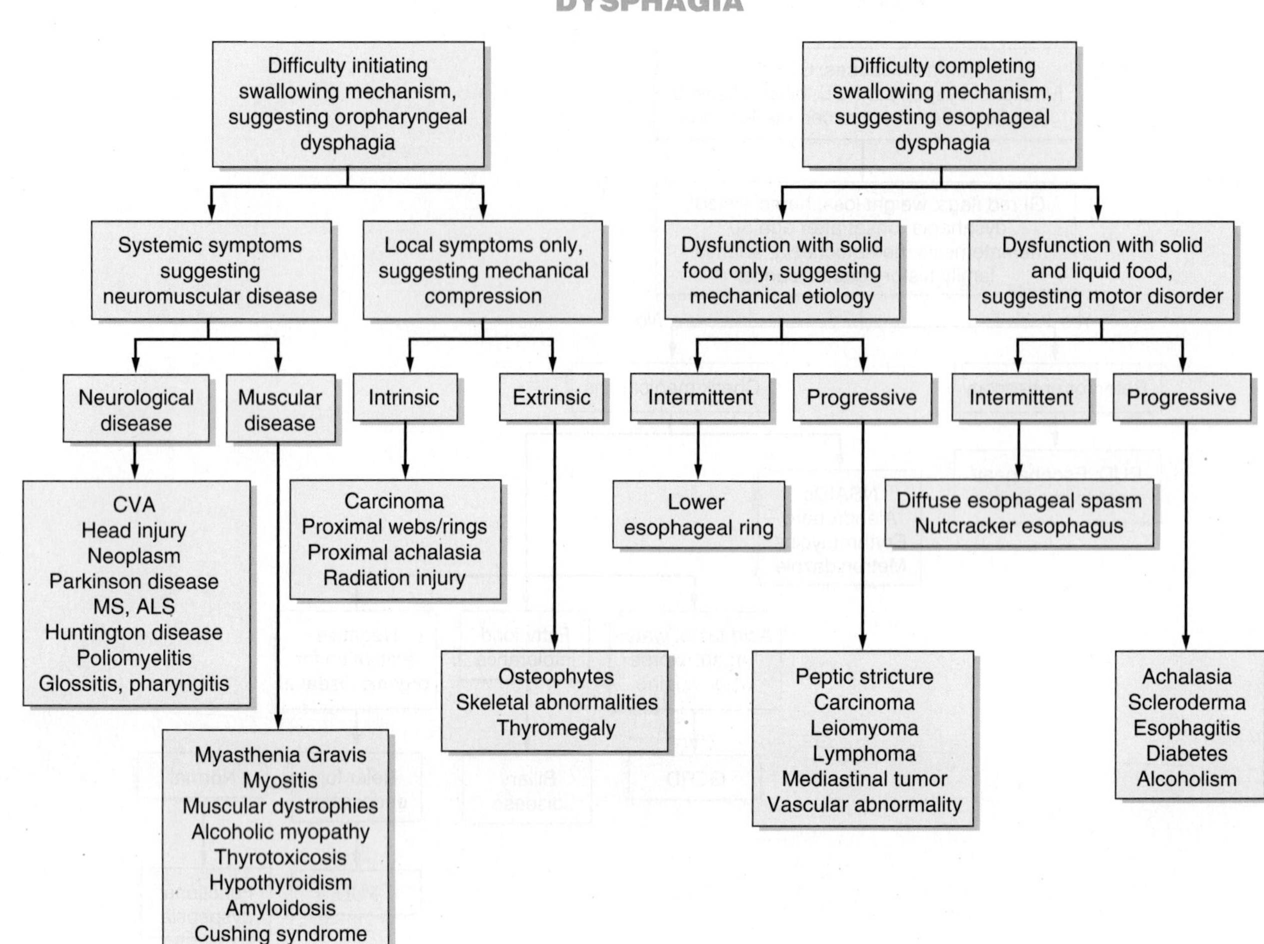
DYSPHAGIA
Difficulty initiating swallowing mechanism, suggesting oropharyngeal dysphagia
Difficulty completing swallowing mechanism, suggesting esophageal dysphagia
Systemic symptoms suggesting neuromuscular disease
Local symptoms only, suggesting mechanical compression
Dysfunction with solid food only, suggesting mechanical etiology
Dysfunction with solid and liquid food, suggesting motor disorder
Neurological disease
Muscular disease
Intrinsic
Extrinsic
Intermittent
Progressive
Intermittent
Progressive
CVA
Head injury
Neoplasm
Parkinson disease
MS, ALS
Huntington disease
Poliomyelitis
Glossitis, pharyngitis
Carcinoma
Proximal webs/rings
Proximal achalasia
Radiation injury
Lower esophageal ring
Diffuse esophageal spasm
Nutcracker esophagus
Osteophytes
Skeletal abnormalities
Thyromegaly
Peptic stricture
Carcinoma
Leiomyoma
Lymphoma
Mediastinal tumor
Vascular abnormality
Achalasia
Scleroderma
Esophagitis
Diabetes
Alcoholism
Myasthenia Gravis
Myositis
Muscular dystrophies
Alcoholic myopathy
Thyrotoxicosis
Hypothyroidism
Amyloidosis
Cushing syndrome

Parag Goyal, MD

Gastroenterol Clin North Am. 2003;32(2):553–75.

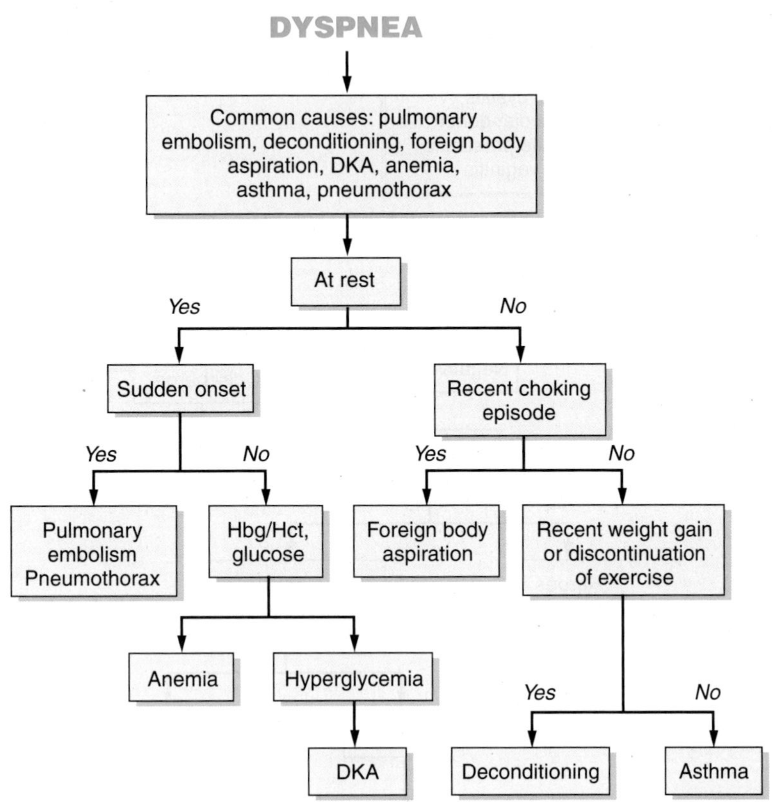

Robert A. Baldor, MD and Alan M. Ehrlich, MD

Am Fam Physician. 1998;57(4):711–6.

DYSURIA

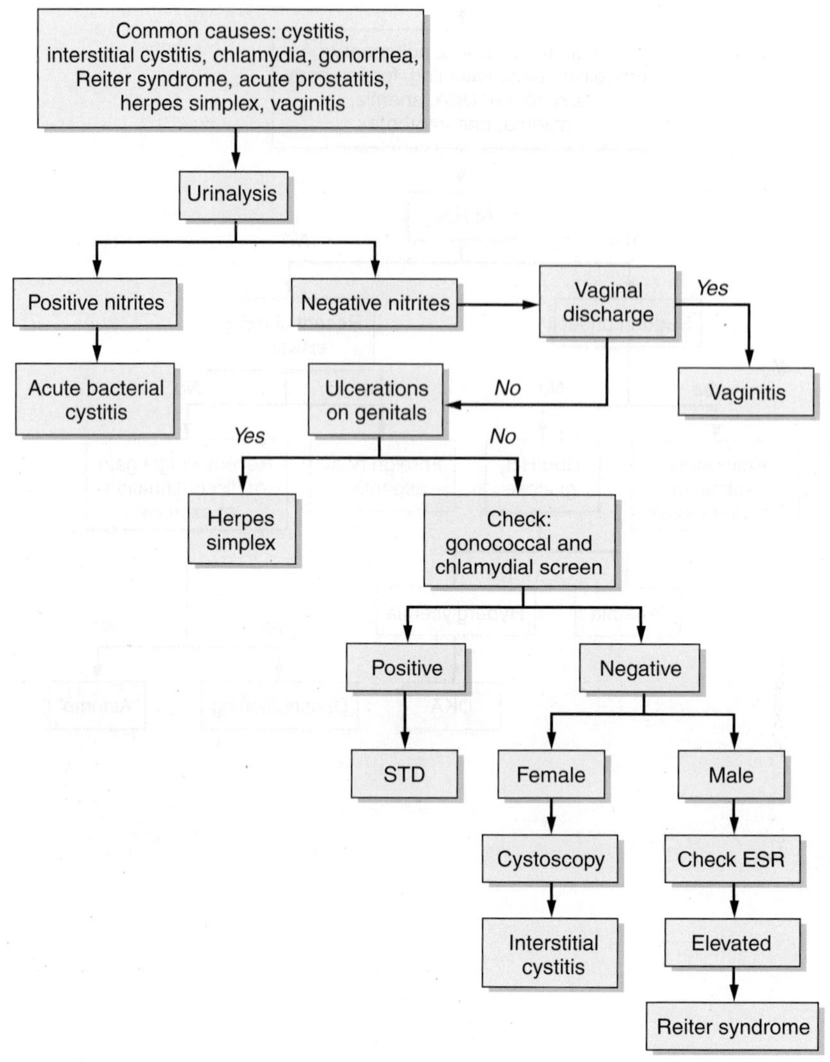

Robert A. Baldor, MD and Alan M. Ehrlich, MD

Am Fam Physician. 2002;65:1589–97.

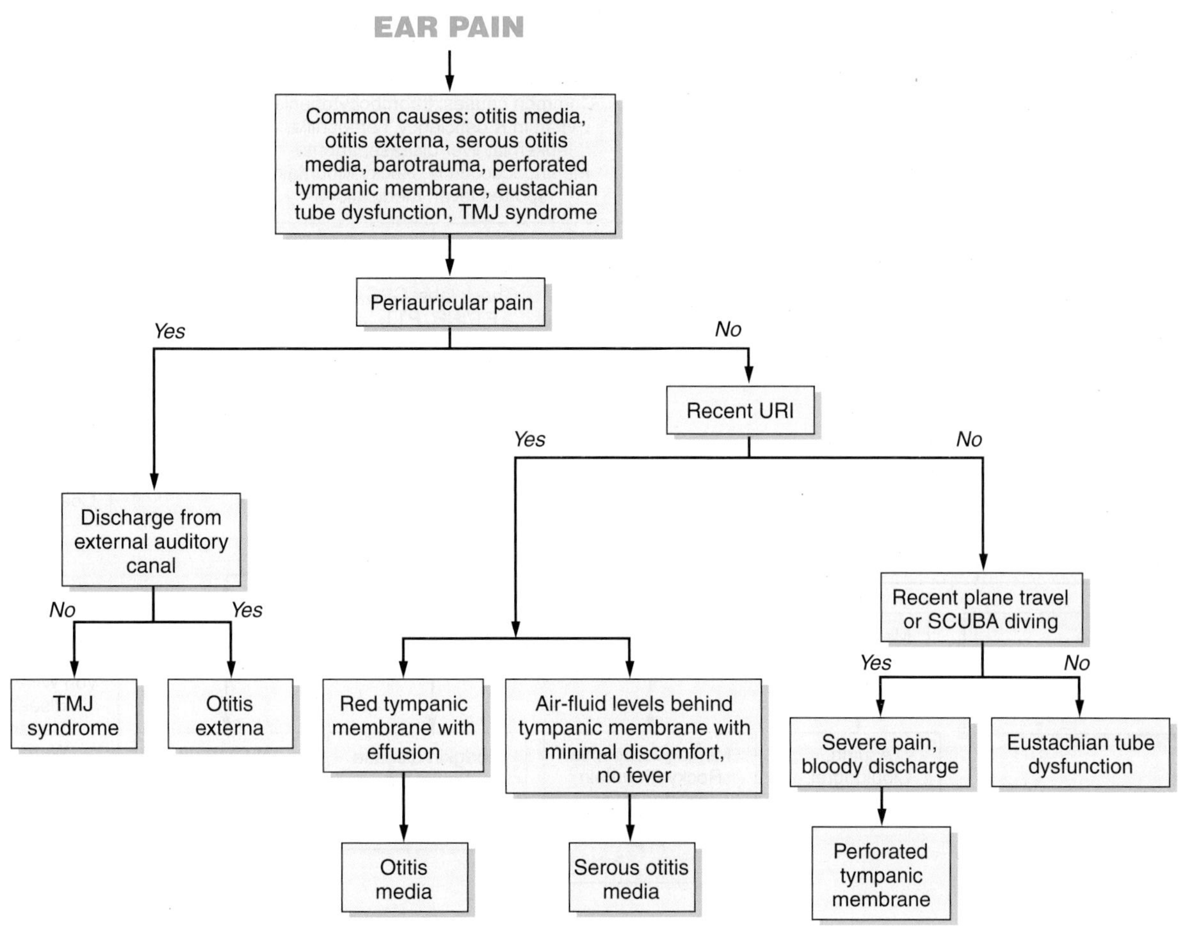

Robert A. Baldor, MD and Alan M. Ehrlich, MD

Am Fam Physician. 2008;77(5):621–8.

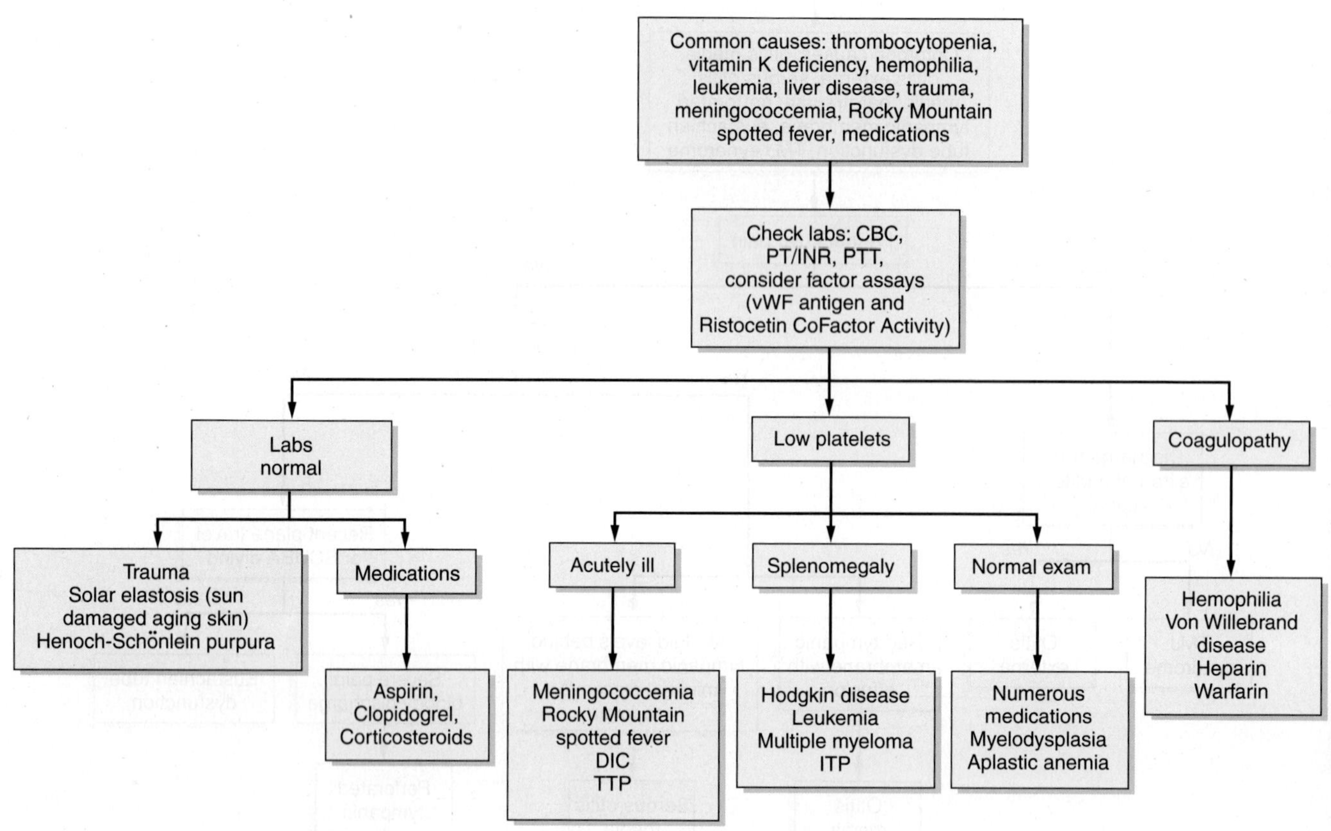
ECCHYMOSIS
Common causes: thrombocytopenia, vitamin K deficiency, hemophilia, leukemia, liver disease, trauma, meningococcemia, Rocky Mountain spotted fever, medications
Check labs: CBC, PT/INR, PTT, consider factor assays (vWF antigen and Ristocetin CoFactor Activity)
Labs normal
Low platelets
Coagulopathy
Trauma
Solar elastosis (sun damaged aging skin)
Henoch-Schönlein purpura
Medications
Aspirin, Clopidogrel, Corticosteroids
Acutely ill
Meningococcemia
Rocky Mountain spotted fever
DIC
TTP
Splenomegaly
Hodgkin disease
Leukemia
Multiple myeloma
ITP
Normal exam
Numerous medications
Myelodysplasia
Aplastic anemia
Hemophilia
Von Willebrand disease
Heparin
Warfarin

Robert A. Baldor, MD and Alan M. Ehrlich, MD

Arch Dermatol. 2010;146(1):94–5.

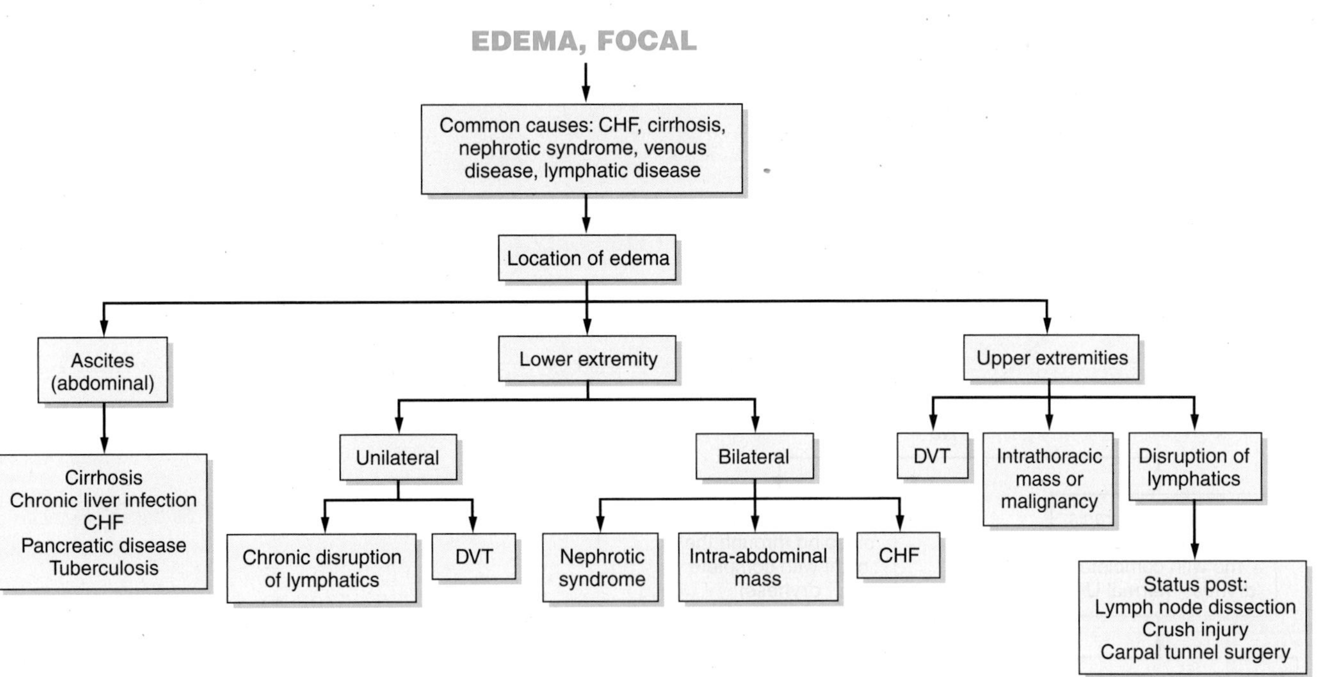

Robert A. Baldor, MD and Alan M. Ehrlich, MD

Am J Med. 2002;113(7):580–6.

ENURESIS

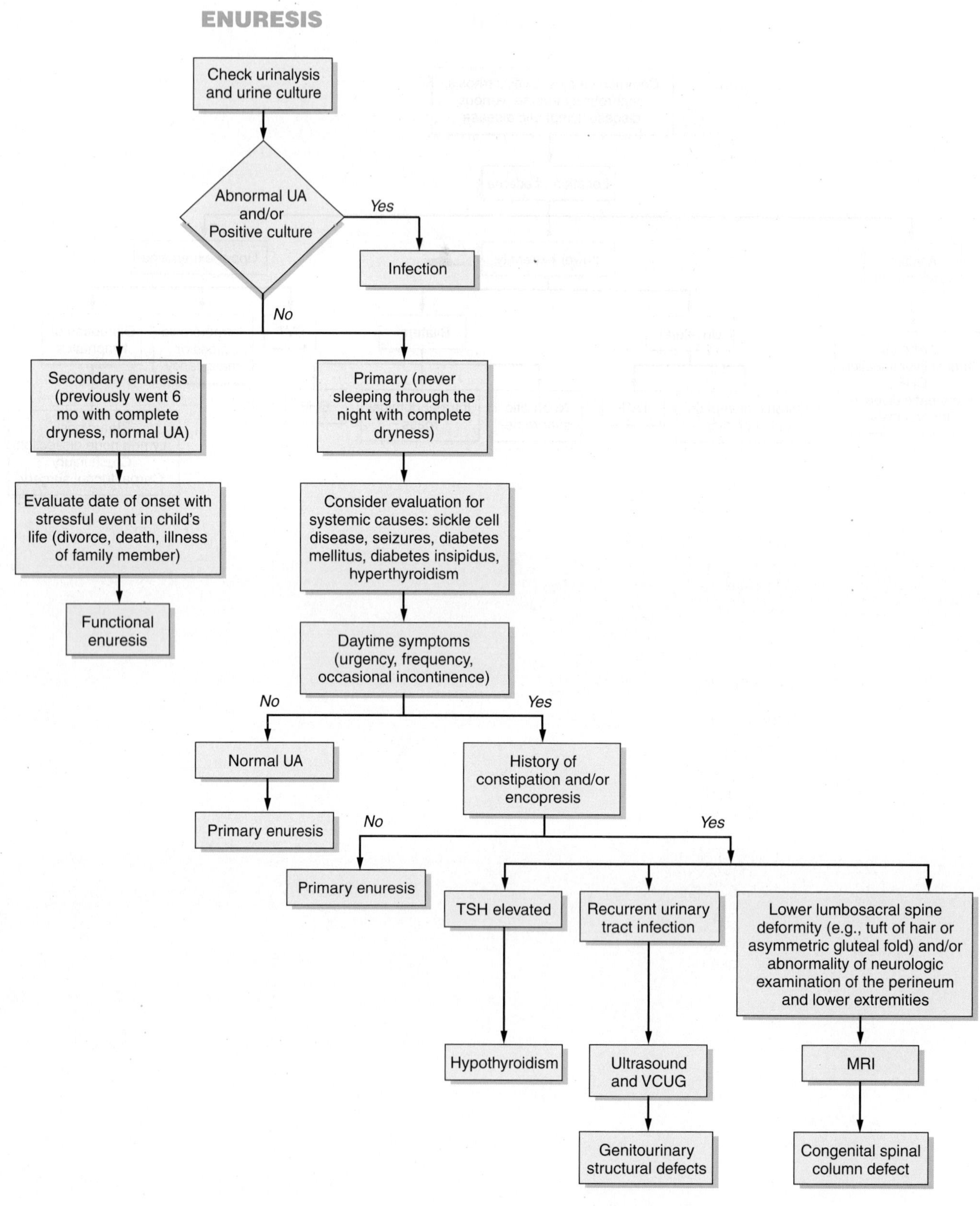

Robert A. Baldor, MD and Alan M. Ehrlich, MD

J Am Acad Child Adolesc Psychiatry. 2004;43(1):123–5.

EPIGASTRIC PAIN

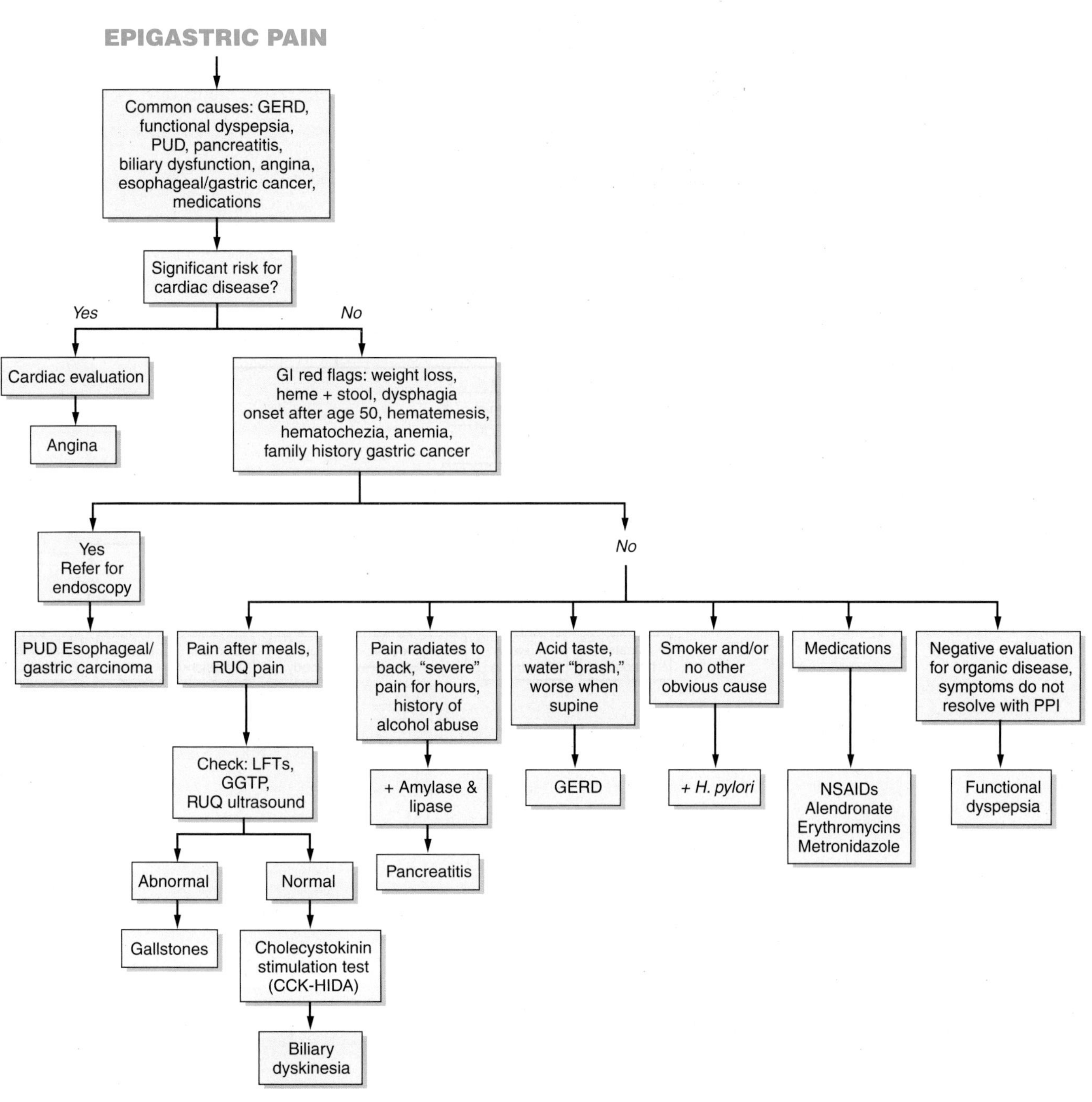

Common causes: GERD, functional dyspepsia, PUD, pancreatitis, biliary dysfunction, angina, esophageal/gastric cancer, medications
Significant risk for cardiac disease?
Yes
No
Cardiac evaluation
Angina
GI red flags: weight loss, heme + stool, dysphagia onset after age 50, hematemesis, hematochezia, anemia, family history gastric cancer
Yes Refer for endoscopy
PUD Esophageal/ gastric carcinoma
No
Pain after meals, RUQ pain
Check: LFTs, GGTP, RUQ ultrasound
Abnormal
Gallstones
Normal
Cholecystokinin stimulation test (CCK-HIDA)
Biliary dyskinesia
Pain radiates to back, "severe" pain for hours, history of alcohol abuse
+ Amylase & lipase
Pancreatitis
Acid taste, water "brash," worse when supine
GERD
Smoker and/or no other obvious cause
+ H. pylori
Medications
NSAIDs Alendronate Erythromycins Metronidazole
Negative evaluation for organic disease, symptoms do not resolve with PPI
Functional dyspepsia

Robert A. Baldor, MD and Alan M. Ehrlich, MD

Curr Gastroenterol Rep. 2009;11(4):288–94.

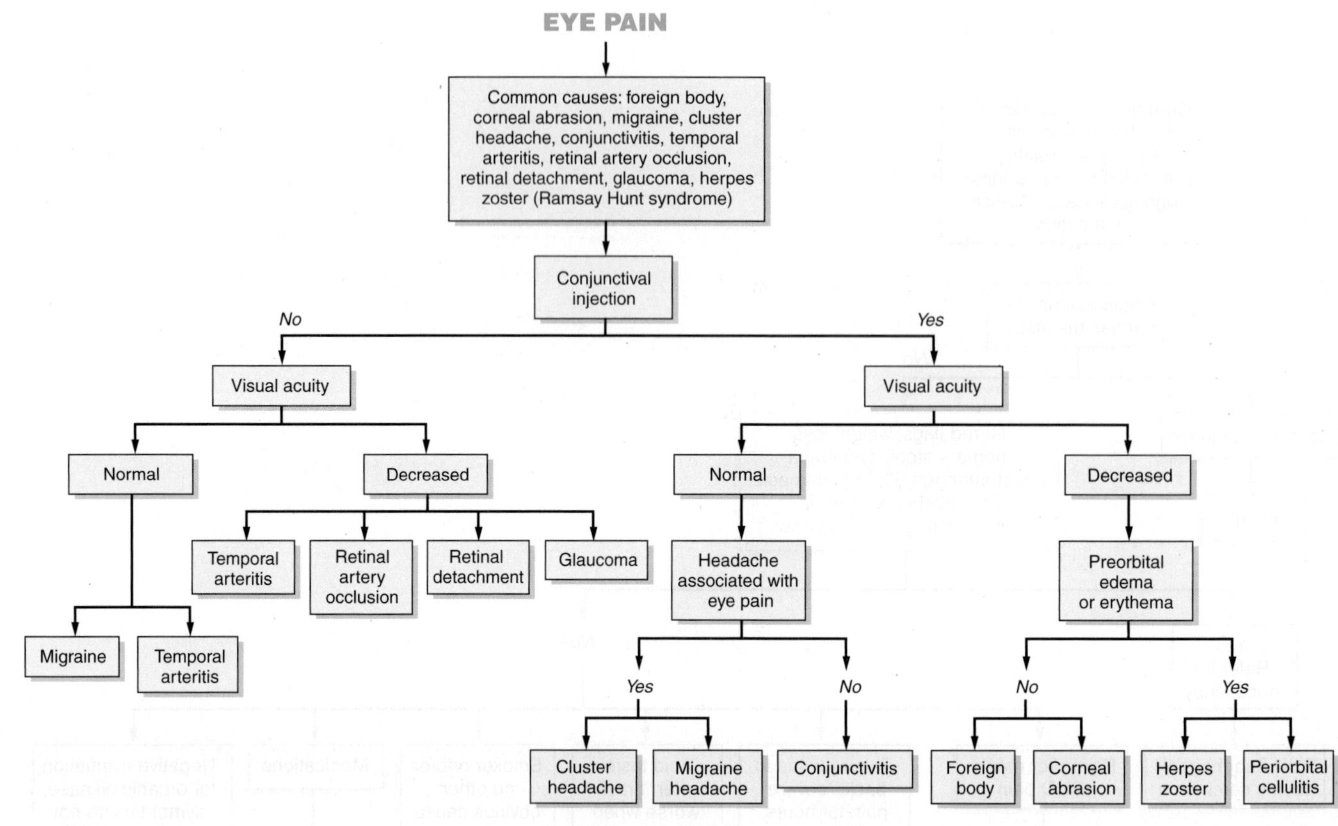

Robert A. Baldor, MD and Alan M. Ehrlich, MD

Curr Pain Headache Rep. 2008;12(4):296–304.

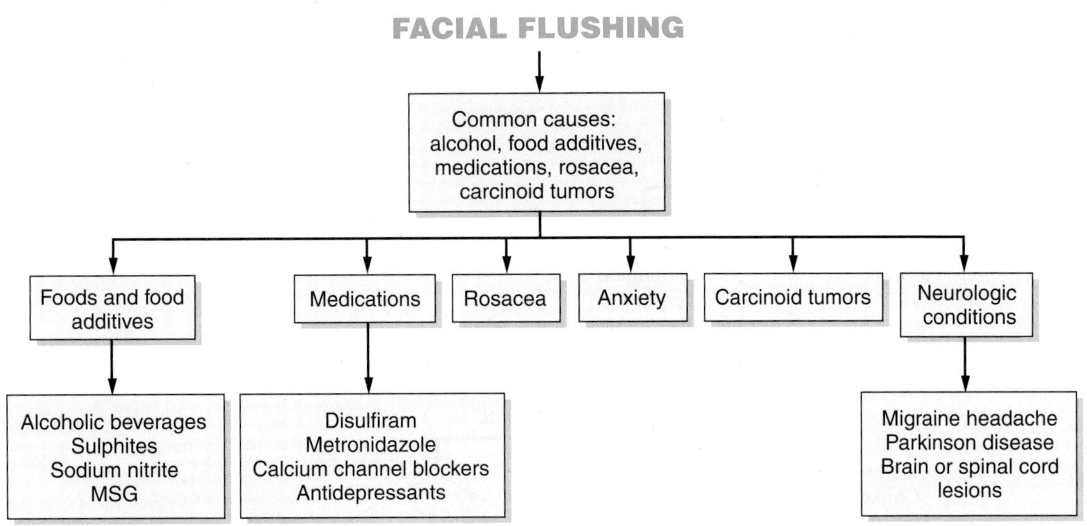

Robert A. Baldor, MD and Alan M. Ehrlich, MD

PLoS Med. 2009;6(3):e50.

FACIAL PARALYSIS

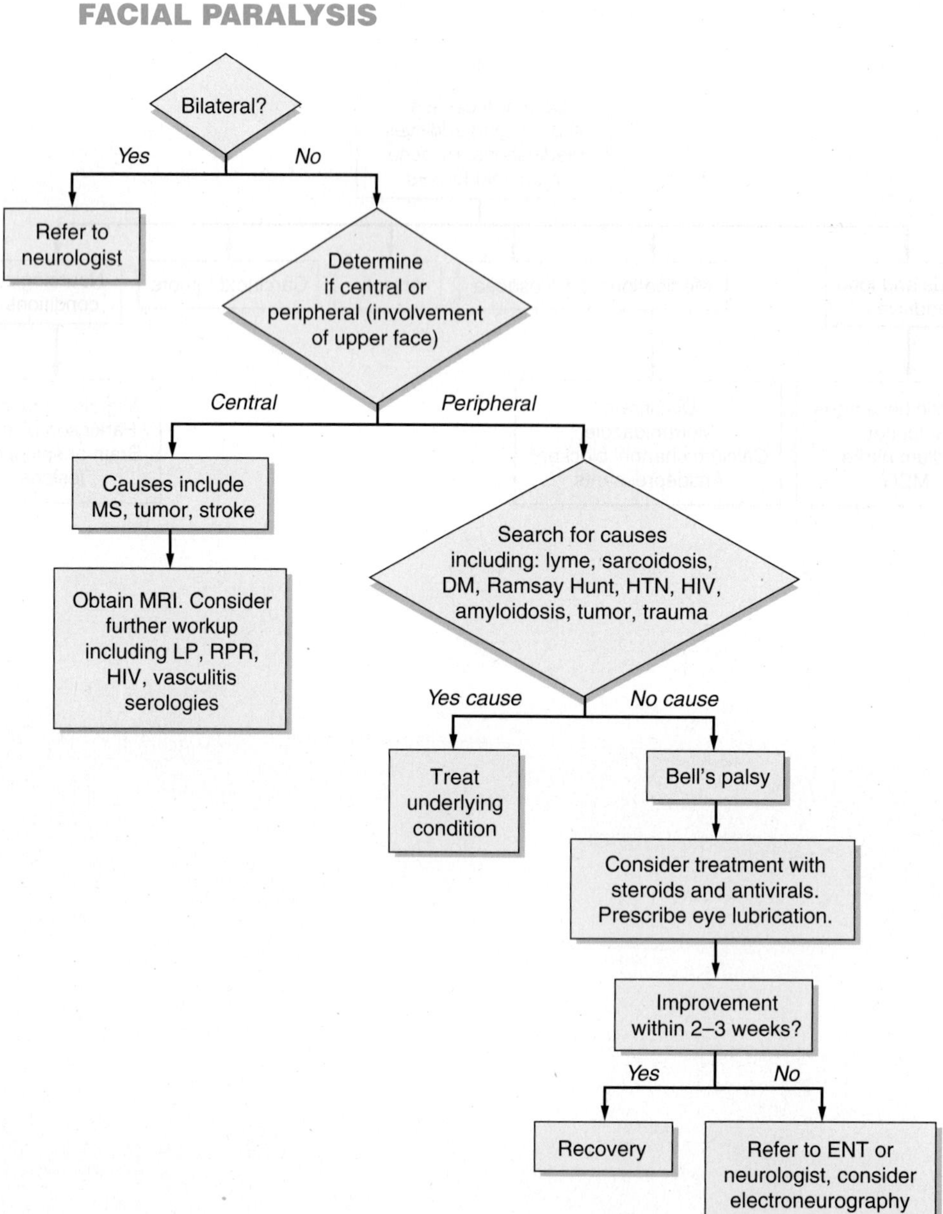

Laura Hagopian, MD and William A. Tosches, MD

Rev Med Intern. 2009;30(9):769–75.

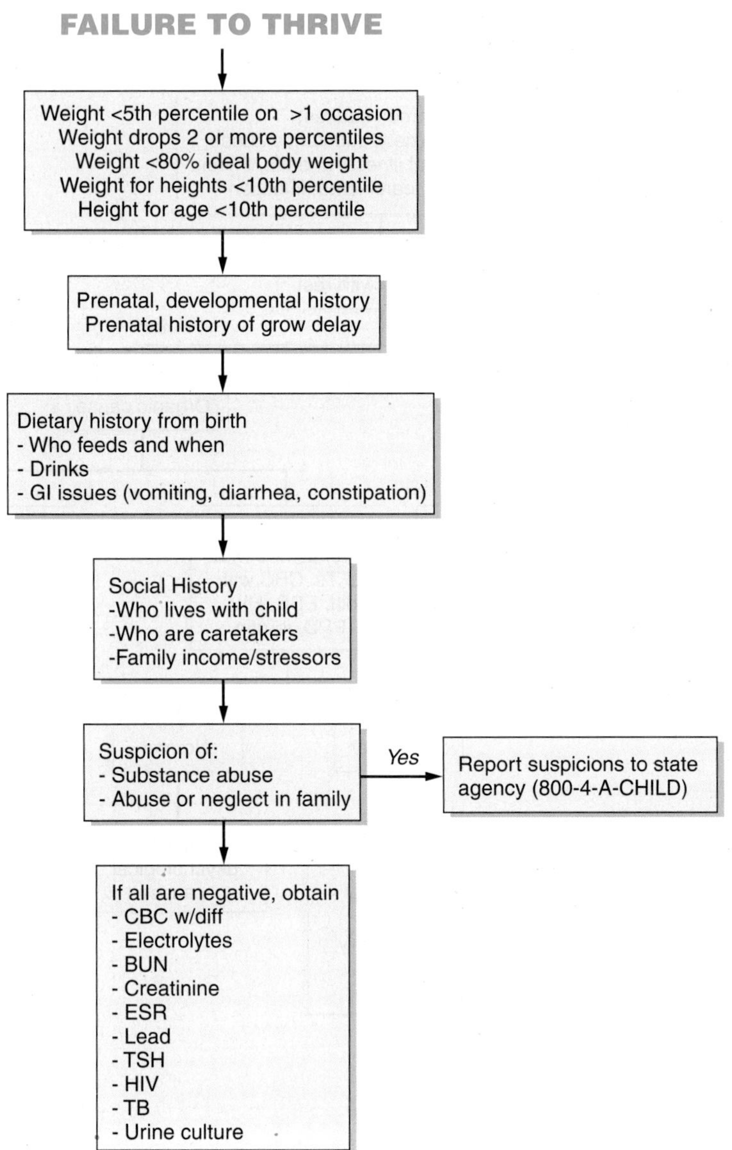
FAILURE TO THRIVE
Weight <5th percentile on >1 occasion
Weight drops 2 or more percentiles
Weight <80% ideal body weight
Weight for heights <10th percentile
Height for age <10th percentile
Prenatal, developmental history
Prenatal history of grow delay
Dietary history from birth
- Who feeds and when
- Drinks
- GI issues (vomiting, diarrhea, constipation)
Social History
-Who lives with child
-Who are caretakers
-Family income/stressors
Suspicion of:
- Substance abuse
- Abuse or neglect in family
Yes
Report suspicions to state agency (800-4-A-CHILD)
If all are negative, obtain
- CBC w/diff
- Electrolytes
- BUN
- Creatinine
- ESR
- Lead
- TSH
- HIV
- TB
- Urine culture

Robert A. Baldor, MD and Alan M. Ehrlich, MD

Eur J Pediatr. 2009;168(7):839–45.

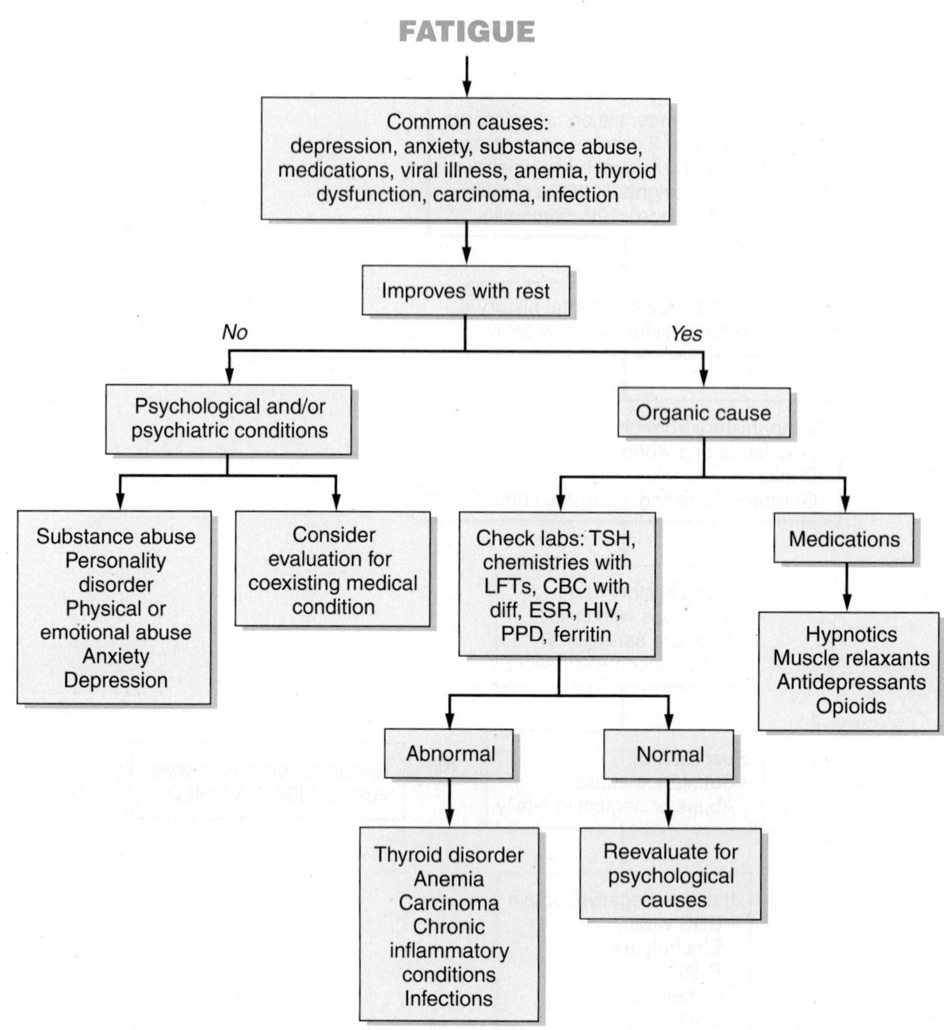
FATIGUE
Common causes: depression, anxiety, substance abuse, medications, viral illness, anemia, thyroid dysfunction, carcinoma, infection
Improves with rest
No
Yes
Psychological and/or psychiatric conditions
Organic cause
Substance abuse Personality disorder Physical or emotional abuse Anxiety Depression
Consider evaluation for coexisting medical condition
Check labs: TSH, chemistries with LFTs, CBC with diff, ESR, HIV, PPD, ferritin
Medications
Hypnotics Muscle relaxants Antidepressants Opioids
Abnormal
Normal
Thyroid disorder Anemia Carcinoma Chronic inflammatory conditions Infections
Reevaluate for psychological causes

Robert A. Baldor, MD and Alan M. Ehrlich, MD

CMAJ. 2009;181(10):683–7.

FEVER IN THE FIRST 3 MONTHS OF LIFE

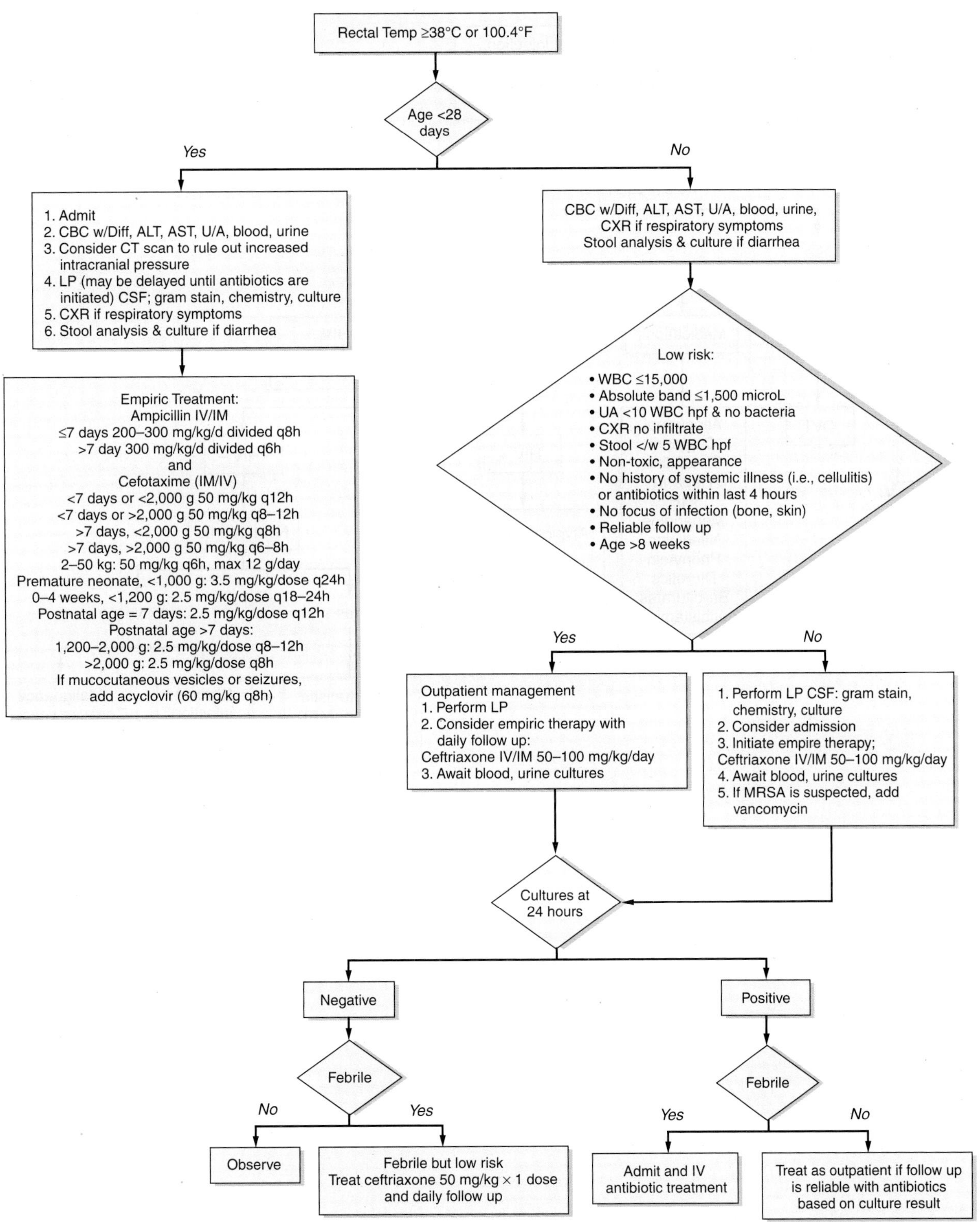

Katharine Tumilty, MD, William J. Durbin, MD, and Mariann Manno, MD

Ann Emerg Med. 2003;42(4):530–45.

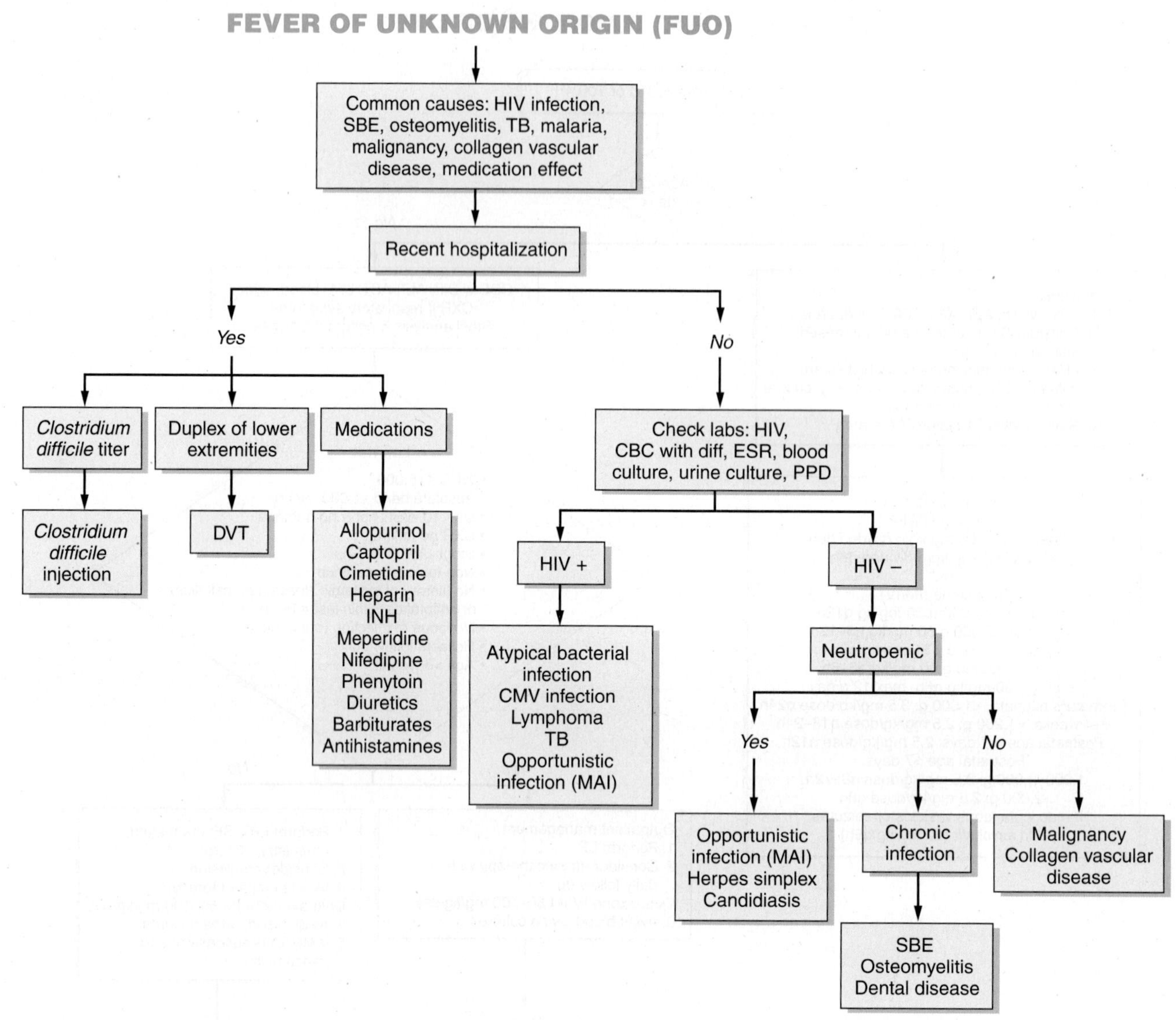

Robert A. Baldor, MD and Alan M. Ehrlich, MD

Pediatr Infect Dis J. 2009;28(11):1026–8.

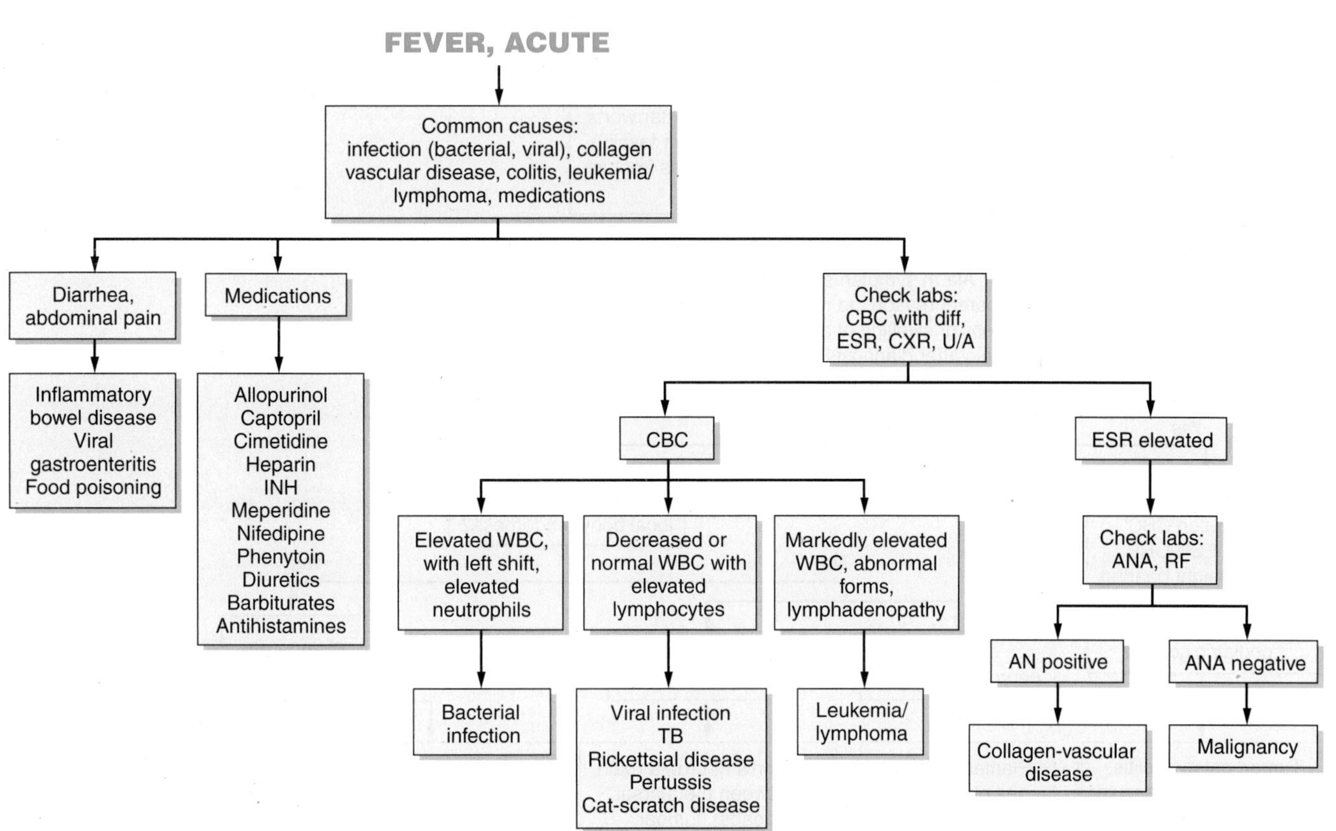

Robert A. Baldor, MD and Alan M. Ehrlich, MD

Crit Care Med. 2010;38(2):457–63.

FOOT PAIN

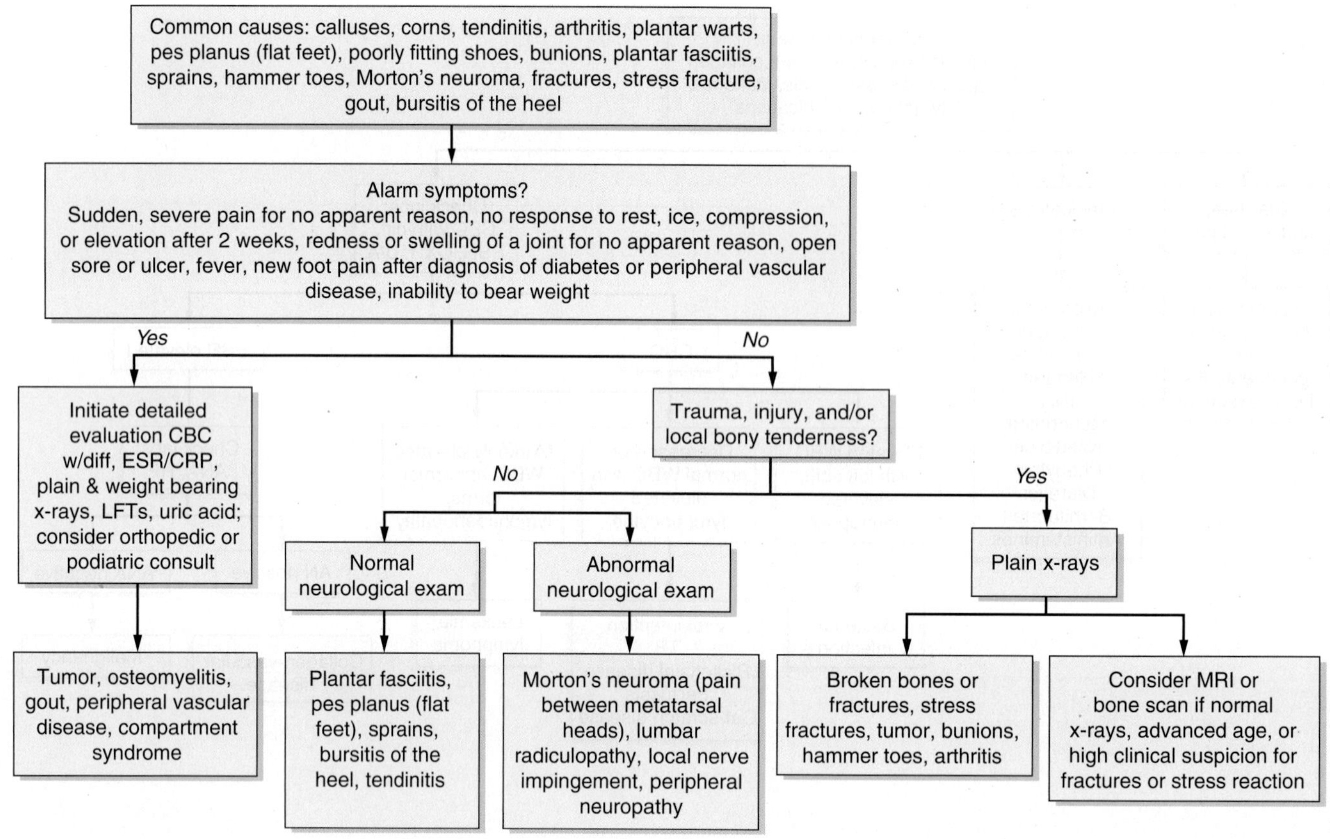
Common causes: calluses, corns, tendinitis, arthritis, plantar warts, pes planus (flat feet), poorly fitting shoes, bunions, plantar fasciitis, sprains, hammer toes, Morton's neuroma, fractures, stress fracture, gout, bursitis of the heel
Alarm symptoms?
Sudden, severe pain for no apparent reason, no response to rest, ice, compression, or elevation after 2 weeks, redness or swelling of a joint for no apparent reason, open sore or ulcer, fever, new foot pain after diagnosis of diabetes or peripheral vascular disease, inability to bear weight
Yes
No
Initiate detailed evaluation CBC w/diff, ESR/CRP, plain & weight bearing x-rays, LFTs, uric acid; consider orthopedic or podiatric consult
Trauma, injury, and/or local bony tenderness?
No
Yes
Normal neurological exam
Abnormal neurological exam
Plain x-rays
Tumor, osteomyelitis, gout, peripheral vascular disease, compartment syndrome
Plantar fasciitis, pes planus (flat feet), sprains, bursitis of the heel, tendinitis
Morton's neuroma (pain between metatarsal heads), lumbar radiculopathy, local nerve impingement, peripheral neuropathy
Broken bones or fractures, stress fractures, tumor, bunions, hammer toes, arthritis
Consider MRI or bone scan if normal x-rays, advanced age, or high clinical suspicion for fractures or stress reaction

George Gunter A. Pujalte, MD

BMJ. 2003;326(7386):417.

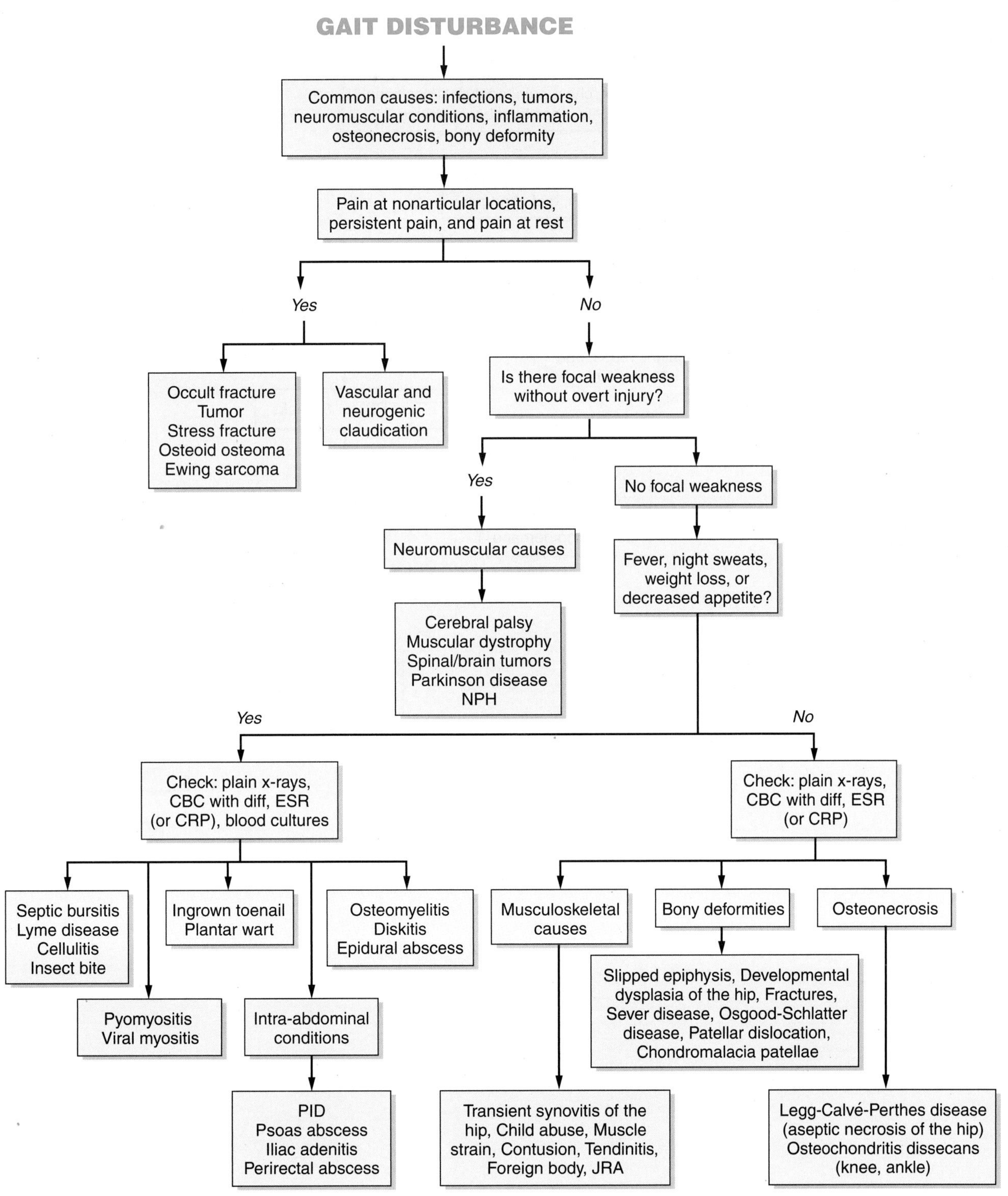
GAIT DISTURBANCE
Common causes: infections, tumors, neuromuscular conditions, inflammation, osteonecrosis, bony deformity
Pain at nonarticular locations, persistent pain, and pain at rest
Yes
No
Occult fracture
Tumor
Stress fracture
Osteoid osteoma
Ewing sarcoma
Vascular and neurogenic claudication
Is there focal weakness without overt injury?
Yes
No focal weakness
Neuromuscular causes
Cerebral palsy
Muscular dystrophy
Spinal/brain tumors
Parkinson disease
NPH
Fever, night sweats, weight loss, or decreased appetite?
Yes
No
Check: plain x-rays, CBC with diff, ESR (or CRP), blood cultures
Check: plain x-rays, CBC with diff, ESR (or CRP)
Septic bursitis
Lyme disease
Cellulitis
Insect bite
Ingrown toenail
Plantar wart
Osteomyelitis
Diskitis
Epidural abscess
Pyomyositis
Viral myositis
Intra-abdominal conditions
PID
Psoas abscess
Iliac adenitis
Perirectal abscess
Musculoskeletal causes
Bony deformities
Osteonecrosis
Slipped epiphysis, Developmental dysplasia of the hip, Fractures, Sever disease, Osgood-Schlatter disease, Patellar dislocation, Chondromalacia patellae
Transient synovitis of the hip, Child abuse, Muscle strain, Contusion, Tendinitis, Foreign body, JRA
Legg-Calvé-Perthes disease (aseptic necrosis of the hip)
Osteochondritis dissecans (knee, ankle)

Robert A. Baldor, MD and Alan M. Ehrlich, MD

Stroke. 2009;40(12):3816–20.

GASTROESOPHAGEAL REFLUX DISEASE (GERD), TREATMENT

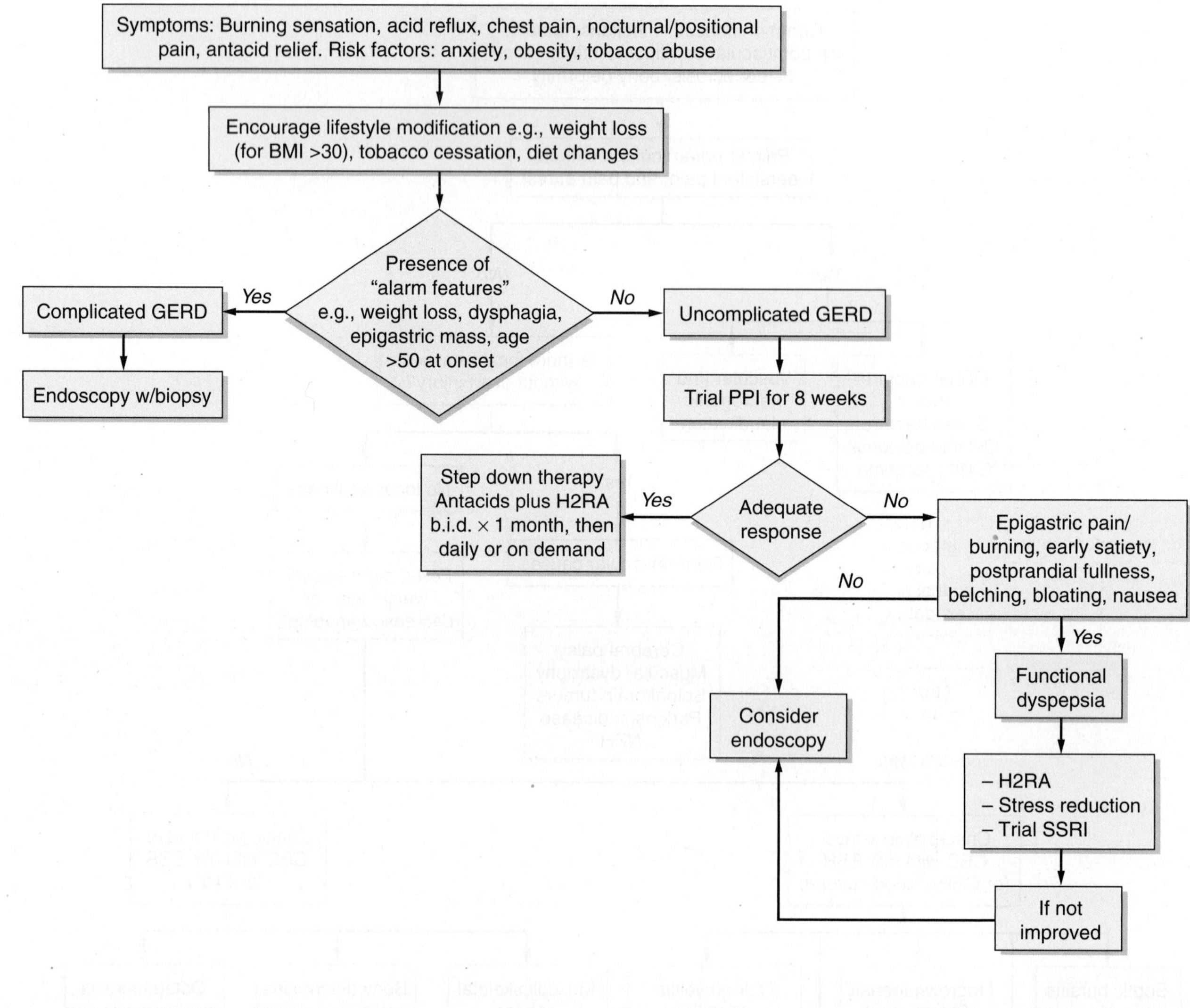

Richard E. Trowbridge, MD and Rebecca A. Frye, DO

Am J Med. 2010;123(7):583–92.

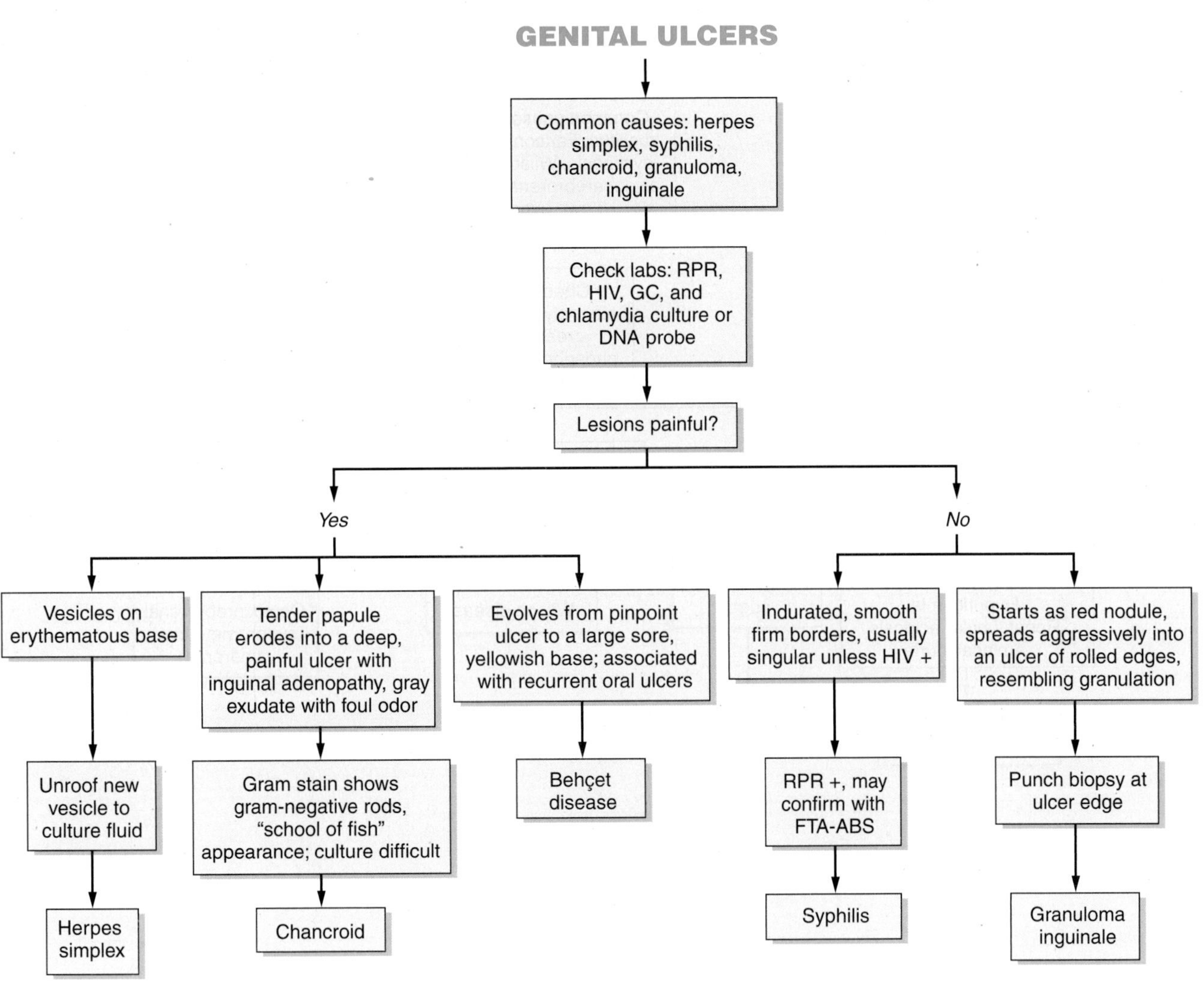

Robert A. Baldor, MD and Alan M. Ehrlich, MD

Sex Transm Dis. 2008;35(6):545–9.

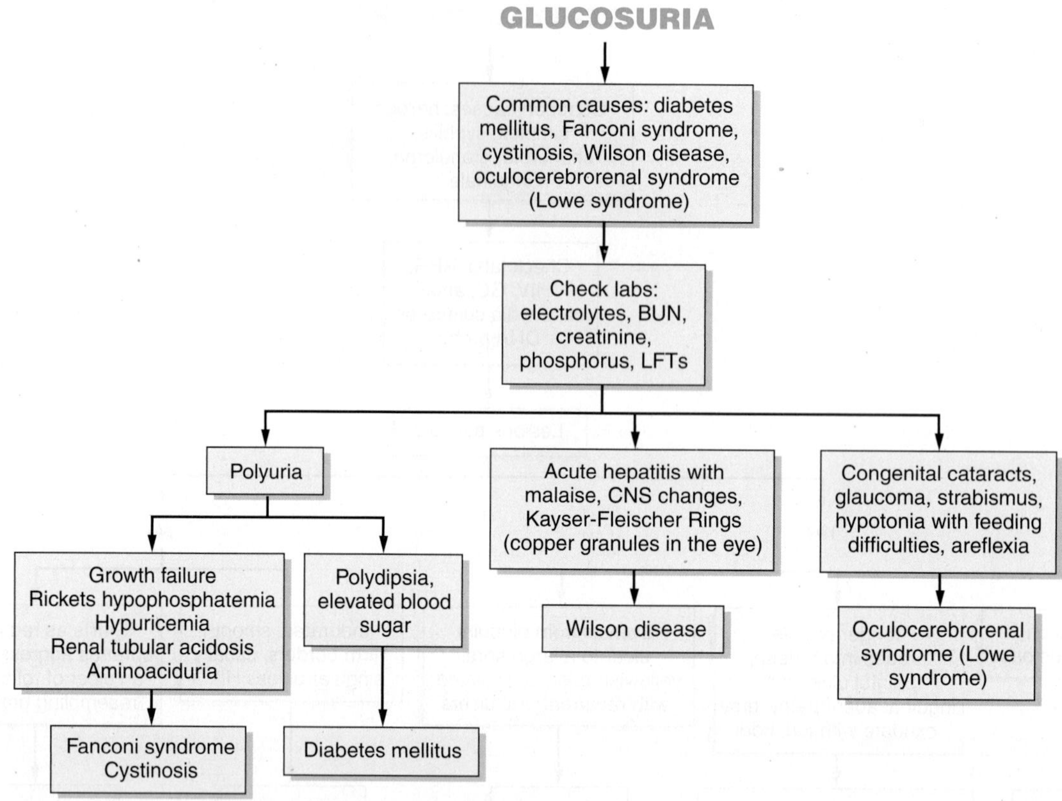

Robert A. Baldor, MD and Alan M. Ehrlich, MD

Scand J Clin Lab Invest. 2009;69(6):662–72.

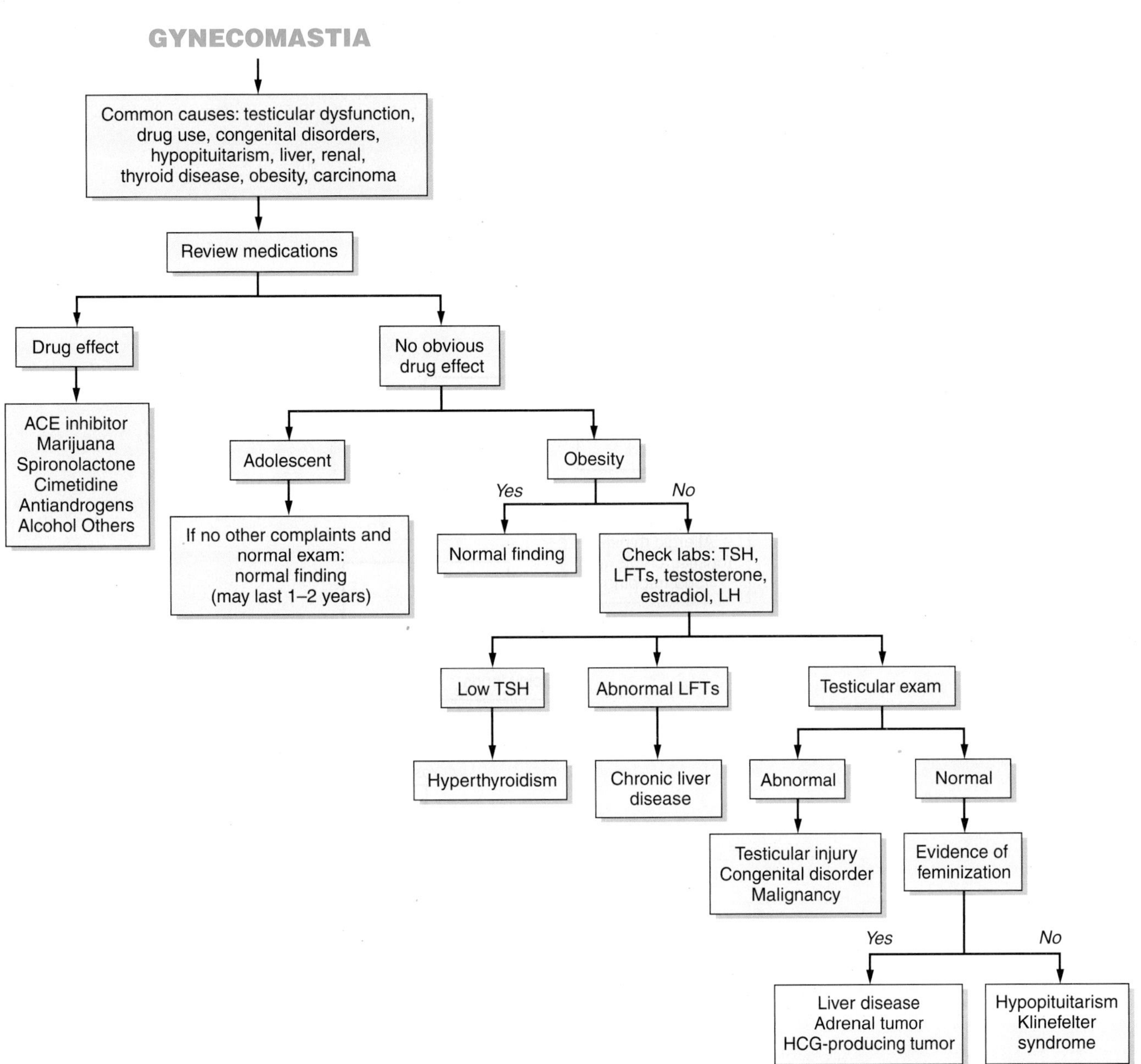
GYNECOMASTIA
Common causes: testicular dysfunction, drug use, congenital disorders, hypopituitarism, liver, renal, thyroid disease, obesity, carcinoma
Review medications
Drug effect
ACE inhibitor
Marijuana
Spironolactone
Cimetidine
Antiandrogens
Alcohol Others
No obvious drug effect
Adolescent
If no other complaints and normal exam: normal finding (may last 1–2 years)
Obesity
Yes
No
Normal finding
Check labs: TSH, LFTs, testosterone, estradiol, LH
Low TSH
Hyperthyroidism
Abnormal LFTs
Chronic liver disease
Testicular exam
Abnormal
Testicular injury
Congenital disorder
Malignancy
Normal
Evidence of feminization
Yes
No
Liver disease
Adrenal tumor
HCG-producing tumor
Hypopituitarism
Klinefelter syndrome

Robert A. Baldor, MD and Alan M. Ehrlich, MD

J Clin Endocrinol Metab. 2009;94(8):2975–8.

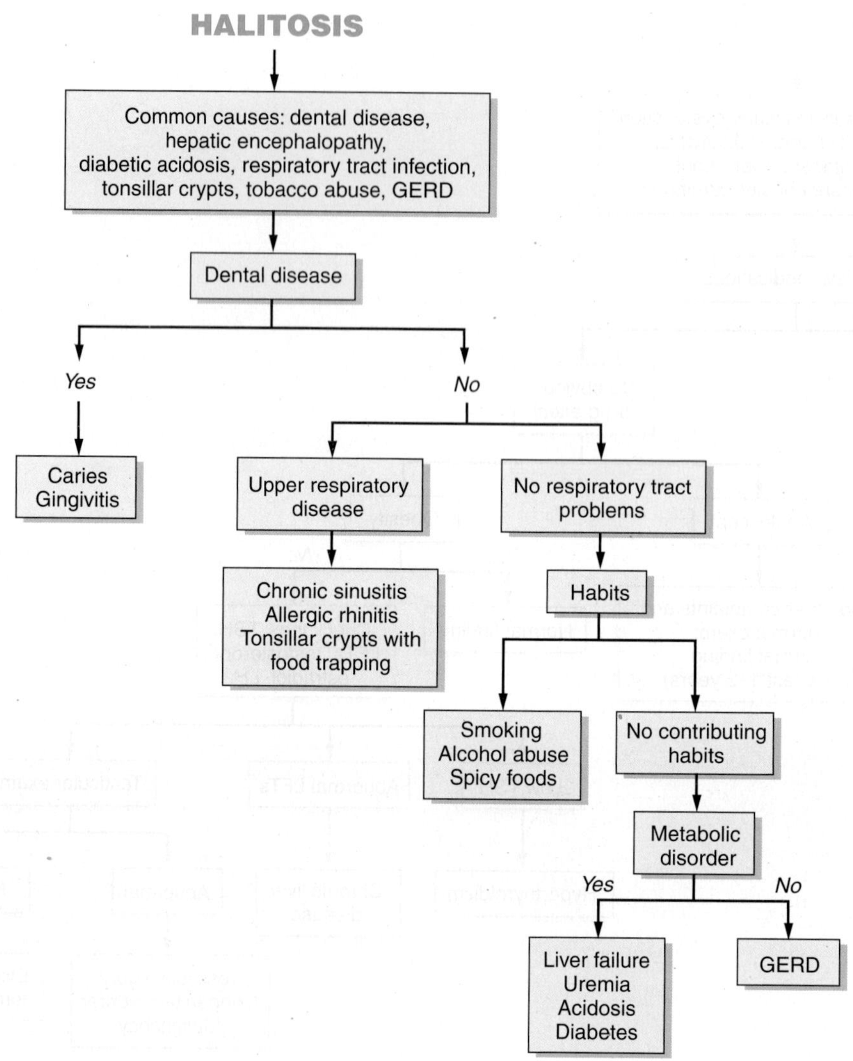

Robert A. Baldor, MD and Alan M. Ehrlich, MD

Oral Surg Oral Med Oral Pathol Oral Radiol Endod. 2008;106(3):384–8.

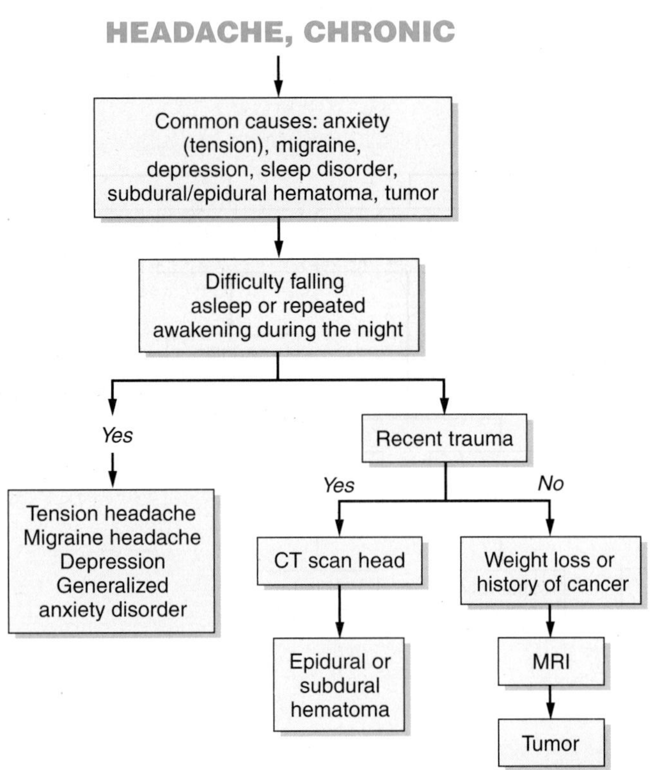

Robert A. Baldor, MD and Alan M. Ehrlich, MD

Acta Neurochir Suppl. 2010;107:65–9.

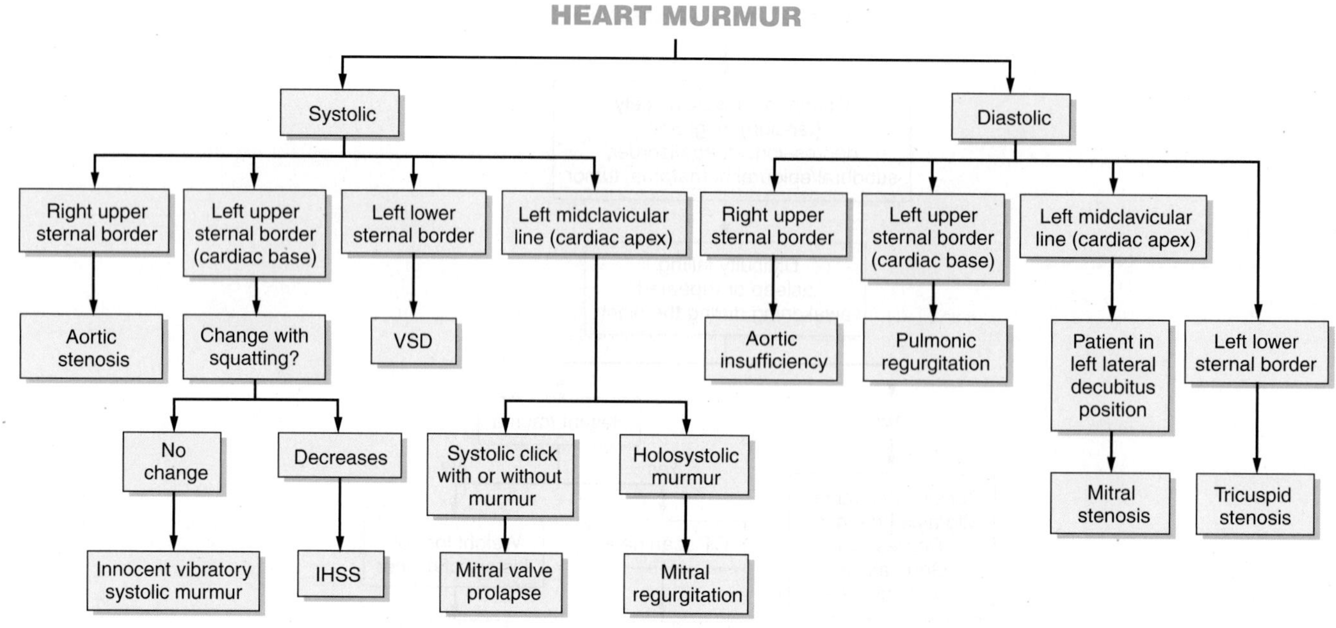

Robert A. Baldor, MD and Alan M. Ehrlich, MD

Pediatr Int. 2008;50(2):145–9.

HEMATEMESIS (BLEEDING, UPPER GI)

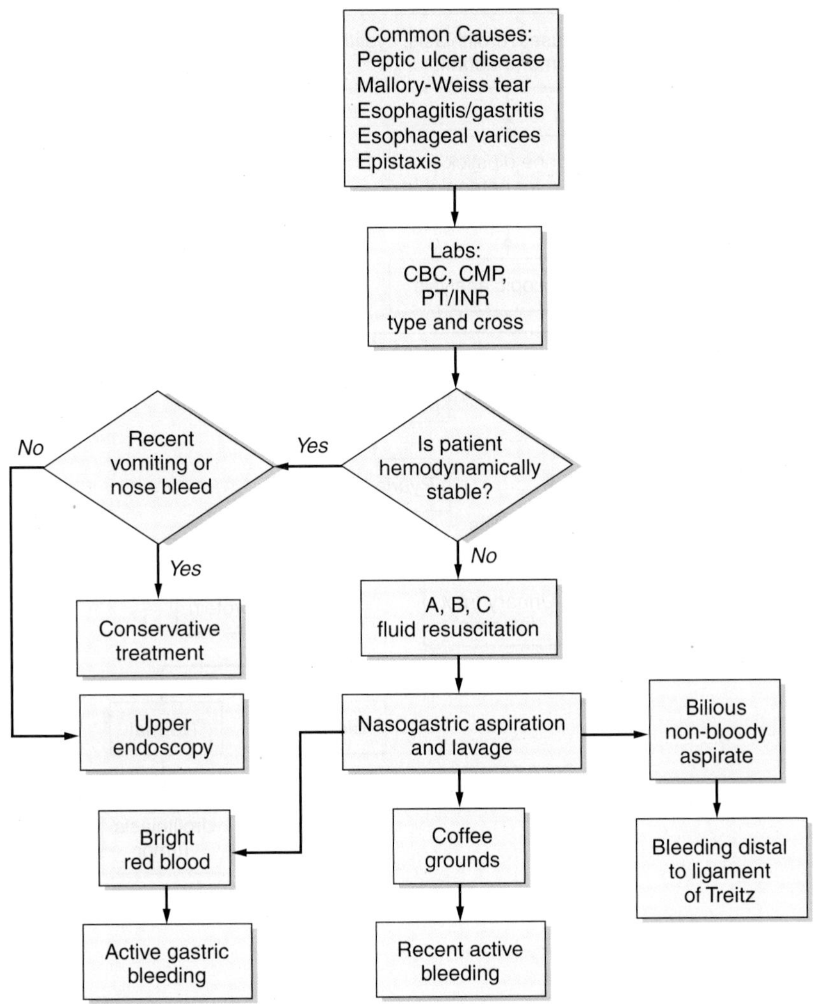

Sanjeev K. Sharma, MD and Kyle V. Contini, MD

Can J Gastroenterol. 2004;18(10):605–9.

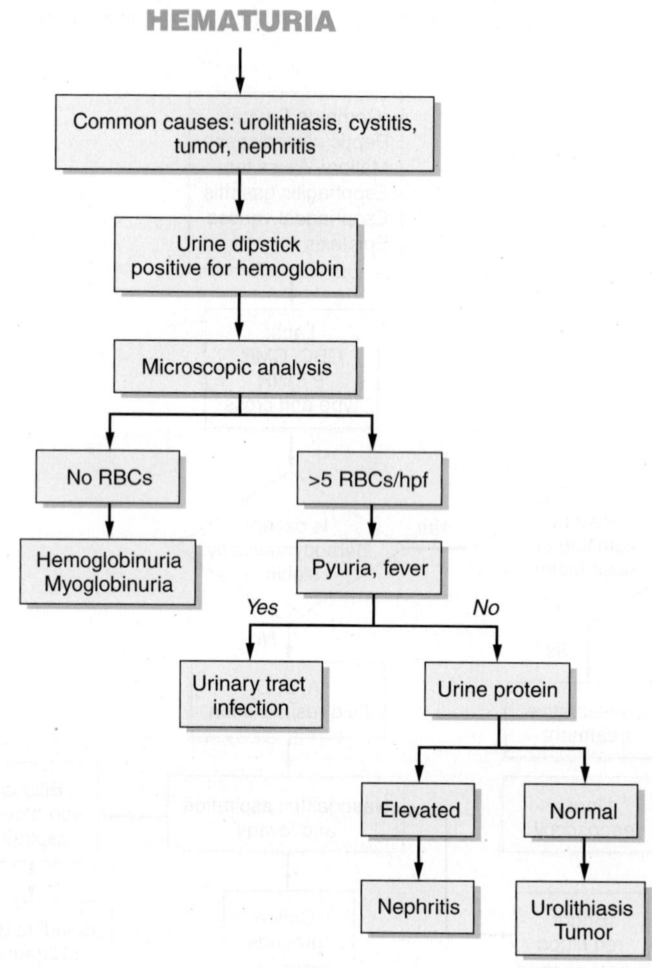

Robert A. Baldor, MD and Alan M. Ehrlich, MD

Med Clin North Am. 2004;88(2):329–43.

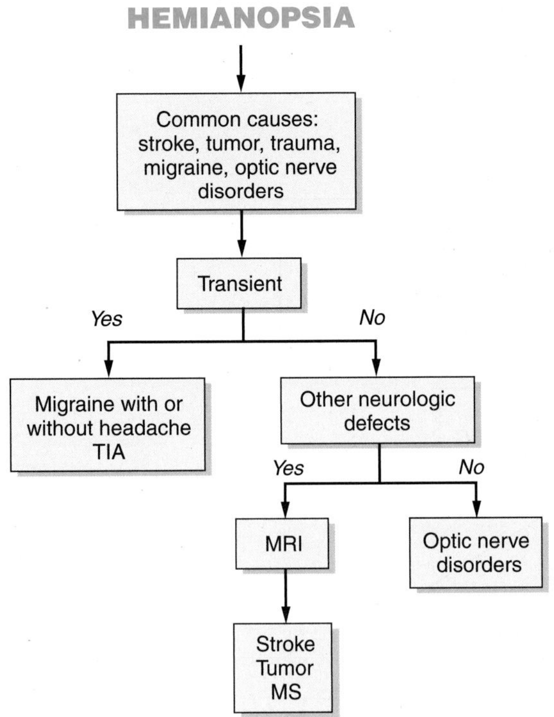

Robert A. Baldor, MD and Alan M. Ehrlich, MD

Stroke. 2010;41(2):e88–90.

HEMOCHROMATOSIS

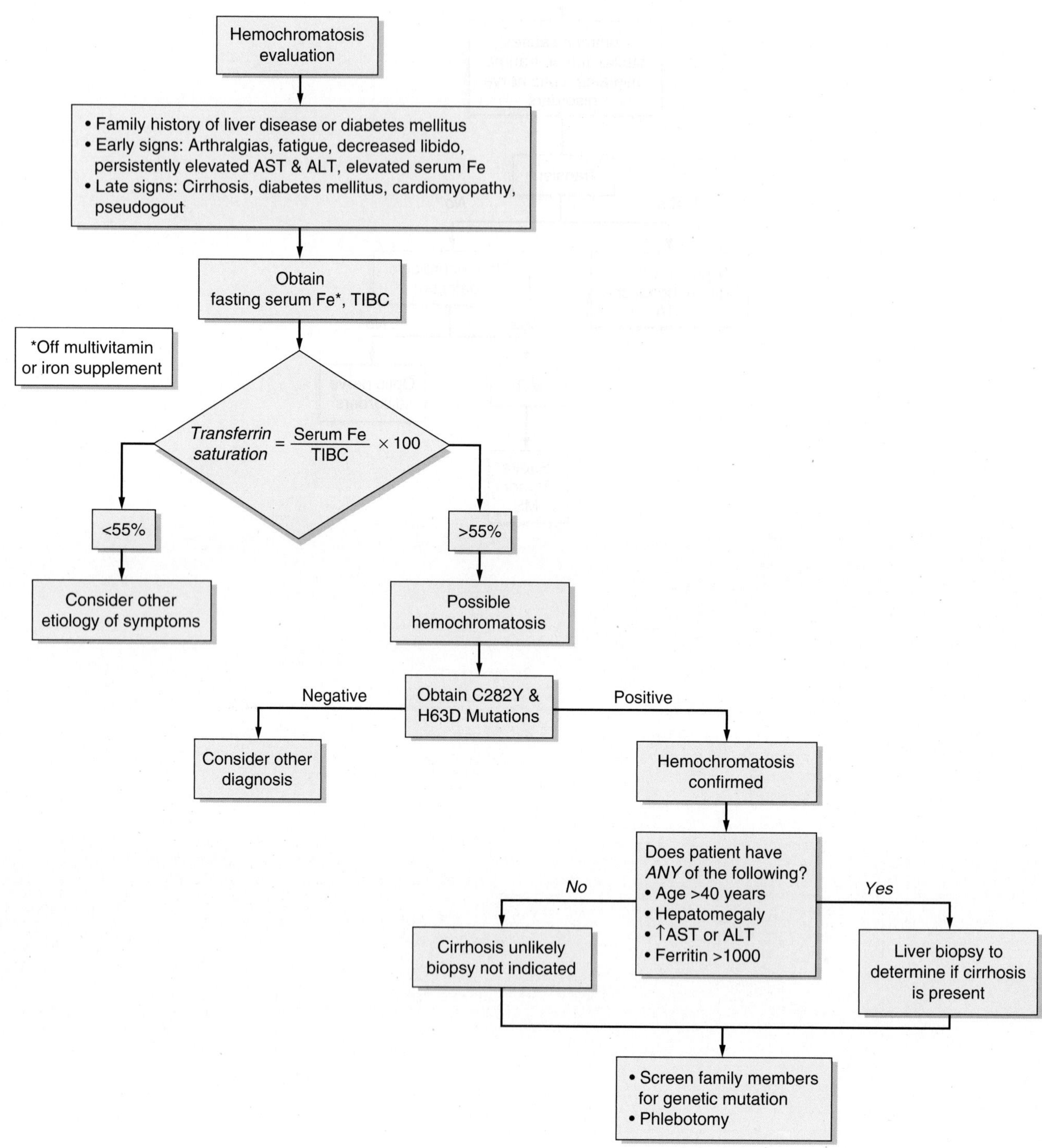

Kristin Burke, MD and Sanjiv Chopra, MBBS, MACP

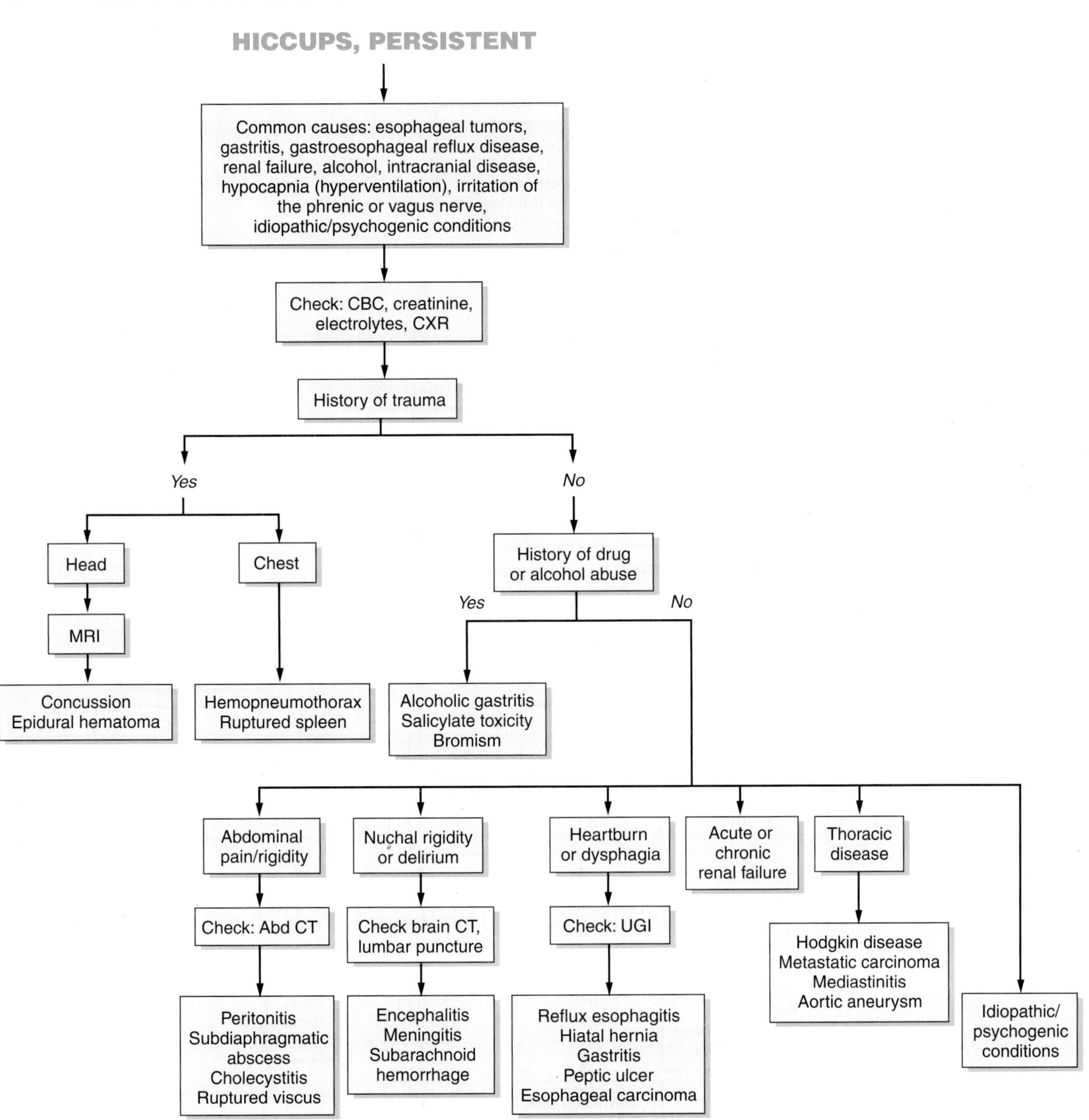

Robert A. Baldor, MD and Alan M. Ehrlich, MD

J Support Oncol. 2009;7(4):122–7, 130.

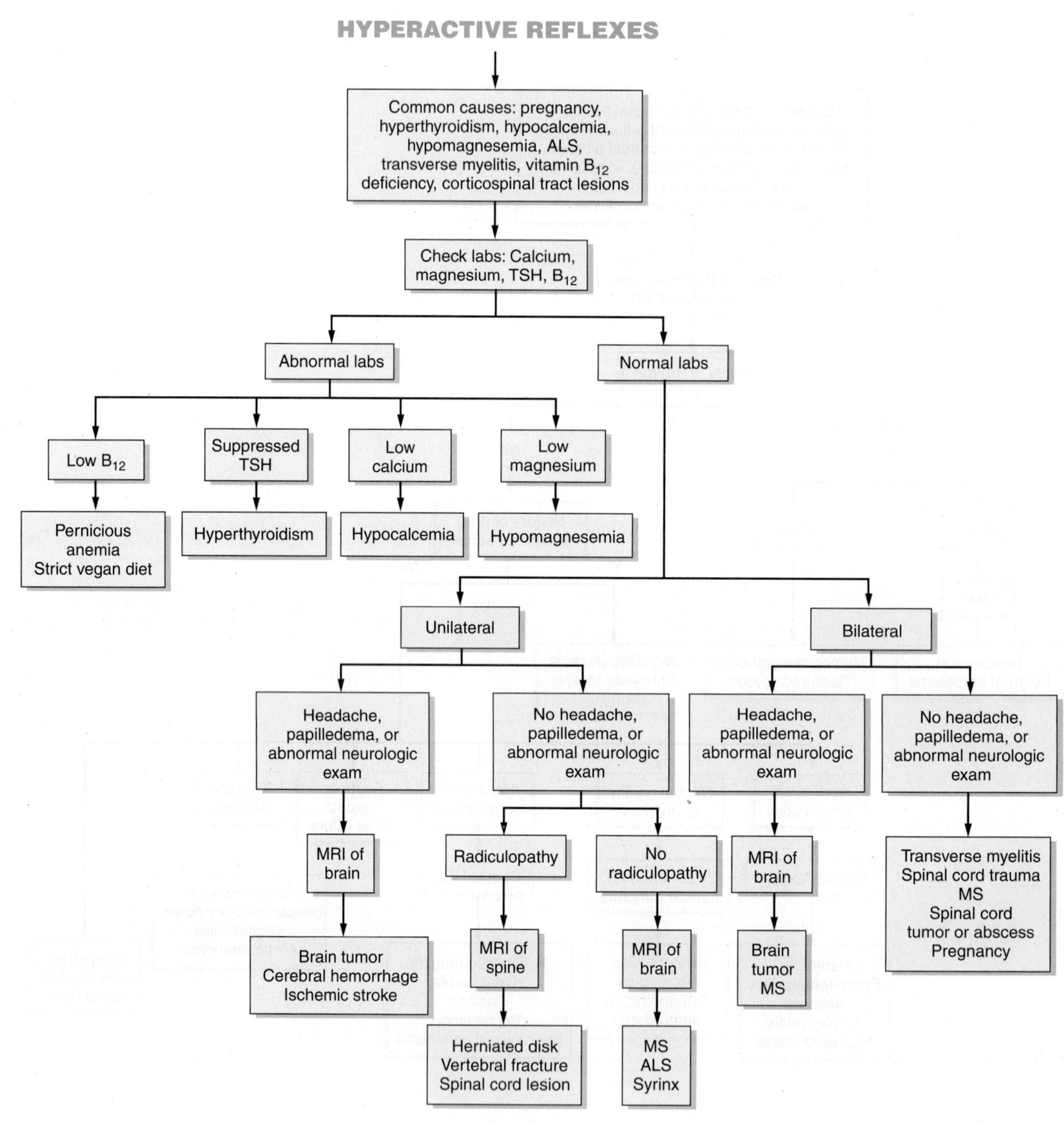

Robert A. Baldor, MD and Alan M. Ehrlich, MD

Dev Med Child Neurol. 2009;51(2):128–35.

HYPERBILIRUBINEMIA

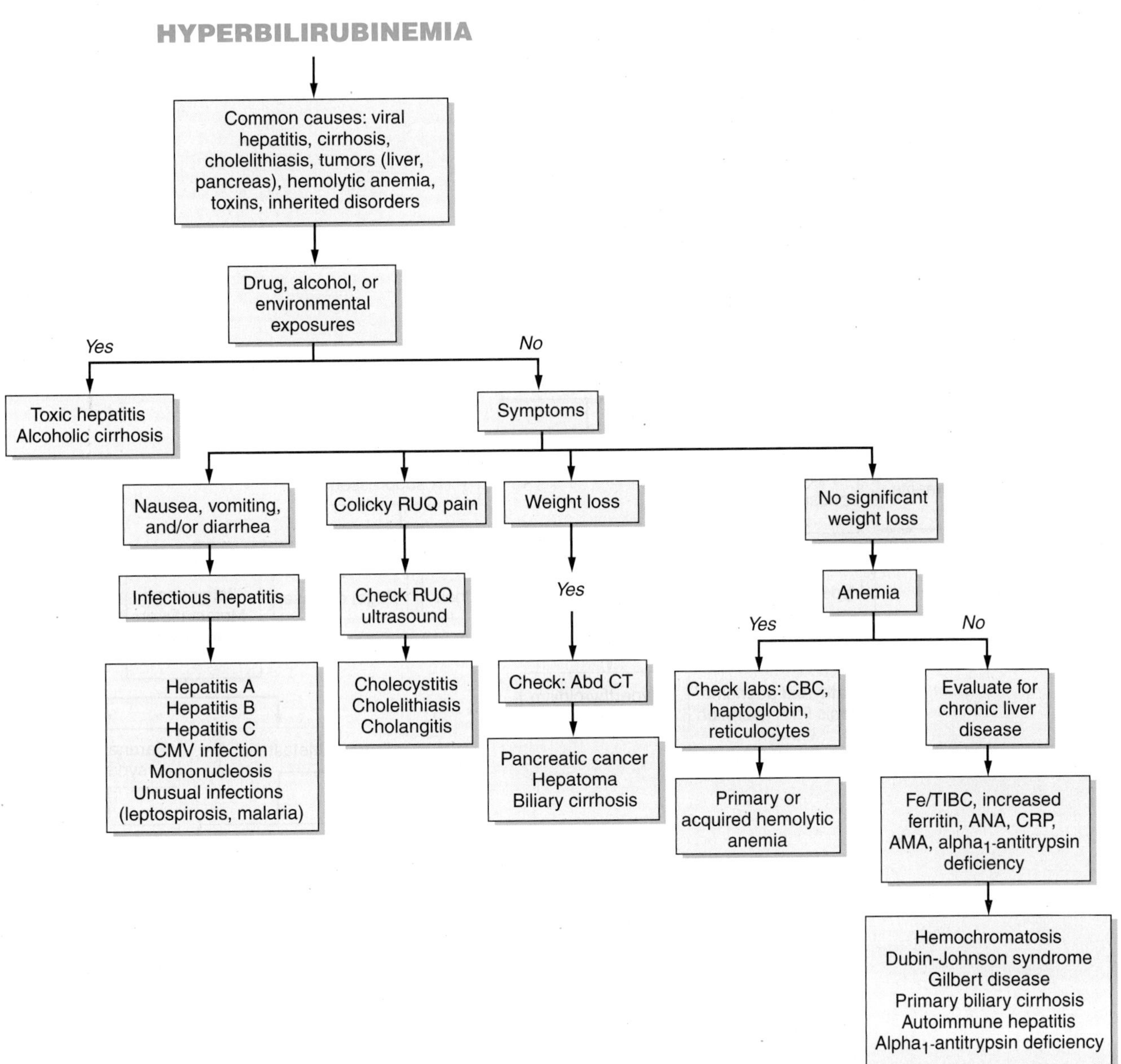

Robert A. Baldor, MD and Alan M. Ehrlich, MD

Am J Surg. 2009;198(2):193–8.

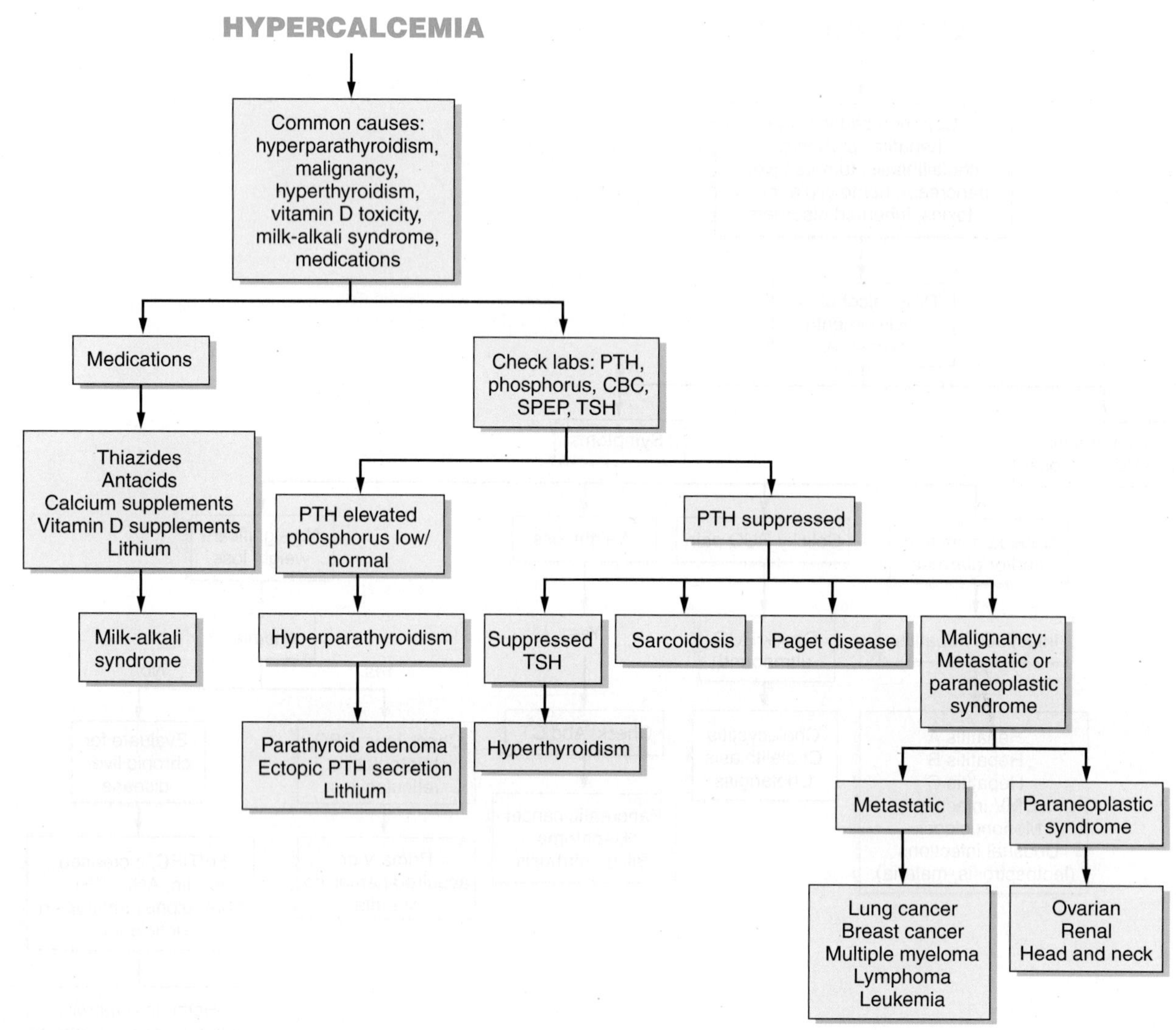

Robert A. Baldor, MD and Alan M. Ehrlich, MD

Iran J Kid. 2009;54(4):19–37.

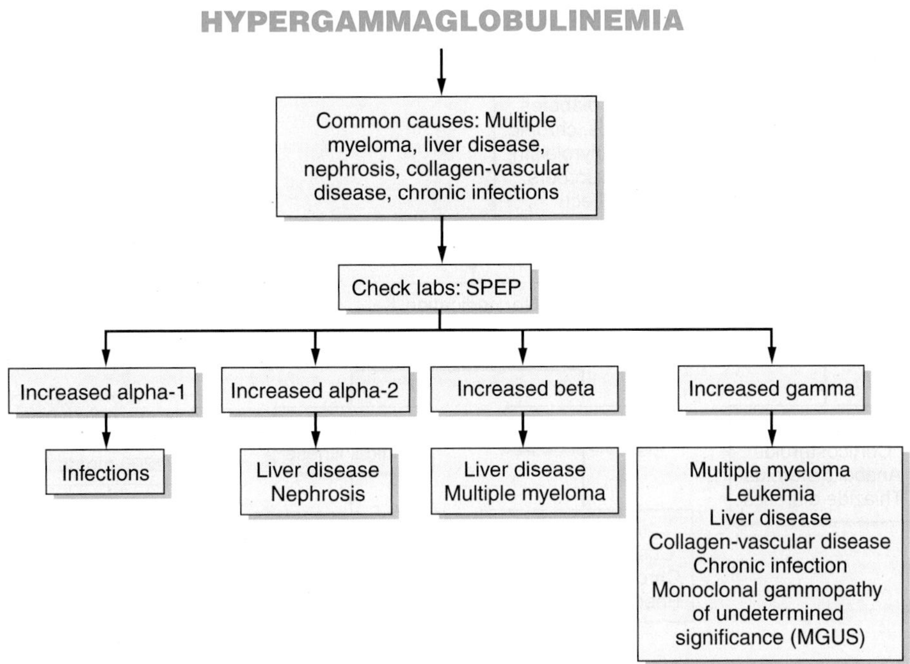

Robert A. Baldor, MD and Alan M. Ehrlich, MD

Medicine (Baltimore). 2009;88(5):284–93.

HYPERGLYCEMIA

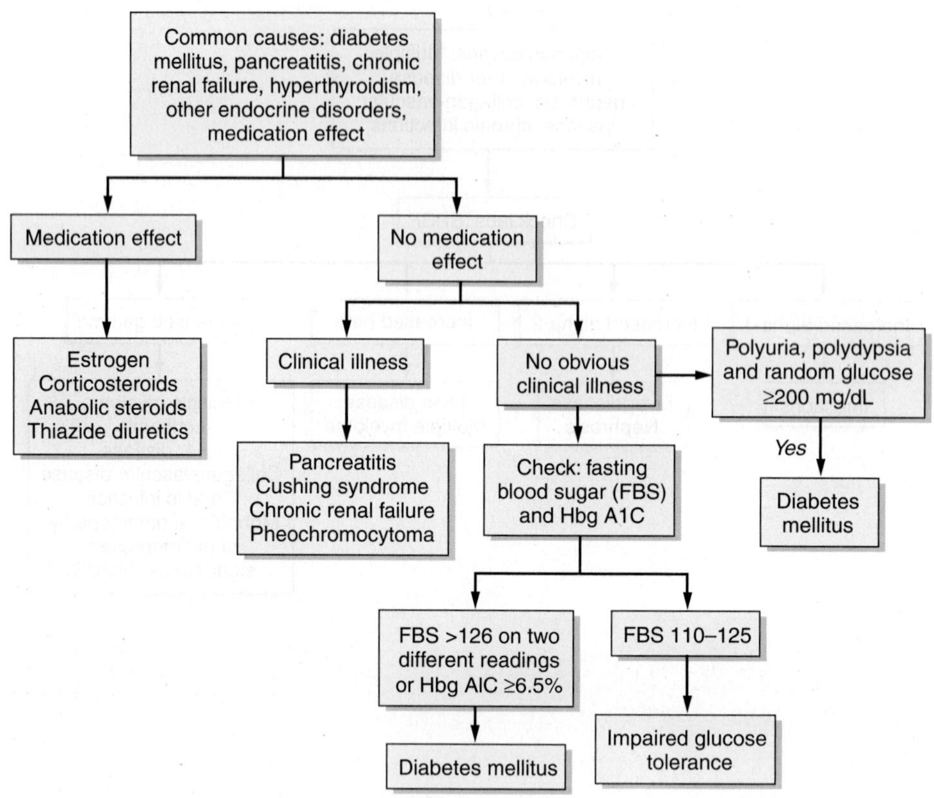

Robert A. Baldor, MD and Alan M. Ehrlich, MD

Crit Care Med. 2009;37(5):1769–76.

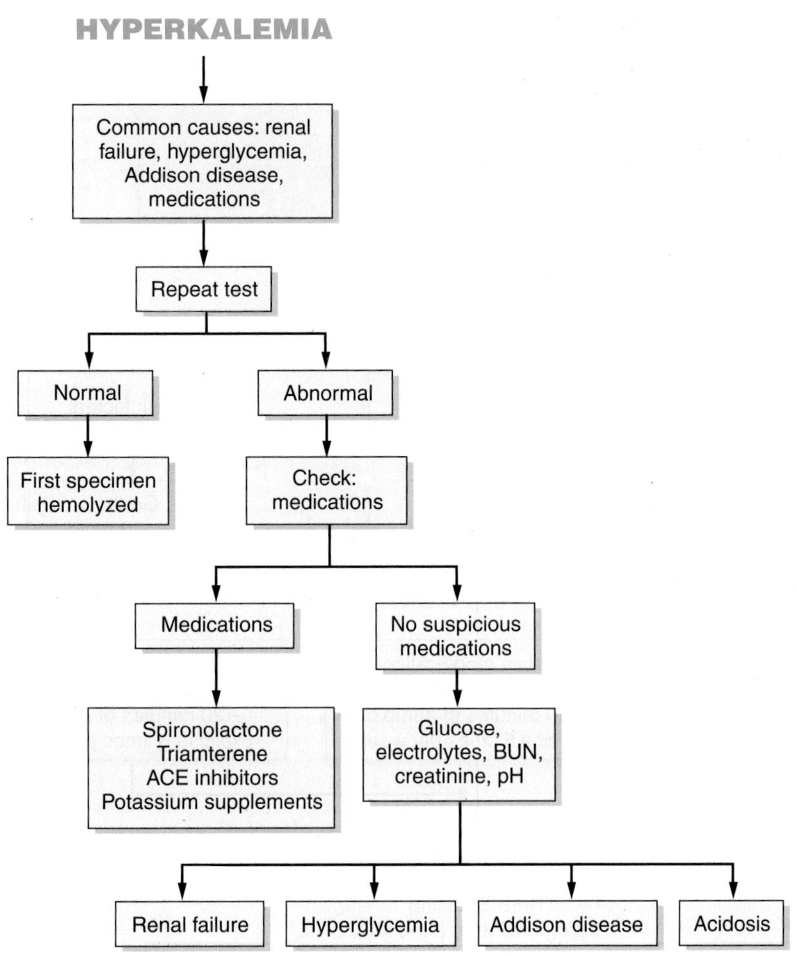

Robert A. Baldor, MD and Alan M. Ehrlich, MD

J Gen Intern Med. 2010;25(4):326–33.

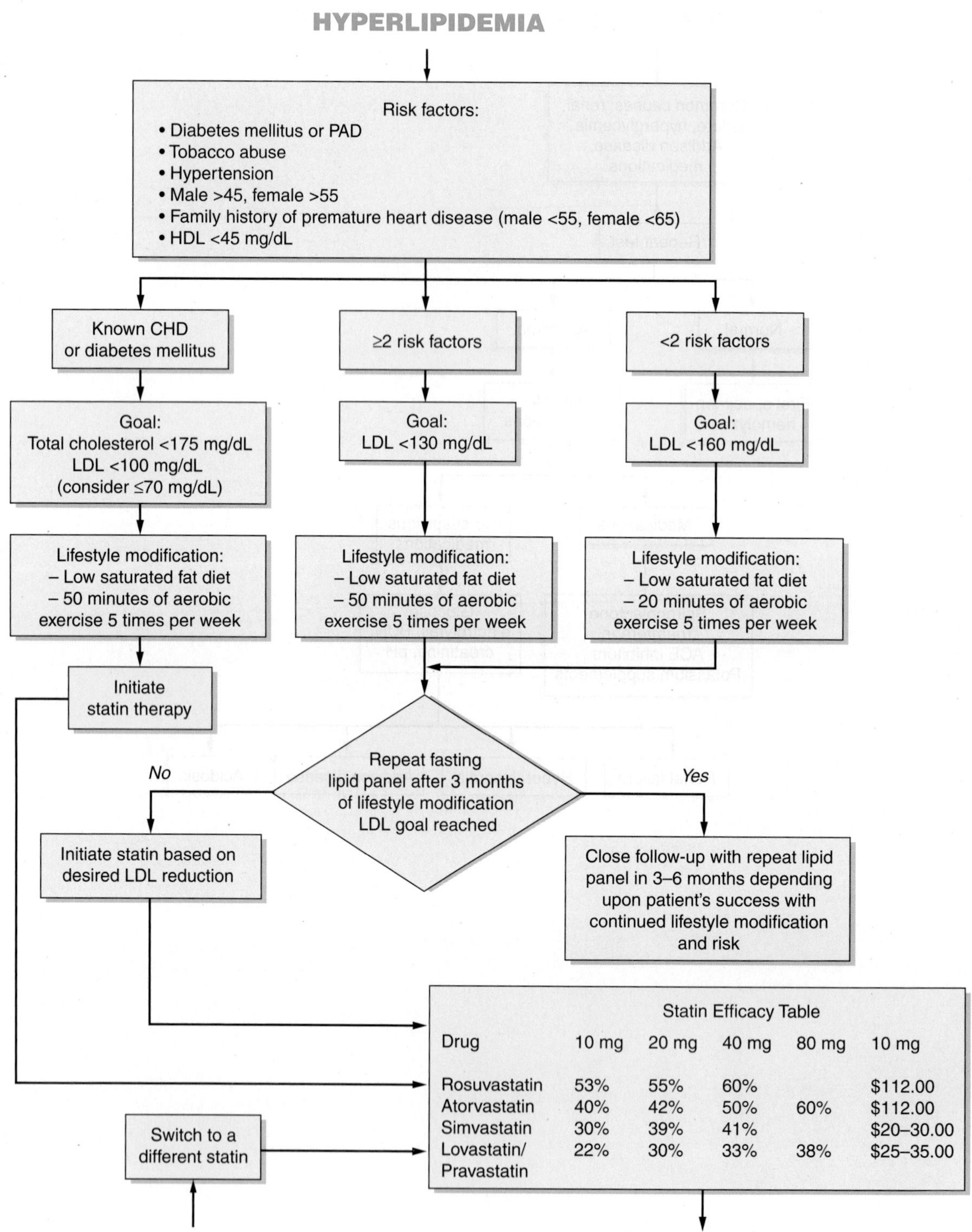
HYPERLIPIDEMIA
Risk factors:
• Diabetes mellitus or PAD
• Tobacco abuse
• Hypertension
• Male >45, female >55
• Family history of premature heart disease (male <55, female <65)
• HDL <45 mg/dL
Known CHD or diabetes mellitus
≥2 risk factors
<2 risk factors
Goal: Total cholesterol <175 mg/dL LDL <100 mg/dL (consider ≤70 mg/dL)
Goal: LDL <130 mg/dL
Goal: LDL <160 mg/dL
Lifestyle modification: – Low saturated fat diet – 50 minutes of aerobic exercise 5 times per week
Lifestyle modification: – Low saturated fat diet – 50 minutes of aerobic exercise 5 times per week
Lifestyle modification: – Low saturated fat diet – 20 minutes of aerobic exercise 5 times per week
Initiate statin therapy
Repeat fasting lipid panel after 3 months of lifestyle modification LDL goal reached
No
Yes
Initiate statin based on desired LDL reduction
Close follow-up with repeat lipid panel in 3–6 months depending upon patient's success with continued lifestyle modification and risk
Switch to a different statin

Statin Efficacy Table

Drug	10 mg	20 mg	40 mg	80 mg	10 mg
Rosuvastatin	53%	55%	60%		$112.00
Atorvastatin	40%	42%	50%	60%	$112.00
Simvastatin	30%	39%	41%		$20–30.00
Lovastatin/ Pravastatin	22%	30%	33%	38%	$25–35.00

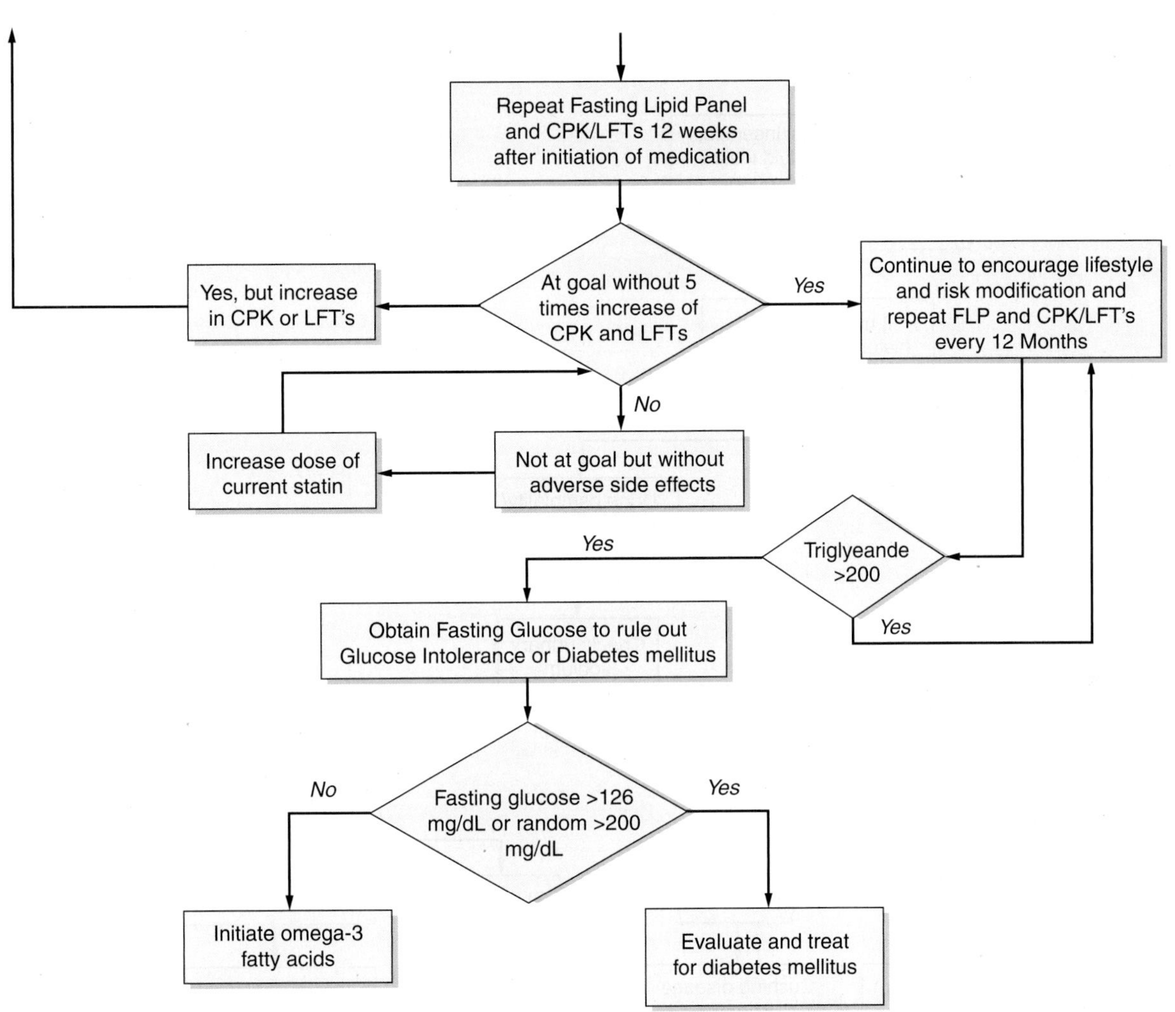

Rade N. Pejic, MD

Adv Ther. 2010;27(6):348–64.

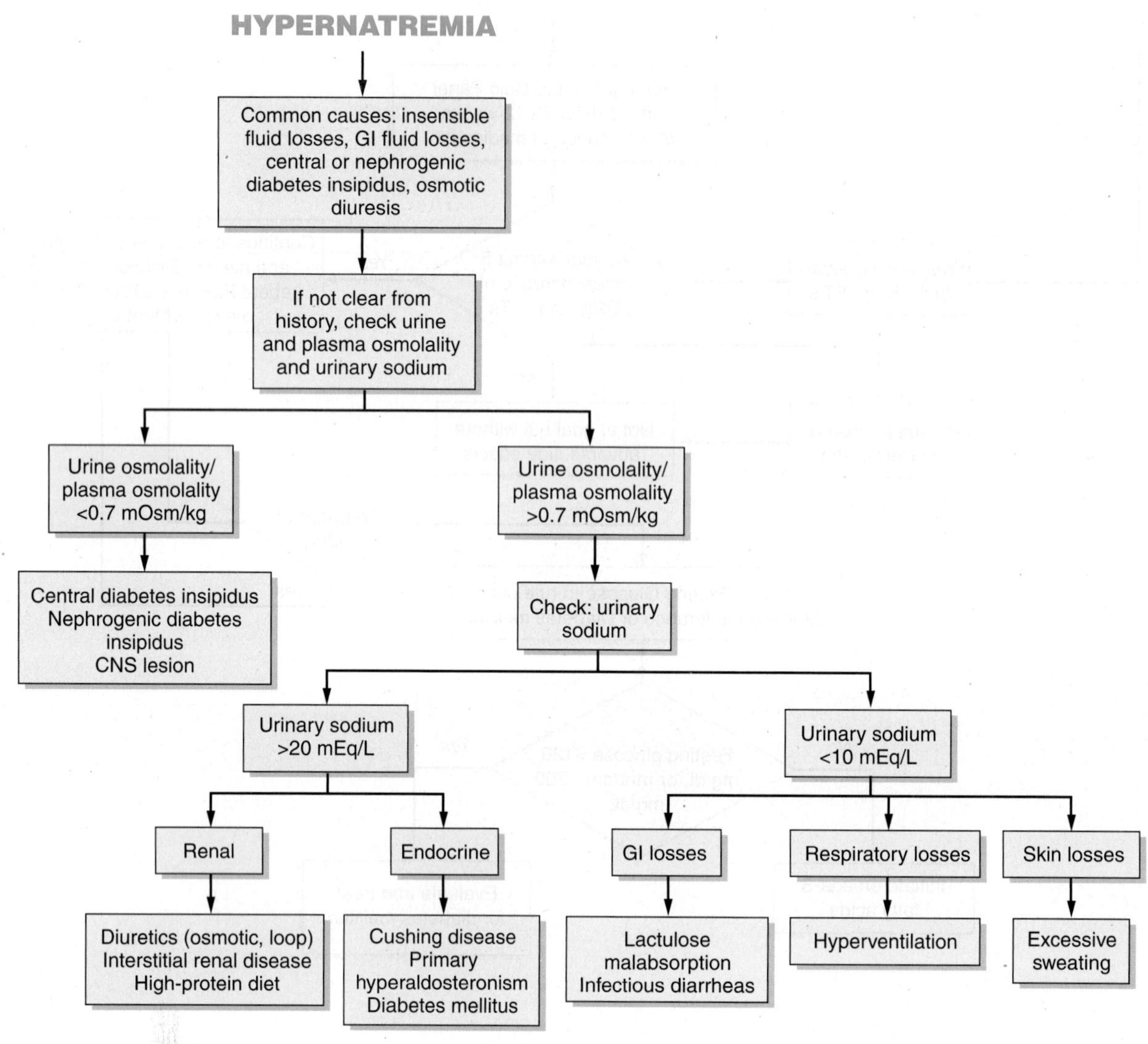

Robert A. Baldor, MD and Alan M. Ehrlich, MD

N Engl J Med. 2000;342(20):1493–9.

HYPERTENSION AND ELEVATED BLOOD PRESSURE, TREATMENT

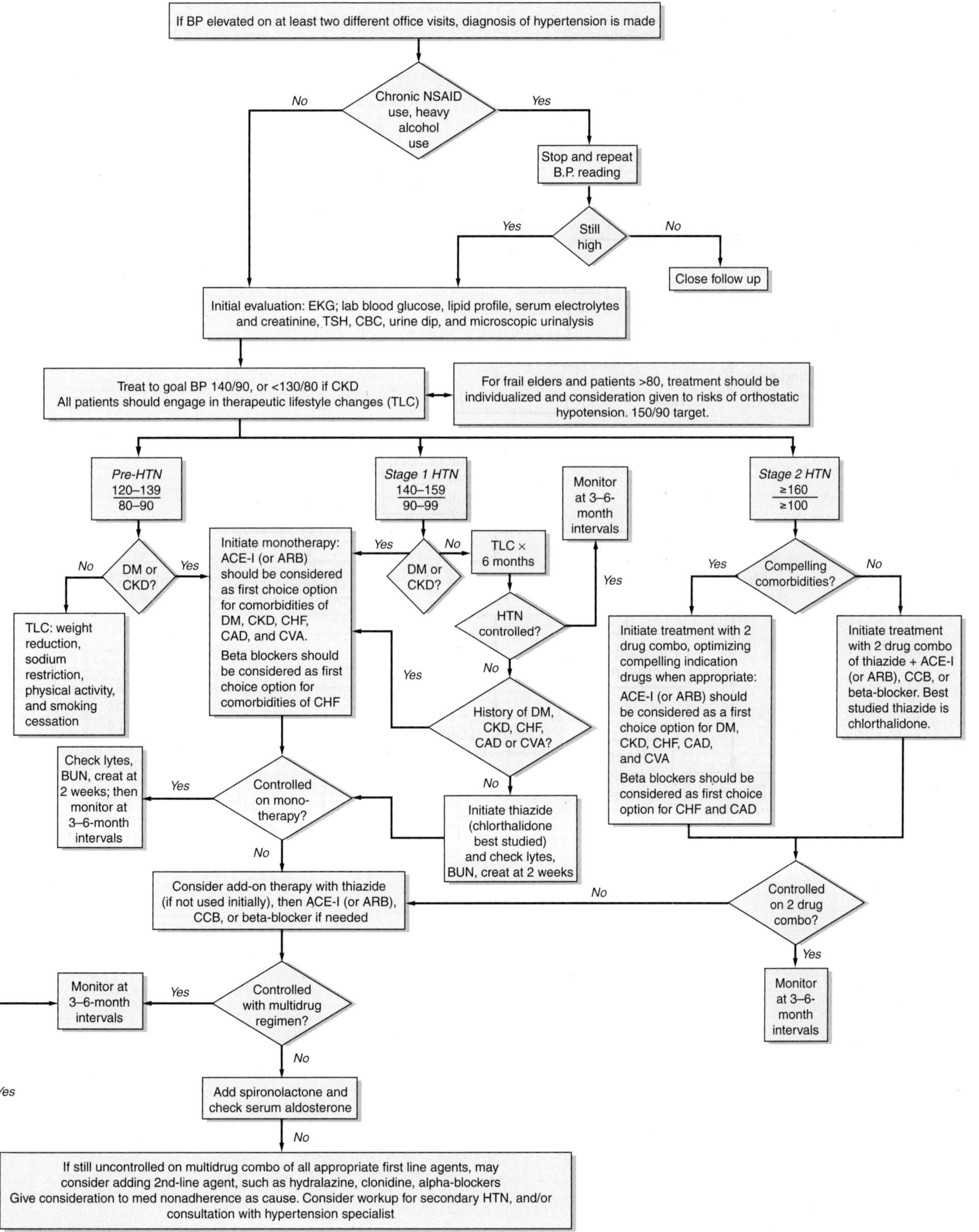

B. Brent Simmons, MD

Hypertension. 2003;42:1206.

HYPERTRIGLYCERIDEMIA

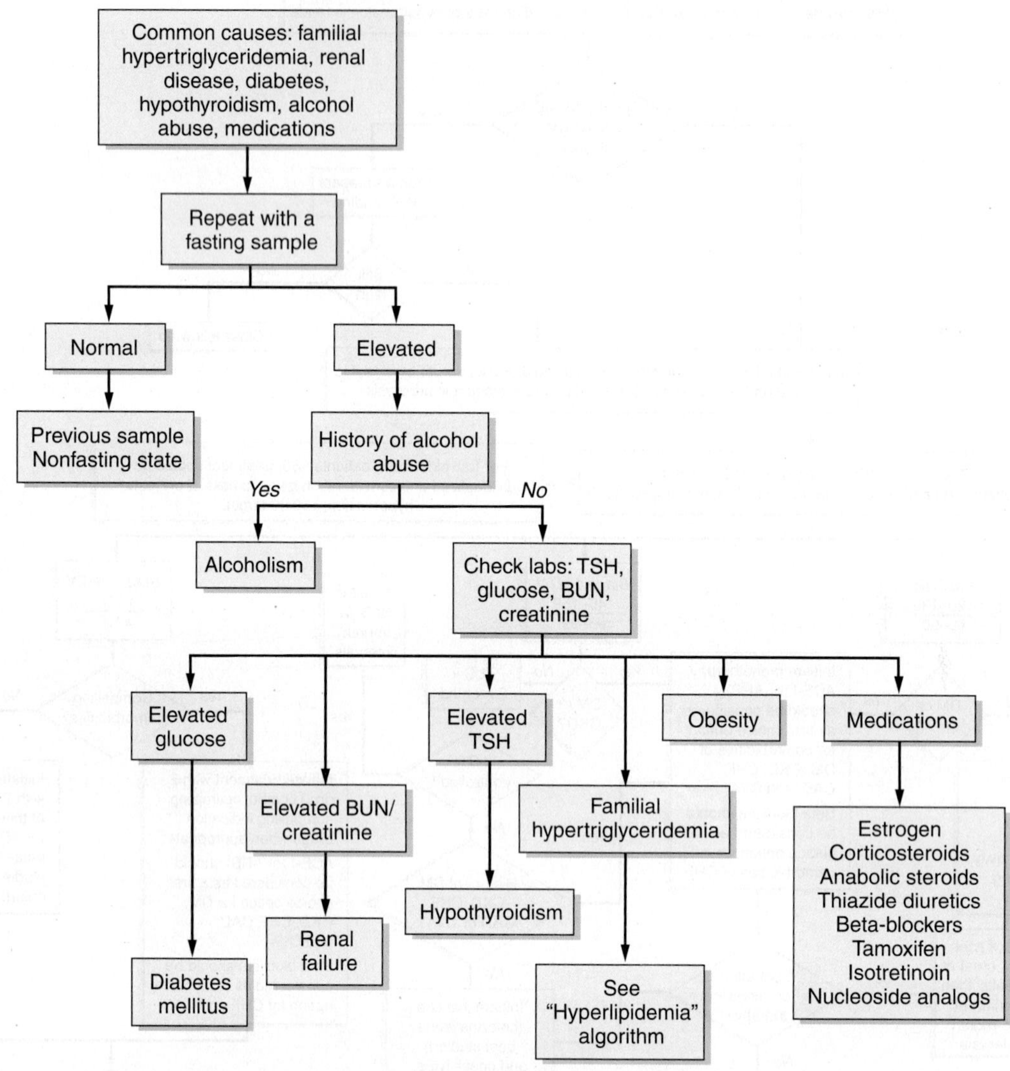

Robert A. Baldor, MD and Alan M. Ehrlich, MD

Am J Cardiol. 2001;87:1174.

HYPOACTIVE REFLEXES

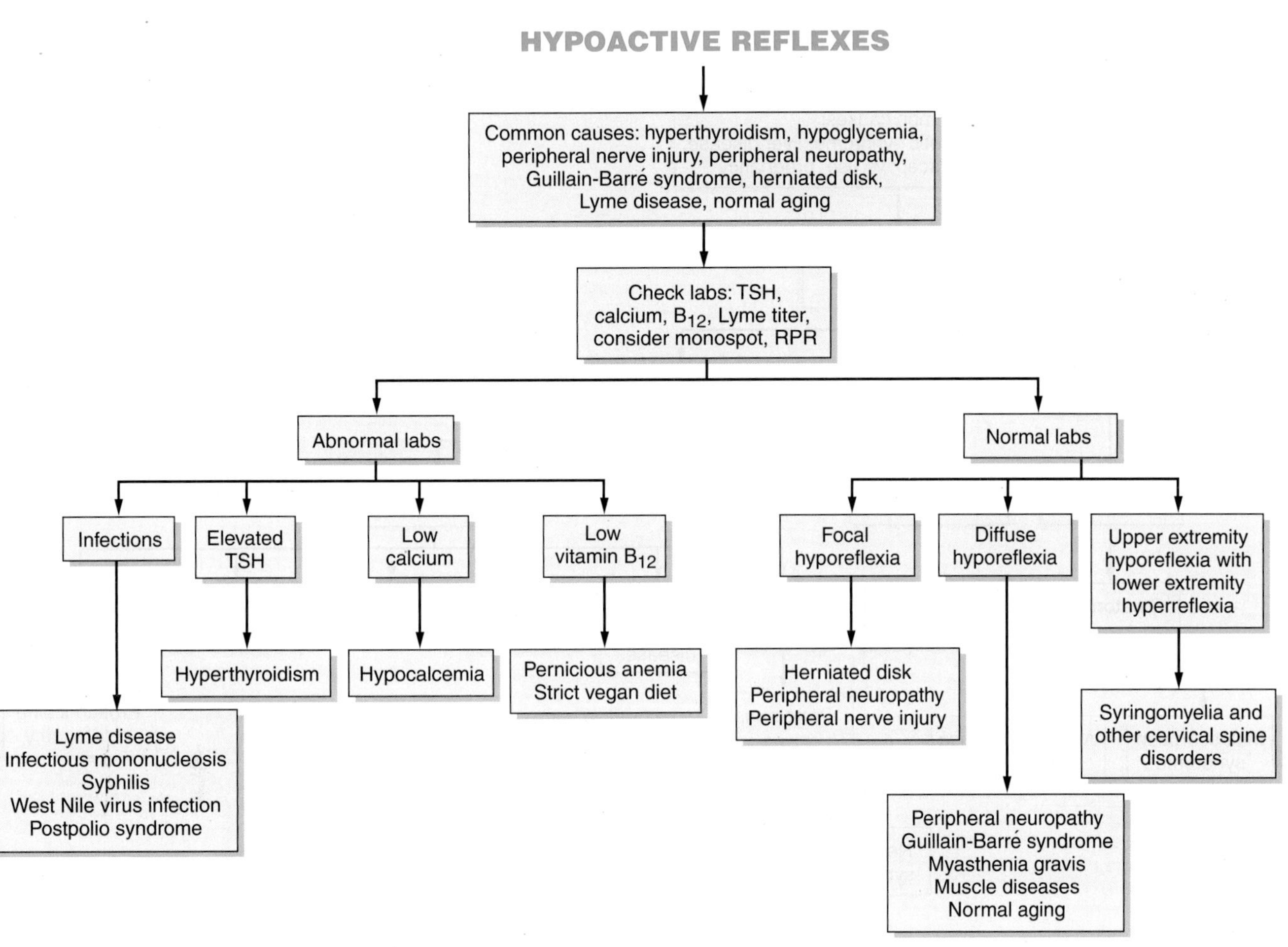

Robert A. Baldor, MD and Alan M. Ehrlich, MD

Med Clin North Am. 2009;93(2):317–42, vii–viii.

HYPOALBUMINEMIA

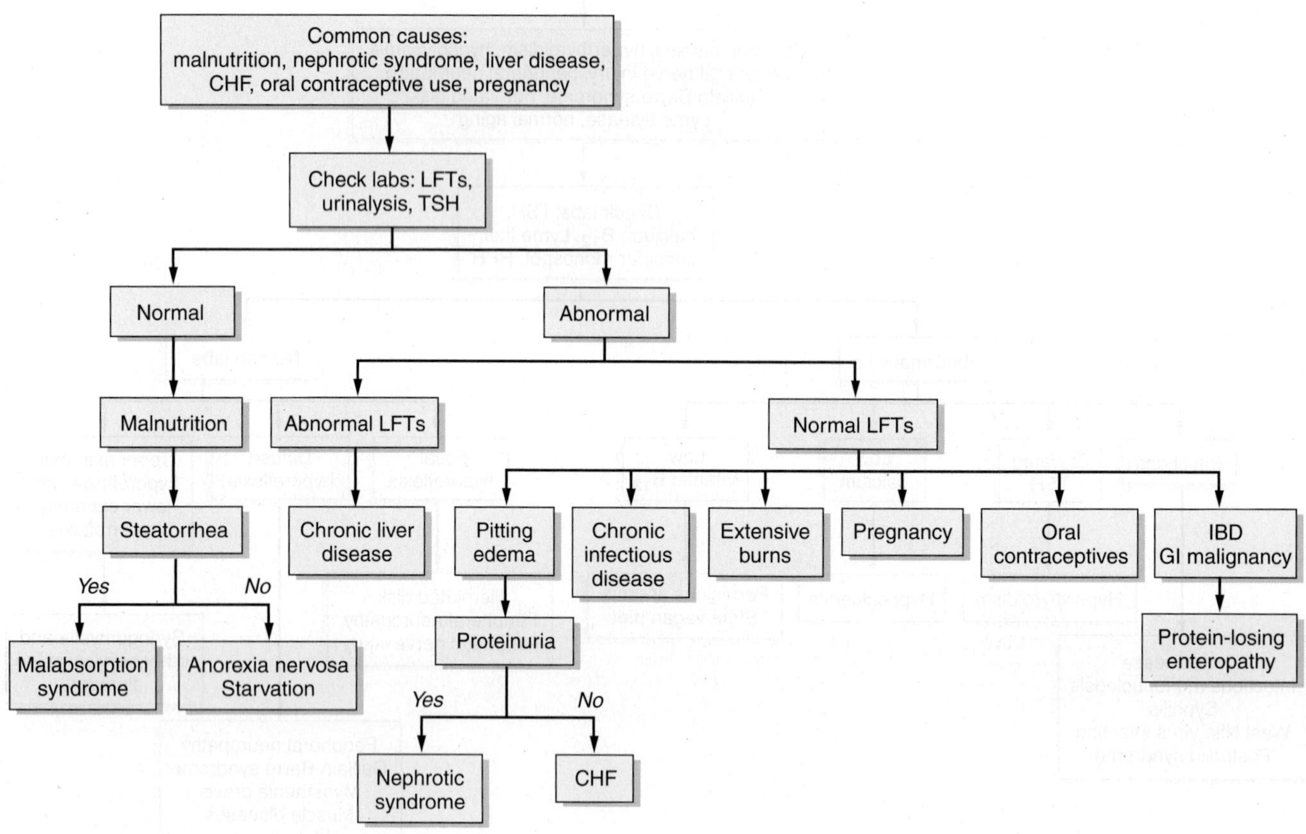

Robert A. Baldor, MD and Alan M. Ehrlich, MD

Am Fam Physician. 2009;80(10):1129–34.

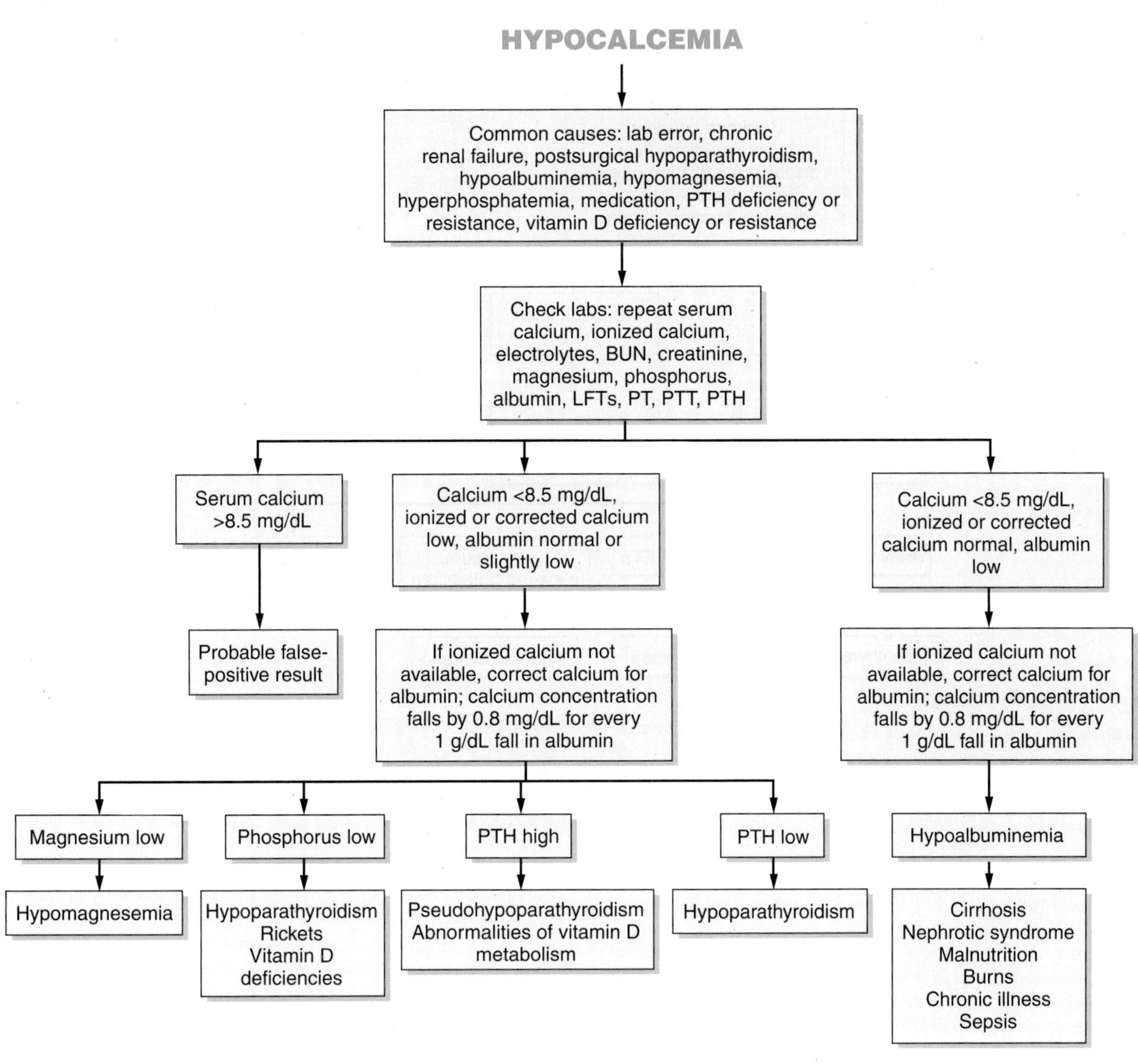

Robert A. Baldor, MD and Alan M. Ehrlich, MD

J Fam Pract. 2008;57(10):677–9.

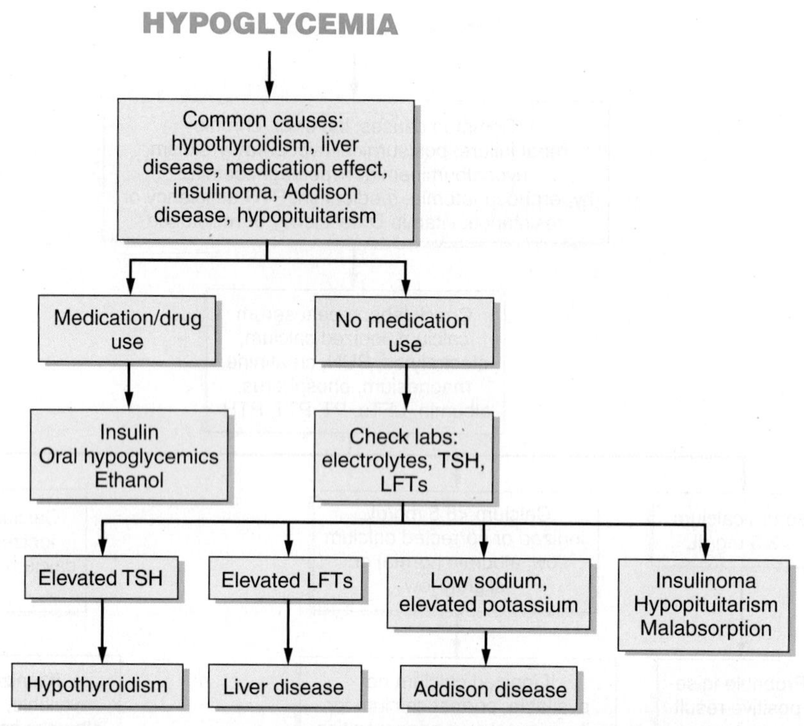

Robert A. Baldor, MD and Alan M. Ehrlich, MD

J Clin Endocrinol Metab. 2009;94(3):741–5.

HYPOKALEMIA

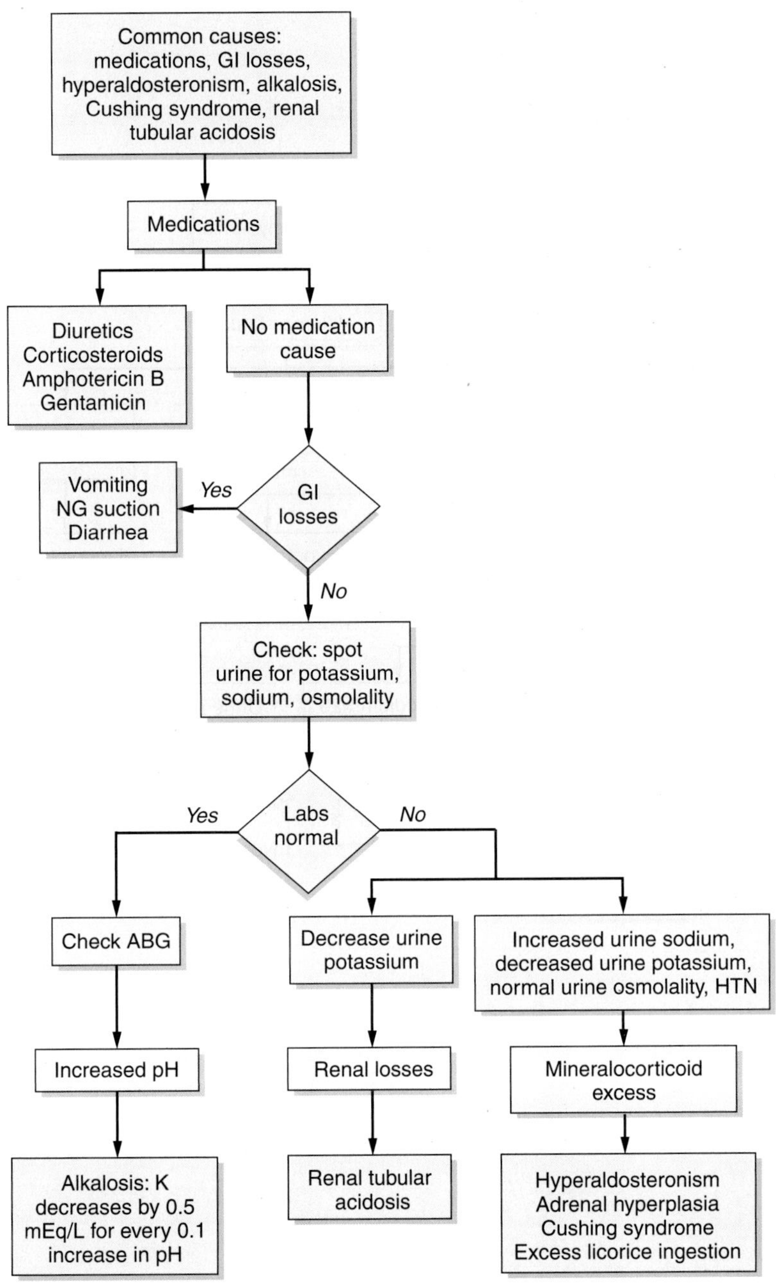

Robert A. Baldor, MD and Alan M. Ehrlich, MD

Ann Intern Med. 2009;150(9):619–25.

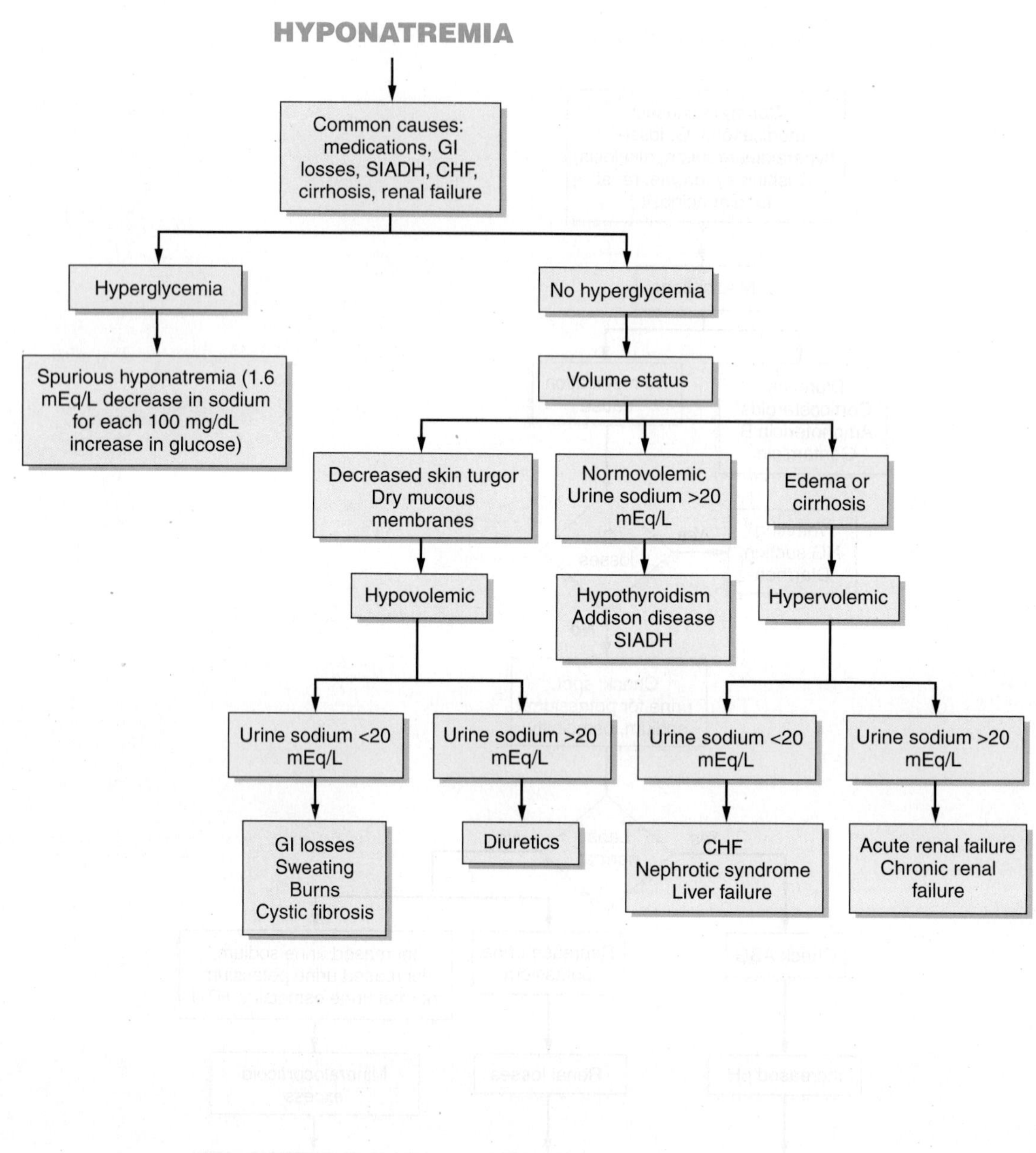

Robert A. Baldor, MD and Alan M. Ehrlich, MD

Am J Med. 2007;120(8):653–8.

HYPOTENSION

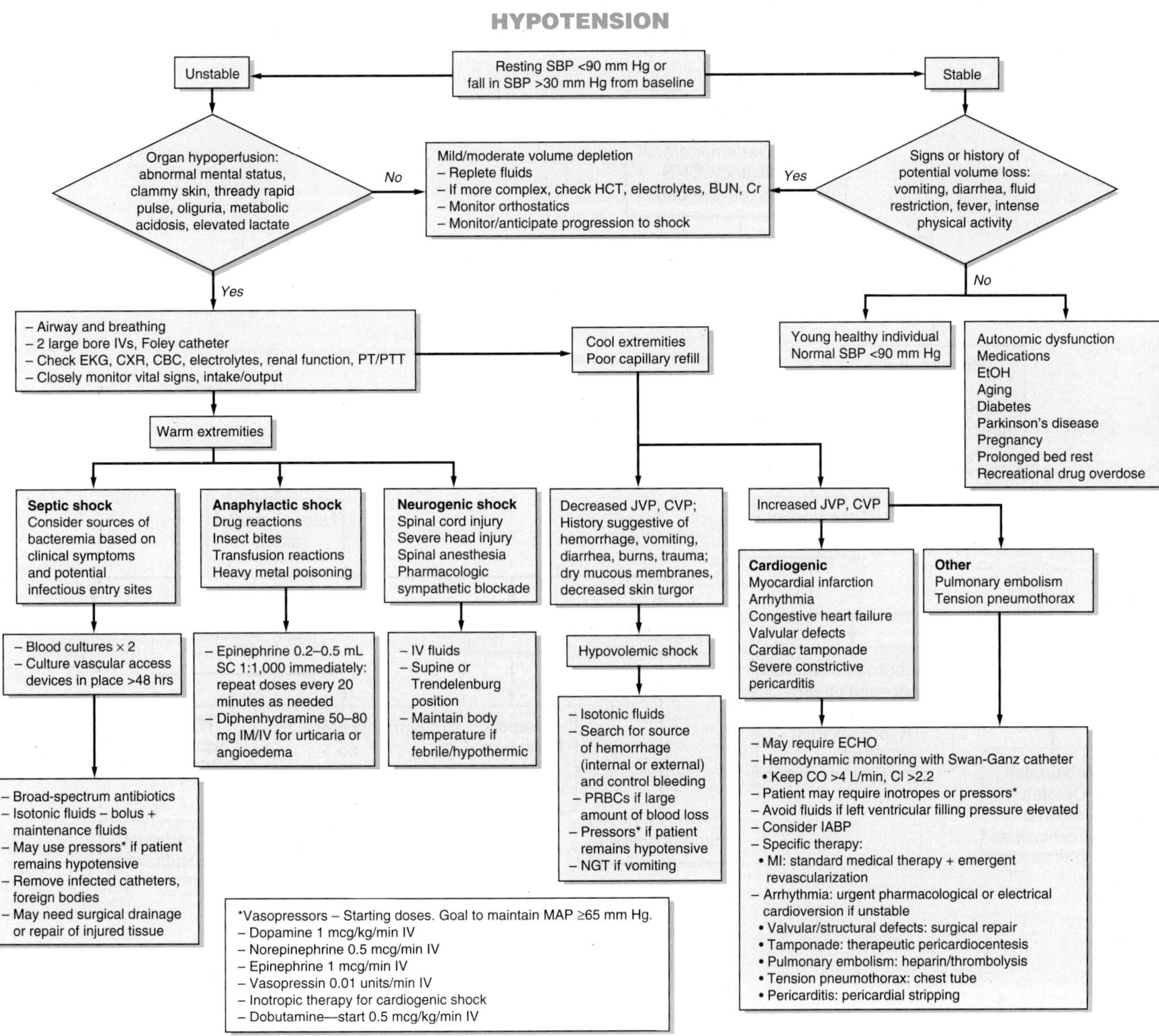

Kristin Burke, MD and Ira S. Ockene, MD

Arch Phys Med Rehabil. 2009;90(5):876–85.

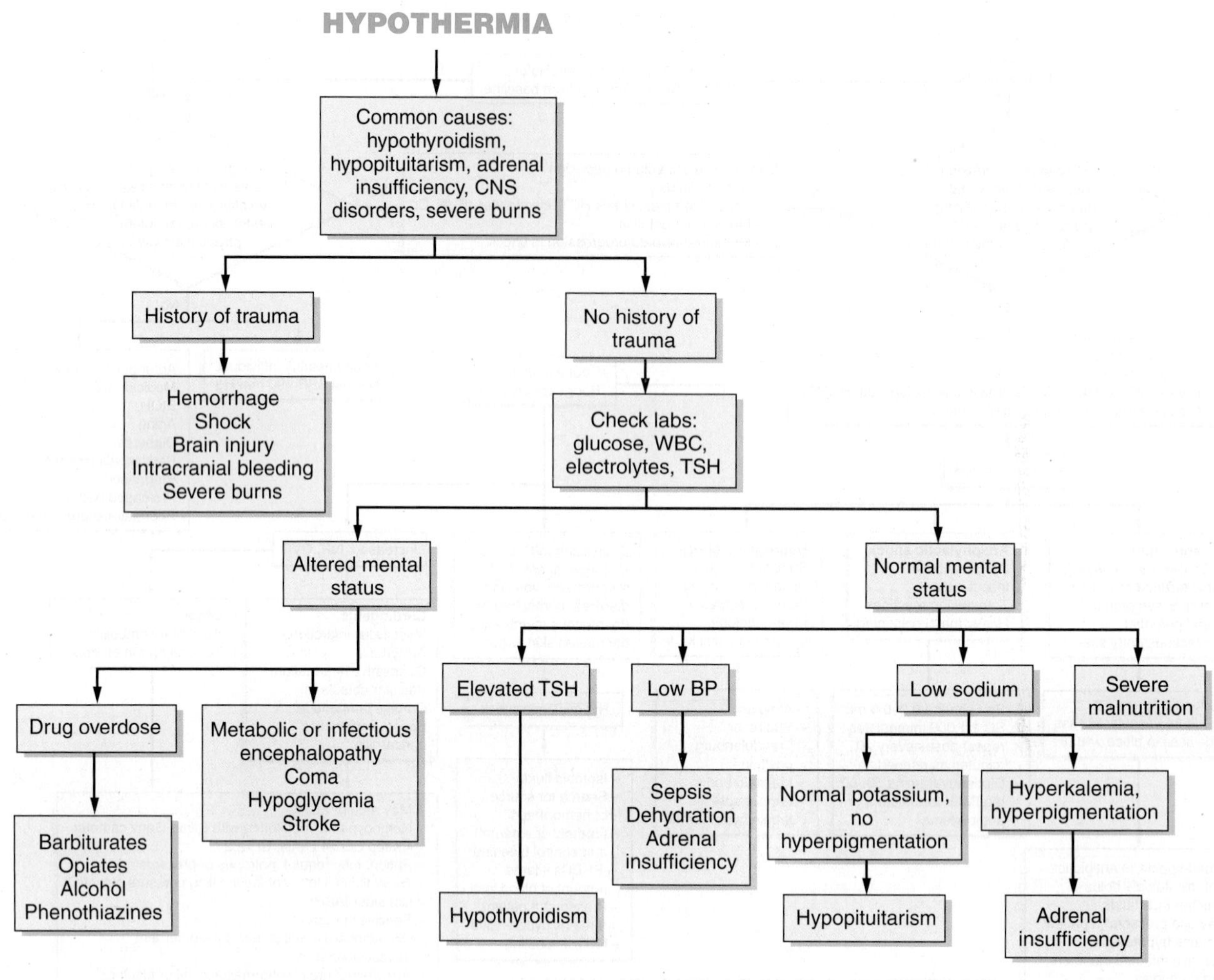
HYPOTHERMIA
Common causes: hypothyroidism, hypopituitarism, adrenal insufficiency, CNS disorders, severe burns
History of trauma
No history of trauma
Hemorrhage
Shock
Brain injury
Intracranial bleeding
Severe burns
Check labs: glucose, WBC, electrolytes, TSH
Altered mental status
Normal mental status
Drug overdose
Metabolic or infectious encephalopathy
Coma
Hypoglycemia
Stroke
Barbiturates
Opiates
Alcohol
Phenothiazines
Elevated TSH
Low BP
Low sodium
Severe malnutrition
Hypothyroidism
Sepsis
Dehydration
Adrenal insufficiency
Normal potassium, no hyperpigmentation
Hyperkalemia, hyperpigmentation
Hypopituitarism
Adrenal insufficiency

Robert A. Baldor, MD and Alan M. Ehrlich, MD

Am J Med. 2006;119(4):297–301.

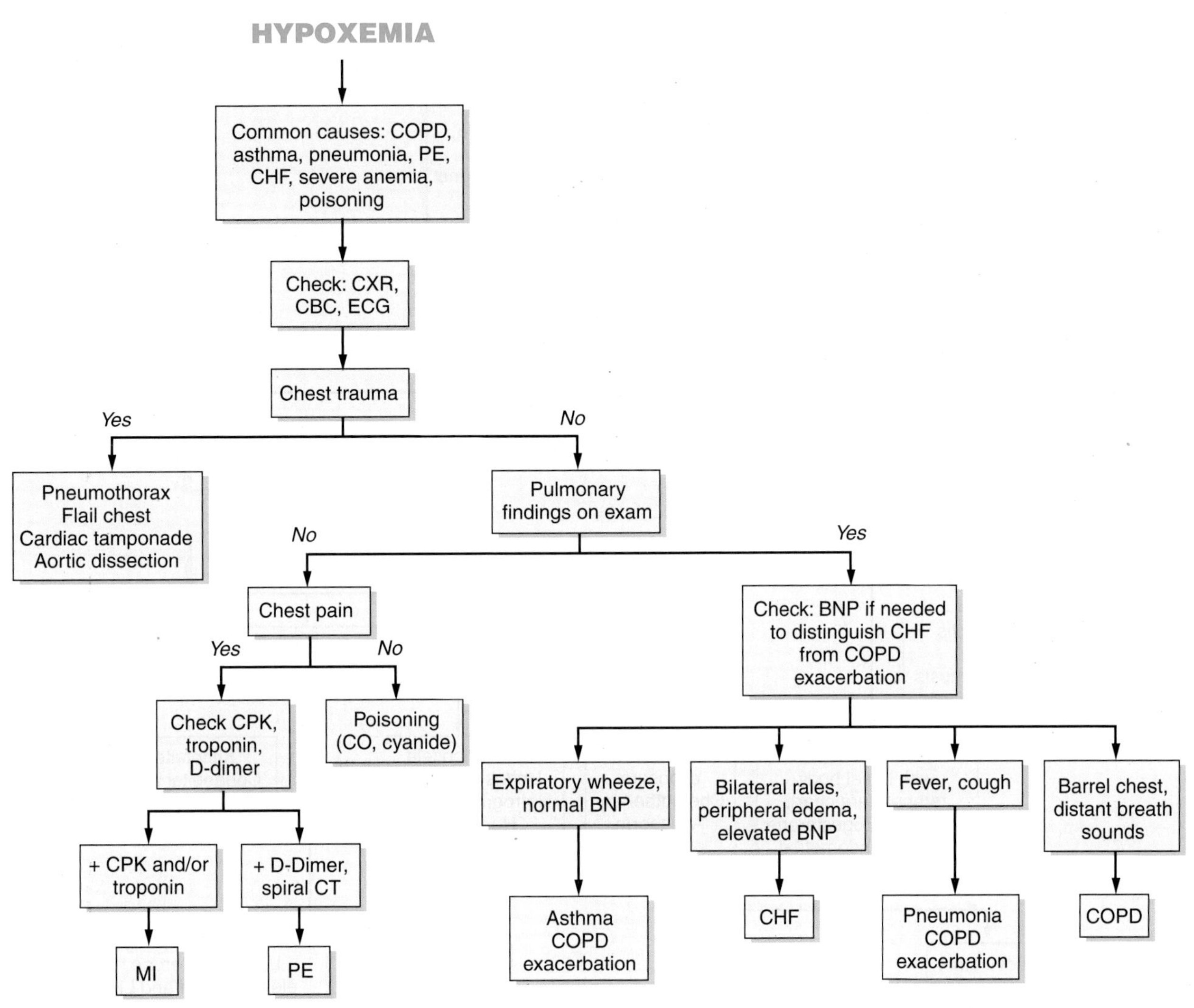

Robert A. Baldor, MD and Alan M. Ehrlich, MD

Lancet. 2009;374(9691):721–32.

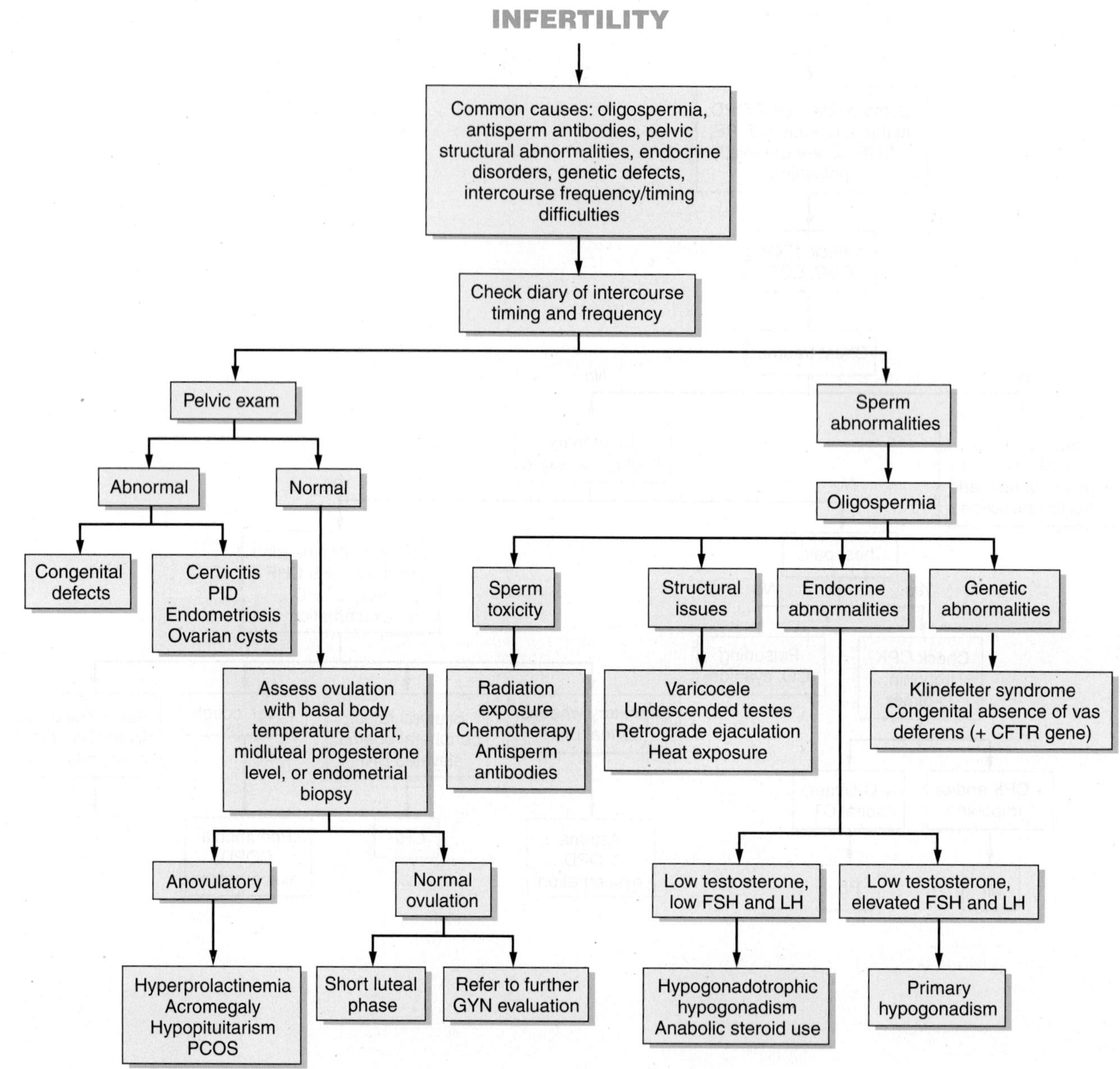

Robert A. Baldor, MD and Alan M. Ehrlich, MD

Med Clin North Am. 2008;92(5):1163–92, xi.

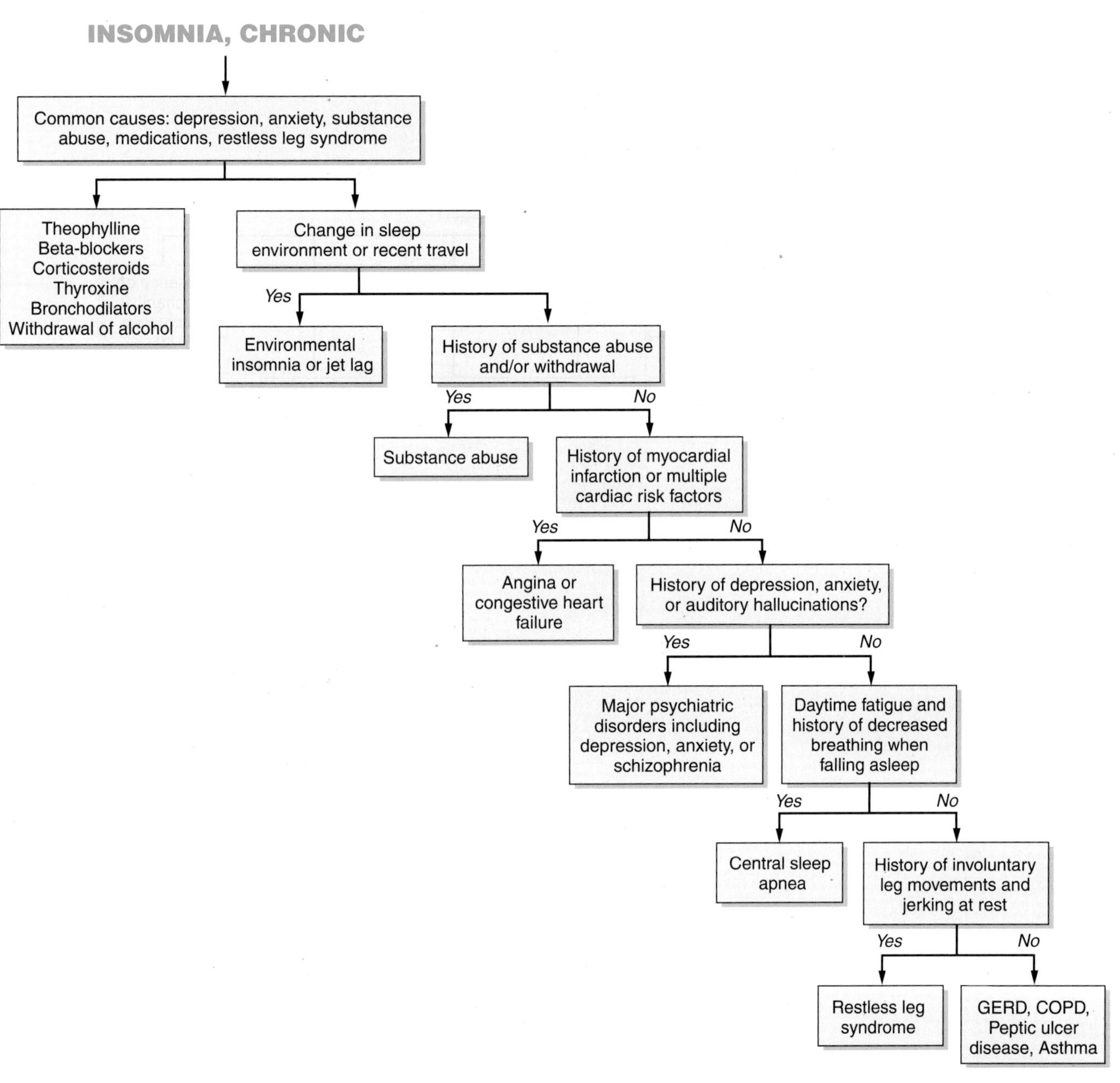

Robert A. Baldor, MD and Alan M. Ehrlich, MD

Am Fam Physician. 2007;76(4):517–26.

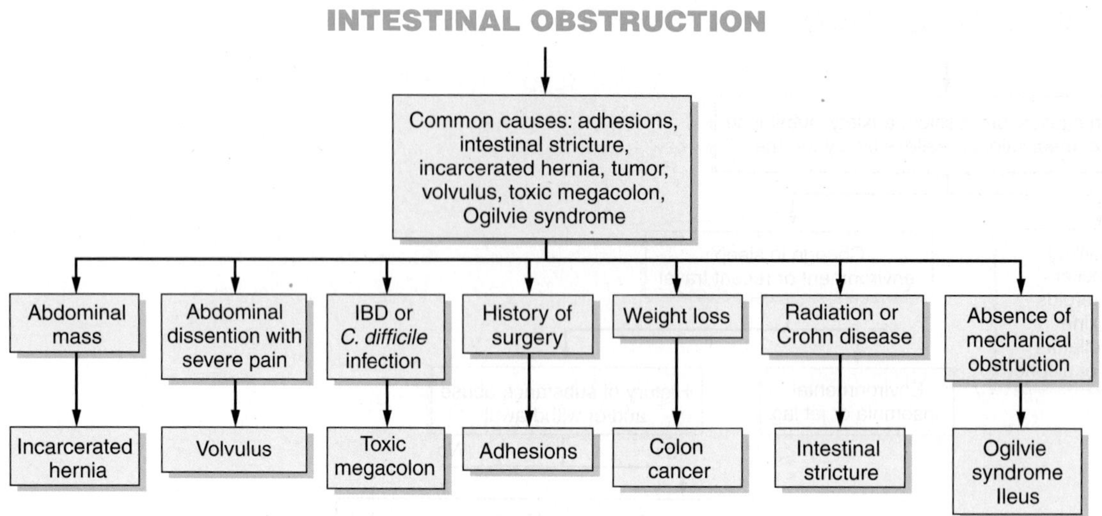

Robert A. Baldor, MD and Alan M. Ehrlich, MD

Med Clin North Am. 2008;92(3):575–97, viii.

JAUNDICE

Jaundice: A yellow discoloration of skin, sclera and mucous membranes by bilirubin, a bile pigment formed by the breakdown of heme rings; detected when the serum bilirubin level >3 mg/dL. Bilirubin results from the breakdown of hemoglobin in spleen. Heme is converted to unconjugated bilirubin, bound to albumin and then sent to the liver where it is then conjugated.

Common causes: Gilbert's syndrome, hemolysis, hepatitis, and choledocholithiasis

CBC with diff, LFTs: ALT, AST, serum alkaline phosphatase (AP), total bilirubin (TB) and direct bilirubin (DB), haptoglobin, hepatitis serologies, amylase, lipase, hCG, urinalysis with urine bilirubin. Ultrasound or CT

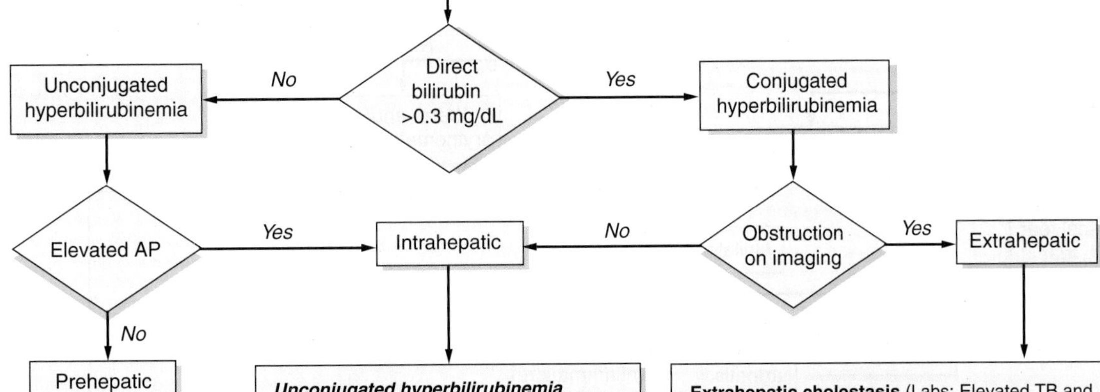

Prehepatic

- **Hemolytic anemia**
- **Reabsorption of large hematoma**

Labs: Anemia, possible reticulocytosis, mild TB elevation (5 mg/dL), increased indirect bilirubin, normal DB levels and negative urine bilirubin. All other LTs are normal.

Unconjugated hyperbilirubinemia

Enzyme defects:

- **Gilbert's syndrome:** Mild defect in UDP glucuronosyltransferase (UGT, responsible for conjugation of bilirubin)
- **Crigler-Najjar syndromes:** More severe defect in UGT, usually presents during infancy
- ***Conjugated hyperbilirubinemia***
- **Dublin-Johnson syndrome:** Defective secretion of conjugated bilirubin
- **Rotor's syndrome**

Both Conjugated & Unconjugated Hepatocellular injury:

- **Hepatitis:** Viral, alcohol, or autoimmune insult leading to inflammation which impedes or prevents transport/secretion of conjugated bilirubin
- **Medication/drug:** Acetaminophen
- **Cirrhosis**
- **Congestive heart failure:** Hypoxia/anoxia of hepatocytes leads to cellular injury.

- **Intrahepatic cholestasis:** Elevated LTs, primarily AP. US shows normal sized bile duct(s).

- **Medication/drug induced**
- **Total parenteral nutrition (TPN)**
- **Sepsis**
- **Sarcoidosis**
- **Pregnancy**

Extrahepatic cholestasis (Labs: Elevated TB and DB, elevated AP and positive urine bilirubin. US shows dilated bile duct(s).

- Choledocholithiasis
- Chronic pancreatitis alcohol
- **Cholangitis:** Fever, pain and jaundice, altered mental status, sepsis
- **Biliary structure:** History of surgical/invasive procedure
- Primary biliary cirrhosis
- Primary sclerosing cholangitis
- **Biliary tract tumor/cholangiocarcinoma:** Hepatomegaly, weight loss, abdominal pain
- **Pancreatic tumor:** Painless jaundice, palpable gallbladder (rare)

Krunal Patel, MD and John K. Zawacki, MD

Am Fam Physician. 2004;60(2):200–305.

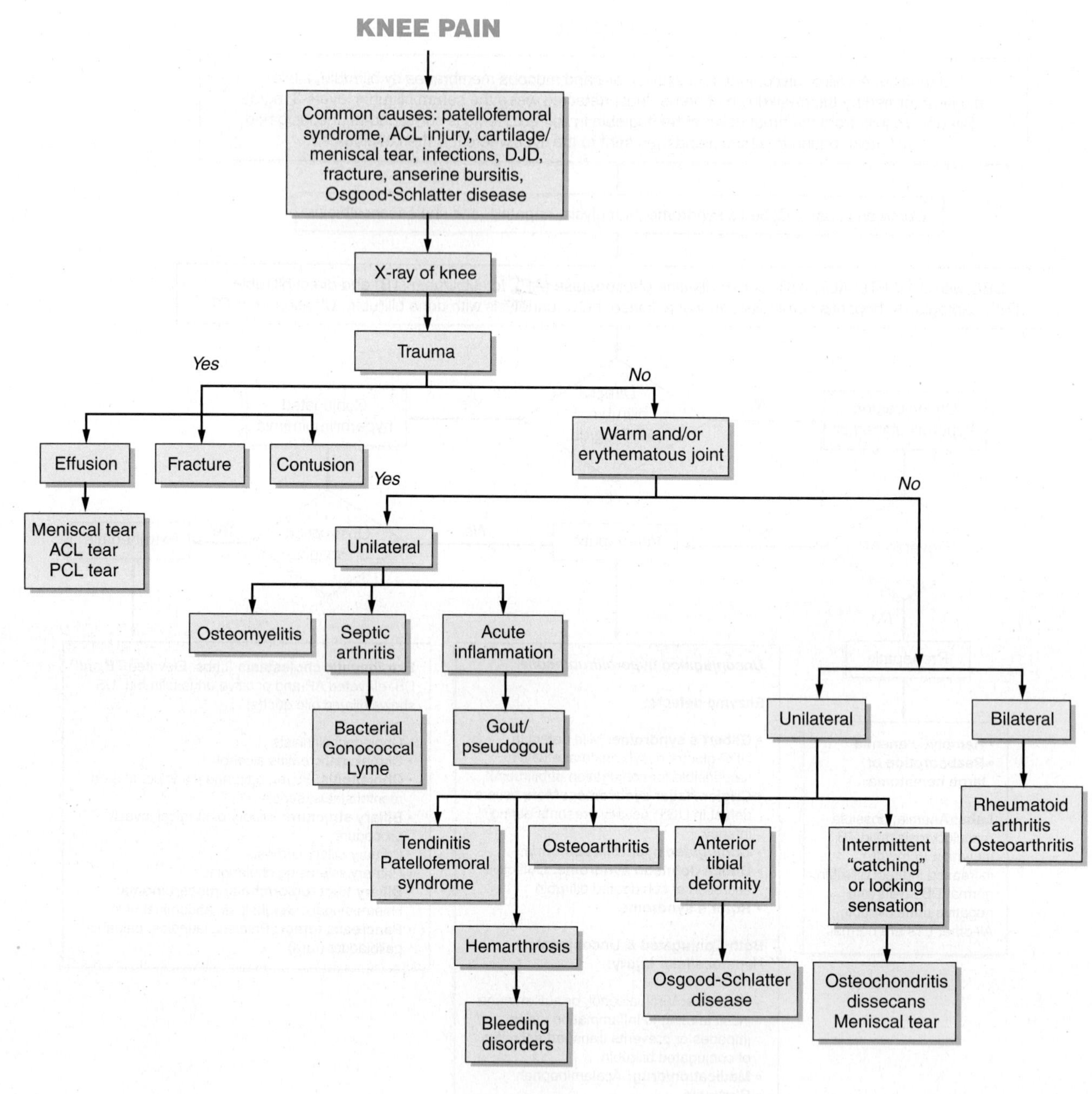
KNEE PAIN
Common causes: patellofemoral syndrome, ACL injury, cartilage/ meniscal tear, infections, DJD, fracture, anserine bursitis, Osgood-Schlatter disease
X-ray of knee
Trauma
Yes
No
Effusion
Fracture
Contusion
Meniscal tear
ACL tear
PCL tear
Warm and/or erythematous joint
Yes
No
Unilateral
Osteomyelitis
Septic arthritis
Acute inflammation
Bacterial
Gonococcal
Lyme
Gout/ pseudogout
Unilateral
Bilateral
Rheumatoid arthritis
Osteoarthritis
Tendinitis
Patellofemoral syndrome
Osteoarthritis
Anterior tibial deformity
Intermittent "catching" or locking sensation
Hemarthrosis
Bleeding disorders
Osgood-Schlatter disease
Osteochondritis dissecans
Meniscal tear

Robert A. Baldor, MD and Alan M. Ehrlich, MD

J Fam Pract. 2008;57(2):116–8.

LACTOSE DEHYDROGENASE ELEVATION

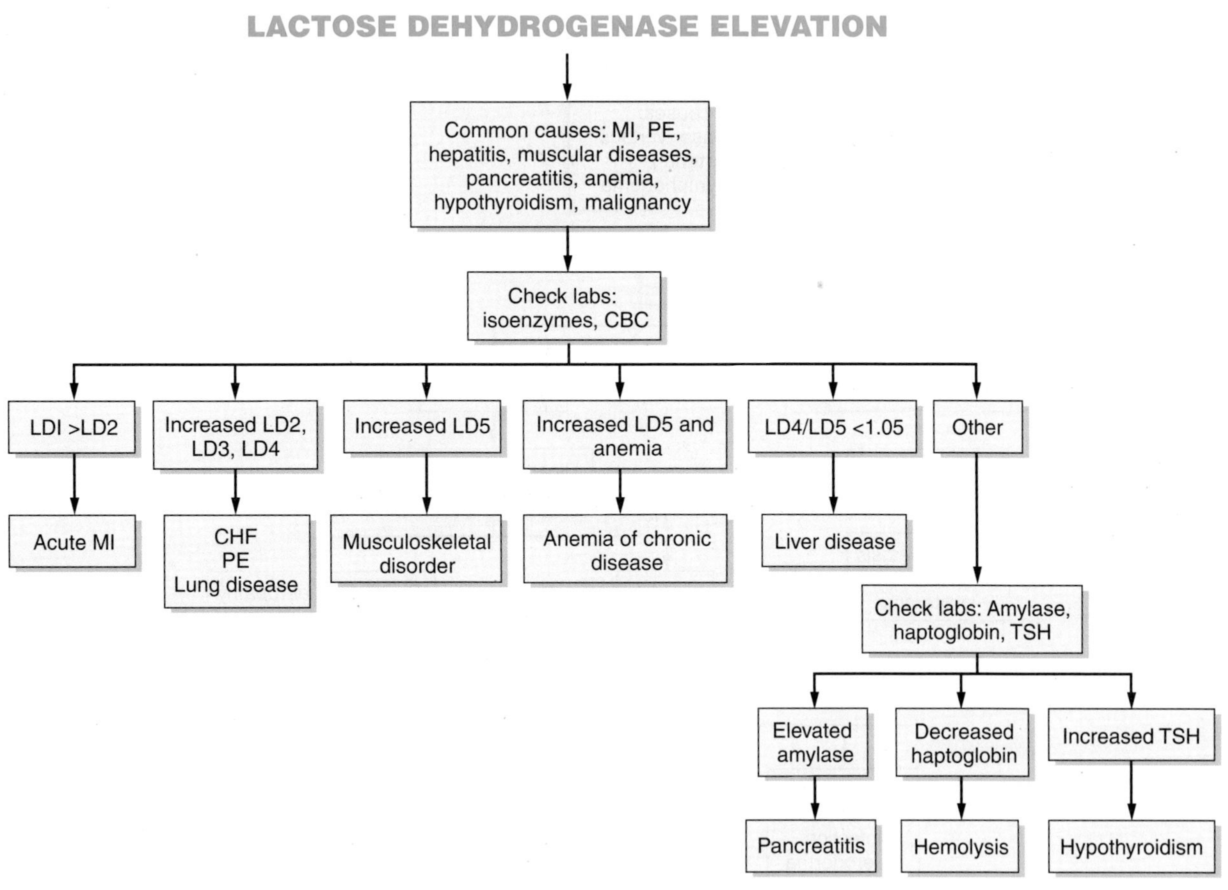

Robert A. Baldor, MD and Alan M. Ehrlich, MD

Ann Int Med. 1991;115(12):931–5.

LEG ULCER

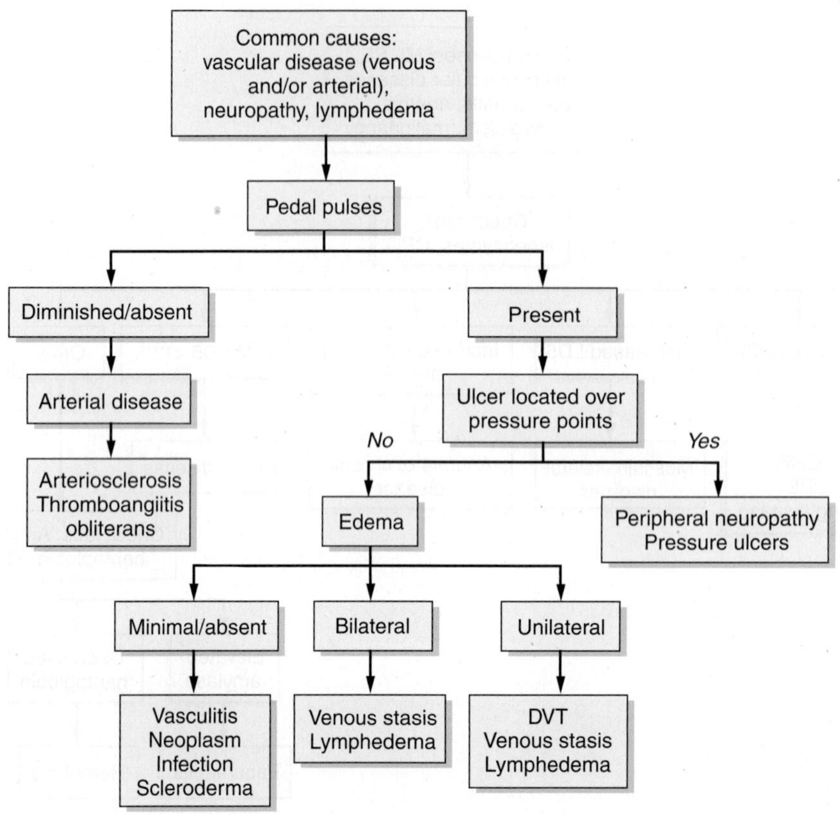

Robert A. Baldor, MD and Alan M. Ehrlich, MD

Surg Clin North Am. 2007;87(5):1149–77, x.

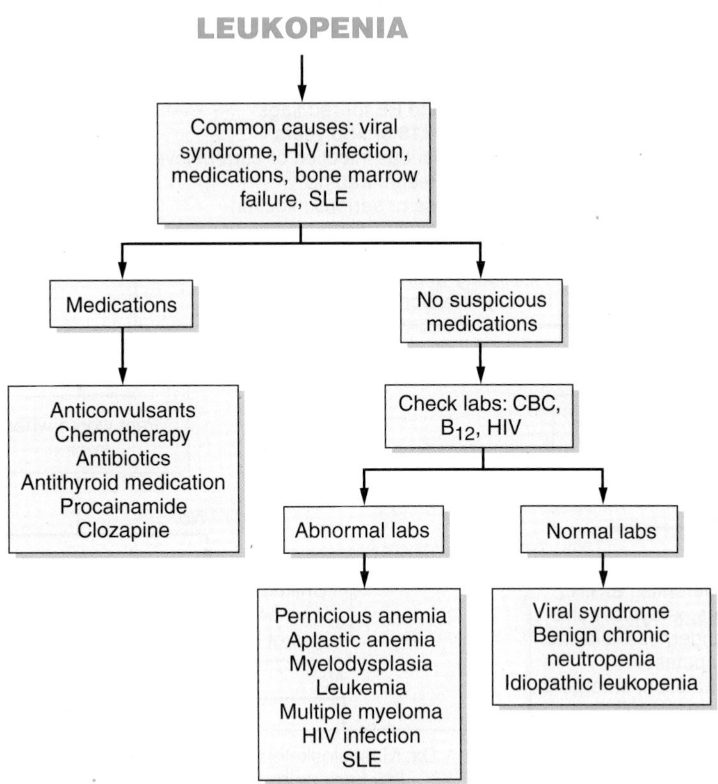

Robert A. Baldor, MD and Alan M. Ehrlich, MD

Mayo Clin Proc. 2005;80(7):923–36.

LOW BACK PAIN, ACUTE

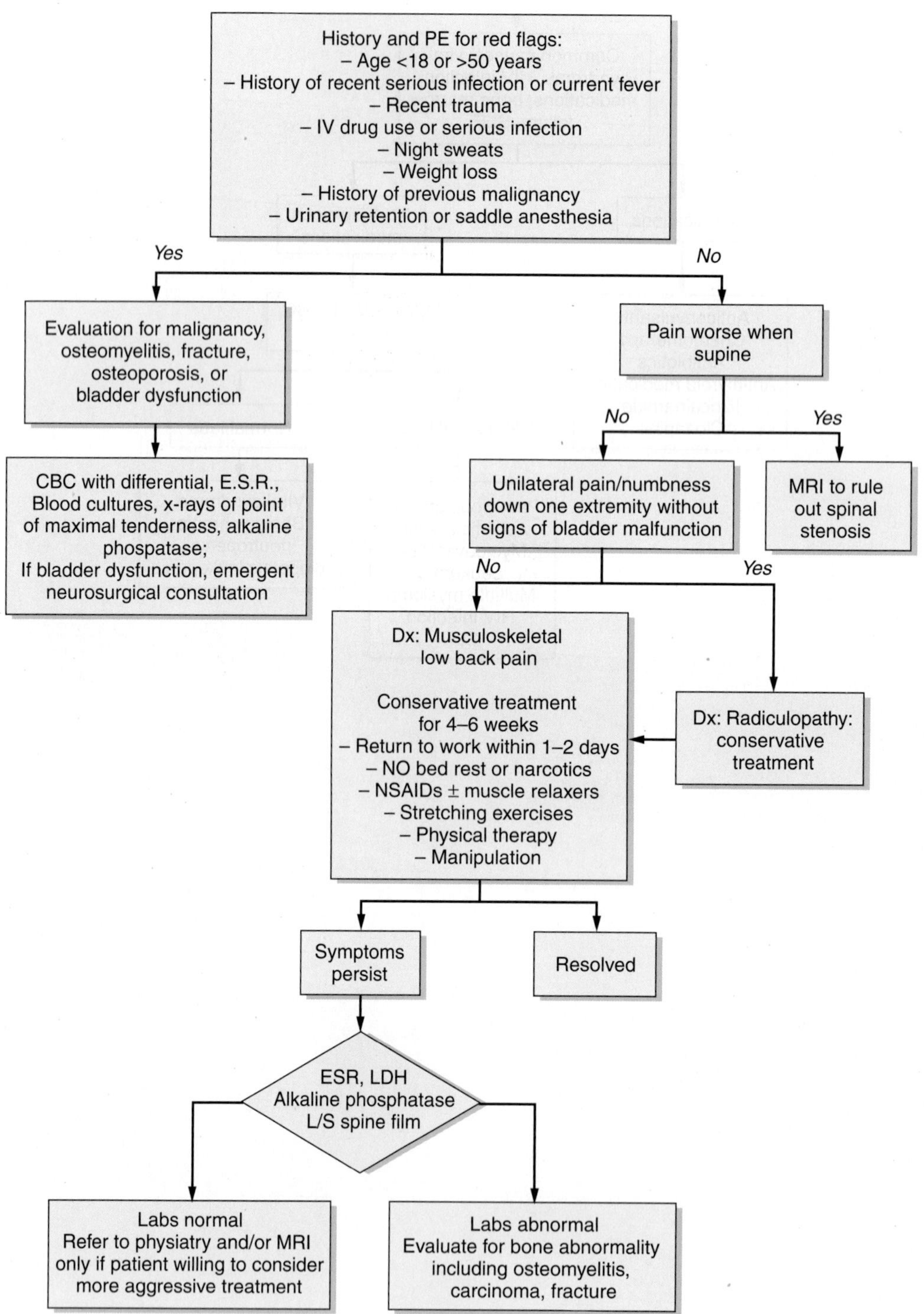
History and PE for red flags:
– Age <18 or >50 years
– History of recent serious infection or current fever
– Recent trauma
– IV drug use or serious infection
– Night sweats
– Weight loss
– History of previous malignancy
– Urinary retention or saddle anesthesia
Yes
No
Evaluation for malignancy, osteomyelitis, fracture, osteoporosis, or bladder dysfunction
CBC with differential, E.S.R., Blood cultures, x-rays of point of maximal tenderness, alkaline phospatase; If bladder dysfunction, emergent neurosurgical consultation
Pain worse when supine
No
Yes
Unilateral pain/numbness down one extremity without signs of bladder malfunction
MRI to rule out spinal stenosis
No
Yes
Dx: Musculoskeletal low back pain
Conservative treatment for 4–6 weeks
– Return to work within 1–2 days
– NO bed rest or narcotics
– NSAIDs ± muscle relaxers
– Stretching exercises
– Physical therapy
– Manipulation
Dx: Radiculopathy: conservative treatment
Symptoms persist
Resolved
ESR, LDH
Alkaline phosphatase
L/S spine film
Labs normal
Refer to physiatry and/or MRI only if patient willing to consider more aggressive treatment
Labs abnormal
Evaluate for bone abnormality including osteomyelitis, carcinoma, fracture

Patricio Bruno, DO

Med Clin North Am. 2009;93(2):477–501, x.

LOW BACK PAIN, CHRONIC

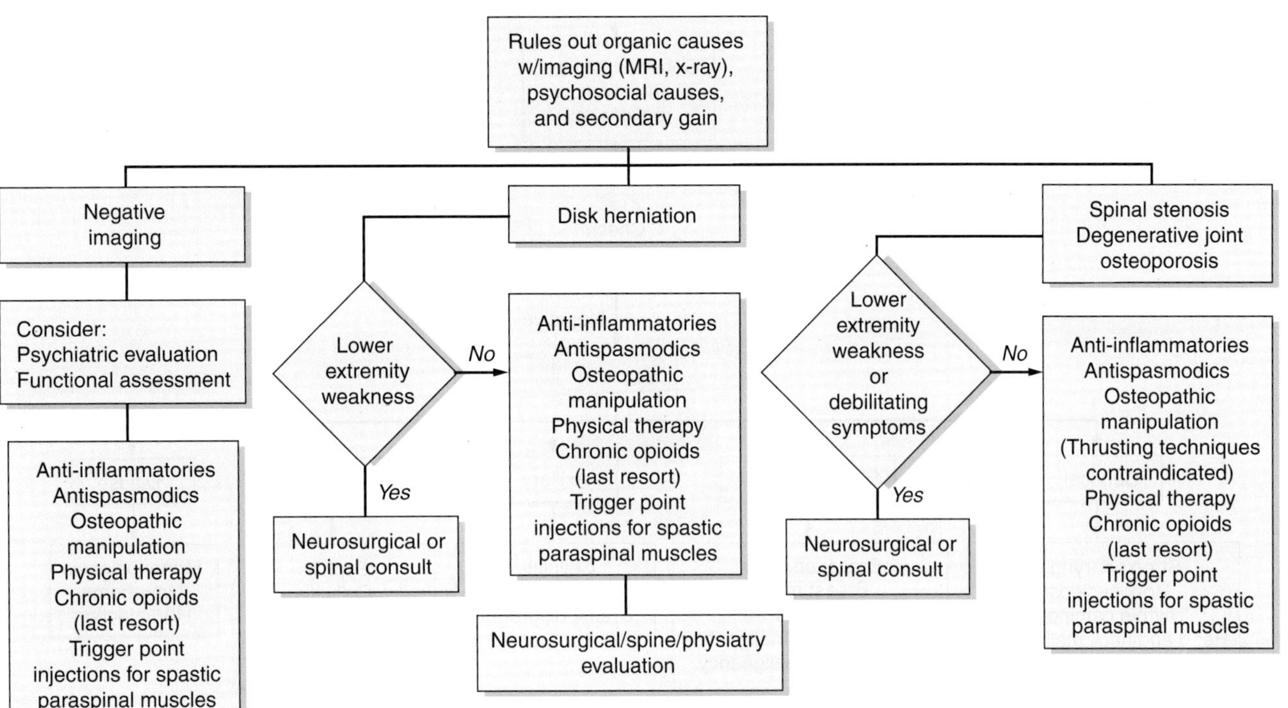

Patricio Bruno, DO

Spine. 2009;34(7):718–24.

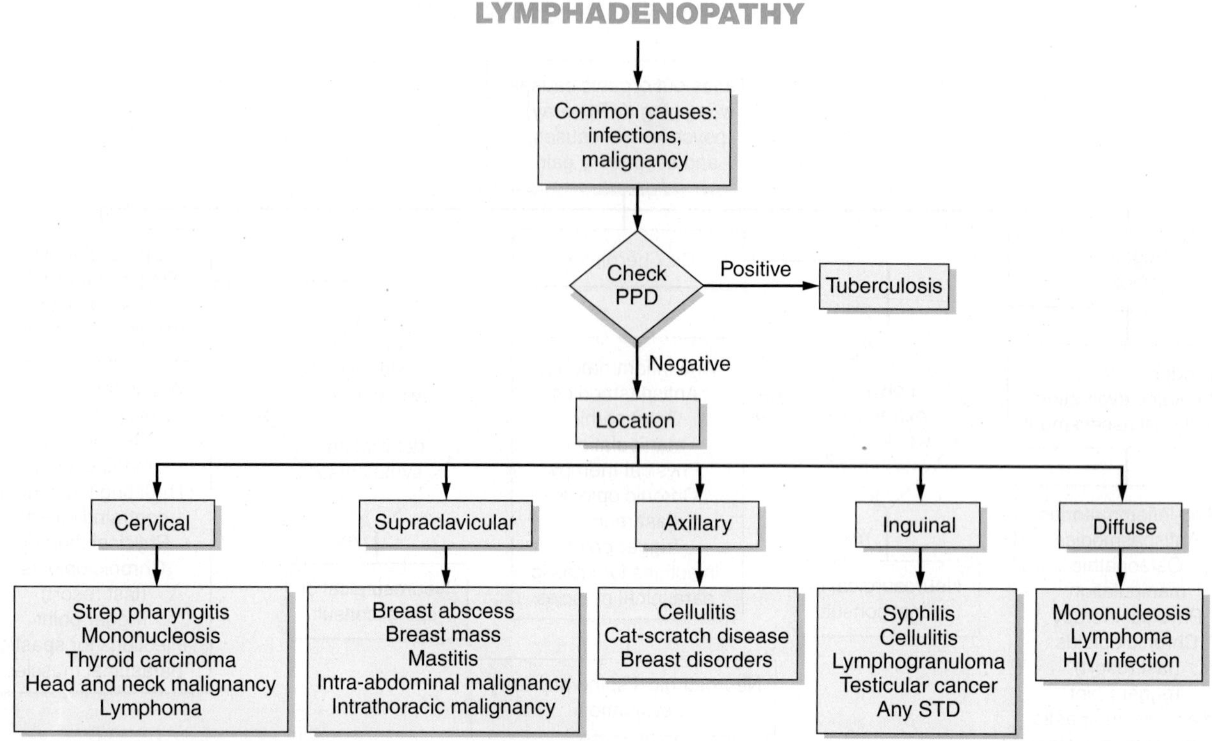

Robert A. Baldor, MD and Alan M. Ehrlich, MD

Radiol Clin North Am. 2008;46(2):175–98, vii.

MALABSORPTION SYNDROME

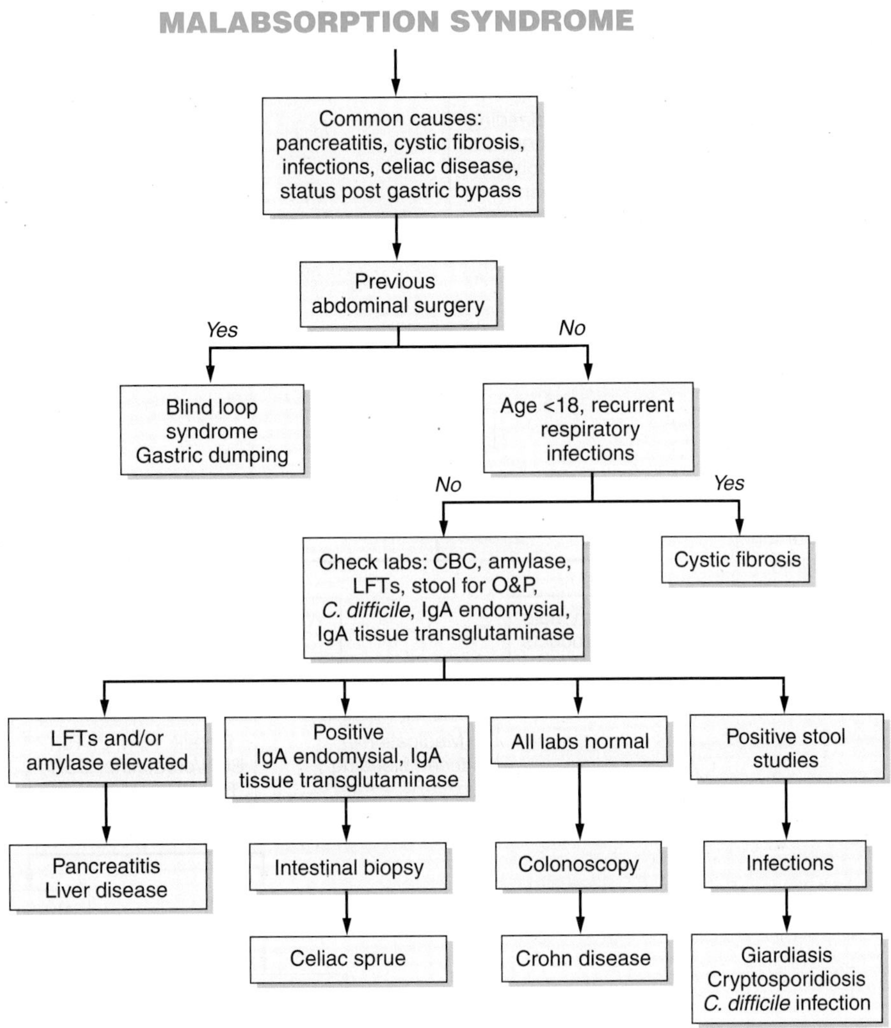

Robert A. Baldor, MD and Alan M. Ehrlich, MD

Pediatr Clin North Am. 2009;56(5):1105–21.

MENORRHAGIA (EXCESSIVE BLEEDING)

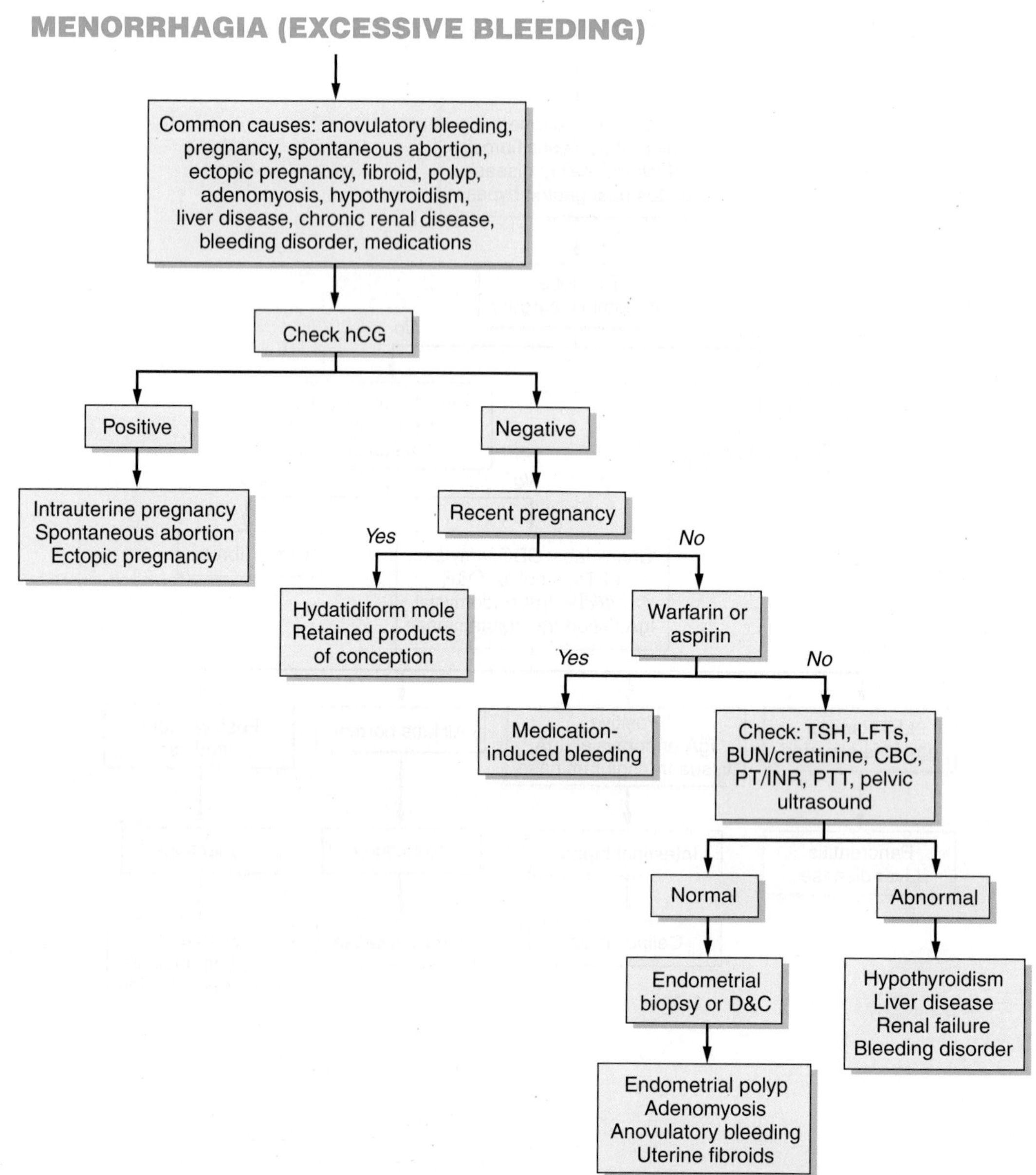

Robert A. Baldor, MD and Alan M. Ehrlich, MD

Am Fam Physician. 2004;69(8):1915–26.

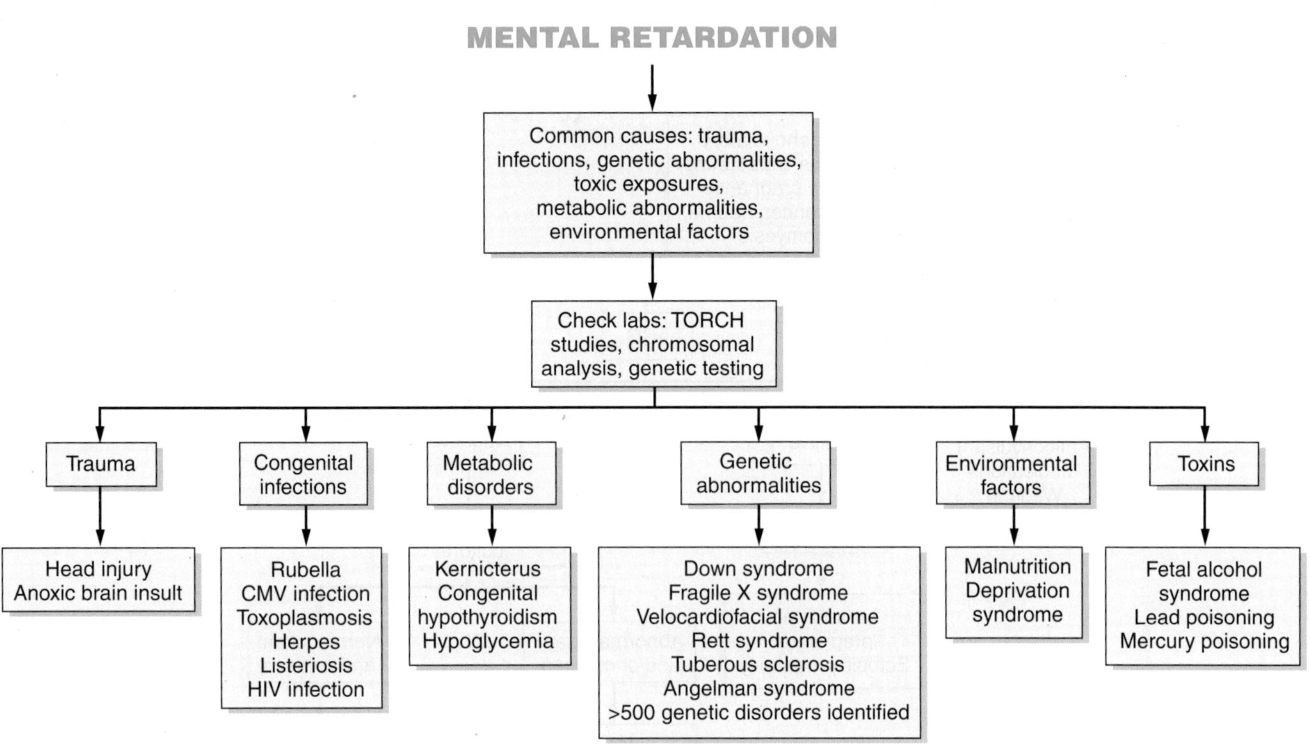

Robert A. Baldor, MD and Alan M. Ehrlich, MD

Pediatr Clin North Am. 2008;55(5):1071–84, xi.

METRORRHAGIA (INTERMENSTRUAL BLEEDING)

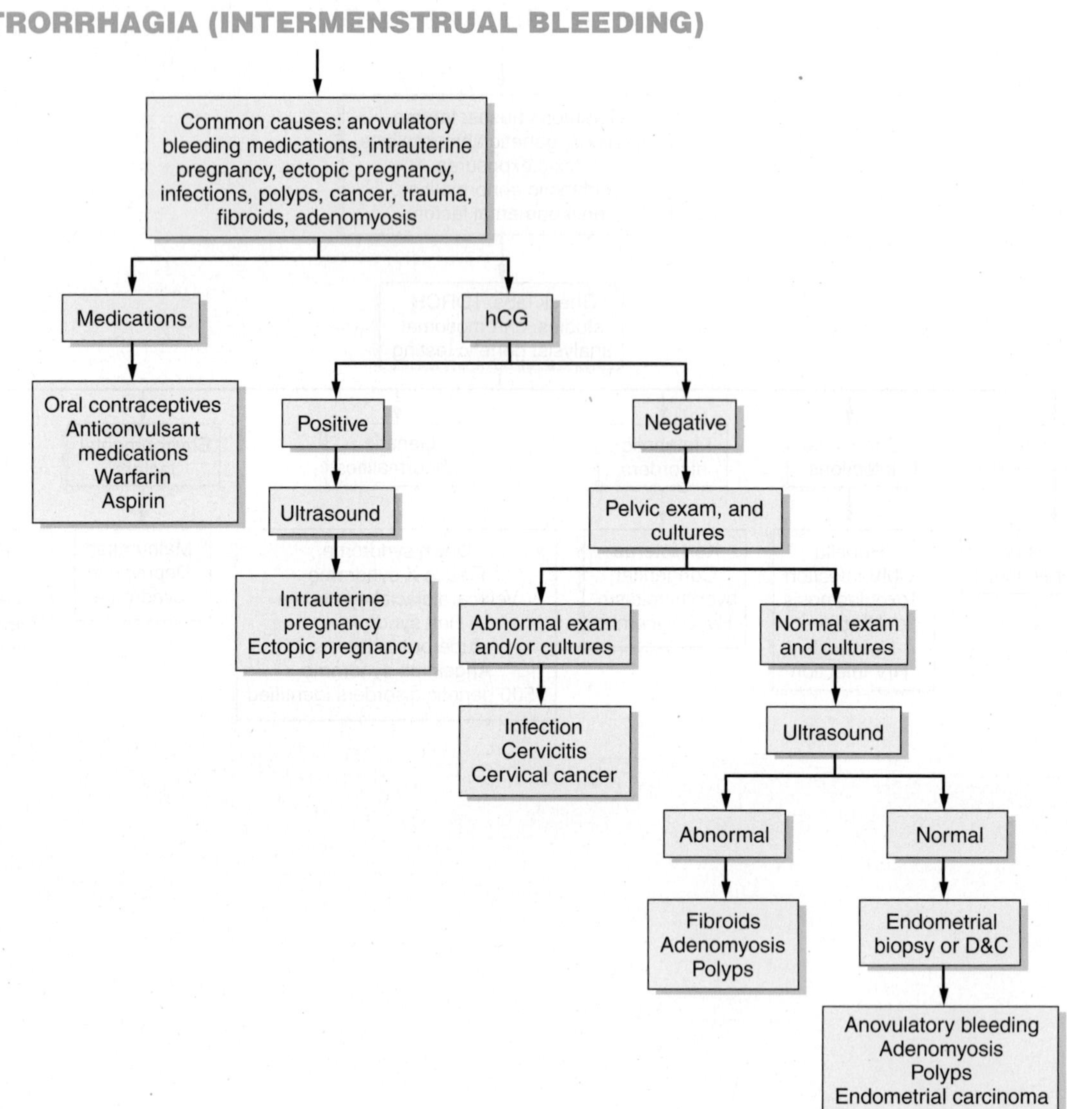

Robert A. Baldor, MD and Alan M. Ehrlich, MD

Am Fam Physician. 2004;69(8):1915–26.

MULTIPLE SCLEROSIS, TREATMENT

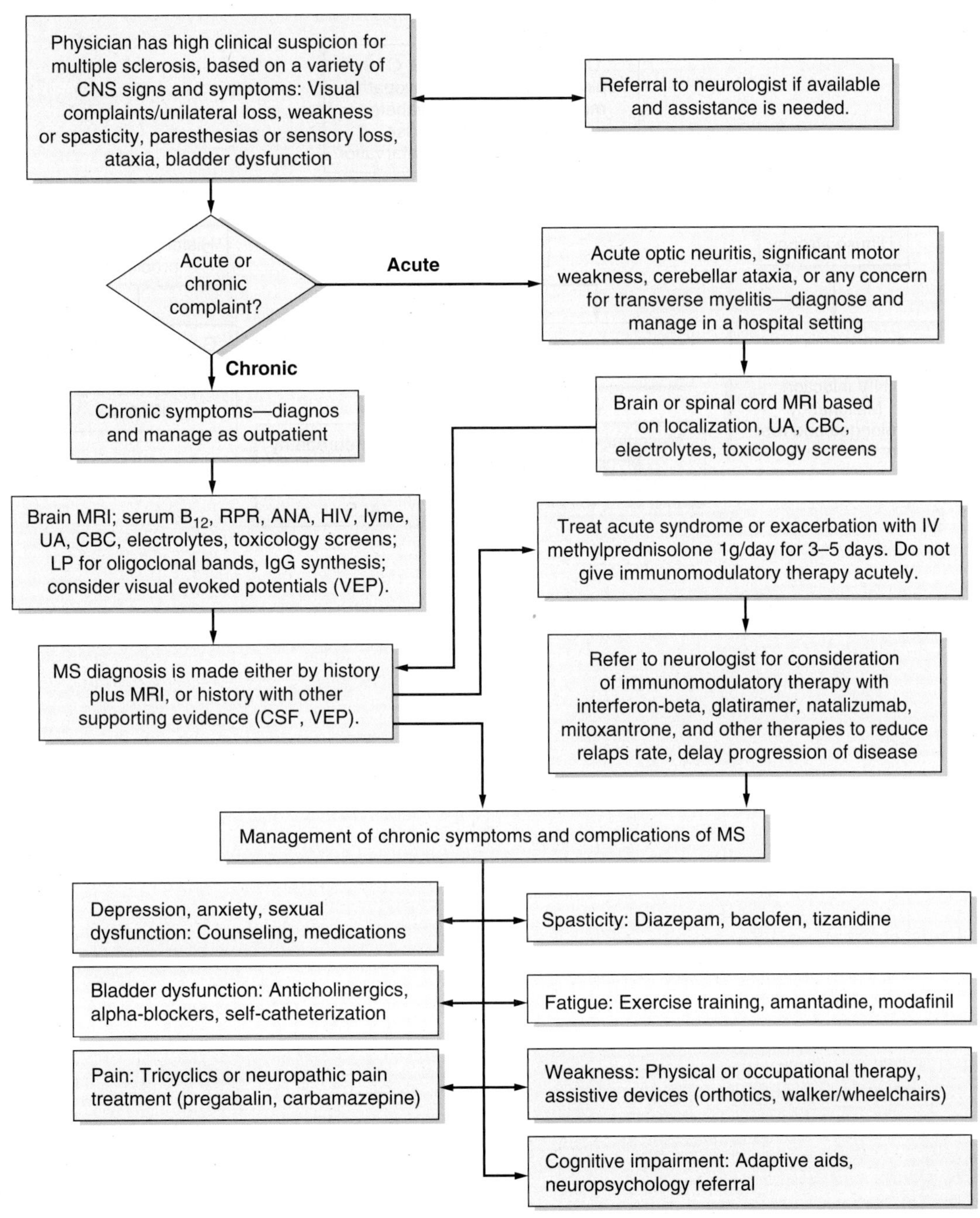
Physician has high clinical suspicion for multiple sclerosis, based on a variety of CNS signs and symptoms: Visual complaints/unilateral loss, weakness or spasticity, paresthesias or sensory loss, ataxia, bladder dysfunction
Referral to neurologist if available and assistance is needed.
Acute or chronic complaint?
Acute
Acute optic neuritis, significant motor weakness, cerebellar ataxia, or any concern for transverse myelitis—diagnose and manage in a hospital setting
Chronic
Chronic symptoms—diagnos and manage as outpatient
Brain or spinal cord MRI based on localization, UA, CBC, electrolytes, toxicology screens
Brain MRI; serum B12, RPR, ANA, HIV, lyme, UA, CBC, electrolytes, toxicology screens; LP for oligoclonal bands, IgG synthesis; consider visual evoked potentials (VEP).
Treat acute syndrome or exacerbation with IV methylprednisolone 1g/day for 3–5 days. Do not give immunomodulatory therapy acutely.
MS diagnosis is made either by history plus MRI, or history with other supporting evidence (CSF, VEP).
Refer to neurologist for consideration of immunomodulatory therapy with interferon-beta, glatiramer, natalizumab, mitoxantrone, and other therapies to reduce relaps rate, delay progression of disease
Management of chronic symptoms and complications of MS
Depression, anxiety, sexual dysfunction: Counseling, medications
Spasticity: Diazepam, baclofen, tizanidine
Bladder dysfunction: Anticholinergics, alpha-blockers, self-catheterization
Fatigue: Exercise training, amantadine, modafinil
Pain: Tricyclics or neuropathic pain treatment (pregabalin, carbamazepine)
Weakness: Physical or occupational therapy, assistive devices (orthotics, walker/wheelchairs)
Cognitive impairment: Adaptive aids, neuropsychology referral

Julie L. Roth, MD

Ann Neurol. 2005;58:840–6.

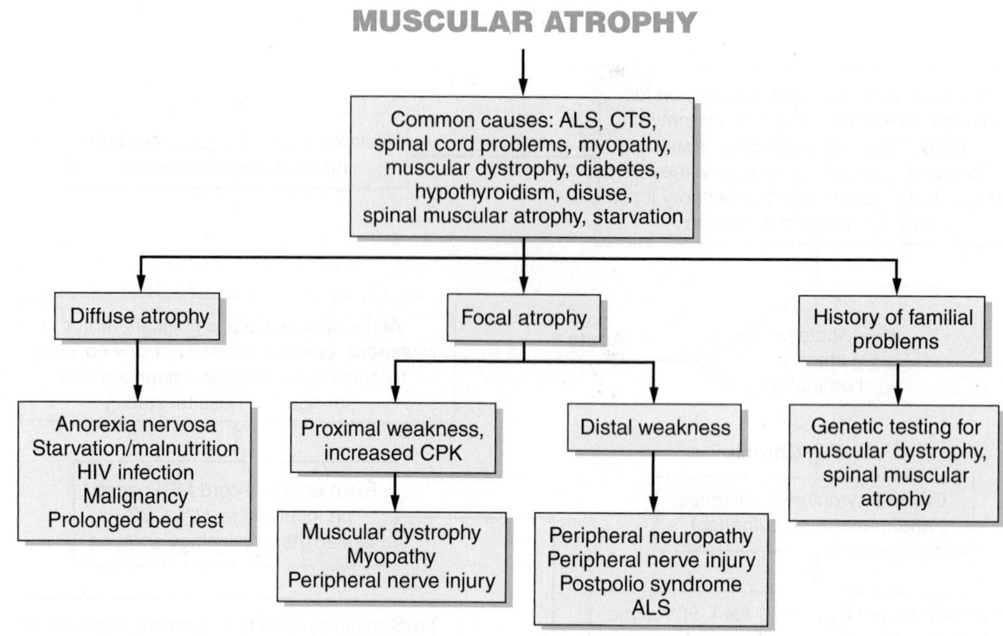

Robert A. Baldor, MD and Alan M. Ehrlich, MD

Lancet. 2007;369(9578):2031–41.

NAIL ABNORMALITIES

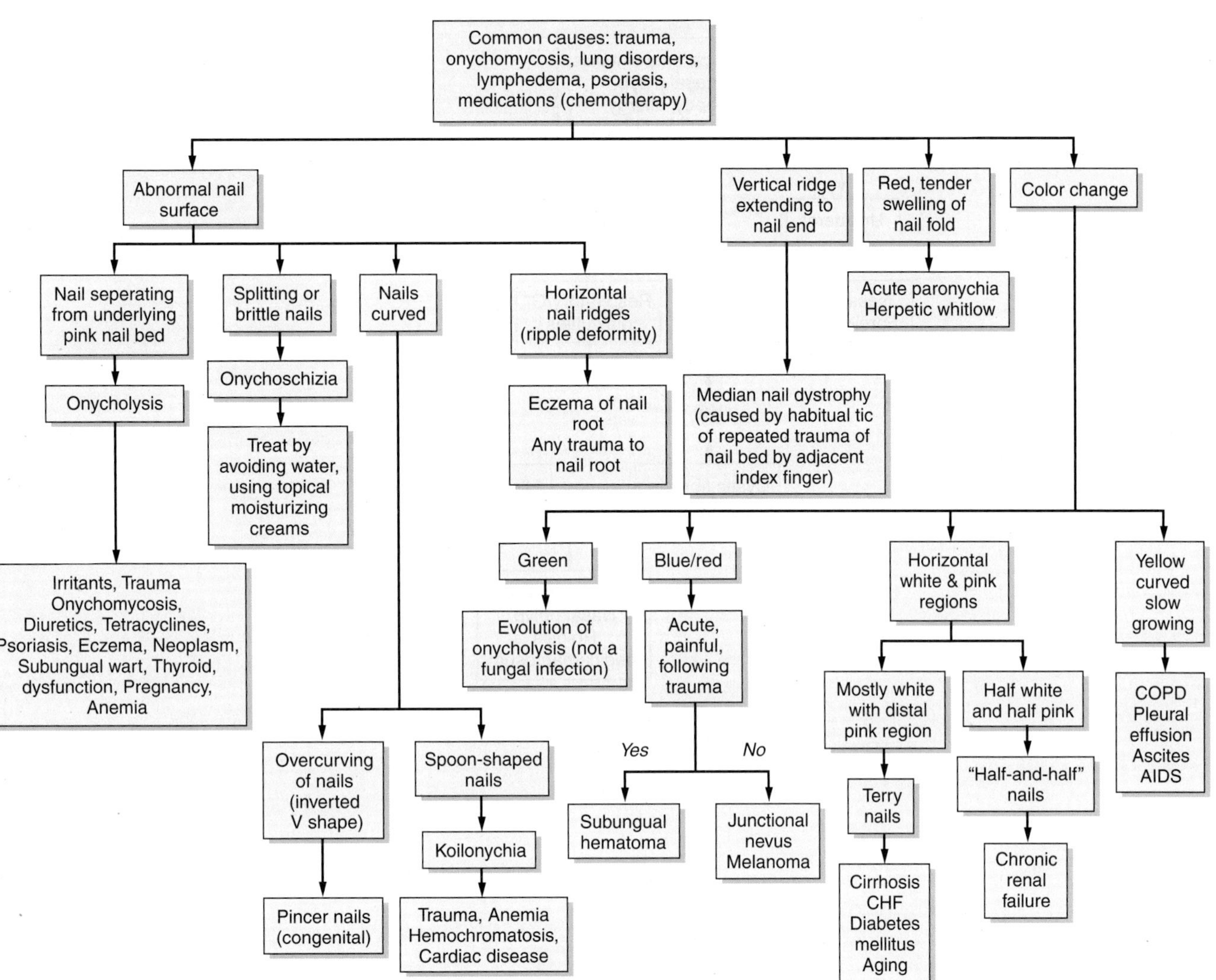

Robert A. Baldor, MD and Alan M. Ehrlich, MD

Am Fam Physician. 2004;69(6):1417–24.

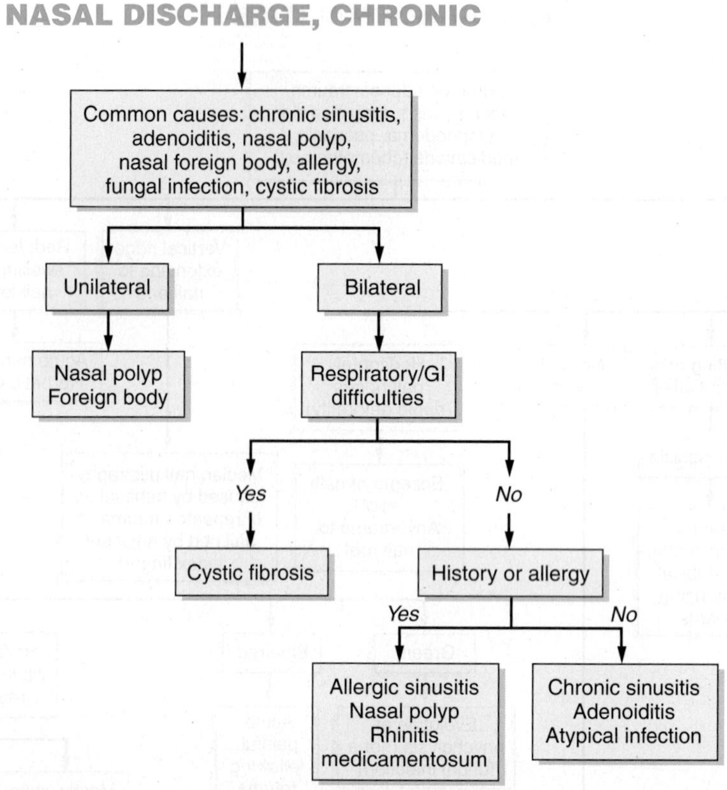

Robert A. Baldor, MD and Alan M. Ehrlich, MD

Postgrad Med. 2009;121(6):121–39.

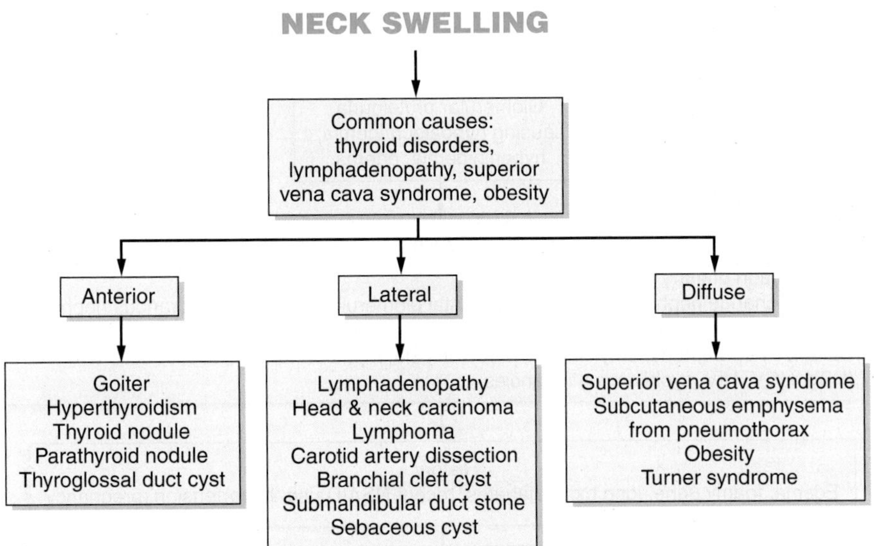

Robert A. Baldor, MD and Alan M. Ehrlich, MD

Am Fam Physician. 1995;51(8):1904–12.

NEPHROTIC SYNDROME

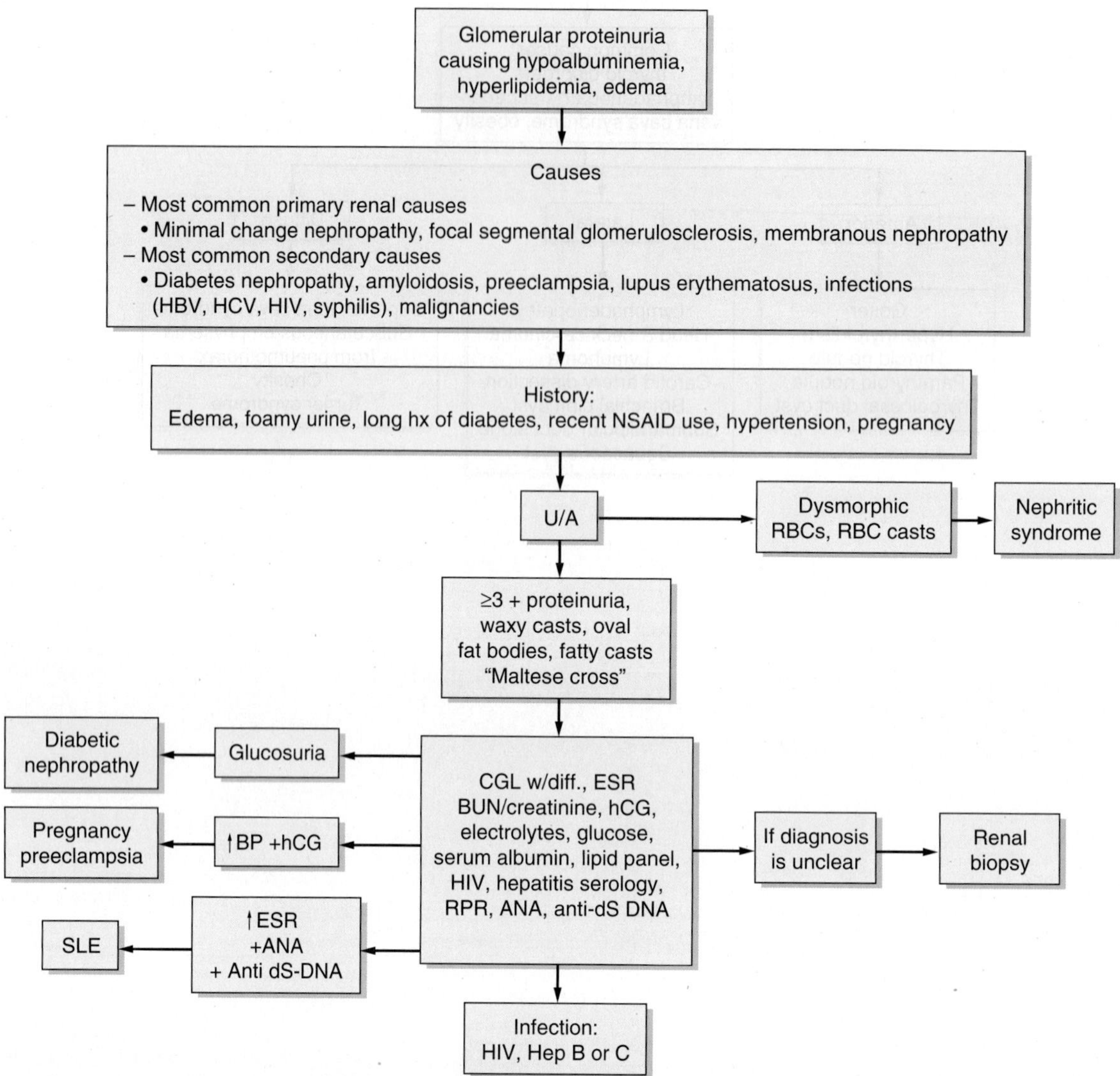

Jonathan Min, MD and Robert M. Black, MD

Cleve Clin J Med. 2006;73(2):161–7.

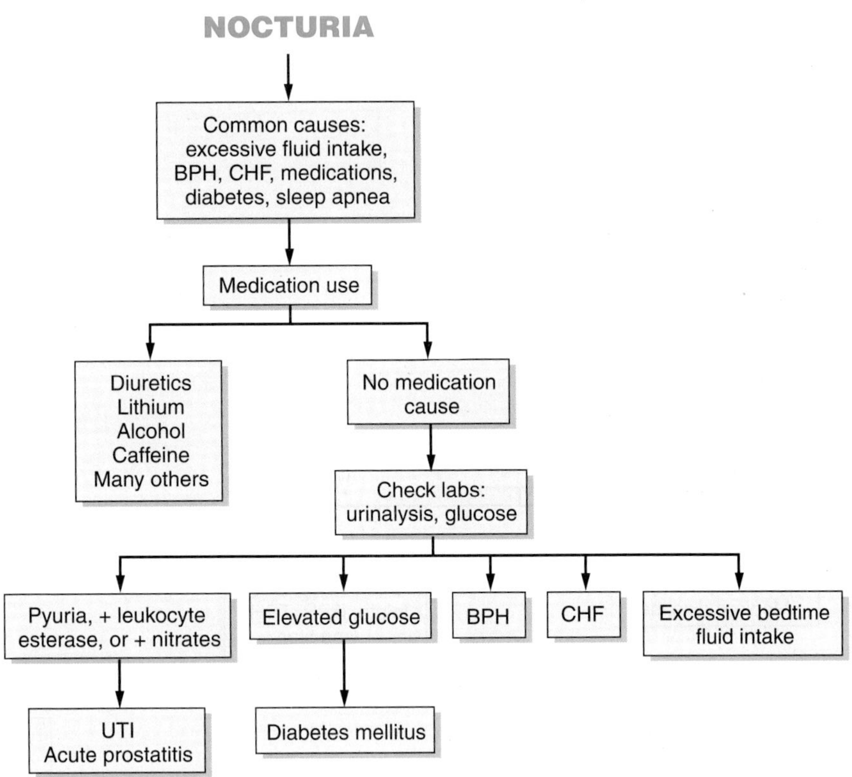

Robert A. Baldor, MD and Alan M. Ehrlich, MD

BMJ. 2004;328(7447):1063–6.

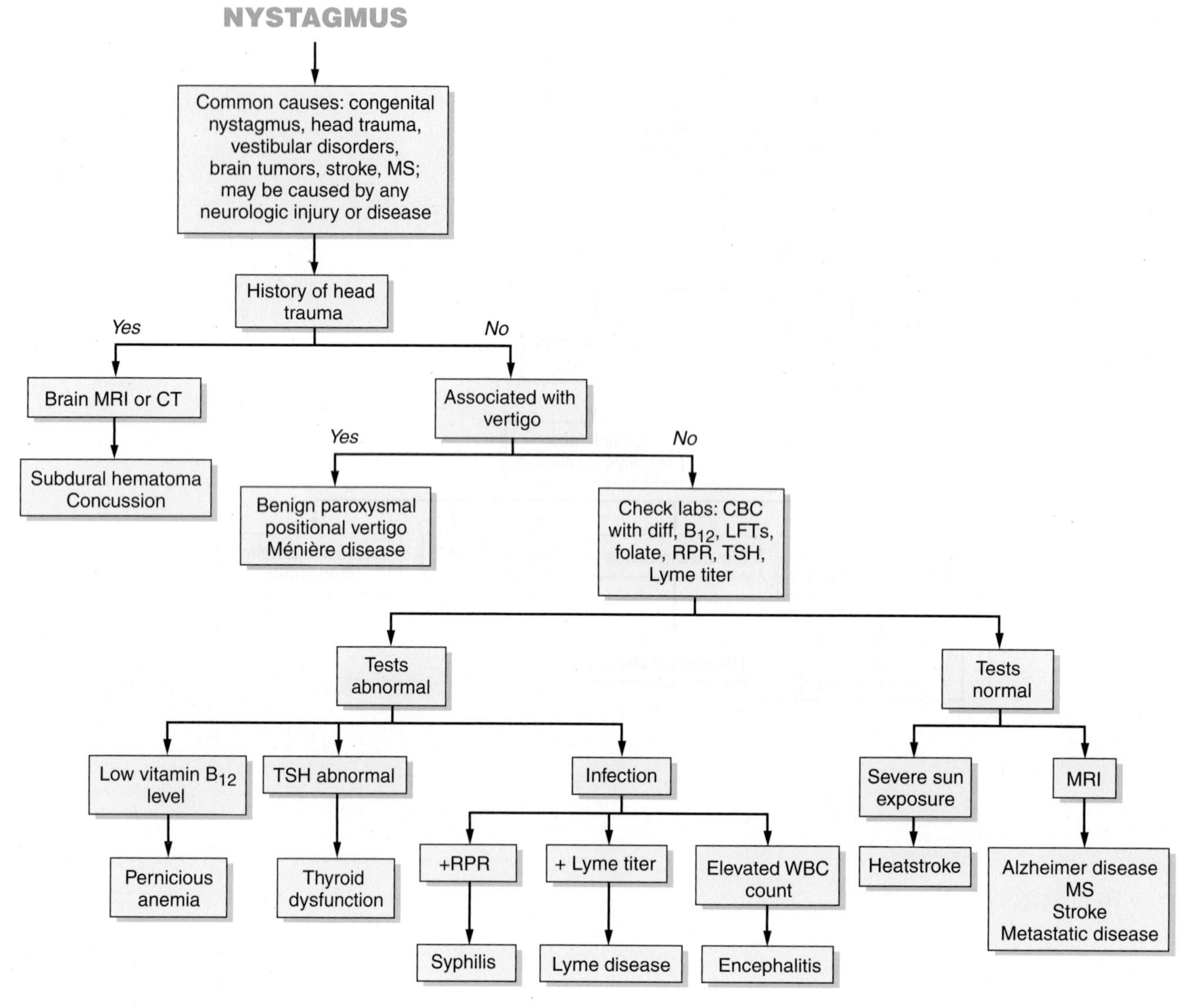

Robert A. Baldor, MD and Alan M. Ehrlich, MD

Med Clin North Am. 2009;93(2):263–71, vii.

PAIN IN UPPER EXTREMITY

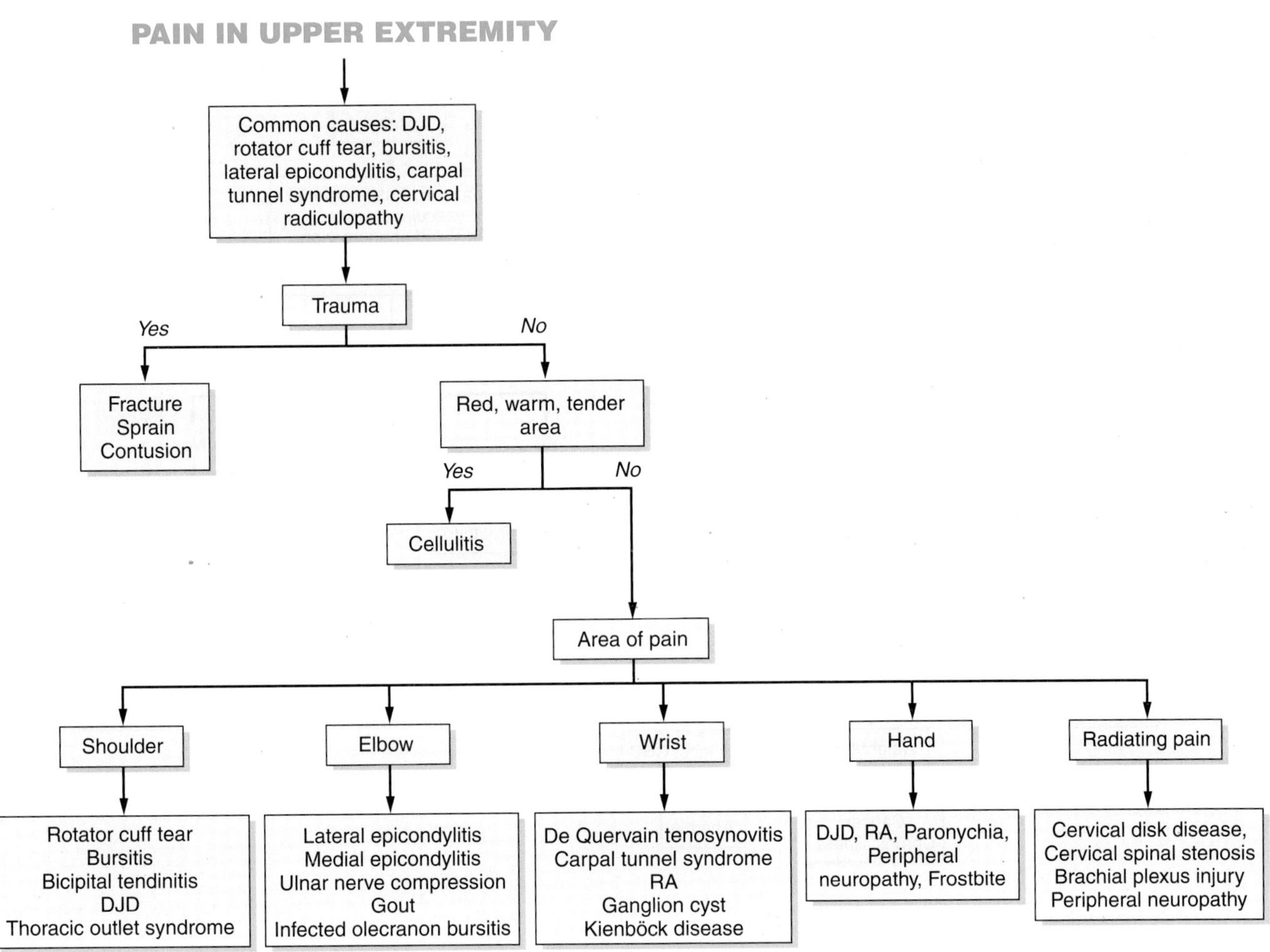

Robert A. Baldor, MD and Alan M. Ehrlich, MD

N Engl J Med. 2008;358(20):2138–47.

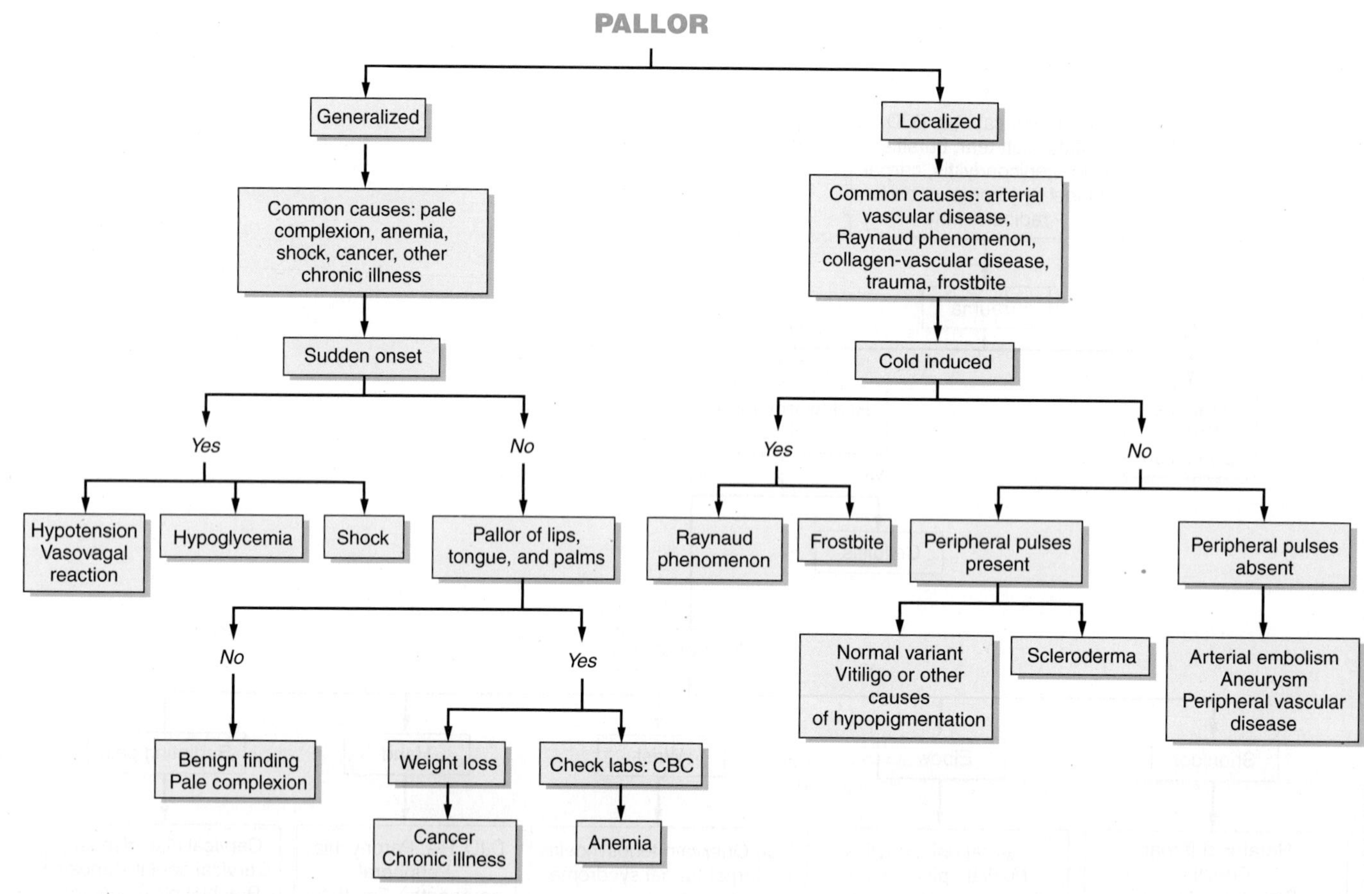

Robert A. Baldor, MD and Alan M. Ehrlich, MD

Am Fam Physician. 2007;75(5):671–8; *South Med J.* 2009;102(11):1141–9.

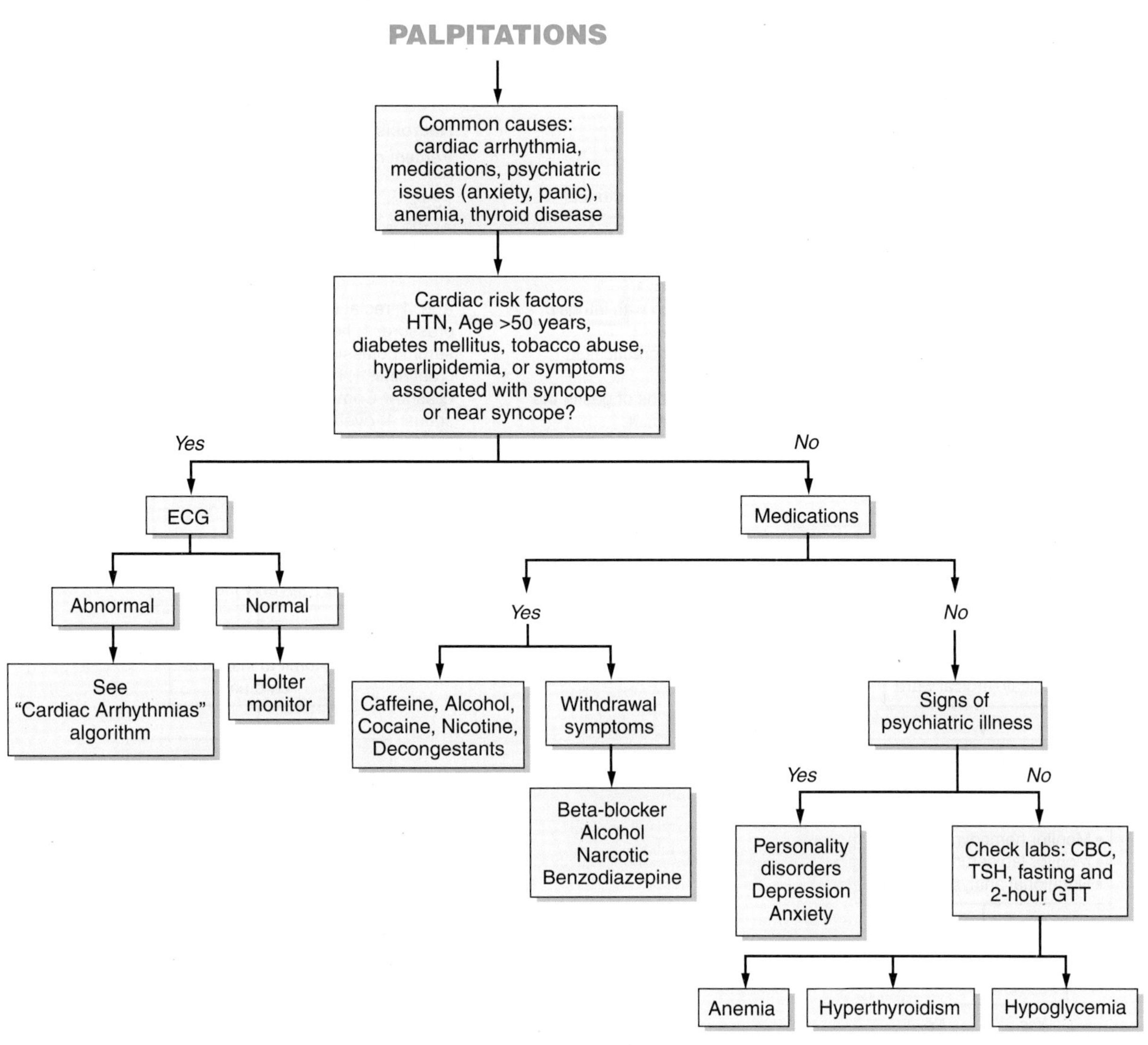

Robert A. Baldor, MD and Alan M. Ehrlich, MD

NEJM. 338(19):1369–73.

PANCREATITIS, ACUTE

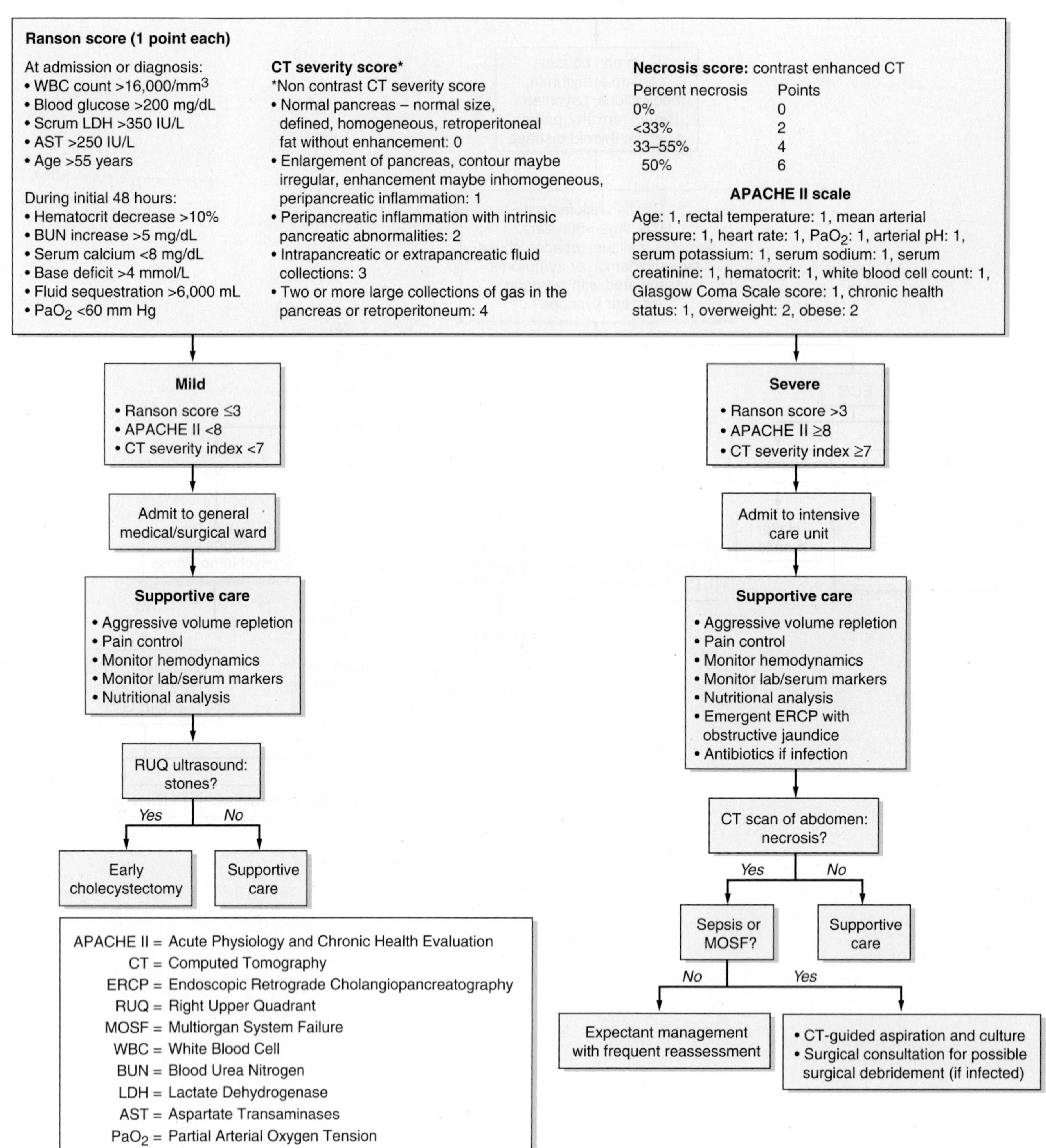
Ranson score (1 point each)
At admission or diagnosis:
• WBC count >16,000/mm3
• Blood glucose >200 mg/dL
• Scrum LDH >350 IU/L
• AST >250 IU/L
• Age >55 years
During initial 48 hours:
• Hematocrit decrease >10%
• BUN increase >5 mg/dL
• Serum calcium <8 mg/dL
• Base deficit >4 mmol/L
• Fluid sequestration >6,000 mL
• PaO2 <60 mm Hg
CT severity score*
*Non contrast CT severity score
• Normal pancreas – normal size, defined, homogeneous, retroperitoneal fat without enhancement: 0
• Enlargement of pancreas, contour maybe irregular, enhancement maybe inhomogeneous, peripancreatic inflammation: 1
• Peripancreatic inflammation with intrinsic pancreatic abnormalities: 2
• Intrapancreatic or extrapancreatic fluid collections: 3
• Two or more large collections of gas in the pancreas or retroperitoneum: 4
Necrosis score: contrast enhanced CT
Percent necrosis Points
0% 0
<33% 2
33–55% 4
50% 6
APACHE II scale
Age: 1, rectal temperature: 1, mean arterial pressure: 1, heart rate: 1, PaO2: 1, arterial pH: 1, serum potassium: 1, serum sodium: 1, serum creatinine: 1, hematocrit: 1, white blood cell count: 1, Glasgow Coma Scale score: 1, chronic health status: 1, overweight: 2, obese: 2
Mild
• Ranson score ≤3
• APACHE II <8
• CT severity index <7
Admit to general medical/surgical ward
Supportive care
• Aggressive volume repletion
• Pain control
• Monitor hemodynamics
• Monitor lab/serum markers
• Nutritional analysis
RUQ ultrasound: stones?
Yes
No
Early cholecystectomy
Supportive care
Severe
• Ranson score >3
• APACHE II ≥8
• CT severity index ≥7
Admit to intensive care unit
Supportive care
• Aggressive volume repletion
• Pain control
• Monitor hemodynamics
• Monitor lab/serum markers
• Nutritional analysis
• Emergent ERCP with obstructive jaundice
• Antibiotics if infection
CT scan of abdomen: necrosis?
Yes
No
Sepsis or MOSF?
Supportive care
No
Yes
Expectant management with frequent reassessment
• CT-guided aspiration and culture
• Surgical consultation for possible surgical debridement (if infected)
APACHE II = Acute Physiology and Chronic Health Evaluation
CT = Computed Tomography
ERCP = Endoscopic Retrograde Cholangiopancreatography
RUQ = Right Upper Quadrant
MOSF = Multiorgan System Failure
WBC = White Blood Cell
BUN = Blood Urea Nitrogen
LDH = Lactate Dehydrogenase
AST = Aspartate Transaminases
PaO2 = Partial Arterial Oxygen Tension

Maurice F. Joyce, III, MD and Mitchell A. Cahan, MD

J Gastrointest Surg. 2005;9(3):440–52.

PAP (ABNORMAL), >21 YEARS OF AGE*

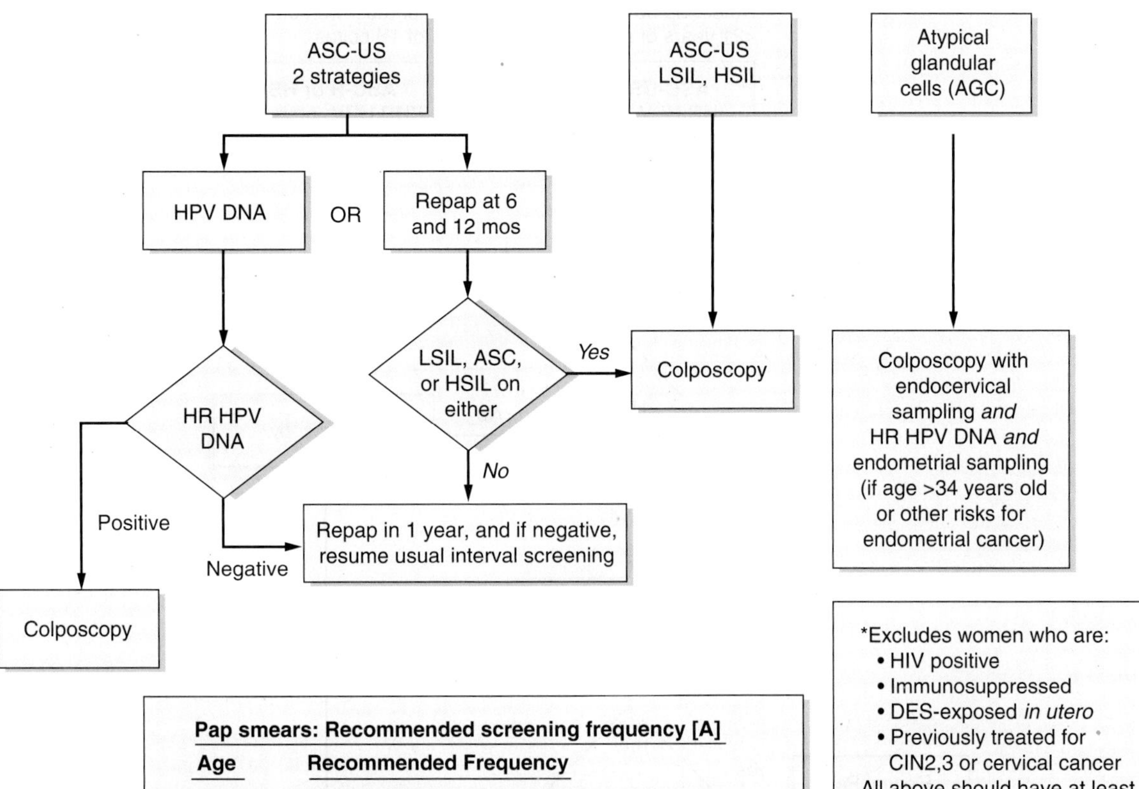

*Excludes women who are:
- HIV positive
- Immunosuppressed
- DES-exposed *in utero*
- Previously treated for CIN2,3 or cervical cancer

All above should have at least an *annual* screening

Pap smears: Recommended screening frequency [A]

Age	Recommended Frequency
<21	Screening not recommended
21–29	Every 2 years, either conventional or liquid-based
30–65	Every 3 years if either • Previous 3 paps (every 1–2 years) all normal *or* • Cytology negative and HR HPV DNA negative
>65	Discontinue screening if 3 previous paps normal and no abnormal results in past 10 years

Women of any age who had total hysterectomy for benign disease (and w/o history of high-grade CIN) do *not* require Pap smears

HR HPV DNA = probe for high-risk HPV strains

Jeremy Golding, MD

ACOG Practice Bulletin Number 109, December 2009.

PAP (ABNORMAL), ADOLESCENTS

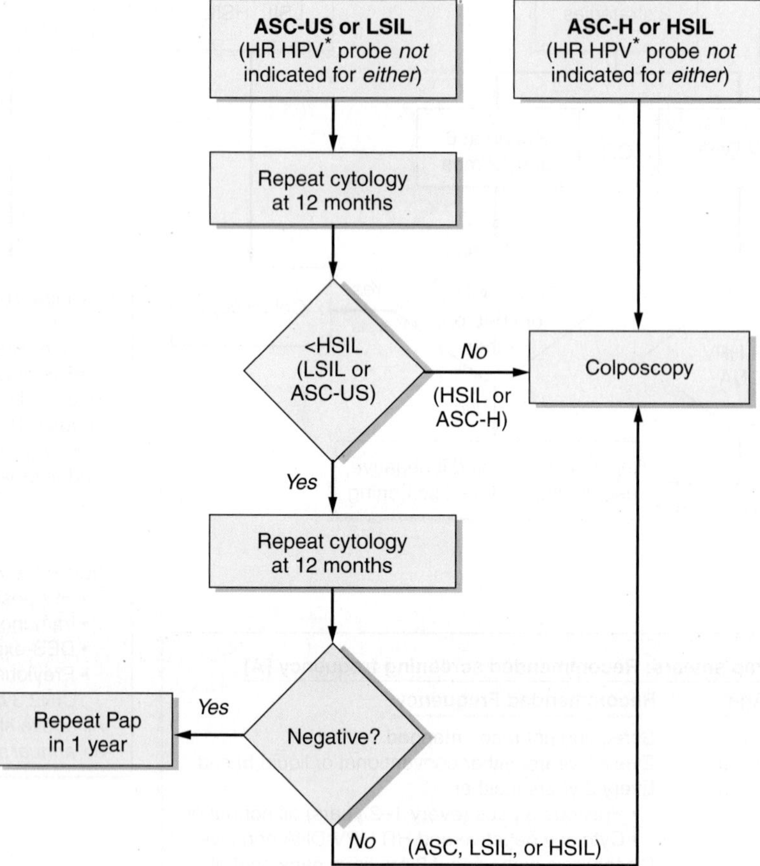

HR HPV DNA = probe for high-risk HPV strains

Jeremy Golding, MD

ACOG Practice Bulletin Number 109, December 2009.

PAP, USE OF HPV DNA TESTING IN WOMEN OVER 30*

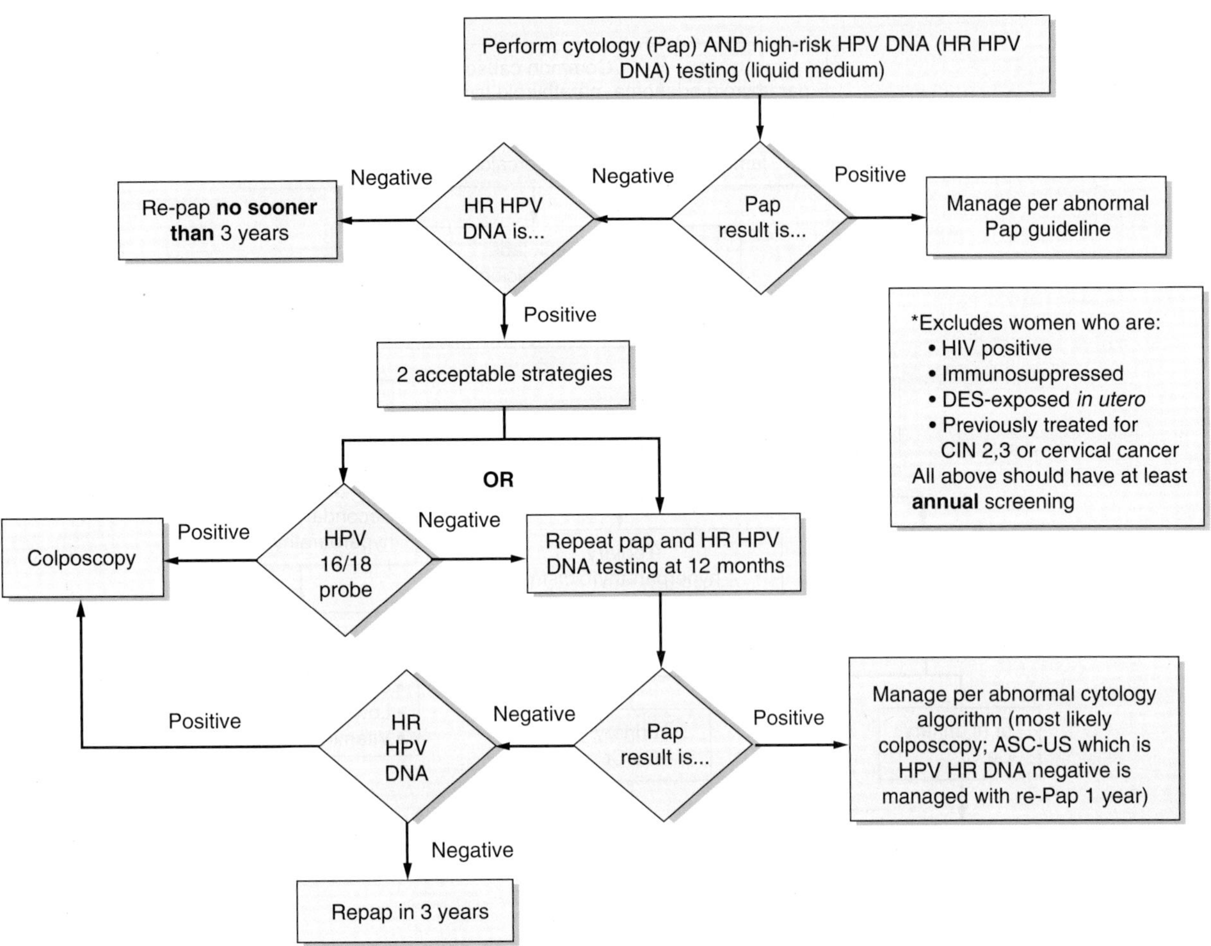

*Excludes women who are:
- HIV positive
- Immunosuppressed
- DES-exposed *in utero*
- Previously treated for CIN 2,3 or cervical cancer

All above should have at least **annual** screening

Jeremy Golding, MD

ACOG Practice Bulletin Number 109, December 2009.

PARATHYROID HORMONE, ELEVATED SERUM

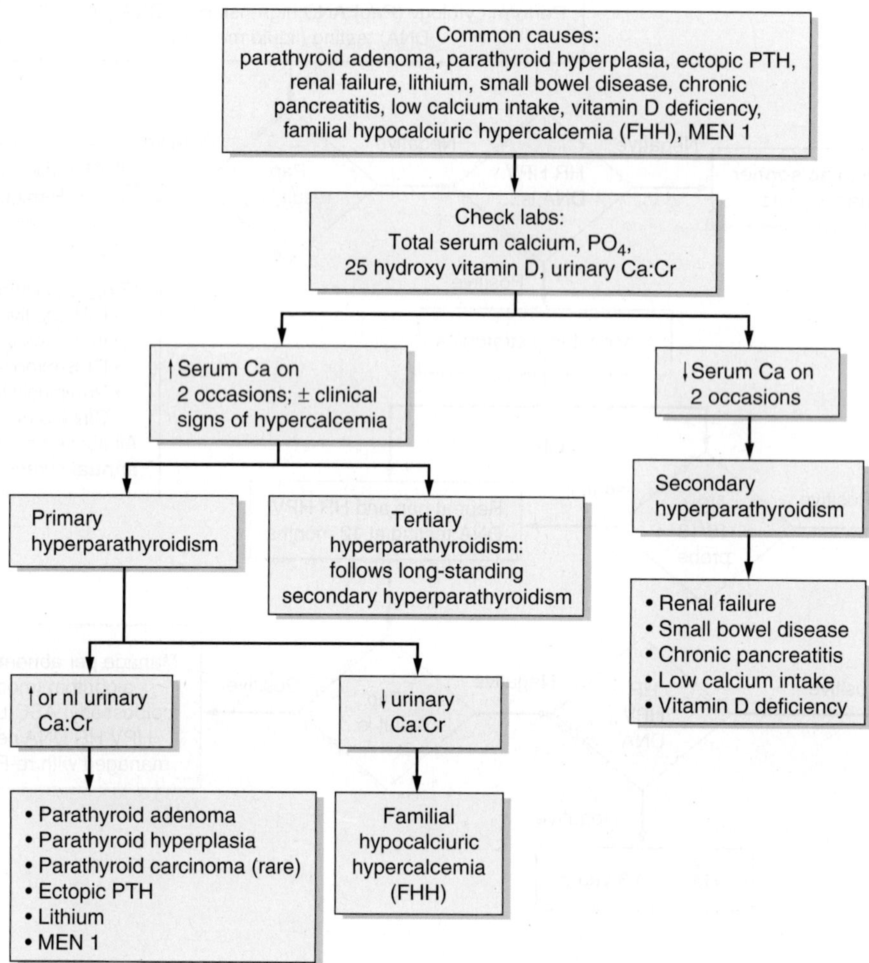

Andrew Gara, MD and Auguste Turnier, MD

JAMA. 2005;294(21):2700.

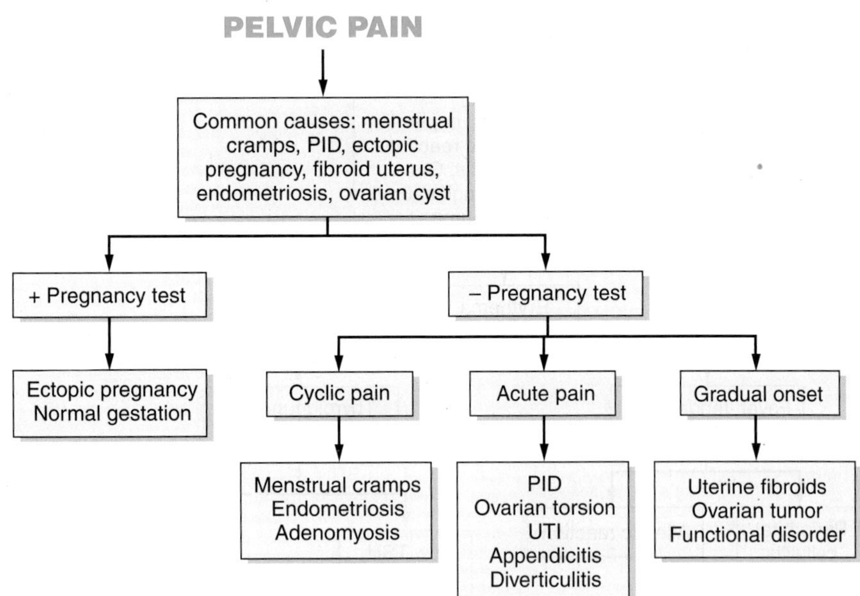

Robert A. Baldor, MD and Alan M. Ehrlich, MD

Am Fam Physician. 2008;77(11):1535–42.

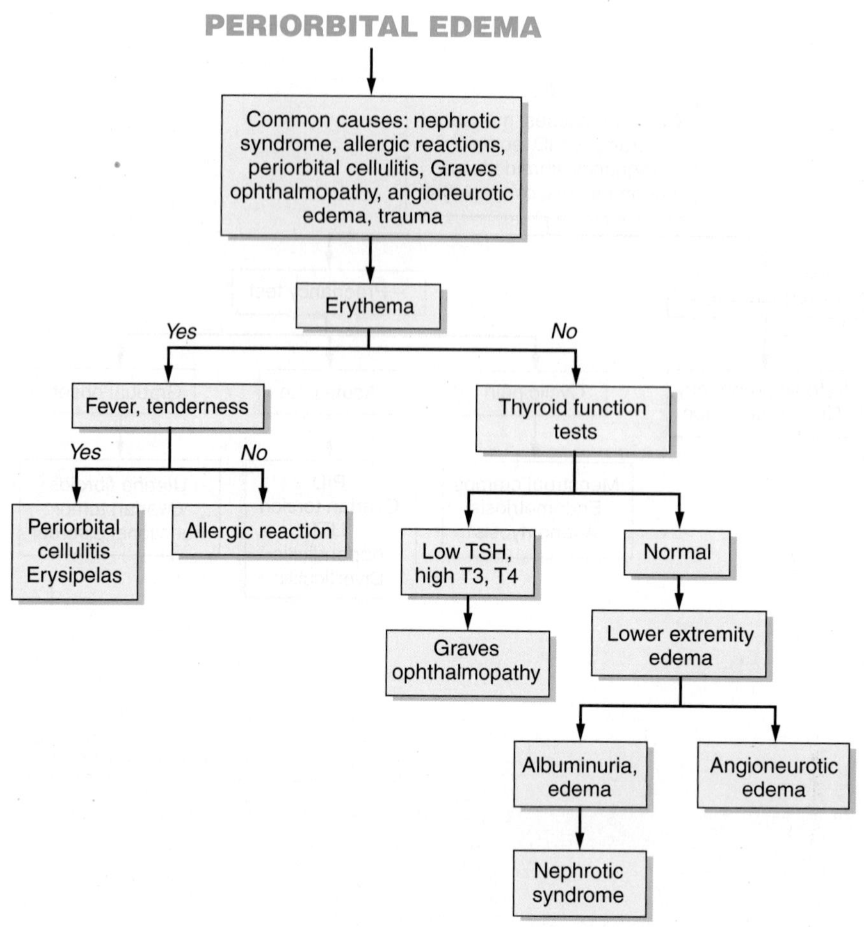

Robert A. Baldor, MD and Alan M. Ehrlich, MD

Infect Dis Clin North Am. 2007;21(2):393–408.

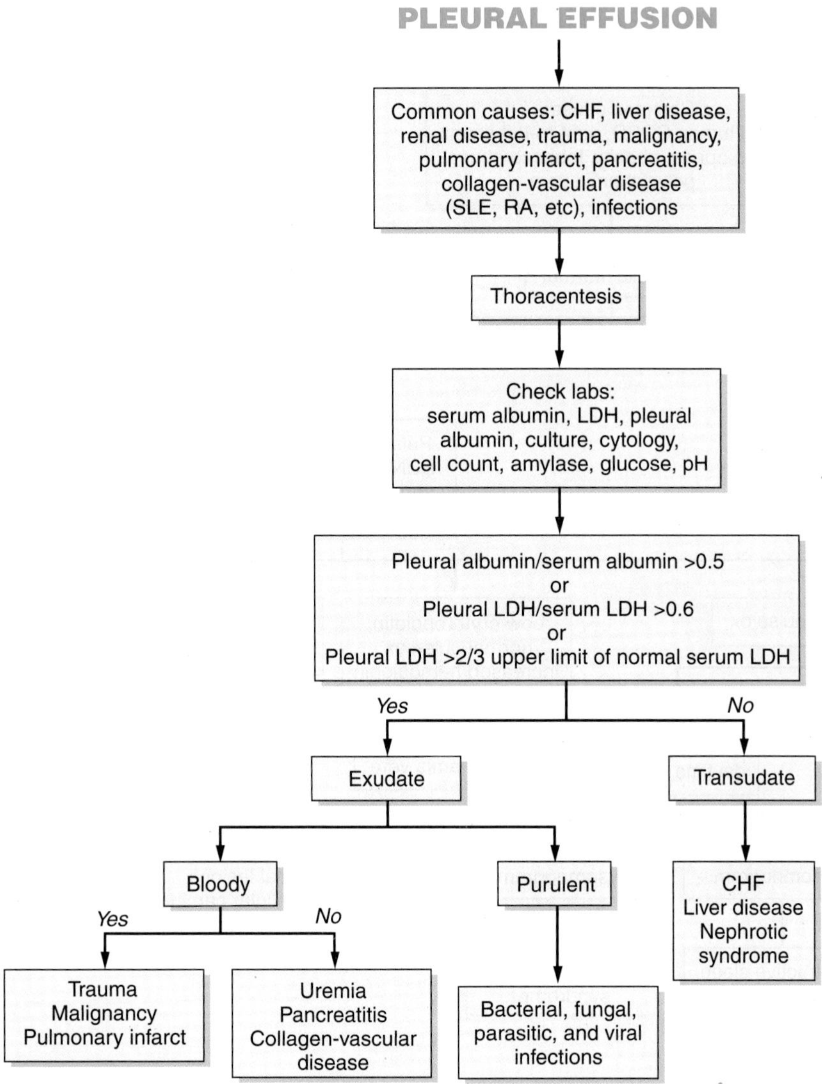

Robert A. Baldor, MD and Alan M. Ehrlich, MD

Am Fam Physician. 2006;73:1211–20.

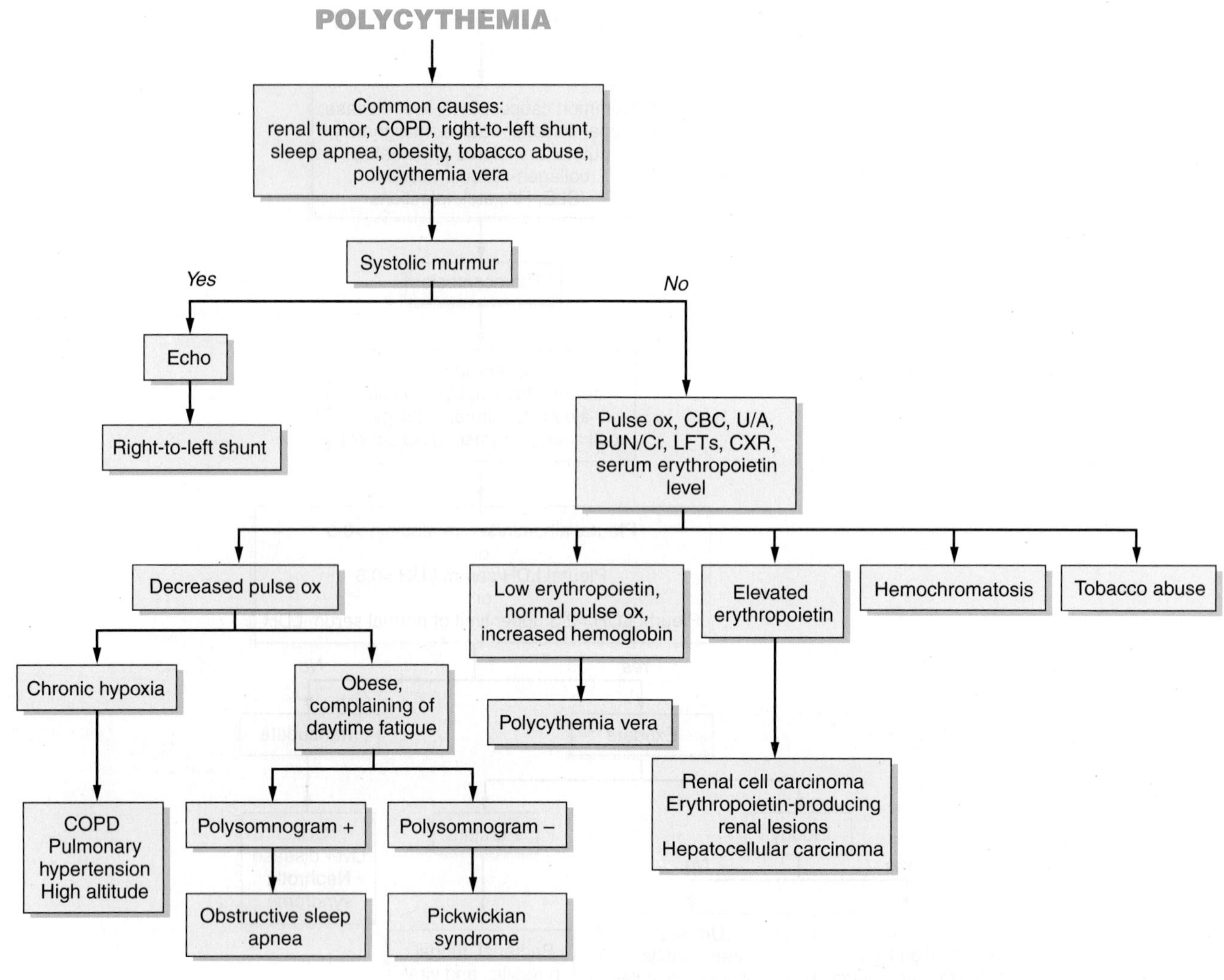
POLYCYTHEMIA
Common causes: renal tumor, COPD, right-to-left shunt, sleep apnea, obesity, tobacco abuse, polycythemia vera
Systolic murmur
Yes
No
Echo
Right-to-left shunt
Pulse ox, CBC, U/A, BUN/Cr, LFTs, CXR, serum erythropoietin level
Decreased pulse ox
Low erythropoietin, normal pulse ox, increased hemoglobin
Elevated erythropoietin
Hemochromatosis
Tobacco abuse
Chronic hypoxia
Obese, complaining of daytime fatigue
Polycythemia vera
Renal cell carcinoma
Erythropoietin-producing renal lesions
Hepatocellular carcinoma
COPD
Pulmonary hypertension
High altitude
Polysomnogram +
Polysomnogram –
Obstructive sleep apnea
Pickwickian syndrome

Robert A. Baldor, MD and Alan M. Ehrlich, MD

Mayo Clin Proc. 2005;80(7):923–36.

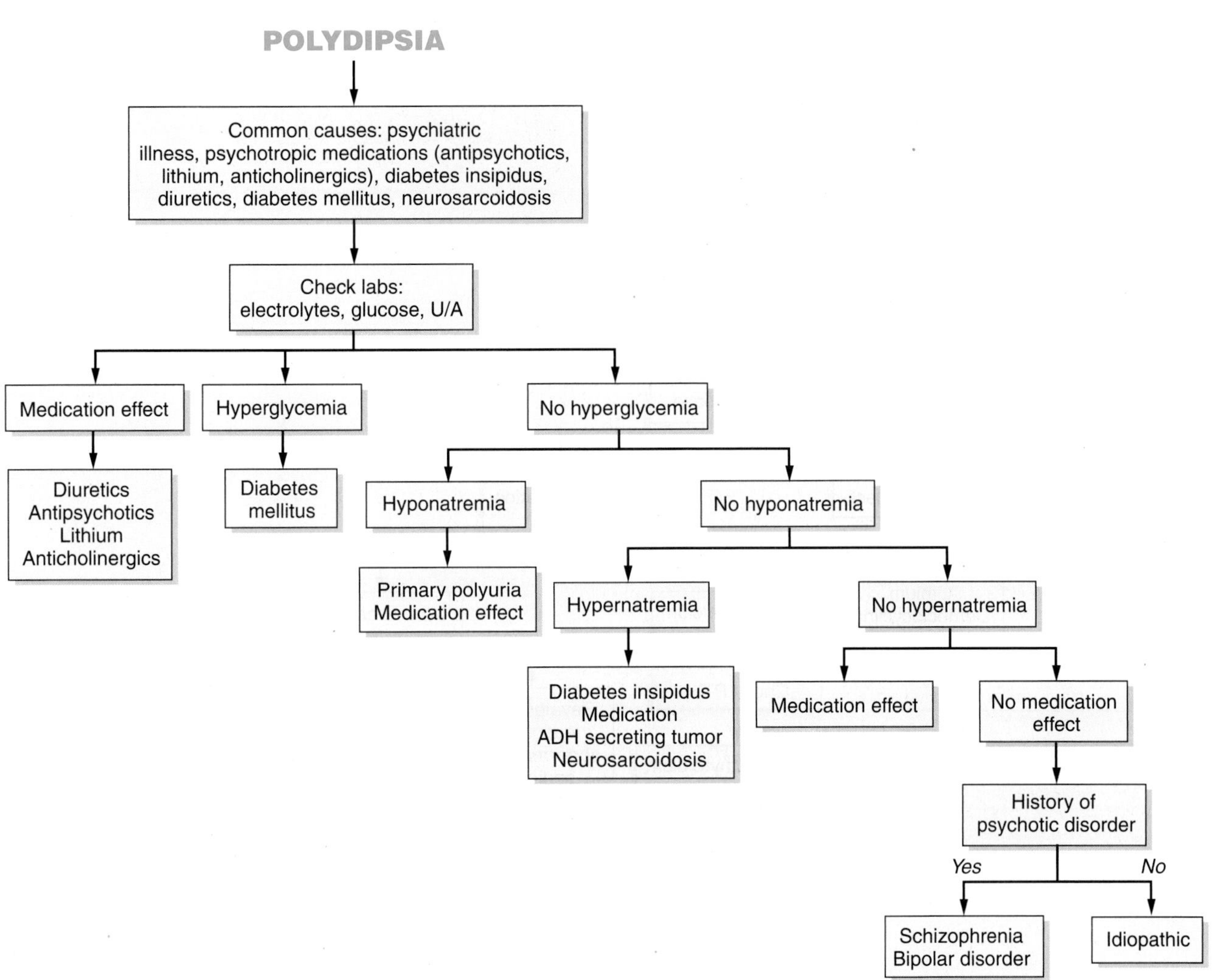

Robert A. Baldor, MD and Alan M. Ehrlich, MD

Nat Clin Proc Nephrol. 2007;3(7):374–82.

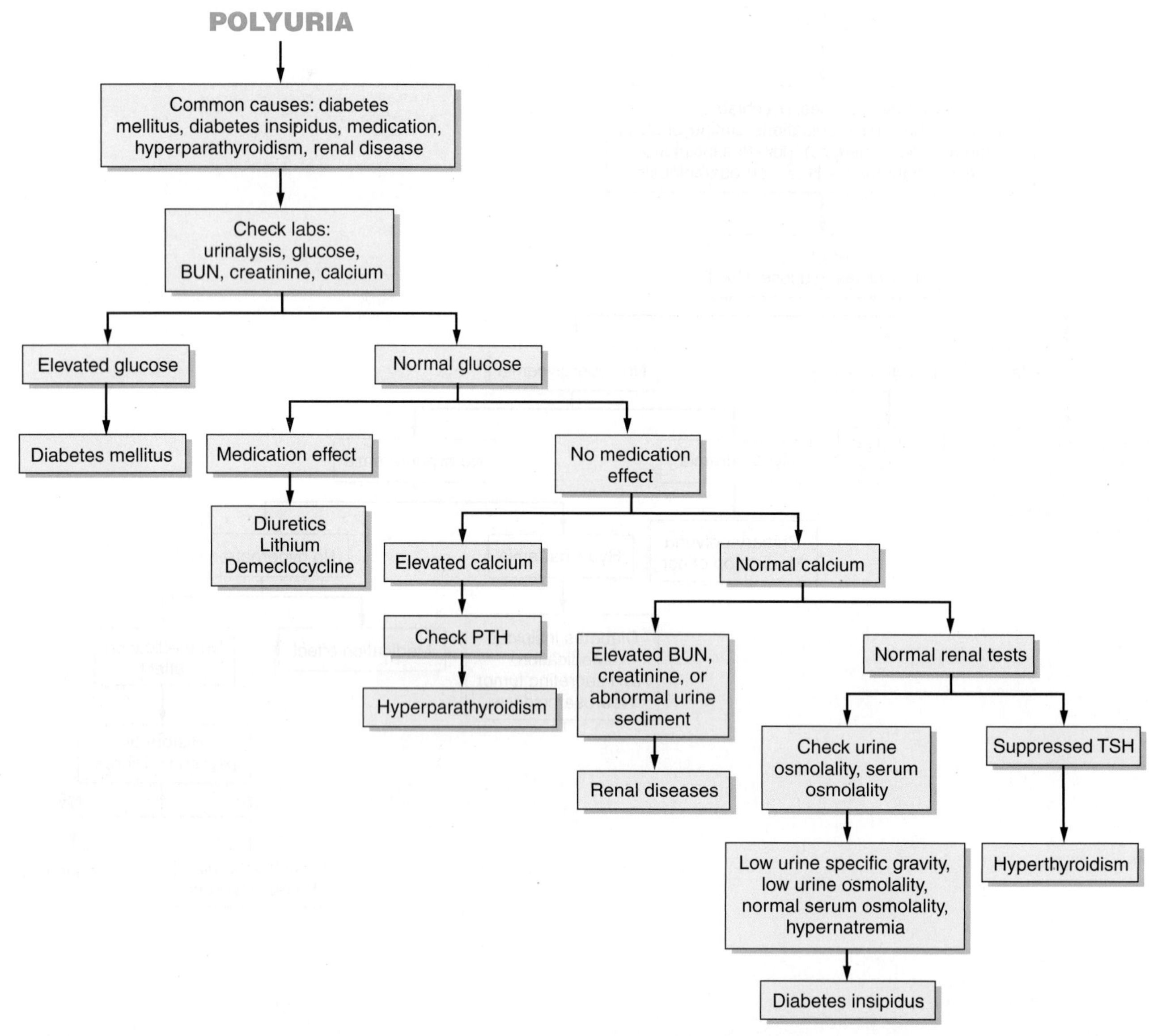

Robert A. Baldor, MD and Alan M. Ehrlich, MD

Nat Clin Pract Nephrol. 2008;4(8):426–35.

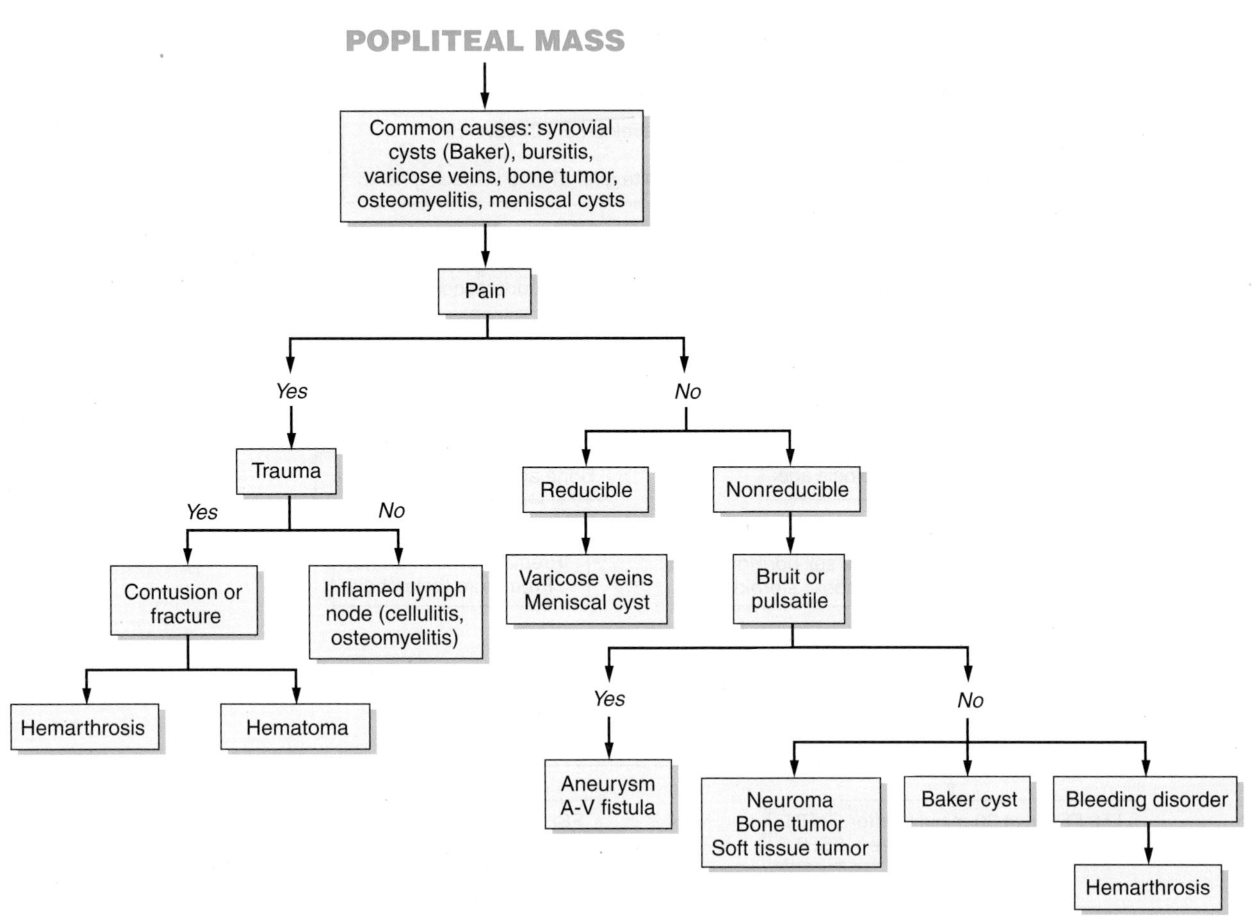

Robert A. Baldor, MD and Alan M. Ehrlich, MD

Am Fam Physician. 2003;68:917–22.

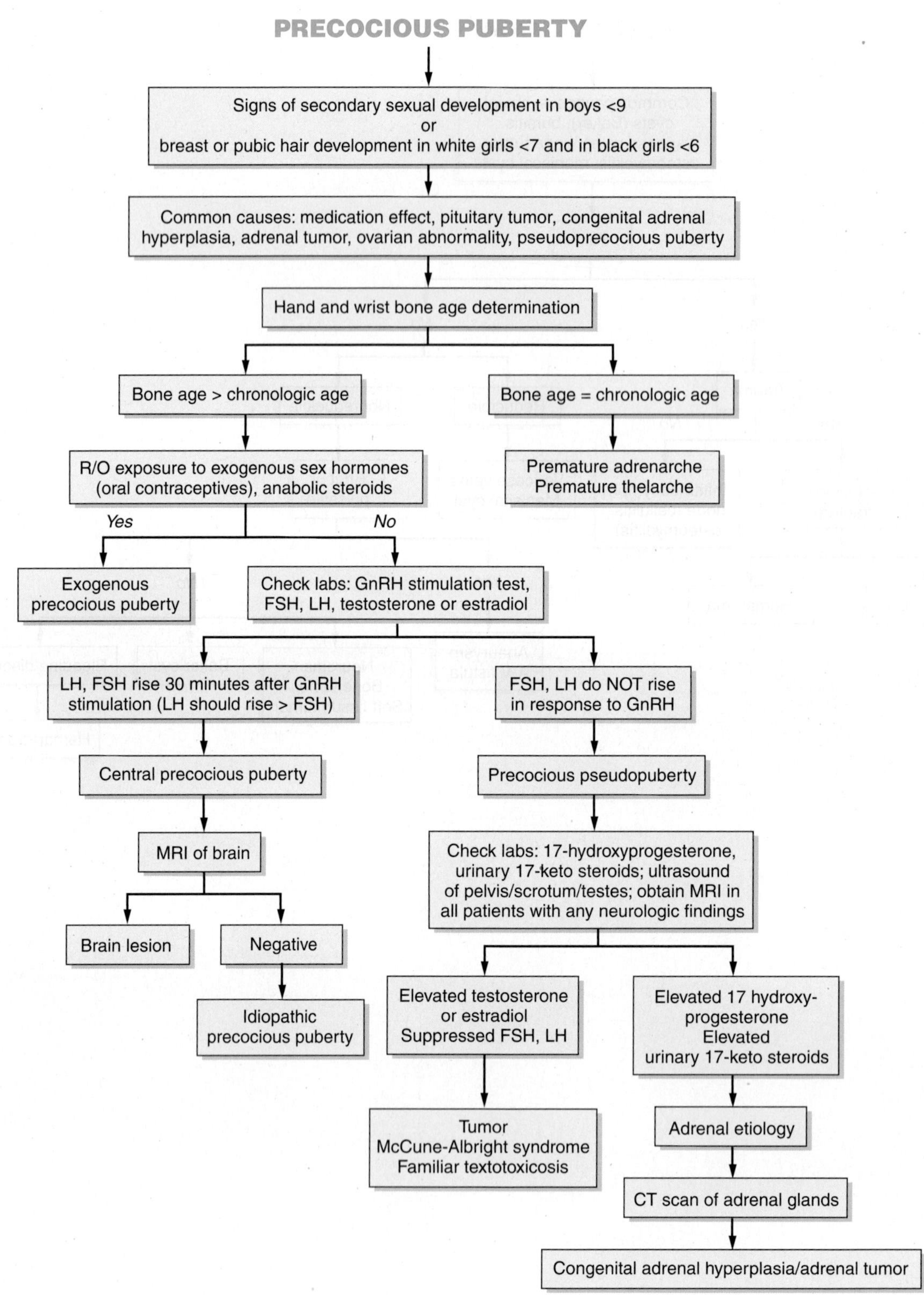
PRECOCIOUS PUBERTY
Signs of secondary sexual development in boys <9
or
breast or pubic hair development in white girls <7 and in black girls <6
Common causes: medication effect, pituitary tumor, congenital adrenal hyperplasia, adrenal tumor, ovarian abnormality, pseudoprecocious puberty
Hand and wrist bone age determination
Bone age > chronologic age
Bone age = chronologic age
R/O exposure to exogenous sex hormones (oral contraceptives), anabolic steroids
Premature adrenarche
Premature thelarche
Yes
No
Exogenous precocious puberty
Check labs: GnRH stimulation test, FSH, LH, testosterone or estradiol
LH, FSH rise 30 minutes after GnRH stimulation (LH should rise > FSH)
FSH, LH do NOT rise in response to GnRH
Central precocious puberty
Precocious pseudopuberty
MRI of brain
Check labs: 17-hydroxyprogesterone, urinary 17-keto steroids; ultrasound of pelvis/scrotum/testes; obtain MRI in all patients with any neurologic findings
Brain lesion
Negative
Idiopathic precocious puberty
Elevated testosterone or estradiol
Suppressed FSH, LH
Elevated 17 hydroxy-progesterone
Elevated urinary 17-keto steroids
Tumor
McCune-Albright syndrome
Familiar textotoxicosis
Adrenal etiology
CT scan of adrenal glands
Congenital adrenal hyperplasia/adrenal tumor

Robert A. Baldor, MD and Alan M. Ehrlich, MD

Am Fam Physician. 2008;78(5):597–604.

PREOPERATIVE EVALUATION OF NONCARDIAC SURGICAL PATIENT

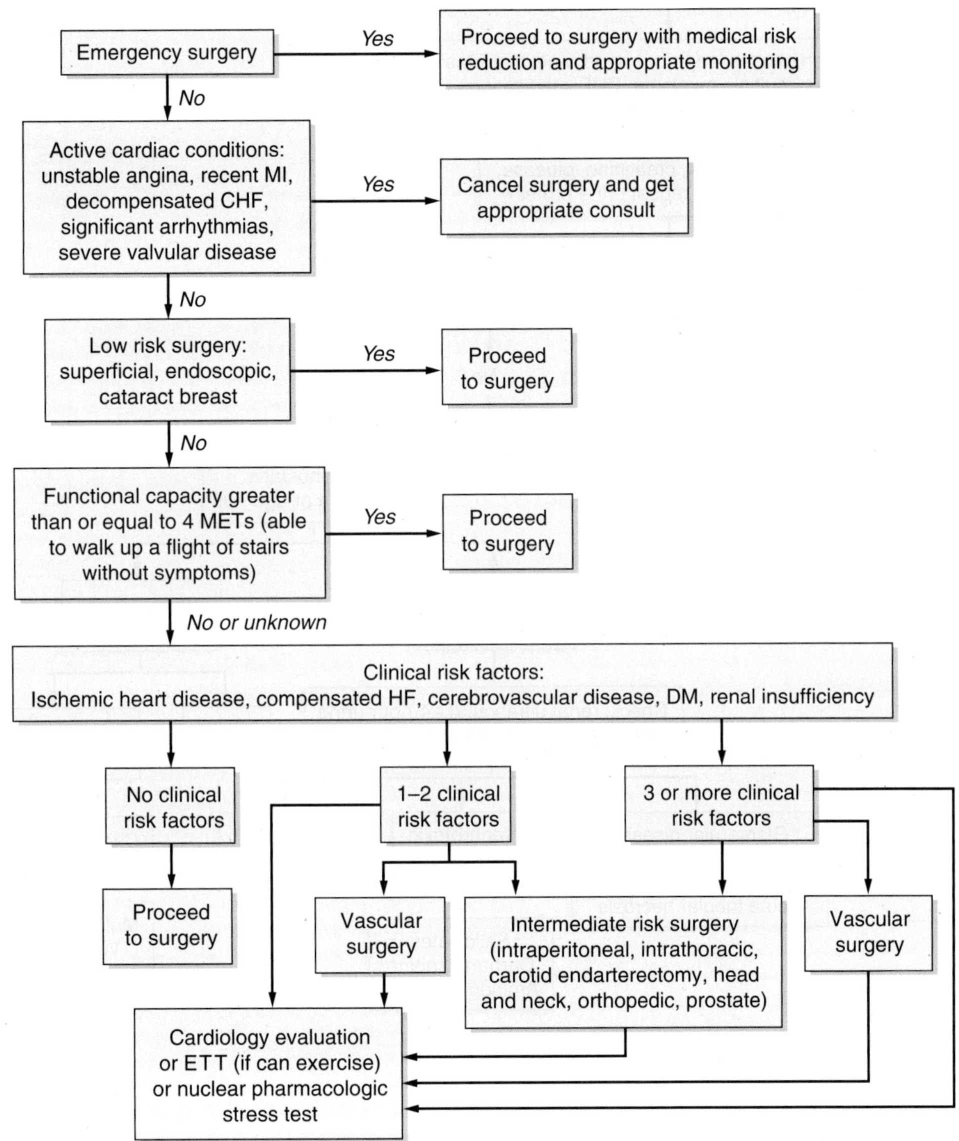

Drew Grimes, MD and Stacy Jones, MD

Circulation. 2007;116(17):e418–99.

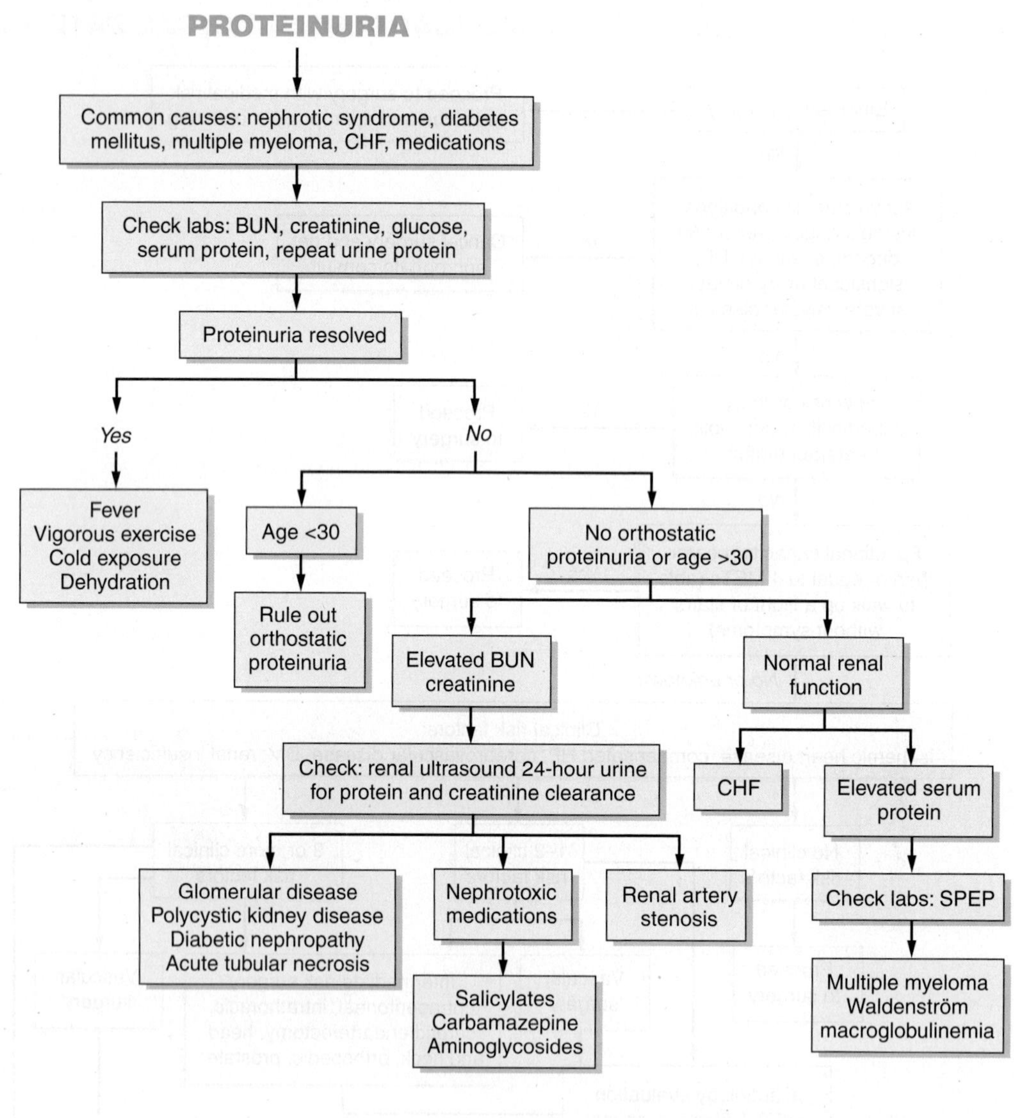
PROTEINURIA
Common causes: nephrotic syndrome, diabetes mellitus, multiple myeloma, CHF, medications
Check labs: BUN, creatinine, glucose, serum protein, repeat urine protein
Proteinuria resolved
Yes
No
Fever
Vigorous exercise
Cold exposure
Dehydration
Age <30
Rule out orthostatic proteinuria
No orthostatic proteinuria or age >30
Elevated BUN creatinine
Normal renal function
Check: renal ultrasound 24-hour urine for protein and creatinine clearance
CHF
Elevated serum protein
Glomerular disease
Polycystic kidney disease
Diabetic nephropathy
Acute tubular necrosis
Nephrotoxic medications
Renal artery stenosis
Check labs: SPEP
Salicylates
Carbamazepine
Aminoglycosides
Multiple myeloma
Waldenström macroglobulinemia

Robert A. Baldor, MD and Alan M. Ehrlich, MD

Am Fam Physician. 2000;62:1333–40.

PULMONARY EMBOLISM, DIAGNOSIS

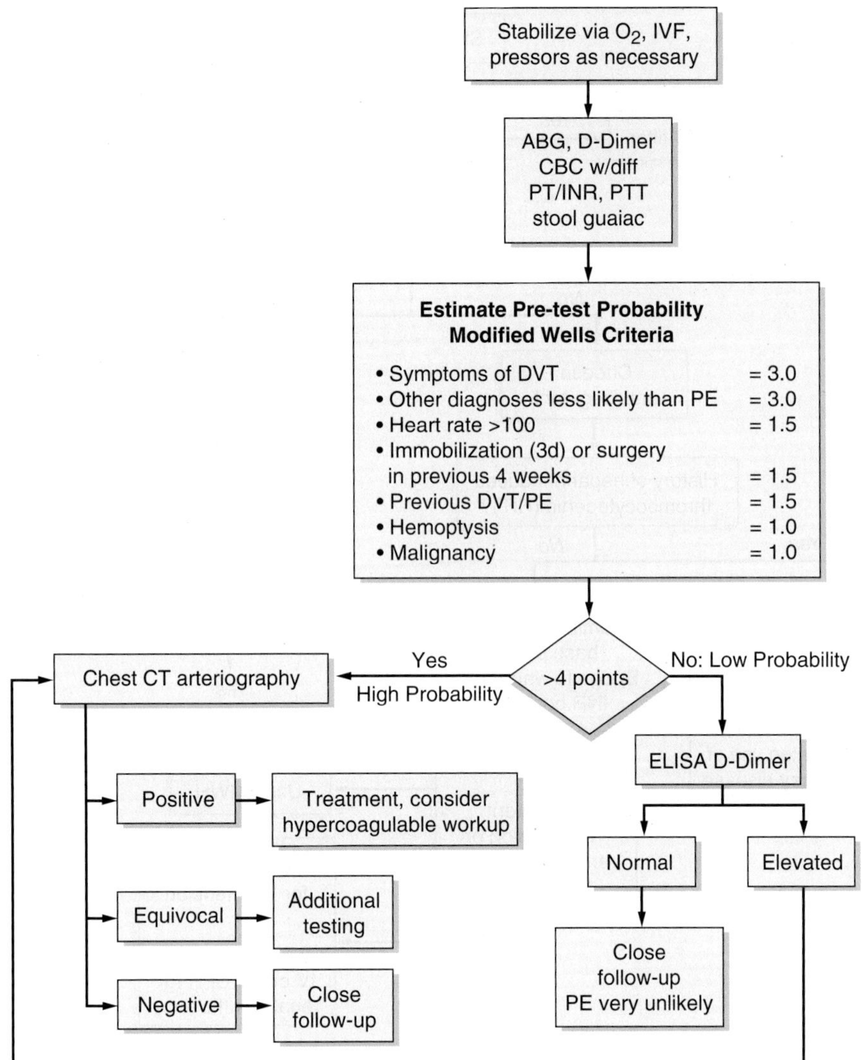

Parag Goyal, MD

Radiol Clin North Am. 2010;48(1):31–50.

PULMONARY EMBOLISM, TREATMENT

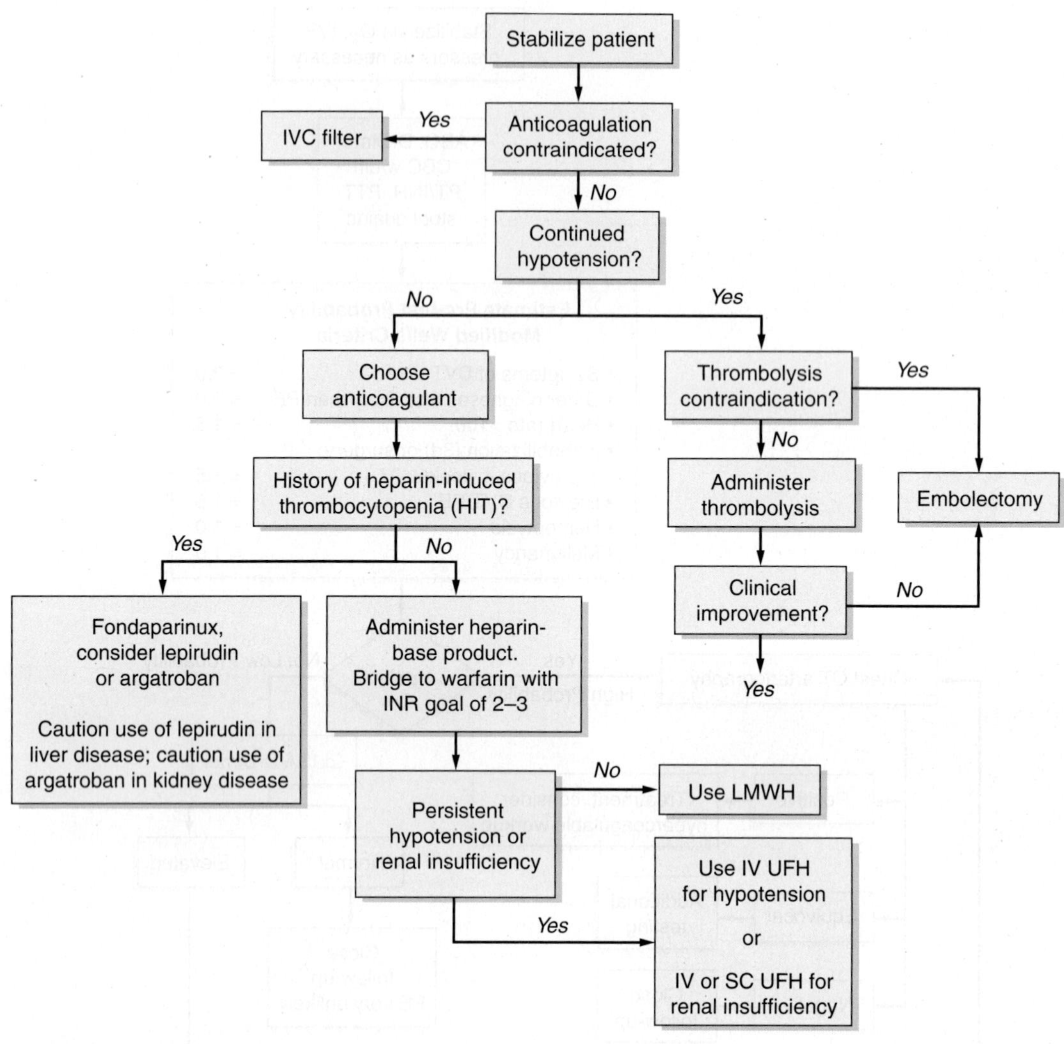

LMWH = Low molecular weight heparin
UFH = Unfractionated heparin

Parag Goyal, MD

NEJM. 2008;358(10):1037–52.

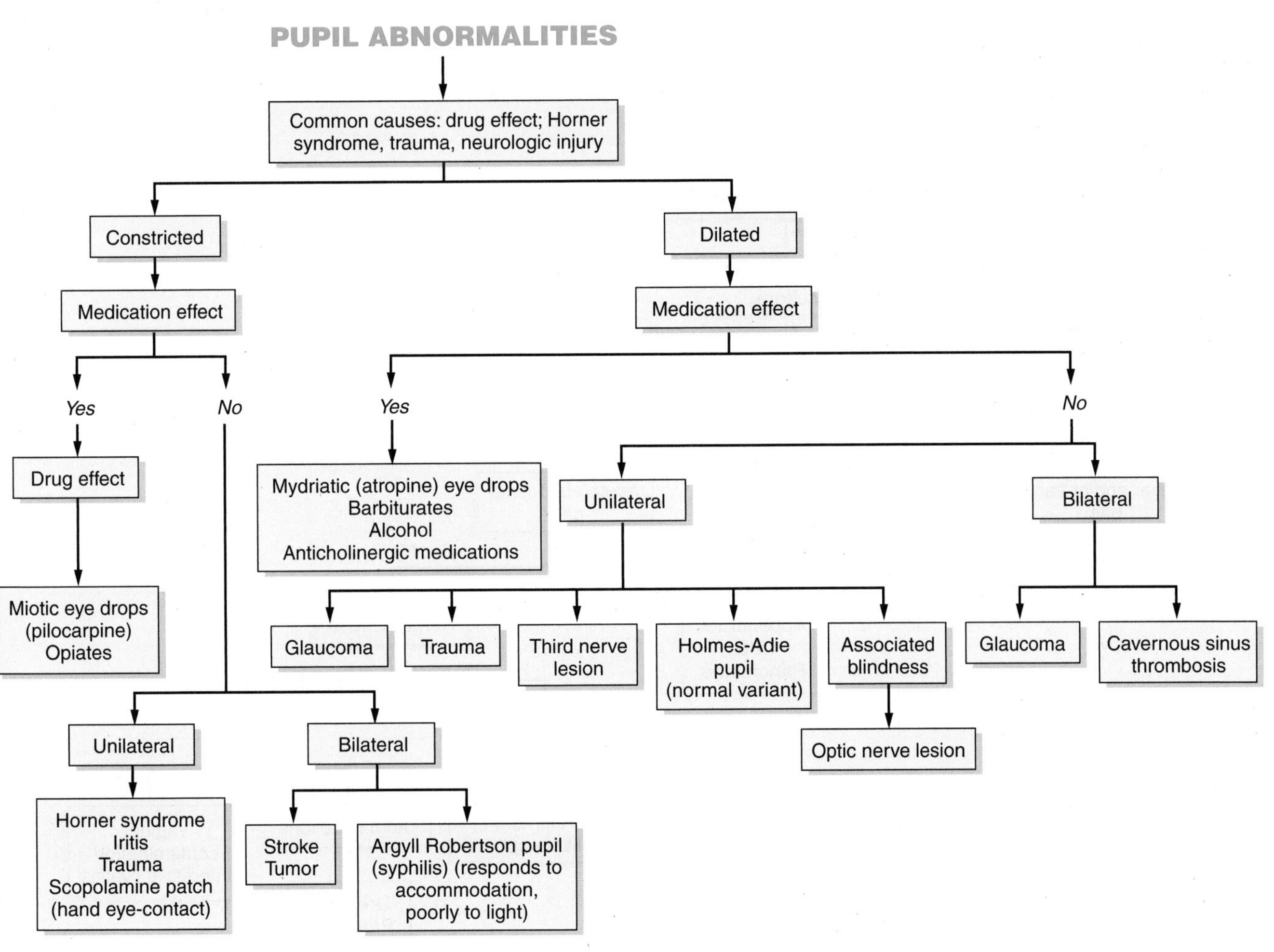

Robert A. Baldor, MD and Alan M. Ehrlich, MD

Vision Res. 2005;45(19):2549–63.

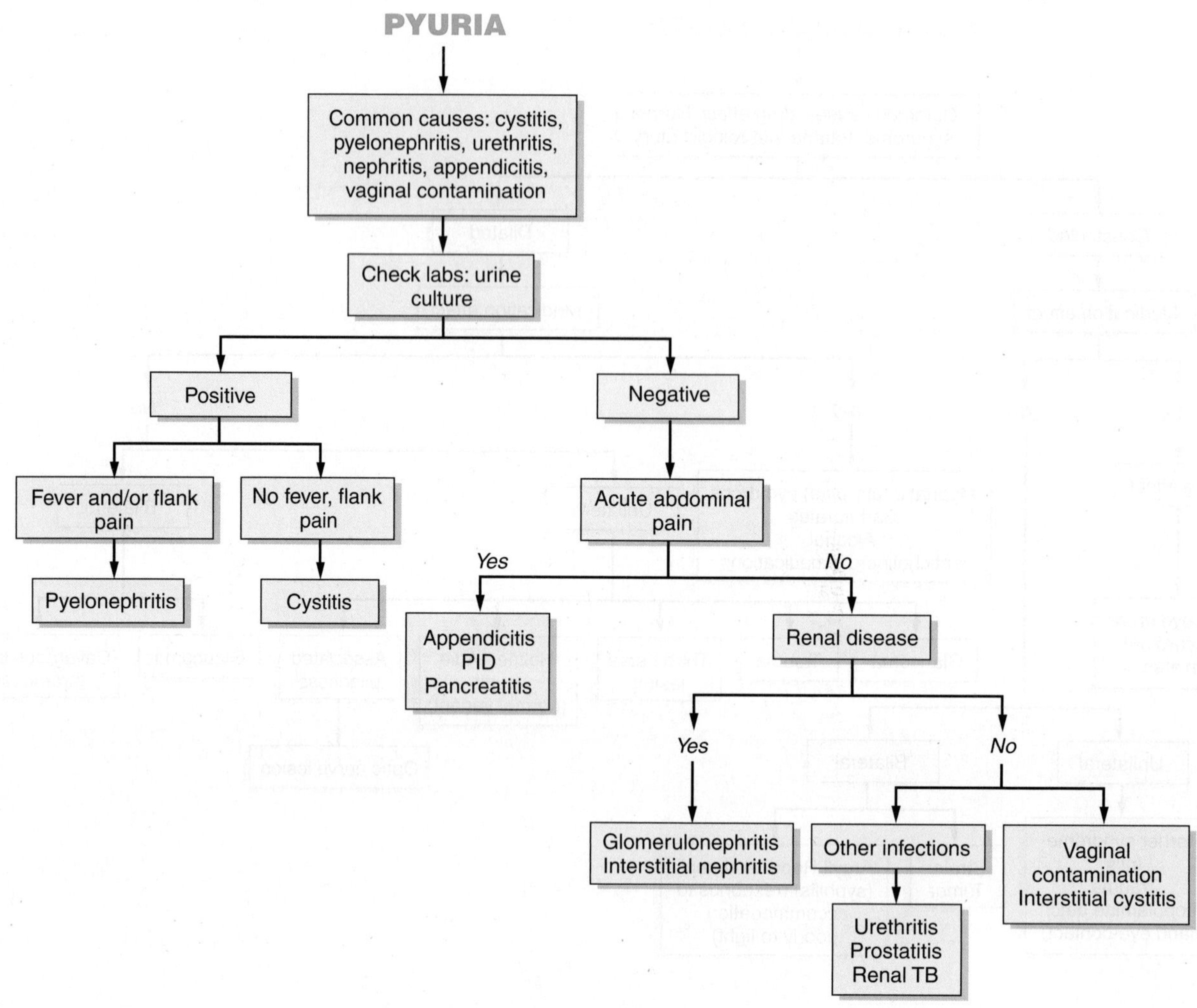

Robert A. Baldor, MD and Alan M. Ehrlich, MD

Am Fam Physician. 2005;71:1153–62.

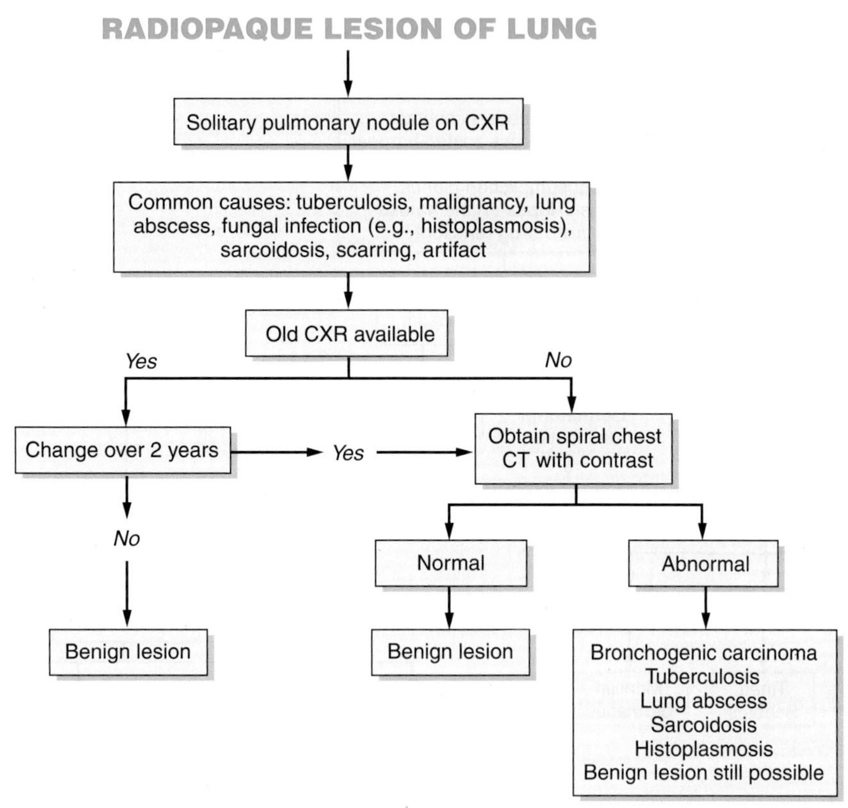

Robert A. Baldor, MD and Alan M. Ehrlich, MD

NEJM. 348(25):2535–42.

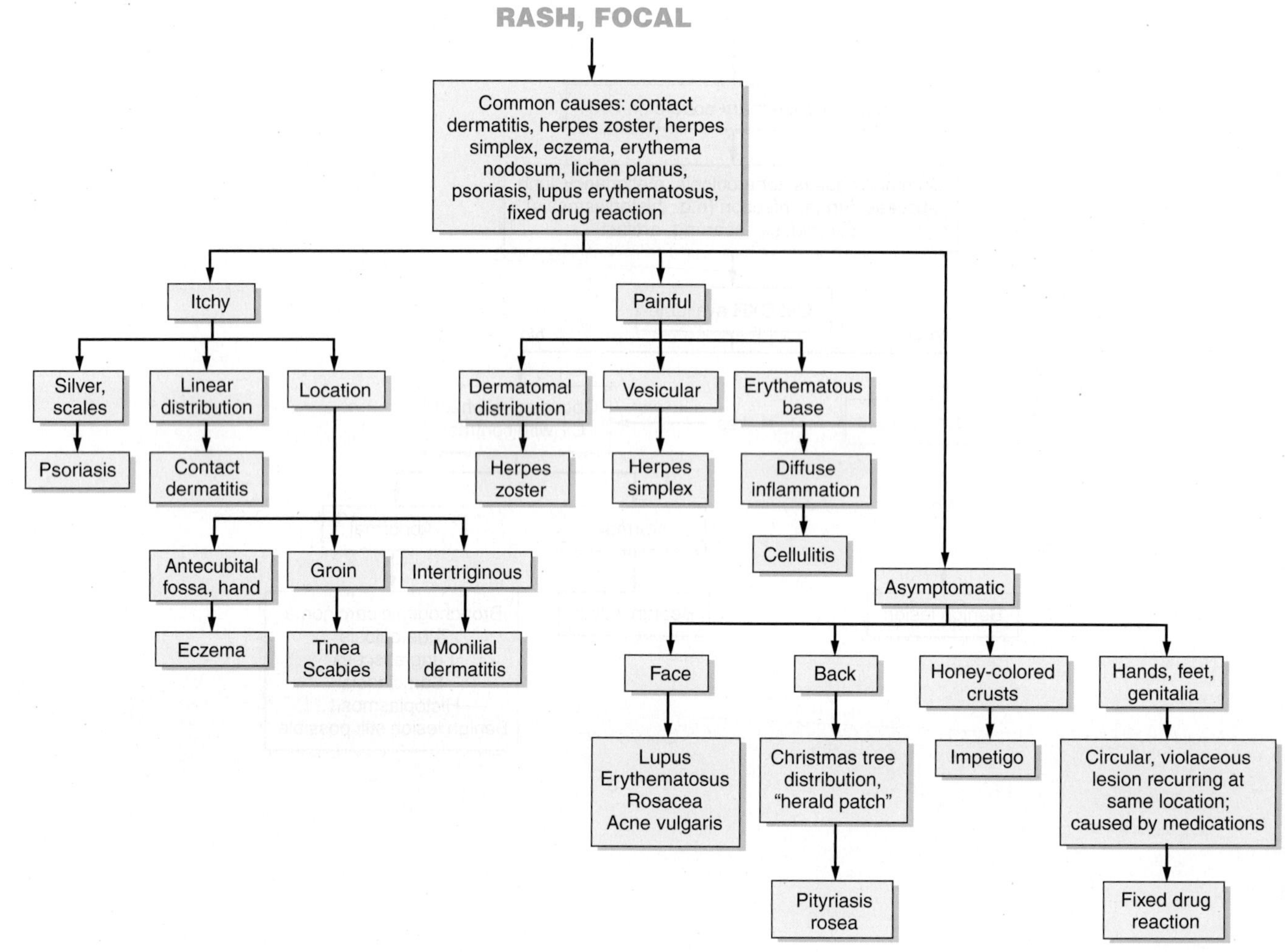

Robert A. Baldor, MD and Alan M. Ehrlich, MD

Arch Dermatol. 2001;137(1):25–9.

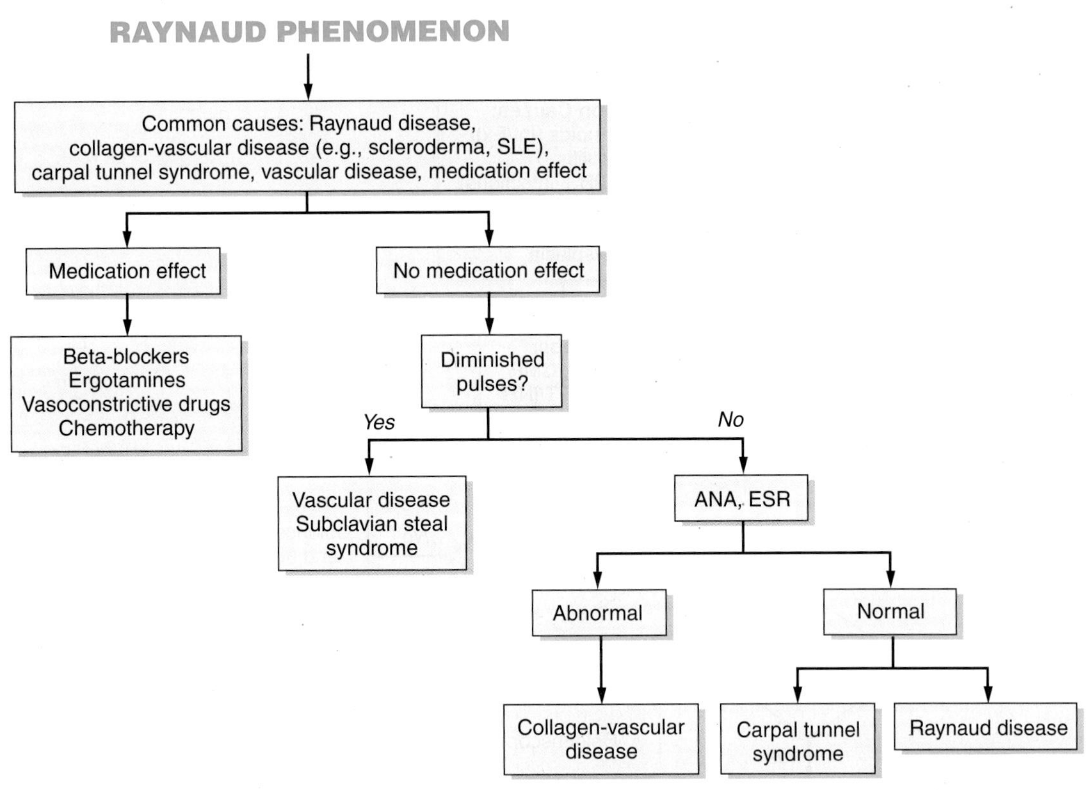

Robert A. Baldor, MD and Alan M. Ehrlich, MD

JFP. 2005;(54:6).

RECTAL BLEEDING AND HEMATOCHEZIA

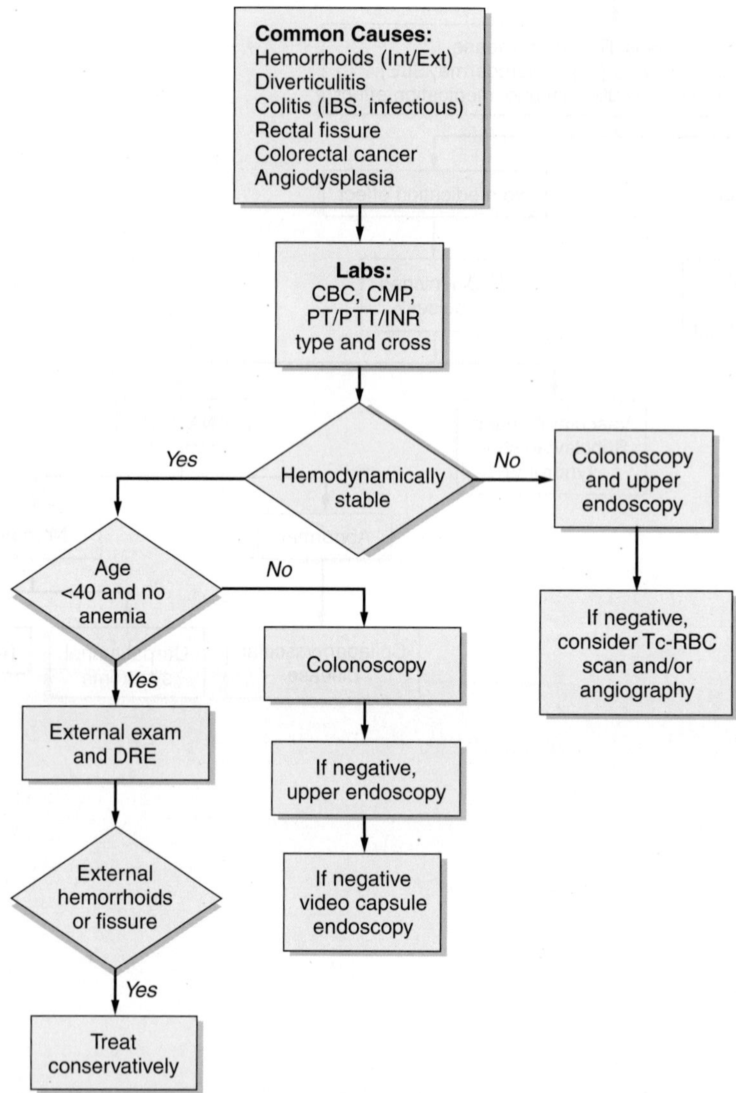

Mohammad Ansar Mughal, MD

Dis Colon Rectum. 2005;48(11):2010–24.

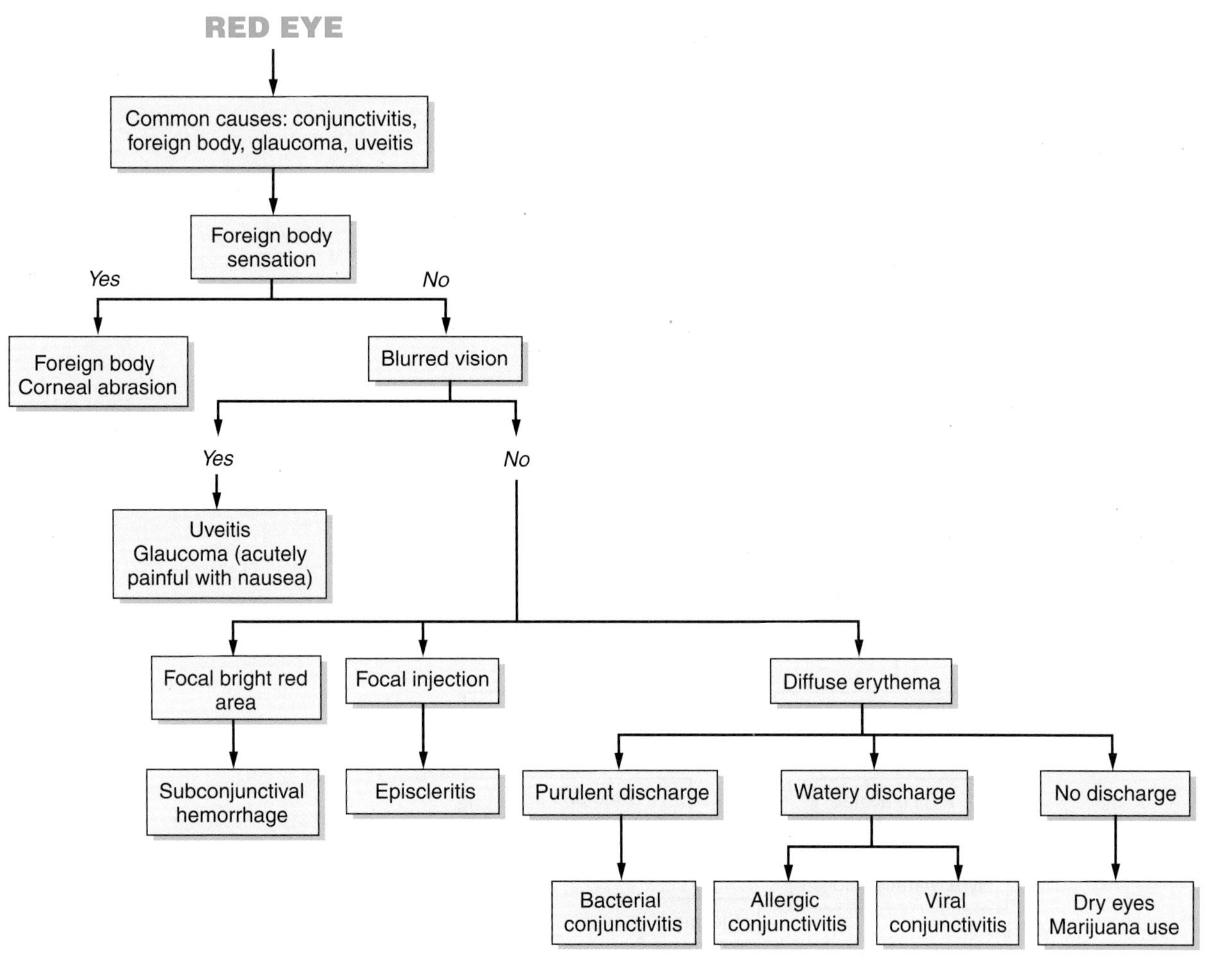

Robert A. Baldor, MD and Alan M. Ehrlich, MD

NEJM. 2000;343(5):345–51.

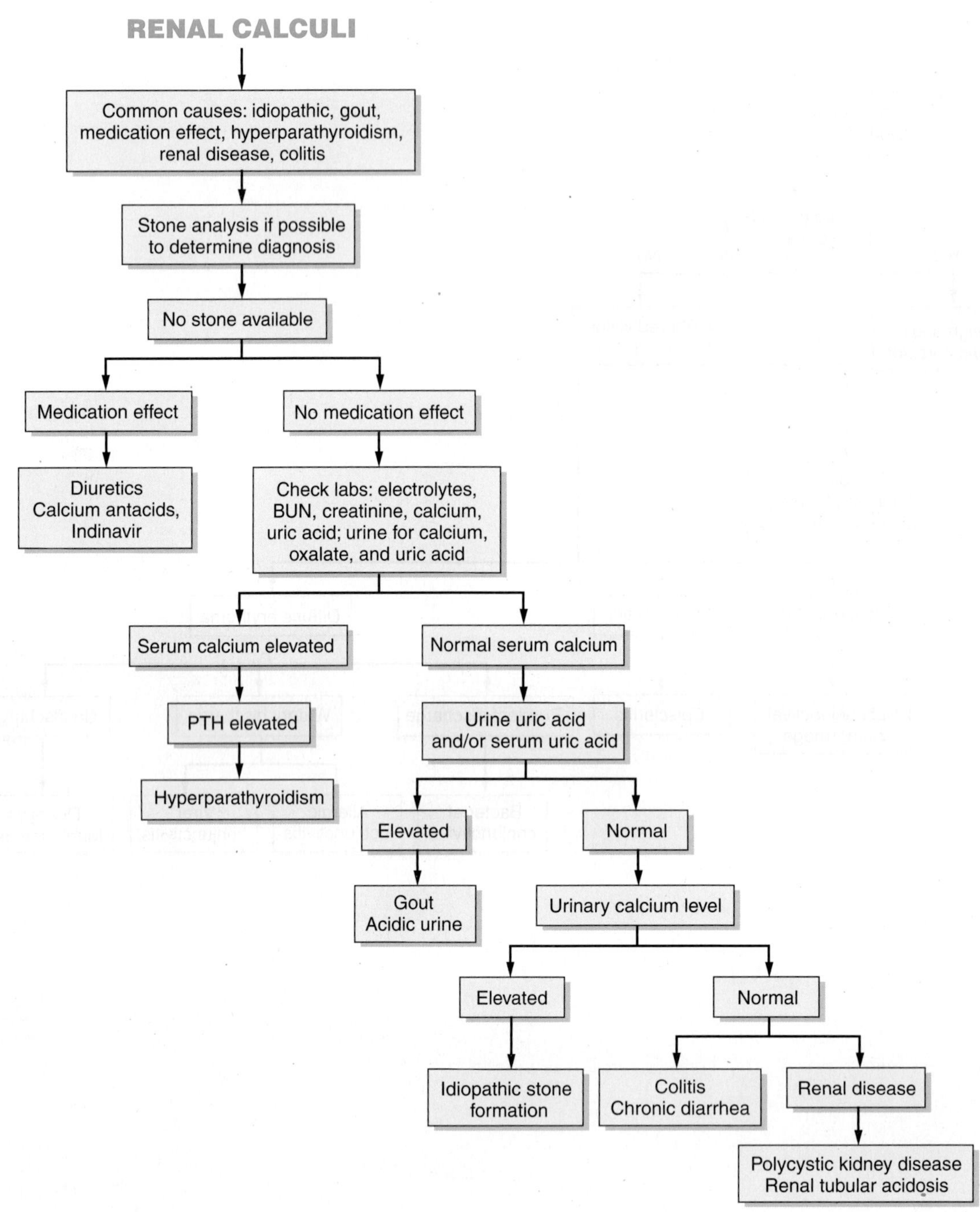
RENAL CALCULI
Common causes: idiopathic, gout, medication effect, hyperparathyroidism, renal disease, colitis
Stone analysis if possible to determine diagnosis
No stone available
Medication effect
No medication effect
Diuretics
Calcium antacids,
Indinavir
Check labs: electrolytes, BUN, creatinine, calcium, uric acid; urine for calcium, oxalate, and uric acid
Serum calcium elevated
Normal serum calcium
PTH elevated
Hyperparathyroidism
Urine uric acid and/or serum uric acid
Elevated
Normal
Gout
Acidic urine
Urinary calcium level
Elevated
Normal
Idiopathic stone formation
Colitis
Chronic diarrhea
Renal disease
Polycystic kidney disease
Renal tubular acidosis

Robert A. Baldor, MD and Alan M. Ehrlich, MD

Prim Care. 2008;35(2):369–91.

RENAL FAILURE, ACUTE

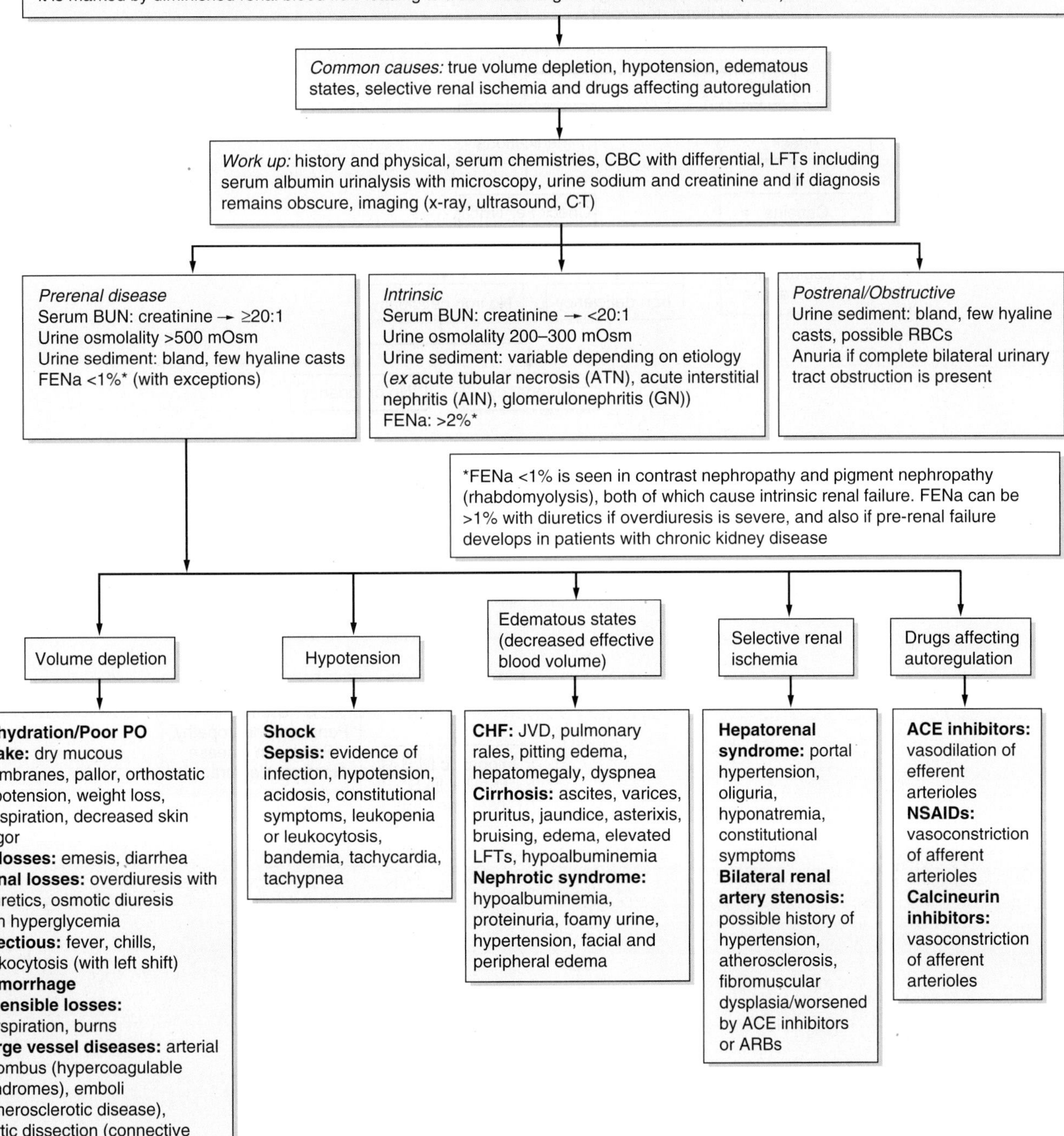

Acute kidney injury (AKI, previously called acute renal failure) is an acute loss of kidney function over days to weeks resulting in an inability to excrete nitrogenous wastes and creatinine. Patients are often asymptomatic, and are recognized by an increase in serum creatinine level (>0.5 mg/dL from baseline). Prerenal disease (PD) is one category of AKI where the injury occurs outside the nephron; it is marked by diminished renal blood flow leading to a decrease in glomerular filtration rate (GFR).
Common causes: true volume depletion, hypotension, edematous states, selective renal ischemia and drugs affecting autoregulation
Work up: history and physical, serum chemistries, CBC with differential, LFTs including serum albumin urinalysis with microscopy, urine sodium and creatinine and if diagnosis remains obscure, imaging (x-ray, ultrasound, CT)
Prerenal disease
Serum BUN: creatinine → ≥20:1
Urine osmolality >500 mOsm
Urine sediment: bland, few hyaline casts
FENa <1%* (with exceptions)
Intrinsic
Serum BUN: creatinine → <20:1
Urine osmolality 200–300 mOsm
Urine sediment: variable depending on etiology (*ex* acute tubular necrosis (ATN), acute interstitial nephritis (AIN), glomerulonephritis (GN))
FENa: >2%*
Postrenal/Obstructive
Urine sediment: bland, few hyaline casts, possible RBCs
Anuria if complete bilateral urinary tract obstruction is present
*FENa <1% is seen in contrast nephropathy and pigment nephropathy (rhabdomyolysis), both of which cause intrinsic renal failure. FENa can be >1% with diuretics if overdiuresis is severe, and also if pre-renal failure develops in patients with chronic kidney disease
Volume depletion
Hypotension
Edematous states (decreased effective blood volume)
Selective renal ischemia
Drugs affecting autoregulation
Dehydration/Poor PO intake: dry mucous membranes, pallor, orthostatic hypotension, weight loss, perspiration, decreased skin turgor
GI losses: emesis, diarrhea
Renal losses: overdiuresis with Diuretics, osmotic diuresis with hyperglycemia
Infectious: fever, chills, leukocytosis (with left shift)
Hemorrhage
Insensible losses: perspiration, burns
Large vessel diseases: arterial thrombus (hypercoagulable syndromes), emboli (atherosclerotic disease), aortic dissection (connective tissue disease, trauma)
Shock
Sepsis: evidence of infection, hypotension, acidosis, constitutional symptoms, leukopenia or leukocytosis, bandemia, tachycardia, tachypnea
CHF: JVD, pulmonary rales, pitting edema, hepatomegaly, dyspnea
Cirrhosis: ascites, varices, pruritus, jaundice, asterixis, bruising, edema, elevated LFTs, hypoalbuminemia
Nephrotic syndrome: hypoalbuminemia, proteinuria, foamy urine, hypertension, facial and peripheral edema
Hepatorenal syndrome: portal hypertension, oliguria, hyponatremia, constitutional symptoms
Bilateral renal artery stenosis: possible history of hypertension, atherosclerosis, fibromuscular dysplasia/worsened by ACE inhibitors or ARBs
ACE inhibitors: vasodilation of efferent arterioles
NSAIDs: vasoconstriction of afferent arterioles
Calcineurin inhibitors: vasoconstriction of afferent arterioles

Krunal Patel, MD and Dagmar Klinger, MD

Am Fam Physician. 2005;72(9):1739–47.

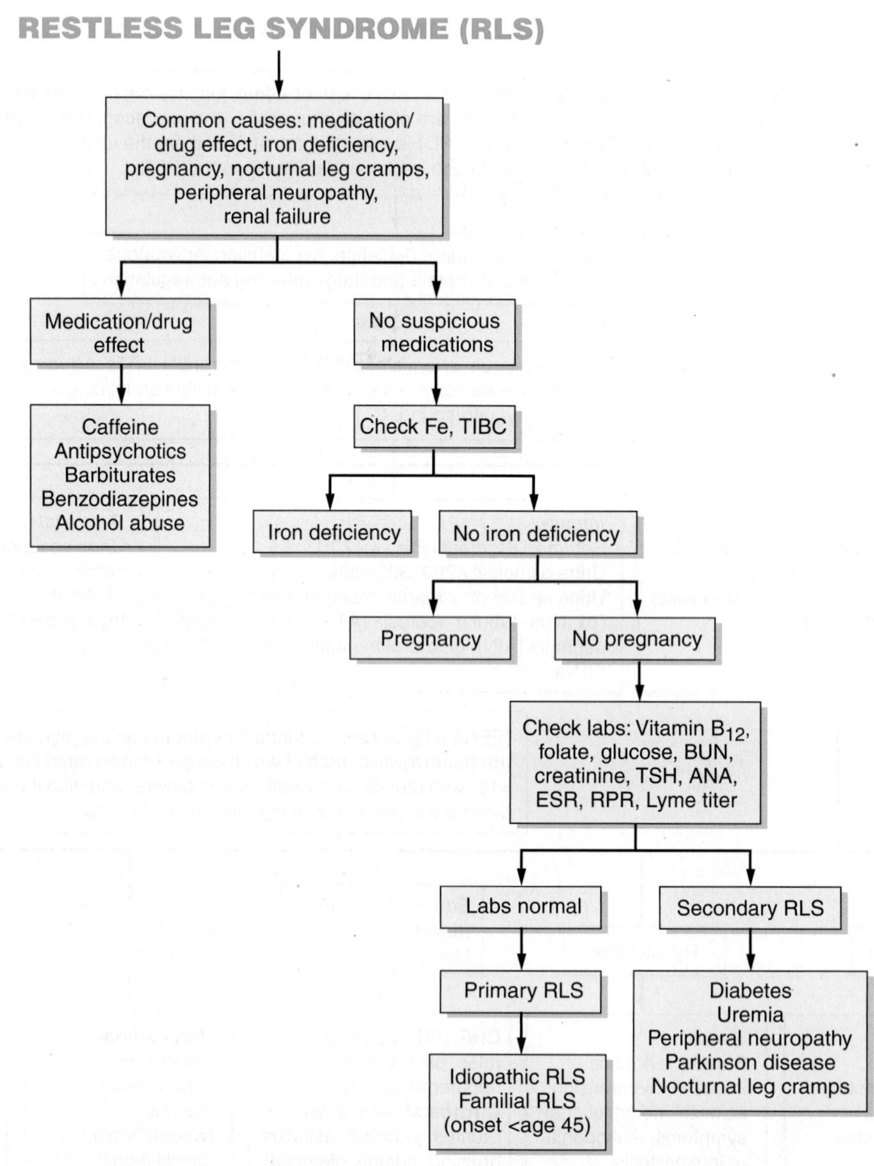

Robert A. Baldor, MD and Alan M. Ehrlich, MD

Am Fam Physician. 2000;62:108–14.

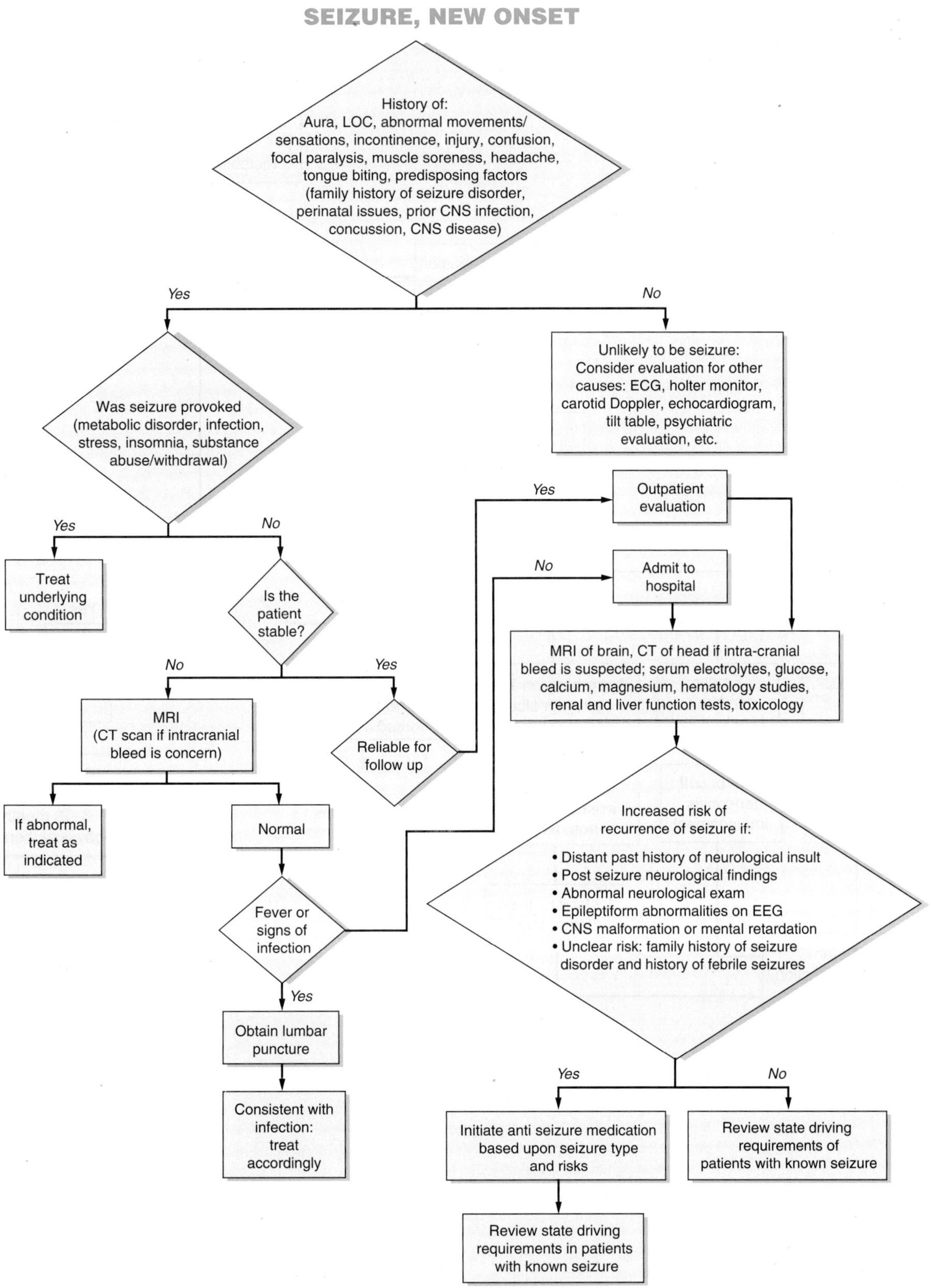

Neepa Patel, MD and Ioannis Karakis, MD

N Engl J Med. 2003;349:1257.

SHOULDER PAIN

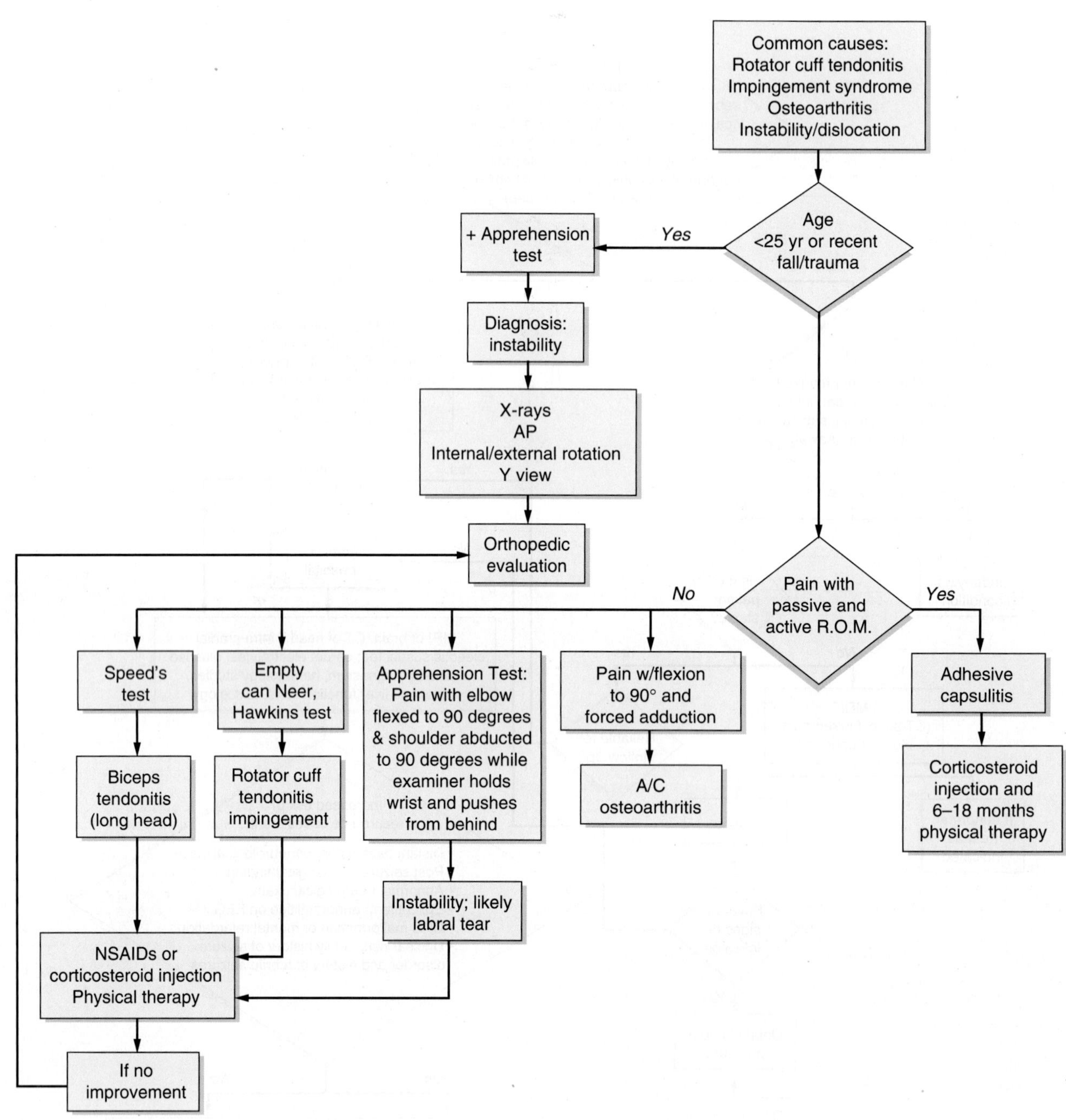

David W. Kruse, MD and Murat Mardirossian, MD

Am Fam Physician. 2000;61:3079–89.

SICKLE CELL ANEMIA, ACUTE COMPLICATIONS

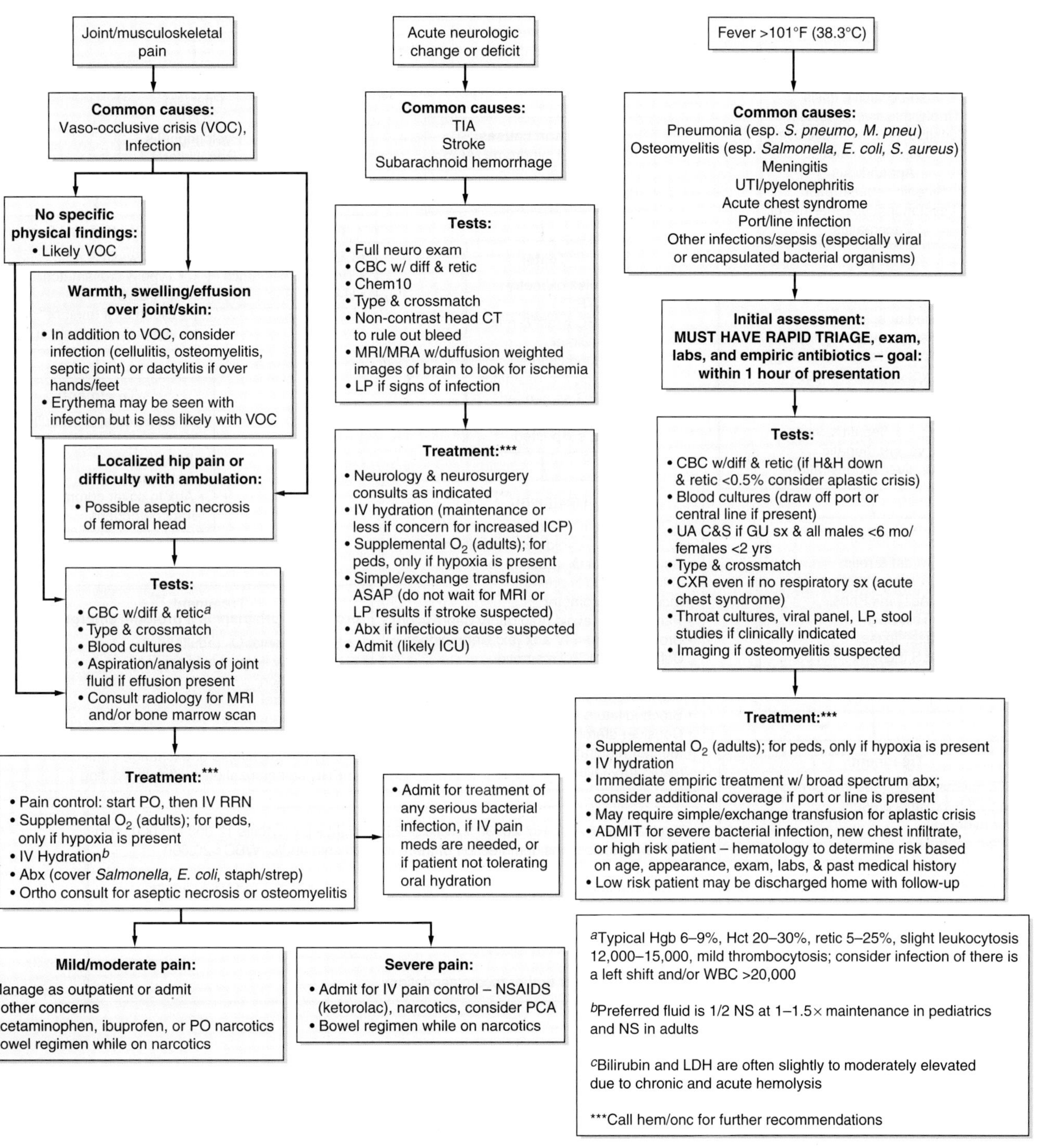

Joint/musculoskeletal pain
Common causes: Vaso-occlusive crisis (VOC), Infection
No specific physical findings:
• Likely VOC
Warmth, swelling/effusion over joint/skin:
• In addition to VOC, consider infection (cellulitis, osteomyelitis, septic joint) or dactylitis if over hands/feet
• Erythema may be seen with infection but is less likely with VOC
Localized hip pain or difficulty with ambulation:
• Possible aseptic necrosis of femoral head
Tests:
• CBC w/diff & retic[a]
• Type & crossmatch
• Blood cultures
• Aspiration/analysis of joint fluid if effusion present
• Consult radiology for MRI and/or bone marrow scan
Treatment:***
• Pain control: start PO, then IV RRN
• Supplemental O_2 (adults); for peds, only if hypoxia is present
• IV Hydration[b]
• Abx (cover *Salmonella*, *E. coli*, staph/strep)
• Ortho consult for aseptic necrosis or osteomyelitis
• Admit for treatment of any serious bacterial infection, if IV pain meds are needed, or if patient not tolerating oral hydration
Mild/moderate pain:
• Manage as outpatient or admit if other concerns
• Acetaminophen, ibuprofen, or PO narcotics
• Bowel regimen while on narcotics
Severe pain:
• Admit for IV pain control – NSAIDS (ketorolac), narcotics, consider PCA
• Bowel regimen while on narcotics
Acute neurologic change or deficit
Common causes: TIA, Stroke, Subarachnoid hemorrhage
Tests:
• Full neuro exam
• CBC w/ diff & retic
• Chem10
• Type & crossmatch
• Non-contrast head CT to rule out bleed
• MRI/MRA w/duffusion weighted images of brain to look for ischemia
• LP if signs of infection
Treatment:***
• Neurology & neurosurgery consults as indicated
• IV hydration (maintenance or less if concern for increased ICP)
• Supplemental O_2 (adults); for peds, only if hypoxia is present
• Simple/exchange transfusion ASAP (do not wait for MRI or LP results if stroke suspected)
• Abx if infectious cause suspected
• Admit (likely ICU)
Fever >101°F (38.3°C)
Common causes: Pneumonia (esp. *S. pneumo, M. pneu*), Osteomyelitis (esp. *Salmonella, E. coli, S. aureus*), Meningitis, UTI/pyelonephritis, Acute chest syndrome, Port/line infection, Other infections/sepsis (especially viral or encapsulated bacterial organisms)
Initial assessment: MUST HAVE RAPID TRIAGE, exam, labs, and empiric antibiotics – goal: within 1 hour of presentation
Tests:
• CBC w/diff & retic (if H&H down & retic <0.5% consider aplastic crisis)
• Blood cultures (draw off port or central line if present)
• UA C&S if GU sx & all males <6 mo/ females <2 yrs
• Type & crossmatch
• CXR even if no respiratory sx (acute chest syndrome)
• Throat cultures, viral panel, LP, stool studies if clinically indicated
• Imaging if osteomyelitis suspected
Treatment:***
• Supplemental O_2 (adults); for peds, only if hypoxia is present
• IV hydration
• Immediate empiric treatment w/ broad spectrum abx; consider additional coverage if port or line is present
• May require simple/exchange transfusion for aplastic crisis
• ADMIT for severe bacterial infection, new chest infiltrate, or high risk patient – hematology to determine risk based on age, appearance, exam, labs, & past medical history
• Low risk patient may be discharged home with follow-up
[a]Typical Hgb 6–9%, Hct 20–30%, retic 5–25%, slight leukocytosis 12,000–15,000, mild thrombocytosis; consider infection of there is a left shift and/or WBC >20,000
[b]Preferred fluid is 1/2 NS at 1–1.5× maintenance in pediatrics and NS in adults
[c]Bilirubin and LDH are often slightly to moderately elevated due to chronic and acute hemolysis
***Call hem/onc for further recommendations

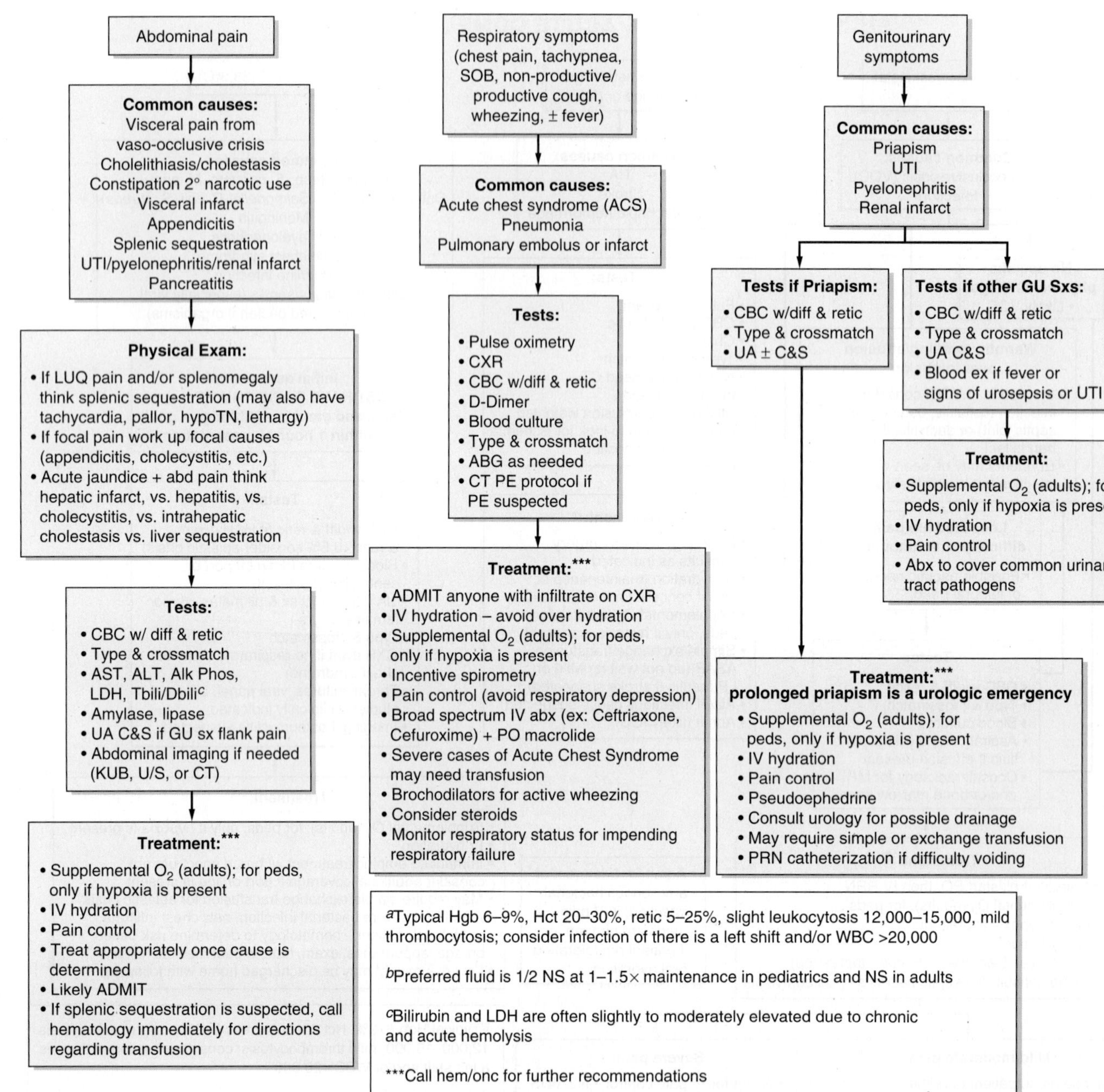
Abdominal pain
Common causes:
Visceral pain from vaso-occlusive crisis
Cholelithiasis/cholestasis
Constipation 2° narcotic use
Visceral infarct
Appendicitis
Splenic sequestration
UTI/pyelonephritis/renal infarct
Pancreatitis
Physical Exam:
• If LUQ pain and/or splenomegaly think splenic sequestration (may also have tachycardia, pallor, hypoTN, lethargy)
• If focal pain work up focal causes (appendicitis, cholecystitis, etc.)
• Acute jaundice + abd pain think hepatic infarct, vs. hepatitis, vs. cholecystitis, vs. intrahepatic cholestasis vs. liver sequestration
Tests:
• CBC w/ diff & retic
• Type & crossmatch
• AST, ALT, Alk Phos, LDH, Tbili/Dbili[c]
• Amylase, lipase
• UA C&S if GU sx flank pain
• Abdominal imaging if needed (KUB, U/S, or CT)
Treatment:***
• Supplemental O_2 (adults); for peds, only if hypoxia is present
• IV hydration
• Pain control
• Treat appropriately once cause is determined
• Likely ADMIT
• If splenic sequestration is suspected, call hematology immediately for directions regarding transfusion
Respiratory symptoms (chest pain, tachypnea, SOB, non-productive/ productive cough, wheezing, ± fever)
Common causes:
Acute chest syndrome (ACS)
Pneumonia
Pulmonary embolus or infarct
Tests:
• Pulse oximetry
• CXR
• CBC w/diff & retic
• D-Dimer
• Blood culture
• Type & crossmatch
• ABG as needed
• CT PE protocol if PE suspected
Treatment:***
• ADMIT anyone with infiltrate on CXR
• IV hydration – avoid over hydration
• Supplemental O_2 (adults); for peds, only if hypoxia is present
• Incentive spirometry
• Pain control (avoid respiratory depression)
• Broad spectrum IV abx (ex: Ceftriaxone, Cefuroxime) + PO macrolide
• Severe cases of Acute Chest Syndrome may need transfusion
• Brochodilators for active wheezing
• Consider steroids
• Monitor respiratory status for impending respiratory failure
Genitourinary symptoms
Common causes:
Priapism
UTI
Pyelonephritis
Renal infarct
Tests if Priapism:
• CBC w/diff & retic
• Type & crossmatch
• UA ± C&S
Tests if other GU Sxs:
• CBC w/diff & retic
• Type & crossmatch
• UA C&S
• Blood ex if fever or signs of urosepsis or UTI
Treatment:
• Supplemental O_2 (adults); for peds, only if hypoxia is present
• IV hydration
• Pain control
• Abx to cover common urinary tract pathogens
Treatment:***
prolonged priapism is a urologic emergency
• Supplemental O_2 (adults); for peds, only if hypoxia is present
• IV hydration
• Pain control
• Pseudoephedrine
• Consult urology for possible drainage
• May require simple or exchange transfusion
• PRN catheterization if difficulty voiding
[a]Typical Hgb 6–9%, Hct 20–30%, retic 5–25%, slight leukocytosis 12,000–15,000, mild thrombocytosis; consider infection of there is a left shift and/or WBC >20,000
[b]Preferred fluid is 1/2 NS at 1–1.5× maintenance in pediatrics and NS in adults
[c]Bilirubin and LDH are often slightly to moderately elevated due to chronic and acute hemolysis
***Call hem/onc for further recommendations

Stephanie Ruest, MD, Neil Grossman, MD and Doreen Brettler, MD

http://www.nepscc.org/index.html.

STROKE

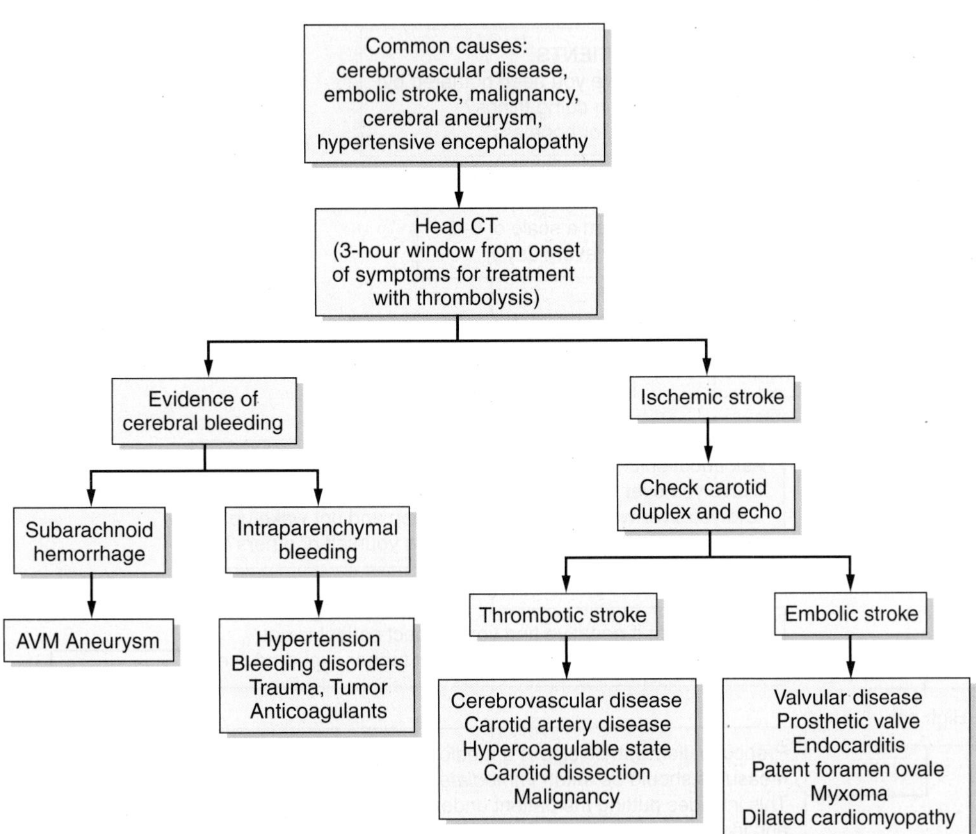

Robert A. Baldor, MD and Alan M. Ehrlich, MD

Stroke. 2007;38:1655–711.

SUICIDE, EVALUATING RISK FOR

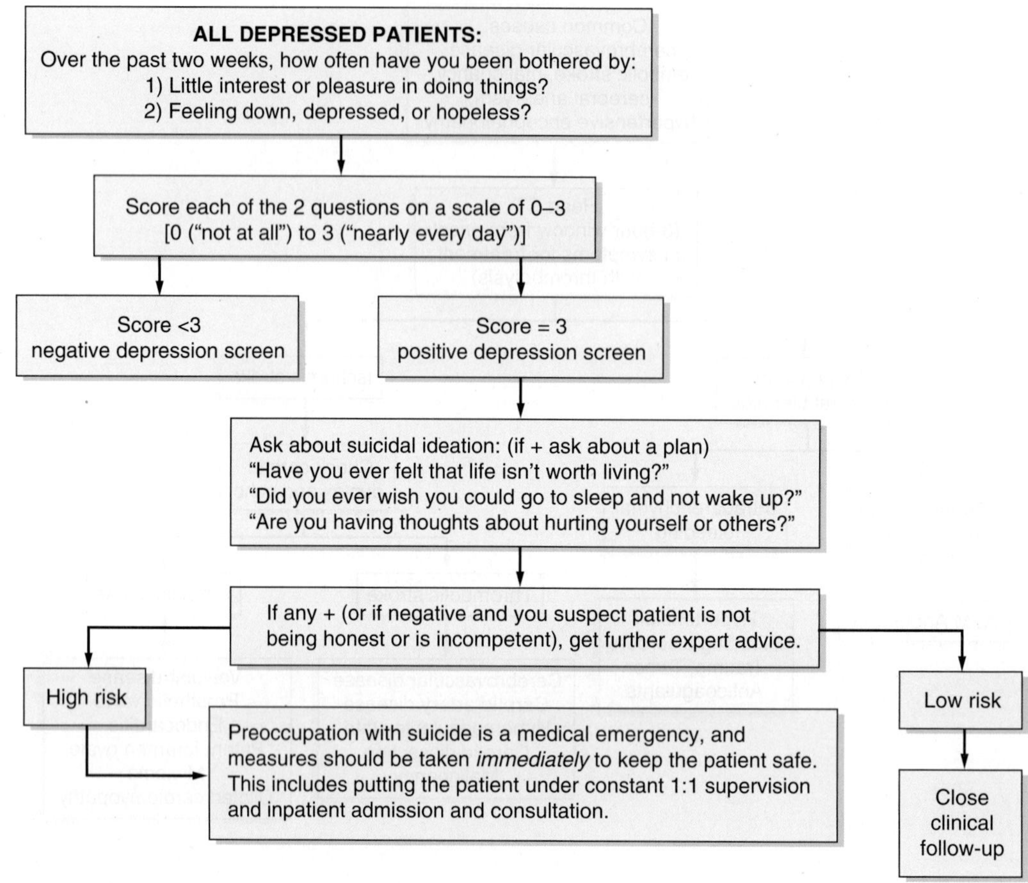

ALL DEPRESSED PATIENTS:
Over the past two weeks, how often have you been bothered by:
1) Little interest or pleasure in doing things?
2) Feeling down, depressed, or hopeless?
Score each of the 2 questions on a scale of 0–3
[0 ("not at all") to 3 ("nearly every day")]
Score <3
negative depression screen
Score = 3
positive depression screen
Ask about suicidal ideation: (if + ask about a plan)
"Have you ever felt that life isn't worth living?"
"Did you ever wish you could go to sleep and not wake up?"
"Are you having thoughts about hurting yourself or others?"
If any + (or if negative and you suspect patient is not being honest or is incompetent), get further expert advice.
High risk
Low risk
Preoccupation with suicide is a medical emergency, and measures should be taken *immediately* to keep the patient safe. This includes putting the patient under constant 1:1 supervision and inpatient admission and consultation.
Close clinical follow-up

Irene C. Coletsos, MD and Harold J. Bursztajn, MD

Am J Psych. 2007;164:1035–43.

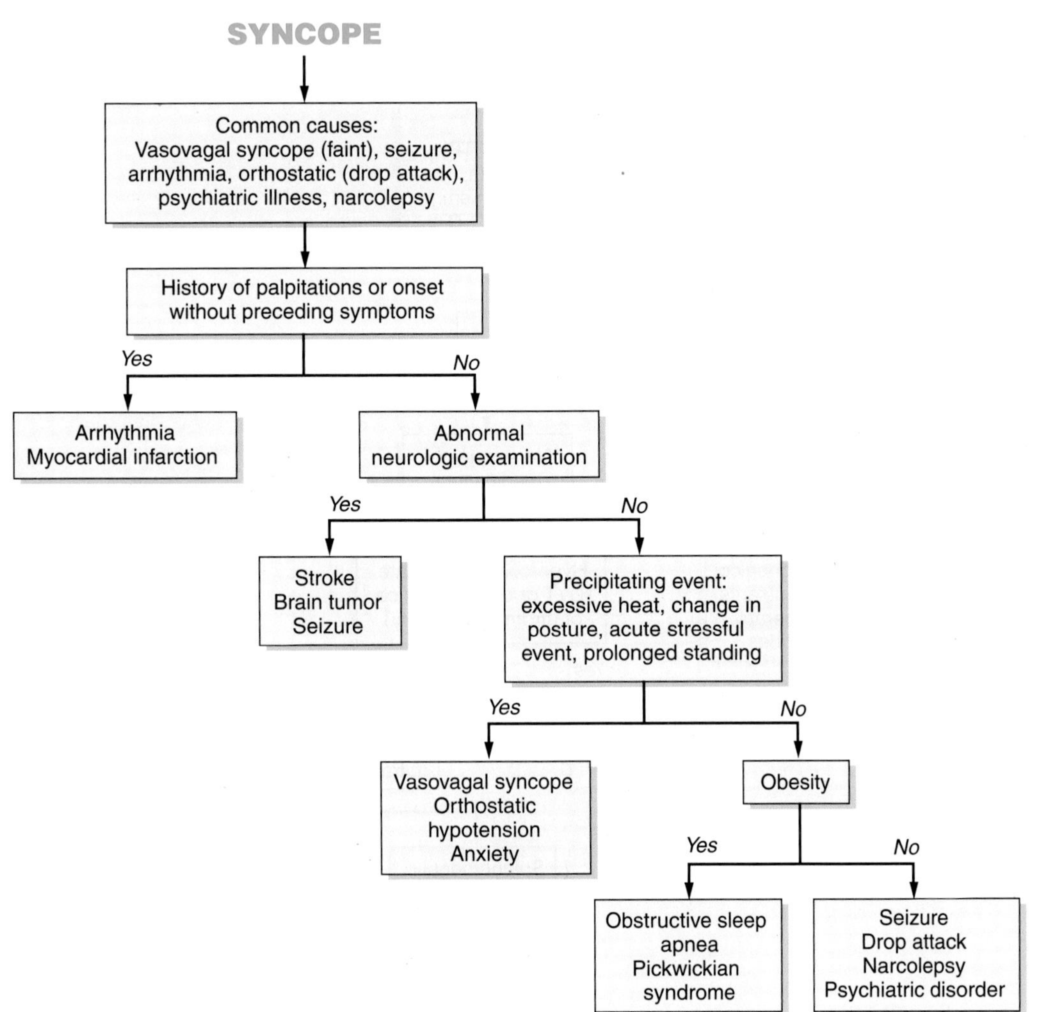

Robert A. Baldor, MD and Alan M. Ehrlich, MD

Med Clin North Am. 1995;79(5):1153–70.

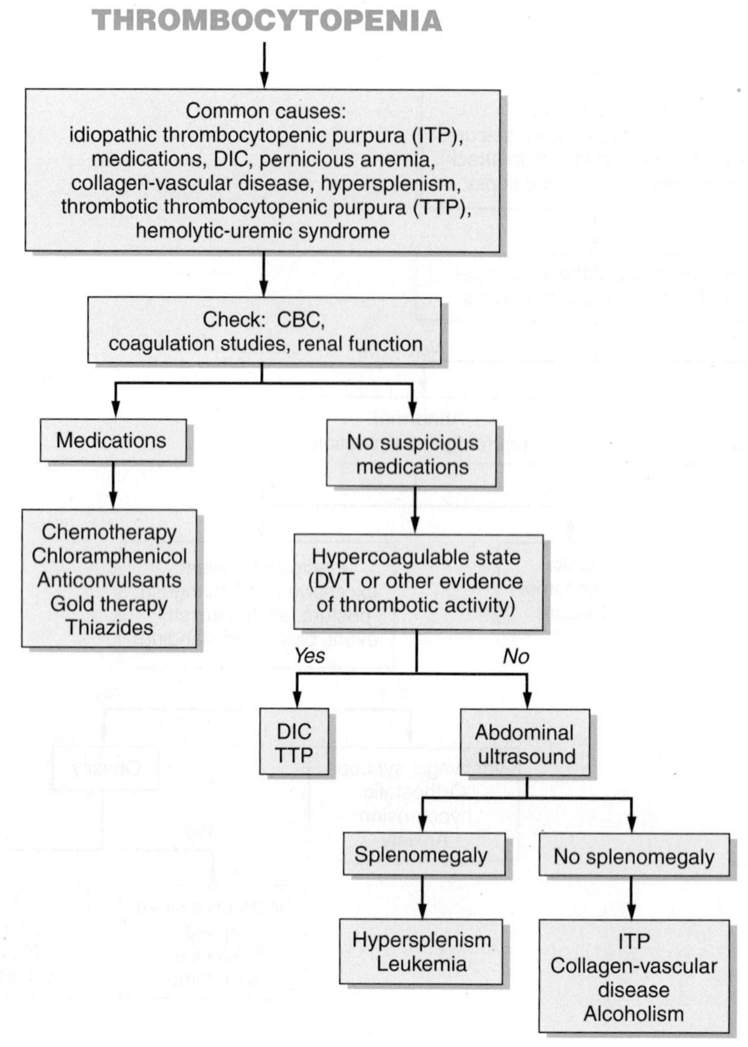
THROMBOCYTOPENIA
Common causes: idiopathic thrombocytopenic purpura (ITP), medications, DIC, pernicious anemia, collagen-vascular disease, hypersplenism, thrombotic thrombocytopenic purpura (TTP), hemolytic-uremic syndrome
Check: CBC, coagulation studies, renal function
Medications
Chemotherapy
Chloramphenicol
Anticonvulsants
Gold therapy
Thiazides
No suspicious medications
Hypercoagulable state (DVT or other evidence of thrombotic activity)
Yes
No
DIC
TTP
Abdominal ultrasound
Splenomegaly
No splenomegaly
Hypersplenism
Leukemia
ITP
Collagen-vascular disease
Alcoholism

Robert A. Baldor, MD and Alan M. Ehrlich, MD

Blood. 2005;106(7):2244–51.

TRANSIENT ISCHEMIC ATTACK AND TRANSIENT NEUROLOGIC DEFICIT

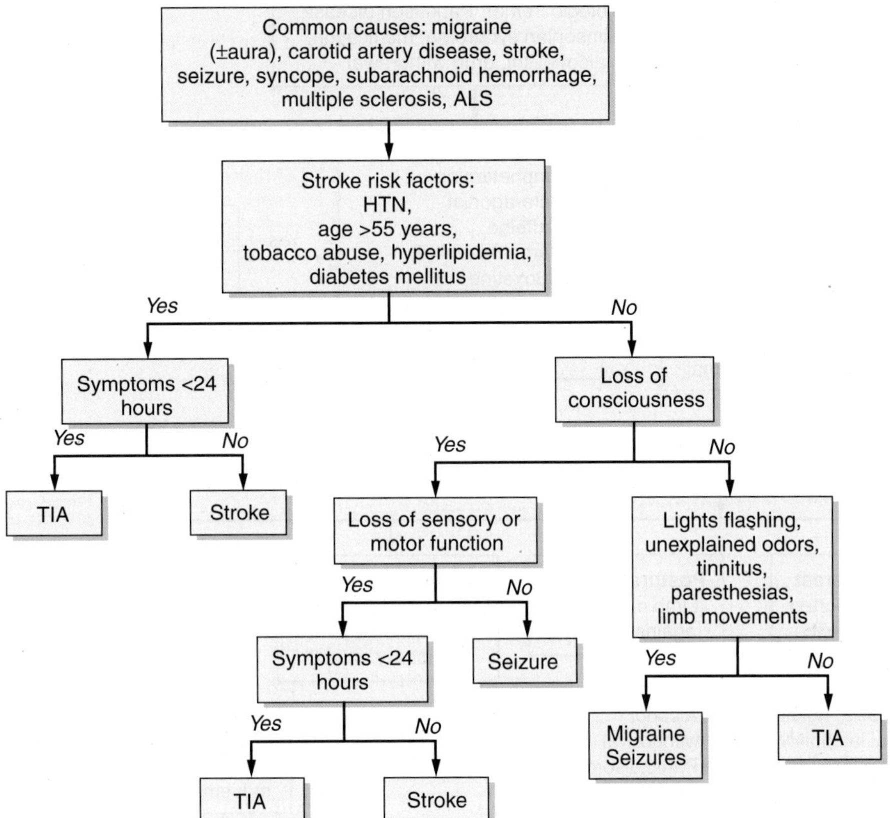

Robert A. Baldor, MD and Alan M. Ehrlich, MD

Am Fam Physician. 2004;69:1665–74, 1679–81.

TREMOR

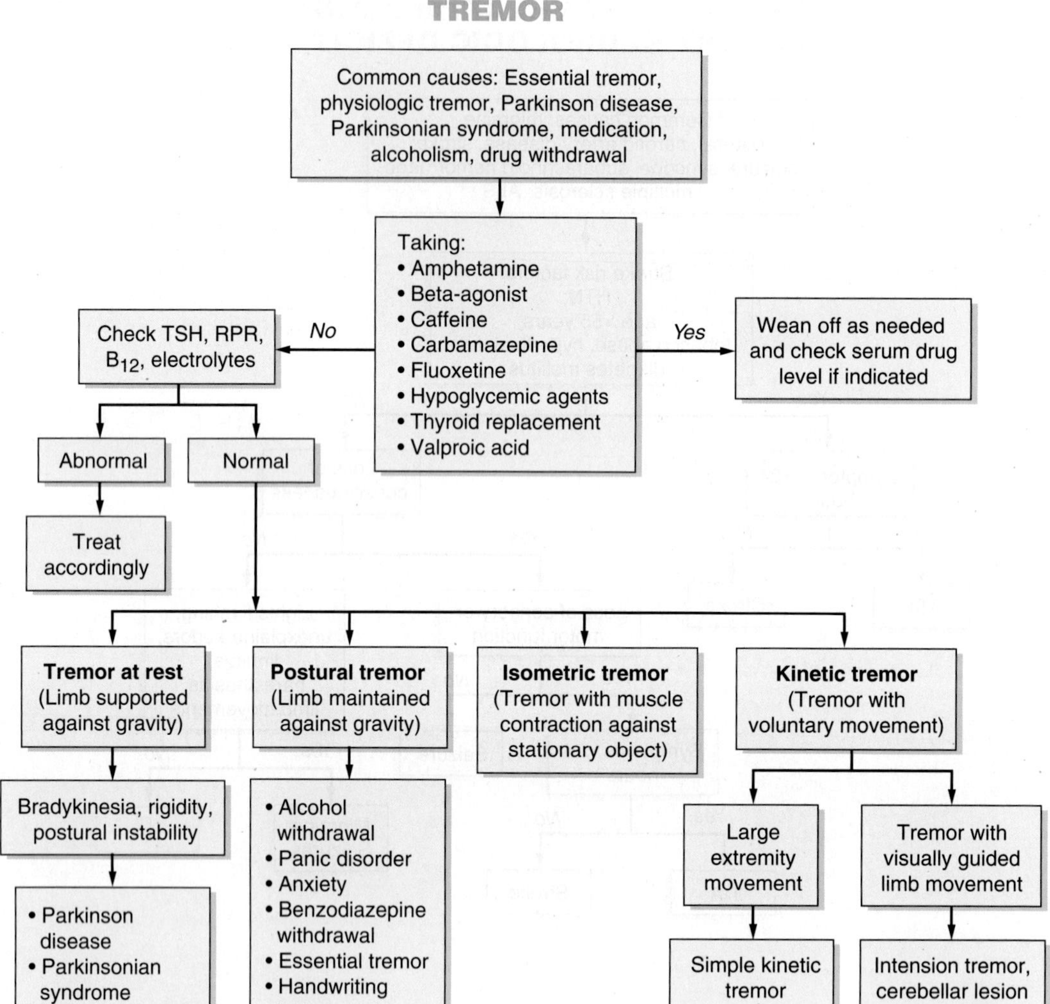

Andrew J. Westwood, MD

Am Fam Physician. 2003;68(8):1545–52.

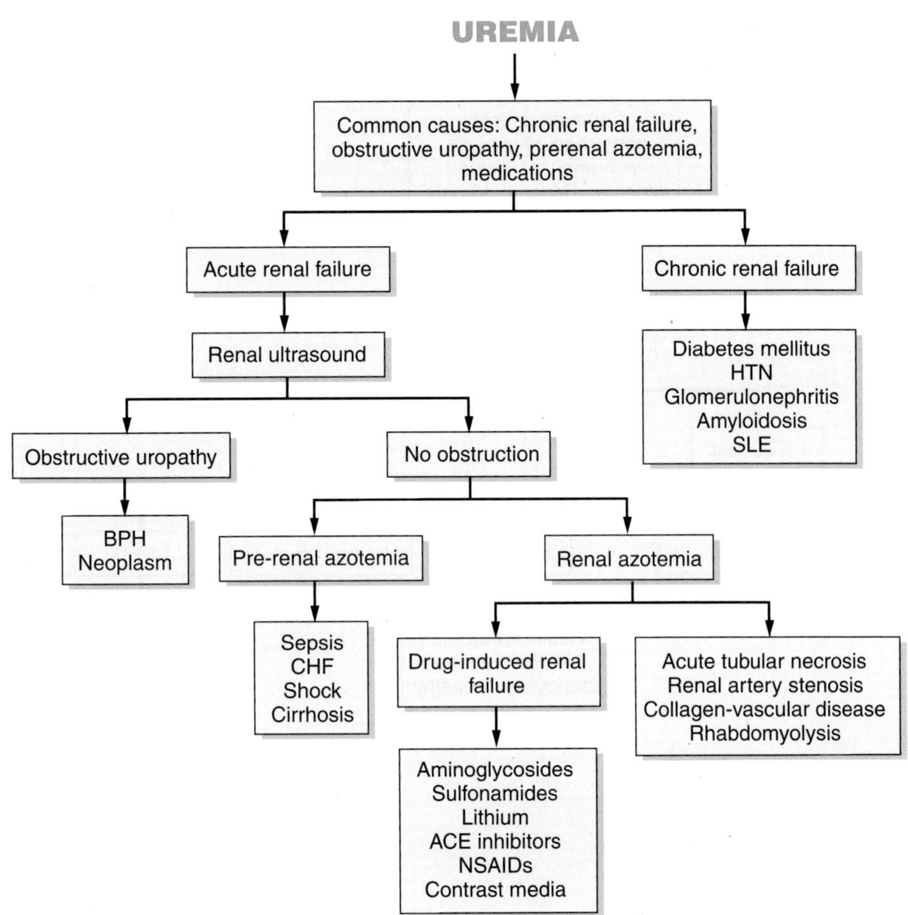

Robert A. Baldor, MD and Alan M. Ehrlich, MD

Diagnosis and management of adults with chronic kidney disease. Michigan Quality Improvement Consortium - Professional Association. 2006 Nov (revised 2008 Nov). 1 page. NGC:007054.

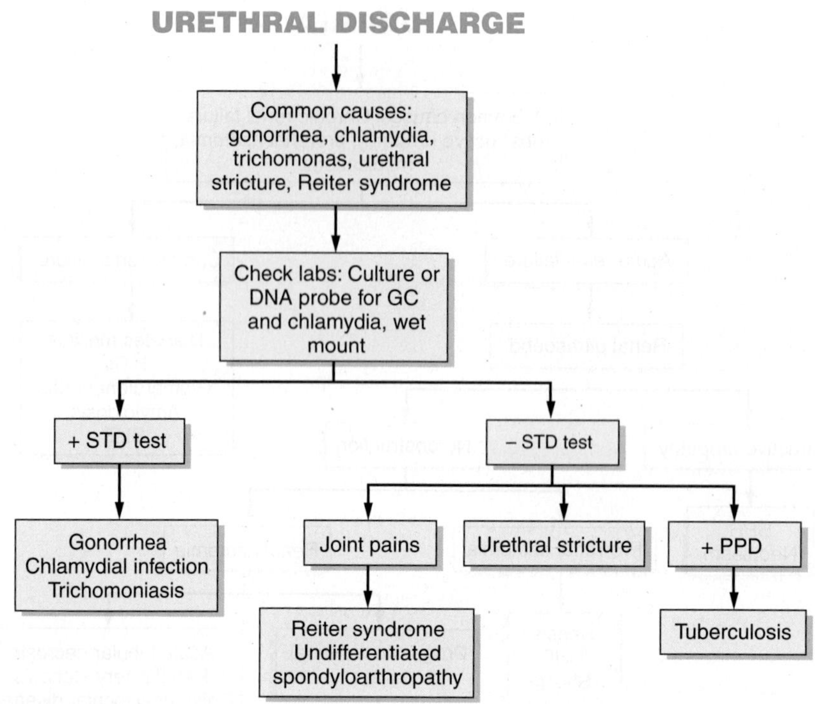

Robert A. Baldor, MD and Alan M. Ehrlich, MD

Sex Transm Infect. 1998;74(Suppl 1):S29–33.

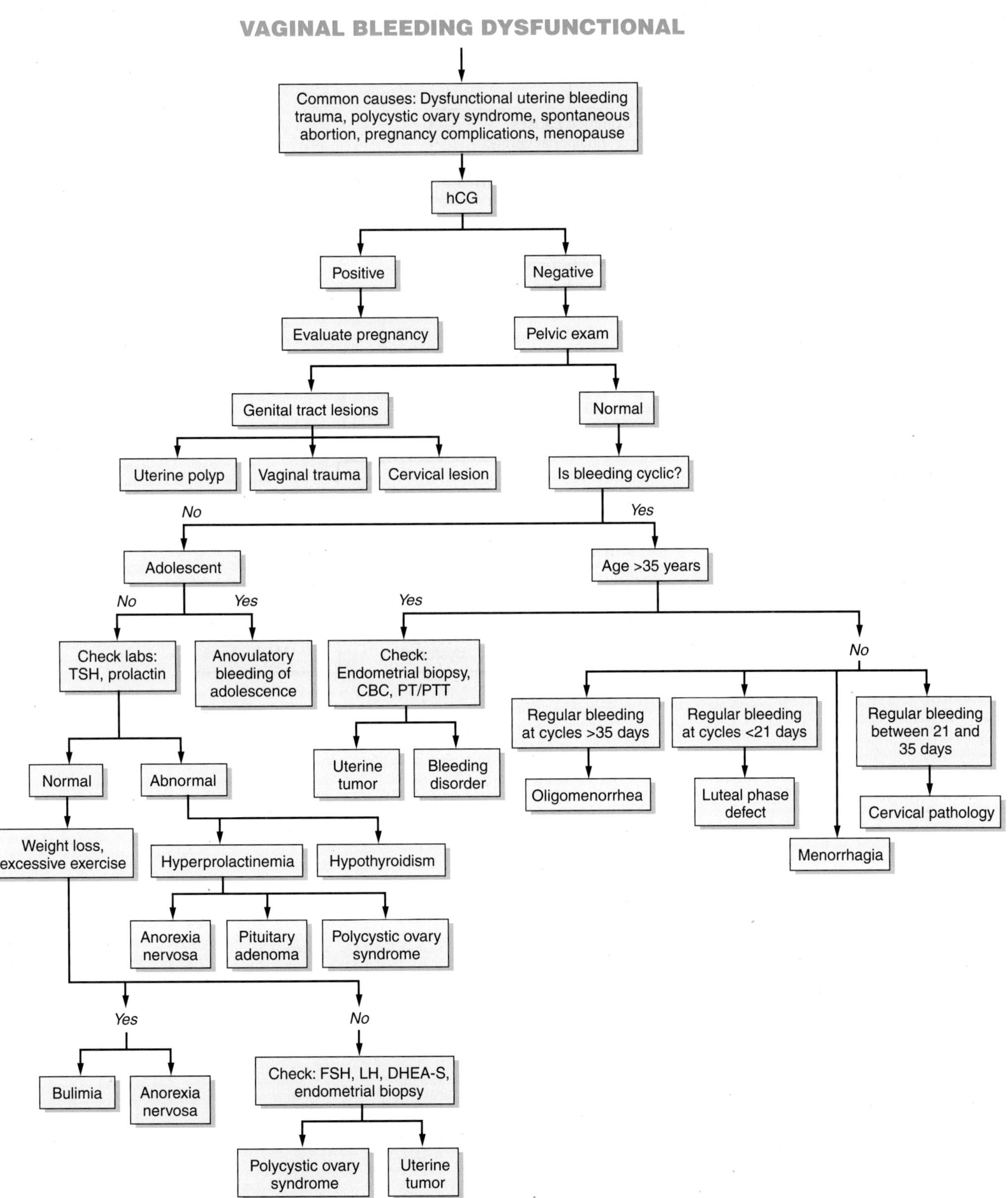

Robert A. Baldor, MD and Alan M. Ehrlich, MD

Am Fam Physician. 2004;69:1915–26;1931–3.

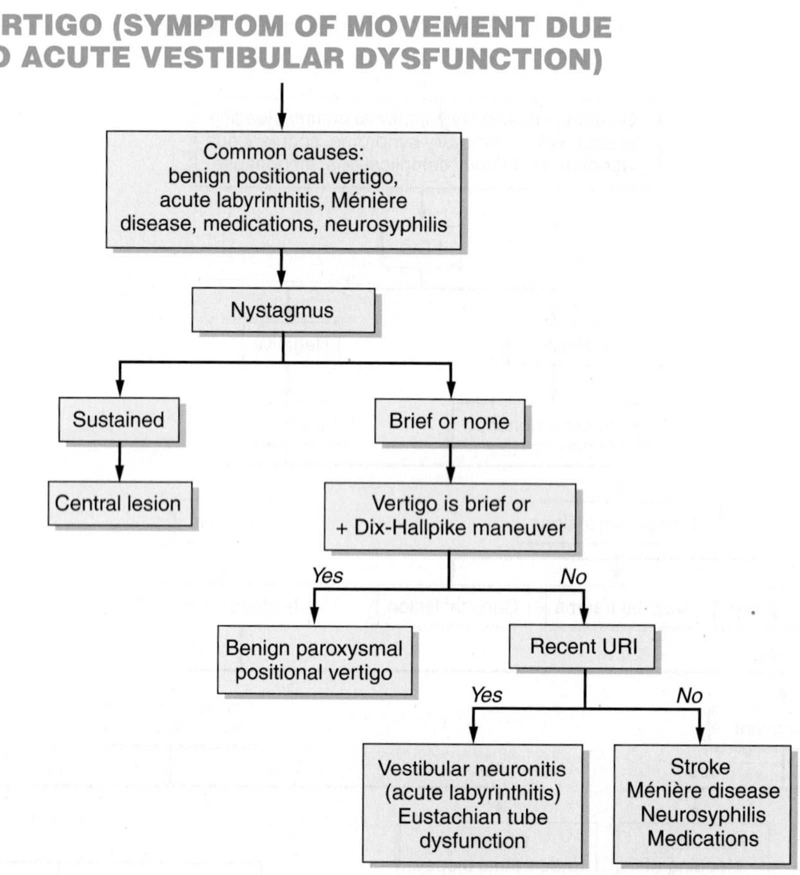

Robert A. Baldor, MD and Alan M. Ehrlich, MD

Am Fam Physician. 2006;73:244–51, 255.

WEIGHT LOSS

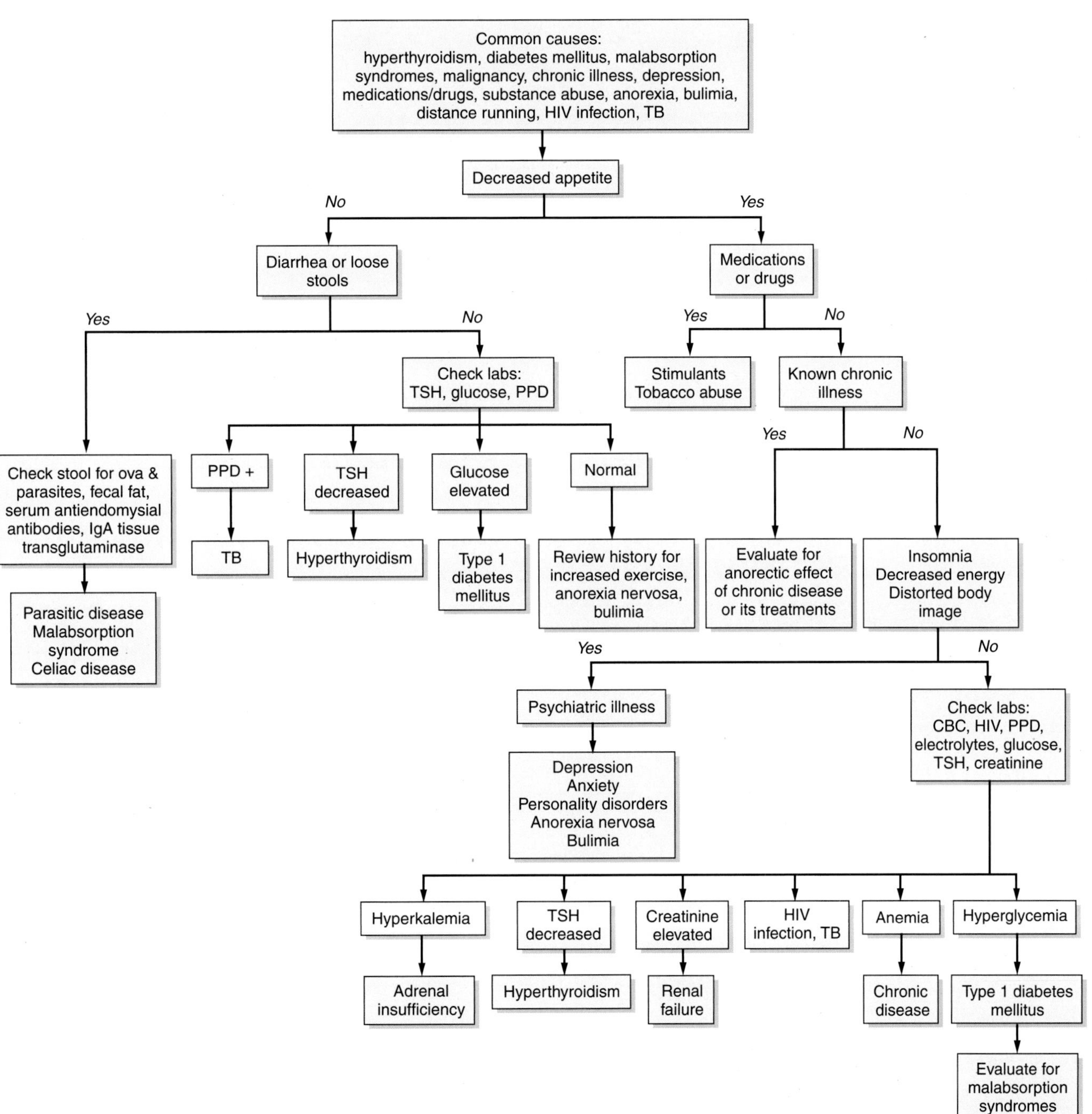

Robert A. Baldor, MD and Alan M. Ehrlich, MD

Am Fam Physician. 2002;65:640–51.

The 5-Minute Clinical Consult 2013

21ST EDITION

ABDOMINAL ADHESIONS

Marina MacNamara, MSIV, MPH
Leslie Roth, MD

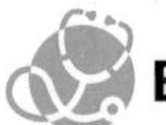

BASICS

Intra-abdominal adhesions are bands of scar tissue that form between 2 previously separated structures. (e.g., bowel to the abdominal wall.)

DESCRIPTION

The majority of adhesions are the result of traumatic injury to abdominal and/or pelvic structures, primarily by surgical procedures.

Although adhesions are asymptomatic for most individuals, for some they can be the cause of significant consequences such as:

- Intestinal obstruction, particularly small bowel
- Chronic pelvic pain and/or reduced fertility in women
- Increased risk of morbidity during colonoscopy (1) and of morbidity and mortality from repeat abdominal surgeries (2):
  - Prolonged surgery due to necessary lysis of adhesions
  - Intraoperative bleeding
  - Trocar injury
  - Conversion of laparoscopy to laparotomy
  - Inadvertent enterotomy or other organ damage
  - Prolonged length of hospital stay

EPIDEMIOLOGY

Incidence

- Postop (93%) (3):
  - The majority of SBO is associated with postoperative adhesion formation. There is an 11% risk of SBO within 1 year of an abdominal operation; 30% at 10 years (3).
- Congenital (4.7%) (4)
- Inflammatory (2.3%) (4)

RISK FACTORS

History of:

- Abdominal inflammation
- Abdominal surgery
- Abdominal adhesions

GENERAL PREVENTION

- Primary prevention: Wherever possible, avoid risk factors for development of abdominal infection or need for abdominal surgery.
- Secondary prevention in abdominal surgery: With no single, effective prevention to date, these barriers are to be considered primarily in high-risk individuals, such as patients with a history of multiple abdominal surgeries, endometriosis.
- Further, a combination of the following options may be the most effective means of prevention available:
  - Surgical technique:
    - Laparoscopy has generally been associated with fewer adhesions compared to laparotomy (with the exception of appendectomies in which the risk is equal) (5)[A].
    - Surgical prevention includes: minimizing tissue trauma, maintaining optimal hemostasis, reducing drying out of tissues (by limiting heat/light, frequent irrigation), minimizing risk of infection, avoiding contaminants, and use of foreign materials (e.g., glove powder) when possible (6)[A].
  - Barrier agents: Including Seprafilm, Gore-Tex, Interceed, Fibrin sheet, fluids/gels (7)[B].

PATHOPHYSIOLOGY

- Congenital: Abnormality formed during organogenesis.
- Postinflammatory and postoperative: Caused by an imbalance of Fibrin deposition and breakdown, induced in part by cytokines such as plasminogen activator inhibitor (PAI1), urokinaselike plasminogen activator (uPA), and transforming growth factor (TGF-β).
  - Morbidity caused by the anchoring of organs to nearby structures thereby impeding normal movement and promoting kinks, deformity, and blockage (8).

ETIOLOGY

- Congenital: Abnormality formed during organogenesis.
- Postinflammatory: From diverticulitis, appendicitis, endometriosis, peritonitis, radiotherapy, long-term peritoneal dialysis.
- Posttrauma: Physical trauma to the abdomen, including surgery

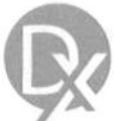

DIAGNOSIS

The presence of adhesions is primarily diagnosed through patient history and/or intraoperatively (either laparoscopically or through a laparotomy).

ALERT

SBO without surgical history should not be blamed on adhesions. Further workup is required in these cases.

HISTORY

- Prior abdominal surgery
- History of abdominal/pelvic inflammatory disease or infection
- If involving the bowel, complaints may include:
  - Crampy abdominal pain
  - Nausea
  - Vomiting
  - Minimal to no flatus.
- If involving a pelvic structure, complaints may include:
  - Lower abdominal pain (either chronic or acute)
  - Nausea
  - Vomiting

PHYSICAL EXAM

- Abdominal scars
- In the case of small bowel obstruction, may see:
  - Abdominal distention
  - Tympany
- Be aware of possible ischemia with signs including:
  - Fever
  - Tachycardia
  - Diffuse abdominal tenderness

DIAGNOSTIC TESTS & INTERPRETATION

Imaging

- No lab or imaging test can demonstrate adhesions.
- However, imaging can diagnose complications to adhesions such as the abdominal x-ray and CT scan for SBO.

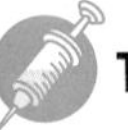

TREATMENT

SURGERY/OTHER PROCEDURES

- Adhesiolysis: Performed for symptomatic complications of adhesions, though criteria for surgery in these cases depends on the specific complication.
  - With adhesiolysis, there is always the risk of induction of new adhesions.
- Laparoscopic: Primarily for pelvic adhesions:
  - May be most effective in removing adhesions to the abdominal wall, and least effective for those affecting the adnexa (9)[B]
  - Helpful in treating chronic pelvic pain only when affected by severe adhesions (10)[B]
- Open: Primarily for peritoneal adhesions.
  - Laparotomy is preferred surgical resolution to SBO related to adhesions in cases of failed conservative management (11)[C].

ONGOING CARE

PROGNOSIS

- Adhesions are typically asymptomatic. However, once present, they cannot be fully removed.
- Possible complications can occur at any time.

COMPLICATIONS

- The most common and significant complication is bowel obstruction (either partial or complete).
- Chronic pelvic pain
- Infertility

REFERENCES

1. Garrett KA, Church J. History of hysterectomy: a significant problem for colonoscopists that is not present in patients who have had sigmoid colectomy. *Dis Colon Rectum*. 2010;53(7):1055–60.
2. van Goor H. Consequences and complications of peritoneal adhesions. *Colorectal Dis*. 2007;9 Suppl 2:25–34.
3. Dijkstra FR, Nieuwenhuijzen M, Reijnen MM, et al. Recent clinical developments in pathophysiology, epidemiology, diagnosis and treatment of intra-abdominal adhesions. *Scand J Gastroenterol Suppl*. 2000;(232):52–9.
4. Menzies D, Ellis H. Intestinal obstruction from adhesions—how big is the problem? *Ann R Coll Surg Engl*. 1990;72(1):60–3.
5. Barmparas G, Branco BC, Schnüriger B, et al. The incidence and risk factors of post-laparotomy adhesive small bowel obstruction. *J Gastrointest Surg*. 2010;14(10):1619–28. Epub 2010 Mar 30.
6. Robertson D, Lefebvre G, Leyland N, et al. Adhesion prevention in gynaecological surgery. *J Obstet Gynaecol Can*. 2010;32(6):598–608.
7. Ahmad G, Duffy JM, Farquhar C, et al. Barrier agents for adhesion prevention after gynaecological surgery. *Cochrane Database Syst Rev*. 2008;16(2):CD000475.
8. Munireddy S, Kavalukas SL, Barbul A. Intra-abdominal healing: Gastrointestinal tract and adhesions. *Surg Clin North Am*. 2010;90(6):1227–36.
9. Luciano DE, Roy G, Luciano AA. Adhesion reformation after laparoscopic adhesiolysis: Where, what type, and in whom they are most likely to recur. *J Minim Invasive Gynecol*. 2008;15(1):44–8.
10. Stones RW, Mountfield J. Interventions for treating chronic pelvic pain in women. *Cochrane Database Syst Rev*. 2000;(4):CD000387.
11. Catena F, Di Saverio S, Kelly MD, et al. Bologna Guidelines for Diagnosis and Management of Adhesive Small Bowel Obstruction (ASBO): 2010 Evidence-Based Guidelines of the World Society of Emergency Surgery. *World J Emerg Surg*. 2011;21(6):5.

ADDITIONAL READING

- Beck DE, Opelka FG, Bailey HR, et al. Incidence of small-bowel obstruction and adhesiolysis after open colorectal and general surgery. *Dis Colon Rectum*. 1999;42(2):241–8
- Brüggmann D, Tchartchian G, Wallwiener M, et al. Intra-abdominal adhesions: definition, origin, significance in surgical practice, and treatment options. *Dtsch Arztebl Int*. 2010;107(44):769–75. Epub 2010 Nov 5.
- Ellis H, Moran BJ, Thompson JN, et al. Adhesion-related hospital readmissions after abdominal and pelvic surgery: A retrospective cohort study. *Lancet*. 1999;353(9163):1476–80.
- Menzies D. Postoperative adhesions: Their treatment and relevance in clinical practice. *Ann R Coll Surg Engl*. 1993;75:147–53.
- Parker MC, Ellis H, Moran BJ, et al. Postoperative adhesions: Ten-year follow-up of 12,584 patients undergoing lower abdominal surgery. *Dis Colon Rectum*. 2001;44(6):822–29; discussion 829–30.
- Prushik SG, Stucchi AF, Matteotti R, et al. Open adhesiolysis is more effective in reducing adhesion reformation than laparoscopic adhesiolysis in an experimental model. *Br J Surg*. 2010;97(3):420–7.
- Sikirica V, Bapat B, Candrilli SD, et al. The inpatient burden of abdominal and gynecological adhesiolysis in the US. *BMC Surg*. 2011 Jun 9;11(1):13. [Epub ahead of print].
- Ward BC, Panitch A. Abdominal adhesions: Current and novel therapies. *J Surg Res*. 2011;165(1):91–111. Epub 2009 Oct 2.

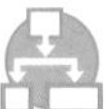

See Also (Topic, Algorithm, Electronic Media Element)

Small Bowel Obstruction; Chronic Pelvic Pain; Infertility

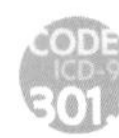

CODES

ICD9

- 568.0 Peritoneal adhesions (postoperative) (postinfection)
- 751.8 Other specified anomalies of digestive system

CLINICAL PEARLS

- Abdominal adhesions result primarily from abdominal infection or trauma, including surgery.
- Although typically asymptomatic, the most common and significant complication is bowel obstruction (either partial or complete).
- Minimizing abdominal inflammation and trauma, including surgery, is the most effective, current means of adhesion prevention.

ABNORMAL PAP AND CERVICAL DYSPLASIA

Patricia Seymour, MD
Jeremy Golding, MD

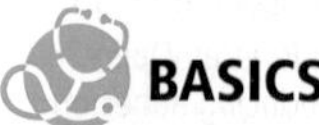

BASICS

DESCRIPTION

Cervical dysplasia: Precancerous epithelial changes in the transformation zone of the uterine cervix almost always associated with human papilloma virus (HPV) infections:

- Mild dysplasia (cervical intraepithelial neoplasia [CIN] I): Cellular changes are limited to the lower 1/3 of the squamous epithelium.
- Moderate dysplasia (CIN II): Cellular changes are limited to the lower 2/3 of the squamous epithelium.
- Severe dysplasia (CIN III or carcinoma in situ): Cellular changes involve the full thickness of the squamous epithelium.
- Pap smear:
  - Screening test for cervical cellular pathology. In many laboratories, automated cervical screening complements the Pap smear or supersedes it.
  - Abnormal cervical smear results can range from benign cellular changes to suggestion of invasive cancer.
- System(s) affected: Reproductive

ALERT

Cervical cancer arises from HPV, which is a sexually transmitted disease. There is good evidence that screening for cervical cancer with Pap smears reduces incidences of, and mortality from, cervical cancer (1)[A].

Geriatric Considerations

Natural progression of cervical dysplasia involves acquisition of HPV at or after first coitus with a small percentage of lesions progressing. One may discontinue screening at age 65 if 3 previous Paps are normal and there are no abnormal results in past 10 years.

Pregnancy Considerations

- Squamous intraepithelial lesions can progress during pregnancy, but often regress postpartum.
- Colposcopy only to rule out invasive cancer in high-risk women (2).

EPIDEMIOLOGY

- Predominant age: Can occur at any age
- Incidence of CIN III peaks between ages 25 and 29; invasive disease peaks 15 years later

Incidence

- Low-grade squamous intraepithelial lesion ranges from 2–3% of all Pap smears.
- High-grade squamous intraepithelial lesion or invasive cancer is present on 1% of Pap smears.
- Other reactive, reparative, and ASC-US (atypical squamous cells of unknown significance) results are difficult to assess because of the lack of reporting mechanisms.

Prevalence

26.8% of women are HPV-positive.

RISK FACTORS

- Cigarette smoking
- Possible deficiency of antioxidants
- Early age at first coitus
- Multiple sexual partners
- Some correlation to low socioeconomic level
- Intercourse with a high-risk male partner
- HPV infection
- Immunosuppression

GENERAL PREVENTION

- HPV immunization of girls and women prior to first intercourse:
  - Gardasil: 3 doses at 0, 2, 6 months, approved for use in ages 9–26, reduces dysplasia due to covered and related HPV strains; Immunization of males ages 9–26 recommended by Advisory Committee on Immunization Practices (ACIP), but controversial.
  - Cervarix: 3 doses at 0, 1, 6 months, approved for use in females ages 10–25. This reduces HPV 16/18 infection and CIN.
  - Immunization decreases high-risk HPV infections and cervical pathology for 5–7 years.
- Help girls to delay first intercourse beyond early adolescence
- Monogamous relationship for both partners
- Smoking cessation
- Adequate antioxidant-rich food intake has been associated with decreased risk
- Obtain routine Pap smears (see guidelines below)
- Use barrier methods of birth control if in nonmonogamous relationship (likely decreases but does not eliminate HPV transmission)
- **Screening:** In the US, many populations may be overscreened (resulting in increased cost and cervical procedures, but not in benefit) because of failure to follow guidelines:
  - Screening indicated for woman beginning at age 21 but not younger
  - Frequency of screening recommendations vary:
    - United States Preventive Services Task Force: Every 3 years
    - American Cancer Society/American Congress of Obstetricians and Gynecologists: Every 2 years until age 30, then every 3 years if normal
    - May be beneficial to do combined cellular screening (Pap) and high-risk HPV test in women younger than 30 (but not before). If normal cytology and high-risk HPV negative, screening should be repeated in no less than 3 years. If cytology is normal, but HPV is positive, repeat both cytology and HPV in 1 year, and if HPV remains positive (or if abnormal cytology), proceed to colposcopy (2,3)
- Screen until age 65–70. May discontinue if 3 or more consecutive, satisfactory normal or negative smears, no abnormal smears in past 10 years, or until total hysterectomy for benign conditions (1,4)

PATHOPHYSIOLOGY

- HPV DNA is found in virtually all cervical carcinomas and precursor lesions worldwide.
- HPV viral types 16, 18, 31, 35, 45, 51, 52, 56, and 58 are common high-risk or oncogenic virus types for cervical cancer.
- HPV viral types 6, 11, 42, 43, and 44 are considered common low-risk types, and may cause genital warts.

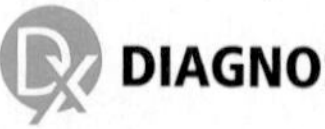

DIAGNOSIS

Frequently there are no symptoms.

HISTORY

- Occasionally vaginal discharge related to sexually transmitted disease
- Rarely vaginal bleeding

PHYSICAL EXAM

Pelvic exam occasionally reveals external HPV lesions.

DIAGNOSTIC TESTS & INTERPRETATION

- ThinPrep is a fluid-based collection and thin-layer preparation for cervical cancer screening.
- Liquid-based and conventional Pap testing are similar in overall performance.
- Sensitivity of a single Pap smear for HSIL ~70%; specificity of ~90%

Lab

Bethesda system for reporting Pap/cervical smear results (*cytologic grading*):

- Specimen adequacy
- Presence of endocervical cells:
  - Negative for intraepithelial lesion or malignancy
- Epithelial cell abnormalities:
  - ASC: Atypical squamous cells
  - ASC-US: Atypical squamous cells of unknown significance
  - ASC-H: Atypical cells cannot exclude high-grade squamous intraepithelial lesion (SIL)
  - LSIL: Low-grade squamous intraepithelial lesion (combines mild dysplasia (CIN I) with HPV)
  - HSIL: High-grade squamous intraepithelial lesion (combines CIN II and III)
  - Squamous cell carcinoma
  - Glandular cells
  - AGC: Atypical glandular cells
  - AGCs of undetermined significance
  - Atypical glandular cells, favor neoplasia
  - Endocervical adenocarcinoma in situ
  - Adenocarcinoma

Diagnostic Procedures/Surgery

- Colposcopy with or without biopsy recommended for the following (2) (and see management algorithms):
  - Initial Pap smear with LSIL (exception for adolescents, although screening of adolescents no longer recommended), HSIL; ASC-US that is + for high-risk HPV types on (reflex) HPV hybrid capture 2 test.
  - ASC-US present on 2 Pap smears 6 months apart if HPV testing not available
  - ASC-H
  - Any abnormal or suspicious lesion of the cervix or vagina that is visualized by the eye
  - Atypical glandular cells (mandate colposcopy and uterine sampling)
- HPV viral typing:
  - Hybrid capture 2 test has 2 viral type probes: A low–risk probe and a high-risk probe.
  - High-risk (HR) probe can be used to identify patients with ASC-US who need colposcopy follow-up.
  - HPV typing may be used in combination with Pap smear for women ≥30.
    - Low-risk women with negative cytology and who are negative for high-risk HPV may be followed every 3 years.
    - Women with negative cytology but positive HR probe may be approached with 1 of 2 strategies (optimal strategy uncertain):

- Repeat Pap and HPV in 1 year. If either Pap abnormal or HPV HR positive, then colposcopy.
- Order an HPV 16/18–specific probe on cytology fluid. If either probe for 16 or 18 is positive, evidence suggests the risk of a high-grade lesion is still similar to the risk for ASC-US/HPV+, and colposcopy is recommended. If HPV 16 and 18 are negative with a negative Pap and a high-risk HPV screen positive, the risk of a high-grade lesion is about 15-fold less, and repeat Pap plus HPV screen in 1 year is recommended. At 1 year, if either the Pap or the HPV test is not negative, then colposcopy is recommended.
- – No utility for low-risk viral type screening and these older probes should not be used
- Loop electrosurgical excision procedure (LEEP):
  - "See and treat" for HSIL in non adolescent age groups acceptable, but not for adolescents (as they should no longer be screened, and most lesions regress in this age group).
- Cone biopsy
- Cervicography: Photographic evaluation of cervix

Pathological Findings
- Atypical squamous or columnar cells
- Coarse nuclear material
- Increased nuclear diameter
- Koilocytosis (HPV hallmark)

DIFFERENTIAL DIAGNOSIS
- Acute or chronic cervicitis
- Cervical squamous intraepithelial neoplasia
- Cervical glandular neoplasia
- Invasive cervical malignancy
- Uterine malignancy (rare)

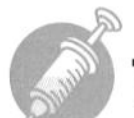

TREATMENT

Evidence-based management algorithms guide Pap smear and post colposcopic diagnostics and therapeutics and are available online (2,3).

MEDICATION
- Infective/reactive Pap smear:
  - Metronidazole 250 mg t.i.d. PO for 7 days
- Condyloma acuminatum:
  - Cryotherapy
  - Podophyllin topically q1–2wk or Podofilox 0.5% applied b.i.d. x 3 days then off 4 days, repeated for 1–4 weeks
  - Trichloroacetic acid, applied topically by a physician and covered for 5–6 days
  - Imiquimod cream 3x/wk at bedtime up to 16 weeks

ADDITIONAL TREATMENT
General Measures
- Office evaluation and observation
- Promote smoking cessation
- Promote protected intercourse
- Promote immunization

SURGERY/OTHER PROCEDURES
- LSILs and HSILs and carcinoma in situ can be treated with outpatient surgery: Cryotherapy, laser ablation, LEEP/large loop excision of transition zone, or cold-knife conization all effective, but require different training and with different side effects for patient
- If cervical malignancy, see "Cervical Malignancy."

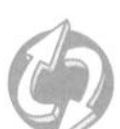

ONGOING CARE

FOLLOW-UP RECOMMENDATIONS
- LSIL/CIN1: Observation with Pap smear repeated every 6 months or high-risk HPV testing every year is appropriate for young women with LSIL, especially with confirmed CIN I.
- HPV-related CIN I typically resolves within 2–3 years.
- LSIL persisting beyond 2–3 years in a young woman is indication for colposcopy.
- After treatment (excision or ablation) for high-grade CIN women may re-enter routine screening only after negative cytology at 6, 12, and 24 months and should be continued for 20 years (5).

DIET
Promote increased intake of antioxidant-rich foods.

PATIENT EDUCATION
- Promote HPV immunization.
- Promote smoking cessation.
- Promote protected intercourse.
- Promote regular Pap smears according to recognized guidelines. Many women need to be educated that this is not usually yearly.
- Ensure adherence to recommended follow-up for any abnormality.

PROGNOSIS
- Generally excellent: <50% of persistent infective, reactive, reparative, or ASC-US Pap/cervical smears will have more advanced lesions.
- Only a small percentage of LSILs will progress to more advanced lesion (80% or more of adolescent and young adult CIN I resolves in 2–3 years). Lesions discovered early are amenable to treatment, with excellent results and few recurrences.

COMPLICATIONS
- Minor abnormalities on Pap/cervical smears can mask more advanced lesions.
- HSIL does progress to invasive cancer. Best estimate of risk of CIN III progression to invasive cervical cancer is >50% (6).
- Aggressive cervical surgery may be associated with cervical stenosis, cervical incompetence, and scarring affecting cervical dilatation in labor.

REFERENCES

1. Guide to Clinical Preventive Services: Report of the US Preventive Services Task Force 2003. Accessed 9/12/2011 at www.ahrq.gov/clinic/3rduspstf/cervcan/cervcanrr.htm
2. Wright TC Jr, Massad LS, Dunton CJ, et al. 2006 Consensus Guidelines for the management of women with abnormal cervical cancer screening tests. *AJOG* 2007;346–56. Accessed 4/22/2009 at http://www.asccp.org/consensus.shtml.
3. ICSI. Management of abnormal Pap smear 2008. Accessed 9/12/2011 at http://guidelines.gov/content.aspx?id=24134&search=icsi+abnormal+pap
4. Saslow D, Runowicz CD, Solomon D, et al. American Cancer Society guideline for the early detection of cervical neoplasia and cancer. *CA Cancer J Clin*. 2002;52:342–62.
5. Kocken M, Helmerhorst TJ, Berkhof J, et al. Risk of recurrent high-grade cervical intraepithelial neoplasia after successful treatment: A long-term multi-cohort study. *Lancet Oncol*. 2011;12(5): 441–50.
6. McCredie MR, Sharples KJ, Paul C, et al. Natural history of cervical neoplasia and risk of invasive cancer in women with cervical intraepithelial neoplasia 3: A retrospective cohort study. *Lancet Oncol*. 2008;5(9):425–34.

ADDITIONAL READING

- Giuliano AR, Palefsky JM, Goldstone S, et al. Efficacy of quadrivalent HPV vaccine against HPV infection and disease in males. *N Engl J Med*. 2011;364(5): 401–11
- Markowitz LE, Dunne EF, Saraiya M, et al. Quadrivalent Human Papillomavirus Vaccine: Recommendations of the Advisory Committee on Immunization Practices (ACIP). *MMWR Recomm Rep*. 2007;56:1–24
- Romanowski B, de Borba PC, Naud PS, et al. Sustained efficacy and immunogenicity of the human papillomavirus (HPV-16/18 AS04-adjuvanted vaccine: Analysis of a randomized placebo-controlled trial up to 6.4 years. *Lancet* 2009;374(9706):1975–85.
- Siebers AG, Klinkhamer PJ, Grefter JM, et al. Comparison of liquid-based cytology with conventional cytology for detection of cervical cancer precursors: A randomized controlled trial. *JAMA*. 2009;302(21):2322

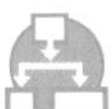

See Also (Topic, Algorithm, Electronic Media Element)

- Cervical Malignancy; Condyloma Acuminata; Failure to Thrive; Trichomoniasis; Vulvovaginitis, Prepubescent
- Algorithm: Pap (Abnormal), >21 Years of Age; Pap (Abnormal), Adolescents; Pap, Use of HPV DNA Testing in Women Over 30

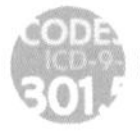

CODES

ICD9
- 622.10 Dysplasia of cervix, unspecified
- 622.11 Mild dysplasia of cervix
- 622.12 Moderate dysplasia of cervix

CLINICAL PEARLS

- A connection exists between HPV infection and abnormal Pap smears. HPV was defined as a "carcinogen" by the World Health Organization in 1996. HPV is present in virtually all cervical cancers (99.7%), but most HPV infections are transient.
- No evidence suggests that offering HPV immunization increases the likelihood of early sexual intercourse and acquisition of sexually transmitted infections.
- Preliminary data suggest that vaccine is much less effective for prevention of cervical dysplasia if offered after women are infected with HPV, and no effect on regression of existing CIN has been seen thus far in trials. Vaccine should, therefore, be offered prior to onset of any sexual activity (even non intercourse activity) for maximum effectiveness.
- Know and adhere to recognized screening guidelines to avoid the harms of over screening.

ABORTION, SPONTANEOUS (MISCARRIAGE)

Elizabeth W. Patton, MD, MPhil
Patricia K. Aronson, MD

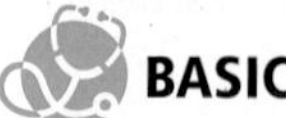

BASICS

DESCRIPTION

- Separation of products of conception from the uterus prior to the potential for fetal survival outside the uterus
- Spontaneous abortion (SAb):
  - Expulsion or extraction from the uterus of an embryo or fetus weighing ≤500 g
- Threatened abortion:
  - Vaginal bleeding early in pregnancy without dilatation of the cervix, rupture of the membranes, or expulsion of products of conception
- Inevitable abortion:
  - Cervical dilatation, rupture of membranes, or expulsion of products in the presence of vaginal bleeding
- Complete abortion:
  - Entire contents of uterus expelled; common before 12 weeks' gestation
- Incomplete abortion:
  - Abortion with retained products of conception, generally placental tissue; more common after 12 weeks' gestation
- Missed abortion:
  - In utero death of embryo/fetus prior to 20 weeks' gestation; products of conception retained
- Induced abortion:
  - Evacuation of uterine contents or products of conception medically or surgically
- Septic abortion:
  - Common complication of illegally performed induced abortions; a spontaneous or therapeutic abortion complicated by pelvic infection
- Habitual spontaneous abortion:
  - 2 or more consecutive pregnancy losses at <15 weeks' gestation
- Synonym(s): Miscarriage; habitual abortion; recurrent abortion; involuntary pregnancy loss

EPIDEMIOLOGY

Predominant age: Increases with advancing age, especially >35 years; at age 40, the loss rate is twice that of age 20

Prevalence

- Between 8% and 20% of all clinically recognized pregnancies end in spontaneous abortion, with 80% of these in the first 12 weeks.
- When both clinical and biochemical (B-HCG detected) pregnancies are considered, up to 50% of pregnancies end in spontaneous abortion.

RISK FACTORS

Most cases of spontaneous abortion occur in patients without identifiable risk factors; however, risk factors listed in order of importance include:

- Chromosomal abnormalities
- Advancing maternal age
- Uterine abnormalities
- Maternal chronic disease (diabetes mellitus, polycystic ovarian syndrome, systemic lupus erythematosus, hypertension, antiphospholipid antibodies, thyroid disease, renal disease)
- Other possible contributing factors include smoking, alcohol, infection, and luteal phase defect, although conclusive data are currently lacking.

Genetics

~50–65% of first-trimester spontaneous abortions have significant chromosomal anomalies, with 50% of these being autosomal trisomies and the remainder being triploidy, tetraploidy, or 45X monosomies.

GENERAL PREVENTION

- Progestogens: Currently, there is no evidence that routine use of oral or IM progestogens prevents miscarriage in early to mid-pregnancy. However, there is some evidence that women with a history of recurrent miscarriage may benefit from this type of treatment (1)[A]. Likewise, there is no evidence that progesterone has utility as a treatment for threatened abortion (2)[A].
- Immunotherapy: There is no current evidence to support use of immunotherapy in patients with a history of recurrent miscarriage (3)[A].

ETIOLOGY

- Chromosomal anomalies
- Congenital anomalies
- Trauma
- Maternal factors: Uterine abnormalities, infection (toxoplasma, other viruses, rubella, cytomegalovirus, herpesvirus), maternal endocrine disorders, hypercoagulable state

DIAGNOSIS

HISTORY

- Consider any reproductive-age woman with vaginal bleeding to be pregnant until proven otherwise.
- Vaginal bleeding:
  - Characteristics (amount, color, consistency, associated symptoms), onset (abrupt or gradual), duration, intensity/quantity, and exacerbating/precipitating factors
  - Document last menstrual period (LMP) if known—allows calculation of estimated gestational age if no prior ultrasound (US) documentation of intrauterine pregnancy (IUP)
- Abdominal pain/uterine cramping, as well as associated nausea/vomiting/syncope
- Rupture of membranes
- Passage of products of conception
- Prenatal course: Toxic or infectious exposures, family or personal history of genetic abnormalities, past history of ectopic pregnancy or spontaneous abortion, endocrine disease, autoimmune disorder, bleeding/clotting disorder

PHYSICAL EXAM

- Estimate hemodynamic stability:
  - Obtain orthostatic vital signs.
- Abdominal exam for tenderness (SAb), guarding, rebound, bowel sounds (peritoneal signs more likely seen with ectopic pregnancy)
- Pelvic exam including speculum exam for visual assessment of cervical dilation, blood, products of conception, and bimanual exam for uterine size/tenderness

DIAGNOSTIC TESTS & INTERPRETATION

Lab

Initial lab tests

- Urine human chorionic gonadotropin (HCG)
- CBC with differential
- Rh type
- Cultures: Gonorrhea/chlamydia
- Serial serum HCG measurements can assess viability of the pregnancy. Serum HCG should rise at least 67% every 48 hours in early pregnancy. An inappropriate rise/plateau of HCG suggests abnormal IUP or possible ectopic pregnancy.

Pregnancy Considerations

HCG levels are particularly useful in cases where an IUP has not been documented by ultrasound.

Follow-Up & Special Considerations

- In the case of vaginal bleeding with no documented IUP, follow serum HCG levels weekly to zero to ensure complete expulsion of all products of conception.
- If levels plateau, suspect ectopic pregnancy or retained products of conception, or rarely, gestational trophoblastic disease.

Imaging

Initial approach

- US exam to evaluate fetal viability and to rule out ectopic pregnancy:
  - HCG >2,000 U/L necessary to detect IUP via transvaginal US (TVUS), >6,500 U/L for abdominal ultrasound
- TVUS criteria for nonviable intrauterine gestation include 5-mm fetal pole without cardiac activity or 16-mm gestational sac without a fetal pole.
- Structures and timing: gestational sac of 2–3 mm generally seen by 4 weeks +1–3 days; yolk sac by 5 weeks estimated gestational age (EGA); fetal pole with + fetal heart tones (FHT) by 5.5–6 weeks EGA → requires high-resolution TVUS

Follow-Up & Special Considerations

- If initial HCG level does not permit documentation of IUP by TVUS, follow serum HCG in 48 hours to ensure appropriate rise.
- Follow HGC and repeat US once HCG at a level commensurate with visualization on US (see above).
- Provide patient with ectopic precautions in interim—worsening abdominal pain, significant vaginal bleeding, dizziness/syncope, and nausea/vomiting.

Diagnostic Procedures/Surgery

- Fetal heart tones can be auscultated with Doppler starting between 10 and 12 weeks' gestation from last menstrual period for a viable pregnancy.
- 90–96% of pregnancies with fetal cardiac activity and vaginal bleeding at 7–11 weeks' gestation result in continued pregnancy.

Pathological Findings

Products of conception, placental villi

DIFFERENTIAL DIAGNOSIS

- Ectopic pregnancy: Potentially life-threatening; must be ruled out with US in any woman of childbearing age with abdominal pain and vaginal bleeding
- Cervical polyps, neoplasias, and/or inflammatory conditions can cause vaginal bleeding.
- Hydatidiform mole pregnancy
- HCG-secreting ovarian tumor
- Physiologic bleeding in normal pregnancy (implantation bleeding)

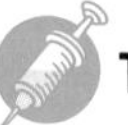

TREATMENT

MEDICATION

- Long-term conception rate and pregnancy outcomes are similar for women who undergo medical or surgical evacuation.
- Postinfection rates are lower with medical versus surgical management.

First Line

- Misoprostol: Most common agent for inducing passage of tissue in missed or incomplete abortion:
  - Not approved by Food and Drug Administration for treatment of early pregnancy failure
  - Efficacy: Complete expulsion of products of conception in 71% by day 3, 84% by day 8
  - Efficacy depends on route of administration, gestational age of pregnancy, and dose.
  - Recommended dose is 800 μg vaginally (4)[A]; alternate regimens exist including the World Health Organization regimen of 800 μg vaginally or 600 μg sublingually q3h for up to 3 doses; multidose regimens and oral dosing (including buccal and sublingual) may result in increased side effects, and pure oral dosing appears somewhat less effective than vaginal/buccal/sublingual routes.
- Common adverse effects include abdominal pain/cramping, nausea, and diarrhea. Pain increases at higher doses but is manageable with analgesia. There is no increase in nausea/diarrhea with a higher dose.
- Recommended for stable patients who decline surgery but do not want to wait for spontaneous passage of products of conception

Second Line

Rh-negative patients should be given Rh immunoglobulin following a spontaneous abortion (5)[C].

ADDITIONAL TREATMENT

General Measures

Evaluate for any 1st-trimester vaginal bleeding.

Issues for Referral

Patients should be monitored for up to 1 year for the development of psychosomatic symptoms such as depression and anxiety (6)[A].

COMPLEMENTARY AND ALTERNATIVE MEDICINE

Vitamin supplementation does not appear to prevent miscarriage (7)[A].

SURGERY/OTHER PROCEDURES

- Uterine aspiration (dilation and curettage or via vacuum aspiration) is the conventional treatment.
- Indications: Septic abortion, heavy bleeding, hypotension, patient choice
- Risks: Anesthesia, uterine perforation, intrauterine adhesions, cervical trauma, infection that may lead to infertility or increased risk of ectopic pregnancy
- When compared with medical management, surgical intervention leads to fewer days of vaginal bleeding, with a lower risk of incomplete abortion and heavy bleeding. It does carry a higher risk of infection (8)[A].
- Vacuum aspiration may be less painful than dilatation and curettage (D&C), and does not require general anesthesia (9)[B].
- Data from induced abortions suggest that antibiotic prophylaxis with doxycycline 100 mg b.i.d. substantially reduces postprocedure infection risk; however, data for incomplete abortions treated surgically are inconclusive (10)[A].
- For patients who desire contraception after completion of a spontaneous abortion, immediate insertion of an intrauterine device is both acceptable and safe (11)[A].

IN-PATIENT CONSIDERATIONS

Initial Stabilization

If the patient has orthostatic vital signs, initiate resuscitation with IV fluids and/or blood products if needed.

IV Fluids

Hemodynamically unstable patients may require IV fluids and/or blood products to maintain BP.

ONGOING CARE

FOLLOW-UP RECOMMENDATIONS

All patients should be seen in 2–6 weeks to monitor for resolution of bleeding, re-establishment of menses, review of contraception plan, and psychosomatic symptoms.

Patient Monitoring

- Identification of products of conception within material expelled from the uterus or D&C specimen (important to distinguish villi and sac from decidua)
- If abortion is complete, observe the patient for further bleeding.
- Pelvic rest until 2 weeks after evacuation
- If spontaneous abortion occurs in setting of previously documented IUP and abortion is completed with resumption of normal menses, it is not necessary to check or follow serum HCG to 0.

DIET

NPO if patient is to undergo D&C

PATIENT EDUCATION

Patient pamphlet (no. AP090) available from the American College of Obstetricians and Gynecologists, 409 12th St., SW, Washington, DC 20090–6290; (800) 762–2264 or online at http://www.acog.org

PROGNOSIS

- If bleeding ceases, prognosis is excellent.
- Habitual abortion:
  - Prognosis depends on etiology.
  - Prognosis is still excellent, with up to 70% rate of success with subsequent pregnancy.

COMPLICATIONS

- Potential complications of D&C include uterine perforation, bleeding, adhesions, cervical trauma, infection that may lead to infertility, or increased risk of ectopic pregnancy.
- Retained products of conception
- Psychological morbidity, including depression, anxiety, and feelings of guilt

REFERENCES

1. Haas DM, Ramsey PS. Progestogen for preventing miscarriage. *Cochrane Database Syst Rev*. 2008; CD003511.
2. Wahabi HA, Abed Althagafi NF, Elawad M, et al. Progestogen for treating threatened miscarriage. *Cochrane Database Syst Rev*. 2011;3:CD005943.
3. Porter TF, LaCoursiere Y, Scott JR. Immunotherapy for recurrent miscarriage. *Cochrane Database Syst Rev*. 2006;CD000112.
4. Neilson JP, Gyte GML, Hickey M, et al. Medical treatments for incomplete miscarriage (less than 24 weeks). *Cochrane Database Syst Rev*. 2010; 1:CD007223.
5. Prevention of Rho(D) alloimmunization. American College of Obstetricians and Gynecologists Practice Bulletin No 4. American College of Obstetricians and Gynecologists, Washington, DC; 1999.
6. Lok IH, Neugebauer R. Psychological morbidity following miscarriage. *Best Pract Res Clin Obstet Gynaecol*. 2007;21:229–47.
7. Rumbold A, Middleton P, Pan N, et al. Vitamin supplementation for preventing miscarriage. *Cochrane Database Syst Rev*. 2011;1:CD004073.
8. Nanda K, Peloggia A, Grimes DA, et al. Expectant care versus surgical treatment for miscarriage. *Cochrane Database Syst Rev*. 2006;2:CD003518.
9. Forna F. Surgical procedures to evacuate incomplete miscarriage. *Cochrane Database Syst Rev*. 2001;1:CD001993.
10. May W, Gülmezoglu AM, Ba-Thike K. Antibiotics for incomplete abortion. *Cochrane Database Syst Rev*. 2007;CD001779.
11. Grimes DA, Lopez LM, Schulz KF, et al. Immediate post-partum insertion of intrauterine devices. *Cochrane Database Syst Rev*. 2010;5:CD003036.

ADDITIONAL READING

Harwood B. Quality of life and acceptability of medical vs. surgical management of early pregnancy. *Br J Obstet Gynaec*. 2008;115(4):501–8.

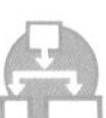

See Also (Topic, Algorithm, Electronic Media Element)

- Ectopic Pregnancy
- Algorithm: Abortion, Recurrent

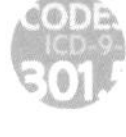

CODES

ICD9

- 632 Missed abortion
- 634.90 Spontaneous abortion, unspecified, without mention of complication
- 640.03 Threatened abortion, antepartum

CLINICAL PEARLS

- Any reproductive-age woman or pregnant woman with abdominal pain and vaginal bleeding must be evaluated to rule out ectopic pregnancy, which is potentially life threatening.
- As all options have similar long-term outcomes, patient preference should determine whether management is medical, expectant, or surgical.
- Assessment of psychological symptoms after spontaneous abortion should be an integral part of follow-up visits, with counseling, medication, and referral as appropriate.

ABRUPTIO PLACENTAE

Mark J. Manning, DO, MsMEL
Amy Ellingson-Itzin, MD

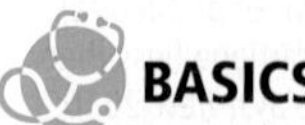

BASICS

DESCRIPTION

- Premature separation of an otherwise normally implanted placenta
- Grades:
  - Grade 1: Minimal or no bleeding; detected as retroplacental clot after delivery of viable fetus. Mild uterine irritability (40% of cases).
  - Grade 2: Viable fetus with bleeding and tender, irritable uterus. Mild-to-moderate bleeding; fibrinogen level decreased (45% of cases).
  - Grade 3: Type A with dead fetus and no coagulopathy; type B with dead fetus and coagulopathy (types A and B = 15% of all cases)

EPIDEMIOLOGY

Incidence

- 0.4–1% of pregnancies are complicated by placental abruption (1)
- 0.5–1.2% of all deliveries
  - Placental abruption is the most common cause of serious vaginal bleeding in late pregnancy (2).
- 15% if 1 prior abruption
- 25% if 2 or more prior abruptions
- 80% of cases occur prior to onset of delivery.
- Peaks at 24–26 weeks, then decreases with increasing gestation
- Rising in the US from 0.8% 1979–1981 to 1.2% 1999–2001

RISK FACTORS

- Prior abruption: Increases 15–20-fold (3)
- Increasing maternal age and parity
- Advanced maternal age
- Maternal smoking: Dose-response relationship (3)
- Cocaine use and abuse
- Factor V Leiden and other thrombophilic disorders
- Hypertensive disorders
- Uterine anomalies
- Multiple-gestation pregnancies (4)[B]
- 1st or 2nd-trimester bleeding
- Preeclampsia: Mild and severe
- Increased risk if hypertension and parity >3
- Preterm rupture of membranes (5)[B]
- Hydramnios
- Severe small-for-gestational-age birth
- Blunt trauma/motor vehicle accident

Genetics

- Genetic predisposition may be the cause of abruption in women with no other inciting factor discovered.
- Placental growth is primarily under control of paternally inherited fetal genes.

GENERAL PREVENTION

Eliminate risk factors when possible: Quit smoking and cocaine use, control hypertension, use seat belts, etc.

PATHOPHYSIOLOGY

Exact cause is unknown: Appears to be the final common clinical event secondary to a variety of causes

ETIOLOGY

- Acute:
  - Trauma of variable amounts, especially blunt abdominal trauma in which external signs of trauma may be incongruent with fetal injury
  - Sudden decompression of overdistended uterus, as in hydramnios or twin gestation
  - Vasospasm secondary to cocaine use
- Chronic (majority of cases):
  - Hypertensive disorders and growth restriction associated with chronic process
  - Early bleeding in pregnancy releases thrombin, which is a potent uterotonic agent

COMMONLY ASSOCIATED CONDITIONS

- Preeclampsia and other forms of hypertension in pregnancy
- Uteroplacental insufficiency
- Postpartum hemorrhage
- Disseminated intravascular coagulation (DIC)
- Rupture of membranes

DIAGNOSIS

HISTORY

- Classic triad of vaginal bleeding, abdominal pain, and contractions
- Abruption in prior pregnancy
- Early trimester bleeding
- Recent trauma
- Cocaine or tobacco use
- Back pain
- Frequent or tetanic contractions
- May present in active labor

PHYSICAL EXAM

- Vital signs: Tachycardia, hypotension
  - Because blood volumes increase in pregnancy, volume lost may exceed 30% before signs of shock or hypovolemia occur.
- Uterine tenderness, hypertonia, or high-frequency contractions
- Vaginal bleeding (not always present):
  - Clinical signs of shock may occur with little vaginal bleeding.
- Fetal distress or demise
- Idiopathic preterm labor with or without fetal distress

DIAGNOSTIC TESTS & INTERPRETATION

Lab

Initial lab tests

- Blood type, Rh, cross-match for possible transfusion:
  - RHoD immunoglobulin administered <12 weeks prior may affect antibody test.
- CBC with platelet count
- Prothrombin time (PT)/partial thromboplastin time (PTT)
- Kleihauer-Betke test checks for evidence of fetal blood in maternal circulation; >30 mL fetal blood indicative of large fetal blood loss:
  - 300 μg dose of RhoGAM will cover up to 30 mL whole fetal blood in maternal circulation
- Bedside clot test: Red-top tube of maternal blood with poor or nonclotting blood after 7–10 minutes indicates coagulopathy.

Follow-Up & Special Considerations

- DIC can result from a large abruption. Best to stabilize patient without waiting for DIC labs. This is typically a clinical diagnosis.
- Can send PT/PTT, fibrinogen levels at clinician discretion when stable or following resolution of DIC:
  - Fibrinogen levels climb to 350–550 mg/dL in 3rd trimester and must fall to 100–150 mg/dL before PTT will rise.
  - Fibrin split or degradation products are elevated in pregnancy and are not specific in assessing DIC.
- There is conflicting evidence that elevated fasting plasma total homocysteine (tHcy) is a risk factor for placental abruption. Prospective, sufficiently powered, studies from preconception/early pregnancy are required to determine whether tHcy is a risk factor for this and other pregnancy complications (6).

Imaging

Initial approach

- Placental abruption is a clinical diagnosis.
- Ultrasound can help to make the diagnosis, but has low sensitivity and is only helpful in cases of a large abruption.

Follow-Up & Special Considerations

Ultrasound: Appearance depends on size and location of the bleed:

- With acute bleed, nothing may be seen.
- Will fail to detect at least 50% of abruptions
- Retroplacental clot is diagnostic of abruption (3):
  - If incidental abruption is found in a patient at term, delivery is reasonable.
  - A preterm patient with an incidental abruption may be managed conservatively if stable.

Diagnostic Procedures/Surgery

- Tocometer often shows elevated baseline pressure and frequent low-amplitude contractions.
- External fetal monitoring may show recurrent late decelerations, variable decelerations, sinusoidal fetal heart tracing, bradycardia, or decreased variability—all indicative of fetal stress.

Pathological Findings

- Placental examination after delivery may show a retroplacental clot, pathologic signs of early separation/inflammation
- Normocytic normochromic anemia with acute bleeding
- Elevated PT/PTT, fibrinogen levels <100–150 mg/dL (1.0–1.5 g/L), platelets 20,000–50,000/μL if DIC is active
- Positive Kleihauer-Betke reaction if fetal–maternal transfusion has occurred
- Positive antibody if RhoD isosensitization has occurred

DIFFERENTIAL DIAGNOSIS

- Placenta previa or vasa previa (2)
- Uterine rupture
- Bloody show associated with labor
- Cervical and vaginal infections (e.g., chlamydia or gonorrhea with bloody, friable cervix)
- Other painful abdominal conditions (e.g., appendicitis, pyelonephritis)
- Fibroid degeneration
- Ovarian pathology: Torsed ovary, ruptured cyst

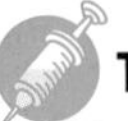

TREATMENT

MEDICATION

First Line

- Tocolytics are generally contraindicated in presence of abruption:
  - Tocolytics, such as nifedipine or terbutaline, may be used in mild noncompromising preterm abruption (specific cases only, such as for fetal lung maturity)
- RhoD immunoglobulin for RhoD-negative mother if undelivered or indicated after delivery if Kleihauer-Betke is positive
- Fluid resuscitation as required for signs of shock

Second Line

- Transfuse packed red blood cells (PRBC) or other factors to stabilize patient as needed.
- Steroids for fetal lung maturation, if fetus is viable

ADDITIONAL TREATMENT

Issues for Referral

- If preterm and hemodynamically stable, refer to tertiary care center.
- Alert anesthesia if delivery via cesarean section is likely.

SURGERY/OTHER PROCEDURES

- May need cesarean delivery after maternal stabilization if fetus is viable, remote from delivery, and non-reassuring fetal heart tracing is present.
- Postpartum hemorrhage/DIC may be treated medically or with uterine packing, embolization, or hysterectomy.

IN-PATIENT CONSIDERATIONS

Initial Stabilization

- History and physical exam with medical history, allergies, prior ultrasounds (present gestation), and time of last meal
- Management depends on presentation, gestational age, and degree of maternal and fetal compromise:
  - In general, severe abruption is best managed by delivery of fetus.
  - Grade 1: Usual labor protocol
  - Grade 2: Rapid delivery, most often by cesarean delivery (if mother stable)
  - Grade 3: Vaginal delivery preferable if mother stable
- In trauma (3)[B], monitor in the inpatient setting for at least 4 hours for evidence of fetal insult, abruption, fetal–maternal transfusion. If contractions or preterm labor occur, patient should be monitored for at least 24 hours. Risk factors for contractions with trauma include:
  - Gestational age >35 weeks
  - Assaults and pedestrian/vehicular collisions, even without direct abdominal trauma
  - Ejections from vehicle or lack of restraints
- Early aggressive restoration of maternal physiology to protect fetus and maternal organs from hypoperfusion/DIC
- Stabilize vitals
- Bed rest with external fetal and labor monitoring, if fetus is viable
- Large-bore, 16–18-gauge IV crystalloid infusion to maintain volume
- Transfusions of whole blood and PRBCs as necessary
- Fresh frozen plasma and platelet transfusions for coagulopathy, with cryoprecipitate and fibrinogen given if indicated
- Follow hemoglobin/hematocrit and coagulation status.
- Consider internal monitoring of fetus if patient is in active labor.
- Role of amniotomy to prevent amniotic fluid embolism is debatable, but may speed delivery
- Positioning on left side may enhance venous return and cardiac output
- Oxygen as needed

Admission Criteria

Patients with suspected placental abruption should be admitted for workup until deemed clinically stable and ready for discharge/outpatient follow-up or delivered for medical indication.

IV Fluids

Saline or Ringer's lactate to restore maternal vascular volume

Nursing

- Bed rest until status defined
- Frequent vital sign monitoring
- Record fluid ins and outs

Discharge Criteria

- 2nd trimester suspected abruption may be managed on outpatient basis if hemodynamically stable
- Viable patients may be discharged if maternal/fetal status is stable.

ONGOING CARE

FOLLOW-UP RECOMMENDATIONS

- Monthly growth ultrasonograms for those patients where conservative management is possible.
- Serial ultrasounds may also be used to follow regression or progression of abruption (3).
- Pelvic rest

Patient Monitoring

Severe cases or unstable patients may require critical care unit admission.

DIET

NPO until status is defined and possibility of immediate cesarean delivery ruled out

PATIENT EDUCATION

- Call physician or proceed to hospital whenever patient experiences vaginal bleeding or if severe uterine or back pain or decreased fetal movement occurs.
- Wear seat belts while in an automobile.
- Discontinue use of cocaine and tobacco.
- Visit Mayo Health: http://mayohealth.org

PROGNOSIS

- 0.5–1% fetal mortality and 30–50% perinatal mortality:
  - 1/2 of perinatal deaths due to preterm delivery
- With trauma and abruption, 1% maternal and 30–70% fetal mortality

COMPLICATIONS

- Maternal complications include anemia, stroke, myocardial infarction, DIC, and Sheehan syndrome, and may include maternal death with severe hemorrhage.
- Surgical interventions and transfusion carry their own morbidity/mortality.
- Amniotic fluid embolism is rare but may present with severe respiratory distress.

REFERENCES

1. Tikkanen M, et al. Placental abruption: Epidemiology, risk factors and consequences. *Acta Obstet Gynecol Scand*. 2011;90:140–9
2. Sakornbut E, Leeman L, Fontaine P. Late pregnancy bleeding. *Am Fam Physician*. 2007;75:1199–206.
3. Ananth CV, Getahun D, Peltier MR, et al. Placental abruption in term and preterm gestations: Evidence for heterogeneity in clinical pathways. *Obstet Gynecol*. 2006;107:785–92.
4. Salihu HM, Bekan B, Aliyu MH, et al. Perinatal mortality associated with abruptio placenta in singletons and multiples. *Am J Obstet Gynecol*. 2005;193:198–203.
5. Ananth CV, Oyelese Y, Srinivas N, et al. Preterm premature rupture of membranes, intrauterine infection, and oligohydramnios: Risk factors for placental abruption. *Obstet Gynecol*. 2004;104: 71–7.
6. Murphy MM, Fernandez-Ballart JD, et al. Homocysteine in pregnancy. *Adv Clin Chem*. 2011;53:105–37

ADDITIONAL READING

- Getahun D, Ananth CV, Peltier MR, et al. Acute and chronic respiratory diseases in pregnancy: Associations with placenta abruption. *Am J Obstet Gynecol*. 2006;195(4):1180–4.
- Oyelese Y, Ananth CV. Placental abruption. *Obstet Gynecol*. 2006;108:1005–16.
- Pressman EV. Imaging of the placenta. *Ultrasound Clin*. 2008;3(1).
- Yang Q, Wen SW, Oppenheimer L, et al. Association of caesarean delivery for first birth with placenta praevia and placental abruption in second pregnancy. *BJOG*. 2007;114:609–13.

CODES

ICD9

- 641.20 Premature separation of placenta, unspecified as to episode of care or not applicable
- 641.21 Premature separation of placenta, delivered, with or without mention of antepartum condition
- 641.23 Premature separation of placenta, antepartum condition or complication

CLINICAL PEARLS

- Placental abruption is the most common cause of serious vaginal bleeding in late pregnancy.
- Abruption is a clinical diagnosis. The classic triad is vaginal bleeding, abdominal pain, and contractions. Ultrasound can help to make the diagnosis, but has low sensitivity and is only helpful in cases of a large abruption.
- Because blood volumes increase in pregnancy, volume lost may exceed 30% before signs of shock or hypovolemia occur.
- Individualize management on a case-by-case basis, depending upon maternal and fetal considerations.

ACETAMINOPHEN POISONING

Lars C. Larsen, MD

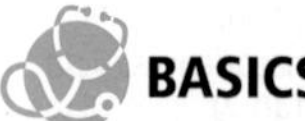

BASICS

DESCRIPTION

- A disorder characterized by hepatic necrosis following large ingestions of acetaminophen. Symptoms may vary from initial nausea, vomiting, diaphoresis, and malaise to jaundice, confusion, somnolence, coma, and death. The clinical hallmark is the onset of symptoms within 24 hours of ingestion of acetaminophen-only or combination products.
- Acetaminophen poisoning is most often encountered following large single ingestions of acetaminophen-containing medications. Usual toxic doses are above 10 g in adults and 150 mg/kg in children. However, poisoning also occurs after acute and chronic ingestions of lesser amounts in susceptible individuals, including those who regularly abuse alcohol, are chronically malnourished, or take medications that affect hepatic metabolism of acetaminophen.
- Therapeutic adult doses are 0.5–1 g q4–6h, up to a maximum of 4 g/d. Therapeutic pediatric doses are 10–15 mg/kg q4–6h, not to exceed 5 doses in 24 hours.
- System(s) affected: Gastrointestinal; Cardiovascular; Renal/Urologic:
  - Multisystem organ failure can occur.
- Synonym(s): Paracetamol poisoning

Geriatric Considerations

Hepatic damage may be increased if taking hepatotoxic medications chronically.

Pediatric Considerations

Hepatic damage at toxic acetaminophen levels is decreased in children <6 years.

Pregnancy Considerations

- Increased incidence of spontaneous abortion, especially with overdose at early gestational age
- Incidence of spontaneous abortion or fetal death appears to be increased when *N*-acetylcysteine (NAC) treatment is delayed.
- IV NAC is generally preferred in pregnancy since it may offer greater bioavailability.

EPIDEMIOLOGY

- Predominant age: Children and adults
- Predominant sex: No reported association

Incidence

- More than 99,800 single-substance ingestions of acetaminophen or acetaminophen combination products reported by poison control centers in 2009
- 144 deaths in 2009; none in children <6 years of age

Prevalence

>47% of single-substance exposures in 2009 were in children <6 years.

RISK FACTORS

- Age >6 years
- Concurrent poisoning with other substances
- Psychiatric illness
- Previous toxic ingestions or suicide attempts
- Regular ingestion of large amounts of alcohol

GENERAL PREVENTION

Parent/caregiver education essential:

- Education during well-child exams regarding poisoning prevention
- Emergency telephone numbers

ETIOLOGY

- Accidental or intentional ingestion of acetaminophen or combination medications containing acetaminophen
- 96% of ingested acetaminophen is metabolized in the liver, with only 2–4% excreted unchanged in the urine. When taken in therapeutic doses, 90–95% of hepatic metabolism occurs via glucuronidation and sulfation and results in the formation of benign metabolites. 5–10% of hepatic metabolism is by oxidation through the cytochrome P_{450} enzyme system (CYP 3A4 and CYP 2E1) and results in the formation of the toxic metabolite *N*-acetyl-*p*-benzoquinoneimine (NAPQI). NAPQI is rapidly conjugated with glutathione to form a nontoxic metabolite. The metabolites are excreted in the urine along with the small amount of unchanged drug. Hepatocellular damage typically occurs when toxic doses of acetaminophen result in saturation of the glucuronidation and sulfation pathways with subsequent production of excessive amounts of NAPQI. Available glutathione stores become depleted, NAPQI accumulates, and hepatocellular damage occurs.

DIAGNOSIS

- Signs and symptoms develop over the first 24 hours following large ingestions, and may last as long as 8 days.
- May develop gradually following long-term ingestion of near maximal-therapeutic amounts of acetaminophen. Such patients may present in stages 1–3, without a history of ingestion of the usual toxic doses.
- Severe symptoms indicate large ingestions or coingestants:
  - Stage 1: First 24 hours after time of ingestion:
    - Nausea
    - Vomiting
    - Diaphoresis
  - Stage 2: 24–48 hours:
    - Right upper quadrant pain
    - Typically less nausea, vomiting, diaphoresis, and malaise than in stage 1
  - Stage 3: 72–96 hours:
    - Nausea, vomiting, and malaise reappear.
    - Severe poisonings may result in jaundice, confusion, somnolence, and coma.
  - Stage 4: 7–8 days:
    - Resolution of clinical signs in survivors
- Fulminant hepatic failure occurs in <1% of adults and is very rare in children <6 years of age.
- Patients with an unexplained rise in liver function tests (LFTs) with negative acetaminophen levels may be overdose patients presenting in stage 3.

HISTORY

Ingestion or suspected ingestion of acetaminophen-containing product

DIAGNOSTIC TESTS & INTERPRETATION

Lab

- Plasma acetaminophen levels should be drawn on all patients 4 hours or more after ingestion (levels prior to 4 hours not helpful).
- Screens for suspected coingestants (aspirin, iron, and others) may be positive (especially when suicide attempt is a possibility).
- With toxic ingestions, aspartate transaminase (AST; serum glutamic-oxaloacetic transaminase), alanine transaminase (ALT; serum glutamic-pyruvic transaminase), and bilirubin levels begin to rise in stage 2 and peak in stage 3. In severe poisonings, the prothrombin time (PT)/international normalized ratio (INR) will parallel these changes and should be monitored.
- AST levels >1,000 IU/L are consistent with the diagnosis, and levels of 20,000 IU/L are not uncommon.
- Laboratory abnormalities usually resolve by stage 4.
- Renal function abnormalities are common in patients with hepatotoxicity.
- Evidence of damage to the pancreas and heart may present following severe poisonings.
- Drugs that may alter lab results: None with clinically significant cross-reactivity with plasma acetaminophen assay
- Disorders that may alter lab results: Diseases or toxic substances that damage the liver, particularly alcohol

Initial lab tests

- Acetaminophen serum concentration: 4 hours or more after ingestion (see above)
- AST, ALT (rise in first 72 hours, then slowly decline), PT/NR, bilirubin, lactate dehydrogenase (LDH)
- Electrolytes, glucose, BUN, creatinine
- Pregnancy screen in females (urine or serum)
- Urinalysis
- Consider arterial blood gas if pH disturbance suspected on clinical or lab grounds.

Follow-Up & Special Considerations

Arterial blood gas after hydration if pH is acidotic

Imaging

No specific imaging required

Pathological Findings

Centrilobular hepatic necrosis

DIFFERENTIAL DIAGNOSIS

- Consider presence of coingestants, especially alcohol and aspirin.
- Other ingested toxins that produce severe acute hepatic injury, including the mushroom *Amanita phalloides* and products containing yellow phosphorus or carbon tetrachloride

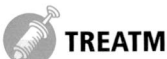

TREATMENT

- Contact a regional poison control center for management recommendations. In the US, a local poison control center can be reached by calling (800) 222-1222.
- NAC should be given when plasma acetaminophen concentrations measured 4 hours or more after ingestion are in the "possible risk" or higher levels on the Rumack-Matthew nomogram. This corresponds to acetaminophen levels >150 μg/mL (993 μmol/L), >75 μg/mL (497 μmol/L), and >37 μg/mL (244 μmol/L) at 4, 8, and 12 hours after ingestion, respectively. See http://www.ars-informatica.ca/toxicity_nomogram.php?calc=acetamin or http://www.merckmanuals.com/professional/sec22/ch346/ch346b.html#v1118627.
- NAC should be started within 8 hours of ingestion for best chance of hepatic protection. Patients presenting near 8 hours should empirically receive NAC while waiting for labs.
- All patients with acetaminophen liver injury (even after 8 hours) should receive NAC.
- NAC therapy may be effective up to 36 hours or more after ingestion.
- Single-dose activated charcoal may be used if given within 1 hour of ingestion (especially in cases of coingestants) (1,2)[C],(3)[A], but not within 1 hour of administration of the antidote NAC. Never delay NAC for activated charcoal.
- NAC should be initiated within 8 hours of ingestion whenever possible.
- Ipecac and gastric lavage are no longer recommended for routine use at home or in health care facilities (4)[C].

MEDICATION

First Line

- Acetylcysteine (NAC, Mucomyst) should be initiated within 8 hours of ingestion whenever possible; single-dose activated charcoal (1 g/kg PO) may be effective if given within 1 hour of ingestion. *Never* delay oral NAC for activated charcoal.
- Acetylcysteine may be given PO or IV, depending on situation and availability:
  - Currently, IV is the recommended form of administration:
    - IV loading dose of Acetadote 150 mg/kg over 60 minutes followed by an infusion of 50 mg/kg over 4 hours (12.5 mg/kg/hr); this is followed by an infusion of 100 mg/kg over the next 16 hours (6.25 mg/kg/hr). Oral loading dose of 140 mg/kg, followed by 70 mg/kg q4h for 17 additional doses.
- Contraindications: Medication allergies
- Precautions:
  - Oral NAC may cause significant nausea and vomiting due to its sulfur content; consider IV administration or by nasogastric tube.
  - Nausea can be treated with metoclopramide (Reglan), 0.5–1 mg/kg IV, or ondansetron (Zofran), 0.15 mg/kg IV (for age >4 years, usually 4 mg/dose).
  - IV NAC (Acetadote) may cause anaphylactoid reactions, including rash, bronchospasm, pruritus, angioedema, tachycardia, or hypotension (higher rates seen in asthmatics and those with atopic history) (5,6)[C].
- Reactions usually occur with loading dose. Slow or temporarily stop the infusion; may concurrently treat with antihistamines.
- Significant possible interactions: Activated charcoal given within 1 hour of oral NAC may adsorb the NAC, limiting its effectiveness.

Second Line

Oral racemethionine (methionine)

ADDITIONAL TREATMENT

Issues for Referral

- Psychiatric and psychological evaluation in emergency room and close follow-up after intentional ingestions
- Consider child abuse reporting if neglect led to overdose.

IN-PATIENT CONSIDERATIONS

Initial Stabilization

Aggressive age- and weight-appropriate IV hydration

Admission Criteria

- Toxic and intentional ingestions
- Any reported ingestion with increased LFTs, acidosis on arterial blood gas (ABG), elevated creatinine, etc.

ONGOING CARE

FOLLOW-UP RECOMMENDATIONS

- All patients should be evaluated at a health care facility.
- Patients with evidence of organ failure, increased LFTs, or coagulopathy should be evaluated for transfer to a site capable of liver transplant.
- Outpatient for nontoxic accidental ingestions
- Activity may be restricted if significant hepatic damage.

Patient Monitoring

Inquire as to possible ingestion by others (i.e., suicide pacts).

DIET

No special diet, except with severe hepatic damage

PATIENT EDUCATION

- Patients should be counseled to avoid Tylenol if already using combination product(s) containing acetaminophen.
- Education of parents/caregivers during well-child visits
- Anticipatory guidance for caregivers, family, and cohabitants of potentially suicidal patients
- Patient brochure (item no. 1515), *Child safety: keeping your home safe for your baby*. American Academy of Family Physicians or: http://familydoctor.org/online/famdocen/home/healthy/safety/kids-family/027.html
- Education of patients taking long-term acetaminophen therapy

PROGNOSIS

- Complete recovery with early therapy
- <1% of adult patients develop hepatic failure. King criteria (pH <7.3, PT >100 s [INR >65], creatinine >3.4 mg/dL [>300 μmol/L]) are associated with a poor prognosis and possible need for liver transplant (7)[C]. Early referral increases the chance for transplant success (8)[A].
- Hepatic failure is very rare in children <6 years of age.

COMPLICATIONS

Rare following recovery from acute poisoning

REFERENCES

1. Gaudreault P. Activated charcoal revisited. *Clin Ped Emerg Med*. 2005;6:76–80.
2. Heard K. Gastrointestinal decontamination. *Med Clin North Am*. 2005;89:1067–78.
3. Brok J, Buckley N, Gluud C. Interventions for paracetamol (acetaminophen) overdose. *Cochrane Database Syst Rev*. 2009;1.
4. American Academy of Pediatrics Committee on Injury, Violence, and Poison Prevention. Poison treatment in the home. American Academy of Pediatrics Committee on Injury, Violence, and Poison Prevention. *Pediatrics*. 2003;112:1182–5.
5. Acetylcysteine (Acetadote) for acetaminophen overdosage. *Med Lett*. 2005;47:70–1.
6. Culley CM, Krenzelok EP. A clinical and pharmacoeconomic justification for intravenous acetylcysteine: A US perspective. *Toxicol Rev*. 2005;24:131–43.
7. O'Grady JG, Alexander GJ, Hayllar KM, et al. Early indicators of prognosis in fulminant hepatic failure. *Gastroenterology*. 1989;97:439–45.
8. Ferner RE, Dear JW, Bateman DN. Management of paracetamol poisoning. *BMJ*. 2011;342.

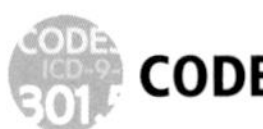

CODES

ICD9

965.4 Poisoning by aromatic analgesics, not elsewhere classified

CLINICAL PEARLS

- Contact a regional poison control center for management recommendations. In the US, a local poison control center can be reached by calling (800) 222-1222.
- NAC should be given when plasma acetaminophen concentrations measured 4 hours or more after ingestion are in the "possible risk" or higher levels on the Rumack-Matthew nomogram. This corresponds to acetaminophen levels >150 μg/mL (993 μmol/L), >75 μg/mL (497 μmol/L), and >40 μg/mL (265 μmol/L) at 4, 8, and 12 hours after ingestion, respectively.
- NAC should be started within 8 hours of ingestion for best chance of hepatic protection. Patients presenting near 8 hours should empirically receive NAC while waiting for labs.
- All patients with acetaminophen liver injury (even after 8 hours) should receive NAC.

ACL INJURY

Chad Beattie, MD
J. Herbert Stevenson, MD

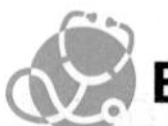

BASICS

DESCRIPTION

- The anterior cruciate ligament (ACL) is one of the major stabilizers of the knee. It prevents excessive anterior translation and internal rotation of the tibia on the femur. During dynamic movement, the ACL and posterior cruciate ligament (PCL) work together to stabilize the knee.
- ACL injuries are common and can occur through noncontact or contact mechanisms. >70% of ACL injuries are caused by noncontact forces (1).
- Partial tears of the ACL can occur, but complete tears are far more common.
- Female athletes are at 2–5 times higher risk of ACL tear, particularly in soccer, basketball, and skiing.
- ACL injury is associated with early onset of knee osteoarthritis, regardless of surgical or nonsurgical treatment (2)[B].

EPIDEMIOLOGY

Incidence

- 250,000 ACL injuries annually in the US (1)
- Female athletes incidence 2–5-fold > male athletes
- Greater incidence of noncontact ACL injuries in sports requiring cutting, pivoting, and rapid deceleration, such as basketball and soccer

Prevalence

- Young athletes aged 15–25 years sustain >50% of all ACL injuries.
- >2/3 of patients with complete ACL tear have associated menisci and/or articular cartilage injury (1).

Pediatric Considerations

- Must be concerned about physeal injuries in the skeletally immature
- The incidence of ACL tears in patients with open physes has increased in recent years.
- ACL injury rates increase for both boys and girls beginning at age 11 years.

RISK FACTORS

- No single risk factor correlates directly with higher ACL injury rates in female athletes. Likely multifactorial etiology:
  - Sex hormones:
    - Increased rate may be due to monthly hormonal fluctuations.
    - No conclusive evidence linking a menstrual cycle phase
  - Anatomic gender differences:
    - Increased Q angle, increased genu valgum, narrower femoral notch size, smaller ACL
    - Neuromuscular imbalances (increased quadriceps activation, decreased hamstring activity during landings)
  - Movement patterns (sudden deceleration, change-of-direction cutting movements, landing from a jump in hyperextension)

Genetics

Familial tendency has been identified.

GENERAL PREVENTION

- Neuromuscular training with proprioceptive, plyometric, and strength exercises may reduce noncontact ACL injuries by 72% in female athletes if performed > once per week for longer than 6 weeks (1,3)[B].
- No evidence that prophylactic knee bracing prevents ACL injuries
- Educate the patient about possible risk factors for ACL injury and provide instruction on neuromuscular training exercises.

ETIOLOGY

- Noncontact mechanisms (torsional or hyperextension forces)
- Direct trauma (player, object on playing field)

COMMONLY ASSOCIATED CONDITIONS

- Meniscal tear
- Collateral ligament tear
- PCL tear
- Tibia or femur fractures
- Osteochondral injury
- Loose bodies
- Early-onset degenerative joint disease

DIAGNOSIS

HISTORY

May recall mechanism:

- Noncontact:
  - Sudden deceleration
  - Cutting, sudden change in direction
  - Landing from a jump in extension
  - Combination of mechanisms
- Contact with player, object
- May recall sudden pop or snap
- Sudden pain and giving way
- Marked effusion/hemarthrosis within 4–12 hours

PHYSICAL EXAM

- Pain
- Effusion
- Decreased range of motion (ROM)
- Joint instability
- Difficulty bearing weight
- Inspect for malalignment (fracture, dislocation)
- Palpate for effusion
- Evaluate extensor mechanism integrity
- Evaluate ROM:
  - Deficits may be secondary to pain, effusion, mechanical blocks (meniscal tear, loose body, torn ACL stump).

DIAGNOSTIC TESTS & INTERPRETATION

- Lachman test: Most sensitive and highly specific diagnostic test for ACL injury, especially in acute setting (4)[A]:
  - Knee placed in 20–30° flexion. Tibia is pulled forward while femur is stabilized with opposite hand. Increased anterior translation compared with uninjured knee indicates injury. Lack of a solid endpoint indicates rupture.
- Pivot shift test: Lower sensitivity, but more specific for ACL tear than Lachman test (4)[B]:
  - Knee placed in extension. Knee is flexed while applying a valgus and internal rotation stress. A positive test is subluxation at 20–40° of flexion.
- Anterior drawer test:
  - Low sensitivity for ACL integrity, especially in acute setting (4)[A]
- Posterior drawer test assesses PCL integrity.
- McMurray test assesses for meniscal tears.
- Valgus/varus stress test for medial collateral ligament/lateral collateral (MCL/LCL) integrity

Imaging

- Radiographs to rule out associated bony injury
- Anterior-posterior (AP), lateral, and tunnel views:
  - Segond fracture: Avulsion fracture of the lateral capsular margin of the tibia
  - Tibial eminence avulsion fracture
  - Fracture of proximal tibia or distal femur
  - Osteochondral injuries
- MRI is the gold standard for imaging ligamentous and intra-articular structures; MRI may show secondary signs of ACL injury.
- Secondary signs include: Bone contusion of the anterior femoral condyle and/or posterior tibial plateau, anterior translation of the tibia, an uncovered or displaced posterior horn of the lateral meniscus, PCL buckling, or a Segond fracture (an avulsion fracture of the lateral tibial condyle)

Diagnostic Procedures/Surgery

Surgical management should be considered in the active population, young or old.

DIFFERENTIAL DIAGNOSIS

- Fracture
- Meniscal injury
- Patellar dislocation/subluxation
- Tendon disruption
- PCL injury
- Collateral ligament injury

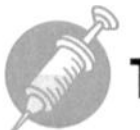

TREATMENT

MEDICATION

First Line

- NSAIDs:
  - Acute ligament sprains:
    - Ibuprofen: 200–800 mg t.i.d.
    - Naproxen: 375–500 mg b.i.d.
    - Indomethacin: 25–50 mg t.i.d.
- Acetaminophen
- Narcotics for severe pain (e.g., acetaminophen-hydrocodone)
- Contraindications/precautions/interactions: Refer to the manufacturer's profile of each drug.

ADDITIONAL TREATMENT

General Measures

- Acute injury: PRICEMM therapy: Protection, Relative rest, Ice, Compression, Elevation, Medications, Modalities
- Crutches may be indicated until patient is able to ambulate without pain.
- Knee immobilizer or brace may be used initially for comfort.
- Aspiration of large effusion may be indicated to alleviate pain and increase ROM.

Geriatric Considerations

Management is based on anticipated activity level, associated injuries, coexisting medical conditions, and acute versus long-standing ACL deficiency.

Issues for Referral

Surgical management should be considered in the active population.

Additional Therapies

- Physical therapy is recommended if an athlete chooses nonsurgical or surgical treatment. Nonsurgical physical therapy (PT) is focused on restoring ROM, strength, and proprioception.
- Preoperative phase:
  - Increase ROM, minimize inflammation
- Early postoperative phase: Weeks 2–4:
  - ROM: Full extension is the most important goal. Rehabilitation begins immediately.
  - Progress to full weightbearing.
- Intermediate postoperative phase: Weeks 4–12:
  - ROM: Full flexion, hyperextension
  - Quadriceps and hamstring strengthening proprioceptive training, normalize gait
- Late postop phase: 2–3 months postop:
  - Straight-line running
  - Increased speed, duration over 6–8 weeks
  - Progress to cutting and sport-specific drills.
  - Strength and proprioceptive training

SURGERY/OTHER PROCEDURES

- Surgical versus conservative management depends on patient's activity level, age, associated injuries, and presence of osteoarthritis (OA).
- Insufficient evidence for ACL reconstructive surgery versus conservative management in the skeletally immature patient
- Insufficient evidence from randomized trials comparing surgical versus nonoperative management of ACL injuries in adults based on studies in the 1980s (5)[A]
- In young, active adults with acute ACL tears, rehabilitation plus early ACL repair was not superior to a strategy of initial rehabilitation with delayed repair if rehab alone failed. In fact, the latter strategy led to an overall reduction of ACL reconstructions (6)[A].
- Reconstruction techniques:
  - Bone-patella tendon-bone autograft
  - Hamstring autograft
  - Allograft tendon (from cadaver)
- No consistent significant differences in outcome between patellar tendon and hamstring tendon autografts (7)[A]
- Concomitant meniscal tears are repaired at the time of ACL reconstruction.

IN-PATIENT CONSIDERATIONS

Initial Stabilization

Outpatient

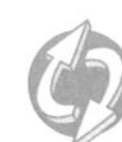

ONGOING CARE

FOLLOW-UP RECOMMENDATIONS

- ROM exercises to regain full flexion and extension
- Advance activity as tolerated

Patient Monitoring

Assess functional status, rehabilitative exercise compliance, and pain control at follow-up visit.

PROGNOSIS

- Athletes typically are out of competitive play for 6–9 months after injury to undergo ACL reconstructive surgery and rehabilitation.
- High prevalence of OA, even in those with early ACL reconstruction (2)[B]
- Delay of surgical reconstruction of torn ACL raises risk of secondary meniscal injury

COMPLICATIONS

- Instability
- Secondary meniscal and articular cartilage injury
- Early-onset degenerative arthritis
- Surgical risks:
  - Infection, pulmonary embolism (PE), subsequent ACL graft rupture, laxity due to failure of graft remodeling

REFERENCES

1. Silvers HJ, Mandelbaum BR. Prevention of anterior cruciate ligament injury in the female athlete. *Br J Sports Med*. 2007;41 (Suppl 1):i52–9.
2. Lohmander LS, Englund PM, Dahl LL, et al. Long term consequences of anterior cruciate ligament and meniscus injuries. *Am J Sports Med*. 2007;35: 1756–69.
3. Hewett TE, Ford KR, Myer GD. Anterior cruciate ligament injuries in female athletes: Part 2, a meta-analysis of neuromuscular interventions aimed at injury prevention. *Am J Sports Med*. 2006;34:490–8.
4. Jackson JL, O'Malley PG, Kroenke K. Evaluation of acute knee pain in primary care. *Ann Intern Med*. 2003;129:575–88.
5. Linko E, Harilainen A, Malmivaara A, et al. Surgical versus conservative interventions for anterior cruciate ligament rupture in adults. *Cochrane Database Syst Rev*. 2005;Issue 4.
6. Frobell RB, Roos EM, Roos HP, et al. A randomized trial of treatment for acute anterior cruciate ligament tears. *N Engl J Med*. 2010;363(4): 331–42.
7. Spindler KP, Kuhn JE, Freedman KB, et al. Anterior cruciate ligament reconstruction autograft choice: bone-tendon-bone versus hamstring: does it really matter? A systematic review. *Am J Sports Med*. 2004;32:1986–95.

ADDITIONAL READING

Cascio BM, Culp L, Cosgarea AJ. Return to play after anterior cruciate ligament reconstruction. *Clin Sports Med*. 2004;23:395–408, ix.

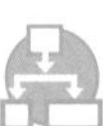

See Also (Topic, Algorithm, Electronic Media Element)

Algorithm: Knee pain

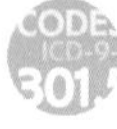

CODES

ICD9

844.2 Sprain of cruciate ligament of knee

CLINICAL PEARLS

- Lachman test: Most sensitive and highly specific diagnostic test for ACL injury, especially in acute setting (4)[A]
- Pivot shift test: Less sensitive but more specific for ACL tear than the Lachman test (4)[B]
- Anterior drawer test: Low sensitivity for ACL integrity, especially in acute setting (4)[A]
- 2/3 of complete ACL tears have associated meniscal or articular injuries.

ACNE ROSACEA

Adarsh K. Gupta, DO, MS

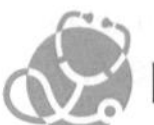

BASICS

DESCRIPTION

- Rosacea is a chronic condition characterized by recurrent episodes of facial flushing, erythema (due to dilatation of small blood vessels in the face), papules, pustules, and telangiectasia (due to increased reactivity of capillaries) in a symmetrical, facial distribution. Sometimes associated with ocular symptoms (ocular rosacea).
- System(s) affected: Skin/Exocrine
- Synonym(s): Rosacea

Geriatric Considerations

- Uncommon >60 years of age
- Effects of aging might increase the side effects associated with oral isotretinoin (at present, data is insufficient due to lack of clinical studies in elderly patients aged 65 and above)

EPIDEMIOLOGY

Prevalence

- Predominant age: 30–50 years
- Predominant sex: Female > Male. However, male will often progress to later stages.

RISK FACTORS

- Exposure to cold, heat, hot drinks
- Environmental trigger factors: Sun, wind, cold

Genetics

People of Northern European and Celtic background commonly afflicted

GENERAL PREVENTION

No preventive measures known

ETIOLOGY

- No proven cause
- Possibilities include:
  - Thyroid and gonadal disturbance
  - Alcohol, coffee, tea, spiced food overindulgence (unproven)
  - Demodex follicular parasite (suspected)
  - Exposure to cold, heat, hot drinks
  - Emotional stress
  - Dysfunction of the GI tract

COMMONLY ASSOCIATED CONDITIONS

- Seborrheic dermatitis of scalp and eyelids
- Keratitis with photophobia, lacrimation, visual disturbance
- Corneal lesions
- Blepharitis
- Uveitis

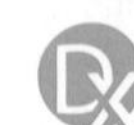

DIAGNOSIS

HISTORY

- Usually have a history of episodic flushing with increases in skin temperature in response to heat stimulus in mouth (hot liquids), spicy foods, alcohol, sun (solar elastosis). Acne may have preceded the onset of rosacea by years; nevertheless, rosacea usually arises de novo without any preceding history of acne or seborrhea.
- Excessive facial warmth and redness are the predominant presenting complaints. Itching is generally absent.

PHYSICAL EXAM

- Rosacea has typical stages of evolution:
  - The rosacea diathesis: Episodic erythema, "flushing and blushing"
  - Stage I: Persistent erythema with telangiectases
  - Stage II: Persistent erythema, telangiectases, papules, tiny pustules
  - Stage III: Persistent deep erythema, dense telangiectases, papules, pustules, nodules; rarely persistent "solid" edema of the central part of the face (Phymatous)
- Facial erythema, particularly on cheeks, nose, and chin. At times, the entire face may be involved.
- Inflammatory papules are prominent, and there may be pustules and telangiectasia.
- Comedones are absent (unlike acne).
- Women usually have lesions on the chin and cheeks, whereas nose is commonly involved in men.
- Ocular findings (mild dryness and irritation with blepharitis, conjunctival injection, burning, stinging, tearing, eyelid inflammation, swelling, and redness) are present in 50% of patients.

DIAGNOSTIC TESTS & INTERPRETATION

Diagnosis is based on physical exam findings.

Pathological Findings

- Inflammation around hypertrophied sebaceous glands, producing papules, pustules, and cysts
- Absence of comedones and blocked ducts
- Vascular dilation and dermal lymphocytic infiltrate

DIFFERENTIAL DIAGNOSIS

- Drug eruptions (iodides and bromides)
- Granulomas of the skin
- Cutaneous lupus erythematosus
- Carcinoid syndrome
- Deep fungal infection
- Acne vulgaris
- Seborrheic dermatitis
- Steroid rosacea (abuse)
- Systemic lupus erythematosus

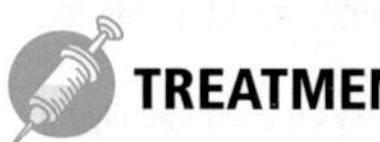

TREATMENT

MEDICATION

First Line

- Azelaic acid (Finacea) with oral doxycycline is very effective as initial therapy and then azelaic acid topical alone is effective for maintenance (1)[A]
- Precautions: Tetracycline may cause photosensitivity; sunscreen is recommended.
- Significant possible interactions:
  - Tetracycline: Avoid concurrent administration with antacids, dairy products, or iron.
  - Broad-spectrum antibiotics: May reduce the effectiveness of oral contraceptives; barrier method is recommended.

Pediatric Considerations

Tetracycline: Not for use in children <8 years

Pregnancy Considerations

- Tetracycline: Not for use during pregnancy
  - Isotretinoin: Teratogenic; not for use during pregnancy or in women of reproductive age who are not using reliable contraception

Second Line

- Topical erythromycin
- Topical clindamycin lotion preferred
- Possible utility of calcineurin inhibitors (tacrolimus 0.1%; pimecrolimus 0.1%)
- Permethrin 5% cream (2)[A] similar efficacy compared to metronidazole
- Topical steroids should not be used, as they may aggravate rosacea.
- For severe cases, isotretinoin PO for 4 months

ADDITIONAL TREATMENT

General Measures

- Use of mild, nondrying soap is recommended; local skin irritants should be avoided.
- Reassurance that rosacea is completely unrelated to poor hygiene
- Treat psychological stress if present.
- Avoid oil-based cosmetics:
  - Others are acceptable and may help women tolerate the symptoms.
- Electrodesiccation or chemical sclerosis of permanently dilated blood vessels
- Possible evolving laser therapy
- Support physical fitness

SURGERY/OTHER PROCEDURES

Laser treatment is an option for progressive telangiectasias or rhinophyma.

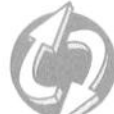

ONGOING CARE

FOLLOW-UP RECOMMENDATIONS

Outpatient treatment

Patient Monitoring

- Occasional and as needed
- Close follow-up for women using isotretinoin

DIET

Avoid alcohol, excessive sun exposure, and hot drinks of any type.

PROGNOSIS

- Slowly progressive
- Subsides spontaneously (sometimes)

COMPLICATIONS

- Rhinophyma (dilated follicles and thickened bulbous skin on nose), especially in men
- Conjunctivitis
- Blepharitis
- Keratitis
- Visual deterioration

REFERENCES

1. Thiboutot DM, Fleischer AB, Del Rosso JQ, et al. A multicenter study of topical azelaic acid 15% gel in combination with oral doxycycline as initial therapy and azelaic acid 15% gel as maintenance monotherapy. *J Drugs Dermatol*. 2009;8:639–48.
2. Koçak M, Yağli S, Vahapooğlu G, et al. Permethrin 5% cream versus metronidazole 0.75% gel for the treatment of papulopustular rosacea. A randomized double-blind placebo-controlled study. *Dermatology*. 2002;205:265–70.

ADDITIONAL READING

- Del Rosso JQ, Webster GF, Jackson M, et al. Two randomized phase III clinical trials evaluating anti-inflammatory dose doxycycline (40-mg doxycycline, USP capsules) administered once daily for treatment of rosacea. *J Am Acad Dermatol*. 2007;56:791–802.
- Liu RH, Smith MK, Basta SA, et al. Azelaic acid in the treatment of papulopustular rosacea: A systematic review of randomized controlled trials. *Arch Dermatol*. 2006;142:1047–52.

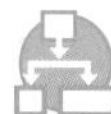

See Also (Topic, Algorithm, Electronic Media Element)

- Acne Vulgaris; Blepharitis; Dermatitis, Seborrheic; Lupus Erythematosus, Discoid; Uveitis
- Algorithm: Acne

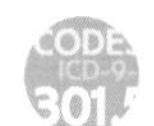

CODES

ICD9

695.3 Rosacea

CLINICAL PEARLS

- Rosacea usually arises de novo without any preceding history of acne or seborrhea.
- Rosacea may cause chronic eye symptoms, including blepharitis.
- Avoid alcohol, sun exposure, and hot drinks.
- Medication treatment resembles that of acne vulgaris with oral and topical antibiotics

ACNE VULGARIS

Gary I. Levine, MD

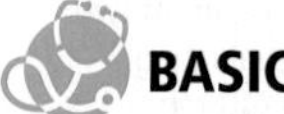

BASICS

DESCRIPTION

- Acne vulgaris is a disorder of the pilosebaceous units. It is a chronic inflammatory dermatosis notable for open/closed comedones and inflammatory lesions, including papules, pustules, or nodules.
- System(s) affected: Skin/Exocrine

Geriatric Considerations

Favre-Racouchot syndrome: Comedones on face and head due to sun exposure

Pregnancy Considerations

- May result in a flare or remission of acne
- Erythromycin can be used in pregnancy; use topical agents when possible.
- Isotretinoin is teratogenic; Class X
- Avoid topical tretinoin, although no good evidence exists that its use is teratogenic.
- Contraindicated: Isotretinoin, tazarotene, tetracycline, doxycycline, minocycline

Pediatric Considerations

Rare in ages 1–7 years:

- Check for hyperandrogenemia of adrenal or ovarian origin.
- Do not use tetracyclines <8 years of age

EPIDEMIOLOGY

- Predominant age: Early to late puberty, may persist into fourth decade
- Predominant sex:
  - Male > Female (adolescence)
  - Female > Male (adult)

Prevalence

- Nearly 80–95% of adolescents affected. A smaller percentage will seek medical advice.
- 8% of adults aged 25–34 years, 3% of those aged 35–44 years

RISK FACTORS

- Increased endogenous androgenic effect
- Oily cosmetics
- Rubbing or occluding skin surface (e.g., sports equipment such as helmets and shoulder pads), telephone, or hands against the skin
- Polyvinyl chloride, chlorinated hydrocarbons, cutting oil, tars
- Numerous drugs, including androgenic steroids (e.g., steroid abuse, some birth control pills)
- Endocrine disorders: Polycystic ovarian syndrome, Cushing syndrome, congenital adrenal hyperplasia, androgen-secreting tumors, acromegaly
- Stress
- High glycemic load diets may exacerbate acne (1).

Genetics

- Familial association in 50%
- If a family history exists, the acne may be more severe and occur earlier.

PATHOPHYSIOLOGY

- Immune changes and inflammatory responses may predate hyperkeratinization.
- Androgens (testosterone and dehydroepiandrosterone [DHEA]) stimulate sebum production and proliferation of keratinocytes in hair follicles.
- Keratin plug obstructs follicle os, causing sebum accumulation and follicular distention.
- *Propionibacterium acnes*, an anaerobe, colonizes and proliferates in the plugged follicle.
- *P. acnes* promotes chemotactic factors and proinflammatory mediators, causing inflammation of follicle and dermis.

COMMONLY ASSOCIATED CONDITIONS

- Acne fulminans
- Pyoderma faciale
- Acne conglobata
- Hidradenitis suppurativa
- Pomade acne
- SAPHO syndrome: Synovitis, acne, pustulosis, hyperostosis, osteitis
- PAPA syndrome: Pyogenic sterile arthritis, pyoderma gangrenosum, cystic acne
- Behçet syndrome
- Apert syndrome
- Dark-skinned patients: 50% keloidal scarring and 50% acne hyperpigmented macules

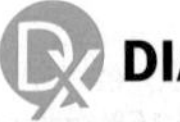

DIAGNOSIS

HISTORY

- Ask duration, medications, cleansing products, stress, smoking, exposures, diet, family history
- Females may worsen prior to menses

PHYSICAL EXAM

- Closed comedones (whiteheads)
- Open comedones (blackheads)
- Nodules or papules
- Pustules ("cysts")
- Scars: Ice pick, rolling, boxcar, atrophic macules, hypertrophic, depressed, sinus tracts
- Grading system (American Academy of Dermatology, 1990):
  - Mild: Few papules/pustules; no nodules
  - Moderate: Some papules/pustules; few nodules
  - Severe: Numerous papules/pustules; many nodules
  - Very severe: Acne conglobata, acne fulminans, acne inversa
- Most common areas affected are: Face, chest, back, and upper arms (areas of greatest concentration of sebaceous glands)

DIAGNOSTIC TESTS & INTERPRETATION

Lab

Labs only indicated if there are additional signs of androgen excess; if so: Free testosterone, dehydroepiandrosterone sulfate (DHEA-S), luteinizing hormone, and follicle-stimulating hormone (2)[A]

DIFFERENTIAL DIAGNOSIS

- Folliculitis: Gram negative and gram positive
- Acne (rosacea, cosmetica, steroid-induced)
- Perioral dermatitis
- Chloracne
- Pseudofolliculitis barbae
- Drug eruption
- Verruca vulgaris and plana
- Keratosis pilaris
- Molluscum contagiosum
- Facial angiofibromas
- Sarcoidosis

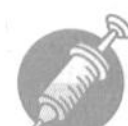

TREATMENT

- Topical retinoid plus a topical antimicrobial agent first-line treatment (3)
- Topical retinoid plus antibiotic (topical or PO) is better than either alone (4,5)[A]
- Topical retinoids first-line agents for maintenance. Avoid long-term antibiotics for maintenance.
- Comedonal acne (grade 1): Keratinolytic agent (4,5)[A]
- Mild inflammatory acne (grade 2): Benzoyl peroxide +/− topical antibiotic. Keratinolytic if needed (5,6)[A].
- Moderate inflammatory acne (grade 3): Add systemic antibiotic to grade 2 regimen.
- Severe inflammatory acne (grade 4): As in grade 3, or isotretinoin (4,5)[A]
- Recommended vehicle type:
  - Cream: Dry or sensitive skin
  - Gel or solution: Oily skin, humid weather
  - Lotion: Hair-bearing areas
- Mild soap daily to control oiliness; avoid abrasives
- Avoid drying agents with keratinolytic agents.
- Use of a gentle cleanser and noncomedogenic moisturizer helps decrease irritation from keratinolytic agents.
- Oil-free, noncomedogenic sunscreens
- Stress management if acne flares with stress

MEDICATION

Keratinolytic agents (side effects include dryness, erythema, scaling, and photosensitivity; start with lower strength; increase as tolerated) (2,4)[A]:

- Tretinoin (Retin-A, Retin A Micro, Avita): Apply at bedtime; wash skin and let skin dry 30 minutes before topical application:
  - Retin-AMicro and Avita are less irritating, less phototoxicity
  - May cause an initial flare of lesions. May be eased by 14-day course of oral antibiotics.
- Adapalene (Differin): 0.1%, apply topically at night:
  - Effective; less irritation than tretinoin or tazarotene (4,6)[A]
  - May be combined with benzoyl peroxide
- Tazarotene (Tazorac): Apply at bedtime:
  - Most effective and most irritating
  - Teratogenic
- Azelaic acid (Azelex, Finevin): 20% topically, b.i.d.:
  - Keratinolytic, antibacterial, anti-inflammatory
  - Reduces postinflammatory hyperpigmentation in dark-skinned individuals
  - Side effects: Erythema, dryness, scaling, hypopigmentation
  - Less effective in clinical use than in studies
- Salicylic acid: Less effective than tretinoin
- Alpha-hydroxy acids: Available over-the-counter
- Topical antibiotics and anti-inflammatories (4)[A]:
  - Topical benzoyl peroxide:
    - Bactericidal through direct toxic effect
    - No *P. acnes* resistance noted
    - 2.5% as effective as stronger preparations
    - When used with tretinoin, apply benzoyl peroxide in morning and tretinoin at night
    - Side effects: Irritation; may bleach clothes

- Topical antibiotics (2,4)[A]:
  - Erythromycin 2%
  - Clindamycin 1%
  - Metronidazole gel or cream: Apply once daily.
  - Azelaic acid (Azelex, Finevin): 20% cream: Enhanced effect and decreased risk of resistance when used with zinc and benzoyl peroxide
  - Benzoyl peroxide-erythromycin (Benzamycin): Especially effective with azelaic acid
  - Benzoyl peroxide-clindamycin (BenzaClin, DUAC, Clindoxyl): Effective combined (6)[A]
  - Benzoyl peroxide-salicylic acid (Cleanse & Treat, Inova): Similar in effectiveness to benzoyl peroxide-clindamycin (7)
  - Sodium sulfacetamide (Sulfacet-R, Novacet, Klaron): Useful in acne with seborrheic dermatitis or rosacea
- Oral antibiotics (2,4)[A]:
  - Tetracycline: 500–2,000 mg/d b.i.d.–q.i.d.; high dose initially, taper in 6 months, as tolerated. Side effects: Photosensitivity, esophagitis:
    - Avoid use with antacids, iron
    - Both antibacterial and anti-inflammatory (8)
  - Minocycline 50–200 mg/d, q.i.d.–b.i.d. Side effects: Photosensitivity, urticaria, gray-blue skin, vertigo, autoimmune hepatitis, pseudotumor cerebri, lupuslike syndrome. May be more effective than tetracycline (2)[A],(9).
  - Doxycycline 50–200 mg/d, given b.i.d.–q.i.d.; side effects include photosensitivity
  - Erythromycin: 500–1,000 mg/d; given b.i.d.–q.i.d.; decreasing effectiveness as a result of increasing *P. acnes* resistance
  - Trimethoprim-sulfamethoxazole (Bactrim DS, Septra DS); 1 daily or b.i.d.
- Oral retinoids:
  - Isotretinoin (Accutane) (2,4)[A]: 0.5–2.0 mg/kg/d b.i.d.; 60–90% cure rate; usually given for 12–20 weeks; maximum cumulative dose = 120–150 mg/kg; 20% of patients relapse and require retreatment:
    - Side effects: Numerous (see package insert). Highly teratogenic.
    - Avoid tetracyclines or vitamin A preparations during isotretinoin therapy.
    - Monitor for pregnancy, CBC, lipids, and liver function tests at baseline and every month.
    - Should be registered member of manufacturer's iPLEDGE program

Pregnancy Considerations

- Isotretinoin is a teratogenic; Class X
- Medications for women only:
  - Oral contraceptives (2,4)[A],(10):
    - Norgestimate/ethinyl estradiol (OrthoTricyclen), norethindrone acetate/ethinyl estradiol (Estrostep), drospirenone/ethinyl estradiol (Yaz, Yasmin) are approved by Food and Drug Administration.
    - Levonorgestrel/ethinyl estradiol (Alesse) is also effective.
  - Spironolactone (Aldactone); 25–200 mg/d; antiandrogen; reduces sebum production
  - Flutamide (Eulexin) 250–500 mg/d; potentially hepatotoxic

ADDITIONAL TREATMENT

Acne hyperpigmented macules:

- Topical hydroquinones (1.5–10%)
- Azelaic acid (20%) topically
- Topical retinoids as above
- Corticosteroids: Low dose, suppresses adrenal androgens (2)[B]
- Dapsone 5% gel (Aczone): Topical, anti-inflammatory use in patients >12 years

Issues for Referral

Consider referral/consultation to dermatologist:

- Refractory lesions despite appropriate therapy
- Consideration of isotretinoin therapy
- Management of acne scars

Additional Therapies

Light-based treatments:

- Ultraviolet A/ultraviolet B (UVA/UVB), blue light, blue/red light, pulse dye laser, KTP laser, infrared laser
- Photodynamic therapy for 30–60 minutes with 5-aminolevulinic acid × 3 sessions is effective for inflammatory lesions:
  - Greatest utility when used as adjunct to medications or in patient who can't tolerate medications

COMPLEMENTARY AND ALTERNATIVE MEDICINE

- Topical tree oil is effective, but has slow onset (2)[B].
- Nicotinamide 4% gel (Nicam): As effective as clindamycin in moderate inflammatory acne (11)

SURGERY/OTHER PROCEDURES

- Comedo extraction after incising the layer of epithelium over comedo (2)[C]
- Incision and drainage for abscesses
- Inject large cystic lesions with 0.05–0.3 mL triamcinolone (Kenalog 2–5 mg/mL); use 30-g needle to inject and slightly distend cyst (2)[C].
- Acne scar treatment: Retinoids, steroid injections, cryosurgery, electrodessication, microdermabrasion, dermabrasion, chemical peels, laser resurfacing, others

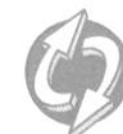

ONGOING CARE

FOLLOW-UP RECOMMENDATIONS

Use oral or topical antibiotics for 3 months; stop if inflammatory lesions resolve. Can switch abruptly from oral to topical without taper. Do not use topical and oral together.

Patient Monitoring

- Pretreatment and monthly lipids, liver function tests, and pregnancy tests when on isotretinoin
- Consider antibiotic resistance (60% overall) or gram-negative folliculitis if treatment fails.

DIET

Special diets do not diminish acne (2)[B].

PATIENT EDUCATION

- There may be a worsening of acne during first 2 weeks of treatment.
- Treatment takes a minimum of 4 weeks to show results.

PROGNOSIS

Gradual improvement over time (usually within 8–12 weeks after beginning therapy)

COMPLICATIONS

- Acne conglobata: Severe confluent inflammatory acne with systemic symptoms
- Facial and psychological scarring
- Gram-negative folliculitis: Superinfection due to long-term oral antibiotic use; treatment with ampicillin, trimethoprim-sulfa, or isotretinoin

REFERENCES

1. Bowe WP, Joshi SS, Shalita AR, et al. Diet and acne. *J. Am. Acad. Dermatol*. 2010;63:124–41.
2. Strauss JS, Krowchuk DP, Leyden JJ, et al. Guidelines of care for acne vulgaris management. *J Am Acad Dermatol*. 2007;56:651–63.
3. Thiboutot D, Gollnick H, Bettoli V, et al. New insights into the management of acne: An update from the Global Alliance to Improve Outcomes in Acne Group. *Journal of the American Academy of Dermatology*. 2009;60(5 suppl).
4. Feldman S, Careccia RE, Barham KL, et al. Diagnosis and treatment of acne. *Am Fam Physician*. 2004;69:2123–30.
5. Webster G. Mechanism-based treatment of acne vulgaris: The value of combination therapy. *J Drugs and Dermatol*. 2005;4(3):281–8.
6. Haider A, Shaw JC. Treatment of acne vulgaris. *JAMA*. 2004;292:726–35.
7. Seider EM, Kimball AB. Meta-analysis comparing efficacy of benzoyl peroxide, clindamycin, benzoyl peroxide with salicylic acid, and combination of benzoyl peroxide/clindamycin in acne. *J Am Acad Dermatol*. 2010;63(1):52–62.
8. Del Rosso JQ, Kim G. Optimizing use of oral antibiotics in acne vulgaris. *Dermatol Clin*. 2009; 27:33–42
9. Leyden JJ, Del Rosso JQ, Webster GF, et al. Clinical considerations in the treatment of acne vulgaris and other inflammatory skin disorders: A status report. *Dermatol Clin*. 2009;27:1–15.
10. Heymann WR. Oral contraceptives for the treatment of acne vulgaris. *J Am Acad Dermatol*. 2007;56:1056–7.
11. Morelli V, Calmet E, Jhingade V, et al. Alternative therapies for common dermatologic disorders, part 2. *Prim Care*. 2010;37:285–96.

See Also (Topic, Algorithm, Electronic Media Element)

- Acne Rosacea
- Algorithm: Acne

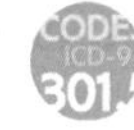

CODES

ICD9

706.1 Other acne

CLINICAL PEARLS

- Expect worsening for the first 2 weeks. Full results take 8–12 weeks.
- Decrease topical frequency from b.i.d. to every day or every day to every other day for irritation; may also use a moisturizing soap and a moisturizer before treatment application.
- Acne resolves with age for most individuals, although 8% of 30-year-olds and 3% of 40-year-olds may have persistent lesions.
- Acne often appears more significant to adolescent than to doctor; may be "entry ticket" for other advice.

ACOUSTIC NEUROMA

Sam Seung Yeol Kim, MBBS, Mmed
Phillip Chang, MBBS

BASICS

DESCRIPTION

- Slow-growing benign tumor, most often arising from the vestibular division of 8th cranial nerve
- Originates from Schwann cells of the nerve sheath ("schwannoma")
- Usually arises in the internal auditory canal near the cerebellopontine angle
- Often has extracanalicular portion into the cerebellopontine angle, but may also stay purely intracanalicular
- Most are unilateral; bilateral only seen in neurofibromatosis type II

EPIDEMIOLOGY

- 6–10% of all intracranial tumors
- 80–90% of cerebellopontine angle tumors
- 95% of cases are unilateral
- Present most commonly in the 5th–6th decade
- Female predominance
- Bilateral acoustic neuroma occurring in neurofibromatosis II present before age 30

Incidence

- 1/100,000 per year
- Asymptomatic lesions may be more common

Prevalence

3,000 diagnosed annually in the US

RISK FACTORS

- Pregnancy and epilepsy may increase risk (1).
- Smoking may decrease the risk (1).

Genetics

- Unknown for unilateral acoustic neuroma (AN)
- Neurofibromatosis type II: Bilateral ANs:
  - Autosomal dominant
  - Gene located on chromosome 22q1

PATHOPHYSIOLOGY

- Exerts pressure on the surrounding structures
- Compression of acoustic and facial nerve when located within internal acoustic canal
- Compression of brainstem, 4th ventricle, and trigeminal nerve when tumor at the cerebellar pontine angle

ETIOLOGY

Unknown

COMMONLY ASSOCIATED CONDITIONS

- Neurofibromatosis type II
- Pregnancy may accelerate the growth of the tumor

DIAGNOSIS

HISTORY

- Common:
  - Sensorineural hearing loss (unilateral), often progressive
  - Loss of speech discrimination
  - Tinnitus
  - Balance problems are common, but vertigo is less common
- Less common:
  - Weakness/loss of facial muscle functions
  - Headache with hydrocephalus and increased intracranial pressure
  - Trigeminal nerve involvement when tumor is large and compressing on cranial nerve (CN) V
  - Ataxia due to cerebellar or brainstem compression from very large tumor

PHYSICAL EXAM

- Examination with otoscope to exclude other causes of hearing loss (e.g., middle-ear effusion, infection, wax, cholesteatoma, or tympanic membrane rupture)
- Detailed neurologic exam concentrating on the cranial nerves
- Weber and Rinne tests to confirm sensorineural hearing loss
- Evaluation of the contralateral ear in patients <30 years; suspect neurofibromatosis type II

DIAGNOSTIC TESTS & INTERPRETATION

Lab

Initial lab tests

- Pure-tone and speech audiometry (asymmetrical, high-frequency sensorineural hearing loss)
- Speech discrimination
- Stacked auditory brainstem response (ABR): 95% sensitivity and 88% specificity. Can detect tumors <1 cm.
- Standard ABR: Can only detect tumors >1 cm

Imaging

Initial approach

- MRI with gadolinium (gold standard):
  - 100% specificity
  - Detects tumors starting at 2 mm
  - Tumor has marked enhancement with gadolinium
- Noncontrast T2-weighted fast spin-echo MRI:
  - 98% specificity
  - Cheaper than MRI with gadolinium
- CT:
  - Detect tumors as small as 1 cm
  - Up to 37% false-negatives
  - Provides good information about surrounding bony structures of the tumor

Pathological Findings

- Well-demarcated and encapsulated mass attached to neural structures without direct invasion
- Can be dense or cystic
- Microscopic: Densely packed spindle cells (Schwann cells) mixed in with myxoid and collagenous matrix:
  - Zones of alternatively dense and sparse areas of Antoni type A and B

DIFFERENTIAL DIAGNOSIS

- Cerebellopontine lesions:
  - Meningioma
  - Glioma
  - Facial nerve schwannoma
  - Epidermoid
  - Hemangioma
  - Arachnoid cyst
- Sensorineural hearing loss:
  - Ménière disease
  - Ototoxicity
  - Presbycusis
  - Cerebellar pathology

TREATMENT

MEDICATION

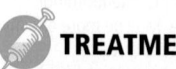

Chemotherapy has not yet been explored sufficiently.

ADDITIONAL TREATMENT

General Measures

- Conservative management is suitable for elderly patients with contraindications to surgery and radiotherapy.
- Up to 57% of acoustic neuromas may show zero growth or shrinkage (2)[B].
- Up to 70% of extracanalicular tumors may never have a growth rate exceeding 2 mm per year (3)[B].
- Growth rate of enlarging acoustic neuromas decreases over time:
  - From 4.9 mm/yr in the 1st year of detected growth to 0.75 mm in 4th year
- Up to 20% of patients eventually may fail conservative management and require intervention.
- It is more likely to preserve hearing than radiotherapy or surgery (4)[C].
- 69% of patients with 100% speech discrimination at diagnosis have maintained good hearing, even after 10 years of observation (5)[B].

Issues for Referral

- Yearly MRI follow-up for slow-growing tumors is advised.
- If an asymptomatic tumor becomes symptomatic, this is often indication for intervention.

Additional Therapies

Stereotactic radiosurgery:

- Gamma knife single-dose stereotactic radiosurgery:
  - Performed on an outpatient basis
  - Alternative for those with smaller tumor (<3 cm) or contraindications to microsurgery
  - No discernible significant difference between growth patterns of untreated tumors and those treated radiosurgically (5)[A]
  - Lower-dose radiation has lower complication rates, but evidence is insufficient whether this is as effective as high-dose radiation in tumor control (6)[A].
  - Higher-dose radiation significantly influences hearing preservation rates (7)[C].
  - Complications include hydrocephalus, trigeminal, and/or facial nerve neuropathy from radiation damage
- Fractionated stereotactic radiosurgery:
  - Conformal radiation delivers a higher dose of radiation within the tumor and less damage to surrounding healthy tissue.
  - Requires multiple treatments and the total dose of radiation is higher compared to the single-dose radiation
  - Suitable for all sizes of tumor

SURGERY/OTHER PROCEDURES

- Recommended definitive treatment (8)[A]
- Lowest rate of recurrence, with up to 97.5% complete tumor removal (8)[A]
- Intraoperative facial nerve monitoring is generally used
- 3 standard approaches, all using operating microscopes:
  - Retromastoid/retrosigmoid: For any size, especially tumors located mostly outside the internal auditory canal and adjacent to the brainstem. May require retraction of cerebellum.
  - Middle cranial fossa: For small tumors with aim of preserving hearing. Involves retraction of temporal lobe and has higher risk of facial nerve injury.
  - Translabyrinthine: For larger tumors. Hearing not preserved. Completely exposes the distal internal auditory canal and has more favorable facial nerve results.
- Endoscopic approach used in some centers
- Surgical complications:
  - Hearing loss
  - CSF leakage
  - Facial nerve injury
  - Headache
  - Meningitis

ONGOING CARE

FOLLOW-UP RECOMMENDATIONS

MRI and audiometric follow-up for those treated by radiotherapy and conservative management

COMPLICATIONS

Due to pressure effect of a large tumor:

- Cranial nerve compression
- Hydrocephalus
- Brainstem compression
- Cerebellar tonsil herniation

REFERENCES

1. Schoemaker MJ, Swerdlow AJ, Auvinen A, et al. Medical history, cigarette smoking and risk of acoustic neuroma: An international case-control study. *Int J Cancer*. 2007;120:103–10.
2. Smouha EE, Yoo M, Mohr K, et al. Conservative management of acoustic neuroma: A meta-analysis and proposed treatment algorithm. *Laryngoscope*. 2005;115:450–4.
3. Stangerup SE, Caye-Thomasen P, Tos M, et al. The natural history of vestibular schwannoma. *Otol Neurotol*. 2006;27:547–52.
4. Lin VY, Stewart C, Grebenyuk J, et al. Unilateral acoustic neuromas: Long-term hearing results in patients managed with fractionated stereotactic radiotherapy, hearing preservation surgery, and expectantly. *Laryngoscope*. 2005;115:292–6.
5. Stangerup SE, Thomsen J, Tos M, et al. Long-term hearing preservation in vestibular schwannoma. *Otol Neurotol*. 2010;31:271–5.
6. Battaglia A, Mastrodimos B, Cueva R. Comparison of growth patterns of acoustic neuromas with and without radiosurgery. *Otol Neurotol*. 2006;27:705–12.
7. Combs SE, Welzel T, Schulz-Ertner D, et al. Differences in clinical results after LINAC-based single-dose radiosurgery versus fractionated stereotactic radiotherapy for patients with vestibular schwannomas. *Int Radiat Oncol Biol Phys*. 2010;76:193–200.
8. Weil RS, Cohen JM, Portarena I, et al. Optimal dose of stereotactic radiosurgery for acoustic neuromas: A systematic review. *Br J Neurosurg*. 2006:195–202.

ADDITIONAL READING

Kaylie DM, Horgan MJ, Delashaw JB, et al. A meta-analysis comparing outcomes of microsurgery and gamma knife radiosurgery. *Laryngoscope*. 2000;110:1850–6.

CODES

ICD9

- 225.1 Benign neoplasm of cranial nerves
- 237.70 Neurofibromatosis, unspecified
- 237.71 Neurofibromatosis, type 1, von Recklinghausen's disease

CLINICAL PEARLS

A bone-anchored hearing aid can restore hearing for those patients with sensorineural hearing loss, which may be present before or after the surgery.

ADDISON DISEASE

Michele L. Matthews, PharmD, CPE, RPh
Rick Kellerman, MD

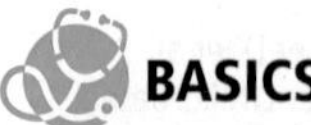

BASICS

DESCRIPTION

- This disease is an adrenal gland insufficiency from partial or complete destruction of the adrenal cells with inadequate secretion of glucocorticoids and mineralocorticoids.
- 80% of cases are caused by an autoimmune process, followed by tuberculosis (TB), AIDS, systemic fungal infections, and adrenoleukodystrophy.
- Addison disease (primary adrenocortical insufficiency) can be differentiated from secondary (pituitary failure) and tertiary (hypothalamic failure) causes because mineralocorticoid function usually remains intact in secondary and tertiary causes.
- Addisonian (adrenal) crisis: Acute complication of adrenal insufficiency (circulatory collapse, dehydration, hypotension, nausea, vomiting, hypoglycemia); usually precipitated by an acute physiologic stressor(s) such as surgery, illness, exacerbation of comorbid process, and/or acute withdrawal of long-term corticosteroid therapy
- System(s) affected: Endocrine/Metabolic
- Synonym(s): Adrenocortical insufficiency; Corticoadrenal insufficiency; Primary adrenocortical insufficiency

EPIDEMIOLOGY

- Predominant age: All ages; mean age at diagnosis in adults is 40 years
- Predominant sex: Females > Males (slight)

Incidence

0.6:100,000

Prevalence

4:100,000

RISK FACTORS

- Forty percent of patients have a 1st- or 2nd-degree relative with associated disorders.
- Chronic steroid use, then experiencing severe infection, trauma, or surgical procedures

Genetics

- Autoimmune polyglandular syndrome (APS) type 2 genetics are complex. It is associated with adrenal insufficiency, type 1 diabetes, and Hashimoto disease. It is more common than APS type 1.
- APS type 1 is caused by mutations of the autoimmune regulator gene. Nearly all have the following triad: Adrenal insufficiency, hypoparathyroidism, and mucocutaneous candidiasis before adulthood.
- Adrenoleukodystrophy is an X-linked recessive disorder resulting in toxic accumulation of unoxidized long-chain fatty acids.
- There is increased risk with cytotoxic T-lymphocyte antigen 4 (CTLA-4).

GENERAL PREVENTION

- No preventive measures known for Addison disease; focus on prevention of complications:
  - Anticipate adrenal crisis and treat before symptoms begin.
- Elective surgical procedures require upward adjustment in steroid dose.

PATHOPHYSIOLOGY

Destruction of the adrenal cortex resulting in deficiencies in cortisol, aldosterone, and androgens

ETIOLOGY

- Autoimmune adrenal insufficiency (80% of cases in the US)
- Infectious causes: TB (most common infectious cause worldwide), HIV (most common infectious cause in the US), Waterhouse-Fredrickson syndrome, fungal disease
- Bilateral adrenal hemorrhage and infarction (for patients on anticoagulants, 50% are in the therapeutic range)
- Antiphospholipid syndrome
- Lymphoma, Kaposi sarcoma, metastasis (lung, breast, kidney, colon, melanoma); tumor must destroy 90% of gland to produce hypofunction
- Drugs (ketoconazole, etomidate)
- Surgical adrenalectomy, radiation therapy
- Sarcoidosis, hemochromatosis, amyloidosis
- Congenital enzyme defects (deficiency of 21-hydroxylase enzyme is most common), neonatal adrenal hypoplasia, congenital adrenal hyperplasia, familial glucocorticoid insufficiency, autoimmune polyglandular syndromes 1 and 2, adrenoleukodystrophy
- Idiopathic

COMMONLY ASSOCIATED CONDITIONS

- Diabetes mellitus
- Graves' disease
- Hashimoto's thyroiditis
- Hypoparathyroidism
- Hypercalcemia
- Ovarian failure
- Pernicious anemia
- Myasthenia gravis
- Vitiligo
- Chronic moniliasis
- Sarcoidosis
- Sjögren's syndrome
- Chronic active hepatitis
- Schmidt's syndrome

DIAGNOSIS

HISTORY

- Weakness, fatigue
- Dizziness
- Anorexia, nausea, vomiting
- Abdominal pain
- Chronic diarrhea
- Depression (60–80% of patients)
- Decreased cold tolerance
- Salt craving

PHYSICAL EXAM

- Weight loss
- Low BP, orthostatic hypotension
- Increased pigmentation (extensor surfaces, hand creases, dental-gingival margins, buccal and vaginal mucosa, lips, areola, pressure points, scars, "tanning," freckles)
- Vitiligo
- Hair loss in females

DIAGNOSTIC TESTS & INTERPRETATION

Lab

Initial lab tests

- Basal plasma cortisol and adrenocorticotropic hormone (ACTH) (low cortisol and high ACTH indicative of Addison disease)
- Standard ACTH stimulation test: Cosyntropin 0.25 mg IV, measure preinjection baseline, and 60-minute postinjection cortisol levels (patients with Addison disease have low-to-normal values that do not rise)
- Insulin-induced hypoglycemia test
- Metapyrone test
- Autoantibody tests: 21-hydroxylase (most common and specific), 17-hydroxylase, 17-alpha-hydroxylase (may not be associated), and adrenomedullin
- Circulating very-long-chain fatty acid levels if boy or young man
- Low serum sodium
- Elevated serum potassium
- Elevated BUN, creatinine, calcium, thyroid-stimulating hormone (TSH)
- Low serum aldosterone
- Hypoglycemia when fasted
- Metabolic acidosis
- Moderate neutropenia
- Eosinophilia
- Relative lymphocytosis
- Anemia, normochromic, normocytic

Follow-Up & Special Considerations

- Plasma ACTH levels do not correlate with treatment and should not be used for routine monitoring of replacement therapy (1)[C].
- TSH: Repeat when condition has stabilized:
  - Thyroid hormone levels may normalize with the treatment of Addison disease.
- Drugs that may alter lab results: Digitalis
- Disorders that may alter lab results: Diabetes

Imaging

Initial approach

- Abdominal CT scan: Small adrenal glands in autoimmune adrenalitis; enlarged adrenal glands in infiltrative and hemorrhagic disorders
- Abdominal radiograph may show adrenal calcifications
- Chest x-ray may show small heart size and/or calcification of cartilage
- MRI of pituitary and hypothalamus if secondary or tertiary cause of adrenocortical insufficiency is suspected

Diagnostic Procedures/Surgery

CT-guided fine-needle biopsy of adrenal masses may identify diagnoses (2)[C].

Pathological Findings

- Atrophic adrenals in autoimmune adrenalitis
- Infiltrative and hemorrhagic disorders produce enlargement with destruction of the entire gland.

DIFFERENTIAL DIAGNOSIS
- Secondary adrenocortical insufficiency (pituitary failure):
  - Withdrawal of long-term corticosteroid use
  - Sheehan's syndrome (postpartum necrosis of pituitary)
  - Empty sella syndrome
  - Radiation to pituitary
  - Pituitary adenomas, craniopharyngiomas
  - Infiltrative disorders of pituitary (sarcoidosis, hemochromatosis, amyloidosis, histiocytosis X)
- Tertiary adrenocortical insufficiency (hypothalamic failure):
  - Pituitary stalk transection
  - Trauma
  - Disruption of production of corticotropic-releasing factor
  - Hypothalamic tumors
- Other:
  - Myopathies
  - Syndrome of inappropriate antidiuretic hormone
  - Heavy-metal ingestion
  - Severe nutritional deficiencies
  - Sprue Syndrome
  - Hyperparathyroidism
  - Neurofibromatosis
  - Peutz-Jeghers syndrome
  - Porphyria cutanea tarda
  - Salt-losing nephritis
  - Bronchogenic carcinoma
  - Anorexia nervosa

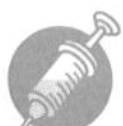

TREATMENT

MEDICATION
First Line
- Chronic adrenal insufficiency:
  - Glucocorticoid supplementation:
    - Dosing: Hydrocortisone 15–20 mg (or therapeutic equivalent) PO each morning upon rising and 10 mg at 4–5 PM each afternoon (3)[C]; dosage may vary and is usually lower in children and the elderly
    - Precautions: Hepatic disease, fluid disturbances, immunosuppression, peptic ulcer disease, pregnancy, osteoporosis
    - Adverse reactions: Immunosuppression, osteoporosis, gastric ulcers, depression, hyperglycemia, weight gain, glaucoma
    - Drug interactions: Concomitant use of rifampin, phenytoin, or barbiturates
  - Mineralocorticoid supplementation:
    - Dosing: Fludrocortisone 0.05–0.2 mg PO per day
  - May require salt supplementation
- Addisonian crisis:
  - Hydrocortisone 100 mg IV followed by 10 mg/hr infusion, or hydrocortisone 100 mg IV bolus q6–8h
  - IV glucose, saline, and plasma expanders
  - Fludrocortisone 0.05 mg/d PO (may not be required; high-dose hydrocortisone is an effective mineralocorticoid)
- Acute illnesses (fever, stress, minor trauma):
  - Double the patient's usual steroid dose, taper the dose gradually over a week or more, and monitor vital signs and serum sodium.
- Supplementation for surgical procedures:
  - Administer hydrocortisone 25–150 mg or methylprednisolone 5–30 mg IV on the day of the procedure in addition to maintenance therapy; taper gradually to the usual dose over 1–2 days.

Second Line
Addition of androgen therapy:

- Dehydroepiandrosterone (DHEA) 25–50 mg PO once daily may be considered in women to improve well-being and sexuality (4)[B].

ADDITIONAL TREATMENT
General Measures
Consider the 5 Ss for the management of adrenal crisis:

- Salt, sugar, steroids, support, and search for a precipitating illness (usually infection, trauma, recent surgery, or not taking prescribed replacement therapy)

IN-PATIENT CONSIDERATIONS
Initial Stabilization
Addisonian crisis:

- Airway, breathing, and circulation management
- Establish IV access; 5% dextrose and normal saline
- Administer hydrocortisone 100 mg IV bolus q6–8h; replacement with fludrocortisone is not necessary (high-dose hydrocortisone is an effective mineralocorticoid)
- Correct electrolyte abnormalities
- BP support for hypotension
- Antibiotics if infection suspected

Admission Criteria
- Presence of circulatory collapse, dehydration, hypotension, nausea, vomiting, hypoglycemia
- Intensive care unit admission for unstable cases

IV Fluids
IV saline containing 5% dextrose and plasma expanders

ONGOING CARE

FOLLOW-UP RECOMMENDATIONS
Patient Monitoring
- Verify adequacy of therapy: Normal BP, serum electrolytes, plasma renin, and fasting blood glucose level
- Periodically assess for the development of long-term complications of corticosteroid use, including screening for osteoporosis, gastric ulcers, depression, and glaucoma
- Lifelong medical supervision for signs of adequate therapy and avoidance of overdose

DIET
Maintain water, sodium, and potassium balance

PATIENT EDUCATION
- For patient education materials, contact: National Adrenal Disease Foundation, 505 Northern Blvd., Suite 200, Great Neck, NY 11021, (516) 487–4992 (http://www.medhelp.org/nadf)
- Patient should wear or carry medical identification about the disease and the need for hydrocortisone or other replacement therapy.
- Instruct patient in self-administering of parenteral hydrocortisone for emergency situations.

PROGNOSIS
Requires lifetime treatment: Life expectancy approximates normal with adequate replacement therapy; without treatment, the disease is 100% lethal.

COMPLICATIONS
- Hyperpyrexia
- Psychotic reactions
- Complications from underlying disease
- Over- or underuse of steroid treatment
- Hyperkalemic paralysis (rare)
- Addisonian crisis

REFERENCES

1. Nieman LK, Chanco Turner ML. Addison's disease. *Clin Dermatol*. 2006;24:276–80
2. Oelkers W. Adrenal insufficiency. *N Engl J Med*. 1996;335:1206–12
3. Coursin DB, Wood KE. Corticosteroid supplementation for adrenal insufficiency. *JAMA*. 2002;287:236–40
4. Arlt W, Callies F, van Vlijmen JC, et al. Dehydroepiandrosterone replacement in women with adrenal insufficiency. *N Engl J Med*. 1999; 341:1013–20

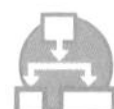

See Also (Topic, Algorithm, Electronic Media Element)

Algorithm: Adrenocortical Insufficiency

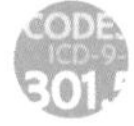

CODES

ICD9
- 017.60 Tuberculosis of adrenal glands, unspecified examination
- 255.41 Glucocorticoid deficiency

CLINICAL PEARLS

- 80% of cases are caused by an autoimmune process, and the average age of diagnosis in adults is 40 years.
- Consider the 5 Ss for the management of Addison disease: Salt, sugar, steroids, support, and search for an underlying cause.
- The goal of steroid replacement therapy should be to use the lowest dose that alleviates patient symptoms while preventing adverse drug events.
- Plasma ACTH levels do not correlate with treatment and should not be used for routine monitoring for efficacy of replacement therapy.
- Long-term use of steroids predisposes patients to the development of osteoporosis; screen accordingly and encourage calcium and vitamin D supplementation.

ADENOMYOSIS

Stanley Sagov, MD

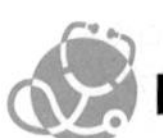

BASICS

- Adenomyosis is uterine thickening that occurs when endometrial tissue, which normally lines the uterus, moves into the muscular wall of the uterus.
- Sometimes adenomyosis may cause a mass or growth within the uterus, which is called an adenomyoma.

DESCRIPTION

Adenomyosis is defined by the presence of endometrial cellular and stromal tissue (endometriosis) within the uterine wall.

EPIDEMIOLOGY

- Adenomyosis is equally common in women who also have fibroids, endometriosis, pelvic pain, or abnormal uterine bleeding, and in women who do not have these conditions (1).
- Adenomyosis is rare but does exist during adolescence (2).

Incidence

- Controversial since definitive diagnosis is usually only possible by uterine biopsy or hysterectomy
- Published findings vary from 8.8% to 61.5% (3)

Prevalence

- Not firmly established
- 40–50% has been reported in studies of perimenopausal women at the time of a hysterectomy.

RISK FACTORS

- Age >30
- Parity
- Previous cesarean section
- Other uterine surgery

PATHOPHYSIOLOGY

Theoretically preeclampsia, fetal growth restriction, and premature delivery are linked together, representing a new, major obstetrical syndrome characterized by a modified uterine environment around the time of nidation (4,5).

ETIOLOGY

All mucosal invasions of abdominal organs used to be considered to be one pathological condition of uncertain origin, termed "adenomyoma" (4).

- In the 1920s, endometriosis and adenomyosis were clearly separated.
- 80 years later, their pathogenesis is reunified.
- 2 current theories:
  - Migration of cells from the endometrium spontaneously, with trauma surgery or disruption during the birth process
  - Possible de novo expression of pluri potentional mesenchymal cells in the uterus undergoing endometrial development

COMMONLY ASSOCIATED CONDITIONS

- Uterine fibroids
- Endometriosis

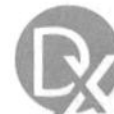

DIAGNOSIS

Pelvic pain, dysmenorrhea, and uteromegaly are the usual cues, which then prompt imaging by US or an MRI with endometrial or uterine biopsies in selected cases to complete the diagnostic pathway.

HISTORY

- Women are often asymptomatic.
- Menorrhagia (6)
- Dysmenorrhea, which gets increasingly worse
- Pelvic pain
- Dyspareunia

PHYSICAL EXAM

Uteromegaly up to 12-week size, usually described as symmetrical and globular

DIAGNOSTIC TESTS & INTERPRETATION

Imaging

A recent systematic review with meta-analysis concluded that a transvaginal ultrasound (TVUS) and an MRI both show high levels of accuracy for the noninvasive diagnosis of adenomyosis (7):

- A TVUS had a pooled sensitivity of 72% (95% CI 65–79%), specificity of 81% (95% CI 77–85%), positive likelihood ratio of 3.7 (95% CI 2.1–6.4) and negative likelihood ratio of 0.3 (95% CI 0.1–0.5).
- An MRI had a pooled sensitivity of 77% (95% CI 67–85%), specificity of 89% (95% CI 84–92%), positive likelihood ratio of 6.5 (95% CI 4.5–9.3), and negative likelihood ratio of 0.2 (95% CI 0.1–0.4). The results show that a correct diagnosis was obtained more often with an MRI.

Initial approach

- Pelvic us
- An MRI can be helpful when an ultrasound does not give definite results.

Diagnostic Procedures/Surgery

- Uterine biopsy
- Posthysterectomy histology

Pathological Findings

Presence of endometrial cells and stromal elements within the uterine muscle (8)

DIFFERENTIAL DIAGNOSIS

- Pregnancy
- Benign uterine tumors
- Malignant uterine tumors

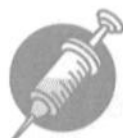

TREATMENT

- Few studies have been performed on medical therapies for adenomyosis (9).
- A dozen different medical or surgical techniques are utilized for the treatment of adenomyosis and novel approaches are currently being tested (4).
- Goals of treatment in the adolescent are toward fertility preservation (2).

MEDICATION

- Systemic hormonal treatments such as continuous combination oral contraceptive pills
- Local hormonal treatment such as the levonorgestrel-releasing intrauterine system (the Mirena IUD) (10)

Second Line

- Gonadotropin-releasing hormone agonists
- Danazol

ADDITIONAL TREATMENT

Angiogenesis inhibitors

SURGERY/OTHER PROCEDURES

- A hysterectomy is curative.
- Minor surgical procedures for therapy include the following (11):
  - Endometrial ablation
  - Laparoscopic myometrial electrocoagulation
  - Adenomyoma excision
  - Uterine artery embolization (12,13)
- Compared with current conservative treatments, a high-intensity focused ultrasound (HIFU) may be a noninvasive approach and may offer complete ablation of adenomyoma, with less trauma, less complication, and a low cost and short hospital stay for treating patients with uterine-localized adenomyosis (14).
- In adolescents, although medical management appears to be a good option for certain types of adenomyosis, surgery may be appropriate in the case of well-circumscribed adenomyotic cysts, adenomyomas, or noncommunicating horns (2).

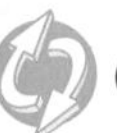

ONGOING CARE

PATIENT EDUCATION

Adenomyosis, PubMed Health, at http://www.ncbi.nlm.nih.gov/pubmedhealth/PMH0002481/

PROGNOSIS

- Symptoms usually resolve after menopause.
- A hysterectomy is curative.

COMPLICATIONS

- Anemia from blood loss associated with heavy periods
- Usual perioperative risks

REFERENCES

1. Weiss G, Maseelall P, Schott LL, et al. Adenomyosis a variant, not a disease? Evidence from hysterectomized menopausal women in the Study of Women's Health Across the Nation (SWAN). *Fertil Steril*. 2009;91:201–6.
2. Dietrich JE. An update on adenomyosis in the adolescent. *Curr Opin Obstet Gynecol*. 2010;22:388–92.
3. Basak S, Saha A. Adenomyosis: Still largely under-diagnosed. *J Obstet Gynaecol*. 2009;29:533–5.
4. Benagiano G, Brosens I, Carrara S, et al. Adenomyosis: New knowledge is generating new treatment strategies. *Womens Health (Lond Engl)*. 2009;5:297–311.
5. Ferenczy A. Pathophysiology of adenomyosis. *Hum Reprod Update*. 1998;4:312–22.
6. Peric H, Fraser IS. The symptomatology of adenomyosis. *Best Pract Res Clin Obstet Gynaecol*. 2006;20:547–55.
7. Champaneria R, Abedin P, Daniels J, et al. Ultrasound scan and magnetic resonance imaging for the diagnosis of adenomyosis: Systematic review comparing test accuracy. *Acta Obstet Gynecol Scand*. 2010;89:1374–84.
8. Hever A, Roth RB, Hevezi PA, et al. Molecular characterization of human adenomyosis. *Mol Hum Reprod*. 2006;12:737–48.
9. Fedele L, Bianchi S, Frontino G, et al. Hormonal treatments for adenomyosis. *Best Pract Res Clin Obstet Gynaecol*. 2008;22:333–9.
10. Sheng J, Zhang WY, Zhang JP, et al. The LNG-IUS study on adenomyosis: A 3-year follow-up study on the efficacy and side effects of the use of levonorgestrel intrauterine system for the treatment of dysmenorrhea associated with adenomyosis. *Contraception*. 2009;79:189–93.
11. Levgur M. Therapeutic options for adenomyosis: A review. *Arch Gynecol Obstet*. 2007;276:1–15.
12. Froeling V, Scheurig-Muenkler C, Hamm B, et al. Uterine artery embolization to treat uterine adenomyosis with or without uterine leiomyomata: Results of symptom control and health-related quality of life 40 months after treatment. *Cardiovasc Intervent Radiol*. 2011 Aug 18. [Epub ahead of print]
13. Popovic M, Puchner S, Berzaczy D, et al. Uterine artery embolization for the treatment of adenomyosis: A review. *J Vasc Interv Radiol*. 2011;22:901–9; quiz 909.
14. Dong X, Yang Z. High-intensity focused ultrasound ablation of uterine localized adenomyosis. *Curr Opin Obstet Gynecol*. 2010;22:326–30.

ADDITIONAL READING

McElin TW, Bird CC. Adenomyosis of the uterus. *Obstet Gynecol Annu*. 1974;3:425.

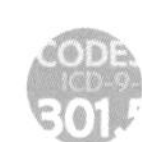

CODES

ICD9

617.0 Endometriosis of uterus

CLINICAL PEARLS

- Adenomyosis is often asymptomatic or difficult to diagnose when managing pelvic pain or menorrhagia.
- Both a TVUS and an MRI are very accurate for the noninvasive diagnosis of adenomyosis.
- Various therapeutic options for adenomyosis, including minimally invasive procedures, are increasingly available but still need further evaluation and improvement.
- Surgical removal of the uterus is curative.

ADENOVIRUS INFECTIONS

Jill SM Omori, MD

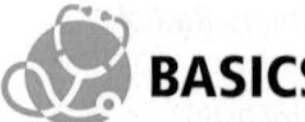

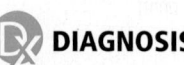

BASICS

DESCRIPTION
- Usually self-limited, febrile illnesses characterized by inflammation of conjunctivae and the respiratory tract
- Adenovirus infections occur in epidemic and endemic situations:
  - Common types:
    - Acute febrile respiratory illness, affecting primarily children
    - Acute respiratory disease, affecting adults
    - Viral pneumonia, affecting children and adults
    - Acute pharyngoconjunctival fever, affecting children, particularly after summer swimming
    - Acute follicular conjunctivitis, affecting all ages
    - Epidemic keratoconjunctivitis, affecting adults
    - Intestinal infections leading to enteritis, mesenteric adenitis, and intussusception
  - Conjunctivitis, sometimes called pink eye
  - System(s) affected: Cardiovascular; Gastrointestinal; Hematologic/Lymphatic/Immunologic; Musculoskeletal; Nervous; Pulmonary; Renal/Urologic; Ophthalmologic

Geriatric Considerations
Complications more likely

Pediatric Considerations
Viral pneumonia in infants and neonates may be fatal.

EPIDEMIOLOGY
- Predominant age: All ages
- Predominant sex: Male = Female
- Occurs worldwide and throughout the year

Incidence
- Very common infection, estimated at 2–5% of all respiratory infections
- More common in infants and children
- Most individuals show evidence of prior adenovirus infection by age 10

RISK FACTORS
- Large number of people gathered in a small area (e.g., military recruits, college students at the beginning of the school year, daycare centers, summer camps, community swimming pools)
- Immunocompromised at risk for severe disease

GENERAL PREVENTION
- Live, oral type 4 and type 7 adenovirus vaccine available for military personnel ages 17–50; reduces incidence of acute respiratory disease (1).
- Frequent handwashing among office personnel and family members
- Decontamination of environmental surfaces; need to use chlorine, bleach, formaldehyde, or heat
- Vigorous handwashing and use of gloves when examining patients with epidemic keratoconjunctivitis or other suspected adenoviral infection
- Health care providers with suspected adenoviral conjunctivitis should avoid direct patient contact for 14 days after onset (in 2nd eye).

PATHOPHYSIOLOGY
- Adenovirus (DNA viruses 60–90 nm in size with 53 known serotypes)
- Transmission:
  - Aerosol droplets, fecal–oral, contact with contaminated fomites
  - Virus can survive long periods on skin and environmental surfaces.
- Most common known pathogens:
  - Types 1, 2, 3, 4, 5, 7, 14, and 21 cause upper respiratory illness and pneumonia.
  - Types 3, 7, and 21 cause pharyngoconjunctival fever.
  - Types 31, 40, and 41 cause infantile gastroenteritis.
  - Types 8, 19, and 37 cause epidemic keratoconjunctivitis.
  - Types 5, 7, 14, and 21 cause the most severe illnesses.

COMMONLY ASSOCIATED CONDITIONS
- Hemorrhagic cystitis and interstitial nephritis
- Otitis media
- Conjunctivitis
- Viral enteritis
- Intussusception and mesenteric adenitis

DIAGNOSIS

HISTORY
Depends on type (see "Differential Diagnosis"). Common symptoms with most respiratory forms (2):

- Headache
- Malaise
- Sore throat
- Cough
- Coryza
- Fever (moderate to high)
- Vomiting
- Diarrhea
- Abdominal pain
- Ear pain
- Urinary symptoms/hematuria
- Eye redness and pain

PHYSICAL EXAM
- Mucosa exhibiting patches of white exudates
- Cervical adenitis
- Otitis media
- Conjunctivitis

DIAGNOSTIC TESTS & INTERPRETATION
Diagnosis only needs to be confirmed in epidemics and severe illnesses.

Lab
- Viral cultures from respiratory, ocular, or fecal sources can establish diagnosis:
  - Pharyngeal isolate suggests recent infection.
- Adenovirus-specific ELISA; more rapid but less sensitive than culture
- Adenovirus DNA detection through polymerase chain reaction (PCR)
- Rapid pathogen screening adeno detector available for detecting adenoviral conjunctivitis (sens 89%, spec 94%); results in 10 minutes (3)
- Antigen detection in stool for enteric serotypes is available.
- Serologic procedures, such as complement fixation, with a 4-fold rise in serum antibody titer, identify recent adenoviral infection.

Imaging
Radiographs: Bronchopneumonia in severe respiratory infections

Diagnostic Procedures/Surgery
Biopsy (lung or other) may be needed in severe or unusual cases; usually only in immunocompromised patients

Pathological Findings
- Varies with each virus:
  - Severe pneumonia may be reflected by extensive intranuclear inclusions.
- Bronchiolitis obliterans may occur.

DIFFERENTIAL DIAGNOSIS
Early diagnosis depends on clinical evaluation. The following are the primary characteristics of the major adenovirus infections:

- **Acute febrile respiratory illness:**
  - Nonspecific coldlike symptoms, similar to other viral respiratory illnesses (e.g., fever, pharyngitis, tracheitis, bronchitis, pneumonitis)
  - Mostly in children
  - Incubation period 2–5 days
  - May be pertussislike syndrome (rarely)
  - DDX: Rhinovirus, influenza, parainfluenza, respiratory syncytial virus (RSV)
- **Acute respiratory disease:**
  - Malaise, fever, chills, headache, pharyngitis, hoarseness, dry cough
  - Fever lasting 2–4 days
  - Illness subsiding in 10–14 days
  - DDX: Rhinovirus, influenza, parainfluenza, RSV
- **Viral pneumonia:**
  - Sudden onset of high fever, rapid infection of upper and lower respiratory tracts, skin rash, diarrhea
  - Occurs in children aged a few days up to 3 years
  - Common; severe illness occurs in subset.
  - DDX: Bacterial pneumonia, RSV, influenza, parainfluenza
- **Acute pharyngoconjunctival fever:**
  - Spiking fever lasting several days, headache, pharyngitis, conjunctivitis, rhinitis, cervical adenitis
  - Conjunctivitis, usually unilateral
  - Subsides in 1 week
  - Highly suspicious for adenovirus
- **Epidemic keratoconjunctivitis:**
  - Usually unilateral onset of ocular redness and edema, periorbital edema, periorbital swelling, local discomfort suggestive of foreign body
  - Lasts 3–4 weeks
  - DDX: Bacterial conjunctivitis, enterovirus, herpes simplex virus

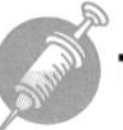

TREATMENT

MEDICATION

- Acetaminophen 10–15 mg/kg PO for analgesia (avoid aspirin)
- Cough suppressants and/or expectorants
- Antihistamine/decongestant combos may decrease cough.
- Antivirals and immunotherapy are reserved for immunocompromised individuals and patients with severe disease. No controlled trials showing benefit of any antiviral agents against human adenovirus infection; however, cidofovir (1 mg/kg every other day) is most commonly used.

ADDITIONAL TREATMENT

General Measures

- Treatment is supportive and symptomatic.
- Infections are usually benign and of short duration.

COMPLEMENTARY AND ALTERNATIVE MEDICINE

Echinacea has not been shown to be better than placebo for treatment of viral upper respiratory infections.

IN-PATIENT CONSIDERATIONS

Admission Criteria

Severely ill infants or immunocompromised with severe illness

Nursing

Hospitalized patients with adenoviral infections should be placed on contact precautions; add droplet precautions for those with respiratory illness.

ONGOING CARE

FOLLOW-UP RECOMMENDATIONS

Rest during febrile phases

Patient Monitoring

For severe infantile pneumonia and conjunctivitis, daily physical exam until well

DIET

No special diet

PATIENT EDUCATION

- Avoid aspirin in children.
- Give instructions for nasal spray, cough preparations, frequent handwashing, and cleaning.

PROGNOSIS

- Self-limited, usually without sequelae
- Severe illness and death in neonates and in immunocompromised hosts can occur.

COMPLICATIONS

Few, if any, recognizable long-term problems

REFERENCES

1. Lyons A, Longfield J, Kuschner R, et al. A double-blind, placebo-controlled study of the safety and immunogenicity of live, oral type 4 and type 7 adenovirus vaccines in adults. *Vaccine*. 2008; 26:2890.
2. Dominguez O, Rojo P, de Las Heras S, et al. Clinical presentation and characteristics of pharyngeal adenovirus infections. *Pediatr Infect Dis J*. 2005; 24:733.
3. Kaufman HE. Adenovirus advances: New diagnostic and therapeutic options. *Curr Opin Ophthalmol*. 2011;22:290–3.
4. Lessler J, Reich NG, Brookmeyer R, et al. Incubation periods of acute respiratory viral infections: A systematic review. *Lancet Infect Dis*. 2009;9: 291–300.
5. Majeed A, Naeem Z, Khan DA, et al. Epidemic adenoviral conjunctivitis report of an outbreak in a military garrison and recommendations for its management and prevention. *J Pak Med Assoc*. 2005;55:273–5.

ADDITIONAL READING

- Barrett BP, Brown RL, Locken K, et al. Treatment of the common cold with unrefined echinacea. A randomized, double-blind, placebo-controlled trial. *Ann Intern Med*. 2002;137:939–46.
- Morris P, Leach A. Antibiotics for persistent nasal discharge (rhinosinusitis) in children. *Cochrane Database Syst Rev*. 2002;(4):CD001094.
- Pratter MR. Cough and the common cold: ACCP evidence-based clinical practice guidelines. *Chest*. 2006;129:72S–74S.
- Smucny J, Fahey T, Becker L, et al. Antibiotics for acute bronchitis. *Cochrane Database Syst Rev*. 2004;(4)CD000245. Review.
- Spurling GKP, Del Mar CB, Dooley L, et al. Delayed antibiotics for symptoms and complications of respiratory infections. *Cochrane Database Syst Rev*. 2004;(4):CD004417.

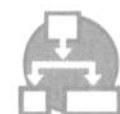

See Also (Topic, Algorithm, Electronic Media Element)

Conjunctivitis, Acute; Intussusception; Pneumonia, Viral

CODES

ICD9

- 008.62 Enteritis due to adenovirus
- 079.0 Adenovirus infection in conditions classified elsewhere and of unspecified site
- 480.0 Pneumonia due to adenovirus

CLINICAL PEARLS

- Can present like strep with pharyngitis, white exudates, and cervical adenitis, but negative strep test. Most common cause of tonsillitis in young children.
- Average incubation time is 5.6 days (4)[A].
- Adenovirus conjunctivitis is highly contagious; cold compresses help relieve symptoms (5)[A].

ADOPTION, INTERNATIONAL

Kara Keating Bench, MD, MPH
James J. Ledwith, Jr., MD

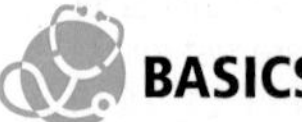

BASICS

DESCRIPTION

Adoption of children from foreign countries into the US has tripled in the past 15 years, and the demographics of those children and their homelands have also shifted significantly during that time. The diverse birth countries, disease exposures, and unknown health histories of these children make them a population that requires special attention (1).

EPIDEMIOLOGY

Incidence

- More than 20,000 international adoptions by US families every year
- >90% are from Asia, Central and South America, and Eastern Europe, with growing numbers from Africa and the Middle East

RISK FACTORS

- Unknown birth history, medical history, and vaccination status
- Possible exposure to toxins and/or inadequate nutrition in utero
- Exposures to infectious diseases not commonly seen in the US
- Previous living conditions:
  - Overcrowding
  - Institutionalization (orphanages)
  - Environmental toxins
- History of neglect, deprivation, or abuse

GENERAL PREVENTION

- Required to be examined by a US State Department physician in their native country before immigration to the US (2)
- Should be examined by a US physician within 3 weeks of arrival
- A follow-up visit 4–6 weeks after their post adoption appointment is recommended.
- All internationally adopted children should be screened for hearing, vision, growth, and developmental delays.

COMMONLY ASSOCIATED CONDITIONS

- Infectious diseases, including (2,3):
  - Hepatitis B
  - Intestinal parasites
  - Tuberculosis
  - Syphilis
- Emotional or behavioral problems
- Developmental delay
- Fetal alcohol syndrome
- Feeding difficulties
- Anemia
- Congenital conditions, including:
  - Cleft lip/palate
  - Orthopedic deformities
- Prematurity or low birth weight
- Malnutrition, rickets
- Inadequate immunizations
- Lead poisoning
- Sensorineural and conductive hearing loss
- Strabismus, blindness

DIAGNOSIS

HISTORY

- Immunization records and titers (most helpful when dates of administration are included) (4)
- Birth/prenatal history
- Known family history of birth parents
- Prenatal and perinatal disease or toxin exposures
- Documented history of emotional or nutritional deprivation, or physical or sexual abuse
- Duration of time, if any, spent in orphanage. (Studies have suggested every 3–5 months spent in orphanage is associated with 1 month delay in developmental milestones, although quality of care can vary widely.)
- Growth charts when available: Failure to gain weight appropriately (or weight loss) is the earliest sign of malnutrition, followed by slowed linear growth, and finally lagging head circumference (brain growth).
- Development, behavior, attachment, parent stress, and parent–child interactions should also be routinely monitored.

PHYSICAL EXAM

- Age-appropriate complete physical exam, particular attention to growth, evaluation for microcephaly (red flag for fetal alcohol syndrome, genetic disorders, or perinatal brain injury), vision, and hearing
- Evaluate for signs of dental decay and refer for prompt treatment.
- Developmental assessment, especially for those with unknown date of birth
- Skin exam for signs of scabies, pediculosis, and tinea

DIAGNOSTIC TESTS & INTERPRETATION

- Developmental screening: Denver II Test and/or PEDS parent questionnaire or other validated developmental screening tools at each visit to screen for potential developmental delay and to assess improvement, decline, and need for additional services
- Age-appropriate hearing screening
- Age-appropriate vision screening

Lab

Initial lab tests

- Obtain (5):
  - Hepatitis B (HBsAg)
  - HIV
  - Rapid plasma reagin (RPR)
  - Tuberculin skin test
  - 3 stool specimens for ova and parasites, and single specimen for *Giardia intestinalis* and *Cryptosporidium parvum* antigens
  - CBC
  - Lead
  - Thyroid-stimulating hormone (TSH)
  - Ca^{++}, PO_4, alkaline phosphate, and 25 vitamin D level (if signs of rickets)
  - Urinalysis
- >6 months old: Measure titers for antibodies to diphtheria and tetanus toxoids and poliovirus (regardless of immunization documentation). If antibody concentrations are protective, complete series appropriate for age.
- >12 months old: Measure titers for antibodies to diphtheria, tetanus toxoids, poliovirus, measles, mumps, rubella, and varicella (regardless of immunization documentation), *Trypanosoma cruzi* serologic testing for adoptees from endemic countries.

Follow-Up & Special Considerations

Follow-up testing (5):

- Hep B: Repeat at 6 months.
- Hep C: Considered in children from China, Russia, Eastern Europe, and Southeast Asia (decision to test children from other countries depends on history & prevalence of infection). Do enzyme immunoassay (EIA).
- HIV: Transplacentally acquired maternal antibody may be present in uninfected infants up to 18 months, so will need to retest those with an initial positive result.
- Tuberculosis (TB): Positive test should NOT be attributed to BCG vaccine, and must be investigated further. Give preventive therapy if known exposures. Consider repeat testing at 6 months because poor nutrition may result in false-negative (anergic) skin test.
- GI tract signs or symptoms occurring years after immigration: Test for intestinal parasites.
- If anemia is detected with a normal lead level, may consider G6PD deficiency in appropriate countries of origin (African, Asian, Mediterranean, Middle Eastern), and can test with rapid fluorescent spot test.
- Eosinophilia: Eosinophilia >450 cells/mm^3 with negative stool ova and parasites, serologic testing for *Schistosoma*; and add *Strongyloides* for adoptees from sub-Saharan African, Latin American, and Southeast Asian countries.
- Developmental screening: Repeat at each visit and follow progress. 50–90% of all internationally adopted children are delayed upon adoption; however, most of them have normal cognition at long-term follow-up.
- Social history screening: Behavioral concerns may first present during adolescence, even for children adopted in infancy (6).

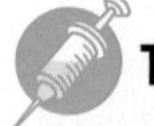

TREATMENT

MEDICATION

- Immunizations per Centers for Disease Control and Prevention schedule with catch-up as needed: http://www.cdc.gov/vaccines/recs/schedules/
- It is recommended that if the child does not have records, or has records that do not comply with the US or World Health Organization guidelines, then he or she should be treated as unimmunized and started on an appropriate catch-up immunization schedule.

ADDITIONAL TREATMENT

General Measures

- Regular diet for children who arrive malnourished should result in rapid weight gain to appropriate weight for height (or length).
- Monitor linear growth.
- If developmental delay is diagnosed, consider early services (e.g., Early Intervention) or referral to developmental specialist, depending on the nature and severity of the delay.
- Recommend local support groups for parents.
- Attention to parental interactions: Post adoption depression may occur.

Issues for Referral

- Many internationally adopted children show sensory-seeking behaviors early on that are sometimes thought to be related to the sensory-depriving orphanage experience of their past. These behaviors typically improve or abate without treatment, but may benefit from work with occupational therapy if the behaviors are significant. Out of context, they may appear quite similar to autistic like features on exam (hand-flapping, rocking, etc.), but as long as the child is otherwise developing normally (socially, emotionally), should not raise significant levels of concern (2).
- If a child continues to have disruptive behaviors, or would rather self-soothe than seek nurturing human interaction, he or she warrants a complete and thorough developmental evaluation with a specialist (developmental/behavioral pediatrician or pediatric psychiatrist).
- Persistent behavioral issues in the parent–child interactions should be evaluated by a pediatric psychologist or psychiatrist.
- Concerns about vision (higher rates of strabismus in international adoptees) should be referred to pediatric ophthalmology for a more extensive vision workup (2).
- Concerns about hearing (higher rates of conductive and sensorineural hearing loss in international adoptees) should be referred to audiology and/or ENT for a more extensive workup for conductive vs. sensorineural hearing loss (2).
- Recommend pediatric dental evaluation by 12 months, sooner if signs of dental pathology. Higher rates of dental disease among international adoptees because of poor hygiene, bottle propping, fluoride deficiency, and rickets (3).

ONGOING CARE

FOLLOW-UP RECOMMENDATIONS

Patient Monitoring

- Regular well-child visits, particularly within first months of entry into the US
- Close monitoring of developmental milestones, behavior, and individual attachment

DIET

- Regular diet
- Weight catch-up will occur with a normal diet, barring other medical conditions, and eating habits should normalize using parenting methods discussed below (7).

PATIENT EDUCATION

- Eating: The recommended approach is to allow access to as much healthy food as the child wants, as often as he or she wants it, so that the child can learn the important self-regulatory behaviors of eating that may not have been learned in an institution (hunger, satiety) and can build trust with the parent(s) who feed him or her.
- Toileting: While some children may simply not be trained yet, others may have accidents in their new home because of regression. Time and positive reinforcement, avoiding punishment, will resolve this issue as the child becomes comfortable with his or her new surroundings.
- Sleeping: Children must learn to trust their new home and parents, and thus this is not a time for aggressive sleep rules (i.e., ferberization). Parents should be present, physically and emotionally, just enough to let the child know he or she is safe, establish a bedtime ritual upon arrival, and then should gently reinforce this ritual.
- Language: As the child experiences a myriad of changes, it may be helpful for the adoptive family to have learned some key phrases in the child's native language for the first few weeks post-adoption. Depending on the child's age and language proficiency, an interpreter may also be useful in the home and at medical appointments until English becomes more comfortably understood and familiar (2).
- Adopted children may experience grieving of lost family, relationships, and culture, which is normal and expected behavior.
- At 3–4 years old, adopted children will begin to recognize physical differences between themselves and adoptive family if they are of different racial origin.
- Children and families should be encouraged to learn about the culture of the birth country and the ethnic group of origin.
- Relationships with others of the same racial or ethnic group may be very helpful to the adopted child.

PROGNOSIS

Long-term issues include (7,8):

- Children who experienced early neglect, deprivation, or loss prior to adoption are more likely to have developmental delay or behavioral or attachment problems.
- These issues decrease with time the child has spent within the adoptive family, although those with significant histories of deprivation are at risk for difficulties that may persist for life.
- Although most adopted children are healthy, as a group, they have been found to have higher rates of moderate to severe physical and mental health problems, hearing and visual impairment, learning disability, developmental delay, and special health care needs when compared with biologic children of the same parents.
- Developmental delay, in particular, is found to be more likely in an internationally adopted child than in his or her nonadopted peers. However, recent studies show marked catch-up development reported after living in adoptive homes, with many children achieving normal-range development later in life (depending on length of time spent in an institution prior to adoption).
- Fortunately, international adoption pairs some of the most vulnerable, potentially high-risk children with the lowest-risk parents (usually financially stable, well educated, with relatively extremely low divorce rates).
- Most families have found the process of international adoption deeply rewarding, while acknowledging the potential challenges.

REFERENCES

1. Dawood F, Serwint JR. International adoption. *Pediatr Rev*. 2008;29:292–4.
2. Schulte EE, Springer SH. Health care in the first year after international adoption. *Pediatr Clin North Am*. 2005;52:1331–49, vii.
3. Johnson DE. Long-term medical issues in international adoptees. *Pediatr Ann*. 2000;29: 234–41.
4. American Academy of Pediatrics Committee on Early Childhood, Adoption & Dependent Care. Initial medical evaluation of an adopted child. *Pediatrics*. 1991;88:642–4.
5. American Academy of Pediatrics. Medical evaluation of internationally adopted children for infectious diseases. In: Pickering LK, ed. *Red Book: 2009 Report of the Committee on Infectious Diseases*, 28th ed. Elk Grove Village, IL: Author.
6. Hawk B, McCall RB, et al. CBCL behavior problems of post-institutionalized international adoptees. *Clin Child Fam Psychol Rev*. 2010;13:199–211
7. Van Ijzendoorn MH, Bakermans-Kranenburg MJ, Juffer F. Plasticity of growth in height, weight, and head circumference: Meta-analytic evidence of massive catch-up after international adoption. *J Dev Behav Pediatr*. 2007;28:334–43.
8. Weitzman C, Albers L. Long-term developmental, behavioral, and attachment outcomes after international adoption. *Pediatr Clin North Am*. 2005;52:1395–419, viii.

ADDITIONAL READING

- Borchers D, American Academy of Pediatrics Committee on Early Childhood, Adoption, and Dependent Care. Families and adoption: The pediatrician's role in supporting communication. *Pediatrics*. 2003;112:1437–41.
- http://www.travel.state.gov/pdf/Prospective_Adoptive_Parents_Guide.pdf.

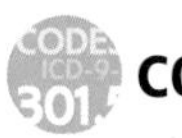

CODES

ICD9

V70.3 Other general medical examination for administrative purposes

CLINICAL PEARLS

- Initial labs: Hepatitis B (HBsAg), HIV, RPR, CBC, TSH, lead, Ca, PO4, 25 OH vitamin D; tuberculin skin test; 3 stool specimens for ova and parasites, and single specimen for *Giardia intestinalis* and *Cryptosporidium parvum* antigens; urinalysis
- $>$6 months old: Measure antibodies to diphtheria and tetanus toxoids and poliovirus (regardless of immunization documentation). If protective antibody concentrations are found, continue series as age appropriate.
- $>$12 months old: Measure antibodies to diphtheria, tetanus toxoids, poliovirus, measles, mumps, rubella, and varicella (regardless of immunization documentation); *Trypanosoma cruzi* serologic testing for adoptees from endemic countries.
- Many internationally adopted children show sensory-seeking behaviors early on that are sometimes thought to be related to the sensory-depriving orphanage experience of their past. These behaviors typically improve or abate without treatment but may benefit from work with occupational therapy if the behaviors are significant. Out of context, they may appear quite similar to autistic-like features on exam (hand-flapping, rocking, etc.), but as long as the child is otherwise developing normally (socially, emotionally), they should not raise significant levels of concern.

ALCOHOL ABUSE AND DEPENDENCE

Gennine M. Zinner, RNCS, ANP

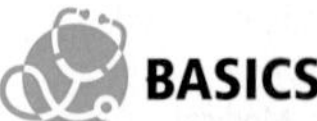

BASICS

DESCRIPTION

- Any pattern of alcohol use causing significant physical, mental, or social dysfunction; key features are tolerance, withdrawal, and persistent use despite problems
- Alcohol abuse: Maladaptive pattern of alcohol use manifested by 1 (or more) of:
  - Failure to fulfill obligations at work, school, or home
  - Recurrent use in hazardous situations
  - Recurrent alcohol-related legal problems
  - Continued use despite related social or interpersonal problems
- Alcohol dependence: Maladaptive pattern of use manifested by 3 (or more) of the following:
  - Tolerance
  - Withdrawal
  - Using more than intended
  - Persistent desire or attempts to cut down/stop
  - Significant amount of time obtaining, using, or recovering from alcohol
  - Social, occupational, or recreational activities sacrificed for alcohol use
  - Continued use despite physical or psychological problems
- National Institute on Alcohol Abuse and Alcoholism criteria for "at-risk" drinking: Men >14 drinks a week or >4 per occasion. Women: >7 drinks a week or >3 per occasion.
- System(s) affected: Nervous; Gastrointestinal
- Synonym(s): Alcoholism; Alcohol abuse; Alcohol dependence

Geriatric Considerations

- Common and underdiagnosed in elderly; less likely to report problem. May exacerbate normal age-related cognitive deficits and disabilities.
- Multiple drug interactions
- Signs and symptoms may be different or attributed to chronic medical problem or dementia.
- Common assessment tools may be inappropriate.

Pediatric Considerations

- Children of alcoholics at high risk
- In 2004, 28% of persons 12–20 years reported use in past month, 1 in 5 binge drink; binge drinkers are 7 times more likely to report illicit drug use.
- Negative effect on maturation and development
- Early drinkers are 4 times more likely to develop a problem than those who begin >21.
- Depression, suicidal or disorderly behavior; family disruption; violence or destruction of property; poor school or work performance; sexual promiscuity; social immaturity; lack of interests; isolation; moodiness

Pregnancy Considerations

- Alcohol is teratogenic, especially during the 1st trimester; women should abstain during conception and throughout pregnancy.
- 10–50% of children born to women who are heavy drinkers will have fetal alcohol syndrome.
- Women experience harmful effects at lower levels and are less likely to report problems.

EPIDEMIOLOGY

- Predominant age: 18–25, but all ages affected
- Predominant sex: Male > Female (3:1)

Prevalence

- Lifetime prevalence: 13.6%
- 20% in primary care setting
- 48.2% of 21-year-olds in the US reported binge drinking in 2004.

RISK FACTORS

- Family history
- Depression (40% with comorbid alcohol abuse)
- Anxiety
- Other substance abuse
- Tobacco
- Male gender
- Low socioeconomic status
- Unemployment
- Peer/social approval
- Family dysfunction or childhood trauma
- Post traumatic stress disorder
- Antisocial personality disorder
- Bipolar disorder
- Eating disorders
- Criminal involvement

Genetics

50–60% of risk is genetic.

GENERAL PREVENTION

Counsel with family history and risk factors

PATHOPHYSIOLOGY

Alcohol is a CNS depressant, facilitating γ-aminobutyric acid (GABA) inhibition and blocking N-methyl-d-aspartate receptors.

ETIOLOGY

Multifactorial: Genetic, environment, psychosocial

COMMONLY ASSOCIATED CONDITIONS

- Cardiomyopathy, atrial fibrillation
- Hypertension
- Peptic ulcer disease/gastritis
- Cirrhosis, fatty liver, cholelithiasis
- Hepatitis
- Diabetes mellitus
- Pancreatitis
- Malnutrition
- Upper GI malignancies
- Peripheral neuropathy, seizures
- Abuse and Violence
- Trauma (falls, motor vehicle accidents [MVAs])
- Severe psychiatric disorders (depression, bipolar, schizophrenia): >50% of patients with these disorders have a comorbid substance abuse problem.

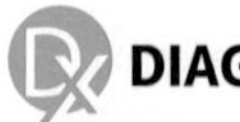

DIAGNOSIS

HISTORY

- Behavioral issues:
  - Anxiety, depression, insomnia
  - Psychological and social dysfunction, marital problems
  - Social isolation/withdrawal
  - Domestic violence
  - Alcohol-related legal problems
  - Repeated attempts to stop/reduce
  - Loss of interest in nondrinking activities
  - Employment problems (tardiness, absenteeism, decreased productivity, interpersonal problems, frequent job loss)
  - Blackouts
  - Complaints about alcohol-related behavior
  - Frequent trauma, MVAs, emergency department visits
- Physical symptoms:
  - Anorexia
  - Nausea, vomiting, abdominal pain
  - Palpitations
  - Headache
  - Impotence
  - Menstrual irregularities
  - Infertility

PHYSICAL EXAM

- Physical exam may be completely normal.
- General: Fever, agitation, diaphoresis
- Head/eyes/ears/nose/throat: Plethoric face, rhinophyma, poor oral hygiene, oropharyngeal malignancies
- Cardiovascular: Hypertension, dilated cardiomyopathy, tachycardia
- Respiratory: Aspiration pneumonia
- GI: Stigmata of chronic liver disease, peptic ulcer disease, pancreatitis, esophageal malignancies, esophageal varices
- Genitourinary: Testicular atrophy
- Musculoskeletal: Poorly healed fractures, myopathy, osteopenia, bone marrow suppression
- Neurologic: Tremors, cognitive deficits (e.g., memory impairment), peripheral neuropathy, Wernicke-Korsakoff syndrome
- Endocrine/metabolic: Hyperlipidemias, cushingoid appearance, gynecomastia
- Dermatologic: Burns (e.g., cigarettes), bruises, poor hygiene, palmar erythema, spider telangiectasias, caput medusa, jaundice

DIAGNOSTIC TESTS & INTERPRETATION

- CAGE Questionnaire: (Cut down, Annoyed, Guilty, and Eye opener): More than 2 "yes" answers is 74–89% sensitive, 79–95% specific for alcohol use disorder; less sensitive for white women, college students, elderly. Not an appropriate tool for less severe forms of alcohol abuse (1)[A].
- AUDIT: Alcohol Use Disorders Identification Test: 10 items, if >4: 70–92% sensitive, better in populations with low incidence of alcoholism (2)[A]: http://www.nams.org.sg/page.aspx/67/self-help-screening-tools/alcohol-the-audit-alcoholism-test
- Single question for unhealthy use screening: "How many times in the last year have you had X or more drinks in one day" (X = 5 for men, 4 for women); 81.8% sensitive, 79% specific for alcohol use disorders (3)

Lab

- CBC, liver function tests (LFTs), electrolytes, BUN/creatinine, lipid panel, thiamine, folate, Hepatitis A, B, C serology
- Serum levels increased in chronic abuse:
  - AST/ALT ratio >2.0
  - γ-glutamyl transferase (GGT)
  - Carbohydrate-deficient transferrin
  - Elevated mean corpuscular volume (MCV)
  - Prothrombin time
  - Uric acid
  - Triglycerides and cholesterol (total)

- Often decreased:
  - Calcium, magnesium, potassium, phosphorus
  - BUN
  - Hemoglobin, hematocrit
  - Platelet count
  - Serum protein, albumin
  - Thiamine, folate
- Blood alcohol concentration:
  - $>$100 mg/dL in outpatient setting
  - $>$150 mg/dL without obvious signs of intoxication
  - $>$300 mg/dL at any time

Imaging
- CAT scan or MRI of brain: Cortical atrophy, lesions in thalamic nucleus and basal forebrain
- Abdominal ultrasound: Ascites, periportal fibrosis, fatty infiltration, inflammation

Pathological Findings
- Liver: Inflammation or fatty infiltration (alcoholic hepatitis), periportal fibrosis (alcoholic cirrhosis occurs in only 10–20% of alcoholics)
- Gastric mucosa: Inflammation, ulceration
- Pancreas: Inflammation, liquefaction necrosis
- Heart: Dilated cardiomyopathy
- Immune system: Decreased granulocytes
- Endocrine organs: Elevated cortisol levels, testicular atrophy, decreased female hormones
- Brain: Cortical atrophy, enlarged ventricles

DIFFERENTIAL DIAGNOSIS
- Other substance use disorders
- Depression
- Dementia
- Cerebellar ataxia
- Cerebrovascular accident (CVA)
- Benign essential tremor
- Seizure disorder
- Hypoglycemia
- Diabetic ketoacidosis
- Viral hepatitis

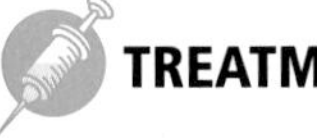

TREATMENT

For management of acute withdrawal, please see "Alcohol Withdrawal."

MEDICATION
First Line
- Adjuncts to withdrawal regimens:
  - Naltrexone 50–100 mg/d PO or 380 mg IM once every 4 weeks: Opiate antagonist reduces craving and likelihood of relapse (IM route may enhance compliance and thus efficacy) (4,5)[A]
  - Acamprosate (Campral) 666 mg PO t.i.d. beginning after completion of withdrawal; reduces relapse risk. If helpful, recommended to use for 1 year (4)[A].
  - Topiramate (Topamax) 25–300 mg/d PO or divided b.i.d.; enhances abstinence (4)[B] (not approved by the Food and Drug Administration [FDA] for use in alcohol dependence, off-label use)
- Supplements to all:
  - Thiamine 100 mg/d (first dose IV prior to glucose to avoid Wernicke encephalopathy)
  - Folic acid 1 mg/d
  - Multivitamin daily
- Contraindications:
  - Naltrexone: Pregnancy, acute hepatitis, hepatic failure
  - Monitor liver function tests.
- Precautions: Organic pain, organic brain syndromes
- Significant possible interactions: Alcohol, sedatives, hypnotics, naltrexone, and narcotics

ALERT

Treat acute symptoms if in alcohol withdrawal; give thiamine 100 mg/d with first dose prior to glucose.

Second Line
- Disulfiram 250–500 mg/d PO: Unproven efficacy; may provide psychologic deterrent
- Selective serotonin reuptake inhibitors may be beneficial if comorbid depression exists.

ADDITIONAL TREATMENT
General Measures
- Brief interventions by primary care clinicians are effective for problem drinking (6)[A].
- Treat comorbid problems (sleep, anxiety, etc.); use caution if prescribing medications with cross-tolerance to alcohol (benzodiazepine).
- Group programs and/or 12-step programs may have benefit in helping patients accept treatment.

Issues for Referral
Addiction specialist, 12-step or long-term program, psychiatrist

IN-PATIENT CONSIDERATIONS
Assess medical and psychiatric condition.

Initial Stabilization
- Correct electrolyte imbalances, acidosis, hypovolemia (treat if in alcohol withdrawal)
- Thiamine 100 mg IM, followed by orally 100 mg, and folic acid 1 mg/d
- Benzodiazepines used to lower risk of alcohol withdrawal, seizures

ONGOING CARE

FOLLOW-UP RECOMMENDATIONS
Patient Monitoring
- Outpatient detoxification: Daily visits
- Early outpatient rehabilitation: Weekly visits
- Detoxification alone is not sufficient.

PATIENT EDUCATION
- American Council on Alcoholism: (800) 527–5344 or http://www.aca-usa.org (treatment facility locator, educational information)
- National Clearinghouse for Alcohol and Drug Information: (800) 729–6686 or http://www.health.org
- Center for Substance Abuse Treatment: (800) 662-HELP or http://www.csat.samhsa.gov
- Alcoholics Anonymous: http://www.aa.org
- Rational Recovery: http://www.rational.org
- Secular Organizations for Sobriety: www.cfiwest.org/sos/index.htm
- http://www.alcoholanswers.org/list: An evidence-based Web site for those seeking credible information on alcohol dependence and online support forums

PROGNOSIS
- Chronic relapsing disease; mortality rate $>$ twice general population, death 10–15 years earlier
- Abstinence benefits survival, mental health, family, employment
- 12-step programs, cognitive behavior, and motivational therapies are effective during first year following treatment (2)[B].

COMPLICATIONS
- Cirrhosis (women sooner than men)
- GI malignancies
- Neuropathy, Dementia, Wernicke-Korsakoff syndrome
- CVA
- Ketoacidosis
- Infection
- Adult respiratory distress syndrome
- Depression
- Suicide
- Trauma

REFERENCES

1. Dhalla S, Kopec JA. The CAGE questionnaire for alcohol misuse: A review of reliability and validity studies. *Clin Invest Med*. 2007;30:33–41.
2. Enoch MA et al. Problem drinking and alcoholism: Diagnosis and treatment. *Am Fam Phys* 2002;65: 441–8.
3. Smith PC, Schmidt SM, Allensworth-Davies D, et al. Primary Care Validation of a Single-Question Alcohol Screening Test. *J Gen Intern Med*. 2009.
4. Williams SH. Medications for treating alcohol dependence. *Am Fam Phys*. 2005;72(pt 9): 1775–80.
5. Pettinati HM, Gastfriend DR, Dong Q, et al. Effect of Extended-Release Naltrexone (XR-NTX) on Quality of Life in Alcohol-Dependent Patients. *Alcohol Clin Exp Res*. 2008.
6. Asplund CA, Aaronson JW, Aaronson HE. 3 regimens for alcohol withdrawal and detoxification. *J Fam Pract*. 2004;53:545–54.

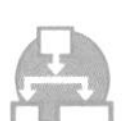

See Also (Topic, Algorithm, Electronic Media Element)

Substance Use Disorders; Alcohol Withdrawal

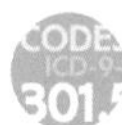

CODES

ICD9
- 303.90 Other and unspecified alcohol dependence, unspecified drinking behavior
- 305.00 Nondependent alcohol abuse, unspecified drinking behavior

CLINICAL PEARLS

- CAGE Questionnaire: (Cut down, Annoyed, Guilty, and Eye opener): More than 2 "yes" answers is 74–89% sensitive, 79–95% specific for alcohol use disorder; less sensitive for white women, college students, elderly. Not an appropriate tool for less severe forms of alcohol abuse
- Single question for unhealthy use screening: "How many times in the last year have you had X or more drinks in one day" (X = 5 for men, 4 for women); 81.8% sensitive, 79% specific for alcohol use disorders
- National Institute on Alcohol Abuse and Alcoholism criteria for "at-risk" drinking: Men $>$14 drinks a week or $>$4 per occasion. Women: $>$7 drinks a week or $>$3 per occasion.

ALCOHOL WITHDRAWAL

Neela Bhajandas, PharmD
Michael C. Barros, PharmD, BCPS
Nathaniel Marchetti, MD

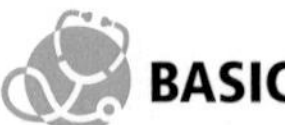

BASICS

DESCRIPTION

Alcohol withdrawal syndrome (AWS) is a spectrum of symptoms that results from abrupt cessation of alcohol in a dependent patient. Symptoms can begin within 5 hours of the last drink and persist for 5–10 days, ranging in severity.

EPIDEMIOLOGY

Each year, 8.2 million Americans meet diagnostic criteria for alcohol dependence. More prevalent among men, whites, Native Americans, younger and unmarried adults, and those with lower socioeconomic status. Only 24% of those with dependence are ever treated. <5% of US adults will experience alcohol withdrawal.

RISK FACTORS

- Older age
- High tolerance, prolonged use, high quantities
- Previous alcohol withdrawal episodes, detoxifications, alcohol withdrawal seizures, and delirium tremens (DTs)
- Serious medical problems
- Concomitant benzodiazepine dependence

Geriatric Considerations

Geriatric populations dependent on alcohol are more susceptible to symptoms of alcohol withdrawal and chronic comorbid conditions place them at higher risk of complications from withdrawal.

Pregnancy Considerations

Hospitalization or inpatient detoxification is usually required for medical treatment and monitoring of acute alcohol withdrawal.

Genetics

There is some evidence for a genetic basis of alcohol dependence.

GENERAL PREVENTION

- Routinely screen all adults for alcohol misuse (1)[B].
- Screen with the **CAGE** or similar questionnaire:
  - Feeling the need to **C**ut down
  - **A**nnoyed by criticism about alcohol use
  - **G**uilt about drinking/behaviors while intoxicated
  - "**E**ye opener" to quell withdrawal symptoms
  - Useful to detect problematic alcohol use, positive screen is ≥2 "yes" responses
- 10-question AUDIT screening test is also useful to identify problem drinking.

PATHOPHYSIOLOGY

- Consumption of alcohol potentiates the effect of the inhibitory neurotransmitter gamma-aminobutyric acid (GABA). With chronic alcohol ingestion, this repeated stimulation down regulates the inhibitory effects of GABA.
- Concurrently, alcohol ingestion inhibits the stimulatory effect of glutamate on the CNS with chronic alcohol use up regulating excitatory NMDA glutamate receptors.
- When alcohol is abruptly stopped, the combined effect of a down regulated inhibitory neurotransmitter system (GABA-modulated) and up regulated excitatory neurotransmitter system (glutamate-modulated) results in brain hyperexcitability when no longer suppressed by alcohol; clinically seen as AWS.

COMMONLY ASSOCIATED CONDITIONS

- General: Poor nutrition, electrolyte abnormalities (hyponatremia, hypomagnesemia, hypophosphatemia), thiamine deficiency, and dehydration
- GI: Hepatitis, cirrhosis, varices, GI bleed
- Heme: Splenomegaly, thrombocytopenia, macrocytic anemia
- Cardiovascular: Cardiomyopathy, hypertension, atrial fibrillation, other arrhythmias
- CNS: Trauma, seizure disorder, generalized atrophy, Wernicke-Korsakoff syndrome
- Peripheral nervous system (PNS): Neuropathy, myopathy
- Pulmonary: Aspiration pneumonitis or pneumonia; increased risk of anaerobic infections
- Psychiatric: Depression, posttraumatic stress disorder, bipolar disease, polysubstance abuse

DIAGNOSIS

- *Diagnostic and Statistical Manual of Mental Disorders* AWS criteria are diagnosed when ≥2 of the following present within a few hours to several days after the cessation or reduction of heavy and prolonged alcohol ingestion:
  - Autonomic hyperactivity (sweating, tachycardia)
  - Increased hand tremor
  - Insomnia
  - Psychomotor agitation
  - Anxiety
  - Nausea
  - Vomiting
  - Grand mal seizures
  - Transient (visual, auditory, or tactile) hallucinations or illusions
  - These should cause clinically significant distress or impair functioning and not be secondary to an underlying medical condition or mental disorder.
  - There are 3 stages to AWS.
- Stage 1 (minor withdrawal; onset 5–8 hours after cessation):
  - Mild anxiety, restlessness, and agitation
  - Mild nausea/GI upset and decreased appetite
  - Sleep disturbance
  - Sweating
  - Mild tremulousness
  - Fluctuating tachycardia and hypertension
- Stage 2 (major withdrawal; onset 24–72 hours after cessation):
  - Marked restlessness and agitation
  - Moderate tremulousness with constant eye movements
  - Diaphoresis
  - Nausea, vomiting, diarrhea, anorexia
  - Marked tachycardia and hypertension
  - Alcoholic hallucinosis (auditory, tactile, or visual); may have mild confusion but can be reoriented
- Stage 3 (delirium tremens; onset 72–96 hours after cessation):
  - Fever
  - Severe hypertension, tachycardia
  - Delirium
  - Drenching sweats
  - Marked tremors
- Alcohol withdrawal–associated seizures are often brief, generalized tonic-clonic seizures and can occur 6–48 hours after last drink.

HISTORY

Essential historical information should be:

- Duration and quantity of alcohol intake, time since last drink
- Previous episodes/symptoms of alcohol withdrawal, prior detox admissions
- Concurrent substance use
- Preexisting medical and psychiatric conditions, prior seizure activity
- Social history: Living situation, social support, stressors, triggers, etc.

PHYSICAL EXAM

Should include assessment of conditions likely to complicate or that are exacerbated by AWS:

- Cardiovascular: Arrhythmias, heart failure, coronary artery disease
- GI: GI bleed, liver disease, pancreatitis
- Neuro: Oculomotor dysfunction, gait ataxia, neuropathy
- Psych: Orientation, memory
- General: Hand tremor, infections

DIAGNOSTIC TESTS & INTERPRETATION

Lab

Initial lab tests

- Blood alcohol level, urine drug screen
- CBC; comprehensive metabolic panel

Imaging

Initial approach

CNS imaging if acute mental status changes

DIFFERENTIAL DIAGNOSIS

- Cocaine intoxication
- Opioid, marijuana, and methamphetamine withdrawal
- Anticholinergic drug toxicity
- Neuroleptic malignant syndrome
- Liver failure
- Sepsis, CNS infection or hemorrhage
- Mania, psychosis
- Thyroid crisis (2)[C]

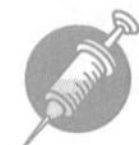

TREATMENT

- The goal is to prevent and treat withdrawal symptoms (i.e., seizures, DTs, cardiovascular events). This is done mainly with benzodiazepines (BZDs), which reduce the duration of symptoms and raise the seizure threshold.
  - Exclude other medical and psychiatric causes.
  - Provide a quiet, protective environment.
  - The Clinical Institute Withdrawal Assessment for Alcohol Scale (CIWA) is useful for determining medication dosing and frequency of evaluation for AWS. The CIWA scale rates the severity of 10 symptoms on a scale from 1–7, 1 being without the symptom and 7 the max score:

- Nausea and vomiting
- Tremor
- Paroxysmal sweats
- Anxiety
- Agitation
- Tactile disturbances
- Auditory disturbances
- Visual disturbances
- Headache or fullness in head
- Orientation and clouding of sensorium

- Frequent reevaluation with CIWA score is crucial.

MEDICATION

First Line

- BZD monotherapy remains the treatment of choice (3)[A], associated with fewer complications compared with neuroleptic agents (4)[A]
- BZD should be chosen by the following considerations:
  - Agents with rapid onset control agitation more quickly (e.g., IV or PO diazepam [Valium])
  - Long-acting BZDs (diazepam, chlordiazepoxide [Librium]) are more effective at preventing breakthrough seizures and delirium management
  - Short-acting BZDs (lorazepam [Ativan], oxazepam [Serax]) are preferable when prolonged sedation is a concern (e.g., elderly patients or other serious concomitant medical illness) and preferable when severe hepatic insufficiency may impair metabolism (4)[A]
- BZD amounts will vary by patients. Given as symptom-triggered or fixed-schedule regimens. Symptom-triggered regimens have been found to require less BZD amounts and reduce hospitalization time (2)[A].
- Symptom-triggered regimen: Start with chlordiazepoxide 50–100 mg PO, repeat CIWA hourly and if score is ≥8, give additional dose of chlordiazepoxide 50 mg PO. Continue to re-evaluate with CIWA hourly until adequate sedation achieved (score <8). May substitute chlordiazepoxide with respective doses of diazepam, lorazepam, or oxazepam (2)[C].

Second Line

- β-blockers (e.g., atenolol [Tenormin]) and $\alpha 2$ agonists (e.g., clonidine [Catapres]) help to control hypertension and tachycardia and can be used with BZDs (2)[C]. Not used as monotherapy, due to their inability to prevent DTs and seizures.
- Carbamazepine: Not recommended as first-line therapy; associated with reduced incidence of seizures but more studies are needed (5,6)[C].
- Thiamine: 100 mg/d IV or IM for at least 3 days (4)[C]:
  - Note that IV glucose administered before treatment with thiamine may precipitate Wernicke encephalopathy and Korsakoff psychosis.
- If the patient exhibits significant agitation and alcoholic hallucinosis, an antipsychotic (haloperidol [Haldol]) can be used, but this requires close observation, as it lowers the seizure threshold (2)[C].

ADDITIONAL TREATMENT

Additional Therapies

Peripheral neuropathy and cerebellar dysfunction merit physical therapy evaluation.

IN-PATIENT CONSIDERATIONS

Patients in withdrawal stages 1 and 2 can be treated as outpatients unless medical comorbidities require in-patient care. A reliable and supportive social environment should be in place with frequent follow-up.

Admission Criteria

- CIWA score >15, or severe withdrawal
- Concurrent acute illness requiring in patient care
- Poor ability to follow up or no reliable social support
- Pregnancy
- Seizure disorder or history of severe alcohol-related seizures
- Suicide risk
- Concurrent BZD dependence
- Age >40 years old
- Prolonged heavy drinking >8 years
- Consumes >1 pint of alcohol or 12 beers per day
- Random blood alcohol level >200 mg/dL
- Elevated MCV, BUN
- Cirrhosis, liver failure

Discharge Criteria

CIWA scores of <10 on 3 consecutive determinations

ONGOING CARE

FOLLOW-UP RECOMMENDATIONS

Discharge arrangements include transfer to a treatment facility (i.e., sober house or residential program), outpatient substance abuse counseling, peer support groups (Alcoholics Anonymous), the use of adjuvant treatment such as disulfiram (Antabuse), acamprosate (Campral), or naltrexone (ReVia, Vivitrol)

- Disulfiram: Irreversibly inhibits aldehyde dehydrogenase, blocking alcohol metabolism, leading to an accumulation of acetaldehyde; therefore, it reinforces the individual's desires to stop drinking by providing a disincentive associated with increase acetaldehyde.
  - 250–500 mg PO daily x 1–2 weeks; maintenance 250 mg PO daily
  - Contraindications: Concomitant use of metronidazole and ethanol-containing products, psychosis, severe myocardial disease
- Acamprosate (666 mg t.i.d.): Glutamate and GABA modulator indicated to reduce cravings
  - Contraindications: Renal impairment (CrCl <30 mL/min)
- Naltrexone (50 mg daily): Opiate receptor antagonist, theorized to attenuate reinforcing pleasurable effects of alcohol and reduce craving
  - Contraindications: Acute hepatitis/liver failure, concomitant opioid therapy

Patient Monitoring

Frequent follow-up to monitor for relapse.

PATIENT EDUCATION

- Alcoholics Anonymous at www.aa.org
- SMART Recovery (Self-Management and Recovery Training) at www.smartrecovery.org (not spiritually based)
- National Institute on Alcohol Abuse and Alcoholism at www.niaaa.nih.gov
- FamilyDoctor.Org: Alcoholism (Spanish resources available)

PROGNOSIS

Mortality from severe withdrawal (DTs) is 1–5%.

COMPLICATIONS

Occurs more frequently in individuals who have prior episodes of withdrawal or concomitant illnesses.

REFERENCES

1. Rockville MD. Screening and Behavioral Counseling Interventions in Primary Care to Reduce Alcohol Misuse, Topic Page. *USPSTF* April. 2004.
2. Mayo-Smith MF. Pharmacological management of alcohol withdrawal: a meta-analysis and evidence-based practice guideline. *JAMA*. 1997; 278:144–51.
3. Ntais C, Pakos E, Kyzas P, Ioannidis JP. Benzodiazepines for alcohol withdrawal. *Cochrane Database Syst Rev*. 2005;20(3):CD005063.
4. Amato L, Minozzi S, Davoli M, et al. Efficacy and safety of pharmacological interventions for the treatment of the Alcohol Withdrawal Syndrome. *Cochrane Database Syst Rev*. 2011;(6): CD008537.
5. Minozzi S, Amato L, Vecchi S, Davoli M, et al. Anticonvulsants for alcohol withdrawal. *Cochrane Database Syst Rev*. 2010;(3):CD005064.
6. Sarff M, Gold JA. Alcohol withdrawal syndromes in the intensive care unit. *Crit Care Med*. 2010;38 (9 Suppl):S494–501.

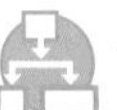

See Also (Topic, Algorithm, Electronic Media Element)

Substance Use Disorders

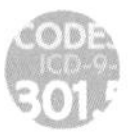

CODES

ICD9

- 291.0 Alcohol withdrawal delirium
- 291.81 Alcohol withdrawal
- 303.90 Other and unspecified alcohol dependence, unspecified

CLINICAL PEARLS

- The Kindling phenomenon has postulated that long-term exposure to alcohol affects neurons, resulting in increased alcohol craving and progressively worse withdrawal episodes.
- The CIWA is a useful tool for managing the symptoms and treatment of alcohol withdrawal.
- Any BZD dose should be patient-specific, sufficient to achieve and maintain a "light somnolence" (e.g., sleeping but easily arousable), and should be tapered off carefully even after AWS resolves.
- Administer thiamine before patient receives glucose, so as not to precipitate Wernicke encephalopathy.
- There should be frequent outpatient follow-up to monitor for relapse.
- Counsel patients taking disulfiram to avoid over-the-counter products that contain alcohol (i.e., mouthwashes)
- IM administration of diazepam and chlordiazepoxide should be avoided because of erratic absorption.

ALOPECIA

Ann M. Rodden, DO, MS

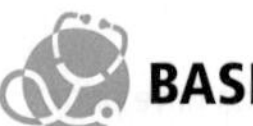

BASICS

DESCRIPTION

- Alopecia: Absence of hair from areas where it normally exists:
  - Anagen phase: Growing hairs
  - Telogen phase: Dead, "resting" hairs
- Androgenic alopecia (male- or female-pattern hair loss): Hair loss and miniaturization of hair follicles:
  - In men: Frontal recession, then vertex affected; over time, only has lateral and occipital hair left (Norwood Hamilton Classification Type I–VII)
  - In women: Thinning across the crown, with frontal hair later affected (Ludwig Classification, Grade I–III)
- Alopecia areata: Patchy, nonscarring hair loss:
  - Alopecia totalis: Hair loss of the entire scalp
  - Alopecia universalis: Loss of all body hair
- Telogen effluvium: Diffuse hair loss that (usually) has temporarily decreased hair density but not complete baldness:
  - Abnormal hair cycling leads to excessive loss of hairs in telogen phase.
  - Usually occurs 3 months after the trigger occurs
- Anagen effluvium: Diffuse shedding of hairs, including growing hairs, that may progress to complete baldness:
  - Growth arrest of hair in anagen phase and sheds
  - Begins days to weeks after inciting incident
- Cicatricial alopecia (scarring alopecia): Slick, smooth scalp without evidence of follicular openings
- Traction alopecia: Patchy, initially nonscarring hair loss usually due to physical stressors on hair:
  - Trichotillomania: Hair loss due to the person pulling hair out
- Tinea capitis: Patches of hair broken off close to the scalp sometimes with inflammation, caused by fungal infection

Pediatric Considerations

Tinea capitis is more common among children.

Pregnancy Considerations

Telogen gravidarum: Hair loss 2–4 months after childbirth

EPIDEMIOLOGY

- Age:
  - Androgenic alopecia: May begin after puberty and increases in prevalence over time
- Predominant sex: Male > Female

Incidence

Alopecia areata: 0.1–0.2% incidence in all races

Prevalence

- Androgenic alopecia:
  - Men: 15% of adolescent males:
    - 50% of white men over 50 years old
  - Women: 6–12% under age of 30 with up to 50% lifetime prevalence
- Alopecia areata:
  - 1.7% of US population

RISK FACTORS

- Physiologic or psychologic stress
- Pregnancy
- Poor nutrition
- Use of certain medications/chemotherapy
- Tight living quarters
- Sharing hair products/supplies

Genetics

- Family history of early hair loss
- Polygenic inheritance of androgenic alopecia

GENERAL PREVENTION

- For traction alopecia: Minimize braids, coloring, bleaching, waving of hair, or hair styles that pull hair.
- For tinea capitis: Avoid sharing hats, combs, hairbrushes, hair ornaments, and pillows.

PATHOPHYSIOLOGY

- All hair follicles pass through anagen and telogen phases.
- When many are in the telogen phase at one time, the hair loss becomes noticeable.
- Activity of hair follicles may diminish due to trauma, medications, or disease.

ETIOLOGY

- Androgenic alopecia:
  - Genetically predisposed
  - Polycystic ovarian syndrome
  - Adrenal hyperplasia
  - Pituitary hyperplasia
  - Drugs (testosterone, progesterone, danazol, adrenocorticosteroids, anabolic steroids)
- Alopecia areata:
  - Autoimmune processes like thyroiditis
- Telogen effluvium:
  - In most cases, no specific etiology is found.
  - Postpartum
  - Adding or changing medications (oral contraceptives, anticoagulants, anticonvulsants, SSRIs, retinoids, β-blockers, ACE inhibitors, colchicine, cholesterol-lowering medications, cimetidine, levodopa, bromocriptine, chemotherapeutic agents, interferon, others)
  - Stress: Physical (fever, trauma, surgery) or psychologic
  - Chronic illness (systemic lupus erythematosus [SLE], syphilis, systemic amyloidosis, hepatic failure, chronic renal failure, inflammatory bowel disease, dermatomyositis, HIV, lymphoproliferative disorders)
  - Hormonal (hypo-/hyperthyroid, pituitary dysfunction)
  - Malnutrition (iron deficiency, zinc deficiency, caloric restriction/eating disorder)
  - Malabsorption (celiac disease, pancreatic disease)
  - Inflammatory skin disorders (psoriasis, seborrheic dermatitis, allergic contact dermatitis)
- Anagen effluvium:
  - Chemotherapy is most common trigger
  - Radiation to the area
  - Drugs (chemotherapeutic agents, allopurinol, colchicine)
  - Poisoning (mercury, thallium, bismuth, arsenic, gold, boric acid)
  - Severe protein malnutrition
- Cicatricial alopecia:
  - Physical agents/trauma (burns, freezing, radiation)
  - Congenital (aplasia cutis congenital, Conradi-Hunermann chondrodysplasia punctata)
  - Lymphocytic (cutaneous discoid lupus erythematous, central centrifugal cicatricial alopecia, lichen planopilaris)
  - Neutrophilic (folliculitis decalvans, dissecting folliculitis)
  - Acne keloidosis
  - Infection (zoster, kerion, folliculitis)
  - Metastatic or primary neoplasm
- Traction alopecia:
  - Trichotillomania (direct self-pulling of the hair, obsessive-compulsive behavior)
  - Tight rollers or braids
- Tinea capitis (*Microsporum, Trichophyton*)

COMMONLY ASSOCIATED CONDITIONS

Alopecia areata:

- Down syndrome
- Autoimmune thyroiditis
- Vitiligo
- Diabetes

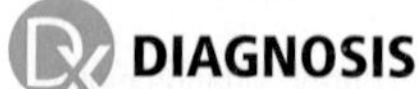

DIAGNOSIS

HISTORY

- Duration of hair loss
- Episodic or continuous
- Pattern of hair loss
- Medications
- Chronic disease, recent illness, surgeries, pregnancy
- Changes in health/medication in past 2–3 months
- Psychological stress
- Dietary history and weight changes
- Menstrual history
- Family history of hair loss or autoimmune disorders
- Radiation or exposure to heavy metals
- Pruritus (in tinea capitis)

PHYSICAL EXAM

- Pattern of hair loss:
  - Is hair loss generalized or local?
  - If local, is it symmetrical at the vertex and/or the hairline at the forehead?
- Scalp scaling, inflammation (in tinea capitis)
- Changes in the hair:
  - Hair-pull test: Pinch 25–50 hairs between thumb and forefinger, and exert slow, gentle traction while sliding fingers up:
    - Normal: 1–2 dislodge
    - Abnormal: $\geq$6 hairs dislodged (in effluvium, alopecia areata)
  - Broken hairs (tinea capitis, traction alopecia)
  - Broken-off hair at the borders of the patch that are easily removable (in alopecia areata)
  - Hair loss in circular pattern (in alopecia areata, tinea capitis)
- Clinical signs of thyroid disease, lupus, or other diseases
- Clinical signs of virilization: Acne, hirsutism, acanthosis nigrans, truncal obesity (in androgenic alopecia)

DIAGNOSTIC TESTS & INTERPRETATION

Lab

- Thyroid-stimulating hormone and free thyroxine (fT_4) (hypo- or hyperthyroidism)
- CBC (anemia)
- Comprehensive metabolic panel (liver and renal disease)
- Free testosterone and dehydroepiandrosterone sulfate (hyperandrogenism)
- Serum ferritin and total iron-binding capacity (iron deficiency)

- Serum zinc (deficiency)
- Rapid plasma reagin test (syphilis)
- Prolactin (pituitary hyperplasia)
- Antinuclear antibody (ANA) (SLE)

Diagnostic Procedures/Surgery

- Light hair-pull test:
  - Pull on 25–50 hairs and ≥6 hairs dislodge is consistent with shedding (effluvium, alopecia areata)
- Direct microscopic exam of the hair shaft:
  - Anagen hairs: Elongated and possibly pigmented bulb with gelatinous root sheath
  - Exclamation point hairs: At periphery of lesion and has club-shaped root with thinner proximal shaft that distally becomes normal in size (alopecia areata)
- Daily hair counts: Collect hair in dated envelopes for 2 weeks, in morning:
  - More than 100 hairs per day is consistent with effluvium
- Ultraviolet light fluorescence and potassium hydroxide prep (to rule out tinea capitis)

Pathological Findings

Scalp biopsy with routine microscopy will aid in the diagnosis if unsure.

DIFFERENTIAL DIAGNOSIS

Search for type of alopecia and then for reversible causes.

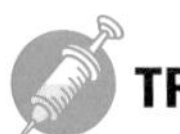

TREATMENT

MEDICATION

- Androgenic alopecia:
  - Minoxidil (Rogaine) 2% topical solution (1 mL b.i.d.) for women, 5% topical solution (1 mL b.i.d.) or foam (daily) for men (1)[A]
  - Finasteride (Propecia), 1 mg/d for men (1)[A]
  - Spironolactone (Aldactone) 100–200 mg/d in hyperandrogenic women (off-label) (1)[C]:
    - Diuretic with antiandrogen actions
  - Oral contraception pills with low levels of androgenic affect in women (Yasmin, Ortho-TriCyclen, Ortho-Cyclen, Ortho-Evra, Mircette) (off-label) (2)[C]
  - Ketoconazole 2% shampoo with minoxidil 2% (1)[C]
- Alopecia areata:
  - Intralesional steroids: Triamcinolone 2.5–10 mg/mL (3,4)[C]:
    - First line in adults if <50% scalp involved
    - Repeat every 4–6 weeks; if no improvement in 6 months, stop treatment
    - 0.5-inch, 30-gauge needle and inject 0.1 mL at each point at 1-cm intervals
  - If >50% scalp involved, refer to dermatologist (3)
  - Children: Topical midpotent corticosteroids (3)[C]
  - Systemic glucocorticoids: May induce regrowth, but alopecia recurs after cessation of medication and risks may outweigh benefits for long-term use (3,)[C]
- Telogen effluvium: Remove offending medication (5)[C].
- Tinea capitis: See appropriate section on tinea.
- Side effects/precautions:
  - Topical minoxidil:
    - Irritant dermatitis or contact allergic dermatitis
    - Hypertrichosis
    - Exacerbation of angina (rare)
  - Intralesional steroids:
    - Local burning/stinging/pruritus/skin atrophy
  - Spironolactone:
    - Menstrual cycle abnormalities
    - Postural hypotension
    - Electrolyte imbalance (hyperkalemia)
  - Finasteride:
    - Caution in known liver disease
    - Sexual side effects
    - Monitor prostate-specific antigen (PSA): Will decrease PSA level by 50%

Pregnancy Considerations

Finasteride not indicated for use in women; pregnancy Category X. Women should not handle crushed or broken pills during childbearing years.

ADDITIONAL TREATMENT

General Measures

- Trial off offending medication may resolve issue. If unsure which medication, may readminister if patient is willing.
- Traction alopecia:
  - Only with discontinuation of the hair pulling will the disorder resolve.
  - Psychological or psychiatric intervention may be necessary.
  - Successful therapeutic approaches have included medications, behavior modification, and hypnosis.

COMPLEMENTARY AND ALTERNATIVE MEDICINE

- Many herbal medications are available but lacking research at this time.
- Androgenic alopecia:
  - Low-energy laser light: HairMax LaserComb (1)[C]: Safe alternative, but lacking research

SURGERY/OTHER PROCEDURES

- Hair transplantation
- Wigs/hairpieces/extensions
- Androgenic alopecia:
  - Surgical (hair transplantation, scalp reduction, transposition flap, and soft tissue expansion)
  - Medical tattooing of eyebrows
- Cicatricial alopecia:
  - The only effective treatment is surgical (graft transplantation, flap transplantation, or excision of the scarred area).

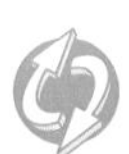

ONGOING CARE

DIET

If nutritional deficit noted, supplementation may be necessary.

PATIENT EDUCATION

National Alopecia Areata Foundation: www.naaf.org

PROGNOSIS

- Androgenic alopecia:
  - Prognosis depends on treatment
- Alopecia areata:
  - Usually regrows within 1 year even without treatment
  - Recurrence common
  - 10% have severe, chronic form
- Telogen effluvium:
  - Maximum shedding 3 months after the inciting event and recovery following correction of the cause
  - Usually subsides in 3–6 months but takes 12–18 months for cosmetically significant regrowth
  - Rarely permanent baldness
  - Chronic effluvium uncommon
- Anagen effluvium:
  - Shedding begins days to a few weeks after the inciting event, with recovery following correction of the cause.
  - Rarely permanent baldness
- Cicatricial alopecia:
  - Hair follicles permanently damaged
- Traction alopecia:
  - Depends on behavior modification
- Tinea capitis:
  - Usually complete recovery

REFERENCES

1. Rogers NE, Avram MR. Medical treatments for male and female pattern hair loss. *J Am Acad Dermatol*. 2008;59:547–66; quiz 567–8.
2. Goh C, Zippin JH. Androgenetic alopecia: Diagnosis and treatment with a focus on recent genetic implications. *J Drugs Dermatol*. 2009;8:185–92.
3. Alkhalifah A, Alsantali A, Wang E, et al. Alopecia areata update: Part II. Treatment. *J Am Acad Dermatol*. 2010;62.
4. Mounsey AL, Reed SW. Diagnosing and treating hair loss. *Am Fam Physician*. 2009;80:356–62.
5. Harrison S, Bergfeld W. Diffuse hair loss: Its triggers and management. *Cleve Clin J Med*. 2009;76: 361–7.

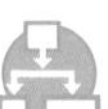

See Also (Topic, Algorithm, Electronic Media Element)

- Tinea (Capitis, Corporis, Cruris); Syphilis; Systemic Lupus Erythematosus; Polycystic Ovarian Syndrome; Lichen Planus; Hyperthyroidism
- Algorithm: Alopecia

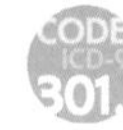

CODES

ICD9

- 704.00 Alopecia, unspecified
- 704.01 Alopecia areata
- 704.02 Telogen effluvium

CLINICAL PEARLS

- History and physical will usually determine type of alopecia.
- Treatment of underlying medical condition or removal of triggering medication in many types of alopecia will reinstate hair growth without the need of further interventions.
- Educating the patient about the nature of the condition and expectations is key to patient care.

ALTITUDE ILLNESS

Robert J. Hyde, MD

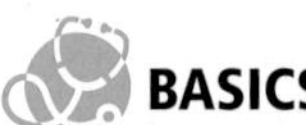

BASICS

DESCRIPTION

Altitude illness is a spectrum of medical problems ranging from mild discomfort to fatal illness that may occur on ascent to higher altitudes (elevations >1,500 m [4,921 feet]). It is divided into 3 categories: high, 1,500–3,500 m; very high, 3,500–5,500 m; and extreme, 5,500–8,850 m (1). Altitude illness can affect anyone, including the most experienced and fit individual (2). For most, it is an unpleasant but self-limiting syndrome that will not require physician intervention.

- Acute mountain sickness (AMS): Symptoms associated with a physiologic response to a hypobaric, hypoxic environment. Onset occurs within 24 hours of arrival at altitude, often within 1–4 hours. Neurologic symptoms are predominant and range from a mild to moderate headache and malaise to severe impairment.
- High-altitude pulmonary edema (HAPE): Noncardiogenic pulmonary edema. Onset 1–4 days at altitude. Rare <8,000 feet (2,438 m).
- High-altitude cerebral edema (HACE): A potentially fatal neurologic syndrome; considered the end stage of AMS. Onset within 3–5 days at elevations as low as 9,022 feet (2,750 m) but may be more abrupt at higher altitudes. Death results from brain herniation.
- System(s) affected: Nervous/Pulmonary
- Synonym(s): Mountain sickness

Geriatric Considerations

- Risk does not increase with age.
- Age alone should not preclude travel to high altitude; allow extra time to acclimate.
- Preexisting medical problems that are made worse are referred to as altitude-exacerbated conditions.

Pediatric Considerations

- Altitude illness seems to have the same incidence in children as in adults, but diagnosis may be delayed in younger children.
- Any child who experiences behavioral symptoms after recent ascent should be presumed to be suffering from altitude illness.

Pregnancy Considerations

- The risk during pregnancy is unknown.
- There is no evidence that exposure to high altitudes (1,500–3,500 m) poses a risk to a pregnancy.
- It may be prudent to advise a low-altitude dwelling for any pregnant woman experiencing complications.

EPIDEMIOLOGY

Most epidemiologic studies are limited to relatively homogeneous populations of men.

Incidence

- AMS: 10–90% of travelers ascending to higher altitudes may experience symptoms.
- HAPE/HACE: These conditions occur in 0.01–1% of sojourner ascents at typical mountain resorts, although incidence increases with rapid and higher ascents (3).

RISK FACTORS

- Rapid rate of ascent
- Maximum altitude attained
- Increased duration at high altitude
- Failure to acclimatize at lower altitude
- Higher altitude during sleep cycle
- Prior history of altitude illness
- Cardiac congenital abnormalities

GENERAL PREVENTION

- General guidelines:
  - Preacclimatization affords some protection against altitude illness.
  - A staged or graded ascent (rest every 600–1,200 m) and a slow ascent rate (maximum 600 m/d) should allow adequate time for acclimatization.
  - Sleeping elevation: "Climb high and sleep low" is a prudent practice for anyone going above 3,500 m.
  - Avoid heavy exertion for the first 1–3 days.
  - Avoid respiratory depressants such as alcohol and soporifics.
  - Preascent physical conditioning is not preventive.
- Drug prophylaxis:
  - Acetazolamide and dexamethasone (see below)
  - For HAPE only:
    - Consider nifedipine and beta agonists (see "Treatment" section).

PATHOPHYSIOLOGY

- Not completely understood
- Hypobaric hypoxia and hypoxemia are the pathophysiologic precursors to altitude illness.
- Symptoms of AMS may be the result of cerebral swelling, either through vasodilatation induced by hypoxia or through cerebral edema.
- Other mechanisms include impaired cerebral autoregulation, release of vasogenic mediators, and alteration of the blood–brain barrier.
- HAPE is a noncardiogenic pulmonary edema characterized by exaggerated pulmonary hypertension leading to vascular leakage through overperfusion, stress failure, or both.

ETIOLOGY

Individuals with a prior episode of HAPE have an increased risk of recurrence (4).

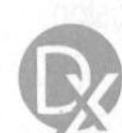

DIAGNOSIS

HISTORY

- AMS, mild to moderate symptoms:
  - Headache, plus at least 1 of the following:
    - Anorexia
    - Nausea or vomiting
    - Dizziness or lightheadedness
    - Insomnia
- AMS, severe symptoms:
  - Increased headache
  - Irritability
  - Marked fatigue
  - Dyspnea with exertion
  - Nausea and vomiting
  - HAPE (Lake Louise diagnostic criteria):
    - At least 2 of the following symptoms: Dyspnea at rest, cough, weakness, decreased exercise performance, chest tightness, congestion
    - AND at least 2 of the following signs: Crackles or wheezing in at least 1 lung field, central cyanosis, tachycardia, tachypnea. (Note: Fatigue may be pulmonary edema.)
  - HACE symptoms: Mental status changes (irrational behavior, lethargy, obtundation, coma)

PHYSICAL EXAM

- HAPE:
  - Lung crackles or wheezing
  - Central cyanosis
  - Tachycardia
  - Tachypnea
- HACE:
  - Abnormal mental status exam (behavioral change, lethargy, obtundation, coma)
  - Truncal ataxia
  - Papilledema, retinal hemorrhage, cranial nerve palsies
  - Focal neurologic deficits (rare)

DIAGNOSTIC TESTS & INTERPRETATION

An electrocardiogram may show sinus tachycardia or right-sided heart strain.

Lab

- AMS: Laboratory studies are nonspecific and rarely required for diagnosis.
- HAPE: Severe hypoxemia demonstrated with oximetry or blood gas analysis.

Imaging

No radiographic feature is specific to HAPE.

DIFFERENTIAL DIAGNOSIS

Onset of symptoms >3 days at a given altitude, the absence of headache, or the lack of rapid response to oxygen or descent suggest other diagnoses.

- AMS/HACE:
  - Subarachnoid hemorrhage, CNS mass, cerebrovascular accident
  - Migraine headache
  - Dehydration
  - Ingestion of toxins, drugs, or alcohol
  - Carbon monoxide exposure
  - CNS infection
  - Acute psychosis
- HAPE:
  - Pneumonia
  - Cardiogenic pulmonary edema
  - Spontaneous pneumothorax
  - Pulmonary embolism
  - Asthma
  - Bronchitis
  - Myocardial infarction
  - Hyperventilation syndrome

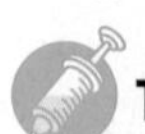

TREATMENT

MEDICATION

First Line

- Oxygen: 2–15 L/min to maintain SaO_2 >90% until symptoms improve
- Acetazolamide: If patient has a history of problems at altitude and/or plans to ascend >500 m/d. Dosage is usually 125–500 mg PO b.i.d. starting 2 days before ascent and continued for 3 days at maximum altitude. Patients with a drug allergy to sulfonamides should avoid acetazolamide.
  - Prevention of AMS: 125–500 mg PO b.i.d. starting 1 day before ascent and continued for 2 days at maximum altitude
  - Treatment of AMS: 125–500 mg PO b.i.d. until symptoms resolve

- Dexamethasone: May significantly reduce the incidence and severity of AMS. Dosage is 2–4 mg PO q6h, begun the day of ascent, continued for 3 days at the higher altitude, and then tapered over 5 days. Adverse side effects are rare:
  - Prevention of AMS: 2 mg PO q6h or 4 mg PO q12h, starting 1 day before ascent and discontinued cautiously after 2 days at maximum altitude
  - Treatment of AMS: 4 mg PO/IV/IM q6h
  - Treatment of HACE: 8 mg PO/IV/IM initially, then 4 mg q6h
- Nifedipine (reduces pulmonary arterial pressure):
  - Prevention of HAPE: 20–30 mg extended-release PO b.i.d. starting 1 day prior to ascent and continued for 2 days at maximum altitude
  - Treatment of HAPE: 10 mg, then 20–30 mg extended-release PO b.i.d.
- Salmeterol:
  - Prevention and possible treatment of HAPE: 125 μg inhaled b.i.d. starting 1 day before ascent and continued for 2 days at maximum altitude
- NSAIDs:
  - Prevention and treatment of headache
  - Aspirin: 325 mg PO q4h for total 3 doses
  - Ibuprofen: 400–600 mg PO
  - Prevention of AMS: Dose unknown. Begin 1–5 days before ascent.
- Antiemetics:
  - Prochlorperazine: 10 mg PO/IM q6–8h
  - Promethazine: 25–50 mg PO/IM/PR q6h

Second Line

Furosemide: Consider for treatment of AMS or HACE, 20–80 mg PO/IV q12h for a total of 2 doses. Currently out of favor; not recommended for prophylaxis; not established for use in HAPE.

ADDITIONAL TREATMENT

General Measures

- Therapy must be tailored to fit disease severity.
- Early recognition is critical.
- Stop ascent, acclimatize at the same altitude, and/or descend if symptoms do not improve over 24 hours. Definitive treatment is to descend to a lower altitude. Dramatic improvement accompanies even modest reductions in altitude.
- Oxygen helps relieve symptoms. Give continuously by cannula or mask initially, and then titrate to SaO_2 >90%.
- AMS:
  - Acetazolamide is effective in reducing mild to moderate symptoms of AMS, but the optimum dosage is unknown. Consider 125–500 mg PO b.i.d. until symptoms resolve.
  - Dexamethasone may also be effective in treating moderate AMS. Consider 4 mg PO/IM/IV q6h.
  - Analgesics and antiemetics as needed for symptomatic relief
- HAPE:
  - Oxygen therapy
  - Minimize exertion and keep patient warm.
  - Immediate descent or evacuation to a lower altitude
  - Portable hyperbaric therapy (2–15 psi), such as the Gamow bag or Chamberlite, is an effective and practical alternative when descent is not possible.
  - Consider nifedipine 10 mg PO, then 20–30 mg extended-release PO b.i.d.
- HACE:
  - Immediate descent
  - Supplemental oxygen (highest flow available; maintain SaO_2 >90%)
  - Dexamethasone: 8 mg IV/IM/PO initially, then 4 mg q6h
  - Hyperbaric therapy if unable to descend

IN-PATIENT CONSIDERATIONS

Initial Stabilization

Outpatient treatment for mild cases

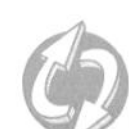

ONGOING CARE

FOLLOW-UP RECOMMENDATIONS

Patient Monitoring

- For mild cases, no follow-up is needed.
- For more severe cases, follow until symptoms subside.

PATIENT EDUCATION

Patients should be counseled about the risks of high-altitude travel and how to recognize high-altitude illnesses.

PROGNOSIS

Most cases of mild to moderate AMS are self-limiting and do not require physician intervention. Patients may resume ascent once the symptoms subside. HAPE and HACE respond well to descent, evacuation, and/or pharmacologic treatment if identified early.

COMPLICATIONS

A patient may experience a high-altitude retinal hemorrhage, which can cause visual changes, but this is usually asymptomatic.

REFERENCES

1. Gallagher SA, Hackett PH. High-altitude illness. *Emerg Med Clin North Am*. 2004;22:329–55, viii.
2. Schoene RB. Illnesses at high altitude. *Chest*. 2008;134:402–16.
3. Maloney JP, Broeckel U. Epidemiology, risk factors, and genetics of high-altitude-related pulmonary disease. *Clin Chest Med*. 2005;26:395–404, v.
4. Basnyat B, Murdoch DR. High-altitude illness. *Lancet*. 2003;361:1967–74.

ADDITIONAL READING

- Imray C, Booth A, Wright A, et al. Acute altitude illnesses. *BMJ*. 2011;343:d4943.
- Luks AM, Swenson ER. Medication and dosage considerations in the prophylaxis and treatment of high-altitude illness. *Chest*. 2008;133:744–55.

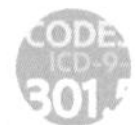

CODES

ICD9

- 348.5 Cerebral edema
- 514 Pulmonary congestion and hypostasis
- 993.2 Other and unspecified effects of high altitude

CLINICAL PEARLS

- Slow ascent and timely descent are important tenets in the prevention and treatment of high-altitude illnesses, respectively.
- High-flow oxygen, followed by oxygen titrated to maintain SaO_2 >90%, is the first-line treatment for all patients with more than a mild illness.

ALVEOLAR PULMONARY PROTEINOSIS

Caitlin M. Connolly, MD
Jerry Balikian, MD

BASICS

DESCRIPTION

- Pulmonary alveolar proteinosis (PAP) is a rare disease characterized by accumulation of lipoproteinaceous (surfactantlike) material in the alveolar spaces, leading to impaired gas exchange. There are 3 recognized categories of PAP (1).
- Congenital PAP (2% of cases):
  - Congenital PAP results from several rare gene mutations (2).
- Secondary PAP (<10% cases):
  - Secondary PAP is associated with environmental exposures, immunodeficiency disorders, and hematologic disorders and malignancies (1).
- Primary or idiopathic PAP (90% of cases):
  - Primary PAP, which is discussed here, has recently been found to be associated with antigranulocyte-macrophage colony-stimulating-factor (GM-CSF) autoantibodies (2).
- Whole lung lavage, the standard treatment for PAP, has improved prognosis (94% 5-year survival) (3).
- Systems affected: Pulmonary

EPIDEMIOLOGY

- Seen worldwide with median age of onset at 39 years old (4)
- 2–3:1 Male:Female incidence; however, may be confounded greater by male smoking, a known association (3)

Incidence

Estimated 0.36 per million annually (5)

Prevalence

Estimated 3.7 per million (5)

RISK FACTORS

- Association between tobacco smoke exposure and primary PAP (3)
- Exposure to environmental dusts, specifically silica, aluminum, cement, titanium dioxide, nitrogen dioxide, and insulation fibers, has been associated with secondary PAP (2).

Genetics

- No genetic predilection in primary or secondary PAP
- Congenital PAP mostly transmitted in autosomal-recessive pattern (1)

Pediatric Considerations

Congenital PAP leads to neonatal respiratory distress syndrome not responsive to surfactant or corticosteroids. Caused by mutation in surfactant protein B or C genes, or GM-CSF receptor beta or alpha chain abnormalities (2). Lung transplant is primary therapy, but prognosis is poor (1)[C].

GENERAL PREVENTION

No specific measure for prevention; avoid tobacco smoke exposure.

PATHOPHYSIOLOGY

Primary PAP has recently been found to be associated with neutralizing anti-GM-CSF autoantibodies causing impaired functioning of alveolar macrophages, resulting in disruption in surfactant homeostasis (6). Surfactant accumulates in alveoli due to reduced clearance.

ETIOLOGY

Primary PAP: Autoimmune

COMMONLY ASSOCIATED CONDITIONS

No conditions commonly associated with primary PAP

DIAGNOSIS

HISTORY

- Diagnosis often delayed due to nonspecific presentation
- Occupational and exposure history to exclude secondary PAP
- Symptoms:
  - Progressive dyspnea with insidious onset (most common presentation)
  - Nonproductive cough (75%):
    - Less common
  - Fatigue
  - Weight loss
  - Low-grade fever (prominent fever should prompt search for complicating infection); hemoptysis or chest pain (<20%)

PHYSICAL EXAM

Often unremarkable:

- Fine crackles (50%)
- Clubbing or cyanosis (<20%)

DIAGNOSTIC TESTS & INTERPRETATION

Lab

Initial lab tests

- CBC, liver and renal function tests to exclude systemic disorders
- Nonspecific:
  - Mild–moderate elevation in serum lactate dehydrogenase (LDH) (82%)
  - Serum levels of carcinoembryonic antigen, cytokeratin 19, and mucin KL-2 can be elevated.
  - Serum levels of surfactant protein-A, -B, and -D can be elevated.
  - Assay for anti-GM-CSF antibodies available at some centers (not commercially available) (2)

Follow-Up & Special Considerations

Serial serum LDH level can correlate with disease activity.

Imaging

Initial approach

- Chest x-ray: Bilateral, symmetric, central lung opacities (often appears worse than clinical symptoms)
- Chest CT: "Crazy-paving" patchy ground-glass opacities with network of thickened reticular lines in a geographic pattern (7) is characteristic of PAP but not specific.

Follow-Up & Special Considerations

Posttherapeutic bronchioalveolar lavage (see "Treatment"), CT shows ground-glass opacities resolve, but thickened septal lines can persist (7).

Diagnostic Procedures/Surgery

Pulmonary function tests:

- Severe reduction of carbon monoxide diffusing capacity
- Restrictive ventilatory defect
- Arterial blood gas: Hypoxemia
- Bronchoalveolar lavage: Milky fluid with large, foamy alveolar macrophages and large, acellular eosinophilic bodies that stain with periodic acid-Schiff

Pathological Findings

Open-lung biopsy is gold standard for diagnosis, but not always required. Can have false negative due to mosaic pattern leading to sampling error (6)[C]:

- Normal alveolar architecture. Alveoli filled with granular, eosinophilic material that stains with periodic acid-Schiff (6)[C].

DIFFERENTIAL DIAGNOSIS

Primary PAP is diagnosis of exclusion; must exclude causes of secondary PAP:

- Differential for material in alveolar space includes pneumonia, cardiogenic pulmonary edema, acute respiratory distress syndrome, sarcoidosis, alveolar hemorrhage, hypersensitivity pneumonitis, bronchiolitis obliterans organizing pneumonia, bronchoalveolar carcinoma.

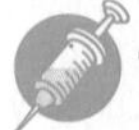

TREATMENT

MEDICATION

No specific medication

First Line

- Whole-lung lavage is the standard treatment for symptomatic PAP; however, there are no randomized controlled trials on any treatment for PAP yet available (2)[C]:
  - Whole-lung lavage is performed under general anesthesia with a dual-lumen endotracheal tube while ventilating the other lung.
  - Large volumes of saline are flushed until returning fluid becomes clear.
  - About 70% of patients with PAP become symptomatic enough to require whole-lung lavage within 5 years of diagnosis.
  - Most patients experience a return to normal exercise capacity after lavage; however, a subset of patients do not respond for unknown reason.
  - Median duration of freedom from symptoms is 15 months, with many patients requiring repeat lavage (2)[C].
- Patients with secondary PAP should have underlying disorder treated, or should avoid exposure to inciting environmental agent. Whole-lung lavage can also be used for symptomatic secondary PAP (4)[C].

ADDITIONAL TREATMENT

General Measures

Supportive measures such as supplemental oxygen, bronchodilators, antibiotics for infection, smoking cessation, and treatment of concurrent diseases that impair respiratory function can improve dyspnea temporarily. Respiratory support should be given when appropriate:

- Steroids should be avoided when possible due to interference with surfactant maturation and secretion (1)[C].
- Pulmonary rehabilitation may be helpful (1)[C].

Issues for Referral

Patients with symptomatic PAP should be referred to centers performing whole-lung lavage, with anesthesiologists skilled in management of double-lumen catheters (4)[C].

Additional Therapies

Clinical trials examining the usefulness of GM-CSF therapy in treating primary PAP are currently ongoing. Initial trials appear to show that high doses of exogenous GM-CSF can overcome anti-GM-CSF neutralizing antibodies. Trials are studying dosage routes of subcutaneous injection for a systemic approach vs. nebulized treatment for a localized approach. These trials are still in the initial stages, and whole-lung lavage remains standard therapy (8)[C]:

- There is no role for GM-CSF therapy in secondary or congenital PAP, as they are not related to anti-GM-CSF antibodies.
- Other immune-modulating therapies are in the early stages of investigation for PAP (9)[C].

SURGERY/OTHER PROCEDURES

Lung transplantation has been used in congenital PAP and for PAP that is not responsive to whole-lung lavage (1)[C].

ONGOING CARE

FOLLOW-UP RECOMMENDATIONS

Patient Monitoring

Respiratory infections are a common complication of PAP, especially with atypical organisms such as *Nocardia*. Any sign of infection should lead to thorough search for organism, including bronchial washings and/or bronchoalveolar lavage (1).

PATIENT EDUCATION

The American Lung Association at http://www.lungusa.org/

PROGNOSIS

Prognosis for those who do not undergo whole-lung lavage is 85% 5-year survival compared to 94% 5-year survival for those who do undergo therapeutic lavage (4). PAP can result in death from respiratory distress (80%) or infection (20%) (1):

- Congenital PAP has an especially poor prognosis.

COMPLICATIONS

Complications from PAP include respiratory failure and increased susceptibility to infection, especially *Nocardia* species:

- Whole-lung lavage complications: Hypoxemia, pneumonia, sepsis, adult respiratory distress syndrome, pneumothorax (1)

REFERENCES

1. Ioachimescu OC, Kavuru MS. Pulmonary alveolar proteinosis. *Chron Respir Dis*. 2006;3:149–59.
2. Huizar I, Kavuru MS. Alveolar proteinosis syndrome: pathogenesis, diagnosis, and management. *Curr Opin Pulm Med*. 2009;15:491–8.
3. Presneill JJ, Nakata K, Inoue Y, et al. Pulmonary alveolar proteinosis. *Clin Chest Med*. 2004;25:593–613, viii.
4. Juvet SC, Hwang D, Waddell TK, et al. Rare lung disease II: Pulmonary alveolar proteinosis. *Can Respir J*. 2008;15:203–10.
5. Seymour JF, Presneill JJ. Pulmonary alveolar proteinosis: Progress in the first 44 years. *Am J Respir Crit Care Med*. 2002;166:215–35.
6. Trapnell BC, Whitsett JA, Nakata K, et al. Pulmonary alveolar proteinosis. *N Engl J Med*. 2003;349:2527–39.
7. Frazier AA, Franks TJ, Cooke EO, et al. From the archives of the AFIP: Pulmonary alveolar proteinosis. *Radiographics*. 2008;28:883–99; quiz 915.
8. Greenhill SR, Kotton DN. Pulmonary alveolar proteinosis: A bench-to-bedside story of granulocyte-macrophage colony-stimulating factor dysfunction. *Chest*. 2009;136:571–7.
9. Kavuru MS, Malur A, Marshall I, et al. An open-label trial of rituximab therapy in pulmonary alveolar proteinosis. *Eur Respir J*. 2011;38(6):1361–7.

ADDITIONAL READING

- Chung MJ, Lee KS, Franquet T, et al. Metabolic lung disease: Imaging and histopathologic findings. *Eur J Radiol*. 2005;54:233–45.
- Khan A, Agarwal R. Pulmonary alveolar proteinosis. *Respir Care*. 2011;56(7):1016–28.
- Wang BM, Stern EJ, Schmidt RA, et al. Diagnosing pulmonary alveolar proteinosis. A review and an update. *Chest*. 1997;111:460–6.

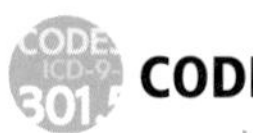

CODES

ICD9

516.0 Pulmonary alveolar proteinosis

CLINICAL PEARLS

- Pulmonary alveolar proteinosis is a rare disease characterized by accumulation of surfactantlike material in the alveolar spaces leading to impaired gas exchange.
- Nonspecific respiratory symptoms and physical exam findings often delay diagnosis.
- Chest CT finding of "crazy paving" is characteristic, but not specific.
- Whole-lung lavage is standard therapy for symptomatic patients. 5-year survival is 94% with treatment.

ALZHEIMER DISEASE

Jill A. Grimes, MD

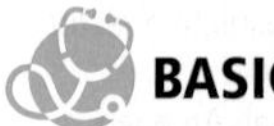

BASICS

DESCRIPTION

- Alzheimer disease (AD) is the most common cause of dementia in the elderly.
- Degenerative neurologic disease with progressive impairment in 2 or more:
  - Memory, executive function, attention, language, or visuospatial skills
  - With significant interference in ability to function in work, home, or social interactions
- New diagnostic criteria released in 2011 that emphasize full spectrum of disease (1)[A]:
  - Preclinical AD (*research purposes only:* Biomarkers present; subtle decline evident to patient but cognitive tests in "normal" range)
  - Mild cognitive impairment (MCI): Social, occupational, and functional skills preserved despite significant decline in cognition
  - Alzheimer dementia
- System(s) affected: Nervous
- Synonym(s): Presenile dementia; Senile dementia of the Alzheimer type

Geriatric Considerations

Asymptomatic screening is not recommended.

EPIDEMIOLOGY

- Predominant age: >65 years
- 2/3 Female, 1/3 Male in US

Incidence

1 in 8 Americans >65 years old; nearly 50% once >85

Prevalence

>5.4 million in US:

- 200,000 younger onset (<65 years old)

RISK FACTORS

- Aging, family history, APOE4, Down syndrome
- Cardiovascular and carotid artery disease
- Smoking (2–4-fold increase) (1)
- Head trauma

Genetics

- Positive family history in 50%, but 90% AD is sporadic:
  - APOE4 increases risk, but full role unclear
- Familial/autosomal-dominant AD accounts for <5% AD:
  - Amyloid precursor protein (APP), presenilin-1 (PS-1), and presenilin-2 (PS-2)

GENERAL PREVENTION

- NSAIDs, estrogen, and vitamin E do NOT delay AD (2)[A].
- Intellectual challenge (puzzles) and regular physical exercise may offer preventive benefit.
- Control vascular risk factors (e.g., hypertension). Statins and lowering cholesterol may retard pathogenesis of AD (4)[A].
- Ginkgo biloba may be beneficial for cognition, but not activities of daily living (5).
- Physical activities and omega-3 fatty acids may help to prevent or delay cognitive decline (6).
- Ultrasound may help to identify asymptomatic patients at increased risk with chronic brain hypoperfusion secondary to cardiovascular or carotid artery pathology (7).

ETIOLOGY

- Unknown, but involves amyloid beta accumulation initially, then synaptic dysfunction, neurodegeneration, and eventual neuronal loss
- Age, genetics, systemic disease, behaviors (smoking), and other host factors may influence the response to amyloid beta and/or the pace of progression toward the clinical manifestations of AD.

COMMONLY ASSOCIATED CONDITIONS

- Down syndrome
- Depression

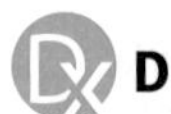

DIAGNOSIS

HISTORY

- Include family members in interview (for accuracy and for behavioral assessment).
- Progressive and disruptive memory loss
- Depression, anhedonia, or apathy
- Intellectual decline, difficulty with calculations, multiple missed appointments
- Loss of interest, social withdrawal
- Date or time confusion
- Occupational dysfunction or personality change
- Restlessness and sleep disturbances

PHYSICAL EXAM

- Neurologic exam to rule out other causes
- Folstein Mini Mental Status Exam (MMSE): Copyrighted, but available (http://www.aafp.org/afp/20010215/703.html)
- Counting coins test: "If I gave you a nickel, quarter, dime, and penny, how much is that?"
- No focal neurologic signs
- Short-term memory loss
- Acalculia (e.g., cannot balance checkbook)
- Agnosia: Inability to recognize objects
- Apraxia: Inability to carry out movements
- Confabulation
- Delusions
- Impaired abstraction
- Decreased attention to hygiene
- Visuospatial distortion
- Late signs: Psychotic features, mutism

DIAGNOSTIC TESTS & INTERPRETATION

Neuropsychologic testing: If clinical picture is confusing, or to help determine level of independence for skills such as balancing checkbooks, driving, or managing medicines

Lab

To help rule out other causes of dementia

Initial lab tests

- CBC, ESR
- Chemistry panel
- Thyroid-stimulating hormone
- Folate and B_{12} levels
- Venereal disease reaction level (VDRL) or rapid plasma reagin (RPR)
- HIV antibody (selected cases)
- *APOE4 or biomarker testing is NOT routine.*

Follow-Up & Special Considerations

Genetic testing for APOE4 or for familial AD types; discuss with genetic counselor (2)[A]

Imaging

Initial approach

- Controversy exists; consider MRI or CT scan if:
  - Cognitive decline is recent and rapid; age <60; history of stroke; gait disturbance or focal neurologic signs
  - Cancer, urinary incontinence, bleeding disorder, or current use of anticoagulants

Single photon emission computed tomography (SPECT) and photon emission tomography (PET): Only if diagnostic uncertainty after CT or MRI; insufficient evidence to use alone

Follow-Up & Special Considerations

- CT scan/MRI: Moderate cortical atrophy, ventricular enlargement
- MRI: Hippocampal volumetry; PET and SPECT not indicated
- Medicare pays for PET to distinguish AD from frontotemporal dementia.

Pathological Findings

- Gross: Diffuse cerebral atrophy in hippocampus, amygdala, and some subcortical nuclei
- Micro:
  - Neuritic senile plaques
  - Neurofibrillary tangles
  - Pyramidal cell loss
  - Decreased cholinergic innervation (other neurotransmitters variably decreased)
  - Degeneration of locus ceruleus and basal forebrain nuclei of Meynert; amyloid angiopathy

DIFFERENTIAL DIAGNOSIS

- *Depression*
- Vascular dementia, multi-infarct dementia
- Lewy body disease
- Dementia associated with Parkinson disease
- Normal-pressure hydrocephalus
- Creutzfeldt-Jakob disease
- End-stage multiple sclerosis
- Brain tumor: Primary or metastatic
- Subdural hematoma
- Progressive multifocal leukoencephalopathy
- Metabolic dementia (hypothyroidism)
- Drug reactions, alcoholism, other addictions
- Dementia pugilistica
- Toxicity from liver and kidney failure
- Vitamin and other nutritional deficiencies
- Vasculitis
- Neurosyphilis

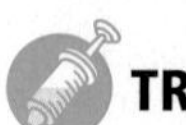

TREATMENT

MEDICATION

First Line

- Delay progression of disease:
  - Cholinesterase inhibitors (9)[A]:
    - Equally effective; all have largely GI side effects
    - Provide only modest benefit for 1–2 years, after which decline continues at somewhat lesser rate than placebo. Number needed to treat (NNT) = 7. No deterioration over 6–12 months is evidence of efficacy.

- Best in mild-to-moderate disease (Folstein MMSE scores 10–24); drugs *may* be effective in Lewy body dementia.
- Donepezil (Aricept): Start at 5 mg PO daily; may increase to 10 mg daily after 1 month:
  - Tablets or orally disintegrating tabs; generic available
  - Caution with digoxin or beta-blockers (can cause 3* heart block)
  - Aricept 23 mg tablet approved in 2010
- Rivastigmine (Exelon): Start 1.5 mg PO b.i.d., increase by 1.5 mg b.i.d. every 2 weeks; maintenance 6–12 mg total daily:
  - Capsule, solution, or patch (patch greatly reduces side effects)
  - *Indicated for both AD and Parkinson dementia*
- Galantamine (Razadyne): Start 4 mg b.i.d. for 4 weeks, then increase by 4 mg b.i.d. every month with goal 16–24 mg daily dose :
  - Tablets, solution, and extended-release (ER) capsule (ER has daily dosing)

– N-methyl-D-aspartate (NMDA) receptor antagonists (*for moderate-to-severe AD; MMSE 5–14)*:
  - Monotherapy or in combination with acetylcholinesterase inhibitors
  - Memantine (Namenda): Start at 5 mg daily, with starter pack titrating to target dose of 10 mg b.i.d. after 4 weeks
  - *Often improves behavioral issues*

- For depression (occurs in 1/3 of patients), use SSRIs
- Insomnia:
  - Trazodone 25–100 mg at bedtime, zolpidem (Ambien) 5 mg at bedtime, zaleplon (Sonata) 5–10 mg at bedtime, ramelteon (Rozerem) 8 mg at bedtime
  - Avoid diphenhydramine in elderly males, which can cause urinary retention.
- Moderate anxiety/restlessness: Consider low-dose, short-acting benzodiazepines, buspirone, or SSRIs (efficacy unproven).
- Severe aggressive agitation:
  - Behavioral techniques and environmental modification help more than medications for wandering, restlessness, uncooperativeness, hoarding, and irritability:
    - Consider changing environment, rewards, behavioral redirection, hearing aids, and bright light therapy.
  - Memantine (Namenda) (9)[A]: Start at 5 mg daily, with starter pack titrating to target dose of 10 mg b.i.d. after 4 weeks
  - *Antipsychotics (both conventional and atypical) are associated with increased mortality and acute care hospital admissions in elderly patients with dementia.*
- Precautions:
  - Avoid anticholinergic drugs, such as tricyclic antidepressants and antihistamines.
  - Ginkgo biloba: Avoid anticoagulants and aspirin.
  - Benzodiazepines may produce paradoxical excitation or daytime drowsiness.
  - Triazolam (Halcion) can produce confusion, memory loss, and psychotic behavior.
  - Benzodiazepines may increase serum phenytoin concentration.
  - Cimetidine may increase benzodiazepine concentration.
  - Donepezil (Aricept): Use with caution with anticholinergic medication or in patients with sick sinus syndrome or a history of peptic ulcers.
  - Paroxetine causes increased donepezil levels.

Second Line

Conflicting efficacy for selegiline 5 mg b.i.d., vitamin E 1,000 mg b.i.d., or NSAIDs in slowing the progression of the disease (2)[A].

ADDITIONAL TREATMENT

General Measures

- Optimize treatment of associated comorbidities (including hearing and vision loss).
- Analyze environment for safety and security, and avoid sudden changes in environment.
- Assess spouse/caregiver burnout.
- Advance directives planning, living will, power of attorney

Issues for Referral

- Assess driving safety (vision, spatial relations, hearing, judgement):
  - http://www.nhtsa.gov/people/injury/olddrive/Driving%20Safely%20Aging%20Web/
- Support groups for patient and family: Alzheimer Association

Additional Therapies

- Exercise to reduce restlessness
- Continued cognitive challenge
- Occupational therapy, music therapy, aroma therapy, pet therapy

COMPLEMENTARY AND ALTERNATIVE MEDICINE

- Huperzine A 400 mg (herbal cholinesterase inhibitors) may improve cognition with minimal side effects
- Ginkgo biloba extracts (120 mg a day) show conflicting efficacy in treatment of AD but may be beneficial (5).
- Coenzyme Q_{10} not effective

ONGOING CARE

FOLLOW-UP RECOMMENDATIONS

Patient Monitoring

- Schedule regular follow-up (3 months) to assess medical complications, provide support for family, and assess need for placement.
- Serial mental status testing is potentially helpful, but bedside tests (Folstein MMSE) offer wide variability and lack of sensitivity.

PATIENT EDUCATION

- Alzheimer Association: http://www.alz.org/
- Explain progressive nature of the disease and start advance directives planning as early as possible.

PROGNOSIS

Poor: Average survival from diagnosis is 4–8 years (*diagnosis is often delayed*).

COMPLICATIONS

- Behavioral: Hostility, agitation, wandering, falls
- Metabolic: Infection, dehydration, drug toxicity
- "Sundowning" (increase full-spectrum lights in evenings/winter)
- Depression (1/3 of patients); suicide

REFERENCES

1. McKhann GM, Knopman DS, Chertkow H, et al. The diagnosis of dementia due to Alzheimer's disease: Recommendations from the National Institute on Aging-Alzheimer's Association workgroups on diagnostic guidelines for Alzheimer's disease. *Alzheimers Dement*. 2011;7(3):263–9.
2. Cataldo JK, Prochaska JJ, Glantz SA. Cigarette smoking is a risk factor for Alzheimer's disease: An analysis controlling for tobacco industry affiliation. *J Alzheimers Dis*. 2010;19:465–480.
3. Patterson C, Feightner JW, Garcia A, et al. Diagnosis and treatment of dementia: 1. Risk assessment and primary prevention of Alzheimer disease. *CMAJ*. 2008;178:548–56.
4. Scott HD, Laake K. Statins for the prevention of Alzheimer's disease and dementia. *Cochrane Database Syst Rev*. 2009:1.
5. Weinmann S, Roll S, Schwarzbach C, et al. Effects of Ginkgo biloba in dementia: Systematic review and meta-analysis. *BMC Geriatr*. 2010;10:14.
6. Daviglus ML, Bell CC, Berrittini W, et al. NIH State-of-the-Science Conference: Preventing Alzheimer's Disease and Cognitive Decline. 2010.
7. de la Torre JC. Vascular risk factor detection and control may prevent Alzheimer's disease. *Ageing Res Rev*. 2010;10.
8. Raina P, Santaguida P, Ismaila A, et al. Effectiveness of cholinesterase inhibitors and memantine for treating dementia: Evidence review for a clinical practice guideline. *Ann Intern Med*. 2008;148:379–97.

ADDITIONAL READING

Hersch EC, Falzgraf S. Management of the behavioral and psychological symptoms of dementia. *Clin Interv Aging*. 2007;2:611–21.

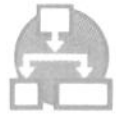

See Also (Topic, Algorithm, Electronic Media Element)

Substance Use Disorders; Hypothyroidism, Adult; Depression

CODES

ICD9

- 290.0 Senile dementia, uncomplicated
- 290.10 Presenile dementia, uncomplicated
- 331.0 Alzheimer's disease

CLINICAL PEARLS

- Daily intellectual stimulation, such as puzzles, and moderate physical exercise may help prevent AD.
- Imaging studies have low yield in patients with a history typical of AD.
- Encourage families to join a chapter of the Alzheimer Association and to pursue advanced directive planning early in the course of the disease.
- Atypical antipsychotic medications increase mortality.

AMBLYOPIA

Robert M. Kershner, MD, MS, FACS

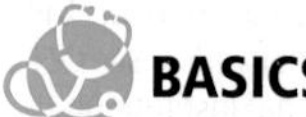

BASICS

DESCRIPTION

- Amblyopia is a reduction in visual acuity resulting from abnormal visual development in the absence of a structural or pathologic abnormality of the eye, which cannot be corrected by eyeglasses or contact lenses.
- The lesion is typically unilateral, although it may be bilateral.
- System(s) affected: Nervous
- Synonym(s): Lazy eye

Pediatric Considerations

More commonly seen in the pediatric age group early in life. The mean age at presentation is 3–6 years old.

EPIDEMIOLOGY

- Predominant age: The onset may be present from birth or in early childhood. The condition may go undiagnosed and be detected at any age.
- Predominant gender: Male = Female

Prevalence

~2–2.5% in the general population

RISK FACTORS

- Pre-existing refractive error, such as myopia, hyperopia, or astigmatism
- More common with occlusion of the visual pathway
- Conditions that cause anisometropia (refractive difference between the eyes) or obstruction to clear vision, i.e., cataract, corneal abnormalities, can lead to permanent amblyopia.

Genetics

Increased incidence in children with 1 parent with a history of amblyopia

PATHOPHYSIOLOGY

- Strabismic amblyopia is a loss of visual acuity in an individual with misalignment of the visual axis in 1 eye, due to suppression of the images from an eye that turns out or in.
- Anisometropic amblyopia is present when 1 eye has a significantly different refractive error from the fellow eye, leading to visual blurring and suppression of the image from that eye.
- Refractive amblyopia is due to uncorrected high refractive error, resulting in visual blurring in either or both eyes.
- Deprivation amblyopia (amblyopia ex anopsia) is due to relatively complete visual deprivation in 1 eye, which may be caused by a congenital abnormality such as a corneal scar or cataract.
- Deficiency amblyopia is also known as nutritional optic neuropathy or tobacco–alcohol amblyopia. Deficiencies of vitamin B_1 or B_{12} or riboflavin may be responsible.
- Amblyopia can only occur early in life:
  - When the brain detects unequal images, for any reason, it is forced to ignore one.
  - The ability of a brain to suppress the unwanted image can only occur when the development of neuroadaptive responses is in a critical "plastic" period, usually the first several years of life.
  - If amblyopia has not developed after that period has passed, the individual will be unable to "suppress" the unwanted image, and diplopia or double vision will result.

ETIOLOGY

- Strabismus causes disparate retinal images whereby one eye sees the object of regard in the fovea and the other in a different part of the retina.
- Inability to fuse the 2 images results in the brain ignoring the less preferred image (this does not necessarily need to be the less clear image).
- Refractive errors such as anisometropia (a difference in refractive error between the 2 eyes) can cause the 2 retinal images to be of unequal clarity.
- An obstruction to the visual axis, such as cataracts, also causes unequal clarity of the retinal image.
- The result of 1 eye seeing better than the other is the interruption of development of fine visual perception, which can contribute to the development of amblyopia.
- Individuals with amblyopia do not have normal degrees of stereo vision and often complain of not appreciating 3D images.

DIAGNOSIS

HISTORY

- Squinting 1 eye in bright light is the most common symptom, hence the alternative term for strabismus, "squint."
- Rubbing the eyes
- Sitting close to television or computer screen
- Problems in sports
- Preference for front-row seating
- Covering or closing an eye
- Eye turns in or out, wandering eye
- Poor vision in 1 eye without apparent explanation or a diagnosable organic cause
- Poor vision that does not correct with glasses

PHYSICAL EXAM

- Ophthalmologic exam to screen for unequal refractive error, outward or inward turning of the eye (strabismic amblyopia), obstruction to the visual pathway. Vision testing of the eye under monocular conditions can reveal dissimilarities.
- All children should have complete visual exams prior to starting school, with each eye tested individually. Children from families with a known history of amblyopia or strabismus should have dilated exams performed by an ophthalmologist.
- The corneal light reflex test (shining a light into the child's eyes and noting the location of the light in relation to the pupil) may be used to assess ocular alignment in young children. An abnormal test should prompt referral to an ophthalmologist.
- When a dilated examination is not possible, evaluation of the "red reflex," such as that seen with flash photography, may indicate an obstruction of vision that would warrant prompt evaluation by an ophthalmologist.
- Any of the above conditions indicate prompt evaluation and referral. In a young child, the earlier the diagnosis, the better the therapeutic outcome:
  - Children with cataract may require cataract surgery.
  - Unequal refractive errors need to be promptly treated with glasses or contact lenses to improve sight before amblyopia sets in.

DIFFERENTIAL DIAGNOSIS

- The diagnosis of amblyopia can be confused with an organic lesion causing decreased visual acuity, and this must always be excluded before the diagnosis of amblyopia is considered.
- Intraocular tumors, glaucoma, and congenital abnormalities can result in and be mistaken for amblyopia.

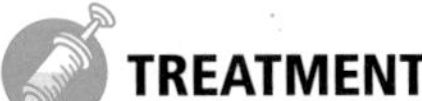

TREATMENT

ADDITIONAL TREATMENT

General Measures

- Correction of the underlying disorder should be instituted promptly, as the condition may become irreversible if the child is more than 4–6 years of age.
- Patching of the stronger eye to encourage visual development of the amblyopic eye is warranted. There may be resistance of the child to the wearing of a patch, which may lessen benefit. Various patching regimens have been studied (from 2–23 hours of patching per day for 4–6 months, and alternate patching). Close follow-up is necessary. Should the "good" eye be patched excessively, the risk of development of amblyopia in that eye increases.
- An alternative therapy to patching is pharmacologic blurring, usually achieved with atropine eye drops. Similar efficacy is achieved compared to patching, with improved compliance. The risk associated with systemic effects from the antimuscarinic effects of the drug cannot be ignored (1)[A].
- Corrective lenses should be prescribed for refractive errors.
- Correction of anatomic obstructions, including cataracts or ptosis, may improve vision and minimize recurrence.
- Amblyopia never corrects itself spontaneously and will always require treatment. Children do not outgrow amblyopia.
- Deficiency amblyopia: Balanced diet, vitamins, and avoidance of alcohol and tobacco

Issues for Referral

Obstruction of vision in the infant or toddler is a potential medical emergency. Failure to refer can result in irreversible loss of vision in an otherwise healthy eye.

COMPLEMENTARY AND ALTERNATIVE MEDICINE

- There are no effective homeopathic remedies for amblyopia.
- Vision training can be an effective adjunct only if the underlying organic causes are addressed and patching therapy instituted.

SURGERY/OTHER PROCEDURES

Surgical correction of an abnormal eye position, or intraocular obstruction may be required.

ONGOING CARE

FOLLOW-UP RECOMMENDATIONS

All children diagnosed with amblyopia need to be followed for years to prevent recurrence.

Patient Monitoring

Once the diagnosis of amblyopia is made, the patient must be seen frequently until complete resolution of the problem occurs.

PATIENT EDUCATION

Advise all parents to have children's eyes examined prior to starting school.

PROGNOSIS

- A treatable condition in most cases if the diagnosis is made early:
  - Patching therapy, pharmacologic blurring, eyeglasses, and surgical correction of abnormal eye positions can result in near-normal vision when instituted early.
  - Visual development occurs during the first several years of life, and amblyopia therapy can be effective until 12 years of age.
- The risk of recurrence is 24% after 1 year; reinstitution of treatment is warranted.

COMPLICATIONS

- Failure to institute early therapy may result in permanent unilateral visual loss:
  - Unilateral amblyopia causes an increased risk of severe visual impairment due to loss of vision in the nonamblyopic eye.
- Psychosocial complications include difficulty in schooling, work, or physical activity, and an increased risk of depression and anxiety.

REFERENCES

1. Kushner BJ. Atropine vs patching for treatment of amblyopia in children. *JAMA*. 2002;287(16): 2145–6.
2. Levi DM, Li RW. Perceptual Learning as a potential treatment for amblyopia: A mini-review. *Vision Res*. 2009.

ADDITIONAL READING

- Li T, Shotton K, et al. Conventional occlusion versus pharmacologic penalization for amblyopia. *Cochrane Database Syst Rev*. 2009;CD006460.
- Schmucker C, Grosselfinger R, Riemsma R, et al. Diagnostic accuracy of vision screening tests for the detection of amblyopia and its risk factors: A systematic review. *Graefes Arch Clin Exp Ophthalmol*. 2009;247(11):1441–54.
- Schmucker C, Kleijnen J, Grosselfinger R, et al. Effectiveness of early in comparison to late(r) treatment in children with amblyopia or its risk factors: a systematic review. *Ophthalmic Epidemiol*. 2010;17:7–17.
- Teed RG, Bui CM, Morrison DG, et al. Amblyopia therapy in children identified by photoscreening. *Ophthalmology*. 2010;117:159–62.

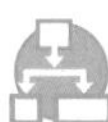

See Also (Topic, Algorithm, Electronic Media Element)

Refractive Errors; Strabismus

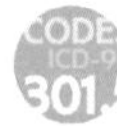

CODES

ICD9

- 368.00 Amblyopia, unspecified
- 368.01 Strabismic amblyopia
- 368.02 Deprivation amblyopia

CLINICAL PEARLS

- Amblyopia typically presents between the ages of 3 and 6 years, but it needs to be diagnosed as soon as possible if treatment is to be effective.
- It is never too early to refer if an inequality in visual appearance of the eyes or function is suspected.
- Due to increased incidence in families where there is a history of amblyopia, all related children should be screened by an ophthalmologist.
- Perceptual learning appears to be beneficial in older youth and adults diagnosed late with amblyopia (2)[A].

AMEBIASIS

Najmul H. Siddiqui, MBBS, MD
Naureen B. Rafiq, MBBS, MD

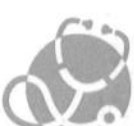

BASICS

Amebiasis is caused by *Entamoeba histolytica*, an intestinal protozoan found worldwide.

DESCRIPTION

- After malaria and schistosomiasis, the 3rd-leading parasitic cause of death all over the world.
- Most common in developing countries, immigrants from or travelers to endemic regions, those who perform anal sex, and immunocompromised individuals
- Most infected patients are asymptomatic or have minimal GI symptoms (about 90%):
  – Severe infection (i.e., amebic colitis) can occur in very young patients, pregnant women, patients on steroid therapy, and malnourished individuals (1,2).
- Infection is spread by the feco–oral route and caused by the ingestion of *E. histolytica* cysts (infective form) in contaminated food (garden vegetables), fecally contaminated soil, or water. Then, excystation in the terminal ileum or colon to form highly motile trophozoites (invasive form). The trophozoites then encyst and are excreted in the feces or invade the intestinal mucosal barrier and spread hematogenously via the portal circulation to the liver or other distant organs. The excreted cysts reach the environment to complete the cycle.
- Amebiasis is primarily an infection of the colon, but extraintestinal (liver, kidney, bladder, skin, lung, brain, male or female genitalia) disease can occur. Amebic liver abscess is the most common complication of invasive amebiasis. It can develop during the acute attack or 1–3 months later.
- The genus *Entamoeba* contains many species, including *E. histolytica, E. dispar, E. moshkovskii, E. polecki, E. coli*, and *E. hartmanni*. Only *E. histolytica* has been clearly associated with disease; the others are considered nonpathogenic (3). *E. dispar* and *E. moshkovskii* are nonpathogenic strains that are morphologically identical to *E. hystolytica*. The previously counted asymptomatic infections by so-called nonpathogenic strains of *E. histolytica* are now evidenced to be due to *E. dispar* and *E. moshkovskii*. Latest availability of sensitive and specific antigen detection and polymerase chain reaction (PCR) can now recognize *E. histolytica* in stool from *E. dispar* and *E. moshkovskii*.
- System(s) affected: Gastrointestinal (GI); Nervous; Renal/Urologic; Reproductive; Skin/Exocrine
- Synonym(s): Amebic colitis; Amebic dysentery

Geriatric Considerations

More severe in elderly

Pediatric Considerations

More severe in neonates

Pregnancy Considerations

More severe in pregnancy

EPIDEMIOLOGY

- Infection can affect patients of all ages.
- Amebic colitis affects both sexes equally (1).
- Amebic liver abscess incidence greater in men than women for unknown reasons

Pediatric Considerations

Very young children seem to be predisposed to fulminant colitis.

Prevalence

- US ~4%; 10% of the world's population. Asymptomatic *E. dispar* infection is 10 times more common than *E. histolytica* infection.
- Entamoeba infection is as high as 50% in areas of Central and South America, Africa, and Asia. Prevalence rates of *E. histolytica,* in asymptomatic persons in developing countries range from 1–21%.

RISK FACTORS

- Low socioeconomic status
- Institutional living
- Male homosexuality
- Immunocompromised
- Severe disease and increased mortality are common in pregnancy, corticosteroid treatment, malignancy, malnutrition, and alcoholism.
- Invasive disease is more common in certain geographic locations, including some parts of Mexico, South Africa, and India.

GENERAL PREVENTION

- Eradication of fecal contamination of food and water through improved sanitation, hygiene, and water treatment.
- Individuals traveling to endemic areas should be advised on proper food and water handling. *Water should be boiled for more than 1 minute and uncooked vegetables washed with a detergent soap or soaked in acetic acid or vinegar for 10–15 minutes before consumption*.
- Avoiding sexual practices that involve fecal–oral contact with potential contamination of infective cysts
- Treatment of patients and close contacts, since reinfection is common
- Amebiasis does not confer lifelong immunity; reinfection possible (4)

PATHOPHYSIOLOGY

- Invasion to the colonic mucosa is mediated by a galactose/N-acetylgalactosamine (GAL/GalNAc)-specific lectin, able to activate lytic and apoptotic pathways, and direct inhibition of the complement system by the trophozoite (4).
- Extraintestinal disease can result from hepatobiliary and/or hematogenous spread.

ETIOLOGY

Infection results from ingestion of *E. histolytica* cysts in contaminated food, water, or by direct fecal–oral transmission.

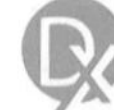

DIAGNOSIS

HISTORY

- Noninvasive infection (symptoms are often nonspecific):
  – Asymptomatic
  – Mild diarrhea
  – Abdominal discomfort
- Invasive infection (amebic colitis):
  – Gradual onset of bloody diarrhea
  – Abdominal pain
  – Fever (10–30%)
  – Weight loss and anorexia
  – Fulminant colitis with severe bloody diarrhea, worsening abdominal pain with peritonitis, and fever. Risk factors include malnutrition, pregnancy, steroid use, and very young age.
- Extraintestinal infection:
  – Amebic liver abscess:
    - Fever (up to 90%), right-upper-quadrant (RUQ) pain <10 days duration
    - Subacute presentation is associated with mild fever, weight loss, and anorexia.
    - Cough can occur. Jaundice is not common.
    - Up to 70% can present without colitis.
    - Symptoms may start years after exposure.
  – Pleuropulmonary amebiasis: Pleuritic chest pain, cough, and respiratory distress after rupture of amebic liver abscess through the diaphragm
  – Cerebral amebiasis: Headache, nausea, vomiting, and rapid mental status change with rapid progression

PHYSICAL EXAM

- Amebic colitis:
  – Diffuse abdominal tenderness (12–85%)
  – Fever (10–30%)
  – Weight loss (40%)
  – Heme-positive stools (70–100%)
- Amebic liver abscess:
  – Fever (85–90%)
  – RUQ tenderness (85–90%)
  – Hepatomegaly (30–50%)
  – Weight loss (30–50%)

DIAGNOSTIC TESTS & INTERPRETATION

Lab

Initial lab tests

- Microscopic stool examination for trophozoites from a single sample is only 33–50% sensitive. *Serial stool sampling × 3 in no more than 10 days increase detection to 85–95% but with poor specificity, as it cannot differentiate E. histolytica from nonpathogenic E. dispar and E. moshkovskii.*
- Antigen detection assays are the best available tool to diagnose intestinal amebiasis. ELISA to detect *E. histolytic*-specific antigens, with an overall sensitivity of 71–100% and specificity of 93–100%. Antigen testing from serum and liver aspirate in amebic liver abscess yields a sensitivity of 96% and 100%, respectively.
- *E. histolytica* infection results in the development of antibodies, whereas *E. dispar* infection does not. Antibodies become usually positive in 5–7 days of acute infection and may persist for years. Cannot differentiate between new and past infection. Indirect hemagglutination (IHA) is 90% sensitive in patients with symptomatic intestinal infection. Serum antilectin antibodies (IgG) are helpful in *E. histolytica* infection with amebic liver abscess with a sensitivity of 97.9% and specificity of 94.8%.
- PCR techniques are more sensitive for detection of *E. histolytica* in fecal or liver aspirate samples but are not routinely available .
- In bladder infections: Amoebae and/or cysts in urine
- Liver enzymes, alkaline phosphatase (80%), and ESR may be elevated, and anemia and leucocytosis without eosinophilia (80%) may be present in amebic liver abscess.

Follow-Up & Special Considerations
Follow-up stool examination after completion of therapy to ensure intestinal eradication

Imaging

Initial approach
Ultrasonography and CT scanning are sensitive but nonspecific for amebic liver abscess. Usually solitary lesions in the right hepatic lobe (70–80%).

Diagnostic Procedures/Surgery

- Ultrasound or CT-guided needle aspiration for suspected amebic abscess with studies of aspirate
- Colonoscopy with biopsy can be performed in highly suspicious cases with negative stool and antigen testing. Contraindicated in fulminant colitis due to increased perforation risk.

Pathological Findings

- Colon biopsy:
  - Amebic invasion through the mucosa and into submucosa is the hallmark of amebic colitis, which gives the classical flask-shaped ulcers.
  - Periodic acid–Schiff-stained trophozoites in magenta color
  - Neutrophils at the periphery
- Liver biopsy:
  - Necrosis surrounded by a rim of trophozoites
- Liver aspirate:
  - Red-brown material (anchovy paste)

DIFFERENTIAL DIAGNOSIS

- Other infectious causes of colitis:
  - Shigellosis
  - *Campylobacter* infection
  - Pseudomembranous colitis
  - Occasionally salmonellosis or *Yersinia* infection
  - Viral hepatitis
- Noninfectious causes of colitis:
  - Ulcerative colitis
  - Crohn colitis
  - Ischemic colitis in elderly
  - Hepatocellular adenoma
- Hepatic amebiasis must be distinguished from pyogenic liver abscess or superinfection of amebic abscess.

TREATMENT

- Mostly treated as an outpatient, but fulminant colitis with hypovolemia and complicated liver abscess requires inpatient management.
- Asymptomatic *E. histolytica* infection should be treated with luminal agent (iodoquinol, paromomycin) alone to eradicate infection, as invasive infection may develop and also continuous shedding of cyst transmits infection through feco–oral route.
- *E. dispar* and *E. moshkovskii* infections do not require treatment, as they are nonpathogenic strains (3,4)[A].

MEDICATION

First Line

- **Noninvasive infection:** Treat with luminal agents only:
  - Paromomycin: Adult: 500–750 mg PO t.i.d. or 25–25 mg/kg/d PO divided t.i.d. for 5–10 days; Pediatric: Administer as in adults
- **Invasive infection:** Treat with nitroimidazole (metronidazole/tinidazole) followed by luminal agent:
  - Metronidazole: Adult: 500–750 mg t.i.d. PO for 10 days, Pediatric: 35–50 mg/kg PO divided t.i.d. for 10 days. IV therapy does not offer significant difference, as metronidazole is well absorbed orally. It is then followed by a paromomycin (for 5–10 days) or diiodohydroxyquin (650 mg PO t.i.d. for 20 days) to eliminate intestinal carriage.
  - Tinidazole: 2 g/d for 3 days with food for intestinal infection and 2 g/d for 3–5 days for liver abscess; better tolerated than metronidazole (2)[A]
- **Contraindications:**
  - Known allergy to given medication
  - Diiodohydroxyquin should be used with caution in patients with thyroid disease. It is contraindicated in renal and hepatic patients, and may cause optic nerve and peripheral neuropathy.
- **Significant possible interactions:**
  - Metronidazole and tinidazole: Disulfiram reaction with concomitant use of ethanol.

Pregnancy Considerations

- Most agents are avoided in pregnancy (especially first trimester) because of concerns of teratogenicity, but invasive disease must still be treated:
  - Paromomycin is sometimes recommended for noninvasive disease because it is not absorbed.
- Infectious disease consultation should be obtained.

Second Line

- Luminal agent for noninvasive infection:
  - Diiodohydroxyquin (also called iodoquinol): Adult: 650 mg t.i.d. PO for 20 days (if available); Pediatric: 10–13 mg/kg PO t.i.d. for 20 days
- Invasive infection:
  - Dehydroemetine (as effective as metronidazole, but cardiotoxic): 1–1.5 mg/kg/d IM for 5 days
  - Chloroquine (less effective): 600 mg base/d PO for 2 days, then 200 mg/d PO for 2–3 weeks (pediatric dose: 10 mg/kg/d up to maximum of 300 mg/d)
  - Treatment for invasive infection should be followed by a luminal agent.

SURGERY/OTHER PROCEDURES

- Surgery may be necessary in severe amebic colitis, peritonitis, and perforated viscus.
- Surgical drainage of uncomplicated amebic liver abscess should be avoided.

ONGOING CARE

FOLLOW-UP RECOMMENDATIONS

Patient Monitoring

Stool studies should be repeated after the completion of therapy to ensure eradication, since no regimen is completely effective.

DIET

As tolerated

PATIENT EDUCATION

Maintain good hygiene and avoid situations of re-exposure.

PROGNOSIS

- Untreated invasive amebiasis is frequently fatal.
- With treatment, improvement usually occurs within a few days.
- Irritable bowel symptoms may persist for weeks after successful treatment, and relapses possible

COMPLICATIONS

- Amebic colitis:
  - Fulminant or necrotizing colitis
  - Toxic megacolon
  - Ameboma
  - Rectovaginal fistula
- Amebic liver abscess:
  - Rupture to intraperitoneal, intrathoracic, or intrapericardial spaces with secondary bacterial infection
  - Direct extension to pleura or pericardium
  - Hematogenous dissemination and formation of brain abscess

REFERENCES

1. Fotedar R, Stark D, Beebe N, et al. Laboratory diagnostic techniques for entamoeba species. *Clin Microbiol Rev*. 2007;20:511–32.
2. Gonzales ML, Dans LF, Martinez EG. Antiamoebic drugs for treating amoebic colitis. *Cochrane Database Syst Rev*. 2009:CD006085.
3. Haque R, Huston CD, Hughes M, et al. Amebiasis. *N Engl J Med*. 2003;348:1565–73.
4. Stanley SL. Amoebiasis. *Lancet*. 2003;361: 1025–34.

ADDITIONAL READING

Haque R, Kabir M, Noor Z, et al. Diagnosis of amebic liver abscess and amebic colitis by detection of *Entamoeba histolytica* DNA in blood, urine, and saliva by a real-time PCR assay. *J Clin Microbiol*. 2010;48: 2798–801.

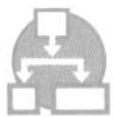

See Also (Topic, Algorithm, Electronic Media Element)

Diarrhea, Acute; Diarrhea, Chronic

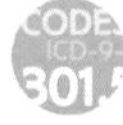

CODES

ICD9

- 006.0 Acute amebic dysentery without mention of abscess
- 006.3 Amebic liver abscess
- 006.4 Amebic lung abscess

CLINICAL PEARLS

- Most infected patients with *E. histolytica* are asymptomatic or have minimal diarrheal symptoms, but they need to be treated with luminal agents.
- Invasive infection is treated by nitroimidazole agents followed by luminal agents.
- Untreated invasive disease is frequently fatal, and treated cases may have relapses.
- Nonpathogenic strains of *Entamoeba* species do not require treatment.
- Irritable bowel symptoms may persist for weeks despite successful treatment of infection.

AMENORRHEA

Heidi L. Gaddey, MD

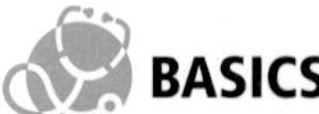

BASICS

DESCRIPTION

- Primary amenorrhea:
  - No menses by age 13–14 with absence of secondary sexual characteristics or
  - No menses by age 15–16 with normal secondary characteristics
- Secondary amenorrhea: Absence of menses for 3 months in a woman with previously normal menstruation or 6 months in a woman with a history of irregular cycles
- System(s) affected: Endocrine/Metabolic; Reproductive

Pregnancy Considerations

Pregnancy is by far the most common cause of secondary amenorrhea.

EPIDEMIOLOGY

Prevalence

- Primary amenorrhea: <1% of female population
- Secondary amenorrhea: 3–5% of female population
- No evidence for race and ethnicity affecting prevalence
- Secondary amenorrhea more common than primary

RISK FACTORS

- Obesity
- Overtraining
- Eating disorders
- Malnutrition
- Anovulatory disorders
- Psychosocial crisis

Genetics

No known genetic pattern

GENERAL PREVENTION

Maintenance of proper body mass index (BMI) and healthy lifestyle with respect to food and exercise

PATHOPHYSIOLOGY

- Pathophysiology varies, depending on etiology.
- Primary amenorrhea should be evaluated in the context of presence or absence of secondary sexual characteristics.
- Can result from dysfunction in hypothalamic–pituitary–gonadal axis, anatomic abnormalities, or another endocrine gland disorder

ETIOLOGY

- Primary amenorrhea:
  - Hypothalamic–pituitary abnormalities:
    - Constitutional delay of puberty
    - Isolated GnRH deficiency
    - Eating disorder
    - Stress/exercise
    - Central lesions (tumors, hypophysitis, granulomas)
    - Hyperprolactinemia
  - Gonadal abnormalities:
    - Chromosomal abnormalities (androgen insensitivity syndrome)
    - Euchromosomal gonadal agenesis or dysgenesis (Turner syndrome, Swyer syndrome, and pure gonadal dysgenesis)
    - Ovarian resistance syndrome
    - Abnormal gonadotropin function
    - Autoimmune gonadal failure
    - Idiopathic gonadal failure
  - Anatomic abnormalities:
    - Imperforate hymen
    - Transverse vaginal septum
    - Congenital absence of the cervix
    - Müllerian agenesis
- Secondary amenorrhea:
  - Pregnancy
  - Thyroid disease
  - Hyperprolactinemia (altered metabolism, ectopic production, breastfeeding/stimulation, hypothyroidism, medications, empty sella syndrome, pituitary adenoma)
  - After pregnancy, thyroid disease, and hyperprolactinemia are ruled out, other causes classified as:
    - Normogonadotropic amenorrhea: Hyperandrogenic anovulation (acromegaly, androgen-secreting tumors, Cushing disease, exogenous androgens, nonclassical congenital adrenal hyperplasia, PCOS); outflow tract obstruction (Asherman syndrome, cervical stenosis, fibroids or polyps)
    - Hypergonadotropic hypogonadism: Postmenopausal ovarian failure; premature ovarian failure (autoimmune, chemotherapy, galactosemia, genetic, 17-hydroxylase deficiency, idiopathic, mumps oophoritis, pelvic radiation)
    - Hypogonadotropic hypogonadism: Eating disorders, CNS tumors, chronic illness, cranial radiation, excessive weight loss/exercise/ malnutrition, hypothalamic or pituitary destruction, Sheehan syndrome

COMMONLY ASSOCIATED CONDITIONS

- Premature ovarian failure may be associated with autoimmune abnormalities (autoimmune thyroiditis, type 1 diabetes).
- Polycystic ovarian syndrome is associated with insulin resistance and obesity.

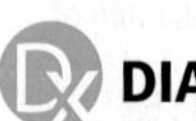

DIAGNOSIS

HISTORY

- Careful review of systems, including recent weight changes, symptoms of early pregnancy or menopause, virilizing changes, cyclic pelvic pain, galactorrhea, headaches, vision changes, fatigue, palpitations
- Growth and pubertal development history, including age of breast development, pubertal growth spurt, and adrenarche
- History of chronic illness, trauma, surgery, medications, prior chemotherapy or radiation
- Psychiatric history
- Social history, including diet and exercise history, drug abuse, and sexual history

PHYSICAL EXAM

- General appearance
- Vital signs, including height and weight, BMI: Hypotension, bradycardia, hypothermia (anorexia nervosa)
- HEENT exam: Evidence of dental erosions, trauma to palate (bulimia), visual field defect, fundoscopic changes, cranial nerve findings (prolactinoma), webbed neck (Turner syndrome), thyromegaly
- Skin exam: Evidence of androgen excess (acne, hirsutism), acanthosis nigricans (PCOS)
- Breast: State of development, evidence of galactorrhea (prolactinoma)
- Pelvic exam: Presence or absence of pubic hair (if sparse: Androgen insensitivity or deficiency); clitoromegaly (androgen excess); distention or bulging of external vagina (imperforate hymen); thin, pale vaginal mucosa without rugae (estrogen deficiency and ovarian failure); presence of cervical mucus (evidence for estrogen production); blind vaginal pouch (müllerian agenesis, androgen insensitivity syndrome); ovarian enlargement (tumors, PCOS, autoimmune oophoritis)

DIAGNOSTIC TESTS & INTERPRETATION

Lab

Initial lab tests

- Primary amenorrhea:
  - Serum prolactin (PRL) and thyroid-stimulating hormone (TSH)
  - If no secondary sexual characteristics, measure serum follicle stimulating hormone (FSH) and luteinizing hormone (LH):
    - FSH/LH <5 IU/L suggests primary hypothalamic or pituitary etiology
    - FSH >20 and LH >40 IU/L suggests gonadal failure, and karyotype analysis should be performed
  - If secondary sexual characteristics present, evaluate for anatomic abnormalities. If uterus is absent or abnormal, perform karyotype analysis.
- Secondary amenorrhea:
  - Exclude pregnancy with HCG
  - Serum TSH: Elevated in hypothyroidism, decreased in hyperthyroidism
  - Serum chemistry, CBC, urinalysis to rule out underlying disease
  - PRL:
    - >100 ng/mL suggests empty sella syndrome or pituitary adenoma. Perform MRI for evaluation.
    - <100 ng/mL: Evaluate for other etiologies of which medications are most common
- If PRL and TSH are normal, perform progestin challenge (see "Treatment"):
  - If withdrawal bleed: Normogonadotropic amenorrhea related to hyperandrogenic chronic anovulation most commonly PCOS
  - If no withdrawal bleed: Follow up with estradiol priming (see "Diagnostic Procedures/Other" and "Treatment") and repeat progestin challenge:
    - If no bleed: Consider outflow tract obstruction.
    - If bleed occurs: Check FSH/LH: Elevated in hypergonadotropic hypogonadism, decreased in pituitary tumors or hypogonadotropic hypogonadism
- If virilizing signs and significant acne present, measure free testosterone, DHEA-S, and 17-OH progesterone levels.

Follow-Up & Special Considerations

- Women <30 with ovarian failure (see below) should have karyotype analysis and be investigated for premutations of FMR1 gene (fragile X syndrome) and for adrenal antibodies.
- If absence of uterus or foreshortened vagina, karyotype analysis should also be performed.

Imaging

- Imaging is not generally indicated as a first-line approach for amenorrhea.
- Ultrasound (US) may show ovarian cysts (PCOS), presence or absence of uterus, and endometrial thickness.

- An MRI of the pelvis can clarify any uterine or vaginal anomalies suggested by US, or if pediatric patient is unable to tolerate transvaginal US probe.
- An MRI of the sella turcica if prolactinoma suspected (elevated PRL >100), and consider with functional hypothalamic amenorrhea (other adenomas)

Follow-Up & Special Considerations
- Laparoscopy: Diagnosis of the streak ovaries of Turner syndrome or PCOS (not often done)
- Hysterosalpingogram: To rule out Asherman syndrome and other etiologies of outflow obstruction

Diagnostic Procedures/Surgery
- If constitutional delay suspected: Obtain bone age
- If hypothalamic amenorrhea from functional suppression suspected: Consider dual-energy x-ray absorptiometry (DEXA) scan to assess for bone loss

DIFFERENTIAL DIAGNOSIS
Includes all causes listed in "Etiology"

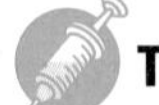

TREATMENT

MEDICATION
- Progesterone challenge and replacement: Medroxyprogesterone (Provera) 10 mg/d for 10 days will result in withdrawal bleed if hypothalamic–pituitary–gonadal axis intact
- Estrogen replacement: Cycling with a combination oral contraceptive (containing 35 or 50 mcg of estrogen) or conjugated estrogen (Premarin) 0.625 mg for 25 days with progesterone added as above for the last 10 days will result in a withdrawal bleed if the uterus and lower genital tract are normal.
- Use of hormonal therapies will not correct the underlying problem. Other drugs might be required to treat specific conditions (e.g., bromocriptine for hyperprolactinemia).
- Use of hormonal replacement therapy is *not* recommended for long-term management of amenorrhea in older women (1)[A]:
  - It may be safe for symptom management in young women (1)[C].
  - Give to maintain secondary sex characteristics and to prevent osteoporosis in adolescents and young women
- Combination estrogen/progesterone contraceptives (oral contraceptive pills [OCPs], patch, ring) replace estrogen and prevent pregnancy:
  - They also have a positive effect on bone mineral density in oligo-/amenorrheic women (2)[B].
  - Can decrease hirsutism in PCOS
- Calcium supplementation 1,500 mg/d if cause is hypoestrogenism
- Because PCOS is related to insulin resistance, metformin (Glucophage) has been used (often starting at 500 mg b.i.d.) in an effort to correct metabolic abnormalities, improve ovulation (3)[A], and restore normal menstrual patterns (3)[B].
- Contraindications to estrogen administration:
  - Pregnancy, thromboembolic disease, previous myocardial infarct or cerebrovascular accident, estrogen-dependent malignancy, severe hepatic impairment or disease
- Precautions:
  - Patients who are amenorrheic and wish to become pregnant should not be given hormone replacement therapy, but should receive treatment for infertility based on the specific cause.

ADDITIONAL TREATMENT

General Measures
- Definitive treatment depends on determining the cause of the amenorrhea.
- May not be necessary to treat all cases, especially if just temporary amenorrhea

Issues for Referral
Many causes of amenorrhea require referral to specialists in ob/gyn, endocrine, surgery, and/or psychiatry.

SURGERY/OTHER PROCEDURES
- A hymenectomy, done as a day surgery, is required for those whose primary amenorrhea is due to imperforate hymen.
- Lysis of adhesions in Asherman syndrome has been shown to be effective in restoring menstrual regularity and fertility.
- In patients with karyotype XY, gonads must be removed due to increased risk of gonadal tumors.
- Patients with müllerian agenesis and other congenital anatomical abnormalities of the vagina can undergo surgery to create a functioning vagina.

ONGOING CARE

FOLLOW-UP RECOMMENDATIONS
If overtraining is suspected, activity level should be reduced by 25% to 50%.

Patient Monitoring
- Depends on the cause and treatment chosen
- If hormonal replacement is used, discontinuation after 6 months is advised to assess spontaneous resumption of menses.

DIET
- Correct overweight or underweight by dietary management and behavior modification.
- If PCOS is the etiology, a weight-loss diet will help restore ovulation.

PATIENT EDUCATION
- Patient education consists of fully informing the patient of your findings, including the presence or absence of pregnancy, and of the underlying cause.
- Specific educational resources can be utilized as necessary (e.g., prenatal classes and menopause support groups).
- Specific information should be given about the expected duration of amenorrhea (temporary or permanent), effect on fertility, and the long-term sequelae of untreated amenorrhea (e.g., osteoporosis, vaginal dryness).
- Appropriate contraceptive advice should be given, as fertility returns before menses.
- Additional support may be needed if the amenorrhea is associated with a reduction in, or loss of, fertility.
- Society for Menstrual Cycle Research, 10559 N. 104th Place, Scottsdale, AZ 85258, (602) 451-9731.

PROGNOSIS
- Reflects the underlying cause
- In secondary amenorrhea from functional suppression of hypothalamic–pituitary–ovarian axis (stress, disordered eating, exercise), 1 study demonstrated 83% reversal rate in presence of obvious contributing factor

COMPLICATIONS
- Estrogen-deficiency symptoms (e.g., hot flashes, vaginal dryness)
- Osteoporosis in prolonged hypoestrogenic amenorrhea
- Increased risk of endometrial cancer in patients whose amenorrhea is secondary to anovulation with estrogen excess (obesity, PCOS)

REFERENCES

1. Farquhar CM, Marjoribanks J, Lethaby A. Long term hormone therapy for perimenopausal and postmenopausal women. *Cochrane Database Syst Rev*. 2005:CD004143.
2. Liu SL, Lebrun CM. Effect of oral contraceptives and hormone replacement therapy on bone mineral density in premenopausal and perimenopausal women: A systematic review. *Br J Sports Med*. 2006;40:11–24.
3. Andy C, Flake D, French L. Clinical inquiries. Do insulin-sensitizing drugs increase ovulation rates for women with PCOS? *J Fam Pract*. 2005;54:156, 159–60.

ADDITIONAL READING

- Gordon CM. Clinical practice. Functional hypothalamic amenorrhea. *N Engl J Med*. 2010;363:365–71.
- Heiman DL. Amenorrhea. *Prim Care*. 2009;36: 1–17, vii.
- Practice Committee of American Society for Reproductive Medicine. Current evaluation of amenorrhea. *Fertil Steril*. 2008;90:S219–25.

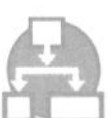

See Also (Topic, Algorithm, Electronic Media Element)

- Diabetes Mellitus, Type 1; Diabetes Mellitus, Type 2; Hyperthyroidism; Hypothyroidism, Adult; Osteoporosis
- Algorithms: Amenorrhea, Primary (Absence of Menarche by Age 16); Amenorrhea, Secondary; Delayed Puberty

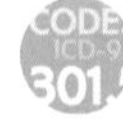

CODES

ICD9
626.0 Absence of menstruation

CLINICAL PEARLS

- There are both physiological and pathological causes of amenorrhea.
- Pregnancy is the most common cause of secondary amenorrhea.
- Among certain women with amenorrhea, a progestin challenge is a useful diagnostic tool.
- The use of hormonal replacement therapy is *not* recommended for long-term management of amenorrhea in older women.

AMNESTIC DISORDER

Sana Syed, MD
Sudha Seshadri, MD

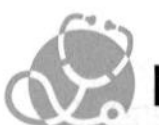

BASICS

- Memory is an arbitrary term that encompasses:
  - Knowledge of facts (*semantic* memory)
  - Knowledge of previous self-experiences (*episodic* memory)
  - Exercise of a learned skill (*procedural* memory)
  - Temporary knowledge for immediate use (*working* memory)
- Coded for by various regions of the brain, with significant involvement of the following:
  - Medial temporal lobe, including:
    - Amygdaloid nucleus
    - Hippocampus
    - Parahippocampal region
  - Thalamus, especially the dorsomedial nuclei
  - Hypothalamus
  - Basal forebrain
- Amnestic disorder is a blanket statement to describe a deficit in any of these various memory types.

DESCRIPTION

- A single disease process can manifest with abnormalities in more than one memory system.
- For example, Alzheimer disease sufferers have a notable deficit in semantic memory but can also have working memory deficits.
- Amnestic disorder, amnestic syndrome, or simply amnesia comes from the Greek for forgetfulness.
- Indicates a loss of, or gap in, one's memory, usually due to brain injury, shock, fatigue, repression, or illness
- Can be categorized based on amnesia for:
  - Events prior to the causative event, as in *retrograde*
  - Events after the causative event, as in *anterograde*
  - Information related to all senses and past experiences, as in *global* amnesia
- Unless otherwise stated, this topic will deal in particular with transient global amnesia (TGA).

EPIDEMIOLOGY

- Incidence and prevalence of amnesia is in direct proportion to the epidemiology of the primary cause.
- In transient global amnesia, incidence is greater among individuals over the age of 50.

Incidence

- In 1 study (1) in Rochester, Minnesota, TGA was found to be 5.2 cases per 100,000.
- The study further estimated 23.5–32 cases per 100,000 per year among those older than 50.
- TGA recurrence rate is low: 4–5% in this study.

RISK FACTORS

- Evidence for and against established risk factors (1)
- Not a symptom of arteriosclerosis
- No higher risk of heart or cerebrovascular disease

Genetics

Recent evidence supports the possibility of a genetic predisposition (2).

PATHOPHYSIOLOGY

- Transient global amnesia is well studied but is not fully understood.
- Thought to have various mechanisms
- Findings from positron emission tomography, diffusion-weighted imaging MRI, single photon emission CT, and MR spectroscopy have demonstrated involvement of known memory-related structures in patients with TGA. In particular, the right hippocampus but in some cases bilateral involvement and even the left hippocampus involvement has been noted.
- Some theorize spreading depression of cortical electrical activity; that is, a wave of cellular depolarization and subsequent cellular edema.
- Others suggest that TGA is the result of:
  - Migraines
  - Venous congestion of the brain
  - Jugular valvular insufficiency

ETIOLOGY

- In general, metabolic or structural changes that cause an imbalance in the memory-related regions of the brain can cause an amnestic disorder
- Common causes:
  - Thiamine deficiency
  - Hypothalamic tumors
  - Vertebrobasilar ischemia
- Less common:
  - Neurodegenerative dementias such as Alzheimer disease
  - Bilateral damage to the medial temporal lobes
  - Head trauma
  - Chronic alcoholism
  - Nutritional disorders
  - In the case of dissociative amnesia, extreme psychological trauma causes the deficit.
- Transient global amnesia has been associated with:
  - Physical exertion
  - Emotional stress
  - Pain
  - Exposure to cold water
  - Sex
  - Valsalva maneuver
  - Malingering and factitious disorder should also be considered.

COMMONLY ASSOCIATED CONDITIONS

- Some relationship has been found between migraines and transient global amnesia.
- TGA patients were found to have a higher frequency of psychiatric disease relative to transient ischemic attack controls in 1 study.

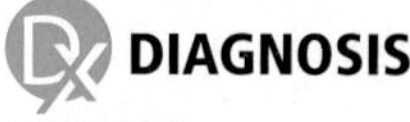

DIAGNOSIS

HISTORY

- In TGA, patients have confusion and global amnesia, usually for 6–12 hours.
- Retrograde, and to a lesser extent anterograde, memory deficits. Anterograde amnesia entails the inability to form new memories but with intact immediate recall.
- The patient retains the ability to perform complex tasks, including cooking, driving, and playing a musical instrument.
- Complete resolution but with amnesic gap for the main episode
- Social history and family history are important.
- There is rarely (<5%) a history of a similar event in the past.
- TGA in women is associated with an emotional precipitating event, a history of anxiety, and a pathological personality.
- TGA in men occurs more after a physical precipitating event.
- There is a history of headaches among younger patients.
- No association with vascular risk factors

PHYSICAL EXAM

- If there are no focal abnormalities on exam, then transient global ischemia can be diagnosed.
- Loss of memory for recent events
- Difficulty with retaining new information
- If neurological exam demonstrates more than memory dysfunction, other differential diagnoses should be further explored.

DIAGNOSTIC TESTS & INTERPRETATION

- TGA is largely a clinical diagnosis.
- Physical exam largely unremarkable

Lab

Initial lab tests

- CBC with differential
- Basic metabolic profile including serum glucose
- Toxicology screen
- Oxygenation level
- Prothrombin time/partial thromboplastin time to rule out hypercoagulable state

Imaging

Initial approach

MRI and/or CT to rule out stroke

Diagnostic Procedures/Surgery

- EEG if seizure is suspected
- ECG if cardiac etiology is suspected

DIFFERENTIAL DIAGNOSIS

- Basilar artery thrombosis
- Cardioembolic stroke
- Complex partial seizures
- Epilepsy of frontal or temporal lobe
- Lacunar syndromes
- Migraine variants
- Posterior cerebral artery stroke
- Syncope

TREATMENT

- Supportive care for TGA
- Reassurance that recurrence of TGA is low (3)
- If there is an underlying disease process present (i.e., Alzheimer disease, herpes encephalitis), it should be treated.

MEDICATION

Patient should receive IV thiamine 100 mg in the ED setting.

ONGOING CARE

Schedule at least 1 follow-up visit to a neurologist for a patient diagnosed with TGA.

FOLLOW-UP RECOMMENDATIONS

Additional neuropsychology testing at follow-up to ensure complete recovery.

DIET

No restrictions on diet

PROGNOSIS

TGA is a benign condition, with low risk of recurrence (3).

REFERENCES

1. Miller JW, Petersen RC, Metter EJ. Transient global amnesia: clinical characteristics and prognosis. *Neurology*. 1987;37:733–7.
2. Segers-van Rijn J, de Brujin SF. Transient global amnesia: a genetic disorder? *Eur Neurol*. 2010; 63:186–7.
3. Hinge HH, Jensen TS, Kjaer M. The prognosis of transient global amnesia. Results of a multicenter study. *Arch Neurol*. 1986;43:673–6.

ADDITIONAL READING

- Agosti C, Akkawi NM, Borroni B, et al. Recurrency in transient global amnesia: A retrospective study. *Eur J Neurol*. 2006;13(9):986–9.
- Budson AE, Price BH. Memory dysfunction. *N Engl J Med*. 2005;352(7):692–9.
- Greer DM, Schaefer PW, Schwamm LH. Unilateral temporal lobe stroke causing ischemic transient global amnesia: Role for diffusion-weighted imaging in the initial evaluation. *J Neuroimaging*. 2001;11:317–9.
- Jenkins KG, Kapur N, Kopelman MD. Retrograde amnesia and malingering. *Curr Opin Neurol*. 2009; 22(6)601–5.
- Piñol-Ripoll G, de la Puerta González-Miró I, Martínez L. A study of the risk factors in transient global amnesia and its differentiation from a transient ischemic attack. *Rev Neurol*. 2005;41: 513–6.
- Quinette P, Guillery-Girard B, Dayan J. What does transient global amnesia really mean? Review of the literature and thorough study of 142 cases. *Brain*. 2006;129(Pt 7):1640–58.
- Sellal F. Transient amnesia in the elderly. *Psychol Neuropsychiatr Vieil*. 2006;4(1):31–8.
- Shekhar R. Transient global amnesia—a review. *Int J Clin Pract*. 2008;62(6):939–42.
- Zorzon M, Antonutti L, Mase G, et al. Transient global amnesia and transient ischemic attack. Natural history, vascular risk factors, and associated conditions. *Stroke*. 1995;26(9):1536–42.

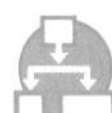

See Also (Topic, Algorithm, Electronic Media Element)

Algorithm: Amnesia

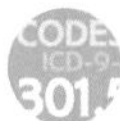

CODES

ICD9

- 291.1 Alcohol-induced persisting amnestic disorder
- 292.83 Drug-induced persisting amnestic disorder
- 294.8 Other persistent mental disorders due to conditions classified elsewhere

CLINICAL PEARLS

- Any patient with possible TGA should be ruled out for stroke, especially if stroke risk factors are present.
- In a patient diagnosed with TGA, reassurance and a follow-up appointment with a neurologist are appropriate management.
- Other than memory problems, the neurological exam of a TGA patient is most often normal.

AMYOTROPHIC LATERAL SCLEROSIS

Mhd Basheer Rahmoun, MD
Dalia Sbat, PharmD

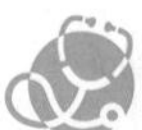

BASICS

Amyotrophic lateral sclerosis (ALS) is a degenerative disease that affects the upper and lower motor neurons (UMN and LMN).

DESCRIPTION

- Sporadic ALS is the most common form of the disease. It includes a number of overlapping syndromes, such as pseudobulbar palsy, progressive bulbar palsy, progressive muscular atrophy, and primary lateral sclerosis.
- Familial ALS is an autosomal-dominant or autosomal-recessive disease, which is clinically similar to sporadic ALS but probably represents a distinct entity pathologically and biochemically.
- Guam ALS and Parkinson-dementia complex are ALS-like syndromes often, but not always, associated with Parkinson syndrome and dementia. Guam ALS is prevalent among the Chamorro Indians of Guam and rare in the US.
- System(s) affected: Nervous
- Synonym(s): Motor neuron disease, MND, Lou Gehrig disease, ALS

ALERT

- Infantile and juvenile spinal muscular atrophies are conditions distinct from ALS, both clinically and pathologically.
- Symptoms of ALS may inappropriately be attributed to age.

Pregnancy Considerations

- Uncommon among affected individuals
- Pregnancy would be unwise in any individual suffering from a disease with poor prognosis.
- If pregnancy did occur, the only foreseeable difficulties would be related to weakness.

EPIDEMIOLOGY

Incidence

In Europe and North America, between 1.47 and 2.7 per 100,000/year

Prevalence

- Estimated prevalence rates range between 2.7 and 7.4 per 100,000.
- Predominant age: Uncommon before age 40
- Predominant sex: Male > Female in sporadic ALS:
  - After 65: Male = Female

RISK FACTORS

- Family history
- Age >40
- Smoking (in women) (1)[A]

Genetics

- Familial ALS (10% of cases) can be autosomal-dominant or autosomal-recessive; X-linked cases have been reported.
- Gene locus has been localized to the long arm of chromosome 21 and encodes the superoxide dismutase (SOD1) enzyme in 20% of familial ALS cases.
- Mutation in the gene encoding fused in sarcoma (FUS) was identified in familial ALS type 6.
- Mutations in the angiogenin gene (ANG) have been recently discovered to be associated with sporadic ALS.
- Mutations in TARDP region encoding TAR DNA-binding protein TDP-43 have also been identified in familial and sporadic ALS.

GENERAL PREVENTION

Genetic counseling is advised if there is a family history of ALS.

PATHOPHYSIOLOGY

Degeneration of the UMN and LMN with their respective axons and with gliosis replacing lost neurons

ETIOLOGY

- Sporadic: Cause is unknown, but elevated levels of glutamate have been found in serum and CSF.
- Familial ALS: A genetically transmitted degenerative disease
- Guam ALS and Parkinson-dementia complex: Possible relationship to ingestion of the cycad nut or to some other environmental toxin

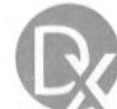

DIAGNOSIS

Diagnosis can be established according to Revised El Escorial World Federation of Neurology criteria.

- The presence of:
  - Evidence of LMN degeneration by clinical, electrophysiological, or neuropathological examination
  - Evidence of UMN degeneration by clinical examination
  - Progressive spread of symptoms or signs within a region or to other regions, as determined by history or examination
- The absence of:
  - Electrophysiological and pathological evidence of other disease processes that might explain the signs of LMN and/or UMN degeneration
  - Neuroimaging evidence of other disease processes that might explain the observed clinical and electrophysiological signs

HISTORY

ALS is suggested when symptoms are consistent with UMN and LMN dysfunction that worsens over time. Symptoms include:

- Loss of muscle strength and coordination
- Difficulty opening and closing the jaw, drooling
- Voice change, hoarseness
- Muscle cramps, difficulty breathing, difficulty swallowing, paralysis

PHYSICAL EXAM

Variable combinations of:

- Unexplained weight loss
- Limb weakness with variable symmetry and distribution
- Gait disorder (steppage-waddling)
- Slurring of speech
- Inability to control affect (inappropriate laughing, crying, yawning)
- Focal atrophy of muscle groups (initially in a myotomal distribution)
- Fasciculations (other than calves)
- Hyperreflexia (including jaw jerk—Hoffmann sign)
- Babinski sign, present in 50% of patients
- Spasticity
- Sialorrhea
- Spares cognitive, oculomotor, sensory, and autonomic functions

DIAGNOSTIC TESTS & INTERPRETATION

Lab

No simple reliable laboratory test is available that confirms the diagnosis.

Initial lab tests

- Elevated levels of glutamate in CSF and serum
- Anti-monosialoganglioside autoantibodies in low titer commonly found (of unclear significance)
- Possibly reduced levels of nerve growth factor

Imaging

Initial approach

MRI: To exclude other possible diagnoses in the evaluation of suspected ALS:

- MRI is usually normal in ALS, although increased signal in the corticospinal tracts on T2-weighted and FLAIR images and hypointensity of the motor cortex on T2-weighted images have been reported.

Diagnostic Procedures/Surgery

- Electromyography: Denervation potentials (fibrillations-positive sharp waves) and often doublets are associated with prominent fasciculations, which suggests anterior horn cell dysfunction. Voluntary motor unit potentials have increased amplitude, long duration, and/or polyphasic pattern. The recruitment pattern is reduced for the force generated, and individual motor units have a high rate of discharge (2).
- Nerve conduction studies: Sensory and motor NCS are most often normal in ALS, although compound motor action potential (CMAP) amplitudes may be reduced in severely atrophic and denervated muscles (2).
- Motor unit number estimation is a nerve conduction–based method that assesses the number of viable motor axons innervating small hand or foot muscles. In ALS, it decreases prior to the onset of clinical weakness.
- Muscle biopsy: Not a routine part of the diagnostic evaluation of ALS but may be performed if myopathy is suspected on clinical, electrodiagnostic, or serological grounds: Muscle biopsy will show groups of shrunken angulated muscle fibers (grouped atrophy) amid other groups of fibers with a uniform fiber type (fiber type grouping).

Pathological Findings

- Loss of Betz cells in the motor cortex
- Atrophic or absent anterior horn cells of spinal cord
- Atrophic or absent neurons within the motor nuclei of the medulla and pons
- Degeneration of the lateral columns of the spinal cord
- Atrophy of the ventral roots
- Grouped atrophy of muscle (motor units)

DIFFERENTIAL DIAGNOSIS

- Multifocal motor neuropathy
- Cervical radiculomyelopathy

- Cervical spondylosis
- Lead intoxication
- Spinal muscular atrophy (adult form)
- Primary lateral sclerosis
- Familial spastic paraparesis
- Benign fasciculations
- Lyme disease
- Spinal multiple sclerosis
- Tropical spastic paraparesis
- Myasthenia gravis

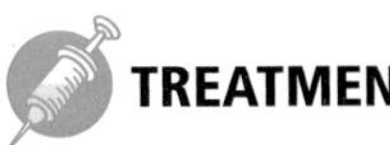

TREATMENT

MEDICATION

Riluzole 50 mg PO b.i.d.: The only FDA-approved drug for ALS. It produces a slight prolongation in life expectancy by decreasing the release of glutamate (3,4), and it slows the disease progression.

ALERT

Riluzole withhold should be considered for patients developing fatigue.

ADDITIONAL TREATMENT

These drugs may be used to relieve severe spasticity:

- Baclofen 5 mg PO t.i.d. initially, followed by gradual increase of 5 mg/d every 4–7 days; not to exceed 80 mg/d divided q.i.d.
- Tizanidine 4–8 mg PO q8h PRN; not to exceed 36 mg/d

General Measures

- Outpatient may ultimately need nursing home placement or hospice.
- Supportive care is necessary for complicating emergencies (aspiration, respiratory failure). Use of a respirator is a major ethical dilemma. Consideration should be given to those with selective respiratory dysfunction.
- Discussion of advance directives, focusing on patient's specific values about which interventions to be used, is critical to meeting the patient's needs.
- Prosthetic devices

Issues for Referral

- Multidisciplinary clinic referral to optimize health care delivery, prolong survival, and enhance quality of life
- Early exam by a neurologist can confirm diagnosis of ALS.
- Tracheostomy or G-tube placement may be performed by surgeon or gastroenterologist.
- Pulmonologist and respiratory therapist for ventilator assistance and management of intercurrent infections and tracheostomy

COMPLEMENTARY AND ALTERNATIVE MEDICINE

- Research offering therapy with stem cells is evolving, providing a new approach in cellular replacement and support for patients (5)[A].
- Therapeutic trials of the efficacy of antioxidants (vitamin E and vitamin C and β-carotene), nerve growth factor, gabapentin, Myotrophin, thyrotropin-releasing hormone, and creatine have been undertaken. Reports are not encouraging (6)[A].

SURGERY/OTHER PROCEDURES

- Treatment for refractory sialorrhea
  - Botulinum toxin B
  - Low-dose radiation therapy to the salivary glands
- Percutaneous endoscopic gastrostomy (PEG) tube should be considered with early signs of malnutrition to stabilize weight and prolong survival.
- Noninvasive ventilation (NIV) can lengthen survival and improve quality of life.
- Elective tracheostomy should be considered in patients with early signs of respiratory difficulty.

ONGOING CARE

FOLLOW-UP RECOMMENDATIONS

Patients should be involved in regular exercise and a physical therapy program.

Patient Monitoring

- Initially every 3 months; frequency to be increased as needed for symptomatic therapy
- Patients with a presumed diagnosis of ALS should have neuroimaging and electrodiagnostic studies.

DIET

- Evaluate swallowing to quantify any dysphagia.
- Modify the patient's diet to prevent aspiration.
- Consider a gastrostomy tube when patient cannot swallow fluids or soft foods (7).

PATIENT EDUCATION

Printed material for patients (and reference lists for physicians) available from:

- The Muscular Dystrophy Association: (520) 529-2000; (800) 572-1717; http://www.mdausa.org
- The ALS Association: (800) 782-4747; http://www.alsa.org
- Families of Spinal Muscular Atrophy: http://www.fsma.org

PROGNOSIS

- ALS usually results in death within 5 years.
- Patients who predominantly manifest progressive muscular atrophy have a better prognosis.
- There have been reports of spontaneous arrest of the disease.

COMPLICATIONS

- Aspiration pneumonia
- Pulmonary embolism
- Nutritional deficiency
- Complications from wheelchair-bound or bedridden states, including decubitus ulcers and skin infections

REFERENCES

1. Alonso A, Logroscino G, Hernán MA. Smoking and the risk of amyotrophic lateral sclerosis: A systematic review and meta-analysis. *J Neurol Neurosurg Psychiatry*. 2010;81(11):1249–52.
2. Daube JR. Electrodiagnostic studies in amyotrophic lateral sclerosis and other motor neuron disorders. *Muscle Nerve*. 2000;23:1488–502.
3. Bensimon G, Lacomblez L, Meininger V. A controlled trial of riluzole in amyotrophic lateral sclerosis. ALS/Riluzole Study Group. *N Engl J Med*. 1994;330:585–91.
4. Riluzole for amyotrophic lateral sclerosis. *Med Lett*. 1995;37:113.
5. Kim SU, de Vellis J. Stem cell-based cell therapy in neurological diseases: A review. *J Neurosci Res*. 2009.
6. Pastula DM, Moore DH, Bedlack RS, et al. Creatine for amyotrophic lateral sclerosis/motor neuron disease. *Cochrane Database Syst Rev*. 2010;6:CD005225.
7. Andersen PM, Borasio GD, Dengler R, et al. Good practice in the management of amyotrophic lateral sclerosis: Clinical guidelines. An evidence-based review with good practice points. EALSC Working Group. *Amyotroph Lateral Scler*. 2007;8:195–213.

ADDITIONAL READING

- Miller RG, Jackson CE, Kasarskis EJ, et al. Practice parameter update: The care of the patient with amyotrophic lateral sclerosis: Drug, nutritional, and respiratory therapies (an evidence-based review): Report of the Quality Standards Subcommittee of the American Academy of Neurology *Neurology*. 2009;73(15):1218–26.
- Practice parameter update: The care of the patient with amyotrophic lateral sclerosis: Multidisciplinary care, symptom management, and cognitive/behavioral impairment (an evidence-based review): Report of the Quality Standards Subcommittee of the American Academy of Neurology. *Neurology*. 2009;73(15):1227–33.

CODES

ICD9

335.20 Amyotrophic lateral sclerosis

CLINICAL PEARLS

- ALS is an upper and lower motor neuron disease.
- Diagnosis is made by history, physical exam, EMG, and NCS.
- Riluzole is the only available treatment that might increase survival.

ANAEROBIC AND NECROTIZING INFECTIONS

Ruben Peralta, MD, FACS

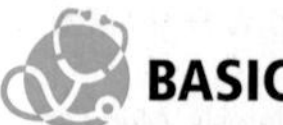

BASICS

DESCRIPTION

- Necrotizing infections of the skin and fascia are called necrotizing cellulitis and necrotizing fasciitis (NF), respectively.
- Necrotizing fasciitis is a rapidly spreading and potentially fatal soft tissue infection located in the fascia, with secondary necrosis of the subcutaneous tissue:
  - Organisms spread from the subcutaneous tissue along the deep fascial planes, presumably facilitated by bacterial enzymes and toxins.
- Type I necrotizing fasciitis is a mixed infection caused by the synergistic effect of *both aerobic and anaerobic bacteria*.
- Type II necrotizing fasciitis is a monomicrobial infection caused by *group A β-hemolytic streptococci* (*Streptococcus pyogenes*).
- Gas gangrene is a subset of necrotizing infection usually caused by the *Clostridium* sp. with gas formation within the tissue (type III), and type IV is *commonly due to fungal infections*.
- Necrotizing skin and soft tissue infections are associated with extensive tissue destruction, systemic toxicity, and loss of limb, and are potentially fatal.
- Synonym(s): Fournier gangrene; Cullen ulcer; Meleney ulcer; Flesh-eating infections

EPIDEMIOLOGY

- Predominant age: Any age
- Predominant sex: Male = Female

Incidence

Incidence of necrotizing fasciitis: 500–1,500 cases annually in the US

RISK FACTORS

Can occur in young, previously healthy persons without predisposing or precipitating risk factors. However, some cases are associated with the following:

- **Predisposing risk factors:**
  - Advanced age
  - Obesity
  - Malnutrition
  - Diabetes mellitus
  - Immune suppression (e.g., HIV, malignancies, alcoholism, steroid exposure)
  - Peripheral vascular disease
  - Inadequate tissue perfusion
- **Precipitating risk factors:**
  - IV drug abuse
  - Trauma
  - Burns
  - Skin ulceration
  - Herpes zoster
- **Prior surgical procedures**
- **Risk factors with patient undergoing surgical procedures includes:**
  - Prior operations
  - Duration of operation
  - Hypoalbuminemia
  - History of chronic obstructive pulmonary disease

GENERAL PREVENTION

- Avoid tight orthopedic casts.
- Routine surgical principles for surgical procedures and skin closure (1)

ETIOLOGY

Most commonly due to polymicrobial infection, including both aerobic and anaerobic bacteria. Bacteria extend from subcutaneous tissue and proliferate along fascial planes. Bacterial toxins and surface proteins facilitate this process and can cause systemic toxicity with serious consequences (such as septic shock).

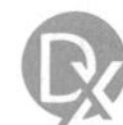

DIAGNOSIS

HISTORY

- Symptoms of malaise, anorexia, and fever progress rapidly over hours; rare cases with slower evolution over days.
- Some cases arise from previous trauma or infection (surgical wound from open or laparoscopic procedure, ulcers, burns, IV drug injection site, abscess).
- *In >20%, a precipitant is never identified.*
- Given the significant risk of delayed diagnosis, keep high index of suspicion if suggestive history but no clear risk factors.

PHYSICAL EXAM

- The diagnosis of necrotizing fasciitis is made clinically:
  - *A high index of suspicion is necessary to make the diagnosis.*
- Not uncommonly, patients report pain out of proportion to physical exam.
- Fever, often low-grade, early in the disease
- Tachycardia
- Hypotension
- Diaphoresis
- Foul odor
- Rapidly spreading skin lesions
- Skin changes, including localized erythema or discoloration, bullae, vesicles, ulceration, necrosis, edema
- Crepitus
- Bacterial toxins may trigger an inflammatory response leading to multiorgan failure or sepsis; in some advanced cases, this may be the presenting concern, and necrotizing infection may not be immediately apparent.

DIAGNOSTIC TESTS & INTERPRETATION

Lab

- Hyponatremia, leukocytosis, anemia, hypocalcemia, acidosis, prolonged prothrombin time, elevated creatine kinase, and serum glucose level
- Elevated liver function tests may result from release of bacterial toxins.
- Renal dysfunction may occur secondary to hypotension and myoglobinuria.
- Cultures and sensitivities are not diagnostic, but may be used to narrow initial broad-spectrum antibiotic treatment.
- Commonly associated pathogens:
  - Gram-positive anaerobes:
    - Cocci: Group A streptococci, *Peptostreptococcus* (anaerobic *Streptococcus*), or *Staphylococcus aureus*
    - Bacilli: *Clostridium perfringens* and other clostridia
  - Gram-negative aerobes: Bacilli: *Escherichia coli, Klebsiella pneumoniae, Enterobacter, Proteus*
- Gram-negative anaerobes: Bacilli: *Bacteroides fragilis* (usually with other gram-negative bacilli)
- Recently reported in salt water contaminated with *Vibrio* species
- In the Far East, the Laboratory Risk Indicator for Necrotizing Fasciitis scoring system has been useful and incorporated in the clinical practice of some centers.

ALERT

Antibiotics given before cultures are performed may alter lab results.

Imaging

- Plain radiographs may show subcutaneous air (a rare finding that is specific but not sensitive).
- CT may reveal soft tissue swelling and presence of gas in tissues.

Pathological Findings

- Only frozen-section biopsy of the fascia is diagnostic. However, treatment should not be delayed while awaiting biopsy.
- Soft tissue necrosis, with polymorphonuclear cells and vascular thrombosis

DIFFERENTIAL DIAGNOSIS

Other soft tissue infection, including abscess and postsurgical wound infection

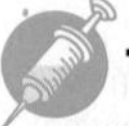

TREATMENT

MEDICATION

- Precautions: Without surgical debridement, antibiotics will not be effective (see "General Measures").
- Important: Do not delay antibiotic treatment, even if smear, cultures, and tests are negative.
- Start with a broad-spectrum antibiotic regimen; then tailor antibiotics to organisms identified by blood and wound cultures and organism sensitivities:
  - Initial broad-spectrum coverage should include penicillin to cover *Streptococcus* and clindamycin, which works synergistically with penicillin when large bacterial load is present and also binds group A streptococci toxin.
  - Aminoglycosides will cover enteric gram-negative organisms.
  - *Metronidazole is an alternative to clindamycin for treatment of anaerobic organisms.*
- Retrospective studies suggest there may be a survival benefit with the use of IV immunoglobulin (IVIG) therapy. IVIG works by binding toxins and superantigens, which suppresses proinflammatory mediators.
- Unlike *C. perfringens* and group A β-hemolytic streptococci, the *Aeromonas* sp. are uniformly resistant to penicillin-G, but are reported to be highly sensitive to 3rd-generation cephalosporins.

ADDITIONAL TREATMENT

General Measures

- Prompt and wide surgical debridement is the cornerstone of treatment.
- Infectious disease consultation, if available
- Hyperbaric oxygen (HBO) is used as an adjunct to antimicrobial agents and aggressive surgical debridement:
  - No survival benefit has been found.
  - The results of studies on the use of HBO therapy in NF are inconsistent.
  - Do not delay surgical intervention for HBO.
- IV fluids with electrolyte repletion, if indicated
- Prophylaxis for tetanus

SURGERY/OTHER PROCEDURES

- Necrotizing soft tissue infections are a surgical emergency. Patients should be taken to the operating room as soon as the diagnosis is made or when there is high clinical suspicion.
- All necrotic tissue should be resected. Dissection should be carried out along all involved fascial planes. Adequate debridement should take priority over preservation of tissue.
- Limb amputation may be necessary because of extensive fascial and subcutaneous soft tissue necrosis and overwhelming systemic toxicity.
- Adequate surgical treatment can rarely be accomplished with a single operation. Repeated daily debridement may be necessary. Debridement should continue until all necrotic tissue is removed.
- Negative-pressure suction dressing (i.e., vacuum-assisted closure dressing) may be utilized to improve wound care and assist with postoperative fluid management.
- Reconstruction can be undertaken once systemic sepsis has been controlled and all nonviable tissue has been removed.

IN-PATIENT CONSIDERATIONS

Nursing

- Following surgical debridement, patients often require intensive care unit (ICU) level of care.
- Close contacts of patients and health care workers do not require chemoprophylaxis with antibiotics.

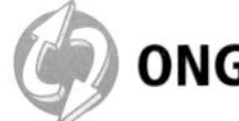

ONGOING CARE

FOLLOW-UP RECOMMENDATIONS

Patient Monitoring

- May require ICU-level critical care
- Diligence required to recognize spreading gangrene that would require repeated debridement
- As clinically indicated; may include following cultures, electrolytes, drug levels

DIET

Depends on clinical scenario; ranges from NPO to diet as tolerated

PROGNOSIS

- Mortality for necrotizing fasciitis ranges from 10–20%, and recent publications document an overall mortality of 17% (ranging between 9% and 25%) (2).
- Mortality for necrotizing soft tissue infections appears to be decreasing, possibly due to improved recognition and earlier delivery of more effective therapy (3).
- Increased mortality associated with: Age >60 years, male, IV drug abuse, malnutrition, significant medical comorbidities (e.g., cardiac or pulmonary disease), carcinoma, presence of bacteremia:
  - Recent study suggests that Fournier gangrene in females has an increased risk for mortality due in part to more aggressive inflammatory manifestations in the retroperitoneum and abdominal cavity (4).
- Independent predictors of mortality include:
  - Admission white blood cell count >30,000
  - Creatinine level >2 mg/dL within 48 hours of admission
  - Presence of clostridial infection
  - Presence of heart disease
- Independent predictors of limb loss include:
  - Shock (systolic pressure <90 mm) on admission
  - Clostridial infection
  - Presence of heart disease

COMPLICATIONS

- Tissue and functional losses
- Amputation
- Septic shock
- Death

REFERENCES

1. Kirby JP, Mazuski JE. Prevention of surgical site infection. *Surg Clin North Am*. 2009;89:365–89.
2. Kao LS, Lew DF, Arab SN, et al. Local variations in the epidemiology, microbiology, and outcome of necrotizing soft-tissue infections: A multicenter study. *Am J Surg*. 2011;202(2):139–45.
3. Ustin JS, Malangoni MA. Necrotizing soft tissue infections. *Critical Care Med*. 2011;39(9):2156–62.
4. Czymek R, Frank P, Limmer S, et al. Fournier's gangrene: Is the female gender a risk factor? *Langenbecks Arch Surg*. 2010;395:173–80.
5. Malangoni MA. Timing is everything. *Ann Surg*. 2009;250:17–8.
6. Steinberg JP, Braun BI, Hellinger WC, et al. Timing of antimicrobial prophylaxis and the risk of surgical site infections: results from the Trial to Reduce Antimicrobial Prophylaxis Errors. *Ann Surg*. 2009;250:10–6.

ADDITIONAL READING

- de Lissovoy G, Fraeman K, Hutchins V, et al. Surgical site infection: Incidence and impact on hospital utilization and treatment costs. *Am J Infect Control*. 2009;37:387–97.
- Morgan MS, et al. Diagnosis and management of necrotising fasciitis: A multiparametric approach. *J Hosp Infect*. 2010;75(4):249–57.

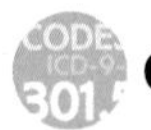

CODES

ICD9

- 041.84 Other specified bacterial infections in conditions classified elsewhere and of unspecified site, other anaerobes
- 728.86 Necrotizing fasciitis
- 785.4 Gangrene

CLINICAL PEARLS

- The symptom most commonly associated with necrotizing soft tissue infection is pain out of proportion to the physical exam.
- A necrotizing infection is a potentially life-threatening condition consisting of a soft tissue infection with rapidly progressive, widespread fascial necrosis.
- Necrotizing fasciitis may be an infection of 1 species of bacteria or may be polymicrobial.
- Prompt diagnosis and treatment are essential (5).
- Surgical debridement and antibiotic therapy are the primary treatment options.
- Be aware of antibiotic-resistant organisms (5,6).

ANAL FISSURE

Michael Rousse, MD, MPH

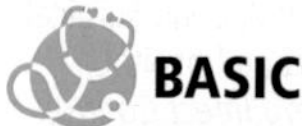

BASICS

DESCRIPTION
Anal fissure is a benign anorectal disease characterized by a knifelike tearing sensation on defecation. An anal fissure is a tear in the lining of the anal canal distal to the dentate line, most commonly in the posterior midline.

EPIDEMIOLOGY
Very common anorectal condition often confused with hemorrhoids

Incidence
Exact incidence is unknown. Patients often treat with home remedies and do not seek medical care.

ALERT
- Common in infants 6–24 months; not common in older children; suspect abuse or trauma. Elderly are spared due to lower resting pressure in the anal canal.
- Predominant sex: Male = Female, but women are more likely to get anterior midline tears (25% vs. 8%).

Prevalence
- 80% of infants, usually self-limited
- 20% of adults, the majority of whom do not seek medical advice, have symptoms referable to the anorectum.

RISK FACTORS
- Constipation
- Passage of hard or large-caliber stool
- High resting tone of internal anal sphincter (prolonged sitting)
- Trauma (anal sex)
- Inflammatory bowel disease (Crohn disease)
- Syphilis
- Tuberculosis

Genetics
None known

GENERAL PREVENTION
Avoid constipation and prolonged sitting on toilet.

PATHOPHYSIOLOGY
High resting pressure within the anal canal can lead to ischemia of the anodermal tissues resulting in splitting of the tissues with passage of stool. Exposed internal sphincter muscle spasms causing the knifelike pain.

ETIOLOGY
Splitting of susceptible anodermal tissue

COMMONLY ASSOCIATED CONDITIONS
Constipation, Crohn disease, tuberculosis, leukemia, and HIV

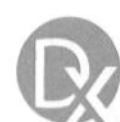

DIAGNOSIS

HISTORY
- Severe rectal pain, often with and following defecation, but can be continuous; some will see bright red blood on the stool or when wiping.
- Occasionally, itch or perianal irritation is the presenting sign.

PHYSICAL EXAM
- Gentle spreading of the buttocks will reveal a tear in the anodermal tissue, typically posterior midline, occasionally anterior midline, rarely eccentric to midline.
- Minimal swelling or bleeding
- Hypertrophic papillae (*sentinel tag*) is seen in chronic fissure.

DIAGNOSTIC TESTS & INTERPRETATION

Diagnostic Procedures/Surgery
- Avoid anoscopy or endoscopy initially unless necessary for other diagnoses.
- Some patients may require exam under anesthesia to diagnose properly.

DIFFERENTIAL DIAGNOSIS
- Thrombosed external hemorrhoid: Swollen, painful mass; no fissure
- Perirectal abscess: Sinus tract with purulent drainage rather than a fissure
- Pruritus ani: Shallow excoriations rather than a fissure

TREATMENT

The goal of treatment is to avoid repeated tearing of the anal mucosa with resultant spasm of the internal anal sphincter.

MEDICATION

First Line
- Stool softeners (docusate)
- Fiber supplements (psyllium)
- Topical analgesics (2% lidocaine gel)
- Warm sitz baths

Second Line
- Topical nitroglycerin ointment 2% diluted to 0.2% applied q.i.d., marginally but significantly better than placebo in healing (48.6% vs. 37%); late recurrence was common (50%) (1)[A]; effect is to reduce resting anal pressure through the release of nitric oxide (2)[B]
- Calcium channel blockers (e.g., nifedipine, diltiazem), oral or topical; no better than nitrates but with fewer side effects (1)[A]; effect is to relax the internal sphincter muscle, thereby reducing the resting anal pressure (3)[A]
- Botulinum toxin 4 mL injected into the internal sphincter muscle; no better than topical nitrates but with fewer side effects (1)[A]; effect is to inhibit the release of acetylcholine from nerve endings to inhibit muscle spasm (4)[B]

ADDITIONAL TREATMENT

General Measures
- Wash area with warm water; high-fiber diet; avoid constipation
- Medical therapy is usually initiated in a stepwise manner: Nitrates–calcium channel blockers–botulinum toxin (5)[B]

Issues for Referral
- Late recurrence is common (50%).
- Medical therapy usually is tried for 90–120 days before referral for surgery (6)[B].

SURGERY/OTHER PROCEDURES

- Reserved for failure of medical therapy; involves division of the internal sphincter muscle
- Lateral internal sphincterectomy appears to be the surgical procedure of choice (7)[B].
- Risk for fecal incontinence: 45% short term, 6–8% long term (8)[B]
- Anal stretching/dilation: Unlikely to benefit (2)[C]

ONGOING CARE

DIET

High fiber; increase fluids

PATIENT EDUCATION

Avoid prolonged sitting during bowel movements; drink plenty of fluids; avoid constipation.

PROGNOSIS

Medical therapy is less likely to be successful for chronic anal fissures; 40% failure rate (9)[A].

COMPLICATIONS

Fecal incontinence and incontinence to flatus; primarily associated with surgery (10)[B]

REFERENCES

1. Nelson RL. Non surgical therapy for anal fissure. *Cochrane Database of Systematic Reviews*. 2006, Issue 4. Art. No.: CD003431. DOI:10.1002/14651858.CD003431.pub2.
2. Madoff RD, Fleshman JW. AGA Technical review on the diagnosis and care of patients with anal fissure. *Gastroenterology*. 2003;124:235–45.
3. Samim M, Twigt B, Stoker L, et al. Topical diltiazem cream versus botulinum toxin A for the treatment of chronic anal fissure: A double-blind randomized clinical trial. *Ann Surg*. 2012;255(1): 18–22.
4. Yiannakopoulou E. Botulinum toxin and anal fissure: Efficacy and safety systematic review. *Int J Colorectal Dis*. 2012;27(1):1–9.
5. Altomare DF, Binda GA, Canuti S, et al. The management of patients with primary chronic anal fissure: A position paper. *Tech Coloproctol*. 2011;15:135–41.
6. Sinha R, Kaiser AM. Efficacy of Management Algorithm for Reducing Need for Sphincterotomy in Chronic Anal Fissures. *Colorectal Dis*. 2011.
7. Mousavi SR, Sharifi M, Mehdikhah Z. A comparison between the results of fissurectomy and lateral internal sphincterotomy in the surgical management of chronic anal fissure. *J Gastrointest Surg*. 2009;13:1279–82.
8. Levin A, Cohen MJ, Mindrul V, et al. Delayed fecal incontinence following surgery for anal fissure. *Int J Colorectal Dis*. 2011;26(12):1595–9.
9. Shao WJ, Li GC, Zhang ZK. Systematic review and meta-analysis of randomized controlled trials comparing botulinum toxin injection with lateral internal sphincterotomy for chronic anal fissure. *Int J Colorectal Dis*. 2009;24:995–1000.
10. Sileri P, Stolfi VM, Franceschilli L, et al. Conservative and surgical treatment of chronic anal fissure: Prospective longer term results. *J Gastrointest Surg*. 2010;14:773–80.

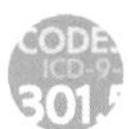

CODES

ICD9

565.0 Anal fissure

CLINICAL PEARLS

- Avoid anoscopy or endoscopy initially unless necessary for other diagnoses:
  - Some patients may require exam under anesthesia to diagnose properly.
- Best chance to prevent recurrence is to avoid prolonged sitting on toilet and avoid constipation.
- No medical therapy approaches the cure rate of surgery.

ANAPHYLAXIS

Bobby X. Peters, MD

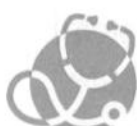

BASICS

DESCRIPTION

- An IgE-mediated, acute systemic reaction following antigen exposure in a sensitized person
- A non–IgE-mediated idiopathic anaphylactoid reaction also may occur. Anaphylactoid reactions are clinically indistinguishable from anaphylaxis and are treated in the same manner.
- System(s) affected: Cardiovascular; Endocrine/Metabolic; Gastrointestinal; Hematologic/Lymphatic/Immunologic; Pulmonary; and Skin/Exocrine
- Synonym(s): Anaphylactoid reactions

EPIDEMIOLOGY

- Predominant age: All ages
- Predominant sex: Male = Female

Incidence

- Up to 40,000 cases of idiopathic anaphylaxis with no identifiable cause occur each year.
- Drug-induced anaphylaxis occurs in 1/2,700 hospitalized patients.
- Anaphylaxis deaths: 0.3–0.7/100,000 per year
- Food allergic reactions constitute 1/3–1/2 of all anaphylactic reactions worldwide.
- Anaphylaxis may occur secondary to allergy skin testing.
- Asthmatics are more prone to anaphylaxis than nonasthmatics. Female asthmatics are at greater risk of anaphylaxis than their male counterparts.

RISK FACTORS

- Previous anaphylaxis
- History of atopy or asthma

Genetics

Genetic predisposition for sensitization to antigens

GENERAL PREVENTION

- Avoid inducing drugs and foods.
- For those with history of anaphylaxis, carry a prefilled epinephrine syringe. Keep a syringe at home, work/school, and in vehicle, although syringe should be protected from temperature extremes.
- Avoid areas where insect exposure is likely. Avoid wearing insect attractants (e.g., perfumes, colored clothing); avoid bare feet outdoors.
- Carry or wear a medical alert ID about the anaphylaxis-causing substance or event.
- When radiologic contrast is unavoidable, use of low osmolar contrast agents (e.g., iothalamate) reduces the risk of contrast reactions to 3.1%:
  - Only 0.22% were considered severe.
  - Stop beta blockers before administering contrast materials.
  - Pretreat with diphenhydramine (50 mg IV) and a steroid (e.g., methylprednisolone 60 mg IV q6h) until procedure. Start methylprednisolone the day before the procedure is scheduled.
  - Those with frequent (>6 per year) episodes of idiopathic anaphylaxis should be treated prophylactically with prednisone (40–60 mg/d in a single morning dose), hydroxyzine (25 mg t.i.d.), and albuterol (2 mg PO t.i.d.). The prednisone should be rapidly tapered to an every-other-day regimen.

ALERT

- Have a latex-free kit (gloves, etc.) available for the treatment of latex-allergic patients. Some latex-allergic patients will react to tropical fruits, such as kiwi, bananas, avocados, and chestnuts.
- Avoid beta-blockers.

ETIOLOGY

- IgE-mediated mast cell degranulation
- Complement activation (C3a, C4a, C5a) by antigen–antibody complexes that contain complement-fixing antibodies
- Other non–IgE-dependent anaphylaxislike syndromes may be caused by modulators of arachidonic acid metabolism, sulfiting agents, exercise-induced anaphylaxis, and idiopathic recurrent anaphylaxis.
- Some important causes of anaphylaxis are:
  - Antimicrobials (e.g., penicillin)
  - Blood products (especially in IgA deficiency)
  - Iodinated contrast media
  - Ethylene oxide gas (dialysis tubing, other sterilized products)
  - Exercise
  - Foods (commonly, peanuts, nuts, fish, crustaceans, mollusks, cow's milk, eggs, and soy)
  - Immunotherapy
  - Insect stings (e.g., honeybees, wasps, kissing bugs, and deer flies)
  - Latex rubber (gloves, catheters)
  - Macromolecules (e.g., chymopapain, insulin, dextran, glucocorticoid, and protamine)
  - Vaccines

COMMONLY ASSOCIATED CONDITIONS

- Asthma
- Atopy

DIAGNOSIS

HISTORY

Rapid progression within minutes to hours of the signs and symptoms of anaphylaxis, with or without an obvious trigger, including but not limited to: Cutaneous symptoms (90% of cases), respiratory symptoms (70%), GI symptoms (40%), and cardiovascular symptoms (35%)

PHYSICAL EXAM

- Pruritus, flushing, urticaria, angioedema
- Dyspnea, cough, rhonchi
- Rhinorrhea, bronchorrhea, wheezing, stridor
- Difficulty swallowing
- Nausea, vomiting, diarrhea, cramps, bloating
- Tachycardia, hypotension, shock, syncope
- Malaise, shivering
- Mydriasis

DIAGNOSTIC TESTS & INTERPRETATION

Lab

- Hypoxemia, hypercarbia, acidosis
- Acidosis may cause apparent hyperkalemia by moving potassium extracellularly
- Elevated serum tryptase, a mast cell enzyme for allergic and anaphylactic reactions (1)[B]
- Drugs that may alter lab results: Epinephrine and albuterol may cause apparent hypokalemia by shifting K+ intracellularly.

DIFFERENTIAL DIAGNOSIS

- Anaphylactoid reactions:
  - May occur after the first contact with substance such as polymyxin, pentamidine, radiographic contrast media, and aspirin
- Carcinoid syndrome
- Globus hystericus:
  - May mimic pharyngeal edema
- Hereditary angioedema:
  - C1q esterase deficiency with painless, pruritus free angioedema without urticaria, flushing, or wheezing
- Pheochromocytoma:
  - Paradoxically, because of beta-2 stimulation, some patients have hypotensive attacks accompanied by tachycardia.
  - Urticaria, angioedema, and wheezing are absent.
- Pseudoanaphylactic reaction:
  - After injection of procaine penicillin:
    - Is a drug effect of procaine and not a penicillin allergy
- Scombroid poisoning:
  - From ingestion of dark meat fish (e.g., tuna, mackerel, and mahi-mahi)
  - Histaminelike mediator: Symptoms include flushing, sweating, nausea, vomiting, diarrhea, headache, palpitations, dizziness, rash, swelling of face and tongue, respiratory distress, and vasodilatory shock.
- Serum sickness:
  - Occurs several days after exposure
- Systemic mastocytosis:
  - Benign or malignant overgrowth of mast cells
  - Urticaria pigmentosa seen in the benign form and the presence of reddish-brown macular–papular cutaneous lesions, which urticate after trauma (Darier sign)
- Vasovagal reactions:
  - Bradycardia and hypotension without tachycardia, flushing, urticaria, angioedema, pruritus, and wheezing
- Pulmonary embolism, foreign body aspiration, and arrhythmia

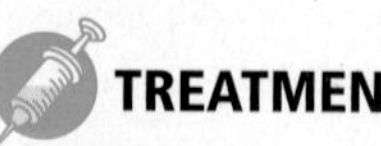

TREATMENT

MEDICATION

First Line

- Epinephrine:
  - Less severe reaction: 0.3–0.5 mg (0.01 mg/kg in children) = (0.3–0.5 mL of a 1:1,000 solution, 0.01 mL/kg in children), SQ q20–30min PRN, up to 3 doses
  - Life-threatening reactions: 0.5 mg (5 mL of a 1:10,000 solution) (for children: 0.05–0.1 mL/kg per dose) IV, slowly: q5–10min as needed. If IV access is not possible, endotracheal or intraosseous may be effective.
- Diphenhydramine: An H_1 blocker: 25–50 mg IV (IM or PO) q6h for 72 hours (children 1.25 mg/kg to 25 mg) (4)[A]
- Cimetidine: An H_2 blocker: 300 mg IV over 3–5 minutes (children 5–10 mg/kg per dose) and then 400 mg PO b.i.d. is helpful and may be more effective than diphenhydramine.

- Corticosteroids: Although routinely used, no immediate effect and no evidence for their use in the emergency department (2)[B]:
  - Hydrocortisone sodium succinate: 250–500 mg IV q4–6h (4–8 mg/kg for children)
  - Prednisone: 1 mg/kg in children, up to 60 mg
  - Methylprednisolone: 60–125 mg IV in adults (1–2 mg/kg in children)
- Bronchodilator, if persistent bronchospasm:
  - Inhaled beta-2 agonists. Continuous nebulized albuterol of 10 mg/hr or 2.5 mg q15–20min is safe, effective, and preferable to aminophylline as a first line.
- Laryngeal edema:
  - Epinephrine: 5 mL 1:1,000 by nebulizer is more effective than racemic epinephrine and is usually available.
- Persistent hypotension:
  - Dopamine: 200 mg in 500 mL of dextrose in water given by infusion pump; titrate to BP (3–20 mcg/kg/min)
  - Glucagon: May be beneficial for resistant hypotension caused by concurrent beta blockade therapy; 50 mcg/kg IV bolus over 1 minute, or alternatively, give as continuous infusion at 5–15 mcg/min
- Normal saline or Ringer's lactate: As necessary to maintain tissue perfusion
- Oral antihistamines for 72 hours

Geriatric Considerations

Epinephrine may induce myocardial ischemia in those with cardiac disease, but is the drug of choice. Be alert for anticholinergic and CNS side effects after giving diphenhydramine or cimetidine.

Pediatric Considerations

Epinephrine could reduce the placental blood flow, but may save the life of the mother and fetus. It also increases the risk of congenital malformation.

Second Line

- Several reports of tranexamic acid: 1,000 mg IV or sigma-aminocaproic acid for refractory anaphylaxis
- These drugs are not standard care; use only in patients who do not respond to other therapy.
- Aminophylline: 5–6 mg/kg IV in 100 cc D_5W over 20 minutes, then maintenance at 1 mg/kg/hr drip
- Anti-IgE monoclonal antibody may have a role in long-term management of food-induced anaphylaxis.
- Venom immunotherapy has been effective in the prevention of sting anaphylaxis, but with a high side-effect risk (2)[A].

ADDITIONAL TREATMENT

General Measures

- Treatment depends on severity.
- Maintain a patent airway:
  - Endotracheal intubation and assisted ventilation may be necessary.
  - Possibly tracheostomy or needle cricothyrotomy in children <12 years
- Oxygen
- IV fluids (normal saline/lactated Ringer's)

Issues for Referral

- Allergist referral if anaphylaxis cause unclear
- Patients with anaphylaxis from insect stings benefit from desensitization immunotherapy.

IN-PATIENT CONSIDERATIONS

Admission Criteria

Moderate–severe anaphylaxis, admit for observation.

Discharge Criteria

Outpatient: Patients with cutaneous angioedema, urticaria, and minimal bronchospasm may be released when symptoms and signs have cleared.

ONGOING CARE

FOLLOW-UP RECOMMENDATIONS

Bed rest until anaphylaxis clears and patient is hemodynamically stable

DIET

NPO until acute symptoms are controlled

PATIENT EDUCATION

- Asthma and Allergy Foundation of America, 1717 Massachusetts Avenue, Suite 305, Washington, DC 20036; (800)-7-ASTHMA or American Allergy Association, P.O. Box 7273, Menlo Park, CA 94026, (415) 322-1663
- Medic-Alert–type tags (Medic-Alert Foundation, Turlock, CA 95381–1009)
- Avoid beta-blockers, if possible.
- Instruct patient in the use of the bee sting kit.

PROGNOSIS

- Good prognosis if treated immediately; worse outcome with a delay of >30 minutes in administration of epinephrine.
- Of those with idiopathic anaphylaxis, 60% are free of anaphylactic episodes at 2.5 years; most others are steroid-free.

COMPLICATIONS

- Hypoxemia
- Cardiac arrest
- Death

REFERENCES

1. Brown SG, Blackman KE, Heddle RJ. Can serum mast cell tryptase help diagnose anaphylaxis? *EMA*. 2004;2:120–4.
2. Choo KJ, Simons E, Sheikh A. Glucocorticoids for the treatment of anaphylaxis. *Allergy*. 2010;65(10):1205–11. Epub 2010.
3. Brown SG, Wiese MD, Blackman KE, et al. Ant venom immunotherapy: A double-blind, placebo-controlled, crossover trial. *Lancet*. 2003;(361)9362:1001–6.
4. Sheikh A, Shehata YA, Brown SGA, Simons FER. Adrenaline (epinephrine) for the treatment of anaphylaxis with and without shock. *Cochrane Database of Systematic Reviews* 2008, Issue 4. Art. No.: CD006312. DOI:10.1002/14651858.CD006312.pub2.

ADDITIONAL READING

- Arias K, Waserman S, Jordana M. Management of food-induced anaphylaxis: Unsolved challenges. *Curr Clin Pharmacol*. 2009;4(2):113–25.
- González-Pérez A, Aponte Z, Vidaurre CF, et al. Anaphylaxis epidemiology in patients with and without asthma: A United Kingdom database review. *J Allergy Clin Immunol*. 2010;125(5): 1098–1104.
- Pitsios C, Dimitriou A, Stefanaki EC, et al. Anaphylaxis during skin testing with food allergens in children. *Eur J Pediatr*. 2010;169:613–5.
- Sheikh A, ten Broek VM, Brown SGA, et al. H1-antihistamines for the treatment of anaphylaxis with and without shock. *Cochrane Database Syst Rev*. 2007, Issue 1. Art. No.: CD006160. DOI:10.1002/14651858.CD006160.pub2.
- Tanus T, Mines D, Atkins PC, et al. Serum tryptase in idiopathic anaphylaxis: a case report and review of the literature. *Ann Emerg Med*. 1994;24:104–7.
- Wittbrodt ET, Spinler A. Prevention of anaphylactoid reactions in high-risk patients receiving radiographic contrast media. *Ann Pharmacother*. 1994;28: 236–41.

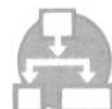

See Also (Topic, Algorithm, Electronic Media Element)

Arthropod Bites and Stings; Food Allergy

CODES

ICD9

- 989.5 Toxic effect of venom
- 995.0 Other anaphylactic reaction
- 995.60 Anaphylactic reaction due to unspecified food

CLINICAL PEARLS

- Allergy to one species of legume (e.g., peanuts) or one type of seafood (e.g., shrimp) doesn't mean allergy to all products in that category. Skin testing is prudent.
- Measles, mumps, rubella (MMR) vaccine can be safely administered to those with a history of egg allergy; most egg allergies are related to the albumin.
- Penicillin-allergic patients can generally tolerate 2nd- and 3rd-generation cephalosporins as well as monobactams (e.g., aztreonam). Generally, they will be allergic to carbapenems (e.g., imipenem) and 1st-generation cephalosporins.
- IgA-deficient patients should have washed red blood cells for transfusion.
- Those allergic to seafood are not allergic to iodine-based radiocontrast. Shellfish allergy is protein related.

ANEMIA, APLASTIC

Muthalagu Ramanathan, MD
Jan Cerny, MD, PhD

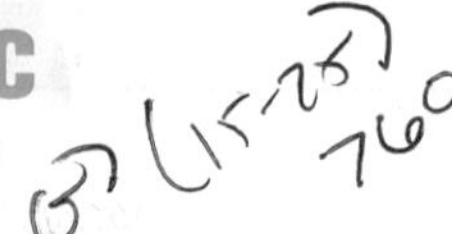

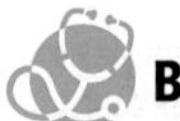

BASICS

DESCRIPTION

- A pancytopenia with hypocellular bone marrow without infiltrates or fibrosis. 2 forms: Acquired (much more common) and congenital
- Acquired aplastic anemia has an insidious onset and is caused by an exogenous insult triggering an autoimmune reaction. This form is usually responsive to immunosuppressive agents.
- The congenital forms are rare and occur mostly in childhood. The exception is an atypical presentation of Fanconi syndrome later in adult life, into the 30s for males and into the 40s for females.
- The identification of specific mutations in genes of the telomere complex in patients with acquired aplastic anemia has blurred the distinction between the congenital and acquired forms.
- System(s) affected: Heme/Lymphatic/Immunologic
- Synonym(s): Hypoplastic anemia; Panmyelophthisis; Refractory anemia; Aleukia hemorrhagica; Toxic paralytic anemia

ALERT

- Early intervention for aplastic anemia greatly improves the chances of treatment success.
- Hematopoietic growth factors should not be used without close monitoring in newly diagnosed patients.

Geriatric Considerations

The elderly are often exposed to large numbers of drugs and, therefore, may be more susceptible to acquired aplastic anemia.

Pediatric Considerations

- Congenital forms of aplastic anemia require different treatment regimens than the acquired forms.
- Acquired aplastic anemia is seen in children exposed to ionizing radiation or treated with cytotoxic chemotherapeutic agents.

Pregnancy Considerations

- Pregnancy appears to be a real but rare cause of aplastic anemia. Symptoms may resolve after delivery and have been shown to disappear with pregnancy termination.
- Complications in pregnant patients appear to be more likely from low platelet counts and paroxysmal nocturnal hemoglobinuria-associated aplastic anemia.

EPIDEMIOLOGY

- Predominant age: Biphasic 15–25 (more common) and over 60
- Predominant sex: Male = Female

Incidence

- 2–3 new cases per million per year in Europe and North America
- The incidence is 3-fold higher in Thailand and China, when compared to the Western world.

RISK FACTORS

- Treatment with high-dose radiation or chemotherapy
- Exposure to toxic chemicals
- Use of certain medications
- Certain blood diseases, autoimmune disorders, and serious infections
- Tumors of thymus (red cell aplasia)
- Pregnancy, rarely

Genetics

- Telomerase mutations have been found in a small number of patients with acquired and congenital forms. These mutations render carriers more susceptible to environmental insults.
- Mutations in genes called TERC and TERT were found in pedigrees of adults with acquired aplastic anemia who lacked the physical abnormalities or a family history typical of inherited forms of bone marrow failure. These genes encode for the RNA component of telomerase.
- HLA-DR2 is twice as frequent as in the normal population.

GENERAL PREVENTION

- Avoid possible toxic industrial agents.
- Use safety measures when working with radiation.

PATHOPHYSIOLOGY

- The immune hypothesis: Bone marrow suppression through activation of T cells with associated cytokine production leading to destruction or injury of hematopoietic stem cells. This leads to a hypocellular bone marrow without marrow fibrosis.
- The activation of T cells likely occurs because of both genetic and environmental factors. Exposure to specific environmental precipitants, diverse host genetic risk factors, and individual differences in characteristics of immune response likely account for variations in its clinical manifestations and patterns of responsiveness to treatment.
- Telomerase deficiency leads to short telomeres. This leads to impaired regenerative capacity and hence a reduction in marrow progenitors and likely a qualitative deficiency in the repair capacity of hematopoietic tissue.
- Reduction of natural killer T cells in the bone marrow

ETIOLOGY

- Idiopathic (~70% of the cases)
- Drugs: Phenylbutazone, chloramphenicol, sulfonamides, gold, cytotoxic drugs, antiepileptics (felbamate, carbamazepine, valproic acid, phenytoin)
- Viral: HIV, Epstein-Barr virus (EBV), nontypeable postinfectious hepatitis (not A, B, or C), parvovirus B19 (mostly in the immunocompromised), atypical mycobacterium
- Toxic exposure (benzene, pesticides, arsenic)
- Radiation exposure
- Immune disorders (systemic lupus erythematosus, eosinophilic fascitis, graft-vs.-host disease)
- Pregnancy (rare)
- Congenital (Fanconi anemia, dyskeratosis congenita, Shwachman-Diamond syndrome, amegakaryocytic thrombocytopenia)

DIAGNOSIS

HISTORY

- Solvent and radiation history, as well as family, environmental, travel, and infectious disease history
- Patients are often asymptomatic, but may complain of frequent infections, fatigue, headache, or bleeding/bruising.

PHYSICAL EXAM

- Mucosal hemorrhage, petechiae
- Pallor
- Fever
- Hemorrhage, menorrhagia, occult stool blood, melena, epistaxis
- Dyspnea
- Palpitations
- Progressive weakness
- Retinal flame hemorrhages
- Systolic ejection murmur
- Weight loss
- Signs of congenital aplastic anemia:
  - Short stature
  - Microcephaly
  - Nail dystrophy
  - Abnormal thumbs
  - Oral leukoplakia
  - Hyperpigmentation (café au lait spots) or hypopigmentation

DIAGNOSTIC TESTS & INTERPRETATION

Screening tests to exclude other etiologies:

- CBC and absolute reticulocyte count
- Blood smear exam
- Cytogenetic studies of peripheral lymphocytes if <35 yrs of age to exclude Fanconi anemia
- Liver function test
- Viral serology: Hepatitis A, B, C; EBV; cytomegalovirus (CMV); HIV
- Vitamin B_{12} and folate levels
- Autoantibody screening antinuclear antibody (ANA) and anti-DNA
- Flow cytometry looking for GPI, negative neutrophils and red blood cells (RBCs) for paroxysmal nocturnal hemoglobinuria
- Fetal hemoglobin in children
- Red cell adenosine deaminase (pure red cell aplasia)
- Cytogenetic analysis of bone marrow

Lab

- CBC: Pancytopenia, anemia (usually normocytic), leucopenia, neutropenia, thrombocytopenia
- Decreased absolute number of reticulocytes
- Increased serum iron secondary to transfusion
- Normal total iron binding capacity (TIBC)
- High mean corpuscular volume (MCV) >104
- CD 34+ cells decreased in blood and marrow
- Urinalysis: Hematuria
- Abnormal liver function tests (hepatitis)
- Increased fetal hemoglobin (Fanconi)
- Increased chromosomal breaks under specialized conditions (Fanconi)
- Molecular determination of abnormal gene (Fanconi)

Imaging

- CT of thymus region if thymoma-associated RBC aplasia suspected
- Radiographs of radius and thumbs (if congenital anemia suspected)
- Renal ultrasound (to rule out congenital anemia or malignant hematologic disorder)
- Chest x-ray to exclude infections such as mycobacterial

Diagnostic Procedures/Surgery

Bone marrow aspiration and biopsy

Pathological Findings

- Normochromic RBC
- Bone marrow:
  - Decreased cellularity (<10%): No fibrosis, no malignant cells seen
  - Decreased megakaryocytes
  - Decreased myeloid precursors
  - Decreased erythroid precursors
  - Prominent fat spaces and marrow stroma, polyclonal plasma cells

DIFFERENTIAL DIAGNOSIS

Includes other causes of bone marrow failure and pancytopenia:

- Marrow replacement:
  - Acute lymphoblastic leukemia
  - Lymphoma
  - Hairy cell leukemia (increased reticulin and infiltration of hairy cells)
  - Large granular lymphocyte leukemia
  - Fibrosis
- Megaloblastic hematopoiesis:
  - Folate deficiency
  - Vitamin B_{12} deficiency
- Paroxysmal nocturnal hemoglobinuria, hemolytic anemia (dark urine), pancytopenia venous thrombosis (classically hepatic veins)
- Systemic lupus erythematosus
- Prolonged starvation or anorexia nervosa (bone marrow is gelatinous with loss of fat cells and increased ground substance)
- Transient erythroblastopenia of childhood
- Drug-induced agranulocytosis that may be reversible on withdrawal of drug
- Overwhelming infection:
  - HIV with myelodysplasia
  - Viral hemophagocytic syndrome

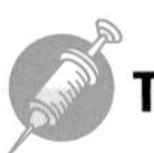

TREATMENT

Early treatment increases the chance of success. 2 major treatment options: Immunosuppressive therapy and hematopoietic stem cell transplantation. Treatment decisions are based on age of the patient, severity of disease, and availability of a human leukocyte antigen (HLA)-matched sibling donor for transplantation.

MEDICATION

First Line

- Immunosuppressive therapy:
  - First-line treatment is a combination of antithymocyte globulin (ATG) plus cyclosporine. ATG lyses lymphocytes, and cyclosporin blocks T cell function (1).
- Antithymocyte globulin (ATG):
  - A horse serum containing polyclonal antibodies against human T cells
  - Treatment for patients >40 years of age and patients without a compatible donor. Consider in patients 30–40 years of age.
  - May be used as a single agent but is more common in combination with cyclosporine
- Cyclosporine following initial ATG therapy for minimum of 6 months:
  - Monitor through blood levels. Normal values for assays vary.
  - Granulocyte colony-stimulating factor (G-CSF):
    - May be used in conjunction with ATG and cyclosporine
    - Shows faster neutrophil recovery, but survival is not improved
    - Treatment is costly and is disputed in 2 randomized trials.
  - Note: Relapses may occur after the initial response to the immunosuppressive therapy if cyclosporine is discontinued too early.
  - Stem cell: Matched sibling allogeneic stem cell transplant for age <20 and absolute neutrophil count (ANC) <500 or age 20–40 and ANC <200

Second Line

- Rabbit ATG + cyclosporine
- Campath
- Androgen in a subset of patients who have anemia predominantly

ADDITIONAL TREATMENT

General Measures

- Supportive measures: RBC and platelet transfusions. Use only irradiated, leukoreduced or CMV-negative blood initially if patient is candidate for hematopoietic stem cell transplantation.
- Antibiotics, antifungals, antivirals when appropriate, especially if ANC <200 cells/μL
- Oxygen therapy for severe anemia
- Good oral hygiene
- Control menorrhagia with norethisterone or oral contraceptive pills.
- Avoid causative agents/isolation if necessary.
- HLA testing on all patients and their immediate families
- Transfusion support (judiciously prescribed RBCs for severe anemia, consider leukocyte-depleted units; platelets for severe thrombocytopenia; white blood cells [WBCs]):
  - Transfuse when platelet count is $<10 \times 10^9$ or if $<20 \times 10^9$ with fever

SURGERY/OTHER PROCEDURES

- First-line hematopoietic stem cell transplantation for patients with an HLA-identical donor and severe aplastic anemia provided age <20 and ANC <500 or age 20–40 and ANC <200. Consider in patients 40–50 in good general medical condition.
- Patients >40 have higher rates of graft-vs.-host disease and graft rejection (2).
- Unrelated donor transplants for patients age <40 without HLA-matched sibling donor who failed second-line immunosuppressive therapy
- Thymectomy for thymoma

IN-PATIENT CONSIDERATIONS

Nursing

If neutropenic, use antiseptic mouthwash such as chlorhexidine.

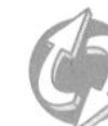

ONGOING CARE

FOLLOW-UP RECOMMENDATIONS

Activity: Isolation procedures if neutropenic

DIET

If neutropenic, give food low in bacterial content.

PATIENT EDUCATION

Printed patient information available from Aplastic Anemia & MDS International Foundation, Inc., 800-747-2828. Web: www.aamds.org/aplastic

PROGNOSIS

- Hematopoietic stem cell transplantation with HLA-matched sibling:
  - Age <16, 91%
  - Age >16, 70–80%
- Immunosuppressive therapy using ATG and cyclosporine: Overall survival of 75%; 90% among responders at 5 years

COMPLICATIONS

- Infection (fungal, sepsis)
- Graft-vs.-host disease in bone marrow transplant recipients (acute 18%; chronic 26%)
- Side effects of immunosuppressant medications
- Hemorrhage
- Transfusion hemosiderosis
- Transfusion hepatitis
- Heart failure
- Development of secondary cancer: Leukemia or myelodysplasia (15–19% risk at 6–10 years)
- Refractory pancytopenia

REFERENCES

1. Bacigalupo A, Passweg J. Diagnosis and treatment of acquired aplastic anemia. *Hematol Oncol Clin N Am*. 2009;23:159–70.
2. Brodsky RA, Jones RJ. Aplastic anaemia. *Lancet*. 2005;365:1647–56

ADDITIONAL READING

Rosenfeld S, Follman D, Nunez O, et al. Antithymocyte globulin and cyclosporine for severe aplastic anemia: Association between hematologic response and long-term outcome. *JAMA*. 2003;289(9):1130–35.

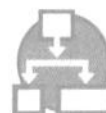

See Also (Topic, Algorithm, Electronic Media Element)

- Myelodysplastic Syndromes; Systemic Lupus Erythematosus (SLE)
- Algorithm: Anemia

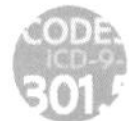

CODES

ICD9

- 284.01 Constitutional red blood cell aplasia
- 284.89 Other specified aplastic anemias
- 284.9 Aplastic anemia, unspecified

CLINICAL PEARLS

- Acquired aplastic anemia has an insidious onset and is caused by an exogenous insult triggering an autoimmune reaction. This form is usually responsive to immunosuppressive therapy.
- Immunosuppressive therapy using ATG and cyclosporine: Overall survival of 75%; 90% among responders at 5 years

ANEMIA, AUTOIMMUNE HEMOLYTIC

Jennifer Gao, MD
Nathan T. Connell, MD

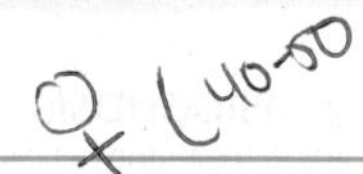

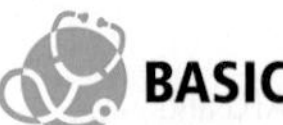

BASICS

DESCRIPTION
- Increased destruction of red blood cells (RBCs) in the presence of anti-RBC autoantibodies (1)
- 3 main types defined by maximal binding temperature of the autoantibodies (1):
  - Warm-reacting [at 37°C or 98.6°F] IgG antibody: Seen in 80–90% of cases
  - Cold-reacting [lower than 37°C or 98.6°F] IgM or IgG antibody
  - Mixed type: Both warm-reacting IgG and cold-reacting C3 antibodies
- Drug-induced: Mostly warm-reacting IgG antibodies
- System(s) affected: Hematopoietic; Lymphatic; Immunologic

EPIDEMIOLOGY
Incidence
- Predominant age: Adults 40–50 years old (2)
- Predominant sex: Female > Male
- Annual incidence of 1–3 per 100,000 individuals (1)
- Cold agglutinin: Primarily affects young patients (2)

RISK FACTORS
- Malignancy
- Autoimmune disorders
- Infection
- Medications
- Prior blood transfusion
- Prior hematopoietic cell transplant

Genetics
No known genetic or familial hereditary component (2)

PATHOPHYSIOLOGY
- Warm autoimmune hemolytic anemia (AIHA): IgG attaches to RBCs, which are then ingested by splenic macrophages .
- Cold AIHA:
  - IgM binding to RBC surfaces activates C3b-mediated phagocytosis by liver Kupffer cells (2).
  - Rare mechanism in setting of low IgM levels: Membrane attack complex insertion causes intravascular hemolysis (2).
- Mixed-antibody AIHA: Warm IgG and cold C3 involved (2)
- Drug-induced:
  - Hapten-induced: Drug attaches to RBC to induce IgG production.
  - Immune complex: Drug–IgM immune complex binds RBC to activate complement.
  - Autoantibody: Drug induces production of anti-RBC IgG.

ETIOLOGY
- Autoantibody most common cause (1):
  - Warm antibody (48–70% of cases):
    - Primary cause: idiopathic
    - Secondary causes:
      - Lymphoproliferative disorders: Chronic lymphocytic leukemia, Hodgkin lymphoma, non-Hodgkin lymphoma
      - Autoimmune disorders: Systemic lupus erythematosus
      - Viral infections: Especially common in children
      - Chronic inflammatory disorders: Crohn disease, ulcerative colitis
  - Cold antibody:
    - Cold agglutinin syndrome (CAS, 16–32% of cases)
      - Acute: Infections (mycoplasma, mononucleosis, viral)
      - Chronic: Lymphoproliferative disorders (lymphoma) (2)
      - Paroxysmal cold hemoglobinuria
  - Alloantibody (2):
    - Post transplant
    - Pregnancy
    - Post transfusion
- Mixed type:
  - Idiopathic
  - Secondary to lymphoproliferative or autoimmune disorders
- Drug-induced (2):
  - Penicillin: Hapten-induced
  - Quinine: Immune complex
  - α-methyldopa: Autoantibody-induced
  - Also seen with cefotetan, ceftriaxone, alemtuzumab, mycophenolate, purine analogs, alkylating agents

COMMONLY ASSOCIATED CONDITIONS
- Evans syndrome (AIHA and idiopathic thrombocytopenic purpura)
- Systemic lupus erythematosus
- Chronic lymphocytic leukemia (CLL): AIHA is the most common autoimmune condition associated with CLL and occurs in 5–37% of patients with CLL (2).
- Diffuse lymphomas

DIAGNOSIS

HISTORY
- Clinical triad: Anemia, splenomegaly, jaundice (2)
- Weakness/fatigue
- Exertional dyspnea
- Dizziness
- Palpitations
- Malaise

PHYSICAL EXAM
- Pallor
- Jaundice
- Splenomegaly
- Hepatomegaly
- Tachycardia
- Flow murmur
- Blue-gray discoloration of acral surfaces (CAS)

DIAGNOSTIC TESTS & INTERPRETATION
Lab

Initial lab tests
- Direct Coombs (direct antiglobulin test [DAT]): Positive test indicates presence of antibodies or complement on RBC surface (4)
- CBC (4):
  - Anemia (normocytic, normochromic); may be sudden and life threatening
  - Mild-to-moderate increase in mean corpuscular volume depending on level of reticulocytosis
  - Increased mean cell hemoglobin concentration
- Peripheral blood smear (4):
  - Spherocytosis
  - Poikilocytosis
  - Anisocytosis
  - Rouleaux
  - Reticulocytosis
  - Nucleated RBCs
  - Large polychromatophilic reticulocytes
- Hyperbilirubinemia (unconjugated)
- Decreased haptoglobin
- Elevated lactate dehydrogenase
- Hemoglobinemia
- Serology:
  - IgG antibody (warm, mixed, drug-induced, paroxysmal hemoglobinuria)
  - IgM antibody (cold)
- Urinalysis: Hemoglobinuria, hemosiderinuria (1)

Pathological Findings
- Peripheral blood smear: Spherocytes, schistocytes
- Bone marrow biopsy: Bone marrow hyperplasia, increased marrow hemosiderin

DIFFERENTIAL DIAGNOSIS
- Other hemolytic anemias
- Evans syndrome
- Microangiopathic hemolytic disorders
- Aplastic anemia
- Megaloblastic anemia

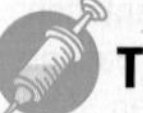

TREATMENT

MEDICATION
First Line
- Warm antibody:
  - Glucocorticoids (4)
    - Use danazol + prednisone for best response.
    - ~80% patients improve within 3 weeks
    - Taper gradually, may require maintenance dose
    - Precautions: Significant side effects with long-term use
- Cold antibody:
  - Malignancy-induced: Chemotherapy
  - Rituximab if concomitant CLL (4)
- Mixed antibody: Glucocorticoids as in warm AIHA

Second Line

- Warm antibody (4):
  - IV immunoglobin (IVIG) controversial
  - Immunosuppressive drugs: If fail splenectomy, relapse status post (s/p) splenectomy, cannot tolerate glucocorticoids, nonsurgical candidate
    - Cyclophosphamide: Monitor for marrow suppression.
    - Azathioprine
    - Cyclosporine
    - Alemtuzumab (anti-CD52 antibody): Use if concomitant CLL
    - Rituximab (anti-CD20 antibody): Median response rate 60%
    - Mycophenolate mofetil
    - Danazol
- Mixed antibody: Immunosuppressives if refractory to steroids and splenectomy

ADDITIONAL TREATMENT

General Measures

- Warm antibody:
  - Folic acid supplementation
  - Mild and moderate: See "Medication."
  - Severe:
    - Controversial: Plasmapheresis or packed RBC transfusion
    - Pregnancy warning: Need adsorption studies to identify alloantibodies (1)
- Cold antibody:
  - Cold agglutinin syndrome:
    - Avoid cold; maintain high temperatures indoors; wear additional clothing outdoors
    - Folic acid supplementation
    - Controversial: Plasmapheresis or packed RBC transfusion
- Paroxysmal cold hemoglobinuria: Supportive care
- Mixed: Same as warm antibody
- Drug-induced:
  - Stop the offending drug.
  - Plasmapheresis/exchange transfusion for severe life-threatening cases

Issues for Referral

Consult an experienced hematologist.

SURGERY/OTHER PROCEDURES

- Warm antibody: Splenectomy second-line treatment if fail glucocorticoids (4):
  - Success rate 38–70% for idiopathic cases
  - May require low-dose maintenance glucocorticoid
  - 2 weeks presplenectomy: Vaccinate against encapsulated organisms.
- Cold antibody: Surgery not recommended
- Mixed antibody: Splenectomy

IN-PATIENT CONSIDERATIONS

Initial Stabilization

If patients start to develop symptoms related to the anemia (i.e., tachycardia, hypotension, chest pain, dyspnea), transfusion may be required.

Admission Criteria

Patients requiring plasmapheresis should be monitored in an intensive care unit (ICU) setting

IV Fluids

ALERT

Use only warmed IV fluids and blood products for cold AIHA in order to prevent further exacerbation of the condition.

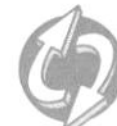

ONGOING CARE

FOLLOW-UP RECOMMENDATIONS

Patient Monitoring

- Monitor carefully if a transfusion is essential.
- Use only warm IV fluids and blood products for cold AIHA.
- Avoid hypothermic surgical procedures for cold AIHA.
- At increased risk for venous thromboembolism, especially if concomitant systemic lupus erythematosus (SLE): Consider prophylactic anticoagulation (5).

PROGNOSIS

- Good with appropriate treatment
- Determined by course of the primary disease if secondary to an underlying disorder

COMPLICATIONS

- Shock (severe anemia)
- Venous thromboembolism
- Thrombocytopenic purpura (Evans syndrome)
- Lymphoproliferative disorders in warm AIHA
- Postsplenectomy sepsis syndrome

REFERENCES

1. Barros M, Blajchman M, Bordin J. Warm autoimmune hemolytic anemia: Recent progress in understanding the immunobiology and treatment. *Transfusion Med Rev*. 2010;24(3):195–210.
2. Lambert F, Nydegger U. Geoepidemiology of autoimmune hemolytic anemia. *Autoimmun Rev*. 2010;9:A350–354.
3. Zent CS, Ding W, Reinalda MS, et al. Autoimmune cytopenia in chronic lymphocytic leukemia/small lymphocytic lymphoma: Changes in clinical presentation and prognosis. *Leuk Lymphoma*. 2009;50:1261–8.
4. Blackall D. How I approach patients with warm-reactive antibodies. *Transfusion*. 2011;51: 14–17.
5. Hoffman PC. Immune hemolytic anemia–selected topics. *Hematology Am Soc Hematol Educ Program*. 2006;13–8.

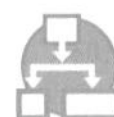

See Also (Topic, Algorithm, Electronic Media Element)

- Lymphoma, Non-Hodgkin's; Leukemia; Systemic Lupus Erythematosus (SLE)
- Algorithm: Anemia

CODES

ICD9

283.0 Autoimmune hemolytic anemias

CLINICAL PEARLS

- Initial workup: CBC, direct Coombs (direct antiglobulin test), fractionated bilirubin, haptoglobin, lactate dehydrogenase (LDH), urinalysis
- Must distinguish between cold and warm antibody disease for proper treatment.
- Hospitalize with ICU care if necessary.
- Consult with experienced hematologist.

ANEMIA, CHRONIC DISEASE

Cheryl L. Gilmartin, PharmD
Claudia M. Lora, MD

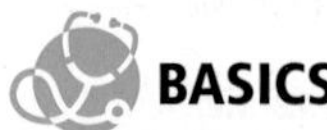

BASICS

DESCRIPTION

Anemia of chronic disease (ACD) is a normocytic, normochromic, hypoproliferative anemia associated with infectious, neoplastic, and inflammatory processes. The chronic immune activation accompanying these processes results in the production of inflammatory cytokines, which in turn create an anemic state by interfering with iron homeostasis and impairing erythropoiesis. ACD is the second most common type of anemia and is the most common anemia found in hospitalized patients (1).

EPIDEMIOLOGY

Incidence

Incidence of anemia in cancer: 30–90% (2)

Prevalence

The estimated reports of ACD prevalence for individual conditions vary widely in the literature.

PATHOPHYSIOLOGY

Inflammatory cytokines (e.g., TNF-α, IFN-γ, IL-6) released by cells of the immune system in the setting of malignant, autoimmune, or infectious disease are the major mediators of anemia in ACD. They exert their effects in three main ways:

- Disrupted iron homeostasis:
  - Chronic inflammation, infection, malignancy → ↑ IFN-γ, LPS, TNF-α → ↑ iron uptake by and ↓ iron release from reticuloendothelial system (RES) cells → ↓ iron availability for heme biosynthesis and RBC production in the bone marrow
  - Chronic inflammation, infection, malignancy → ↑ IL-6, LPS → ↑ hepatocyte production of hepcidin, a major negative iron regulator → ↓ iron absorption in duodenum and ↓ iron release from RES cells → ↓ iron availability for RBC production
- Impaired erythropoiesis:
  - ↑ IFN-γ, TNF-α, IL-1 → down regulation of erythropoietin (EPO) receptors on erythroid precursors, cytokine-induced apoptosis of erythroid precursors, ↓ hematopoietic growth factors in the marrow → impaired function, proliferation, and differentiation of erythroid cells → ↓ RBC production
  - ↑ IFN-γ, TNF-α, IL-1 → ↓ synthesis and diminished effect of EPO → ↓ RBC production
- RBC destruction:
  - ↑ TNF-α, IL-1 → ↑ phagocytosis of RBCs by RES cells → ↓ RBC half-life
  - ↑ IFN-γ, TNF-α, IL-1 → ↑ free radical formation → ↑ RBC destruction

ETIOLOGY

Inflammatory cytokines (e.g., TNF-α, IFN-γ, IL-6) released by cells of the immune system in the setting of infectious, inflammatory, or neoplastic diseases cause anemia by interfering with iron metabolism and RBC production.

COMMONLY ASSOCIATED CONDITIONS

- Autoimmune disease:
  - Rheumatoid arthritis
  - Systemic lupus erythematosus
  - Inflammatory bowel disease
  - Sarcoidosis
  - Vasculitis
- Infectious disease:
  - HIV and other viral infections
  - Chronic or subacute bacterial, fungal, parasitic infection
- Neoplastic disease:
  - Both solid and hematologic tumors
- Chronic kidney disease (CDK)
- Chronic rejection post solid-organ transplantation

DIAGNOSIS

HISTORY

History or symptoms of an acute or chronic inflammatory, infectious, or neoplastic process and no clinical evidence for occult bleeding

PHYSICAL EXAM

Findings related to the underlying disease

DIAGNOSTIC TESTS & INTERPRETATION

Lab

Initial lab tests

- Hemoglobin: Mild (Hgb <10–12 g/dL) or moderate (Hgb 8–10 g/dL) or severe (Hgb <8 g/dL) anemia
  - Assess patients with CKD: Hgb <11 g/dL
  - Assess patients with cancer: Hgb <11 g/dL or a drop from baseline >2 g/dL
- MCV: Normal, 80–100 fL (in the absence of coexistent additional cause of anemia)
- Peripheral smear: No evidence of other hematologic disorders
- Reticulocyte count (production index): Inappropriately low or normal, <2%
- Serum iron: Low (M: <65 μg/dL, F: <50 μg/dL)
- Transferrin or TIBC: Low
  - CKD or patients with cancer TSAT >20%
- Ferritin: Normal (M: 215–365 mg/dL, F: 250–380 mg/dL) or high in the absence of coexisting iron deficiency
- Elevated levels ESR, CRP, fibrinogen, cytokines
- Rule out other causes of anemia: TSH, Hgb electrophoresis, B_{12} and folate levels, direct and indirect Coombs tests, bone marrow aspiration.

DIFFERENTIAL DIAGNOSIS

- Iron deficiency anemia
- Thalassemia
- Myelodysplastic syndromes
- Hyperthyroidism or hypothyroidism
- Hypopituitarism
- Hyperparathyroidism

TREATMENT

- Treat the underlying disease (1).
- RBC transfusion may be considered in severe (< 8.0 g/dL) or life threatening (< 6.5 g/dL) anemia (1).
- The erythropoietic stimulating agents (ESA), recombinant erythropoietin (rEPO), and darbepoetin (DARB) decrease the need for transfusions, increase hemoglobin levels, and may improve quality of life in patients with CKD. The Food and Drug Administration recommends therapy should be initiated when hemoglobin levels (Hgb) are <10 g/dL and TSAT >20%. The National Kidney Foundation Kidney Disease Outcomes Quality Initiatives (KDOQI) recommend individual evaluation of the benefit of ESA utilization and maintaining the Hgb between 11 and 12 g/dL, TSAT >20% and ferritin >100 ng/mL in nondialysis CKD patients, and >200 ng/mL in dialysis-treated CKD patients (4)[A]. The FDA, however, recommends Hgb be maintained at levels <11 g/dL in CKD stage 5 and at ≤10 g/dL in CKD stage 3–4 (9).
- rEPO also increases Hgb levels in patients with ACD from HIV and CKD.
- DARB has a simpler dosing schedule than rEPO (6).
- Iron therapy given prior to or concurrently with ESA improves response to ESA. IV iron is recommended for hemodialysis-treated CKD patients. Iron indices should be evaluated prior to and during ESA use (4).
- Target Hgb levels in patients treated with ESA should not exceed 12 g/dL because of the increased risk of thromboembolic events at higher levels.
- Treatment with ESA should be reserved for symptomatic chemotherapy-induced anemia (CIA) in cancer treatment without curative intent (i.e., palliative treatment). ESA therapy should not be continued beyond 6–8 weeks after completion of chemotherapy (5)[A].
- Iron studies and IV iron supplementation are recommended for absolute iron deficiency (ferritin <30 ng/mL and TSAT <15%) and considered for functional iron deficiency (ferritin <800 ng/mL and TSAT <20%) in patients receiving ESA for palliative treatment (5).
- ESA therapy in patients with cancer has been associated with increased risk of venous thromboembolism and mortality (6).
- CIA symptomatic and asymptomatic patients with comorbidities receiving myelosuppressive chemotherapy with curative intent should be evaluated for red blood cell transfusions to maintain an Hgb between 8 and 10 g/dL (5).

MEDICATION

- Epoetin α:
  - CKD start at 50–100 U/kg IV or SC 3 times a week (TIW). ESA dosage should be adjusted according to the patient's Hgb level and response (4).
  - Cancer patients on chemotherapy start at 150 U/kg SC TIW or 40,000 U SC weekly; if no rise in Hgb >1 g/dL in 4 weeks, may increase to 300 U/kg TIW or 60,000 U SC weekly, respectively (5). Decrease dose by 25% if a rise in Hgb >1 g/dL in any 2-week period.

- Darbepoetin α:
  - CKD start at 0.45 μg/kg IV or SC weekly; alternative for CKD not on dialysis 0.75 μg/kg SC every 2 weeks. Dose adjustments are made similar to epoetin α (4).
  - Cancer patients on chemotherapy start with 2.25 μg/kg weekly or 500 μg/kg every 3 weeks SC. If Hgb rise $\leq$1 g/dL in 4 weeks, increase to 4.5 μg/kg SC weekly (5). Decrease dose by 40% if an increase in Hgb >1 g/dL in any 2-week period.
- ESA dosing should be titrated to the lowest Hgb level to avoid transfusion.
- With EPO/DARB use:
  - CKD: Increased risk for death, stroke, and serious cardiovascular events when dosed to Hgb $\geq$13 g/dL
  - Cancer-related anemia and CIA with curative intent: ESA therapy is not indicated, except in CIA without curative intent.
  - ESA therapy should be avoided in CKD patients with cancer who are:
    - Not receiving chemotherapy
    - Actively treated with chemotherapy for curable solid tumors. After chemotherapy risk/benefit assessment for ESA use considering residual neoplastic disease (5)
  - The FDA has included ESA therapy in CIA without curative intent in the Risk Evaluation and Mitigation Strategy (REMS) to assess the risk vs benefit for ESA use in this indication. To utilize ESA therapy physicians need to enroll in the **A**ssisting **P**roviders and cancer **P**atients with **R**isk **I**nformation for the **S**afe use of **E**SAs (APPRISE). Enrollment in the ESA Oncology APPRISE Program may be found at www.esa-apprise.com or by calling 1-866-284-8089.

ADDITIONAL TREATMENT

- IV iron is recommended to treat iron deficiency in CKD patients receiving hemodialysis and CIA patients receiving ESA (4,5).
- The FDA recommends the following iron indices prior to ESA use:
  - TSAT >20% and ferritin >100 ng/mL
- To calculate an iron repletion dose for CIA patients receiving ESA:
  - Dose = 0.0442 (desired Hgb–observed Hgb) x lean body weight (LBW) + (0.26 × LBW)
- Test doses are required for iron dextran:
  - 25 mg slow IVP then wait 1 hour prior to administering dose
- Low-molecular-weight iron dextran (INFed) is preferred for CIA patients receiving ESA due to decreased adverse events (5).
- Ferric gluconate, iron sucrose, and ferumoxytol are indicated for CKD. Ferric gluconate and iron sucrose may be utilized in CIA (5). Test doses are not required for the aforementioned iron products.
- Iron dextran administration 100 mg IV over 5 minutes may repeat per treatment or total dose infusion over several hours.
- Ferric gluconate 125 mg slow IVP or 125 mg IVPB over 60 minutes or 200 mg over 3–4 hours.
- Iron sucrose 100–200 mg IVP or 2–5 minutes or 100–200 mg IVPB over 1 hour.
- Ferumoxytol 510 mg IVP over 17 seconds.

General Measures

- Most patients with ACD have asymptomatic anemia. If anemia becomes severe (Hgb <8 g/dL) or patient is symptomatic, transfuse with PRBCs, especially if concurrent bleeding.
- Long-term transfusion therapy is not recommended in ACD patients with chronic kidney disease (1).

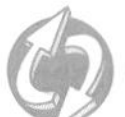

ONGOING CARE

FOLLOW-UP RECOMMENDATIONS

To minimize the risks of thromboembolic events, the lowest dose needed to avoid RBC transfusion should be utilized (5).

Patient Monitoring

- Hgb or hematocrit levels should be checked biweekly until a stable dose, then monthly.
- TSAT and ferritin should be >20% and >100 ng/mL respectively, prior to initiating ESA therapy.
- Iron indices for patients with CKD should be obtained prior to initiating ESA therapy and then every 3 months or more often if clinically needed.
- For patients with CIA receiving palliative ESA treatment: ferritin <800 ng/mL and TSAT<20%; consider IV iron supplementation.

PATIENT EDUCATION

- Patients treated with CIA without curative intent should be advised ESA may cause:
  - Tumor progression
  - Early mortality in some patients
  - Blood clots which may precipitate a heart attack, stroke, or heart failure
- Patients treated with CIA without curative intent are required to read an ESA medication guide and understand the risks and benefits of ESA use.
- Patients treated with CIA without curative intent need to give signed informed consent prior to ESA use.
- Medication guides may also be provided to CKD patients treated with ESA.
- Medication guides for ESA are available at:
  - http://pi.amgen.com/united_states/aranesp/ckd/aranesp_mg_hcp_english.pdf
  - http://pi.amgen.com/united_states/epogen/epogen_mg_hcp_english.pdf
  - http://www.procrit.com/sites/default/files/shared/OBI/PI/MedGuide.pdf

PROGNOSIS

Although ACD is chronic, it is usually not progressive.

COMPLICATIONS

- Anemia is associated with a worse prognosis in cardiovascular, chronic renal, and neoplastic disease (1).
- Treating anemia with ESA in these conditions improves quality of life (1) but may not improve length of life (and may shorten in some circumstances).

REFERENCES

1. Weiss G. Anemia of chronic disease. *N Engl J Med*. 2005;52:1011–23.
2. Knight K, Wade S, Balducci L. Prevalence and outcomes of anemia in cancer: a systematic review of the literature. *Am J Med*. 2004;116(Suppl 7A): 11S–26S.
3. KDOQI, National Kidney Foundation. KDOQI Clinical Practice Guidelines and Clinical Practice Recommendations for Anemia in Chronic Kidney Disease. *Am J Kidney Dis*. 2006;47:S11–145.
4. Vanrenterghem Y, Bárány P, Mann JF, et al. Randomized trial of darbepoetin alfa for treatment of renal anemia at a reduced dose frequency compared with rHuEPO in dialysis patients. *Kidney Int*. 2002;62:2167–75.
5. National Comprehensive Cancer Network (NCCN.org). Jenkintown: NCCN Clinical Practice Guidelines in Oncology. Cancer- and Chemotherapy-Induced Anemia. V.2.2011. Accessed June 6, 2011 Fort Washington: National Comprehensive Cancer Network; 2011, at http://www.nccn.org/professionals/physician_gls/PDF/anemia.pdf.
6. Bennett CL, Silver SM, Djulbegovic B, et al. Venous thromboembolism and mortality associated with recombinant erythropoietin and darbepoetin administration for the treatment of cancer-associated anemia. *JAMA*. 2008;299: 914–24.

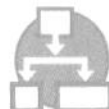

See Also (Topic, Algorithm, Electronic Media Element)

Algorithm: Anemia

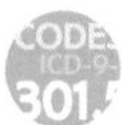

CODES

ICD9

- 285.21 Anemia in chronic kidney disease
- 285.22 Anemia in neoplastic disease
- 285.29 Anemia of other chronic disease

CLINICAL PEARLS

- ACD and iron-deficiency anemia (IDA) may coexist. The following parameters can generally distinguish them:
  - ACD-normocytic, ↓ or normal transferrin, ↑ or normal ferritin, normal soluble transferrin receptor levels (sTfR), ratio sTfRods:log ferritin <1
  - IDA-microcytic, ↑ transferrin, ↓ ferritin, ↑ sTfR levels, ratio sTfR:log ferritin >2
- Anemia in ACD is usually symptomatic, although anemia is often mild or moderate. Patients with ACD always have an underlying disease, such as RA, cancer, or CKD. These diseases will usually limit the patient's mobility, exercise capacity, or energy level, and typical symptoms of anemia (e.g., exertional dyspnea, fatigue, weakness) are attributed to the underlying disease.
- Iron sequestration and anemia may be an adaptive response when inflammation, infection, or neoplasia is present. When iron is hoarded in RES cells in ACD, rapidly proliferating microorganisms or tumor cells do not have access to it, thereby limiting their growth. These rapidly proliferating cells also have increased oxygen demand, which is more difficult to meet in an anemic state.

ANEMIA, IRON DEFICIENCY

Jennifer O'Brien, MD
Fred Schiffman, MD

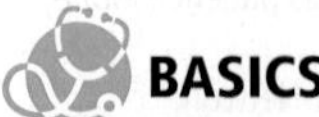

BASICS

DESCRIPTION

- Deficiency in red blood cells, hemoglobin, or blood volume due to decreased iron stores
- Onset may be acute with rapid blood loss or chronic, with nutrition derangement or slow blood loss.
- System(s) affected: Hemi, Lymphatic, Immunologic
- Synonym(s): Anemia of chronic blood loss; Hypochromic; Microcytic anemia; Chlorosis

Geriatric Considerations

60% of anemias occur in people >65 years of age.

Pediatric Considerations

Frequent problem in infants whose major source of nutrition is unfortified cow's milk and/or juices

Pregnancy Considerations

Common during pregnancy unless iron supplements are included in the diet

EPIDEMIOLOGY

- Iron deficiency anemia (IDA) is the most common cause of anemia in the US.
- Predominant age: All ages, but especially among toddlers and menstruating women
- Predominant sex: Female > male
- More likely in the poor and in underimmunized children

Incidence

- Adults: Men 2%, women 15–20% annually
- Infants and toddlers: 3–5% annually
- Pregnant patients: 20%

Prevalence

- Infants and children <12 years old: 4–7% (1)
- Men: 2–5% (1)
- Women: 9–16% (18–50% in menstruant blood donors) (1,2)

RISK FACTORS

- Premenopausal woman
- Frequent blood donor
- Pregnancy and breast-feeding
- Strict vegan diet
- Use of NSAIDs

GENERAL PREVENTION

- Screen asymptomatic pregnant women (3)[B].
- Supplementation in asymptomatic children aged 6–12 months if at increased risk for IDA (3)[B]

PATHOPHYSIOLOGY

Depletion of iron stores leads to decrease in reticulocyte count and decrease in production of hemoglobin.

ETIOLOGY

- Blood loss (e.g., menses, GI bleeding, trauma)
- Poor iron intake
- Poor iron absorption (e.g., atrophic gastritis, postgastrectomy, celiac disease)
- Increased demand for iron (e.g., infancy, adolescence, pregnancy and breast-feeding)

COMMONLY ASSOCIATED CONDITIONS

- GI tract malignancy, peptic ulcer disease (PUD), *Helicobacter pylori* infection, irritable bowel disease
- Hookworm or other parasitic infestations
- Hypermetrorrhagia
- Pregnancy

DIAGNOSIS

HISTORY

- Asymptomatic in most cases
- Weakness, fatigue, and/or malaise
- Exertional dyspnea
- Palpitations
- Angina in patients with coronary artery disease
- Headaches or inability to concentrate
- Melena
- Pica

PHYSICAL EXAM

- Pallor
- Cheilosis
- Tachycardia
- Tachypnea
- Koilonychia (spoon-shaped, brittle nails)

DIAGNOSTIC TESTS & INTERPRETATION

Lab

Initial lab tests

- Hemoglobin: <13 g in men and <12 g in women (4). Patients with higher premorbid hemoglobin (such as those with chronic hypoxemia, smokers, those who live at high altitudes) may be anemic at higher hemoglobin levels.
- Mean corpuscular volume (MCV): <80 fL
- Ferritin: <41 ng/mL (98% sensitivity and specificity); gold standard noninvasive test for diagnosis in adults, but may miss some deficient patients (e.g., cirrhosis) because ferritin is an acute-phase reactant.
- Total iron-binding capacity (TIBC): Increased
- Transferrin saturation: <9%
- CBC with differential, peripheral smear, reticulocyte count, and index. A peripheral smear usually shows hypochromia and microcytosis, but may be normal, and reticulocyte production index is low.
- Iron/TIBC (transferrin ratio) is usually not recommended because it is less sensitive and less specific than ferritin.
- Consider testing for G6PD deficiency: Assay at least 6 weeks after the last drop in hemoglobin.
- Rule out thalassemia:
  - Review prior CBCs for persisting mild anemia and marked micro-ovalocytosis, elevated hemoglobin A2 or hemoglobin F, family history, and especially high or high normal red blood cell (RBC) count
  - A low RBC count in patients with chronic bleeding helps to distinguish it from the thalassemia trait, where the count is high or high-normal.
  - Microcytosis with ovalocytosis and anemia unresponsive to iron suggests the thalassemia trait.
- MCV may be normal in mild anemia or hidden by the population of larger cells (e.g., reticulocytes or macrocytes). Red cell distribution width will be increased if a mixed population of cells is present (e.g., mixed iron deficiency anemia and B_{12} deficiency)
- An empiric trial of iron at 3 mg/kg/d may be the best way to diagnose decreased iron stores in infants and children; reticulocytes become elevated in 7–10 days or hemoglobin increases >1.0 g/dL weekly, indicating iron deficiency.
- Drugs that may alter lab results: Iron supplements or multivitamin–mineral preparations that contain iron
- Disorders that may alter lab results:
  - Elevated ferritin: Acute or chronic liver disease, Hodgkin disease, acute leukemia, solid tumors, fever, acute inflammation, renal dialysis
  - Elevated hemoglobin: Smoking, chronic hypoxemia, long-term residency at high altitude
  - Stool guaiac (2)[C]; if high index of suspicion of GI bleed, perform GI endoscopy. Under appropriate circumstances, check stool for ova and parasites.
  - Rule out poor reutilization: Trial of iron, bone marrow aspiration, and iron stain
  - Rule out colorectal cancer and gastric carcinoma, especially in the elderly.

Diagnostic Procedures/Surgery

- GI endoscopy to evaluate for bleeding sites
- Bone marrow aspiration confirms diagnosis, but is rarely performed

Pathological Findings

- Absent marrow iron stores
- Marrow: Hyperplastic, micronormoblastic

DIFFERENTIAL DIAGNOSIS

- GI bleeding (e.g., gastritis, PUD, carcinoma, varices)
- Chronic intravascular hemolysis (e.g., paroxysmal nocturnal hemoglobinuria, malfunctioning prosthetic valve)
- Defective iron utilization (e.g., thalassemia trait, sideroblastosis, G6PD deficiency)
- Defective iron reutilization (e.g., infection, inflammation, cancer, other chronic diseases)
- Hypoproliferation (e.g., decreased erythropoietin from hypothyroidism, renal failure)

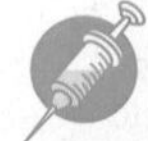

TREATMENT

MEDICATION

- Ferrous sulfate 325 mg 3 times per day on an empty stomach 1 hour before meals provides 180 mg of elemental iron per day:
  - Reduce dose as needed for GI symptoms, which affect 25% of patients receiving standard iron therapy; or, the dose can be taken with meals, which may reduce the delivery of iron by 50%. Constipation will occur in ~1 in 4 patients using various iron formulations (5).
  - Drugs that increase gastric pH (e.g., proton pump inhibitors, H_2 antagonists) also reduce iron absorption (6).
  - Individuals with moderate anemia (mercury = 10 g/dL) need only a total of 1,500–2,000 mg of elemental iron replacement; reducing the iron per dose as much as necessary to abate adverse effects will make parenteral iron therapy unnecessary in almost all cases.

– Special oral iron formulations (including enteric-coated iron) and compounds are expensive and reduce symptoms only to the degree that they reduce the delivery of iron.
- Liquid iron preparations are useful for children, with a recommended dose of 3 mg/kg/d; can also be used in adults when tablets are not absorbed or low tolerance requires a dose reduction.
- Foods and beverages containing ascorbic acid (vitamin C) enhance iron absorption when taken simultaneously with the iron.
- Continued bleeding and untreated hypothyroidism are causes for "failure to respond" to iron.
- Consider parenteral iron for patients with an hemoglobin level <6 g/dL, malabsorption, or if higher oral doses and use of vitamin C fail:
  – Anaphylaxis to parenteral iron therapy has occurred; ferric gluconate or iron sucrose may be safer alternatives to iron dextran (7,8)[B]. Dimercaprol increases risk of nephrotoxicity.
  – Iron sucrose 200 mg IV, 5 doses over 2 weeks, or 500 mg IV, 2 doses every 2 weeks (less experience with this regimen); total dose is 1,000 mg, then re-evaluate. 1 mL = 20 mg elemental iron. Hemodialysis-dependent patients should receive 100 mg 1–3 times per week for total of 10 doses.
- Reserve blood transfusion for severe acute blood loss or severely symptomatic patients (e.g., demand ischemia due to anemia). Hemoglobin threshold varies by risk factors and clinical scenario.
- Contraindications (oral iron):
  – Antacids concomitantly
  – Dairy products concomitantly
  – Tetracycline concomitantly
- Significant possible interactions (oral iron):
  – Allopurinol
  – Antacids
  – Penicillamine
  – Quinolones
  – Tetracyclines
  – Vitamin E
- Precautions:
  – Iron preparations may cause black bowel movements and constipation.
  – Iron overdose is highly toxic; patients should be instructed to keep tablets and liquids out of the reach of small children.

ADDITIONAL TREATMENT

General Measures

- Search for the cause and correct it.
- Occult GI malignancy should be suspected in all men and postmenopausal women with iron deficiency.
- Avoid transfusions except in rare cases.

Issues for Referral

- Pregnant women with a hemoglobin (Hgb) level <9 g/dL or failure to respond to a 4–6-week trial or oral iron therapy
- Nonpregnant women or other patients with an Hgb level <6 g/dL

IN-PATIENT CONSIDERATIONS

Initial Stabilization

Outpatient

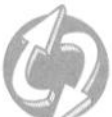

ONGOING CARE

FOLLOW-UP RECOMMENDATIONS

Patient Monitoring

- Regularly after Hgb returns to normal (to detect recurrences)
- Hgb increases 1 g/dL every 2–3 weeks.
- Iron stores may take up to 4 weeks to correct after Hgb returns to normal.

DIET

- Do not consume milk or other dairy products, antacids, quinolones, or tetracycline within 2 hours of iron supplement ingestion.
- Limit tea, coffee, and caffeinated beverages.
- Limit milk to 16 ounces per day (adults).
- Emphasize protein and iron-containing foods (meat, beans, and leafy green vegetables).
- Taking iron with orange juice or ascorbic acid increases absorption but decreases GI tolerability.
- Increase fluid and dietary fiber to decrease likelihood of constipation during iron replacement therapy.

PATIENT EDUCATION

National Heart, Lung & Blood Institute, Communications & Public Information Branch, National Institutes of Health, Building 31, Room 41-21, 9000 Rockville Pike, Bethesda, MD 20892; (301) 251-1222.

PROGNOSIS

- Can be resolved with iron therapy if the underlying cause can be discovered and appropriately treated
- Treat subclinical hypothyroidism and iron deficiency anemia together when these conditions coexist. Failure to treat hypothyroidism results in poor response to iron therapy (9)[B].

COMPLICATIONS

- Neglecting to identify hidden bleeding points, particularly a bleeding malignancy
- Maternal iron deficiency negatively affects mother–child interactions. Iron supplementation protects against these negative effects (10).

REFERENCES

1. Iron Deficiency—United States, 1999–2000. *MMWR Morb Mortal Wkly Rep*. 2002;51:897–9.
2. Dubois RW, Goodnough LT, Ershler WB, et al. Identification, diagnosis, and management of anemia in adult ambulatory patients treated by primary care physicians: Evidence-based and consensus recommendations. *Curr Med Res Opin*. 2006;22:385–95.
3. U.S. Preventative Services Task Force (USPSTF). Screening for iron deficiency anemia—including iron supplementation for children and pregnant women. Rockville (MD): Agency for Healthcare Research and Quality (AHRQ); 2006. 12p.
4. de Benoist B, McLean E, Egli I, Cogswell M, eds. Worldwide prevalence of anaemia 1993–1995. WHO Global Database on Anaemia. Geneva: World Health Organization; 2008. http://whqlibdoc.who.int/publications/2008/9789241596657_eng.pdf. Accessed October 19, 2011.
5. Melamed N, Ben-Haroush A, Kaplan B, et al. Iron supplementation in pregnancy–does the preparation matter? *Arch Gynecol Obstet*. 2007;276:601–4.
6. Killip S, Bennett JM, Chambers MD. Iron deficiency anemia. *Am Fam Physician*. 2007;75:671–8.
7. Chertow GM, Mason PD, Vaage-Nilsen O, et al. On the relative safety of parenteral iron formulations. *Nephrol Dial Transplant*. 2004;19:1571–5.
8. Chertow GM, Mason PD, Vaage-Nilsen O, et al. Update on adverse drug events associated with parenteral iron. *Nephrol Dial Transplant*. 2006;21:378–82.
9. Cinemre H, Bilir C, Gokosmanoglu F, et al. Hematologic effects of levothyroxine in iron-deficient subclinical hypothyroid patients: A randomized, double-blind, controlled study. *J. Clin. Endocrinol. Metab*. 2009;94:151–6
10. Murray-Kolb LE, Beard JL. Iron deficiency and child and maternal health. *Am J Clin Nutr*. 2009;89:946S–950S.

ADDITIONAL READING

- Baker WF. Iron deficiency anemia in pregnancy, obstetrics and gynecology. *Hematol Oncol Clin North Am*. 2000;64(4):231–6.
- Steensma DP, Tefferi A. Anemia in the elderly: How should we define it, when does it matter, and what can be done? [Review]. *Mayo Clinic Proc*. 2007;82(8):958–66.
- Tefferi A, Hanson CA, Inwards DJ. How to interpret and pursue an abnormal complete blood cell count in adults. *Mayo Clin Proc*. 2005;80:923–36.
- Zhu A, Kaneshiro M, Kaunitz JD. Evaluation and treatment of iron deficiency anemia: A gastroenterological perspective. *Dig Dis Sci*. 2010;55(3):548–59.

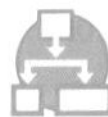

See Also (Topic, Algorithm, Electronic Media Element)

Algorithm: Anemia

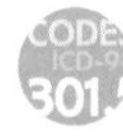

CODES

ICD9

- 280.0 Iron deficiency anemia secondary to blood loss (chronic)
- 280.9 Iron deficiency anemia, unspecified

CLINICAL PEARLS

- IDA is the most common type of anemia in the US and in the world.
- Blood loss and reduced iron stores due to malabsorption or poor utilization are major factors for IDA.
- Premenopausal women and children are at the greatest risk for IDA.
- Oral iron supplementation is the standard treatment option for patients with IDA.

ANEMIA, SICKLE CELL

Erica Braverman, MSIV
Liberto Pechet, MD, FACP

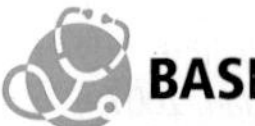

BASICS

DESCRIPTION

- Chronic hemoglobinopathy marked by chronic hemolytic anemia, periodic acute episodes of painful "crises," and increased susceptibility to intercurrent infections. Hereditary, generally manifesting in first 6–12 months of life
- The heterozygous condition (Hb A/S), sickle cell trait, is usually asymptomatic without anemia.
- Among the compound heterozygotes, sickle-hemoglobin C disease (HbSC) and $S\beta+$ thalassemia are clinically similar to the heterozygous condition, whereas $S\beta^{\circ}$ thalassemia is clinically similar to the homozygous condition.
- Synonym(s): Sickle cell disease (SCD); Hb SS disease

Pediatric Considerations

- Sequestration crises and hand–foot syndrome seen typically in infants/young children
- Adolescence/young adulthood:
  - Frequency of complications and organ/tissue damage increases with age (except for strokes, which occur mostly in childhood).
  - Psychological complications: Body image, interrupted schooling, restriction of activities; stigma of disease; low self-esteem

Pregnancy Considerations

- Usually complicated and hazardous, especially 3rd trimester and delivery:
  - Fetal survival is >90% if the fetus reaches the 3rd trimester.
- Increased risk of pain, toxemia, infection, pulmonary infarction, phlebitis
- Fetal mortality 35–40%
- Partial exchange transfusion in 3rd trimester may reduce maternal morbidity and fetal mortality, but this is controversial.
- Chronic transfusions have been effective in diminishing pain episodes in pregnant women. However, this method should be used with caution due to risk of alloimmunization.

EPIDEMIOLOGY

Prevalence

- ~90,000 Americans have SCA and 10% of African Americans carry trait. ~1/500 African Americans and 1/1,000 Hispanics have homozygous sickle cell anemia. Each year in the US, about 1/400 African-American infants are born with sickle cell disease.
- Lesser risk: Middle East, Mediterranean area, and populations in India may be affected.

RISK FACTORS

- For vaso-occlusive crisis ("painful crisis"): Pain results from tissue ischemia and necrosis: Hypoxia, dehydration, fever, infection, acidosis, cold, anesthesia, strenuous physical exercise, smoking
- For aplastic crisis (suppression of RBC production): Severe infections, human parvovirus B19 infection, folic acid deficiency
- Hyperhemolytic crisis (accelerated hemolysis with reticulocytosis) (existence is controversial): Acute bacterial infections, exposure to oxidant drugs

Genetics

Autosomal recessive. Homozygous presence of Hb S, or sickle hemoglobin (genotype SS). Heterozygous condition Hb AS. The heterozygote condition can also be combined with other hemoglobinopathies, the most common of which are HbC and β thalassemia.

GENERAL PREVENTION

- Prevention of crises:
  - Avoid hypoxia, dehydration, cold, infection, fever, acidosis, and anesthesia.
  - Prompt management of fever, infections, pain
  - Hydration
  - Avoid alcohol and smoking.
  - Avoid high-altitude areas.
- Minimizing trauma: Aseptic technique is imperative.

PATHOPHYSIOLOGY

- Sickle cells are abnormally shaped, fragile red blood cells. Increased red cell destruction causes an inability to maintain adequate hemoglobin levels and results in anemia and fatigue.
- Sickle cells exhibit increased adhesion and decreased ability to maneuver small vessels, leading to vaso-occlusion.

ETIOLOGY

- Substitution of valine for glutamic acid in 6th amino acid of hemoglobin β-chain. Mutation → red blood cells (RBCs) change from biconcave to sickle shape when deoxygenated due to poor solubility of mutated hemoglobin chain.
- Sickle RBCs are inflexible, causing increased blood viscosity, stasis, obstruction of small arterioles and capillaries, and ischemia. Sickle RBCs are fragile, leading to hemolysis.
- Chronic anemia; crises:
  - Vaso-occlusive crisis ("painful crisis"): Tissue ischemia and necrosis; progressive organ failure/tissue damage from repeated episodes
  - Hand–foot syndrome: Vessel occlusion/ischemia affects small blood vessels in hands or feet
  - Aplastic crisis: Suppression of RBC production by severe infection (e.g., parvoviral and other viral infections)
  - Suppression of RBC production
  - Hyperhemolytic crisis: Accelerated hemolysis with reticulocytosis; increased RBC fragility/shortened lifespan
  - Sequestration crisis: Splenic sequestration of blood (only in young children as spleen is later lost to autoinfarction
- Susceptibility to infection: Impaired/absent splenic function leading to decreased ability to clear infection; defect in alternate pathway of complement activation

DIAGNOSIS

A chronic hemolytic anemia. Increased infection risk (e.g., pneumococcal sepsis, *Salmonella* osteomyelitis), with functional asplenia by ~5–6 years of age, and delayed physical/sexual maturation. Diagnosis now often made by newborn screening programs.

HISTORY

- Often asymptomatic in early months of life due to presence of fetal hemoglobin.
- >6 months of age, earliest symptoms are irritability and painful swelling of the hands and feet (hand–foot syndrome). May also see pneumococcal sepsis or meningitis, severe anemia and acute splenic enlargement (splenic sequestration), acute chest syndrome, pallor, jaundice, or splenomegaly.
- Major manifestations in older children include anemia, severe or recurrent musculoskeletal or abdominal pain, aplastic crisis, acute chest syndrome, splenomegaly or splenic sequestration, and cholelithiasis.
- Painful crises in bones, joints, abdomen, back, and viscera account for 90% of all hospital admissions.
- Acute chest syndrome: Tachycardia, fever, bilateral infiltrates caused by pulmonary infarctions

PHYSICAL EXAM

Fever, pale skin and nail beds, mild jaundice

DIAGNOSTIC TESTS & INTERPRETATION

Lab

- Screening test: Sickledex test
  - Hb electrophoresis (diagnostic test of choice). Sickle cell anemia (FS pattern):
  - 80–100% Hb S, variable amounts of Hb F and no Hb A1
  - Sickle cell trait (FS pattern): 30–45% Hb S, 50–70% Hb A1, minimal Hb F
- Hemoglobin ~5–10 g/dL; RBC indices: MCV normal to increased; MCHC increased; HgSS, reticulocytes 3–15%
- Leukocytosis; bands in absence of infection, platelets elevated; peripheral smear: sickled RBCs, nucleated RBCs, Howell-Jolly bodies
- Serum bilirubin mildly elevated (2–4 mg/dL); Ferritin very elevated in multiply transfused patients; serum lactate dehydrogenase (LDH) elevated
- Fecal/urinary urobilinogen high
- Haptoglobin absent or very low

Imaging

Need for imaging depends on clinical circumstances:

- Bone scan to rule out osteomyelitis
- CT/MRI to rule out CVA; high index of suspicion required for any acute neurological symptoms other than mild headache
- Chest x-ray: May show enlarged heart; diffuse alveolar infiltrates in acute chest syndrome
- Transcranial Doppler: Start at age 2; repeat yearly (1,2)[B]. Transcranial Doppler ultrasound identifies children age 2–16 at higher risk of stroke.
- ECG to detect pulmonary hypertension (2)[C] and echocardiogram every other year from age 15 on.

Pathological Findings

Hyposplenism due to autosplenectomy is common; hypoxia/infarction in multiple organs

DIFFERENTIAL DIAGNOSIS
Anemia: Other hemoglobinopathies

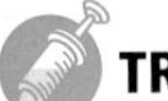

TREATMENT

MEDICATION
First Line
- Supplemental oxygen
- Painful crises (mild, outpatient):
  - Nonnarcotic analgesics (ibuprofen, tramadol) (1,2)[C]
- Painful crises (severe, hospitalized) (1,2)[B]:
  - Parenteral narcotics (e.g., morphine on fixed schedule); patient-controlled analgesia (PCA) pump may be useful.
  - Hydroxyurea is indicated for prevention of painful crises, acute chest syndrome, vaso-occlusive episodes, and very severe anemia. Start with 15 mg/kg/d single daily dose; titrate upward every 12 weeks if blood counts satisfactory (avoid severe neutropenia):
    - Increase in 5 mg/kg increments to maximum of 35 mg/kg/d. Long-term safety unknown
    - Contraindicated in pregnancy (3)[A]
    - Inhaled nitric oxide, arginine butyrate (may enhance availability of nitric oxide), and combination of erythropoietin with hydroxyurea (3)[B]
- Acute chest syndrome
  - May deteriorate quickly; aggressive management with oxygen, analgesics, antibiotics, simple or exchange transfusion (1)
- Empiric antibiotics (2) to cover *S. pneumoniae*, *H. influenzae*, *Mycoplasma pneumoniae*, and *Chlamydia pneumoniae* (cephalosporins or azithromycin). If osteomyelitis, cover for *Staphylococcus aureus* and *Salmonella* (e.g., ciprofloxacin). If apparent pneumonia not promptly responding to antibiotics, consider diagnosis of acute chest syndrome and initiate simple or exchange transfusion.
- Prophylactic penicillin is indicated in all infants and children starting at 2 months (1,3)[A]: 2–6 months of age: 62.5 mg b.i.d.; 6 months–3 years: 125 mg b.i.d.; 3–5 years: 250 mg b.i.d. If no pneumococcal infections, stop at 6 years; if high risk remains, continue until puberty. Rising pneumococcal resistance to penicillin may change future recommendations.
- Precautions: Avoid high-dose estrogen oral contraceptives; consider Depo-Provera.

Second Line
Folic acid (1,2)[C]: 0–6 months: 0.1 mg/d; 6–12 months: 0.25 mg/d; 1–2 years: 0.5 mg/d; >2 years of age 1 mg/d

ADDITIONAL TREATMENT
- Transfusions and additional therapies
  - Transfusion for aplastic crises, severe complications (i.e., CVA), prophylactically before surgery, and treatment for acute chest syndrome.
  - Transfusions carry risk of iron overload, resulting in damage to heart, liver, and other organs. Avoid blood hyperviscosity.
  - Prophylactic transfusions for primary or secondary stroke prevention in children
  - Consider chelation with Deferasirox, an oral agent, if the patient is multiply transfused (after age 2).

General Measures
- Painful crises: Hydration, analgesics; oxygen regardless of whether the patient is hypoxic
- Retinal evaluation starting at school age to detect proliferative sickle retinopathy
- Occupational therapy, cognitive and behavioral therapies, support groups
- Special immunizations (1,2)[B]:
  - Influenza vaccine yearly starting at age 2
  - Heptavalent conjugated pneumococcal vaccine at 2, 4, 6 months; booster at 15 months, 2 years, 5 years
  - 23-valent pneumococcal vaccine at 2 years; booster at age 5; always separate this by 8 weeks from heptavalent vaccine
- Meningococcal vaccine >2 years of age
- H1N1 vaccination

SURGERY/OTHER PROCEDURES
- Experimental gene therapy: Replace normal gene and inactivate Hgb S while reactivating Hgb F (fetal hemoglobin).
- Hematopoietic stem cell transplant (HSCT): Curative, but with significant morbidity and mortality

IN-PATIENT CONSIDERATIONS
Admission Criteria
Severe pain, suspected infection or sepsis, evidence of acute chest syndrome

IV Fluids
The preferred maintenance IV fluid is 1/2 NS, as NS may theoretically increase the risk of sickling.

ONGOING CARE

FOLLOW-UP RECOMMENDATIONS
Patient Monitoring
- Treat infections early. Parents/patients: Any temperature of ≥101°F (38.3°C) requires immediate medical attention.
- For patients who receive chronic transfusions, monitor for hepatitis and hemosiderosis.
- Periodic eye evaluations: Starting age 5 to detect proliferative sickle retinopathy (1,2)[C].
- Bi-annual examination for hepatic, renal, and pulmonary dysfunction

DIET
Folic acid supplementation; avoid alcohol (leads to dehydration); maintain hydration

PATIENT EDUCATION
- Sicklecellkids.org—Education Web site for children with sickle cell anemia: http://www.sicklecelldisease.org
- American Sickle Cell Anemia Association: http://www.ascaa.org

PROGNOSIS
- In 2nd decade of life, fewer crises, but more complications. Median age of death is 42 for men and 48 for women. Causes: Infections, thrombosis, pulmonary emboli, pulmonary hypertension, and renal failure
- Children become anemic in infancy and begin to have sickle cell crises at 1–2 years of age; some children die in their 1st year.

COMPLICATIONS
- Alloimmunization, bone infarct and osteomyelitis, aseptic necrosis of femoral head
- CVA (peak age 6–7), impaired mental development, even without history of stroke
- Cholelithiasis/abnormal liver function
- Chronic leg ulcers, poor wound healing
- Impotence, priapism, hematuria/hyposthenuria, renal concentrating, and acidifying defects
- Retinopathy, splenic infarction (by 10 years of age)
- Acute chest syndrome (infection/infarction) leading to chronic pulmonary disease
- Infections (pneumonia, osteomyelitis, meningitis, pyelonephritis); sepsis (leading cause of morbidity and mortality)
- Hemosiderosis (secondary to multiple transfusions). Substance abuse related to chronic pain

REFERENCES

1. Section on Hematology/Oncology Committee on Genetics, American Academy of Pediatrics. Health supervision for children with sickle cell disease. *Pediatrics*. 2002;109:526–35.
2. National Institutes of Health. *The management of sickle cell disease*, 4th ed. 2002. NH Publ No. 02-2117.
3. Bonds DR. Three decades of innovation in the management of sickle cell disease: The road to understanding the sickle cell disease clinical phenotype. *Blood Rev*. 2005;19:99–110.

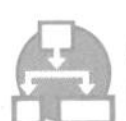

See Also (Topic, Algorithm, Electronic Media Element)

Algorithm: Anemia

CODES

ICD9
- 282.60 Sickle cell disease, unspecified
- 282.61 Hb SS disease without crisis
- 282.62 Hb SS disease with crisis

CLINICAL PEARLS
- Almost 90,000 Americans have SCA, ~1/500 African Americans have SCA; 10% carry the trait
- The preferred maintenance IV fluid is 1/2 NS, as NS may theoretically increase the risk of sickling.
- Painful crises in bones, joints, abdomen, back, and viscera account for 90% of all hospital admissions.
- Acute chest syndrome: Tachycardia, fever, bilateral infiltrates caused by pulmonary infarctions

ANEMIA, SIDEROBLASTIC

Pia Prakash, MD
Neha Jakhete, MD
Marie L. Borum, MD, EdD, MPH

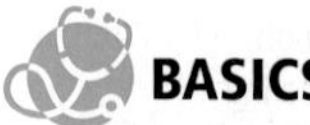

BASICS

DESCRIPTION

- Sideroblastic anemia is a defect in heme synthesis affecting red blood cell production resulting in anemia. It is characterized by the presence of ringed sideroblasts in the bone marrow. This disease process can be congenital or acquired.
- Although the body has available iron stores, iron cannot be incorporated into the hemoglobin, resulting in granules of iron that accumulate in the mitochondria where heme is produced.

EPIDEMIOLOGY

- Sideroblastic anemias (SAs) are uncommon. Incidence and prevalence are not well studied.
- Acquired forms are more common than hereditary forms (1) and usually occur in older adults; present in 25–30% of alcoholics with anemia, most commonly with folate and B_6 deficiency.
- Hereditary forms vary in severity, usually manifesting in childhood.

RISK FACTORS

- Male gender (X-linked SA)
- Family history of hereditary SA
- Chronic alcohol abuse

Genetics

- Congenital form can arise from multiple gene defects:
  - Defect in aminolevulinic acid synthase (ALAS-2 mutation): The first and rate-limiting enzyme in heme biosynthesis
  - Defect in mitochondrial amino acid transporter (SLC25A38)
  - Defect in ferrochelatase
  - Defect in glutaredoxin 5
  - Defect in thiamine transporter 1
  - Defect in mitochondrial proteins and exporters
- Can be X-linked or autosomal recessive

GENERAL PREVENTION

Pyridoxine should be given to all patients on isoniazid to avoid anemia.

PATHOPHYSIOLOGY

- Inability to utilize iron for the production of hemoglobin due to inherited or acquired impairment
- Ineffective erythropoiesis despite abundance of iron in the body
- Increased GI absorption of iron leading to iron overload
- The inability to utilize iron for heme synthesis results in sideroblasts, which are abnormal erythroblasts with granules of iron accumulated in the mitochondria, forming a ring around the nucleus.

ETIOLOGY

- Congenital SAs are inherited forms of SA resulting from genetic defects:
  - X-linked sideroblastic anemia is caused by mutation in 5-aminolevulinate synthase, which is the first enzyme in the heme biosynthesis pathway. This is the most common congenital form. More prevalent in males.
  - X-linked sideroblastic anemia with spinocerebellar ataxia results from defect in ABCB7 gene.
  - Mitochondrial defects:
    - Defect of mitochondrial transporter SLC25A38. Usually autosomal recessive.
    - Deficiency in mitochondrial GXRL5, which effects iron-sulfur cluster synthesis
  - Deficiency of ferrochelatase, a necessary enzyme in the heme biosynthesis pathway
  - Roger syndrome results from defect in thiamine transporter protein, usually improved with administration of thiamine
  - Pearson syndrome results from defect in mitochondria of erythroblasts.
- Acquired SA is usually reversible when the inciting factor is removed. Acquired SA is more common than congenital SA. Acquired SA can be caused by:
  - Alcohol
  - Isoniazid
  - Pyrazinamide
  - Pyridoxine deficiency
  - Chloramphenicol
  - Cycloserine
  - Azathioprine
  - D-penicillamine
  - Copper deficiency
  - Zinc toxicity leading to copper deficiency
  - Lead poisoning
  - Hypothermia affecting mitochondrial functions
- Refractory anemia with ring sideroblasts (RARS) and pure SA (PSA) are subtypes of the myelodysplastic syndromes related to clonal overproliferation of hematopoietic cell lines:
  - RARS is more commonly associated with acute leukemia than is PSA.

COMMONLY ASSOCIATED CONDITIONS

- Iron overload or secondary hemochromatosis from transfused blood products
- Transformation into acute leukemia is rare.
- Alcohol abuse

DIAGNOSIS

Moderate-to-severe anemia with symptoms of fatigue, dizziness, and dyspnea should prompt an evaluation for sideroblastic anemia.

HISTORY

- Symptoms of anemia, including fatigue, dizziness, and dyspnea
- Alcohol or drug exposures as listed above
- Toxin exposures
- Developmental delays in children
- Symptoms of iron overload
- Cardiac arrhythmias or heart failure related to iron overload
- Family history of anemia or myopathy, especially in men
- Patients can present with peripheral neuropathy or dermatitis if SA related to pyridoxine deficiency.

PHYSICAL EXAM

- No pathognomonic physical findings
- Signs of anemia, including tachycardia, conjunctival pallor, etc.
- Mild-to-moderate hepatosplenomegaly may be present.

DIAGNOSTIC TESTS & INTERPRETATION

Lab

Initial lab tests

CBC with diff, ferritin, serum Fe, transferrin saturation, serum transferrin, TIBC, LFTs

Follow-Up & Special Considerations

- CBC:
  - Microcytosis with low mean corpuscular volume (MCV) in most cases
  - Hypochromia with low mean corpuscular hemoglobin (MCH)
  - Increased red cell distribution width (RDW)
  - Normal leukocytes and platelets
  - It is important to note that in SA related to myelodysplastic syndromes, normocytosis or macrocytosis may be seen.
  - Peripheral smear showing siderocytes. Anisocytosis and poikilocytosis may be present:
    - Basophilic stippling may be seen in lead poisoning.
  - Iron studies are consistent with iron overload:
    - Ferritin increased
    - Serum iron levels increased
    - Transferrin saturation increased
    - Serum transferrin decreased
    - Total iron binding capacity (TIBC) normal
- Serum copper, ceruloplasmin, serum zinc if suspected as cause
- Bone marrow evaluation reveals ringed sideroblasts, which is diagnostic for SA. Prussian blue staining also reveals ringed sideroblasts. Electron micrograph shows iron-filled mitochondria clustered around the nucleus.
- Abnormal liver function tests may be seen if cause is related to alcohol, cirrhosis, or iron overload.
- Molecular studies may be done to identify specific mutations causing hereditary SA syndromes.
- Serum erythrocyte protoporphyrin is low in X-linked SA. This level is increased in X-linked SA with ataxia.
- Liver biopsy is helpful to assess degree of iron overload.

Diagnostic Procedures/Surgery

Bone marrow biopsy confirms the diagnosis of sideroblastic anemia.

Pathological Findings

- Bone marrow exam is the key diagnostic modality (1)[C]:
  - Normoblastic erythroid hyperplasia
  - Prussian blue iron stain showing ringed sideroblasts, >10% of erythroblasts with increased number of abnormally large granules ringing the nucleus
  - Electron microscopy reveals iron-overloaded mitochondria within erythroblasts.
  - Iron-laden macrophages
- Liver biopsy:
  - Iron deposition indistinguishable from hereditary hemochromatosis

DIFFERENTIAL DIAGNOSIS

- Thalassemias
- Iron deficiency anemia
- Folate or B_{12} deficiency
- Anemia of chronic disease
- Myelodysplastic syndromes
- Lead toxicity with anemia

TREATMENT

MEDICATION

First Line

- Treatment is largely supportive.
- Pyridoxine (1)[B]:
  - Will only improve anemia in X-linked SA and alcohol-related SA
  - Initial dose should be 50–100 mg PO daily.
  - Supplement folate to compensate for increased erythropoiesis if pyridoxine is effective.
  - Positive clinical response if reticulocytosis is seen within 2 weeks followed by increase in hemoglobin level over several months
- Combination therapy with erythropoietin and G-CSF can be helpful in acquired SA (1)[B].
- Blood transfusion based on symptoms of anemia. May worsen iron overload and create need for iron chelation therapy (1)[C]
- Treatment for iron overload:
  - Therapeutic phlebotomy can be considered.
  - Iron chelation therapy (2)[A]:
    - Deferoxamine 40 mg/kg daily in continuous 12–24-hour daily infusions (2)[B]:
      - Iron removal improved with addition of ascorbate. Due to cardiac, visual, auditory toxicity, limit ascorbate intake to 200 mg or less per day (3)[C].
    - Deferasirox is an oral once-daily iron chelator (4)[B]:
      - Recommended dose 20–30 mg/kg daily
      - Long-term safety profile not well studied
      - Side effects include skin rash, GI symptoms, and acute kidney injury.
    - Goal of chelation therapy is to maintain serum ferritin <500 μg/L (2)[A,B].
- Removal of causative factors such as alcohol, drugs, or toxins should fully reverse SA.
- Repletion of copper in patients with copper deficiency

Second Line

Chemotherapeutic agents may have a role.

ADDITIONAL TREATMENT

Issues for Referral

- Hematology consultation
- Genetic counseling is important for patients with heritable cause of SA.

Additional Therapies

Allogeneic stem cell transplantation has been successful in a few cases in younger patients with myelodysplastic syndromes.

SURGERY/OTHER PROCEDURES

Splenectomy is contraindicated due to frequent postoperative thromboembolic complications.

IN-PATIENT CONSIDERATIONS

Admission Criteria

Most patients without cardiac complications can be managed in the outpatient setting.

ONGOING CARE

FOLLOW-UP RECOMMENDATIONS

Patient Monitoring

- Yearly ferritin and transferrin saturation to monitor for Fe overload.
- Patients given pyridoxine should be followed for response to treatment. As above, lab results should show reticulocytosis within 2 weeks and improved hemoglobin within 1–2 months.
- Correction of nutritional deficiency
- Ensure withdrawal of reversible cause.

DIET

- Patients may need to avoid excessive alcohol intake.
- Patients with copper deficiency may need oral copper repletion.

PROGNOSIS

- 75% of X-linked SA with ALAS-2 mutations are pyridoxine-responsive.
- Prognosis is better if iron overload is prevented.
- RARS: Median survival 3–6 years, $<10\%$ progression to leukemia
- When only the erythroid line is affected (PSA), progression to acute leukemia is not usually seen.
- If SA follows treatment for malignancy, leukemic transformation is common.

COMPLICATIONS

- Iron overload may cause organ damage:
  - Cardiac arrhythmia or CHF
  - Hepatic dysfunction
- Complication may arise from blood transfusions.

REFERENCES

1. Alcindor T, Bridges KR. Sideroblastic anaemias. *Br J Haematol*. 2002;116:733–43.
2. Olivieri NF, Brittenham GM. Iron-chelating therapy and the treatment of thalassemia. *Blood*. 1997;89:739–61.
3. Thalassemia major: Molecular and clinical aspects. NIH Conference. *Ann Intern Med*. 1979;91:883–97.
4. Porter J, Galanello R, Saglio G, et al. Relative response of patients with myelodysplastic syndromes and other transfusion-dependent anaemias to deferasirox (ICL670): A 1-yr prospective study. *Eur J Haematol*. 2008;80:168–76.

ADDITIONAL READING

- Camaschella C. Hereditary sideroblastic anemias: pathophysiology, diagnosis, and treatment. *Semin. Hematol*. 2009;46:371–7.
- Cuijpers ML, van Spronsen DJ, Muus P, et al. Need for early recognition and therapeutic guidelines of congenital sideroblastic anaemia. *Int J Hematol*. 2011;94:97–100.
- Müller-Berndorff H, Haas PS, Kunzmann R, et al. Comparison of five prognostic scoring systems, the French-American-British (FAB) and World Health Organization (WHO) classifications in patients with myelodysplastic syndromes: Results of a single-center analysis. *Ann Hematol*. 2006;85:502–13.
- Rovó A, Stüssi G, Meyer-Monard S, et al. Sideroblastic changes of the bone marrow can be predicted by the erythrogram of peripheral blood. *Int J Lab Hematol*. 2010;32(3):329–35.

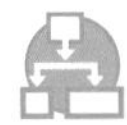

See Also (Topic, Algorithm, Electronic Media Element)

Algorithms: Anemia, Sideroblastic; Anemia

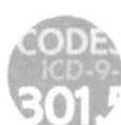

CODES

ICD9

- 285.0 Sideroblastic anemia
- 980.0 Toxic effect of ethyl alcohol

CLINICAL PEARLS

- Sideroblastic anemia results from inability to incorporate iron during heme synthesis in the mitochondria, leading to microcytic anemia and sideroblasts in the bone marrow.
- There are multiple inherited forms linked to genetic mutations as well as acquired forms of SA.
- Patients may present with symptomatic anemia, with blood tests revealing iron overload.
- Bone marrow biopsy is required for diagnosis. Prussian blue staining reveals ringed sideroblasts.
- Treatment includes blood transfusions for symptomatic anemia, chelation therapy for iron overload, pyridoxine in X-linked SA and alcohol-related SA, and removal of causative factors if present.

ANEURYSM OF THE ABDOMINAL AORTA

Michael J. Gray, MD

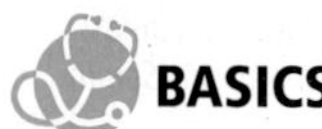

BASICS

DESCRIPTION
- An infrarenal aorta 3 cm in diameter or larger is considered aneurysmal.
- Types:
  - Fusiform aneurysm: Involves the whole circumference or wall of the artery
  - Saccular aneurysm: Does not involve the full circumference, often appears as an asymmetrical bleb or blister on the side of the aorta. Clinical presentation relates to aneurysm location, size, type, and comorbid factors affecting the patient. The majority are asymptomatic. May present with rupture, embolism, or thrombosis. Treatment and indications for surgical repair dictated by risk of rupture, risk of surgical repair, and estimated patient life expectancy.
- System(s) affected: Cardiovascular; Neurologic; Heme/Lymphatic/Immunologic
- Synonym(s): Aortic aneurysms; AAA

Geriatric Considerations
Incidence of AAA, risk of rupture, and operative morbidity and mortality all rise with age.

Pediatric Considerations
AAA in children is rare and may be associated with umbilical artery catheters, connective tissue diseases, arteritides, or congenital abnormalities.

EPIDEMIOLOGY
- Frequency increases >50 years of age
- Predominant sex: Male > Female (5:1) (1)

Incidence
- >15,000 deaths per year in US
- 10th leading cause of death in men 65–75
- 8% of men age >65

Prevalence
- Depends on risk factors associated with AAA
- Prevalence of AAAs 2.9–4.9 cm in diameter ranges from 1.3% for men aged 45–54 to up to 12.5% for men aged 75–84 years of age. Data for women are 0% and 5.2%, respectively (2); however, when detected, women presented at an older age and were more likely to present with a ruptured AAA. Female sex is an independent risk factor for *death* from AAA (3).

RISK FACTORS
Older age, male, Northern European ethnicity, family history, smoking, hypertension (HTN), hyperlipidemia, peripheral vascular disease, peripheral aneurysms, chronic obstructive peripheral disease (COPD), obesity (3)

Genetics
- Familial aggregations exist: Aneurysms may develop at an earlier age.
- 2 times risk of AAA if 1st-degree relative with AAA (1)
- Marfan syndrome
- Ehlers-Danlos syndrome
- Polycystic kidney disease
- Tuberous sclerosis

GENERAL PREVENTION
- Address cardiovascular disease risk factors.
- Follow screening guidelines: Ultrasound screening for detection of AAA in male patients, ages 65–75, who have ever smoked and men >60 who are siblings or offspring of patients with AAA (4)

PATHOPHYSIOLOGY
- Vascular inflammatory degenerative disease with major role of matrix metalloproteinases and inflammatory markers that result in aortic medial degeneration (2)
- Gradual and/or sporadic expansion of aneurysm and accumulation of mural thrombus
- Mural thrombus can contribute to an area of localized hypoxia, thus further weakening the aneurysm.
- Aneurysms tend to expand over time. (Laplace law: T (wall tension) = pressure × radius. Wall tension directly related to BP and the radius of the artery.) When wall tension exceeds wall tensile strength, rupture occurs (3).
- Average small AAA (<5.5 cm) grows at a rate of 2.6–3.2 mm/yr. Larger aneurysms grew at a faster rate, as did aneurysms in current smokers, but otherwise no identifiable risk factors to assess which small AAAs will advance to require further intervention.
- 60–80% of AAAs between 40 and 49 mm will enlarge and require surgery in 5 years.

ETIOLOGY
- Degenerative: Atherosclerotic (80%)
- Other causes: Inflammatory diseases (5%); trauma; connective tissue disorders; infection (Brucella, Salmonella, staph, tuberculosis)

COMMONLY ASSOCIATED CONDITIONS
- HTN, myocardial infarction (MI), heart failure, carotid artery, and/or lower extremity peripheral arterial disease
- Screening for thoracic aneurysm should also be considered.

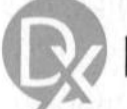

DIAGNOSIS

Screening: Recommended 1-time ultrasound for AAA in men 65–75 years of age who have ever smoked. Men >60 years old who are siblings or offspring of patients with AAA should undergo physical exam and ultrasound screening (2)[B]. US Preventive Services Task Force has recommended against routine screening for women (4):
- Most often asymptomatic: Discovered during exams for other complaints
- Symptomatic: Embolization, thrombosis, vague abdominal or back pain, syncope, lower extremity paralysis
- Rupture

ALERT
- The triad of shock, pulsatile mass, and abdominal pain always suggests rupture of AAA:
  - Shock may be absent if rupture is contained.
  - Palpable pulsatile mass may be absent in up to 50% of patients with rupture.
  - Pain may radiate to the back, groin, flank, buttocks, or legs.
- Unusual presentations:
  - Primary aortoenteric fistula: Erosion/rupture of AAA into duodenum
  - Aortocaval fistula: Erosion/rupture of AAA into vena cava or left renal vein: 3–6%
  - Inflammatory aneurysm: Encasement by thick inflammatory rind; can cause chronic abdominal pain, weight loss, and elevated erythrocyte sedimentation rate. Surrounding viscera densely adherent.

HISTORY
Abdominal or back pain; AAA risk factors

PHYSICAL EXAM
- Pulsatile supraumbilical mass
- Only 30–40% of AAA detected by physical exam
- 14% of AAA associated with femoral or popliteal aneurysms (1)
- Vague abdominal tenderness: May radiate to the back or flank
- Encroachment by aneurysm:
  - Vertebral body erosion; gastric outlet obstruction; ureteral obstruction
  - Lower extremity ischemia secondary to embolization of mural thrombus
- Rupture leads to tachycardia, hypotension, evidence of shock and anemia, and possible flank contusion (Grey-Turner sign).

DIAGNOSTIC TESTS & INTERPRETATION

Lab

Initial lab tests

If rupturing AAA being considered: Complete blood chemistry, chemistries, coags, type and cross, electrocardiogram.

Follow-Up & Special Considerations

Evaluation for coronary artery disease is appropriate prior to elective AAA repair (i.e., cardiac clearance), including stress test, echocardiography, and ECG if appropriate (1).

Imaging

Initial approach
- Ultrasonography: Simplest and least expensive diagnostic procedure
- Multiple studies have demonstrated high sensitivity (94–100%) and specificity (98–100%) of ultrasonographic diagnosis of AAA by emergency physicians.
- Although effective in detecting AAA, it is a poor test to show leakage or rupture if bleeding is into the retroperitoneal space.
- Surveillance of asymptomatic aneurysm (1)[C]:
  - 2.6–2.9 cm: Screen at 5-year intervals.
  - 3.0–3.4 cm: Screen at 3-year intervals.
  - 3.5–4.4 cm: Screen every 12 months.
  - 4.4–5.4 cm: Screen every 6 months.
- CT scans are the preferred preoperative study (caution with IV contrast in renal failure).
- MRI/MRA can also visualize AAA, but is often not possible in emergent situations.
- Aortography: Does not define outer dimensions of aneurysm
- Abdominal x-rays can be diagnostic if calcifications exist; not a diagnostic tool of choice
- Ongoing research into exploring alternative diagnostic measurements, including measurement of total aortic volume compared to a single axial diameter measurement as well as measurement of total thrombus burden associated with AAA since this appears to have a greater risk association (3).

Diagnostic Procedures/Surgery

ALERT

Use clinical judgment: Patients with known AAA having abdominal or back pain symptoms may be rupturing despite a negative CT scan.

DIFFERENTIAL DIAGNOSIS

- Other abdominal masses
- Other causes of abdominal or back pain (e.g., peptic ulcer disease, renal colic, diverticulitis, appendicitis, incarcerated hernia, GI hemorrhage, arthritis, metastatic disease)

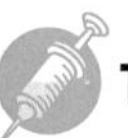

TREATMENT

- Emergent treatment in unstable or symptomatic patients is immediate vascular surgery consultation, adequate IV access and resuscitation, type and cross for multiple units, and rapid bedside ultrasound.
- Less acute treatment of AAA and prevention of rupture is elective repair and risk factor modification.

MEDICATION

- Beta-blockers may be initiated to reduce the rate of aneurysm expansion (2)[C].
- Beta-blockers should be used perioperatively in absence of contraindications (2)[A]; bronchodilators should be used for 2 weeks prior to repair for patients with COPD (1)[C].
- Statins may be beneficial perioperatively, but have not been shown to inhibit future expansion despite initial reports. Research on this topic is ongoing (5).
- Aspirin may inhibit expansion by inhibiting thrombus growth (5)[C].
- Doxycycline may also inhibit expansion, but further studies are needed. Early animal studies indicate a possible role for angiotensin-converting enzyme (ACE)-I/angiotensin receptor blockers (ARBs), mast cell stabilizers, prostaglandin inhibitors, and novel gene therapy (2).

ADDITIONAL TREATMENT

General Measures

- Treat atherosclerotic risk factors (2,5,6)[C].
- Medical optimization of cardiac, renal, and pulmonary conditions
- Smoking cessation (increased rate of expansion of 20–25% with continued smoking) and exercise (6)

SURGERY/OTHER PROCEDURES

Current recommendations (6)[C]:

- Elective:
  - 5.5-cm diameter is the threshold for repair in "average" patient.
  - Younger, low-risk patients with long life expectancy may prefer early repair.
  - Women or AAA with high risk of rupture: Consider elective repair at 4.5–5 cm
  - Consider delayed repair in high-risk patients.
  - 5% perioperative mortality for open elective repair (3)
- High risk of rupture:
  - Expansion >0.6 cm/yr
  - Smoking/COPD severe/steroids
  - Family history; multiple relatives
  - Hypertension poorly controlled
  - Shape nonfusiform
- High-risk patients for elective repair:
  - Risk factors for open repair include age >70 years, COPD, chronic renal insufficiency (CRI), suprarenal clamp site, with 1-year mortality if 0 risk factors present of 1.2% and 67% for all 4 risk factors present.
  - Other poor prognostic factors include inactive/poor stamina, congestive heart failure, significant coronary artery disease, liver disease, and family history of AAA.
  - Consider coronary revascularization prior to aneurysm repair if coronary artery disease (CAD) (1)[B]
  - Discontinue thienopyridine (clopidogrel and others) use 10 days prior to AAA repair and restart immediately postoperatively (1)[C].
  - Transfusion to hematocrit >28.0 if elective open repair planned (1)[C]
- Emergent/symptomatic repair:
  - Traditionally has been open repair; however, candidates with appropriate anatomy can have endovascular repair, with an estimated mortality of 32% for endovascular vs. 44% open
- Open repair vs. endovascular repair (EVAR):
  - Open repair indicated in patients who are good or average surgical candidates (2)[B]
  - EVAR for patients at high risk of complication based on cardiopulmonary or other comorbid illness: Periodic long-term surveillance indicated to monitor for endoleak, status of aneurysmal sac, and need for further intervention (2)[B]

IN-PATIENT CONSIDERATIONS

Risk of abdominal compartment syndrome after repair 4–12%; usually associated with large fluid resuscitation

ONGOING CARE

FOLLOW-UP RECOMMENDATIONS

See surveillance recommendations.

Patient Monitoring

BP and fasting lipid values: Control as would for atherosclerotic disease (2)[C]

DIET

Low-fat, low-salt, and low-caffeine diet; nutrition optimized prior to elective repair; and parenteral nutrition started within 7 days postoperatively if unable to have enteral feeds (1)[B]

PATIENT EDUCATION

Smoking cessation (2)[B], aerobic exercise

PROGNOSIS

- Annual risk of rupture (6):
  - <4 cm diameter: ~0%
  - 4–4.9 cm: ~0.5–5%
  - 5–5.9 cm: ~3–15%
  - 6–6.9 cm: ~10–20%
  - 7–7.9 cm: ~20–40%
  - >8 cm: 30–50%
- Patients with AAAs measuring 5.5 cm or larger should undergo repair (2)[B], as should all patients with symptomatic AAA (2)[C].
- Only ~18% of patients with ruptured AAA survive.
- Although there is a 5:1 ratio of AAA between males and females, women have a higher mortality and morbidity associated with AAA, regardless of open or endovascular repair (3).
- Recommended routine surveillance at 1 year and every 5 years following repair (3)

COMPLICATIONS

- Nonoperative: Rupture, dissection, thromboembolization
- Elective operative (conventional): Death 2–8%, all cardiac 10–12% (MI 2–8%)
- Pulmonary 5–10%; renal 5–7%; wound infection >5%; colon ischemia 1%; spinal cord ischemia <1%

REFERENCES

1. Chaikof EL, Brewster DC, Dalman RL, et al. The care of patients with an abdominal aortic aneurysm: The Society for Vascular Surgery practice guidelines. *J Vasc Surg*. 2009;50:S2–49.
2. Hirsch AT, Haskal ZJ, Hertzer NR, et al. ACC/AHA 2005 Practice Guidelines for the management of patients with peripheral arterial disease: A collaborative report. *Circulation*. 2006;113: e563–e601.
3. Moxon JV, Parr A, Emeto TI, et al. Diagnosis and monitoring of abdominal aortic aneurysm: Current status and future prospects. *Curr Probl Cardiol*. 2010;35:512–48.
4. U.S. Preventive Services Task Force. Screening for abdominal aortic aneurysm. *Ann Intern Med*. 2005;142:198–202.
5. Golledge J, Norman PE. Current status of medical management for abdominal aortic aneurysm. *Atherosclerosis*. 2011;217(1):57–63.
6. Aggarwal S, Qamar A, Sharma V, et al. Abdominal aortic aneurysm: A comprehensive review. *Exp Clin Cardiol*. 2011;16:11–5.

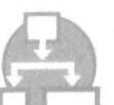

See Also (Topic, Algorithm, Electronic Media Element)

Aortic Dissection; Ehlers-Danlos; Giant Cell Arteritis; Marfan Syndrome; Polyarteritis Nodosa; Turner Syndrome

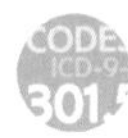

CODES

ICD9

- 441.3 Abdominal aneurysm, ruptured
- 441.4 Abdominal aneurysm without mention of rupture

CLINICAL PEARLS

- Major risk factors: Smoking, HTN, hyperlipidemia, family history, male gender, age
- Ultrasound is procedure of choice for screening for AAA in any male older than 65 with any history of tobacco use.
- Suspect AAA for any elderly patient with back, abdominal, or groin pain. Triad of hypotension/shock, pulsatile abdominal mass, and abdominal/back pain always suggests rupture, which requires emergent evaluation for surgery.
- 5.5 cm is the threshold diameter for elective surgical treatment (with some exceptions).

ANGINA PECTORIS, STABLE

Balakumar Pandian, MD

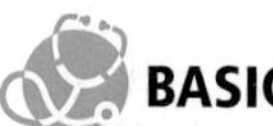

BASICS

DESCRIPTION

- Predictable and reproducible chest discomfort that occurs in a consistent pattern at a certain level of exertion or emotional stress and is relieved with rest or sublingual nitroglycerin
- Definitions:
  - Typical angina: A sense of choking or of pressure or heaviness deep to the precordium, frequently radiating to the jaw, arms, or epigastrium; usually brought on by exertion or anxiety and relieved by rest. Discomfort may be described with a clenched fist over the sternum (Levine sign).
  - Anginal equivalent: Patients with angina may present without chest discomfort, but with nonspecific symptoms such as dyspnea, fatigue, belching, nausea, lightheadedness, indigestion
- Unstable angina: Anginal symptoms that are new or are changed in character to become more frequent, more severe, or both. Considered an acute coronary syndrome in the same continuum as non–ST segment elevation myocardial infarction (NSTEMI).
- System(s) affected: Cardiovascular

Geriatric Considerations

Elderly patients may present with atypical anginal symptoms. Maintain a high degree of suspicion during evaluation. They may also be very sensitive to the side effects of medications.

Pregnancy Considerations

Other diagnoses should be excluded and the patient managed closely by an obstetrician or family physician and cardiologist; the metabolic demands of pregnancy can exacerbate symptoms and directly interfere with treatment.

EPIDEMIOLOGY

- Predominant age: Most common in middle-age and older men, postmenopausal women
- Predominant sex: Male > Female

Incidence

~500,000 new cases of stable angina occur yearly in patients ≥45 years old (1).

Prevalence

More than 10 million people ≥20 years old suffer from angina in the US (1).

RISK FACTORS

Risk factors for coronary artery disease include:

- Family history of premature coronary artery disease (CAD) in first-degree relatives (in male relatives <55 years old or female relatives <65 years old)
- Obesity
- Hypercholesterolemia
- Elevated BP
- Cigarette smoking
- Diabetes mellitus
- Male gender
- Advanced age

GENERAL PREVENTION

- Stop smoking.
- Low-fat/low-cholesterol diet
- Regular aerobic exercise program
- Weight loss (goal BMI <25)
- BP control (goal BP <140/90)
- Antilipidemics if indicated by current ATP guidelines or a risk-based approach
- Optimize glycemic control in those with diabetes mellitus.

PATHOPHYSIOLOGY

- Anginal symptoms occur during times of myocardial ischemia caused by a mismatch between coronary artery perfusion and myocardial oxygen demand. Sensory nerves from the heart travel up the sympathetic chain and enter the spinal cord at levels C7–T4, causing diffuse referred pain/discomfort in the associated dermatomes.
- Atherosclerotic narrowing of the coronary arteries (stenosis of >70%) is the most common pathology. Angina may occur in those with significant aortic valve disease or hypertrophic cardiomyopathy, even with normal coronary arteries.

ETIOLOGY

- Atherosclerosis of the coronary arteries (most common)
- Aortic stenosis
- Hypertrophic cardiomyopathy
- Aortic insufficiency
- Primary pulmonary hypertension (HTN)

COMMONLY ASSOCIATED CONDITIONS

- Hypercholesterolemia
- Peripheral vascular disease
- Hypertension
- Overweight
- Diabetes mellitus

DIAGNOSIS

- Predictable and reproducible anginal symptoms lasting 3–15 minutes brought on by exertion, emotional stress, meals, cold air, or smoking; symptoms relieved by rest or nitrates
- Careful history is important in eliciting symptoms of angina as listed above.
- Dyspnea on exertion may present as the only symptom.
- Atypical symptoms are more likely in women, elderly, and diabetic patients.
- Canadian Cardiovascular Society grading of chronic stable angina severity:
  - Class 1: Ordinary physical activity does not cause angina; angina with strenuous or rapid or prolonged exertion
  - Class 2: Slight limitation of ordinary activity (walking rapidly or >2 blocks, climbing >1 flight of stairs, emotional stress)
  - Class 3: Marked limitation of ordinary physical activity
  - Class 4: Inability to carry on any physical activity without discomfort. Angina may occur at rest.

HISTORY

- Quality of any previous anginal episodes and pattern over time
- Underlying history of heart disease or valvular disease
- Family history of myocardial infarction, CAD, sudden death

PHYSICAL EXAM

- Measure vital signs such as BP, heart rate, respiratory rate, and oxygen saturation.
- Cardiac exam may reveal dysrhythmias, heart murmurs indicative of valvular disease, signs of ventricular hypertrophy, gallops, or signs of congestive heart failure.
- Vascular exam may show signs of peripheral vascular disease (diminished pulses, bruits, abdominal aneurysm)
- Pulmonary exam may reveal signs of obstructive or restrictive diseases, pulmonary edema
- May see signs of dyslipidemia (xanthomas, xanthelasma)
- Normal physical exam should not exclude cardiac causes of anginal symptoms.

DIAGNOSTIC TESTS & INTERPRETATION

- ECG:
  - May show evidence of prior myocardial infarction. However, ECG is frequently unremarkable when asymptomatic. May show signs of myocardial ischemia during symptomatic episodes.
  - Bundle branch block, Wolff Parkinson White syndrome, or intraventricular conduction delay may make stress ECG interpretation unreliable.
- Stress testing (exercise testing preferable):
  - Exercise testing for those who can physically exercise (≥5 metabolic equivalents [METS]):
    - Standard exercise ECG for those with normal baseline ECG
    - Exercise stress testing with echocardiography or perfusion imaging for those with abnormal baseline ECG or in premenopausal women
  - In patients who cannot tolerate exercise, pharmacologic stress testing with adenosine, regadenoson, or dipyridamole. Dobutamine preferred if asthma or heart block (2° or 3°).
- Coronary angiography is the gold standard for confirmation and delineation of coronary disease and direction of interventional therapy or surgery.

Lab

- Total cholesterol and low-density lipoprotein (LDL) may be elevated, and high-density lipoprotein (HDL) cholesterol may be reduced.
- C-reactive protein (CRP): Most useful for those individuals at intermediate risk of developing coronary artery disease (10–20% over 10 years by Framingham risk criteria) in whom an elevated CRP may suggest an increased likelihood of benefit from statin therapy)

Initial lab tests

Hematocrit, fasting lipid profile, fasting blood sugar, basic metabolic panel

Imaging

- Consider echocardiogram if valvular disease or hypertrophic cardiomyopathy is suspected.
- Stress imaging with echocardiogram or perfusion imaging (see section on stress testing)
- Consider chest radiography if signs of pulmonary disease.

DIFFERENTIAL DIAGNOSIS

- Pulmonary disease
- Deconditioning

TREATMENT

MEDICATION

First Line

- Anti-ischemic (antianginal) medications:
  - Beta blockers decrease heart rate, BP, and myocardial contractility:
    - Atenolol (25–100 mg/d), metoprolol (25–100 mg b.i.d.)
    - Adjust doses according to clinical response. Aim to maintain resting heart rate of 50–60 beats per minute.
    - Side effects may include fatigue, exercise intolerance, erectile dysfunction, bradycardia, or heart block.
    - Contraindications include decompensated congestive heart failure (CHF), severe bradycardia, advanced arterioventricular (AV) block, or severe lung disease.
  - Nitrates dilate systemic veins and arteries (including coronary vessels) and cause decreased afterload and increased myocardial flow:
    - Sublingual nitroglycerin 0.4 mg SL. For acute anginal episodes. Repeat 2–3 times over a 10–15-minute period; if no relief, immediate medical attention must be sought.
    - Long–acting nitrates: Should be used with a drug–free interval of 8–12 hours to prevent tolerance. Side effects such as headaches and hypotension tend to clear with continued usage.
    - Concurrent use of phosphodiesterase inhibitors for erectile dysfunction (e.g. sildenafil, vardenafil, tadalafil) may cause life-threatening hypotension and are contraindicated.
  - Calcium channel blockers (CCBs) cause arterial vasodilation, decrease myocardial oxygen demand, and improve coronary blood flow. Only long-acting CCBs should be used:
    - Dihydropyridine CCBs such as nifedipine (30–90 mg/d), amlodipine (5–10 mg/d), or felodipine (2.5–10 mg/d) cause more vasodilation. Nondihydropyridine CCBs such as diltiazem (120–480 mg/d) or verapamil (120–480 mg/d). Amlodipine preferred in patients with low ejection fraction.
    - Side effects include constipation and peripheral edema. The nondihydropyridine CCBs may also cause bradycardia, heart block, and precipitate heart failure in those with severe systolic dysfunction.
  - Ranolazine (500–1,000 mg b.i.d.) likely works by improving left ventricular function, although the exact mechanisms are unclear:
    - Use as adjunctive therapy in those who are still symptomatic on optimal doses of β-blockers, nitrates, or amlodipine
    - Side effects may include nausea, constipation, dizziness, and headache.
    - Contraindications include combination with nondihydropyridine CCBs, prolonged QT, and medications that inhibit cytochrome P-450 system.
- Vasculoprotective therapies:
  - Antiplatelet therapy is indicated in all patients:
    - Aspirin (81–325 mg/d) is preferred.
    - Clopidogrel (75 mg/d) may be used in patients with contraindications to aspirin.
    - Combination of aspirin and clopidogrel is indicated for those with stent placement to reduce rate of stent thrombosis (1 month for bare metal stents and ≥12 months for drug eluting stents)
  - Statins (e.g., simvastatin, atorvastatin, pravastatin, lovastatin) for hypercholesterolemia:
    - Most beneficial as secondary prevention in those with CAD. Decrease incidence of symptomatic CAD and reduce both myocardial infarction (MI) and death from MI.
    - LDL target <100 mg/dL for established CAD. Consider target <70 in high-risk patients.
    - Current ATP guidelines support using lipid-lowering drugs for those with suspected or documented CAD.
    - Side effects may include elevated transaminases, myalgias. May rarely cause myositis or rhabdomyolysis. Monitor labs with any changes in medication doses.
  - ACE inhibitors have been shown to reduce both cardiovascular death and MI. Indicated in patients with CAD or other vascular disease, particularly in those with diabetes or left ventricular (LV) systolic dysfunction. Angiotensin receptor blockers may be used in patients intolerant of ACE inhibitors.

ADDITIONAL TREATMENT

General Measures

Lifestyle modifications are very important:

- BP control
- Smoking cessation
- Minimize emotional stress.
- Weight reduction in obese patients (2)[C]
- Daily physical activity (30–60 minutes) (3)[C]
- Annual influenza vaccination (3)[C]

COMPLEMENTARY AND ALTERNATIVE MEDICINE

Relaxation/stress reduction therapy may help reduce anginal episodes.

SURGERY/OTHER PROCEDURES

- Revascularization therapies: Consider if optimal medication management is inadequate in controlling symptoms:
  - Percutaneous coronary intervention (PCI):
    - Balloon angioplasty
    - Stent placement (with drug eluting or bare metal stent)
    - Although patients may become symptom-free faster, PCI does not decrease mortality or myocardial infarction compared to optimal medical management in those with stable angina (4).
  - Coronary artery bypass grafting (CABG)
- For refractory angina (5):
  - Spinal cord stimulation
  - Enhanced external counterpulsation
  - Myocardial laser revascularization therapy

IN-PATIENT CONSIDERATIONS

Admission Criteria

Inpatient evaluation is warranted in any patient with new changes in their angina symptoms.

ONGOING CARE

FOLLOW-UP RECOMMENDATIONS

Lifestyle modifications should be stressed at every visit.

Patient Monitoring

Changes in severity or frequency of anginal symptoms need further evaluation.

DIET

Low-fat, low-cholesterol, low-salt diet

PROGNOSIS

Variable; depends on severity of symptoms, the extent of CAD, and LV function

COMPLICATIONS

- Unstable angina or MI
- Arrhythmia
- Cardiac arrest
- CHF

REFERENCES

1. Lloyd-Jones D, Adams RJ, Browm TM, et al. Heart Disease and Stroke Statistics–2010 Update: A report from the American Heart Association. *Circulation*. 2010;121:3.46–e.215.
2. Gibbons RJ, Abrams J, Chatterjee K, et al. ACC/AHA 2002 guideline update for the management of patients with chronic stable angina—summary article: A report of the American College of Cardiology/American Heart Association Task Force on Practice Guidelines (Committee on the Management of Patients with Chronic Stable Angina). *Circulation*. 2003;107:149–58.
3. Fraker TD, Fihn SD writing on behalf of the 2002 Chronic Stable Angina Writing Committee. 2007 Chronic Angina Focused Update of the ACC/AHA 2002 Guidelines for the Management of Patients with Chronic Stable Angina. *Circulation*. 2007; 116:2762–2772.
4. William B, O'Rourke RA, Teo KK, et al. Optimal medical therapy with or without PCI for stable coronary disease. *N Engl J Med*. 2007; 356(15): 1503–16.
5. Khan SN, Dutka DP. A systematic approach to refractory angina. *Curr Opin Support Palliat Care*. 2008;2:247–251.

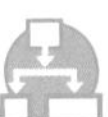

See Also (Topic, Algorithm, Electronic Media Element)

Algorithms: Chest Pain; Chest Pain/Acute Coronary Syndrome

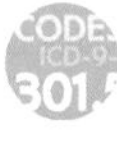

CODES

ICD9

- 411.1 Intermediate coronary syndrome
- 413.9 Other and unspecified angina pectoris

CLINICAL PEARLS

- Careful history taking is important in diagnosis, especially in the elderly.
- Maximize antianginal therapy by combining β-blockers, CCB, and nitrates in those still symptomatic with monotherapy.
- Exercise testing may be useful diagnostically and to assess effectiveness of antianginal therapy.

ANGIOEDEMA

Michelle T. Martin, PharmD
Jamie Berkes, MD

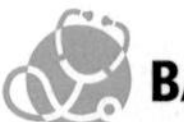

BASICS

DESCRIPTION

- Angioedema (AE) is an acute, localized swelling of skin, mucosa, and submucosa caused by extravasation of fluid into the affected tissues.
- Often resolves in hours to days, but can be life-threatening if the upper airway is involved
- Usually involves the face, tongue, larynx, GI tract, and extremities
- Causes: Idiopathic; medications such as ACE inhibitors; allergens such as foods, latex, or venom; physical elements such as vibration or cold
- Hereditary AE (HAE) and acquired AE (AAE) are diseases of the complement cascade that result in recurrent episodes of AE of the skin, upper airway, and GI tract.
- Synonym(s): Angioneurotic edema; Quincke edema

EPIDEMIOLOGY

- Predominant age:
  - Allergen, medication, or other triggers can affect all ages.
  - HAE: Infancy to second decade of life
  - AAE: Typically patients in 4th decade of life
- Predominant gender: Male = Female (except type III HAE affects more women than men)

Prevalence

- AE occurs in about 15% of the population over a lifetime.
- AE: 0.1–2.2% of patients receiving ACE inhibitors: African Americans have a 4–5 times greater risk of ACE inhibitor–induced AE than Caucasians.
- HAE: 1:10,000–50,000 population in US

RISK FACTORS

- Consuming medications and foods that can cause allergic reactions
- Pre-existing diagnosis of HAE or AAE

Genetics

- HAE types I and II are autosomal dominant, whereas type III is dominant X-linked.
- HAE occurs in 25% of patients as a result of spontaneous genetic mutations.

GENERAL PREVENTION

- Avoid known triggers.
- Avoid ACE inhibitors if history of AE.
- Do not use ACE inhibitors in patients with C1 esterase inhibitor (C1 INH) deficiency.

PATHOPHYSIOLOGY

- Type 1 hypersensitivity reaction
- Increase in vascular permeability secondary to IgE-mediated mast cell–stimulated histamine release or from activation of the complement system and an elevation in bradykinin (HAE)
- Attacks of HAE are triggered by prolonged mechanical pressure, cold, heat, trauma, emotional stress, menses, illness, and inflammation:
  - Type I HAE is the most common form, caused by decreased production of C1 esterase inhibitor (C1 INH), and has autosomal-dominant inheritance.
  - Type II HAE has functionally impaired C1 INH and autosomal-dominant inheritance.
  - Type III (HAE-FXII) involves mutations in coagulation factor XII gene (occurs more frequently in women, often estrogen-dependent, associated with estrogen administration); also type III HAE-unknown exists.
- AAE is a rare condition:
  - Type I is associated with lymphoproliferative diseases or paraneoplastic diseases.
  - Type II is due to autoimmune disorders (anti-C1 INH antibody).
  - Affected patients have circulating antibodies directed either against specific immunoglobulins expressed on B cells (type I) or against C1 INH (type II).

ETIOLOGY

- Idiopathic
- Medication-induced:
  - ACE inhibitors cause 10–25% of AE cases, mostly occurring within the 1st month of use. However, onset may be delayed by years.
  - Angiotensin-receptor blockers (ARBs) also can cause AE, but more rarely than ACE inhibitors.
- Allergic triggers:
  - Food allergens such as shellfish, nuts, eggs, milk, wheat, soy
  - Medications such as aspirin, NSAIDs, antibiotics, narcotics, and oral contraceptives
- Physically induced: Cold, heat, pressure, vibration, trauma, emotional stress, ultraviolet light
- Hereditary or acquired C1 INH deficiency
- Thyroid autoimmune disease–associated AE

COMMONLY ASSOCIATED CONDITIONS

- Quincke disease (AE of the uvula)
- Urticaria

DIAGNOSIS

HISTORY

- Identify potential triggers, including medication history, recent exposure to allergens, physical elements, or trauma (1)[C].
- In comparison with urticaria, AE typically is nonpruritic, but it can cause a burning sensation.
- Family history

PHYSICAL EXAM

- Acute onset of asymmetric localized swelling, usually of the face (eyelids, lips, ears, nose), and less often of the extremities or genitalia
- GI tract involvement may manifest as intermittent unexplained abdominal pain.

ALERT

10–35% of patients present with severe respiratory compromise requiring endotracheal intubation.

DIAGNOSTIC TESTS & INTERPRETATION

Lab

Initial lab tests

- If AE with urticaria and/or anaphylaxis, check for allergen-specific IgE to verify suspected trigger. Serum tryptase is elevated during acute AE (1)[C].
- Without a clear etiology and recurrence in AE and urticaria, check CBC and ESR:
  - Macrocytosis implies a pernicious anemia.
  - Eosinophilia may imply atopy or, rarely, a parasitic infection.
  - Elevated ESR may imply systemic disorders (1)[C].
- In recurrent AE without a clear etiology and without urticaria, consider ordering serum C4 level for determination:
  - Low serum C4 is a sensitive but nonspecific screening test for hereditary and acquired C1 INH deficiency.
  - If C4 is normal, determine C1 INH level and function, and recheck C4 during an acute attack.
  - If C4 level and C1 INH level and function are still normal, consider other causes (i.e., medications or HAE type III) for AE (2)[C].
  - If C4 level, C1 INH level, and C1 INH function are low, this indicates HAE type I.
  - HAE type II is characterized by low C4 and low C1 INH function, but C1 INH level can be normal or elevated (2)[C].
  - C1q is decreased in ~75% of AAE but is usually normal in all types of HAE (2)[C].
  - AAE typically presents later in life (over age 40), and patients lack family history of AE.

Follow-Up & Special Considerations

If C4 and C1q are low (as in AAE), neoplastic and autoimmune workup is warranted. CBC, a peripheral smear, protein electrophoresis, immunophenotyping of lymphocytes, and imaging studies are often undertaken to rule out hematologic malignancies or cancer (1)[C].

Imaging

Initial approach

- Abdominal radiographs and CT scan can demonstrate GI AE or ileus.
- C1 INH deficiency may occur in association with internal malignancy, so AE rarely can be a paraneoplastic disease. Imaging (CT scan, radiography, etc.) then would be done as part of a neoplastic workup for patients with AAE.

Diagnostic Procedures/Surgery

Skin biopsy (may be nonspecific)

Pathological Findings

- Edema of deep dermis and SC tissue
- Variable perivascular and interstitial infiltrate

DIFFERENTIAL DIAGNOSIS

Urticaria (with AE in 40–50% of patients); allergic contact dermatitis; connective-tissue disease: Lupus, dermatomyositis; anaphylaxis; cellulitis, erysipelas; lymphedema; diffuse SC infiltrative process

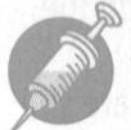

TREATMENT

MEDICATION

First Line

- Acute allergic AE (with airway compromise):
  - Epinephrine 1:1,000, 0.3 mL IV or SC (1)[C]
  - Glucocorticoids (hydrocortisone 200 mg IV or Solu-Medrol 40 mg IV) (1)[C]
  - Diphenhydramine 50 mg IV
  - If medication-induced, stop the causative agent.
- Idiopathic recurrent AE:
  - 1st-generation antihistamines for acute AE (cause drowsiness)
  - Older children and adults: Hydroxyzine (Vistaril 5 mg/5 mL, 25-mg tablets) 10–25 mg t.i.d., or diphenhydramine (Benadryl) 25–50 mg q6h (3)[C]
  - Children <6 years of age: Diphenhydramine 12.5 mg (elixir) q6–8h (5 mg/kg/d) (2)[C]

- 2nd-generation H_1 blockers: Fexofenadine (Allegra) 180 mg/d b.i.d., loratadine (Claritin) 10 mg/d, cetirizine (Zyrtec) 10 mg/d, desloratadine (Clarinex) 5 mg/d (3)[C]; use with caution in pregnancy and in the elderly.
- HAE chronic prophylaxis:
  - A nanofiltered plasma-derived C1 INH (pdC1 INH) concentrate (Cinryze) dosed at 1,000 units/10 mL IV, rate of 1 mL/min (for 10 min) q3–4d. Administration setting options include clinic, home health care, and after proper training, home self-administration (4,5)[B].
  - Attenuated androgens increase hepatic production of C1 INH: Oral Danazol 50–200 mg/d or oral stanozolol 2 mg/d; use lowest effective dose. Side effects include but are not limited to headache, weight gain, liver dysfunction, hirsutism, and menstrual disturbances. Monitor CBC, liver function tests, creatinine kinase, lactic dehydrogenase, fasting lipid profile, and urinalysis at baseline and q6mo. Abdominal ultrasound to be performed annually or q6mo. if dose of danazol >200 mg/d. Danazol is not to be used in children, during first 2 trimesters of pregnancy, during lactation, and in patients with hepatitis or cancer (2)[C].
- HAE short-term prophylaxis:
  - Minor procedures (dental work): If C1 INH is available, no prophylaxis; otherwise: Danazol 2.5–10 mg/kg/d (maximum 600 mg/d), stanozolol 4–6 mg/d, for 5 days prior to and 2–5 days after event (2)[C].
  - Major procedures (including intubation): C1 INH 1 (max 6) hour prior with additional dose on hand during procedure. If unavailable, danazol 2.5–10 mg/kg/d (max 600 mg/d) and solvent/detergent treated plasma (SDP). If SDP unavailable, use fresh-frozen plasma (FFP) 10 mL/kg; 2–4 units (400–800 mL) for an adult 1–6 hours prior.
- Acute HAE treatment:
  - C1 INH concentrate IV, dosed at 1,000 units if <50 kg; 1,500 units if 50–100 kg; 2,000 units if >100 kg (2)[C]; a pasteurized human pdC1 INH (Berinert), dosed at 20 units/kg (available in 500 units/10 mL, max infusion rate of 4 mL/min IV via peripheral vein. DO NOT SHAKE (will denature the protein). Worsening of HAE pain was reported as the most severe adverse event (4,6)[B].
  - Kalbitor (Ecallantide), a kallikrein inhibitor, is dosed in patients ≥16 years old at 30 mg SC with 3 separate 10 mg/mL injections in the abdomen, thigh, or upper arm, and a second 30-mg dose may be repeated within 24 hours if needed. Injection-site rotation not necessary but must be 2 inches away from attack site. A black box warning of anaphylaxis (potential adverse event) mandates administration in health care setting (4,7)[B].
  - Antihistamines and glucocorticoids typically do not benefit HAE patients. Epinephrine can offer transient stabilization/improvement in laryngeal AE, but is not sufficient for full treatment.
- New therapies are in phase 3 clinical trials for acute HAE treatment:
  - A bradykinin receptor-2 antagonist (icatibant), dosed SC and supplied in a prefilled 3-mL syringe for home administration; received favorable Food and Drug Administration (FDA) Advisory Committee review in June 2011. It was approved in the European Union (EU) as Firazyr (4,8)[B,C].
  - Other C1 INH replacement therapy: A recombinant human C1 INH isolated from the milk of transgenic rabbits (Rhucin), dosed IV, studied at 50 or 100 units/kg. Treatment is approved in Europe: Ruconest (9)[B],(10)[C].
  - Cinryze is awaiting FDA approval for use during acute attacks (4)[C].
- Acute AAE treatment:
  - C1 INH concentrate and FFP
  - Treatment of underlying lymphoproliferative disease is often curative in AAE type I.
  - Immunosuppressive therapy to suppress antibody production
  - Clinical trials underway with recombinant human C1 INH (Rhucin) (4)[C]

Second Line

- HAE chronic prophylaxis: If patient cannot tolerate attenuated androgens, antifibrinolytic agents (plasmin inhibitors), such as tranexamic acid (not approved by the FDA in US) 25–50 mg/kg/d divided b.i.d. or t.i.d. (3–6 g/d maximum) or ϵ-aminocaproic acid could be used. They are less effective than attenuated androgens and have many side effects. On rare occasions, they have been linked to (but not proven to cause) thrombophlebitis, embolism, or myositis (2)[C],(10).
- Acute HAE: FFP if C1 INH concentrate is not available, but it can potentially worsen attack (10)
- Idiopathic AE: Oral Doxepin (Sinequan) may be effective for AE (10–25 mg at bedtime).
- H2RA: Oral Ranitidine (Zantac) 150 mg/d b.i.d.

ADDITIONAL TREATMENT

General Measures

Intubation if airway is threatened

SURGERY/OTHER PROCEDURES

Tracheostomy if progressive laryngeal edema prevents endotracheal intubation

IN-PATIENT CONSIDERATIONS

Initial Stabilization

Ensure patent airway. If anaphylaxis, epinephrine (1:1,000) SC 0.3–0.5 mg q10–15min

IV Fluids

Given if needed to stabilize patient

ONGOING CARE

FOLLOW-UP RECOMMENDATIONS

Patient Monitoring

- Diagnostic workup if symptoms are severe, persistent, or recurrent
- Protect airway if mouth, tongue, or throat is involved.

DIET

Avoid known dietary allergens.

PATIENT EDUCATION

Educate on avoidance of triggers (i.e., food, medication, other physical stimuli), types of treatment, when to seek emergency care, and wearing Medic Alert bracelet.

PROGNOSIS

- AE symptoms often resolve in hours to 2–4 days. If airway is compromised, AE can be life threatening.
- Patients with HAE have an average of 20 attacks/year; each may last 3–5 days. Prophylaxis can decrease the frequency of events and number of missed days of school or work.

COMPLICATIONS

Anaphylaxis

REFERENCES

1. Temiño VM, Peebles RS. The spectrum and treatment of angioedema. *Am J Med.* 2008; 121:282–6.
2. Bowen T, Cicardi M, Farkas H, et al. 2010 International consensus algorithm for the diagnosis, therapy and management of hereditary angioedema. *Allergy Asthma Clin Immunol.* 2010;6(1):24.
3. Frigas E, Park M. Idiopathic recurrent angioedema. *Immunol Allergy Clin North Am.* 2006;26:739–51.
4. Levy JH, Freiberger DJ, Roback J, et al. Hereditary angioedema: Current and emerging treatment options. *Anesth Analg.* 2010;110:1271–80.
5. Zuraw BL, Busse PJ, White M, et al. Nanofiltered C1 inhibitor concentrate for treatment of hereditary angioedema. *N Engl J Med.* 2010; 363(6):513–22.
6. Craig TJ, Levy RJ, Wasserman RL, et al. Efficacy of human C1 esterase inhibitor concentrate compared with placebo in acute hereditary angioedema attacks. *J Allergy Clin Immunol.* 2009;124:801–8.
7. Cicardi M, Levy RJ, McNeil DL, et al. Ecallantide for the treatment of acute attacks in hereditary angioedema. *N Engl J Med.* 2010;363(6): 523–31.
8. Cicardi M, Banerji A, Bracho F, et al. Icatibant, a new bradykinin-receptor antagonist, in hereditary angioedema. *N Engl J Med.* 2010;363(6): 532–41.
9. Zuraw B, Cicardi M, Levy RJ, et al. Recombinant human C1-inhibitor for the treatment of acute angioedema attacks in patients with hereditary angioedema. *J Allergy Clin Immunol.* 2010; 126(4):821–827.e14.
10. Craig T, Riedl M, Dykewicz MS, et al. When is prophylaxis for hereditary angioedema necessary? *Ann Allergy Asthma Immunol.* 2009;102:366–72.

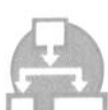

See Also (Topic, Algorithm, Electronic Media Element)

Urticaria; Anaphylaxis

CODES

ICD9

995.1 Angioneurotic edema, not elsewhere classified

CLINICAL PEARLS

- Trigger identification and avoidance are key in the prevention of AE.
- New AE treatments are in development.
- Patients with a history of allergies and AE should be prescribed an epinephrine autoinjector.

ANKLE FRACTURES

Francesca L. Beaudoin, MS, MD
Kimberly Pringle, MD

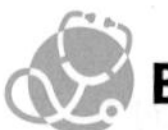

BASICS

- Bones: Tibia, fibula, talus. Mortise: Tibial plafond (horizontal surface of the tibia), medial malleolus, and lateral malleolus.
- Ligaments:
  - Syndesmotic ligaments: Anterior, posterior, and transverse tibiofibular ligaments and interosseous ligament (strongest)
  - Lateral collateral ligaments: Posterior tibiofibular, calcaneofibular, lateral talocalcaneal, anterior talofibular
  - Medial collateral ligaments; "deltoid ligament": Medial support via 4 ligaments that attach the tibia to the talus, navicular, and calcaneus: Posterior tibiotalar, anterior tibiotalar, tibiocalcaneal, tibionavicular

DESCRIPTION

- Fractures involving the distal fibula (lateral malleolus) and/or distal tibia (medial malleolus and plafond)
- Fractures that commonly occur with ligamentous injury:
  - Maisonneuve fracture: Proximal fibular fracture and rupture of the deltoid ligament with avulsion of medial malleolus
  - Osteochondral fracture of the talar dome
  - Avulsion fracture of the 5th metatarsal
- 2 common classification systems useful for describing fractures, but neither addresses ankle stability or reliably describes prognosis (1)[B]:
  - Danis-Weber system: Type A, B, C based on the location of the fibular fracture in relationship to the syndesmosis:
    - Type A: Below the level of syndesmosis (of tibiofibular joint); type B: At the level of the syndesmosis; both usually stable
    - Type C: Above syndesmosis; usually unstable
  - Lauge Hansen (theorized the type of fracture based on foot position and applied force): Based on pronation/supination, abduction/adduction, and internal/external forces that were applied to the foot at the time of injury
- The most basic nomenclature refers to the number of fractures:
  - Unimalleolar:
    - Lateral malleolus if type C, unstable
    - Medial malleolus fracture usually occurs in conjunction with ligamentous or lateral/posterior malleolus injury.
  - Bimalleolar: Most commonly the medial and lateral malleolus; usually unstable
  - Trimalleolar: Lateral, medial, and posterior malleoli; unstable
- Pilon fracture: Fracture of the talar dome and the tibial plafond; usually axial loading mechanism; unstable

Pediatric Considerations

- The distal tibial and fibial physis 3rd most common fracture in children
- Distal tibia most common site of pathologic fracture
- Injuries more likely to affect the growth plate
- Salter-Harris classification of fractures
- Juvenile Tillaux: Isolated fracture of anterolateral portion of the distal tibia epiphysis
- Triplane fracture: 2-, 3-, and 4-part fractures:
  - Most commonly epiphyseal fragment anteriorly and metaphyseal fragment posteriorly

EPIDEMIOLOGY

- Predominant ages: Even age distribution
- Predominant sex:
  - Age <50: Male > Female
  - Age >50: Female > Male
- Unimalleolar (fibular fractures) = 60–70%; bimalleolar = 15–20%; trimalleolar = 7–12%

Incidence

- 1–2 cases per 1,000 people per year
- Highest incidence in elderly women (2)[B]

RISK FACTORS

- Increased body mass index
- History of smoking or osteoporosis

GENERAL PREVENTION

- Proper shoe wear (i.e., flat, supportive shoes)
- Avoid, or use caution for, activities on uneven or slick surfaces.
- Avoid physical activity when fatigued.

PATHOPHYSIOLOGY

- The location and pattern of injury depend on foot position and the direction of force applied.
- Most commonly the foot is plantar flexed and inverted, and the force is external rotation.
- Axial loading can cause a tibial plafond or pilon fracture, an intra-articular fracture of the distal tibia with talus

ETIOLOGY

- Fall or twisting injury to the ankle
- Alcohol involved in 1/3 injuries
- Slippery surfaces involved in 1/3 cases

COMMONLY ASSOCIATED CONDITIONS

- Ligamentous injury (sprains):
  - Lateral collateral sprains are the most common (85–90%); medial collateral sprains and distal syndesmotic are uncommon.
- Syndesmosis injury
- Ankle or subtalar dislocation
- Fractures of metatarsals, talus, or calcaneus
- Osteochondral fractures
- Posterior ankle impingement (os trigonum)
- Peroneal tendon dislocation
- Compartment syndrome (rare)
- Neurovascular injury (rare)
- Other axial loading or shearing injuries:
  - Vertebral compression fractures
  - Contralateral pelvic fractures

DIAGNOSIS

HISTORY

- Location of pain
- Timing/mechanism of injury
- Weightbearing status at scene of injury
- Past history of ankle injuries or surgery
- Comorbidities (diabetes, coagulopathy)

Geriatric Considerations

Assess for safety and fall risk.

PHYSICAL EXAM

- Pain, swelling, and ecchymosis
- Inability to bear weight
- Possible deformity
- Find point of maximal tenderness.
- Skin integrity: Tenting, lacerations, or blistering
- Neurovascular status: Motor/sensory exam of foot/ankle; check dorsalis pedis and posterior tibial pulses:
  - If equivocal vascular exam, use a Doppler.
- Capillary refill
- Evaluate for compartment syndrome:
  - Swelling and pain with passive extension
- Palpate ankle, foot, leg, and knee.
- Examine for other associated injuries (i.e., pilon fractures: Vertebral injuries, contralateral tibial plateau).

DIAGNOSTIC TESTS & INTERPRETATION

Imaging

- Plain radiographs are the standard.
- Ottawa Ankle Rules (OAR) has a sensitivity 96.4–99.6% in adults (3)[B]:
  - X-rays indicated when malleolar pain AND:
    - Bone tenderness at the posterior edge or tip of the medial malleolus, or
    - Bone tenderness at the posterior edge or tip of the lateral malleolus, or
    - Inability to bear weight both immediately and in the emergency department, or
    - Pain at navicular or along 5th metatarsal
  - If OAR criteria not met for immediate x-ray, but symptoms persist beyond 48–72 hours, obtain films
  - OAR performs well in children (missing ~1% of fractures) (3), but some experts have proposed alternate rules.
  - OAR is not valid in intoxicated patients, patients with multiple injuries, or sensory deficits (diabetics with neuropathy).
- 3 standard views:
  - Anteroposterior (AP)
  - Lateral: Instability depicted by talar dome and distal tibia incongruity
  - Mortise (15–25° internal rotation view): Look for parallel lines between joint spaces, and space between the medial malleolus and talus should not exceed 4 mm.
- CT useful for Tillaux, triplane, and pilon fractures or fractures with intra-articular involvement:
  - Newer 3D reconstruction technology shows relationships between ligaments and bones.
- MRI sometimes used to explore Salter-Harris fractures or ligamentous injuries

Diagnostic Procedures/Surgery

- Arthroscopy is an option in cases of persistent pain or suspicion of any cartilaginous lesions.
- Surgery is definitive in cases of instability (see "Treatment").

DIFFERENTIAL DIAGNOSIS

- Stress fracture
- Ankle sprain
- Osteochondral fracture
- Talus fracture
- 5th metatarsal fracture
- Calcaneus fracture

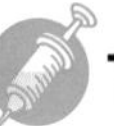

TREATMENT

Medication, joint support, consultation, surgical repair, physical therapy

MEDICATION

In general, ankle fractures are painful, particularly in the first 5–7 days following an injury. As the swelling decreases, so does the pain.

First Line

- Acetaminophen 1,000 mg q.i.d.
- NSAIDs
- Opioid analgesics

Second Line

Nonopioid analgesics (i.e., tramadol)

ADDITIONAL TREATMENT

General Measures

- Assess the extent of all injuries.
- Immobilization:
  - If there is a suspected open fracture, remove any debris from the wound and place a moist (Betadine) dressing over the wound.
  - Noncircular cast; short leg posterior splint stirrup
  - Jones compression bandage
  - Crutches
  - For suspected open fractures, tetanus booster, broad-spectrum cephalosporin and aminoglycoside penicillin G for farm injuries at risk for *Clostridium perfringens*
  - Do not reduce the fracture or dislocation unless neurovascular compromise is apparent.
- Ice and elevate the extremity.

Issues for Referral

- Send to emergency department for surgical evaluation:
  - Neurovascular compromise
  - Tenting of skin/open fracture
  - Displaced fracture of malleoli
  - Intra-articular fracture
  - Bi- or trimalleolar
  - Pilon fracture
  - Unstable fracture
  - Signs of compartment syndrome
  - Pediatric Salter types III, IV, V
  - Maisonneuve fracture
- All other fractures orthopedic follow-up within 1 week and be non–weight-bearing EXCEPT:
  - Isolated avulsion fractures of the tip of the lateral malleolus may be weight-bearing as tolerated.
  - Pediatric Salter I, II of the distal fibula

SURGERY/OTHER PROCEDURES

- Surgical options:
  - Open reduction internal fixation
  - External fixation for comminuted distal tibia fractures
- Timing of surgery:
  - Within 6–8 hours for emergent cases (i.e., open fractures)
  - After swelling decreased in all other cases (preferably not >1 week)
- Circular cast or protective boot:
  - Isolated nondisplaced medial malleolar: Non–weight-bearing 3 weeks + 6–8 weeks in a cast
  - Posterior malleolar with no instability: 6-week cast
  - Bimalleolar: Surgery vs. cast; orthopedic follow-up
- Length of recovery:
  - In general, 6–8 weeks for healing
  - 6–8 weeks in a cast or splint (longer if fracture involves both medial and lateral malleoli)
  - 2–4 months for syndesmotic injury
  - Orthopedist may allow range of motion after 4 weeks and place in removable cast boot (fracture pattern and surgeon dependent)

IN-PATIENT CONSIDERATIONS

Admission Criteria

Admit to the hospital if:

- Patient will require emergency surgery (e.g., open fracture, neurovascular injury, compartment syndrome)
- Cannot maintain non–weight-bearing status and requires physical therapy consultation
- Concern of mechanism of injury (i.e., syncope, myocardial infarction [MI], head injury)

Nursing

- Apply ice.
- Instruct patient to keep leg elevated.

Discharge Criteria

When patient has completed the following:

- Able to ambulate with walker/crutches
- Medical workup (if needed) is completed
- Appropriate orthopedic follow-up is arranged
- Elderly patients may require a short stay in a rehabilitation facility.

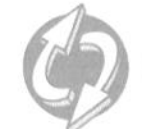

ONGOING CARE

FOLLOW-UP RECOMMENDATIONS

If the fracture does not require emergent orthopedic consultation, most ankle fractures require an orthopedic consultation within 1 week and close follow-up.

Patient Monitoring

- Orthopedic follow-up:
  - Serial x-rays should be performed weekly for 4 weeks if there is any question about stability.
  - Otherwise, x-rays should be performed at 2 weeks, 4 weeks, and 8 weeks or until the fracture is healed.
- Physical therapy: Once begins healing:
  - Encourage toe and knee motion as soon as possible.
  - Start ankle range of motion (ROM).
  - Physical therapy for strength and proprioception critical for full recovery

DIET

NPO if surgery is being considered

PATIENT EDUCATION

- Ice and elevate the affected leg for 2–3 weeks following the injury to decrease swelling.
- Prevent splint/cast from getting wet.
- Use crutches/cane as instructed.
- Call physician if:
  - Swelling increases
  - Toes become numb or painful
  - Burning pain under the cast
  - Pain increases and is not helped by elevation and pain medication

PROGNOSIS

- Good results can be achieved in many ankle fractures without surgery, provided the ankle mortise is maintained (4)[B]:
  - Back to normal activities, except for sports, in 3–4 months
- Long term, 30% of patients may develop ankle arthritis; timing is unpredictable.
- Effusion or pain can persist for up to 1 year.

COMPLICATIONS

Nonoperative and operative:

- Displacement of the fracture
- Malunion or nonunion
- Skin breakdown or necrosis (early)
- Deep venous thrombosis (DVT) (rarely pulmonary embolism)
- Complex regional pain syndrome
- Infection (osteomyelitis)
- Loss of fixation (postop)
- Osteoarthritis (late)

REFERENCES

1. Michelson JD, Maqid D, McHale K. Clinical utility of a stability-based ankle fracture classification system. *J Orthop Trauma*. 2007;21:301–307.
2. Court-Brown CM, McBirnie J, Wilson G. Adult ankle fractures–an increasing problem? *Acta Orthop Scand*. 1998;69:43–7.
3. Bachmann LM, Kolb E, Koller MT, et al. Accuracy of Ottawa ankle rules to exclude fractures of the ankle and mid-foot: Systematic review. *BMJ*. 2003; 326:417.
4. Michelson JD. Ankle fractures resulting from rotational injuries. *J Am Acad Orthop Surg*. 2003;11:403–12.

ADDITIONAL READING

- Bible J, Smith B. Ankle fractures in children and adolescents. *Techniques in Orthopaedics* 2009;24(3):211–9.
- Bucholz RW, Heckman JD, eds. *Rockwood and Green's Fractures in Adults*, 5th ed. Philadelphia: Lippincott Williams & Wilkins; 2001.
- Stielll G, Greenberg GH, McKnight RD, et al. Decision rules for the use of radiography in acute ankle injuries: Refinement and prospective validation. *JAMA*. 1993;269:1127–32.

CODES

ICD9

- 824.1 Fracture of medial malleolus, open
- 824.8 Unspecified fracture of ankle, closed
- 824.9 Unspecified fracture of ankle, open

CLINICAL PEARLS

- OAR has a near 100% sensitivity in adults for identifying significant ankle fractures.
- Ankle fractures mandating immediate surgical consultation include: Signs of compartment syndrome, neurovascular compromise, or skin compromise (open or tenting).

ANKYLOSING SPONDYLITIS

Sangeetha Balasubramanian, MD
Nancy Y. Liu, MD

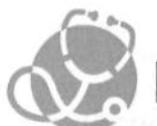

BASICS

DESCRIPTION

- Ankylosing spondylitis (AS) is a chronic inflammatory seronegative arthritis affecting mainly the axial skeleton and sacroiliac (SI) joints, but hips and shoulders may also be involved.
- System(s) affected: Musculoskeletal; Eyes; Cardiac; Neurological; Pulmonary
- Synonym: Marie-Strümpell disease

EPIDEMIOLOGY

- Predominant age: Onset usually in early 20s, rarely occurs after age 40
- Predominant sex: Male > female (2–3:1)

Incidence

Age- and gender-adjusted rate of 6.3–7.3 per 100,000 person-years

Prevalence

~0.1–1% in US

RISK FACTORS

- HLA-B27 (but only 1–8% of HLA-B27–positive adults have AS)
- Positive family history: A HLA-B27–positive child of a parent with AS has a 10–30% risk of developing the disease.

Genetics

About 90–95% of Caucasian patients with AS are HLA-B27–positive.

PATHOPHYSIOLOGY

Inflammation at the insertion of tendons (enthesitis), ligaments and fasciae to bone, causing inflammation, erosion, and new bone formation

ETIOLOGY

Interaction between genetic factors and unknown trigger(s)

COMMONLY ASSOCIATED CONDITIONS

- Uveitis/iritis (up to 40%)
- Aortitis
- Cardiac conduction defects
- Spondylitis and sacroiliitis also seen in psoriatic arthritis, reactive arthritis, and arthropathy associated with inflammatory bowel disease

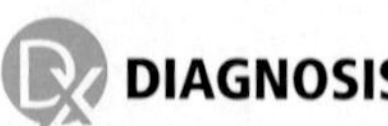

DIAGNOSIS

HISTORY

- Insidious onset of back pain
- Duration >3 months
- Morning stiffness in spine lasting more than 1 hour
- Frequent awakenings at night secondary to back pain
- Increased pain and stiffness with rest and improvement with activity
- Alternating buttock pain is a common symptom.
- Constitutional symptoms (fatigue, weight loss, low-grade fever)

PHYSICAL EXAM

- Sacroiliac joint tenderness, loss of lumbar lordosis, and cervical spine rotation
- Diminished range of motion in the lumbar spine in all 3 planes of motion
- Modified Wright-Schober test for lumbar spine flexion is abnormal or <5 cm:
  - Mark the patient's back over the L5 spinous process (or at dimples of Venus) and measure 10 cm above and 5 cm below this point. Have the patient bend forward. The normal exam is at least 5 cm of expansion between these 2 marks.
- Thoracocervical kyphosis (rarely occurs before 10 years of symptoms)
- Chest pain with inspiration due to enthesitis at costochondral junction and chest wall expansion
- Measurement of respiratory excursion of chest wall:
  - Normal is >5 cm of maximal respiratory excursion of chest wall measured at fourth intercostal space
  - <2.5 cm is virtually diagnostic of ankylosing spondylitis.
- Aortic regurgitation murmur (1%)
- Acute anterior uveitis (usually unilateral on initial presentation but can recur on contralateral side)
- Achilles tendonitis
- Plantar fasciitis
- Peripheral oligoarthritis rare; seen mostly with psoriatic arthropathy, reactive arthritis, and arthropathy associated with inflammatory bowel disease
- Cauda equina syndrome is rare but well recognized late in the disease.

DIAGNOSTIC TESTS & INTERPRETATION

Lab

- Since up to 10% of Caucasian population and 4% of African American population is HLA-B27–positive, gene testing is not recommended as part of initial evaluation.
- ESR and C-reactive protein (CRP) may be mildly elevated or normal; if high, correlate poorly with disease activity and prognosis
- Absent rheumatoid factor
- Mild normochromic anemia (15%)
- Synovial fluid: Mild leukocytosis

Imaging

- SI joints: Preferred position for imaging the SI joints with plain films is oblique projection:
  - X-ray changes may not be apparent for up to 10 years after disease onset. MRI is more sensitive in documenting changes; increased signal from the bone and bone marrow suggesting osteitis and edema.
  - Sequential plain radiographic changes with time: Widening, erosions, sclerosis on both sides of joint not extending >1 cm from articular surface and finally ankylosis of sacroiliac joint
- Spine:
  - Early plain radiograph changes include "shiny corners" due to osteitis and sclerosis at site of annulus fibrosus attachments to the corners of vertebral bodies and "squaring" due to erosion and remodeling of vertebral body; contrast-enhanced MRI imaging is more sensitive in revealing these early changes
  - Late changes include ossification of annulus fibrosis resulting in bony bridging between vertebral bodies (syndesmophytes) to give the classic "bamboo spine" appearance; ankylosis of apophyseal joints, ossification of spinal ligaments, and/or spondylodiscitis also occurs
- Peripheral joints:
  - Rare; asymmetric involvement of joints of lower extremities
  - Pericapsular ossification, sclerosis, loss of joint space, and erosions may occur.

Diagnostic Procedures/Surgery

- ECG: Conduction defects; echocardiogram: Aortic valvular abnormalities
- Dual-energy x-ray absorptiometry scan may reveal osteopenia/osteoporosis.

Pathological Findings

- Erosive changes coupled with new bone formation at the attachment of the tendons and ligaments to the bone, resulting in ossification of periarticular soft tissues
- Synovial hypertrophy and pannus formation, mononuclear cell infiltrate into subsynovium and subchondral bone marrow inflammation in the SI joint with erosions is followed by granulation tissue formation, and finally, obliteration of joint space by fusion of joint and sclerosis of para-articular bone

DIFFERENTIAL DIAGNOSIS

- Osteoarthritis of the axial spine
- Diffuse idiopathic skeletal hypertrophy (DISH)
- Psoriatic arthritis
- Reactive arthritis
- Spondylitis associated with inflammatory bowel disease
- Osteitis condensans illi: Benign sclerotic changes in the iliac portion of the SI joint found in women after pregnancies
- Infectious arthritis or discitis, especially unilateral sacroiliitis: Tuberculosis, brucellosis, bacterial (in IV drug users)

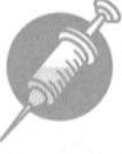

TREATMENT

Aggressive physical therapy, with referral to a physical therapist for daily home exercises, as well as group programs, is the most important nonpharmacological management.

MEDICATION

First Line

- Anti-inflammatory drugs:
  - NSAIDs provide rapid and dramatic symptomatic relief, which can be virtually diagnostic of AS. NSAIDs chosen empirically but most importantly, in high doses
  - Injection of intra-articular corticosteroids into SI joints and estheses can provide relief, but systemic corticosteroids are usually ineffective.
- Precautions:
  - All patients on long-term NSAIDs should have their hepatic and renal function monitored.
  - NSAIDs may aggravate peptic ulcer disease or cause gastritis; such patients and all patients >60 years of age should receive prophylactic proton pump inhibitors (PPIs) or misoprostol while on NSAIDs.
  - NSAIDs should be used with caution in patients with a bleeding diathesis or patients receiving anticoagulants.

Second Line

- Disease-modifying agents:
  - Used in those patients who have persistently high disease activity, fail, or become intolerant of NSAIDs
  - Biologic disease-modifying agents: Anti-TNF-α-blocking agents that are approved by FDA for AS include Etanercept (recombinant TNF receptor fusion protein) (1)[A], infliximab (chimeric monoclonal IgG1 antibody to TNF-α) (2)[A], adalimumab (fully humanized IgG1 monoclonal antibody to TNF-α) (3), and golimumab (human IgG1 kappa monoclonal antibody to TNF-α) (4).
  - Pamidronate may also help function and decrease disease activity.
  - Nonbiologic disease-modifying antirheumatic drugs such as methotrexate and sulfasalazine are ineffective for axial disease; sulfasalazine may be effective for peripheral arthritis (5).
- Precautions:
  - Anti-TNFs increase the risk for serious and even fatal, bacterial, mycobacterial, fungal, opportunistic, and viral infections.
  - It is imperative to screen for latent tuberculosis before initiation of treatment.
  - Screening for hepatitis B is also required.
  - Monitoring for reactivation of tuberculosis in all patients and invasive fungal infections like histoplasmosis, especially with travel to, or residence in, endemic areas
  - Lymphomas, skin cancers, and other malignancies have been reported in patients receiving anti-TNFs.
  - Immunizations should be updated before initiation of anti-TNFs since live vaccines are contraindicated in patients receiving anti-TNFs.

ADDITIONAL TREATMENT

General Measures

- Posture training and range-of-motion exercises for the spine are essential.
- Firm bed, sleep in supine position without a pillow
- Breathing exercises 2–3 times a day
- Smoking cessation

Issues for Referral

Confirmation of diagnosis before initiating any type of second-line therapy

Additional Therapies

- May need treatment with antiresorptive medications if osteopenia or osteoporosis is present
- Monitoring and management of cardiovascular risk factors and comorbidities

SURGERY/OTHER PROCEDURES

- Crucial to evaluate for C-spine ankylosis/instability before intubation
- Total hip replacement should be considered to restore mobility and to control pain.
- Vertebral osteotomy can improve posture for those patients with severe cervical or thoracolumbar flexion

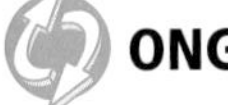

ONGOING CARE

FOLLOW-UP RECOMMENDATIONS

- Maintaining physical activity and posture is critical in preventing disability.
- Swimming, tai chi, walking, and maintenance of active lifestyle are recommended.
- Avoid trauma/contact sports.
- Appropriate work ergonomics

Patient Monitoring

- Visits every 6–12 months to monitor posture and range of motion
- Counsel about risk of spinal fracture.

PATIENT EDUCATION

- Arthritis Foundation: http://www.arthritis.org
- Spondylitis Association of America: http://www.spondylitis.org

PROGNOSIS

- Extent and rapidity of progression of ankylosis are highly variable.
- Progressive limitation of spinal mobility necessitates lifestyle modification.

COMPLICATIONS

- Spine:
  - Spinal fusion causing kyphosis
  - Cervical spine fracture carries high mortality rate; fracture can occur at any level of ankylosed spine
  - C1–C2 subluxation
  - Cauda equina syndrome (rare)
- Pulmonary:
  - Restrictive lung disease
  - Upper lobe fibrosis (rare)
- Cardiac:
  - Conduction defects at atrioventricular (AV) node
  - Aortic insufficiency
  - Aortitis
  - Pericarditis (extremely rare)
- Uveitis and cataracts
- Renal:
  - IgA nephropathy
  - Amyloidosis (<1%)
- GI: Microscopic, subclinical ileal, and colonic mucosal ulcerations in up to 50% of patients, mostly asymptomatic

REFERENCES

1. Davis JC, van der Heijde DM, Braun J. Sustained durability and tolerability of etanercept in ankylosing spondylitis for 96 weeks. *Ann Rheum Dis*. 2005;64:1557–62.
2. Baraliakos X, Listing J, Brandt J. Radiographic progression in patients with ankylosing spondylitis after 4 yrs of treatment with the anti-TNF-alpha antibody infliximab. *Rheumatology (Oxford)*. 2007;46:1450–3.
3. Haibel H, Rudwaleit M, Brandt HC. Adalimumab reduces spinal symptoms in active ankylosing spondylitis: Clinical and magnetic resonance imaging results of a fifty-two-week open-label trial. *Arthritis Rheum*. 2006;54:678–81.
4. Inman RD, Davis JC, Heijde DV. Efficacy and safety of golimumab in patients with ankylosing spondylitis: Results of a randomized, double-blind, placebo-controlled, phase III trial. *Arthritis Rheum*. 2008;58:3402–12.
5. Braun J, Zochling J, Baraliakos X, et al. Efficacy of sulfasalazine in patients with inflammatory back pain due to undifferentiated spondyloarthritis and early ankylosing spondylitis: A multicentre randomised controlled trial. *Ann Rheum Dis*. 2006;65:1147–53.
6. Sieper J, Rudwaleit M. Early referral recommendations for ankylosing spondylitis (including pre-radiographic and radiographic forms) in primary care. *Ann Rheum Dis*. 2005;64:659–63.

ADDITIONAL READING

- van der Heijde D, Maksymowych WP. Spondyloarthritis: State of the art and future perspectives. *Ann Rheum Dis*. 2010;69:949–54.
- Zochling J, van der Heijde D, Burgos-Vargas R, et al. ASAS/EULAR recommendations for the management of ankylosing spondylitis. *Ann Rheum Dis*. 2006;65:442–52.

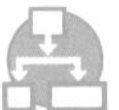

See Also (Topic, Algorithm, Electronic Media Element)

Arthritis, Psoriatic; Arthritis, Rheumatoid (RA); Crohn Disease; Reiter Syndrome; Ulcerative Colitis

CODES

ICD9

720.0 Ankylosing spondylitis

CLINICAL PEARLS

- HLA-B27 antigen exists in 8–10% of Caucasians and 4% of African Americans in the general US population.
- Diagnosis is based on history of inflammatory back pain and morning stiffness for more than an hour, alternating buttock pain, and evidence of limitation of chest wall expansion and spinal movements in all planes; evidence of sacroiliitis and response to NSAIDs (6).
- HLA-B27 testing is an expensive and unnecessary test when clinical diagnosis is clear, but it may help support the diagnosis when clinical features are less definitive.
- Plain radiography may fail to reveal changes of sacroiliitis or axial changes for up to 10 years.
- MRI is sensitive for detecting early changes of sacroiliitis or enthesitis in the axial spine.
- Physical therapy to maintain posture and mobility remains the most important nonpharmacological intervention.
- NSAIDs and TNF-α blockers are the mainstay of treatment and improve symptoms and function, but unfortunately, there is no current evidence that the latter treatment prevents bony ankylosis.

ANORECTAL FISTULA

Timothy L. Black, MD

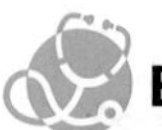

BASICS

DESCRIPTION

- Inflammatory tract with 1 opening in the anal canal and another in perianal skin.
- Fistulas occur spontaneously or secondary to perirectal abscess. Most fistulas originate in the anal crypts at the anorectal junction:
  - Goodsall rule:
    - If external opening is anterior to an imaginary line drawn horizontally through anal canal, fistula usually runs directly into anal canal. Positive predictive value (PPV) is ~70%.
    - If external opening is posterior to line, fistula usually curves to posterior midline of anal canal. PPV is ~40%.
    - In children, tract is usually straight.
  - Classification:
    - Intersphincteric: Fistula is confined to the intersphincteric plane (most common).
    - Trans-sphincteric: Fistula connects intersphincteric plane with ischiorectal fossa by perforating the external sphincter.
    - Suprasphincteric: Fistula connects intersphincteric plane with ischiorectal fossa but loops over external sphincter.
    - Extrasphincteric: Fistula connects rectum to perineal skin but passes external to sphincter.
- System(s) affected: Gastrointestinal; Skin/Exocrine
- Synonym(s): Fistula-in-ano; Anal fistula

Geriatric Considerations

Constipation is a common complication.

Pediatric Considerations

- Most common in infants
- More frequent in males

EPIDEMIOLOGY

- Predominant age: All ages
- Predominant sex: Male > Female

Incidence

Common

RISK FACTORS

- Injection of internal hemorrhoids, puncture wound from eggshells or fish bones, foreign objects, enema tip injuries
- Ruptured anal hematoma
- Prolapsed internal hemorrhoid
- Acute appendicitis, salpingitis, diverticulitis
- Inflammatory bowel disease (chronic ulcerative colitis, Crohn disease)
- Previous perirectal abscess
- Radiation treatment to perineum/pelvis
- Trauma, either internal or external
- Carcinoma

GENERAL PREVENTION

Prevention or prompt treatment of anorectal abscess

ETIOLOGY

- Erosion of anal canal
- Extension from infection from a tear in lining of anal canal
- Infecting organism is commonly *Escherichia coli* (other enteric pathogens may also contribute to infection)

COMMONLY ASSOCIATED CONDITIONS

- Possibly associated with penetrating injury, intestinal tuberculosis, ulcerative colitis
- Hidradenitis suppurativa
- Crohn disease

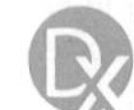

DIAGNOSIS

HISTORY

- History of perianal drainage
- History of perianal pain
- History of perianal abscesses in 26–37% (may be higher in recurrent abscesses) (1)[A]

PHYSICAL EXAM

- Constant or intermittent drainage or discharge (drainage may be purulent, bloody, or fecal)
- Firm, tender perianal mass
- External anal sphincter pain during and after defecation
- Spasm of external anal sphincter during and after defecation
- Anal bleeding
- Discoloration of skin surrounding fistula
- Fistulous opening frequently granulose or scarred
- Possible fever (uncommon)
- Perineal or perianal draining orifice
- Recurrent perianal abscesses in identical location
- Small palpable lesion sometimes identified on rectal exam at level of anal crypts

DIAGNOSTIC TESTS & INTERPRETATION

Lab

- CBC (usually not indicated)
- Serologic testing using perinuclear antineutrophil cytoplasmic antibody and anti-*Saccharomyces cerevisiae* antibody if inflammatory bowel disease (i.e., Crohn disease) suspected
- Consider rapid plasma reagin for recurrent fistulas in sexually active patients to rule out syphilis.

Imaging

- Lower GI series if inflammatory bowel disease suspected
- Pelvic MRI or endorectal ultrasound may be useful in complex or recurrent fistulas.

Diagnostic Procedures/Surgery

- Proctoscopy or sigmoidoscopy
- Colonoscopy and esophagogastroduodenoscopy if Crohn disease suspected
- Probe inserted into tract to determine its course (be careful not to create an artificial opening); best done at time of surgery
- Injection of dilute methylene blue into abscess cavity at time of surgery may be helpful in demonstrating fistula

Pathological Findings

- Fistulous tract may be simple or multiple
- Fistulous tract has primary opening in anal crypt; secondary opening in anal skin, para-anal skin, perineal skin, or in rectal mucous membrane
- Anal sinus: Opens in anal crypt
- Termination of sinus is blind and located in para-anal or pararectal tissue.

DIFFERENTIAL DIAGNOSIS

- Pilonidal sinus
- Perianal abscess
- Urethroperineal fistulas
- Ischiorectal abscess
- Submucous or high muscular abscess
- Pelvirectal abscess (rare)
- Rule out: Crohn disease, carcinoma, retrorectal tumors

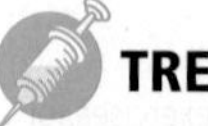

TREATMENT

MEDICATION

- Broad-spectrum antibiotic if active infection:
  - Cephalexin (Keflex)
  - Cefadroxil (Duricef)
  - Ampicillin-sulbactam (Unasyn)
  - Amoxicillin-clavulanate (Augmentin)
  - Cefoxitin or piperacillin/tazobactam (Zosyn) for IV use
- Stool-softening laxative

ADDITIONAL TREATMENT

General Measures

- Appropriate health care: Outpatient surgery
- Sitz baths 3–4 times per day until definitive surgery

SURGERY/OTHER PROCEDURES

- Fistulotomy:
  - Surgical incision of entire length of fistula (unroofing) (2)[A]
  - Mucosal tract should be cauterized or curetted.
  - Consider fistulotomy at time of initial abscess drainage if fistula tract can be identified.
  - Sphincterotomy
- Fistulectomy:
  - Complete excision of tract (rarely indicated because of extensive tissue loss)
  - Sphincterotomy
- Consider Seton stitch placement (especially for suprasphincteric or trans-sphincteric fistulas) (2)[A].
- Endorectal advancement flap closure for complex fistulas (2)[A]
- General anesthesia or regional anesthesia usually required (usually done as outpatient procedure in children)
- Consider use of fibrin glue in selected cases of anal fistulas (2)[A],(3)[A]:
  - There is slightly lower healing rate in fibrin glue-treated patients.
  - Very low incontinence rate following fibrin glue
  - Repeat applications of fibrin glue improve results.
- Fistulas in Crohn disease (2)[A],(4)[B]:
  - Asymptomatic fistulas may not need treatment.
  - Simple fistulas treated with unroofing
  - Complex fistulas treated with advancement flap or long-term Setons
  - Fibrin glue may be of benefit in patients with complex fistulae or Crohn disease (1)[A].
  - May require a diverting stoma
  - Occasional patients may require proctectomy.
  - Aggressive treatment of Crohn disease
- Postoperative: Sitz baths several times per day
- Avoid constipation.

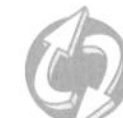

ONGOING CARE

FOLLOW-UP RECOMMENDATIONS

Resume work and normal activity as soon as possible.

Patient Monitoring

Frequent follow-up examinations following surgery to ensure complete healing and assess continence

DIET

Clear liquid diet until GI function returns

PROGNOSIS

- Surgical results usually excellent
- No major difference between the various techniques used as far as recurrence rates are concerned (5)[A]
- Postoperative healing:
  - 4–5 weeks for perianal fistulas
  - 12–16 weeks for deeper fistulas
  - $<1/3$ of patients with Crohn disease who have active proctitis demonstrate significant healing following surgical intervention (4)[B].
- Postoperative healing may occur within 2–3 weeks in children.
- Recurrence rates 2–9% in simple fistulas (2)[A]
- Healing may be significantly delayed in patients with Crohn disease.

COMPLICATIONS

- Constipation (urge to defecate may be suppressed due to pain)
- Rectovaginal fistula
- Partial incontinence of fecal material if sphincter is divided
- Delayed wound healing
- Low-grade carcinoma may develop in long-standing fistulas.
- Recurrent anorectal fistula if fistula is incompletely opened or excised
- Chronic intermittent infections
- Sepsis (rarely)

REFERENCES

1. Malik AI, Nelson RL. Surgical management of anal fistulae: A systematic review. *Colorectal Dis.* 2008;10:420–30.
2. Whiteford MH, Kilkenny J, Hyman N, et al. Practice parameters for the treatment of perianal abscess and fistula-in-ano (revised). *Dis Colon Rectum.* 2005;48:1337–42.
3. Cirocchi R, Farinella E, La Mura F, et al. Fibrin Glue in the treatment of anal fistula: A systematic review. *Ann Surg Innov Res.* 2009;3:12.
4. Lewis RT, Maron DJ. Anorectal Crohn's disease. *Surg Clin North Am.* 2010;90:83–97, Table of Contents
5. Jacob TJ, Perakath B, Keighley MR. Surgical intervention for anorectal fistula. *Sao Paulo Med J.* 2011;129(2):120–1. PMID: 2160379

ADDITIONAL READING

Hammond TM, Grahn MF, Lunniss PJ. Fibrin glue in the management of anal fistulae. *Colorectal Dis.* 2004;6:308–19.

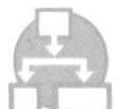

See Also (Topic, Algorithm, Electronic Media Element)

Anorectal Abscess; Crohn Disease

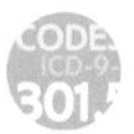

CODES

ICD9

565.1 Anal fistula

CLINICAL PEARLS

- Suspect anorectal fistula when patient complains of constant or intermittent perianal drainage or discharge (drainage may be purulent, bloody, or fecal).
- Surgery is the definitive treatment and usually produces excellent results.
- Antibiotics should be reserved for acute infection.

ANOREXIA NERVOSA

Pamela M. Williams, MD, Lt Col, USAF, MC
Jeffrey L. Goodie, PhD

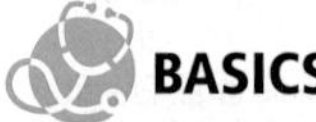

BASICS

DESCRIPTION
- Refusal to maintain normal body weight, with associated fear of weight gain, body-image disturbance, and amenorrhea
- Restricting and binge eating/purging subtypes
- System(s) affected: Cardiovascular; Endocrine; Metabolic; Gastrointestinal; Nervous; Reproductive

EPIDEMIOLOGY
- Predominant age: 13–20 years
- Predominant sex: Female > Male (20:1)
- Global distribution

Incidence
8–19 women/2 men per 100,000 population per year

Prevalence
- 0.9% in women
- 0.3% in men (higher in gay and bisexual men)

RISK FACTORS
- Female gender
- Adolescence
- Body dissatisfaction
- Perfectionism, obsessionality, rigidity
- Negative self-evaluation
- Academic and other achievement pressure
- Severe life stressors
- Participation in sports or artistic activities that emphasize leanness or involve subjective scoring: Ballet, running, wrestling, figure skating, gymnastics, cheerleading, weight lifting
- Type I diabetes mellitus
- Family history of substance abuse, affective disorders, or eating disorder

Genetics
- Underlying genetic vulnerability likely but not well understood
- 1st-degree female relative with eating disorder increases risk 6–10 fold.

GENERAL PREVENTION
Prevention programs can reduce risk factors and future onset of eating disorders (1)[C]:
- Target adolescents and young women 15 years of age or older.
- Encourage realistic and healthy weight-management strategies and attitudes.
- Decrease body dissatisfaction.
- Promote self-esteem.
- Reduce focus on thin as ideal.
- Moderate overly high self-expectations.
- Decrease anxiety/depressive symptoms.
- Improve stress management.

PATHOPHYSIOLOGY
- Complex relationship between genetic, biological, environmental, psychological, and social factors that results in an unrealistic perception of fatness
- Subsequent malnutrition leads to disorder of multiple organs.

ETIOLOGY
- Serotonin neuronal systems are implicated.
- Multifactorial with psychological, biologic, genetic, environmental, and social factors

COMMONLY ASSOCIATED CONDITIONS
- Mood disorder
- Social phobia, obsessive-compulsive disorder
- Substance abuse disorder
- High rates of cluster C personality disorders

DIAGNOSIS

- *Diagnostic and Statistical Manual of Mental Disorders, Fourth Edition, Text Revision* (2) criteria:
  - Refusal to maintain body weight at or above a minimally normal weight for age and height
  - Intense fear of gaining weight even though underweight
  - A disturbance in the way body weight/shape is experienced; undue influence of body on self-evaluation or denial of seriousness of low body weight
  - Specific types:
    - Restricting type: Not engaged in binge eating or purging behaviors
    - Binge eating/purging type: Regularly engages in binge eating or purging behaviors (see bulimia information related to these behaviors)
- Psychological self-report screening tools:
  - Eating Attitudes Test
  - Eating Disorder Inventory
  - Eating Disorder Screen for Primary Care
  - SCOFF (Sick, Control, One, Fat, Food) Questionnaire

HISTORY
- Patient unlikely to self-identify problem; corroborate with family or friends
- Fear of weight gain and/or distorted body image
- Report feeling fat even when emaciated
- Preoccupation with body size, weight control
- Onset may be insidious or stress-related.
- Elaborate food preparation and eating rituals
- Extensive exercise
- Amenorrhea (primary or secondary)
- Weakness, fatigue, cognitive impairment
- Cold intolerance
- Constipation, bloating, early satiety
- Growth arrest, delayed puberty
- Decreased bone density, fractures

PHYSICAL EXAM
- Often normal
- Vital signs: Hypothermia, bradycardia, orthostatic hypotension, body weight <85% of expected
- Cardiac: Dysrhythmias, midsystolic click of mitral valve prolapse
- Skin/extremities: Dry skin; lanugo hair on extremities, face, and trunk; hair loss; edema
- Neurologic and abdominal exams: To rule out other causes of weight loss and vomiting

DIAGNOSTIC TESTS & INTERPRETATION

Lab
- No specific test for anorexia nervosa (AN)
- Most findings are related directly to starvation and/or dehydration.
- All findings may be within normal limits.

Initial lab tests
- Low serum leuteinizing hormone, follicle-stimulating hormone; low serum testosterone in men
- Thyroid function tests: Low thyroid-stimulating hormone with normal T_3/T_4
- Liver function tests: Abnormal liver enzymes
- Chem 7: Altered BUN, creatinine clearance; electrolyte disturbances
- Hypoglycemia, hypercholesterolemia, hypercortisolemia, hypophosphatemia
- Low sedimentation rate
- CBC: Anemia, leukopenia, thrombocytopenia
- 12-lead electrocardiogram to assess for prolonged QT interval

Imaging
Dual-energy x-ray absorptiometry of bone to assess for diminished bone density, only if underweight for >6 months

Pathological Findings
- Osteoporosis/osteopenia, pathologic fractures
- Sick euthyroid syndrome
- Cardiac impairment

DIFFERENTIAL DIAGNOSIS
- Hyperthyroidism, adrenal insufficiency
- Inflammatory bowel disease, malabsorption
- Immunodeficiency, chronic infections
- Diabetes
- CNS lesion
- Bulimia; body dysmorphic disorder
- Depressive disorders with loss of appetite
- Anxiety disorder, food phobia
- Conversion disorder, schizophrenic disorder

ALERT
AN may exist concurrently with chronic medical disorders such as diabetes and cystic fibrosis.

TREATMENT

- Most patients should be treated as outpatients using an interdisciplinary team (3,4)[C].
- Behavioral therapies (e.g., cognitive-behavioral, interpersonal, or family therapy) should be offered (3,5,6,7)[C].
- Pharmacotherapy should not be used as the sole treatment modality (3,4,8)[C].

MEDICATION

First Line
- No medications are available that effectively treat patients with AN, but pharmacotherapy may be used as an adjuvant to cognitive-behavioral therapies (3,4,7,8)[C].
- SSRIs may:
  - Help to prevent relapse after weight gain
  - Treat comorbid depression or obsessive–compulsive disorder (3,4,7,8)[C]
- Studies using atypical antipsychotics are underway, with some early promising results.
- Attend to black-box warnings concerning antidepressants, and conduct appropriate informed consent if they are prescribed.

Second Line
- Management of osteopenia:
  – Primary treatment is weight gain (4)[C].
  – Elemental calcium 1,200–1,500 mg/d plus multiple vitamin injection containing 800 IU of vitamin D (4)[C]
  – No indication for bisphosphonates in AN (4)[C]
  – Weak evidence for use of hormone-replacement therapy (4)[C]
- Psyllium (Metamucil) preparations (1 T) to prevent constipation

ADDITIONAL TREATMENT
General Measures
- Initial treatment goal geared to weight restoration; most managed as outpatients
- Outpatient treatment:
  – Interdisciplinary team (primary care physician, mental health provider, nutritionist) (3,4)[C]
  – Average weekly weight gain goal: 0.5–1.0 kg (3,4)[C], with stepwise increase in calories
  – Cognitive-behavioral therapy, interpersonal psychotherapy, family-based therapy (3,5,6,7)[C]
  – Focus on health, not weight gain alone.
  – Build trust and a treatment alliance.
  – Involve the patient in establishing diet and exercise goals.
  – Challenge fear of uncontrolled weight gain; help the patient to recognize feelings that lead to disordered eating.
  – In chronic cases, goal may be to achieve a safe weight rather than a healthy weight.
- Inpatient treatment:
  – If possible, admit to a specialized eating disorders unit (4)[C].
  – Assess risk for refeeding syndrome (weight loss >10% in 2–3 months; current weight <70% ideal body weight).
  – Monitor vital signs, electrolytes, cardiac function, edema, and weight gain.
  – Initial bed rest with supervised meals may be necessary.
  – Stepwise increase in activity
  – Tube feeding or total parenteral nutrition is used only as a last resort.
  – Supportive symptomatic care as needed

Issues for Referral
Patients with AN require an interdisciplinary team (primary care physician, mental health provider, nutritionist).

IN-PATIENT CONSIDERATIONS
Admission Criteria
- Suggested physiologic values: Heart rate, <40 beats/min; BP, <90/60 mmHg; symptomatic hypoglycemia; potassium, <3 mmol/L; temperature, <97.0°F (36.1°C); dehydration; other cardiovascular abnormalities; weight, <75% of expected; rapid weight loss; lack of improvement while in outpatient therapy
- Suggested psychological indications: Poor motivation/insight, lack of cooperation with outpatient treatment, inability to eat, need for nasogastric feeding, suicidal intent or plan, severe coexisting psychiatric disease, problematic family environment

Pediatric Considerations
- Children often present with nausea, abdominal pain, fullness, and inability to swallow.
- Additional indications for hospitalization: Heart rate, <50 beats/min; orthostatic BP; hypokalemia or hypophosphatemia; rapid weight loss even if weight not <75% below normal
- Children and adolescents should be offered family-based treatment.

Geriatric Considerations
Late-onset AN (>50 years of age) may be long-term disease or triggered by death of loved one, marital discord, or divorce.

Discharge Criteria
Lower relapse rate when discharged at expected healthy weight

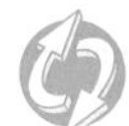

ONGOING CARE

FOLLOW-UP RECOMMENDATIONS
- Close follow-up until patient demonstrates forward progress in care plan
- Focus on enjoyable activities rather than goal-oriented ones.
- Emphasize importance of moderate activity for health, not thinness.

Patient Monitoring
- Level of exercise activity
- Weigh weekly until stable, then monthly.
- Depression, self-esteem, suicidal ideation

DIET
- Importance of adherence to prescribed diet
- Goal is stabilization at a healthy weight on a balanced diet with a normal eating pattern.
- Diminished ruminations about calories, weight; increased enjoyment

PATIENT EDUCATION
- Provide patients and families with information about the diagnosis and its natural history, health risks, and treatment strategies.
- The National Alliance on Mental Illness has information at www.nami.org/helpline/anorexia.htm
- See also: familydoctor.org

PROGNOSIS
- Prognosis: ~50% recover; 30% improve; 20% are chronically ill.
- Outcomes in men likely better than for women.
- Mortality: 3%

COMPLICATIONS
- Refeeding syndrome
- Cardiac arrhythmia, cardiac arrest
- Cardiomyopathy, congestive heart failure
- Delayed gastric emptying, necrotizing colitis
- Seizures, Wernicke encephalopathy, peripheral neuropathy, cognitive deficits
- Osteopenia, osteoporosis

Pregnancy Considerations
- Fertility may be affected.
- Behaviors may persist, decrease, or recur during pregnancy and the postpartum interval.
- Increased risk for preterm labor, operative delivery, and infants with low birth weight, smaller head circumference, and/or microcephaly; anemia; genitourinary infections; and labor induction; should be managed as high risk

REFERENCES

1. Stice E, Shaw H, Marti CN. A meta-analytic review of eating disorder prevention programs: Encouraging findings. *Ann Rev Clin Psychol.* 2007;3:207–31.
2. American Psychiatric Association. *Diagnostic and Statistical Manual of Mental Disorders DSM-IV-TR*, 4th ed. Arlington, VA: American Psychiatric Publishing, Inc; 2000.
3. NICE. Eating disorders—core interventions in the treatment and management of anorexia nervosa, bulimia nervosa and related eating disorders. NICE Clinical Guideline no 9. London: NICE, 200.
4. American Psychiatric Association. *Practice Guideline for the Treatment of Patients with Eating Disorders*, 3rd ed. Arlington, VA: American Psychiatric Publishing; 2006.
5. Hay P, Bacaltchuk J, Claudino A, et al. Individual psychotherapy in the outpatient treatment of adults with anorexia. *Cochrane Database Syst Rev.* 2003;4:CD003909.
6. Fisher CA, Hetrick SE, Rushford N, et al. Family therapy for anorexia nervosa. *Cochrane Database Syst Rev.* 2010;4:CD004780.
7. Bulik CM, Berkman ND, Brownley KA, et al. Anorexia nervosa treatment: A systematic review of randomized controlled trials. *Int J Eat Disord.* 2007;40:310–20.
8. Claudino A, Hay P, Lima M, et al. Antidepressants for anorexia nervosa. *Cochrane Database Syst Rev.* 2006;1:CD04365.

ADDITIONAL READING

- Dalle Grave R. Eating disorders: progress and challenges. *Eur J Intern Med.* 2011;22:153–60.
- Mehler PS, Cleary BS, Gaudiani JL. Osteoporosis in anorexia nervosa. *Eat Disord.* 2011;19:194–202.

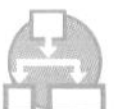

See Also (Topic, Algorithm, Electronic Media Element)
- Amenorrhea; Osteoporosis; Bulimia Nervosa
- Algorithm: Weight Loss

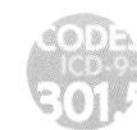

CODES

ICD9

307.1 Anorexia nervosa

CLINICAL PEARLS
- Particularly for young women with a risk factor, asking, "Are you satisfied with your eating patterns?" and/or "Do you worry that you have lost control over how you eat?" may help to screen those with an eating problem.
- In AN, there is a sustained and determined pursuit of weight loss, resulting in a body weight <85% of expected.
- To care for a patient with AN, an interdisciplinary team that includes a medical provider, a dietician, and a behavioral health professional is the most accepted approach.

ANTHRAX

Gregory D. Gutke, MD, MPH
Richard J. Thomas, MD, MPH
Jill A. Grimes, MD

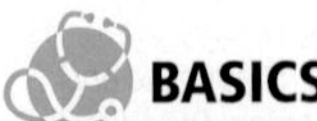

BASICS

DESCRIPTION

- Anthrax is a highly infectious disease of animals, especially ruminants (hooved animals such as cows, goats, and sheep) that is caused by the bacteria *Bacillus anthracis*. Cutaneous (95% of US cases), inhalational, and GI forms can be transmitted to humans by contact with the animals or their products (typically hair or hides).
- Synonym(s) for cutaneous anthrax: Charbon; malignant pustule; Siberian ulcer; malignant edema; splenic fever; milzbrand
- Synonym(s) for inhalational anthrax: Ragpicker disease; woolsorter disease

EPIDEMIOLOGY

- Total of 235 anthrax cases (224 cutaneous and 11 inhalational) occurred in the US between 1955 and 1994, resulting in 20 fatalities.
- Cutaneous: 95% of cases in the US; cases of cutaneous anthrax without occupational risk should raise concern for bioterrorism.
  - ~5–20% of untreated cases result in death; case fatality rate is <1% with antibiotic therapy.
- GI: Very rare in the US (no documented case in the 20th century).
- Inhalational anthrax is rare in the US; must be considered a bioterrorist event in US until proven otherwise (the last US occupational case occurred in 1976):
  - Death results in 99% of untreated cases and in 45–80% of patients with severe symptoms who are treated in a state-of-the-art facility.
- Anthrax is most common in agricultural regions, where it occurs in animals. These regions include the Middle East, Asia, Southern and Eastern Europe, Africa, South and Central America, and the Caribbean.

RISK FACTORS

- Contact with infected animals or their products
- Bioterrorist event

GENERAL PREVENTION

- Anthrax vaccine protects against all forms of anthrax and is as safe as other vaccines, according to the FDA, CDC, and the National Academy of Sciences.
- A 2009 review by the Cochrane Infectious Disease Group concluded that the anthrax vaccine is effective in reducing the risk of contracting anthrax and has a low rate of adverse effects (1)[A].
- Anthrax vaccine should be effective against all known strains of *B. anthracis* as well as against any strains that might be bioengineered by terrorists or others.
- Vaccine schedule and route changed in late 2008: Route is now IM (previously SC) and schedule is decreased from 6 doses to 5 doses (0 and 4 weeks, and 6, 12, and 18 months) plus annual boosters. IM versus SC injection greatly reduces the incidence of injection-site adverse events (2)[A]:
  - Anthrax vaccine adsorbed (trade name BioThrax) is FDA approved for ages 18 through 65 and is pregnancy category D.
  - If you get behind schedule, do not start the series over; begin where you left off (delays do not reduce the resulting protection).
  - Individuals are not considered protected until they have completed the full vaccination series.
  - The most common (>10%) local (injection-site) adverse reactions observed in clinical studies were tenderness, pain, erythema, and arm motion limitation. The most common (>5%) systemic adverse reactions were muscle aches, fatigue, and headache.
  - The Advisory Committee on Immunization Practices recommends vaccination for the following groups:
    - Persons who work directly with the organism in the laboratory
    - Persons who work with imported animal hides or furs in areas where standards are insufficient to prevent exposure to anthrax spores
    - Persons who handle potentially infected animal products in high-incidence areas
    - Military personnel deployed to areas with high risk for exposure to organisms (when used as a biologic warfare weapon)
    - Pregnant women should be vaccinated for anthrax only if absolutely necessary.
- Patients with a likely inhalational exposure history but no symptoms are candidates for postexposure prophylaxis with either ciprofloxacin 500 mg PO b.i.d. or doxycycline 100 mg PO b.i.d. for 60 days. Levofloxacin is also FDA approved for patients age 18 or older. CDC guidelines state patients should also receive 3 doses of anthrax vaccine (0, 2 weeks, 4 weeks), but since BioThrax is not licensed for postexposure prophylaxis or for a 3-dose series, this would need to be conducted under an Investigational New Drug application. Prophylactic medications are not indicated for prevention of cutaneous anthrax.

PATHOPHYSIOLOGY

- *B. anthracis* is a spore-forming, gram-positive bacterium found in the soil worldwide. The word *anthracis* is derived from a Greek word meaning "coal," which is used to describe the cutaneous form of the disease that leads to a characteristic black lesion.
- *B. anthracis* has 3 known virulence factors: An antiphagocytic capsule and 2 protein toxins (known as edema factor and lethal factor):
  - The capsule provides resistance to phagocytosis.
  - Lethal factor and edema factor are named for the effects they induce when injected into experimental animals.
  - A protein called *protective antigen* binds to the host cell's surface; when cleaved by a protease on the cell surface it creates a site to which the lethal factor and edema factor can bind; protective antigen is required for the action of the 2 protein toxins.
- *B. anthracis* spores introduced into the host are ingested at the exposed site by macrophages and then germinate into vegetative forms that produce the virulence factors.

ETIOLOGY

- Cutaneous: Occurs when *B. anthracis* enters the skin through a cut or abrasion during the handling of animal products (e.g., meat, wool, or hides infected with *B. anthracis*)
- GI: Ingestion of bacillus-contaminated meat
- Inhalational: Inhalation of aerosolized *B. anthracis* spores

DIAGNOSIS

- Cutaneous: Incubation period is usually immediate up to 1 day. Begins as a pruritic spot, followed by a red-brown papule that enlarges with peripheral erythema, vesiculation, and induration, followed by black eschar formation within 7–10 days of the initial lesion:
  - The papule, blister, and eschar are painless, and cutaneous symptoms may be accompanied by fever, malaise, and headache.
  - A black eschar with massive edema is nearly pathognomonic for cutaneous anthrax.
- GI: Incubation period is usually 1–7 days. Presents as 1 of 2 distinct syndromes—oropharyngeal and abdominal:
  - Oropharyngeal syndrome presentation can include fever, edema, ulcer, severe sore throat, and lymphadenopathy, resulting in marked unilateral or bilateral neck swelling.
  - Abdominal syndrome may present with fever, malaise, hematemesis, anorexia, severe abdominal pain, and hematochezia or melena. 2–4 days after onset of symptoms, pain begins to subside and ascites develops, with shock and death within just a few days.
- Inhalational: Incubation period is usually <1 week, but may be up to 60 days. Biphasic presentation, with initial phase featuring nonspecific influenzalike symptoms (e.g., low-grade fever, chills, headache, nonproductive cough, diaphoresis, malaise, chest discomfort, nausea, vomiting, diarrhea, abdominal pain):
  - This initial phase is followed by a 2nd fulminant phase that begins 1–5 days after onset of the initial phase symptoms. Signs and symptoms of the fulminant phase include abrupt onset of high fever, severe dyspnea, hypoxia, hypotension, and death within 24–36 hours.

HISTORY

- Cutaneous: Crucial clinical clues are rapid evolution of symptoms, lack of pain, occasional massive edema, and the near pathognomonic black eschar. Incubation period is usually immediate but may last up to 1 day.
- GI: Incubation period usually 1–7 days; 2–4 days after onset of symptoms, ascites develops as abdominal pain decreases. Shock and death occur within 2–5 days after onset of symptoms.
- Inhalational: Incubation period is usually <1 week but may be as long as 2 months. 2nd portion of the biphasic presentation begins 1–5 days after onset of initial symptoms. There may be a 1–3 day period of improvement after the 1st phase and before the 2nd phase begins. Shock and death occur within 24–36 hours after onset of the 2nd phase.

PHYSICAL EXAM
- Cutaneous: Red-brown papule, vesicles, or black eschar
- GI: Acute abdomen with rebound tenderness may occur. Ascites presents later in course.
- Inhalational: Rhonchi may be present.

DIAGNOSTIC TESTS & INTERPRETATION
Lab
Gram stain and culture. Obtain specimens for culture before initiating antimicrobial therapy. *B. anthracis* is easily isolated from blood cultures in <24 hours. A presumptive diagnosis can be made if gram-positive rods are present that are nonmotile, nonhemolytic, and encapsulated (usually seen with India ink). If antibiotics have been given for >24 hours, perform immunohistochemical staining and/or PCR.

Imaging
- Inhalational: Widened mediastinum on chest x-ray (CXR) may be present; pleural effusions frequently present; infiltrates are rare.
- CXR is indicated for suspected inhalational anthrax (3)[A].
- CT chest for patients with suspected anthrax but normal CXR (3)[A]
- GI: Mesenteric adenopathy on CT scan is likely.

DIFFERENTIAL DIAGNOSIS
- Skin cellulitis
- Brown recluse spider bite
- Cat-scratch disease
- Rat bite fever
- Rickettsial spotted fever
- Carbuncle
- Cowpox
- Bullous erysipelas
- Tularemia vasculitides
- Ecthyma gangrenosum
- Orf (a transmissible viral disease of goats and sheep)

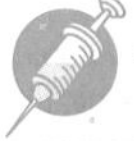

TREATMENT

MEDICATION
First Line
- Cutaneous: Ciprofloxacin 500 mg PO b.i.d. or doxycycline 100 mg PO b.i.d. for 7–10 days for localized or uncomplicated cases of naturally acquired cutaneous anthrax. Treat for 7–10 days with IV instead for severe cases of naturally acquired cutaneous anthrax with signs of systemic involvement, extensive edema, or lesions of the head and neck.
  - If cutaneous case is localized or uncomplicated but is bioterrorism-related, the patient must be treated for 60 days with PO ciprofloxacin or doxycycline because they are at risk for inhalational anthrax.
  - Patients with bioterrorism-related cutaneous anthrax who show signs of systemic involvement, massive edema, or lesions on the head or neck should be treated per inhalational anthrax recommendation (below) (4,5)[C].
- Inhalational and GI: IV ciprofloxacin 400 mg q12h (1st line) or doxycycline 100 mg q12h (2nd line) and 1 or 2 additional antimicrobials such as rifampin, vancomycin, penicillin, ampicillin, chloramphenicol, imipenem, clindamycin, and clarithromycin
  - May switch to PO when clinically appropriate.
  - Must complete 60-day course (combined PO and IV) (4)[C].
  - Early and aggressive pleural fluid drainage is recommended for all inhalational anthrax patients (5)[C].

Second Line
Patients being treated for anthrax may also benefit from vaccination as part of their regimen.

ADDITIONAL TREATMENT
General Measures
- Inhalational and GI anthrax are not known to spread from person to person, so communicability concerns are not an issue during management of the patient.
- Although cutaneous anthrax is also considered noncontagious, avoidance of contact with the wound or wound drainage seems prudent.

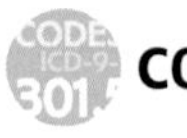

ONGOING CARE

FOLLOW-UP RECOMMENDATIONS
Patient Monitoring
Must monitor patient for 60 days to ensure completion of the treatment course.

PROGNOSIS
- Cutaneous: Death in 5–20% of untreated cases, but the case fatality rate is <1% with antibiotic therapy
- GI: Mortality rates as high as 50% reported
- Inhalational: Death in 45–80% of patients with severe symptoms who are treated in a state-of-the-art facility; case fatality rate approaches 99% in untreated cases.

REFERENCES

1. Donegan S, Bellamy R, Gamble CL. Vaccines for preventing anthrax. *Cochrane Database Syst Rev.* 2009;2:CD006403.
2. Wright JG, Quinn CP, Shadomy S, et al. Use of anthrax vaccine in the United States: Recommendations of the Advisory Committee on Immunization Practices (ACIP), 2009. *MMWR Recomm Rep.* 2010;59:1–30.
3. Kirsch J, Ramirez J, Mohammed TL, et al. ACR Appropriateness Criteria®acute respiratory illness in immunocompetent patients. *J Thorac Imaging.* 2011;26:W42–4.
4. Centers for Disease Control and Prevention. Update: Investigation of bioterrorism-related anthrax and interim guidelines for exposure management and antimicrobial therapy, October 2001. *MMWR Morb Mortal Wkly Rep.* 2001; 50:909–19.
5. Stern EJ, Uhde KB, Shadomy SV, et al. Conference report on public health and clinical guidelines for anthrax. *Emerg Infect Dis.* 2008;14.

ADDITIONAL READING

- Centers for Disease Control and Prevention, Emergency Preparedness and Response. http://www.bt.cdc.gov/agent/anthrax/
- Durning SJ, Roy MJ. Anthrax. In: Roy MJ, ed. *Physician's Guide to Terrorist Attack*. Totowa, NJ: Humana, 2003.
- Marano N, Plikaytis BD, Martin SW, et al. Effects of a reduced dose schedule and intramuscular administration of anthrax vaccine adsorbed on immunogenicity and safety at 7 months: A randomized trial. *JAMA*. 2008;300:1532–43.
- Schwartz MN. Recognition and management of anthrax—an update. *N Engl J Med*. 2001;345: 1621–1626.
- The anthrax vaccine immunization program. http://www.anthrax.mil

CODES

ICD9
- 022.0 Cutaneous anthrax
- 022.1 Pulmonary anthrax
- 022.9 Anthrax, unspecified

CLINICAL PEARLS

- Anthrax vaccine (only recommended for high-risk groups) protects against all forms of anthrax and is as safe as other vaccines, according to the FDA, CDC, and the National Academy of Sciences.
- Inhalational anthrax is rare in US; must be considered a bioterrorist event until proven otherwise (last US occupational case occurred in 1976):
  - Death results in 99% of untreated cases and in 45–80% of patients with severe symptoms who are treated in a state-of-the-art facility.
- Widened mediastinum on CXR may be present; pleural effusions frequently present; infiltrates are rare.

ANTIPHOSPHOLIPID ANTIBODY SYNDROME

Liberto Pechet, MD, FACP

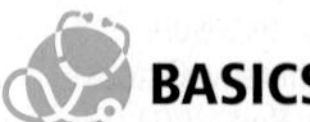

BASICS

DESCRIPTION

Antiphospholipid antibody syndrome (APS) is an autoimmune syndrome characterized by the presence of antiphospholipid antibodies (APAs) in association with either recurrent venous or arterial thromboembolic events or repeated fetal loss (1). The antiphospholipid antibodies are directed against phospholipid-binding plasma proteins and cause an increased risk of clot formation.

- Types:
  - Primary (50%): Occurs in patients without clinical evidence of another autoimmune disease
  - Secondary: Most commonly systemic lupus erythematosus (SLE). APAs may be transient in certain infections or the result of drugs.
  - Catastrophic APS (<1%):
    - Differs from primary and secondary types in caliber of vessels affected. Venous or arterial thrombosis of large vessels is less common, and patients present with acute thrombotic microangiopathy, the kidneys being the most commonly affected organ.
    - DIC, which does not occur in primary or secondary forms, is seen in up to 25% of patients with the catastrophic type.
    - Has a high mortality death due to multiorgan system failure if not treated aggressively
  - Possible APS: Related clinical manifestations without a clear relationship to APS, such as livedo reticularis

Pregnancy Considerations

- Increased risk of ischemic stroke, especially in young adults, and of deep vein thrombosis (DVT)
- Increased frequency of recurrent fetal loss
- Increased risk of premature delivery due to pregnancy-related hypertension and uteroplacental insufficiency

EPIDEMIOLOGY

- No specific age or race predilection
- Female predilection for both primary and secondary forms because of inclusion of pregnancy-related events in the classification criteria and because of the female predominance in autoimmune diseases such as SLE, respectively.

Incidence

- 15% of women with recurrent pregnancy loss have APS; 50% of pregnancy losses occur beyond the 10th week of gestation.
- 10–25% of patients with DVT have antiphospholipid antibodies.

Prevalence

APAs are present in 1–15% of the general population and in up to 70% of those with SLE. Primary APS rarely evolves into SLE.

RISK FACTORS

The following may increase the likelihood of thrombosis in patients with APAs:

- Smoking
- Oral contraceptive use
- Surgery
- Immobilization
- Pregnancy

Genetics

Increased risk in relatives of individuals with APS; however, no specific genetic patterns isolated

GENERAL PREVENTION

- Modification of secondary risk factors includes control of HTN, diabetes, hyperlipidemia, and smoking cessation
- Avoidance of oral contraceptives in patients with known APAs

PATHOPHYSIOLOGY

APAs may promote thrombosis in any organ by the following hypotheses:

- Increased platelet adhesion and aggregation due to interactions of the antibodies with platelet membrane phospholipids
- Annexin V disruption by anti-β2 GP1 results in loss of protection of vascular endothelium.
- Interference with the natural anticoagulant pathways involved in the regulation of coagulation

ETIOLOGY

- The mechanism by which APAs become generated is speculative; complement activation may have a pathogenetic role (2).
- The presence of APAs alone may not generate thrombosis, but the occurrence of a "second hit" via environmental factors or comorbidities may be required for activation.

COMMONLY ASSOCIATED CONDITIONS

- SLE (most common autoimmune disease associated with APAs)
- Cardiac valvular disease, renal thrombotic microangiopathy, thrombocytopenia, hemolytic anemia, cognitive impairment
- Thrombotic thrombocytopenic purpura (TTP), especially in the catastrophic APS
- Hemolytic-uremic syndrome (HUS)
- Malignant hypertension
- Acute renal failure
- Nephrotic syndrome
- HELLP syndrome (hemolysis, elevated liver enzymes, and low platelet count in association with pregnancy)
- DVT/pulmonary embolism (PE)
- Valvular disease
- Sneddon syndrome (APS variant syndrome in which livedo reticularis is associated with HTN and stroke)
- Malignant neoplasms
- Multiple bacterial, viral, and parasitic infections may result in transient increases in APAs.
- Certain medications may be associated with APA production, including phenothiazines, hydralazine, procainamide, and phenytoin, but they usually do not result in thrombotic events.

DIAGNOSIS

Sapporo criteria, revised 2006 (1)[A]:

- The presence of at least 1 of the following clinical criteria:
  - Vascular thrombosis:
    - $\geq$1 clinical episodes of arterial, venous, or small vessel thrombosis, occurring within any tissue or organ, confirmed by imaging studies, Doppler studies, or histopathology
  - Complications of pregnancy (up to 15% of women with recurrent miscarriages have APL antibodies:
    - $\geq$3 consecutive spontaneous abortions before the 10th week of pregnancy, unexplained by maternal or paternal chromosomal abnormalities or maternal anatomic or hormonal causes
    - $\geq$1 unexplained deaths of morphologically normal fetuses at or after the 10th week of gestation OR
    - $\geq$1 premature births of morphologically normal neonates at or before the 34th week of pregnancy due to severe preeclampsia, eclampsia, or placental insufficiency OR
    - Intrauterine growth retardation and premature birth
- AND the presence of at least 1 of the following 3 on $\geq$2 occasions at least 12 weeks apart:
  - Lupus anticoagulant (LAC) detected in the blood
  - Anticardiolipin IgG or IgM antibodies present at moderate or high levels in the blood via a standardized ELISA
  - Anti-β2 GP1 IgG or IgM antibodies in blood at a titer >99th percentile via a standardized ELISA
  - Valid lab findings should occur no more than 5 years prior to clinical manifestations.

HISTORY

- Personal history of thrombosis (DVT, PE, stroke)
- Obstetric history (especially pregnancy losses)
- Bleeding from thrombocytopenia if severe, or acquired factor II deficiency
- Family history of rheumatologic illness
- Vaso-occlusive events can occur in any organ system, so perform thorough review of systems.

PHYSICAL EXAM

- DVT of the legs (most common manifestation of APS)
- Skin exam may include findings of livedo reticularis (lacy, erythematous rash in net-like pattern, typically on wrists and knees), purpuric lesions, or ulcerations
- Insufficiency murmur of aortic or mitral valve
- Diverse neurologic symptoms: Paresthesias, weakness, tremors, cognitive deficits, stroke/TIA

DIAGNOSTIC TESTS & INTERPRETATION

- May result in false-positive VDRL/RPR
- The risk of thrombosis may increase with the level of APA detected and the number of APA types present in one individual.
- The antibodies directed against β2-glycoprotein 1 (GP1) express high LAC activity and highest risk of thrombotic events.
- The clinical significance of other autoantibodies, including those directed against annexin V, phosphatidylserine, and phosphatidylinositol, remains unclear.

Lab

"Lupus anticoagulant" (LAC) is a misnomer; it results in an increased risk of thrombus, not an anticoagulant effect (except for anti–factor II antibodies), and is found in >50% patients without SLE. Antibodies cause an increase in the aPTT while paradoxically are associated with a hypercoagulable state in vivo.

Initial lab tests

- CBC, PT/INR, aPTT, lupus anticoagulant, anticardiolipin antibodies, anti-β_2 GP1 antibodies

- Clotting test for LAC (3)[A]. Use 2 coagulation-based tests because LAC activity is heterogeneous: 1. One on inhibition of the PTT clotting using an LAC-sensitive reagent; 2. Dilute Russell viper venom time (dRVVT).
- Testing positive for anti–factor II, although a risk factor for both thrombosis and bleeding, is not a laboratory criterion for the diagnosis of APS.
- ELISA test for anticardiolipin antibodies
- ELISA test for anti-β_2 GP1 antibodies; the antibodies that associate with the APS clinical phenotype are predominantly of the IgG isotype.
- CBC to determine if thrombocytopenia or hemolytic anemia are present

Follow-Up & Special Considerations

The results of LAC are difficult to interpret in patients treated with Warfarin. Unfractionated heparin (if <1 unit/mL) or low-molecular-weight heparin and fondaparinux do not affect the LAC assay.

Imaging

- Doppler ultrasonography of lower extremities to look for DVT
- If PE suspected, CT angiography
- Echocardiography with cardiac involvement
- MRI may demonstrate CNS involvement
- Arteriography in patients with arterial thrombotic events

Diagnostic Procedures/Surgery

Biopsy of the affected organ system may be necessary to distinguish the vasculopathy from vasculitis.

Pathological Findings

- Usual finding is microangiopathic process with bland thrombosis and minimal vascular or perivascular inflammation:
  - Acute changes: Capillary congestion and noninflammatory fibrin thrombi
  - Chronic changes: Ischemic hypoperfusion
- Atrophy and fibrosis

DIFFERENTIAL DIAGNOSIS

- Conditions that cause thrombotic microangiopathy, such as hemolytic-uremic syndrome or TTP
- Thrombophilic conditions, such as:
  - Deficiency of protein C, protein S
  - Deficiency of antithrombin III
  - Mutation of factor V Leiden
  - Prothrombin gene mutation
  - Neoplastic and myeloproliferative disorders
  - Hyperviscosity syndromes
- Embolic disease secondary to atrial fibrillation, marked LV dysfunction, endocarditis, cholesterol emboli
- Heparin-induced thrombocytopenia
- Homocystinemia
- Atherosclerosis

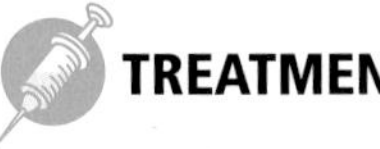

TREATMENT

MEDICATION

First Line

- Asymptomatic carriers of APAs should be followed; they do not require anticoagulation but may benefit from low-dose aspirin (2)[C].
- In symptomatic nonpregnant individuals with APS, the following secondary thromboprophylaxis is recommended: Initial therapy for venous thrombosis is with both unfractionated or LMW heparin and warfarin, then continuing on only warfarin to achieve INR between 2.0 and 3.0 (2)[A].
  - Higher intensity
  - Warfarin (to achieve INR 3.0–4.0) may be required in patients with an initial arterial thrombotic event or recurrent venous thromboembolic event despite anticoagulation.
  - Lifelong anticoagulation is recommended by most authors for patients on oral anticoagulants.
  - Other therapies to be considered may include combinations of ASA with clopidogrel or dipyridamole, statins, hydroxychloroquine, new oral anticoagulants, and rituximab to suppress the autoimmune process (2).
- In pregnant individuals with APS:
  - For women with no prior history of thrombosis and ≥ 2 early pregnancy losses or ≥ 1 later pregnancy loss, or previous early delivery, consider ASA (81 mg daily) with attempted conception and add low-dose unfractionated heparin 5,000–10,000 units SC b.i.d. or LMW heparin in usual prophylactic doses when a viable intrauterine pregnancy is documented (4)[B].
  - The use of prednisolone has been largely discarded as a therapeutic option (except in the presence of associated LSE), although more recently its use in low doses (10 mg daily) for the refractory APS-related 1st-trimester pregnancies has been shown to be beneficial, despite a relative high incidence of complications (5).
  - Treatment should continue until at least the third trimester (rate of fetal loss may exceed 90% in untreated patients, whereas therapies such as aspirin and heparin can reduce the rate to 25%), and consider the same therapy throughout delivery and for a few weeks postpartum.
- For the catastrophic APS, aggressive therapy with high-dose steroids, anticoagulants, and plasma exchange with or without IVIG has improved the prognosis in otherwise a frequently fatal condition.

SURGERY/OTHER PROCEDURES

Patients with thrombosis may require thrombectomy or an IVC filter for those with lower extremity DVT for whom anticoagulation is contraindicated.

IN-PATIENT CONSIDERATIONS

Patients with APS-related events should be hospitalized in the following situations:

- Massive DVT, PE, high risk of bleeding on anticoagulation therapy, comorbid conditions, and the APA catastrophic syndrome

ONGOING CARE

FOLLOW-UP RECOMMENDATIONS

Patient Monitoring

Warfarin therapy is lifelong; patients need monitoring to maintain INR of 2.0–3.0. Pregnant patients on prolonged heparin (especially UFH) should be closely monitored for heparin-induced thrombocytopenia (HIT).

DIET

- Those on anticoagulation should maintain a diet of foods containing steady amounts of vitamin K.
- Healthy diet to prevent obesity and dyslipidemia to decrease risk of atherothrombotic events

PATIENT EDUCATION

Avoid use of oral hormonal contraceptives.

PROGNOSIS

- Pulmonary HTN, neurologic involvement, myocardial ischemia, nephropathy, gangrene of extremities, and catastrophic APS are associated with a worse prognosis.
- Most patients experience recurrences months or years after the initial event.

COMPLICATIONS

Discontinuation of warfarin results in increased risk of thrombosis (even death), particularly in the 1st 6 months after stopping treatment.

REFERENCES

1. Miyakis S, Lockshin MD, Atsumi T, et al. International consensus statement on an update of the classification criteria for definite antiphospholipid syndrome (APS). *J Thromb Haemost*. 2006;4:295–306.
2. Ruiz-Irastorza G, Crowther M, Branch W, et al. Antiphospholipid syndrome. *Lancet*. 2010; 376:1498–1509.
3. Pengo V, Tripodi I, Reber G, et al. Update of the guidelines for lupus anticoagulant detection. *J Thrombosis and Haemostasis*. 2009;7: 1737–40.
4. Ziakas PD, Pavlou M, Voulgarelis M, et al. Heparin treatment in antiphospholipid syndrome with recurrent pregnancy loss: A systematic review and meta-analysis. *Obstet Gynecol*. 2010;115: 1256–62.
5. Branham K, Thomas M, Nelson-Piery C, et al. First-trimester low-dose prednisolone in refractory antiphospholipid antibody-related pregnancy loss. *Blood*. 2011;117:6948–51.

ADDITIONAL READING

Derksen RHWM, de Groot PG. Towards evidence-based treatment of thrombotic antiphospholipid syndrome. *Lupus*. 2010;19: 470–74.

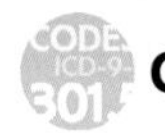

CODES

ICD9

- 289.81 Primary hypercoagulable state
- 289.82 Secondary hypercoagulable state

CLINICAL PEARLS

- APS can be either primary or secondary (associated with another underlying illness [e.g., SLE])
- The diagnosis of APS requires both clinical and laboratory criteria.
- Thrombosis is the most common clinical manifestation of APS, either venous or arterial. The most common site of arterial thrombosis is the brain.
- Treatment for nonobstetrical APS is with lifelong warfarin, but may vary, depending on the underlying condition.
- Patients with APS and recurrent fetal loss should be considered for combination heparin and ASA treatment during pregnancy.

ANTITHROMBIN DEFICIENCY

Marc Jeffrey Kahn, MD, MBA
Rebecca Kruse-Jarres, MD, MPH

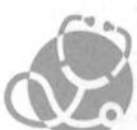

BASICS

DESCRIPTION

Antithrombin is a protease that inhibits thrombin by forming an irreversible thrombin-antithrombin complex. Antithrombin can also inhibit factors Xa, IXa, and XIa. This process is catalyzed by the presence of heparin. Patients deficient in antithrombin have an increased incidence of venous thrombosis, including deep vein thrombosis (DVT) of the lower extremity. Arterial thrombosis is much less common in patients deficient in antithrombin:

- System(s) affected: Cardiovascular; Nervous; Pulmonary; Reproductive; Hemic/Lymphatic/Immunologic
- Synonym(s): Antithrombin III deficiency

EPIDEMIOLOGY

- Predominant age: Mean age of 1st thrombosis is in 2nd decade.
- Predominant sex: Male = Female

Incidence

4% of patients with thrombophilia

Prevalence

0.16% of normal individuals

RISK FACTORS

- Oral contraceptives, pregnancy, and the use of hormone replacement therapy (HRT) increase the risk of venous thrombosis in patients with antithrombin deficiency.
- Patients with antithrombin deficiency and another prothrombotic state, such as factor V Leiden or the prothrombin 20210 mutation, have increased rates of thrombosis.
- Heterozygotes have an odds ratio of venous thrombosis of 10–20.

Pregnancy Considerations

Increases thrombotic risk in patients with antithrombin deficiency

Genetics

Autosomal dominant

GENERAL PREVENTION

Patients with antithrombin deficiency without a history of thrombosis do not require prophylactic treatment.

PATHOPHYSIOLOGY

- Type I deficiency is characterized by low levels of antigen. Type II deficiency is found when the antithrombin molecule is dysfunctional.
- Type II deficiencies are due to mutations in either the active center of antithrombin that binds the target enzyme or the heparin-binding site.
- No patients homozygous for defects in the active center have been described, suggesting that this is a lethal condition. Patients heterozygous for mutations in the heparin-binding site rarely have thrombotic episodes.

ETIOLOGY

Many mutations in the antithrombin gene have been identified.

COMMONLY ASSOCIATED CONDITIONS

Venous thromboembolism

DIAGNOSIS

HISTORY

- Previous thrombosis
- Family history of thrombosis
- Family history of antithrombin deficiency

PHYSICAL EXAM

Deep or superficial venous thrombosis

DIAGNOSTIC TESTS & INTERPRETATION

Lab

Initial lab tests

- For evaluation of new clot in patient at risk: CBC with peripheral smear, PT/INR, aPTT, thrombin time, lupus anticoagulant, antiphospholipid antibodies, factor VIII, anticardiolipin antibody, anti-B2 glycoprotein I antibody, activated protein C resistance, protein S antigen and resistance, antithrombin III assay, fibrinogen, factor V Leiden, prothrombin G20210A, homocysteine
- Specific testing depends on the clinical setting, and standard coagulation tests should be obtained as necessary in the setting of thrombosis and to rule out other coagulopathies, such as protein C and S deficiencies (see "Differential Diagnosis").
- Testing should be done off heparin.
- 2 tests useful in the workup of antithrombin deficiency include:
  - Antithrombin-heparin cofactor assay, which measures the ability of heparin to bind to antithrombin, which neutralizes the action of thrombin and factor Xa. This is an indirect measure of factor Xa inhibition.
  - Antithrombin activity assay
- Drugs that may alter lab results: Heparin, estrogen, and asparaginase can lower antithrombin levels.

Follow-Up & Special Considerations

- The role of family screening for antithrombin deficiency is unclear, because most patients with this mutation do not have thrombosis. Screening may be considered for women considering using oral contraceptives or for pregnant women with a family history of factor protein S deficiency (1)[C].
- Antithrombin levels are low in:
  - DIC
  - Sepsis
  - Burns
  - Severe trauma
  - Acute thrombosis
  - Pregnancy
  - Liver disease
- Antithrombin levels could be elevated by oral contraceptive pills.

Imaging

Initial approach

- Ultrasound to diagnose DVT if clinically indicated
- Spiral CT or V/Q scan to diagnose pulmonary embolism (PE) if clinically indicated

Follow-Up & Special Considerations

- Ultrasound may not show DVT acutely; repeat in 1–2 days if strong suspicion.
- V/Q scan may be difficult to interpret in patients with other lung disease.

Pathological Findings

Venous thrombosis

DIFFERENTIAL DIAGNOSIS

- Factor V Leiden
- Protein C deficiency
- Protein S deficiency
- Dysfibrinogenemia
- Dysplasminogenemia
- Homocystinemia
- Prothrombin 20210 mutation
- Elevated factor VIII levels

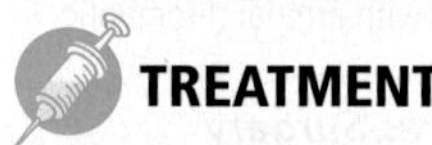

TREATMENT

MEDICATION

First Line

- Patients with antithrombin deficiency and a 1st thrombosis should be anticoagulated initially with unfractionated heparin followed by oral anticoagulation with warfarin (1)[A].
- After the INR is 2–3, heparin can be stopped after 5 total days of therapy (1)[A].
- Oral anticoagulant following the initial administration of heparin. Warfarin (Coumadin) 5 mg/d PO and adjusted to INR of 2–3. Patients should be maintained on warfarin for at least 6 months (1)[A].
- Recurrent thrombosis requires indefinite anticoagulation (1)[A].
- Contraindications:
  - Active bleeding precludes anticoagulation; risk of bleeding is a relative contraindication to long-term anticoagulation.
- Precautions:
  - Observe patient for signs of embolization, further thrombosis, or bleeding.
  - Avoid IM injections.
  - Periodically check stool and urine for occult blood, and monitor CBCs, including platelets.
  - Heparin-thrombocytopenia and/or paradoxical thrombosis with thrombocytopenia

- Significant possible interactions:
  - Agents that intensify the response to oral anticoagulants: Alcohol, allopurinol, amiodarone, anabolic steroids, androgens, many antimicrobials, cimetidine, chloral hydrate, disulfiram, all NSAIDs, sulfinpyrazone, tamoxifen, thyroid hormone, vitamin E, ranitidine, salicylates, acetaminophen
  - Agents that diminish the response to oral anticoagulants: Aminoglutethimide, antacids, barbiturates, carbamazepine, cholestyramine, diuretics, griseofulvin, rifampin, oral contraceptives

Second Line

- Argatroban 0.4–0.5 μg/kg/min. Case reports describing the use of the direct thrombin inhibitor in patients with antithrombin deficiency have been published (2)[C].
- Antithrombin III (ATnativ, Thrombate III) 50–100 IU/min IV titrated to antithrombin level desired. Precise role in therapy remains unclear (1)[C].
- LMWH is difficult to manage in this population (1)[C].

ADDITIONAL TREATMENT

General Measures

Routine anticoagulation for asymptomatic patients with antithrombin deficiency is not recommended (1)[A].

Issues for Referral

- Recurrent thrombosis on anticoagulation
- Difficulty anticoagulating
- Genetic counseling

Additional Therapies

- Patients with severe antithrombin deficiency may require plasma replacement of thrombin in order for heparin to be effective (3)[C].
- Compression stockings for prevention

SURGERY/OTHER PROCEDURES

Thrombectomy may be indicated in complicated cases.

IN-PATIENT CONSIDERATIONS

Initial Stabilization

Heparin initial bolus of 80 U/kg followed by infusion of 18 U/kg/hr. Frequent monitoring of the partial thromboplastin time (PTT) is important, as nearly 50% of patients deficient in antithrombin require more than 40,000 U of heparin daily to adequately prolong PTT (1)[C].

Admission Criteria

Complicated thrombosis, such as pulmonary embolus

Discharge Criteria

Stable on anticoagulation

ONGOING CARE

FOLLOW-UP RECOMMENDATIONS

Patient Monitoring

Warfarin use requires periodic INR measurements (monthly after initial stabilization) with a goal of 2–3 (1)[A].

DIET

Foods high in vitamin K may interfere with anticoagulation on warfarin. Consider nutrition consultation.

PATIENT EDUCATION

- Patients should be educated about:
  - Use of oral anticoagulant therapy
  - Avoidance of NSAIDs while on warfarin
- The role of family screening is unclear, as most patients with this mutation do not have thrombosis. In a patient with a family history of factor V Leiden, consider screening during pregnancy or if considering oral contraceptive use.

PROGNOSIS

- The odds ratio of thrombosis in a patient with antithrombin deficiency is much higher than in patients with other thrombophilic conditions. The recurrence rate is similarly high.
- There is no difference in clinical severity between patients with type I defects and type II mutations.
- Overall, prognosis is good, if appropriately anticoagulated.

COMPLICATIONS

Recurrent thrombosis (requires indefinite anticoagulation)

REFERENCES

1. Vinazzer H. Hereditary and acquired antithrombin deficiency. *Semin Thromb Hemost*. 1999;25: 257–63.
2. Dager WE, Gosselin RC, Owings JT. Argatroban therapy for antithrombin deficiency and mesenteric thrombosis: Case report and review of the literature. *Pharmacotherapy*. 2004;24:659–63.
3. Maclean PS, Tait RC. Hereditary and acquired antithrombin deficiency: Epidemiology, pathogenesis and treatment options. *Drugs*. 2007;67:1429–40.

ADDITIONAL READING

- Bates SM, Greer IA, Pabinger I, et al. Venous thromboembolism, thrombophilia, antithrombotic therapy, and pregnancy: American College of Chest Physicians Evidence-Based Clinical Practice Guidelines (8th Edition). *Chest*. 2008;133: 844S–86S.
- Kottke-Marchant K, Duncan A. Antithrombin deficiency: issues in laboratory diagnosis. *Arch Pathol Lab Med*. 2002;126:1326–36.
- Vossen CY, Conard J, Fontcuberta J, et al. Risk of a first venous thrombotic event in carriers of a familial thrombotic defect. The European Prospective Cohort on Thrombophilia (EPCOT). *J Thromb Heamost*. 2005;3:459–64.

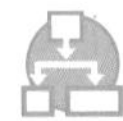

See Also (Topic, Algorithm, Electronic Media Element)

Deep Vein Thrombophlebitis (DVT)

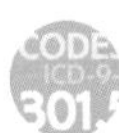

CODES

ICD9

289.81 Primary hypercoagulable state

CLINICAL PEARLS

- Antithrombin levels will be low on heparin and during acute thrombosis.
- Diagnosis can be difficult, and conditions causing low levels of antithrombin III, such as pregnancy, liver disease, sepsis, and DIC, must be ruled out.
- Both antepartum and postpartum prophylaxis for pregnant women with no prior history of venous thromboembolism, but antithrombin deficiency is indicated

ANXIETY

Mary K. Flynn, MD
Margo L. Kaplan Gill, MD

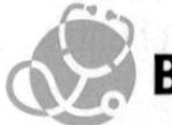

BASICS

DESCRIPTION

- Persistent, excessive, and difficult-to-control worry associated with significant symptoms of motor tension, autonomic hyperactivity, and/or disturbances of sleep or concentration
- System(s) affected: Nervous (resulting in increased sympathetic tone and increased catecholamine release)

EPIDEMIOLOGY

Prevalence

- 12-month prevalence rate: 3.1%
- Lifetime prevalence rate: 5.7%
- Onset can occur any time in life, from adolescence to adulthood; median age of onset in US is 31 years.
- Predominant sex: Female > male (2:1)
- Anxiety accounts for 5–8% of primary care office visits.

RISK FACTORS

- Caucasian race
- Adverse life events: Stress, medical illness, disability, unemployment, childhood physical and mental abuse
- Family history
- Lack of social support
- Lesbian/bisexual women at increased risk above heterosexual women; no increased risk found for homosexual/bisexual men
- Depression

Genetics

- Strongly linked to depression in heritability studies
- A variant of the serotonin transporter gene (*5HT1A*) may contribute to both conditions; other genes (such as that for glutamic acid decarboxylase) also may play a role.

GENERAL PREVENTION

Regular exercise is associated with decreased anxiety and depression.

PATHOPHYSIOLOGY

- fMRI studies display decreased amygdala connectivity bilaterally
- Neuroreceptors such as γ-aminobutyric acid, serotonin, and cholecystokinin

ETIOLOGY

Mediated by abnormalities of neurotransmitter systems (i.e., serotonin, norepinephrine, and γ-aminobutyric acid [GABA])

COMMONLY ASSOCIATED CONDITIONS

- Major depressive disorder (>60%), dysthymia, bipolar disorder
- Alcohol/drug abuse (37.6%/27.6%)
- Cigarette smoking in adolescence
- Panic disorder; agoraphobia, simple phobia; social anxiety disorder

DIAGNOSIS

HISTORY

History and evaluation should carefully identify generalized anxiety disorder (GAD) from other anxiety disorders. In GAD:

- Symptoms of excessive anxiety and worry must occur more often than not for at least 6 months.
- At least 3 additional criteria are required for diagnosis of GAD in adults; only 1 is required in children:
  - Restlessness or feeling keyed up or on edge
  - Easily fatigued
  - Difficulty concentrating or mind going blank
  - Irritability
  - Muscle tension
  - Sleep disturbances (difficulty falling or staying asleep)
  - Difficulty controlling worry
- Persistent worry must cause significant distress or impairment in social, occupational, or other areas of functioning.
- Focus of anxiety and worry is not consistent with or limited to the occurrence of other types of psychiatric disorders and is not directly related to posttraumatic stress disorder (PTSD).
- All other causes of anxiety and worry have been eliminated (see "Differential Diagnosis") (1).
- Patient may report symptoms of dyspnea, palpitations, diaphoresis, nausea, or diarrhea, or may experience tremor.

PHYSICAL EXAM

No specific physical findings, but patient may be noted to be irritable or easily startled and observable findings of bitten nails, a tremor, or clammy hands may also be present.

DIAGNOSTIC TESTS & INTERPRETATION

Lab

Initial lab tests

- Laboratory tests are normal. Initial tests should include the following: Thyroid-stimulating hormone, CBC, basic metabolic panel, and ECG
- See "Differential Diagnosis" for other conditions to rule out.

Diagnostic Procedures/Surgery

Psychological testing:

- GAD-2: 2-question self-reporting scale (22% positive predictive value [PPV]/78% negative predictive value [NPV]) (2)
- GAD-7: 5 additional questions; provides more detailed information for treatment (29% PPV/71% NPV); also may be indicative of panic disorder (GAD-7: 29% PPV/71% NPV).
- Hamilton's Anxiety Scale (HAM-A), Anxiety Disorders Interview Schedule (ADIS-IV)
- In pediatric populations: ADIS-IV Parent and Child Version, Multidimensional Anxiety Scale for Children (MASC), Screen for Child Anxiety Related Emotional Disorders (SCARED)

DIFFERENTIAL DIAGNOSIS

- Cardiovascular: Ischemic heart disease, valvular heart disease (mitral valve prolapse), cardiomyopathies, myocarditis, arrhythmias, congestive heart failure
- Respiratory: Asthma, chronic obstructive pulmonary disease, pulmonary embolism, pneumonia
- CNS: Stroke, seizures, dementia, migraine, vestibular dysfunction, encephalitis, neoplasms
- Metabolic and hormonal: Hyper- or hypothyroidism, pheochromocytoma, adrenal insufficiency, Cushing syndrome, hypokalemia, hypoglycemia, hyperparathyroidism
- Nutritional: Thiamine, pyridoxine, or folate deficiency; iron-deficiency anemia
- Drug-induced anxiety: Alcohol, sympathomimetics (cocaine, amphetamine, caffeine), corticosteroids, herbals (ginseng)
- Withdrawal: Alcohol, sedative-hypnotics
- Psychiatric: Other disorders (e.g., panic disorder, obsessive-compulsive disorder, PTSD, social phobia, adjustment disorder, and somatization disorder)

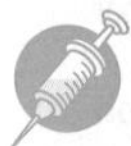

TREATMENT

MEDICATION

First Line

Antidepressants take longer to have effect (2–4 weeks) but outperform benzodiazepines in the long term.

- SSRIs (2,3):
  - Escitalopram (Lexapro): Initially 10 mg/d; may titrate to a maximum of 20 mg/d
  - Paroxetine (Paxil): Initially 10–20 mg/d; may titrate to a maximum of 50 mg/d (no added benefit above 20 mg/d)
  - Sertraline (Zoloft): Initially 25 mg/d; may titrate to a maximum of 200 mg/d
- Selective-norepinephrine reuptake inhibitors (SNRIs) (2,3):
  - Duloxetine (Cymbalta): Initially 30 mg/d; may titrate to a maximum of 120 mg/d
  - Venlafaxine XR (Effexor XR): Initially 37.5–75 mg; may titrate up by 75 mg every 4 days to a maximum of 225 mg/d
- Tricyclic antidepressants (TCAs): Imipramine (Tofranil): Initially 25–50 mg/d; maximum of 300 mg/d, 100 mg/d in the elderly (2,3)[A]
- Azapirones: Buspirone (BuSpar): 15 mg/d divided b.i.d. to t.i.d. initially; maximum of 60 mg/d divided b.i.d. to t.i.d. (2,3)[A]

Second Line

- Benzodiazepines (best for short-term use) (2,3)[A]:
  - Alprazolam (Xanax): 0.25–0.5 mg b.i.d. to t.i.d.; may increase by 0.25 mg to 4 mg/d
  - Clonazepam (Klonopin): 0.25 mg b.i.d.; may increase to 4 mg/d divided b.i.d.
  - Diazepam (Valium): 2–5 mg b.i.d. to q.i.d.; may increase to a maximum of 40 mg/d
  - Lorazepam (Ativan): 0.5 mg b.i.d. to t.i.d.; may increase to 6 mg/d divided t.i.d.
- Hydroxyzine (Vistaril, Atarax): CNS depressant, antihistamine, anticholinergic; decreased risk of dependence compared with benzodiazepines: Usual dose: 50–100 mg PO q.i.d.
- Pregabalin (Lyrica) and quetiapine (Seroquel): Preliminary promise as treatments, but further investigation is needed into safety and efficacy

Geriatric Considerations
Avoid TCAs and long-acting benzodiazepines. Benzodiazepines may cause delirium.

Pediatric Considerations
- Black box warning (SSRIs): Antidepressants increase the risk of suicidal thinking and behavior in children, adolescents, and young adults.
- Anxiety often comorbidly exists with attention deficit hyperactivity disorder (ADHD).

Pregnancy Considerations
- Buspirone: Category B: Secreted in breast milk; inadequate studies to assess risk
- Benzodiazepines: Category D: May cause lethargy and weight loss in nursing infants; avoid breastfeeding if the mother is taking chronically or in high doses.
- SSRIs: If possible, taper and discontinue. After 20 weeks' gestation, there is increased risk of pulmonary hypertension; mild transient neonatal syndrome of CNS; and motor, respiratory, and GI signs. Most are Category C.
  - Paroxetine: Category D: Conflicting evidence regarding the risk of congenital cardiac defects and other congenital anomalies.
- Hydroxyzine: Category C: Case reports of neonatal withdrawal exist.

ALERT
Precautions:
- Benzodiazepines: Age >65 years, hepatic insufficiency, respiratory disease/sleep apnea, renal insufficiency, suicidal tendency, contraindicated with narrow-angle glaucoma, precaution with open-angle glaucoma. Sudden discontinuation, especially of alprazolam, increases seizure risk. Long-term use has potential for tolerance and dependence; use with caution in patients with history of substance abuse.
- Buspirone: Hepatic and/or renal dysfunction; monoamine oxidase inhibitor (MAOI) treatment
- TCAs: Advanced age, glaucoma, benign prostate hypertrophy, hyperthyroidism, cardiovascular disease, liver disease, urinary retention, MAOI treatment
- SSRIs: Use caution when treating anxiety symptoms in those with comorbid bipolar disorder; may trigger mania.

ADDITIONAL TREATMENT

Additional Therapies
Psychological:
- Cognitive-behavioral therapy (CBT): Has shown comparable benefit to medical management; may improve comorbid conditions such as depression
- Mindfulness-based cognitive therapy and stress-reduction studies have been limited. A 2010 meta-analysis showed promise in reducing acute symptoms of anxiety in individuals diagnosed with anxiety disorders and in other populations with high anxiety (i.e., the chronically ill) (4).
- Relaxation training: Historically, treatment of choice for GAD but limited evidence for objective benefit
- Psychodynamic psychotherapy: Treatment is focused on patient discovering and verbalizing unconscious content of the psyche.

General Measures
- At increased risk for suicidal ideation and attempts; risk increases with comorbid conditions.
- Identify and treat coexisting substance abuse and other psychiatric conditions.

Issues for Referral
Concomitant depression may warrant a psychiatric evaluation in light of increased suicide risk.

COMPLEMENTARY AND ALTERNATIVE MEDICINE
- Yoga and meditation may help; additional studies are needed, but few adverse effects are known. Small studies have shown increased GABA levels and decreased anxiety after yoga.
- Kava: Evidence for benefit over placebo in mild to moderate anxiety, but concern regarding potential hepatotoxicity.
  - May consider for short-term use (up to 24 weeks) (5,6)
  - Studied doses 70–240 mg/d; up to 330 mg/d appears to be safe (7).
  - Must avoid concomitant use of alcohol or other medications metabolized via the liver (CYP 450 inhibitor); other adverse effects include dermatopathy (usually reversible), ataxia, hearing loss, and loss of appetite.
- St. John's wort: There are some reports of benefit in adults, but little evidence for use with anxiety in randomized controlled trials
  - Drug interactions: CYP 450 3A4, 1A2, or 2E1 inducer; may activate P-glycoprotein (may reduce oral contraceptive efficacy)
  - In combination with SSRI or buspirone, may lead to serotonin syndrome; otherwise, benign side-effect profile (rare photosensitivity or triggering of mania)
- Passionflower, valerian: Little evidence to support use; benign side-effect profile
- Inositol: Evidence for efficacy in panic disorder and obsessive-compulsive disorder; not studied in GAD

ONGOING CARE

FOLLOW-UP RECOMMENDATIONS

Patient Monitoring
- Monitor for development of comorbid conditions.
- Monitor mental status on benzodiazepines, and avoid drug dependence.
- Monitor BP, heart rate, and anticholinergic side effects of TCAs.
- Monitor all patients for suicidal ideation, but especially those on SSRIs, SNRIs, and imipramine.

DIET
- Limit caffeine intake.
- Avoid alcohol (drug interactions, high rate of abuse, potential for increased anxiety).

PATIENT EDUCATION
- Regular exercise, especially yoga, may be beneficial for both anxiety and comorbid conditions.
- Continue with meditation, CBT, and other therapies that provide relief.
- www.familydoctor.org
- National Institute of Mental Health (NIMH): www.nimh.nih.gov/health/publications/index.shtml

PROGNOSIS
- A chronic disease, with many patients experiencing continued symptoms or relapse.
- Successful treatment is possible but must be carried out over the long term.
- Relapse is more likely with the discontinuation of medications, particularly in the 1st year of treatment and during periods of increased stress.

REFERENCES

1. American Psychiatric Association. *Diagnostic and Statistical Manual of Mental Disorders*, 4th ed. Washington, DC: American Psychiatric Association; 2000:429–84.
2. Kavan MG, Elsasser GN, Barone EJ. Generalized anxiety disorder: Practical assessment and management. *Am Fam Physician*. 2009;79: 785–91.
3. Davidson JR. First-line pharmacotherapy approaches for generalized anxiety disorder. *J Clin Psychiatry*. 2009;70(Suppl 2):25–31.
4. Hofmann SG, Sawyer AT, Witt AA, et al. The effect of mindfulness-based therapy on anxiety and depression: A meta-analytic review. *J Consult Clin Psychol*. 2010;78:169–83.
5. Saeed SA, Bloch RM, Antonacci DJ. Herbal and dietary supplements for treatment of anxiety disorders. *Am Fam Physician*. 2007;76:549–56.
6. Pittler MH, Ernst E. Kava extract for treating anxiety. *Cochrane Database Syst Rev*. 2003;(1):CD003383.
7. Ernst E. The risk-benefit profile of commonly used herbal therapies: Ginkgo, St. John's Wort, Ginseng, Echinacea, Saw Palmetto, and Kava. *Ann Intern Med*. 2002;136:42–53.

ADDITIONAL READING

- Gorman JM. Treating generalized anxiety disorder. *J Clin Psychiatry*. 2003;64(Suppl 2):24–9.
- Shearer SL. Recent advances in the understanding and treatment of anxiety disorders. *Prim Care*. 2007;34:475–504.
- Ströhle A. Physical activity, exercise, depression and anxiety disorders. *J Neural Transm*. 2009;116(6): 777–84.
- Weisberg RB. Overview of generalized anxiety disorder: Epidemiology, presentation, and course. *J Clin Psychiatry*. 2009;70(Suppl 2):4–9.

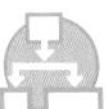

See Also (Topic, Algorithm, Electronic Media Element)

Algorithms: Depression, Adult; Anxiety

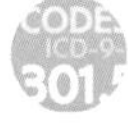

CODES

ICD9
- 300.00 Anxiety state, unspecified
- 300.02 Generalized anxiety disorder
- 300.09 Other anxiety states

CLINICAL PEARLS
- Psychiatric comorbidities, especially depression, are extremely common with GAD; patients are at increased risk for suicidality and should be screened accordingly.
- Antidepressants are the treatment of choice, though they require up to 4 weeks for full effect.
- Benzodiazepines may be used initially but should be tapered and withdrawn if possible.
- CBT is comparable with medical management; mindfulness meditation and yoga have shown initial promise.

AORTIC DISSECTION

Mia D. Sorcinelli, MD

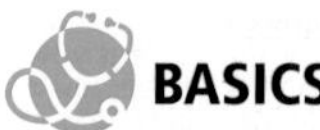

BASICS

DESCRIPTION

Intimal tear in the aorta resulting in hematoma formation. Accumulating blood in false lumen of arterial wall leads to propagation of a dissection (1):

- Stanford classification (most widely used):
  - Type A: Involves ascending aorta and aortic arch regardless of site of intimal tear
  - Type B: Involves descending aorta
- DeBakey classification (based on origin site):
  - Type 1: Originates in ascending aorta, propagates at least as far as aortic arch
  - Type 2: Involves only ascending aorta
  - Type 3: Originates in descending aorta, may propagate proximately or distally
- Svensson:
  - Class 1: Classic dissection with true and false lumen
  - Class 2: Intramural hematoma or hemorrhage
  - Class 3: Subtle dissection without hematoma
  - Class 4: Atherosclerotic plaque rupture and ulceration
  - Class 5: Iatrogenic
- Synonym(s): Dissecting aneurysm

EPIDEMIOLOGY

- Predominant age varies with cause
- Type A dissection occurs in patients with an average age of 60.
- Type B dissection occurs in patients generally older.
- Patients with Marfan syndrome have a mean age of 36.
- ~2/3 of patients are male.
- Studies indicate the peak time of day between 8 and 9 AM.
- Some studies also report a slightly higher incidence in winter months.

Incidence

About 3 cases per 100,000 people per year

Prevalence

US:

- Diagnosed in 1 in 10,000 patients admitted to hospital
- Found in 1 in 350 patients at autopsy
- Numbers may be slightly higher due to unexplained deaths at home or in hospital without autopsy

RISK FACTORS

- Most common associated factors:
  - Hypertension (about 70% of patients)
  - Old age
  - Atherosclerosis
  - Previous cardiovascular surgery, particularly repair of aneurysm or dissection
- Collagen abnormalities:
  - Marfan syndrome
  - Ehlers-Danlos syndrome
- Recreational drug use:
  - Smoking
  - Cocaine
- Inflammatory vasculitis:
  - Takayasu arteritis
  - Giant cell arteritis
- Chest trauma
- Turner syndrome
- Bicuspid aortic valve
- Uncommonly seen in infants following infection
- Also seen in infants during balloon dilation of aortic coarctation
- Reports of dissection in patients with untreated coarctation of the aorta

Genetics

Up to 20% of patients with thoracic aneurysm or dissection were found to have 1st-degree relatives with aneurysm or dissection. Studies have found that the TGFBR1 and TGFBR2 genes are related to aneurysm and dissection in isolated cases and in patients with Marfan syndrome. Other research has found ACTA2 gene mutations to be involved in isolated and familial dissections and aneurysms.

GENERAL PREVENTION

- Rigorous medical management of precipitating risk factors, such as hypertension
- Surveillance of aortic root and replacement when appropriate in patients with collagen disorders (e.g., Marfan, Ehlers-Danlos)

PATHOPHYSIOLOGY

In most cases, dissection develops in the absence of an aneurysm, but the false lumen that can be created during dissection can later expand to form an aneurysm. In patients with inherited connective tissue disease, abnormal and/or deficient proteins lead to the weakening of vessel walls. Bicuspid aortic valves may also lead to an acquired dysfunction of vascular walls and smooth muscle cells. Histological investigations of postmortem and biopsy specimens reveal cystic medial necrosis, especially in those patients with known preexisting aneurysms.

ETIOLOGY

Although the exact sequence of events is controversial, an aortic dissection is likely the result of multiple pathological processes. Stress on the aortic wall from hypertension; intimal damage with subsequent tear, rupture, or ulceration of atherosclerotic plaques; and the involvement of vasa vasorum and intramural hematoma may be contributory.

COMMONLY ASSOCIATED CONDITIONS

See "Risk Factors."

DIAGNOSIS

HISTORY

- A high level of clinical suspicion is the key to a correct and prompt diagnosis.
- A typical patient is a hypertensive man aged 60–80.
- A positive family history raises index of suspicion.
- Subjective complaints: 85% of patients report abrupt onset of pain. Pain was more often described as sharp, less often as tearing or ripping. 90% of patients stated that the pain was "severe" or "worst ever." Patients with type A dissections more often report chest pain. Patients with type B dissections more often report back and abdominal pain. Symptoms overlap between type A and type B dissections.

PHYSICAL EXAM

- Hypotension and shock are more common with type A dissections.
- Hypertension is more common with type B dissections.
- Syncope or cerebrovascular accident symptoms
- Pulse deficit
- Auscultation of aortic regurgitation
- Signs of congestive heart failure
- Limb ischemia
- Acute myocardial infarction (MI)/angina
- Spinal cord syndromes/deficits (2)
- Features of tamponade

DIAGNOSTIC TESTS & INTERPRETATION

- It is important to use easily available testing to assist in prompt diagnosis.
- Blood testing, EKG, chest x-rays, CT scans, and echocardiograms can all assist in diagnosis.
- A normal EKG and chest x-ray cannot be used to rule out the diagnosis if clinical suspicion is high.
- An EKG may show the following:
  - Normal findings in up to 1/3 of patients
  - Nonspecific ST-T changes (about 40%), left ventricular hypertrophy (about 25%)
  - Ischemic changes (about 15%), acute MI (about 3%), old MI with Q waves (about 7%)

Lab

Possible novel markers for aortic dissection include a combination of D-dimer, elastin fragments, and smooth-muscle myosin heavy-chain protein. Presently, none of these tests are used routinely as diagnostic tools, and several authors debate the use of D-dimer alone, with research being inconclusive as to its sensitivity and specificity.

Imaging

- A chest X-ray may show the following:
  - Normal findings in about 15% of patients
  - Widening of the mediastinum (about 60%), abnormal aortic outline (about 50%)
  - Abnormal cardiac silhouette (about 25%), calcified or displaced aorta (about 15%)
  - Pleural effusion (about 19%)
- Studies suggest that a CT scan with IV contrast, transesophageal echocardiography, and MRI imaging all provide around 95% sensitivity and specificity for diagnosis:
  - An MRI may be better for patients where clinical suspicion and pretest probability for aortic dissection are already high.
  - A CT scan may be better to rule out dissection in those patients where clinical suspicion and pretest probability are both low.
  - Transesophageal echocardiography can be done at the bedside of an unstable patient in 15–20 minutes, and it can offer additional information about heart function (3).
  - In reality, the ready availability and speed with which CT scans can be performed in many hospitals may outweigh the above considerations.
- Both MRI and CT scans can be used by clinicians to assess the extent, size, and location of the dissection, as well as involvement of the branches off the aorta, although some sources suggest an MRI as the preferred modality for precise anatomic definition.

Diagnostic Procedures/Surgery

Contrast angiography can be used specifically as a diagnostic tool, especially when visceral perfusion defects are suspected. Angiography may also be used as an entry point into endovascular treatment of dissection.

Pathological Findings

- About 60% of intimal tears occur in the proximal ascending aorta. The remaining incidence of tears occur between the origin of the left subclavian artery and ligamentum arteriosum, descending aorta (20%), aortic arch (10%), and abdominal aorta.

- Although medial necrosis is found in aging aortas, it is more extensive in patients who develop aortic dissections.
- Cystic medial necrosis is seen in patients with defects in elastin and connective tissue organization (e.g., Marfan, Ehlers-Danlos).
- Death usually is due to rupture and tamponade.

DIFFERENTIAL DIAGNOSIS

Myocardial infarction, pericarditis, pericardial tamponade not from aortic dissection, angina or atherosclerotic embolism, pulmonary embolism, pneumonia, pleurisy, acute pancreatitis or cholecystitis, penetrating duodenal ulcer, Mallory-Weiss tear or esophageal rupture, mediastinal pathology, musculoskeletal pain

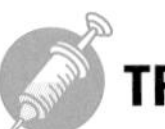

TREATMENT

Due to the acute nature of an aortic dissection, there are no randomized controlled trials related to treatment and management.

MEDICATION

For an uncomplicated dissection of descending aorta (Stanford B), medical therapy is indicated.

First Line

The cornerstone of medical management is BP control by using beta blockers, including propranolol, metoprolol, labetalol, and esmolol.

Second Line

- For patients with severe asthma, calcium-channel blockers may be used.
- If hypertension is refractory to initial therapies, nitroprusside can be considered, but the patient should be evaluated for a possible surgical intervention at that time.

ADDITIONAL TREATMENT

General Measures

- Patients should be monitored in intensive care units.
- Arterial BP monitoring is preferred, particularly in less stable patients.
- Pain control should involve the use of morphine.
- If surgical repair of aneurysm is indicated, do not delay repair to evaluate for CAD and valvular dysfunction.
- Prompt correction of hypotension and identification of the cause are essential.
- Hemodynamically unstable patients will likely require intubation and mechanical ventilation.

SURGERY/OTHER PROCEDURES

- Stanford A type dissection:
  - Surgery is the treatment of choice for dissections of the ascending aorta (80% treated surgically) to prevent aortic rupture and cardiac tamponade, while relieving any aortic regurgitation that may be present.
  - Patients who are inappropriate surgical candidates (comorbid medical conditions, patient choice, very advanced age) have an in-hospital mortality of 50% after 30 days.
  - Surgical correction aims to resect the ascending aorta and arch and to replace them with a graft.
  - Other procedures, including repair/replacement of aortic valves and coronary arteries, may be indicated depending on the extent of the dissection.
  - Many different surgical options exist and depend on the extent of the dissection.
- Stanford B type dissection:
  - A surgical resection of the aorta for type B is generally associated with worse outcomes than medical management.
  - Surgical indications for Stanford B include the following (4):
    - Continued aortic expansion
    - Impending aortic rupture
    - Occlusion of major aortic branch to renal, mesenteric, or iliac arteries
    - Persistent and recurrent chest pain
    - Periaortic or mediastinal hematoma
- Poor prognostic factors for surgical success:
  - Age >70 years
  - Abrupt-onset chest pain
  - Hypotension, shock, or tamponade at presentation
  - Renal failure
  - Pulse deficit
  - Abnormal ECG, ST-segment elevation
  - History of aortic valve replacement
  - Renal and/or visceral ischemia
- Stenting of complicated type B dissections seems to be a reasonable and safe alternative to surgical management, although further follow-up is needed (5).

IN-PATIENT CONSIDERATIONS

Initial Stabilization

- Admit to ICU
- Intubate hemodynamically unstable patients
- Control BP:
  - Systolic 100–120 mm Hg
  - IV beta blocker to achieve HR 60
  - Determine etiology of hypotension: Blood loss, tamponade, heart failure
- Pain control

Admission Criteria

Low threshold for admission in presence of thoracic or abdominal pain, radiographic corroboration, or pulse deficit

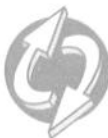

ONGOING CARE

FOLLOW-UP RECOMMENDATIONS

Patient Monitoring

- Maintain systolic BP at 120 mm Hg (16 kPa) or below, as tolerated.
- Routine chest films and/or a chest CT may be helpful for a patient treated medically in the long term.
- During follow-up, pay careful attention to signs and symptoms of aortic insufficiency, chest or back pain, and development of saccular aneurysms as displayed on chest films.

DIET

NPO until surgical evaluation is complete and patient is classified as medical therapy only

PATIENT EDUCATION

Depending on etiology, emphasis must be placed on risk factors and prevention of recurrence:

- Smoking cessation
- BP control with beta blockers
- Diabetic control

PROGNOSIS

- Hospital survival estimate, treated medically and surgically: 70% (4)
- Data for type A dissections treated surgically show a 90% survival rate at 3 years (6).
- Survival at 10 years is similar for both medically and surgically treated patients.
- Redissection risk: 5 years: 13%; 10 years: 23%

COMPLICATIONS

Redissection, localized saccular aneurysm, cardiac tamponade, aortic valvular insufficiency, progressive aortic enlargement. Stent placement risks include paraplegia, stroke, embolization, side-branch occlusion, and infection.

REFERENCES

1. Golledge J, Eagle KA. Acute aortic dissection. *Lancet*. 2008;372:55–66.
2. Gaul C, Dietrich W, Friedrich I. Neurological symptoms in type A aortic dissections. *Stroke*. 2007;38:292–7.
3. Nair HC. Transesophageal echocardiography evaluation of thoracic aorta. *Ann Card Anaesth*. 2010;13:186.
4. Hagan PG, Nienaber CA, Isselbacher EM. The International Registry of Acute Aortic Dissection (IRAD): New insights into an old disease. *JAMA*. 2000;283:897–903.
5. Nienaber CA, Kische S, Ince H, et al. Thoracic endovascular aneurysm repair for complicated type B aortic dissection. Journal of vascular surgery: Official publication, the Society for Vascular Surgery [and] International Society for Cardiovascular Surgery, North American Chapter. 2011.
6. Tsai TT, Evangelista A, Nienaber CA, et al. Long-term survival in patients presenting with type A acute aortic dissection: Insights from the International Registry of Acute Aortic Dissection (IRAD). *Circulation*. 2006;114:I350–6.

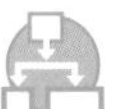

See Also (Topic, Algorithm, Electronic Media Element)

Hypertension, Essential; Hypertension, Secondary and Resistant; Ehlers-Danlos Syndrome; Marfan Syndrome

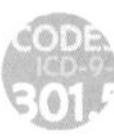

CODES

ICD9

- 441.00 Dissection of aorta, unspecified site
- 441.01 Dissection of aorta, thoracic

CLINICAL PEARLS

- Acute pain is reported by 90% of patients with aortic dissections. The pain is more often sharp than tearing, and is located in the chest, abdomen, or back.
- Maintain a high level of suspicion and act quickly if the diagnosis of aortic dissection is suspected.
- Survival at 10 years is similar for both medically and surgically treated patients.

AORTIC VALVULAR STENOSIS

Ajar Kochar, MD
Dawn Abbott, MD

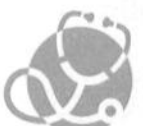

BASICS

DESCRIPTION

Aortic stenosis (AS) is a narrowing of the aortic valve area that causes an obstruction to left ventricular outflow. The disease has a long asymptomatic latency period, but development of severe obstruction or onset of symptoms such as syncope and angina are associated with a high mortality rate if surgical intervention is not accomplished promptly.

EPIDEMIOLOGY

- Most common valvular disease in developed countries
- >50% of patients with isolated AS also have a congenitally malformed valve (1).
- Predominant age:
  - <30 years: Congenital
  - 30–70 years: Congenital or rheumatic fever
  - >70 years: Degenerative calcification of aortic valve

Prevalence

- 1.3% at 65–74 years old, 2.4% at 75–84 years old, 4% at >84 years old (1)
- Bicuspid aortic valve: 1–2% of population (1)

RISK FACTORS

- Congenital (1):
  - Bicuspid valve
    - Men > Women
    - AS occurs at younger age
    - Associated with coarctation of aorta
  - Unicommissural valve
- Acquired (1):
  - Rheumatic fever (RF)
  - Degenerative (coronary artery disease–related RF): Hypercholesterolemia (elevated LDL, lipoprotein [a]), smoking, male gender, age, hypertension, diabetes mellitus

PATHOPHYSIOLOGY

- Progressive stiffening of aortic valve results in left ventricular (LV) outflow obstruction.
- Obstruction causes increased afterload and decreased forward flow.
- Increased afterload is compensated for by development of concentric left ventricular hypertrophy (LVH).
- LVH preserves ejection fraction but adversely affects heart functioning:
  - LVH impairs coronary blood flow reserve by compression of coronary arteries and reduced capillary ingrowth into hypertrophied muscle.
  - LVH results in diastolic dysfunction by reducing ventricular compliance.
- Diastolic dysfunction mandates stronger left atrial (LA) contraction to augment preload and maintain stroke volume. Loss of LA contraction by atrial fibrillation (AFib) can induce acute deterioration.
- Angina: Myocardial demand is elevated due to increased LV pressure. Myocardial supply is compromised due to LVH.
- Syncope (exertional): Ventricular contraction cannot augment cardiac output enough to match increase demands of exercise due to the fixed obstruction to LV outflow.
- Heart failure: Eventually LVH cannot compensate for increasing afterload, resulting in high LV pressure and volume, which are accompanied by an increase in LA and pulmonary pressures.

ETIOLOGY

- Calcific aortic stenosis (2): Initiating insult is mechanical stress to valve leaflets:
  - Note bicuspid valves are at higher risk for shear stress.
  - Early lesions: Subendothelial accumulation of oxidized LDL and macrophages and T-lymphocytes (inflammatory response)
  - Disease progression: Fibroblasts undergo transformation into osteoblasts. Protein production of osteopontin, osteocalcitonin, and BMP-2, which modulate calcification of leaflets
- Congenital: Unicuspid valve. Tricuspid valve with fusion of commissures, hypoplastic annulus
- Rheumatic fever: Fusion of commissures and scarring

COMMONLY ASSOCIATED CONDITIONS

- Coronary artery disease (50% of patients)
- Hypertension (40% of patients): Results in "double-loaded" left ventricle (dual source of obstruction from AS and hypertension).
- Aortic regurgitation (common in calcified bicuspid valves and rheumatic disease)
- Mitral valve disease: 95% of patients with AS from RF also have mitral valve disease.
- LV dysfunction and congestive heart failure (CHF)
- Atrial fibrillation associated with CHF
- Acquired von Willebrand disease: Impaired platelet function and decreased vWF results in bleeding (ecchymosis and epistaxis) in 20% of AS patients. Severity of coagulopathy is directly related to severity of AS.
- Rarely: Calcific embolization to systemic organs

DIAGNOSIS

HISTORY

- Primary symptoms: Angina, syncope, and heart failure (3). Angina is most frequent symptom. Syncope is often exertional. Heart failure symptoms include fatigue, exertional dyspnea, orthopnea, paroxysmal nocturnal dyspnea, shortness of breath.
- Palpitations
- Neurological events (transient ischemic attack or cerebrovascular accident) owing to embolization
- Geriatric patients may have subtle symptoms such as fatigue and exertional dyspnea.
- Note: Symptoms do not always correlate with valve area (severity of AS) but most commonly occur when AV area is <1.0 cm^2.

PHYSICAL EXAM

- Auscultation (3):
  - Harsh, systolic crescendo-decrescendo murmur (grade 4/6):
    - Best heard at 2nd right sternal border
    - Radiates into carotid arteries
    - Peak of murmur correlates with severity of stenosis: Earlier peaking murmur suggests less severe narrowing
  - High-pitched diastolic blow, suggests associated aortic regurgitation
  - Paradoxically split S2 or absent A2
  - Note: Normally split S2 reliably excludes severe AS.
  - S4
- Other associated signs (3): Thrill (denotes more severe narrowing); Parvus et Tardus: Carotid upstrokes decreased in volume, delayed in rate. LV heave

DIAGNOSTIC TESTS & INTERPRETATION

Lab

BNP may be elevated (no cutoffs exist) (1). Values altered by obesity, pulmonary hypertension, renal disease.

Imaging

Initial approach

- Chest x-ray (CXR) (1)
  - May be normal in compensated, isolated valvular aortic stenosis.
  - Boot-shaped heart reflective of concentric hypertrophy
  - Post-stenotic dilatation of ascending aorta
  - Calcification of aortic valve (seen on lateral PA CXR)
- ECG:
  - Often normal ECG (ECG is nondiagnostic)
  - LV hypertrophy
  - Left atrial enlargement
  - Nonspecific ST and T-wave abnormalities
- Echo indications:
  - Initial workup:
    - Doppler echocardiogram is mainstay of diagnosis.
    - Severity of AS
    - Assess left ventricular wall thickness, size, function.
  - In known AS and changing signs/symptoms
  - In known AS and pregnancy due to hemodynamic changes of pregnancy
- Echo findings:
  - Aortic valve morphology, thickening, calcifications
  - Decreased aortic valve excursion
  - Aortic valve area
  - LV hypertrophy
  - LV ejection fraction
  - Chamber dimensions will often be normal.
  - Wall-motion abnormalities suggesting CAD
  - Evaluate for concomitant mitral valve disease.
- Doppler echo adds information on:
  - Transvalvular gradient
  - Valve area
  - Diastolic function
  - Associated aortic regurgitation
- Aortic stenosis severity based on echo values (assumes normal cardiac output):
  - Normal: Area: 3–4 cm gradient: 0 mm Hg jet vel. <2.5 m/s
  - Mild: Area: 1.5–2 cm gradient: <25 mm Hg jet vel. 2.5–2.9 m/s
  - Mod: Area: 1–1.5 cm gradient: 25–40 mm Hg jet vel. 3–4 m/s
  - Severe: Area: <1 cm gradient: >40 mm Hg jet vel. >4 m/s
- Patients with severe AS and low cardiac output may have a relatively low transvalvular pressure gradient (i.e., mean gradient <30 mm Hg).

Diagnostic Procedures/Surgery

- Exercise stress testing:
  - Asymptomatic patients (4)[B]: Helpful to uncover subtle symptoms or changes, abnormal BP (increase <20 mm Hg), and ECG changes (ST depressions). 1/3 of patients develop symptoms with exercise testing; STOP testing at this point.
  - Symptomatic patients (4)[B]: DO NOT perform exercise stress testing as may induce hypotension or ventricular tachycardia.
  - CHF patients (4)[B]: Dobutamine stress echocardiography is reasonable to evaluate patients with low-flow/low-gradient AS and LV dysfunction.
- Cardiac catheterization: Perform prior to AVR in patients with suspected CAD (4)[B]. Determines need for coronary artery bypass graft (CABG). If unambiguous diagnosis of AS, perform only coronary angiography.
- Perform as diagnostic adjunct:
  - Catheterization is gold standard for diagnosis.
  - Use if noninvasive testing is inconclusive.
  - Use if discrepancy in severity of symptoms and findings on echo
  - Perform complete right and left heart catheterization.
  - Measure: Transvalvular flow, transvalvular pressure gradient, and effective valve area
  - Hemodynamic measurements with infusion of dobutamine can be useful for evaluation of patients with low-flow/low-gradient AS and LV dysfunction.

Pathological Findings

- Aortic valve: Nodular calcification on valve cusps (initially at bases), cusp rigidity, cusp thickening, and fibrosis.
- LV hypertrophy
- Myocardial interstitial fibrosis
- 50% incidence of concomitant CAD

DIFFERENTIAL DIAGNOSIS

- Mitral regurgitation: Either primary or secondary to underlying coronary artery disease or dilated cardiomyopathy. Usually an apical, high-frequency, pansystolic murmur, often radiating to axilla.
- Hypertrophic obstructive cardiomyopathy: Also systolic crescendo-decrescendo murmur, but best heard at left sternal border and may radiate into axilla. Murmur intensity increases by changing from squatting to standing and/or by Valsalva maneuver.
- Discrete fixed subaortic stenosis: 50–65% have associated cardiac deformity (PDA, VSD, coarctation of aorta).
- Aortic supravalvular stenosis: Williams syndrome, homozygous familial hypercholesterolemia

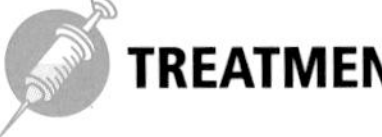

TREATMENT

MEDICATION

- NO medical therapy for severe or symptomatic aortic stenosis
- Prevention: Currently no recommended medical therapy. Statins may have a role if initiated during mild disease. Antibiotic prophylaxis against recurrent RF is indicated for patients with rheumatic AS (Penicillin G 1,200,000 U IM every 4 weeks, duration varies with age and history of carditis). Antibiotic prophylaxis is no longer indicated for prevention of infective endocarditis (4).
- Complications: Decompensated heart failure responds rapidly to IV nitroprusside (dose titrated to MAP of 60–70); can be used as bridge therapy until surgery.
- Comorbidities: Hypertension: ACE inhibitors, start with low dose and increase cautiously. Be cautious of vasodilators, which may cause hypotension.

ADDITIONAL TREATMENT

Percutaneous balloon aortic valvotomy or valvuloplasty (BAV):

- Percutaneous prosthetic valve implantation is under development and improves outcomes in patients who are not candidates for surgery. Poor surgical candidates: Advanced age, left ventricular dysfunction, numerous comorbidities
- In young adults and others without significantly calcified aortic valves and no AR, BAV is indicated in the following patients:
  - Symptoms of angina, syncope, dyspnea on exertion, and peak-to-peak gradients at catheterization >50 mm Hg
  - Asymptomatic adolescents or young adults who demonstrate ST or T-wave abnormalities in the left precordial leads on ECG at rest or with exercise and a peak-to-peak catheter gradient >60 mm Hg (4)[C]
  - Asymptomatic adolescent or young adult with AS and a peak-to-peak gradient on catheterization >50 mm Hg when the patient is interested in playing competitive sports or becoming pregnant (4)[C]
- In older adults with rheumatic or degenerative AS, BAV may be considered as a bridge to surgery in hemodynamically unstable adults with AS, adults at high risk for AVR, or when AVR cannot be performed secondary to significant comorbidities (4)[C].

SURGERY/OTHER PROCEDURES

Indications for aortic valve replacement (AVR):

- Symptomatic and severe AS (4)[B]; should be performed rapidly due to high risk of sudden cardiac death
- Asymptomatic, severe AS and
  - Requires aortic root surgery or other valvular surgery (4)[C]
  - Requires CABG (4)[C]
  - Ejection fraction (EF) (<50%) (4)[C]
  - Positive exercise stress testing findings (4)[C]
  - Risk of rapid progression (moderate-severe calcification, age, CAD) (4)[C]
- Asymptomatic, extremely severe AS (4)[C]: Aortic valve area <0.6 cm, gradient >60 mm Hg, or jet velocity >5 m/s
- Moderate stenosis and undergoing CABG or valvular surgery (4)[B]
- Mild AS and CABG and high risk of rapid progression (4)[C]. Note if AV Area >1.5 cm and gradient <15 mm Hg no benefit from AVR.

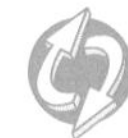

ONGOING CARE

FOLLOW-UP RECOMMENDATIONS

- Advise patient to immediately report symptoms referable to AS.
- Asymptomatic patients: Yearly history and physical (4)[C]
- Serial echo: Recommendation (4)[B]: Yearly for severe AS, every 1–2 years for moderate AS, every 3–5 years for mild AS

PATIENT EDUCATION

Physical activity limitations:

- Asymptomatic mild AS: No restrictions, competitive sports are okay.
- Asymptomatic moderate-to-severe AS: Avoid competitive sports that have high muscle demand. Milder exercise can be done safely. Consider exercise stress test prior to starting exercise program.

PROGNOSIS

- 25% mortality/yr in symptomatic patients who do not undergo valve replacement; average survival is 2–3 years without AVR surgery.
- Median survival in symptomatic AS (3): Heart failure: 2 years; syncope: 3 years; angina: 5 years
- After AVR, a patient's lifespan returns to near that of an unselected population.
- Perisurgical mortality: AVR surgery has 4% mortality rate; AVR + CABG has 6.8% mortality rate.
- Adverse postoperative prognostic factors: Age, HF NYHA III/IV, cerebrovascular disease, renal dysfunction, CAD

REFERENCES

1. Carabello BA, Paulus WJ. Aortic stenosis. *Lancet*. 2009;373:956–66
2. Otto CM. Calcific aortic stenosis–time to look more closely at the valve. *N Engl J Med*. 2008;359: 1395–8.
3. Grimard BH, Larson JM. Aortic stenosis: Diagnosis and treatment. *Am Fam Physician*. 2008; 78:717–24.
4. Bonow RO, Carbello BA, Chatterjee K, et al. ACC/AHA 2006 guidelines for the management of patients with valvular heart disease: A report of the American College of Cardiology/American Heart Association Task Force on Practice. Guidelines. *Circulation*. 2006;114:e84–231.

ADDITIONAL READING

Kurtz CE, Otto CM. Aortic stenosis: Clinical aspects of diagnosis and management, with 10 illustrative case reports from a 25-year experience. *Medicine (Baltimore)*. 2010;89:349–79.

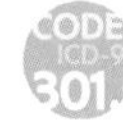

CODES

ICD9

- 395.0 Rheumatic aortic stenosis
- 424.1 Aortic valve disorders
- 746.3 Congenital stenosis of aortic valve

CLINICAL PEARLS

- Aortic stenosis is diagnosed on physical exam by a systolic crescendo-decrescendo murmur, and delayed and diminished pulses.
- Symptomatic AS most commonly presents as angina, syncope, and heart failure.
- Symptomatic AS has a very poor prognosis unless treated with surgical intervention.

APPENDICITIS, ACUTE

Francesca L. Beaudoin, MS, MD
Reagan J. Herrington, MD

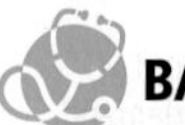

BASICS

DESCRIPTION

- Acute inflammation of the vermiform appendix, first described by Reginald Fitz in 1886
- Arising from the base of the cecum in right lower quadrant (RLQ); can be localized anterior, posterior, medial, lateral to the cecum, as well as in the pelvis. Vascular supply by appendicular artery, a branch of the ileocolic artery.
- Most common cause of the acute surgical abdomen

EPIDEMIOLOGY

- Predominant age: 10–30 years: Rare in infancy
- Predominant sex: Slight male predominance:
  - Ages 10–30: Male > Female (3:2)
  - Age >30: Male = Female

Incidence

- 1 case per 1,000 people per year
- Lifetime incidence 1 in every 15 persons (7%)

Pregnancy Considerations

- Most common extrauterine surgical emergency
- No more common in pregnant vs. nonpregnant women
- Higher rate of perforation; more likely to present with peritonitis

RISK FACTORS

Adolescent males, familial tendency, Intra-abdominal tumors

Genetics

1st-degree relative with history of appendicitis increases risk, although no direct genetic link has been found

PATHOPHYSIOLOGY

The initial event inciting appendicitis is thought to be obstruction of the appendiceal lumen. This leads to distention, ischemia, and bacterial overgrowth. Without intervention, most cases of appendicitis will lead to perforation and subsequently abscess formation or generalized peritonitis.

ETIOLOGY

Causes of obstruction:

- Fecaliths (most common)
- Lymphoid tissue hyperplasia (in children)
- Vegetable, fruit seeds, and other foreign bodies
- Intestinal worms (ascarids)
- Strictures, fibrosis, neoplasms

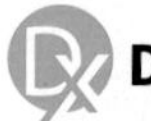

DIAGNOSIS

Diagnosis of acute appendicitis relies on the clinical integration of history, physical exam, and often laboratories and imaging. Scoring systems, including the Alvarado Score and the Pediatric Appendicitis Score, have been developed to help predict the likelihood of acute appendicitis, although diagnosis is still considered a clinical decision.

HISTORY

- The classic history is vague periumbilical pain, followed by anorexia/nausea/vomiting. Over the next 4–48 hours, pain then migrates to the right lower quadrant.
- Only 50% of patients present with this classic history.
- Pain before vomiting (~100% sensitive), abdominal pain (~100%), pain migration
- Anorexia (~100%), nausea (90%), vomiting (75%), obstipation
- Atypical symptoms and pain associated with a retrocecal or pelvic appendix

PHYSICAL EXAM

- Fever; temp >100.4°F (may be absent). Tachycardia.
- RLQ tenderness. Maximal tenderness at McBurney point (1/3 the distance from the anterior superior iliac spine to the umbilicus)
- Voluntary and involuntary guarding
- Rovsing sign: RLQ pain with palpation of left lower quadrant. Psoas sign: Pain with right thigh extension (retrocecal appendix)
- Obturator sign: Pain with internal rotation of flexed right thigh (pelvic appendix). Local and suprapubic pain on rectal exam (pelvic appendix).
- Pelvic and rectal exams are necessary to rule out other causes of lower abdominal pain (pelvic inflammatory disease, prostatitis, etc.).
- Serial exams can be useful in indeterminate cases.

Pediatric Considerations

- Decreased diagnostic accuracy of history and physical
- Higher fever, more vomiting and diarrhea

Pregnancy Considerations

- Difficult diagnosis
- Normal response to infection/inflammation is suppressed.
- Appendix displaced out of pelvis by gravid uterus

Geriatric Considerations

Decreased diagnostic accuracy, more likely to be atypical presentation

DIAGNOSTIC TESTS & INTERPRETATION

Lab

- Leukocytosis: White blood cells (WBC) $>10{,}000/\text{mm}^3$ (70%)
- Polymorphonuclear predominance or "left shift" (>90%)
- Human chorionic gonadotropin (hCG) (if negative, rules out ectopic pregnancy)
- Urinalysis: Hematuria, pyuria (~30%)
- C-reactive protein: Nonspecific inflammatory marker. When paired with an elevated WBC can increase the likelihood of appendicitis.
- Drugs that may alter lab results: Antibiotics, steroids

Imaging

- Used in cases of suspected appendicitis when the diagnosis is not clear
- Helpful to detect complications (abscess, perforation)
- CT scan: Sensitivity ~91–98%; specificity 95–99%; imaging modality of choice. However, growing concern regarding radiation dose, particularly in young patients.
- CT scan with IV contrast alone provides equivalent information to CT scan with rectal or oral contrast (1)[A].
- Ultrasound: Viable alternative in pregnant patients, children, and in women with suspected gynecologic pathology. Sensitivity ~86%; specificity ~81%. Starting with an initial ultrasound and, if negative, obtaining a CT scan has been shown to be an effective workup strategy for all patients (2)[B].
- Plain films: Little utility, nonspecific findings, may visualize fecalith
- MRI: Growing in popularity for diagnosing pregnant patients, but also may be useful for patients with contrast allergies and/or renal failure patients. Limitations include cost, availability, and time required to complete study.
- Radioisotope-labeled WBC scans: May be used in patients with indeterminate CT scans and suspected appendicitis as an alternative to observation or surgery. Limitations include availability and time required to complete study.

Diagnostic Procedures/Surgery

Diagnostic laparoscopy may be useful in establishing a diagnosis in equivocal cases in fertile women, but more studies are needed.

Pathological Findings

- Acute appendiceal inflammation, local vascular congestion, obstruction
- Gangrene, perforation with abscess (15–30%), fecalith

DIFFERENTIAL DIAGNOSIS

- GI:
  - Gastroenteritis, Inflammatory bowel disease
  - Diverticulitis, ileitis
  - Cholecystitis, pancreatitis
  - Intussusception, volvulus
- Gynecologic:
  - Pelvic inflammatory disease, ectopic pregnancy
  - Ovarian cyst, ovarian torsion, tubo-ovarian abscess
  - Endometriosis
  - Ruptured graafian follicle
- Urologic:
  - Testicular torsion, epididymitis
  - Kidney stones, prostatitis, cystitis, pyelonephritis
- Systemic:
  - Diabetic ketoacidosis
  - Henoch Schönlein purpura
  - Sickle cell crisis
  - Porphyria
- Other:
  - Acute mesenteric lymphadenitis
  - No organic pathologic condition
  - Hernias
  - Psoas abscess
  - Rectus sheath hematoma
  - Epiploic appendagitis
  - Pneumonia (basilar)

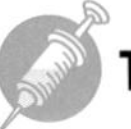

TREATMENT

MEDICATION

First Line

- Uncomplicated acute appendicitis: Perioperative dose of broad-spectrum antibiotic (3)[A]: Cefoxitin (Mefoxin); cefotetan (Cefotan)
- Gangrenous or perforating appendicitis:
  - Broadened antibiotic coverage for aerobic and anaerobic enteric pathogens
  - Fluoroquinolone and metronidazole or ampicillin and gentamicin and metronidazole typically used
  - Adjust dosage and choice of antibiotic based on intraoperative cultures.
  - Continue antibiotics for 7 days postoperatively or until patient becomes afebrile with normal WBC count.

Second Line

- Ampicillin-sulbactam (Unasyn)
- Ticarcillin-clavulanate (Timentin)
- Piperacillin-tazobactam (Zosyn)

ADDITIONAL TREATMENT

General Measures

Surgery (appendectomy) is still the standard of care for acute uncomplicated appendicitis (4,5). However, nonoperative management with antibiotics has been studied as an alternative. Some literature suggests that antibiotic therapy alone may be initially as successful as appendectomy, but this approach carries recurrent appendicitis rates of 14–20% in the 1st year. The possibility of recurrence or progression to perforation must be weighed against the potential complications of surgery. In the case of acute appendicitis complicated by abscess formation or phlegmon in pediatric patients, some studies show initial conservative management with antibiotics alone to carry fewer risks and complications than emergent appendectomy (6).

Issues for Referral

All cases of appendicitis require emergent surgical consultation.

SURGERY/OTHER PROCEDURES

- Inpatient surgery is indicated
- Patients presenting within 72 hours of onset:
  - Immediate appendectomy; laparoscopic favored unless perforation (7)[A]
  - Drainage of abscess, if present
- Patients who present late (>4–5 days after symptom onset) may be treated initially with antibiotics, bowel rest, and drainage of any abscess. Later (4–10 weeks) appendectomy can then be performed in this subgroup only.

IN-PATIENT CONSIDERATIONS

Admission Criteria

All patients with appendicitis should be admitted.

IV Fluids

Fluid resuscitation with normal saline (NS) or lactated Ringer's (LR). Correct fluid and electrolyte deficits.

Nursing

Preoperative preparation

Discharge Criteria

Tolerating PO; return of bowel function; afebrile; normal WBC

ONGOING CARE

FOLLOW-UP RECOMMENDATIONS

- Return to work is usually possible 1–2 weeks following most uncomplicated appendicitis.
- Restrict activity for 4–6 weeks after surgery: No heavy lifting (>10 lbs) or strenuous physical activity.

Patient Monitoring

Routine visits at 2 and 6 weeks after surgery

DIET

NPO before surgery

PATIENT EDUCATION

Contact physician for postoperative development of:

- Anorexia, nausea, vomiting
- Abdominal pain, fever, chills
- Signs or symptoms of wound infection

PROGNOSIS

- Generally uncomplicated course in young adults with unruptured appendicitis
- Factors increasing morbidity and mortality: Extremes of age, presence of appendiceal rupture
- Morbidity rates:
  - Nonperforated appendicitis: 3%
  - Perforated appendicitis: 47%
- Mortality rates:
  - Unruptured appendicitis: 0.1%
  - Ruptured appendicitis: 3%
  - Patients >60 years of age make up 50% of total deaths from appendicitis.
  - Older patients with ruptured appendix: 15%

Pediatric Considerations

- Rupture earlier
- Rupture rate: 15–60%

Pregnancy Considerations

- Rupture rate: 40%
- Fetal mortality rate: 2–8.5%

Geriatric Considerations

Rupture rate: 67–90%

COMPLICATIONS

- Wound infection, intra-abdominal abscess; lower rate with antibiotic prophylaxis (3)[A], intestinal fistulas
- Intestinal obstruction, paralytic ileus, incisional hernia
- Liver abscess (rare), pyelophlebitis

REFERENCES

1. Mun S, Ernst RD, Chen K, et al. Rapid CT diagnosis of acute appendicitis with IV contrast material. *Emerg Radiol*. 2006;12:99–102.
2. Poortman P, Oostvogel HJ, Bosma E, et al. Improving diagnosis of acute appendicitis: Results of a diagnostic pathway with standard use of ultrasonography followed by selective use of CT. *J Am Coll Surg*. 2009;208:434–41.
3. Andersen BR, Kallehaue FL, Andersen HK. Antibiotics versus placebo for prevention of postoperative infection after appendectomy. *Cochrane Database Syst Rev*. 2006;(1).
4. Varadhan KK, Humes DJ, Neal KR, et al. Antibiotic therapy versus appendectomy for acute appendicitis: A meta-analysis. *World J Surg*. 2010;34:199–209.
5. Vons C, Barry C, Maitre S, et al. Amoxicillin plus clavulanic acid versus appendicectomy for treatment of acute uncomplicated appendicitis: An open-label, non-inferiority, randomised controlled trial. *Lancet*. 2011;377:1573–9.
6. Simillis C, Symeonides P, Shorthouse AJ, et al. A meta-analysis comparing conservative treatment versus acute appendectomy for complicated appendicitis (abscess or phlegmon). *Surgery*. 2010;147:818–29.
7. Sauerland S, Lefering R, Neugebauer EAM. Laparoscopic versus open surgery for suspected appendicitis. *Cochrane Database Syst Rev*. 2005;(1).

ADDITIONAL READING

- Bauer T, Vennits B, Holm B, et al. Antibiotic prophylaxis in acute nonperforated appendicitis. The Danish Multicenter Study Group III. *Ann Surg*. 1989;209:307–11.
- Domínguez LC, Sanabria A, Vega V, et al. Early laparoscopy for the evaluation of nonspecific abdominal pain: A critical appraisal of the evidence. *Surg Endosc*. 2011;25:10–8.
- Hansson J, Körner U, Khorram-Manesh A, et al. Randomized clinical trial of antibiotic therapy versus appendectomy as primary treatment of acute appendicitis in unselected patients. *Br J Surg*. 2009;96:473–81.
- Hlibczuk V, Dattaro JA, Jin Z, et al. Diagnostic accuracy of noncontrast computed tomography for appendicitis in adults: A systematic review. *Ann Emerg Med*. 2010;55:51–59.e1.
- Singh AK, Desai H, Novelline RA, et al. Emergency MRI of acute pelvic pain: MR protocol with no oral contrast. *Emerg Radiol*. 2009;16:133–41.

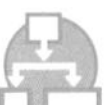

See Also (Topic, Algorithm, Electronic Media Element)

Algorithm: Abdominal Rigidity

CODES

ICD9

- 540.0 Acute appendicitis with generalized peritonitis
- 540.9 Acute appendicitis without mention of peritonitis
- 541 Appendicitis, unqualified

CLINICAL PEARLS

- Classic history of anorexia with periumbilical pain localizing to RLQ is the cornerstone of diagnosis for acute appendicitis.
- Diagnosis is much more challenging in children, pregnant patients, and the elderly due to varying symptoms and signs.
- CT of abdomen and pelvis is the diagnostic test of choice, although ultrasound in experienced hands has good sensitivity and avoids radiation exposure, as does MRI.
- Acute appendicitis is the most common surgical emergency during pregnancy.

ARTERIAL EMBOLUS AND THROMBOSIS

Edward Pokorny, MSIV
Gina M. DeFranco, DO

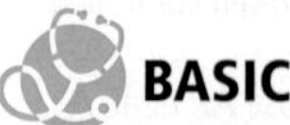

BASICS

DESCRIPTION

- Acute loss of perfusion distal to occlusion of major artery due to: An embolus that migrates to point of occlusion (air, fat, and amniotic fluid embolism) or a clot (thrombosis) intrinsic to point of occlusion (most common). Both are true emergencies.
- Following obstruction of artery, soft coagulum forms both proximally and distally in areas of stagnant flow.
- As clot extends, collateral pathways become involved, and process becomes self-propagating. Ultimately, venous circulation can become involved.
- Extent of vascular compromise is critical and determines "golden" period of 4–6 hours, depending on involved organ. After this time, the profound ischemia leads to irreversible cellular death.
- Distribution of emboli: Femoral artery: 30%; iliac artery: 15%; aortic bifurcation: 10%; popliteal artery: 10%; brachial: 10%; mesenteric arteries: 5–7%; cerebral (estimated): 15–20%
- Classic presentations:
  - Blue toe syndrome: Sudden painful, cool, blue toe in the presence of palpable distal pulses
  - Mesenteric ischemia: Pain out of proportion to abdominal component of physical exam, typically begins periumbilical then becomes diffusely painful.
- System(s) affected: Cardiovascular; Hematologic/Lymphatic/Immunologic

EPIDEMIOLOGY

Incidence

50–100/100,000 hospital admissions annually

Prevalence

- Predominant age: Elderly (over age 65)
- Predominant sex: Male > Female
- A leading cause of limb loss in elderly
- More common in African Americans

RISK FACTORS

Atherosclerotic disease, tobacco abuse, endocarditis, diabetes, drug abuse, cardiac arrhythmia, trauma

Genetics

Sometimes associated with inheritable hypercoagulable and premature atherosclerotic syndromes

GENERAL PREVENTION

Anticoagulation in atrial arrhythmia, reduction of atherosclerosis risk factors, smoking cessation

PATHOPHYSIOLOGY

Initiation of thrombosis in arterial circulation based on platelet aggregation and adhesion, not fibrin clot formation, as in venous thrombosis

ETIOLOGY

- Emboli:
  - Arise from degenerative, stenotic, and ulcerative atherosclerotic plaques
  - Bilateral lower extremity disease signifies proximal aortic source.
  - Unilateral embolic disease signifies disease distal to aortic bifurcation.
  - More commonly ,lodge in areas of bifurcation
- Cardiac:
  - Atrial flutter/fibrillation
  - Valve disease
  - Myocardial infarction
  - Cardiomyopathy (low ejection fraction)
  - Endocarditis
- Aortic atheroembolism
- Secondary to angiographic procedures
- Aneurysms: Cardiac, aortic, peripheral
- Thrombosis:
  - Atherosclerotic occlusive disease
  - Aortic and peripheral aneurysms (i.e., popliteal)
  - Hypercoagulable states
  - Venous gangrene
  - Drug abuse
  - Heparin allergy (heparin-induced thrombocytopenia)
  - Vascular bypass
- Trauma:
  - Blunt or penetrating
  - Vascular/cardiac interventional procedures
- Venous thrombosis with patent foramen ovale (paradoxical embolus)

COMMONLY ASSOCIATED CONDITIONS

- Acute mesenteric ischemia
- Renal infarction
- Carotid/cerebrovascular accident
- Multiple emboli
- Digital microembolization
- Systemic vasculitis
- Atrial fibrillation
- Atrial myxoma
- Aneurysmal disease
- Hypercholesterolemia

DIAGNOSIS

HISTORY

- The 5 *Ps*: If any one is present, frequent re-evaluations indicated. Proximal occlusions lead to more rapid progression of findings. Occlusion at aortic bifurcation can produce bilateral findings:
  - Pain: Diffuse distally. Crescendo in nature. Most common symptom in embolism. Not alleviated by change of position.
  - Pulselessness: Mandatory for diagnosis of embolism or thrombosis. Pedal pulses subject to observer error. Always compare to opposite limb.
  - Pallor: Skin color pale early, cyanotic later. Check extremity temperature left to right and top to bottom. Signs of chronic ischemia: Skin atrophy, hair loss, thick nails.
  - Paresthesia: Numbness early with thrombosis. Proprioception and light touch 1st to be lost. Not reliable in diabetics. Loss of pain and pressure indicate advanced ischemia.
  - Paralysis: Motor defect occurs after sensory and indicates profound ischemia.
- Later symptoms include: Blisters, skin erosion (ulcer), tissue death/necrosis

PHYSICAL EXAM

- To estimate occlusion location:
  - Symptoms typically start 1 joint below occlusion.
  - Palpable pulses may be absent below occlusion and accentuated above.
- In acute mesenteric ischemia: Painful periumbilical abdomen initially, which later becomes diffusely painful

DIAGNOSTIC TESTS & INTERPRETATION

Lab

Initial lab tests

For preoperative evaluation, elucidation of cause, or documentation of ischemia severity:

- Myocardial/muscle isoenzymes
- Coagulation parameters
- Blood pH/bicarbonate
- Urine myoglobin
- Electrolytes
- Amylase

Diagnostic Procedures/Surgery

- Arteriography:
  - Rarely indicated preoperatively for embolus
  - Standard of care is to perform intraoperative arteriography after an embolectomy
  - May help differentiate thrombosis from embolus in nonthreatened limb
  - Useful with occluded grafts or thrombosis
  - Crescent-shaped (meniscus sign) or multiple filling defects within an otherwise normal artery implicates an embolus.
  - Along with thrombolytic therapy may depict the causative factor (e.g., anastomotic stricture) and allow for more directed operative care
- Abdominal CT with contrast for acute mesenteric ischemia
- ECG
- Noninvasive/indirect:
  - Doppler: Presence or absence of flow
  - Ankle/arm index (AAI; aka ankle/brachial index [ABI]) = dorsal pedal/posterior tibial pressure divided by brachial pressure
- AAI >0.30 favorable (normal >1)

Pathological Findings

Mucosal infarction of the small bowel will show mucosal hemorrhage and loss of epithelial layer.

DIFFERENTIAL DIAGNOSIS

- Emboli vs. thrombosis
- Emboli:
  - Myocardial diseases: Infarction, arrhythmias (e.g., atrial fibrillation), aneurysms
  - Pain as 1st symptom
- Thrombosis:
  - Absence of heart disease: Infarction, arrhythmias
  - Chronic vascular history
  - Bilateral changes of chronic ischemia
  - Numbness rather than pain as 1st symptom
  - Vascular procedures: Bypass/interventional
- Other conditions:
  - Acute aortic dissection (chest or back pain with rapid clinical deterioration)
  - Acute deep vein thrombosis (massive swelling and warm skin)
- Low flow states

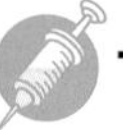

TREATMENT

Treatment must first be centered on hemodynamic stabilization, including volume resuscitation, maintenance of end organ perfusion, and correction of cardiac arrhythmias.

MEDICATION

First Line

- Heparin (1): Goal to prevent distal and proximal extension of thrombus, anti-inflammatory effects:
  - 80–100 U/kg IV loading (5,000–10,000 U)
  - Continuous infusion sufficient to double partial thromboplastin time, generally 18 U/kg/hr
  - Transition to 3–6-month period of warfarin therapy indicated if below-knee bypass performed with synthetic graft
  - Contraindications: Heparin: Allergy, bleeding diathesis, trauma (e.g., head injury), hematuria/hemoptysis, acute aortic dissection
- t-PA/urokinase 0.5 mg/hr:
  - Urokinase (1):
    - Loading dose: 4,400 IU/kg at a rate of 90 mL/hr over 10 minutes; then 4,400 IU/kg at a rate of 15 mL/hr over 12 hours; may be repeated as needed
  - Had been off the market, currently widely available
  - Equivalent results to t-PA
  - Do not use thrombolytic agents for >72 hours; risk of systemic/intracranial bleeding increases at this point:
    - Contraindications: Nonsalvageable ischemia, recent myocardial infarction, aneurysm, aortic dissection, trauma, uncontrolled hypertension
- In pediatric femoral artery thrombosis: IV unfractionated heparin for 5–7 days, surgery if life or limb threatened

ADDITIONAL TREATMENT

For chronic PAD with intermittent claudication, aspirin is preferred to clopidogrel unless aspirin allergy is present. Lifelong 75–100 mg/d of aspirin is the recommended treatment.

General Measures

Revascularization of an ischemic area results in return of blood with a low pH and high potassium. This must be closely monitored after treatment.

Issues for Referral

- Mesenteric ischemia: Immediate GI follow-up/ endoscopy (mortality of 70%)
- Renal infarction/nephrotic syndrome: Nephrology follow-up

SURGERY/OTHER PROCEDURES

- Angioplasty, thromboembolectomy, thromboaspiration (clot aspiration). These less invasive procedures are used when the ischemic limb is not imminently threatened. These techniques are more often utilized at a tertiary center where access to angiography equipment/specially trained practitioners is more readily available.
- Arterial bypass
- Extended embolic time may require bypass secondary to intimal damage/fibrosis.
- IV UFH at therapeutic levels is considered recommended treatment prior to vascular bypass cross-clamp application.

IN-PATIENT CONSIDERATIONS

Initial Stabilization

- Time is of the essence:
  - Unless contraindicated, systemic heparinization to decrease clot propagation and prophylaxis against further emboli
  - Resuscitation and stabilization of patient to extent permitted by time
  - Triage, based on detailed exam, history, and Doppler examination, determines appropriate therapy.
- Early subcritical stenosis criteria:
  - Mild ischemic pain
  - Normal neurologic exam
  - Capillary refill present
  - Arterial signals present by Doppler in distal extremity
  - Ankle/arm index >0.30
  - Treatment:
    - Heparin (see "Medications")
    - Arteriography
  - Embolism:
    - Surgical removal if acceptable operative risk, for example, balloon embolectomy (Fogarty catheter)
    - Anticoagulation vs. intra-arterial thrombolytics if prohibitive risk
  - Thrombosis:
    - Trial of thrombolytics and correction of arterial defect if good risk
    - Anticoagulation if poor risk or thrombolytics contraindicated
- Critical stenosis criteria: Ischemic pain, mild neurologic deficit, weakness of ankle dorsiflexion, minimal sensory loss: Light touch and/or vibratory, no pulsatile flow by Doppler, venous flow present. Treatment:
  - Time to intervention is critical.
  - Arteriography
  - Individualize thrombolysis and/or operative procedure (depending on extent of thrombosis and amenability for surgical removal)
  - Thrombolysis to optimize alternatives
  - Adjunctive operative therapy
  - Intraoperative lytic therapy: Bypass, patch angioplasty
- Late (nonsalvageable) criteria: Profound sensory loss, muscle paralysis, absent capillary refill, skin mottling, muscle rigor, no arterial or venous signals by Doppler. Treatment:
  - Arteriography usually not warranted
  - Attempts at reperfusion contraindicated
  - Anticoagulation
  - Definitive amputation, if possible

Admission Criteria

If embolus/thrombosis is suspected, admission is required.

IV Fluids

IVF to manage dehydration and increase blood volume is essential: IV pain management also important.

Pregnancy Considerations

- Pregnancy is a contraindication to thrombolytic therapy.
- Pregnancy is a contraindication to warfarin use (teratogenic).

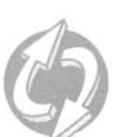

ONGOING CARE

FOLLOW-UP RECOMMENDATIONS

After definitive treatment of an embolus, patients should be evaluated for other systemic complications of atherosclerosis, including carotid stenosis, aortic aneurysm, peripheral vascular disease, and coronary arterial disease.

Patient Monitoring

Postoperative monitoring: Anticoagulation, establish brisk diuresis, continued resuscitation and diagnosis, including echocardiography and other studies (see "Causes" and "Risk Factors"), monitor perfusion stability, treat/eliminate causative factors

PATIENT EDUCATION

Quit smoking, use appropriate cholesterol-lowering medications, discuss antithrombotic or anticoagulant therapy

PROGNOSIS

- 90% good outcome with prompt treatment. Delayed/untreated associated with high mortality and limb loss.
- 20–30% hospital mortality associated with causative factors

COMPLICATIONS

- Acidosis, myoglobinuria, and acute renal failure, hyperkalemia
- Recurrent occlusion or failure to remove clot/obstruction
- Compartment syndromes/reperfusion syndrome, delayed or acute. Predisposing factors include: Combined arterial injury, profound and prolonged ischemia, hypotension
- Clinical findings of compartment syndrome: Severe pain, pain with passive muscle movement, hypesthesias of nerves in compartment, paralysis of nerves, especially peroneal foot drop, tender, tense edema, compartment pressure >30–45 mm Hg
- Consequences of unrecognized compartment syndrome:
  - Acute: Amputation, sepsis, myoglobin renal failure, shock, multiple organ failure
  - Delayed: Ischemic contracture, infection, causalgia, gangrene

REFERENCES

1. Clagett GP, Sobel M, Jackson MR, et al. Antithrombotic therapy in peripheral arterial occlusive disease: The Seventh ACCP Conference on Antithrombotic and Thrombolytic Therapy. *Chest*. 2004;126:609S–26S.

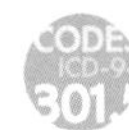

CODES

ICD9

- 444.22 Arterial embolism and thrombosis of lower extremity
- 444.81 Embolism and thrombosis of iliac artery
- 444.9 Embolism and thrombosis of unspecified artery

CLINICAL PEARLS

5 *Ps* of occlusion history: Pain, pallor, paresthesia, pulselessness, and paralysis

ARTERIOSCLEROTIC HEART DISEASE

Jonathan Liu, MD
James Arrighi, MD

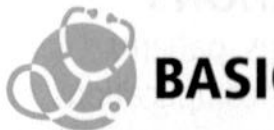

BASICS

DESCRIPTION

- Arteriosclerosis progressively blocks coronary arteries and their branches, limiting blood flow to the myocardium.
- Synonyms include atherosclerotic heart disease, coronary artery disease (CAD).

EPIDEMIOLOGY

- Leading cause of death in the US and Europe
- Predominant sex: Male > Female
- Prevalence increases with age. Predominant age for peak clinical manifestations: Men: 50–60 years; Women: 60–70 years
- In postmenopausal women, the risk for incident coronary disease is tripled compared with premenopausal women.
- Mortality from coronary heart disease (CHD) has decreased over the past 4 decades.

Incidence

Framingham data suggest that the age-adjusted annual incidence for men aged 35–64 is 12 per 1,000 per year, and for women, 5 per 1,000 per year. For men >65, the incidence is 27 per 1,000 per year, and for women, 16 per 1,000 per year.

Prevalence

The 2011 Heart Disease and Stroke Statistics update of the American Heart Association reported that 16.3 million persons in the US have CHD, including 7.9 million with myocardial infarction (MI) and 9 million with angina pectoris.

RISK FACTORS

- Nonmodifiable risk factors:
  - Age: Males > 45; Females > 55; Male gender
  - Family history of premature CHD (1st-degree relative: Male <55 years; female <65 years)
- Modifiable risk factors:
  - Diabetes mellitus
  - BP >140/90
  - Active cigarette abuse
  - Obesity
  - Hyperlipidemia (elevated LDL-C and HDL-C <40 mg/dL; HDL >60 mg/dL is a protective factor)
  - Sedentary lifestyle
- Other risk factors: Depression and stress, cocaine use, chronic inflammation and inflammatory conditions, ESRD, estrogen deficiency
- Emerging risk factors or markers for increased risk: Elevated highly sensitive C-reactive protein (hs-CRP), elevated homocysteine, elevated lipoprotein(a), elevated fibrinogen

GENERAL PREVENTION

- Lifestyle changes are indicated when lifestyle-related factors (obesity, physical inactivity, increased triglycerides, decreased HDL, metabolic syndrome) are present, regardless of LDL.
- Obtain a global risk assessment in all adults using the Framingham Risk Score at http://hp2010.nhlbihin.net/atpiii/calculator.asp or Reynolds Risk Score at http://www.reynoldsriskscore.org. Calculation modified for diabetes http://www.mdcalc.com/framingham-cardiac-risk-score

ETIOLOGY

- Atherosclerosis, inflammation, including autoimmunity
- Embolism compromising coronary arteries
- Subintimal atheromas in large and medium vessels

COMMONLY ASSOCIATED CONDITIONS

Cerebrovascular disease (ischemic stroke); carotid artery disease (TIA); peripheral arterial disease (claudication); aortic atherosclerosis (abdominal aortic aneurysm); metabolic syndrome

DIAGNOSIS

HISTORY

- Substernal chest pain, diaphoresis, palpitations
- Exertional dyspnea, orthopnea, paroxysmal nocturnal dyspnea (PND)

Consideration: Advanced obstructive CHD can exist with minimal or no symptoms, and can progress rapidly.

PHYSICAL EXAM

- HEENT exam (corneal arcus, xanthelasmas)
- Cardiac exam (arrhythmias, murmurs, S3, S4 gallop)
- Pulmonary exam (crackles)
- Abdominal exam (HJR, ascites, hepatomegaly, AAA)
- Vascular exam (JVD, clubbing, bruits, aneurysms)
- Musculoskeletal exam (pedal edema)
- Skin exam (xanthomas)

Consideration: Physical exam in a patient with CHD may be completely normal.

DIAGNOSTIC TESTS & INTERPRETATION

Lab

When workup is indicated for clinical reasons:

- 12-Lead ECG (ST elevation/depression, T-wave inversion, Q-waves from old infarct. 10–20% of acute MIs have an initially normal ECG).
- Stress testing (in selected patients, preferably based on guidelines and appropriate use criteria)
- Modality: ECG, echocardiogram, nuclear
- Stressor: Exercise (treadmill or bicycle) or pharmacologic (dobutamine, dipyridamole, adenosine)
- Fasting glucose, lipid profile
- hs-CRP (optional; independent marker of prognosis for those with stable CHD or ACS. USPSTF Grade Indeterminate)
- Lipoprotein(a) (optional; USPSTF Grade Indeterminate)

Follow-Up & Special Considerations

- Follow-up dependent on patient presentation, risk factor profile, and the severity of abnormality on diagnostic tests.
- Options include follow-up exams, additional diagnostic testing, or therapeutic interventions.

Imaging

- Chest x-ray: Rule out other causes of chest pain (e.g., pneumonia).
- Echocardiography: Especially useful for suspected valvular disease, assessment of LV function, and other structural heart abnormalities
- Angiography (cath): Gold standard for the anatomic diagnosis of CAD; diagnostic and therapeutic
- Nuclear myocardial perfusion imaging (MPI): Quantifies extent and severity of myocardial ischemia and/or scar
- Cardiac CT: Detection of coronary artery calcification and/or noninvasive coronary angiography. For asymptomatic patients, coronary artery calcium scoring may be useful only in those with intermediate CHD risk (10–20% 10-year risk of coronary event). It should not be used to screen the general population or in those with low or high CHD risk (1).
- Cardiac MRI: Predominately used for research purposes

Pathological Findings

- Fibrotic, lipid-laden plaques protruding into lumen of coronary arteries.
- When fibrous cap weakens by enzymatic digestion, a "vulnerable" plaque may rupture, leading to thrombus and possibly ACS.

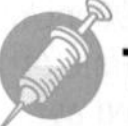

TREATMENT

MEDICATION

Primary Prevention:

- Aspirin (ASA):
  - The use of aspirin for primary prevention is controversial because benefits of reduction in risk of stroke and MI must be balanced against risk of hemorrhage.
  - USPSTF recommends aspirin for primary prevention in women 55–79 years (when the potential benefit of a reduction in ischemic stroke outweighs the risk of an increase in GI bleed) and men 45–79 (when the potential benefit of a reduction in the rate of MI outweighs the risk of an increase in GI bleed) (2,3)[A].
  - AHA recommendations are gender based:
    - Men: Consideration of 75–160 mg/d ASA for patients with a 10-year risk of CHD ≥10% (4).
    - Women: If high risk, use 75–325 mg/d ASA unless contraindicated, in which case consider clopidogrel (5)[A]. If "other at-risk" or healthy and ≥65 years, consider 81 mg/d (or 100 mg every other day) if BP is controlled and benefit of stroke and MI prevention outweighs GI bleed risk and hemorrhagic stroke risk. And if <65 years, use when stroke prevention outweighs GI bleed risk (5)[B]. Stroke risk calculator available at: http://www.westernstroke.org/personalstrokerisk1.xls
  - ADA recommends ASA 75–162 mg/d for primary prevention in diabetics at increased risk including those >40 years old or who have additional risk factors such as FHx, HTN, smoking, dyslipidemia, albuminuria (6).
- Statins:
  - A 2011 Cochrane Review showed primary prevention with statins reduced all-cause mortality with the caveat of selective reporting of outcomes and other study limitations. They conclude there is only limited evidence that statins are cost effective and improve quality of life and caution providers when prescribing for primary prevention, especially for low-risk individuals (7).

- WHO Cooperative Trial (clofibrate), Lipid Research Clinics Coronary Primary Prevention Trial (cholestyramine), and the Helsinki Heart Study (gemfibrozil) did not demonstrate a reduction in coronary mortality. The ASCOT-LLA trial (atorvastatin) did not show statistically significant reductions in cardiovascular mortality.

Secondary Prevention:

- Aspirin: 75–162 mg/d (or Clopidogrel 75 mg/d if contraindicated):
  - Aspirin is recommended for secondary prevention of CVD after acute MI, unstable angina, stable angina, occlusive stroke, TIA, and coronary artery bypass surgery to reduce risk of MI, stroke, and vascular death (8)[A].
- Statins:
  - Atorvastatin (10–80 mg/d PO), initial dose 10–20 mg/d; fluvastatin (20–80 mg/d), initial dose 20–40 mg/dL; lovastatin (10–80 mg/d), initial dose 10–20 mg/dL; pravastatin (maintenance 10–80 mg/d), initial dose 40 mg/dL; simvastatin (20–40 mg/d), maintenance 5–80 mg/dL; rosuvastatin (5–40 mg/d), initial dose 10–20 mg/dL
  - Statins reduce mortality and MI in adults with CHD (8)[A]. Lipid-lowering therapy (primarily with statins) is recommended for most patients with diabetes. Statins also have anti-inflammatory and immunomodulatory effects, and effects on vascular tone and thrombogenicity.
  - Average reduction % in LDL is dose-dependent: Atorvastatin 35–60%, fluvastatin 22–35%, lovastatin 21–42%; pravastatin 22–37%, rosuvastatin 45–63%, simvastatin 26–47%.
- Beta-blockers:
  - Starting dose: Atenolol 25 mg/d or Metoprolol 25 mg b.i.d.
  - Shown to decrease mortality and should be used in all post-MI and systolic heart failure patients unless contraindicated (9)[A]
- ACE inhibitors/angiotensin receptor blockers (ARBs):
  - Starting dose: Captopril 6.25 mg/d, Enalapril 2.5 mg/d, Lisinopril 2.5 mg/d
  - Start in patients with EF ≤40%, HTN, DM, or CKD unless contraindicated (9)[A]. Shown to decrease mortality in post-MI patients.
- Fish oil and other omega-3 acid ethyl esters:
  - Consume at least 1–2 servings/wk of oily fish or take a 1 g daily supplement containing both EPA and DHA.

ADDITIONAL TREATMENT

General Measures

Smoking cessation; Control BP (<140/90; <130/80 if DM or renal disease); consume a healthy diet (see "Diet" section); optimal lipid management including LDL-C goal <100 mg/dL (optionally <70 mg/dL) for known CHD or CHD risk equivalents. Raise HDL-C via exercise or medication. Physical activity (at least 30 minutes of moderate-intensity activity at least 5 days/wk). Weight management via diet and exercise. Management of diabetes (HbA1c <7%) in newly diagnosed diabetics possibly helpful; HgbA1c <7.5% target in patients long-standing diabetes or those with comorbidity likely harmful). Annual influenza vaccine.

ONGOING CARE

FOLLOW-UP RECOMMENDATIONS

Patient Monitoring

- Monitor fasting lipid panel every 5 years for men 35 years and older and women 45 and older; younger if risk factors for CAD or dyslipidemia
- Preventive programs (weight loss, smoking cessation, diabetes nutritional education)
- For patients with type 2 diabetes taking statins, routine monitoring of liver function test or muscle enzymes is not recommended.

DIET

- Low fat: 20–30 g/d, and eliminate or reduce trans fats
- Weight loss diet if obesity a problem
- Increase soluble fiber and plant stanols.
- Reduce consumption of red meat; increase fish, olive oil, and nuts.
- Individuals who consume a healthy diet have significantly lower risks of CVD, including both CHD and stroke:
  - High intake of fruits and vegetables, high fiber intake, including cereals, low glycemic index, and low glycemic load
  - Monounsaturated fats rather than trans fatty acids or saturated fats; limited intake of red or processed meats
  - Omega-3 fatty acids (from fish, fish oil supplements, or plant sources)

PATIENT EDUCATION

For patient education literature, quizzes, risk calculators, and more, visit the AHA Patient Portal: www.hearthub.org

PROGNOSIS

- In (observational) population studies, lower cholesterol correlates with lower CHD and lower total mortality: for every 10% reduction in serum cholesterol, CHD was reduced by 15%; and total mortality risk, by 11%.
- The incidence of a MI is increased 6-fold in women and 3-fold in men who smoke at least 20 cigarettes per day.
- Current smoking was associated with a 50% increase in the progression of atherosclerosis versus nonsmokers.

COMPLICATIONS

Unstable angina/STEMI, ventricular fibrillation CHF, sudden cardiac death

REFERENCES

1. Greenland P, Bonow RO, Brundage BH, et al. ACCF/AHA 2007 clinical expert consensus document on coronary artery calcium scoring. *J Am Coll Cardiol*. 2007;49:378–402
2. Aspirin for the prevention of cardiovascular disease: U.S. Preventive Services Tasks Force recommendation statement. *Ann Intern Med*. 2009;150(6):396–404.
3. Wolff T, Miller T, Ko S. Aspirin for the primary prevention of cardiovascular events: An update of the evidence for the U.S. Preventive Services Task Force. *Ann Intern Med*. 2009;150(6):405–10.
4. AHA Guidelines for Primary Prevention of Cardiovascular Disease and Stroke: 2002 Update: Consensus Panel Guide to Comprehensive Risk Reduction for Adult Patients Without Coronary of Other Atherosclerotic Vascular Diseases. American Heart Association Science Advisory and Coordinated Committee. *Circulation*. 2002;106(3): 388–91.
5. Evidence-based guidelines for cardiovascular disease prevention in women: 2007 update. *Circulation*. 2007;115(11):1481–501.
6. Buse JB, Ginsberg HN, Bakris GL, et al. Primary prevention of cardiovascular diseases in people with diabetes mellitus: A scientific statement from the American Heart Association and the American Diabetes Association. *Diabetes Care*. 2007;30: 162–72.
7. Taylor F, Ward K, Moore TH, et al. Statins for the primary prevention of cardiovascular disease. *Cochrane Database Syst Rev*. 2011(1):CD004816.
8. Becker RC, Meade TW, Berger PB, et al. The primary and secondary prevention of coronary artery disease: American College of Chest Physicians Evidence-Based Clinical Practice Guidelines (8th Edition). *Chest*. 2008;133:776S.
9. AHA; ACC; National Heart, Lung, and Blood Institute, et al. AHA/ACC guidelines for secondary prevention for patients with coronary and other atherosclerotic vascular disease: 2006 update endorsed by the National Heart, Lung, and Blood Institute. *J Am Coll Cardiol*. 2006;47:2130–9.

ADDITIONAL READING

- Aspirin for the prevention of cardiovascular disease. U.S. Preventive Services Task Force recommendation statement. *Ann Intern Med*. 2009;150(6):396–404.
- Framingham risk estimates: http://www.nhlbi.nih.gov/guidelines/cholesterol/index.htm
- Reynolds risk score: http://www.reynoldsriskscore.org.

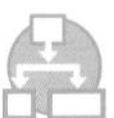

See Also (Topic, Algorithm, Electronic Media Element)

- Angina; Atherosclerosis; Myocardial Infarction; ST-Segment Elevation (STEMI)
- Algorithm: Chest_Pain/Acute Coronary Syndrome

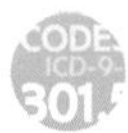

CODES

ICD9

414.00 Coronary atherosclerosis of unspecified type of vessel, native or graft

CLINICAL PEARLS

- Net benefit of aspirin increases with increasing cardiovascular risk.
- Aspirin significantly reduced the relative risk of subsequent vascular events (nonfatal MI, nonfatal stroke, and vascular death) by ~22%.
- The CHD death rate increases at higher plasma concentrations of total and LDL-cholesterol. Statins for patients with known CAD reduce morbidity and mortality.

ARTERITIS, TEMPORAL

Prachaya Nitichaikulvatana, MD

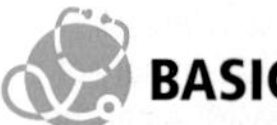

BASICS

DESCRIPTION

- Also known as giant cell arteritis (GCA)
- Systemic immune-mediated vasculitis affects large and middle-sized blood vessels with predisposition to the involvement of cranial branches derived from the carotid artery.

EPIDEMIOLOGY

- Age of onset >50 years
- Incidence increases in individuals 70 years of age and older
- Mean age at diagnosis is ~72 years.
- Female > Male (2–6:1)

Incidence

- More common in Northern Europe, especially Scandinavia (20 per 100,000 per year) vs. Southern Europe (10 per 100,000 per year).
- In the US, incidence in a largely white Minnesota cohort was 19 per 100,000 per year.
- Incidence is lower in Hispanic, Asian, and African American populations (1).

RISK FACTORS

- Increasing age
- Polymyalgia rheumatica
- Atherosclerosis and smoking in women but not men

Genetics

- Some family clusters have been documented.
- HLA-DR4 and HLA-DRB1 are associated with temporal arteritis.
- Polymorphism of the gene for intercellular adhesion molecule-1 (ICAM-1)

ETIOLOGY

Unclear, involves cell-mediated immune response and IL-6 production

COMMONLY ASSOCIATED CONDITIONS

Polymyalgia rheumatica

DIAGNOSIS

HISTORY

Usually gradual in onset, but may be abrupt:

- New or changed headache (usually unilateral temporal, but may be generalized)
- Scalp and facial tenderness
- Jaw and tongue claudication with chewing (most specific symptom for temporal arteritis)
- Visual changes:
  - Amaurosis fugax (transient monocular loss of vision)
  - Diplopia
  - Scotoma
  - Blindness
- Upper respiratory tract symptoms such as nonproductive cough (10% of patients), sore throat, hoarseness
- Arm claudication
- Constitutional symptoms :
  - Fever
  - Weight loss
  - Fatigue
  - Malaise
- Polymyalgia rheumatica (stiffness and aching in shoulder and hip girdles). Present in 50% in GCA patients. GCA is found in about 15% of patients with polymyalgia rheumatica.
- Peripheral joint pain and distal extremity swelling with edema

PHYSICAL EXAM

- Thickened, tender, with reduced or absent pulsation in temporal artery
- Scalp tenderness
- Cranial nerve palsies
- Visual field defect
- Fundoscopic examination shows pale and edema of the optic disk, scattered cotton-wool patches, and small hemorrhages
- Proximal muscle tenderness but no weakness
- Bruits or diminished pulses in carotid, brachial, radial, femoral, and pedal pulses
- Aortic regurgitation (signal the development of an ascending aortic aneurysm)
- Peripheral synovitis and pitting edema in distal extremities

DIAGNOSTIC TESTS & INTERPRETATION

Lab

- ESR/C-reactive protein (CRP); usually very elevated (ESR >50). <10% have a normal ESR. If both ESR and CRP are normal, consider alternative diagnoses.
- Normocytic, normochromic anemia; usually mild
- Elevated acute-phase reactants (platelets, liver function tests [LFTs], albumin)

Follow-Up & Special Considerations

Development of aortic aneurysms (late and potentially serious complication of GCA) that can lead to aortic dissection

Imaging

- Ultrasonography of the temporal artery with concentric hypoechogenic mural thickening, halo sign, has sensitivity of 68% and a specificity of 91% for the unilateral halo sign, as well as 43% and 100%, respectively, for the bilateral halo sign. It is quite operator-dependent. It does not replace biopsy for definitive diagnosis (2).
- MRI/magnetic resonance angiography (MRA) in patients with arm claudication or other evidence of aortic branch involvement. It also should be considered, especially in patients with an aortic insufficiency murmur to evaluate for presence of aortic aneurysm.
- 18 fluorodeoxyglucose (FDG)-positron emission topography (PET) may be useful to detect large vessel arteritis in the setting of GCA, which can involve the larger thoracic, abdominal, and peripheral arteries (3).
- Chest x-ray to screen ascending aortic aneurysm

Diagnostic Procedures/Surgery

Temporal artery biopsy: The gold standard for the diagnosis of temporal arteritis:

- Treatment prior to biopsy is unlikely to affect the biopsy results. Histopathologic findings can persist for at least 2–6 weeks following steroid initiation.
- A segment 3–5 cm long is needed, as there are often skip lesions.
- Serial sections should be done.
- Routine biopsy of both temporal arteries is not necessary; however, if the first biopsy is negative and clinical suspicion remains high, a contralateral biopsy could be considered.

Pathological Findings

- Granulomatous inflammation and inflammatory cells (macrophages, lymphocytes, fibroblasts, multinucleated giant cell) surrounding the internal elastic lamina in medium and large vessel with resultant disruption of the internal elastic lamina
- Lesions may be isolated (e.g., skip lesions).

DIFFERENTIAL DIAGNOSIS

- Migraine headache, cluster headache, tension headache, intracranial mass or bleed in patients with headache
- CNS vasculitis
- Cerebrovascular accident (CVA), embolic disease
- Temporomandibular joint syndrome
- Retinal disease
- Leukemia, multiple myeloma, and other neoplasms should be ruled out in patient with fever, weight loss, and elevated ESR.

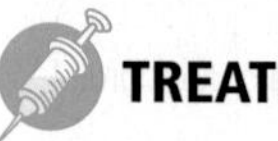

TREATMENT

MEDICATION

First Line

Prednisone:

- Due to the risk of irreversible vision loss, treatment with high-dose steroids should be started on strong clinical suspicion of temporal arteritis, prior to the temporal biopsy being done.
- The initial dose of prednisone is 60 mg/d (or 1 mg/kg/d). Steroids should not be in the form of alternate day therapy, as this is more likely to lead to a relapse of vasculitis.
- Pulsed-dose IV methylprednisolone (1 g/d for 3 days) may be of benefit to patients who present with recent onset of visual symptoms (4)[C]. This is followed by prednisone 60 mg/d as above.

- The initial dose of steroids is continued for 2–4 weeks or until symptoms have resolved and a normal ESR is achieved; then the dose can be tapered.
- Tapering is done with a gentle reduction of 10% of the total daily dose every 2 weeks until a dose of 10 mg/d is reached. After that, the prednisone is very gradually weaned by 1 mg every month. Dose reduction should be considered only in the absence of clinical symptoms, signs, and laboratory abnormalities suggestive of active disease. Many patients may require a slower taper.
- Consider low-dose aspirin for all patients with giant cell arteritis (5)[B].
- Patients on corticosteroids should be on bone protection therapy unless they have contraindications.

Second Line

Methotrexate (10–15 mg/wk) has a modest effect in temporal arteritis and could be considered in patients who have not responded to glucocorticoids or who have significant side effects from steroids (6)[B].

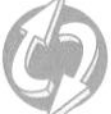

ONGOING CARE

FOLLOW-UP RECOMMENDATIONS

- Follow up in clinic at least monthly initially. When stable and steroids are being tapered, every 2–3 months.
- Disease relapse should be suspected in patients with new headaches, visual changes, fever, myalgias. A rise in ESR/CRP is usually seen with relapse. An increase in steroids by 10 mg/d is usually significant to control a relapse.

Patient Monitoring

- Check ESR/CRP with each visit to monitor disease activity.
- Consider yearly chest x-ray (CXR) (to evaluate for aortic aneurysm) and biannual dual energy x-ray absorptiometry (DEXA) scans.

DIET

Calcium and vitamin D supplementation

PATIENT EDUCATION

- Consequences of discontinuing steroids abruptly (adrenal insufficiency, disease relapse)
- Risks of long-term steroid use (infection, hyperglycemia, weight gain, impaired wound healing, osteoporosis, hypertension)
- Importance of reporting new headaches and vision changes to provider immediately

PROGNOSIS

- Prior vision loss is unlikely to be recovered, but treatment resolves the other symptoms and prevents future vision loss and stroke.
- Average disease duration is 1–2 years, but may be up to 5 years.

COMPLICATIONS

- Sequelae of long-term steroid use
- Blindness
- Stroke
- Aortic aneurysm/dissection

REFERENCES

1. Gonzalez-Gay MA, Vazquez-Rodriguez TR, Lopez-Diaz MJ, et al. Epidemiology of giant cell arteritis and polymyalgia rheumatica. *Arthritis Rheum*. 2009;61:1454–61
2. Arida A, Kyprianou M, Kanakis M, et al. The diagnostic value of ultrasonography-derived edema of the temporal artery wall in giant cell arteritis: A second meta-analysis. *BMC Musculoskelet Disord*. 2010;11:44.
3. Blockmans D, de Ceuninck L, Vanderschueren S et al. Repetitive 18F-fluorodeoxyglucose positron emission tomography in giant cell arteritis: A prospective study of 35 patients. *Arthritis Rheum* 2006;55:131–7.
4. Hayreh SS, Zimmerman B, Kardon RH, et al. Visual improvement with corticosteroid therapy in giant cell arteritis. Report of a large study and review of literature. *Acta Ophthalmol Scand*. 2002;80: 355–67.
5. Lee MS, Smith SD, Galor A, et al. Antiplatelet and anticoagulant therapy in patients with giant cell arteritis. *Arthritis Rheum*. 2006;54:3306–9.
6. Mahr AD, Jover JA, Spiera RF, et al. Adjunctive methotrexate for treatment of giant cell arteritis: An individual patient data meta-analysis. *Arthritis Rheum*. 2007;56:2789–97.

ADDITIONAL READING

- Hunder GG, Bloch DA, Michel BA, et al. The American College of Rheumatology 1990 criteria for the classification of giant cell arteritis. *Arthritis Rheum*. 1990;33:1122–8.
- Mukhtyar C, Guillevin L, Cid MC, et al. EULAR recommendations for the management of large vessel vasculitis. *Ann Rheum Dis*. 2009;68:318–23.

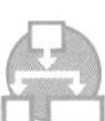

See Also (Topic, Algorithm, Electronic Media Element)

Depression; Fibromyalgia; Headache, Cluster; Headache, Tension; Polymyalgia Rheumatica; Polymyositis/Dermatomyositis

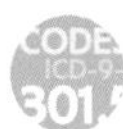

CODES

ICD9

446.5 Giant cell arteritis

CLINICAL PEARLS

- Due to the risk of irreversible vision loss, treatment with high-dose steroids (prednisone 60 mg/d) should be started immediately in patients suspected of temporal arteritis.
- Temporal artery biopsy is the gold standard for diagnosis. Temporal artery biopsy is not likely to be affected by a few weeks of treatment.
- Treatment consists of a very slow steroid taper. Bone protection therapy and low-dose aspirin should be considered.
- Normal ESR level = value of age/2 for men and (age + 10)/2 for women

ARTHRITIS, INFECTIOUS, BACTERIAL

Christopher J. Scola, MD
Raul Davaro, MD

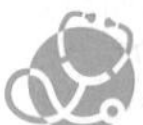

BASICS

DESCRIPTION

- Invasion of joints by pyogenic microorganisms. One of the curable causes of arthritis. May be part of systemic infection/disease.
- System(s) affected: Musculoskeletal
- Synonym(s): Suppurative arthritis; septic arthritis; pyarthrosis; pyogenic arthritis; bacterial arthritis

EPIDEMIOLOGY

- Predominant age:
  - Neisserial: Especially 15–40 years of age; can occur at any age
  - Nonneisserial (approximate):
    - Years <2: 60% *Staphylococcus*, 20% *Streptococcus*, 10% gram-negative rods, <5% miscellaneous
    - Years 2–14: 60% *Staphylococcus*, 30% *Streptococcus*, 5% *Haemophilus*, 5% other gram-negative rods, 5% miscellaneous
    - Adult: 60% *Staphylococcus*, 25% *Streptococcus*, <1% *Haemophilus*, and 15% other gram-negative rods
- Predominant gender:
  - Neisserial: Female > Male (4:1)
  - Nonneisserial: Male > Female (2:1)

Prevalence

- Neisserial:
  - Responsible for 50% of all types of infectious arthritis
  - 0.6% of women with gonorrhea
  - 0.1% of men with gonorrhea
  - Arthritis occurs in 7% of individuals with *Neisseria meningitidis*.
- Nonneisserial: Half as frequent as neisserial
- The prevalence of nongonococcal septic arthritis in ED patients with a single acutely painful joint is ~27% (1).

RISK FACTORS

- Sexual exposure: Neisserial
- Inflammatory arthritis (e.g., rheumatoid arthritis)
- Concurrent extra-articular infection
- Prior arthritis in affected joint
- Trauma
- Joint puncture or surgery
- Prosthetic joint (2)[A]
- Prior corticosteroid or immunosuppressive therapy
- Serious chronic systemic illness (e.g., diabetes, liver disease, malignancy, immunodeficiency)
- Defective phagocytic mechanisms (e.g., chronic granulomatous disease)
- Injection drug use
- Sickle cell anemia
- Complement deficiency
- Systemic infection; infection elsewhere
- Immunodeficiency; immunosuppression
- Dental procedures; poor dental/gingival hygiene
- Advanced age >80 years

GENERAL PREVENTION

- Prompt treatment of skin and soft tissue infections
- Condoms and limiting number of sexual partners for sexually transmitted disease protection

ETIOLOGY

- Hematogenous invasion (80–90%)
- Contiguous spread (10–15%)
- Direct penetration of microorganisms secondary to trauma or joint infection (5%)

COMMONLY ASSOCIATED CONDITIONS

- Serious chronic illness (e.g., rheumatoid arthritis, diabetes, liver disease, malignancy, primary immunodeficiency, complement deficiencies)
- Immunosuppressive therapy (disease-modifying antirheumatic drugs [DMARDs] agents, glucocorticoids, chemotherapy)
- Systemic infection associated with bacteremia, especially endocarditis

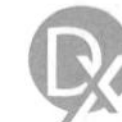

DIAGNOSIS

HISTORY

- Nongonococcal:
  - Predominantly monoarticular (90%)
  - Recent joint surgery or cellulitis overlying a prosthetic hip or knee increase risk (1)[A]
- Fever: In 90% during course of infection
- Malaise
- Back pain: Subacute bacterial endocarditis
- Neisserial:
  - Bacteremic phase: Migratory polyarthritis, tenosynovitis, high fever, chills, pustules
  - Localized phase: Usually monoarticular with low-grade fever

PHYSICAL EXAM

- Limited or loss of joint use/motion
- Joint effusion, tenderness
- Joint warmth and redness: Present intenosynovitis; pustular skin lesions common for neisserial infection
- Hip and shoulder involvement may reveal severe pain on range of motion with less obvious joint swelling on exam.

DIAGNOSTIC TESTS & INTERPRETATION

Lab

Initial lab tests

- Synovial fluid (3)[A]:
  - Arthrocentesis prior to starting antibiotics increases diagnostic yield.
  - Synovial fluid is usually cloudy with >50,000 white blood cells (WBC)/HPF.
    - Caveat: To be valid, cell count must be performed within 1 hour of obtaining specimen.
    - WBC count alone is insufficient to rule in or rule out septic arthritis (4)[A].
  - Polymorphonuclear leukocytes usually predominate in synovial fluid, >90%.
  - Crystals (e.g., urate or calcium pyrophosphate) do not exclude infectious arthritis.
  - Joint fluid: For Gram stain (positive in 50%); culture (positive in 50–70%); usually negative in neisserial
- Cervical culture or urethral culture highest diagnostic yield for disseminated gonococcal infection in young adults
- There is insufficient evidence to support the routine use of serum procalcitonin in the differentiation of septic and non-septic arthritis (5)[A].

Pediatric Considerations

- There is no single lab test that can distinguish septic arthritis from transient synovitis (6)[A].
- The combination of fever, non–weight-bearing, C-reactive protein >20 or ESR >40, and a WBC >12 is suspicious of septic arthritis (6)[B].

Follow-Up & Special Considerations

- Bedside culture is recommended to enhance isolation of fastidious organisms.
- All cultures should be maintained and observed for 3 days to 2 weeks (3,7)[A].
- Neisserial infection generally requires use of special media (e.g., chocolate or Thayer Martin).
- Drugs that may alter lab results: Antibiotics

Imaging

Initial approach

- X-ray (7)[A]:
  - Soft tissue swelling
  - Juxta-articular osteoporosis
  - Radiolucent area (gas) in a joint space from gas-forming organisms (Caveat: May be normal as a "vacuum phenomenon")
  - Effacement of obturator fat pad (with hip involvement)
  - X-ray changes usually a late phenomenon
  - Rarefaction of subchondral bone may occur.
  - Joint-space loss (secondary to cartilage destruction) may occur in 4–10 days.
  - Erosions
  - Joint destruction with ankylosis may occur.
- Other imaging techniques:
  - Technetium joint scans: Reveal distribution of inflammation; sensitive, not specific
  - Gallium WBC scan, indium scans: Reveal inflammation as well as infection
  - CT: To identify sequestration
  - MRI: Effusion, perhaps early cartilage damage, osteomyelitis

Diagnostic Procedures/Surgery

Arthrocentesis with Gram stain and culture: Positive in 50–70% (8)[A]:

- Shoulder or hip joints may require image-guided aspiration.
- Must always be done when possibility of infectious arthritis is considered
- Arthrocentesis should be performed prior to initiation of antibiotics whenever possible. Arthrocentesis approach must avoid contaminated tissue (e.g., overlying cellulitis) when possible.

Pathological Findings

Synovial biopsy will reveal polymorphonuclear leukocytes and possibly the causative organism, if synovial fluid and blood cultures are negative.

DIFFERENTIAL DIAGNOSIS
- Gout
- Pseudogout (calcium pyrophosphate deposition disease)
- Spondyloarthropathy (Reiter syndrome, psoriatic arthritis, ankylosing spondylitis, arthritis of inflammatory bowel disease)
- Juvenile rheumatoid arthritis
- Foreign-body synovitis
- Rheumatoid arthritis
- Rheumatic fever
- Cellulitis
- Palindromic rheumatism
- Neuropathic arthropathy
- Lyme arthritis
- Granulomatous arthritis

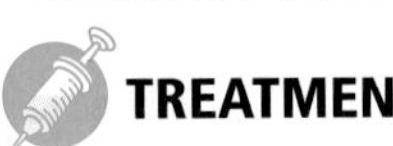

TREATMENT

MEDICATION
First Line
- Neisserial (7)[A]:
  - Ceftriaxone 1 g IM or IV every day for 14 days (and at least 7 days after symptoms resolve)
  - Fluoroquinolone for 14 days; caveat resistance
  - Concomitant treatment for *Chlamydia*
- Nonneisserial (7)[A]:
  - Gram-positive cocci in clusters: Empiric therapy: Vancomycin or linezolid IV. If methicillin-sensitive *Staphylococcus aureus* (MSSA), nafcillin or cefazolin IV
  - Gram-positive cocci in chains: Ceftriaxone
  - Gram-negative bacilli: Neonates: Cefotaxime, and gentamicin; ages 6 months to 4 years: 3rd-generation cephalosporin; adult: 3rd-generation cephalosporin plus gentamicin. No bacteria seen on smear: Vancomycin or linezolid plus 3rd-generation cephalosporin.
- Precautions:
  - Observe for allergic reactions
- Significant possible interactions:
  - Broad-spectrum antibiotics: May reduce effectiveness of oral contraceptives; barrier method recommended

Second Line
Fluoroquinolones (e.g., ciprofloxacin)

ADDITIONAL TREATMENT
General Measures
- Hospitalization for parenteral therapy
- Outpatient treatment rarely possible for extremely compliant patient with known organism.
- Repeat (once) arthrocentesis if fluid reaccumulates. Next step is arthroscopic debridement and irrigation.
- Avoid anti-inflammatory therapy to allow assessment of therapeutic response to antibiotic.
- If joint prosthesis is present in an infection, orthopedic surgery, to include possible removal of the prosthesis, must be considered.
- Continue treatment for 1–2 weeks after total resolution of all signs of inflammation, for a total of 4–6 weeks for most organisms, except neisserial (2–3 weeks).
- Intra-articular antibiotics are not required.

Issues for Referral
Infectious disease and orthopedic consults strongly advised to supplement rheumatologist.

SURGERY/OTHER PROCEDURES
- Arthroscopy indicated if fluid accumulated is loculated and/or not amenable to needle drainage.
- Surgical drainage typically is required for shoulder or hip involvement.

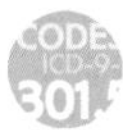

ONGOING CARE

FOLLOW-UP RECOMMENDATIONS
Patient Monitoring
- Repeat arthrocentesis (once) if fluid reaccumulates to verify sterilization of joint and reversion of inflammatory signs to normal.
- If no improvement within 24 hours, re-evaluate and consider arthroscopy.
- CBC, liver and kidney function, and urinalysis twice a week while on antibiotics (with creatinine when gentamicin used)
- Aminoglycoside levels
- Follow-up 1 week and 1 month after stopping antibiotics to detect any relapse

PROGNOSIS
- Early treatment should allow cure.
- Delayed recognition/treatment complicated by morbidity and mortality

COMPLICATIONS
- Death (9–33% in elderly)
- Limited joint range of motion
- Secondary osteoarthritis
- Flail or fused or dislocated joint
- Septic necrosis
- Sinus formation
- Ankylosis
- Osteomyelitis
- Postinfectious synovitis
- Shortening of limb (in children)

REFERENCES

1. Carpenter CR, Schuur JD, Everett WW, et al. Evidence-based diagnostics: Adult septic arthritis. *Acad Emerg Med*. 2011;18:781–96
2. Zimmerli W, Trampuz A, Ochsner PE. Prostheticjoint infections. *N Engl J Med*. 2004;351:1645–54.
3. Mathews CJ, Weston VC, Jones A, et al. Bacterial septic arthritis in adults. *Lancet*. 2010;375(9717): 846–55.
4. O'Malley A, Svinos H. Towards evidence based emergency medicine: Best BETs from the Manchester Royal Infirmary. BET 3: Is the white cell count of the joint aspirate sufficiently sensitive/specific to rule in/out septic arthritis? *Emerg Med J*. 2009;26:435–7.
5. Wang CH, Yen ZS. Best Evidence Topic report. BET 3. Is there a role for serum procalcitonin in the differentiation between septic and non-septic arthritis. *Emerg Med J*. 2010;27:144–5.
6. Taekema HC, Landham PR, Maconochie I. Towards evidence based medicine for paediatricians. Distinguishing between transient synovitis and septic arthritis in the limping child: How useful are clinical prediction tools? *Arch Dis Child*. 2009;94: 167–8.
7. Margaretten ME, Kohlwes J, Moore D, et al. Does this adult patient have septic arthritis? *JAMA*. 2007;297:1478–88.
8. Khachatourians AG, Patzakis MJ, Roidis N, et al. Laboratory monitoring in pediatric acute osteomyelitis and septic arthritis. *Clin Orthop Relat Res*. 2003;186–94.

ADDITIONAL READING

- Clerc O, Prod'hom G, Greub G, et al. Adult native septic arthritis: A review of 10 years of experience and lessons for empirical antibiotic therapy. *J Antimicrob Chemother*. 2011;66:1168–73.
- García-De La Torre I, Nava-Zavala A. Gonococcal and nongonococcal arthritis. *Rheum. Dis. Clin. North Am*. 2009;35:63–73
- Mathews CJ, Coakley G. Septic arthritis: Current diagnostic and therapeutic algorithm. *Curr Opin Rheumatol*. 2008;20:457–62.
- Ross JJ, Hu LT. Bacterial and Lyme arthritis. *Curr Infect Dis Rep* 2004;5:380–7.

CODES

ICD9
- 041.10 Staphylococcus infection in conditions classified elsewhere and of unspecified site, staphylococcus, unspecified
- 711.00 Pyogenic arthritis, site unspecified
- 711.40 Arthropathy, site unspecified, associated with other bacterial diseases

CLINICAL PEARLS
- Neisseria is the most common cause of septic arthritis in young adults.
- Acute onset of joint pain with redness and warmth is typical of nonneisserial infection.
- Crystalline process can mimic septic arthritis.
- Aspiration of joint prior to the initiation of antibiotics will optimize diagnostic yield.
- Synovial fluid appears inflammatory and is typically purulent.

ARTHRITIS, JUVENILE IDIOPATHIC

Marri K. Brackman, DO
Bodie Correll, MD

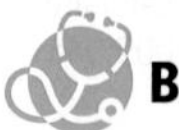

BASICS

DESCRIPTION

- Most common chronic rheumatic illness in children and a significant cause of short- and long-term disability
- General characteristics:
  - Age of onset <16 years
  - Signs of arthritis: Joint swelling, limitation of motion, pain, heat, or tenderness
  - >6 weeks of symptoms
- 7 subtypes exist, according to the International League of Associations for Rheumatology, determined by clinical characteristics seen in first 6 months of illness (1):
  - Systemic (Still's): 10–20%; usually characterized by febrile onset and evanescent rash with multiple physical and laboratory abnormalities
  - Polyarticular rheumatoid factor (RF) (+): 5–10%; multiple (≥5) joint involvement; large and small joints affected. RF positive 2x on tests at least 3 months apart.
  - Polyarticular RhF (–): 30%; ≥5 joint involvement, large and small joints affected; RF negative
  - Oligoarticular: 40–50%; involvement of ≤4 joints, usually larger joints, especially of lower extremities; risk for chronic uveitis in young girls and axial skeletal involvement in older boys
  - Psoriatic arthritis: 2–15%; arthritis with psoriasis or arthritis with at least 2 of following: dactylitis, nail pitting or onycholysis, psoriasis in first-degree relative
  - Enthesitis arthritis: 1–7%; includes ankylosing spondylitis and inflammatory bowel disease–related arthritis. Peripheral and axial involvement.
  - Undifferentiated arthritis: Arthritis that does not fulfill above categories or fills 2 or more categories
- System(s) affected: Hematologic/Lymphatic/Immunologic; Musculoskeletal
- Synonym(s): Juvenile chronic arthritis; Juvenile arthritis; Juvenile rheumatoid arthritis (JRA); Still disease

EPIDEMIOLOGY

- General: Age of onset most predominantly ages 1–3 years (1)
- Systemic: Girls = Boys; onset is throughout childhood (1)
- Polyarticular RF (+): Girls:Boys 2.8:1; age of onset 1–4 years and again 9–14 years (1)
- Polyarticular (–): Girls:Boys 2.8:1; age of onset 1–4 years and again 9–14 years
- Oligoarticular: Girls:Boys 3;1; age of onset 1–4 years and again 9–14 years
- Psoriatic: Age of onset 1–3 years (1)
- Enthesitis: Male > Female; age of onset 10–12 years (1)

Incidence

1–22 per 100,000 children <16 years per year

Prevalence

8–150 per 100,000 children <16 years

RISK FACTORS

Genetics

- Certain human leukocyte antigen (HLA) class I and II alleles
- HLA-A2 in early-onset oligoarthritis in girls
- HLA-DRB1*11 confers increased risk of systemic and oligo-JIA.
- HLA-B27 risk of enthesitis-related arthritis
- HLA-DR4 associated with RF (+) polyarticular disease

GENERAL PREVENTION

No known preventive measures

ETIOLOGY

Multifactorial, including:

- Immunodysregulation
- Genetic predisposition
- Environmental triggers, possibly infectious:
  - Rubella or parvovirus B19 (2)
  - Heat shock proteins (2)
- Immunoglobulin or complement deficiency

COMMONLY ASSOCIATED CONDITIONS

Other autoimmune disorders, chronic anterior uveitis (iridocyclitis), nutritional impairment, growth disturbances (2)

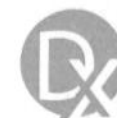

DIAGNOSIS

Clinical diagnostic criteria: Age of onset <16 years and >6 weeks duration of objective arthritis in ≥1 joints, defined as swelling or limitation of motion of a joint accompanied by heat, pain, or tenderness

HISTORY

- Arthralgias, fever, fatigue, malaise, myalgias, weight loss, morning stiffness, rash, limp in patients with lower extremity involvement
- Arthritis for at least 6 weeks
- Behavioral and compliance problems frequent in toddlers and teenagers

PHYSICAL EXAM

- Arthritis: Swelling, effusion, limitation of motion, tenderness, pain on motion, warmth
- Rash, rheumatoid nodules, lymphadenopathy, hepato- or splenomegaly, enthesitis, dactylitis

DIAGNOSTIC TESTS & INTERPRETATION

Lab

Initial lab tests

- CBC:
  - Leukocyte count normal or markedly elevated (systemic), lymphopenia, reactive thrombocytosis, anemia
- Joint-fluid aspiration and analysis helpful in excluding infection
- Inflammatory markers: ESR and C-reactive protein may be elevated
- Antinuclear antibodies (ANA) positive (>1:80): 40% (polyarticular or oligoarticular): Increased risk of uveitis
- RF positive: 2–10% (usually polyarticular): Poor prognosis
- HLA-B27 positive: Enthesitis-related arthritis

Follow-Up & Special Considerations

- In polyarticular RF-positive variant, positivity should be confirmed at least twice, 3 months apart (3).
- RF and ANA may be present in mixed connective tissue disease.

Imaging

Diagnostic radiography, MRI, ultrasonography, and CT, all play an important role in diagnosing or monitoring juvenile idiopathic arthritis (JIA); no one modality has evidence for superior diagnostic value (4)[A].

Initial approach

- Radiograph of affected joint(s); Early radiographic changes: Soft tissue swelling, periosteal reaction, juxta-articular demineralization; later changes include joint-space loss, articular surface erosions, subchondral cyst formation, sclerosis, joint fusion
- ECG (pericarditis)
- Radionuclide scans (infection, malignancy)
- MRI can assess synovial hypertrophy, cartilage degeneration, and clinical responsiveness to treatment in peripheral joints in JIA.

Follow-Up & Special Considerations

In interpreting results of dual energy x-ray photon absorptiometry scans, it is important to use pediatric, not adult, controls as normative data.

Diagnostic Procedures/Surgery

- Synovial biopsy occasionally indicated
- Arthrocentesis

Pathological Findings

Synovium shows hyperplasia of synovial cells, hyperemia, and infiltration of small lymphocytes and mononuclear cells.

DIFFERENTIAL DIAGNOSIS

- Other rheumatic diseases:
  - Systemic lupus erythematosus, dermatomyositis, mixed connective tissue disease, sarcoidosis
- Musculoskeletal:
  - Legg-Calve-Perthes, toxic synovitis, growing pains
- Infectious:
  - Septic arthritis, osteomyelitis, Lyme disease
- Reactive arthritis:
  - Postinfectious, rheumatic fever, Reiter syndrome
- Inflammatory bowel disease:
  - Crohn disease and ulcerative colitis
- Hemoglobinopathies
- Malignancy:
  - Leukemia, bone tumors (osteoid osteoma), neuroblastoma
- Vasculitis, Kawasaki disease

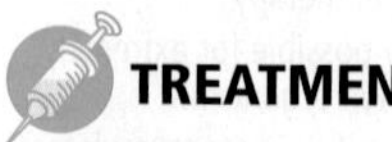

TREATMENT

MEDICATION

First Line

- NSAIDs are adequate in ~50% of patients, symptoms often improve within days, full efficacy 2–3 months
- Drugs for children include:
  - Ibuprofen (Motrin, Advil, Nuprin): 30–40 mg/kg/d, divided q.i.d., max 800 mg t.i.d.
  - Naproxen (Naprosyn, Aleve): 10–20 mg/kg/d divided b.i.d., max dose of 500 mg b.i.d.
  - Tolmetin sodium: 15–30 mg/kg/d; t.i.d. or q.i.d., max dose 600 mg t.i.d.
  - Diclofenac 2–3 mg/kg, divided t.i.d., max of 50 mg t.i.d.
  - Indomethacin 3 mg/kg/d, max of 200 mg/d
- Contraindications to NSAIDs: Known allergies

- Precautions: May worsen bleeding diatheses; use caution with all NSAIDs in renal insufficiency and hypovolemic states
- Significant possible interactions: NSAIDs may lower serum levels of digitalis and anticonvulsants and blunt the effect of loop diuretics. NSAIDs may increase serum methotrexate levels.
- Intra-articular long-acting corticosteroids especially for oligo-JIA. Immediately effective, local treatment. Improve synovitis, joint damage, contractures, and prevent leg length discrepancy (3)[B]:
  - Triamcinolone hexacetonide
- Glucocorticoids: Only in patients with extreme pain and functional limitation, while waiting for a 2nd-line agent to show some effect

Second Line

- 30–40% of patients will require addition of disease-modifying antirheumatic drugs (DMARDs), including methotrexate, sulfasalazine, leflunomide, and tumor necrosis factor (TNF) antagonists (etanercept, infliximab, adalimumab). Newer biologic therapies, including IL-1 and IL-6 receptor antagonists, currently under investigation.
- Methotrexate: Standard dose 8–12.5 mg/m^2/wk PO or SC. 10 mg/m^2/wk is most frequently used (3)[B]:
  - Plateau of efficacy reached with 15 mg/m^2/wk; further increase in dosage is not associated with therapeutic benefit (5)
- Sulfasalazine: Oligoarticular and HLA B27 spondyloarthritis
- Leflunomide: Not Food and Drug Administration–approved for JIA
- Etanercept (Enbrel): 0.4 mg/kg, max of 25 mg, given SC twice weekly (3)[B]
- Infliximab: 3–6 mg/kg q6–8wk
- Adalimumab: 40 mg SC q2wk
- Tocilizumab: IL-6 antibody demonstrating efficacy in phase III open label trials, ongoing studies to evaluate efficacy and appropriate dosing regimen (3)
- Anakinra: IL-1 receptor antibody under investigation with phase II and III clinical trials for systemic JIA (3)
- Analgesics for pain control, including narcotics

ADDITIONAL TREATMENT

General Measures

- Treatment goal: Control active disease and extra-articular manifestations to maintain musculoskeletal function as normal as possible.
- Begin treatment with TNF-α inhibitors in children with a history of arthritis in 4 or fewer joints and significant active arthritis despite treatment with methotrexate, or arthritis in 5 or more joints and any active arthritis following an adequate trial of methotrexate (1).
- Beginning treatment with anakinra in children with systemic arthritis and active fever whose treatment requires a second medication in addition to systemic glucocorticoids (1)
- All patients require regular (every 3–4 months for oligo-JIA and in ANA-positive patients) ophthalmic exams to uncover asymptomatic eye disease, at least for first 3 years.
- Moist heat, sleeping bag, or electric blanket to relieve morning stiffness
- Splints for contractures

Issues for Referral

- In general, a pediatric rheumatologist is best suited to manage juvenile idiopathic arthritis.
- Orthopedic surgeon: Need for surgery (joint replacement)
- Ophthalmologist: Uveitis
- Physical therapist for joint protection, to maintain range of motion, improve muscle strength, prevent deformities
- Occupational therapist to maintain and improve the normal life function
- Psychologists for coping

SURGERY/OTHER PROCEDURES

- Total hip and/or knee replacement may be needed for severe disease.
- Soft tissue release, if splinting, traction unsuccessful
- Limb length or angular deformity corrections
- Synovectomy is rarely performed.

IN-PATIENT CONSIDERATIONS

Admission Criteria

- Patient loses ambulatory ability
- Signs/symptoms of pericarditis
- Persistent fever

Discharge Criteria

Resolution of fever and swelling or serositis

ONGOING CARE

FOLLOW-UP RECOMMENDATIONS

Patient Monitoring

Determined by medication:

- NSAIDs: Periodic CBC, urinalysis, liver function tests (LFTs), renal function tests
- Aspirin and/or other salicylates: Transaminase and salicylate levels, weekly for 1st month, then every 3–4 months
- Methotrexate: Monthly LFTs, CBC, BUN, creatinine

DIET

Regular diet with special attention to adequate calcium, iron, protein, and caloric intake

PATIENT EDUCATION

- Ongoing education of patients and families with attention to: Psychosocial needs; school issues, educational needs; behavioral strategies for dealing with pain and noncompliance; use of health care resources
- Printed and audiovisual information available from local arthritis foundation

PROGNOSIS

- 50–60% ultimately remit, but functional ability depends on adequacy of long-term therapy (disease control, maintaining muscle and joint function).
- Poor prognosis: Active disease at 6 months, polyarticular disease ,extended pauciarticular disease course, female gender, (+) RF and ANA, persistent morning stiffness, rapid appearance of erosions, hip involvement

COMPLICATIONS

- Blindness, band keratopathy, glaucoma, short stature, micrognathia if temporomandibular joint involvement, debilitating joint disease, disseminated intravascular coagulation; hemolytic anemia
- Patient on NSAIDs: Peptic ulcer, GI hemorrhage, CNS reactions, renal disease, leukopenia
- Patient on DMARD: Bone marrow suppression, hepatitis, renal disease, dermatitis, mouth ulcers, retinal toxicity (antimalarials, rare)
- Patients on tumor necrosis factor antagonists: Higher risk of infection
- Osteoporosis, avascular necrosis
- Macrophage activation syndrome:
  - Decreased blood cell precursors secondary to histiocyte degradation of marrow

REFERENCES

1. Beukelman T, Patkar N, Saag K, et al. 2011 American College of Rheumatology recommendation for the treatment of Juvenile Idiopathic Arthritis: Initiation and safety monitoring of therapeutic agents for the treatment of arthritis and systemic features. *Arthritis Care and Research*. 2011;63(4):465–482.
2. Weiss JE, Ilowite NT. Juvenile idiopathic arthritis. *Rheum Dis Clin N Am*. 2007;33:441–70.
3. Kahn P. Juvenile idiopathic arthritis–current and future therapies. *Bull NYU Hosp Jt Dis*. 2009;67: 291–302.
4. McKay GM, Cox LA, Long BW, et al. Imaging juvenile idiopathic arthritis: Assessing the modalities. *Radiol Technol*. 2010;81:318–27.
5. Takken T, van der Net J, Helders P. Methotrexate for treating juvenile idiopathic arthritis. *Cochrane Database Syst Rev*. 2001;(4):CD003129.
6. Shigemura T, Yamazaki T, Hara Y, et al. Monitoring serum IL-18 levels is useful for treatment of a patient with systemic juvenile idiopathic arthritis complicated by macrophage activation syndrome. *Pediatr Rheumatol Online J*. 2011;9:15.

ADDITIONAL READING

- Benitze JL. *Juvenile Idiopathic Arthiris*. Tufts OpenCourseWare. 2007. http://ocw.tufts.edu/Content/19/lecturenotes/303181/303190.
- Miller E, Uleryk E, Doria AS. Evidence-based outcomes of studies addressing diagnostic accuracy of MRI of juvenile idiopathic arthritis. *AJR Am J Roentgenol*. 2009;192:1209–18.

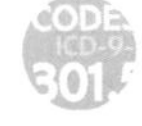

CODES

ICD9

- 714.30 Chronic or unspecified polyarticular juvenile rheumatoid arthritis
- 714.31 Acute polyarticular juvenile rheumatoid arthritis
- 714.32 Pauciarticular juvenile rheumatoid arthritis

CLINICAL PEARLS

- High-titer RF correlates with severity, and positive titers confer poorer prognosis.
- ANA confers risk of uveitis.
- No specific biomarker or test, but there is research pointing to using interleukin 18 as a marker of disease and severity (6).
- Diagnosis is one of exclusion; consult pediatric rheumatologist.

ARTHRITIS, OSTEO

Patrick W. Joyner, MD, MS
Jill A. Grimes, MD

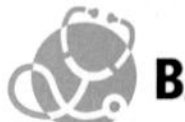

BASICS

DESCRIPTION

- A common joint disease that involves progressive loss of articular cartilage and reactive changes at joint margins and in subchondral bone
- Primary:
  - Idiopathic: Divided into subsets by clinical features (localized, generalized, erosive)
- Secondary:
  - Posttraumatic
  - Childhood anatomic abnormalities (e.g., congenital hip dysplasia, SCFE, Legg-Calvé-Perthes disease)
  - Inheritable metabolic disorders (e.g., Wilson disease, alkaptonuria, hemochromatosis)
  - Neuropathic arthropathy (Charcot joints)
  - Hemophilic arthropathy
  - Endocrinopathies: Acromegalic arthropathy, hyperparathyroidism, hypothyroidism
  - Paget disease
  - Noninfectious inflammatory arthritis (e.g., rheumatoid arthritis [RA], spondyloarthropathies)
  - Gout, calcium pyrophosphate deposition disease (pseudogout)
  - Septic or tuberculous arthritis
- System(s) affected: Musculoskeletal
- Synonym(s): Osteoarthrosis; degenerative joint disease

EPIDEMIOLOGY

- Symptomatic disease: >40 years old
- Leading cause of disability in those >65 years old
- Radiographic evidence (estimates): 33% to almost 90% in those >65 years old
- Predominant sex: Male = Female
- 90% of hip osteoarthritis is primary and predominantly found in Caucasians.

Prevalence

- ~60 million patients
- Increases with age, almost universal >65 (by x-ray study but not clinically)
- Moderate to severe hip osteoarthritis is 3–6% in Caucasians; <1% in East Indians, blacks, Chinese, and Native Americans.

RISK FACTORS

- Increasing age: >50 years old
- Obesity (weight-bearing joints)
- Prolonged occupational or sports stress
- Injury to a joint from trauma, infection, or preexisting inflammatory arthritis
- Female gender (knee and hand osteoarthritis [OA])

Genetics

- Up to 65% of OA may occur on a genetic basis.
- The heritability of end-stage hip OA has been estimated, by one study, to be 27%.
- Twin studies in women show heritability rates of OA: knee, 49%; hand, 65%; hip, 50%.
- The genetic contribution may involve a combination of effects on structure (collagen), cartilage, or bone metabolism or inflammation.

PATHOPHYSIOLOGY

Failure of chondrocytes to maintain the balance between degradation and synthesis of extracellular matrix

ETIOLOGY

Biomechanical, biochemical, inflammatory, and immunologic factors all implicated in pathogenesis

DIAGNOSIS

HISTORY

- Slowly developing joint pain that typically follows use of a joint
- Transient stiffness (especially after awakening in morning and after sitting) which tends to lessen 10–15 minutes after some movement and mobility of the joint.

PHYSICAL EXAM

- Joint bony enlargement (Heberden nodules of distal interphalangeal joints; osteophytes can be palpated in many joints with severe OA)
- Decreased range of motion with pain at the end of the range
- Tenderness usually absent; may occur along joint margin associated with synovitis
- Crepitation is a late sign.
- Weakness and wasting of muscles around the joint
- Local pain and stiffness with OA of spine, with radicular pain (if compression of nerve roots)
- Changes in overall joint alignment (i.e., genu varus [bow-legged] and genu valgum [knock-kneed])

DIAGNOSTIC TESTS & INTERPRETATION

Lab

Initial lab tests

Usually not helpful in diagnosis (sedimentation rate not increased)

Follow-Up & Special Considerations

- May be useful in monitoring treatment with NSAIDs (renal insufficiency and GI bleeding)
- In secondary OA, underlying disorder may have abnormal lab results, e.g., hemochromatosis (abnormal iron studies).

Imaging

Initial approach

- X-ray films usually normal early
- Later often show:
  - Narrowed, asymmetric joint space
  - Osteophyte formation
  - Subchondral bony sclerosis
  - Subchondral cyst formation
  - In the hip may appreciate changes in anatomical shape of the femoral head, especially in later stages of avascular necrosis
- Erosions may occur on surface of distal and proximal interphalangeal joints when OA is associated with inflammation (erosive OA).

Diagnostic Procedures/Surgery

- Joint aspiration:
  - May be helpful in distinguishing from chronic inflammatory arthritis
  - OA: Cell count usually <500 cells/mm^3, predominantly mononuclear
  - Inflammatory: Cell count usually >2,000 cells/mm^3, predominantly neutrophils
- Calcium pyrophosphate dihydrate and/or apatite crystals may be seen in effusions.

Pathological Findings

- Characterized macroscopically by patchy cartilage damage and bony hypertrophy
- Histological phases:
  - Edema of the extracellular matrix and cartilage microcracks
  - Fissuring and pitting of the subchondral bone
  - Erosion and osteocartilaginous loose bodies
- Subchondral bone trabecular microfractures and sclerosis with osteophyte formation
- Degradation response produced by release of proteolytic enzymes, collagenolytic enzymes, prostaglandins, and immune responses

DIFFERENTIAL DIAGNOSIS

- Distinguish from other types of arthritis by:
  - Absence of systemic findings
  - Minimal articular inflammation
  - Distribution of involved joints (e.g., distal and proximal interphalangeal joints, not wrist and metacarpophalangeal joints)
- In spine, distinguish from osteoporosis, metastatic disease, multiple myeloma, or other bone diseases.

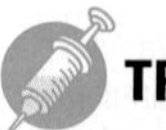

TREATMENT

MEDICATION

First Line

Management of pain and inflammation:

- **Acetaminophen** up to 1,000 mg q.i.d.: Good evidence as most effective for pain relief in OA of knee and hip (1)[A]
- A number of studies, mainly of OA of knee, have shown short-term (<4 weeks) benefits from topical NSAID gels, creams, and ointments when compared with placebo. Topical NSAIDs should be a core treatment for knee and hand OA.
- If acetaminophen or topical NSAIDs are insufficient, then the addition or substitution by an oral NSAID/COX-2 inhibitor should be considered. Use at the lowest effective dose for the shortest time possible. Prolonged use is associated with renal insufficiency, hypertension, leg edema, and GI bleeding.
- May use nonacetylated salicylates (e.g., salsalate, choline-magnesium salicylate) or low-dose ibuprofen ≤1,600 mg/d.
- Topical NSAIDs and capsaicin can be effective as adjunctives and alternatives to oral analgesic/anti-inflammatory agents in knee OA (1)[A].
- Other NSAIDs have similar efficacy.
- Contraindications:
  - All oral NSAIDs/COX-2 inhibitors have analgesic effects of a similar magnitude but vary in their potential GI and cardio-renal toxicity.
  - NSAIDs are contraindicated in patients with renal disease, CHF, HTN, active peptic ulcer disease, and previous hypersensitivity to an NSAID or aspirin (asthma, nasal polyps, hypotension, urticaria/angioedema).
  - Combinations of NSAIDs or concomitant aspirin are contraindicated due to risk of adverse reactions.
  - If cardiovascular risk: Combination of a nonselective NSAID and low-dose aspirin is recommended.
  - Oral or parenteral corticosteroids are contraindicated.

- Precautions:
  - If oral NSAID/COX-2 inhibitor is necessary for a patient aged >65 or a patient <65 with any increased GI risk factors, offer a proton-pump inhibitor.
  - Significant possible interactions:
    - NSAIDs reduce effectiveness of ACE inhibitors and diuretics.
    - Aspirin and NSAIDs (except COX-2 inhibitors) may increase effects of anticoagulants.
    - Increased hypoglycemic effects of oral hypoglycemics with aspirin
    - Salicylates reduce effectiveness of spironolactone (Aldactone) and uricosurics.
    - Corticosteroids and some antacids increase salicylate excretion, whereas ascorbic acid and ammonium chloride reduce salicylate excretion and may cause toxicity.

Pregnancy Considerations

- ASA and NSAIDs: Some risk to fetus during 1st and 3rd trimesters of pregnancy
- Compatible with breastfeeding

Second Line

- A number of studies, mainly of knee OA, have shown short-term (<4 weeks) benefits from topical NSAID gels, creams, and ointments when compared with placebo. Topical NSAIDs should be a core treatment for knee and hand OA (2)[B].
- Topical capsaicin should be considered as an adjunct therapy for knee and hand OA; may cause local burning.
- Rubefacients are not recommended.
- Opioid analgesics (e.g., codeine, oxycodone, propoxyphene): Evidence supporting use in OA is extremely poor; restrict for treatment of acute episodes.
- Judiciously use intra-articular injections of corticosteroids for selected acute flare-ups of joints (no more than 4 per year up to a maximum of 12 injections per joint). If used excessively, can accelerate joint deterioration.
- Intra-articular viscosupplementation with hyaluronic acid preparations into a painful knee may provide relief of pain and improve function at earlier stages, though not statistically significant over injections with saline (placebo) (3)[B]. Definitive evidence is lacking in other joints. However, there are few randomized head-to-head comparisons of different products.

ADDITIONAL TREATMENT

General Measures

- Weight reduction with a fitness program if overweight is essential (1,4)[A].
- Walking aids and proper footwear (1)[A]
- Heat (e.g., local, tub baths) or cold applications
- Physical therapy to maintain or regain joint motion and muscle strength. Quadriceps-strengthening exercises can relieve knee pain and disability.
- Muscle strengthening exercises are specific for impairment-related outcomes (i.e., pain).
- Aerobic exercise contributes to better long-term functional outcomes.
- At 12-month follow-up, the best results are achieved in patients that supplement a home exercise program with supervised exercise classes (i.e., physical therapy).
- Maintain exercise; all benefits gained are lost 6 months after cessation of the program.
- Protect joints from overuse; ambulatory aides are beneficial (e.g., cane, crutches, walker).
- Assessment for bracing, joint supports, or insoles in those with biomechanical joint pain or instability. Bracing is more beneficial in patients with unicompartmental disease of the knee, and in higher-demand patients.

Additional Therapies

Address psychosocial factors (i.e., self-efficacy, coping skills). Prevent or treat anxiety and depression. Improve social support.

COMPLEMENTARY AND ALTERNATIVE MEDICINE

- Nutritional supplements such as glucosamine and chondroitin sulfate may symptomatically benefit some patients and have low toxicity, but studies lack standardized case definition and outcome assessments. *If no response is apparent within 6 months, treatment should be discontinued.*
- A 2010 meta-analysis shows glucosamine, chondroitin, and their combination do not reduce joint pain or have an impact on narrowing of joint space compared with placebo (5)[A].
- TENS units and acupuncture may be beneficial (1)[A].

SURGERY/OTHER PROCEDURES

May be indicated in advanced disease (e.g., osteotomy, debridement, removal of loose bodies, joint replacement, fusion)

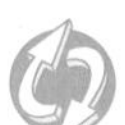

ONGOING CARE

FOLLOW-UP RECOMMENDATIONS

Patient Monitoring

- Follow range of motion and functional status at regular intervals.
- Watch for GI blood loss and follow cardiac, renal, and mental status in older patients on NSAIDs or aspirin.
- Periodic CBC, renal function tests, stool for occult blood

PATIENT EDUCATION

- American College of Rheumatology patient education overviews: http://www.rheumatology.org/public/factsheets/index.asp?aud=pat
- Arthritis Foundation: http://www.arthritis.org

PROGNOSIS

- Progressive disease: Early in course, pain relieved by rest; later, pain may occur at rest and at night.
- Joint effusions and enlargement may occur, especially in knees.
- Osteophyte (spur) formation, especially at joint margins
- Advanced stage with full-thickness loss of cartilage down to bone

COMPLICATIONS

- Leading causes of pain and disability
- Decompensated CHF, GI bleeding, decreased renal function on NSAIDs or aspirin
- Infection or accelerated cartilage loss with intra-articular corticosteroids

REFERENCES

1. Zhang W, Moskowitz RW, Nuki G, et al. OARSI recommendations for the management of hip and knee osteoarthritis, Part II: OARSI evidence-based, expert consensus guidelines. *Osteoarthr Cartil*. 2008;16:137–62.
2. Altman R, Barkin RL. Topical therapy for osteoarthritis: Clinical and pharmacologic perspectives. *Postgrad Med*. 2009;121:139–47.
3. Kul-Panza E, Berker N. Is hyaluronate sodium effective in the management of knee osteoarthritis? A placebo-controlled double-blind study. *Minerva Med*. 2010;101:63–72.
4. Jiang L, Tian W, Wang Y, et al. Body mass index and susceptibility to knee osteoarthritis: A systematic review and meta-analysis. *Joint Bone Spine*. 2011.
5. Wandel S, Jüni P, Tendal B, et al. Effects of glucosamine, chondroitin, or placebo in patients with osteoarthritis of hip or knee: Network meta-analysis. *BMJ*. 2010;341:c4675.

ADDITIONAL READING

- Ernst E, Posadzki P. Complementary and alternative medicine for rheumatoid arthritis and osteoarthritis: An overview of systematic reviews. *Curr Pain Headache Rep*. 2011;15(6):431–7.
- Harvey WF, Hunter DJ. Pharmacologic intervention for osteoarthritis in older adults. *Clin Geriatr Med*. 2010;26:503–15.
- Wallis JA, Taylor NF. Pre-operative interventions (non-surgical and non-pharmacological) for patients with hip or knee osteoarthritis awaiting joint replacement surgery - a systematic review and meta-analysis. *Osteoarthritis Cartilage*. 2011; 19(12):1381–95.
- Walsh NE, Hurley MV. Evidence based guidelines and current practice for physiotherapy management of knee osteoarthritis. *Musculoskeletal Care*. 2009; 7:45–56.

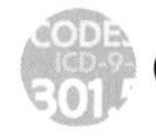

CODES

ICD9

- 715.10 Osteoarthrosis, localized, primary, involving unspecified site
- 715.20 Osteoarthrosis, localized, secondary, involving unspecified site
- 715.90 Osteoarthrosis, unspecified whether generalized or localized, involving unspecified site

CLINICAL PEARLS

- Morning stiffness lasts <15 minutes (vs. 1 hour in rheumatoid arthritis).
- Distal predominance in hands
- Limit intra-articular steroid injections to 4 per year.

ARTHRITIS, PSORIATIC

Michael S. Krathen, MD
Amit Garg, MD

BASICS

Psoriatic arthritis (PsA) is a chronic, destructive, seronegative arthropathy seen most commonly in patients with long-standing psoriasis.

DESCRIPTION

- PsA is a seronegative spondyloarthropathy characterized by inflammatory arthritis and enthesitis.
- 5 patterns of arthritis in PsA include:
  - Asymmetric oligoarthritis: Usually involves large joints
  - Distal interphalangeal (DIP) joint predominant: Often associated with nail psoriasis
  - Symmetric polyarthritis: May be indistinguishable from rheumatoid arthritis (RA)
  - Spondyloarthritis: Asymmetric and discontinuous, unlike ankylosing spondylitis (AS)
  - Arthritis mutilans: Destructive, resorptive arthritis; produces so-called opera-glass or telescoping digit
- Although psoriasis generally is present, it may be limited in extent:
  - Course of arthritis and extent of psoriasis do not appear to correlate.
  - Other extra-articular features, such as iritis, are less common.
  - Damaging joint disease may occur in 40–57%. Characteristic radiologic changes include joint erosions that begin marginally and move centrally ("pencil-in-cup deformity") and periostitis.
- Rheumatoid factor (RF) and cyclic citrullinated peptide (anti-CCP) antibody are usually negative. HLA-B27 may be positive.

EPIDEMIOLOGY

- Peak onset age: 35–40 years
- Predominant gender: Female = Male
- Polyarthritis is more common in women.
- Spondylitis in up to 25%, more common in males
- Psoriasis precedes arthritis in the majority by an average of 12 years. Arthritis may precede psoriasis in up to 15%, and this occurs more often in children. Arthritis and psoriasis also may present simultaneously.
- Psoriasis occurs in 2–3% of the US population; 6–42% of these individuals develop PsA (1).

Prevalence

Prevalence: 1–2/1,000 population (1)

RISK FACTORS

- Psoriasis
- Family history of PsA

Genetics

- 30–40% concordance in identical twins
- HLA-B27 in 15–50% with PsA (spondylitis pattern) vs. 90% in AS
- Other HLA associations in psoriatic arthritis: HLA-B7, HLA-B38, HLA-B39, HLA-Cw6

GENERAL PREVENTION

There are no currently available prevention strategies. It is unknown if early systemic treatment of psoriasis prevents the onset of PsA.

PATHOPHYSIOLOGY

- CD4+/CD8+ T cells; tumor necrosis factor α (TNF-α); interleukins 1 (IL-1), 6, 8, and 10; and matrix metalloproteases present in synovial fluid (1)
- Osteoclast precursor cell upregulation

ETIOLOGY

Unknown. Probably multifactorial: Immunologic, genetic, environmental factors

COMMONLY ASSOCIATED CONDITIONS

Psoriasis

DIAGNOSIS

- Establishing a history of inflammatory arthritis, dactylitis, or enthesitis in a patient with existing psoriasis is usually adequate to establish the diagnosis. Nonetheless, differentiation from other inflammatory arthropathies such as RA can be difficult.
- The CASPAR criteria (2) comprise a validated instrument that may be used to screen patients for the presence of PsA. The sensitivity and specificity of the CASPAR criteria are 91.4% and 98.7%, respectively. To establish the presence of PsA, a patient must have inflammatory articular disease (joint, spine, or entheseal) with ≥3 points from the following 5 categories: (i) evidence of current psoriasis, a personal history of psoriasis, or family history of psoriasis (2 points); (ii) typical psoriatic nail dystrophy, including onycholysis, pitting, and hyperkeratosis (1 point); (iii) a negative rheumatoid factor, preferentially analyzed by ELISA (1 point); (iv) current dactylitis or a history of dactylitis (1 point); and (v) radiologic evidence of new bone formation (excluding osteophyte formation) on plain radiographs of the hand or foot (1 point).

HISTORY

- Long-standing (most often) psoriasis
- Morning stiffness of hands, feet, or low back for >45 minutes
- Discomfort or pain of involved joints
- Swelling or redness of peripheral joints
- Low back or buttock pain
- Ankle or heel pain
- Dactylitis, or uniform swelling of an entire digit

PHYSICAL EXAM

- Affected peripheral joints may have overlying erythema, warmth, and swelling:
  - Synovitis
  - Dactylitis
  - Swelling of tendons (e.g., Achilles tendon) and tenderness at insertion sites (e.g., calcaneus)
  - Limited range of motion of axial skeleton
  - Pain with stress on the sacroiliac joint
- Well-demarcated pink-to-red erythematous plaques with a white silvery scale; common locations include scalp, ears, trunk, buttocks, elbows and forearms, knees and legs, and palms and soles
- Nails may be dystrophic with pits, oil spots, crumbling, leukonychia, and red lunulae.

DIAGNOSTIC TESTS & INTERPRETATION

History and physical examination may provide adequate data to establish the diagnosis of PsA. Plain radiographs may demonstrate characteristic changes and aid in the diagnosis of PsA. Imaging allows assessment of current damage, disease progression, and response to therapy.

Lab

There is no specific blood test for PsA. Autoantibodies associated with RA or systemic lupus erythematosus, for example, generally are not found.

Initial lab tests

- Serum RF is usually negative.
- Anti-CCP is usually negative.
- Antinuclear antibodies are usually negative.
- Acute-phase reactants (ESR and C-reactive protein) may be elevated.
- HLA-B27 is noted in 50–70% with axial disease and <15% with peripheral disease.

Imaging

Juxta-articular new bone formation (periostitis) and marginal joint erosions that may progress centrally to form the "pencil-in-cup" erosions are the most characteristic plain radiographic features.

Initial approach

Baseline plain radiographs of affected joints

Follow-Up & Special Considerations

Follow-up radiographs; interval based on severity

Diagnostic Procedures/Surgery

Diagnosis is clinical.

Pathological Findings

Diagnosis is clinical, and biopsy of either skin or synovium is not usually required.

DIFFERENTIAL DIAGNOSIS

- Reactive arthritis
- Psoriasis and RA
- Psoriasis and osteoarthritis
- Psoriasis and polyarticular gout
- Psoriasis and AS

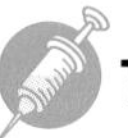

TREATMENT

- Treatment algorithms in PsA are based on severity of joint symptoms, extent of structural damage, and extent and severity of psoriasis (3)[A].
- It is essential that the psychological burden of skin disease not be underestimated or discounted.
- NSAIDs may be considered for control of symptoms. Intra-articular glucocorticoid injections may be given judiciously to control symptoms for persistent mono- or oligoarthritis.
- Combination therapy (at least 2 drugs from the following: Analgesics, NSAIDs, opioids, opioidlike drugs, and neuromodulators [antidepressants, anticonvulsants, and muscle relaxants]) no more effective than monotherapy for adults (4)[A]
- All patients with severe or moderate peripheral arthritis should be started on disease-modifying antirheumatic drugs (DMARDs). DMARDs have the potential to reduce or prevent joint damage and preserve joint integrity and function.
- DMARDs recommended as 1st-line therapy are sulfasalazine, leflunomide, methotrexate, and cyclosporine. No evidence supports the use of combination DMARD therapy.
- Patients who fail to respond to at least 1 standard DMARD drug should be considered for anti-TNF-α therapy. Patients with poor prognosis could be considered for anti-TNF-α therapy even if they have not failed a standard DMARD (5)[A].

MEDICATION

First Line

NSAIDs (6)[A]

Second Line

- Sulfasalazine (6)[A]
- Methotrexate (6)[B]
- Cyclosporine (6)[B]
- Azathioprine (6)[B]
- TNF-α inhibitors:
  - Adalimumab (6)[A]
  - Etanercept (6)[A]
  - Infliximab (6)[A]
- IL-12/23 inhibitor: Ustekinumab (7)[A]

ALERT

Anti-TNF agents should not be used in the setting of active infection, including patients with tuberculosis and hepatitis B infection, with concurrent live vaccinations, with New York Heart Association (NYHA) class III–IV congestive heart failure, with malignancy, or with history of demyelinating disease.

Pregnancy Considerations

- Avoid teratogenic medications (e.g., methotrexate, gold, antimalarials, sulfasalazine, acitretin) during pregnancy.
- Adalimumab, etanercept, and infliximab are currently listed as Category B medications.

ADDITIONAL TREATMENT

General Measures

Physical therapy may be beneficial in all stages of disease.

Issues for Referral

- Rheumatology
- Dermatology

SURGERY/OTHER PROCEDURES

Joint fusion or replacement for advanced destruction

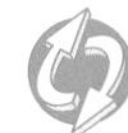

ONGOING CARE

FOLLOW-UP RECOMMENDATIONS

Epidemiologic evidence suggests a relationship between psoriasis, the metabolic syndrome, myocardial infarction, and stroke. Periodic measurement of BP, fasting lipids and glucose, cholesterol, and body mass index is recommended (8).

PATIENT EDUCATION

- Stress noncontagious nature of condition.
- For a listing of sources for patient education materials favorably reviewed on this topic, physicians may contact:
  - American Academy of Family Physicians Foundation, P.O. Box 8418, Kansas City, MO 64114, (800) 274–2237, ext. 4400. Also see http://www.familydoctor.org.
  - National Psoriasis Foundation, 6600 SW 92nd Ave., Suite 300, Portland, OR 97223–7195. Also see http://www.psoriasis.org/about/psa.
  - Arthritis Foundation, 1314 Spring Street N.W., Atlanta, GA 30309, (404) 872–7100 or http://www.arthritis.org/conditions/diseasecenter/psoriatic_arthritis.asp.

PROGNOSIS

- Course: Insidious and chronic joint disease and recurring and remitting chronic skin disease
- More favorable than for RA (except for patients who develop arthritis mutilans)

COMPLICATIONS

- Chronicity
- Disability
- Psychosocial impact of psoriasis

REFERENCES

1. Gottlieb A, Korman NJ, Gordon KB, et al. Guidelines of care for management of psoriatic arthritis. *J Am Acad Dermatol*. 2008;58:851–64.
2. Taylor W, Gladman D, Helliwell P, et al. Classification criteria for psoriatic arthritis: development of new criteria from a large international study. *Arthritis Rheum*. 2006;54(8): 2665–73.
3. Menter A, Gottlieb A, Fedman SR, et al. American Academy of Dermatology. Links Guidelines of care for the management of psoriasis and psoriatic arthritis. Section 3. Guidelines of care for the management and treatment of psoriasis with topical therapies. *J Am Acad Dermatol*. 2009;60(4): 643–59.
4. Ramiro S, Radner H, van der Heijde D, et al. Combination therapy for pain management in inflammatory arthritis (rheumatoid arthritis, ankylosing spondylitis, psoriatic arthritis, other spondyloarthritis). *Cochrane Database Syst Rev*. 2011;10:CD008886.
5. Ash Z, Gaujoux-Viala C, Gossec L, et al. A systematic literature review of drug therapies for the treatment of psoriatic arthritis: Current evidence and meta-analysis informing the EULAR recommendations for the management of psoriatic arthritis. *Ann Rheum Dis*. 2011.
6. Kavanaugh AF, Ritchlin CT, GRAPPA Treatment Guideline Committee. Systematic review of treatments for psoriatic arthritis: An evidence based approach and basis for treatment guidelines. *J Rheumatol*. 2006;33:1417–21.
7. Gottlieb A, Menter A, Mendelsohn A, et al. Ustekinumab, a human interleukin 12/23 monoclonal antibody, for psoriatic arthritis: Randomised, double-blind, placebo-controlled, crossover trial. *Lancet*. 2009;373:633–40.
8. Gottlieb AB, Dann F. Comorbidities in patients with psoriasis. *Am J Med*. 2009;122:1150.e1–9.
9. Prey S, Paul C, Bronsard V, et al. Assessment of risk of psoriatic arthritis in patients with plaque psoriasis: a systematic review of the literature. *J Eur Acad Dermatol Venereol*. 2010;24(Suppl 2):31–5.

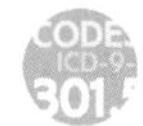

CODES

ICD9

696.0 Psoriatic arthropathy

CLINICAL PEARLS

- Severity of psoriasis may correlate with the likelihood of developing arthritis; however, severity of psoriasis does not correlate with severity of arthritis; 24% of psoriasis patients develop PsA (9)[A].
- Often overlooked locations of psoriasis include scalp, ears, umbilicus, and gluteal cleft.
- Other conditions may mimic or coexist with PsA: Osteoarthritis and polyarticular gout
- The polyarticular pattern of PsA may mimic RA; however, the presence of enthesitis and recognition of psoriasis characterize PsA.
- Axial skeleton in PsA is asymmetric and discontinuous, in contrast to axial involvement in AS.

ARTHRITIS, RHEUMATOID (RA)

Sergio A. Leon, MD

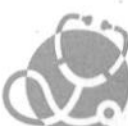

BASICS

DESCRIPTION

- RA is a chronic systemic inflammatory disease (typically joint-involving) of unknown cause.
- Articular inflammation may be remitting, but if continued, it may result in joint damage and disability.
- Characteristic extra-articular manifestations include the following:
  - Rheumatoid nodules, vasculitis, neuropathy, scleritis, pericarditis, splenomegaly
- System(s) affected: Musculoskeletal; Skin; Hematologic; Lymphatic; Immunologic; Muscular; Renal; Cardiovascular; Neurologic; Pulmonary

Geriatric Considerations

- Increased contribution/interaction of age-related comorbidities; pericarditis, septic arthritis, Sjögren syndrome are more common
- Less tolerance to drugs; increased incidence of hydroxychloroquine-associated maculopathy, D-penicillamine rash, and sulfasalazine-induced nausea/vomiting

Pregnancy Considerations

- Use effective contraception with disease-modifying antirheumatic drugs (DMARDs). Modify regimen with pregnancy or breastfeeding.
- Labor/delivery pose no serious problems, unless there is severe mechanical joint disease.
- >75% improve during pregnancy, but relapse in 6 months. First episodes may occur in pregnancy.

EPIDEMIOLOGY

Incidence

- Predominant age: 3rd–6th decades
- Predominant sex:
  - Female > Male (2–3:1; overall incidence and prevalence of articular manifestations)
  - Male > Female (systemic disease)

Prevalence

- US population: 0.5–1.5%
- Native Americans: >3.5–5.3%

RISK FACTORS

- HLA genes contribute to 30–50% genetic risk.
- Family history
- Native American ethnicity

Genetics

- 1st-degree relatives have 1.5-fold higher risk than the general population of developing RA.
- Twin studies show heritability of 60%.
- Seropositive RA aggregates in families.
- HLA-DR4+ persons have increased relative risk of 4–5 times.

PATHOPHYSIOLOGY

Antibody-complement complex results in intra-articular inflammation

ETIOLOGY

- Genetic factors
- Host factors: Hormonal, immunologic, obesity
- Environmental: Socioeconomic, smoking

COMMONLY ASSOCIATED CONDITIONS

- Sjögren syndrome, Felty syndrome, amyloidosis
- Increased incidence of infections, lymphomas, and renal and cardiovascular disease

DIAGNOSIS

HISTORY

- The 2010 American College of Rheumatology/European League Against Rheumatism classification criteria: *Who should be screened?* (1)
  - Patients who have at least 1 joint with definite clinical synovitis (swelling), which is not better explained by another disease
- A score of ≥6 is needed for the classification of a patient as having definite RA.
- Joint involvement: Any swollen or tender joint at exam
  - Score 1 large joint: 0
  - 2–10 large joints: 1
  - 1–3 small joints (with or without large joints): 2
  - 4–10 small joints (with or without large joints): 3
  - >10 joints (at least 1 small joint): 5
- Serology: At least 1 test is needed: Negative RF (rheumatoid factor) and negative ACPA (anti-citrullinated protein antibody): 0; low positive RF or low positive ACPA: 2; high positive RF or high positive ACPA: 3
- Acute phase reactants: At least 1 result is needed. Normal CRP (C-reactive protein) and normal ESR: 0; abnormal CRP or ESR: 1
- Duration of symptoms:(self-reported) <6 weeks: 0; ≥6 weeks: 1
- Small joints include MCP, PIP, wrist, 2nd to 5th MTP, and thumb IP. Large joints include shoulders, elbows, hips, knees, and ankles. (DIP, first MCP and first MTP joints are excluded from assessment.)
- Although patients with a score <6/10 are not classifiable as having RA, their status can be reassessed and the criteria might be fulfilled cumulatively over time
- Important clinical data not included in the classification criteria are prolonged morning stiffness (>1 hour), SC nodules, and radiographic changes consistent with RA
- Systemic symptoms: Fatigue, depression, malaise, anorexia, rheumatoid nodules, ocular disease, lymphadenopathy, splenomegaly, entrapment neuropathies, osteoporosis

PHYSICAL EXAM

Evaluate for swollen or tender joints, especially in the following:

- Small joints: MCP, PIP, wrist, 2nd–5th MTP, and thumb IP joints
- Large joints: Shoulders, elbows, hips, knees, and ankles. DIP, 1st MCP, and 1st MTP joints are excluded from assessment.
- Abdomen: Splenomegaly
- Skin: SC nodules

DIAGNOSTIC TESTS & INTERPRETATION

Lab

Initial lab tests

- Hematocrit: Mild anemia (of chronic disease)
- ESR: Usually elevated
- CRP: Unspecific, direct measure of impact of IL-6 on liver cells
- Rheumatoid factor (RF): >1:80 in 70–80% of patients with RA (most commonly IgM Ab):
  - Poor screening tool
  - Disorders that may yield false-positive RF results: Sjögren syndrome, mixed cryoglobulinemia, parasitic infections (e.g., malaria), liver disease, endocarditis, acute viral infections
- *Anticyclic citrullinated peptide antibodies (anti-CCP antibodies) are highly specific and present early.* (2)[A] Linked to erosive RA.
- Antinuclear antibody: Present in 20–30%
- Electrolytes, creatinine, liver function, and urinalysis to assess comorbid states

Follow-Up & Special Considerations

RF is not useful for monitoring the course of the illness.

Imaging

Initial approach

- Radiographic abnormalities are very useful in diagnosis and treatment.
- Periarticular osteopenia is the earliest change.
- More typical findings are juxta-articular bone erosions and symmetrical joint space narrowing.
- A CT/MRI and ultrasound are useful in specific situations such as cervical-spine symptoms or detection of early joint erosions.
- Bone scan if suspected aseptic necrosis

Follow-Up & Special Considerations

Radiographs of the hands, wrists, and feet can be repeated to follow disease progression.

Diagnostic Procedures/Surgery

Synovial fluid:

- No pathognomonic findings
- Yellowish-white, turbid, poor viscosity
- WBC increased (3,500–50,000)
- Protein: ~4.2 g/dL (42 g/L)
- Serum-synovial glucose difference ≥30 mg/dL (≥1.67 mmol/L)

Pathological Findings

Synovial tissue is expanded by the recruitment and retention of inflammatory cells, with formation of villous projections and pannus that invades and destroys cartilage and bone.

DIFFERENTIAL DIAGNOSIS

- Other systemic connective tissue diseases: Sjögren syndrome, systemic lupus erythematosus, systemic sclerosis, adult Still disease, mixed
- Psoriatic arthritis
- Viral-induced arthritis: Parvovirus B19, hepatitis C (with cryoglobulinemia)
- Occult malignancy
- Vasculitis: Behçet syndrome
- Seronegative polyarthritis
- Erosive osteoarthritis
- Chronic infections: Lyme disease

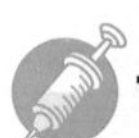

TREATMENT

Goals: Controlling disease activity, relieving pain, maintaining or improving function, preventing or correcting impairments, and promoting self-management

MEDICATION

DMARDs are usually administered in combination following four general strategies: sequential monotherapy, step-up therapy, induction therapy, or individualized targeted "tight" control.

First Line

- Nonbiologic DMARDs:
  - Start DMARDs within 2 months of diagnosis if patient has ongoing active disease despite appropriate dose of aspirin or other NSAIDs.
  - Precautions: Offer proton pump inhibitors (PPIs) for chronic NSAID therapy; avoid NSAIDs.
  - Due to their greater convenience, lower toxicity profiles, and quicker onset of action, the initial therapy is a nonbiologic DMARD: Methotrexate, sulfasalazine, or leflunomide have shown evidence of comparable efficacy. Hydroxychloroquine is less potent.
  - Combination DMARDs may be more effective than individual drugs.
  - Bridging and/or low-dose corticosteroids, NSAIDs, and simple analgesics are often required to maximize symptom management.
  - Prednisone: 5–15 mg/d for severe disease or to minimize disease activity. Use only for short periods, or intermittently. Low-dose prednisolone is more effective than NSAIDs (3)[A].
  - Methotrexate (MTX) (Rheumatrex): 7.5–25 mg/wk PO. It is the DMARD with the most predictable benefit. Many significant side effects, but the addition of folate reduces toxicity. 3–6-month trial. Monitor CBC, renal, and liver function every 8–12 weeks. Contraindicated in renal disease.
  - Sulfasalazine (SSZ): 500 mg/d, increase to 2 g/d over 1 month; max: 2–3 g/d; 6-month trial (4)[A]. Monitor CBC, liver enzymes every 8–12 weeks. Screen for G6PD deficiency.
  - Leflunomide (Arava): Dose: 10–20 mg/d. Modifies T-cell function to decrease autoimmune activity, reduce structural damage. Response rate similar to SSZ and MTX. GI side effects and potentially teratogenic (5)[A]. Contraindicated in pregnancy.
  - Antimalarials: Hydroxychloroquine (HCQ) (Plaquenil) 400 mg qhs for 2–3 months, then 200 mg at bedtime; 6-month trial is usual (6)[A]. Usually to treat milder forms or in combination with other DMARDs. Yearly ophthalmologic exam. Adjust dose in renal insufficiency.
- Biological DMARDs:
  - Tumor necrosis factor (TNF) inhibitors: IV infliximab (Remicade), SC adalimumab (Humira), and SC etanercept (Enbrel). No evidence that one is superior. The combination with MTX appears to be the most effective. Optimal dosage and duration of treatment unclear. Low toxicity. Costly. Check PPD prior to treatment and periodic CBC. Risk of lymphoma, CHF.
  - Anakinra (Kineret), an IL-1 receptor antagonist. Injection site reaction, neutropenia, bacterial infections. Fewer clinical benefits than TNF inhibitors.
  - Abatacept (Orencia) and rituximab (Rituxan) are approved for active moderate-to-severe RA with inadequate response to other DMARDs or failed anti-TNF agent.
  - 2 long-acting anti-TNF agents, Certolizumab pegol (Cimzia) and golimumab (Simponi), have been also approved in moderate to severe disease.
- Other older nonbiologic DMARDs have been virtually abandoned in developed countries for the treatment of RA:
  - Minocycline: In active mild/moderate disease.
  - Auranofin (Ridaura): 6–10 mg/d PO. Slow onset of action. Poor GI tolerability.
  - Injectable gold (Aurolate): Seldom used because of frequent toxicity.
  - D-Penicillamine: 250–1,000 mg/d. Has dose-related side effects. Close monitoring.
  - Protein A immunoadsorption (Prosorba): Removes antibodies. Costly.
  - Cyclosporine: Inhibition of T-cell response. Incremental benefit combined with MTX.
  - Azathioprine: Because of toxicity, reserved for persons not responsive to other DMARDs.

Second Line

- Intra-articular steroids: If disease is well controlled except for a single joint or 2, after establishing that the joint is not infected
- Hyaluronate (Hyalgan): Hyaluronic acid substitute. For pain relief; exact role in RA unclear.

ADDITIONAL TREATMENT

Interdisciplinary care and management to minimize the consequences of loss of function, joint damage, maladaptive coping, and social isolation

General Measures

- The complete remission of disease activity should be the ultimate goal.
- Early, aggressive treatment is desirable to prevent structural damage and disability.
- Key elements include periodical evaluation of disease activity and extent of synovitis.
- Arthritis self-management education is a proven effective intervention.

COMPLEMENTARY AND ALTERNATIVE MEDICINE

Acupuncture and fish oil supplements may relieve pain (7)[A]

SURGERY/OTHER PROCEDURES

Surgical treatment, including synovectomy, tendon reconstruction, joint fusion, and joint replacement are powerful treatment modalities to prevent disability in advanced RA.

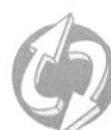

ONGOING CARE

The goals of comprehensive, interdisciplinary care are to stop the disease process, reduce pain, manage symptoms such as fatigue and stiffness, preserve joint integrity and function, and maintain social and occupational roles and quality of life.

FOLLOW-UP RECOMMENDATIONS

- Encourage full activity, but avoid heavy work or exercise during active phases.
- Emphasize exercise, mobility, and reduction of joint stress.
- Promote general health care and psychosocial functional status.

Patient Monitoring

- Address risk factors and evaluate for osteoporosis, a major comorbidity that can result from the disease itself or corticosteroids.
- Cardiovascular disease is the number one cause of death. Evaluate and manage CV risk factors; use low-dose aspirin as a preventive.

DIET

No specific diet recommended

PATIENT EDUCATION

- American College of Rheumatology patient education overviews: www.rheumatology.org/public/factsheets/index.asp?aud=pat
- American Academy of Family Physicians Foundation: www.familydoctor.org
- Arthritis Foundation: www.arthritis.org

PROGNOSIS

- Poor prognostic findings:
  - Persistent moderate-to-severe disease
  - Inheritance of shared epitope
  - Early or advanced age at disease onset
- 50% cannot function in their primary jobs within 10 years of onset.

COMPLICATIONS

Extra-articular involvement: Pulmonary disease, vasculitis, pericarditis, nephropathy, nerve entrapment, muscle atrophy, eye disease, Felty syndrome, chronic anemia

REFERENCES

1. Aletaha D, Neogi T, Silman AJ. Rheumatoid arthritis classification criteria: An American College of Rheumatology/European League against Rheumatism collaborative initiative. *Ann Rheum Dis*. 2010;69:1580–8.
2. Taylor P, Gartemann J, Hsieh J, et al. A systematic review of serum biomarkers anti-cyclic citrullinated Peptide and rheumatoid factor as tests for rheumatoid arthritis. *Autoimmune Dis*. 2011; 2011:815038.
3. Gøtzsche PC, Johansen HK. Short-term low-dose corticosteroids vs. placebo and nonsteroidal antiinflammatory drugs in rheumatoid arthritis. *Cochrane Database Syst Rev*. 2005;(1):CD000189.
4. Suarez-Almazor ME, Belseck E, Shea B, et al. Sulfasalazine for treating rheumatoid arthritis. *Cochrane Database Syst Rev*. 1998;(2):CD000958.
5. Osiri M, Shea B, Robinson V, et al. Leflunomide for treating rheumatoid arthritis. *Cochrane Database Syst Rev*. 2003;(1):CD002047.
6. Suarez-Almazor ME, Belseck E, Shea B, et al. Antimalarials for treating rheumatoid arthritis. *Cochrane Database Syst Rev*. 2000;(4):CD000959.
7. Ernst E, Posadzki P. Complementary and alternative medicine for rheumatoid arthritis and osteoarthritis: An overview of systematic reviews. *Curr Pain Headache Rep*. 2011;15(6):431–7.

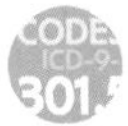

CODES

ICD9

- 714.0 Rheumatoid arthritis
- 714.1 Felty's syndrome
- 714.2 Other rheumatoid arthritis with visceral or systemic involvement

CLINICAL PEARLS

- Females have more articular disease and males have more systemic presentations.
- Morning stiffness with symmetrical joint involvement of wrists and proximal interphalangeal and metacarpophalangeal joints.
- Start DMARDs early if the patient is still having symptoms despite adequate doses of NSAIDS or aspirin, and use a combination of DMARDs.

ARTHROPOD BITES AND STINGS

James Powers, DO, FACEP

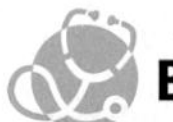

BASICS

DESCRIPTION

Arthropods make up the largest division of the animal kingdom. 2 classes, insects and arachnids, have the greatest medical impact on humans. Arthropods affect humans by inoculating poison or irritative substances through a bite or sting, by invading tissue, or by contact allergy to their skin, hairs or secretions. The greatest medical importance is transmission of infectious microorganisms that may occur during insect feeding. Sequelae to arthropod bites, stings, or contact may include:

- Local redness with itch, pain, and swelling: Common, usually immediate and transient
- Large local reactions increasing over 24–48 hours
- Systemic reactions with anaphylaxis, neurotoxicity, organ damage, or other systemic toxin effects
- Tissue necrosis or secondary infection
- Infectious disease transmission: Presentation may be delayed weeks to years

EPIDEMIOLOGY

Incidence

- Difficult to estimate, as most encounters unreported
- ~50 deaths/yr in the US from fatal anaphylactic reaction to *Hymenoptera* stings
- Unrecognized anaphylactic reactions to *Hymenoptera* stings may be cause of 1/4 of sudden and unexpected deaths outdoors (1).

Prevalence

Widespread, with regional and seasonal variations

RISK FACTORS

- Previous sensitization is key to most severe allergic reactions, but exposure history may not be recalled.
- While most arthropod contact is inadvertent, certain activities, occupations, and travel increase risk.
- Greater risk for adverse outcome in young, elderly, immune compromised, or those with unstable cardiac or respiratory status

Genetics

Family history of atopy may be a factor in the development of more severe allergic reactions.

GENERAL PREVENTION

- Avoidance of common arthropod habitats where possible
- Insect repellents (not effective for bees, spiders, scorpions, caterpillars, bedbugs, fleas, ants):
  - DEET:
    - Most effective broad-spectrum repellent against biting arthropods (2)
    - Formulations with higher concentrations (20–50%) are 1st-line choice when visiting areas where arthropodborne diseases are endemic (2)
    - Apply to skin or outer clothing.
    - Concentrations >30% give longer duration of effect (5+ hours)
    - Appears safe for children >2 months of age at lower concentrations
  - Icaridin (formerly known as Picaridin):
    - Use of concentrations <20% may require more frequent application to maintain effectiveness
    - Less toxic effects on humans than DEET
  - PMD: Component of lemon eucalyptus extract:
    - Recommended alternative repellent to DEET at concentrations >20% (2)
    - Not studied for use in children under age 3
  - IR3535: Less effective in most studies
  - Citronella: Not for disease-endemic areas (2)
  - Other botanical oils: Less effective than DEET
  - Barrier methods: Clothing, bed nets:
    - Use of light-colored pants, long-sleeved shirts, and hats may reduce arthropod impact.
    - Permethrin: Synthetic insecticide derived from Chrysanthemum plant. Should not be applied to skin, but permethrin-impregnated clothing provides good protection against arthropods.
    - Mosquito nets: Insecticide-treated nets advised for all travelers visiting disease-endemic areas at risk from biting arthropods (2)
- Desensitization 75–95% effective for *Hymenoptera*-specific venom:
  - Skin tests are needed to determine sensitivity.
  - Refer to allergist/immunologist if candidate
- Fire ant control (but not elimination) possible:
  - Baits; sprays, dusts, aerosols; biologic agents
- Tickborne diseases prevented by prompt removal of ticks within 24 hours of attachment

PATHOPHYSIOLOGY

4 general categories of pathophysiological effects: toxic, allergic, infectious, traumatic:

- Toxic effects of venom: Local (tissue inflammation or destruction) vs. systemic (neurotoxic or organ damage)
- Allergic: Antigens in saliva may cause local inflammation. Exaggerated immune responses may result in anaphylaxis, serum sickness.
- Trauma: Mechanical injury from biting or stinging causes pain, swelling, and portal of entry for bacteria and secondary infection. Retention of arthropod parts can cause a granulomatous reaction.
- Infection: Arthropods are vectors and can transmit bacterial, viral, and protozoal diseases.

ETIOLOGY

Arthropods: 4 medically important classes:

- Insects: *Hymenoptera* (bees, wasps, hornets, fire ants), mosquitoes, bed bugs, flies, lice, fleas, beetles, caterpillars and moths
- Arachnids: Spiders, scorpions, mites, and ticks
- Chilopods (centipedes)
- Diplopods (millipedes)

DIAGNOSIS

HISTORY

- Sudden onset of pain or itching with visualization of arthropod
- Many cases unknown to patient or asymptomatic initially (bed bugs, lice, scabies, ticks). Consider in patients presenting with localized erythema, urticaria, wheals, papules, pruritus, or bullae.
- May identify insect by its habitat or by remnants brought by patient
- History of prior exposure useful, but not always available or reliable
- Travel, occupational, social, and recreational history important

PHYSICAL EXAM

- If stinger still present in skin, remove by flicking or scraping away from skin.
- Essential to examine for signs and symptoms of anaphylaxis:
  - Erythema, urticaria, angioedema
  - Itching/edema of lips, tongue, uvula; drooling
  - Persistent vomiting
  - Respiratory distress, wheeze, repetitive cough, stridor, dysphonia
  - Hypotension, dysrhythmia, syncope, chest pain
- If anaphylaxis not present, exam focuses on the sting or bite itself. Common findings include local erythema, swelling, wheals, urticaria, papules, or bullae. Excoriations from scratching.
- Thorough exam to look for arthropod infestation (lice, scabies) or attached ticks. Body lice usually found in seams of clothing.
- Signs of secondary bacterial infection after 24–48 hours: Increasing erythema, pain, fever, lymphangitis, or abscess
- Delayed manifestations of insect-borne diseases

DIAGNOSTIC TESTS & INTERPRETATION

Lab

Initial lab tests

Seldom needed; basic lab parameters usually normal. Some findings may help confirm diagnosis of anaphylaxis:

- Plasma histamine levels elevated briefly (5–60 minutes) after mast cell activation
- Metabolite *N*-methyl-histamine elevated in urine for a number of hours (do 24-hour collection)
- Serum tryptase levels peak in 1 hour after anaphylaxis and stay up for 6 hours.

Follow-Up & Special Considerations

- Severe envenomations may affect organ function and require monitoring of lab values.
- Labs for arthropod-borne diseases as indicated:
  - Ticks: Lyme disease, RMSF, relapsing fever, ehrlichiosis, babesiosis, tularemia
  - Flies: Tularemia, leishmaniasis, African trypanosomiasis, bartonellosis, loiasis
  - Chigger mites: Scrub typhus
  - Body lice: Epidemic typhus, relapsing fever
  - Kissing bugs: Chagas disease
  - Mosquitoes: Malaria, yellow fever, dengue fever, West Nile virus, equine encephalitis
- Refer to allergist for formal testing with history of anaphylaxis, significant systemic symptoms, progressively severe reactions

Diagnostic Procedures/Surgery

Various skin tests and immunologic tests available to try to predict anaphylactic risk

DIFFERENTIAL DIAGNOSIS

- Urticaria and localized dermatologic manifestations:
  - Contact dermatitis, drug eruption, mastocytosis, bullous diseases, dermatitis herpetiformis, tinea, eczema, vasculitis, pityriasis, erythema multiforme, viral exanthem, cellulitis, abscess, impetigo, folliculitis
- Anaphylactic-type reactions:
  - Cardiac, hemorrhagic, or septic shock; acute respiratory failure, asthma; angioedema, urticarial vasculitis; flushing syndromes (catecholamines, vasoactive peptides); panic attacks, syncope
- Clinical pearl: Differential diagnosis of the acute abdomen should include black widow spider bite.

TREATMENT

ALERT
- The more rapidly anaphylaxis develops, the more likely the reaction is to be severe and potentially life threatening (3). Most deaths due to anaphylaxis occur within 30–60 minutes of sting.
- Epinephrine should be given as soon as diagnosis of anaphylaxis is suspected (3). Delayed injection of epinephrine is associated with fatal anaphylaxis (4).
- Antihistamines do not replace epinephrine in anaphylaxis, and no direct outcome data regarding their effectiveness in anaphylaxis (3).
- Airway management critical if angioedema

MEDICATION
First Line
- **For arthropod bites/stings with anaphylaxis:**
  - Order of treatment importance: Epinephrine, patient position, oxygen, IV fluids, nebulized therapy, vasopressors, antihistamines, corticosteroids (3)
  - Epinephrine: Most important: IM injection in midanterolateral thigh (vastus lateralis muscle)
    - IM injection: Epinephrine 1:1,000: Give 0.01mg/kg of a 1 mg/mL (1:1,000) dilution to a maximum dose of 0.5 mg in an adult and 0.3 mg in a child. Can repeat every 5–15 minutes (4)[A].
    - IV infusion of epinephrine: For patients poorly responsive to IM epinephrine. No clear dosing regimen in anaphylaxis recognized (3). 1 regimen suggests adding 1 mg (1 mL) of 1:1,000 epinephrine to a 250-cc bag of D5W to produce a 4 mcg/mL concentration. Infuse at 2–10 mcg/min (3)[C].
  - Positioning: Supine with legs elevated (3)
  - Oxygen 6–8 L/min to 100% as needed
  - IV fluids: Establish 1–2 large-bore IV lines. Normal saline rapid bolus 1–2 L IV; repeat as needed (pediatrics 20–30 mL/kg)
  - H1 antihistamines: Diphenhydramine 25–50 mg IV (pediatrics 1–2 mg/kg)
  - B2 agonists: Albuterol for bronchospasm nebulized 2.5–5 mg in 3 mL
  - Emergency treatment of refractory cases: Consider epinephrine infusion, dopamine, glucagon, vasopressin, large-volume crystalloids
- **Arthropod bites/stings without anaphylaxis:**
  - Tetanus booster as indicated
  - Oral antihistamines:
    - Diphenhydramine 25–75 mg q6h (pediatrics 5 mg/kg/d divided q4–6h)
    - Cetirizine 5–10 mg/d age >6 years. 2.5 mg/d if 6 months–2 years; 2.5–5 mg/d if 2–6 years
    - H2 blockers: Ranitidine 150 mg PO b.i.d.; peds 2–4 mg/kg PO b.i.d. no more than 300 mg/d
  - Oral steroids: Consider short course for severe pruritus. Prednisone or prednisolone 1–2 mg/kg once daily
  - Topical intermediate-potency steroid cream or ointment × 3–5 days:
    - Desoximetasone 0.05%
    - Triamcinolone 0.1%
    - Fluocinolone 0.025%
  - Wound care: Antibiotics *only* if infected
  - **Other specific therapies:**
    - Scorpion stings: Treat excess catecholamine release (nitroprusside, prazosin, beta-blockers). Diazepam for muscle spasms. Atropine for hypersalivation. Scorpion antivenom no longer made in US.
    - Black widow bites: Treat muscle spasms with diazepam, opioid analgesics PO or IV. Antivenom: Available for black widow, but should be administered in conjunction with toxicologist. Poison control 1-800-222-1222.
  - Fire ants: Characteristically cause sterile pustules. Leave intact: Do not open or drain.
  - Brown recluse spider: Pain control, supportive treatment. Surgical consult if debridement needed.
  - Ticks: Early removal. Review guidelines for disease prophylaxis.
  - Pediculosis: Head, pubic, and body lice:
    - 1st line: Permethrin 1% (Nix) topical lotion. Apply to affected area, wash off in 10 minutes.
    - Alternatives: Pyrethrin or malathion 0.5% lotion, ivermectin orally
    - Repeat above in 7–10 days
    - For eyelash infestation: Apply ophthalmic-grade petroleum jelly 2 times a day for 10 days.
  - *Sarcoptes scabii* scabies:
    - Permethrin 5% cream: Apply to entire body. Wash off after 8–14 hours. Repeat in 1 week.
    - Ivermectin: 200 mcg/kg PO once; repeat in 2 weeks (not FDA approved for this use)
    - Crotamiton 10% cream or lotion less efficacious; apply daily for 2 days after bathing

Second Line
2nd-line options for anaphylaxis:
- Ranitidine 150 mg IV (pediatrics 1–2 mg/kg)
- Methylprednisolone 125 mg IV (pediatrics 2 mg/kg)

ADDITIONAL TREATMENT
General Measures
Local wound cleansing, ice, elevation

Issues for Referral
Refer to allergist with history of anaphylaxis, severe systemic symptoms, or progressively severe reactions

COMPLEMENTARY AND ALTERNATIVE MEDICINE
- Some stings may be treated with a paste of 3 teaspoons of baking soda and 1 teaspoon water.
- None well tested

SURGERY/OTHER PROCEDURES
Debridement and delayed skin grafting may be needed for brown recluse spider and other bites.

IN-PATIENT CONSIDERATIONS
Admission Criteria
Anaphylaxis, vascular instability, neuromuscular events, pain, GI symptoms, renal damage/failure

ONGOING CARE

FOLLOW-UP RECOMMENDATIONS
- Immunotherapy as recommended by allergist/consultant for anaphylaxis or serious reactions; antivenom therapy is available for *Hymenoptera*.
- Patient-administered epinephrine must be provided to patients with anaphylaxis. Consider med-alert identifiers.

Patient Monitoring
- Monitor for delayed effects, including infectious diseases from arthropod vectors.
- Serum sickness reactions, vasculitis (rare)

PATIENT EDUCATION
Avoidance and prevention. See above.

PROGNOSIS
- Excellent for local reactions
- For systemic reactions, best response with early intervention to prevent cardiorespiratory collapse

COMPLICATIONS
- Scarring
- Secondary bacterial infection
- Arthropod-associated diseases as above
- Psychological effects, phobias

REFERENCES

1. Diaz JH. Recognition, management, and prevention of hymenopteran stings and allergic reactions in travelers. *J Travel Med*. 2009;16(5):357–364.
2. Goodyer LI, Croft AM, Frances SP, et al. Expert review of the evidence base for arthropod bite avoidance. *J Travel Med*. 2010;17(3):182–192.
3. Lieberman P, Nicklas RA, Oppenheimer J, et al. The diagnosis and management of anaphylaxis practice parameter: 2010 update. *J Allergy Clin Immunol*. 2010;126(3):477–80.
4. Simons FER. Anaphylaxis. *J Allergy Clin Immunol*. 2010;125:S161–81.

ADDITIONAL READING

- Demain JG, Minaei AA, Tracy JM. Anaphylaxis and Insect Allergy. *Curr Opin Allergy Clin Immunol*. 2010;10:318–322.
- http://cdc.gov/travel/yellowBookCh2-InsectsArthropods.
- Insect Repellent Use: www.cdc.gov/ncidod/dvbid/westnile/qa/insect_repellent.htm
- Leonard EA, Sheldon IV. Ectoparasitic infections. *Clin Fam Practice*. 2005;7(1):97–104.
- Saucier JR. Arachnid envenomation. *Emerg Med Clin N Am*. 2004;22:405–22.
- Swanson DL, Vetter RS. Bites of brown recluse spiders and suspected necrotic arachnidism. *N Eng J Med*. 2005;352:700–7.

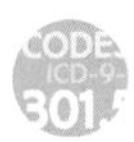

CODES

ICD9
- 919.4 Insect bite, nonvenomous, of other, multiple, and unspecified sites, without mention of infection
- 989.5 Toxic effect of venom

CLINICAL PEARLS
- Urgent administration of epinephrine is key to anaphylaxis treatment.
- Local treatment and symptom management are sufficient in most insect bites and stings.

ASBESTOSIS

Ruben Peralta, MD, FACS

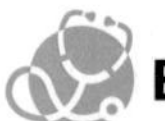

BASICS

DESCRIPTION

- Slowly progressive lung disease caused by inhalation of dust from fibrous silicate asbestos used in insulation, cement, and other building and construction materials
- Nodular interstitial fibrotic lung disease caused by cascade of inflammatory responses to inhaled asbestos fibers:
  - Pleural fibrosis, pleural plaques, and interstitial fibrosis develop.
  - Lung cancer risk is increased.
- Synonym(s): Asbestos pneumoconiosis

EPIDEMIOLOGY

- In the US, an estimated 1.3 million people who work in maintenance and construction are at risk for exposure.
- In a very large part of the world, data on mesothelioma are not available.
- Predominant age: Middle age (40–75 years)
- Predominant sex: Male > Female, due to exposure pattern

RISK FACTORS

- Professional exposures most common in construction workers; those who mine, mill, or remove asbestos; ship builders; textile workers; railroad workers
- Office workers, teachers, and students in buildings with asbestos in place have exposure significantly lower than those of construction workers.
- Dose-response phenomenon: Higher amounts of asbestos exposure are associated with higher risk of asbestosis.
- Cigarette smoking markedly increases risk of radiographic changes and eventual lung cancer risk:
  - Likely mechanism: Decreased clearance of asbestos fibers

Genetics

- Genetic polymorphisms have been implicated (1).
- Familial mesothelioma has been reported.

GENERAL PREVENTION

- In the US, asbestos is federally regulated by the Occupational Health and Safety Administration.
- Primary responsibility of employers is to provide safe work environment (2)
- Exposure control: Substitution of safer materials or adoption of control technologies
- During high-exposure periods, such as building repair, use fit-tested personal respirators for workers.
- To limit exposure to others in their household, those who work with asbestos should leave their clothing at work, if possible. Work clothes should be washed and stored separately from other clothing.

ETIOLOGY

- Asbestos fibers are inhaled. Macrophages engulf the fibers and release inflammatory mediators. Inflammatory mediators cause fibroblast proliferation, leading to fibrosis and remodeling of interstitial lung tissue, including intra-alveolar fibrosis and loss of alveolar capillary units.
- Disease continues to slowly progress over the course of years, even if exposure is not ongoing (2).
- Symptoms may be related to impaired gas exchange and/or a pattern of restrictive lung disease.

COMMONLY ASSOCIATED CONDITIONS

In addition to asbestosis, inhalation of asbestos is associated with several lung problems (3), including:

- Benign plaques
- Benign pleural effusions
- Lung cancer
- Malignant mesothelioma

DIAGNOSIS

HISTORY

- Credible history of exposure (usually occupational) to asbestos fibers (4,5):
  - Ask about intensity and duration of exposure.
  - Aircraft or electrical maintenance
  - Shipyard workers
  - Those exposed to cement or building materials
  - Asbestos mining
  - People exposed to asbestos when it is disrupted during building maintenance
  - Family members of those who work with asbestos
- In addition to job type and activities and length of exposure, ask patients whether there was visible dust in air or on surfaces, visible dust in sputum, personal protective equipment used, and whether the workplace was cleaned during or after a shift.
- Common symptoms include:
  - Dyspnea upon exertion
  - Nonproductive cough
- Delay from exposure to detection typically becomes clinically apparent 10–15 years after exposure.

PHYSICAL EXAM

- Insidious onset
- Progressive dyspnea is the most common symptom.
- Dry cough
- Progressive exercise intolerance
- Pleuritic chest pain
- Inspiratory crackles (may be best heard laterally)
- Wheeze with forced exhalation
- Digital clubbing and cyanosis in advanced disease
- Right-sided heart failure

DIAGNOSTIC TESTS & INTERPRETATION

Pulmonary function testing:

- Not diagnostically specific
- Mainly restrictive pattern unless a smoker (6)
- Decreased total lung capacity and vital capacity
- Reduction in diffusing capacity to carbon monoxide
- Useful for following level of impairment

Lab

No pathognomonic lab findings

Imaging

- Chest x-ray (CXR) (sensitivity 90%, specificity 93%):
  - Most common findings are bilateral pleural thickening and circumscribed calcified pleural plaques
  - Pleural plaques usually posterior-lateral, may also involve diaphragm
  - As disease progresses, small, irregular, linear opacities with a fine reticular pattern are seen.
  - Less common: Rounded atelectasis (Blesovsky syndrome) when fibrosis of visceral pleura extends into parenchyma
- Classification scheme available through International Labour Office (http://www.ilo.org)
- High-resolution CT may increase sensitivity to near 100%:
  - Improves detection of interstitial fibrosis
  - May show honeycombing in later stages of the disease
- Gallium scan with higher uptake even if the CXR and CT are normal

Pathological Findings

- Lung biopsy or bronchoalveolar lavage (BAL) can reveal asbestos fibers or asbestos bodies:
  - May help diagnostically in cases with history of minimal exposure or with atypical clinical or radiographic features
  - Transbronchial biopsy is less reliable than BAL or open-lung biopsy in establishing diagnosis.
- Pleural plaques are found in parietal pleura; made up of collagen bundles with rare inflammatory cells. Pleural thickening involves the visceral pleura.
- Asbestos bodies may be seen with iron staining in intra-alveolar macrophages.

DIFFERENTIAL DIAGNOSIS

Other pneumoconioses:

- Idiopathic pulmonary fibrosis
- Hypersensitivity pneumonitis
- Sarcoidosis
- Other pneumoconiosis, including mixed exposures

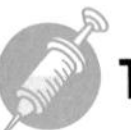

TREATMENT

MEDICATION

First Line

- No specific pharmacologic treatment
- Oxygen
- Bronchodilators for pulmonary toilet

Second Line

- Antibiotics for respiratory infections
- Diuretics if cor pulmonale develops

ADDITIONAL TREATMENT

General Measures

- As of now, there is no effective treatment to reverse the course of the disease.
- Clinical approach is directed at amelioration of symptoms, elimination of progression, and reduction of risk of associated disorders.
- Withdrawal from exposure:
  - Workers with no symptoms and only radiographic changes may make an informed choice to continue employment using maximum environmental and personal protection.
- Smoking cessation:
  - Cigarette smokers have more radiographic signs of disease and have a significantly increased risk for lung cancer.
- Pneumococcal and influenza vaccines
- Chest physiotherapy as needed
- Home oxygen as needed

Issues for Referral

All new cases must be reported to health authorities.

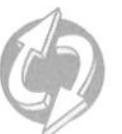

ONGOING CARE

Follow World Health Organization (WHO) recommendations for regular health screening of exposed workers:

- CXR film at baseline
- For workers with <10 years since 1st exposure: CXR every 3–5 years
- >10 years: CXR every 1–2 years
- >20 years: CXR annually
- All workers: Annual respiratory symptom questionnaire, physical exam, and spirometry (alternatively can be done on CXR schedule)

FOLLOW-UP RECOMMENDATIONS

Patient Monitoring

- CXR
- Occasional pulmonary function tests
- Prompt treatment of infections

DIET

High-calorie, high-protein with advanced disease

PATIENT EDUCATION

- Smoking cessation counseling as needed
- In the US, asbestos has been federally regulated by the Occupational Health and Safety Administration since 1972: http://www.osha.gov.
- Printed patient information available from the National Cancer Institute: http://www.cancer.gov/cancertopics/factsheet/Risk/asbestos
- Agency for Toxic Substances and Disease Registry: http://www.atsdr.cdc.gov

PROGNOSIS

- Severity depends on duration and intensity of exposure (5).
- Lung disease is irreversible.
- Increased risk for lung cancer (synergistic increase with cigarette smoking) and mesothelioma

COMPLICATIONS

- Mesothelioma:
  - Related to dose, time elapsed from exposure (usually 25–40 years after exposure)
  - Risk is higher with exposure to amphibole fibers rather than chrysotile fibers.
  - Pleural effusion in 80–95%
  - Insidious but progressive. Median survival for mesothelioma is 8–18 months.
- Lung cancer risk is associated with asbestos exposure, whether asbestosis is present or not; synergistically increased risk in asbestos workers who smoke.
- GI cancer risk may also be increased with asbestos exposure.

REFERENCES

1. Helmig S, Belwe A, Schneider J. Association of transforming growth factor beta1 gene polymorphisms and asbestos-induced fibrosis and tumors. *J Investig Med*. 2009;57(5):655–61.
2. Centers for Disease Control and Prevention (CDC). Asbestosis-related years of potential life lost before age 65 years—United States, 1968–2005. *MMWR Morb Mortal Wkly Rep*. 2008;57:1321–5.
3. Toyokuni S. Mechanisms of asbestos-induced carcinogenesis. *Nagoya J Med Sci*. 2009;71:1–10.
4. Banks DE, Shi R, McLarty J, et al. American College of Chest Physicians consensus statement on the respiratory health effects of asbestos. Results of a Delphi study. *Chest*. 2009;135:1619–27.
5. Deng Q, Wang X, Wang M, et al. Exposure-response relationship between chrysotile exposure and mortality from lung cancer and asbestosis. *Occup Environ Med*. 2011.
6. Abejie BA, Wang X, Kales SN, et al. Patterns of pulmonary dysfunction in asbestos workers: A cross-sectional study. *J Occup Med Toxicol*. 2010;5:12.

ADDITIONAL READING

- Antonescu-Turcu AL, Schapira RM. Parenchymal and airway diseases caused by asbestos. *Curr Opin Pulm Med*. 2010;16:155–61.
- Brody AR. Asbestos and lung disease. *Am J Respir Cell Mol Biol*. 2010;42:131–2.
- Kamp DW. Asbestos-induced lung diseases: An update. *Transl Res*. 2009;153:143–52.

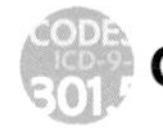

CODES

ICD9

- 501 Asbestosis
- 515 Postinflammatory pulmonary fibrosis

CLINICAL PEARLS

- Associations between asbestos and all histologic subtypes of lung cancer have been observed.
- Detection of asbestosis due to asbestos exposure does not typically become clinically apparent until 10–15 years after exposure.
- Higher amounts of asbestos exposure are associated with higher risk of asbestosis.
- Smoking cessation is particularly important, because cigarette smokers have more radiographic signs of asbestosis and are at a synergistically increased risk for lung cancer.
- For those who work with asbestos, to limit exposure to others in their household, clothing should either be left at work or should be washed and stored separately from other clothing.

ASCITES

Mohammed A. Razvi, BA
Marie Borum, MD, EdD, MPH

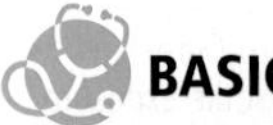

BASICS

DESCRIPTION

Pathologic accumulation of fluid in the peritoneal cavity; may occur in any condition that causes generalized edema

EPIDEMIOLOGY

- Children: Nephrotic syndrome and malignancy most common
- Adults: Cirrhosis, heart failure, nephrotic syndrome, peritonitis most common
- ~85% of all cases of ascites are caused by liver cirrhosis.

Incidence

~50% of patients with cirrhosis will develop ascites within 10 years.

RISK FACTORS

Remote or current alcohol ingestion, history of IV drug use

ETIOLOGY

- **Acute liver failure**
- **Hepatitis** (alcoholic, viral, autoimmune, drugs)
- **Peritoneal infection and inflammation:**
  - Bacterial infection (foreign body, fistula)
  - Tuberculosis
  - Fungal disease
  - Parasitic infection
  - Perforated viscus
  - Granulomatous peritonitis (e.g., sarcoidosis)
- **Metabolic diseases:**
  - Cirrhosis
  - Prehepatic and posthepatic portal hypertension
  - Nephrotic syndrome
  - Myxedema
  - Dialysis-related
  - Protein malnutrition (hypoalbuminemia <2 g/dL)
- **Cardiac congestion:**
  - Congestive heart failure (CHF)
  - Constrictive pericarditis
- **Trauma:**
  - Pancreatic or biliary fistula
  - Lymphatic tear (chylous ascites)
  - Hemoperitoneum (trauma, ectopic pregnancy, tumor)
- **Malignancy:**
  - Peritoneal seeding: Ovarian, colon, pancreas, others
  - Primary peritoneal carcinoma
  - Leukemia, lymphoma
- **Mixed** (more than 1 of the above causes, e.g., cirrhosis and cancer)

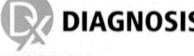

DIAGNOSIS

HISTORY

- Abdominal or flank pain
- Enlarged abdomen
- Anorexia
- Nausea
- Early satiety
- Heartburn
- Weight gain
- Dyspnea/orthopnea
- Edema

PHYSICAL EXAM

- Abdominal distention
- Bulging flanks
- Abdominal fluid wave
- Shifting dullness or "puddle sign" (dullness over dependent abdomen)
- Edema (penile/scrotal, pedal)
- Umbilical/inguinal herniae
- Pleural effusion
- Rales
- Peripheral stigmata of cirrhosis/liver disease (palmar erythema, spider angiomata, gynecomastia)

DIAGNOSTIC TESTS & INTERPRETATION

Lab

Ascitic fluid should be sampled in all new-onset, new-to-treat, or hospitalized cases (1)[B]:

- Obtain in all:
  - Total cell count :
    - Polymorphonuclear leukocytes: ≥250 mm^3 suggests infection (even if culture is negative) requiring antibiotics
  - Albumin in both serum and ascites: Calculate serum-to-ascites albumin gradient (SAAG):
    - <1.1 g indicates exudate (i.e., inflammatory, biliary/pancreatic, carcinomatosis)
    - ≥1.1 g indicates transudate/portal hypertension
  - Protein: >2 g (some sources cite 2.5 g) indicates exudate
- Of use in specific circumstances:
  - Culture if infection suspected (fever, abdominal pain, hypotension, etc.)
  - Amylase, triglycerides, glucose
  - Lactate dehydrogenase
  - Gram stain, acid-fast stain, or fungal cultures/smears
  - Cytology to evaluate for peritoneal carcinomatosis; three 20–50 cc fluid samples should be processed immediately
- Blood tests:
  - BUN/creatinine
  - Electrolytes
- Urine tests:
  - Sodium levels in single sample:
    - <10 mEq/L (<10 mmol/L) diuretic response unlikely
    - >10–70 mEq/L (>10–70 mmol/L) diuretic response likely
    - >70 mEq/L (>70 mmol/L) diuretics unnecessary
- Other labs as indicated by underlying condition (liver enzymes, tumor markers, etc.)

Imaging

Initial approach

- Abdominal US highly sensitive, cost-effective, no radiation, available at bedside (2)[A]
- CT scan to rule out intra-abdominal pathology
- MRI best for evaluation of liver disease and presence of hepatoma

Diagnostic Procedures/Surgery

- Diagnostic paracentesis: Complication rate of 1% despite high prevalence of abnormal coagulation parameters, no benefit to use of plasma or platelet transfusions (2)[A]
- Laparoscopic peritoneal biopsy needed for definitive diagnosis of tuberculosis peritonitis

Pathological Findings

- Peritoneal biopsy may reveal tuberculosis or malignancy; of no value in other types of fluid
- Cytology may reveal malignant cells: Typically adenocarcinoma (ovary, breast, GI tract); rarely primary peritoneal carcinoma

DIFFERENTIAL DIAGNOSIS

- If transudate (SAAG ≥1.1 g), likely causes include:
  - Cirrhosis
  - Congestive heart failure
  - Constrictive pericarditis
  - Budd-Chiari syndrome
  - Nephrotic syndrome
  - Protein malnutrition/hypoalbuminemia
- If exudate (SAAG <1.1 g), likely causes include:
  - Neoplasm
  - Tuberculosis
  - Pancreatitis
  - Biliary pathology
  - Myxedema

TREATMENT

- Outpatient or inpatient, depending on physical condition
- For all patients:
  - Daily record of weight to monitor gains and losses
  - Sodium restriction required (1)[A]:
    - 2 g/d until renal excretion improves, usually required 3–6 months
  - Water restriction generally not helpful, only necessary if serum sodium <120 mEq/L
  - Creatinine >2.0 mg/dL: Decrease diuretic doses, peritoneal paracentesis

MEDICATION

ALERT

Carefully approach diuresis; too aggressive diuresis can induce hepatorenal syndrome. Monitor creatinine and electrolytes closely.

First Line

- Diuretics needed in nearly all patients:
  - Spironolactone 100–400 mg daily PO in single dose best for minimal ascites in outpatient setting; typical initial dose is 100–200 mg given in A.M.
  - Furosemide 20–160 mg daily PO best for refractory ascites; typical initial dose is 40 mg given in A.M.
  - May use spironolactone and furosemide together for max efficacy, maintains normokalemia, most patients will require combination therapy eventually
  - Dose should be sufficient to obtain net sodium loss in urine.
  - Discontinue NSAIDs except 81-mg dose of aspirin.
  - Follow body weight daily. If there is a <2-pound loss in the next 4 days, increase either spironolactone by 100 mg or furosemide by 40 mg. If the 2-pound weight loss continues in the next 4 days, continue with the same dose. Emphasize sodium restriction.
  - Spot Na in mEq/L × estimated urine output (1 L if no information) should equal estimated dietary Na. Increase diuretics daily until this goal is attained. Measure serum electrolytes before each dose change.

- Precautions:
  - In hospital or in rapid diuresis, observe creatinine and electrolytes closely. NSAIDs may worsen or initiate oliguria or azotemia.
  - Spironolactone or amiloride may cause hyperkalemia; monitor serum potassium
  - Observe patients closely for signs of volume depletion, encephalopathy, and renal insufficiency.
- Significant possible interactions: Avoid concomitant potassium supplements if spironolactone used alone.

Second Line

Alternative diuretics unlikely to succeed if combinations of spironolactone and furosemide fail or result in increased BUN/creatinine:

- Most commonly used in cases of GI intolerance or allergic reactions
- Alternatives to spironolactone: Amiloride up to 10 mg/d; triamterene up to 200 mg/d in divided doses
- Alternatives to furosemide: Torsemide up to 100 mg/d; ethacrynic acid 50 mg IV (may be effective when oral drugs cannot be used)

ADDITIONAL TREATMENT

General Measures

- For ascites with edema:
  - Salt restriction and diuretics usually effective
  - Maximum weight loss of 5 lb/d
  - Draw weekly serum electrolytes during rapid weight loss.
- For ascites without edema:
  - Dietary restrictions and diuretics as above
  - Maximum weight loss of 2 lb/d
- Refractory ascites:
  - Confirm patient compliance with adequate Na restriction (most common cause)
- Diuretic-intractable ascites (10% of patients): Worse despite max doses spironolactone (400 mg/d) and furosemide (160–200 mg/d) and sodium restriction OR progressive rise in creatinine to 2.0:
  - Serial large volume paracentesis, performed every 10–14 days, 5–10 L per session:
    - Complications: Infection, hemodynamic collapse, renal failure
    - Replace albumin IV for all removals >5 L at rate of 8 g albumin for each liter removed; has been shown to decrease renal dysfunction and overall morbidity (2)[A]
  - Continue diuretics at 1/2 previous dose.

Issues for Referral

Referral to liver transplant center in patients with cirrhosis and ascites may be appropriate (2)[B].

COMPLEMENTARY AND ALTERNATIVE MEDICINE

Caution patients to avoid herbs and other supplements unless approved by health care provider (risk drug interactions, hepatotoxicity, coagulopathy).

SURGERY/OTHER PROCEDURES

- Transjugular intrahepatic portosystemic shunt (TIPS):
  - Transjugular conduit from the liver to the hepatic vein used for intractable ascites; placed by interventional radiologists under fluoroscopy (3)[A]:
    - At time of placement, measure portal pressure; should drop ≥20 mm Hg or to <12 mm Hg, and ascites should be readily controlled with diuretics. Conduct yearly US study to confirm functional shunt; evaluate with increased ascites.
    - Dilation/replacement may be required after >2 years.
    - Encephalopathy is a known complication; superior to paracentesis in control of ascites, no difference in mortality (2)[A]
- Surgical portacaval shunt: An 8–10-mm mesenteric caval shunt often is effective:
  - Significant operative mortality, morbidity, encephalopathy; most experts prefer TIPS, rarely used in the US due to greater risks (3)[C]
- When recurrent pleural effusion is present in patient with chronic ascites, fusing of pleural surfaces is sometimes performed. Alternative is TIPS.
- Liver transplant referral should be considered in patients with decompensated liver disease, whether or not ascites is present/controlled; definitive treatment of portal HTN

ONGOING CARE

FOLLOW-UP RECOMMENDATIONS

Patient Monitoring

- Daily body weight
- Closely follow creatinine and electrolytes when initiating diuresis and 1 week after change in dose/type of diuretic
- Mental status to assess for encephalopathy

DIET

Consultation with dietician helpful:

- Sodium restriction, 2 g/d, monitored
- Fluid restriction (1–1.5 L/d) only if dilutional hyponatremia (Na <120 mEq/L)
- Complete abstinence from alcohol and adequate nutrition if liver disease

PROGNOSIS

- Varies depending on underlying cause
- Rarely life-threatening in itself, but may be a sign of life-threatening disease (e.g., cancer, end-stage liver disease):
  - Conservative therapy usually successful if cause is reversible or treatable (e.g., infection)

COMPLICATIONS

- Spontaneous bacterial peritonitis (SBP):
  - Ascitic fluid cell count ≥250, polymorphonuclear leukocytes, fever, clinical deterioration. Treat with 3rd-generation cephalosporin or comparable antibiotic; combined antibiotic treatment plus IV albumin results in improved survival in some patients (4)[B].
  - Lifetime antibiotic prophylaxis with norfloxacin or similar antibiotic is indicated in some patients who survive an episode of SBP (1)[A].
  - No antibiotic prophylaxis is necessary for patients with cirrhotic ascites and no GI bleeding, as there is concern of developing resistant pathogens and transplant complication (1)[B].
  - GI bleeding and cirrhosis: IV ceftriaxone for 7 days to prevent bacterial infection (1)[A]
- Overly aggressive diuresis may lead to hypokalemia, encephalopathy; intravascular volume depletion may lead to azotemia, hepatorenal syndrome
- Hepatorenal syndrome:
  - Acute renal failure secondary to decreased intravascular volume in ascites
  - May be induced by aggressive diuresis or paracentesis
  - Urine volume <500 mL/d, decreasing urine sodium, rising BUN, and creatinine >1.5 mg/dL
  - Stop all diuretics; IV fluid challenge of 1.5 L plasma expander after 1 day if no improvement. Vasopressors (e.g., terlipressin IV every 4–6 hours) may resolve renal failure in 50% of patients (5)[B].
- Hydrothorax: Always on right side; cell and lab properties same as ascites. Treat ascites vigorously; if hydrothorax does not disappear, consider TIPS. Chest tube rarely helpful in acute setting.

REFERENCES

1. Runyon BA, Practice Guidelines Committee, American Association for the Study of Liver Diseases (AASLD). Management of adult patients with ascites due to cirrhosis. *Hepatology*. 2009;49:2087–2107.
2. Reshamwala PA. Management of ascites. *Crit Care Nurs Clin North Am*. 2010;22(3):309–14.
3. Salerno F, Guevara M, Bernardi M, et al. Refractory ascites: pathogenesis, definition and therapy of a severe complication in patients with cirrhosis. *Liver Int*. 2010;30(7):937–47.
4. Hou W, Sanyal AJ. Ascites: Diagnosis and management. *Med Clin North Am*. 2009;93(4): 801–17, vii.
5. European Association for the Study of the Liver. EASL Clinical Practice Guidelines on the management of ascites, spontaneous bacterial peritonitis, and hepatorenal syndrome in cirrhosis. *J Hepatol*. 2010;53(3):397–417.

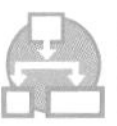

See Also (Topic, Algorithm, Electronic Media Element)

- Cirrhosis of the Liver; Congestive Heart Failure; Nephrotic Syndrome; Hepatorenal Syndrome
- Algorithm: Cirrhosis

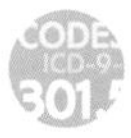

CODES

ICD9

- 789.51 Malignant ascites
- 789.59 Other ascites

CLINICAL PEARLS

- Diuretics are used for clinically significant ascites; spironolactone, alone or in combination with furosemide, is a highly effective treatment.
- US is highly sensitive to detect ascites, but use CT to rule-out intra-abdominal pathology and MRI if evaluating liver disease.
- Most common cause of "refractory ascites" is noncompliance with dietary sodium restriction.
- SAAG <1.1 g indicates exudate (i.e., inflammatory, biliary/pancreatic, carcinomatosis); ≥1.1 g indicates transudate/portal HTN.

ASTHMA

Fozia A. Ali, MD

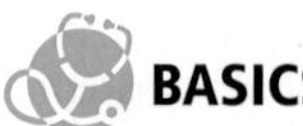

BASICS

DESCRIPTION

- Chronic, reversible inflammatory airway disease
- 4 major classifications of asthma severity used primarily to initiate therapy (1,2):
  - Intermittent: Symptoms ≤2 days/week, nighttime awakenings ≤2×/month, short-acting β-agonist use ≤2 days/week, no interference with normal activity, and normal FEV1 between exacerbations with FEV1 (predicted) >80% and FEV1/FVC >85%
  - Mild persistent: Symptoms >2 days/week but not daily, nighttime awakenings 1–4×/month, short-acting β-agonist use >2 days/week but not daily, minor limitations in normal activity, and FEV1 (predicted) >80% and FEV1/FVC >80%
  - Moderate persistent: Daily symptoms, nighttime awakenings 3–4×/month or ≥1×/week but not nightly, depending on age, daily use of short-acting β-agonist, some limitation in normal activity, and FEV1 (predicted) 60–80% and FEV1/FVC 75–80%
  - Severe persistent: Symptoms throughout the day, nighttime awakenings >1×/week, short-acting β-agonist use several times a day, extremely limited normal activity, and FEV1 (predicted) <60% and FEV1/FVC <75%

EPIDEMIOLOGY

Prevalence

- One of the most common chronic diseases of childhood, affecting 6 million children
- In children, more common in boys than girls
- In adults, more common in women than men

Pregnancy Considerations

- In the US, 3.7–8.4% of pregnant women are affected. Maternal asthma complicates approximately 4–8% of all pregnancies.

Geriatric Considerations

Prevalence of asthma in seniors (>age 65) is 5.3%

RISK FACTORS

- Host factors: Genetic predisposition, gender, race, body mass index
- Environmental exposures: Viral infections, airborne allergens, tobacco smoke, etc.
- Patients with food allergies and asthma are at increased risk for fatal anaphylaxis from those foods.

Genetics

- Inheritable component with complex genetics
- Active area of research: Treatments may be directed to specific genotypes.

GENERAL PREVENTION

- Eliminate or modify exposure to asthma triggers.
- Consider allergen immunotherapy when indicated.
- Treat comorbidities such as allergic rhinitis.
- Annual influenza vaccine (inactivated influenza vaccine) is recommended for all patients <6 months (3).
- Patients at risk for anaphylaxis should carry an EpiPen.

PATHOPHYSIOLOGY

- Inflammatory cell infiltration, sub-basement fibrosis, mucus hypersecretion, epithelial injury, smooth muscle hypertrophy, angiogenesis
- Remodeling of airways may occur (1).

ETIOLOGY

Host and environmental factors

COMMONLY ASSOCIATED CONDITIONS

- Atopy: Eczema, allergic conjunctivitis, allergic rhinitis
- Obesity (associated with higher asthma rates)
- Sinusitis
- Gastroesophageal reflux disease (GERD)
- Obstructive sleep apnea (OSA)
- Allergic bronchopulmonary aspergillosis (rare)
- Stress/depression

DIAGNOSIS

It is important to classify asthma severity.

HISTORY

Symptoms include:

- Cough (particularly if worse at night)
- Wheeze
- Chest tightness
- Difficulty breathing

PHYSICAL EXAM

- May be normal
- Focus on:
  - General appearance: Signs of respiratory distress such as use of accessory muscles
  - Upper respiratory tract: Rhinitis, nasal polyps, swollen nasal turbinates
  - Lower respiratory tract: Wheezing, prolonged expiratory phase
  - Skin: Eczema

DIAGNOSTIC TESTS & INTERPRETATION

Lab

Initial lab tests

- Spirometry: Does not rule out disease
- Peak expiratory flow rates are inappropriate for diagnosis.

Follow-Up & Special Considerations

- Bronchoprovocation (methacholine, histamine, cold air, or exercise) is the only definitive diagnostic test.
- Asthma Action Plan: Patients monitor their own symptoms and/or peak flow measurements.

Imaging

Initial approach

Chest x-ray is used to exclude alternative diagnoses and to evaluate patients for complicating cardiopulmonary processes.

Diagnostic Procedures/Surgery

- Allergy skin testing may be considered to evaluate atopic triggers.
- Sweat testing if diagnosis of cystic fibrosis
- Arterial blood gases is indicated for patients with respiratory distress and hypoxia.

Pathological Findings

Inflammatory cell infiltration, edema, goblet cell hyperplasia, smooth muscle hyperplasia, thickened basement membrane

DIFFERENTIAL DIAGNOSIS

- In children:
  - Upper airway diseases (allergic rhinitis or sinusitis)
  - Large airway obstruction (foreign-body aspiration, vocal cord dysfunction, vascular ring or laryngeal web, laryngotracheomalacia, lymph nodes or tumor)
  - Small airway obstruction (viral bronchiolitis, cystic fibrosis, bronchopulmonary dysplasia, heart disease)
  - Other causes (recurrent cough *not* due to asthma, aspiration/GERD)
- In adults:
  - Chronic obstructive pulmonary disease, congestive heart failure, pulmonary embolism, benign or malignant tumor, pulmonary infiltration with eosinophilia, drugs such as an ACE inhibitor, vocal cord dysfunction

TREATMENT

MEDICATION

First Line

Short-acting β-agonist (SABA) for quick relief of acute symptoms and for prevention of exercise-induced bronchospasm

ALERT

- Delivery of SABA and other inhaled agents via "spacer" or holding chamber (AeroChamber, OptiChamber, others) provides increased efficacy with decreased side effects when compared to nebulized delivery. Reserve nebulized delivery of medication for those unable to use spacer (infants, those intubated, etc.).
- All short-acting agents are pregnancy Category C.
- Specific medicines include albuterol, levalbuterol (Xopenex), metaproterenol (Alupent) Pirbuterol (Maxair) (4)
- Anticholinergic agent:
  - Ipratropium bromide: Used in combination with SABA for added benefit in emergency situations
- Systemic corticosteroids can be used:
  - In moderate-to-severe asthma as adjunct
  - In patients with all but the mildest of acute asthma exacerbations (5)[A]
  - Steroids should be prescribed for up to 7 days in adults and for 3 days in children with no need for tapering.
  - Use corticosteroid doses of prednisolone 1–2 mg/kg/d or equivalent.

Second Line

For long-term control (4):

- Inhaled corticosteroids (ICS):
  - Preferred long-term controller therapy for children and adults with persistent asthma and persistent asthma during pregnancy

Pregnancy Considerations

- Most ICS agents are pregnancy Category C, except budesonide, which is Category B.
- Long-acting β_2-agonists (LABA):
  - Should not be used as monotherapy
  - Salbutamol or formoterol
- Combination products, including a LABA and ICS, are available and offer additional control over ICS alone; preferred in moderate persistent asthma.
- Leukotriene receptor agonists: Alternative, not preferred for mild persistent asthma:
  - Montelukast or
  - Zafirlukast (patients ≥7 years)

- Lipoxygenase pathway inhibitor: Alternative not preferred for adjunctive treatment in adults:
  - Zileuton (patients ≥12 years)
- Theophylline alternative not preferred as adjunctive therapy with inhaled corticosteroids
- Cromolyn sodium and nedocromil are alternatives, but not a preferred option.
- Immunomodulators:
  - Omalizumab: Adjunctive not preferred therapy for patients ≥12 years with allergies and severe persistent asthma

ADDITIONAL TREATMENT

General Measures

- Identify triggers and control exposures.
- Identify patients at risk for reactions to aspirin and NSAIDs, and avoid exposure.

Issues for Referral

Referral to an asthma specialist (either a pulmonologist or an allergist) should be considered:

- Diagnosis unclear
- Additional asthma education needed
- Comorbidities: Rhinitis, GERD, sinusitis, OSA
- Specialized testing (bronchoprovocation, skin testing, etc.)
- Specialized treatments (e.g., immunotherapy, anti-IgE therapy)
- Moderate-to-severe persistent asthma in adults
- Moderate-to-persistent asthma in children
- Not well-controlled or very poorly controlled asthma: Multiple emergency room visits for asthma

Additional Therapies

- Allergen immunotherapy
- Omalizumab (Xolair): Anti-IgE therapy

COMPLEMENTARY AND ALTERNATIVE MEDICINE

Patients should be cautioned regarding the potential for harmful ingredients and for interactions with recommended asthma medications.

IN-PATIENT CONSIDERATIONS

Initial Stabilization

- Supplemental oxygen to correct hypoxemia
- Repeated doses or continuous administration of SABA (1)[A]
- Ipratropium bromide may be used in the emergency room, but is not recommended for inpatient treatment (1)[B].
- Systemic corticosteroids for moderate or severe exacerbations or poor response to SABA (1)[A]
- Adjunctive therapy with $MgSO_4$ or Heliox may be considered in severe cases, but not routinely (1,6)[B].

Admission Criteria

No single measure is predictive:

- Dyspnea
- Hypoxia
- Poor or no response to SABA
- Peak expiratory flow rate (PEFR) or FEV_1 <40%
- Decision for admission should be based on duration and severity of symptoms, severity of airflow obstruction, response to emergency department treatment, course and severity of prior exacerbations, access to medical care and medication, and adequacy of home condition (1).

IV Fluids

- Avoid aggressive hydration in older children and adults.
- Monitor electrolytes.

Nursing

- Careful respiratory monitoring, including vital signs, pulse oximetry, response and duration of response to SABA, and, when possible, an objective measure of lung function such as PEF or FEV1
- Asthma education

Discharge Criteria

- Minimal or absent asthma symptoms
- Hypoxia has resolved
- FEV1 or PEF ≥70% predicted or personal best
- Bronchodilator response sustained ≥60 minutes

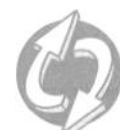

ONGOING CARE

FOLLOW-UP RECOMMENDATIONS

Smoking cessation counseling or elimination of secondhand smoke, if applicable

Patient Monitoring

- Quality-of-life measures: Impact on activities, sleep, emergency visits, hospitalizations, etc.
- Pharmacotherapy: Efficacy, compliance, side effects, technique
- Lung function: Peak flow is an inexpensive and easily available monitoring device once the diagnosis of asthma has been established.

DIET

Food allergies and sulfites (in food and wine) can precipitate symptoms for some patients. GERD precautions may be helpful with both symptomatic reflux and in those who are asymptomatic for reflux but with poorly controlled or nocturnal asthma.

PATIENT EDUCATION

- Patients' technique for using inhaled medications should be reviewed at every visit.
- American Academy of Allergy, Asthma & Immunology: 1-800-822-2762 or http://www.aaaai.org
- American Lung Association: http://www.lungusa.org
- Food Allergy & Anaphylaxis Network: http://www.foodallergy.org
- Asthma and Allergy Foundation of America: 1-800-727-8462 or http:www.aafa.org

PROGNOSIS

- Risk factors for persistent asthma (in children <3 years of age with ≥4 episodes of wheezing in preceding year): Either history of asthma in ≥1 parent or documented atopic dermatitis or aeroallergen sensitivity
- Alternatively, ≥2 of the following will also place these children at increased risk:
  - Food sensitivity
  - ≥4% peripheral eosinophilia
  - Wheezing episodes unrelated to upper respiratory tract infections
- Asthma worsens in 1/3 of women during pregnancy and improves in another 1/3.

COMPLICATIONS

- Atelectasis
- Pneumonia
- Air leak syndromes: Pneumomediastinum, pneumothorax
- Medication-specific side effects/adverse effects/interactions
- Respiratory failure
- Death: ~50% of asthma deaths occur in the elderly (age >65 years), and mortality is increasing in that population (7).

REFERENCES

1. National Asthma Education and Prevention Program Expert Panel Report 3, Guidelines for the Diagnosis and Management of Asthma. No. 08-5846 Washington DC: NIH, 2007.
2. Reddel HK, Taylor DR, Bateman ED, et al. An official American Thoracic Society/European Respiratory Society statement: Asthma control and exacerbations: standardizing endpoints for clinical asthma trials and clinical practice. *Am J Respir Crit Care Med*. 2009;180:59–99.
3. Centers for Disease Control and Prevention. Recommended adult immunization schedule – United States 2009. *MMWR*. 2008;57(53).
4. Fanta CH. Asthma. *N Engl J Med*. 2009;360: 1002–14.
5. Doherty S. Prescribe systemic corticosteroids in acute asthma. *BMJ*. 2009;338:b1234.
6. McGarvey JM, Pollack CV. Heliox in airway management. *Emerg Med Clin North Am*. 2008;26:905–20, viii.
7. Stupka E, deShazo R. Asthma in seniors: Part 1 evidence for underdiagnosis, undertreatment and increasing morbidity and mortality. *Am J Med*. 2009;122(1):6–11.

ADDITIONAL READING

- American Lung Association. http://www.lungusa.org
- Dombrowski M, Schatz M; ACOC Committee on Practice Bulletins-Obstetrics. ACOG practice bulletin: Clinical management guidelines for obstetrician-gynecologists number 90, February 2008: Asthma in pregnancy. *Obstet Gynecol*. 2008;111(2 Part 1): 457–64.
- Global Strategy for Asthma Management and prevention, 2006. At: http://www.ginasthma.org

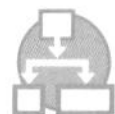

See Also (Topic, Algorithm, Electronic Media Element)

Algorithm: Asthma Exacerbation, Pediatric Acute

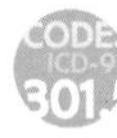

CODES

ICD9

- 493.00 Extrinsic asthma, unspecified
- 493.90 Asthma, unspecified
- 493.92 Asthma, unspecified, with (acute) exacerbation

CLINICAL PEARLS

- Asthma is a chronic, reversible inflammatory airway disease whose exacerbations are characterized by reversible bronchoconstriction, airway hyper-responsiveness, and airway edema.
- Short-acting β-agonist (SABA) is the most effective rescue therapy for acute asthma symptoms.
- ICSs are the preferred long-term control therapy for patients of all ages.
- Peak flow is an inexpensive and easily available monitoring device once the diagnosis of asthma has been established.

ATELECTASIS

Matthew C. Plosker, MD
Felix B. Chang, MD

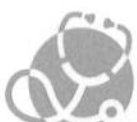

BASICS

DESCRIPTION

- Atelectasis: Loss of lung volume due to collapse of lung tissue
  - Obstructive: Blockage of an airway
  - Non-obstructive: Loss of contact between the parietal and visceral pleurae, replacement of lung tissue by scarring or infiltrative disease, surfactant dysfunction, and parenchymal compression.
- Symptoms and signs are determined by the rapidity with which the bronchial occlusion occurs, the size of the lung area affected, and the presence, or absence, of lung disease and comorbidities.
- Reduced respiratory gas exchange, leading to hypoxemia if severe

EPIDEMIOLOGY

- Predominant age: All ages
  - The mean age of presentation is 60 years.
- Male = Female. No racial predilection.

Incidence

- Round atelectasis (see "Imaging") is high in asbestos workers (65–70%).
- Incidence of lobar atelectasis is dependent on the collateral ventilation within each individual lung lobe.

Prevalence

Postoperative atelectasis is extremely common.

RISK FACTORS

- General anesthesia (1)
- Prolonged immobilization, as with bed rest
- Common postoperatively, particularly following thoracic or upper abdominal surgery, prolonged or emergency surgery, and vascular surgery (1,2)
- Risk factors for developing atelectasis after surgery:
  - Age >60, ASA class II+ functional dependence in activities of daily living (ADL), heart failure, smoking (1)
- Intensive care and prolonged immobilization (3)
- Brock syndrome: Recurrent right-middle lobe collapse secondary to airway disease, infection, or a combination thereof. The right-middle lobe airway is long and thin and has the poorest drainage of clearance of all the lobes, resulting in trapped mucus.

GENERAL PREVENTION

Encourage activity and mobilization.

PATHOPHYSIOLOGY

- Obstructive atelectasis:
  - There are three collateral ventilation systems in each lobe, the pores of Kohn, canals of Lambert, and fenestrations of Boren. The patency and formation of the systems is dependent on multiple factors including age, lung disease, and fraction of inspired oxygen (FiO_2).
  - Age: Due to the late development of collaterals in children, atelectasis is frequently diagnosed after foreign body aspiration.
  - Emphysema: The fenestra of Boren in emphysematous patients often become enlarged, it's this enlargement that can lead to a delay in atelectasis despite an obstructing lesion or mass.
  - FiO_2: Oxygen rapidly dissociates from the alveoli to deoxygenated vessels in a obstructed airway. The 79% nitrogen in atmospheric air has a much slower rate of dissociation from the alveoli, and thereby prevents collapse by maintaining a positive pressure inside the alveoli. With increased FiO_2, the concentration of nitrogen is decreased, predisposing the patient to a rapid development of atelectasis at the onset of obstruction.

ETIOLOGY

- Obstructive (resorptive) atelectasis (most common): Intrinsic respiratory blockage.
  - Due to luminal blockage (foreign body, mucous plug, asthma, cystic fibrosis, trauma, tumor) or airway wall abnormality (congenital malformation, emphysema)
  - Distal to the obstruction, air is reabsorbed from the alveoli into the deoxygenated venous system causing complete collapse of the alveolar tissue.
- Non-obstructive atelectasis:
  - Passive atelectasis: Results from pleural membrane separation of the visceral and parietal layers
    - Pleural effusion, pneumothorax
  - Compression atelectasis: Alveoli compression leading to diminished resting volume (FRC)
    - Space occupying lesions, lymphadenopathy, cardiomegaly, abscess, chest-wall pressure
  - Adhesive atelectasis: Surfactant dysfunction, resulting in increased surface tension and alveoli collapse
    - Respiratory distress syndrome, acute respiratory distress syndrome (ARDS), radiation exposure, smoke inhalation, uremia
  - Cicatrization: Pleural or parenchymal scarring
    - Granulomatous disease, toxic inhalation, drug-induced fibrosis (e.g., Amiodarone), radiation exposure
  - Replacement atelectasis: Diffuse tumor manifestation resulting in complete lobar collapse
    - Bronchioalveolar cell carcinoma
  - Rounded atelectasis: Distinct form of atelectasis following asbestosis exposure
- Other:
  - Hypoxemia due to pulmonary embolus
  - Muscular weakness (anesthesia, neuromuscular disease)

COMMONLY ASSOCIATED CONDITIONS

- Chronic obstructive pulmonary disease and asthma
- Trauma
- ARDS, neonatal respiratory distress syndrome, pulmonary edema, pulmonary embolism
- Neuromuscular disorders (muscular dystrophy, spinal muscular atrophy, spinal cord injury), cystic fibrosis
- Respiratory syncytial virus (RSV), bronchiolitis
- Bronchial stenosis, pulmonic valve disease, pulmonary hypertension
- Pneumonia, pleural effusion, pneumothorax

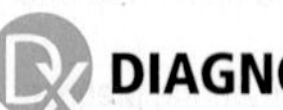

DIAGNOSIS

HISTORY

- Frequently asymptomatic
- Tachypnea and sudden-onset dyspnea
- Nonproductive cough
- Pleuritic pain on affected side
- History of smoking, radiation, asbestos, or other air pollutants

PHYSICAL EXAM

- Hypoxia, cyanosis
- Tracheal or precordial impulse displacement toward the affected side
- Bronchial breathing if airway is patent or absent breath sounds if airway is occluded
- Diminished chest expansion
- Wheezing may be heard with focal obstruction, dullness to percussion over the involved area

DIAGNOSTIC TESTS & INTERPRETATION

Lab

Initial lab tests

- CBC and sputum culture if infection is suspected
- ABG: Despite hypoxemia, the partial pressure of carbon dioxide in ($PaCO_2$) level is usually normal or low.

Follow-Up & Special Considerations

Albumin level: Low serum albumin level (<3.5 g/L) is a powerful marker of increased risk for postoperative pulmonary complications, including atelectasis (1)[A].

Imaging

Initial approach

- Chest x-ray (CXR), posterior-anterior and lateral:
  - Raised diaphragm, flattened chest wall, movement of fissures and mediastinal structures toward the atelectatic region
  - Unaffected lung may show compensatory hyperinflation.
  - Wedge-shaped densities: Obstructive atelectasis
  - Small, linear bands (Fleischner lines) often at lung bases: Discoid (subsegmental or plate) atelectasis
  - Lobar collapse:
    - Direct signs: Displacement of fissures and opacification of the collapse lobe
    - Indirect signs: Displacement of the hilum, mediastinal shift toward the side of collapse, loss of volume on ipsilateral hemithorax, elevation of ipsilateral diaphragm, crowding of the ribs, compensatory hyperlucency of the remaining lobes, and silhouetting of the diaphragm or the heart border.
  - Air bronchograms: Evidence of pleural fluid or air may indicate compressive atelectasis.
  - Adhesive atelectasis may present as a diffuse reticular granular pattern progressing to a pulmonary edemalike pattern and finally to bilateral opacification in severe cases.
  - Pleural-based round density on CXR: Round atelectasis
  - Complete atelectasis of an entire lung: Opacification of the entire hemithorax and an ipsilateral shift of the mediastinum.

Follow-Up & Special Considerations

- Chest CT or MRI may be indicated to visualize airway and mediastinal structures and to identify cause of atelectasis.
- Pulmonary function tests (PFTs) may detect restrictive disease, decreased respiratory muscle pressures, or airflow obstruction.

Diagnostic Procedures/Surgery

- Bronchoscopy to assess airway patency in unexplained or refractory cases
- Echocardiography to assess cardiac status in cardiomegaly
- Barium swallow to assess mediastinal vascular compression

Pathological Findings

Pathology varies with underlying cause.

DIFFERENTIAL DIAGNOSIS

The differential is found under "Etiology."

TREATMENT

MEDICATION

First Line

Therapies directed at basic cause:

- Antibiotics for infection
- Chemo/radiation therapy for tumor
- Steroids for asthma
- Analgesia for pain control to permit deep inspiration and coughing

Pediatric Considerations

- RhDNase may be effective in clearing mucinous secretions in persistent atelectasis in children (4)[C].
- Chest physiotherapy including percussion, drainage, deep insufflation, and saline lavage is a common treatment in the prevention and treatment of atelectasis in the hospital setting. However, caution is required when interpreting the possible positive effects of chest physiotherapy of a reduction in the use of reintubation and the trend for decreased postextubation atelectasis as the numbers of babies studied are small, the results are not consistent across trials, data on safety are insufficient, and applicability to current practice may be limited (5)[C].
- Good tolerance and physiologic short-term benefit with mechanical insufflation-exsufflation has been seen in children with neuromuscular disease. However further studies, including a larger number of patients, are clearly needed to validate the efficacy of this treatment (6)[C]. Evidence from a single randomized control trial exhibited that tracheal gas insufflation may reduce the duration of mechanical ventilation in preterm infants. However, tracheal gas insufflation is a new technique to supplement mechanical ventilation in neonatal intensive care, and benefit and safety have not been proven (7)[B].
- The application of continuous distending pressure (CDP) has been shown to have some benefits in the treatment of preterm infants with respiratory distress syndrome (RDS). CDP has the potential to reduce lung damage particularly if applied early before atelectasis has occurred (8)[A].

Second Line

Bronchofibroscopy in aspiration of inspissated secretions in atelectasis has been efficacious in several studies. However, counter-evidence continues to question its efficacy in the treatment of atelectasis.

Pediatric Considerations

In obstructive atelectasis, bronchoscopy remains controversial (9)[B]. In the presence of a mucus plug or cast, bronchoscopy may be beneficial (10)[C].

ADDITIONAL TREATMENT

General Measures

- If known, treat the underlying cause.
- Ensure patient is lying on the unaffected side to promote drainage
  - Maximize patient mobility and encourage frequent coughing and deep breathing every hour (physical therapy).
- Incentive spirometry
  - Evidence has not shown that incentive spirometry prevents postoperative pulmonary complications in CABG (11)[A].
- Initiate intubation and mechanical ventilation with positive end-expiratory pressure (PEEP) in severe respiratory distress or hypoxemia:
  - Lower tidal volume (6 mL/kg) and lower end-inspiratory values (<30 mm Hg) associated with reduced mortality (12)[B]
  - PEEP 15–20 mL may be necessary to maintain arterial O_2 saturation in surfactant-impaired states (12)[B].
- Postsurgical measures include positive airway pressure, continuous or intermittent.

Issues for Referral

As needed for underlying etiology

Additional Therapies

As listed under "General Measures"

SURGERY/OTHER PROCEDURES

Only for resectable underlying disease (e.g., tumor, severe lymphadenopathy), bronchoscopy

IN-PATIENT CONSIDERATIONS

Initial Stabilization

Ensure adequate oxygenation (may start with 100% FiO_2 then taper) and humidification.

Admission Criteria

As determined by underlying etiology

ONGOING CARE

FOLLOW-UP RECOMMENDATIONS

Patient Monitoring

- Varies with cause and patient status
- In simple atelectasis associated with asthma or infection, outpatient visits are adequate.

DIET

No special diet

PATIENT EDUCATION

Maximize patient mobility and encourage frequent coughing and deep breathing every hour.

PROGNOSIS

- Spontaneous resolution
- The prognosis of lobar atelectasis secondary to endobronchial obstruction depends on treatment of the underlying malignancy.
- Surgical therapy needed only for resectable causes or if chronic infection and bronchiectasis supervene.

COMPLICATIONS

- Pneumonia
- Acute atelectasis:
  - Hypoxemia and respiratory failure
  - Postobstructive drowning of the lung
  - Pneumonia
- Chronic atelectasis:
  - Bronchiectasis
  - Pleural effusion and empyema

REFERENCES

1. Qaseem A, Snow V, Fitterman N, et al. Risk assessment for and strategies to reduce perioperative pulmonary complications for patients undergoing noncardiothoracic surgery: A guideline from the American College of Physicians. *Ann Intern Med*. 2006;144:575–80.
2. Ferreyra G, Long Y, Ranieri VM, et al. Respiratory complications after major surgery. *Curr Opin Crit Care*. 2009;15:342–8.
3. Brower RG. Consequences of bed rest. *Crit. Care Med*. 2009;37:S422–8.
4. Hendriks T, de Hoog M, Lequin MH, et al. DNase and atelectasis in non-cystic fibrosis pediatric patients. *Crit Care*. 2005;9:R351–6.
5. Flenady V, Gray PH. Chest physiotherapy for preventing morbidity in babies being extubated from mechanical ventilation. *Cochrane Database Syst Rev*. 2002;(2):CD000283.
6. Fauroux B, Guillemot N, Aubertin G, et al. Physiologic benefits of mechanical insufflation-exsufflation in children with neuromuscular diseases. *Chest*. 2008;133:161–8.
7. Davies MW, Woodgate PG. Tracheal gas insufflation for the prevention of morbidity and mortality in mechanically ventilated newborn infants. *Cochrane Database Syst Rev*. 2002;(2): CD002973.
8. Ho JJ, Henderson-Smart DJ, Davis PG. Early versus delayed initiation of continuous distending pressure for respiratory distress syndrome in preterm infants. *Cochrane Database Syst Rev*. 2002;(2):CD002975.
9. Wu KH, Lin CF, Huang CJ, et al. Rigid ventilation bronchoscopy under general anesthesia for treatment of pediatric pulmonary atelectasis caused by pneumonia: A review of 33 cases. *Int Surg*. 2006;91:291–4.
10. Deng J, Zheng Y, Li C, et al. Plastic bronchitis in three children associated with 2009 influenza A(H1N1) virus infection. *Chest*. 2010;138: 1486–8.
11. Freitas ERFS, Soares B, Cardoso JRosa, et al. Incentive spirometry for preventing pulmonary complications after coronary artery bypass graft. *Cochrane Database Syst Rev*. 2007;(3): CD004466.
12. McCunn M, et al. Guidelines for management of mechanical ventilation in critically injured patients. *Trauma Care*. 2004;14(4):147–51.

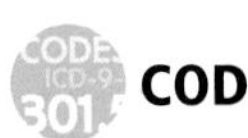

CODES

ICD9

518.0 Pulmonary collapse

CLINICAL PEARLS

- Bronchogenic carcinoma, which may present with atelectasis, must be excluded in all patients older than 35 years.
- In complete atelectasis of an entire lung, the mediastinal ipsilateral shift separates atelectasis from massive pleural effusion.

ATHEROSCLEROSIS

Angela Y. Higgins, MD
Frank J. Domino, MD

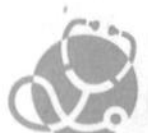

BASICS

DESCRIPTION

- Atherosclerosis is a common and chronic inflammatory disease characterized by deposits of yellowish plaques (atheromas) containing cholesterol, lipoid material, and lipophages within the intima and inner media of large and medium-sized arteries.
- Manifestations most commonly include coronary artery disease, cerebrovascular disease, and peripheral artery disease.

ALERT

- Atherosclerosis happens to all who live long enough.
- Effects and complications can be minimized and/or delayed by treating all risk factors possible.

EPIDEMIOLOGY

- 1/3 of all deaths globally are attributed to coronary artery disease (CAD) according to the World Health Organization.
- More common in males and with increasing age

Incidence

- In 2010, it is estimated that 785,000 Americans will have a new coronary event, and 470,000 will have a recurrent episode (1).
- Each year, 795,000 people experience a new or recurrent stroke. ~610,000 of these are first attacks, and 185,000 are recurrent attacks (1).

Prevalence

- Total coronary heart disease (CHD) prevalence is 7.9% in US adults 20 years of age (9.1% for men and 7.0% for women). Prevalence increases with age (1).
- During 2006, it is estimated that 400,000 Americans have had a stroke. Overall stroke prevalence during this period is an estimated 2.9% (1).

RISK FACTORS

- Diabetes mellitus is considered a CAD equivalent.
- Modifiable:
  - Hypertension: BP 140/90 or on antihypertensive medications
  - Tobacco smoking: Dose-dependent risk
  - Physical inactivity and obesity
  - Decreased high-density lipoprotein (HDL) cholesterol <40 mg/dL
  - Increased low-density lipoprotein (LDL) cholesterol >160 mg/dL
- Nonmodifiable:
  - Male gender
  - Increasing age: Male >45 years of age, female >55 years of age
- Family history of *premature* atherosclerosis: MI/sudden death in 1st-degree male relative <55 years of age or 1st-degree female relative <65 years of age
- Negative risk factors: HDL >60 mg/dL is protective.

Genetics

Development of atherosclerosis is multifactorial, but there is likely a genetic link. Twin studies have shown that 30–60% of individual variation of atherosclerosis is genetic. There are many ongoing studies, and to date 17 loci have been identified as associated with atherosclerosis (2).

GENERAL PREVENTION

Treat or control modifiable risk factors as listed above.

PATHOPHYSIOLOGY

- Early changes (simple), potentially reversible:
  - Accumulation of lipid-laden macrophages in the intimal layer of the artery
  - Fatty streaks in aorta and coronary arteries
- Late changes (complicated) usually reversible:
  - Atheromatous plaques with necrosis, fibrosis, calcification
  - Weakening of elastic lamella, neovascularization, arterial obstruction or thrombosis
- Oxidized LDL induces vascular smooth-muscle cell apoptosis and cell death.
- Alteration of endothelial function involving mostly nitrous oxide pathways promotes platelet adhesion and aggregation, local clotting, and vascular growth and alters vascular tone.
- Vulnerable plaques have a thin fibrous cap, large lipid core, and high macrophage content and are not necessarily seen by typical angiography.

ETIOLOGY

Biochemical, physiologic, and environmental factors in association with risk factors lead to inflammation, thickening, and occlusion of the lumen of arteries. Some degree of atherosclerosis is universal with aging.

COMMONLY ASSOCIATED CONDITIONS

Hypertension, diabetes, dyslipidemia, hypothyroid, obesity, cerebrovascular accident

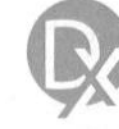

DIAGNOSIS

- Characteristically silent until atheromas produce stenosis, thrombosis, aneurysm, or embolus
- Symptoms vary and are further described in other sections:
  - Cardiac: Angina, myocardial infarction, CHF, arrhythmias, essential hypertension, dissecting aneurysm
  - Neurologic: Cerebrovascular accident, transient ischemic attack
  - Renal: Renal failure
  - GI: Ischemic colitis
  - Extremities: Claudication, weakness, difficulty walking, infection, hair loss

HISTORY

Question patients regarding diet and exercise habits. Always ask patients about smoking and encourage smoking cessation. Inquire about family history and personal history of premature heart disease, stroke, peripheral artery disease, sudden death, and diabetes.

PHYSICAL EXAM

- Vitals: Height and weight to calculate BMI and BP:
  - U.S. Preventive Services Task Force (USPSTF) recommends screening all adults for obesity and offering intensive counseling and behavioral interventions.
  - Screen children aged 6 years and older for obesity and offer or refer them to comprehensive, intensive behavioral interventions to promote weight loss.
  - Screen all adults 19 and older for hypertension.
- Physical exam: Heart, lungs, aorta, carotids, extremities

DIAGNOSTIC TESTS & INTERPRETATION

Lab

Initial lab tests

- USPSTF recommendations on lipid screening:
  - Screen all men 35 and older for lipid disorder
  - Screen men ages 20–35 who are at increased risk of CHD.
  - Screen women ages 45 and older if at increased risk of CHD.
  - Screen women 20–45 if at increased risk of CHD.
- Many, including the National Cholesterol Education program, advocate screening all patients with fasting lipid profile every 5 years starting at age 20 and screening patients at increased risk earlier and more frequently.
- USPSTF recommendations on diabetes screening:
  - Screen for type 2 diabetes in asymptomatic adults with sustained BP (either treated or untreated) >135/80 mm Hg.
  - Current evidence is insufficient for screening for type 2 diabetes in asymptomatic adults with a BP of 135/80 mm Hg or lower.
- Other laboratory tests: HS-CRP, leukocyte count, homocysteine level, lipoprotein A level. According to the USPSTF, there is insufficient evidence for screening with these nontraditional risk factors.

Imaging

- Coronary computed tomographic angiography (CCTA): High negative predictive value (near 100%) for major cardiac events in patients with known or suspected CAD (3)[B]
- Coronary Artery Calcium score (CAC): CAC scoring may be appropriate for intermediate-risk patients with a 10–20% 10-year risk. CAC varies by age, ethnicity, and sex. Patients >75th percentile may warrant more aggressive risk factor management.
- Arterial Doppler studies (carotid, renal): For diagnostic purposes; it is not recommended to screen asymptomatic patients for carotid artery stenosis.
- Evidence for general screening with noninvasive imaging is limited (4)[A].

Diagnostic Procedures/Surgery

- Framingham Risk Score: Uses age, gender, total cholesterol, HDL cholesterol, tobacco use, BP, and antihypertensive medication use to calculate 10-year risk.
- Arterial Doppler studies (carotid, renal), angiography, ankle–brachial index, cardiac stress test depending on clinical assessment

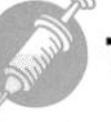

TREATMENT

MEDICATION

First Line

HMG-CoA reductase inhibitors (statins): Primary lipid-lowering medication:

- Pleiotropic effects: Decrease CRP independent of lowering LDL, plaque stabilization via antiproliferative action, decrease in collagen formation, increased tPA expression, antioxidant effects (5)
- Debate continues over whether pleiotropic effects are LDL dependent or independent (5).
- For patients currently on statins, residual risk factors include: Waist circumference, homocysteine, coronary artery calcification, and large artery elasticity (6)
- 2011: FDA issued warning about increased risk of myopathy with simvastatin 80 mg.
- Requires liver function test monitoring monthly for 3 months then every 3–6 months
- Goal LDL <100 mg/dL for patients with CHD or CHD equivalents, <130 mg/dL for patients without CHD but with 2 or more risk factors, <160 for no CHD and 0–1 risk factors

Second Line

- Niacin: 1st line for hypertriglyceridemia with TG >500 mg/dL
- Bile acid binding resins such as cholestyramine and colestipol
- Fibrates such as gemfibrozil
- Ezetimibe (lowers LDL effectively, but no outcomes data currently support use)

ADDITIONAL TREATMENT

General Measures

Treat all modifiable risk factors and encourage healthy lifestyle as recommended by AHA.

COMPLEMENTARY AND ALTERNATIVE MEDICINE

Evidence is lacking to recommend the following alternative treatments: Omega-3 fatty acids, vitamin E, lowering homocysteine level, chelation therapy, acupuncture (7)[B]

SURGERY/OTHER PROCEDURES

- Angioplasty (8)[A], stent (9)[A], coronary artery bypass
- Carotid endarterectomy: For symptomatic patients, NNT 15 if severe (>70%) blockage, NNT 21 if blockage less severe (50–69%) (10)[A]

IN-PATIENT CONSIDERATIONS

Initial Stabilization

Inpatient management of complications. See specific chapter for detailed information.

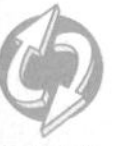

ONGOING CARE

DIET

2006 American Heart Association (AHA) diet and lifestyle recommendations to reduce cardiovascular disease risk (11)[B]:

- Balance calorie intake and physical activity to maintain or achieve a healthy BMI:
  - 30 minutes or more of exercise on most days for adults and 60 minutes of exercise on most days for children and adults trying to lose weight
- Consume a diet rich in vegetables and fruits, and choose whole-grain and high-fiber foods.
- Limit intake of saturated fat to <7%, trans-fat to <1%, and cholesterol to <300 mg/d:
  - This may be achieved by choosing lean meats and vegetables; selecting fat-free, low fat, or 1% milk; and minimizing partially hydrogenated fat intake.
- Minimize intake of beverages and foods with added sugars. Choose or prepare foods with little or no salt. Consume fish, especially oily fish, at least twice per week.
- If you choose to consume alcohol, do so in moderation. For men, no more than 2 drinks per day and for women, no more than 1 drink per day.
- When eating food that is prepared outside the home, follow AHA recommendations.

PATIENT EDUCATION

Crucial parts of preventing and treating atherosclerosis involve nutrition, fitness, and smoking cessation and treating modifiable risk factors.

PROGNOSIS

Prognosis is variable and based on extent of disease and vulnerability of plaques. The Framingham Risk Score provides an assessment of 10-year cardiovascular risk.

COMPLICATIONS

Coronary artery disease, renal failure, cerebrovascular accidents, dissecting or ruptured aneurysms, arterial thrombosis, gangrene, sudden death

REFERENCES

1. WRITING GROUP MEMBERS, Lloyd-Jones D, Adams RJ, Brown TM, et al. Heart disease and stroke statistics–2010 update: A report from the American Heart Association. *Circulation*. 2010; 121:e46–e215.
2. Sivapalaratnam S, Motazacker MM, Maiwald S, et al. Genome-wide association studies in atherosclerosis. *Curr Atheroscler Rep*. 2011;13: 225–32.
3. Min JK, Feignoux J, Treutenaere J, et al. The prognostic value of multidetector coronary CT angiography for the prediction of major adverse cardiovascular events: A multicenter observational cohort study. *Int J Cardiovasc Imaging*. 2010;26: 721–8.
4. Rodondi N, Auer R, de Bosset Sulzer V, et al. Atherosclerosis screening by noninvasive imaging for cardiovascular prevention: A systematic review. *J Gen Intern Med*. 2011.
5. Mizuno Y, Jacob RF, Mason RP, et al. Inflammation and the development of atherosclerosis. *J Atheroscler Thromb*. 2011;18:351–8.
6. Afonso L, Veeranna V, Zalawadiya S, et al. Predictors of residual cardiovascular risk in patients on statin therapy for primary prevention. *Cardiology*. 2011;119:187–90.
7. Pittler MH, Ernst E. Complementary therapies for peripheral arterial disease: Systematic review. *Atherosclerosis*. 2005;181:1–7.
8. Fowkes G, Gillespie IN. Angioplasty (versus non surgical management) for intermittent claudication. *Cochrane Database Syst Rev*. 1998;(2):CD000017.
9. Bachoo P, Thorpe PA, Maxwell H, et al. Endovascular stents for intermittent claudication. *Cochrane Database Syst Rev*. 2010;(1): CD003228.
10. Cina C, Clase C, Haynes RB. Carotid endarterectomy for symptomatic carotid stenosis. *Cochrane Database Syst Rev*. 1999;(3): CD001081.
11. American Heart Association Nutrition Committee, Lichtenstein AH, Appel LJ, et al. Diet and lifestyle recommendations revision 2006: A scientific statement from the American Heart Association Nutrition Committee. *Circulation*. 2006;114: 82–96.

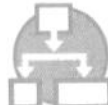

See Also (Topic, Algorithm, Electronic Media Element)

- Aortic Dissection; Arterial Embolus and Thrombosis; Atherosclerotic Heart Disease; Congestive Heart Failure; Hypertension, Essential; Renal Failure, Acute; Stroke, Acute
- Algorithm: Chest Pain/Acute Coronary Syndrome

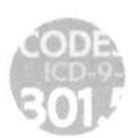

CODES

ICD9

- 414.00 Coronary atherosclerosis of unspecified type of vessel, native or graft
- 414.01 Coronary atherosclerosis of native coronary artery
- 440.9 Generalized and unspecified atherosclerosis

CLINICAL PEARLS

- Atherosclerosis is a generalized condition affecting multiple organ systems.
- It is very likely that improvement in diet and exercise, control of hypertension, and elimination of risk factors like smoking can delay the development of this condition.
- Statins control atherosclerosis via multiple mechanisms in addition to lipid-lowering effects.

ATRIAL FIBRILLATION AND ATRIAL FLUTTER

Matthew McGuiness, MD
Samuel Joffe, MD

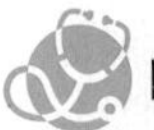

BASICS

This topic covers both atrial fibrillation (AFib) and atrial flutter (AFlut).

DESCRIPTION

- AFib: Continuous or paroxysmal arrhythmia characterized by rapid, chaotic atrial electrical activity and an irregularly irregular ventricular response. In most patients, the ventricular rate is accelerated because the AV node is bombarded with nearly continuous atrial electrical impulses.
- AFlut: Continuous or paroxysmal arrhythmia with rapid but organized atrial electrical activity. The atrial rate is typically between 250 and 350 bpm and is often manifested as "sawtooth" flutter waves on the ECG, particularly in the inferior leads. 2:1 or 3:1 conduction through the AV node to the ventricle is common, so the ventricular response may be regular and often at a rate of around 150 bpm.
- AFib and AFlut are related rhythms, sometimes seen in the same patient. Atrial fibrillation can appear electrically organized in some instances, particularly in lead V1 of the ECG, thus appearing flutter-like. Distinguishing the 2 is important, however, as it may have implications for management.
- Clinical pattern:
  – Paroxysmal: Self-terminating episodes, usually <7 days
  – Persistent: Sustained >7 days, usually requiring pharmacologic or DC cardioversion to restore sinus rhythm
  – Permanent: Sinus rhythm cannot be restored; cardioversion has failed or has not been attempted.
- So-called "lone" atrial fibrillation occurs in patients under the age of 60 who have no clinical or echocardiographic evidence of cardiovascular disease, including the absence of hypertension (HTN). Such patients are thought to often have a genetic predisposition towards the development of AFib.

EPIDEMIOLOGY

- Incidence/prevalence increases significantly with age.
- Young patients with atrial fibrillation, particularly "lone AFib," are most commonly male.

Incidence

- AFib: Age <40, <0.1%/year; >80, >1.5%/year.
- Lifetime risk: 25% for those ≥40 years.
- Atrial flutter is less common.

Prevalence

- Estimated 0.4–1% of general population <60.
- ~2–5%, 7th decade; 5–10%, 8th decade.

RISK FACTORS

Age and HTN are the most important risk factors for both atrial fibrillation and atrial flutter. See "Etiology."

Genetics

Familial forms are rare but do exist. There are ongoing efforts to identify the genetic underpinnings of such cases.

GENERAL PREVENTION

Adequate control of HTN may prevent development of AFib due to hypertensive heart disease and is the most significant modifiable risk factor for AFib. Ethanol consumption may trigger AFib in some.

PATHOPHYSIOLOGY

- In patients with no/minimal structural heart disease, premature atrial beats and/or bursts of tachycardia emanating from the pulmonary venous ostia or other sites may trigger atrial fibrillation or flutter (1).
- Many patients with atrial fibrillation are thought to have some degree of atrial fibrosis or scarring. This is often subclinical and usually not detectable with current cardiac imaging techniques, but it plays an important role in the pathogenesis of the dysrhythmia (1).
- In patients with a heavier burden of atrial fibrillation, the atria can undergo electrical and structural remodeling that can further sustain the dysrhythmia. This phenomenon has lead to the notion that "AFib begets AFib."

ETIOLOGY

- Cardiac: Hypertensive heart disease, valvular/rheumatic disease, CAD, acute myocardial infarction (MI), cardiomyopathy, congestive heart failure (CHF), pericarditis, infiltrative heart disease
- Pulmonary: Pulmonary embolism, chronic obstructive pulmonary disease (COPD), obstructive sleep apnea, pneumonia
- Ingestion: Ethanol, digoxin toxicity
- Endocrine: Hyperthyroidism or hypothyroidism
- Postoperative: For example, cardiothoracic surgery
- Idiopathic: Including lone AF (<60 without clinical or ECG evidence of cardiopulmonary disease, including HTN)

COMMONLY ASSOCIATED CONDITIONS

HTN

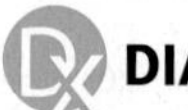

DIAGNOSIS

HISTORY

Symptoms vary from none to mild (palpitations, lightheadedness, fatigue, poor exercise capacity) to severe (angina, dyspnea, syncope).

PHYSICAL EXAM

- AFib: Irregularly irregular pulse, frequently tachycardic.
- AFlut: Usually regular pulse, frequently tachycardic.

DIAGNOSTIC TESTS & INTERPRETATION

- AFib: The ECG is diagnostic with findings of low-amplitude fibrillatory waves without discrete P waves and an irregularly irregular pattern of QRS complexes. There is often tachycardia in the absence of heart rate–controlling medications.
- AFlut: The ECG is again diagnostic. Sawtooth P-waves are the classic sign, generally best seen in the inferior leads. QRS complexes may be regular or irregular; there is usually tachycardia.
- Holter monitor and event monitor helpful in diagnosing paroxysmal AFib or AFlut and monitoring for recurrence.

Lab

Initial lab tests

TSH, electrolytes, CBC, PT/INR (if anticoagulation is contemplated); digoxin level (if appropriate).

Follow-Up & Special Considerations

Occasional Holter monitoring and/or exercise stress testing to assess for adequacy of rate and/or rhythm control.

Imaging

- Chest x-ray (CXR) for cardiopulmonary disease.
- ECG for structural heart disease, signs of ischemia and/or other dysrhythmias.
- Transesophageal echocardiogram to detect left atria appendage thrombus if cardioversion planned.

Pathological Findings

- Atrial dilatation and fibrosis
- Atrial thrombus, especially in atrial appendage
- Valvular/rheumatic disease
- Cardiomyopathy

DIFFERENTIAL DIAGNOSIS

- Multifocal atrial tachycardia
- Sinus tachycardia with frequent atrial premature beats
- Atrial flutter/atrial fibrillation

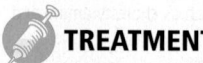

TREATMENT

MEDICATION

- There are two primary issues in the management of AFib and/or AFlut: (i) protection against thromboembolism (primarily stroke) and (ii) control of ventricular rate or restoration of sinus rhythm.
- Of note, ventricular rate control can often be difficult to achieve in AFlut, due to the more organized nature of the atrial electrical activity. For this reason, conversion to sinus rhythm, once issues related to anticoagulation have been addressed, is often the preferred strategy.
- Anticoagulation guidelines (same for AFib and AFlut):
  – Unless contraindicated, patients with AFib or AFlut with any high-risk factors for stroke (prior transient ischemic attack [TIA]/cerebrovascular accident [CVA]/thromboembolism, mitral stenosis, prosthetic valve) should receive long-term warfarin therapy to maintain an INR of 2.0–3.0 (patients with mechanical valves should maintain an INR >2.5). Dabigatran (Pradaxa), a direct thrombin inhibitor, has recently been approved as an alternative to warfarin for patients with nonvalvular atrial fibrillation. It offers the advantage of not requiring regular INR monitoring. Clinical experience with this agent continues to accumulate. Rivaroxaban and apixaban, factor Xa inhibitors, will likely also soon be approved for use in AFib, although Rivaroxaban may be approved as a 2nd- or 3rd-line agent (1,2).
  – CHADS2 score: Patients with ≥2 moderate risk factors (**C**HF, **H**TN, **A**ge >75, and/or **D**M), should receive anticoagulation unless contraindicated. Patients with a CHADS2 score of 0 (including most patients with "lone" AFib) should not be anticoagulated as risk likely exceeds benefit (1,2).

- Patients with one moderate risk factor should be treated with anticoagulation or aspirin (162–325 mg/d) (1,2).
- Patients at low risk of thromboembolic complications or in whom warfarin is contraindicated should receive aspirin (162–325 mg/d) or clopidogrel (1).
- Anticoagulation recommendations are independent of AF pattern (paroxysmal, persistent, permanent) (1).

- 3 classes of medications are available to achieve control of ventricular response rate. These include beta-blockers (i.e., metoprolol), nondihydropyridine calcium channel blockers (i.e., diltiazem) and digoxin. The optimal target for ventricular rate has not been firmly established, though there is evidence that aggressive control of the ventricular rate offers no benefit beyond more modest rate control (i.e., resting heart rate <110 bpm) (3).
- Restoration of sinus rhythm using electrical or pharmacologic cardioversion may significantly reduce the symptom burden of AFib or AFlut in many patients and may also be useful for controlling the ventricular rate. Cardioversion does not impact the long-term risk/benefit ratio of anticoagulation.
  - Cardioversion is most often performed electrically, but may also be achieved using antiarrhythmic drug therapy in some instances by experienced clinicians (4,5).
  - If duration of AF is >24–48 hours or unknown, anticoagulate for ≥3 weeks before cardioversion to reduce the risk of stroke. Alternatively, once anticoagulation is established, a transesophageal echocardiogram may be performed to exclude the presence of left atrial thrombus, allowing cardioversion to proceed. After cardioversion, anticoagulation should be continued for ≥4 weeks in all patients where the duration of AFib/AFlut is >24–48 hours, as the postcardioversion period is a time of increased stroke risk (1).
- Chronic oral antiarrhythmic therapy to suppress recurrence of AFib is available for appropriately selected patients. Such medication should generally be started with expert consultation owing to the complexities of safe antiarrhythmic drug selection.

ADDITIONAL TREATMENT

Issues for Referral

Management of AFib or AFlut refractory to standard medical therapy (i.e., unable to achieve adequate rate control with medication or development of significant bradycardia with treatment) may require the use of more aggressive treatments. These may include pacemaker implantation (to allow for more intensive pharmacologic blocking of the AV node) or an ablation procedure. AFlut in particular is often very amenable to ablation; thus, consideration should be given to early expert referral in appropriate patients. Antiarrhythmic drug therapy can often be very effective but should be prescribed by experienced practitioners.

SURGERY/OTHER PROCEDURES

- Electrophysiologic study and ablation may be considered for patients with either AFib or AFlut. In the case of AFlut, ablation is often a relatively straightforward procedure that is generally viewed as a 1st-line therapy due to its high rate of success in appropriate candidates. Ablation of atrial fibrillation is a much more complex procedure with a more variable success rate that continues to evolve.
- Cardiac surgery (e.g., the maze procedure, ligation of the left atrial appendage) may be considered in patients planned to undergo cardiac surgery for other reasons. Surgical therapy in isolation is rarely indicated for AFib or AFlut.

IN-PATIENT CONSIDERATIONS

Initial Stabilization

Acute therapy for symptomatic or hemodynamically compromised patients with AFib or AFlut:

- IV β- or calcium channel blocker for control of ventricular rate if BP is adequate. If successful, it is essential to follow this treatment with the prompt administration of oral medication, as the duration of IV drugs is generally short (1).
- Commonly utilized therapies in the acute setting include:
  - Metoprolol: 5-mg IV boluses every 5 minutes, followed by oral metoprolol.
  - Diltiazem: In most adult patients, this may be administered as a 10-mg IV bolus, which can be repeated in 15 minutes as tolerated. Alternatively, weight-based dosing may be employed (0.25 mg/kg followed by 0.35 mg/kg in 15 minutes). If there is an appropriate response to diltiazem, oral administration or an IV infusion (5–15 mg/hr) may be initiated.
  - Some patients will be far more responsive to one class of agents than another. For this reason, if rate control is difficult to achieve, switching drug classes may be useful.
- Urgent cardioversion should be performed in hemodynamically unstable patients. It is somewhat unusual for AFib or AFlut alone to cause marked hemodynamic insult; thus, the possibility of a concurrent process should be considered in this setting (1).
- Consider the initiation of oral anticoagulation therapy. Inpatients may be "bridged" with IV or SC heparin while waiting for warfarin to become effective.

Admission Criteria

- Patients with any of the following features likely require admission to the hospital for a period of stabilization:
  - Significant symptoms
  - Extremely rapid ventricular rate
  - Initiating antiarrhythmic therapy
  - AF triggered by an acute process (acute MI, CHF, pulmonary embolus)
- Outpatient management is reasonable for low-risk patients with controlled ventricular rates

Discharge Criteria

Adequate rate or rhythm control without symptoms. Long-term plan for anticoagulation established.

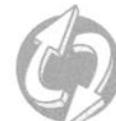

ONGOING CARE

Given the increasing array of therapies available for the management of AFib and AFlut, many patients may benefit from elective expert consultation. Alternatively, in patients where there are no significant symptoms, the ventricular rate control or sinus rhythm is easily achieved, and the choice of thromboembolic protection is clear, management in a primary care setting may be appropriate.

FOLLOW-UP RECOMMENDATIONS

Patient Monitoring

Adequate anticoagulation levels (if warfarin is employed) and control of the ventricular rate should be assessed on a regular basis.

DIET

Patients on warfarin should attempt to consume a stable amount of vitamin K to help keep the effect of the drug stable.

PROGNOSIS

Anticoagulation reduces the annual embolic stroke rate to 1–2% for most patients. AFib and AFlut may increase morbidity and mortality, but the overall prognosis is a function of underlying heart disease and adherence with therapy.

COMPLICATIONS

- Embolic stroke
- Peripheral arterial embolization
- Bleeding with anticoagulation
- Tachycardia-induced cardiomyopathy with prolonged periods of inadequate rate control

REFERENCES

1. Fuster V, Rydén LE, Cannom DS. ACC/AHA/ESC 2006 guidelines for the management of patients with atrial fibrillation. *Circulation*. 2006; 114:e257–354.
2. Singer D, Albers G, Dalen J, et al. Antithrombotic therapy in atrial fibrillation: American College of Chest Physicians Evidence-Based Clinical Practice Guidelines (8th edition). *Chest*. 2008;133: 546S–92S.
3. Wann L, Curtis A, January C, et al. 2011 ACCF/AHA/HRS focused update on the management of patients with atrial fibrillation. *J Am Coll Cardiology*. 2011;57(2):233.
4. Mead GE, Elder AT, Flapan AD, et al. Electrical cardioversion for atrial fibrillation and flutter. *Cochrane Database Sys Rev*. 2005;CD002903.
5. Cordina J, Mead G. Pharmacological cardioversion for atrial fibrillation and flutter. *Cochrane Database Sys Rev*. 2005;CD003713.

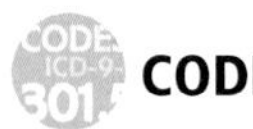

CODES

ICD9

- 427.31 Atrial fibrillation
- 427.32 Atrial flutter

CLINICAL PEARLS

- The 2 primary issues in management of atrial fibrillation are rate control and anticoagulation.
- Atrial fibrillation may be the manifestation of intrinsic heart disease, or of pulmonary disease, endocrine disease, or toxins.

ATRIAL SEPTAL DEFECT (ASD)

Daniel Stein, BA
Stephen K. Lane, MD, FAAFP

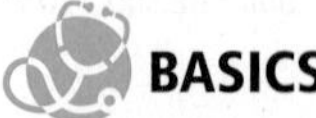

BASICS

DESCRIPTION

- Anatomy:
  - Opening in the atrial septum allowing flow of blood between the 2 atria
  - Patent foramen ovale is similar, but is not open the majority of the time, causes no hemodynamic disturbance, and is not considered an atrial septal defect (ASD) (no tissue defect)
- Types (by location in the interatrial septum) (1):
  - 75%: Ostium secundum defect occurs in the fossa ovalis region.
  - 15%: Ostium primum defect occurs in the inferior septum; often associated with cleft mitral valve and failure of endocardial cushion development.
  - 10%: Sinus venosus defect occurs in the superior-posterior septum near the orifice of the superior vena cava; usually associated with partial anomalous right upper pulmonary venous return.
- Hemodynamic effects:
  - Left-to-right shunting in late ventricular systole and early diastole
  - Degree depends on size of the defect and relative pressures of the 2 ventricles
  - Causes excessive blood flow through the right-sided circulation, ultimately leading to reactive pulmonary hypertension and possibly heart failure
- Management (1):
  - Symptomatic patients or patients with a high degree of shunt flow should undergo closure to reduce subsequent morbidity and mortality.
  - Ostium primum and sinus venosus defects are treated surgically.
  - Percutaneous closure is an alternative to surgical repair for many patients with secundum ASD.
- Systems affected: Cardiovascular; Pulmonary

Pediatric Considerations

- Most cases of ASD are detected and corrected in the pediatric population.
- The smaller the defect and the younger the age of the child, the greater the chance of spontaneous closure.

EPIDEMIOLOGY

Incidence

- Predominant age: Newborn, but may be diagnosed at any age
- Predominant sex: Female > Male (2:1)
- No race predilection
- 4 per 10,000 births

Prevalence

Accounts for 10% of congenital heart defects, and 25–30% of congenital heart defects detected in adulthood

RISK FACTORS

- Other congenital heart defects
- Family history (~7–10% recurrence)
- Thalidomide, alcohol exposure in utero

Genetics

- Most cases are spontaneous.
- 5% with chromosomal abnormalities, other rare mutations exist
- ~25% prevalence in Down syndrome

PATHOPHYSIOLOGY

- Flow across ASD usually left-to-right shunt because of higher left-sided pressures:
  - There can be minimal right-to-left shunting in early ventricular systole, especially during inspiration
  - Increased right-sided pressure/pulmonary hypertension can cause reversal of shunt flow (Eisenmenger syndrome) with resulting cyanosis and clubbing.
- Symptoms typically occur due to right ventricular and pulmonary vascular volume overload and right heart failure.

COMMONLY ASSOCIATED CONDITIONS

- ASDs may occur as a component of other complex cardiac structural defects
- Important to exclude anomalous pulmonary venous return
- Occasionally can indicate underlying genetic syndromes, e.g.:
  - Holt-Oram syndrome: Secundum defect with bony abnormalities of forearms + hands (0.95 per 100,000)
  - Ellis-von-Creveld syndrome: Chondroectodermal dysplasia + ASD
  - VACTERL (vertebral, anorectal, cardiac, tracheoesophageal, renal/urinary and limb defects)

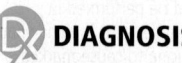

DIAGNOSIS

HISTORY

- May be initially asymptomatic
- Infants/children may be small for their age, even in the absence of other symptoms. Will generally improve with surgical treatment.
- Most common symptoms are dyspnea on exertion, palpitations, and easy fatigability
- Consider if history of right heart failure (more advanced, only 10% at diagnosis), frequent respiratory tract infections, stroke, or unexplained end-organ infarcts due to paradoxical emboli

PHYSICAL EXAM

Signs vary according to extent of shunting:

- Cardiac auscultation:
  - Fixed, widely split S2 (key physical finding)
  - May also have:
    - Systolic ejection murmur (pulmonic flow murmur)
    - Low-pitched diastolic rumble (tricuspid flow murmur)
    - Diastolic murmur (pulmonic regurgitation)
    - Systolic murmur (mitral regurgitation)
- Right ventricular heave
- Palpable pulmonary artery pulse at left upper sternal border
- If heart failure has developed, may hear a 4th heart sound (right-sided)
- Signs of Eisenmenger syndrome:
  - Cyanosis and clubbing
  - Jugular venous distention and edema

DIAGNOSTIC TESTS & INTERPRETATION

Lab

Oximetry: Cyanosis may suggest Eisenmenger syndrome (right-to-left shunting).

Initial lab tests

ECG findings:

- Right axis deviation
- Right atrial enlargement
- Right ventricular conduction delay
- Q wave in lead V1
- Mild PR prolongation
- Leftward axis, inverted P wave in lead III (sinus venosus)
- Leftward axis (ostium primum)

Imaging

Initial approach

- Echocardiography: 1st-line is transthoracic color Doppler imaging of the entire atrial septum
- Sensitivity is ~89% of secundum, ~100% of primum, and ~44% of sinus venosus ASDs. Patient with right ventricular overload by transthoracic echocardiography (TTE), but an otherwise negative study should have further testing

Follow-Up & Special Considerations

- "Bubble" contrast enhancement may be helpful.
- Transesophageal echocardiography (TEE) may be required to define ASD morphology and to locate the pulmonary veins; often used prior to percutaneous closure. TEE has excellent sensitivity and specificity.

Diagnostic Procedures/Surgery

- Cardiac catheterization:
  - Demonstrates right ventricle enlargement, location/fraction of the shunt, size of the ASD, any valvular disease, and overall anatomy
  - Used to assess pulmonary vascular resistance if pulmonary hypertension is suspected, particularly if surgery is planned
  - Generally not used in young patients for initial diagnosis, more often reserved for use when:
    - Part of a planned interventional (device) closure
    - Evaluating other disease simultaneously (e.g., coronary artery disease in older individuals)
    - Visualization by other methods insufficient
- Cardiac magnetic resonance: A noninvasive follow-up to echo that allows viewing the defect/pulmonary veins and measurement of shunt fraction and right ventricular (RV) function
- Exercise testing: Useful to quantify symptoms not consistent with clinical findings or to document change over time
- Chest x-ray: May demonstrate right ventricular and pulmonary artery enlargement, increased pulmonary vascular markings
- Ultrafast CT scans can also define ASDs, but with significant radiation exposure.

DIFFERENTIAL DIAGNOSIS

- Other congenital heart disease
- Right bundle branch block (for widely split S2)

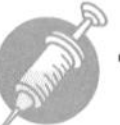

TREATMENT

MEDICATION

First Line

- Treatment of secondary atrial fibrillation/supraventricular tachycardia with anticoagulation and cardioversion, followed by anticoagulation with maintenance of sinus rhythm if possible, or rate control if this fails
- Respiratory tract infections should be treated promptly.
- Treatment of heart failure (diuretics, oxygen, digoxin, etc.)

Second Line

- No antibiotic prophylaxis is recommended for unrepaired ASDs.
- Antibiotic prophylaxis against infective endocarditis during dental or other oral procedures is recommended for 6 months by the American Heart Association (AHA) after a device or patch is placed (2)[B]:
  - In patients with repaired ASD who have a residual defect at or adjacent to the device, prophylaxis is recommended indefinitely.
  - Generally, for dental procedures, amoxicillin 2 g (adults) or 50 mg/kg (children). Other options include cephalosporins (e.g., ceftriaxone 1 g [adults] or 50 mg/kg [children] IM or IV) or clindamycin 600 mg PO (adults) or 20 mg/kg PO (children) in patients who are penicillin-sensitive (3).
- To prevent thrombus formation after device deployment, aspirin 325 mg daily for 6 months and clopidogrel 75 mg for at least a month

ADDITIONAL TREATMENT

General Measures

75% of small ASDs (<8 mm) will close spontaneously by 18 months of age; however, close follow-up is warranted (4)[B]. Likelihood of spontaneous closure mainly determined by diameter of defect: >10 mm at time of diagnosis are unlikely to spontaneously close (5)[B].

Issues for Referral

Appropriate health care: Referral to a cardiologist for evaluation

SURGERY/OTHER PROCEDURES

- In adults, closure via percutaneous transcatheter device or surgery if:
  - Right heart enlargement regardless of symptoms
  - Pulmonary systemic flow ratio is ≥2:1 (or >1.5:1 and under 21 years old according to the AHA)
  - Symptoms, such as documented orthodeoxia/platypnea, or paradoxical embolism (1)[C]
- Flow ratio can be measured with Doppler echo (lab-specific) or cardiac catheterization.
- Surgical repair is standard for a sinus venosus, coronary sinus, or primum ASD.
- Percutaneous transcatheter device closure of secundum atrial septal defects is standard and has largely replaced surgery except when other interventions are planned or anatomy is not favorable (6)[A]. Secundum ASDs that are suitable for percutaneous closure should be 35 mm or less in stretched balloon diameter and should have a sufficient rim of surrounding atrial tissue.
- Closure is not indicated for patients who have developed irreversible severe pulmonary hypertension without continued shunting or those who never develop symptoms and have an ASD <5 mm.
- In children, closure is usually delayed until preschool age (2–4 years), except for symptomatic defects (poor growth or exercise intolerance) because of the high rate of spontaneous closure.
- Closing small asymptomatic ASDs is controversial and not often done.

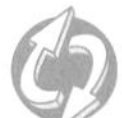

ONGOING CARE

FOLLOW-UP RECOMMENDATIONS

Echocardiography can be used to monitor both repaired and unrepaired ASDs.

Patient Monitoring

- In otherwise asymptomatic healthy children, follow until defect has closed or become negligible in size.
- Appropriate evaluation and management for atrial tachyarrhythmias in patients with long-term follow-up
- If ASD repaired as an adult, periodic long-term follow-up indicated.
- ASDs repaired in childhood generally do not have late complications.
- In female patients with unrepaired ASD and Eisenmenger syndrome, pregnancy is not recommended due to increased risk of maternal and fetal mortality.
- Pregnancy is well tolerated in patients with repaired ASD and small unrepaired ASDs.

PATIENT EDUCATION

For patient education materials on this topic, consult:

- American Heart Association: http://www.heart.org
- Mayo Clinic information: http://www.mayoclinic.com/health/atrial-septal-defect/DS00628

PROGNOSIS

- ASD closure in asymptomatic or minimally symptomatic adults reduces morbidity but not mortality (7)[A].
- ASD closure before age 25 in symptomatic adults improves morbidity and likely reduces mortality.
- ASD repair deferred until after adolescence may not decrease long-term risk of future atrial arrhythmias.
- Up to 50% mortality by age 50 in untreated symptomatic patients with large defects

COMPLICATIONS

- Unrepaired:
  - Pulmonary infections
  - Congestive heart failure
  - Stroke
  - Pulmonary hypertension/Eisenmenger syndrome
  - Atrial arrhythmias
  - Cerebral abscess
  - Infective endocarditis
- Surgically repaired:
  - Late-onset arrhythmias 10–20 years after surgery (5%)
  - Perioperative atrial tachyarrhythmias in 10–13% of patients
- Device closure: Device embolization (1%), cardiac perforation, thrombus formation, endocarditis, supraventricular arrhythmias

REFERENCES

1. Warnes CA, Williams RG, Bashore TM, et al. ACC/AHA 2008 guidelines for the management of adults with congenital heart disease. *J Am Coll Cardiol*. 2008;52:e1–121.
2. Nishimura RA, Carabello BA, Faxon DP, et al. ACC/AHA 2008 guideline update on valvular heart disease: Focused update on infective endocarditis. *Circulation*. 2008;118:887–96.
3. Wilson et al. Prevention of infective endocarditis: guidelines from the American Heart Association. *Circulation*. 2007;116:1736–54.
4. McMahon CJ, Feltes TF, Fraley JK, et al. Natural history of growth of secundum atrial septal defects and implications for transcatheter closure. *Heart*. 2002;87:256–9.
5. Hanslik A, Pospisil U, Salzer-Muhar U, et al. Predictors of spontaneous closure of isolated secundum atrial septal defect in children: A longitudinal study. *Pediatrics*. 2006;118:1560–5.
6. Holzer R, Hijazi ZM. Interventional approach to congenital heart disease. *Curr Opin Cardiol*. 2004;19:84–90.
7. Attie F, Rosas M, Granados N, et al. Surgical treatment for secundum atrial septal defects in patients >40 years old. A randomized clinical trial. *J Am Coll Cardiol*. 2001;38:2035–42.

ADDITIONAL READING

- Lindsey JB, Hillis LD. Clinical update: atrial septal defect in adults. *Lancet*. 2007;369:1244–6.
- Tubman TR, Shields MD, Craig BG, et al. Congenital heart disease in Down's syndrome: Two year prospective early screening study. *BMJ*. 1991;302:1425–7.

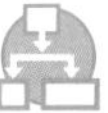

See Also (Topic, Algorithm, Electronic Media Element)

Aortic Valvular Stenosis; Coarctation of the Aorta; Patent Ductus Arteriosus; Pulmonary Valvular Stenosis; Tetralogy of Fallot; Ventricular Septal Defect

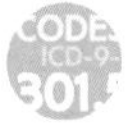

CODES

ICD9

- 745.5 Ostium secundum, type atrial septal defect
- 745.60 Endocardial cushion defect, unspecified type
- 745.61 Ostium primum defect

CLINICAL PEARLS

- ASD is often missed due to subtle clinical presentation.
- Ideally, hemodynamically significant ASDs should be closed in early childhood, though some benefit from closure is present in older patients.
- Many ASDs can be treated by catheter-directed percutaneous closure, rather than open-heart surgery.
- Routine endocarditis prophylaxis is not recommended for unrepaired ASDs.
- Patent foramen ovales, unlike large ASDs, are very common and generally require no treatment in asymptomatic individuals.

ATTENTION DEFICIT/HYPERACTIVITY DISORDER

Laura L. Novak, MD

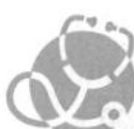

BASICS

DESCRIPTION

- Attention deficit hyperactivity disorder (ADHD) is a behavior problem characterized by a short attention span, distractibility, low frustration tolerance, impulsivity, and hyperactivity.
- ADHD is divided into 3 subsets: Predominantly hyperactivity-impulsive (ADHD-HI), predominantly inattentive (ADHD-I), or combined (ADHD-C).
- System(s) affected: Nervous
- Synonym(s): Attention deficit disorder; Hyperactivity

EPIDEMIOLOGY

- Predominant age: Onset <7 years old; lasts into adolescence and adulthood; 50% meet diagnostic criteria by age 4 years
- Predominant sex: Male > Female (5:1); predominantly inattentive type may be more common in girls

Incidence

5% of school-aged children

RISK FACTORS

- Family history
- Comorbid conditions (associated with, but not caused by):
  - Learning disabilities
  - Mood disorders
  - Oppositional defiant disorder; conduct disorder

Genetics

Familial pattern

GENERAL PREVENTION

- Children are at risk for abuse, depression, and social isolation.
- Parents need regular support and advice.
- Parents should establish contact with teacher each school year.

COMMONLY ASSOCIATED CONDITIONS

See "Risk Factors."

DIAGNOSIS

- American Academy of Pediatrics (AAP) guidelines recommend using the *DSM-IV* criteria to establish the diagnosis.
- Children undergoing extreme stress (divorce, illness, homelessness, abuse) may demonstrate ADHD behaviors secondary to stress. This can be assessed using the American Academy of Child and Adolescent Psychiatry (AACAP) screening tool, if needed.
- If diagnostic behaviors are noted in only 1 setting, explore the stressors in that setting.
- The diagnostic behaviors are more noticeable in tasks that require concentration or boredom tolerance than in free play or office situations.
- *DSM-IV* criteria: 6 or more inattention criteria and/or 6 or more hyperactivity/impulsivity criteria. Symptoms must begin by age 7 years, be present for >6 months, and be noticed in 2 settings (e.g., home and school). Teachers and caretakers should fill out assessments in addition to parents.
- Inattention:
  - Careless mistakes in tasks
  - Difficulty in sustaining attention
  - Does not seem to listen
  - Does not follow through or finish tasks
  - Difficulty in organizing tasks
  - Avoids tasks that require sustained mental effort
  - Loses things
  - Easily distracted
  - Forgetful
- Hyperactivity/impulsivity:
  - Fidgets
  - Difficulty in remaining seated
  - Runs or climbs excessively
  - Difficulty in playing quietly
  - Acts as if "driven by a motor"
  - Talks excessively
  - Blurts out answers before question is complete
  - Has difficulty in awaiting turn
  - Interrupts others

HISTORY

- Birth and development history
- Comprehensive psychosocial evaluation of home environment
- School performance history

DIAGNOSTIC TESTS & INTERPRETATION

Behavioral testing:

- Behavior rating scales (Connors, others) should be completed by parents and teachers. They are repeated after therapy is started to gauge differences (*DSM-IV* criteria can be used).
- An ADHD toolkit with forms is available from www.nichq.org/adhd.html.
- Testing for learning disability (e.g., dyslexia) through the school

Lab

Rarely needed; check lead level if high risk

Diagnostic Procedures/Surgery

Electroencephalogram not needed unless symptoms are highly suggestive of seizure disorder (e.g., absence seizures)

Pathological Findings

Motor tics can be present (e.g., cough, noises, twitching).

DIFFERENTIAL DIAGNOSIS

- Activity level appropriate for age
- Hearing or vision disorder
- Lead poisoning
- Medication reaction (decongestant, antihistamine, theophylline, phenobarbital)
- Dysfunctional family situation
- Learning disability (e.g., dyslexia)
- Pervasive developmental delay (autism)
- Asperger syndrome: High-functioning autism
- Oppositional/defiant disorder (see *DSM-IV*)
- Conduct disorder (see *DSM-IV*)
- Tourette syndrome: Motor and verbal tics
- Absence seizures (inattentive type ADHD only)

TREATMENT

MEDICATION

First Line

The 2001 AAP guideline recommends (1)[C] the use of stimulant medications as 1st-line in treatment. A second type of stimulant should be tried if the 1st treatment fails.

ALERT

The Food and Drug Administration (FDA) has considered applying a "black box" warning to stimulants based on some reported cases of sudden death seen in patients using stimulant medications. It recommends that patients with a personal or family history of congenital heart disease or sudden death be screened with an EKG and possible cardiology consultation before beginning stimulant medication.

- Stimulant:
  - Methylphenidate (Ritalin, Concerta, Metadate CD, Ritalin LA, others):
    - Short-acting: Ritalin 5–20 mg in the morning, at noon, and at 4 P.M.; maximum dose, 60 mg/d
    - Long-acting: Concerta 18, 36, 54 mg in the morning; Metadate CD 40 mg in the morning; Ritalin LA 20, 30, 40 mg in the morning
    - Methylphenidate patch (Daytrana): Apply to hip for up to 9 hours daily. Begin at 10 mg and titrate upward weekly as needed. Available as 10, 15, 20, and 30 mg.
    - Methylphenidate hydrochloride (Methylin): Available as liquid or chewable tab
  - Lisdexamfetamine (Vyvanse) 30–70 mg every morning, pediatric (ages 6–17 years) and adult
  - Dextroamphetamine: Short-acting 5–20 mg b.i.d. Long-acting, 40 mg daily.
  - Mixed amphetamine salts:
    - Adderall: 2.5–20 mg q4–6h
    - Adderall XR: 5–30 mg every morning; ≥6 years
- Precautions:
  - If not responding, check compliance and consider another diagnosis (1)[C].
  - Some children experience withdrawal (tearfulness, agitation) after a missed dose or when medication wears off.
  - Stimulants are drugs of abuse and should be monitored carefully.
  - Drug holidays should be given only if family/peer relationships are not harmed.
- Significant possible interactions:
  - Stimulants may increase levels of anticonvulsants, SSRIs, tricyclics, and warfarin.

Pregnancy Considerations

Medications used in ADHD are Category C: Caution in pregnancy.

Second Line

- Nonstimulant:
  - Atomoxetine carries a "black box" warning regarding potential exacerbation of suicidality (similar to SSRIs). Close follow-up recommended: Weekly visits for 1st month, then every-other-week visits for 4 sessions, then every-12-weeks visits:
    - Atomoxetine associated with hepatic injury in a small number of cases; check liver enzymes if symptoms (jaundice, fatigue, malaise) develop

- Atomoxetine (Strattera): Selective norepinephrine reuptake inhibitor; 0.5–2 mg/kg/d every morning (10 mg, 18 mg, 25 mg, 40 mg, 60 mg). Maximum dose, 1.4 mg/kg/d or 100 mg/d, whichever is less:
  - Slower onset of efficacy; GI side effects and sedation. Not addictive.
- Atomoxetine interacts with paroxetine (Paxil), fluoxetine (Prozac), and quinidine.
- Alpha$_2$ agonists:
  - Guanfacine (Intuiv): 1–4 mg once daily. Very sedating, expensive.
  - Clonidine (Kapvay): 0.1–0.4 mg divided. Very sedating, expensive.
- Other nonstimulant drugs (e.g., clonidine, tricyclic antidepressants, SSRIs): Due to the mixed efficacy and high side effects of these drugs, they are not recommended for use without a consultant.

ADDITIONAL TREATMENT

- Medication alone or combined with behavioral therapy produced better results than behavioral therapy alone.
- Behavioral therapy may be useful in cases where parents object to medication (2).

General Measures

- Parent/school/patient education (2)
- Work closely with teacher.
- Avoid unproven therapies.

Issues for Referral

Specialist referral should be considered for children younger than age 6, for psychological or medical complications, or poor response to medication.

COMPLEMENTARY AND ALTERNATIVE MEDICINE

- Surveys have shown that parents of children with ADHD use herbals and complementary treatments frequently (20–60%) (3,4).
- Many herbals have been assessed for efficacy, but studies are small and brief and, therefore, difficult to translate into clinical recommendations.
- Dietary and nutritional supplements have also been assessed:
  - Omega-3 fatty acids (found in fish oil and some supplements) showed improvement in rating scales in 2 double-blind, placebo-controlled studies of 116 and 130 patients.
- Rapid eye training and biofeedback have contradictory results and can be costly.

ONGOING CARE

The "toolkit for physicians" may be useful: http://www.nichq.org/adhd.html

FOLLOW-UP RECOMMENDATIONS

Patient Monitoring

- Parent/teacher rating scales initially, 2 weeks after an intervention such as starting medication, and regularly
- Office visits to monitor side effects and efficacy: Endpoints are improved grades, improved rating scales, acceptable family interactions, and improved peer interactions.
- Monitor growth (especially weight gain) and BP.

DIET

"Insufficient evidence exists to suggest that dietary interventions improve the symptoms of ADHD in children" (5).

PATIENT EDUCATION

- Excellent reference: www.parentsmedguide.org
- Key points for parents:
  - 50% of children with ADHD have 1 parent with ADHD; modify education sessions with parents accordingly.
  - Behavioral interventions such as token systems may be helpful (1)[A].
  - Find things child is good at and emphasize these.
  - Reinforce good behavior (with rewards and attention).
  - Make eye contact with each request.
  - Give 1 task at a time.
  - Stop behavior before it escalates with quiet discipline.
  - Organize home and schoolwork.
  - Some families benefit from "parent training" and family therapy.
  - Coordinate homework with teachers using daily assignment notebook.
  - Refer to advocacy and support groups.
- Schools are required by law to provide necessary testing and Individualized Educational Plans (IEPs) or 504 plans to accommodate the child's educational needs.
- Support groups:
  - Children and Adults with Attention Deficit Disorder (CHADD): chadd.org; 800-233-4050
  - Attention Deficit Disorder Warehouse: addwarehouse.com; 800-233-9273
  - Learning Disabilities Association (LDA): LDAlearning.com
  - National Information Center for Children and Youth with Disabilities: www.nichcy.org

PROGNOSIS

- May last into adulthood
- The hyperactivity component may become easier to control with increasing age.
- Encourage career choices that allow autonomy and mobility.
- Prognosis data is derived from small studies and may not apply to all patients.
- 2–4 times increase in automobile accidents and injuries. Improves with medication.
- Encourage parents to subtract 2 years from their child's chronological age when allowing privileges (e.g., treat a 16-year-old like a 14-year-old, delay driving until age 18).

COMPLICATIONS

- Untreated ADHD can lead to failing school, parental abuse, social isolation, and poor self-esteem.
- Some children experience withdrawal (tearfulness, agitation) after a missed medication dose or when medication wears off.
- Monitor growth with stimulant use. If appetite is poor as a side effect of stimulant medication, eat before the medication is given and after it wears off.
- Increased risk of substance abuse is controversial and may be related to comorbid conditions (conduct disorder).

REFERENCES

1. American Academy of Pediatrics. Subcommittee on Attention-Deficit/Hyperactivity Disorder and Committee on Quality Improvement. Clinical practice guideline: Treatment of the school-aged child with attention-deficit/hyperactivity disorder. *Pediatrics*. 2001;108:1033–44.
2. Laforett DR, Murray DW, Kollins SH. Psychosocial treatments for preschool-aged children with attention-deficit hyperactivity disorder. *Dev Disabil Res Rev*. 2008;14:300–10.
3. Sawni A. Attention-deficit/hyperactivity disorder and complementary/alternative medicine. *Adolesc Med State Art Rev*. 2008;19:313–26, xi.
4. Weber W, Newmark S. Complementary and alternative medical therapies for attention-deficit/hyperactivity disorder and autism. *Pediatr Clin North Am*. 2007;54:983–1006; xii.
5. Sinn N. Nutritional and dietary influences on attention deficit hyperactivity disorder. *Nutr Rev*. 2008;66:558–68.

ADDITIONAL READING

- American Psychiatric Association. *Diagnostic and Statistical Manual of Mental Disorders*, 4th ed. Revised. Washington, DC: American Psychiatric Association; 2000.
- Another extended release alpha$_2$ agonist for ADHD. *Med Lett*. 2011;53(1357).
- Barkley RA. *ADHD: A Handbook for Diagnosis and Treatment*, 2nd ed. New York: Guilford Press, 1998.
- Brown RT, Amler RW, Freeman WS, et al. Treatment of attention deficit/hyperactivity disorder: Overview of the evidence. *Pediatrics*. 2005;115(6): e749–e757.
- Ghuman JK, Arnold LE, Anthony BJ. Psychopharmacological and other treatments in preschool children with attention-deficit/ hyperactivity disorder: Current Evidence and Practice. *J Child Adolesc Psychopharmacol*. 2008;18(5):413–47.
- Pliszka S, AACAP Work Group on Quality Issues. Practice parameter for the assessment and treatment of children and adolescents with attention-deficit/hyperactivity disorder. *J Am Acad Child Adolesc Psychiatry*. 2007;46:894–921.
- Rader R, McCauley L, Callen EC. Current strategies in the diagnosis and treatment of childhood attention-deficit/hyperactivity disorder. *Am Fam Physician*. 2009;79:657–65.
- Rappley MD. attention deficit-hyperactivity disorder. *N Engl J Med*. 2005;352(2):165–73.
- Rostain AL. Attention-deficit/hyperactivity disorder in adults: Evidence-based recommendations for management. *Postgrad Med*. 2008;120:27–38.
- Soileau EJ. Medications for adolescents with attention-deficit/hyperactivity disorder. *Adolesc Med State Art Rev*. 2008;19:254–67, viii–ix.

CODES

ICD9

- 314.00 Attention deficit disorder of childhood without mention of hyperactivity
- 314.01 Attention deficit disorder of childhood with hyperactivity

CLINICAL PEARLS

- Children undergoing extreme stress (divorce, illness, homelessness, abuse) may demonstrate ADHD behaviors secondary to stress.
- 50% of ADHD children have a parent with ADHD.
- AAP recommends the use of stimulant medications as the 1st-line treatment.

AUTISM SPECTRUM DISORDERS

Macario C. Corpuz, Jr., MD, FAAFP
Alphonsus W. Kung, MD

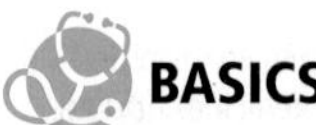

BASICS

DESCRIPTION

Group of neurodevelopmental disorders of early childhood:

- Includes autistic disorder, Rett syndrome, childhood disintegrative disorder, Asperger's disorder, and pervasive developmental disorder not otherwise specified (PDD-NOS)
- Autistic disorder includes classic autism and childhood autism.
- Rett syndrome involves mutations in the MECP2 gene, mostly in females with initial normal development until ~18 months of age with microcephaly and dementia.
- Childhood disintegrative disorder: Regression after at least 2 years of normal development.
- Asperger's disorder: Better development with mechanics of verbal expression, higher levels of cognition and interest in social activity.
- PDD-NOS: Meets some, but not all of *Diagnostic and Statistical Manual of Mental Disorders-Fourth Edition (Text Revision) DSM-IV-TR* criteria for autistic disorder.
- Characterized by:
  - Impairment of effective social skills
  - Absent or impaired communication skills
  - Repetitive and/or stereotyped behaviors and interests, especially in inanimate objects
  - System(s) affected: Nervous

EPIDEMIOLOGY

- Predominant age: Onset in early childhood
- Predominant sex: Male > Female (4:1) except for Rett syndrome

Pediatric Considerations

Symptom onset seen in children <3 years (except for childhood disintegrative disorder)

Prevalence

Estimated 1/100 to 1/500 children

RISK FACTORS

Siblings with autism have shown to have a 5-times greater risk of developing autism. Prevalence ranging from 2–8%.

Genetics

- High concordance in monozygotic twins
- Increased recurrence risk (3–7%) in subsequent siblings

GENERAL PREVENTION

- Early screening for early treatment means a better prognosis.
- Some autism spectrum disorders (ASDs) such as Rett syndrome are known to be caused by genetic mutations.

PATHOPHYSIOLOGY

Pathophysiology is incompletely understood.

ETIOLOGY

- No single cause has been identified.
- General consensus: A genetic abnormality leads to altered neurologic development.
- Research continues to investigate the links between heredity, genetics, and medical problems.
- No documented scientific evidence exists that proves vaccines or thimerosal cause ASDs.

COMMONLY ASSOCIATED CONDITIONS

- Mental retardation
- ADHD
- Phenylketonuria (PKU), tuberous sclerosis, fragile X syndrome, Angelman syndrome, and fetal alcohol syndrome (rare)
- Anxiety
- Depression
- Obsessive behavior
- Seizures (increased risk if severe mental retardation)
- Maternal use of SSRIs during pregnancy (1)

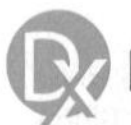

DIAGNOSIS

HISTORY

- Impairment in social interaction:
  - Impairment in nonverbal behaviors such as eye-to-eye gaze, facial expression
  - Unable to develop peer relationships
  - Does not smile nor share emotions
  - Loss of social or emotional reciprocity
- Communication impairment:
  - Delay or lack of development in language skills
  - Inability to initiate or sustain conversation
  - Stereotyped and repetitive use of language
  - Preoccupation with parts of toys or body parts
- Repetitive and stereotyped patterns of behavior:
  - Excessively lines up toys or other objects
  - Unusually attached to one particular toy or object
  - Repetitive odd movements (toe walking, hand flapping)
  - Adherence to specific routines or rituals
- Asperger's disorder does not have clinically significant delays in cognitive development, language acquisitions, nor learning/adaptive skills.
- Rett syndrome is predominantly in females without macrocephaly.
- Childhood disintegrative disorder with normal development until 2 years of age
- PDD-NOS does not meet DSM-IV-TR criteria for autism.
- Prenatal, neonatal, and developmental history
- Seizure disorder
- Family history of autism, genetic disorders, learning disabilities, psychiatric illness, neurological disorders, genetic disorders, or mental retardation
- Commonly associated with sleep disorders (2,3)

PHYSICAL EXAM

- Macrocephaly in 25% (except in Rett syndrome); head circumference growth peaks at age 6 months and begins to decline by 1 year.
- Dysmorphic features consistent with genetic disorder (fragile X syndrome)
- Hypotonia can occur in autism, but neurological deficit is a sign that imaging may be needed.
- Wood lamp skin exam to rule out tuberous sclerosis

DIAGNOSTIC TESTS & INTERPRETATION

- Checklist for Autism in Toddlers (CHAT) to screen for ASDs at 18 months of age. (To order: http://www.autism.org.uk/working-with/health/screening-and-diagnosis/checklist-for-autism-in-toddlers-chat.aspx)
- The Pervasive Developmental Disorders Screening Test-II (PDDST-II) to screen for ASDs beginning at 18 months
- Modified Checklist for Autism in Toddlers (M-CHAT) to screen for ASDs at 16–30 months
- Social Communication Questionnaire (SCQ) (formerly Autism Screening Questionnaire)—used with children age 4 years and older—the gold-standard diagnostic interview used in research studies

Lab

- Lead screening
- PKU screening
- Karyotype and DNA analysis (fragile X, PKU, tuberous sclerosis, and others)
- Metabolic testing if signs of:
  - Lethargy, limited endurance
  - Hypotonia
  - Recurrent vomiting and dehydration
  - Developmental regression
  - Unusual habits
  - Specific food intolerance

Follow-Up & Special Considerations

- Hearing tests: Audiometry and brainstem auditory evoked response (BAERS)
- Comprehensive speech and language evaluation
- Evaluation by multidisciplinary team: Includes a psychiatrist, neurologist, psychologist, speech therapist, and other autism specialists
- Intellectual level needs to be established and monitored, as it is one of the best measures of prognosis.
- Test used to follow autism are:
  - Autism Behavior Checklist (ABC)
  - Gilliam Autism Rating Scale (GARS)
  - Childhood Autism Rating Scale (CARS)
  - Autism Diagnosis Interview-Revised (ADI-R)
  - Autism Diagnostic Observation Schedule-Generic (ADOS-G) Imaging

Imaging

Initial approach

MRI is useful only if focal neurologic symptoms

Diagnostic Procedures/Surgery

Electroencephalogram (EEG) only if history of seizures or spells

DIFFERENTIAL DIAGNOSIS

Other mental and CNS disorders:

- Obsessive-compulsive disorder
- Elective mutism
- Language disorder/hearing impairment
- Intellectual disability/global developmental delay
- Stereotyped movement disorder
- Severe early deprivation/reactive attachment disorder
- Anxiety disorder
- Developmental language disorder

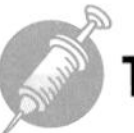

TREATMENT

MEDICATION

Medical causes of autisticlike behavior should be excluded with behavioral management maximized prior to considering medication with symptom-specific therapy, as pharmacological therapy data are scant.

First Line

- No true first-line medical therapy
- Stimulant medications (such as methylphenidate): Efficacious in treating concomitant symptoms of attention deficit disorder, such as impulsiveness, hyperactivity, and inattention; however, the magnitude of response is less than in typically developing children, and adverse effects are more frequent.
- SSRIs have shown some help in reducing ritualistic behavior and improving mood and language skills. Initial choice for anxiety and depressive mood. Also administered for dysregulated mood (4).
- Risperidone (an atypical antipsychotic) has been shown to be effective for short-term treatment of tantrums, aggression, and self-injurious behavior. Improvements in stereotyped behavior, hyperactivity, irritability, repetitious behaviors, and social withdrawal have also been noted (5)[A]. Precautions: Causes weight gain as an adverse effect. Associated with sedation, dry mouth, agitation enuresis, dyspepsia, diarrhea, constipation, and tremor.
- Melatonin used for patients with concomitant sleep disorders.

Second Line

Vitamin B6 and magnesium with inconclusive evidence in improving speech and language (6,7)[C].

ADDITIONAL TREATMENT

General Measures

- Comprehensive structured educational programming of a sustained and intensive design, most commonly applied behavioral analysis therapy
- Core features of a successful education program:
  - High staff–student ratio 1:2, or less
  - Individualized programming
  - Specialized teacher training with ongoing evaluation of teachers and programs
  - 25 hours a week minimum of specialized services
  - A structured routine environment that emphasizes attention, imitation, communication, socialization, and play interactions
  - Functional analysis of behavioral problems
  - Transition planning and involvement of the family
- Currently no cure for ASDs. Early diagnosis and initiation of multidisciplinary intervention help enhance functioning in later life.
- Early intervention for ages 3 and under
- School-based special education for older children
- Find alternative methods of communication: Sign language; picture exchange communication system

Issues for Referral

- Refer early to:
  - Early learning for evaluation of behavior and language
  - Genetic counseling
  - Audiology
- Consider referrals to psychiatry, ophthalmology, otolaryngology, neurology, and nutrition
- Refer family members to parent support groups and respite programs

COMPLEMENTARY AND ALTERNATIVE MEDICINE

- Music therapy has been shown to improve communication skills in autistic patients with limited data (8)[B].
- Auditory integration training is used for autistic children with sound sensitivity (9)[B].
- Osteopathic manipulative treatment (OMT) has been shown to improve sensory and motor performance with neurological problems, including autism. Treatment that starts before the age of 2 years showed the greatest effect.

ONGOING CARE

FOLLOW-UP RECOMMENDATIONS

Patient Monitoring

- Constant monitoring by caregivers
- Reevaluation every 6–12 months by physician for seizures, sleep and nutritional problems, and prescribed medical management
- Intellectual and language testing every 2 years in childhood

DIET

Gluten- and casein-free diets show some reduction in autistic traits; however, large-scale, good-quality randomized controlled trials are needed (10).

PATIENT EDUCATION

- Autism Society of America: http://www.autismsociety.org
- Autism and vaccines: http://www.aap.org/immunization/families/faq/VaccineStudies.pdf

PROGNOSIS

- Those who begin treatment at a young age (2–4 years) have significantly better outcomes.
- Prognosis is closely related to initial intellectual abilities, with only 20% functioning above the mentally retarded level.
- Communicative language development before 5 years is also associated with a better outcome.
- The general expected course is for a lifelong need for supervised structured care.

COMPLICATIONS

- Increasing incidents of seizure disorders in up to 1 in 4 children.
- Increased risk for physical and sexual abuse
- With pica, increased risk of lead poisoning
- Limited variety of food consumed due to dietary obsessions
- Increased risk for GI symptoms, including weight abnormalities and abnormal stool patterns

REFERENCES

1. Croen LA, Grether JK, Yoshida CK, et al. Antidepressants use during pregnancy and childhood autism spectrum disorders. *Arch Gen Psychiatry*. 2011;68(11)1104–12.
2. Vriend JL, Corkum PV, Moon EC, et al. Behavioral interventions for sleep problems in children with autism spectrum disorders: Current findings and future directions. *J Pediatr Psychol*. 2011;36(9):1017–29.
3. Reynolds AM, Malow BA. Sleep and austim spectrum disorders. *Pediatr Clin Am*. 2011;58(3):685–98.
4. Williams K, Wheeler DM, Silove N, et al. Selective serotonin reuptake inhibitors (SSRIs) for autism spectrum disorders (ASD). *Cochrane Database Syst Rev*. 2010;(8):CD004677.
5. Jesner OS, Aref-Adib M, Coren E. Risperdone for autistic spectrum disorder. *Cochrane Database Syst Rev*. 2007;(1):CD005040.
6. Malouf R, Grimley Evans J. Vitamin B6 for cognition. *Cochrane Database Syst Rev*. 2003;(4):CD004393.
7. Nye C, Brice A. Combined vitamin B6-magnesium treatment in autism spectrum disorder. *Cochrane Database Syst Rev*. 2005;(4):CD003497.
8. Gold C, Wigram T, Elefant C. Music therapy for autistic spectrum disorder. *Cochrane Database of Syst Rev*. 2006;(2):CD004381.
9. Sinha Y, Silove N, Wheeler D, et al. Auditory integration training and other sound therapies for autism spectrum disorders. *Cochrane Database Syst Rev*. 2004;(1):CD003681.
10. Millward C, Ferriter M, Calver S, et al. Gluten- and casein-free diets for autistic spectrum disorder. *Cochrane Database Syst Rev*. 2008;(2):CD003498.

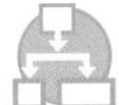

See Also (Topic, Algorithm, Electronic Media Element)

Algorithm: Mental Retardation

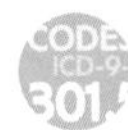

CODES

ICD9

- 299.00 Infantile autism, current or active state
- 299.10 Disintegrative psychosis, current or active state
- 299.80 Other specified early childhood psychoses, current or active state

CLINICAL PEARLS

ALARM mnemonic from the American Academy of Pediatrics (AAP):

- Autism spectrum disorder is prevalent (screen ALL children between 18 and 24 months).
- Listen to parents when they feel something is wrong.
- Act early: Screen all children who fall behind in language and social developmental milestones (use early learning to help with evaluation).
- Refer to multidisciplinary teams (speech and language evaluation, genetic screening, social support groups).
- Monitor support for patient and families.

BACK PAIN, LOW

Richard Hinds, MD
Christopher Garofalo, MD

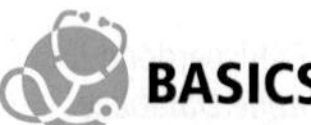

BASICS

DESCRIPTION

- Mechanical low back pain (LBP) is a common, benign, and self-limiting condition responsive to conservative treatment, including maintenance of activity and short-term use of analgesics.
- Patients typically present with pain, muscle soreness, or stiffness at the posterior lower back. The symptoms may be unilateral or bilateral and may radiate to the buttocks and/or posterior thighs. Symptoms are often the result of the mechanical stress and increased functional demand.
- For most patients, pain is of short duration. Complete recovery is expected within 4–6 weeks.
- The primary goal in the evaluation is to rule out red-flag signs or symptoms that may be indicative of more serious etiologies. When one of these red-flag signs or symptoms is present, further investigation is required.
- System(s) affected: Musculoskeletal; Nervous
- Synonym(s): Low back syndrome; Lumbar strain/sprain; Lumbago

Geriatric Considerations

Tumors, degenerative conditions, fractures, and spinal stenosis are possible etiologies.

Pediatric Considerations

The presence of LBP is considered a red-flag symptom. A thorough workup is imperative.

Pregnancy Considerations

LBP is commonly associated with pregnancy, and treatment is conservative.

EPIDEMIOLOGY

Prevalence

- 90% of Americans experience mechanical LBP at some time in their lives.
- LBP is one of the most common primary care complaints.
- Repetitive episodes are common.
- Predominant age: ≥25 years
- Predominant sex: Male = Female

RISK FACTORS

- Increasing age
- Activity (e.g., heavy lifting, bending, twisting)
- Smoking
- Obesity
- Vibration (e.g., driving motor vehicles)
- Sedentary lifestyle
- Psychosocial factors such as increased stress, anxiety, or depressed mood

GENERAL PREVENTION

- Maintaining physical fitness
- Weight loss
- Smoking cessation
- Stress reduction
- Avoidance of aggravating tasks

ETIOLOGY

- Underlying degenerative joint and disc disease involving the lumbosacral spine
- Acute event that exacerbates the degenerative process
- In primary care setting, <15% of LBP patients have identifiable significant disease.

COMMONLY ASSOCIATED CONDITIONS

- Deconditioning, obesity
- Psychosocial disease
- Compression fracture

DIAGNOSIS

HISTORY

- Onset of pain may either be acute or insidious.
- Occasional radiation of pain to buttocks and/or posterior thighs
- Pain can be aggravated by back motion, sitting, standing, lifting, bending, and twisting.
- Pain is often relieved by rest.
- Back pain is greater than lower extremity pain.
- Bowel and bladder function are preserved.
- Psychosocial stressors at work and/or home may be present.
- Medical history and previous injuries should be reviewed.
- Red flags:
  - Age >50 years or <20 years (neoplastic)
  - History of cancer (recurrence or metastatic)
  - Night sweats or weight loss (neoplastic, rheumatologic)
  - Urinary or bowel incontinence or saddle anesthesia (neurologic compromise/cauda equina syndrome)
  - Recent bacterial infection
  - Pain worse when supine (rheumatologic, neurologic, neoplastic)
  - History of trauma

PHYSICAL EXAM

- Observation reveals preferred posture and pain behaviors.
- Decreased lumbar range of motion, paraspinous musculature tenderness, and spasm
- Motor, sensory, and reflex examinations are normal.
- Straight-leg raise test may worsen LBP, but a positive test suggests sciatica.

DIAGNOSTIC TESTS & INTERPRETATION

Lab

Initial lab tests

- Not typically indicated on initial presentation.
- For patients with red flags, pain that worsens, persists for >6 weeks, or is refractory to conservative treatment, consider:
  - CBC with differential
  - ESR
  - Alkaline and acid phosphatase
  - Serum calcium
  - Serum protein electrophoresis
- Special tests: System-directed investigation

Imaging

Initial approach

Plain radiographs:

- Not recommended in the absence of red flags (1)[B]
- Indicated for persistent symptoms (>6 weeks), age < 20 or >50 years, systemic symptoms, presence of neurologic deficits, trauma, history of cancer, use of immunosuppressants, IV drug abuse, or if abnormalities such as ankylosing spondylitis are suspected
- Anteroposterior, lateral, spot lateral of L5–S1, and oblique films are included in routine lumbosacral series.

Diagnostic Procedures/Surgery

- MRI and CT scan indicated only for persistent symptoms, neurologic deficits, and/or suspected infection or malignancy:
  - MRI is useful for visualization of soft tissue.
  - CT scan is useful for visualization of bony anatomy.
- Bone scan (scintigraphy): Technetium-99m-labeled phosphorus to rule out fractures, infections, or metastases

DIFFERENTIAL DIAGNOSIS

- Structural:
  - Lumbar strain/sprain
  - Herniated lumbar intervertebral disk
  - Degenerative disk disease
  - Degenerative segmental instability
  - Spinal stenosis
  - Spondylolisthesis
  - Congenital disease: Severe kyphosis, severe scoliosis
  - Fractures
- Inflammatory:
  - Ankylosing spondylitis and related inflammatory spondylopathies
  - Rheumatoid arthritis
- Infectious: Vertebral osteomyelitis
- Neoplastic:
  - Primary tumors
  - Metastatic disease
- Referred pain:
  - Orthopedic: Osteoarthritis of hip
  - GI: Duodenal ulcer, chronic pancreatitis, cholecystitis, irritable bowel syndrome, diverticulitis
  - Genitourinary: Pyelonephritis, nephrolithiasis, prostatitis
  - Gynecologic: Pregnancy, endometriosis, ovarian cystic disease, pelvic inflammatory disease
  - Cardiovascular: Abdominal aortic aneurysm, vascular claudication

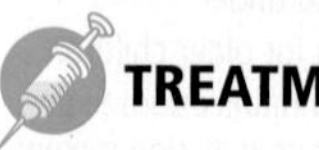

TREATMENT

MEDICATION

First Line

- NSAIDs: Agents are considered equally effective (2)[A]:
  - Ibuprofen (Motrin): 800 mg PO q6h × 10 days, then as needed (maximum 2,400 mg/d)
  - Naproxen (Naprosyn): 500 mg PO b.i.d. × 10 days, then as needed (maximum 1,500 mg/d)

- Celecoxib (Celebrex): 200 mg PO daily:
  - Adverse reactions: GI discomfort, dizziness, tinnitus, GI bleeding, hypertension, acute renal failure
  - Contraindications: Coronary artery bypass grafting perioperative pain, aspirin allergy, third trimester of pregnancy
  - Precautions: Increased risk of cardiovascular event, high risk of GI bleeding, history of GI ulcer, renal disease, elderly patients
  - Possible interactions: Antiplatelet agents, ACE inhibitors, lithium, warfarin, low-molecular-weight heparin
  - Note: Naproxen is associated with lower risk of cardiovascular dysfunction as compared to ibuprofen.
- Muscle relaxants. Comparative efficacy to NSAIDs is unknown (3):
  - Cyclobenzaprine (Flexeril): 10 mg PO at bedtime or q8h (maximum 60 mg/d)
  - Metaxalone (Skelaxin): 800 mg PO t.i.d.–q.i.d.
    - Adverse reactions: Sedation, GI discomfort, dry mouth, confusion
    - Contraindications:
      - Cyclobenzaprine: Arrhythmias, congestive heart failure, hyperthyroidism, concomitant monoamine oxidase inhibitors
      - Metaxalone: Anemia, severe renal/hepatic impairment
    - Precautions: Elderly, urinary retention, glaucoma
    - Possible interactions:
      - Cyclobenzaprine: Antihistamines, benzodiazepines, anticholinergics, SSRIs
      - Metaxalone: Antihistamines, benzodiazepines, antipsychotics

ALERT

Avoid alcohol, driving, or operating heavy machinery.

ALERT

Some muscle relaxants have a high potential for abuse.

Second Line

- Short-acting combination opioid analgesic products should be considered only for moderate–severe pain refractory to NSAIDs and muscle relaxants (4)[A].
- Antidepressants are not effective treatments for LBP in the general population. However, depressed patients with LBP may benefit from antidepressant treatment (5)[A].

ALERT

Use of narcotics in acute LBP may increase risk of progression to chronic LBP.

ADDITIONAL TREATMENT

General Measures

- Outpatient management is appropriate.
- Activity modification as appropriate
- Short-term nonopioid analgesics at fixed time intervals
- Use of opioid analgesics does not improve return-to-work status.

Issues for Referral

Refer patients with progressive motor and sensory signs or symptoms or evidence of infection, tumor, or fracture for emergent or specialist evaluation.

Additional Therapies

There is strong evidence that an intensive individual education session is as effective as other interventions in short- and long-term return to work.

COMPLEMENTARY AND ALTERNATIVE MEDICINE

- Chiropractic manipulation may be helpful.
- Behavioral therapy has not been shown to be more effective than group exercises for pain or depressive symptoms (6)[A].
- Devil's claw, white willow bark, and capsaicin have demonstrated efficacy vs. placebo for acute episodes of chronic LBP (7)[B].

IN-PATIENT CONSIDERATIONS

Admission Criteria

Limit to patients who require surgical procedures for underlying red flag etiologies

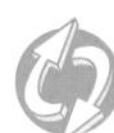

ONGOING CARE

FOLLOW-UP RECOMMENDATIONS

- Bed rest is *not* recommended.
- Activities of daily living should be resumed as soon as possible.
- Consider restrictions on more strenuous activities until symptoms have resolved.

Patient Monitoring

- Estimated duration of care is 1–6 weeks:
  - Schedule follow-up at 2–4 weeks.
  - Assess the following at each follow-up visit: Pain, functional status, and medication-related adverse effects.
- Re-evaluate for possible underlying causes if improvement does not occur.
- Patients should be encouraged to maintain normal levels of activity.
- Consider ongoing physical therapy.

DIET

Weight reduction, if appropriate

PATIENT EDUCATION

Advise the patient to stay active, use medication as prescribed, and discuss adverse drug effects.

PROGNOSIS

- Usually self-limiting; recovery is expected within 6 weeks in 90% of patients (3)
- Symptoms can recur in 50–80% of patients within the first year.
- Adverse psychosocial factors to resolving back pain:
  - Pending litigation or compensation
  - Prolonged use of habit-forming medications or alcohol
  - Poor coping strategies, depressed or hostile patient
  - Job dissatisfaction

COMPLICATIONS

- Chronic LBP
- Persistent psychosocial impairment

REFERENCES

1. Flynn TW, Smith B, Chou R. Appropriate use of diagnostic imaging in low back pain: A reminder that unnecessary imaging may do as much harm as good. *J Orthop Sports Phys Ther*. 2011;41(11): 838–46.
2. Roelofs PDDM, Deyo RA, Koes BW, et al. Non-steroidal antiinflammatory drugs for low back pain. *Cochrane Database Syst Rev*. 2008;1: CD000396.
3. van Tulder MW, Touray T, Furlan AD, et al. Muscle relaxants for non-specific low back pain. *Cochrane Database Syst Rev*. 2006;(3).
4. Deshpande A, Furlan A, Mailis-Gagnon A, et al. Opioids for chronic low-back pain. *Cochrane Database Syst Rev*. 2007;(3):CD004959.
5. Urquhart DM, Hoving JL, Assendelft WW, et al. Antidepressants for non-specific low back pain. *Cochrane Database Syst Rev*. 2008;(1):CD001703.
6. Henschkle N, Ostelo RW, van Tulder MW, et al. Behavioral treatment for chronic low-back pain. *Cochrane Database Syst Rev*. 2010;(7):CD002014.
7. Dahm KT, Brurberg KG, Jamtvedt G, et al. Advice to rest in bed versus advice to stay active for acute low-back pain and sciatica. *Cochrane Database Syst Rev*. 2010;(6):CD007612.

ADDITIONAL READING

- Engers AJ, Jellema P, Wensing M, et al. Individual patient education for low back pain. *Cochrane Database Syst Rev*. 2008;(1):CD004057.
- Gagnier JJ, van Tulder MW, Berman B, et al. Herbal medicine for low back pain. *Cochrane Database Syst Rev*. 2006;(2).
- Shiri R, Koskimäki J, Häkkinen J, et al. Effect of nonsteroidal anti-inflammatory drug use on the incidence of erectile dysfunction. *J Urol*. 2006;175(5):1812–5; discussion 1815–6.
- Walker BF, French SD, Grant W, et al. A Cochrane review of combined chiropractic interventions for low-back pain. *Spine*. 2011:36(3):230–42.

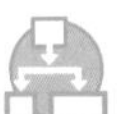

See Also (Topic, Algorithm, Electronic Media Element)

- Lumbar (Intervertebral) Disk Disorders
- Algorithm: Low Back Pain, Acute.

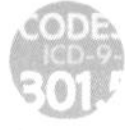

CODES

ICD9

724.2 Lumbago

CLINICAL PEARLS

- Red flags include age <20 years or >55 years, nonmechanical pain, night sweats and/or weight loss, temperature >38°C, history of cancer, history of trauma, presence of neurologic deficits, and pain worse when supine.
- Bed rest is not recommended; patients are encouraged to maintain activity.
- NSAIDs are beneficial and should be considered as first-line therapy.

BAKER CYST

Chris Wheelock, MD

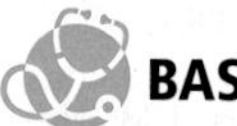

BASICS

DESCRIPTION

- A fluid-filled synovial sac arising in the popliteal fossa
- Distention of the gastrocnemial-semimembranous bursa
- Can be unilateral or bilateral
- Most frequent cystic mass around the knee (1)
- Primary cysts are a distention of the bursa arising independently without an intra-articular disorder.
- Secondary cysts occur if a communication exists between the bursa and knee joint, allowing articular fluid to fill the cyst. Pathologic joint processes can also be transmitted in this manner.
- Associated with synovial inflammation
- Synonym(s): Popliteal cyst

EPIDEMIOLOGY

Incidence

- Bimodal distribution: Children ages 4–7, and adults increasing with age
- Primary cysts usually seen in children under 15 years of age
- Secondary cysts seen in the adult population

Prevalence

- Varies by study
- Studies report a prevalence of 19–47% in symptomatic knees, 2–5% in asymptomatic knees
- In children, 6.3% in symptomatic knees, 2.4% in asymptomatic knees

RISK FACTORS

- Osteoarthritis of knee (most common) (2)[B]
- Rheumatoid arthritis
- Meniscal degeneration or tear
- Advancing age
- Ligamentous insufficiency

PATHOPHYSIOLOGY

- Extension or herniation of synovial membrane of the knee joint capsule or connection of normal bursa with the joint capsule
- May be the result of increased intra-articular pressure
- Commonly seen with knee effusions
- Direct trauma to the bursa likely the primary cause in children because there is no communication between the bursa and the joint in children
- A valvelike mechanism allowing 1-way passage of fluid from the joint to the bursal connection has been described.

ETIOLOGY

Associated intra-articular pathological findings include:

- Meniscal tears, posterior horn
- Anterior cruciate ligament (ACL) insufficiency
- Degenerative articular cartilage lesions
- Rheumatoid arthritis
- Osteoarthritis
- Osteochondritis
- Other potential factors: Infectious arthritis, polyarthritis, villonodular synovitis, lymphoma, sarcoidosis, and connective tissue diseases

COMMONLY ASSOCIATED CONDITIONS

Any condition causing knee joint effusion

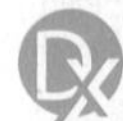

DIAGNOSIS

HISTORY

- Painless mass arising in the popliteal fossa
- Most cysts are asymptomatic.
- Painful if cyst ruptures
- May report restricted range of motion or tightness with knee flexion
- Large cysts may cause entrapment neuropathy of the tibial nerve.
- Vascular compression, most commonly of the popliteal vein, may produce claudication or thrombophlebitis.
- Activity will alter the cyst size.

PHYSICAL EXAM

- Examine in full extension and 90° of flexion.
- Foucher sign: Mass increases with extension and disappears with flexion.
- Most commonly found in medial aspect of popliteal fossa lateral to the head of the gastrocnemius and medial to the neurovascular bundle
- Mass may be fluctuant or tender.
- Transillumination can distinguish cyst from solid mass.
- Ruptured cyst typically painful with associated swelling over calf and medial malleolus, pseudothrombophlebitis

DIAGNOSTIC TESTS & INTERPRETATION

Lab

Initial lab tests

- CBC, sedimentation rate if suspicious of septic arthritis
- Send aspirate for cell count to determine nature of effusion: Infectious, inflammatory, or mechanical

Follow-Up & Special Considerations

In children, consider observation before invasive testing.

Imaging

Initial approach

- Ultrasound confirms presence and size; with Doppler can differentiate Baker cysts from popliteal vessel aneurysms or soft tissue tumors (3)[B].
- MRI is useful to assess for causal derangements of internal joint structures and to identify cyst leakage or rupture.
- Radiographs may show soft tissue density posteriorly.
- Arthrography may demonstrate communication with joint capsule or rupture.
- CT–arthrography together is superior in visualizing cystic details and can help separate lipomas, aneurysms, and malignancies from cysts.

B

DIFFERENTIAL DIAGNOSIS

- Infection/abscess
- Lipoma
- Liposarcoma
- Fibroma
- Fibrosarcoma
- Hematoma
- Deep venous thrombosis
- Vascular tumor
- Popliteal vein varices
- Xanthoma
- Aneurysm (rare)
- Ganglion cyst
- Any condition causing synovitis
- Thrombophlebitis
- Muscular herniation (rare, related to trauma)

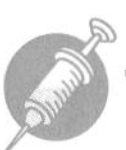

TREATMENT

MEDICATION

- Once etiology is identified from cellular fluid examination, treat the underlying condition.
- Analgesics, NSAIDs for symptomatic relief

ADDITIONAL TREATMENT

General Measures

- No treatment if cyst is asymptomatic
- Compressive wrap or sleeve may be used for comfort.

Additional Therapies

- Physical therapy improves knee range of motion and strength, particularly with coexisting pathology.
- Temporary relief with needle aspiration; recurrence common
- Improvement in joint range of motion, knee pain, swelling, accompanied reduction in bursa size has been shown after intra-articular or intracystic corticosteroid injection (3)[B]
- Sclerotherapy injections of ethanol or dextrose/ sodium morrhuate shown to have good results in studies with small sample sizes (4)[B]

SURGERY/OTHER PROCEDURES

- Consider excision when symptoms persist despite treatment or no etiology is found.
- Recurrence after standard surgery is common and is highest when chondral lesions are present (5)[B].
- A modified surgical technique in children has been proven effective without recurrence (6)[B].
- Excision via arthroscopy or open procedure often requires concomitant treatment of underlying pathology (7)[B].

ONGOING CARE

PROGNOSIS

- Variable
- Many cysts remain asymptomatic.
- Some will regress or resolve with treatment of underlying etiology.
- In children, most resolve without treatment because there is rarely internal derangement.

COMPLICATIONS

- Compartment syndrome in ruptured cyst
- Thrombophlebitis from compression of the popliteal vein
- Infection of popliteal cyst
- Hemorrhage into cyst if on anticoagulants

REFERENCES

1. Marra MD, Crema MD, Chung M, et al. MRI features of cystic lesions around the knee. *Knee*. 2008;15:423–38.
2. Chatzopoulos D, Moralidis E, Markou P, et al. Baker's cysts in knees with chronic osteoarthritic pain: a clinical, ultrasonographic, radiographic and scintigraphic evaluation. *Rheumatol Int*. 2008.
3. Acebes JC, Sanchez-Pernaute O, Diaz-Oca A, et al. Ultrasonographic Assessment of Baker's Cysts after Intra-articular Corticosteroid Injection in Knee Osteoarthritis. *J Clin Ultrasound*. 2006;34:113–7.
4. Centeno CJ, Schultz J, Freeman M, et al. Sclerotherapy of Baker's cyst with imaging confirmation of resolution. *Pain Physician*. 2008;11:257–61.
5. Rupp S, Seil R, et al. Popliteal cysts in adults: Prevalence, associated intraarticular lesions, and results after arthroscopic treatment. *Am Sport Med*. 2002;30(1):112–5.
6. Chen J-C, Cheng-Chang L, Lu Y-M, et al. A modified surgical method for treating Baker's cyst in children. *The Knee*. 2008;15:9–14.
7. Handy JR. Popliteal cysts in adults: A review. *Semin Arthritis Rheu*. 2001;31(2):108–18.

ADDITIONAL READING

- Fritschy D, Fasel J, Imbert J, et al. The popliteal cyst. *Knee Surg Sports Traumatol Arthosc*. 2006;14:623–8.
- Seil R, Rupp S, et al. Prevalence of popliteal cysts in children: A sonographic study and review of the literature. *Arch Ortho Traum Su*. 1999;119:73–5.
- Van Rhijn L, Jansen E, Pruijs H. Long-term follow-up of conservatively treated popliteal cysts in children. *Journal of Pediatric Orthopedics Part B*. 2000;9: 62–4.

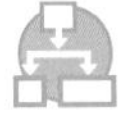

See Also (Topic, Algorithm, Electronic Media Element)

Algorithm: Knee Pain

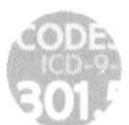

CODES

ICD9

727.51 Synovial cyst of popliteal space

CLINICAL PEARLS

- In children, it is acceptable to wait and observe Baker cysts.
- Treat underlying cause.
- Pain and swelling over the medial malleolus is classic for cyst rupture, also known as pseudothrombophlebitis.

BALANITIS

James P. Miller, MD
Timothy L. Black, MD

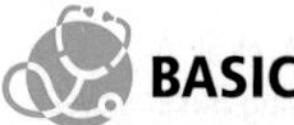

BASICS

DESCRIPTION
- Balanitis is an inflammation of the glans penis.
- Posthitis is an inflammation of the foreskin.
- Balanitis xerotica obliterans (BXO) is lichen sclerosis of the glans penis (uncommon).
- System(s) affected: Reproductive; skin/exocrine

Geriatric Considerations
Condom catheters can predispose to balanitis.

Pediatric Considerations
Oral antibiotics predispose male infants to *Candida balanitis*.

EPIDEMIOLOGY
- Predominant age: Adult
- Predominant gender: Male only

RISK FACTORS
- Presence of foreskin
- Morbid obesity
- Poor hygiene
- Diabetes
- Nursing home environment

GENERAL PREVENTION
- Proper hygiene and avoidance of allergens
- Circumcision

ETIOLOGY
- Allergic reaction (condom latex, contraceptive jelly)
- Infections (*C. albicans, Borrelia vincentii*, streptococci, *Trichomonas*)
- Fixed-drug eruption (sulfa, tetracycline)
- Plasma cell infiltration (Zoon balanitis)
- Autodigestion by activated pancreatic transplant exocrine enzymes

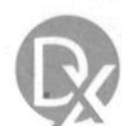

DIAGNOSIS

HISTORY
- Pain
- Drainage
- Dysuria

PHYSICAL EXAM
- Erythema
- Edema
- Discharge
- Ulceration
- Plaque

DIAGNOSTIC TESTS & INTERPRETATION

Lab
- Microbiology culture
- Wet mount
- Serology for syphilis
- Serum glucose

Initial lab tests
- Gram stain
- Wet prep

Diagnostic Procedures/Surgery
Biopsy, if persistent

Pathological Findings
Plasma cells infiltration with Zoon balanitis

DIFFERENTIAL DIAGNOSIS
- Leukoplakia
- Lichen planus
- Psoriasis
- Reiter syndrome
- Lichen sclerosus et atrophicus
- Erythroplasia of Queyrat
- BXO

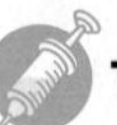

TREATMENT

MEDICATION
- Antifungal:
  - Clotrimazole (Lotrimin), 1% b.i.d.
  - Nystatin (Mycostatin), b.i.d.–q.i.d.
  - Fluconazole, 150-mg single dose (1)[B]
- Antibacterial:
  - Bacitracin, q.i.d.
  - Neomycin-polymyxin B-bacitracin (Neosporin), q.i.d.
  - If cellulitis, cephalosporin or sulfa drug PO or parenteral:
    - Dermatitis: Topical steroids q.i.d.
    - Zoon balanitis: Topical steroids q.i.d.
- BXO:
  - 0.05% betamethasone b.i.d. (2)[B]
  - 0.1% tacrolimus b.i.d. (3)[C]

ADDITIONAL TREATMENT

General Measures

- Appropriate health care: Outpatient
- Warm compresses or sitz baths
- Local hygiene

Issues for Referral

Recurrent infections or development of meatal stenosis

SURGERY/OTHER PROCEDURES

Consider circumcision as preventive measure.

IN-PATIENT CONSIDERATIONS

Admission Criteria

- Uncontrolled diabetes
- Sepsis

Nursing

Appropriate hygiene if condom catheters are used

Discharge Criteria

Resolution of problem

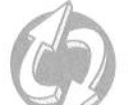

ONGOING CARE

FOLLOW-UP RECOMMENDATIONS

Patient Monitoring

- Every 1–2 weeks until etiology has been established
- Persistent balanitis may require biopsy to rule out malignancy or BXO.

DIET

Weight reduction, if obese

PATIENT EDUCATION

- Need for appropriate hygiene
- Avoidance of known allergens

PROGNOSIS

Should resolve with appropriate treatment

COMPLICATIONS

- Meatal stenosis
- Premalignant changes from chronic irritation
- UTIs

REFERENCES

1. Stary A, Soeltz-Szoets J, Ziegler C, et al. Comparison of the efficacy and safety of oral fluconazole and topical clotrimazole in patients with candida balanitis. *Genitourin Med*. 1996;72:98–102.
2. Kiss A, Csontai A, Pirót L, et al. The response of balanitis xerotica obliterans to local steroid application compared with placebo in children. *J Urol*. 2001;165:219–20.
3. Pandher BS, Rustin MH, Kaisary AV. Treatment of balanitis xerotica obliterans with topical tacrolimus. *J Urol*. 2003;170:923.

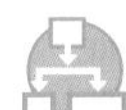

See Also (Topic, Algorithm, Electronic Media Element)

Reiter Syndrome

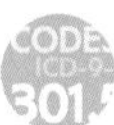

CODES

ICD9

- 112.2 Candidiasis of other urogenital sites
- 607.1 Balanoposthitis

CLINICAL PEARLS

- Balanitis is an inflammation of the glans penis. Posthitis is an inflammation of the foreskin. BXO is lichen sclerosis of the glans penis.
- With recurrent infections and a plaque, a biopsy should be done to rule out BXO or malignancy.
- If there is a true phimosis that interferes with appropriate hygiene, treatment of the phimosis with steroids or circumcision should be performed to help with hygiene.

BAROTRAUMA OF THE MIDDLE EAR, SINUSES, AND LUNG

Ryung Suh, MD, MPP, MBA, MPH

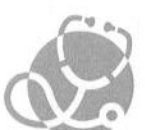

BASICS

DESCRIPTION

- Physical damage to tissue lining an enclosed body cavity resulting from rapid or extreme changes or imbalance between ambient pressure and pressure within the cavity
- Cavities at greatest risk for barotrauma include the middle ear (otic barotrauma), paranasal sinuses (sinus barotrauma), and lungs (pulmonary barotrauma).
- Otic and sinus barotrauma are associated with rapid or extreme changes in environmental pressure, as might result from air travel, mountain climbing, or scuba diving, especially in the presence of nasal congestion or eustachian tube dysfunction of any etiology:
  - Pressure changes with failure of eustachian tube to equilibrate pressure may distort the tympanic membrane (TM), causing discomfort and injury.
  - Rupture of round or oval membrane may cause inner ear barotrauma, vertigo, and sensorineural hearing loss.
- Pulmonary barotrauma:
  - An iatrogenic complication of mechanical ventilation
  - Also a complication of scuba diving
- Dental barotrauma is seen occasionally in scuba divers in whom small pockets of air trapped in dental work can cause rupture of teeth
- System(s) affected: Ear/Nose/Throat (ENT); Pulmonary
- Synonym(s): Dysbarism; Aerotitis; Otitic barotrauma; Middle ear barotrauma

ALERT

- Dizziness and sensorineural hearing loss warrant immediate ENT referral for inner ear involvement.
- Valsalva maneuver can spread nasopharyngeal infection into the middle ear.
- Vertigo and hearing loss may cause disorientation.

EPIDEMIOLOGY

- Predominant age: All ages
- Predominant sex: Male = Female

Incidence

- Pulmonary barotrauma is the second-leading cause of death among divers.
- Otic barotrauma is common in air travel, especially among flight personnel.
- Pulmonary barotrauma is noted in 3% of mechanically ventilated patients.

Pediatric Considerations

- Children have difficulty opening the eustachian tube and have frequent upper respiratory infections. This combination results in higher risk for otic or sinus barotraumas at small pressure changes, as compared with adults.
- Mechanical ventilation of neonates is associated with barotrauma and contributes to bronchopulmonary dysplasia.

Pregnancy Considerations

Increased nasal congestion in pregnancy increases risk of barotitis media.

RISK FACTORS

- Otic or sinus:
  - Participation in high-risk activities without adequate pressure equilibration:
    - Scuba diving, especially with rapid ascent or breath-holding
    - Airplane flight (especially high performance)
    - Sky diving
    - High-altitude travel or elevator rides
    - Underwater employment
    - High-impact sports: Boxing, soccer, water skiing
  - Upper respiratory infection: Sinusitis, rhinitis, tonsillitis, adenoiditis, otitis media
  - Nasal congestion or allergic rhinitis
  - Any cause of eustachian tube dysfunction
  - Exposure to blasting
  - Pregnancy (associated nasal congestion)
  - Anatomic obstruction in the nasopharynx:
    - Deviated nasal septum
    - Nasal polyps
    - Congenital anomalies, including cleft palate
  - Trauma to ear
- Pulmonary:
  - Iatrogenic:
    - Mechanical ventilation, especially in the presence of asthma, chronic interstitial lung disease, acute respiratory distress syndrome
    - Hyperbaric oxygen therapy
  - Scuba diving or other underwater activities
  - Air travel in people with pre-existing pulmonary pathology

GENERAL PREVENTION

- Pulmonary barotrauma:
  - Judicious use of mechanical ventilation and hyperbaric oxygen therapy
  - In scuba diving, avoidance of breath-holding during ascent
- Otic barotrauma:
  - Avoidance of altitude changes or scuba diving when at risk for eustachian tube dysfunction
  - Treatment of upper respiratory congestion
- Equilibration of pressure by Valsalva, yawning, swallowing, drinking, chewing gum

ETIOLOGY

- For any gas at a constant temperature, the volume of the gas varies inversely with the pressure. When gas is trapped in a confined space such as the middle ear, paranasal sinus, or lungs, a sudden decrease in ambient pressure causes expansion of the gas within the cavity.
- Otalgia and hearing loss occur as a result of stretching and deformation of the TM.
- Sudden pressure differential between middle and inner ear may lead to rupture of round or oval window and consequent labyrinthine fistula and leakage of perilymph. Damage to inner ear may be permanent.
- When transalveolar pressure disrupts the structural integrity of the alveolus, the alveolar wall ruptures, leading to interstitial emphysema, followed by pneumothorax, pneumomediastinum.

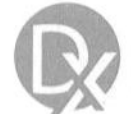

DIAGNOSIS

- Otic (middle ear) barotrauma:
  - Otalgia, sensation of fullness or pressure in ear
  - Conductive hearing loss
  - Vertigo secondary to cold water entering middle ear
  - Transient facial paralysis
  - With TM rupture, discharge of fluid from ear
  - Abnormality of TM
- All patients with middle ear barotrauma should be evaluated for inner ear barotrauma:
  - Sensorineural hearing loss
  - Tinnitus
  - Vertigo
  - Disorientation
- Sinus barotrauma: Facial pain, sensation of fullness or pressure
- Pulmonary barotrauma:
  - Chest pain, dyspnea
  - Hypoxia, hypotension

HISTORY

- Otic barotrauma: History of high-risk activity
- Pulmonary barotrauma: Scuba diving, mechanical ventilation, air travel with pre-existing lung disease

PHYSICAL EXAM

- Otic barotrauma:
  - Otoscopic exam
  - Assess patient's balance and hearing.
  - Palpate eustachian tube for tenderness.
- Pulmonary barotrauma:
  - Auscultation, percussion
- Assessment of respiratory distress

DIAGNOSTIC TESTS & INTERPRETATION

Lab

Initial lab tests

Pulmonary: Arterial blood gas

Imaging

Initial approach

- Otic or sinus: Imaging to rule out nasopharyngeal tumor or sinusitis, if indicated
- Pulmonary:
  - Chest radiograph
  - Chest CT if chest x-ray (CXR) not informative
- Ultrasound

Diagnostic Procedures/Surgery

- Otic barotrauma:
  - Tympanometry
  - Audiometry: Conductive (middle ear) vs. sensorineural (inner ear) hearing loss
  - Surgical exploration to rule out inner ear involvement if suspected
- Pulmonary barotrauma: Chest tube insertion if indicated for pneumothorax

Pathological Findings
- TM retraction or bulging:
  - Teed 0: No visible damage
  - Teed 1: Congestion around umbo (2 psi)
  - Teed 2: Congestion of entire TM (2–3 psi)
  - Teed 3: Hemorrhage into middle ear
  - Teed 4: Extensive middle ear hemorrhage; TM may rupture
  - Teed 5: Entire middle ear filled with deoxygenated blood
- Inner ear involvement with rupture of the round or oval windows, perilymphatic fistula, and leakage of perilymph into the middle ear
- Pulmonary barotrauma:
  - Alveolar rupture may progress to interstitial emphysema, pneumoperitoneum, pneumothorax
- Petechial hemorrhages in area covered by diver's mask, as well as subconjunctival hemorrhages

DIFFERENTIAL DIAGNOSIS
- Acute and chronic otitis media
- Otitis externa
- Temporomandibular joint syndrome
- Pulmonary: Other causes of decompensation on mechanical ventilation

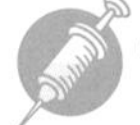

TREATMENT

MEDICATION
- Treatment of predisposing conditions, upper respiratory congestion prior to air travel:
  - Oral decongestants
  - Nasal decongestants
  - Antihistamines
- Antibiotics are not indicated for middle ear effusion secondary to barotrauma.
- Analgesics for pain control
- Tinnitus can be treated with high-dose steroids if given within 3 weeks of onset (1)[C].

ADDITIONAL TREATMENT
General Measures
- Prevention/avoidance is best: Avoid flying or diving when risk factors are present.
- Autoinflate the eustachian tube during pressure changes:
  - Valsalva method (2)[B] during ascent and descent in air travel
  - Infants: Breast-feeding or sucking on pacifier or bottle
  - ≥4 years: Chewing gum
  - ≥8 years: Blowing up a balloon
  - Adults: Chewing gum, sucking hard candy, swallowing, or yawning
- Nasal balloon (2)[B]
- For inner ear barotrauma:
  - Bed rest with head elevated to avoid leakage of perilymph
  - Tympanotomy and repair of round or oval window may be necessary.
- Treatment of pneumothorax:
  - Removal of air from pleural space
- Adjustment of iatrogenic cause (adjustment of mechanical ventilation)

Issues for Referral
- Refer to otolaryngology if inner ear is exposed, perilymphatic fistula, or sensorineural hearing loss.
- Chest tube placement

SURGERY/OTHER PROCEDURES
- If necessary, myringotomy or tympanoplasty
- Tympanotomy and repair of round or oval window may be necessary in inner ear barotrauma.
- Tube thoracostomy for persistent pneumothorax

IN-PATIENT CONSIDERATIONS
Admission Criteria
- Patients with complicating emergencies (e.g., incapacitating pain requiring myringotomy, large tympanic perforation requiring tympanoplasty)
- Inner ear barotrauma with hearing loss
- Management of pneumothorax

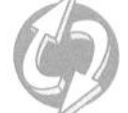

ONGOING CARE

FOLLOW-UP RECOMMENDATIONS
- No flying or diving until complete resolution of all signs and symptoms, and Valsalva succeeds in equalizing pressure.
- Complete bed rest for inner ear barotrauma
- No high-risk activities or air travel until pneumothorax is completely resolved.

Patient Monitoring
- Otoscopic exams until symptoms clear
- In severe cases, audiograms

PATIENT EDUCATION
- Teach Valsalva maneuver.
- Educate on how to create allergy-free environment.
- American Academy of Pediatrics Travel Safety Tips: http://www.aap.org
- Divers Alert Network of Duke University Medical Center information line: (919) 684-2948

PROGNOSIS
- Mild barotitis media may resolve spontaneously.
- Tympanic rupture: Recovery within weeks–months
- Hearing loss may be permanent in barotitis externa.
- Prognosis of pulmonary barotrauma depends on underlying pathology.

COMPLICATIONS
- Permanent hearing loss
- Ruptured TM
- Chronic tinnitus, vertigo
- Fluid exudate in middle ear
- Perilymphatic fistula
- Sensorineural hearing loss

REFERENCES

1. Duplessis C, Hoffer M. Tinnitus in an active duty navy diver: A review of inner ear barotrauma, tinnitus, and its treatment. *Undersea Hyperbaric Med*. 2006;33(4):223–30.
2. Stangerup SE. Point prevalence of barotitis and its prevention and treatment with nasal balloon inflation: A prospective, controlled study. *Otol Neurol*. 2004;25(2):89–94.

ADDITIONAL READING

- Arts HA. Sensorineural hearing loss in adults. In: Cummings CW, Flint PW, Haughey BH, et al., eds. *Otolaryngology: Head and Neck Surgery*, 5th ed. Philadelphia, PA: Mosby Elsevier; 2010.
- Mirza S, Richardson H. Otic barotrauma from air travel. *J Laryngol Otol*. 2005;119:366–70.
- Plötz FB, Slutsky AS, van Vught AJ. Ventilator-induced lung injury and multiple system organ failure: A critical review of facts and hypotheses. *Intensive Care Med*. 2004;30:1865–72.
- Zadik Y, Drucker S. Diving dentistry: A review of the dental implications of scuba diving. *Aust Dent J*. 56(3):265–71.

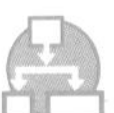

See Also (Topic, Algorithm, Electronic Media Element)

Algorithm: Ear Pain

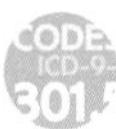

CODES

ICD9
- 993.0 Barotrauma, otitic
- 993.1 Barotrauma, sinus
- 993.8 Other specified effects of air pressure

CLINICAL PEARLS
- Small children can equalize eustachian tube pressure by sucking on bottles or pacifiers. Crying also serves as autoinflation.
- Pulmonary barotrauma is the 2nd-leading cause of death among divers.
- Otic barotrauma is common in air travel, especially among flight personnel.
- Pulmonary barotrauma is noted in 3% of mechanically ventilated patients.

BARRETT'S ESOPHAGUS

Jonathan T. Lin, MD
Harlan Rich, MD

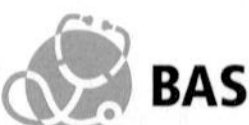

BASICS

DESCRIPTION

- Replacement of the normal distal esophageal stratified squamous epithelium with abnormal columnar (intestinalized) epithelium, most likely as a consequence of chronic GERD
- Predisposes to the development of adenocarcinoma of the esophagus

EPIDEMIOLOGY

- Predominant age: >50 years old
- May occur in children (rare <5 years)

Incidence

- 10–15% of patients undergoing endoscopy for evaluation of reflux symptoms (1)
- 39/100,000 person-years among non-Hispanic white men in a large community-based study (2)
- Esophageal adenocarcinoma incidence rising faster than any other malignancy in the US:
  - From 1975–2001, nearly a 6-fold increase from 4 to 23 cases per million person-years
  - Attributed to trends in smoking and obesity rather than reclassification or overdiagnosis

Prevalence

- Difficult to ascertain because of asymptomatic cases, different populations studied, and varying definitions used
- 131/100,000 person-years in a large community-based study (2)
- As many as 1.5–2.0 million adults in the US based on a 1.6% prevalence of the general population in Sweden (1)

RISK FACTORS

- Chronic reflux (>5 years)
- Hiatal hernia
- Age >50
- Male gender
- White or Hispanic ethnicity
- Smoking history
- Obesity
- Intra-abdominal body fat distribution

Genetics

- Familial predisposition to GERD and familial aggregation of Barrett esophagus have been described, although a discrete genetic marker has not yet been described (1,3,4)[B].
- Multiple acquired genetic changes in the genome lead to progression to adenocarcinoma; some are under active investigation for use as biomarkers for risk stratification and early detection (1,3)[B].

GENERAL PREVENTION

- Case-controlled studies have shown that aspirin and NSAIDs may prevent progression to esophageal cancer due to the inhibition of COX-2 (6)[A]:
  - Administration of the COX-2 selective inhibitor celecoxib was not shown to affect progression of Barrett dysplasia to adenocarcinoma (7)[A].
  - The use of aspirin and a proton pump inhibitor (PPI) for chemoprevention of esophageal cancer is being investigated in a randomized, controlled trial (1,7).
  - Low-dose aspirin may be considered in patients with Barrett's who also have risk factors for cardiovascular disease (6,7).
- Weight loss, smoking cessation, eating fruits and vegetables, and wine consumption may decrease risk of both Barrett esophagus and progression to cancer (5,8)[C].

ALERT

Neither suppression of gastric acid production via high-dose PPIs, nor reduction in esophageal acid exposure via antireflux surgery, has been shown to decrease cancer risk (5,6)[A].

PATHOPHYSIOLOGY

- Reflux of gastric contents injures mature cells and triggers metaplastic transformation from squamous cells to more resistant columnar cells.
- Columnar cells in the esophagus have higher malignant potential than squamous cells.
- Elevated levels of COX-2, a mediator of inflammation and regulator of epithelial cell growth, have been associated with Barrett esophagus (7).
- Normal epithelium → esophagitis → metaplasia (Barrett's) → low-grade dysplasia → high-grade dysplasia → adenocarcinoma

ETIOLOGY

Caused by chronic GERD

COMMONLY ASSOCIATED CONDITIONS

GERD, obesity, hiatal hernia

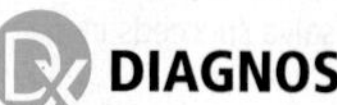

DIAGNOSIS

HISTORY

- Common in GERD: Heartburn, regurgitation, or dysphagia
- Less common: Chest pain, odynophagia, chronic cough, water brash, globus sensation, laryngitis, or asthma
- Suggestive of complicated GERD or cancer: Weight loss, anorexia, dysphagia, odynophagia, or bleeding

ALERT

Up to 25% of patients with Barrett esophagus are asymptomatic (7)[B].

PHYSICAL EXAM

No specific abnormal findings

DIAGNOSTIC TESTS & INTERPRETATION

- Endoscopy with multiple biopsies for histologic exam are required to diagnose Barrett esophagus.
- Screening for Barrett esophagus remains controversial because of the lack of demonstrated impact on mortality. The 2011 American Gastroenterological Association (AGA) guidelines suggest individualized screening for patients with multiple risk factors (8)[C].

Lab

Initial lab tests

None:

- *H. pylori* testing is not indicated. In fact, such infection may decrease the amount of acid produced by the stomach. A systematic review and meta-analysis revealed an inverse relationship between *H. pylori* infections and Barrett esophagus when compared to endoscopically normal controls and no association when compared to blood donors (9)[A].
- No biomarkers currently effective for diagnosis (1,5,8)[B].

Diagnostic Procedures/Surgery

- Endoscopy: Visual identification of columnar epithelium (reddish, velvety appearance) replacing the squamous lining of the distal esophagus:
  - PPI therapy may be initiated prior to endoscopy to reduce confusing reactive esophagitis/atypia with low-grade dysplasia on biopsy (5)[C].
  - Extent of disease may be characterized:
    - As long-segment (≥3 cm) vs. short-segment (<3 cm)
    - Via Prague C (circumference) and M (maximum extent) criteria (1,7)[B]
  - White light endoscopy remains the standard of care (8)[C]:
    - Advanced imaging techniques such as narrow band imaging (NBI) may help identify dysplasia but are still under preliminary evaluation (1,5,8)[A].
- Systematic biopsies of columnar epithelium taken at endoscopy:
  - Seattle Protocol: 4-quadrant biopsies at regular intervals with additional biopsies of visible mucosal irregularities:
    - More time-consuming but higher diagnostic yield than random biopsies (8)[A]
- Capsule endoscopy is still under development and currently has poor sensitivity compared to conventional endoscopy (5)[B].

Pathological Findings

Specialized intestinal metaplasia (also called specialized columnar epithelium) is diagnostic:

- Dysplasia (low-grade or high-grade) should be confirmed by an expert pathologist before treatment (5,8)[B].
- Cardiac-type columnar epithelium may predispose to malignancy but with an unclear magnitude of risk; the AGA currently does not recommend including this type of epithelium in the definition of Barrett esophagus (8)[B].

DIFFERENTIAL DIAGNOSIS

- Erosive esophagitis: Should be treated prior to endoscopy (5)[B]
- Gastric fundic-type epithelium: May be found on pathology, but does not have clear malignant potential and may reflect sampling error (8)[B]
- Specialized intestinal metaplasia at the gastroesophageal junction (GEJ): Carries risk of cancer, but difficult to characterize due to varying definitions of the GEJ landmarks (8)[B]

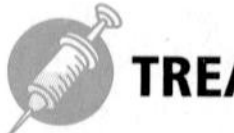

TREATMENT

MEDICATION

- The goal of medical therapy is to control GERD to reduce esophagitis and maintain a healed mucosa (1,5)[A].
- Therapy usually does **not** result in reversal of Barrett esophagus or progression to cancer (1,5,7)[B].

First Line

Unlike the stepwise management of GERD without evidence of Barrett esophagus, patients with Barrett esophagus and GERD symptoms should be treated initially with a once-daily PPI (1,5,8)[A]:

- PPIs should be dosed 30 minutes before a meal (ideally, the first meal of the day).
- Therapy should be titrated to symptoms; pH monitoring is **not** recommended (1,7)[C].

Second Line

If once-daily PPI does not control symptoms, b.i.d. dosing is recommended (5)[A].

ADDITIONAL TREATMENT

Issues for Referral

- Patients should be treated with a PPI prior to endoscopy to reduce esophagitis.
- Patients considering esophagectomy should be referred to a high-volume institution; mortality and morbidity rates are inversely related to volume (5,8)[A].

Additional Therapies

- Low-grade dysplasia: Additional treatment controversial:
  - Endoscopic eradication therapy may be offered with shared decision-making; a long-term benefit has not been clearly established (8)[B].
- High-grade dysplasia: Endoscopic eradication therapy is recommended (1,7,8)[B]. Methods include:
  - Photodynamic therapy (PDT): Eradication rate 77–100%, but with strictures in roughly 40%
  - Radiofrequency ablation (RFA): Eradication rate 54–90%, comparable efficacy to PDT, fewer adverse effects
  - Endoscopic mucosal resection (EMR): Eradication rate 86–100%, involves excision to submucosa, allows staging, preferred for visible irregularities:
    - EMR may be coupled with RFA or PDT to attempt to eliminate all Barrett epithelium.
  - Other ablative procedures such as cryotherapy: Additional studies still required before this can be recommended

COMPLEMENTARY AND ALTERNATIVE MEDICINE

A prospective study of 339 men and women with Barrett esophagus found those taking either a multivitamin, vitamin C, or vitamin E once a day were less likely to develop esophageal adenocarcinoma (10)[B].

SURGERY/OTHER PROCEDURES

- Fundoplication may control GERD symptoms, but it has not been convincingly shown to reverse Barrett esophagus, decrease risk of cancer, or be more effective than medical therapy (1)[A].
- Esophagectomy is definitive therapy and should be offered as an alternative to endoscopic eradication therapy to patients with high-grade dysplasia (1,8)[B]:
  - Added benefit of removing lymph nodes with potential metastases
  - Mortality rate: 8–23%, but <5% among patients with high-grade dysplasia who are otherwise healthy
  - Serious postoperative complications: 30–50%
  - Ideally should be performed by an experienced surgeon in a high-volume medical center

ALERT

Available data suggest that antireflux surgery does **not** decrease risk of esophageal cancer.

Geriatric Considerations

- If the patient is a poor operative candidate for endoscopic eradication therapy or esophagectomy, surveillance or no treatment may be preferable.
- Treatment must be individualized.

ONGOING CARE

FOLLOW-UP RECOMMENDATIONS

- Surveillance (to detect high-grade dysplasia or early carcinoma) remains controversial due to the lack of high-quality prospective studies.
- Recommended surveillance intervals depend on the grade of dysplasia (5,8)[B].

Patient Monitoring

2011 AGA guidelines for surveillance intervals in Barrett esophagus (8)[C]:

- No dysplasia: 3–5 years
- Low-grade dysplasia: 6–12 months
- High-grade dysplasia without eradication therapy: 3 months

ALERT

- Adherence to recommended surveillance protocols may improve the rate of dysplasia and cancer detection.
- Surveillance should continue even if the patient has had endoscopic ablation therapy, antireflux surgery, or esophagectomy.

DIET

Patients should avoid foods that can trigger reflux: Caffeine, alcohol, chocolate, peppermint, carbonated drinks, garlic, onions, spicy foods, fatty foods, citrus, and tomato-based products.

PATIENT EDUCATION

- Lifestyle modifications:
  - Smoking cessation
  - Weight loss
  - Avoiding supine position after eating
  - Avoiding tight-fitting clothes
  - Head of bed elevation
- *No evidence suggests that treating GERD will reverse Barrett esophagus or prevent esophageal cancer.*
- Ongoing research:
  - Biomarkers and screening measures
  - Chemoprevention with NSAIDs and aspirin
  - Capsule endoscopy as a screening tool in high-risk individuals
  - Advanced endoscopic imaging techniques and endoscopic eradication modalities
  - Multivitamin and antioxidant supplements in preventing disease progression

PROGNOSIS

Annual incidence of esophageal cancer in patients with Barrett esophagus is 0.5% per year (5,8)[B]:

- Low-grade dysplasia: May be transient; cancer risk 0.6% per year
- High-grade dysplasia: Cancer risk 5–7% per year

COMPLICATIONS

Same as GERD: Stricture, bleeding, ulceration

REFERENCES

1. Sharma P, et al. Clinical practice. Barrett's esophagus. *N Engl J Med*. 2009;361:2548–56.
2. Corley DA, Kubo A, Levin TR, et al. Race, ethnicity, sex and temporal differences in Barrett's oesophagus diagnosis: A large community-based study, 1994-2006. *Gut*. 2009;58:182–8.
3. Reid BJ, Kostadinov R, Maley CC, et al. New strategies in Barrett's esophagus: Integrating clonal evolutionary theory with clinical management. *Clin Cancer Res*. 2011;17:3512–9.
4. Ash S, Vaccaro BJ, Dabney MK, et al. Comparison of endoscopic and clinical characteristics of patients with familial and sporadic Barrett's esophagus. *Dig Dis Sci*. 2011;56:1702–6.
5. Wang KK, Sampliner RE, Practice Parameters Committee of the American College of Gastroenterology. Updated guidelines 2008 for the diagnosis, surveillance and therapy of Barrett's esophagus. *Am J Gastroenterol*. 2008;103:788–97.
6. Corley DA, Kerlikowske K, Verma R, et al. Protective association of aspirin/NSAIDs and esophageal cancer: A systematic review and meta-analysis. *Gastroenterology*. 2003;124: 47–56.
7. Spechler SJ, Sharma P, Souza RF, et al. American Gastroenterological Association technical review on the management of Barrett's esophagus. *Gastroenterology*. 2011;140:e18–52; quiz e13.
8. American Gastroenterological Association, Spechler SJ, Sharma P, et al. American Gastroenterological Association medical position statement on the management of Barrett's esophagus. *Gastroenterology*. 2011;140: 1084–91.
9. Wang C, Yuan Y, Hunt RH, et al. Helicobacter pylori infection and Barrett's esophagus: A systematic review and meta-analysis. *Am J Gastroenterol*. 2009;104:492–500; quiz 491, 501.
10. Dong LM, et al. Dietary supplement use and risk of neoplastic progression in esophageal adenocarcinoma: A prospective study. *Nutrition Cancer*. 2008;60:39–48.

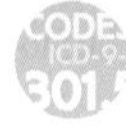

CODES

ICD9

530.85 Barrett's esophagus

CLINICAL PEARLS

- The incidence of esophageal carcinoma is rising faster than any other malignancy. Barrett esophagus is a known precursor.
- Highest incidence is among white males >50 years old.
- Medical or surgical treatment of GERD in patients with Barrett esophagus does **not** decrease cancer rates or mortality.
- Endoscopic eradication therapy is now the preferred treatment for high-grade dysplasia. However, esophagectomy is an alternative that offers definitive therapy.
- Promising areas of research include: Biomarkers for risk stratification, chemoprevention, capsule endoscopy for screening, advances in endoscopic imaging and endoscopic eradication therapy, and the benefit of vitamins and antioxidants.

BASAL CELL CARCINOMA

K. John Burhan, MD

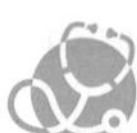

BASICS

Incidence in US: ~1,000,000 cases/yr and is increasing about 10% each year

DESCRIPTION

Basal cell carcinoma (BCC) is the most common cancer, originating from the basal cell layer of the skin appendages:

- Rarely metastasizes, but capable of local tissue destruction

Geriatric Considerations

- Greater frequency in geriatric patients (ages 55–75 have 100 times incidence of age <20)
- The incidence is rapidly increasing in 20–40-year-olds.

Pediatric Considerations

Rare in children, but childhood sun exposure is important in adult disease.

EPIDEMIOLOGY

Worldwide, the most common form of cancer.

Incidence

- Incidence in US: 1,000,000 cases/yr and is increasing about 10% each year
- Predominant age: Generally >40, but incidence is increasing in younger populations
- Predominant sex: Male > Female (although incidence is increasing in females)
- Lifetime risk of white North Americans: 30%

RISK FACTORS

- Chronic sun exposure (UV radiation)
- Most common in the following phenotypes:
  - Light complexion: Skin type I (burns but does not tan) and skin type II (usually burns, sometimes tans)
  - Red or blond hair
  - Blue or green eyes
- Tendency to sunburn
- Male sex, although increasing risk in women due to lifestyle changes such as tanning beds
- History of nonmelanoma skin cancer:
  - After initial diagnosis of skin cancer, 35% risk of new nonmelanoma skin cancer at 3 years and 50% at 5 years
- Family history of skin cancer
- 3–4 decades after chronic arsenic exposure
- 2 decades after therapeutic radiation
- Chronic immunosuppression: Transplant recipients (10 times higher incidence), patients with HIV or lymphomas

Genetics

Several genetic conditions increase the risk of developing BCC:

- Albinism (recessive alleles)
- Xeroderma pigmentosum (autosomal recessive)
- Bazex syndrome (rare, x-linked dominant)
- Nevoid basal cell carcinoma syndrome/Gorlin syndrome (rare, autosomal dominant)
- Cytochrome P-450 CYP2D6 and glutathione S-transferase detoxifying enzyme gene mutations (especially in truncal BCC, marked by clusters of basal cell carcinomas and a younger age of onset)

GENERAL PREVENTION

- Use broad-spectrum sunscreens of at least SPF 30 daily and reapply after swimming or sweating.
- Avoid overexposure to the sun by seeking shade between 10 a.m. and 4 p.m. and wearing wide-brimmed hats and long-sleeved shirts.
- Avoid tanning and sunburns (including tanning salons).

PATHOPHYSIOLOGY

- UV-induced inflammation and cyclooxygenase activation in skin
- Mutation of PTCH1 (patched homolog 1), a tumor-suppressor gene that inhibits the hedgehog signaling pathway
- Mutation of the SMO (smoothened homolog) gene, which is also involved in the hedgehog signaling pathway
- UV-induced mutations of the TP53 (tumor protein 53), a tumor-suppressor gene
- Activation of BCL2, an antiapoptosis proto-oncogene

COMMONLY ASSOCIATED CONDITIONS

- Cosmetic disfigurement since head and neck most often affected
- Loss of vision with orbital involvement
- Loss of nerve function due to perineural spread or extensive and deep invasion
- Ulcerating neoplasms are prone to infections.

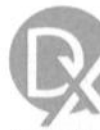

DIAGNOSIS

HISTORY

Exposure to risk factors, family history

PHYSICAL EXAM

- 80% on face and neck, 20% on trunk and lower limbs (mostly women) (1)[B]
- Nodular: Most common (60%); presents as pinkish, pearly papule, plaque, or nodule often with telangiectatic vessels, ulceration, and a rolled periphery usually on face:
  - Pigmented: Presents as a translucent papule with "floating pigment"; more commonly seen in darker skin types
- Superficial: (30%); light red, scaly papule or plaque with atrophic center, ringed by translucent micropapules, usually on trunk or extremities; more common in men
- Morpheaform: (5–10%); firm, smooth, flesh-colored, scarlike papule or plaque with ill-defined borders

DIAGNOSTIC TESTS & INTERPRETATION

Diagnostic Procedures/Surgery

- Clinical diagnosis and histological subtype are confirmed through skin biopsy and pathological examination.
- Shave biopsy is typically sufficient; however, punch biopsy is more useful to assess depth of tumor and perineural invasion.
- If a genetic disorder is suspected, additional tests may be needed to confirm it.

Pathological Findings

- Nodular BCC:
  - Extending from the epidermis are nodular aggregates of basaloid cells.
  - Tumor cells are uniform; rarely have mitotic figures; and have large, oval, hyperchromatic nuclei with little cytoplasm, surrounded by a peripheral palisade.
  - Early lesions are usually connected to the epidermis, unlike late lesions.
  - Increased mucin in dermal stroma:
    - Cleft formation (retraction artifact) common between BCC "nests" and stroma due to mucin shrinkage during fixation and staining
- Superficial BCC:
  - Appear as buds of basaloid cells attached to undersurface of epidermis
  - Peripheral palisading

- Morpheoform BCC:
  - Thin cords and strands of basaloid cells, embedded in dense, fibrous, "scarlike" stroma
  - Less peripheral palisading and retraction, greater subclinical involvement
- Infiltrating BCC:
  - Like morpheoform BCC, but no "scarlike" stroma and thicker, more spiky, irregular strands
  - Less peripheral palisading and retraction, greater subclinical involvement
- Micronodular BCC:
  - Small, nodular aggregates of tumor cells
  - Less retraction artifact and higher subclinical involvement than nodular BCC

DIFFERENTIAL DIAGNOSIS

- Sebaceous hyperplasia
- Epidermal inclusion cyst
- Intradermal nevi (pigmented and nonpigmented)
- Molluscum contagiosum
- Squamous cell carcinoma
- Nummular dermatitis
- Psoriasis
- Melanoma (pigmented lesions)
- Atypical fibroxanthoma
- Rare adnexal neoplasms

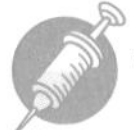

TREATMENT

MEDICATION

- May be especially useful in those who cannot tolerate surgical procedures and in those who refuse to have surgery
- 5-fluorouracil cream inhibits thymidylate synthetase, interrupting DNA synthesis for superficial lesions in low-risk areas; primary treatment only 5% applied b.i.d. for 3–10 weeks.
- Imiquimod (Aldara) cream approved for treatment of low-risk superficial BCC; daily dosing for 6–12 weeks; 90% histologic cure

ADDITIONAL TREATMENT

- Radiation therapy:
  - Useful for patients who cannot or will not undergo surgery
  - Used following surgery, particularly if margins of tumor were not cleared
  - Cure rate is ~90%.
  - Tumors that recur in areas previously treated with radiation are harder to treat, and the area is more difficult to reconstruct.
- Photodynamic therapy (PDT) (2)[A]:
  - 5-aminolevulinic acid, a photosensitizer, is activated by specific wavelengths of light, creating singlet oxygen radicals that destroy local tissue (no damage to surrounding or deep tissues).
  - Useful in areas where tissue preservation is cosmetically or functionally important

SURGERY/OTHER PROCEDURES

- Generally first choice; specific treatment selection varies with extent and location of lesion as well as tumor border demarcation (3)[A]
- High-risk areas:
  - Inner canthus, nasolabial sulcus, philtrum, preauricular area, retroauricular sulcus, lip, temple
- Curettage and electrodesiccation:
  - If nodular lesion <1 cm, in low-risk area, not deeply invasive
- Excision:
  - Useful for lesions in high-risk areas
  - Not as dependent on lesion size
- Cryosurgery:
  - Reserved for small lesions in low-risk areas
  - May want pre- and posttreatment biopsies
- Mohs surgery:
  - Preferred microsurgically controlled surgical treatment for lesions in high-risk areas, recurrent lesions, and lesions exhibiting an aggressive growth pattern
  - Requires referral to appropriately trained dermatologic surgeon

IN-PATIENT CONSIDERATIONS

Outpatient unless extensive lesion

ONGOING CARE

FOLLOW-UP RECOMMENDATIONS

- Avoid sun exposure.
- Oral retinoids may prevent the development of new BCCs in patients with Gorlin syndrome, renal transplant patients, and patients with severe actinic damage.

Patient Monitoring

- Every month for 3 months, then twice yearly for 5 years; yearly thereafter
- Increased risk of other skin cancers (4)[C]

PATIENT EDUCATION

- Teach patient appropriate sun-avoidance techniques, sunscreens, etc.
- Monthly skin self-exam
- Educate patients concerning adequate calcium and vitamin D intake.

PROGNOSIS

- Proper treatment yields 90–95% cure.
- Most recurrences happen within 5 years.
- Development of new BCCs: Patients (36%) will develop a new lesion within 5 years.

COMPLICATIONS

- Local recurrence and spread
- Usually, recurrences will appear within 5 years.
- Metastasis: Rare (<0.1%), but metastatic disease usually fatal within 8 months

REFERENCES

1. Wong CS, Strange RC, Lear JT. Basal cell carcinoma. *BMJ*. 2003;327:794–8.
2. Soler AM, Angell-Petersen E, Warloe T, et al. Photodynamic therapy of superficial basal cell carcinoma with 5-aminolevulinic acid with dimethylsulfoxide and ethylenediaminetetraacetic acid: a comparison of two light sources. *Photochem Photobiol*. 2000;71:724–9.
3. Bath FJ, Bong J, Perkins W, et al. Interventions for basal cell carcinoma of the skin. *Cochrane Database Syst Rev*. 2003;CD003412.
4. Friedman GD, Tekawa IS. Association of basal cell skin cancers with other cancers (United States). *Cancer Causes Control*. 2000;11:891–7.

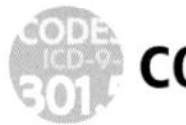

CODES

ICD9

- 173.01 Basal cell carcinoma of skin of lip
- 173.81 Basal cell carcinoma of other specified sites of skin
- 173.91 Basal cell carcinoma of skin, site unspecified

CLINICAL PEARLS

- Use diagnostic keys above to differentiate between BCC and cutaneous squamous cell carcinoma (SCC). SCC arises from actinic keratosis in 60% of cases and generally presents as an asymptomatic hyperkeratotic lesion. If unsure, biopsy or refer to a specialist.
- Some hyperpigmented BCCs may appear similar to melanoma. Remember the ABCDEs of melanoma recognition: *A*symmetry, *B*order irregularities, *C*olor variability, *D*iameter >6 mm, *E*nlargement. If unsure, refer to a specialist.
- The USPSTF concludes there is insufficient evidence to recommend for or against routine total body skin exams for melanoma, BCC, or SCC. Exams should be based on risk factors, including exposures and family and prior medical history. All patients may receive education about risks and self-exam.

BEHAVIORAL PROBLEMS, PEDIATRIC

Jerry Friemoth, MD

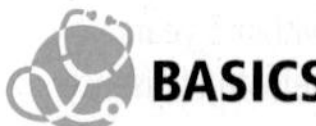

BASICS

DESCRIPTION

Behavior that disrupts ≥1 area of psychosocial functioning but not seriously enough to receive an official *DSM-IV* diagnosis. Most commonly reported behavioral problems are:

- Noncompliance: Purposeful refusal (active/passive) to do what is requested by parent or other adult authority figure
- Temper tantrums: Loss of internal control believed to be provoked by overtiredness, physical discomfort, or fear that leads the child to exhibit behaviors such as crying, whining, breath holding, or in extreme cases, acts of aggression
- Sleep problems: Sleep patterns that are distressing to parents, child, or physician; difficulty going to sleep or staying asleep at night, nightmares, night terrors. These can be further broken down into 2 categories based on polysomnography:
  - Primary: Abnormal polysomnogram: Sleepwalking, night terrors
  - Secondary: Normal polysomnogram (more common): Resistance to bedtime, insomnia (difficulty falling asleep or staying asleep), and nighttime awakenings
- Nocturnal enuresis: Enuresis that occurs only at night in children >5 years of age with no medical problems:
  - Primary: Nocturnal enuresis in a child who has never been dry at night
  - Secondary: Nocturnal enuresis in a child who has been dry at night for at least 6 months
- Eating problems: "Picky eating," difficult mealtime behaviors

EPIDEMIOLOGY

- Noncompliance: More common in children <1 year of age, especially as they develop autonomy; boys have a modestly greater likelihood of being noncompliant. Noncompliant behavior decreases with age.
- Temper tantrums: 70% of 18–24-month-old children; 75.3% of 3–5-year-old children; in children with severe tantrums, 52% have other nontantrum-related behavioral/emotional problems (1).
- Sleep disorders:
  - Night wakings in 25–50% of infants 6–12 months
  - Bedtime refusal in 10–30% of toddlers
  - Nightmares in 10–30% preschoolers and peak at ages 6–10
  - Night terrors in 1–6.5% early childhood and peaks between ages 4 and 12
  - Sleepwalking at least once in 15–40% of children, frequently in 3–5% with peak between ages 4 and 8 (2)
- Nocturnal enuresis:
  - At least 20% of children in the first grade wet the bed occasionally, and 4% wet 2 or more times per week.
  - More common in boys than in girls (3):
    - Enuresis in boys aged 7 and 10 years is 9% and 7%, respectively.
    - Enuresis in girls aged 7 and 10 years is 6% and 3%, respectively.
- "Picky eating":
  - Prevalence increases from 19% to 50% from 4–24 months of age
  - No relation to sex, ethnicity, or household income (4)

COMMONLY ASSOCIATED CONDITIONS

- Temper tantrums: Difficult child temperament, stress
- Oppositional behavior: Normal developmental issue when behavior is mild and is limited in time and specific situations only
- Sleep problems: Often with inconsistent bedtime routine or sleep schedule, stimulating bedtime environment; can be associated with hyperactive behavior, poor impulse control, and poor attention in young children (2)
- Enuresis: Secondary often with medical problems, especially constipation, and frequent behavior problems, especially attention-deficit hyperactivity disorder (ADHD)

DIAGNOSIS

HISTORY

- Noncompliance: Complete history taken from parents and teachers; direct observation of child or child–parent interaction:
  - Criteria: Is problematic for at least some adults in child's life, leading to stressful/difficult interactions for minimum period of 6 months
  - Reduces child's ability to take part in structured activities
  - Creates stressful interactions and relationships with compliant children
  - Disrupts academic progress; places child at risk for physical injury
- Temper tantrums: History with focus on development, family depression, or violence:
  - Criteria: May consist of stiffening limbs and arching back, dropping to the floor, shouting, screaming, crying, pushing/pulling, stamping, hitting, kicking, throwing, or running away (1)
- Sleep disorders: Screening questions about sleep during well-child visit such as the BEARS screen (Bedtime problems, Excessive daytime sleepiness, Awakenings during the night, Regularity and duration of sleep, and Snoring); bedtime routine, any behavioral or developmental disorders (2)[C]
- Nocturnal enuresis: Severity, onset, and duration; daytime wetting or any associated genitourinary symptoms, family history of enuresis, medical and psychosocial history, constipation, child's motivation for treatment (5)[C]
- "Picky eating": Review of child's diet, growth curves, nutritional needs, and parent's response to behavior (4)[C]

PHYSICAL EXAM

- Nocturnal enuresis: Physical exam should focus on abdomen, spine, genitalia, and perineum, followed by a neurologic exam. Specifically, evaluate for:
  - Abdomen: Enlarged bladder, kidneys, or fecal masses
  - Spine: Dimpling or tufts of hair on sacrum
  - Genital urinary exam:
    - Males: Meatal stenosis, hypospadias, epispadias, phimosis
    - Females: Vulvitis, vaginitis, labial adhesions, ureterocele at introitus; wide vaginal orifice with scar or healed laceration may be evidence of abuse.
- Rectal exam: Consider if history of constipation.
- Neurologic exam: Focus on the lower extremities.

DIAGNOSTIC TESTS & INTERPRETATION

Lab

Initial lab tests

- For nocturnal enuresis: Urinalysis (dipstick test OK) and if abnormal, consider urine culture
- For secondary enuresis: Serum glucose, creatinine, thyroid-stimulating hormone (TSH) (6)[C]

Follow-Up & Special Considerations

Sleep studies should be performed in children if there is a history of snoring and daytime ADHD–type symptoms (2).

Imaging

Urinary tract imaging and urodynamic studies if significant daytime symptoms with history or diagnosis of UTI, or history of structural renal abnormalities (6)[C]

Diagnostic Procedures/Surgery

- General screening tools: Child Behavioral Checklist
- Pediatric Symptom Checklist (www.brightfutures.org/mentalhealth/pdf/professionals/ped_symptom_chklst.pdf)
- National Initiative for Children's Healthcare Quality (NICHQ) Vanderbilt Assessment (ADHD screen; www.myadhd.com/vanderbiltparent6175.html)

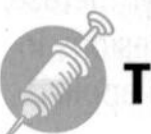

TREATMENT

- General: Educate parent about the specific behavioral problem (3).
- Noncompliance: In the case of extreme child disobedience, consider parent training programs. Child may need to be formally screened for ADHD, oppositional defiant disorder (ODD), or conduct disorder (CD).
- Temper tantrums: Remind parent(s) that this is a normal aspect of childhood:
  - If tantrum is set off by external factors such as hunger or overtiredness, then correct.
  - Other methods for dealing with a tantrum include 1 of the following:
    - Ignoring the tantrum
    - Removing the child and placing him or her in time-out (1 minute for each year of age)
    - Holding child/restraining child until he or she calms down
    - Giving child clear, firm, and consistent instructions as well as enough time to obey
- Sleep disorders: Aside from parent education, other interventions include (2)[A]:
  - Extinction: Child goes to bed at designated time, and cries/tantrums are ignored while monitoring child for safety.
  - Graduated extinction: Parent ignores cries/tantrums for specified period. Parent can check at a fixed time or check at increasing intervals.
  - "Fading": Gradual decrease in direct contact with the child as he falls asleep; goal is for parent to exit the room and allow child to fall asleep independently.

- Nocturnal enuresis:
  - Bedwetting alarm: First-line therapy for child/families with motivation to use. Continue for at least 2–3 months, or until 14 consecutive dry nights are achieved. About 2/3 of children respond while using the alarm, and if enuresis recurs after use, it will often resolve with a second trial (5)[A].
  - Little evidence from clinical trials, but good empirical evidence for behavioral training, including positive reinforcement (small reward for each dry night), or responsibility training (if old enough, child is responsible for changing or washing sheets), encouraging daily bowel movements, and frequent bladder emptying during the day (3)
  - If behavioral therapy fails: Desmopressin if child >6 years of age
  - If either alarm or desmopressin fails, can try using the other alternative (5).
  - If behavioral and medical therapy fail, then refer to a specialist.
- "Picky eating":
  - Avoid punishment, prodding, or rewards.
  - Offer a variety of healthy foods at every meal; limit milk to 24 oz/d, and limit serving juice (4)[C].

MEDICATION

Most pediatric behavioral issues respond well to nonpharmacologic therapy:

- Sleep disorders:
  - For certain delayed sleep-onset disorders, after behavioral methods are exhausted, melatonin at low doses can be tried while behavior modification is continued (7). However, this is not approved by the Food and Drug Administration (FDA) for pediatric patients.
  - Melatonin has been used in pediatric patients in doses of 0.5–10 mg PO given at night.
- Nocturnal enuresis (also see topic "Enuresis"):
  - If behavioral therapy fails: Desmopressin is the only medicine approved as first-line therapy if child >6 years of age (5)[A]:
    - As of 2007, the FDA recommends against use of intranasal formulations in children due to reports of severe hyponatremia resulting in seizures and death in children using intranasal formulations of desmopressin.
    - Oral desmopressin (DDAVP): Dose-dependent; begin with 0.2-mg tablet taken at least 1 hour before bedtime on empty stomach; may titrate to 0.6 mg. Combine with fluid restriction from 1 hour before medication until the next morning.
    - Maximally effective in 1 hour; cleared within 9 hours
    - Give nightly for 6 months, then stop for 2 weeks for test of dryness.
    - Suspend dose in children who experience acute condition affecting fluid/electrolyte balances (i.e., fever, vomiting, diarrhea, vigorous exercise).
    - Potential risks include water intoxication with hyponatremia.
    - 10–60% success; safe even when used for >12 months; high relapse rate after discontinuation without a structured withdrawal program. Many families use only on "important nights" like sleepovers or on camping trips (5)[A].

ADDITIONAL TREATMENT

Issues for Referral

- A patient who exhibits self-injurious behaviors, slow recovery time from tantrums, more tantrums in the home than outside the home, or more aggressive behaviors toward others (including oral aggression) may require referral to a neurodevelopmental or psychiatric specialist.
- A child with loud nightly snoring with observed apnea spells, daytime excessive sleeping, and neurobehavioral signs such as mood changes, ADHD-like symptoms, or academic problems, should be referred for sleep studies (2).
- A child with enuresis and obstructive sleep apnea symptoms should be referred for sleep studies, since surgical correction of airway obstruction often improves or cures enuresis and daytime wetting (6).

COMPLEMENTARY AND ALTERNATIVE MEDICINE

Observational studies suggest efficacy of acupuncture/pressure, biofeedback, and hypnosis (8)[B].

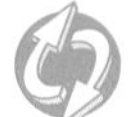

ONGOING CARE

DIET

Nutrition is very important in behavioral issues. Avoiding high-sugar foods and caffeine, and providing balanced, whole meals have been shown to decrease aggressive and noncompliant behaviors in children.

PATIENT EDUCATION

- A few examples of parent training programs are:
  - The Oregon Social Learning Center program: www.oslc.org
  - Forehand and McMahon program: Helping the Noncompliant Child (ages 3–8 years): www.strengtheningfamilies.org/html/programs_1999/02_HNCC.html
  - The BASIC program by Webster-Stratton: www.incredibleyears.com
  - A good review of these programs is "Parent Training Programs: Insight for Practitioners" at www.cdc.gov/violenceprevention/pdf/Parent_Training_Brief-a.pdf
- Also check local community organizations for parenting classes.

REFERENCES

1. Potegal M, Davidson RJ. Temper tantrums in young children: 1. Behavioral composition. *J Dev Behav Pediatr*. 2003;24:140–7.
2. Bhargava S. Diagnosis and management of common sleep problems in children. *Pediatr Rev*. 2011;32;91–8.
3. Robson WL. Clinical practice. Evaluation and management of enuresis. *N Engl J Med*. 2009;360:1429–36.
4. Tseng AG, Biagioli FE. Counseling on early childhood concerns: Sleep issues, thumb sucking, picky eating, and school readiness. *Am Fam Physician*. 2009;80(2):139–42.
5. Neveus T. Nocturnal enuresis-theoretical background and practical guidelines. *Pediatr Nephrol*. 2011;26:1207–1214.
6. Ramakrishnan K. Evaluation and treatment of enuresis. *Am Fam Physician*. 2008;78(4):489–96.
7. Gringras P. When to use drugs to help sleep. *Arch Dis Child*. 2008.
8. Adams D, Vohra S. Complementary, holistic, and integrative medicine: Nocturnal enuresis. *Pediatr Rev*. 2009;30;396–400.
9. Banks FB. Childhood discipline: Challenges for clinicians and parents. *Am Fam Physician*. 2002;66:1447–1452.

ADDITIONAL READING

- Arnell H, Hjälmås K, Jägervall M, et al. The genetics of primary nocturnal enuresis: Inheritance and suggestion of a second major gene on chromosome 12q. *J Med Genet*. 1997;34:360–5.
- Belden AC, Thomson NR, Luby JL. Temper tantrums in healthy versus depressed and disruptive preschoolers: Defining tantrum behaviors associated with clinical problems. *J Pediatr*. 2008;152:117–22.
- Hamilton SS, Armando J. Oppositional defiant disorder. *Am Fam Physician*. 2008;78(7):861–6.
- Luby JL, Heffelfinger A, Koenig-McNaught AL, et al. The preschool feelings checklist: A brief and sensitive screening measure for depression in young children. *J Am Acad Child Adolesc Psychiatry*. 2004;43:708–17.
- Miller JW. Screening children for developmental behavioral problems: Principles for the practitioner. *Prim Care Clin Office Pract*. 2007;34:177–201.
- Mindell FA, Khun B, Lewin DS, et al. Behavioral treatment of bedtime problems and night wakings in infants and young children. *Sleep*. 2006;29(10):1263–76.
- Zahrt DM, Melzer-Lange MD. Aggressive behavior in children and adolescents. *Peds Rev*. 2011;32:325–31.

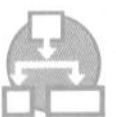

See Also (Topic, Algorithm, Electronic Media Element)

Enuresis

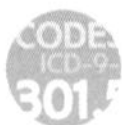

CODES

ICD9

- V40.3 Other behavioral problems
- 312.9 Unspecified disturbance of conduct
- 313.81 Oppositional defiant disorder

CLINICAL PEARLS

- Most commonly reported pediatric behavioral problems are noncompliance, temper tantrums, sleep disorders, nocturnal enuresis, and picky eating.
- Well-child visits provide opportunities to systematically screen for these common conditions.
- Parental education, including a review of age-appropriate discipline, is a key component of treatment (9).

BEHÇET SYNDROME

Prachaya Nitichaikulvatana, MD
Sangeetha Balasubramanian, MD

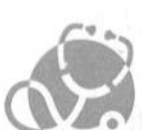

BASICS

DESCRIPTION

- Multisystem, chronic disease characterized by oral and genital mucocutaneous ulcerations, skin rashes, arthritis, thrombophlebitis, uveitis, colitis, and neurologic symptoms
- Rare in the US and northern Europe; endemic in Japan, the Middle East, and the Mediterranean region (along the former Silk Route)
- Rare in pediatric and geriatric populations
- Synonym(s): Mucocutaneous ocular syndrome; Franceschetti-Valero syndrome, Adamantiades' syndrome

Pregnancy Considerations

- Thalidomide for treatment contraindicated in pregnancy
- Possible increase in thrombosis and fetal demise

EPIDEMIOLOGY

- Predominant age: 3rd–4th decades
- Predominant gender: Male = Female, with males affected more severely and more in the Middle East.

Prevalence

- 1/100,000 population in the US
- In other countries, per 100,000:
  - Japan: 10
  - Islamic Republic of Iran: 16–100
  - Northern Europe: 0.3
  - Kingdom of Saudi Arabia: 20

RISK FACTORS

HLA-B51-positive; HLA B5 positivity also marker of eye disease

Genetics

One report of a mother and newborn

ETIOLOGY

Unknown: Classified as systemic vasculitis; associated with HLA-B51; possible immune response to ubiquitous heat-shock protein; possible infectious causes: Herpes simplex virus (HSV), *Streptococcus*; report associated with HIV infection; possible environmental toxin: heavy metals, pesticides, possibly English walnuts or ginkgo nuts

COMMONLY ASSOCIATED CONDITIONS

- Amyloid
- Myelodysplastic syndrome and trisomy 8

DIAGNOSIS

HISTORY

- GI: Recurrent painful stomatitis or aphthous ulcers (nearly all cases); at least 3 crops in 12 months; spontaneous healing without scar, abdominal pain, melena
- Genital: Recurrent, painful ulcers with scarring
- Musculoskeletal: Myositis (rare), morning stiffness (1/3 of patients), arthralgias
- Ocular: Painful, red eyes
- Neurologic: Headache, weakness, numbness, cranial nerve palsy, seizures

PHYSICAL EXAM

- GI: Painful, shallow, or deep oral ulcers with central yellowish necrotic base and punched-out, clean margin; commonly on tongue, lips, buccal mucosa, and gingivae; ulceration in terminal ileum, cecum, ascending colon
- Genital: Painful, scarring ulcers
- Dermal: Papulopustular (acneiform) lesions, erythema nodosum, pyoderma
- Musculoskeletal: Self-limited, nonerosive arthritis mostly mono- or oligoarthritis predominantly affecting lower extremities, rarely polyarthritis
- Ocular: Anterior uveitis with hypopyon, iridocyclitis, chorioretinitis, retinal vasculitis, vitreous hemorrhage, papilledema, secondary glaucoma, optic atrophy
- Thrombophlebitis: Peripheral, pulmonary, cerebral, Budd-Chiari syndrome
- Neurologic: Parenchymal involvement, common in brain stem; cranial nerve palsy, hemiplegia, intracranial hypertension, meningoencephalitis and recurrent meningitis, cerebral venous sinus thrombosis, confusional state (1)
- Pulmonary infiltrates, possibly related to thrombosis, noncavitating mass lesion
- Vascular: Peripheral gangrene, aneurysms
- Renal: Glomerulonephritis, epididymitis (rare)

DIAGNOSTIC TESTS & INTERPRETATION

- Pathergy phenomenon: Hallmark of this condition: Nonspecific cutaneous hypersensitivity reaction—formation of sterile pustules and/or papules along sites of puncture or needle track
- Normal to mildly elevated ESR and C-reactive protein (CRP)
- Circulating immune complexes detected by Raji cell and C1q solid-phase assays and elevated interleukin 1 (IL-1), IL-8, and tumor necrosis factor α (TNF-α), but not clinically useful
- Hypergammaglobulinemia
- Depression of plasma antithrombin III levels with active disease
- Increased fibrinolytic activity during attacks; demyelinating antibodies in neurologic Behçet syndrome
- Anticardiolipin antibodies (rare), lupus anticoagulants
- Antiendothelial antibodies

Lab

Initial lab tests

- ESR and CRP
- If elevated or high clinical suspicion, order additional tests noted earlier.

Follow-Up & Special Considerations

- Periodic ophthalmologic examinations
- A careful history and examination, with attention to the vascular and neurologic systems

Diagnostic Procedures/Surgery

- Careful history and physical examination, with frequent re-evaluations
- Synovial fluid: Inflammatory effusion
- Arteriography: For aneurysms or thrombosis

Pathological Findings

- May be no recognizable changes; neutrophilic perivascular infiltration ± fibrinoid necrosis
- Picture of leukocytoclastic vasculitis in older lesions
- Neutrophilic dermatitis (Sweet's syndrome) (rarely)

DIFFERENTIAL DIAGNOSIS

- Reactive arthritis and other forms of seronegative spondyloarthropathy
- Inflammatory bowel disease (Crohn disease and ulcerative colitis)
- Syphilis and other venereal diseases
- Multiple sclerosis
- Aphthous stomatitis
- Herpes simplex
- Stevens-Johnson syndrome
- Other systemic vasculitides
- Relapsing polychondritis (mouth and genital ulcers with inflamed cartilage [MAGIC] syndrome)
- Coxsackievirus and echovirus infection
- Mollaret meningitis
- Sarcoidosis

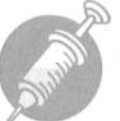

TREATMENT

MEDICATION

First Line

- Colchicine: 0.6 mg b.i.d. for mucocutaneous and joint symptoms
- Topical steroids for ocular and genital lesions Prednisone: 1 mg/kg for severe involvement, especially CNS
- Dapsone: 50–150 mg/d (2)[B]
- Azathioprine: 2–3 mg/kg/d PO
- Methotrexate: Use lowest possible dose; perhaps 7.5 mg/wk. Monitor LFT.
- Cyclosporine: 1–4 mg/kg, but monitor liver function, creatinine, magnesium, and lipids every 2 weeks for 3 months, then every month
- Sulfasalazine 2–6 g/d for GI involvement
- Resistant cases may require:
  - Tacrolimus (FK 506) 0.09–0.15 mg/kg/d
  - Thalidomide 100 mg/d or 300 mg/d (3)[A]: Regulated prescription, teratogenic, refer to manufacturer's literature
  - Interferon alpha for severe ocular and mucocutaneous syndrome (4)[A] and GI manifestations
  - Anticoagulants for patients with anticardiolipin antibodies: Warfarin (Coumadin) to establish PT international normalized ratio 3.0–3.5
  - Precautions: Absorption of drugs such as amitriptyline, diazepam, carbamazepine, phenytoin, and acetaminophen may be reduced in Behçet syndrome

Second Line

- Cyclophosphamide: 2–2.5 mg/kg/d PO for severe cutaneous, arterial, pulmonary vasculitic or aneurysmal manifestations, risk of hemorrhagic cystitis with drug
- Tumor necrosis factor inhibitors: Infliximab (5)[A] etanercept (6)[A]
- Topical sucralfate suspension
- Topical Pimecrolimus (7)

ADDITIONAL TREATMENT

Issues for Referral

Ophthalmologic, neurological, GI, vascular surgery referrals as appropriate

IN-PATIENT CONSIDERATIONS

Initial Stabilization

- Usually outpatient
- Inpatient usually required for neurologic complication or GI perforation

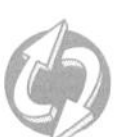

ONGOING CARE

FOLLOW-UP RECOMMENDATIONS

Patient Monitoring

Depends on severity of system involvement and medication monitoring

DIET

No special diet

PATIENT EDUCATION

American Behçet's Association, 421 21st Avenue SW, Rochester, MN 55902; (507) 281-3059

PROGNOSIS

- Normal life expectancy, except with neurologic involvement, ruptured aneurysms, and catastrophic GI involvement. Most serious morbidity is blindness.
- Remissions and exacerbations of disease activity, with severity abating over time

COMPLICATIONS

- Death
- Blindness (most serious morbidity)
- Paralysis
- Embolism/thrombosis (pulmonary, vena cava, peripheral, intracardiac [rare])
- Aneurysms
- Amyloidosis
- Thrombotic events, especially when anticardiolipin antibodies present
- Intestinal perforation

REFERENCES

1. Al-Araji A, Kidd DP, et al. Neuro-Behçet's disease: Epidemiology, clinical characteristics, and management. *Lancet Neurol*. 2009;8:192–204.
2. Lin P, Liang G, et al. Behçet disease: Recommendation for clinical management of mucocutaneous lesions. *J Clin Rheumatol*. 2006;12:282–6.
3. Hamuryudan V, Mat C, Saip S, et al. Thalidomide in the treatment of the mucocutaneous lesions of the Behçet syndrome. A randomized, double-blind, placebo-controlled trial. *Ann Intern Med*. 1998; 128:443–50.
4. Alpsoy E, Durusoy C, Yilmaz E, et al. Interferon alfa-2a in the treatment of Behçet disease: A randomized placebo-controlled and double-blind study. *Arch Dermatol*. 2002;138:467–71.
5. Tugal-Tutkun I, Mudun A, Urgancioglu M, et al. Efficacy of infliximab in the treatment of uveitis that is resistant to treatment with the combination of azathioprine, cyclosporine, and corticosteroids in Behçet's disease: An open-label trial. *Arthritis Rheum*. 2005;52:2478–84.
6. Melikoglu M, Fresko I, Mat C, et al. Short-term trial of etanercept in Behçet's disease: A double blind, placebo controlled study. *J Rheumatol*. 2005;32: 98–105.
7. Chams-Davatchi C, Barikbin B, et al. Pimecrolimus versus placebo in genital aphthous ulcers of Behcet's disease: A randomized double-blind controlled trial. *Int J Rheum Dis*. 2010;13(3):253–8.

ADDITIONAL READING

- Alpsoy E, Akman A, et al. Behçet's disease: An algorithmic approach to its treatment. *Arch Dermatol Res*. 2009;301:693–702.
- Hatemi G, Silman A, EULAR Expert Committee, et al. EULAR recommendations for the management of Behcet disease. *Ann Rheum Dis*. 2008;67(12): 1656–62.

CLINICAL PEARLS

- Nonsuperficial oral or genital ulcers suggest Behçet syndrome rather than reactive arthritis (previously called *Reiter syndrome*). The combination of oral and genital ulcers is especially suggestive.
- The pathergy phenomenon (a cutaneous hypersensitivity reaction—formation of sterile pustules and/or papules along sites of puncture or needle track) is helpful if present but is insufficiently sensitive to rule out Behçet syndrome, if absent.
- Colchicine is the first line of therapy for Behçet syndrome.
- IgG, IgM, and IgA assays for anticardiolipin antibody tests are indicated for vascular complications in Behçet syndrome.

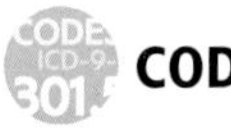

CODES

ICD9

136.1 Behcet's syndrome

BELL PALSY

Serena Mak, MD
Dylan C. Kwait, MD

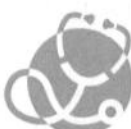

BASICS

DESCRIPTION

A peripheral lower motor neuron facial palsy, usually unilateral, which arises secondary to inflammation and subsequent swelling and compression of cranial nerve VII (facial) and the associated vasa nervorum.

EPIDEMIOLOGY

- Affects 0.02% of the population annually (1)
- Most patients recover, but as many as 30% are left with facial disfigurement and pain (2).
- Accounts for 60–75% of all cases of unilateral facial paralysis (3)
- Median age of onset is 40 years, but it affects all ages (4).
- Predominant sex: Equal occurrence in men and women (4)
- Occurs with equal frequency on the left and right sides of the face (4)

Incidence

- 20–30 cases per 100,000 people in the US per year (4)
- Lowest in children ≤10 years of age; highest in people ≥70 years of age (4)
- Higher among pregnant women (3)

Prevalence

Affects 40,000 Americans every year (5)

RISK FACTORS

- Pregnancy
- Diabetes mellitus
- Age >30 years
- Exposure to cold temperatures
- Upper respiratory infection (e.g., coryza, influenza)

Genetics

A genetic predisposition may be associated with Bell palsy, but it is unclear which factors are inherited.

ETIOLOGY

- Results from damage to the facial cranial nerve (VII)
- Inflammation of cranial nerve VII causes swelling and subsequent compression of both the nerve and the associated vasa nervorum.
- May arise secondary to reactivation of latent herpes virus (herpes simplex virus [HSV] type 1 and herpes zoster virus) in cranial nerve ganglia (3)[A] or because of ischemia from arteriosclerosis associated with diabetes mellitus (4)[A]

COMMONLY ASSOCIATED CONDITIONS

- HSV
- Lyme disease
- Diabetes mellitus
- Hypertension
- Herpes zoster virus
- Ramsay-Hunt syndrome
- Sjögren syndrome
- Sarcoidosis
- Eclampsia
- Amyloidosis

DIAGNOSIS

HISTORY

- Time course of the illness (rapid onset)
- Any predisposing factors (e.g., recent viral infection, trauma, new medications, hypertension, diabetes mellitus)
- Presence of hyperacusis or history of recurrent Bell palsy (both associated with poor prognosis)
- Any associated rash (suggestive of herpes zoster, Lyme disease, or sarcoid)
- Weakness on affected side of face, often sudden in onset
- Pain in or behind the ear in 50% of cases (may precede the palsy in 25% of cases) (4)
- Subjective numbness on the ipsilateral side of the face
- Alteration of taste on the ipsilateral anterior 2/3 of the tongue (chorda tympani branch of the facial nerve)
- Hyperacusis (nerve to the stapedius muscle)
- Decreased tear production

PHYSICAL EXAM

- Neurologic:
  - Determine if the weakness is caused by a problem in either the central or peripheral nervous systems.
  - Flaccid paralysis of muscles on the affected side, *including the forehead:*
    - Impaired ability to raise the ipsilateral eyebrow
    - Impaired closure of the ipsilateral eye
    - Bell phenomenon: Upward diversion of the eye with attempted closure of the lid
    - Impaired ability to smile, grin, or purse the lips
  - Patients may complain of numbness, but on sensory testing, no deficit is present.
  - Examine for involvement of other cranial nerves
- Head, ears, eyes, nose, and throat:
  - Carefully examine head, neck, and oropharynx to exclude masses.
  - Perform pneumatic otoscopic exam.
- Skin: Examine for erythema migrans (Lyme disease) and vesicular rash (herpes zoster virus).

DIAGNOSTIC TESTS & INTERPRETATION

Lab

Initial lab tests

- Lyme titer ELISA and Western blot for immunoglobulin (Ig) M, IgG for *Borrelia burgdorferi*
- In appropriate circumstances, consider titers for varicella zoster virus, cytomegalovirus, rubella, hepatitis A, hepatitis B, and hepatitis C (none is routinely indicated).
- ESR
- Blood glucose level (if diabetes a consideration)
- Consider CBC
- Consider rapid plasma reagin test
- Consider HIV test

Follow-Up & Special Considerations

- CSF analysis:
  - Not routinely indicated
  - CSF protein is elevated in 1/3 of cases.
  - CSF cells show mild elevation in 10% of cases with a mononuclear cell predominance.
- Salivary polymerase chain reaction for HSV1 or herpes zoster virus (these tests are largely reserved for research purposes) (3)

Imaging

Initial approach

- If trauma, facial radiograph to rule out fractures
- Consider CT to:
  - Rule out fractures.
  - Rule out stroke if stroke remains in differential.
- Brain MRI:
  - Not routinely indicated
  - Rule out central pontine, temporal bone, and parotid neoplasms (4).

Diagnostic Procedures/Surgery

- Electromyograph: Nerve conduction on affected and nonaffected sides can be compared to determine the extent of nerve injury, especially if there is dense palsy or no recovery after several weeks.
- Electroneurography: Evoked potentials of affected and nonaffected sides can be compared.

Pathological Findings

Invasive diagnostic procedures are not indicated because biopsy could further damage cranial nerve XII.

DIFFERENTIAL DIAGNOSIS

- Infectious:
  - Acute or chronic otitis media
  - Malignant otitis externa
  - Osteomyelitis of the skull base
  - Leprosy
- Trauma:
  - Temporal bone fracture
  - Mandibular bone fracture
- Neoplastic (onset of palsy is usually slow and progressive and accompanied by additional cranial nerve deficits and/or headache) (3):
  - Tumors of the parotid gland
  - Cholesteatoma
  - Skull-base tumor
  - Carcinomatous meningitis
  - Leukemic meningitis
- Cerebrovascular:
  - Brainstem stroke involving anteroinferior cerebellar artery
  - Aneurysm involving carotid, vertebral, or basilar arteries
- Other:
  - Multiple sclerosis
  - Myasthenia gravis (should be considered in cases of recurrent or bilateral facial palsy) (4)[A]
  - Guillain-Barré syndrome (may also present with bilateral facial palsy) (4)[A]
  - Sjögren syndrome
  - Sarcoidosis
  - Amyloidosis
  - Melkersson-Rosenthal syndrome
  - Mononeuritis or polyneuritis

TREATMENT

MEDICATION

- Recent randomized control trials demonstrate definitively that corticosteroids decrease inflammation and limit nerve damage, thereby reducing the number of patients with residual facial weakness (6)[A].
- Routine use of antiviral medication is not recommended. However, evidence suggests that antiviral agents targeting herpes simplex, when administered concurrently with corticosteroids, may further reduce the risk of unfavorable outcomes in patients with a dense Bell palsy (7,8)[A].
  - Antivirals alone are less likely to produce full recovery than corticosteroids (1)[B].
  - A combination of valacyclovir and steroids provides only minimal added benefit over steroid use alone (1)[B].
- Corticosteroids:
  - Prednisone: Total of 410 mg over 10 days to 760 mg PO over 16 days, tapering dose (adults only)
    - Treatment should begin immediately after onset and should not be instituted if symptoms have been present for >7 days.
    - May reduce edema around cranial nerve XII.
  - Prednisolone (9)[B]: Total of 500 mg over 10 days, 25 mg PO b.i.d.:
    - Prednisolone alone may be an effective treatment.
    - Should be instituted within 72 hours of symptom onset
- Antivirals in combination with corticosteroids:
  - Valacyclovir (1)[B]: 1,000 mg × 5 days plus prednisone 60 mg/d × 5 days then 30 mg/d × 3 days then 10 mg/d × 2 days
- Contraindications:
  - Documented hypersensitivity
  - Pre-existing infections, including tuberculosis (TB) and systemic mycosis
- Precautions: Use with discretion in pregnant patients and those with peptic ulcer disease and diabetes.
- Significant possible interactions: Measles-mumps-rubella, oral polio virus vaccine, and other live vaccines

Pregnancy Considerations

Steroids should be used cautiously during pregnancy; consult with an obstetrician.

ADDITIONAL TREATMENT

General Measures

- Artificial tears should be used to lubricate the cornea.
- The ipsilateral eye should be patched and taped shut at night to avoid drying and infection.

Issues for Referral

Patients may need to be referred to an ear, nose, and throat specialist or a neurologist.

Additional Therapies

- Physical therapy: No evidence of significant benefit or harm, but there is a possibility that facial exercises may reduce time to recover and/or sequelae (10)[C]
- Electrostimulation has limited evidence of effect; more studies are needed (11)[C].

SURGERY/OTHER PROCEDURES

- Surgical treatment of Bell palsy remains controversial and is reserved for intractable cases (3)[A].
- There is insufficient evidence to decide whether surgical intervention in beneficial or harmful in the management of Bell palsy (12)[B].
- In those cases where surgical intervention is performed, cranial nerve XII is surgically decompressed at the entrance to the meatal foramen where the labyrinthine segment and geniculate ganglion reside (4)[A].
- Decompression surgery should not be performed >14 days after the onset of paralysis because severe degeneration of the facial nerve is likely irreversible after 2–3 weeks (4)[A].

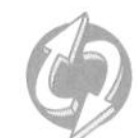

ONGOING CARE

FOLLOW-UP RECOMMENDATIONS

Patient Monitoring

- Patients should start treatment immediately, and it should be followed for 12 months.
- Patients who do not recover complete facial nerve function should be referred to an ophthalmologist for tarsorrhaphy.

DIET

No restrictions

PROGNOSIS

- Most achieve complete spontaneous recovery within 2 weeks, and 85% of untreated patients will experience the first signs of recovery within 3 weeks of onset (5).
- More than 80% recover within 3 months (5).
- 16% are left with a partial palsy, motor synkinesis, and autonomic synkinesis (3).
- 5% experience severe sequelae, and a small number of patients experience permanent facial weakness and dysfunction (3).
- Poor prognostic factors include:
  - Age >60 years
  - Complete facial weakness
  - Hypertension
  - Ramsay-Hunt syndrome
- Absence of recovery at 3 weeks

COMPLICATIONS

- Corneal abrasion or ulceration
- Steroid-induced psychological disturbances; avascular necrosis of the hips, knees, and/or shoulders
- Steroid use can unmask subclinical infection (e.g., TB)

REFERENCES

1. Worster A, Keim SM, Sahsi R, et al. Do either corticosteroids or antiviral agents reduce the risk of long-term facial paresis in patients with new-onset Bell's palsy? *J Emerg Med*. 2010;38: 518–23.
2. De Diego-Sastre JI, Prim-Espada MP, Fernández García F. [The epidemiology of Bell's palsy.] *Rev Neurol*. 2005;41:287–90.
3. Holland NJ, et al. Recent developments in Bell's palsy. *Br Med J*. 2004;329:553–7.
4. Gilden DH. Clinical practice. Bell's Palsy. *N Engl J Med*. 2004;351:1323–31.
5. Holten KB. How should we manage Bell's palsy? *J Fam Pract*. 2004;53:797–8.
6. Salinas RA, Alvarez G, Daly F, et al. Corticosteroids for Bell's palsy (idiopathic facial paralysis). *Cochrane Database Syst Rev*. 2010;3: CD001942.
7. Lockhart P, Daly F, Pitkethly M, et al. Antiviral treatment for Bell's palsy (idiopathic facial paralysis). *Cochrane Database Syst Rev*. 2009;CD001869.
8. Thaera GM, Wellik KE, Barrs DM, et al. Are corticosteroid and antiviral treatments effective for bell palsy? A critically appraised topic. *Neurologist*. 2010;16:138–40.
9. Madhok V, Falk G, Fahey T, et al. Prescribe prednisolone alone for Bell's palsy diagnosed within 72 hours of symptom onset. *BMJ*. 2009;338:b255.
10. Teixeira LJ, et al. Physical therapy for Bell's palsy (idiopathic facial paralysis). *Cochrane Database Syst Rev*. 2008;16(3):CD006283.
11. Alakram P, Puckree T, et al. Effects of electrical stimulation on House-Brackmann scores in early Bell's palsy. *Physiother Theory Pract*. 2010;26: 160–6.
12. McAllister K, Walker D, Donnan PT, et al. Surgical interventions for the early management of Bell's palsy. *Cochrane Database Syst Rev*. 2011: CD007468.

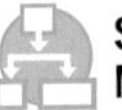

See Also (Topic, Algorithm, Electronic Media Element)

Amyloidosis; Herpes Simplex; Herpes Zoster; Sarcoidosis; Lyme Disease; Diabetes Mellitus Type 1; Diabetes Mellitus Type 2; Ramsay-Hunt Syndrome; Sjögren Syndrome; Melkersson-Rosenthal Syndrome

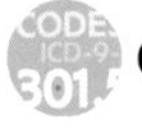

CODES

ICD9

351.0 Bell's palsy

CLINICAL PEARLS

- Steroids must be initiated immediately after the onset of symptoms.
- Look closely at the voluntary movement on the upper part of the face on the affected side; in Bell palsy, all of the muscles are involved (weak or paralyzed), whereas in a stroke, the upper muscles are spared (because of bilateral innervation).
- Remember to protect the affected eye with lubrication and taping.
- In areas with endemic Lyme disease, Bell palsy should be considered to be Lyme disease until proven otherwise.

BIPOLAR I DISORDER

Laurie A. Carrier, MD

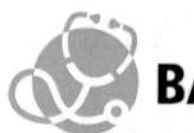

BASICS

DESCRIPTION

- Bipolar I (BP-I) is a mood disorder characterized by at least 1 manic or mixed episode, often alternating with episodes of major depression, that causes marked impairment and/or hospitalization.
- Symptoms are not caused by a substance (e.g., drug), a general medical condition, or a medication.

Geriatric Considerations

New onset in older patients (>50 years of age) requires a workup for organic or chemically induced pathology.

Pediatric Considerations

There is overlap with symptoms of attention-deficit hyperactivity disorder (ADHD) and oppositional defiant disorder (ODD). Children and adolescents experience more rapid cycling and mixed states. Depression often presents as irritable mood.

Pregnancy Considerations

- Potential teratogenic effects of commonly used medications (e.g., lithium, valproic acid)
- Symptoms may be exacerbated in the postpartum period.

EPIDEMIOLOGY

- Onset usually between 15 and 30 years of age
- More common in single and divorced persons
- Less common in college graduates
- Higher-than-average incidence in higher socioeconomic groups

Prevalence

- 1.0–1.6% lifetime prevalence
- Equal among men and women (manic episodes more common in men; depressive episodes more common in women)
- Equal among races; however, clinicians tend to misdiagnose schizophrenia in African American patients with BP-I.

RISK FACTORS

Genetics, major life stressors (especially loss of parent or spouse), or substance abuse

Genetics

- Monozygotic twin concordance 40–70%
- Dizygotic twin concordance 5–25%
- 50% of patients have at least 1 parent with a mood disorder.
- First-degree relatives of people with BP-I are ~7× more likely to develop BP-I than the general population.

GENERAL PREVENTION

Treatment adherence and education can help to prevent relapses.

PATHOPHYSIOLOGY

Dysregulation of biogenic amines or neurotransmitters (particularly serotonin, norepinephrine, and dopamine). MRI findings suggest abnormalities in prefrontal cortical areas, striatum, and amygdala that predate illness onset (1).

ETIOLOGY

Genetic predisposition and major life stressors can trigger initial and subsequent episodes.

COMMONLY ASSOCIATED CONDITIONS

Substance abuse (60%), ADHD, anxiety disorders, and eating disorders

DIAGNOSIS

- The diagnosis of BP-I requires at least 1 manic or mixed episode (simultaneous mania and depression). Although a depressive episode is not necessary for the diagnosis, 80–90% of people with BP-I also experience depression.
- Manic episode, *DSM-IV-TR* criteria:
  - Distinct period of abnormally and persistently elevated, expansive, or irritable mood lasting at least 1 week (or any duration if hospitalization is necessary)
  - During the period of mood disturbance, 3 or more of the "DIG FAST" symptoms must persist (4 if the mood is only irritable) and must be present to a significant degree:
    - *D*istractibility (attention too easily drawn to unimportant or irrelevant external stimuli)
    - *I*nsomnia, decreased need for sleep (e.g., feels rested after only 3 hours of sleep)
    - *G*randiosity or inflated self-esteem
    - *F*light of ideas or subjective experience that thoughts are racing
    - *A*gitation or increase in goal-directed activity (socially, at work or school, or sexually)
    - *S*peech pressured/more talkative than usual
    - *T*aking risks: Excessive involvement in pleasurable activities that have a high potential for painful consequences (e.g., financial or sexual)
- Mixed episode: Criteria are met for both a manic and major depressive episode nearly every day during at least a 1-week period, and the mood disturbance causes significant impairment in functioning.
- Signs and symptoms more likely in bipolar than in unipolar depression (2): Agitation/restlessness, suicidal ideation/planning, increased frequency of depressive episodes, melancholia, psychomotor retardation, younger age of onset, hyperphagia, hypersomnia, family history of bipolar disorder, subsyndromal hypomanic symptoms (particularly increased goal-directed activity)

HISTORY

- Collateral information makes diagnostics more complete and is often necessary for a clear history.
- History: Safety concerns (e.g., Suicide/homicide ideation? Safety plan? Psychosis present?); Physical well-being (e.g., Number of hours of sleep? Appetite? Substance abuse?); Personal history (e.g., Told life of the party? Talkative? Speeding? Spending sprees or donations? Credit-card or gambling debt? Promiscuous? Other risk-taking behavior? Legal trouble? Religious infatuation?)

PHYSICAL EXAM

- Mental status exam in acute mania:
  - General appearance: Bright clothing, excessive makeup, disorganized or discombobulated, psychomotor agitation
  - Speech: Pressured, difficult to interrupt
  - Mood/affect: Euphoria, irritability/expansive, labile
  - Thought process: Flight of ideas (streams of thought occur to patient at rapid rate), easily distracted
  - Thought content: Grandiosity, paranoia, hyperreligious
  - Perceptual abnormalities: 3/4 of manic patients experience delusions, grandiose or paranoid
  - Suicidal/homicidal ideation: Irritability or delusions may lead to aggression toward self or others; suicidal ideation is common with mixed episode.
  - Insight/judgment: Poor/impaired
- See "Bipolar II Disorder" for an example of a mental status exam in depression.
- With mixed episodes, patients may exhibit a combination of manic and depressive mental states.

DIAGNOSTIC TESTS & INTERPRETATION

- BP-I is a clinical diagnosis.
- The Mood Disorder Questionnaire is a self-assessment screen for bipolar disorders (sensitivity 73%, specificity 90%) (3).
- Patient Health Questionnaire-9 helps to determine the presence and severity of a depressive episode.

Lab

- Thyroid-stimulating hormone, CBC, comprehensive metabolic panel (CMP), liver function tests, antinuclear antibody, rapid plasma reagent (RPR), HIV, ESR
- Drug/alcohol screen with each presentation
- Dementia workup if new onset in seniors

Imaging

Consider brain imaging (CT, scan, MRI) with initial onset of mania to rule out organic cause (e.g., tumor, infection, or stroke), especially with onset in elderly and if psychosis is present.

Diagnostic Procedures/Surgery

Consider electroencephalogram if presentation suggests temporal lobe epilepsy (hyperreligiosity, hypergraphia).

DIFFERENTIAL DIAGNOSIS

- Other psychiatric considerations: Unipolar depression ± psychotic features, schizophrenia, schizoaffective disorder, personality disorders (particularly antisocial, borderline, histrionic, and narcissistic), attention-deficit disorder ± hyperactivity, substance-induced mood disorder
- Medical considerations: Epilepsy (e.g., temporal lobe), brain tumor, infection (e.g., AIDS, syphilis), stroke, endocrine (e.g., thyroid disease), multiple sclerosis
- In children, consider ADHD and ODD.

TREATMENT

- Ensure safety.
- Medication management
- Psychotherapy (e.g., cognitive-behavioral therapy, social rhythm therapy)
- Stress reduction
- Patient and family education

MEDICATION

First Line

- Treatment may consist of 1–4 of the following mood stabilizers or other psychotropic medications. When combining these agents, consider adding different classes (e.g., an atypical antipsychotic and/or an antiseizure medication and/or lithium).

- Lithium (Lithobid, Eskalith, generic): *Dosing:* 600–1,200 mg/d divided b.i.d.–q.i.d.; start 600 mg PO t.i.d. in acute mania, and titrate based on blood levels. *Warning:* Use caution in kidney and heart disease; use can lead to diabetes insipidus, thyroid disease. Use caution in sodium-depleted patients (e.g., those using diuretics or ACE inhibitors); dehydration can lead to toxicity (seizures, encephalopathy, arrhythmias). Pregnancy Category D (Ebstein anomaly). *Monitor:* Check ECG >40 years, thyroid-stimulating hormone (TSH), BUN, creatine, lytes at baseline and every 6 months; check level 5 days after initiation or dose change, then every 1–2 weeks ×3, then every 2–3 months (Goal: 0.8–1.2 mmol/L).
- Antiseizure medications:
  - Divalproex sodium, valproic acid (Depakote, Depakene, generic): *Dosing:* Start 250–500 mg b.i.d.–t.i.d.; maximum 60 mg/kg/d. *Black box warnings:* Hepatotoxicity, pancreatitis, thrombocytopenia, pregnancy Category D (neural tube defects). Monitor: CBC, liver function tests (LFTs) at baseline and every 6 months; check valproic acid (VPA) level 5 days after initiation and dose changes (Goal: 50–125 μg/mL).
  - Carbamazepine (Carbatrol, Equetro, Tegretol, generic): *Dosing:* 800–1,200 mg/d PO divided b.i.d.–q.i.d.; start 100–200 mg PO b.i.d. and titrate to lowest effective dose. *Warning:* Do not use with tricyclic acid or within 14 days of a monoamine oxidase inhibitor. Use caution with kidney/heart disease; risk of aplastic anemia/agranulocytosis, enzyme inducer; pregnancy Category D. *Monitor:* CBC, LFTs at baseline and every 3–6 months; check level 4–5 days after initiation and dose changes (Goal: 4–12 μg/mL).
  - Lamotrigine (Lamictal): *Dosing:* 200 mg/d; start 25 mg/d × 2 weeks, then 50 mg/d × 2 weeks, then 100 mg/d × 1 week (*Note:* Use different dosing if adjunct to valproate). *Warning:* Titrate slowly (risk of Stevens-Johnson syndrome); use caution with kidney/liver/heart disease; pregnancy Category C.
  - Oxcarbazepine (Trileptal), gabapentin (Neurontin), and topiramate (Topamax) are also used in BP-I, but are not approved by the Food and Drug Administration (FDA).
- Atypical antipsychotics (AAs):
  - Side effects of AAs: Orthostatic hypotension, metabolic side effects (glucose and lipid dysregulation, weight gain), tardive dyskinesia, neuroleptic malignant syndrome (NMS), prolactinemia (except Abilify), increased risk of death in elderly with dementia-related psychosis, pregnancy Category C
  - Monitor: LFTs, lipids, glucose at baseline, 3 months, and annually; check for extrapyramidal symptoms (EPS) with Abnormal Involuntary Movement Scale (AIMS) and assess weight (with abdominal circumference) at baseline, at 4, 8, and 12 weeks, and then every 3–6 months; monitor for orthostatic hypotension 3–5 days after starting or changing dose.
  - Aripiprazole (Abilify): *Dosing:* 15 mg/d, max. 30 mg/d; less likely to cause metabolic side effects
  - Olanzapine (Zyprexa, Zydis): *Dosing:* 5–20 mg/d; most likely to cause metabolic side effects (weight gain, diabetes)
  - Symbyax (olanzapine + fluoxetine): *Dosing:* 6/25 mg, FDA approved for BP depression
  - Quetiapine (Seroquel): *Dosing:* In mania, 200–400 mg b.i.d.; in bipolar depression, 50–300 mg qhs. *Caution:* Cataracts.
  - Risperidone (Risperdal): *Dosing:* 1–6 mg/d divided q.i.d.–b.i.d. Generic and every 2 weeks IM preparations available.
  - Ziprasidone (Geodon): *Dosing:* 40–80 mg b.i.d.; less likely to cause metabolic side effects. *Caution:* QTc prolongation (>500 ms) has been actual weight (a/w) use (0.06%). Consider ECG at baseline.

Second Line
- Antidepressants (in addition to mood stabilizers)
- Benzodiazepines (for acute agitation with mania, associated anxiety)
- Sleep medications

ADDITIONAL TREATMENT
General Measures
- Psychotherapy (e.g., cognitive-behavioral therapy, social rhythm therapy) in conjunction with medications is key (4).
- Regular exercise, a healthy diet, and sobriety have been shown to help prevent worsening of symptoms.

Issues for Referral
Comfort level of doctor, stability of patient; patients benefit from a multidisciplinary team, including a primary care physician and a psychiatrist.

Additional Therapies
- Electroconvulsive therapy can be helpful in acute mania and depression.
- Light therapy for seasonal component to depressive episodes (use with caution because it can precipitate manic episode)

IN-PATIENT CONSIDERATIONS
Admit if acutely dangerous to self or others.

Admission Criteria
To admit a patient (>18 years of age) to a psychiatric unit involuntarily, the patient must have a psychiatric diagnosis (e.g., BP-I) or present a danger to him- or herself or others, or their mental disease must be inhibiting them from obtaining their basic needs (e.g., food, clothing, etc.).

Nursing
Alert staff to potentially dangerous or agitated patients. Acute suicidal threats need continuous observation.

Discharge Criteria
Determined by safety

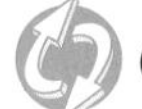

ONGOING CARE

FOLLOW-UP RECOMMENDATIONS
- Regularly scheduled visits support adherence with treatment.
- Frequent communication among primary care doctor, psychiatrist, and therapist

Patient Monitoring
Mood charts are helpful to monitor symptoms.

PATIENT EDUCATION
- National Alliance on Mental Illness (NAMI): http://www.nami.org/
- National Institutes of Mental Health (NIMH): http://www.nimh.nih.gov

PROGNOSIS
- Frequency and severity of episodes are related to medication adherence, consistency with therapy, amount of sleep, and support systems.
- 40–50% of patients experience another manic episode within 2 years of the first episode.
- 25–50% attempt suicide, and 15% die.
- Substance abuse, unemployment, psychosis, depression, and male sex are associated with a worse prognosis.

REFERENCES

1. Fornito A, Yücel M, Wood SJ, et al. Anterior cingulate cortex abnormalities associated with a first psychotic episode in bipolar disorder. *Br J Psychiatry*. 2009;194:426–33.
2. Perlis RH, Brown E, Baker RW, et al. Clinical features of bipolar depression versus major depressive disorder in large multicenter trials. *Am J Psychiatry*. 2006;163:225–31.
3. Hirschfeld RM, Holzer C, Calabrese JR, et al. Validity of the mood disorder questionnaire: A general population study. *Am J Psychiatry*. 2003;160: 178–80.
4. Depp CA, Moore DJ, Patterson TL, et al. Psychosocial interventions and medication adherence in bipolar disorder. *Dialogues Clin Neurosci*. 2008;10:239–50.

ADDITIONAL READING

- American Psychiatric Association. Practice guideline for the treatment of patients with bipolar disorder (revision). *Am J Psychiatry*. 2002;159:1–50.
- McAllister-Williams RH. Relapse prevention in bipolar disorder: A critical review of current guidelines. *Psychopharmacol*. 2006;20(2 Suppl): 12–6.

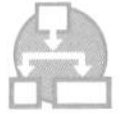

See Also (Topic, Algorithm, Electronic Media Element)

Algorithm: Depressive Episode, Major

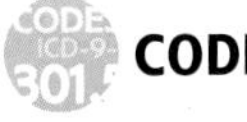

CODES

ICD9
- 296.7 Bipolar I disorder, most recent episode (or current) unspecified
- 296.40 Bipolar affective disorder, manic, unspecified degree
- 296.50 Bipolar affective disorder, depressed, unspecified degree

CLINICAL PEARLS

- Bipolar I is characterized by at least 1 manic or mixed episode, often alternating with episodes of major depression, that causes marked impairment.
- 25–50% of BP-I patients attempt suicide, and 15% die by suicide.
- There is no way to prevent the onset of BP-I, but treatment adherence and education can help to prevent further episodes.

BIPOLAR II DISORDER

Laurie A. Carrier, MD

BASICS

DESCRIPTION

Bipolar II (BP-2) is a mood disorder characterized by at least 1 episode of major depression and at least 1 episode of hypomania, a milder form of mania.

Geriatric Considerations

New onset in older patients (>50) requires a workup for organic or chemically induced pathology.

Pediatric Considerations

- Large overlap with symptoms of attention deficit hyperactivity disorder (ADHD) and oppositional defiant disorder (ODD)
- Depression often presents as irritable mood.

Pregnancy Considerations

- Counsel women of childbearing age about potentially teratogenic effects of commonly used medications (e.g., lithium, valproic acid).
- Symptoms may be exacerbated in the postpartum period.

EPIDEMIOLOGY

More common in women

Prevalence

0.5–1.1% lifetime prevalence

RISK FACTORS

Genetics

Heritability estimate: >77%

GENERAL PREVENTION

There is no way to prevent the onset of BP-2, but treatment adherence and education can help to prevent further episodes.

PATHOPHYSIOLOGY

Dysregulation of biogenic amines or neurotransmitters (particularly serotonin, norepinephrine, and dopamine)

ETIOLOGY

- Genetics
- Major life stressors (especially loss of parent or spouse)

COMMONLY ASSOCIATED CONDITIONS

Substance abuse or dependence, ADHD, anxiety disorders, and eating disorders

DIAGNOSIS

- *DSM-IV-TR* criteria: Patient must experience at least 1 hypomanic episode and at least 1 major depressive episode. The symptoms have caused *some* distress or impairment in social, occupational, or other areas of functioning. There can be no history of full manic or mixed episodes.
- Hypomania is a distinct period of persistently elevated, expansive, or irritable mood, different from usual nondepressed mood, lasting at least 4 days:
  - The episode must include at least 3 of the "DIG FAST" symptoms below (4 if the mood is only irritable):
    - **D**istractibility
    - **I**nsomnia, decreased need for sleep
    - **G**randiosity or inflated self-esteem
    - **F**light of ideas or subjective experience that thoughts are racing
    - **A**gitation or increase in goal-directed activity (socially, at work or school, or sexually)
    - **S**peech pressured/more talkative than usual
    - **T**aking risks: Excessive involvement in pleasurable activities that have high potential for painful consequences (e.g., sexual or financial)
  - The symptoms are not severe enough to cause *marked* impairment in functioning or hospitalization, and there is no associated psychosis as with BP-1.
- Major depression:
  - Depressed mood or diminished interest and 4 or more of the "SIG E CAPS" symptoms are present during the same 2-week period:
    - **S**leep disturbance (e.g., trouble falling asleep, early morning awakening)
    - **I**nterest: Loss or anhedonia
    - **G**uilt (or feelings of worthlessness)
    - **E**nergy, loss of
    - **C**oncentration, loss of
    - **A**ppetite changes, increase or decrease
    - **P**sychomotor changes (retardation or agitation)
    - **S**uicidal/homicidal thoughts
  - BP-2 with rapid cycling is diagnosed when a patient experiences at least 4 episodes of a mood disturbance in a 12-month period (either major depression or hypomania).
- Signs, symptoms, and history seen more often in BP-2 than in unipolar depression (1):
  - Agitation, hyperphagia, hypersomnia, melancholia, psychomotor retardation, suicidal ideation/planning, increased frequency of depressive episodes, younger age of onset, family history of bipolar disorder, subsyndromal hypomanic symptoms (especially overactivity) (2)
- Note: If symptoms have *ever* met criteria for a full manic episode or hospitalization was necessary secondary to manic/mixed symptoms or psychosis was present, then the diagnosis changes to bipolar I disorder (BP-1).

HISTORY

Collateral information makes diagnostics more complete and is often necessary for a clear history.

PHYSICAL EXAM

- Mental status exam in hypomania:
  - General appearance: Usually appropriately dressed, with psychomotor agitation
  - Speech: May be pressured, talkative, difficult to interrupt
  - Mood/affect: Euphoria, irritability/congruent or expansive
  - Thought process: May be easily distracted, difficulty concentrating on 1 task
  - Thought content: Usually positive with "big" plans
  - Perceptual abnormalities: None
  - Suicidal/homicidal ideation: Low incidence of homicidal or suicidal ideation
  - Insight/judgment: Usually stable/may be impaired by their distractibility
- Mental status exam in acute depression:
  - General appearance: Unkempt, psychomotor retardation, poor eye contact
  - Speech: Low, soft, monotone
  - Mood/affect: Sad, depressed/congruent, flat
  - Thought process: Ruminating thoughts, generalized slowing
  - Thought content: Preoccupied with negative or nihilistic ideas
  - Perceptual abnormalities: 15% of depressed patients experience hallucinations or delusions.
  - Suicidal/homicidal ideation: Suicidal ideation is very common.
  - Insight/judgment: Often impaired

DIAGNOSTIC TESTS & INTERPRETATION

- BP-2 is a clinical diagnosis.
- Mood disorder questionnaire, self-assessment screen for BP, sensitivity 73%, specificity 90% (3)
- Hypomania checklist-32 distinguishes between BP-2 and unipolar depression (sensitivity 80%, specificity 51%) (4)
- Patient health questionnaire-9 helps to determine the presence and severity of depression.

Lab

- Rule out organic causes of mood disorder during initial episode.
- Drug/alcohol screen is prudent with each presentation.
- Dementia workup if new onset in seniors

Initial lab tests

With initial presentation: Consider CBC, chem 7, thyroid-stimulating hormone (TSH), liver function tests, antinuclear antibody, rapid plasma reagent (RPR), HIV, ESR

Imaging

Consider brain imaging with initial onset of hypomania to rule out organic cause, especially with onset in elderly.

DIFFERENTIAL DIAGNOSIS

- Other psychiatric considerations:
  - Bipolar 1 disorder, unipolar depression, personality disorders (particularly borderline, antisocial, and narcissistic), attention-deficit disorder +/– hyperactivity, substance-induced mood disorder
- Medical considerations:
  - Epilepsy (e.g., temporal lobe), brain tumor, infection (e.g., AIDS syphilis), stroke, endocrine (e.g., thyroid disease), multiple sclerosis
- In children, consider ADHD and ODD.

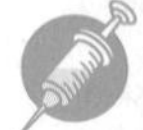

TREATMENT

- Ensure safety.
- Medication management
- Psychotherapy (e.g., cognitive-behavioral therapy [CBT], social rhythm therapy)
- Stress reduction
- Patient and family education

MEDICATION

- Less research has been conducted on the appropriate treatment of BP-2, but current consensus is to treat with the same medications as BP-1.
- Antidepressant medications must be used with caution during depressive episodes, as they may precipitate hypomanic episodes (less common than with BP-1).

First Line

- American Psychological Association guidelines state lithium or lamotrigine as first-line treatment for bipolar depression.
- Treatment may consist of 1–4. When combining mood stabilizers, consider adding different classes (e.g., an atypical antipsychotic and/or an antiseizure medication and/or lithium).
- Lithium (Lithobid, Eskalith, generic): Dosing 600–1,200 mg/d divided b.i.d.–q.i.d., titrate based on blood levels:
  - Caution in kidney or heart disease; use can lead to diabetes insipidus, thyroid disease; caution sodium-depleted patients (diuretics, ACE inhibitors); dehydration can lead to toxicity, which may cause seizures, encephalopathic syndrome, arrhythmias, pregnancy Category D (Ebstein anomaly with first trimeter use)
  - Monitor electrocardiogram >40 years, TSH, BUN, creatinine, lytes at baseline and q6mo; check level 5 days after initiation or dose change, then q1–2wk × 3, then q2–3mo (goal: 0.8–1.2 mmol/L)
- Anticonvulsants:
  - Valproic acid, divalproex sodium: Dosing: Start 250–500 mg b.i.d.–t.i.d., max 60 mg/kg/d. Warnings: Hepatotoxicity, pancreatitis, thrombocytopenia, pregnancy Category D (neural tube defects). Monitor: CBC, liver function tests (LFTs) at baseline and q6mo; check valproic acid level 5 days after initiation and dose changes (goal: 50–125 mcg/mL).
  - Carbamazepine: Dosing: 800–1,200 mg/d PO divided b.i.d.–q.i.d., start 100–200 mg PO b.i.d. and titrate to lowest effective dose. Do not use with tricyclic antidepressants or within 14 days of monoamine oxidase inhibitor; caution with kidney or heart disease, may cause aplastic anemia/agranulocytosis, pregnancy Category D. Monitor: CBC, LFTs at baseline and q3–6mo; check level 4–5 days after initiation and dose changes (goal: 4–12 mcg/mL).
  - Lamotrigine: Dosing: 200 mg/d start 25 mg × 2 weeks, then 50 mg × 2 weeks, then 100 mg × 1 week (Note: Different dosing if adjunct to valproate). Selected warnings: Titrate slowly (risk of Stevens-Johnson syndrome); caution with kidney, liver, or heart impairment; pregnancy Category C. Monitor: Patient to monitor for rash.
  - Oxcarbazepine, gabapentin, and topiramate are also used in BP but are not Food and Drug Administration (FDA) approved.
- Atypical antipsychotics (AAs):
  - Side effects of AAs: Orthostatic hypotension, negative metabolic side effects (effect glucose and lipid regulation, weight gain), tardive dyskinesia, neuroleptic malignant syndrome, prolactinemia (except Abilify), increased risk of mortality in elderly with dementia-related psychosis, pregnancy Category C
  - Monitor: LFTs, lipids, glucose at baseline, 3 months and annually; check for extrapyramidal symptoms with Abnormal Involuntary Movement Scale (AIMS) and assess weight (with abdominal circumference) at baseline, then 4, 8, and 12 weeks, then q3–6mo; monitor for orthostatic hypotension 3–5 days after starting or changing dose
  - Aripiprazole: Dosing: 15 mg/d, max 30 mg/d, less likely to cause metabolic side effects
  - Olanzapine: Dosing: 5–20 mg/d, most likely AA to cause metabolic side effects (weight gain, diabetes mellitus)
  - Symbyax (olanzapine + fluoxetine): Dosing: 6/25 mg, FDA approved for bipolar depression
  - Quetiapine: Dosing: Hypomania 200–400 mg b.i.d. Depression 50–300 mg qhs Caution: Cataracts, sedation.
  - Risperidone: Dosing: 1–6 mg/d every day-b.i.d. Generic and q2wk IM preparations available.
  - Ziprasidone: Dosing: 40–80 mg b.i.d. Less likely to cause metabolic side effects, Warnings: QTc prolongation (>500 ms) has been associated with use (0.06%), consider EKG at baseline.

Second Line

- Antidepressants (in addition to mood stabilizers)
- Benzodiazepines (for acute agitation, anxiety)
- Sleep medications

ADDITIONAL TREATMENT

General Measures

- Psychotherapy (e.g., CBT, social rhythm therapy) in conjunction with medications is key.
- Regular exercise, a healthy diet, and sobriety have shown to help prevent worsening of symptoms.

Issues for Referral

Patients may benefit from care by a multidisciplinary team, including a primary care physician and a psychiatrist.

Additional Therapies

- Electroconvulsive therapy with severe depression (may precipitate hypomania)
- Light therapy if there is seasonal component to depressive episodes (may precipitate hypomania)

IN-PATIENT CONSIDERATIONS

If hypomanic symptoms are severe enough to necessitate hospitalization, the patient automatically meets criteria for mania and BP-1.

Admission Criteria

To admit a patient (>18) to a psychiatric unit involuntarily, they must have a psychiatric diagnosis (e.g., major depression) and present a danger to themselves or others, or their mental disease must be inhibiting them from providing their basic needs (e.g., food, clothing, and/or shelter).

Nursing

Acute suicidal threats need closer observation.

Discharge Criteria

Determined by safety

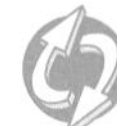

ONGOING CARE

FOLLOW-UP RECOMMENDATIONS

- Regularly scheduled visits support treatment adherence.
- Frequent communication between primary care doctor, psychiatrist, and therapist ensures comprehensive care.

Patient Monitoring

Mood charts are helpful adjuncts to care.

PATIENT EDUCATION

- Support groups for patients and families are recommended.
- National Alliance on Mental Illness: http://www.nami.org/

PROGNOSIS

- Frequency and severity of problematic episodes are related to medication adherence, consistency with psychotherapy, sleep, support systems, regularity of daily activities, and social history.
- Substance abuse, unemployment, persistent depression, and male sex are associated with a worse prognosis.
- Although data are limited, evidence indicates that patients with BP-2 may be at greater risk of both attempting and completing suicide than with BP-1 and unipolar depression.

REFERENCES

1. Perlis RH, Brown E, Baker RW, et al. Clinical features of bipolar depression versus major depressive disorder in large multicenter trials. *Am J Psychiatry*. 2006;163:225–31.
2. Benazzi F. A prediction rule for diagnosing hypomania. *Prog Neuropsychopharmacol Biol Psychiatry*. 2009;33:317–22.
3. Hirshfeld RM. Validation of the mood disorder questionnaire. *Bipolar Depression Bulletin*. 2004.
4. Angst J, Adolfsson R, Benazzi F, et al. The HCL-32: Towards a self-assessment tool for hypomanic symptoms in outpatients. *J Affect Disord*. 2005;88: 217–33.

ADDITIONAL READING

Benazzi F. Bipolar disorder–focus on bipolar II disorder and mixed depression. *Lancet*. 2007;369:935–45.

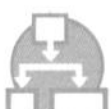

See Also (Topic, Algorithm, Electronic Media Element)

Algorithm: Depressive Episode, Major

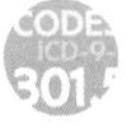

CODES

ICD9

296.89 Other manic-depressive psychosis

CLINICAL PEARLS

- BP-2 is characterized by at least 1 episode of major depression and 1 episode of hypomania.
- Patients are often resistant to treatment during a hypomanic episode, as they enjoy the elevated mood and productivity.
- Evidence indicates that patients with BP-2 may be at greater risk of both attempting and completing suicide than with BP-1 and unipolar depression.

BITES

Jennifer S. Daly, MD

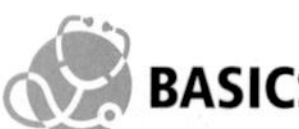

BASICS

DESCRIPTION

- Animal bites to humans from dogs (85–90%), cats (5–10%), rodents (2–3%), humans (2–3%), and other animals, including snakes
- System(s) affected: Potentially any

Pediatric Considerations

Young children are more likely to sustain bites and 50% may have bites to the face.

EPIDEMIOLOGY

- Predominant age: All ages, but children > adults
- Predominant gender: Dog bites: Male > Female; cat bites: Female > Male

Incidence

- 4–5 million dog bites per year in the US
- Account for 1% of all emergency room visits
- 20% of bites will require medical attention, 10,000 will require hospital admission, and an average of 19 victims will die from the bites annually (1).

RISK FACTORS

- Male dogs and older dogs are more likely to bite.
- Clenched-fist human bites are frequently associated with the use of alcohol.
- Patients presenting >8 hours following the bite are at greater risk of infection.

GENERAL PREVENTION

- Instruct children and adults about animal hazards and strongly enforce animal control laws.
- Educate dog owners.

PATHOPHYSIOLOGY

- Animal bites can cause tears, punctures, scratches, avulsions, or crush injuries.
- Contamination of wound with flora from the mouth of the biting animal or from the broken skin of the victim can lead to infection.

ETIOLOGY

- Most bite wounds are from a domestic pet known to the victim.
- 89% of cat bites are provoked.
- Pit bull terriers, German shepherds, Rottweilers, and mixed breeds are most commonly associated with bites (2).
- Human bites are often the result of 1 person striking another in the mouth with a clenched fist.
- Bites can also occur incidentally in the case of paronychia due to nail biting, or thumb sucking, or "love nips" to the face, breasts, or genital areas.

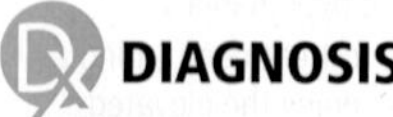

DIAGNOSIS

HISTORY

- Obtain detailed history of the incident (provoked or unprovoked).
- Type of animal
- Vaccine status
- Site of the bite
- Geographic setting

PHYSICAL EXAM

- Dog bites (85–90% of bites):
  - Hands and face most common site of injury in adults and children, respectively
  - More likely to have associated crush injury
- Cat bites (5–10% of bites):
  - Predominantly involve the hands, followed by lower extremities, face, and trunk
- Human bites (2–3% of bites):
  - Intentional bite: Semicircular or oval area of erythema and bruising, with or without break in skin
  - Clenched-fist injury: Small wounds over the metacarpophalangeal joints from striking the fist against another's teeth
- Signs of wound infection include fever, erythema, swelling, tenderness, purulent drainage, lymphangitis.

ALERT

Cat bites (often puncture wounds) are twice as likely to cause infection as dog bites, with higher risks of osteomyelitis, tenosynovitis, and septic arthritis.

Pediatric Considerations

If human bite mark on child has intercanine distance >3 cm, bite probably came from an adult and should raise concerns about child abuse.

DIAGNOSTIC TESTS & INTERPRETATION

Lab

Initial lab tests

- Drainage from infected wounds should be Gram-stained and cultured:
  - If wound fails to heal, perform cultures for atypical pathogens(fungi, nocardia. and mycobacteria) and ask lab to keep bacterial cultures for 7–10 days (some pathogens are slow-growing).
- 85% of bite wounds will yield a positive culture, with an average of 5 pathogens.
- Blood cultures should be obtained before starting antibiotics if bacteremia suspected (e.g., fever or chills).

Follow-Up & Special Considerations

Previous antibiotic therapy may alter culture results.

Imaging

Initial approach

- If bite wound is near a bone or joint, a plain radiograph is needed to check for bone injury and to use for comparison later if osteomyelitis is subsequently suspected.
- Radiographs are needed to check for fractures in clenched-fist injuries.

Follow-Up & Special Considerations

Subsequent suspicion of osteomyelitis warrants comparison plain radiograph or MRI.

Diagnostic Procedures/Surgery

Surgical exploration may be needed to ascertain extent of injuries, or drain deep infections (such as tendon sheath infections) especially in serious hand wounds.

Pathological Findings

- Dog bites (3,4):
  - *Pasteurella* sp. is present in 50% of bites.
  - Also found: Viridans streptococci, *Staphylococcus aureus, Staphylococcus intermedius, Bacteroides, Capnocytophaga canimorsus, Fusobacterium*
- Cat bites:
  - *Pasteurella* sp. is present in 75% of bites.
  - Also found: *Streptococcus* spp. (including *Streptococcus pyogenes*), *Staphylococcus* spp. (including methicillin-resistant *Staphylococcus aureus* [MRSA]), *Fusobacterium* spp., *Bacteroides* spp., *Porphyromonas* spp., *Moraxella* spp.
- Human bites:
  - *Streptococcus* species, *S. aureus, Eikenella corrodens*, and various anaerobic bacteria (e.g., *Fusobacterium, Peptostreptococcus, Prevotella*, and *Porphyromonas* spp.)
  - Although rare, case reports have suggested transmission of viruses such as hepatitis, HIV, and herpes simplex (5)[C].
- Reptile bites:
  - If from a venomous snake, need to use antivenom. Bacteria: *P. aeruginosa, Proteus* spp., *Salmonella, Bacteroides fragilis*, and *Clostridium* spp.
- Rodent bites:
  - *Streptobacillus moniliformis* or *Spirillum minor*, which cause rat-bite fever

ALERT

Asplenic patients and those with underlying hepatic disease are at risk of bacteremia and fatal sepsis after dog bites infected with *Capnocytophaga canimorsus* (gram-negative rod).

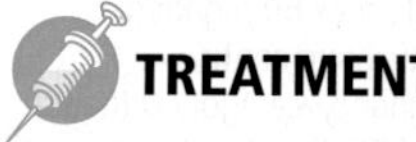

TREATMENT

MEDICATION

- Consider need for antirabies therapy: Rabies immunoglobulin and human diploid cell rabies vaccine for those bitten by wild animals (in US, primary vector is bat bite), rabid pets, or unvaccinated pets, or if animal cannot be quarantined for 10 days (6)[A].
- Tetanus toxoid for those previously immunized, but >5 years since their last dose and tetanus immunoglobulin and tetanus vaccination in patients without a full primary series of immunizations (7)[A]
- A patient negative for anti-HBs antibodies and bitten by an HBsAg-positive individual should receive both hepatitis B immunoglobulin (HBIG) and hepatitis B vaccine.
- HIV postexposure prophylaxis is generally not recommended for human bites, given the extremely low risk for transmission.
- Prophylactic antibiotics are only recommended for human bites and all penetrating animal bites to the hand (8,9)[A].
- For prophylaxis and for empiric treatment of established infection, amoxicillin-clavulanate is first line (6)[B]:
  - Adults: 500 mg PO t.i.d. or 875 mg PO b.i.d.
  - Children: <3 months: 30 mg/kg/d PO q12h; ≥3 months and <40 kg: 45 mg/kg/d q12h; >40 kg, use adult dosing
    - Adverse reaction: Amoxicillin-clavulanate should be given with food to decrease GI side effects.
    - Precautions: Dose antibiotics by body weight and renal function.
    - Significant possible interactions: Antibiotics may decrease efficacy of oral contraceptives.

- Duration of therapy: Prophylaxis: 3–5 days; treatment: Cellulitis/skin abscess: 5–10 days; bacteremia: 10–14 days. Antibiotic and duration of therapy should be adjusted based on culture results and clinical improvement:
  - Adults: Clindamycin (300 mg PO q.i.d.) plus either:
    - TMP-SMX (1 DS tablet PO b.i.d.–t.i.d.) or
    - ciprofloxacin (500 mg PO b.i.d.) (6)[B] for 7–21 days
  - Children: Clindamycin (5–10 mg/kg IV [to a maximum of 600 mg] followed by 10–30 mg/kg/d in 3–4 divided doses to a maximum of 300 mg per dose) plus
    - Trimethoprimsulfamethoxazole (8–10 mg/kg of trimethoprim) or
    - Cefoxitin IM/IV until culture results obtained
- Avoid: first-generation cephalosporins (e.g., cephalexin), penicillinase-resistant penicillins (e.g., dicloxacillin), macrolides (e.g., erythromycin), and clindamycin (when not administered with another agent) as they lack activity against *P. multocida* (dog/cat bites) and *Eikenella corrodens* (human bites) (6)[B].

Pregnancy Considerations

- Penicillin-allergic pregnant women:
  - Azithromycin 250–500 mg PO every day (6)[B]
- Observe closely and note potential increased risk of failure.

ALERT

Consider community-acquired MRSA as possible pathogen (from human skin or colonized pet). If high suspicion, doxycycline or trimethoprim-sulfamethoxazole provide good coverage (7)[A].

ADDITIONAL TREATMENT

General Measures

- Elevation of the injured extremity to prevent swelling
- Contact the local health department regarding the prevalence of rabies in the species of animal involved (highest in bats).
- Snake bite: If venomous, patient needs rapid transport to facility capable of definitive evaluation. If envenomation has occurred, patient should receive antivenom. Be sure patient is stable for transport; consider measuring and/or treating coagulation and renal status along with any anaphylactic reactions before transport.

Issues for Referral

Deep wounds to the hand and face should be referred to a hand surgeon or plastic surgeon, respectively.

SURGERY/OTHER PROCEDURES

- Copious irrigation of the wound with normal saline via a catheter tip is needed to reduce risk of infection.
- Devitalized tissue needs debridement.
- Debridement of puncture wounds is not advised.
- Primary closure can be considered if the wound is clean after irrigation and bite is <12 hours old, and in bites to the face (cosmesis) (10)[B].
- Infected wounds and those at risk of infection (cat bites, human bites, bites to the hand, crush injuries, presentation >12 hours from injury) should be left open (11)[B].
- Delayed primary closure in 3–5 days is an option for infected wounds.
- Splint hand if it is injured.
- Large, gaping wounds should be reapproximated with widely spaced sutures or Steri-Strips.

IN-PATIENT CONSIDERATIONS

Initial Stabilization

ABCs for associated trauma or severe infection

Admission Criteria

- Patients with deep or severe wound infections, systemic infections requiring IV antibiotics, those requiring surgery, and the immunocompromised
- If hospitalized with established infection (animal or human bite):
  - Adults: Ampicillin/sulbactam 1.5–3 g IV q6h or piperacillin/tazobactam 3.375 g q6h or 4.5 g IV q8h or ticarcillin/clavulanate 3.1 g IV q4–6h (6)[B]
  - Alternative: Ciprofloxacin 400 mg IV q12h or levofloxacin 500 mg IV every day with metronidazole 500 mg IV q8h
  - Children: Ampicillin/sulbactam 100–200 mg/kg/d IV given in 4 divided doses to maximum of 3 g per dose

Discharge Criteria

Pending clinical improvement

ONGOING CARE

FOLLOW-UP RECOMMENDATIONS

Patient Monitoring

- Patient should be rechecked in 24–48 hours if not infected at time of first encounter (12)[B].
- Daily follow-up is warranted for infections.
- Subsequent revisions of empiric antibiotic therapy should be based on the culture results and the clinical response.

PATIENT EDUCATION

- Educate parents at well-child checks about how to avoid animal bites.
- AAFP: http://familydoctor.org/online/famdocen/home/healthy/safety/kids-family/668.html
- CDC: http://www.cdc.gov/homeandrecreationalsafety/dog-bites/biteprevention.html

PROGNOSIS

Wounds should steadily improve and close over by 7–10 days.

COMPLICATIONS

- Septic arthritis
- Osteomyelitis
- Extensive soft tissue injuries with scarring
- Hemorrhage
- Gas gangrene
- Sepsis
- Meningitis
- Endocarditis
- Posttraumatic stress disorder
- Death

REFERENCES

1. Langley RL. Human fatalities resulting from dog attacks in the United States, 1979–2005. *Wilderness Environ Med*. 2009;20(1):19–25.
2. Rovetta G, Sessarego P, Monteforte P, et al. Stretching exercises for costochondritis pain. *G Ital Med Lav Ergon*. 2009;31:169–71.
3. Bini JK, Cohn SM, Acosta SM, et al. Mortality, mauling, and maiming by vicious dogs. *Ann Surg*. 2011;253:791–7.
4. Abrahamian FM, Goldstein EJ, et al. Microbiology of animal bite wound infections. *Clin Microbiol Rev*. 2011;24:231–46.
5. Bartholomew CF, Jones AM. Human bites: A rare risk factor for HIV transmission. *AIDS*. 2006;20: 631–2.
6. Stevens DL, Bisno AL, Chambers HF, et al. Practice guidelines for the diagnosis and management of skin and soft-tissue infections. *Clin Infect Dis*. 2005;41:1373–406.
7. Oehler RL, Velez AP, Mizrachi M, et al. Bite-related and septic syndromes caused by cats and dogs. *Lancet Infect Dis*. 2009;9:439–47.
8. Medeiros I, et al. Antibiotic prophylaxis for mammalian bites. *Cochrane Database Syst Rev*. 2008;2:CD001738.
9. Rittner AV, Fitzpatrick K, Corfield A. Best evidence topic report. Are antibiotics indicated following human bites? *Emerg Med J*. 2005;22:654.
10. Stefanopoulos PK, Tarantzopoulou AD. Facial bite wounds: Management update. *Int J Oral Maxillofac Surg*. 2005;34:464–72.
11. Benson LS, Edwards SL, Schiff AP, et al. Dog and cat bites to the hand: Treatment and cost assessment. *J Hand Surg [Am]*. 2006;31:468–73.
12. Okonkwo U, et al. Animal bites: Practical tips for effective management. *J Emerg Nursing*. 2008;34(3):225–6.

ADDITIONAL READING

Daly JS, Scharf MJ. Bites and stings of terrestrial and aquatic life. In Fitzpatrick TB, Eisen AZ, Wolff K, et al. (eds). *Dermatology in General Medicine*, 7th ed. New York: McGraw Hill; 2011.

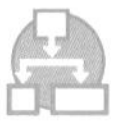

See Also (Topic, Algorithm, Electronic Media Element)

Cellulitis; Rabies; Snake Envenomations; Bartonella Infections

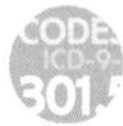

CODES

ICD9

- 879.8 Open wound(s) (multiple) of unspecified site(s), without mention of complication
- 879.9 Open wound(s) (multiple) of unspecified site(s), complicated

CLINICAL PEARLS

- Wound cleansing, debridement, and culture are essential. Most wounds should be left open.
- Prophylaxis is recommended for human bites and bites to the hand.
- Consider rabies and tetanus vaccination.
- Patients bitten by animals or humans require close follow-up to monitor for infection.

BLADDER CANCER

Margaret E. Thompson, MD

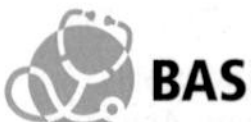

BASICS

DESCRIPTION

- Primary malignant neoplasms arising in the urinary bladder
- Most common type is transitional cell carcinoma (90%)
- Other types include adenocarcinoma, small cell carcinoma, squamous cell carcinoma
- Rhabdomyosarcoma of the bladder may occur in children.

EPIDEMIOLOGY

Incidence

- Increases with age (median age at diagnosis is 73 years)
- More common in Caucasians than in Asians or African Americans
- Male > Female (4:1), but in smokers, risk is 1:1
- 37.2 per 100,000 men per year (1)
- 9.2 per 100,000 women per year (1)
- 21.1 per 100,000 men and women per year (1)

Prevalence

As of January 1, 2007, 535,236 cases in US (1)

RISK FACTORS

- Smoking is the single greatest risk factor (increases risk 4-fold) (2) and increases risk equally for men and women (3).
- Other risk factors:
  - Occupational carcinogens in dye, rubber, paint, plastics, metal, and automotive exhaust
  - Schistosomiasis in Mediterranean (squamous cell) cancer
  - Arsenic in well water
  - History of pelvic irradiation
  - Chronic lower UTI
  - Chronic indwelling urinary catheter
  - Cyclophosphamide exposure
  - High-fat diet
  - Chronic low fluid intake
  - Slight increase in risk with prostate cancer

ALERT

Any patient who smokes and presents with microscopic or gross hematuria, or irritative voiding symptoms such as urgency and frequency not clearly due to UTI, should be evaluated by cystoscopy for the presence of a bladder neoplasm.

Genetics

Hereditary transmission is unlikely, although transitional cell carcinoma pathophysiology is related to oncogenes.

GENERAL PREVENTION

- Avoid smoking and other risk factors.
- The US Preventive Services Task Force notes that there is insufficient evidence to recommend screening for bladder cancer (4).

PATHOPHYSIOLOGY

- 70–80% is superficial (in lamina propria or mucosa):
  - Usually highly differentiated with long survival
  - Initial event seems to be activation of an oncogene on chromosome 9 in superficial cancers
- 20% of tumors are invasive (deeper than lamina propria) at presentation:
  - Tend to be high grade with worse prognosis
  - Associated with other chromosome deletions

ETIOLOGY

Unknown, other than related to risk factors

DIAGNOSIS

HISTORY

- Painless hematuria is most common symptom
- Urinary symptoms (frequency, urgency)
- Abdominal or pelvic pain in advanced disease
- Exposures (see "Risk Factors")

PHYSICAL EXAM

- Normal in early cases
- Pelvic or abdominal mass in advanced disease
- Wasting in systemic disease

DIAGNOSTIC TESTS & INTERPRETATION

Lab

Initial lab tests

- Urinalysis is the initial test in patients presenting with gross hematuria or urinary symptoms such as frequency, urgency, and dysuria.
- Macroscopic hematuria (55% sensitivity, positive predictive value [PPV] 0.22 for urologic cancer) (5)[C]

Follow-Up & Special Considerations

- Urine cytology 54% sensitivity overall (lower in less advanced tumors), 94% specific (6)[A]
- Other urine markers:
  - NMP22: 67% sensitive, 78% specific (6)[A]
  - Bladder tumor-associated antigen stat: 70% sensitive, 75% specific (6)[A]
  - Fluorescent in situ hybridization assay: 69% sensitive, 78% specific (PPV 27.1, negative predictive value 95.3) for all tumors, more sensitive and specific for higher grade (7)[B]
- Bottom line: None of the urine markers are sensitive enough to rule out bladder cancer on its own.
- Liver function tests, alkaline phosphatase if metastasis suspected

Imaging

Initial approach

- Done for staging and evaluating extent of disease, but not for diagnosis itself:
  - CT urogram replacing IV to image upper tracts if there is suspicion of disease there
  - Diffusion-weighted MRI and multidimensional CT scan are undergoing study for use in diagnosis and staging of bladder tumors.
  - For invasive disease, metastatic workup should include chest x-ray.
  - Bone scan should be performed if the patient has bone pain or if alkaline phosphatase is elevated (8)[B].
- Urologic CT scan (abdomen, pelvis, with and without contrast) or MRI 40–98% accurate, with MRI slightly more accurate (8)[B], is recommended if metastasis is suspected.

Follow-Up & Special Considerations

Regular cystoscopy (initiated at 3 months postprocedure) indicated after TURBT and intravesical chemotherapy for superficial bladder cancers

Diagnostic Procedures/Surgery

- Cystoscopy with biopsy is the gold standard for diagnosis, but 1 study showed that 33% of patients had residual tumor after transurethral resection of superficial tumor (TURBT) (8)[B].
- TURBT with bladder washings: Sensitivity of cytology on bladder washings for carcinoma in situ is nearly 100%.

Pathological Findings

- Characterized as superficial or invasive
- 70–80% present as superficial lesion
- Superficial lesions:
  - Carcinoma in situ: Flat lesion, high grade
  - Ta: Noninvasive papillary carcinoma
  - T1: Extends into submucosa, lamina propria
- Invasive cancer:
  - T2: Invasion into muscle:
    - pT2a: Invasion into superficial muscle
    - pT2b: Invasion into deep muscle
  - T3: Invasion into perivesical fat:
    - pT3a: Microscopic
    - pT3b: Macroscopic
  - T4: Invasion into adjacent organs:
    - aT4a: Invades prostate, uterus, or vagina
    - aT4b: Invades abdominal or pelvic wall
  - N1–N3: Invades lymph nodes
- M: Metastasis to bone or soft tissue

DIFFERENTIAL DIAGNOSIS

- Other urinary tract neoplasms
- UTI
- Prostatism
- Bladder instability
- Interstitial cystitis
- Urolithiasis
- Interstitial nephritis
- Papillary urothelial hyperplasia

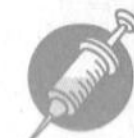

TREATMENT

For superficial bladder cancer, the treatment is generally removal via cystoscopic surgery. For muscle-invasive cancer, a radical cystectomy is preferred.

MEDICATION

First Line

- There is insufficient evidence to show that cisplatin-based neoadjuvant chemotherapy in patients with locally advanced bladder cancer improves survival (9)[A].
- Intravesical bacillus Calmette-Guérin (BCG) after TURBT in high-grade lesions has been shown to decrease recurrence in Ta and T1 tumors (10)[A].
- Intravesical BCG has been shown to be superior in efficacy to intravesical epirubicin in preventing recurrence of tumor in Ta and T1 tumors (11)[B].

Second Line
- Chemotherapy is the first-line treatment for metastatic bladder cancer: Methotrexate-vinblastinedoxorubicin-cisplatin (MVAC) is the preferred regimen.
- A recent review showed that gemcitabine plus cisplatin may be better tolerated and result in equivalent survival to MVAC, making it a possible first choice in metastatic bladder cancer (12)[A].

ADDITIONAL TREATMENT
Issues for Referral
Patients with microscopic or gross hematuria not otherwise explained or resolving should be referred to a urologist for cystoscopy.

Additional Therapies
Radiotherapy:
- In the US, used for patients with muscle-invasive cancer who are not surgical candidates
- Preoperative (radical cystectomy) radiotherapy also an option
- Treatment of choice for muscle-invasive cancer in some European and Canadian centers:
  - 65–70 Gy over 6–7 weeks is standard.

SURGERY/OTHER PROCEDURES
- Surgery is definitive therapy for superficial and invasive cancer:
  - Superficial cancer: TURBT sometimes followed by intravesical therapy
- Invasive cancer:
  - Radical cystectomy for invasive disease that is confined to the bladder is more effective than radical radiotherapy (13)[A]. Urine is diverted via an ileal loop with ostomy or neobladder constructed with intestine.

IN-PATIENT CONSIDERATIONS
Admission Criteria
Need for surgery or intensive therapy

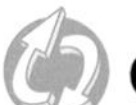

ONGOING CARE

FOLLOW-UP RECOMMENDATIONS
- Superficial cancers:
  - Urine cytology alone has not been shown to be sufficient for follow-up.
  - Cystoscopy every 3 months for 18–24 months, every 6 months for the next 2 years, then annually
- Follow-up for invasive cancers depends on the approach to treatment.
- Patients treated with BCG require lifelong follow-up.

DIET
Continue adequate fluid intake.

PATIENT EDUCATION
Smoking cessation

PROGNOSIS
- 5-year relative survival rates:
  - Localized: 93.7%
  - Regional metastasis: 46.0%
  - Distant metastasis: 6.2%
- Superficial bladder cancer:
  - BCG treatment prevents recurrence vs. TURBT alone; difference 30%, NNT 3.3 (13)[A]
  - BCG prevents progression vs. TURBT alone, difference 8%
- Invasive cancer:
  - T2 disease: Radical cystectomy results in 60–75% 5-year survival.
  - T3 or T4 disease: Radical cystectomy results in 20–40% 5-year survival.
  - Neoadjuvant chemotherapy with cystectomy has led to varying degrees of increased survival.
  - Radiation with chemotherapy has led to varying degrees of increased survival.
- Metastatic cancer:
  - MVAC resulted in mean survival of 12.5 months.

COMPLICATIONS
- Superficial bladder cancer:
  - Local symptoms:
    - Dysuria, frequency, nocturia, pain, passing debris in urine
    - Bacterial cystitis
    - Perforation
  - General symptoms:
    - Flulike symptoms
    - Systemic infection
- Invasive cancer:
  - Symptoms related to definitive treatment, including incontinence, bleeding
  - Patients with neobladder at risk for azotemia and metabolic acidosis

REFERENCES

1. Altekruse SF, Kosary CL, Krapcho M, et al., eds. *SEER Cancer Statistics Review, 1975–2007*, National Cancer Institute. Bethesda, MD. http://seer.cancer.gov/csr/1975_2007/, based on November 2009 SEER data submission, posted to the SEER web site, 2010.
2. Kaplan M, Cologlu M. Bladder tumors. In *Essential Evidence Plus*, John Wiley and Sons, Ltd, 2011, http://www.essentialevidenceplus.com/content/eee/480, accessed 7/16/2011.
3. Freedman N, et al. Association between smoking and risk of bladder cancer among men and women. *JAMA*. 2011;306(7):737–45.
4. Chou R, Dana T. Screening adults for bladder cancer: A review of the evidence for the U.S. Preventive Services Task Force. *Ann Intern Med*. 2010;153(7):461–8.
5. Buntinx F, Wauters H. The diagnostic value of macroscopic haematuria in diagnosing urological cancers: A meta-analysis. *Fam Pract*. 1997;14:63–8.
6. Glas AS, Roos D, Deutekom M, et al. Tumor markers in the diagnosis of primary bladder cancer. A systematic review. *J Urol*. 2003;169:1975–82.
7. Sarosdy MF, Kahn PR, Ziffer MD, et al. Use of a multitarget fluorescence in situ hybridization assay to diagnose bladder cancer in patients with hematuria. *J Urol*. 2006;176:44–7.
8. Kirkali Z, Chan T, Manoharan M, et al. Bladder cancer: Epidemiology, staging and grading, and diagnosis. *Urology*. 2005;66:4–34.
9. Advanced Bladder Cancer Meta-analysis Collaboration. Neoadjuvant Cisplatin for advanced bladder cancer (Cochrane Review). In *the Cochrane Library Issue* 1, 2009. Chichester, UK: John Wiley and Sons, Ltd.
10. Shelley M, Court JB, Kynaston H, et al. Intravesical Bacillus Calmette-Guerin in Ta and T1 bladder cancer (Cochrane Review). In: *The Cochrane Library*, Issue 3, 2010. Chichester, UK: John Wiley and Sons, Ltd.
11. Shang PF, Kwong J, Chang CP, et al. Intravesical Bacillus Calmette-Guerin versus epirubicin for Ta and T1 bladder cancer. *Cochrane Database Syst Rev*. 2011;11:5.
12. Shelley M, Cleves A, Wilt TJ, et al. Gemcitabine for unresectable, locally advanced or metastatic bladder cancer. *Cochrane Database Syst Rev*. 2011;13(4).
13. Shelley MD, et al. Surgery versus radiotherapy for muscle invasive bladder cancer (Cochrane Review). In: *The Cochrane Library*, Issue 4, 2005. Chichester, UK: John Wiley and Sons, Ltd.
14. U.S. Preventive Services Task Force. Screening for bladder cancer in adults: Recommendation statement. Rockville, MD: Agency for Healthcare Research and Quality; 2004.

ADDITIONAL READING

- Sharma S, Ksheersagar P, Sharma P. Diagnosis and treatment of bladder cancer. *Am Fam Physician*. 2009;80(7):717–23.
- Vale C. Neoadjuvant chemotherapy for invasive bladder cancer (Cochrane Review). In: *The Cochrane Library* Issue 1, 2007. Chichester, UK: John Wiley and Sons, Ltd.

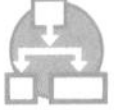

See Also (Topic, Algorithm, Electronic Media Element)

- Hematuria
- Algorithm: Hematuria

CODES

ICD9
- 188.0 Malignant neoplasm of trigone of urinary bladder
- 188.1 Malignant neoplasm of dome of urinary bladder
- 188.9 Malignant neoplasm of bladder, part unspecified

CLINICAL PEARLS

- Gross hematuria in smokers should be evaluated with complete urologic workup.
- The US Preventive Services Task Force recommends against routine screening for bladder cancer (14)[A].

BLADDER INJURY

Kyle D. Wood, MD
Ilya Gorbachinsky, MD

BASICS

DESCRIPTION

- Bladder injury can result from one of these situations:
  - Blunt or penetrating trauma
  - Bladder rupture secondary to a full bladder or blunt injury
  - Surgical complication (iatrogenic injury)
- Classified as either intraperitoneal or extraperitoneal rupture
- Bladder contusion is injury to the mucosa or muscularis without full-thickness loss; without urine extravasation.
- Often associated with ureter/urethral injury and/or other nonurological injuries

EPIDEMIOLOGY

Incidence

- ~0.5% of civilian trauma patients (1)
- 12% of civilian injuries in Iraq, mostly due to gunshot wounds (2)
- Blunt trauma with bladder injury is associated with other injuries 94% of the time (3); pelvic fracture is the most common, followed by lower abdominal impact in the presence of a full bladder (4).
- During pelvic surgery, it is the most commonly damaged organ (5).

Pediatric Considerations

Children are more prone to rupture and are more likely to have intraperitoneal ruptures than adults do (1).

RISK FACTORS

- High-energy mechanism (fall, motor vehicle accident [MVA])
- Pelvic fracture
- Penetrating wound
- Prior bladder/pelvic surgery
- Pelvic radiotherapy

GENERAL PREVENTION

Seat belts:

- Voiding prior to automobile travel

PATHOPHYSIOLOGY

- The bladder is often protected by its deep location in the bony pelvis.
- Contusion: Damage sustained to bladder mucosa and muscularis without loss of wall continuity (5)
- Intraperitoneal rupture: Increases in intravesical pressure can lead to rupture at the most weak and mobile portion, the bladder dome (6,7)
- Extraperitoneal rupture: Disruption of bony pelvis can tear bladder at fascial attachments while this or other bony protrusions can perforate the bladder (6).

Pediatric Considerations

Children <6 years old are more prone to bladder injury as the organ still lacks protection from the pubic symphysis (7).

ETIOLOGY

- The cause of injury is usually high-energy trauma (MVAs, falls).
- Rupture due to increased pressure in nondistensible (full) bladder
- Laceration due to bone fragment or penetrating object (knife, bullet)
- Surgical complications: Gynecologic, general surgery, and urologic operations are the most common reported causes of iatrogenic bladder injury, in decreasing order of frequency (8).

ALERT

Rare instances of intravesical vascular graft erosion have recently been reported up to 8 years postopertively (9).

COMMONLY ASSOCIATED CONDITIONS

- Pelvic fracture
- Urethral injury; almost exclusively males

DIAGNOSIS

HISTORY

- Isolated bladder injury is rare. Typically, the patient has other serious injuries.
- High mechanism deceleration injury (fall, MVA)
- Penetrating trauma
- Recent abdominal/pelvic surgery
- Urinary retention
- Pre-existing bladder outlet obstruction
- Anatomical abnormalities
- Inability to void or oliguria
- Pain in the genital area or abdomen

PHYSICAL EXAM

- Abdominal exam: Suprapubic tenderness to palpation, guarding, distention, decreased bowel sounds, bruising
- Genitourinary exam: Blood at meatus, gross hematuria, clots in the urine, scrotal/urethral hematoma, free-floating or high-riding prostate, unstable pelvis

ALERT

Peritonitis is unusual in bladder injury.

DIAGNOSTIC TESTS & INTERPRETATION

Lab

Initial lab tests

- Immediate catheterization will likely demonstrate gross hematuria (3).
- Urinalysis will demonstrate blood.
- Basic metabolic panel: Serum BUN, creatinine, chloride, and potassium levels may be elevated, and sodium and bicarbonate may be decreased in intraperitoneal ruptures secondary to peritoneal absorption. An increase in the BUN/creatinine ratio may also be observed (5).
- Serum labs are unchanged in extraperitoneal ruptures (6).

Follow-Up & Special Considerations

If blood is at the meatus or if the catheter does not pass easily, consider urethral injury and the need for retrograde urethrography.

Imaging

Initial approach

- 2 types of imaging are acceptable:
  - Plain film cystography: Fill bladder until patient has sense of discomfort or fill with 350 mL. Use 3-film technique capturing before filling, when full, and after drainage.
    - Contusion: No extravasation but may see distortion of bladder outline with contrast.
    - Intraperitoneal: Contrast may be seen in cul-de-sac and paracolic gutters. Bowel loops may also be outlined.
    - Extraperitoneal: Flame-shaped perivesical stranding of contrast (5)
  - CT cystography: High-resolution CT cystogram is also acceptable. CT or radiology with only excreted contrast is not sensitive (6). Dilute contrast material.
- Absolute indication for immediate cystography: Gross hematuria with pelvic fracture as 29% of these patients will have a bladder injury (10).
- Relative indications: Gross hematuria without pelvic fracture, microhematuria with pelvic fracture, isolated microscopic hematuria (10)

ALERT

During plain film cystography, a postvoid view is mandatory as contrast in the bladder may mask extravasation. This is not required with a CT cystogram.

Follow-Up & Special Considerations

- Retrograde urethrography must be performed before placing a Foley catheter when urethral injury is suspected.
- Other signs of bladder injury can include free intraperitoneal fluid on CT scan or ultrasound

Pathological Findings

- Perivesicular hematoma
- Perforation at dome of bladder (in trigone, near urachus)
- Jagged tear in bladder
- Intraoperative clues (11):
  - Appearance of Foley catheter/balloon or urine in the operative field
  - Presence of gas in catheter bag (during laparoscopy)

DIFFERENTIAL DIAGNOSIS

- Isolated urethral injury
- Isolated pelvic fracture
- Isolated ureteral injury
- Other visceral rupture

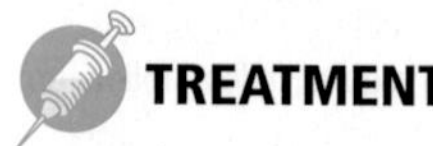

TREATMENT

- Contusion: Observation or 20–22 French Foley catheter for 10–14 days (6)[B]
- Intraperitoneal rupture: Immediate surgical repair (6)[C]
  - Often intraoperative damage falls under this heading and can also be treated immediately.
- Extraperitoneal rupture: 20–22 French Foley catheter for 10–14 days (6)

MEDICATION

- Analgesics
- Antibiotics
- Antispasmodics

B

First Line

- Narcotic pain control (i.e., morphine, hydromorphone); titrate to effect
- Broad-spectrum antibiotics like ciprofloxacin 500 mg b.i.d.
- Oxybutynin 5–10 mg t.i.d. for spasm

Second Line

- Broad-spectrum antibiotics
- Antispasmodics (i.e., flavoxate)

ALERT

There is concern about fluoroquinolones causing damage to cartilage in children.

ADDITIONAL TREATMENT

- If an uncomplicated extraperitoneal bladder rupture:
  - Can be treated with urethral catheter alone (use large-bore catheter [22 French])
  - Exception: In pediatric patients, consider placing a suprapubic catheter as small catheters through the urethra will clot and larger catheters through the urethra risk future urethral stricture
  - A catheter should remain in place for 2 weeks. Cystography is necessary prior to removal of a catheter.
  - Antibiotics should be given on day of injury and continued for 3 days after catheter removal.
- If a complicated extraperitoneal bladder rupture:
  - Needs to be treated with open repair
  - Complicated rupture is considered when there is coexisting bladder neck injury, vaginal injury, or rectal injury. Also if an open pelvic fracture or bone fragments are present.
  - Consider open repair if patient is scheduled for exploratory laparotomy or internal fixation of pelvic fracture (prevents urine leak on hardware).
- If an intraperitoneal bladder rupture or penetrating injury:
  - Urgent operative management is necessary.
  - Cystography should be repeated 7–10 days after surgery.
  - Antibiotics are needed for 3 days.
  - No need for suprapubic catheter as urethral catheter is sufficient, except in pediatric population (3)
- During pelvic surgery, iatrogenic full thickness defects are likely to be intraperitoneal, so they can be fixed immediately with 2-layer (mucosa and muscularis) closure via absorbable sutures
  - Prior to repair, be sure to confirm that ureters were not damaged concomitantly either with IV indigo carmine administration and visualization of blue dye expulsion from the ureteral orifices (UO) or by confirming easy placement of ureteral catheters through the UO (11).

General Measures

- Place Foley catheter
- Pain control
- Antibiotics
- Antispasmodics (Ditropan)
- Obtain imaging diagnosis

Issues for Referral

A urologist or trauma surgeon should be involved with all bladder injury management.

SURGERY/OTHER PROCEDURES

- Urgent surgery is indicated for intraperitoneal or bladder neck rupture
- Extraperitoneal rupture is usually manageable with 10–14 days of catheter drainage (20–22 French).

IN-PATIENT CONSIDERATIONS

Initial Stabilization

- Cervical spine precautions
- Stabilize hemodynamics
- Stabilize pelvis
- Follow advanced trauma life support protocols

Admission Criteria

All bladder injuries require admission for monitoring renal function and hemodynamic stability.

IV Fluids

Lactated Ringer's for initial resuscitation, unless contraindicated (i.e., concomitant head injury)

Nursing

- Foley to gravity
- Hourly urine output recorded

Discharge Criteria

- Stable for transfer to rehabilitation or home if the patient can perform activities of daily living
- Extraperitoneal ruptures controlled with in-dwelling Foley catheter if rupture not healed
- Able to void if no catheter in place
- No evidence of infection
- Pain is controlled

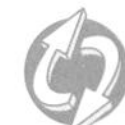

ONGOING CARE

FOLLOW-UP RECOMMENDATIONS

Patient Monitoring

- Hourly urine output
- Hemodynamic monitoring
- Progressive abdominal distention

DIET

No restrictions

PATIENT EDUCATION

- Regular lifestyle is expected
- Use of seatbelts
- No special instructions needed

PROGNOSIS

Full return to normal function

COMPLICATIONS

- Infection
- Urine leak and/or urinoma
- Abscess formation
- Peritonitis or sepsis
- Bladder calculi
- Vesicocutaneous or other fistulas
- Stricture is a rare complication.
- Death; usually from other injuries

REFERENCES

1. Inaba K, McKenney M, Munera F. Cystogram follow-up in the management of traumatic bladder disruption. *J Trauma*. 2006;60:23–8.
2. Ramani AP, Ryndin I, Veetil RT. Novel technique for removal of misdirected laparoscopic Weck clips. *Urology*. 2007;70:168–9.
3. Parry NG, Rozycki GS, Feliciano DV, et al. Traumatic rupture of the urinary bladder: Is the suprapubic tube necessary? *J Trauma*. 2003;54:431–6.
4. Tezval H, Tezval M, von Klot C, et al. Urinary tract injuries in patients with multiple trauma. *World J Urol*. 2007;25:177–84.
5. Gomez RG, Ceballos L, Coburn M, et al. Consensus statement on bladder injuries. *BJU Int*. 2004;94:27–32.
6. Corriere JN, Sandler CM. Diagnosis and management of bladder injuries. *Urol Clin North Am*. 2006;33:67–71, vi.
7. Kessler DO, Francis DL, Esernio-Jenssen D. Bladder rupture after minor accidental trauma: Case reports and a review of the literature. *Pediatr Emerg Care*. 2010;26:43–5.
8. Armenakas NA, Pareek G, Fracchia JA. Iatrogenic bladder perforations: Long-term follow-up of 65 patients. *J Am Coll Surg*. 2004;198:78–82.
9. Nakamura LY, Ferrigni RG, Stone WM, et al. Urinary bladder injuries during vascular surgery. *J Vasc Surg*. 2010;52:453–5.
10. Morey AF, Iverson AJ, Swan A, et al. Bladder rupture after blunt trauma: Guidelines for diagnostic imaging. *J Trauma*. 2001;51:683–6.
11. Sharp HT, Swenson C. Hollow viscus injury during surgery. *Obstet Gynecol Clin North Am*. 2010;37:461–7.

ADDITIONAL READING

- ATLS Protocol from the Committee on Trauma of the American College of Surgeons, http://www.facs.org/trauma/atls/.
- Eastern Association for the Surgery of Trauma, Management of Genitourinary Trauma, 2004, http://www.east.org/tpg/GUmgmt.pdf.

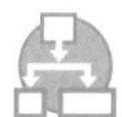

See Also (Topic, Algorithm, Electronic Media Element)

Algorithm: Hematuria

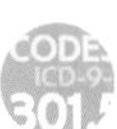

CODES

ICD9

- 596.9 Unspecified disorder of bladder
- 867.0 Injury to bladder and urethra without mention of open wound into cavity
- 867.1 Injury to bladder and urethra, with open wound into cavity

CLINICAL PEARLS

- The Foley should remain in place for 10–14 days. After this point, 85% of patients have healed all injuries.
- A cystogram must be performed before Foley removal to verify no extravasation of fluid. If extravasation continues, recheck every 3–5 days.
- An intraoperative consult to urology is indicated if an inadvertent bladder perforation occurs during another procedure. If urology is not available, the bladder must be examined intravesically, generally by increasing the size of the wound and searching for another occult injury. Do not delay repair.
- Repair bladder injuries in 2 layers with absorbable sutures and place a Foley catheter.

BLEPHARITIS

Joshua J. Spooner, PharmD, MS
A. Raquel Mateo-Bibeau, MD

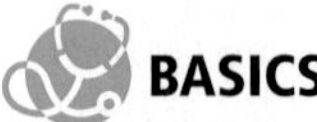

BASICS

DESCRIPTION

- An inflammatory reaction of the eyelid margin (1,2):
  - Usually occurs as seborrheic or staphylococcal blepharitis
  - Multiple types may coexist.
- System(s) affected: Skin/Exocrine
- Synonym(s): Granulated eyelids

EPIDEMIOLOGY

Incidence

- One of the most common ocular disorders
- Predominant age: Adult
- Predominant sex: Male = Female

RISK FACTORS

- Seborrheic dermatitis
- Contact dermatitis
- Herpes simplex dermatitis
- Varicella-zoster dermatitis
- Acne rosacea
- Diabetes mellitus
- Immunocompromised state (e.g., AIDS, chemotherapy)
- Isotretinoin use
- Dry eye syndromes

ETIOLOGY

- Seborrheic:
  - Accelerated shedding of skin cells with associated sebaceous gland dysfunction
  - *Malassezia furfur* (formerly *Pityrosporum ovale*) yeasts often colonize.
- Staphylococcal:
  - Superinfection of Zeis glands of lid margin and meibomian glands posterior to lashes with *Staphylococcus aureus*
  - Usually part of mixed blepharitis
- Meibomian gland dysfunction: Obstruction and inflammation of the meibomian glands; associated with acne rosacea, acne vulgaris, and oral retinoid therapy
- Other types of blepharitis:
  - Ulcerative blepharitis: More severe blepharitis with small marginal ulceration and destruction of the hair follicles
  - Contact dermatitis/blepharitis:
    - Develops from type IV hypersensitivity; common causes include ocular medications, topical anesthetics, antivirals, and cosmetics
    - May occur with secondary *Staphylococcus* infection
  - Eczematoid blepharitis:
    - Caused by hypersensitivity reaction to exotoxins and antigens from local flora
    - Strong association with eczema, asthma
    - Staphylococcal infection common
  - Angular blepharitis: Often caused by *Staphylococcus* or *Moraxella* infection

COMMONLY ASSOCIATED CONDITIONS

See "Risk Factors" and "Differential Diagnosis."

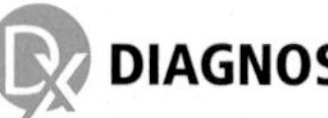

DIAGNOSIS

HISTORY

- Duration of symptoms
- Unilateral or bilateral presentation
- Note any exacerbating conditions (e.g., smoke, allergens, wind, contact lenses, etc.).
- Symptoms related to systemic diseases
- Current and recent medication use
- Recent exposure to infected individuals
- Frequently reported in all types of blepharitis:
  - Burning
  - Itching
  - Eyelid erythema
  - Conjunctival infection (red eyes)
  - Lacrimation, tearing
  - Tear deficiency
  - Foreign-body sensation
  - Photophobia (light sensitivity)
  - Impaired vision

PHYSICAL EXAM

- Test of visual acuity
- External exam (skin and eyelids):
  - Staphylococcal:
    - Recurrent stye (external or internal hordeolum)
    - Missing, broken, or misdirected eyelashes (trichiasis)
    - Eyelid deposits: Matted, hard scales; collarettes (ringlike formation around the lash shaft)
    - Ulcerations at base of eyelashes (rare)
    - Eyelid scarring may occur
  - Seborrheic blepharitis:
    - Eyelid deposits: Dry flakes, oily or greasy secretions on lid margins and/or lashes
    - Associated dandruff of scalp, eyebrows
  - Meibomian gland dysfunction:
    - Eyelash misdirection may occur with long-standing disease
    - Eyelid deposits: Fatty deposits; may be foamy
    - Eyelid margin thickening
    - Plugged meibomian gland orifices
    - Chalazion (sometimes multiple)
    - Eyelid scarring with long-term disease
  - Mixed blepharitis: Signs and symptoms of >1 type of blepharitis may be present.

DIAGNOSTIC TESTS & INTERPRETATION

Lab

Follow-Up & Special Considerations

- Cultures in atypical blepharitis
- Biopsy in atypical cases for carcinoma

Imaging

Initial approach

Slit-lamp biomicroscopy:

- Examine tear film, eyelid margins, eyelashes, tarsal and bulbar conjunctivae, and cornea.
- Reveals loss of lashes (madarosis), whitening of the lashes (poliosis), trichiasis, crusting, eyelid margin ulcers, and lid irregularities

DIFFERENTIAL DIAGNOSIS

Masquerade syndrome:

- Persistent inflammation and thickening of eyelid margin may indicate squamous cell, basal cell, or sebaceous cell carcinoma masquerading as blepharitis. These carcinomas also may mimic styes or chalazia.
- Sebaceous carcinoma of the eyelid has a 22% fatality rate. Up to 1/2 of these potentially fatal sebaceous cell carcinomas may resemble benign inflammatory diseases, particularly chalazia and chronic blepharoconjunctivitis.
- Consider this in all cases of recurrent, persistent, or atypical chalazion; chronic unilateral unresponsive blepharoconjunctivitis; diffuse or nodular tumors of the eyelid; orbital mass developing after removal of an eyelid or caruncular tumor; and any tumor developing in a person with a history of ocular radiotherapy (3)[C].

TREATMENT

MEDICATION

First Line

- Topical treatment to lid, if *Staphylococcus* likely: Bacitracin 500 μg/g or (second choice) erythromycin 0.5% ophthalmic ointment:
  - Apply with a cotton-tipped applicator.
  - The frequency and duration of treatment are guided by the severity (4)[C].
- Topical corticosteroids (short term) may be useful for eyelid or ocular surface inflammation. The minimum effective dose should be used; long-term use should be avoided if possible (4,5)[C].
- For patients with meibomian gland dysfunction inadequately controlled with eyelid hygiene, consider doxycycline 100 mg/d or tetracycline 1,000 mg/d in divided doses, tapered after clinical improvement (2–4 weeks) to doxycycline 50 mg/d or tetracycline 250–500 mg/d (4)[C].

- Since aqueous tear deficiency is common in blepharitis, use twice-daily artificial tears in addition to eyelid hygiene and medications.
- Contraindications: Allergy to medication; tetracyclines are not for use in pregnancy, nursing women, or children <8 years of age.
- Precautions: Tetracyclines may cause photosensitivity; sunscreen is recommended. Corticosteroids may increase intraocular pressure and risk of cataract.

Second Line

- Topical fluoroquinolones (e.g., gatifloxacin 0.3%, levofloxacin 0.5%, or moxifloxacin 0.5%) may be helpful for persistent or recurrent staphylococcal blepharitis or for those patients who prefer a solution.
- Seborrheic blepharitis may respond to antifungal agents such as a short course of itraconazole (6)[C].

ADDITIONAL TREATMENT

General Measures

- Promote proper eyelid hygiene (4,7)[C]:
  - Apply warm compresses for several minutes once daily to soften adherent encrustations.
  - The eyelid margins then are scrubbed gently with eyelid cleanser or diluted baby shampoo twice a day to remove adherent material and clean the meibomian gland orifices (8)[C].
- Brief, gentle massage of the eyelids can help to express meibomian secretions in patients with meibomian gland dysfunction (4)[C].
- Discontinue soft contact lenses use during an acute case of blepharitis (9).

Issues for Referral

Chronic recurrent blepharitis requires referral to an ophthalmologist for evaluation as to whether patient should continue soft lens use.

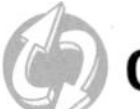

ONGOING CARE

FOLLOW-UP RECOMMENDATIONS

Patient Monitoring

- Patients should schedule a return visit if their condition worsens despite treatment.
- Return visit intervals for patients with severe disease vary.
- If corticosteroid is prescribed, re-evaluate within a few weeks to measure intraocular pressure and determine response to therapy.

PATIENT EDUCATION

- "Blepharitis Fact Sheet" from the American Academy of Ophthalmology
- Advise patient that blepharitis is a chronic condition, prone to recurrence if eyelid hygiene is not maintained after antibiotic treatment is discontinued (7).

PROGNOSIS

- Symptoms frequently can be improved, but rarely are eliminated.
- Long-term eyelid hygiene is required for control.

COMPLICATIONS

- Stye and chalazion
- Scarring of eyelid margin
- Corneal infection

REFERENCES

1. Bernardes TF, Bonfioli AA, et al. Blepharitis. *Semin Ophthalmol*. 2010;25:79–83.
2. Jackson WB, et al. Blepharitis: Current strategies for diagnosis and management. *Can J Ophthalmol*. 2008;43:170–9.
3. Tsai T, O'Brien JM. Masquerade syndromes: Malignancies mimicking inflammation in the eye. *Int Ophthalmol Clin*. 2002;41:115–31.
4. American Academy of Ophthalmology Cornea/External Disease Panel, Preferred Practice Patterns Committee. Preferred Practice Pattern: *Blepharitis*. San Francisco: AAO. 2003.
5. Abelson MB, et al. Blepharitis hiding in plain sight. *Rev Ophthalmol*. May 15, 2004.
6. Ninomiya J, Nakabayashi A, Higuchi R, et al. A case of seborrheic blepharitis: Treatment with itraconazole. *Nippon Ishinkin Gakkai Zasshi*. 2002;43:189–91.
7. Eyelid hygiene for blepharitis. *Insight*. 2011;36:24.
8. McCulley JP, Shine WE. Changing concepts in the diagnosis and management of blepharitis. *Cornea*. 2000;19:650–8.
9. Lemp MA, Bielory L. Contact lenses and associated anterior segment disorders: Dry eye disease, blepharitis, and allergy. *Immunol Allergy Clin North Am*. 2008;28:105–17, vi–vii.

ADDITIONAL READING

- Lemp MA. Contact lenses and associated anterior segment disorders: Dry eye, blepharitis, and allergy. *Ophthalmol Clin North Am*. 2003;16:463–9.
- McCulley JP, Shine WE. Eyelid disorders: The meibomian gland, blepharitis, and contact lenses. *Eye Contact Lens*. 2003;29:S93–5; discussion S115–8, S192–4.

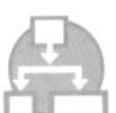

See Also (Topic, Algorithm, Electronic Media Element)

Conjunctivitis, Acute; Dry Eye Syndrome (Keratoconjunctivitis Sicca)

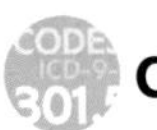

CODES

ICD9

- 373.00 Blepharitis, unspecified
- 373.01 Ulcerative blepharitis
- 373.02 Squamous blepharitis

CLINICAL PEARLS

- Blepharitis is often a chronic condition; symptoms frequently can be improved, but rarely are eliminated.
- Promote proper eyelid hygiene.
- Bacitracin ophthalmic ointment is the first-line treatment if *Staphylococcus* is suspected.

BODY DYSMORPHIC DISORDER

Katherine M. Callaghan, MD
Dawn S. Tasillo, MD

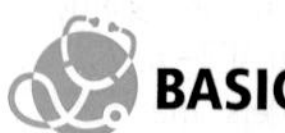

BASICS

DESCRIPTION

Body dysmorphic disorder (BDD) is a somatoform disorder in which patients have a pervasive subjective feeling of ugliness of an aspect of their appearance despite a normal or near-normal appearance.

- Diagnostic criteria according to the *DSM-IV*:
  - Preoccupation with an imagined defect in appearance. If there is a minor physical anomaly, the concern is excessive.
  - The preoccupation causes clinically significant distress or impairment in social, occupational, or other important areas of function.
  - The preoccupation is not accounted for by another mental disorder.

EPIDEMIOLOGY

- High comorbidity with depressive disorders
- Usually begins during adolescence, with an average age of onset between 15 and 30 years.
- Women are affected more often than men.
- Affected patients are likely to be unmarried.
- Different cultural beliefs may influence or amplify preoccupations:
  - Adolescents usually present similar to adults.
  - Can present in childhood, often with refusing to attend school or planning suicide
- Onset can be gradual or abrupt.
- Often a delay in diagnosis until 10–15 years after the onset

Prevalence

- ~1% in general population
- More common in women than men.
- More common in individuals with anxiety or depressive disorders
- 6–15% in cosmetic surgery patients and in dermatologic clinics (1)

RISK FACTORS

- Genetic predisposition
- Shyness, perfectionism, or anxious temperament
- Childhood adversity:
  - Teasing or bullying
  - Poor peer relationships
  - Social isolation
  - Lack of support of family
  - Sexual abuse
- History of dermatologic or other physical stigmata
- Being more aesthetically sensitive than average
- Low self-esteem

PATHOPHYSIOLOGY

- Not well understood
- A cognitive behavioral model has been described in which an external representation of the person's appearance (i.e., a photograph or mirror reflection) creates a distorted mental image. Through selective attention, awareness of the image and its specific features is increased. The affected individual becomes preoccupied by the distorted image; this is maintained by various safety and submissive behaviors meant to decrease scrutiny by others, but which may increase the individual's abnormal self-image and thus reinforces the behavior.
- MRI studies note left cerebral hemisphere hyperactivity, which may imply abnormal visual information processing, leading to selective recall of details and perception of distortions that do not exist (2).

ETIOLOGY

Not known, but likely multifactorial involving genetic, biological, and environmental factors

COMMONLY ASSOCIATED CONDITIONS

- Depression
- Social phobia
- Bipolar disorder
- Eating disorders
- Obsessive-compulsive disorder
- Suicide
- Delusional disorder

DIAGNOSIS

HISTORY

- Determine the patient's concern.
- Determine the severity of the disorder.
- Quantify the amount of time spent worrying about the "distorted" appearance.
- Determine what is done to hide or eliminate the problem.
- Determine the degree to which the defect affects school, job, or social life.
- Rule out other psychiatric disorders.
- Signs and symptoms may include:
  - Preoccupation that $\geq$1 features are unattractive, ugly, or deformed
  - Can involve any part of the body, but usually involves the skin, hair, or facial features:
    - Women are more likely to be preoccupied with their weight, hips, legs, and breasts.
    - Men are more likely to be preoccupied with their height, body hair, body build, and genitals.
- Nature of the preoccupation can change with time.
- Patient may have little insight.
- Patient tends to display delusions of reference.
- Large amounts of time are consumed by behaviors to examine the perceived defect repeatedly, disguise it, or improve it:
  - Mirror gazing
  - Excessive grooming
  - Camouflaging the "defect"
  - Skin picking
  - Reassurance seeking
  - Dieting
  - Pursuing dermatologic treatment or cosmetic surgery
- Tendency to avoid social interactions
- Trouble staying in school, maintaining a job, or maintaining significant relationships:
  - Tend to be unhappy with results of dermatologic and cosmetic procedures

PHYSICAL EXAM

- Important to do a mental status examination:
  - Look for:
    - Depression
    - Suicidal ideation
    - Anxiety
  - Rule out organic factors by reviewing:
    - Orientation
    - Memory
    - Ability to concentrate
- Rule out actual physical pathology.

DIAGNOSTIC TESTS & INTERPRETATION

- Several modules have been developed to assist with the diagnosis and severity rating of BDD (2).
- Administered by a trained clinician, these include:
  - The BDD Examination
  - Yale-Brown Obsessive Compulsive Scale modified for BDD

DIFFERENTIAL DIAGNOSIS

- Normal concerns about appearance
- Eating disorders: BDD differs from an eating disorder in that an eating disorder involves a preoccupation with overall body shape and weight, and with BDD, the preoccupation is with only a specific body part.
- Obsessive compulsive disorder (OCD): While BDD may be a version of OCD, the diagnosis differs in that in OCD, the obsessions and compulsions are not just restricted to appearance, as they are in BDD.
- Gender identity disorder
- Major depressive episode
- Narcissistic personality disorder
- Avoidant personality disorder
- Social phobia
- Schizophrenia
- Trichotillomania
- Hypochondriasis
- Delusional disorder, somatic type
- Koro: A culture-related syndrome seen in Southeast Asia that involves a preoccupation that the genitals (penis, labia, nipples, or breast) are shrinking and disappearing into the abdomen

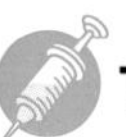

TREATMENT

- In any patient with a coexisting mental disorder, such as a depressive or anxiety disorder, the coexisting disorder should be treated with the appropriate psychotherapy or pharmacotherapy.
- Cognitive behavior therapy has been shown to be very effective (3,4)[A]:
  - Behavioral experiments
  - Graded exposure tasks
  - Imagery rescripting
  - Cognitive restructuring
  - Reverse role-playing
  - Relaxation
- Support groups
- Psychotherapy may be effective.
- Therapy with and for family members, spouses, or significant others

MEDICATION

First Line

- SSRIs are currently considered the medication of choice for BDD (5).
  - Not an approved use by the FDA
- Results from the small number of available randomized controlled trials suggest that SSRIs may be useful in treating patients with BDD (3)[A].
- Patients with and without a delusional disorder did equally well with SSRIs.
- Maximum tolerated dose should be taken for at least 12–16 weeks.
- Dosages may need to be higher than typically recommended for an eating disorder.

Second Line

Add a low-dose antipsychotic drug to an SSRI if there is failure to respond to ≥2 SSRIs.

ADDITIONAL TREATMENT

Issues for Referral

- Referral to a psychiatrist for diagnosis and therapy can be helpful and necessary for difficult cases.
- Regular counseling

SURGERY/OTHER PROCEDURES

- Studies investigating the rate of BDD among persons who seek appearance-enhancing treatments suggest that ~5–15% of individuals who seek these treatments suffer from BDD (6).
- Retrospective reports suggest that persons with BDD rarely experience improvement in their symptoms following these treatments, leading some to suggest that BDD is a contraindication to cosmetic surgery and other treatments (6).

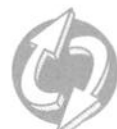

ONGOING CARE

FOLLOW-UP RECOMMENDATIONS

Patient Monitoring

Many patients have substantial improvement in core BDD symptoms, psychosocial functioning, quality of life, suicidality, and other aspects of BDD when treated with appropriate pharmacotherapy that targets BDD symptoms (5).

PATIENT EDUCATION

- Phillips KA. *The Broken Mirror: Understanding and Treating Body Dysmorphic Disorder*. Revised and expanded. New York: Oxford University Press, 2005.
- Butler Hospital Body Dysmorphic Disorder and Body Image Program at http://www.butler.org/body.cfm?id=123

PROGNOSIS

- Continuous course with periods of waxing and waning in the intensity of symptoms
- The longer the duration and the more severe the symptoms, the less the chance of partial or full remission.

COMPLICATIONS

- Repeated surgical or dermatologic procedures
- Inability or limited ability to function in society
- Poor social relations
- Poor self-esteem
- Suicide

REFERENCES

1. Sarwer DB, Crerand CE, Magee L, et al. Body dysmorphic disorder in patients who seek appearance-enhancing medical treatments. *Oral Maxillofac Surg Clin North Am*. 2010;22:445–53.
2. Feusner JD, Moody T, Hembacher E, et al. Abnormalities of visual processing and frontostriatal systems in body dysmorphic disorder. *Arch Gen Psychiatry*. 2010;67(2):197–205.
3. Ipser JC, Sander C, Stein DJ. Pharmacotherapy and psychotherapy for body dysmorphic disorder. *Cochrane Database Syst Rev*. 2009;CD005332.
4. Buhlmann U, Winter A. Perceived ugliness: An update on treatment-relevant aspects of body dysmorphic disorder. *Curr Psychiatry Rep*. 2011; 13(4):283–8.
5. Phillips KA, Hollander E. Treating body dysmorphic disorder with medication: Evidence, misconceptions, and a suggested approach. *Body Image*. 2008;5(1):13–27.
6. Shridharani SM, Magarakis M, Manson PN, et al. Psychology of plastic and reconstructive surgery: A systematic clinical review. *Plast Reconstr Surg*. 2010;126(6):2243–51.

ADDITIONAL READING

- *American Psychiatric Association: Diagnostic and Statistical Manual of Mental Disorders*, 4th Edition, *Text Revision*. Washington, DC: American Psychiatric Association; 2000:507–10.
- Philips KA, et al. Predictors of remission from body dysmorphic disorder: A prospective study. *J Ner Ment Dis*. 2005;193:564–7.
- Phillips KA. *The Broken Mirror: Understanding and Treating Body Dysmorphic Disorder. Revised and expanded*. New York: Oxford University Press; 2005.
- Phillips KA. The presentation of body dysmorphic disorder in medical settings. *Prim Psychiatry*. 2006;13:51–9.
- Phillips KA, Rogers J, et al. Cognitive-behavioral therapy for youth with body dysmorphic disorder: Current status and future directions. *Child Adolesc Psychiatr Clin N Am*. 2011;20:287–304.
- Sadock BJ, Sadock VA. *Kaplan & Sadock's Synopsis of Psychiatry*, 9th ed. Philadelphia: Lippincott Williams & Wilkins; 2003:653–5.
- Slaughter JR, Sun AM. In pursuit of perfection: A primary care physician's guide to body dysmorphic disorder. *Am Fam Physician*. 1999;60:1738–42.

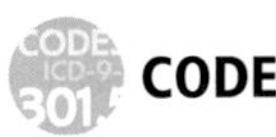

CODES

ICD9

300.7 Hypochondriasis

CLINICAL PEARLS

- BDD is characterized by the patient's preoccupation with a subjective feeling of ugliness, despite normal appearance, of one body part/area.
- An eating disorder involves a preoccupation with overall body shape and weight, while in BDD, the preoccupation is with only a specific body part (4).
- In obsessive-compulsive disorder, the obsessions and compulsions are not just restricted to appearance, as in BDD.
- BDD is a lifelong condition and treatment requires a combination of medication, therapy, and social support.
- If the patient insists there is a physical defect and wants it surgically corrected, but a physical defect isn't appreciated, refer to a psychiatrist for further evaluation before performing the procedure. Most patients with BDD are not content after the procedure, and their concerns persist.

BORDERLINE PERSONALITY DISORDER

Heath A. Grames, PhD
W. Jeff Hinton, PhD

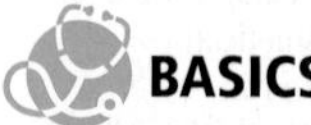

BASICS

DESCRIPTION

Beginning no later than adolescence or early adulthood, borderline personality disorder (BPD) is a consistent and pervasive pattern of an unstable affect and sense of self, impulsivity, and volatile interpersonal relationships (1):

- Common behaviors and variations:
  - Self-mutilation: Pinching, scratching, cutting
  - Suicide: Ideation, history of attempts, plans
  - Splitting: Idealizing then devaluing people and relationships
  - Presentation of helplessness or victimization
  - Emotional pain: May look for physical diagnoses
  - May be high utilizer of medical services
  - High rate of associated mental disorders (see "Associated Conditions")
- Patients with this disorder typically display little insight into their behavior.

Geriatric Considerations

Illness (both acute and chronic) may exacerbate BPD behaviors and may lead to intense feelings of fear and helplessness. Manifestations may decrease with age.

Pediatric Considerations

Diagnosis is rarely made in children. Must first rule out Axis I disorders and behavior related to a general medical condition or to the developmental cycle of the child.

Pregnancy Considerations

Physical and social changes may induce stress or increased fears, resulting in possible escalation of borderline behaviors.

EPIDEMIOLOGY

- Predominant age: Onset no later than adolescence or early adulthood (may go undiagnosed for years)
- Predominant sex: Female > Male

Prevalence

- General population: 2%
- Estimated lifetime prevalence: 10%–13%
- 20–30% of patients in primary care outpatient settings have a personality disorder.
- 20% of patients in psychiatry inpatient settings have BPD.

RISK FACTORS

- Biological relatives with the disorder
- Childhood sexual and/or physical abuse and neglect
- Disrupted family life
- Physical illness and external social factors may exacerbate borderline personality behaviors
- Poor family communication

Genetics

First-degree relatives are at greater risk for this disorder (undetermined if due to genetic or psychosocial factors).

GENERAL PREVENTION

- Tends to be a multigenerational problem
- Children, caregivers, and significant others should have some time and activities away from the borderline individual, which may protect them.

ETIOLOGY

Undetermined, but generally accepted that PDs are due to a combination of the following:

- Hereditary temperamental traits
- Environment (i.e., history of childhood sexual and/or physical abuse, history of childhood neglect, ongoing conflict in home)
- Developmental traits

COMMONLY ASSOCIATED CONDITIONS

Other psychiatric disorders, including:

- Co-occurring personality disorders, frequent
- Mood disorders, common
- Anxiety disorders, common
- Substance-related disorders, common
- Eating disorders, common
- Posttraumatic stress disorder, common

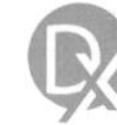

DIAGNOSIS

- The comprehensive evaluation should focus on (2):
  - Comorbid conditions
  - Functional impairments
  - Needs/goals
  - Adaptive/maladaptive coping styles
  - Psychosocial stressors
  - Patient strengths
- Initial assessment should focus on determining treatment setting (2):
  - Establish treatment agreement with patient and outline treatment goals.
  - Assess suicide ideation and self-harm behavior.
  - Assess for psychosis.
  - Hospitalization is necessary if patient presents a threat of harm to self or others.

HISTORY

- Clinic visits for problems that do not have biological findings
- Problems with medical staff members
- Idealizing or unexplained anger at physician
- History of unrealistic expectations of physician (e.g., "I know you can take care of me." "You're the best, unlike my last provider.")
- Obtain collateral information (i.e., from family, partner) about patient behaviors.

PHYSICAL EXAM

Possible scarring from self-mutilation (look on arms and legs where hidden by clothing, but can occur on other parts of the body)

DIAGNOSTIC TESTS & INTERPRETATION

- Consider age of onset. To meet criteria for BPD, borderline pattern will be present from adolescence or early adulthood.
- Formal psychological testing.
- Rule out personality change due to a general medical condition (GMC) (1):
  - Traits may emerge due to the effect of a GMC on the CNS.
- Rule out symptoms related to chronic substance use.
- If symptoms begin later than early adulthood or are related to trauma (e.g., after a head injury), a GMC, or substance use, then consider other diagnoses.
- The Structured Clinical Interview for DSM-IV Axis II disorders (SCID-II). The SCID-II may facilitate a more accurate diagnosis.

Diagnostic Procedures/Surgery

Patient must meet at least 5 of the following criteria (1):

- Attempt to avoid abandonment
- Volatile interpersonal relationships
- Identity disturbance
- Impulsive behavior:
  - In ≥2 areas
  - Impulsive behavior is self-damaging.
- Suicidal or self-mutilating behavior
- Mood instability
- Feeling empty
- Is unable to control anger, or finds it difficult
- Paranoid or dissociative when under stress

DIFFERENTIAL DIAGNOSIS

- Mood disorders:
  - Look at baseline behaviors when considering BPD vs. mood disorder.
  - BPD symptoms increase the likelihood of misdiagnosing bipolar disorder (3).
- Psychotic disorder:
  - With BPD, only occurs under intense stress and is not characteristic of disorder
- Other PD:
  - Consider patient's thoughts, feelings, and behavior to differentiate borderline from other PDs.
  - High co-occurrence of borderline and other PDs
- GMC:
  - Traits may emerge due to the effect of a GMC on the central nervous system.
- Chronic substance abuse

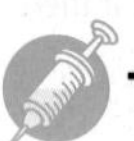

TREATMENT

- Outpatient psychotherapy for BPD is the preferred treatment
  - Referral for psychotherapy, including talk/behavioral therapy may amend some of the problems for patients with BPD (4)
- Patient may need to be placed on suicide watch.
- Inpatient hospitalization is ineffective in changing Axis II disorder behaviors.
- Inpatient hospital services for conditions related to Axis II disorder should be limited and of short duration to decrease dependence. Hospitalization should be considered for:
  - Adjusting medications
  - Implementing psychotherapy for crisis intervention
  - Stabilizing patient (psychosocial stressors)
- Extended inpatient hospitalization should be considered for the following reasons (2)[C]:
  - Persistent/severe suicidal ideation or risk to others
  - Nonadherence to outpatient or partial hospitalization treatments
  - Comorbid Axis I disorders that may increase threat to life for the patient (i.e., eating disorders, mood disorders)
  - Comorbid substance abuse or dependence that is unresponsive to outpatient or partial hospitalization treatments

MEDICATION

- While there are no specific medications approved by the US Food and Drug Administration (FDA) to treat BPD, American Psychiatric Association (APA) guidelines recommend pharmacotherapy to manage symptoms (2)[B].
- Treat individual symptoms (5)[C].
- Treat Axis I disorders (2)[B].
- Consider high rate of self-harm and suicidal behavior in patients with BPD when prescribing (6)[C].
  - Use of olanzapine with BPD patients may increase self-harming behavior (7)
- Depression/anxiety (8)[A]:
  - SSRIs
- Impulsive, aggressive, or history of bipolar disorder (5)[C]:
  - Mood stabilizer
- Psychosis, paranoid or hostile behavior, debilitating anxiety (5)[C]:
  - Atypical antipsychotic
- APA guideline recommendations (2)[B]:
  - Affective dysregulation: SSRI and monoamine oxidase inhibitors (MAOIs)
  - Impulsive-behavioral control: SSRIs and mood stabilizers
  - Cognitive-perceptual symptoms: Antipsychotics
- Cochrane review summary (7):
  - Second-generation antipsychotics, mood stabilizers, and omega-3 fatty acid dietary supplementation have shown beneficial effects.

ADDITIONAL TREATMENT

General Measures

- Focus on patient management rather than on "fixing" behaviors.
- Schedule consistent appointment follow-ups to relieve patient anxiety.
- Meet with and rely on treatment team to avoid splitting of team by patient, and to provide opportunity for team to discuss issues with patient.
- Psychotherapy (referral to mental health therapist) is considered treatment of choice (2,9,10)[A].

Issues for Referral

- If hospitalized, probably for suicide risk, mood or anxiety disorders, or substance-related disorders
- Urgency for scheduled follow-up depends on community resources (i.e., Do outpatient day programs for suicidal patients exist? What substance abuse programs are available?):
  - With increased risk for self-harm or self-defeating behaviors and low community resources, the patient can/will use increased need for frequent visits.
- Treatment of Axis II disorder should include psychotherapy and/or psychiatry (2)[B].

Additional Therapies

Consider referring patient for specialty mental health behavioral services, including (2,4):

- Dialectic behavioral therapy (DBT)
- Psychoanalytic-oriented day hospital therapy
- Transference-focused psychotherapy

IN-PATIENT CONSIDERATIONS

Hospitalization is necessary if patient presents a threat of harm to self or others.

Initial Stabilization

- Assess suicidal ideation.
- Consider inpatient treatment if crisis intervention is warranted.
- If psychotic, consider antipsychotic medications (5)

Admission Criteria

- Refer to inpatient or outpatient psychiatry services if harm to self or others is expressed.
- Call police or admit for inpatient services immediately if patient is psychotic and/or presents risk of harm to self or others

Nursing

Nurses can be helpful in managing patient and calling the patient as needed (contact with the patient helps relieve patient stress).

Discharge Criteria

- Patient should not present risk of harm to self or others.
- Patient should have safety plan.
- Routine follow-up should be scheduled with psychiatrist, mental health therapist, or primary care provider.

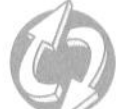

ONGOING CARE

FOLLOW-UP RECOMMENDATIONS

- Schedule routine follow-up with patient: Relieves patient anxiety about medical care relationship with physician
- Focus primarily on medical conditions and comorbid Axis I disorders.
- Exercise to decrease stress
- Find time to relax: Remove self from daily problems (teaches self-management)

Patient Monitoring

Monitor for suicidal or other self-harm behaviors.

PATIENT EDUCATION

As appropriate, provide patient education about the disorder, treatment, and self-care (2).

PROGNOSIS

- Borderline behaviors may decrease with age (1) and over time (10).
- Treatment is complex and takes time.
- Medical focus is on patient management and caring for medical and Axis I disorders.

REFERENCES

1. American Psychiatric Association. *Diagnostic and Statistical Manual of Mental Disorders-Text Revision*. 4th ed. Washington, DC: American Psychiatric Association; 2000.
2. American Psychiatric Association: *Practice Guideline for the Treatment of Patients with Borderline Personality Disorder*. Arlington, VA: American Psychiatric Association; 2001.
3. Ruggero CJ, Zimmerman M, Chelminski I, et al. Borderline personality disorder and the misdiagnosis of bipolar disorder. *J Psychiatr Res*. 2010;44:405–8.
4. Binks CA, Fenton M, McCarthy L et al. Psychological therapies for people with borderline personality disorder. *Cochrane Database Syst Rev*. 2006;1:CD005652.
5. Ward RK. Assessment and management of personality disorders. *Am Fam Phys*. 2004;70: 1505–12.
6. Makela EH, Moeller KE, Fullen JE, et al. Medication utilization patterns and methods of suicidality in borderline personality disorder. *Ann Pharmacother*. 2006;40:49–52.
7. Stoffers J, Völlm BA, Rücker G, et al. Pharmacological interventions for borderline personality disorder. *Cochrane Database Syst Rev*. 2010;CD005653.
8. Binks CA, Fenton M, McCarthy L, et al. Pharmacological interventions for people with borderline personality disorder. *Cochrane Database Syst Rev*. 2006;1:CD005653.
9. Kraus G, Reynolds DJ. The "A-B-C's" of the cluster B's: identifying, understanding, and treating cluster B personality disorders. *Clin Psychol Rev*. 2001;21:345–73.
10. Oldham JA. *Guideline Watch: Practice Guideline for the Treatment of Patients with Borderline Personality Disorder*. Arlington, VA: American Psychiatric Association; 2005.

ADDITIONAL READING

First MB, Gibbon M, Spitzer RL, et al. *Structured Clinical Interview for DSM-IV Axis II Personality Disorders, (SCID-II)*. Washington, DC: American Psychiatric Press, Inc.; 1997.

CODES

ICD9

301.83 Borderline personality disorder

CLINICAL PEARLS

- BPD should be viewed as a chronic condition.
- BPD patients are at increased risk for suicide attempts.
- If there are problems with the patient disrespecting the physician or support staff, clear guidelines should be established with the treatment team and then with the patient.
- If you are considering terminating your relationship with the patient, the patient may improve if he or she is warmly confronted about certain behaviors and is given clear guidelines on how to behave in the clinic. As it is the patient's job to follow the guidelines, it is you and your team's job to enforce the guidelines. Finally, designate a case management nurse or well-trained support staff person who can be the primary contact person for the patient.
- Have an agenda when you visit with BPD patients. Be cordial—they deserve the same professionalism any patient gets. Help your patient understand that she can have 1–2 issues discussed per clinic visit. Frequently scheduled visits can help with this.
- Patients will benefit from regularly scheduled psychotherapy treatment, in conjunction with or in addition to, regularly scheduled office visits. Psychotherapy can help maximize physician performance by becoming the "home" for mental health treatment, leaving the physician to focus on the patient's immediate physical/medical issues.

BOTULISM

Payal S. Patel, DO

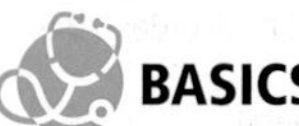

BASICS

DESCRIPTION

- Botulism is a muscle-paralyzing illness caused by a neurotoxin made by the bacterium *Clostridium botulinum*.
- Characterized by acute onset of bilateral cranial nerve involvement (diplopia, difficulty swallowing or speaking) associated with symmetric descending weakness, intact mental state, no fever, and no sensory dysfunction
- 7 types of *C. botulinum* (A–G) are distinguished by their antigenic characteristics. Types A, B, E, and, in rare cases, F, cause disease in humans.
- Forms include:
  - Foodborne: Caused by ingestion of preform toxin
  - Infant botulism: Caused by ingestion of *C. botulinum* that produce toxin in the GI tract
  - Wound: Caused by wound infection with *C. botulinum* that secretes the toxin
  - Aerosolized/inhalational botulinum: Bioterrorism attack potential because of high toxicity; $<1\ \mu g$ is lethal human dose
  - Injection related: Rare
  - Adult colonization botulism: Rare
- Diagnosis is made through history and clinical exam.
- Laboratory confirmation demonstrates presence of toxin in serum, stool, or wound or culturing *C. botulinum* from stool, wound, or food
- Treatment should not wait for laboratory confirmation.
- A purified and diluted form of type A neurotoxin is used to produce Botox injections.
- System(s) affected: Neuromuscular; Respiratory; GI
- Synonym(s): Sausage poisoning; Kerner disease

EPIDEMIOLOGY

Incidence

- Average of 110 cases of botulism reported annually in US
- ~20% of cases are foodborne; 30–40% wound-related; 65% infant botulism
- Wound botulism incidence increasing due to IV heroin use and cocaine abuse
- Hidden or intestinal: More common in disorders of the GI tract, such as prior surgery, Crohn disease, or recent antibiotic use
- Inhalation: Only a single incident involving 3 laboratory workers has been described.

Prevalence

- Predominant age:
  - Foodborne: Mean age is 46 years; range of 3–78 years
  - Infantile: Mean age of onset 13 weeks, with range of 1–63 weeks
  - Wound: Median age is 41 years with a range of 23–58 years
- Predominant gender:
  - Foodborne and infantile: Male = Female
  - Wound: Female > Male

RISK FACTORS

- Foodborne: Ingestion of home-canned or prepared contaminated foods
- Infantile: From ingestion of honey or corn syrup; breastfeeding (controversial)
- Wound: IV drug use (black tar heroin; IM/SC) or "skin popping"

GENERAL PREVENTION

- Foodborne: Proper handling, processing, preparation (heating), and storage of food; avoid eating food from bulging cans and food that smells/looks spoiled.
- Infant: Avoid honey before 1 year of age.
- Wound: Proper wound care
- Health care providers: Standard precautions
- If meningitis is suspected in patients with flaccid paralysis, medical personnel should use droplet precautions.
- Heat potentially contaminated food or drink to an internal temperature of 85°C for at least 5 minutes.
- After exposure to *C. botulinum* toxin, clothing and skin should be cleaned with soap and water.
- Contaminated objects or surfaces should be cleaned with 0.1% bleach solution. All food suspected of contamination should be promptly removed from potential consumers.

PATHOPHYSIOLOGY

- Disease results from hematogenous spread of toxin from mucosal surface (stomach, small intestine) or from an infected wound.
- The toxin prevents acetylcholine release at presynaptic membranes, blocking neuromuscular transmission in cholinergic nerve fibers.

ETIOLOGY

- Toxin produced by *C. botulinum*, an encapsulated, anaerobe, gram-positive, spore-forming, rod-shaped bacillus
- Ingestion of *C. botulinum* neurotoxins (A, B, and E most common)
- Foodborne, usually from home-canned vegetables, prepared foods, or foods incubated in anaerobic conditions
- Infantile from ingestion of spores in environment or occasionally in honey
- Wound due to contamination with toxin-producing *C. botulinum*
- Inadvertent: IM injections of botulinum toxin

DIAGNOSIS

HISTORY

- Foodborne:
  - Incubation: Typically 12–36 hours after toxin ingestion. Rare case as late as 10 days after ingestion.
  - Wound and infant botulism: Incubation time cannot be ascertained.
  - Inhalational: Same as foodborne botulism
- Adults: Acute onset of symmetric neuropathies. Difficulty in swallowing or speaking, dry mouth. Diplopia, blurred vision, dilated or nonrelated ptosis (drooping eyelids).
- Symmetric descending, flaccid paralysis in oriented, afebrile patient
- Respiratory dysfunction
- Infant botulism: Disease presentation and severity variable:
  - Constipation, shortly followed by weakness, feeding difficulties, descending or global hypotonia, drooling, anorexia, irritability, and weak cry
- Ask about diet, travel, drug use, and other persons with same symptoms.

PHYSICAL EXAM

- General appearance: Oriented, flaccid; may complain of malaise, dizziness, nausea, vomiting
- Vital signs, afebrile (fever may occur in wound botulism due to secondary infection), normal BP
- Head, eyes, ears, nose, throat: Dry mouth
- Chest/lungs: Respiratory muscle weakness, respiratory dysfunction, paralysis
- Heart: Normal or slow rate
- Abdomen: Distention, constipation (early sign in infant form); may be absent in wound form
- Genitourinary: Urinary retention
- Neurologic:
  - Symmetric descending weakness beginning with the cranial nerves
  - Ptosis; extraocular muscle paresis; fixed, dilated pupils; dysphagia
  - Infant botulism: Poor muscle tone (loss of head control and facial expression), poor feeding (loss of suck), drooling, feeding difficulties, weak cry
  - Diminished or absent deep tendon reflexes

DIAGNOSTIC TESTS & INTERPRETATION

Lab

Initial lab tests

- Laboratory confirmation is done by demonstrating the presence of toxin in serum or stool, or by culturing *C. botulinum* from stool, wounds, or food.
- Mouse neutralization assay confirmation:
  - Standard method of diagnosis (1)[B]
  - Available from Centers for Disease Control and some state laboratories; takes ~4 days for results
- Routine tests (CBC, electrolytes, liver function tests, urinalysis) generally not helpful/show no characteristic abnormalities
- CSF testing: Normal helps differentiate from Guillain-Barré syndrome. Occasionally a borderline elevation in protein is seen.
- Toxin detected in gastric contents, serum, stool, and suspected food and containers:
  - Polymerase chain reaction (PCR) tests are also available for rapid detection of clostridia in food samples (2)[B].
- A normal Tensilon test helps to differentiate botulism from myasthenia gravis; borderline can occur in botulism

Imaging

CT or MRI to rule out neurologic pathology

Diagnostic Procedures/Surgery

Electrophysiology testing:

- Presumptive evidence in patients with negative bioassay studies (3)[C]
- Brief, small-amplitude motor potential with incremental response on repetitive nerve stimulation

DIFFERENTIAL DIAGNOSIS

- Adult botulisms:
  - Guillain-Barré syndrome
  - Encephalitis, meningitis
  - Tick paralysis
  - Myasthenia gravis
  - Eaton Lambert myasthenic syndrome
  - Cerebrovascular accident: Basilar artery stroke
  - Congenital neuropathy or myopathy

B

- Sepsis
- Hypokalemic periodic paralysis
- Poliomyelitis
- Other poisonings (organophosphate, shellfish, *Amanita* mushrooms, atropine, and aminoglycosides)
- Miller-Fisher variant of Guillain-Barré syndrome
- Diphtheritic neuropathy
- Carbon monoxide intoxication
- Hypermagnesemia
- Infant botulism:
  - Sepsis
  - Meningitis
  - Electrolyte–mineral imbalance
  - Reye syndrome
  - Congenital myopathy
  - Leigh disease
  - Werdnig-Hoffman disease

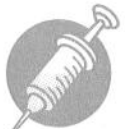

TREATMENT

MEDICATION

First Line

- Antitoxin therapy with trivalent A-B-E antitoxin:
  - Call Centers for Disease Control (CDC) Assistance: (770) 488-7100
  - Initiating botulinum antitoxin therapy is primarily based on symptoms and physical examination findings that are consistent with botulism (4)[B].
  - Early administration is important (4)[B].
  - Horse serum derived: Up to 20% reaction incidence. Consider skin testing or pretreatment with steroids or antihistamines.
- Infantile:
  - Treatment with human botulism immunoglobulin (BIG-IV or Baby BIG) for botulism types A and B (5)[A]
  - Available only through the California State Health Department: (510) 540-2646 or (510) 231-7600
- Wound:
  - Antitoxin therapy with trivalent A-B-E antitoxin, 1 vial IV and 1 vial IM, repeat in 2–4 hours if persistent symptoms
  - Antibiotics unproven by clinical trial, but widely used and recommended:
    - Penicillin G (3 million units IV q4h in adults)
    - Metronidazole (500 mg IV q8h) for penicillin-allergic patients
  - Vaccine: Pentavalent vaccine available:
    - Efficiency in terrorist attack is unknown
    - Newer vaccines being developed

Second Line

Supportive care, including mechanical ventilation (6)[C]

Pregnancy Considerations

Safety of botulism antitoxin during pregnancy and breastfeeding unknown or controversial (6)

ADDITIONAL TREATMENT

Issues for Referral

- Nutrition: For hyperalimentation, and later, tube feeding
- Physical/occupational therapy: Including swallow evaluation

Additional Therapies

- Stress ulcer and deep vein thrombosis prophylaxis
- Pulmonary and physical rehabilitation

SURGERY/OTHER PROCEDURES

Wound excision/debridement

IN-PATIENT CONSIDERATIONS

Initial Stabilization

Hospital admission with meticulous airway management

Admission Criteria

All suspected cases must be admitted.

IV Fluids

Keep patient well hydrated.

Nursing

- Prevent decubitus ulcer, IV line infections, other nosocomial infections
- Before administration of antitoxin, skin testing should be performed for sensitivity.

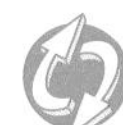

ONGOING CARE

FOLLOW-UP RECOMMENDATIONS

Outpatient follow-up with physical/occupational therapy, nutrition specialist, and psychiatry as needed

Patient Monitoring

- Pulmonary function testing
- Cardiorespiratory monitoring

DIET

Nasogastric feedings, if needed

PATIENT EDUCATION

- Spores destroyed by pressure cooking at 250°F (120°C) for 30 minutes
- Toxin destroyed by boiling for 10 minutes or cooking at 175°F (80°C) for 30 minutes
- Avoid honey in first year of life.
- Avoid IV drug use.
- Do not eat/sample foods that look and smell rotten or come from bulging cans.

PROGNOSIS

- Delay in administering antitoxin: Most important factor affecting clinical course and outcome (4)[B]
- Mortality: Overall 7–10%; <5% if infection is treated, but approaches 60% if untreated (6)
- Mortality for patients >60 years is twice that of younger patients
- Full recovery may take months.
- Significant health, functional, and social limitations several years after infection (7)[C]:
  - Recovery follows the regeneration of new neuromuscular connections.
  - 2–8 weeks of ventilator support may be required in more severe cases.
- Dyspnea with severe ptosis and pupil abnormality has been shown to correlate with severe illness and respiratory failure (8)[C].
- Increased incubation time has been shown to correlate with better outcomes (8)[C].

COMPLICATIONS

- Nosocomial infections, including aspiration pneumonia and ventilator-associated pneumonia
- Hypoxic tissue damage
- Death

REFERENCES

1. Lindström M, Korkeala H. Laboratory diagnostics of botulism. *Clin Microbiol Rev.* 2006;19:298–314.
2. Fach P, Micheau P, Mazuet C, et al. Development of real-time PCR tests for detecting botulinum neurotoxins A, B, E, F producing *Clostridium botulinum, Clostridium baratii* and *Clostridium butyricum. J Appl Microbiol.* 2009;107:465–73.
3. Bayrak A, et al. Electrophysiologic findings in a case of severe botulism. *J Neurol Sci.* 2006;23:49–53.
4. Dembek ZF, Smith LA, Rusnak JM. Botulism: Cause, effects, diagnosis, clinical and laboratory identification, and treatment modalities. *Disaster Med Public Health Prep.* 2007;1:122–34.
5. Chalk C, Benstead TJ, Keezer M. Medical treatment for botulism. *Cochrane Database Syst Rev.* 2011;3: CD008123.
6. O'Brien KK, Higdon ML, Halverson JJ. Recognition and management of bioterrorism infections. *Am Fam Physician.* 2003;67:1927–34.
7. Gottlieb SL, Kretsinger K, Tarkhashvili N, et al. Long-term outcomes of 217 botulism cases in the Republic of Georgia. *Clin Infect Dis.* 2007;45: 174–80.
8. Witoonpanich R, Vichayanrat E, Tantisiriwit K, et al. Survival analysis for respiratory failure in patients with food-borne botulism. *Clin Toxicol (Phila).* 2010;48:177–83.
9. Botulism Facts for Healthcare Providers. Accessed 5/30/2010 at http://emergency.cdc.gov/agent/botulism/hcpfacts.asp.

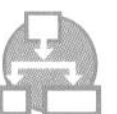

See Also (Topic, Algorithm, Electronic Media Element)

Food Poisoning, Bacterial

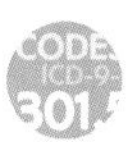

CODES

ICD9

- 005.1 Botulism food poisoning
- 040.41 Infant botulism
- 040.42 Wound botulism

CLINICAL PEARLS

- Botulinum antitoxin should be administered as soon as possible; don't wait for lab results.
- Medical care providers who suspect botulism in a patient should immediately call their state health department's emergency 24-hour telephone number.
- A helpful mnemonic to recall progression of symptoms is the "dozen D's": Dry mouth, diplopia, dilated pupils, droopy eyes, droopy face, diminished gag reflex, dysphagia, dysarthria, dysphonia, difficulty lifting head, descending paralysis, and diaphragmatic paralysis (9)

BRAIN ABSCESS

Nathan Weldon, MD

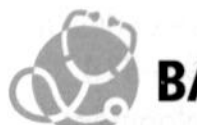

BASICS

DESCRIPTION

- Single or multiple abscesses within the brain, usually occurring secondary to a focus of infection outside the CNS
- May mimic brain tumor but generally evolves more rapidly (over days to weeks)
- Starts as a cerebritis, becomes necrotic, and subsequently becomes encapsulated
- Synonym(s): Cerebral abscess

Geriatric Considerations

Age does not affect outcome as much as the abscess size and state of neurologic dysfunction at presentation.

Pediatric Considerations

- About 1/3 of total cases occur in the pediatric age group
- Rarely found in infants <1 year of age
- Cyanotic congenital heart disease frequently associated

EPIDEMIOLOGY

- Predominant age: Median age 30–40 years, although brain abscess occurs at all ages
- Predominant sex: Male > Female (2:1)

Incidence

Infrequent, but increasing due to increase in immune-suppressed individuals, opportunistic pathogens, and resistance to antibiotics (1)

RISK FACTORS

- HIV/AIDS
- Immunocompromised state
- IV drug abuse

Genetics

No known genetic pattern

GENERAL PREVENTION

- Adequate treatment of otitis media, mastoiditis, sinusitis, dental abscess, other ear/nose/throat (ENT) infections
- Prophylactic antibiotics after compound skull fracture or penetrating head wound

ETIOLOGY

- Hematogenous source is most common overall for single or multiple cerebral abscesses.
- Direct extension from otitis, mastoiditis, sinusitis, or dental infection
- Cranial osteomyelitis
- Penetrating skull trauma
- Prior craniotomy
- Bacteremia from lung abscess, pneumonia
- Bacterial endocarditis
- Fungal infection of the nasopharynx
- *Toxoplasma gondii* (in AIDS patients)
- Cyanotic congenital heart disease
- IV drug use
- No source found in 20%.
- Most common infective organisms: Streptococci, staphylococci (especially after neurosurgery), enteric gram-negative bacilli and anaerobes (usually same as source of infection), *Nocardia*
- Amebic brain abscess, amebiasis, amebic dysentery
- The frontal lobe of the brain is the most common site for an abscess.

COMMONLY ASSOCIATED CONDITIONS

- AIDS
- Congenital heart disease

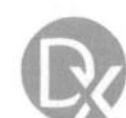

DIAGNOSIS

HISTORY

- Recent onset of headache becoming severe
- New focal neurological deficit
- Altered mental status progressing to stupor and coma
- Nausea and vomiting
- Seizures

PHYSICAL EXAM

- Afebrile or low-grade fever
- Papilledema
- Neck stiffness
- Focal neurologic signs depending on location

DIAGNOSTIC TESTS & INTERPRETATION

Abscess culture: Predominant organisms include *Toxoplasma* (AIDS), *Staphylococcus* (trauma), aerobic or anaerobic bacteria, fungi (rare).

ALERT

- Lumbar puncture often contraindicated
- Prior administration of antibiotics may alter lab results.

Lab

Initial lab tests

- White blood cell (WBC) count may be normal or mildly elevated.
- Blood studies: Mild PMN leukocytosis; elevated ESR
- Culture and susceptibilities of the abscess material
- If available, consider broad-range bacterial rDNA polymerase chain reaction with DNA sequencing (2)

Imaging

- Search for primary source of infection, depending on suspected source.
- Solitary intracerebral abscess suggests a direct contiguous source such as sinus or ear infection.
- Multiple cerebral abscesses suggest hematological spread.
- Head CT and MRI are the diagnostic methods of choice. Specific findings are dependent on stages of the abscess (3)[B].
- CT provides sufficient diagnostic information in most cases (4)[B], including skull fracture, sinus infection, or otic source.
- Consider cardiac echo, chest x-ray, and chest CT if cardiac or pulmonary source suspected.
- Radionuclide ^{117}In-labeled leukocytes may distinguish abscess from neoplasm.

Diagnostic Procedures/Surgery

- Lumbar puncture often contraindicated
- Surgical burr hole with aspiration to make a specific bacteriologic diagnosis

Pathological Findings

- Suppuration, liquefaction, or encapsulation, depending on stage of evolution
- Fibrosis

DIFFERENTIAL DIAGNOSIS

- Brain tumors
- Cysticercosis
- Stroke
- Resolving intracranial hemorrhage
- Subdural empyema
- Extradural abscess
- Encephalitis

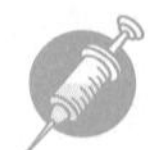

TREATMENT

Immediate neurosurgical consult is indicated for suspected CNS abscess.

MEDICATION

- Antibiotics according to organism and sensitivities, if known
- Initial empiric treatment according to suspected source
- Hematogenous sources should cover MRSA initially, and should include vancomycin, and may be broadened to include metronidazole and a third-generation cephalosporin.
- For dental source, penicillin G and metronidazole are reasonable initial choices.
- For otogenic or sinus source, coverage should include metronidazole and either ceftriaxone or cefotaxime.
- For GI or genitourinary source, consider a third-generation cephalosporin such as cefotaxime to cover gram negatives.
- For traumatic source, consider vancomycin plus either ceftriaxone or cefotaxime.
- Hospital-acquired sources, including postsurgical abscess, consider vancomycin and cefepime or ceftazidime
- If MSSA is isolated, change vancomycin to oxacillin or nafcillin.
- Use vancomycin in penicillin-sensitive patients.
- Generally a 6–8-week course of parenteral antibiotics is required.
- If brain abscess is associated with HIV/AIDS:
  - Daily doses of sulfadiazine and pyrimethamine
  - Lifelong therapy in AIDS patients
- Anticonvulsants:
  - Phenytoin until abscess resolves or perhaps longer
  - Monitor anticonvulsant levels.
- Following a neurosurgical procedure, use corticosteroids such as dexamethasone to reduce edema. Taper rapidly. Use is usually limited to 1 week.
- Contraindications: Sensitivity or allergy to any prescribed medications
- Precautions:
  - Sulfadiazine is poorly water-soluble. Patients must maintain adequate hydration or risk developing crystalluria.
  - Decrease dosage of penicillin in patients with renal dysfunction.
  - Monitor serum levels of anticonvulsants.
  - A dose of pyrimethamine is required for the treatment of toxoplasmosis, which may approach toxic levels. The patient should be observed for folic acid deficiency and treated with folinic acid (leucovorin) 5–15 mg (PO, IM, IV) if necessary.

ADDITIONAL TREATMENT

General Measures

- Palliative and supportive
- Treatment of brain abscess requires a combination of antimicrobial agents, surgical intervention, and eradication of the primary foci of infection (5)[A].
- Initial medical therapy includes broad-spectrum antibiotics pending determination of the causative organism.
- Determination of point of entry and source of infection is critical to effective treatment (6).
- Medical therapy only may be indicated:
  - For surgically inaccessible lesions or multiple abscesses
  - For abscesses in early cerebritis stage
  - For small (<2.5 cm) abscesses
- Antibiotic therapy may be directed toward most likely organism if no specific organism is identified.
- Monitor clinical response to antibiotic therapy.

Issues for Referral

Neurosurgical referral for all patients. Consider infectious disease and neurology consultations if available.

SURGERY/OTHER PROCEDURES

- Mandatory when neurologic deficits are severe or progressive
- Often used when the abscess is in the posterior fossa or is the result of trauma
- Type of surgical treatment used depends on the patient's clinical status, the neuroradiographic characteristics of the abscess, and the experience of the surgeon(s) carrying out the procedure (5).
- Abscess drainage via a needle under stereotactic CT guidance through a burr hole under local anesthesia is the most rapid and effective surgical method of treatment and may be repeated if needed.
- Craniotomy: If abscess is large or multilocular
- In general, similar outcomes for stereotactic-guided drainage or craniotomy (7)

IN-PATIENT CONSIDERATIONS

Initial Stabilization

Inpatient care for close observation, diagnostic evaluation, and specialty consultation (neurology, neurosurgery, or infectious disease)

Admission Criteria

Upon diagnosis for close monitoring, IV antibiotics, and possible surgery. A brain abscess often requires admission to an intensive care unit, or may be a complication of intensive care unit patients with neurologic injury, contributing significantly to morbidity and mortality (8)[B].

IV Fluids

IV fluids if nausea and vomiting present

Discharge Criteria

When patient is asymptomatic, afebrile, and responding to therapy as determined by serial imaging studies

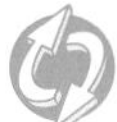

ONGOING CARE

FOLLOW-UP RECOMMENDATIONS

- Bed rest until infection controlled and abscess evacuated or resolving, then as tolerated
- May need long-term rehabilitative care

Patient Monitoring

- Postsurgical monitoring as needed
- Serial CT or MRI for at least 3 months to evaluate the therapeutic response, confirm progressive resolution, detect new lesions, and manage complications.

DIET

IV fluids if significant nausea and vomiting

PATIENT EDUCATION

- Brain Research Foundation, 208 S. LaSalle Street, Suite 1426, Chicago, IL 60604; (312) 782-4311.
- Pri-Med Patient Education Center: Brain Abscess at http://www.patienteducationcenter.org/aspx/HealthELibrary/HealthETopic.aspx?cid=210320

PROGNOSIS

- The route of spread, the type and virulence of the organism, thickness of the capsule, location and number of abscesses in the brain, and immune status of the host are important determinants of outcome (1).
- Survival: >80% with early diagnosis and treatment
- In 1 retrospective analysis, 80% of patients recovered fully or had minimal incapacity and 10% died (4)[B].
- Patients with underlying cranial neoplasms or medical conditions have worse outcomes than those with a contiguous focus of infection or posttraumatic abscess (4)[B].

COMPLICATIONS

- Permanent neurologic deficits
- Surgical complications
- ICU-related complications
- Recurrent abscess
- Seizures
- Death

REFERENCES

1. Sundaram C, Lakshmi V. Pathogenesis and pathology of brain abscess. *Indian J Pathol Microbiol*. 2006;49:317–26.
2. Al Masalma M, Armougom F, Scheld WM, et al. The expansion of the microbiological spectrum of brain abscesses with the use of multiple 16S ribosomal DNA sequencing. *Clin Infect Dis*. 2009; 48(9):1169–78.
3. Foerster BR, Thurnher MM, Malani PN. Intracranial infections: clinical and imaging characteristics. *Acta Radiol*. 2007;48:875–93.
4. Carpenter J, Stapleton S, Holliman R. Retrospective analysis of 49 cases of brain abscess and review of the literature. *Eur J Clin Microbiol Infect Dis*. 2007;26:1–11.
5. Lu CH. Strategies for the management of bacterial brain abscess. *J Clin Neurosci*. 2006;13(10): 979–85. Epub 2006 Oct 23.
6. Bernardini GL. Diagnosis and management of brain abscess and subdural empyema. *Curr Neurol Neurosci Rep*. 2004;4:448–56.
7. Smith SJ, Ughratdar I, MacArthur DC. Never go to sleep on undrained pus: A retrospective review of surgery for intraparenchymal cerebral abscess. *Br J Neurosurg*. 2009;23:412–7.
8. Ziai WC, Lewin JJ. Update in the diagnosis and management of central nervous system infections. *Neurol Clin*. 2008;26:427–68, viii.

ADDITIONAL READING

- Alangaden G, Chandrasekar PH. Case 10-2010: A woman with weakness and a mass in the brain. *N Engl J Med*. 2010;363:395; author reply 395–6.
- Chang YT, Lu CH, Chuang MJ, et al. Supratentorial deep-seated bacterial brain abscess in adults: Clinical characteristics and therapeutic outcomes. *Acta Neurol Taiwan*. 2010;19:174–9.
- Mace SE. Central nervous system infections as a cause of an altered mental status? What is the pathogen growing in your central nervous system? *Emerg Med Clin North Am*. 2010;28:535–70.
- Patron V, Orsel S, Caire F, et al. Transethmoidal drainage of frontal brain abscesses. *Surg Innov*. 2010;17(4):300–5.
- Shachor-Meyouhas Y, Bar-Joseph G, Guilburd JN, et al. Brain abscess in children—epidemiology, predisposing factors and management in the modern medicine era. *Acta Paediatr*. 2010;99: 1163–7.

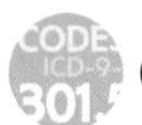

CODES

ICD9

324.0 Intracranial abscess

CLINICAL PEARLS

- Headache and altered mental status are common presenting symptoms of a brain abscess.
- Determination of point of entry and source of infection is essential for adequate treatment.
- Treatment of a brain abscess may require a combination of antimicrobial agents for 6–8 weeks, surgical intervention, and eradication of the primary focus of infection.
- Serial head CTs for at least 3 months can help to evaluate a patient's response to therapies.

BRAIN INJURY, TRAUMATIC

Dana M. Collaguazo, MD

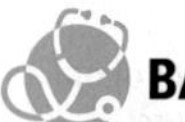

BASICS

DESCRIPTION

- A dynamic process with penetrating or blunt injury to the brain with initial bleeding followed by secondary injury due to cerebral edema and/or continued bleeding
- Frequently related to rapid deceleration, as in motor vehicle or diving accidents, or blunt trauma
- System(s) affected: Cardiovascular, Endocrine/Metabolic, Nervous
- Synonym(s): Head injury

EPIDEMIOLOGY

Incidence

- 1.7 million per year
- 1,365,000 hospital emergency-room visits per year
- 275,000 hospitalizations per year
- 52,000 deaths per year

Prevalence

- Predominant age: 0–4, 15–19, and over 65 years
- Predominant gender: Male > Female

RISK FACTORS

Alcohol, prior head injury, contact sports; "heading" soccer balls may cause long-term cognitive loss.

Geriatric Considerations

Subdural hematomas are common after fall or blow in elderly; symptoms may be subtle.

GENERAL PREVENTION

- Safety education
- Seat belts, bicycle, and motorcycle helmets
- Protective headgear for contact sports

PATHOPHYSIOLOGY

Initial brain dysfunction from direct trauma (bleeding, laceration) followed by secondary injury due to cerebral edema, continued bleeding, decreased blood flow

ETIOLOGY

- Motor vehicle accidents (17%)
- Falls (35%)
- Assault

Pediatric Considerations

Child abuse: Consider if dropped or fell <4 feet (e.g., off bed, couch) and significant injury present or any retinal hemorrhages

COMMONLY ASSOCIATED CONDITIONS

Alcohol and drug abuse

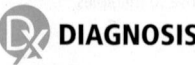

DIAGNOSIS

HISTORY

- Loss of consciousness (LOC)
- Headache
- Vomiting
- Amnesia
- Epidural hemorrhage from blunt trauma is generally acute, 30% with a "lucid interval" (initial LOC followed by recovery of consciousness, then LOC recurs and persists)

Geriatric Considerations

Subdural hemorrhage usually has a slower onset and may present weeks after the initial injury, especially in the elderly.

PHYSICAL EXAM

- Focal neurologic signs and symptoms
- Evidence of increased intracranial pressure (ICP) (elevated BP, decreased pulse rate, or slow or irregular breathing [Cushing triad]—only 30% have all 3)
- Decorticate or decerebrate posturing (bad prognostic signs)
- Seizures
- Signs of basilar skull fracture: Raccoon eyes, battle sign, hemotympanum, CSF rhinorrhea or otorrhea (see "Diagnostic Procedures")
- Unilateral dilated pupil in an alert patient is not consistent with impending herniation, as these patients are always unconscious.

DIAGNOSTIC TESTS & INTERPRETATION

Lab

Initial lab tests

- Evaluate for coagulopathy.
- Type and screen for possible surgical intervention.
- Perform drug and alcohol screening.

Imaging

Initial approach

CT, noncontrast, is study of choice to review bone windows, tissue windows, and subdural space:

- NEXUS II study (1)[B] demonstrated that if all 8 clinical criteria are absent, there is a low likelihood of significant TBI:
  - Evidence of significant skull fracture (depressed, basilar, or diastatic)
  - Altered level of alertness
  - Neurologic deficit
  - Persistent vomiting
  - Presence of scalp hematoma
  - Abnormal behavior
  - Coagulopathy
  - Age >65

Follow-Up & Special Considerations

Pediatric Considerations

Skull radiographs are not helpful in most cases but can be done to document child abuse.

Diagnostic Procedures/Surgery

- CSF rhinorrhea:
  - Contains glucose; nasal mucus does not
  - Check for the double-halo sign: If nasal discharge contains CSF and blood, 2 rings appear when placed on filter paper—a central ring followed by a paler ring.
- Placement of ICP monitor when indicated
- Serial neurologic exams
- Neuropsychometric testing when able

Pathological Findings

- Epidural, subdural, or intraparenchymal hemorrhage
- Coup or contrecoup injury
- Evolving, diffuse axonal injury is a principal cause of neurologic sequelae with mild head trauma.

DIFFERENTIAL DIAGNOSIS

Other causes of altered mental status (e.g., toxicologic, infectious, metabolic, vascular causes)

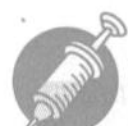

TREATMENT

MEDICATION

First Line

- Pain: Morphine 1–2 mg IV PRN with caution as can depress mental status further and alter serial neurologic evaluations.
- Increased ICP:
  - Mannitol: 0.25–2 g/kg (0.25–1 g/kg in children) given over 30–60 minutes in patients with adequate renal function; should not be used unless there is evidence of increased ICP; prophylactic use is associated with worse outcomes.
  - Lasix: 20–40 mg IV to promote diuresis:
    - Neither furosemide nor mannitol should be given to a hypotensive patient.
  - Hypertonic saline: 2 mL/kg IV decreases ICP without adverse hemodynamic status and may have beneficial effects on immune system and excitatory neurotransmitters (2)[B].
- Sedation:
  - Propofol: Preferred due to short duration of action, which allows serial neurologic exams
- Seizures:
  - Phenytoin (Dilantin): 15 mg/kg IV (1 mg/kg/min IV, not to exceed 50 mg/min). Stop infusion if QT interval increases by >50%.
  - Lorazepam (Ativan): 1–2 mg (0.1 mg/kg in children) IV
  - Fosphenytoin (Cerebyx): 15 mg/kg IV, not to exceed 150 mg/min. May give IM.
  - Levetiracetam (Keppra): May be desirable; lower complication rates, but prospective studies are needed. Use at neurosurgeon's instruction.
- Contraindications: Allergy

Second Line

- Diuretics and IV β-blockers (e.g., esmolol or labetalol) can be used to maintain a Central Cerebral Pressure (CCP = MAP − ICP) between 50–70 mm Hg.
- Nitrates may be helpful; however, may increase ICP
- Antibiotics (e.g., cefazolin): Given if penetrating trauma is present; prophylactic antibiotics are not useful in basilar skull fractures.

ADDITIONAL TREATMENT

General Measures

- Acute management depends on severity of injury. Most patients need no interventions.
- Immediate goal: Determine who needs further therapy, imaging studies (CT), and hospitalization to prevent further injury.
- For the severely injured patient:
  - Avoid hypotension or hypoxia. Head injury causes increased ICP secondary to edema, and perfusion pressure must be maintained.
  - 30° head elevation decreases ICP and improves cerebral perfusion pressure (3)[B]
  - Hyperventilation (hypocapnia) use should be limited to patients with impending herniation while preparing for definitive treatment or intraoperatively. It should never be used prophylactically or accidentally as it can cause and/or worsen cerebral ischemia and injure other organs (4)[B].

- Mild Hypothermia (32°–34°C) in severe TBI (GCS ≤8) decreases mortality and improves functional outcome (5)[B].
- Seizure prophylaxis does not change outcomes (such as death rates) but may prevent seizures. Consider phenytoin or levetiracetam for 1 week postinjury.

- Manage breakthrough seizures with lorazepam.
- Brain tissue oxygen monitors measure brain tissue hypoxia associated with mortality and poor outcome. Combined use with ICP monitoring is associated with better outcome than ICP monitors alone (6)[B].

Issues for Referral

Consult neurosurgery for:

- All penetrating head trauma
- All abnormal head CTs

SURGERY/OTHER PROCEDURES

Depends on neurosurgical consult

IN-PATIENT CONSIDERATIONS

Initial Stabilization

- ABCs take priority over head injury.
- C-spine immobilization should be considered in all head trauma.

Admission Criteria

- Abnormal CT
- Abnormal Glasgow Coma Scale
- Clinical evidence of basilar skull fracture
- Persistent neurologic deficits (e.g., confusion, somnolence)
- Patient with no competent adult at home for observation
- Possibly admit: LOC, amnesia, etc.

IV Fluids

Use normal saline for resuscitation fluid.

Discharge Criteria

Normal CT with return-to-normal mental status and responsible adult to observe patient at home (see "Patient Monitoring")

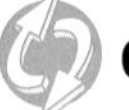

ONGOING CARE

FOLLOW-UP RECOMMENDATIONS

- Schedule regular follow-up within a week to determine return to activities.
- Rehabilitation indicated following a significant acute injury. Set realistic goals.

Patient Monitoring

Any patient discharged should have head-injury instructions to use to watch for symptoms indicating need for further intervention (e.g., changing mental status, worsening headache, focal findings). Give to a competent adult who will observe the patient. A patient who deteriorates is not likely to remember or act on any instructions.

DIET

As tolerated

PATIENT EDUCATION

Proper counseling, symptomatic management, and gradual return to normal activities are essential to prevent a posttraumatic neurosis that can become refractory to treatment.

PROGNOSIS

- Gradual improvement for many
- 30–50% of severe head injuries may be fatal.
- Prolonged coma may be followed by satisfactory outcome.
- Predicting outcome is difficult, and patients may improve for years.

Geriatric Considerations

Poorer prognosis with increasing age. Patients 75 and older have the highest rate of TBI hospitalizations and death.

Pediatric Considerations

Outcome is more positive in pediatric patients, except in severe TBI.

COMPLICATIONS

- Delayed hematomas
- Chronic subdural hematoma, which may follow even "mild" head injury, especially in the elderly. Often presents with headache and decreased mentation.
- Delayed hydrocephalus
- Emotional disturbances and psychiatric disorders resulting from head injury may be refractory to treatment.
- Seizure disorders: In 50% of penetrating head injuries, in 20% of severe closed head injuries, and in <5% of head injuries overall. Hematomas significantly increase risk of epilepsy.
- The postconcussion syndrome can follow mild head injury without LOC and includes headaches, dizziness, fatigue, and subtle cognitive or affective changes.
- Second-impact syndrome occurs when the CNS loses autoregulation. An individual with a minor head injury is returned to a contact sport and, following even minor trauma (e.g., whiplash), the patient loses consciousness and may quickly herniate, with a 50% mortality. A similar syndrome of malignant edema can occur in children with even a single injury.
- Increased risk for Alzheimer's disease, Parkinson's disease, and other brain disorders whose prevalence increases with age

REFERENCES

1. Mower WR, Hoffman JR, Herbert M, et al. Developing a decision instrument to guide computed tomographic imaging of blunt head injury patients. *J Trauma*. 2005;59:954–9.
2. Meyer MJ, Megyesi J, Meythaler J, et al. Acute management of acquired brain injury part II: An evidence-based review of pharmacological interventions. *Brain Inj*. 2010;24:706–21.
3. Meyer MJ, Megyesi J, Meythaler J, et al. Acute management of acquired brain injury part I: An evidence-based review of non-pharmacological interventions. *Brain Inj*. 2010;24:694–705.
4. Curley G, Kavanagh BP, Laffey JG, et al. Hypocapnia and the injured brain: more harm than benefit. *Crit. Care Med*. 2010;38:1348–59.
5. Fox JL, Vu EN, Doyle-Waters M, et al. Prophylactic hypothermia for traumatic brain injury: A quantitative systematic review. *CJEM*. 2010;12: 355–64.
6. Nangunoori R, Maloney-Wilensky E, Stiefel M, et al. Brain tissue oxygen-based therapy and outcome after severe traumatic brain injury: A systematic literature review. *Neurocritical Care*. 2011.

ADDITIONAL READING

Faul M, Xu L, Wald MM, et al. *Traumatic Brain Injury in the United States: Emergency Department Visits, Hospitalizations, and Deaths*. Atlanta GA: Centers for Disease Control and Prevention, National Center for Injury Prevention and Control; 2010.

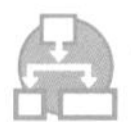

See Also (Topic, Algorithm, Electronic Media Element)

Brain Injury–Post Acute Care Issues; Postconcussive Syndrome; Seizure Disorders

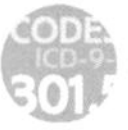

CODES

ICD9

- 852.00 Subarachnoid hemorrhage following injury, without mention of open intracranial wound, with state of consciousness unspecified
- 853.00 Other and unspecified intracranial hemorrhage following injury, without mention of open intracranial wound, with state of consciousness unspecified
- 854.00 Intracranial injury of other and unspecified nature, without mention of open intracranial wound, with state of consciousness unspecified

CLINICAL PEARLS

- Head injury is a dynamic process: Initial bleeding followed by secondary injury due to cerebral edema, continued bleeding, etc.
- Patients with history of head injury should have imaging if any of the following are present: Evidence of skull fracture, altered consciousness, neurologic deficit, persistent vomiting, scalp hematoma, abnormal behavior, coagulopathy, age >65.
- Patient with normal head CT who has returned to normal mental status may be discharged to home with a competent adult observer for 24 hours.
- Strict criteria exist for patients to return to normal sport activity following head injury to avoid the second-impact syndrome, which has 50% mortality.
- Predicting outcome is difficult, and patients may improve for years.

BRAIN INJURY–POST ACUTE CARE ISSUES

Maria I. Aguilar, MD

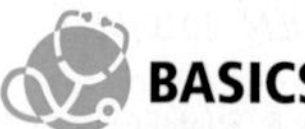

BASICS

DESCRIPTION

Traumatic brain injury (TBI) is a brain injury due to externally inflicted trauma; may result in significant impairment of an individual's physical, cognitive, and psychosocial functioning. TBI: Leading mortality cause in North America for ages 1–45.

EPIDEMIOLOGY

- Predominant age: Highest incidence in the very young (ages 0–4), in persons 15–24 years of age, and those >75 years old
- Predominant sex: Male > Female (2:1)

Incidence

- 1.2-1.7 million Americans sustain a TBI per year.
- 50,000 deaths per year
- 80,000–90,000 sustain long-term disabilities.

Prevalence

5.3 million Americans are living with TBI-related disabilities for which they require long-term assistance with activities of daily living.

RISK FACTORS

- High risk: Male, age 15–34
- Moderate risk <5 years and >60 years
- Lower socioeconomic status (head injury)

GENERAL PREVENTION

Improved safety standards and programs designed to minimize injury from vehicular-related events (motor vehicle, motorcycle, bicycle, pedestrian), falls, violence, sports, and recreation provide best prevention against TBI (1)[C].

PATHOPHYSIOLOGY

- Cortical contusions due to coup-contrecoup injuries. While axonal rupture from shear and tensile forces can occur at the time of severe head injury, milder degrees of axonal damage may play a role in mild TBI.
- Disruption of axonal neurofilament organization impairs axonal transport, leading to axonal swelling, Wallerian degeneration, and transection.
- Release of excitatory neurotransmitters acetylcholine, glutamate, and aspartate, and generation of free radicals may contribute to secondary injury.

ETIOLOGY

Leading causes of TBI: Falls and motor vehicle accidents (MVAs). Violence-related TBI has increased during the past decade and accounts for about 10% of all cases. Sports and recreation injuries are also an important cause of TBI, especially in teenagers and young adults.

COMMONLY ASSOCIATED CONDITIONS

- Psychosis
- Suicide attempts
- Substance abuse
- Attention deficit disorder

DIAGNOSIS

HISTORY

- Nonneurologic complications: Pulmonary, metabolic and endocrinologic, nutritional, GI, musculoskeletal, genitourinary, dermatologic, chronic pain
- Most neurologic complications are apparent within the first days following injury. Long-term sequelae include seizures, headache, hydrocephalus, visual defects, neuroendocrine abnormalities, and movement and sleep disorders.
- Cognitive consequences: Memory impairment, difficulties in attention and concentration, language deficits, visual perception problems, and poor problem-solving, reasoning, insight, judgment, and information processing
- Behavioral problems: Decreased ability to initiate responses, verbal and physical aggression, agitation, learning difficulties, shallow self-awareness, altered sexual functioning, impulsivity, social disinhibition
- Psychological consequences: Mood disorders, personality changes, altered emotional control, depression, anxiety
- Disruption of normal sleep
- Social consequences: Risk of suicide, divorce, unemployment, economic strain, alcohol/substance abuse

Pediatric Considerations

Interactions of physical, cognitive, and behavioral sequelae interfere with new learning. Effects of early TBI may not become apparent until later in the child's development.

PHYSICAL EXAM

- TBI's severity is classified based on the Glasgow Coma Scale (GCS) as follows: Mild injury GCS 13–15; moderate injury GCS 9–12; severe injury GCS 8 or less.
- GCS: For all 3 categories, score best response:

Verbal response	Score
Oriented	5
Confused	4
Inappropriate words	3
Incomprehensible speech	2
No response	1
Eye opening	
Spontaneous	4
To speech	3
To pain	2
No response	1
Motor response	
Obeys commands	6
Localizes pain	5
Withdraws from pain	4
Abnormal flexion to pain	3
Abnormal extension to pain	2
No response	1

DIAGNOSTIC TESTS & INTERPRETATION

- Evoked potentials (auditory, visual, somatosensory)
- Behavioral assessment, neuropsychological testing, vocational assessment
- Cognitive test for orientation and arousal; use Western Neurosensory Stimulation Profile or Galveston Orientation Amnesia Test
- Electroencephalograph (EEG)

Lab

Initial lab tests

As needed for suspected metabolic complications

Imaging

Initial approach

- Bone scan: Heterotopic ossification
- CT: Hydrocephalus, atrophy, hematoma
- Video fluoroscopic swallowing study
- MRI to evaluate diffuse axonal injury
- EEG: To evaluate subclinical seizure activity. Limited predictive value in the setting of acute TBI.

Pathological Findings

- Evidence of microscopic axonal injury, axon retraction bulbs, and microglial clusters
- Hydrocephalus with periventricular edema
- Joint contractures result in collagen cross-linking: Decreased range of motion
- Heterotopic ossification: Disorganized osteoid calcification in soft tissue

DIFFERENTIAL DIAGNOSIS

- The diagnosis of pain following TBI can be difficult in light of limitations imposed by cognitive, language, and behavioral deficits.:
  - Dysautonomia: Tachypnea, hypertension, painful posturing/contractions, diaphoresis
  - Neuropathic pain: Burning, shocklike, or pins and needles; allodynia/hyperpathia. 3 most common: Complex regional pain syndrome, central pain syndrome, and peripheral neuropathy.
  - Spasticity or spastic dystonia
  - Headache: Posttraumatic headache, hydrocephalus, increased intracranial pressure
  - Myofascial pain syndrome
  - Neurogenic heterotopic ossification: Bone formation in soft tissue
  - Deep vein thrombosis
  - Constipation and urinary retention
  - Trauma: Fractures, musculoskeletal injuries
  - Shoulder: Subluxation, acromioclavicular separation, rotator cuff tendonitis/tear
- Chronic infection, depression, hypothyroidism, hydrocephalus, intracerebral hemorrhage, seizures, fractures, tracheal stricture, pain, alcohol, drugs, polypharmacy, and/or CNS depressant

TREATMENT

MEDICATION

- Psychostimulants may affect speed of cognitive processing, mood, and behavior:
  - Methylphenidate 20–40 mg/d in 2 divided doses; dextroamphetamine
  - Also likely to improve memory, attention, concentration, and mental processing in children/adults (2)[A]
- Agitation:
  - Treat epilepsy or depression first.
  - Minimize the use of antipsychotics and benzodiazepines, as they worsen cognition.
  - β-blockers have best evidence for efficacy in agitation/aggression (3)[A].

- Antidepressants (SSRIs) and antiepileptic drugs (AEDs) in the context of an affective disorder or epilepsy, respectively, may help agitation/aggression (4)[B]
  - If necessary, use antipsychotics of the atypical class (clozapine, olanzapine, quetiapine, risperidone, and ziprasidone) (5)[B].
- Abulia (lack of initiative): Amantadine (Symmetrel), bromocriptine, methylphenidate, levodopa (5)[C]
- Epilepsy: American Academy of Physical Medicine and Rehabilitation does not recommend AEDs for preventing late (>7 days post-TBI) posttraumatic seizures (6)[B]. If epilepsy occurs, avoid phenobarbital; too sedating (6).
- Spasticity caution: Be aware of potential negative consequences of all agents:
  - Use dantrolene sodium 25–200 mg/d divided t.i.d.; baclofen; intrathecal baclofen; diazepam, clonidine, tizanidine, and gabapentin; botulinum toxin injections for focal spasticity (7)[B]
- Neurogenic bladder: Oxybutynin 2.5 mg t.i.d.–10 mg q.i.d. if bladder pressures low and/or postvoid residuals low (1)[B]
- Bowel routine: Stool softener such as docusate sodium (daily) combined with laxative (night-before suppository), high-fiber diet, and suppository (every other day) (1)[C]
- Heterotopic ossification: Indomethacin 25–50 mg t.i.d. If severe, progressive, or history of GI ulceration, then etidronate (Didronel) 20 mg/kg for 6 months or alendronate 20 mg/d (1)[C].
- Neurobehavioral problems: Weak evidence supports psychostimulants as effective in treatment of inattention, apathy, and slowness; high-dose β-blockers in treatment of agitation and aggression; and anticonvulsants and antidepressants in treatment of agitation and aggression with an affective disorder (4)[B].
- Precautions: Medications may have significant adverse effects in persons with TBI and can impede rehabilitation progress.
- Insomnia: Nonpharmacologic interventions (relaxation, cognitive behavioral therapy, sleep hygiene education); pharmacologic interventions (zopiclone, lorazepam, melatonin, tricyclic antidepressants) (8)

ADDITIONAL TREATMENT

General Measures

- Diminished level of arousal: Identify best modality for communication, assess functional skills (proper seating, hand function) with behaviorist/neuropsychologist.
- Social work (family education and long-term planning) and nursing
- Reduce sedatives.
- Neurogenic bladder: Treat UTI:
  - If postvoid residual <50 mL, then try regular voiding routine q2h.
  - If still incontinent, add oxybutynin.
  - If still incontinent, try condom catheter during the day; incontinence pads at night.
  - If high postvoid residuals or high-pressure bladder or dyssynergic bladder on urodynamics: Intermittent catheter q4–6h
- Neurogenic bowel: Regular bowel routine
- Contractures and spasticity; stretching:
  - If no progress after 4 weeks, consider serial casting or custom-made orthotic
  - Contractures >45°: Consider tendon release.
- Heterotopic ossification: Stretch soft tissue to decrease maturation of osteoid, consider orthotics/splinting, bone scan at baseline
- Skin: Turn patient q2h; avoid sitting such as in bed at 45°, observe for erythema around tube sites, and rule out latex allergy.
- Respiratory: Night humidification for tracheotomy
- Endocrine: Monitor fluid balance
- Rehabilitative practices: Rehabilitative programs should be interdisciplinary, comprehensive, and include cognitive and behavioral assessment and intervention (1)[C].

Issues for Referral

- Refer to multidisciplinary rehabilitation programs.
- Suicide attempts and ideation (SI) are more prevalent in people with TBI, even after controlling for psychiatric disorders (9)[C]. Assess hopelessness and SI proactively.

COMPLEMENTARY AND ALTERNATIVE MEDICINE

- Cognitive exercises (including computer-assisted strategies), compensatory devices (memory books, paging systems), psychotherapy, behavior modification, vocational rehabilitation, school rehabilitation, nutritional support, music and art therapy, therapeutic recreation
- Hyperbaric oxygen therapy (HBOT) cannot be routinely recommended for patients with TBI because of few trials, methodologic shortcomings, and poor reporting (10)[A].

ONGOING CARE

FOLLOW-UP RECOMMENDATIONS

Patient Monitoring

Patients make slow, steady gains; review medical status monthly.

DIET

- Ensure adequate hydration; 2-2.5 L/D of water.
- Bolus feeds preferred if fed by gastrostomy
- Upright and quiet for 30 minutes following feeds, as aspiration can occur even with a g-tube
- Early feeding is associated with trend toward better survival and disability outcomes (11)[A].

PATIENT EDUCATION

- For information and family support groups:
  - Brain Injury Information Network: www.tbinet.org
  - Brain Injury Association of America: www.biausa.org
- Families need support, advocacy, education, information (verbally and written), opportunity to have input regarding priorities and treatment plans, and to discuss limits of treatment for patient (advance directive).

PROGNOSIS

- Most rapid return of function is during first 2 years, but some improve slowly for 5–10 years
- Highly variable (80% of individuals with severe injuries become independent in dressing and self-care at 1 year)
- Negative prognostic factors:
  - Age >40 years old
  - Abnormal pupillary responses or extraocular eye movements
  - Prolonged coma
- Abnormal evoked potentials
- Accurate prediction of return to work is not feasible, with rates in the 12–70% range.

COMPLICATIONS

Major affective disorder (depression, psychosis) in up to 50% of patients, family and caregiver burnout, substance abuse, social isolation, dental caries, osteoporosis, aspiration pneumonia, pressure ulcers, dysphagia, esophagitis, bladder incontinence, contractures/spasticity

REFERENCES

1. Consensus conference. Rehabilitation of persons with traumatic brain injury. NIH Consensus Development Panel on Rehabilitation of Persons With Traumatic Brain Injury. *JAMA*. 1999;282:974–83.
2. Siddall OM. Use of methylphenidate in traumatic brain injury. *Ann Pharmacother*. 2005;39:1309–13.
3. Fleminger S, et al. Pharmacological management for agitation and aggression in people with acquired brain injury. *Cochrane Database Syst Rev*. 2003/2006;(1):CD003299.
4. Deb S, Crownshaw T. The role of pharmacotherapy in the management of behaviour disorders in traumatic brain injury patients. *Brain Inj*. 2004;18:1–31.
5. Elovic EP, et al. The use of atypical antipsychotics in traumatic brain injury. *J Head Trauma Rehab*. 2003;18(2):177–95.
6. Bushnik T, et al. Medical and social issues related to posttraumatic seizures in persons with traumatic brain injury. *J Head Trauma Rehab*. 2004;19(4):296–304.
7. Zafonte R, et al. Acute care management of post-TBI spasticity. *J Head Trauma Rehab*. 2004;19(2):89–100.
8. Zeiter JM, Friedman L, O'Hara R. Insomnia in the context of traumatic brain injury. *J Rehabil Res Dev*. 2009;6:827–36.
9. Simpson G, Tate R, et al. Suicidality in people surviving a traumatic brain injury: Prevalence, risk factors and implications for clinical management. *Brain Inj*. 2007;21:1335–51.
10. Bennett M, Heard R. Hyperbaric oxygen therapy for multiple sclerosis. *Cochrane Database Syst Rev*. 2004:CD003057.
11. Perel P, Yanagawa T, Bunn F, et al. Nutritional support for head-injured patients. *Cochrane Database Syst Rev*. 2006:CD001530.

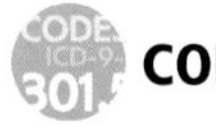

CODES

ICD9

- 854.00 Intracranial injury of other and unspecified nature without mention of open intracranial wound, unspecified state of consciousness
- 907.0 Late effect of intracranial injury without mention of skull fracture
- 908.6 Late effect of certain complications of trauma

CLINICAL PEARLS

- TBI can cause both neurologic and nonneurologic manifestations.
- Best approach to treatment includes multi- and interdisciplinary team member participation.
- TBI can lead to devastating sequelae; prevention is key.

BREAST ABSCESS

Lisa M. Schroeder, MD
Sabrina Mia, MD

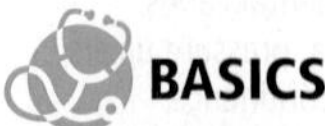

BASICS

DESCRIPTION

- Collection of pus, usually localized
- Can be associated with lactation or fistulous tracts secondary to squamous epithelial neoplasm or duct occlusion
- System(s) affected: Skin/Exocrine
- Synonym(s): Mammary abscess; Peripheral breast abscess; Subareolar abscess; Puerperal abscess

Pregnancy Considerations

Most commonly associated with postpartum lactation

EPIDEMIOLOGY

- Predominant age:
  - Puerperal abscess: Lactational
  - Subareolar abscess: Postmenopausal
- Predominant sex: Female
- African American higher incidence

Incidence

- 0.1–0.5% of breastfeeding women
- Puerperal abscess rare after first 6 weeks of lactation

RISK FACTORS

- **Puerperal mastitis**:
  - 5–11% go on to abscess (most often due to inadequate therapy).
  - Risk factors for mastitis are those that result in milk stasis (infrequent feeds, missing feeds).
- Poor latch, damaged nipple, illness in mother or baby, rapid weaning, breast pressure, blocked nipple pore or duct, maternal stress or fatigue, maternal malnutrition
- General factors: Smoking, diabetes, rheumatoid arthritis, obesity
- Steroids, silicone/paraffin implants, lumpectomy with radiation
- Nipple retraction
- Nipple piercing for mastitis (1)[A]
- Higher recurrence rate if multiorganism abscess

GENERAL PREVENTION

- Prevention of mastitis
- Early treatment of mastitis with milk expression and cold compresses
- Early treatment with antibiotics

ETIOLOGY

- Delayed treatment of mastitis
- Puerperal abscesses: Blocked lactiferous duct
- Subareolar abscess: Squamous epithelial neoplasm with keratin plugs or ductal extension with associated inflammation
- Peripheral abscess: Stasis of the duct
- Other bacteria: Nonlactational abscess and recurrent abscesses associated with anaerobic bacteria:
  - *Escheria coli*, *Proteus*, mixed bacteria less common

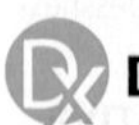

DIAGNOSIS

- Tender breast lump, fluctuant, usually unilateral
- Systemic malaise (though usually less malaise than with mastitis)
- Fever

HISTORY

Tender breast lump, usually unilateral

PHYSICAL EXAM

- Erythema
- Draining pus
- Local edema
- Nipple and skin retraction
- Proximal lymphadenopathy

DIAGNOSTIC TESTS & INTERPRETATION

Lab

- Leukocytosis
- Elevated ESR
- Culture and sensitivity of drainage to identify pathogen, usually *Staphylococci* or *Streptococci*.
- Methicillin-resistant *Staphylococcus aureus* (MRSA) is a recent increasingly important pathogen in both lactational and nonlactational abscesses.

Imaging

- Ultrasound
- Mammogram

Diagnostic Procedures/Surgery

- Aspiration for culture
- Fine-needle aspiration not accurate to exclude carcinoma

Pathological Findings

- Squamous metaplasia of the ducts
- Intraductal hyperplasia
- Epithelial overgrowth
- Fat necrosis
- Duct ectasia

DIFFERENTIAL DIAGNOSIS

- Carcinoma (inflammatory or primary squamous cell)
- Engorgement
- Galactocele
- Tuberculosis (may be associated with human immunodeficiency [HIV] infection)
- Actinomycosis
- Typhoid
- Sarcoid
- Granulomatous disease
- Syphilis
- Foreign body reactions (e.g., to silicone and paraffin)
- Mammary duct ectasia
- Hydatid cyst
- Sebaceous cyst

TREATMENT

MEDICATION

- **Combine antibiotics with drainage for cure.**
- Culture midstream sample of milk for mastitis
- Culture abscess fluid for breast abscess
- NSAIDs
- Dicloxacillin 500 mg q.i.d. for 10–14 days
- If no response in 24–48 hours, switch to cephalexin 500 mg q.i.d. for 10–14 days:
  - Or amoxicillin-clavulanate (Augmentin) 250 mg t.i.d.
- Clindamycin 300 mg t.i.d. if anaerobes suspected
- If MRSA a concern TMP-SMZ 2 PO bid for 10–14 days, or clindamycin
- *Contraindications*: Allergy to the antibiotic
- Precautions: Refer to manufacturer's profile for each drug
- New techniques include percutaneous intracavitary urokinase irrigation for large abscesses in nonlactating women (2)[C]

ADDITIONAL TREATMENT

General Measures

- Cold compresses for pain control
- *Important to continue to breastfeed or express milk*

COMPLEMENTARY AND ALTERNATIVE MEDICINE

- Lecithin supplementation
- Acupuncture may help with breast engorgement, and possibly with breast abscess prevention (3)[A].

SURGERY/OTHER PROCEDURES

- Aspiration under ultrasound (2,4)[B],(5)[C]
- Serial aspirations under ultrasound (U/S) may be necessary (q2–3 d) (6)[C].
- Needle aspiration alone (without antibiotics) may be effective for small breast abscesses (7)[A].
- If aspiration and antibiotics fail, incision and drainage with removal of loculations
- Biopsy of all nonpuerperal abscesses to rule out carcinoma
- Open all fistulous tracts, especially in nonlactating abscesses.

IN-PATIENT CONSIDERATIONS

Initial Stabilization

- Outpatient, unless systemically immunocompromised or septic
- Aggressive glycemic control important (5)[B]

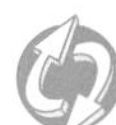

ONGOING CARE

FOLLOW-UP RECOMMENDATIONS

Patient Monitoring

Ensure resolution to exclude carcinoma.

PATIENT EDUCATION

- Care of wound
- Breastfeeding precautions

PROGNOSIS

- Complete healing expected in 8–10 days
- Subareolar abscesses frequently recur, even after incision and drainage (I&D) and antibiotics; may require surgical removal of ducts.

COMPLICATIONS

- Fistula
- Poor cosmetic outcome

REFERENCES

1. Gollapalli V, Liao J, Dudkavic A, et al. Risk factors for developmet and recurrence of primary breast abscess. *J Am Coll Surg*. 2010;211:41–8.
2. Schwarz RJ, Shrestha R. Needle aspiration of breast abscesses. *Am J Surgery*. 2001;182:117.
3. Mangesi L, Dowswell T. Treatments for breast engorgement during lactation. *Cochrane Database Syst Rev*. 2010;CD006946.
4. Dener C, Inan A. Breast abscesses in lactating women. *World J Surgery*. 2003;27:130.
5. Christensen AF, Al-Suliman N, Nielsen KR, et al. Ultrasound-guided drainage of breast abscesses: Results in 151 patients. *Br J Radiol*. 2005;78: 186–8.
6. Elder E, Brennan M. Nonsurgical management should be first-line therapy for breast abscess. *World J Surg*. 2010;34:2257–8.
7. Thirumalaikumar S, Kommu S, et al. Best evidence topic reports. Aspiration of breast abscesses. *Emerg Med J*. 2004;21:333–4.

ADDITIONAL READING

- Berná-Serna JD, Berná-Mestre JD, Galindo PJ, et al. Use of urokinase in percutaneous drainage of large breast abscesses. *J Ultrasound Med*. 2009;28: 449–54.
- Dabbas N, Chand M, Pallett A, et al. Have the organisms that cause breast abscess changed with time?–Implications for appropriate antibiotic usage in primary and secondary care. *Breast J*. 2010;16: 412–5.
- Jahanfar S, Ng CJ, Teng CL, et al. Antibiotics for mastitis in breastfeeding women. *Cochrane Database Syst Rev*. 2009;CD005458.
- Rizzo M, Gabram S, Staley C, et al. Management of breast abscesses in nonlactating women. *Am Surg*. 2010;76:292–5.

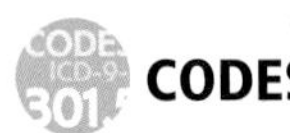

CODES

ICD9

- 611.0 Inflammatory disease of breast
- 675.14 Postpartum abscess of breast

CLINICAL PEARLS

- 5–11% of cases of puerperal mastitis go on to abscess (most often due to inadequate therapy for mastitis). Risk factors for mastitis are those that result in milk stasis (infrequent feeds, missing feeds).
- Abscess not associated with lactation should prompt coverage with antibiotics that cover anaerobic bacteria.
- Treatment is antibiotic and aspiration, with I&D, with breakup of loculations reserved for those failing more conservative management.

BREAST CANCER

Bethany Gentilesco, MD
Komal Talati, MD

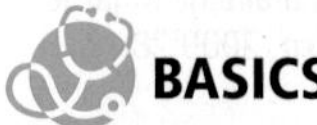

BASICS

DESCRIPTION

- Common malignant tumor that originates from breast epithelial cells, glandular cells, or connective tissue (rare)
- Types: Ductal carcinoma in situ (DCIS—a precursor to invasive disease), invasive infiltrating ductal carcinoma, invasive lobular carcinoma, inflammatory breast cancer, Paget disease of the nipple, phyllodes tumor, angiosarcoma

EPIDEMIOLOGY

Incidence

- 123 cases per 100,000 women per year in 2006
- Invasive cancer new cases in 2009: Women: 194,280
- In situ cancer new cases in 2009: 62,280 (85% ductal carcinoma in situ)
- Breast cancer (BC) deaths: 40,480; lifetime risk BC: 1 in 8 (12.5%); lifetime risk BC death: 1 in 35
- Most common malignancy in US women, second only to lung cancer as cause of cancer death (1)

Prevalence

2.5 million women in the US (1)

RISK FACTORS

- Female, family history (FH), genetics, nulliparity or older age at first live birth, early menarche, delayed menopause, increasing patient age, personal history of BC or ovarian cancer, obesity, heavy alcohol intake
- Benign/at risk breast disease: Atypical hyperplasia (ductal/lobular), lobular carcinoma in situ increases risk for bilateral BC
- Prior chest radiation (lymphoma), DES (diethylstilbestrol)
- Prolonged hormone replacement therapy, high ethyl alcohol use, high body mass index, physical inactivity
- Men less at risk for BC, but at increased risk with Klinefelter syndrome, testicular pathology, FH, or *BRCA2* mutations

Genetics

- *BRCA1* and *BRCA2*
- Other genes: *AR, ATM, BARD1, BRIP1, CDH1, PTEN, STK11, CHEK2, p53, ERBB2, DIRAS3, NBN, RAD50, RAD51*
- Cowden syndrome (PTEN): Hamartomas skin, intestine, oral mucosa (trichilemmoma), BC, microencephaly, endometrial cancer, nonmedullary thyroid cancer, benign thyroid lesions
- Li-Fraumeni syndrome (TP53): Autosomal dominance, cancer (CA) in CNS, leukemia, sarcoma, osteosarcoma, adrenal cortex, breast
- Ataxia-telangiectasia (ATM): Autosomal recessive, ataxia, telangiectasia, lymphoma, leukemia, CA of breast, stomach, ovary
- Peutz-Jeghers (STK11): Autosomal dominance, hamartomatous polyps of GI tract, mucocutaneous melanin in lips, buccal mucosa, fingers, toes, CA in GI, lung, breast, uterus, ovary
- Criteria for additional risk evaluation/gene testing in affected individual (2):
  - BC at age $\leq$50 years
  - Triple-negative BC (ER-, PR-, Her2-)
  - 2 breast primaries in single patient
  - Ovarian/fallopian tube/primary peritoneal CA
  - $\geq$1 family member BC at $\leq$50 years or $\geq$1 family member with ovarian/fallopian tube/primary peritoneal CA any age
  - $\geq$2 family members BC and/or pancreatic CA any age
  - BC with thyroid CA, sarcoma, adrenal cortex, endometrial, pancreas, CNS, diffuse gastric, leukemia/lymphoma same side of family
  - Male BC
- Criteria for additional risk evaluation/gene testing in unaffected individual with FH (2):
  - $\geq$2 breast primaries from same side of family
  - $\geq$1 ovarian primary from same side of family
  - Clustering of BC with thyroid CA, sarcoma, adrenal cortex, endometrial, pancreas, CNS, diffuse gastric, leukemia/lymphoma same side of family
  - FH BC susceptibility gene (*BRCA1* , *BRCA2*)
  - Ashkenazi Jewish with breast/ovary cancer at any age
  - Male BC (2)

GENERAL PREVENTION

- General population screening (3):
  - Risk assessment tool at http://www.cancer.gov/bcrisktool/
  - Clinical Breast Exam (CBE) 1–3 years (controversial; no evidence CBE improves outcomes, but may decrease in patient anxiety)
  - Mammography: Age 40 controversial, on patient request; age 50: Mammography every 1–2 years
  - Folate supplementation (controversial) (4)[A]
- For hereditary breast and/or ovarian CA:
  - Begin at age 25 or age of earliest family diagnosis: Monthly self-breast exam, semiannual CBE, annual mammogram and breast MRI; if *BRCA2* consider yearly skin exam/pancreatic CA screening
  - Starting at age 30: Semiannual transvaginal ultrasound (US) and CA125 until salpingo-oophorectomy
  - Selective estrogen receptor modulators in premenopausal women, aromatase inhibitors in postmenopausal women
  - Discuss risk-reducing mastectomy and salpingo-oophorectomy done after 35 or after child-bearing

PATHOPHYSIOLOGY

- Genetic mutations such as *BCRA1* and *BRCA2* can cause hereditary breast and ovarian cancer. These genes function as tumor suppressor genes, and a mutation leads to cell cycle progression and limitations in DNA repair.
- Mutations in estrogen/progesterone receptors through genetic changes can cause BC by inducing cyclin D1 and c-myc expression downstream leading to cell cycle progression (5).
- ~1/3 of BC do not express estrogen receptor (ER) mutations; however, many of these tumors may display cross-talk with ER receptor and epidermal growth factors (EGFR).

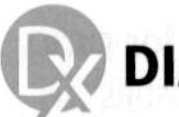

DIAGNOSIS

HISTORY

FH

PHYSICAL EXAM

- Visualize breasts with patient sitting for skin dimpling, peau d'orange, asymmetry
- Palpation of breast and regional lymph node exam: Supraclavicular, infraclavicular, axillary

DIAGNOSTIC TESTS & INTERPRETATION

Lab

Initial lab tests

- Mammography BI-RADS: Breast Imaging-Reporting and Data System is a quality assurance (QA) method published by the American Radiology Society.
- BI-RADS interpretation: 0: Incomplete; 1: Negative; 2: Benign finding(s); 3: Probably benign; 4: Suspicious abnormality; 5: Highly suggestive of malignancy; 6: Known biopsy—proven malignancy
- All newly diagnosed BC: CBC, comprehensive metabolic profile, serum calcium

Imaging

Initial approach

- Clinical sign (3):
  - Palpable mass $\geq$30 years: Obtain diagnostic mammography
    - If BI-RADS 1–3 then get US $\pm$ biopsy
    - If BI-RADS 4–6 then get core needle biopsy $\pm$ surgical excision
  - Palpable mass <30 years: Obtain US $\pm$ mammogram $\pm$ biopsy, or if low clinical suspicion observe for 1 menstrual cycle for resolution
  - Spontaneous, reproducible nipple discharge: Obtain mammogram, $\pm$ US:
    - If BI-RADS 1–3 then get ductogram
    - If BI-RADS 4–6 then surgical excision
  - Asymmetric thickening/nodularity $\geq$30 years: Obtain mammogram + US $\pm$ biopsy
  - Asymmetric thickening/nodularity <30 years: Obtain US $\pm$ mammogram $\pm$ biopsy
  - Skin changes, peau d'orange: Obtain mammogram $\pm$ US $\pm$ biopsy
- Obtain MRI + BRCA1 or 2, has lifetime BC risk of $\geq$20% (BRCAPRO model), history of prior chest radiation
- MRI commonly used to define extent of disease such as multifocal/multicentric disease
- Lymph node scintigraphy for sentinel lymph node assessment (3)

Follow-Up & Special Considerations

- Advanced disease (stage IIIA or higher):
  - Chest imaging, bone scan, abdominal $\pm$ pelvis CT, positron emission tomography (PET) scan
- Most common metastasis sites for BC are lungs, liver, bone, brain:
  - Bone scan: Localized pain, elevated alk phos
  - Abdominal $\pm$ pelvis CT: Abdominal symptoms, elevated alk phos, abnormal liver function tests
  - Chest imaging: Pulmonary symptoms
  - MRI: CNS/spinal cord symptoms (6)

Diagnostic Procedures/Surgery
- Primary tumor: Fine-needle aspiration, US-guided core needle biopsy, stereotactic-guided core needle biopsy ± wire localization, sentinel lymph node, surgical excision, sentinel lymph node biopsy, post biopsy may get inflammatory changes/hematoma
- Genomic assay on formalin-fixed tissue for select +ER, -HER2, node negative tumor to assess chemotherapy responsiveness (6)

Pathological Findings
- Histology:
  - Ductal/lobular/other, tumor size, inflammatory component, invasive/noninvasive, margins, nodal involvement
  - Nodal micrometastases: Increased risk of disease recurrence
- ER, progesterone receptor, HER-2 assay

DIFFERENTIAL DIAGNOSIS
- Benign breast disease: Fibrocystic disease, fibroadenoma, intraductal papilloma (presents with bloody nipple discharge), duct ectasia, cyst, sclerosing adenosis, fat necrosis (s/p breast trauma)
- Infection: Abscess, cellulitis, mastitis

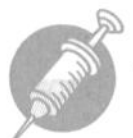

TREATMENT

MEDICATION
- Secondary prevention:
  - Chemoprevention/hormone therapy:
    - Risk reduction for ER-positive tumors
- Hormone therapy for ER-positive tumors (6):
  - Tamoxifen: Premenopausal women; 5-year treatment; avoid during lactation, pregnancy, or in patients with history of deep venous thrombosis/ pulmonary embolism
  - Ovarian ablation or suppression with luteinizing hormone-releasing hormone agonists: Premenopausal women
  - Aromatase inhibitors: Postmenopausal women, 5-year treatment
- Anti-HER2/neu antibody in select HER2/neu-positive patients (6):
  - Monitor cardiac toxicity via EKG, especially with anthracycline.
- Neoadjuvant chemotherapy (pre op) (6):
  - Locally advanced, inoperable advanced BC (stage III)
  - Early operable BC for breast conservation surgery
  - Triple negative BC
  - Cytotoxic therapy:
    - Anthracyclines, taxanes, alkylating agents, antimetabolites
    - Combinations of above
- Adjuvant chemotherapy (post op):
  - Higher-risk patients with nonmetastatic operable tumors
  - Patients with high risk of recurrence after local treatment (serial/parallel [s/p] surgery ± radiation)
  - Online tool to estimate recurrence risk and benefits of adjuvant chemotherapy (http://www.adjuvantonline.com/online.jsp)
  - Cytotoxic therapy (6):
    - Anthracyclines, alkylating agents, taxanes, antimetabolites
    - Combinations of above
    - Dose-dense chemotherapy demonstrates overall survival advantage in early BC (7).
- Advanced disease (6):
  - Hormone therapy
  - Cytotoxic therapy
  - Bisphosphonates to decrease skeletal complications
  - Antivascular endothelial growth factor antibody
  - Anti-HER2/neu antibody in select HER2/neu-positive patients

SURGERY/OTHER PROCEDURES
- Secondary prevention (6):
  - Risk-reducing mastectomy and bilateral salpingo-oophorectomy for breast and ovary CA syndromes
- Breast-conserving partial mastectomy/lumpectomy if possible (6):
  - Negative margins; tumor usually <5 cm
  - No prior breast radiation, relative contraindication: Lupus, scleroderma
- Modified radical mastectomy (6):
  - Large tumors; multicentric disease; young women with known BRCA; consider immediate or delayed reconstruction
- Radiation therapy should be initiated without delay (6):
  - After breast-conserving therapy (BCT), stage I, IIA, IIB treatable with BCT + radiation
  - Postmastectomy in select high-risk patients; palliation of metastatic disease; cord compression
- Pregnancy and BC:
  - Surgical: Mastectomy or breast conservation: Mastectomy preferred due to limitations of radiation during pregnancy
  - Sentinel lymph node biopsy: Safe to use with lymphoscintigraphy
  - Chemotherapy: Appropriate in second and third trimesters
  - Radiation therapy: Avoid until after delivery

IN-PATIENT CONSIDERATIONS
Discharge Criteria
Postmastectomy:
- Complications: Seroma, phantom breast syndrome, cellulitis, chest wall/axilla/arm pain, long thoracic nerve damage leading to winged scapula sign
- At risk for lymphedema, avoid having BP taken on side of surgery

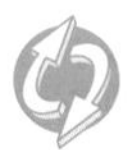

ONGOING CARE

FOLLOW-UP RECOMMENDATIONS
- Interval history/physical every 3–6 months for 3 years after primary therapy, and 6–12 months for years 4 and 5, then annually
- No evidence to support the use of routine CBC, liver function test, "tumor markers" for BC, routine bone scan, chest x-ray, liver US, CT scans, MRI, (PET, ultrasound in the asymptomatic patient
- Mammogram/imaging 1 year after initial mammo, but 6 months postradiation, then annually
- Annual gynecologic exam for women with uterus and on tamoxifen

COMPLICATIONS
- Spinal cord compression, hypercalcemia, visceral metastatic disease, postoperative lymphedema
- Emotional issues, especially depression and body-image alteration

REFERENCES

1. National Cancer Institute, US National institutes of Health. 2009/2010 Update http://progressreport.cancer.gov/doc_detail.asp?pid=1&did=2009&chid=93&coid=920&mid=.
2. NCCN Guidelines: Breast and/or Ovarian Cancer Genetic Assessment (Version1.2011) © 2011 Breast Cancer National Comprehensive Cancer Network, Inc. Accessed 7/20/2011 at http://www.nccn.org.
3. NCCN Clinical Practice Guidelines In Oncology: Breast Cancer Screening and Diagnosis (Version 1.2011)©2011 Breast Cancer National Comprehensive Cancer Network, Inc. Accessed 7/22/2011 at http://www.nccn.org.
4. Larsson SC, Giovannucci E, Wolk A. Folate and risk of breast cancer: A meta-analysis. *J Natl Cancer Inst*. 2007;99:64.
5. Sutherland RL, Prall OW, Watts CK, et al. Estrogen and progestin regulation of cell cycle progression. *J Mammary Gland Biol Neoplasia*. 1998;3:63–72.
6. NCCN Clinical Practice Guidelines In Oncology: Breast Cancer (Version 2.2011)©2011 Breast Cancer National Comprehensive Cancer Network, Inc. Accessed 7/21/2011 at http://www.nccn.org.
7. Lyman GH, Barron RL, Natoli JL, et al. Systematic review of efficacy of dose-dense versus non-dose-dense chemotherapy in breast cancer, non-Hodgkin lymphoma, and non-small cell lung cancer. *Crit Rev Oncol Hematol*. 2011.

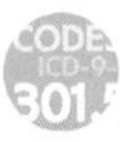

CODES

ICD9
- 174.0 Malignant neoplasm of nipple and areola of female breast
- 174.1 Malignant neoplasm of central portion of female breast
- 174.9 Malignant neoplasm of breast (female), unspecified site

CLINICAL PEARLS
- BC is most common malignancy in the US women, with lifetime risk of 1 in 8.
- High alcohol use, high BMI, and physical inactivity are modifiable risk factors.
- Pursue/refer all abnormal breast physical exam/ imaging findings.
- If patient ≥30 years with palpable mass, obtain mammogram, if <30 years obtain US.
- Normal mammography does not exclude possibility of CA with a palpable mass.
- Most common metastasis sites for BC are lungs, liver, bone, and brain.
- If on selective estrogen receptor modulator (tamoxifen) patient at risk for endometrial cancer
- Postmastectomy patient at increased risk for lymphedema on affected side; avoid BP measurement on that side

BREASTFEEDING

Deborah Ikhena, MD
Julie Scott Taylor, MD, MSc

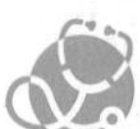

BASICS

- Breastfeeding is the natural process of feeding an infant human milk directly from the breast.
- "Breast milk feeding" is the process of feeding a child human milk that has been expressed, either by hand or by pump.
- The American Academy of Pediatrics (AAP), the American Academy of Family Physicians (AAFP), and other medical organizations recommend breastfeeding for 1–2 years with the gradual introduction of solid foods starting at 6 months (1).

DESCRIPTION

- Maternal benefits (as compared to mothers who do not breastfeed) include (2):
  - Decreased postpartum bleeding (due to oxytocin release)
  - Decreased risk of postpartum depression
  - Easier postpartum weight loss
  - Delayed postpartum fertility
  - Decreased risk of breast and ovarian cancer
  - Decreased risk of type 2 diabetes
  - Increased bonding
  - Convenience
  - Cost
- Infant benefits (as compared with children who are formula-fed) include (2):
  - Ideal food: Easily digestible, nutrients well absorbed, less constipation
  - Lower rates of virtually all infections via maternal antibody protection:
    - Fewer respiratory and GI infections
    - Decreased incidence of otitis media
    - Decreased risk of bacterial meningitis and sepsis
  - Decreased incidence of obesity
  - Decreased incidence of allergies and atopic dermatitis in childhood
  - Decreased incidence of type 1 and 2 diabetes
  - Decreased risk of childhood leukemia
  - Decreased risk of sudden infant death syndrome (SIDS)
  - Decreased mortality
  - Increased attachment between mother and baby

EPIDEMIOLOGY

Incidence

According to the most recent National Immunization Survey, for births in the US in 2007 (3):

- Any breastfeeding: 75.0%
- Breastfeeding at 6 months: 43.0%
- Breastfeeding at 12 months: 22.4%
- Exclusive breastfeeding at 3 months: 33.0%
- Exclusive breastfeeding at 6 months: 13.3%

RISK FACTORS

- Breast surgery, especially reduction surgery, prior to pregnancy may disrupt breast milk production in the future.
- Severe postpartum hemorrhage may lead to Sheehan syndrome, which is associated with difficulty breastfeeding due to poor milk production.

GENERAL PREVENTION

Maternal avoidance diets during lactation not usually recommended to prevent allergic disease

PATHOPHYSIOLOGY

The overarching mechanism of milk production is based on supply and demand:

- Stimulation of areola causes secretion of oxytocin.
- Oxytocin is responsible for let-down reflex when milk is ejected from cells into milk ducts.
- Sucking stimulates secretion of prolactin, which triggers milk production. Thus, milk is made in response to breastfeeding and increases supply:
  - Endocrine/metabolic: Thyroid dysfunction may cause delayed lactation or decreased milk production.

COMMONLY ASSOCIATED CONDITIONS

- Breast milk jaundice should be considered if jaundice persists for >1 week in an otherwise healthy, well-hydrated newborn. It peaks at 10–14 days.
- Other causes, such as hypothyroidism and infection, should be considered.

DIAGNOSIS

PHYSICAL EXAM

- Examine breasts, ideally during pregnancy, looking for scars or inverted nipples.
- Breast cancer incidence low but possible in premenopausal women

ALERT

A breast lump should be followed to complete resolution or worked up if present and not just attributed to changes from lactation.

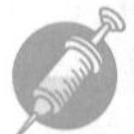

TREATMENT

ADDITIONAL TREATMENT

General Measures

- Flat or inverted nipples:
  - When stimulated, inverted nipples will retract inward, flat nipples remain flat; check for this on initial prenatal physical.
  - Nipple shells, a doughnut-shaped insert, can be worn inside the bra during the last month of pregnancy to gently force the nipple through the center opening of the shell.
  - Babies can nurse successfully even if the shell does not correct the problem before birth.
- Contraindications to breastfeeding are few:
  - Maternal HIV or human T-cell leukemia virus (HTLV) infection
  - Active tuberculosis
  - Active herpes simplex virus (HSV) lesions on the breast
  - Substances of abuse and some medications that will pass into human milk (4)[B]
  - Infants with galactosemia should not be fed with breast milk.
  - Maternal hepatitis is not a contraindication to breastfeeding.

Issues for Referral

- Refer to trained physician, nurse, or lactation consultant for inpatient and/or outpatient teaching.
- Frequent follow-up if having problems with latching, sore nipples, or inadequate milk production

COMPLEMENTARY AND ALTERNATIVE MEDICINE

Fenugreek may increase breast milk production. Suggested dose: 3 tablets t.i.d. Safety is not established.

IN-PATIENT CONSIDERATIONS

Initial Stabilization

- Initiate breastfeeding immediately after birth, ideally placing the infant at the mother's breast in the delivery room.
- Get mother in a comfortable position, usually sitting or reclining with the baby's head in crook of her arm:
  - Side-lying position often useful following cesarean-section delivery
- Bring baby to mother to decrease stress on mother's back.
- Baby's belly and mother's belly should face each other or touch ("belly to belly"). Initiate the rooting reflex by tickling baby's lips with nipple or finger. As baby's mouth opens wide, mother guides her nipple to back of her baby's mouth while pulling the baby closer. This will ensure that the baby's gums are sucking on the areola, not the nipple (5)[C].
- Feed every 2–4 hours, 20 minutes per side.
- Rooming-in to encourage on-demand feeding (5)
- Observation of a nursing session by an experienced physician, nurse, or lactation consultant
- Avoid supplementation with formula or water.
- Review expectations, techniques, and feeding cues.

ONGOING CARE

FOLLOW-UP RECOMMENDATIONS

See mother and baby within a few days of hospital discharge, especially if first time breastfeeding, and frequently thereafter.

Patient Monitoring

- Monitor infant's weight and output closely.
- Supplementation with infant formula recommended only if infant has lost 7% or more of birth weight, shows signs of dehydration such as decreased urine output, or has fewer than 3 small stools a day.
- Supplementation without persistent and regular breast stimulation with frequent feedings or breast pump use will decrease milk production and decrease breastfeeding success.

DIET

- For mothers:
  - Continue prenatal vitamins.
  - Drink plenty of fluids: 12.5 cups or 3 L of fluids per day.
  - Breastfeeding mothers require 1,800–2,300 calories per day; ~500 more than prepregnancy needs.
  - Gassy foods such as cabbage may cause baby to have colic.
  - Limit caffeine to 300 mg/d.
  - Alcohol should be avoided. 1–2 drinks/wk of alcohol may be okay, but mothers should avoid nursing 2–3 hours after a drink. Only <2% of alcohol is passed to baby via breast milk.

- For infants:
  - In 2008, the AAP increased its recommended daily intake of vitamin D in infants from 200 to 400 IU. For exclusively breastfed babies, this will require taking a vitamin supplement such as Poly-Vi-Sol or Vi-Daylin vitamin drops, 0.5 cc/d, beginning in the first few days of life (6).
  - In 2010, the AAP recommended adding supplementation for breastfed infants with oral iron 1 mg/kg/d beginning at age 4 months (7):
    - Preterm infants fed human milk should receive an iron supplement of 2 mg/kg/d by 1 month of age, and this should be continued until the infant is weaned to iron-fortified formula or begins eating complementary foods that supply the 2 mg/kg of iron.
  - Fluoride supplement unnecessary until 6 months of age.

PATIENT EDUCATION

- Primary care-initiated interventions to promote breastfeeding have been shown to be successful with respect to child and maternal health outcomes (8):
  - The US Preventive Services Task Force (USPSTF) recommends structured breastfeeding education and behavioral counseling programs to promote breastfeeding.
  - Regular promotion of the advantages of breastfeeding/risks of not breastfeeding
  - Emphasize importance of exclusive breastfeeding for first 4 weeks of life to allow adequate buildup of sufficient milk supply
- Milk usually comes in around postpartum day #3.
- Frequent nursing (8–12 feedings per 24 hours)
- Baby should have 5–8 wet diapers per day and 2–5 bowel movements per day.
- After day 4 of life, baby should gain 4–7 oz per week.
- Signs of adequate nursing:
  - Breasts become hard before and soft after feeding.
  - 6 or more wet diapers in 24 hours
  - Baby satisfied; appropriate weight gain (average 1 oz/d in first few months)
- Growth spurts: Anticipate these ~10 days, 6 weeks, 3 months, and 4–6 months. Baby will nurse more often at these times for several days. This will increase milk production to allow for further adequate growth.
- Weaning:
  - Exclusive breast milk is optimal food for first 6 months
  - Solid food may be introduced at 6 months.
  - For mothers going to work, start switching the baby to breast milk feeding (or formula feeding) during the hours mother will be gone about a week ahead of time. Do this by dropping a feeding every few days and substituting pumped breast milk or formula, preferably given by another caregiver.
- Family planning:
  - Lactational amenorrhea method (LAM): Breastfeeding may be used as effective birth control option if (i) infant is <6 months old, (ii) infant is exclusively breastfeeding, and (iii) mother is amenorrheic (9).
  - Other options include barrier methods, implants, Depo-Provera, oral contraception, and intrauterine devices (IUDs). The Centers for Disease Control (CDC) recommends that progesterone-only pills, Depo-Provera, IUDs, and Implanon can be used within 1 month postpartum if breastfeeding. However, they recommend delaying the use of combined oral contraceptives until after 1 month postpartum (10):
    - Most providers use progesterone-only birth control pills in the early postpartum period.
- The Academy of Breastfeeding Medicine (ABM), a worldwide organization of physicians dedicated to the promotion, protection, and support of breastfeeding and human lactation: www.bfmed.org
- La Leche League at www.llli.org
- Protecting, Promoting and Supporting Breastfeeding: The Special Role of Maternity Services, a joint World Health Organization/United Nations Children's Fund (WHO/UNICEF) statement published by the World Health Organization: http://www.unicef.org/newsline/tenstps.htm
- Thomas Hale's *Medications and Mother's Milk: A Manual of Lactational Pharmacology*

COMPLICATIONS

- Plugged duct:
  - Mother is well except for sore lump in 1 or both breasts without fever
  - Use moist, hot packs on lump prior to and during nursing.
  - More frequent nursing on affected side; ensure good technique
- Mastitis (see topic "Mastitis"):
  - Sore lump in 1 or both breasts plus fever and/or redness on skin overlying lump
  - Use moist, hot packs on lump prior to and during nursing; more frequent nursing on affected side
  - Antibiotics covering for *Staphylococcus aureus* (the most common organism) for at least 7 days (11)
  - Other possible sources of fever should be ruled out, endometritis, pyelonephritis in particular
  - Mother should get increased rest; use acetaminophen (Tylenol) as necessary.
  - Fever should resolve within 48 hours or consider changing antibiotics. Lump should also resolve. If it continues, an abscess may be present, requiring surgical drainage.
- Milk supply inadequate:
  - Check infant weight gain.
  - Review signs of adequate supply; technique, frequency, and duration of nursing.
  - Check to see if mother has been supplementing with formula, thereby decreasing her own milk production.
- Sore nipples:
  - Check technique
  - Baby should be taken off the breast by breaking the suction with a finger in the mouth.
  - Air-dry nipples after each nursing and/or coat with expressed breast milk.
  - Do not wash nipples with soap and water.
  - Check for signs of thrush in baby and on mother's nipple. If affected, treat both.
- Engorgement:
  - Usually develops after milk first comes in (day 3 or 4 postpartum)
  - Signs are warm, hard, sore breasts.
  - To resolve, offer baby more frequent nursing:
    - May have to hand express a little milk to soften areola enough to let baby latch on
    - Breastfeed long enough to empty breasts.
  - Generally resolves within a day or 2

REFERENCES

1. http://www.aap.org/advocacy/releases/feb05breastfeeding.htm.
2. *Breastfeeding and Maternal and Infant Health Outcomes in Developed Countries [Structured Abstract]*. Rockville, MD: Agency for Healthcare Research and Quality, 2007. Available at: http://www.ahrq.gov/clinic/tp/brfouttp.htm.
3. http://www.cdc.gov/breastfeeding/pdf/BreastfeedingReportCard2010.pdf.
4. Berlin CM, Briggs GG. Drugs and chemicals in human milk. *Semin Fetal Neonatal Med*. 2005;10:149–59.
5. Sinusas K, Gagliardi A. Initial management of breast-feeding. *Am Fam Phys*. 2001;15;64:981–8.
6. Wagner CL, Greer FR; Section on Breastfeeding and Committee on Nutrition. Prevention of rickets and vitamin D deficiency in infants, children, and adolescents. *Pediatrics*. 2008;122(5);1142–1152.
7. Greer FR; Committee on Nutrition American Academy of Pediatrics. Diagnosis and prevention of iron deficiency and iron-deficiency anemia in infants and young children (0-3 years of age). *Pediatrics*. 2010;126(5):1040–50.
8. Chung M, Raman G, Trikalinos T, et al. Interventions in primary care to promote breastfeeding: An evidence review for the U.S. Preventive Services Task Force. *Ann Intern Med*. 2008;149:565–82.
9. http://www.llli.org/ba/Aug93.html.
10. http://www.cdc.gov/mmwr/preview/mmwrhtml/rr5904a2.htm.
11. Jahanfar S, Ng CJ, Teng CL, et al. Antibiotics for mastitis in breastfeeding women. *Cochrane Database Syst Rev*. 2009;CD005458.

ADDITIONAL READING

- Casey CF, Slawson DC, Neal LR, et al. VItamin D supplementation in infants, children, and adolescents. *Am Fam Physician*. 2010;81:745–8.
- Cramton R, Zain-Ul-Abideen M, Whalen B, et al. Optimizing successful breastfeeding in the newborn. *Curr Opin Pediatr*. 2009;21:386–96.
- Grummer-Strawn LM, Shealy KR, et al. Progress in protecting, promoting, and supporting breastfeeding: 1984–2009. *Breastfeed Med*. 2009;4(Suppl 1):S31–9.

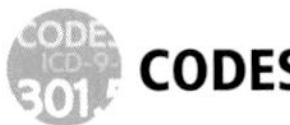

CODES

ICD9

V24.1 Postpartum care and examination of lactating mother

CLINICAL PEARLS

- Breast milk is the optimal food for infants, with myriad health benefits for mothers and children.
- USPSTF recommends regular, structured education during pregnancy to promote breastfeeding.
- Vitamin D and iron supplementation should begin at birth and 4 months of age, respectively, for exclusively breastfed infants.

BREECH BIRTH

Erin Marchand, MD
Jerry Michael Cline, MD

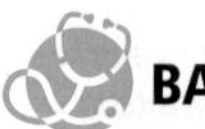

BASICS

DESCRIPTION

At time of delivery, the buttocks or lower limbs are the presenting fetal part:

- Frank breech: Fetal hips flexed and knees extended with feet near the face. Buttocks presents first (40–60% of breech presentations at term)
- Footling or incomplete breech: Foot or knee presents first (25–35%)
- Complete breech: Hips and knees flexed. Feet and buttocks present together (5–15%)

EPIDEMIOLOGY

Prevalence

Early gestational age is highly associated with breech presentation and risk decreases as gestational age advances:

- 22% of fetuses prior to 28 weeks are breech
- 3–4% of singleton term fetuses

RISK FACTORS

- Early gestational age is #1 risk factor
- History of breech birth
- Low-birth-weight infant
- Fetal anomalies (9% of term breech and 17% of preterm breech)
- Oligohydramnios, polyhydramnios
- Grand multiparity, multiple gestation
- Uterine anomalies, fibroids, bicornuate uterus, pelvic tumors
- Pelvic contractures or irregularly shaped pelvis, such as android or platypelloid
- Little evidence to support abnormal placentation (placenta previa, cornual-fundal) as a risk factor

Genetics

Fetal anomalies including anencephaly, head or neck tumors, hydrocephalus, trisomy 21 and 18, Potter syndrome, myotonic dystrophy

GENERAL PREVENTION

- Prenatal folate therapy to decrease risk of neural tube defects
- Tight first trimester glucose control in diabetics
- Prenatal screening to diagnose chromosomal or fetal anomalies
- Routine assessment of fetal presentation at 36 weeks to afford time for trial of external cephalic version

COMMONLY ASSOCIATED CONDITIONS

- Increased risk of cord prolapse (0.4% in cephalic presentation, compared to 0.5% in frank breech, 4–6% in complete breech, and 15–18% in footling breech)
- Congenital hip dislocation has higher incidence in infants with breech presentation at term.

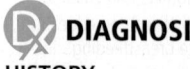

DIAGNOSIS

HISTORY

- Often asymptomatic and discovered on exam or US
- Often found emergently in PPROM
- May be discovered late in labor

PHYSICAL EXAM

- Anus/buttocks/genitals/feet palpable on vaginal exam
- Leopold maneuver or US reveals head in fundal region
- Terminal meconium found during vaginal exam after rupture of membranes

DIAGNOSTIC TESTS & INTERPRETATION

Imaging

Initial approach

US confirms presenting part. Can also potentially reveal fetal anomalies and be used to determine the attitude of the fetal head (flexed, neutral, or extended).

Diagnostic Procedures/Surgery

- All women should be examined at 36 weeks to determine fetal lie. In some practices, US is routinely done at 36 weeks to verify cephalic presentation.
- In breech presentation, the greater trochanters and anus form a straight line. In facial presentation, the malar bones and mouth form a triangle.

DIFFERENTIAL DIAGNOSIS

Facial, compound, asynclitic presentation on vaginal exam

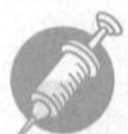

TREATMENT

ADDITIONAL TREATMENT

General Measures

- The options of external cephalic version (ECV), elective trial of labor (TOL), or elective C-section should be discussed with the patient:
  - Favorable characteristics for successful ECV may include: Adequate AFI, normal EFW, normal BMI, multiparity, adequate anesthesia (e.g., spinal/epidural), use of terbutaline prior to trial of ECV.
  - Favorable characteristics for successful TOL may include: Multiparity, estimated fetal weight of current fetus less than that of previous infant who delivered vaginally, flexed/neutral position of fetal head
- Continuous electronic fetal monitoring during labor
- Cord gasses should be obtained following delivery, whether vaginal or by C-section.
- The Term Breech Trial was a large international, multicenter randomized clinical trial published in 2000, comparing a policy of planned C-section with planned vaginal delivery (1).
  - Perinatal mortality, neonatal mortality, and serious neonatal morbidity were significantly lower in the planned C-section group compared to the vaginal delivery group (1.6% compared to 5%) with no difference in maternal morbidity or mortality (1)[B].
  - A 2-year follow-up study showing no significant difference in the risk of death or neurodevelopmental delay between the 2 modes of delivery (2)[B].
  - These later findings, with several other recent studies, bring into question the routine practice of planned C-section for breech presentation.
- Currently, several international obstetrical societies are advocating the consideration of TOL for appropriate candidates when skilled staff is present and the hospital has appropriate institutional guidelines for management of vaginal breech delivery.
  - With careful case selection and labor management, perinatal mortality occurs in ~0.2% and serious short-term neonatal morbidity in ~2% of breech births (3)[A].
  - Planned vaginal delivery is reasonable in selected women with a term singleton breech fetus (3)[A].
- ACOG 2006 Opinion on Mode of Term Singleton Breech Delivery recommends (4):
  - Obstetricians should offer and perform ECV whenever possible (5)[A]
  - Decision for delivery mode should depend on the experience of the health care provider. Cesarean delivery will be the preferred mode of delivery for most physicians because of the diminishing expertise in vaginal breech delivery.
  - Planned vaginal delivery of a term singleton breech fetus may be reasonable under hospital-specific protocol guidelines for both eligibility and labor management.
  - There are no recent data to support recommendation of cesarean delivery to patients whose second twin is in a nonvertex presentation, although a large multicenter randomized controlled trial is in progress.

Additional Therapies

ECV should be offered to all women with breech presentation after 36 weeks (5,6)[B]:

- Fetal assessment before and after the procedure is recommended.
- Success rate ranges from 35–86% (average 58%), depending on provider skill and patient characteristics.
- RhoGHAM should be given to all Rh-negative mothers prior to attempted ECV.
- Use of tocolytics and epidural anesthesia is associated with an increased rate of successful version, especially in nulliparas.
- ECV should only be attempted in settings where emergency cesarean delivery services are available.
- Contraindications to ECV (vary depending on the institution) include: Any contraindication to TOL (e.g., classic cesarean scar, placenta previa, active HSV), abnormal FHR tracing, major uterine anomaly, ruptured membranes, multiple pregnancy, major fetal anomaly, evidence of uteroplacental insufficiency (IUGR, oligohydramnios).
- Nulliparity, advanced dilation, fetal weight <2,500g, anterior placenta, and low station are all thought to be poor predictors of successful ECV, but no studies have validated this assumption.

SURGERY/OTHER PROCEDURES

Breech delivery is accomplished either vaginally or by C-section.

- C-section:
  - Elective C-section is usually planned for the 39th week of pregnancy.
  - Delivery is typically accomplished via low transverse uterine incision

- Vaginal delivery—labor management:
  - Consultation with a provider experienced in breech vaginal delivery should be obtained. Health care professionals skilled in neonatal resuscitation and C-section should be in attendance at the time of delivery.
  - Pre- or early-labor US should be performed to assess type of breech presentation, estimated fetal weight, and attitude of fetal head. A flexed head is reassuring against anterior neck mass, which could cause fetal head entrapment. If US is not available, C-section is recommended.
  - Clinical pelvic examination should be performed to rule out pathological pelvic contraction. Radiologic pelvimetry is not recommended. Good progress in labor is the best indicator of adequate fetal-pelvic proportions.
  - When membranes rupture, immediate vaginal examination is recommended to rule out cord prolapse.
  - In the absence of adequate progress in labor, C-section is advised.
  - Induction of labor is usually not recommended for breech presentation.
  - Oxytocin augmentation is acceptable in the presence of labor dystocia.
  - A passive second stage without active pushing for up to 90 minutes allows the breech to descend well into the pelvis. Once active pushing commences, if delivery is not imminent after 60 minutes, C-section is recommended.
  - The active second stage of labor should take place in or near an operating room with equipment and personnel available to perform a timely C-section if necessary.
- Vaginal delivery—delivery techniques:
  - The delivering provider should have a rehearsed plan of action with the delivery team, especially the critical stage of delivering the fetal head.
  - Avoid pulling traction on the fetus. Instead, support the body and, if necessary, use side-to-side gentle rotation to assist with body descent.
  - Effective maternal pushing efforts are essential to safe delivery and should be encouraged once delivery is imminent.
  - Maintain fetal body temperature with warm towels while body is exposed and head has not yet delivered.
  - When umbilicus is delivered, gently reduce 3–4 cm of umbilical cord to avoid cord traction. The neonatal provider should palpate umbilical cord pulse and communicate fetal heart rate to team, as Doppler tones become very difficult to obtain at this point.
  - Nuchal arms may be delivered by the Løvset or Bickenback maneuvers.
  - At the time of delivery of the after-coming head, an assistant should be present to apply suprapubic pressure to favor flexion and engagement of the fetal head.
  - For the rare circumstance of a trapped after-coming head or irreducible nuchal arms, nitroglycerine or general anesthesia with isoflurane to relax the uterus, generous episiotomy, pubic symphysiotomy, or emergency abdominal rescue can be life saving.
  - The fetal head often delivers spontaneously with the assistance of suprapubic pressure, by Mauriceau-Smellie-Veit maneuver, or with the assistance of piper forceps.
- Contraindications to vaginal breech delivery:
  - Any presentation other than a frank or complete breech (e.g., footling breech or cord presentation)
  - Fetal growth restriction or macrosomia (<2,500 g or >4,000 g)
  - Any fetal head attitude other than flexed or neutral
  - Inadequate maternal pelvis
  - Any usual contraindication to vaginal delivery such as some fetal anomalies

IN-PATIENT CONSIDERATIONS

Admission Criteria

Admit to labor and delivery for rupture of membranes, labor, or elective C-section

IV Fluids

Maintain IV access and hydration status with lactated Ringer's or normal saline solution.

Discharge Criteria

Postpartum stay is generally 1–4 days depending on method of delivery

ONGOING CARE

FOLLOW-UP RECOMMENDATIONS

Bilateral hip US of the neonate at 6 weeks of life to rule out developmental dysplasia of the hip.

Patient Monitoring

Continuous electronic fetal monitoring during labor and continuous measurement of maternal pulse, ideally displayed on the same graph.

DIET

NPO prior to delivery

PATIENT EDUCATION

- In the absence of a contraindication to vaginal delivery, a woman with a breech presentation should be informed of the risks and benefits of a trial of labor vs. elective C-section, and informed consent should be obtained.
- Theoretical and hands-on breech birth training simulation should be a part of basic obstetrical skills training programs such as Advanced Life Support in Obstetrics (ALSO) to prepare health providers for unexpected vaginal breech births.

PROGNOSIS

- Successful ECV at term significantly lowers cesarean rate.
- For infants <1,500 g or <32 weeks gestational age, a higher rate of cerebral hemorrhage and perinatal death is associated with vaginal compared to cesarean delivery. This is due, in large part, to delivery of the fetal body through an incompletely dilated cervix and subsequent entrapment of fetal head.
- Careful case selection and labor management in a modern obstetrical setting may achieve a level of safety similar to elective C-section (4)[B].
- Planned C-section is not associated with a reduction in risk of death or neurodevelopmental delay.

COMPLICATIONS

- Complications associated with breech presentation:
  - Fetal asphyxia secondary to cord prolapse or compression
  - Congenital hip dislocation
- Complications of ECV:
  - Abnormal FHR pattern (5.7%), persisting pathological FHR pattern (0.37%), vaginal bleeding (0.47%), placental abruption (0.12%), perinatal mortality (0.16%), emergency C-section (0.43%) (6)[B].
- Complications of vaginal delivery:
  - Trauma to the head, soft tissue, brachial plexus, and spinal cord; not always prevented by C-section
  - Entrapment of fetal head
- Complications of C-section:
  - Bleeding, infection, damage to maternal bowel or bladder, increased risk of placenta previa or accreta in future pregnancies, and hysterectomy.
  - Increased risk of maternal mortality compared to vaginal delivery
  - Maternal recovery time is often longer following a C-section

REFERENCES

1. Hannah ME, Hannah WJ, Hewson SA, et al. Planned caesarean section versus planned vaginal birth for breech presentation at term: A randomised multicentre trial. Term Breech Trial Collaborative Group. *Lancet*. 2000;356:1375–83.
2. Whyte H, Hannah ME, Saroj S, et al. Outcomes of children at 2 years after planned cesarean birth versus planned vaginal birth for breech presentation at term: The international randomized Term Breech Trial. *Am J Obstet Gynecol*. 2004;191(3):864–71.
3. The Society of Obstetricians and Gynaecologists of Canada. Vaginal Delivery of Breech Presentation Clinical Practice Guideline No. 226. June 2009.
4. American College of Obstetricians and Gynecologists, Committee on Obstetric Practice. ACOG committee opinion. Mode of term singleton breech delivery. Practice Bulletin No. 340. July, 2006. American College of Obstetricians and Gynecologists.
5. American College of Obstetricians and Gynecologists. External cephalic version. Practice Bulletin No. 13. February, 2000.
6. Collaris RJ, Oei SG. External cephalic version: a safe procedure? A systematic review of version-related risks. *ACTA Obstetricia et Gynecologia Scandinavica*. 2004;83(6):511–8.

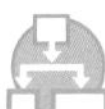

See Also (Topic, Algorithm, Electronic Media Element)

Placenta Previa; Preterm Labor

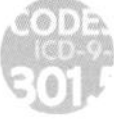

CODES

ICD9

- 652.10 Breech or other malpresentation successfully converted to cephalic presentation, unspecified as to episode of care or not applicable
- 652.11 Breech or other malpresentation successfully converted to cephalic presentation, delivered, with or without mention of antepartum condition
- 652.13 Breech or other malpresentation successfully converted to cephalic presentation, antepartum condition or complication

CLINICAL PEARLS

- External cephalic version should be offered to all women without contraindications with a breech presentation, ideally at 37 weeks.
- Planned vaginal delivery by an experienced provider is reasonable in selected women with a term singleton fetus using a specific protocol for labor and delivery management.
- Long-term outcomes of neonatal death or neurodevelopmental delay are not reduced by planned C-section.

BRONCHIECTASIS

Dylan C. Kwait, MD

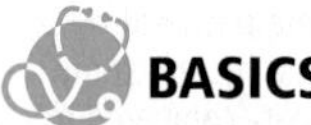

BASICS

DESCRIPTION

- Bronchiectasis is an irreversible dilation of 1 or more airways accompanied by recurrent transmural bronchial infection/inflammation and chronic mucopurulent sputum production.
- Generally classified into cystic fibrosis (CF) and noncystic fibrosis (non-CF) bronchiectasis.

EPIDEMIOLOGY

- Predominant age: Most commonly presents in sixth decade of life (1)
- Predominant sex: Female > Male (1)

Incidence

Incidence has decreased in the US for 2 reasons:

- Widespread childhood vaccination against pertussis (2)
- Effective treatment of childhood respiratory infections with antibiotics (1)

Prevalence

- Prevalence in adult US population estimated to be >110,000 affected individuals (1)
- Internationally, prevalence increases with age from 4.2 per 100,000 persons aged 18–34 years to 271.8 per 100,000 among those aged 75 years or older (3).

RISK FACTORS

- Nontuberculous mycobacterial infection is both a cause and a complication of non-CF bronchiectasis (4).
- Severe respiratory infection in childhood (measles, adenovirus, influenza, pertussis, or bronchiolitis)
- Systemic diseases (e.g., rheumatoid arthritis and connective tissue disorders)
- Chronic rhinosinusitis
- Recurrent pneumonia
- Aspirated foreign body
- Immunodeficiency

GENERAL PREVENTION

- Routine immunizations against pertussis, measles, *Haemophilus influenza* type B, influenza, and pneumococcal pneumonia
- Genetic counseling where congenital condition may increase likelihood of bronchiectasis
- Smoking cessation counseling

PATHOPHYSIOLOGY

Vicious circle hypothesis: Transmural infection, generally by bacterial organisms, causes inflammation and obstruction of airways. Damaged airways and dysfunctional cilia foster bacterial colonization, which leads to further inflammation and obstruction (2)[A].

ETIOLOGY

- CF bronchiectasis: Bronchiectasis due to CF
- Non-CF bronchiectasis:
  - Most cases are idiopathic.
  - Most commonly associated with non-CF bronchiectasis is childhood infection (2).

COMMONLY ASSOCIATED CONDITIONS

- Mucociliary clearance defects:
  - Primary ciliary dyskinesia
  - Young syndrome (secondary ciliary dyskinesia)
  - Kartagener syndrome
- Other congenital conditions:
  - α1-Antitrypsin deficiency
  - Marfan syndrome
  - Cartilage deficiency (Williams-Campbell syndrome)
- Chronic obstructive pulmonary disease
- Postinfectious conditions:
  - Bacteria (*H. influenzae* and *Pseudomonas aeruginosa*)
  - Mycobacterial infections (tuberculosis [TB] and *Mycobacterium avium* complex [MAC])
  - Whooping cough
  - *Aspergillus* species
  - Viral (HIV, adenovirus, measles, influenza virus)
- Immunodeficient conditions:
  - Primary: Hypogammaglobulinemia
  - Secondary: Allergic bronchopulmonary aspergillosis, posttransplantation
- Sequelae of toxic inhalation or aspiration (e.g., chlorine, luminal foreign body)
- Rheumatic/chronic inflammatory conditions:
  - Rheumatoid arthritis
  - Sjögren syndrome
  - Systemic lupus erythematosus
  - Inflammatory bowel disease
- Miscellaneous:
  - Yellow nail syndrome

DIAGNOSIS

- Typical symptoms include chronic productive cough, wheezing, and dyspnea.
- Symptoms are often accompanied by repeated respiratory infections (5).
- Once diagnosed, investigation of possible causes and associated conditions is essential.

HISTORY

- Time course of illness
- Any predisposing factors (congenital, infectious, and/or exposure-related)
- Immunization history

PHYSICAL EXAM

Symptoms are commonly present for many years and include the following (1,2):

- Chronic cough (90%)
- Sputum may be copious and purulent (90%).
- Rhinosinusitis (60–70%)
- Fatigue may be a dominant symptom (70%).
- Dyspnea (75%)
- Chest pain may be pleuritic (20–30%).
- Hemoptysis ((20–30%)
- Wheezing (20%)
- Bibasilar crackles (60%)
- Rhonchi (44%)
- Digital clubbing (3%)

DIAGNOSTIC TESTS & INTERPRETATION

- Spirometry:
  - Limited use in diagnosis
  - Characterized by moderate airflow obstruction and hyperresponsive airways (1)
  - FEV1: <80% predicted and FEV1/FVC <0.7 (6)
- Special tests:
  - Ciliary biopsy by electron microscopy

Lab

- Sputum culture (1):
  - *H. influenzae*, nontypeable form (42%)
  - *P. aeruginosa* (18%)
  - Cultures may also be positive for *S. pneumoniae*, *Moraxella catarrhalis*, MAC, and *Aspergillus*.
  - Of all isolates, 30–40% will show no growth.
- Special tests:
  - Sweat test for CF
  - PPD test for TB
  - Skin test for *Aspergillus*
  - HIV
  - Serum immunoglobulins to test for humoral immunodeficiency

Imaging

- Chest radiograph:
  - Nonspecific findings; sensitivity and specificity are too low to confirm the diagnosis (6).
  - Increased lung markings (1)
  - May appear normal
- Chest CT:
  - Noncontrast high-resolution chest CT is the most important diagnostic tool (2).
  - Bronchi are dilated and do not taper.
  - Varicose constrictions and balloon cysts may also be appreciated (2).

Diagnostic Procedures/Surgery

Interventional bronchoscopy may be used to obtain cultures and evacuate sputum.

Pathological Findings

Bronchoscopy findings include the following (2):

- Dilation of airways
- Thickened bronchial walls with necrosis of bronchial mucosa
- Peribronchial scarring

DIFFERENTIAL DIAGNOSIS

- CF
- Chronic obstructive pulmonary disease
- Asthma
- Chronic bronchitis
- Pulmonary TB
- Allergic bronchopulmonary aspergillosis

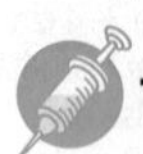

TREATMENT

- Non-CF bronchiectasis: Determining cause of exacerbations, promoting good bronchopulmonary hygiene via daily airway clearance, and surgical resection of damaged lung if necessary
- Medical management: Reduce morbidity by controlling symptoms and preventing disease progression.
- Patients with non-CF bronchiectasis may not respond to CF treatment regimens in the same way as patients with CF do (4)[A].

MEDICATION

- There is insufficient evidence in the current literature to make reasonable conclusions about the efficacy of short-course antibiotics in the management of adults and children with bronchiectasis (7)[A].
- Frequent exacerbations may be treated with prolonged and aerosolized antibiotics (5)[A].
- The role of mucolytics, anti-inflammatory agents, and bronchodilators is still unclear (5)[A].

First Line
- Antibiotics:
  - Potentially useful in acute exacerbations
  - Chronic therapy decreases sputum volume and purulence, but it does not diminish the frequency of exacerbations (8)[A].
  - Patients may require twice the usual dose and longer treatment (7–14 days) (6)[B].
  - Sputum culture and sensitivity should direct therapy; antibiotic selection is complicated by a wide range of pathogens and resistant organisms.
  - Should be administered IV in cases of severe infection:
    - Augmentin (6)[B]: 500 mg PO q8–12h for 7–10 days. Pediatric: Base dosing on amoxicillin content.
    - Trimethoprim/sulfamethoxazole (6)[B]: 160 mg TMP/800 mg SMX PO q12h for 10–14 days. Pediatric: $\geq$2 months, 8 mg/kg TMP and 40 mg/kg SMX PO per 24 hours, administered in 2 divided doses q12h for 10 days
    - Doxycycline and cefaclor given PO are also effective (6)[B].
    - Nebulized aminoglycosides (tobramycin): 300 mg by aerosol b.i.d. (9)[B]
    - Macrolides: Appear to have immunomodulatory benefits (1)[A]
- Bronchodilators:
  - Chronic use of β_2–agonists (e.g., albuterol) reverses airflow obstruction (1)[A].
- Inhaled corticosteroids:
  - There is insufficient evidence to recommend use of inhaled steroids in adults with stable-state bronchiectasis (10)[A].
  - A therapeutic trial of inhaled steroids may be justified in adults with difficult-to-control symptoms and in certain subgroups (10)[A].
  - Decrease sputum and tend to improve lung function (6)[B]:
    - Fluticasone: 110–220 μg inhaled b.i.d.

Second Line
Other broad-spectrum antimicrobials, including antipseudomonals

ADDITIONAL TREATMENT
General Measures
- Dry powder mannitol improves tracheobronchial clearance (1)[A].
- Maintain hydration (nebulized saline may be used) (2)[A].
- Noninvasive positive-pressure ventilation (2)[A]

Issues for Referral
May require pulmonologist for bronchoscopy and/or long-term management

Additional Therapies
Sputum clearance techniques, including physiotherapy (percussion and postural drainage) and pulmonary rehabilitation (improves exercise tolerance) (1)[A]

SURGERY/OTHER PROCEDURES
- Surgery if area of bronchiectasis is localized and symptoms remain intolerable despite medical therapy or if disease is life threatening (5)[A]
- Surgery effectively improves symptoms in 80% of these cases (1)[A].

IN-PATIENT CONSIDERATIONS
For non-CF bronchiectasis, determine cause of exacerbations, promoting good bronchopulmonary hygiene via daily airway clearance, and surgical resection when necessary.

Initial Stabilization
Hemoptysis, although rare, may occur and can be life threatening.

ONGOING CARE

Long-term outpatient treatment recommendations for bronchiectasis in children (11)[B]:
- Children with CF- and non–CF-related bronchiectasis should be treated by comprehensive interdisciplinary chronic disease management programs.
- Pathogen-directed aerosolized tobramycin treatment should be used long term on a regular basis to improve the course of CF-related bronchiectasis.
- Oral macrolide antibiotic use short term (up to 6 months) improves lung function among children with CF-related bronchiectasis.
- Long-term antibiotic use (oral or aerosolized) in children with non–CF-related bronchiectasis has not been studied enough to warrant routine use.
- Hypertonic saline administered by inhalation used long term (48 weeks) improves lung function and is safer when used with pretreatment bronchodilator therapy among children who have CF.
- Nebulized dornase improves multiple pulmonary outcomes of children who have CF and is indicated for long-term use.
- The risks for long-term oral corticosteroid use outweigh pulmonary benefits in the treatment of CF-related bronchiectasis.
- High-dose ibuprofen therapy reduces the rate of decline among children with mild CF-related bronchiectasis and is indicated for long-term use.
- Mucolytic agents, airway hydrating treatments, anti-inflammatory therapy, CPT, and bronchodilator therapy have not been studied sufficiently long term in children with non–CF-related bronchiectasis to merit their routine use.

FOLLOW-UP RECOMMENDATIONS
Regular exercise is recommended.

Patient Monitoring
- Serial spirometry, every 2–5 years, to monitor the course of the disease (1)[A]
- Routine microbiological sputum analysis (1)[A]

PATIENT EDUCATION
American Lung Association, 1740 Broadway, New York, NY 10019; (212) 315-8700, http://www.lungusa.org

PROGNOSIS
- The mortality rate (death due directly to bronchiectasis) is 13% (1).
- *Pseudomonas* infection is associated with poorer prognosis (1).

COMPLICATIONS
- Hemoptysis
- Recurrent pulmonary infections
- Pulmonary hypertension
- Cor pulmonale
- Lung abscess

REFERENCES

1. King P, Holdsworth S, Freezer N. Bronchiectasis. *Intern Med J*. 2006;36:729–37.
2. Barker AF. Bronchiectasis. *N Engl J Med*. 2002;346:1383–93.
3. Pappalettera M, Aliberti S, Castellotti P, et al. Bronchiectasis: an update. *Clin Respir J*. 2009;3:126–34.
4. Bilton D. Update on non-cystic fibrosis bronchiectasis. *Curr Opin Pulm Med*. 2008;14:595–9.
5. ten Hacken NH, Wijkstra PJ, Kerstjens HA. Treatment of bronchiectasis in adults. *BMJ*. 2007;335:1089–93.
6. Bradley J, Lavery K, Rendall J. Managing bronchiectasis. *Practitioner*. 2006;250:194, 197, 199–200 passim.
7. Wurzel D, Marchant JM, Yerkovich ST, et al. Short courses of antibiotics for children and adults with bronchiectasis. *Cochrane Database Sys Rev*. 2011;CD008695.
8. Evans DJ, Bara AI, Greenstone M. Prolonged antibiotics for purulent bronchiectasis. *Cochrane Database Sys Rev*. 2006;4:CD00284.
9. Lobue PA. Inhaled tobramycin: Not just for cystic fibrosis anymore? *Chest*. 2005;127:1098–101.
10. Kapur N, Bell S, Kolbe J. Inhaled steroids for bronchiectasis. *Cochrane Database Sys Rev*. 2009:CD000996.
11. Redding GJ. Bronchiectasis in children. *Pediatr Clin North Am*. 2009;56:157–71, xi.

ADDITIONAL READING

Pasteur MC, Bilton D, Hill AT, et al. British Thoracic Society guideline for non-CF bronchiectasis. *Thorax*. 2010;65(Suppl 1):i1–58.

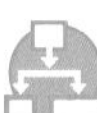

See Also (Topic, Algorithm, Electronic Media Element)

Cystic Fibrosis; Chronic Obstructive Pulmonary Disease and Emphysema; Asthma; Tuberculosis; Aspergillosis; Kartagener Syndrome

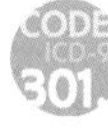

CODES

ICD9
- 494.0 Bronchiectasis without acute exacerbation
- 494.1 Bronchiectasis with acute exacerbation
- 748.61 Congenital bronchiectasis

CLINICAL PEARLS

- Symptoms of bronchiectasis include chronic productive cough, wheezing, and dyspnea, often accompanied by repeated respiratory infections.
- A chest x-ray has poor sensitivity and specificity for the diagnosis; a noncontrast high-resolution chest CT is the most important diagnostic tool.
- Current practice guidelines recommend treating acute exacerbations with short courses of antibiotics, even though the evidence is currently insufficient to support this strategy; frequent exacerbations may be treated with prolonged and aerosolized antibiotics.

BRONCHIOLITIS

Dennis E. Hughes, DO

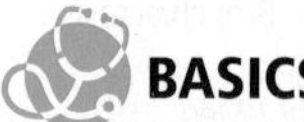

BASICS

DESCRIPTION

- Inflammation and obstruction of small airways and reactive airways generally affecting infants and young children
- May be seasonal (November–April) and often occurs in epidemics
- Usual course: Insidious, acute, progressive
- Leading cause of hospitalizations in infants and children
- Predominant age: Newborn–2 years (peak age <6 months). Neonates are not protected despite transfer of maternal antibody
- Predominant sex: Male > Female

EPIDEMIOLOGY

Incidence

- 21% in North America
- 18.8% (90,000 annually) of all pediatric hospitalizations (excluding live births) in children <2 years of age
- Incidence increasing since 1980

RISK FACTORS

- Smoking exposure
- Low birth weight
- Immunodeficiency
- Formula feeding (not breastfed)
- Contact with infected person (primary mode of spread)
- Children in daycare environment
- Heart-lung transplantation patient (immune compromise)
- Adults: Exposure to toxic fumes, connective tissue disease (respiratory epithelial damage)

GENERAL PREVENTION

- Hand washing
- Contact isolation of infected babies
- Persons with colds should keep contact with infants to a minimum
- Palivizumab (Synagis), a monoclonal product, administered monthly, October–May, 15 mg/kg IM; used for respiratory syncytial virus prevention in high-risk patients (1):
  - 32–35-week gestation and <3 months old at the start of RSV season with at least 1 risk factor: Either attending daycare or with a sibling <5 years old at home
  - 28–32-weeks gestation and <6 months old
  - <28 weeks gestation and <12 months old
  - Moderately severe bronchopulmonary dysplasia and up to 2 years old
  - Hemodynamically significant congenital heart disease (until age 6 months)
  - Once begun, continue through end of season regardless of age attained.
- Respiratory syncytial virus immunoglobulin, a human blood product, can also be used in at-risk patients. Monthly infusions of 750 mg/kg, October–May

PATHOPHYSIOLOGY

- Infection results in necrosis and lysis of epithelial cells and subsequent release of inflammatory mediators.
- Edema and mucus secretion which, combined with accumulating necrotic debris and loss of cilia clearance, results in luminal obstruction.
- Ventilation-perfusion mismatching resulting in hypoxia
- Air trapping is due to dynamic airways narrowing during expiration, which increases work of breathing

ETIOLOGY

Respiratory syncytial virus accounts for 70–85% of all cases, but parainfluenza virus, adenovirus, rhinovirus, influenza virus, *Mycoplasma pneumoniae*, and *Chlamydophila pneumoniae* have all been implicated.

Pediatric Considerations

Prior infection does not seem to confer subsequent immunity.

COMMONLY ASSOCIATED CONDITIONS

- Upper respiratory congestion
- Conjunctivitis
- Pharyngitis
- Otitis media
- Diarrhea

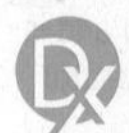

DIAGNOSIS

Consensus is that history and physical examination should be the basis for the diagnosis of bronchiolitis (2).

HISTORY

- Irritability
- Anorexia
- Fever
- Noisy breathing (due to rhinorrhea)
- Cough
- Grunting
- Cyanosis
- Apnea
- Vomiting

PHYSICAL EXAM

- Tachypnea
- Retractions
- Rhinorrhea
- Wheezing
- Upper respiratory findings: Pharyngitis, conjunctivitis, otitis

DIAGNOSTIC TESTS & INTERPRETATION

Routine laboratory and other ancillary testing not warranted

Lab

Initial lab tests

- Arterial oxygen saturation by pulse oximetry (<94% significant)
- Rapid respiratory viral antigen testing (not usually necessary during respiratory syncytial virus [RSV] season because the disease is managed symptomatically, but may be useful for epidemiologic, hospital cohorting, or in the very young to reduce unnecessary other work-up)
  - Sensitivity 87–91%; specificity 96–100% (2)

Imaging

Initial approach

Chest x-ray (CXR):

- Increased anteroposterior diameter
- Flattened diaphragm
- Air trapping
- Patchy infiltrates
- Focal atelectasis: Right upper lobe common
- Peribronchial cuffing

Pathological Findings

- Abundant mucous exudate
- Mucosal: Hyperemia, edema
- Submucosal lymphocytic infiltrate, monocytic infiltrate, plasmacytic infiltrate
- Small airway debris, fibrin, inflammatory exudate, fibrosis
- Peribronchiolar mononuclear infiltrate

DIFFERENTIAL DIAGNOSIS

- Other pulmonary infections such as pertussis, croup, or bacterial pneumonia
- Aspiration
- Vascular ring
- Foreign body
- Asthma
- Heart failure
- Gastroesophageal reflux
- Cystic fibrosis

TREATMENT

Mainstay of therapy is supportive to prevent hypoxia and dehydration.

MEDICATION

First Line

- Oxygen
- Nebulized albuterol (0.15 mg/kg) is often tried for acute symptoms; a trial of therapy may be reasonable in the presence of a bronchospastic component, but no benefit noted in several high-quality studies (3)[B]
- Epinephrine aerosols (0.5 mL of 2.25% solution in 3 mL NS) also may be tried. Benefit remains unproved, but some studies support short-term improvement in outpatient settings (4,5)[B].
- Corticosteroids:
  - Oral dexamethasone (1 mg/kg loading dose, then 0.6 mg/kg b.i.d. for 5 days) reduced subsequent hospitalization. A recent multiple-center trial found no difference in admission rates or respiratory assessment scores in children treated with 1 mg/kg dexamethasone (6)[B].
  - Nebulized dexamethasone (2–4 mg in 3 mL NS) may have anecdotal benefit; studies show mixed results.

Second Line

- Antibiotics only if secondary bacterial infection present (rare) (7)[B]
- Heliox therapy (70% helium–30% oxygen) may be of benefit early in moderate-to-severe bronchiolitis to reduce amount of respiratory distress, but Cochrane review found little evidence of sustained benefit at 24 hours (8).
- Ribavirin (palivizumab):
  - Updated AAP guidelines for use (for prevention in high-risk children)
  - Inhaled antiviral agent active against RSV
  - Nebulize via small-particle aerosol generator.
  - Pregnant women should not be exposed.

ADDITIONAL TREATMENT

- Nebulized hypertonic (3%) saline has recently been studied and may decease LOS in hospitalized patients (5).
- Positive-pressure ventilation (PPV) in the form of CPAP can be used in cases of respiratory failure. There is limited clinical evidence other than observational studies (5).
- Leukotriene receptor antagonists currently show no sustained benefit (5).

IN-PATIENT CONSIDERATIONS

Bronchiolitis can be associated with apnea in children <6 weeks of age.

Initial Stabilization

Supplemental oxygen for pulse oximetry <94% on room air

Admission Criteria

- Respiratory rate >45/min with respiratory distress or apnea
- Hypoxia is common; evidence-based cut-off requiring admission is not available (only D-level expert opinion), so clinical criteria are more helpful (pulse oximetry <94% used by many as cutoff).
- Ill or toxic appearance
- Underlying heart, respiratory condition, or immune suppression
- High risk for apnea (<30 days of age, preterm birth [<37 weeks]) (7)[B]
- Dehydrated or unable to feed
- Uncertain home care
- Use of Respiratory Distress Assessment Instrument may aid in determining admission vs. discharge. Scoring based on quantification and quality of wheezes, retractions, and respiratory rate (6).

IV Fluids

Indicated only if tachypnea precludes oral feeding. Weight-based maintenance rate plus insensible losses.

Discharge Criteria

Normal respiratory rate and no oxygen requirement. Recent small studies suggest that after a period of observation, children can be safely discharged on home oxygen.

ONGOING CARE

FOLLOW-UP RECOMMENDATIONS

Patient Monitoring

- Hospitalization is usually only required if oxygen is a requirement or unable to feed/drink.
- For a hospitalized patient, monitor as needed depending on the severity of the infection.
- If the patient is receiving home care, follow daily by telephone for 2–4 days; the patient may need frequent office visits.

PATIENT EDUCATION

- American Academy of Pediatrics: http://www.aap.org
- American Academy of Family Physicians: http://www.familydoctor.org

PROGNOSIS

- In most cases, recovery is complete within 7–14 days.
- Mortality statistics differ, but probably <1%
- High-risk infants (bronchopulmonary dysplasia, congenital heart disease) may have a prolonged course.

COMPLICATIONS

- Bacterial superinfection
- Bronchiolitis obliterans
- Apnea
- Respiratory failure
- Death
- Increased incidence of development of reactive airway disease (asthma)

REFERENCES

1. *REDBOOK: Report of the Committee on Infectious Disease*. Elk Grove Village, IL: American Academy of Pediatrics; 2009.
2. Cincinnati Children's Hospital Medical Center. Evidence-based clinical practice guideline for medical management of bronchiolitis in children less than 1 year of age presenting with a first time episode. Cincinnati (OH): Cincinnati Children's Hospital Medical Center; 2006. May. 13p (85 references).
3. Patel H, et al. A randomized, controlled trial of the effectiveness of nebulized therapy with epinephrine compared with albuterol and saline in infants hospitalized for acute viral bronchiolitis. *J Ped*. 2002;141(6):818–24.
4. Mull CC, Scarfone RJ, Ferri LR, et al. A randomized trial of nebulized epinephrine vs albuterol in the emergency department treatment of bronchiolitis. *Arch Pediatr Adolesc Med*. 2004;158:113–8.
5. Petruzella FD, Gorelick MH, et al. Current therapies in bronchiolitis. *Pediatr Emerg Care*. 2010;26: 302–7.
6. Corneli HM, Zorc JJ, Majahan P, et al. A multicenter, randomized, controlled trial of dexamethasone for bronchiolitis. *N Engl J Med*. 2007;357:331–9.
7. Spurling GKP, et al. Antibiotics for bronchiolitis in children. *Cochrane Database Syst Rev*. 2007;1: CD005189.
8. Liet JM, Ducruet T, Gupta V, et al. Heliox inhalation therapy for bronchiolitis in infants. *Cochrane Database Syst Rev*. 2010;4:CD006915.

ADDITIONAL READING

- Bush A, Thomson AH. Acute bronchiolitis. *BMJ*. 2007;335:1037–41.
- Everard ML. Acute bronchiolitis and croup. *Pediatr Clin North Am*. 2009;56:119–33, x–xi.
- Worrall G. Bronchiolitis. *Can Fam Physician*. 2008;54:742–3.
- Yanney M, Vyas H. The treatment of bronchiolitis. *Arch Dis Child*. 2008;93:793–8.

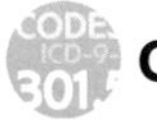

CODES

ICD9

466.19 Acute bronchiolitis due to other infectious organisms

CLINICAL PEARLS

- Bronchiolitis is the leading cause of hospitalizations in infants and children.
- Treatment is primarily supportive.
- Antibiotics are not helpful in the majority of cases.
- Parental education of expected course of illness is important.
- Be aware of new Synagis treatment guidelines for premature infants.

BRONCHIOLITIS OBLITERANS AND ORGANIZING PNEUMONIA

Gretchen M. Dickson, MD, MBA
Caleb Bowers, MD

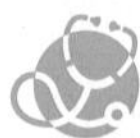

BASICS

DESCRIPTION

- A primary or secondary process of the lungs characterized by granulationlike tissue involving the distal airways and alveoli
- First described in 1985
- A specific reaction of lung tissue to a variety of injuries
- It may occur as patchy infiltrates, or it may be nodular or secondary to another lung disease.
- May also appear to be a migrating process
- May have a gradual or sudden onset
- Lungs show a pattern of multiple patchy pneumonia, which are seen on the chest X-ray (CXR) as patchy alveolar or ground-glass. opacifications, with or without interstitial infiltrates; there may be air bronchograms as well.
- Most cases will respond to corticosteroids, which may have to be given for a year or more.
- Synonym(s): Intraluminal fibrosis of distal airways; Idiopathic bronchiolitis obliterans and organizing pneumonitis (BOOP); Cryptogenic organizing pneumonia; Obliterative bronchiolitis

Geriatric Considerations

More common than originally thought and may be sudden and very severe

Pediatric Considerations

- Rare, but has been reported after viral pneumonia (adenovirus influenza):
  - Characteristics include delayed recovery, persistent cough, crackles, or wheezing after pneumonia.
  - Laboratory findings generally not helpful
  - Imaging shows: Ventilation-perfusion ratio-matched defects; high-resolution CT, bronchiectasis, bronchogram, pruned tree appearance
  - Diagnosis confirmed by biopsy
- Treatment includes steroids: 1 mg/kg q24h for 1 month, followed by weaning over several months

EPIDEMIOLOGY

- Incidence/prevalence in the US: Estimated at 0.01%, but may be underdiagnosed.
- Predominant age: Reported cases range age 0–70; most commonly seen in ages 40–60s

Prevalence

Unknown

RISK FACTORS

- AIDS
- Immunocompromised patients, including transplant patients
- Smoking

Genetics

No known genetic component

GENERAL PREVENTION

Except for prevention of relapse, none known

ETIOLOGY

Idiopathic: A complex response to a variety of injuries such as toxic inhalation, postmycoplasma, viral and bacterial infection, aspiration, immunologic factors, drugs

Pediatric Considerations

In the nontransplant pediatric population, adenovirus infection is the most common cause of bronchiolitis obliterans (1).

COMMONLY ASSOCIATED CONDITIONS

- Drug-induced pneumonitis:
  - Paraquat poisoning
  - Amiodarone toxicity
  - Acebutolol toxicity
  - Amphotericin B
  - Bleomycin
  - Carbamazepine
  - Cephalosporins
  - Gold
  - Minocycline
  - Nitrofurantoin
  - Phenytoin
  - Sulfamethoxypyridazine
  - Sulfasalazine
  - Ticlopidine
  - Freebase cocaine pulmonary toxicity
  - Overdose of L-tryptophan
- Infections:
  - Chronic infectious pneumonia
  - Malaria
  - Chlamydia
  - *Legionella*
  - *Mycoplasma*
  - *Pneumocystis*
  - *Cryptococcus*
- Immunocompromise: Bone marrow, lung, renal, transplantation
- Connective tissue diseases:
  - Rheumatic lung
  - Sjögren syndrome
  - Polymyositis
  - Scleroderma
  - Essential mixed cryoglobulinemia
- Miscellaneous:
  - Cystic fibrosis
  - Bronchopulmonary dysplasia
  - Renal failure
  - Congestive heart failure (CHF)
  - Adult respiratory distress syndrome
  - Chronic eosinophilic pneumonia
  - Hypersensitivity pneumonitis
  - Histiocytosis X
  - Sarcoidosis
  - Pneumoconioses
- Radiation pneumonitis

DIAGNOSIS

Think of the possibility in patients presenting with (2):

- Flulike illness that lasts 4–10 weeks or longer. Most have been treated with antibiotics without success.
- Fatigue, fever, and weight loss
- Dry cough
- Dyspnea may be severe.
- Bilateral crackles

HISTORY

- Fatigue
- Fever
- Weight loss
- Dry cough
- Dyspnea may be severe.

PHYSICAL EXAM

- Hypoxia
- Respiratory distress
- Bilateral crackles

DIAGNOSTIC TESTS & INTERPRETATION

- May have normal or nonspecific laboratory findings
- Leukocytosis with a normal differential
- Elevated ESR
- Negative cultures
- Negative serology for mycoplasma, *Coxiella*, *Legionella*, psittacosis, and fungus
- Negative viral studies

Imaging

- CXR: Often appears more normal than the physical exam
- CXR may show bilateral patchy alveolar opacities, often in the middle or upper lung area, a ground-glass pattern that may have air bronchograms
- Throughout the disease, new infiltrates may appear or may seem to migrate.
- Effusions and cavitary lesions are rare on x-ray.
- Patients with linear opacities at lung bases may have a poorer prognosis.
- CT scans more accurately define the distribution and extent of the patchy alveolar opacities with areas of hyperlucency (3).
- Up to 90% of CT scans may show airspace consolidation with air bronchograms.

Initial approach

- Pulmonary function shows a restrictive/obstructive pattern.
- Flow-volume loop shows terminal airway obstruction.
- The involved area may seem to migrate.
- Ventilation-perfusion ratio scan: Matched patchy defects

Diagnostic Procedures/Surgery

- Open lung biopsy
- Transbronchial biopsy
- It may be wise to use a trial of steroids as a diagnostic trial, although not all would agree.
- If a diagnostic trial is successful, be prepared to treat the patient for at least 1 year.

Pathological Findings

- Intraluminal fibrosis of distal airspaces is the major pathologic feature.
- Fibroblasts and plugs of inflammatory cells and loose connective tissue fill these distal airways.
- Inflammatory cells are mainly lymphocytes and plasma cells.
- Interstitial fibrosis is present.
- Plugs of edematous granulation tissue in the terminal and respiratory bronchioles and alveolar ducts do not cause permanent damage.

DIFFERENTIAL DIAGNOSIS

- Usual interstitial pneumonitis
- Noninfectious diseases
- Tuberculosis
- Sarcoidosis
- Histoplasmosis
- Berylliosis
- Goodpasture syndrome
- Neoplasm
- Polyarteritis nodosa
- Systemic lupus erythematosus
- Wegener granulomatosis
- Sjögren syndrome
- Chronic eosinophilic pneumonia
- Cryptogenic bronchiolitis

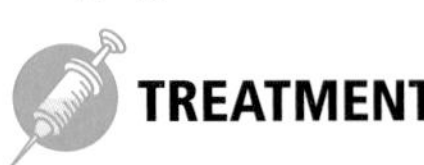

TREATMENT

Inpatient care may be required.

MEDICATION

First Line

Prednisone:

- 1 mg/kg (up to 60mg/d) for 1–3 months, then 40 mg/d for 3 months, then 10–20 mg/d for up to 1 year
- May consider a 6-months-only taper or alternate day dosing for 1 year to limit steroid exposure
- Increase length of taper for patients on long-term therapy to avoid precipitating addisonian crisis.
- Treatment may be needed for 1 year or more.
- Contraindications: Refer to the manufacturer's literature.
- Precautions: Be aware of the patient's Mantoux status and history of peptic ulcer disease. Long-term steroid treatment is associated with significant adverse effects, including Cushing syndrome, fluid retention, osteoporosis, hyperkalemia, and poor wound healing.
- Significant possible interactions: Refer to the manufacturer's literature.

Second Line

- Steroids other than prednisone may be used.
- 1 paper reported the use of erythromycin 600 mg/d for 3–4 months after initial control with prednisone.
- Prescribe antimicrobials if the original infection is persistent. The proper choice depends on the pathogen.
- Anecdotal use of inhaled triamcinolone and cyclophosphamide has been reported.

ADDITIONAL TREATMENT

General Measures

- Monitor blood gases or pulse oximetry.
- Oxygen as necessary

Issues for Referral

Patients should be followed by a pulmonologist.

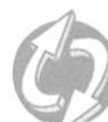

ONGOING CARE

FOLLOW-UP RECOMMENDATIONS

Patient Monitoring

- Frequent visits, weekly at first
- Prednisone must be continued because of the chance of relapse.
- Monitor the lung disease and the side effects of prednisone therapy:
  - Annual Mantoux/purified protein derivative
  - Monthly CBC
  - Funduscopic exam every 3–6 months
  - Serial dual-energy x-ray absorptiometry (DEXA) scans for osteoporosis

DIET

No special diet

PATIENT EDUCATION

- Compliance: Emphasize the need to continue prednisone because of the chance of a relapse.
- Recurrence can occur in up to 1/3 who do not complete full steroid treatment.

PROGNOSIS

Typically complete recovery, but individual case management is mandatory.

COMPLICATIONS

- Bronchiectasis
- Most people recover completely without permanent sequelae if full course of steroids completed
- Death occurs in up to 7%, but usually in individuals who are elderly or have pre-existing comorbid conditions.

REFERENCES

1. Moonnumakal SP, Fan LL. Bronchiolitis obliterans in children. *Curr Opin Pediatr*. 2008;20:272–8.
2. Cordier JF, Loire R, Brune J. Idiopathic bronchiolitis obliterans organizing pneumonia. Definition of characteristic clinical profiles in a series of 16 patients. *Chest*. 1989;96:999–1004.
3. Müller NL, Staples CA, Miller RR. Bronchiolitis obliterans organizing pneumonia: CT features in 14 patients. *AJR Am J Roentgenol*. 1990;154:983–7.

ADDITIONAL READING

- Drakopanagiotakis F, Polychronopoulos V, Judson MA. Organizing pneumonia. *Am J Med Sci*. 2008;335:34–9.
- Epler GR, Colby TV, McLoud TC, et al. Bronchiolitis obliterans organizing pneumonia. *N Engl J Med*. 1985;312:152–8.
- Hardy KA, Schidlow DV, Zaeri N. Obliterative bronchiolitis in children. *Chest*. 1988;93:460–6.
- http://www.epler.com/boop1.html.
- Lynch DA. Imaging of small airways diseases. *Clin Chest Med*. 1993;14:623–34.
- Ruth-Sahd LA, White KA, et al. Bronchiolitis obliterans organizing pneumonia. *Dimens Crit Care Nurs*. 2009;28:204–8.
- Schlesinger C, Koss MN. The organizing pneumonias: An update and review. *Curr Opin Pulm Med*. 2005;11:422–30.
- St John RC, Dorinsky PM. Cryptogenic bronchiolitis. *Clin Chest Med*. 1993;14:667–75.
- White KA, Ruth-Sahd LA. Bronchiolitis obliterans organizing pneumonia. *Crit Care Nurse*. 2007;27:53–66.

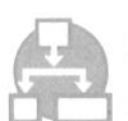

See Also (Topic, Algorithm, Electronic Media Element)

Sjögren Syndrome

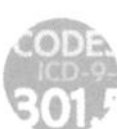

CODES

ICD9

516.8 Other specified alveolar and parietoalveolar pneumonopathies

CLINICAL PEARLS

- Bronchiolitis obliterans and organizing pneumonia and bronchiolitis obliterans are very different.
- Bronchiolitis obliterans and organizing pneumonia are restrictive problems that are completely reversible.
- Bronchiolitis obliterans is an obstructive problem that causes permanent lung damage.

BRONCHITIS, ACUTE

Alan J. Cropp, MD

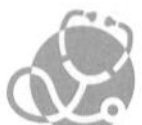

BASICS

DESCRIPTION

- Inflammation of trachea, bronchi, and bronchioles resulting from a respiratory tract infection or chemical irritant (1,2)
- Cough is the predominant symptom and may last as long as 10–20 days (1,3).
- Generally self-limited, with complete healing and full return of function
- Most infections are viral if no underlying cardiopulmonary disease is present.
- Synonym(s): Tracheobronchitis, Chest cold

Geriatric Considerations

Can be serious, particularly if part of influenza, with underlying chronic obstructive pulmonary disease (COPD) or congestive heart failure (CHF) (3)

Pediatric Considerations

- Usually occurs in association with other conditions of upper- and lower-respiratory tract (trachea usually involved) (4).
- If repeated attacks occur, child should be evaluated for anomalies of the respiratory tract, including immune deficiencies, or for chronic asthma.
- When acute bronchitis is caused by respiratory syncytial virus (RSV), it may be fatal.

EPIDEMIOLOGY

- Predominant age: All ages
- Predominant gender: Male = Female

Incidence

- ~5% of adults per year (3)
- A common cause of infection in children (4)

Prevalence

Results in 10–12 million office visits per year (3)

RISK FACTORS

- Infants
- Elderly
- Air pollutants
- Smoking
- Second-hand smoke
- Environmental changes
- Chronic bronchopulmonary diseases
- Chronic sinusitis
- Tracheostomy
- Bronchopulmonary allergy
- Hypertrophied tonsils and adenoids in children
- Immunosuppression:
  - Immunoglobulin deficiency
  - HIV infection
  - Alcoholism
- Gastroesophageal reflux disease (GERD)

Genetics

No known genetic pattern

GENERAL PREVENTION

- Avoid smoking.
- Control underlying risk factors (i.e., asthma, sinusitis, and reflux).
- Avoid exposure, especially day care.
- Pneumovax, influenza immunization

PATHOPHYSIOLOGY

Acute bronchitis causes an injury to the epithelial surfaces, resulting in an increase in mucous production (2) and thickening of the bronchiole wall (1).

ETIOLOGY

- Viral infections, such as adenovirus, influenza A and B, parainfluenza virus, coxsackievirus, RSV, rhinovirus, coronavirus (types 1–3), herpes simplex virus
- Bacterial infections, such as *Chlamydia pneumoniae* (Taiwan acute respiratory [TWAR] agent), *Mycoplasma, Bordetella pertussis, Haemophilus influenzae, Streptococcus pneumoniae, Moraxella catarrhalis,* and *Mycobacterium tuberculosis*
- Secondary bacterial infection as part of an acute upper respiratory infection
- Possibly fungal infections
- Chemical irritants

COMMONLY ASSOCIATED CONDITIONS

- Allergic rhinitis
- Sinusitis
- Pharyngitis
- Epiglottitis (rare but can be rapidly fatal)
- Coryza
- Croup
- Influenza
- Pneumonia
- Asthma
- COPD/emphysema
- GERD

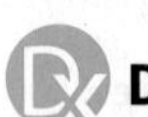

DIAGNOSIS

HISTORY

- Sudden onset of cough and no evidence of pneumonia, asthma, exacerbation of COPD, or the common cold (3)
- Cough is initially dry and unproductive, then productive; later, mucopurulent sputum, which may indicate secondary infection
- Dyspnea, wheeze, fever, and fatigue may occur.
- Possible contact with others who have respiratory infections (1)

PHYSICAL EXAM

- Fever
- Tachypnea
- Pharynx injected
- Rales, rhonchi, wheezing
- No evidence of pulmonary consolidation

DIAGNOSTIC TESTS & INTERPRETATION

Lab

Initial lab tests

- White blood cell (WBC)
- Procalcitonin level (5)[B]
- Sputum culture/sensitivity if chest x-ray is abnormal (3)
- Influenza titers (if appropriate for time of year)

Follow-Up & Special Considerations

- Arterial blood gases: Hypoxemia (rarely)
- Pulmonary function tests (seldom needed during acute stages): Increased residual volume, decreased maximal expiratory rate (2)

Imaging

Initial approach

Chest radiograph (CXR):

- Lungs normal if uncomplicated
- Helps to rule out other diseases (pneumonia) or complications

DIFFERENTIAL DIAGNOSIS

- Common cold
- Acute sinusitis
- Bronchopneumonia
- Influenza
- Bacterial tracheitis
- Bronchiectasis
- Asthma
- Reactive airways dysfunction syndrome (RADS)
- Allergy
- Eosinophilic pneumonitis
- Aspiration
- Retained foreign body
- Inhalation injury
- Cystic fibrosis
- Bronchogenic carcinoma
- Heart failure
- GERD

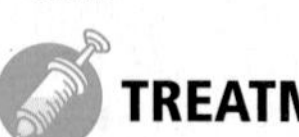

TREATMENT

MEDICATION

ALERT

Antibiotics are usually not recommended (1,3,6)[A] unless a treatable pathogen has been identified or significant comorbidities are present.

First Line

- Amantadine or rimantadine therapy if influenza A is suspected; most effective if started within 24–48 hours of development of symptoms (also consider oseltamivir [Tamiflu] or zanamivir [Relenza])
- Decongestants if accompanied by sinus condition (1)
- Antipyretic analgesic, such as aspirin, acetaminophen, or ibuprofen
- Antibiotics if a treatable cause (i.e., pertussis) is identified (6)[A]:
  - Amoxicillin 500 mg q8h or trimethoprim-sulfamethoxazole DS q12h for routine infection
    - Penicillins and trimethoprim-based regimens seem to be equivalent in terms of effectiveness and toxicity for acute bacterial exacerbations of chronic bronchitis (ABECB) (7)[B].
    - Clarithromycin (Biaxin) 500 mg q12h or azithromycin (Zithromax) Z-pack for penicillin allergy or *Mycoplasma* infection: In patients with acute bronchitis of a suspected bacterial cause, azithromycin tends to be more effective in terms of lower incidence of treatment failure and adverse events than amoxicillin or amoxycillin-clavulanic acid (8)[B].

– Doxycycline 100 mg/d × 10 days if *Moraxella, Chlamydia*, or *Mycoplasma* suspected
– Quinolone for more serious infections or other antibiotic failure or in elderly or patients with multiple comorbidities
– Macrolide for pertussis (1)[A]
- Cough suppressant for troublesome cough (not with COPD); guaifenesin with codeine or dextromethorphan (3)[A]
- Mucolytic agents are not recommended (3)[B].
- Inhaled beta agonist (e.g., albuterol) or in combination with steroids for cough with bronchospasm (2,3)[B]
- Consider steroids for bronchospasm
- Contraindication(s): Doxycycline should not be used during pregnancy or in children.
- Precautions:
  – Watch for theophylline toxicity with macrolides and quinolones.
  – Multiple antibiotics have the potential to interfere with the effectiveness of oral contraceptives.

Second Line
- Other antibiotics if indicated by sputum culture (*Moraxella* needs a different set of antibiotics)
- Antivirals
- Other macrolides or quinolones based on pathogen and sensitivity

ADDITIONAL TREATMENT
General Measures
- Rest
- Stop smoking or avoid smoke.
- Steam inhalations
- Vaporizers
- Adequate hydration
- Antitussives
- Antibiotics are usually not recommended (1,3,6)[A].
- Treat associated illnesses (e.g., GERD).

Issues for Referral
- Complications, such as pneumonia or respiratory failure
- Comorbidities, such as COPD
- Cough lasting longer than 3 months

Additional Therapies
Antipyretic for fever (e.g., acetaminophen, aspirin, or ibuprofen)

COMPLEMENTARY AND ALTERNATIVE MEDICINE
Throat lozenges for pharyngitis

IN-PATIENT CONSIDERATIONS
Initial Stabilization
- Outpatient, unless elderly or complicated by severe underlying disease
- May require supplemental oxygen in selected patients
- Bronchodilators if patient is bronchospastic

Admission Criteria
- Hypoxia
- Severe bronchospasm
- Exacerbation of underlying disease

IV Fluids
May be helpful if patient is dehydrated

Nursing
- Ensure patient comfort and monitor for signs of deterioration, especially if underlying lung disease exists.
- May need to follow oxygen saturation in patients with underlying lung disease

Discharge Criteria
Improvement in symptoms and comorbidities

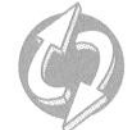

ONGOING CARE

FOLLOW-UP RECOMMENDATIONS
- Usually a self-limited disease not requiring follow-up
- Cough may linger for several weeks.
- In children, if recurrent, need to consider other diagnoses, such as asthma (4)

Patient Monitoring
- Oximetry until no longer hypoxemic
- Recheck for chronicity.

DIET
Increased fluids (3–4 L/d) while febrile

PATIENT EDUCATION
- For patient education materials favorably reviewed on this topic, contact the American Lung Association, 1740 Broadway, New York, NY 10019, (212) 315-8700; www.lungusa.org.
- American Academy of Family Physicians: www.familydoctor.org

PROGNOSIS
- Usual: Complete resolution
- Can be serious in the elderly or debilitated
- Cough may persist for several weeks after an initial improvement (1,2).
- Postbronchitic reactive airways disease (rare)
- Bronchiolitis obliterans and organizing pneumonia (rare)

COMPLICATIONS
- Superinfection such as bronchopneumonia
- Bronchiectasis
- Hemoptysis
- Acute respiratory failure
- Chronic cough

REFERENCES

1. Wenzel RP, Fowler AA. Clinical practice. Acute bronchitis. *N Engl J Med*. 2006;355:2125–30.
2. Knutson D, Braun C. Diagnosis and management of acute bronchitis. *Am Fam Physician*. 2002;65:2039–44.
3. Braman SS. Chronic cough due to acute bronchitis: ACCP evidence-based clinical practice guidelines. *Chest*. 2006;129:95S–103S.
4. Fleming DM, Elliot AJ. The management of acute bronchitis in children. *Expert Opin Pharmacother*. 2007;8:415–26.
5. Briel M, Schuetz P, et al. Procalcitonin-guided antibiotic use vs a standard approach for acute respiratory tract infections in primary care. *Arch Intern Med*. 2008;168(18):2000–7.
6. Fahey T, et al. Antibiotics for acute bronchitis. *Cochrane Database Syst Rev*. 2004;4:CD000245.
7. Korbila IP, Manta KG, Siempos II, et al. Penicillins vs trimethoprim-based regimens for acute bacterial exacerbations of chronic bronchitis: Meta-analysis of randomized controlled trials. *Can Fam Physician*. 2009;55:60–7.
8. Panpanich R, Lerttrakarnnon P, Laopaiboon M. Azithromycin for acute lower respiratory tract infections. *Cochrane Database Syst Rev*. 2008;CD001954.

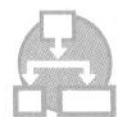

See Also (Topic, Algorithm, Electronic Media Element)

- Asthma; Chronic Obstructive Pulmonary Disease and Emphysema
- Algorithm: Cough, Chronic

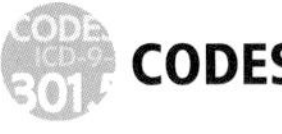

CODES

ICD9
- 041.5 Haemophilus influenzae [H. influenzae] infection in conditions classified elsewhere and of unspecified site
- 079.6 Respiratory syncytial virus (RSV)
- 466.0 Acute bronchitis

CLINICAL PEARLS

- Acute bronchitis is a common and generally self-limited disease.
- Usually does not require treatment with antibiotics
- Cough may linger for several weeks.
- Recurrent or seasonal episodes may suggest another disease process, such as asthma.

BULIMIA NERVOSA

Jeffrey L. Goodie, PhD
Pamela M. Williams, MD, Lt Col, USAF, MC

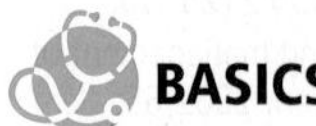

BASICS

DESCRIPTION
- A pattern of discrete periods of uncontrolled eating, followed by compensatory behaviors
- System(s) affected: Oropharyngeal; endocrine/metabolic; gastrointestinal; dermatologic; cardiovascular; nervous

EPIDEMIOLOGY
- Predominant age: Adolescents and young adults
- Mean age of onset: 18–21 years
- Predominant sex: Female > Male (10–20:1)

Incidence
28.8 women, 0.8 men per 100,000 per year

Prevalence
- 1–3% in women 16–35 years old
- 0.5% in young men (higher among gay and bisexual men)

RISK FACTORS
- Female gender
- History of obesity and dieting
- Body dissatisfaction
- Critical comments by family or others about weight, body shape, or eating
- Severe life stressor
- Low self-esteem
- Perceived pressure to be thin
- Perfectionist or obsessive thinking
- Poor impulse control, alcohol misuse
- History of anorexia nervosa (AN)
- Environment stressing high achievement, competition, thinness, or physical fitness (e.g., armed forces, ballet, cheerleading, gymnastics, or modeling)
- Family history of substance abuse, affective disorders, eating disorder, or obesity
- Early feeding problems
- Low birth weight for gestational age
- Hyporeactivity at birth
- Type I diabetes
- Sexual abuse is not causally related to bulimia.

GENERAL PREVENTION
- Prevention programs can reduce risk factors and future onset of eating disorders (1)[C].
- Target adolescents and young women 15 years or older.
- Encourage realistic and healthy weight management strategies and attitudes.
- Decrease body dissatisfaction.
- Promote self-esteem.
- Reduce focus on thin as ideal.
- Moderate overly high self-expectations.
- Decrease anxiety/depressive symptoms.
- Improve stress management.

ETIOLOGY
Combination of biological, psychological, environmental, and social factors. Unique contribution of any specific factor remains unclear.

COMMONLY ASSOCIATED CONDITIONS
- Major depression and dysthymia
- Anxiety disorders
- Substance abuse/dependence
- Bipolar disorder
- Obsessive-compulsive disorder
- Borderline personality disorder
- Schizophrenic disorder

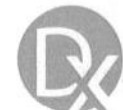

DIAGNOSIS

DSM-IV-TR criteria:
- Recurrent episodes of binge eating (2 times per week for 3 months):
  - Eating in a discrete period more than most people would eat during that time
  - Perceived lack of control during binges
- Recurrent inappropriate compensatory behavior (2 times per week for 3 months)
- Purging and nonpurging subtypes:
  - Purging: Often by self-induced vomiting, laxatives, diuretics
  - Nonpurging: Binges followed by sharply restricted diet and/or vigorous exercise
- Body shape and weight significantly affect self-evaluation.
- Does not occur during AN episodes
- Psychological self-report screening tests:
  - Eating Attitudes Test
  - Eating Disorder Inventory
  - Eating Disorder Screen for Primary Care
  - Bulimia Test (revised)
  - Bulimia Investigatory Test Edinburgh
  - SCOFF (sick, control, one, fat, food)

HISTORY
- Patients unlikely to self-identify binge eating or purging behaviors; corroborate with parent/relative
- Unhappiness and/or preoccupation with weight and diet attempts
- Pattern of restricting diet, binge eating, and purging behaviors:
  - Binge is context-specific; amount can vary
  - Vomiting (often with little effort)
  - Vigorous aerobic exercise
  - Distress/shame related to loss of control
- Depressed mood and self-depreciation following the binges
- Relief and increased ability to concentrate following the purges
- Other possible signs and symptoms:
  - Requesting weight loss help and mildly underweight to overweight
  - Diet pill, diuretic, laxative, ipecac, and thyroid medication use/abuse
  - Menstrual disturbance
  - Fatigue and lethargy
  - Abdominal pain, bloating, constipation, diarrhea, rectal prolapse
  - Sore throat
  - Thermal tooth sensitivity
  - Frequent fluctuations in weight
  - Omission/underdosing insulin in diabetes patients

PHYSICAL EXAM
- Often normal
- Bradycardia
- Eroded tooth enamel
- Perimylolysis
- Cheilosis
- Gingivitis
- Sialadenosis
- Asymptomatic, noninflammatory parotid gland enlargement
- Epigastric tenderness to palpation
- Calluses, abrasions, bruising on hand, thumb
- Peripheral edema

DIAGNOSTIC TESTS & INTERPRETATION
All lab results may be within normal limits and are not necessary for diagnosis.

Lab
- Blood work:
  - Hypokalemia, hypochloremia
  - Hypomagnesemia, hyponatremia, hypocalcemia, hypophosphatasemia
  - Serum amylase levels
  - Alkalosis
  - Elevated BUN
  - Hypoglycemia
- Urinalysis:
  - Increased urine-specific gravity

Diagnostic Procedures/Surgery
Electrocardiogram:
- Bradycardia or arrhythmias
- Conduction defects
- Depressed ST segment due to hypokalemia

Pathological Findings
- Esophagitis
- Acute pancreatitis
- Cardiomyopathy and muscle weakness due to ipecac abuse
- Melanosis coli
- Cathartic colon syndrome
- Delayed or arrested skeletal growth
- Stress fracture
- Irreversible dental erosions
- Osteopenia/osteoporosis

DIFFERENTIAL DIAGNOSIS
- Anorexia, binge eating/purging type
- Major depressive disorder
- Anxiety disorders
- Psychogenic vomiting
- Malabsorption
- Addison disease
- Celiac disease
- Diabetes mellitus
- Hyperthyroidism, hypothyroidism
- Hyperpituitarism
- Hypothalamic brain tumor
- Kleine-Levin syndrome
- Body dysmorphic disorder
- Borderline personality disorder

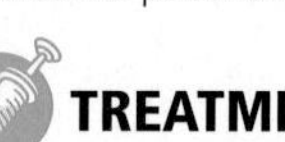

TREATMENT

- Cognitive-behavioral therapy (CBT) should be considered as first-line treatment (2,3,4)[A].
- Guided self-help therapies may be effective (3,4)[B].

B

MEDICATION

First Line

- SSRIs, particularly fluoxetine (Prozac) at 60 mg, are effective in reducing symptoms with relatively few side effects. Higher doses than standard doses for depression are often needed (3,5,6)[B]:
  - Combination of medication and CBT has been shown to have added benefit over medication or therapy alone (6).
- To prevent relapse, maintain antidepressant at full therapeutic dose for at least 1 year.
- Bupropion not recommended due to its association with seizures in patients who purge.
- Misrepresentation and nonadherence may be more likely in this population.
- Precautions:
  - Serious toxicity following overdose is common.
  - Patients may vomit medications.

Second Line

- Ondansetron (Zofran) 4–8 mg t.i.d. between meals can help prevent vomiting.
- Psyllium (Metamucil) preparations, 1 Tbs q.h.s. with glass of water, can prevent constipation during laxative withdrawal.

ADDITIONAL TREATMENT

Most patients can be treated as outpatients.

General Measures

- Psychotherapies should be employed as first-line treatments.
- Multidisciplinary team:
  - Primary care physician, behavioral health provider, nutritionist
- Build trust; increase motivation for change.
- Assess psychological and nutritional status.
- Consider evidence-based self-help program.
- Cognitive behavioral therapy for bulimia nervosa (2,3,4,5)[A]:
  - 16–20 50-minute appointments
  - Involve patient in establishing goals.
  - Self-monitoring of food intake, frequency of binges/purges, related antecedents, consequences, thoughts, and emotions
  - Self-monitoring of weight once per week
  - Educate about ineffectiveness of purging for weight control and adverse outcomes.
  - Establish prescribed eating plan to develop regular eating habits; realistic weight goal.
  - Gradually introduce feared foods into diet.
  - Problem-solve how to cope with triggers.
  - Decrease ruminations about calories, weight, and purging.
  - Challenge fear of loss of control.
  - Establish relapse prevention plan.
  - Gradual laxative withdrawal
- Interpersonal therapy (2,3)[B]:
  - May act more slowly than CBT
- Transdiagnostic cognitive-behavioral therapy
- Dialectical behavior therapy
- Family therapy for adolescents
- Nutritional education, relaxation techniques
- Educate patient to brush teeth and use baking soda to rinse mouth after vomiting.

Issues for Referral

Patients with bulimia require a multidisciplinary team, including a primary care physician, behavioral health provider, and a nutritionist.

COMPLEMENTARY AND ALTERNATIVE MEDICINE

Bright light therapy may help (3).

IN-PATIENT CONSIDERATIONS

- If possible, admit to a specialized eating disorders unit.
- Supervised meals and bathroom privileges
- Monitor weight and physical activity.
- Monitor electrolytes.
- Gradually shift control to patients as they demonstrate responsibility.

Admission Criteria

Hospitalize if severe malnutrition, dehydration, electrolyte disturbances, cardiac dysrhythmia, uncontrolled binging and purging, psychiatric emergency, or if outpatient treatment failed.

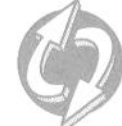

ONGOING CARE

FOLLOW-UP RECOMMENDATIONS

Patient Monitoring

- Binge-purge activity, including antecedents and consequences
- Level of exercise activity
- Self-esteem, comfort with body and self
- Ruminations and depressive symptoms
- Repeat any abnormal lab values weekly or monthly until stable.

DIET

- Balanced diet, normal eating pattern
- Reintroduce feared foods.

PATIENT EDUCATION

The following books may be useful for guided self-help treatment programs:

- Fairburn CG. *Overcoming Binge Eating*. New York: Guilford Press; 1995.
- McCabe RE, McFarlane TL, Olmstead MP. *Overcoming Bulimia: Your Comprehensive, Step-by-Step Guide to Recovery*. Oakland, CA: New Harbinger; 2003.

PROGNOSIS

- After effective cognitive behavioral treatment:
  - In the short term, 50% of treated individuals do not meet criteria for diagnosis.
  - In the long term (2–10 years), 70% may be asymptomatic.
  - Symptomatic individuals may demonstrate remissions, relapses, subclinical, or other eating disorder-related behaviors.
- Untreated:
  - Likely to remain chronic/relapsing problem
- Greater weight fluctuations, other impulsive behaviors, childhood obesity, low self-esteem, family history of alcohol abuse, psychiatric comorbidity, and personality disorder diagnoses (e.g., avoidant personality disorder) may predict poor prognosis.
- Mortality rate: 0–2%

COMPLICATIONS

- Drug and alcohol abuse
- Osteopenia/osteoporosis
- Stress fracture
- Gastric dilatation
- Boerhaave syndrome
- Mallory-Weiss tears
- Pseudo-Bartter syndrome
- Spontaneous pneumomediastinum
- Potassium depletion, cardiac arrhythmia, cardiac arrest
- Suicide

Pregnancy Considerations

Maternal and fetal problems if pregnant:

- Binging/purging behaviors may persist, increase, or decrease with pregnancy.
- Increased risk for preterm delivery, operative delivery, and infants with low birth weight, smaller head circumference, and/or microcephaly; should be managed as high risk

REFERENCES

1. Stice E, Shaw H, Marti CN. A meta-analytic review of eating disorder prevention programs: Encouraging findings. *Annu Rev Clin Psychol*. 2007;3:207–31.
2. Hay PP, Bacaltchuk J, Stefano S, et al. Psychological treatments for bulimia nervosa and binging. *Cochrane Database Syst Rev*. 2009;CD000562.
3. Shapiro JR, Berkman ND, Brownley KA, et al. Bulimia nervosa treatment: A systematic review of randomized controlled trials. *Int J Eat Disord*. 2007;40:321–36.
4. NICE. *Eating Disorders–Core Interventions in the Treatment of Anorexia Nervosa, Bulimia Nervosa, and Related Eating Disorders*. NICE Clinical Guideline no 9. London: NICE, 2004: Available at: http://www.nice.org.uk. Accessed July 17, 2008.
5. *Practice Guideline for the Treatment of Patients with Eating Disorders*, 3rd ed. American Psychiatric Association. Available at http://www.psych.org. Accessed February 22, 2007.
6. Bacaltchuk J, Hay P, Trefiglio R. Antidepressants versus psychological treatments and their combination for bulimia nervosa. *Cochrane Database Sys Rev*. 2001(4):CD003385.

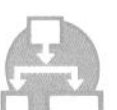

See Also (Topic, Algorithm, Electronic Media Element)

- Anorexia Nervosa; Hyperkalemia; Laxative Abuse; Salivary Gland Tumors
- Algorithm: Weight Loss

CODES

ICD9

307.51 Bulimia nervosa

CLINICAL PEARLS

- Particularly among young women with a risk factor, asking "Are you satisfied with your eating patterns?" and/or "Do you worry that you have lost control over how much you eat?" may help to screen for an eating problem. A brief, standardized screening measure (e.g., SCOFF, ESP, EAT) will help to identify those who may need a broader assessment.
- Binging and purging behaviors can be seen in anorexia nervosa as well.
- Consider using a stepped-care approach. Start with a guided self-help program using instructional aids; next, begin cognitive behavioral therapy (e.g., 16–20 sessions over 4–5 months).
- SSRIs, particularly fluoxetine (60 mg daily), may be helpful as a first step or as an adjunctive treatment.

BUNION

Linda Sinclair, MD
Jason M. Kittler, MD, PhD, JD

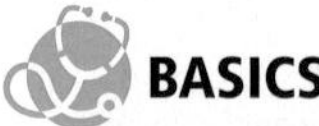

BASICS

DESCRIPTION

- Commonly known as a bunion, a hallux valgus deformity consists of a lateral deviation of the great toe (hallux) with medial deviation of the first metatarsal
- This results in a medial prominence of the first metatarsophalangeal (MTP) joint and a potentially painful and/or debilitating deformity.
- Progressive subluxation of the first MTP joint is common.
- There is often lateral rotation of the toe such that the nail faces medially (eversion) (1)[A].
- System(s) affected: Musculoskeletal/Skin

EPIDEMIOLOGY

- Predominant age: More common in adults (2)[A]:
  - Estimated 23% in adults aged 18–65
  - Estimated 35.7% in elderly over age 65
- Predominant sex: Female > Male by about 50%
- Prevalence increases with age.

RISK FACTORS

- Familial predisposition
- Abnormal anatomy/mechanics
- Joint hypermobility or laxity
- Pronation of hindfoot
- Achilles tendon contracture
- Pes planus (fallen arches)
- Metatarsus primus varus
- Amputation of second toe
- Inflammatory joint disease
- Neuromuscular disorders
- Exacerbated by improper footwear, especially tight-fitting or pointed shoes

GENERAL PREVENTION

No known effective prevention exists, given that the etiology is poorly understood.

PATHOPHYSIOLOGY

- Pressure at the head of the first metatarsal forces it to move medially. The hallux is forced laterally, and a misalignment between the first metatarsal and the hallux develops.
- Strain on the medial collateral ligament along the MTP joint leads to loss of tensile strength, and eventually rupture, which decreases the medial stabilization and causes progressive subluxation of the first MTP joint (3)[B].
- Changes in muscle positioning and tightening of the lateral collateral ligament can allow for the adductor hallucis muscle to pull unopposed, which can lead to lateral rotation and eversion of the hallux (1)[A].

ETIOLOGY

The exact etiology of hallux valgus is unknown, but the disease is thought to be multifactorial. The risk factors listed above may all contribute to the development of the disease.

COMMONLY ASSOCIATED CONDITIONS

- Medial bursitis of the first MTP joint (most common)
- Hammertoe deformity of the second phalanx
- Plantar callus
- Central metatarsalgia
- Metatarsalgia of MTP joint
- Degeneration of first metatarsal head cartilage
- Pronated feet
- Ankle equinus
- Ingrown toenail
- Entrapment of the medial dorsal cutaneous nerve
- Synovitis of the MTP joint (1)[A]

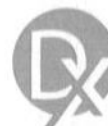

DIAGNOSIS

- Most often made on clinical exam
- Radiography for staging purposes

PHYSICAL EXAM

- Pain or deformity at the first digit (great toe)
- Increased valgus angle at the first MTP joint
- Medial eminence of first metatarsal
- Bursal inflammation/ulceration over medial surface
- Painful callus development on second toe
- Displacement of the first digit above/below second digit
- Lateral deviation of other digits
- Impaired gait
- To perform a complete exam, the physician should:
  - Observe the patient in sitting and standing positions, as weightbearing often accentuates the deformity.
  - Assess the magnitude of hallux valgus deformity, including any rotation of the first digit.
  - Measure the active/passive range of motion of the first MTP joint.
  - Assess the congruency of the first MTP joint by passive correction of the deformity.
  - Assess for pain and/or crepitus with movement of first MTP joint (may indicate degenerative osteoarthritis and change management).
  - Assess the neurovasculature of the foot.
  - Assess the gait of the patient.

DIAGNOSTIC TESTS & INTERPRETATION

Imaging

Weightbearing anteroposterior, lateral, and oblique radiographs may be obtained. The radiographs are used to make the following measurements:

- Hallux abductus (HA) angle: Created by the bisection of the longitudinal axis of the hallux and the longitudinal axis of the first metatarsal:
  - A normal angle is <20° (1)[A].
  - Deformity is considered severe when the HA angle is >40° (3)[B].
- Intermetatarsal (IM) angle: Created by the bisection of the longitudinal axes of the first and second metatarsals:
  - A normal angle is <9° (1)[A].
  - Deformity is considered severe when the IM angle is >16° (3)[B].
- Medial prominence of the first metatarsal head: Note erosions or squaring.
- MTP joint congruency: A congruent joint displays no lateral subluxation of the proximal phalanx on the metatarsal head.

DIFFERENTIAL DIAGNOSIS

- Trauma:
  - Turf toe
  - Sesamoiditis
  - Stress fracture
- Infection:
  - Osteomyelitis
  - Septic arthritis
- Joint disorder:
  - Osteoarthritis
  - Rheumatoid arthritis
  - Gout
- Tendon disorder:
  - Tendinosis
  - Tenosynovitis
  - Tendon rupture
- Other:
  - Bursitis
  - Ganglia
  - Foreign-body granuloma

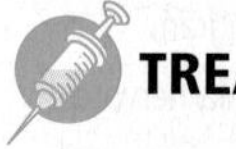

TREATMENT

Hallux valgus deformity will not resolve without treatment. Surgical treatment is more effective in improving patient outcomes than conservative therapy, although evidence is limited.

MEDICATION

While no medication is available to treat the underlying cause of hallux valgus, nonsteroidal anti-inflammatory agents can be used for relief of pain and swelling. As with the use of any medication, patients should be evaluated for contraindications and monitored for adverse reactions.

ADDITIONAL TREATMENT

Conservative treatments (e.g., orthoses and night splints) did not appear to be any more beneficial in improving outcomes and preventing progression than no treatment (4)[A]. Evidence suggests that custom-made orthoses are a safe intervention that may slightly decrease pain at 6 and 12 months (but no continued decrease in pain after 12 months) compared to no treatment; however, this improvement is less than that seen with surgical interventions (see below) (5)[A].

General Measures

Despite the lack of strong evidence supporting the clinical efficacy of conservative therapy, a number of nonoperative modalities have been recommended to attempt to alleviate symptoms and decrease the rates of progression of hallux valgus deformity before surgical referral:

- Shoe modification: Low-heeled, wide shoes to alleviate pressure on MTP joint and friction over the medial eminence
- Orthoses: Shoe inserts may alter abnormal foot rotation and can temporarily alleviate foot pain; may be used in patients awaiting surgical treatment and can also help pes planus.
- Night splinting: May help balance supporting ligaments by stretching the soft tissue around the joint that has become contracted; improvement only seen with continued use
- Manual and manipulative therapy (MMT): Stretches contracted soft tissue
- Foot exercises and stretching: To improve intrinsic foot muscle strength
- Bunion pads: To decrease friction on the medial eminence/MTP joint
- Ice: To reduce inflammation

COMPLEMENTARY AND ALTERNATIVE MEDICINE

Marigold ointment may reduce pain and soft tissue swelling over an 8-week period (6)[C].

SURGERY/OTHER PROCEDURES

Surgery is indicated if patient has severe pain, dysfunction, or symptoms that do not improve with conservative therapy. Surgery is shown to be more beneficial than conservative therapy, and patient should be referred to a foot and ankle surgeon. There are over 150 different surgical techniques to treat hallux valgus; however, none have been proven to be superior, and there is no universally accepted standard for selecting one procedure over another. Choice of surgical technique will depend on the severity of disease, the HA and the IM angles, congruency and subluxation of the MTP joint, patient-specific factors, and the pathologic element the surgeon determines needs correcting. Examples include:

- Arthrodesis: Fusion of the first MTP joint; reserved for severe and/or recurrent hallux valgus
- Arthroplasty: Removing the joint or replacing it with a prosthesis
- Exostectomy/bunionectomy: Removing the medial bony prominence of the MTP joint
- Soft tissue realignment: Alters the function of surrounding ligaments and tendons
- Osteotomy and realignment: Can correct large deformities, but evidence of long-term outcome is lacking

Surgery has been shown to decrease pain and improve foot function subjectively in a larger proportion of patients. However, it is important that patients have realistic expectations about surgical outcomes. Patients may not be able to fit into smaller shoes after surgery, the great toe may not appear straight, and there is chance of recurrence.

ONGOING CARE

FOLLOW-UP RECOMMENDATIONS

Activity after surgery is indicated to decrease joint stiffness. Postoperative treatment may include physical therapy, physiotherapy, use of supportive shoe, continuous passive motion or manual manipulation. Although there is little evidence to support clinical efficacy, physical therapy and gait training after surgery may improve ability to bear weight and ambulate after surgery, and passive motion may improve time to recovery and range of motion of MTP. Early weightbearing has not been found to be detrimental to final outcome. Refer to specific recommendation made by the patient's surgeon.

PROGNOSIS

Patient outcome varies depending on individual factors, severity, and treatment modality used. The radiologic HA angle is a predictor of surgical correction; patients with an HA angle $<37°$ have a higher chance of having the deformity corrected with surgery compared to patients with an HA angle $>37°$ (7)[B].

COMPLICATIONS

- All surgery carries the risk of wound infection or poor wound healing.
- Additional complications may include:
  - Early swelling
  - Hallux varus
  - Recurrence of bunion
  - Decreased sensation over the first metatarsal or phalanx

REFERENCES

1. Ferrari J, et al. Hallux valgus deformity (bunion). *Article from UpToDate*. Lasted updated 2/22/2010.
2. Nix S, et al. Prevalence of hallux valgus in the general population: A systemic review and meta-analysis. *J Foot Ankle Res*. 2010;3:21.
3. Glasoe WM, Nuckley DJ, Ludewig PM, et al. Hallux valgus and the first metatarsal arch segment: A theoretical biomechanical perspective. *Phys Ther*. 2010;90:110–20.
4. Ferrari J, et al. Interventions for treating hallux valgus (abductovalgus) and bunions. *Cochrane Database Syst Rev*. 2009.
5. Hawke F, et al. Custom-made foot orthoses for the treatment of foot pain. *Cochrane Database Syst Rev*. 2009.
6. Khan MT. The podiatric treatment of hallux abducto valgus and its associated condition, bunion, with Tagetes patula. *J Pharm Pharmacol*. 1996;48: 768–70.
7. Deenik AR, de Visser E, Louwerens JW, et al. Hallux valgus angle as main predictor for correction of hallux valgus. *BMC Musculoskelet Disord*. 2008; 9:70.

ADDITIONAL READING

- Ashman CJ, Klecker RJ, Yu JS. Forefoot pain involving the metatarsal region: Differential diagnosis with MR imaging. *Radiographics*. 2001;21:1425–40.
- Coughlin MJ. Hallux valgus. *J Bone Joint Surg Am*. 1996;78:932–66.
- Du Plessis M, et al. Manual and manipulative therapy compared to night splint for symptomatic hallux abducto valgus: An exploratory randomized clinical trial. *Foot (Edinb)*. 2011.
- Klosok JK, Pring DJ, Jessop JH, et al. Chevron or Wilson metatarsal osteotomy for hallux valgus. A prospective randomised trial. *J Bone Joint Surg Br*. 1993;75:825–9.
- Schuh R, Hofstaetter SG, Adams SB, et al. Rehabilitation after hallux valgus surgery: Importance of physical therapy to restore weight bearing of the first ray during the stance phase. *Phys Ther*. 2009;89:934–45.
- Spruce MC, et al. A longitudinal study of hallux valgus surgical outcomes using a validated patient centered outcome measure. *J Foot*. 2011.
- Thomas NJ, et al. Decision making in the treatment of hallux valgus. *Bull NYU Hosp Jt Dis*. 2007;65(1): 19–23.
- Torkki M, et al. Surgery vs orthosis vs watchful waiting for hallux valgus: A randomized control trial. *JAMA*. 2001;285:2474–80.
- Vanore JV, Christensen JC, Kravitz SR, et al. Diagnosis and treatment of first metatarsophalangeal joint disorders. Section 1: Hallux valgus. *J Foot Ankle Surg*. 2003;42:112–23.

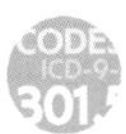

CODES

ICD9

727.1 Bunion

CLINICAL PEARLS

- When bunions occur in children or adolescents, the condition may be termed juvenile or adolescent hallux valgus, respectively, and is thought to have an etiology different from that in the adult population.
- Also known as a bunionette, a tailor's bunion is a lateral prominence of the fifth metatarsal head.
- Patients should avoid any footwear with high heels, pointed toe boxes, or inadequate space for the toes to reduce the risk of bunions. Women's high-heeled shoes and cowboy boots often fall into this category.

BURNS

Timothy L. Black, MD
James P. Miller, MD

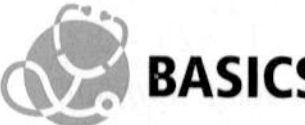

BASICS

DESCRIPTION

- Tissue injuries caused by application of heat, chemicals, electricity, or irradiation to the tissue
- Extent of injury (depth of burn) is result of intensity of heat (or other exposure) and duration of exposure.
  - First degree involves superficial layers of epidermis.
  - Second degree involves varying degrees of epidermis (with blister formation) and part of the dermis.
  - Third degree involves destruction of all skin elements (full thickness) with coagulation of subdermal plexus.
- System(s) affected: Endocrine/Metabolic; Skin/Exocrine

Geriatric Considerations

- Prognosis is poorer for severe burns.
- Patients >60 years of age account for 11% of burns.

Pediatric Considerations

Consider child abuse or neglect when dealing with hot-water burns in children.

EPIDEMIOLOGY

- Predominant age: 30 years; 13% infants; 11% >60 years of age
- Predominant gender: Males account for 70%

Incidence

Per year in US:

- 1.2–2 million burns; 700,000 emergency room visits; 45,000–50,000 hospitalizations; 3,900 deaths owing to burn-related complications
- In children: 250,000 burns; 15,000 hospitalizations; 1,100 deaths
- Estimated total cost of $2 billion annually for burn care
- House fires cause 75% of deaths.

RISK FACTORS

- Water heaters set too high
- Workplace exposure to chemicals, electricity, or irradiation
- Young children and older adults with thin skin are more susceptible to injury.
- Carelessness with burning cigarettes: Related to 18% of fatal fires in 2006
- Inadequate or faulty electrical wiring
- Lack of smoke detectors: Lacking or nonfunctioning smoke alarms are implicated in 63% of residential fires.
- Arson: Cause of 27% of fires that resulted in fatalities in 2006

GENERAL PREVENTION

- Home safety education should be a key mechanism for injury prevention.
  - Home education families were more likely to have safe hot-water temperatures.
  - Home education results in more families having functioning smoke alarms and increased use of fire guards.
  - There is no evidence that home education results in increasing the chance of possessing a fire extinguisher.
  - Home education did not improve the odds of keeping hot drinks or food out of reach of children and did not increase the safe storage of matches.
  - There is a lack of evidence that home safety education with or without the provision of safety equipment results in a reduction of thermal injuries.
- Skin grafts or newly epithelialized skin is highly sensitive to sun exposure and thermal extremes.

ETIOLOGY

- Open flame and hot liquid are the most common causes of burns (heat usually ≥45°C): Flame burns more common in adults; scald burns more common in children.
- Caustic chemicals or acids (may show little signs or symptoms for the first few days)
- Electricity (may have significant injury with very little damage to overlying skin)
- Excess sun exposure

COMMONLY ASSOCIATED CONDITIONS

Smoke inhalation syndrome:

- May involve thermal burn to respiratory mucosa (e.g., trachea, bronchi) as well as carbon monoxide inhalation
- Occurs within 72 hours of burn
- Should be suspected in all burns occurring in an enclosed space

DIAGNOSIS

HISTORY

- History of source of burn
- In children, check for consistency between the history and the burn's physical characteristics.

PHYSICAL EXAM

- First degree:
  - Erythema of involved tissue
  - Skin blanches with pressure.
  - Skin may be tender.
- Second degree:
  - Skin is red and blistered.
  - Skin is very tender.
- Third degree:
  - Burned skin is tough and leathery.
  - Skin is not tender.
- Rule of 9s (1)[C]:
  - Each upper extremity: Adult and child 9%
  - Each lower extremity: Adult 18%; child 14%
  - Anterior trunk: Adult and child 18%
  - Posterior trunk: Adult and child 18%
  - Head and neck: Adult 10%; child 18%
- Careful documentation of extent of burn and the estimated depth of burn
- Check for any signs suggestive of potential airway involvement: Singed nasal hair, facial burns, carbonaceous sputum, progressive hoarseness, or tachypnea.

DIAGNOSTIC TESTS & INTERPRETATION

- Children: Glucose (hypoglycemia may occur in children because of limited glycogen storage)
- Smoke inhalation: Arterial blood gas, carboxyhemoglobin
- Electrical burns: ECG, urine myoglobin, creatine kinase isoenzymes

Lab

- Hematocrit
- Type and cross
- Electrolytes, including BUN and creatinine
- Urinalysis

Imaging

- Chest radiograph
- Xenon scan useful in suspected smoke inhalation

Diagnostic Procedures/Surgery

Bronchoscopy may be necessary in smoke inhalation to evaluate lower respiratory tract.

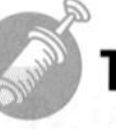

TREATMENT

- Prehospital care (1)[C]:
  - Remove the patient from the source of burn.
  - Extinguish and remove all burning clothing.
  - Remove all rings, watches, and jewelry.
  - Room-temperature water may be poured onto burn, but only in the first 15 minutes following burn exposure.
  - Wrap patient to prevent hypothermia.
  - All patients to receive 100% O_2 via face mask
- Hospitalization for all serious burns:
  - Second-degree burns >10% of body surface area (BSA)
  - Any third-degree burn
  - Burns of hands, feet, face, or perineum
  - Electrical or lightning burns
  - Inhalation injury
  - Chemical burns
  - Circumferential burn
- Transfer to burn center for (1)[C]:
  - Second- and third-degree burns >10% of BSA in patients <10 years and >50 years of age
  - Second-degree burns >20% of BSA and full-thickness burns >5% BSA in any age range
  - Burns of hands, feet, face, or perineum
  - Electrical or lightning burns
  - Inhalation injury
  - Chemical burns
  - Circumferential burn

MEDICATION

First Line

- Morphine: Small, frequent IV doses (0.1 mg/kg per dose in children; 2.5–20 mg q2–6h in adults)
- Silver sulfadiazine (Silvadene): Apply topically to burn site (can cause leukopenia).
- Neosporin or bacitracin ointment: Apply to facial burns.

B

- Mupirocin: Has potent inhibitory activity against methicillin-resistant *Staphylococcus aureus* (MRSA) (2)[B]
- Acticote A.B. (a dressing consisting of 2 sheets of high-density polyethylene mesh coated with nanocrystalline silver) has a more controlled, prolonged release of silver, allowing less frequent dressing changes (2)[B].
- Electrical burn with myoglobinuria will require alkalinization of urine and mannitol.
- Consider H_2 blockers or proton-pump inhibitors (e.g., cimetidine, ranitidine, famotidine, lansoprazole, or nizatidine) for stress ulcer prophylaxis in severely burned patients.
- Tetanus toxoid/tetanus immunoglobulin
- There is no clear indication for prophylactic systemic antibiotics (2)[B].
- Use of VAC system may result in a low-protease environment with higher levels of angiogenic factor (vascular endothelial growth factor [VEGF]) during wound healing, leading to more chaotic, hyperkeratinized, thickened epidermis when compared with a standard hydrocolloid dressing (3)[C].

Second Line

- Mafenide (Sulfamylon) for full-thickness burn (*Caution:* Metabolic acidosis)
- Silver nitrate 0.5% (messy, leaches electrolytes from burn, causes water toxicity)
- Povidone–iodine (Betadine) may result in iodine absorption from burn and "tan eschar." Makes débridement more difficult.
- Travase (enzymatic débridement)

ADDITIONAL TREATMENT

General Measures

- Based on depth of burns and accurate estimate of total BSA involved (rule of 9s)
- Quick estimate (for smaller burns): The surface area of the patient's hand is ~1% of the BSA.
- Tetanus prophylaxis (if not current)
- Remove all rings, watches, and other items from injured extremities to avoid tourniquet effect.
- Remove clothing, and cover all burned areas with dry sheets.
- Flush area of chemical burn (for ~2 hours).
- For all major burns, use 100% oxygen administration; consider early intubation.
- Do not apply ice to burn site.
- Nasogastric tube (high risk of paralytic ileus)
- Foley catheter
- Pain relief:
  - IV meperidine (Demerol), morphine, or methadone for severe pain
  - Oral analgesics, such as acetaminophen (Tylenol) with codeine, acetaminophen with oxycodone (Percocet), or acetaminophen with hydrocodone (Lortab) for moderate pain
- ECG monitoring in first 24 hours following electrical burn
- Whirlpool hydrotherapy followed by silver sulfadiazine (Silvadene) occlusive dressings in severe burns
- Daily or b.i.d. cleansing with dressing changes
- Epilock or Elasto-Gel may be used as dressing in selected patients (especially useful for outpatient treatment of minor burns).

- Burn fluid resuscitation (1)[C]:
  - Calculate fluid resuscitation from time of burn, not from time treatment begins.
  - 2–4 mL Ringer's lactate × body weight (kg) × % BSA burn (1/2 given in first 8 hours, in second 8 hours, and in third 8 hours); in children, this is given in addition to maintenance fluids and is adjusted according to urine output and vital signs.
  - Colloid solutions are not recommended during the first 12–24 hours of resuscitation (1)[C],(4)[A].
- Other: Use of biologic membranes or skin substitutes may be indicated for burn coverage.
- Inhalation injury:
  - Intubation, ventilation with positive end-expiratory pressure assistance
  - Hyperbaric oxygen treatment may be useful in patients with carbon monoxide levels >25%, patients with coma, focal neurologic deficit, ischemic ECG changes, and pregnant patients (1)[C].

SURGERY/OTHER PROCEDURES

- Escharotomy may be necessary in constricting circumferential burns of extremities or chest.
- Tangential excision with split-thickness skin grafts
- Early excision of burns results in a significant reduction in mortality (excluding patients with inhalational injury) and a significant decrease in hospital length of stay (5)[B].

ONGOING CARE

FOLLOW-UP RECOMMENDATIONS

Early mobilization is the goal.

DIET

- High-protein, high-calorie diet when bowel function resumes
- Nasogastric tube feedings may be required in early postburn period.
- Total parenteral nutrition if NPO expected for >5 days

PATIENT EDUCATION

- Use of sunscreen
- Access to electrical cords/outlets
- Isolate household chemicals
- Use low-temperature setting for water heater (below 54°C)
- Household smoke detectors with special emphasis on maintenance
- Family/household evacuation plan
- Proper storage and use of flammable substances
- Burn management: www.aafp.org/afp/20001101/2029ph.html
- Burn prevention: www.aafp.org/afp/20001101/2032ph.html

PROGNOSIS

- First-degree burn: Complete resolution
- Second-degree burn: Epithelialization in 10–14 days (deep second-degree burns probably will require skin graft)
- Third-degree burn: No potential for re-epithelialization; skin graft required
- Length of hospital stay and need for ICU care depend on extent of burn, smoke inhalation, and age.
- A 50% survival rate can be expected with a 62% burn in patients aged 0–14 years, 63% burn in patients aged 15–40 years, 38% burn in patients aged 40–65 years, and 25% burn in patients >65 years of age (1)[C].
- 90% of survivors can be expected to return to an occupation as remunerative as their preburn employment.

COMPLICATIONS

- Gastroduodenal ulceration (curling ulcer)
- Marjolin ulcer: Squamous cell carcinoma developing in old burn site
- Burn wound sepsis: Most commonly *S. aureus* (including MRSA), vancomycin-resistant enterococci, and gram-negative organisms (2)[B]
- Pneumonia
- Decreased mobility with possibility of future flexion contractures
- Hypertrophic scarring common with burns

REFERENCES

1. Teague H, Sweneki SA, Tang A. The burned patient: assessment, diagnosis, and management in the ED. *Trauma Reports*. 2005;6:1–12.
2. Church D, Elsayed S, Reid O, et al. Burn wound infections. *Clin Microbiol Rev*. 2006;19:403–34.
3. Caulfield RH, Tyler MP, Austyn JM. The relationship between protease/anti-protease profile, angiogenesis and re-epithelialisation in acute burn wounds. *Burns*. 2008;34:474–86.
4. Roberts I, Alderson P, Bunn F. Colloids versus crystalloids for fluid resuscitation in critically ill patients (Review). *Cochrane Database Syst Rev*. 2007;(4):CD000567.
5. Ong YS, Samuel M, Song C. Meta-analysis of early excision of burns. *Burns*. 2006;32:145–50.

ADDITIONAL READING

Kessides MC, Skelsey MK. Management of acute partial-thickness burns. *Cutis*. 2010;86:249–57.

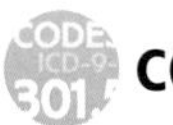

CODES

ICD9

- 949.0 Burn of unspecified site, unspecified degree
- 949.1 Erythema [first degree], unspecified site
- 949.2 Blisters, epidermal loss [second degree], unspecified site

CLINICAL PEARLS

- First degree:
  - Erythema of involved tissue
  - Skin blanches with pressure.
  - Skin may be tender.
- Second degree:
  - Skin is red and blistered.
  - Skin is very tender.
- Third degree:
  - Burned skin is tough and leathery.
  - Skin is not tender.

BURSITIS

Chad Beattie, MD
J. Herbert Stevenson, MD

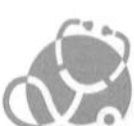

BASICS

DESCRIPTION

A *bursa* is a sac that is formed or found in areas subject to friction, such as locations where tendons pass over bony landmarks. Most common sites are subdeltoid/subacromial, olecranon, prepatellar, trochanteric, and radiohumeral. Bursae essentially lubricate the region with synovial fluid:

- Large bursae usually communicate with joints and are responsible for retaining the synovial fluid in place.
- Bursae are fluid-filled sacs that serve as a cushion between tendons and bones.
- E.G. Bywaters, an English rheumatologist, found at least 78 bursae symmetrically placed on each side of the body.
- System(s) affected: Musculoskeletal

Pediatric Considerations

Bursitis is less common in the pediatric population.

EPIDEMIOLOGY

Predominant age:

- 15–50 years (most common in skeletally mature)
- Traumatic bursitis more likely in patients <35 years of age

Incidence

- Common
- Trochanteric pain: 1.8/1,000 per year

RISK FACTORS

Individuals who engage in repetitive and vigorous training or others who suddenly increase their level of activity (e.g., "weekend warriors")

GENERAL PREVENTION

- Appropriate warm-up and cool-down maneuvers, avoidance of overuse or inadequate rest between workouts
- Range-of-motion exercises
- Maintain high level of fitness and general good health

ETIOLOGY

- Bursitis may be acute or chronic.
- Many types of bursitis, including infectious, traumatic, inflammatory, and gouty
- Less often rheumatoid disease or tuberculosis, as well as gout and pseudogout

COMMONLY ASSOCIATED CONDITIONS

- Tendinitis
- Sprains, strains
- Associated stress fractures

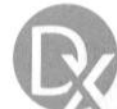

DIAGNOSIS

PHYSICAL EXAM

- Pain/tenderness
- Decreased range of motion of affected region (rare except at shoulder)
- Erythema if infection present
- Swelling
- Crepitus sometimes found

DIAGNOSTIC TESTS & INTERPRETATION

Consider ECG (if left shoulder pain mimics cardiac pain).

Lab

- The following may help in differentiating soft tissue disease from rheumatic and connective tissue disease, but are not usually necessary for routine evaluation:
  - CBC
  - ESR
  - Serum protein electrophoresis
  - Rheumatoid factor
  - Serum uric acid
  - Phosphorus
  - Alkaline phosphatase
  - Blood testing for syphilis
  - Joint fluid analysis and culture (when indicated)
  - Send joint fluid for: Gram stain, culture, cell count, crystal analysis
- Drugs that may alter lab results:
  - ESR may be increased with coexistent use of methyldopa, methysergide, penicillamine, theophylline, vitamin A.
  - ESR may be decreased with coexistent use of quinine, salicylates, and drugs that cause a high glucose level.

Imaging

- MRI may prove beneficial if diagnosis is unclear.
- Calcific deposits may be seen on plain radiograph.
- Ultrasound (1)[B]

Diagnostic Procedures/Surgery

- Aspiration of swollen bursa and evaluation of synovial fluid; the clinician must differentiate infected from inflammatory bursitis:
  - Fluid white blood cell (WBC) 2,000–5,000/μL imply inflammatory, whereas >5,000 imply infectious cause
  - Fluid analysis, Gram stain, culture, and crystal analysis are required to make the diagnosis.
- If the Gram stain and culture yield an infective cause, treat with appropriate antibiotics. If the etiology is inflammatory, give local care.

Pathological Findings

- Acute with early inflammation: Bursa is distended with watery or mucoid fluid.
- Infection: Purulent fluid on aspiration
- Chronic:
  - Bursal wall is thickened, and inner surface is shaggy and trabeculated.
  - The space is filled with granular, brown, inspissated blood admixed with gritty, calcific precipitations.
  - Upper extremity tendinitis and bursitis are usually the result of repetitive microtrauma, probably resulting in disruption of fibers, leading to pain, spasm, and disability.

DIFFERENTIAL DIAGNOSIS

- Septic arthritis
- Gout, pseudogout
- Rheumatic disorders
- Osteoarthritis
- Tendinitis, strains, and sprains
- Lyme arthritis

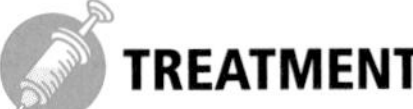

TREATMENT

Outpatient; refer only difficult cases

MEDICATION

First Line

- NSAIDs or aspirin (2)[C]
- Antibiotic therapy if infection present; cover for staph and strep species (most common)

Second Line

- Injectable corticosteroids once infectious etiology ruled out (2)[C],(3)[C],(4)[B]
- Systemic steroids provide limited short-term benefit (5)[B].
- A recent study showed local corticosteroid injection may be used in the management of prepatellar and olecranon bursitis; however, steroid injection into the retrocalcaneal bursa may adversely affect the biomechanical properties of the Achilles tendon (6)[C].

ADDITIONAL TREATMENT

General Measures

- Conservative therapy consists of rest, ice, and local care; elevation, gentle compression (often referred to as RICE therapy [rest-ice-compression-elevation]).
- Compression with Ace wrap or neoprene sleeve
- Bursa aspiration
- Corticosteroid injection if infectious etiology ruled out
- Treatment of any underlying infection

SURGERY/OTHER PROCEDURES

- Surgical excision in severe cases unresponsive to conservative treatments
- Outpatient arthroscopic bursectomy under local anaesthesia is an effective procedure for the treatment of posttraumatic prepatellar bursitis after failed conservative treatments.

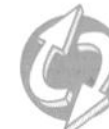

ONGOING CARE

FOLLOW-UP RECOMMENDATIONS

Rest and elevation of affected extremity

Patient Monitoring

- Discontinue NSAIDs as soon as possible to avoid side effects.
- Some patients may require repeated injections (usually no more than 3) of a corticosteroid and lidocaine (2,3)[C].

DIET

Consider changes if bursitis is directly related to obesity/crystalline deposition.

PROGNOSIS

- Most bouts of bursitis heal without sequelae.
- Repetitive acute bouts may lead to chronic bursitis, necessitating repeated joint/bursal aspirations or, eventually, surgical excision of involved bursa.
- While multiple aspirations may not be curative, they can provide significant symptom relief while awaiting a more definitive treatment (i.e., surgery).

COMPLICATIONS

- Septic bursitis may extend to the nearby joint.
- Acute bursitis may progress to chronic.
- Severe long-range limitation of motion

REFERENCES

1. Finlay K, Friedman L. Ultrasonography of the lower extremity. *Orthop Clin North Am.* 2006;37: 245–75, v.
2. Talia AH, Cardone D. Diagnostic and therapeutic injection of the shoulder region. *Am Fam Phys.* 2003;67(6):1271–8.
3. Cardone D, Tallia AH. Diagnostic and therapeutic injection of the hip and knee. *Am Fam Phys.* 2003;67(10):2147–53.
4. Buchbinder R, et al. Corticosteroid injection for shoulder pain. *Cochrane Database Sys Rev.* 2003;(1):CD004016.
5. Buchbinder R, Hoving JL, Green S, et al. Short course prednisolone for adhesive capsulitis (frozen shoulder or stiff painful shoulder): A randomised, double blind, placebo controlled trial. *Ann Rheum Dis.* 2004;63:1460–9.
6. Aaron DL, Patel A, Kayiaros S, et al. Four common types of bursitis: Diagnosis and management. *J Am Acad Orthop Surg.* 2011;19:359–67.

ADDITIONAL READING

- Cardone D, Tallia AH. Diagnostic and therapeutic injection of the elbow. *Am Fam Phys.* 2002;66(11): 2097–3100.
- McFarland EG, Gill HS, Laporte DM, et al. Miscellaneous conditions about the elbow in athletes. *Clin Sports Med.* 2004;23:743–63, xi–xii.

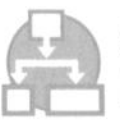

See Also (Topic, Algorithm, Electronic Media Element)

- Tendinitis
- Video: Olecranon Bursitis Aspiration

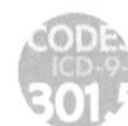

CODES

ICD9

727.3 Other bursitis disorders

CLINICAL PEARLS

Remember RICE acronym for conservative therapy:

- Rest affected area.
- Ice inflamed bursa.
- Compression (with Ace wrap or neoprene sleeve)
- Elevate joint.

BURSITIS, PES ANSERINE

Thomas W. Mahoney, MD
Alan Williamson, MD

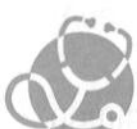

BASICS

DESCRIPTION
- The pes anserinus is formed by the confluence of the tendons of the gracilis, sartorius, and semitendinosus muscles at their insertion on the proximal medial tibia. The pes anserine bursa lies just deep to the tendons.
- Pes anserine bursitis is characterized by medial knee pain not involving the joint line, usually located 4–6 cm distal on the medial aspect of the tibia at the insertion of the pes anserinus.

EPIDEMIOLOGY
Incidence
Common

RISK FACTORS
- Obesity
- Knee joint laxity/ligamentous injury

PATHOPHYSIOLOGY
Friction, whether from dysfunction (valgus deformity) or overuse, causing inflammation and pain

ETIOLOGY
Pes anserine bursitis occurs secondary to:
- Direct trauma
- Overuse injury
- Excessive valgus and rotary stresses

COMMONLY ASSOCIATED CONDITIONS
- Osteoarthritis
- Valgus knee deformity
- Obesity
- Female sex
- Diabetes mellitus (questionable association)

DIAGNOSIS

HISTORY
- Medial knee pain is the most common complaint.
- Pain located distal to the joint line
- Pain exacerbated by active knee flexion, such as climbing or descending stairs

PHYSICAL EXAM
- **Common findings:**
  - Tenderness to palpation over the medial tibia slightly posterior to and 4–6 cm distal to the joint line
  - Pain worsened with active flexion and extension against resistance
  - Possible localized swelling over the pes anserine insertion
- **Findings that should prompt investigation of alternate diagnosis:**
  - Joint effusion
  - Tenderness directly over the joint line
  - Locking of the knee
  - Erythema or warmth
  - Systemic signs such as fever

DIAGNOSTIC TESTS & INTERPRETATION
Lab
Lab work is not indicated unless there is suspicion for infection, in which case consider a:
- CBC
- ESR
- C-reactive protein (CRP)
- Aspirate fluid analysis

Imaging
- Imaging is not indicated unless there is concern for:
  - Bony injury/fracture
  - Ligamentous injury of the knee, such as medial collateral ligament (MCL) injury
  - Meniscal injury
- Ultrasound: Mixed results when evaluated for diagnosis:
  - Can demonstrate focal edema within the pes anserine bursa but poor correlation to clinical findings.
- MRI: Demonstrates inflammation of the bursa well and delineates the pes anserine bursa from other structures:
  - No large studies evaluating correlation between clinical diagnosis and radiographic evidence on MRI

DIFFERENTIAL DIAGNOSIS
- Medial collateral ligament injury
- Medial meniscal injury
- Medial plica syndrome
- Medial compartment osteoarthritis
- Tibial stress fracture

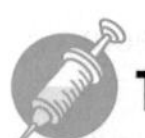

TREATMENT

Conservative therapy is the most common approach to treating pes anserine bursitis:
- Rest: Relative rest; avoiding offending activities is recommended while still performing range of motion, stretching, and other strengthening exercises that do not cause pain.
- Ice can be employed acutely for pain relief and to decrease inflammation.
- Physical therapy
- NSAIDs
- Corticosteroid injection

MEDICATION

First Line

NSAIDs such as ibuprofen (800 mg PO t.i.d.) or naproxen (500 mg PO b.i.d.) are considered the first-line therapy.

Second Line

- Corticosteroid injection combined with local anesthetic has been shown to provide relief in many patients (1)[C].
- Ultrasound-guided injection appears to be superior to blind injection (2)[C].
- The injection is usually performed at the point of maximal tenderness. The area is prepared with standard aseptic practices. 3–5 mL of 1% lidocaine mixed with 20–40 mg of methylprednisolone or triamcinolone is injected in the bursa with a small-gauge needle such as a 22–25-guage 1.5" needle. Care should be taken to avoid injecting directly into the tendon (3)[C].

ADDITIONAL TREATMENT

Physical therapy

- Hamstring and Achilles stretching
- Quadriceps strengthening
- Adductor strengthening

SURGERY/OTHER PROCEDURES

No role for surgery in routine isolated pes anserine bursitis

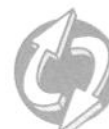

ONGOING CARE

Home exercise program focusing on flexibility and strength

DIET

Consider dietary changes as part of a comprehensive weight-loss program if obesity is a contributing factor.

PROGNOSIS

Most cases of pes anserine bursitis respond to conservative therapy. Recurrence is common, and multiple treatments may be required.

REFERENCES

1. Yoon HS, Kim SE, Suh YR, et al. Correlation between ultrasonographic findings and the response to corticosteroid injection in pes anserinus tendinobursitis syndrome in knee osteoarthritis patients. *J Korean Med Sci*. 2005;20:109–12.
2. Finoff JT, et al. Accuracy of ultrasound-guided versus unguided pes anserinus bursa injections. *PM&R*. 2010;2:732–9.
3. Wittich CM, Ficalora RD, Mason TG, et al. Musculoskeletal injection. *Mayo Clin Proc*. 2009;84:831–6; quiz 837.

ADDITIONAL READING

- Alvarez-Nemegyei J. Risk factors for pes anserine tendinitis/bursitis syndrome: A case control study. *J Clin Rheumatol*. 2007;13–2:63–65.
- Butcher JD, Salzman KL, Lillegard WA, et al. Lower extremity bursitis. *Am Fam Physician*. 1996;53:2317–24.
- Calmbach WL, Hutchens M, et al. Evaluation of patients presenting with knee pain: Part II. Differential diagnosis. *Am Fam Physician*. 2003;68:917–22.
- Rennie WJ, Saifuddin A. Pes anserine bursitis: incidence in symptomatic knees and clinical presentation. *Skeletal Radiol*. 2005;34:395–398.
- Stephens MB, Beutler AI, O'Connor FG, et al. Musculoskeletal injections: A review of the evidence. *Am Fam Physician*. 2008;78:971–6.
- Uson J, Aguado P, Bernad M, et al. Pes anserinus tendino-bursitis: What are we talking about? *Scand J Rheumatol*. 2000;29:184–6.
- Valley VT, Shermer CD. Use of musculoskeletal ultrasonography in the diagnosis of pes anserine tendinitis: A case report. *J Emerg Med*. 2001;201:43–45.

CODES

ICD9

727.3 Other bursitis

CLINICAL PEARLS

- Consider pes anserine bursitis/tendinitis in patients presenting with "knee" pain.
- Physical examination reveals tenderness over the insertion of the pes anserine tendon on the medial aspect of the tibia 4–6 cm distal to the joint line, and (usually) absence of other knee pathology.

B

CANDIDIASIS, INVASIVE

Amimi S. Osayande, MD

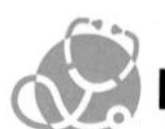

BASICS

DESCRIPTION

Candida albicans and related species cause a variety of infections:

- Cutaneous syndromes include erosio interdigitalis blastomycetica, folliculitis, balanitis, intertrigo, paronychia, onychomycosis, diaper rash, perianal candidiasis, and the syndromes of chronic mucocutaneous candidiasis.
- Mucous membrane infections include oral candidiasis (thrush), esophagitis, and vaginitis.
- This topic addresses the most serious manifestations of candidiasis: Candidemia and hematogenously disseminated invasive candidiasis.

EPIDEMIOLOGY

- Predominant age: All ages are susceptible to hematogenously disseminated candidiasis; premature neonates are at particularly high risk.
- Predominant sex: Male = Female (hematogenously disseminated candidiasis)

Incidence

≥20/100,000 persons per year

Prevalence

Data not available

RISK FACTORS

- Indwelling intravascular access devices
- Immunocompromised states: HIV, neutropenia, chronic corticosteroid treatment
- Diabetes mellitus
- Mucocutaneous colonization/infection
- Broad-spectrum antibacterial chemotherapy
- Recent chemotherapy or radiation
- Cardiothoracic or abdominal surgery
- Parenteral nutrition
- Prolonged hospital stay
- ICU stay
- Burns
- End-stage renal disease
- Bone marrow or solid organ transplant recipient
- Cancer
- Premature birth
- Mechanical ventilation
- Urinary catheter
- Multiple blood transfusions

GENERAL PREVENTION

- Adult ICU: Preemptively treat high-risk patients in ICUs that have a high incidence of invasive candidiasis with fluconazole (1)[B].
- Postoperative prophylaxis with fluconazole or liposomal amphotericin B is recommended in solid organ transplant recipients with a high risk of candidiasis (1)[A].
- Patients with chemotherapy-induced neutropenia or stem cell transplant patients with risk for neutropenia should be treated with echinocandins or azoles (1)[A].

PATHOPHYSIOLOGY

Systemic fungal infection caused by candidal species, usually as a result of decreased polymorphonuclear host defenses

ETIOLOGY

- *Candida albicans* is the most frequent pathogen. Other important human pathogens include *C. tropicalis, C. krusei, C. stellatoidea, C. pseudotropicalis, C. guilliermondi, C. parapsilosis, C. lusitaniae, C. rugosa, C. lambica*, and *C. glabrata*.
- *Candida* species colonize human mucocutaneous surfaces; most infections are endogenously acquired from this reservoir.
- Human-to-human transmission of *Candida* occurs in some settings.

COMMONLY ASSOCIATED CONDITIONS

See "Risk Factors."

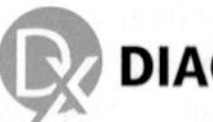

DIAGNOSIS

- Blood or tissue cultures (1)[A]
- Plasma 1,3-beta-D-glucan assay (1)[B]

HISTORY

- Several days of fever that is unresponsive to broad-spectrum antibiotics
- Prolonged IV catheterization
- A history of several key risk factors
- Be alert to organ system dysfunction.

PHYSICAL EXAM

- Fever
- Malaise
- Tachycardia
- Hypotension
- Altered mental status
- Hepatosplenomegaly
- Maculopapular or nodular skin rash

Pediatric Considerations

- For an infant with thrush, be sure to also check for candidal diaper dermatitis. Also, there is often a concomitant infection.
- Fever
- Macronodular skin lesions (10%)
- Candidal endophthalmitis (10–28%)
- Generally, patients are ill and may manifest septic shock.

DIAGNOSTIC TESTS & INTERPRETATION

- The diagnosis is established by isolating the causative organism from blood cultures or other normally sterile body sites or by demonstration of organisms in histopathologic specimens of normally sterile tissues.
- Isolation of *Candida* from multiple sites should raise the diagnostic suspicion of hematogenously disseminated invasive candidiasis.
- *Candida* species isolated from a normally sterile site should be identified to the species level (2)[A].
- Because fluconazole-resistant *C. albicans* and particularly nonalbicans species are reported with increasing frequency, fluconazole susceptibility testing should be performed before treatment with fluconazole (2)[B].
- Plasma 1,3-beta-D-glucan assay has sensitivity of 80–90% in patients with candidemia (1)[B].

Lab

Initial lab tests

- CBC may show leukocytosis.
- Blood cultures may sometimes be negative.

Imaging

- Generally not specifically useful in diagnosis of hematogenously invasive disseminated candidiasis. However, multisite metastasis of infection is common.
- In the syndrome of hepatosplenic candidiasis (chronic systemic candidiasis), imaging of the liver and spleen by liver scan, ultrasound, CT, or MRI may suggest this syndrome as the cause of persistent fever and liver dysfunction in patients who have recently recovered from neutropenia.

Diagnostic Procedures/Surgery

- If blood cultures remain consistently negative, aspiration or excisional biopsy of sites of focal infection may be useful in diagnosis.
- Aspiration and biopsy of skin lesions occasionally seen with hematogenously disseminated candidiasis are also useful.

Pathological Findings

Characteristic histopathology of lesions of *Candida* invasion of visceral organs is microabscess formation.

DIFFERENTIAL DIAGNOSIS

Includes a variety of cryptic bacterial infections and, in the neutropenic host, multiple opportunistic infections

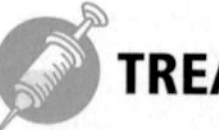

TREATMENT

Inpatient for hematogenously disseminated invasive candidiasis

MEDICATION

- Echinocandins:
  - An initial therapy of choice for moderately severe-to-severe candidemia, neutropenic patients, or patients with prior azole exposure (1)[A]
  - Preferred for use in patients with *Candida glabrata* (1)[B]
  - Caspofungin: Administer 70-mg IV dose on day 1 followed by 50 mg/d IV for 2 weeks after last positive sterile site culture if no evident metastatic infection. Monitor for hepatic impairment.
  - The echinocandins anidulafungin and micafungin have similar efficacy.
  - Transition from an echinocandin to fluconazole is recommended for patients who have isolates that are likely to be susceptible to fluconazole (e.g., *Candida albicans*) and who are clinically stable (1)[A].
  - Duration of treatment for neutropenic patients without metastatic complications is 14 days after first negative blood culture result and resolution of signs and symptoms in patients, plus resolution of neutropenia (1)[B].
  - Echinocandins are pregnancy Category C.
- Triazoles: Fluconazole, itraconazole, voriconazole:
  - Fluconazole is the initial therapy of choice for nonneutropenic patients (1)[A].
  - May also use in neutropenic patients who are less critically ill and who have had no recent azole exposure (1)[B]
  - Also recommended for infections due to *Candida parapsilosis* (1)[B]

- Not recommended for treatment of *Candida glabrata*; however, for patients who initially received fluconazole that are clinically improved and whose follow-up culture results are negative, continuing an azole to completion is acceptable (1)[B].
- Fluconazole 800 mg (12 mg/kg) PO or IV loading dose, then 400 mg (6 mg/kg) PO or IV once daily. Fluconazole oral dose has ~90% bioavailability of IV dosing.
- Duration of treatment for nonneutropenic candidemia is 14 days after first negative blood culture result and resolution of signs and symptoms in patients without obvious metastatic complications (1)[C].
- Other azole antifungals, depending on activity and safety (itraconazole and voriconazole)

- Liposomal amphotericin B (L-AmB):
  - Can be used as an initial therapy for any patient with candidemia (2)[A]. Only recommended if there is intolerance to or limited availability of other antifungal medications. Cautious use is indicated given relative risks of toxicity compared to alternative therapies.
  - There are different lipid formulations of amphotericin B. L-AmB is only one of such. These should not be used interchangeably. Toxicity is less common than with other amphotericin B preparations but may still be formidable. Amphotericin B also exists in the deoxycholate preparation.
  - Usual dosage of L-AmB is 3–5 mg/kg/d IV.
  - Consider higher doses for *C. krusei* or *C. glabrata* (5–10 mg/kg/d).
- Contraindications:
  - The safety of amphotericin B therapy in pregnant patients has not been established.
- Precautions:
  - Liposomal amphotericin B:
    - Acute reactions (fever, rigors, and hypotension) may occur during the initiation of therapy. Ameliorate or eliminate by premedication with acetaminophen or ibuprofen. Use meperidine if needed to abort rigors.
    - Azotemia may occur. Maintenance of optimal fluid status and prevention of dehydration help minimize the risk of azotemia. "Sodium loading" with 1 L half-normal saline daily may decrease renal toxicity.
    - Significant hypokalemia and renal tubular acidosis may develop. Significant hypomagnesemia may worsen hypokalemia.
    - Anemia commonly develops in patients on protracted therapy, but is almost always reversible.
    - Headache and phlebitis are common. Use central venous access for administration.
    - Leukopenia, thrombocytopenia, and liver function abnormalities are rare.
- Significant possible drug–drug interactions:
  - Echinocandins:
    - Potentially important interactions with carbamazepine, phenytoin, cyclosporine, tacrolimus, sirolimus, nonnucleoside reverse transcriptase inhibitors, and rifampin.
  - Liposomal amphotericin B:
    - Concomitant therapy with cyclosporine or other nephrotoxic agents, such as aminoglycosides or vancomycin, may increase the risk of amphotericin-induced nephrotoxicity.
  - Fluconazole and other azoles:
    - Potentially important drug-drug interactions may occur in patients receiving oral hypoglycemics, coumarin-type anticoagulants, phenytoin, cyclosporine, rifampin, theophylline, or terfenadine or astemizole.
    - These drug–drug interactions are more likely with itraconazole and voriconazole than with fluconazole.

ADDITIONAL TREATMENT

General Measures

- Remove all IV catheters if possible (1)[B].
- Fluid and electrolyte therapy are often required.
- Hemodynamic and respiratory support may be required in seriously ill patients.
- All patients with candidemia should undergo a dilated ophthalmological evaluation to exclude *Candida* endophthalmitis (1)[B].

Issues for Referral

Invasive *Candida* infections should be managed with the assistance of an infectious disease specialist.

SURGERY/OTHER PROCEDURES

Drainage of abscess (by any means clinically feasible) is necessary for resolution. Removal of any indwelling contaminated device or catheter is necessary.

IN-PATIENT CONSIDERATIONS

IV Fluids

Generally necessary in critically ill patients

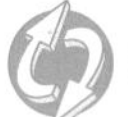

ONGOING CARE

FOLLOW-UP RECOMMENDATIONS

Patients should receive follow-up visit ~6 weeks after end of therapy and be screened for metastatic infection complications by history and physical exam.

Patient Monitoring

- Evaluate CBC, serum electrolytes, and serum creatinine at least twice weekly in patients on liposomal amphotericin B therapy.
- Follow-up blood cultures should be obtained for all patients with candidemia to ensure clearance of *Candida* from the bloodstream.
- Blood cultures be performed daily or every other day until they no longer yield yeast (1)[C].

DIET

Popular literature has reports of diet being linked to yeast overgrowth and subsequent chronic fatigue; randomized controlled trials suggest following a low-sugar, low-yeast diet has no benefit over general healthy eating for symptoms of fatigue (3)[B].

PATIENT EDUCATION

Advise patients of the nature of the infection and the toxicities associated with therapy.

PROGNOSIS

All-cause mortality in adult patients with candidemia is estimated at 47% within 3 months of diagnosis; however, mortality may not always be directly due to candidemia. About 10% of patients with candidemia have mortality attributed to *Candida* (4).

COMPLICATIONS

- Systemic inflammatory response syndrome
- Pyelonephritis
- Endophthalmitis
- Endocarditis, myocarditis, pericarditis
- Arthritis, chondritis, osteomyelitis
- Pneumonitis
- CNS infection

REFERENCES

1. Pappas PG, Kauffman CA, Andes D, et al. Clinical practice guidelines for the management of candidiasis: 2009 update by the Infectious Diseases Society of America. *Clin Infect Dis*. 2009;48:503–35.
2. Spellberg BJ, Filler SG, Edwards JE. Current treatment strategies for disseminated candidiasis. *Clin Infect Dis*. 2006;42:244–51.
3. Hobday RA, Thomas S, O'Donovan A, et al. Dietary intervention in chronic fatigue syndrome. *J Hum Nutr Diet*. 2008;21:141–9.
4. Pappas PG, Rex JH, Lee J, et al. A prospective observational study of candidemia: Epidemiology, therapy, and influences on mortality in hospitalized adult and pediatric patients. *Clin Infect Dis*. 2003;37:634–43.

ADDITIONAL READING

- Kale-Pradhan PB, Morgan G, Wilhelm SM, et al. Comparative efficacy of echinocandins and nonechinocandins for the treatment of Candida parapsilosis Infections: A meta-analysis. *Pharmacotherapy*. 2010;30(12):1207–13.
- Ostrosky-Zeichner L, Pappas PG. Invasive candidiasis in the intensive care unit. *Crit Care Med*. 2006;34:857–63.

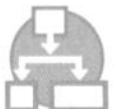

See Also (Topic, Algorithm, Electronic Media Element)

Candidiasis, vulvovaginal

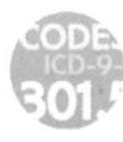

CODES

ICD9

- 112.0 Candidiasis of mouth
- 112.1 Candidiasis of vulva and vagina
- 112.9 Candidiasis of unspecified site

CLINICAL PEARLS

- Antifungal therapy should be started on all candidemic patients within 24 hours after a blood culture positive for yeast. Delays are associated with increased mortality (1)[A].
- Treat for 14 days after first negative blood culture result, resolution of signs and symptoms, and resolution of neutropenia, if any (1)[B].
- Fluconazole prophylaxis in high-risk ICU patients reduces the incidence of invasive candidiasis.

CANDIDIASIS, MUCOCUTANEOUS

Hugh J. Silk, MD, MPH
Sheila O. Stille, DMD, MAGD
Stacy Temple, DMD

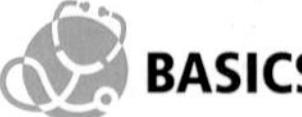

BASICS

DESCRIPTION

- A mucocutaneous disorder caused by infection with various *Candida* spp.
- Areas include:
  - GI:
    - Oropharyngeal candidiasis: Mouth, pharynx
    - Angular cheilitis: Fissures at mouth corners
    - Candida esophagitis: Esophagus
    - GI candidiasis: Gastritis and/or ulcers, associated with thrush; in tract or perianal
  - Non-GI:
    - Candida vulvovaginitis: Vaginal mucosa and/or cutaneous aspects of the vulva
    - Candidal balanitis: Glans penis
    - Candidal paronychia: Nail bed of a digit
    - Folliculitis: Hair follicles
    - Interdigital candidiasis: Webs of the digits
- System(s) affected: Oropharynx, GI, skin/exocrine, genitourinary
- Synonym(s): Monilia; thrush; yeast

ALERT
Vaginal antifungal creams and suppositories can weaken condoms and diaphragms.

Pregnancy Considerations

No known fetal complications of maternal *Candida*

EPIDEMIOLOGY

- Common in the US; very common with immunodeficiency and/or uncontrolled diabetes
- Predominant age: None
  - Infants and seniors: Thrush and cutaneous infections (infant diaper rash)
  - Women of childbearing age: Vaginitis
  - Prepubertal or postmenopausal: Yeast vaginitis uncommon
  - Predominant sex: Female > Male (because of vaginitis)

Incidence

Not well studied, but some estimate 50 per 100,000 annually

Prevalence

Candida colonization: >50% of US population

RISK FACTORS

- Immunosuppression
- Hormonal fluctuations in women
- Antibacterial therapy, especially broad-spectrum antibiotics
- Douches, chemical irritants, and other vaginitides can predispose to yeast vaginitis
- Dentures
- Birth control pills
- Hyperglycemia; diabetes

Genetics

Chronic mucocutaneous candidiasis is a heterogeneous, genetic syndrome; it usually presents during childhood, but the mode of inheritance has not been clarified.

GENERAL PREVENTION

- Minimize antibiotic use.
- Minimize inhaled and systemic steroid use; rinse mouth after inhaled steroid use.
- Avoid douching and use of chemicals (i.e., spermicides).
- Treat other vaginitides.
- Minimize moist environments (e.g., wear cotton underwear).
- Clean dentures appropriately; have new, well-fitting dentures fabricated.
- Control diabetes (if present).

ETIOLOGY

Candida albicans predominant (responsible for 80–92% vulvovaginal candidiasis and 70–80% oral isolates)

COMMONLY ASSOCIATED CONDITIONS

- HIV and other leukopenias
- Diabetes mellitus
- Cancer and other immunosuppressive disorders
- Disorders requiring corticosteroids (1) or other immunosuppressive chemotherapy

DIAGNOSIS

NOTE: *Candida* is normal flora and occurs in very small amounts in the oral cavity, GI tract, and female genital tract.

HISTORY

Symptoms are site specific; see "Physical Exam."

PHYSICAL EXAM

- Children:
  - Oral: White, raised, painless, distinct patches within the mouth; can be wiped off to reveal red base, sometimes with pinpoint bleeding
  - Perineal: Erythematous maculopapular rash with satellite pustules or papules
  - Angular cheilitis: Painful fissures in mouth corners, often cracked and bleeding
- Adults:
  - Vulvovaginal lesions; thin to thick, whitish, cottage cheese–like discharge; red patches in vagina or perineum; symptoms range from none to intense pruritus/burning
- Immunocompromised hosts:
  - Oral: White, raised, painless, distinct patches; red, slightly raised patches; thick, dark-brownish coating; deep fissures
  - Esophagitis: Dysphagia, odynophagia, retrosternal pain; usually with thrush
  - GI symptoms: Ulcerations, pain
  - Balanitis: Erythema, linear erosions, scaling; possible dysuria
  - Angular cheilitis (see "Description.")
  - Folliculitis: Follicular pustules
  - Interdigital: Redness, itchiness at base of fingers and/or toes susceptible to maceration

DIAGNOSTIC TESTS & INTERPRETATION

Imaging

Barium swallow: Esophageal candidiasis may reveal a cobblestone appearance, fistulas, or esophageal dilatation (from denervation)

Diagnostic Procedures/Surgery

- Potassium hydroxide (KOH) prep: A sample of the discharge or coating of the infected area or ulcer is needed.
- Esophagitis may require biopsy.
- Oral hyperplastic candidiasis should be biopsied to rule out carcinoma.
- HIV seropositivity plus thrush with dysphagia relieved by antifungal treatment are acceptable criteria for diagnosis of *Candida* esophagitis.
- Perform culture for rare types of fungal/yeast infections or alternative infection if first-line treatment fails.

Pathological Findings

- Slide preparation: Mycelia (hyphae) or pseudomycelia (pseudohyphae) yeast forms; *Candida* does not induce an increased polymorphonuclear (PMN) leukocyte response.
- pH paper <4.5
- Biopsy: Epithelial parakeratosis with PMN leukocytes in superficial layers; periodic acid Schiff staining reveals presence of candidal hyphae.

DIFFERENTIAL DIAGNOSIS

- For oral candidiasis:
  - Leukoplakia
  - Lichen planus
  - Geographic tongue
  - Herpes simplex
  - Erythema multiforme
  - Pemphigus
- Baby formula or breast milk can mimic thrush.
- Hairy leukoplakia: Does not rub off to erythematous base; usually on lateral tongue
- Angular cheilitis from vitamin B or iron deficiency, staph infection, or edentulous over closure
- *Bacterial vaginosis* and *Trichomonas vaginalis* tend to have more odor, itch, and have a different discharge, but symptoms that are similar to those of *Candida vaginalis* include:
  - Marked vulvar irritation
  - Labial erythema
  - External dysuria
  - Vaginal tenderness

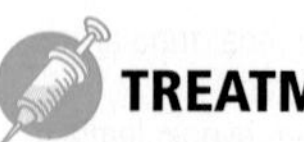

TREATMENT

MEDICATION

First Line

- Vaginal (choose 1):
  - Miconazole (Monistat) 2% cream: 1 applicator or one 100–200-mg suppository, intravaginally q.h.s. for 7 days
  - Clotrimazole (Gyne-Lotrimin, Mycelex): Intravaginal tablets (100 mg q.h.s. for 6–7 days; 200 mg q.h.s. for 3 days; 500 mg daily for 1 day) or 1% cream (1 applicator q.h.s. for 6–7 days)
  - Fluconazole 150 mg PO in 1 dose.
  - Nystatin (Mycostatin, Nilstat): 100,000 U/g cream (1 applicator) or 100,000-U tablets (1 tablet) intravaginally once a day for 7–14 days

- Oropharyngeal:
  - Mild disease:
    - Clotrimazole (Mycelex): 10 mg troche, suck on over 20 minutes 5 times a day for 7–14 days, or
    - Nystatin suspension: 100,000 U/mL given 4–6 times daily, or
    - Nystatin pastilles: 200,000 U each, administered q.i.d. daily for 7–14 days (2)[B]
    - Denture wearers:
      - Nystatin ointment: 100,000 U/g on fitting surfaces of denture and corners of mouth for 3 weeks
      - Remove dentures at night; clean twice weekly with diluted (1:20) bleach.
  - Moderate to severe disease:
    - Fluconazole: 100–200 mg (3 mg/kg) daily for 7–14 days
- Esophagitis:
  - Fluconazole: 100 mg/d for 14–21 days, load with 200 mg
  - Itraconazole (Sporanox):
    - Solution: 1–200 mg daily for 7–14 days
    - Capsules: 200 mg/d (take with food) for 2–3 weeks
- GI: Therapy not well defined
- Any site during pregnancy

Pregnancy Considerations

Miconazole is usually the drug of choice.

Second Line

- Vaginal:
  - Terconazole (Terazol): Recurrent cases: 0.4% cream (1 applicator q.h.s. for 10–14 days of induction therapy); 0.8% cream/80-mg suppositories (1 applicator or 1 suppository q.h.s. for 3 days)
  - Prophylaxis: fluconazole, 150 mg once per week for 6 months to prevent recurrent infections
- Oropharyngeal:
  - Clotrimazole troches at a dosage of 10 mg 5 times daily
  - Nystatin oral suspension (100,000 U/mL):
    - Children: 5–10 mL q.i.d. daily for 10 days; apply directly to oral lesions
    - Infants: 0.5 mL in each cheek q.i.d. daily for 10 days
    - Adults: Swish for as long as reasonable and swallow 5–10 mL q.i.d. daily for 14 days; prophylaxis is achieved with the same dosages 2–5 times a day.
  - Fluconazole: 100 mg/d for 7–14 days (load immunocompromised patient with 200 mg)
  - Itraconazole (Sporanox) suspension: 200 mg (20 mL) daily; swish and swallow for 7–14 days; capsules: 200 mg/d (take with food) for 2–4 weeks
  - Miconazole oral gel (20 mg/mL): q.i.d., swish for as long as reasonable and swallow
  - Amphotericin B (Fungizone) oral suspension (100 mg/mL): 1 mL q.i.d. daily, swish for as long as reasonable and swallow; use between meals
  - Ketoconazole: 200–400 mg PO daily for 14–21 days
- Esophagitis:
  - Oral fluconazole at a dosage of 200–400 mg (3–6 mg/kg) daily for 14–21 days
  - Amphotericin B (variable dosing) IV dose of 0.3–0.7 mg/kg daily; an echinocandin should be used for patients who cannot tolerate oral therapy
- Continue all treatments until 2 days after disappearance of infection:
  - Contraindications:
    - Ketoconazole, itraconazole, or nystatin (if swallowed): Severe hepatotoxicity
    - Amphotericin B: Renal failure
  - Precautions:
    - Miconazole: Can potentiate the effect of warfarin, but drug of choice in pregnancy
    - Fluconazole: Renal excretion; rare hepatotoxicity; resistance frequent
    - Itraconazole: Doubling the dosage results in ~3-fold increase in itraconazole plasma concentrations
- Possible interactions (rarely seen with creams, lotions, or suppositories):
  - Fluconazole:
    - Rifampin: Decreased fluconazole concentrations
    - Tolbutamide: Decreased tolbutamide concentrations
    - Warfarin, phenytoin, cyclosporine: Altered metabolism; check levels
  - Itraconazole: Potent CYP 3A4 inhibitor. Carefully assess all coadministered medications.

ADDITIONAL TREATMENT

General Measures

Screen severely immunodeficient patients at routine visits.

Issues for Referral

- Patients without obvious reasons for recurrent superficial candidal infections
- GI candidiasis

Additional Therapies

- For infants with thrush: Boil pacifiers and bottle nipples; assess mother's breasts/nipples for candida infections as well
- For denture-related candidiasis, disinfection of the denture, in addition to antifungal therapy

COMPLEMENTARY AND ALTERNATIVE MEDICINE

Probiotics: *Lactobacillus* and *Bifidobacterium* may inhibit *Candida* spp (3).

IN-PATIENT CONSIDERATIONS

Nursing

Staff caring for elderly patients should be properly trained in oral hygiene. Protocols for brushing, proper denture care, and moistening the oral cavity can reduce candidal infections among the elderly.

ONGOING CARE

FOLLOW-UP RECOMMENDATIONS

Patient Monitoring

Immunocompromised persons may benefit from regular symptom evaluation plus routine KOH preps during vaginal and oral exams.

DIET

Active-culture yogurt or other live lactobacillus may decrease colonization; indeterminate evidence

PATIENT EDUCATION

- Advise patients at risk for recurrence about antibacterial therapy overgrowth (1)[B].
- "Zole-type" medications are category C

PROGNOSIS

- For immunocompetent individuals: Benign course, excellent prognosis
- For immunosuppressed persons: *Candida* may become an AIDS-defining illness, and chronicity may cause much morbidity.

COMPLICATIONS

In immunosuppressed persons, complications depend on the severity of the immune status. In HIV infection, moderate immunosuppression (e.g., CD4 200–500 cells/mm^3) may be associated with chronic candidiasis. In severe immunosuppression (e.g., CD4 <100 cells/mm^3), thrush may lead to esophagitis, then a full systemic infection involving every organ system, particularly renal.

REFERENCES

1. Kyrmizakis DE, Papadakis CE, Lohuis PJ, et al. Acute candidiasis of the oro- and hypopharynx as the result of topical intranasal steroids administration. *Rhinology*. 2000;38:87–9.
2. Pappas PG, Kauffman CA, Andes D, et al. Clinical practice guidelines for the management of candidiasis: 2009 update by the Infectious Diseases Society of America. *Clin Infect Dis*. 2009;48:503–35.
3. Strus M, Kucharska A, Kukla G, et al. The in vitro activity of vaginal Lactobacillus with probiotic properties against Candida. *Infect Dis Obstet Gynecol*. 2005;13:69–75.

ADDITIONAL READING

- Achkar JM, Fries BC. Candida infections of the genitourinary tract. *Clin Microbiol Rev*. 2010;23:253–73.
- Laudenbach JM, Epstein JB. Treatment strategies for oropharyngeal candidiasis. *Expert Opin Pharmacother*. 2009;10:1413–21.
- Ray A, Ray S, George AT, et al. Interventions for prevention and treatment of vulvovaginal candidiasis in women with HIV infection. *Cochrane Database Syst Rev*. 2011;CD008739.
- Terai H, Shimahara M. Tongue pain: Burning mouth syndrome vs Candida-associated lesion. *Oral Dis*. 2007;13:440–2.

See Also (Topic, Algorithm, Electronic Media Element)

Candidiasis, Invasive; Candidiasis, Mucocutaneous; HIV Infection and AIDS

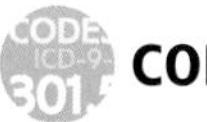

CODES

ICD9

- 112.0 Candidiasis of mouth
- 112.1 Candidiasis of vulva and vagina
- 112.9 Candidiasis of unspecified site

CLINICAL PEARLS

- The diagnosis of candidiasis is generally made clinically, but may include KOH. Rarely, a culture of skin scrapings or even a biopsy is needed for resistant strains or to explore the differential.
- Transmission from person to person is rare. Rarely, *Candida* vaginitis may be sexually transmitted.
- If tongue pain continues after treatment, consider burning mouth syndrome.
- Topical antifungals rarely cause problems, but oral medications may have hepatic side effects.
- Amphotericin B can cause nephrotoxicity.

CARBON MONOXIDE POISONING

Kimberly Snyder, MD

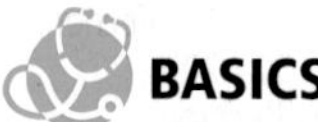

BASICS

DESCRIPTION

Carbon monoxide (CO) is a leading cause of poisoning death in the US. CO is an odorless, tasteless, colorless gas produced by combustion of carbon-containing compounds such as wood, charcoal, oil, and gas:

- CO inhalation leads to displacement of oxygen from binding sites on hemoglobin.
- Detrimental effects are related to tissue hypoxia from decreased oxygen content and a shift of the oxyhemoglobin dissociation curve to the left.
- CO also binds to mitochondrial cytochrome oxidase, impairing adenosine triphosphate (ATP) production, and to myoglobin, affecting muscle function.
- System(s) affected: Cardiovascular; Musculoskeletal; Nervous

Pregnancy Considerations

Tissue hypoxia includes the fetus. CO poisoning may cause significant fetal abnormalities, depending on the developmental stage. Also, adult hemoglobin holds oxygen less tightly than does fetal hemoglobin. Therefore, a pregnant mother potentially may be unaffected while the fetus is affected.

EPIDEMIOLOGY

Incidence

- 40,000 emergency department visits annually
- 5,000–6,000 deaths annually in the US
- Unintentional CO poisoning likely causes 450 deaths annually.
- Intentional CO poisoning is ~10 times higher.
- Unintended poisoning is most common during winter months in cold climates, but can also occur in warm climates with use of generators, boats, etc.
- 10,000 individuals miss 1 or more days of work due to CO poisoning.

RISK FACTORS

- Smoke inhalation
- Being in a closed space with a faulty furnace or stove or running engine
- Cigarette smoking
- Children riding in the back of enclosed pickup trucks
- Employment in a coal mine, as an auto mechanic, paint stripper, or in the solvent industry
- Improperly vented fuel-burning devices:
  - Kerosene heaters, charcoal grills, camping stoves, gasoline-powered generators, wood stoves
  - Open-air exposure to motorboat exhaust, especially swimming too close to the site of exhaust
- Underground utility electrical cable fires produce large amounts of CO, which can seep into adjacent buildings and homes.

GENERAL PREVENTION

- Appropriate ventilation, especially where there are fuel-burning devices
- Use of CO monitors
- Public education
- Determining the mechanism of exposure is critical in cases of accidental poisoning in order to limit future risk

PATHOPHYSIOLOGY

- CO is rapidly absorbed in lungs.
- CO has ~220 times the affinity for hemoglobin that oxygen has.
- CO binds to hemoglobin to form carboxyhemoglobin (COHb), resulting in impaired oxygen-carrying capacity, utilization, and delivery:
  - Leftward shift of the oxyhemoglobin dissociation curve occurs.
  - CO interferes with peripheral oxygen utilization by inactivating cytochrome oxidase.
- Delayed neurologic sequelae, probably due to lipid peroxidation by toxic oxygen species generated by xanthine oxidase.
- The half-life of CO while the patient is breathing room air is ~300 minutes, while breathing 100% oxygen via a tight-fitting, nonrebreathing face mask is ~60 minutes, and with 100% hyperbaric oxygen is ~20 minutes.

ETIOLOGY

- CO inhalation
- Inhaled or ingested methylene chloride (from paint remover [dichloromethane]) is metabolized to CO by the liver, causing CO toxicity in the absence of ambient CO.

COMMONLY ASSOCIATED CONDITIONS

CO and cyanide poisoning can occur simultaneously following smoke inhalation (synergistic effect).

DIAGNOSIS

- Acute CO poisoning is suggested by history, physical examination, and an elevated COHb.
- Chronic CO intoxication is difficult to diagnose.
- The newest pulse CO-oximeters *can* screen for CO exposure using different lengths of infrared light.
- Older pulse oximeters do *not* differentiate carboxyhemoglobin from oxyhemoglobin.

HISTORY

- Headaches
- Dizziness
- Nausea, vomiting, or diarrhea
- Weakness or fatigue
- Confusion or impaired judgement
- Chest pain
- Syncope

PHYSICAL EXAM

- "Cherry red" appearance of the lips and skin
- In absence of trauma or burns, look for altered mental status.
- Respiratory depression, arrhythmias, hypotension
- Cyanosis or tachypnea
- A careful neurologic examination is crucial.
- Visual-field defects, blindness, papilledema, or nystagmus
- CNS depression
- Ataxia
- Seizures
- Coma
- Tachycardia or cardiac dysrhythmias
- Cardiopulmonary arrest

DIAGNOSTIC TESTS & INTERPRETATION

Lab

Initial lab tests

- Measurement of COHb
- Check CO level via co-oximetry of arterial or venous blood (some authors question their accuracy).
- Check acid-base status on blood gas.
- EKG in all patients
- Cardiac enzymes in:
  - ≥65 years
  - Patient with cardiac risk factors or anemia

Follow-Up & Special Considerations

Think of CO poisoning in younger patients with chest pain or symptoms suggestive of ischemia.

Imaging

Head CT scan is helpful to rule out other causes of neurologic decompensation.

DIFFERENTIAL DIAGNOSIS

- Cyanide toxicity
- Acute viral syndrome
- Other causes of mental status changes:
  - Infectious: Meningitis, gastroenteritis
  - Metabolic
  - Drugs: Alcohol (ETOH) intoxication, opiates, acetylsalicylic acid (ASA) overdose
  - Trauma

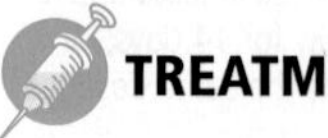

TREATMENT

MEDICATION

- Prompt removal from the source of CO: Important to leave area without looking for a source of the poisoning!
- Institution of 100% oxygen by high-flow mask or endotracheal tube
- 100% normobaric oxygen for all suspected victims of CO poisoning, regardless of pulse oximetry or arterial PO_2 (1)[B]

ADDITIONAL TREATMENT

General Measures

- Removal from source
- Rapid reduction in tissue hypoxia with 100% oxygen to reduce the half-time of elimination of CO to 60 minutes
- Supportive care as necessary
- Intubation and mechanical ventilation may be necessary for severe intoxication. All patients who are comatose or have severely impaired mental status should be intubated and mechanically ventilated without delay (1)[B].
- Volume resuscitation

Additional Therapies

- 100% oxygen by tight-fitting nonrebreathing mask
- Hyperbaric oxygen for severe poisoning or in the following conditions (2)[B]:
  - CO level >15% in a pregnant patient
  - Loss of consciousness
  - Severe metabolic acidosis (pH <7.1)
  - Possible end-organ ischemia (EKG changes, chest pain, altered mental status)
- For mild poisoning (carboxyhemoglobin levels <30%); no signs or symptoms of cardiovascular or neurologic dysfunction:
  - Treatment: Admission if carboxyhemoglobin >25%
  - Symptomatic medication for headache
  - 100% oxygen by nonrebreathing mask until carboxyhemoglobin <5%
  - Patients with underlying heart disease should be admitted, regardless of level of carboxyhemoglobin
- For moderate poisoning (carboxyhemoglobin 30–40%); no signs or symptoms of cardiovascular or neurologic dysfunction:
  - Treatment: Admission
  - Cardiovascular status should be followed closely, even in the absence of clear cardiac effects
  - Determination of acid–base status: Corrected by oxygen
  - 100% oxygen by nonrebreathing mask until carboxyhemoglobin <5%
- For severe poisoning (carboxyhemoglobin >40%); cardiovascular or neurologic functional impairment at any carboxyhemoglobin level:
  - Treatment: Admission
  - Cardiovascular function monitoring
  - Acid–base status monitoring
  - 100% oxygen by nonrebreathing mask until carboxyhemoglobin <5%
  - Hyperbaric oxygen immediately if available; if unavailable, treat as in moderate poisoning
- If no improvement occurs in cardiovascular or neurologic function within 4 hours, transport the patient to the nearest facility with hyperbaric oxygen, regardless of distance.

IN-PATIENT CONSIDERATIONS

Patients often present in clusters, with similar symptoms and a common environment.

Initial Stabilization

- Emergency department (ED) for mild poisoning
- Inpatient treatment for moderate or severe poisoning

Admission Criteria

Patients whose symptoms do not resolve, who demonstrate EKG or laboratory evidence of severe poisoning, or who have other medical or social cause of concern should be hospitalized.

Discharge Criteria

Patients with mild symptoms from accidental poisoning can be managed in the ED and safely discharged.

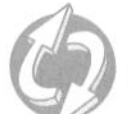

ONGOING CARE

FOLLOW-UP RECOMMENDATIONS

Rest until carboxyhemoglobin reduced and symptoms abate

Patient Monitoring

- Measurement of carboxyhemoglobin levels
- Arterial blood gases
- Psychiatric evaluation and follow-up for intentional exposure

PATIENT EDUCATION

- Professional installation and maintenance of combustion devices: 1-800-638-2772; Consumer Products Safety Commission hotline
- CO detector installation in homes, especially near bedrooms and potential sources

PROGNOSIS

Most survivors recover completely, with only a minority developing chronic neuropsychiatric impairment.

COMPLICATIONS

- Myocardial infarction
- Pulmonary edema (congestive heart failure)
- Pneumonia (aspiration)
- Anoxic encephalopathy
- Long-term neuropsychiatric complications:
  - Intellectual deterioration
  - Memory impairment
- Dysrhythmia
- Shock
- Rhabdomyolysis
- Personality changes:
  - Irritability
  - Aggressiveness
  - Violence
  - Moodiness

Geriatric Considerations

- Higher incidence of cardiovascular and neurologic disease, increasing complications
- Atherosclerosis with chronic exposure

REFERENCES

1. Hampson NB, Scott KL, Zmaeff JL. Carboxyhemoglobin measurement by hospitals: Implications for the diagnosis of carbon monoxide poisoning. *J Emerg Med*. 2006;31:13–6.
2. Kao LW, Nañagas KA. Carbon monoxide poisoning. *Emerg Med Clin North Am*. 2004;22:985–1018.

ADDITIONAL READING

- CDC. Carbon monoxide–related deaths—United States, 1999–2004. *MMWR*. 2007;56:1309–12.
- Insufficient evidence to establish usefulness of hyperbaric oxygen for carbon monoxide poisoning. *Cochrane Library*. 2005;1:CD002041.
- Internet resources available at: http://www.cpsc.gov, http://www.cdc.gov/co, and http://www.epa.gov/iaq/co.html.
- Juurlink DN, Buckley NA, Stanbrook MB, et al. Hyperbaric oxygen for carbon monoxide poisoning. *Cochrane Database Syst Rev*. 2005:CD002041.
- Satran D, Henry CR, Adkinson C, et al. Cardiovascular manifestations of moderate to severe carbon monoxide poisoning. *J Am Coll Cardiol*. 2005;45:1513–6.
- Wolf SJ, Lavonas EJ, Sloan EP, et al. Clinical policy: Critical issues in the management of adult patients presenting to the emergency department with acute carbon monoxide poisoning. *Ann Emerg Med*. 2008;51:138–52.
- World Health Organization's List of International Poison Control Centers: www.who.int/ipcs/poisons/centre/directory/en.

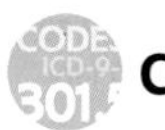

CODES

ICD9

986 Toxic effect of carbon monoxide

CLINICAL PEARLS

- The most appropriate intervention in the management of a CO-poisoned patient is a prompt removal from the source of CO and institution of 100% oxygen by high-flow face mask or endotracheal tube.
- A pregnant woman may appear normal, while her fetus is severely affected.
- Consider CO poisoning in younger patients with chest pain or ischemia.

CARCINOID SYNDROME (NEUROENDOCRINE TUMOR)

JL Godwin, MD
Edward Feller, MD

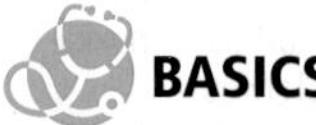

BASICS

DESCRIPTION

- Carcinoid tumors encompass a diverse range of neoplasms and clinical characteristics depending on the site of origin, hormone production, and level of differentiation (1).
- Most common form of neuroendocrine tumors
- Most commonly found in the GI tract and bronchi
- Carcinoid syndrome:
  - Cluster of symptoms related to release of bioactive humoral mediators by carcinoid tumors, including primarily:
    - Cutaneous flushing
    - Diarrhea
    - Bronchospasm
- Tumors can arise almost anywhere:
  - Usually cause a classic carcinoid syndrome, only if liver metastasis has occurred
- Liver inactivates bioactive tumor products, but metastases can release these amines, peptides and prostaglandins directly into hepatic veins and then to the systemic circulation.
- The term carcinoid has fallen out of favor due to lack of specificity; use of neuroendocrine tumor (NET) is more common (e.g., small intestine NET).

EPIDEMIOLOGY

Incidence

- Incidence rates for gastroenteropancreatic (GEP) NETs are roughly 2.5–5 cases per 100,000.
- About 0.46% of all malignant diseases are carcinoid tumors originating in the GI or bronchopulmonary systems.
- Incidence and prevalence has increased substantially since the 1970s; change may be due to advances in imaging.

Prevalence

True prevalence rates of carcinoid tumors are difficult to determine because they are often asymptomatic.

RISK FACTORS

- African Americans: Higher incidence
- Almost all cases of carcinoid syndrome are diagnosed in patients >50 years of age.
- Carcinoid syndrome: More common in intestinal tumors with rates as high as 50%; less common with bronchial carcinoids

Genetics

Multiple genes may be associated: Point mutations, deletions, methylation, chromosomal loss and gain (2,3)

PATHOPHYSIOLOGY

- Common symptoms are linked to bioactive products secreted by tumors:
  - Common products include serotonin, kallikrein, prostaglandins, and histamine, among others.
- Serotonin contributes to diarrhea (stimulating motility and inhibiting GI absorption), flushing, and bronchospasm; may also contribute to right-sided cardiac findings (tricuspid valve or pulmonary valve dysfunction secondary to endocardial plaques) by stimulating fibroblasts.
- Cardiac findings; typically right-sided because the lungs can inactivate many of these mediators. Kallikrein can also contribute to flushing by generating bradykinin, a vasodilator.
- Histamine can cause flushing, pruritus, and possibly peptic ulcers.
- Prostaglandins can cause bronchospasm and affect GI motility.
- Wide variability in types of products secreted by tumors, encompassing biogenic amines (e.g., serotonin, histamine), peptides (e.g., substance P, vasoactive intestinal polypeptide (VIP), atrial natriuretic peptide), tachykinins (e.g., kallikrein, neuropeptide K), and prostaglandins.

COMMONLY ASSOCIATED CONDITIONS

- GEP NETs are associated with multiple endocrine neoplasia (MEN) type 1 syndrome.
- May also be seen in conjunction with familial syndromes such as von Hippel-Landau and neurofibromatosis type 1

DIAGNOSIS

HISTORY

- Most carcinoid tumors are nonfunctioning and asymptomatic, discovered incidentally at imaging, endoscopy, surgery, or autopsy.
- If symptomatic, common presentations include flushing, abdominal pain, diarrhea, bowel obstruction, pulmonary complaints, or symptoms of carcinoid heart disease (especially right-sided heart failure).
- Flushing: Sudden onset on face and upper trunk, lasts 5–10 minutes, intermittent throughout the day, especially after stress or tyramine-containing foods.
- History includes timing and frequency of events, potential precipitating factors. Flushing and diarrhea, the most common symptoms, are very nonspecific. High threshold of suspicion must be present before a full carcinoid-specific investigation.

PHYSICAL EXAM

- Often, no significant findings, since carcinoid syndrome usually features intermittent symptoms
- Full skin exam looking for flushing or telangiectasia, with severe metastatic carcinoid, pellagra (which includes dermatitis) may be found, because tryptophan is a precursor for both serotonin and niacin; tumors take up nearly all available tryptophan, causing niacin (vitamin B_3) deficiency.
- Cardiopulmonary exam should assess for murmurs suggestive of right-sided valvular damage, or evidence of bronchospasm.

DIAGNOSTIC TESTS & INTERPRETATION

Lab

Initial lab tests

- Initial diagnostic test for suspected carcinoid syndrome is a measurement of 24-hour urinary excretion of 5-hydroxyindoleacetic acid (5-HIAA), the final product of serotonin metabolism. (Specificity nearly 100% but sensitivity is only ~75%).
- Many foods (e.g., avocado, chocolate, tomatoes, bananas, nuts) and medications (e.g., acetaminophen, nicotine, caffeine) can alter test results; full list should be reviewed with patients before ordering the test (1).
- Plasma chromogranin A concentration has a reported sensitivity of 75–85% and specificity of 84–95%. This test may be an independent predictor of prognosis, with higher plasma CgA levels associated with poorer prognosis.
- Serum serotonin concentration can be useful if results of 24-hour-urine-5-HIAA test are nondiagnostic.
- Epinephrine provocation test can also be considered. This test must be performed in a highly controlled, monitored environment; it has a reported sensitivity of nearly 100%.

Imaging

- Imaging for tumor localization usually follows a positive lab test result. Abdominal CT is often the first choice, although sensitivity is low (44–55%) (4).
- ^{111}Indium-labeled octreotide scintigraphy scans are often more helpful. Sensitivity for small intestine NETs with symptoms has been reported as >90%.
- Other modalities, including MRI and endoscopic ultrasound are occasionally used; PET scans with targeted tracers (e.g., 18F-DOPA) have shown promise but are not readily available .

Initial approach

- Upper- and lower-GI endoscopies are vital in gastroduodenal and ileo-colonic tumors, respectively; frequent ileal submucosal location limits endoscopic detection and biopsy.
- Small bowel visualization is difficult. Small bowel enteroscopy, MR enterography and video capsule endoscopy are increasingly utilized for localization.
- Liver metastases: Evaluated by CT or MRI

Pathological Findings

- Historically, carcinoid tumors were classified by embryologic site of origin (e.g., foregut, midgut, hindgut), affinity for silver staining, and morphology.
- More recently, the WHO released classification guidelines based on criteria including degree of differentiation and site of origin. Active debate persists regarding classification.
- Improved ability to identify genetic markers in tumors may help.

DIFFERENTIAL DIAGNOSIS

Differential diagnosis for common symptoms of carcinoid syndrome is broad:

- Flushing: Alcohol, alcohol plus disulfiram, menopause, hot drinks, spicy foods, emotional distress, medications (e.g., niacin, nitrates), pheochromocytoma, VIPoma, mastocytosis, renal cell carcinoma, among many others
- Diarrhea: Gastroenteritis, infectious colitis, laxative use/abuse, irritable bowel, inflammatory bowel disease, malabsorption, among many others
- Bronchoconstriction/wheezing: Asthma, pulmonary edema, foreign body, post nasal drip syndrome, COPD, among many others.

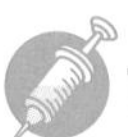

TREATMENT

Rarity has resulted in a lack of large, well-designed, and randomized controlled trials.

MEDICATION

- Primary medications to treat severe symptoms of carcinoid syndrome are somatostatin analogs, most commonly octreotide (others include lanreotide and, more recently, pasireotide).
- Interferon alfa can be added for symptoms refractory to somatostatin analogs; often provides benefits (in terms of risk of progressive disease and median survival), but adverse effects are common.
- Chemotherapy: For poorly differentiated, rapidly progressive metastatic carcinoid tumors; no consensus on a standardized regimen. Agents used include fluorouracil, doxorubicin, etoposide, cisplatin, and streptozocin. Studies are currently looking for benefits of tyrosine kinase inhibitors and VEGF-antibodies (5).
- For patients with milder symptoms due to a carcinoid tumor, initial therapy may be aimed at symptom control: Antidiarrheals, avoiding triggers for flushing (e.g., alcohol, spicy foods), using albuterol for bronchoconstriction. Antihistamines may also provide some relief for a histamine-secreting tumor.

SURGERY/OTHER PROCEDURES

- Surgery is the focus of treatment for solitary tumors localized via imaging. If the disease is more extensive (i.e., metastatic), surgery may still play a role depending on the extent and location of the metastases (6,7).
- Hepatic metastases may be treated with hepatic artery embolization, chemoembolization, radioembolization, radiofrequency ablation, and cryoablation.
- Liver transplant may be required for extensive hepatic disease, but this is rare.
- Ongoing investigations: Peptide-receptor radionuclide therapy with radiolabeled somatostatin analogs, which could deliver radioactivity directly to SSTR-expressing tissues, such as carcinoid metastases. This therapy is not yet readily available to clinicians.

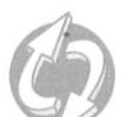

ONGOING CARE

FOLLOW-UP RECOMMENDATIONS

Carcinoid tumors can be associated with development of a second primary tumor, hypothesized to occur due to tumorigenic activity of bioactive products released by the tumor. There is no clear consensus on screening; clinicians should be aware of this possibility and consider surveillance.

DIET

Patients should be counseled to avoid food and drink which may provoke symptoms (e.g., alcohol, caffeine, spicy foods) prior to treatment.

PATIENT EDUCATION

The following Web site sponsored by Novartis that discusses many aspects of carcinoid syndrome: http://www.carcinoid.com

PROGNOSIS

- Prognosis varies widely depending on the site of origin, histologic features, and the extent (stage) of the disease.
- 5-year survival for early stage disease >90%; with distant metastases, 5-year survival: 40–50% (6)
- Presence of the carcinoid syndrome itself is a negative prognostic factor; estimated median survival rates: 5–8 years for these patients.

COMPLICATIONS

- Carcinoid crisis is a cardiovascular collapse due to massive release of bioactive products from a carcinoid tumor; the hallmarks are hypertension or hypotension, tachycardia/arrhythmias, profound flushing and altered mental status.
- Carcinoid crisis can be induced by surgical manipulation of the tumor, anesthesia, chemotherapy, or hepatic artery embolization. Treatment must be immediate, usually by an infusion of plasma and octreotide.

REFERENCES

1. Srirajaskanthan R, Shanmugabavan D, Ramage JK. Carcinoid syndrome. *Easily missed? BMJ*. 2010;341:603–11.
2. Kidd M, Modlin IM. Small intestinal neuroendocrine cell pathobiology: 'Carcinoid' tumors. *Curr Opin Oncol*. 2011;23:45-52.
3. Robertson RG, Geiger WJ, Davis NB, et al. Carcinoid tumors. *Am Fam Physician*. 2006;74:429–34.
4. Heller MT, Shah AB. Imaging of neuroendocrine tumors. *Radiol Clin N Am*. 2011;49:528–48.
5. Lawrence B, Gustafsson BI, Kidd M, et al. New pharmacologic therapies for gastropancreatic neuroendocrine tumors. *Gastroenterol Clin N Am*. 2010;39:615–628.
6. Modlin IM, Oberg K, Chung DC, et al. Gastroenteropancreatic neuroendocrine tumours. *Lancet Oncol*. 2008;9:61–72.
7. Pasieka JL. Carcinoid tumors. *Surg Clin N Am*. 2010;89:1123–37.

ADDITIONAL READING

- Modlin IM, Moss SF, Chung DC, et al. Priorities for improving the management of gastroenteropancreatic neuroendocrine tumors. *J Natl Cancer Inst*. 2008;100:1282–9.
- Pinchot SN, Holen K, Sippel RS, et al. Carcinoid tumors. *Oncologist*. 2008;13:1255–69.
- Rorstad O, et al. Prognostic indicators for carcinoid neuroendocrine tumors of the gastrointestinal tract. *J Surg Oncol*. 2005;89:151–60.

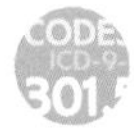

CODES

ICD9

- 239.7 Neoplasm of unspecified nature of endocrine glands and other parts of nervous system
- 259.2 Carcinoid syndrome

CLINICAL PEARLS

- Delay in diagnosis is common due to nonspecific symptoms mimicking more common disorders.
- <10% of carcinoid tumors produce symptoms; incidental diagnosis is common.
- Major symptoms include diarrhea, flushing, wheezing, and bronchoconstriction.
- Diagnosis is established by detecting elevated 5-HIAA by 24-hour urine collection.

CARDIAC ARREST

Marc Grossman, MD, FACEP, CPHM

BASICS

DESCRIPTION

- The absence of effective mechanical cardiac activity
- This section is not a substitute for an AHA-approved Advanced Cardiac Life Support (ACLS) course and is intended only as a quick reference.
- Synonym(s): Code blue in many institutions

Geriatric Considerations

This condition has a low rate of survival and a poor long-term outcome. Be aware of Do Not Resuscitate orders on patients at risk.

Pediatric Considerations

Bradycardia is linked to hypoxia. Bradycardia is the most common initial form of cardiac arrest and is often the response to hypoxia. Adequate oxygenation and ventilation are critical.

Pregnancy Considerations

- Displace the uterus to the left either manually or by placing a rolled towel under the right hip. If the patient cannot be resuscitated within 5–15 minutes, consider an emergency C-section to relieve uterine obstruction and increase blood return to the heart. This may also be done to save the fetus if the fetus has reached gestational age of viability.
- Consider amniotic fluid embolism or eclampsia-related seizures as precipitating factors.

EPIDEMIOLOGY

- Predominant age: Risk increases with age.
- Predominant sex: Male > Female

Incidence

0.5–1.5/1,000 persons per year

RISK FACTORS

- Male gender
- Advanced age
- Hypercholesterolemia
- HTN
- Cigarette smoking
- Family history of atherosclerosis
- Diabetes
- Cardiomyopathy
- Prolonged QT

ETIOLOGY

- Asystole (confirm in 2 leads)
- Ventricular fibrillation (VF)
- Pulseless ventricular tachycardia (VT)
- Pulseless electrical activity (PEA, previously known as electrical mechanical dissociation [EMD])
- Consider possible reversible causes (5 Hs and 4 Ts):
  - Hypoxia, severe hypovolemia, hyper- and hypokalemia [H+] (acidosis), hypothermia
  - Cardiac tamponade, tension pneumothorax, thrombosis (pulmonary embolism, myocardial infarction), tablets (medications and overdoses)

COMMONLY ASSOCIATED CONDITIONS

- Coronary artery disease/acute coronary syndrome (ACS) (cardiac arrest may be presenting symptom)
- Valvular heart disease
- HTN

DIAGNOSIS

- Loss of consciousness secondary to CNS hypoperfusion
- Absence of pulses in large arteries
- Apnea or agonal breathing
- Cyanosis or pallor

HISTORY

- Witnessed or unwitnessed
- Seizure activity
- History or risk factors
- Associated trauma

PHYSICAL EXAM

- Check pupils: May indicate drug overdose. Cannot interpret if patient has received atropine.
- Check pulse.
- Check lungs (i.e., did patient have respiratory decline prior to cardiac decline?).
- Check for dialysis shunt: Patients on dialysis are at increased risk for an electrolyte imbalance that can cause arrest (especially hyperkalemia).

DIAGNOSTIC TESTS & INTERPRETATION

Lab

- Fingerstick glucose
- ABG
- Cardiac enzymes (troponin, CK, CK-MB) every 8 hours for 24 hours
- Chemistry and/or electrolyte panel
- CBC with platelets
- Drug levels (toxicology screen, acetaminophen/aspirin levels, history of specific medication (e.g., digoxin, antiepileptics)
- Blood type and cross, if indicated

Imaging

- Chest x-ray for endotracheal tube (ET) placement, pneumothorax; consider emergency echocardiogram for pericardial effusion and assessment of cardiac motion.
- Once stabilized, consider a CT scan of the brain.

Diagnostic Procedures/Surgery

- ECG
- 2-dimensional echocardiogram
- Airway management/intubation
- Peripheral IV access as close to central circulation as possible; intraosseous if no venous access. Avoid placement of central line during CPR. If it must be placed during CPR, use the femoral approach. Many medications may be administered by endotracheal tube if access is otherwise unobtainable (double dose and flush with saline).
- Pericardiocentesis for cardiac tamponade
- Needle decompression/chest tube for pneumothorax

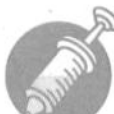

TREATMENT

- New order is C-A-B (Circulation, Airway, Breathing). Use compressions first, then check airway and breathing.
- Prompt initiation of CPR, particularly chest compressions (push hard, push fast, and don't interrupt!), and immediate defibrillation (in witnessed VF and pulseless VT but not in PEA) are first priority (1)[A]:
  - In unwitnessed arrest, complete 1–2 minutes of CPR before attempting defibrillation (2)[A].
- Establishing IV access, intubation, and medications are second priority.
- Continue CPR for 1–2 minutes following the return of a potentially perfusing rhythm before stopping for a pulse check, except for witnessed arrest with a prompt return of rhythm following defibrillation.
- Patients with a return of spontaneous circulation (ROSC) should be strongly considered for Primary Coronary Intervention. If not available in your facility, then consider a transfer to a hospital with this capacity. Early 12 lead may not demonstrate myocardial infarction but this may develop late. Intervention should not be delayed in the appropriate setting.

MEDICATION

First Line

- Vascular access for medications: IV or intraosseous
- Consider medications after initiation of CPR and defibrillation attempt. Medications should be administered during CPR as soon as possible following a rhythm check.
- Epinephrine: 1 mg IV q3–5 min (1)[B] *OR* vasopressin 40 U IV single dose (1)[B] (can be used once in lieu of the first or second dose of epinephrine in VT or VF, but not in PEA):
  - Vasopressin is not recommended in children.
  - Pediatric dose of epinephrine: 0.01 mg/kg
- Atropine for asystole; consider in PEA with absolute bradycardia: 1 mg q3–5 min IV push to total dose of 3 mg (1)[C]:
  - Pediatric dose: 0.02 mg/kg
  - Minimum dose: 0.1 mg; maximum single dose is 0.5 mg in child, 1.0 mg in adolescent
- Magnesium sulfate: 1–2 g diluted in 10 mL D_5W IV push in suspected torsades de pointes (1)[B]:
  - Magnesium is relatively contraindicated in renal failure, but given the consequences of not correcting this rhythm, contraindication is only relative in this setting.

- Antiarrhythmics:
  - Consider if VT/VF is unresponsive to 2–3 shocks and the first dose of vasopressor.
  - Amiodarone is the drug preferred by the AHA. Dosing: 300 mg IV push followed by second dose of 150 mg IV (1)[B]
  - Amiodarone for perfusing tachyarrhythmias: Loading dose of 5 mg/kg IV or IO over 20–60 minutes, maximum dose, 15 mg/kg/d
  - Lidocaine: Initial dose, 1–1.5 mg/kg IV; a repeat loading dose of 1–1.5 mg/kg can be given at 5–10-minute intervals if VT/VF persist to maximum dose of 3 mg/kg (1)[C], then followed by drip if perfusing rhythm recovered
- Endotracheal medications (NAVEL): Narcan, atropine, vasopressin (and Valium), epinephrine, or lidocaine. Each may be placed in 5–10 mL of normal saline or sterile water and given by ET followed by bagging. Dosage should be 2–2.5 times the recommended IV dose. IV or IO is preferred.

Second Line
- Dopamine 2–10 mcg/kg/min IV for bradycardia
- Procainamide: 30 mg/min IV in refractory VF/VT (maximum dose: 17 mg/kg) is permissible. However, because the time to a useful level by infusion is so long, it is unlikely to be of benefit in cardiac arrest, but it may be useful in perfusing tachycardias (1)[C].
- Calcium: May be useful in hyperkalemia, ionized hypokalemia secondary multiple transfusions, and Ca+ channel blocker toxicity; otherwise, no clear benefit is shown.
- High-dose epinephrine: No survival benefit is seen with a high dose (0.1 mg/kg), but it may be considered in exceptional situations, such as β-blocker or calcium channel blocker overdoses.
- Bicarbonate: 1 mEq/kg IV only in known pre-existing bicarbonate-responsive acidosis, hyperkalemia, or to alkalinize the urine in known responsive overdoses (i.e., tricyclics, aspirin). Also may be considered in patients with prolonged or unknown down-time (1)[C].

ADDITIONAL TREATMENT
General Measures
- Perform CPR: Fast (100/min) and hard, with minimal interruptions (1)[B]
- 80–100 bpm without interruption of CPR
- Sequence should be:
  - CPR
  - Rhythm check
  - Resume CPR
  - Shock/meds (charge defibrillator and administer drugs during CPR)
  - Continue CPR (after shocking) for 5 cycles before rechecking rhythm (repeat as needed) (1)[B]
- In VF/pulseless VT, 1 shock should be delivered, and continue sequence above (1)[B]:
  - Monophasic automatic external defibrillators (AEDs) initial and subsequent shocks at 360 J
  - Biphasic AEDs:
    - 150–200 J for biphasic truncated exponential waveform
    - 120 J for rectilinear biphasic waveform
    - If not specified on the biphasic defibrillator, use default of 200 J.
  - Subsequent shocks should be the same or at a higher energy.
  - Pediatric manual defibrillation energy should be 2 J/kg for the first attempt and 4 J/kg for following attempts.
- Consider possible causes of VT/VF, including hypoxia, hyperkalemia, hypokalemia, pre-existing acidosis, drug overdose, and hypothermia.
- Administer 100% oxygen by bag-valve-mask or ET.
- IV and IO are the preferred methods of medication administration, followed by ET.
- Start IV lines as close to the heart as possible. Large-bore peripheral lines can deliver fluid more quickly than a triple-lumen catheter (avoid central line placement during CPR).
- Use an end-tidal CO_2 monitor to assess gas exchange, if available. Esophageal intubation will produce a very low end-tidal CO_2 and requires proper reintubation (1). The use of sodium bicarbonate will increase ET-CO_2 levels.
- Consider a termination of efforts if no reversible underlying cause is found.

Issues for Referral
- Consider communication with the medical examiner's office.
- Consider communication with an organ/tissue bank.

Additional Therapies
Mild therapeutic hypothermia after resuscitation (to 32–34°C for 12–24 hours if initial rhythm was VF) is now strongly suggested and is standard of care in many situations. The greatest benefit is seen in VF as initial rhythm and short down-time (<25 minutes) but it may be considered with any patient that has an ROSC and coma state.

IN-PATIENT CONSIDERATIONS
Initial Stabilization
- Decreasing the EMS response interval increases survival (1)[A].
- The home use of automatic external defibrillators does not improve survival (3).

ONGOING CARE

FOLLOW-UP RECOMMENDATIONS
Patient Monitoring
Admit to ICU or CCU on continuous monitoring.

PROGNOSIS
- The outcome is related to underlying disease, age, duration of arrest, and other factors.
- The outcome is poor with the following indicators:
  - >4 minutes to CPR or >8 minutes to ACLS
  - Arrest occurs out of hospital
  - Resuscitation effort >30 minutes
- ~17% survive in-hospital arrest.
- ~1–10% survive to leave the hospital in out-of-hospital arrest, varying by geographic region.
- ~10–15% of those with VF survive.
- If the arrest is out of hospital without a return of vital signs from ALS prehospital care, the patient is unlikely to respond to ED resuscitation efforts.
- If the patient has an ROSC with coma, strongly consider induced hypothermia to improve the neurologic outcome (number needed to treat in VF = 6).

COMPLICATIONS
- Significant neurologic, hepatic, renal, or cardiac ischemic injury
- Rib fractures, hemopneumothorax, abdominal organ injury from CPR

REFERENCES

1. Hypothermia after Cardiac Arrest Study Group. Mild therapeutic hypothermia to improve the neurologic outcome after cardiac arrest. *N Engl J Med*. 2002;346:549–56.
2. Wik L, Hansen TB, Fylling F. Delaying defibrillation to give basic cardiopulmonary resuscitation to patients with out-of-hospital ventricular fibrillation: A randomized trial. *JAMA*. 2003;289:1389–95.
3. Bardy GH, Lee KL, Mark DB. Home use of automated external defibrillators for sudden cardiac arrest. *N Engl J Med*. 2008;358:1793–804.

ADDITIONAL READING

2005 American Heart Association Guidelines for Cardiopulmonary Resuscitation and Emergency Cardiovascular Care. *Circulation*. 2005;112(Suppl I): IV-1–IV-203.

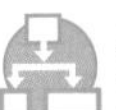

See Also (Topic, Algorithm, Electronic Media Element)

Algorithm: Coronary Syndrome, Acute

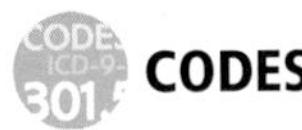

CODES

ICD9

427.5 Cardiac arrest

CLINICAL PEARLS
- C-A-B replaces ABCs for the priority of approach to a patient with a suspected cardiac arrest.
- Prompt initiation of CPR, particularly chest compressions (push hard, push fast, and don't interrupt!), and immediate defibrillation (in witnessed VF and pulseless VT but not in PEA) are first priority.
- For an unwitnessed arrest, complete 1–2 minutes of CPR before attempting defibrillation.
- Get an ECG following the return of circulation to evaluate for acute coronary syndrome.
- Epinephrine is the first drug to give in any case requiring CPR: Avoid the use of central lines during CPR; intraosseous and endotracheal routes are preferred if peripheral access is not attainable.

CARDIAC TAMPONADE

Parag Goyal, MD
James Horowitz, MD

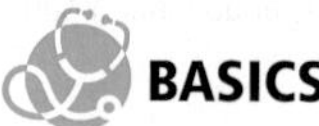

BASICS

DESCRIPTION

- An accumulation of fluid within the pericardium that causes compression of the chambers of the heart, impairing diastolic filling and ultimately leading to cardiovascular collapse
- Tamponade can be acute or subacute, depending on the etiology:
  - Acute: Rapid accumulation (usually blood) within a stiff, noncompliant pericardium
  - Subacute: Gradual increase of a pre-existing effusion, overwhelming normal accommodative pericardial stretch

EPIDEMIOLOGY

Incidence

Difficult to assess due to absence of population-based studies

Prevalence

Difficult to assess due to absence of population-based studies

PATHOPHYSIOLOGY

- As a pericardial effusion accumulates, it overcomes the pericardium's intrinsic compliance, yielding increased intrapericardial pressure. This pressure eventually exceeds intracardiac diastolic pressures, compresses the chambers of the heart, and limits diastolic filling with a subsequent reduction of cardiac output.
- Diastolic filling is decreased first in the more compliant right-sided chambers—right atrium (RA), then right ventricle (RV)—followed by decrease of the left side. Tamponade is defined as the critical point at which diastolic equalization of the left and right ventricles occurs, total venous return drops, and cardiac output falls.
- The hemodynamic significance of the effusion depends on:
  - Rate of accumulation
  - Compliance of the pericardium to accommodate the enlarging effusion

ETIOLOGY

- Acute tamponade (most commonly from a rapidly accumulating hemopericardium, with sometimes as little as 50–100 mL of fluid):
  - Penetrating or blunt trauma
  - Iatrogenic instrumentation (1. cardiac surgery, 2. pacer wire migration or electrophysiological study, 3. central venous catheterization)
  - Aortic dissection
  - Rupture of cardiac free wall, ventricular aneurysm, or coronary artery. These most commonly occur during the post–myocardial infarction (MI) period.
- Subacute tamponade most commonly associated with development of pericardial effusion) (1):
  - Idiopathic pericarditis (20% of subacute tamponade)
  - Iatrogenic effusions (16%) (see above)
  - Malignancy (13%): Breast, lung, lymphoma, leukemia, or radiation pericarditis
  - Idiopathic effusion (9%)
  - Acute MI (8%) (1)
  - End-stage renal disease (ESRD) (6%): Usually BUN >60 mg/dL, but hemodialysis is an independent risk factor
  - Congestive heart failure (CHF) (5%)
  - Collagen vascular disease (5%): Systemic lupus erythematosus, rheumatoid arthritis (RA)
  - Infection (4%):
    - HIV
    - Bacterial infection: *Staphylococcus aureus*, *Mycobacterium tuberculosis*, *Streptococcus pneumoniae* (rare)
    - Fungal infection: *Histoplasmosis capsulatum*
    - Viral infection: Coxsackie group B, influenza, enteric cytopathogenic human orphan, herpes
  - Hypothyroidism with myxedema
  - Massive fluid resuscitation
  - Coagulopathies
- Low-pressure tamponade (when left- and right-sided pressures equalize at lower pressures)
  - Patients with pre-existing effusions who receive hemodialysis or diuretics, thus reducing intravascular volume
  - A decrease in intravascular volume makes an unchanged pre-existing effusion hemodynamically significant (2)
- Regional tamponade (when a loculation or hematoma limits diastolic filling)
  - Loculations are associated with tuberculosis.
  - Localized hematomas are associated with cardiac surgery or post-MI.

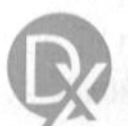

DIAGNOSIS

HISTORY

- Dyspnea: Most sensitive symptom (88%) (1)
- Vague chest pain or an overall subjective sense of discomfort
- Syncope or presyncopal symptoms
- Altered mentation from poor perfusion
- Nausea or abdominal pain from hepatic venous engorgement
- In acute presentations, look for history of recent trauma, surgery, vascular instrumentation
- In subacute presentations, patients may have histories of known pre-existing effusions with new or worsening exertional dyspnea.

PHYSICAL EXAM

- Beck's triad: Distant heart sounds, hypotension, distended neck veins:
  - Pertains specifically to acute tamponade
  - Subacute tamponade: Beck's triad is often absent, and BP may be normal or elevated (1).
- Most sensitive physical findings on exam (1):
  - Pulsus paradoxus (82%)
  - Tachypnea (80%)
  - Tachycardia (77%)
  - Jugular venous distention (76%)
- Pulsus paradoxus: Defined as an exaggerated drop in systolic blood pressure (SBP) (usually >10 mm Hg) during inspiration:
  - In normal physiology: With inspiration, there is a relative decrease in the pressures across the pulmonary vascular bed with a relatively fixed left atrial pressure. This leads to decreased pulmonary venous drainage into the left atrium and therefore a decrease in left-sided stroke volume with inspiration (3).
  - In cardiac tamponade physiology: Normal transmission of pressure from the intrapleural to intrapericardial cavity does not occur. Therefore, increased pressure in the right ventricle with filling occurs at the expense of left ventricle filling, causing a further reduction in cardiac output and a greater drop in SBP than usual.
  - Likelihood ratio (LR) for >12 mm Hg: 5.9; LR for >10 mm Hg: 3.3
  - Can be absent in the settings of hypovolemia, severe aortic insufficiency, severe left ventricular dysfunction, atrial septal defect, or in patients with positive-pressure ventilation (4)
  - Can also be seen in the setting of acute pulmonary embolus, right ventricular infarction, chronic obstructive pulmonary disease (COPD), asthma, and severe lung disease
  - Performed best via sphygmomanometer by the following steps:
    - Insufflate cuff >20 mm Hg beyond systolic pressure.
    - Slowly deflate cuff and record pressure at which Korotkoff sounds are slightly audible at expiration only.
    - Further deflate cuff and record pressure at which Korotkoff sounds are equally audible at inspiration and expiration.
    - If these pressures differ by >10 mm Hg, pulsus paradoxus is present.
- Respiratory distress, but with surprisingly little or no pulmonary edema
- Jugular venous distention with a rapid systolic (X) descent and absent diastolic (Y) descent
- Narrow pulse pressure (due to limited stroke volume and increased peripheral vascular resistance)
- Signs of cardiogenic shock: Low BP with poor mentation and cool, poorly perfused extremities
- Kussmaul's sign (elevation of jugular venous distention with inspiration caused by increased right-sided pressure)
- Increased peripheral (right-sided) edema due to impaired venous return
- Right upper quadrant tenderness due to hepatic engorgement
- Increased area of cardiac dullness outside the apical point of maximum impulse
- Only sign may be pulseless electrical activity

DIAGNOSTIC TESTS & INTERPRETATION

ECG:

- Sinus tachycardia
- Low-voltage QRS, defined as <5 mm in limb leads and <10 mm in precordial leads; sensitivity of 42%
- Signs of pericarditis (except in uremic pericarditis): Initially diffuse ST-segment elevation and PR-segment depression of pericarditis; later stages exhibit T-wave inversions that may be transient or permanent
- Electrical alternans (QRS and/or P-wave beat-to-beat variation in axis and/or amplitude) is only seen in 10–20% of cases of tamponade. However, it is the most specific ECG finding for tamponade (4).

Lab

Initial lab tests

- Acute tamponade (trauma and preoperative labs): CBC, serum chemistries, coagulation panel, ethanol, drugs of abuse, urinalysis
- Subacute tamponade (evaluate cause of the effusion):
  – CBC, serum chemistries, ESR, cardiac enzymes, antinuclear antibodies (ANA), rheumatoid factor (RF)
  – Fluid analysis of glucose, protein, cell count, lactate dehydrogenase (LDH), amylase, cholesterol, cytology, complement levels, Gram stain, and cultures (including bacterial, viral, acid-fast bacilli, and fungal cultures)

Imaging

Initial approach

- Chest radiograph: Utility is limited. May show enlargement of cardiac shadow (if >200 mL fluid present). Cardiomegaly is 89% sensitive, with very poor specificity
- Echocardiography (5):
  – Diastolic chamber collapse: RA collapse in late diastole (more sensitive 55–60%, less specific 50–68%) and RV collapse in early diastole (less sensitive 38–48%, more specific 84–100%) (3)
  – Doppler flow evidence of pulsus paradoxus: An exaggerated increase through tricuspid valve (>40% variation) and exaggerated decrease (>25% variation) through mitral valve. High sensitivity (75%) and specificity (91%).
  – Inferior vena cava (IVC) distention with <50% collapse during inspiration (3)
  – Compression of pulmonary trunk
  – Paradoxical motion of interventricular septum
  – Swinging heart
- CT: May be helpful in evaluating cause (i.e., aortic dissection) and characterizing the effusion (i.e., blood, pus, serous). A pericardial effusion with any of the following is suggestive of tamponade (3):
  – IVC diameter ≥ aorta diameter x 2
  – Reflux of contrast into IVC and/or azygous vein
  – Compression of coronary sinus
  – Flattening of anterior surface of heart and concave chamber deformity
  – Bowing of the interventricular septum into the left ventricle
- MRI (3): Use is limited due to emergent nature of tamponade. Can detect fluid collection as small as 30 mL. Highly effective in evaluating the composition of pericardial effusion.

Diagnostic Procedures/Surgery

Right heart catheterization:

- Diastolic pressures of RA and RV are increased and eventually equalize with the left-sided chambers and the intrapericardial pressure (usually at 15–20 mm Hg) (4).
- The dip and plateau pattern of constriction or restriction pericardial disease is absent.

DIFFERENTIAL DIAGNOSIS

- Any condition causing obstructive or cardiogenic shock, such as massive pulmonary embolism, tension pneumothorax, anterior wall MI, MI with valve rupture or dysfunction, or constrictive/restrictive pericarditis
- Of note, effusive-constrictive pericarditis can be especially difficult to distinguish from tamponade because it involves an effusion that is present with chamber collapse but is not the reason for the collapse. Differentiation can be made on echo by close examination of the diastolic filling patterns:
  – In tamponade, chamber filling is decreased but continuous throughout diastole.
  – In constrictive pericarditis, there is a surge of filling at the beginning of diastole, but is minimal during the rest of the diastolic cycle.

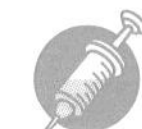

TREATMENT

MEDICATION

First Line

Fluid resuscitation:

- Fluid bolus is temporizing in acute setting.
- In subacute tamponade, most agree that while all patients do not universally benefit from fluid, those with hypotension do (6)[B].

Second Line

Vasopressors if necessary: Dobutamine is thought to maintain better cardiac output and delivery of oxygen than does norepinephrine, although benefit of inotropes is unclear. Treat underlying cause if apparent.

ADDITIONAL TREATMENT

General Measures

Maintain hemodynamic stability until definitive drainage. Intensive care unit monitoring. May consider Swan-Ganz catheter if time allows.

Additional Therapies

- Hemodialysis for ESRD if patient is not in extremis (volume overload can be a cause for increasing pericardial effusions in ESRD)
- Minimize positive end-expiratory pressure and pressure support if mechanically ventilated to preserve cardiac filling (4)[A].

SURGERY/OTHER PROCEDURES

Drainage is the definitive treatment (7)[A]:

- Acute tamponade: Requires surgical intervention. Pericardiocentesis may be performed as a temporizing measure in the setting of hypotension despite fluid resuscitation. However, pericardiocentesis is NOT the definitive treatment, as coagulated blood within the pericardium makes aspiration limited and hemorrhage from the cardiac injury usually refills the sac immediately.
- Subacute tamponade: Pericardiocentesis is usually sufficient for definitive treatment. May be guided by CT (98% success rate), fluoroscopy (93%), or ultrasound (93% for effusions >10 mm). Blind approach may be necessary in sudden cardiovascular collapse (73% success rate). If pericardiocentesis is unsuccessful in the setting of cardiovascular collapse, an immediate thoracotomy may be indicated (8)[B].

IN-PATIENT CONSIDERATIONS

Admission Criteria

Requires ICU-level monitoring

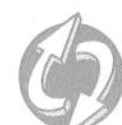

ONGOING CARE

FOLLOW-UP RECOMMENDATIONS

Follow-up echocardiogram may be used to evaluate for recurrence of effusions (7)[A].

PROGNOSIS

Acute traumatic tamponade: 70–80% survival rate at level-1 trauma centers (8).

COMPLICATIONS

- Chamber lacerations
- Pneumothorax
- Ventricular tachycardia

REFERENCES

1. Roy CL, Minor MA, Brookhart MA. Does this patient with a pericardial effusion have cardiac tamponade? *JAMA*. 2007;297:1810–8.
2. Sagristà-Sauleda J, Angel J, Sambola A. Low-pressure cardiac tamponade: Clinical and hemodynamic profile. *Circulation*. 2006;114: 945–52.
3. Restrepo CS, Lemos DF, Lemos JA. Imaging findings in cardiac tamponade with emphasis on CT. *Radiographics*. 2007;27:1595–610.
4. Spodick DH. Acute cardiac tamponade. *N Engl J Med*. 2003;349:684–90.
5. Wann S, Passen E. Echocardiography in pericardial disease. *J Am Soc Echocardiogr*. 2008;21:7–13.
6. Sagristà-Sauleda J, Angel J, Sambola A. Hemodynamic effects of volume expansion in patients with cardiac tamponade. *Circulation*. 2008;117:1545–9.
7. Cheitlin MD, Armstrong WF, Aurigemma GP. ACC/AHA/ASE 2003 guideline update for the clinical application of echocardiography: Summary article: A report of the American College of Cardiology/American Heart Association Task Force on Practice Guidelines (ACC/AHA/ASE Committee to Update the 1997 Guidelines for the Clinical Application of Echocardiography). *Circulation*. 2003;108:1146–62.
8. Fitzgerald M. Definitive management of acute cardiac tamponade secondary to blunt trauma. *Emerg Med Australasia*. 2005;17:494–9.

ADDITIONAL READING

Hoit BD. Pericardial disease and pericardial tamponade. *Crit Care Med*. 2007;35:S355–64.

CODES

ICD9

423.3 Cardiac tamponade

CLINICAL PEARLS

- Pericardial tamponade is a potentially reversible cause of pulseless electrical activity: Perform emergent pericardiocentesis as a diagnostic and therapeutic maneuver.
- Checking for pulsus paradoxus may be a useful bedside maneuver with reasonable sensitivity in most cases, although nonspecific.
- Acute tamponade from trauma or intrapericardial rupture presents with much more rapid clinical deterioration than does subacute tamponade due to sudden rises in pericardial pressure and inability of the pericardium to stretch to accommodate the effusion.

CARDIOMYOPATHY, END STAGE

Timothy P. Fitzgibbons, MD
Theo E. Meyer, MD, DPhil

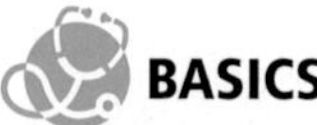

BASICS

DESCRIPTION

In 1995, the World Health Organization (WHO) defined cardiomyopathy as a "disease of the myocardium associated with cardiac dysfunction." The WHO proposed a classification system based on pathophysiology (1). Each class may be caused by many disorders, and some disorders may overlap classes:

- Classification of cardiomyopathy:
  - Dilated (systolic):
    - Characterized by dilation and reduced systolic function of 1 or both ventricles
  - Hypertrophic (diastolic):
    - Left and/or right ventricular hypertrophy with normal to reduced end diastolic volumes
    - May include asymmetric septal hypertrophy
    - Cause of sudden cardiac death in young athletes
  - Restrictive (diastolic):
    - Restrictive filling and reduced diastolic volume of either or both ventricles
    - Systolic function may be near normal.
    - Etiology: Idiopathic, amyloidosis, etc.
  - Arrhythmogenic right ventricular (RV) dysplasia:
    - Fibrofatty replacement of the RV
    - May present with arrhythmia or sudden cardiac death in the young
  - Unclassified:
    - Cases that do not fit easily into 1 group (i.e., noncompacted myocardium)
  - Specific: Includes patients with cardiomyopathy in association with a known systemic disorder:
    - Ischemic
    - Valvular
    - Hypertensive
    - Inflammatory
    - Metabolic
    - Peripartum
- End-stage cardiomyopathy patients have stage D heart failure or severe symptoms at rest refractory to standard medical therapy.
- System(s) affected: Cardiovascular; Renal

Pediatric Considerations

Etiology: Idiopathic, viral, congenital heart disease, and familial

Pregnancy Considerations

May occur in women postpartum

EPIDEMIOLOGY

Predominant age: Ischemic cardiomyopathy is the most common etiology; predominantly in patients >50 years. Consider uncommon causes in young.

Incidence

- 60,000 patients <65 die each year from end-stage heart disease.
- 35,000–70,000 people might benefit from cardiac transplant or chronic support.

Prevalence

Most rapidly growing form of heart disease

RISK FACTORS

- Hypertension
- Hyperlipidemia
- Obesity
- Diabetes mellitus
- Smoking
- Physical inactivity
- Excessive alcohol intake
- Dietary sodium
- Obstructive sleep apnea
- Chemotherapy

Genetics

Hypertrophic, dilated cardiomyopathy, and arrhythmogenic RV dysplasia may present as familial syndromes with autosomal-dominant inheritance.

GENERAL PREVENTION

Reduce salt and water intake; home BP and daily weight measurement

ETIOLOGY

The most frequent causes are in bold:

- **Ischemic heart disease: Most common etiology; up to 66% of patients**
- **Hypertension**
- **Familial cardiomyopathies**
- Congenital heart disease
- Peripartum/postpartum
- Toxic/metabolic causes:
  - **Alcoholism**
  - Radiation
  - Beriberi
  - Cobalt
  - Selenium deficiency
  - Thyrotoxicosis
- Infectious causes:
  - **Viral** (e.g., HIV, Coxsackie virus)
  - Diphtheria
  - Toxoplasmosis
  - Trichinosis
  - Trypanosomiasis
  - Acute rheumatic fever
- Inherited disorders of metabolism:
  - Glycogen storage disease
  - Pompe disease
  - Hurler syndrome
  - Hunter syndrome
  - Fabry disease
- Inherited neuromuscular disorders:
  - Duchenne muscular dystrophy
  - Friedreich ataxia
- Drugs:
  - Chemotherapy: Anthracyclines, cyclophosphamide, Herceptin
- Inflammatory/infiltrative causes:
  - Giant cell myocarditis
  - Loeffler eosinophilia
  - Sarcoidosis
  - Amyloidosis
  - Hemochromatosis
- Idiopathic
- Other causes:
  - **Tachycardia-mediated cardiomyopathy**
  - Valvular heart disease
  - Endomyocardial fibrosis

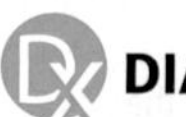

DIAGNOSIS

HISTORY

- Dyspnea at rest or with exertion
- Paroxysmal nocturnal dyspnea
- Orthopnea
- Postprandial dyspnea
- Right upper quadrant pain or bloating
- Fatigue
- Syncope
- Edema

PHYSICAL EXAM

- Tachypnea
- Low pulse pressure
- Cool extremities
- Jugular venous distention
- Bibasilar rales
- Tachycardia
- Displaced point of maximal impulse (PMI)
- S3 gallop
- Blowing systolic murmur
- Hepatosplenomegaly
- Ascites
- Edema

DIAGNOSTIC TESTS & INTERPRETATION

- ECG: Left ventricular (LV) hypertrophy, interventricular conduction delay, atrial fibrillation, evidence of prior Q-wave infarction
- Cardiopulmonary exercise testing: Maximal oxygen consumption <10 mL/kg/min correlates with 50% 1-year mortality, and >18 mL/kg/mm correlates with >90% 1-year survival. Used in stable outpatients to estimate prognosis and prior to cardiac transplant referral.

Lab

- Hyponatremia
- Prerenal azotemia
- Anemia
- Mild elevation in troponin
- Elevated B-type natriuretic peptide (BNP) or pro-BNP
- Mild hyperbilirubinemia
- Elevated liver function tests
- Elevated uric acid

Imaging

- Chest radiograph:
  - Cardiomegaly
  - Increased vascular markings to the upper lobes
  - Pleural effusions may or may not be present.
- Echocardiography:
  - In dilated cardiomyopathy, 4-chamber enlargement and global hypokinesis are present.
  - In hypertrophic cardiomyopathy, severe left ventricular (LV) hypertrophy is present.
  - Segmental contraction abnormalities of the LV are indicative of previous localized myocardial infarction.
- Cardiac MRI:
  - May be useful to characterize certain nonischemic cardiomyopathies
- Myocardial stress perfusion imaging (MPI)
  - Recommended in those with new onset LV dysfunction or when ischemia is suspected

Diagnostic Procedures/Surgery

Cardiac catheterization:

- Helpful to rule out ischemic heart disease
- Characterize hemodynamic severity
- Pulmonary artery catheters may be reasonable in patients with refractory heart failure (HF) to help guide management (2)[C].

DIFFERENTIAL DIAGNOSIS

- Severe pulmonary disease
- Primary pulmonary hypertension
- Recurrent pulmonary embolism
- Constrictive pericarditis
- Hypothyroidism
- Some advanced forms of malignancy
- Anemia
- Chronic illness

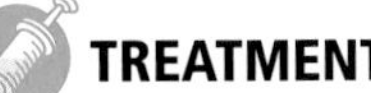

TREATMENT

See "Congestive Heart Failure" for detailed treatment protocols.

MEDICATION

First Line

- Systolic failure syndromes:
  - ACE inhibitors:
    - Lisinopril, 5–40 mg/d or captopril, 6.25–50 mg t.i.d. (2)[A]
  - Loop diuretics:
    - May need to be given IV initially and then orally as patient stabilizes
    - Furosemide, 40–120 mg/d or t.i.d. (2)[A]
  - β-blockers:
    - Use with caution in acutely decompensated or low cardiac output states.
    - Metoprolol succinate, 12.5–200 mg/d; carvedilol, 3.125–25 mg b.i.d.; or bisoprolol, 1.25–10 mg/d (2)[A]
  - Aldosterone antagonists:
    - Patients with New York Heart Association (NYHA) II–IV congestive heart failure (CHF), ejection fraction (EF) <35%, on standard therapy; spironolactone, 12.5–25 mg/d (2)[A]
  - Digoxin, 0.125–0.250 mg/d for symptomatic patients on standard therapy (2)[A]
  - Combination hydralazine/isosorbide dinitrate is first-line treatment in African American patients with class III–IV symptoms (2)[A] already on standard therapy, and for all patients with reduced EF and symptoms incompletely responsive to ACE inhibitor and β-blocker.
- Diastolic failure:
  - Few evidence-based therapies for diastolic heart failure. Empiric management goals include:
    - Management of hypertension
    - Reduction of congestive states (i.e., diuretics)
    - Prevention of progression of left ventricular hypertrophy (i.e., renin-angiotensin-aldosterone system blockade)
    - Maintenance of sinus rhythm
- Contraindications:
  - β-blockers: Low cardiac output, first- or second-degree heart block
  - Ca-blockers (nondihydropyridine): Low cardiac output, heart block
  - Aldosterone antagonists: Oliguria, anuria, renal dysfunction
  - Loop diuretics: Hypokalemia, hypomagnesemia
  - ACE inhibitors: Pregnancy, angioedema
- Precautions:
  - In patients with chronic kidney disease, digoxin dosage should be ≤0.125 mg/d and drug levels followed carefully to avoid toxicity.
  - Closely monitor electrolytes.
  - ACE inhibitors: Initiate with care if BP is low. Begin with low-dose captopril, such as 6.25 mg t.i.d.
  - β-blockers: Avoid in patients with evidence of poor tissue perfusion; they may further depress systolic function.
  - Milrinone, amrinone: Contraindicated for long-term use due to increased mortality

Second Line

- Angiotensin receptor blockers as an alternative to, or (rarely) in addition to, ACE inhibitors
- Inotropic therapy (e.g., dobutamine or milrinone) for support prior to surgery or cardiac transplantation

ADDITIONAL TREATMENT

General Measures

- Reduction of filling pressures
- Treatment of electrolyte disturbances

Issues for Referral

Management by a heart failure team improves outcomes and facilitates early transplant referral.

Additional Therapies

- Prophylactic implantable cardioverter defibrillator (ICD) should be considered for patients with an LVEF <35% and mild to moderate symptoms (2)[A].
- Biventricular pacing should be considered for patients with QRS interval >120 ms, LVEF <35%, and class III CHF despite medical therapy (2)[A]. MADIT-CRT data suggests patients with class II and possibly class I may also benefit (3)[A].
- Patients with severe, refractory HF with no reasonable expectation of improvement should not be considered for an ICD (2)[C].
- Consideration of an LV assist device as "permanent" or destination therapy is reasonable in selected stage D patients.

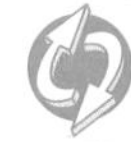

ONGOING CARE

DIET

Low fat, low salt, fluid restriction

PROGNOSIS

~20–40% of patients in NYHA functional class IV die within 1 year. With a transplant, a 1-year survival is as high as 94%.

COMPLICATIONS

Worsening CHF, syncope, renal failure, arrhythmias, or sudden death

REFERENCES

1. Richardson P, McKenna W, Bristow M. Report of the 1995 World Health Organization/International Society and Federation of Cardiology Task Force on the Definition and Classification of cardiomyopathies. *Circulation*. 1996;93:841–2.
2. Lindenfield J, et al. HFSA 2010 Comprehensive Guidelines. *J Cardiac Failure*. 2010;16:e1–e194.
3. Moss AJ, Hall WJ, Cannom DS. Cardiac-resynchronization therapy for the prevention of heart-failure events. *N Engl J Med*. 2009;361(14):1329–38.

ADDITIONAL READING

Nohria A, Lewis E, Stevenson LW. Medical management of advanced heart failure. *JAMA*. 2002;287:628–40.

See Also (Topic, Algorithm, Electronic Media Element)

Alcohol Abuse and Dependence; Alcohol Withdrawal; Amyloidosis; Congestive Heart Failure; Diabetes Mellitus, Type 1; Diabetes Mellitus, Type 2; Hypertension, Essential; Hypothyroidism, Adult; Idiopathic Hypertrophic Subaortic Stenosis; Protein Energy Malnutrition; Rheumatic Fever; Sarcoidosis

CODES

ICD9

- 425.4 Other primary cardiomyopathies
- 425.5 Alcoholic cardiomyopathy
- 425.8 Cardiomyopathy in other diseases classified elsewhere

CLINICAL PEARLS

- Cardiomyopathy represents the end-stage of a large number of disease processes involving the heart muscle.
- Ischemic, hypertensive, postviral, familial, alcoholic, and incessant tachycardia-induced are the most common varieties seen in the US.
- Core therapy for heart failure applies: Salt-restriction, diuretics, ACE inhibitors, β-blockers, digoxin, and electrical treatments such as cardiac resynchronization and implantable defibrillators, as appropriate.

CAROTID SINUS HYPERSENSITIVITY

Adam P. Vasconcellos, MD

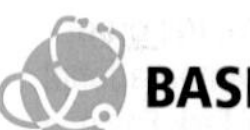

BASICS

DESCRIPTION

- The carotid sinus, located at the bifurcation of the internal and external carotid arteries, contains baroreceptors that are responsive to increases or decreases in arterial pressure. An endogenous increase in BP or external pressure placed on the carotid sinus causes an increase in the baroreceptor firing rate and activates vagal efferents, resulting in a slowing of the heart rate and/or drop in BP.
- In carotid sinus hypersensitivity (CSH), stimulation of one or both carotid sinuses causes an exaggerated baroreceptor response that can result in dizziness or syncope.
- CSH is defined as asystole of at least 3 seconds and/or a drop in systolic BP of at least 50 mm Hg during carotid sinus massage.
- CSH is generally divided into 3 subtypes:
  - Cardioinhibitory (70–75%): Carotid sinus massage resulting in asystole of at least 3 seconds
  - Vasodepressor (5–10%): Carotid sinus massage resulting in a fall in systolic BP of at least 50 mm Hg.
  - Mixed (20–25%): Includes both cardioinhibitory and vasodepressor components

EPIDEMIOLOGY

- Average patient: older men, usually with a history of coronary artery disease and hypertension, with right CSH greater than left CSH
- An estimated 35–100 patients per million have CSH complicated by symptoms of dizziness or syncope. Note that "carotid sinus syndrome" implies a patient who has CSH as diagnosed by carotid sinus massage testing (see below) *and* has had a history of symptoms potentially attributable to this, such as syncope, dizziness, or unexplained falls (1). Both terms, however, are often used interchangeably in the literature (2).
- Estimated prevalence of CSH in persons with a history of recurrent syncope is 13–42% (3).

RISK FACTORS

- Male gender (twice as likely in men as in women)
- Advanced age
- Coronary artery disease or hypertension

PATHOPHYSIOLOGY

- Numerous theories exist regarding the mechanism of CSH, although no single proposed theory is universally accepted:
  - An abnormality of the afferent limb of the baroreflex (neuronal projections from the carotid sinus to the nucleus tractus solitarius)
  - Atherosclerotic disease at the carotid sinus, resulting in carotid ischemia induced by carotid sinus massage
  - Increased sensitivity of the baroreflex arc secondary to chronic loss of innervation of the sternocleidomastoid muscles
- Resultant efferent manifestations are mediated by the vagus nerve in the cardioinhibitory subtype, with sympathetic withdrawal causing the vasodilatation and arterial hypotension observed in the vasodepressor and mixed subtypes.

ETIOLOGY

- Idiopathic
- Carotid body tumors
- Inflammatory and malignant lymph nodes in the neck
- Extensive scarring from prior neck surgery in the area of the carotid sinus
- Metastatic cancer

COMMONLY ASSOCIATED CONDITIONS

- Sick sinus syndrome
- Atrioventricular block
- Coronary artery disease
- Hypertension
- Orthostatic hypotension
- Vasovagal syncope

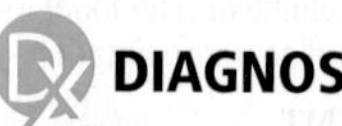

DIAGNOSIS

HISTORY

- Syncope: Usually sudden, of short duration, seemingly spontaneous, and with complete recovery
- Unexplained falls: Evidence of a causal relationship is suggested between falls and the cardioinhibitory subgroup.
- Dizziness: Manifests as transient lightheadedness to presyncope, not usually as a true vertigo; more associated with vasodepressor and mixed subtypes.
- Causative or exacerbating factors:
  - Any carotid sinus massage–like maneuver such as shaving, wearing tight collars, or turning one's head sharply
  - Certain medications can potentiate symptoms associated with carotid sinus hypersensitivity:
    - Digoxin or beta blockers (especially with cardioinhibitory subtype)
    - Physostigmine, morphine, methacholine: Sensitizers of carotid sinus reflex

PHYSICAL EXAM

- Bradycardia
- Hypotension
- Pallor
- Diaphoresis
- Orthostatic vital signs (exclude orthostatic hypotension)

DIAGNOSTIC TESTS & INTERPRETATION

ECG

Imaging

Carotid duplex scan (if needed, see below)

Diagnostic Procedures/Surgery

- Carotid sinus massage: Correct technique for accurate diagnosis:
  - Patient supine for 5 minutes with continuous BP monitoring and ECG (on footplate type tilt table for increased diagnostic accuracy); baseline BP and ECG recorded
  - For 5–10 seconds, apply firm longitudinal massage at right carotid sinus (between the superior border of the thyroid and the angle of the mandible) over the site of maximal pulsation:
    - Note that light pressure over the carotid sinus will not reliably produce a hypersensitivity response.
    - Record symptoms, BP, and note ECG changes.
    - Discontinue if asystole $\geq$3 seconds.
    - Positive response defined per criteria listed above (asystole $\geq$3 seconds and/or drop in BP $\geq$50 mm Hg), although specificity of the carotid sinus massage technique increases if reproduction of a patient's syncope is demonstrated during a test (4)
  - If nondiagnostic, repeat in left supine position, right and left at 70° head-up tilt, allowing the patient time to adjust hemodynamically.
  - Evidence behind the testing strategy:
    - Right side first: Up to 66% with CSH have positive response on the right. If a positive right response, no need to repeat test on the left side.
    - 30% of carotid sinus massage exams are found to be nondiagnostic via the supine position but diagnostic in the 70° position (5).
    - Positive predictive value increases from 77% to 96% with a specificity of 93% by also performing carotid sinus massage in 60–70° tilt position if nondiagnostic in supine position (6)
  - Absolute contraindications for carotid sinus massage testing:
    - Carotid bruit present: Must examine via carotid ultrasound with Doppler first:
      - No testing if >70% stenosis
      - Supine only testing if 50–70% stenosis
    - Myocardial infarction, transient ischemic attack, or stroke within the past 3 months
  - Relative contraindications to carotid sinus massage testing:
    - History of ventricular tachycardia or ventricular fibrillation

DIFFERENTIAL DIAGNOSIS

- Neurocardiogenic syncope
- Postural hypotension
- Primary autonomic insufficiency
- Hypovolemia
- Dysrhythmias
- Sick sinus syndrome
- Cerebrovascular insufficiency
- Other causes of syncope

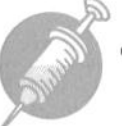

TREATMENT

MEDICATION

First Line

No single agent has demonstrated long-term effectiveness for treatment of recurrent and symptomatic carotid sinus hypersensitivity.

Second Line

- Fludrocortisone or midodrine may be used to improve orthostatic symptoms in patients with vasodepressor subtype.
- Atropine may be used in the acute setting in patients with cardiogenic subtype with bradycardia.

ADDITIONAL TREATMENT

General Measures

- No treatment is required for asymptomatic individuals.
- High dietary salt intake and increased fluid intake may be helpful to maintain intravascular volume in patients with vasodepressor subtype and absence of other cardiovascular disease.

SURGERY/OTHER PROCEDURES

- **Permanent pacing**: Treatment of choice for CSH patients with recurrent syncope:
  - Class I indication for patients with recurrent syncope caused by carotid sinus massage and who are not taking a drug that slows atrioventricular conduction
  - Class IIa indication for patients with recurrent syncope, cardioinhibitory subtype on carotid sinus massage testing, and absence of known precipitating event for syncope
  - Dual-chamber pacing preferred:
    - Meta-analysis of studies testing pacemaker vs. no pacemaker in CSH patients with recurrent syncope suggested syncope recurrence rates of 0–20% in individuals who were given a pacemaker vs. 20–60% in those who were not given a pacemaker (4).
- Carotid sinus denervation by surgery or radiation therapy is no longer recommended because of the high rate of complications.
- Surgery for patients with CSH secondary to mass effect from tumor burden

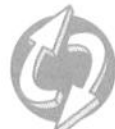

ONGOING CARE

PATIENT EDUCATION

- Avoid precipitating maneuvers (as described above) that place pressure on the neck, such as tight collars and neckties.
- With syncope, restrict driving or other potentially hazardous activities until the patient is cleared by the physician.
- Avoid precipitating medications.

PROGNOSIS

The presence of CSH has not been demonstrated to confer an independent mortality risk.

REFERENCES

1. Humm AM, Mathias CJ. Unexplained syncope–is screening for carotid sinus hypersensitivity indicated in all patients aged >40 years? *J Neurol Neurosurg Psychiatry*. 2006;77:1267–70.
2. Kerr SR, Pearce MS, Brayne C, et al. Carotid sinus hypersensitivity in asymptomatic older persons: Implications for diagnosis of syncope and falls. *Arch Intern Med*. 2006;166:515–20.
3. Kapoor WN, et al. Current evaluation and management of syncope. *Circulation*. 2002;106: 1606–9.
4. Brignole M, Menozzi C, et al. The natural history of carotid sinus syncope and the effect of cardiac pacing. *Europace*. 2011;13:462–4.
5. Parry SW, Richardson DA, O'Shea D, et al. Diagnosis of carotid sinus hypersensitivity in older adults: Carotid sinus massage in the upright position is essential. *Heart*. 2000;83:22–3.
6. Kapoor JR, et al. Carotid sinus hypersensitivity: A diagnostic pearl. *J Am Coll Cardiol*. 2009;54:1633; author reply 1633–4.

ADDITIONAL READING

- ACC/AHA/NASPE 2002 Guideline update for implantation of cardiac pacemakers and antiarrhythmia devices: Summary article. A report of the American College of Cardiology/American Heart Association task force on practice guidelines (ACC/AHA/NASPE committee to update the 1998 pacemaker guidelines).
- Alboni P, Brignole M, Menozzi C, et al. Diagnostic value of history in patients with syncope with or without heart disease. *J Am Coll Cardiol*. 2001;37: 1921–8.
- Bartoletti A, Fabiani P, Bagnoli L, et al. Physical injuries caused by a transient loss of consciousness: Main clinical characteristics of patients and diagnostic contribution of carotid sinus massage. *Eur Heart J*. 2008;29:618–24.
- Davies AJ, Kenny RA. Frequency of neurologic complications following carotid sinus massage. *Am J Cardiol*. 1998;81:1256–7.
- Kenny RA, Richardson DA, Steen N, et al. Carotid sinus syndrome: A modifiable risk factor for nonaccidental falls in older adults (SAFE PACE). *J Am Coll Cardiol*. 2001;38:1491–6.
- Krediet CT, Parry SW, Jardine DL, et al. The history of diagnosing carotid sinus hypersensitivity: Why are the current criteria too sensitive? *Europace*. 2011; 13:14–22.
- Mathias CJ, Deguchi K, Schatz I. Observations on recurrent syncope and presyncope in 641 patients. *Lancet*. 2001;357:348–53.
- Parry SW, Steen N, Bexton RS, et al. Pacing in elderly recurrent fallers with carotid sinus hypersensitivity: A randomised, double-blind, placebo controlled crossover trial. *Heart*. 2009;95:405–9.
- Tan MP, Kenny RA, Chadwick TJ, et al. Carotid sinus hypersensitivity: Disease state or clinical sign of ageing? Insights from a controlled study of autonomic function in symptomatic and asymptomatic subjects. *Europace*. 2010;12:1630–6.

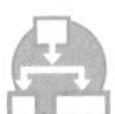

See Also (Topic, Algorithm, Electronic Media Element)

Syncope

CODES

ICD9

337.01 Carotid sinus syndrome

CLINICAL PEARLS

- Consider CSH as a potential cause for syncope, dizziness, or unexplained falls, especially in the elderly.
- Diagnose CSH via carotid sinus massage (using firm pressure for 5–10 seconds), producing asystole of at least 3 seconds and/or a drop in systolic BP of at least 50 mm Hg.
- Consider dual-chamber pacemaker in patients with CSH and recurrent syncope.
- The finding of CSH does not exclude other causes of syncope.

C

CAROTID STENOSIS

Alfonso J. Tafur, MD, RPVI
Angeline Opina, MD

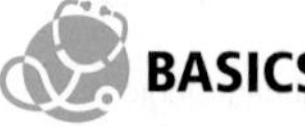

BASICS

Carotid stenosis may be caused by atherosclerosis, intimal fibroplasia, vasculitis, adventitial cysts, or vascular tumors; atherosclerosis is the most common etiology.

DESCRIPTION

- Narrowing of carotid artery lumen is typically due to atherosclerotic changes in the vessel wall. Atherosclerotic plaques are responsible for 90% of extracranial carotid lesions and up to 30% of all ischemic strokes.
- A "hemodynamically significant" carotid stenosis produces a drop in pressure, reduction in flow, or both and corresponds approximately to a 60% diameter-reducing stenosis (1).
- Carotid lesions are classified by:
  - Symptom status:
    - Asymptomatic: Tend to be homogenous and stable
    - Symptomatic (stroke, transient cerebral ischemic event): Tend to be heterogeneous and unstable
  - Degree of stenosis:
    - High grade: 80–99% stenosis
    - Moderate grade: 50–79% stenosis
    - Low grade: <50% stenosis

EPIDEMIOLOGY

More common in men and with increasing age (see "Risk Factors")

Incidence

Unclear (asymptomatic patients often go undiagnosed)

Prevalence

- Of patients aged >50 years, 4.8% of men and 2.2% of women have moderate (≥50%) stenosis (2).
- Of patients aged >70 years, moderate stenosis affects 12.5% of men and 6.9% of women (2).

RISK FACTORS

- Nonmodifiable factors: Advanced age, male sex, family history, cardiac disease, congenital arteriopathies (1)
- Modifiable factors: Smoking, hyperlipidemia, sedentary lifestyle, obesity, hypertension (HTN), diabetes mellitus

Genetics

- Increased incidence among family members
- Genetically linked factors:
  - Diabetes mellitus, race, HTN, family history, obesity
  - In a recent single nucleotide polymorphism study, the following genes were strongly associated with worse carotid plaque: TNFSF4, PPARA, TLR4, ITGA2, and HABP2.

GENERAL PREVENTION

- Antihypertensive treatment to maintain BP <140/90 mm Hg
- Patients should quit smoking and be offered smoking cessation interventions to reduce the risks of atherosclerosis progression and stroke.
- Diet, exercise, and glucose-lowering drugs can be useful for patients with diabetes mellitus.

PATHOPHYSIOLOGY

Atherosclerosis formation begins during adolescence, consistently at carotid bifurcation. The carotid bulb has unique blood-flow dynamics. Hemodynamic disturbances cause endothelial injury and dysfunction. Plaque formation in vessel wall results, and stenosis then ensues.

ETIOLOGY

Initial cause not well understood, but certain risk factors are frequently present (see "Risk Factors"). Tensile stress on the vessel wall, turbulence, and arterial wall shear stress seem to be involved.

COMMONLY ASSOCIATED CONDITIONS

- Transient ischemic attack (TIA)/stroke
- Coronary artery disease (CAD)/myocardial infarction (MI)
- Peripheral vascular disease (PVD)
- HTN
- Diabetes mellitus
- Hyperlipidemia

DIAGNOSIS

Screening for carotid stenosis is not recommended. However, in the setting of symptoms suggestive of stroke or TIA, workup for this condition may be indicated.

HISTORY

- Identification of modifiable and nonmodifiable comorbidities (see "Risk Factors")
- History of cerebral ischemic event
- Stroke, TIA, amaurosis fugax (monocular blindness), aphasia
- Coronary artery disease/MI
- Peripheral arterial disease
- Full review of systems, with focus on risk factors for:
  - Cardiovascular disease
  - Stroke (HTN and arrhythmia)

PHYSICAL EXAM

- Lateralizing neurologic deficits:
  - Contralateral motor and/or sensory deficit
- Monocular blindness (amaurosis fugax):
  - Hollenhorst plaques on retinal examination
- Cerebellar abnormalities:
  - Binocular vision loss, falls without syncope, vertigo, loss of coordination
- Carotid bruit (low sensitivity and specificity)

DIAGNOSTIC TESTS & INTERPRETATION

Lab

Initial lab tests

Workup for suspected TIA/stroke may include:

- CBC with differential
- Basic metabolic panel
- ESR (if temporal arteritis a consideration)
- Glucose/HbA1c
- Fasting lipid profile

Follow-Up & Special Considerations

Proceed to imaging if there is suggestion of stenosis from history or physical examination.

Imaging

Initial approach

Duplex ultrasound identifies ≥50% stenosis, with 98% sensitivity and 88% specificity (3)[A]. Doppler ultrasound determines degree of stenosis by assessing velocity of blood flow through stenotic vessel. Although findings should be confirmed by angiogram (MR or CT) ultrasound is increasingly used to screen prior to surgical assessment.

Follow-Up & Special Considerations

Other noninvasive imaging techniques can add detail to duplex results:

- CT angiography:
  - 88% sensitivity and 100% specificity
  - Requires contrast load with risk for subsequent renal morbidity
- MR angiography:
  - 95% sensitivity and 90% specificity
  - Evaluates cerebral circulation (extracranial and intracranial) as well as aortic arch and common carotid artery
  - The presence of unstable plaque can be determined if the following characteristics are seen (4):
    - Presence of thin/ruptured fibrous cap
    - Presence of lipid-rich necrotic core
  - Tends to overestimate degree of stenosis

Diagnostic Procedures/Surgery

Contrast angiography is the traditional gold standard for diagnosis:

- Delineates anatomy pertaining to aortic arch and proximal vessels
- However, procedure is invasive and has multiple risks:
  - Contrast-induced renal dysfunction (1–5% complication rate)
  - Thromboembolic-related complications (1–2.6% complication rate)
  - Should be used only when other tests are not conclusive

Pathological Findings

- Stenosis consistently occurs at carotid bifurcation, with plaque formation most often at proximal internal carotid artery:
  - Plaque is thickest at the carotid bifurcation.
  - Plaque occupies the intima and inner media, and avoids outer media and adventitia.
- Plaque histology:
  - Homogenous (stable) plaques seldom hemorrhage or ulcerate:
    - Fatty streak and fibrous tissue deposition
    - Diffuse intimal thickening
  - Heterogenous (unstable) plaques may hemorrhage or ulcerate:
    - Presence of lipid-laden macrophages, necrotic debris, cholesterol crystals
    - Ulcerated plaques
  - Soft and gelatinous clots with platelets, fibrin, and red and white blood cells

DIFFERENTIAL DIAGNOSIS

- Aortic valve stenosis
- Aortic arch atherosclerosis
- Arrhythmia with cardiogenic embolization
- Migraine

- Brain tumor
- Metabolic disturbances
- Functional/psychological deficit
- Seizure

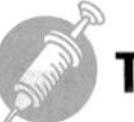

TREATMENT

Smoking cessation, BP control, use of antiplatelet medication, and statin medication are the primary treatments for both asymptomatic and symptomatic carotid stenosis (5).

MEDICATION

- Antihypertensives: Type of therapy appears less important than the response (5)[A]
- Statin initiation is recommended to reduce low-density lipoprotein (LDL) cholesterol below 100 mg/dL.
- Aspirin, 75–325 mg daily
- If patient has sustained ischemic stroke or transient ischemic attack (TIA), antiplatelet therapy with:
  - Aspirin alone (75–325 mg daily)
  - Clopidogrel alone (75 mg daily), or
  - Aspirin plus extended-release dipyridamole (25 and 200 mg b.i.d.)

ADDITIONAL TREATMENT

General Measures

- Lifestyle modifications: Dietary control and weight loss, exercise of 30 minutes/day least 5 days/week
- Control of hypertension (HTN), generally with target BP <140/90 mm Hg
- Avoidance of cigarettes

Issues for Referral

- For acute symptomatic stroke, order imaging and contact neurology.
- For known carotid stenosis, some suggest duplex imaging every 6 months if stenosis is >50% and patient is a surgical candidate.

SURGERY/OTHER PROCEDURES

Goal: Prevention of stroke:

- Patients at average or low surgical risk, with nondisabling ischemic stroke or TIA should undergo carotid endarterectomy (CEA) or carotid artery stenting (CAS) if the diameter of the lumen of the ipsilateral internal carotid artery is reduced more than 70% or more than 50% (5). The anticipated rate of perioperative stroke or mortality must be <6%.
- The selection of asymptomatic patients for carotid revascularization should be guided by an assessment of comorbid conditions, life expectancy, and other individual factors. Should include a thorough discussion of the risks and benefits of the procedure with an understanding of patient preferences (5):
  - It is reasonable to perform CEA in asymptomatic patients who have >70% stenosis of the internal carotid artery if the risk of perioperative stroke, MI, and death is low (5).
  - It is reasonable to choose CEA over CAS when revascularization is indicated in older patients, particularly when arterial pathoanatomy is unfavorable for endovascular intervention (5).
  - It is reasonable to choose CAS over CEA when revascularization is indicated in patients with neck anatomy unfavorable for arterial surgery (5).
- Use of embolic protection devices is now recommended during CAS (6).
- Regional anesthesia may be preferable to general (fewer strokes, arrhythmias, and MIs).

IN-PATIENT CONSIDERATIONS

Initial Stabilization

Rapid evaluation for symptoms compatible with TIA should be obtained in the emergency department or inpatient setting.

Admission Criteria

Any patient with presentation of acute symptomatic carotid stenosis should be hospitalized for further diagnostic workup and appropriate therapy.

IV Fluids

Not necessary

Discharge Criteria

24–48 hours post-CEA, if ambulating, taking adequate PO intake, and neurologically intact

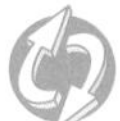

ONGOING CARE

FOLLOW-UP RECOMMENDATIONS

Patient Monitoring

After CEA, overnight in postanesthesia care unit or step-down:

- Duplex at 2–6 weeks postop
- Duplex every 6–12 months
- Reoperative CEA or CAS is reasonable if there is rapidly progressive restenosis (5).

DIET

- NPO postop (in case return to operating room)
- Low-fat, low-cholesterol, low-salt diet at discharge

PATIENT EDUCATION

- Signs and symptoms of TIA/stroke:
  - Lateralizing neurologic deficits, monocular blindness, aphasia
- Diet and lifestyle modification

COMPLICATIONS

- Untreated:
  - TIA/stroke
- Postoperative (s/p CEA):
  - Perioperative (within 30 days):
    - Stroke/death, cranial nerve injury, hemorrhage, hemodynamic instability, MI (because of comorbid CAD)
  - Late (>30 days postop):
    - Recurrent stenosis, false aneurysm at surgical site

REFERENCES

1. Goldstein LB, Bushnell CD, Adams RJ, et al. Guidelines for the primary prevention of stroke: A guideline for healthcare professionals from the American Heart Association/ American Stroke Association. *Stroke*. 2011;42(2):517–84.
2. de Weerd M, Greving JP, de Jong AW, et al. Prevalence of asymptomatic carotid artery stenosis according to age and sex. Systematic Review and metaregression analysis. *Stroke*. 2009.
3. Jahromi AS, Cinà CS, Liu Y, et al. Sensitivity and specificity of color duplex ultrasound measurement in the estimation of internal carotid artery stenosis: A systematic review and meta-analysis. *J Vasc Surg*. 2005;41:962–72.
4. DeMarco JK, Ota H, Underhill HR, et al. MR carotid plaque imaging and contrast-enhanced MR angiography identifies lesions associated with recent ipsilateral thromboembolic symptoms: An in vivo study at 3T. *AJNR Am J Neuroradiol*. 2010; 31(8):1395–402.
5. Brott TG, Halperin JL. 2011 ASA/ACCF/AHA/ AANN/AANS/ACR/ASNR/CNS/SAIP/SCAI/SIR/SNIS/ SVM/SVS guideline on the management of patients with extracranial carotid and vertebral artery disease: executive summary. *J Am Coll Cardiol*. 2011;57(8):1002–44.
6. Margey R, Drachman D. Carotid artery disease and stenting: Insights from recent clinical trials. *Curr Treat Options Cardiovasc Med*. 2011;13:129–45.
7. Murad MH, Shahrour A, Shah ND, et al. A systematic review and meta-analysis of randomized trials of carotid endarterectomy vs stenting. *J Vasc Surg*. 2011;53(3):792–7.

C

ADDITIONAL READING

- Fluri F, Engelter S, Lyrer P. Extracranial-intracranial arterial bypass surgery for occlusive carotid artery disease *Cochrane Database Syst Rev*. 2010;(2): CD005953.
- Sacco RL, Adams R, Albers G, et al. Guidelines for prevention of stroke in patients with ischemic stroke or transient ischemic attack: A statement for healthcare professionals from the American Heart Association/American Stroke Association Council on Stroke: Co-sponsored by the Council on Cardiovascular Radiology and Intervention: The American Academy of Neurology affirms the value of this guideline. *Stroke*. 2006;37:577–617.

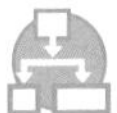

See Also (Topic, Algorithm, Electronic Media Element)

Algorithms: Transient ischemic attack; Stroke; Hypercholesterolemia

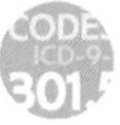

CODES

ICD9

- 433.10 Occlusion and stenosis of carotid artery without mention of cerebral infarction
- 433.11 Occlusion and stenosis of carotid artery with cerebral infarction

CLINICAL PEARLS

- Atherosclerosis is responsible for 90% of all cases of carotid artery stenosis.
- The greater the degree of stenosis, the greater the risk of embolism and stroke.
- Duplex ultrasound is the best initial imaging modality.
- Medical management is the cornerstone of treatment, with surgical management in carefully selected cases and situations.
- Compared with CEA, CAS increases the risk of any stroke and decreases the risk of MI. For every 1,000 patients opting for stenting rather than endarterectomy:
  - 19 more patients would have strokes
  - 10 fewer would have MIs (7)

CARPAL TUNNEL SYNDROME

Jay U. Howington, MD

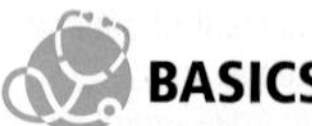

BASICS

DESCRIPTION

- Carpal tunnel syndrome is the most common cause of peripheral nerve compression.
- The median nerve is compressed as it traverses the carpal tunnel in the wrist and hand.
- The tunnel is composed of the carpal bones dorsally and the transverse carpal ligament ventrally. It contains flexor tendons and the median nerve.
- Symptoms tend to affect the dominant hand, but >50% of patients experience bilateral symptoms.
- System(s) affected: Musculoskeletal; Nervous

Pregnancy Considerations

Common during pregnancy

EPIDEMIOLOGY

- Predominant age: 40–60
- Predominant sex: Female > Male (3:1–10:1)

Incidence

- 2 peaks: Late 50s in women, and late 70s when the sex ratio is more equal
- Older patients tend to have more severe carpal tunnel syndrome (59% >65 have thenar atrophy) (1).

Prevalence

Most common entrapment neuropathy. Most recent estimates of prevalence indicate that the disorder occurs in 346/100,000 population.

RISK FACTORS

- There is no clear evidence that repetitive flexion and extension of the wrist may influence the development of carpal tunnel syndrome.
- Occupation as a seamstress or computer operator may exacerbate carpal tunnel syndrome. There is, however, no universal agreement that carpal tunnel syndrome is job-related.
- Obesity is a risk factor in younger patients.

Genetics

Unknown; however, a familial type has been reported.

GENERAL PREVENTION

Take a break once an hour when doing repetitive work involving hands.

ETIOLOGY

- Disorders affecting the musculoskeletal system in the region of the wrist, including the following:
  - Trauma or Colles fracture
  - Degenerative joint disease
  - Rheumatoid arthritis
  - Ganglion cyst
  - Scleroderma
- Hypothyroidism and diabetes are frequently associated with this condition, which also occurs with increased frequency during pregnancy.
- Other miscellaneous causes include the following:
  - Acromegaly
  - Lupus erythematosus
  - Leukemia
  - Pyogenic infections
  - Sarcoidosis
  - Primary amyloidosis
  - Paget disease
- Hyperparathyroidism, hypocalcemia

COMMONLY ASSOCIATED CONDITIONS

- Diabetes
- Obesity
- Pregnancy

DIAGNOSIS

HISTORY

- Burning pain and/or tingling in the fingers, particularly at night (acroparesthesias):
  - The altered sensation (tingling or prickling) is characteristically confined to the thumb and the index and middle fingers, but many patients do not distinguish this localization and feel the entire hand is affected.
- Arm pain
- Symptoms characteristically are relieved by shaking or rubbing the hands.
- During waking hours, symptoms occur when driving the car, reading the newspaper, and occasionally when using the hands for repetitive maneuvers.

PHYSICAL EXAM

- Positive Tinel sign: Tapping of the wrist proximal to the carpal tunnel may produce an electric sensation perceived by the patient, a sign of nerve compression (50% sensitivity and 77% specificity) (2).
- Positive Phalen sign: Holding the wrist flexed for 60 seconds may precipitate the paresthesias experienced by the patient (68% sensitivity and 73% specificity) (2).
- Finger sensory loss
- Wasting of the thenar and hypothenar muscles is a late sign.
- Weakness of the hand, however, for such tasks as opening jars is often noted by the patient early in the disorder.

DIAGNOSTIC TESTS & INTERPRETATION

Lab

- No laboratory test is diagnostic.
- Normal serum TSH and normal serum glucose may be helpful in excluding conditions associated with carpal tunnel syndrome.

Initial lab tests

- Special tests:
  - Electromyography:
    - Will be abnormal in >85% of cases
    - Prolonged distal latency of the median motor nerves may be seen.
    - The most sensitive indicator is the median sensory distal latency, which is prolonged. Further, the sensory nerve action potential may be reduced or unobtainable.
    - Not required as a diagnostic test where clinical symptoms are well defined or to predict surgical outcome (2)[A]
- Stimulation of the ulnar nerve should be done as well to exclude generalized polyneuropathy.

Imaging

Initial approach

- Special radiographic views of the carpal tunnel may be obtained. These are of limited usefulness unless heterotopic calcification can be identified.
- Magnetic resonance neurography may be used to confirm compression of the median nerve in the carpal tunnel and to assess the success of surgical decompression.

Diagnostic Procedures/Surgery

A BP tourniquet to cut off circulation to the arm may precipitate symptoms promptly.

DIFFERENTIAL DIAGNOSIS

- Cervical spondylosis (carpal tunnel may also occur with cervical spine disease; so-called "double crush")
- Generalized peripheral neuropathy
- Brachial plexus lesion
- Pronator syndrome
- Anterior interosseous syndrome

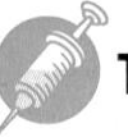

TREATMENT

MEDICATION

First Line

NSAIDs such as ibuprofen, 800 mg b.i.d. or t.i.d., or naproxen sodium, 500 mg b.i.d., may provide significant relief of symptoms in many patients:

- Contraindications: GI intolerance
- Precautions: GI side effects of NSAIDs may preclude their use in selected patients.

Second Line

Oral steroid

ADDITIONAL TREATMENT

General Measures

- Splinting of the wrist in mild extension while sleeping may provide significant relief of symptoms. Prolonged use of splinting, if possible, may allow some symptoms to resolve.
- Injection of the carpal tunnel with a steroid may provide significant temporary relief. This is particularly useful during pregnancy. This can be expected to provide relief for up to 1 month or longer.
- The combination of splinting and steroid injections provides long-term relief in only 10% of cases and is not better than either treatment in isolation (3,4)[A].

COMPLEMENTARY AND ALTERNATIVE MEDICINE

Despite studies, no data exist to support the use of vitamin B_6 in the prevention or treatment of carpal tunnel syndrome.

SURGERY/OTHER PROCEDURES

- Surgical decompression of the carpal tunnel by dividing the transverse carpal ligament completely provides almost total relief of symptoms in >95% of patients.
- Surgical decompression is usually done as an outpatient procedure under local anesthesia.
- Healing of the incision generally takes 2 weeks; an additional 2 weeks of recuperation may be required before the hand can be fully used for tasks requiring strength.
- Recent randomized controlled studies indicate that surgery is more effective than splinting at 18 months (5,6)[A].
- Open vs. endoscopic procedures produce similar outcomes at 1 year and the approach should be driven based on surgeon and patient preference (7)[A].

IN-PATIENT CONSIDERATIONS

Initial Stabilization

- Outpatient
- Outpatient surgery

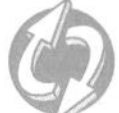

ONGOING CARE

FOLLOW-UP RECOMMENDATIONS

Patient Monitoring

- Patients treated with wrist splints or other palliative measures such as cortisone injections will require follow-up in the ensuing 4–12 weeks to assess the success of treatment modalities.
- Patients treated surgically rarely experience recurrence of the disorder. Routine follow-up once healing of the incision has occurred is not necessary.

PATIENT EDUCATION

Carpal Tunnel Syndrome Foundation. For patient education materials favorably reviewed on this topic, contact: American Academy of Family Physicians Foundation, P.O. Box 8418, Kansas City, MO 64114, (800) 274-2237, Ext. 4400.

PROGNOSIS

Untreated, more severe cases of the condition can be expected to lead to numbness and weakness in the hand, with atrophy of hand muscles and permanent loss of function of the extremity.

COMPLICATIONS

- Postoperative infection (rare)
- Injury to recurrent branch of the nerve

REFERENCES

1. Blumenthal S, Herskovitz S, Verghese J. Carpal tunnel syndrome in older adults. *Muscle Nerve*. 2006;34:78–83.
2. Jordan R, Carter T, Cummins C. A systematic review of the utility of electrodiagnostic testing in carpal tunnel syndrome. *Br J Gen Pract*. 2002;52:670–3.
3. Graham RG. A prospective study to assess the outcome of steroid injections and wrist splinting for the treatment of carpal tunnel syndrome. *Plas Reconst Surg*. 2004;113:550–6.
4. Marshall S, Tardif G, Ashworth N. Local corticosteroid injection for carpal tunnel syndrome. *Cochrane Database Syst Rev*. 2007;CD001554.
5. Verdugo RJ, Salinas RA, Castillo JL. Surgical versus non-surgical treatment for carpal tunnel syndrome. *Cochrane Database Syst Rev*. 2008;CD001552.
6. Gerritsen AA, de Vet HC, Scholten RJ. Splinting vs. surgery in the treatment of carpal tunnel syndrome: A randomized controlled trial. *JAMA*. 2002;288: 1245–51.
7. Scholten RJ, Mink van der Molen A, Uitdehaag BM, et al. Surgical treatment options for carpal tunnel syndrome. *Cochrane Database Syst Rev*. 2007; CD003905.

ADDITIONAL READING

- Cudlip SA, Howe FA, Clifton A. Magnetic resonance neurography studies of the median nerve before and after carpal tunnel decompression. *J Neurosurg*. 2002;96:1046–51.
- Nordstrom DL, DeStefano F, Vierkant RA. Incidence of diagnosed carpal tunnel syndrome in a general population. *Epidemiology*. 1998;9:342–5.

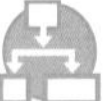

See Also (Topic, Algorithm, Electronic Media Element)

- Arthritis, Rheumatoid; Hypoparathyroidism; Scleroderma; Systemic Lupus Erythematosus (SLE)
- Algorithms: Carpal Tunnel Syndrome; Pain in Upper Extremity

CODES

ICD9

354.0 Carpal tunnel syndrome

CLINICAL PEARLS

- The altered sensation (tingling or prickling) in carpal tunnel syndrome is characteristically confined to the thumb and the index and middle fingers, but many patients do not distinguish this localization and feel that the entire hand is affected.
- Tinel and Phalen signs have poor sensitivity and specificity.
- Normal serum TSH and normal serum glucose may be helpful in excluding conditions associated with carpal tunnel syndrome.
- Strongly consider surgical treatment for moderate and severe cases. Atrophy is a late finding indicating severe disease.

C

CATARACT

Yasir Ahmed, MD
Peter Fay, MD

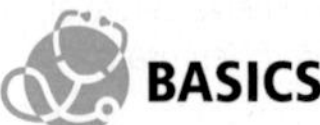

BASICS

DESCRIPTION

A cataract is any opacity or discoloration of the lens, localized or generalized; the term is usually reserved for changes that affect visual acuity:

- Etymology: From Latin *catarractes*, for "waterfall"; named after foamy appearance of opacity
- Leading cause of blindness worldwide, an estimated 20 million people
- Types include:
  - Age-related ("senile"): 90% of total
  - Metabolic (diabetes via accelerated sorbitol pathway, hypocalcemia, Wilson disease)
  - Congenital (1/250 newborns; 10–38% of childhood blindness)
  - Systemic disease associated (myotonic dystrophy, atopic dermatitis)
  - Secondary to associated eye disease, so-called complicated (e.g., uveitis associated with juvenile rheumatoid arthritis or sarcoid, tumor such as melanoma or retinoblastoma)
  - Traumatic (e.g., heat, electric shock, radiation, concussion, perforating eye injuries, intraocular foreign body)
  - Toxic/nutritional (e.g., corticosteroids, medications)
- Morphologic classification:
  - Nuclear: Exaggeration of normal aging changes of *central* lens nucleus, often associated with myopia due to increased refractive index of lens (some elderly patients consequently may be able to read again *without spectacles*, so-called second sight of the aged)
  - Cortical: Outer portion of lens; may involve anterior, posterior, or equatorial cortex; radial, spokelike opacities
  - Subcapsular: Posterior subcapsular cataract has more profound effect on vision than nuclear or cortical cataract; patients particularly troubled under conditions of miosis; near vision frequently impaired more than distance vision
- System(s) affected: Nervous

Geriatric Considerations

Some degree of cataract formation is expected in all people >70 years of age

Pediatric Considerations

See "Congenital Cataracts"; may present as leukocoria

Pregnancy Considerations

See "Congenital Cataracts" (i.e., medications, metabolic dysfunction, intrauterine infection, and malnutrition)

EPIDEMIOLOGY

Incidence

- Nearly 48% of the 37 million cases of blindness worldwide result from cataracts.
- Leading cause of treatable blindness and vision loss in developing countries
- Predominant age: Depends on type of cataract
- Predominant sex: Male ≈ Female

Prevalence

- Cataract type and prevalence highly variable based on population demographic
- It is estimated that 50% of people 65–74 years of age and 70% of people >75 years of age have age-related cataract change.

RISK FACTORS

- Aging
- Cigarette smoking
- Ultraviolet B (UVB) sunlight exposure
- Diabetes
- Prolonged high-dose steroids
- Positive family history
- Alcohol

Genetics

- Congenital sometimes associated (e.g., heredofamilial systemic disorders [Laurence-Moon-Biedl syndrome], chromosomal disorders [Down syndrome]) (1)[A]
- Genetics of age-related cataract not yet established, but likely multifactorial contribution (2)

GENERAL PREVENTION

- Use of UVB protective glasses (2,3)[A]
- Avoidance of tobacco products (2,3)[A]
- Effective control of diabetes (2,3)[A]
- Care with high-dose, long-term steroid use (systemic therapy > inhaled treatment) (2)[B]
- Protective methods using pharmaceutical intervention (e.g., antioxidants, acetylsalicylic acid (ASA), hormone replacement therapy [HRT]) show no proven benefit to date (2,3)[C].

ETIOLOGY

- Age-related cataract:
  - Continual addition of layers of lens fibers throughout life creates hard, dehydrated lens nucleus that impairs vision (nuclear cataract)
  - Aging alters biochemical and osmotic balance required for lens clarity; outer lens layers hydrate and become opaque, adversely affecting vision
- Congenital:
  - Usually obscure cause
  - Drugs (corticosteroids in first trimester, sulfonamides)
  - Metabolic (diabetes in mother, galactosemia in fetus)
  - Intrauterine infection during first trimester (e.g., rubella, herpes, mumps)
  - Maternal malnutrition
- Other cataract types:
  - Common feature is a biochemical/osmotic imbalance that disrupts lens clarity
  - Local changes in lens protein distribution lead to light scattering (lens opacity).

COMMONLY ASSOCIATED CONDITIONS

- Diabetes (especially with poor control)
- Myotonic dystrophy (90% of patients develop visually innocuous change in third decade; becomes disabling in fifth decade)
- Atopic dermatitis (AD) (10% of patients with severe AD develop cataracts in second–fourth decades, often bilateral)
- Neurofibromatosis type 2
- Associated ocular disease or "secondary cataract" (e.g., chronic anterior uveitis, acute [or repetitive] angle-closure glaucoma or high myopia)
- Drug-induced (e.g., steroids, chlorpromazine)
- Trauma

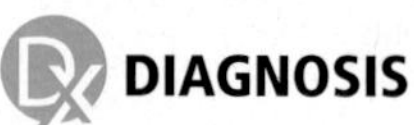

DIAGNOSIS

HISTORY

- Age-related cataract:
  - Decreased visual acuity, blurred vision, distortion, or "ghosting" of images
  - Problems with visual acuity in any lighting condition
  - Falls or accidents; injuries (e.g., hip fracture)
- Congenital: Often asymptomatic, leukocoria, parents noticing child's visual inattention or strabismus
- Other types of cataract:
  - May also present with decreased visual acuity
  - Appropriate clinical history or signs to help in diagnosis

PHYSICAL EXAM

- Visual acuity assessment for all cataracts
- Age-related cataract: Lens opacity on eye examination
- Congenital:
  - Lens opacity present at birth or within 3 months of birth
  - Leukocoria (white pupil), strabismus, nystagmus, signs of associated syndrome (as with Down or rubella syndrome)
  - *Note:* Always must rule out ocular tumor; early diagnosis and treatment of retinoblastoma may be lifesaving
- Other types of cataract: May present with decreased visual acuity associated with characteristic physical findings (e.g., metabolic, trauma)

DIAGNOSTIC TESTS & INTERPRETATION

- Visual quality assessment: Glare testing, contrast sensitivity sometimes indicated
- Retinal/macular function assessment: Potential acuity meter testing

Lab

Workup of underlying process

Pathological Findings

Consistent with lens changes found in the type of cataract; however, diagnosis is made by clinical examination

DIFFERENTIAL DIAGNOSIS

An opaque-appearing eye may be due to opacities of the cornea (e.g., scarring, edema, calcification), lens opacities, tumor, or retinal detachment. Biomicroscopic examination (slit lamp) or careful ophthalmoscopic exam should provide diagnosis:

- In the elderly, visual impairment is often due to multiple factors, such as cataract and macular degeneration, both contributing to visual loss.
- Age-related cataract is significant if symptoms and ophthalmic exam support cataract as a major cause of vision impairment

- Congenital lens opacity in the absence of other ocular pathology may cause severe amblyopia.
- *Note:* Cataract *does not* produce a relative afferent pupillary reaction defect. Abnormal pupillary reactions mandate further evaluation for other pathology.

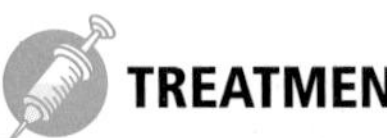

TREATMENT

- Outpatient (usually) (4)[A] or inpatient surgery
- ~1.64 million cataract extractions in US yearly

MEDICATION

There is currently no medication to prevent or slow the progression of cataracts.

ADDITIONAL TREATMENT

General Measures

Eye protection from ultraviolet (UV) light

Issues for Referral

If patient has cataract and symptoms do not seem to support recommended surgery, a second opinion by another ophthalmologist may be indicated.

SURGERY/OTHER PROCEDURES

- Age-related cataract:
  - Surgical removal is indicated if visual impairment–producing symptoms are distressing to the patient, interfering with lifestyle or occupation, or posing a risk for fall or injury.
  - Because significant cataract may develop gradually, the patient may not be aware of how it has changed his or her lifestyle. Physician may note a significant cataract, and patient reports "no problems." Thus, evaluation requires effective physician–patient exchange of information.
  - Surgical technique: Cataract extraction via small incisions, followed by implantation of a prosthetic intraocular lens; lenses have power calculated based on size of the eye and curvature of cornea usually to correct for distance vision; surgery performed on 1 (worse) eye, with contralateral surgery only after recovery and if deemed necessary; generally takes <1 hour depending on surgical technique
  - Anesthesia: Usually local with sedation and monitoring of vital signs
  - Preoperative evaluation: By the primary care physician:
    - Patients on anticoagulants may need to be temporarily discontinued 1–2 weeks before surgery if possible (but not always necessary; thus, need to discuss with ophthalmologist)
    - Patients who have ever taken an α-blocker such as tamsulosin (Flomax) should alert their ophthalmologist (increased risk of intraoperative floppy iris syndrome (IFIS) even in patients who no longer use these drugs).
  - Postoperative care: Usually protective eye shield as directed, topical antibiotic, and steroid ophthalmic medications; avoid lifting or bending over for a few weeks.
- Congenital cataract:
  - Treatment is surgical removal of cataract. Newborn may require surgery within days to reduce risk of severe amblyopia. Use of lens implants is controversial.
  - Postoperative care: Long-term patching program for good eye to combat amblyopia; refractive correction of operative eye, with multiple repeat examinations; challenging for physician and parents

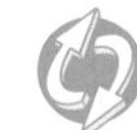

ONGOING CARE

FOLLOW-UP RECOMMENDATIONS

Patient Monitoring

- As cataract progresses, an ophthalmologist may change spectacle correction to maintain vision. When this is no longer successful and interferes with patient's activities of daily living, surgery is indicated.
- Following surgery, spectacle correction may be required to maximize near and/or far visual acuity. Refraction is usually prescribed several weeks after surgery.

PATIENT EDUCATION

Medline Plus on Cataracts at: http://www.nlm.nih.gov/medlineplus/cataract.html

PROGNOSIS

- Ocular prognosis good after cataract removal if no prior ocular disease: 95% of otherwise healthy eyes achieve best corrected visual acuity of 20/40 or better (90% when all eyes are considered, including comorbidity such as diabetes and glaucoma)
- In congenital cataracts, prognosis often is poorer because of the high risk of amblyopia.

COMPLICATIONS

- Vary widely from delay in visual recovery or protracted visual discomfort to blindness and loss of eye
- Nearly all reported complications occur rarely (<2% of eyes) except for posterior capsule opacification (14.7–42.7% of eyes, usually treated with Nd-YAG laser capsulotomy in office with a rate of 4–25.3%) (5,6)[A].

REFERENCES

1. Tasman W, ed. *Duane's Ophthalmology.* Philadelphia: JB Lippincott Co; 2002.
2. Abraham AG, Condon NG, West Gower E. The new epidemiology of cataract. *Ophthalmol Clin North Am.* 2006;19:415–25.
3. Asbell PA, Dualan I, Mindel J, et al. Age-related cataract. *Lancet.* 2005;365:599–609.
4. Fedorowicz Z, Lawrence D, Gutierrez P. Day care versus in-patient surgery for age-related cataract. *Cochrane Database Syst Rev.* 2005;(1):CD004242.
5. Findl O, Buehl W, Bauer P, et al. Interventions for preventing posterior capsule opacification. *Cochrane Database Syst Rev.* 2010;(2):CD003738.
6. Biber JM, Sandoval HP, Trivedi RH, et al. Comparison of the incidence and visual significance of posterior capsule opacification between multifocal spherical, monofocal spherical, and monofocal aspheric intraocular lenses. *J Cataract Refract Surg.* 2009;35(7):1234–8.

C

ADDITIONAL READING

- Harper RA, ed. *Basic Ophthalmology*, 9th ed. San Francisco: American Academy of Ophthalmology; 2010.
- Riaz Y, Mehta JS, Wormald R, et al. Surgical interventions for age-related cataract. *Cochrane Database Syst Rev.* 2006;(4):CD001323.

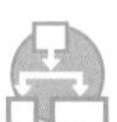

See Also (Topic, Algorithm, Electronic Media Element)

Algorithm: Cataracts

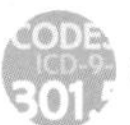

CODES

ICD9

- 366.9 Unspecified cataract
- 366.10 Senile cataract, unspecified
- 743.30 Congenital cataract, unspecified

CLINICAL PEARLS

- Cataracts are the leading cause of blindness worldwide, 90% of which are age-related or "senile."
- For congenital cataracts, must always rule out ocular tumor, since early diagnosis and treatment of retinoblastoma may be lifesaving.
- Before prescribing an α-blocker for an older adult with hypertension or a prostate or urinary retention problem, consider whether the patient has cataracts (due to increased risk of intraoperative floppy iris syndrome).
- Primary indication for cataract surgery is visual impairment leading to significant lifestyle changes for the patient.

CELIAC DISEASE

Brandi Kelly, PharmD
Gary Mark McWilliams, MD
Jill A. Grimes, MD

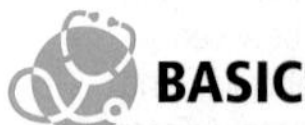

BASICS

DESCRIPTION

- Celiac disease is a chronic diarrheal illness characterized by intestinal malabsorption of virtually all nutrients and precipitated by eating gluten-containing foods.
- Nondiarrheal, often asymptomatic form may actually be more common (intestinal villous atrophy produces vitamin and mineral malabsorption)
- System(s) affected: Gastrointestinal
- Synonym(s): Sprue; Gluten enteropathy; Celiac sprue

EPIDEMIOLOGY

Incidence

- Disease primarily of individuals of Northern European ancestry
- Predominant sex: Female > Male (3:2)

Prevalence

- ~1 in 133–160 persons in US (1)
- An estimated 3 million Americans have celiac disease.

RISK FACTORS

- First-degree relatives: 10% incidence
- 71% in monozygotic twins

Genetics

HLA-DQ2 and/or DQ8 closely associated (testing may be indicated if indeterminate small bowel pathology)

GENERAL PREVENTION

Avoid all gluten-containing products (wheat, barley, rye, and possibly oat products).

ETIOLOGY

Sensitivity to gluten, specifically gliadin fraction

COMMONLY ASSOCIATED CONDITIONS

- *Dermatitis herpetiformis*: Very strong association with celiac disease (2)
- May have secondary lactase deficiency
- Extraintestinal manifestation may include marked decrease in bone density.
- Autoimmune thyroiditis
- Diabetes, type 1 (prevalence of celiac disease in type 1 diabetes is 3–8%)
- Elevated AST and ALT
- Recurrent fetal loss or infertility
- Irritable bowel syndrome (IBS) (3)[A]
- Restless leg syndrome (4)
- GI lymphoma: Celiac disease is associated with both Hodgkin and non-Hodgkin lymphomas:
  - Recent studies show the risk of lymphoproliferative malignancies in celiac disease is dependent on small intestinal histopathology.
  - There appears to be little to no increased risk in latent celiac disease (seropositive but normal biopsy) (5)[C].

Pregnancy Considerations

- Celiac disease may be an underappreciated cause of male and female infertility.
- Consider celiac disease in pregnant women with severe anemia.

DIAGNOSIS

HISTORY

- Diarrhea, cramping, and gas pains
- Steatorrhea (fatty stools)
- Muscle cramps
- Iron-deficiency anemia
- Nervousness
- Weight loss
- Failure to thrive (slowing velocity of weight gain)
- Weakness, fatigue, lassitude
- Explosive flatulence
- Abdominal pain, nausea; rarely vomiting
- Recurrent aphthous stomatitis
- Abdominal distention
- Migraines

Pediatric Considerations

Failure to thrive and delayed growth with short stature may be early manifestations. A few children may outgrow intolerance to wheat after prolonged gluten-free diets, but should be cautioned to watch for signs of recurrence in middle age.

PHYSICAL EXAM

Often normal, but look for:

- Oropharynx: Aphthous stomatitis
- Skin: Dermatitis herpetiformis (excoriations, symmetrical erythematous papules and blisters on elbows, knees, buttocks, and back)
- Abdomen: Distention

DIAGNOSTIC TESTS & INTERPRETATION

Lab

Initial lab tests

Positive IgA antiendomysial antibodies and IgA tissue transglutaminase (sensitivity 90–98%, specificity 98%) when on normal (nongluten-free) diet

Follow-Up & Special Considerations

- IgA-deficient patients have false-negative IgA antiendomysial and IgA antitransglutaminase antibodies.
- Selective IgA deficiency is 10–15 times more prevalent in patients with celiac (vs. the general population):
  - This can delay diagnosis due to "negative" IgA antiendomysial antibody testing
- tTG (the tissue transglutaminase antibody test) is the preferred test (over the deamidated gliadin peptide [DGP] antibody) (6,7)[A].
- 72-hour fecal fat showing >7% fat malabsorption
- Elevated liver function tests
- d-Xylose test showing malabsorption
- Decreased calcium
- Increased prothrombin time (PT)
- Decreased neutral fats
- Decreased cholesterol
- Decreased vitamin A
- Decreased vitamin B_{12} (rare)
- Decreased vitamin D
- Decreased vitamin C
- Decreased folic acid
- Decreased iron (common)
- Decreased total protein
- Decreased hemoglobin (common)

Imaging

Initial approach

Upper GI series showing flocculation of barium, edema, and flattening of mucosal folds

Follow-Up & Special Considerations

Evaluate for osteoporosis

Diagnostic Procedures/Surgery

Endoscopy with diagnostic biopsy of the duodenal mucosa with repeat endoscopy and normal biopsy on a gluten-free diet is necessary before a firm diagnosis can be made:

- *In general, diagnosis should not be made based on serology alone.*

Pathological Findings

Small bowel biopsy:

- Flattened villi, hyperplasia and lengthening of crypts, infiltration of plasma cells, and lymphocytes in lamina propria

DIFFERENTIAL DIAGNOSIS

- Short bowel syndrome
- Pancreatic insufficiency
- Crohn disease
- Whipple disease
- Hypogammaglobulinemia
- Tropical sprue
- Lymphoma
- AIDS
- Acute enteritis
- Giardiasis
- Eosinophilic gastroenteritis
- Pancreatic disease

TREATMENT

MEDICATION

First Line

Usually no medications: Gluten-free diet is treatment.

Second Line

- In refractory disease, consider:
  - Steroids (prednisone, 40–60 mg/d PO in cases of refractory sprue)
  - Azathioprine (immunosuppressants should be used with caution; use may lead to lymphoma in celiac disease)
  - Cyclosporine
  - Infliximab
  - Cladribine
- Patients may require supplemental calcium, calcium carbonate, 500 mg PO b.i.d., and vitamin D (ergocalciferol)

ADDITIONAL TREATMENT

General Measures

- Removal of gluten from the diet:
  - Rice, corn, and soybean flour are safe, palatable substitutes.
- Levels of IgA antigliadin normalize with gluten abstinence.

Issues for Referral

- Additional nutritional support
- Refractory disease

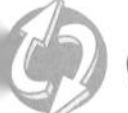

ONGOING CARE

FOLLOW-UP RECOMMENDATIONS

- Consultation with registered dietitian
- Screening for osteoporosis

Patient Monitoring

- Repeat endoscopy after 6–8 weeks on a gluten-free diet (in selected cases).
- IgA antigliadin assay may be used to monitor response to gluten-free diet.

DIET

- Removal of gluten: Wheat, rye, barley, and those with gluten additives.
- This can be a challenging diet (especially learning sources of "hidden" gluten) and should be coordinated with a skilled registered dietitian.

PATIENT EDUCATION

- Discuss importance of recognizing gluten in various products.
- Highlight potential complications and outcomes of failing to follow a gluten-free diet.

PROGNOSIS

- Good with correct diagnosis and adherence to gluten-free diet
- *Patient should feel better in 7 days.*
- All symptoms usually disappear in 4–6 weeks.
- It is unknown whether strict dietary adherence decreases cancer risk.

COMPLICATIONS

- Malignancy: <10% of patients (50% of whom have small bowel lymphoma)
- Refractory sprue:
  - May respond to prednisone 40–60 mg/d PO
  - Refractory sprue unresponsive to corticosteroid therapy raises the specter of adult-onset autoimmune enteropathy or cryptic T-cell lymphoma. In this circumstance, screening for antienterocyte autoantibodies and careful scrutiny of the small intestine, including retroperitoneal lymph node biopsy with full-thickness small bowel biopsy, may be needed.
- Chronic ulcerative jejunoileitis:
  - Associated with multiple ulcers, intestinal bleeding, strictures, perforation, obstruction, and peritonitis
  - 7% mortality
- Osteoporosis secondary to decreased vitamin D and calcium absorption
- Dehydration
- Electrolyte depletion
- Refractory cases may need total parenteral nutrition.

REFERENCES

1. Biagi F, Klersy C, Balduzzi D, et al. Are we not over-estimating the prevalence of coeliac disease in the general population? *Ann Med*. 2010;42:557–61.
2. Bolotin D, Petronic-Rosic V, et al. Dermatitis herpetiformis. Part II. Diagnosis, management, and prognosis. *J Am Acad Dermatol*. 2011;64:1027–33.
3. Ford AC, Chey WD, Talley NJ, et al. Yield of diagnostic tests for celiac disease in individuals with symptoms suggestive of irritable bowel syndrome: Systematic review and meta-analysis. *Arch Intern Med*. 2009;169:651–8.
4. Weinstock L, Walters A, Mullin G, et al. Celiac disease is associated with restless legs syndrome. *Dig Dis Sci*. 2010;55:1667–73.
5. Elfström P, Granath F, Ekström Smedby K, et al. Risk of lymphoproliferative malignancy in relation to small intestinal histopathology among patients with celiac disease. *J Natl Cancer Inst*. 2011;103:436–44.
6. Lewis NR, Scott BB, et al. Meta-analysis: Deamidated gliadin peptide antibody and tissue transglutaminase antibody compared as screening tests for coeliac disease. *Aliment Pharmacol Ther*. 2010;31:73–81.
7. van der Windt DA, Jellema P, Mulder CJ, et al. Diagnostic testing for celiac disease among patients with abdominal symptoms: A systematic review. *JAMA*. 2010;303:1738–46.

ADDITIONAL READING

- AGA Institute. AGA Institute Medical Position Statement on the Diagnosis and Management of Celiac Disease. *Gastroenterology*. 2006;131:1977–80.
- Celiac Disease Foundation. *Guidelines for a Gluten-free Lifestyle*, 3rd ed. http://www.celiac.org.
- Celiac Sprue Association (CSA) http://www.csaceliacs.org.
- Green PHR, Jones R. *Celiac Disease: A Hidden Epidemic*. New York: HarperCollins; 2006.
- Katz KD, Rashtak S, Lahr BD, et al. Screening for celiac disease in a North American population: Sequential serology and gastrointestinal symptoms. *Am J Gastroenterol*. 2011;106:1333–9.
- Quick Start Diet Guide: Celiac Disease Foundation (CDF) & Gluten Intolerance Group (GIG): http://www.celiac.org,http://www.gluten.net.

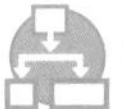

See Also (Topic, Algorithm, Electronic Media Element)

Algorithms: Diarrhea, Chronic; Malabsorption Syndrome

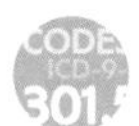

CODES

ICD9

579.0 Celiac disease

CLINICAL PEARLS

- Common condition (1 in 133) and may not be associated with diarrhea.
- Definitive treatment is gluten-free diet.
- Test for celiac disease in patients with presumed IBS.
- Test IgA levels along with IgA antiendomysial AB and tTG
- Positive serology alone is not enough to ascertain diagnosis; must have biopsy via endoscopy.

CELLULITIS

David R. Norris, MD
Sridevi Alla, MD

facial - HIB

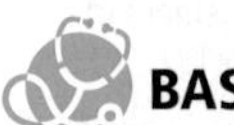

BASICS

DESCRIPTION

- An acute inflammatory condition of the skin and soft tissue characterized by pain, erythema, warmth, and swelling
- There are several anatomic variants:
  - Erysipelas is a superficial form affecting the dermis and lymphatics, classically involving the face and ears.
  - Periorbital cellulitis is a bacterial infection of the eyelid and surrounding tissues. It is more common than orbital cellulitis and occurs in children more often than adults.
  - Orbital cellulitis is infection of the eye posterior to the septum; sinusitis is the most common risk factor.
  - Facial cellulitis, preceded by upper respiratory or middle ear infection, is usually unilateral.
  - Buccal cellulitis is a mild-appearing infection of the cheek in children with a high incidence of bacteremia.
  - Peritonsillar cellulitis is most common in children; presents with fever, sore throat, and "hot potato" speech.
  - Abdominal wall cellulitis is more common in morbidly obese individuals.
  - Perianal cellulitis presents as a sharply demarcated, bright, perianal erythema 2–3 cm around the anal verge.
  - Gangrenous cellulitis is caused by gas-producing bacteria in the lower extremities; common in diabetics.
- System(s) affected: Skin/Exocrine

EPIDEMIOLOGY

- Cellulitis can affect any part of body, but commonly affects the extremities or head.
- Predominant age: Cellulitis in the middle-aged and elderly; erysipelas in children and the elderly
- Predominant sex: Male = Female (perianal cellulitis more common in boys)

Incidence

200 cases per 100,000 patient-years

Prevalence

Unknown

RISK FACTORS

- Disruption to skin barrier: Trauma, infection, inflammation, edema, and lymphatic obstruction
- Recurrent cellulitis: Immunocompromised, diabetes, chronic venous stasis, saphenous vein surgery

Genetics

No genetic pattern

GENERAL PREVENTION

- Avoid trauma, including human or animal bites. Maintain good skin hygiene, especially with minor cuts.
- Wear support stockings to decrease edema.
- Maintain tight glycemic control and proper foot care for diabetics.

PATHOPHYSIOLOGY

Cellulitis is caused by bacterial penetration through a break in the skin. Hyaluronidase mediates SC spread.

ETIOLOGY

- According to site (*Staphylococcus aureus* most common overall) (1)[B]:
  - Cellulitis of the extremities: Group A streptococcus, *S. aureus*
  - Recurrent cellulitis of the leg: Non–group A β-hemolytic streptococci (groups C, G, and B)
  - Facial cellulitis in adults: *Haemophilus influenzae* type B
  - Facial cellulitis in children: *H. influenzae* type B, Staphylococcus and streptococcus
  - Synergistic necrotizing cellulitis: Mixed aerobic-anaerobic flora
  - IV drug use: Methicillin-resistant *Staphylococcus aureus* (MRSA), streptococci, Enterobacteriaceae, *Pseudomonas aeruginosa*, fungi
- Specific diseases:
  - Diabetes mellitus: *S. aureus*, streptococci, gram-negative bacilli, anaerobes
  - Human bites: *Eikenella corrodens*.
  - Animal bites: *Pasteurella multocida, Capnocytophaga canimorsus*.
- Patient groups:
  - Neonates: Group B streptococcus
  - Immunocompromised:
    - Bacteria (e.g., *Serratia, Proteus*, and other Enterobacteriaceae)
    - Fungi (e.g., *Cryptococcus neoformans*)
    - Atypical mycobacterium
  - Cirrhotics:
    - *Campylobacter fetus, Coliforms, Vibrio vulnificus*
  - Environmental and occupational exposures:
    - *Erysipelothrix rhusiopathiae* in patients handling fish, shellfish, meat, and poultry
    - *Vibrio* sp: Saltwater exposure
    - *Aeromonas hydrophila*: Freshwater exposure
    - *Pseudomonas aeruginosa:* Hot-tub exposure
- Microbiology:
  - Most common pathogens are beta-hemolytic streptococci (groups A, B, C, G, and F), *Staphylococcus aureus*, including MRSA and gram-negative aerobic bacilli
  - *Staphylococcus aureus:* Periorbital and orbital cellulitis and IV drug users
  - *Pseudomonas aeruginosa*: Diabetics and other immunocompromised patients
  - *Aeromonas hydrophila* and *Vibrio vulnificus:* Cellulitis caused by waterborne pathogens
  - *Haemophilus influenzae:* Buccal cellulitis
  - Clostridia and non spore-forming anaerobes: Crepitant/gangrenous cellulitis
  - *Streptococcus agalactiae:* Cellulitis following lymph node dissection
  - *Pasteurella multocida* and *Capnocytophaga canimorsus:* Cellulitis preceded by bites
  - *Streptococcus iniae:* Immunocompromised hosts
  - Rare causes: Mycobacterium, fungal (mucormycosis, aspergillosis, syphilis)

COMMONLY ASSOCIATED CONDITIONS

- Facial cellulitis in children associated with upper respiratory infection and otitis media
- Perianal cellulitis may be preceded by pharyngitis.

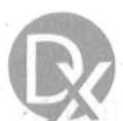

DIAGNOSIS

HISTORY

Previous trauma, surgery, or animal/human bites

PHYSICAL EXAM

- Localized pain and tenderness (2)[A], erythema, induration, itching, or burning
- Peau d' orange appearance
- Fever, chills, and malaise
- Regional lymphadenopathy of the face, periorbital region, neck, or extremities
- Purulent drainage from abscesses
- Orbital cellulitis: Proptosis, globe displacement, limitation of ocular movements, vision loss, diplopia
- Facial cellulitis: Malaise, anorexia, vomiting, pruritus, burning, anterior neck swelling

DIAGNOSTIC TESTS & INTERPRETATION

Diagnosis based on skin appearance and clinical setting, but laboratory, pathology, and imaging modalities can confirm diagnosis.

Lab

Initial lab tests

- For patients with signs of systemic disease (fever or hypothermia, hear rate [HR] >100 bpm, or systolic blood pressure [SBP] <90 mm Hg) include blood cultures, drug susceptibility, CBC, creatinine, bicarbonate, CPK, and CRP levels (3)[C]
- Aspirates from point of maximum inflammation yield 45% positive culture compared with 5% from leading edge; recommended in systemic toxicity, immunocompromise, recurrent cellulitis, or progression while on antibiotics (2)[B]
- Blood cultures: Pathogens isolated in <5% of patients. Better yield in patients with systemic symptoms. Blood cultures in children are more likely to show a contaminant than a true positive (4)[C].
- Blood cultures indicated if lymphedema present, buccal or periorbital cellulitis, infection originating from salt or freshwater, patient has chills and high fever, immunocompromised patients, progression while on antibiotics, unusual exposures

Imaging

Initial approach

- Plain radiographs, CT, or MRI useful if osteomyelitis, fracture, or necrotizing fasciitis is suspect. Ultrasonography is helpful in detecting SC accumulation of pus, and aids in aspiration.
- Gallium^{67} scintillography is helpful for detecting cellulitis superimposed on recently increasing chronic lymphedema of a limb.

Diagnostic Procedures/Surgery

- Skin biopsy is not indicated in immunocompetent patients with mild cellulitis.
- Lumbar puncture should be considered for children with *H. influenzae* type B or if meningeal signs and facial cellulitis.
- Gram stain of cellulitis aspirate may be useful for making preliminary microbial diagnosis to direct specific antibiotic therapy.

Pathological Findings

Biopsy of skin shows marked infiltration of the dermis with eosinophils and inflammatory changes.

DIFFERENTIAL DIAGNOSIS

- Toxic shock syndrome
- Bursitis
- Acute dermatitis or intertrigo
- Herpes zoster or herpetic Whitlow
- Deep vein thrombosis or thrombophlebitis
- Acute gout or pseudogout
- Necrotizing fasciitis or myositis
- Gas gangrene
- Osteomyelitis
- Erythema chronicum migrans or malignancy
- Drug reaction, sunburn, or insect stings

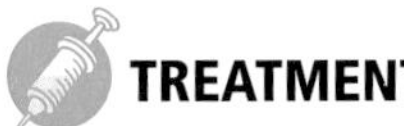

TREATMENT

MEDICATION

First Line

Treat 5–15 days or longer, depending on response, and guided by culture when possible. 5-day therapy is as effective as (10 days) in patients with uncomplicated cellulitis (5)[B]. Empiric therapy should be guided by local resistance patterns. Use IV therapy for rapidly spreading infection or significant comorbidities:

- Empiric therapy for mild cellulitis infection (activity against β-hemolytic streptococci and methicillin-susceptible *S. aureus*): Oral dicloxacillin, cephalexin, clindamycin, or IV cefazolin, oxacillin, or nafcillin.
- Parenteral therapy if severely ill or unable to tolerate oral therapy: Include penicillinase-resistant penicillins, a first-generation cephalosporin; if penicillin-allergic, use clindamycin or vancomycin.
- Necrotizing fasciitis and gas gangrene: Parenteral clindamycin and penicillin.
- In patients with recurrent infection underlying predisposing conditions, previous episode of proven MRSA infection, or systemic toxicity, use agents with activity against MRSA: Parenteral vancomycin, daptomycin, linezolid or oral trimethoprim-sulfamethoxazole (TMP/SMX), doxycycline or minocycline, or clindamycin (3)[C].
- Mild early-suspected streptococcal etiology: Penicillin G, 600,000 U, then IM procaine penicillin at 600,000 U q8h–12h.
- Freshwater exposure: Penicillinase-resistant: Penicillin plus gentamicin or fluoroquinolone. In saltwater exposure: Doxycycline 200 mg IV in divided doses.
- Bites: Oral amoxicillin-clavulanate or IV ampicillin-sulbactam or ertapenem. If mild allergy to penicillin, use cefoxitin or carbapenems. For severe penicillin reactions, use doxycycline, TMP/SMX, or a fluoroquinolone plus clindamycin.
- Facial cellulitis in adults and children (*H. influenza* B): Cefotaxime IV (2)[B]
- Diabetic foot infection: Ampicillin/sulbactam 3 g IV q6h or imipenem/cilastatin, or meropenem. Alternative: Combinations targeting anaerobes as well as gram-positive and gram-negative aerobes.
- Severe infection, toxicity, immunocompromised patients, or worsening infection despite empirical therapy: Consider agents effective against MRSA (i.e., vancomycin, linezolid, tigecycline, quinupristin/dalfopristin, or daptomycin). Switch to oral dicloxacillin, cephradine, cephalexin, or cefadroxil when symptoms begin to resolve (6)[A].
- Recurrent streptococcal cellulitis: Penicillin IV 250 mg b.i.d., or if penicillin-allergic, use erythromycin 250 mg b.i.d.

ALERT

If community-acquired MRSA is a concern, treatment options (7–14 days) include trimethoprim/sulfamethoxazole: DS (160 mg TMP and 800 mg of SMX) 1–2 PO b.i.d. daily; doxycycline: 100 mg PO b.i.d., *or* clindamycin: 300–600 mg PO t.i.d.

Pediatric Considerations

- Avoid doxycycline in children ≤8 years old and during pregnancy.
- Now that children are HIB-vaccinated, the most common predisposing conditions are conjunctivitis or an infected wound near the eye, rather than bacteremia (7)[A].

Second Line

Mild infection:

- Penicillin allergy: Erythromycin 500 mg PO q6h
- Cephalexin remains a cost-effective therapy for outpatient management of cellulitis at current estimated MRSA levels.

ADDITIONAL TREATMENT

General Measures

- Immobilization and elevation of the involved limb to reduce swelling
- Sterile saline dressings or cool aluminum acetate compresses for pain relief
- Edema: Compression stocking, pneumatic pumps, and diuretic therapy
- Steroids (prednisone 0.5 mg/kg/d for 5–8 days) if partial response to antibiotics in hemorrhagic or bullous cellulitis

Issues for Referral

Consider consulting infectious disease if patient is immunocompromised, not responding to treatment, or infection is severe.

SURGERY/OTHER PROCEDURES

- Debridement for gas and purulent matter collections
- Intubation or tracheotomy may be needed for cellulitis of the head or neck.

IN-PATIENT CONSIDERATIONS

Admission Criteria

- Severe infection, suspicion of deeper or rapidly spreading infection, tissue necrosis, or severe pain
- Marked systemic toxicity or worsening symptoms that do not resolve after 24–48 hours of therapy
- Patients with underlying risk factors or severe comorbidities

Nursing

- Ambulate patient in mild infection
- Bed rest in severe infection

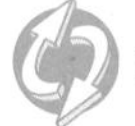

ONGOING CARE

FOLLOW-UP RECOMMENDATIONS

Patient Monitoring

- Repeat blood count if patient is toxic. Repeat lumbar puncture in case of meningitis.
- Consider prophylaxis of deep vein thrombosis.
- Cutaneous inflammation may worsen in first 24 hours due to release of bacterial antigens. Symptomatic improvement usually occurs in 24–48 hours, but visible improvement may take up to 72 hours.

PATIENT EDUCATION

- Practice good skin hygiene, especially with minor cuts.
- Report early skin changes to physician.

PROGNOSIS

With adequate antibiotic treatment, prognosis is good.

COMPLICATIONS

- Local abscess or bacteremia
- Superinfection with gram-negative organisms
- Lymphangitis, especially in recurrent cellulitis
- Thrombophlebitis or venous thrombosis
- Bacterial meningitis
- Gangrenous disorder

REFERENCES

1. Chira S, Miller LG, et al. Staphylococcus aureus is the most common identified cause of cellulitis: A systematic review. *Epidemiol Infect*. 2010;138:313–7.
2. Swartz MN. Clinical practice. Cellulitis. *N Engl J Med*. 2004;350:904–12.
3. Stevens DL, Bisno AL, Chambers HF, et al. Practice guidelines for the diagnosis and management of skin and soft-tissue infections. *Clin Infect Dis*. 2005;41(10):1373–406.
4. Sadow KB, Chamberlain JM. Blood cultures in the evaluation of children with cellulitis. *Pediatrics*. 1998;101;e4.
5. Hepburn MJ, Skidmore PJ, Starnes WF. Comparison of short-course (5 days) and standard (10 days) treatment for uncomplicated cellulitis. *Arch Intern Med*. 2004;164:1669–74.
6. Daum RS. Clinical practice. Skin and soft-tissue infections caused by methicillin-resistant *Staphylococcus aureus*. *N Engl J Med*. 2007;357:380–90.
7. Rimon A, Hoffer V, Prais D, et al. Periorbital cellulitis in the era of Haemophilus influenzae type B vaccine: Predisposing factors and etiologic agents in hospitalized children. *J Pediatr Ophthalmol Strabismus*. 2008;45:300–4.

ADDITIONAL READING

Wells RD, Mason P, Roarty J, et al. Comparison of initial antibiotic choice and treatment of cellulitis in the pre- and post-community-acquired methicillin-resistant *Staphylococcus aureus* eras. *Am J Emerg Med*. 2009;27:436–9.

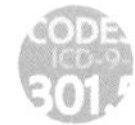

CODES

ICD9

- 682.0 Cellulitis and abscess of face
- 682.8 Cellulitis and abscess of other specified sites
- 682.9 Cellulitis and abscess of unspecified sites

CLINICAL PEARLS

- Most common overall causes of cellulitis are *Staphylococcus aureus* and group A *Streptococcus*.
- Consider MRSA if cellulitis is not responding to antibiotics in the first 48 hours.
- Rapid expansion of infected area with red/purple discoloration and severe pain may suggest necrotizing fasciitis requiring urgent surgical evaluation.

CELLULITIS, ORBITAL

E. Anderson Penno, MD, MS

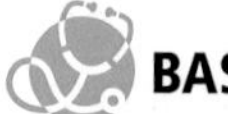

BASICS

DESCRIPTION

- Acute infection of orbital contents posterior to orbital septum with edema and erythema of the conjunctiva and eyelids
- Synonym(s): Postseptal cellulitis

ALERT

- Differentiating orbital from preseptal cellulitis is a difficult but critical step in prompt diagnosis.
- Orbital cellulitis needs immediate IV antibiotics; ophthalmology referral; and monitoring for vision loss, cavernous sinus thrombosis, abscess, and meningitis.
- Intraorbital foreign body (FB) may cause delayed orbital cellulitis.

EPIDEMIOLOGY

- More common in winter due to increased incidence of sinusitis (1,2)[C]
- No frequency difference between the sexes in adults
- More common in children, with a median age of 7–12 years in hospitalized children
- *Haemophilus influenzae* type B (Hib) was the most common organism prior to the Hib vaccine. Other common organisms include *Staphylococcus* and *Streptococcus* species.

Incidence

Orbital cellulitis incidence has declined since the Hib vaccine was introduced in 1985. The reported incidence of orbital cellulitis per 100,000 in California was 3.5 in whites, 6.1 in blacks, and 3.2 in Hispanics in 2000, compared to 6.5 in whites, 10.2 in blacks, and 5.5 in Hispanics in the same population in 1990 (3)[C].

RISK FACTORS

- Sinusitis accounts for up to 80–90% of cases (1,4)[C].
- Orbital trauma or retained orbital FB
- Dental, periorbital, skin, or intracranial infection
- Acute dacryocystitis and acute dacryoadenitis
- Ophthalmic surgery

Genetics

No known genetic predisposition

GENERAL PREVENTION

- Appropriate treatment of bacterial sinusitis
- Proper wound care and perioperative monitoring of orbital surgery and trauma
- Hib vaccine
- High index of suspicion in patients with eyelid and conjunctival erythema with fever

PATHOPHYSIOLOGY

- Sinusitis is the major risk factor for orbital cellulitis due to the thin medial orbital wall. Risk factors include upper respiratory infections, orbital trauma, orbital FB, orbital and periorbital surgery, and seeding from bacteremia.
- Cellulitis within the closed bony orbit can cause proptosis, globe displacement, orbital apex syndrome, optic nerve compression, and vision loss.
- Orbital cellulitis can lead to orbital abscess (along medial wall most common), meningitis, and cavernous sinus fibrosis.

ETIOLOGY

- Cultures in adults often grow multiple organisms
- Most common organisms (2,4)[C]:
  - *Staphylococcus aureus*
  - *Streptococcus pneumoniae*
- Less common organisms:
  - *Moraxella catarrhalis*
  - *Haemophilus influenza*
  - Group A β-hemolytic streptococcus
  - *Pseudomonas aeruginosa*
  - Anaerobes
  - Phycomycosis (mucormycosis)
  - Aspergillosis
  - *Mycobacterium tuberculosis*
  - *Mycobacterium avium* complex
  - Trichinosis and echinococcosis
- Since the introduction of routine vaccination, *Haemophilus influenzae* B is no longer a leading cause of orbital cellulitis (2,4)[B].

COMMONLY ASSOCIATED CONDITIONS

- More than 80% of orbital cellulitis cases result from contiguous sinusitis.
- Trauma and intraorbital FB
- Preseptal cellulitis
- Orbital cellulitis may lead to orbital apex syndrome, vision loss, abscess, meningitis, or cavernous sinus thrombosis.

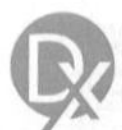

DIAGNOSIS

- Differentiating preseptal cellulitis and orbital cellulitis by examination and imaging are the key to management, as well as frequent monitoring for signs of abscess, meningitis, orbital apex syndrome, or cavernous sinus thrombosis.
- *Chandler staging of orbital cellulitis is less widely used today due to the availability of imaging* (1,4)[C]. Stages are I: Preorbital cellulitis (considered a different entity) (1,4)[B]; II: Edema of orbital lining, chemosis, proptosis, limitation of extraocular movement, fever, III: Include stage II with a subperiosteal abscess and occasional vision loss; IV: Orbital abscess, ophthalmoplegia with visual loss; and V: Extension of the infection to cavernous sinus, subdural space, meninges, or brain

HISTORY

- Malaise and fever
- History of surgery, trauma, sinus or upper respiratory infection, dental infection
- Stiff neck, vision loss, double vision, pain with eye movement, mental status changes
- Systemic immunosuppression or diabetes

ALERT

Ophthalmoplegia, mental status changes, contralateral cranial nerve palsy, or bilateral orbital cellulitis may indicate CNS involvement.

PHYSICAL EXAM

- Examination should include:
  - Vital signs
  - Vision (with glasses if required)
  - Lid examination and palpation of the orbit
  - Pupil check for afferent papillary defect
  - Extraocular movements
  - Red desaturation: Ask patient to view a red object with 1 eye and compare to the other; reduction in the red color may indicate optic nerve involvement.
  - Confrontation visual field
  - Critically ill patients may not be able to do more involved testing.
  - Consult ophthalmology for slit lamp and dilated funduscopic exam, exophthalmometry measurement for proptosis, color vision, and automated visual field.
- Signs of orbital cellulitis include:
  - Proptosis
  - Double vision
  - Vision loss (or decreased field of vision)
  - Pain with eye movement
  - Decreased color vision
- See "Differential Diagnosis" for further diagnostic tips.

DIAGNOSTIC TESTS & INTERPRETATION

Lab

- CBC with differential, C-reactive protein, and ESR
- Cultures obtained from sinus aspirates and abscesses may grow multiple organisms.
- Cultures of eye secretions or nasopharyngeal aspirates are often contaminated by normal flora, but may identify antibiotic-resistant organisms.
- Cultures from orbital and sinus abscesses more often yield positive results, but should be limited to cases where invasive procedures are clinically indicated.
- Blood cultures should be obtained prior to initiation of antibiotic therapy (more often positive in children <5 years old) (4)[C] and lumbar puncture when indicated.

Follow-Up & Special Considerations

A full septic evaluation, including lumbar puncture, should be considered before antibiotic administration in toxic patients, or if any signs or symptoms suggestive of meningitis (4)[C].

Imaging

CT scan of orbits and sinuses with axial and coronal views, with and without contrast, for diagnosis and screening for sinus disease, orbital FB, and abscess

Initial approach

- Contrast CT is most widely used for evaluating orbital cellulitis (5)[B]:
  - Consider CT imaging if concern for stage III or IV disease (5)[C]
  - Thin sections (2 mm) CT, coronal and axial views with bone windows to differentiate preorbital from orbital cellulitis, confirm extension of inflammation into orbit, detect coexisting sinus disease, and identify orbital or subperiosteal abscesses
  - Deviation of medial rectus on the affected side indicates intraorbital involvement.
- MRI offers superior resolution of soft tissue infections for identification of cavernous sinus thrombosis.
- U can be used to rule out orbital myositis, locate FBs or abscesses, and follow progression of a drained abscess.

Follow-Up & Special Considerations

Frequent monitoring of eye examination and vitals is essential for early diagnosis and treatment of associated conditions such as meningitis or abscess.

Diagnostic Procedures/Surgery

Neurology consult may be necessary in cases of suspected meningitis.

DIFFERENTIAL DIAGNOSIS

- Preseptal cellulitis:
  - Eyelid erythema with or without conjunctival erythema, afebrile, no pain on eye movement, no diplopia, normal eye examination
- Idiopathic orbital inflammatory disease (orbital pseudotumor) (4)[C]:
  - Afebrile, normal WBCs, can be acute, may have pain, responds to steroids
- Orbital foreign body
- Arteriovenous fistula (carotid-cavernous fistula):
  - Spontaneous or due to trauma; bruit may be present
- Cavernous sinus thrombosis:
  - Signs of orbital cellulitis with cranial nerve 3, 4, 5, and 6 signs; often bilateral and acute
- Acute thyroid orbitopathy:
  - Afebrile; patient may have other signs of thyroid disease
- Orbital tumor:
  - Rhabdomyosarcoma in children may present acutely, acute lymphoblastic leukemia, or metastatic
- Trauma, including insect bite
- Ruptured dermoid cyst

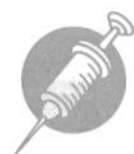

TREATMENT

Orbital cellulitis patients should be admitted to a hospital for treatment and careful monitoring of ocular status, vitals, and signs of CNS involvement and IV broad-spectrum antibiotic treatment for gram-positive, gram-negative, and anaerobic organisms for at least 1 week followed by oral antibiotics.

MEDICATION

- Empiric antibiotic therapy at all ages should provide coverage for pathogens associated with acute sinusitis (*S. pneumoniae*, *H. influenzae*, *M. catarrhalis*, *S. pyogenes*), as well as for *S. aureus* and anaerobes.
- IV antibiotic treatment should be modified when microbiological sensitivities return. Duration of IV therapy is usually a week, based on clinical picture.
- Oral antibiotic therapy should continue for 2–3 wks or longer (3–6 wks) is recommended for patients with severe sinusitis and bony destruction.

First Line

- Mainstay of therapy is broad-spectrum IV antibiotics for at least 1 week: Ampicillin/sulbactam (Unasyn) or ceftriaxone plus metronidazole or clindamycin if concurrent anaerobic infection is suspected (2)[C]:
  - Ampicillin/sulbactam 3 g IV q6h for adult; 200–300 mg/kg/d divided q6h for children
  - Ceftriaxone 1–2 g IV q12 hours for adults or 100 mg/kg/d divided b.i.d. in children with maximum 4 g/d
  - Clindamycin 300 mg IV q6h for adults; 20–40 mg/kg/d IV q6–8h for children
  - Metronidazole 30–35 mg/kg/d divided q8h
- In severe, culture-proven methicillin-resistant *Staphylococcus aureus* infection, vancomycin remains parenteral drug of choice (2)[C]:
  - Vancomycin 1g IV q12h for adults; 40 mg/kg/d IV divided q8–12h, max daily dose 2 g for children

ADDITIONAL TREATMENT

- *Steroid use is controversial*. Short-term systemic steroid may be recommended for orbital cellulitis secondary to sinusitis (4)[C]. Topical erythromycin or nonmedicated ophthalmic ointment may be indicated to protect against exposure in cases with severe proptosis. Nasal decongestants may be indicated.
- Oral antibiotics for 2 weeks or longer are recommended following IV treatment. Children may be treated with amoxicillin/clavulanate 20–40 mg/kg/d divided t.i.d. or in adults 250–500 mg t.i.d. Cefaclor may be used 20–40 mg/kg/d divided t.i.d. in children or 250–500 mg t.i.d. in adults.

Issues for Referral

- Early consultation with ophthalmology and otolaryngology when orbital cellulitis is suspected
- Infectious disease consultation should be considered if available.
- Neurology or neurosurgery consultation if intracranial spread is suspected (4,6)[B]

SURGERY/OTHER PROCEDURES

- IV antibiotic therapy is the best initial therapy.
- Surgical intervention is warranted when a patient has visual loss, complete ophthalmoplegia, or well-defined large abscess (>10 mm) on presentation or no clinical improvement after 24 hours of antibiotic therapy.
- Trauma cases may need wound debridement or FB removal.
- Orbital abscess may need surgical drainage, and treatment of choice for brain abscess is surgical excision or drainage with 4–8 weeks of antibiotics.
- Surgical interventions may include external ethmoidectomy, endoscopic ethmoidectomy, uncinectomy, antrostomy, and subperiosteal drainage (1)[C].

IN-PATIENT CONSIDERATIONS

Patients with orbital cellulitis should be admitted for IV antibiotics and repeated eye examination to evaluate progression of infection or involvement of optic nerve (1,2,4)[A]:

- Careful monitoring with temperature, WBC, visual acuity, papillary reflex, ocular motility, and degree of proptosis measurement should be done q24h or more frequently in severe/progressive cases.
- Repeat CT, surgical intervention, neurology consult with lumbar puncture may be required for worsening orbital cellulitis cases.

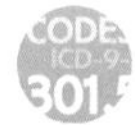

ONGOING CARE

FOLLOW-UP RECOMMENDATIONS

Patient Monitoring

Visual acuity testing and slit lamp examination daily

ALERT

Close monitoring is indicated, as complications can develop rapidly.

PATIENT EDUCATION

- Maintain proper hand washing and good skin hygiene.
- Avoid skin or lid trauma.
- See a health care provider promptly for periorbital swelling and/or erythema.

COMPLICATIONS

- Complications can develop rapidly and include permanent vision loss, CNS involvement, and death.
- Permanent vision loss:
  - Corneal exposure
  - Optic neuritis
  - Endophthalmitis
  - Septic uveitis or retinitis
  - Exudative retinal detachment
  - Retinal artery or vein occlusions
  - Globe rupture due to significantly increased intraocular pressure
  - Orbital compartment syndrome, compression of orbital soft tissues and optic nerve
- CNS complications:
  - Intracranial abscess
  - Meningitis
  - Cavernous sinus thrombosis (2,4,6)[B]

REFERENCES

1. Botting AM, McIntosh D, Mahadevan M. Paediatric pre- and post-septal peri-orbital infections are different diseases. A retrospective review of 262 cases. *Int J Pediatr Otorhinolaryngol*. 2008;72(3): 377–83.
2. Hauser A, Fogarasi S, et al. Periorbital and orbital cellulitis. *Pediatr Rev*. 2010;31:242–9.
3. Soroudi A, Casey R, Pan D, et al. An epidemiologic survey of orbital cellulitis. *Invest Ophthalmol Vis Sci*. 2003;44: E-Abstract 786.
4. Kloek CE, Rubin PA. Role of inflammation in orbital cellulitis. *Int Ophthalmol Clin*. 2006;46:57–68.
5. Rudloe TF, Harper MB, Prabhu SP, et al. Acute periorbital infections: who needs emergent imaging? *Pediatrics*. 2010;125:e719–26.
6. Brook I, et al. Microbiology and antimicrobial treatment of orbital and intracranial complications of sinusitis in children and their management. *Int J Pediatr Otorhinolaryngol*. 2009;73:1183–6.

ADDITIONAL READING

Cannon PS, Mc Keag D, Radford R, et al. Our experience using primary oral antibiotics in the management of orbital cellulitis in a tertiary referral centre. *Eye (Lond)*. 2009;23:612–5.

CODES

ICD9

376.01 Orbital cellulitis

CLINICAL PEARLS

- Most of orbital cellulitis cases result from sinusitis.
- Patients should be admitted to the hospital for monitoring and IV antibiotic treatment if orbital cellulitis is diagnosed.
- Ophthalmoplegia, mental status changes, contralateral cranial nerve palsy, or bilateral orbital cellulitis may herald intracranial involvement.
- Ophthalmology and otolaryngology should be consulted early when orbital cellulitis is suspected.

CELLULITIS, PERIORBITAL

Fozia A. Ali, MD

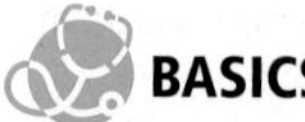

BASICS

DESCRIPTION

- An acute, spreading infection of the skin and SC tissue of the area surrounding the eye, usually secondary to external inoculation, but the inflammation does not extend into the bony orbit
- Synonym(s): Preseptal cellulitis

ALERT

It is important to distinguish periorbital cellulitis from orbital cellulitis (restricted extraocular mobility, diplopia, proptosis, and globe displacement vision loss), which is a potentially life-threatening condition.

EPIDEMIOLOGY

Occurs more commonly in children, with mean age 21 months

Incidence

Increased incidence in the winter months (due to increased number of cases of sinusitis)

RISK FACTORS

- Contiguous spread from upper respiratory infection
- Sinusitis
- Local skin trauma
- Insect bite
- Puncture wound
- Bacteremia

Genetics

No known genetic predisposition

GENERAL PREVENTION

- Avoid dermatologic trauma.
- Avoid swimming in fresh or salt water with skin abrasion.

PATHOPHYSIOLOGY

- An understanding of the anatomy of the eyelid is important in distinguishing preseptal from orbital cellulitis:
  - The orbital septum is a sheet of connective tissue that extends from the orbital bones to the margins of the upper and lower eyelids, and it acts as a barrier to infection deep in the orbital structures.
  - Infection of the tissues superficial to the orbital septum is called preseptal cellulitis, whereas infection deep in the orbital septum is termed orbital cellulitis.
- Periorbital cellulitis classically arises from a contiguous infection of soft tissues of the face, secondary to:
  - Sinusitis (via lamina papyracea)
  - Local trauma
  - Insect or animal bites
  - Foreign bodies

ETIOLOGY

- Common organisms:
  - *Streptococcus pneumoniae*
  - *Staphylococcus aureus*
  - *Streptococcus pyogenes*
- Atypical organisms:
  - *Acinetobacter* sp.
  - *Nocardia brasiliensis*
  - *Bacillus anthracis*
  - *Pseudomonas aeruginosa*
  - *Neisseria gonorrhoeae*
  - *Proteus* sp.
  - *Pasteurella multocida*
  - *Mycobacterium tuberculosis*
  - *Trichophyton* sp. (ringworm)
- Since the introduction of routine vaccination in 1990, *Haemophilus influenzae* B is no longer a leading cause of orbital cellulitis.

DIAGNOSIS

HISTORY

- Induration, erythema, warmth, and/or tenderness of periorbital soft tissues
- Chemosis (conjunctival swelling), proptosis, pain with extraocular eye movements
- Fever (although not necessary for diagnosis)

ALERT

Pain with eye movement and conjunctival swelling can occur, although both should raise the suspicion for orbital cellulitis.

PHYSICAL EXAM

- Thorough inspection of the eye and surrounding structures is a key part in physical exam.
- Erythema, swelling, and tenderness of lids without orbital congestion:
  - Violaceous discoloration of eyelid is more commonly associated with *Haemophilus influenza*.
- Also look for any break in skin if history of trauma causing periorbital cellulitis.
- Look for vesicle to rule out herpetic infection.
- Inspection of nasal vaults and sinus palpation for signs of acute sinusitis
- Ocular motility and visual acuity testing to rule out orbital cellulitis

DIAGNOSTIC TESTS & INTERPRETATION

Lab

- CBC with differential
- Blood cultures

Follow-Up & Special Considerations

- Children with periorbital or orbital cellulitis often have underlying sinusitis.
- If the child is febrile and appears toxic, blood cultures should be performed and lumbar puncture considered.

Imaging

If suspicious for orbital involvement, CT scan can be used to evaluate the extent of infection and detect orbital inflammation or abscess (1)[B]:

- The classic sign of orbital cellulitis on CT scan is bulging of the medial rectus.
- CT should be performed with contrast, thin sections (2 mm), coronal and axial views with bone windows.

DIFFERENTIAL DIAGNOSIS

- Orbital cellulitis: Orbital cellulitis may have the same signs and symptoms in the periorbital tissue, but also results in proptosis, edema of the conjunctiva, ophthalmoplegia, or decreased visual acuity.
- Abscess
- Dacryocystitis
- Hordeolum
- Allergic inflammation
- Orbital or periorbital trauma
- Idiopathic orbital inflammatory syndrome
- Rapidly progressive tumors:
  - Rhabdomyosarcoma
  - Retinoblastoma
  - Lymphoma
- Leukemia

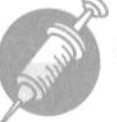

TREATMENT

MEDICATION

- Empiric antibiotic treatment regimens are based on coverage of the most likely organisms, paying attention to local resistance patterns and the pathogens usually associated with sinusitis.
- Uncomplicated posttraumatic:
  - Usually due to skin flora, including *Staphylococcus* and *Streptococcus*
  - Cephalexin
  - Dicloxacillin
  - Clindamycin
- Extension from sinusitis:
  - Amoxicillin
  - Clavulanate
  - Third-generation cephalosporin
- Bacteremic cellulitis:
  - May be associated with meningitis
  - Ceftriaxone plus vancomycin to cover methicillin-resistant *Staphylococcus aureus*
- Duration of therapy should be 7–10 days:
  - If symptoms do not improve within 24 hours, IV antibiotic therapy is indicated (2)[B].

ADDITIONAL TREATMENT

Issues for Referral

Although treatment may consist of IV antibiotics alone, management should be in consultation with otolaryngologists and ophthalmologists, especially when there is concern of orbital cellulitis.

SURGERY/OTHER PROCEDURES

Orbital surgery is indicated if the patient:

- Fails to respond
- No improvement by 24–48 hours
- Visual impairment
- Complete ophthalmoplegia
- Well-defined periosteal abscess (1,2)
- Deteriorates clinically despite treatment
- Has worsening visual acuity or pupillary changes
- Develops an abscess, except in selected pediatric cases of medial subperiosteal abscess, which may be successfully treated medically.
- Abscess formation necessitates incision and drainage.
- Endoscopic and transcaruncular surgery has been successfully employed to treat subperiosteal and intraorbital abscesses.

IN-PATIENT CONSIDERATIONS

- Mild cases in adults and children >1 year can be managed on an outpatient basis, provided the patient is stable and without systemic signs of toxicity.
- Preseptal cellulitis in children <4 years may warrant hospitalization and the use of IV antibiotics.

Admission Criteria

Consider hospitalization and IV antibiotics:

- For children <1 year
- Patients who have not been immunized for *S. pneumoniae* or *H. influenza*
- If no signs of clinical improvement are apparent after 24 hours of oral antibiotics

Discharge Criteria

- There are no strict guidelines to indicate when to switch therapy from parenteral to oral agents.
- Generally, we switch to oral therapy after the patient is afebrile and the skin findings have begun to resolve, which usually takes 3–5 days.
- Once we switch to oral therapy, it should be continued for 2–3 weeks.
- The longer duration is recommended for those patients with severe ethmoid sinusitis associated with bony destruction.

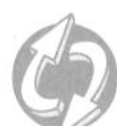

ONGOING CARE

FOLLOW-UP RECOMMENDATIONS

Patient Monitoring

The patient should be monitored for signs of orbital involvement, including decreased visual acuity or painful/limited ocular motility.

PATIENT EDUCATION

- Maintain good skin hygiene.
- Avoid skin trauma.
- Report early skin changes to health care professional.

PROGNOSIS

With adequate antibiotic treatment, outlook is good. Response to antibiotics in children with periorbital cellulitis usually is rapid, and a 10-day course of treatment generally is sufficient.

COMPLICATIONS

- Orbital cellulitis
- Abscess formation
- Scarring
- Delay in diagnosis and adequate treatment may result in serious complications, including blindness.

REFERENCES

1. Beech T, Robinson A, McDermott AL, et al. Paediatric periorbital cellulitis and its management. *Rhinology*. 2007;45:47–9.
2. Hennemann S, et al. Clinical inquiries. What is the best initial treatment for orbital cellulitis in children? *J Fam Prac*. 2007;56(8):662–4.
3. Georgakopoulos CD, Eliopoulou MI, Stasinos S, et al. Periorbital and orbital cellulitis: A 10-year review of hospitalized children. *Eur J Ophthalmol*. 2010;20(6):1066–72.

ADDITIONAL READING

- Chaudhry IA, Shamsi FA, Elzaridi E, et al. Inpatient preseptal cellulitis: Experience from a tertiary eye care centre. *Br J Ophthalmol*. 2008;92:1337–41 doi:10.1136/bjo.2007.128975.
- Goldstein SM, Shelsta HN. Community-acquired methicillin-resistant *Staphylococcus aureus* periorbital cellulitis: A problem here to stay. *Ophthal Plast Reconstr Surg*. 2009;25:77.
- http://emedicine.medscape.com/article/798397-overview.

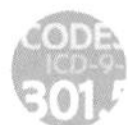

CODES

ICD9

682.0 Cellulitis and abscess of face

CLINICAL PEARLS

- Preseptal and orbital cellulitis occur most commonly in children.
- A multidisciplinary approach is needed in managing children with this condition, and CT scan of the patient's sinuses is essential to differentiate from orbital cellulitis.
- Early detection of periorbital cellulitis is important to prevent complications.
- The 2 most important factors for periorbital cellulitis are upper respiratory infection and eyelid trauma; sinusitis is more associated with orbital cellulitis (3)[C].

CEREBRAL PALSY

Beverly L. Nazarian, MD

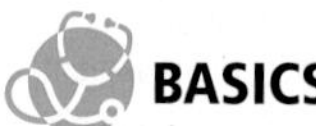

BASICS

DESCRIPTION

Cerebral palsy (CP): A group of permanent disorders of the development of movement and posture causing activity limitation, that are attributed to *nonprogressive* disturbances that occurred in the developing fetal or infant brain. The motor disorders of CP are often accompanied by disturbances of sensation, perception, cognition, communication, and behavior, by epilepsy and by secondary musculoskeletal problems (1).

EPIDEMIOLOGY

Incidence

- Overall, 1.5–2.5 per 1,000 live births
- Incidence increases as gestational age (GA) at birth decreases (2):
  - 146/1,000 for GA of 22–27 weeks
  - 62/1,000 for GA of 28–31 weeks
  - 7/1,000 for GA of 32–36 weeks
  - 1/1,000 for GA of 37+ weeks

Prevalence

3–4/1,000 of the population

RISK FACTORS

- Prenatal: Congenital anomalies, multiple gestation, in utero stroke, intrauterine infection (CMV, varicella), intrauterine growth retardation (IUGR), chorioamnionitis, antepartum bleeding, maternal factors (cognitive impairment, seizure disorders, hyperthyroidism), abnormal fetal position (e.g., breech)
- Perinatal: Preterm birth, low birth weight, periventricular leukomalacia, perinatal hypoxia/asphyxia, intracranial hemorrhage/intraventricular hemorrhage, neonatal seizure or stroke, hyperbilirubinemia
- Postnatal: Traumatic brain injury or stroke, sepsis, meningitis, encephalitis, asphyxia

Genetics

There are reports of associations between CP and candidate genes: Thrombophilic, cytokines, and apolipoprotein E

GENERAL PREVENTION

- Magnesium sulfate administration to mothers at risk for preterm delivery has a neuroprotective effect and reduces CP risk (3).
- Improved management of hyperbilirubinemia with decrease in kernicterus has greatly reduced dyskinetic CP.
- Prevention or reduction of chorioamnionitis and premature births

PATHOPHYSIOLOGY

- Multifactorial; CP results from static injury or lesions in the developing brain, occurring prenatally, perinatally, or postnatally.
- Cytokines and free radicals and inflammatory response are likely contributing factors.

ETIOLOGY

- 50% of cases: Etiology is not established; most likely multifactorial.
- Spastic CP is most common, usually related to premature birth, with either periventricular leukomalacia or germinal matrix hemorrhage.
- Dystonic or athetotic CP, often resulting from kernicterus, is now rare due to improved management of hyperbilirubinemia.

COMMONLY ASSOCIATED CONDITIONS

- Seizure disorder (22–40%)
- Intellectual impairment (23–44%)
- Behavioral problems
- Speech and language impairment (42–81%)
  - May have an impact on expressive and/or receptive language
  - May be nonverbal
- Sensory impairments:
  - Hearing deficits
  - Visual (62–71%): Poor visual acuity, strabismus (50%), or hemianopsia
- Feeding impairment, swallowing dysfunction, and aspiration: When severe, may require gastrostomy feedings
- Poor dentition, excessive drooling
- GI conditions: Constipation (59%), vomiting (22%), gastroesophageal reflux
- Decreased linear growth and weight abnormalities (under- and overweight)
- Osteopenia
- Bowel and bladder incontinence
- Orthopedic: Contractures, hip subluxation/dislocation, scoliosis (60%)

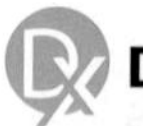

DIAGNOSIS

- A clinical diagnosis including:
  - Delayed motor milestones
  - Abnormal tone
  - Abnormal neurological exam suggesting a cerebral etiology
  - Absence of regression
  - Absence of underlying syndromes or alternative explanation for etiology
- Although the pathological lesion is static, clinical presentation may change as the infant grows and develops.
- Accurate early diagnosis remains difficult. Neurologic abnormalities observed in the first 1–2 years of life may resolve. Caution against diagnosis of CP before age 2.

HISTORY

- Presentation: Concerns over movements or motor development
- Ask about:
  - Prenatal, perinatal, and postnatal risk factors
  - Neurobehavioral signs:
    - Poor feeding/frequent vomiting
    - Irritability
  - Timing of motor milestones: Delay in milestones is not sensitive or specific until after 6 months of age.
  - Abnormal spontaneous general movements
  - Asymmetry of movements, such as early hand preference
  - Symptoms of other conditions
- Regression of motor skills does not occur with CP.

PHYSICAL EXAM

- Assess for 1 or more types of neurological impairment:
  - Spasticity: Increased tone/reflexes/clonus
  - Dyskinesia: Abnormal movements
  - Hypotonia: Decreased tone
  - Ataxia: Abnormal balance/coordination
- Areas of exam:
  - Tone: May be increased or decreased
  - Trunk and head control: Often poor, but may be advanced due to high tone
  - Reduced strength and motor control
  - Persistence of primitive reflexes
  - Asymmetry of movement or reflexes
  - Decreased joint range of motion and contractures
  - Brisk DTRs
  - Clonus
  - Delayed motor milestones: Serial exams most effective
  - Gait abnormalities: Scissoring, toe-walking
- CP should be classified by (1):
  - The primary disorder of tone or movement:
    - Spasticity:
      - Hemiplegic (unilateral)
      - Diplegic (bilateral with LE > UE involvement)
      - Quadriplegic (bilateral with UE > or = LE involvement)
    - Dystonia: Hypertonia and reduced movement
    - Choreoathetosis: Irregular spasmodic involuntary movements of the limbs or facial muscles
    - Ataxia: Loss of orderly muscular coordination
    - Additional disorders of tone or movement; these should be listed as secondary components
  - Level of motor functioning:
    - The Gross Motor Function Classification System (GMFCS) is often used:
      - A score of I indicates ability to walk without limitation.
      - A score of IV or V indicates more severe involvement.
    - The Manual Ability Classification System (MACS) can be used to assess upper extremity function (4).

DIAGNOSTIC TESTS & INTERPRETATION

CP is a clinical diagnosis based on history, physical, and risk factors. Diagnostic tests rule out other conditions.

Lab

- Laboratory testing is not needed to make diagnosis, but can sometimes help to exclude other etiologies.
- Testing for metabolic and genetic syndromes (5):
  - Not routinely obtained in the evaluation for CP
  - If no specific etiology is identified by neuroimaging, or if there are atypical features in clinical presentation, genetic or metabolic testing may be useful.
  - Detection of certain brain malformations may warrant genetic or metabolic testing to identify syndromes.
- Screening for coagulopathies: Diagnostic testing for coagulopathies should be considered in children with hemiplegic CP with cerebral infarction identified on neuroimaging (5)[C].

Imaging

- Neuroimaging is not essential, but it is recommended in children with CP for whom the etiology has not been established (5)[C].
- MRI is preferred to CT scanning (5)[C].
- Abnormalities in 80–90% of patients: Brain malformation, cerebral infarction, intraventricular or other intracranial hemorrhage, periventricular leukomalacia, ventricular enlargement, or other CSF space abnormalities

Diagnostic Procedures/Surgery
- The Communication Function Classification System has recently been developed as another means of assessing function.
- Screening for comorbid conditions: Developmental delay/intellectual impairment, vision/hearing impairments, speech and language disorders, or feeding/swallowing dysfunction

Pathological Findings
Perinatal brain injury may include:
- White matter damage:
  - Most common in premature infants
  - Periventricular leukomalacia: Gliosis with or without focal necrosis with resulting cysts and scarring. May be multiple lesions of various ages. Necrosis can lead to cysts/scarring.
  - Germinal matrix hemorrhage: May lead to intraventricular hemorrhage
- Grey matter damage: More common in term infants. Cortical infarcts, focal neuronal damage, myelination abnormalities

DIFFERENTIAL DIAGNOSIS
Benign congenital hypotonia, brachial plexus injury, familial spastic paraplegia, dopa-responsive dystonia, transient toe-walking, muscular dystrophy, metabolic disorders (e.g., glutaric aciduria type 1), mitochondrial disorders, genetic disorders (e.g., Rett syndrome)

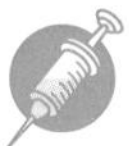

TREATMENT

Focuses on control of symptoms: Reduction in spasticity, management of comorbid conditions, maximization of functioning and quality of life

MEDICATION
First Line
- Diazepam (6)[B]:
  - A $GABA_A$ agonist, facilitating CNS inhibition at spinal and supraspinal levels to reduce spasticity
  - Adult dose: 2–12 mg/dose PO q6–12h.
  - Pediatric dose (<12 years): 0.12–0.8 mg/kg/d. PO, divided q6–8h
- Botulinum toxin type A (6)[A]:
  - Injected directly into muscles of interest
  - Acts at neuromuscular junction to inhibit the release of acetylcholine
  - Chemically denervates muscles, reducing tone
  - Lasts for 12–16 weeks, following injection

Second Line
- Baclofen (6):
  - γ-aminobutyric acid B ($GABA_B$) agonist, facilitates presynaptic inhibition of mono- and polysynaptic reflexes
  - Adults: Initial dose is 5 mg t.i.d. and increase dosage every 3 days to an average maintenance dose of 20 mg t.i.d. 80 mg/d maximum
  - Pediatric dose (>2 years old): Initial 10–15 mg/d. Titrate to effective dose. <8 years old = 40 mg/d maximum. >8 years old 60 mg/d maximum.
- Intrathecal Baclofen (Baclofen Pump) (6):
  - Continuous intrathecal route allows greater maximal response with smaller dosage
  - Significantly reduces spasticity in children with CP
  - Multiple adverse effects due to catheter placement and medication side effects
- Dantrolene (6):
  - Limits calcium release from muscles, reducing spasticity
  - Adult dosing: 25 mg PO daily titrated to effective dose, maximum 100 mg PO q.i.d.
  - Pediatric dosing: 0.5 mg/kg PO daily titrated to effective dose, maximum 12 mg/kg/d.
- Tizanidine and other α-adrenergic agents:
  - α-adrenergic agonist, presynaptically inhibits motor activation, reducing spasticity
  - Adult dosing: 4 mg/d PO, titrate to effective dose, up to 8 mg PO q4–6h, 36 mg/d maximum

ADDITIONAL TREATMENT
- Care needs to be multidisciplinary, usually including specialists from orthopedics, neurology, ophthalmology, and physiatry, as well as physical, occupational, and speech therapists.
- "Medical home" with primary care physician (7) which requires:
  - Identification of patient's and family's needs for support, respite, and community resources
  - Care coordination among medical providers and with community agencies
  - Collaboration with schools
  - Transition to adult care

General Measures
- Referral to early intervention for children ages 0–3 is essential.
- Various therapy modalities enhance functioning:
  - Physical therapy: Posture stability and gait, motor strength and control, contracture prevention
  - Occupational therapy: Functional activities of daily living and other fine motor skills
  - Speech therapy: Verbal and nonverbal speech and aid in feeding
- Equipment optimizes participation in activities:
  - Orthotic splinting: Maintains functional positioning and prevents contractures: Ankle-foot orthosis, and dynamic ankle-foot orthosis
  - Spinal bracing (body jacket) may slow scoliosis.
  - Augmentative communication: Pictures, switches, or computer systems for nonverbal individuals
  - Electrical stimulation: Therapeutic and functional
  - Use of adaptive equipment such as standers to allow weight bearing, and for mobility: Crutches, walkers, gait trainers, wheelchairs

COMPLEMENTARY AND ALTERNATIVE MEDICINE
Hyperbaric oxygen: Conflicting results. Hippotherapy: Therapeutic horse riding to improve posture and balance. Aquatic therapy.

SURGERY/OTHER PROCEDURES
- Dorsal root rhizotomy: Selectively cutting dorsal rootlets from L1–S2: Best for patients with normal intelligence with spastic diplegia. Minimizes spasticity in lower limbs, but associated with adverse effects. Evidence lacking as to long-term outcomes.
- Surgical treatment of joint dislocations/subluxation, scoliosis management, tendon lengthening, gastrostomy, etc.

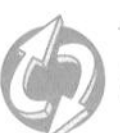

ONGOING CARE

PROGNOSIS
Reduced lifespan in those with most severely affected.

REFERENCES

1. Rosenbaum P, Paneth N, Leviton A, et al. A report: the definition and classification of cerebral palsy April 2006. *Dev Med Child Neurol Suppl*. 2007; 109:8–14.
2. Himpens E, Van den Broeck C, Oostra A, et al. Prevalence, type, distribution, and severity of cerebral palsy in relation to gestational age: A meta-analytic review. *Dev Med Child Neurol*. 2008;50:334–40.
3. Doyle LW, Crowther CA, Middleton P, et al. Magnesium sulphate for women at risk of preterm birth for neuroprotection of the fetus. *Cochrane Database Syst Rev*. 2009:CD004661.
4. Eliasson AC, Krumlinde-Sundholm L, Rösblad B, et al. The Manual Ability Classification System (MACS) for children with cerebral palsy: Scale development and evidence of validity and reliability. *Dev Med Child Neurol*. 2006;48:549–54.
5. Ashwal S, Russman BS, Blasco PA, et al. Practice parameter: diagnostic assessment of the child with cerebral palsy: Report of the Quality Standards Subcommittee of the American Academy of Neurology and the Practice Committee of the Child Neurology Society. *Neurology*. 2004;62:851–63.
6. Quality Standards Subcommittee of the American Academy of Neurology and the Practice Committee of the Child Neurology Society, Delgado MR, et al. Practice parameter: Pharmacologic treatment of spasticity in children and adolescents with cerebral palsy (an evidence-based review): Report of the Quality Standards Subcommittee of the American Academy of Neurology and the Practice Committee of the Child Neurology Society. *Neurology*. 2010; 74:336–43.
7. Cooley WC, American Academy of Pediatrics Committee on Children With Disabilities. Providing a primary care medical home for children and youth with cerebral palsy. *Pediatrics*. 2004;114:1106–13.

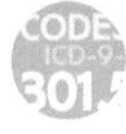

CODES

ICD9
- 343.0 Congenital diplegia
- 343.1 Congenital hemiplegia
- 343.2 Congenital quadriplegia

CLINICAL PEARLS

- Management should focus on maximizing functioning and quality of life with multidisciplinary team approach.
- Regression of motor skills does not occur with CP.

CERVICAL HYPEREXTENSION INJURIES

Francesca L. Beaudoin, MS, MD
Stephanie Carreiro, MD

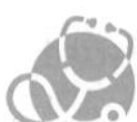

BASICS

DESCRIPTION

- Group of injuries involving the neck that result from a rapid, forceful, backwards motion
- May involve:
  - Injury to vertebral and paravertebral structures: Fractures, dislocations, ligamentous tears, and disc disruption/subluxation
  - Spinal cord injury: Traumatic central cord syndrome (CCS) secondary to cord compression or vascular insult
  - Blunt cerebrovascular injury (BCVI): Vertebral artery or carotid artery dissection
  - Soft tissue injury around cervical spine: Cervical strain/sprain

EPIDEMIOLOGY

- Predominant age: Trauma and sports injuries more common in young adults (average age 29.4 years); however, CCS mostly seen in older population (average age 53 years)
- Predominant sex: Male > Female

Incidence

In the US:

- Cervical fractures: 2–5/100 blunt trauma patients
- Central cord syndrome: 3.6/100,000 people/yr
- BCVI: Estimated 1/1,000 of hospitalized trauma patients; incidence increased with known cervical/petrous bone fracture, LeFort II/III facial fractures, or diffuse axonal injury (1)
- Cervical strain: 3–4/1,000 people/yr

RISK FACTORS

- Fractures: Osteoporosis, conditions predisposing to spinal rigidity, such as ankylosing spondylitis
- CCS: Pre-existing spinal stenosis is present in >50% of cases, which may be:
  - Acquired: Prior trauma, spondylosis
  - Congenital: Klippel-Feil syndrome (congenital fusion of any 2 cervical vertebra) with cervical stenosis

GENERAL PREVENTION

Seat belts and use of proper safety equipment in sports activities can prevent/minimize injury.

ETIOLOGY

Blunt trauma due to motor vehicle accidents, sports injuries, falls, and assaults

COMMONLY ASSOCIATED CONDITIONS

Closed head injuries (concussion, cerebral contusions, intracranial hemorrhage), facial fractures, thoracic/lumbar spinal injury

DIAGNOSIS

HISTORY

Usually acute presentation with mechanism of cervical hyperextension (see "Etiology") and complaints of neck pain, stiffness, or headaches +/− neurologic symptoms

PHYSICAL EXAM

- External signs of trauma on the head and neck such as abrasions, lacerations, ecchymoses, or contusions are clues to mechanism.
- Presence, severity, and location of neck tenderness localize involved structure(s):
  - Posterior midline, bony point tenderness concerning for bony injury
  - Paraspinal or lateral soft tissue tenderness suggestive of muscular/ligamentous injury
  - Anterior tenderness concerning for carotid injury
- Carotid bruit suggestive of carotid dissection
- Neurologic exam: Paresthesias/numbness, weakness suggests spinal cord injury:
  - CCS often presents as:
    - Distal > proximal symptom distribution, upper extremity > lower extremity
    - Extremity weakness/paralysis predominates
    - Variable sensory changes below level of lesion (including paresthesias and dysesthesia)
    - Bladder/bowel dysfunction may occur.

DIAGNOSTIC TESTS & INTERPRETATION

Imaging

Initial approach

- Low-risk patients can be cleared clinically (without radiographic evaluation) using either the Canadian C-Spine Rule (CCR) or the National Emergency X-ray Utilization Study (NEXUS) Criteria:
  - CCR: Clinically clear a stable, adult patient with no history of cervical spine disease/surgery if all of the following conditions are met:
    - Glasgow Coma Scale (GCS) = 15
    - Nonintoxicated patients without a distracting injury
    - No dangerous mechanism or extremity paresthesias
    - At least 1 "low-risk factor" (i.e., simple rear-end motor vehicle accident [MVA], ambulation at the accident scene, no midline cervical tenderness, delayed onset of neck pain, or sitting position at the time of exam)
  - NEXUS: Clinically clear if all of the following are met:
    - No alteration of mental status or intoxication
    - No focal/neuro deficits
    - No distracting injury
    - No posterior, midline C-spine tenderness
  - Reported sensitivity/specificity: CCR (99.4%/45.1%), NEXUS (90.7%/36.8%) (2)[A]
- In patients with high-risk mechanism or any concerning historical/physical exam elements, imaging should strongly be considered. Choose from the following options based on the suspected injury and level of clinical suspicion:
  - Plain radiographs: Recommended by some in patients who cannot be cleared clinically but still are in low-suspicion category: Sensitivity for C-spine injury as low as 39% (3)[B]:
    - Static: Lateral, anterior-posterior (A-P), and odontoid views; in addition to bony abnormalities, may show prevertebral soft tissue swelling
    - Dynamic: Flexion/extension, only if asymptomatic and no neurologic deficits or mental impairment. Of limited utility in the acute setting.
  - CT: Axial CT from occiput to T1 with coronal and sagittal reconstructions: Rapidly replacing plain radiography as the test of choice for cases with moderate-to-high clinical suspicion of C-spine injury given high sensitivity (90–100%) (3)[B]
  - MRI: Diagnostic test of choice in CCS with direct visualization of traumatic cord lesions (edema or hematomyelia), soft tissue compressing cord, and/or stenosis of canal. Also detects ligamentous injury and abnormalities of intervertebral discs and soft tissues, but modality is poor with fractures and is prone to false-positive results due to nonspecific findings. Some authors suggest that an MRI is required to screen for occult injury in obtunded/noncommunicative patients with a negative CT scan; however, this recommendation is controversial and evidence is limited (4)[B].
  - CT angiography: Visualization of cervical and cerebral vascular structures to detect BCVI, with reported sensitivity approaching 100% when a 16 slice or greater CT scanner is used. MR angiography is an alternative modality, although reported sensitivities of 47–50% limit its utility (1)[B].

Pathological Findings

- Vertebral fractures: See "General Measures."
- CCS: Currently thought to be due to axonal disruption within the white matter of the lateral column, particularly the corticospinal tracts
- BCVI: Intimal disruption, leading to thrombosis and embolization
- Acute cervical strain/sprain: Models based on animal, cadaver, and postmortem studies show myofascial tearing, edema, and inflammation, but facet joint capsular pain may also play a role.

DIFFERENTIAL DIAGNOSIS

- Acute or chronic disc pathology (including herniation or internal disruption)
- Osteoarthritis
- Cervical radiculopathy
- For CCS:
  - Bell cruciate palsy
  - Bilateral brachial plexus injuries
  - Carotid or vertebral artery dissection

Geriatric Considerations

Degenerative disease of C-spine may be confused with acute traumatic change on imaging, particularly on plain radiographs; CT imaging is more helpful to distinguish the 2.

Pediatric Considerations

Consider spinal cord injury without radiographic abnormality (SCIWORA), which has a high incidence at <9 years old and accounts for up to 50% of all pediatric cervical spine injuries. MRI may help detect the injury.

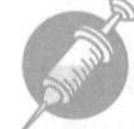

TREATMENT

MEDICATION

- Fractures: Pain control as needed with opiate analgesics
- CCS: Methylprednisolone 30 mg/kg IV over 15 minutes, then continuous infusion 5.4 mg/kg/h IV for 24 hours. Further improvement in motor function recovery may be seen if infusion is continued for 48 hours, especially if initial bolus administration is delayed by 3–8 hours after injury (5)[A].

- BCVI: Anticoagulation with IV heparin, followed by warfarin therapy for 3–6 months, then long-term antiplatelet therapy is common practice. However, an antiplatelet agent is used as the sole initial therapy in patients with contraindications to anticoagulation (1)[B]. To date, there are no randomized controlled trials comparing the efficacy of antiplatelets versus anticoagulant therapy, so evidence-based recommendations are not available (6)[A].
- Cervical strain: Muscle relaxants, acetaminophen/NSAIDs +/– opiate analgesics are commonly used

ADDITIONAL TREATMENT

General Measures

- Fractures:
  - Stability determined by imaging; decompression and stabilization are indicated in:
    - Incomplete spinal cord injuries (SCIs) with spinal canal compromise
    - Clinical deterioration or failure to improve despite conservative management
  - Hangman fracture: Traumatic spondylolisthesis of C2 (the "axis") with bilateral fractures through C2 pedicles, often with anterior subluxation of C2 over C3: Can be unstable:
    - Managed with halo vest immobilization for 12 weeks until repeated flexion/extension films normalize
  - Odontoid (dens) fractures: Treated according to type:
    - I: Through apex; usually stable; external immobilization with a cervical collar or (less often halo vest) for up to 12 weeks
    - II: Most common, at base of dens, usually unstable; nonunion rates of up to 67% with halo immobilization alone, especially with dens displacement >6 mm or age >50 years
    - III: Through C2 body, usually stable; immobilization in halo or cervical collar for 12–20 weeks
  - Hyperextension teardrop fractures:
    - If stable, rigid collar or cervicothoracic brace for 8–14 weeks
    - If unstable, halo brace for up to 3 months
- CCS: Neck immobilization with cervical collar, physical therapy/occupational therapy (PT/OT)
- Cervical strain: No evidence of different outcomes with active (PT) versus passive (immobilization, rest) treatment (7)[A], but may use soft cervical collar for up to 10 days for symptomatic relief, then mobilization and activity as tolerated

Issues for Referral

- When cervical spine injury is suspected, the patient should be immobilized and sent to the emergency department for evaluation.
- Emergent consultation from a spinal surgeon (neurosurgery and/or orthopedics) is indicated if there is any concern for unstable fracture or spinal cord injury.

SURGERY/OTHER PROCEDURES

- Fractures:
  - Hangman's fracture: Consider surgical fixation in cases of excessive angulation or subluxation, disruption of intervertebral disc space or failure to obtain alignment with external orthosis.
  - Odontoid fractures:
    - Type II: Early surgical stabilization recommended in setting of age >50 years old, dens displacement >5 mm, and in certain fracture patterns
    - Type III: Surgical intervention often reserved for cases of nonunion/malunion after trial of external immobilization
  - Hyperextension teardrop fractures: Consider surgical repair if unstable with neurologic deficit
- CCS: Surgical decompression/fixation is indicated if occurs in setting of unstable injury and/or herniated disc, or when neurologic function plateaus/deteriorates
- BCVI: Surgical and/or angiographic intervention may be required if there is evidence of pseudoaneurysm, total occlusion, or transection of the vessel (1)[B].

IN-PATIENT CONSIDERATIONS

Initial Stabilization

Advanced Trauma Life Support (ATLS) protocol with backboard and collar

Admission Criteria

Varies by injury; clinical judgment, radiographic findings, concomitant injuries, and need for operative intervention influence decision

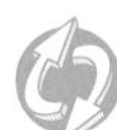

ONGOING CARE

FOLLOW-UP RECOMMENDATIONS

Patient Monitoring

Patients with known injuries will often be followed with serial radiographs under the care of a specialist.

PATIENT EDUCATION

For patient instruction on prevention: THINK FIRST Foundation at: http://www.thinkfirst.org

PROGNOSIS

- Overall, the most important prognostic factor is the initial neurologic status.
- Fractures:
  - Hangman fracture: 93–100% fusion rate after 8–14 weeks external immobilization
  - Odontoid fracture, fusion rate by type: Type I ~100% with external immobilization alone; type III, 85% with external immobilization, 100% with surgical fixation
- BCVI: With early diagnosis and initiation of antithrombotic therapy, patients may have fewer neurologic sequelae.
- CCS:
  - Spontaneous recovery of motor function in >50% of cases over several weeks, with younger patients more likely to regain function
  - Leg, bowel, and bladder functions return first, followed by upper extremities.
- Cervical strain: Up to 50% of patients continue to have neck pain at 1 year:
  - Prognostic factors for development of late whiplash syndrome (>6 months of symptoms affecting normal activity) include increased initial pain intensity, pain-related disability, and cold hyperalgesia.

COMPLICATIONS

- Fractures: Nonunion/malunion of fractures or persistent instability requiring second procedure, reactions, and infection related to orthosis
- BCVI: Embolic ischemic events and pseudoaneurysm formation

REFERENCES

1. Bromberg WJ, et al. Blunt cerebrovascular injury practice management guidelines: The Eastern Association for the Surgery of Trauma. *J Trauma*. 2010;68(2):471–7.
2. Stiell IG, Clement CM, McKnight RD, et al. The Canadian C-spine rule versus the NEXUS low-risk criteria in patients with trauma. *N Engl J Med*. 2003;349:2510–8.
3. Cain G, et al. Imaging suspected cervical spine injury: plain radiography or computed tomography? Systematic review (Structured abstract). *Radiography*. 2010;68–77.
4. Schoenfeld AJ, et al. Computed tomography alone versus computed tomography and magnetic resonance imaging in the identification of occult injuries to the cervical spine: A meta-analysis (Structured abstract). *J Trauma*. 2010; 109–114.
5. Bracken MB. Steroids for acute spinal cord injury. Cochrane injuries group. *Cochrane Database Syst Rev*. 2008;3.
6. Lyrer P, Engelter S. Engelter Antithrombotic drugs for carotid artery dissection. *Cochrane Database Syst Rev*. 2010. DOI:10.1002/14651858. CD000255.pub2.
7. Verhagen AP, Scholten-Peeters GGGM, van Wijngaarden S, et al. Conservative treatments for whiplash. *Cochrane Database Syst Rev*. 2007;2: CD003338.

ADDITIONAL READING

Pryputniewicz DM, Hadley MN, et al. Axis fractures. *Neurosurgery*. 2010;66:68–82.

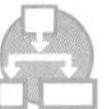

See Also (Topic, Algorithm, Electronic Media Element)

Cervical Spine Injury

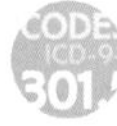

CODES

ICD9

- 847.0 Neck sprain
- 952.00 C1-C4 level spinal cord injury, unspecified
- 952.03 C1-C4 level with central cord syndrome

CLINICAL PEARLS

- Follow NEXUS or Canadian Cervical Spine rules on every patient with potential neck injury to determine imaging needs, but use clinical judgment!
- Inquire about pre-existing cervical spine injuries or conditions, especially in the elderly, as they may increase risk of injury or alter radiographic interpretation.
- Suspect spinal cord injury until exam and imaging suggest otherwise.
- Consider BCVI when neurologic deficits are inconsistent with level of known injury or significant mechanism exists.

CERVICAL MALIGNANCY

Benjamin P. Brown, MD
Trevor Tejada-Berges, MD

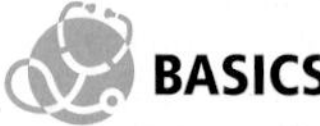

BASICS

DESCRIPTION

- Invasive cancer of the uterine cervix
- Commonly involves the vagina, parametria, and pelvic side walls
- Invasion of bladder, rectum, and other pelvic sites in advanced disease
- Disease prognosis differs with tumor stage.

EPIDEMIOLOGY

Incidence

- Worldwide, cervical cancer ranks second among all malignancies for women (1).
- There is a higher incidence of cervical cancer in developing countries, contributing up to 83% of reported cases annually.
- In the US, it is the third most common gynecologic cancer and the sixth most common solid malignant neoplasm among women.
- The disease has a bimodal distribution, with highest risk among women ages 40–59 and >70.

Prevalence

- In 2010, the American Cancer Society (ACS) estimated there were 12,200 new US cases with 4,210 deaths from the malignancy.
- African Americans and women in lower socioeconomic groups have the highest age-standardized cervical cancer death rates.
- Hispanic and Latina women have the highest incidence rate of the malignancy.

RISK FACTORS

- Causative agent in the majority of cases is persistent human papillomavirus (HPV) infection.
- Other risk factors include:
  - Lack of regular Pap smears
  - Early coitarche
  - Multiple sexual partners
  - Unprotected sex
  - A history of sexually transmitted diseases (STDs)
  - Low socioeconomic status
  - High parity
  - Cigarette smoking
  - Immunosuppression
  - DES exposure in utero

Genetics

Not an inherited disease, except in very rare cases of Peutz-Jeghers syndrome

GENERAL PREVENTION

- Patient education regarding safer sex, decreasing number of sexual partners
- Smoking cessation
- Gardasil vaccine: Quadrivalent vaccine containing proteins from HPV strains 6, 11, 16, and 18. Food and Drug Administration (FDA)-approved in females and in males (for prevention of genital warts). Cervarix vaccine: Bivalent vaccine against oncogenic HPV strains 16 and 18.
- Recommended age of vaccination is 11–12 years (prior to initiation of coitus), but Gardasil can be given at any time from 9–26 and Cervarix can be given at any time from 10–25 (2)[C].
- Both vaccines are series of 3 IM injections, with the second and third following 1–2 and 6 months after the first, respectively.
- Regular Pap smears and pelvic exams at appropriate intervals according to American College of Obstetricians and Gynecologists (ACOG). Current ACOG guidelines recommend starting annual Pap smear testing at age 21, regardless of age at coitarche.
- The International Federation of Gynecology and Obstetrics (FIGO) recommends visual inspection with acetic acid (VIA) or visual inspection with Lugol's iodine (VILI) as reasonable alternatives to Pap smear screening in resource-poor settings. A 3–5-year screening interval is currently recommended (3)[B].
- Despite HPV vaccination, cervical cancer screening will remain the main preventive measure for both vaccinated and nonvaccinated women, but the nature of screening and management of women with cervical disease are being adapted to the new technologies.

PATHOPHYSIOLOGY

- Arise from pre-existing dysplastic lesions usually following persistent HPV infection
- Pattern of local growth may be exophytic or endophytic.
- Lymphatic spread typically through cervical lymphatic drainage
- Local tumor extension involving the bladder, ureters, rectum, and distant metastasis from hematogenous spread

ETIOLOGY

- Epidemiologic and experimental evidence supports oncogenic strains of HPV 16 and 18 as etiologic agents in ~70% of cervical cancers.
- Association with the E6 and E7 oncogenic proteins responsible for malignant cell transformation by inactivation of the p53 and Rb tumor suppressor genes.
- Slow progression from dysplasia to invasive cancer allows sufficient time for effective screening and treatment of preinvasive disease.

COMMONLY ASSOCIATED CONDITIONS

- Condyloma acuminata
- Preinvasive/invasive lesions of the vulva and vagina

DIAGNOSIS

HISTORY

- May be asymptomatic
- Most common symptom is vaginal bleeding, often postcoital
- Other gynecologic symptoms include intermenstrual or postmenopausal bleeding and vaginal discharge.
- Other less common symptoms include low back pain with radiation down posterior leg, lower extremity edema, vesicovaginal and rectovaginal fistula, and urinary symptoms.

PHYSICAL EXAM

- Thorough external genitalia and internal vaginal exam is needed to look for lesions:
  - Most patients have a normal exam, especially with microinvasive disease.
  - Lesions may be exophytic, endophytic, polypoid, papillary, ulcerative, or necrotic.
  - Watery, purulent, or bloody discharge
- Bimanual and rectovaginal examination for uterine size, vaginal wall, rectovaginal septum, parametrial, uterosacral, and pelvic sidewall involvement
- Enlarged supraclavicular or inguinal lymphadenopathy, lower extremity edema, ascites, or decreased breath sounds with lung auscultation may indicate metastases.
- Examination under anesthesia for extent of pelvic tumor spread

DIAGNOSTIC TESTS & INTERPRETATION

Lab

Initial lab tests

- Biopsy of gross lesions and colposcopically directed biopsies are the definitive means of diagnosis.
- CBC may show anemia.
- Urinalysis may show hematuria.
- In advanced disease, BUN, creatinine, and liver function tests (LFTs) may be helpful.

Follow-Up & Special Considerations

Prompt follow-up for test results and treatment plans

Imaging

Initial approach

- Initially, a CT scan of the chest, abdomen, and pelvis and/or a positron emission tomography (PET) scan.
- Apart from chest x-ray (CXR) and intravenous pyelogram (IVP), use of imaging is discouraged when establishing clinical stage.
- MRI may be helpful in evaluating parametrial involvement in patients who are primary surgical candidates.

Follow-Up & Special Considerations

- Prompt multidisciplinary plan of care
- Disease is staged clinically, not surgically.

Diagnostic Procedures/Surgery

- Exam under anesthesia may help in determining clinical stage and disease extent.
- Biopsy of gross lesion
- If no gross lesion identified, colposcopy with biopsy of abnormal blood vessels, irregular surface contour with loss of surface epithelium is indicated
- Endocervical curettage and cervical conization as indicated to determine depth of invasion and presence of lymphovascular involvement
- Cystoscopy to evaluate bladder invasion
- Proctoscopy for invasion into rectum

Pathological Findings

- Majority of cases (80%) are invasive squamous cell types usually arising from the ectocervix.
- Adenocarcinomas comprise 10–15% of cervical cancer arising from endocervical mucus-producing glandular cells.
- Other cell types that may be present include rare mixed cell types, neuroendocrine tumors, sarcomas, lymphomas, and melanomas.

DIFFERENTIAL DIAGNOSIS

- Marked cervicitis and erosion
- Glandular hyperplasia
- Sexually transmitted infection (STI)
- Cervical condyloma, leiomyoma, or polyp
- Metastasis from endometrial carcinoma or gestational trophoblastic disease

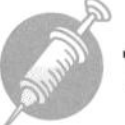

TREATMENT

MEDICATION

- Chemoradiation with cisplatin-containing regimen has been associated with superior survival rates compared with pelvic and extended-field radiation alone (4)[A].
- Neoadjuvant chemotherapy followed by surgery has not been shown to have a survival benefit for patients who are not initially surgical candidates due to tumor stage (5)[A].

ADDITIONAL TREATMENT

General Measures

Improve nutritional state, correct any anemia, and treat any vaginal and/or pelvic infections.

Issues for Referral

Multidisciplinary management of patients as needed and in a timely fashion

Additional Therapies

- Chemoradiation (without surgery) is the first-line therapy for tumors stage IIB and higher (gross lesions with obvious parametrial involvement) and for most bulky stage IB2 tumors (6)[A].
- Combination of external beam pelvic radiation and brachytherapy is usually employed.
- If para-aortic nodal metastases are evident, then extended-field radiation can be added to treat affected lymph nodes. Alternatively, lymph node dissection prior to radiation therapy may be performed.

SURGERY/OTHER PROCEDURES

- Surgical management is an option for patients with early-stage tumors.
- Removal of precursor lesions (cervical intraepithelial neoplasia [CIN]) by loop electrosurgical excision procedure (LEEP), cold knife conization, laser ablation, or cryotherapy (7)[A]
- Stage IA1 (lesions with <3 mm invasion from basement membrane) without lymphovascular space invasion: Option of conization and simple extrafascial hysterectomy (6)[B]
- Stage IA2 (lesions with >3 mm but <5 mm invasion from basement membrane): Option of radical hysterectomy with lymph node dissection or chemoradiation, depending on clinical setting (6)[B]
- Stage IA2–IB1: Fertility-sparing radical trachelectomy may be considered in selected patients.
- Stages IB1–IIA (gross lesions without obvious parametrial involvement): Option of radical hysterectomy with lymph node sampling or primary chemoradiation with brachytherapy and teletherapy (6)[A]
- Stage IVA (lesions limited to central metastasis to the bladder and/or rectum): Pelvic exenteration may be feasible.
- Stage IVB disease has poor prognosis and is treated with goal of palliation.

Pregnancy Considerations

- Management of cervical dysplasia in pregnancy is guided by consideration of stage of lesion, gestational age, and maternal assessment of risks and benefits from treatment (6)[C].
- Abnormal cytology is best followed up by colposcopy and biopsy.
- Intraepithelial lesions (CIN): Colposcopy every 8 weeks during pregnancy and follow up at the 6-week postpartum visit.
- Microinvasive carcinoma: Conization or wedge biopsy. If depth of invasion ≤3mm, follow up at the 6-week postpartum visit.
- Invasive carcinoma: Definitive therapy, with timing determined by maternal preference

IN-PATIENT CONSIDERATIONS

Initial Stabilization

- Active vaginal bleeding can be controlled with timely vaginal packing and radiation therapy.
- Recognition of ureteral blockage, hydronephrosis, urosepsis, and timely intervention

Admission Criteria

- Signs of active bleeding
- Urinary symptoms
- Dehydration
- Complications from surgery, chemotherapy, or radiation

Discharge Criteria

- Discharge criteria based on multidisciplinary assessment, including physicians, physical therapists
- Discharge to home, long- or short-term rehabilitation, home nursing care, or hospice as appropriate

ONGOING CARE

FOLLOW-UP RECOMMENDATIONS

Patient Monitoring

- With completion of definitive therapy, each patient is evaluated with physical/pelvic examinations and Pap smears:
  - Every 3–4 months for 1–2 years
  - Every 6 months until the fifth year
  - Yearly thereafter
- Signs of cancer recurrence may include vaginal bleeding, unexplained weight loss, leg edema, and pelvic or thigh pain.

PATIENT EDUCATION

Patient education material available through the American Cancer Society at www.cancer.org and the National Cancer Institute at www.cancer.gov.

PROGNOSIS

After commonly accepted surgical and radiation treatments, 5-year survival:

Stage	5-yr Survival (%)
1	75–98
2	66–73
3	40–42
4	9–22

COMPLICATIONS

- Loss of ovarian function from radiotherapy or indication for bilateral oophorectomy
- Hemorrhage
- Pelvic infection
- Genitourinary fistula
- Bladder dysfunction
- Sexual dysfunction
- Ureteral obstruction with renal failure
- Bowel obstruction
- Pulmonary embolism
- Lower extremity lymphedema

REFERENCES

1. Scarinci IC, Garcia FA, Kobetz E, et al. Cervical cancer prevention: New tools and old barriers. *Cancer*. 2010;116:2531–42.
2. CDC. FDA licensure of human papilloma virus vaccine (HPV2, Cervarix) for use in females and updated HPV vaccination recommendations from the Advisory Committee on Immunization Practices (ACIP). *MMWR*. 2010;59(20);626-629.
3. Bhatla N, et al. Global Guidance for Cervical Cancer Prevention and Control. Rep. FIGO, 2009 Oct. http://www.rho.org/files/FIGO_cervical_cancer_guidelines_2009.pdf.
4. Chemotherapy for Cervical Cancer Meta-analysis Collaboration (CCCMAC). Reducing uncertainties about the effects of chemoradiotherapy for cervical cancer: Individual patient data meta-analysis. *Cochrane Database Syst Rev*. 2010:1.
5. Rydzewska L, Tierney J, Vale CL, et al. Neoadjuvant chemotherapy plus surgery versus surgery for cervical cancer. *Cochrane Database Syst Rev*. 2010:1.
6. ACOG Committee on Practice Bulletins-Gynecology. ACOG practice bulletin: Diagnosis and treatment of cervical carcinomas, number 35, May 2002. *Obstet Gynecol*. 2002;99(5 Pt 1):855-67.
7. Martin-Hirsch PL, et al. Surgery for cervical intraepithelial neoplasia. Cochrane Gynaecological Cancer Group. *Cochrane Database Syst Rev*. 2007:3.

ADDITIONAL READING

- ACOG Committee on Practice Bulletins-Gynecology. ACOG practice bulletin: Cervical cytology screening. *Obstet Gynecol*. 2009;114:1409–1420.
- Grce M, Matovina M, Milutin-Gasperov N, et al. Advances in cervical cancer control and future perspectives. *Coll Antropol*. 2010;34:731–6.
- Jemal A, Siegel R, Xu J, et al. Cancer Statistics, 2010. *CA Cancer J Clin*. 2010;60(5):277.
- Quinn MA, Benedet JL, Odicino F, et al. Carcinoma of the cervix uteri. *Int J Gynaecol Obstet*. 2006;95: S43.

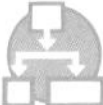

See Also (Topic, Algorithm, Electronic Media Element)

Abnormal Pap and Cervical Dysplasia

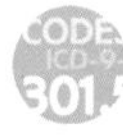

CODES

ICD9

- 180.0 Malignant neoplasm of endocervix
- 180.1 Malignant neoplasm of exocervix
- 180.8 Malignant neoplasm of other specified sites of cervix

CLINICAL PEARLS

- Worldwide, cervical cancer ranks second among all malignancies for women.
- Women with cervical cancer may be asymptomatic and have a normal physical exam.
- Surgical management is an option for patients with early-stage tumors.
- Chemoradiation is the first-line therapy for higher-stage tumors.

CERVICAL SPINE INJURY

Caroline Tschibelu, MD
Joao Tavares, MD

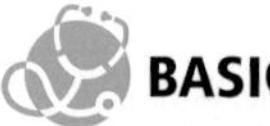

BASICS

DESCRIPTION

- Cervical spine injuries can result in vertebral fracture, ligamentous injury, or spinal cord injury.
- Vertebral and ligamentous injuries can cause cervical spine instability leading to cord injury.

EPIDEMIOLOGY

Incidence

- There are an estimated 12,000 new cases of spinal cord injury per year in the US, with >50% involving the cervical spine.
- Primarily affects young adults with active lifestyles, but the elderly are also affected due to prevalence of degenerative joint disease and increased risk of falls
- Average age at time of injury: 39.5
- Male-to-female ratio: 4:1

RISK FACTORS

Anatomic irregularities:

- Degenerative joint disease (particularly the elderly)
- Osteoporosis
- Spinal canal stenosis
- Spina bifida

Genetics

Inherited connective tissue disorders (e.g., familial cervical spondylosis, a spondylitis)

GENERAL PREVENTION

- Use seat belts and child safety seats.
- Avoidance of high-risk activities such as driving while intoxicated
- Treatment of osteoporosis (e.g., calcium and vitamin D supplement, hormone replacement therapy [HRT], bisphosphonates)
- Fall prevention for the elderly

PATHOPHYSIOLOGY

4 major vertebral and ligamentous injuries are classified by mechanism:

- Flexion:
  - Simple wedge compression fracture:
    - Anterior compression fracture of vertebrae
    - Nuchal ligament stretch but not disruption
    - Diminished vertebral body height on x-ray
    - Stable fracture
  - Flexion teardrop fracture:
    - Anteroinferior vertebral body fracture
    - Displaced anterior fragment ("teardrop")
    - Posterior and anterior ligamentous disruption
    - Extremely unstable, high risk of cord injury
  - Anterior subluxation:
    - Posterior ligament rupture without fracture
    - Rarely associated with neurologic deficit
    - Seen on flexion-extension views
    - Treated as unstable due to risk while in flexion, but not unstable by definition
  - Bilateral facet dislocation:
    - More severe anterior subluxation
    - Includes disruption of annulus, anterior, and posterior ligaments
    - Inferior facets move superior and anterior to the superior facets, causing displacement.
    - Neurologic injury related to disk herniation
  - Clay shoveler fracture:
    - Oblique fracture at base of spinous process
    - Occurs with abrupt flexion with simultaneous contraction of lower neck and upper body
    - Also occurs with blunt trauma
    - Avulsed fragment seen on lateral views
    - Stable fracture, low risk for neurologic deficit
- Flexion–rotation:
  - Unilateral facet dislocation:
    - Less anterior displacement than bilateral
  - Rotary atlantoaxial dislocation (C1–C2):
    - Specific type of unilateral facet dislocation
    - Asymmetry of the lateral masses of C1 seen
    - Considered unstable due to location
- Extension:
  - Hangman fracture:
    - Traumatic spondylolisthesis of C2
    - Bilateral fractures through C2 pedicles
    - Unstable fracture, but cord injury rare
  - Extension teardrop fracture:
    - Avulsion fracture from stretch on anterior longitudinal ligament, causing anteroinferior bony fragment
    - Commonly found at lower cervical levels
    - Cord injury possible due to ligamenta flava encroaching into spinal canal
    - Unstable fracture in extension
  - Fracture of C1 posterior arch:
    - Stable fracture
  - Posterior atlantoaxial dislocation (C1–C2):
    - Cord injury possible
- Vertical compression (from axial load):
  - Jefferson fracture:
    - Burst fracture of C1 ring
    - Instability determined by severity of transverse ligamentous disruption
    - Unstable if more than 25% loss of height
  - Occipital condyle fracture:
    - Can be avulsion or compression fracture
    - Associated with cranial nerve deficits
- Unclear mechanisms:
  - Odontoid (dens) fracture, part of C2 (axis):
    - Type I: Involving tip of dens
    - Type II: Involving base of dens
    - Type III: Extends into body of axis
    - Types II and III can become unstable.
  - Atlanto-occipital dislocation:
    - Brainstem stretch may cause immediate respiratory arrest and death.
- Spinal cord injury (SCI):
  - Complete cord injury: Characterized by complete loss of sensory and motor functions below injury through S4–S5. Can also present with priapism, urinary retention, and bladder distention.
  - Incomplete deficits: Sensory and motor functions partially preserved below injury. Sensory preserved to a greater degree because sensory tracts peripherally located. Incidence of incomplete cord injury has increased compared to complete injury with implementation of Advanced Trauma Life Support protocols for all trauma patients (1). Most SCI are mixed injuries, but there are some specific syndromes:
    - Central cord syndrome: Most common incomplete injury; motor deficits greater in upper than lower extremities. Sensory loss in the distribution of a "cape" and due to watershed injury affecting long fiber tracts; may be due to hyperextension.
    - Anterior cord syndrome: Posterior columns spared; affects spinothalamic, corticospinal, anterior, and lateral columns; loss of pain, temperature, motor with preserved vibration and position sense below the lesion
    - Posterior cord syndrome: Sensory deficits more pronounced than motor, due to contusion of posterior columns
    - Brown-Sequard syndrome: Ipsilateral motor loss and vibration sensation deficits with contralateral loss of pain and temperature sensation; hemisection of cord most often due to penetrating trauma

ETIOLOGY

Traumatic injury to the head or neck from:

- Motor vehicle accidents (MVAs) or falls
- Violence, commonly gunshot wounds
- High-risk or high-impact sports

COMMONLY ASSOCIATED CONDITIONS

- Intracranial hemorrhage
- Skull and facial fractures
- Thoracolumbar spine injury
- Other: Visceral/extremities injuries in polytrauma

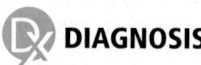

DIAGNOSIS

HISTORY

- History of traumatic injury to head or neck
- Neck pain or neurologic symptoms
- Past medical history, including medications
- Substance abuse or intoxication

PHYSICAL EXAM

- Midline cervical tenderness on palpation
- Limited or painful cervical range of motion
- Weakness, paresthesias, or numbness on complete neurologic exam
- Abnormal rectal tone

DIAGNOSTIC TESTS & INTERPRETATION

Lab

Initial lab tests

- CBC, basic metabolic panel
- Urine toxicology, blood alcohol level

Imaging

Initial approach

- Standard trauma series includes 5 x-ray views. However, if high suspicion for C-spine injury, consider CT as first-line imaging.
- Use Canadian C-spine Rules (CCR) or NEXUS Low-Risk Criteria (LRC) to decide when not to radiograph:
  - CCR, no imaging needed if (2)[A]:
    - Patient is alert (GCS = 15) and stable
    - No high-risk factors, no dangerous mechanism of injury, no paresthesias, age <65
    - A low-risk factor (simple rear-end MVA, ambulatory, delayed pain, absence of midline tenderness) in a patient who can rotate neck 45° left and right
  - NEXUS LRC, no imaging needed if (3)[A]:
    - No posterior midline cervical tenderness
    - Alert, without evidence of intoxication
    - No focal neurologic deficit
    - No painful distracting injury
- 2003 prospective cohort of 8,283 patients found CCR superior to NEXUS LRC.
- CT is superior to radiography in higher-risk patients with decreased mentation.
- If C7–T1 cannot be visualized, consider CT.

C

Geriatric Considerations
In the geriatric population, avoid sedating medications. Strongly consider CT of cervical spine due to degenerative disease.

Pediatric Considerations
- Subluxation more likely than fracture
- Larger head size increases risk of cord injury
- C1-C3 more likely affected in children under 8
- Some sources support CT scan as first-line in children under 14, but risk of radiation outweighs the benefits in asymptomatic children (4)[B].
- Spinal cord injury without radiographic abnormality (SCIWORA): Neurologic deficits without signs of bony or ligamentous injury on adequate radiographs or CT. SCIWORA primarily seen in children due to ligamentous laxity and incomplete ossification of the spine. Consider MRI to better visualize ligamentous injury in this population.

Follow-Up & Special Considerations
- If negative cervical spine CT with persistent midline tenderness, consider MRI in 72 hours.
- If there is persistent concern for ligamentous cervical spine injury not seen on standard x-rays, MRI should be used for its ability to detect those injuries. Flexion–extension radiographs used to be considered if the patient was alert and cooperative, but they are falling out of favor because they may worsen spinal injury.
- MRI has negative predictive value (NPV) of 100% for noninjury, including injuries not seen on x-rays or CT (5)[A].

Diagnostic Procedures/Surgery
CT angiography of carotid or vertebral arteries if concerned for associated vascular injury

Pathological Findings
- Vertebral fractures on x-rays or CT
- Ligamentous tear or soft tissue edema on MRI
- Spinal cord entrapment on MRI

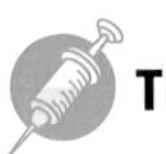

TREATMENT

MEDICATION
- Pain control
- Steroid treatment controversial for cord injury because effectiveness uncertain:
  - Methylprednisolone: Bolus: 30 mg/kg, then 5.4 mg/kg/h for the next 23 hours if within 3 hours of injury; if within 3–8 hours of injury, treat for total of 48 hours (6)[A]
- Increased risk of infection, GI bleeding, and steroid myopathy with steroid use (7)[C]

ADDITIONAL TREATMENT
General Measures
Long-term cervical collar or halo-style orthosis if evidence of vertebral, ligamentous, or cord injury

Issues for Referral
Orthopedics and/or neurosurgery

COMPLEMENTARY AND ALTERNATIVE MEDICINE
Massage therapy for residual muscular pain or spasm

SURGERY/OTHER PROCEDURES
Surgical stabilization used for a minority of cases

IN-PATIENT CONSIDERATIONS
Initial Stabilization
Follow the Advanced Trauma Life Support (ATLS) algorithm.

ALERT
- Immediately place patient in cervical collar if:
  - High-impact accident
  - Facial trauma, head injury, or direct cervical injury
  - Altered consciousness
- Presents from home after recent injury, despite functional status or time elapsed
- If transporting, use a backboard with stabilizing blocks to maintain neutral position.
- Keep oxygen saturation normal to prevent further cord injury from hypoxia.

Admission Criteria
- Respiratory: Oxygen requirements
- Cardiovascular: Hemodynamic instability
- Neurologic: Focal neurologic findings, limited independent function, or concern for delayed intracranial bleed
- Surgical: Awaiting surgical stabilization

IV Fluids
Volume resuscitation or pressors as needed

Nursing
Frequent neurologic checks and use of appropriate, well-fitted collar

Discharge Criteria
Patient can be discharged if:
- Cleared according to NEXUS or CCR criteria or after neurology/orthopedic consults
- Ligamentous injury is present or suspected and sent home in cervical orthosis
- Stable vertebral fracture present and sent home in a cervical orthosis
- In permanent halo device and placed in a rehabilitation facility

ONGOING CARE

FOLLOW-UP RECOMMENDATIONS
Follow-up required if discharged with a collar

Patient Monitoring
If spinal cord injury, high cervical fracture, respiratory failure, or hemodynamic instability, critical care monitoring required

DIET
- NPO until alert and protecting airway
- Early nutrition due to hypermetabolic state related to trauma and injury

PATIENT EDUCATION
- The National Spinal Cord Injury Association: http://www.spinalcord.org 1-800-962-9629
- National Institute of Neurological Disorders and Stroke (NINDS) spinal cord injury information page: http://www.ninds.nih.gov/disorders/sci/sci.htm

PROGNOSIS
Function after 1 year postinjury indicates long-term function.

COMPLICATIONS
- Common complications of cervical trauma:
  - Chronic musculoskeletal pain
  - Herniated discs
  - Chronic radiculopathy
- Common complications of spinal cord injury:
  - Pneumonia
  - Deep vein thrombosis
  - Pulmonary embolus
  - Pressure ulcers
  - Wound infections
  - UTIs
  - Chronic pain
  - Depression
  - Renal failure
- Death in cord injury patients usually related to pneumonia, pulmonary embolus, or sepsis

REFERENCES

1. O'Dowd JK, et al. Basic principles of management for cervical spine trauma. *Eur Spine J*. 2010; 19 Suppl 1:S18–22.
2. Stiell IG, Wells GA, Vandemheen KL, et al. The Canadian C-spine rule for radiography in alert and stable trauma patients. *JAMA*. 2001;286:1841–8.
3. Hoffman JR, Mower WR, Wolfson AB, et al. Validity of a set of clinical criteria to rule out injury to the cervical spine in patients with blunt trauma. National Emergency X-Radiography Utilization Study Group. *N Engl J Med*. 2000;343(2):94–9.
4. Jimenez RR, DeGuzman MA, Shiran S, et al. CT versus plain radiographs for evaluation of c-spine injury in young children: Do benefits outweigh risks? *Pediatr Radiol*. 2008;38:635–44.
5. Muchow RD, Resnick DK, Abdel MP. Magnetic resonance imaging (MRI) in the clearance of the cervical spine in blunt trauma: A meta-analysis. *J Trauma*. 2008;64(1):179–89.
6. Bracken MB. Steroids for acute spinal cord injury. *Cochrane Database Syst Rev*. 2002:CD001046.
7. Wuermser L, Ho CH, Chiodo AE, et al. Spinal cord injury medicine: Acute care management of traumatic and nontraumatic injury. *Arch Phys Med Rehabil*. 2007;88(1):S55–S61.

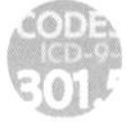

CODES

ICD9
- 806.00 Closed fracture of C1-C4 level with unspecified spinal cord injury
- 952.00 C1-C4 level spinal cord injury, unspecified
- 952.05 C5-C7 level spinal cord injury, unspecified

CLINICAL PEARLS

- Suspect cervical injury in any patient with facial or head trauma, especially if obtunded or intoxicated.
- Follow clear imaging guidelines, such as the Canadian C-spine Rules.
- Leave the collar on until patient has been cleared by appropriate imaging studies and a comprehensive neurologic exam.
- Although controversial, consider early steroids if spinal cord injury suspected.

CERVICAL SPONDYLOSIS

Eric J. Kujawski, DO
Kenneth M. Bielak, MD
Brian K. Linn, MD

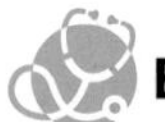

BASICS

DESCRIPTION

Considered the most common progressive disorder of the cervical spine due to the process of noninflammatory degeneration of the facet joints and intervertebral discs and osteophyte formation:

- Seen as a natural process of aging; most people remain asymptomatic.
- Symptomatic patients fall into 3 groups: Axial neck pain, cervical radiculopathy, and cervical myelopathy
- System(s) affected: Musculoskeletal; Neurological
- Synonym(s): Cervical arthritis; Cervical myelopathy; Cervical osteophyte; Cervicalgia

Geriatric Considerations

- Patients <55 usually present due to a herniated disc.
- Patients >55 usually have osteophyte formation with canal or foraminal stenosis.
- Rule out myelopathy before considering conservative treatment.

Pediatric Considerations

Symptoms are less common, but radiographic changes can be seen as early as skeletal maturity.

EPIDEMIOLOGY

Incidence

Predominant sex: Male > Female (3:2)

Prevalence

- 10% by age 25
- 95% by age 65

RISK FACTORS

- Aging
- Smoking
- Laborers
- Congenital spinal canal narrowing

PATHOPHYSIOLOGY

- Loss of disc height:
  - Desiccation leads the nucleus pulposus to lose elasticity and become smaller and more fibrous.
  - The annulus fibrosus takes on more weight and can bulge into the spinal canal.
  - Loss of height begins ventrally, leading to loss of cervical lordosis and a resulting focal kyphosis.
- Osteophyte formation:
  - Bare edges of the vertebral bodies
  - Uncovertebral joints
  - Facet joints (C5–C7 most common)
- Thickened laminae
- Thickened or ossified posterior longitudinal ligament
- Thickened or buckling ligamentum flavum
- Vertebral artery involvement

COMMONLY ASSOCIATED CONDITIONS

See "Etiology."

DIAGNOSIS

HISTORY

- Gradual chronic onset is more common than acute presentation. Radiculopathy can be acute, subacute, or chronic.
- Generally worse with movement. Common complaint of neck being "stiff."
- Pain in the posterior neck and trapezius muscle associated at times with radiation into the arms.
- Scapular pain
- Arm pain usually on the outer aspect of the arm at least to the elbow (coronary heart pain is almost always on the inner aspect of the arm)
- Radicular pain may be present without neck pain.
- Loss of neck extension
- Lateral flexion is limited while erect, but improves while lying down.
- Tenderness of biceps and pectoralis major in C5–C6 segment disease
- Tenderness of triceps in C6–C7 disease
- Long tract signs and positive Babinski may develop in severe cases with myelopathy.

PHYSICAL EXAM

- Tenderness over the affected segments
- Palpation occasionally reproduces radicular pain.
- Coughing, sneezing, Valsalva, and certain cervical movements can increase radicular pain.
- The "shoulder abduction sign" relieves pain in some patients. The patient holds the arm over their head and rests the wrist or forearm on top of the head.

DIAGNOSTIC TESTS & INTERPRETATION

Lab

Initial lab tests

Only if diagnosis is in question:

- ESR
- Rheumatoid factor
- CBC with differential

Imaging

Initial approach

X-rays of cervical spine, anteroposterior (AP), lateral, open-mouth odontoid, and obliques. Osteophytes and/or joint space narrowing will be evident (1).

Follow-Up & Special Considerations

- CT or MRI scans are valuable in cases where surgery is contemplated or the diagnosis is in doubt.
- Degenerative changes and disc herniations are commonly seen in asymptomatic patients, so correlation with neurologic exam is needed.
- MRI better depicts cord changes, enlargement, compression, or atrophy.
- CT shows bony changes better, especially foraminal stenosis (2)[B].
- CT myelography in place of MRI in patients with metal hardware or pacemaker (3)[C]

Diagnostic Procedures/Surgery

Electromyogram (EMG) and nerve conduction studies may be needed to rule out other neurologic causes. These studies are usually not needed in most patients with well-defined radiculopathy and correlating radiology findings.

DIFFERENTIAL DIAGNOSIS

- Cervical strain
- Rheumatoid arthritis
- Polymyalgia rheumatica
- Bone metastases
- Thoracic outlet syndrome
- With radiculopathy or myelopathy symptoms:
  - Multiple sclerosis
  - Syringomyelia
  - Tumor
  - Epidural abscess
  - Amyotrophic lateral sclerosis
  - Cervical herniated disc
  - Herpes zoster
  - Lyme radiculopathy
  - Diabetic polyradiculopathy

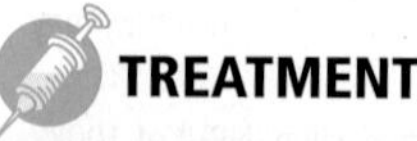

TREATMENT

MEDICATION

First Line

- NSAIDs (ibuprofen 800 mg t.i.d. 7–14 days or naproxen 500 b.i.d. 7–14 days) (4)[C]:
  - Contraindications: GI bleeding or ulcer
  - Precautions in patients with renal disease, hepatic disease, or coagulation disorders
- Acetaminophen 650 mg/dose 5 × per 24 hours or maximum of 3,250 mg/d
- Muscle relaxants (up to 2 weeks) (4)[C]
- Topical pain relief cream (ketoprofen 20%, cyclobenzaprine 2%, lidocaine 10%; apply sparingly 2–3 × daily)
- Lidocaine or diclofenac patches
- Anticonvulsants for radiculopathy (gabapentin, pregabalin, tiagabine, or oxcarbazepine) (4)[C]

Second Line

- Short course of oral corticosteroids may benefit patients with acute radicular pain
- Facet joint steroid injections (3)[B]
- Opioids in patients who do not improve with other conservative treatments and are not surgical candidates

ADDITIONAL TREATMENT

General Measures

- Avoidance of any provocative activities
- Physical therapy with exercise and gradual mobilization (5)[C]
- Return to normal activities as soon as possible.
- Conservative treatment for patients with only axial pain:
  - Oral analgesics (NSAIDS)
  - A short course of oral corticosteroids
  - Referral to physical therapy
  - Use of a cervical pillow
  - Soft cervical collar (up to 2 weeks)
  - Isometric exercises
- Patients with radicular pain with only paresthesia or numbness and no specific weakness:
  - Conservative treatment for 6–12 weeks
  - Facet joint injections if continued symptoms after conservative treatment
  - Epidural steroid injections (4)[C]
- Patients with myelopathy:
  - Surgical decompression is indicated (6)[B].

Issues for Referral

Immediate referral to an orthopedic surgeon for symptoms of myelopathy (gait disturbances, frequent falls, bowel or bladder dysfunction, loss of dexterity, Babinski sign, clonus, hyperreflexia)

Additional Therapies

- Cervical traction unit: 8–12 lbs at 24° angle of flexion for 15–20-minute intervals (3)[C]
- Avoid high-velocity manual manipulative therapy.

SURGERY/OTHER PROCEDURES

- Surgical decompression for myelopathy can be beneficial in early cases (5,6)[B].
- Cervical arthroplasty (artificial disks) are being used in some studies, but there are no long-term randomized trials yet that may differentiate improved outcomes of arthroplasty versus arthrodesis as currently practiced. The incidence of adjacent segment disease must decrease in order for cervical arthroplasty to become the standard of care (7)[C].
- One preliminary study of 269 patients followed for 2 years finds that cervical total disc replacement allows for neural decompression and clinical results comparable to anterior cervical discectomy and fusion. The cervical arthroplasty was associated with a significantly greater overall success rate than fusion while maintaining motion at the index level. Furthermore, there were significantly fewer patients showing severe adjacent-level radiographic changes at the 2-year follow-up (8)[C].

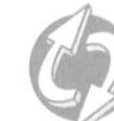

ONGOING CARE

FOLLOW-UP RECOMMENDATIONS

Referral indicated for continued severe pain with conservative treatment, significant or progression of neurologic deficits, or any sign/symptoms of myelopathy

Patient Monitoring

Follow-up visit in 3–4 weeks for evaluation of neurologic status. If no change, follow at intervals of 3–6 months, depending on severity of symptoms.

PATIENT EDUCATION

Patients should immediately report any weakness, eye symptoms, bladder or bowel incontinence, gait disturbance, loss of dexterity, or fine motor control.

PROGNOSIS

75% of patients have complete or significant relief of symptoms with nonoperative approach (4)[B].

REFERENCES

1. Pateder DB, Berg JH, Thal R, et al. Neck and shoulder pain: differentiating cervical spine pathology from shoulder pathology. *J Surg Orthop Adv*. 2009;18:170–4.
2. Binder AI. Cervical spondylosis and neck pain. *BMJ*. 2007;334:527–31.
3. Eubanks JD. Cervical radiculopathy: Nonoperative management of neck pain and radicular symptoms. *Am Fam Physician*. 2010;81(1):33–40.
4. Mazanec D, Reddy A. Medical management of cervical spondylosis. *Neurosurgery*. 2007;60: S43–50.
5. Rao RD, Currier BL, Albert TJ, et al. Degenerative cervical spondylosis: Clinical syndromes, pathogenesis, and management. *J Bone Joint Surg Am*. 2007;89:1360–78.
6. Hsu W, Dorsi MJ, Witham TF, et al. Surgical management of cervical spondylotic myelopathy. *Neurosurg Q*. 2009;19:302–7.
7. Richards O, Choi D, Timothy J, et al. Cervical arthroplasty: The beginning, the middle, the end? *British journal of neurosurgery*. 2011.
8. Coric D, Nunley PD, Guyer RD, et al. Prospective, randomized, multicenter study of cervical arthroplasty: 269 patients from the Kineflex|C artificial disc investigational device exemption study with a minimum 2-year follow-up. *J Neurosurg Spine*. 2011.

ADDITIONAL READING

- Robinson J, Kothari M. Treatment of cervical radiculopathy. Retrieved July 6, 2008, from http://www.utdol.com.
- Röllinghoff M, Zarghooni K, Groos D, et al. Multilevel spinal fusion in the aged: Not a panacea. *Acta Orthop Belg*. 2011;77:97–102.
- Shedid D, Benzel EC. Cervical spondylosis anatomy: Pathophysiology and biomechanics. *Neurosurgery*. 2007;60(1 Suppl 1):S7–13.
- Woiciechowsky C, et al. Degenerative spondylolisthesis of the cervical spine. *Eur Spine J*. 2004;13:680–4.
- Young WF. Cervical spondylotic myelopathy: A common cause of spinal cord dysfunction in older persons. *Am Fam Physician*. 2000;62:1064–70, 1073.

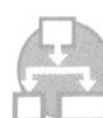

See Also (Topic, Algorithm, Electronic Media Element)

See videos: Neck Stretch with a Towel; Neck Extension in Prone; Neck Stretches - Chin Tucks; Neck Trigger Point Massage - Trapezius

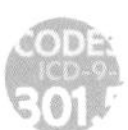

CODES

ICD9

- 721.0 Cervical spondylosis without myelopathy
- 721.1 Cervical spondylosis with myelopathy

CLINICAL PEARLS

- Spondylosis is a noninflammatory degeneration of the facet joints and intervertebral discs.
- Considered a natural process of aging, most people remain asymptomatic. Symptomatic patients fall into 3 groups: Axial neck pain, cervical radiculopathy, and cervical myelopathy.
- Patients <55 usually present due to herniated disc, whereas patients >55 usually present due to radicular symptoms related to osteophyte formation or foraminal stenosis.
- Diagnosis via x-rays of cervical spine, AP, lateral, open-mouth odontoid, and obliques
- Referral indicated for continued severe pain with conservative treatment, significant or progression of neurologic deficits, or any sign/symptoms of myelopathy
- 75% of patients have complete or significant relief of symptoms with nonoperative approach.
- Not to be confused with spondylolysis, which is a stress fracture of the pars interarticularis most common at L5. Bilateral spondylolysis with anterior slippage of vertebral segment is spondylolisthesis.

C

CERVICITIS, ECTROPION, AND TRUE EROSION

Marie Ellen Caggiano, MD, MPH

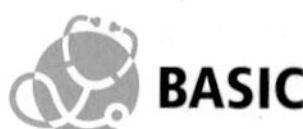

BASICS

DESCRIPTION

Cervicitis refers to any inflammatory changes of the cervix:

- Ectropion: Presence of cervical columnar cells on the vaginal portion of the cervix (portio); often seen during adolescence and during pregnancy
- True erosion: Loss of overlying cervical epithelium due to trauma (e.g., forceful insertion of vaginal speculum in patient with atrophic mucosa)
- System(s) affected: Reproductive

Geriatric Considerations

- Chronic cervicitis in postmenopausal women may be related to lack of estrogen.
- The possibility of infectious cervicitis should not be overlooked in geriatric patients, because many remain sexually active.

Pregnancy Considerations

Screen all pregnant women for infectious cervicitis because of risk of pregnancy complications and potential for transmission to the fetus.

Pediatric Considerations

Infectious cervicitis in children should lead to an investigation for possible sexual abuse.

EPIDEMIOLOGY

Incidence

- Cervicitis: Cervicitis-specific data are not available:
  - Chlamydia incidence: 1,244,180 cases were reported to the Centers for Disease Control (CDC) in 2009, although it is estimated that as many as 4 million new cases of chlamydia occur in the US annually. The total number of reported cases has been rising.
  - Gonorrhea: Next to chlamydia, gonorrhea is the second-most common reported notifiable disease in the US, with 301,174 cases reported to the CDC in 2009. The number of reported cases has decreased in recent years, although higher rates persist among certain populations.
  - Trichomoniasis: Case reporting data are not available. National Health and Nutrition Examination Survey (NHANES) data estimate an overall prevalence in the US of 3.1% (1).
- Ectropion: Common with oral contraceptive use; very common in pregnant women
- True erosion: Occasionally seen in postmenopausal women
- Predominant age: 15–19 years
- Predominant sex: Women, especially sexually active women

RISK FACTORS

- Cervicitis:
  - Multiple sexual partners
  - Adolescence and young adulthood
  - Unprotected sex
  - History of sexually transmitted disease (STD)
  - Smoking
  - Other reproductive tract infections: Vaginitis, pelvic inflammatory disease (PID)
  - Foreign objects: Pessary, diaphragm, cervical cap, etc.
- Ectropion: Adolescence, pregnancy
- True erosion: Estrogen deficiency, trauma

GENERAL PREVENTION

- Sexually transmitted infection (gonorrhea, chlamydia, trichomoniasis):
  - Follow CDC-recommended screening measures: The US Preventive Services Task Force recommends screening for chlamydial infection in all sexually active nonpregnant young women $\leq$24 years and for older nonpregnant women who are at increased risk, but no routine screening for women >24 years not at increased risk (2)[C].
  - Treat sexual partners of infected women.
  - Advise use of condom during coitus.
- Estrogen deficiency: Estrogen replacement therapy

ETIOLOGY

- Often, no specific etiology is identified.
- Cervicitis: *C. trachomatis*, *N. gonorrhoeae*, *T. vaginalis*, herpes simplex virus (HSV; especially primary infections of HSV-2), mycoplasmas (e.g., *M. genitalium*), *Ureaplasma*, cytomegalovirus
- Nonsexually transmitted infectious cervicitis can be caused by overgrowth of β-hemolytic streptococcus or *E. coli*.
- Noninfectious causes include chemical irritation (e.g., from douching or latex exposure) and local trauma from vaginal foreign bodies such as diaphragms or cervical caps.
- Ectropion:
  - Hormonal changes with oral contraceptive use (especially with progesterone) or pregnancy
  - Resulting from cervical laceration during childbirth
- True erosion: Injury to atrophic epithelium:
  - Estrogen-deficient states such as menopause

DIAGNOSIS

HISTORY

- Patient may be asymptomatic.
- Vaginal discharge
- Dyspareunia
- Bleeding/spotting following intercourse

PHYSICAL EXAM

- Cervicitis: Purulent vaginal discharge, cervical friability, erythema, ulceration (HSV); punctate hemorrhage causes "strawberry" cervix appearance in trichomoniasis.
- Ectropion: Cervix appears red due to the color of the columnar epithelium.
- True erosion: Vaginal bleeding, sharply defined ulcers of cervix
- Cervical motion tenderness may be appreciated on bimanual pelvic exam (suggests PID).

DIAGNOSTIC TESTS & INTERPRETATION

Lab

- Saline and KOH preparation of cervical and vaginal smears may show leukorrhea (endocervical sample with >10 WBC/hpf suggests cervicitis)
- Nucleic acid amplification tests: More sensitive and also may be used on urine, self-obtained vaginal swabs, and endocervical specimens (3)[A]. (Sensitivity and specificity between 95% and 99% for both gonorrhea and chlamydia.)
- Vaginal wet mount for *T. vaginalis*:
  - Sensitivity for microscopy is low (~50%).
  - Culture, antigen assays, and nucleic acid amplification tests are available and have higher sensitivity for the detection of trichomoniasis. These should be considered in cases where microscopy is unavailable or inconclusive.
- If ulcerations are present, culture for HSV.
- Pap smear of cervix

Diagnostic Procedures/Surgery

Colposcopy may be helpful in cases of chronic inflammation with a biopsy of suspicious areas.

Pathological Findings

- Cervicitis: Acute and chronic inflammatory changes, presence of infective organisms
- Ectropion: None/squamous metaplasia
- True erosion: Sharply defined ulcer borders, loss of epithelium

DIFFERENTIAL DIAGNOSIS

- Cervical dysplasia
- Carcinoma of the cervix
- Bacterial vaginosis (discharge is noninflammatory)

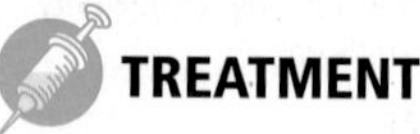

TREATMENT

MEDICATION

First Line

- If infectious cervicitis suspected, treat without awaiting culture results: Ceftriaxone (Rocephin) 125 mg single dose IM, followed by either doxycycline (Vibramycin) 100 mg PO b.i.d. × 7 days or azithromycin (Zithromax) 1 g single dose (4)[A]. Option of ceftriaxone and azithromycin removes patient-compliance factor because they are 1-time doses.
- Trichomoniasis: Metronidazole 2 g once or 500 mg b.i.d. × 7 days or 1 g b.i.d. × 2 doses
- Known or suspected chlamydial infection: For nonpregnant women, azithromycin 1 g PO once or doxycycline 100 mg b.i.d. PO × 7 days; for pregnant women, azithromycin 1 g once or erythromycin base 500 mg q.i.d. PO × 7 days or erythromycin ethylsuccinate 800 mg q.i.d. × 7 days
- Ectropion: None, unless patient is extremely symptomatic with copious discharge. In that case, acid-buffered vaginal jelly can be used to decrease discharge. Cautery can be used, but generally is considered overly invasive.
- True erosion: Conjugated estrogen cream applied vaginally daily for 1–2 weeks, followed by maintenance dosing twice weekly or oral hormone replacement therapy (HRT)

- Contraindications:
  - Metronidazole: Older references state that metronidazole is relatively contraindicated during first trimester of pregnancy. More recent meta-analyses suggest absence of teratogenicity. Treatment of trichomoniasis may be deferred until second trimester if clinician remains concerned by product labeling.
  - Doxycycline: Pregnancy or lactation
  - Estrogen: See extended list of contraindications to estrogen use in standard texts.
- Precautions:
  - Metronidazole: See above; disulfiram reaction with ethanol ingestion
  - Doxycycline: Possible fetal harm if used during pregnancy; staining of the infant's teeth if used during breastfeeding; allergy; photosensitization
  - Erythromycin: Nausea or vomiting
  - Estrogens: History of estrogen-dependent neoplasms; history of thromboembolic diseases. See extended list of contraindications to estrogen therapy in standard texts.
- Significant possible interactions:
  - Metronidazole: Ethanol
  - Doxycycline: Dairy products, iron preparations, warfarin, and oral contraceptives (advise use of alternative contraceptive method)
  - Erythromycin: Theophylline (elevated theophylline level)
  - Estrogen: N/A

Pregnancy Considerations

Doxycycline should be avoided in pregnancy.

Second Line

- Cefixime 400 mg PO single dose is an acceptable alternative to ceftriaxone.
- Quinolones are no longer recommended for primary management due to the rise of quinolone-resistant *N. gonorrhoea*. The exception to this recommendation occurs only if the patient is penicillin-allergic and the organism is known to be sensitive to quinolones. The lack of availability of spectinomycin in the US creates a problem for patients with gonorrhea and true penicillin allergy. It seems reasonable to treat with a quinolone as below, with follow-up testing to ensure eradication in this case (4):
  - Ofloxacin (Floxin) 400 mg PO single dose
  - Ciprofloxacin (Cipro) 500 mg PO single dose
  - Levofloxacin (Levaquin) 250 mg PO single dose
- Alternative to metronidazole for trichomoniasis: Tinidazole 2 g PO × 1 dose
- Estrogen deficiency: A number of estrogen vaginal preparations are available commercially.

Pregnancy Considerations

Quinolones are also contraindicated in pregnancy.

SURGERY/OTHER PROCEDURES

- Chronic cervicitis with negative cultures that does not respond to empirical medical treatment may be treated with cryosurgery, electrocautery, or loop excision.
- Adverse effects of cautery or cryosurgery can include cervical stenosis, which may affect fertility.

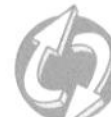

ONGOING CARE

FOLLOW-UP RECOMMENDATIONS

Patient Monitoring

- Test of cure is recommended in pregnant patients to document eradication of infection and should be performed ~4 weeks following treatment.
- Reinfection with gonorrhea and chlamydia is common, and repeat screening should be performed routinely for all patients 3–4 months following treatment.
- Estrogen deficiency: Re-examine in 1 month to confirm healing.

ALERT

Test of cure with nucleic acid amplification tests should not be done <3 weeks after treatment because of false-positive results due to dead organisms.

PATIENT EDUCATION

If the etiology of a patient's cervicitis is confirmed to be an STI, educate patient on the necessity of treating her sexual partners to avoid reinfection.

PROGNOSIS

- Cervicitis: Excellent after infection is eradicated
- Ectropion: Spontaneous regression postpartum and with cessation of use of oral contraceptives
- True erosion: Spontaneous healing

COMPLICATIONS

- Cervicitis due to *C. trachomatis* or *N. gonorrhoeae* is associated with an 8–10% risk of developing subsequent PID. Adolescents are a high-risk group for reinfection with sexually transmitted organisms, and screening frequency should be once/twice yearly in this population.
- Among women who are positive for HIV, the presence of cervicitis increases the risk of viral shedding and transmission to sexual partners (4).

REFERENCES

1. Sutton M, Sternberg M, Koumans EH, et al. The prevalence of *Trichomonas vaginalis* infection among reproductive-age women in the United States, 2001–2004. *Clin Infect Dis*. 2007;45: 1319–26.
2. US Preventive Services Task Force. Screening for chlamydial infection: U.S. Preventive Services Task Force recommendation statement. *Ann Intern Med*. 2007;147:128–34.
3. Cook RL, Hutchison SL, Østergaard L, et al. Systematic review: Noninvasive testing for *Chlamydia trachomatis* and *Neisseria gonorrhoeae*. *Ann Intern Med*. 2005;142:914–25.
4. Workowski KA, Berman S, Centers for Disease Control and Prevention (CDC), et al. Sexually transmitted diseases treatment guidelines, 2010. *MMWR Recomm Rep*. 2010;59:1–110.

ADDITIONAL READING

- Gaydos C, Maldeis NE, Hardick A, et al. Mycoplasma genitalium as a contributor to the multiple etiologies of cervicitis in women attending sexually transmitted disease clinics. *Sex Transm Dis*. 2009;36:598–606.
- Gülmezoglu AM, Azhar M, et al. Interventions for trichomoniasis in pregnancy. *Cochrane Database Syst Rev*. 2011;5:CD000220.
- Hosenfeld CB, Workowski KA, Berman S, et al. Repeat infection with Chlamydia and gonorrhea among females: A systematic review of the literature. *Sex Transm Dis*. 2009;36:478–89.
- Johnson LF, Lewis DA. The effect of genital tract infections on HIV-1 shedding in the genital tract: A systematic review and meta-analysis. *Sex Transm Dis*. 2008.
- Taylor-Robinson D, Jensen JS, et al. *Mycoplasma genitalium*: From chrysalis to multicolored butterfly. *Clin Microbiol Rev*. 2011;24:498–514.
- Wilson JF, et al. In the clinic. Vaginitis and cervicitis. *Ann Intern Med*. 2009;151.

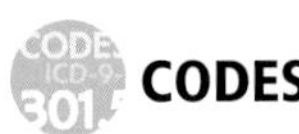

CODES

ICD9

- 616.0 Cervicitis and endocervicitis
- 622.0 Erosion and ectropion of cervix

CLINICAL PEARLS

- If infectious cervicitis is suspected, treatment of choice is ceftriaxone 125 mg IM plus azithromycin 1 g PO × 1 dose. Do not wait for test results.
- Encourage patient to have sexual partner(s) treated.
- Quinolones are no longer recommended to treat gonorrhea.
- Lubricants (e.g., KY Jelly) do not alter Pap smear results, so small quantities may be used when performing Pap smears.
- Positive results for *N. gonorrhoeae* or chlamydia should be reported to local or state health department.

CHANCROID

Jeffery T. Kirchner, DO, FAAFP, AAHIVS

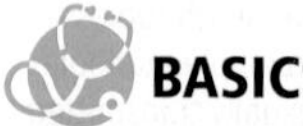

BASICS

DESCRIPTION

An STD characterized by painful genital ulcerations and inflammatory inguinal adenopathy. Although uncommon in the US, it is found worldwide. Chancroid is endemic in developing countries, especially sub-Saharan Africa, and is a cofactor for HIV transmission.

EPIDEMIOLOGY

Incidence

- <50 cases reported to Centers for Disease Control (CDC) in 2004–2009
- Actual numbers are considered higher due to lack of testing and thus underreporting.

Prevalence

- Endemic in developing countries, annual estimated global prevalence of 4–6 million, but actual prevalence is unknown due to lack of testing
- Thought to be extremely common in sub-Saharan Africa, southeast Asia, Latin America

RISK FACTORS

- Multiple sexual partners
- Uncircumcised men
- Prostitutes may be carriers.
- Patients presenting with other genital ulcerative diseases

GENERAL PREVENTION

Condom use should be demonstrated and promoted.

PATHOPHYSIOLOGY

- Involves entry of the bacteria through abraded skin, followed by attachment of the bacteria to susceptible cells
- Cytotoxin is secreted, which may play a role in epithelial injury and ulcer formation.
- Dendritic cells and natural killer cells respond to *H. ducreyi*, and this innate host response determines bacterial clearance versus disease progression.

ETIOLOGY

Haemophilus ducreyi (gram-negative rod) thought to be strictly a human pathogen

COMMONLY ASSOCIATED CONDITIONS

- Syphilis: Concurrent in 10% of patients
- Herpes simplex virus (HSV) or HIV infection

DIAGNOSIS

HISTORY

- Exposure to infected individual, but often not helpful or obtained
- Incubation period typically lasts 4–10 days.

PHYSICAL EXAM

- Tender erythematous genital papule that progresses into a pustule that erodes into an ulcer:
  - Infected persons commonly have >1 ulcer.
- Typical ulcer is 1–2 cm, but size is variable.
- Ulcers are painful, with erythematous base and ragged edges, which are sometimes undermined:
  - Common sites for ulcers in men include the penile shaft, glans, and meatus.
  - Common sites for ulcers in women include labia, introitus, and perianal areas.
- Inguinal lymphadenitis with abscess (bubo) formation occurs in ~50% of men but less common in women.
- Buboes arise 1–2 weeks after ulceration, are typically painful
- Buboes may spontaneously rupture if the primary disease is untreated.
- Atypical presentations include folliculitis and foreskin abscess.

DIAGNOSTIC TESTS & INTERPRETATION

Lab

CDC criteria for presumptive diagnosis:

- Definite: Isolation of *H. ducreyi* from a lesion
- Probable: Clinical findings including genital ulcer and regional adenopathy *plus* negative darkfield exam, negative serologic test for syphilis, negative cultures for HSV, or a clinical presentation not typical for HSV.

Initial lab tests

- "School of fish" pattern on Gram stain with organisms clumped in long parallel strands
- Serologic testing for antibody to *H. ducreyi* with ELISA (although may not be diagnostic of acute infection)
- Culture of the organism on Mueller-Hinton agar with incorporated vancomycin but sensitivity is <80%
- Multiplex polymerase chain reaction (PCR) has sensitivity of 95–98%, but no Food and Drug Administration–approved tests in the US; available from some commercial labs

Follow-Up & Special Considerations

All patients should also concurrently be tested for syphilis and HSV.

Diagnostic Procedures/Surgery

Gram stain and culture of exudate (1):

- Aspiration of inguinal bubo (lymph node)
- PCR testing of ulcer exudate for *H. ducreyi* DNA
- Darkfield examination of exudate to rule out *Treponema pallidum* infection
- Culture or PCR testing for HSV

DIFFERENTIAL DIAGNOSIS

- Syphilis (*Treponema pallidum*)
- Genital herpes (HSV-1 and -2)
- Lymphogranuloma venereum (*Chlamydia trachomatis*)
- Granuloma inguinale (donovanosis)
- Drug eruption; Behçet disease

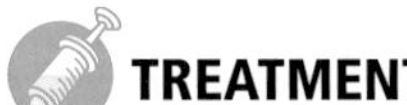

TREATMENT

MEDICATION

First Line

- Azithromycin: 1 g PO single dose (2,3)[A], OR
- Ceftriaxone 250 mg IM single dose

Second Line

- Ciprofloxacin 500 mg PO b.i.d. for 3 days (2,3,4)[A]
- Erythromycin base 500 mg t.i.d. for 7 days (2,3,4)[A]
- Contraindications:
  - Allergy to the medication
  - Ciprofloxacin during pregnancy and lactation and in patients <18 years

ADDITIONAL TREATMENT

General Measures

- Outpatient treatment
- Saline or Burrow's solution to soak ulcers
- Aspiration of buboes if >5 cm; approached through adjacent skin. Also consider incision and drainage for larger lesions.

ALERT

HIV may affect treatment response.

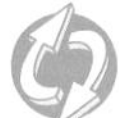

ONGOING CARE

FOLLOW-UP RECOMMENDATIONS

Patient Monitoring

- Avoid sexual activity until ulcers are resolved.
- Clinical improvement usually occurs within 48 hours.
- Patients should be re-examined 3–7 days after initiation of therapy and followed closely until all clinical signs of infection are resolved.
- Baseline syphilis serology and at 3 months
- Baseline HIV testing and at 3 months posttreatment

PATIENT EDUCATION

- Sexual counseling
- Use of condoms
- Local wound care
- Treatment of all sexual partners with same regimen as index
- HIV testing

PROGNOSIS

- Full clinical resolution with appropriate treatment
- Failure to respond may be due to incorrect diagnosis, coinfection with syphilis or HIV, medication nonadherence, or resistant *H. ducreyi*.
- 5% relapse after treatment.

COMPLICATIONS

- Phimosis
- Balanoposthitis
- Rupture of buboes with fistula formation and scarring

REFERENCES

1. Alfa M, et al. The laboratory diagnosis of *Haemophilus ducreyi*. *Can J Infect Dis Med Microbiol*. 2005;16:31–4.
2. Lewis DA. Chancroid: Clinical manifestations, diagnosis, and management. *Sex Transm Inf*. 2003;79:68–71.
3. Kemp M, Christensen JJ, Lautenschlager S, et al. European guideline for the management of chancroid, 2011. *Int J STD AIDS*. 2011;22:241–4.
4. Centers for Disease Control and Prevention. Sexually transmitted diseases treatment guidelines—2010. *MMWR*. 2010;59:19–20.

ADDITIONAL READING

- Centers for Disease Control and Prevention [Summary of notifiable diseases - United States 2009], published May 13, 2011 for *MMWR*. 2009;58(53):85.
- Janowicz DM, Li W, Bauer ME, et al. Host-pathogen interplay of *Haemophilus ducreyi*. *Curr Opin Infect Dis*. 2010;23:64–9.
- Janowicz DM, Ofner S, Katz BP, et al. Experimental infection of human volunteers with Haemophilus ducreyi: Fifteen years of clinical data and experience. *J Infect Dis*. 2009;199:1671–9.

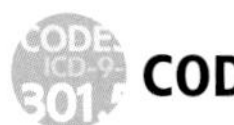

CODES

ICD9

099.0 Chancroid

CLINICAL PEARLS

- Chancroid is a rare disorder in the US but more common elsewhere.
- Characterized by genital papules that progress to pustules that open, producing painful ulcers
- Treatment of choice is azithromycin 1 g once.
- Treat sexual partners (from prior 3 months) even in the absence of signs or symptoms of disease.

CHARCOT JOINT

Patrick W. Joyner, MD, MS
David M. Joyner, MD

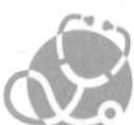

BASICS

In 1703, Dr. William Musgrave first reported swollen, inflamed joints in a paralyzed patient. French neurologist, Jean Martin Charcot, first described rapid joint deterioration in patients with tabes dorsalis in 1868. In 1936, Dr. William Jordan described an association of diabetes mellitus (DM) neuropathic changes in the foot and ankle.

DESCRIPTION

- A progressive destructive arthritis secondary to peripheral neuropathy and loss of pain sensation. The affected joints are subjected to repeated stress that is unrecognized by the patient, therefore causing continuous damage to the underlying bone and cartilage.
- Most often seen in tarsal and tarsometatarsal joints, less in metatarsophalangeal and talotibial joints. May also be seen in knee, hip, spine.
- Upper extremity joints rarely are involved.
- DM is the most common cause in the US.
- 3 stages are identified:
  - Fragmentation/destruction
  - Coalescence
  - Consolidation/resolution
- Patients suspected of having a Charcot neuropathy should be referred to an orthopedic foot and ankle surgeon or podiatrist for follow-up and treatment.
- System(s) affected: Musculoskeletal; Endocrine; Neurological
- Synonym(s): Neuropathic joint disease; neuropathic arthropathy

EPIDEMIOLOGY

- Primarily seen in the fifth and sixth decades
- Male = Female
- Bilateral involvement in 9–35% of cases
- 80% have had diabetes for at least 10 years

Incidence

3–11.7/1,000 patients per year

Prevalence

- 0.1% in all patients, up to 13% in high-risk diabetes foot clinics
- 0.8–8% in patients with DM
- 5–10% of patients with peripheral neuropathy

RISK FACTORS

- >15-year history of diabetes
- Poor blood sugar control: DM is the most common cause in the US.
- Poor foot hygiene; ill-fitting shoes, socks
- Globally, other medical conditions, such as syphilis and leprosy, are also risk factors.

Genetics

Family history of DM

GENERAL PREVENTION

- Excellent control of blood sugar in type I diabetes; not clearly established for type II
- Good diabetic foot care, with frequent exams of feet for signs of pressure sores or ulcerations and good foot hygiene
- Well-fitting footwear with adequate support

PATHOPHYSIOLOGY

Exact cause unknown, 3 major theories:

- Autonomic neuropathy: Autonomic neuropathy leads to local increase in blood flow, which leads to osteopenia secondary to increased osteoclastic activity, and increased bone resorption.
- Neurotraumatic: Repetitive microtrauma not sensed by the patient leads to osseous destruction and progressive damage to ligaments, articular surfaces, and may lead to fractures and subluxation. This is in part secondary to loss of protective sensation as a result of peripheral neuropathy.
- Neurovascular: Underlying medical disorder creates hypervascularity; this in conjunction with increased osteoclastic resorption and osteoporosis. Both mechanisms in the setting of microfractures and subchondral collapse will lead to joint destruction.

ETIOLOGY

Many causes of peripheral neuropathy:

- DM
- Multiple sclerosis
- Raynaud disease
- Any connective tissue disease (i.e., scleroderma, rheumatoid arthritis)
- Syphilis/tabes dorsalis
- Syringomyelia, upper extremity disease
- Meningomyelocele
- Frequent intra-articular steroid injections
- Alcoholism
- Pernicious anemia
- Charcot-Marie-Tooth disease
- Leprosy (Hansen disease)
- Renal dialysis
- Amyloidosis

DIAGNOSIS

- Findings frequently confused with cellulitis
- Symptoms usually unilateral
- Significant swelling:
  - Early: Large effusion
  - Late: Swelling usually resolved
- Local increased warmth: 2–7°C higher than unaffected extremity
- Skin erythema: Classically will resolve with elevation; helps to differentiate from infection (erythema from infection would not be affected by elevation)
- Loss of distal sensation; decreased pain and proprioception in affected limb
- Skin intact
- Laxity/instability of joint: May lead to calluses and/or ulcerations

HISTORY

- Long-standing diabetes
- May recall predisposing trauma, such as ankle twist/sprain, object dropped on foot
- May present with pain; however, proportionally less pain than expected by appearance
- Limited motion
- Can affect any number of joints. Charcot joint has been reported in the following anatomic locations: spine, shoulder, elbow, wrist, hand, hip, knee, ankle, and foot.

PHYSICAL EXAM

- Localized warmth, swelling, erythema
- Brodsky test: Elevating the foot should resolve swelling.
- Neurological exam:
  - Findings normally symmetric, sensory, and distal.
  - Absent sensation on 4/10 sites using 5.07 g monofilament
  - Decreased or absent reflexes
  - Loss of pain, proprioception, and vibratory sensation
- Foot deformities:
  - Corns/calluses
  - Collapse of arch
  - Collapse of tarsal bones causing rocker-bottom foot
  - Protruding osteophytes
  - Plantar ulcer
- Peripheral circulation often normal

DIAGNOSTIC TESTS & INTERPRETATION

Resolution of erythema with elevation of affected extremity

Lab

Initial lab tests

- Blood sugar, hemoglobin A1c
- White blood cells may be elevated in osteomyelitis.
- ESR: Elevated in osteomyelitis
- Basic metabolic panel: BUN, creatinine to rule out renal disease
- B_{12}/folate, hematocrit, mean corpuscular volume
- Rapid plasma reagin, FTA-ABS to rule out syphilis
- Elevated alkaline phosphatase, calcium, parathyroid hormone, and low phosphate to rule out metabolic bone disease

Imaging

- Radiographs:
  - Initially may be negative, for the first few days and up to 3 weeks. All that may be appreciated initially is soft tissue swelling.
  - Early changes:
    - Slight fracture with joint subluxation
    - Joint effusion
    - Joint space narrowing
    - Sclerosis of subchondral bone
    - Bone fragmentation
  - Late changes:
    - Marked articular destruction
    - Fractures
    - Hypertrophic changes: Periarticular new bone, osteophytes, osseous debris, may look like severe arthritis
    - Bone resorption
    - Subluxation
    - Intra-articular loose bodies
    - Osteolysis
    - Large osteophytes
    - Atrophic changes: Massive bone resorption, joint disintegration, may look like chronic infection
    - In the forefoot, a "pencil and cup" deformity of the metatarsophalangeal joint may be appreciated as well as fragmentation of the metatarsal heads
    - In the midfoot, the Lisfranc joint can dislocate, as well as develop fragmentation of the tarsal-metatarsal joints and loss of the longitudinal arch

- In the hindfoot, talocalcaneal dislocation with collapse of the talus and atypical fragmentation/fractures of the calcaneus can occur
- May be difficult to differentiate radiograph findings from those of osteomyelitis
- MRI: Assists in ruling out osteomyelitis, but can be difficult because joint will most likely have increased signal secondary to edema, especially in the setting of acute Charcot osteoarthropathy
- Bone scan in conjunction with a tagged WBC scan: Assists in ruling out osteomyelitis:
  - Indium^{111} more specific than technetium^{99}
  - Combination of both Indium^{111} and technetium^{99}may improve sensitivity (93–100%) and specificity (almost 80%).

Initial approach

Rule out underlying neurological disorder.

Diagnostic Procedures/Surgery

Arthrocentesis: Fluid for culture and sensitivity if osteomyelitis is suspected. Presence of WBC, calcium pyrophosphate dihydrate (CPPD) crystals. Rule out malignancy of any cause for concern.

DIFFERENTIAL DIAGNOSIS

- Cellulitis, osteomyelitis
- Osteonecrosis
- Advanced osteoarthritis
- Calcium pyrophosphate dihydrate crystal deposition disease
- Acute gout
- Neoplasm
- Trauma or acute injury (i.e., sprain)
- Deep vein thrombosis

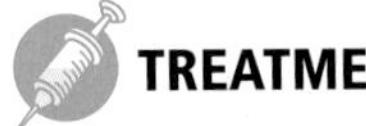

TREATMENT

- Early recognition of diabetic foot pathology
- No weight-bearing on affected extremity
- Total contact cast (gold standard), for 2–4 months until the fragmentation stage is complete and normal skin temperature is observed
- Reconstruction of foot to help prevent ulceration if conservative management fails. However, cannot be performed until erythema has resolved (i.e., late phase)
- If reconstruction fails or ulceration/osteomyelitis does not resolve, amputation is often the treatment of choice. It is estimated that 2.7% of Charcot deformities annually lead to amputation.

MEDICATION

Because pathophysiology is thought to involve increased osteoclastic activity, bisphosphonates have been used to halt progression of disease: Pamidronate, alendronate shown to give clinical improvement (1)[B].

ADDITIONAL TREATMENT

General Measures

- Goal of treatment is to restore joint stability and limit progression of disease.
- After casting, various braces are used to protect affected extremity: Ankle-foot orthotic, rocker-bottom shoes, Charcot restraint orthotic walker, prefabricated pneumatic walking brace, custom prescription footwear
- Good blood sugar control might help limit progression of peripheral neuropathy.

Additional Therapies

Protective treatment with bracing, orthotics. Radiotherapy does not appear to benefit healing of acute Charcot feet in people with diabetes (2)[B].

SURGERY/OTHER PROCEDURES

- Surgical treatment is reserved for severe cases and/or failure of conservative treatment.
- Surgery is indicated when a risk of skin ulceration, unstable fracture, or dislocation is present, or failure of medical therapy.
- Procedures performed vary, depending on joints involved and surgeon experience:
  - Exostosectomy of bony projections
  - Open reduction internal fixation
  - Osteotomy
  - Arthrodesis, with or without tendon lengthening
  - Amputation
  - Use of external fixation if poor skin quality or increase risk of postoperative healing complications
- Any surgical treatment should be delayed until after early fragmentation and inflammatory stages.
- Patients treated surgically often have long healing times.

IN-PATIENT CONSIDERATIONS

Initial Stabilization

- Immobilization of joint is initial treatment:
  - Casting:
    - Provides full immobilization. Casts must be checked weekly for correct fit, especially if underlying ulceration of skin.
    - Casts should be changed every 1–2 weeks.
    - Time in cast determined by clinical and radiographic measures.
    - Total-contact cast better disperses pressure. Ensure pressure points are well padded, as these patients frequently have severely limited to no sensation and will likely not be aware of the development of pressure ulcer.
  - Brace/orthotic: Alternative to casting, removable. Patients may be noncompliant, and may not be able to sense a poor-fitting brace.
- Immobilization needed for minimum of 6 months; possibly 1 year or longer
- Also necessary to reduce stress on affected joint by limiting pressure: Non–weight-bearing preferred, partial weight-bearing at minimum

Admission Criteria

Foot ulceration, suspicion of associated osteomyelitis, fractures

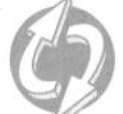

ONGOING CARE

FOLLOW-UP RECOMMENDATIONS

Activity: Non- or partial weight-bearing initially. Regular follow-up with podiatrist to maintain strict foot care

Patient Monitoring

After initial radiographs, repeat films should be obtained in 4–6 weeks.

Geriatric Considerations

Because most cases occur in patients >50, diabetic patients in this age group should be counseled about the symptoms and signs of neuropathic joint disease.

PATIENT EDUCATION

Multidisciplinary team approach

PROGNOSIS

- Patients often are immobilized for several months.
- Usually non–weight-bearing of extremity for an average of 6 months if surgery is required. Total healing may take years to achieve.
- Patients must be vigilant about preventing further injury, receiving regular footcare, examining feet daily, and noting swelling and/or temperature of joints.
- Maintain good diabetic control: Especially critical if patient to undergo surgery. Increased likelihood of nonunion, wound healing complications, and postoperative infection if diabetes not well controlled.

COMPLICATIONS

- Unidentified fractures can lead to debilitating joint deformities and skin ulcerations, increasing risk of infection.
- Collapse and inversion of arch into clubfoot or rocker-bottom foot
- Amputation

REFERENCES

1. Anderson JJ, et al. Bisphosphonates for the treatment of Charcot neuroarthropathy. *J Foot Ankle Surg*. 2004;43(5):285–9.
2. Chantelau E, et al. Palliative radiotherapy for acute osteoarthropathy of diabetic feet: A preliminary study. *Pract Diabetes Int*. 1997;14(6):154–6.

ADDITIONAL READING

- Gouveri E, Papanas N, et al. Charcot osteoarthropathy in diabetes: A brief review with an emphasis on clinical practice. *World J Diabetes*. 2011;2:59–65.
- Jude EB. Medical treatment of Charcot's arthropathy. *J Am Podiatric Med Assoc*. 2002;92(7): 381–3.

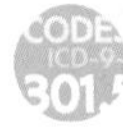

CODES

ICD9

- Neuropathic joint disease (Charcot's joints):
  - 094.0 Tabes dorsalis
  - 250.60 Diabetes mellitus with neurological manifestations, Type II or unspecified type, not stated as uncontrolled
- 713.5 Arthropathy associated with neurological disorders

CLINICAL PEARLS

- The most common presenting symptoms of Charcot joint are significant unilateral swelling, warmth, and erythema, usually in the feet. Patients may or may not recall minor preceding trauma.
- The goal of early prolonged immobilization is to prevent repetitive trauma and progression of arthropathy. Significant complications, such as severe foot deformities, ulcerations leading to infections, and amputation, can result if treatment is delayed.

CHICKENPOX (VARICELLA ZOSTER)

Kay A. Bauman, MD, MPH

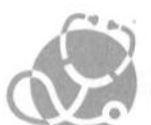

BASICS

DESCRIPTION

- Common, highly contagious generalized exanthem characterized by the development of crops of pruritic vesicles on the skin and mucous membranes
- Fever in up to 70% of persons
- Virus is spread by respiratory (airborne) droplets, direct contact with varicella vesicles, or rarely zoster lesions.
- Virus establishes latency in the dorsal root ganglia; reactivation results in herpes zoster or "shingles."
- Outbreaks tend to occur late winter to early spring in temperate climates.
- The usual incubation period is 14–16 days (range, 10–21). Patients are infectious from ~48 hours before appearance of the rash until the final lesions have crusted. Historically, most people acquire chickenpox during childhood and develop lifelong immunity:
  – *Now it is an immunizable disease.*
- Systems affected: Nervous; Skin/Exocrine
- Synonym: Varicella

EPIDEMIOLOGY

- Predominant age: Peak incidence preschoolers to 9 years, but may occur at any age
- Predominant gender: Male = Female

Incidence

- Decreasing incidence since vaccine available: Estimated at 3.5 million cases annually prior to vaccine introduction with an incidence rate of 8–9% in children 1–9 years of age. Reported US varicella cases 1991: 147,076; reported for 2008: 30,386, reported for 2009: 20,480 cases (1,2).
- Prior to vaccine availability, ~100 deaths in the US/year were reported; for 2009, only 2 deaths were reported (1).
- US rates: 1994, prior to vaccine: 135.76/100,000 persons; 2009: 8.71/100,000 persons (1,2)
- Rates in the US had dropped continuously after vaccine development until mid-2000s when they evened out; 2nd dose of vaccine recommended in 2006, and rates again have declined year by year (1).

RISK FACTORS

- No prior history of varicella infection
- Immunosuppressed patients (especially children with leukemia/lymphoma in remission or receiving high-dose corticosteroids)

Geriatric Considerations

- Infection more severe in adults than in children
- Latent varicella infection may reactivate and cause the exanthem known as shingles or zoster.
- Herpes zoster vaccine, a live attenuated vaccine licensed in 2006, is now recommended for persons ≥60 to prevent zoster (shingles) (3):
  – 1-time dose. Recommended for those previously infected with varicella (chickenpox); those never infected should receive regular varicella vaccine. Dose: 0.65 mL SQ, available as single-dose vial.
  – ACIP recommends routine vaccination of all persons aged >60 years with 1 dose of zoster vaccine. It is not necessary to ask patients about their history of varicella (chickenpox) or to conduct serologic testing for varicella immunity.
  – Most common cause of death: Primary viral pneumonia

Pediatric Considerations

- Neonates born to mothers who develop chickenpox from 5 days before to 2 days after delivery are at risk for serious disease. Must give varicella-zoster immune globulin.
- Varicella bullosa seen mainly in children <2 years. Lesions appear as bullae instead of vesicles. The clinical course does not change.
- Most common cause of death: Septic complications and encephalitis
- Avoid aspirin/acetylsalicylic acid in children because of link to Reye syndrome.

Pregnancy Considerations

- Risk of transplacental infection after maternal infection is 25%.
- Congenital malformations are seen in 2% of patients when the fetus is infected during the first or second trimesters, characterized by limb atrophy and scarring of the skin of the extremities and occasional CNS and eye manifestations.
- Morbidity is increased in women infected during pregnancy (e.g., pneumonia).

GENERAL PREVENTION

- Exposed, susceptible people should be considered at risk and potentially infectious for 21 days.
- Isolate hospitalized patients.
- Passive immunization with IM varicella-zoster immune globulin given within 96 hours (preferably within 72 hours) of exposure to ensure efficacy:
  – Recommended for people exposed to chickenpox or shingles within 96 hours who are immunocompromised, ≥15 years old without prior history of chickenpox, newborns of mothers with onset of chickenpox <5 days before delivery or <2 days after delivery. Exposure criteria: Continued household contact, prolonged face-to-face contact (same room), or indoor playmate >1 hour.
- Active immunization after exposure: Shown to prevent or reduce significantly the severity of varicella if given within 72 hours postexposure
- Active immunization: Varicella virus vaccine (Varivax): Live attenuated vaccine approved by FDA in 1995 for pediatrics immunization and recommended by Advisory Committee on Immunization Practices for immunization of healthy patients ≥12 months who have not had chickenpox:
  – 12 months–12 years old: Initial dose 0.5 mL SC at age 12–15 months; second dose age 4–6 years. Prelicensure studies showed efficacy rates: 70–90% against any disease and 95% against severe disease 7–10 years after vaccination. Other studies showed 100% efficacy at 1 year and 98% at 2 years after vaccination. More recent studies show rates of 85–94% effectiveness, the higher end for the prevention of severe disease. The 2-dose regimen is even more effective, with rates of 96–98% effectiveness. Breakthrough disease generally has <50 lesions, shorter duration of illness, and lower incidence of fever (4)[A].
  – ≥13 years: Two 0.5 mL SC doses 4–8 weeks apart, seroconversion rates 78–82% after 1 dose, 99% after 2 doses. Adults have efficacy rates in the lower end of this range.
  – Estimated 2-dose vaccine coverage in US for 2009 in children ages 19–35 months: 89.6%
  – Vaccine side effects are pain and redness at vaccine site.
  – Vaccine contraindications (5):
    ○ Severe allergic reaction (e.g., anaphylaxis) to a previous dose or vaccine component
    ○ Severe immunodeficiency (ex. severely immunocompromised HIV patients, on chemotherapy, congenital immunodeficiency, or long-term immunosuppressive therapy)
    ○ Pregnancy
- The newly approved MMRV vaccine, which combines the measles, mumps, and rubella vaccine with varicella, is equally effective. There are rare reports of an increased risk of febrile seizures 5–12 days after vaccination in 1 per 2,300–2,600 patients (6)[A].
- May be considered for a subset of HIV-positive children in CDC class I with CD4 >25%:
  – Vaccine recipients should avoid contact with immunocompromised people and pregnant women who have never had chickenpox and their newborns, for up to 6 weeks after vaccination.
  – Children needing catch-up vaccination need at least 3 months between doses 1 and 2.

PATHOPHYSIOLOGY

- Skin lesions identical histologically to those of herpes simplex virus.
- In fatal cases, intranuclear inclusions can be found in the endothelium of blood vessels and most organs.

ETIOLOGY

- Varicella-zoster virus is a member of the α-Herpesviridae subfamily; a double-stranded DNA virus.
- Reservoir is humans

DIAGNOSIS

HISTORY

- Prodromal symptoms: Fever, malaise, anorexia, mild headache
- Malaise, muscle aches, arthralgias, and headache more common in adults
- Subclinical in ~4% of cases

PHYSICAL EXAM

- Characteristic rash: Crops of "teardrop" vesicles on erythematous bases
- Lesions erupt in successive crops.
- Progress from macule to papule to vesicle, then begin to crust
- Pruritic rash is present in various stages of development.
- Lesions may be present on mucous membranes, both oral and vaginal.

DIAGNOSTIC TESTS & INTERPRETATION

Generally used for complicated cases and epidemiologic studies

Lab

Initial lab tests

- Leukocyte count may be normal, low, or mildly increased.
- Marked leukocytosis suggests secondary infection.
- Multinucleated giant cells visible on Tzanck smear from scrapings of vesicles
- Isolated virus from human tissue culture

Follow-Up & Special Considerations

- Visualization of the virus by electron microscopy, tissue culture (costly), and various methods of acute and convalescent sera collection: Latex agglutination (most available), enzyme immunoassay, indirect immunofluorescence antibody, fluorescent antibody to membrane assay, or PCR assay, which can detect wild from vaccine viral strains
- Vaccine-modified cases can be more difficult to diagnose; consider PCR testing of skin lesions (7)[B].

DIFFERENTIAL DIAGNOSIS

- Herpes simplex virus infection
- Herpes zoster
- Impetigo
- Coxsackievirus infection
- Scabies
- Dermatitis herpetiformis
- Drug rash
- Rickettsial pox infection

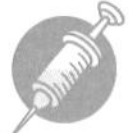

TREATMENT

Outpatient except for complicating emergencies

MEDICATION

First Line

- Supportive: Antipyretics for fever; avoid aspirin in children
- Local and/or systemic antipruritic agents for itching
- In immunocompromised patients: Varicella-zoster immunoglobulin available for passive immunization. Varicella-zoster immunoglobulin must be given within 96 hours after exposure to be beneficial. After fourth day postexposure, wait for rash to develop, then give acyclovir 500 mg/m^2/d q8h for 7 days.
- Acyclovir: Decreases duration of fever and shortens time of viral shedding. Recommended for adolescents, adults, and high-risk patients. Most beneficial if initiated early in the disease ($\leq$24 hours):
  - 2–16-year-old patients: 20 mg/kg/dose (max. 800 mg/dose), q.i.d. for 5 days
  - Adults: 800 mg, 5 times daily
- Contraindications:
  - Hypersensitivity to the drug
- Precautions:
  - Possible renal insufficiency with acyclovir
  - Significant possible interactions
  - Concurrent administration of probenecid increases half-life; increased effects with zidovudine (e.g., drowsiness, lethargy)

Second Line

- Famciclovir: 500 mg t.i.d. for 7–10 days (adults)
- Valacyclovir: 1 g t.i.d. for 7–10 days (adults)

ADDITIONAL TREATMENT

General Measures

- Supportive/symptomatic treatment
- Antihistamines and/or Aveeno or oatmeal baths as needed for itch
- Acetaminophen and/or ibuprofen as needed
- Nail clipping in children to prevent scarring or secondary infection from itching

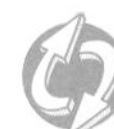

ONGOING CARE

FOLLOW-UP RECOMMENDATIONS

Patient Monitoring

- Usually none needed in mild cases. If complications occur, intensive supportive care may be required.
- Activity as tolerated. Children may return to school when lesions have scabbed.

DIET

No special diet

PATIENT EDUCATION

- In the healthy child, chickenpox is rarely serious and recovery is complete.
- Confers lifelong immunity
- Second attack rare, but subclinical infection can occur; happens occasionally after vaccination in children
- Infection latent and may recur years later as herpes zoster in adults (and sometimes in children)
- Fatalities rarely occur from complications.

COMPLICATIONS

- Although only 2% of cases are reported after second decade, 35% of deaths occur in this age group.
- Secondary bacterial infection: Cellulitis, abscess, erysipelas, sepsis, septic arthritis/osteomyelitis, or staphylococcal pyomyositis
- Pneumonia: 20–30% of adults with chickenpox have lung involvement; 1/400 are hospitalized.
- Encephalitis (the most common CNS complication)
- Meningitis
- Reye syndrome
- Purpura
- Thrombocytopenia
- Glomerulonephritis
- Arthritis
- Hepatitis

REFERENCES

1. Centers for Disease Control and Prevention, Summary of notifiable diseases, US, 2009. *MMWR*. 2011;58(53).
2. Centers for Disease Control and Prevention, Summary of notifiable diseases, US, 2008. *MMWR*. 2010;57(54).
3. *The Medical Letter*. 2006;48:73–4.
4. Marin M, Güris D, Chaves SS, et al. Prevention of varicella: Recommendations of the Advisory Committee on Immunization Practices (ACIP). *MMWR Recomm Rep*. 2007;56:1–40.
5. General Recommendations on Immunization. *MMWR*. 2011;60(2).
6. Marin M, Broder KR, Temte JL, et al. Use of combination measles, mumps, rubella, and varicella vaccine: Recommendations of the Advisory Committee on Immunization Practices (ACIP). *MMWR Recomm Rep*. 2010;59:1–12.
7. Leung J, Harpaz R, Baughman AL, et al. Evaluation of laboratory methods for diagnosis of varicella. *Clin Infect Dis*. 2010;51:23–32.

ADDITIONAL READING

- Centers for Disease Control and Prevention (CDC). Varicella-related deaths–United States, January 2003-June 2004. *MMWR*. 2005;54:272–4.
- Centers for Disease Control and Prevention, Summary of Notifiable Diseases, US, 1991. *MMWR*. 1992;40(53).
- Galea SA, Sweet A, Beninger P, et al. The safety profile of varicella vaccine: A 10-year review. *J Infect Dis*. 2008;197(Suppl 2):S165–9.

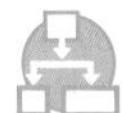

See Also (Topic, Algorithm, Electronic Media Element)

Herpes Zoster

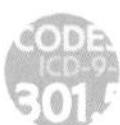

CODES

ICD9

- 052.1 Varicella (hemorrhagic) pneumonitis
- 052.9 Varicella without mention of complication

CLINICAL PEARLS

- Infection is more likely to produce serious illness in adults than in children.
- All people being immunized should receive 2 doses of vaccine, preferably at least 3 months but no fewer than 28 days apart.
- Herpes zoster vaccine (Zostavax) recommended for persons $\geq$60 years of age to prevent shingles (zoster).

C

CHILD ABUSE

Karen A. Hulbert, MD

BASICS

DESCRIPTION

- Types of abuse: Neglect (most common and highest mortality), physical abuse, emotional/psychological abuse, sexual abuse
- Child Welfare Information Gateway (sponsored by US Dept of Health & Human Services): http://www.childwelfare.gov/responding/reporting.cfm
- System(s) affected: Gastrointestinal (GI); Endocrine/Metabolic; Musculoskeletal; Nervous; Renal; Reproductive; Skin/Exocrine; Psychiatric
- Synonym(s): Suspected nonaccidental trauma; Child maltreatment; Child neglect

EPIDEMIOLOGY

Prevalence

- In 2009 more than 3.6 million children in the US were subjects of at least 1 report for alleged child maltreatment (1).
- Cases of abuse and neglect considered together, the US victimization rate in 2009 was 10.1 for every 1,000 children; with those aged <1 year having the highest rate (1).
- Nationally, the number and rate of fatalities have been increasing in the past 5 years (national rate of 2.34 per 100,000 children). 4/5 of fatalities are in children <4 years old and 3/4 are caused by 1 or more parents (1).
- Neglect leads to more child deaths than physical abuse.
- It is estimated that the actual number of victims may be 3× greater than number reported.

RISK FACTORS

- All ages; Male = Female:
  - Risk of physical abuse increases with age
  - Risk of fatal abuse more common <2 years of age
  - Physical abuse 2.1× higher among children with disabilities (2)
- Poverty, drug abuse, lower educational status, parental history of abuse, mentally ill parent/maternal depression, poor support network, and domestic violence:
  - Child abuse may be 4.9 times more likely in family with spouse abuse (2).
  - Children in households with unrelated adults 50 times more likely to die of inflicted injuries (2)
  - Adults who were abused as children are at much higher risk of becoming abusers than those not raised with abuse.

GENERAL PREVENTION

- Know your patients and document their family situations; have increased suspicion to screen for risk factors at prenatal, postnatal, pediatric visit.
- Physicians can educate parents on range of normal behaviors to expect in infants and children:
  - Anticipatory guidance on ways to handle crying infants; methods of discipline for toddlers
- Train first responders—teachers, childcare workers—to look for signs of abuse.
- Early childhood home visitation programs recommended to reduce maltreatment in high-risk families (3)[A]
- More research urgently needed to assess effectiveness of interventions such as parenting programs on ability to reduce abuse and neglect

COMMONLY ASSOCIATED CONDITIONS

- Failure to thrive
- Prematurity
- Developmental deficits
- Poor school performance
- Poor social skills
- Low self-esteem, depression

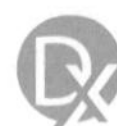

DIAGNOSIS

Documentation:

- Information in the medical record is an important piece of evidence for investigation and litigation (4)[C].
- Critical elements include (4)[C]:
  - Brief statement of child's disclosure or caregiver's explanation, including any alternate explanations offered
  - Time the incident occurred and date/time of disclosure
  - Whether witnesses were present
  - Developmental abilities of child
  - Objective medical findings
  - Interpretation of the findings
- DO NOT use terms such as "rule out," "R/O," and "alleged." They may cause ambiguity; clearly state physician opinion (4)[C].
- Documentation should include disposition of patient and record any report made to child protective services (4)[C].

HISTORY

- Use nonjudgmental, open-ended questions (ask: Who, what, when, and where; NEVER why).
- Use quotes whenever possible.
- Document past medical and developmental history, child's temperament, and interactions among family members.
- Suggestive of intentional trauma:
  - No explanation or vague explanation (2)
  - Important detail of explanation changes dramatically (2)
  - Explanation is inconsistent with pattern, age, or severity (2).
  - Explanation is inconsistent with child's physical or developmental abilities (2).
  - Different witnesses provide markedly different history (2).
  - Considerable delay in seeking treatment
- Nonspecific symptoms of abuse:
  - Behavior changes; self-destructive behavior
  - Anxiety and/or depression
  - Sleep disturbances, night terrors
  - School problems

PHYSICAL EXAM

- General assessment for signs of physical abuse, neglect, self-injurious behaviors (5)[C]
- Thorough physical exam:
  - Skin, head, eyes, ears, nose, and mouth
  - Chest/abdomen
  - Genital (consider exam under sedation) or refer to emergency department (ED)
  - Extremities with focus on inner arms and legs
  - Growth data
- Maintain high index of suspicion for occult head, chest, and abdominal trauma
- Physical abuse:
  - Skin markings (e.g., lacerations, burns, ecchymoses, linear/shaped contusions, bites)
  - Immersion injuries with clearly distinguished outlines (e.g., from boiling water)
  - Oral trauma (e.g., torn frenulum, loose teeth)
  - Ear trauma (e.g., signs of ear pulling)
  - Eye trauma (e.g., hyphema, hemorrhage)
  - Head/abdominal blunt trauma
  - Fractures
- Sexual abuse:
  - Unexplained penile, vaginal, hymenal, perianal, or anal injuries/bleeding/discharge
  - Pregnancy or sexually transmitted infections (STIs)
  - Sperm is a definitive finding of child abuse.
- Neglect:
  - Child may be low weight for height, unclean, or unkempt.
  - Rashes
  - Fearful or too trusting
  - Clinging to or avoiding caregiver
  - Flat or balding occiput
  - Abnormal development or growth parameters
- Measurements, photographs, and careful descriptions are critical for accurate diagnosis.
- Collaboration with specialist and child abuse assessment team (2)[C]

DIAGNOSTIC TESTS & INTERPRETATION

Lab

Initial lab tests

- Lab testing should be directed by history and physical exam:
  - Urinalysis (e.g., abdominal/flank/back/genital trauma), urine DNA probe for STIs
  - Complete blood chemistry. Consideration of coagulation studies and platelet count (e.g., rule out bleeding disorder, abdominal trauma) as appropriate.
  - Electrolytes, creatinine, BUN, glucose
  - Liver and pancreatic function tests (e.g., abdominal trauma)
  - Guaiac stool (abdominal trauma)
- In cases of suspected neglect:
  - Stool exam, calorie count, purified protein derivative and anergy panel, sweat test, lead and zinc levels
- In cases of suspected sexual abuse:
  - STI testing: Gonorrhea, chlamydia, trichomonas; also consider HIV, herpes simplex virus (HSV), hepatitis panel, syphilis (5)[C]
  - Serum pregnancy test (5)[C]

Follow-Up & Special Considerations

- Bruising is a common presenting feature:
  - Bruising in babies that are not independently mobile is very uncommon (<1%) (6)[A].
- Patterns suggestive of abuse (6)[A]:
  - Bruises seen away from bony prominences
  - Bruises to face, back, abdomen, arms, buttocks, ears, hands
  - Multiple bruises in clusters or uniform shape
  - Patterned injuries (such as bite marks or the imprint of an object like a belt or cord) should be considered inflicted until proven otherwise.

- Red flags (7)[B]:
  - History that is inconsistent with the injury
  - No explanation offered for the injury, or injury blamed on sibling or another child
  - History that is inconsistent with the child's developmental level

Imaging

Initial approach

Imaging should be directed by history and injury/condition:

- All children with fractures and children with suspicious injuries under age 2:
  - Skeletal survey (2)[B]: X-rays include 2 views of each extremity; skull: Anteroposterior (AP) and lateral; spine: AP and lateral, chest x-ray, and/or rib (posterior), abdomen, pelvis, hands, and feet
  - Consider bone scan for acute rib fractures and subtle long bone fractures (2)[B].
- Intracranial and extracranial injury:
  - CT scan of head (2)[B]
  - Consider MRI of head/neck for better dating of injuries, looking at subtle findings, intercerebral edema, or hemorrhage (2)[B].
- Intra-abdominal injuries:
  - CT scan of abdomen

Diagnostic Procedures/Surgery

Sexual abuse:

- Consider photocolposcopy.
- <72 hours from time of abuse: Collect samples for the forensic laboratory (contact authorities for appropriate protocol) (5)[C].

Pathological Findings

- Spiral fractures in nonambulatory patients (children that are not walking or cruising should not have bruising or fractures from "falls")
- Chip or bucket-handle fractures
- Epiphyseal/metaphyseal rib fractures in infants
- Rupture of liver/spleen in abdominal blunt trauma
- Retinal hemorrhages in shaken baby syndrome

DIFFERENTIAL DIAGNOSIS

- Physical trauma (including but not limited to):
  - Accidental injury; toxic ingestion
  - Bleeding disorders (e.g., classic hemophilia)
  - Metabolic diseases; congenital conditions
  - Conditions with skin manifestations (e.g., mongolian spots, Henoch-Schönlein purpura, meningococcemia, erythema multiforme, hypersensitivity, car seat burns, staphylococcal scalded skin syndrome, chickenpox, impetigo)
  - Cultural practices (e.g., cupping, coining)
- Neglect (including but not limited to):
  - Endocrinopathies (e.g., diabetes mellitus)
  - Constitutional
  - GI (clefts, malabsorption, irritable bowel)
  - Seizure disorder
  - Sudden infant death syndrome (SIDS)
- Skeletal trauma (including but not limited to):
  - Obstetrical trauma
  - Nutritional (scurvy, rickets)
  - Infection (congenital syphilis, osteomyelitis)
  - Osteogenesis imperfecta
- Neoplasm

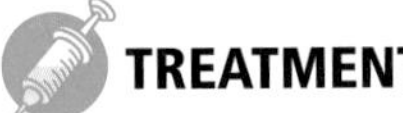

TREATMENT

MEDICATION

First Line

Antibiotics as indicated for treatment of documented STIs or infection

Second Line

Consider antidepressants if needed.

ALERT

Emergency contraception reduces rate of pregnancy after sexual assault if given within 5 days: Levonorgestrel 1.5 mg as a single dose as effective as 2 split doses (0.75 mg each) 12 hours apart (8)[A]

ADDITIONAL TREATMENT

General Measures

- Always explain what the physical exam will involve and why certain procedures are necessary.
- Examine child in a comfortable setting.
- Allow child to choose who will be in the room.
- Use appropriate positions to examine the anal and genital areas of young children (5)[C].
- Test for STIs before treatment (5)[C].

Issues for Referral

- Consider managing in ED to collect forensic specimens and maintain chain of evidence.
- Mandatory reporting to child protective authorities

SURGERY/OTHER PROCEDURES

As clinically indicated

IN-PATIENT CONSIDERATIONS

Initial Stabilization

As clinically indicated

Admission Criteria

- Moderate-to-severe injuries or unstable
- Acute psychological trauma
- If safety of child outside the hospital cannot be guaranteed

IV Fluids

As clinically indicated

Nursing

As clinically indicated

Discharge Criteria

- Child should be sent to another relative or into foster care if the suspected abuser lives with the child.
- Counseling for individual and family
- After initial evaluation, consider referral to sexual assault center.

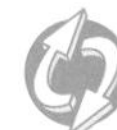

ONGOING CARE

FOLLOW-UP RECOMMENDATIONS

As clinically indicated

Patient Monitoring

- Refer to the state protective services.
- Monitor injury healing over time.
- Follow-up assessment for STIs that may not present acutely (e.g., HPV, herpes) (5)[C]

DIET

Routine

PATIENT EDUCATION

As clinically indicated

PROGNOSIS

Without intervention, child abuse is often a chronic and escalating phenomenon.

COMPLICATIONS

Growing evidence that sexual, physical, and emotional abuse in childhood are risk factors for poorer adult mental and physical health (10)[A]

REFERENCES

1. Department of Health & Human Services. Administration on Children, Youth & Families. Children's Bureau. Child Maltreatment 2009 Report. Http://www.acf.hhs.gov/programs/cb/pubs/cm09/.
2. Kellogg ND, American Academy of Pediatrics Committee on Child Abuse and Neglect. Evaluation of suspected child physical abuse. *Pediatrics*. 2007;119(6):1232–41.
3. Hahn RA, Bilukha OO, Crosby A, et al. First reports evaluating the effectiveness of strategies for preventing violence: Early childhood home visitation. Findings from the Task Force on Community Preventive Services. *MMWR Recomm Rep*. 2003;52(RR-14):1–9.
4. Jackson A, et al. Let the record speak: Medicolegal documentation in cases of child maltreatment. *Clin Ped Emerg Med*. 2006;7:181–5.
5. Kellogg N and the Committee on Child Abuse and Neglect. The evaluation of sexual abuse in children. *Pediatrics*. 2005;116:506–12.
6. Maguire S, Mann MK, Sibert J, et al. Are there patterns of bruising in childhood which are diagnostic or suggestive of abuse? A systematic review. *Arch Dis Child*. 2005;90:182–6.
7. Harris T. Bruises in children: Normal or child abuse? *J Pediatr Health Care*. 2010;24(4):216–21.
8. Cheng L, Gülmezoglu AM, Van Oel CJ, et al. Interventions for emergency contraception. *Cochrane Database Syst Rev*. 2004:(3).
9. Greenfield EA. Child abuse as a life-course determinant of adult health. *Maturitas* 2010;66:51–55.

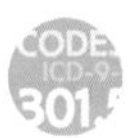

CODES

ICD9

- 995.50 Child abuse, unspecified
- 995.51 Child emotional/psychological abuse
- 995.59 Other child abuse and neglect

CLINICAL PEARLS

- High index of suspicion important for both prevention (knowing risk factors, ways to intervene) and recognition of abuse.
- Neglect is the most common and lethal form of abuse and should be aggressively reported.
- Detailed exam with documentation is key.
- Mandated reporting is required for suspected child abuse and neglect (reasonable suspicion); the physician does not have to prove abuse before reporting.
- Child Abuse Hotline by state: http://www.childwelfare.gov/responding/reporting.cfm

CHLAMYDIA PNEUMONIAE

Lawrence M. Hwang, MD
Daniel T. Lee, MD
Jeremy Golding, MD

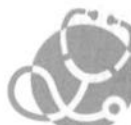

BASICS

DESCRIPTION

- *Chlamydia pneumoniae*, an obligate intracellular, gram-negative bacterium, has been established as an important cause of adult and pediatric respiratory disease and is capable of causing persistent latent infection.
- Humans are the only known reservoir.
- First recognized as a respiratory pathogen in 1989
- System(s) affected: Respiratory; Cardiovascular; Neurologic
- Synonym(s): Taiwan acute respiratory agent; *Chlamydophila pneumoniae*

EPIDEMIOLOGY

- The incubation period is ~30 days.
- Predominant age: More common in elderly; less common in children 2 months–5 years
- Serologic evidence of acute and chronic infection found in 1/3 of patients with acute chronic obstructive pulmonary disease (COPD) exacerbation, often together with other concurrent bacterial infection

Incidence

- Overall incidence rate of *C. pneumoniae* is unknown.
- No particular seasonal variation
- Outbreaks have occurred among military recruits, university students, and nursing home residents.

Prevalence

- Accounts for 5–20% of community-acquired pneumonia in adults and children. Greatly varied rates exist between study locations.
- Most cases occur sporadically, although intrafamilial spread also occurs.

Pediatric Considerations

Uncommon in children 2 months–5 years of age

GENERAL PREVENTION

- As transmission is via contact with respiratory secretions, advise hand washing and avoid exposure to infected persons.
- Flu and pneumococcal vaccines for high-risk groups

PATHOPHYSIOLOGY

Infection with *C. pneumoniae* and resultant host responses may lead to mucus production in the nasal passages, sinuses, bronchial tree, and alveoli, along with nasopharyngeal and airway inflammation and bronchospasm.

COMMONLY ASSOCIATED CONDITIONS

- COPD
- Asthma
- HIV infection
- Cystic fibrosis
- Diabetes mellitus
- Atherosclerosis
- Multiple sclerosis
- Alzheimer disease

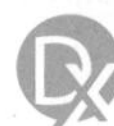

DIAGNOSIS

HISTORY

- Spectrum of illness may vary from mild and self-limited to severe pneumonia.
- Onset often gradual with delayed presentation
- Sore throat and hoarseness may precede cough by a week or more, giving biphasic appearance to illness (uncommon in *Legionella*, less common in *Mycoplasma*, *Streptococcus pneumoniae*, and *Haemophilus influenzae*).
- Dry cough
- Low-grade fever (usually early in illness)
- Chills
- Rhinitis
- Headache
- Malaise
- Myalgias
- Sinus congestion
- Nausea
- Altered mental status

PHYSICAL EXAM

- General appearance usually nontoxic, unless extremely ill
- Fever
- Tachypnea
- Tachycardia
- Diminished breath sounds
- Crackles or wheezing
- Bronchial breath sounds
- Percussion dullness and egophony less sensitive but more specific for pneumonia
- Pharyngeal erythema (without exudates)
- Retropharyngeal lymphoid granulation

Geriatric Considerations

- Usually more severe disease in older adults, and more common in the elderly who also have concomitant medical problems
- Elderly patients are less likely to exhibit respiratory symptoms with pneumonia and may present with altered mental status or history of falls.

DIAGNOSTIC TESTS & INTERPRETATION

Lab

Initial lab tests

- Multiple unreliable laboratory methods for diagnosis including culture, antigen detection, serology, PCR
- Leukocyte count usually normal or low, but may be mildly elevated
- Blood cultures recommended if toxic and requiring ICU admission; otherwise not likely to be helpful
- Culture has traditionally been the gold standard diagnostic method (1):
  - Many limitations include technical complexity, limited availability, and variable yield (1)
  - Most easily cultured in HL or HEp2 cells (culture is 10–80% sensitive and >95% specific) (2)
- Testing with microimmunofluorescence (MIF) is recommended by the Centers for Disease Control (CDC), as enzyme immunoassay testing is less specific. However, MIF testing is not standardized for *C. pneumoniae* and may also lack specificity and sensitivity (2):
  - 4-fold increase in IgG titer diagnostic of acute infection (10–100% sensitivity) (2)
  - Presence of IgM antibody (≥1:16) (1)
  - Single IgG titers are discouraged (1)
- Complement fixation for *Chlamydia* is widely available but cannot distinguish *C. pneumonia* from *Chlamydophila psittaci*.
- PCR from pharyngeal swab or bronchioalveolar lavage specimen (30–95% sensitivity, >95% specificity) (2)

Imaging

Initial approach

- Patients with suspected community-acquired pneumonia (CAP) who are more than mildly ill should be evaluated with a chest x-ray (CXR) (2)[A]. The CXR may be abnormal even in clinically mild disease.
- Variable radiographic abnormalities include unilateral and bilateral infiltrates and pleural effusions. Single, subsegmental funnel-shaped or circumscribed infiltrate is common.

Diagnostic Procedures/Surgery

Although serology is 95% specific, definitive diagnosis requires a positive culture or PCR testing (2)[A].

C

DIFFERENTIAL DIAGNOSIS

- Other causes of atypical pneumonia, including *M. pneumoniae* and *L. pneumophila*
- Other bacterial causes of pneumonia, including *S. pneumoniae. H. influenzae, Moraxella catarrhalis*, and *Staphylococcus aureus*
- Respiratory viruses: Adenovirus, influenza A, influenza B, parainfluenza virus, and respiratory syncytial virus
- Endemic fungal pathogens: Blastomycosis, coccidioidomycosis, histoplasmosis
- Bioterrorism agents: Anthrax, plague, tularemia
- Conditions that mimic CAP: Acute respiratory disease syndrome, atelectasis, idiopathic pulmonary fibrosis, neoplasm, pulmonary embolus, sarcoidosis, congestive heart failure

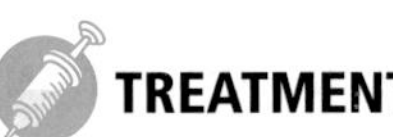

TREATMENT

MEDICATION

- β-Lactam antibiotics and sulfasoxazole not effective for *C. pneumoniae*.
- An advantage in clinical efficacy or mortality by empiric coverage of atypical pathogens in patients with CAP has not been shown (3)[A].
- The treatment course may be extended by several weeks in certain patients whose symptoms have not resolved.

First Line

- Azithromycin: 500 mg on day 1, then 250 mg on days 2–5 *OR*
- Clarithromycin: 500 mg q12h for 10–14 days *OR*
- Doxycycline: 100 mg q12h for at least 14 days:
  - Tetracycline not for use during pregnancy or in children <8 years
  - Tetracycline may cause photosensitivity; sunscreen is recommended.
    - Tetracyclines may increase the anticoagulant effect of warfarin.

Second Line

- Alternative drugs: Erythromycin base, 250–500 mg q.i.d. for 14–21 days
- Levofloxacin: 250–500 mg/d (PO or IV) or other respiratory fluoroquinolones have good bioavailability and the convenience of once-daily dosing, but are recommended for use only when patients have failed treatment with a first-line drug or have had recent antibiotics, significant comorbidities, or allergies to alternatives.

Pregnancy Considerations

Tetracyclines and fluoroquinolones are contraindicated.

COMPLEMENTARY AND ALTERNATIVE MEDICINE

In small studies, manipulative treatment was shown to reduce duration of IV antibiotic treatment and days in the hospital for hospitalized elderly patients with pneumonia (4)[C].

IN-PATIENT CONSIDERATIONS

- Usually outpatient care for most. Those with severe pneumonia or coexisting illness may require hospitalization.
- Pneumonia severity index or other validated prediction rule can assist in predicting those patients with CAP with higher morbidity and those requiring hospitalization (5)[A].

Initial Stabilization

Infection in debilitated or hospitalized patients can be severe. Stabilize respiratory distress as per advanced cardiac life support protocol.

IV Fluids

Increased fluids generally recommended

Discharge Criteria

Reversal of any respiratory distress, with the patient tolerating oral medications, otherwise stable medically, and stable for discharge per the clinical judgment of the physician

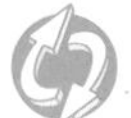

ONGOING CARE

FOLLOW-UP RECOMMENDATIONS

Patient Monitoring

- Weekly patient monitoring until well
- Follow-up CXR for resolution
- Reinfection is possible
- Some reports of individuals who are persistently culture-positive despite antibiotic treatment

PROGNOSIS

- Pneumonia is especially life threatening in older adults and patients with other illnesses that affect the lungs (e.g., asthma, COPD) or the immune system (e.g., diabetes), with an overall 0.5–29% mortality rate.
- Estimated mortality rate from *C. pneumoniae* is 9%, but this may be an overestimate due to the number of subclinical cases.
- Death usually from secondary infection or underlying comorbidity

COMPLICATIONS

- Reactive airway disease
- Erythema nodosum
- Otitis media
- Endocarditis
- Pericarditis or myocarditis
- Meningoencephalitis
- Associated with atherosclerotic disease: *C. pneumoniae* has been cultured from atherosclerotic plaque in patients with coronary artery disease, but treatment has not been shown to affect mortality.

REFERENCES

1. Kumar S, Hammerschlag MR. Acute respiratory infection due to *Chlamydia pneumoniae:* Current status of diagnostic methods. *Clin Infect Dis*. 2007;44:568–76.
2. Lutfiyya MN. Diagnosis and treatment of community-acquired pneumonia. *AFP*. 2006;73(3): 442–50.
3. Shefet D. Empiric antibiotic coverage of atypical pathogens for community acquired pneumonia in hospitalized adults. *Cochrane Database Sys Rev*. 2006;1:CD004418.
4. Noll DR, Shores JH, Gamber RG. Benefits of osteopathic manipulative treatment for hospitalized elderly patients with pneumonia. *J Am Osteopath Assoc*. 2000;100:776–82.
5. Fine MJ, Auble TE, Yealy DM. A prediction rule to identify low-risk patients with community-acquired pneumonia. *N Engl J Med*. 1997;336:243–50.

ADDITIONAL READING

- Blasi F, Tarsia P, Aliberti S. *Chlamydophila pneumoniae. Clin Microbiol Infect*. 2009;15:29–35.
- Miyashita N. Clinical presentation of community-acquired *Chlamydia pneumonia* in adults. *Chest*. 2002;121:1176–81.
- Thibodeau KP. Atypical pathogens and challenges in community-acquired pneumonia. *AFP*. 2004;69(7): 1701–6.

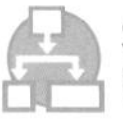

See Also (Topic, Algorithm, Electronic Media Element)

Algorithm: Cough, Chronic

CODES

ICD9

483.1 Pneumonia due to chlamydia

CLINICAL PEARLS

- *C. pneumoniae* is a significant cause of adult and pediatric pneumonias.
- Formal and accurate diagnosis of *C. pneumoniae* is difficult due to lack of standardized diagnostic tests. Culture remains the gold standard.
- Initial treatment should include tetracyclines, macrolides, and quinolones.

CHLAMYDIAL SEXUALLY TRANSMITTED DISEASES

Rachel Sagor, MD
Jeremy Golding, MD

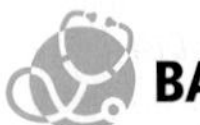

BASICS

DESCRIPTION

- An obligate, intracellular membrane-bound prokaryotic organism, *C. trachomatis* is the most common bacterial STI in the US.
- Transmitted through vaginal, anal, or oral sex. May also occur vertically from mother to infant during vaginal birth.
- Screening has increased over the last 20 years, but remains suboptimal with annual screening rates of only 41–45% among sexually active females ages 16–25 in 2009 (1). Majority of cases are asymptomatic (75–90% females, 50–75% males).
- If untreated, may lead to pelvic inflammatory disease, ectopic pregnancies, and infertility.
- System(s) affected: Reproductive

Pregnancy Considerations

Perinatal acquisition may result in neonatal pneumonia and/or conjunctivitis.

EPIDEMIOLOGY

Incidence

- Mandatory reporting started in 1985 with national data showing steady increase in incidence since.
- 1.2 million *reported* cases in 2009, with an estimated 2.8 million cases yearly in the US. Increasing incidence reflects greater screening and improved testing modalities.

Prevalence

- 409 per 100,000 people in the US in 2009. This was an 11.5% increase from 2007.
- Populations most affected: Young females, particularly those of ethnic minority groups in the US
- Peak incidence: Late teens, early 20s. Predominant sex: Females have 3 times higher reported incidence and prevalence than males, but this likely reflects increased testing in females.
- Minorities bear the highest burden, with infection rates among blacks in 2009 8 times that of whites. Rates among American Indian/Alaska natives and Hispanics were 4.3 and 2.8 times higher than whites, respectively. Rates higher in US southern states as compared with the Northeast.

RISK FACTORS

Risk correlates with:

- Number of lifetime sexual partners and number of concurrent sexual partners
- Lack of barrier contraception during sexual intercourse
- Younger age (highest in females 15–19 years, males 20–24 years)
- Black/Hispanic/American Indian and Alaskan native ethnicity (2)

GENERAL PREVENTION

- Populations with prevalence >5% should be screened at least annually (3). Screen if: New or >1 sex partner in past 6 months, attending an adolescent or family-planning clinic or a STD or abortion clinic, attending a jail or other detention-center clinic, rectal pain, discharge or tenesmus, testicular pain, testing of any individual with urethral or cervical discharge.
- *All sexually active women ≤25 years of age should be screened at least yearly*, and repeat testing in ∼3 months is recommended for those who screen positive, not as test of cure but because reinfection rate is high regardless of whether the sexual partner is treated (3)[A].
- Screening sexually active men ≤25 years controversial but should be strongly considered in high-risk populations (4)[A]
- United States Preventative Services Task Force (USPSTF) recommends that pregnant women ≤25 years of age and those engaging in high-risk sexual behaviors be screened (5).

ETIOLOGY

C. trachomatis serotypes D–K

COMMONLY ASSOCIATED CONDITIONS

- Females:
  - Pelvic inflammatory disease (PID): As many as 40% of untreated women will develop PID.
  - Infertility and ectopic pregnancies
  - Chronic pelvic pain
  - Mucopurulent cervicitis with cervical edema and propensity to bleed during speculum exam
  - Urethral syndrome (common in women with dysuria, frequency, and pyuria in the absence of infection with uropathogen)
  - Arthritis (rare)
- Males:
  - Epididymitis and nongonococcal urethritis
  - Reiter syndrome (HLA-B27)
  - Proctitis (men who have sex with men)
- Neonates:
  - Inclusion conjunctivitis (occurs in ∼40% of exposed neonates) (3)
  - Otitis media
  - Pneumonia
  - Pharyngitis
- Diseases caused by other chlamydial species:
  - Lymphogranuloma venereum: *C. trachomatis* serotypes L1–L3
  - Trachoma: *C. trachomatis* serotypes A–C

DIAGNOSIS

- *Majority of patients are asymptomatic.* Of those with symptoms, the most common are as follows:
  - In females: Mucopurulent vaginal discharge, dysuria (urethral syndrome), bartholinitis, abdominopelvic pain (endometritis, salpingitis/PID), right-upper-quadrant pain (Fitz-Hugh-Curtis perihepatitis syndrome)
  - In males: Dysuria, urethral discharge (urethritis), scrotal pain (epididymitis), rectal pain or discharge (proctitis), acute arthritis (Reiter syndrome)
  - In infants: Conjunctivitis, pneumonitis, carriage in pharynx/GI tract
- Lymphogranuloma venereum (LVG) (*C. trachomatis* serovars L1, L2, or L3): Primary lesion is a small genital or rectal papule that may ulcerate at the site of transmission after an incubation period of 3–30 days. Most common manifestation in heterosexuals is unilateral tender lymphadenopathy. With rectal transmission, LGV causes an invasive proctocolitis, which may be scarring and cause strictures.

HISTORY

- Complete sexual history, including number of sex partners lifetime and past year, prior history of STIs, use of barrier protection, exchange of money or drugs for sex, oral or anal receptive intercourse, partner fidelity
- Symptom history, with onset date for each symptom

PHYSICAL EXAM

- Men and women: External genitalia (rash? lesions?), urethra (discharge?), inguinal lymph nodes, pharynx and perianal area, if history indicates
- In addition, for women: Cervix (discharge? motion tenderness?), uterus, ovaries, adnexae

DIAGNOSTIC TESTS & INTERPRETATION

Lab

- *Test of choice: Nucleic acid amplification tests (NAAT)*: Amplified molecular testing (e.g., polymerase chain reaction [PCR], ligase chain reaction, specific dynamic action, human chorionic somatotropin, thyroid microsomal antigen): Sensitivity >95%; specificity >99%. Urine equally as sensitive as cervical swab. Patient self-collected vaginal swabs have also been shown to be effective. Lab tests may remain positive for as long as 3 weeks after successful treatment.
- Chlamydial cell culture: Sensitivity 50–80%; specificity >99%
- Enzyme immunoassay: Sensitivity 40–60%; specificity >99%
- Direct fluorescent antibody detection: Sensitivity 50–70%; specificity >99%
- Specimens should contain cell scrapings rather than inflammatory discharge because the organism lives only inside the epithelial cells.

Imaging

Imaging not indicated for initial screening; consider pelvic ultrasound/CT if high clinical suspicion for PID or tubo-ovarian abscess.

Initial approach

Offer testing for other STDs, including gonorrhea, HIV, syphilis, and perform Pap if appropriate

Follow-Up & Special Considerations

See "Patient Monitoring."

DIFFERENTIAL DIAGNOSIS

- *N. gonorrhoeae:* Urethritis, proctitis, epididymitis, cervicitis, PID, Bartholin abscess, perihepatitis
- *Mycoplasma* or *U. urealyticum*: Urethritis, epididymitis, Reiter disease, PID
- *C. trachomatis* (serotypes L1–L3): LGV, proctitis

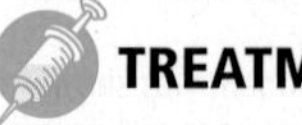

TREATMENT

MEDICATION

First Line

Treatment of chlamydial urethritis, cervicitis (including sexual partners of infected persons) (3):

- Azithromycin 1 g PO single dose, *or*
- Doxycycline: 100 mg PO b.i.d. × 7 days

- First-line PID treatment (outpatient) (3):
  - Ceftriaxone 250 mg IM × 1 *plus* doxycycline 100 mg PO × 14 days with or without metronidazole 500 mg PO b.i.d. × 14 days, *or*
  - Cefoxitin 2 g IM × 1 with probenecid 1 g PO × 1 *PLUS* doxycycline 100 mg PO × 14 days with or without metronidazole 500 mg PO b.i.d. × 14 days
- First-line PID treatment parenteral therapy: See "Pelvic Inflammatory Disease."
- First-line treatment of LGV: Doxycycline 100 mg b.i.d. × 21 days *or* erythromycin base 500 mg PO q.i.d. × 21 days
- Tetracyclines may cause photosensitivity; sunscreen is recommended. Avoid concurrent administration of tetracyclines with antacids, dairy products, or iron.
- Practitioners may elect to give azithromycin and ceftriaxone together to the patient in the office to reduce patient noncompliance.

Pregnancy Considerations

- Tetracyclines (e.g., doxycycline) and quinolones (e.g., ofloxacin, levofloxacin) are contraindicated in pregnant women.
- Consider azithromycin or amoxicillin:
  - Azithromycin as above, or
  - Amoxicillin 500 mg PO t.i.d. × 7 day

ALERT

- In children: Tetracyclines and quinolones are contraindicated in children:
  - <45 kg: Erythromycin base ethinyl succinate 500 mg/kg/d PO q.i.d x 14 days
  - >45 kg: Adult dosing

Pediatric Considerations

Tetracyclines and quinolones are contraindicated in children. Must rule out sexual abuse if child presents with *Chlamydia* infection.

Second Line

- Second-line therapy for chlamydial urethritis/cervicitis
- Erythromycin base: 500 mg PO q.i.d. × 7 days
- Levofloxacin: 500 mg PO daily × 7 days

ADDITIONAL TREATMENT

Expedited partner therapy (EPT) is the practice of physicians delivering medications or prescriptions to sexual partners of persons infected with STIs without clinical assessment of the partners:

- Treatment of sexual partners is a key component to STI control. EPT has been shown to be more effective than traditional partner referral in reducing recurrence rates. 80% of partners received treatment if partner-delivered, compared to only 25% of partners getting the medication if needing to access it independently.
- EPT is currently legal in 27 states, "potentially allowable" in 15 states, and illegal in 8. The logistics of this practice differ from state to state and continue to evolve.
- For an updated review on the legal status of EPT, please refer to the Centers for Disease Control (CDC) Web site on this subject: http://www.cdc.gov/std/ept/legal/default.htm.

General Measures

- All patients with known or suspected chlamydia should be tested for gonorrhea, HIV (the latter requires individual counseling and consent), and possibly syphilis (3)[C]. Also, ensure females are up to date with Pap smears.
- Some experts recommend that all patients treated for chlamydia should be treated empirically for gonorrhea simultaneously, unless they are known to be negative for gonorrhea by sensitive lab testing.
- All partners (most recent partner and all partners within the past 60 days) of patients treated for chlamydia should be tested, if possible. They should be treated empirically rather than waiting for test results. They should also be treated empirically even if they were not tested.

IN-PATIENT CONSIDERATIONS

Treatment of PID: Continuing trend toward outpatient treatment. However, decision to hospitalize made on case-by-case basis. Those falling into the following categories recommended for inpatient treatment: Pregnancy, lack of response or intolerance to oral meds, suspicion of poor compliance/nonadherence to therapy, severe clinical illness (fevers, severe vomiting, or abdominal pain), pelvic abscess, possible need for surgical intervention.

Initial Stabilization

Outpatient treatment, unless patient is moderately or severely ill with PID or other complications

Admission Criteria

As outlined above

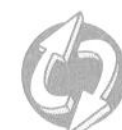

ONGOING CARE

FOLLOW-UP RECOMMENDATIONS

Patient and all partners should abstain from sexual contact until at least 7 days after treatment with a single dose of azithromycin or after completion of multiple-day course of another medication, whichever is longer.

Patient Monitoring

- It is not routine to test the patient to see if a cure has been obtained, except in pregnancy. However, retesting of infected women at 3 months is indicated because of high risk of reinfection (3,6)[A].
- Sexual partners must be evaluated and treated empirically, if necessary, to prevent passing the disease back and forth between partners. Partnerships with local public health departments should be fostered to assist with partner tracing.
- Lack of resolution or recurrence of symptoms must be reported immediately to the physician, and severe cases of urethritis/cervicitis, as well as the chlamydial syndromes, should be seen in follow-up after completion of therapy.
- Up to 25% of asymptomatic patients screened for chlamydia may not return for treatment after chlamydia culture results. Strategies must be developed to ensure treatment can be instituted.

PATIENT EDUCATION

- Suggest risk-reduction counseling and encourage delay of initiation of sexual activity, especially in younger adolescents.
- Encourage safe-sex practices, such as barrier protection (condoms particularly).
- Stress the need to finish entire course of antibiotics.

PROGNOSIS

Prognosis is good with early and compliant therapy; however, because of the asymptomatic nature of the early disease and the population affected, symptomatic PID still accounts annually for 2.5 million outpatient visits and >250,000 hospitalizations.

COMPLICATIONS

Both sexes: Enhancement of transmission of and susceptibility to HIV. Males: Transient oligospermia and postepididymitis urethral stricture (rare). Females: Tubal infertility (most common cause of acquired infertility), tubal (ectopic) pregnancy, chronic pelvic pain

REFERENCES

1. National Committee for Quality Assurance. The state of healthcare quality 2010. Washington (DC): National Committee for Quality Assurance; 2010:43–4.
2. http://www.cdc.gov/std/stats09/chlamydia.htm.
3. Centers for Disease Control and Prevention (CDC). Sexually transmitted diseases treatment guidelines, 2010. *MMWR*. 2010;59.
4. Turner CF, Rogers SM, Miller HG, et al. Untreated gonococcal and chlamydial infection in a probability sample of adults. *JAMA*. 2002;287:726–33.
5. Meyers DS, Halvorson H, Luckhaupt S. Screening for chlamydial infection: An evidence update for the U.S. Preventive Services Task Force. *Ann Intern Med*. 2007;147;117–22.
6. Hosenfeld CB, Workowski KA, Berman S, et al. Repeat infection with chlamydia and gonorrhea among females: A systematic review of the literature. *Sex Transm Dis*. 2009;36:478–89.

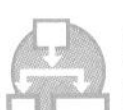

See Also (Topic, Algorithm, Electronic Media Element)

Cervicitis, Ectropion, and True Erosion; Epididymitis; Gonococcal Infections; HIV Infection and AIDS; Pelvic Inflammatory Disease (PID); Syphilis; Urethritis

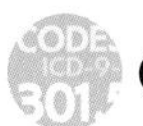

CODES

ICD9

099.55 Other venereal diseases due to chlamydia trachomatis, unspecified genitourinary site

CLINICAL PEARLS

- *C. trachomatis* infection is common in sexually active teens and young adults. Perhaps 40% of untreated chlamydial infections progress to PID, and 1 in 5 cases of PID lead to infertility. To prevent recurrence, treat patients and their partners concurrently.
- If all eligible women were screened, we would *annually* prevent an estimated 60,000 cases of PID, 8,000 cases of chronic pelvic pain, and over 7,000 cases of infertility. False positives do occur, and are especially likely in screening very low-risk populations. Patients should be advised of the possibility that the test is falsely positive, but should be treated anyway.

CHOLANGITIS, ACUTE

Wesley Wu, MD
Edward Feller, MD

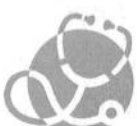

BASICS

DESCRIPTION

- Bacterial infection of the biliary tree due to partial or complete obstruction, most commonly caused by migration of a gallstone from the gallbladder into the common bile duct (CBD) stones.
- Classically presents as:
  - Clinical triad of fever, jaundice, and right upper quadrant (RUQ) pain *(Charcot triad)* OR
  - Pentad of fever, jaundice, RUQ pain, mental status changes, and hypotension (*Reynolds pentad*)
- Severity may range from mild to life threatening.
- Management includes medical and/or surgical interventions.
- System(s) affected: Gastrointestinal (GI); Hepatobiliary; Other systems via hematogenous spread of infection

EPIDEMIOLOGY

- Any age, but more common in adults after age 40; incidence increases with age:
  - Rare in children (except in hemolytic disorders)
- Although gallstones are more frequent in females, cholangitis occurs equally among men and women.
- Occurs more commonly in Native Americans, Asians, and African Americans with sickle cell disease or any cause of hemolysis
- 1–3% of patients undergoing endoscopic retrograde cholangiopancreatography (ERCP) develop cholangitis.

Prevalence

- CBD stones discovered incidentally during evaluation of gallstones: 5–12%
- Acute cholangitis occurs in 6–9% of patients hospitalized with gallstone disease.
- Blood cultures positive with CBD stones: 20–30%

RISK FACTORS

- Cholelithiasis (see "Cholelithiasis, Risk Factors")
- CBD gallstones, more frequent in Asians, the elderly, chronic bile duct inflammation due to sclerosing cholangitis, infection, and possibly hypothyroidism
- Advanced age >70 years old
- Neurologic disease
- Periampullary diverticula
- Cirrhosis
- Ileal Crohn disease
- Hepatobiliary infections (*Ascaris lumbricoides, Clonorchis sinensis, Schistosomiasis mansoni, Opisthorchis viverrini*)
- Conditions that predispose to biliary stasis, including diabetes mellitus, obesity, pregnancy, rapid weight loss, prolonged fasting
- Narrowing or obstruction of the biliary tree by strictures or neoplasms, including pancreatic masses that compress the duct; chronic pancreatitis with inflammatory CBD stricture
- Endoscopic or surgical manipulation; biliary stent
- Immunosuppression

Genetics

Increased risk with positive family history of gallstones

GENERAL PREVENTION

- Moderate physical activity
- Avoid diet rich in saturated fatty acids
- Prophylactic use of ursodeoxycholic acid in rapid weight loss and in patients using longer-term somatostatin therapy or parenteral nutrition
- Statins may have a protective effect against gallstones (not recommended for prevention).
- If cholecystectomy (CCY) is performed, ensure patency of biliary tree with endoscopic or intraoperative cholangiography.
- Prophylactic antibiotics before (endoscopic retrograde cholangiopancreatography (ERCP) (1)[A]

PATHOPHYSIOLOGY

- Bacteria may gain access to the biliary tree via retrograde ascent from the duodenum and trapped by a stone migrating from the gallbladder into the CBD.
- Rarely, infection may enter from portal venous system, periportal lymphatics, or an eroding hepatic abscess or infected pancreatic fluid collection.
- Obstruction of biliary flow via choledocholithiasis (90%), infection, neoplasms, and/or strictures promotes bile stasis and spread of bacteria through the biliary tree into hepatic ducts.
- Increased intraluminal pressure (>20 cm H_2O) decreases intrabiliary IgA secretion, disrupts the hepatocellular tight junction, and pushes the bacteria into the hepatic veins, biliary canaliculi, and perihepatic lymphatics, leading to bacteremia (25–40%).
- Pyogenic cholangitis in Asia is characterized by intrahepatic stones and recurrent attacks, most commonly due to parasitic infection.

ETIOLOGY

- Most commonly *Escherichia coli, Klebsiella pneumonia*, and *Enterococcus*
- Also frequently isolated: *Bacteroides fragilis, Streptococcus faecalis, Enterobacter*, and *Pseudomonas*
- Anaerobic bacteria, including *Clostridium* and *Bacteroides* species, are more frequently isolated in polymicrobial infections and prior biliary-enteric surgery.
- Hospitalized patients are prone to methicillin-resistant *Staphylococcus aureus, Pseudomonas* species, and vancomycin-resistant *Enterococcus* (VRE).
- Cytomegalovirus, *Cryptosporidium*, *Monoavium intracellulare*, herpes simplex virus are common isolates in AIDS cholangiopathy. In AIDS, acute cholecystitis may be acalculous without visualized gallstones due to infection, inflammation, or ischemia of the gallbladder wall.

COMMONLY ASSOCIATED CONDITIONS

- Biliary pancreatitis
- Inflammatory bowel disease
- Malignancy (periampullary)
- AIDS

DIAGNOSIS

HISTORY

- Charcot's triad is present in <2/3 of patients.
- RUQ pain is variable from mild to severe, and generally less than that in patients with pain from CBD stone without infection.
- Pain may be intermittent when stones or sludge ball-valve within the CBD causing transient, intermittent obstruction.
- Weight loss and anorexia possible

Geriatric Considerations

Elderly may present atypically with later stages of the disease and sudden decompensation from sepsis with features of Reynolds pentad (5–7%) or not have leukocytosis or fever.

PHYSICAL EXAM

Patient may have only some of the following symptoms; the abdominal exam may be unrevealing:

- Chills and fever (90%)
- RUQ or epigastric tenderness (70%), with or without cessation of inspiration on palpation (Murphy sign); atypical locations can occur
- Jaundice (60%)
- Hypotension (30%)
- CNS depression (10–20%)
- Palpable nontender gallbladder (Courvoisier sign) rarely
- Signs of underlying pathology, such as chronic liver disease

DIAGNOSTIC TESTS & INTERPRETATION

Lab

- CBC: Elevated white blood cell count (WBC), neutrophil predominance
- Liver enzyme tests usually have a cholestatic pattern with elevated direct bilirubin, alkaline phosphatase, gamma glutamyl transpeptidase, and aminotransaminases generally <400 IU/L, but may increase acutely >2,000 IU/L in acute CBD stone impaction and microabscess formation in liver, with subsequent sharp decline)
- Serum amylase and lipase
- Blood cultures positive in 21–71%.
- WBC ≥20,000 and total bilirubin ≥10 mg/dL are selective predictors of adverse outcomes (2)[B].
- Prothrombin time (PT) and partial thromboplastin time (PTT) for possible chronic liver disease or disseminated intravascular coagulopathy

Imaging

See "Diagnostic Procedures."

Diagnostic Procedures/Surgery

- Transabdominal ultrasound (TUS) is the initial imaging study of choice, but sensitivity for CBD stones is <60%; TUS is a sensitive tool to detect gallstones.
- CT is indicated for most patients with abdominal pain, jaundice, and fever. However, unenhanced CT is insensitive in detecting gallstones, but may document biliary dilatation or suppurative cholangitis (3)[C], pancreatic disease, local complications such as a liver abscess, and exclude other causes of obstruction.

- IV contrast-enhanced CT with a helical cholangiography protocol has high sensitivity and specificity for gallstones and is the preferred CT strategy.
- Magnetic resonance cholangiopancreatography (MRCP) is a noninvasive method of imaging the bile, useful in confirming biliary pathology prior to ERCP (92% sensitivity), and has a high specificity for primary sclerosing cholangitis (4)[A]. However, MRCP has no potential to remove CBD stones.
- ERCP is the most definitive diagnostic test, and permits therapeutic intervention such as biliary sphincterotomy, stone extraction, or stent placement.
- Endoscopic ultrasound (US) may be helpful to differentiate neoplasms vs. inflammatory processes in periampullary masses.
- Percutaneous transhepatic cholangiography (PTC) is an invasive, second-line procedure, largely supplanted by the aforementioned modalities.

DIFFERENTIAL DIAGNOSIS
- Acute cholecystitis
- Mirizzi syndrome
- Biliary leaks
- Liver abscess
- Hepatitis
- Infected choledochal cysts
- Acute pancreatitis
- Perforated duodenal ulcer
- Pelvic inflammatory disease
- Kidney stones
- Acute mesenteric ischemia
- Abdominal aortic aneurysm rupture
- Right lower-lobe pneumonia
- Septic shock

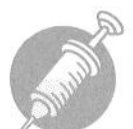

TREATMENT

- Monitor airway, breathing, hydration, circulation, and resuscitate as needed; IV crystalloid
- Make patient NPO; if vomiting, place nasogastric tube.
- Medical treatment is effective in 80% for symptomatic control, but removal of obstruction is the definitive curative method.

MEDICATION
Management consists of IV antibiotics, fluid resuscitation, oxygen supplementation, coagulopathy correction, and biliary drainage:
- Initial empiric antibiotic therapy should be broad spectrum until results of blood cultures are obtained and therapy modified accordingly.
- Biliary excretion of some antibiotics is compromised when biliary obstruction is present.
- Antibiotics in mild disease for 5–7 days and if blood culture positive, treat for 10–14 days
- Incomplete data is available on the best initial antibiotic regimen, but sample initial broad-spectrum regimens are listed below in no particular order:
  – Monotherapy with a beta-lactam/beta-lactamase inhibitor, such as ampicillin-sulbactam (3 g q6h) OR piperacillin/tazobactam (4.5 g q6h) OR ticarcillin-clavulanate (3.1 g q4h)
  – Metronidazole (500 mg IV q8h) PLUS a third-generation cephalosporin, such as ceftriaxone (1 g q12h)
  – Metronidazole (500 mg IV q8h) PLUS a fluoroquinolone (ciprofloxacin 400 mg IV q12h or levofloxacin 500 mg IV daily)
  – Monotherapy with meropenem (1 g q6h)

ADDITIONAL TREATMENT
General Measures
- Most respond to antibiotics and conservative management, and should undergo biliary drainage with timing dependent on clinical urgency.
- ~1/5 of patients require urgent biliary decompression within 24–48 hours, including ERCP with sphincterotomy, percutaneous biliary drainage, open surgical decompression, or T-tube placement.
- Indications for urgent decompression include: Persistent abdominal pain, mental status changes, fever >39°C, refractory hypotension

SURGERY/OTHER PROCEDURES
Removal of obstruction is the primary treatment goal:
- For high-risk patients, decompression by ERCP with prophylactic antibiotics is first-line treatment with potential for endoscopic sphincterotomy, stone extraction, and/or biliary stenting (5)[B].
- For lower-risk, noninvasive, evaluation may be preferred. Secondary options include surgery with intraoperative cholangiography (IOC). Controversy exists concerning routine IOC in all patients undergoing laparoscopic cholecystectomy.
- Interval cholecystectomy for CBD-related cholangitis or percutaneous drainage in nonsurgical patients after stabilization and in gallstone-associated pancreatitis

IN-PATIENT CONSIDERATIONS
- See "Treatment."
- Immediately consult surgeon and gastroenterologist.

ONGOING CARE

FOLLOW-UP RECOMMENDATIONS
Some patients with recurrent symptoms indicative of cholangitis may require maintenance antibiotics and imaging to exclude liver abscess or undetected residual stones.

DIET
NPO until acute phase is terminated

PATIENT EDUCATION
For patient education materials favorably reviewed on this topic, contact National Digestive Diseases Information Clearinghouse, Box NDDIC, Bethesda, MD 20892, (301) 468-6344

PROGNOSIS
- Mortality with current interventions: 5%, especially in patients with relevant comorbidities
- Mortality with Reynolds pentad: As high as 50%
- Coexistent cardiac or kidney impairment, malignancies, and hepatic abscesses worsen the prognosis.
- 4–24% recurrence even after cholecystectomy, related to residual increased intrabiliary pressure, biliary tract ectasias, focal strictures, intrahepatic pigment stones, and parasitic infections

COMPLICATIONS
- Hepatic abscess
- Sepsis
- Hepatic dysfunction and atrophy
- Bile peritonitis, portal vein thrombosis, gallstone ileus
- Pneumobilia
- Cholangiocarcinoma

REFERENCES

1. Brand M, Bizos D, O'Farrell P, et al. Antibiotic prophylaxis for patients undergoing elective endoscopic retrograde cholangiopancreatography. *Cochrane Database Syst Rev*. 2010;CD007345.
2. Rosing DK, De Virgilio C, Nguyen AT, et al. Cholangitis: Analysis of admission prognostic indicators and outcomes. *Am Surg*. 2007;73: 949–54.
3. Lee NK, Kim S, Lee JW, et al. Discrimination of suppurative cholangitis from nonsuppurative cholangitis with computed tomography (CT). *Eur J Radiol*. 2008.
4. Dave M, Elmunzer BJ, Dwamena BA, et al. Primary sclerosing cholangitis: Meta-analysis of diagnostic performance of MR cholangiopancreatography. *Radiology*. 2010;256:387–96.
5. Yoo K-S, Lehman GA. Endoscopic management of biliary duct stones Gastroenterol *Clin N Am*. 2010;39:209–227.

ADDITIONAL READING

- Attasaranya S, Fogel EL, Lehman GA. Choledocholithiasis, ascending cholangitis, and gallstone pancreatitis. *Med Clin N Am*. 2008;92: 925–60.
- Catalano OA, et al. Biliary infections: Spectrum of imaging findings and management. *Radiographics*. 2009;29:2059–80.

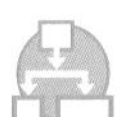

See Also (Topic, Algorithm, Electronic Media Element)

Cholelithiasis

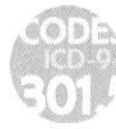

CODES

ICD9
576.1 Cholangitis

CLINICAL PEARLS

- The complete Charcot triad is present in only 2/3 of patients.
- Serum bilirubin is typically <15 mg/dL because it is most commonly intermittent and incomplete.
- Jaundice may be absent and bilirubin normal when only partial obstruction exists. Clue is marked alkaline phosphatase elevation.
- Ultrasound helps with diagnosis, but ERCP is both diagnostic and therapeutic.
- Malignant obstruction rarely presents with cholangitis because biliary obstruction is slow and progressive rather than abrupt as in CBD stones (which trap bacteria above the obstruction).

CHOLELITHIASIS

Hongyi Cui, MD, PhD
John J. Kelly, MD

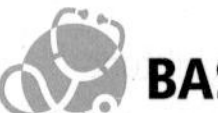

BASICS

DESCRIPTION

Cholelithiasis manifests in cholesterol, pigment, or mixed stones formed and contained in the gallbladder:

- Synonym(s): Gallstones

Pediatric Considerations

- Uncommon at <10 years of age
- Associated with blood dyscrasia
- Most gallstones in pediatric population are pigment stones.

EPIDEMIOLOGY

Incidence

- Increased in Native Americans and Hispanics
- Increases with age by 1–3% per year; peaks at seventh decade
- 2% of the US population develops gallstones annually.

Prevalence

- Population: 8–10% of US
- Predominant sex: Female > Male (2–3:1)

RISK FACTORS

- Age (peak in 60–70s)
- Female gender
- Caucasian, Hispanic, or Native American descent
- Cholestasis or impaired gallbladder motility in association with prolonged fasting, long-term total parenteral nutrition, and rapid weight loss following bariatric surgery
- Hereditary (such as patients carrying the p.D19H variant for the hepatocanalicular cholesterol transporter ABCG5/ABG8 have an increased risk for gallstones)
- Metabolic syndrome (i.e., obesity, dyslipidemia, and type 2 diabetes)
- Pregnancy and multiparity
- Metabolic changes in association with short gut syndrome, terminal ileal resection, and inflammatory bowel disease
- Hemolytic disorders (e.g., hereditary spherocytosis and sickle cell anemia) and cirrhosis (for black or pigment stones)
- Medications (such as early use of birth control pills; estrogen replacement therapy at high doses)
- Biliary tract infection (such as liver flukes) and stricture (for intraductal formation of brown pigment stones)

GENERAL PREVENTION

- Ursodiol (Actigall) taken during rapid weight loss prevents gallstone formation (1)[A]
- Regular exercise and dietary modification may reduce the incidence of gallstone formation.

PATHOPHYSIOLOGY

Gallstone formation is a complex process mediated by genetic, metabolic, immune, and environmental factors. Gallbladder sludge (a mixture of cholesterol crystals, calcium bilirubinate granules, and mucin gel matrix) serves as the nidus for gallstone formation.

ETIOLOGY

- Production of bile supersaturated with cholesterol (cholesterol stones)
- Decrease in bile content of either phospholipid (lecithin) or bile salts
- Biliary stasis or impaired gallbladder motility
- Generation of excess unconjugated bilirubin in patients with hemolytic diseases; passage of excess bile salt into the colon with subsequent absorption of excess unconjugated bilirubin in patients with inflammatory bowel disease or after distal ileal resection (black or pigment stones)
- Hydrolysis of conjugated bilirubin or phospholipid by bacteria in patients with biliary tract infection or stricture (brown stones or primary bile duct stones; rare in the Western world and common in Asia)

COMMONLY ASSOCIATED CONDITIONS

90% of people with gallbladder carcinoma have gallstones.

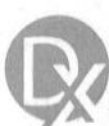

DIAGNOSIS

HISTORY

- Mostly asymptomatic (80%):
  - 5–10% become symptomatic each year.
  - Over their lifetime, <1/2 of the patients with gallstones develop symptoms.
- Episodic right upper quadrant or epigastric pain lasting longer than 15 minutes and sometimes radiating to the back (biliary colic), usually postprandially; the majority of patients will develop recurrent symptoms after the first episode.
- Nausea, vomiting
- Fatty food intolerance
- Indigestion or bloating sensation

PHYSICAL EXAM

- Physical exam is *usually normal* in patients with cholelithiasis.
- Epigastric and/or right upper quadrant tenderness (Murphy sign) when in association with cholecystitis
- Fever and jaundice in patients with choledocholithiasis and cholangitis; jaundice can also be caused by extrinsic compression of the bile duct by a stone in the gallbladder or cystic duct (Mirizzi syndrome)
- Flank and periumbilical ecchymoses (Cullen sign and Grey-Turner sign) in patients with acute hemorrhagic pancreatitis
- In patients with concomitant acute calculus cholecystitis and gallbladder cancer, a mass in the right upper quadrant may be palpated.

DIAGNOSTIC TESTS & INTERPRETATION

Lab

- No lab study is specific for cholelithiasis.
- Leukocytosis and elevated C-reactive protein level are associated with acute calculus cholecystitis.

Imaging

- Ultrasound (best technique to diagnose gallstones and differentiate from cholecystitis). Ultrasound can detect gallstones in 97–98% of patients. Thickening of the gallbladder wall (5 mm or greater), pericholecystic fluid, and direct tenderness when the probe is pushed against the gallbladder (sonographic Murphy sign) are all radiographic signs of acute calculus cholecystitis.
- Ct scan (no advantage over ultrasound except in detecting distal common bile duct stones)
- Magnetic resonance cholangiopancreatography is reserved for cases of suspected common bile duct stones due to high cost.
- Endoscopic ultrasound has been shown to be as sensitive as endoscopic retrograde cholangiopancreatography (ERCP) for detection of common bile duct stones in patients with gallstone pancreatitis.
- Hepatobiliary iminodiacetic acid (HIDA) scan is useful in differentiating acalculous cholecystitis from other causes of abdominal pain. False-positive results can arise from fasting status, insufficient resistance of the sphincter of Oddi and gallbladder agenesis:
  - Cholecystokinin (CCK)-HIDA is specifically used to diagnose gallbladder dysmotility disorder (i.e., biliary dyskinesia).
- 10–30% of gallstones are radiopaque calcium or pigment-containing gallstones and are more likely to be visible on plain x-ray. A "porcelain gallbladder" is a calcified gallbladder, visible by x-ray; associated with gallbladder cancer (25%).

Pathological Findings

- Pure cholesterol stones have a white or slightly yellow color.
- Pigment stones may be black or brown. Black stones contain polymerized calcium bilirubinate, most often secondary to cirrhosis or hemolysis, and almost always form in the gallbladder. Brown stones are associated with biliary tract infection, caused by bile stasis, and as such may form either in the bile ducts or gallbladder.

DIFFERENTIAL DIAGNOSIS

- Peptic ulcer diseases
- Gastritis
- Hepatitis
- Pancreatitis
- Cholangitis
- Gallbladder cancer
- Gallbladder polyps
- Acalculous cholecystitis
- Biliary dyskinesia
- Choledocholithiasis
- Choledochocyst

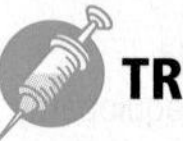

TREATMENT

Geriatric Considerations

Age alone should not alter the therapy plan.

MEDICATION

First Line

- Analgesics for pain relief
- Antibiotics are indicated in patients with signs of acute cholecystitis.
- Prophylactic antibiotics in low-risk patients do not prevent infections for laparoscopic cholecystectomies (2)[A].

Second Line

NSAIDs may have a role in pain relief, given that prostaglandins are important in the development of pain.

ADDITIONAL TREATMENT

General Measures

- Treat only symptomatic gallstones and observe asymptomatic stones.

- Attempt conservative therapy during pregnancy. If necessary, perform surgery preferentially in the second trimester.
- Prophylactic cholecystectomy for patients with calcified (porcelain) gallbladder (risk for gallbladder cancer), and patients with recurrent pancreatitis due to microlithiasis
- In morbidly obese patients, simultaneous cholecystectomy may be performed in combination with bariatric procedures (3) in an effort to reduce later stone-related complications.

Issues for Referral

Patients with retained or recurrent bile duct stones following cholecystectomy should be referred to gastroenterology for ERCP.

SURGERY/OTHER PROCEDURES

- Surgical intervention should be considered for patients who have symptomatic cholelithiasis or gallstone-related complications such as cholecystitis, or in asymptomatic patients with immune suppression, calcified gallbladder, or family history of gallbladder cancer (4)[A].
- Open, small incision, or laparoscopic cholecystectomy (LC), have similar mortality and complication rates (5)[A]. The minimally invasive techniques offer quicker recovery. In well-selected patients, single-incision LC (SILC) is a novel method for the treatment of symptomatic cholelithiasis. Natural orifice transluminal endoscopic surgery (NOTES) is still at an experimental stage, and NOTES cholecystectomy is only available in a limited number of specialized centers:
  - Surgery-related complications include common bile duct injury (0.5%), right hepatic duct/artery injury, retained stones, cystic duct or duct of Luschka leak, biloma formation, or bile duct stricture in the long term.
  - Conversion to open procedure based on the judgment of the operating surgeon
  - In 10–15% patients with symptomatic cholelithiasis, common bile duct (CBD) stones are detected during LC with intraoperative cholangiogram (IOC). CBD stone(s) can be removed via either laparoscopic CBD exploration or postoperative ERCP depending on surgeon expertise and GI availability.
  - IOC may help delineate bile duct anatomy when dissection proves difficult. Selective or routine use of IOC is a topic of debate, but may be associated with earlier recognition and decreased incidence of bile duct injury (6)[B].
- Percutaneous cholecystostomy (PC) in high-risk patients with cholecystitis or gallbladder empyema. PC may also be used in patients with symptoms of cholecystitis for >72 hours in which altered anatomy might significantly increase the surgical risk. Interval cholecystectomy is usually advisable after the resolution of cholecystitis and optimization of associated medical conditions to prevent recurrent cholecystitis.

IN-PATIENT CONSIDERATIONS

For patients with symptomatic cholelithiasis, laparoscopic cholecystectomy has become an outpatient procedure; for patients who developed gallstone-related complications (i.e., cholecystitis, cholangitis, and pancreatitis), inpatient care is necessary.

Initial Stabilization

- Acute phase: NPO, IV fluids, and antibiotics
- Adequate pain control with narcotics and/or NSAIDs

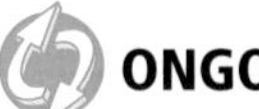

ONGOING CARE

FOLLOW-UP RECOMMENDATIONS

Patient Monitoring

- Medical attention if asymptomatic stones become symptomatic
- Patients on oral dissolution agents should be followed up with liver enzyme, serum cholesterol, and imaging studies.

DIET

A low-fat diet may be helpful.

PATIENT EDUCATION

- Change in lifestyle (e.g., regular exercise) and dietary modification (low-fat diet and reduction of total calorie intake) may reduce gallstone-related hospitalizations.
- Patients with asymptomatic gallstones should be educated about the typical symptoms of biliary colic and gallstone-related complications.

PROGNOSIS

- <1/2 of patients with gallstones become symptomatic.
- Cholecystectomy: Mortality <0.5% elective, 3–5% emergency; morbidity <10% elective, 30–40% emergency
- ~10–15% of the patients will have associated choledocholithiasis.
- After cholecystectomy, stones may recur in the bile duct.

COMPLICATIONS

- Acute cholecystitis (90–95% secondary to gallstones)
- Gallstone pancreatitis
- Acute cholangitis
- Common bile duct stones with obstructive jaundice
- Biliary-enteric fistula and gallstone ileus
- Gallbladder perforation, peritonitis, and sepsis
- Gallbladder cancer
- Mirizzi syndrome (bile duct obstruction caused by gallstones lodged in gallbladder or cystic duct)

REFERENCES

1. Uy MC, Talingdan-Te MC, Espinosa WZ, et al. Ursodeoxycholic acid in the prevention of gallstone formation after bariatric surgery: A meta-analysis. *Obes Surg.* 2008.
2. Zhou H, Zhang J, Wang Q, et al. Meta-analysis: Antibiotic prophylaxis in elective laparoscopic cholecystectomy. *Aliment Pharmacol Ther.* 2009;29:1086–95.
3. Sakcak I, Avsar FM, Cosgun E, et al. Management of concurrent cholelithiasis in gastric banding for morbid obesity. *Eur J Gastroenterol Hepatol.* 2011.
4. Society for Surgery of the Alimentary Tract, et al. SSAT patient care guidelines. Treatment of gallstone and gallbladder disease. *J Gastrointest Surg.* 2007;11:1222–4.
5. Keus F, Gooszen HG, van Laarhoven CJ, et al. Open, small-incision, or laparoscopic cholecystectomy for patients with symptomatic cholecystolithiasis. An overview of Cochrane Hepato-Biliary Group reviews. *Cochrane Database Syst Rev.* 2010; CD008318.
6. Connor S, Garden OJ. Bile duct injury in the era of laparoscopic cholecystectomy. *Br J Surg.* 2006;93: 158–68.

ADDITIONAL READING

- Bogue CO, Murphy AJ, Gerstle JT, et al. Risk factors, complications, and outcomes of gallstones in children: A single-center review. *J Pediatr Gastroenterol Nutr.* 2010;50:303–8.
- Brown LM, Rogers SJ, Cello JP, et al. Cost-effective treatments of patients with symptomatic cholelithiasis and possible common bile duct stones. *J Am Coll Surg.* 2011;212(6):1049–60.
- Gurusamy KS, Samraj K, et al. Cholecystectomy versus no cholecystectomy in patients with silent gallstones. *Cochrane Database Syst Rev.* 2007; CD006230.
- Sakorafas GH, Milingos D, Peros G, et al. Asymptomatic cholelithiasis: Is cholecystectomy really needed? A critical reappraisal 15 years after the introduction of laparoscopic cholecystectomy. *Dig Dis Sci.* 2007;52:1313–25.

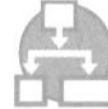

See Also (Topic, Algorithm, Electronic Media Element)

Cholangitis, Acute; Choledocholithiasis

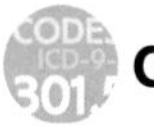

CODES

ICD9

- 574.00 Calculus of gallbladder with acute cholecystitis, without mention of obstruction
- 574.01 Calculus of gallbladder with acute cholecystitis, with obstruction
- 574.10 Calculus of gallbladder with other cholecystitis, without mention of obstruction

CLINICAL PEARLS

- Laparoscopic cholecystectomy has become the most frequently used procedure; lithotripsy and oral dissolution therapy may be considered in rare circumstances.
- Acute acalculous cholecystitis is associated with bile stasis and gallbladder ischemia.
- Prophylactic cholecystectomy is not indicated in patients with diabetes and asymptomatic gallstones. There is no evidence that asymptomatic diabetics are at increased risk of developing complications of gallstone disease.
- The best imaging modality for the diagnosis of gallstones is transabdominal ultrasound (sensitivity of 97% and specificity of 95%); not sensitive for occult gallstones or microlithiasis (stones smaller than 5 mm).
- Think of gallstones in the postbariatric surgery patient complaining of "gas pains" as they are adjusting to their new diet.

CHRONIC COUGH

Jacqueline L. Olin, MS, PharmD, BCPS, CPP, CDE
Susan Ziglar, MD

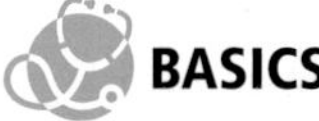

BASICS

DESCRIPTION

- Chronic cough is defined as a cough that persists for >8 weeks in adults.
- Subacute cough describes a cough lasting 3–8 weeks.
- In children, chronic cough is defined as a cough for >4 weeks in duration.
- Patients present because of fear of the causative illness (e.g., cancer), as well as annoyance, self-consciousness, and hoarseness.
- Patients with stress urinary incontinence may find cough particularly troubling.
- At the primary care level, chronic obstructive pulmonary disease (COPD) and smoking-related cough are common causes of chronic cough.
- System(s) affected: Gastrointestinal; Pulmonary

EPIDEMIOLOGY

- Predominant age: All age groups
- Predominant sex: Male = Female

Incidence

Recurrent cough has been reported at 3–40% by various population estimates.

Prevalence

Chronic cough is one of the most common reasons for primary care visits.

RISK FACTORS

Although various conditions may contribute to chronic cough, the main causes include smoking and pulmonary diseases.

PATHOPHYSIOLOGY

Varies with findings and disorders implicated

ETIOLOGY

- Often multiple etiologies, but most are related to bronchial irritation. Most frequent etiologies (account for >90% of cases) in nonsmokers include:
  - Upper airway cough syndrome (UACS) (formerly referred to as postnasal drip syndrome) and other upper airway abnormalities including rhinitis syndromes
  - Asthma
  - Nonasthmatic eosinophilic bronchitis (NAEB)
  - Gastroesophageal reflux disease (GERD)
- Other causes:
  - Chronic smoking or exposure to smoke or pollutants
  - Aspiration
  - Bronchiectasis
  - ACE inhibitors
  - Infections (e.g., pertussis, tuberculosis)
  - Cystic fibrosis
  - Sleep apnea
  - Restrictive lung diseases (e.g., chronic interstitial lung disease)
  - Neoplasms: Lung or laryngeal cancer, other
  - Psychogenic (habit cough)
- Cough reflex hypersensitivity or cough hypersensitivity syndrome are new labels attempting to define a syndrome of cough with characteristic trigger symptoms but are not adequately explained by other medical conditions (1).

COMMONLY ASSOCIATED CONDITIONS

Patients with UACS, asthma, and GERD may present with chronic cough as the only symptom and not the usual symptoms associated with the diagnoses.

DIAGNOSIS

HISTORY

- The age of the patient, presence of associated signs/symptoms, medical history, medication history (especially use of ACE inhibitors), environmental and occupational exposures, potential for aspiration, and smoking history may make some causes more likely.
- The character of cough or description of sputum quality is rarely helpful in predicting the underlying cause.
- Cough diaries have not correlated well with objective measures.
- Various ambulatory systems for recording cough are under development.
- Hemoptysis or signs of systemic illness preclude empiric therapy.

PHYSICAL EXAM

- Signs and symptoms are variable and related to the underlying cause; usually a nonproductive cough with no other signs or symptoms.
- Possible signs and symptoms of UACS, sinusitis, GERD, congestive heart failure
- Absence of additional signs/symptoms of a particular condition not necessarily helpful:
  - For example, 5% of GERD patients have no other signs or symptoms and sometimes have poor response to empiric proton pump inhibitor trials.

DIAGNOSTIC TESTS & INTERPRETATION

- Often evaluation starts with empiric therapy directed at likely underlying etiology and/or simple testing such as a chest x-ray (CXR).
- Extensive testing only if indicated by the history and physical

Pediatric Considerations

Children with chronic cough not responsive to an inhaled β-agonist should undergo, at a minimum, spirometry (if age-appropriate) and CXR.

Lab

Initial lab tests

Evaluation will be dictated by findings in the comprehensive history and physical.

Follow-Up & Special Considerations

- Examples:
  - If considering COPD, asthma, or restrictive lung disease: Spirometry
  - If suspect cystic fibrosis: Sweat chloride testing
  - If suspect hypereosinophilic syndrome, tuberculosis, or malignancy: Sputum for eosinophils and cytology

Imaging

Initial approach

- If considering neoplasm, heart failure, or infectious etiologies, CXR may be indicated
- In cases of failure to respond to initial trial of empiric therapy, CXR may also be beneficial

Follow-Up & Special Considerations

- If abnormal CXR, suspected neoplasm, or underlying pulmonary disorder, consider a chest CT.
- Consider pulmonary consultation.
- Refer to gastroenterologist for endoscopy.

Diagnostic Procedures/Surgery

If diagnosis suspected and inadequate response to initial measures, other procedures can be considered:

- Pulmonary function testing
- Purified protein derivative (PPD) skin testing
- Allergen testing
- 24-hour esophageal pH monitor
- Bronchoscopy if necessary
- Endoscopic or video fluoroscopic swallow evaluation or barium esophagram
- Sinus CT
- Ambulatory cough monitoring and cough challenge with citric acid or capsaicin (at specialized cough clinic)
- Echocardiogram

Pathological Findings

Specific to underlying cause

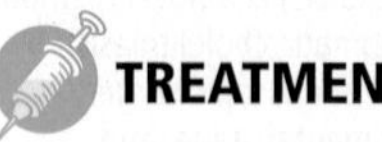

TREATMENT

- With chronic cough, empiric treatment should be directed at the most common causes (UACS, asthma, GERD, NAEB) (2)[C].
- Oral antihistamine/decongestant therapy with a first-generation antihistamine should be initial empiric treatment (2)[C].
- In patients with cough associated with the common cold, nonsedating antihistamines were not found to be effective in reducing cough (2)[C].
- In stable patients with chronic bronchitis, therapy with ipratropium bromide may reduce chronic cough (3)[C].
- Centrally acting antitussive drugs (codeine, dextromethorphan) are recommended for short-term symptomatic relief of coughing in patients with chronic bronchitis (3)[C]:
  - These agents have limited efficacy in cough due to upper respiratory infections (3)[C].
- For cough associated with lung cancer, the use of narcotic cough suppressants is recommended (3)[C].
- The FDA issued a public health advisory stating that OTC cough and cold medicines, including antitussives, expectorants, nasal decongestants, antihistamines, or combinations should not be given to children <2 years.
- The American Academy of Pediatrics does not recommend central cough suppressants for treating any kind of cough (2)[B].
- In children <14 years old, when pediatric recommendations are not available, adult recommendations should be used with caution (2)[C].
- Some children with recurrent cough and no evidence of airway obstruction may benefit from an inhaled β-agonist (4)[C].
- In infants and children with nonspecific chronic cough, trials of empiric proton pump inhibitor therapy were not effective (5)[C].

MEDICATION

- Treatments (antacids, bronchodilators, inhaled corticosteroids, proton pump inhibitors, antibiotics) should be directed at the specific cause of cough.
- The FDA issued a public health advisory stating that OTC cough and cold medicines should not be given to children <2 years.
- Consumer Healthcare Products Association (CHPA) members have changed OTC cough expectorant and suppressant product labels to state "do not use" in children <4 years old.

First Line

- In adults, oral antihistamine/decongestant therapy should be empiric treatment. Multiple formulations are available OTC in combination with other ingredients. Advise patients to review labels carefully or consult pharmacist:
  - Chlorpheniramine 2 mg/phenylephrine 5 mg/ Acetaminophen 325 mg (Tylenol Allergy Multi-Symptom) 2 caplets or gelcaps PO q4h (Maximum 12 caplets or gelcaps in 24 hours: Age >12 years)
- Central cough suppressants for short-term symptomatic relief of nonproductive cough:
  - Dextromethorphan 10–20 mg PO q4h: Age >12 years. Use 5–10 mg PO q4h for age 6–12 years:
    - Concomitant use of dextromethorphan and agents with serotonergic activity (such as SSRIs) should be avoided due to risk of serotonin syndrome.
  - Narcotics: Codeine 15–30 mg PO q6h; hydrocodone (Vicodin) 5 mg PO q6h; hydrocodone (Tussionex Pennkinetic) 10 mg (5 mL) PO q12h for ages 12 or over

Second Line

- A peripherally acting antitussive agent has been used:
  - In patients > age 10, Benzonatate (Tessalon Perles) 100–200 mg PO t.i.d. as needed (maximum 600 mg daily)
- Results from a small randomized placebo-controlled trial (*n* = 27) demonstrated subjective cough score improvement in patients using slow-release morphine sulfate. Patients had failed with other antitussive therapies. Side effects included constipation and drowsiness and there were no discontinuations due to adverse events (6)[C]:
  - Morphine was administered 5–10 mg PO b.i.d.
- For patients with cystic fibrosis, amiloride may improve cough clearance of sputum.

ADDITIONAL TREATMENT

General Measures

- In patients with chronic cough, considerations for potential etiology should include asthma (2)[B] or UACS (2)[C].
- With concomitant complaints of heartburn and regurgitation, GERD should be considered as a potential etiology (2)[C].
- 90% of patients will have resolution of cough after smoking cessation (2)[A].
- When indicated, ACE inhibitor therapy should be switched in patients in whom intolerable cough occurs (2)[A].
- Empiric treatment of postnasal drip and GERD.
- Consider nonpharmacological options such as warm fluids, hard candy, or nasal drops. In infants and children, can try clearing secretions with a bulb syringe.
- Attempt maximal therapy for single most-likely cause for several weeks, then search for coexistent etiologies.

Issues for Referral

- Refer as needed based on specific suspected diagnosis for cough.
- Patients with chronic cough may benefit from evaluation by pulmonary, gastroenterology, ear-nose-and-throat (ENT), and/or allergy specialists.

SURGERY/OTHER PROCEDURES

Fundoplication may be effective for cough secondary to refractory GERD.

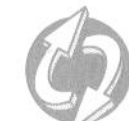

ONGOING CARE

FOLLOW-UP RECOMMENDATIONS

Consider stepwise withdrawal of medications after resolution of cough.

Patient Monitoring

Frequent follow-up is necessary to assess the effectiveness of the treatment and the addition of other medications as needed.

DIET

Dietary modification: Patients with GERD may benefit by avoiding ethanol, caffeine, nicotine, citrus, tomatoes, chocolate, and fatty foods.

PATIENT EDUCATION

- Reassure patient that most cases of chronic cough do not have life-threatening causes and that the condition can usually be managed effectively.
- Counsel that several weeks to a month may be needed for significant reduction or total elimination of cough.
- Prepare the patient for the possibility of multiple diagnostic tests and therapeutic regimens, because the treatment is very often empiric.

PROGNOSIS

- >80% of patients can be effectively diagnosed and treated using a systematic approach.
- Cough from any cause may take weeks to months until resolution, and resolution depends greatly on efficacy of treatment directed at underlying etiology.

COMPLICATIONS

- Cardiovascular: Arrhythmias, syncope
- Stress urinary incontinence
- Abdominal and intercostal muscle strain
- GI: Emesis, hemorrhage, herniation
- Neurologic: Dizziness, headache, seizures
- Respiratory: Pneumothorax, laryngeal, or tracheobronchial trauma
- Skin: Petechiae, purpura, disruption of surgical wounds
- Medication side effects
- Other: Negative impact on quality of life

REFERENCES

1. Chung KF. Chronic 'cough hypersensitivity syndrome': A more precise label for chronic cough. *Pulm Pharmacol Ther*. 2011:24:267–71.
2. Irwin RS, Baumann MH, Bolser DC, et al. Diagnosis and management of cough executive summary: ACCP evidence-based clinical practice guidelines. *Chest*. 2006;129:1S–23S.
3. Bolser DC. Cough suppressant and pharmacologic protussive therapy: ACCP evidence-based clinical practice guidelines. *Chest*. 2006;129:238S–249S.
4. Gupta A, et al. Management of chronic non-specific cough in childhood: An evidence-based review. *Arch Dis Child Educ Pract Ed*. 2007;92:ep33–ep39.
5. Chang AB, Lasserson TJ, Gaffney J, et al. Gastro-oesophageal reflux treatment for prolonged non-specific cough in children and adults. *Cochrane Database Syst Rev*. 2011;CD004823.
6. Morice AH, Menon MS, Mulrennan SA, et al. Opiate therapy in chronic cough. *Am J Respir Crit Care Med*. 2007;175:312–5.

ADDITIONAL READING

- Birring SS. Controversies in the evaluation and management of chronic cough. *Am J Respir Crit Care Med*. 2011;183:708–15.
- Pavord ID, Chung KF. Management of chronic cough. *Lancet*. 2008;371:1375–84.

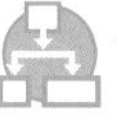

See Also (Topic, Algorithm, Electronic Media Element)

- Asthma; Bronchiectasis; Congestive Heart Failure; Eosinophilic Pneumonias; Gastroesophageal Reflux Disease; Laryngeal Cancer; Lung, Primary Malignancies; Pertussis; Pulmonary Edema; Rhinitis, Allergic; Sinusitis; Tuberculosis
- Algorithm: Cough, Chronic

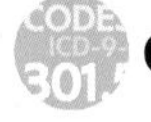

CODES

ICD9

- 496 Chronic airway obstruction, not elsewhere classified
- 786.2 Cough

CLINICAL PEARLS

- Chronic cough is defined as a cough that persists for >8 weeks in adults.
- In patients with chronic cough, most frequent etiologies include a history of smoking, asthma, UACS, and GERD.
- The FDA issued a public health advisory stating that OTC cough and cold medicines should not be given to children <2 years.
- Consumer Healthcare Products Association (CHPA) members have changed OTC cough expectorant and suppressant product labels to state "do not use" in children <4 years old.

CHRONIC FATIGUE SYNDROME

Joan M. Stachnik, PharmD, BCPS
Anthony Valdini, MD, MS, FACP, FAAFP

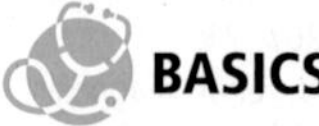

BASICS

DESCRIPTION

- A condition characterized by profound mental and physical exhaustion, with at least 6 months presence of multiple systemic and neuropsychiatric symptoms. At least 4 of 8 associated conditions are required per Centers for Disease Control and Prevention (CDC) definition:
  - Impaired memory
  - Sore throat
  - Tender lymph nodes
  - Persistent muscle or joint pain
  - New headaches
  - Unrefreshing sleep
  - Postexertion malaise
- Must have a new or definite onset (not lifelong). Fatigue is not relieved by rest and results in >50% reduction in previous activities (occupational, educational, social, and personal). Other potential medical causes must be ruled out.
- Exclusions:
  - Patients are excluded from chronic fatigue syndrome (CFS) definition until 2 years after resolution of substance/alcohol abuse and 5 years after resolution of anorexia nervosa or bulimia.

EPIDEMIOLOGY

- Predominant age: 20–50 years
- Predominant sex: Male < Female
- All socioeconomic groups
- Because of cultural differences in presentation, doctors in less developed countries may not recognize the syndrome, making an accurate prevalence difficult to determine (1).
- Various associations between ethnicity and incidence have been reported. Higher rates found in ethnic minorities (Native Americans, Latinos, and African Americans) compared with white populations, based on population studies. Service-based studies (tertiary care) have reported higher rates among whites, or no association between incidence and ethnicity (2).

Prevalence

Estimates vary widely and depend on case definition and population studied, but a reasonable estimate using a strict case definition is 100 cases per 100,000 population. Community-based studies have reported prevalence rates of 0.23% and 0.42%.

RISK FACTORS

Possible predisposing factors include (3,4):

- Personality characteristics (neuroticism and introversion)
- Lifestyle:
  - Childhood inactivity or overactivity
  - Inactivity in adulthood after infectious mononucleosis
  - Familial predisposition
  - Comorbid mood disorders of depression and anxiety
- Long-standing medical conditions in childhood
- Childhood trauma (emotional, physical, sexual abuse)

Genetics

- Higher concordance has been reported among monozygotic twins compared with dizygotic twins.
- Gender may be a significant predictor.

ETIOLOGY

- Unknown and likely multifactorial:
  - Possible interaction between genetic predisposition, environmental factors, an initiating stressor, and perpetuating factors
- Physiologic or environmental stressor could be precipitant.
- Many patients with chronic fatigue recall significant stressors (e.g., major medical procedure, loss of a loved one, loss of employment) in months before symptoms began.
- Systems hypothesized to contribute to physiology include:
  - Neuroendocrine (e.g., diminished cortisol response to increased corticotropin concentrations)
  - Immune (e.g., increased C-reactive protein and beta-2 microglobulin) (5)
  - Neuromuscular (e.g., dysfunction of oxidative metabolism) (5)
  - Automatic (or thosfatic hypothesized is reported in a proportion of CFS sufferers)
- Serotonergic (e.g., hyperserotonergic mechanisms or upregulation of serotonin receptors)

COMMONLY ASSOCIATED CONDITIONS

Common comorbidities include:

- Fibromyalgia
- Irritable bowel syndrome
- Temporomandibular joint disorder
- Anxiety disorders
- Major depression
- Posttraumatic stress disorder (including physical and/or sexual past abuse)
- Domestic violence

DIAGNOSIS

HISTORY

See "Description" for CFS historical features.

PHYSICAL EXAM

Complete physical examination to rule out other medical causes for symptoms. Note: Tender adenopathy is one of the defining criteria.

ALERT

Detailed mental status examination (or referral to psychiatrist) to rule out both other primary etiologies or comorbidities

DIAGNOSTIC TESTS & INTERPRETATION

No single diagnostic test available

Lab

Standard laboratory tests are recommended to rule out other causes for symptoms (6):

- Chemistry panel
- CBC
- Urinalysis
- Thyroid-stimulating hormone (TSH)
- ESR or C-reactive protein
- Liver function
- Screen for drugs of abuse
- Age-/gender-appropriate cancer screening
- Additional studies, if clinical findings are suggestive or patient at risk (6):
  - Antinuclear antibodies (if +ESR)
  - Rheumatoid factor (if +ESR)
  - Creatine kinase
  - Tuberculin skin test
  - Serum cortisol
  - HIV
  - VDRL or RPR
  - Lyme serology
  - Gluten sensitivity (IgA tissue transglutaminase)

Follow-Up & Special Considerations

- Assessment for comorbid psychiatric disorders
- Assessment for personality and psychosocial factors and maladaptive coping styles
- In patients with sleep disturbance, polysomnography may reveal a treatable comorbid disease

Imaging

No applicable imaging tests available

DIFFERENTIAL DIAGNOSIS

- Insomnia: Primary (no clear etiology) vs. secondary (e.g., due to anxiety, depression, environmental factors, poor sleep hygiene)
- Idiopathic chronic fatigue (i.e., fatigue of unknown cause for >6 months without meeting criteria for CFS)
- Morbid obesity, body mass index (BMI) >40
- Malignancy
- Autoimmune disease
- Localized infection (e.g., occult abscess)
- Chronic or subacute bacterial disease (e.g., endocarditis)
- Lyme disease
- Fungal disease (e.g., histoplasmosis, coccidioidomycosis)
- Parasitic disease (e.g., amebiasis, giardiasis, helminth infestation)
- HIV or related disease
- Psychiatric disorders:
  - Major depression
  - Somatization disorder
- Chronic inflammatory disease (sarcoidosis, Wegener granulomatosis)
- Neuromuscular disease (multiple sclerosis, myasthenia gravis)
- Endocrine disorder (hypothyroidism, Addison disease, Cushing syndrome, diabetes mellitus)
- Iatrogenic (e.g., medication side effects)
- Toxic agent exposure
- Other known or defined systemic disease (chronic pulmonary, cardiac, hepatic, renal, or hematologic disease)
- Pregnancy until 3 months postpartum
- Physiologic fatigue (inadequate or disrupted sleep, menopause)
- *Weakness* and *sleepiness* can indicate a different etiology.

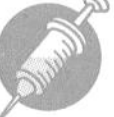

TREATMENT

Focus on changes in lifestyle and insight, with a goal to not use complicating treatments (e.g., addicting medications, invasive testing), or interventions that support secondary gain.

MEDICATION

- No established pharmacologic treatment recommendations
- Studies have been conducted with antidepressants, immunoglobulins, hydrocortisone, and modafinil. None have shown clear benefit (6).
- If insomnia is present, use of nonaddicting sleep aids (hydroxyzine, trazodone, doxepin, etc.) may improve outcomes.

ADDITIONAL TREATMENT

General Measures

ALERT

Treatment cornerstones include BOTH cognitive behavioral therapy and graded exercise therapy. Medications of little value

2 treatments have been shown effective, often used in combination (7,8,9):

- Individual cognitive-behavioral therapy (CBT): Challenge fatigue-related cognition. Plan social and occupational rehabilitation.
- Graded exercise therapy (GET): Track amount of exercise patient can do without exacerbating symptoms and gradually increase the intensity and duration. Both involve a carefully planned balance between activity and rest.
- Patients learn how to gradually increase activity in a way that will not exacerbate their illness. Vigorous exercise can trigger relapse, perhaps related to immune dysregulation; therefore, activity plan must be carefully monitored (8).
- Improves functional capacity and diminishes sense of fatigue (9).
- GET is more effective when delivered with educational interventions, explaining symptoms, and encouragement with telephone reminders (9).
- The duration of illness does not predict treatment outcome, so this approach can be applied to patients with chronic symptoms.

Issues for Referral

- Psychiatrist to assist in managing comorbid disorders if needed
- Rehabilitative medicine

COMPLEMENTARY AND ALTERNATIVE MEDICINE

- Although complementary and alternative medicines have been suggested, data are insufficient to recommend their use (10)[A].
- Social support groups have not proven to be effective.

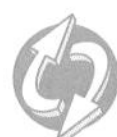

ONGOING CARE

FOLLOW-UP RECOMMENDATIONS

- Gradual increase in physical exercise with scheduled rest periods.
- Avoid extended periods of rest.

Patient Monitoring

Although no consensus exists, periodic re-evaluation is appropriate for support, relief of symptoms, and assessment for other possible causes of symptoms.

DIET

- No diet has been shown to be effective for treatment of CFS.
- A BMI of 40 has been associated with fatigue in general. Whether weight loss improves symptoms in such patients has yet to be tested.

PATIENT EDUCATION

- Patient education is an important part of treatment of CFS, such as education on the benefits of cognitive therapies, lifestyle changes, and pharmacologic therapy directed at specific associated symptoms.
- Chronic Fatigue and Immune Dysfunction Syndrome Association of America: www.cfids.org
- CDC Chronic Fatigue Syndrome: www.cdc.gov

PROGNOSIS

- Fluctuating course
- Generally, improvement is slow, with a course of months to years.
- An estimated 5% fully recover.

COMPLICATIONS

- Depression
- Unemployment. Although studies document improvement with treatment, fewer than 1/3 of patients in trials return to work (11).
- Polypharmacy

REFERENCES

1. Cho HJ, Menezes PR, Hotopf M, et al. Comparative epidemiology of chronic fatigue syndrome in Brazilian and British primary care: Prevalence and recognition. *Br J Psychiatry*. 2009;194:117–22.
2. Dinos S, Khoshaba B, Ashby D, et al. A systematic review of chronic fatigue, its syndromes and ethnicity: Prevalence, severity, co-morbidity and coping. *Int J Epidemiol*. 2009;38:1554–70.
3. Viner R, Hotopf M. Childhood predictors of self reported chronic fatigue syndrome/myalgic encephalomyelitis in adults: National birth cohort study. *BMJ*. 2004;329:941.
4. Heim C, Wagner D, Maloney E, et al. Early adverse experience and risk for chronic fatigue syndrome: Results from a population-based study. *Arch Gen Psychiatry*. 2006;63:1258–66.
5. Fulle S, Pietrangelo T, Mancinelli R, et al. Specific correlations between muscle oxidative stress and chronic fatigue syndrome: A working hypothesis. *J Muscle Res Cell Motil*. 2007;28:355–62.
6. Baker R, Shaw EJ. Diagnosis and management of chronic fatigue syndrome or myalgic encephalomyelitis (or encephalopathy): Summary of NICE guidance. *BMJ*. 2007;335:446–8.
7. White PD, Goldsmith KA, Johnson AL, et al. Comparison of adaptive pacing therapy, cognitive behaviour therapy, graded exercise therapy, and specialist medical care for chronic fatigue syndrome (PACE): A randomised trial. *Lancet*. 2011;377:823–36.
8. Nijs J, Paul L, Wallman K. Chronic fatigue syndrome: An approach combining self-management with graded exercise to avoid exacerbations. *J Rehabil Med*. 2008;40:241–7.
9. Price JR, Mitchell E, Tidy E, et al. Cognitive behaviour therapy for chronic fatigue syndrome in adults. *Cochrane Database Syst Rev*. 2008: CD001027.
10. Adams D, Wu T, Yang X, et al. Traditional Chinese medicinal herbs for the treatment of idiopathic chronic fatigue and chronic fatigue syndrome. *Cochrane Database Syst Rev*. 2009;CD006348.
11. Cairns R, Hotopf M. A systematic review describing the prognosis of chronic fatigue syndrome. *Occup Med-Oxford*. 2005;55:20–31.

C

ADDITIONAL READING

- Baker R, Shaw EJ, et al. Diagnosis and management of chronic fatigue syndrome or myalgic encephalomyelitis (or encephalopathy): Summary of NICE guidance. *BMJ*. 2007;335:446–8.
- Margo KL, Margo GM. Two therapies lift mood in chronic fatigue syndrome. *Current Psychiatry*. 2006;5:91–100.
- Prins JB, van der Meer JW, Bleijenberg G, et al. Chronic fatigue syndrome. *Lancet*. 2006;367:346–55.
- Rimes KA, Chalder T, et al. Treatments for chronic fatigue syndrome. *Occup Med (Lond)*. 2005;55:32–9.

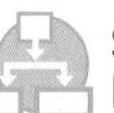

See Also (Topic, Algorithm, Electronic Media Element)

Algorithm: Fatigue

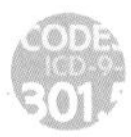

CODES

ICD9

780.71 Chronic fatigue syndrome

CLINICAL PEARLS

- CFS and depression can be comorbid. However, to differentiate between the 2, sore throat, tender lymph nodes, and postexercise fatigue are much more characteristic of CFS.
- Although a number randomized controlled trials on various pharmacologic agents (e.g., antidepressants, immune modulators) have been conducted, no single agent has been shown to be consistently effective.
- About 70% of patients show improvement with cognitive behavioral therapy, compared to 55% with graded exercise therapy; in many cases, these 2 treatments can be undertaken in combination.
- There are many more patients with idiopathic chronic fatigue than true CFS. To diagnose CFS, CDC criteria need to be met; standardized instruments (SF-36, symptom index) have been shown to be of use in the empirical diagnosis of CFS.

CHRONIC KIDNEY DISEASE

Lisa Pelunis-Messier, PharmD
Mhd Basheer Rahmoun, MD

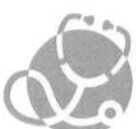

BASICS

Chronic kidney disease (CKD) is defined as:

- Kidney damage for ≥3 months, defined by structural or functional abnormalities of the kidney, with or without decrease in glomerular filtration rate (GFR), by either pathologic abnormalities or markers of damage, including abnormalities in blood or urine tests or imaging studies, *or*
- GFR <60 mL/min/1.73 m^2 for ≥3 months, with or without kidney damage

DESCRIPTION

- CKD is classified into 5 stages by GFR estimated by Modification of Diet in Renal Disease (MDRD) equation:
  - Stage 1: Kidney damage with GFR ≥90 mL/min/1.73 m^2
  - Stage 2: Kidney damage with mild ↓ GFR 60–89 mL/min/1.73 m^2
  - Stage 3: Moderate ↓ GFR 30–59 mL/min/1.73 m^2
  - Stage 4: Severe ↓ GFR 15–29 mL/min/1.73 m^2
  - Stage 5: Kidney failure: GFR <15 mL/min/1.73 m^2 or dialysis
- System(s) affected: Renal/Urinary; Cardiovascular; Skeletal; Endocrine; Metabolic; Hematologic; Lymphatic; Immune; Neurologic
- Synonym(s): Chronic renal failure; Chronic renal insufficiency

Geriatric Considerations

GFR normally decreases with age, despite normal creatinine (Cr).

ALERT

Adjust renally cleared drugs for GFR in elderly.

Pediatric Considerations

CKD definition is not applicable for children <6 years; lower GFR even when corrected for body surface area.

Pregnancy Considerations

- Renal function in CKD may deteriorate during pregnancy.
- Cr >1.5 and hypertension are major risk factors for worsening renal function.
- Increased risk of premature labor, preeclampsia, and/or fetal loss
- ACE inhibitors and angiotensin receptor blockers (ARBs) are contraindicated due to teratogenicity.
- Use diuretics with caution.

EPIDEMIOLOGY

- Majority of people with CKD in stages 1–3
- African Americans are 4 times more likely to develop chronic kidney failure than Caucasians.
- Predominant sex: For the CKD stages, was similar in both sexes; however, incidence rate of end-stage renal disease (ESRD) is males 409/million > females 276/million (USRDS 2004).

Incidence

- An estimated annual incidence of CKD was 1,700/million population.
- Estimated ESRD patients by 2010: 129,200 ± 7,742 new patients; 651,330 ± 15,874 long-term ESRD; 520,240 ± 25,609 dialysis; 178,806 ± 4,349 with functioning transplants; and 95,550 ± 5,478 patients on waiting lists

Prevalence

The unadjusted prevalence and incidence rates of ESRD (stage 5) are 1,585 and 350.7/million, respectively. These numbers do not reflect the burden of earlier stages of CKD (1–40), which are estimated to affect 13.2% of the population nationwide, or 26.3 million Americans (1).

RISK FACTORS

- Type 1 or 2 diabetes mellitus (most common)
- Age >60 years
- Cardiovascular disease (e.g., hypertension [HTN] [common], renal artery stenosis)
- Acute kidney injury
- Previous kidney transplant
- Urinary tract obstruction (e.g., benign prostatic hyperplasia)
- Autoimmune disease, vasculitis/connective tissue disorder
- Family history of CKD
- Nephrotoxic drugs (lithium, salicylate, high-dose NSAIDs)
- Congenital anomalies; obstructive uropathy; renal aplasia/hypoplasia/dysplasia; reflux nephropathy
- Hyperlipidemia
- Low income/education/ethnic minority status
- Obesity/smoking
- Neoplasia

Genetics

- Alport syndrome, Fabry disease, sickle cell anemia, systemic lupus erythematosus (SLE), and autosomal-dominant polycystic kidney disease can lead to CKD.
- Polymorphisms in gene that encodes for podocyte mom muscle myosin IIA are more common in African Americans than Caucasians and appear to increase risk for nondiabetic ESRD

GENERAL PREVENTION

- Treat reversible causes: Hypovolemia, infections, diuretics, drugs (NSAIDS, aminoglycosides, IV contrast).
- Treat risk factors: Diabetes mellitus, HTN, hyperlipidemia, smoking, and obesity.
- Adjust medication doses to prevent renal toxicity.

PATHOPHYSIOLOGY

Progressive destruction of kidney nephrons; GFR will drop gradually, and plasma Cr values will approximately double with 50% reduction in GFR and 75% loss of functioning nephrons mass.

ETIOLOGY

- Renal parenchymal/glomerular:
  - Nephritic: Hematuria, red blood cell (RBC) casts, HTN, variable proteinuria:
    - Focal proliferative: IgA nephropathy, SLE, Henoch-Schöenlein purpura, Alport syndrome; proliferative glomerulonephritis; crescentic glomerulonephritis
    - Diffuse proliferative: Membranoproliferative glomerulonephritis, SLE, cryoglobulinemia, rapidly progressive glomerulonephritis (RPGN), Goodpasture syndrome
  - Nephrotic: Proteinuria (>3.5 g/d), hypoalbuminemia, hyperlipidemia, and edema:
    - Minimal change disease, membranous nephropathy, focal segmental glomerulosclerosis
    - Amyloidosis, diabetic nephropathy
- Vascular: HTN, thrombotic microangiopathies, vasculitis (Wegener), scleroderma
- Interstitial-tubular: Infections, obstruction, toxins, allergic interstitial nephritis, multiple myeloma, connective tissue disease, cystic disease
- Postrenal: Obstruction (benign prostatic hyperplasia), neoplasm, neurogenic bladder

COMMONLY ASSOCIATED CONDITIONS

HTN, diabetes mellitus, cardiovascular disease

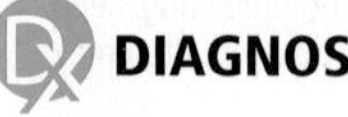

DIAGNOSIS

HISTORY

- Oliguria, nocturia, polyuria, hematuria, change in urinary frequency
- Bone disease
- Edema
- Fatigue, depression, weakness
- Pruritus
- Metallic taste in mouth, anorexia, nausea, vomiting
- Dyspnea
- Hypertension
- Poorly controlled diabetes with retinopathy, neuropathy
- Hyperlipidemia
- Claudication, restless legs

PHYSICAL EXAM

- Volume status (pallor, BP/orthostatics; edema; jugular venous distention; weight)
- Skin: Sallow complexion, uremic frost
- Ammonialike odor (uremic fetor)
- Cardiovascular: Assess for murmurs, bruits, pericarditis
- Chest: Pleural effusion
- Rectal: Enlarged prostate
- CNS: Asterixis, confusion, seizures, coma, peripheral neuropathy

DIAGNOSTIC TESTS & INTERPRETATION

Lab

Initial lab tests

- GFR can be estimated by MDRD equation:
  - GFR(mL/min/1.73 m^2) = 186 × {[serum Cr μmol/1/88.4] − 1.154} × {age (years) − 0.203} × 0.742 for females, or 1.21 for males
- Cr clearance (CrCl) can be calculated using Cockroft-Gault formula:
  - CrCl (male) = ([140 − age] × weight(kg)/(serum Cr × 72)
  - CrCl (female) = CrCl (male) × 0.82
- Urine analysis:
  - Urine microscopy: White blood cell/RBC casts, dysmorphic RBCs
  - Urine electrolytes: Sodium, Cr, urea (if on loop diuretics)
  - Proteinuria/albuminuria:
    - 24-hour urine collection: >20–200 μg/min
    - Spot urine sample: >30–300 mg/L
    - Albumin/Cr ratio (ACR): ≥3.5 mg/mmol (females); 2.5 mg/mmol (males)
- Hematology:
  - Normochromic, normocytic anemia, increased bleeding time

- Chemistry:
  - Elevated BUN, Cr, hyperkalemia
  - Increased parathyroid hormone, decreased 25-(OH) vitamin D
  - Hypocalcemia, hyperphosphatemia
  - Hyperlipidemia
  - Metabolic acidosis
  - Decreased albumin

ALERT

Drugs that may alter lab result:

- Cimetidine: Inhibits Cr secretion
- Trimethoprim: Inhibits Cr secretion
- Cefoxitin and flucytosine: Increases serum Cr
- Diltiazem and verapamil: Have significant antiproteinuric effects in patients with >300 mg/d of proteinuria

Follow-Up & Special Considerations

- Serology: ANA; antineutrophil cytoplasmic antibody; complements (C3, C4, CH50); anti-GBM antibodies; hepatitis B, C; and HIV screening
- If proteinuria in patient >45 years, serum and urine immunoelectrophoresis

Imaging

- Ultrasound: Small, echogenic kidneys; may see obstruction (e.g., hydronephrosis); cysts; kidneys may be enlarged with HIV and diabetic nephropathy
- Doppler ultrasound to assess for renovascular disease, thrombosis
- Noncontrast CAT scan: Obstruction; calculi; cysts; neoplasm; renal artery stenosis
- MRI/MRA; avoid gadolinium because of the risk of nephrogenic systemic fibrosis.
- Renal arteriogram for renal artery stenosis can be therapeutic (angioplasty or stenting).
- Renal scan to screen for differential function between kidneys

Diagnostic Procedures/Surgery

Biopsy: Hematuria, proteinuria, acute/progressive renal failure, nephritic or nephrotic syndrome

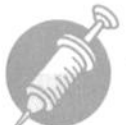

TREATMENT

MEDICATION

- Hypertension: Goal is BP <130/80 (in nonhemodialysis patients) and <150/90 (in patients on hemodialysis):
  - ACE inhibitors or ARBs for BP control and antiproteinuric effect:
    - Potential for hyperkalemia
    - Can tolerate up to 30% rise in serum Cr unless hyperkalemia develops
    - If goal not reached, add diuretic (thiazides, then loop diuretic), followed by diltiazem or verapamil or a β-blocker
    - Aldosterone antagonists for antiproteinuric effect; hyperkalemia potential
- Secondary hyperparathyroidism:
  - Cinacalcet, paricalcitol (decrease PTH levels)
  - Recommended serum phosphate maintenance levels for CKD patients (2)

Stage	mg/dL	mmol/L
Normal range *may vary by institution*	2.5–4.5	0.81–1.45
Stage 3 and 4 CKD (not on dialysis)	2.7–4.6	0.87–1.49
Stage 5 and ALL stages on dialysis	3.0–5.0	1.13–1.78

  - Stages 3–5 CKD (not on dialysis): Restrict dietary phosphate to 900 mg/d :
    - Calcium-containing phosphate binders (with meals): Calcium carbonate, calcium acetate—risk of hypercalcemia
    - Noncalcium phosphate binders (to be taken with meals): Sevelamer, lanthanum
    - Vitamin D: Inactive vitamin D 25 (ergocalciferol or cholecalciferol), calcitriol (active vitamin D 1,25 [OH]):
      - Vitamin D may increase absorption of phosphate by intestines and should not be started until serum phosphate concentration is controlled.
- Anemia: Ferrous sulfate, erythropoietin:
  - Indication: Start when Hgb <10 g/dL; goal range 11–12 g/dL—not to exceed 13 g/dL
- Hyperlipidemia: Statins
- Glycemic control: Goal HbA1c <7; avoid metformin due to the risk of metabolic acidosis.
- Metabolic acidosis: Start treatment when bicarb <20 mEq/L; goal >23 mEq/L:
  - Sodium bicarbonate: Daily dose of 0.5–1 mEq/kg/d
  - Sodium citrate: Should be avoided in patients taking aluminum-containing antacid

ADDITIONAL TREATMENT

General Measures

- Minimize radiocontrast exposure; prehydrate; N-acetylcysteine use is controversial.
- Renal replacement: Prepare for dialysis or transplant when GFR <30 mL/min/1.73 m^2.
- Vaccines: Pneumococcal; influenza
- Encourage smoking cessation.
- Encourage weight loss (if applicable).
- Limit alcohol consumption.

Issues for Referral

- Nephrology consultation early to slow progression
- If GFR <15 immediate referral; 15 < GFR < 29 urgent referral; 30 < GFR < 59 routine referral in presence of risk factors; 60 < GFR < 89 no referral required unless other problem present

SURGERY/OTHER PROCEDURES

Placement of dialysis access or transplantation for ESRD

IN-PATIENT CONSIDERATIONS

Admission Criteria

Uremia: Nausea/vomiting, fluid overload, pericarditis, uremic encephalopathy, resistant hypertension, hyperkalemia, metabolic acidosis, hyperphosphatemia (consider dialysis)

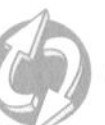

ONGOING CARE

DIET

Nutrition consult for CKD diet:

- For GFR <60 mL/min/1.73 m^2, assess protein intake; important to maintain adequate nutrition.
- Restricted intake of phosphates
- Sodium restriction
- Potassium restriction if hyperkalemic

PATIENT EDUCATION

National Kidney Federation patient Web site at: http://www.kidney.org/patients

PROGNOSIS

Patients with CKD gradually progress to ESRD.

COMPLICATIONS

HTN, anemia, 2° hyperparathyroidism, renal osteodystrophy, sleep disturbances, infections, malnutrition, electrolyte imbalances, platelet dysfunction/bleeding, pseudogout, gout, metabolic calcification, sexual dysfunction

REFERENCES

1. Coresh J, Selvin E, Stevens LA, et al. Prevalence of chronic kidney disease in the United States. *JAMA*. 2007;298:2038–47.
2. KDIGO Clinical Practice guidelines for the diagnosis, evaluation, and treatment of chronic kidney disease-mineral and bone disorder (CKD-MBD). *Kidney Int*. 2009;76(Suppl 113):S1.

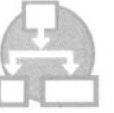

See Also (Topic, Algorithm, Electronic Media Element)

- Hydronephrosis; Nephrotic Syndrome; Polycystic Kidney Disease; Proteinuria
- Algorithm: Anuria or Oliguria

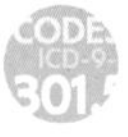

CODES

ICD9

- 585.1 Chronic kidney disease, Stage I
- 585.2 Chronic kidney disease, Stage II (mild)
- 585.9 Chronic kidney disease, unspecified

CLINICAL PEARLS

- Patient education is important in slowing the progression of CKD.
- Maintaining BP <130/80 is crucial (in patients not on dialysis).
- Prevent and treat reversible causes of renal dysfunction.

CHRONIC OBSTRUCTIVE PULMONARY DISEASE AND EMPHYSEMA

Alan J. Cropp, MD

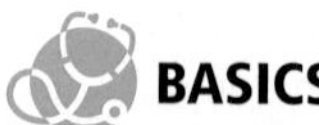

BASICS

DESCRIPTION

- Chronic obstructive pulmonary disease (COPD) encompasses several diffuse pulmonary diseases, including chronic bronchitis, asthma, cystic fibrosis, bronchiectasis, and emphysema:
  - The term usually describes a mixture of chronic bronchitis and emphysema.
  - Characterized by airflow limitation that is not fully reversible, is progressive, and is inflamed (1,2,3)
- Chronic bronchitis is defined clinically by increased mucus production and recurrent cough present on most days for at least 3 months during at least 2 consecutive years.
- Emphysema is the destruction of interalveolar septa; it occurs in the distal or terminal airways and involves both airways and lung parenchyma.

EPIDEMIOLOGY

Incidence

Affects ~10–20% of adults; >100,000 deaths/year in US

Prevalence

- 14 million people have chronic bronchitis; 2 million people have emphysema.
- Fourth leading cause of death in US

RISK FACTORS

- Smoking
- Passive smoking, especially adults whose parents smoked
- Cannabis use (1 joint is equivalent to 2.5–5 cigarettes) (4)
- Severe viral pneumonia early in life
- Aging
- Alcohol consumption
- Airway hyperactivity
- Pollution (indoor such as heating or outdoor) (4)

Genetics

- Chronic bronchitis is not a genetic disorder.
- Antiprotease deficiency (due to α_1 antitrypsin deficiency) is an inherited, rare disorder due to 2 autosomal-codominant alleles.

GENERAL PREVENTION

- Avoidance of smoking is the most important preventive measure.
- Early detection through pulmonary function tests (PFTs) in high-risk patients may be useful in preserving remaining lung function.

PATHOPHYSIOLOGY

- Impaired gas (CO_2 and O_2) exchange
- Chronic bronchitis: Airway obstruction (1)
- Emphysema: Destruction of lung parenchyma

ETIOLOGY

Cigarette and/or cannabis smoking, air pollution, antiprotease deficiency (α_1 antitrypsin), occupational exposure (firefighters), infection possibly (viral), occupational pollutants (cadmium, silica)

COMMONLY ASSOCIATED CONDITIONS

- Pulmonary: Lung cancer, chronic respiratory failure, acute bronchitis, sleep apnea
- Cardiac: Coronary artery disease
- Ear, nose, and throat (ENT): Chronic sinusitis, laryngeal carcinoma
- Miscellaneous: Malnutrition, osteoporosis, muscle dysfunction, depression

DIAGNOSIS

HISTORY

- Patient's habits with regard to tobacco should be discussed. Also review possible causes of exacerbation (e.g., recent infection) and history of cough, sputum, and dyspnea (1).
- Chronic bronchitis: Cough, sputum production, frequent infections, intermittent dyspnea, wheeze, hemoptysis, morning headache, pedal edema
- Emphysema: Minimal cough, scant sputum, dyspnea, weight loss, occasional infections

PHYSICAL EXAM

- Rarely diagnostic for COPD (3)
- Chronic bronchitis: Cyanosis, wheezing, weight gain, diminished breath sounds, distant heart sounds
- Emphysema: Barrel chest, minimal wheezing, accessory muscles used, pursed lip breathing, cyanosis slight or absent, breath sounds diminished

DIAGNOSTIC TESTS & INTERPRETATION

Lab

Initial lab tests

- Chronic bronchitis:
  - Arterial blood gases (ABGs) may show hypercapnia and hypoxia.
  - Hemoglobin may be increased.
- Emphysema:
  - Normal serum hemoglobin or polycythemia
  - Normal $PaCO_2$ on ABGs unless forced expiratory volume in 1 second (FEV1) <1 L, in which case it can be elevated.
  - Mild hypoxia

Follow-Up & Special Considerations

- Consider checking continuous overnight oximetry in selected patients.
- α_1-antitrypsin screening for those with COPD who are <45 years old or have a blood relative with this disease

Imaging

Initial approach

- Chronic bronchitis chest x-ray (CXR): Increased bronchovascular markings and cardiomegaly
- Emphysema CXR: Small heart, hyperinflation, flat diaphragms, and possibly bullous changes

Follow-Up & Special Considerations

Chest CT may show diffuse bullous changes or upper lobe predominance.

Diagnostic Procedures/Surgery

- PFTs:
  - Not indicated during acute exacerbation
  - Decreased FEV_1 and resulting reduction in FEV_1/FVC (forced vital capacity) ratio
  - Poor or absent reversibility to bronchodilator
  - Normal or reduced FVC
  - Normal or increased total lung capacity
  - Increased residual volume and functional residual capacity
  - Diffusing capacity is normal or reduced.
- Nocturnal oximetry

Pathological Findings

- Chronic bronchitis: Bronchial mucous gland enlargement, increased number of secretory cells in surface epithelium, thickened small airways from edema and inflammation, smooth muscle hyperplasia, mucus plugging, bacterial colonization of airways
- Emphysema: Entire lung affected, bronchi usually clear of secretions, anthracotic pigment, alveoli enlarged with loss of septa, cartilage atrophy, bullae

DIFFERENTIAL DIAGNOSIS

- Asthma
- Bronchiectasis
- Lung cancer
- Acute viral infection
- Normal aging of lungs
- Occupational asthma
- Chronic pulmonary embolism
- Sleep apnea
- Primary alveolar hypoventilation
- Chronic sinusitis
- Reactive airways dysfunction syndrome
- Congestive heart failure (CHF)
- Bronchiolitis obliterans
- Gastroesophageal reflux disease

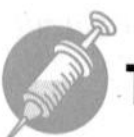

TREATMENT

MEDICATION

Medications help to reduce symptoms and exacerbations (3) and may prevent progression of disease (5,6)[A].

First Line

- Patients should have a short-acting β-agonist (Albuterol) to use as a rescue drug if necessary.
- Anticholinergics (2)[A]:
  - Ipratropium (Atrovent), tiotropium (Spiriva): 1 inhalation daily (7)[A]

AND/OR

- Long-acting β-agonists:
  - Salmeterol (Serevent), formoterol (Foradil), 1 inhalation q12h; or arformoterol (Brovana), formoterol (Perforomist), nebulized q12h (7)[A]

Second Line

- Trial of inhaled corticosteroids for moderate or severe disease (5)[A]; 10–20% of patients may have salutary response. Discontinue if no benefit in symptoms or objective measures in 6–8 weeks:
  - May initiate earlier if suggestion of asthmatic component to disease
  - Systemic corticosteroids; prednisone (Deltasone) can be given orally 7.5–15 mg/d
  - Consider pulse dosing (40 mg/d) with taper depending on length of therapy. Most useful in bronchitis with some reversibility (1)[A].
  - Among patients with COPD, inhaled corticosteroid use for at least 24 weeks is associated with a significantly increased risk of serious pneumonia, without a significantly increased risk of death (8)[A].
- Theophylline (1)[A]: 400 mg/d; increase by 100–200 mg in 1–2 weeks, if necessary:
  - Reduce dosage in patients with impaired renal or liver function, age >55, or CHF.
  - Monitor serum level. Therapeutic range is 8–13 μg/mL (1)[A].
- Combination of inhaled corticosteroid, long-acting β-agonist, and anticholinergic indicated for severe disease (7)[A]

- Mucolytic agents may improve secretions but do not improve outcomes.
- Low-dose macrolides (clarithromycin, azithromycin, or erythromycin) to decrease inflammation (9)[A]
- α1-antitrypsin, if deficient: 60 mg/kg weekly to maintain level exceeding 80 mg/dL
- Precautions:
  – Sympathomimetics: Excessive use may be dangerous. May need to reduce dosage or use levalbuterol (Xopenex) in patients with cardiovascular disease, hypertension (HTN), hyperthyroidism, diabetes, or convulsive disorders.
  – Anticholinergics: Narrow-angle glaucoma, benign prostatic hyperplasia, bladder-neck obstruction
  – Corticosteroids: Multiple potential side effects including masked infection, worsening diabetes (see manufacturer's insert)
- Sympathomimetics may be aerosolized.
- Anticholinergics: Ipratropium (Atrovent) may be aerosolized or combined with albuterol (Combivent).

ADDITIONAL TREATMENT

General Measures

- Smoking cessation: This is the most important intervention to decrease risk (3).
- Mucolytic agents
- Aggressive treatment of infections (3)[A]
- Treat any reversible bronchospasm.
- Home oxygen: May improve survival in hypoxemia and cor pulmonale, and should be initiated early in these conditions if oxygen <89% (9)[A]
- Influenza and pneumococcal immunizations

Issues for Referral

Severe exacerbation, frequent hospitalizations, age <40, rapid progression, weight loss, severe disease, or surgical evaluation

Additional Therapies

- Adequate hydration and pulmonary hygiene
- Consider postural drainage, flutter valve, or other devices to assist mucus clearance.
- Pulmonary rehabilitation may be of benefit (10).
- Intermittent noninvasive ventilation may help with severe chronic respiratory failure (5)[A]
- A short course of antibiotics (5 days) for acute exacerbations is as effective and safer than longer courses of antibiotics (11)[A].

SURGERY/OTHER PROCEDURES

- Lung reduction surgery (selected cases)
- Lung transplantation (selected cases)

IN-PATIENT CONSIDERATIONS

Initial Stabilization

- Outpatient treatment is usually adequate.
- Supplemental oxygen and short-acting bronchodilators should be given in the emergency room (3)[A].
- Acute respiratory failure may require intensive care unit and mechanical ventilation.
- A short course of antibiotics for change in sputum volume, purulence, and increased dyspnea (4)[B]

Admission Criteria

- Exacerbation with acute decompensation (hypoxemia, hypercarbia) due to infection
- Potential need for mechanical ventilation
- Serious comorbidities, such as decompensated CHF

Nursing

- Teach proper inhaler use.
- Monitor fluid balance.

Discharge Criteria

- Not waking at night due to dyspnea (3)
- Ability to ambulate
- Patient should have adequate gas exchange.
- Hypoxia can be treated with home O_2 (may only be temporary) (2)[A].
- Inhaled β-agonist therapy no more frequently than q4h (3).

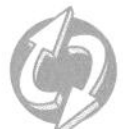

ONGOING CARE

FOLLOW-UP RECOMMENDATIONS

- May taper oral steroids as outpatient
- If pneumonia caused exacerbation, need to follow CXR until clear.
- Pulmonary rehabilitation will help to improve muscle function

Patient Monitoring

- Severe or unstable patients should be seen monthly. When stable, see every 6 months.
- Check theophylline level with dose adjustment, then check every 6–12 months.
- With home O_2, check ABGs yearly or with change in condition. Monitor O_2 saturation (pulse oximetry) more frequently.
- Some patients only desaturate at night, thus only need nocturnal O_2.
- Avoid travel at high altitude.
- Discuss advance directive and health care proxy.
- Yearly PFTs

DIET

A high-protein diet is suggested. Decreased carbohydrates may benefit those with hypercarbia.

PATIENT EDUCATION

Printed material available from National Jewish Hospital in Denver, CO. The local branch of American Lung Association also has informational material.

PROGNOSIS

- Patient's age and postbronchodilator FEV_1 are the most important predictors of prognosis. Young age and FEV_1 >50% predicted to have a good prognosis. Older patients do worse.
- Supplemental O_2, when indicated, is shown to increase survival (may only need at night).
- Smoking cessation improves prognosis.
- Malnutrition, cor pulmonale, hypercapnia, and pulse >100 indicate a poor prognosis.

COMPLICATIONS

- Malnutrition, poor sleep quality, infections, secondary polycythemia
- Acute or chronic respiratory failure, bullous lung disease, pneumothorax
- Arrhythmias, cor pulmonale, pulmonary HTN

REFERENCES

1. Braman SS. Chronic cough due to chronic bronchitis: ACCP evidence-based clinical practice guidelines. *Chest*. 2006;129:104S–15S.
2. Celli BR. Update on the management of COPD. *Chest*. 2008;133:1451–62.
3. Wilt TJ, Niewoehner D, MacDonald R. Management of stable chronic obstructive pulmonary disease: A systematic review for a clinical practice guideline. *Ann Intern Med*. 2007;147:639–53.
4. Abdool-Gaffar MS, Ambaram A, et al. Guideline for the management of chronic obstructive pulmonary disease-2011 update. *S Afr Med J*. 2011;101:61–73.
5. Maclay JD, Rabinovich RA, MacNee W. Update in chronic obstructive pulmonary disease 2008. *Am J Respir Crit Care Med*. 2009;179:533–41.
6. Rubins JB, Raci E, Kunisaki KM. Managing stable COPD in 2009: Incorporating results from recent clinical studies into a goal-directed approach for clinicians. *Postgrad Med*. 2009;121:104–12.
7. Rabe KF, Hurd S, Anzueto A. Global strategy for the diagnosis, management, and prevention of chronic obstructive pulmonary disease: GOLD executive summary. *Am J Respir Crit Care Med*. 2007;176:532–55.
8. Singh S, Amin AV, Loke YK. Long-term use of inhaled corticosteroids and the risk of pneumonia in chronic obstructive pulmonary disease: A meta-analysis. *Arch Intern Med*. 2009;169:219–29.
9. Cosio BG, Agustí A. Update in chronic obstructive pulmonary disease 2009. *Am J Respir Crit Care Med*. 2010;181:655–60.
10. Casaburi R, ZuWallack R. Pulmonary rehabilitation for management of chronic obstructive pulmonary disease. *N Engl J Med*. 2009;360:1329–35.
11. Anzueto A. Short-course fluoroquinolone therapy in exacerbations of chronic bronchitis and COPD. *Resp Med*. 2010;104:1396–403.

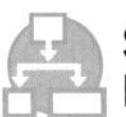

See Also (Topic, Algorithm, Electronic Media Element)

- Bronchitis, Acute
- Algorithms: Clubbing; Cyanosis

CODES

ICD9

- 492.8 Other emphysema
- 493.20 Chronic obstructive asthma, unspecified
- 496 Chronic airway obstruction, not elsewhere classified

CLINICAL PEARLS

- Screening PFTs should be done on all high-risk patients.
- Check overnight oximetry when daytime saturation is borderline.
- Influenza and pneumococcal vaccines should be kept up to date.

CHRONIC PAIN MANAGEMENT: AN EVIDENCE-BASED APPROACH

Jennifer Reidy, MD

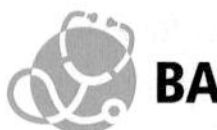

BASICS

- Chronic pain is pain persisting beyond the time of normal tissue healing, usually >3 months.
- Over time, neuroplastic changes in the CNS transform pain into a chronic disease itself. Pain levels can exceed observed pathology on exam or imaging.
- Pain experience is inherently related to emotional, psychological, and cognitive factors.
- An epidemic of undertreated pain coexists with an epidemic of prescription drug abuse in the US.

EPIDEMIOLOGY

Incidence

Incidence is rising, but exact rate is unclear. The annual economic cost of chronic pain in the US is estimated at $560–635 billion (1).

Prevalence

In the US, an estimated 116 million adults live with chronic pain—more than the total affected by heart disease, cancer, and diabetes combined.

RISK FACTORS

- Traumatic: Motor vehicle accidents, repetitive-motion injuries, sports injuries, work-related injuries, falls
- Postsurgical: Any surgery, but especially back surgeries, amputations, thoracotomies
- Medical conditions: See "Commonly Associated Conditions" below.
- Psychiatric comorbidities: Substance abuse, depression, posttraumatic stress disorder (PTSD), personality disorders
- Aging: Increased incidence with age, but should not be considered a "normal" part of aging

Genetics

Current research suggests genetic polymorphism in opioid receptors, which may affect patient's response and/or side effects to individual opioids.

GENERAL PREVENTION

- Avoidance of work-related injuries through the use of ergonomically correct workplace design
- Exercise and physical therapy to help prevent work-related low back pain
- Varicella vaccine and rapid treatment of shingles to lower risk of postherpetic neuralgia
- Tight glycemic control for diabetic patients, alcohol cessation for alcoholics, smoking cessation

PATHOPHYSIOLOGY

With intense, repeated, or prolonged stimulation of damaged or inflamed tissues, the threshold for activating primary afferent pain fibers is lowered, the frequency of firing is higher, and there is increased response to noxious and/or normal stimuli (central sensitization). The amygdala, prefrontal cortex, and cortex are thought to relay emotions and thoughts that create the pain experience, and these areas may undergo structural and functional changes with chronic pain.

ETIOLOGY

Many patients have an identifiable etiology (most commonly musculoskeletal problems or headache), but pain levels can be worse than observable tissue injury. A significant percentage of patients have no obvious cause of chronic pain.

COMMONLY ASSOCIATED CONDITIONS

Any chronic disease and/or its treatment can cause chronic pain, including diabetes, cardiovascular disease, HIV, progressive neurologic conditions, lung disease, cirrhosis, autoimmune disease, cancer, renal failure, depression, and mental illness.

DIAGNOSIS

Chronic pain can be divided into 3 general categories:

- Nociceptive pain (2 types):
  - Somatic: Skin, bone, soft tissue disease; described as well localized, sharp, stabbing, aching
  - Visceral: Visceral inflammation/injury; described as poorly localized, dull, aching; may refer to sites remote from lesion
- Neuropathic pain: Damaged peripheral or central nerves; described as burning, tingling, and/or numbness.
- Sympathetically mediated pain: Peripheral nerve injury can cause severe burning pain, swelling of the affected limb, and focal changes in sweat production and skin appearance. Example: Complex regional pain syndrome.

HISTORY

- Obtain pain history: Location, onset, severity, duration, quality, temporal pattern, exacerbators, alleviators, prior treatments
- Assess and document how pain affects patient's functioning and quality of life, and what they expect from treatment.
- Screen for personal or family history of substance abuse (including tobacco addiction), mental health conditions, domestic violence, or sexual abuse.
- Screening: A single question: "How many times in the past year have you used an illegal drug or used a prescription medication for nonmedical reasons?": In primary care setting, resulted in sensitivity of 100% and specificity of ~75%
- Use standardized tools: Pain severity—Brief Pain Inventory (short form); mood—Patient Health Questionnaire-9 (PHQ-9); substance abuse—Screener and Opioid Assessment for Patients with Pain (SOAPP), multiple versions

PHYSICAL EXAM

Exam is guided by history, and should include functional and mental assessments.

DIAGNOSTIC TESTS & INTERPRETATION

Lab

Testing is based on differential diagnosis of pain syndrome to elucidate etiology.

Initial lab tests

If suspect substance abuse, order urine drug screen. Most tests are immunoassays, which usually detect morphine and heroin but often not other opioids. Laboratory-based chromatography/spectrometry can identify specific drugs. Clinicians should be aware of uses and limitations of local laboratory testing (http://www.aafp.org/afp/2010/0301/p635.html).

Follow-Up & Special Considerations

If patient taking chronic opioid therapy, order random urine drug screens as part of the "universal precautions" approach (see "Ongoing Care").

Diagnostic Procedures/Surgery

- Consider interventional pain clinic for facet joint injections, nerve root blocks, sacroiliac joint injection, or intrathecal trial.
- If complex regional pain syndrome is suspected, a sympathetic block can be diagnostic and possibly prevent chronic pain.

DIFFERENTIAL DIAGNOSIS

- The causes of pain are numerous and clinic presentations are protean, depending on the individual patient.
- There is a spectrum of aberrant drug-taking behaviors, and differential diagnosis includes:
  - Inadequate analgesia ("pseudoaddiction"), disease progression, opioid-resistant pain, opioid-induced hyperalgesia, addiction, opioid tolerance, self-medication of nonpain symptoms, criminal intent (diversion)

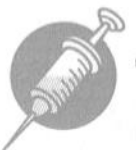

TREATMENT

- Goals of treatment are pain relief and restoring function, while balancing risks and benefits of therapies.
- Intradisciplinary teams offer most effective approach to chronic pain, including its physical, emotional, and psychological aspects. These teams may include the patient, family, primary care doctor, pain management specialist, psychologist, psychiatrist, physical and occupational therapists, physiatrist, complementary medicine practitioners, and (if needed) addiction medicine specialist.
- Treatment should always include nonpharmacologic therapies such as exercise, yoga, patient and family education, massage, transcutaneous electrical nerve stimulation (TENS), relaxation techniques, cognitive behavioral therapies, support groups, meditation, and acupuncture.

MEDICATION

Sequential time-limited trials of medications, starting at low doses and gradually increasing until either effect or dose-limiting side effects are reached. Rational polypharmacy may be indicated (such as an opioid + neuropathic agent):

- For mild-to-moderate chronic pain:
  - Acetaminophen: Daily dose not to exceed total 4 g in healthy adults and 2 g in the elderly or those with hepatic disease or active or past history of alcohol use
  - NSAIDs: Patients taking aspirin for cardiovascular protection should avoid the added GI toxicity of NSAIDs. Cox-2 selective inhibitors should be used with caution because of cardiac risks.
  - "Weak" opioids, including codeine, hydrocodone, and tramadol. Caution: Opioid-analgesic combinations can lead to serious acetaminophen or NSAID toxicities if patients exceed safely prescribed doses.
  - Avoid tramadol and propoxyphene in elderly or patients at risk for seizures.
  - Topical agents: NSAIDs, lidocaine, ketamine, capsaicain

- For neuropathic pain:
  - Classes of medications include: (i) tricyclic, SSRI, and selective serotonin-norepinephrine reuptake inhibitor (SSNRI) antidepressants; (ii) anticonvulsants; (iii) antiarrhythmics; (iv) opioids, particularly methadone. Example: Combination of amitriptyline or duloxetine + gabapentin.
  - See "Neuropathic Pain" topic.
- For moderate-to-severe chronic pain:
  - Strong opioids, including morphine, oxycodone, hydromorphone, oxymorphone, fentanyl. Check opioid equianalgesic tables for dosing by route of administration. Note: No evidence supports any of these strong opioids as superior or having improved side-effect profile. Morphine should be avoided in patients with significant renal insufficiency:
    - Methadone: The only opioid that also acts as N-methyl-D-aspartate receptor antagonist; may be uniquely effective in neuropathic pain. Methadone has many drug interactions, and it is easy to cause overdose. Methadone can contribute to potentially fatal cardiac arrhythmias. To find mentor for prescribing methadone for pain, see Physician Clinical Support System (www.pcssmentor.org).
    - Buprenorphine: A mixed opioid agonist and antagonist; growing interest for pain management but complicated pharmacology
  - Once stable dose of opioids is established, change to sustained-release formulations. Short-acting formulations only for breakthrough or episodic pain.
  - Common side effects: Constipation: Senna and docusate should be prescribed at time opioids are started. Also: Nausea, sedation, mental status changes, pruritus.

ALERT
Patients on chronic opioid therapy must agree to monitoring. Clinicians should use "universal precautions" and systems-based practice, including written agreements, random urine drug screens, pill/patch counts, and other measures (see "Ongoing Care").

ADDITIONAL TREATMENT

General Measures

Keep a "pain diary" to record pain, better or worse, and how much medication is taken.

COMPLEMENTARY AND ALTERNATIVE MEDICINE

- Acupuncture: Efficacy in chronic neck, back pain, and fibromyalgia
- Exercise: Efficacy in low back pain and fibromyalgia
- Improved mood and coping skills with behavioral and cognitive-behavioral therapies (CBT). CBT may also decrease disability from chronic pain.
- Mind–body interventions: Yoga, tai chi, hypnosis, progressive muscle relaxation
- Children with chronic headaches, abdominal pain, etc: Biofeedback, CBT, hypnosis, and relaxation exercises

SURGERY/OTHER PROCEDURES

Consider interventional procedures, including joint injections, nerve blocks, ablative procedures, and spinal cord stimulation among others, as needed.

ONGOING CARE

FOLLOW-UP RECOMMENDATIONS

Patient Monitoring

- It can be difficult to identify appropriate pain-relief seeking behavior from inappropriate drug-seeking, but consistent patient–clinician relationships over time can often discern the difference.
- Always maintain a risk–benefit stance and avoid judging a patient.
- At each visit, assess and document benefits, pain levels, functioning, and quality of life. In general, patients successfully taking opioids for pain become more engaged (better relationships and productive work).
- At each visit, assess and document harm, using "universal precautions" approach. This systems-based practice includes:
  - Informed consent for opioid therapy
  - Written or electronic agreement between patient and clinician (sample at http://www.ohsu.edu/ahec/pain/med_contractlf.pdf)
  - 1 prescribing clinician (or designee) and 1 pharmacy
  - No after-hours prescriptions or early refills
  - Mandatory police reports for medication thefts
  - Random urine drug tests, pill/patch counts
  - Requirements for patient to continue with physical therapy, counseling, psychiatric medications, or other necessary treatments
  - Participate in state's prescription drug monitoring program: See www.pmpalliance.org
  - Taper and discontinue medications if patient does not benefit, if side effects outweigh benefits, or if medications are abused or diverted. If addiction suspected, always offer treatment for substance abuse (2).

PATIENT EDUCATION

American Chronic Pain Association: http://www.theacpa.org

COMPLICATIONS

Rate of addiction in chronic pain patients is unclear (3–19% in published literature), but may reflect rate in the general population. Definitions:

- Addiction: Impaired control over drug use, compulsive use, and continued use despite harm. Taking drug for nonprescribed reasons.
- Physical dependence: Withdrawal syndrome produced by abrupt cessation or rapid dose reduction; is not addiction but a physiologic phenomenon
- Tolerance: State of adaptation when a drug induces changes that diminish 1 or more of its effects over time
- Diversion: Selling drugs or giving them to persons other than for whom they are prescribed

ALERT
Caution: From 1999–2007, the rate of unintentional overdose death increased by 124%, largely due to prescription opioid overdoses (especially methadone). However, the absolute risk of opioid overdose appears low (0.04% in 155,434 Veterans Administration patients treated with opioids) (3).

REFERENCES

1. Institute of Medicine, Committee on Advancing Pain Research, Care and Education. Relieving Pain in America: A Blueprint for Transforming Prevention, Care, Education and Research. Washington, DC: The National Academies Press; 2011.
2. Chou R, Fanciullo GJ, Fine PG, et al. Clinical guidelines for the use of chronic opioid therapy in chronic noncancer pain. *J Pain*. 2009;10:113–30.
3. Bohnert AS, Valenstein M, Bair MJ, et al. Association between opioid prescribing patterns and opioid overdose-related deaths. *JAMA* 2011; 305(13):1315–21.

C

ADDITIONAL READING

- American Society of Anesthesiologists Task Force on Chronic Pain Management, American Society of Regional Anesthesia and Pain Medicine, et al. Practice guidelines for chronic pain management: an updated report by the American Society of Anesthesiologists Task Force on Chronic Pain Management and the American Society of Regional Anesthesia and Pain Medicine. *Anesthesiology*. 2010;112:810–33.
- Federation of State Medical Boards of the United States, Inc. Model Policy for the Use of Controlled Substances for the Treatment of Pain: www.painpolicy.wisc.edu/domestic/model04.pdf
- Passik SD. Issues in long-term opioid therapy: Unmet needs, risks and solutions. *Mayo Clin Proc*. 2009;84(7):593–601.

CODES

ICD9

- 338.21 Chronic pain due to trauma
- 338.22 Chronic post-thoracotomy pain
- 338.29 Other chronic pain

CLINICAL PEARLS

- Start with the presumption the patient's pain is *real*, even if pathophysiological evidence for it cannot be found.
- Emphasize that being pain-free may not be possible, but that better function and quality of life can be shared goals.
- Use "universal precautions" and systems-based practice to safely and effectively prescribe opioids for chronic pain.

CIRRHOSIS OF THE LIVER

Najmul H. Siddiqui, MBBS, MD

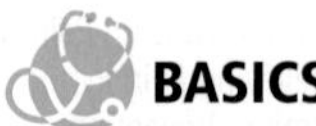

BASICS

DESCRIPTION

A chronic disease in which liver cell injury causes inflammation, necrosis, and stellate cell activation, leading to liver failure and/or cancer.

EPIDEMIOLOGY

- Predominant age: 40–50 years old
- Predominant sex: Male > Female; but more women get cirrhosis from alcohol abuse.
- Ninth leading cause of death among all US adults

RISK FACTORS

Alcohol abuse; IV drug abuse; obesity; blood transfusion

Genetics

Hemochromatosis, Wilson disease, and alpha-1-antitrypsin deficiency in adults

GENERAL PREVENTION

- Counsel patients to prevent risk factors for chronic liver disease (e.g., alcohol abuse); *more than 80% of chronic liver disease is preventable*.
- Limit alcohol consumption to <2 drinks/d and advise weight loss for obesity:
  - Raised BMI and alcohol both are linked to liver disease, with evidence of a supra-additive interaction between the 2 (1)[A].

ETIOLOGY

- Chronic hepatitis C (26%)
- Alcohol abuse (21%)
- Hepatitis C with alcohol liver disease (15%)
- Nonalcoholic steatohepatitis/obesity (~10%)
- Hepatitis B + hepatitis D infection (15%)
- Other: Hemochromatosis; autoimmune hepatitis; primary biliary cirrhosis; secondary biliary cirrhosis; primary sclerosing cholangitis; Wilson disease; alpha-1 antitrypsin deficiency; granulomatous disease (e.g., sarcoidosis); drug-induced liver disease (e.g., methotrexate, alpha methyldopa, amiodarone); venous outflow obstruction (e.g., Budd-Chiari syndrome, veno-occlusive disease); chronic right-sided heart failure; tricuspid regurgitation; and rare genetic, metabolic, and infectious causes

COMMONLY ASSOCIATED CONDITIONS

Diabetes, alcoholism, drug abuse, depression, obesity

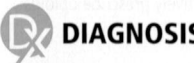

DIAGNOSIS

HISTORY

- Review risk factors (alcohol abuse, viral hepatitis; family history of primary liver cancer, other liver disease, or autoimmune disease)
- Symptoms:
  - Fatigue, malaise, weakness
  - Anorexia, weight loss (gain if ascites/edema)
  - Right upper abdominal pain
  - Absent/irregular menses
  - Diminished libido, erectile dysfunction
  - Tea-colored urine, clay-colored stools
  - Edema, abdominal swelling/bloating
  - Bruising, bleeding, hematemesis, hematochezia, melena, pruritus
  - Night blindness

PHYSICAL EXAM

Physical exam may be normal until end-stage disease:

- Skin changes: Spider angiomata, palmar erythema, jaundice, scleral icterus, ecchymoses, caput medusa, hyperpigmentation
- Hepatomegaly (small liver in end-stage disease)
- Splenomegaly if portal hypertension
- Central obesity
- Abdominal fluid wave, shifting dullness if ascites
- Gynecomastia
- Dupuytren contractures
- Pretibial, presacral pitting edema and clubbing (especially in hepatopulmonary syndrome)
- Asterixis; mental status changes
- Muscle wasting, weakness

DIAGNOSTIC TESTS & INTERPRETATION

Lab

- ALT and AST: Mildly elevated; typically AST > ALT; enzymes normalize as cirrhosis progresses
- Elevated alkaline phosphatase (ALP), gamma-glutamyl transpeptidase (GGT), and total/direct bilirubin indicates cholestasis.
- Anemia from hemolysis, folate deficiency, and splenomegaly
- Decreased platelet count from portal hypertension with splenomegaly
- Impaired synthetic liver function:
  - Low albumin and cholesterol
  - Prolonged prothrombin (PT), international normalized ratio (INR), partial thromboplastin time (PTT)
- Progressive cirrhosis:
  - Elevated ammonia level; decreased BUN, sodium, and potassium
- Alpha-fetoprotein level at diagnosis to screen for hepatocellular carcinoma (HCC)

Follow-Up & Special Considerations

To determine specific etiology, consider:

- Hepatitis B surface antigen (HBsAg), core antibody (HBcAb), and surface antibody (HBsAb)
- Hepatitis C antibody
- Serum ethanol and GGT if suspected ongoing alcohol abuse
- Antimitochondrial antibody to screen for primary biliary cirrhosis
- Antismooth muscle and antinuclear antibodies to screen for chronic active (autoimmune) hepatitis
- Iron saturation (>50%) and ferritin (markedly increased) to screen for hemochromatosis; if abnormal, check hemochromatosis (HFE) genetics/mutation analysis
- Alpha-1-antitrypsin phenotype to screen for deficiency
- Ceruloplasmin level to screen for Wilson disease; if low, check copper excretion (serum copper plus 24-hour urine copper)

Imaging

- Abdominal ultrasound (US) every 6–12 months to screen for hepatocellular carcinoma
- Doppler US of hepatic/portal veins
- MRI to clarify patency of blood vessels and collaterals; best follow-up test for HCC if alpha-fetoprotein elevated and/or liver mass found on US
- Noninvasive modalities such as elastography are being researched as an alternative to liver biopsy (2).

Diagnostic Procedures/Surgery

- Liver biopsy: Percutaneous if INR <1.5 and no ascites; otherwise, transjugular biopsy
- Liver–spleen scan to diagnose portal hypertension if patient cannot be biopsied
- Endoscopy if portal hypertension, R/O esophageal varices/portal hypertensive gastropathy (3)[C]

Pathological Findings

- Fibrosis and regenerative nodules are general features of cirrhosis on biopsy
- Other histologic findings vary with etiology:
  - Alcoholic liver disease: Steatosis, polymorphonuclear (PMN) leukocyte infiltrate, ballooning degeneration of hepatocytes, Mallory bodies, giant mitochondria
  - Chronic hepatitis B and C: Periportal lymphocytic inflammation
  - Nonalcoholic steatohepatitis (NASH): Identical to alcoholic liver disease and confirmed by history. Steatosis may be absent in advanced disease ("burned-out NASH")
  - Biliary cirrhosis: PMN infiltrate in wall of bile ducts, inflammation increased in portal spaces, progressive loss of bile ducts in portal spaces
  - Hemochromatosis: Intrahepatic iron stores increased (iron stain or weighted biopsy tissue)
  - Alpha-1-antitrypsin deficiency: Positive periodic acid-Schiff (PAS) bodies in hepatocytes

DIFFERENTIAL DIAGNOSIS

Diffuse hepatic parenchymal disease (e.g., fatty liver); other causes of portal hypertension (e.g., portal vein thrombosis, lymphoma); metastatic or multifocal cancer in the liver; vascular congestion (e.g., cardiac cirrhosis); reversible (e.g., acute alcoholic hepatitis)

TREATMENT

Outpatient care except for major GI bleeding, altered mental status, sepsis/infection, rapidly progressing hepatic decompensation, renal failure

MEDICATION

First Line

As indicated to treat the underlying cause (*note prescribing precautions in decompensated cirrhosis*):

- Hepatitis C: Goal of treatment is to eradicate HCV RNA. (See "Hepatitis C" for details.)
- Hepatitis B: Goal of treatment is to achieve HBeAg seroconversion. Lamivudine, 100 mg PO daily; adefovir, 10 mg PO daily; entecavir, 0.5–1 mg PO daily; or telbivudine, 600 mg PO daily for minimum of 1 year, or continue for at least 6 months after HBeAg seroconversion; alternatively, peginterferon alpha 2a, 180 μg SC weekly for 48 weeks
- Biliary cirrhosis: Ursodeoxycholic acid (Ursodiol) 13–15 mg/kg PO daily, indefinitely (4)[A]; bile acid sequestrants (BAS) are first-line therapy for pruritus. Rifampicin 150–300 mg b.i.d. or oral opiate antagonists such as naltrexone 50 mg daily can be used for pruritus if ursodiol is refractory.
- Wilson disease: Initial treatment with penicillamine 1,000–1,500 mg/d PO b.i.d.–q.i.d. or trientine 750-1,500 mg PO b.i.d.–t.i.d. Trientine (Syprine) is better tolerated. After 1 year, zinc acetate 75–300 mg PO b.i.d.–t.i.d. for maintenance. Zinc is a drug of choice for presymptomatic, pregnant, and pediatric populations.

- Autoimmune (chronic active) hepatitis: Prednisone 30–60 mg/d initially, maintenance 5–20 mg/d with or without azathioprine (Imuran) 0.5–1 mg/kg; adjust to keep transaminase levels normal. The combination regime is preferred. Maintenance therapy can be discontinued after at least 24 months of treatment and continued normal AST and ALT.
- Esophageal varices: Propranolol 40–160 mg or nadolol 40 mg daily, to lower portal pressure by 20 mm Hg, systolic pressure to 90–100 mm Hg, and pulse rate by 25% (3)[A].
- Ascites/edema: Low-sodium (<2 g/d) diet and spironolactone 100–400 mg daily with or without furosemide 40–160 mg PO daily; torsemide may substitute for furosemide.
- Encephalopathy: Lactulose 15 mL b.i.d., titrate to induce 3 loose bowel movements daily. Combination therapy with rifaximin (550 mg PO b.i.d.) is superior to prevent recurrent hepatic encephalopathy (5).
- Pruritus: Ursodiol and antihistamines (e.g., hydroxyzine)
- Renal insufficiency: Stop diuretics and nephrotoxic drugs, normalize electrolytes, and hospitalize for plasma expansion or dialysis.
- Prophylactic antibiotics for invasive procedures, GI bleeding, or history of spontaneous bacterial peritonitis (3)[A]
- Proton pump inhibitor for esophageal varices requiring banding or portal hypertensive gastropathy (6)[A]
- Recombinant factor VIIa to correct bleeding shows no survival benefit (7).

ADDITIONAL TREATMENT

General Measures

- Patients *must* abstain from alcohol, drugs, liver toxic medications, and herbs.
- Immunize for pneumococcal disease, hepatitis A and B, and influenza.
- NASH: Weight reduction, exercise, optimal control of lipids/glucose

Issues for Referral

Liver transplant evaluation at first onset of complications (ascites, variceal bleed, encephalopathy), jaundice, or liver lesion suggestive of hepatocellular carcinoma and/or when evidence of hepatic dysfunction develops (Child-Turcotte-Pugh >7 and MELD >10) (8)[C].

COMPLEMENTARY AND ALTERNATIVE MEDICINE

- Milk thistle (silymarin) may lower transaminases and improve symptoms.
- Hepatotoxicity and drug interactions are common with many herbal medications (9)[A].

SURGERY/OTHER PROCEDURES

- Varices: Endoscopic ligation, typically 4–6 treatments (if acute bleed, use pre-esophagogastroduodenoscopy [EGD] octreotide as vasoconstrictor); transjugular intrahepatic shunt (TIPS) second-line or salvage therapy for acute bleed (3)
- Ascites: If tense, therapeutic paracentesis every 2 weeks PRN; caution if pedal edema absent.
- Fulminant hepatic failure: Liver transplantation
- Hepatocellular carcinoma: Curable if small with radiofrequency ablation or resection and transplant

IN-PATIENT CONSIDERATIONS

Admission Criteria

Major GI bleeding, altered mental status, sepsis/infection, rapidly progressing hepatic decompensation, renal failure

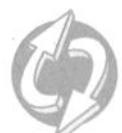

ONGOING CARE

FOLLOW-UP RECOMMENDATIONS

Regular conditioning may help fatigue.

Patient Monitoring

- Once stable, monitor liver enzymes, platelets, and PT every 6–12 months.
- Patients >55 years old with chronic hepatitis B or C, elevated INR, or low platelets are at highest risk for HCC. Check alpha-fetoprotein and liver ultrasound every 6–12 months for screening in patients with cirrhotics (7)[A].
- Endoscopy at diagnosis and every 3 years in compensated and every 1 year in decompensated cirrhotic patients to screen for varices (3)[C]

DIET

Protein (1–1.5 g/kg body weight), high fiber, daily multivitamin (without iron), and sodium (<2 g/d, essential if ascites/edema). A high-protein diet may precipitate encephalopathy, but protein restriction is no longer recommended (7). Coffee consumption has a graded and inverse association with liver cancer (10)[B].

PATIENT EDUCATION

- Educate caregivers about when to seek emergency care (e.g., hematemesis, altered mental status).
- Maintain sobriety/recovery/smoking cessation (includes no cannabis).
- Hepatitis A/B immunization and hepatitis C transmission precautions

PROGNOSIS

- At diagnosis of cirrhosis, expect 5–20 years of asymptomatic disease.
- At onset of complications, expect death within 5 years without transplant:
  - 5% per year develop HCC
  - 50% of cirrhotics develop ascites over 10 years; 50% 5-year survival if ascites develop
  - Acute variceal bleed most common fatal complication; carries 30% mortality
  - Median survival at onset decompensation (ascites, variceal bleed, encephalopathy) is 1.5 years (7).
  - With transplant, 85% survive 1 year; deaths after transplant, ~5% per year
- Fewer than 25% of eligible patients receive a transplant because of donor organ shortage.

COMPLICATIONS

Ascites; edema; infections; encephalopathy; GI bleed; esophageal varices, gastropathy, colopathy; hepatorenal syndrome; hepatopulmonary syndrome; hepatocellular carcinoma; fulminant hepatic failure; complications after transplant (e.g., surgical, rejection, infections)

REFERENCES

1. Hart CL, Morrison DS, Batty GD, et al. Effect of body mass index and alcohol consumption on liver disease: Analysis of data from two prospective cohort studies. *BMJ*. 2010;340:c1240.
2. Tsochatzis EA, Gurusamy KS, Ntaoula S, et al. Elastography for the diagnosis of severity of fibrosis in chronic liver disease: A meta-analysis of diagnostic accuracy. *J Hepatol*. 2011;54:650–9.
3. Garcia-Tsao G, Sanyal AJ, Grace ND, et al. Prevention and management of gastroesophageal varices and variceal hemorrhage in cirrhosis. *Hepatology*. 2007;46:922–38.
4. Lindor KD, Gershwin ME, Poupon R, et al. Primary biliary cirrhosis. *Hepatology*. 2009;50:291–308.
5. Sharma P, Sharma BC, et al. Rifaximin treatment in hepatic encephalopathy. *N Engl J Med*. 2010; 362:1071–81.
6. Leontiadis GI, Sharma VK, Howden CW. Proton pump inhibitor therapy for peptic ulcer bleeding: Cochrane collaboration meta-analysis of randomized controlled trials. *Mayo Clin Proc*. 2007;82(3):286–96.
7. Garcia-Tsao G. Managing the Complications of Cirrhosis, Hepatitis Annual Update 2008, Clinical Care Options Hepatitis, http://clinicaloptions.com/Hepatitis/Annual%20Updates/2008%20Annual%20Update.aspx.
8. Murray KF, Carithers RL, AASLD. AASLD practice guidelines: Evaluation of the patient for liver transplantation. *Hepatology*. 2005;41:1407–32.
9. Verma S, Thuluvath PJ, et al. Complementary and alternative medicine in hepatology: Review of the evidence of efficacy. *Clin Gastroenterol Hepatol*. 2007;5:408–16.
10. Hu G, Tuomilehto J, Pukkala E, et al. Joint effects of coffee consumption and serum gamma-glutamyltransferase on the risk of liver cancer. *Hepatology*. 2008;48:129–36.

ADDITIONAL READING

Bota S, Sporea I, Popescu A, et al. Response to standard of care antiviral treatment in patients with HCV liver cirrhosis: A systematic review. *J Gastrointestin Liver Dis*. 2011;20:293–8.

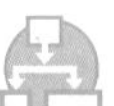

See Also (Topic, Algorithm, Electronic Media Element)

Algorithm: Cirrhosis

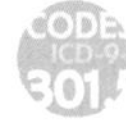

CODES

ICD9

- 571.2 Alcoholic cirrhosis of liver
- 571.5 Cirrhosis of liver without mention of alcohol

CLINICAL PEARLS

- 80% of chronic liver disease that leads to cirrhosis is preventable (primarily alcoholic).
- Check abdominal US every 6 months for early detection of hepatocellular carcinoma.

CIRRHOSIS, PRIMARY BILIARY

Lauren Michal de Leon, MD
Edward Feller, MD

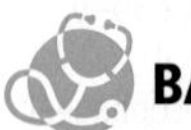

BASICS

Primary biliary cirrhosis (PBC) should be suspected in patients with unexplained pruritus or cholestatic pattern of liver enzymes.

DESCRIPTION

- PBC is a chronic immune-mediated disease that leads to fibrosis and destruction of small intrahepatic bile ducts.
- If untreated, PBC can lead to cirrhosis and possibly the need for liver transplantation.
- At diagnosis, 60% are asymptomatic.

EPIDEMIOLOGY

- PBC primarily affects women (95%).
- Peak age: 40–60 years

Prevalence

- Rare, but present universally; more common in Northern European countries and the northern US
- Prevalence ranges from 7–400 cases/million

RISK FACTORS

Smoking increases risk of disease development:

- Data also indicates that pregnancy may be a trigger for PBC; hormone replacement therapy is a possible, yet unproven precipitating factor.
- Diverse autoimmune diseases are associated with PBC.

Genetics

PBC is believed to result in individuals with susceptible genetic makeup (multiple inherited defects in immune tolerance) exposed to specific environmental triggers; concordance rate is as high as 63% in monozygotic twins.

PATHOPHYSIOLOGY

- PBC is caused by a T-cell–mediated attack on intralobular bile ducts.
- The T cells are targeted against mitochondrial antigens responsible for oxidative phosphorylation.
- The autoimmune attack is isolated to the liver for unknown reasons.
- This destruction causes cholestasis, which can lead to cirrhosis and liver failure.
- The retained bile acids from bile duct destruction leads to foamy degeneration of hepatocytes.

COMMONLY ASSOCIATED CONDITIONS

- PBC can be associated with diverse autoimmune diseases, including Sjögren syndrome, scleroderma, rheumatoid arthritis, lupus erythematosus, Hashimoto thyroiditis, and ulcerative colitis.
- Overlap syndrome with autoimmune hepatitis exists in 5–15%.

DIAGNOSIS

HISTORY

- More than 60% are asymptomatic at diagnosis, identified by incidental finding of elevated serum alkaline phosphatase (ALP), gamma-glutamyl transpeptidase (GGTP), total serum cholesterol, or investigation of an autoimmune disease such as scleroderma; unexpected hepatomegaly is present in some.
- Common complaints include:
  - Fatigue: Does not correlate with age, duration, or severity of disease
  - Pruritus: Correlates with fatigue
  - Hyperpigmentation of the skin (not jaundice)
  - Musculoskeletal complaints (often a peripheral arthropathy)
- If patient has a liver workup for other reasons, important information to obtain includes:
  - Medication history (cholestatic-causing drugs)
  - Family history of liver disease, autoimmune disorders
  - Sexual history (assess risk of hepatitis, HIV)

PHYSICAL EXAM

Physical exam findings usually correlate with severity of disease:

- Skin: Hyperpigmentation, excoriations secondary to pruritus, jaundice (late finding)
- Abdomen: Hepatosplenomegaly (may be present in asymptomatic patients), spider nevi (late)
- Evidence of decompensated portal hypertension in advanced cirrhosis (ascites, encephalopathy)
- Psych: Fatigue, depression

DIAGNOSTIC TESTS & INTERPRETATION

- Diagnostic evaluation should begin based on clinical suspicion or if liver enzymes are suspicious for cholestasis.
- The American Association for the Study of Liver Disease (AASLD) requires 2 of the 3 following for diagnosis of PBC:
  - Serum antimitochondrial antibody (AMA) positive
  - Cholestasis based on lab results
  - Histologic evidence of bile duct destruction

Lab

Initial lab tests

- Liver enzymes reflect a cholestatic picture:
  - Elevated alkaline phosphatase
  - Elevated bilirubin (more severe disease)
  - Aminotransaminase elevations, if present, are mild. If they are, causes of cholestatic hepatitis may be considered (e.g., autoimmune hepatitis, drugs, viral hepatitis).
- Antimitochondrial antibodies: Positive in 95% of those with PBC:
  - AMA-positive and AMA-negative patients have the same natural history and have same response rates to treatment.
  - AMA titers do not correlate with disease progression or response to treatment.
- Antismooth muscle antibodies: Rule out autoimmune hepatitis.
- Lipid levels: Mild elevations in low-density lipoprotein (LDL) and very low-density lipoprotein (VLDL); marked elevation in high-density lipoprotein (HDL)

Follow-Up & Special Considerations

- AMA-negative patients: Occurs in 5% with biopsy-proven PBC:
  - These patients commonly have antinuclear antibody (ANA) positivity (particularly anti-GB210 and anti-SP100) and/or antismooth muscle antibody (SMA) positivity.
- Drugs can cause a cholestatic picture that resembles PBC: Phenothiazines, synthetic androgenic steroids, trimethoprim-sulfamethoxazole, among others
- Women of childbearing age should have a pregnancy test, as symptoms can vary with pregnancy.

Imaging

- Imaging of hepatobiliary system required to rule out obstruction. Modalities include:
  - Right upper quadrant ultrasound
  - Abdominal CT
  - Magnetic resonance cholangiopancreatography (MRCP) preferred to endoscopic retrograde cholangiopancreatography (ERCP) to visualize biliary system because it is noninvasive; ERCP useful if a therapeutic intervention is considered likely (stone removal, stent placement, biopsy)
  - Esophageal ultrasound (EUS)
- If any of these modalities are negative, proceed with serologic studies as above.

Diagnostic Procedures/Surgery

- Liver biopsy is important for diagnosis and staging and should be considered if AMA is negative or aspartate aminotransferase (AST) 5× > normal.
- ERCP considered if AMA is negative or if there is suspicion of bile duct or pancreatic carcinoma

Pathological Findings

- Florid bile duct destruction is the pathognomonic finding for PBC, but is uncommon.
- Atypical bile duct hyperplasia with lymphocyte infiltration can be seen as well.

DIFFERENTIAL DIAGNOSIS

Includes, but is not limited to:

- Cholestasis secondary to medications or pregnancy; nonalcoholic steatohepatitis; alcoholic liver disease
- Other autoimmune-related hepatobiliary conditions: Autoimmune hepatitis, primary sclerosing cholangitis, etc.
- Pancreatobiliary carcinoma

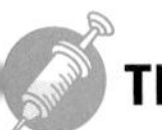

TREATMENT

MEDICATION

- Ursodeoxycholic acid (UDCA) is the only Food and Drug Administration (FDA)-approved treatment for PBC.
- Dosing: 13–15 mg/kg/d is recommended for patients with abnormal liver enzymes regardless of histologic stage.

ADDITIONAL TREATMENT

- Supplemental treatment includes symptomatic relief.
- Pruritus: Bile acid sequestrants (cholestyramine). If refractory, rifampicin 150–300 mg/d, opioid antagonist (e.g., naltrexone 50 mg daily), sertraline 75–100 mg daily can be tried.
- Fatigue: No suggested therapy. Can resolve with treatment of underlying condition or associated conditions (hypothyroidism)
- Although methotrexate may benefit other outcomes (pruritus score, serum alkaline phosphatase, IgM levels), there is no sufficient evidence to support methotrexate for patients with primary biliary cirrhosis (1)[A].
- Tetrathiomolybdate therapy in primary biliary cirrhosis shows promise, but further studies are needed (2)[A].

SURGERY/OTHER PROCEDURES

Liver transplant may be indicated for patients with progressive or nonresponsive disease and decompensated cirrhosis. Posttransplant, 5-year survival is as high as 77%; recurrent PBC post-transplant: 15% at 3 years, 30% at 5 years.

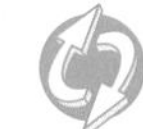

ONGOING CARE

FOLLOW-UP RECOMMENDATIONS

- Patients with PBC should be given the same counseling as patients with other liver disorders (e.g., decreased alcohol intake, weight management, smoking cessation).
- Also, pregnant women may need closer monitoring due to the increased incidence of symptoms and complications that can occur during pregnancy.

Patient Monitoring

- Liver tests every 3–6 months; monitor cholesterol
- Thyroid-stimulating hormone (TSH) annually
- Bone mineral density every 2–4 years
- Vitamin A, D, and K levels yearly
- If bilirubin >2.0, thrombocytopenia, then upper endoscopy every 1–2 years
- If cirrhosis or Mayo risk score >4.1, alpha-fetoprotein
- Ultrasound in patients with known cirrhosis

PROGNOSIS

- Varies widely between individual patients. Prognostic factors include histologic stage, UDCA therapy, bilirubin level, presence of thrombocytopenia, poor hepatic protein synthesis (albumin, prothrombin time)
- Antibodies to the nuclear rim pore protein, gp210 have shown the most promise as prognostic markers in primary biliary cirrhosis, as they have been associated with severe interface hepatitis, lobular inflammation, and progression to liver failure (3)[A].

COMPLICATIONS

- Hepatocellular carcinoma
- Portal hypertension
- Varices
- Osteopenia/osteoporosis
- Intense pruritus, fatigue

REFERENCES

1. Giljaca V, Poropat G, Stimac D, et al. Methotrexate for primary biliary cirrhosis. *Cochrane Database Syst Rev*. 2010;5:CD004385.
2. Askari F, Innis D, Dick RB, et al. Treatment of primary biliary cirrhosis with tetrathiomolybdate: Results of a double-blind trial. *Transl Res*. 2010;155:123–30.
3. Czaja AJ, et al. Autoantibodies as prognostic markers in autoimmune liver disease. *Dig Dis Sci*. 2010;55:2144–61.

ADDITIONAL READING

Lindor KD, Gershwin ME, Poupon R, et al. Primary biliary cirrhosis. *Hepatology*. 2009;50:291–308.

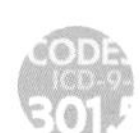

CODES

ICD9

571.6 Biliary cirrhosis

CLINICAL PEARLS

Diagnostic algorithm:

- Elevated alkaline phosphatase
- Exclude other causes of liver disease.
- Imaging to rule out obstruction
- AMA, ANA, antismooth muscle antibody titers
- Consider liver biopsy if AMA negative or AST >5× normal.

CLAUDICATION

Zarna J. Dahya, MD

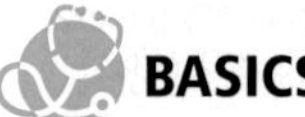

BASICS

DESCRIPTION
- Reproducible, exercise-induced cramping pain in a defined group of muscles that is relieved by rest.
- Most patients with peripheral arterial disease (PAD) have atherosclerotic disease of the lower extremity and therefore compromised blood flow most commonly felt in the calves, but it also can affect the feet, thighs, hips, and/or buttocks.
- 10–35% of patients with PAD report classic claudication symptoms.

EPIDEMIOLOGY
- Strongly associated with smoking and diabetes mellitus
- Predominant sex: Male > Female (<2:1 ratio)
- Increases progressively with age (estimated 6% in those older than 70 years)

Incidence
- Incidence is related to age: 0.07% of men 35–44 years old and 1.4% of men >65 years old develop the disease per year.
- Diabetic patients have an incidence 4–6 times greater than nondiabetic patients.

Prevalence
- 2–3% of men >60 years of age have symptomatic PAD compared with 1–2% of women of the same age.
- Noninvasive testing shows that the true prevalence of PAD is at least 5 times higher than the reported prevalence of intermittent claudication.

RISK FACTORS
- Cigarette smoking:
  - 90% of all patients with claudication
- Diabetes mellitus
- Hypertension
- Hyperlipidemia
- Family history
- Pre-existing heart disease (15% of congestive heart disease [CHD] patients have vascular disease in other beds)
- Advanced age

GENERAL PREVENTION
- Frequent walking exercises
- Smoking cessation
- Control of BP, lipids, and glucose levels

PATHOPHYSIOLOGY
- Atherosclerotic stenosis or occlusion of arterial flow diminishes BP to the muscles of an extremity.
- Symptoms generally are exacerbated by exercise when blood flow demand exceeds supply distal to the area of stenosis or occlusion and reduces tissue perfusion.

ETIOLOGY
- Usually defined by clinical history (e.g., history of atherosclerosis, migraines, vasculitis, radiation exposure, limb trauma)
- Sites affected depend upon the area of arterial supply involved: Symptoms occur distal to the area of arterial stenosis or occlusion.
- Superficial-femoral artery: Most common area associated with claudication; pain in the upper 2/3 of the calf
- Aortoiliac disease: Pain may extend from buttock to thigh (if impotence also is present, consider Leriche syndrome)
- Aortoiliac or common femoral artery: Pain in the thigh
- Popliteal artery: Pain in lower 1/3 of calf.
- Tibial or peroneal artery: Pain in the feet (if isolated foot claudication, consider thromboangiitis obliterans)
- Subclavian, axillary, and brachial disease: Pain may extend to the upper extremities.

COMMONLY ASSOCIATED CONDITIONS
- Other manifestations of atherosclerosis:
  - Myocardial infarction
  - Carotid artery occlusive disease
  - Renovascular occlusive disease
  - Hypertension
- Of all patients with PAD, 25–68% have concurrent coronary artery disease and 34–50% have a concomitant cerebrovascular disease.

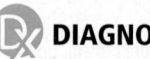

DIAGNOSIS

- Patients will limit their walking based on their symptoms (calf muscle fatigue to severe cramps and pain)
- Pain occurs at rest as PAD worsens.
- Cold feet are an early warning symptom.
- Paresthesias or numbness are later symptoms (diabetics are less likely to report pain).
- Rubor in dependent limb; leg color may darken to a dusky crimson when in a lowered position
- Nonhealing ulcer is associated with poor circulation.
- Can lead to marked limitation of daily activities

HISTORY
- Reproducible pain associated with restricted walking distance and relieved by rest.
- The Edinburgh is a questionnaire with the following criteria required for peripheral vascular disease (PVD) diagnosis (sensitivity, 99%; specificity, 91%) (1):
  - Leg pain occurs when walking.
  - Pain does not occur while standing or sitting.
  - Pain occurs while walking fast or uphill.
  - Pain resolves within 10 minutes of standing still.
- Modifiers:
  - Pain occurring even at a normal pace on level ground suggests severe claudication.
  - Classic pain location is in the calf; thigh or buttock pain without calf pain is atypical.

PHYSICAL EXAM
- Signs of PVD: Abnormal skin coloration (pallor, rubor), cool feet, atrophy of nails, prolonged capillary refill, poor wound healing over affected area. The absence of hair is not a clinical predictor of the presence of PAD.
- Diminished or absent femoral, popliteal, posterior tibial, or dorsalis pedis pulses (2)[B] with occasional bruits

DIAGNOSTIC TESTS & INTERPRETATION

Lab

Initial lab tests
- Fasting lipid panel, fasting glucose
- BP readings in both arms
- Arterial Brachial Index (ABI)
- Measuring fibrinogen and homocysteine if elevated have not led to improved outcomes, so it is not recommended.

Imaging
- Digital-subtraction angiography: The gold standard
- Contrast-enhanced magnetic resonance angiography: Highly accurate and reliable in identifying >50% stenosis (sensitivity, 95%; specificity, 97%)
- CT angiography (sensitivity 91%, specificity 91%)
- Duplex ultrasound (sensitivity, 88%; specificity, 96%) (3): Recommended initial screen to check blood flow

Diagnostic Procedures/Surgery
- The ABI is the systolic BP taken by a Doppler at the dorsalis pedis divided by the systolic pressure taken in the brachial artery: Sensitivity, 95%; specificity, 90%
- Normal value is minimally ≥1. ABI <0.9 correlates with at ≥50% stenosis of at least 1 vessel (4)[B]:
  - ABI between 0.4 and 0.9 suggests stenosis and correlates with clinical claudication.
  - ABI <0.5 suggests multisegmental arterial stenoses.
  - ABI of <0.3 correlates with probable tissue death and/or rest pain.
- Photoplethysmography is another diagnostic option to evaluate BP in the lower extremities.

DIFFERENTIAL DIAGNOSIS
- Osteoarthritis: Weight bearing worsens pain.
- Pseudoclaudication: Attributed to spinal cord impingement or spinal stenosis. Relieved by sitting or squatting:
  - Neither pseudoclaudication nor osteoarthritis affects the ABI.
- Thromboarterial occlusive disease (Buerger)
- Cystic adventitial disease
- Extraluminal compression (e.g., popliteal artery entrapment syndrome)
- Leriche syndrome: Lower extremity claudication, absence of femoral pulse, impotence, buttock muscle wasting
- Compartment syndrome
- Venous congestion

TREATMENT

- Smoking cessation (most important); aggressive blood sugar control might reduce the risk of microvascular complications; control hypertension to reduce morbidity from cardiovascular and cerebrovascular complications, and use statin therapy because it has been show in many studies to reduce disease progression:
  - HMG-CoA reductase inhibitor with a low-density lipoprotein goal of ≤100 mg/dL (≤70 for high-risk patients) (5)
- Supervised exercise rehabilitation programs are a mainstay of therapy. There was a greater benefit (walking distance) seen with this therapy than with the angioplasty at 6 months.
- Recommended exercise regimen:
  - Improve walking distance by 150% over 3–12 months.
  - Recommend treadmill walking until pain is elicited (5).
  - Then, briefly rest until symptoms subside, then resume.
  - Goal is 30–60 minutes per day, minimally 3 days per week for 3 months.

MEDICATION

First Line

- Lifelong antiplatelet therapy is recommended for patients with symptomatic disease (6):
  - Aspirin should be considered for all patients. It has no proven benefit for decreasing lower extremity claudication, but it may be beneficial as secondary prevention for coronary disease and stroke. Dose: Aspirin 75–325 mg/d PO
  - Clopidogrel (Plavix) can be used if aspirin is not tolerated. There is no evidence supporting dual antiplatelet therapy (6).
  - Aspirin plus dipyridamole has mixed benefits according to different studies.
  - Ticlopidine (Ticlid) has best evidence of efficacy, but because of its side effect profile, is not preferred.
- Cilostazol (Pletal) slightly improves maximal and pain-free walking distance. It is recommended for moderate to severe disabling intermittent claudication that is unresponsive to exercise regimens in patients who are not candidates for surgical or percutaneous intervention (6):
  - Dose: 100 mg PO b.i.d.
  - Precautions: Headache occurs in >30% of patients taking cilostazol.
  - Contraindication: Patients with symptoms of congestive heart failure
  - Significant possible drug–drug interactions: Use caution when combining with drugs metabolized by the cytochrome-P450 3A4 isoenzyme.

Second Line

- Pentoxifylline (Trental): There is conflicting evidence regarding its efficacy in improving walking distance; 400 mg PO t.i.d. (6).
- Arginine: 3 g PO t.i.d.
- Propionyl levocarnitine: 1–2 g PO b.i.d.
- Ginkgo biloba: 120–160 mg PO b.i.d.
- Vitamin E: 50 mg/d PO
- Naftidrofuryl
- Prostaglandin analogues and stimulants continue to be investigated (7).

ADDITIONAL TREATMENT

General Measures

- Eliminate risk factors whenever possible.
- Smoking cessation is critical to success and is the single most important intervention.
- Optimize diet with a low-fat and low-cholesterol regimen.
- Exercise is essential to management, significantly improving maximal walking time, distance to claudication, and calf blood flow.

COMPLEMENTARY AND ALTERNATIVE MEDICINE

Naftidrofuryl (unavailable in US; Cochrane review found clinical benefit to its use)

SURGERY/OTHER PROCEDURES

- Revascularization is reserved for a minority of patients:
  - Indications:
    - Severe claudication in which symptoms limit lifestyle or job performance
    - Unresponsive to exercise and medical management
- Angioplasty is preferred for patients with favorable anatomic features and younger patients (≤50 years old).
- Arterial bypass surgery is recommended for patients ≥50 years old or those with less certain anatomical features.
- Stenting modalities continue to be investigated (5).

ONGOING CARE

FOLLOW-UP RECOMMENDATIONS

- Recommend continued, frequent exercise.
- Consider referral to vascular surgeon or cardiologist for follow-up of unresponsive or advanced cases.
- Peripheral noninvasive vascular studies every 6 months
- Findings that suggest condition of patient is worsening are an indication for surgery.

DIET

A cardiovascular diet (low-fat, low-cholesterol) is recommended.

PATIENT EDUCATION

- Encourage an exercise program, smoking cessation, healthy dietary choices, management of blood glucose levels in diabetic patients, and BP control.
- Reassure that most patients improve walking distance over time and symptoms generally improve

PROGNOSIS

- Patients should experience gradual improvement with an intense walking program, appropriate medical therapy, as well as modification of risk factors.
- Disease progression may include pain at rest, tissue loss, and gangrene.
- Select patients may require revascularization.

COMPLICATIONS

- Severe cases can result in tissue loss and gangrene, possibly requiring amputation of affected area.
- Largely affects patients with advanced, uncontrolled diabetes mellitus.
- Risk of venous thrombosis is increased due to the low-flow state indicated by claudication.

REFERENCES

1. Leng GC, Fowkes FG. The Edinburgh Claudication Questionnaire: An improved version of the WHO/Rose Questionnaire for use in epidemiological surveys. *J Clin Epidemiol*. 1992;45:1101–9.
2. Khan NA, Rahim SA, Anand SS, et al. Does the clinical examination predict lower extremity peripheral arterial disease? *JAMA*. 2006;295: 536–46.
3. Collins R, Burch J, Cranny G, et al. Duplex ultrasonography, magnetic resonance angiography, and computed tomography angiography for diagnosis and assessment of symptomatic, lower limb peripheral arterial disease: Systematic review. *BMJ*. 2007;334:1257.
4. Feringa HHH, et al. The long-term prognostic value of the resting and postexercise ankle brachial index. *Arch Int Med*. 2006;166:529–35.
5. White C. Clinical practice. Intermittent claudication. *N Engl J Med*. 2007;356:1241–50.
6. Sobel M, Verhaeghe R. Antithrombotic therapy for peripheral artery occlusive disease: American College of Chest Physicians Evidence-Based Clinical Practice Guidelines (8th Edition). *Chest*. 2008;133:815S–843S.
7. Reiter M, Bucek RA, Stümpflen A, et al. Prostanoids for intermittent claudication. *Cochrane Database Syst Rev*. 2004:CD000986.

ADDITIONAL READING

- Brueske TJ, Macrino S, et al. Lack of lower extremity hair is not a predictor for peripheral arterial disease. *Arch Dermatol*. 2009;145:1456.
- Robless P, Mikhailidis DP, Stansby GP. Cilostazol for peripheral arterial disease. *Cochrane Database Syst Rev*. 2008:CD003748.
- Watson L, Ellis B, Leng GC. Exercise for intermittent claudication. *Cochrane Database Syst Rev*. 2008:CD000990.

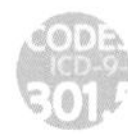

CODES

ICD9

- 440.21 Atherosclerosis of native arteries of the extremities with intermittent claudication
- 443.9 Peripheral vascular disease, unspecified

CLINICAL PEARLS

- Mainstay of treatment involves gradual increase in exercise in supervised setting and maximizing reduction of CHD risk factors: Smoking cessation, low-density lipoprotein reduction, glucose control in diabetes, and controlling BP.
- Available revascularization techniques include catheter-based balloon dilation with or without luminal stenting, endarterectomy, arterial reconstruction with an anatomically placed bypass graft, or with an extra-anatomically placed bypass prosthesis. Selection is based on patient risk, surgeon experience, and pattern of occlusions.
- Indications for revascularization are critical limb ischemia, patients with repeated atheroembolism, or severe lifestyle-limiting symptoms.

CLOSTRIDIUM DIFFICILE INFECTION

Marc Grossman, MD, FACEP, CPHM

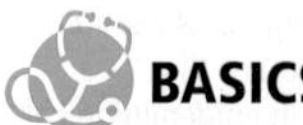

BASICS

DESCRIPTION

- *Clostridium difficile* is a gram-positive, spore-forming anaerobic bacillus.
- Infection caused by *C. difficile* is usually linked to broad-spectrum antibiotic use.
- Severity of infection can range from diarrhea to colitis to perforation to death.
- System(s) affected: GI
- Synonyms(s): *C. difficile*–associated disease or diarrhea (CDAD); antibiotic-associated diarrhea; *C. diff*

EPIDEMIOLOGY

Incidence

- Most cases of *C. difficile* infection occur in hospitals or long-term care facilities at a rate of 25–80 per 100,000 occupied bed-days (1).
- For outpatient setting, the rate is ~7.7 cases per 100,000 person-years.

Prevalence

- *C. difficile* causes ~25% of all cases of antibiotic-associated diarrhea.
- C. *difficile* infections account for ~25% of all nosocomial antibiotic associated infections (1).

RISK FACTORS

- Exposure to all antimicrobial agents (except aminoglycosides) is associated with *C. difficile* infection.
- Patients in health care settings have a higher risk of developing *C. difficile* infection.
- Age >65 years
- Duration of stay in the hospital
- Nasogastric intubation
- Previous *C. difficile* infection
- Severe primary illness
- Controversial: Use of antiulcer medications
- Chemotherapy
- Perioperative antibiotic prophylaxis:
  - Even if patients receive no antibiotics other than perioperative prophylaxis, they are still at risk for developing *C. difficile* infection (2).

Geriatric Considerations

C. difficile is the most common cause of acute diarrheal illness in long-term care facilities. These patients are older and receive more antibiotics and antacids than the general public; thus, it is difficult to determine which factors contribute most to this increased risk.

Pediatric Considerations

Neonates have a higher rate of *C. difficile* colonization (25–80%), yet they are much less likely to be symptomatic than adults, possibly due to immature toxin receptors.

Genetics

No known genetic factors

GENERAL PREVENTION

- Implementation of a comprehensive infection-control program has resulted in a decrease in the incidence of *C. difficile* infection.
- Disinfection with hypochlorite solution
- Hand washing with soap and water:
  - Alcohol-based hand gels do not kill spores.
- Reduction in the use of rectal thermometers
- Reduction of unnecessary broad-spectrum antibiotic use
- Isolation of infected patients and use of contact precautions
- Education of hospital personnel

PATHOPHYSIOLOGY

- *C. difficile* can thrive in the colon and cause infection if disruption of the normal flora and ingestion of *C. difficile* occur.
- *C. difficile* spores can survive for months.
- Host factors such as the presence of antibodies to *C. difficile* toxins can reduce the severity and prevent recurrences of infection.
- *C. difficile* produces toxins that are essential for disease to occur:
  - Toxins A (enterotoxin) and B (cytotoxin) attract neutrophils and monocytes, and degrade colonic epithelial cells, causing colitis, pseudomembrane colitis, and watery diarrhea.
  - BI/NAP1 strain of *C. difficile* has been shown to produce more virulent characteristics (3).
  - Binary toxin produces a virulent form of disease (different from toxin A or B); this may result in increased rates of colectomies and mortality.
  - Binary toxin has been identified in ~6% of clinical *C. difficile* isolates obtained in the US and Europe.

ETIOLOGY

- Altered colonic mucosa
- *C. difficile* spore ingestion
- Active toxin release

DIAGNOSIS

HISTORY

- Recent antibiotic use (especially broad-spectrum fluoroquinolones and cephalosporins)
- Diarrhea that is watery, foul-smelling
- Fever (typically <10%)
- Recent hospitalization or stay at nursing facility

PHYSICAL EXAM

- Mild disease:
  - Mild lower abdominal cramping pain
- Moderate disease:
  - Fever
  - Nausea and vomiting
- Severe disease:
  - Peritonitis
  - Ileus
  - Hypovolemia
- Mild abdominal tenderness to peritonitis, depending on severity
- Hypovolemia

DIAGNOSTIC TESTS & INTERPRETATION

Markers of severe or fulminant infection include hypotension, sepsis, markedly elevated white blood cell count, and bandemia. Other signs include obstruction, perforation, toxic megacolon, colonic-wall thickening, and ascites.

Lab

- ELISA for toxins:
  - Available within several hours
  - Sensitivity 63–99%
  - Specificity 75–100%
  - Some labs test only for toxin A, others test for A and B.
- Tissue culture cytotoxicity assay:
  - Takes 24–48 hours for results; labor-intensive
  - Sensitivity 67–100%
  - Specificity 85–100%
- Microbiology culture:
  - Nontoxin-producing strains also detected
  - Mostly used to evaluate epidemiology studies
- PCR-based testing is currently research-based.
- Repeat testing during the same episode of diarrhea is discouraged (3).

Imaging

- Plain films may show thumbprinting and colonic distension.
- CT radiography may show mucosal wall thickening, thickened colonic wall, and pericolonic inflammation.

Diagnostic Procedures/Surgery

- Endoscopy can be used to evaluate for pseudomembranes and exclude other conditions.
- Flexible sigmoidoscopy may miss 15–20% of pseudomembranes that may be more proximal in the colon.
- Colonoscopy evaluates the entire colon: Used when diagnosis is in doubt or severity demands rapid diagnosis

Pathological Findings

Pseudomembranes consist of inflammatory and cellular debris that forms visible exudates that can obscure the underlying mucosa. These exudates have a yellow to grayish color.

DIFFERENTIAL DIAGNOSIS

- Food poisoning
- Enteric infections
- Antibiotic-associated diarrhea

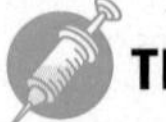

TREATMENT

MEDICATION

- If clinically indicated (i.e., moderate-to-severe diarrhea, fever, significant leukocytosis, abdominal pain), consider antimicrobial against *C. difficile* (4)[A].
- Current evidence leads to uncertainty whether mild CDAD needs to be treated (5)[A].

First Line

- Metronidazole is the drug of choice for mild-to-moderate *C. difficile* infection due to low cost and prevention of the emergence of vancomycin-resistant organisms (3)[A]:
  - 500 mg PO t.i.d. a day for 10–14 days
  - If patient is unable to take oral medications, then IV metronidazole or intraluminal vancomycin can be used.
- Vancomycin is first-line therapy in patients with severe or fulminant *C. difficile* infection. Vancomycin is also first-line therapy for the third and subsequent relapse in fewer than 6 months (3):
  - 125 mg PO q.i.d. for 10–14 days
  - Vancomycin retention enema if unable to take PO or there is evidence of poor GI motility.
  - No statistically significant difference in efficacy between vancomycin and other antibiotics, including metronidazole, fusidic acid, nitazoxanide, or rifaximin (5)[A].
- For the first recurrence of *C. difficile* infection, the treatment is the same as the initial treatment, although current severity of illness should be taken into account. For subsequent relapses, use oral vancomycin as treatment in a pulse-taper format. Consultation with an infectious diseases specialist is recommended.

ALERT

When using vancomycin for treatment of *C. difficile* infection, oral or rectal formulations must be used because IV formulations are not excreted into the colonic lumen.

Second Line

- Vancomycin (4,6)[A]:
  - 125 mg PO q.i.d. for 10–14 days
  - Indicated for patients who cannot tolerate or have failed metronidazole therapy, and for those who are pregnant
- IV immunoglobulin (IVIG) has been used in special cases.
- Nitazoxanide, teicoplanin, and fidaxomicin may be considered as alternatives to traditional treatment.
  - Clinical experience is limited with these agents for this indication (7)[A].

ADDITIONAL TREATMENT

General Measures

- Avoid antimotility agents and opiates (4,8)[A].
- Avoid use of proton pump inhibitors (PPIs) unless absolutely necessary, as they have been associated with a 42% increased risk of recurrence if used concurrently with treatment for *C. difficile* colitis (9).

COMPLEMENTARY AND ALTERNATIVE MEDICINE

- Probiotics (*Lactobacilli* and *Saccharomyces)* have shown conflicting data, and have been associated with increased bacteremia (3):
  - Use oral *Lactobacilli* with caution if also using vancomycin, since the latter antibiotic is active against *Lactobacilli*.
- Fecal transplant in severe or relapsing disease

SURGERY/OTHER PROCEDURES

If *C. difficile* infection progresses to toxic megacolon, peritonitis, or sepsis after initiation of treatment, other therapeutic options should be explored, including a surgical consult (4,6)[A].

IN-PATIENT CONSIDERATIONS

Initial Stabilization

- Current nonessential antibiotic therapy should be discontinued if possible (3,4)[A].
- Institute supportive therapy with fluids and electrolytes if needed (3,4)[A].

Admission Criteria

- Hypovolemia
- Comorbid conditions
- Inability to keep up with enteric losses
- Hematochezia
- Electrolyte disturbances

IV Fluids

- Infuse to keep patient euvolemic
- Once over acute phase, patient can be weaned off IV fluids.

Nursing

See "General Prevention."

Discharge Criteria

- Improved diarrhea severity and frequency
- Tolerating both medications and PO
- Afebrile

ONGOING CARE

FOLLOW-UP RECOMMENDATIONS

- Many patients can be treated as outpatients.
- Bed rest during acute phase

Patient Monitoring

- Relapses of colitis will occur in 15–30%.
- Relapses typically occur 2–10 days after discontinuation of antibiotics.
- Repeat treatment with 14-day course of antibiotics will result in 40% cure rate.
- The management of the first relapse following therapy for *C. difficile* diarrhea and colitis does not differ substantially from treatment of the initial episode.
- Administration of vancomycin or metronidazole every other day or every third day allows spores to germinate on the off days and then be killed when the antibiotics are taken again.
- For multiple relapses, some success has been reported with the following PO vancomycin taper regimen:
  - Week 1: 125 mg q.i.d.
  - Week 2: 125 mg b.i.d.
  - Week 3: 125 mg/d
  - Week 4: 125 mg every other day
  - Weeks 5 and 6: 125 mg every 3 days
- If continued infection, consider pulse therapy with vancomycin in consultation with an infectious disease specialist.

DIET

No restrictions; as tolerated

PATIENT EDUCATION

Patients should be kept informed of the progress of disease and taught to practice good hygiene (i.e., hand washing).

PROGNOSIS

- Majority of patients will improve with conservative management and antibiotics.
- 1–3% of patients will develop severe colitis requiring emergency colectomy.

REFERENCES

1. McDonald LC, Owings M, Jernigan DB. *Clostridium difficile* infection in patients discharged from US short-stay hospitals, 1996–2003. *Emerg Infect Dis.* 2006;12:409–15.
2. Carignan A, Allard C, Pépin J, et al. Risk of *Clostridium difficile* infection after perioperative antibacterial prophylaxis before and during an outbreak of infection due to a hypervirulent strain. *Clin Infect Dis.* 2008;46:1838–43.
3. Cohen SH, Gerding DN, Johnson S, et al. Clinical practice guidelines for *Clostridium difficile* infection in adults: 2010 update by the society for healthcare epidemiology of America (SHEA) and the infectious diseases society of America (IDSA). *Infect Control Hosp Epidemiol.* 2010;31:431–55.
4. Bartlett JG. Narrative review: The new epidemic of *Clostridium difficile*-associated enteric disease. *Ann Intern Med.* 2006;145:758–64.
5. Nelson RL, Kelsey P, Leeman H, et al. Antibiotic treatment for *Clostridium difficile*-associated diarrhea in adults. *Cochrane Database Syst Rev.* 2011;9:CD004610.
6. McFarland LV. Alternative treatments for *Clostridium difficile* disease: What really works? *J Med Micro.* 2005;54:101–11.
7. Venuto C, Butler M, Ashley ED, et al. Alternative therapies for *Clostridium difficile* infections. *Pharmacotherapy.* 2010;30:1266–78.
8. Koo HL, Koo DC, Musher DM, et al. Antimotility agents for the treatment of *Clostridium difficile* diarrhea and colitis. *Clin Infect Dis.* 2009;48:598–605.
9. Linsky A, Gupta K, Lawler EV, et al. Proton pump inhibitors and risk for recurrent *Clostridium difficile* infection. *Arch Intern Med.* 2010;170:772–8.

ADDITIONAL READING

- Larson KC, Belliveau PP, Spooner LM, et al. Tigecycline for the treatment of severe *Clostridium difficile* infection. *Ann Pharmacother.* 2011; 45:1005–10.
- McFarland LV. Meta-analysis of probiotics for the prevention of antibiotic associated diarrhea and the treatment of *Clostridium difficile* disease. *Am J Gastroenterol.* 2006;101:812–22.

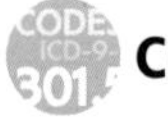

CODES

ICD9

008.45 Intestinal infection due to clostridium difficile

CLINICAL PEARLS

- Treatment of asymptomatic patients is not recommended.
- Therapeutic response should be based on clinical signs and symptoms. Patients may shed organism or toxin for weeks after treatment.

COLIC, INFANTILE

Daniel T. Lee, MD
Leanne Zakrzewski, MD

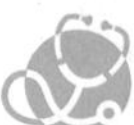

BASICS

DESCRIPTION

- Colic is defined as excessive crying in an otherwise healthy baby.
- A commonly used criteria is the Wessel criteria, or the Rule of Three: Crying lasts for:
  - >3 hours a day
  - >3 days a week
  - Persists >3 weeks
- Many clinicians no longer use the criterion of persistence for >3 weeks because few parents or clinicians will wait that long before evaluation or intervention.
- Some clinicians feel that colic represents the extreme end of the spectrum of normal crying, whereas most feel that colic is a distinct clinical entity.

EPIDEMIOLOGY

Incidence

- Predominant age: Between 2 weeks and 4 months of age
- Predominant sex: Male = Female

Prevalence

- Probably between 10% and 25% of infants
- Range is somewhere between 8% and 40% of infants.

Pediatric Considerations

This is a problem during infancy.

RISK FACTORS

Physiologic predisposition in infant, but no definitive risk factors have been established.

GENERAL PREVENTION

Colic is generally not preventable.

ETIOLOGY

The cause is unknown. Factors that may play a role include:

- Infant gastroesophageal reflux disease
- Allergy to cow's milk, soy milk, or breast milk protein
- Fruit juice intolerance
- Swallowing air during the process of crying, feeding, or sucking
- Overfeeding or feeding too quickly; underfeeding also has been proposed
- Inadequate burping after feeding
- Family tension
- Parental anxiety, depression, and/or fatigue
- Parent–infant interaction mismatch
- Baby's inability to console his/herself when dealing with stimuli
- Increased gut hormone motilin, causing hyperperistalsis
- Tobacco smoke exposure
- Disorder of impaired synchronization between infant arousal and environment (1)[C]

DIAGNOSIS

HISTORY

- Evaluation for Wessel criteria: Crying lasts for >3 hours per day, >3 days per week, and persists >3 weeks.
- The colicky episodes may have a clear beginning and end.
- The crying is generally spontaneous, without preceding events triggering the episodes.
- The crying is typically different from normal crying. Colicky crying may be louder, more turbulent, variable in pitch, and appear more like screaming.
- The infant may be difficult to soothe or console regardless of how the parents try to help.
- The infant acts normally when not colicky.
- Assess the support system of caregivers and families, including coping skills.

PHYSICAL EXAM

- A comprehensive physical exam is normal.
- Since excessive crying may be a risk factor for shaken baby syndrome or other forms of child abuse (2)[B], be sure to examine the child carefully for signs of shaken baby syndrome or other types of child abuse.

DIAGNOSTIC TESTS & INTERPRETATION

Diagnostic Procedures/Surgery

A thorough history and physical examination should be performed to rule out other causes. Otherwise, no diagnostic procedures or imaging is indicated.

DIFFERENTIAL DIAGNOSIS

Any organic cause for excessive or qualitatively different crying in infants such as:

- Infections, e.g., meningitis, sepsis, otitis media, or UTI
- GI issues, such as gastroesophageal reflux, intussusception, lactose intolerance, constipation, anal fissure, or strangulated hernia
- Trauma, which includes foreign bodies, corneal abrasion, occult fracture, digit or penile hair tourniquet, or child abuse

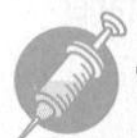

TREATMENT

MEDICATION

- Dicyclomine (Bentyl) has been proven beneficial, but the potential serious adverse effects such as apnea, seizures, and syncope have precluded its use. Further, the manufacturer has made the medication contraindicated for infants <6 months of age (3,4)[B].
- Simethicone has not been shown to be beneficial (3,4)[B].

ADDITIONAL TREATMENT

General Measures

- Soothe by holding and rocking the baby (3)[C].
- Use a pacifier (3)[C].
- Use of gentle rhythmic motion (e.g., strollers, infant swings, car rides) (3)[C].
- Place near white noise (e.g., vacuum cleaner, clothes dryer, white-noise machine) (3)[C].
- Crib vibrators or car-ride simulators have not proven to be helpful (3,5)[B].
- Increased carrying or use of infant carrier has not been shown to improve colic (3,5)[B].
- Employ the 5-Ss (need to be done concurrently):
  - Swaddling: Tight wrapping with blanket; may be especially beneficial in infants <8 weeks of age (6)[B]
  - Side/stomach: Laying baby on side or stomach
  - Shushing: Loud white noise
  - Swinging: Rhythmic, jiggly motion
  - Sucking: Sucking on anything (e.g., nipple, finger, pacifier) (3)[C]

Issues for Referral

Excessive vomiting, poor weight gain, recurrent respiratory diseases, or bloody stools should prompt referral to a specialist.

COMPLEMENTARY AND ALTERNATIVE MEDICINE

- A recent RCT of 50 full-term infants diagnosed with colic evaluated the safety and effectiveness of *Lactobacillus reuteri* supplementation. Infants were exclusively breastfed, and mothers were instructed to avoid cow's milk during the 21-day study. Infants were randomized to receive *L. reuteri* or placebo 30 minutes before the first feed of each day. Parents kept diaries. Crying times decreased in both groups, but infants in the *L. reuteri* group had significantly reduced median daily crying times throughout the study (370 to 35 min/d vs. 300 to 90 min/d in placebo group). Weight gain, stooling frequency, and incidence of regurgitation were similar in both groups (7)[B]:
  - *L. reuteri* is available as over-the-counter drops, but it is not regulated by the FDA.
- Herbal teas and supplements may help but are not recommended because of limited, inconclusive evidence. Examples:
  - One study concluded that herbal teas containing mixtures of chamomile, vervain, licorice, fennel, and balm-mint used up to t.i.d. may be beneficial (4)[C]. However, the study used high dosages, raising clinical concerns that this therapy may impair needed milk consumption in infants and be impractical to administer. In addition, preparations used in the study may not be commercially available in the US.
  - A second double-blind, randomized trial of 0.1% fennel seed oil emulsion vs. placebo demonstrated a decrease in colic symptoms according to the Wessel criteria. However, this preparation of fennel seed oil is not commercially available in the US, and the long-term health effects are unknown (8).

- A home-based intervention focusing on reducing infant stimulation and synchronizing infant sleep–wake cycles with the environment, as well as parental support, has been shown to be effective (1)[B].
- Use of music may help (9,10)[C].
- Chiropractic treatment has shown no benefit over placebo (3)[C].
- Infant massage has not been shown to be helpful (3)[B].

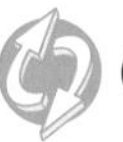

ONGOING CARE

FOLLOW-UP RECOMMENDATIONS

Frequent outpatient visits as needed for parental reassurance, education, and monitoring and to ensure the health of the infant and parents.

Patient Monitoring

Follow for proper feeding, growth, and development

DIET

- If breastfeeding:
  - Continue breastfeeding. Switching to formula probably will not help (3)[C].
  - Possible therapeutic benefit from eliminating milk products, eggs, wheat, and nuts from the diet of breastfeeding mothers (3,5)[B].
  - Along with eliminating the preceding foods from the maternal diet, removing soy, nuts, and fish may be beneficial.
- If formula feeding:
  - Feeding the infant in a vertical position using a curved bottle or bottle with collapsible bag may help to reduce air swallowing.
  - Consider a 1-week trial of hypoallergenic formulas, such as whey hydrolysate (e.g., Good Start) or casein hydrolysate (e.g., Alimentum, Nutramigen, Pregestimil) (4,5)[B].
  - The American Academy of Pediatrics concluded that there is no proven role for soy formula in the treatment of colic (11)[C].
  - Adding fiber to formula also has not been shown to be helpful (5,9)[B].
- Supplementing with sucrose solution may be helpful, but the effect may be short-lived (<1 hour) (4,5)[B].
- Use of lactase enzymes in formula or breast milk or given directly to the infant has no therapeutic benefit (5)[B].

PATIENT EDUCATION

- Reassure parents that colic is not the result of bad parenting, and advise parents about having proper rest breaks, adequate sleep, and help in caring for the infant.
- Explain the spectrum of crying behavior.
- Avoid overfeeding or underfeeding.
- Instruct in better feeding techniques such as improved bottles (low air, curved) and sufficient burping after feeding.
- Colic information at American Family Physician: www.aafp.org/afp/2004/0815/p741.html

PROGNOSIS

- Usually subsides by 3–6 months of age, often on its own.
- Despite apparent abdominal pain, colicky infants eat well and gain weight normally.
- A handful of studies indicate that temper tantrums may be more common among formerly colicky infants, as studied in toddlers up to 4 years of age (12,13).
- Colic has no bearing on the baby's intelligence or future development.

COMPLICATIONS

Colic is self-limiting and does not result in lasting effects to infant or maternal mental health (14)[C].

REFERENCES

1. Keefe MR, Lobo ML, Froese-Fretz A, et al. Effectiveness of an intervention for colic. *Clin Pediatr (Phila)*. 2006;45:123–33.
2. Reijneveld SA, van der Wal MF, Brugman E, et al. Infant crying and abuse. *Lancet*. 2004;364: 1340–2.
3. Roberts DM, Ostapchuk M, O'Brien JG. Infantile colic. *Am Fam Physician*. 2004;70:735–40.
4. Wade S, Kilgour T. Extracts from "clinical evidence": Infantile colic. *BMJ*. 2001;323: 437–40.
5. Garrison MM, Christakis DA. A systematic review of treatments for infant colic. *Pediatrics*. 2000; 106:184–90.
6. van Sleuwen BE, L'hoir MP, Engelberts AC, et al. Comparison of behavior modification with and without swaddling as interventions for excessive crying. *J Pediatr*. 2006;149:512–7.
7. Savino F, Cordisco L, Tarasco V, et al. Lactobacillus reuteri DSM 17938 in infantile colic: A randomized double-blind placebo controlled trial. *Pediatrics*. 2010;126(3):e526–33.
8. Alexandrovich I, Rakovitskaya O, Kolmo E, et al. The effect of fennel (Foeniculum Vulgare) seed oil emulsion in infantile colic: a randomized, placebo-controlled study. *Altern Ther Health Med*. 2003;9(4):58–61.
9. Clemons RM. Issues in newborn care. *Prim Care*. 2000;27:251–67.
10. McCollough M, Sharieff GQ. Common complaints in the first 30 days of life. *Emerg Med Clin North Am*. 2002;20:27–48, v.
11. O'Connor NR. Infant formula. *Am Fam Physician*. 2009;79:565–70.
12. Canivet C, Jakobsson I, Hagander B, et al. Infantile colic. Follow-up at four years of age: Still more "emotional". *Acta Paediatr*. 2000;89:13–7.
13. Rautava P, Lehtonen L, Helenius H, et al. Infantile colic: Child and family three years later. *Pediatrics*. 1995;96:43–7.
14. Clifford TJ, Campbell MK, Speechley KN, et al. Sequelae of infant colic: Evidence of transient infant distress and absence of lasting effects on maternal mental health. *Arch Pediatr Adolesc Med*. 2002;156:1183–8.

ADDITIONAL READING

- Hill DJ, Roy N, Heine RG, et al. Effect of a low-allergen maternal diet on colic among breastfed infants: A randomized, controlled trial. *Pediatrics*. 2005;116:e709–15.
- Savino F, Pelle E, Palumeri E, et al. Lactobacillus reuteri (American Type Culture Collection Strain 55730) versus simethicone in the treatment of infantile colic: A prospective randomized study. *Pediatrics*. 2007;119:e124–30.

CODES

ICD9

789.7 Colic

CLINICAL PEARLS

- Colic is defined as excessive crying in an otherwise healthy baby.
- Excessive crying may be a risk factor for shaken baby syndrome or other forms of child abuse.
- Usually subsides spontaneously by 3–6 months of age.
- Provide advice, support, and reassurance to parents (3)[B].
- Prevent caregiver burnout by advising parents to get proper rest breaks, sleep, and help in caring for the infant.

COLITIS, ISCHEMIC

Neha Jakhete, MD
Pia Prakash, MD
Marie L. Borum, MD, EdD, MPH

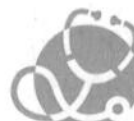

BASICS

Ischemic colitis results from decreased blood flow and secondary inflammation of the colon from a variety of underlying etiologies.

DESCRIPTION

- Associated with the elderly, but can affect patients of all ages
- Patients can present with:
  - *Nonacute ischemic colitis* from a chronic process with irreversible ischemic injury and associated sequelae such as persistent bacteremia or sepsis
  - *Acute process* with self-limited transient mucosal ischemia
- Illness is self-limited and reversible in 80% of patients:
  - 20% of patients progress to full-thickness necrosis and require surgical intervention.
- Most commonly, ischemia is related to nonocclusive reduction in blood flow:
  - Occlusive events are less common.
- Presentation may vary, but patients with acute ischemic colitis present with localized abdominal pain and palpable tenderness and frequent loose bloody stool within 12–24 hours of onset.
- Laboratory and radiographic findings are nonspecific and must be correlated closely with clinical presentation.
- Colonoscopy is the gold standard diagnostic test in patients with suspected ischemic colitis.
- In the absence of complications, most patients require supportive care, including IV fluids, bowel rest, and close monitoring for clinical decompensation. Empiric broad-spectrum antibiotics should be considered in moderate-to-severe cases.

EPIDEMIOLOGY

- Data describing the incidence and prevalence of ischemic colitis are limited, as it is uncommon in the general population.
- Females may be at increased risk.
- Patients with inflammatory bowel disease or COPD have an increased risk.

Geriatric Considerations

Rarely seen in those <60 years old, with average age at diagnosis being 70 years of age

Incidence

- 4.5–44 cases per 100,000 in the general population
- 1 case per 2,000 in hospitalized patients
- True incidence may be underestimated due to nonspecific clinical manifestations.

Prevalence

19 cases per 100,000 in the general population

RISK FACTORS

- Age >60 (90% of patients)
- Hypertension
- Diabetes mellitus
- Rheumatologic disorders/vasculitis
- Cerebrovascular disease (history of stroke or heart attack)
- Ischemic heart disease
- Recent abdominal surgery
- Constipation-inducing medications
- History of vascular surgery
- Irritable bowel syndrome
- Hypoalbuminemia
- Hemodialysis
- Smoking
- Hypercoagulable state

PATHOPHYSIOLOGY

- Results from reduction in blood flow compromising ability of colonic tissue to meet metabolic demands
- Most commonly, this is an acute, self-limited process resulting in ischemia to segments of colon.
- The colon is perfused by both the superior and inferior mesenteric arteries and branches of the internal iliac arteries. With extensive collateral circulation, occlusion of branches of the SMA or IMA rarely leads to ischemic consequences.
- Watershed areas of the colon, the splenic flexure, and rectosigmoid junction are most susceptible to ischemic damage. Blood is carried by narrow branches of the SMA and IMA to these areas, putting them at increased risk for ischemia. The splenic flexure is supplied by the terminal branches of the SMA, and the rectosigmoid junction is supplied by the terminal branches of the IMA.
- The left colon is more commonly affected than the right.
- The rectum is often spared because of the additional blood supply from the internal iliac arteries.
- Poor perfusion may result from systemic etiologies, local vascular compromise, and anatomic or functional changes in the colon itself. An occluding lesion of the large vessels is usually not identified.
- Acute ischemic colitis is largely self-limited and often resolves without long-term complications.
- Repeated episodes of ischemia and inflammation may result in a chronic colonic ischemia, possibly resulting in stricture formation, recurrent bacteremia, and sepsis. These patients may have unresolving areas of colitis requiring segmental colonic resection.

ETIOLOGY

- Hypoperfusion from shock
- Embolic occlusion of mesenteric vessels
- Hypercoagulable states
- Sickle cell disease
- Arterial thrombosis
- Venous thrombosis
- Vasculitis
- Mechanical colonic obstruction (e.g., tumor, adhesions, hernia, volvulus, prolapse, diverticulitis)
- Surgical complications (e.g., related to abdominal aortic aneurism repair)
- Trauma
- Medications (intestinally active vasoconstrictive substances, medications that induce hypotension and thus hypoperfusion)
- Cocaine abuse
- Aortic dissection
- Strenuous physical activity (e.g., long-distance running)

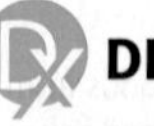

DIAGNOSIS

Diagnosis is based on history, risk factors, and physical examination. Laboratory values and radiographic findings are usually nonspecific. Colonoscopy may reveal suggestive findings.

HISTORY

- Symptoms vary depending on severity of ischemic colitis.
- Sudden-onset, mild-to-moderate abdominal pain with tenderness over the affected segment of bowel
- Loose, bloody bowel movements are common. Usually occurs within 12–24 hours of abdominal pain onset. Hematochezia is rarely associated with hemodynamic compromise.
- Nausea, vomiting, and abdominal distention may develop if ileus or stricture is present. This finding is more common in chronic ischemic colitis.
- It is important to differentiate ischemic colitis from mesenteric ischemia. Patient may describe lateral mild abdominal pain in ischemic colitis vs. intense periumbilical pain out of proportion to physical exam findings in mesenteric ischemia.

PHYSICAL EXAM

- In nonacute cases, physical exam may be relatively benign.
- Tenderness to palpation over the involved segment of bowel (21% sensitivity) (1)
- Abdominal distention
- Hypoactive or absent bowel sounds
- Peritoneal signs, including involuntary guarding and rebound tenderness, may suggest transmural ischemia or bowel perforation, which may require surgical intervention.

DIAGNOSTIC TESTS & INTERPRETATION

- Diagnosis is mostly clinical.
- Colonoscopy is the gold standard diagnostic test.
- Radiographic tests and laboratory values are nonspecific but may increase clinical suspicion.

Lab

There are no specific laboratory markers of ischemia.

Initial lab tests

- CBC for leukocytosis
- BMP to evaluate for metabolic acidosis
- Lactate
- CPK
- Alkaline phosphatase
- Lactate dehydrogenase (LDH)
- Amylase

Follow-Up & Special Considerations

- Stool cultures, fecal leukocytes, stool ova and parasites should be sent to rule out infectious etiologies.
- *Clostridium difficile* should also be excluded in patients with recent antibiotic use.

Imaging

Imaging is nonspecific.

Initial approach

- Abdominal plain film should be obtained:
  - Nonspecific findings include generalized bowel distention, air-filled bowel loops, and mural thickening.
  - Thumbprinting of the colonic wall is a more specific finding; however, it is only seen in a small portion of patients.
  - Pneumatosis and pneumoperitoneum suggest advanced ischemia.
  - Abdominal plain film is necessary to rule out bowel perforation.
- Abdominal CT scan with contrast should also be obtained with abdominal pain in suspected ischemic colitis:
  - The most common CT finding is segmental circumferential thickening of the bowel wall, which is nonspecific, as it can be seen in other intestinal diseases.
  - Pneumatosis or pneumoperitoneum may also be seen, suggesting advanced ischemia.

Follow-Up & Special Considerations

Patients who have undergone aortic surgery should be closely monitored for postoperative ischemic colitis.

Diagnostic Procedures/Surgery

Colonoscopy is gold standard. Sigmoidoscopy may also be used:

- Visualization of cyanotic hemorrhagic tissue and edematous mucosa is suggestive of ischemia.
- Segmental distribution (watershed) and rectal sparing can be seen during colonoscopy in patients with ischemic colitis.
- Biopsies should be obtained during colonoscopy.

Pathological Findings

Biopsies may reveal pathologic changes, including distorted crypt architecture, hemorrhage, intramural leukocyte infiltrates, capillary thrombosis, granulation tissue, and necrosis.

DIFFERENTIAL DIAGNOSIS

- Infectious colitis
- Inflammatory bowel disease (ulcerative colitis, Crohn disease)
- Colon cancer
- Diverticulitis
- Radiation enteritis
- Toxic megacolon

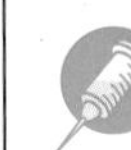

TREATMENT

- Treatment is dependent on the severity of disease.
- Continuous monitoring of clinical status, including vital signs and serial abdominal exams, is necessary.
- In the absence of colonic necrosis or perforation, most patients respond to supportive care, including (2)[A]:
  - Bowel rest
  - IV fluids
  - Oxygenation
  - Maintenance of hemodynamic stability
  - Broad-spectrum antibiotics covering aerobic and anaerobic bacteria to avoid bacterial translocation secondary to colonic mucosal damage
  - Avoidance of intestinally active vasoconstrictive medications
  - Avoidance of oral cathartics
  - Avoidance of systemic corticosteroids, as it may worsen ischemic damage
  - If ileus is present, nasogastric tube should be placed
- If radiographic findings are present, serial abdominal x-rays may be helpful.
- If signs of clinical deterioration are present despite supportive care, including increased abdominal pain, peritoneal signs, persistent diarrhea or bleeding, or sepsis, lapartomy or surgery must be considered.

MEDICATION

Broad-spectrum antibiotics as above

SURGERY/OTHER PROCEDURES

- 20% of patients progress to full-thickness necrosis and require surgical intervention.
- Surgery is indicated if patient has peritonitis and pneumoperitoneum (3)[A].
- Surgery may be indicated for patients with:
  - Development of peritoneal signs or increased abdominal tenderness
  - Persistent diarrhea
  - Persistent leukocytosis or fever, or clinical signs of sepsis
  - Bleeding for more than 2 weeks
- Most common surgical intervention is colectomy with end ileostomy (4):
  - If the margins appear ischemic, more bowel should be resected until well-perfused margins are achieved.
- Generally, the patient may undergo reversal of their ostomy after several months as their clinical condition allows.
- Mortality ranges from 30–60% in patients who require surgery (2,5).

ONGOING CARE

DIET

- Bowel rest until symptoms resolve
- Parenteral nutrition can be considered for patients who have contraindications to surgery, therefore needing prolonged bowel rest (2).

PROGNOSIS

- In most patients, symptoms of ischemic colitis resolve within 24–48 hours.
- Radiographic or endoscopic resolution is seen within 2 weeks (2).
- Follow-up colonoscopy may be performed to ensure complete resolution.

COMPLICATIONS

20–30% of patients go on to develop chronic ischemic colitis with persistent diarrhea or stricture formation requiring surgical intervention (4).

REFERENCES

1. Huguier M, Barrier A, Boelle PY, et al. Ischemic colitis. *Am J Surg*. 2006;192:679–84.
2. Theodoropoulou A, Koutroubakis IE, et al. Ischemic colitis: Clinical practice in diagnosis and treatment. *World J. Gastroenterol*. 2008;14:7302–8.
3. Paterno F, McGillicuddy EA, Schuster KM, et al. Ischemic colitis: Risk factors for eventual surgery. *Am J Surg*. 2010;200:646–50.
4. Sun MY, Maykel JA, et al. Ischemic colitis. *Clin Colon Rectal Surg*. 2007;20:5–12.
5. Feuerstadt P, Brandt LJ, et al. Colon ischemia: recent insights and advances. *Curr Gastroenterol Rep*. 2010;12:383–90.

CODES

ICD9

- 557.0 Acute vascular insufficiency of intestine
- 557.1 Chronic vascular insufficiency of intestine
- 557.9 Unspecified vascular insufficiency of intestine

CLINICAL PEARLS

- Ischemic colitis should be diagnosed promptly using clinical symptoms and examination, as surgical intervention may be required in 20% of cases.
- Suspicion for ischemic colitis should be high in patients with multiple risk factors presenting with abdominal and loose bloody stools.
- Imaging yields nonspecific findings in most cases.
- Colonoscopy is the diagnostic modality of choice.
- Most often, ischemic colitis is a self-limited disease that responds to conservative management with IV fluids, bowel rest, and empiric broad-spectrum antibiotics.
- Peritoneal signs or lack of clinical improvement is suggestive of extensive ischemia and requires surgical intervention.

COLONIC POLYPS

Macario C. Corpuz, Jr., MD, FAAFP
Pamela L. Grimaldi, DO, FAAFP

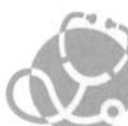

BASICS

DESCRIPTION

- A colonic polyp is an intraluminal outgrowth arising from the large intestinal epithelial lining, and is usually benign.
  - The potential for malignant transformation necessitates close evaluation and monitoring (See "Colorectal Malignancy").
- 3 types:
  - Adenomatous: May become malignant:
    - Villous: Polyps tend to be larger, most likely to become malignant (10%)
    - Tubular (75%)
    - Tubulovillous (15%)
  - Hyperplastic: Rarely become malignant
  - Inflammatory: No malignant potential

EPIDEMIOLOGY

- Varies considerably worldwide:
  - Industrialized countries are generally at greater risk compared to the rest of the world.
- Age is an important determinant in the US and other high-risk countries.
- Adenomas more common in men than women.

Incidence

- Estimated 5% of the US population
- ~20% of middle-aged and older adults
- 50% seen in ≥50 years

Prevalence

Average prevalence of 25% before age 40 to as high as 55% at age 80

RISK FACTORS

- Advancing age
- Male
- Obesity
- Family history of polyposis, polyps, or colorectal cancer (CRC)
- Inflammatory bowel disease
- Current cigarette smoking
- Excessive alcohol intake: >8 drinks of beer or spirits a week (1)
- Sedentary lifestyle

Genetics

May occur in the setting of genetic syndromes that are associated with gene mutations

GENERAL PREVENTION

- Diet: High-fiber diet has been a controversial risk. 2 recent studies stressed that doubling fiber intake can significantly reduce CRC risk (2,3).
- Avoid smoking.
- Limit alcohol intake.
- Calcium supplement: Shown reduction of colorectal adenoma recurrence (4)
- Vitamin D, folic acid, vitamin B_6
- Aspirin. 3 randomized controlled trials revealed that ASA caused significant reduction in the recurrence of sporadic adenomatous polyps after 1–3 years, while short-term studies support regression of colorectal adenomas in familial adenomatous polyposis (FAP) (5).

PATHOPHYSIOLOGY

- Adenomatous polyps:
  - Formed from abnormal proliferation and from dysplasia
- Nonadenomatous polyps:
  - Result from abnormal mucosal maturation, inflammation, or architecture

ETIOLOGY

Unknown. May be related to environmental and genetic factors.

COMMONLY ASSOCIATED CONDITIONS

Associated with several hereditary disorders:

- FAP
- Peutz-Jeghers syndrome
- Gardner syndrome
- Hereditary nonpolyposis colon cancer (HNPCC)

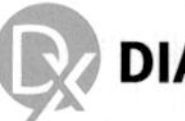

DIAGNOSIS

HISTORY

- Asymptomatic
- Hematochezia
- Melena
- Diarrhea or constipation
- Anemia
- Fatigue
- Abdominal pain

PHYSICAL EXAM

- Usually normal
- Rectal lesions may be felt by digital examination.

DIAGNOSTIC TESTS & INTERPRETATION

Lab

Initial lab tests

- CBC: Anemia
- Electrolyte abnormalities: In villous adenoma

Diagnostic Procedures/Surgery

- Colonoscopy (6): Gold standard:
  - Most sensitive test available, but its sensitivity is a concern.
  - Chromoscopy enhances the detection of neoplastic lesions in the colon and the rectum that could be missed with conventional colonoscopy (7).
- Chromoscopy: Studies are examining narrow-band imaging for histologic differentiation between adenomatous and hyperplastic polyps (8,9).
- CT colonography (formerly known as "virtual colonoscopy")
- Sigmoidoscopy
- Air-contrast barium enema: Misses small lesions
- Fecal occult blood test (FOBT): Many false-positive results
- Fecal DNA testing
- Some polyps are more likely to become malignant; hence, they require histopathologic evaluation.

Pathological Findings

- Villous adenoma:
  - Gross: Velvety, multiple-frond projections
  - Micro: Glands proliferate in fingerlike projections, malignant degenerations
- Tubular adenoma:
  - Gross: Smooth, firm, pink surface; microlobulated; fissures; pedunculated
  - Glands proliferate in tubular fashion, nuclei elongated, hyperchromatic

TREATMENT

SURGERY/OTHER PROCEDURES

- Endoscopic polypectomy: Major risks include perforation and bleeding
- Colonic resection: For multiple intestinal polyps associated with FAP

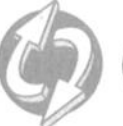

ONGOING CARE

FOLLOW-UP RECOMMENDATIONS

Benign polyps should have follow-up colonoscopy every 3–5 years.

Patient Monitoring

Offer CRC screening for average-risk patients beginning at age 50, earlier for at-risk patients:

- Most guidelines recommend to stop screening if life expectancy is <10 years.

DIET

Calcium supplementation might contribute a moderate degree to the prevention of colorectal adenomatous polyps (4).

PROGNOSIS

- Curable with polypectomy
- Projection estimates suggested that 50% of postpolypectomy patients will have a recurrence within 7.6 years; hence, need follow-up (10).
- Adenomatous polyps may undergo malignant transformation if not removed.
- Multiple polyps are particularly at increased risk of developing into CRC.

COMPLICATIONS

Perforation with colonoscopy is rare.

REFERENCES

1. Anderson JC, Alpern Z, Sethi G, et al. Prevalence and risk of colorectal neoplasia in consumers of alcohol in a screening population. *Am J Gastroenterol*. 2005;100:2049–55.
2. Asano TK, McLeod RS. Dietary fibre for the prevention of colorectal adenomas and carcinomas. *Cochrane Database Syst Rev*. 2002;1:CD003430.
3. Peters U, et al. Dietary fibre and colorectal adenoma in a colorectal cancer early detection programme. *Lancet*. 2003;361(9368):1491–5.
4. Weingarten MA, Zalmanovici A, Yaphe J. Dietary calcium supplementation for preventing colorectal cancer and adenomatous polyps. *Cochrane Database Syst Rev*. 2008:CD003548.
5. Asano T, McLeod R. Nonsteroidal anti-inflammatory drugs (NSAID) and aspirin for preventing colorectal adenomas and carcinomas *Cochrane Database Syst Rev*. 2010;2:CD004079.
6. Kim DH, Pickhardt PJ, Taylor AJ, et al. CT colonography versus colonoscopy for the detection of advanced neoplasia. *N Engl J Med*. 2007;357:1403–12.
7. Brown SR, Baraza W. Chromoscopy versus conventional endoscopy for the detection of polyps in the colon and rectum. *Cochrane Database Syst Rev*. 2011;1:CD006439.
8. Brown SR, et al. Chromoscopy versus conventional endoscopy for the detection of polyps in the colon and rectum. *Cochrane Database Syst Rev*. 2007;4:CD006439.
9. Rastogi A, et al. Recognition of surface mucosal and vascular patterns of colon polyps by using narrow-band imaging: Interobserver and intraobserver agreement and prediction of polyp histology. *Gastrointest Endosc*. 2009;69(Suppl 3):716–22.
10. Yood MU, et al. Colon polyp recurrence in a managed care population. *Arch Intern Med*. 2003;163(4):422–6.

ADDITIONAL READING

- Elwood PC, Gallagher AM, Duthie GG, et al. Aspirin, salicylates, and cancer. *Lancet*. 2009;373:1301–9.
- Larsen IK, Grotmol T, Almendingen K, et al. Lifestyle as a predictor for colonic neoplasia in asymptomatic individuals. *BMC Gastroenterol*. 2006;6:5.
- Seong-Eun K, et al. An association between obesity and the prevalence of colonic adenoma according to age and gender. *J Gastroenterol*. 2007;42(8).

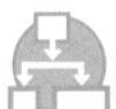

See Also (Topic, Algorithm, Electronic Media Element)

Algorithm: Bleeding, Upper GI

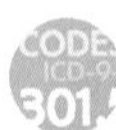

CODES

ICD9

211.3 Benign neoplasm of colon

CLINICAL PEARLS

- Villous adenomatous polyps are the "villains" (most likely to become malignant).
- Hyperplastic polyps rarely become cancer.
- Up to 50% of patients who have polyps removed have recurrent polyps.

COLORECTAL CANCER

Stephen M. Scott, MD, MPH

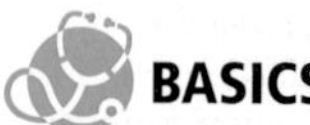

BASICS

DESCRIPTION

- Colorectal cancer (CRC) denotes a neoplasm that develops in the colon or rectum.
- CRC is the second most commonly diagnosed cancer and is the second leading cause of cancer deaths in the US.
- Screening for CRC reduces the incidence of and mortality from CRC.

EPIDEMIOLOGY

Incidence

In 2007, 142,672 new cases of CRC were diagnosed, and 53,219 deaths occurred from CRC.

Prevalence

- The overall lifetime risk for developing CRC in the US is about 1 in 19 (5.4%).
- Death rates have been declining due to improved screening, prevention, and treatment.

RISK FACTORS

- Age: >90% of people diagnosed with CRC are >50 years old.
- Personal history of colorectal polyps:
  - Risks increase with multiple polyps, villous polyps, and larger polyps.
- Personal history of cancer:
  - Rectal cancer has a higher incidence of local recurrence than proximal cancers (20–30% vs. 2–4%).
- History of inflammatory bowel disease:
  - The prevalence of CRC in ulcerative colitis and Crohn disease is about 3%, with a cumulative risk of CRC of 2% at 10 years, 8% at 20 years, and 18% at 30 years (1,2).
- Family history of CRC (although most CRCs occur in people without a family history):
  - The risk doubles in those who have a single first-degree relative with a history of CRC.
  - The risk is > double for those who have a history of CRC or polyps in:
    - Any first-degree relative <60 years old
    - ≥2 first-degree relatives, regardless of age
- Inherited syndromes:
  - Familial adenomatous polyposis (FAP):
    - Affected individuals develop hundreds to thousands of polyps in colon and rectum.
    - CRC usually present by age 40
    - Accounts for about 1% of CRCs
  - Hereditary nonpolyposis colon cancer (HNPCC, also called Lynch syndrome):
    - Often develops at a relatively young age
    - Lifetime risk of CRC 70–80%
    - Accounts for about 3–4% of all CRCs
  - Peutz-Jeghers syndrome:
    - Individuals may have freckles (mouth, hands, feet) and large polyps in GI tract.
    - Greatly increased risk for CRC and cancers
- Race and ethnicity:
  - African Americans have highest CRC incidence and mortality rates in US.
  - Several different gene mutations have been identified among Ashkenazi Jews.
- Miscellaneous:
  - *Streptococcus bovis* bacteremia is associated with CRC.
  - Patients with acromegaly are at increased risk.

Genetics

- Most result from acquired DNA mutation.
- There does not seem to be a single genetic pathway to CRC, although mutations are frequently seen in APC, K-Ras, p53, and SMAD4.
- A small percentage of colon cancers are known to be caused by inherited gene mutations:
  - APC, a tumor suppressor gene, is altered in FAP.
  - Genes encoding DNA repair enzymes implicated in HNPCC: MLH1, MSH2, MSH6, PMS1, PMS2, and others
  - STK11, a tumor suppressor gene, is altered in Peutz-Jeghers syndrome.

GENERAL PREVENTION

- Diets high in fruits and vegetables have been linked with decreased risk; those high in red and processed meats may increase CRC risk.
- People who are physically inactive are at higher risk for CRC.
- Long-term smokers are more likely than nonsmokers to develop and die from CRC.
- CRC has been linked to heavy alcohol consumption; may be related to low folic acid.
- Some studies suggest that vitamin D, calcium, and folate may lower CRC risk.
- NSAIDs may reduce risk in some groups; however, experts do not recommend NSAID use as a cancer prevention strategy in people at average risk for CRC.
- Colon cancer screening is one of the most powerful tools in preventing colon cancer.

ALERT

The United States Preventive Services Task Force (USPSTF) strongly recommends that clinicians screen men and women between the ages of 50 and 75 for CRC using one of the following: Fecal occult blood testing, sigmoidoscopy, or colonoscopy (3)[A]

- The less evidence-based American Cancer Society recommendations include completing one of the following tests (1)[C]:
  - Fecal occult blood testing (FOBT) annually
  - Fecal immunochemical test (FIT) annually
  - Stool DNA test (sDNA), interval uncertain
  - Flexible sigmoidoscopy every 5 years
  - Double-contrast barium enema every 5 years
  - Colonoscopy every 10 years
  - CT colonography every 5 years (colonoscopy completed if positive)
  - The USPSTF does not recommend barium enema as a screening test and concludes the evidence is insufficient to assess the benefits and harms of CT colonography and stool DNA testing as screening modalities for CRC (2)[A].
  - Digital rectal exam (DRE), alone or in combination with a 1-sample FOBT or FIT test, is not an acceptable method for CRC screening.
- Screening in high-risk groups (3):
  - People with a personal history of polyps need more frequent colonoscopy screening, depending on risk (i.e., 1 or 2 <1 cm polyps with low-grade dysplasia is deemed low-risk and may warrant repeat colonoscopy in 5–10 years; decision is influenced by family history, age, quality of initial colonoscopy, and patient comorbidities).
  - People who have a family history of CRC should begin colonoscopy at age 40 or 10 years younger than the age of relative at cancer diagnosis, whichever is earlier.
  - People with a family history of polyps should begin colonoscopy screening at age 40.
  - People with inflammatory bowel disease (IBD) should have regular surveillance colonoscopy with biopsies to detect dysplasia; guidelines for timing and location vary by professional society, but generally indicate starting surveillance by about 8 years of onset of disease followed by surveillance every 1–2 years.
  - Genetic testing may be appropriate for individuals with a strong family history of CRC or polyps:
    - Family members of a person affected by HNPCCC should start colonoscopy screening during their early 20s.
    - Individuals who test positive for the gene linked to FAP should start colonoscopy screening in their teens.

PATHOPHYSIOLOGY

- The progression from the first abnormal cells to the appearance of CRC usually occurs over 10–15 years, a disease characteristic that contributes to the effectiveness of prevention.
- High-risk polyp findings include multiple polyps, villous polyps, and larger polyps; hyperplastic polyps are less likely to evolve into colorectal cancer.

ETIOLOGY

Multiple genetic and environmental factors have been linked to the development of CRC.

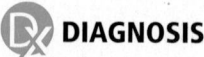

DIAGNOSIS

HISTORY

- Many patients with CRC are asymptomatic.
- Common presenting symptoms and signs in symptomatic patients include:
  - Abdominal pain or cramping
  - Change in bowel habits (constipation, diarrhea, narrowing of stool)
  - Rectal bleeding, dark stools, or blood in stool
  - Weakness or fatigue
  - Weight loss
  - Anemia
- Other presentations may include symptoms due to the presence of metastatic lesions (lymph nodes, liver, lung, peritoneum), fever of unknown origin, and *S. bovis* or *Clostridium septicum* sepsis.

PHYSICAL EXAM

- Weight loss
- Palpable abdominal mass
- Signs of anemia (i.e., conjunctival pallor)

DIAGNOSTIC TESTS & INTERPRETATION

Lab

Initial lab tests

- CBC (to evaluate anemia)
- Liver function (CRC may spread to the liver)

Imaging

Initial approach

- CT scanning to evaluate the presence of metastatic disease
- Chest x-ray may be used to evaluate the presence of chest metastases.

- Endoscopic ultrasound (EUS) may be used to evaluate the extent of rectal cancers; endorectal MRI may also provide further detail.
- Intraoperative ultrasound may be used to evaluate solid organs (e.g., the liver) after tumor resection.

Follow-Up & Special Considerations
- X-ray, CT, and/or MRI examinations may be used to monitor the presence or absence of CRC.
- Positron emission tomography (PET) may be used in some cases to detect metastatic disease.

Diagnostic Procedures/Surgery
- Biopsy is usually performed (most often during colonoscopy) if CRC is suspected.
- CT needle-guided biopsy may be needed to evaluate a suspected tumor or metastasis.

Pathological Findings
- The American Joint Committee on Cancer (AJCC) TNM criteria and Duke's criteria are most often used for staging. TNM staging for CRC is:
  - Stage 0: Limited to the mucosa (*carcinoma in situ* or *intramucosal carcinoma*, Tis, N0, M0)
  - Stage I: Through the muscularis mucosa into the submucosa or muscularis propria; no invasion of lymph nodes or distant sites (T1, N0, M0 or T2, N0, M0)
  - Stage IIA: Invades serosa; no lymph nodes or distant sites (T3, N0, M0)
  - Stage IIB: Through the wall of the colon or rectum and into adjacent tissues or organs; no lymph nodes or distant sites (T4, N0, M0)
  - Stage IIIA: Through mucosa into submucosa or muscularis propria with spread to 1–3 lymph nodes; no distant sites (T1, N1, M0 or T2, N1, M0)
  - Stage IIIB: Through colon or rectum with or without invasion of adjacent tissues or organs plus spread to 1–3 lymph nodes; no distant sites (T3, N1, M0, or T4, N1, M0)
  - Stage IIIC: Through colon or rectum and spread to 4 or more nearby lymph nodes; no distant sites (any T, N2, M0)
  - Stage IV: Any level of invasion with spread to distant site (any T, any N, M1)
- CRCs are graded on a 4-point scale from G1–G4. G1–G2 may be called low-grade and G3–G4 high-grade.

DIFFERENTIAL DIAGNOSIS
- >95% of CRCs are adenocarcinomas.
- Other colonic tumors include carcinoid tumors, lymphomas, and Kaposi sarcoma in HIV.
- Many conditions can mimic CRC, including other cancers, hemorrhoids, inflammatory bowel disease, infection, and extrinsic masses (i.e., cysts, abscesses).

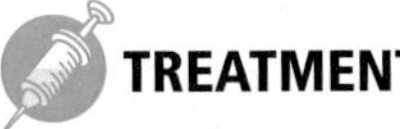

TREATMENT

MEDICATION
Surgical resection is the primary treatment for CRC. Chemotherapeutic regimens for metastatic disease may extend overall survival from 6 months to ~2 years. Adjuvant chemotherapy is most clearly beneficial for stage III (node-positive) disease, in which reductions of ~30% may be achieved in both disease recurrence and overall survival, compared with nontreated controls.

First Line
Chemotherapeutic agents include fluorouracil (5-FU), capecitabine (Xeloda, which is available in oral tablet form and is converted by body to 5-FU), irinotecan (Camptosar), and oxaliplatin (Eloxatin).

Geriatric Considerations
Elderly patients tend to tolerate CRC chemotherapy fairly well and should be considered for treatment when appropriate.

Second Line
Targeted therapies may be used alongside first-line agents or by themselves if first-line agents are ineffective:
- Bevacizumab (Avastin) is a monoclonal antibody that targets vascular endothelial growth factor (VEGF); inhibits angiogenesis.
- Cetuximab (Erbitux) and panitumumab (Vectibix) are monoclonal antibodies that target epidermal growth factor receptor (EGFR).

COMPLEMENTARY AND ALTERNATIVE MEDICINE
- May serve as an adjunct to treatment for CRC
- 70–75% of cancer survivors report using at least 1 type of complementary and alternative medicine (CAM), and almost all report that the alternative therapy improved their well-being.

SURGERY/OTHER PROCEDURES
- Surgery is the primary treatment for CRC:
  - May involve segmental resection, hemicolectomy, or colectomy, as well as resection of nodes, depending on size and invasion
  - Laparoscopic-assisted colectomy is an emerging option for earlier-stage tumors.
  - Surgery for rectal cancer may include local transanal, low anterior, or abdominoperineal resection, or pelvic exenteration.
- Radiation therapy is most often used for peritoneal or rectal cancers; it is rarely used for metastatic disease due to side effects.

ONGOING CARE

FOLLOW-UP RECOMMENDATIONS

Patient Monitoring
- People with a personal history of proximal cancer (nonrectal) should have follow-up colonoscopy in 1 year, and if normal, in 3 and 5 years subsequently.
- Carcinoembryonic antigen (CEA) and/or CA 19-9 are used to detect recurrence in people treated for CRC. (Note: CEA levels may be elevated in ulcerative colitis, nonmalignant GI tumors, liver disease, lung disease, and in smokers.)

PATIENT EDUCATION
- NCI: What You Need to Know About Cancer of the Colon and Rectum: http://www.cancer.gov/cancertopics/wyntk/colon-and-rectal
- AAFP: Colorectal Cancer Screening (includes Spanish): http://familydoctor.org/online/famdocen/home/common/cancer/risk/556.html

PROGNOSIS
5-year relative survival rate is determined by stage (adjusted for patients dying of other diseases): Stage I: 92%; stage II: 73%; stage III: 56%; stage IV: 8% (2)[A]

COMPLICATIONS
- Colorectal surgery: Pain, deep vein thrombosis, anastomotic leaks, infection, scarring, bowel obstruction
- Chemotherapy: Hair loss, nausea, vomiting, bruising, fatigue, increased risk for infections
- Radiation therapy: Skin irritation, nausea, rectal pain, incontinence, bladder irritation, fatigue, and sexual problems

C

REFERENCES

1. American cancer society guidelines for the early detection of cancer. Available at: http://www.cancer.org/docroot/PED/content/PED_2_3X_ACS_Cancer_Detection_Guidelines_36.asp?sitearea=PED. Accessed 9/30/2008.
2. O'Connell JB, Maggard MA, Ko CY. Colon cancer survival rates with the new American Joint Committee on Cancer sixth edition staging. *J Natl Cancer Inst*. 2004;96:1420–5.
3. Konda A, Duffy MC. Surveillance of patients at increased risk of colon cancer: Inflammatory bowel disease and other conditions. *Gastroenterol Clin North Am*. 2008;37:191–213, viii.

ADDITIONAL READING

- National Cancer Institute. At: http://www.cancer.gov/cancertopics/types/colon-and-rectal.
- National Colorectal Cancer Roundtable. At: http://www.nccrt.org.
- US Preventive Services Task Force: http://www.uspreventiveservicestaskforce.org/uspstf/uspscolo.htm.

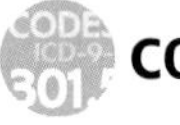

CODES

ICD9
- 153.9 Malignant neoplasm of colon, unspecified site
- 154.0 Malignant neoplasm of rectosigmoid junction
- 154.1 Malignant neoplasm of rectum

CLINICAL PEARLS
- The USPSTF recommends screening beginning at age 50, and notes that evidence supports fecal occult blood testing (yearly), sigmoidoscopy or colonoscopy (every 10 years).
- High-risk polyp findings include multiple polyps, villous polyps, and larger polyps; hyperplastic polyps are less likely to evolve into CRC.
- 10% of cases of CRC occur in people younger than age 50. People who have a family history of CRC should begin colonoscopy at age 40, or 10 years younger than the age of relative at cancer diagnosis, whichever is earlier.
- Iron deficiency anemia in the elderly should prompt a search for CRC, and should not be attributed to normal aging.

COMPLEMENTARY AND ALTERNATIVE MEDICINE

Jennifer A. Caragol, MD
D. Matthew Ziegler, MD
Andrew Bentley, MS

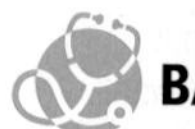

BASICS

- Complementary and alternative medicine (CAM) are medical and health care systems, practices, and products not presently considered part of conventional medicine.
- The National Center for Health Statistics (NCHS) 2007 survey reports 38% of adult Americans and 12% of children use some form of CAM, and this percentage is increasing.
- Medical professionals who incorporate CAM into their medical practice will often refer to their health care model as "integrative medicine."

DESCRIPTION

- Definitions and additional terms:
  - Complementary medicine is used with conventional medicine to address a health concern. For example, massage plus physical therapy to address low back pain, or medication plus osteopathic manipulation to address recurrent headaches.
  - Alternative medicine is used in place of conventional medicine to promote healing of conditions that cannot be explained by the conventional biomedical model or for which the effectiveness of therapy is not yet established by clinical research.
  - Integrative medicine is the combination of allopathic medicine with CAM, and may be provided to the patient by a single licensed medical professional versed in CAM or by a group of diverse health care providers. For example, a nurse on the oncology unit who integrates healing touch into the care of the patient.
  - Holistic is a descriptive term for a practitioner's approach to patient care. A holistic practitioner assesses the emotional, spiritual, mental, and physical state of wellness of the client and then works to provide comprehensive care. A holistic practice may include practitioners of different disciplines to best address all aspects of wellness or illness.
- Biologically based therapies: Diets, herbals, vitamins, supplements, flower essences
- Manipulative and body-based methods:
  - Massage therapy is the manipulation of the soft tissues of the body whereby the licensed practitioner uses knowledge of anatomy and physiology to restore function, promote relaxation, and relieve pain. There are several different types of massage.
  - Osteopathic manipulative medicine focuses on the musculoskeletal system. It includes indirect techniques, e.g., muscle energy, myofascial release, osteopathy in the cranial field, and strain-counterstrain approach, as well as direct action techniques (high-velocity thrusts).
  - Craniosacral therapy is a gentle manual treatment focusing on the release of bony and fascial restrictions in the craniosacral system, which includes the cranium, sacrum, spinal cord, meninges, and CSF.
  - Chiropractic therapy is a discipline that focuses on the musculoskeletal and nervous systems and how imbalances in these systems can affect general health. It is most often used to treat back pain, neck pain, and joint pain. Doctors of chiropractic (DCs) complete 4–5 years of intensive training in anatomy, physiology, and manipulation.
- Mind–body medicine:
  - Meditation is a practice of detachment in which a person sits quietly, generally focusing on the breath while releasing all thoughts from the mind with the intention to center the self, restore balance, and enhance well-being.
  - Spiritual practices/prayer
  - Yoga is an exercise of mindfulness, meditation, strength, and balance. It is composed of asanas (postures) and pranayamas (focused breathing). The discipline of yoga originated in India and has been practiced for thousands of years.
  - Aromatherapy utilizes highly concentrated plant extracts to stimulate physical, emotional, and energetic healing processes. These aromatic oils are rubbed on the skin, aerosolized, or used in compresses.
  - Tai chi and qi gong are Chinese exercise systems that combine meditation, regulated breathing, and flowing dancelike movements to enhance and balance chi (qi), or life force energy.
- Alternative medical systems:
  - Traditional Chinese medicine incorporates Chinese herbs and acupuncture. Acupuncture is the practice of regulating chi by inserting hair-thin needles at specific points along meridian pathways of the body. Chi movement is responsible for animating and protecting the body; relieving pain; and regulating blood, oxygen, and nourishment to every cell.
  - Ayurvedic medicine originated in India and is one of the world's oldest medical systems. It utilizes healing modalities and herbs to integrate and balance the body, mind, and spirit.
  - Homeopathy is a system of therapy based on the concept that very dilute quantities of an offending agent can stimulate the body's own immune system to produce a reaction against this offense, thereby healing itself. In general, homeopathic remedies are considered safe and unlikely to cause serious adverse reactions.
  - Naturopathy is based on providing natural and minimally invasive options for prevention and treatment of disease. Treatment regimens can include herbs, vitamins, supplements, dietary counseling, homeopathic remedies, manipulative therapies, acupuncture, and hydrotherapy. 4-year doctoral training programs are available; however, because only 16 states have licensing laws for naturopathic physicians, patients are encouraged to research their prospective naturopath's credentials.
- Energy therapies:
  - Reiki, which means source energy, is a healing practice from Japan. Laying hands lightly on the patient or holding the hands just above the body, the Reiki practitioner facilitates spiritual and physical healing by stimulating a patient's life force energy.
  - Healing touch was designed by a registered nurse. Practitioners use their hands to clear, energize, and balance a patient's energy field to enhance well-being.
- Common reasons patients choose CAM:
  - Additive therapy to address aspects of healing not provided for in conventional medical treatment
  - Conventional medicine has been unsuccessful in fully addressing ailment
  - Preventative health care
  - Desire for a holistic and natural approach to well-being
  - Preference for noninvasive treatment options
  - Concern about side effects of prescription medication
  - Desire for spiritual support to be incorporated into healing practice
  - Cultural or familial belief system may be more aligned with "natural" solutions not provided for or supported by the standard allopathic model of health care

EPIDEMIOLOGY

- All ages use CAM, but it is most prevalent among adults aged 30–69 years (1).
- Gender ratio: Female predominance (1)
- College graduates and residents from Western states are more likely to use CAM (1).
- Cancer survivors are more likely than the general population to use CAM.
- 11 most-utilized CAM therapies based on the NCHS 2007 survey; prayer is also reported. These CAM therapies were used by the indicated percentage of survey participants:
  - Prayer/self (43%); prayer/others (24.4%); prayer group (9.6%)
  - Natural products (17.7%)
  - Deep breathing (12.7%)
  - Meditation (9.4%)
  - Chiropractic and osteopathic (8.6%)
  - Massage (8.3%)
  - Yoga (6.1%)
  - Diet-based therapies (3.6%)
  - Progressive relaxation (2.9%)
  - Guided imagery (2.2%)
  - Homeopathic treatment (1.8%)

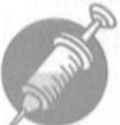

TREATMENT

- Evidence supports both safety and efficacy:
  - Meditation for lowering BP (2)[A]
  - Acupuncture for chronic low back pain (3)[A]
  - Spinal manipulative therapy for prophylactic treatment of headaches
  - Manipulation, massage, and mobilization for acute low back and posterior neck pain
  - Massage therapy to promote weight gain in preterm infants
  - Acupuncture for nausea and vomiting
  - Tai chi for improving balance and decreasing the risk of and fear of falling in elderly
  - Aromatherapy massage for temporary relief of anxiety or depression in cancer patients (4)
  - Mind–body techniques for migraines, chronic pain, and insomnia

- Homeopathic remedy for the treatment of chemotherapy-induced stomatitis in children
- Riboflavin for migraine prophylaxis
- Horse chestnut seed extract to improve lower leg venous tone, pain, and edema
- Glucosamine and chondroitin sulfate for osteoarthritis and knee pain
- Yoga and meditation appear to improve endothelial function in patients with CAD and can have potential beneficial effects on depressive disorders.
- Omega-3 fatty acids may reduce inflammation and anxiety in young healthy adults (5).
- Vitamin D 800 IU/d may reduce falls and fractures in the elderly (6).
- Evidence supports safety, but evidence regarding efficacy is inconclusive:
  - Saw palmetto for benign prostatic hyperplasia
  - Acupuncture for recurrent headache
  - Homeopathy for induction and augmentation of labor
  - Dietary fat reduction for certain types of cancer
  - Mind–body techniques for metastatic cancer
  - Copper and magnetic bracelets for pain
  - Vitamin D levels >30 ng/mL may prevent certain types of cancer. Adequate vitamin D intake may prevent atopy and asthma symptoms and ameliorate autoimmune disease (6).
- Evidence supports efficacy, but evidence regarding safety is inconclusive:
  - St. John's wort extract for short-term treatment of depression in adults
  - Ginkgo biloba for cognitive function in dementia
- Evidence indicates serious risk:
  - Delay in seeking medical care or replacement of curative conventional treatment
  - Use of toxic herbs or substances
  - Known herb–drug interactions

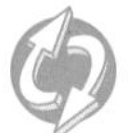

ONGOING CARE

PATIENT EDUCATION

The National Center for Complementary and Alternative Medicine (nccam.nih.gov)

COMPLICATIONS

- Potentially toxic herbs:
  - Serious adverse events from herbal remedies remain extremely rare.
  - Some ethnic medicines, as those prescribed by practitioners of Ayurveda or traditional Chinese medicine, may intentionally contain heavy metals or other toxic substances. These are usually listed by their pharmacopeial names, e.g., *qian dan* = lead oxide.
  - Bitter orange (*Citrus sinensis*): Sympathomimetic; increases heart rate (HR), BP
  - California poppy (*Eschscholzia californica*): May cause respiratory depression, drowsiness; contains opioids
  - Cascara sagrada (*Frangula purshiana*): Depletes serum potassium
  - Chaparral (*Larrea tridentata*): Hepatotoxic
  - Ephedra (*Ephedra* species): Sympathomimetic; increases HR, BP; insomnia, gastric distress
  - Ginkgo (*Ginkgo biloba*): Extravasation, increased bleeding time
  - Guarana (*Paullinia cupana*): Tachycardia, hypertension; contains caffeine
  - Kava (*Piper methysticum*): Decreases utilization of niacin; possibly hepatotoxic
  - Licorice (*Glycyrrhiza* species): Long-term use depletes serum potassium.
  - Lily of the valley (*Convallaria majalis*): Contains cardiac glycosides
  - Poke root (*Phytolacca* species): Strong gastric irritant, may cause sedation
  - Senna (*Cassia senna*): Depletes serum potassium
  - Snakeroot (*Aristolochia* species): Nephrotoxic
  - Wormwood (*Artemisia absinthium*): Elevates serotonin level, may raise BP
  - Yohimbe (*Pausinystalia yohimbe*): Elevates BP
- Important herbal–medication interactions:
  - Ginkgo and St. John's wort account for most herb–drug interactions described in the medical literature.
  - Angelica, dong quai (*Angelica* species): Additive effect with calcium channel blockers
  - Bitter melon (*Momordica charantia*): Additive effect with other hypoglycemic agents
  - Cascara sagrada (*Frangula purshiana*): Shortens transit time of intestinally absorbed drugs; potential for causing hypokalemia may potentiate digoxin toxicity
  - Chamomile (*Anthemis, Matricaria* species): Antagonistic interaction with benzodiazepines
  - Echinacea (*Echinacea* species): May counteract immunosuppressants
  - Garlic (*Allium sativum*): Modest anticoagulant effect; decreases levels of saquinavir
  - Guarana (*Paullina cupana*): Contains caffeine; may inhibit platelet aggregation
  - Ginkgo (*G. biloba*): Dangerous synergistic effect with anticoagulants (2)
  - Ginseng (*Panax* species): Potentiates dopaminergic drugs; counteracts phenothiazines
  - Kava (*Piper methysticum*): Additive effect with sedatives
  - Kelp (*Laminaria* species): May interfere with thyroxine and liothyronine
  - Lemon balm (*Melissa officinalis*): Additive effect with sedatives; binds TSH and may interfere with thyroid testing and function
  - Licorice (*Glycyrrhiza* species): Increases potential for digoxin toxicity; depletes potassium
  - Lobelia (*Lobelia* species): Potentially counteracts β_2 adrenergic bronchodilators
  - Meadowsweet (*Filipendula ulmaria*): Increased anticoagulant effect; contains salicylates
  - Motherwort (*Leonurus cardiaca*): Can potentiate digoxin; contains cardiac glycosides
  - Milk thistle (*Silybum marianum*): Might accelerate clearance of liver-metabolized drugs
  - Pumpkin seed (*Cucurbita pepo*): Elevates levels of androgenic drugs
  - Red clover (*Trifolium pratense*): Partial agonistic/antagonistic interaction with estrogens
  - Saw palmetto (*Serenoa repens*): May potentiate or antagonize androgenic drugs
  - Soy isoflavones (*Glycine max*): Partial agonistic/antagonistic interaction with estrogens
  - St. John's wort (*Hypericum perforatum*): Induces CYP450 pathways, reducing levels of many drugs (3)
  - Tobacco (*Nicotiana tabacum*): May counteract β-blockers
  - Uva ursi (*Arctostaphylos uva-ursi*): Interferes with action of other diuretics; may cause faster clearance of renally metabolized drugs
  - Valerian (*Valeriana officinalis*): Potential for interference with valproic acid derivatives
  - Willow bark (*Salix alba*): Additive effect with anticoagulants; contains salicylates
- Vitamins and minerals with potential toxicity:
  - Iron is a leading cause of accidental poisoning in children under 6. Minerals (i.e., potassium, calcium, magnesium, zinc, copper, and selenium) may cause toxicity.
  - Fat-soluble vitamins have the potential to cause hypervitaminosis:
    - Vitamin A is most common cause of hypervitaminosis.
    - β-carotene may have a limited potential for overdose.
  - Vitamin A: Pseudotumor cerebri, hepatic damage, loss of appetite, osteomalacia
  - Vitamin D: Constipation, hypercalcemia. Recommended dose for children is 400 IU/d and for adults is 800 IU/d.
  - Vitamin E: Coagulopathy, fatigue, pain in extremities

REFERENCES

1. Barnes PM, Bloom B, Nahin RL, et al. Complementary and alternative medicine use among adults and children: United States, 2007. *Natl Health Stat Report*. 2008;1–23.
2. Anderson JW, Liu C, Kryscio RJ. Blood pressure response to transcendental meditation: A meta-analysis. *Am J Hypertens*. 2008;21:310–6.
3. Manheimer E, White A, Berman B, et al. Meta-analysis: Acupuncture for low back pain. *Ann Intern Med*. 2005;142:651–63.
4. Wilkinson SM, Love SB, Westcombe AM, et al. Effectiveness of aromatherapy massage in the management of anxiety and depression in patients with cancer: A multicenter randomized controlled trial. *J Clin Oncol*. 2007;25:532–9.
5. Kiecolt-Glaser JK, Belury MA, Andridge R, et al. Omega-3 supplementation lowers inflammation and anxiety in medical students: A randomized controlled trial. *Brain Behav Immun*. 2011;25(8): 1725–34.
6. Makariou S, Liberopoulos EN, Elisaf M, et al. Novel roles of vitamin D in disease: What is new in 2011? *Eur J Intern Med*. 2011;22:355–62.

ADDITIONAL READING

Bent S, et al. Herbal medicine in the United States: Review of efficacy, safety, and regulation: Grand rounds at University of California, San Francisco Medical Center. *J Gen Intern Med*. 2008;23:854–9.

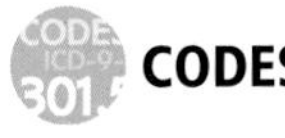

CODES

CLINICAL PEARLS

- CAM are medical and health care systems, practices, and products not presently considered part of conventional medicine.
- Medical professionals who incorporate CAM into their medical practice will often refer to their health care model as "integrative medicine."

COMPLEX REGIONAL PAIN SYNDROME

Dennis E. Hughes, DO

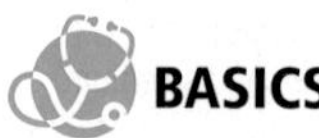

BASICS

Multidisciplinary approach with physical, occupational, and recreational therapy involvement

DESCRIPTION

- Pain syndrome after injury to bone and soft tissue; pathogenesis is obscure. Evidence suggests that these syndromes involve areas of the brain and nervous system:
  - Type I: No nerve injury (reflex sympathetic dystrophy [RSD])
  - Type II: Associated with a demonstrable nerve injury (causalgia)
- System(s) affected: Nervous
- Synonym(s): Traumatic erythromelalgia; Weir Mitchell causalgia; Causalgia; Reflex sympathetic dystrophy; Posttraumatic neuralgia; Sympathetically maintained pain

EPIDEMIOLOGY

- Predominant age: Mean age 36–46 years
- Predominant gender: Female > Male (3:1, 60–81%)
- Extremely rare in children

Incidence

26.2/100,000 person-years, but may be higher due to misdiagnosis initially

Prevalence

~6 million in the US

RISK FACTORS

- Minor or severe trauma (upper extremity fracture noted in 44%)
- Surgery (particularly carpal tunnel release)
- Lacerations
- Burns
- Frostbite
- Casting/immobilization after extremity injury
- Penetrating injury
- Polymyalgia rheumatica
- Myocardial infarction
- Cerebral vascular accident

Genetics

No known genetic pattern

GENERAL PREVENTION

- Early mobilization after fracture, stroke, and myocardial infarction has proven benefit in reducing incidence of complex regional pain syndrome (CRPS).
- 1 study of wrist fractures found that addition of 500 mg/d of vitamin C lowered rates of CRPS.
- There is evidence that limited use of tourniquets, regional anesthetic use, and ensuring adequate perioperative analgesia can reduce the incidence of CRPS-I (1)[A].

PATHOPHYSIOLOGY

Poorly understood activation of abnormal sympathetic reflex that lowers pain threshold

ETIOLOGY

Other than known nerve injury (type II or causalgia), no known definitive pathogenesis

COMMONLY ASSOCIATED CONDITIONS

- Serious injury to bone and soft tissue
- Herpes zoster
- Postherpetic neuralgia results from partial or complete damage to afferent nerve pathways.
- Pain occurs in dermatomes as a sequela of herpes zoster.

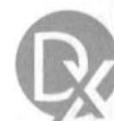

DIAGNOSIS

Unprovoked pain is the hallmark of the condition.

HISTORY

- Inciting injury ranges from minor sprains to major trauma.
- Hyperhydrosis
- Thermal hypersensitivity
- Hair loss
- Burning paroxysms of pain
- Increased symptoms during emotional stress
- Muscle spasms
- Hypersensitivity to light touch
- Mottled skin
- Partial motor paralysis

PHYSICAL EXAM

- Early: Area usually edematous; may be either hyper- or hypothermic; decreased hair; diminished nail growth
- Established: Skin is indurated, cool, hyperhydrotic; notable hair loss and nail changes; SC tissue atrophy
- Late: Skin appears thin and shiny; may see contractures of extremity

DIAGNOSTIC TESTS & INTERPRETATION

Lab

Initial lab tests

- CBC
- ESR

Imaging

Initial approach

- Plain radiographs may show patchy demineralization within 3–6 weeks of onset of CRPS and more pronounced than one would see from disuse alone.
- 3-phase bone scanning has varying sensitivity but is most accurate for support of the diagnosis when there is diffuse activity (especially on phase 3).
- Bone densometry

Diagnostic Procedures/Surgery

- Electromyelography (EMG) shows nerve injury with type II CRPS.
- Sudomotor function testing (resting sweat testing, resting skin temperature, quantitative sudomotor axon reflex testing—all related to increased autonomic activity of the affected limb)

Pathological Findings

- Partial or complete damage to afferent nerve pathways and probably reorganized central pain pathways
- Nerves most commonly involved are median and sciatic.
- Atrophy in affected muscles
- Incomplete nerve plexus lesion

DIFFERENTIAL DIAGNOSIS

- Infection
- Hypertrophic scar
- Bone fragments
- Neuroma
- CNS tumor or syrinx
- Deep vein thrombosis or thrombophlebitis
- Thoracic outlet syndrome

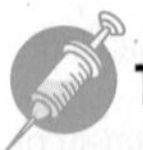

TREATMENT

MEDICATION

First Line

- No single drug or combination of drugs has produced consistent results; early therapy is crucial. There is no scientific support for the use of narcotic pain relievers, and this approach should be avoided.
- The following have literature support of either limited or suggestive benefit in treatment of CRPS-I (1)[A]:
  - Gabapentin 600–1,800 mg q24h for 8 weeks following diagnosis
  - 50% DMSO cream applied to affected extremity up to 5 times daily
  - N-acetylcysteine 600 mg t.i.d.
  - Bisphosphonates (alendronate) at 40 mg daily (however, optimal dose uncertain)
  - Nifedipine 20 mg daily showed benefit early in the course of the condition
  - Corticosteroids seemed to be beneficial, but dosing is uncertain. Prednisone 30 mg daily for 2–3 weeks with a tapering dose over the following 2–4 weeks has been used.
- Although many have advocated the use of tricyclic antidepressants in the treatment of CRPS, there is no credible evidence of improvement of pain. They may be helpful in controlling depressive symptoms that develop with disease progression.
- No evidence currently exists that supports the use of oral muscle relaxants (1)[A].

Second Line
Subanesthetic doses of IV ketamine

ADDITIONAL TREATMENT
General Measures
Discourage maladaptive behaviors (pain-medication seeking, secondary gain).

Issues for Referral
- After 2 months of the illness, psychological evaluation generally is indicated to identify and treat any comorbid conditions.
- Identifying local resources and early referral for expert management give increased likelihood of long-term success in controlling condition.

Additional Therapies
Type I:
- Physical therapy (beneficial to the overall prognosis for recovery):
  - Should be started early
  - "Mirror therapy" has shown good results (2)[A].
- Transcutaneous nerve stimulation
- Psychotherapy

COMPLEMENTARY AND ALTERNATIVE MEDICINE
- Vitamin C (500 mg/d) may help to prevent CRPS in those with wrist fracture.
- Briskly rub the affected part several times per day.
- Acupuncture
- Hypnosis can be suggested.
- Relaxation training (alternate muscle relaxing and contracting)
- Biofeedback

SURGERY/OTHER PROCEDURES
- Type II responds more favorably to nerve-directed treatment:
  - Sympathetic blocks
  - Cervicothoracic or lumbar sympathectomies have little data to support their use and should be used judiciously and after all therapies have failed (3)[A].
- Anesthetic blockade (chemical or surgical) of sympathetic nerve function:
  - Transient relief suggests that chemical or surgical sympathectomy will be helpful.
  - Little in the way of quality clinical trials exist to support local sympathetic blockage as the "gold standard" of therapy.
- IV regional sympathetic block with guanethidine or reserpine by pain specialist or anesthetist
- Transcutaneous electric nerve stimulation (controversial)
- Inject myofascial painful trigger points
- Spinal cord stimulation (quality of life improved only with implanted system)
- Intrathecal analgesia
- Amputation as a last resort in severe cases with patients reporting improved quality of life

IN-PATIENT CONSIDERATIONS
Admission Criteria
Only for proposed surgical therapy

ONGOING CARE

FOLLOW-UP RECOMMENDATIONS
Weekly to monitor progress and initiate additional modalities as needed

PATIENT EDUCATION
- Stress need to remain active physically.
- Instruct carefully about any prescribed medications.
- Reflex Sympathetic Dystrophy Syndrome Association, www.rsds.org, (203) 877-3790 or American RSD Hope Group, www.rsdhope.org, (207) 583-4589

PROGNOSIS
Most improve with early treatment, but symptoms may be lifelong if there is limited response to initial treatments.

COMPLICATIONS
- Depression
- Disability
- Opioid dependence

REFERENCES

1. Perez RS, Zollinger PE, Dijkstra PU, et al. Evidence based guidlines for complex regional pain syndrome type I. *BMC Neurol*. 2010;10:20.
2. Ezendam D, Bongers RM, Jannink MJ, et al. Systematic review of the effectiveness of mirror therapy in upper extremity function. *Disabil Rehabil*. 2009;31:2135–49.
3. Straube S, Derry S, Moore RA, et al. Cervical-thorasic or lumbar sympathectomy for neuropathic pain and complex regional pain syndrome. *Cochran Database Syst Rev*. 2010;7:CD002918.

ADDITIONAL READING

- Brunner F, Schmid A, Kissling R, et al. Biphosphonates for the therapy of complex regional pain syndrome I—Systematic review. *Eur J Pain*. 2008.
- Lang L. Living with RSDS. *Your Guide to Coping with Reflex Sympathetic Dystrophy Syndrome*. Oakland CA: New Harbinger; 2003.
- Tran de QH, Duong S, Bertini P, et al. Treatment of complex regional pain syndrome: A review of the evidence. *Can J Anaesth*. 2010;57(2):149–66.

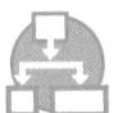

See Also (Topic, Algorithm, Electronic Media Element)

Algorithm: Pain in Upper Extremity

CODES

ICD9
- 337.20 Reflex sympathetic dystrophy, unspecified
- 337.21 Reflex sympathetic dystrophy of the upper limb
- 337.22 Reflex sympathetic dystrophy of the lower limb

CLINICAL PEARLS
- Pain control and early mobility are key to recovery.
- Avoidance of narcotic analgesics
- Use multidisciplinary approach.

CONCUSSION

J. Herbert Stevenson, MD

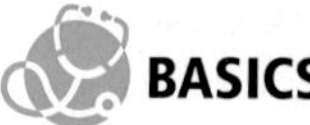

BASICS

DESCRIPTION

- A complex pathophysiologic process affecting brain function, induced by traumatic biomechanical forces, that generally resolves over 7–10 days
- Concussion severity can only be determined in retrospect.
- System(s) affected: Cardiovascular; Endocrine/Metabolic; Nervous; Psychiatric
- Synonym(s): Mild traumatic brain injury (TBI)

Pediatric Considerations

Children (ages 5–18) should not be allowed to return to training or play that same day and not until completely symptom-free. Resolution of symptoms and clinical findings often take longer in the pediatric athlete.

EPIDEMIOLOGY

- Predominant age: 12–24 years
- Predominant sex: Male > Female
- Usually related to accidents, sometimes sports related

Incidence

- 0.14–3.66 injuries/100 players each season at high school level
- 0.5–3.0 injuries/1,000 athlete exposures at college level (1)
- Average annual incidence 503:100,000
- ~1.5 million cases of TBI in US annually, 85% of which are considered mild TBI
- ~10% of TBIs are related to sports or cycling injuries.
- Among the 5–14 age group, 26.4% of mild TBI is related to sports or cycling (2).

RISK FACTORS

Contact sports, particularly football, and history of recent concussion

GENERAL PREVENTION

- Educate athletes, coaches, parents, and officials on signs and symptoms of concussions.
- Rule enforcement in sports (e.g., penalties for spearing or head-to-head contact)
- Consideration of rule changes in sports to decrease dangerous plays
- Current protective headgear for contact sports decreases facial injuries but has not been shown to decrease the overall concussion risk.
- Useful Web site: www.thinkfirst.ca/default.asp

PATHOPHYSIOLOGY

Concussion represents a functional brain injury rather than a structural brain injury. The neurobiologic cascade has been shown to include excitatory amino acid release, ionic flux, hyperglycolysis, and reduced cerebral blood flow.

ETIOLOGY

- Falls
- Sports related
- Motor vehicle accidents

DIAGNOSIS

HISTORY

- Cognitive symptoms:
  - Confusion
  - Posttraumatic amnesia (PTA)
  - Retrograde amnesia (RGA)
  - Loss of consciousness (LOC)
  - Disorientation
  - Feeling "in a fog," "zoned out"
  - Inability to focus
  - Delayed verbal and motor responses
  - Slurred/incoherent speech
  - Excessive drowsiness
- Somatic:
  - Headache
  - Fatigue
  - Disequilibrium, dizziness
  - Visual disturbances
  - Phonophobia
- Affective:
  - Emotional lability
  - Irritability
- Sleep disturbance

PHYSICAL EXAM

Variable and dependent on degree of injury:

- ABCs if seen acutely
- External evidence of major trauma
- Focal neurologic signs and symptoms
- Musculoskeletal: Evaluate for possible C-spine injury and stability.
- Detailed neurologic exam, including:
  - State of alertness
  - Orientation
  - 3- or 5-word recall at 5 minutes
  - Concentration/attention (serial 3s or 7s)
  - Cerebellar function and postural stability assessment

DIAGNOSTIC TESTS & INTERPRETATION

- The validated sideline assessment of concussion (SAC) scale score has been shown in studies to drop from baseline after a concussion and return to baseline once symptoms clear.
- Serial cognitive evaluations should be done by an experienced health care provider using the neurologic exam listed above or by using other assessment tools, such as the sport concussion assessment tool (SCAT) (3)[C].
- Computerized neurocognitive testing to date lacks sufficient evidence on validity, cost effectiveness, and improved management to warrant global usage (4)[B].
- Current gold standard is evaluation and treatment by a trained physician. Until improved outcomes, validity, and cost-effectiveness of computerized testing are established, use should be limited to experimental situations or possibly in management of complex concussions.

Lab

Generally not necessary

Imaging

- Structural neuroimaging is usually normal in the setting of concussion.
- Consider MRI or CT with prolonged LOC, focal neurologic deficit, or overall worsening symptoms.
- Role of functional MRI is largely experimental and unvalidated at this time.
- Consider C-spine films.

Diagnostic Procedures/Surgery

Serial neurologic exams at least every 10–15 minutes until symptoms are clearing and patient is stabilizing or patient has been transported to hospital for further evaluation.

DIFFERENTIAL DIAGNOSIS

- Concussion
- Subdural hematoma
- Epidural hematoma
- Cerebral contusion
- Facial or skull fracture

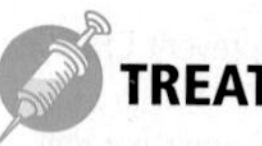

TREATMENT

MEDICATION

- Ibuprofen or acetaminophen may be used as adjunct pain management for headache once structural brain injury ruled out.
- Prolonged symptoms, such as sleep disturbance, depression, or anxiety, may benefit from appropriate pharmacologic treatment for symptom relief.

ADDITIONAL TREATMENT

General Measures

- Acute management depends on severity of injury. Most patients need only physical and cognitive rest, serial clinical evaluations to include neurologic checks, and a plan for follow-up evaluation (1)[C].
- Prolonged LOC, abnormal neurologic exam, or deteriorating symptoms necessitate urgent or emergent referral to the hospital for further evaluation (1)[C].

Issues for Referral

- Most concussions can be managed by primary care physicians using the standard guidelines for return to play; generally, referral to a specialist is not needed.
- Patients with a complex or atypical concussion, or who have suffered recurrent concussions, should be referred to a sports medicine physician or neurologist for management and clearance prior to returning to sports activities.

SURGERY/OTHER PROCEDURES

Generally not indicated, unless signs of more severe TBI present, with increased intracranial pressure or large bleed

IN-PATIENT CONSIDERATIONS

Initial Stabilization

- ABCs take priority over head injury and concussion.
- C-spine immobilization should be considered in all head trauma.

Admission Criteria

- Progressive neurologic symptoms, including deterioration of mental status, seizures, and focal neurologic signs
- No competent adult at home

Discharge Criteria

- Improving mental status at or near baseline
- Competent adult at home for patient observation (see "Patient Monitoring")

ONGOING CARE

FOLLOW-UP RECOMMENDATIONS

- Any athlete with a suspected concussion should be withheld that day from sports participation and not returned until a concussion has been ruled out or a diagnosed concussion has been appropriately treated as noted below (3).
- Current recommendation on treatment involves an asymptomatic graduated return to play as follows (3)[C]:
  - Complete rest until symptom-free, including cognitive rest (e.g., video games and potentially scholastic activities)
  - May then begin gradual reintroduction of activity as long as symptom-free. Each step should be generally done 24 hours apart:
    - Light aerobic exercise
    - Sport-specific exercise
    - Noncontact training drills
    - Full-contact training
    - Game play
- If postconcussive symptoms occur (exertional headache, visual disturbance, or disequilibrium), decrease level of activity until again asymptomatic, and progress again in 24 hours.
- High-risk athletes for more prolonged recovery include pediatric athletes, athletes with mood disorders, athletes with learning disabilities, and athletes with migraine headaches. These athletes should have a slower return to play progression and may require more intensive evaluation (formal neuropsychologic, balance, symptom testing).
- Athletes with multiple concussions should have slower return to play and may benefit from sports medicine consultation or neurology referral.

Patient Monitoring

- Written instructions regarding postconcussion management should be given to a competent adult describing signs to watch for and when to bring the patient back for further evaluation.
- Have a follow-up plan prior to discharge to home, ideally to be seen within a few days.
- Instruct patients and families regarding postconcussive symptoms, including the cognitive, somatic, and affective symptoms listed earlier.
- Ensure adequate rest and symptom-free return to both school and sports-related activities.

DIET

As tolerated

COMPLICATIONS

- Delayed hematomas, including subdural hematomas, can present minutes to hours after initial injury, necessitating serial neurologic checks and close observation.
- Postconcussion syndrome occurs when symptoms of concussion, such as headache, fatigue, memory changes, or emotional lability, are persistent and last >1–3 months.
- Second-impact syndrome describes a rare, but life-threatening, cerebral edema that occurs after repeated head injury, before the brain has had adequate time to completely recover. The etiology is thought to be due to loss of regulation of either cerebral circulation or glucose metabolism in the concussed brain.
- Recurrent concussions can lead to second-impact syndrome or can occur with less and less impact force. Symptoms can persist longer than after the first concussion, and progression to chronic cognitive and psychiatric symptoms is possible.
- Chronic TBI with chronic cognitive, mood, and potential Parkinson-type symptoms (5) "dementia pugilistica."

REFERENCES

1. Concussion (mild traumatic brain injury) and the team physician: A consensus statement. *Med Sci Sports Exerc*. 2006;38:395–9.
2. Bazarian JJ, McClung J, Shah MN, et al. Mild traumatic brain injury in the United States, 1998–2000. *Brain Inj*. 2005;19:85–91.
3. McCrory P, Meeuwisse W, Johnston K, et al. Consensus Statement on Concussion in Sport: The 3rd International Conference on Concussion in Sport held in Zurich, November 2008. *Br J Sports Med*. 2009;42(Suppl 1):i76–90.
4. Randolph C, McCrea M, Barr W. Is neuropsychological testing useful in the management of sport-related concussion? *J Athletic Train*. 2005;40(3):136–51.
5. Guskiewicz KM, Marshall SW, Bailes J, et al. Association between recurrent concussion and late-life cognitive impairment in retired professional football players. *Neurosurgery*. 2005;57.

ADDITIONAL READING

- Halstead ME, Walter KD, Council on Sports Medicine and Fitness, et al. American Academy of Pediatrics. Clinical report–sport-related concussion in children and adolescents. *Pediatrics*. 2010;126:597–615.
- Mayers L. Return-to-play criteria after athletic concussion: A need for revision. *Arch Neurol*. 2008;65:1158–61.

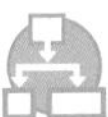

See Also (Topic, Algorithm, Electronic Media Element)

Brain Injury, Post Acute Care Issues; Brain Injury, Traumatic; Postconcussive Syndrome; Seizure Disorders

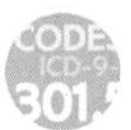

CODES

ICD9

- 780.93 Memory loss
- 850.0 Concussion with no loss of consciousness
- 850.9 Concussion, unspecified

CLINICAL PEARLS

- Most symptoms resolve completely within 7–10 days, but each person recovers at a different rate, and some symptoms may continue for weeks to months.
- Some athletes notice worsening symptoms, such as headache or nausea, while concentrating. If symptoms worsen while in class, the student should stay home from school until symptoms clear.
- Generally, patients who have been observed for at least 1–2 hours and are stable or improving do not need to be roused from sleep.
- When symptom-free at rest, the athlete may begin a gradual ramp-up of activity over 3–5 days, as listed above. If symptoms recur during any level of play, the athlete should postpone further activity for at least another 24 hours.

CONDYLOMATA ACUMINATA

Meredith Ulmer, DO
Sabrina A. Indyk, MD
William J. Moran, DO

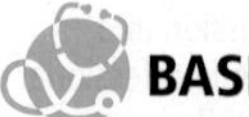

BASICS

DESCRIPTION

Condylomata acuminata are soft, skin-colored, fleshy lesions (commonly called genital warts) that are caused by human papillomavirus (HPV):

- HPV types 6, 11, 16, 18, 31, 33, and 35 associated with condylomata acuminata
- Highly contagious; incubation period may be from 1–8 months.
- Most infections are transient and clear within 2 years.
- Warts appear singly or in groups, small or large; on the vagina, cervix, around the external genitalia and rectum, and in the urethra and anus. Reports of conjunctival, nasal, oral, and laryngeal warts and occasionally the throat.
- System(s) affected: Skin/Exocrine; Reproductive

Pediatric Considerations

- Consider sexual abuse if seen in children, although they can be infected by other means (e.g., transfer from wart on another child's hand). It has also been suggested that condyloma in children younger than age 4 may still be due to nonsexual route of transmission due to the possibility of a prolonged latency period.
- American Academy of Pediatrics recommends all school-aged children who present with lesions be evaluated for abuse and screened for other STDs (1).

Pregnancy Considerations

- Warts often grow larger during pregnancy and regress spontaneously after delivery.
- Virus does not cross the placenta. Treatment during pregnancy is somewhat controversial. Cesarean section is not absolutely indicated.
- Cervical infection has been found to be a risk factor for preterm birth (2).
- There have been a few documented cases of laryngeal papillomas due to HPV transmission at the time of delivery. While rare, the condition is life threatening.
- HPV vaccination is contraindicated in pregnancy.

EPIDEMIOLOGY

- Most common viral sexually transmitted infection (STI) in the US
- More than half of sexually active women have been shown to harbor the virus.
- Predominant age: 15–30 years old
- Predominant sex: Male = Female

Incidence

- Venereal warts are increasing in an ever-younger population. A recent study indicated that 50% of new cases occur in adolescent females ages 15–34.
- Increased size and number in immunocompromised patients

Prevalence

- Peak prevalence in ages 17–33
- 10–20% of sexually active women may be infected with HPV. Studies in men suggest a similar prevalence.
- Pregnancy and immunosuppression favor recurrence and increasing growth of lesions.

RISK FACTORS

- Young adults and adolescents
- Multiple sexual partners
- Not using condoms
- Young age of commencing sexual activity
- Tobacco smoke has been shown to reduce cellular protection by decreasing cervical keratinocyte production.
- Poor hygiene
- Immunosuppression
- Short interval between meeting new sex partner and first intercourse

GENERAL PREVENTION

- Use of condoms (preventive effects not adequately evaluated; 40% of infected men have scrotal warts)
- Abstinence until treatment completed
- Circumcision may prevent recurrence in some men.
- Quadrivalent HPV vaccine available against genital warts and cervical cancer. This vaccination is targeted to adolescents before the period of their greatest risk for exposure to HPV. The vaccine does not treat previous infections:
  - Immunity has been documented to last at least 5 years after HPV vaccination.
  - The use of 4 HPV-specific virion protein capsids addresses the 2 most common HPV serotypes to be contracted in 6 and 11, and the 2 most cancer-promoting types in 16 and 18 (Gardasil) (3)[A].
  - HPV quadrivalent vaccine protects against some types of condyloma-producing virus.
  - Quadrivalent vaccine, females and males (3)[A] ages 9–26: Vaccine is administered IM; 3 doses to achieve optimal seroconversion
  - Vaccination: 0.5 mL IM first dose and at months 2 and 6
- Bivalent HPV vaccine is available, but does not cover the common viruses that cause condyloma lesions (Cervarix).
- Quadrivalent vaccine has recently been proven effective in prevention of external lesions in males 16–26 years of age (4).

ETIOLOGY

HPV is a circular, double-stranded DNA molecule. There are >70 HPV subtypes. Types 6 and 11 cause common venereal warts. Cervical dysplasia and carcinoma in situ associated with types 16, 18, 31, 33, and 35.

COMMONLY ASSOCIATED CONDITIONS

- >90% of cervical cancer associated with HPV
- 60% oropharyngeal carcinomas and anogenital squamous cell carcinomas are associated with HPV (5).
- STIs (i.e., gonorrhea, syphilis, chlamydia); AIDS

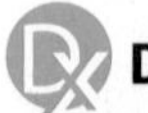

DIAGNOSIS

HISTORY

Explore sexual history, contraception use, and other lifestyle issues:

- Pruritus
- Vaginal discharge
- Irritation (burning and redness)

PHYSICAL EXAM

- Multiple fingerlike projections; soft, sessile; smooth or rough
- Perianal condylomata acuminata usually rough and cauliflowerlike
- Male sites include frenulum, corona, glans, prepuce, meatus, shaft, and scrotum:
  - Penile lesions often smooth and papular; occur in groups of 3 or 4
- Female sites include labia, clitoris, periurethral area, perineum, vagina, and cervix (flat lesions).
- Bleeding (result of trauma)
- Perianal area (both sexes)

DIAGNOSTIC TESTS & INTERPRETATION

Acetowhitening test: Subclinical lesions can be visualized by wrapping the penis with gauze soaked with 5% acetic acid for 5 minutes. Using a 10× hand lens or colposcope, warts appear as tiny white papules. A shiny white appearance of the skin represents foci of epithelial hyperplasia (subclinical infection); not highly specific, low positive predictive value.

Lab

- Serologic tests for syphilis negative
- Pap smear

Diagnostic Procedures/Surgery

Biopsy with highly specialized identification techniques rarely useful. HPV DNA detected through polymerase chain reaction:

- Colposcopy
- Antroscopy, anoscopy, urethroscopy may be required

Pathological Findings

- Possible cervical dysplasia
- Sometimes difficult to differentiate from squamous cell carcinoma

DIFFERENTIAL DIAGNOSIS

- Condylomata lata (flat warts of syphilis)
- Lichen planus
- Normal sebaceous glands
- Seborrheic keratosis
- Molluscum contagiosum
- Keratomas, micropapillomatosis
- Scabies
- Crohn disease
- Skin tags
- Melanocytic nevi
- Vulvar intraepithelial neoplasia
- Buschke-Lowenstein tumor

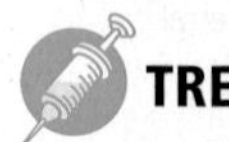

TREATMENT

MEDICATION

First Line

- Imiquimod (Aldara): Self-treatment with a 5% cream applied overnight 3 times weekly until warts resolve for up to 16 weeks. Wash off with soap and water 6–10 hours after application (1,6):
  - Precautions: Imiquimod has been noted to weaken condoms and diaphragms; therefore, patients should refrain from sexual contact while the cream is on the skin (6).
- Cryotherapy: Liquid nitrogen applied to warts for two 10-second bursts; usually requires 2–3 weekly sessions (6):

- Recent study shows that addition of ALA-photodynamic therapy increased efficacy of treatment (7)[B].
- Podophyllin in tincture of benzoin. Apply directly to warts. Leave on for 1–4 hours, then wash off. Repeat every 7 days in office until gone (6,8).
- Podofilox (Condylox): Apply to warts q12h (allowing to dry) for 3 consecutive days at home. May repeat after 4 days (6,8).
- Trichloroacetic acid: 25–85%. Apply only to warts. Use powder/talc to remove unreacted acid. Repeat in office at weekly intervals. Ideal for isolated lesions in pregnancy.
- Intralesion interferon has been shown to be effective in refractory cases and should be reserved for such cases (9).
- Oral cimetidine: 30–40 mg/kg divided t.i.d. for 3 months in children with genital and perigenital condyloma. Used as primary and adjunctive therapy (10).
- Contraindications:
  - Podophyllin: Do not use in pregnant patients or on oral, cervical, urethral, or perianal warts. Can use on limited number of vaginal warts with careful drying after application. It is recommended that no more than 0.5 mL be used.
  - Cryotherapy: Cryoglobulinemia
- Precautions:
  - Electrocautery: Do not use in patients with pacemaker.

Second Line
- External (penile and perianal):
  - Podophyllin (6)
  - Podofilox (Condylox) self-treatment (6)
  - Intralesional interferon
  - Cidofovir 1% topical applied once daily for 5 contiguous days per week for 6 cycles (11)
- Urethral meatus:
  - Podophyllin (6)
  - Cryotherapy (6)
- Anal:
  - Trichloroacetic acid: Apply weekly (12).
  - Topical fluorouracil is no longer recommended.
- Uterine/cervix:
  - Trichloroacetic acid and cryrotherapy are treatment options (6).
  - Oral isotretinoins can be used for the treatment of recalcitrant condyloma acuminata of the cervix (note special prescription monitoring for this class of medications) (13).

ADDITIONAL TREATMENT
Pregnancy Considerations
- Podophyllin, podofilox, and fluorouracil should not be used in pregnancy due to possible teratogenicity (6).
- Surgical excision, trichloroacetic acid, cryotherapy, and electrocautery are treatment options during pregnancy to minimize neonatal exposure to the virus (6).

General Measures
- May resolve spontaneously
- Change therapy if no improvement after 3 treatments, no complete clearance after 6 treatments, or therapy's duration or dosage exceeds manufacturer's recommendations.
- Appropriate screening/counseling of partners

SURGERY/OTHER PROCEDURES
- Larger warts require laser treatment or electrocoagulation, including infrared therapy (14):
  - Precaution: Laser treatment may create smoke plumes that contain HPV; it is recommended that masks be worn while performing this procedure.
- Surgical excision for large warts
- Intraurethral, external (penile and perianal), anal, and oral lesions can be treated with fulgurating CO_2 laser. Oral or external penile/perianal lesions can also be treated with electrocautery or surgery (6).

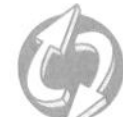

ONGOING CARE

FOLLOW-UP RECOMMENDATIONS
No restrictions, except for sexual contact

Patient Monitoring
- Patients seen every 2 weeks until lesions resolve and have annual Pap test.
- Patients should also follow up 3 months after completion of treatment.
- Persistent warts require biopsy.
- Sexual partners require monitoring.
- Treatment does not decrease transmissible infectivity.

PATIENT EDUCATION
- Provide pamphlets on HPV, STI prevention, and condom use.
- Emphasize the need for women to get regular Pap smears.

PROGNOSIS
- Warts will clear with treatment or resolve spontaneously, but recurrences are frequent and may necessitate repeated treatment.
- Some studies identified 3 independent risk factors for condylomatous relapse: Positive HIV status, male gender, and Langerhans cell level: Cell level per millimeter of anal tissue (15 vs. 30)
- Asymptomatic infection persists indefinitely.

COMPLICATIONS
- Cervical dysplasia
- Malignant change: Progression to cancer rarely, if ever, occurs.
- Male urethral obstruction
- The prevalence of high-grade dysplasia and cancer in anal canal is higher in HIV-positive than in HIV-negative patients, probably because of HPV activity.

REFERENCES

1. Culton DA, Morrell DS, Burkhart CN, et al. The management of condyloma acuminata in the pediatric population. *Pediatr Ann*. 2009;38: 368–72.
2. Zuo Z, Goel S, Carter JE, et al. Association of cervical cytology and HPV DNA status during pregnancy with placental abnormalities and preterm birth. *Am J Clin Pathol*. 2011;136:260–5.
3. Centers for Disease Control and Prevention (CDC), et al. FDA licensure of quadrivalent human papillomavirus vaccine (HPV4, Gardasil) for use in males and guidance from the Advisory Committee on Immunization Practices (ACIP). *MMWR Morb Mortal Wkly Rep*. 2010;59:630–2.
4. Giuliano AR, Palefsky JM, Goldstone S, et al. Efficacy of quadrivalent HPV vaccine against HPV Infection and disease in males. *N Engl J Med*. 2011;364:401–11.
5. van Monsjou HS, Balm AJ, van den Brekel MM, et al. Oropharyngeal squamous cell carcinoma: A unique disease on the rise? *Oral Oncol*. 2010;46: 780–5.
6. Charles M, Kodner MD, Soraya Nasraty MD. University of Louisville School of Medicine, Louisville, Kentucky. *Am Fam Physician*. 2004; 70(12):2335–2342.
7. Mi X, Chai W, Zheng H, et al. A randomized clinical comparative study of cryotherapy plus photodynamic therapy vs. cryotherapy in the treatment of multiple condylomata acuminata. *Photodermatol Photoimmunol Photomed*. 2011; 27:176–80.
8. Lacey CJ, et al. Randomised controlled trial and economic evaluation of podophyllotoxin solution, podophyllotoxin cream, and podophyllin in the treatment of genital warts. *Sex Transm Infect*. 2003;79:270.
9. Welander CE, Homesley HD, Smiles KA, et al. Intralesional interferon alfa-2b for the treatment of genital warts. *Am J Obstet Gynecol*. 1990;162: 348–54.
10. Franco I. Oral cimetidine for the management of genital and perigenital warts in children. *J Urol*. 2000;164:1074–5.
11. Snoeck R, Bossens M, Parent D, et al. Phase II double-blind, placebo-controlled study of the safety and efficacy of cidofovir topical gel for the treatment of patients with human papillomavirus infection. *Clin Infect Dis*. 2001;33:597–602.
12. Sobhani I, Vuagnat A, Walker F, et al. Prevalence of high-grade dysplasia and cancer in the anal canal in human papillomavirus-infected individuals. *Gastroenterology*. 2001;120:857–66.
13. Georgala S, Katoulis AC, Georgala C, et al. Oral isotretinoin in the treatment of recalcitrant condylomata acuminata of the cervix: A randomised placebo controlled trial. *Sex Transm Infect*. 2004;80:216–8.
14. Bekassy Z, Weström L, et al. Infrared coagulation in the treatment of condyloma acuminata in the female genital tract. *Sex Transm Dis*. 1987;14: 209–12.

ADDITIONAL READING

Workowski KA, Berman SM. Sexually transmitted diseases treatment guidelines, 2006. *MMWR Recomm Rep*. 2006;55:1–94.

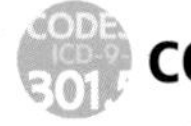

CODES

ICD9
078.11 Condyloma acuminatum

CLINICAL PEARLS
- Condylomata acuminata are soft, skin-colored, fleshy lesions caused by human papillomavirus (HPV) subtypes 6, 11, 16, 18, 31, 33, and 35
- Quadrivalent HPV vaccine available against genital warts and cervical cancer
- The use of 4 HPV-specific virion protein capsids addresses the 2 most common HPV serotypes to be contracted in 6 and 11, and the 2 most cancer-promoting types in 16 and 18 (Gardasil)
- Vaccine: 0.5 mL IM first dose and at months 2 and 6

C

CONGESTIVE HEART FAILURE

Jeremy Golding, MD

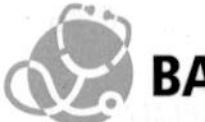

BASICS

DESCRIPTION

Congestive heart failure (CHF) (better term: Heart failure [HF], because not all heart failure is *congestive*) affects both the cardiovascular and pulmonary systems. It is the principal complication of heart disease. The heart is unable to fill and/or pump blood sufficiently to meet tissue metabolic needs. HF may involve the left heart, the right heart, or be biventricular. New York Heart Association (NYHA) Classification is a fundamental descriptive system used for classifying patients with HF: NYHA I—Asymptomatic; NYHA II—Symptomatic with moderate exertion; NYHA III—Symptomatic with mild exertion and may limit activities of daily living; NYHA IV—Symptomatic at rest.

EPIDEMIOLOGY

Medicare spends more to diagnose and treat HF than any other medical condition. In 2008, the total cost of HF approached $28 billion.

Incidence

In the US, 550,000 new cases annually with 250,000 deaths per year

Prevalence

- About 5.7 million people in the US have HF. <1% in those <50, increasing to 10% of those older than age 80.
- Primarily a disease of the elderly; 75% of hospital admissions for HF are in persons >65.

RISK FACTORS

- For development of HF: Coronary artery disease (CAD) and myocardial infarction (MI), hypertension (HTN) (80% of cases of HF in the US caused by either CAD or HTN), valvular heart disease, diabetes mellitus, cardiotoxic medications
- For HF exacerbation: Sodium intake and/or fluid excess; nonadherence to medication regimen; arrhythmia (e.g., atrial fibrillation); ischemic ventricular dysfunction; negative inotropic drugs (e.g., calcium blocker, introduction of beta-blocker); excessive physical, emotional, or environmental stress; thyrotoxicosis; pregnancy; or increased metabolic demand

Genetics

Familial cardiomyopathy predisposes to development of HF (rare).

GENERAL PREVENTION

Control BP and other risk factors. Thiazide diuretics and ACE inhibitors are superior to other agents in preventing development of HF.

PATHOPHYSIOLOGY

2 physiologic components explain most of the clinical findings of CHF:

- Systolic dysfunction: An *inotropic* abnormality, often due to MI or dilated or ischemic cardiomyopathy, resulting in diminished systolic emptying (ejection fraction <45%)
- Diastolic dysfunction: A *compliance* abnormality, often due to hypertensive cardiomyopathy, in which the ventricular relaxation is impaired (ejection fraction >45%)
- Patients with systolic dysfunction may also have diastolic dysfunction.

ETIOLOGY

- Coronary artery disease and ischemia, myocardial infarction
- Myocarditis and cardiomyopathy: Alcoholic, viral, longstanding HTN, drugs (e.g., chemotherapeutic agents), muscular dystrophy, amyloidosis (infiltrative), sarcoidosis (infiltrative), postpartum state, infectious (e.g., Chagas disease), HIV
- Valvular and vascular abnormalities: Aortic stenosis or regurgitation, rheumatic heart disease (mitral and aortic valvular disease). Renal artery stenosis, usually bilateral, may cause recurrent "flash" pulmonary edema, especially in setting of severe chronic HTN.
- Chronic lung disease and pulmonary HTN (right HF)
- Volume overload (requires extreme overload in patients with normal hearts and kidneys)
- Arrhythmias (atrial fibrillation and other tachyarrhythmias, high-grade heart block)
- Misc: High-output states: Hyperthyroidism, anemia, cardiac depressants (beta-blocker overdose)

COMMONLY ASSOCIATED CONDITIONS

Dysrhythmia, followed by pump failure, are the leading causes of death in this condition. Most patients have more than 5 comorbid medical conditions and take >5 medications.

DIAGNOSIS

HISTORY

- Dyspnea on exertion: *Cardinal sign of left HF*. Deteriorating exercise capacity: Easy fatigue, general weakness.
- Nocturnal nonproductive cough, orthopnea, and paroxysmal nocturnal dyspnea; sometimes frothy or pink sputum
- Wheezing, especially nocturnal, in absence of history of asthma or infection (cardiac asthma). Cheyne-Stokes breathing
- Anorexia/cachexia and/or fullness or dull pain in right upper quadrant (hepatic distension in right HF)
- Edema often with cool extremities due to peripheral vasoconstriction. Abdominal bloating (ascites) or anasarca. Cyanosis.

PHYSICAL EXAM

Rales (crackles) and sometimes wheezing, peripheral edema, S3 gallop, hepatomegaly, hepatojugular reflux, ascites, hypotension

DIAGNOSTIC TESTS & INTERPRETATION

Diagnosis of HF or HF exacerbation should be primarily clinical, with laboratory data as adjunctive and indicative of complications.

Lab

Initial lab tests

- β-type natriuretic peptide (BNP) and N-type pro-BNP (NT-BNP) may be helpful in:
  - Emergency department (ED) setting to help differentiate the cause of dyspnea (BNP <100 essentially rules out HF as cause of dyspnea with negative predictive value (NPV) of ~99%. Most dyspneic patients with HF have BNP >400.)
  - Titrating treatment, because its value changes rapidly with left ventricular (LV) functional status (unclear, however, that BNP- or NT-BNP guided therapy improves outcomes) (1)
  - BNP values of 100–400 are most problematic, as they may indicate HF or may be due to conditions like pulmonary embolism, renal failure, acute coronary syndromes, and pulmonary HTN.
  - Patients may have BNP elevation due to HF, but acute dyspnea may be from another cause (like pneumonia or pulmonary embolism).
- Lab findings in early and mild-to-moderately severe CHF include respiratory alkalosis, mild azotemia, decreased ESR, proteinuria (usually <1 g/24 h), elevated creatinine, dilutional hyponatremia (poor prognosis), and rarely hyperbilirubinemia.

Imaging

Initial approach

Chest x-ray (CXR) (changes lag clinical symptoms by up to 6 hours): Increased heart size, vascular redistribution (cephalization) with "butterfly" pattern of pulmonary edema, interstitial and alveolar edema, Kerley B lines, pleural effusions

Diagnostic Procedures/Surgery

Determination of ejection fraction is critical to proper diagnosis and management:

- Echocardiographic study is most-useful single test to determine ejection fraction and valvular abnormalities. May be repeated if change suspected in underlying cardiac status.
- Nuclear imaging to estimate left and right ventricular size, perfusion, and systolic function

Pathological Findings

- Cardiac pathology depends on underlying process (etiology) of HF.
- Noncardiac findings: Liver is engorged, firm, and fluid-filled. Microscopic analysis reveals dilated central hepatic veins and sinusoids. Late/chronic findings include hemosiderin deposits in lungs and "nutmeg" liver with centrilobular necrosis.

DIFFERENTIAL DIAGNOSIS

Simple dependent edema, pulmonary embolism, exertional asthma, cardiac ischemia with angina, chronic obstructive pulmonary disease (COPD), constrictive pericarditis, nephrotic syndrome, cirrhosis, venous occlusive disease with subsequent peripheral edema, high-output states: Anemia, sepsis, hyperthyroidism

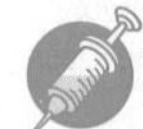

TREATMENT

MEDICATION

Diuretics are used initially in fluid-overload acute HF, with nitrates added if needed. Nitrates are primary therapy in ischemic acute HF (flash pulmonary edema), with diuretics secondary. Once acute HF is stabilized, an ACE inhibitor or beta-blocker should be started. Instruct patients not to use NSAIDs, which markedly worsen HF. Avoid use of diltiazem and verapamil in patients with systolic dysfunction.

First Line

The following is all [A]-level evidence unless otherwise noted:

- ACE inhibitors: Used to decrease afterload: Shown to increase survival, improve general symptomatology and overall exercise capacity in patients in all NYHA classifications; benefit greatest for patients with systolic dysfunction and post-MI. Number needed to treat (NNT) ~25/yr for mortality (2).

- β-blockers used in systolic or diastolic HF (Note: Initiate in hospital or outpatient setting in hemodynamically stable patients at low dose and titrate upward slowly); NNT = 25 for mortality. Evidence mounting for titration to heart rate rather than specific dose:
  - Carvedilol: 3.125 mg b.i.d. to a maintenance of 25 mg b.i.d.; metoprolol succinate extended release: 12.5 mg/d to a maximum of 200 mg/d (Note: Metoprolol tartrate may be equivalent but is taken b.i.d.) or bisoprolol 1.25–10 mg once daily
- Digoxin reduces symptoms, but has not shown any effect on mortality (2):
  - In patients with preserved renal function (creatinine clearance >50 mL/min), the recommended dose is 0.125 mg/d.
  - Levels lower than used for atrial fibrillation are effective and safer
- Diuretics helpful to manage volume overload. Continuous infusion is not better than bolus, and high-dose not significantly better than low-dose (3):
  - Furosemide (Lasix): 20–320 mg IV/IM/PO
  - Metolazone (Zaroxolyn): 2.5–20 mg/d PO
  - Spironolactone, eplerenone (only diuretics to reduce mortality when added to standard therapy in NYHA Class II, III, and IV) (4): Spironolactone 12.5–25 mg/d PO; maximum 50 mg/d PO Eplerenone 25–50 mg/d. Caution regarding hyperkalemia (2).
- Vasodilators:
  - IV nitroglycerin may be of short-term benefit to decrease preload, afterload, and systemic resistance, especially in acute heart failure.
  - The combination of hydralazine (75 mg/d divided b.i.d. or t.i.d.) and isosorbide dinitrate (40 mg q.i.d.) is effective for African Americans (2) or if unable to take ACE inhibitors or an angiotensin receptor blocker (ARB).
- Fish oil/omega-3 fatty acids: 1 g daily of n-3 polyunsaturated fatty acid (PUFA) reduced mortality and time to hospitalization (NNT ~170/yr) (5).

Second Line

- Angiotensin receptor blockers (ARBs) *have fewer side effects than ACE inhibitors, but are less effective than ACE inhibitors* and are, therefore, not first-line treatment.
- Dobutamine in outpatient basis with intermittent infusions. Despite improving quality of life, it reduces short-term survival.
- Nesiritide is approved for short-term use in decompensated HF. It is a recombinant form of human brain-type natriuretic peptide. Should not be used in ED, and is not appropriate for use in most patients with acute HF.

ADDITIONAL TREATMENT

Device therapy for HF increasingly successful, especially biventricular pacing for ventricular dyssynchrony and implantable cardiac defibrillators (automatic implantable cardioverter defibrillators [AICDs]):

- Biventricular pacing/cardiac resynchronization therapy (CRT) indicated for NYHA II, III (especially), or IV with low ejection fraction (EF) who are on optimal management for at least 3 months (2), with QRS >0.120 ms and who remain significantly symptomatic. Improves symptoms and all-cause mortality. Therapy likely indicated for most systolic dysfunction patients with wide QRS, even those with mild HF (6).
- AICD: Improve survival in dilated cardiomyopathy (7) and are recommended for: Primary prevention in patients with *ischemic* heart disease (HD) who are post-MI, LVEF<30%, Class 2 or 3 HF on optimal medical therapy, and >1 year estimated survival (2)[A], as well as for *nonischemic* HF EF<30%. Not indicated in Stage D (end-stage) HF.
- Treat anemia. Target minimum hematocrit (Hct) at least 30 and possibly somewhat higher. Improves quality of life and may reduce mortality.

Additional Therapies

Home oxygen for pulse oximetry <89% (resting or with activity)

SURGERY/OTHER PROCEDURES

- Heart valve surgery if defective heart valve is responsible; mitral valve repair especially helpful if mitral regurgitation is aggravating condition
- Cardiac transplantation to be considered in patients <55 and without other disqualifying medical problems who are developing CHF unresponsive to other therapeutic maneuvers, and who are considered to have a life expectancy of >1 year

IN-PATIENT CONSIDERATIONS

Initial Stabilization

Sublingual nitroglycerin is rapid-onset and reduces both pre- and afterload. Bilevel positive airway pressure (BiPap) may help delay or avoid intubation, and often gives rapid symptomatic relief. Morphine titrated to reduce anxiety/air hunger.

Admission Criteria

Acute change in HF, with pulmonary edema accompanied by decreased oxygenation, change in mental status, with acute renal insufficiency, or significant hyponatremia

IV Fluids

Limit. Avoid sodium-containing fluids unless necessary to urgently correct hyponatremia. Fluid restriction is best for nonurgent correction of hyponatremia.

Discharge Criteria

Subjective improvement, resting heart rate (HR) <100, systolic BP >80 mm Hg, HF outpatient education performed

ONGOING CARE

FOLLOW-UP RECOMMENDATIONS

Critical patient education performed at all outpatient and inpatient physician visits "MAWDS":

- **M**edications: Take every day; don't skip. **A**ctivity: A little every day; don't overdo.
- **W**eight: Daily. If gain >2 lb in a day or 5 lb above ideal, CALL **D**iet: Eat <2,000 mg Na+ daily.
- **S**ymptoms: Know the signs of worsening HF (cough, weight gain, worsening or rest dyspnea, swelling) and call the doctor early! Quit smoking, if a smoker!

Patient Monitoring

Rapid office follow-up after hospitalization and home health monitoring by specially trained nurses have both been shown to decrease frequency of hospitalizations.

DIET

Reduce sodium load (2 g).

PATIENT EDUCATION

- American Heart Association, 7320 Greenville Avenue, Dallas, TX 75231, (214) 373-6300

PROGNOSIS

After diagnosis 1-year survival ~75%, 5-year survival <50%, 10 year<25%

COMPLICATIONS

Sudden death (arrhythmic), acute pulmonary edema, death

REFERENCES

1. Porapakkham P, Porapakkham P, Zimmet H, et al. B-type natriuretic peptide-guided heart failure therapy: A meta-analysis. *Arch Intern Med*. 2010; 170:507–14.
2. Hunt SA, Abraham WT, Chin MH, et al. 2009 Focused update incorporated into the ACC/AHA 2005 Guidelines for the Diagnosis and Management of Heart Failure in Adults A Report of the American College of Cardiology Foundation/American Heart Association Task Force on Practice Guidelines. *J Am Coll Cardiol*. 2009;53:e1–e90.
3. Felker GM, Lee KL, Redfield MM, et al. Diuretic strategies in patients with acute decompensated heart failure. *N Engl J Med*. 2011;64:797.
4. Zannad F, et al. Eplerenone in patients with systolic heart failure and mild symptoms. *N Engl J Med*. 2011;364:11–21.
5. Gissi-Hf Investigators. Effect of n-3 polyunsaturated fatty acids in patients with chronic heart failure (the GISSI-HF trial): a randomised, double-blind, placebo-controlled trial. *Lancet*. 2008.
6. Al-Majed NS, et al. Meta-analysis: Cardiac resynchronization therapy for patients with less symptomatic heart failure. *Ann Intern Med*. 2011; 154(6):401–12.
7. Moss AJ, Hall WJ, Cannom DS, et al. Cardiac-resynchronization therapy for the prevention of heart-failure events. *N Engl J Med*. 2009.

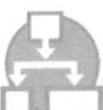

See Also (Topic, Algorithm, Electronic Media Element)

Algorithms: Congestive Heart Failure; Congestive Heart Failure, Treatment

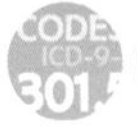

CODES

ICD9

428.0 Congestive heart failure, unspecified

CLINICAL PEARLS

- Have patients weigh themselves daily and report weight gains of >2 lb in a day or 5lb above dry weight.
- Beta-blockers, ACE inhibitors, and mineralocorticoid antagonists are the core medications for management of this condition.
- Consider referral for biventricular pacing in patients with bundle branch block, and AICD in those with low EF.

C

CONJUNCTIVITIS, ACUTE

Frances Y. Wu, MD

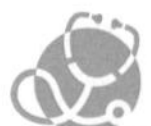

BASICS

DESCRIPTION

- Inflammation of the bulbar and/or palpebral conjunctiva of <4 weeks duration
- System(s) affected: Nervous, skin/exocrine
- Synonym(s): Pink eye

Geriatric Considerations

Suspect autoimmune, systemic, or irritative conditions

Pediatric Considerations

- Neonatal conjunctivitis may be gonococcal, chlamydial, irritative, or related to dacryocystitis.
- Pediatric emergency room study; 78% positive bacterial cult, mostly *H. influenzae*; 13% no growth; other studies showed greater than 50% adenovirus
- Daycare regulations sometimes require any child with presumed conjunctivitis to be treated with a topical antibiotic despite the lack of evidence.

EPIDEMIOLOGY

- Predominant age:
  - Pediatric: Viral, bacterial
  - Adult: Viral, bacterial, allergic
- Predominant sex: Male = Female

Incidence

In the US: Variable, but accounts for 1–2% of all ambulatory office visits

RISK FACTORS

- History of contact with infected persons
- Sexually transmitted disease (STD) contact: Gonococcal, chlamydial, syphilis, or herpes
- Contact lenses: Pseudomonal or acanthamoeba keratitis
- Epidemic bacterial (streptococcal) conjunctivitis reported in school settings

GENERAL PREVENTION

- Wash hands frequently.
- Demonstrate eye dropper technique: Eye is closed and head back, several drops at nasal margin; open eyes to allow liquid to enter. Never touch tip of dropper to skin or eye.

ETIOLOGY

- Viral:
  - Adenovirus (common cold) or coxsackie
  - Enterovirus (acute hemorrhagic conjunctivitis)
  - Herpes simplex
  - Herpes zoster or varicella
  - Measles, mumps, or influenza
- Bacterial:
  - *Staphylococcus aureus* or *epidermidis*
  - *Streptococcus pneumoniae*
  - *Haemophilus influenzae* (children)
  - *Pseudomonas* species or anaerobes (in contact lens users)
  - *Acanthamoeba* from contaminated contact lens solution may cause keratitis.
  - *Neisseria gonorrhoeae* and *meningitidis*
  - *Chlamydia trachomatis*: Gradual onset >4 weeks
- Allergic:
  - Hay fever, seasonal allergies, atopy
- Nonspecific:
  - Irritative: Topical medications, wind, dry eye, ultraviolet light exposure, smoke
  - Autoimmune: Sjögren's syndrome, pemphigoid, Wegener granulomatosis
  - Rare: Rickettsial, fungal, parasitic, tuberculosis, syphilis, Kawasaki disease, chikungunya, Graves, gout, carcinoid, sarcoid, psoriasis, Stevens-Johnson, Reiter syndrome

COMMONLY ASSOCIATED CONDITIONS

- Viral infection (e.g., common cold)
- STD

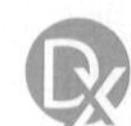

DIAGNOSIS

HISTORY

- Red flag: Any decrease in visual acuity is not consistent with conjunctivitis alone; must document normal vision for diagnosis of isolated conjunctivitis.
- Viral: Contact or travel:
  - May start with 1 eye, then both
  - If herpetic, recurrences or vesicles on skin
- Bacterial: Difficult to distinguish from viral, unless contact-lens user. Assume bacterial in contact lens wearer unless cultures negative. If recent STD, suspect chlamydia or GC
- Allergic: Itching, atopy, seasonal, dander
- Irritative: Feels dry, exposure to wind, tear film deficit may persist 30 days after acute conjunctivitis, chemicals, or drug: Atropine, aminoglycosides, iodide, phenylephrine, antivirals, bisphosphonates, retinoids, topiramate, chamomile, COX-2 inhibitors
- Foreign body: Redness may persist 24 hours after removal.

PHYSICAL EXAM

- General: Common to all types of conjunctivitis:
  - Red eye, conjunctival injection
  - Foreign body sensation
  - Eyelid sticking or crusting, discharge
  - Normal visual acuity and pupillary reactivity
- Viral:
  - Palpable preauricular lymphadenopathy may be present.
  - Severe viral: Herpes simplex or zoster:
    - Burning sensation, rarely itching
    - Unilateral, herpetic skin vesicles in herpes zoster
    - Palpable preauricular node
- Bacterial (non-STD): May be epidemic:
  - Mild pruritus, discharge mild to heavy
  - Conjunctival chemosis/edema
  - If contact lens user, must rule out pseudomonal (or other bacterial) keratitis
- Bacterial: Gonococcal (or meningococcal) hyperacute infection:
  - Rapid onset 12–24 hours
  - Severe purulent discharge
  - Chemosis/conjunctival/lid edema
  - Rapid growth of superior corneal ulceration
  - Preauricular adenopathy
  - Signs of STDs (chlamydia, GC, HIV, etc.)
- Allergic:
  - Itching predominant
  - Seasonal or dander allergies
  - Chemosis/conjunctival/eyelid edema
- Nonspecific irritative:
  - Dry eyes, intermittent redness, chemical/drug exposure
  - Foreign body: May have redness and discharge 24 hours after removal
- Must document normal visual acuity
- Cornea should be clear and without fluorescein uptake. If cloudy or signs of keratitis, consult ophthalmologist.
- Recommend fluorescein exam: Evert lid to inspect for foreign bodies.
- Skin: Look for herpetic vesicles, nits on lashes (lice), scaliness (seborrhea), or styes
- Limbal flush at corneal margin if uveitis
- If pupil is irregular (i.e., penetrating foreign body), emergent referral
- Discharge but no conjunctival injection: Blepharitis

DIAGNOSTIC TESTS & INTERPRETATION

Lab

- Usually not needed initially for the most common causes
- Culture swab if STD suspected, very severe symptoms, or patient is a contact lens user

Diagnostic Procedures/Surgery

- Fluorescein exam for ulcer or abrasion on cornea
- Small superficial foreign bodies may be removed with irrigation or moistened swab.

DIFFERENTIAL DIAGNOSIS

- Uveitis (iritis, iridocyclitis, choroiditis): Limbal flush (red band at corneal margin), hazy anterior chamber, and decreased visual acuity
- Penetrating ocular trauma: Emergently hospitalize
- Acute glaucoma (emergency): Headache, corneal clouding, poor visual acuity
- Corneal ulcer(s) or foreign body: Lesions on fluorescein exam
- Dacryocystitis: Tenderness and swelling over tear sac (below medial canthus)
- Scleritis and episcleritis: Red injected vessels radially oriented, sectoral (pie wedge), nodularity of sclera
- Pingueculitis: Inflammation of a yellow nodular or wedge-like area of chronic conjunctival degeneration (pinguecula)
- Ophthalmia neonatorum: Neonates in first 2 days of life (gonococcal; 5–12 days of life): Chlamydial, HSV, very rare *Neisseria meningitidis*. Consider specialty consultation for required systemic therapy.
- Blepharitis: Lid margins inflamed and producing itching, scale, or discharge, but no conjunctival injection.

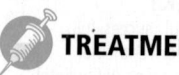

TREATMENT

MEDICATION

First Line

- Viral (nonherpetic):
  - Artificial tears for symptomatic relief
  - Vasoconstrictor/antihistamine (e.g., naphazoline/pheniramine) q.i.d. for severe itching
  - May consider topical antibiotic (see bacterial below) if return to daycare requires treatment (1)[C]

- Viral (herpetic) (by ophthalmologist):
  - Trifluridine: 1% drops 1 q2h (2)[C]
  - Acyclovir oral: 400 mg 5 × day for herpes simplex virus (HSV) (use 800 mg for zoster) × 7 days
- Bacterial (non-STD) is self-limited (5–7 days), so treatment is optional (and should take cost and bacterial resistance-production factors into consideration), although it may shorten the symptoms by half a day (3)[A]. Alternative strategy: Delay treatment until third day (using simple warm moist towel cleansing of closed eye), same duration of symptoms (4)[B]. Contact lens wearers should be referred for evaluation of possible keratitis:
  - Trimethoprim/polymyxin (Polytrim) ophthalmic: 1 drop q4h (while awake) for 5 days *or*
  - Erythromycin ophthalmic ointment: 1/2 inch b.i.d.–q.i.d. for 5 days *or*
  - Sodium sulfacetamide (10% solution) (Bleph-10) 2 drops q4h (while awake) for 5 days *or*
  - Tobramycin 0.3% ophthalmic drops/ointment q4h (drops) to q8h (ointment)
- Bacterial (gonococcal) hospitalize for IV ceftriaxone:
  - If no corneal lesions, ceftriaxone 1 g IM as single dose and topical bacitracin ophthalmic ointment 1/2 inch q.i.d. Chlamydial in neonates requires oral erythromycin ethylsuccinate 30 mg/kg daily q6h PO × 14 d, max 3 g/d.
- Allergic and atopic (listed by approximate, increasing cost, from lowest to highest: All are efficacious, but evidence favoring one over another is inconclusive):
  - Ketotifen (Zaditor; Alaway and other generics) 0.25% 1 drop b.i.d. (5)[A]
  - Cromolyn (Opticrom) 4%, q.i.d. (4)[A]
  - Epinastine (Elestat) 0.05% b.i.d. (5)[A]
  - Ketorolac (Acular) 0.1% 1 drop q.i.d. (5)[A]
  - Emedastine 0.05% 1 drop q.i.d. (5)[A]
  - Azelastine (Optivar) 0.05% 1 drop b.i.d. (4)[A]
  - Olopatadine (Patanol) 0.1% 1 drop b.i.d. or 0.2% 1 drop daily (5)[A]
  - Oral nonsedating antihistamines (Zyrtec [cetirizine] 10 mg/d, Allegra [fexofenadine] 60 mg b.i.d.), etc., to treat nasal and urticarial symptoms
  - Oral antihistamine (e.g., diphenhydramine 25 mg t.i.d.) in severe cases
- Contraindications: Avoid topical steroids unless able to monitor intraocular pressure. Also case report of HSV keratitis presenting without distinguishing findings from viral conjunctivitis would discourage initial use of steroids.
- Precautions:
  - Do not allow dropper to touch the eye.
  - Vasoconstrictor/antihistamine: Rebound vasodilation after prolonged use

Second Line

- Viral and allergic: Numerous over-the-counter products
- Bacterial: Polymyxin-gramicidin, ciprofloxacin (Ciloxan), moxifloxacin (Vigamox)

ADDITIONAL TREATMENT

General Measures

- Appropriate health care: Outpatient
- Eyelid cleansing with wet cloth up to q.i.d.
- Stop use of contact lenses while red
- Patching of eye not beneficial
- Avoid irritants such as smoke, wind, and sun

Issues for Referral

Any significantly decreased visual acuity, herpetic keratitis, or contact lens-related bacterial conjunctivitis: Ophthalmologic consultation

COMPLEMENTARY AND ALTERNATIVE MEDICINE

As condition is usually benign and self-limited, saline flushes and other placebos would be expected to appear to work.

SURGERY/OTHER PROCEDURES

No surgery for this condition. Other eye surgeries may be delayed until resolution of this condition.

IN-PATIENT CONSIDERATIONS

Acute gonococcal conjunctivitis (or very rare case of meningococcal conjunctivitis) would require inpatient treatment with ceftriaxone 50 mg/kg IV every day (pediatric), 1 g IM × 1 (adult) along with ophthalmologic consultation.

Admission Criteria

Penetrating ocular trauma, GC

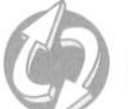

ONGOING CARE

FOLLOW-UP RECOMMENDATIONS

- If not resolved within 5–7 days, alternate diagnoses should be considered or consultation obtained, although epidemic keratoconjunctivitis and other adenoviral conjunctivitis typically lasts 1–2 weeks.
- Children may be excluded from school until eye is no longer red, if viral or bacterial, depending on school policy. Allergic conjunctivitis should be able to return to school with doctor's note.

Patient Monitoring

Referral if worse in 24 hours

PATIENT EDUCATION

- Patients should not wear contacts until their eyes are fully healed (typically 1 week).
- Patients should discard current pair of contacts.
- Patients should discard any eye makeup that they have been using, especially mascara.
- Cool, moist compresses can ease irritation and itch.

PROGNOSIS

- Viral: 5–10 days for pharyngitis with conjunctivitis, 2 weeks with adenovirus
- Herpes simplex: 2–3 weeks
- Bacterial: Self-limited; treated, 2–5 days; untreated, 5–7 days

COMPLICATIONS

- Corneal scars with herpes simplex
- Lid scars or entropion with varicella zoster
- Corneal ulcers or perforation, very rapid with gonococcal
- Hypopyon: Pus in anterior chamber
- Chlamydial neonatal ophthalmia: Could have concomitant pneumonia
- Otitis media may follow *H. influenzae* conjunctivitis.
- The very rare *Neisseria meningitidis* conjunctivitis may be followed by meningitis.

REFERENCES

1. David SP. Should we prescribe antibiotics for acute conjunctivitis? *Am Fam Physician*. 2002;66: 1649–50.
2. Greenberg MF, Pollard ZF. The red eye in childhood. *Pediatr Clin North Am*. 2003;50:105–24.
3. Sheikh A, Hurwitz B. Antibiotics vs. placebo for acute bacterial conjunctivitis. *Cochrane Database Syst Rev*. 2006;2:CD001211.
4. Bielory L, Lien KW, Bigelsen S. Efficacy and tolerability of newer antihistamines in the treatment of allergic conjunctivitis. *Drugs*. 2005;65:215–28.
5. Chigbu DI, et al. The management of allergic eye diseases in primary eye care. *Cont Lens Anterior Eye*. 2009;32:260–72.

C

ADDITIONAL READING

- Everitt HA, Little PS, Smith PW. A randomised controlled trial of management strategies for acute infective conjunctivitis in general practice. *BMJ*. 2006;333:321.
- Gupta R, Levent F, Healy CM, et al. Unusual soft tissue manifestations of *Neisseria meningitidis* infections. *Clin Pediatr (Phila)*. 2008;47:400–3.
- Hamerlynck JV, Rietveld RP, Hooft L. [From the Cochrane Library: Marginally higher chance of cure by antibiotic treatment in acute bacterial conjunctivitis] *Ned Tijdschr Geneeskd*. 2007; 151:594–6.
- Richards A, Guzman-Cottrill JA, et al. Conjunctivitis. *Pediatr Rev*. 2010;31:196–208.
- Rose PW, Harnden A, Brueggemann AB, et al. Chloramphenicol treatment for acute infective conjunctivitis in children in primary care: A randomised double-blind placebo-controlled trial. *Lancet*. 2005;366:37–43.

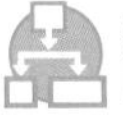

See Also (Topic, Algorithm, Electronic Media Element)

- Rhinitis, Allergic
- Algorithm: Eye Pain

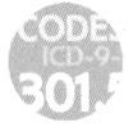

CODES

ICD9

- 372.00 Acute conjunctivitis, unspecified
- 372.30 Conjunctivitis, unspecified
- 771.6 Neonatal conjunctivitis and dacryocystitis

CLINICAL PEARLS

- Conjunctivitis does not alter visual acuity; decreased acuity or photophobia should prompt consideration of more serious ophthalmic disorders.
- Culture discharge in all contact lens wearers, consider referral and remind patient to throw away current contacts and avoid contacts until eyes fully healed.
- Antibiotic therapy is of no value in viral conjunctivitis (most cases of infectious conjunctivitis), and does not significantly alter the course of most types of bacterial conjunctivitis (therefore, is optional in these cases).

CONSTIPATION

Robert A. Baldor, MD

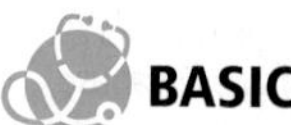

BASICS

A group of syndromes with similar findings that include unsatisfactory defecation characterized by infrequent stools, difficult stool passage, or both. Characteristics include fewer than 3 bowel movements a week, hard stools, excessive straining, prolonged time spent on the toilet, a sense of incomplete evacuation, and abdominal discomfort/bloating.

DESCRIPTION

- System(s) affected: Gastrointestinal (GI)
- Synonym(s): Obstipation

Geriatric Considerations

Increased incidence of colorectal neoplasms with age may be associated with constipation; thus, new onset of constipation after 50 years of age is considered a "red flag."

Pediatric Considerations

Consider Hirschsprung disease (absence of colonic ganglion cells): 25% of all newborn intestinal obstructions, milder cases diagnosed in older children with chronic constipation, abdominal distension, decreased growth. 5:1 Male:Female ratio. Associated with inherited conditions such as Down syndrome.

EPIDEMIOLOGY

- Predominant age: May affect all ages, but more pronounced in children and elderly
- Predominant sex: Female > Male (2:1)
- Nonwhites > Whites

Incidence

- 5 million office visits annually
- 100,000 hospitalizations

Prevalence

~15% of population affected

RISK FACTORS

- Extremes of life (very young and very old)
- Polypharmacy
- Sedentary lifestyle or condition
- Improper diet and inadequate fluid intake

Genetics

Unknown, but condition may be familial

GENERAL PREVENTION

High-fiber diet, adequate fluids, exercise, and bowel training to "obey the urge" to defecate are useful preventive strategies.

PATHOPHYSIOLOGY

- As food leaves the stomach, the ileocecal valve relaxes (gastroileal reflex) and chyme enters the colon (1–2 L/d). Peristaltic contractions move the chyme through the colon into the rectum. In the colon, sodium is actively absorbed in exchange for potassium and bicarb—water follows because of the generated osmotic gradient. The chyme is converted into feces (200–250 mL).
- Normal transit time for a meal to reach the cecum is 4 hours, and to the pelvic colon 8 hours later. Transit then slows to the anus. Rectal distention initiates the defecation reflex.
- Defecation follows as a reflex that can be inhibited by voluntarily contracting the external sphincter or facilitated by straining to contract the abdominal muscles while voluntarily relaxing the anal sphincter. The urge to defecate occurs as rectal pressures increase. Distention of the stomach by food also initiates rectal contractions and a desire to defecate.

ETIOLOGY

- **Primary constipation:**
  - Slow colonic transit time (13%)
  - Pelvic floor/anal sphincter dysfunction (25%)
  - Functional—normal transit time and sphincter function, yet problems (bloating, abdominal discomfort, perceived difficulty going, presence of hard stools) (69%)
- **Secondary constipation:**
  - Irritable bowel syndrome (IBS)
  - Endocrine dysfunction (diabetes mellitus, hypothyroid)
  - Metabolic disorder (increased calcium, decreased potassium)
  - Mechanical (obstruction, rectocele)
  - Pregnancy
  - Neurologic disorders (Hirschsprung, multiple sclerosis, spinal cord injuries)
- **Medication effect:**
  - Anticholinergic effects (antidepressants, narcotics, antipsychotics)
  - Antacids (calcium, aluminum)
  - Calcium channel blockers

COMMONLY ASSOCIATED CONDITIONS

- Debility, either general as in the aged or that imposed by specific underlying illness
- Dehydration
- Hypothyroidism
- Hypokalemia
- Hypercalcemia

DIAGNOSIS

A group of syndromes with similar findings that include unsatisfactory defecation characterized by infrequent stools, difficult stool passage, or both

ALERT

Red flags:

- New onset after age of 50
- Hematochezia/melena
- Unintentional weight loss
- Anemia
- Neurologic defects

HISTORY

Ask about the Rome III criteria (1)[C]:

- At least 2 of the following, for 12 weeks, in the previous 6 months:
  - Fewer than 3 stools/week
  - Straining at least 1/4 of the time
  - Hard stools at least 1/4 of the time
  - Need for manual assist at least 1/4 of the time
  - Sense of incomplete evacuation at least 1/4 of the time
  - Sense of anorectal blockade at least 1/4 of the time
- Loose stools rarely seen without use of laxatives

PHYSICAL EXAM

- Digital rectal exam (masses, pain, stool, fissures, hemorrhoids, anal tone)
- Abdominal/gynecologic exam (masses, pain)
- Neurologic exam

DIAGNOSTIC TESTS & INTERPRETATION

For the most part, this is a clinical diagnosis, as evidence to support the use of routine labs/x-rays/scoping is lacking in the workup of constipation (2)[B].

Lab

Initial lab tests

However, the American Gastroenterological Association guidelines suggest CBC, glucose, TSH, calcium, and creatinine routinely and sigmoid/colonoscopy if red flags are present (3)[C].

Imaging

Initial approach

If condition is refractory to empiric approach, pursue further testing:

- Colonoscopy
- Barium enema to look for obstruction and/or megarectum, megacolon, or Hirschsprung disease

Follow-Up & Special Considerations

Measure colonic transit time by ingesting radiopaque (Sitz-Mark) markers:

- Plain abdominal film obtained 5 days later (120 hours): Retention >20% markers indicates slow transit
- Markers seen exclusively in distal colon/rectum suggests defecatory disorder.

Diagnostic Procedures/Surgery

Consider referral to evaluate defecation:

- Balloon expulsion
- Defecography using a barium paste
- Anorectal manometry with a rectal catheter

Pathological Findings

- None in common, functional constipation
- Paucity or absence of intramural enteric ganglia in certain cases of congenital or acquired megacolon
- Neuromuscular abnormalities in certain cases of pseudo-obstruction

DIFFERENTIAL DIAGNOSIS

- Congenital:
  - Hirschsprung disease/syndrome
  - Hypoganglionosis
  - Congenital dilation of the colon
  - Small left colon syndrome
- Meconium ileus
- Other causes of abdominal pain

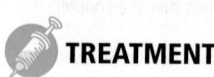

TREATMENT

Address immediate concerns:

- Bloating/discomfort/straining: Osmotic agents
- Postop, childbirth, hemorrhoids, fissures: Stool softener to make defecation easier
- Stimulants and suppositories
- Manual disimpaction as needed, then approach the chronic condition

MEDICATION

- In patients with no known secondary causes of constipation, conservative nonpharmacologic treatment measures generally are recommended, including:
  - Regular exercise
  - Increased fluid intake
  - Bowel habit training
- Other nonpharmacologic therapies include:
  - Biofeedback therapy
  - Behavior therapy
  - Electric stimulation

First Line

Bulking agents (need to be accompanied by adequate amounts of liquid to be useful):

- Hydrophilic colloids (bulk-forming agents):
  - Psyllium (Konsyl, Metamucil, Perdiem Fiber): 1 rounded tsp in liquid PO daily up to t.i.d.
  - Bran methylcellulose (Citrucel): 1 rounded tsp in 8 oz cold water PO daily up to t.i.d.
  - Polycarbophil (Mitrolan, FiberCon): 1 g PO q.i.d.
- Stool softeners:
  - Docusate sodium (Colace): 100 mg b.i.d.
- Osmotic laxatives:
  - Polyethylene glycol (MiraLax) (0.8 mg/kg/d) 17 g daily (current evidence shows PEG to be superior to lactulose) (4)[A]
  - Saccharines lactulose (Chronulac) 15–60 mL q.h.s. (flatulence, bloating, cramping side effects)
  - Sorbitol 15–60 mL q.h.s. (as effective as lactulose)
  - Magnesium salts (Milk of Magnesia) avoid in renal insufficiency

Second Line

- Stimulants (irritate bowel causing muscle contraction; usually combined with a softener; work in 8–12 hours):
  - Senna/docusate (Senokot-S, Ex-lax) 1–2 capsules or 15–30 mL at bedtime
  - Bisacodyl/docusate (Dulcolax, Correctol) 2–3 tablets daily
  - Casanthranol/docusate (Peri-Colace) lubricants (contain mineral oil, coating the stool)
- Lubricants (soften stool and facilitate passage of the feces by its lubricating oily effects):
  - Mineral oil (15–45 mL/d)
  - Short-term use only. Can bind fat-soluble vitamins with the potential for deficiencies. May similarly decrease absorption of some drugs.
  - Avoid in those at risk for aspiration (lipid pneumonia).
- Suppositories:
  - Osmotic: Sodium phosphate
  - Lubricant: Glycerin
  - Stimulatory: Bisacodyl
  - Enemas: Sodium phosphate (Fleet enema)
- Lubiprostone (Amitiza): A selective chloride channel activator; 24 mcg b.i.d.:
  - Avoid in pregnancy and breastfeeding
- Methylnaltrexone (Relistor) a peripherally acting mu-opioid receptor (PAM-OR) antagonist; 12 mg SC every other day PRN:
  - Indicated for short-term palliative care use (<4 months)
  - Side effects: Abdominal pain and flatulence
- Prokinetic agents (partial 5-HT4 agonists): Have been withdrawn due to cardiac side effects (tegaserod [Zelnorm], cisapride [Propulsid])
- Other agents not approved by the Food and Drug Administration:
  - Misoprostol (Cytotec): A prostaglandin that increases colonic motility (5)[C]
  - Colchicine: Neurogenic stimulation to increase colonic motility (6)[C]

ADDITIONAL TREATMENT

General Measures

- Attempt to eliminate medications that may cause or worsen constipation.
- Increase fluid intake.
- Increase fiber in diet.
- Enemas if other methods fail

Additional Therapies

Biofeedback with artificial silicon stool

SURGERY/OTHER PROCEDURES

Surgery rarely indicated

IN-PATIENT CONSIDERATIONS

Nursing

Manual disimpaction occasionally required in difficult chronic situations

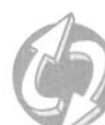

ONGOING CARE

FOLLOW-UP RECOMMENDATIONS

Encourage exercise and physical activity.

Patient Monitoring

If what seems to be simple, functional constipation persists, further investigate for a possible organic cause.

DIET

Increase fiber, but bloating and gas can be problematic:

- Gradually increase intake to 25 g/d over a 6-week period.
- Insoluble, less fermentable fiber, like wheat bran, tends to be better tolerated.
- Bran (hard outer layer of cereal grains)
- Vegetables and fruits
- Whole-grain foods
- Encourage liberal intake of fluids.

PATIENT EDUCATION

- Occasional mild constipation is normal.
- Instruction in consistent bowel training; the best time to move bowels is in the morning, after eating breakfast, when the normal bowel transit and defecation reflexes are typically functioning to move the bowels.

PROGNOSIS

- Constipation that is only occasional, brief, and responsive to simple measures is harmless.
- That which is habitual can be a lifelong nuisance.
- Those with neurologic compromise can suffer from ill effects such as obstipation and impaction to toxic megacolon.
- No evidence for dependence
- No evidence for harm from stimulant use; melanosis coli may develop, but it is a benign condition (7)[B].

COMPLICATIONS

- Volvulus
- Toxic megacolon
- Acquired megacolon: In severe, long-standing cases
- Fluid and electrolyte depletion: Laxative abuse
- Rectal ulceration (stercoral ulcer) related to recurrent fecal impaction
- Anal fissures

REFERENCES

1. Longstreth GF, Thompson WG, Chey WD, et al. Functional bowel disorders. *Gastroenterology*. 2006;130:1480–91.
2. American College of Gastroenterology Chronic Constipation Task Force. An evidence-based approach to the management of chronic constipation in North America. *Am J Gastroenterol*. 2005;100 (Suppl 1):S1–4.
3. Locke GR, Pemberton JH, Phillips SF. American Gastroenterological Association Medical Position Statement: guidelines on constipation. *Gastroenterology*. 2000;119:1761–6.
4. Lee-Robichaud H, Thomas K, Morgan J, et al. Lactulose versus polyethylene glycol for chronic constipation. *Cochrane Database Syst Rev*. 2010;7:CD007570.
5. Roarty TP, Weber F, Soykan I, et al. Misoprostol in the treatment of chronic refractory constipation: Results of a long-term open label trial. *Aliment Pharmacol Ther*. 1997;11:1059–66.
6. Verne GN, Davis RH, Robinson ME, et al. Treatment of chronic constipation with colchicine: Randomized, double-blind, placebo-controlled, crossover trial. *Am J Gastroenterol*. 2003;98: 1112–6.
7. Müller-Lissner SA, Kamm MA, et al. Myths and misconceptions about chronic constipation. *Am J Gastroenterol*. 2005;100:232–42.

ADDITIONAL READING

- Spinzi G, Amato A, Imperiali G, et al. Constipation in the elderly: Management strategies. *Drugs Aging*. 2009;26:469–74.
- van Dijk M, Benninga MA, Grootenhuis MA, et al. Chronic childhood constipation: A review of the literature and the introduction of a protocolized behavioral intervention program. *Patient Educ Couns*. 2007.

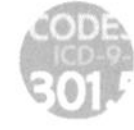

CODES

ICD9

- 564.00 Constipation, unspecified
- 564.01 Slow transit constipation
- 564.09 Other constipation

CLINICAL PEARLS

- Constipation can be characterized as unsatisfactory defecation, with infrequent stools, difficult stool passage, or both, for 3 months.
- Functional constipation (normal transit time and sphincter function) seen most often
- Workup is necessary in the presence of red flags: Onset >50 years hematochezia/melena, unintentional weight loss, anemia, neurologic defects
- Best evidence for effectiveness is for osmotic agents (polyethylene glycol [PEG]) (4)[A].

CONTRACEPTION

AuTumn Davidson, MD
Jeremy Golding, MD

BASICS

DESCRIPTION

- Methods to prevent pregnancy, including prevention/delay of ovulation, inhibition of sperm entry into the uterus, or interference with implantation of fertilized ovum
- The most effective methods of reversible contraception are the long-acting reversible contraceptive (LARC) methods—including the intrauterine system and progesterone implant—and permanent sterilization of both males and females.

EPIDEMIOLOGY

Incidence

- 50% of all pregnancies in the US are unintended. 50% of these occur in women using a form of reversible contraception. 50% of all unintended pregnancies in the US result in termination.
- The most frequently used form of contraception in the US (in order of prevalence) are oral contraceptives, female sterilization, male condom, male sterilization, and depot injectables. Despite their proven safety, effectiveness, and cost-effectiveness, LARC methods (intrauterine devices [IUDs] and the subdermal implant) are underused in the US. Efforts to increase use of LARC methods remain a focus of family planning experts in the US (1).

RISK FACTORS

- Unintended pregnancy: Women ages 18–24, and 35–44 years old, unmarried/cohabitating women, women with less than a college education, minority women, pregnancy ambivalence
- Contraception nonuse: Being dissatisfied with one's method of contraception, believing that contraceptive service providers were not available to answer method-related questions

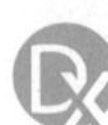

DIAGNOSIS

DIAGNOSTIC TESTS & INTERPRETATION

Lab

- No routine testing is needed prior to initiating oral contraception except reassurance that the patient is not pregnant (by history or laboratory). Testing for gonorrhea and chlamydia may be performed but is not required prior to IUD insertion. In high-risk populations, active infection should be ruled out prior to IUD insertion.
- If family history of thrombophilia, consider testing for the specific defect (if known) or common disorders (factor V Leiden, prothrombin gene G20210A mutation) prior to initiation of combined oral contraceptive pills (OCPs).

Follow-Up & Special Considerations

Routine 2–3 month follow-up after initiation of all methods of contraception to assess patient tolerance and acceptability of contraceptive method. BP should be checked within 3 months of initiation in all patients on combined OCPs due to the rare occurrence of hypertension in this population.

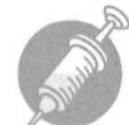

TREATMENT

The CDC issued comprehensive, highly useful guidelines in 2010 for selection of contraceptive methods in patients with comorbid medical conditions (2).

MEDICATION

- Spermicides: All contain nonoxynol-9; may alter vaginal flora and mucosal barrier
- Sponge: 2-inch circular disk that contains nonoxynol-9. Moisten with water before insertion in vagina; effective for 24 hours.
- Oral Contraceptive Pills:
  - Combined estrogen/progestin pills (COCs) should be used for nonbreastfeeding patients without a contraindication to exogenous estrogen therapy (see below):
    - Pills may be started at any time after pregnancy has been ruled out. Some providers prefer a "Sunday Start" because they feel this is less confusing for patients. One study found better compliance at 3 months among patients assigned to start pills the day they were prescribed ("Quick Start").
    - All COCs contain the same type of estrogen (ethinyl estradiol). COCs differ in the level of estrogen (range of 20–50 μg), and the type of progestin. Newer progestogens are less androgenic and have less effect on lipoproteins (clinical significance unknown).
    - Patient response to any one type of COC is unpredictable. A starting pill is one that is inexpensive (generic), contains an average amount of estrogen (30–35 μg), and a well-studied, second-generation progestin. Sprintec or Necon are reasonable starting pills.
    - Patients should be instructed to take the pill every day and use backup birth control for the first 2 weeks after the initiation of pills. If a pill is missed, she should take 2 pills the following day. If 2 pills are missed, she should take 3 pills the following day and use a backup method for 7 days. If 3 or more pills are missed, the patient should be instructed to restart a new pack and use a backup for 2 weeks.
    - Most pills have a 21/7 regimen (21 active days and 7 placebo). Newer preparations have 24/4 combinations. It is reasonable for patients to skip the placebo pills and begin a new pack immediately on the active pill so as to avoid a period (continuous dosing). All women should have a withdraw bleed at least 4 times a year to reduce breakthrough bleeding.
    - The most common side effects include nausea, bloating, headaches, and mastalgia. These symptoms tend to decrease over time. Nausea can be reduced by taking the pill at nighttime. Women who experience headaches can be counseled that these usually decrease over time.
  - Breastfeeding women desiring oral contraceptive medications should be prescribed progestin-only pills (Ortho Micronor), especially for the first months. Patients should be instructed to take these pills at the same time every day.
- Weekly hormonal patch (Ortho-Evra): The "patch" contains 20 μg ethinyl estradiol and 150 μg norelgestromin. It is applied transdermally and changed weekly. Produces higher serum estrogen levels than oral 20 μg pill, and may be associated with a slightly increased risk of blood clot. Patch may cause local skin irritation. Not as reliable in women >90 kg.
- Vaginal contraceptive ring (NuvaRing): A flexible polymer ring containing 15 μg ethinyl estradiol and 120 μg etonogestrel; inserted into vagina for 3 weeks per cycle (also may be used for continuous cycling for 4 weeks [off label])
- Contraindications to estrogen-containing hormonal contraception (see WHO Medical Eligibility Criteria for Contraceptive Use) (2):
  - History of coronary artery disease (CAD) or multiple risk factors (age >55, smoking, high BP, diabetes mellitus)
  - History of deep vein thrombosis (DVT)/pulmonary embolism (PE) or personal history of cerebrovascular accident (CVA)
  - History of migraines at age >35 or migraine at any age with aura
  - Current or past breast cancer, active liver disease, or hepatic tumor
  - Pregnancy, unexplained abnormal uterine bleeding without further investigation
  - Relative contraindication to estrogen-containing hormonal contraception: Smokers >35. Healthy nonsmokers may use oral contraceptives until menopause.
- Medroxyprogesterone (Depo-Provera), also known as depot-medroxyprogesterone acetate (DMPA): 150 mg IM *or* 104 mg/0.65 mL SC, both are given every 3 months. Contraceptive levels of hormone persist for up to 4 months (2–4-week margin of safety). Major side effects include irregular bleeding and weight gain. Potential for decreased bone mineral density if used for >2 years, so recommend that women take 1,300 mg of calcium and 400 IU of vitamin D when using DMPA (3).
- Intrauterine systems (IUs): These are highly effective, long-acting reversible contraceptive methods with few side effects. 5-year failure rates are ~0.5%. IUD may be inserted anytime pregnancy is ruled out. May also be inserted immediately postpartum (within 10 minutes of removal of placenta) as well as postabortion (4). IUDs are commonly used in adolescents and other nulliparous women. Contraindications to IUs include pregnancy, active uterine infection, malignancy in the uterus or cervix, an inability to place or retain the device, unexplained abnormal bleeding, and adverse reaction to product ingredients. 2 types of IUs are currently available in the US:
  - ParaGard (Copper T): Interferes with sperm transport and ova fertilization; approved for up to 10 years, but likely remains effective for longer. May increase menstrual blood loss. Also effective as postcoital contraceptive up to 5 days from intercourse.
  - Mirena (Levonorgestrel intrauterine system): A T-shaped IUD that releases 20 μg of levonorgestrel per day (very low serum levels). Approved for use up to 5 years; has been used off label for up to 7. Safe and effective for use in adolescents and nulliparous women. Side effects include irregular menstrual spotting for the first 3–6 months that usually resolves after 6 months of use.

- Etonogestrel implant (Implanon): A small, single, plastic rod that is implanted into the superficial SC tissue of the upper arm and provides continuous contraception via progestin hormone. This prevents ovulation and thickens cervical mucus to halt fertilization. Effective for up to 3 years. The device may be inserted only by trained and certified providers, as improper placement may result in unintended pregnancy, pain, infection, and difficult removal. Menstrual irregularities are common the first 6–12 months (and beyond); some will not have menses after 1 year, although others may have continuing irregular spotting for years.
- **Emergency contraception**: Start within 72 hours for maximum effectiveness, but evidence supports up to 120 hours:
  - Levonorgestrel: 1.5 mg taken as two 0.75 mg tablets (Plan B) or one 1.5 mg tablet (Plan B 1-Step). Less nausea and slightly more effective than the "Yuzpe regimen" (see below) (5)[A]: Available over the counter, but may be less expensive for many women if prescribed. Prescription is needed for women under age 17.
  - Estradiol/levonorgestrel (Preven, Ovral, Ogestrel): "Yuzpe regimen" 50 μg/0.25 mg, 2 tablets q12h (4 tablets total). Other OCs may be used as long as dose of estrogen component $\geq$100 μg/dose. *Note*: Antinausea medication (e.g., Phenergan) should be given 1–2 hours before the doses.
  - Copper-bearing IUD (Paragard): Insert up to 5 days after intercourse; over 99% effective in preventing pregnancy and continues to provide contraception for up to 10 years.
  - Ulipristal acetate (Ella): 30 mg; approved by FDA in 2010. Selective progesterone modulator, approved for use up to 5 days following unprotected intercourse.

ADDITIONAL TREATMENT

General Measures

Nondrug methods: Latex condom (benefit: reduces risk of sexually transmitted disease [STD]), diaphragm (needs fitting), periodic abstinence:

- Calendar method: Track length of last 6 cycles; fertility period is calculated by subtracting 18 from the number of days of shortest cycle and 11 from number of days in longest cycle. Example: If shortest cycle is 28 days and longest cycle is 31 days, fertile period is from days 10–20.
- Symptothermal method: Calculate the first day of abstinence by subtracting 21 from the length of the shortest menstrual cycle in the previous 6 months, or the first day cervical mucus is detected, whichever comes first. End calculated as 3 days after body temperature rises 1°C.
- Withdrawal method: Male partner withdraws from vagina before ejaculation. Failure occurs if withdrawal is not timed accurately or if the pre-ejaculatory fluid contains sperm.
- Lactation delays resumption of ovulation postpartum due to prolactin-induced inhibition of gonadotropin-releasing hormone (GNRH) release. Breastfeeding is effective contraception only if (i) the infant is <6 months old, (ii) the infant is exclusively breastfeeding, and (iii) the mother has not resumed her regular menses (lactational amenorrhea method, or LAM).

SURGERY/OTHER PROCEDURES

- Permanent sterilization in the female: Tubal ligation or hysteroscopic sterilization via polyester fibers (Essure): Polyester fibers with a coiled spring are introduced into each fallopian tube by transcervical route. Requires another contraceptive to be used for 3 months after procedure.
- Permanent sterilization in the male: Vasectomy

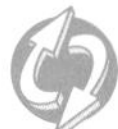

ONGOING CARE

FOLLOW-UP RECOMMENDATIONS

Patient Monitoring

- Pelvic exam, Pap smear, and STD testing per guidelines
- Check for IUD strings 1 month after insertion. Spontaneous expulsion rate highest in first month. The patient should monitor presence of the string monthly following menses.
- OC users: Monitor BP 3 months after starting, then annual follow up

DIET

Vitamin C and some herbals such as St. John's wort may alter estrogen levels, reducing efficacy or causing breakthrough bleeding.

PATIENT EDUCATION

- Condoms: Water-based lubricants (inside and outside) reduce the risk of breakage. Withdraw penis before it becomes flaccid.
- IUD: Check string periodically.
- Diaphragm: Refit after childbirth or if weight changes by more than 10%. Before inserting, 1 Tbs of water-soluble spermicidal jelly or cream should be placed in the dome. Leave in at least 6 hours after coitus. If coitus is repeated before 6 hours, insert another teaspoon of spermicidal jelly into the vagina without removing the diaphragm.
- Female condom: A new condom is required for each sex act.
- OCP: Pill should be taken at approximately the same time each day. If a pill is missed, see above instructions.
- Emergency contraception prevents pregnancy via several proposed mechanisms, including inhibition of sperm motility, alterations in tubal transport, unfavorable uterine receptivity, and/or fertilization inhibition. Emergency contraception does not affect an established pregnancy: 1-888-NOT-2-LATE or http://www.planbonestep.com/

COMPLICATIONS

- Hormonal contraceptives, serious: Thromboembolism, hypertension, myocardial infarction, stroke
- Hormonal contraceptives, minor: Nausea and vomiting: take after eating. Breakthrough bleeding: Usually self-limiting after 3 months; if persists, change pill. Amenorrhea: Pregnancy must be ruled out. Cyclic weight gain: Use smallest dose of estrogen available. Breast tenderness: Rare with low-dose pill. Depression: Rare with low-dose pill. Chloasma: Stop pill or cover with makeup. Acne or hirsutism: Change to a less androgenic progesterone. Cholestatic jaundice: Stop pill; do not restart. Weight gain throughout cycle: Use triphasic pill to minimize dose of progesterone or use newer progesterone.
- Injectable contraceptive (Depo-Provera): Irregular bleeding: No treatment needed; NSAID may help. Weight gain: Average of 5 lbs per year of use. Amenorrhea: Common after 1 year of use. Possible ↑ bone resorption and ↓ bone mineral density, but rapid recovery following discontinuation. Food and Drug Administration recommends BMD for use >2 years and to consider periodic estrogen.
- Progesterone implant: Irregular bleeding: Counsel patients extensively prior to insertion.
- Sponge and diaphragm: Associated with toxic shock syndrome (rare)
- IUD: Pelvic inflammatory disease (PID) or salpingitis: Device removal is not necessary for mild PID treated as outpatient. For infections requiring hospitalization: Remove device. For heavy bleeding and cramps: Remove device. Although absolute risk is no higher than without IUD, pregnancy, when it occurs, is more likely to be ectopic.

C

REFERENCES

1. Blumenthal PD, Voedisch A, Gemzell-Danielsson K, et al. Strategies to prevent unintended pregnancy: Increasing use of long-acting reversible contraception. *Hum Reprod Update*. 2011;17:121–37.
2. Division of Reproductive Health, National Center for Chronic Disease Prevention and Health Promotion, Centers for Disease Control and Prevention (CDC), Farr S, et al. US Medical Eligibility Criteria for Contraceptive Use, 2010: Adapted from the WHO Medical Eligibility Criteria for Contraceptive Use, 4th ed. *MMWR Recomm Rep*. 2010;59:1–86.
3. Schrager SB. DMPA's effect on bone mineral density: A particular concern for adolescents. *J Fam Pract*. 2009;58:E1–8.
4. Shimoni N. Intrauterine contraceptives: A review of uses, side effects and candidates. *Semin Reprod Med*. 2010;28(2):118–25.
5. Cheng L, Gülmezoglu AM, Piaggio G. Interventions for emergency contraception. *Cochrane Database Syst Rev*. 2008;CD001324.

ADDITIONAL READING

http://www.guttmacher.org/pubs/journals/3809006.html.

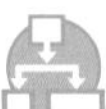

See Also (Topic, Algorithm, Electronic Media Element)

Factor V Leiden; Prothrombin 20210 (Mutation); Thrombophilia and Hypercoagulable States

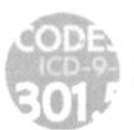

CODES

ICD9

- V25.01 General counseling on prescription of oral contraceptives
- V25.02 General counseling on initiation of other contraceptive measures
- V25.03 Encounter for emergency contraceptive counseling and prescription

CLINICAL PEARLS

- Hormonal and IUD contraceptives may be initiated immediately ("Quick-Start") if the likelihood of pre-existing pregnancy is low.
- Clearly established benefits of OCPs include reduction in ovarian cancer, endometrial cancer, ectopic pregnancies, and PID; less dysmenorrhea and anemia; reduced number of functional ovarian cysts, a regular menstrual cycle; improvement in acne.

COR PULMONALE

Parag Goyal, MD
Oscar Starobin, MD

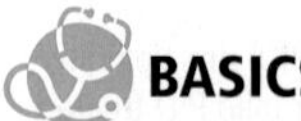

BASICS

DESCRIPTION
- Enlargement and subsequent dysfunction and failure of the right ventricle (RV) in the presence of pulmonary arterial hypertension secondary to abnormalities of the lungs, thorax, pulmonary ventilation, or circulation
- May occur in acute or chronic setting:
  - Acute: Rapid increase of pulmonary arterial pressure causing RV overload and resulting dysfunction/failure
  - Chronic: Progressive hypertrophy and dilation of RV over months to years, with eventual dysfunction/failure

EPIDEMIOLOGY
- ~6–7% of all types of adult heart disease in US
- Between 10% and 30% of heart failure admissions in the US are the result of cor pulmonale (1).

Incidence
Difficult to assess. Best estimate is 1/10,000 or 3/10,000 per year (2).

Prevalence
Difficult to assess. Best estimate is 2/1,000 or 6/1,000 (2).

RISK FACTORS
- Acute cor pulmonale is most commonly caused by massive pulmonary embolism (PE):
  - Risk factors associated with PE include:
    - Vessel injury
    - Stasis
    - Hypercoagulable states
- Chronic cor pulmonale is most commonly caused by chronic obstructive pulmonary disease (COPD) and/or pulmonary arterial hypertension (PAH).
  - Risk factors associated with COPD and/or PAH include:
    - Tobacco use
    - Living at high altitudes
    - Industrial exposures such as asbestos
    - Alpha-1-antitrypsin deficiency
    - Connective tissue disease

GENERAL PREVENTION
- Prevention of pulmonary embolism via deep venous thrombosis prophylaxis when necessary
- Early detection and timely management of COPD to delay its progression
- Management of underlying disease, including aggressive correction of hypoxia and acidosis, that may contribute to worsening pulmonary hypertension

PATHOPHYSIOLOGY
- Acute: A sudden event, such as large pulmonary embolism, increases resistance to blood flow in the pulmonary vasculature, causing a quick and significant increase of pressure proximally. The RV is unable to overcome this pressure, leading to low cardiac output and RV failure.
- Chronic: PAH develops from many possible etiologies, although predominantly from alveolar hypoxia. The RV is initially able to compensate for this increased pressure through concentric hypertrophy. However, worsening pulmonary hypertension eventually overcomes the RV's accommodative abilities, leading to dilation of the RV. This results in both systolic and diastolic dysfunction, causing reduced cardiac output and right-sided heart failure.

ETIOLOGY
- Lung disease: COPD including emphysema and chronic bronchitis (80–90%) (3), cystic fibrosis, restrictive and interstitial lung disease, including scleroderma and sarcoidosis, pulmonary thromboembolism, tumor emboli, idiopathic pulmonary arterial hypertension
- Hematological abnormalities: Sickle cell anemia, polycythemia vera
- Neuromuscular disease: Amyotrophic lateral sclerosis, myasthenia gravis, Guillain-Barré syndrome, polio, spinal cord injuries
- Disorders of ventilator control: Primary central hypoventilation, sleep apnea syndromes
- Thoracic cage deformities: Kyphoscoliosis
- Collagen vascular disease
- Left ventricular failure is not considered to be a cause of cor pulmonale.

COMMONLY ASSOCIATED CONDITIONS
PAH is classically defined as the presence of a resting mean pulmonary artery pressure (PAP) >20 mm Hg, though some sources define it as >25 mm Hg at rest and >30 mm Hg with exercise

DIAGNOSIS

HISTORY
- Dyspnea, orthopnea
- Fatigue, lethargy, syncope
- Cyanosis, pallor, diaphoresis
- Pleuritic chest pain, cough, hemoptysis
- Exertional angina
- Hoarseness secondary to compression of the left recurrent laryngeal nerve by enlarged pulmonary vessels
- Anorexia and/or right upper quadrant discomfort from hepatic congestion
- Cardiovascular collapse, shock, and/or cardiac arrest may occur in acute setting or advanced chronic setting.

PHYSICAL EXAM
- Peripheral edema is the most common sign of right heart failure (RHF), though it is nonspecific.
- Tachypnea, wheeze
- Increased intensity of pulmonic component of second heart sound (P2)
- Splitting of S2 over the cardiac apex with inspiration
- Audible S3 or S4
- Pansystolic murmur heard best at right midsternal border increasing with inspiration, consistent with tricuspid regurgitation (typically a late sign).
- Early diastolic murmur heard best at left upper sternal border, consistent with pulmonary regurgitation
- Right ventricular heave
- Jugular venous distension with inspiration (Kussmaul sign)
- Prominent a and v waves on jugular venous pulse tracing
- Hepatomegaly
- Signs of deep vein thrombosis (DVT), such as tenderness or unilateral swelling, may or may not be present.

DIAGNOSTIC TESTS & INTERPRETATION
ECG (poor sensitivity; up to 67% of patients will have normal findings) (1):
- Rightward P-wave axis deviation
- Peaked P waves anteriorly and in inferior leads (i.e., "P pulmonale")
- $S_1S_2S_3$ pattern, or $S_1Q_3T_3$, inverted pattern (McGinn-White pattern)
- RV hypertrophy (high specificity, low sensitivity)
- Right bundle-branch block
- Low-voltage QRS

Lab
Initial lab tests
- CBC and serum chemistries may be obtained to rule out other conditions:
  - Lab findings such as polycythemia and hypercapnia may be present due to COPD.
  - LFTs may be elevated due to hepatic congestion secondary to RV failure.
- Pulmonary function testing may show airflow obstruction with reduced PO_2, or other findings associated with COPD.
- Arterial blood gas, indicated for acute respiratory distress, may show hypercapnic acidosis and hypoxemia.
- BNP and cardiac troponins may be elevated secondary to RV stretch.

Imaging
- Chest x-ray:
  - Cardiomegaly
  - Increased width of right descending pulmonary artery
  - Left main pulmonary artery prominence below the aortic knob
- 2-dimensional echocardiogram:
  - RV mid-wall hypokinesis/akinesis plus normokinesis/hyperkinesis of RV apex (McConnell sign) are associated with acute cor pulmonale caused by acute pulmonary embolism.
  - RV dilatation and/or hypertrophy may be indicative of chronic cor pulmonale.
  - Doppler echocardiography with saline contrast to estimate tricuspid regurgitation is the most reliable noninvasive estimation of PAP.
- Spiral CT scan of chest:
  - Most accurate modality for diagnosing emphysema and interstitial lung disease
  - Test of choice for assessment of acute pulmonary embolism
- V/Q scan may be used to assess for pulmonary embolism in acute cor pulmonale.
- MRI commonly used, as it can characterize right ventricular size, mass morphology, and gross function

Diagnostic Procedures/Surgery
- Right heart catheterization is the gold standard for quantitation of ventricular and pulmonary pressures, and exclusion of congenital heart disease as etiology. Right heart catheterization is also recommended to assess vasoreactivity prior to implementing calcium channel blocker (CCB) therapy.
- Pulmonary function tests should be performed in patients with a suggestive history of underlying lung disease and in those with normal cardiac function.

DIFFERENTIAL DIAGNOSIS
- Right-sided heart failure secondary to left-sided heart failure
- Right-sided cardiomyopathy, ischemic or nonischemic
- Tricuspid valvulopathy
- Severe congenital pulmonary hypertension secondary to congenital heart disease with left-to-right shunting, most frequently from unrepaired nonrestrictive ventricular septal defect (VSD)

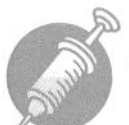

TREATMENT

Reduce disease burden via oxygenation, preservation of cardiac function, and attenuation of PAH (4).

MEDICATION
- Oxygenation:
  - Oxygen:
    - Long-term continuous oxygen therapy improves the survival of hypoxemic patients with COPD and cor pulmonale.
    - All patients with pulmonary hypertension whose PaO_2 is consistently <55 mm Hg or saturation ≤88% at rest, during sleep, or with ambulation should be prescribed oxygen to keep O_2 >90 mm Hg (5)[A].
- Preservation of cardiac function:
  - Diuretics: Decrease RV filling pressures; also improves peripheral edema secondary to RHF:
    - Furosemide: Starting at 20–80 mg PO/IV, titrate and increase dose per diuresis.
    - Excessive volume depletion should be avoided.
    - Monitor closely for metabolic alkalosis, as this may suppress ventilatory drive and contribute to hypoxia.
  - Cardiac glycosides:
    - Impact of digoxin on cor pulmonale alone is unclear
    - Digoxin may be appropriate in the presence of coexistent left ventricular systolic failure.
    - Digoxin may also be appropriate in the presence of atrial fibrillation as adjunct for rate control.
- Amelioration of PAH:
  - CCBs (4):
    - May be used as adjunctive therapy in those with low to moderate disease
    - Vasodilator therapy to reduce pulmonary vascular resistance has been shown to be effective in a small subset of patients (10%).
    - Vasoreactivity trial should be attempted with short-acting vasodilator at cardiac catheterization to determine likelihood of response. Reduction of >20% PAP without reduction of cardiac output should prompt adding CCB such as nifedipine, diltiazem, amlodipine to treatment regimen.
    - Repeat vasoreactivity trial via cardiac catheterization is recommended at 3–6 months following initiation of CCB therapy to assess sustained response. For nonsustained response, discontinue CCB and pursue alternative medications (6).
  - For nonresponse or unsustained response to CCB, treatment with phosphodiesterase inhibitors, endothelin receptor antagonists, and/or prostanoids may be appropriate based on World Health Organization (WHO) classification (6):
    - WHO Class I: Supportive therapy.
    - WHO Class II: Monotherapy is recommended with either phosphodiesterase inhibitor or endothelin receptor antagonist.
    - WHO Class III: Combination therapy may be used with phosphodiesterase inhibitor, endothelin receptor antagonist, or prostanoids. There is currently little randomized data on which combination is most efficacious (7).
    - WHO Class IV: Epoprostenol IV is first-line therapy in critically ill patients; other classes of drugs may also be added for combination therapy.
    - Phosphodiesterase inhibitors: Vasodilates by increasing cAMP and therefore increasing nitric oxide, an endogenous vasodilator. Sildenafil, tadalafil: Endothelin receptor antagonists: Vasodilates by blocking the function of endothelin, a potent vasoconstrictor. Bosentan, Ambrisentan, Sitaxsentan.
    - Prostanoids: Vasodilates by mimicking endogenous vasodilators. Iloprost Inhaled. IV may also be used; evidence to date limited to expert opinion. Treprostinil SC. IV may also be used; evidence to date limited to expert opinion. Beraprost PO Epoprostenol IV: Currently recommended for WHO Class IV only.
  - Anticoagulation:
    - Recommended for patients with underlying thromboembolic disease
    - Recommended for patients with cor pulmonale in association with idiopathic PAH (5)[B]
    - Use in secondary causes of PAH is widely accepted, though little supportive evidence to date (8)
    - In general, warfarin is recommended unless contraindications. Target international normalized ratio (INR) for prophylaxis is 2–3.

ADDITIONAL TREATMENT
General Measures
- Treat underlying disease.
- Supportive therapy as necessary:
  - Continuous positive airway pressure or bilevel positive airway pressure may be used for hypoxia/sleep disorders.
  - Ventilation using positive-pressure masks, negative-pressure body suits, or mechanical ventilation is suggested for patients with neuromuscular disease.
  - Phlebotomy may be indicated for severe polycythemia (hematocrit >55%).

Issues for Referral
Patients with cor pulmonale should be referred to a cardiologist or pulmonologist for expert consultation.

SURGERY/OTHER PROCEDURES
Moderate to severe disease refractory to medication may require atrioseptostomy and/or lung transplantation.

ONGOING CARE

Referral of patients with PAH to a specialized center with close follow-up is strongly recommended.

DIET
Salt and fluid restriction

PATIENT EDUCATION
- Smoking cessation and avoidance of exposure to secondary smoke is strongly recommended.
- Exertional activity should be limited.
- Pregnancy should be avoided in PAH.

PROGNOSIS
- Patients with cor pulmonale resulting from COPD have a greater likelihood of dying than do similar patients with COPD alone.
- The PAP is a reliable indicator of prognosis; higher pressure is associated with a worse prognosis.
- In patients with COPD and mild disease (PAP 20–35 mm Hg), 5-year survival is 50%.

REFERENCES

1. Han MK, McLaughlin VV, Criner GJ, et al. Pulmonary diseases and the heart. *Circulation*. 2007;116:2992–3005.
2. Naeije R, et al. Pulmonary hypertension and right heart failure in chronic obstructive pulmonary disease. *Proc Am Thorac Soc*. 2005;2:20–2.
3. Weitzenblum E, Chaouat A, et al. Cor pulmonale. *Chron Respir Dis*. 2009;6:177–85.
4. Hoeper MM, et al. Drug treatment of pulmonary arterial hypertension: Current and future agents. *Drugs*. 2005;65:1337–54.
5. Badesch DB, Abman SH, Simonneau G, et al. Medical therapy for pulmonary arterial hypertension: Updated ACCP evidence-based clinical practice guidelines. *Chest*. 2007;131: 1917–28.
6. Barst RJ, Gibbs JS, Ghofrani HA, et al. Updated evidence-based treatment algorithm in pulmonary arterial hypertension. *J Am Coll Cardiol*. 2009;54: S78–84.
7. Benedict N, Seybert A, Mathier MA, et al. Evidence-based pharmacologic management of pulmonary arterial hypertension. *Clin Ther*. 2007;29:2134–53.
8. Alam S, Palevsky HI. Standard therapies for pulmonary arterial hypertension. *Clin Chest Med*. 2007;28:91–115, viii.

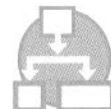

See Also (Topic, Algorithm, Electronic Media Element)

Chronic Obstructive Pulmonary Disease and Emphysema; Congestive Heart Failure; Pulmonary Arterial Hypertension; Pulmonary Embolism

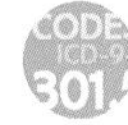

CODES

ICD9
- 415.0 Acute cor pulmonale
- 416.9 Chronic pulmonary heart disease, unspecified

CLINICAL PEARLS

- Continuous, long-term oxygen therapy improves life expectancy and quality of life in cor pulmonale.
- Referral of patients with PAH to a specialized center is strongly recommended.

C

CORNEAL ABRASION AND ULCERATION

Ravinder Singh, MD

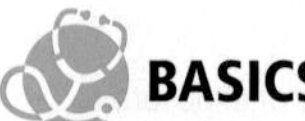

BASICS

DESCRIPTION

- Corneal abrasions result from scratching, denuding, abrading, or cutting of the outermost layer of the eye. They are usually traumatic and accidental, but can occur spontaneously as well.
- Corneal ulcers usually represent an infection of the cornea by bacteria, viruses, or fungi as a result of breakdown in the protective epithelial barrier.
- Both corneal abrasions and ulcerations can result in scarring, which may impair vision.
- Both lesions can occur centrally or marginally.

EPIDEMIOLOGY

Incidence

- Corneal abrasion is the most common ophthalmologic visit to the emergency department and is a commonly seen problem in urgent care:
  - 64% of cases are caused by direct minor trauma to eye
  - 12% of cases are due to contact lens–related problems
- Ulceration is also common in the US.

RISK FACTORS

- Any abrasive injury
- Contact lenses (especially soft lenses)
- Blepharitis
- Dry eye syndrome
- Entropion (with lashes scratching cornea)
- Chronic topical steroid use
- Abuse of topical anesthetics
- Autoimmune disorders
- Vitamin A deficiency
- Chronic corneal exposure (e.g., Bell's palsy, exophthalmos)
- Recent eye surgery
- Immunosuppression and trigeminal nerve abnormalities

GENERAL PREVENTION

- Eye protection to avoid injury during work, crafts, and sports
- Proper contact lens handling:
  - Do not sleep while wearing contact lens
- Artificial tears for those with inability to blink or known dry eyes

ETIOLOGY

- Corneal abrasions typically result from accidental trauma (e.g., fingernail scratch, makeup brush):
  - Dirt, sand, sawdust, or some other foreign body gets caught under eyelid.
- Corneal ulcers result from presence of an entryway to the external eye through dry eye, burns, abrasion, contact lenses, inappropriate use of topical anesthetics, antibiotics, or antiviral drops, immunosuppressant drugs, diabetes, or immunodeficiency:
  - Causative agents of ulceration:
    - Gram-positive organisms ~29–53% (*Staphylococcus aureus* and coag neg streptococcus are common ones)
    - Gram-negative organisms ~47–50% (*Pseudomonas* being most common followed by *Serratia marcescens*, *Proteus mirabilis*, and gram-negative enteric bacilli)
    - Viruses, such as herpes
    - Fungal organisms (*Candida, Aspergillus, Fusarium, Acanthamoeba*) in agricultural workers or associated with ocular corticosteroid use
    - Peripheral ulcerative keratitis usually caused by autoimmune disorders such as rheumatoid arthritis (RA), systemic lupus erythematosus (SLE), scleroderma.
    - Vitamin A deficiency may cause corneal necrosis or keratomalacia.

COMMONLY ASSOCIATED CONDITIONS

- Chronic ulcerations may be associated with neurotrophic keratitis due to lack of fifth nerve innervation of the cornea. Individuals with thyroid disease, diabetes, or immunosuppressive conditions are particularly at risk.
- Any cause of fat malabsorption may be associated with vitamin A deficiency.

DIAGNOSIS

HISTORY

- History remarkable for contact lens use, dry eyes, rubbing eye, history of trauma from foreign body or chemical burn
- History of connective tissue disorder
- Sudden onset of eye pain, photophobia, tearing, foreign-body sensation, blurring of vision, and/or conjunctival injection
- Abrasions and ulcerations are usually unilateral.

PHYSICAL EXAM

- Visual acuity may be decreased if abrasion or ulcer is centrally located.
- Conjunctival injection
- Increased lacrimation on affected side
- Photophobia
- Blepharospasm
- Lesion seen on slit lamp exam and area of damage shows fluorescein uptake; staining seen using Wood lamp or cobalt blue slit lamp.

DIAGNOSTIC TESTS & INTERPRETATION

Lab

Initial lab tests

Culture ulcer and contact lens if applicable.

ALERT

Pretreatment with topical antibiotics may alter culture results.

Diagnostic Procedures/Surgery

Scrapings of the corneal ulcer for culture and sensitivity ideally should be done before beginning local antibiotics. The sample should be plated directly onto the culture medium.

Pathological Findings

Scrapings for Gram and Giemsa stain may demonstrate bacteria, yeast, or intranuclear inclusions that may aid in the diagnosis.

DIFFERENTIAL DIAGNOSIS

- Foreign bodies
- Unilateral iritis
- Acute or chronic glaucoma
- Keratitis
- Scleritis
- Herpes simplex or zoster
- Bilateral or true idiopathic lesions may suggest basement membrane dystrophy.

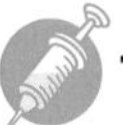

TREATMENT

MEDICATION

First Line

- Eye patching does not reduce pain, might make pain worse, and results in loss of binocular vision.
- Topical NSAIDS have been proven to reduce eye pain (1),(2)[A]:
  - Ophthalmic NSAIDs: Diclofenac 0.1% q.i.d. helps relieve moderate pain:
    - Alternatives include ketorolac 0.5% and bromfenac 0.09%.
- Ophthalmic antibiotics may help prevent further infection and ulceration of corneal abrasions (1)[C],(3).
- Some ophthalmic antibiotics include ciprofloxacin 0.3%, ofloxacin 0.3%, gentamicin 0.3%, erythromycin 0.5%, tobramycin 0.3%:
  - Ointment preparations may be more soothing to the eye than solutions.
  - They should be continued until eye feels better.
  - Chloramphenicol should not be used due to high risk of toxicity and Steven Johnson syndrome.
- Large corneal abrasions (>4 mm) or very painful abrasion should be treated with combination of topical antibiotic, topical NSAID, and topical cycloplegic:
  - Cycloplegic may cause blurring of vision, so these patients should not drive.
  - Re-evaluate in 24 hours and if improving, there is no need for further follow-up (1)[C].
- Fungal keratitis is treated with a protracted course of topical antifungal agents.
- Herpetic keratitis should be treated initially with trifluridine:
  - Vidarabine and acyclovir are alternatives (4)[A].

Second Line

- Oral analgesic medication if topical analgesia not adequate
- Supplemental topical cycloplegia (i.e., homatropine 5% and cyclopentolate 1%) has not been found to be beneficial (5)[B].

ADDITIONAL TREATMENT

General Measures

- Simple corneal abrasions can be managed by primary care physicians (6)[C]. See indications for referral below.
- All patients with corneal ulceration should be referred immediately to an ophthalmologist, as they need corneal cultures directly on media plates before starting antibiotics. If immediate referral is not possible, it is reasonable to start antibiotics without delay.
- Cycloplegics should be used with extra caution, especially in children and older patients, as they can impair vision significantly. Avoid driving.

Issues for Referral

- Consultation with an ophthalmologist is recommended for all ulcers to help determine appropriate therapy (1)[C]. Moreover, ulcers need corneal cultures to be taken directly onto culture media. If stat ophthalmologist consult or referral is not available, it is reasonable to start antibiotics without delay.
- Also refer to ophthalmologist if there is history of (1)[C]:
  - Significant ocular trauma
  - Corneal infection is suspected
  - Recurrent or nonhealing abrasion is encountered despite standard treatment.

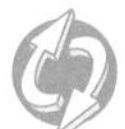

ONGOING CARE

FOLLOW-UP RECOMMENDATIONS

Patient Monitoring

- Contact lens wearer should be monitored daily with slit lamp for signs of secondary infection (1)[C].
- Minor abrasion should be re-evaluated only if becomes more painful (1)[C].
- Large abrasion (>4 mm) should be re-evaluated in 24 hours, and if improving, no need to follow further unless symptoms worsen again (1)[C].

PATIENT EDUCATION

Prevention of abrasions and proper handling of contact lenses can prevent recurrence of corneal ulcers.

PROGNOSIS

- Corneal abrasions and ulcerations should improve daily and heal with appropriate therapy.
- If healing does not occur within 24–48 hours or the lesion extends, obtain an ophthalmology consultation.

COMPLICATIONS

- Recurrence
- Scarring of the cornea
- Loss of vision
- Corneal perforation

REFERENCES

1. Fraser S, et al. Corneal abrasion. *Clin Ophthalmol*. 2010;4:387–90.
2. Turner A, Rabiu M, et al. Patching for corneal abrasion. *Cochrane Database Syst Rev*. 2006;CD004764.
3. Upadhyay MP, Karmacharya PC, Koirala S, et al. The Bhaktapur eye study: Ocular trauma and antibiotic prophylaxis for the prevention of corneal ulceration in Nepal. *Br J Ophthalmol*. 2001;85:388–92.
4. Wilhelmus KR, et al. Therapeutic interventions for herpes simplex virus epithelial keratitis. *Cochrane Database Syst Rev*. 2008;CD002898.
5. Carley F, Carley S, et al. Towards evidence based emergency medicine: Best BETs from the Manchester Royal Infirmary. Mydriatics in corneal abrasion. *Emerg Med J*. 2001;18:273.
6. Wirbelauer C, et al. Management of the red eye for the primary care physician. *Am J Med*. 2006; 119:302–6.

ADDITIONAL READING

- Ehler JP, Shah CP, Fenton GL. *The Wills Eye Manual: Office and Emergency Room Diagnosis and Treatment of Eye Disease*. Baltimore: Lippincott Williams & Wilkins; 2008.
- Kaiser PK, Pineda R, et al. A study of topical nonsteroidal anti-inflammatory drops and no pressure patching in the treatment of corneal abrasions. Corneal Abrasion Patching Study Group. *Ophthalmology*. 1997;104:1353–9.
- Morden NE, Berke EM. Topical fluoroquinolones for eye and ear. *Am Fam Physician*. 2000;62:1870–6.
- Watson SL, Barker NH. Interventions for recurrent corneal erosions. *Cochrane Database Syst Rev*. 2007;CD001861.

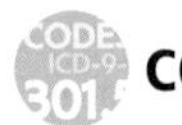

CODES

ICD9

- 370.00 Corneal ulcer, unspecified
- 370.03 Central corneal ulcer
- 918.1 Superficial injury of cornea

CLINICAL PEARLS

- Contact lens use should be discontinued until corneal abrasion or ulcer is healed and pain is fully resolved.
- Eye patching is not recommended.
- Prescribe topical and/or oral analgesic medication for symptom relief and consider ophthalmic antibiotics.
- Prompt referral to an ophthalmologist should be made for suspicion of an ulcer, recurrence of abrasion, retained foreign body, or lack of improvement despite therapy.

CORNS AND CALLUSES

Neil J. Feldman, DPM

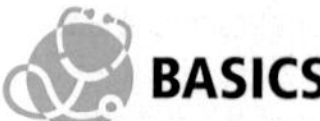

BASICS

DESCRIPTION

- A callus (tyloma) is a diffuse area of hyperkeratosis, usually without a distinct border.
- Typically the result of exposure to repetitive forces, including friction and mechanical pressure. Tend to occur on the palms of hands and soles of feet (1).
- A corn (heloma) is a circumscribed hyperkeratotic lesion with a central conical core of keratin that causes pain and inflammation. The conical core in a corn is a thickening of the stratum corneum.
- Hard corn or heloma durum (more common): More often on toe surfaces, especially fifth toe (proximal interphalangeal [PIP]) joint
- Soft corn (heloma molle): Commonly in the interdigital space (1)
- Digital corns are also known as clavi.
- Intractable plantar keratosis is usually located under a metatarsal head (first and fifth most common), is typically more difficult to resolve, and resistant to usual conservative treatments.

EPIDEMIOLOGY

Corns and calluses have the largest prevalence of all foot disorders.

Incidence

Incidence of corns and calluses increases with age. Less common in pediatric patients. Women affected more often than men. Blacks report corns and calluses 30% more often than whites.

Prevalence

- 9.2 million Americans
- Nearly 38/1,000 people affected

RISK FACTORS

- Extrinsic factors producing pressure, friction, and local stress:
  - Ill-fitting shoes
  - Not using socks, gloves
  - Manual labor
  - Walking barefoot
  - Activities that increase stress applied to skin of hands or feet (running, walking, sports)
- Intrinsic factors:
  - Bony prominences: Bunions
- Enlarged bursa or abnormal foot function/structure: Hammertoe, claw toe, or mallet toe deformity

Genetics

No true genetic basis identified, since most corns and calluses are due to mechanical stressors on the foot/hands.

GENERAL PREVENTION

External irritation is by far the most common cause of calluses and corns. General measures to reduce friction on the skin are recommended to reduce incidence of callus formation. Examples include wearing shoes that fit well and using socks and gloves.

Geriatric Considerations

In elderly patients, especially those with neurologic or vascular compromise, skin breakdown from calluses/corns may lead to increased risk of infection/ulceration. 30% of foot ulcers in the elderly arise from eroded hyperkeratosis. Regular foot exams are emphasized for these patients, as well as diabetic patients.

PATHOPHYSIOLOGY

Increased activity of keratinocytes in superficial layer of skin leading to hyperkeratosis. This is a normal response to excess friction, pressure, or stress.

ETIOLOGY

- Calluses typically arise from repetitive friction, motion, or pressure to skin.
- Soft corns arise from increased moisture from perspiration leading to maceration of the skin, along with mechanical irritation, especially between toes.
- Hard corns are an extreme form of callus with a keratin-based core. Often found on the digital surfaces and commonly linked to bony protrusions causing skin to rub against shoe surfaces.

COMMONLY ASSOCIATED CONDITIONS

- Foot ulcers, especially in diabetic patients or patients with neuropathy or vascular compromise
- Infection; look for warning signs of:
  - Spreading or redness around sore
  - Puslike drainage
  - Increased pain/swelling
  - Fever
  - Change in color of fingers or toes
- Signs of gangrene

DIAGNOSIS

- Most commonly a clinical diagnosis based on visualization of the lesion
- Examination of footwear may also provide clues.

HISTORY

- Careful history can usually pinpoint cause
- Ask about neurologic and vascular history and diabetes. These may be risk factors for progression of corns/calluses to frank ulcerations and infection.

PHYSICAL EXAM

- Calluses:
  - Thickening of skin without distinct borders
  - Often on feet, hands; especially over palms of hands, soles of feet
  - Colors from white to gray–yellow, brown, red
  - May be painless or tender
  - May throb or burn
- Corns:
  - Hard corns: Commonly on dorsum of toes or dorsum of fifth PIP joint:
    - Varied texture: Dry, waxy, transparent to a hornlike mass
    - Distinct borders
    - More common on feet
    - Often painful
  - Soft corns:
    - Often between toes, especially between fourth and fifth digits at the base of the webspace
    - Often yellowed, macerated appearance
    - Often extremely painful

DIAGNOSTIC TESTS & INTERPRETATION

Imaging

Initial approach

- Radiographs may be warranted if no external cause found. Look for abnormalities in foot structure, bone spurs.
- Use of metallic radiographic marker and weightbearing films often highlight the relationship between the callus and bony prominence.

Diagnostic Procedures/Surgery

Biopsy with microscopic evaluation in rare cases

Pathological Findings

Abnormal accumulation of keratin in epidermis, stratum corneum

DIFFERENTIAL DIAGNOSIS

- Plantar warts (typically a loss of skin lines within the wart)
- Porokeratoses (blocked sweat gland)

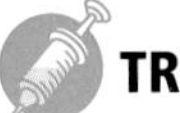

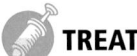

TREATMENT

MEDICATION

- Most therapy for corns and calluses can be done as self-care in the home (1).
- Use bandages, soft foam padding, or silicone sleeve over the affected area to decrease friction on the skin and promote healing with digital clavi.
- Use socks or gloves regularly.
- Use lotion/moisturizers for dry calluses and corns.
- Keratolytic agents such as urea or ammonium lactate can be applied safely.
- Use sandpaper discs or pumice stones over hard, thickened areas of skin.

Geriatric Considerations

Use of salicylic acid corn plasters can cause skin breakdown and ulceration in patients with thin, atrophic skin; diabetes; and those with vascular compromise. The skin surrounding the callus will often turn white and can become quite painful.

ADDITIONAL TREATMENT

General Measures

- Debridement of affected tissue and use of protective padding
- Low-heeled shoes, soft upper with deep and wide toebox
- Extra-width shoes for fifth-toe corns
- Avoidance of activities that contribute to painful lesions
- Prefabricated or custom orthotics

Issues for Referral

- May benefit from referral to podiatrist if use of topical agents and shoe changes are ineffective.
- Abnormalities in foot structure may require surgical treatment.
- Diabetic, vascular, and neuropathic patients may benefit from referral to podiatrist for regular foot exams to prevent infection or ulceration.

COMPLEMENTARY AND ALTERNATIVE MEDICINE

- Many over-the-counter topical ointments and lotions available for calluses (Keralac, Callex, urea, Lac-Hydrin). Do not use on broken skin.
- Epsom salt soaks for 5–10 minutes at a time

SURGERY/OTHER PROCEDURES

- Surgical treatment of areas of protruding bone where corns and calluses form
- Rebalancing of foot pressure through functional foot orthotics
- Shaving or cutting off hardened area of skin using a chisel or 15-blade scalpel. For corns, remove keratin core and place pad over area during healing.

IN-PATIENT CONSIDERATIONS

Admission Criteria

- Admission usually not necessary, unless progression to ulcerated lesion with signs of severe infection, gangrene
- May require aggressive debridement in operating room should an abscess or deep-space infection be suspected.

Nursing

Wound care, dressing changes for infected lesions

ONGOING CARE

PATIENT EDUCATION

- General information available at: http://www.mayoclinic.com/health/corns-and-calluses/DS00033/DSECTION=9
- American Podiatric Medical Association. Available at: http://www.apma.org

PROGNOSIS

Complete cure is possible once factors causing injury are eliminated.

COMPLICATIONS

Ulceration, infection

REFERENCE

1. Freeman DB. Corns and Calluses Resulting from Mechanical Hyperkeratosis. *Am Fam Physician*. 2002;65(11):2277–80.

ADDITIONAL READING

- Freeman DB. Corns and calluses resulting from mechanical hyperkeratosis. *Am Fam Physician*. 2002;65:2277–80.
- Pinzur MS, Slovenkai MP, Trepman E, et al. Guidelines for diabetic foot care: Recommendations endorsed by the Diabetes Committee of the American Orthopaedic Foot and Ankle Society. *Foot Ankle Int*. 2005;26:113–9.
- Theodosat A. Skin diseases of the lower extremities in the elderly. *Dermatol Clin*. 2004;22:13–21.

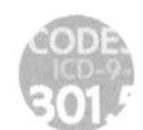

CODES

ICD9

700 Corns and callosities

CLINICAL PEARLS

Most therapy for corns and calluses can be done as self-care in the home using padding over the affected area to decrease friction; however, if simple home care is not helpful, then removal of the lesions is often immediately curative.

COSTOCHONDRITIS

Scott A. Fields, MD

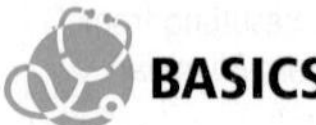

BASICS

DESCRIPTION
- Anterior chest wall pain associated with pain and tenderness of the costochondral and costosternal regions
- System(s) affected: Musculoskeletal
- Synonym(s): Costosternal syndrome; Parasternal chondrodynia; Anterior chest wall syndrome; Tietze disease and syndrome; Chondrocostal junction syndrome

Pediatric Considerations
Pay special attention to psychogenic chest pain in children who perceive family discord.

EPIDEMIOLOGY
- Predominant age: 20–40 years
- Predominant gender: Female

Incidence
~10% of chest pain complaints; 15–20% of teenagers with chest pain may have costochondritis.

RISK FACTORS
- Unusual physical activity or overuse
- Recent trauma (e.g., including motor vehicle accident, domestic violence) or new activity (1)
- Recent upper respiratory infection (URI)

ETIOLOGY
- Not fully understood
- Trauma
- Overuse

COMMONLY ASSOCIATED CONDITIONS
- URI
- Acute onset of cough
- Trauma to chest (MVA, sports)

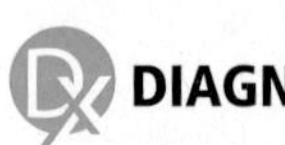

DIAGNOSIS

- Insidious onset
- Pain, usually sharp, sometimes pleuritic
- Pain involves multiple locations, the second to fifth costal cartilages are most often involved.
- Pain worsens with movement and breathing.
- Heat often relieves pain.
- Chest tightness is often associated with the pain.
- Pain sometimes radiates into arm.
- Nonsuppurative edema and tenderness at rib articulations
- Redness and warmth at sites of tenderness

HISTORY
- A complete and thorough history is mandatory for the diagnosis, with special emphasis on cardiac risk factor evaluation.
- Social history: Careful screening and evaluation for domestic violence and substance abuse

PHYSICAL EXAM
- A physical exam to exclude more serious conditions that may present with chest pain is necessary for the diagnosis.
- Tenderness elicited over the costochondral junctions is necessary to establish the diagnosis, but does not completely exclude other causes of chest pain.
- Palpation of epigastric region to evaluate for GERD and deep palpation in right upper quadrant of abdomen to evaluate gall bladder
- Mental status exam with focus on vegetative symptoms to evaluate for anxiety and panic disorders

Geriatric Considerations
Often presents with multiple problems capable of causing chest pain, making a thorough history and physical exam imperative.

DIAGNOSTIC TESTS & INTERPRETATION

Lab
- The diagnosis of costochondritis is primarily based on a thorough history and physical exam.
- Laboratory exams should be used only if concern exists regarding other elements of the differential diagnosis.
- ESR is inconsistently elevated.

Imaging
No imaging is indicated for the diagnosis of costochondritis; chest x-ray and rib films are often normal.

Diagnostic Procedures/Surgery
- None indicated for the diagnosis of costochondritis
- Consider ECG if any concern for cardiac involvement (myocardial infarction, cardiac contusion, recent URI/viral pericarditis).
- Consider chest x-ray if clinical concern is pneumothorax.
- Consider spiral CT for pulmonary embolism and D-dimer if history or risk factors are present.

Pathological Findings
Costochondral joint inflammation

DIFFERENTIAL DIAGNOSIS
- Cardiac (2):
  - Coronary artery disease
  - Cardiac contusion from trauma
  - Aortic aneurysm
  - Mitral valve prolapse
  - Pericarditis
  - Myocarditis
- GI:
  - Gastroesophageal reflux
  - Peptic esophagitis
  - Esophageal spasm
  - Gastritis
- Musculoskeletal:
  - Fibromyalgia
  - Slipping rib syndrome involves the lower ribs
  - Costovertebral arthritis
  - Painful xiphoid syndrome
  - Rib trauma with swelling
  - Thoracic disc compression
  - Ankylosing spondylitis
  - Epidemic myalgia
  - Precordial catch syndrome
- Psychogenic:
  - Anxiety disorder
  - Panic attacks
  - Hyperventilation
- Respiratory:
  - Asthma
  - Pulmonary embolism
  - Pneumonia
  - Chronic cough
  - Pneumothorax
- Other:
  - Domestic violence and abuse
  - Herpes zoster
  - Spinal tumor
  - Metastatic cancer
  - Substance abuse (cocaine)

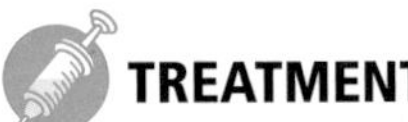

TREATMENT

Reassurance of benign nature of condition and potential for long, slow recovery from pain

MEDICATION

First Line

NSAIDs (aspirin, ibuprofen, naproxen, or diclofenac). Narcotics not indicated (3,4)[C].

Second Line

Acetaminophen (3,4)[C]

ADDITIONAL TREATMENT

General Measures

- Patient reassurance, rest, and heat (or ice massage, whichever makes the patient feel better)
- For ice massage, freeze a small paper cupful of water, then peel away a small amount of cup; massage should go from the patient's experience of cold, then burning, until numb, about 15 minutes 3 times per day, until symptoms improve.
- Stretching exercises (5, 6)

Issues for Referral

Consider referral to osteopathy or physical therapy if any concern rib is partially dislocated.

COMPLEMENTARY AND ALTERNATIVE MEDICINE

Limited data on use of manipulation or ice massage, but may be safely tried if patient interested

IN-PATIENT CONSIDERATIONS

Admission Criteria

Only indicated if differential diagnosis is unclear and cardiac or other more serious etiology of chest pain is being considered (7)[C]

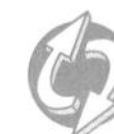

ONGOING CARE

FOLLOW-UP RECOMMENDATIONS

Follow-up within 1 week if diagnosis is unclear or symptoms do not improve with conservative treatment.

PATIENT EDUCATION

- Educate the patient in regard to the self-limited (although potentially recurrent) nature of the illness.
- Instruct patient on proper physical activity regimens to avoid overuse syndromes.
- Stress importance of avoiding sudden, significant changes in activity.

PROGNOSIS

- Self-limited illness, although sometimes chronic
- Often recurs

COMPLICATIONS

Incomplete attention to differential diagnosis or overly aggressive interventions to ensure a more life-threatening diagnosis is not missed

REFERENCES

1. Gregory PL, Biswas AC, Batt ME. Musculoskeletal problems of the chest wall in athletes. *Sports Med*. 2002;32:235–50.
2. Disla E, Rhim HR, Reddy A, et al. Costochondritis. A prospective analysis in an emergency department setting. *Arch Intern Med*. 1994;154:2466–9.
3. Freeston J, Karim Z, Lindsay K, et al. Can early diagnosis and management of costochondritis reduce acute chest pain admissions? *J Rheumatol*. 2004;31:2269–71.
4. Jensen S. Musculoskeletal causes of chest pain. *Aust Fam Physician*. 2001;30:834–9.
5. Aspegren D, Hyde T, Miller M, et al. Conservative treatment of a female collegiate volleyball player with costochondritis. *J Manipulative Physiol Ther*. 2007;30:321–5.
6. Rovetta G, Sessarego P, Monteforte P, et al. Stretching exercises for costochondritis pain. *G Ital Med Lav Ergon*. 2009;31:169–71.
7. Mukamel M, Kornreich L, Horev G, et al. Tietze's syndrome in children and infants. *J Pediatr*. 1997;131:774–5.

See Also (Topic, Algorithm, Electronic Media Element)

Algorithm: Chest Pain/Acute Coronary Syndrome

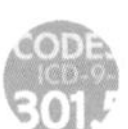

CODES

ICD9

733.6 Tietze's disease

CLINICAL PEARLS

- A very common disorder, accounting for perhaps 10% of all cases of chest pain, and a greater percentage in teenagers and young adults
- Educate the patient in regard to the self-limited (although potentially recurrent) nature of the illness. Instruct patient on proper physical activity regimens to avoid overuse syndromes. Also stress importance of avoiding sudden, significant changes in activity.
- Consider an anxiety disorder as a contributor to all cases of persistent chest pain, whether musculoskeletal or cardiac.

COUNSELING TYPES

William T. Garrison, PhD

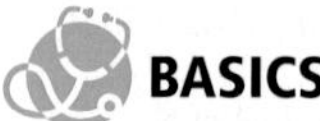

BASICS

DESCRIPTION

- Psychotherapeutic and counseling interventions play an important role in the management of chronic- and acute-onset diseases and disorders. They are typically the primary initial mode of evaluation and/or treatment for most mild-to-moderate psychiatric disorders that reach criteria using the DSM or ICD diagnostic classification systems. Treatment and successful control of either medical or psychological conditions require some form of professional counseling experience. Best outcomes occur when they are employed by a skilled practitioner. However, psychotherapy differs from generic counseling, which can take many forms and is delivered commonly in nonmedical settings with mixed results.
- Counseling approaches are usually tailored to the specific presenting problem or issue, and serve educational and emotional support functions. Typically, such counseling in medical settings will be time-limited and problem-focused, and is often not intended to lead to major medical symptom relief or major behavioral changes.
- The goals of psychotherapy range from increasing individual psychological insight and motivation for change, to reduction of interpersonal conflict in the marriage or family, reduction of chronic or acute emotional suffering, and reversal of dysfunctional or habitual behaviors. There are several general types of psychotherapy, starting with individual, marital, or family approaches. In addition, a number of psychological theories guide various methods and treatment philosophies. The following is a brief overview of commonly used psychotherapeutic and counseling methods.
- Psychodynamic therapy: Unconscious conflict manifests as patient's symptoms/problem behaviors:
  - Short-term (4–6 months) and long-term (≥1 year)
  - Focus is on increasing insight of underlying conflict or processes to initiate symptomatic change.
  - Therapist actively helps patient identify patterns of behavior stemming from existence of an unconscious conflict, or motivations that may not be accurately perceived.
- Cognitive-behavioral therapy (CBT): Patterns of thoughts and behaviors can lead to development and/or maintenance of symptoms. Thought patterns may not accurately reflect reality and may lead to psychological distress:
  - Therapy aims at modifying thought patterns by increasing cognitive flexibility and changing dysfunctional behavioral patterns.
  - Encourages patient self-monitoring of symptoms, and the precursors or results of maladaptive behavior
  - Uses therapist-assisted challenges to patient's basic beliefs/assumptions
  - May utilize *exposure*, a procedure derived from basic learning theories, which encourages gradual steps toward change
  - Can be offered in group or individual formats
  - Therapist role is suggestive and supportive.
- Dialectical behavior therapy (DBT): Techniques such as social skills training, mindfulness, and problem solving are used to modulate impulse control and affect management:
  - Derivative of CBT
  - Originally used in treatment of patients with self-destructive behaviors (e.g., cutting, suicide attempts)
  - Seeks to change rigid patterns of cognitions and behaviors that have been maladaptive
  - Utilizes both individual and group treatment modalities
  - Therapist takes an active role in interpretation and support.
- Interpersonal psychotherapy: Interpersonal relationships in a patient's life are linked to symptoms. Therapy seeks to alleviate symptoms and improve social adjustment through exploration of patient's relationships and experiences. Focus is on 1 of 4 potential problem areas:
  - Grief
  - Interpersonal role disputes
  - Role transitions
  - Interpersonal deficits: Therapist works with the patient in resolving the problematic interpersonal issues to facilitate change in symptoms
- Family therapy: Focuses on the family as a unit of intervention:
  - Uses psychoeducation to increase patient's and family's insight
  - Trains in communication and problem-solving skills
- Motivational interviewing: Focuses on motivation as a key to successful change process:
  - Short-term and problem-focused
  - Focuses on identifying discrepancies between goals and behavior
  - "5 A's" model is a brief counseling framework developed specifically for physicians to effect behavioral change in patients:
    - Assess for a problem.
    - Advise making a change.
    - Agree on action to be taken.
    - Assist with self-care support to make the change.
    - Arrange follow-up to support the change.
- Counseling (heterogeneous treatment):
  - Often focuses on situational factors maintaining symptoms
  - Often encourages utilization of community resources
- Behavioral therapy: Relatively nontheoretical approach to behavioral change or symptom reduction/eradication through application of principles of stimulus and response

Pediatric Considerations

- Important distinctions are made between psychotherapy and counseling for children/teens compared to adults/couples.
- The focus of evaluation must include attention to parent and family processes and factors. Interventions typically include interactions and sessions with parents, as well as collateral work with teachers and other school personnel.
- Younger children will often be evaluated and diagnosed through behavioral descriptions provided by parents and other adults who know them well, as well as through direct observation and/or play techniques. Children of all ages should be screened using behavioral checklists that are norm-referenced for age.
- Any child or teenager who requests counseling should be interviewed initially by the primary care provider and referred appropriately. Most referrals will be in response to parental request, however.
- Psychotherapeutic interventions with the strongest empirical basis with children include behavior therapy/modification, CBT, and family/parenting therapy. Play therapy has the least empirical support, and insight-oriented therapies appear to be more effective with older children (>11 years).
- There is controversy regarding the efficacy of psychopharmacologic treatment in preadolescents, although clear benefits have been demonstrated in some studies. Treatment guidelines for mild-to-moderate depressed mood and/or anxiety disorders typically recommend pediatric CBT initially, and studies have typically supported this approach in preteen and milder cases.

EPIDEMIOLOGY

- ~18.8 million adults suffer from clinical depression, and 20 million suffer from a diagnosable anxiety disorder.
- 1 in 4 Americans report seeking some form of mental health treatment in their adult life. This includes generic counseling in nonmedical settings such as work, clergy, or school settings, but also includes visits to primary care providers. It is estimated that between 3.5% and 5% of adults in the US actually participate in formal mental health psychotherapy annually.
- Public health experts report that the majority of those adults with diagnosable psychiatric disorders, however, do not receive professional mental health services. This is due to multiple factors, including failure to identify, noncompliance with psychiatric referral, regional shortages of providers, economic barriers, and excessive time duration from referral to available service.
- A large study conducted between 1987 and 1997 concluded that the percentage of adults in psychotherapy remained relatively stable over that decade, the use of psychopharmacology doubled, and older adults (ages 55–64) increasingly sought psychotherapy services. In that same study, it was found that psychotherapy duration (number of sessions) decreased substantially and about 1/3 of psychotherapy patients only attended 1 or 2 sessions.

RISK FACTORS

The need for psychotherapy or counseling services is directly and indirectly associated with a host of socioeconomic and biogenetic factors, including the general effects of poverty, family or marital dysfunction, life stressors, medical diseases or conditions, and individual biologic predisposition to mental health disorders.

GENERAL PREVENTION

It is generally assumed that early identification and intervention of child and adolescent psychopathology increases the likelihood of reducing the risk for adult psychopathology, but this has not been sufficiently validated in all categories of psychological disorders. Data support such claims in disorders such as childhood ADHD, anxiety disorders, and habit disorders of childhood, however.

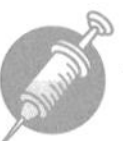

TREATMENT

MEDICATION

- Psychotherapy is most likely to be accompanied by use of pharmaceutical adjuncts in moderate-to-severe cases of psychological dysfunction that do not respond to other therapies, or in cases of extremely poor quality of life or high risk. The most common examples are in cases of clinical depression or anxiety that clearly incapacitates the patient or significantly reduces their quality of life. Patients at risk for suicide or who represent a danger to others are also candidates for acute psychopharmacotherapy. Studies suggest that verbal and behaviorally oriented therapies can add efficacy to medication treatment in both depression and anxiety.
- There is controversy in the research field regarding the efficacy of medication alone vs. psychotherapy alone vs. combined treatments. The most recent consensus has been that combined treatments in moderate-to-severe psychological dysfunction are most likely to render positive short-term results and increase the likelihood such effects can be sustained over time.

ADDITIONAL TREATMENT

General Measures

There is evidence of a "dose effect" in psychotherapy outcomes research, with some investigators suggesting that 6–8 sessions are necessary to yield positive initial effects, and upwards of 15–20 sessions for longer-term, sustainable therapeutic effects. This dose effect may not be applicable to counseling services with primarily informational or emotional/supportive functions.

Additional Therapies

- Anxiety disorders:
  - Panic disorder with and without agoraphobia (1)[A]: CBT, psychodynamic therapy
  - Generalized anxiety disorder: CBT (2)[A]
  - Obsessive-compulsive disorder: CBT (3)[A]
  - Posttraumatic stress disorder: CBT
  - Specific phobia: CBT
  - Social phobia: CBT (4)[A]
- Mood disorders:
  - Unipolar depression: CBT, interpersonal therapy, psychodynamic therapy (5)[A]
  - Bipolar disorder: Family therapy, interpersonal therapy, CBT
  - Schizophrenia: Psychodynamic therapy, family therapy, CBT
- Eating disorders:
  - Binge eating disorder: CBT, interpersonal therapy
  - Bulimia nervosa: CBT, interpersonal therapy
- Personality disorders:
  - Borderline: DBT, CBT
- Substance-use disorders:
  - Alcohol: Counseling, CBT, motivational interviewing
  - Cocaine: CBT, counseling
  - Heroin: CBT, counseling
  - Smoking: 5 A's
- Somatoform disorders:
  - Hypochondriasis: CBT
  - Body dysmorphic disorder: CBT

COMPLEMENTARY AND ALTERNATIVE MEDICINE

A host of nonempirically based psychological and nutritional therapies can be found outside of mainstream medicine and psychological science. Very little or no evidence exists to support such experimental therapies, but all have the considerable power of the placebo effect fueling their anecdotal supports or claims. Placebo effects are also thought to be further enhanced by the use of ingested or applied substances that create perceived or real physiologic changes in the patient.

REFERENCES

1. Furukawa TA, et al. Combined psychotherapy plus antidepressants for panic disorder with or without agoraphobia. *Cochrane Database Sys Rev.* 2007;2: CD004364.
2. Hunot V, et al. Psychological therapies for generalized anxiety disorder. *Cochrane Database Sys Rev.* 2007;2.
3. Eddy KT, Dutra L, Bradley R, et al. A multidimensional meta-analysis of psychotherapy and pharmacotherapy for obsessive-compulsive disorder. *Clin Psychol Rev.* 2004;24:1011–30.
4. Rodebaugh TL, Holaway RM, Heimberg RG. The treatment of social anxiety disorder. *Clin Psychol Rev.* 2004;24:883–908.
5. Bortolotti B, Menchetti M, Bellini F, et al. Psychological interventions for major depression in primary care: A meta-analytic review of randomized controlled trials. *Gen Hosp Psychiatry.* 2008;30: 293–302.

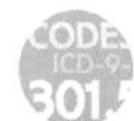

CODES

ICD9

- V65.49 Other specified counseling
- V65.8 Other reasons for seeking consultation

CLINICAL PEARLS

- Combined medication and psychotherapeutic treatments in moderate-to-severe psychological dysfunction are most likely to render positive short-term results and increase the likelihood such effects can be sustained over time. Relapse is common over time and/or as treatments are discontinued. Children under 10 may benefit significantly from counseling or psychotherapy alone for symptom relief. Older children and those with more severe symptoms typically require psychopharmacologic options in concert with counseling or verbal therapy approaches.
- There is evidence of a "dose effect" in psychotherapy outcomes research, with some investigators suggesting that 6–8 sessions are necessary to yield positive initial effects, and upwards of 15–20 sessions for longer-term, sustainable therapeutic effects. This dose effect may not be applicable to counseling services with primarily informational or emotional/supportive functions. Since many patients cease attendance to psychotherapy sessions after 1 or a few sessions, most interventions of this type cannot be accurately evaluated by the referring provider.

C

CROHN DISEASE

Tracey G. Simon, MD
Samir A. Shah, MD
Edward Feller, MD

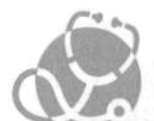

BASICS

DESCRIPTION

Crohn disease (CD) is a chronic, relapsing inflammatory disorder affecting the GI tract, most often terminal ileum (80%).

Hallmark Features:

- Transmural inflammation, which can result in fibrosis and stricture formation, as well as fissures leading to sinus tracts, abscesses, or fistulas.
- Noncaseating granulomas (50%), crypt abscesses
- Skip lesions: Patchy, segmental distribution of disease; lesions may affect multiple bowel segments, interspersed with areas of normal mucosa; however, disease can also be continuous, potentially mimicking ulcerative colitis (UC).
- Diverse presentations: 50% with ileocolitis, 20% have isolated colitis; of the latter, 10% involve the rectum. 1/3 have anorectal disease; <5% have upper GI disease.

Early Disease:

- Ulcerations: Initially focal with surrounding edema, resembling aphthous ulcers
- Perianal disease (pain, anal fissures, perirectal abscess) may precede intestinal disease.
- May present as wasting illness or anorexia

Developed Disease:

- Cobblestoning of mucosa
- Stenotic lumen
- Creeping fat
- Fissures develop between mucosal folds, resulting in strictures/adhesions and/or fistulae.

EPIDEMIOLOGY

Incidence

- In the US, 6–8 cases per 100,000 adults. Incidence is rising in US and Western Europe
- Bimodal age distribution: Predominant age is 15–25 years, with a second smaller peak at 50–70
- Females slightly > males; increased incidence among patients in northern climates
- 2–5 times increased risk in white patients vs. nonwhites
- 3–5 times increased risk in Ashkenazi Jewish patients

Prevalence

US adults: 100–200 cases per 100,000

RISK FACTORS

Environmental factors:

- Cigarette smoking (double the risk of developing CD); smoking cessation may reduce frequency of flares, relapse after surgery
- Dietary factors: Higher incidence in diets high in refined sugars, protein (meat, fish)
- Acute bacterial gastroenteritis: Salmonella or Campylobacter associated with increased risk of developing inflammatory bowel disease (IBD) (highest in 1 year).

Immunological abnormalities: Not yet established whether the immune responses in IBD are directed against self-antigens of the intestinal epithelium or to foreign, bacterial antigens:

- TNF: Up-regulation of inflammatory Th1 cytokines
- Recent studies indicate that tissue inflammation may result from increased secretion of cytokine IL-17, by Th17 subset of CD4+ T cells.

Genetics

Of CD patients, 15% have a first-degree relative with IBD; first-degree relative of an IBD patient has 3–30 times the increased risk of developing IBD by age 28:

- Mutations in susceptibility loci:
  - Ileal CD: IBD1 gene (chrom 16) encodes protein NOD2 (CARD15), which is expressed in Paneth cells; aberrant forms of NOD2 may have a dysfunctional response to bacterial pathogens.
  - Early-onset CD (age <15): Mutations in 5q31-33 (IBD5), 21q22, and 20q13
  - North American white males with CD: 30% have HLA-DR7 and DQ4
  - Extra-intestinal manifestations of CD: Mutations in HLA-A2, HLA-DR1, HLA-DQw5
  - Others: IL-10, IL-23 receptors; ATG16L1; IRGM
- Genetic syndromes associated with IBD risk:
  - Turner syndrome, Hermansky-Pudlak syndrome, Glycogen Storage Disease type 1b

PATHOPHYSIOLOGY

- General: Clinical manifestations result from activation of inflammatory cells, whose by-products produce nonspecific tissue injury
- Mechanism of diarrhea: Excess fluid secretion and impaired fluid absorption; bile salt malabsorption in inflamed ileum, with subsequent steatorrhea; bacterial overgrowth

ETIOLOGY

Multifactorial: Genetic, environmental triggers and immunological abnormalities result in inflammation and tissue injury, in genetically predisposed individuals.

COMMONLY ASSOCIATED CONDITIONS

- Extraintestinal manifestations:
  - Arthritis (20% of patients): Seronegative, primarily involving large joints; axial arthritis or ankylosing spondylitis (AS) and sacroiliitis (SI).
  - Skin disorders (10%): Erythema nodosum, pyoderma gangrenosum, psoriasis
  - Ocular disease (5%): Uveitis, iritis, episcleritis
  - Kidney stones: Calcium oxalate stones (from steatorrhea and diarrhea) or uric acid stones (from dehydration and metabolic acidosis)
  - Vitamin deficiencies: Fat-soluble vitamins (A, D, E, K), B_{12}
  - Osteopenia and osteoporosis; hypocalcemia
  - Hypercoagulability: Venous thromboembolism prophylaxis critical in hospitalized patients
  - Gallstones: Cholesterol stones, resulting from impaired bile acid reabsorption
  - Primary sclerosing cholangitis (5%): More common with UC; asymptomatic, elevated alkaline phosphatase
  - Autoimmune hemolytic anemia
- Conditions that correlate with increased disease activity in the bowel:
  - Peripheral arthropathy (but not SI and AS)
  - Episcleritis (but not uveitis)
  - Oral aphthous ulcers and erythema nodosum
  - SI, AS, and uveitis are associated with HLA-B27
- Potentially devastating complications: GI bleed, toxic megacolon, bowel perforation/peritonitis, malignancy, sclerosing cholangitis

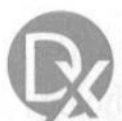

DIAGNOSIS

HISTORY

Hallmarks: Fatigue, fever, weight loss, prolonged diarrhea; perianal disease, with crampy abdominal pain, with or without gross bleeding. Children may present with growth failure:

- Factors that exacerbate CD: Concurrent infection, smoking, NSAIDs, and possibly stress

PHYSICAL EXAM

Presentation varies with location of disease:

- General: Signs of sepsis/disease activity (fever, tachycardia, hypotension) or wasting/malnutrition
- Abdominal: Focal or diffuse tenderness, distension, rebound/guarding
- Perianal: Fistulae, fissures
- Extraintestinal manifestations (see above)

DIAGNOSTIC TESTS & INTERPRETATION

Lab

Initial lab tests

- CBC; Chem10; LFTs; ESR/CRP; serum iron, vitamin B12, vitamin D-25 OH
- If diarrhea, stool specimen for routine culture, fecal leukocytes, *C. difficile*, and ova and parasites.
- In hospitalized patients with severe flare-ups, KUB to rule out toxic megacolon.

Follow-Up & Special Considerations

Evidence of complications:

- Stricture: Results in obstructive signs: nausea, vomiting, abdominal pain, weight loss, diarrhea, or inability to pass gas or feces
- Abscess/phlegmon: Localized abdominal peritonitis with fever and abdominal pain; diffuse peritonitis suggests intestinal perforation or abscess rupture (but may be masked by steroids, narcotics)
- Fistulae (seen in 33–50% of patients, after 10 and 20 years of disease, respectively):
  - Enteroenteric: Asymptomatic, or a palpable, commonly indolent abdominal mass
  - Enterovesical: Pneumaturia, recurrent polymicrobial UTI
  - Retroperitoneal: Psoas abscess, ureteral obstruction
  - Enterovaginal: Vaginal passage of gas or feces; clear, nonfeculent drainage from ileal fistula may be misdiagnosed as primary vaginal infection

Imaging

- Colon: A colonoscopy with ileoscopy provides the greatest sensitivity and specificity.
- Small bowel: CT or MR enterography have sensitivity that surpasses SBFT and visualize extraluminal disease. MR enterography: Added benefit of no radiation exposure. Capsule endoscopy allows small bowel visualization but not biopsy:
  - Signs of small bowel disease: Narrowed lumen with nodularity and/or the string sign; cobblestone appearance, fistula and abscess formation, separation of bowel loops (due to transmural inflammation with bowel-wall thickening)
- Gastroduodenal: Upper GI endoscopy

- Signs of gastroduodenal disease: Antral narrowing and segmental duodenal stricturing; inflammatory mucosal disease on endoscopy
- Perirectal complications: Optimal results from combination of endoscopic ultrasound (EUS) or MRI, with exam under anesthesia (EUA)
- Contraindications to endoscopy: Perforated viscus, recent myocardial infarction, severe diverticulitis, toxic megacolon, or inability to undergo appropriate bowel preparation (although, in most cases, unprepped limited sigmoidoscopy allows adequate visualization to assess endoscopic severity, extent, and aspirate of stool for *C. difficile*, obtain biopsies to assess histologic severity, and exclude other disorders, such as CMV)

Diagnostic Procedures/Surgery

How to distinguish CD from UC:

- CD: Small bowel involvement, rectal sparing; granulomas, perianal disease and/or fistulae; absence of gross bleeding; focal gross/microscopic lesions.
  - Commercially available antibody tests (overall 70% sensitive): ASCA, Cbir-1, OmpC, I2
  - Not yet available: ALCA, AMCA, ACCA
- UC: Diffuse, continuous lesions involving the rectum; loss of normal vascularity with friable tissue; pANCA
- Note: CD can mimic UC, with continuous, rather than intermittent, involvement. 10–15% of cases will be difficult to differentiate and will receive a diagnosis of IBDU (IBD undetermined).

DIFFERENTIAL DIAGNOSIS

- Acute, severe abdominal pain: Perforated viscus; pancreatitis; appendicitis; diverticulitis; bowel obstruction; kidney stones; gynecologic emergency in women
- Chronic diarrhea with crampy pain (colitis-like): UC, radiation colitis, infection, drugs, ischemia, microscopic colitis, IBD, celiac disease, malignancy (lymphoma, carcinoma), carcinoid
- Wasting illness: Malabsorption, malignancy, psychiatric illness

TREATMENT

- Assessment of disease severity: Clinical trials use formal grading systems such as the Crohn's Disease Activity Index (CDAI). Others include HBI, IBDQ, CDEIS, and MAYO scores. Improved methods to assess disease severity, incorporating endoscopic findings, are currently in development.
  - Asymptomatic remission (CDAI <150)
  - Mild to moderate CD: Ambulatory patients able to tolerate PO intake without dehydration, obstruction or >10% weight loss. No abdominal tenderness, toxicity, or mass (CDAI 150–220)
  - Moderate to severe CD: Patients who have failed initial treatment, or who continue to have mild symptoms such as fever, weight loss, and abdominal pain (CDAI 220–450)
  - Severe: Persistent symptoms despite outpatient therapy with glucocorticoids and/or biologics, or evidence of fulminant disease (peritoneal signs, cachexia, intestinal obstruction, or abscess) (CDAI >450)
- General strategies:
  - Step-up approach: Begin treatment with milder therapy (5-ASA, antibiotics) followed by more aggressive agents (steroids, immunomodulators, anti-TNF agents), as needed (1)[A]
  - Top-down approach: Early management with immunomodulators and/or anti-TNF agents, before patients receive steroids, become steroid-dependent, or require surgery (1)[A]

MEDICATION

First Line

- Asymptomatic patients: Observation Mild CD:
  - Induction: Controversial: Slow-release oral 5-ASA agent (1.6–4.8 g/d). Evidence does not support this approach, but clinical practice suggests that some patients respond; therefore, it is commonly used as first-line therapy (2)[B]
  - Mesalamine preferred for ileitis. For ileocolitis, sulfasalazine (2–4 g/d) or mesalamine.
  - Antibiotics use is also controversial.
  - Glucocorticoid therapy: Controlled ileal release budesonide (9 mg/d for 8–16 weeks, then discontinued over 2–4 week taper).
  - Consider adjunctive therapy: Antidiarrheals (loperamide); bile-acid binding resin (cholestyramine 4–12 g/d); probiotics (selected species either alone or in combination may prevent recurrent intestinal inflammation and improve symptoms in acute CD) (1)[B].
  - Maintenance: 5-ASA 1.6–4.8 g/d. Controlled ileal release budesonide, 6 mg/d, effective for maintenance for up to 6 months (2)[A]
- Moderate-to-severe CD:
  - Induction: Prednisone 40–60 g/d, or controlled-release budesonide (for patients with isolated, moderate ileitis), or anti-TNF agents (see below) (1)[A]
  - Maintenance: Little role for mesalamine. If steroids required for induction, then use immunomodulator +/– biologic (anti-TNF agent) for maintenance. Except for budesonide, do not use steroids for maintenance (1)[A].
- Severe disease: Immunomodulators +/– anti-TNF agents +/– steroids.
  - Azathioprine and 6-mercaptopurine: Thiopurine methyltransferase (TPMT) and LFTs, prior to initiation. Check CBC, LFTs every 2–3 months.
  - Methotrexate: Effective for steroid-dependent and steroid-refractory CD (1)[B]
    - Folic acid supplements 1 mg/d; follow LFTs
  - Anti-TNF therapies: Active disease, perianal fistula, steroid sparing, some extraintestinal disease. Check for TB, HBV, prior to initiation; continue to monitor for infection (3)[A]
    - Infliximab, adalimumab, certolizumab pegol
- Combination Therapy:
  - Azathioprine + infliximab more effective than either alone in patients not previously treated with either
  - Rare: Hepatosplenic T cell lymphoma (fatal)
- Antiadhesion molecules: Reserved for patients who fail anti-TNF therapy. These agents prevent inflammatory cells from entering the GI tract.
  - Natalizumab: Risk of PML (1/1,000)
  - Others currently in clinical trials

ADDITIONAL TREATMENT

General Measures

Additional therapies depend on location of disease:

- Oral lesions: Hydrocortisone and carboxymethyl-cellulose or topical sucralfate for aphthous ulcers, cheilitis, and/or granulomatous sialadenitis.
- Gastroduodenal CD: No clinical trials, although the slow-release form of mesalamine may be of benefit, as it is partially released in the proximal small bowel. Case reports detail success with anti-TNF therapies. Otherwise, symptomatic relief may be obtained from proton pump inhibitors, H2-receptor antagonists, and/or sucralfate.
- Ileitis: Patients often require supplementation of fat-soluble vitamins, as well as iron, B_{12}, and/or folate, and calcium to prevent bone loss.
- Treatment toxicity: Pancreatitis, bone marrow toxicity, lymphoma, nonmelanoma skin cancer, infections (TB, histoplasmosis, others), malignancy

Additional Therapies

Complications:

- Peritonitis: Bowel rest and antibiotic therapy (7–10 days parenteral antibiotics, followed by 2–4 week course of PO ciprofloxacin and metronidazole); surgery as indicated:
  - Consider holding steroids, which mask sepsis.
- Abscess: Antibiotics, percutaneous drainage, or surgery with resection of affected segments.
- Small bowel obstruction: IV hydration, NG suction, TPN for malnutrition, with resolution typically in 24–48 hours. Surgery for nonresponders.

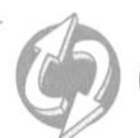

ONGOING CARE

FOLLOW-UP RECOMMENDATIONS

Patient Monitoring

- Vaccinations in CD:
  - Check titers; avoid live vaccines (MMR, varicella, zoster) in immunosuppression (steroids, 6MP, AZA, MTX, or anti-TNF)
  - Regardless of immunosuppression: HPV, influenza, pneumococcal, meningococcal, Hepatitis A, B; Tdap
- Pregnancy and Pediatrics
  - Please refer to Mahadevan U, et al. *Am J Gastroenterol*. 2011;106:214–23.

PATIENT EDUCATION

Crohn and Colitis Foundation of America, (800) 343-3637, www.ccfa.org

REFERENCES

1. Lictenstein GR, Hanauer SR, Sandborn WJ, et al. ACG Practice Guidelines. Management of Crohn's disease in adults. *Am J Gastroenterol*. 2009; 104:465–83.
2. Talley N, Abreu M, Achkar J-P, et al. An evidence-based systematic review on medical therapies for inflammatory bowel disease. *Am J Gastroenterol*. 2011;106:S2–S25.
3. Colombel J-F, Sandborn W, Reinisch W, et al. Infliximab, azathioprine, or combination therapy for Crohn's disease. *NEJM*. 2010;362(15):1383–95.

CODES

ICD9

- 555.0 Regional enteritis of small intestine
- 555.1 Regional enteritis of large intestine
- 555.9 Regional enteritis of unspecified site

CLINICAL PEARLS

- MRe allows assessment of luminal and extraluminal CD without radiation exposure.
- Assess for TB and HBV prior to anti-TNF therapy.

CROUP (LARYNGOTRACHEOBRONCHITIS)

Garreth C. Debiegun, MD

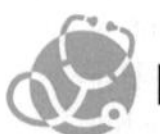

BASICS

DESCRIPTION

- Croup is a subacute viral illness characterized by upper-airway symptoms such as barking cough, stridor, and fever. "Croup" is used to refer to viral laryngotracheitis or laryngotracheobronchitis (LTB), though it is sometimes used for LTB with pneumonitis, bacterial tracheitis, or spasmodic croup.
- Most common cause of upper-airway obstruction or stridor in children
- System(s) affected: Pulmonary and respiratory
- Synonym(s): Croup; infectious croup; viral croup; LTB
- Spasmodic croup: Noninfectious form with sudden resolution:
  - No fever or radiographic changes
  - Initially treated as croup
  - Usually self-limiting and resolves with mist therapy at home
  - Often recurs on same night or in 2–3 nights

EPIDEMIOLOGY

- Predominant age (1):
  - Common among children aged 7 months to 3 years
  - Most common during the second year of life
  - Rare among those >6 years
- Predominant sex: Male > Female (1.5:1) (1)
- Timing:
  - Possible during any time of year but is most common in autumn and winter (with parainfluenza 1 and respiratory syncytial virus [RSV])

Incidence

- 6 cases of croup per year per 100 children <6 years old
- 1.5–6% of cases require hospitalization.
- 2–6% of those require intubation.
- Decreasing incidence in the US and Canada

RISK FACTORS

- History of croup
- Recurrent upper respiratory infections
- Atopic disease increases the risk of spasmodic croup.

PATHOPHYSIOLOGY

- Subglottic region/larynx is entirely encircled by the cricoid cartilage.
- Inflammatory edema and subglottic mucus production decrease airway radius.
- Small children have small airways with more compliant walls.
- Negative-pressure inspiration pulls airway walls closer together.
- Small decrease in airway radius causes significant increase in resistance (Poiseuille law: Resistance proportional to 1/radius^4).

ETIOLOGY

- Usually viruses that initially infect oropharyngeal mucosa and then migrate inferiorly
- Parainfluenza virus:
  - Most common pathogen: 75% of cases
  - Type 1 is most common, causing 18% of all cases of croup.
  - Types 2, 3, and 4 are also common.
  - Type 3 may cause a particularly severe illness.
- Other viruses:
  - RSV
  - Paramyxovirus
  - Influenza virus type A or B
  - Adenovirus
  - Rhinovirus
  - Enteroviruses (Coxsackie and Echo)
  - Reovirus
  - Measles virus where vaccination not common
- *Haemophilus influenzae* type B now rare with routine immunization (2)
- May have bacterial cause: *Mycoplasma pneumoniae* has been reported.

COMMONLY ASSOCIATED CONDITIONS

If recurrent (>2 episodes in a year) or during first 90 days of life, consider host factors:

- Underlying anatomic abnormality (e.g., subglottic stenosis)
- Paradoxical vocal cord dysfunction
- Gastroesophageal reflux disease
- Prolonged neonatal intubation

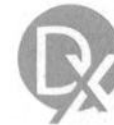

DIAGNOSIS

- Most children who present with acute onset of barky cough, stridor, and chest-wall indrawing have croup.
- Croup is a clinical diagnosis; lab tests and imaging serve only ancillary purposes (3).
- Classic "seal-like" barking, spasmodic cough
- May have biphasic stridor
- Low-grade to moderate fever
- Upper respiratory infection prodrome lasting 1–7 days
- Severity usually is determined by clinical observation for signs of respiratory effort: Nasal flaring, retractions, tripoding, sniffing position, abdominal breathing, tachypnea. Later symptoms: Hypoxia/cyanosis or fatigue.
- Westley Croup Scale (≤2 mild; 3–7 moderate; ≥8 severe):
  - Level of consciousness: Normal, including sleep = 0; disoriented = 5
  - Cyanosis: None = 0; with agitation = 4; at rest = 5
  - Stridor: None = 0; with agitation = 1; at rest = 2
  - Air entry: Normal = 0; decreased = 1; markedly decreased = 2
  - Retractions: None = 0; mild = 1; moderate = 2; severe = 3
- Child who appears nontoxic: Normal voice, no drooling
- No change in stridor with positioning
- Nontender larynx
- Inflamed subglottic region with normal-appearing supraglottic region

HISTORY

- 2–3 days of nonspecific prodromal syndrome with low-grade fever, coryza, and rhinorrhea
- Onset and recurrence at night when child is sleeping
- Symptoms often resolve en route to the hospital as the child is exposed to cool night air.
- Lack of prodrome indicates spasmodic croup.

PHYSICAL EXAM

- Pulse oximetry often is normal because there is no disturbance of alveolar gas exchange.
- Overall appearance: Is the child comfortable or struggling?
- Work of breathing: Labored or comfortable?
- Sound of breathing and voice: Hoarse, stridor, inspiratory wheezing, short sentences?
- Observed/subjective tidal volume: Sufficient for child's size?

DIAGNOSTIC TESTS & INTERPRETATION

Lab

- No laboratory abnormality is diagnostic.
- White blood cells may be low, normal, or elevated.
- Lymphocytosis is expected but not required.
- Rapid antigen or viral culture tests are available in some centers:
  - Guide isolation precautions not management.

Imaging

- Posteroanterior and lateral neck films show funnel-shaped subglottic region with normal epiglottis: "Steeple," "hour glass," or "pencil point" sign (present in 40–60% of children with LTB).
- CT may be more sensitive for defining etiology of obstruction in a confusing clinical picture.
- Patient should be monitored during imaging; progression of airway obstruction may be rapid.

Pathological Findings

- Inflammatory reaction of respiratory mucosa
- Loss of epithelial cells
- Thick mucoid secretions

DIFFERENTIAL DIAGNOSIS

- Epiglottitis: Currently rare
- Foreign-body aspiration
- Subglottic stenosis (congenital or acquired)
- Bacterial tracheitis
- Simple upper respiratory infection
- Retropharyngeal or peritonsillar abscess
- Trauma
- Allergic reaction (acute angioneurotic edema)
- Airway anomalies (e.g., tracheo/laryngomalacia)
- Subglottic hemangioma

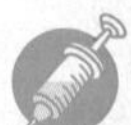

TREATMENT

MEDICATION

First Line

- Well established in the literature; cornerstones of treatment are immediate nebulized epinephrine and dexamethasone (4)[A]
- Racemic or L-epinephrine (equal efficacy and side-effect profiles (5); L-epinephrine is used for most other hospital purposes and is less expensive):
  - Racemic epinephrine: 0.05 mL/kg/dose (max, 0.5 mL) of 2.25% solution nebulized in normal saline total volume 3 mL (6)[A],(7)[B]
  - L-epinephrine: 0.5 mL/kg/dose (max, 5 mL) of a 1:1,000 dilution
  - Onset in 1–5 minutes, duration of 2 hours
  - Repeat as necessary if side effects are tolerated.
  - Must observe child for 3–4 hours.

- Corticosteroids (8)[A]:
  - Dexamethasone (cheapest, most literature, easiest), 0.15–0.6 mg/kg; higher doses have been traditional care, but studies have proven 0.15 mg/kg has equal efficacy (9). Single dose, IV/IM/PO have proven equal efficacy (10)[A]
  - Nebulized budesonide also has been proven effective (11)[B].
  - Other steroids (betamethasone and prednisolone) seem to be beneficial but not as good as dexamethasone (5).
  - Onset by 6 hours
- Heli-Ox: A helium-oxygen mixture:
  - Smaller, lower-mass helium molecule (compared with nitrogen) theoretically maintains laminar flow in narrower airways and serves as bridge therapy to steroids.
  - Minimum of 60% helium must be used; 70% is preferable; 79% if patient has no O_2 requirement
  - There is limited data. Anecdotal reports and 1 case series support its use, but 2 prospective studies showed no benefit (12,13). Also, a Cochrane review found insufficient evidence to support the use of Heliox in croup (14).
- Antibiotics not indicated in this viral illness:
  - Antecedent or subsequent bacterial infection is possible but uncommon.
- Oxygen as needed
- Contraindications, precautions, and significant possible interactions: Refer to the manufacturer's literature.

Second Line

Amantadine for influenza A: 100 mg PO b.i.d. for 3–5 days

ADDITIONAL TREATMENT

General Measures

- Minimize lab tests, imaging, and other procedures that upset the child; agitation that worsens tachypnea is more detrimental than accepting a clinical diagnosis.
- ECG monitoring and pulse oximetry:
  - Frequent checks are more sensitive to worsening disease than is pulse oximetry.

COMPLEMENTARY AND ALTERNATIVE MEDICINE

- Mist therapy often helps with symptoms. Do not use high-temperature misters (e.g., teakettles) because of a risk of burns. A hot shower running in a bathroom is a good steam generator.
- Some children respond well to cold, dry air.
- Probiotics may decrease the incidence of upper respiratory tract infections (15).

SURGERY/OTHER PROCEDURES

- Intubation rarely is required; tube 0.5–1 mm smaller than normal:
  - After trial of medical management, intubation is for fatigue caused by work of breathing or beginning total obstruction; not secondary to low oxygen saturation.
  - Extubate in 3–5 days when there is an appropriate air leak around the endotracheal tube.
- Tracheotomy: Rarely; maintenance 3–7 days

IN-PATIENT CONSIDERATIONS

Initial Stabilization

- Outpatient care in mild cases
- Admit patients who do not respond to therapy or who have O_2 requirement, pneumonia, or congestive heart failure
- In most cases, observation in the emergency department after medical management is sufficient.

Admission Criteria

Minor cases need no visit to a hospital or primary care physician (PCP):

- No stridor at rest, no difficulty breathing
- Child able to tolerate liquids PO
- No underlying medical condition
- Caretakers able to assess changes to clinical picture and reaccess medical care

Discharge Criteria

Patients who maintain a good response to medical therapy for 3–4 hours (after epinephrine dose) may be safely discharged as long as they have reliable caretakers and good access to medical services if symptoms return (16)[C].

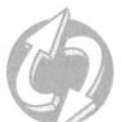

ONGOING CARE

FOLLOW-UP RECOMMENDATIONS

Patient Monitoring

Most patients will be seen in an ED or PCP office setting. Some will be overnight by telephone.

DIET

- NPO and IV fluids for severe cases
- Frequent small feedings with increased fluids for mild cases

PATIENT EDUCATION

- Must keep the patient quiet; crying may exacerbate symptoms.
- Educate parents about when to seek emergency care if mild cases progress.
- Provide emotional support and reassurance for the patient.

PROGNOSIS

- Up to 1/3 of patients will have a recurrence.
- Recovery is usually full and without lasting effects.
- If multiple recurrences, consider referral to ear, nose, and throat specialist to evaluate for possible anatomic etiology (17).

COMPLICATIONS

- Rare
- Subglottic stenosis in intubated patients
- Bacterial tracheitis
- Cardiopulmonary arrest
- Pneumonia

REFERENCES

1. Cherry JD. Clinical practice. Croup. *N Engl J Med*. 2008;358:384–91.
2. Sobol SE, Zapata S. Epiglottitis and croup. *Otolaryngol Clin North Am*. 2008;41:551–66, ix.
3. Everard ML. Acute bronchiolitis and croup. *Pediatr Clin North Am*. 2009;56:119–33, x–xi.
4. Johnson DW, Jacobson S, Edney PC, et al. A comparison of nebulized budesonide, intramuscular dexamethasone, and placebo for moderately severe croup. *N Engl J Med*. 1998; 339:498–503.
5. Bjornson C, Russell KF, Vandermeer B, et al. Nebulized epinephrine for croup in children. *Cochrane Database Syst Rev*. 2011;CD006619.
6. Westley CR, Cotton EK, Brooks JG. Nebulized racemic epinephrine by IPPB for the treatment of croup: a double-blind study. *Am J Dis Child*. 1978;132:484–7.
7. Waisman Y, Klein BL, Boenning DA, et al. Prospective randomized double-blind study comparing L-epinephrine and racemic epinephrine aerosols in the treatment of laryngotracheitis (croup). *Pediatrics*. 1992;89:302–6.
8. Russell KF, Liang Y, O'Gorman K, et al. Glucocorticoids for croup. *Cochrane Database Syst Rev*. 2011;CD001955.
9. Dobrovoljac M, Geelhoed GC, et al. 27 years of croup: An update highlighting the effectiveness of 0.15 mg/kg of dexamethasone. *Emerg Med Australas*. 2009;21:309–14.
10. Geelhoed GC, Turner J, MacDonald WB. Efficacy of a small single dose of oral dexamethasone for outpatient croup: A double-blind placebo controlled clinical trial. *Br Med J*. 1996;313(7050): 140–2.
11. Cetinkaya F, Tüfekçi BS, Kutluk G. A comparison of nebulized budesonide, and intramuscular, and oral dexamethasone for treatment of croup. *Int J Pediatr Otorhinolaryngol*. 2004;68:453–6.
12. Vorwerk C, Coats TJ. Use of helium-oxygen mixtures in the treatment of croup: A systematic review. *Emerg Med J*. 2008;25:547–50.
13. Gupta VK, Cheifetz IM. Heliox administration in the pediatric intensive care unit: An evidence-based review. *Pediatr Crit Care Med*. 2005;6:204–11.
14. Vorwerk C, Coats T, et al. Heliox for croup in children. *Cochrane Database Syst Rev*. 2010;2:CD006822.
15. Hao Q, Lu Z, Dong BR, et al. Probiotics for preventing acute upper respiratory tract infections. *Cochrane Database Syst Rev*. 2011;9:CD006895.
16. Klassen TP. Croup. A current perspective. *Pediatr Clin North Am*. 1999;46:1167–78.
17. Jabbour N, Parker NP, Finkelstein M, et al. Incidence of operative endoscopy findings in recurrent croup. *Otolaryngol Head Neck Surg*. 2011;144:596–601.

ADDITIONAL READING

Bjornson CL, Johnson DW. Croup. *Lancet*. 2008;371:329–39.

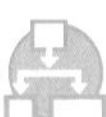

See Also (Topic, Algorithm, Electronic Media Element)

Bronchiolitis; Epiglottitis; Tracheitis, Bacterial

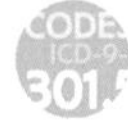

CODES

ICD9

464.4 Croup

CLINICAL PEARLS

- Parainfluenza virus is the most common pathogen.
- Also caused by RSV, paramyxovirus, influenza virus type A or B, adenovirus, rhinovirus, enteroviruses (Coxsackie and Echo)
- Established efficacy of inhaled epinephrine and corticosteroids
- Lateral neck films show funnel-shaped subglottic region with normal epiglottis: "Steeple," "hour glass," or "pencil point" sign (present in 40–60% of children with laryngotracheobronchitis)

CRYPTORCHIDISM

Pamela I. Ellsworth, MD

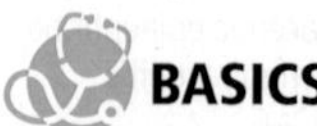

BASICS

DESCRIPTION

- Incomplete or improper descent of one or both testicles; normally, descent is in the seventh to eighth month of gestation. The cryptorchid testis may be palpable or nonpalpable.
- Types of cryptorchidism:
  - Abdominal: Located inside the internal ring
  - Canalicular: Located between the internal and external rings
  - Ectopic: Located outside the normal path of testicular descent from abdominal cavity to scrotum; may be ectopic to perineum, femoral canal, superficial inguinal pouch (most common), suprapubic area, or opposite hemiscrotum
  - Retractile: Fully descended testis that moves freely between the scrotum and the groin
  - Iatrogenic: Previously descended testis becomes undescended secondary to scar tissue after inguinal surgery, such as an inguinal hernia repair or hydrocelectomy.
  - Also may be referred to as *palpable* versus *nonpalpable*
- System(s) affected: Reproductive
- Synonym(s): Undescended testes (UDT)

EPIDEMIOLOGY

Incidence

- Predominant age: Premature newborns
- Predominant sex: Male only

Prevalence

- In the US, cryptorchidism occurs in 3% of full-term, and 33% of premature newborn males.
- Spontaneous testicular descent occurs by age 1–3 months in 50–70% of full-term males with cryptorchidism.
- Descent at 6–9 months of age is rare.

RISK FACTORS

- Family history of cryptorchidism: Boys with UDTs: 4% of their fathers and 6.2–9.8% of their brothers have UDTs (2).
- Low birth weight, prematurity, and small for gestational age are associated with a substantial increase in incidence of cryptorchidism, which may reach 20–25% in infants with birth weight <2.5 kg (4).

Genetics

Occurrence of UDT in siblings as well as fathers suggests a genetic etiology.

ETIOLOGY

- Not fully known
- May involve alterations in:
  - Mechanical factors (gubernaculum, length of vas deferens and testicular vessels, groin anatomy, epididymis, cremasteric muscles, and abdominal pressure), hormonal factors (gonadotropin, testosterone, dihydrotestosterone, and müllerian inhibiting substance) and neural factors (ilioinguinal nerve and genitofemoral nerve)
  - Major regulators of testicular descent from intraabdominal location into the bottom of the scrotum are the Leydig cell–derived hormones testosterone and insulinlike growth factor 3 (IGF-3).
  - Mutations in the gene for IGF-3 and in the androgen receptor gene have been recognized as causes of cryptorchidism as well as chromosomal alterations.
  - Environmental factors acting as endocrine disruptors of testicular descent also may contribute to the etiology of cryptorchidism (5).

COMMONLY ASSOCIATED CONDITIONS

- Inguinal hernia/hydrocele
- Abnormalities of vas deferens and epididymis
- Intersex abnormalities
- Hypogonadotropic hypogonadism
- Germinal cell aplasia
- Prune-belly syndrome
- Meningomyelocele
- Hypospadias
- Wilms' tumor
- Prader-Willi syndrome
- Kallmann syndrome
- Cystic fibrosis

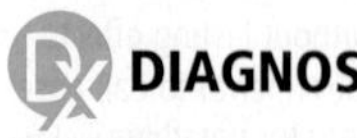

DIAGNOSIS

HISTORY

- ≥1 testicles in a site other than the scrotum
- May be an isolated defect or associated with other congenital anomalies

PHYSICAL EXAM

- Performed with warm hands, with child in sitting, standing, and squatting position
- A Valsalva maneuver and applied pressure to lower abdomen may help to identify the testes, especially a gliding testis.
- Failure to palpate a testis after repeated exams suggests an intra-abdominal or atrophic testis.
- An enlarged contralateral testis in the presence of a nonpalpable testis suggests testicular atrophy/absence.

DIAGNOSTIC TESTS & INTERPRETATION

Lab

Initial lab tests

- In boys ≤3 months of age with bilateral nonpalpable UDTs, hormone levels are helpful to determine whether the testes are present:
  - Luteinizing hormone (LH)
  - Follicle-stimulating hormone (FSH)
  - Testosterone
- >3 months of age, a human chorionic gonadotropin (hCG) stimulation test to determine presence/absence of testicular tissue (hCG 2,000 IU/d × 3 days, and check testosterone before and after stimulation)

Follow-Up & Special Considerations

In newborns and children <6–12 months of age, periodic examination to determine if testis is palpable and descended prior to considering further intervention

Imaging

Initial approach

- Ultrasound has a sensitivity of 45% (95% confidence interval [CI]: 29–61) and a specificity of 78% (95% CI: 43–94) (5):
  - Ultrasound does not reliably localize nonpalpable testes and does not rule out an intraabdominal testis. A recent meta-analysis therefore concluded that eliminating the use of ultrasound will not change management of nonpalpable cryptorchidism but will decrease health care expenditures (5,6).
  - In earlier studies, ultrasonography had a sensitivity of 76%, a specificity of 100%, and an accuracy of 84% in the diagnosis of nonpalpable UDT (6).
- MRI has a sensitivity of 86%, a specificity of 79%, and an accuracy of 85% (6)[C].
- CT scan findings in children are inconsistent.

Diagnostic Procedures/Surgery

Laparoscopy is useful in a child with nonpalpable cryptorchidism to accurately confirm testicular absence or presence and to determine the feasibility of performing a standard orchiopexy (7)[C].

Pathological Findings

- Higher incidence of carcinoma in UDT and alterations in spermatogenesis
- Histologic changes occur by 1.5 years of age and include smaller seminiferous tubules, fewer spermatogonia, and more peritubular tissue.

DIFFERENTIAL DIAGNOSIS

- Retractile testis (hypermobile testis): A normally descended testis that ascends into the inguinal canal because of an active cremasteric reflex (more common in males 4–6 years of age)
- Atrophic testis: May occur as a result of neonatal torsion
- Vanished testis may be the result of a lack of development or in utero torsion.

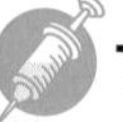

TREATMENT

MEDICATION

- The International Health Foundation recommends biweekly hCG injections for 5 weeks: 250 (IU) for infants, 500 IU for children ≤6 years of age, and 1,000 IU for children ≥6 years of age. This is an off-label use of hCG.
- Success rates for descent into the scrotum range from 0–55% (8)[B]:
  - The more distal the testis, the more likely the descent.
  - A systematic review with a meta-analysis of randomized clinical trials concluded that the evidence for the use of hCG versus gonadotropin-releasing hormone (GnRH) shows advantages for hCG, but noted that the evidence was based on few trials (9)[B].
- Contraindications: hCG therapy is contraindicated in patients with a clinically apparent inguinal hernia, those with a history of previous ipsilateral groin surgery, or those with ectopic testicles. Also refer to manufacturer's literature.
- Precautions: (i) May induce precocious puberty; discontinue drug; effects should reverse in 4 weeks; (ii) premature epiphyseal closure
- Significant possible interactions: Refer to manufacturer's literature.
- GnRH is approved for use in Europe, and neoadjuvant GnRH therapy may improve fertility index in UDT (10)[C].

ADDITIONAL TREATMENT

General Measures

- Rule out retractile testis.
- Appropriate health care: Outpatient until surgery performed
- Administration of chorionic gonadotropin may cause testicular descent in some boys. Reports of efficacy are inconsistent.

Issues for Referral

- Bilateral nonpalpable UDTs
- ≥1 testes not descended by 6 months to 1 year of age

SURGERY/OTHER PROCEDURES

- Reasons to consider: Avoids torsion, averts trauma, decreases but does not eliminate risk of malignancy, and prevents further alterations in spermatogenesis
- Orchiopexy should be performed by age 1. Alterations in germ cell count in the cryptorchid testis have been identified by age 2.
- Laparoscopy is performed first if testis is nonpalpable.
- If palpable, an inguinal approach is usually performed. Prepubertal approach is considered in select situations, but may increase the risk of hernia (11)[C].

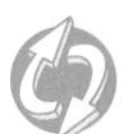

ONGOING CARE

FOLLOW-UP RECOMMENDATIONS

Initial follow-up within 1 month of surgery and periodically thereafter to assess testicular size/growth

Patient Monitoring

- Patients should be followed after surgery to evaluate testicular growth.
- Testicular tumors occur mainly during or after puberty; thus, these children should be taught self-examination when they are older.

DIET

No restrictions

PATIENT EDUCATION

Discuss with parents about causes, available treatments, and possible effects on patient's reproductive potential; also increased risk for testicular cancer and need for regular self-examination.

PROGNOSIS

- Disorder is usually corrected with medical or surgical therapy; however, possible lifelong consequences.
- If testicle is absent or orchiectomy is required, may consider placement of testicular prosthesis.
- Early orchidopexy may decrease risk of testicular damage and risk of malignancy.

COMPLICATIONS

- Progressive failure of spermatogenesis, if left untreated; even with orchiopexy, the fertility rate is still reduced, especially with bilateral UDTs.
- Spermatogenesis is related to the duration of cryptorchidism and the location of the testis.
- Formerly bilaterally cryptorchid men have a greater decrease in fertility compared with unilateral cryptorchid male and the general male population.
- Abnormalities also have been identified in the contralateral descended testis, although less severe.

REFERENCES

1. Lee PA. Fertility after cryptorchidism: Epidemiology and other outcome studies. *Urology*. 2005;66: 427–31.
2. Cortes D. Cryptorchidism: Aspects of pathogenesis, histology and treatment. *Scan J Nephrol*. 1998;9:54.
3. Cryptorchidism: A prospective study of 7500 consecutive male births, 1984–8. John Radcliffe Hospital Cryptorchidism Study Group. *Arch Dis Child*. 1992;67(7):892–9.
4. Foresta C, Zuccarello D, Garolla A, et al. Role of hormones, genes, and environment in human cryptorchidism. *Endocr Rev*. 2008;29:560–80.
5. Tasian GE, Copp HL et al. Diagnostic performance of ultrasound in nonpalpable cryptorchidism: a systematic review and meta-analysis. *Pediatrics*. 2011;127:119–28.
6. Tasian GE, Yiee JH, Copp HL, et al. Imaging use and cryptorchidism: Determinants of practice patterns. *J Urol*. 2011;185:1882–7.
7. Kanemoto K, Hayashi Y, Kojima Y, et al. Accuracy of ultrasonography and magnetic resonance imaging in the diagnosis of non-palpable testis. *Int J Urol*. 2005;12:668–72.
8. Patil KK, et al. Laparoscopy for impalpable testis. *Br J Urol*. 2005;95:704–8.
9. Henna MR, Del Nero RG, Sampaio CZ, et al. Hormonal cryptorchidism therapy: Systematic review with metanalysis of randomized clinical trials. *Pediatr Surg Int*. 2004;20:357–9.
10. Henna MR, Del Nero RG, Sampaio CZ, et al. Hormonal cryptorchidism therapy: Systematic review with metanalysis of randomized clinical trials. *Pediatr Surg Int*. 2004;20:357–9.
11. Schwentner C, Oswald J, Kreczy A, et al. Neoadjuvant gonadotropin-releasing hormone therapy before surgery may improve the fertility index in undescended testes: A prospective randomized trial. *J Urol*. 2005;173:974–7.
12. Al-Mandil M, Khoury AE, El-Hout Y, et al. Potential complications with the prescrotal approach for the palpable undescended testis? A comparison of single prescrotal incision to the traditional inguinal approach. *J Urol*. 2008;180:686–9.

ADDITIONAL READING

Hutson JM, Balic A, Nation T, et al. Cryptorchidism. *Semin Pediatr Surg*. 2010;19:215–24.

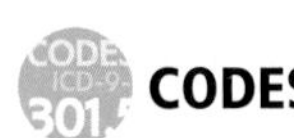

CODES

ICD9

752.51 Undescended testis

CLINICAL PEARLS

- If testicular descent does not occur by 6–9 months of age, it is unlikely to occur. Therefore, refer patients to a urologist if a testes has not descended by 6 months to 1 year of age.
- Children with bilateral nonpalpable UDTs require laboratory evaluation to determine if viable testicular tissue is present.
- Limiting the use of ultrasound may not change management of nonpalpable cryptorchidism.
- The risk of infertility is increased with bilateral UDTs.

CUBITAL TUNNEL SYNDROME

James Winger, MD

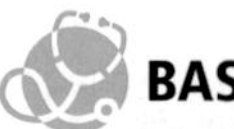

BASICS

DESCRIPTION

- Compression of the ulnar nerve on the medial aspect of the elbow where it enters the cubital tunnel. Often resulting in elbow pain and paresthesias of the forearm, wrist, fourth and fifth fingers.
- Synonym(s): Ulnar neuropathy

EPIDEMIOLOGY

- Predominant sex: Male > Female (3–8 times more common)
- Elbow is most common site of compression of ulnar nerve. Less common sites of entrapment include the arcade of Struthers, the medial intermuscular septum, the medial epicondyle, and the deep flexor pronator aponeurosis (1).
- Second most common nerve compression of upper extremity (behind median nerve compression in carpal tunnel) (2)

RISK FACTORS

- Patients who sleep or position themselves with their elbows bent, their arms overhead, or both
- Patients with occupations demanding prolonged time with elbows bent (8)[A]
- Athletes in throwing sports, racquet sports, weightlifting, and skiing
- Pre-existing polyneuropathy
- Patients with end-stage renal disease on hemodialysis
- Patients placed in dependent positioning (surgery, ICU)

GENERAL PREVENTION

- Avoid long periods with elbows bent or pressure on elbows.
- Sleep with elbows straight and avoid sleeping with arms overhead.
- Keep proper posture when working at a desk.

PATHOPHYSIOLOGY

- The ulnar nerve is the terminal branch of the medial cord of the brachial plexus and is composed of portions of the C8 and T1 nerve roots.
- The ulnar nerve becomes more superficial as it enters the ulnar sulcus ~3.5 cm proximal to the medial epicondyle. The nerve courses posterior to the medial epicondyle and medial to the olecranon, then enters the cubital tunnel (2).
- The cubital tunnel is a fibro-osseous canal. The roof is defined by the arcuate ligament of Osborne. The floor consists of the medial collateral ligament of the elbow, the joint capsule, and the olecranon.
- Elbow flexion increases distance from medial epicondyle to olecranon 5 mm for every 45°.
- Elbow flexion places stress on medial (ulnar) collateral ligament, overlying retinaculum, and ulnar nerve.
- Shape of cubital tunnel changes from circular to ovoid, losing 2.5-mm of height with elbow flexion.
- Loss of height of cubital tunnel with elbow flexion decreases tunnel volume by 55%, which doubles intraneural pressure on the ulnar nerve.
- Maximal pressure on the ulnar nerve in cubital tunnel is created by shoulder abduction, elbow flexion, and wrist extension.

ETIOLOGY

- Elbow flexion decreases volume of cubital tunnel, causing compression of ulnar nerve.
- Compression of ulnar nerve causes pain at medial aspect of elbow and symptoms at forearm and hand.
- Caused by constricting fascial bands, subluxation of ulnar nerve over medial epicondyle, cubitus valgus, bony spurs, hypertrophied synovium, tumors, ganglia, or direct compression of ulnar nerve as it crosses cubital tunnel

COMMONLY ASSOCIATED CONDITIONS

- Ulnar nerve subluxation
- Ulnar collateral ligament laxity
- Osteoarthritis of elbow joint

DIAGNOSIS

HISTORY

- Nocturnal elbow pain
- Medial elbow pain
- Paresthesias along medial forearm, wrist, and fourth and fifth digits
- Paresthesias may be intermittent at first and then become more constant.
- History of trauma over the area
- Repetitive elbow flexion and extension activities (such as in hammering)
- Overhead throwing athlete with repetitive elbow motion
- Chronic symptoms: Loss of grip strength and loss of fine motor skills in hand

PHYSICAL EXAM

- Inspect carrying angle of both elbows.
- Palpate medial epicondyle and cubital tunnel for areas of tenderness or ulnar nerve subluxation.
- Assess elbow range of motion.
- Positive Hoffman-Tinel test (percussion at ulnar nerve) (2)
- Pain on palpating over ulnar nerve
- Atrophy of intrinsic hand muscles
- Loss of sensation at fifth digit and medial side of fourth digit
- Wasting of hypothenar muscles and flexion contracture of fourth and fifth digits (ulnar claw)
- Wartenberg sign is clawing or abduction of the fifth digit with extension.
- Assess ability to cross second and third digits.
- Evaluate grip and pinch strength for weakness.
- Froment's sign describes hyperflexion of thumb interphalangeal joint when trying to maintain a sheet of paper between the thumb and first finger as the examiner pulls the paper away (3)
- Assess vibration and light touch sensation.
- Recently, the scratch-collapse test has been described. The patient faces the examiner with arms adducted, elbows flexed, hands outstretched, and wrists at neutral. The patient resists bilateral shoulder adduction and internal rotation as examiner applies these forces to the forearm. The examiner "scratches" or swipes fingertips over course of compressed ulnar nerve. The force is then reapplied to the forearm. A positive result occurs when the patient has a temporary loss of external rotation resistance tone.
- Sensitivity for the scratch collapse was 69% compared with 54% and 46% for Tinel test and elbow flexion-compression test, respectively. Tinel test, however, had the highest negative predictive value (98%) of all tests for cubital tunnel (4).

DIAGNOSTIC TESTS & INTERPRETATION

McGowan grades quantify the degree of physical exam findings and are specific for cubital tunnel syndrome:

- McGowan grade I: No wasting or weakness of intrinsic muscles, feeling of clumsiness in affected hand, mild paresthesias in ulnar nerve distribution
- McGowan grade II: Intermediate lesions with weak interossei and muscle wasting
- McGowan grade III: Severe lesions with paralysis of interossei and a marked weakness of the hand

Imaging

Initial approach

- X-rays may reveal osteophytes impinging on the area. Include anterior posterior (AP) lateral, and cubital tunnel views (1). Radiographs may also show signs of instability, deformity from old trauma, or presence of a supracondylar process (which can cause median nerve compression).
- Cubital tunnel view: Elbow is maximally flexed and x-ray beam is shot as an AP view of the distal humerus.

Follow-Up & Special Considerations

- Chest x-ray if patient has history of smoking and ulnar nerve symptoms (to exclude Pancoast tumor in apical lung)
- MRI shows inflammation and irritation of ulnar nerve.
- High-resolution ultrasound

Diagnostic Procedures/Surgery

- Corticosteroid injection into ulnar groove
- Electromyogram (EMG) is not essential when diagnosis is obvious on clinical exam. Use to determine the efficacy of conservative treatment or when the diagnosis is unclear.
- EMG is considered positive if motor conduction delay across the elbow is <50 m/s or difference between motor velocity across elbow and below the elbow is >10 m/s.
- Nerve conduction studies

Pathological Findings

Inflammation and swelling of ulnar nerve

DIFFERENTIAL DIAGNOSIS

- Cervical radiculopathy
- Thoracic outlet syndrome
- Carpal tunnel syndrome
- Medial epicondylosis
- Ulnar collateral ligament injury
- Pancoast syndrome
- Metabolic disorders creating peripheral neuropathies
- Multiple sclerosis and other myelopathies

TREATMENT

Mild cubital tunnel syndrome can often be treated without surgery. If provocative causes can be identified and avoided, there is tendency for recovery. In mild cases, nonoperative treatment is utilized for 3 months. Patients with constant symptoms and/or muscle atrophy typically require surgical intervention (1).

MEDICATION

First Line

NSAIDs and activity modification to limit elbow flexion

Second Line

Corticosteroid injection into the cubital tunnel

ADDITIONAL TREATMENT

General Measures

- Active rest
- Avoidance of aggravating activities
- Conservative treatment is initial approach if no motor weakness
- Instruct patient to avoid periods of prolonged elbow flexion.
- Instruct patient to avoid long periods of pressure and compression on ulnar nerve at elbow.
- Ice for symptom relief
- Splint or brace while sleeping to keep affected elbow in extension and take pressure off cubital tunnel (e.g., wrap towel around elbow and hold in place with tape; use a small size soft knee splint but wear it backward on the elbow, tie a scarf around waist then around wrist)
- Physical therapy (nerve mobilization techniques and forearm and wrist stretching)
- Workplace/ergonomic modifications (e.g., correct posture, avoid long periods with elbows bent)
- Otherwise activity as tolerated

Issues for Referral

Failure of 3–6 months of conservative treatment, loss of grip strength, flexion contracture of fourth and fifth digits, positive EMG for motor conduction delay

Additional Therapies

- Use 1 mL lidocaine and 20–40 mg methylprednisolone injected into ulnar groove, parallel to ulnar nerve (5).
- Hand therapy and custom-splint prescription

COMPLEMENTARY AND ALTERNATIVE MEDICINE

Vitamin B_6 (100 mg/d) not found to be effective in randomized trials

SURGERY/OTHER PROCEDURES

- Goal of surgery is to create more space for the ulnar nerve (6).
- Many surgical treatments exist for the treatment of cubital tunnel syndrome. In situ decompression, transposition of the ulnar nerve into the SC, IM, or submuscular plane, or medial epicondylectomy have all been shown to be effective in the treatment of this disease process. Comparative studies have shown some short-term advantages to one or another technique, but overall results between the treatments have essentially been equivocal. The choice of surgical treatment is based on multiple factors, and a single surgical approach cannot be applied to all clinical situations (2,9)[A].

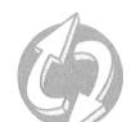

ONGOING CARE

FOLLOW-UP RECOMMENDATIONS

Patient Monitoring

- In severe cases, the nerve damage may be permanent and the patient may not recover.
- Patients with symptoms lasting longer than 6 months have a worse prognosis.

DIET

No restrictions

PATIENT EDUCATION

- Use correct posture; avoid putting pressure on your elbows, and place padding under your elbows.
- Inability to straighten fingers is often a sign of severe ulnar nerve damage. Patients with this level of irritation usually do not recover, even with surgery.

PROGNOSIS

- Both conservative and surgical methods result in 85–90% good-to-excellent results.
- For McGowan grade III: Anterior IM transposition has best outcome (7)[C].

COMPLICATIONS

Anterior transposition and simple decompression may have recurrent subluxation of the ulnar nerve.

REFERENCES

1. Hariri S, McAdams TR, et al. Nerve injuries about the elbow. *Clin Sports Med*. 2010;29:655–75.
2. Palmer BA, Hughes TB, et al. Cubital tunnel syndrome. *J Hand Surg Am*. 2010;35:153–63.
3. Anderton M, Webb M, et al. Cubital tunnel syndrome. *Br J Hosp Med (Lond)*. 2010;71: M167–9.
4. Cheng CJ, Mackinnon-Patterson B, Beck JL, et al. Scratch collapse test for evaluation of carpal and cubital tunnel syndrome. *J Hand Surg Am*. 2008;33:1518–24.
5. Rampen AJ, Wirtz PW, Tavy DL, et al. Ultrasound-guided steroid injection to treat mild ulnar neuropathy at the elbow. *Muscle Nerve*. 2011;44:128–30.
6. Mowlavi A, Andrews K, Lille S, et al. The management of cubital tunnel syndrome: A meta-analysis of clinical studies. *Plast Reconstr Surg*. 2000;106:327–34.
7. Mitsionis GI, Manoudis GN, Paschos NK, et al. Comparative study of surgical treatment of ulnar nerve compression at the elbow. *J Shoulder Elbow Surg*. 2010;19:513–9.
8. van Rijn RM, Huisstede BM, Koes BW, et al. Associations between work-related factors and specific disorders at the elbow: A systematic literature review. *Rheumatology (Oxford)*. 2009;48(5):528–36.
9. Shi Q, Macdermid JC, Santaguida PL, et al. Predictors of surgical outcomes following anterior transposition of ulnar nerve for cubital tunnel syndrome: A systematic review. *J Hand Surg Am*. 2011;36(12):1996–2001.

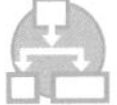

See Also (Topic, Algorithm, Electronic Media Element)

Epicondylitis

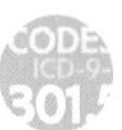

CODES

ICD9

354.2 Lesion of ulnar nerve

CLINICAL PEARLS

- Elbow flexion decreases depth of cubital tunnel, thus compressing the ulnar nerve.
- Sleeping with elbow bent and arm overhead can cause symptoms.
- Improper posture when working at a desk can cause symptoms.
- Conservative treatment consists of ice, rest, hand therapy, splint fabrication, and activity modifications for 3 months in selected patients.
- Both conservative and surgical methods result in good-to-excellent results 85–90% of the time.

CUSHING DISEASE AND CUSHING SYNDROME

Linda Paniagua, MD
Geetha Gopalakrishnan, MD

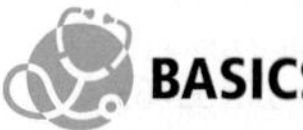

BASICS

DESCRIPTION

- Clinical abnormalities associated with chronic exposure to excessive amounts of cortisol (the major adrenocorticoid)
- Cushing disease is defined as glucocorticoid excess due to excessive adrenocorticotropic hormone (ACTH) secretion from a pituitary tumor. This is the most common cause of primary Cushing syndrome.
- Cushing syndrome is defined as excessive corticosteroid exposure from exogenous sources (medications) or endogenous sources (pituitary, adrenal, pulmonary, etc., or tumor).
- System(s) affected: Endocrine/Metabolic; Musculoskeletal; Skin/Exocrine; Cardiovascular; Neuropsychiatric

Pediatric Considerations

- Rare in infancy and childhood
- Most cases in children <8 years are a result of malignant adrenal tumors.

Pregnancy Considerations

Pregnancy may exacerbate disease.

EPIDEMIOLOGY

Incidence

Uncommon: 0.7–2.4 per million per year

Prevalence

2–5% prevalence reported in difficult-to-control diabetics with obesity and hypertension

RISK FACTORS

- Female:Male ratio is 3:1.
- Most often occurs between age 25 and 40
- Pituitary tumor
- Adrenal mass
- Neuroendocrine tumor (e.g., bronchial carcinoid)
- Prolonged use of corticosteroids

Genetics

- Multiple endocrine neoplasia type I
- Carney complex (an inherited multiple neoplasia syndrome)
- McCune-Albright syndrome (mutation of GNAS1 gene)
- Familial isolated pituitary adenomas (mutations in the aryl hydrocarbon receptor interacting protein gene)

GENERAL PREVENTION

Avoid corticosteroid exposure when possible.

PATHOPHYSIOLOGY

- Disease: Pituitary tumor causing excess ACTH (corticotropin)
- Syndrome: Excessive corticosteroid exposure from exogenous sources (medications) or endogenous sources (pituitary, adrenal, pulmonary, etc., or tumor)

ETIOLOGY

- Exogenous glucocorticoids or ACTH
- Endogenous ACTH-dependent hypercortisolism: 80–85%:
  - ACTH-secreting pituitary tumor: 75%
  - Ectopic ACTH production (e.g., small-cell carcinoma of lung, bronchial carcinoid): 20%
- Endogenous ACTH-independent hypercortisolism: 15–20%:
  - Adrenal adenoma
  - Adrenal carcinoma
  - Macronodular or micronodular hyperplasia
- Pediatric/adolescent (1):
  - Adrenal hyperplasia secondary to McCune-Albright: Mean age 1.2 years
  - Adrenocortical tumors: Mean age 4.5 years
  - Ectopic ACTH syndrome: Mean age 10.1 years
  - Primary pigmented nodular adrenocortical disease: Mean age 13.0 years
  - Cushing disease: Mean age 14.1 years
- Pregnancy (*Lindsay*):
  - Pituitary-dependent Cushing syndrome: 33%
  - Adrenal causes: 40–50%
  - ACTH-independent adrenal hyperplasia: 3%

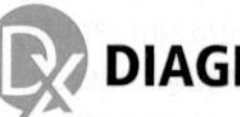

DIAGNOSIS

HISTORY

- Weight gain: 95% (2)[B]
- Decreased libido: 90%
- Menstrual irregularity: 80%
- Hirsutism: 75%
- Depression/emotional lability: 50–80%
- Easy bruising: 65%
- Proximal muscle weakness: 60%
- Diabetes or glucose intolerance: 60%

PHYSICAL EXAM

- Obesity (usually central): 95%
- Facial plethora: 90%
- Moon face (facial adiposity): 90%
- Thin skin: 85%
- Hypertension: 75%
- Skeletal growth retardation in children (epiphyseal plates remain open): 70–80%
- Purple striae on the skin
- Increased adipose tissue in neck and trunk
- Acne
- RECENT GUIDELINES (3)[C]:
  - The Endocrine Society published new guidelines in 2008. They currently recommend against widespread testing for Cushing syndrome except in patients with:
    - Adrenal incidentaloma
    - Multiple progressive features suggestive of Cushing syndrome
    - Unusual features for their age, such as osteoporosis and hypertension
    - Abnormal growth (children)

DIAGNOSTIC TESTS & INTERPRETATION

Lab

Initial lab tests

- Late-night salivary cortisol, 24-hour urinary-free cortisol or low-dose dexamethasone suppression testing:
  - Elevated late-night salivary cortisol: Obtain at least 2 measurements. Cortisol secretion is highest in the morning and lowest between 11 p.m. and midnight. The nadir of serum cortisol is maintained in pseudo-Cushing (e.g., obesity, alcoholism, depression), but not in Cushing syndrome. Sensitivity and specificity are >90–95% (4,5)[B].
  - 24-hour urinary-free cortisol level: Obtain ≥2 samples to rule out intermittent hypercortisolism if results are normal and suspicion is high. Also measure 24-hour urinary creatinine excretion to verify adequacy of collection. Results may be falsely low if glomerular filtration rate <30 mL/min. Overall sensitivity and specificity varies , 90–97% and 85–96%, respectively (4)[B]. Avoid drinking excessive amounts of water due to risk of false-positive values. False-positive values can be seen in the presence of pseudo-Cushing states.
  - Low-dose dexamethasone suppression testing: Dexamethasone 1 mg is given between 11 p.m. and midnight, and fasting plasma cortisol is measured between 8 and 9 a.m. the following morning. A serum cortisol level below 1.89 μg/dL excludes Cushing syndrome, but specificity is limited. The presence of pseudo-Cushing states (depression, obesity, etc.), hepatic or renal disease, or any drug that induces cytochrome P-450 enzymes may cause a false result.
- If the initial results are positive or if clinical suspicion is high, perform 1 or 2 more studies to confirm the diagnosis. Other tests to consider include:
  - Awake midnight plasma cortisol: Obtain samples on 3 consecutive nights. A late-evening serum cortisol >7.5 μg/dL has a sensitivity of 96% and a specificity of 100% (6)[B]. Persistently elevated serum cortisol implies Cushing syndrome; nadir of serum cortisol is maintained in obese patients, but not in Cushings.
  - Corticotropin-releasing hormone (CRH) after dexamethasone: Used to distinguish Cushing syndrome from pseudo-Cushing syndrome. Dexamethasone 0.5 mg is given q6h for 48 hours starting at noon. CRH (1 μg/kg) is given 2 hours after the last dose of dexamethasone. Plasma cortisol is >1.4 μg/dL 15 minutes after CRH in patients with Cushing syndrome but not in those with pseudo-Cushing (7)[B].

ALERT

- Antiepileptic drugs, progesterone, oral contraceptives (withdraw estrogen-containing drugs 6 wk before testing), rifampin, and spironolactone may cause a false-positive dexamethasone suppression test.
- Pregnancy (3)[C]: Urine-free cortisol is recommended instead of dexamethasone testing in the initial evaluation of pregnant women. Only urine-free cortisol in the second or third trimester >3 times the upper limit of normal can be taken to indicate Cushing's syndrome.
- Epilepsy (3)[C]: It is recommended to use measurements of nonsuppressed cortisol in blood, saliva, or urine instead of the dexamethasone testing. There is no data to guide the length of time needed after withdrawal of such medication to allow dexamethasone metabolism to return to normal, and such a medication change may not be clinically possible.

Follow-Up & Special Considerations

- Once the diagnosis of Cushing syndrome is confirmed, localization is the next step:

- ACTH level: Elevated in ACTH-dependent Cushing syndrome (e.g., pituitary and ectopic tumor) and low in ACTH-independent Cushing syndrome (e.g., adrenal tumors and exogenous glucocorticoids)
- High-dose dexamethasone suppression testing: This test is used to distinguish between an ACTH-secreting pituitary tumor and an ectopic ACTH-secreting tumor. 0.5 mg dexamethasone is given q6h for 8 doses, with serum cortisol measured at 2 and 6 hours after last dose (sensitivity 79%, specificity 74%).

- The diagnosis of Cushing syndrome is complicated by the nonspecificity and high prevalence of clinical symptoms in patients without the disorder and involves a variety of biochemical tests of variable sensitivity and specificity. Efficient screening and confirmatory procedures are, therefore, essential before considering therapy.

Imaging

Initial approach

- Pituitary MRI scan if pituitary tumor suspected
- Abdominal CT scan if adrenal disease is suspected
- Chest CT scan if ectopic ACTH secretion is suspected (8)[C]
- Octreotide scintigraphy to look for occult ACTH-secreting tumor
- DXA to evaluate for osteoporosis

Diagnostic Procedures/Surgery

Diagnostic procedure depends on circumstances and clinical judgment. Inferior petrosal sinus sampling with CRH stimulation can be considered if ACTH-dependent tumor is suspected but not localized (8)[C].

Pathological Findings

- Thyroid function suppressed
- Hypertension
- Dyslipidemia
- Polycystic ovarian syndrome/hyperandrogenism
- Oligomenorrhea/hypogonadism
- Myopathy/cutaneous wasting
- Neuropsychiatric problems
- Nodular adrenal disease
- Hypercoagulable state
- Osteoporosis
- Nephrolithiasis
- Growth hormone reduced

DIFFERENTIAL DIAGNOSIS

- Obesity
- Diabetes mellitus
- Hypertension
- Metabolic syndrome X
- Polycystic ovarian disease
- Hypercortisolism secondary to alcoholism (pseudo-Cushing)
- Severe major depression
- Physical stress (e.g., severe bacterial infection)

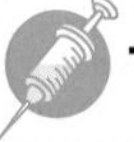

TREATMENT

MEDICATION

- Drugs are not usually effective as the primary long-term treatment; primarily used in preparation for surgery or as adjunctive treatment after surgery, pituitary radiotherapy, or both.
- Metyrapone, ketoconazole, and mitotane all lower cortisol by directly inhibiting synthesis and secretion in the adrenal gland. As initial treatment, remission rates up to 85% (8,9)[C].

SURGERY/OTHER PROCEDURES

- Tumor-specific surgery:
  - Transsphenoidal surgery for Cushing disease (remission rate 60–80%)
  - Resection of the ACTH-producing ectopic tumor
  - Adrenal surgery:
    - For unilateral adrenal adenomas, laparoscopic surgery is the treatment of choice.
    - For nodular hyperplasia, bilateral adrenalectomy is usually recommended.
    - For patients with Cushing disease, bilateral laparoscopic adrenalectomy can be considered if the patient has persistent disease even after pituitary surgery and radiotherapy.
- Pituitary radiotherapy can be used to treat persistent hypercortisolism after transsphenoidal surgery.
- Note: Treatment decision should be weighed carefully in patients with mild or intermittent hypercortisolism because the benefits of surgery have not been established definitively in this population.

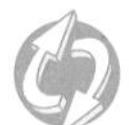

ONGOING CARE

PATIENT EDUCATION

- Comprehensive teaching to help patient cope with lifelong treatment may be needed:
  - Diet and monitoring weight daily
  - Early treatment of infections
  - Emotional lability prevention
- Refer to National Adrenal Disease Foundation: NADF 505 Northern Blvd. Great Neck, NY 11021; (516) 407-4992

PROGNOSIS

- Guardedly favorable prognosis with surgery for Cushing disease. Generally chronic course with cyclic exacerbations and rare remissions.
- Better prognosis following surgery for benign adrenal tumors. Long-term recurrence rate is 20%.
- Poor with small-cell carcinoma of the lung producing ectopic hormone; neuroendocrine tumors (bronchial carcinoid) have much better prognosis (6)[C].

COMPLICATIONS

- Osteoporosis
- Increased susceptibility to infections
- Metastases of malignant tumors
- Increased cardiovascular risk even after treatment
- Lifelong glucocorticoid dependence following treatment with bilateral adrenalectomy
- Nelson syndrome (pituitary tumor) after treatment with bilateral adrenalectomy (can occur in 8–38% of patients)

REFERENCES

1. Storr HL, Chan LF, Grossman AB, et al. Pediatric Cushing's syndrome: epidemiology, investigation and therapeutic advances. *Trends Endocrinol Met.* 2007;18:167–74.
2. Newell-Price J, Bertagna X, Grossman AB, et al. Cushing's syndrome. *Lancet.* 2006;367:1605–17.
3. Nieman LK, Biller MK, Findling JW, et al. The diagnosis of Cushing's syndrome: An endocrine society clinical practice guideline. *J Clin endocrinol Metab.* 2008:1526–40.
4. Putignano P, et al. Midnight salivary cortisol versus urinary free and midnight serum cortisol as screening tests for Cushing's syndrome. *J Clin Endocrinol Metabol.* 2003;88(9):4153–7.
5. Yaneva M, Mosnier-Pudar H, Dugué MA, et al. Midnight salivary cortisol for the initial diagnosis of Cushing's syndrome of various causes. *J Clin Endocrinol Metab.* 2004;89:3345–51.
6. Isidori AM, et al. The ectopic adrenocorticotropin syndrome: Clinical features, diagnosis, management and long term follow up. *J Clin Endocrinol Metabol.* 2006;91(2):371–7.
7. Yanovski JA, Cutler GB, Chrousos GP, et al. Corticotropin-releasing hormone stimulation following low-dose dexamethasone administration. A new test to distinguish Cushing's syndrome from pseudo-Cushing's states. *JAMA.* 1993;269: 2232–8.
8. Findling JF, et al. Cushing's syndrome: Important issues in diagnosis and management. *J Clin Endocrinol Metabol.* 2006;10:3746–53.
9. Nieman LK, Ilias I. Evaluation and treatment of Cushing's syndrome. *Am J Med.* 2005;118: 1340–6.

ADDITIONAL READING

- Davies JH, Storr HL, Davies K, et al. Final adult height and body mass index after cure of paediatric Cushing's disease. *Clin Endocrinol (Oxf).* 2005; 62:466–72.
- Lindsay JR, Nieman LK. Adrenal disorders in pregnancy. *Endocrinol Metab Clin North Am.* 2006;35:1–20.

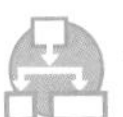

See Also (Topic, Algorithm, Electronic Media Element)

Algorithm: Cushing Syndrome

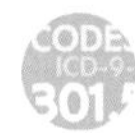

CODES

ICD9

255.0 Cushing's syndrome

CLINICAL PEARLS

- Cushing disease is due to excessive ACTH secretion from a pituitary tumor, resulting in corticosteroid excess.
- Cushing syndrome is due to excessive corticosteroid exposure from exogenous sources (medications) or endogenous sources (pituitary, adrenal, pulmonary, etc., or tumor).
- Depression, alcoholism, medications, eating disorders, and other conditions can cause mild clinical and laboratory findings similar to those in Cushing syndrome (termed "pseudo-Cushing syndrome").

CUTANEOUS DRUG REACTIONS

Adam J. Tinklepaugh, MD
Alison Ehrlich, MD

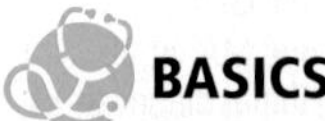

BASICS

DESCRIPTION

- An adverse cutaneous reaction in response to administration of a drug. Cutaneous eruptions are the most common negative reactions to medications.
- Reactions are divided into immunologic and nonimmunologic reaction types.
- Morbilliform and urticarial eruptions are most common, but multiple morphologic types may occur.
- System(s) affected: Skin/Mucosa/Exocrine; Hematologic/Lymphatic/Immunologic

EPIDEMIOLOGY

- Predominant age: Geriatric, but all ages affected
- Predominant sex: Female > Male

Incidence

- In the US, seen in 2–3% of inpatients, most commonly secondary to antibiotic use.
- 2–28% of all hospital admissions are related to adverse drug eruptions. Most are mild and resolve after removal of the agent, but severe and potentially fatal reactions may affect 1 in 1,000.

RISK FACTORS

Concurrent infections, immunocompromise, metabolic disorders, multiple medications, and HLA haplotype

Genetics

Genetic predisposition may play a role, as certain HLA antigens have been associated with specific cutaneous drug eruptions:

- HLA-B*5801 and HLA-B*1502 have been linked to allopurinol-induced and carbamazepine-induced Stevens-Johnson syndrome (SJS), respectively.
- HLA class I antigens such as HLA-B12 and HLA-B22 have been linked to toxic epidermal necrolysis (TEN) and fixed drug eruptions, respectively.

GENERAL PREVENTION

- Always query patients about prior adverse drug events.
- Be aware of any potential drug cross-reactions.

PATHOPHYSIOLOGY

- Most drug reactions are nonimmunologic. Mechanisms include drug accumulation, idiosyncratic reactions, direct release of mast-cell mediators, Jarisch-Herxheimer phenomenon, overdosage, phototoxic dermatitis, intolerance, or adverse effects.
- Reactions may be immunologically mediated, IgE-dependent, immune complex–dependent (type 3 hypersensitivity), cytotoxic, or most commonly delayed-type (type 4 hypersensitivity).

ETIOLOGY

- More than 700 drugs are known to cause a dermatologic reaction. Temporal relationship and type of reaction may elucidate the causative agent:
  - Acneiform: OCPs, corticosteroids, iodinated compounds, hydantoins, lithium
  - Erythema multiforme/SJS/TEN: Sulfonamides, penicillins, barbiturates, hydantoins, NSAIDs, cephalosporins, tetracycline, terbinafine
  - Fixed drug eruptions: OCPs, barbiturates, salicylates, tetracycline, sulfonamides
  - Lichenoid: Sildenafil, gold, antimalarials, thiazides, captopril
  - Photosensitivity: Doxycycline, thiazides, sulfonylureas, quinolones
  - Vasculitis: Thiazides, gold, sulfonamides, NSAIDs, tetracycline
  - Drug rash with eosinophilia and systemic symptoms (DRESS) syndrome: Anticonvulsants, sulfonamides, dapsone, minocycline, allopurinol
  - Acute generalized exanthematous pustulosis (AGEP): Penicillins, cephalosporins, macrolides, calcium channel blockers, antimalarials, carbamazepine, acetaminophen, terbinafine, nystatin, vancomycin
  - Sweet syndrome (acute febrile neutrophilic dermatosis): Sulfa drugs, G-CSF, GM-CSF
  - Serum sicknesslike reaction: Penicillins, propranolol, bupropion, minocycline
  - Morbilliform/urticarial/exfoliative erythroderma: Numerous medications, including penicillins, cephalosporins, sulfonamides, tetracyclines, ibuprofen, naproxen, acetylsalicylic acid, radiocontrast media

DIAGNOSIS

HISTORY

- New medications within past month: All oral, parenteral, and topical agents; all OTC drugs; vitamins, homeopathic, and herbal remedies
- Inquire about previous adverse reactions to medications.
- Consider other etiologies, including bacterial infections and viral exanthems.

PHYSICAL EXAM

May present as a number of different eruption types, including but not limited to:

- Acneiform eruptions:
  - Folliculocentric, monomorphous pustules typically involving the face, chest, and back
  - Distinguished from acne vulgaris by absence of comedones grossly and microscopically
  - Often become secondarily infected
- EM:
  - Most commonly associated with herpes simplex virus; also due to result of preceding drug exposure (1)[A]:
    - Possible viral etiologies: Orf, vaccinia, varicella zoster, adenovirus, Epstein–Barr, cytomegalovirus, hepatitis, coxsackievirus, parvovirus, and HIV
    - Possible bacterial etiologies: *Mycoplasma*, *Chlamydia*, *Salmonella*, and *Mycobacterium*
  - 3 zone target lesions and raised atypical 2-zone targets (1)[A]
  - Lesions predominantly on acral surfaces with localized erythema and occasional mucosal involvement
  - <10% epidermal detachment
- SJS/TEN:
  - Classification and distinction between SJS and TEN are determined by affected body surface area (BSA):
    - SJS: <10% BSA
    - SJS-TEN overlap: 10–30% BSA
    - TEN: >30% BSA
  - Strong association with preceding drug exposure; less commonly associated with underlying disease
  - Typical onset 1–3 weeks after starting offending agent
  - Flat atypical 2-zone target lesions and macules (1)[A]
  - Lesions predominantly generalized and truncal with diffuse erythema and mucosal involvement
  - May develop confluent areas of necrosis, significant risk for secondary infections and sepsis
  - SJS: 5–15% mortality (2)[C]
  - TEN: 30% mortality
- Fixed drug eruptions:
  - Single or multiple, round, sharply defined, violaceous plaques with gray center that leave postinflammatory hyperpigmentation
  - Appear shortly after drug exposure and recur in identical location after re-exposure
  - Lesions may occur on any body site.
  - Onset usually 48 hours after ingestion of drug (3)[B]
  - Some patients have a refractory period during which the drug fails to activate lesions.
- Lichenoid eruptions:
  - Violaceous, pruritic papules on extensor surfaces
  - Reticular pattern, buccal mucosa
- Photosensitivity reaction:
  - Phototoxic reactions within 24 hours of light exposure with exaggerated sunburn reaction
  - Photoallergic reactions; less common, more pruritic than painful, caused by UVA exposure
- Vasculitis:
  - Petechiae or purpura concentrated on lower extremities and dependent areas
  - Fever, myalgias, arthritis, and abdominal pain may also be present.
- DRESS syndrome:
  - Classic triad of fever, exanthem, and internal organ involvement. May also present with pharyngitis and lymphadenopathy.
  - Internal organ involvement: 80% hepatic, 40% renal, 33% pulmonary (4)[C]
  - Atypical lymphocytosis with prominent eosinophilia and elevated liver function tests
  - Onset 2–8 weeks after drug exposure; may develop 3 months or later into therapy
- AGEP:
  - Fever with multiple small, sterile, nonfollicular pustules on erythematous background with desquamation after 7–10 days
  - Appears similar to pustular psoriasis, but AGEP has more marked leukocytosis with neutrophilia and eosinophilia
  - Short time to onset (24 hours to 2 weeks)
- Sweet syndrome:
  - Fever, neutrophilia, tender reddish-blue or violet papules, plaques, or nodules, with or without pustules or vesicles that spontaneously resolve
  - May have oral ulcers or ocular manifestations such as conjunctivitis
  - Classically seen in young women after a mild respiratory illness, but 7–56% associated with malignancy
  - Serum sicknesslike reaction:
    - Fever, nonspecific cutaneous eruption, arthralgias
    - Onset 7–14 days
    - May have bullous lesions

- Morbilliform eruptions (exanthems):
  - Most frequent cutaneous reaction (28–95%)
  - May be indistinguishable from viral exanthem
  - Erythematous macules and papules; confluent, symmetric, and pruritic
  - Most common on trunk and in dependent areas
  - Onset 7–21 days after initiation of drug
- Urticaria:
  - Pruritic erythematous wheals distributed anywhere on the body, including mucous membranes
  - May progress to angioedema, appearing as nonpitting edema without erythema or margins
  - May be annular in pediatric patient
  - Individual lesions fade within 24 hours, but new lesions may develop.
- Exfoliative erythroderma:
  - Generalized erythema with exfoliation and/or eczema over 90% of body surface
  - Difficult to distinguish between drug etiology, inflammatory etiology, cutaneous lymphoma etiology
  - Lymphadenopathy, hepatosplenomegaly, leukocytosis, eosinophilia, or anemia may be present.
  - Potentially life threatening if associated with systemic symptoms

DIAGNOSTIC TESTS & INTERPRETATION

Lab

Initial lab tests

- Routine laboratory tests generally are nonspecific and not helpful.
- CBC with differential; significant eosinophilia may be related to more severe disease in allergic reactions. Significant eosinophilia in DRESS syndrome; consider LFTs to check hepatic function.
- Special tests dependent on suspected mechanism:
  - Type I: Skin testing, RAST, serum tryptase
  - Type II: Direct or indirect Coombs test
  - Type III: ESR, C-reactive protein, ANA, antihistone antibody, tissue biopsy for immunofluorescence studies
  - Type IV: Patch testing, lymphocyte proliferation assay (investigational)
- Cultures may be useful to exclude an infectious etiology.

Imaging

For vasculitic eruptions, chest radiography and urinalysis

Diagnostic Procedures/Surgery

- Withdrawal of suspected offending agent and observation for resolution; Develop a timeline for start date and stop date of all medications to determine possible suspect agents of all medications preceding cutaneous lesions.
- Punch biopsy sometimes helpful for fixed drug eruptions, vasculitis, EM

Pathological Findings

Nonspecific histologic findings are superficial infiltrates composed variably of lymphocytes, neutrophils, and eosinophils (5)[A].

DIFFERENTIAL DIAGNOSIS

- Viral exanthem: Presence of fever, lymphocytosis, and other systemic findings may help differentiate
- Primary dermatosis: Correlation of drug withdrawal to rash resolution may clarify diagnosis; skin biopsy may be helpful.

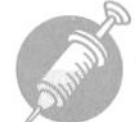

TREATMENT

MEDICATION

- Withdrawal of offending drug. Depending on the type of eruption, symptomatic treatment may be useful, but most require no additional therapy except cessation of offending drug.
- Anaphylaxis or widespread urticaria: Epinephrine 1:1,000, 0.01 mL/kg (0.3 mL maximum) SC
- Acute urticaria (<6 weeks) and chronic urticaria (>6 weeks):
  - First-generation antihistamines: Diphendydramine 10–25 mg q.h.s., hydroxyzine 10–25 mg t.i.d., doxepin 10–50 mg q.h.s.
  - Second-generation antihistamines: Cetirizine 10 mg daily, loratadine 10 mg daily, fexofenadine 180 mg daily, levocetirizine 5 mg daily
  - H2 antagonists: Cimetidine 400 mg b.i.d., ranitidine 150 mg b.i.d.
- Anaphylaxis, severe urticaria: Prednisone PO 1 mg/kg in tapering doses
- Erythema multiforme:
  - Treatment is generally supportive with management of suspected underlying infection.
  - HSV-associated: Prophylaxis with acyclovir 10 mg/kg/d, valacyclovir 500–1,000 mg/d, or famciclovir 250 mg b.i.d.
  - "Magic mouthwash" b.i.d. or t.i.d. is helpful for mucosal erosion. Consider ophthalmology consult for severe ocular involvement.
- SJS/TEN: Treatment is supportive. Consider consultation with a dermatologist. Systemic corticosteroids use remains controversial. Consider IVIG 2–3 g/kg/d for severe disease (6)[A].

ADDITIONAL TREATMENT

General Measures

- Monitor for signs of impending cardiovascular collapse:
  - Urticaria or bullous lesions, angioedema, and generalized erythroderma are all potentially more serious.
  - Anaphylactic reactions, SJS/TEN, and extensive bullous reactions: Consider inpatient treatment.
- Do not rechallenge with drugs causing urticaria, bullae, angioedema, anaphylaxis, or erythema multiforme.

ONGOING CARE

FOLLOW-UP RECOMMENDATIONS

Patient Monitoring

- For urticarial, bullous, or erythema multiforme spectrum lesions, close follow-up is needed.
- Patients with anaphylaxis or angioedema should be given EpiPen for secondary prevention and a Med Alert bracelet.
- Label the patient's medical record with the suspected agent and type of reaction.

PROGNOSIS

- Eruptions generally begin fading within days after removing offending agent.
- Anaphylaxis, angioedema, and bullous reactions are potentially fatal.

COMPLICATIONS

Anaphylaxis, bone marrow suppression, hepatitis (dapsone, hydantoin), cross-reaction to chemically similar agents

REFERENCES

1. Hughey LC. Approach to the hospitalized patient with targetoid lesions. *Dermatol Ther*. 2011;24(2): 196–206.
2. Hazin R, Ibrahimi OA, Hazin MI, et al. Stevens-Johnson syndrome: pathogenesis, diagnosis, and management. *Ann Med*. 2008;40: 129–38.
3. Brahimi N, Routier E, Raison-Peyron N, et al. A three-year-analysis of fixed drug eruptions in hospital settings in France. *Eur J Dermatol*. 2010; 20:461–4.
4. Chen YC, Chiu HC, Chu CY, et al. Drug reaction with eosinophilia and systemic symptoms: A retrospective study of 60 cases. *Arch Dermatol*. 2010.
5. Gerson D, et al. Cutaneous drug eruptions: A 5-year experience. *J Am Acad Dermatol*. 2008;59(6): 995–9.
6. Worswick S, Cotliar J. Stevens–Johnson syndrome and toxic epidermal necrolysis: A review of treatment options. *Dermatol Ther*. 2011;24: 207–18.

ADDITIONAL READING

- Hung SI, Chung WH, Liou LB, et al. Version: HLA-B*5801 allele as a genetic marker for severe cutaneous adverse reactions caused by allopurinol. *Proc Natl Acad Sci USA*. 2005;102:4134–9.
- Knowles SR, Shear NH. Recognition and management of severe cutaneous drug reactions. *Dermatol Clin*. 2007;25:245–53.

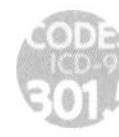

CODES

ICD9

- 693.0 Dermatitis due to drugs and medicines taken internally
- 708.0 Allergic urticaria
- 709.8 Other specified disorders of skin

CLINICAL PEARLS

- Virtually any drug can cause a rash; antibiotics are the most common culprits causing cutaneous drug reactions.
- Focus on drug history with new suspicious skin eruptions.
- Morbilliform rashes are the most frequent.
- Usually self-limited after withdrawal of offending agent
- Symptoms such as tongue swelling/angioedema, skin necrosis, blisters, high fever, dyspnea, and mucous membrane erosions signify more severe drug reactions.

CUTANEOUS SQUAMOUS CELL CARCINOMA

Herbert P. Goodheart, MD

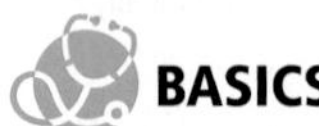

BASICS

- Squamous cell carcinoma (SCC) is a malignant epithelial tumor arising from keratinocytes of the epidermis. Cutaneous (nonmucous membrane) SCC is the second most common form of skin cancer.
- Lesions most frequently occur on sun-exposed sites of elderly, fair-skinned individuals. The majority of SCCs arise in solar keratoses *(actinic keratoses)*. Such actinically derived SCCs that develop from solar keratoses are slow-growing, minimally invasive, unaggressive; and the prognosis is usually excellent because distant metastases that arise from these lesions are extremely rare.
- An SCC may also appear de novo without a preceding solar keratosis. SCCs may also develop from causes other than sun exposure. For example, from an old burn scar or from sites previously exposed to ionizing radiation. An SCC may also emerge from pre-existing human papilloma virus infection *(verrucous carcinoma)*.
- When metastases from SCC do occur, they often appear on the ears or on the vermilion border of the lips or from tumors >2 cm in diameter. Other risks for metastasis include lesions that arise on mucous membranes, from sites that received ionizing radiation, on the skin of organ transplant recipients, in chronic inflammatory lesions (e.g., discoid lupus erythematosus (1)[C]), and in long-standing scars or cutaneous ulcers (e.g., venous stasis ulcers) or other nonhealing wounds.
- System(s) affected: Skin/Exocrine
- Synonym(s): Squamous cell carcinoma of the skin; epidermoid carcinoma; prickle cell carcinoma

EPIDEMIOLOGY

- Predominant age: Elderly population
- Predominant sex: Males > Females
- In the US, there are 200,000 new cases each year

Incidence

- The escalating incidence in the US is due to an increase in sun exposure in the general population, aging of the population, earlier and more frequent diagnosis of SCC, and the increase of immunosuppressed patients.
- The incidence is highest in Australia and in the Sun Belt of the US.

ALERT

- Bowen disease (SCC in situ) and frank SCC are 2 of the few skin cancers that should be considered in blacks. Such non–sun-related SCCs tend to arise on the extremities de novo, in an old scar, or in a lesion of discoid lupus erythematosus.

RISK FACTORS

- Older age
- Male sex: However, incidence is increasing in females due to lifestyle changes (e.g., suntan parlors, shorter dresses, etc.)
- Chronic sun exposure: SCC is noted more frequently in those with a greater degree of outdoor activity (e.g., farmers, sailors, gardeners).
- Patients with multiple solar keratoses
- Personal or family history of skin cancer
- Northern European descent
- Fair complexion, fair hair, light eyes
- Poor tanning ability, with tendency to burn
- Organ transplant recipients, chronic immunosuppression
- Exposure to chemical carcinogens (e.g., arsenic, tar) or ionizing radiation
- Therapeutic UV and ionizing radiation exposure
- Defects in cell-mediated immunity related to lymphoproliferative disorders (CLL, lymphoma)
- Human papillomavirus (HPV) infection (certain subtypes)
- Chronic scarring and inflammatory conditions
- Specific genodermatoses (e.g., xeroderma pigmentosum)

Genetics

- Persons of Irish or Scottish ancestry have the highest prevalence of SCC.
- SCC is rare in people of African and Asian descent, although it is the most common form of skin cancer in these populations.
- Patients with oculocutaneous albinism are at greater risk.

GENERAL PREVENTION

- Sun-avoidance measures: Sunscreens, hats, sunglasses with UV protection; tinted windshields and side windows in cars; sun-protective garments

ETIOLOGY

- Exact mechanisms are not established; however, ultraviolet radiation damages skin cell nucleic acids (DNA), resulting in a mutant clone of the gene p53. This leads to an uncontrolled growth of skin cells. Ultraviolet radiation also suppresses the immune response preventing recovery from this damage.
- Epidemiologic and experimental evidence suggests the following as causative agents: Sunlight (solar radiation), radiation exposure, tanning parlors, PUVA phototherapy exposure, inorganic arsenic exposure, coal tar, and other oil derivatives.
- Immunosuppression by medications or disease such as HIV/AIDS

COMMONLY ASSOCIATED CONDITIONS

- Solar keratosis (some investigators consider a solar keratosis to be an early SCC, although relatively few ultimately are found to develop into an SCC)
- Actinic cheilitis (solar keratoses of the mucous membranes of the lips) and leukoplakia of lip
- Keratoacanthoma
- Cutaneous horn
- Xeroderma pigmentosum, albinism, and vitiligo
- Immunosuppression
- Chronic skin ulcers, pre-existing scars, and thermal burns

DIAGNOSIS

PHYSICAL EXAM

Lesions occur chiefly on chronically sun-exposed areas:

- The face and the backs of the forearms and hands
- Bald areas of the scalp and top of ears in men
- The sun-exposed "V" of the neck, as well as the posterior neck below the occipital hairline
- In elderly females, lesions tend to occur on the legs and other sun-exposed locations.
- In blacks, equal frequency in sun-exposed and unexposed areas
- Clinical appearance:
  - Generally slow-growing, firm, hyperkeratotic papules, nodules, or plaques
  - Most SCCs are asymptomatic, although bleeding, pain, and tenderness may be noted.
  - Lesions may have a smooth, verrucous, or papillomatous surface.
  - Varying degrees of ulceration, erosion, crust, or scale
  - Color is often red to brown, tan, or pearly (indistinguishable from basal cell carcinoma)
- Clinical variants of SCC:
  - Bowen disease (SCC in situ): Solitary lesion that resembles a scaly psoriatic plaque.
  - Invasive SCC: Often presents as a raised, firm papule, nodule, or plaque. Individual lesions may be smooth, verrucous, or papillomatous with varying degrees of ulceration, erosion, crust, or scale.
  - Cutaneous horn: SCC with an overlying cutaneous horn. A cutaneous horn represents a fingernail platelike keratinization produced by the SCC. Bowen disease may also produce a cutaneous horn on its surface.
  - Erythroplasia of Queyrat refers to Bowen disease of the glans penis, which manifests as one or more velvety red plaques.
  - Subungual SCC (2)[C]: Such lesions typically mimic warts.
  - Marjolin ulcer: An SCC evolving from a new area of ulceration or elevation at site of a scar or ulcer
  - HPV-associated SCC: Virally induced SCC most commonly manifests as a new or enlarging warty growth on the penis, vulva, perianal area, or periungual region.
  - Verrucous carcinoma: Subtype of SCC that is extremely well differentiated, can be locally destructive but rarely metastasizes. Lesions are "cauliflowerlike" verrucous nodules or plaques.
  - Basaloid SCC: Less common than typical SCC, is seen more often in men aged 40–70 years.

ALERT

Subungual SCC (2)[C]: Such lesions typically mimic warts.

DIAGNOSTIC TESTS & INTERPRETATION

Imaging

Patients with lymphadenopathy should be evaluated for metastases either with CT scanning, MRI, ultrasound, or PET.

Diagnostic Procedures/Surgery

- Surgical biopsy to ensure diagnosis: Shave biopsy, punch biopsy, excisional biopsy, incisional biopsy
- Sentinel lymph node biopsy rarely used to identify micrometastases in patients with high-risk SCC and clinically negative nodes. Whether the early detection of lymph node metastasis leads to enhanced survival in SCC is unknown.

Pathological Findings

- Noninvasive SCC is characterized by an intraepidermal proliferation of atypical keratinocytes. Hyperkeratosis, acanthosis, and confluent parakeratosis are seen within the epidermis. Cellular atypia, including pleomorphism, hyperchromatic nuclei and mitoses, are prominent. Atypical keratinocytes may be found in the basal layer and often extend deeply down the hair follicles, but they do not invade the dermis.

- In the in situ type of SCC (Bowen disease), atypia involves the full thickness of the epidermis. The basement membrane remains intact.
- An invasive SCC penetrates through the basement membrane into the dermis. It has various levels of anaplasia and may manifest relatively few to multiple mitoses and display varying degrees of differentiation, such as keratinization.
- Poorly differentiated tumors are clinically more aggressive. SCCs proliferate first by local invasion. Metastases, when they do occur, spread via local lymph ducts to local lymph nodes.

DIFFERENTIAL DIAGNOSIS

- Solar keratosis: Early SCC lesions may be clinically difficult, if not impossible, to distinguish from a precursor solar keratosis.
- Basal cell carcinoma may be indistinguishable from an SCC, particularly if the lesion is ulcerated.
- Keratoacanthoma: This lesion also may be clinically and histopathologically impossible to differentiate from an SCC; considered by some to be a low-grade variant of an SCC.
- Verruca vulgaris: The appearance of common warts is often similar to that of SCC lesions.
- Seborrheic keratosis
- Pyoderma gangrenosum
- Venous stasis ulcer
- Chemical or thermal burn

ALERT

Melanoma: An amelanotic melanoma and ulcerated melanoma may also be impossible to distinguish from an SCC.

TREATMENT

MEDICATION

First Line

- Total excision: The preferred method of therapy for SCCs, permitting histologic diagnosis of the tumor margins
- Electrocautery (electrodesiccation) and curettage (ED&C)
  - Best for small lesions (generally <1 cm) on flat surfaces (e.g., forehead, cheek) and SCC in situ (Bowen disease). ED&C may be used to treat superficially invasive SCCs without high-risk characteristics, but it is not appropriate for certain high-risk anatomic locations.
- Cryosurgery with LN_2 in selected lesions, such as SCC in situ
- Micrographic (Mohs) surgery is a microscopically controlled method of removing skin cancers that allows for controlled excision and maximum preservation of normal tissue. It has the highest cure rate (94–99%) of all surgical treatments. Mohs surgery may be indicated for the following:
  - Large, recurrent or invasive SCCs (e.g., to bone or cartilage)
  - Lesions with a poorly delineated clinical border
  - Locations where preservation of normal tissue is extremely important (e.g., tip of the nose, eyelids, ala nasi, ears, lips, and glans penis)
- Radiation therapy is a primary treatment option that is generally restricted to older patients who are physically debilitated or are unable to undergo, or refuse to undergo, excisional surgery.

Second Line

- Immunotherapy with topical imiquimod (Aldara) (3)[A] 5% cream, approved for the treatment of solar keratoses, genital warts, and superficial basal cell carcinomas, is now being used "off-label" for SCC in situ (Bowen disease).
- Topical chemotherapy: Topical formulations of 5-fluorouracil (5-FU)
- Intralesional 5-FU has also been used to successfully treat keratoacanthomas.
- Photodynamic therapy (PDT): Treatment with PDT involves the application of a photosensitizer (given topically or systemically) followed by exposure to a light source. PDT is used primarily to treat large numbers of solar keratoses and is not recommended for treatment of invasive SCCs.
- In patients with multiple or recurrent SCCs, chemoprevention with systemic retinoids (4) such as acitretin may be effective for reducing the number of new SCCs; shown to be beneficial in treating existing SCCs or at reducing the risk of recurrence after treatment.

ADDITIONAL TREATMENT

Various chemotherapeutic agents have been used to treat metastatic SCC (e.g., oral 5-FU, used alone or in combination with SC interferon).

SURGERY/OTHER PROCEDURES

- Complete lymphadenectomy of the draining nodal basin for high-risk tumors
- Metastatic disease requires aggressive management by a multidisciplinary team, involving plastic, ENT/maxillofacial, and general surgeons, or a surgical oncologist.

ONGOING CARE

FOLLOW-UP RECOMMENDATIONS

Patient Monitoring

Skin exam every month for 3 months, 6 months after treatment, and then yearly

PATIENT EDUCATION

Skin self-exam, encourage sun-avoidance techniques, protective clothing, sunscreens, etc. Artificial tanning devices should be avoided.

PROGNOSIS

- For low risk SCCs, there is a 90–95% cure rate with appropriate treatment.
- Overall, head and neck lesions have better prognosis (5); however, lip and ear lesions metastasize more frequently when compared to other sites.
- The ability to produce scale (*keratinization)* indicates a tendency for a lesion to be more differentiated and less likely to metastasize.
- Softer, nonkeratinizing lesions are not as well differentiated and thus are more likely to spread.
- Lesions ≥2 cm more prone to recur
- SCCs that arise in areas of non–sun-exposed skin or those that originate de novo on areas of sun-exposed skin have a greater tendency to metastasize.
- An SCC arising on a mucous membrane, one arising from a chronic ulcer, or one arising in an immunocompromised patient should be regarded as potentially metastatic.
- SCCs that are deeply invasive in SC fat or deeper, or those that have perineural involvement, are more likely to metastasize.
- When SCC does metastasize, it usually occurs within several years from the time of diagnosis and involves draining lymph nodes.
- Once nodal metastasis of cutaneous SCC has occurred, the overall 5-year survival rate has historically been in the range of 25–35%.

COMPLICATIONS

- Untreated, an SCC becomes indurated, with a tendency to ooze, ulcerate, or bleed.
- Local recurrence
- Metastatic disease

REFERENCES

1. Harper JG, Piltcher MF, Szlam S, et al. Squamous cell carcinoma in an African American with discoid lupus erythematosus: A case report and review of the literature: *South Med J*. 2010;103(30):256–9.
2. Riddel C, Rashid R, Thomas V. Ungual and perungual human papillomavirus-associated squamous cell carcinoma: A review. *J Am Acad Dermatol*. 2011;64:1147–53.
3. Patel GK, Goodwin R. Imiquimod 5% cream monotherapy for cutaneous *squamous cell carcinoma in situ* (Bowen's disease): A randomized, double-blind, placebo-controlled trial. *J Am Acad Dermatol*. 2006;54(1):25–32.
4. Harwood CA, Leedham-Green M, Leigh IM. Low-dose retinoids in the prevention of cutaneous squamous cell carcinomas in organ transplant recipients: A 16-year retrospective study. *Arch Dermatol*. 2005;141:456–64.
5. Clayman GL, Lee JJ, Holsinger FC. Mortality risk from squamous cell skin cancer. *J Clin Oncol*. 2005;23:759–65.

ADDITIONAL READING

Jennings L, Schmults CD. Management of high-risk cutaneous squamous cell carcinoma. *J Clin Aesthetic Dermatol*. 2010;3(4):39–48.

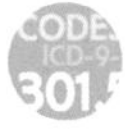

CODES

ICD9

- 173.02 Squamous cell carcinoma of skin of lip
- 173.82 Squamous cell carcinoma of other specified sites of skin
- 173.92 Squamous cell carcinoma of skin, site unspecified

CLINICAL PEARLS

- SCCs that develop from solar keratoses are generally unaggressive.
- Unlike most basal cell carcinomas, SCCs of the skin are associated with a risk of metastasis, especially those arising on mucous membranes, chronic ulcers, or in immunocompromised patients.
- A subungual SCC can easily be mistaken for a wart.

CUTANEOUS T-CELL LYMPHOMA, MYCOSIS FUNGOIDES

Sandra Cuellar, PharmD, BCOP
Kelly Valla, PharmD
Amber Seba, MD

BASICS

Cutaneous T-cell lymphomas are a rare group of mature T-cell lymphomas presenting primarily in the skin. These diseases involve overlap of the disciplines of dermatology, medical oncology, and radiation oncology. Other than allogeneic stem cell transplant, there are no curative therapies for this disease (1,2).

DESCRIPTION

- A heterogeneous group of relatively uncommon extranodal non-Hodgkin's lymphomas
- This section focuses on mycosis fungoides (MF), the most common type of cutaneous lymphoma. For other subtypes, please consult the reference section (3).

EPIDEMIOLOGY

- Median age at diagnosis is 55–60; however, it can occur in children and young adults (4).
- Male:Female = 2:1 (4)
- African American incidence greater compared to Whites (4)

Incidence

- 0.6 cases per 100,000 per year
- ~4% of all non-Hodgkin's lymphoma cases

RISK FACTORS

No compelling evidence that mycosis fungoides is caused by viral infection or chemical exposure

Genetics

- Clonal T-cell receptor gene rearrangements are detected in most cases (5).
- No recurrent, mycosis fungoides-specific chromosomal translocations have been identified (4).
- Loss at chromosome 10q and abnormalities in the tumor suppressor genes p15, p16, and p53 are common (1,4).

PATHOPHYSIOLOGY

- Malignancy of $CD4^{+}$ helper T cells
- Malignant cells have a high affinity to the epidermis
- Malignant T cells are also activated T cells ($CD45RO^{+}$) and produce cytokines, such as IL-4 and IL-5, which can lead to eosinophilia and atopylike symptoms

ETIOLOGY

Unknown

DIAGNOSIS

- Diagnostic algorithm for MF is a point-based system. Points are scored for clinical, histopathologic, molecular biological, and immunopathological categories. A diagnosis of MF is made when a total of 4 points or more are determined (6)
- Clinical criteria: Patient has persistent and/or progressive patches and plaques plus lesions in a non–sun-exposed location, size/shape variation of lesions, poikiloderma (6)
- Histopathologic criteria: Superficial lymphoid infiltrate present plus epidermotropism without spongiosis, lymphoid atypia (6)
- Molecular biological criteria: Clonal TCR gene rearrangement is present (6)
- Immunopathologic criteria: <50% of T cells express CD2, CD3, CD5; <10% of T cells express CD 7; there is discordance of the epidermal and dermal cells with regard to expression of CD2, CD3, CD5, or CD7 (6)

PHYSICAL EXAM

- Examination of the entire skin, with assessment of percent of involved body surface area (%BSA), and lesions found, is critical.
- Pink scaly patches and plaques, typically in sun-protected areas such as the buttocks, thighs, and breasts
- Cutaneous tumors and ulcerations
- Exfoliative erythroderma
- Palmoplantar keratoderma (thickened scaly skin on palms and soles)
- Lymphadenopathy can be present in later stages
- Hepatosplenomegaly can be present at late stages

DIAGNOSTIC TESTS & INTERPRETATION

Lab

- CBC with differential and platelets and Sézary screen
- Polymerase chain reaction (PCR) of peripheral blood to detect clonal rearrangement of the T-cell receptor
- Flow cytometric studies to establish the presence of Sézary cells. Markers for CD3,4,7,8,26 need to be analyzed
- If the CD4:CD8 ratio of >10, a circulating clonal T-cell population is identified, a positive Sézary cell count of over 1,000 cells/mm^3 is found, this is consistent with Sézary syndrome (see below)
- Comprehensive metabolic profile
- LDH

Imaging

- CT of the neck, chest, abdomen or CT-PET for T2 disease or greater (see staging system described below)
- Chest x-ray should be used in limited disease without any palpable lymphadenopathy

Diagnostic Procedures/Surgery

- Skin biopsy: Diagnostic procedure of choice
- Lymph node biopsy if there is clinical adenopathy or advanced disease
- Bone marrow biopsy for unexplained hematologic abnormality: Not normally done

Pathological Findings

- Skin biopsy shows superficial bandlike infiltrate, epidermotropism of lymphocytes, Pautrier microabscesses, and dermal infiltrates of atypical cells in tumors (6)
- Cells are usually CD3+, CD4+, CD45RO+, CD8–, CD 30–
- Loss of T-cell antigens such as CD2, CD3, CD5, and CD7 is often seen
- Sézary syndrome is diagnosed when Sézary cells are found in the peripheral circulation. Sézary cells are defined as atypical lymphocytes with cerebriform nuclei. Generalized erythroderma and lymphadenopathy usually accompanies this blood finding to complete the syndrome (4):
  - Sézary syndrome (leukemic phase of cutaneous T-cell lymphoma) is defined by the following: If the CD4:CD8 ratio >10, a circulating clonal T-cell population is identified, a positive Sézary cell count >1,000 cells/mm^3, a CD4/CD26- ≥30% of all of the lymphocytes in the presence of a clonal T-cell population (4)
- Large cell transformation of cutaneous T-cell lymphoma is a rare and lethal event. If 25% of large cells are found on a biopsy taken from an MF lesion, this represents a transformation from an indolent lymphoma, MF, to a very aggressive form of cutaneous T-cell lymphoma. It is refractory to most chemotherapies, and overall survival is limited to months (1,2,3).
- The treatment of the disease and prognosis (see "Prognosis" section below) is determined by the stage (3):
  - Staging is done based on physical exam and pathology. Bone marrow biopsy is not needed for staging of the disease. The TNMB staging system ([T]umor, [N]ode, [M]Visceral, and [B]lood involvement with Sézary cells):
    - T1: Patches or plaques involving <10% of total BSA
    - T2: Patches, papules, and/or plaques involving ≥10% of total BSA
    - T3: 1 or more cutaneous tumors (≥1 cm in diameter)
    - T4: Generalized erythroderma (>80% of total BSA)
    - N0: Lymph nodes clinically uninvolved
    - N1: Lymph nodes clinically enlarged but not histologically involved
    - N2: Lymph nodes clinically normal but histologically involved
    - N3: Lymph nodes clinically enlarged and histologically involved
    - M0: No visceral organ involvement
    - M1: Visceral involvement with pathological confirmation

- B0: No circulating atypical cells (<1,000 Sézary cells (CD 4+/7-)/μL)
- B1: Circulating atypical cells present (>1,000 Sézary cells (CD 4+/7-)/μL)
- Stage groups:
  - IA: T1N0M0
  - IB: T2N0M0
  - IIA: T1-2N1M0
  - IIB: T3N0-1M0
  - IIIA: T4N0M0
  - IIIB: T4N1M0
  - IVA: T1-4N2-3M0
  - IVB: T1-4N0-3M1

DIFFERENTIAL DIAGNOSIS

- Patches and plaques seen in MF resemble lesions of:
  - Eczema
  - Parapsoriasis
  - Atopic dermatitis
  - Photodermatitis
  - Drug eruptions
  - Psoriasis
  - Contact dermatitis
- Cutaneous tumors:
  - Similar to other cutaneous lymphomas
- Erythroderma, though rare, can present like:
  - Atopic dermatitis
  - Contact dermatitis
  - Drug eruptions
  - Erythrodermic psoriasis

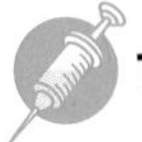

TREATMENT

MEDICATION

Treatment must be individualized, and ranges from skin-directed therapies to systemic cytotoxic or systemic biologic therapy. No universally accepted standard approach exists to treat this disease. The stage of disease dictates the aggressiveness and type of therapy (1,2):

- T1 and T2 disease:
  - Topical potent corticosteroids
  - Topical mechlorethamine (nitrogen mustard)
  - Topical bischloronitrosourea (aka: BCNU, carmustine) (alkylating agent)
  - Topical bexarotene (retinoid)
  - Topical tacrolimus (immunosuppressant)
  - Topical imiquimod (immune modulator)
  - Phototherapy: Psoralen ultraviolet A light (PUVA) or narrow-band ultraviolet B (UVB)
  - Oral bexarotene (retinoid)
  - Oral methotrexate
  - Radiation therapy (Total skin electron beam therapy [TSEBT]) (See "Issues for Referral" section below.)
- T3 disease:
  - Oral bexarotene (retinoid)
  - Interferon α-2b (immune modulator)
  - Denileukin diftitox
  - Chemotherapy: If the disease progresses on the above therapies, gemcitabine or pegylated doxorubicin is usually used first-line. If the disease continues to progress, low-dose methotrexate, bortezomib, cyclophosphamide, and fludarabine are used as second-line therapy. Stem cell transplantation can also be used in certain cases; see below.
- T4 disease and Sézary syndrome:
  - Oral bexarotene (retinoid)
  - Interferon α-2b (immune modulator)
  - Denileukin diftitox (immune modulator, combination of IL-2 and diphtheria toxin)
  - Phototherapy
  - Vorinostat (oral histone deacetylase inhibitor)
  - Romidepsin (injectable histone deacetylase inhibitor)
  - Alemtuzumab (humanized monoclonal antibody targeting CD52)
  - Pralatrexate (antifolate analogue)
  - Lenalidomide (immune modulator)
  - Extracorporeal photopheresis
  - Radiotherapy
  - Additional chemotherapy agents (used upon disease progression despite above therapies):
    - First line: Gemcitabine or pegylated doxorubicin
    - Second line: Low-dose methotrexate, bortezomib, cyclophosphamide, and fludarabine
  - Stem cell transplantation (reserved for extensive and/or refractory disease)

ADDITIONAL TREATMENT

General Measures

- Most patients are managed on an outpatient basis
- Treatment should be individualized for each patient, based on their extent of disease and side effects of possible therapies (1,2).
- Skin lesions commonly become infected, and treatment with antibiotic may be necessary.

Issues for Referral

- Dermatology manages early disease.
- Hematology-oncology is involved for later-stage diseases.
- Radiation oncology can be referred for limited disease or to treat extensive or painful skin lesions when refractory to chemotherapy.

Additional Therapies

Localized or total skin electron-beam therapy can be used in most stages of disease, either as monotherapy or in combination with other agents.

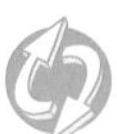

ONGOING CARE

FOLLOW-UP RECOMMENDATIONS

Patient Monitoring

Must be individualized

PATIENT EDUCATION

Patient information can be found at:

- American Academy of Dermatology Web site: http://www.aad.org
- Cutaneous Lymphoma Foundation Web site: http://www.clfoundation.org

PROGNOSIS

- MF is a chronic disease, though early-stage disease is curable.
- Survival by stage:
  - Stage 1A: Survival similar to age-/sex-matched individuals without disease
  - Stage IB and IIA: 11 years
  - Stage IIB: 3.2 years
  - Stage III: 4.6 years
  - Stage IVA or B: 13 months

COMPLICATIONS

- Immunosuppression from the disease and treatments can lead to infections.
- Skin lesions commonly become infected and can lead to sepsis.
- Long-term use of topical corticosteroids may lead to skin atrophy.
- High-potency topical corticosteroids may be systemically absorbed leading to numerous adverse effects.

REFERENCES

1. Horwitz SM, Olsen EA, Duvic M, et al. Review of the treatment of mycosis fungoides and Sézary syndrome: A stage-based approach. *J Natl Compr Canc Netw*. 2008;6:436–42.
2. Prince HM, Whittaker S, Hoppe RT, et al. How I treat mycosis fungoides and Sézary syndrome. *Blood*. 2009;114:4337–53.
3. Willemze R, Jaffe ES, Burg G, et al. WHO-EORTC classification for cutaneous lymphomas. *Blood*. 2005;105:3768–85.
4. Hwang ST, Janik JE, Jaffe ES, et al. Mycosis fungoides and Sézary syndrome. *Lancet*. 2008;371:945–57.
5. Girardi M, Heald PW, Wilson LD. The pathogenesis of mycosis fungoides. *N Engl J Med*. 2004;350:1978–88.
6. Pimpinelli N, Olsen EA, Santucci M, et al. Defining early mycosis fungoides. *J Am Acad Dermatol*. 2005;53(6):1053–63.

ADDITIONAL READING

- Akilov O, Geskin L Therapeutic advances in cutaneous t cell lymphoma. *Skin Therapy Lett* 2011;16(2)1–5.
- Galper S, Smith BD, Wilson LD. Diagnosis and management of mycosis fungoides. *Oncology*. 2010;24(6):491–501.

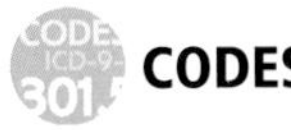

CODES

ICD9

- 202.10 Mycosis fungoides, unspecified site, extranodal and solid organ sites
- 202.80 Other malignant lymphomas, unspecified site, extranodal and solid organ sites

CLINICAL PEARLS

- Mycosis fungoides: various treatments are available, and choice depends on staging of disease
- Most treatment options affect immune function; therefore, patients are at higher risk for infection.
- Bexarotene is a vitamin A analog (retinoid) used primarily for the treatment of cutaneous T-cell lymphoma; therefore, some pertinent clinical pearls are as follows:
  - Dietary vitamin A should be limited to <15,000 IU/d.
  - This medication should be taken after a high-fat meal.
  - This medication is contraindicated in combination with gemfibrozil.

CYST, SEBACEOUS

K. John Burhan, MD
M. Keenan Mak, MD

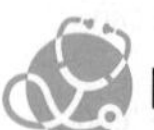

BASICS

Synonym(s): Epidermoid cysts; Epidermal cysts; Epidermal inclusion cysts; Keratin cyst

DESCRIPTION

A benign encapsulated subepidermal lesion that is filled with keratin

EPIDEMIOLOGY

- Most common cutaneous cyst
- Male:Female ratio is 2:1.
- Most common in third to fourth decade of life

RISK FACTORS

Genetics

- Gardner syndrome (autosomal dominant)
- Gorlin syndrome (autosomal dominant)
- Pachyonychia congenita type II (autosomal dominant)

PATHOPHYSIOLOGY

Pilosebaceous follicles that are either obstructed or ruptured resulting in the accumulation of keratin in the subepidermis or dermis layer of the skin

ETIOLOGY

- Spontaneous
- Trauma
- Congenital

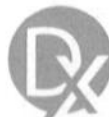

DIAGNOSIS

HISTORY

- Mass slowly growing over time
- Recent trauma
- "Cheeselike" material from cyst

PHYSICAL EXAM

- Firm to fluctuant, mobile, dome-shaped, flesh-to-yellow colored
- Commonly located on face, neck, upper back, and chest; if due to trauma, on buttocks, palms, or plantar side of feet
- Varying in size (few millimeters to centimeters)
- Cyst with or without comedo
- Signs of rupture or inflammation (erythema, tenderness, swelling)

DIAGNOSTIC TESTS & INTERPRETATION

Diagnosis is by clinical examination

Diagnostic Procedures/Surgery

Histologic examination of excised mass is debatable (1)[C].

Pathological Findings

- Stratified, squamous lining
- Granular layer
- Eosinophilic keratinaceous debris

DIFFERENTIAL DIAGNOSIS

- Trichilemmal cyst (Pilar cyst)
- Lipoma
- Steatocystoma

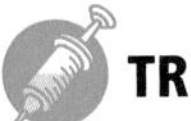

TREATMENT

Sebaceous cysts are generally benign and do not require excision.

SURGERY/OTHER PROCEDURES

- Indications:
  - Cosmetic reasons
  - Inflamed cyst (must wait until inflammation subsides) (2)[C]
  - Cyst impairing patient's functioning
- For 1–2-cm uncomplicated cysts, a punch biopsy is superior to a elliptical incision to allow for its expulsion by lateral pressure (3)[B].
- No published data on effectiveness of minimal excision technique
- Must ensure that entire cyst wall has been removed to prevent recurrence

ONGOING CARE

FOLLOW-UP RECOMMENDATIONS

- Uncomplicated sebaceous cysts do not require follow-up.
- Any recurrence of cysts should be excised using an elliptical incision.
- Solid or atypical masses noted in excision should be followed up with histologic analysis.

PROGNOSIS

Overall recurrence rate after excision is <3% (less with elliptical incision vs. punch biopsy).

COMPLICATIONS

- Rupture of sebaceous cyst resulting in foreign-body giant cell reaction
- Secondary polymicrobial infection
- Rare: Transition into malignancy (squamous cell carcinoma, basal cell carcinoma)

REFERENCES

1. Zuber TJ, et al. Minimal excision technique for epidermoid (sebaceous) cysts. *Am Fam Physician*. 2002;65:1409–12, 1417–8, 1420.
2. Moore RB, Fagan EB, Hulkower S, et al. Clinical inquiries. What's the best treatment for sebaceous cysts? *J Fam Pract*. 2007;56:315–6.
3. Lee HE, Yang CH, Chen CH, et al. Comparison of the surgical outcomes of punch incision and elliptical excision in treating epidermal inclusion cysts: A prospective, randomized study. *Dermatol Surg*. 2006;32:520–5.

CODES

ICD9

706.2 Sebaceous cyst

CLINICAL PEARLS

- Sebaceous cysts are generally benign and do not require excision.
- For 1–2-cm uncomplicated cysts, a punch biopsy is superior to a elliptical incision to allow for its expulsion by lateral pressure (3)[B].
- Must ensure that entire cyst wall has been removed to prevent recurrence
- Solid or atypical masses noted in excision should be followed up with histologic analysis.

CYSTIC FIBROSIS

Michael S. Stalvey, MD
Christian Müller, PhD
Terence R. Flotte, MD

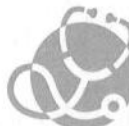

BASICS

DESCRIPTION
- Cystic fibrosis (CF) is an autosomal-recessive genetic condition that most prominently affects the lungs and pancreas.
- The intestinal tract, liver, endocrine system, reproductive organs, and skin can all be involved.
- Initially a pediatric disease, CF has become a chronic pediatric and adult medical condition as improvements in medical care have led to a dramatic increase in long-term survival.

EPIDEMIOLOGY
CF is the most common lethal inherited disease in Caucasians and is found in every racial group.

Incidence
- Prevalence varies according to country and ethnic background.
- Number of infants born with CF in relation to the total number of live births in the US:
  - 1 in 3,000 Caucasians
  - 1 in 4,000–10,000 Latin Americans
  - 1 in 15,000–20,000 African Americans
  - Uncommon in Africa and Asia, with reported frequency in Japan of 1 in 350,000 (1)[A]

Prevalence
- As per the 2009 CF Foundation Patient Registry, there are 30,000 patients with CF living in the US (2)[A].
- ~1,000 new diagnoses are made annually (2)[A].

RISK FACTORS
CF is a single-gene disorder. The severity of the phenotype can be affected by the specific CFTR mutation (most predictive of pancreatic disease), other modifier genes (CFTM1 for meconium ileus), and environmental factors, such as environmental tobacco smoke exposure, gastroesophageal reflux, and severe respiratory virus infections.

Genetics
CFTR gene (cystic fibrosis transmembrane conductance regulator). More than 1,500 mutations exist that can cause phenotypic CF, all of which are recessively inherited. Most common is loss of the phenylalanine residue at 508th position (deltaF508), which accounts for ~2/3 of affected alleles in the CF population in the US (1)[A].

GENERAL PREVENTION
- ACOG recommends genetic analysis for all North American couples planning a pregnancy, with appropriate counseling to identified carriers. Genetic analysis of siblings of known CF patients is highly recommended.
- Newborn screening for CF is offered throughout the US. Identification of an affected newborn in a family has resulted in a reduction in the incidence of new cases, allowing genetic counseling prior to the birth of subsequent siblings.
- Prevention or amelioration of complications of CF can be accomplished through early diagnosis (by newborn screening or otherwise) followed by referral to an accredited regional CF center.

PATHOPHYSIOLOGY
- Abnormal CFTR function leads to abnormally viscous secretions that alter organ function.
- The lungs; obstruction, infection, and inflammation negatively affect lung growth, structure, and function:
  - Decreased mucociliary clearance
  - Infection is accompanied by an intense neutrophilic response.
  - Degradation of supporting tissues causes bronchiectasis and eventual failure.

COMMONLY ASSOCIATED CONDITIONS
- The GI tract:
  - Pancreatic exocrine insufficiency (85–90%) (1)[A]:
    - Malabsorption of fat, protein, and fat-soluble vitamins (A, D, E, and K)
  - Hepatobiliary disease (10.8%) (2)[A]:
    - Focal biliary cirrhosis
    - Cholelithiasis
  - Meconium ileus at birth (10–15%) (1)[A]
  - Distal intestinal obstruction syndrome (DIOS): Intestinal blockage that typically occurs in older children and adults
- Endocrine:
  - CF-related diabetes (CFRD):
    - May present as steady decline in weight, lung function, or increased frequency of exacerbation
    - Leading comorbid complication (21.5%) (2)[A]
    - Result of progressive insulin deficiency
    - Early screening and treatment may improve reduced survival found in CFRD (3)[A].
  - Bone mineral disease (10.2%) (2)[A]
  - Hypogonadism:
    - Frequent low testosterone levels in men
    - Menstrual irregularities are common.
- Reproductive organs:
  - Congenital absence of the vas deferens: Obstructive azoospermia in 98% of males
- Depression in adults (21.6%) (2)[A]

Pregnancy Considerations
- Originally considered too dangerous for women with CF, successful pregnancies occur more frequently (2)[A].
- Pulmonary disease may worsen during pregnancy.

DIAGNOSIS
- General (any age):
  - Family history
  - Chronic/recurrent respiratory symptoms, including airway obstruction and infections
  - Persistent infiltrates on chest x-rays
  - Hypochloremic metabolic acidosis
- Neonatal:
  - Meconium ileus
  - Prolonged jaundice
- Infancy:
  - Failure to thrive
  - Chronic diarrhea
  - Anasarca/hypoproteinemia
  - Pseudotumor cerebri (vitamin A deficiency)
  - Hemolytic anemia (vitamin E deficiency)
- Childhood:
  - Recurrent endobronchial infection
  - Bronchiectasis
  - Recurrent sinusitis
  - Steatorrhea
  - Rectal prolapse
  - Distal intestinal obstruction syndrome (DIOS)
  - Poor growth
  - Allergic bronchopulmonary aspergillosis
- Adolescence and adulthood:
  - Recurrent endobronchial infection
  - Bronchiectasis
  - Allergic bronchopulmonary aspergillosis
  - Chronic sinusitis
  - Hemoptysis
  - Pancreatitis
  - Portal hypertension
  - Azoospermia
  - Delayed puberty

HISTORY
Suspected in any child with failure to thrive, steatorrhea, and recurrent respiratory problems

PHYSICAL EXAM
- Respiratory:
  - Rhonchi and/or crackles
  - Hyperresonance on percussion
  - Nasal polyps
- GI: Hepatosplenomegaly when cirrhosis present
- Other: Digital clubbing, growth retardation, and pubertal delay

DIAGNOSTIC TESTS & INTERPRETATION
Lab
Initial lab tests
- Newborn screening (49.8% of new cases) (2)[A]
- Sweat test (gold standard):
  - Sweat chloride:
    - >60 mmol/L is positive for CF.
    - <40 mmol/L is normal.
- CFTR mutation analysis:
  - Limited panel testing: Allele-specific PCR identifies >90% of mutations; finite chance of false negative. Full-sequence testing more costly and time-consuming. Greater sensitivity than PCR in patients of non-European descent.

Follow-Up & Special Considerations
- Sputum culture (common CF organisms)
- Pulmonary function tests (PFTs)
- 72-hour fecal fat
- Stool elastase
- Oral glucose tolerance test (OGTT)

Imaging
Initial approach
Chest x-ray:
- Hyperinflation early in disease
- Bronchial thickening and plugging
- Nodular densities, patchy atelectasis, and confluent infiltrates
- Bronchiectasis

Follow-Up & Special Considerations
- Head CT: Abnormal sinus CT findings are nearly universal in CF and may include mucosal thickening, intraluminal sinus polyps, and sinus effusions. Many children with CF never develop aerated frontal sinuses.

- Chest CT (not routine): Useful when unusual findings noted on CXR

Diagnostic Procedures/Surgery

- Flexible bronchoscopy
- Bronchoalveolar lavage

DIFFERENTIAL DIAGNOSIS

- Pulmonary:
  - Difficult-to-manage asthma
  - Chronic bronchitis
  - Recurrent pneumonia
  - Chronic/recurrent sinusitis
- GI:
  - Celiac disease
  - Protein-losing enteropathy
  - Pancreatitis of unknown etiology
  - Shwachman-Diamond syndrome

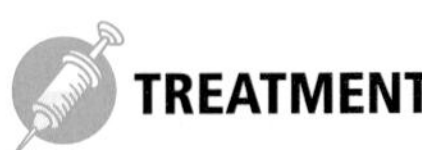

TREATMENT

MEDICATION

- Pulmonary:
  - Antibiotics, oral:
    - *S. aureus*: Bactrim or cephalexin
    - *P. aeruginosa*: Fluoroquinolones
    - Azithromycin (anti-inflammatory properties)
  - Antibiotics, inhaled:
    - TOBI (tobramycin 300 mg/dose via nebulizer)
    - Colistin (more commonly used in Europe)
    - Cayston (aerosolized aztreonam) 75 mg t.i.d. following bronchodilator use for 28 days
  - Antibiotics, IV:
    - *S. aureus*: Zosyn or nafcillin
    - MRSA: Vancomycin or linezolid
    - *P. aeruginosa*: Zosyn or ceftazidime plus aminoglycoside (tobramycin)
    - *B. cepacia*: $\geq$3 drugs based on synergy studies
  - Inhalation therapy:
    - β-agonist in conjunction with chest physiotherapy
    - Recombinant human DNAse
    - Hypertonic saline
  - Anti-inflammatory agents:
    - Oral steroids (useful in setting of ABPA)
    - Ibuprofen (high dose)
  - CFTR modulation therapy:
    - VX770: A small molecule, investigational CFTR potentiator. Although non-FDA approved, it is available to all CF patients with the G551D-*CFTR* mutation on at least 1 allele and critical need (FEV1 <40% predicted or patient is on lung transplant list) (4)[B].
- GI:
  - Pancreatic enzymes:
    - Use in pancreatic-insufficient patients.
  - Vitamin supplementation:
    - Fat-soluble vitamins (A, D, E, and K)
  - Liver disease (cholestasis):
    - Ursodeoxycholic acid

ADDITIONAL TREATMENT

General Measures

- Yearly influenza vaccination for all CF patients >6 months of age (2)[A]
- Avoidance of smoke

Issues for Referral

All patients should be followed in a CF center (accredited sites are listed at www.cff.org).

Additional Therapies

- Airway clearance techniques (5)[A]
- Routine chest physiotherapy with postural drainage is critical in prevention of pulmonary exacerbations:
  - VEST (airway clearance system)
  - Flutter valve or acapella
- Endocrine:
  - CFRD: Insulin is the primary therapy, and dietary restrictions should be avoided (3)[A].
  - CF-related bone disease: Consider bisphosphonate therapy.

SURGERY/OTHER PROCEDURES

- Lung transplantation reserved for patients with limited life expectancy (FEV_1 <30% predicted):
  - 212 patients with CF underwent lung transplantation during 2009 (2)[A].
  - 5-year posttransplant survival is up to 62% (6)[A].
- Liver transplantation is reserved for progressive liver failure and/or portal hypertension with GI bleeding.

IN-PATIENT CONSIDERATIONS

Initial Stabilization

Nasal cannula oxygen when the patient is hypoxic (SaO_2 <90%)

Admission Criteria

- Pulmonary exacerbation (most common reason for admission):
  - Increased cough, sputum production, and decreased pulmonary function
  - Change in lung examination (rales, retractions, tachypnea)
  - New abnormalities on CXR
  - Decreased energy level, appetite, and weight loss
  - Fever, leukocytosis, elevation of acute-phase reactants
- Bowel obstruction (due to distal intestinal obstruction syndrome, or DIOS, previously known as meconium ileus equivalent or MIE)
- Pancreatitis (in pancreatic-sufficient patients)

IV Fluids

- Increased salt loss increases risk of hyponatremic hypochloremic dehydration.
- Cautious use of IV fluids with worsening lung disease

Nursing

Nursing assignments should involve only 1 CF patient per nurse for isolation purposes.

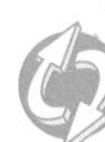

ONGOING CARE

FOLLOW-UP RECOMMENDATIONS

- Upon discharge for a pulmonary exacerbation, follow up with their CF provider within 2–4 weeks
- Routine clinic visits every 3 months, with airway cultures and pulmonary function testing (2)[A]
- Annual comprehensive nutritional evaluation with morphometric analysis
- Yearly OGTT after 10 years of age (3)[A]
- Bone densitometry after age 18 (2)[A]

DIET

High-calorie, high-fat diet with added salt

PATIENT EDUCATION

Cystic Fibrosis Foundation: www.cff.org

PROGNOSIS

- Most recent median survival is 35.9 years, as of 2009 CF Foundation Patient Registry (2)[A].
- Progression of lung disease usually determines length of survival.

REFERENCES

1. O'Sullivan BP, Freedman SD, et al. Cystic fibrosis. *Lancet*. 2009;373:1891–904.
2. *Cystic Fibrosis Foundation Patient Registry, 2009 Annual Data Report*. Bethesda, MD: Cystic Fibrosis Foundation; 2011.
3. Moran A, Brunzell C, Cohen RC, et al. Clinical care guidelines for cystic fibrosis-related diabetes: A position statement of the American Diabetes Association and a clinical practice guideline of the Cystic Fibrosis Foundation, endorsed by the Pediatric Endocrine Society. *Diabetes Care*. 2010;33:2697–708.
4. Accurso F, et al. Effect of VX-770 in persons with cystic fibrosis and the G551D-*CFTR* mutation. *NEJM*. 2010;363:1991–2003.
5. Main E, et al. Conventional chest physiotherapy compared to other airway clearance techniques for cystic fibrosis. *Cochrane Database Sys Rev*. 2005;(1):CD002011.
6. Meachery G, De Soyza A, Nicholson A, et al. Outcomes of Lung transplantation for Cystic Fibrosis in a large United Kingdom cohort. *Thorax*. 2008.

ADDITIONAL READING

Mueller C, Flotte TR, et al. Gene therapy for cystic fibrosis. *Clin Rev Allergy Immunol*. 2008;35:164–78.

CODES

ICD9

- 277.00 Cystic fibrosis without mention of meconium ileus
- 277.01 Cystic fibrosis with meconium ileus
- 277.09 Cystic fibrosis with other manifestations

CLINICAL PEARLS

- CF must be considered in *any* child with chronic diarrhea, especially if associated with poor growth or failure to thrive.
- All children with nasal polyps should be evaluated.
- Children with CF may present with generalized edema due to protein/calorie malnutrition.
- The presence of digital clubbing or bronchiectasis should always trigger consideration of CF.
- A rapid decline in pulmonary function suggests the acquisition of resistant organisms (such as *B. cepacia*), CF-related diabetes, ABPA, or GE reflux disease.

CYTOMEGALOVIRUS INCLUSION DISEASE

Penelope H. Dennehy, MD

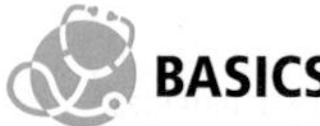

BASICS

Cytomegalovirus (CMV) is a ubiquitous virus that commonly infects people across all ages, ethnic and socioeconomic groups, and geographic areas. Although most CMV infections are asymptomatic or cause mild disease, the virus can cause serious disease in neonates and immunocompromised people. Because of its ubiquity, it is often difficult to define the role of CMV in a disease process. A thorough knowledge of CMV virology, epidemiology, clinical manifestations, diagnostic testing, and indications for treatment is required to appropriately manage patients with suspected CMV infections.

DESCRIPTION

- CMV is a DNA virus in the *Herpesvirus* family. It is a member of the β herpesvirus subfamily, which also includes HHV-6 and -7.
- Primary infection: Often asymptomatic; may remain latent throughout a person's life if not immunocompromised
- Severe disease can result from primary infection of the fetus and newborn or reactivation in setting of immunocompromise or organ transplantation.
- Name derives from the infected cells, which are large and contain intranuclear inclusions, described as "owl's eye" inclusions
- Not highly contagious:
  - Spread via close contact with persons shedding virus from saliva, urine, blood, breast milk, or semen
  - Also acquired via infected transplant organs
  - Any organ can be affected.
- Categories of CMV infections:
  - Congenital:
    - ~1% (0.2–2.5%) of newborns are congenitally infected with CMV.
    - Most infected newborns appear normal and are asymptomatic.
    - As many as 15% of these children may later develop progressive hearing loss, which is most often unilateral.
    - ~10% (5–15%) of congenitally infected newborns will be symptomatic at birth with manifestations including small size for gestational age, hepatosplenomegaly, petechial or purpuric rash, and jaundice.
  - Perinatal: Exposure to CMV in maternal cervicovaginal secretions, breast milk, or from blood product transfusions. Often asymptomatic.
  - Acute infection in a normal host: Symptomatic infection commonly presents with acute mononucleosis syndrome (1).
  - Latent infection: Higher IgG titers may contribute to development of atherosclerotic disease (4).
  - Infection in bone marrow and solid organ transplant patients:
    - Heart transplant: Early myocarditis followed by late atherosclerosis
    - Lung and bone marrow transplant: Interstitial pneumonia
    - Liver transplant: Hepatitis and colitis
    - Kidney transplant: Graft loss
  - Infection in patients with AIDS: Most commonly retinitis, second most common is colitis, followed by esophagitis and neurologic disease (3)
  - Infections in other immunocompromised patients: Pulmonary, GI, or renal disease
- System(s) affected: Ophthalmic; Pulmonary; GI; Neurologic; Renal; Skin/Exocrine
- Synonym(s): Giant cell inclusion disease; CID CMV

Pregnancy Considerations

- CMV infection in pregnancy may cause illness in the newborn ranging from asymptomatic infection to severe disease or even death.
- Infection may occur in utero, intrapartum, or postnatally.
- Pre-existing maternal CMV seropositivity substantially decreases, but does not completely eliminate fetal infection.

Pediatric Considerations

Breastfeeding can transmit virus to high-risk preterm infants. However, there is low risk of symptomatic disease and no evidence of long-term sequelae from transmission from breastfeeding. Currently, there are no recommendations for avoidance or treated breast milk (6).

EPIDEMIOLOGY

Incidence

- Common, but frequently asymptomatic
- <2–3 cases of end-organ disease per 100 person-years in HIV patients
- CMV infection is even more prevalent in populations at higher risk for HIV infection (IV drug users 75%, homosexual males 90%).
- Predominant age: All ages, peaks at <3 months, 16–40 years, and 40–75 years
- Predominant sex: Male > Female

Prevalence

- Occurs worldwide
- 40–100% of the general US population is seropositive from prior exposure during childhood or early adulthood (5).
- 20% of children in the US are seropositive before reaching puberty (5).
- Most common perinatally transmitted infection: 0.2–2.2% of births in the US (6)

RISK FACTORS

- HIV infection with specific risks, including:
  - CD4 count <50 cells/μL (3)[B]
  - Absence of treatment with or failure to respond to ART (3)[B]
  - Previous opportunistic infections (3)[B]
  - HIV viral load >100,000 (3)[B]
- Organ transplantation
- Blood transfusion
- Immunocompromise
- Living in closed population
- Corticosteroid therapy
- Daycare environment, infant, or geriatric
- For congenital infection, maternal infection during pregnancy
- Low socioeconomic status (6)[C]
- Critically ill immunocompetent adults in intensive care unit settings (up to 1/3 develop CMV, primarily between days 4 and 12 after admission) (7)[A]

GENERAL PREVENTION

- Hand washing/basic hygiene
- Avoid immunosuppression.
- Highly active antiretroviral therapy (HAART) is the best method for high-risk HIV patients (5)[A].
- Chronic maintenance therapy for life in HIV patients with CMV end-organ disease unless successfully treated with ART (1)[A]
- Options include:
  - Parenteral or oral ganciclovir (1)[A]
  - Parenteral foscarnet (1)[A]
  - Combined parenteral ganciclovir and foscarnet (1)[A]
  - Parenteral cidofovir (1)[A]
  - Ganciclovir via intraocular implant or repetitive intravitreous injection of fomivirsen (1)[A]
- CMV antibody+, HIV+ children who are severely immunosuppressed require oral ganciclovir 30 mg/kg t.i.d.
- Antiviral suppression of CMV reactivation in CMV+ transplant recipients or recipients of CMV+ organs:
  - Solid organ transplant: Prophylactic or preemptive treatment with oral ganciclovir, valganciclovir (8)[A]
  - Bone marrow transplant: IV ganciclovir
- CMV immunoglobulins decrease rate of severe disease after liver transplant (9)[A] and decrease incidence of disease after renal transplant.

ETIOLOGY

- Primary infection
- Reinfection with different CMV strains
- Reactivation of latent virus in patients who are immunosuppressed

COMMONLY ASSOCIATED CONDITIONS

AIDS, corticosteroid therapy, transplantation, or immunosuppression

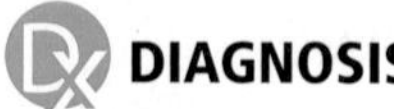

DIAGNOSIS

HISTORY

- Congenital:
  - Asymptomatic cytomegaloviremia
  - Symptomatic: Small for gestational age, purpura/petechiae, jaundice, hepatosplenomegaly, chorioretinitis, microcephaly, intracranial calcifications, hearing impairment
  - 90% have late complications: Sensorineural hearing loss occurs in 14%; 3–5% moderate to severe (9)[A]
  - Mental retardation, chorioretinitis, optic atrophy, seizures, learning disabilities (6)
- Acquired: Acute infection in a normal host (1):
  - Usually asymptomatic
  - Mononucleosis syndrome: Fever, malaise, sore throat, headache, antibiotic rash
  - Less common: Exudative pharyngitis, splenomegaly, cervical adenopathy, rash
- Infections in AIDS patients (3):
  - Retinitis: Usually unilateral, floaters, scotomata, peripheral field defects. Diagnosis made when characteristic retinal changes noted by ophthalmologist on funduscopic exam.
  - Colitis: Fever, weight loss, anorexia, abdominal pain, diarrhea, malaise; hemorrhage or perforation rare but serious
  - Esophagitis: Fever, odynophagia, nausea, abdominal discomfort
  - Pneumonitis: Dyspnea with or without exertion, nonproductive cough, hypoxemia

- Neurologic disease: Dementia, lethargy, confusion, fever, focal neurologic signs
- Infections in transplant recipients:
  - Persistent fever (most common)
  - Bone marrow transplant: Interstitial pneumonia (8)
  - Liver transplant: Hepatitis (8)
  - Kidney transplant: CMV syndrome (fever, leucopenia, atypical lymphocytes, hepatomegaly, myalgia, arthralgia)

PHYSICAL EXAM

See "History."

DIAGNOSTIC TESTS & INTERPRETATION

Lab

- Acute infection in a normal host:
  - Elevated liver transaminases in 92%, although transaminases rarely increase to >5 times normal ranges (1)
  - Anemia (1)
  - Thrombocytopenia (1)
  - Positive cold agglutinins (1)
  - Lymphocytosis with >10% atypical (1)
  - Negative heterophil antibody test (rules out Epstein-Barr virus mononucleosis) (1)
  - Positive CMV IgM antibodies; may not peak until 4–7 weeks after acute infection (1)
  - CMV IgG should increase 4-fold during acute infection (1).
- Congenital:
  - Isolation of the virus in urine or saliva samples collected within the first 3 weeks of life
  - Direct hyperbilirubinemia >3 mg/dL
  - Thrombocytopenia (<75,000/mL) (6)
  - Elevated liver transaminases (6)
- Immunocompromised:
  - Viremia: PCR, antigen assays (pp65 lower-matrix protein in leukocytes), blood culture, although viremia can be present without CMV disease (3)[A]
  - Serum CMV antibodies not useful; can be falsely negative due to immunosuppression (3)[C]
  - Neurologic disease: CMV detected in CSF or brain tissue clinches diagnosis. Enhanced by PCR analysis (3)[A].
  - Recovery of virus from tissue in symptomatic patient (GI or pulmonary tissue) indicates infection, although 1–6 weeks are required for distinctive cytopathic events to occur.
  - Quantitative DNA polymerase chain reaction (PCR) evidences disease and can be used to monitor therapy.

Imaging

- Head CT or MRI: Periventricular enhancement (CMV neurologic disease in neonate)
- Chest x-ray: Interstitial infiltrates (CMV pneumonitis)

Diagnostic Procedures/Surgery

- Bronchoscopy: Identification of CMV inclusion bodies in lung tissue in context of pulmonary infiltrates (pneumonitis)
- Endoscopic exam of GI tract: Mucosal ulcerations and colonoscopic, rectal, or esophageal biopsy (colitis, esophagitis) (3)[B]

Pathological Findings

Giant cells with basophilic inclusion bodies (owl's eye)

DIFFERENTIAL DIAGNOSIS

- Congenital: Toxoplasmosis or rubella
- Acquired in immunocompetent: Epstein-Barr virus (EBV) mononucleosis, viral hepatitis
- Acquired immunocompromised: Other viral, bacterial, fungal opportunistic infections

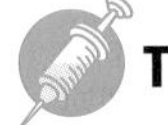

TREATMENT

MEDICATION

First Line

- Congenital disease: Ganciclovir 12 mg/kg IV q12h for 6 weeks (6)[B]
- Pediatric disseminated disease: IV ganciclovir (1)[A]
- CMV mononucleosis/asymptomatic viremia: No treatment (3)
- Retinitis: Effective treatments include the following and should be chosen in consultation with a specialist:
  - Oral valganciclovir (for peripheral lesions) (3)[A]
  - IV ganciclovir followed by oral valganciclovir (3)[A]
  - IV foscarnet (3)[A]
  - IV cidofovir (3)[A]
  - Ganciclovir intraocular implant with oral or IV valganciclovir (3)[A]
  - Treat until CD4 >100 for 3–6 months (3)[A]
- Colitis or esophagitis: IV ganciclovir or foscarnet for 21–28 days or until symptom resolution (3)[B]
- Neurologic disease: Prompt treatment with ganciclovir and foscarnet (3)[B]
- CMV disease in transplant patients: IV ganciclovir for 2–4 weeks (8)[B]

Second Line

- Adult CMV retinitis: Fomivirsen (6)[A]
- Pediatric disseminated disease: Foscarnet 60 mg/kg q8h for 14–21 days (6)[A], combination ganciclovir and foscarnet (6)[B]
- CMV disease in transplant patients: Valganciclovir (8)[C]
- CMV in bone marrow transplant patients:
  - Prophylaxis: Valacyclovir (8)[B]
  - Preemptive: Foscarnet (8)[B]

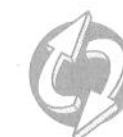

ONGOING CARE

FOLLOW-UP RECOMMENDATIONS

Bed rest

Patient Monitoring

- CMV urine culture at birth for all HIV-infected or -exposed and annual testing for CMV seronegative/HIV+ children
- Patients with CD4 counts <50 should have ophthalmologic screening every 3–6 months.
- Patients on therapy should be followed for neutropenia, anemia, and thrombocytopenia.

PROGNOSIS

Severe disease with primary infection in newborns and reactivation in immunocompromised

COMPLICATIONS

- Congenital: Hearing loss, mental retardation, optic atrophy, seizures, learning disabilities
- Colitis: Hemorrhage and perforation

REFERENCES

1. Taylor GH. Cytomegalovirus. *Am Fam Phys*. 2003;67(3):519–24.
2. Crumpacker CS. Invited commentary: Human cytomegalovirus, inflammation, cardiovascular disease, and mortality. *Am J Epidemiol*. 2010; 172(4):372–4.
3. Benson CA, Kaplan JE, Masur H, et al. Treating opportunistic infections among HIV-infected adults and adolescents: Recommendations from CDC, the National Institutes of Health, and the HIV Medicine Association/Infectious Diseases Society of America. *MMWR Recomm Rep*. 2004;53:1–112.
4. Kurath S, Halwachs-Baumann G, Müller W, et al. Transmission of cytomegalovirus via breast milk to the prematurely born infant: A systematic review. *Clin Microbiol Infect*. 2010;16:1172–8.
5. Salzberger B, Hartmann P, Hanses F, et al. Incidence and prognosis of CMV disease in HIV-infected patients before and after introduction of combination antiretroviral therapy. *Infection*. 2005;33:345–9.
6. Mofenson LM, Oleske J, Serchuck L, et al. Treating opportunistic infections among HIV-exposed and infected children: recommendations from CDC, the National Institutes of Health, and the Infectious Diseases Society of America. *MMWR Recomm Rep*. 2004;53:1–92.
7. Osawa R, Singh N. Cytomegalovirus infection in critically ill patients: A systematic review. *Crit Care*. 2009;13:R68.
8. Razonable RR, Emery VC, 11th Annual Meeting of the IHMF (International Herpes Management Forum). Management of CMV infection and disease in transplant patients. 27–29 February 2004. *Herpes*. 2004;11:77–86.
9. Grosse SD, Ross DS, Dollard SC. Congenital cytomegalovirus (CMV) infection as a cause of permanent bilateral hearing loss: A quantitative assessment. *J Clin Virol*. 2008;41:57–62.

ADDITIONAL READING

Yinon Y, Farine D, Yudin MH, et al. Cytomegalovirus infection in pregnancy. *J Obstet Gynaecol Can*. 2010;32:348–54.

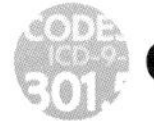

CODES

ICD9

- 078.5 Cytomegaloviral disease
- 771.1 Congenital cytomegalovirus infection

CLINICAL PEARLS

- CMV mono has much less cervical adenopathy and/or splenomegaly than EBV mono in adults.
- CMV is a major cause of sensorineural hearing loss in young children.

DE QUERVAIN TENOSYNOVITIS

Chad Beattie, MD
J. Herbert Stevenson, MD

BASICS

DESCRIPTION

De Quervain tenosynovitis is a stenosis of the first dorsal compartment of the wrist, including the extensor pollicis brevis (EPB) and abductor pollicis longus (APL). It is an inflammation or thickening of the tendon sheath that surrounds the EPB and the APL, which leads to pain with certain movements of the thumb.

EPIDEMIOLOGY

- Predominant age: 30–50 years old
- Predominant sex: Female > Male (women 6–10× more likely than men)

Incidence

Common condition

RISK FACTORS

- Women age 30–50
- Pregnancy (primarily third trimester and postpartum)
- Individuals participating in golf, fly fishing, and racquet sports
- Repetitive motions with the hand/thumb requiring forceful grasping or wrist ulna/radial deviation; often seen in carpenters and machine operators

GENERAL PREVENTION

Avoidance of repetitive actions of the thumb associated with forceful grasping or repetitive wrist ulna/radial deviation (e.g., hammering)

PATHOPHYSIOLOGY

Repetitive actions of the wrist and the thumb result in microtrauma and thickening of the surrounding tendon and tendon sheath (EPB, APL). This thickening causes inflammation and pain with movements of the thumb and wrist, and may elicit pain over the radial styloid as they rub over the prominence.

ETIOLOGY

- Repetitive movements of the wrist and thumb and activities that require forceful grasping
- Trauma
- Systemic diseases (e.g., rheumatoid arthritis)

DIAGNOSIS

HISTORY

- Patients may complain of gradual worsening pain along their thumb and radial aspect of their wrist with certain movements, including ulnar deviation of the wrist.
- Usually insidious in onset
- Usually no associated trauma

PHYSICAL EXAM

- Pain and swelling are present over the radial styloid, which may be exacerbated when patients move their thumb or make a fist.
- Crepitus with movement of the thumb may be felt or heard.
- Occasionally, slight swelling at the base of the thumb and wrist is noted.
- Decreased range of motion of the thumb
- Swelling and tenderness may be appreciated over the distal radius.
- Pain over the first extensor compartment on resisted thumb abduction or extension
- Crepitus may be associated with movement of the thumb.

DIAGNOSTIC TESTS & INTERPRETATION

Finkelstein test is pathognomonic for De Quervain tenosynovitis. This test involves the patient flexing thumb in palm, while the examiner ulnar-deviates the wrist. The test is positive if patient's symptoms are reproduced.

Lab

No labs are indicated.

Imaging

- This disease is primarily a clinical diagnosis, but if the diagnosis is questionable, then radiographs of the wrist may be indicated to rule out other pathology. Radiographs may rule out CMC arthritis, which can be misdiagnosed as De Quervain. MRI is the test of choice to rule out coexisting soft tissue injury or wrist joint pathology.
- Ultrasound has also been shown to be a helpful tool, especially in detecting anatomic variations in the first dorsal extensor compartment of the wrist. Awareness of anatomic variations may aid in improving outcomes of corticosteroid injections (1)[C],(2)[C].

Pathological Findings

Inflamed and thickened retinacular sheath of the tendon

DIFFERENTIAL DIAGNOSIS

- Fracture of the scaphoid
- Dorsal wrist ganglion
- Osteoarthritis of the first carpometacarpal joint
- Flexor carpi radialis tendonitis
- Infectious tenosynovitis
- Tendonitis of the wrist extensors
- Intersection syndrome
- Trigger thumb

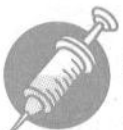

TREATMENT

- Rest and immobilization may be helpful early in the disease process. This is achieved with the use of a thumb spica splint.
- NSAIDs may help along with the splint to decrease the inflammation.

MEDICATION

First Line

Immobilization and NSAIDs

Second Line

- Corticosteroid injection of the tendon sheath has shown significant cure rates. An 83% success rate after single injection has been reported (3)[B]. Additional injections are sometimes required.
- A recent study has shown some evidence that a newer, 4-point injection technique may yield more favorable results compared to older, 1- and 2-point injection techniques in high-resistance training athletes (4)[B].

ADDITIONAL TREATMENT

General Measures

- If full relief is not being achieved, a corticosteroid injection of the tendon sheath has been shown to result in 83% cure rate (3)[B].
- Anatomic variants may complicate treatment, including 2 tendon sheaths in the first compartment or the EPB tendon may travel in a separate compartment. Ultrasound has been shown to be useful in helping distinguish these variants (1)[C],(2)[C].
- Surgery is indicated for cases not responding to 3–6 months of conservative treatment. Surgery has been found to result in 91% cure rate (5)[B].

Issues for Referral
Referral to a hand surgeon is indicated if no improvement is noted after conservative treatments.

Additional Therapies
- Hand therapy along with iontophoresis/phonophoresis may help improve outcomes for moderate cases.
- Patients may incorporate thumb-stretching exercises into their rehabilitation.

SURGERY/OTHER PROCEDURES
Only indicated for patients who have failed conservative treatment. Surgical release has shown cure rates of up to 91% (5)[B].

IN-PATIENT CONSIDERATIONS
Initial Stabilization
- Splinting of the thumb (thumb spica splint or dorsal hood splint)
- Rest
- Ice (15–20 minutes 5–6× a day)
- Anti-inflammatory medications

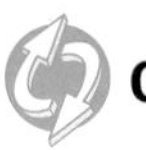

ONGOING CARE

FOLLOW-UP RECOMMENDATIONS
- Additional corticosteroid injection may be performed at 4–6 weeks if symptoms are not significantly reduced.
- Avoid repetitive activities and motions that aggravate the pain.

DIET
As tolerated

PATIENT EDUCATION
Modification of activities eliciting pain, such as repetitive movement of the wrist and thumb, and forceful grasping.

PROGNOSIS
Prognosis is extremely good with conservative treatments. 95% success rates have been shown with conservative therapy over 1 year, although up to 1/3 of patients will have recurrence (6)[A]. Surgery has shown success in 91% of patients who did not improve with conservative therapy.

COMPLICATIONS
- Most complications are secondary to the treatment modalities. This includes GI, renal, and hepatic injury secondary to NSAIDs.
- Nerve damage may occur during surgery.
- Hypopigmentation, fat atrophy, bleeding, and infection are potential adverse events from corticosteroid injections.
- If not treated correctly, loss of flexibility of the thumb due to fibrosis may occur.

REFERENCES

1. Choi SJ, Ahn JH, Lee YJ, et al. De Quervain disease: US identification of anatomic variations in the first extensor compartment with an emphasis on subcompartmentalization. *Radiology*. 2011;260(2): 480–6.
2. Kwon BC, Choi SJ, Shin DJ, et al. Sonographic identification of the intracompartmental septum in de Quervain's disease. *Clin Orthop Relat Res*. 2010;468(8):2129–34.
3. Richie CA, Briner WW. Corticosteroid injection for treatment of de Quervain's tenosynovitis: A pooled quantitative literature evaluation. *J Am Board Fam Pract*. 2003;16:102–6.
4. Pagonis T, Ditsios K, Toli P, et al. Improved corticosteroid treatment of recalcitrant de Quervain's tenosynovitis with a novel 4-point injection technique. *Am J Sports Med*. 2011;39(2): 398–403.
5. Ta KT, Eidelman D, Thomson JG. Patient satisfaction and outcomes of surgery for de Quervain's tenosynovitis. *J Hand Surg Am*. 1999;24:1071–7.
6. Jirarattanaphochai K, Saengnipanthkul S, Vipulakorn K, et al. Treatment of de Quervain disease with triamcinolone injection with or without nimesulide. A randomized, double-blind, placebo-controlled trial. *J Bone Joint Surg Am*. 2004;86-A:2700–6.

ADDITIONAL READING

- Rettig AC. Athletic injuries of the wrist and hand. Part II overuse injuries of the wrist and traumatic injuries of the hand. *Am J Sport Med*. 2004;32: 262–73.
- Rossi R, et al. De Quervain disease in volleyball players. *Am J Sport Med*. 2005;33:424–7.
- Tallia AF, Cardone DA. Diagnostic and therapeutic injection of the wrist and hand region. *Am Fam Physician*. 2003;67:745–50.

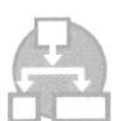

See Also (Topic, Algorithm, Electronic Media Element)

Algorithm: Pain in Upper Extremity

CODES

ICD9
727.04 Radial styloid tenosynovitis

CLINICAL PEARLS

- Repetitive movements of the wrist and thumb and activities that require forceful grasping are the most common causes of De Quervain tenosynovitis.
- De Quervain tenosynovitis is a stenosis of the first dorsal compartment of the wrist, including the EPB and APL. It is an inflammation or thickening of the tendon sheath that surrounds the EPB and the APL, which leads to pain with certain movements of the thumb.
- It is diagnosed via the Finkelstein test, which is pathognomonic for De Quervain tenosynovitis. This test involves the patient flexing the thumb in the palm, while the examiner ulnar deviates the wrist. The test is positive if patient's symptoms are reproduced.
- Activity can be as-tolerated, using pain as a threshold; however, most people require modification of their activities to assist with rehabilitation and improvement.

DEEP VEIN THROMBOPHLEBITIS (DVT)

Alfonso J. Tafur, MD, RPVI
Denisse Tafur Chang, MD

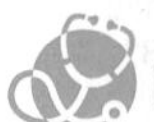

BASICS

DESCRIPTION
- Development of blood clot within the deep veins, usually accompanied by inflammation of the vessel wall.
- The major clinical consequences are embolization (usually to the lung) and postphlebitic syndrome.
- System(s) affected: Cardiovascular

EPIDEMIOLOGY
- The age- and gender-adjusted incidence of venous thromboembolism (VTE) is 100 times higher in the hospital than in the community.
- 1/3 of VTE cases die within 30 days, 1/5 will have sudden death due to pulmonary embolism (PE). The 28-day DVT fatality rate is 9%.

Incidence
- In the US, VTE occurs for the first time in 100 persons per 100,000 per year.
- ~2/3 of the new VTE cases are deep vein thrombophlebitis (DVT) alone.
- Higher incidence among Caucasians and African Americans relative to Hispanics and Asians
- Complicates ~1 in 1,000 pregnancies

Prevalence
Variable; dependent on medical condition or procedure:
- 22–52% of the patients with PE have DVT.
- 25% of patients with superficial venous thrombosis (1)
- Present in 11% of patients with acquired brain injury entering to neurorehabilitation

RISK FACTORS
- Acquired: Age, previous thrombosis, immobilization, major surgery, orthopedic surgery, malignancy, oral contraceptives, hormonal replacement therapy, antiphospholipid syndrome, polycythemia vera, paroxysmal nocturnal hemoglobinuria, prolonged travel, pregnancy/puerperium
- Inherited: Antithrombin deficiency, protein C deficiency, protein S deficiency, factor V Leiden R506Q, prothrombin G20210A, dysfibrinogenemia
- Mixed/unknown: Hyperhomocysteinemia, high levels of factor VIII, activated protein C resistance not factor V Leiden, high levels of factor IX, high levels of thrombin activatable fibrinolysis inhibitor (TAFI), high levels of factor XI

Genetics
- Factor V Leiden is found in 5% of the population and in 20% of all VTE events. It is the most common thrombophilia. Homozygosity is found in 1 per 5,000 persons. It increases the risk of VTE 3–8-fold in heterozygous carriers and 50–80-fold in homozygous.
- PT20210A is found in 3% of Caucasians. Increases the risk of thrombosis about 3-fold.

GENERAL PREVENTION
- Mechanical thromboprophylaxis is recommended in patients with high bleeding risk and as an adjunct to anticoagulant-based thromboprophylaxis. Mechanical measures include early ambulation, graduated compression stockings, venous foot pump, and intermittent pneumatic compression.
- Level of risk :
  - With minor surgery in mobile patient or fully mobile medical patients, risk of VTE <10%; early ambulation recommended
  - With medical patients on bed rest, general, and gynecologic or urologic surgeries, risk of VTE 10–40%; prophylactic low molecular weight heparin (LMWH), low-dose unfractioned heparin (UFH) or fondaparinux recommended
- Hip or knee arthroplasty, major trauma, spinal cord injury, or hip fracture surgery, risk of VTE is 40–80%; LMWH, fondaparinux, or oral vitamin K antagonist (international normalized ratio [INR] 2–3) recommended

ETIOLOGY
Factors involved may include venous stasis, endothelial injury, and abnormalities of coagulation.

DIAGNOSIS

- Wells criteria:
  - **Wells score or criteria**: (Possible score −2 to 9) Active cancer (treatment within last 6 months or palliative) +1 point. Calf swelling >3 cm compared to other calf (measured 10 cm below tibial tuberosity) +1 point. Collateral superficial veins (nonvaricose) +1 point. Pitting edema (confined to symptomatic leg) +1 point. Previous documented DVT +1 point. Swelling of entire leg +1 point. Localized pain along distribution of deep venous system +1 point. Paralysis, paresis, or recent cast immobilization of lower extremities +1 point. Recently bedridden >3 days, or major surgery requiring regional or general anesthetic in past 4 weeks +1 point. Alternative diagnosis at least as likely −2 points. Interpretation: Score 0–1 DVT unlikely. Score 2 or higher: Moderate-to-high probability.

HISTORY
- Establish pretest probability based on Wells criteria.
- Classify as "Provoked" or "Idiopathic." Determine the presence of risk factors, including family history.
- Clinical assessment of bleeding risk: Bleeding with previous history of anticoagulation, history of liver disease, recent interventions, history of GI bleed

PHYSICAL EXAM
Physical exam is only 30% accurate for DVT. Resistance to dorsiflexion of the foot (Homan sign) is unreliable. Palpable tender cords are helpful if present but are often not present. Erythema over area of thrombosis (often not present). Fever is occasionally present. Swelling of collateral veins. Massive edema with cyanosis is a medical emergency (phlegmasia cerulea dolens, rare). Pain on medial tibia percussion (Lisker sign). Pain on compression of calf against tibia in the anteroposterior plane (Bancroft or Moses sign). Thoracic outlet maneuvers in upper extremity DVT. Attention to signs of possible malignancy.

DIAGNOSTIC TESTS & INTERPRETATION
Lab
- D-dimer (sensitive but not specific; has a high negative predictive value [NPV]); most protocols are used to rule out DVT in low pretest probability cases: If D-dimer negative, DVT is ruled out with low pretest probability cases. Do not order D-dimer if pretest probability is moderate or high:
  - Repeated D-dimer testing after anticoagulation suspension may help tailor the individual duration of treatment after a first unprovoked VTE.
- CBC, platelet count, activated partial thromboplastin time (aPTT), prothrombin time (PT)/INR
- In young patients with idiopathic or recurrent VTE consider:
  - Factor V Leiden, G20210A prothrombin, serum homocysteine, factor VIII level, and lupus anticoagulant
  - Protein C and S levels, antithrombin activity, anticardiolipin antibodies.
- Testing for genetic polymorphisms CYP2C9 and VKORC1 (www.warfarindosing.org for current recommendations)
- Thrombosis lowers antithrombin; workup for deficiency performed after therapy completed. Secondary antithrombin deficiency is more common than primary.

Follow-Up & Special Considerations
In specific scenarios an underlying malignancy is more likely: Recurrent VTE, risk: 3.2 (95% CI 2.0–4.8), Unprovoked VTE, 4.6 times higher (vs secondary), upper extremity DVT, not catheter associated. OR 1.8 (2), abdominal DVT, OR 2.2 (2), bilateral lower extremity DVT, OR 2.1 (2)

Imaging
- Compression ultrasound (US): Noninvasive; sensitive and specific for popliteal, femoral thrombi, but has poor ability to detect calf vein thrombi
- Contrast venography: Gold standard, is technically difficult, risk of morbidity
- Impedance plethysmography: As accurate as duplex US, less operator dependency, but poor at detecting calf vein thrombi; not widely available
- Magnetic resonance venography: As accurate as contrast venography; may be useful for patients with contraindications to IV contrast
- ^{125}I-fibrinogen scan: Detects only active clot formation; very good at detecting ongoing calf thrombi; takes 4 hours for results

DIFFERENTIAL DIAGNOSIS
Cellulitis, fracture, ruptured synovial cyst (Baker cyst), lymphedema, muscle strain/tear, extrinsic compression of vein (e.g., by tumor or enlarged lymph nodes), compartment syndrome, localized allergic reaction, filariasis (in developing countries)

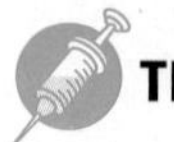

TREATMENT

MEDICATION
- All DVTs should receive treatment. Consider starting therapy even before confirmation in patients with high pretest probability.
- 2008 American College of Chest Physicians Guidelines recommend LMWH, UFH (IV, fixed-dose, or adjusted-dose SC heparin), or fondaparinux and warfarin for at least 5 days until the INR is 2–3 for 24 hours (3)[A].

First Line

- UFH:
  - IV drip: Initial dose of 80 units/kg or 5,000 units followed by continuous infusion of 18 units/kg/hr. Target an aPTT ratio >1.5. The aPTT prolongation shall correspond to a 0.3–0.7 anti-Xa level.
  - SC UFH: Monitored: 17,500 units or 250 units/kg b.i.d. with aPTT adjustment to an equivalent to 0.3–0.7 anti-Xa. Alternatively, fixed dose: 333 units/kg followed by b.i.d. dose 250 units/kg.
- Enoxaparin (Lovenox): 1 mg/kg/dose SC q12h or 1.5 mg/kg/dose/d
- Dalteparin (Fragmin): 200 IU/kg SC q24h
- Fondaparinux (Arixtra): 5 mg (body weight <50 kg), 7.5 mg (body weight = 50–100 kg), or 10 mg (body weight >100 kg) SC once daily
- Maintenance therapy:
  - Warfarin (Coumadin): 5 mg/d for 3 days, then adjust to a target INR of 2–3
- Adverse effects:
  - Heparin or LMWH: Bleeding, edema, injection site irritation, skin eruptions, hematoma, thrombocytopenia
  - Fondaparinux: Bleeding, injection site irritation, rash, fever, anemia
  - Warfarin: Bleeding, skin necrosis, teratogenicity
- Contraindications:
  - Heparin or LMWH: Bleeding, heparin hypersensitivity, heparin-induced thrombocytopenia (HIT), ITP, infants/neonates
  - Fondaparinux: Bleeding, endocarditis, renal failure, thrombocytopenia
  - Warfarin: Current bleeding, alcoholism, preeclampsia, pregnancy, surgery, high fall risk

Second Line

If warfarin is contraindicated, heparin can be given by intermittent SC self-injection.

Pregnancy Considerations

- Warfarin (Coumadin) is a teratogen; treat with full-dose heparin initially, followed by subcutaneous heparin starting at 15,000 units every 12 hours.
- Warfarin is safe with breastfeeding.
- LMWH, dalteparin, and fondaparinux are pregnancy Category B.

ADDITIONAL TREATMENT

- Dabigatran as a fixed oral dose is as effective as warfarin for the treatment of acute venous thromboembolism. However, this is not yet an approved indication in the US (4).
- Rivaroxaban has not been approved for VTE treatment in US, but it has shown to be noninferior to conventional anticoagulation for the treatment of acute VTE.

Additional Therapies

Discharge with compression stockings 30–40 mm Hg. Stress use to prevent postphlebitic syndrome. Continue compression therapy for 2 years. Intermittent pneumatic compression may be tried in patients with significant edema.

SURGERY/OTHER PROCEDURES

- In selected patients with proximal DVT (iliofemoral DVT, <2 weeks of symptoms, good functional status, >1 year of life expectancy), catheter-directed thrombolysis or open thrombectomy may be considered.
- When anticoagulants have failed or are contraindicated, filtering devices are recommended.

IN-PATIENT CONSIDERATIONS

Admission Criteria

Admission for respiratory distress, proximal VTE, candidates for thrombolysis, active bleeding, renal failure, phlegmasia cerulea dolens, history of heparin-induced thrombocytopenia

Nursing

Limb elevation

Discharge Criteria

Medically stable and properly anticoagulated; overlap of anticoagulation and warfarin monitoring may be done as an outpatient

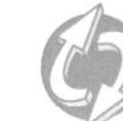

ONGOING CARE

FOLLOW-UP RECOMMENDATIONS

- Gradual resumption of normal activity, with avoidance of prolonged immobility
- Duration of warfarin treatment after DVT:
  - 3 months for treatment of a DVT secondary to a reversible risk factor
  - Patients with unprovoked DVT shall be considered for prolonged secondary prophylaxis:
    - In patients who have completed 3 months of anticoagulation after an unprovoked VTE, a positive D-dimer 1 month after discontinuation of therapy correlates with the risk of VTE recurrence (5).
    - Tailoring the anticoagulation duration base on recanalization US evidence may reduce the rate of recurrent VTE (6).
  - Consider prolonged secondary prophylaxis (1 year or indefinitely): Recurrent DVT; PE; active cancer (LMWH preferred over warfarin); life-threatening event (large pulmonary embolism, limb-threatening DVT); cerebral or visceral vein thrombosis; antithrombin deficiency with event; homozygous for factor V Leiden; combined clotting disorders (e.g., combined heterozygous factor V Leiden and PT20210A); antiphospholipid syndrome

Patient Monitoring

- Monitor platelet count while on heparin.
- Monitoring with LMWH and fondaparinux: Periodic platelet count. An anti-factor Xa activity level may help guide titration of therapy.
- Investigate significant bleeding (e.g., hematuria or GI hemorrhage) because anticoagulant therapy may unmask a pre-existing lesion (e.g., cancer, peptic ulcer disease, or arteriovenous malformation).

PATIENT EDUCATION

- Patients should wear compression stockings post-DVT; these can be cumbersome and uncomfortable; however, they can reduce the risk of DVT recurrence and postphlebitic syndrome.
- Dietary habits should be discussed when warfarin is initiated to ensure that intake of vitamin K-rich foods are identified.

PROGNOSIS

- 20% of untreated proximal (e.g., above the calf) DVTs progress to pulmonary emboli, and 10–20% of those are fatal; with anticoagulant therapy, mortality is decreased 5–10-fold.
- DVT confined to the infrapopliteal veins has a small risk of embolization but can propagate into the proximal system. Best treatment uncertain, but most recommend 6–12 weeks of anticoagulation.

COMPLICATIONS

- Pulmonary embolism (fatal in 10–20%), arterial embolism (paradoxical embolization) with arteriovenous (AV) shunting, chronic venous insufficiency, postphlebitic syndrome (pain and swelling in affected limb without new clot formation), treatment-induced hemorrhage, soft tissue ischemia associated with massive clot and high venous pressures: phlegmasia cerulea dolens (rare, but a surgical emergency)

REFERENCES

1. Decousus H, Quéré I, Presles E, et al. Superficial venous thrombosis and venous thromboembolism: A large, prospective epidemiologic study. *Ann Intern Med*. 2010;152:218–24.
2. Tafur AJ, Kalsi H, Wysokinski WE, et al. The association of active cancer with venous thromboembolism location: A population-based study. *Mayo Clin Proc*. 2011;86(1):25–30.
3. Kearon C, Kahn SR, Agnelli G, et al. Antithrombotic therapy for venous thromboembolic disease: American College of Chest Physicians Evidence-Based Clinical Practice Guidelines (8th Edition). *Chest*. 2008;133:454S–545S.
4. Schulman S, Kearon C, Kakkar AK, et al. Dabigatran versus warfarin in the treatment of acute venous thromboembolism. *N Engl J Med*. 2009;361(24): 2342–52.
5. Palareti G, Cosmi B, Legnani C, et al. D-dimer testing to determine the duration of anticoagulation therapy. *N Engl J Med*. 2006;355:1780–9.
6. Prandoni P, Prins MH, Lensing AW, et al. Residual thrombosis on ultrasonography to guide the duration of anticoagulation in patients with deep venous thrombosis: A randomized trial. *Ann Intern Med*. 2009;150:577–85.

ADDITIONAL READING

Kyrle PA, Rosendaal FR, Eichinger S. Risk assessment for recurrent venous thrombosis. *Lancet*. 2010; 376(9757):2032–9.

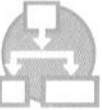

See Also (Topic, Algorithm, Electronic Media Element)

Antithrombin Deficiency; Factor V Leiden; Protein C Deficiency; Protein S Deficiency; Prothrombin 20210 (Mutation); Pulmonary Embolism

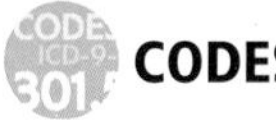

CODES

ICD9

- 451.19 Phlebitis and thrombophlebitis of deep veins of lower extremities, other
- 453.40 Acute venous embolism and thrombosis of unspecified deep vessels of lower extremity
- 453.42 Acute venous embolism and thrombosis of deep vessels of distal lower extremity

CLINICAL PEARLS

- Many cases are asymptomatic and are diagnosed after embolization.
- 25% of the patients with superficial thrombophlebitis will have DVT at presentation.
- Heparin and warfarin should overlap for a minimum of 5 days or longer to achieve target INR.

DEHYDRATION

Nitin Aggarwal, MD
Julie Scott Taylor, MD, MSc

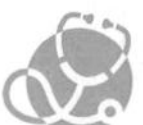

BASICS

DESCRIPTION

- Dehydration is a state of negative fluid balance.
- There are 2 types of dehydration:
  - Water loss dehydration (hyperosmolar, associated with either increased sodium or glucose)
  - Salt and water loss dehydration (hyponatremia)

EPIDEMIOLOGY

- The cause of 10% of all pediatric hospitalizations in the US
- Gastroenteritis, one of its leading causes, leads to hospital admissions for 13 out of 1,000 children <5 years annually in the US (1).

Incidence

- There are more than a half-million hospital admissions annually in the US for dehydration.
- Of hospitalized older persons, 7.8% have the diagnosis of dehydration (2).
- Worldwide, ~3–5 billion cases of acute gastroenteritis occur each year in children <5 years, resulting in nearly 2 million deaths (1).

RISK FACTORS

- Children <5 years old at highest risk
- Elderly
- Decreased cognition

Genetics

Some underlying causes of dehydration have a genetic component (diabetes), while others do not (gastroenteritis).

GENERAL PREVENTION

- Patient/parent education on the early signs of dehydration
- Regular hand washing decreases the spread of contagious viral gastroenteritis.

Geriatric Considerations

A systematic approach in assessing risk factors is necessary for early prevention and management of dehydration in the elderly, especially those in long-term care facilities.

PATHOPHYSIOLOGY

- Negative fluid balance occurs when ongoing fluid losses exceed fluid intake.
- Fluid losses can be insensible (sweat, respiration), obligate (urine, stool), or abnormal (diarrhea, vomiting, osmotic diuresis in diabetic ketoacidosis).
- Negative fluid balance can ultimately lead to severe intravascular volume depletion and ultimately end-organ damage from inadequate perfusion.
- The elderly are at increased risk as kidney function, urine concentration, thirst sensation, aldosterone secretion, release of vasopressin, and renin activity are all significantly lowered with age.

ETIOLOGY

- Decreased intake
- Increased output: Vomiting, diarrheal illnesses, sweating, frequent urination
- Third-spacing of fluids: Effusions, ascites, capillary leaks from burns or sepsis

Clinical Finding (3)	Mild	Moderate	Severe
% Dehydration: Children	5–10%	10–15%	>15%
% Dehydration: Adults	3–5%	5–10%	>10%
General Condition: Infants	Thirsty, alert, restless	Lethargic or drowsy	Limp, cold, cyanotic extremities, may be comatose
General Condition: Older Children	Thirsty, alert, restless	Alert, postural dizziness	Apprehensive, cold, cyanotic extremities, muscle cramps
Quality of Radial Pulse	Normal	Thready or weak	Feeble or impalpable
Quality of Respiration	Normal	Deep	Deep and rapid/tachypnea
BP	Normal	Normal to low	Low (shock)
Skin Turgor	Normal skin turgor	Reduced skin turgor, cool skin	Skin tenting, cool, mottled, acrocyanotic skin
Eyes	Normal	Sunken	Very sunken
Tears	Present	Absent	Absent
Mucous Membranes	Moist	Dry	Very dry
Urine Output	Normal	Reduced	None passed in many hours
Anterior Fontanelle	Normal	Sunken	Markedly sunken

COMMONLY ASSOCIATED CONDITIONS

- Hypo-/hypernatremia
- Hyperkalemia
- Hyperglycemia
- Hypovolemic shock
- Renal failure

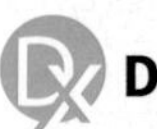

DIAGNOSIS

Calculate % dehydration = (preillness weight – illness weight)/preillness weight × 100.

HISTORY

- Fever
- Intake (including description and amount)
- Diarrhea (including duration, frequency, consistency, ± mucus or blood)
- Vomiting (including duration, frequency, consistency, ± bilious/nonbilious)
- Urination pattern
- Sick contacts
- Medication history (e.g., diuretics, laxatives)

PHYSICAL EXAM

- Vitals: Pulse, BP, temperature
- Weight loss: <5%, 10%, or >15%
- Mental status
- Head: Sunken anterior fontanelle (for infants)
- Eyes: Sunken, ± tear production
- Mucous membranes: Tacky, dry, or parched
- Capillary refill: Ranges from brisk to >3 seconds

DIAGNOSTIC TESTS & INTERPRETATION

Lab

For mild dehydration: Generally not necessary

Pediatric Considerations

Infants and the elderly may not concentrate urine maximally, so a nonelevated specific gravity should not be reassuring.

Initial lab tests

For moderate to severe dehydration:

- Blood work, including electrolytes, BUN, creatinine, and glucose
- Urinalysis (specific gravity, hematuria, glucosuria)

Imaging

Imaging does not play a role in the diagnosis of dehydration, unless diagnosis of the specific medical condition causing the dehydration requires imaging.

DIFFERENTIAL DIAGNOSIS

- Decreased intake: Ineffective breastfeeding, inadequate thirst response, anorexia, malabsorption, metabolic disorder, obtunded state
- Excessive losses: Gastroenteritis, diarrhea, febrile illness, diabetes/diabetic ketoacidosis (DKA)/hyperosmolar hyperglycemic state (HHS), diabetes insipidus, intestinal obstruction, inadequate intravascular volume, sepsis

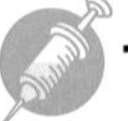

TREATMENT

MEDICATION

First Line

- If the patient is experiencing excessive vomiting, consider using an antiemetic.
- Antiemetic medications that are currently available include ondansetron, granisetron, tropisetron, dolasetron, ramosetron, promethazine, dimenhydrinate, metoclopramide, domperidone, droperidol, prochlorperazine, and trimethobenzamide.
- One randomized controlled trial (RCT) showed that a single oral dose of ondansetron reduced gastroenteritis-related vomiting and facilitated oral rehydration therapy (ORT) without significant adverse events (4)[B].

Second Line

- Loperamide may reduce the duration of diarrhea compared with placebo in children with mild to moderate dehydration (2 RCTs yes, 1 RCT no) (4)[B].
- In children ages 3–12 with mild diarrhea and minimal dehydration, loperamide improves diarrhea duration and frequency when used with oral rehydration (5)[A].

Pediatric Considerations

Given a higher risk for serious adverse events, loperamide is not indicated for children <3 years old with acute diarrhea (5)[A].

ADDITIONAL TREATMENT

Issues for Referral

- For severe dehydration, critical care referral and intensive care unit (ICU)-level care may be warranted.
- Surgical consultation for acute abdominal issues

SURGERY/OTHER PROCEDURES

For specific underlying causes of dehydration, such as intestinal obstruction or appendicitis

IN-PATIENT CONSIDERATIONS

Initial Stabilization

- Stabilize ABCs.
- If mild dehydration, try oral rehydration therapy (ORT): See "Oral Rehydration."
- If excessive vomiting or severe dehydration with shock, start IV access and IV fluids immediately.

Admission Criteria

- Intractable vomiting or diarrhea
- Electrolyte abnormalities
- Hemodynamic instability
- Inability to tolerate ORT

IV Fluids

- Stage I:
  - For moderate to severe dehydration in children: Isotonic saline or Ringer's lactate solution bolus of 10–20 mL/kg. May repeat up to 60 mL/kg; if still hemodynamically unstable, consider colloid replacement (blood, albumin, fresh frozen plasma) and address other causes for shock.
  - For moderate to severe dehydration in adults: Isotonic saline or Ringer's lactate 20 mL/kg/hr until normal state of consciousness returns or vital signs stabilize. Also consider colloid replacement if continued fluids required beyond 3 L.
- Stage II: Replace fluid deficit along with maintenance over 48 hours. Fluid deficit = preillness weight – illness weight.
- An alternative IVF treatment option for moderate (10%) dehydration in children (6):
  - Bolus with NS/LR at 20 mL/kg for 1 hour
  - Replete fluid deficit with D5 1/2NS + 20 mEq KCl/L at 10 mL/kg for 8 hours (hours 2–9)
  - Replete 1.5× maintenance fluids with D5 1/4NS + 20 mEq/L of KCl for 16 hours (hours 10–24)
- An alternative to IV fluids is hypodermoclysis, the SC infusion of fluids into the body:
  - Indications: Hydration of patients with mild to moderate dehydration who do not tolerate oral intake because of cognitive impairment, severe dysphagia, advanced terminal illness, or intractable vomiting. It is also indicated to prevent dehydration, especially in frail elderly residents living in long-term care settings who reject the oral route for any reason. Useful technique for patients with difficult IV access.
  - Contraindications: Severe dehydration or shock, patients with coagulopathy or receiving full anticoagulation, patients with severe generalized edema (anasarca) or congestive heart failure, and those with fluid overload (7).

Nursing

Strict intake and outputs: Oral and IV intake and output of urine and stool, which may include weighing wet diapers

Discharge Criteria

- Intake > Output
- Underlying etiology treated and improving

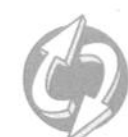

ONGOING CARE

FOLLOW-UP RECOMMENDATIONS

Activity as tolerated:

- If mild-to-moderate dehydration, the patient may be mobile without restrictions, although watch for orthostasis/falls.
- If moderate to severe dehydration, bed rest.

Patient Monitoring

Ongoing surveillance for recurrence

DIET

- Bland food such as a BRAT diet (bananas, rice, apples, toast)
- If diarrhea, avoid dairy for 48 hours after symptoms resolve. One review of weak RCTs and 3 of 5 subsequent RCTs found that lactose-free feeds reduced the duration of diarrhea in children with mild to severe dehydration, compared with lactose-containing feeds. However, 2 subsequent RCTs found no difference between lactose-free and lactose-containing feeds in duration of diarrhea (1)[A].
- Small frequent sips of room-temperature liquids
- For children, Pedialyte (liquid or Popsicles)
- Continue breastfeeding ad lib.

PATIENT EDUCATION

- Patients should go to the nearest emergency facility or call 911 if they or their child feels faint or dizzy when rising from a sitting or lying position, becomes lethargic and/or confused, or complains of a rapid heart rate.
- Patients should call their physician if they are unable to keep down any fluids, vomiting has been going on >24 hours in an adult or >12 hours in a child, diarrhea has lasted >2 days in an adult or child, or an infant or child is much less active than usual or is very irritable.
- Patient information on dehydration: http://www.mayoclinic.com/health/dehydration/DS00561
- Additional patient information: http://familydoctor.org/online/famdocen/home/children/parents/common/stomach/196.html

PROGNOSIS

Self-limited if treated early; potentially fatal

COMPLICATIONS

- Seizures
- Renal failure
- Cardiovascular arrest

REFERENCES

1. Dalby-Payne J. Clinical evidence concise: gastroenteritis in children. *Am Fam Physician*. 2008;77(3):353. Available at: http://www.aafp.org/afp/20080201/bmj.html.
2. Thomas DR, Cote TR, Lawhorne L, et al. Understanding clinical dehydration and its treatment. *J Am Med Dir Assoc*. 2008;9:292–301.
3. Gorelick MH, Shaw KN, Murphy KO. Validity and reliability of clinical signs in the diagnosis of dehydration in children. *Pediatrics*. 1997;99:E6.
4. Leung AK, Robson WL. Acute gastroenteritis in children: role of anti-emetic medication for gastroenteritis-related vomiting. *Paediatr Drugs*. 2007;9:175–84.
5. Barclay L. Adjunctive loperamide therapy reduces acute diarrhea in children. Available at: http://www.medscape.com/viewarticle/554475.
6. Holliday MA, Ray PE, Friedman AL. Fluid therapy for children: facts, fashions and questions. *Arch Dis Child*. 2007;92:546–50.
7. Lopez JH, Reyes-Ortiz CA. Subcutaneous hydration by hypodermoclysis. *Rev Clin Gerontol*. 2010;20(2):105–13.

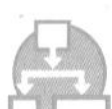

See Also (Topic, Algorithm, Electronic Media Element)

Oral Rehydration

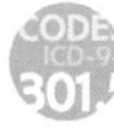

CODES

ICD9

- 276.1 Hyposmolality and/or hyponatremia
- 276.51 Dehydration

CLINICAL PEARLS

- Dehydration is the result of a negative fluid balance and is a common cause of hospitalization in both children and the elderly.
- Begin by assessing the level of dehydration and determining the underlying cause.
- Treatment is directed at restoring fluid balance via oral rehydration therapy or IV fluids and treating underlying causes.

D

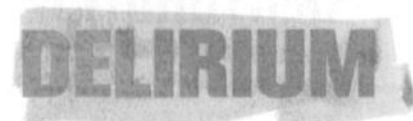

DELIRIUM

Jonathan M. Flacker, MD

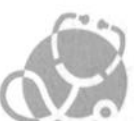

BASICS

DESCRIPTION
- A neurologic complication of illness and/or medication(s) especially common in older patients manifested by confusion and disorientation
- A medical emergency requiring immediate evaluation to decrease morbidity and mortality
- System(s) affected: Nervous
- Synonym(s): Acute confusional state; Altered mental status; Organic brain syndrome; Acute mental status change

EPIDEMIOLOGY
- Predominant age: Older persons
- Predominant sex: Male = Female

Incidence
>50% in high-risk older patients

Prevalence
- 10% in older emergency room patients
- 10–40% in hospitalized older patients
- 25% in older post–acute care patients
- Highest rates (>50%) in intensive care unit (ICU), posthip fracture repair, postcardiothoracic surgery

RISK FACTORS
- Predisposing risk factors:
  - Advanced age
  - Prior cognitive impairment
  - Functional impairment
  - High BUN: Creatinine ratio
  - Dehydration
  - Malnutrition
  - Hearing or vision impairment
  - Frailty
- Precipitating risk factors:
  - Severe illness in any organ system(s)
  - Need for a urinary catheter
  - >3 medications
  - Specific medications, especially long-acting sedative hypnotics (e.g., diazepam and flurazepam), narcotics (especially meperidine), and anticholinergics (especially diphenhydramine)
  - Pain
  - Any adverse iatrogenic event

GENERAL PREVENTION
Follow treatment approach.

PATHOPHYSIOLOGY
- Believed to be a manifestation of homeostenosis (decline in physiologic reserves with aging) resulting in the inability to manage acute and chronic stress (1)
- Neuropathophysiology is not clearly defined; cholinergic deficiency is a leading hypothesis.
- Multicomponent approach addressing contributing factors can reduce incidence and complications.

ETIOLOGY
- Usually multifactorial
- Often interaction between predisposing and precipitating risk factors
- With more predisposing factors (i.e., frail patients), fewer precipitating factors needed to produce delirium
- If few predisposing factors (e.g., very robust patients), more precipitating factors needed to manifest delirium

COMMONLY ASSOCIATED CONDITIONS
Multiple, but most common are:
- New medicine or medicine changes
- Infections (especially lung and urine, but meningitis needs consideration as well)
- Toxic-metabolic (especially low sodium, elevated calcium, renal failure, and hepatic failure)
- Heart attack
- Stroke
- Alcohol or drug withdrawal
- Pre-existing cognitive impairment increases risk.

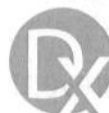

DIAGNOSIS

The Confusion Assessment Method (CAM) is the most well-validated and tested tool, and has been adapted for ICU setting in adults (CAM-ICU) and children (pCAM-ICU).

ALERT
- Key diagnostic features of the CAM (2):
  - Acute change in mental status that fluctuates
  - Abnormal attention and either disorganized thinking or altered level of consciousness
- Any of the following nondiagnostic symptoms may be present:
  - Short- and long-term memory problems
  - Sleep–wake cycle disturbances
  - Hallucinations and/or delusions
  - Emotional lability
  - Tremors and asterixis
- Subtypes based on level of consciousness:
  - Hyperactive delirium (15%): Patients are loud, rambunctious, and disruptive.
  - Hypoactive delirium (20%): Quietly confused; may sit and not eat, drink, or move
  - Mixed delirium (50%): Features of both hyperactive and hypoactive delirium
  - Normal consciousness delirium (15%): Still display disorganized thinking, along with acute onset, inattention, and fluctuation

HISTORY
- Time course of mental status changes
- Recent medication changes
- Symptoms of infection
- New neurologic signs

PHYSICAL EXAM
- Comprehensive cardiorespiratory exam is essential.
- Focal neurologic signs usually absent
- Formal mini mental state exam is not diagnostic, but is helpful as structured interview and followed serially over time.

DIAGNOSTIC TESTS & INTERPRETATION
ECG as necessary

Lab
Guided by history and physical exam

Initial lab tests
- CBC
- Electrolytes, BUN, and creatinine
- Urinalysis, urine culture
- Medication levels (digoxin, theophylline where applicable)

Follow-Up & Special Considerations
If the above does not indicate a precipitator of delirium, consider:
- Arterial blood gases
- Troponin
- Toxicology screen
- Liver panel
- Thyroid-stimulating hormone

Imaging
Guided by history and physical exam

Initial approach
- Chest radiograph for most
- Other if indicated by history and exam

Follow-Up & Special Considerations
Noncontrast-enhanced head CT scan if:
- Unclear diagnosis
- Recent fall
- Receiving anticoagulants
- New focal neurologic signs
- Need to rule out increased intracranial pressure before lumbar puncture

Diagnostic Procedures/Surgery
- Lumbar puncture:
  - Rarely necessary
  - Perform if clinical suspicion of a CNS bleed or infection is high
- EEG:
  - Rarely necessary; consider after above evaluation if:
    - Diagnosis remains unclear
    - Suspicion of seizure activity

DIFFERENTIAL DIAGNOSIS
- Depression (slow onset, disturbance of mood, normal level of consciousness, and fluctuates over weeks to months)
- Dementia (insidious onset, memory problems, normal level of consciousness, and fluctuates over days to weeks)
- Psychosis (rarely sudden onset in older adults)

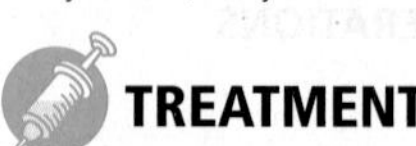

TREATMENT

- Stabilize vitals if needed.
- Ensure immediate evaluation. Addressing 6 risk factors (i.e., cognitive impairment, sleep deprivation, dehydration, immobility, vision impairment, and hearing impairment) in at-risk hospitalized patients can reduce the incidence of delirium by 33%.

MEDICATION
- Nonpharmacologic approaches are preferred for initial treatment, but may be needed for behavioral management, especially in the ICU setting.
- Medications often treat only the symptoms and do not address the underlying cause.

First Line
- Neuroleptics:
  - Haloperidol (Haldol): Initially, 0.25–0.5 mg PO/IM/IV unless urgent sedation needed; re-evaluate and potentially redose hourly
  - Quetiapine (Seroquel): 25–50 mg PO b.i.d.
  - Risperidone (Risperdal): 0.25–0.5 mg/d PO
- Short-acting benzodiazepines if neuroleptics do not work or should be avoided:
  - Lorazepam (Ativan): Initially, 0.25–0.5 mg PO/IM/IV q6–8h; may need to adjust to effect (caution in patients with impaired liver function)

- Contraindications: Avoid neuroleptics in patients with parkinsonism or Parkinson disease.
- Precautions: Neuroleptics may cause extrapyramidal effects, and benzodiazepines may lead to sedation. Both increase the risk of falls.

Second Line

- Olanzapine (Zyprexa): 2.5–5.0 mg/d PO
- Despite multiple trials, there is no evidence to support the use of cholinesterase inhibitors in the prevention or treatment of delirium.

ADDITIONAL TREATMENT

General Measures

- Postoperative patients should be monitored and treated for the following:
  - Myocardial infarction/ischemia
  - Pulmonary complications/pneumonia
  - Pulmonary embolism
  - Urinary or stool retention (attempt catheter removal by postoperative day 2)
- Anesthesia route (general epidural) does not affect the risk of delirium.
- Multifactorial treatment: Identify contributing factors and provide preemptive care to avoid iatrogenic problems (2)[A], with special attention to:
  - CNS oxygen delivery (attempt to attain the following):
    - $SaO_2 > 90\%$ with goal of $SaO_2 > 95\%$
    - Systolic BP $< 2/3$ of baseline or > 90 mm Hg
    - Hematocrit $> 30\%$
- Fluid/electrolyte balance:
  - Sodium, potassium, and glucose normal (glucose < 300 mg/dL in diabetics)
  - Treat fluid overload or dehydration.
- Treat pain:
  - Schedule acetaminophen (1 g q.i.d.) if daily pain
  - Morphine or oxycodone for breakthrough pain if acetaminophen ineffective

ALERT

- Avoid meperidine (Demerol).
- Eliminate unnecessary medications:
  - Investigate new symptoms as potential medication side effects.
- Regulate bowel/bladder function:
  - Bowel movement at least every 48 hours
  - Screen for urinary retention or incontinence, especially after catheter removal.
- Prevent major hospital-acquired problems:
  - 6-inch-thick foam mattress overlay or a pressure-reducing mattress
  - Avoid urinary catheter.
  - Incentive spirometry, if bed-bound
  - SC heparin 5,000 U b.i.d., if bed-fast
  - Environmental stimulation:
    - Glasses and hearing aids
    - Clock and calendar
    - Soft lighting
    - Radio, tapes, and television, if desired
  - Sleep:
    - Quiet environment
    - Soft music
    - Therapeutic massage
- Restraints do not reduce risk of falls/injury:
  - Use only in the most difficult-to-manage patients, as briefly as possible.

Issues for Referral

Psychiatric and/or neurologic assessment helpful if delirium is not easily explainable after full evaluation

Additional Therapies

Early mobilization critical:

- Out of bed on hospital day 2 (or postoperative day 1) if no contraindications
- Out of bed several hours daily if able
- Daily therapy if not ambulating independently
- Daily therapy if not functionally independent

IN-PATIENT CONSIDERATIONS

General measures described above are also applicable to delirium prevention.

Admission Criteria

New delirium is a medical emergency and requires admission, except in the setting of palliative home care.

IV Fluids

As needed for dehydration

Nursing

- Institute skin care program for patients with established incontinence.
- Turning regimen if at risk of pressure ulcers
- Soft restraints are acceptable for a short time only if needed for protection of patient and others.

Discharge Criteria

- Resolution of precipitating factor(s)
- Safe discharge site if still delirious

ONGOING CARE

FOLLOW-UP RECOMMENDATIONS

- If delirium at discharge, will usually be followed in postacute facility
- If no delirium at discharge, follow up with primary care physician in 1–2 weeks.
- As tolerated
- Early physical therapy consultation to prevent deconditioning

Patient Monitoring

- Evaluate and assess mental status daily.
- Depends on specific conditions present

DIET

- Nutritional supplements (1–3 cans daily) if intake is poor
- Temporary nasogastric tube if unable to eat and bowels working

PROGNOSIS

- Usually improves with treatment of underlying condition, but may become chronic
- Delirium complicating medical illness significantly increases a person's chance of dying from that illness

COMPLICATIONS

- Falls
- Pressure ulcers
- Malnutrition
- Functional decline
- Oversedation
- Polypharmacy

REFERENCES

1. Jones RN, Fong TG, Metzger E, et al. Aging, brain disease, and reserve: Implications for delirium. *Am J Geriatr Psychiatry*. 2010;18(2):117–27.
2. Fong TG, Tulebave SR, Inouye SK. Delirium in elderly adults: Diagnosis, prevention, and treatment. *Nat Rev Neurol*. 2009;5:210–20.

ADDITIONAL READING

- van Eijk MM, van Marum RJ, Klijn IA, et al. Comparison of delirium assessment tools in a mixed intensive care unit. *Crit Care Med*. 2009;37:1881–5.
- Yang FM, Marcantonio ER, Inouye SK, et al. Phenomenological subtypes of delirium in older persons: Patterns, prevalence, and prognosis. *Psychosomatics*. 2009;50:248–54.

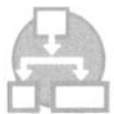

See Also (Topic, Algorithm, Electronic Media Element)

- Dementia; Depression; Substance Use Disorders
- Algorithm: Delirium

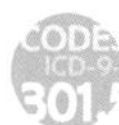

CODES

ICD9

- 293.0 Delirium due to conditions classified elsewhere
- 293.1 Subacute delirium
- 293.9 Unspecified transient mental disorder in conditions classified elsewhere

CLINICAL PEARLS

- The Confusion Assessment Method (CAM) criteria for delirium are acute onset of fluctuating mental status, inattention, disorganized thinking, and either disorganized thinking or altered level of consciousness.
- In the absence of active monitoring, the hypoactive subtype of delirium can easily be missed.
- Addressing 6 risk factors (i.e., cognitive impairment, sleep deprivation, dehydration, immobility, vision impairment, and hearing impairment) in at-risk hospitalized patients can reduce the incidence of delirium by 33%.
- Delirium may not resolve as soon as the treatable contributors are fixed; resolution may take weeks or months. Rarely will become chronic.
- Avoid diphenhydramine in older patients. Nonpharmacologic measures are preferable as a sleep aid, but if needed, zolpidem (5 mg at bedtime) or trazodone (25 mg at bedtime) are reasonable alternatives.

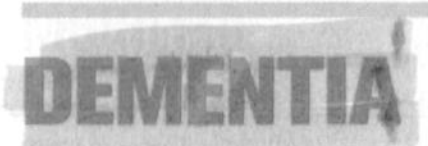

DEMENTIA

Alicia R. Desilets, PharmD
Karen Bryant, MD
Jill A. Grimes, MD

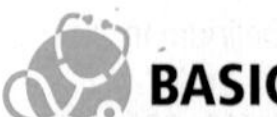

BASICS

DESCRIPTION

Dementia is a decline in cognitive function caused by a number of disorders:

- Alzheimer dementia (AD):
  - Progressive deterioration of higher cortical functioning
- Vascular dementia (VaD):
  - Usually correlated with a cerebrovascular event and/or cerebrovascular disease
  - Stepwise deterioration with periods of clinical plateaus
- Lewy body dementia:
  - Fluctuating cognition associated with parkinsonism, hallucinations and delusions, gait difficulties, and falls
- Frontotemporal dementia:
  - Language difficulties, personality changes, and behavioral disturbances
- Creutzfeldt-Jacob disease (CJD):
  - Very rare; rapid onset

EPIDEMIOLOGY

Prevalence

- In patients ≥71 years old:
  - AD: 70%
  - VaD: 17%
  - Other: 13%
- AD 60–64 years: <1%, approximately doubles every 5 years after age 60
- Estimated 5.4 million Americans had AD in 2010:
  - 5 million >65 years old; 200,000 <65 years

RISK FACTORS

- Increasing age
- Female > Male
- Lower educational status
- Genetic predisposition
- Head injury early in life
- Sedentary lifestyle
- Hypertension: AD; VaD
- Hypercholesterolemia: AD; VaD
- Diabetes: VaD
- Cigarette smoking: VaD

Genetics

- AD: Positive family history in 50%, but 90% AD is sporadic:
  - APOE4 increases risk, but full role unclear
- Familial/autosomal dominant AD accounts for <5% AD
  - Amyloid precursor protein (APP), presenilin-1 (PS-1), and presenilin-2 (PS-2)

GENERAL PREVENTION

Data supporting specific preventative measures are limited and not conclusive:

- Smoking cessation
- Physical and mental activity
- Treatment of hypertension, hypercholesterolemia, and diabetes

- There is no evidence for statins (or any other specific medication) to prevent onset of dementia (1)[A].

ETIOLOGY

- AD: Unknown, but involves amyloid beta accumulation initially, then synaptic dysfunction, neurodegeneration, and eventual neuronal loss
  - Age, genetics, systemic disease, behaviors (smoking), and other host factors may influence the response to amyloid beta and/or the pace of progression toward the clinical manifestations of AD.
- VaD:
  - Cerebral atherosclerosis or emboli with clinical or subclinical infarcts

COMMONLY ASSOCIATED CONDITIONS

- Anxiety and depression
- Delirium
- Behavioral disturbances (agitation, aggression)
- Sleep disturbances
- Caregiver stress

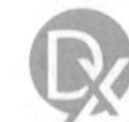

DIAGNOSIS

HISTORY

Probable diagnosis AD (2)[A]:

- Age between 40 and 90 (usually >65)
- Progressive cognitive decline of insidious onset
- No disturbances of consciousness
- Deficits in >2 areas of cognition
- No other explainable cause of symptoms
- Specifically, rule out thyroid disease, vitamin deficiency (B_{12}), grief reaction
- Supportive factors: Family history

PHYSICAL EXAM

- No disturbances of consciousness
- Cognitive decline demonstrated by standardized instruments, including:
  - Mini-Mental Status Exam
  - ADAS-Cog
  - Clock draw test
  - Change test
  - Although caution in relying solely on cognition scores, especially in those with learning difficulty, language barriers, or similar limitations (3)[A]
- Deficits in >2 areas of cognition

DIAGNOSTIC TESTS & INTERPRETATION

Lab

Initial lab tests

- Used to rule out other causes (2)[A]:
  - Comprehensive metabolic profile
  - CBC
  - Thyroid-stimulating hormone
  - Vitamin B_{12} level
  - Neuroimaging (preferably MRI of brain)
- Select patients:
  - HIV
  - Rapid plasma reagin
  - ESR
  - Folate
  - Heavy metal screen
  - Toxicology screen
- Biomarkers: In research settings only, may prove helpful in differential dx of dementia types; CSF Tau proteins very increased in CJD (4)[A]

Imaging

Tests that support the diagnosis:

- Cerebral atrophy on neuroimaging
- Normal lumbar puncture

Initial approach

- Early age of onset (<65 years old), rapid progression, focal neurologic deficits, cerebrovascular disease risk, or atypical symptoms: Neuroimaging (MRI or CT) to rule out other causes (2)[A]
- Important findings:
  - AD: Diffuse cerebral atrophy starting in association areas, hippocampus, amygdala
  - VaD: Old infarcts, including lacunes

Diagnostic Procedures/Surgery

Positron emission tomography (PET) scan not routinely recommended; has been approved to differentiate between Alzheimer disease and frontotemporal dementia (5)[A]

Pathological Findings

AD:

- Neurofibrillary tangles: Abnormally phosphorylated tau protein
- Senile plaques: Amyloid precursor protein derivatives
- Microvascular amyloid

DIFFERENTIAL DIAGNOSIS

- Mild cognitive impairment
- Major depression
- Medication side effect
- Chronic alcohol use
- Delirium
- Subdural hematoma
- Normal pressure hydrocephalus
- Brain tumor
- Thyroid disease
- Parkinson disease
- Vitamin B_{12} deficiency
- Toxins (aromatic hydrocarbons, solvents, heavy metals, marijuana, opiates, sedative-hypnotics)

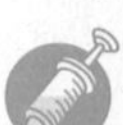

TREATMENT

MEDICATION

First Line

- Cognitive dysfunction, mild (5)[A]:
  - Cholinesterase inhibitors: Donepezil (Aricept), 5–10 mg/d; rivastigmine (Exelon), 1.5–6 mg b.i.d., transdermal system 4.6 mg/24 hours and 9.5 mg/24 hours; galantamine (Razadyne), 4–12 mg b.i.d., extended release 8–24 mg/d:
    - Adverse events: Nausea, vomiting, diarrhea, anorexia, nightmares
    - Galantamine warning: Associated with mortality in patients with mild cognitive impairment in clinical trial
    - Start drug with lowest acquisition cost; also consider adverse event profile, adherence, medical comorbidity, drug interactions, and dosing profiles (3)
- Cognitive dysfunction, moderate to severe (5)[A]:
  - Cholinesterase inhibitors OR

- Memantine (Namenda), 5–20 mg/d:
    - Adverse events: Dizziness, confusion, headache, constipation
- OR combination cholinesterase inhibitor and memantine

- Commonly associated conditions:
    - Psychosis and agitation/aggressive behavior:
        - Antipsychotics: Initiate low doses, haloperidol 0.25–0.5 mg/d; risperidone 0.25–1 mg/d; clozapine 12.5 mg/d; olanzapine 1.25–5 mg/d; quetiapine 12.5–50 mg/d; aripiprazole 5 mg/d; ziprasidone 20 mg/d (5)[A]
        - Atypical antipsychotics associated with a better side effect profile; quetiapine and aripiprazole often first-line due to decreased extrapyramidal side effects

ALERT

- Black box warning on atypical antipsychotics due to increased mortality found when used in elderly patients with dementia
- Depression:
    - SSRIs: Initiate low doses, citalopram (Celexa) 10 mg/d; escitalopram (Lexapro) 5 mg/d; sertraline (Zoloft) 25 mg/d (5)[A]
    - Adverse events: Nausea, vomiting, agitation, parkinsonian effects, sexual dysfunction, hyponatremia
    - Fluoxetine (Prozac) and paroxetine (Paxil) should be avoided in elderly patients.
- Sleep disturbances:
    - Mirtazapine (7.5–60 mg) or trazodone (25–100 mg) at bedtime if patient also has depression (5)[A]
    - Atypical antipsychotics if psychotic symptoms present (5)[A]
    - Zolpidem (5–10 mg); zaleplon (5–10 mg) (5)[A]
    - Benzodiazepines only for short term if anxiety or as needed: Lorazepam 0.5–1.0 mg; oxazepam 7.5–15 mg (5)[A]

Second Line

Associated conditions:

- Depression: Venlafaxine, mirtazapine, and bupropion (5)[A]
- Psychosis and agitation/aggressive behavior:
    - Some data for SSRIs (5)[A]
    - Benzodiazepines if agitation with anxiety; in elderly, use as needed (5)[A]

Geriatric Considerations

- Initiate pharmacotherapy at low doses and titrate slowly up if necessary.
- If benzodiazepines indicated for anxiety, choose drug with short half-life
- Watch decreased renal function and hepatic metabolism.

ADDITIONAL TREATMENT

Behavioral modification:

- Socialization such as adult day care to prevent isolation and depression
- Sleep hygiene program as alternative to pharmaceuticals for sleep disturbance
- Scheduled toileting to prevent incontinence

General Measures

- Daily schedules and written directions
- Emphasis on nutrition, personal hygiene, accident-proofing the home, safety issues, sleep hygiene and supervision
- Socialization (adult day care)
- Sensory stimulation (display of clocks and calendars) in the early to middle stages
- Discussion with the family concerning support and advance directives

Issues for Referral

- Neuropsychiatric evaluation particularly helpful in early stages or mild cognitive impairment
- Assessment and management of the following:
    - Cognitive problems
    - Mood disorders (e.g., depression, anxiety)
    - Psychosis
    - Behavioral problems (e.g., agitation, aggression)

COMPLEMENTARY AND ALTERNATIVE MEDICINE

- Vitamin E is no longer recommended due to lack of evidence and possible association with an increase in mortality (5)[A].
- Ginkgo biloba not recommended due to lack of evidence (5)[A].
- Huperzine-A appears to have potential in small trials; however, clinical evidence lacking to recommend.
- NSAIDs, selegiline, and estrogen lack efficacy and safety data (5)[A].

IN-PATIENT CONSIDERATIONS

Admission Criteria

- Patients who cannot be treated in an outpatient setting
- Patients who may require geropsychiatry admission for aggressive behaviors

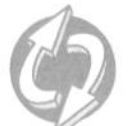

ONGOING CARE

FOLLOW-UP RECOMMENDATIONS

Patient Monitoring

- Progression of cognitive impairment by use of standardized tool (e.g., MMSE, ADAS-Cog)
- Development of behavioral problems
- Adverse events of pharmacotherapy
- Nutritional status
- Caregiver evaluation of stress
- Evaluate issues that may affect quality of life.

PATIENT EDUCATION

- Safety concerns
- Long-term issues: Management of finances, medical decision making, possible placement when appropriate
- Advance directives

PROGNOSIS

- AD: Progressive disease (variable rates) leading to profound cognitive impairment:
    - Without treatment, average decline on MMSE of 2 points per year
- VaD: Less likely to be progressive, but cognitive improvement is unlikely
- Secondary dementias: Treatment of the underlying condition may lead to improvement.

COMPLICATIONS

- Wandering
- Falls with injury:
    - Hip fracture
    - Head trauma
    - Subdural hematoma
- Aspiration pneumonia in end stage
- Caregiver burnout

REFERENCES

1. McGuinness B, Craig D, Bullock R, et al. Statins for the prevention of dementia. *Cochrane Database Syst Rev*. 2009;CD003160.
2. Blass DM, Rabins PV. In the clinic. Dementia. *Ann Intern Med*. 2008;148:ITC4–1-ITC4-16.
3. National Institute for Health and Clinical Excellence. Dementia: Supporting people with dementia and their carers in health and social care. 2011.
4. van Harten AC, Kester MI, Visser PJ, et al. Tau and p-tau as CSF biomarkers in dementia: A meta-analysis. *Clin Chem Lab Med*. 2011;49:353–66.
5. APA Work Group on Alzheimer's Disease and Other Dementias, Rabins PV, Blacker D. American Psychiatric Association practice guideline for the treatment of patients with Alzheimer's disease and other dementias. 2nd ed. *Am J Psychiatry*. 2007;164:5–56.

ADDITIONAL READING

- Birks J. Cholinesterase inhibitors for Alzheimer's disease. *Cochrane Database Syst Rev*. 2006;CD005593.
- Blennow K, de Leon MJ, Zetterberg H. Alzheimer's disease. *Lancet*. 2006;368:387–403.
- Burns A, Iliffe S. Alzheimer's disease. *BMJ*. 2009;338:b158.
- Lleó A, Greenberg SM, Growdon JH. Current pharmacotherapy for Alzheimer's disease. *Annu Rev Med*. 2006;57:513–33.
- Lyketsos CG, Colenda CC, Beck C. Position statement of the American Association for Geriatric Psychiatry regarding principles of care for patients with dementia resulting from Alzheimer disease. *Am J Geriatr Psychiatry*. 2006;14:561–72.

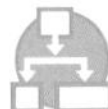

See Also (Topic, Algorithm, Electronic Media Element)

Algorithm: Dementia

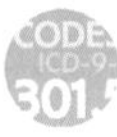

CODES

ICD9

- 290.0 Senile dementia, uncomplicated
- 290.40 Vascular dementia, uncomplicated
- 331.0 Alzheimer's disease

CLINICAL PEARLS

- Dementia is loss of cognitive function in multiple areas.
- Time is diagnostic; AD is a progressive disease that will manifest with continual decline over time.
- Medications for AD show a small, statistically significant improvement in some cognitive measures, but it remains unclear if the improvement is clinically significant.

DEMENTIA, VASCULAR

Birju B. Patel, MD, FACP
N. Wilson Holland, MD

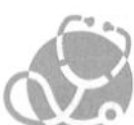

BASICS

Vascular dementia is a heterogeneous disorder caused by the sequel of cerebrovascular disease that manifests in cognitive impairment affecting memory, thinking, language, behavior, and judgment.

DESCRIPTION

- Vascular dementia (previously known as multi-infarct dementia) was first mentioned by Thomas Willis in 1672. It was later further described in the late 19th century by Binswanger and Alzheimer as a separate entity from dementia paralytica caused by neurosyphillis. This concept has evolved tremendously since the advent of neuroimaging modalities.
- Synonym(s): Vascular cognitive impairment (VCI); Vascular cognitive disorder (VCD); Arteriosclerotic dementia; Post-stroke dementia; Senile dementia due to hardening of the arteries; Binswanger disease.

EPIDEMIOLOGY

- It is the second most common cause of dementia after Alzheimer dementia in the elderly.
- After careful consideration of the difficulties in diagnosing vascular dementia, and the many geographical and methodological differences, there is a lack of agreement in terms of its prevalence and epidemiology.

Incidence

About 6–12 cases per 1,000 person years >70

Prevalence

- About 1.2–4.2% in those >65
- 14–32% prevalence of dementia after a stroke (7)

RISK FACTORS

- Age
- Previous stroke
- Smoking
- Diabetes
- Hypertension
- Atrial fibrillation
- Peripheral vascular disease (PVD)
- Hyperlipidemia
- Metabolic syndrome
- Coronary atherosclerotic heart disease

Genetics

- Cerebral autosomal dominant arteriopathy (CADASIL) is caused by a mutation in the NOTCH3 gene on chromosome 19 that results in leukoencephalopathy and subcortical infarcts. This is clinically manifested in recurrent strokes and associated cognitive decline (1).
- Apolipoprotein E gene type: Those with ApoE4 subtypes are at higher risk of developing both vascular and Alzheimer dementia.
- Amyloid precursor protein (APP) gene: Leads to a form of vascular dementia called heritable cerebral hemorrhage with amyloidosis (2).

GENERAL PREVENTION

- Optimization and aggressive treatment of vascular risk factors such as hypertension, diabetes, and hyperlipidemia
- Hypertension is the single most modifiable risk factor and must be optimized.
- Lifestyle modification: Weight loss, physical activity, smoking cessation
- Medication management for vascular risk reduction: Aspirin usage, statin therapy for hyperlipidemia, antihypertensive therapy

PATHOPHYSIOLOGY

Upon autopsy of those with dementia, 1/3 have significant vascular pathology present but this is not necessarily correlated clinically with vascular dementia (3). There are no set pathological criteria for the diagnosis of vascular dementia such as those that exist for Alzheimer dementia:

- Large vessel disease: Cognitive impairment that follows a stroke
- Small vessel disease: Includes white matter changes (leukoaraiosis), subcortical infarcts, and incomplete infarction. This is usually the most common cause of multi-infarct dementia.
- Subcortical ischemic vascular disease: Due to small vessel involvement within cerebral white matter, brainstem, and basal ganglia. Lacunar infarcts and deep white matter changes are typically included in this category (4).
- Noninfarct ischemic changes and atrophy (5)

ETIOLOGY

- Transient ischemic attack (TIA)/stroke
- Vascular, demographic, genetic factors
- Vascular disease (i.e., hypertension, PVD, atrial fibrillation, hyperlipidemia, diabetes, etc.)

COMMONLY ASSOCIATED CONDITIONS

- CADASIL
- Cerebral amyloid angiopathy (CAA): Accumulation of amyloid in cerebral vasculature resulting in infarctions and hemorrhages

DIAGNOSIS

Differentiation between Alzheimer dementia and vascular dementia can be difficult, and there can be significant overlap in the clinical presentation of these 2 dementias. The diagnosis of vascular dementia is a clinical diagnosis.

HISTORY

- Gradual, stepwise progression is typical.
- Ask about onset and progression of cognitive impairment and the specific cognitive domains involved.
- Ask about vascular risk factors and previous attempts to control these risk factors.
- Ask about medication compliance.
- Ask about urinary incontinence and gait disturbances.
- Look for early symptoms including difficulty performing cognitive tasks, memory, mood, and assessment of instrumental activities of daily living (IADLs) (5).
- Past history may include TIAs, cerebrovascular accidents, coronary atherosclerotic heart disease, atrial fibrillation, hyperlipidemia, and/or peripheral vascular disease.

PHYSICAL EXAM

- Screen for hypertension.
- Focal neurological deficits may be present.
- Gait assessment is important especially looking at gait initiation, gait speed, and balance.
- Check for carotid bruits as well as abdominal bruits and assess for presence of peripheral vascular disease.
- Check body mass index and waist circumference.
- Do a thorough cardiac evaluation that includes looking for arrhythmias (i.e., atrial fibrillation).

DIAGNOSTIC TESTS & INTERPRETATION

- Cognitive testing, such as Mini-Cog, mini-mental status exam (MMSE), Saint Louis University Mental Status (SLUMS), and Montreal Cognitive Assessment (MOCA), provides more definitive information in terms of cognitive deficits, especially executive function, which may be lost earlier in vascular dementia (5).
- Neuropsychological testing may also be beneficial especially in evaluating multiple cognitive domains and their specific involvements and deficits.

Lab

As appropriate, consider: CBC, comprehensive metabolic profile, lipid panel, thyroid function, hemoglobin A1C, vitamin B_{12}.

Imaging

- Imaging is used in conjunction with history and physical examination to support a clinical diagnosis of vascular dementia.
- Cognitive deficits observed clinically do not always have to correlate with findings found on neuroimaging studies.
- MRI is best in terms of evaluation of subtle subcortical deficits.

DIFFERENTIAL DIAGNOSIS

- Alzheimer dementia
- Depression
- Drug intoxication
- CNS tumors
- Hypothyroidism
- Vitamin B_{12} deficiency

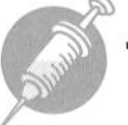

TREATMENT

Prevention is the real key to treatment:

- Control of risk factors including hypertension, hyperlipidemia, and diabetes
- Avoidance of tobacco and smoking cessation
- Healthy, low-cholesterol diet

MEDICATION

- Acetylcholinesterase inhibitors may be used but are of limited benefit in vascular dementia (6).
- The clinical evidence for use of memantine is not as strong as for acetylcholinesterase inhibitors and, therefore, the clinical benefit is likely modest.
- Controlling BP with any antihypertensive medications, treatment of dyslipidemia (e.g., statins), and treatment of diabetes are very important (7).

ADDITIONAL TREATMENT

- Limit alcohol intake to ≤1 drink per day in women and 2 per day in men.
- Heavy sustained alcohol use contributes to hypertension.
- Aspirin and/or clopidogrel may be useful in some cases.

COMPLEMENTARY AND ALTERNATIVE MEDICINE

Ginkgo biloba should be avoided due to increased risk of bleeding especially in cerebral amyloid angiopathy.

SURGERY/OTHER PROCEDURES

Carotid endarterectomy or stenting if evidence of significant internal carotid artery stenosis (i.e., >70–80%).

IN-PATIENT CONSIDERATIONS

- Remain sensitive to functional assessment and avoidance of pressure ulcers after cerebrovascular accidents (CVAs).
- Urinary incontinence treatment may be needed after CVA.
- Avoid Foley catheter usage unless absolutely necessary due to increased risk of infection.

Nursing

- Nonpharmacological approaches to behavior management should be attempted prior to medication usage.
- Providing optimal sensory input to patients with cognitive impairment is important during hospitalizations to avoid delirium and confusion. Patients should be given frequent cues to keep them oriented to place and time. They should be informed of any changes in the daily schedule of activities and evaluations. Family and caregivers should be encouraged to be with patients with dementia as much as possible to further help them from becoming confused during hospitalization. Recreational, physical, occupational, and music therapy can be beneficial during hospitalization in avoiding delirium and preventing functional decline.
- Particular emphasis has to be placed on screening for and optimizing the mood of the patient. Depression is very common in older patients especially those that have had strokes and have become hospitalized. Depression in itself can present as "pseudodementia" with worsening confusion during hospitalization and is a treatable condition.

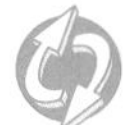

ONGOING CARE

Vascular dementia is a condition that should be followed with multiple visits in the office setting with goals of optimizing cardiovascular risk profiles for patients. Future planning and advanced directives should be addressed early. Family and caregiver evaluation and burden should also be evaluated.

FOLLOW-UP RECOMMENDATIONS

Perform regular follow-up with a primary care provider or geriatrician for risk-factor modification and education on importance of regular physical and mental exercises as tolerated.

Patient Monitoring

Appropriate evaluation and diagnosis of this condition, need for future planning, optimizing vascular risk factors, lifestyle modification counseling, therapeutic interventions

DIET

- The American Heart Association diet and dietary approaches to stop hypertension (DASH) diet is recommended for optimal BP and cardiovascular risk factor control.
- Low-fat, decreased concentrated sweets and carbohydrates, especially in those with metabolic syndrome

PATIENT EDUCATION

- Lifestyle modification is important in vascular risk reduction (smoking cessation, exercise counseling, dietary counseling, weight-loss counseling).
- Optimizing vascular risk factors via medications (i.e., hypertension, diabetes, atrial fibrillation, PVD, heart disease)
- Avoiding smoking, including second-hand smoke.
- Home BP monitoring and glucometer testing of blood sugars if hypertension, impaired glucose tolerance and/or diabetes is present
- Instruct patients to call 911 for any TIA type symptoms.

PROGNOSIS

- Lost cognitive abilities that persist after initial recovery of deficits from stroke do not usually return. Some individuals can have intermittent periods of self-reported improvement in cognitive function.
- Risk factors for progression of cognitive and functional impairment poststroke include age, prestroke cognitive abilities, depression, polypharmacy, and decreased cerebral perfusion during acute stroke.

COMPLICATIONS

- Physical disability from stroke
- Severe cognitive impairment
- Death

REFERENCES

1. Pinkston JB, Alekseeva N, González Toledo E, et al. Stroke and dementia. *Neurol Res*. 2009;31:824–31.
2. Russell MB, et al. Genetics of dementia. *Acta Neurol Scand Suppl*. 2010:58–61.
3. OBrien RJ, et al. Vascular dementia: Atherosclerosis, cognition and Alzheimer disease. *Curr Alzheimer Res*. 2011;8(4):341–4.
4. Chui HC, et al. Subcortical ischemic vascular dementia. *Neurol Clin*. 2007;25:717–40, vi.
5. Moorhouse P, Rockwood K, et al. Vascular cognitive impairment: Current concepts and clinical developments. *Lancet Neurol*. 2008;7:246–55.
6. Kavirajan H, Schneider LS, et al. Efficacy and adverse effects of cholinesterase inhibitors and memantine in vascular dementia: A meta-analysis of randomised controlled trials. *Lancet Neurol*. 2007;6:782–92.
7. Gorelick PB, et al. Vascular contributions to cognitive impairment and dementia: A statement for healthcare professionals from the American Heart Association/American Stroke Association. *Stroke*. 2011;42(9):2672–713.

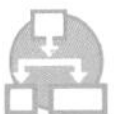

See Also (Topic, Algorithm, Electronic Media Element)

Alzheimer Disease; Depression; Mild Cognitive Impairment

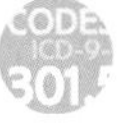

CODES

ICD9

290.40 Vascular dementia, uncomplicated

CLINICAL PEARLS

- Executive dysfunction and gait abnormalities are often seen early and are more pronounced in vascular dementia as opposed to Alzheimer dementia (1,5).
- Memory is relatively preserved in vascular dementia when compared to Alzheimer dementia in the early stages of this disease (1).
- Stepwise progression, as opposed to progressive decline in Alzheimer dementia, is typical.
- There is a considerable overlap between vascular dementia and Alzheimer dementia in clinical practice and classification into one of these categories is often difficult.

DENTAL INFECTION

Hugh J. Silk, MD, MPH
Sheila O. Stille, DMD, MAGD
Amy Li, DMD

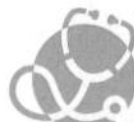

BASICS

DESCRIPTION

- Very painful area ± swelling in the head and neck region arising from the teeth and supporting structures. If left untreated, can lead to serious and potentially life-threatening illnesses.
- Assume any head and neck infection or swelling to be odontogenic in origin until proven otherwise.

EPIDEMIOLOGY

Incidence

- Caries is a contagious bacterial infection that is transmitted vertically from caregivers.
- The introduction of fluoride has dramatically decreased dental caries.

Prevalence

25% of children between ages of 5 and 17 years account for 80% of caries in the US (1).

RISK FACTORS

- Low socioeconomic status
- Poor access to dental and health care
- Fear of dentist
- Poor oral hygiene
- Poor nutrition including high level of sugary foods and drinks
- Prior trauma to the teeth or jaws
- Heavily restored dentition
- Inadequate fluoride
- Gingival recession (increased risk of root caries)
- Physical and mental disabilities
- Decreased salivary flow (e.g., use of anticholinergic medications)

GENERAL PREVENTION

- Prevent caries and contagious bacterial infection (*Streptococcus mutans*)
- Majority of dental problems can be avoided through flossing, brushing with fluoride toothpaste, systemic fluoride (water or supplements), fluoride varnish for high-risk patients, and biannual cleaning (2,3)[A,B].
- Consider prevention of transmission of *S. mutans* from mother to infant by improving mother's dentition and bacterial load through proper dental care, xylitol gum
- Avoid smoking; linked to severe periodontal disease
- Good control of systemic diseases (e.g., diabetes)

PATHOPHYSIOLOGY

Caries or trauma can lead to pulpal death, which in turn leads to infection of pulp and/or abscess of adjacent tissues via direct or hematogenous bacterial colonization.

ETIOLOGY

- *S. mutans* vertically transmitted to newly dentate infants from caregivers
- Acidic secretions from *S. mutans* are implicated in early caries.
- Often polymicrobial
- Anaerobes, including *Pepto streptococci*, *Bacteroides*, *Prevotella*, and *Fusobacterium*, have been implicated. *Lactobacilli* may subsequently be involved.

COMMONLY ASSOCIATED CONDITIONS

- Rampant caries throughout dentition; multiple missing teeth
- Periodontal abscess
- Soft tissue cellulitis
- Pericoronitis (inflamed ± infection of gum flap over molar)
- Periodontitis (deep inflammation ± infection of gingiva and ligaments)

DIAGNOSIS

HISTORY

- Pain at infected site or referred to ears, jaw, cheek, or sinuses
- Sensitivity to hot or cold stimuli
- Unprovoked, intermittent, or constant throb along nerve pathway
- Pain on biting
- Trismus (inability to open mouth)
- Bleeding or purulent drainage from gingival tissues
- When severe infection (systemic):
  - Fever
  - Difficulty breathing or swallowing
  - Death
- Children <4 years with stiff neck, sore throat, and dysphagia should be worked up for retropharyngeal abscess secondary to molar infection.

PHYSICAL EXAM

- Gingival edema and erythema
- Cheek or intraoral swelling
- Presence of fluctuant mass
- Suppuration of gingival margin or tooth
- Lymphadenopathy
- Severe infection may present with dysphagia, fever, and signs of airway compromise.

DIAGNOSTIC TESTS & INTERPRETATION

Lab

Initial lab tests

- No initial labs needed, unless patient looks acutely ill
- If acutely ill:
  - Consider CBC with differential.
  - Culture and sensitivity; if abscess present, aspirate pus. Test for aerobes and anaerobes.
  - Note: Multiple organisms involved, most likely anaerobic gram-negative rods and anaerobic gram-positive cocci (2).

Imaging

Initial approach

- Individual dental films of suspected teeth
- Panoramic film of the teeth and jaw for evaluation of the extent of infection

Follow-Up & Special Considerations

CT scan can be used to determine the extent and density of the swelling, locating the abscess within the soft tissue and bone. This aids in determining treatment course.

DIFFERENTIAL DIAGNOSIS

- Bacterial or viral throat infection
- Otitis media
- Sinusitis
- Viral or aphthous stomatitis
- Temporomandibular joint (TMJ) dysfunction (myofascial pain)
- Parotitis
- Cyst
- Jaw pain can be anginal equivalent, especially in women, and especially lower-left portion of the jaw.

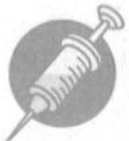

TREATMENT

- Place patient on appropriate antibiotic, if indicated (if systemic). Or if localized, incision and drainage may be warranted.
- Tend to appropriate pain control: Anti-inflammatory agents
- Refer to dentist as soon as possible for definitive treatment: Root canal or extraction
- If infection is severe, consider hospitalization with IV antibiotics until stabilized. Patient may need incision and drainage of abscess.

MEDICATION

First Line

- Penicillin VK loading dose of 1,000 mg, followed by 500 mg q.i.d. for 7–10 days. In children, 40–60 mg/kg/d divided q.i.d.
- Amoxicillin loading dose of 1,000 mg, followed by 500 mg t.i.d. for 7–10 days. In children, 40–60 mg/kg/d divided t.i.d.
- If penicillin-allergic, use clindamycin.

Second Line

If long-standing infection or previously treated infection that does not respond to first-line treatment:

- Clindamycin 300 mg PO t.i.d. for 7–10 days
- If severe infection, load with clindamycin 600 mg, 900 mg IV, then 300 mg q6h; consider double coverage with metronidazole.

ADDITIONAL TREATMENT

General Measures

- Ibuprofen 600–800 mg (or 10 mg/kg) q6h, or acetaminophen 650–1,000 mg (10–15 mg/kg) q4–6h
- For more severe pain, consider acetaminophen or ibuprofen + opioids.
- Can consider local anesthetic nerve block with long-acting anesthetic (bupivacaine) as adjunct; avoid penetrating infection with needle to avoid tracking infection.

Issues for Referral

A dentist should be consulted and follow-up definitive care appointment should be secured prior to discharge from medical office, emergency room, or hospital unit.

SURGERY/OTHER PROCEDURES

- Incision and drainage of abscess should be performed if abscess is large and fluctuant.
- Root canal or extraction should be performed as definitive treatment.

IN-PATIENT CONSIDERATIONS

Initial Stabilization

- Secure airway, if compromised, with either endotracheal intubation or tracheotomy.
- IV fluid resuscitation with normal saline may be indicated in acutely ill patients.

Admission Criteria

Criteria for hospital admission include swelling involving deep spaces of the neck, unstable vital signs, fever, chills, confusion or delirium, or evidence of invasive infection or cellulitis.

Nursing

- Ensure good oral hygiene.
- Rinse mouth with chlorhexidine gluconate 2 times per day.
- Use warm salt water rinses several times per day to encourage drainage, especially after incision and drainage.

Discharge Criteria

Discharge patient if:

- Airway not compromised
- Abscess and sepsis eliminated
- Able to take PO intake and ambulate

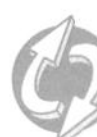

ONGOING CARE

Educate patient in need for proper oral hygiene, need for follow-up dental care, need for routine dental care, and stress medical complications that can and have occurred due to lack of dental care.

FOLLOW-UP RECOMMENDATIONS

- Follow-up with dentist within 24 hours.
- Ensure adequate PO intake, including protein.

DIET

- Maintain a healthy diet. Bacteria thrive on refined sugar and starch.
- Avoid sugary foods that stick between the teeth.

Pediatric Considerations

In children, limit the frequency of sugary drinks, and advise against sleeping with a bottle to decrease the chance of dental caries.

PATIENT EDUCATION

- Biannual dental visits
- Nutritional education
- Limit the frequency of sugar/carbonated drinks and sugary or sticky foods.
- In young children, avoid sleeping with a bottle to decrease the chance of dental caries.
- Brush and floss daily.
- Caretakers should tend to their personal oral hygiene, ± chlorhexidine rinses in first 3 years of the child's life to decrease the risk of transmission of the caries-causing microorganisms.

PROGNOSIS

Prognosis is excellent with proper treatment.

COMPLICATIONS

- Ludwig angina
- Retropharyngeal and mediastinal infection
- Osteomyelitis
- Endocarditis
- Submental infection
- Submandibular infection
- Can cause unstable diabetes in diabetics/worsen pre-existing heart disease
- Possible link to preterm labor
- Brain abscess/death

REFERENCES

1. Kaste LM, Selwitz RH, Oldakowski RJ, et al. Coronal caries in the primary and permanent dentition of children and adolescents 1–17 years of age: United States, 1988–1991. *J Dent Res*. 1996;75:631–41.
2. Lockhart PB, ed. *Dental Care of the Medically Complex Patient*, 5th ed. New York: Elsevier; 2004.
3. Marinho VCC, et al. Topical fluoride (toothpastes, mouthrinses, gels or varnishes) for preventing dental caries in children and adolescents. Cochrane Oral Health Group. *Cochrane Database Syst Rev*. 2007;(4):CD002781.

D

ADDITIONAL READING

- Cliff K, et al. An evidence-based update of the use of analgesics in dentistry. *Periodontology*. 2008;46(1): 143–64.
- Matijevi S, Lazi Z, Kulji-Kapulica N, et al. Empirical antimicrobial therapy of acute dentoalveolar abscess. *Vojnosanit Pregl*. 2009;66:544–50.
- Stefanopoulos PK, Kolokotronis AE. Controversies in antibiotic choices for odontogenic infections. *Oral Surg Oral Med Oral Pathol Oral Radiol Endod*. 2006;101:697–8.
- Stefanopoulos PK, Kolokotronis AE. The clinical significance of anaerobic bacteria in acute orofacial odontogenic infections. *Oral Surg Oral Med Oral Pathol Oral Radiol Endod*. 2004;98:398–408.
- Vargas CM, Crall JJ, Schneider DA. Sociodemographic distribution of pediatric dental caries: NHANES III, 1988–1994. *J Am Dent Assoc*. 1998;129:1229–38.
- Vellappally S, Fiala Z, Smejkalová J, et al. Smoking related systemic and oral diseases. *Acta Medica (Hradec Kralove)*. 2007;50:161–6.

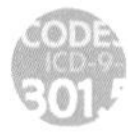

CODES

ICD9

- 521.00 Dental caries, unspecified
- 522.4 Acute apical periodontitis of pulpal origin
- 522.5 Periapical abscess without sinus

CLINICAL PEARLS

- Do not ignore toothache pain.
- Treat patients with facial swelling aggressively, as infections can spread quickly.
- Promote prevention (oral hygiene, fluoride, dental visits) to avoid infections.

DENTAL TRAUMA

Hugh J. Silk, MD, MPH
Sheila O. Stille, DMD, MAGD
Amy Li, DMD

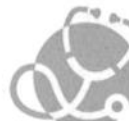

BASICS

DESCRIPTION

Loss or fracture of a tooth and/or supporting bone due to trauma. Trauma can result in shifting of remaining teeth, loss of teeth, loss of alveolar bone, displaced or nonunion of maxilla and/or mandible, resulting in functional and aesthetic deformities that may become difficult to correct.

EPIDEMIOLOGY

- Dental injuries of the teeth, supporting bone, and surrounding soft tissue constitute 7% of all physical injuries.
- Causes: Falls/sports, 63%; assault, 17%; auto or motorcycle accidents, 2%
- Male > Female (2–3:1)

Prevalence

- Prevalence: 5% of all school-age children; 7–13% in primary dentition, 1–16% in permanent dentition
- Affects 13% of population <12 years

RISK FACTORS

- Physical and mental disabilities
- Contact sports without wearing proper protective equipment (i.e., helmets, mouth guards)
- High-risk sports include football, boxing, wrestling, soccer, baseball, hockey, bicycling, and skateboarding
- Age: Youth <12 years
- Tongue/mouth piercings
- Prior dental trauma
- Male gender

GENERAL PREVENTION

- Mouth guards and helmets may prevent traumatic dental injuries. Custom mouth guards are better than boil and bite, which are better than stock guards.
- Avoid tongue piercings.
- Wear seat belts while in the car.
- Monitor home for slippery areas.
- Childproof house with gates and pad sharp table edges.

PATHOPHYSIOLOGY

Direct force sufficient to overcome the bond between the tooth and periodontal ligament within the alveolar socket or disruption of enamel and dentin. Force against maxilla or mandibular arch great enough to cause fracture.

COMMONLY ASSOCIATED CONDITIONS

- Tooth loss can cause loss of space in dental arch.
- Malocclusion causing functional problems
- Trauma to dentition resulting in pulpitis, which causes necrosis of the pulp
- Child abuse: Be alert for history inconsistent with injuries.

DIAGNOSIS

HISTORY

- Assess ABCs.
- Determine nature, time of injury; associated injuries
- Dental fractures:
  - Ask patient if they have possession of missing tooth pieces or swallowed/aspirated teeth.
- Concussion of teeth; subluxed; intruded; extruded
- Tooth avulsion:
  - Time out of socket (critical to management and prognosis)
  - Location of tooth when recovered
  - Type of tooth transfer medium (i.e., milk, water, towel)
- Jaw or facial pain (maxilla or mandibular fracture)
- other systemic injuries; neurologic status
- Consider child abuse in patients with dental fractures.
- Most recent tetanus vaccine

PHYSICAL EXAM

- Irrigate if blood, clots, or debris.
- Inspect the surrounding tissue for laceration, ecchymosis, embedded tooth fragments, or foreign bodies.
- Classify fracture by Ellis classification:
  - Ellis I fracture involves only the enamel.
  - Ellis II fracture includes enamel and dentin (pale yellow material underlying the enamel).
  - Ellis III fracture involves enamel, dentin, and pulp (red material under dentin).
- Check for sensitivity to hot/cold/percussion.
- Check if the tooth is mobile: Palpate tooth and surrounding bone.
- Check for mandibular fracture: Percuss/twist with tongue blade to evaluate. Pain suggests possible fracture.
- Bimanual palpation for maxilla fracture/alveolar fracture
- If tooth missing, investigate for intrusion of tooth or root fragment in socket.

DIAGNOSTIC TESTS & INTERPRETATION

Lab

Initial lab tests

No initial labs needed, unless patient appears acutely ill.

Imaging

Initial approach

Panoramic radiograph of the teeth and jaw for evaluation of the extent of injury (note there can be fractures of nonerupted teeth or jaw fractures that are not evident); CT scan only needed if other associated head trauma.

Follow-Up & Special Considerations

Chest x-ray may be needed for lost avulsed teeth: May be in trachea, lungs, esophagus, or stomach

DIFFERENTIAL DIAGNOSIS

- Crown fracture
- Root fracture
- Subluxation of tooth
- Extrusion/intrusion of tooth
- Trismus

TREATMENT

Assess ABCs and neurologic exam for other problems associated with the traumatic injury.

MEDICATION

First Line

- Pain management:
  - Ibuprofen 600–800 mg (or 10 mg/kg) q6h, or acetaminophen 650–1,000 mg (10–15 mg/kg) q4–6h
  - For more severe pain, consider acetaminophen or ibuprofen, + opioids.
  - Can consider local anesthetic nerve block with long-acting anesthetic (bupivacaine) as adjunct.
- Antibiotics for fractures or avulsions to prevent complications:
  - Penicillin VK 500 mg q.i.d. for 7 days in adults. For children, 10 mg/kg/dose q.i.d.
  - Clindamycin 150–300 mg t.i.d. (or 5–7.5 mg/kg/dose) in penicillin-allergic patients

Second Line

- Phenoxymethyl penicillin 200–500 mg PO q6h for children <12 years
- Clindamycin 150–300 mg t.i.d. (or 5–7.5 mg/kg/dose) in penicillin-allergic patients

ADDITIONAL TREATMENT

General Measures

- Fractured teeth:
  - Ellis I: Smooth edges with emery board or dental drill; cosmetic repair can be done by dentist in follow-up.
  - Ellis II and III: Cover exposed area with calcium hydroxide paste (Dycal). Tooth must be dry before adding Dycal. If not available, Coe-Pak (zinc oxide preparation) can be used. Wrap preparation around fractured tooth edge. Follow up with dentist within 24 hours, if other injuries permit.
- Primary goal of reimplantation/repositioning is to protect periodontal ligament; tooth pulp may die, but tooth can be saved by root canal.
- Subluxation (abnormal mobility) of teeth:
  - Patient should be referred to dentist as soon as possible to evaluate for possible repositioning and splinting.
  - Nonrigid splint should be placed ASAP.
- Intrusion (apical displacement of tooth into the alveolar bone):
  - Primary teeth should be left alone to allow for spontaneous re-eruption after dental follow-up.
  - For permanent teeth, do not reposition; refer to oral surgeon ASAP. Attempts to reposition may cause compromise of blood supply to supporting bone and nerve. Alveolar bone may have necrosis, causing bony defect. Tooth usually needs to be extracted when bone heals.
- Avulsed teeth: Dental emergency:
  - Time is of the essence when reimplanting teeth.
  - If primary tooth: Do not reimplant. If unsure, consult dentist.
  - If permanent tooth: Avoid touching tooth root, handle only by the crown; rinse with normal saline. Minimize trauma to socket. If dirt or large clot in socket, perform gentle irrigation of the socket with normal saline and light aspiration of blood clot before implantation.

- After implantation, have patient bite down on gauze while transporting to dentist.
- If unable to implant at scene, transport in Hanks, milk, or saline (not water) or the buccal sulcus if patient is alert and age appropriate.
- If tooth is outside of socket <20 minutes, attempt implantation of tooth and stabilize with resin/metal splint, or, if not available, zinc oxide (Coe-Pak) splint.
- If tooth is outside of socket 20–60 minutes, soak tooth in Hanks solution for 30 minutes to preserve pH. If Hanks is not available, use saline. Attempt implantation and stabilization.
- If tooth is outside of socket >60 minutes, soak tooth in citric acid and fluoride for 30 minutes; attempt reimplantation and stabilization. If citric acid/fluoride not available, use Hanks or saline.
- Consult dentist for follow-up and for any questions.

- Soft foods only for 10–14 days, depending on injury.
- Jaw fracture:
  - Assess for displacement.
  - If nerve impingement, immediate surgery needed. Contact oral surgeon ASAP.
  - If not displaced or no indication of nerve impingement, have patient see oral surgeon within 24 hours for fixation.

Issues for Referral
- All patients should be referred to a dentist for follow-up. Often, x-rays will be performed to be sure that permanent nonerupted teeth were not damaged in children
- Splints are typically maintained in place for 7–10 days for subluxed teeth and 2–8 weeks for avulsed teeth. Alveolar fractures should be splinted for 4–6 weeks and can take up to 6 months to heal.
- Avulsed teeth continue to deteriorate up to 36 months after injury and typically require root canal therapy. Warn patient of this possibility.
- Oral surgeon should follow jaw fractures in consultation with general dentist.

Additional Therapies
Tetanus booster should be considered if tetanus coverage is uncertain or if tooth has been in contact with soil or deep lacerations present.

COMPLEMENTARY AND ALTERNATIVE MEDICINE
- Acupuncture (1)[C]
- Clove oils (2)[C]

SURGERY/OTHER PROCEDURES
Oral surgeon referral within 1 hour if patient has alveolar bone fracture or jaw fracture. Reduction is easier before swelling.

IN-PATIENT CONSIDERATIONS
Initial Stabilization
Secure airway if compromised with either endotracheal intubation or tracheotomy.

Admission Criteria
Criteria for hospital admission include swelling compromising airway, mental status change due to concussion or hypoxia, after aspiration of teeth, or unstable vital signs.

IV Fluids
IV fluid resuscitation with normal saline may be indicated in septic patients.

Nursing
Ensure excellent oral hygiene. Rinse mouth with chlorhexidine gluconate to minimize bacterial load in oral cavity.

Discharge Criteria
Discharge patient when:
- Abscess and sepsis have been eliminated
- Patient able to take in adequate PO and ambulation
- Cleared from concussion

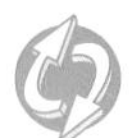

ONGOING CARE

FOLLOW-UP RECOMMENDATIONS
Follow-up with dentist or oral surgeon within 24 hours after any dental trauma:
- Restrict use of pacifiers if dental injuries are involved.
- Ellis III fractures in children <12 years are likely to get infected; clinicians should consider antibiotic coverage.

Patient Monitoring
Biannual cleaning and follow-up. First 36 months most critical to long-term prognosis.

DIET
Avoid any solid food before following up with dentist, and maintain diet as directed by dentist.

PATIENT EDUCATION
- Use a soft toothbrush and soft diet for 10–14 days after dental trauma. Rinse with chlorhexidine 0.1% b.i.d. for 1 week to prevent plaque and debris accumulation (3)[A].
- If tooth avulsion occurs, handle tooth only by the crown.
- Cold milk is the best transportation medium before coming to the emergency room, as it maintains the periodontal ligament for about 3 hours and has pH and osmolarity to maintain vitality of the cells. Saline or saliva is a good substitute. Water is the least desirable transport medium because it is a hypotonic solution that can lyse the cells.

PROGNOSIS
- <20 minutes of tooth separation from socket: Good prognosis
- >60 minutes of tooth separation: Poor prognosis for tooth reattachment
- Alveolar fracture: Poor prognosis for teeth involved
- Jaw fracture: Good prognosis with proper reduction/fixation

COMPLICATIONS
- Tooth loss
- Infection
- Cosmetic and/or functional deformity
- Anesthesia/paraesthesia of nerve entrapment with fractured jaw, especially mandibular fracture

REFERENCES

1. NIH Consensus Conference. Acupuncture. *JAMA*. 1998;280:1518–24.
2. Alan S. Marathon man lessons for dental pain. *Emerg Med News*. 2005;27(9):20–21.
3. Flores MT, Andersson L, Andreasen JO, et al. Guidelines for the management of traumatic dental injuries. II. Avulsion of permanent teeth. *Dent Traumatol*. 2007;23:130–6.

ADDITIONAL READING

- Andreasen JO, Lauridsen E, Christensen SS. Development of an interactive dental trauma guide. *Pediatr Dent*. 2009;31:133–6.
- Celenk S, Sezgin B, Ayna B, et al. Causes of dental fractures in the early permanent dentition: A retrospective study. *J Endod*. 2002;28:208–10.
- Evidence-based review of clinical studies on trauma. *J Endod*. 2009;35:1160–2.
- Flores MT, Andersson L, Andreasen JO, et al. Guidelines for the management of traumatic dental injuries. I. Fractures and luxations of permanent teeth. *Dent Traumatol*. 2007;23:66–71.
- Flores MT, Andreasen JO, Bakland LK, et al. Guidelines for the evaluation and management of traumatic dental injuries. *Dent Traumatol*. 2001;17:193–8.
- Ong CKS, et al. An evidence-based update of the use of analgesics in dentistry. *Periodontology*. 2008;46(1):143–64.
- Vellappally S, Fiala Z, Smejkalová J, et al. Smoking related systemic and oral diseases. *Acta Medica (Hradec Kralove)*. 2007;50:161–6.
- Wilson S, et al. Epidemiology of dental trauma treated in an urban pediatric emergency department. *Pediatr Emerg Care*. 1997;13:12–5.

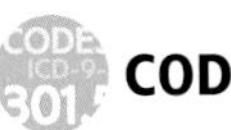

CODES

ICD9
- 802.20 Closed fracture of unspecified site of mandible
- 873.63 Open wound of internal structures of mouth, tooth (broken) (fractured) (due to trauma), uncomplicated
- 873.73 Open wound of internal structures of mouth, tooth (broken) (fractured) (due to trauma), complicated

CLINICAL PEARLS
- Do not reimplant primary teeth.
- Avulsed permanent teeth are a medical emergency. Reimplant permanent teeth ASAP.
- Milk is the best transportation medium before coming to emergency room, as it maintains the periodontal ligament for about 3 hours and has protective pH and osmolarity. Saline or saliva is a good substitute. Water is the least desirable transport medium because it is a hypotonic solution.
- Consider child abuse in younger patients.
- Young children are more likely to get infection after Ellis fractures; consider antibiotic coverage.
- Ensure tetanus vaccination is updated.

D

DEPRESSION

Robert A. Baldor, MD

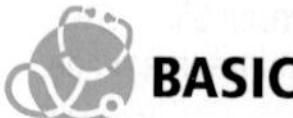

BASICS

DESCRIPTION

- Depression is a primary mood disorder characterized by a depressed mood and/or decreased interest in things that used to give pleasure (anhedonia), which represents a change from previous functioning.
- Synonym(s): Unipolar affective disorder
- System(s) affected: Nervous

EPIDEMIOLOGY

Incidence

Affects >18 million in the US

Prevalence

- 15% lifetime risk of having major depressive disorder (MDD)
- Fourth most common reason to visit a physician

RISK FACTORS

- Female > Male (2:1)
- Predominant age: First onset usually in late 20s (earlier in women than men)
- Elderly (≥65)
- History of behavioral disorders
- Presence of chronic disease(s)
- Recent myocardial infarction/stroke
- Peptic ulcer disease
- Strong family history (depression, bipolar, suicide, alcoholism, other substance abuse)
- Domestic abuse or violence
- Substance abuse and dependence
- Losses and stressors
- Single, divorced, or unhappily married

Genetics

Multiple gene loci place a person at increased risk when faced with environmental stressors.

PATHOPHYSIOLOGY

- Changes in receptor–neurotransmitter relationship in the limbic system:
  - Serotonin and norepinephrine are the primary neurotransmitters involved; dopamine, acetylcholine, and γ-aminobutyric acid have also been involved.
- As action potential is passed on, the neurotransmitter is:
  - Reabsorbed into the neuron, where it is either destroyed by an enzyme or actively removed by a reuptake pump and stored until needed or
  - Destroyed by monoamine oxidase in the mitochondria
- Symptoms related to decreased levels of norepinephrine (dullness and lethargy) and serotonin (irritability, hostility, and suicidal ideation)

ETIOLOGY

- Impaired synthesis of neurotransmitters
- Increased metabolism of neurotransmitters
- Environmental factors and learned behavior may affect neurotransmitters and/or have an independent influence on depression.

COMMONLY ASSOCIATED CONDITIONS

- Manic depression (bipolar disorder)
- Cyclothymic and grief reactions
- Anxiety disorders
- Schizophrenia/schizoaffective disorders
- Psychophysiologic disorders
- Physical disorders
- Substance abuse

DIAGNOSIS

HISTORY

- The Patient Health Questionnaire-2 (PHQ-2) is a validated screening test, which asks how often the patient has been bothered by the following during the past 2 weeks (1)[A]:
  - Little interest or pleasure in doing things?
  - Feeling down, depressed, or hopeless?
- Depressed mood most of the day, nearly every day
- Anhedonia
- Depression is probable when at least 4 of the following exist in addition to depressed mood or anhedonia:
  - Appetite: Significant weight gain or loss when not dieting (change of >5% of body weight in 1 month)
  - Sleep disturbance: Insomnia or hypersomnia nearly every day
  - Fatigue: Out of proportion to the amount of energy expended
  - Psychomotor retardation or agitation: Restlessness, irritability, or withdrawal
  - Poor self-image: Worthlessness, excessive or inappropriate guilt
  - Concentration: Diminished thinking or concentration, poor memory, indecisiveness
  - Suicidal ideation: Recurrent thoughts of death; sometimes, as patients begin to recover, they gain enough energy to think about and sometimes attempt suicide.

Geriatric Considerations

- Can present with pseudodementia
- More common in elderly and difficult to precisely diagnose due to medical comorbidities (highest rates of depression are associated with stroke, coronary artery disease, cancer, Parkinson disease, and Alzheimer disease)

Pediatric Considerations

Depression occurs in children and can present with somatic complaints, irritability (versus depressed mood), and social withdrawal.

PHYSICAL EXAM

Vital signs and complete physical exam with special attention paid to:

- Thyroid
- Cardiac exam, listening for arrhythmias
- Mental status, including affect

DIAGNOSTIC TESTS & INTERPRETATION

Lab

Initial lab tests

Labs may not be necessary, but they are sometimes used to rule out other diagnoses:

- Thyroid-stimulating hormone
- CBC
- Comprehensive metabolic panel

Imaging

Follow-Up & Special Considerations

- EEG, CT, MRI of brain to rule out organic brain disease if suspected
- ECG

Diagnostic Procedures/Surgery

- Depression is primarily a clinical diagnosis made by eliciting personal, family, social, and psychosocial factors.
- Validated standard rating scales can assist:
  - Clinical Global Impressions Scale
  - Montgomery-Asberg Depression Rating Scale
  - Hamilton Rating Scale for Depression
  - Beck Depression Inventory

DIFFERENTIAL DIAGNOSIS

- Dysthymic disorder
- Bipolar disorder
- Organic brain diseases
- Endocrine/thyroid disorders, diabetes
- Metabolic abnormalities (hypercalcemia)
- Adrenal disease (Cushing)
- Liver/renal failure
- Malignancy
- Chronic fatigue syndrome
- Lupus
- Nutritional: Pernicious anemia, pellagra
- Medications: Abuse, side effects, overdose
- Substances: Abuse, dependence, withdrawal

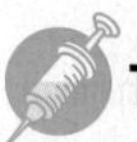

TREATMENT

- Medication is recommended as initial therapy for mild to moderate major depressive disorder and especially for those with severe major depressive disorder (2)[A].
- However, psychotherapy alone is also recommended as an initial treatment choice for mild to moderate depression, especially cognitive-behavioral therapy, interpersonal psychotherapy, psychodynamic therapy, and problem-solving therapy (2)[A].
- The decision should be based on patient preference and the availability of skilled psychotherapy services.

MEDICATION

First Line

Effectiveness of antidepressant medications is generally comparable between and within classes of medications; selection should be based on provider familiarity and patient characteristics/preferences (2)[A]:

- SSRIs:
  - Fluoxetine (Prozac): 20–80 mg/d
  - Sertraline (Zoloft): 50–200 mg/d
  - Paroxetine (Paxil): 10–50 mg/d
  - Paroxetine CR (Paxil CR): 12.5–62.5 mg/d
  - Citalopram (Celexa): 20–60 mg/d
  - Escitalopram (Lexapro): 10–20 mg/d

- Others:
  - Venlafaxine (Effexor): 75–375 mg/d (divided doses)
  - Venlafaxine XR (Effexor XR): 75–225 mg/d
  - Bupropion (Wellbutrin): 100–450 mg/d (divided doses, t.i.d.)
  - Bupropion SR (Wellbutrin SR): 100–450 mg/d (divided doses, b.i.d.)
  - Bupropion XL (Wellbutrin XL): 150–300 mg/d
  - Duloxetine (Cymbalta): 30–60 mg/d

Second Line

- Tricyclic antidepressants (TCAs) with sedating properties *condensed list*:
  - Amitriptyline (Elavil): 50–150 mg at bedtime (max 300)
  - Nortriptyline (Pamelor): 75–150 mg at bedtime
  - Doxepin (Prudoxin, Zonalon): 75–150 mg at bedtime
- TCAs with activating properties *condensed list*:
  - Imipramine (Tofranil, Tofranil-PM): 150–200 mg at bedtime
  - Desipramine (Norpramin): 150–300 mg/d
- α_2-antagonists (sedating):
  - Mirtazapine (Remeron): 15–45 mg at bedtime
- SSRI/antagonists:
  - Trazodone: 150 mg/d (divided doses), maximum 600 mg/d (divided doses)
- Precautions:
  - Bupropion: Increased risk of seizures
  - TCAs: Advanced age, glaucoma, benign prostate hypertrophy, hyperthyroidism, cardiovascular disease, liver disease, urinary retention, MAOI treatment, potential for fatal overdose
  - SSRIs: Abrupt discontinuation may result in withdrawal symptoms (i.e., dizziness), may raise serum levels of other drugs
- Significant potential interactions:
  - TCAs: Amphetamines, barbiturates, clonidine, epinephrine, ethanol, norepinephrine, MAOIs: Allow 14-day washout period before starting MAOIs, propoxyphene
  - SSRIs and MAOIs: 14-day washout before instituting therapy
  - Venlafaxine may cause fatal serotonin syndrome.
  - MAOIs: Significant drug and food interactions limit use, but they can be useful in refractory cases.

ALERT

Black box warning: Increased risk of suicidality in children, adolescents, and young adults up to age 25 who are treated with SSRIs. Although this has not been extended to adults, suicide risk assessments are warranted for all patients.

Geriatric Considerations

Reduce dosage of medications (1/2 usual starting dose); may need to treat longer than younger adults.

Pediatric Considerations

Reduce dosage of medications in adolescents; also see "Alert."

Pregnancy Considerations

SSRIs: If possible, taper and discontinue. (Paroxetine is Category D; the rest of SSRIs are Category C.)

ADDITIONAL TREATMENT

Additional Therapies

Electroconvulsive therapy for refractory cases

COMPLEMENTARY AND ALTERNATIVE MEDICINE

Use in mild depression; conflicting evidence regarding effectiveness:

- Hypericum perforatum (St. John's wort) (3)[A]: Be aware of multiple drug interactions.
- SAM-e (S-adenosyl methionine): 400–1,600 mg/d (4)[A]

IN-PATIENT CONSIDERATIONS

Admission Criteria

In-patient care is indicated for severely depressed, psychotic, or suicidal patients.

Discharge Criteria

Depressive symptoms improving, no longer suicidal

ONGOING CARE

FOLLOW-UP RECOMMENDATIONS

Patient Monitoring

- See within 2 weeks after starting medication.
- During follow-up, evaluate the side effects, dosage, and effectiveness of the medication.
- Follow up every 2 weeks until improvement.
- Follow up every 3 months thereafter.
- Explain treatment must continue for at least 6 months to 2 years; longer with family history, severe depression, and in the very young.

PATIENT EDUCATION

- Depression is a medical illness, not a character defect.
- Stress the need for long-term treatment and follow-up, which includes lifestyle changes.
- Healthy adults need to perform 30 minutes of moderate-intensity exercise on 3–5 days per week (5)[A].

PROGNOSIS

- 70% show significant improvement.
- Of patients with a single depressive episode, 50% develop a recurrent episode.

COMPLICATIONS

- Suicide
- Lower quality of life

REFERENCES

1. Kroenke K, Spitzer RL, Williams JB, et al. The Patient Health Questionnaire-2: Validity of a two-item depression screener. *Med Care*. 2003;41:1284–92.
2. http://www.psychiatryonline.com/pracGuide/pracGuideChapToc_7.aspx.
3. Keller MB. Issues in treatment-resistant depression. *J Clin Psychiatry*. 2005;66(Suppl 8):5–12.
4. Institute for Clinical Systems Improvement. *Major Depression in Adults in Primary Care*. Bloomington, MN: Institute for Clinical Systems Improvement; 2006.
5. American Psychiatric Association. *Diagnostic and Statistical Manual of Mental Disorders DSM-IV-TR*. 4th ed. [text revision]. Washington, DC: American Psychiatric Publishing; 2000.

ADDITIONAL READING

- Adams SM, Miller KE, Zylstra RG. Pharmacologic management of adult depression. *Am Fam Physician*. 2008;77:785–92.
- Halfin A. Depression: The benefits of early and appropriate treatment. *Am J Manag Care*. 2007;13:S92–7.
- Kessler RC, Berglund P, Demler O. The epidemiology of major depressive disorder: Results from the National Comorbidity Survey Replication (NCS-R). *JAMA*. 2003;289:3095–105.
- Maurer D, Colt R. An evidence-based approach to the management of depression. *Prim Care*. 2006;33:923–41.
- Skultety KM, Rodriguez RL. Treating geriatric depression in primary care. *Curr Psychiatry Rep*. 2008;10:44–50.
- Thase ME. Treatment of severe depression. *J Clin Psychiatry*. 2000;61(Suppl 1):17–25.

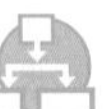

See Also (Topic, Algorithm, Electronic Media Element)

Algorithms: Depressed Mood Resulting from Medical Illness; Depressive Episode, Major

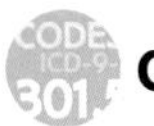

CODES

ICD9

- 296.20 Major depressive affective disorder, single episode, unspecified
- 296.30 Major depressive affective disorder, recurrent episode, unspecified
- 311 Depressive disorder, not elsewhere classified

CLINICAL PEARLS

- The PHQ-2 is a validated screening test, which asks how often the patient has been bothered by the following during the past 2 weeks (1)[A]:
  - Little interest or pleasure in doing things?
  - Feeling down, depressed, or hopeless?
- The relationship (therapeutic alliance) between the patient and health care provider is important to the success of treatment.
- Given the high recurrence rates, long-term treatment is often necessary.

DEPRESSION, ADOLESCENT

Rebecca Sills, MD
Bruce B. Peters, DO

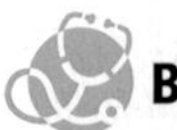

BASICS

DESCRIPTION

- Primary mood disorder characterized by sadness or irritability with impairment of functioning, abnormal psychological development, and a loss of self-worth and interest in typically pleasurable activities
- Dysthymic disorder is differentiated from major depression by less intense symptoms that are more persistent, lasting at least 1 year.
- The depressive disorder NOS is diagnosed when an adolescent presents with depressive symptoms but does not meet the criteria for other diagnoses.
- Treatment-resistant depression is a failure of treatment with 2 antidepressants administered in adequate dosage for at least 6 weeks.
- Adolescents with depression are likely to suffer broad functional impairment across social, academic, family, and occupational domains along with a higher risk for substance abuse and other psychiatric comorbidities.

EPIDEMIOLOGY

Incidence

During adolescence, 15–20%; an estimated 70–80% do not receive appropriate care.

Prevalence

~4–8% of adolescents; at least twice as common in females

RISK FACTORS

- Increased 3–6 times if first-degree relative has a major affective disorder; 3–4 times in offspring of parents with depression
- Prior depressive episodes
- History of low self-esteem, anxiety disorders, attention-deficit/hyperactivity disorder (ADHD), and/or learning disabilities
- Hormonal changes during puberty
- Female gender
- General stressors: Socioeconomic deprivations, adverse life events, difficulties with peers, loss of a loved one, academic difficulties, abuse, chronic illness, and tobacco abuse

Genetics

There is a 76% concordance rate in monozygotic twins reared together and a 67% concordance rate among those reared apart, along with a 19% concordance rate in dizygotic twins reared together.

GENERAL PREVENTION

Insufficient evidence supports the universal implementation of depression prevention programs (psychological and social) (1)[B]. There may be a small benefit to regular exercise in preventing episodes of depression (2)[B]:

- There is some evidence that child and adolescent mental health can be improved by successfully treating maternal depression (3).

PATHOPHYSIOLOGY

Unclear, but low functional levels of neurotransmitters (serotonin, norepinephrine) may produce symptoms, and decreased functioning of the dopamine system also contributes.

ETIOLOGY

External factors may affect neurotransmitters or independently affect depression.

COMMONLY ASSOCIATED CONDITIONS

- Eating disorders (especially bulimia)
- Substance abuse
- Anxiety and somatization disorders
- Behavioral disorders (i.e., ADHD, oppositional defiant disorder, conduct disorder)
- Learning disorders
- Headaches

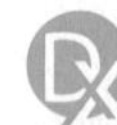

DIAGNOSIS

HISTORY

- According to the *DSM-IV*, adolescents must display EITHER (i) depressed or irritable mood OR (ii) loss of interest or pleasure (anhedonia) for most of the day, nearly every day, for at least 2 weeks, causing significant distress or functional impairment.
- In addition, 4 or more of the following symptoms must be present during the same 2-week period:
  - Change in appetite with weight loss or gain (change of >5% of body weight in 1 month)
  - Insomnia or hypersomnia nearly every day
  - Psychomotor agitation or retardation
  - Fatigue or loss of energy
  - Feelings of excessive guilt or worthlessness: Adolescents may be extremely self-critical, unable to identify positive self-attributes, or feel they deserve to be punished for things that are not their fault.
  - Indecisiveness or impaired thinking or concentration: School performance may decline significantly.
  - Recurring thoughts of death or suicide or actual attempts at suicide
- Symptoms must not meet the criteria for a mixed manic episode (suggestive of bipolar disorder), be due to the effects of a drug or other condition, or be secondary to bereavement.
- In adolescents, depression may present as behavioral problems, school refusal, physical complaints, academic difficulties, anxiety, and substance abuse (3).

PHYSICAL EXAM

- Psychomotor retardation or agitation may be present.
- Clinicians should carefully assess patients for signs of self-injury (wrist lacerations) or abuse.

DIAGNOSTIC TESTS & INTERPRETATION

Lab

Initial lab tests

May be used to rule out other diagnoses (i.e., CBC, TSH/T4, glucose, mono spot, and urine drug)

Follow-Up & Special Considerations

No test has sufficient sensitivity or specificity to assist in the diagnostic assessment of depression.

Diagnostic Procedures/Surgery

- Depression is primarily diagnosed after conducting a formal clinical interview with the adolescent, combined with supporting information obtained from caregivers and teachers.
- The following standardized tests can be useful as screening tools and to monitor response to treatment, but should not be used as the sole basis for diagnosis:
  - Beck Depression Inventory (BDI): All ages
  - Child Depression Inventory (CDI): Ages 7–17
  - Reynolds Adolescent Depression Scale (RADS): Teenagers in grades 7–12
  - Mood and Feelings Questionnaire (MFQ) (3)
  - Patient Health Questionnaire-9 (PHQ-9): Ages 13–17 with ideal cut point of 11 or higher (instead of 10 used for adults) (4)
- Suicide risk assessment should be performed.
- Office-based screening/case-finding questionnaires have minimal impact on the detection, management, or outcome of depression by clinicians (5)[A].

DIFFERENTIAL DIAGNOSIS

- Normal bereavement
- Substance-induced mood disorder
- Bipolar disorder
- Mood disorder secondary to a medical condition
- Endocrine diseases (hypo- or hyperthyroidism)
- Organic CNS diseases
- Malignancy
- Infectious mononucleosis
- Anemia or vitamin deficiency
- Chronic diseases (diabetes)
- ADHD, posttraumatic stress disorder (PTSD), eating disorders, and anxiety disorders

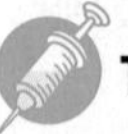

TREATMENT

Pediatric depression is often managed by primary care providers rather than psychiatrists (6). Response rate to first antidepressant tried is 40–50%. If no response to first medication, response rate to second antidepressant used is 40–50%. Adequate duration of antidepressant trial is 8–10 weeks at therapeutic dose (7). However, new research finds that lack of response to medication after only 6 weeks may be a reliable predictor of failure to remit and could suggest switching to an alternative medication (8).

MEDICATION

First Line

- Fluoxetine: Starting dose 5–10 mg/d. Effective dose 20–60 mg/d: Fluoxetine is approved by the FDA for the treatment of depression in age >8. (9)[B].
- Escitalopram: Starting dose 5 mg/d. Effective dose 10–20 mg/d. FDA approved for treatment of depression age >12 (7).
- Careful monitoring of the patient for suicidal thoughts and behavior is required, given the possible increased risk while taking any antidepressant. However, there is no evidence proving causality and there may be a decrease in suicidal ideation, while completed suicide rates are higher in areas where SSRIs are not prescribed to adolescents. However, paroxetine has a higher association with suicidality than other SSRIs and is therefore not recommended (7),(9)[C].

Second Line

- The following SSRIs are NOT approved by the FDA for treatment of adolescent depression but may be tried as second-line agents at the clinician's discretion (9)[B]:
  - Citalopram: Starting dose 5–10 mg/d. Effective dose 20–40 mg/d.
  - Sertraline: Starting dose 25 mg/d. Effective dose 50–200 mg/d.
  - Fluvoxamine: Starting dose 12.5–50 mg/d. Effective dose 150–300 mg/d (shorter half-life).
- Other antidepressants (less studied but reasonable if failed 2 SSRIs):
  - Venlafaxine: 37.5–225 mg/d (consider if comorbid anxiety or if failed 2 SSRIs).
  - Desvenlafaxine: 50–400 mg/d
  - Bupropion: 37.5–400 mg/d (consider if comorbid ADHD).
  - Duloxetine: 20–60 mg/d (although no randomized controlled trials in minors) (7).
- Antidepressants not recommended in adolescents:
  - Tricyclic antidepressants have not been proven to be effective in adolescents and should NOT be used (9,10)[A].
    - Mirtazapine has not been shown to be effective in adolescents (7).
    - Paroxetine (SSRI): Contraindicated due to short half-life, associated withdrawal symptoms, and higher association with suicidal ideation (7)

ADDITIONAL TREATMENT

General Measures

- Evidence for the effectiveness of cognitive-behavioral therapy (CBT) alone is mixed but may be effective in the treatment of mild to moderate adolescent depression and shown to be useful adjunct to SSRIs in some studies though overall may be most effective for decreasing impairment in the short term with limited evidence for long-term benefit or short-term symptom reduction (9)[A](3,11):
  - The goal is to alter a patient's negative thoughts and behaviors to improve his or her mood by encouraging pleasurable activities (behavioral activation), reducing negative thoughts (cognitive restructuring), and improving assertiveness and problem-solving skills to reduce feelings of hopelessness.
  - Interpersonal psychotherapy (IPT) has been shown to be effective for adolescent depression. The treatment targets a patient's interpersonal problems to improve both interpersonal functioning and his or her mood (3).
- Regular exercise may help reduce depressive symptoms (2)[B].

Issues for Referral

Referral to a child psychiatrist is recommended for adolescents with severe, recurrent, or treatment-resistant depression; if the patient has comorbidities or if clinician is uncomfortable prescribing complex therapies.

COMPLEMENTARY AND ALTERNATIVE MEDICINE

No evidence supports the use of St. John's wort or acupuncture.

IN-PATIENT CONSIDERATIONS

Admission Criteria

Indicated if severely depressed, psychotic, suicidal, or homicidal; 1-on-1 supervision may be needed

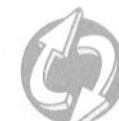

ONGOING CARE

Treatment for at least 6 months reduced the likelihood of suicide attempts compared with treatment for <8 weeks (10).

FOLLOW-UP RECOMMENDATIONS

- Systematic and regular tracking of goals and outcomes from treatment should be performed, including assessment of depressive symptoms and functioning in home, school, and peer settings (10).
- Monitor for the emergence of adverse events during antidepressant treatment.
- Diagnosis and initial treatment should be reassessed if no improvement is noted after 6–8 weeks of treatment.

Patient Monitoring

- Once started on antidepressants, patients should be seen weekly for the first month, biweekly for the second month, and again at least at 12 weeks and as needed thereafter: Careful monitoring for suicidal thoughts or behavior is required, particularly in the first 2 months after initiation or dose increase. It is also important to monitor for signs of antidepressant-induced mania, especially between the first and fourth weeks (7).
- Length of medication treatment:
  - First episode: Minimum 6–9 months followed by a slow taper over 6–8 weeks (risk of discontinuation syndrome highest with paroxetine and fluvoxamine)
  - Second episode: At least 1 year
  - Third episode: 1–3 years
  - >3 episodes: Lifelong
- Adverse effects (i.e., nausea, headaches, behavioral activation, etc.) occur in up to 93% of patients treated with SSRIs and tend to occur earlier than therapeutic response. Therefore, routine monitoring and discussion of possible medication side effects is critical for depressed youth who are treated with antidepressants. While it is rare, serotonin syndrome can occur with multiple medications or high doses of SSRIs (7).

PATIENT EDUCATION

Educate patients and parents about mental health and the fact that depression is a medical illness, not a character defect.

PROGNOSIS

- If left untreated, major depressive episode in adolescents typically lasts 7–9 months, with 90% resolving within 2 years.
- Combination therapy of CBT with fluoxetine results in improvement in 71% of patients.
- Recurrence is 40% by 2 years and 50–70% by 5 years.
- Persistent and severe depression in adulthood is more likely with an earlier onset of disease (3).
- Patients with family conflict, drug and alcohol use, and anxiety disorders are less likely to achieve remission (8).

COMPLICATIONS

- Treatment-induced mania, aggression, or lack of improvement in symptoms
- School failure or refusal
- Suicide
- Low self-esteem, substance abuse (nicotine, etc.)

REFERENCES

1. Merry S. Psychological and/or educational interventions for the prevention of depression in children and adolescents. *Cochrane Database Syst Rev.* 2007:4.
2. Larun L. Exercise in prevention and treatment of anxiety and depression among children and young people. *Cochrane Database Syst Rev.* 2007:4.
3. Thapar A, et al. Managing and preventing depression in adolescents. *BMJ.* 2010;340:c209.
4. Richardson LP, et al. Evaluation of the Patient Health Questionnaire-9 item for detecting major depression among adolescents. *Pediatrics.* 2010;126:1117–23.
5. Gilbody S. Screening and case finding instruments for depression. *Cochrane Database Syst Rev.* 2007:4.
6. Cheung AH, Dewa CS, Levitt AJ, et al. Pediatric depressive disorders: Management priorities in primary care. *Curr Opin Pediatr.* 2008;20:551–9.
7. Smiga SM, Elliott GR. Psychopharmacology of depression in children and adolescents. *Pediatr Clin N Am.* 2011;58:155–71.
8. Emslie GJ, et al. Treatment of resistant depression in adolescents (TORDIA): Week 24 outcomes. *Am J Psychiatry.* 2010;167:782–91.
9. Bhatia SK, Bhatia SC. Childhood and adolescent depression. *Am Fam Physician.* 2007;75:73–80.
10. Hazell P. Tricyclic drugs for depression in children and adolescents (review). *Cochrane Database Syst Rev.* 2007:4.
11. Dubicka B, et al. Combined treatment with cognitive behavioural therapy in adolescent depression. *Br J Psychiatry.* 2010;197:433–40.

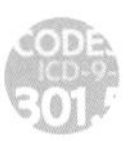

CODES

ICD9

- 296.20 Major depressive affective disorder, single episode, unspecified
- 296.30 Major depressive affective disorder, recurrent episode, unspecified degree
- 311 Depressive disorder, not elsewhere classified

CLINICAL PEARLS

- Adolescent depression is underdiagnosed and often presents with irritability and anhedonia.
- Fluoxetine and escitalopram are FDA approved for treatment of adolescent depression.
- CBT combined with fluoxetine is efficacious for adolescents with major depression.
- Paroxetine, TCAs, and mirtazapine should not be used to treat adolescent depression. Referral to a child psychiatrist is appropriate for complex cases or treatment-resistant depression.
- All adolescents with depression should be monitored for suicidality, especially during the first month of treatment with an antidepressant.

DEPRESSION, GERIATRIC

Anna Mirk, MD

BASICS

DESCRIPTION

Depression is a primary mood disorder characterized by a depressed mood and/or a markedly decreased interest or pleasure in normally enjoyable activities for at least 2 weeks and causing significant distress or impairment in daily functioning.

EPIDEMIOLOGY

Prevalence rates among the elderly vary, largely depending on the specific diagnostic instruments used and their current health and/or home environment:

- 1–3% of community-dwelling elderly
- 7.5% seen in primary care clinics
- 10–21% of hospitalized elderly patients
- 12–27% of nursing-home residents

RISK FACTORS

- General:
  - Chronic physical health condition(s)
  - History of mental health problems
  - Death of a loved one
  - Caregiving
  - Social isolation
  - Lack or loss of social support
  - Significant loss of independence
  - Uncontrolled pain
  - Insomnia/sleep disturbance
- Prevalence of depression in medical illness:
  - Stroke (22–50%)
  - Cancer (18–50%)
  - Myocardial infarction (15–45%)
  - Parkinson's disease (10–39%)
  - Rheumatoid arthritis (13%)
  - Diabetes mellitus (5–11%)
  - Alzheimer dementia (5–15%)
- Suicide:
  - Suicide is the 11th leading cause of death in the US for all ages.
  - Suicide rates are higher for Americans age >65 compared to the general population (~15 per 100,000 people).
  - Suicide rates are highest for males aged >75 (rate 38.5 per 100,000).

PATHOPHYSIOLOGY

- There are still significant gaps in the understanding of the underlying pathophysiology.
- Ongoing research has identified several possible mechanisms, including:
  - Monoamine transmission and associated transcriptional and translational activity
  - Epigenetic mechanisms and resilience factors
  - Neurotrophins, neurogenesis, neuroimmune systems, and neuroendocrine systems

ETIOLOGY

Depression appears to be a complex interaction between heritable and environmental factors.

DIAGNOSIS

HISTORY

- Depressed mood most of the day, nearly every day, and/or loss of interest or pleasure in life
- Other common symptoms include:
  - Feeling hopeless, helpless, or worthless
  - Insomnia and loss of appetite/weight (alternatively, hypersomnia with increased appetite/weight in atypical depression)
  - Fatigue and loss of energy
  - Somatic symptoms (headaches, chronic pain)
  - Neglect of personal responsibility or care
  - Psychomotor retardation or agitation
  - Diminished concentration, indecisiveness
  - Thoughts of death or suicide
- Screening with **SIGECAPS:**
  - **S**LEEP: Changes in sleep habits from baseline, including excessive sleep, early waking, or inability to fall asleep
  - **I**NTEREST: Loss of interest in previously enjoyable activities
  - **G**UILT: Guilt that may or may not focus on a specific problem or circumstance
  - **E**NERGY: Perceived lack of energy
  - **C**ONCENTRATION: Inability to concentrate on specific tasks
  - **A**PPETITE: Increase or decrease in appetite
  - **P**SYCHOMOTOR: Restlessness and agitation, or the perception that everyday activities are too strenuous to manage
  - **S**UICIDALITY: Desire to end life or hurt oneself, harmful thoughts directed internally, or thoughts of homicidality

DIAGNOSTIC TESTS & INTERPRETATION

Lab

Initial laboratory evaluation is done primarily to rule out potential medical factors that could be causing symptoms.

Initial lab tests

- Thyroid-stimulating hormone (TSH)
- CBC with differential
- Comprehensive metabolic panel, including liver function
- Urine drug screen
- Vitamin B_{12}

Follow-Up & Special Considerations

Additional testing for possible confounding medical and cognitive disorders as warranted

Diagnostic Procedures/Surgery

Validated screening tools and rating scales:

- Geriatric Depression Scale: 15- or 30-point scales
- Patient Health Questionnaire (PHQ-2 or PHQ-9)
- The Hamilton Depression Rating Scale
- The Beck Depression Inventory

DIFFERENTIAL DIAGNOSIS

Concurrent medical conditions, cognitive disorders, and medications may produce neurovegetative symptoms that may mimic depression:

- Medical conditions: e.g., hypothyroidism, vitamin B_{12} deficiency, liver or renal failure, cancers, stroke
- Medication induced: e.g., interferon-b1, β_2-blockers, isotretinoin
- Dementia and neurodegenerative disorders
- Delirium
- Psychiatric disorders: e.g., bipolar disorder, dysthymic disorder, anxiety disorders, substance abuse-related mood disorders, psychotic disorders

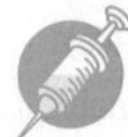

TREATMENT

Although response alone, usually interpreted as a 50% reduction in symptoms, can be clinically meaningful, the goal is to treat patients to the point of remission (i.e., essentially the absence of depressive symptoms).

MEDICATION

- Typically more conservative initial dosing and titration of antidepressants in the elderly, starting with 1/2 of the usual initiation dose and increasing within a couple of weeks if tolerated
- Continue titrating dose every 2–4 weeks as appropriate. It is important to reach an adequate treatment dose.

First Line

- SSRIs have been found to be effective in treating depression in the elderly (1,2)[A].
- No single SSRI clearly outperforms others in the class; choice of medication often reflects side effect profile or practitioner familiarity:
  - Citalopram: Start at 10 mg/d. Treatment range 20–40 mg/d.
  - Sertraline: Start at 25 mg/d. Treatment range 50–200 mg/d.
  - Escitalopram: Start at 5–10 mg/d. Treatment range 10–20 mg/d.
  - Fluoxetine: Start at 10 mg/d. Treatment range 20–60 mg/d.
  - Paroxetine: Start at 10 mg/d. Treatment range 20–60 mg/d.
- SSRIs should not be used concomitantly with monoamine oxidase inhibitors (MAOIs).

Second Line

- Atypical antidepressants: More effective than placebo in treatment of depression in the elderly, although additional studies are needed to better delineate patient factors that determine response (3)[A]:
  - Bupropion (immediate, sustained/twice a day, and extended/once daily available): Start at 100 mg/d. Increase dose in 3 days. Treatment range 200–300 mg/d. Avoid in patients with elevated seizure risk.
  - Venlafaxine (immediate and sustained release available): Start at 37.5 mg and titrate weekly. Treatment range 75–300 mg/d. May be associated with elevated BP at higher doses.
  - Duloxetine: Start at 30 mg/d. Treatment range 30–60 mg/d. Also may be associated with elevated BP.
  - Mirtazapine: Start at 7.5–15 mg/nightly. Treatment range 15–45 mg/d. Can produce problems with weight gain, sedation, and cognitive dysfunction.

- For patients who have not responded to initial SSRI trial:
  - Switch to a different SSRI medication, switch to an atypical antidepressant, or augment initial antidepressant with bupropion (4,5,6)[B].

ADDITIONAL TREATMENT

- Tricyclic antidepressants (TCAs) have been shown to be effective in treating depression in the elderly (1,2)[A]. However, they are difficult for elderly patients to tolerate due to side effect profile and are potentially lethal in overdose, limiting their use as initial treatment agents.
- Although not FDA approved, buspirone, lithium, or triiodothyronine are sometimes used off-label to augment a primary antidepressant (6)[B].
- MAOIs also appear more effective than placebo in the treatment of depression in the elderly (1)[A]. They are not used frequently in clinical practice due to potential side effects and necessary dietary restrictions.

General Measures

Psychotherapy: Studies do show some benefit in depressed elderly patients (7)[B]:

- Cognitive-behavioral therapy
- Problem-solving therapy
- Interpersonal therapy
- Psychodynamic psychotherapy

Issues for Referral

Depression with suicidal ideation, psychotic depression, bipolar disorder, comorbid substance-abuse issues, severe or refractory illness

Additional Therapies

- Electroconvulsive therapy (ECT): Has been shown to produce remission of depressive symptoms in the elderly (8)[B]. It should be considered as an initial option for patients with severe or psychotic depression.
- Exercise: May be beneficial for depression in the elderly population (9,10)[B].

COMPLEMENTARY AND ALTERNATIVE MEDICINE

- St. John's wort may have minimal benefit (11)[A].
- Tryptophan and hydroxytryptophan: 150–300 mg/d; possible efficacy, additional investigation required (12)[B],(13)[C]

IN-PATIENT CONSIDERATIONS

Inpatient care indicated for imminent safety risk (e.g., acutely suicidal patients) or for those patients unable to care adequately for themselves due to depression.

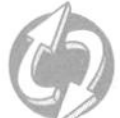

ONGOING CARE

FOLLOW-UP RECOMMENDATIONS

Due to the delay of benefit following initiation of antidepressant therapy (2–4 weeks), it is necessary to ensure open communication with the patient to prevent premature discontinuation of therapy. An adequate explanation of potential side effects with instructions to call the office before discontinuing therapy is imperative.

Patient Monitoring

- A patient with severe depression who exhibits suicidality may require admission to an appropriate facility.
- Monitor for worsening anxiety symptoms or increase in suicidality.

DIET

No dietary restrictions are necessary, except for patients taking MAOIs, which necessitate dietary restriction of foods high in tyramine.

PATIENT EDUCATION

- Depression is a treatable illness.
- Medications may need to be taken for at least 2–4 weeks before any beneficial effect is noted.
- Depression is often a recurring illness.
- National Suicide Prevention Lifeline at 1-800-273-TALK (8255) is a free, 24-hour hotline available to anyone in suicidal crisis or emotional distress. Calls will be routed to the nearest crisis center.

PROGNOSIS

- Treatment outcomes in the elderly may be worse than in the general population, possibly mediated by physical comorbidities and other factors.
- Depending on the population studied and specific clinical measures used, estimates vary for initial clinical response and remission (between 30% and 70%).

COMPLICATIONS

- Impairment in social, occupational, or interpersonal functioning
- Difficulty performing activities of daily living and self-care
- Increase in medical services utilization and increased costs of care
- Suicide

REFERENCES

1. Wilson K, Mottram PG, Sivananthan A, et al. Antidepressants versus placebo for the depressed elderly. *Cochrane Database Syst Rev*. 2009;1.
2. Mottram PG, Wilson K, Strobl JJ. Antidepressants for depressed elderly. *Cochrane Database Syst Rev*. 2009;1.
3. Nelson JC, Delucchi K, Schneider LS, et al. Efficacy of second generation antidepressants in late-life depression: A meta-analysis of the evidence. *Am J Geriatr Psychiatry*. 2008;16:558–67.
4. Ruhe HG, Huyser J, et al. Switching antidepressants after a first selective serotonin reuptake inhibitor in major depressive disorder: A systematic review. *J Clin Psychiatry* 2006;67(12): 1836–55.
5. Rush AJ, Trivedi MH, et al. Bupropion-SR, sertraline, or venlafaxine-XR after failure of SSRIs for depression. *N Engl J Med*. 2006;354(12): 1231–42.
6. Trivedi MH, Fava M, et al. Medication augmentation after the failure of SSRIs for depression. *N Engl J Med*. 2006;354(12): 1243–52.
7. Wilson KC, Mottram PG, Vassilas CA, et al. Psychotherapeutic treatments for older depressed people. *Cochrane Database Syst Rev*. 2008; CD004853.
8. Van der Wurff FB, et al. Electroconvulsive therapy for the depressed elderly. *Cochrane Database Sys Rev*. 2003;CD003593.
9. Blake H, Mo P, Malik S, et al. How effective are physical activity interventions for alleviating depressive symptoms in older people? A systematic review. *Clin Rehabil*. 2009.
10. Sjösten N, Kivelä SL, et al. The effects of physical exercise on depressive symptoms among the aged: A systematic review. *Int J Geriatr Psychiatry*. 2006;21:410–8.
11. Linde K, et al. St. John's wort for depression. *Cochrane Database Sys Rev*. 2005;CD000448.
12. Shaw K, Turner J, DelMar C. Tryptophan and 5-hydroxytryptophan for depression. *Cochrane Database Sys Rev*. 2002;CD003198.
13. Sarris J, Schoendorfer N, Kavanagh DJ. Major depressive disorder and nutritional medicine: A review of monotherapies and adjuvant treatments. *Nutr Rev*. 2009;67:125–31.

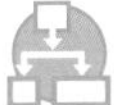

See Also (Topic, Algorithm, Electronic Media Element)

Algorithms: Depressed Mood Resulting from Medical Illness; Depressive Episode, Major

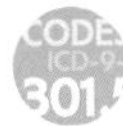

CODES

ICD9

- 290.21 Senile dementia with depressive features
- 311 Depressive disorder, not elsewhere classified

CLINICAL PEARLS

- Depression is not a normal part of aging.
- Depression in the elderly may be difficult to precisely diagnose due to medical and cognitive comorbidities.
- Depression may present primarily with cognitive dysfunction. Cognitive function may improve with treatment of the depression.
- A multidisciplinary approach to the treatment of depression is often most efficacious.
- SSRIs are considered first-line therapy for safety and tolerability. A full remission may take upward of 12 weeks of treatment. Long-term treatment may be needed to prevent recurrence.

DEPRESSION, POSTPARTUM

Nancy Byatt, DO, MBA

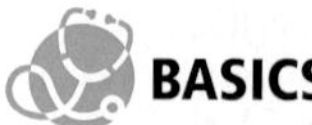

BASICS

DESCRIPTION

- Major depressive disorder (MDD) that recurs or has its onset in the postpartum period. May also occur in mothers adopting a baby or in fathers (1).
- Post Partum Depression is similar to non-pregnancy depression (sleep disorders, anhedonia, psychomotor changes, etc.), has its onset within 4–12 weeks postpartum, and affects 13% of pregnancies.
- Contrast to Post-partum "Blues" (sadness and emotional lability) which is experienced by 30–70% of women; onset and resolution within first by 10 days postpartum

EPIDEMIOLOGY

Incidence

10–15% of mothers within first year of giving birth (2)

Prevalence

- Controversial; assessments range from 10–20% during the early postpartum weeks
- Investigators have reported elevated depressive symptoms in 30–50% of women during the early postpartum period with continued symptoms throughout the first postpartum year (3).

RISK FACTORS

- Previous episodes of postpartum depression
- History of MDD
- MDD during pregnancy
- Anxiety during pregnancy (4)
- History of premenstrual dysphoria
- Family history of depression (5)
- Unwanted pregnancy
- Socioeconomic stress
- Low self-esteem
- Young maternal age
- Alcohol abuse
- Marital conflict
- Multiple births (6)
- Lack of social and family support system (7)
- Postpartum pain, sleep disturbance, and fatigue
- Assisted reproductive technology pregnancy (8)
- Recent immigrant status
- Increased stressful life events
- History of childhood sexual abuse
- Decision to decrease antidepressants during pregnancy

GENERAL PREVENTION

- Universal screening during pregnancy to diagnose depression and risk factors for depression and to allow initiation of treatment before or immediately after delivery (9)[A]
- Postpartum screening using Edinburgh Postnatal Depression Scale within 4–6 weeks after delivery (9)[A] http://www.testandcalc.com/etc/tests/edin.asp
- Continuation of antidepressants in high-risk women during pregnancy may prevent postnatal depression.
- Provide postnatal visits and psychotherapy and/or education for high-risk women.
- Use of depression care manager who provides education, routine telephone contact, and follow-up to engage women in treatment

PATHOPHYSIOLOGY

May be related to sensitivity in hormonal fluctuations, including estrogen, progesterone, and other gonadal hormones, as well as neuroactive steroids; cytokines; HPA axis hormones; and altered fatty acid, oxytocin, and arginine vasopressin levels (4)

ETIOLOGY

Multifactorial, including biologic–genetic predisposition in terms of neurobiologic deficit, destabilizing effects of hormone withdrawal at birth, inflammation, and psychosocial stressors (2)

COMMONLY ASSOCIATED CONDITIONS

- Bipolar mood disorder
- Depressive disorder not otherwise specified
- Dysthymic disorder
- Cyclothymic disorder
- MDD (10)

DIAGNOSIS

HISTORY

- Increased/decreased sleep
- Decreased interest in formerly compelling or pleasurable activities
- Guilt, low self-esteem
- Decreased energy
- Decreased concentration
- Increased/decreased appetite
- Psychomotor agitation or retardation
- Suicidal ideation

DIAGNOSTIC TESTS & INTERPRETATION

Lab

Initial lab tests

Thyroid-stimulating hormone (TSH) (11)[A]

Diagnostic Procedures/Surgery

- Edinburgh Postnatal Depression Scale is the primary screening tool.
- Beck, Hamilton, and Zung depression inventories may provide information about the severity of the depression and suicidal risks.
- Edinburgh Postnatal Depression Scale (Partner Version). To be completed by mother's partner to obtain his/her view of mother's depression.

DIFFERENTIAL DIAGNOSIS

- Baby blues: Not a psychiatric disorder, mood lability, resolves within days
- Postpartum psychosis: A psychiatric emergency
- Postpartum anxiety/panic disorder
- Postpartum obsessive-compulsive disorder
- Hypothyroidism
- Postpartum thyroiditis: Can occur in up to 7.5% of patients and can present as depression (12)[A]
- Sleep apnea

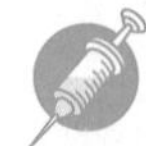

TREATMENT

MEDICATION

First Line

- SSRIs are generally effective and safe:
  - Fluoxetine (Prozac): 20–80 mg/d PO (most activating of all SSRIs); less expensive
  - Sertraline (Zoloft): 50–200 mg/d PO (sedating)
  - Paroxetine (Paxil): 20–60 mg/d PO (sedating)
  - Citalopram (Celexa): 20–60 mg/d PO
- Tricyclic antidepressants (TCAs) effective and less expensive, yet are lethal in overdose and have unfavorable side effects:
  - Avoid TCAs in mothers with a history of suicide attempts.
- Bupropion (Wellbutrin): 150–450 mg/d PO in patients with depression plus psychomotor retardation, hypersomnia, and with weight gain. Bupropion is less likely to cause weight gain or sexual dysfunction and is highly activating.
- Mirtazapine (Remeron): 15–45 mg/d PO at bedtime. May assist with sleep restoration and weight gain; no sexual dysfunction
- Venlafaxine (Effexor XR): A dual-action antidepressant that blocks the reuptake of serotonin in doses of up to 150 mg/d and then blocks the reuptake of norepinephrine in doses of 150–450 mg/d PO
- Bipolar disorder requires treatment with mood stabilizer.
- Among breastfeeding mothers:
  - Weigh potential efficacy of treatment with antidepressant, risks of exposure to infant, and known negative effects of not treating on child development.
  - All antidepressants are excreted in breast milk, but are generally compatible with lactation.
  - Paroxetine and sertraline offer best safety profile during lactation.
  - Start with low doses and increase slowly. Monitor infant for adverse side effects.
  - Minimize infant exposure to medication by avoiding breastfeeding at time of peak concentration.
  - Consider continuing medication that is efficacious while monitoring infant carefully, rather than switching antidepressants (4,13)[B].
  - For further information: *Medications and Mother's Milk* by Thomas Hale, PhD

Second Line

Electroconvulsive therapy (ECT): May be indicated in patients who cannot tolerate antidepressant medication, are actively engaged in suicidal self-destructive behaviors, or have a previous history of response to ECT (14)[C]

ADDITIONAL TREATMENT

General Measures

- Most patients respond to outpatient individual psychotherapy in combination with pharmacotherapy.
- Support/therapy groups may be helpful.
- Assess suicidal ideation.
- Assess homicidal ideation and thoughts of harming baby. Thoughts of harming baby require immediate hospitalization.
- Visiting nurse services can provide direct observations of the mother about safety issues and mother–child bonding (10)[A].

Issues for Referral

- Obtain psychiatric consultation for patients with psychotic symptoms.
- Immediate hospitalization is mandatory if delusions or hallucinations are present.
- Hospitalization is indicated if mother's ability to care for self and/or infant is significantly compromised.

Additional Therapies
- Psychoeducation, including providing reading material for the patient and family (10)[C]
- Psychotherapy: Interpersonal psychotherapy, cognitive-behavioral therapy, and psychodynamic psychotherapy shown to be effective (4)[C]

COMPLEMENTARY AND ALTERNATIVE MEDICINE
- Breastfeeding is effective in reducing stress and protecting maternal mood (11)[A].
- Infant massage, infant sleep intervention, exercise, and bright light therapy may be beneficial (4)[B],(15)[A].

IN-PATIENT CONSIDERATIONS

ALERT

Obtain psychiatric consultation for patients with psychotic symptoms. If delusions or hallucinations are present, immediate hospitalization is mandatory. The psychotic mother should *not* be left alone with the baby.

Admission Criteria
Presence of suicidal or homicidal ideation and/or psychotic symptoms and/or thoughts of harming baby and/or inability to care for self or infant, severe weight loss

Discharge Criteria
- Absence of suicidal or homicidal ideation and/or psychotic symptoms and/or thoughts of harming baby
- Mother must be able to care for self and infant.

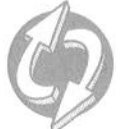

ONGOING CARE

FOLLOW-UP RECOMMENDATIONS
Patient Monitoring
- Collaborative care approach, including primary care visits and case manager follow-ups
- Consultation with the infant's doctor, particularly if mother is breastfeeding while taking psychotropic medications

DIET
- Good nutrition and hydration, especially when breastfeeding
- The addition of a multivitamin with minerals and omega-3 fatty acids may be helpful.

PATIENT EDUCATION
- *This Isn't What I Expected: Overcoming Postpartum Depression*, by Karen R. Kleinman and Valerie Davis Radkin
- *Down Came the Rain: My Journey Through Postpartum Depression*, by Brooke Shields, 2005
- *Behind the Smile: My Journey Out of Postpartum Depression*, by Marie Osmond, Marcie Wilkie, and Judith Morre, 2001
- *A Medication Guide for Breastfeeding Moms*, by Thomas Hale and Ghia Mcafee, 2008
- Web resources:
  - Postpartum support international: http://www.postpartum.net
  - http://www.4women.gov
  - La Leche League: http://www.lalecheleague.org
  - http://toxnet.nlm.nih.gov
  - www.mededppd.org
  - www.womensmentalhealth.org
  - www.motherrisk.org

PROGNOSIS
- Treatment of maternal depression to remission has been shown to have a positive impact on children's mental health (13)[B].
- Some patients, particularly those with undertreated or undiagnosed depression, may develop chronic depression requiring long-term treatment (16)[A].
- Untreated maternal depression is linked to impaired child development, including poor cognitive functioning and emotional maladjustment in infants and children (4,13)[B].
- Postpartum psychosis associated with tragic outcomes, such as maternal suicide and infanticide (2,16)[C]

COMPLICATIONS
- Suicide
- Self-injurious behavior
- Psychosis
- Neglect of baby
- Harm to the baby (12)[A]

REFERENCES

1. Paulson JF, Dauber S, Leiferman JA. Individual and combined effects of postpartum depression in mothers and fathers on parenting behavior. *Pediatrics*. 2006;118:659–68.
2. Brett K, et al. Prevalence of self-reported postpartum depressive symptoms: 17 Sate, 2004–2005. *MMWR Weekly*. 2008;361–6.
3. Mayberry J, et al. Depression symptom prevalence and demographic risk factors among U.S. women during the 1st 2 years postpartum. *J Obstet Gynecol Neo Nurs*. 2007:542–9.
4. Pearlstein T, Howard M, Salisbury A, et al. Postpartum depression. *Am J Obstet Gynecol*. 2009;200:357–64.
5. Davey HL, Tough SC, Adair CE, et al. Risk factors for sub-clinical and major postpartum depression among a community cohort of Canadian women. *Matern Child Health J*. 2011;15(7):866–75.
6. Choi Y, Bishai D, Minkovitz CS. Multiple births are a risk factor for postpartum maternal depressive symptoms. *Pediatrics*. 2009;123:1147–54.
7. Lee AM, et al. Prevalence, course, risk factors for antenatal anxiety and depression. *Obstet Gyn*. 2007;5:1102–12.
8. Monti F, et al. Depressive symptoms during late pregnancy and early adulthood following assisted reproductive technology. *Fertility Sterility*. 2008;1–7.
9. Jomeen J, et al. Replicability and stability of the multidimensional model of the Edinburgh Postnatal Depression Scale I late pregnancy. *J Psychiatr Mental Health Nurs*. 2007;14:319–24.
10. Howard LM, et al. Antidepressant prevention of postnatal depression. *PLoS Medicine*. 2006;3: 1741–2.
11. Kendall-Tackett K. A new paradigm for depression in new mothers: The central role of inflammation and how breastfeeding and anti-inflammatory treatments protect maternal health. *Intl Breastfeeding J*. 2007;2:6.
12. Harrington AR, Greene-Harrington CC. Healthy Start screens for depression among urban pregnant, postpartum and interconceptional women. *J Natl Med Assoc*. 2007;99:226–31.
13. Freeman MP. Breastfeeding and antidepressants: Clinical dilemmas and expert perspectives. *J Clin Psychiatry*. 2009;70:291–2.
14. Forray A, Ostroff RB. The use of electroconvulsive therapy in postpartum affective disorders. *J ECT*. 2007;23:188–93.
15. Daley AJ, Macarthur C, Winter H. The role of exercise in treating postpartum depression: A review of the literature. *J Midwifery Womens Health*. 2007;52:56–62.
16. Tammentie T, Tarkka MT, Astedt-Kurki P, et al. Family dynamics and postnatal depression. *J Psychiatr Ment Health Nurs*. 2004;11:141–9.
17. Musters C, McDonald E, Jones I. Management of postnatal depression. *BMJ*. 2008;337:a736.

D

ADDITIONAL READING

- Gjerdingen D, et al. Stepped care treatment of postpartum depression. *Women's Health Issues*. 2007;18:44–52.
- Hirst KP, Moutier CY, et al. Postpartum major depression. *Am Fam Physician*. 2010;82:926–33.
- Ng RC, Hirata CK, Yeung W, et al. Pharmacologic treatment for postpartum depression: A systematic review. *Pharmacotherapy*. 2010;30:928–41.
- Sit DK, Wisner KL, et al. Identification of postpartum depression. *Clin Obstet Gynecol*. 2009;52:456–68.
- Edinborough Postnatal depression scale: http://www.testandcalc.com/etc/tests/edin.asp

CODES

ICD9
- 296.20 Major depressive affective disorder, single episode, unspecified
- 296.30 Major depressive affective disorder, recurrent episode, unspecified
- 648.44 Postpartum mental disorders of mother

CLINICAL PEARLS
- PPD is a common, debilitating medical condition that impairs a mother's ability to function and interact with her infant and family.
- Universal screening for PPD is recommended during the third trimester and at regular intervals during the postpartum period.
- Early diagnosis and treatment are vital, as untreated PPD can lead to developmental difficulties for the infant and prolonged disability and suffering for the mother (4,17)[B].
- Breastfeeding is recommended for maternal and child health. There are several medication options for treating depression in mothers that are safe for breastfeeding infants.

DEPRESSION, TREATMENT RESISTANT

Michelle Magid, MD

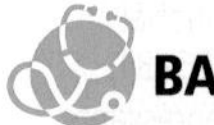

BASICS

DESCRIPTION

- Major depressive disorder (MDD) that has failed to respond to 2 or more adequate trials of antidepressant therapy
- Antidepressant therapy must be given for 6 weeks at standard doses before being considered a failure.

EPIDEMIOLOGY

- Depression affects >18 million people in the US and >340 million people worldwide.
- 16% lifetime risk of MDD
- Of those with MDD, ~1/3 will become treatment-resistant.

RISK FACTORS

- Severity of disease
- Mislabeling patients with depression who are bipolar
- Comorbid medical disease
- Comorbid personality disorder
- Comorbid anxiety disorder
- Substance abuse
- Familial predisposition to poor response to antidepressants

Genetics

Limited studies have shown that a genetic abnormality in the serotonin transporter gene (5-HTTLPR) may increase risk for treatment-resistant depression (1).

GENERAL PREVENTION

- Medication adherence in combination with psychotherapy
- Maintenance electroconvulsive therapy (ECT) may prevent relapse.

PATHOPHYSIOLOGY

- Unclear. Low levels of neurotransmitters (serotonin, norepinephrine, dopamine) have been indicated.
- Serotonin has been linked to irritability, hostility, and suicidal ideation.
- Norepinephrine has been linked to low energy.
- Dopamine may play a role in low motivation and depression with psychotic features.

ETIOLOGY

- Impaired synthesis and/or metabolism of neurotransmitters
- Environmental stressors such as abuse and neglect may affect neurotransmission.

COMMONLY ASSOCIATED CONDITIONS

- Suicide
- Bipolar disorder
- Substance abuse
- Anxiety disorders
- Dysthymia
- Eating disorders
- Somatization disorders

DIAGNOSIS

HISTORY

- Symptoms are the same as in MDD. However, patients do not respond to standard form of treatment. Severity and duration are extreme.
- Especially important to screen for suicidality in treatment-resistant depression
- Screening with SIGECAPS:
  - SLEEP: Too much or too little
  - INTEREST: Failure to enjoy activities
  - GUILT: Excessive and uncontrollable
  - ENERGY: Poor energy
  - CONCENTRATION: Inability to focus on tasks
  - APPETITE: Too much or too little
  - PSYCHOMOTOR CHANGES: Restlessness/agitation or slowing/lethargy
  - SUICIDALITY: Desire to end life

PHYSICAL EXAM

Mental status exam may reveal poor hygiene, poor eye contact, blunted affect, tearfulness, weight loss or gain, psychomotor retardation, or agitation.

DIAGNOSTIC TESTS & INTERPRETATION

Lab

Used to rule out medical factors that could be causing/contributing to treatment resistance

Initial lab tests

- CBC
- Complete metabolic profile, including liver tests, calcium, and glucose
- Urine drug screen
- Thyroid-stimulating Hormone (TSH)
- Vitamin D level (25 OH Vit D)

Follow-Up & Special Considerations

Delirium and dementia may often look like depression.

Imaging

CT or MRI of the brain if neurologic disease, tumor, or dementia is suspected

Diagnostic Procedures/Surgery

- Depression is a clinical diagnosis
- Validated depression rating scales can assist:
  - Beck Depression Inventory
  - Hamilton Rating Scale for Depression
  - Patient Health Questionnaire 9 (PHQ-9)

DIFFERENTIAL DIAGNOSIS

- Bipolar disorder
- Dysthymia
- Dementia
- Early-stage Parkinson disease
- Personality disorder
- Medical illness such as malignancy, thyroid disease, HIV
- Substance abuse

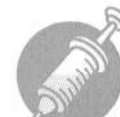

TREATMENT

MEDICATION

First Line

- Please see "Depression" topic. When those fail, augmentation and combination strategies are as follows:
  - Antidepressant + lithium:
    - Tricyclic antidepressant (TCA): Nortriptyline (start 50 mg at bedtime. Max dose 200 mg at bedtime) + lithium (start 300 mg at bedtime. Max dose 900 mg b.i.d.) (2,3,4)
    - SSRI: Citalopram (start 20 mg daily Max dose 80 mg every day) + lithium (start 300 mg at bedtime. Max dose 900 mg b.i.d.) (2,3,5)
  - Antidepressant + thyroid supplementation:
    - Citalopram (start 20 daily. Max dose 80 daily) + triiodothyronine (T3) (12.5–50 mcg daily) (3,5,6)
  - Antidepressants in combination:
    - Citalopram (start 20 daily. Max dose 80 daily) + bupropion (start 100 mg b.i.d. Max dose 450 mg/every day) (5,7)
    - TCAs and SSRIs may be used in combination. Proceed with caution, due to risk of serotonin syndrome. Citalopram (start 20 daily. Max dose 80 daily) + nortriptyline (start 50 at bedtime. Max dose 200 at bedtime)
  - Antidepressants + antipsychotics:
    - Citalopram (start 20 daily. Max dose 80 daily) + aripiprazole (start 2–5 mg, titrate to 15–20 mg daily) (3,8)
    - Citalopram (start 20 daily. Max dose 80 daily + olanzapine (start 2.5 mg at bedtime. Max dose 20 mg at bedtime) (3,8). Citalopram (start 20 daily. Max dose 80 daily) + quetiapine (start 25 at bedtime. Titrate to 100–300 at bedtime) (3,8).
- In above combinations, citalopram (Celexa) can be replaced with other SSRIs such as fluoxetine (Prozac) 20–80 mg/d, sertraline (Zoloft) 50–200 mg/d, and escitalopram (Lexapro) 10–20 mg/d or with serotonin-norepinephrine reuptake inhibitor (SNRI) duloxetine (Cymbalta) 30–120 mg/d
- Maximum doses for medication in treatment-resistant cases are higher than in treatment-responsive cases.

Second Line

MAOI:

- Tranylcypromine (Parnate) (start 10 mg t.i.d. Increase 10 mg/d every 1–3 weeks. Max dose: 60 mg/d)
- Selegiline transdermal (Emsam patch) (apply 6 mg patch daily, increase 3 mg/d. Max dose 12 mg/d)
- Side-effect profile (e.g., hypertensive crisis), drug–drug interactions, and dietary restrictions make MAOIs less appealing. Patch version does not require dietary restrictions at lower doses.
- High risk of serotonin syndrome, if combined with another antidepressant. 2-week washout period is advised.

ADDITIONAL TREATMENT

- First line:
  - Electroconvulsive therapy (ECT): Safe and effective treatment for treatment-resistant and life-threatening depression, with a 50–80% success rate (9,10)[A]:
    - Known to rapidly relieve suicidality, psychotic depression, and catatonia
    - Controversy due to cognitive side effects during the treatment
    - 4 types of lead placements:
      - Bitemporal: Most effective, most cognitive side effects. Usually need 610 treatments at 1.5 times seizure threshold
      - Right unilateral: May be slightly less effective but fewer cognitive side effects. Usually need 8–12 treatments at 4–6 times seizure threshold
      - Ultrabrief right unilateral and bifrontal lead placements are newer techniques being studied.
- Second line:
  - Deep brain stimulation (DBS): Surgical implantation of intracranial electrodes, connected to an impulse generator implanted in the chest wall (11,12)[C]:
    - Reserved for those who have failed medications, psychotherapy, and ECT
    - Preliminary data is promising, showing 53% response rate and 35% remission rate, but further trials are warranted (11).
  - Transmagnetic stimulation (TMS): Noninvasive brain stimulation technique that is generally safe. A few case reports on efficacy in treatment-resistant depression, but thus far used for less severe forms of the illness (12)[C].
  - Vagus nerve stimulation (VNS): Surgical implantation of electrodes onto left vagus nerve. Its use in treatment-resistant depression has become limited in recent years (12)[C].

Issues for Referral

Treatment-resistant depression should be managed by a psychiatrist.

IN-PATIENT CONSIDERATIONS

Admission Criteria

Inpatient care is indicated for severely depressed, psychotic, catatonic, or suicidal patients.

Discharge Criteria

Symptoms improving, no longer suicidal, psychosocial stressors addressed

ONGOING CARE

FOLLOW-UP RECOMMENDATIONS

- Frequent visits, i.e., every month
- During follow-up, evaluate side effects, dosage, and effectiveness of medication, as well as need for referral to ECT.
- Patients who have responded to ECT may need maintenance treatments (q4–8wk) to prevent relapse.
- Combination of lithium/nortriptyline after ECT appears to be as effective as maintenance ECT in reducing relapse

DIET

Patients on MAOIs need dietary restriction.

PATIENT EDUCATION

- Educate patients that depression is a medical illness, not a character defect.
- Review signs and symptoms of worsening depression and when patient needs to come in for further evaluation.
- Discuss safety plan to address suicidal thoughts.

PROGNOSIS

With medication adherence, close follow-up, improved social support, and psychotherapy, prognosis improves.

COMPLICATIONS

- Suicide
- Disability
- Poor quality of life

REFERENCES

1. Arias B, et al. 5-HTTLPR polymorphism of the serotonin transporter gene predicts non-remission in major depression patients treated with citalopram in a 12-week follow-up study. *J Clin Psychopharmacol*. 2003;23(6):563–7.
2. Keller MB. Issues in treatment-resistant depression. *J Clin Psychiatry*. 2005;66(suppl 8): 5–12.
3. Hicks P, et al. How to best manage treatment-resistant depression? *J Fam Pract*. 2010;59;490–7.
4. Kellner CH, et al. Continuation electroconvulsive therapy vs pharmacotherapy for relapse prevention in major depression: A multisite study from the Consortium for Research in Electroconvulsive Therapy (CORE). *Arch Gen Psychiatry*. 2006;63:1337–44.
5. Rush AJ, et al. Acute and longer term outcomes in depressed patients who require one or several treatment steps: A STAR*D report. *Am J Psych*. 2006;163:1905–17.
6. Nierenberg AA, et al. A comparison of Lithium and T3 augmentation following two failed medication treatments for depression: A STAR*D report. *Am J Psych*. 2006;163:1519–30.
7. Trivedi MH, et al. Medication augmentation after the failure of SSRIs for depression. *N Engl J Med*. 2006;354:1243–52.
8. Chen J, et al. Second-generation antipsychotics in major depressive disorder: Update and clinical perspective. *Curr Opin in Psych*. 2011;24:10–17.
9. Lisanby S. Electroconvulsive therapy for depression. *N Engl J Med*. 2007;357:1939–45.
10. Fink M, Taylor MA. Electroconvulsive therapy evidences and challenges. *JAMA*. 2007;298: 330–2.
11. Malone DA. Use of deep brain stimulation in treatment-resistant depression. *Cleveland Clinic J Med*. 2010;77(suppl 3):S77–S80.
12. Holtzheimer PE, Mayberg HS. Deep brain stimulation for treatment-resistant depression. *Am J Psychiatry*. 2010;167:14377–444.

ADDITIONAL READING

American Psychiatric Association: Practice Guideline for the Treatment of Patients with Major Depressive Disorder, Third Edition. *Am J Psychiatry*. 2010; 167(10):1–118.

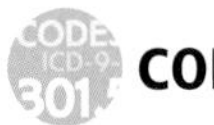

CODES

ICD9

311 Depressive disorder, not elsewhere classified

CLINICAL PEARLS

- Treatment-resistant depression is common, affecting 1/3 of those with MDD.
- Combination and augmentation strategies with antidepressants, mood stabilizers, and antipsychotics can be helpful.
- ECT should be considered in severe and life-threatening cases.

D

DERMATITIS, ATOPIC

Dennis E. Hughes, DO

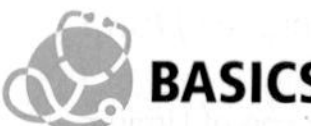

BASICS

DESCRIPTION

- A chronic, relapsing, pruritic eczematous condition affecting characteristic sites
- Although called atopic, the majority of children with the typical clinical presentation will not have a measurable IgE-mediated sensitivity to allergens.
- System(s) affected: Skin/Exocrine

EPIDEMIOLOGY

Environmentally triggered in susceptible individuals

Incidence

- 45% of all cases begin in the first 6 months of life.
- 70% of affected children will have a spontaneous remission before adolescence.

Prevalence

- Mainly childhood disease; affects 10% of all children
- Also may have late-onset dermatitis in adults
- Visits for the condition have been rising over the last 10 years.
- Asians and blacks affected more often than whites
- 60% if 1 parent affected; rises to 80% if both parents affected

RISK FACTORS

- "Itch-scratch cycle"(stimulates histamine release)
- Skin infections
- Emotional stress
- Irritating clothes and chemicals
- Excessively hot or cold climate
- Food allergy in children (in some cases)
- Exposure to tobacco smoke
- Family history of atopy:
  - Asthma
  - Allergic rhinitis

Genetics

- Arises from gene–gene and gene–environment interactions
- Both epidermal and immune coding likely involved

PATHOPHYSIOLOGY

- Alteration in stratum corneum results in transepidermal water loss.
- Epidermal adhesion is reduced either as a result of genetic mutation or as a result of inflammatory response.
- Interleukin-31 (IL-31) upregulation is thought to be a major factor in pruritus rather than histamine excess.

COMMONLY ASSOCIATED CONDITIONS

- Food sensitivity/allergy in many cases
- Asthma
- Allergic rhinitis
- Hyper-IgE syndrome (Job syndrome):
  - Atopic dermatitis
  - Elevated IgE
  - Recurrent pyodermas
  - Decreased chemotaxis of mononuclear cells

DIAGNOSIS

HISTORY

Pruritus is the most common symptom.

PHYSICAL EXAM

- Distribution of lesions:
  - Infants: Trunk, face, and flexural surfaces; diaper-sparing
  - Children: Antecubital and popliteal fossae
  - Adults: Hands, feet, face, neck, upper chest, and genital areas
- Morphology of lesions:
  - Infants: Erythema and papules; may develop oozing, crusting vesicles
  - Children and adults: Lichenification and scaling are typical with chronic eczema as a result of persistent scratching and rubbing (lichenification rare in infants).
- Associated signs:
  - Facial erythema, mild to moderate
  - Perioral pallor
  - Infraorbital fold (Dennie sign/Morgan line)
  - Dry skin
  - Increased palmar linear markings
  - Pityriasis alba (hypopigmented asymptomatic areas on face and shoulders)
  - Keratosis pilaris

DIAGNOSTIC TESTS & INTERPRETATION

Lab

Initial lab tests

- No test is diagnostic.
- Serum IgE levels are elevated in as many as 80% of affected individuals.
- Eosinophilia tends to correlate with disease severity.

Pathological Findings

- Epidermis thickened and hyperkeratotic
- Perivascular inflammation of dermis

DIFFERENTIAL DIAGNOSIS

- Photosensitivity rashes
- Contact dermatitis (especially if only the face is involved)
- Scabies
- Seborrheic dermatitis (especially in infants)
- Psoriasis or lichen simplex chronicus if only localized disease is present in adults
- Rare conditions of infancy:
  - Histiocytosis X
  - Wiskott-Aldrich syndrome
  - Ataxia-telangiectasia syndrome
- Ichthyosis vulgaris

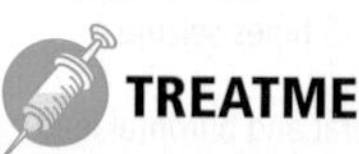

TREATMENT

Pediatric Considerations

Chronic potent fluorinated corticosteroid use may cause striae, hypopigmentation, or atrophy, especially in children.

MEDICATION

First Line

- Frequent systemic lubrication with thick emollient creams (e.g., Eucerin, Vaseline) over moist skin is the mainstay of treatment before any other intervention is considered.
- Infants and children: 0.5–1% topical hydrocortisone creams or ointments (1)[C]
- Adults: Higher-potency topical corticosteroids in areas other than face and skin folds
- Short-course higher-potency corticosteroids for flares; then return to the lowest potency (creams preferred) that will control dermatitis (2)[C]. Hypopigmentation can occur even with short-term use.
- Antihistamines for pruritus (e.g., Hydroxyzine 10–25 mg at bedtime and as needed)

Second Line

- Topical immunomodulators (tacrolimus or pimecrolimus) for episodic use for children >2 years of age. There is a black box warning from the Food and Drug Administration regarding potential cancer risk (3).
- Plastic occlusion in combination with topical medication to promote absorption
- For severe atopic dermatitis, consider systemic steroids × 1–2 weeks (e.g., Prednisone 2 mg/kg/d PO [maximum 80 mg/d] initially, tapered over 7–14 days).
- Topical tricyclic doxepin as a 5% cream may decrease pruritus.
- Modified Goeckerman regimen (tar and ultraviolet light)
- Immune modifiers (methotrexate, azathioprine, cyclosporine)

ADDITIONAL TREATMENT

General Measures

- Decrease stress if possible.
- Avoid agents that may cause irritation (e.g., wool, perfumes).
- Minimize sweating.
- Lukewarm (not hot) baths
- Minimize use of soap (superfatted soaps best).
- Frequent systemic lubrication with thick emollient creams (e.g., Eucerin) over moist skin
- Sun exposure may be helpful.
- Humidify the house.
- Avoid excessive contact with water.
- Avoid lotions that contain alcohol.
- If very resistant to treatment, search for a coexisting contact dermatitis.

Issues for Referral

- Ophthalmology evaluation for persistent vernal conjunctivitis
- If using topical steroids around eyes for extended periods, ophthalmology follow-up for cataract evaluation

Additional Therapies

- Methods to reduce house mite allergens (micropore filters on heating, ventilation, and air-conditioning systems; impermeable mattress covers) (4)[C]
- Behavioral relaxation therapy to reduce scratching (4)[B]

COMPLEMENTARY AND ALTERNATIVE MEDICINE

- Evening primrose oil (includes high content of fatty acids):
  - May decrease prostaglandin synthesis
  - May promote conversion of linoleic acid to omega-6 fatty acid
- Probiotics may reduce the severity of the condition, reducing medication use (4)[C].

ONGOING CARE

FOLLOW-UP RECOMMENDATIONS

Patient Monitoring

Evaluate to ensure that secondary bacterial or fungal infection does not develop as a result of disruption of the skin barrier. There is little evidence for the routine use of antimicrobial interventions to reduce skin bacteria.

DIET

- Trials of elimination may find certain "triggers" in some patients.
- Breastfeeding in conjunction with maternal hypoallergenic diets may decrease the severity in some infants.

PATIENT EDUCATION

- http://www.add.org/public/publications/pamplets/eczemaatopicdermatitis.htm
- National Eczema Association: www.nationaleczema.org

PROGNOSIS

- Chronic disease
- Declines with increasing age.
- 90% of patients have spontaneous resolution by puberty.
- Localized eczema (e.g., chronic hand or foot dermatitis, eyelid dermatitis, or lichen simplex chronicus) may continue in some adults.

COMPLICATIONS

- Cataracts are more common in patients with atopic dermatitis.
- Skin infections (usually *Staphylococcus aureus*); sometimes subclinical
- Eczema herpeticum:
  - Generalized vesiculopustular eruption caused by infection with herpes simplex or vaccinia virus
  - Causes acute illness requiring hospitalization
- Atrophy and/or striae if fluorinated corticosteroids are used on face or skin folds
- Systemic absorption may occur if large areas of skin are treated, particularly if high-potency medications and occlusion are combined.

REFERENCES

1. Bieber T. Atopic dermatitis. *N Engl J Med*. 2008; 358:1483–94.
2. Williams HC. Clinical practice. Atopic dermatitis. *N Engl J Med*. 2005;352:2314–24.
3. Trammell S, Shakil A, Wilder L, et al. Clinical inquiries. What is the role of tacrolimus and pimecrolimus in atopic dermatitis? *J Fam Pract*. 2005;54:714–6.
4. Weston S, et al. Effects of probiotics on atopic dermatitis: A randomized controlled trial. *Arch Disease Child*. 2005;90:892–7.

ADDITIONAL READING

Hill DJ, Hosking CS. Food allergy and atopic dermatitis in infancy: An epidemiological study. *Padiatr Allergy Immunol*. 2004;15(5):421–7.

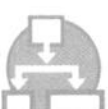

See Also (Topic, Algorithm, Electronic Media Element)

Algorithm: Rash, Focal

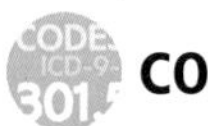

CODES

ICD9

691.8 Other atopic dermatitis and related conditions

CLINICAL PEARLS

- Institute early and proactive treatment to reduce inflammation.
- Monitor for secondary bacterial infection.
- Frequent systemic lubrication with thick emollient creams (e.g., Eucerin, Vaseline) over moist skin is the mainstay of treatment before any other intervention is considered.
- Use the lowest-potency topical steroid that controls symptoms.

D

DERMATITIS, CONTACT

Aamir Siddiqi, MD

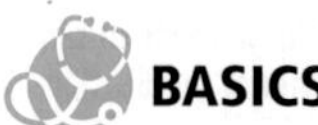

BASICS

DESCRIPTION

- The cutaneous reaction to an external substance
- Primary irritant dermatitis is due to direct injury of the skin. It affects individuals exposed to specific irritants and generally produces discomfort immediately after exposure.
- Allergic contact dermatitis (ACD) affects only individuals previously sensitized to the substance. It represents a delayed hypersensitivity reaction, requiring several hours for the cascade of cellular immunity to be completed to manifest itself.
- System(s) affected: Skin/Exocrine
- Synonym(s): Dermatitis venenata

EPIDEMIOLOGY

Common

Incidence

Occupational contact dermatitis: 20.5/100,000 workers

Prevalence

- Contact dermatitis represents >90% of all occupational skin disorders.
- Predominant sex: Male = Female:
  - Variations due to differences in exposure to offending agents, as well as normal cutaneous variations between male and female (eccrine and sebaceous gland function and hair distribution)

Geriatric Considerations

Increased incidence of irritant dermatitis secondary to skin dryness

Pediatric Considerations

Increased incidence of positive patch testing due to better delayed hypersensitivity reactions

RISK FACTORS

- Occupation
- Hobbies
- Travel
- Cosmetics
- Jewelry

Genetics

Increased frequency of ACD in families with allergies

GENERAL PREVENTION

- Avoid causative agents.
- Use of protective gloves (with cotton lining) may be helpful (1)[A].

PATHOPHYSIOLOGY

Hypersensitivity reaction to a substance generating cellular immunity response

ETIOLOGY

- Plants:
  - Rhus-urushiol: Poison ivy, oak, sumac
  - Primary contact: Plant (roots/stems/leaves)
  - Secondary contact: Clothes/fingernails (not blister fluid)
- Chemicals:
  - Nickel: Jewelry, zippers, hooks, and watches
  - Potassium dichromate: Tanning agent in leather
  - Paraphenylenediamine: Hair dyes, fur dyes, and industrial chemicals
  - Turpentine: Cleaning agents, polishes, and waxes
  - Soaps and detergents
- Topical medicines:
  - Neomycin: Topical antibiotics
  - Thimerosal (Merthiolate): Preservative in topical medications
  - Anesthetics: Benzocaine
  - Parabens: Preservative in topical medications
  - Formalin: Cosmetics, shampoos, and nail enamel

DIAGNOSIS

HISTORY

- Itchy rash
- Assess for prior exposure to irritating substance.

PHYSICAL EXAM

- Acute:
  - Papules, vesicles, bullae with surrounding erythema
  - Crusting and oozing
  - Pruritus
- Chronic:
  - Erythematous base
  - Thickening with lichenification
  - Scaling
  - Fissuring
- Distribution:
  - Where epidermis is thinner (eyelids, genitalia)
  - Areas of contact with offending agent (e.g., nail polish)
  - Palms and soles more resistant
  - Deeper skin folds spared
  - Linear arrays of lesions
  - Lesions with sharp borders and sharp angles are pathognomonic.
- Well-demarcated area with a papulovesicular rash

DIAGNOSTIC TESTS & INTERPRETATION

Diagnostic Procedures/Surgery

Consider patch tests for suspected allergic trigger (systemic corticosteroids or recent, aggressive use of topical steroids may alter results) (2)[B].

Pathological Findings

- Intercellular edema
- Bullae

DIFFERENTIAL DIAGNOSIS

- Based on clinical impression:
  - Appearance, periodicity, and localization
- Groups of vesicles:
  - Herpes simplex
- Diffuse bullous or vesicular lesions:
  - Bullous pemphigoid
- Photodistribution:
  - Phototoxic/allergic reaction to systemic allergen
- Eyelids:
  - Seborrheic dermatitis
- Scaly eczematous lesions:
  - Atopic dermatitis
  - Nummular eczema
  - Lichen simplex chronicus
  - Stasis dermatitis
  - Xerosis

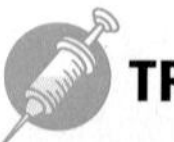

TREATMENT

MEDICATION

First Line

- Topical medications:
  - Lotion of zinc oxide, talc, menthol 0.25%, phenol 0.5% (Gold Bond, others)
  - Corticosteroids for allergic contact dermatitis as well as irritant dermatitis (1)[A]:
    - High-potency steroids: Fluocinonide (Lidex) 0.05% ointment t.i.d.–q.i.d.
    - Use high-potency steroids only for a short time and then switch to low- or medium-potency steroid cream or ointment.
    - Caution regarding face/skin folds: Use lower-potency steroids and avoid prolonged usage. Switch to lower-potency topical steroid once the acute phase is resolved.
- Calamine lotion for symptomatic relief
- Topical antibiotics for secondary infection (bacitracin, erythromycin)

- Systemic:
  - Antihistamine:
    - Hydroxyzine: 25–50 mg PO q.i.d., especially useful for itching
    - Diphenhydramine: 25–50 mg PO q.i.d.
  - Corticosteroids:
    - Prednisone: Taper starting at 60–80 mg/d PO, over 10–14 days
    - Used for moderate-to-severe cases
    - May use burst dose of steroids for up to 5 days
  - Antibiotics for secondary skin infections:
    - Dicloxacillin: 250 mg PO q.i.d. for 7–10 days
    - Amoxicillin-clavulanate (Augmentin): 500 mg PO b.i.d. for 7–10 days
    - Erythromycin: 250 mg PO q.i.d. in penicillin-allergic patients
- Precautions:
  - Antihistamines may cause drowsiness.
  - Prolonged use of potent topical steroids may cause local skin effects (atrophy, stria, telangiectasia).
  - Use tapering dose of oral steroids if using more than 5 days.

Second Line
Other topical or systemic antibiotics, depending on organisms and sensitivity

Pregnancy Considerations
Usual cautions with medications

ADDITIONAL TREATMENT
General Measures
- Removal of offending agent:
  - Avoidance
  - Work modification
  - Protective clothing
  - Barrier creams, especially high-lipid content moisturizing creams (e.g., Keri lotion, petrolatum, coconut oil) (3)[A]
- Topical soaks with cool tap water, Burow solution (1:40 dilution), saline (1 tsp/pint water), or silver nitrate solution (25.5%)
- Lukewarm water baths
- Aveeno oatmeal baths
- Emollients (white petrolatum, Eucerin)

Issues for Referral
May need referral to a dermatologist or allergist if refractory to conventional treatment

COMPLEMENTARY AND ALTERNATIVE MEDICINE
The use of complementary and alternative treatment is a supplement and not an alternative to conventional treatment (4).

IN-PATIENT CONSIDERATIONS
Admission Criteria
Rarely will need hospital admission

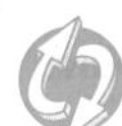

ONGOING CARE

FOLLOW-UP RECOMMENDATIONS
Stay active, but avoid overheating.

Patient Monitoring
- As necessary for recurrence
- Patch testing for etiology after resolved

DIET
No special diet

PATIENT EDUCATION
- Avoidance of irritating substance
- Cleaning of secondary sources (nails, clothes)
- Fallacy of blister fluid spreading disease

PROGNOSIS
- Self-limited
- Benign

COMPLICATIONS
- Generalized eruption secondary to autosensitization
- Secondary bacterial infection

REFERENCES

1. Saary J, Qureshi R, Palda V, et al. A systematic review of contact dermatitis treatment and prevention. *J Am Acad Dermatol*. 2005;53:845.
2. Saripalli YV, Achen F, Belsito DV. The detection of clinically relevant contact allergens using a standard screening tray of twenty-three allergens. *J Am Acad Dermatol*. 2003;49:65–9.
3. Hachem JP, De Paepe K, Vanpée E, et al. Efficacy of topical corticosteroids in nickel-induced contact allergy. *Clin Exp Dermatol*. 2002;27:47–50.
4. Noiesen E, Munk MD, Larsen K, et al. Use of complementary and alternative treatment for allergic contact dermatitis. *Br J Dermatol*. 2007.

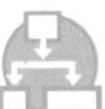

See Also (Topic, Algorithm, Electronic Media Element)
Algorithm: Rash, Focal

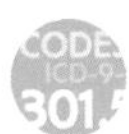

CODES

ICD9
- 692.0 Contact dermatitis and other eczema due to detergents
- 692.3 Contact dermatitis and other eczema due to drugs and medicines in contact with skin
- 692.4 Contact dermatitis and other eczema due to other chemical products

CLINICAL PEARLS
- Anyone exposed to irritants or allergic substances is predisposed to contact dermatitis, especially in occupations that have high exposure to chemicals.
- The most common allergens causing contact dermatitis are plants of the *Toxicodendron* genus (poison ivy, poison oak, poison sumac).
- The usual treatment for contact dermatitis is avoidance of the allergen or irritating substance and temporary use of topical steroids.
- A contact dermatitis rash presents in a nondermatomal geographic fashion, due to the skin being in contact with an external source.

DERMATITIS, DIAPER

Dennis E. Hughes, DO

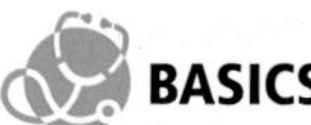

BASICS

DESCRIPTION

- Diaper dermatitis is a rash occurring under the covered area of a diaper. The rash may be a direct result of wearing the diaper, aggravated by the diaper, or coincidental with a rash that appears elsewhere on the body.
- System(s) affected: Skin/Exocrine
- Synonym(s): Diaper rash

Geriatric Considerations

Incontinence is a significant cofactor.

EPIDEMIOLOGY

Incidence

- The most common dermatitis found in infancy
- Peak incidence: 7–12 months of age, then decreases

Prevalence

Prevalence has been variably reported from 4–35% in the first 2 years of life.

RISK FACTORS

- Infrequent diaper changes
- Waterproof diapers
- Improper laundering (cloth diapers)
- Family history of dermatitis
- Hot, humid weather
- Recent treatment with oral antibiotics
- Diarrhea (>3 stools per day increases risk)
- Dye allergy
- Prior history of eczema may increase risk.

GENERAL PREVENTION

Attention to hygiene during bouts of diarrhea

PATHOPHYSIOLOGY

- Fecal proteases and lipases are irritants.
- Superhydrase urease enzyme found in the stratum corneum liberates ammonia from cutaneous bacteria.
- Fecal lipase and protease activity is increased by acceleration of GI transit; thus, a higher incidence of irritant diaper dermatitis is observed in babies who have had diarrhea in the previous 48 hours.
- Once the skin is compromised, secondary infection by *Candida albicans* is common. 40–75% of diaper rashes that last >3 days are colonized with *C. albicans*.
- Bacteria may play a role in diaper dermatitis through reduction of fecal pH and resulting activation of enzymes.
- Allergy is exceedingly rare as a cause in infants.

ETIOLOGY

- Wet skin from prolonged contact with urine or feces resulting in susceptibility to chemical, enzymatic, and physical injury; wet skin is also penetrated more easily.
- Some have raised the possibility of contact allergy from the dye in disposable diapers.

COMMONLY ASSOCIATED CONDITIONS

- Contact (allergic or irritant) dermatitis
- Seborrheic dermatitis
- Psoriasis
- Candidiasis
- Atopic dermatitis

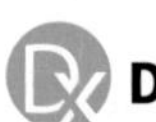

DIAGNOSIS

HISTORY

- Onset, duration, and change in the nature of the rash
- Presence of rashes outside the diaper area
- Associated scratching or crying
- Contact with infants with a similar rash
- Recent illness, diarrhea, or antibiotic use
- Fever
- Pustular drainage
- Lymphangitis

PHYSICAL EXAM

- Mild forms consist of shiny erythema ± scale.
- Margins are not always evident.
- Moderate cases have areas of papules, vesicles, and small superficial erosions.
- It can progress to well-demarcated ulcerated nodules that measure 1 cm or more in diameter.
- It is found on the prominent parts of the buttocks, medial thighs, mons pubis, and scrotum.
- Skin folds are spared or involved last.
- *Tidemark dermatitis* refers to the bandlike form of erythema of irritated diaper margins.
- Diaper dermatitis can cause an id (autoeczematous) reaction outside the diaper area.

DIAGNOSTIC TESTS & INTERPRETATION

Lab

Initial lab tests

Rarely needed

Follow-Up & Special Considerations

- Consider a culture of lesions or a potassium hydroxide (KOH) preparation.
- The finding of anemia in association with hepatosplenomegaly and the appropriate rash may suggest a diagnosis of Langerhans cell histiocytosis or congenital syphilis.
- Finding mites, ova, or feces on a mineral oil preparation of a burrow scraping can confirm the diagnosis of scabies.

Pathological Findings

- Biopsy is rare.
- Histology may reveal acute, subacute, or chronic spongiotic dermatitis.

DIFFERENTIAL DIAGNOSIS

- Contact dermatitis
- Seborrheic dermatitis
- Candidiasis
- Atopic dermatitis
- Scabies
- Acrodermatitis enteropathica
- Letterer-Siwe disease
- Congenital syphilis
- Child abuse
- Streptococcal infection
- Kawasaki disease
- Biotin deficiency
- Psoriasis
- HIV infection

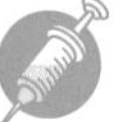

TREATMENT

See "General Measures" for first-line approach.

MEDICATION

First Line

- For a pure contact dermatitis, a low-potency topical steroid (hydrocortisone 0.5–1% t.i.d.) and removal of the offending agent should suffice.
- If candidiasis is suspected or diaper rash persists, use an antifungal such as miconazole nitrate 2% cream, miconazole powder, econazole (Spectazole), clotrimazole (Lotrimin), or ketoconazole (Nizoral) cream at each diaper change (1)[B].
- If inflammation is prominent, consider a very low-potency steroid cream such as hydrocortisone 0.5–1% t.i.d. along with an antifungal cream ± a combination product such as clioquinol-hydrocortisone (Vioform–hydrocortisone) cream (1)[B].
- If a secondary bacterial infection is suspected, use an antistaphylococcal oral antibiotic or mupirocin (Bactroban) ointment topically.
- Precautions: Avoid high- or moderate-potency steroids often found in combination steroid antifungal mixtures (1)[B].

Second Line

Sucralfate paste for resistant cases

ADDITIONAL TREATMENT

General Measures

- Expose the buttocks to air as much as possible (1)[B].
- Avoid waterproof pants during treatment (day or night); they keep the skin wet and subject to rash or infection.
- Change diapers frequently, even at night, if the rash is extensive (2)[B].
- Superabsorbable diapers are beneficial (1,2)[B].
- Discontinue using baby lotion, powder, ointment, or baby oil (except zinc oxide).
- Disposable baby wipes may contain substances that induce or worsen contact or irritant dermatitis, such as fragrance, benzalkonium chloride, and isothiazolinone or alcohol.
- Apply zinc oxide ointment or other barrier cream to the rash at the earliest sign and b.i.d. or t.i.d. (e.g., Desitin or Balmex). Thereafter, apply to clean, thoroughly dry skin (1)[B].
- Use mild soap, and pat dry.
- Cornstarch can reduce friction. Talc powders that do not enhance the growth of yeast can provide protection against frictional injury in diaper dermatitis, but do not form a continuous lipid barrier layer over the skin and obstruct the skin pores. These treatments are not recommended.

Issues for Referral

Consider if a systemic disease such as Langerhans cell histiocytosis, acrodermatitis enteropathica, or HIV infection is suspected.

IN-PATIENT CONSIDERATIONS

Admission Criteria

- Febrile neonates
- Recalcitrant rash suggestive of immunodeficiency
- Toxic-appearing infants

Nursing

Assist first-time parents with hygiene education.

ONGOING CARE

FOLLOW-UP RECOMMENDATIONS

Patient Monitoring

Recheck weekly until clear; then at times of recurrence.

PATIENT EDUCATION

Patient education is vital to the treatment and prevention of recurrent cases.

PROGNOSIS

- Quick, complete clearing with appropriate treatment
- Secondary candidal infections may last a few weeks after treatment is begun.

COMPLICATIONS

- Secondary bacterial infection (consider community-acquired methicillin-resistant *Staphylococcus aureus* [MRSA] in pustular dermatitis that does not respond to normal therapy)
- Rare complication is inoculation with group A β-hemolytic *Streptococcus* resulting in necrotizing fascitis.
- Secondary yeast infection

REFERENCES

1. Scheinfeld N. Diaper dermatitis: A review and brief survey of eruptions of the diaper area. *Am J Clin Derm*. 2005;6:273–81.
2. Janniger CK, Thomas I. Diaper dermatitis: An approach to prevention employing effective diaper care. *Cutis*. 1993;52:153–5.

ADDITIONAL READING

- Alberta L, et al. Diaper dye dermatitis. *Pediatrics*. 2005;116(3):450–2.
- Kazaks EL, et al. Diaper dermatitis. *Pediatr Clin North Am*. 2000;47(4):909–19.

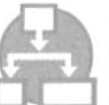

See Also (Topic, Algorithm, Electronic Media Element)

Algorithm: Rash, Focal

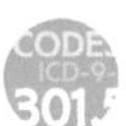

CODES

ICD9

- 112.3 Candidiasis of skin and nails
- 691.0 Diaper or napkin rash

CLINICAL PEARLS

- Hygiene is the main preventative measure.
- Look for secondary infection in persistent cases.

DERMATITIS, EXFOLIATIVE

Herbert P. Goodheart, MD

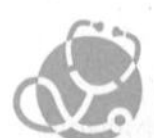

BASICS

- Exfoliative dermatitis (ED), or erythroderma, is a rare disorder characterized by a generalized scaling eruption of most, if not all, of the skin.
- It arises secondary to an underlying cutaneous or systemic disease, as a reaction to medications, or it may develop idiopathically.
- ED may appear suddenly or gradually, occasionally accompanied by fever, chills, and lymphadenopathy.
- When fulminant, ED is potentially life threatening.

DESCRIPTION

- Cutaneous involvement consists of redness and/or scaling of most of the skin.
- System(s) affected: Skin/Exocrine
- Synonym(s): Erythroderma; Exfoliative erythroderma; Red man syndrome (*homme rouge*); Pityriasis rubra

EPIDEMIOLOGY

The vast majority of patients are older than 40 years of age and are mostly males.

Incidence

- In the US: Rare; estimated 1% of hospitalizations for skin disease
- Predominant age: >40 years, except when it results from atopic dermatitis, seborrheic dermatitis, staphylococcal scalded-skin syndrome, or hereditary ichthyosis, all of which are most common in the pediatric age group.
- Predominant sex: Male > Female (2–4:1)
- No racial predilection

RISK FACTORS

- Underlying diseases as noted below
- Male sex
- Age >40 years

PATHOPHYSIOLOGY

Arises idiopathically or secondary to an underlying cutaneous or systemic disease, or as a reaction to medications

COMMONLY ASSOCIATED CONDITIONS

- The most commonly associated conditions or diseases that have been reported to present with or develop into exfoliative dermatitis include:
  - In adults, psoriasis most frequently
  - In children, most often secondary to severe atopic dermatitis
  - Drug reactions
  - Idiopathic in up to 20–30% of cases
- Less commonly, ED has been noted as a finding in the following skin disorders:
  - Allergic contact dermatitis
  - Stasis dermatitis with secondary autoeczematization
  - Pityriasis rubra pilaris (a rare disorder of keratinization)
  - Graft-versus-host disease
  - Seborrheic dermatitis (Leiner disease) in infants
  - Ichthyosiform dermatoses
  - Pemphigus foliaceus
  - Papulosquamous dermatitis of AIDS
  - Fungal disease with id reaction
- Other rare reported associations include:
  - Reiter syndrome
  - Systemic lupus erythematosus (SLE)
  - Hailey-Hailey disease
  - Norwegian scabies
  - Sarcoidosis
  - Lichen planus
  - Dermatomyositis
- Medications: May occur as a reaction to the following drugs: Allopurinol, antimalarials, aspirin, barbiturates, captopril, codeine, cefoxitin, cimetidine, dapsone, gold salts, hydantoin, isoniazid, lithium, NSAIDs, omeprazole, para-aminosalicylic acid, penicillin, phenylbutazone, phenothiazine, St. John's wort, sulfonamide, sulfonylurea, thalidomide, and vancomycin
- May occur as a complication or presenting symptom of the following malignancies:
  - Mycosis fungoides (cutaneous T-cell lymphoma)
  - Sézary syndrome (leukemic variant of mycosis fungoides)
  - Hodgkin disease
  - Non-Hodgkin lymphoma and leukemia

DIAGNOSIS

- Diagnosis is made on a clinical basis.
- Determination of the cause is often elusive, but history is the most important aid in finding the underlying etiology of ED.

HISTORY

- Patients may have a history of the primary disease (e.g., psoriasis, atopic dermatitis).
- Elicit a comprehensive drug history, including over-the-counter drugs.

PHYSICAL EXAM

- Patients often present with generalized erythema followed by extensive scaling that appears in 2–6 days after the onset of erythema.
- Alopecia: Hair may shed.
- Nail dystrophy in 40%: Nails may become ridged, dystrophic, thickened, and also may shed.
- Fever in 40–50%
- Chills
- Malaise/weakness
- Eosinophilia (30%)
- Hepatomegaly (20%)
- Splenomegaly when underlying lymphoma/leukemia is present
- Hypoproteinemia
- Dehydration
- High-output cardiac failure
- Tachycardia (40%)
- In time, lichenification may occur.
- Postinflammatory dyspigmentation (hyper- or hypopigmented areas of the skin)
- Eliciting a history of drug ingestion or a pre-existing dermatosis or disease may be valuable.
- Infrequently, the characteristic lichenification of atopic dermatitis or the nail pitting that suggests psoriasis or islands of sparing in pityriasis rubra pilaris may be found.
- There is marked generalized erythema followed by scaling.
- Pruritus may be severe.
- Edema and increased warmth of the skin
- Pedal or pretibial edema; periorbital skin may be inflamed and edematous, resulting in ectropion.
- Lymphadenopathy, usually a reactive type (*dermatopathic lymphadenopathy*) may be present. A lymph node biopsy is advised when lymph nodes exhibit lymphomatous characteristics (e.g., large size, rubbery consistency) and the cause of exfoliative dermatitis is undetermined.
- Most often, primary lesions that might offer clues to making an etiologic diagnosis are obscured or lacking.

DIAGNOSTIC TESTS & INTERPRETATION

Multiple serial skin biopsies may be necessary to exclude cutaneous T-cell lymphoma.

Lab

- None are diagnostic; however, may have elevated WBC count with eosinophilia, anemia, elevated ESR, decreased albumin, and electrolyte abnormalities
- Increased IgE may be observed in when caused by atopic dermatitis.
- Search for occult tumors or cancers. Perform chest radiography and routine cancer screenings appropriate for age and sex.
- Immunophenotyping, flow cytometry, and particularly B- and T-cell gene rearrangement analysis may be helpful in confirming the diagnosis if lymphoma is suspected.

Imaging

Chest x-ray (CXR) and other imaging procedures as indicated to investigate any underlying disease process

Diagnostic Procedures/Surgery

- Laboratory testing can provide serologic evidence of Sézary syndrome or leukemia.
- Patch testing during a period of remission may uncover a contact allergen.
- Skin biopsy (lymph node or bone marrow) as indicated to investigate an underlying disease process
- Further tests are performed if suggested by the review of systems and physical examination.

Pathological Findings

- May have characteristics of an underlying cutaneous disease; however, findings are most often nonspecific and consist of hyperkeratosis, parakeratosis, and acanthosis in the epidermis and edema, vasodilation, and perivascular infiltrates with lymphocytes, histiocytes, and eosinophils in the dermis
- Repeated or multiple biopsies are sometimes helpful in finding an underlying cause.

DIFFERENTIAL DIAGNOSIS

- Extensive acute eczematous dermatoses, such as contact dermatitis and drug eruptions
- Toxic epidermal necrolysis
- Staphylococcal scalded-skin syndrome
- Erythema multiforme major
- Acute generalized exanthematous pustulosis (AGEP)

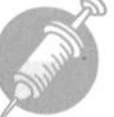

TREATMENT

- Cool tap water dressings
- Application of intermediate-strength topical steroids (e.g., triamcinolone cream 0.025–0.1%) beneath wet dressings
- Cool colloid baths with oatmeal (e.g., Aveeno)
- Local bland moisturizing ointments/lotions
- Systemic antibiotics if signs of secondary infection are observed
- Antihistamines act primarily as sedatives.

ALERT

Systemic steroids may be helpful in some cases, but should be avoided in suspected cases of psoriasis.

MEDICATION

First Line

- Midpotency topical steroids
- In addition, treatment specific to any underlying infection or disease should be provided.
- Systemic steroids: Initial dosage equivalent to prednisone 40 mg/d with increases in dosage by 20 mg/d if there is no response after 3–4 days. Subsequently, dosage should be tapered as symptoms are controlled.
- Oral retinoids: If psoriasis is determined to be the underlying cause of the ED, an oral retinoid such as isotretinoin probably is a better choice than systemic steroids, which may exacerbate psoriasis.

Second Line

- When psoriasis is the underlying cause, cyclosporine, methotrexate, etretinate, phototherapy, photopheresis, photochemotherapy, as well as monoclonal antibodies such as infliximab and alemtuzumab may be effective.
- Photochemotherapy also may be useful therapy for treating ED associated with mycosis fungoides.
- Oral acitretin and isotretinoin have been used when pityriasis rubra pilaris is the underlying cause.
- Antimetabolites/cytotoxic drugs
- Bexarotene
- Infliximab (1)
- Etanercept (2)

ADDITIONAL TREATMENT

General Measures

- Outpatient care except in patients with complications of secondary infection, dehydration, or heart failure
- Withdrawal of any implicated medications or treatment of any identified underlying infection/disease
- Protection from development of hypothermia
- When ED evolves rapidly, the patient frequently requires hospitalization, where measures such as fluid replacement, temperature control, and expert topical skin care are available.

IN-PATIENT CONSIDERATIONS

Admission Criteria

- Impending or actual heart failure
- Inability to control ED on an outpatient basis
- The very young and elderly with fulminant disease are more apt to develop complications such as septicemia and high output failure are best managed in hospital (3,4).

Nursing

Bed rest, cool compresses, lubrication with emollients, antipruritic therapy with oral antihistamines, and low- to intermediate-strength topical steroids

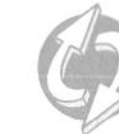

ONGOING CARE

DIET

- Increased fluid intake
- Ensure adequate nutrition with emphasis on sufficient protein intake.

PROGNOSIS

- The prognosis of ED depends largely on underlying etiology.
- In patients with an identified underlying cause, the course and prognosis generally will parallel those of the primary disease. For example, in patients who have underlying psoriasis or atopic dermatitis, the progression of disease generally is gradual.
- ED due to a drug eruption usually clears after the drug is discontinued.
- In patients with idiopathic ED, the prognosis is poor, and recurrences are not uncommon.

Geriatric Considerations

Acute, severe episodes, particularly in elderly persons or in persons with pre-existing heart disease, also have a more guarded prognosis.

Pediatric Considerations

A study of erythrodermic pediatric patients indicated that age <3 years, fever, ill appearance, hypotension, and elevated creatinine levels are poor prognostic signs, and the possibility of toxic shock syndrome should be considered.

COMPLICATIONS

- Secondary infection, sepsis due to loss of effective barrier
- A marked loss of exfoliated scales (uncontrolled mitosis and desquamation) and an increase in cutaneous blood perfusion may contribute to:
  - Dehydration/electrolyte disturbances
  - Hypoalbuminemia
  - Edema
  - Heat loss and hypothermia
  - Possible high-output cardiac failure and death
- Depending on the underlying cause and possible complications, the overall mortality ranges from 20–40%.
- Complications in ED depend on underlying disease. Secondary infection, dehydration, electrolyte imbalance, temperature dysregulation, and high-output cardiac failure are all potential complications.

REFERENCES

1. Rongioletti F, Borenstein M, Kirsner R, et al. Erythrodermic, recalcitrant psoriasis: Clinical resolution with infliximab. *J Dermatolog Treat*. 2003;14:222–5.
2. Querfeld C, Guitart J, et al. Successful treatment of recalcitrant, erythroderma-associated pruritus with etanercept. *Arch Dermatol*. 2004;140(12):1539–40.
3. Byer RL, Bachur RG. Clinical deterioration among patients with fever and erythroderma. *Pediatrics*. 2006;118:2450–60.
4. Pruszkowski A, Bodemer C, Fraitag S, et al. Neonatal and infantile erythrodermas: A retrospective study of 51 patients. *Arch Dermatol*. 2000;136:875–80.

ADDITIONAL READING

- Heald P. The treatment of cutaneous T-cell lymphoma with a novel retinoid. *Clin Lymphoma*. 2000:1S45–9.
- Okoduwa C, Lambert WC, Schwartz RA, et al. Erythroderma: Review of a potentially life-threatening dermatosis. *Indian J Dermatol*. 2009;54(1):1–6.
- Ott H, Hütten M, Baron JM, et al. Neonatal and infantile erythrodermas. *J Dtsch Dermatol Ges*. 2008;6:1070–85; quiz 1086.
- Tomi NS, Kränke B, Aberer E. Staphylococcal toxins in patients with psoriasis, atopic dermatitis, and erythroderma, and in healthy control subjects. *J Am Acad Dermatol*. 2005;53:67–72.

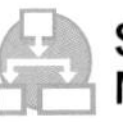

See Also (Topic, Algorithm, Electronic Media Element)

Algorithm: Rash, Focal

CODES

ICD9

695.89 Other specified erythematous conditions

CLINICAL PEARLS

- In its more severe manifestations, ED is a medical and dermatologic emergency.
- In many cases, the underlying cause is never established.
- Prednisone is generally contraindicated in exfoliative dermatitis secondary to psoriasis, while an oral retinoid (acitretin) or an immunosuppressant such as (cyclosporine) may be appropriate choices for this disease.

DERMATITIS HERPETIFORMIS

Anne M. Mahoney, MD

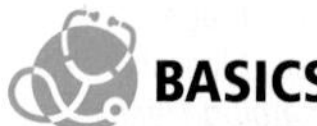

BASICS

DESCRIPTION

- Dermatitis herpetiformis (DH) is a chronic, intensely pruritic, papulovesicular eruption involving primarily extensor skin surfaces (elbows, knees, buttocks, back) and the scalp.
- DH is distinguished from other bullous diseases by characteristic histologic and immunologic findings, as well as associated gluten-sensitive enteropathy.
- System(s) affected: Skin
- Synonym(s): Duhring disease

EPIDEMIOLOGY

- Occurs most frequently in those of Northern European origin
- Rare in persons of Asian or African American origin
- Predominant age: Most common between the ages of 30 and 40 years, but may occur in children
- Predominant sex: Male > Female (1.4:1 in the US, 2:1 worldwide)

Incidence

1/100,000 persons per year in US

Prevalence

11/100,000 persons in US population; as high as 39/100,000 persons worldwide

RISK FACTORS

- Gluten-sensitive enteropathy (GSE): >90% of those with DH will have GSE, which may be asymptomatic.
- Family history of DH or CD

Genetics

- High incidence of human leukocyte antigen A1, B8, DR3, and DQ2 (1)
- Strong association with combination of alleles DQA1*0501 and DQB1*02 *or* DQA1*03 and DQB1*0302 (2)

GENERAL PREVENTION

Gluten-free diet (GFD) results in improvement of DH and reduces dependence on medical therapy. GFD also may prevent complications associated with DH.

PATHOPHYSIOLOGY

- Evidence suggests that epidermal transglutaminase (eTG) 3, a keratinocyte enzyme involved in cell envelope formation, is the autoantigen in DH (3).
- eTG is highly homologous with tissue transglutaminase (tTG), which is the antigenic target in celiac disease (2).
- The initiating event for DH is presumed to be the interaction of wheat peptides with TTGs, which results in activation of T cells and the humoral immune system.
- IgA antibodies against tTGs cross-react with eTG and result in IgA-eTG immune complexes that are deposited in the papillary dermis. Subsequent activation of complement and recruitment of neutrophils to the area result in inflammation and blistering.
- Skin eruption may be delayed 5–6 weeks after exposure to gluten.
- Gluten applied directly to the skin does not result in the eruption, whereas gluten taken by mouth or rectum does. This implies necessary processing by the GI system (4).

ETIOLOGY

Thought to be autoimmune or immune complex–mediated (2)

COMMONLY ASSOCIATED CONDITIONS

- Gluten-sensitive enteropathy
- Gastric atrophy, hypochlorhydria, pernicious anemia
- GI lymphoma, non-Hodgkin lymphoma
- Hyperthyroidism, hypothyroidism, thyroid nodules, thyroid cancer
- Down syndrome
- Glomerulopathy
- Autoimmune disorders, including systemic lupus erythematosus, dermatomyositis, Sjögren syndrome, rheumatoid arthritis, Raynaud phenomenon, insulin-dependent diabetes mellitus, myasthenia gravis, Addison disease, vitiligo, alopecia, and psoriasis

DIAGNOSIS

Diagnosis of DH involves a clinicopathologic correlation among clinical presentation, histologic and direct immunofluorescence evaluation, serology, and response to therapy or dietary restriction.

HISTORY

- Waxing and waning, intensely pruritic eruption with papules and tiny vesicles
- Eruption may worsen with gluten intake.
- GI symptoms may be absent or may not be reported until prompted.

PHYSICAL EXAM

- Symmetric, grouped, erythematous papules and vesicles
- Only erosions, excoriations, and hyperpigmentation secondary to scratching may be apparent on presentation (5).
- Areas involved include extensor surfaces of elbows (90%), knees (30%), shoulders, buttocks, and sacrum. The scalp is also frequently affected. Oral lesions are rare. Palms and soles are spared (5).
- The eruption in children is similar to that in adults (4).
- Adults with associated enteropathy are most often asymptomatic, with <10% complaining of bloating, diarrhea, or steatorrhea.
- Children with associated enteropathy may present with abdominal pain, diarrhea, iron deficiency, and reduced growth rate (5).

DIAGNOSTIC TESTS & INTERPRETATION

Lab

Initial lab tests

- IgA TTG antibodies: Detection of tTG antibodies was noted to be 94.4% sensitive and 92.3% specific for DH in patients on unrestricted diets (6).
- IgA eTG antibodies: Antibodies to eTG, the primary autoantigen in DH, were shown to be more sensitive than antibodies to tTG in the diagnosis of patients with DH on unrestricted diets (95% vs. 79%) (7).
- IgA endomysial antibodies: Have a sensitivity between 50% and 100% and a specificity close to 100% in patients on unrestricted diets (5)

Follow-Up & Special Considerations

Serologic assessment of anti-tTG and antiendomysial antibodies (EMA) may be useful in monitoring major deviations from GFD (5).

Diagnostic Procedures/Surgery

The "gold standard" for diagnosing DH is a skin biopsy evaluated via direct immunofluorescence, which demonstrates granular IgA deposited in dermal papillae (5)[A].

Pathological Findings

- Direct immunofluorescence of skin reveals a granular pattern of IgA deposition in the dermal papillae (5).
- Histopathology with routine staining reveals neutrophilic microabscesses in dermal papillae and also may show subepidermal blistering (4).

DIFFERENTIAL DIAGNOSIS

- In adults (5):
  - Bullous pemphigoid: Linear deposition of C3 and IgG at the basement membrane zone
  - Linear IgA disease: Homogeneous and linear deposition of IgA at the basement membrane zone, absence of GSE
  - Transient acantholytic dermatosis
  - Urticaria: Wheals, angioedema, dermal edema
  - Erythema multiforme
- In children (5):
  - Atopic dermatitis: Face and flexural areas
  - Scabies: Interdigital areas, axillae, genital region
  - Papular urticaria: Dermal edema
  - Impetigo

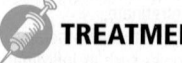

TREATMENT

MEDICATION

- Disease control is achieved with dietary modification, medication, or both.
- Medication is useful for immediate symptom management.
- A GFD is necessary for long-term management of underlying gluten sensitivity.

First Line

- Dapsone is the only medication approved by the Food and Drug Administration for use in DH and the most widely used (4)[A]. Adult doses range from 25–400 mg/d, which result in improvement of symptoms within 24–48 hours. Use minimum effective dose. Average maintenance dose is 1 mg/kg/d. Minor outbreaks on the face and scalp are common even with treatment.
- Dapsone works by inhibiting neutrophil recruitment, inhibiting the respiratory burst of neutrophils, and protecting cells from neutrophil-mediated injury, thereby suppressing the skin reaction. It has no role in preventing IgA deposition or mitigating the immune reaction in the gut (4).
- Precautions:
  - Common side effects include nausea, vomiting, headache, dizziness, and weakness.
  - A drop in hemoglobin of 1–2 g is characteristic with dapsone 100 mg/d.
  - G6PD deficiency increases severity of hemolytic stress. Dapsone should be avoided if possible in those who are G6PD-deficient.

- Dose-related methemoglobinemia may occur, typically with doses >100 mg/d.
- Other adverse events include toxic hepatitis, cholestatic jaundice, hypoalbuminemia, sensory and motor neuropathy, psychosis, infectious mononucleosis syndrome with fever and lymphadenopathy, agranulocytosis, aplastic anemia, leukopenia, exfoliative dermatitis, erythema multiforme, erythema nodosum, and urticaria.
- The drug is secreted in breast milk and will produce hemolytic anemia in infants.

ALERT
- Monitor for potentially fatal sulfone syndrome: Fever, jaundice and hepatic necrosis, exfoliative dermatitis, lymphadenopathy, methemoglobinemia, and hemolytic anemia.
- Can occur 48 hours or 6 months after treatment, most often 5 weeks after initiation

Pediatric Considerations
- <2 years: Dosing not established
- >2 years: 0.5–1.0 mg/kg/d

Pregnancy Considerations
- Category C: Safety during pregnancy is not established
- Adherence to a strict GFD 6–12 months before conception should be considered with the hope of eliminating need for dapsone during pregnancy.

Second Line
Sulfasalazine (1–2 g/d), sulphamethoxypyridazine (0.25–1.5 g/d): Side effects include nausea, vomiting, anorexia, hypersensitivity reactions, hemolytic anemia, proteinuria, and crystalluria (5).

ALERT
- Prior to treatment, monthly for the first 3 months of treatment and biannually thereafter, CBC with differential and urinalysis with urine microscopy should be done (5).
- Colchicine, prednisone, tetracycline plus nicotinamide, minocycline, cyclosporine, and topical steroids are third-line medications.

ADDITIONAL TREATMENT
GFD:
- Average of 2 years is often necessary for diet to completely eliminate skin eruptions, and lesions usually recur within 12 weeks of gluten reintroduction (5).
- Fundamentals of the GFD (8):
  - Grains that should be avoided:
    - Wheat (includes spelt, kamut, semolina, and triticale)
    - Rye
    - Barley (including malt)
  - Safe grains (gluten-free):
    - Rice
    - Amaranth
    - Buckwheat
    - Corn
    - Millet
    - Quinoa
    - Sorghum
    - Teff (an Ethiopian cereal grain)
    - Oats
  - Sources of gluten-free starches that can be used as flour alternatives:
    - Cereal grains: Amaranth, buckwheat, corn, millet, quinoa, sorghum, teff, rice (white, brown, wild, basmati, jasmine), and montina
    - Tubers: Arrowroot, jicama, taro, potato, and tapioca
    - Legumes: Chickpeas, lentils, kidney beans, navy beans, pea beans, peanuts, and soybeans
    - Nuts: Almonds, walnuts, chestnuts, hazelnuts, and cashews
    - Seeds: Sunflower, flax, and pumpkin

Issues for Referral
Interdisciplinary treatment involves a dermatologist, gastroenterologist, and a registered dietician.

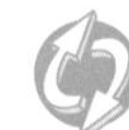

ONGOING CARE

FOLLOW-UP RECOMMENDATIONS
Patient Monitoring
Follow safety monitoring protocols if treating with dapsone.

DIET
- 87% of patients showed complete remission of skin manifestations after 18 months of a GFD (9)[C].
- Improvement in cutaneous disease and normalization of small bowel mucosa result from strict compliance with a GFD in most patients (5)[C].

PATIENT EDUCATION
- Patient should be made aware of potential hemolytic anemia and the signs associated with methemoglobinemia.
- American Academy of Dermatology, 930 N. Meacham Road., P.O. Box 4014, Schaumberg, IL 60168-4014; (708) 330-0230
- Gluten Intolerance Group of North America, 31214–124 Ave. SE, Auburn, WA 98092; phone (206) 246-6652; fax (206) 246-6531; www.gluten.net
- The Celiac Disease Foundation, 13251 Ventura Blvd., #1, Studio City, CA 9160; phone (818) 990-2354; fax (818) 990-2379

PROGNOSIS
- Lifelong disease
- Remission in 10–20%
- Skin disease responds readily to dapsone.
- Strict adherence to a GFD improves clinical symptoms and decreases dapsone requirement. GFD is the only sustainable method of eliminating cutaneous and GI disease. Dapsone does not alter GI mucosal pathology.
- Occasional new lesions (2–3 per week) are to be expected and are not an indication for altering daily dosage.
- Risk of lymphoma may be decreased in those who maintain a GFD.

COMPLICATIONS
- Malnutrition, weight loss
- Abdominal pain, dyspepsia
- Nutritional deficiencies (folate, B_{12}, iron)
- Osteoporosis
- Chronic fatigue
- Autoimmune diseases
- Lymphomas

REFERENCES

1. Patrício P, Ferreira C, Gomes MM, et al. Autoimmune bullous dermatoses: A review. *Ann N Y Acad Sci*. 2009;1173:203–10.
2. Kárpáti S, et al. Dermatitis herpetiformis: Close to unravelling a disease. *J Dermatol Sci*. 2004;34: 83–90.
3. Sárdy M, Kárpáti S, Merkl B, et al. Epidermal transglutaminase (TGase 3) is the autoantigen of dermatitis herpetiformis. *J Exp Med*. 2002;195: 747–57.
4. Nicolas ME, Krause PK, Gibson LE, et al. Dermatitis herpetiformis. *Int J Dermatol*. 2003;42:588–600.
5. Caproni M, Antiga E, Melani L, et al. Guidelines for the diagnosis and treatment of dermatitis herpetiformis. *J Eur Acad Dermatol Venereol*. 2009.
6. Caproni M, Cardinali C, Renzi D, et al. Tissue transglutaminase antibody assessment in dermatitis herpetiformis. *Br J Dermatol*. 2001;144:196–7.
7. Rose C, Armbruster FP, Ruppert J, et al. Autoantibodies against epidermal transglutaminase are a sensitive diagnostic marker in patients with dermatitis herpetiformis on a normal or gluten-free diet. *J Am Acad Dermatol*. 2009;61:39–43.
8. Green PH, Cellier C. Celiac disease. *N Engl J Med*. 2007;357:1731–43.
9. Nino M, Ciacci C, Delfino M. A long-term gluten-free diet as an alternative treatment in severe forms of dermatitis herpetiformis. *J Dermatolog Treat*. 2007;18:10–2.

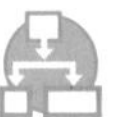

See Also (Topic, Algorithm, Electronic Media Element)
- Celiac Disease
- Algorithm: Rash, Focal

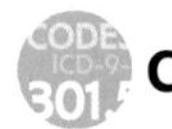

CODES

ICD9
694.0 Dermatitis herpetiformis

CLINICAL PEARLS

- DH is a chronic, intensely pruritic papulovesicular eruption involving primarily extensor skin surfaces symmetrically as well as the scalp.
- Strong association with gluten-sensitive enteropathy
- Diagnosed by skin biopsy with direct immunofluorescence
- First-line treatment: Dapsone

DERMATITIS, SEBORRHEIC

Juan Qiu, MD, PhD

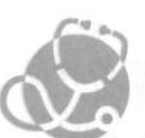

BASICS

DESCRIPTION

Chronic, superficial, recurrent inflammatory rash affecting sebum-rich, hairy regions of the body, especially scalp, eyebrows, and face

EPIDEMIOLOGY

Incidence

- Predominant age: Infancy, adolescence, and adulthood
- Predominant sex: Male > Female

Prevalence

Seborrheic dermatitis: 3–5%

RISK FACTORS

- Parkinson disease
- AIDS (disease severity correlated with progression of immune deficiency)
- Emotional stress
- Medications may flare or induce seborrheic dermatitis: Auranofin, aurothioglucose, buspirone, chlorpromazine, cimetidine, ethionamide, gold, griseofulvin, haloperidol, interferon alfa, lithium, methoxsalen, methyldopa, phenothiazine, psoralen, stanozolol, thiothixene, trioxsalen

Genetics

Positive family history; no genetic marker identified to date

GENERAL PREVENTION

Seborrheic skin should be washed more often than usual.

PATHOPHYSIOLOGY

Helper T cells, phytohemagglutinin and concanavalin stimulation, and antibody titers are depressed compared with those of control subjects.

ETIOLOGY

- Skin surface yeasts *Malassezia* (formerly *P. ovale*) may be a contributing factor (1).
- *Malassezia* spp. may have a role in T-cell suppression and complement activation.
- The mite *D. folliculorum* may have a direct or indirect role.
- Genetic and environmental factors: Flares are common with stress or illness.
- Parallels increased sebaceous gland activity in infancy and adolescence or as a result of some acnegenic drugs

COMMONLY ASSOCIATED CONDITIONS

- Parkinson disease
- AIDS

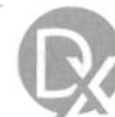

DIAGNOSIS

The diagnosis of seborrheic dermatitis usually can be made by history and physical examination.

HISTORY

- Intermittent active phases manifest with burning, scaling, and itching, alternating with inactive periods; activity is increased in winter and early spring, with remissions commonly occurring in summer.
- Infants:
  - Cradle cap: Greasy scaling of scalp, sometimes with associated mild erythema
  - Diaper and/or axillary rash
  - Age at onset typically ~1 month
  - Usually resolves by 8–12 months
- Adults:
  - Red, greasy, scaling rash in most locations consisting of patches and plaques with indistinct margins
  - Red, smooth, glazed appearance in skin folds
  - Minimal pruritus
  - Chronic waxing and waning course
  - Bilateral and symmetric
  - Most commonly located in hairy skin areas: Scalp and scalp margins, eyebrows and eyelid margins, nasolabial folds, ears and retroauricular folds, presternal area, middle to upper back, buttock crease, inguinal area, genitals, and armpits

PHYSICAL EXAM

- Scalp appearance varies from mild, patchy scaling to widespread, thick, adherent crusts. Plaques are rare.
- Seborrheic dermatitis can spread onto the forehead, the posterior part of the neck, and the postauricular skin, as in psoriasis.
- Skin lesions manifest as branny or greasy scaling over red, inflamed skin.
- Hypopigmentation is seen in blacks.
- Infectious eczematoid dermatitis, with oozing and crusting, suggests secondary infection.
- Seborrheic blepharitis may occur independently.

DIAGNOSTIC TESTS & INTERPRETATION

Diagnostic Procedures/Surgery

Consider biopsy if:

- Usual therapies fail
- Petechiae noted
- Histiocytosis X suspected
- Fungal cultures in refractory cases or when pustules and alopecia are present

Pathological Findings

Nonspecific changes:

- Hyperkeratosis, acanthosis, accentuated rete ridges, focal spongiosis, and parakeratosis are characteristic.
- Parakeratotic scale around hair follicles and mild superficial inflammatory lymphocytic infiltrate

DIFFERENTIAL DIAGNOSIS

- Atopic dermatitis: Distinction may be difficult in infants.
- Psoriasis:
  - Usually knees, elbows, and nails are involved.
  - Scalp psoriasis will be more sharply demarcated than seborrhea, with crusted, infiltrated plaques rather than mild scaling and erythema.
- *Candida*
- Tinea cruris or capitis: Suspect these when usual medications fail or if hair loss occurs.
- Eczema of auricle or otitis externa
- Rosacea
- Discoid lupus erythematosus: Skin biopsy will be beneficial.
- Histiocytosis X: May appear as seborrheic-type eruption
- Dandruff: Scalp only, noninflammatory

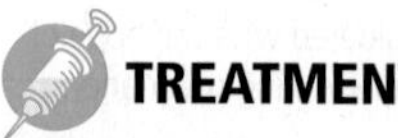

TREATMENT

MEDICATION

First Line

- Cradle cap: Use a coal tar shampoo or ketoconazole (Nizoral) shampoo if the nonmedicated shampoo is ineffective (2).
- Adults:
  - Topical antifungal agents:
    - Ketoconazole 2% foam or shampoo twice a week for clearance, then once a week or every other week for maintenance
    - Ketoconazole (Nizoral) cream may be used to clear scales in other areas.
    - Ciclopirox 1% shampoo twice weekly (1)[B]

- Topical corticosteroids:
  - Begin with 1%hydrocortisone, and advance to more potent (fluorinated) steroid preparations as needed.
  - Avoid continuous use of the more potent steroids to reduce the risk of skin atrophy, hypopigmentation, or systemic absorption (especially in infants and children).
  - Precautions: Fluorinated corticosteroids and higher concentrations of hydrocortisone (e.g., 2.5%) may cause atrophy or striae if used on the face or on skin folds.
- Other topical agents:
  - Coal tar 1% shampoo twice a week
  - Selenium sulfide 2.5% shampoo twice a week
  - Zinc pyrithione shampoo twice a week
  - Lithium succinate ointment twice a week
- Once controlled, washing with zinc soaps or selenium lotion with periodic use of steroid cream may help to maintain remission.

Second Line

- Calcineurin inhibitors:
  - Pimecrolimus 1% cream b.i.d.
  - Tacrolimus 0.1% ointment b.i.d.
- Systemic antifungal therapy:
  - Data are limited.
  - For moderate-to-severe seborrheic dermatitis:
    - Ketoconazole 200 mg/d
    - Itraconazole 200 mg/d
    - Daily regimen for 1–2 months followed by twice-weekly dosing for chronic treatment
    - Monitor potential hepatotoxic effects.

ADDITIONAL TREATMENT

General Measures

- Increase frequency of shampooing.
- Sunlight in moderate doses may be helpful.
- Cradle cap:
  - Frequent shampooing with a mild, nonmedicated shampoo
  - Remove thick scale by applying warm mineral oil, and then wash off 1 hour later with a mild soap and a soft-bristle toothbrush or terrycloth washcloth (2).
- Adults: Wash all affected areas with antiseborrheic shampoos. Start with over-the-counter brands (Tegrin, Selsun Blue), and increase to more potent preparations (containing coal tar, sulfur, selenium, or salicylic acid) if no improvement is noted (2).
- For dense scalp scaling, 10% liquor carbonic detergens in Nivea oil may be used at bedtime, covering the head with a shower cap. This should be done nightly for 1–3 weeks.

Issues for Referral

No response to first-line therapy and concerns regarding systemic illness (HIV, etc.)

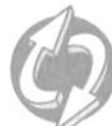

ONGOING CARE

FOLLOW-UP RECOMMENDATIONS

Patient Monitoring

Every 2–12 weeks as necessary depending on disease severity and degree of patient sophistication

PATIENT EDUCATION

http://familydoctor.org/online/famdocen/home/common/skin/disorders/157.html

PROGNOSIS

- In infants, seborrheic dermatitis usually remits after 6–8 months.
- In adults, seborrheic dermatitis is usually chronic and unpredictable, with exacerbations and remissions. Disease is usually easily controlled with shampoos and topical steroids.

COMPLICATIONS

- Skin atrophy or striae are possible from fluorinated corticosteroids, especially if used on the face.
- Glaucoma can result from use of fluorinated steroids around the eyes.
- Photosensitivity is caused occasionally by tars.
- Herpes keratitis is a rare complication of herpes simplex: Instruct patient to stop eyelid steroids if herpes simplex develops.

REFERENCES

1. Shuster S, Meynadier J, Kerl H, et al. Treatment and prophylaxis of seborrheic dermatitis of the scalp with antipityrosporal 1% ciclopirox shampoo. *Arch Dermatol*. 2005;141:47–52.
2. Johnson BA, Nunley JR. Treatment of seborrheic dermatitis. *Am Fam Physician*. 2000;61:2703–10, 2713–4.

ADDITIONAL READING

- Darabi K, Hostetler SG, Bechtel MA, et al. The role of Malassezia in atopic dermatitis affecting the head and neck of adults. *J Am Acad Dermatol*. 2009; 60(1):125–36.
- Karincaoglu Y, Tepe B, Kalayci B, et al. Is Demodex folliculorum an aetiological factor in seborrhoeic dermatitis? *Clin Exp Dermatol*. 2009;34(8): e516–20.
- Naldi L, Rebora A. Clinical practice. Seborrheic dermatitis. *N Engl J Med*. 2009;360:387–96.
- Shemer A, Kaplan B, Nathansohn N, et al. Treatment of moderate to severe facial seborrheic dermatitis with itraconazole: An open non-comparative study. *Isr Med Assoc J*. 2008;10:417–8.
- Shin H, Kwon OS, Won CH, et al. Clinical efficacies of topical agents for the treatment of seborrheic dermatitis of the scalp: A comparative study. *J Dermatol*. 2009;36:131–7.

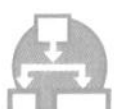

See Also (Topic, Algorithm, Electronic Media Element)

Algorithm: Rash, Focal

CODES

ICD9

- 690.10 Seborrheic dermatitis, unspecified
- 690.11 Seborrhea capitis
- 690.12 Seborrheic infantile dermatitis

CLINICAL PEARLS

- Search for an underlying systemic disease in a patient who is unresponsive to usual therapy.
- In adults, seborrheic dermatitis is usually chronic and unpredictable, with exacerbations and remissions. Disease is usually easily controlled with shampoos and topical steroids.

D

DERMATITIS, STASIS

Joseph A. Florence, MD

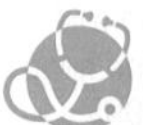

BASICS

DESCRIPTION

- Chronic, eczematous, erythremic, scaling, and noninflammatory edema of the lower extremities accompanied by cycle of scratching, excoriations, weeping, crusting, and inflammation in patients with chronic venous insufficiency, due to impaired circulation and other factors (nutritional edema) (1)
- Clinical skin manifestation of chronic venous insufficiency usually appears late in the disease
- May present as a solitary lesion (2)
- System(s) affected: Skin/Exocrine
- Synonym(s): Gravitational eczema; Varicose eczema; Venous dermatitis

EPIDEMIOLOGY

Incidence

- In the US: Common in patients >50 (6–7%)
- Predominant age: Adult, geriatric
- Predominant sex: Female > Male

Geriatric Considerations

Common in this age group:

- Estimated to affect 15–20 million patients >50 years in the US

RISK FACTORS

- Atopy
- Superimposition of itch–scratch cycle
- Trauma
- Previous deep vein thrombosis (DVT)
- Previous pregnancy
- Prolonged medical illness
- Obesity
- Secondary infection
- Low-protein diet
- Old age
- Deposition of fibrin around capillaries
- Microvascular abnormalities
- Ischemia
- Genetic propensity
- Edema
- Tight garments that constrict the thigh
- Vein stripping
- Vein harvesting for coronary artery bypass graft surgery
- Previous cellulitis

Genetics

Familial link probable

GENERAL PREVENTION

- Use compression stockings to avoid recurrence of edema and to mobilize the interstitial lymphatic fluid from the region of stasis dermatitis.
- Topical lubricants twice a day to prevent fissuring and itching

ETIOLOGY

- Incompetence of perforating veins causing blood to backflow to the superficial venous system leading to venous hypertension (HTN) and cutaneous inflammation
- Continuous presence of edema in ankles, usually present because of venous valve incompetency (varicose veins)
- Weakness of venous walls in lower extremities
- Trauma to edematous, eczematized skin
- Itch may be caused by inflammatory mediators (from mast cells, monocytes, macrophages, or neutrophils) liberated in the microcirculation and endothelium
- Abnormal leukocyte–endothelium interaction is proposed to be a major factor.
- A cascade of biochemical events leads to ulceration.
- Is associated with amlodipine therapy
- Elevated homocysteine has been noted in patients with stasis dermatitis.

COMMONLY ASSOCIATED CONDITIONS

- Varicose veins
- Venous insufficiency
- Other eczematous disease
- Homocystine levels are elevated (3)[C].

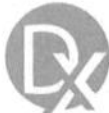

DIAGNOSIS

HISTORY

- Erythema, scaling, edema of lower extremities
- Pruritus
- Excoriations
- Weeping, crusting, inflammation of the skin
- Noninflammatory edema precedes the skin eruption and ulceration.
- Edema initially develops around the ankle.
- Itching, pain, and burning may precede skin signs, which are aggravated during evening hours (4)[B].
- Insidious onset
- Usually bilateral
- Description may include aching/heavy legs.

PHYSICAL EXAM

- Evaluation of the lower extremities characteristically reveals:
  - Bilateral scaly, eczematous patches, papules, and/or plaques
  - Violaceous (sometimes brown), erythematous-colored lesions due to deoxygenation of venous blood (postinflammatory hyperpigmentation and hemosiderin deposition within the cutaneous tissue)
- Distribution: Medial aspect of ankle with frequent extension onto the foot and lower leg
- Brawny induration
- Stasis ulcers (frequently accompany stasis dermatitis) secondary to cuts, bruises, and excoriations to the weakened skin around the ankle
- Mild pruritus, pain (if ulcer present)
- Varicosities are often associated with ulcers.
- Clinical inspection reveals erythematous color with increased pigmentation, swelling, and warmth.
- Skin changes are more common in the lower 1/3 of the extremity and medially.
- Early signs include prominent superficial veins and pitting ankle edema.
- May present as a solitary lesion mimicking a neoplasm (2)[C]

DIAGNOSTIC TESTS & INTERPRETATION

Lab

Initial lab tests

Culture stasis ulcers if bacterial infection is suspected.

Imaging

Initial approach

Duplex ultrasound imaging is helpful in diagnosis (5)[C].

Diagnostic Procedures/Surgery

Rule out arterial insufficiency (check peripheral pulses, leg BPs).

Pathological Findings

Chronic inflammation, characterized histologically by proliferation of small blood vessels in the papillary dermis

DIFFERENTIAL DIAGNOSIS

- Other eczematous diseases:
  - Atopic dermatitis
  - Uremic dermatitis
  - Contact dermatitis (due to topical agents used to self-treat)
  - Neurodermatitis
  - Arterial insufficiency
  - Sickle cell disease causing skin ulceration
  - Cellulitis (6)
  - Erysipelas
- Tinea dermatophyte infection
- Pretibial myxedema
- Nummular eczema
- Lichen simplex chronicus
- Xerosis
- Asteatotic eczema
- Amyopathic dermatomyositis

TREATMENT

MEDICATION

First Line

- Use of antibiotics topically or systemically is controversial, as stasis ulcer may not be infected.
- Antibiotics are indicated if bacterial infection is present, or may be used empirically if bacterial infection is suspected.
- If ulcer is present, local povidone-iodine treatment is as effective as systemic antibiotics (7)[B].
- If secondary infection, treat with oral antibiotics for *Staphylococcus* or *Streptococcus* organisms (e.g., dicloxacillin 250 mg q.i.d., cephalexin 250 mg q.i.d. or 500 mg b.i.d., or levofloxacin 250 mg q.i.d.).
- Gram-negative colonization: Treat with topical antimicrobial agents (e.g., benzoyl peroxide, acetic acid, silver nitrate, or Hibiclens) or broad-spectrum topical antibiotics (e.g., neomycin or bacitracin-polymyxin B [Polysporin]).
- 5% Aluminum acetate (Burow solution) wet dressings and cooling pastes
- Topical triamcinolone 0.1% (Kenalog, Aristocort) cream/ointment t.i.d. or topical betamethasone
- Betamethasone valerate (Valisone) 0.1% cream/ointment/solution t.i.d. (8)[A]
- Topical antipruritic: Pramoxine, camphor, menthol, and doxepin

- Systemic steroids for severe cases
- Calcium dobesilate has been shown to be an effective adjuvant therapy (9)[B].
- Vitamin supplementation in patients with hyperhomocysteinemia (10)[C]
- Evidenced-based treatment options for associated venous ulcers include aspirin and pentoxifylline (11)[B].

Second Line

- Consider antibiotics on basis of culture results of exudate from ulcer craters.
- Lubricants when dermatitis is quiescent
- Chronic stasis dermatitis can be treated with topical emollients (e.g., white petroleum, lanolin, Eucerin).
- Antipruritic medications (e.g., diphenhydramine, cetirizine hydrochloride, desloratadine)

ADDITIONAL TREATMENT

If the patient is on amlodipine therapy, consider discontinuing amlodipine (12)[B].

General Measures

Primary role of treatment is to reverse effects of venous HTN. Appropriate health care:

- Outpatient:
  - Reduce edema (11)[B]:
    - Leg elevation: Heels higher than knees, knees higher than hips
    - Compression therapy: Elastic bandage wraps: Ace bandages or Unna paste boot (zinc gelatin) if lesions are dry or compression stockings (Jobst or nonfitted type) (13,14)[A]
    - Pneumatic compression devices
    - Diuretic therapy
  - Treat infection:
    - Débride the ulcer base of necrotic tissue.
    - Improvement of lipodermatosclerosis
  - Activity:
    - Avoid standing still.
    - Stay active and exercise regularly.
    - Elevate foot of bed unless contraindicated.
- Inpatient for vein stripping, sclerotherapy, or skin grafts:
  - Venous ulcer treatment includes autolytic, biologic, chemical, mechanical, and surgical:
    - Autolytic: Hydrogels, alginates, hydrocolloids, foams, and films
    - Biologic: Topical application of granulocyte macrophage colony-stimulating factor promotes healing of ulcers.
    - Chemical: Enzyme débriding agents
    - Mechanical: Wet to dry dressings, hydrotherapy, and irrigation
    - Surgical modifying cause of venous HTN, treat ulcer by graft

Issues for Referral

Consider referral for:

- Nonhealing ulcer
- Uncertain diagnosis
- Associated disease (e.g., arterial insufficiency, symptomatic varicose veins)

SURGERY/OTHER PROCEDURES

Sclerotherapy and surgery may be required for associated disease.

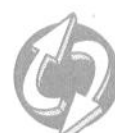

ONGOING CARE

FOLLOW-UP RECOMMENDATIONS

Patient Monitoring

If Unna boot compression is used: Cut off and reapply boot once a week (restricts edema and prevents scratching).

DIET

Lose weight, if overweight

PATIENT EDUCATION

- Stress staying active to keep circulation and leg muscles in good condition. Walking is ideal.
- Keep legs elevated while sitting or lying.
- Don't wear girdles, garters, or pantyhose with tight elastic tops.
- Don't scratch.
- Elevate foot of bed with 2–4-inch blocks.

PROGNOSIS

- Chronic course with intermittent exacerbations and remissions
- The healing process for ulceration is often prolonged and may take months.

COMPLICATIONS

- Sensations of itching, pain, and burning have negative impact on the quality of life
- Secondary bacterial infection
- DVT
- Bleeding at dermatitis sites
- Squamous cell carcinoma in edges of long-standing stasis ulcers
- Scarring, which in turn leads to further compromise to blood flow and increased likelihood of minor trauma

REFERENCES

1. Antignani PL. Classification of chronic venous insufficiency: A review. *Angiology*. 2001; 52(Suppl 1):S17–26.
2. Weaver J, Billings SD, et al. Initial presentation of stasis dermatitis mimicking solitary lesions: A previously unrecognized clinical scenario. *J Am Acad Dermatol*. 2009;61:1028–32.
3. Durmazlar SPK, Akgul A, Eskioglu F. Hyperhomocysteinemia in patients with stasis dermatitis and ulcer: A novel finding with important therapeutic implications. *J Dermatolog Treat*. 2009;20:3;1–4.
4. Duque MI, Yosipovitch G, Chan YH, et al. Itch, pain, and burning sensation are common symptoms in mild to moderate chronic venous insufficiency with an impact on quality of life. *J Am Acad Dermatol*. 2005;53:504–8.
5. Coleridge-Smith P, Labropoulos N, Partsch H, et al. Duplex ultrasound investigation of the veins in chronic venous disease of the lower limbs–UIP consensus document. Part I. Basic principles. *Eur J Vasc Endovasc Surg*. 2006;31:83–92.
6. Bailey E, Kroshinsky D, et al. Cellulitis: Diagnosis and management. *Dermatol Ther*. 2011;24: 229–39.
7. Daróczy J. Quality control in chronic wound management: The role of local povidone-iodine (Betadine) therapy. *Dermatology*. 2006; 212(Suppl 1):82–7.
8. Weiss SC, Nguyen J, Chon S, et al. A randomized controlled clinical trial assessing the effect of betamethasone valerate 0.12% foam on the short-term treatment of stasis dermatitis. *J Drugs Dermatol*. 2005;4:339–45.
9. Kaur C, Sarkar R, Kanwar AJ, et al. An open trial of calcium dobesilate in patients with venous ulcers and stasis dermatitis. *Int J Dermatol*. 2003;42: 147–52.
10. Kartal Durmazlar SP, Akgul A, Eskioglu F, et al. Hyperhomocysteinemia in patients with stasis dermatitis and ulcer: A novel finding with important therapeutic implications. *J Dermatolog Treat*. 2009;1–4.
11. Collins L, Seraj S, et al. Diagnosis and treatment of venous ulcers. *Am Fam Physician*. 2010;81: 989–96.
12. Gosnell AL, Nedorost ST, et al. Stasis dermatitis as a complication of amlodipine therapy. *J Drugs Dermatol*. 2009;8:135–7.
13. Partsch H, Flour M, Coleridge Smith P. Indications for compression therapy in venous and lymphatic disease consensus based on experimental data and scientific evidence. Under the auspices of the IUP. *Int Angiol*. 2008;27:193–219.
14. Coleridge-Smith PD. Leg ulcer treatment. *J Vasc Surg*. 2009;49:804–8.

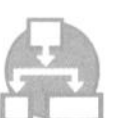

See Also (Topic, Algorithm, Electronic Media Element)

- Varicose Veins
- Algorithm: Rash, Focal

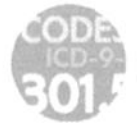

CODES

ICD9

- 454.1 Varicose veins of lower extremities with inflammation
- 454.9 Asymptomatic varicose veins
- 459.81 Venous (peripheral) insufficiency, unspecified

CLINICAL PEARLS

Treatment of edema associated with stasis dermatitis via elevation and/or compression stockings is essential for optimal results.

DIABETES INSIPIDUS

Erik J. Garcia, MD

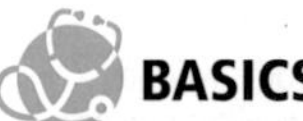

BASICS

DESCRIPTION

- A condition of intense thirst (polydipsia) and excessive urination (polyuria) owing to the kidneys' inability to conserve water as they filter blood.
- Most commonly, this results from decreased pituitary secretion of vasopressin (central diabetes insipidus [DI]) or failure of response to vasopressin (nephrogenic DI).
- Rarely, DI can be induced by pregnancy (gestational DI)
- System(s) affected: Endocrine/Metabolic

EPIDEMIOLOGY

Incidence

- 1 in 25,000 persons
- May occur in 18.3% after transsphenoidal microsurgery

Prevalence

- Vasopressin deficiency may occur at any age.
- Nephrogenic DI usually manifests during infancy.
- Nephrogenic DI is encountered in men more commonly, reflecting its X-linked mode of inheritance.

RISK FACTORS

- Intracranial neoplasm
- Infection
- Following surgery
- Drug induced (amphotericin B, colchicine, demeclocycline, foscarnet, gentamicin, lithium, loop diuretics, methoxyflurane)
- Head trauma
- Genetic predisposition

Genetics

- Central DI: Familial cases of vasopressin deficiency have been reported (commonly autosomal dominant; >20 mutations have been identified), but the disease usually is isolated and often secondary to other disorders.
- Nephrogenic DI:
  - Most common is an X-linked defect in the V_2 receptor that binds antidiuretic hormone (ADH).
  - Autosomal dominant or recessive defects in the aquaporin-2 gene that encodes an ADH-responsive water channel

PATHOPHYSIOLOGY

- Central DI:
  - Inadequate secretion of vasopressin may be due to loss or malfunction of the neurosecretory neurons that make up the neurohypophysis (posterior pituitary) and the pituitary stalk.
  - Posterior pituitary lesions rarely cause DI because ADH is produced in the hypothalamus and, therefore, still would be secreted.
- Nephrogenic DI:
  - Inadequate response of kidney to vasopressin
  - A disorder of renal tubular function resulting in inability to respond to vasopressin in absorption of water

ETIOLOGY

- Central DI (inadequate secretion of vasopressin; may be idiopathic or familial):
  - Idiopathic
  - Trauma/head injury: A study of 89 patients with traumatic brain injury found that primary hormonal dysfunction (including DI) occurred in 21% of patients and tended to occur in patients with the lowest Glasgow Outcome Scale scores (1).
  - Neurosurgery
  - Tumors (e.g., craniopharyngioma, lymphoma, metastasis)
  - Infections (e.g., meningitis, encephalitis)
  - Granulomas (e.g., sarcoid, histiocytosis)
  - Hypoxic encephalopathy
  - Vascular disorders
  - Inheritable defects (rare, occurs in 1–2%)
- Nephrogenic DI (inadequate response of kidneys to vasopressin):
  - Familial genetic defect in resorption of water in renal collecting ducts, including X-linked V_2 receptor mutation and autosomal recessive aquaporin-2 mutation
  - Drug induced (amphotericin B, colchicine, demeclocycline, foscarnet, gentamicin, lithium, loop diuretics, methoxyflurane)

COMMONLY ASSOCIATED CONDITIONS

- Potassium depletion
- Chronic hypercalcemia
- Tumors
- Infection:
  - Encephalitis
  - Tuberculosis
  - Syphilis
- Xanthomatosis
- Pyelonephritis
- Renal amyloidosis
- Sjögren syndrome
- Sickle-cell anemia
- Multiple myeloma
- Wolfram syndrome (DIDMOAD: *DI*, *d*iabetes *m*ellitus, *o*ptic *a*trophy, *d*eafness)

DIAGNOSIS

The diagnosis of DI may be difficult to make because the clinical presentation depends on the cause, severity, and other medical conditions that may or may not be present. The course of DI not associated with brain injury tends to be indolent and, as long as water is available, may be hard to detect. Polyuria is highly variable, as is tolerance for dehydration.

HISTORY

- Thirst/polydipsia (with a particular preference for cold or iced drinks)
- Polyuria (3–20 L/d)
- Nocturia, bed wetting
- Dehydration
- Headache
- Visual disturbances
- Rate of onset of polydipsia is more rapid in central DI than in nephrogenic DI.
- Family history of polyuria
- In children, enuresis, anorexia, linear growth defects, and frequent fatigue may be found.
- In infants, crying, irritability, poor growth, hyperthermia, and weight loss are often found.

PHYSICAL EXAM

Signs of dehydration and an enlarged bladder may be present, but otherwise the exam is usually unremarkable.

DIAGNOSTIC TESTS & INTERPRETATION

Lab

- Low urine specific gravity and osmolality alone are indicative of DI.
- Urine/plasma osmolality ratio and plasma vasopressin concentration results may be difficult to interpret; low ratios may be found in patients with primary polydipsia.
- Water deprivation test (Miller-Moses test) to evaluate the ability to concentrate urine; aids in determining etiology
  - Water is withheld, and urine and plasma osmolality are measured at hourly intervals.
  - A rise in urine osmolality indicates an intact ADH response.
  - A rise in plasma osmolality or stable urine osmolality indicates poor ADH response.
  - Perform the test during the day, not overnight, to avoid serious volume depletion/hyponatremia; patients with DI will continue to urinate even when dehydrated.
  - If the results support the diagnosis, desmopressin should be administered to test renal concentrating ability.

Initial lab tests

- Serum electrolyte levels (hypernatremia)
- Serum glucose to rule out diabetes mellitus
- Urine osmolality
- Urine specific gravity
- Urine electrolytes; hypokalemia and hypercalcemia alter the ability to concentrate urine.
- Plasma vasopressin or urinary vasopressin following osmotic stimulus, such as fluid restriction or administration of hypertonic saline
- Drugs that may alter lab results: Lithium, demeclocycline, and methoxyflurane may induce vasopressin insensitivity.

Imaging

Head MRI

Initial approach

If the diagnosis of DI is made, appropriate studies for cause, including MRI of the brain, must be performed.

Pathological Findings

Degeneration of neurosecretory neurons in the neurohypophysis

DIFFERENTIAL DIAGNOSIS
- Diabetes mellitus and other causes of polydipsia and polyuria
- Increased solute load for excretion, as occurs with high salt intake; osmotic diuresis
- Psychogenic polydipsia (ultimately impairs vasopressin secretion)

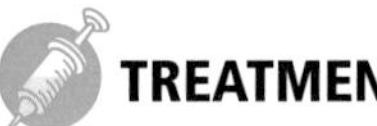

TREATMENT

MEDICATION
- Therapy depends on type of DI.
- Central DI (2,3):
  - Desmopressin (DDAVP), a derivative of vasopressin, may be given orally; parenterally (IV, IM, SC); or intranasally.
    - Intranasally (100 μg/mL solution): Recommended initial dose is 10 μg at bedtime to relieve nocturia; may dose twice daily if symptoms persist in daytime.
    - Orally available as 0.1–0.2-mg tablets; recommended initial dose in children >4 years of age is 0.05 mg b.i.d.
  - Thiazide diuretic dosed once or twice daily
- Nephrogenic DI (2,3):
  - Does not respond to desmopressin (DDAVP)
  - Remove offending agent(s).
  - Correct electrolyte imbalances (i.e., hypokalemia, hypocalcemia).
  - Pitressin has vasopressor and ADH activity, increasing water resorption at collecting ducts.
    - Adults: 5–10 units SC q3–6h; children: 2.5–10 units SC b.i.d.–q.i.d.
    - Major side effect is coronary artery constriction.
    - Contraindicated in patients with hypertension, angina, coronary heart disease
    - Pregnancy category B
  - Chlorpropamide (Diabinese) promotes renal response to ADH:
    - Adult 125–250 mg PO b.i.d.; not recommended for pediatric patients
    - Contraindicated in type I diabetes mellitus, severe renal or hepatic impairment, thyroid dysfunction
    - Pregnancy category C
    - Hypoglycemia may occur.
- Contraindications: Use desmopressin with caution during the immediate postoperative period for intracranial lesions because of possible cerebral edema.
- Precautions: An overdose of desmopressin may produce water intoxication and hyponatremia in patients with excessive water intake.

First Line
- Desmopressin is the treatment of choice in patients with central DI or gestational DI (pregnancy category B).

ADDITIONAL TREATMENT

General Measures
- Control fluid balance and prevent dehydration.
- Careful follow-up and management of electrolytes
- Check weight daily.
- Provide good skin and mouth care.
- Nephrogenic DI: Correct hypercalcemia and hypokalemia, and discontinue causative medications (2)[A].

Issues for Referral
- Dilatation of urinary tract (may be secondary to large urine volumes)
- Complications of primary disease (tumor, histiocytosis, etc.)
- In congenital nephrogenic DI, an associated retardation of mental development may occur in some patients.
- Subnormal growth rate

ONGOING CARE

FOLLOW-UP RECOMMENDATIONS
Continuing care is provided on an outpatient basis with self-medication.

Patient Monitoring
- Regular follow-up at 2–3-week intervals initially and 3–4 months later
- Adjust treatment on the basis of urine and electrolyte concentrations.
- Following moderate to severe traumatic brain injury, testing should done 6 and 12 months after injury.

DIET
- Normal, with free access to fluids
- Young infants with nephrogenic DI may benefit from low-solute formula.
- A low-sodium, low-protein diet may reduce urine output in nephrogenic DI.

PATIENT EDUCATION
- Reassurance of good prognosis
- Monitor medications/urinary pattern.
- Special precautions during travel, hot weather, exertion, and times of vomiting or diarrhea to avoid dehydration

PROGNOSIS
- Most reversible cases of nephrogenic DI are caused by medications, and patient symptoms improve with removal of the offending agent (4)[A]. Lithium may cause irreversible DI (4)[A].
- Generally good prognosis depending on underlying disorder

COMPLICATIONS
- Dilatation of the urinary tract has been observed (probably secondary to large volume of urine).
- Complications of the primary disease (tumor histiocytosis, etc.) should be anticipated. In congenital nephrogenic DI, an associated retardation of mental development may occur in some patients (cause undetermined).
- Without treatment, dehydration can lead to confusion, stupor, and coma.
- Subnormal growth rate

REFERENCES

1. Karhulik D, Zapletalova J, Frysak Z, et al. Dysfunction of hypothalamic-hypophysial axis after traumatic brain injury in adcults. *J Neurosurg*. 2009:1–4.
2. Makaryus AN, McFarlane SI. Diabetes insipidus: Diagnosis and treatment of a complex disease. *Cleve Clin J Med*. 2006;73:65–71.
3. http://www.diabetesinsipidus.net/.
4. Garofeanu CG, Weir M, Rosas-Arellano MP, et al. Causes of reversible nephrogenic diabetes insipidus: A systematic review. *Am J Kidney Dis*. 2005;45:626–37.

ADDITIONAL READING

- Fukuda I, Hizuka N, Takano K. Oral DDAVP is a good alternative therapy for patients with central diabetes insipidus: Experience of five-year treatment. *Endocr J*. 2003;50:437–43.
- Nemergut EC, Zuo Z, Jane JA, et al. Predictors of diabetes insipidus after transsphenoidal surgery: A review of 881 patients. *J Neurosurg*. 2005;103:448–54.

CODES

ICD9
253.5 Diabetes insipidus

CLINICAL PEARLS
- To distinguish primary polydipsia from DI in a patient with polyuria, a patient with primary polydipsia will have a normal response to a water restriction test and normal levels of plasma ADH.
- Vasopressin (IM) had been used previously but has been replaced by desmopressin, which provides the antidiuretic but not the vasoconstrictive activity of vasopressin for the treatment of central DI.
- The goal for adult patients with congenital nephrogenic DI is to prevent dehydration by ensuring proper fluid intake. Genetic testing should be recommended for access to genetic counseling and to facilitate newborn screening.

DIABETES MELLITUS, TYPE 1

Alfred Chege Gitu, MD

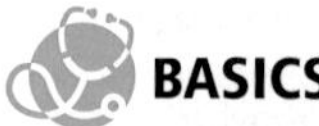

BASICS

DESCRIPTION

- Chronic disease caused by pancreatic insufficiency (deficiency) of insulin production
- Results in hyperglycemia and end-organ complications (e.g., accelerated atherosclerosis, neuropathy, nephropathy, and retinopathy)
- Features include:
  - Patients are insulinopenic and require insulin.
  - Ketosis
  - Usually rapid onset
  - Nutritional status: Normal or thin physique
- System(s) affected: Endocrine/Metabolic

Pregnancy Considerations

- During embryogenesis, hyperglycemia increases the incidence of congenital malformations. Tight control of blood sugar prior to conception is important.
- Women with microalbuminuria during the first trimester are at increased risk for preeclampsia and preterm delivery.
- A safe pregnancy is possible with vaginal delivery of a term baby. Close monitoring of blood sugar during labor is important.

EPIDEMIOLOGY

- Mean age of onset 8–12 years, peaking in adolescence
- Onset 1.5 years earlier in girls than boys
- Rapid decline in incidence after adolescence
- Overall incidence increasing worldwide
- Age of presentation has a bimodal distribution, being highest at ages 4–6 and 10–14 years.

Incidence

- 15/100,000 per year
- Racial predilection for whites
- African Americans have lowest overall incidence.

Pediatric Considerations

- Although onset is usually before the age of 19 years, true type 1 diabetes can occur for the first time in patients who are well into their 30s.
- Young children are more likely to present in diabetic ketoacidosis (DKA) due to atypical presentation, and because they may not express thirst or obtain fluids as readily as older children or adults.

RISK FACTORS

- Certain human leukocyte antigen (HLA) types
- Presence of a specific 64,000 mw protein may be responsible for antibody formation.
- Family history: Insulin-dependent or noninsulin-dependent diabetes in any first-degree relatives
- Dietary factors: Breastfeeding may provide a degree of protection against the disease, whereas exposure to cow's milk at an early age is associated with an increased risk of the disease.
- Maternal age at birth may play a role (1).
- Slightly greater risk for a child if the father has type 1 diabetes

Genetics

- Mode of genetic expression not clear
- Genes located on major histocompatibility complex on chromosome 6
- HLA DR3 and DR4 are individually associated with an increased risk; if a person is carrying both susceptibility genes, the relative risk is increased.
- HLA B8 and B15 also associated with increased risk

PATHOPHYSIOLOGY

- Alteration in immunologic integrity, placing the β-cell at special risk for inflammatory damage, accounts for most cases
- Autoantibodies to islet cells, glutamic acid decarboxylase (GAD), tyrosine phosphatase antibodies, and insulin identified in certain cases (type 1A diabetes)
- Some idiopathic cases (type 1B) have no evidence of autoimmune or other reason for beta cell damage.

ETIOLOGY

- Inherited defect
- Associated environmental triggers: None have been verified:
  - Viruses (e.g., mumps, coxsackie, cytomegalovirus, and hepatitis viruses)
  - Diet high in nitrosamines
  - Environmental toxins
- Emotional and physical stress

COMMONLY ASSOCIATED CONDITIONS

- Autoimmune diseases, such as celiac disease, hypothyroidism, and Addison disease:
  - Screening regularly for hypothyroidism is particularly important in females.
- Diabetes mellitus can also be seen as part of multiple endocrine adenomatosis.

DIAGNOSIS

DIAGNOSTIC TESTS & INTERPRETATION

Lab

- Criteria for the diagnosis of diabetes:
  - Fasting glucose >126 mg/dL (7.0 mmol/L) OR
  - Random of >200 mg/dL (11.1 mmol/L) in a patient with classic symptoms of hyperglycemia OR
  - Oral glucose tolerance test; plasma glucose ≥200 mg/dL 2 hours after a glucose load of 1.75 g/kg (max dose 75 g) OR
  - Glycated hemoglobin (HbA1c) level ≥6.5% (2)[C]
- Other tests to consider:
  - Serum electrolytes, especially in sicker patients who may have ketoacidosis
  - Urinalysis for glucose and ketones and microalbuminuria
  - Pancreatic autoantibodies (to diagnose type 1A diabetes):
    - Islet cells, insulin, GAD, tyrosine phosphatase antibodies
  - CBC (WBC count and hemoglobin may be elevated)
- C-peptide insulin level if needed to differentiate from type 2 diabetes

Pathological Findings

Inflammatory changes, lymphocytic infiltration around the islets of Langerhans, or islet cell loss

HISTORY

- Polyuria and polydipsia:
  - Polyuria may present as nocturia, bedwetting, or incontinence in a previously continent child.
  - Polyuria may be difficult to appreciate in diaper-clad children.
- Weight loss 10–30%:
  - Often almost devoid of body fat at diagnosis
  - Due to hypovolemia and increased catabolism
- Prolonged or recurrent candidal infection, usually in the diaper area
- Increased fatigue, lethargy, muscle cramps
- Irritability and emotional lability, headaches, abdominal discomfort, nausea
- Vision changes, such as blurriness
- Altered school or work performance
- Anxiety attacks

DIFFERENTIAL DIAGNOSIS

- Benign renal glycosuria
- Glucose intolerance
- Type 2 noninsulin-dependent diabetes:
  - Obese children might have maturity-onset diabetes of the young (MODY)
- Secondary diabetes:
  - Pancreatic disease (chronic pancreatitis, cystic fibrosis, hereditary hemochromatosis)
  - Hormonal disorders (pheochromocytoma, multiple endocrine adenomatosis)
  - Inborn errors of metabolism (glycogen storage disease, type 1)
  - Hereditary neuromuscular disease
  - Progeroid syndromes
  - Obesity (Prader-Willi syndrome)
  - Cytogenetic syndromes (trisomy 21, Klinefelter, and Turner syndromes)
  - Drug- or chemical-induced glucose intolerance: Glucocorticosteroids, HIV protease inhibitors, atypical antipsychotics, tacrolimus, cyclosporine
- Acute poisonings (salicylate poisoning can cause hyperglycemia and glycosuria, and may mimic diabetic ketoacidosis)

TREATMENT

MEDICATION

- All type 1 diabetes patients will require some form of insulin supplementation.
- Types of insulin:
  - Long-acting insulin analogues (insulin glargine [Lantus] and insulin detemir [Levemir]). These should not be mixed with other insulins in the same syringe.
  - Intermediate-acting insulin (NPH)—Humulin N or Novolin N—can be mixed with other insulins.
  - Short-acting (regular) insulin: Novolin R or Humulin R
  - Very rapid-acting insulin analogues (insulin lispro [Humalog], insulin aspart [Novolog], and insulin glulisine [Apidra])

First Line

- Flexible intensive insulin therapy is the gold standard.
- Frequent daily injections (FDI) or continuous SC insulin infusion (CSII) have equal efficacy.

- Total initial dose is 0.2–0.4 units/gg/day for insulin-naïve patients.
- 40–60% of total dose given as basal insulin, and the rest as bolus insulin
- FDI regime:
  - Basal, long-acting insulin once or twice a day
  - Prandial, short-acting insulin based on number of carbohydrate portions (e.g., 1:10, meaning 1 unit of insulin for every 10 g of carbohydrate to be eaten)
  - Correctional short-acting mealtime insulin based on premeal blood glucose level (e.g., BS-100/50, meaning if the blood glucose is >150, subtract 100 from the BG level, and divide that number by 50)
  - Administration of the mealtime insulin before a meal may be more efficacious than during or after the meal.
- CSII regime:
  - May use regular insulin or rapid-acting insulin analogues
  - Basal insulin is infused continuously at a preset rate, and bolus doses are given with meals as above.

Second Line

- Conventional insulin therapy
- Once- to twice-daily injections with NPH mixed with regular or rapid-acting insulin in the same syringe
- Not physiologic, but lower cost and fewer injections may improve compliance in the less motivated patient.
- Premixed insulin available as NPH/regular (Novolin or Humulin 70/30) or NPH/rapid-acting insulin (e.g., Novolog 75/25 Mix or Humulin 75/25 Mix)
- Pancreatic transplantation is usually reserved for patients with end-stage renal failure, who may receive kidney-pancreatic transplants at the same time.
- Oral hypoglycemics not indicated in type 1 diabetes (except in obese patients, who may have MODY, or a combination of type 1 and type 2): Metformin (Glucophage)

ADDITIONAL TREATMENT

General Measures

- Overall control of carbohydrate metabolism for the very young child:
  - Normoglycemia (adjusted for age): Strive for blood glucose levels in range of 80–150 mg/dL (4.4–8.3 mmol/L) all the time (80–120 in older patients)
  - Very tight control might be dangerous in young children due to risk of repeated hypoglycemia.
  - Hemoglobin A1c target levels:
    - Children <6 years: 7.5–8.5%
    - Children 6–12 years: <8.0%
    - Adolescents 13–19: <7.5% (<7.0% if achieved without excessive hypoglycemia)
    - Nonpediatric patients: <6.0%
- Normal growth and development and overall good health (asymptomatic):
  - Reach optimal height for genetic potential
  - Appropriate and timely pubertal maturation
  - Coping psychosocial development: Normal school or work attendance and performance; normal goals/career plans. Screen adolescents annually for depression.
- Prevent acute complications, including:
  - Hypoglycemic insulin reactions
  - Ketoacidosis
- Delay or prevent chronic complications.

IN-PATIENT CONSIDERATIONS

Newly diagnosed type 1 diabetics may require hospitalization during initiation of insulin therapy.

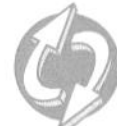

ONGOING CARE

FOLLOW-UP RECOMMENDATIONS

- Normal; full participation in sports activities
- Regular aerobic exercise is recommended.

Patient Monitoring

- BP monitoring at every office visit (3)[C]
- Monitor height, weight, and sexual maturation (in children).
- Daily home blood glucose monitoring with home blood glucose meter: Blood tests should be done at least 4–6 times daily (more frequently in pump patients) for optimal monitoring.
- Quarterly measurement of hemoglobin A1c
- Annual screenings after 5 years of diabetes, sooner if glycemic control is suboptimal:
  - Microalbuminuria for earliest signs of possible nephropathy
  - If elevated, depending on level, even if BP is normal, consider an ACE inhibitor (such as Vasotec [enalapril])
  - Ophthalmology exam (after 3–5 years of diabetes, also depending on glycemic control); regularly thereafter
  - Yearly lipid profile, thyroid levels, blood chemistries, CBC
  - Annual influenza vaccine

DIET

- American Diabetic Association diet: http://www.diabetes.org/food-and-fitness/food/
- Carbohydrate counting using insulin-to-carbohydrate ratio with all meals and snacks. Allows patient flexibility of eating and ability to eat almost anything.

PROGNOSIS

- Initial remission or honeymoon phase with decreased insulin needs and easier control, usually 3–6 months and rarely beyond a year
- Progression to total diabetes when endogenous insulin is insignificant; usually is gradual, but stress or illness initiate it suddenly
- Current prognosis:
  - Increasing longevity and quality of life with careful blood glucose monitoring and improvement in insulin delivery regimens
- At this time, reduced life expectancy, but has improved greatly over the past 20 years

COMPLICATIONS

- Microvascular disease (retinopathy, nephropathy, neuropathy)
- Hyperlipidemia
- Macrovascular disease (coronary and cerebral artery disease)
- Chronic foot ulcers/amputations
- Hypoglycemia
- Diabetic ketoacidosis
- Excessive weight gain
- Increased risk for preeclampsia and preterm delivery (4)
- Driving mishaps (5)
- Psychological problems of chronic disease

REFERENCES

1. Cardwell CR, Stene LC, Joner G, et al. Maternal age at birth and childhood type 1 diabetes: A pooled analysis of 30 observational studies. *Diabetes*. 2010;59:486–94.
2. International Expert Committee, et al. International Expert Committee report on the role of the A1C assay in the diagnosis of diabetes. *Diabetes Care*. 2009;32:1327–34.
3. American Diabetes Association (ADA). Standards of medical care in diabetes. V. Diabetes care. *Diabetes Care*. 2006;29(Suppl 1):S8–17.
4. Jensen DM, Damm P, Ovesen P, et al. Microalbuminuria, preeclampsia, and preterm delivery in pregnant women with type 1 diabetes: Results from a nationwide Danish study. *Diabetes Care*. 2010;33:90–4.
5. Cox DJ, Ford D, Gonder-Frederick L, et al. Driving mishaps among individuals with type 1 diabetes: A prospective study. *Diabetes Care*. 2009;32: 2177–80.

ADDITIONAL READING

Silverstein J, Klingensmith G, Copeland K, et al. Care of children and adolescents with type 1 diabetes: A statement of the American Diabetes Association. *Diabetes Care*. 2005;28:186–212.

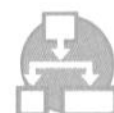

See Also (Topic, Algorithm, Electronic Media Element)

Diabetes Mellitus, Type 2; Diabetic Ketoacidosis (DKA)

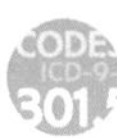

CODES

ICD9

- 250.01 Diabetes mellitus without mention of complication, type I (juvenile type), not stated as uncontrolled
- 250.03 Diabetes mellitus without mention of complication, type I (juvenile type), uncontrolled
- 250.11 Diabetes with ketoacidosis, type I [juvenile type], not stated as uncontrolled

CLINICAL PEARLS

- Polyuria may present as nocturia, bedwetting, or incontinence in a previously continent child.
- Young children are more likely to present in DKA because they may not express thirst or obtain fluids as readily as older children or adults.
- Onset usually before the age of 19 years, but type 1 diabetes can present in patients who are well into their 30s.
- Obese children might have MODY.

DIABETES MELLITUS, TYPE 2

Ramothea L. Webster, MD, PhD

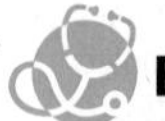

BASICS

DESCRIPTION
- Diabetes mellitus (DM) type 2 manifests in nonketotic hyperglycemia due to insulin resistance and relative impairment in insulin secretion.
- System(s) affected: Endocrine/Metabolic; Nervous; Renal/Urologic; Cardiovascular

Geriatric Considerations
- Significant contributing factor to blindness, renal failure, and lower limb amputations.
- Dietary restrictions for elderly patients with DM in long-term facilities is not warranted; give regular diet.

Pediatric Considerations
- Incidence increasing dramatically.
- Prevalence: About 1/400 under 20 years

Pregnancy Considerations
First-line drug is insulin (class B), but may consider glyburide (class B) only after the first trimester or metformin (class B)

EPIDEMIOLOGY
Incidence
1.9 million new cases reported in 2010 within US age >20 years

Prevalence
- 18.8 million diagnosed; 7 million undiagnosed
- Age >20 years, Men 13 million (11.8%); Women 12.6 million (10.8%)
- Race: 7.1% whites, 11.8% Hispanics, 12.6% blacks, 8.4% Asian Americans, and 35% Pima Indians
- If diagnosed <40 years, average reduction in life-years is 12 years (male) and 19 years (female).
- Lifetime risk of developing diabetes if born in 2000 is 33% (male) and 39% (female)

RISK FACTORS
- Family history: First-degree relative
- Gestational diabetes (GDM)
- Obesity: BMI ≥25; induces resistance to insulin-mediated peripheral glucose uptake
- Hypertriglyceridemia
- Ethnicity: African American, Latino, Native American, Asian American, and Pacific Islander
- Impaired fasting glucose (IFG) or impaired glucose tolerance (IGT)

Genetics
- Strong polygenic familial susceptibility with strong association with variations in TCF7L2 gene
- Concordance nearly complete in identical twins

GENERAL PREVENTION
- Lose 5–10% body weight, exercise 150 min/wk, and decrease fat and caloric intake.
- Protein increases insulin response, but not to exceed 15% of caloric intake

PATHOPHYSIOLOGY
- Decrease in peripheral insulin effects ("insulin resistance") and resultant progressive loss of β-cell function and mass
- Cellular damage due to inability of cells to regulate uptake of glucose during hyperglycemic events via mitochondrial superoxide production to capillary endothelial cells in retina, mesangial cells in renal glomerulus, and to neurons and Schwann cells in peripheral nerves (1)[A]

ETIOLOGY
- Genetic factors (β-cell dysfunction, defects in insulin action, diseases of the exocrine pancreas [e.g., cystic fibrosis])
- Obesity, immune-mediated, infection, hemochromatosis
- Drug- or chemical-induced (e.g., medications used for psychosis, HIV, or transplant recipients)

COMMONLY ASSOCIATED CONDITIONS
Hypertension, hyperlipidemia, impotence, stroke, peripheral neuropathy, metabolic syndrome, renal insufficiency, cardiovascular disease, retinopathy, infertility, pancreatic cancer, polycystic ovary syndrome, acanthosis nigricans

DIAGNOSIS

HISTORY
Polyuria, polydipsia, polyphagia, weight loss, weakness, fatigue, and frequent infections

PHYSICAL EXAM
Complications of hyperglycemia: Retinopathy, neuropathy, and poor wound healing

DIAGNOSTIC TESTS & INTERPRETATION
Lab
- Criteria for diagnosis:
  - HbA1c ≥6.5% on 2 or more occasions is diagnostic; HbA1c between 5.7% and 6.4% is prediabetes (2)[A].
  - Symptoms of diabetes plus random plasma glucose ≥200 mg/dL (11.1 mmol/L), *or*
  - Fasting plasma glucose (FPG) ≥126 mg/dL (7.0 mmol/L) on 2 occasions, *or*
  - 2-hour plasma glucose ≥200 mg/dL (11.1 mmol/L) during oral glucose tolerance test (GTT) with 75-g glucose load (3)[A]
- HbA1c has advantages over FPG for diagnosis and analysis (2)[A].
- GTT is usually not necessary, except when diagnosing gestational diabetes.
- Drugs that may alter lab results: Atypical antipsychotics, pentamidine, nicotinic acid, glucocorticoids, thyroid hormone, diazoxide, beta-adrenergic agonists, thiazides, Dilantin, alpha-interferon, and some fluoroquinolones

Follow-Up & Special Considerations
- A1c <8.5% is mostly due to postprandial hyperglycemia and less fasting hyperglycemia
- A1c ≥8.5% is mostly due to fasting hyperglycemia and less by postprandial hyperglycemia (1)[A].

DIFFERENTIAL DIAGNOSIS
- Type 1 DM
- GDM
- IFG and/or IGT

TREATMENT

- Goals are controversial: Recent recommendations include the following A1c targets (4)[A]:
  - A1C <7.0: for those with a long life expectancy and no cardiovascular, who have had DM for a short duration and no history of hypoglycemia
  - A1C >7.0: for those with a limited life expectancy, advanced micro- or macrovascular complications, extensive comorbidities, a history of hypoglycemia or long-standing DM in whom the general goal is difficult to attain
- FPG goal is <110 mg/dL (5.5 mmol/L)
- If HbA1c >8%, consider starting 2 oral agents (3)[A]:
  - Use drugs from different classes to achieve adequate control.
  - Insulin might be the next best addition if uncontrolled by oral agents.

MEDICATION
First Line
- Biguanides:
  - Metformin (Glucophage, Fortamet, Riomet, Glumetza): Preferred first medication because of its effects on weight loss and insulin resistance: 500–1,000 mg b.i.d.–t.i.d. or ER 1,000–2,000 mg every evening, max 2,550 mg/d, except Glumetza, 2,000 mg/d
  - Avoid situations that increase risk for lactic acidosis: Renal insufficiency, radiocontrast agents, surgery, or acute illnesses (e.g., liver disease, cardiogenic shock, pancreatitis, hypoxia)
  - Caution with congestive heart failure (CHF), alcohol abuse, elderly, or with tetracycline
- Sulfonylureas:
  - Glipizide (Glucotrol): 2.5–40 mg/d; dosage >10 mg/d given b.i.d., take 30 minutes before meals
  - Glipizide extended-release: 5–20 mg/d
  - Glyburide (DiaBeta, Glynase, Micronase): 1.25–20 mg/d, Glynase 0.75–12 mg/d
  - Glimepiride (Amaryl): 1–8 mg/d
  - Caution with renal, liver, or thyroid disease, sulfa allergy, Cr CL <50, late pregnancy
  - Chlorpropamide (Diabinese): 100–500 mg/d, max 750 mg/d
- Thiazolidinediones:
  - Pioglitazone (Actos): 15–45 mg/d
  - Monitor serum transaminase every 2 months for the first year; contraindicated for liver disease and symptomatic heart failure patients
  - May cause or exacerbate CHF, myocardial infarction, and bladder cancer.
- Alpha-glucosidase inhibitors:
  - Acarbose (Precose): 25–100 mg t.i.d.
  - Miglitol (Glyset): 25–100 mg t.i.d.
  - Take at beginning of meals to decrease postprandial glucose peaks.
  - Poor patient compliance due to GI symptoms
  - Avoid in renal insufficiency, inflammatory bowel disease, colonic ulceration, or partial bowel obstruction.

- Dipeptidyl peptidase-4 inhibitor:
  - Sitagliptin (Januvia): 100 mg/d
  - Sitagliptin/Metformin (Janumet): Start 50/500 mg b.i.d.; max 100 mg/2,000 mg/d; give with meals hold for iodinated contrast studies
  - Saxagliptin (Onglyza): 2.5 mg/d; max 5 mg/d
  - Saxagliptin/Metformin XR (Kombiglyze XR): Start 5/500 mg/d, given with evening meals, max 5/2,000 mg, hold for iodinated contrast studies
  - Linagliptin (Tradjenta): 5 mg/d
  - Alogliptin (in Japan only)
  - Renally excreted; therefore, adjust dosage for renal patients.
  - Increased risk of acute pancreatitis
- Precautions: Warn patients of signs of hypo- and hyperglycemia:
  - Combination of metformin and sulfonylurea may increase patient's relative risk of cardiovascular hospitalization or mortality.
- Significant possible interactions:
  - Drugs that may potentiate sulfonylureas: Salicylates, clofibrate, warfarin (Coumadin), ethanol, and ACE inhibitors
  - Thiazides can cause IGT.
  - Gatifloxacin can cause either severe hypo- or hyperglycemia.
  - TZD pioglitazone may decrease effectiveness of oral contraceptives.
  - Drug binders, such as cholestyramine resin, should be taken at least 2 hours apart from alpha-glucosidase inhibitors.

ALERT

Avandia: Associated with an increased risk of heart attack, stroke, PE, and CHF. As of fall 2010, Avandia has been suspended in Europe; and in the US, is restricted for use only when other medicines have failed and patients are aware of the drug's cardiovascular risks.

Second Line

- Insulin: Rapid (Aspart, Lispro, Glulisine), short (regular insulin), intermediate (NPH), and long/peakless (Glargine) or long/peak (Detemir):
  - Can be given up to t.i.d.
  - May be used in combination with oral agents, or with an insulin of a different half-life
  - Most often required in late stages of type 2 DM, when oral agents fail to control glucose levels
  - Insulin detemir (Levemir) or insulin glargine (Lantus): 0.5–1 U/kg/d, onset 1 hour, no true peak, duration 6–23 hours, given at bedtime or b.i.d.; start with 10 units SC at bedtime, then increase by 1 unit daily until FPG <100.
  - Long-acting insulins have a lower risk of hypoglycemia and lower variability than other insulins.
- Amylinomimetic:
  - Pramlintide (Symlin): 60–120 μg SC before every meal
  - When used with insulin, may cause severe hypoglycemia
  - Preprandial insulins, short-acting or rapid-acting, should be reduced by 50% at initiation of drug.
  - Contraindicated in patients with gastroparesis
  - Drug interactions: Anticholinergic drugs or agents that slow intestinal absorption of nutrients
- GLP-1 (glucagonlike peptide-1) receptor agonist:
  - Exenatide (Byetta): 5–10 μg SC b.i.d. within 60 minutes before meals and at least 6 hours apart
  - Liraglutide (Victoza): 0.6 mg/d SC for 1 week, then increase to 1.2; max 1.8 mg/d; less expensive and better tolerated than exenatide; should not be used in patients with history or family history of medullary thyroid cancer or MEN type II (black box warning) (5)[A]
  - Increased risk of acute pancreatitis and kidney disease
- Promotes weight loss, increases high-density lipoprotein cholesterol, and decreases diastolic BP
- Sulfonylureas should be decreased to reduce the chance of hypoglycemia. Patients should be advised to take other oral medications 1 hour before injecting Exenatide.
- Meglitinides:
  - Repaglinide (Prandin): 0.5–4 mg before meals; may be useful in patients with sulfa allergy or renal impairment
  - Nateglinide (Starlix): 60–120 mg before meals t.i.d.

ADDITIONAL TREATMENT

General Measures

- Foot exam every visit for neuropathy (monofilament), arterial insufficiency, and ulcers
- Nephropathy: Urinalysis to check microalbumin yearly
- Retinopathy: Yearly eye exams
- NCEP guidelines recommend a low-density lipoprotein cholesterol goal of <70 mg/dL in patients with existing cardiovascular disease (CVD) or risk factors for CVD
- Hypertension control (goal BP <130/80 mm Hg)
- Low-dose aspirin for all adults, unless there is a contraindication
- ACEI/ARB first-line hypertension drug (3)[A]; if contraindicated, consider a calcium channel blocker

COMPLEMENTARY AND ALTERNATIVE MEDICINE

- Cinnamon not shown to improve A1c or, but has shown improvements with FBG in DM types 1 or 2. Its role in preventing DM is unknown.
- Chromium shown to reduce A1c and FBG; further studies needed to fully understand its role in diabetes treatment and prevention.

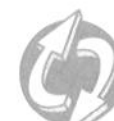

ONGOING CARE

FOLLOW-UP RECOMMENDATIONS

Patient Monitoring

- Office visits every 2–4 months
- Monitor glucose, HbA1c, lipids, BP, body weight, and renal function.
- HbA1c twice a year for glycemic-controlled patients and quarterly for uncontrolled or change-in-therapy patients (3)[A]

DIET

Mild caloric restriction to achieve weight loss. Carbohydrates <45–65% of caloric consumption per day; fat <30%; protein <15%; and fiber 50 g/d (3)[A].

PATIENT EDUCATION

- Regular aerobic exercise (150 min/wk) can improve glucose tolerance and decrease medication requirements (3)[A].
- Lifestyle modifications with pharmacotherapy can delay progression from prediabetes to diabetes (1)[A].

PROGNOSIS

In susceptible individuals, complications begin to appear 10–15 years after onset, but can be present at time of diagnosis since disease may go undetected for years.

COMPLICATIONS

Damage of macro- and microvascular arterial cell walls, peripheral neuropathy, proliferative retinopathy, nephropathy and chronic renal failure, atherosclerotic CVD and peripheral vascular disease, hyperosmolar coma, gangrene of extremities, blindness, glaucoma, cataracts, skin ulceration, Charcot joints

REFERENCES

1. Blonde L, et al. Current antihyperglycemic treatment guidelines and algorithms for patients with type 2 diabetes mellitus. *Am J Med.* 2010;123:S12–8.
2. The International Expert Committee. International Expert Committee Report on the Role of the A1C Assay in the Diagnosis of Diabetes. *Diabetes Care.* 2009.
3. American Diabetes Association, et al. Standards of medical care in diabetes–2011. *Diabetes Care.* 2011;34(Suppl 1):S11–61.
4. Skyler JS, Bergenstal R, Bonow RO, et al. Intensive glycemic control and the prevention of cardiovascular events: Implications of the ACCORD, ADVANCE, and VA diabetes trials: A position statement of the American Diabetes Association and a scientific statement of the American College of Cardiology Foundation and the American Heart Association. *Diabetes Care.* 2009;32:187–92.
5. Fakhoury WK, Lereun C, Wright D, et al. A meta-analysis of placebo-controlled clinical trials assessing the efficacy and safety of incretin-based medications in patients with type 2 diabetes. *Pharmacology.* 2010;86:44–57.

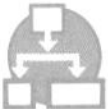

See Also (Topic, Algorithm, Electronic Media Element)

- Diabetes Mellitus, Type 1; Diabetic Ketoacidosis (DKA); Hypertension, Essential
- Algorithm: Diabetes Mellitus, Type 2

CODES

ICD9

- 250.00 Diabetes mellitus without mention of complication, type II or unspecified type, not stated as uncontrolled
- 250.02 Diabetes mellitus without mention of complication, type II or unspecified type, uncontrolled

CLINICAL PEARLS

- Screening: ≥45 years with a body mass index (BMI) ≥25 kg/m^2 or <45 years, overweight (BMI >25 kg/m^2), and other risk factors. Repeat every 3 years; if IFG or IGT, check every 1–2 years
- Metformin preferred first medication

DIABETIC KETOACIDOSIS (DKA)

Francesca L. Beaudoin, MS, MD
Nadine T. Himelfarb, MD

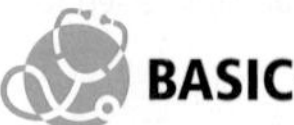

BASICS

DESCRIPTION
- A true medical emergency secondary to severe insulin deficiency and characterized by hyperglycemia, ketosis, and metabolic acidosis
- System(s) affected: Endocrine/Metabolic

EPIDEMIOLOGY
Incidence
- In US: 46 episodes/10,000 diabetic patients; 2/100 patient-years of type 1 diabetes mellitus (DM)
- Predominant age: 0–19 years
- Predominant sex: Male = Female

RISK FACTORS
- Type 1 > Type 2 DM
- Younger patients at higher risk

GENERAL PREVENTION
- Close monitoring of glucose during periods of stress, infection, and trauma
- Careful insulin control and monitoring of the blood glucose level
- "Sick day" management instructions

PATHOPHYSIOLOGY
A relative or absolute deficiency of insulin, exacerbated by an increase in counterregulatory hormones (e.g., catecholamines, cortisol, glucagon, and growth hormone) leading to a hyperglycemic crisis

ETIOLOGY
- Noncompliance/insufficient insulin: 25%
- Infection: 30–40%
- First presentation of DM: 10–20%
- Myocardial infarction (MI): 5–7%
- No cause identified: 10–30%
- Cerebrovascular accident (CVA)
- Medications (corticosteroids, thiazides)
- Drugs (cocaine)
- Trauma
- Surgery
- Emotional stress
- Pregnancy

COMMONLY ASSOCIATED CONDITIONS
Complications of chronic DM such as nephropathy, neuropathy, and retinopathy

DIAGNOSIS

HISTORY
- Recent illness
- Changes in diet or medications
- Missed insulin doses
- Polyuria, nocturia
- Polydipsia
- Generalized weakness
- Malaise, lethargy
- Anorexia or increased appetite
- Nausea, vomiting
- Abdominal pain
- Decreased perspiration
- Fever
- Confusion
- Coma

PHYSICAL EXAM
- Hypotension
- Tachycardia
- Hypothermia or fever
- Tachypnea, Kussmaul respirations
- Fruity odor to breath (acetone smell)
- Decreased reflexes
- Abdominal tenderness
- Decreased bowel sounds
- Dry mucous membranes, poor skin turgor
- Decreased perspiration
- Confusion
- Coma
- Attempt to find precipitating cause (i.e., source of infection).

DIAGNOSTIC TESTS & INTERPRETATION
- ECG:
  - Usually shows sinus tachycardia
  - Look for changes consistent with electrolyte abnormalities and ischemia/MI.
- Urine and blood cultures
- Consider lumbar puncture (meningitis).

Lab

ALERT
- Hyponatremia: Hyperglycemia or hypertriglyceridemia may cause an artificially low or very low sodium concentration. The measured sodium is suppressed by 1.6 mg/dL for every 100 mg/dL of glucose over normal.
- Hyperglycemia (usually 250–800 mg/dL)
- Serum ketosis: Check β-hydroxybutyrate (β-HB) instead of ketones to evaluate ketosis (1)[B]. With concomitant lactic acidosis, acetoacetate production may be inhibited in the presence of high levels of β-HB. Nitroprusside reaction, which measures only acetoacetate, may not be strongly positive.
- Urine ketosis (may be falsely negative initially; urinalysis (UA) may only identify acetoacetate and not β-HB)
- Glycosuria
- Hyperamylasemia, hyperlipasemia
- Hypertriglyceridemia/hypercholesterolemia
- Increased creatinine and BUN: Markedly increased serum ketones may cross-react and cause a falsely high serum creatinine.
- HCO_3 (usually $\leq$15 mEq/L)
- Decreased calculated total-body K^+: Severe acidosis gives an artificially high K^+ level.
- Metabolic acidosis on arterial blood gases
- Increased serum osmolality
- Increased anion gap
- Elevated base deficit

Initial lab tests
- CBC, electrolytes, BUN, creatinine
- Serum β-HB or ketones
- Arterial blood gases; venous blood gases (VBGs) also may be used (VBG pH 0.03 lower).

Imaging
- Chest x-ray to rule out pulmonary infection
- Head CT scan if suspected CVA or cerebral edema

Diagnostic Procedures/Surgery
Only if surgical problem is the underlying precipitant (e.g., appendicitis)

DIFFERENTIAL DIAGNOSIS
- Hyperosmolar nonketotic coma
- Alcoholic ketoacidosis
- Starvation ketosis
- Toxic ingestions (e.g., salicylates)
- Lactic acidosis
- Acute hypoglycemic coma
- Uremia/chronic renal failure

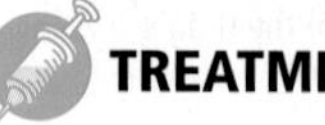

TREATMENT

- Oxygen and airway management as needed
- Establish IV access.
- Cardiac monitoring
- Start isotonic crystalloid solution (0.9% saline).
- Fingerstick glucose testing
- Empirical naloxone if altered mental status

MEDICATION
First Line
- Insulin: IV infusion of regular insulin at 0.1 unit/kg/h; may use IM or SC route, but IV is recommended for moderate-to-severe DKA (1,2)[B]
- Potassium: Falsely elevated due to acidosis; start replacement when K^+ $\leq$5.0 mg/dL and urine output is adequate. Start 30–40 mEq/L IV fluids. Increase rate (up to 60 mEq/L) if K^+ $\leq$3.5 mg/dL (1,2)[A]:
  - Hold insulin if K^+ $\leq$2.5 mg/dL; give IV potassium 1 mEq/kg over 1 h.
  - For each 0.1 unit of pH, serum K^+ will change by ~0.6 mEq in opposite direction.

- Phosphorus: Routine replacement may lead to hypocalcemia; if very low (<1.0), give 1/3 of K^+ replacement as KPhos.
- Sodium bicarbonate: No demonstrable benefit with a pH >7.0 (1,2)[B]; rehydration usually leads to resolution of acidosis. Consider its use in patients with arterial pH <6.9 or patients with life-threatening hyperkalemia.
- Magnesium: If Mg ≤1.8 mg/dL and the patient is symptomatic, consider replacement.
- Precautions:
  - If the patient is on an insulin pump, it should be stopped.
  - Double insulin if no response in serum glucose over first 2 hours.
  - If blood glucose does not fall by ~75 mg every 2 hours, increase insulin rate.
  - If using bicarbonate, add 50–100 mEq $NaHCO_3$ to 1 L 0.45% saline *or* 150 mEq $NaHCO_3$ to 1 L D_5W and give over 1 hour. Once a pH of 7.1 has been reached, infusion should be stopped.

Second Line

Insulin, SC or IM: Load with 0.3 unit/kg SC, followed by 0.1 unit/kg/h. Space dosing to q2h once glucose <250 mg/dL.

ADDITIONAL TREATMENT

General Measures

- All but mild cases require inpatient management; severe DKA requires an ICU setting.
- Goals:
  - Fluid resuscitation
  - Insulin therapy
  - Resolution of anion-gap acidosis
  - Correction of electrolytes
- Laboratory testing during management:
  - Serum glucose q1–2h until stable
  - Electrolytes, phosphorous, and venous pH q2–6h as needed

Pediatric Considerations

- Children with moderate-to-severe DKA should be transferred to the nearest pediatric critical-care hospital.
- In 0.3–1% of children/adolescents, fluid resuscitation and treatment may result in marked mental deterioration, including development of coma 4–6 hours after therapy has begun; death is 21–24%:
  - Think of cerebral edema secondary to rapid IV hydration.
  - Diagnose by CT scan.
  - Treat with IV bolus of mannitol 1 g/kg in 20% solution.
  - If no response, hyperventilation to a pCO_2 of 28 mm Hg.

Geriatric Considerations

Must be careful with impaired renal function or congestive heart failure when correcting fluid and electrolyte abnormalities

Pregnancy Considerations

- Pregnancy itself is diabetogenic. It also results in a compensated respiratory alkalosis (HCO_3 19–20 mEq/L) with theoretically reduced buffering capacity. Therefore, pregnant patients are more susceptible to DKA.
- Euglycemic DKA
- Increased risk of preeclampsia and fetal death
- β-tocolytics and corticosteroids can trigger DKA.
- Perinatal death: 9–35%

IN-PATIENT CONSIDERATIONS

Admission Criteria

ADA admission guidelines: Blood glucose >250 mg/dL; pH <7.3; HCO_3 ≤15 mEq/L; ketones in urine; ICU setting for severe DKA (3)

IV Fluids

- 10–20 mL/kg over the first hour then 500 mL/h (~0.7 mL/kg/h) for 4 hours or until hemodynamics improve; then 250 mL/h (3.5 mL/kg/h) until tolerating PO
- Switch to 5% dextrose in 0.45% saline at maintenance rate when serum glucose <250 mg/dL. Maintain blood glucose between 150 and 250 mg/dL. Too rapid correction of fluid balance may precipitate cerebral edema (1)[C]. If the blood glucose level is falling too rapidly, consider using a 10% dextrose solution instead.

Pediatric Considerations

Bolus 10–20 mL/kg initially; 4-hour fluid total should be <50 mL/kg to reduce chance of cerebral edema

Discharge Criteria

Discharge when DKA has resolved: Glucose <200 mg/dL; pH >7.3; bicarbonate >18 mEq/L; additionally, patients must be tolerating PO intake and able to resume home medication regimen, and the underlying precipitant (e.g., infection) must be identified and treated.

ONGOING CARE

FOLLOW-UP RECOMMENDATIONS

Bed rest

Patient Monitoring

- Monitor mental status, vital signs, and urine output q30–60min until improved, then q2–4h every 24 hours.
- Monitor blood sugar q1h until <300 mg/dL, then q2–6h.
- Monitor electrolytes (Na, K, HCO_3) q2h.
- Monitor phosphate, calcium, and magnesium q4–6h.

DIET

- NPO initially
- Advance to preketotic diet when nausea and vomiting are controlled.
- Avoid foods with high glycemic index (e.g., soft drinks, white bread, etc.).

PROGNOSIS

- 16% of all diabetes-related fatalities
- Death 1–2%
- In children <10 years of age, DKA causes 70% of diabetes-related fatalities.

COMPLICATIONS

- Cerebral edema
- Pulmonary edema
- Vascular thrombosis
- Hypokalemia
- Cardica dysrhythmia
- MI
- Acute gastric dilatation
- Late hypoglycemia
- Erosive gastritis
- Infection, mucormycosis
- Respiratory distress

REFERENCES

1. Agus MS, Wolfsdorf JI. Diabetic ketoacidosis in children. *Pediatr Clin North Am*. 2005;52: 1147–63, ix.
2. Kitabchi AE, Umpierrez GE, Murphy MB, et al. Hyperglycemic crises in diabetes. *Diabetes Care*. 2004;27(Suppl 1):S94–102.
3. American Diabetes Association. Hospital admission guidelines for diabetes. *Diabetes Care*. 2004; 27(Suppl 1):S103.

ADDITIONAL READING

- Carroll MA, Yeomans ER. Diabetic ketoacidosis in pregnancy. *Crit Care Med*. 2005;33:S347–53.
- Trachtenbarg DE. Diabetic ketoacidosis. *Am Fam Physician*. 2005;71:1705–14.

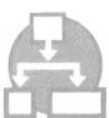

See Also (Topic, Algorithm, Electronic Media Element)

Diabetes Mellitus, Type 1

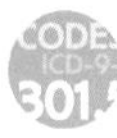

CODES

ICD9

- 250.12 Diabetes mellitus with ketoacidosis, type ii or unspecified type, uncontrolled
- 250.13 Diabetes mellitus with ketoacidosis, type I (juvenile type), uncontrolled

CLINICAL PEARLS

- Admit if blood glucose >250 mg/dL, pH <7.3, HCO_3 ≤15 mEq/L, and ketones in urine.
- Potassium is falsely elevated due to acidosis; start replacement when K^+ ≤5.0 mg/dL and urine output is adequate.

DIABETIC POLYNEUROPATHY

Samir Malkani, MD

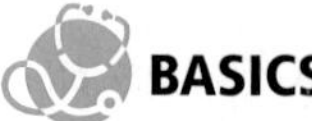

BASICS

DESCRIPTION

Peripheral nerve dysfunction seen in diabetes; several patterns described:

- Symmetric polyneuropathy:
  - Distal sensory or sensorimotor
  - Proximal lower extremity polyneuropathy
- Focal and multifocal neuropathy:
  - Cranial neuropathy
  - Focal limb neuropathy
  - Diabetic amyotrophy
  - Truncal neuropathy
- Autonomic neuropathies
- Chronic inflammatory demyelinating polyneuropathy (CIDP)

EPIDEMIOLOGY

Prevalence

- Prevalence increases with diabetes duration
- Generalized polyneuropathy:
  - 10% at diabetes diagnosis
  - 50% at 25 years
  - Cross-sectional prevalence: 15% by symptoms; 50% by nerve conduction
- Autonomic neuropathy: 16.7% in a UK study

RISK FACTORS

- Poor glycemic control
- Duration of diabetes
- Older age
- Presence of retinopathy

GENERAL PREVENTION

Maintenance of normal blood sugar

PATHOPHYSIOLOGY

- >1 pathogenetic factor may operate
- Metabolic derangement due to hyperglycemia:
  - Aldose reductase converts excess glucose to sorbitol, which causes nerve damage.
  - Nonenzymatic glycation of neural proteins and lipids forms damaging advanced glycosylation end products.
  - Protein kinase C activation causes vascular endothelial changes.
  - Oxidative stress from excessive production of reactive oxygen species
- Vasculopathy causing nerve ischemia: Likely in mononeuropathies

ETIOLOGY

Diabetes mellitus (type 1 and 2)

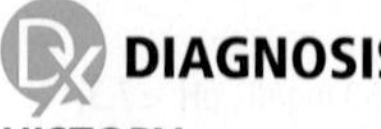

DIAGNOSIS

HISTORY

- Most common form: Symmetric distal sensory or sensorimotor polyneuropathy:
  - Distressing numbness, tingling, pain of legs/feet, usually worse at night; allodynia; hyperalgesia
  - Sometimes silent and unnoticed by patient
  - Ataxia due to proprioceptive loss
  - Neuropathic foot ulcers due to analgesia and repetitive injury
  - Neuropathic degeneration of foot joints
  - Hands involved late
  - Distal muscle involvement, usually mild
- Symmetric proximal polyneuropathy:
  - Proximal leg weakness and wasting
  - Muscles of shoulder girdle rarely involved
  - Pain and sensory changes less prominent
- Focal cranial or limb mononeuropathy:
  - May involve third, fourth, sixth, or seventh cranial nerve
  - Femoral, sciatic, or peroneal neuropathy: Weakness or pain in nerve distribution
  - Any major peripheral nerve can be involved.
- Truncal neuropathies: Painful radiculopathy over dermatomes
- Diabetic amyotrophy (this term is used for a lumbar radiculoplexopathy):
  - Unilateral hip, thigh pain
  - Pelvic girdle, thigh weakness, atrophy
  - Recovery over months
- Diabetic autonomic neuropathy:
  - GI: Nocturnal diarrhea, sometimes alternating with constipation; gastroparesis with postprandial fullness; nausea and vomiting
  - Cardiovascular: Postural dizziness; increased risk for coronary event; exercise intolerance
  - Urogenital: Urinary hesitancy, overflow incontinence; erectile dysfunction; vaginal dryness; sexual dysfunction
  - Sudomotor: Anhidrosis or hyperhydrosis; gustatory sweating of head and upper body
- CIDP: Progressive, severe motor loss
- Diabetic cachexia: Weight loss and depression with polyneuropathy

PHYSICAL EXAM

- Symmetric distal polyneuropathy:
  - "Stocking-and-glove" distal sensory loss
  - Large-fiber neuropathy: Loss of vibratory perception and light touch (10-G monofilament)
  - Small-fiber involvement: Loss of temperature and pinprick
  - Absent ankle reflexes
  - Wasting, weakness of small muscles in foot; changes to arch of foot or clawing of toes
  - With small-fiber involvement, there may be lack of objective sensory deficit despite pain
- Symmetric proximal polyneuropathy:
  - Proximal leg, arm wasting, and weakness
  - Loss of patellar reflexes
- Focal cranial or limb mononeuropathy:
  - Third cranial nerve palsy: Painful ophthalmoplegia and ptosis; preserved pupillary reflexes (in contrast to compressive palsies)
  - Sixth cranial nerve: Lateral gaze palsy
  - Femoral neuropathy: Weakness of lower leg extension, hip flexion, quadriceps wasting, absent patellar reflex, sensory loss in anterior thigh
  - Sciatic neuropathy: Pain or sensory loss in back of thigh and leg; weakness of hamstrings, lower leg muscles
  - Peroneal neuropathy: Foot drop
- Truncal neuropathies: Sensory loss along dermatome
- Lumbar radiculoplexopathy (amyotrophy):
  - Weakness and wasting pelvic girdle and thigh
  - Sensory loss in L2–L3
  - Absent patellar reflex
- Autonomic neuropathy:
  - Cardiovascular: Resting tachycardia; orthostatic hypotension
  - Gastroparesis: Postprandial distension; gastric splash
- CIDP: Motor weakness

DIAGNOSTIC TESTS & INTERPRETATION

Lab

Initial lab tests

- Fasting plasma glucose, 2-hour glucose tolerance test or hemoglobin A1c for diagnosis and to assess glycemic control
- Serum B_{12} levels
- Thyroid function
- Creatinine and BUN
- Syphilis testing
- Serum protein electrophoresis
- In mononeuropathy/mononeuritis multiplex, test for vasculitis, paraproteinemia, and sarcoid.

Imaging

Initial approach

In radiculopathy or mononeuropathy, imaging studies to exclude compressive lesions

Diagnostic Procedures/Surgery

- Quantitative sensory testing for vibratory and thermal thresholds:
  - Standardized measures for assessing severity and risk of foot ulceration
- Electromyogram nerve conduction velocity (1):
  - Useful to confirm mononeuropathy and entrapment syndromes
  - Sensitive but nonspecific index of presence and severity of diabetic polyneuropathy
  - In small unmyelinated fiber painful neuropathy, test may be normal
- Lumbar puncture:
  - In CIDP, elevation of spinal fluid protein
- Skin biopsy (2):
  - Enables direct study of small nerve fibers that are difficult to assess electrophysiologically
- Corneal confocal microscopy (2):
  - Noninvasive approach based on examination of corneal innervation

Pathological Findings

- In peripheral nerve, Wallerian degeneration, focal axonal swellings containing neurofilaments, axonal atrophy, and demyelination are seen.
- Thick neural capillary basement membrane
- Obliterative microvascular lesions and perivascular inflammation

DIFFERENTIAL DIAGNOSIS

- Uremic polyneuropathy
- Drug-induced:
  - Antineoplastic drugs: Cisplatin, vincristine
  - Isoniazid
  - Amiodarone
- Toxic:
  - Chronic arsenic poisoning
  - n-hexane, methyl-*n*-butyl ketone
- Nutritional deficiency:
  - Usually associated with alcoholism
- Paraneoplastic polyneuropathy
- Hypothyroidism

TREATMENT

MEDICATION

First Line

- Management of pain and sensory neuropathy:
  - Tricyclic antidepressants (TCAs) (1,3)[A] (off-label):
    - Analgesia may be related to effects on sodium channels.
    - Amitriptyline 25–150 mg at bedtime
    - Nortriptyline (25–150 mg); desipramine (25–200 mg) less sedating than amitriptyline, but limited trial data
    - Anticholinergic side effects may occur.
  - Calcium channel modulators: Gabapentin (1,3)[A] (off-label):
    - Binds Ca^{2+} channel-associated protein $b1_2$-b4, inhibits neurotransmitter release
    - Dose titration is from 300–1,200 mg t.i.d.
    - Reduce dose in renal insufficiency
    - Adverse effects: Dizziness, fatigue, edema
    - Fewer side effects than TCA
  - Calcium channel modulators: Pregabalin (1,3)[A]:
    - Binds same calcium channel as gabapentin
    - Linear pharmacokinetics unlike gabapentin
    - Usual dose 150–600 mg
    - Adverse effects are dizziness and edema.
  - Duloxetine (1,3)[A]:
    - Selective serotonin and norepinephrine uptake inhibitor
    - Usual dose is 60–120 mg/d
    - Adverse effects are nausea and dizziness.
- Management of autonomic neuropathy (4):
  - Orthostatic hypotension:
    - Fludrocortisone (off-label)
    - Midodrine (off-label)
  - Gastroparesis:
    - Metoclopramide or domperidone
    - Erythromycin (off-label)
  - Diabetic diarrhea:
    - Loperamide
    - Clonidine (off-label)
    - Octreotide (off-label)
    - Antibiotics for bacterial overgrowth
  - Erectile dysfunction:
    - Phosphodiesterase-5 inhibitors
    - Prostaglandin E_1 injection
    - Mechanical devices
  - Hyperhidrosis:
    - Propantheline (off-label)

Geriatric Considerations

Anticholinergic effects of TCAs may cause urinary retention, arrhythmias

Second Line

- Antidepressants:
  - Venlafaxine (75–225 mg daily) (3)[B] (off-label):
    - Serotonin norepinephrine reuptake inhibitor
  - SSRIs:
    - Paroxetine and citalopram (off-label) demonstrate some efficacy.
- Anticonvulsants:
  - Sodium valproate (3)[B] (off-label):
    - Blocks sodium channels and gamma-aminobutyric acid (GABA) transmission
    - Dose 500–1,000 mg/d
- Topical therapies:
  - Capsaicin 0.075% cream applied t.i.d. (3)[B]:
    - Depletes C fibers in skin of substance P
  - Lidocaine 5% (700 mg) patches applied daily to feet (1,3)[C] (off-label):
    - Causes sodium channel blockade
- Opiate analgesia:
  - Tramadol 100–400 mg daily (1)[B]:
    - Nonnarcotic medication; binds opiate receptors; fewer opiate side effects
  - Oxycodone (1,3)[B]:
    - Controversial due to dependence potential
- b1-lipoic acid (3)[C]:
  - Antioxidant properties may limit free radical-mediated damage.
  - 600-mg PO daily dose; showed benefit in small studies

ADDITIONAL TREATMENT

General Measures

- Maintain blood glucose close to normal.
- Provide appropriate footwear to prevent pressure damage to insensate feet.

Issues for Referral

If CIDP suspected, refer to neurologist for investigation and treatment.

Additional Therapies

- Transcutaneous electrical nerve stimulation
- Percutaneous nerve stimulation (3)
- Electrical spinal cord stimulation (1)

COMPLEMENTARY AND ALTERNATIVE MEDICINE

Acupuncture, Reiki, electromagnetic field treatment (3): No convincing trial data

SURGERY/OTHER PROCEDURES

Electrical spinal cord stimulation (1)

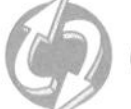

ONGOING CARE

PROGNOSIS

- Generalized symmetric polyneuropathies:
  - Usually slow chronic progression
  - Insensitive but painless foot as pain lessens
- Focal neuropathies:
  - Recovery over months to years

COMPLICATIONS

- Claw foot deformity
- Neurotropic ulceration:
  - Painless ulcers on weightbearing area
  - Callus formation is a precursor to ulceration.
- Neuropathic arthropathy:
  - Results in complete disorganization of joint structure in foot, Charcot joint

REFERENCES

1. Tesfaye S, Boulton AJ, Dyck PJ, et al. Diabetic neuropathies: Update on definitions, diagnostic criteria, estimation of severity, and treatments. *Diabetes Care*. 2010;33:2285–93.
2. Zochodne DW. Diabetic Neuropathy: An update. *Curr Opin Neurol*. 2008;21(5):527–33.
3. Bril V, England J, Franklin GM, et al. Evidence-based guideline: Treatment of painful diabetic neuropathy: Report of the American Academy of Neurology, the American Association of Neuromuscular and Electrodiagnostic Medicine, and the American Academy of Physical Medicine and Rehabilitation. *Neurology*. 2011;76:1758–65.
4. Unger J, Cole BE, et al. Recognition and management of diabetic neuropathy. *Prim Care*. 2007;34:887–913, viii.

ADDITIONAL READING

- Dworkin RH, O'Connor AB, Audette J, et al. Recommendations for the pharmacological management of neuropathic pain: An overview and literature update. *Mayo Clin Proc*. 2010;85:S3–14.
- Finnerup NB, Sindrup SH, Jensen TS, et al. The evidence for pharmacological treatment of neuropathic pain. *Pain*. 2010;150:573–81.
- Habib AA, Brannagan TH, et al. Therapeutic strategies for diabetic neuropathy. *Curr Neurol Neurosci Rep*. 2010;10:92–100.
- Saarto T, Wiffen PJ, et al. Antidepressants for neuropathic pain: A Cochrane review. *J Neurol Neurosurg Psychiatr*. 2010;81:1372–3.
- Zilliox L, Russell JW, et al. Treatment of diabetic sensory polyneuropathy. *Curr Treat Options Neurol*. 2011;13:143–59.

See Also (Topic, Algorithm, Electronic Media Element)

Diabetes Mellitus, Type 1; Diabetes Mellitus, Type 2

CODES

ICD9

- 250.60 Diabetes with neurological manifestations, type II or unspecified type, not stated as uncontrolled
- 250.61 Diabetes with neurological manifestations, type I [juvenile type], not stated as uncontrolled
- 250.62 Diabetes with neurological manifestations, type II or unspecified type, uncontrolled

CLINICAL PEARLS

- Occasionally, when glycemic control improves dramatically, as can occur when treatment for diabetes is initiated, there may be a worsening of neuropathy symptoms. Symptoms usually stabilize and gradually improve as glycemic control is maintained.
- It is common to combine agents with different mechanisms of action in the management of neuropathic pain. Topical therapies can also be combined with systemic therapies.

DIARRHEA, ACUTE

Fernando A. Hernandez, MD
Dillon Savard, MD

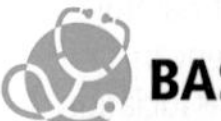

BASICS

DESCRIPTION

- Abnormal increase in stool frequency (3 or more in 24 hours) or liquidity in an otherwise healthy individual
- Often self-limiting; <14 days duration
- Acute viral diarrhea (50–70%):
  - Most common form; usually occurs for 1–3 days; self-limited
- Bacterial diarrhea (15–20%):
  - Develops 6–24 hours after infected food ingested
  - Suspect if simultaneous illness is present in others who have shared contaminated food
- Protozoal infections (10–15%):
  - Cause prolonged, watery diarrhea (travelers from areas with contaminated water supply)
- Traveler's diarrhea typically begins 3–7 days after arrival in foreign location; often quite acute.
- System(s) affected: Endocrine/Metabolic; Gastrointestinal

EPIDEMIOLOGY

Predominant age: All ages

Prevalence

- Fifth leading cause of death worldwide
- 11% of the general population
- Highest in children <5 years old

RISK FACTORS

- Individual from an industrialized country visiting a developing country
- Immunocompromised host
- Antibiotic use
- Daycare attendance; nursing home residency
- Pregnancy (20-fold increase for *Listeriosis*)

GENERAL PREVENTION

- Frequent handwashing; proper hygiene
- Rotavirus vaccine
- Strict food handling
- Care during foreign travel to avoid brushing teeth with contaminated water, ingesting ice cubes, or eating cold salads or meats
- Probiotics may be used to help prevent traveler's diarrhea (1)[A].

ETIOLOGY

- Bacterial:
  - *Escherichia coli*
  - *Salmonella*
  - *Shigella*
  - *Campylobacter jejuni*
  - *Vibrio parahaemolyticus*
  - *Vibrio cholerae*
  - *Yersinia enterocolitica*
  - *Clostridium difficile*
  - *Staphylococcus aureus*
  - *Bacillus cereus*
  - *Clostridium perfringens*
- Viral:
  - Rotavirus
  - Norwalklike virus (Norovirus)
  - Cytomegalovirus (HIV, immunocompromised)
- Protozoal:
  - *Giardia lamblia*
  - *Cryptosporidium*
  - *Entamoeba histolytica*
  - *Isospora belli*
  - *Cyclospora*

Pediatric Considerations

- Rotavirus is a common cause of viral diarrhea in the winter months and is accompanied by vomiting.
- Other etiologies include overfeeding, medications, cystic fibrosis, and malabsorption.

COMMONLY ASSOCIATED CONDITIONS

- Diabetes mellitus
- Ileal resection
- Gastrectomy
- Hyperthyroidism
- Inflammatory bowel disease

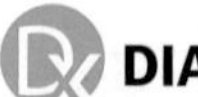

DIAGNOSIS

HISTORY

- Anorexia ± vomiting
- Malaise
- Headache
- Myalgia
- Fever
- Immunocompromised or pregnancy
- Recently hospitalized or antibiotic use
- Assess stool characteristics: Frequency and quantity, presence of mucus or blood, consistency (2)[A]
- Travel history, daycare attendance, ingestion of raw or undercooked meat, raw seafood, unpasteurized milk, sick contacts (2)[A]
- With *Giardia*: Cramping; pale, greasy stools; fatigue; weight loss; chronicity

PHYSICAL EXAM

- Loose liquid stools ± blood or mucus
- Fever
- Abdominal pain and distension
- Determine hydration status; look for decreased skin turgor, dry mucous membranes, hypotension, or decreased urination:
  - In children: Absence of tears, depressed fontanelles, dry diapers
- Abdominal exam to rule out potential surgical causes of diarrhea, such as appendicitis or pelvic abscess

Geriatric Considerations

Watery diarrhea with chronic constipation may be caused by fecal impaction or obstructing neoplasm.

Pregnancy Considerations

Dehydration may lead to preterm labor.

DIAGNOSTIC TESTS & INTERPRETATION

Lab

Initial lab tests

- Consider testing if diarrhea is prolonged, in severe illness, bloody diarrhea, and in high-risk patients.
- CBC:
  - Increased WBCs with a left shift may indicate an infectious process.
  - A decreased hemoglobin/hematocrit may indicate anemia from blood loss.
- Serum electrolytes:
  - Increased sodium from dehydration
  - Decreased potassium from diarrhea
- BUN, creatinine: Elevated in dehydration
- pH: Hyperchloremic acidosis
- Stool sample:
  - Occult blood present in inflammatory bowel disease, bowel ischemia, bacterial infections
  - Fecal leukocytes present in diarrhea caused by *Salmonella, Campylobacter, Yersinia*
  - For community-acquired or traveler's diarrhea >1 day or accompanied by fever or bloody stools: Culture or test for *Salmonella, Shigella, Campylobacter, E. coli* O157:H7. If antibiotics or chemotherapy in recent weeks, *C. difficile* toxin A and B (2)[B].
  - For nosocomial diarrhea (onset ≥3 days in hospital): Test for *C. difficile* toxins A and B. Also consider bacterial cultures listed above in patients with bloody stools or infants (2)[B].
  - For diarrhea >7 days: Stool ova and parasites (O&P) plus bacterial cultures if immunocompromised (2)[B]
  - *Giardia* ELISA: >90% sensitive in at-risk population, consider prior to O&P

Imaging

Abdominal radiographs (flat plate and upright) indicated with severe abdominal pain or evidence of obstruction to rule out toxic megacolon and bowel ischemia

Diagnostic Procedures/Surgery

Sigmoidoscopy may be helpful in distinguishing between bloody diarrhea caused by inflammatory bowel disease and infectious diarrhea.

Pathological Findings

- Viral diarrhea: Changes in small intestine cell morphology that include villous shortening, increased number of crypt cells, and increased cellularity of the lamina propria
- Bacterial diarrhea: Bacterial invasion of colonic wall leads to mucosal hyperemia, edema, and leukocytic infiltration.

DIFFERENTIAL DIAGNOSIS

- Inflammatory bowel disease
- Drugs (cholinergic agents, magnesium-containing antacids)
- Pseudomembranous colitis secondary to antibiotic use
- Diverticulitis
- Spastic (irritable) colon
- Fecal impaction
- Malabsorption
- Zollinger-Ellison syndrome
- Ischemic bowel
- Gastrinoma

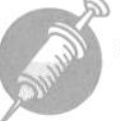

TREATMENT

MEDICATION

First Line

- Loperamide: 4 mg followed by 2-mg capsule after each unformed stool (see "Precautions" below) (3)[A]
- Bismuth subsalicylate: 30 mL q30min until 8 doses; not superior to loperamide
- If diarrhea persists and a bacterial or parasitic organism is identified, antibiotic therapy should be started:
  - *Giardia*: Metronidazole 250 mg t.i.d. for 5 days
  - *E. histolytica*: Metronidazole 750 mg t.i.d. for 10 days
  - *Shigella*: Trimethoprim-sulfamethoxazole (Bactrim DS) 160 mg/800 mg b.i.d. for 5 days, or ciprofloxacin 500 mg b.i.d. for 3 days
  - *Campylobacter*: Erythromycin 500 mg q.i.d. for 5 days or ciprofloxacin 500 mg b.i.d. for 3 days
  - *C. difficile*: Discontinue antibiotics if possible. Consider metronidazole 500 mg t.i.d. for 10–14 days if diarrhea persists or worsens.
  - Traveler's diarrhea: Ciprofloxacin 750 mg 1 dose or, if severe, 500 mg divided PO b.i.d. for 3 days *or* TMP/SMX (Bactrim DS) 1 tab b.i.d. for 3 days (3)[A]
- Contraindications:
  - Antibiotics are contraindicated in *Salmonella* infections unless caused by *S. typhosa* or the patient is severely ill.
  - Avoid alcoholic beverages with metronidazole due to the possibility of a disulfiram reaction.
  - Antibiotics are not indicated in foodborne toxigenic diarrhea.
- Precautions:
  - Antiperistaltic agents (e.g., loperamide) should be used with caution in patients suspected of having infectious diarrhea (especially if *E. coli* 0157:H7 suspected) or antibiotic-associated colitis.
  - Antiperistaltic agents may speed recovery from traveler's diarrhea when used in combination with an antibiotic.
  - Doxycycline, sulfamethoxazole-trimethoprim, and ciprofloxacin may cause photosensitivity; use sunscreen.
- Significant possible interactions:
  - Salicylate absorption from bismuth subsalicylate can cause toxicity in patients already taking aspirin-containing compounds and may alter anticoagulation control in patients taking Coumadin.
  - Ciprofloxacin and erythromycin increase theophylline levels.

Second Line

- Doxycycline: 100 mg b.i.d. for 3 days
- Diphenoxylate-atropine in nonpregnant adults
- Tinidazole or secnidazole for *E. histolytica*
- Oral vancomycin for *C. difficile* infections

ADDITIONAL TREATMENT

General Measures

Replace lost fluid and electrolytes (3)[A]:

- Clear liquids at room temperature, such as tea, broth, carbonated beverages (without caffeine), and rehydration fluids (e.g., Gatorade) to replace lost fluid
- Packets of rehydration salts (1 packet to be diluted in 1 quart of water); drink until thirst is quenched (helps replace electrolytes); treatment of choice for pediatric patients
- Oral rehydration solutions (ORS): Polymer-based ORS may be superior to glucose-based ORS in watery diarrhea (3)[A].
- IV fluids if patient cannot tolerate oral rehydration

COMPLEMENTARY AND ALTERNATIVE MEDICINE

- In children with acute infectious diarrhea, treatment with probiotics appears to be safe and effective for reducing the duration and frequency of diarrhea (4)[A].
- In patients being treated with antibiotics, administration of a probiotic at levels above 10^{10}/g may prevent diarrhea (5)[A].
- Zinc supplementation can decrease diarrhea-related morbidity and mortality (6)[A].

IN-PATIENT CONSIDERATIONS

Initial Stabilization

Outpatient health care except for complicating emergencies (dehydration)

ONGOING CARE

DIET

- Early refeeding is encouraged.
- During periods of active diarrhea, avoid coffee, alcohol, dairy products, most fruits, vegetables, red meats, and heavily seasoned foods.
- Begin by eating clear soup with rice, salted crackers, dry toast or bread, and sherbet.
- As stooling rate decreases, slowly add to diet baked potato and chicken soup with noodles.
- As stool begins to retain shape, add to diet baked fish, poultry, applesauce, and bananas.
- The traditional bananas, rice, applesauce, toast diet has little evidence-based support despite heavy clinical use.

PATIENT EDUCATION

See guidelines in "Prevention" section.

PROGNOSIS

This common problem is rarely life threatening if adequate hydration is maintained.

COMPLICATIONS

- Dehydration
- Sepsis
- Shock
- Anemia

REFERENCES

1. Szajweska H, Mrukowicz JZ. Probiotics in the treatment and prevention of acute infectious diarrhea in infants and children: A systematic review of published randomized, double-blind, placebo-controlled trials. *J Pediatr Gastroenterol Nutr*. 2001;33(Supple 2):S17.
2. Pawlowski SW, Warren CA, Guerrant R. Diagnosis and treatment of acute or persistent diarrhea. *Gastroenterology*. 2009;136(6):1874–86.
3. DuPont HL. Clinical Practice. Bacterial diarrhea. *N Engl J Med*. 2009;361(16):1560–9.
4. Chen CC, Kong MS, Lai MW, et al. Probiotics have clinical, microbiologic, and immunologic efficacy in acute infectious diarrhea. *Pediatr Infect Dis J*. 2010;29:135–8.
5. McFarland LV, et al. Evidence-based review of probiotics for antibiotic-associated diarrhea and *Clostridium difficile* infections. *Anaerobe*. 2009;15:274–80.
6. Walker CL, Black RE, et al. Zinc for the treatment of diarrhoea: Effect on diarrhoea morbidity, mortality and incidence of future episodes. *Int J Epidemiol*. 2010;39(Suppl 1):i63–9.

ADDITIONAL READING

- Dupont HL. Systematic review: The epidemiology and clinical features of travellers' diarrhoea. *Aliment Pharmacol Ther*. 2009.
- Gottlieb T, Heather CS. Diarrhea in adults (acute). *Clin Evid* (Online). 2011;2011. pii: 0901.
- Marcos LA, DuPont HL. Advances in defining etiology and new therapeutic approaches in acute diarrhea. *J Infect*. 2007;55:385–93.

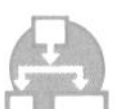

See Also (Topic, Algorithm, Electronic Media Element)

Botulism; Cholera; Food Poisoning, Bacterial

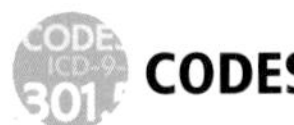

CODES

ICD9

- 005.9 Food poisoning, unspecified
- 009.2 Infectious diarrhea
- 787.91 Diarrhea

CLINICAL PEARLS

- Viruses, especially norovirus, are the most common causes of acute diarrheal illness in the US:
  - Antibiotics are not generally needed for routine bacterial causes of gastroenteritis.
- Early refeeding and use of probiotics is encouraged.
- Loperamide and bismuth are useful antidiarrheal medications.
- Bismuth can cause transient black tongues and stools.

DIARRHEA, CHRONIC

Morgan Sendzischew, MD
Mia Souheil Hindi, MD
Amar Deshpande, MD

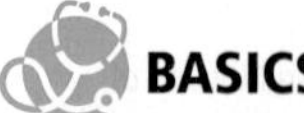

BASICS

DESCRIPTION
- Chronic diarrhea refers to an increase in frequency of defecation or decrease in stool consistency (typically >3 loose stools per day) for >6 weeks:
  - Etiologies include osmotic, secretory, fat-losing, and inflammatory
  - Infectious is possible, but in a chronic setting it is less common.
- System(s) affected: Gastrointestinal

EPIDEMIOLOGY
Prevalence
Variable depending on etiology, but overall ~5% of US population is affected.

RISK FACTORS
- Osmotic:
  - Excessive ingestion of sorbitol or fructose
  - Lactose intolerance
- Secretory:
  - Extensive small bowel resection/ileal surgery
  - History of neuroendocrine disease
  - History of laxative abuse
  - Dysmotility syndromes
- Fat-losing:
  - Cystic fibrosis
  - Chronic alcohol abuse
  - Chronic pancreatitis/pancreatic insufficiency
- Inflammatory:
  - Family history of inflammatory bowel disease (IBD)
  - Use of NSAIDs
  - Thoracoabdominal radiation
  - HIV/AIDS

ALERT
Diabetes mellitus and history of cholecystectomy can cause both secretory and osmotic diarrhea.

Genetics
- Celiac disease is associated with HLA-DQ2 and HLA-DQ8 haplotypes on MHC Class II antigen-presenting cells.
- IBD is polygenic and new genome-wide association studies continue to demonstrate new polymorphisms.

GENERAL PREVENTION
- Variable depending on etiology of the diarrhea
- Treating the underlying disorder.

PATHOPHYSIOLOGY
Also variable depending on etiology, but in all causes it is the result of disturbances in luminal water and electrolyte balance

ETIOLOGY
- Osmotic:
  - Carbohydrate malabsorption:
    - Humans cannot absorb disaccharides.
    - Sorbitol is found in gums and candies as a sugar substitute.
    - Fructose is absorbed through a different transporter than glucose and galactose.
  - Substances including magnesium, phosphate, sulfate
- Secretory:
  - Laxative ingestion
  - Postcholecystectomy (1):
    - Leads to excessive bile salts in intestinal lumen causing cholerheic diarrhea; often resolves in 6–12 months
  - Ileal bile acid malabsorption:
    - Ileal resection of <100 cm leads to cholerheic diarrhea due to excessive presentation of bile salts to colon
  - Disordered motility (2):
    - Postvagotomy
    - Diabetic autonomic neuropathy
    - Hyperthyroidism
    - IBS
  - Neuroendocrine tumors:
    - VIPoma
    - Gastrinoma
    - Somatostatinoma
    - Carcinoid syndrome
  - Metastatic medullary carcinoma of the thyroid
  - Systemic mastocytosis
  - Protein-losing enteropathy
- Fatty:
  - Malabsorption:
    - Whipple disease
    - Short bowel syndrome:
      - Ileal resection of >100 cm leads to insufficient bile salt concentrations in the duodenum for optimal fat absorption, leading to fat and fat-soluble vitamin malabsorption.
    - Small intestinal bacterial overgrowth
  - Maldigestion:
    - Pancreatic exocrine insufficiency (cystic fibrosis, chronic pancreatitis)
- Inflammatory:
  - Ulcerative colitis
  - Crohn disease
  - Celiac disease
  - Microscopic colitis (lymphocytic or collagenous)
  - HIV/AIDS
  - Vasculitis
  - Radiation enterocolitis
  - Eosinophilic enterocolitis
- Drugs: NSAIDs, colchicine, metformin, digoxin, SSRIs
- Herbal products: St. John's wort, echinacea, garlic, saw palmetto, ginseng, cranberry extract, aloe vera
- Infectious:
  - Bacterial: *Clostridium difficile*, *Mycobacterium avium intracellulare*
  - Parasites: *Giardia lamblia*, *Isospora*
  - Helminths: *Strongyloides*

COMMONLY ASSOCIATED CONDITIONS
- Extraintestinal manifestations of IBD include arthralgias, aphthous stomatitis, uveitis/episcleritis, erythema nodosum, pyoderma gangrenosum, perianal fistulas, ankylosing spondylitis, and primary sclerosing cholangitis.
- Celiac disease is associated with dermatitis herpetiformis.

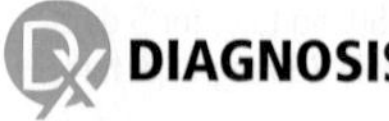

DIAGNOSIS

HISTORY
- Detailed history of symptoms, including:
  - Onset
  - Pattern and frequency
  - Stool volume and quality (including presence of blood or mucus)
  - Presence of nocturnal symptoms
  - Travel history
  - Antibiotic exposure
  - Dietary habits
  - Current medications
- Evaluate for aggravating or alleviating factors, including changes with oral intake or improvement with selective food avoidance (e.g., wheat).
- Evaluate for unintentional weight loss within the recent past.
- Complete review of systems, including rashes, ocular problems, heat intolerance, polyuria/polydypsia, headache, fever, flushing, alcohol intake
- Evaluate for IBS or functional diarrhea by Rome III criteria:
  - IBS: Recurrent abdominal pain or discomfort ≥3 times/month in the last 3 months (symptoms >6 months) with 2 or more of the following:
    - Improvement with defecation
    - Change in frequency of stool
    - Change in form of stool
  - Functional diarrhea: Loose or watery stools ≥75% of the time without pain for >3 months (symptoms >6 months)

PHYSICAL EXAM
- General: Assess for volume depletion, nutritional status
- Neck: Thyromegaly, lymphadenopathy
- Cardiovascular: Tachycardia, systolic ejection murmur
- Pulmonary: Wheezing
- Abdomen: Hepatosplenomegaly, palpable mass, ascites
- Anorectal: Sphincter competence
- Extremities: Peripheral edema, flushing, rashes

DIAGNOSTIC TESTS & INTERPRETATION
Lab
Initial lab tests
- Blood: CBC with differential, electrolytes (Mg, P, Ca), total protein, albumin, thyroid-stimulating hormone (TSH), free T4
- Stool: WBCs, electrolytes (stool gap), fecal occult blood, qualitative fecal fat (Sudan stain), culture, ova and parasites, *Giardia* stool antigen

Follow-Up & Special Considerations

- Tests by differential:
  - Celiac disease: Antiendomysial antibody IgA, antitissue transglutaminase (TTG) IgA, antigliadin (AGA) IgA, serum IgA (10× increase in IgA deficiency). Can check genetics (DQ2/DQ8) to rule out celiac disease.
  - Chronic pancreatic insufficiency: Fecal elastase
  - Protein-losing enteropathy: Fecal b1-1 antitrypsin
  - Carbohydrate malabsorption: Fecal pH
  - Prior history of hospitalization or antibiotics: *C. difficile* toxin
  - Neuroendocrine tumor:
    - Serum: Chromogranin A, VIP, gastrin
    - Urine: 5-HIAA, histamine
  - HIV ELISA, special stains for *Isospora* and *Cryptosporidium*
  - Allergy testing

Imaging

Initial approach

- Plain film abdomen: Rule out dilation or obstruction.
- CT to rule out chronic pancreatitis if abnormal pancreatic enzymes or evidence of malabsorption

Diagnostic Procedures/Surgery

- Flexible sigmoidoscopy: Especially if pregnant, with comorbidities, or if left-sided symptoms predominate (tenesmus and urgency) (3)[A]
- Colonoscopy with ileal intubation and biopsies: To diagnose IBS, microscopic inflammatory disorders, and colorectal neoplasia (3)[A]
- Esophagogastroduodenoscopy (EGD) with small bowel biopsies if malabsorption disorder suspected:
  - Celiac, *Giardia* infection, Crohn disease, eosinophilic gastroenteropathy, Whipple disease, intestinal amyloid, and pancreatic insufficiency (3)[A]
- Wireless capsule endoscopy
- Upper GI series with small bowel follow-through
- CT or magnetic resonance (MR) enterography

Pathological Findings

- Celiac disease: Marsh classification:
  - Intraepithelial lymphocytosis, increased ratio of crypt to villous height, villous blunting
- IBD: Crypt abscesses, granulomas, lymphoplasmacytic infiltrate
- Melanosis coli suggests cathartic abuse.

DIFFERENTIAL DIAGNOSIS

See above.

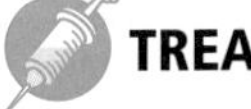

TREATMENT

MEDICATION

First Line

- **Symptom relief:**
  - Loperamide (Imodium) 2 mg after loose bowel movement; maximum 16 mg daily
  - Diphenoxylate-atropine (Lomotil) 5–20 mg daily
- **Based on underlying cause:**
  - Lactose intolerance: Lactose-free diet and lactase supplementation
  - Cholecystectomy or ileal resection: Cholestyramine (Questran) or other bile acid resin 4–8 g q8h
  - Diabetes: Aggressive diabetes management and glucose control
  - Hyperthyroidism: Methimazole, propylthiouracil (PTU), thyroid ablation
  - *C. difficile*: Vancomycin or metronidazole (Flagyl)
  - *Giardia lamblia*: Metronidazole (Flagyl) or nitazoxanide
  - Whipple disease: Ceftriaxone IV or Bactrim PO
  - Small intestinal bacterial overgrowth: Rifaximin, fluoroquinolones, metronidazole, penicillins
  - Pancreatic insufficiency: Pancreatic enzyme replacement
  - HIV/AIDS: Antiretroviral therapy
  - Microscopic colitis: Budesonide, mesalamine, Pepto-Bismol
  - IBD: Mesalamine, corticosteroids (short-term only), antibiotics (short-term only), immunomodulators (azathioprine, methotrexate), biologic therapy (antitumor necrosis factor [TNFs])
  - Neuroendocrine tumor: Octreotide
  - Celiac disease: Wheat/barley/rye avoidance; corticosteroids in rare refractory cases

ADDITIONAL TREATMENT

General Measures

- If the patient presents volume depleted, first-line therapy is to restore euvolemia with IV fluids (normal saline) and electrolyte replacement if indicated.
- If the patient is euvolemic, therapy is generally outpatient.

COMPLEMENTARY AND ALTERNATIVE MEDICINE

Many homeopathic and naturopathic formulations are available to treat diarrhea; most have not been subject to the scrutiny of controlled clinical trials.

SURGERY/OTHER PROCEDURES

Resection of neuroendocrine tumors, intestinal resection for medically refractory IBD

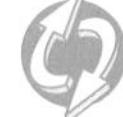

ONGOING CARE

DIET

Abstain from gluten products, sorbitol, lactose-containing products, and food allergens.

PATIENT EDUCATION

- Reassurance that there is a wide variation in what is accepted as "normal" bowel habits
- Restrict colon stimulants.
- Dietary consult when appropriate

PROGNOSIS

Depends on etiology

COMPLICATIONS

- Fluid and electrolyte abnormalities
- Malnutrition
- Anemia
- Malignancy (colon cancer in ulcerative colitis, small bowel cancer in celiac disease and Crohn disease, lymphoma with IBD therapies)
- Infection with immunomodulator, biologic, and corticosteroid therapies for IBD

REFERENCES

1. Sauter GH, Moussavian AC, Meyer G, et al. Bowel habits and bile acid malabsorption in the months after cholecystectomy. *Am J Gastroenterol.* 2002;97.
2. Longstreth GF, Thomson WG, Chey WD, et al. Functional bowel disorders. *Gastroenterology.* 2006;130:1480–91.
3. ASGE Standards of Practice Committee. The role of endoscopy in the management of patients with diarrhea. *Gastrointest Endosc.* 2010;71(6):887.

ADDITIONAL READING

- Fan X, Sellin JH. Review article: Small intestinal bacterial overgrowth, bile acid malabsorption and gluten intolerance as possible causes of chronic watery diarrhea. *Aliment Pharmacol Ther.* 2009; 29(10):1069–77.
- Fine KD, Seidel RH, Do K. The prevalence, anatomic distribution, and diagnosis of colonic causes of chronic diarrhea. *Gastrointest Endosc.* 2000; 51(3):318.
- Thomas PD. Forbes A, Green J, et al. Guidelines for the investigation of chronic diarrhea, 2nd edition. *Gut.* 2003;52(Suppl 5):v1–15.
- Zins BJ, Tremaine WJ, Carpenter HA. Collagenous colitis: Mucosal biopsies and association with fecal leukocytes. *Mayo CLin Proc.* 1995;70(5):430.

See Also (Topic, Algorithm, Electronic Media Element)

Algorithm: Diarrhea, Chronic

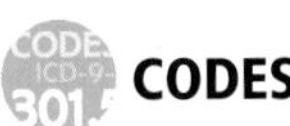

CODES

ICD9

787.91 Diarrhea

CLINICAL PEARLS

- IBS, IBD, malabsorption syndromes (such as lactose intolerance), celiac disease, and chronic infections (particularly in patients who are immunocompromised).
- A thorough medical history can guide appropriate evaluation.
- The selection of specific tests should be performed depending upon the likelihood of specific diagnoses.
- Consider over-the-counter medications and herbal products as potential causative agents.

DIFFUSE INTERSTITIAL LUNG DISEASE

Jacqueline L. Olin, MS, PharmD, BCPS, CPP, CDE
Julie Scott Taylor, MD, MSc

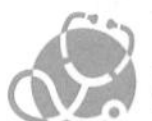

BASICS

DESCRIPTION

- Interstitial lung diseases (ILDs) represent a diverse group of chronic progressive lung diseases associated with alveolar inflammation and/or potentially irreversible pulmonary fibrosis.
- >200 individual diseases may present with similar characteristics, making ILD difficult to classify.
- A classification scheme proposed by the American Thoracic Society and European Respiratory Society includes these subtypes:
  - Known causes (environmental, occupational, or drug-associated disease)
  - Systemic disorders (sarcoidosis, Wegener granulomatosis, collagen vascular disease, etc.)
  - Rare lung diseases (pulmonary histiocytosis, lymphangioleiomyomatosis, etc.)
  - Idiopathic interstitial pneumonias (IIPs)
- Based on clinical, radiologic, and histologic features, IIPs are further subclassified into the following diagnoses:
  - Idiopathic pulmonary fibrosis (IPF), characterized by progressive dyspnea, cough, restrictive lung disease, and a specific histopathologic pattern
  - IIPs other than IPF (including nonspecific interstitial pneumonia [NSIP], respiratory bronchiolitis-associated ILD [RBILD], acute interstitial pneumonia [AIP], bronchiolitis obliterans with organizing pneumonia [BOOP], etc.)
- The classification of IIPs and relationships between the subtypes continue to be areas of clinical controversy.

Pediatric Considerations

ILD in infants and children represents a heterogeneous group of respiratory disorders that are mostly chronic and associated with high morbidity and mortality. Like with adults, diseases result from a variety of processes involving genetic factors and inflammatory or fibrotic responses (1). Some diseases result from developmental disorders and growth abnormalities in infancy (1). Classification can center around whether disease is primarily a pulmonary process or if symptoms occur as a result of a systemic disorder.

EPIDEMIOLOGY

Incidence

- Due to lack of consistency in disease presentation and definition, epidemiologic data are not well defined. Exact incidence has been difficult to determine because of differences in case definitions and procedures used in diagnosis.
- Ranges cited for incidence of IPF: 4.6–10.7 per 100,000 (2)
- According to the National Heart, Lung, and Blood Institute, about 50,000 new cases of IPF are diagnosed each year in the US.

Prevalence

- Exact prevalence has been difficult to determine because of differences in case definitions and procedures used in diagnosis.
- Ranges cited for prevalence of IPF: 2–29 cases per 100,000 in the general population (2)

RISK FACTORS

- Environmental or occupational exposure to inorganic or organic dusts
- 66–75% of patients with ILD have a history of smoking.
- Due to diversity of diseases, age is not a reliable predictor of pathology:
  - Most patients with connective tissue disease–related pathology and inherited subtypes present between ages 20 and 40.
  - Patients with IPF are typically age 50 or older.

Genetics

- Some studies suggest that some subtypes of ILD may be associated with specific predisposing genes and environmental exposures; however, the role of genetic factors is unknown at this time.
- About 10% of IPF cases are inherited (3).

GENERAL PREVENTION

Avoiding environmental/occupational exposure to organic or inorganic dust and smoking cessation may reduce incidence or improve clinical course in patients with established ILD.

PATHOPHYSIOLOGY

- Alveolar inflammation may progress into irreversible fibrosis.
- Varying degrees of ventilatory dysfunction occur among the ILD subtypes.
- ILD associated with collagen vascular disease and systemic connective disorders can manifest involvement of skin, joints, muscular, and ocular systems.

ETIOLOGY

Some types of ILD are associated with specific exposures:

- Medications (amiodarone, antibiotics [especially nitrofurantoin], chemotherapy agents, gold, illicit drugs)
- Inorganic dusts (silicates, asbestos, talc, mica, coal dust, graphite)
- Organic dusts (moldy hay, inhalation of fungi, bacteria, animal proteins)
- Metals (tin, aluminum, cobalt, iron, barium)
- Gases, fumes, vapors, aerosols

COMMONLY ASSOCIATED CONDITIONS

Many systemic disorders and primary diseases are associated with ILD. A partial list includes:

- Collagen vascular disease
- Sarcoidosis
- Amyloidosis
- Goodpasture syndrome
- Churg-Strauss syndrome
- Wegener granulomatosis

DIAGNOSIS

- Diagnosis should be based on clinical, radiologic, and histologic data.
- A multidisciplinary consensus is recommended for diagnosis, since even among experts, diagnostic criteria are subject to interpretation.
- The diagnosis of IPF requires exclusion of other known ILD causes, the presence of a UIP pattern on high-resolution computed tomography (HRCT), and/or surgical lung biopsy pattern (2).

HISTORY

- Symptoms may include progressive exertional dyspnea and nonproductive cough.
- Patients may also present with hemoptysis (due to idiopathic alveolar hemosiderosis) or fatigue.
- Obtaining a history of illness duration (acute vs. chronic), potential environmental/occupational exposures, travel, and medical conditions (including systemic diseases) is important in assessing the cause of the ILD.
- Some cases of lung disease may occur weeks to years after discontinuation of an offending agent.

PHYSICAL EXAM

Physical findings are usually nonspecific. Some common features include:

- Rales
- Inspiratory "squeaks"
- Clubbing of the digits
- Cyanosis in advanced disease

DIAGNOSTIC TESTS & INTERPRETATION

Lab

Initial lab tests

- Arterial blood gas (ABG)
- If a systemic disorder is suspected, consider obtaining an antinuclear antibody (ANA), rheumatoid factor (RF), ESR, and antineutrophil cytoplasmic antibodies (ANCA).

Follow-Up & Special Considerations

If indicated, hypersensitivity pneumonitis panel, plasma ACE concentration (sarcoidosis)

Imaging

Patients may also present initially with an abnormal chest x-ray (CXR) as compared with previous imaging.

Initial approach

CXR

Follow-Up & Special Considerations

HRCT of the chest is the most useful tool for distinguishing among ILD subclasses, especially in those patients with normal CXRs.

Diagnostic Procedures/Surgery

- Pulmonary function testing (PFT; spirometry, lung volumes, carbon monoxide diffusing capacity):
  - Commonly demonstrates a restrictive defect (decreased vital capacity and total lung capacity)
- Bronchoscopy:
  - Bronchoalveolar lavage (BAL) cellular analysis studies may be useful in distinguishing some subtypes (including sarcoidosis, hypersensitivity pneumonitis, cancer), but its role in diagnosis, prognostication, and assessment of disease progression is not clear (4).
  - Bronchoscopic transbronchial lung biopsy may help diagnose sarcoidosis and, on occasion, is sufficiently supportive of other ILD diagnoses.
- Thoracoscopic surgery for lung biopsy has the greatest diagnostic specificity for ILDs, but is less frequently used given improved specificity of HRCT. It may be indicated if a specific diagnosis cannot be determined from transbronchial biopsy, HRCT, etc., or if deemed necessary prior to further treatment.

Pathological Findings
- The diagnostic classifications of IIPs are based on histopathologic patterns seen on lung biopsy.
- The major histologies include an inflammation and fibrotic and granulomatous patterns.
- Characteristic changes on HRCT may help to distinguish between subtypes:
  - Reticulonodular, ground-glass opacities, and, in later stages, honeycombing may be seen.
  - Associated hilar and mediastinal adenopathy are characteristic of stage I and II sarcoidosis.
- No specific test is the "gold standard," which emphasizes the importance of a multidisciplinary consensus for diagnosis with clinical, radiologic, and pathologic findings.

DIFFERENTIAL DIAGNOSIS
- Acute pulmonary edema
- Diffuse hemorrhage
- Atypical pneumonia
- Diffuse bronchoalveolar cell carcinoma or lymphatic spread of tumor

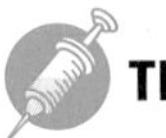

TREATMENT

- Evidence does not support the routine use of any specific therapy for ILD in general, and especially IPF (2).
- A single randomized-controlled trial did not demonstrate survival benefit of home oxygen use in ILD (5).
- There is no evidence that any pharmacologic therapies improve survival or quality of life (2,6)[B].
- Corticosteroids have a role in some ILD subtypes (7)[A].
- Current evidence does not clearly support routine use of noncorticosteroid anti-inflammatory agents for IPF, including cyclosporine, azathioprine, colchicines, cyclophosphamide, cytokines, bosentan, etanercept, methotrexate, or interferon (2,8,9).

MEDICATION
First Line
- In general, corticosteroids are most effective for certain ILDs, especially exacerbations of sarcoidosis, NSIP, BOOP, and hypersensitivity pneumonitis. However, response rates have been variable across and within subtypes. The optimal dose and duration of therapy are unknown.
- Common starting dose of prednisone is 0.5–1 mg/kg/d for 4–12 weeks, with potential up-titration to 0.5 mg/kg based on patient response.

Second Line
- Second-line agents have been used for IPF alone or in combination with steroids, with limited success rates:
  - Azathioprine was studied at 2–3 mg/kg/d (not to exceed 200 mg/d; adjusted to the nearest 25-mg dose increment) in combination with prednisone and ultimately as a steroid-sparing agent.
  - Cyclosporine has been studied in a limited number of patients.
  - The addition of acetylcysteine (1,800 mg/d for 12 months) to therapy with azathioprine and prednisone in IPF was studied in a double-blind, placebo-controlled trial. Improvements in vital capacity and carbon monoxide diffusing capacity were noted in the acetylcysteine-treated patients.
  - Pirfenidone, an orally active antifibroblast agent, decreased the rate of decline in vital capacity in 1 study in 275 patients with IPF (10). In 2011, it was approved for use in Europe, but has not yet been approved in the US. The FDA has requested more information.
- Several second-line agents have been used in Wegener granulomatosis:
  - Cyclophosphamide is commonly used in treatment of Wegener granulomatosis. It is given 1.5–2 mg/kg/d PO for 3–6 months.
  - Methotrexate has been used in treatment of mild Wegener granulomatosis in combination with corticosteroids. A studied dosing regimen consisted of an initial methotrexate dose of 0.3 mg/kg (maximum dose of 15 mg) once weekly, with 2.5 mg titration each week (maximum dose of 25 mg/wk).
  - Other second-line agents that have been studied include mycophenolate mofetil and rituximab.

ADDITIONAL TREATMENT
General Measures
- Avoid/minimize offending environmental/occupational exposures.
- Smoking cessation
- Discontinue culprit medications.
- Supplemental oxygen, if indicated

Issues for Referral
Patients benefit from ongoing care by a pulmonary specialist.

SURGERY/OTHER PROCEDURES
Single- or double-lung transplantation may be a treatment of last resort in some patients. However, some ILDs associated with systemic disease may recur in the recipient lung.

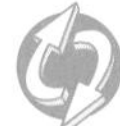

ONGOING CARE

FOLLOW-UP RECOMMENDATIONS
Follow-up testing should include PFTs, cardiopulmonary stress test, pulse oximetry, and CXR.

Patient Monitoring
Patients must be carefully monitored for objective response to treatments and adverse effects.

PATIENT EDUCATION
- Wide degree of prognostic variation occurs among ILD subtypes.
- National Heart, Lung, and Blood Institute at http://www.nhlbi.nih.gov/health/dci/Diseases/ipf/ipf_whatis. html

PROGNOSIS
Overall prognosis is varied among subtypes. IPF confers the worst prognosis (50–80% mortality in 5 years). Some entities, including hypersensitivity pneumonitis, nonspecific interstitial pneumonia, and cryptogenic organizing pneumonia, have a good prognosis.

COMPLICATIONS
- Cor pulmonale
- Pneumothorax
- Progressive respiratory failure

REFERENCES

1. Das S, Langston C, Fan LL. Interstitial lung disease in children. *Curr Opin Pediatr*. 2011;23:325–31.
2. Raghu G, Collard HR, Egan JJ, et al. An official ATS/ERS/JRS/ALAT statement: Idiopathic pulmonary fibrosis: Evidence-based guidelines for diagnosis and management. *Am J Respir Crit Care Med*. 2011;183:788–824.
3. Markart P, Wygrecka M, Guenther A, et al. Update in diffuse parenchymal lung disease 2010. *Am J Respir Crit Care Med*. 2011;183:1316–21.
4. Reynolds HY, et al. Present status of bronchoalveolar lavage in interstitial lung disease. *Curr Opin Pulm Med*. 2009;15:479–85.
5. Crockett AJ, Cranston JM, Antic N, et al. Domiciliary oxygen for interstitial lung disease. *Cochrane Database Syst Rev*. 2001;CD002883.
6. King TE. Clinical advances in the diagnosis and therapy of the interstitial lung diseases. *Am J Respir Crit Care Med*. 2005;172:268–79.
7. Richeldi L, Davies HR, Ferrara G, et al. Corticosteroids for idiopathic pulmonary fibrosis. *Cochrane Database Syst Rev*. 2003;CD002880.
8. Spagnolo P, Del Giovane C, Luppi F, et al. Non-steroid agents for idiopathic pulmonary fibrosis. *Cochrane Database Syst Rev*. 2010; CD003134.
9. Davies HR, et al. Immunomodulatory agents for idiopathic pulmonary fibrosis. *Cochrane Database Syst Rev*. 2006;(3).
10. Taniguchi H, Ebina M, Kondoh Y, et al. Pirfenidone in idiopathic pulmonary fibrosis. *Eur Respir J*. 2010;35:821–9.

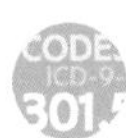

CODES

ICD9
- 515 Postinflammatory pulmonary fibrosis
- 516.30 Idiopathic interstitial pneumonia, not otherwise specified
- 516.31 Idiopathic pulmonary fibrosis

CLINICAL PEARLS

- ILD differs from COPD; anatomically, ILD involves the lung parenchyma (i.e., alveoli) and COPD involves both airways and alveoli.
- In some cases, for ILD due to organic or inorganic dust or drug-related ILD, avoiding or minimizing offending environmental/occupational exposures, medications, and smoking may alter the severity of disease, but other general preventative measures are not known at this time.
- A wide degree of prognostic variation occurs among different subtypes of ILD. For example, death is rare with cryptogenic organizing pneumonia, but acute interstitial pneumonia has 60% mortality in <6 months.

DIGITALIS TOXICITY

Ziad Alnabki, MD
Arka Chatterjee, MD
Frederick C. Weitendorf, RPH, RN

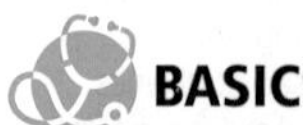

BASICS

DESCRIPTION

- A life-threatening condition resulting from intoxication by digitalis (digoxin) when used for chronic therapy, from accidental or intentional overdose, or from ingestion of naturally occurring compounds containing cardiac glycosides (e.g., foxglove, oleander)
- Can be acute or chronic
- System(s) affected: Cardiovascular; Gastrointestinal; Ocular; Central Nervous System

EPIDEMIOLOGY

Incidence

About 1.1% of outpatients on digitalis glycosides per year develop toxicity, with as many as 10–20% of nursing home residents annually experiencing some degree of digoxin-related toxicity.

Prevalence

- In 2009, the American Association of Poison Control Centers' National Poison Data System reported 2,550 cases of cardiac glycoside overdose, including 651 cases of plant cardiac glycoside exposure (1).
- Digitalis toxicity is the fourth most common adverse drug reaction in hospitals.

RISK FACTORS

- Advanced age
- Renal failure
- Hypoxemia
- Electrolyte disturbances:
  - Hypokalemia
  - Hypomagnesemia
  - Hypernatremia
  - Hypercalcemia
- Acid–base disturbances
- Decompensating congestive heart failure
- Myocardial infarction
- Myocarditis
- Recent cardiac surgery
- Hypothyroidism
- Cor pulmonale

GENERAL PREVENTION

- Use caution when prescribing digitalis if the patient is taking medications that interfere with digoxin metabolism or clearance.
- Adjust dosing when there are circumstances that increase total body levels of the drug (e.g., acute or chronic renal failure), increase cardiac sensitivity (e.g., ischemia, myocarditis), or increase bioavailability by altering gut flora (e.g., macrolides).
- Prescribe lower doses of digoxin (0.125 mg/d instead of 0.25 mg/d) (2). Digoxin is effective in heart failure at much lower levels than necessary for rate control in atrial fibrillation.

PATHOPHYSIOLOGY

- Digitalis inhibits Na^+-K^+-ATPase in myocytes, resulting in an increase in intracellular sodium and a decrease in the transmembrane sodium gradient.
- The loss of the sodium gradient decreases the drive of the Na^+-Ca^{2+} transporter, leading to increased intracellular calcium and thus increased inotropy.
- At high/toxic digoxin concentrations, elevated intracellular calcium generates small depolarizations, and the additive effects of these depolarizations produce dysrhythmias.
- Digitalis also acts on the parasympathetic system resulting in increased vagal tone and slowing atrioventricular (AV) node conduction.
- The combination of these effects can cause tachyarrhythmias and conduction block, which can present simultaneously.

ETIOLOGY

- Chronic therapy
- Intentional overdose (suicide attempt)
- Accidental overdose (children)
- Prescription/administration error
- Electrolyte disturbances—predominantly potassium balance
- Renal failure or any condition that decreases clearance of the drug
- Poisoning with plants containing cardiac glycosides (e.g., oleander, foxglove, lily of the valley)
- Concurrent use of medications:
  - Antibiotics: Rifampin, tetracycline, macrolides
  - SSRIs
  - Calcium channel blockers: Diltiazem, verapamil
  - Antiarrhythmics: Quinidine, amiodarone
  - Diuretics: Spironolactone
  - β-blockers

COMMONLY ASSOCIATED CONDITIONS

- Renal failure
- Congestive heart failure
- Dehydration
- Syncope

DIAGNOSIS

HISTORY

- For patients at risk for toxicity from chronic use, ask about new medications or new or worsened cardiac or renal disease.
- For suspected accidental overdose in children, a careful history of childproofing and available medications should be obtained.
- As with all suspected or confirmed intentional ingestions, ask about timing of ingestions and coingestions.
- Signs and symptoms generally nonspecific:
  - Anorexia
  - Nausea
  - Vomiting
  - Diarrhea
  - Visual disturbances (e.g., yellow halos)
  - Mydriasis
  - Confusion
  - Fatigue
  - Restlessness
  - Weakness
  - Headache
  - Depression
  - Hallucinations
  - Neuralgias
  - Vertigo

DIAGNOSTIC TESTS & INTERPRETATION

Lab

Initial lab tests

- Na^+, K^+, Cl^-, $HCO3^-$, Mg^+, Ca^+, BUN, Cr, and cardiac enzyme biomarkers
- Blood glucose to look for hypoglycemia as a potential cause of altered mental status
- Serum (total) digoxin level:
  - The upper accepted therapeutic range in serum is 2.0 ng/mL, with toxicity more common above 2.5 ng/mL (2)[B].
  - Toxicity may occur with plasma digoxin levels within therapeutic range, especially in chronic overdose (3)[C].
  - Digoxin level may be falsely high if measured <6 hours after acute ingestion or last dose (2)[C].
  - Nondigoxin cardiac glycoside (e.g., foxglove, oleander) may cross-react and generate a positive/elevated level; a negative level does not rule out exposure.
- Free serum digoxin level:
  - Free levels are useful for monitoring response to therapy after digoxin-specific Fab antibody fragments are given (Fab bound to digoxin increases the total digoxin level).
- Potassium:
  - In acute toxicity, hyperkalemia can predict poor outcome/death (2)[B].
  - Hypokalemia potentiates digoxin toxicity and is more of a concern in chronic use. Concurrent diuretic use is a common precipitating factor.
  - Hypomagnesemia and hypercalcemia also predispose to digoxin toxicity.

Diagnostic Procedures/Surgery

- EKG:
  - Digoxin has been reported to cause a wide variety of rhythm disturbances, so consider the diagnosis with any sudden change in cardiac rhythm. Look for rhythms that suggest increased automaticity and/or delayed conduction (3)[C].
  - Characteristic EKG changes ("digitalis effect") can occur at therapeutic levels:
    - Prolonged PR segment
    - T-wave changes, prolonged QT interval, scooping of ST segment
  - EKG changes relatively specific for digitalis toxicity:
    - Accelerated junctional rhythm
    - Bidirectional ventricular tachycardia/premature ventricular contractions (PVC)
    - New-onset Mobitz type I AV block
    - Nonparoxysmal atrial tachycardia with variable AV block (very specific, but uncommon)
  - Other associated rhythms:
    - PVCs
    - High-degree heart block
    - Sinus bradycardia
    - Sinus bradycardia with junctional tachycardia
    - Ventricular fibrillation or tachycardia
    - Atrial flutter
  - Digoxin toxicity is less likely to cause supraventricular tachycardia, rapid atrial fibrillation, or Mobitz type II AV block

DIFFERENTIAL DIAGNOSIS

- Conduction abnormalities:
  - Sick sinus syndrome
  - AV nodal dysfunction
- Toxicity with beta blockers, calcium channel blockers, and alpha agonists (e.g., clonidine).
- Electrolyte disturbances
- Other causes of life-threatening arrhythmia

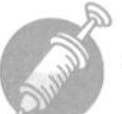

TREATMENT

MEDICATION

First Line

- Digoxin-specific Fab antibody fragments (Digibind)
- Indications:
  - Treatment of severe, life-threatening arrhythmias due to digitalis toxicity (4)[A]:
    - Sustained ventricular arrhythmias
    - Advanced AV block
    - Asystole
  - Hemodynamic instability
  - Plasma potassium concentration >5 mEq/L in the setting of acute overdose
  - Plasma digoxin concentration above 10 ng/mL (at steady state)
  - Acute ingestion of >10 mg digoxin in adults or >4 mg in children
- Dosage of Digibind:
  - If possible, obtain a total digoxin level before administration.
  - Use free levels to monitor treatment response.
  - To calculate Digibind dosage (2)[A]:
    - If serum digoxin level unknown: No. of vials = Total body load/0.5
    - Total body load = Dose ingested (mg)/ Bioavailability (digoxin 0.8, digitoxin 1)
    - If serum digoxin level known: No. of vials = [(Serum digoxin concentration in ng/mL) (patient's weight in kg)/100]
  - Unknown acute ingestion or drug level:
    - Empiric dose is 10 vials (5)[C].
  - Dosing for children is the same as for adults.
  - Slow administration increases the efficiency and elimination of digoxin (6)[C].
  - Onset of action for reversal of digoxin toxicity is rapid (minutes) (2)[C].
- Adverse reactions:
  - Hypokalemia: Monitor potassium carefully, since rapid development of hypokalemia can occur after Digibind therapy (2)[A].
  - Exacerbation of heart failure, increased ventricular response in atrial fibrillation, and hypersensitivity reactions can occur (2)[A].

Second Line

- Activated charcoal (2)[C]:
  - Consider in acute or overdose settings.
  - Increases GI elimination and systemic clearance
- Magnesium: 2 g IV initially, consider maintenance infusion (4)[C]
- Temporary pacing if no Digibind available (4)[C]
- Hemodialysis can be used to treat hyperkalemia, but is not effective for reversal of toxicity because of the extensive tissue distribution of digoxin (2)[C].

ADDITIONAL TREATMENT

General Measures

- Discontinue digoxin and other medications that interact with digoxin or exacerbate dysrhythmias.
- Correct electrolyte abnormalities and monitor potassium levels:
  - Maintain potassium in high–normal range.
  - Treat hyperkalemia; however, monitor for hypokalemia.
  - Do not use calcium salts, which can worsen ventricular arrhythmias by further increasing intracellular calcium (3)[C].
- For chronic toxicity, treat the underlying cause.

IN-PATIENT CONSIDERATIONS

Initial Stabilization

- Manage airway
- IV access/fluid resuscitation
- Supplemental oxygen
- Atropine for symptomatic bradycardia (2)[C]
- Temporary cutaneous pacing (2)[C]
- Hemodynamically unstable patients should receive Digibind as soon as possible (4)[A].

Admission Criteria

All patients with suspected digoxin toxicity who have cardiac dysrhythmias, toxic digoxin levels, or hyperkalemia should be admitted for continuous cardiac monitoring.

IV Fluids

Administration of appropriate IV fluids depends on underlying etiology for toxicity (e.g., decompensated congestive heart failure vs. acute renal failure secondary to dehydration).

Discharge Criteria

Patients should remain in the hospital until the signs and symptoms have resolved and the serum digoxin level ≤2 ng/mL.

ONGOING CARE

FOLLOW-UP RECOMMENDATIONS

- Psychiatric referral is indicated for all intentional overdoses.
- In chronic toxicity, close follow-up by a primary care physician or cardiologist is recommended if digoxin therapy is continued after discharge.

Patient Monitoring

- Digoxin levels should be monitored in acute toxicity. However, Digibind administration can interfere with the assay and give unreliable results.
- Electrolytes, especially potassium, should be carefully monitored.
- Medications that may have precipitated or contributed to digoxin intoxication should be discontinued and restarted when clinical symptoms have resolved.
- EKG and cardiac monitoring should continue until resolution of dysrhythmias.

PROGNOSIS

Moderate/major morbidity or death has been reported from 20–25% of exposures treated in hospitals (7).

REFERENCES

1. Bronstein AC, Spyker DA, Cantilena LR Jr, et al. 2008 Annual Report of the American Association of Poison Control Centers' National Poison Data System (NPDS): 26th *Annual Report*. 2009;47(10): 911–1084.
2. Bauman JL, Didomenico RJ, Galanter WL. Mechanisms manifestations, and management of digoxin toxicity in the modern era. *Am J Cardiovasc Drugs*. 2006;6:77–86.
3. Hauptman PJ, Kelly RA. Digitalis. *Circulation*. 1999;99:1265–70.
4. ACC/AHA/ESC 2006 guidelines for management of patients with ventricular arrhythmias and the prevention of sudden cardiac death-executive summary: A report of the American College of Cardiology/American Heart Association Task Force and the European Society of Cardiology Committee for Practice Guidelines. *Circulation*. 2006;114: 1088–132.
5. Brubacher JR, Heller MB, Ravikumar PR, et al. Treatment of toad venom poisoning with digoxin-specific Fab fragments. *Chest*. 1996;110: 1282–8.
6. Lapostolle F, Borron S, Verdier C, et al. Digoxin-specific Fab fragments as single first-line therapy in digitalis poisoning. *Crit Care Med*. 2008;36(11):3014–8.
7. Lapostolle F, Borron SW, Verdier C, et al. Assessment of digoxin antibody use in patients with elevated serum digoxin following chronic or acute exposure. *Intensive Care Med*. 2008;34: 1448–53.

ADDITIONAL READING

- Rajapakse S. Management of yellow oleander poisoning. *Clin Toxicol*. 2009;47(3):206–12.
- Roberts DM, Buckley N. Antidotes for acute cardenolide (cardiac glycoside) poisoning (Review). *Cochrane Database Syst Rev*. 2006;4.

CODES

ICD9

972.1 Poisoning by cardiotonic glycosides and drugs of similar action

CLINICAL PEARLS

- The onset of vague symptoms accompanied by dysrhythmia should raise suspicion of toxicity by digitalis or other cardiac glycosides (e.g., foxglove, oleander).
- Toxicity may develop even when digoxin serum levels are within normal therapeutic range.
- Digoxin-specific Fab antibody fragments are the treatment of choice for severe, life-threatening arrhythmias due to digitalis toxicity.

DIPHTHERIA

Richard Kent Zimmerman, MD, MPH

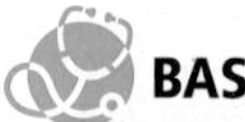

BASICS

DESCRIPTION

- Acute respiratory tract infection caused by *Corynebacterium diphtheriae*, usually producing a membranous pharyngitis
- Incubation period 2–5 days typically (range 1–10)
- Infection usually occurs during fall and winter in temperate regions.
  - In the tropics, seasonal trends are less distinct.
- Transmission by respiratory route from infected person or carrier.
  - Humans are the only reservoir.
  - Rarely directly from skin lesions or contaminated fomites.
- Several forms occur:
  - Membranous pharyngotonsillar diphtheria: The membrane is gray, adheres to the pharynx, and is surrounded by erythema. The underlying mucosa bleeds when the membrane is removed.
  - Nasal diphtheria: Unilateral discharge
  - Obstructive laryngotracheitis: Complication when membrane descends into larynx or bronchial tree. When it breaks up in young children, total obstruction of the airway may occur.
  - Cutaneous diphtheria: Punched-out ulcer covered by gray membrane (particularly in tropics and among homeless). Peaks August–October in southern US.
- System(s) affected: Cardiovascular; Nervous; Skin/Exocrine; Respiratory

EPIDEMIOLOGY

- Predominant age: Children <15 years old and poorly immunized adults
- Predominant sex: Male = Female

Incidence

In the US: For noncutaneous form, 1.6 in 100 million:

- Diphtheria is a rare condition in the US today.
- Fairly recent outbreaks have occurred in the independent states of the former Soviet Union.

RISK FACTORS

- Crowded living conditions
- Inadequate immunization
- Lower socioeconomic status
- Native Americans
- Alcoholism
- Travelers: Outbreaks have occurred in various countries; see CDC's travel Web site.

GENERAL PREVENTION

Prevention is by immunization:

- Children age 6 weeks up to 7 years of age should receive doses at 2, 4, 6, and 15–18 months and 4–6 years of age with 0.5 mL of DTaP vaccine IM. If the pertussis component is contraindicated, then pediatric diphtheria tetanus (DT) should be used. A booster dose of adult Tdap should be given at age 11–12 years.
- Unimmunized persons ≥7 years should receive 2 doses of adult Td 4–8 weeks apart with a third dose 6–12 months later. 0.5 mL of Td should be given. Subsequently, booster doses with Td should be given every 10 years to all individuals without a contraindication. CDC currently recommends that Tdap substitute for 1 of the recommended decennial Td boosters.
- Immunized individuals may develop diphtheria, but their course is milder; immunization protects against the toxin, not infection or microbial carriage in the nose, pharynx, or skin. Disinfect all articles in contact with patient.
- Close contacts should be cultured and given antibiotic prophylaxis, regardless of immunization status.
- Contacts should receive an age-appropriate diphtheria toxoid-containing vaccine unless given a booster within the past 5 years.
- Contacts should receive a diphtheria toxoid-containing vaccine unless vaccinated within the past 5 years.

PATHOPHYSIOLOGY

Toxigenic strains produce an exotoxin that inhibits protein synthesis in all cell types. Toxin causes local damage and results in the membrane, leading to the name, translated as "leather hide." Toxin is absorbed and disseminated hematogenously. Toxin can lead to myocarditis and neuritis.

ETIOLOGY

C. diphtheriae infection

DIAGNOSIS

- Membranous pharyngotonsillar diphtheria:
  - Initially, bluish white membrane, which is easily removed
  - Adherent, whitish gray, leathery membrane on tonsils or pharynx, which may turn gray-green or black
  - Removing membrane causes bleeding of mucosa.
  - Injected pharynx
  - Membrane may become black due to hemorrhage.
  - Sore throat
  - Cervical adenopathy with swelling
  - Malaise and prostration
  - Enlarged, tender cervical and submandibular lymph nodes
  - May progress to edematous, swollen neck (bull neck)
  - Paralysis of soft palate
  - Low-grade fever of 37.8–38.8°C (100–100.9°F)
  - Thrombocytopenia and purpura
- Nasal diphtheria:
  - Serosanguineous or seropurulent discharge and excoriations
  - Often, discharge is unilateral.
  - Often chronic, mild course
- Obstructive laryngotracheitis:
  - Hoarseness
  - Croupy cough
  - Progresses to dyspnea and stridor
  - Labored breathing
  - Thick speech
- Cutaneous diphtheria:
  - On skin, conjunctiva, vulva, vagina, and penis
  - Primary cutaneous diphtheria: Starts as tender pustule on lower extremity and becomes deep, round, punched-out ulcer covered by grayish membrane
  - Secondary infection of pre-existing wound, purulent exudate, partial membrane

HISTORY

Membranous pharyngotonsillar diphtheria:

- Sore throat
- Malaise and prostration

Nasal diphtheria:

- Often, discharge is unilateral.
- Often chronic, mild course

Obstructive laryngotracheitis:

- Hoarseness
- Cough progressing to dyspnea
- Labored breathing

Cutaneous diphtheria:

- Initially tender pustule on skin, conjunctiva, vulva, vagina, and penis

PHYSICAL EXAM

- Membranous pharyngotonsillar diphtheria:
  - Initially, bluish white membrane, which is easily removed
  - Adherent, whitish gray, leathery membrane on tonsils or pharynx which may turn gray-green or black
  - Removing membrane causes bleeding of mucosa.
  - Injected pharynx
  - Membrane may become black due to hemorrhage.
  - Cervical adenopathy with swelling
  - Enlarged, tender cervical and submandibular lymph nodes
  - May progress to edematous, swollen neck (bull neck)
  - Paralysis of soft palate
  - Low-grade fever of 37.8–38.8°C (100–100.9°F)
  - Thrombocytopenia and purpura
- Nasal diphtheria:
  - Serosanguineous or seropurulent discharge and excoriations
- Obstructive laryngotracheitis:
  - Croupy cough
  - Stridor
  - Labored breathing
  - Thick speech
- Cutaneous diphtheria:
  - On skin, conjunctiva, vulva, vagina, and penis
  - Primary cutaneous diphtheria: Starts as tender pustule on lower extremity and becomes deep, round, punched-out ulcer covered by grayish membrane
  - Secondary infection of pre-existing wound, purulent exudate, partial membrane

DIAGNOSTIC TESTS & INTERPRETATION

Lab

- Gram-positive rods in the pathognomonic Chinese character configuration
- Moderate leukocytosis
- Thrombocytopenia
- Transient albuminuria
- In experienced hands, methylene-blue stains can assist in a presumptive diagnosis.
- Culture from nose and throat beneath membrane and plate on special media; inform lab that diphtheria is suspected.
- Should test for toxigenicity of strain
- Serial ECGs and cardiac enzymes to detect myocarditis

- Delayed peripheral nerve conduction velocities
- Culture on special media (cystine-tellurite blood agar or modified Tinsdale agar) is positive in 8–12 hours if not previously treated with an antibiotic. Laboratory must be alerted to use special media.
- Toxin production confirmed by modified Elek test.
- Polymerase chain reaction
- Drugs that may alter lab results:
  - If an antibiotic was used, then ≥5 days may be required for the culture to grow on medium.

Pathological Findings

- Pleomorphic gram-positive rods
- Necrotic epithelium
- Hyaline degeneration

DIFFERENTIAL DIAGNOSIS

- Bacterial pharyngitis including group A Streptococcus
- Viral pharyngitis
- Mononucleosis
- Oral syphilis
- Candidiasis
- Vincent angina
- Acute epiglottitis

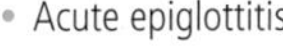
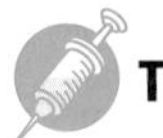

TREATMENT

MEDICATION

First Line

- Both antitoxins and antibiotics are needed for noncutaneous diphtheria.
- Diphtheria antitoxin, equine: Use 20,000–40,000 U of antitoxin for laryngeal or pharyngeal disease of <48 hours' duration; 40,000–60,000 U for nasopharyngeal lesions; 80,000–120,000 U for extensive disease ≥3 days or swelling of the neck (bull neck) (1)[B].
- Some experts recommend treating cutaneous disease with 20,000–40,000 U of antitoxin, while others doubt its value when there are no signs of systemic disease.
- Antitoxin is obtained from the CDC under Investigation New Drug protocol at 770-488-7100.
- Erythromycin parenterally or PO, 40–50 mg/kg/d; maximum of 2 g/d for 14 days (2)[B], or penicillin G IM or IV for 14 days, or penicillin G procaine IM for 14 days. For cutaneous diphtheria, 10 days of one of these antibiotics.
- Precautions:
  - Equine antitoxin: 7% of patients are sensitive to equine antitoxin and need desensitization. Always test for hypersensitivity to antitoxin prior to its administration:
    - First, a drop of 1:100 dilution of antitoxin is placed on a scratch on the forearm, read at 15–20 minutes. If negative, an intradermal skin test is done with 1:1,000 dilution (0.02 mL). A positive reaction is the development of urticaria within 20 minutes of injection.
    - If no reaction to first intradermal, then repeat test with a 1:100 dilution
    - If the person has a negative history for animal allergy, has not previously received animal serum, and had a negative scratch test, then 1:100 dilution may be used initially.

Second Line

DL-carnitine 100 mg/kg/d b.i.d. PO in children for 4 days in myocarditis is experimental.

ADDITIONAL TREATMENT

Antibiotics recommended for close contacts (oral erythromycin for 7–10 days or single IM penicillin G benzathine [600,000 U if <6 years, otherwise 1,200,000 U]). Contacts should receive an age-appropriate diphtheria toxoid-containing vaccine unless given a booster within the past 5 years. Contacts who are children <7 years and who lack their fourth dose of DTaP should be vaccinated. Antibiotics recommended for carriers.

General Measures

- Appropriate health care:
  - Inpatient, initially hospitalized in unit that can monitor cardiac and respiratory status (must act on presumptive diagnosis because therapy cannot wait for culture confirmation)
  - Droplet isolation for pharyngeal diphtheria until cultures on 2 consecutive days are negative. The first culture must be taken at least 24 hours after the cessation of antibiotic therapy.
  - Contact precautions for cutaneous diphtheria.
- Have intubation or tracheostomy readily available. For laryngeal disease, laryngoscopy is desirable. Intubation or tracheostomy should be considered early for laryngeal disease.
- Avoid hypnotics and sedatives while monitoring respiratory status.

Additional Therapies

Physical therapy in convalescence for range-of-motion exercises to prevent contractions

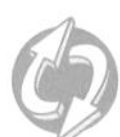

ONGOING CARE

FOLLOW-UP RECOMMENDATIONS

Rest for at least 3 weeks until risk of developing myocarditis has passed.

Patient Monitoring

- ECG, cardiac enzymes, and respiratory status. Serial ECG 2–3 times per week for 4–6 weeks to detect myocarditis
- Elimination of the organism should be documented by 2 negative cultures 24 hours apart. The first culture should be 24 hours after the completion of antimicrobial therapy.
- During convalescence, patients should be immunized against diphtheria, because infection does not necessarily confer immunity.

DIET

Liquid to soft as tolerated

PATIENT EDUCATION

Explain aspects of illness and complications.

PROGNOSIS

- <5% mortality rate unless respiratory form, for which case-fatality rate is 5–10%
- Prognosis guarded until recovery
- In convalescing patients, 5–10% persistence in nasopharynx
- Worse prognosis if myocarditis

COMPLICATIONS

- Myocarditis (10–25%) may occur early.
- Cranial and peripheral neuropathy (2–6 weeks after onset)
- ECG abnormalities in 2/3 of patients, including bundle branch block, tachycardia, atrial or ventricular fibrillation, and extrasystoles
- Right-sided heart failure
- Local paralysis of soft palate and posterior pharynx demonstrated by regurgitation of fluids through the nares
- Peripheral and cranial neuropathy affecting primarily motor nerve functions. Motor dysfunction starts proximally and extends distally. It usually resolves slowly.
- Syndrome resembling Guillain-Barré

REFERENCES

1. Hrobjartsson A, et al. The controlled clinical trial turns 100 years: Fibiger's trial of serum treatment of diphtheria. *Br Med J*. 1998;317:1243–5.
2. Kneen R, Pham NG, Solomon T, et al. Penicillin vs. erythromycin in the treatment of diphtheria. *Clin Infect Dis*. 1998;27:845–50.

ADDITIONAL READING

- American Academy of Pediatrics. Diphtheria. In Pickering LK, Baker CJ, Kimberlin DW, et al., eds. *Red Book: 2009 Report of the Committee on Infectious Diseases*, 28th ed. Elk Grove Village, IL: American Academy of Pediatrics, 2009:280–3.
- Karam AG, Cherry JD. Hypotonic and hyporesponsive episodes after diptheria-tetanus-acellular pertussis vaccination. *Pediatr Infect Dis J*. 2007;26:966–7.
- The original streptomycin trial paper: Fibiger J. Om Serumbehandling af Difteri. *Hospitalstidende*. 1898;6:309–25, 337–50.
- http://www.cdc.gov/vaccines/vpd-vac/diphtheria
- http://wwwnc.cdc.gov/travel/yellowbook/2010/chapter-2/diphtheria.aspx

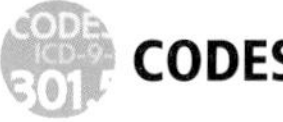

CODES

ICD9

- 032.0 Faucial diphtheria
- 032.2 Anterior nasal diphtheria
- 032.9 Diphtheria, unspecified

CLINICAL PEARLS

- Close contacts should be cultured, checked for immunization status, and considered for antimicrobial prophylaxis (penicillin or erythromycin).
- Past infection does not necessarily confer immunity.
- Alert lab if sending a culture because *C. diphtheriae* requires a special media to grow.

DISSECTION, CAROTID AND VERTEBRAL ARTERY

Deepak K. Ozhathil, MD
Andres Schanzer, MD, FACS

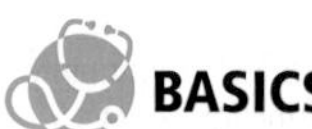

BASICS

DESCRIPTION

A cervical artery dissection occurs when a tear develops between one or more of the 3 layers of the internal carotid artery or the vertebral artery. As a result, an intramural thrombus or pseudoaneurysm is formed. Together, carotid artery dissections (CAD) and vertebral artery dissections (VAD) make up a significant portion of ischemic strokes among young and middle-aged adults.

EPIDEMIOLOGY

The incidence of cervical artery dissection in the general population is quite low (2.6 cases in 100,000 per year; 95% CI 1.9–3.3) and likely underestimated due to the unknown number of asymptomatic cases (1). However, CAD occurs more frequently than VAD.

Incidence

- CAD was first described in 1959, a case study of a spontaneous internal CAD.
- Spontaneous CADs account for 14–20% of ischemic strokes in patients younger than 50 years old and 0.6–32% of ischemic strokes in all age groups (2). In total, nearly 1/4 of ischemic strokes affecting young adult patients can be attributed to CAD.
- CAD occurs 1.7 times in 100,000 people per year (95% CI 0.5–1.4) (1)
- VAD occurs 1.0 times in 100,000 people per year (95% CI 1.1–2.3) (1)
- CAD and VAD occur simultaneously in 13–16% of cases
- Peak incidence occurs in the fifth decade of life, with women being affected on average 5 years earlier than men.

Prevalence

- Although cross-sectional North American studies have not shown any gender-predominance (50–52% female), their European counterparts have demonstrated a male predominance (53–57% male).
- Seasonal patterns suggest higher rates of occurrence during the autumn and winter months, which may correlate with the incidence of weather-related confounding variables like infection rates and seasonal sports (3).

RISK FACTORS

- Recent studies have proposed a number of potential risk factors, including infection, hyperhomocysteinanemia, low folate levels, oral contraceptives, migraines, and arterial hypertension, as potential predisposing risk factors. However, the literature on this topic is composed of isolated case studies and single-institution trials limited by small sample size, selection bias, and confounding variables.

Genetics

- Concomitant occurrence with genetic disorders like Ehlers-Danlos type IV (most common), Marfan syndrome, osteogenesis imperfecta type I, syphilis, autosomal-dominant polycystic kidney disease, α1-antitrypsin deficiency, hereditary hemochromatosis, Turner syndrome, and Williams syndrome have all been published in case reports. The rarity of these genetic conditions, however, makes it difficult to evaluate the clinical significance of their associations:
  - About 20% of CAD and 25% of VAD are considered to be associated with a connective tissue disorder (4).
- Polymorphisms: ICAM-1 (intracellular adhesion molecule-1) and MTHFR (methylene-tetrahydrofolate reductase) have been implicated as well, but studies are underpowered (4).

GENERAL PREVENTION

No specific prevention measures are known.

PATHOPHYSIOLOGY

- Dissection can occur as a result of intimal tearing caused by traumatic shearing forces. Expansion of the intramural hematoma that develops eventually results in the stenosis of the vascular lumen.
- Dissection can also occur through intramural bleeding directly from the rupture of penetrating vasa vasorum vessels. In this case, adventitial expansion results in an aneurysmal dilation of the injured artery.
- Extracranial arterial segments are more vulnerable than their intracranial counterparts. This is a result of neck mobility exceeding vascular elasticity:
  - The internal carotid artery is tethered at the carotid canal, its entry point into the skull.
  - The vertebral artery is at risk as it tortuously passes through the transverse foramina of C2 to C1.
- Embolism of intraluminal thrombi at the site of intimal tearing make up 92% of the ischemic strokes following cervical artery dissection. Other mechanisms of CNS hypoperfusion include stenosis, occlusion, and pseudoaneurysmal rupture.
- Subarachnoid hemorrhages can occur when arterial dissections extend beyond the base of the skull. This is because intracranial arterial walls are thinner and less elastic than their cervical counterparts.

ETIOLOGY

- Roughly classified as traumatic and spontaneous mechanisms:
  - Traumatic: Significant penetrating or blunt trauma. Occurs in 1–2% of trauma patients, especially those who have endured skull fractures. CAD in particular is associated with major thoracic injuries, whereas VAD occurs more often with cervical spine fractures.
  - Spontaneous: Unprovoked lesions associated with a wide variety of physical activities, otherwise presumed to be benign, involving sudden or sustained neck hyperextensions or rotations including coughing, sneezing, vomiting, swimming, chiropractic manipulation, and yoga.

COMMONLY ASSOCIATED CONDITIONS

- Retinal ischemia and ischemic optic neuropathy (CAD)
- Spinal cord ischemia and cervical radiculopathies (VAD)
- Horner syndrome (CAD more often than VAD)

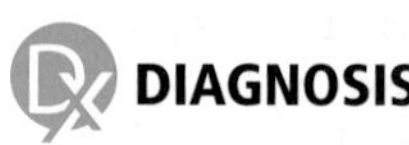

DIAGNOSIS

HISTORY

- Symptoms preceding cerebral ischemia:
  - Headaches: The most common finding. Gradual to sudden onset that precedes ischemic symptoms by minutes to days.
    - CAD: Ipsilateral and frontotemporal discomfort with stereotypic headache features.
    - VAD: Occipital and posterior location, and more challenging to identify.
  - Neck pain: More common in VAD (46%) than CAD (26%)
  - Horner syndrome (oculosympathetic palsy): Presents as ipsilateral miosis and ptosis without anhidrosis (the sympathetic innervation of facial sweat glands is located on the external carotid artery). More common in CAD (28–58%) than VAD (27%).
  - Cranial nerve palsy: Relatively rare (7% incidence) and most commonly affects the hypoglossal nerve (12%), presenting as taste impairment and pulsatile tinnitus, followed by the glossopharyngeal and the vagus nerves.
  - Transient monocular blindness may also precede an ischemic stroke.
- Manifestations of cerebral transient ischemic attacks: Occur in 67% of cervical artery dissections and can vary in onset from minutes to up to a month before the stroke itself (1). 20% of patients have no warning signs prior to their strokes.

PHYSICAL EXAM

- Horner syndrome: Ptosis and miosis without anhidrosis; innervation to the sweat glands is from the sympathetic plexus around the external carotid artery.
- Cerebral ischemia:
  - CAD: Most commonly affects the middle cerebral artery perfusion territory, which includes most of the outer cortex of the brain, the basal ganglia, and the posterior and anterior internal capsules. Therefore, sequelae of an ischemic injury include a wide range of motor and/or sensory deficits.
  - VAD: Typically affects the brain stem, cerebellum, and occipital lobes, resulting in a range of medullary syndromes, ataxias, and visual impairments.

DIAGNOSTIC TESTS & INTERPRETATION

Lab

No specific labs

Imaging

Imaging is crucial in the diagnosis and monitoring of CADs. Angiographic images facilitate high-resolution visualization of intramural and intraluminal hematoma development.

Initial approach

- CT angiography is the test of choice ("string and pearl sign"), though digital subtraction arteriography is the gold standard.
- CT angiography is a noninvasive method using contrast and providing useful information about the arterial lumen and the vessel wall, with a sensitivity approaching 100% and specificity approaching 96–98% when compared with conventional angiography (4).
- Conventional angiography is no longer recommended because of the associated risks of a more invasive procedure and poor visualization of intramural lesions.
- MRI/MRA is rapidly replacing CT angiography in many centers as the image quality continues to improve. Benefits include no radiation exposure, renoprotective doses of contrast, better intramural visualization, and T1-weighted fat-suppression techniques detect smaller lesions (5).

Diagnostic Procedures/Surgery

Color duplex ultrasound is noninvasive and has a sensitivity of 96%, specificity of 94% for patients with CAD who have symptoms of carotid territory ischemia. However, it is highly operator-dependent, and findings always require confirmation by CT angiography or MRI/MRA.

DIFFERENTIAL DIAGNOSIS

- Migraine, cluster, or tension headaches
- Neck trauma and cervical spine fracture
- Ischemic stroke, hemorrhagic stroke
- Retinal artery or vein occlusion

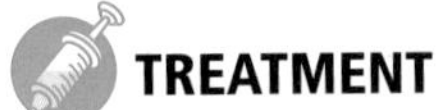

TREATMENT

MEDICATION

- Anticoagulation therapy, short-acting (acute phase)
- Antiplatelet therapy (acute phase)
- Anticoagulation therapy, long-acting (subacute phase)
- Antiplatelet therapy (chronic phase)

First Line

- Anticoagulation or antiplatelet therapy should be initiated in the acute phase of a CAD to reduce the incidence of primary or recurrent ischemic stroke. Despite being standard practice, a randomized control trial comparing the efficacy of each treatment modality is not yet available (6)[A].
- Anticoagulation is sometimes preferred over antiplatelet therapy when there is a severe stenosis, or there is evidence of a free-floating thrombus or a cerebral embolism.
- Antiplatelet therapy is favored when a large infarction or hemorrhage has occurred. In addition, antiplatelet therapy should be used when the dissection affects the intracranial portion of the vessels, which significantly increases the risk of subarachnoid hemorrhage.
- Patients who undergo antiplatelet therapy have a 1.8–3.8% risk of stroke, while anticoagulation has a 1.2% risk of stroke and a 0.5% risk of intracranial hemorrhage.
- Despite expressed concerns, available data show that IV thrombolysis (tPA) should not be withheld in cases where CAD is associated with acute ischemic stroke (6)[A].

Second Line

See "Surgery/Other Procedures."

SURGERY/OTHER PROCEDURES

- Surgical therapies include thrombectomy, vessel ligation, primary dissection, and repair. However, surgical interventions are often technically challenging and more risky than endovascular techniques.
- Endovascular therapy includes stenting, coiling, stent-assisted coiling, and embolization and occlusion of the vascular lesion along with the parent vessel:
  - Endovascular therapy is recommended in patients who fail medical therapy after 6 months of anticoagulation therapy or for whom anticoagulation is contraindicated.
  - Failure of medical therapy is defined as a new ischemic event, worsening neurological findings, or enlargement of the pseudoaneurysm.
  - Data on endovascular interventions are limited and lacking homogeneity between surgical technique and equipment types; however, overall outcomes analysis suggests impressive results (98.4% technical success with only a 1.3% complication rate) (7).

ONGOING CARE

FOLLOW-UP RECOMMENDATIONS

- Follow-up with a neurologist is highly recommended.
- After initiating a short course of anticoagulation or antiplatelet therapy, patients should be bridged to Warfarin for 3 months.
- Repeat imaging is useful to guide further treatment decisions. Another 3 months of Warfarin therapy may be considered if persistent stenosis is detected.
- Anticoagulants usually maintained for no longer than 6 months. Following this period, anticoagulation is either stopped or substituted by antiplatelet therapy, which can be continued for 2 years.

Patient Monitoring

Closer follow-up for an extended period of time is recommended in patients with underlying connective tissue disorders, as they are at a higher risk of recurrence.

PROGNOSIS

- Highest risk of death occurs during the acute phase (<5%); however, among patient subgroups symptomatic for ischemic stroke, risk of mortality can rises to 23%.
- Recurrence rates for ischemic events within the first year varied from 0% to 13.3%; however, most occurred in the initial weeks after dissection.
- Overall good long-term prognosis with low rates of recurrence and complications and high rates of favorable outcome (4)

REFERENCES

1. Lee VH, Brown RD, Mandrekar JN, et al. Incidence and outcome of cervical artery dissection: A population-based study. *Neurology*. 2006; 67:1809–12.
2. Chandra A, Suliman A, Angle N, et al. Spontaneous dissection of the carotid and vertebral arteries: The 10-year UCSD experience. *Ann Vasc Surg*. 2007; 21:178–85.
3. Paciaroni M, Georgiadis D, Arnold M, et al. Seasonal variability in spontaneous cervical artery dissection. *J Neurol Neurosurg Psychiatr*. 2006;77: 677–9.
4. Kim YK, Schulman S, et al. Cervical artery dissection: Pathology, epidemiology and management. *Thromb. Res*. 2009;123:810–21.
5. Provenzale JM, et al. MRI and MRA for evaluation of dissection of craniocerebral arteries: Lessons from the medical literature. *Emerg Radiol*. 2009;16: 185–93.
6. Menon R, Kerry S, Norris JW, et al. Treatment of cervical artery dissection: A systematic review and meta-analysis. *J Neurol Neurosurg Psychiatr*. 2008;79:1122–7.
7. Pham MH, Rahme RJ, Arnaout O, et al. Endovascular stenting of extracranial carotid and vertebral artery dissections: A systematic review of the literature. *Neurosurgery*. 2011;68:856–66; discussion 866.

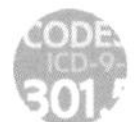

CODES

ICD9

- 443.21 Dissection of carotid artery
- 443.24 Dissection of vertebral artery

CLINICAL PEARLS

- CAD and VAD are common causes of ischemic stroke in young and middle-aged adults.
- Neck pain, headache, and/or Horner syndrome followed by manifestations of cerebral ischemia should prompt evaluation for CAD.
- The mechanism of cerebral ischemia is, in the vast majority of cases, embolic and less commonly thrombotic or hemorrhagic.
- CT angiography is the test of choice ("string and pearl sign").
- Anticoagulation and/or antiplatelet therapy are the mainstays of treatment. Patients refractory to conservative treatment after 6 months should be re-evaluated for invasive interventions including angioplasty, stenting, surgical ligation, or primary vascular repair.

DISSEMINATED INTRAVASCULAR COAGULATION (DIC)

Jan Cerny, MD, PhD
Eva Medvedova, MD

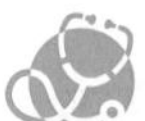

BASICS

DESCRIPTION

- Acquired syndrome characterized by diffuse activation of intravascular coagulation. It can originate from and cause damage to the microvasculature, which, if sufficiently severe, can produce organ dysfunction.
- Occurs as a complication of pregnancy (e.g., abruptio placentae, fetus retention, amniotic fluid embolism), infection (especially gram-negative), malignancy (uncontrolled, metastatic tumor or leukemia), trauma, and other severe illnesses
- System(s) affected: Hematologic/Lymphatic/Immunologic
- Synonym(s): Consumptive coagulopathy; DIC

EPIDEMIOLOGY

Incidence

Unknown

Prevalence

- Predominant age: None
- Predominant sex: Male = Female

RISK FACTORS

See "Etiology."

GENERAL PREVENTION

Aggressive interventions aimed at early treatment of the underlying clinical conditions

PATHOPHYSIOLOGY

- Systemic formation of fibrin is the result of the simultaneous coexistence of:
  - Increased thrombin generation via tissue factor/factor VII mediated pathway
  - Suppression of the physiologic anticoagulant pathways:
    - Antithrombin due to consumption, degradation, and impaired synthesis
    - Proteins C and S due to decreased levels of thrombomodulin
  - Impaired fibrinolysis (early on):
    - Sustained increase in plasminogen activator inhibitor, type 1
- Increased fibrinolysis (late during the process) leads to bleeding.

ETIOLOGY

Causes can be classified as acute or chronic, systemic or localized:

- Sepsis/severe infection (any microorganism)
- Trauma (polytrauma, neurotrauma)
- Obstetric complications (amniotic fluid embolism, abruptio placentae)
- Solid tumors and leukemias (especially acute promyelocytic leukemia)
- Vascular disorders, such as Kasabach-Merritt syndrome, large vascular aneurysms, and thrombosis
- Organ destruction (severe pancreatitis, severe liver failure)
- Severe toxic or immunologic reactions:
  - Snake bite
  - Recreational drugs
  - Transfusion reactions
  - Transplant rejection
  - Thermal injury
- Infant and adult respiratory distress syndrome
- Neonatal purpura fulminans

COMMONLY ASSOCIATED CONDITIONS

Thromboembolic phenomena are associated with venous thrombosis, thrombotic vegetations on the aortic heart valve, arterial emboli, and neonatal purpura fulminans (homozygous protein C or protein S deficiency).

Pediatric Considerations

Neonatal purpura fulminans is associated with DIC and protein C or protein S deficiency (homozygous).

DIAGNOSIS

Symptoms and signs are related to the underlying disease process and disseminated intravascular coagulation.

HISTORY

Symptoms of microvascular thrombosis (e.g., renal failure), as well as diffuse bleeding

PHYSICAL EXAM

- Bleeding manifestations:
  - Skin (petechiae, purpura, ecchymosis, generalized oozing from venipuncture sites and wounds)
  - Renal (hematuria)
  - GI (mucous membranes and intestinal bleeding)
  - Neurologic (hemorrhagic infarction, massive intracerebral bleeding)
  - Respiratory (epistaxis, pulmonary hemorrhage)
- Microvascular thrombosis:
  - Skin (skin infarction, digital gangrene)
  - GI (mucosal ulcerations, bowel infarction)
  - Renal (oliguria, anuria, uremia)
  - Pulmonary (hypoxemia, acute respiratory distress syndrome)
  - Neurologic (convulsions, delirium, coma, multifocal cortical infarction)

DIAGNOSTIC TESTS & INTERPRETATION

No single laboratory test is sensitive and specific enough to allow a definitive diagnosis of DIC.

Lab

- Thrombocytopenia
- Increased partial thromboplastin time (PTT)
- Increased prothrombin test (PT)
- Decreased fibrinogen (serial levels)
- Increased fibrin degradation product (FDP)
- Positive D-dimer
- Decreased antithrombin III, decreased protein C
- Microangiopathic hemolytic anemia (schistocytes, increased lactate dehydrogenase levels, low hemoglobin)

Initial lab tests

Diagnostic algorithm for overt DIC (International Society on Thrombosis and Haemostasis) (1):

- Assess if underlying disease is known to be associated with DIC:
  - YES: Proceed with this algorithm.
  - NO: Do not use this algorithm.
- Order global coagulation tests (PT, PTT, fibrinogen, soluble fibrin monomers, or FDPs)
- Score global coagulation test results:
  - Platelet count ($>100 = 0$, $<100 = 1$, $<50 = 2$)
  - Elevated fibrin-related markers (no increase = 0, moderate increase = 2, strong increase = 3)
  - Prolonged PT (<3 seconds = 0, >3 but <6 seconds = 1, >6 seconds = 2)
  - Fibrinogen level (>1 g/L = 0, <1 g/L = 1)
- Calculate score:
  - If ≥ 5: Compatible with DIC, repeat scoring daily. If <5: Suggestive of nonovert DIC: Repeat in 1–2 days (2)

Follow-Up & Special Considerations
Frequent follow-up of initially abnormal laboratory tests to see effect of therapeutic interventions

DIFFERENTIAL DIAGNOSIS

- Fulminant liver failure or massive hepatic necrosis
- Vitamin K deficiency
- Thrombotic thrombocytopenic purpura
- Hemolytic–uremic syndrome
- Heparin-induced thrombocytopenia
- Primary fibrinolysis
- HELLP syndrome in pregnancy (hemolysis, elevated liver function, and low platelets)

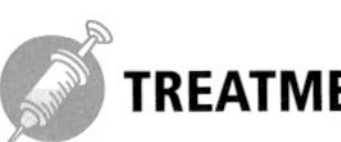

TREATMENT

Heterogeneity of the underlying disorders and the clinical presentations makes the therapeutic approach to DIC difficult:

- Appropriate health care: Inpatient and often intensive care unit (depending on underlying condition)
- Treat underlying condition (e.g., evacuation of uterus in abruptio placentae; broad-spectrum antibiotics for gram-negative sepsis)
- Supportive care with transfusions in patients who are bleeding, going for surgery, or at high risk of bleeding. Do not treat abnormal laboratory parameters:
  - Fresh frozen plasma
  - Platelet concentrates
  - Cryoprecipitate or fibrinogen concentrates (3)
- Anticoagulants remain very controversial. Deep venous thrombosis prophylaxis is recommended in patients who are not bleeding.
- Restoration of anticoagulant pathways:
  - Recombinant human-activated protein C (benefit only in carefully selected patients at high risk of death from sepsis. The drug should only be administered in an intensive care unit (ICU) when patient is monitored by trained personnel) (4)[A].
  - Activated factor VII use remains controversial.

MEDICATION

- Broad-spectrum antibiotics for sepsis
- Recombinant human-activated protein C in severe sepsis (4)

SURGERY/OTHER PROCEDURES

Surgical treatment or procedures should be considered, especially if they are treating the underlying condition (e.g., evacuation of uterus in abruptio placentae; some trauma or bleeding situations).

IN-PATIENT CONSIDERATIONS

Initial Stabilization

- Treat underlying disorder.
- Frequent monitoring of clinical and laboratory response

Admission Criteria

Usually dictated by severity of underlying condition. Some cases can be managed on a standard ward, but ICU care is typical.

Discharge Criteria

Once clinical and laboratory criteria are significantly improved and underlying reason for DIC is under control

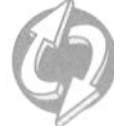

ONGOING CARE

FOLLOW-UP RECOMMENDATIONS

Patient Monitoring

- Monitor closely until much improved
- Serial platelet count, coagulation tests, and fibrinogen levels to see effect of therapeutic interventions

PROGNOSIS

- Related to the severity of cause
- Decreased antithrombin level is a poor prognostic factor in DIC.

COMPLICATIONS

- Acute renal failure
- Shock
- Cardiac tamponade
- Hemothorax
- Intracerebral hematoma
- Various thrombotic complications, including myocardial infarction, stroke, gangrene, and loss of digits

REFERENCES

1. Voves C, Wuillemin WA, Zeerleder S, et al. International Society on Thrombosis and Haemostasis score for overt disseminated intravascular coagulation predicts organ dysfunction and fatality in sepsis patients. *Blood Coagul. Fibrinolysis*. 2006;17:445–51.
2. Levi M, Toh CH, Thachil J, et al. Guidelines for the diagnosis and management of disseminated intravascular coagulation. British Committee for Standards in Haematology. *Br J Haematol*. 2009; 145:24–33.
3. Franchini M, Lippi G, Manzato F. Recent acquisitions in the pathophysiology, diagnosis and treatment of disseminated intravascular coagulation. *Thromb J*. 2006;4:4.
4. Vincent JL, Bernard GR, Beale R, et al. Drotrecogin alfa (activated) treatment in severe sepsis from the global open-label trial ENHANCE: Further evidence for survival and safety and implications for early treatment. *Crit Care Med*. 2005;33:2266–77.

ADDITIONAL READING

- Levi M. Disseminated intravascular coagulation. *Crit Care Med*. 2007;35:2191–5.
- Taylor FB, Toh CH, Hoots WK, et al. Towards definition, clinical and laboratory criteria, and a scoring system for disseminated intravascular coagulation. *Thromb Haemost*. 2001;86:1327–30.

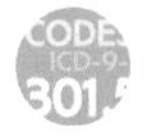

CODES

ICD9

286.6 Defibrination syndrome

CLINICAL PEARLS

- Treat underlying condition(s); transfusions represent supportive measures.
- Transfusions are not indicated in patients with abnormal laboratory parameters without clinical bleeding.

DIVERTICULAR DISEASE

Dennis M. Dimitri, MD

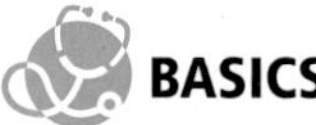

BASICS

DESCRIPTION

- Diverticular disease includes asymptomatic diverticulosis, symptomatic uncomplicated diverticulitis, symptomatic complicated diverticulitis, and diverticular bleeding
- Diverticula: Saclike protrusion of the mucosal and submucosal wall of the colon
  - Diverticulosis has a higher prevalence in societies that consume a low-fiber diet.
  - In Western societies, 90–95% of diverticulosis is left-sided, whereas Asian populations have more right-sided disease.
  - Prevalence of diverticulosis and number of diverticulae increase with age.
- Diverticular hemorrhage: Occurs in 3–5% of patients with diverticular disease:
  - Accounts for >40% of lower GI bleeds and 17–40% of cases of hematochezia in general
  - Bleeding is more common from right-sided diverticula.
- Uncomplicated diverticulitis: Typical presentation, affects 10–25% of patients with diverticulosis
- Complicated diverticulitis includes associated abscess, perforation, fistula, or stricture.
- System(s) affected: Gastrointestinal

EPIDEMIOLOGY

Incidence

- Diverticulosis is present in up to 20% general population, but increases progressively with age reaching up to 2/3 of people by the eighth decade
- Diverticulitis: 2,400–3,800/100,000
- Yearly mortality rate: 2.5/100,000

Prevalence

- 5% by age 40; 30% by age 60; 65% by age 85
- Male = Female overall, but more male <65 and more female >65 years old

RISK FACTORS

- Age >40
- Low-fiber diet
- Sedentary lifestyle, obesity
- Previous diverticulitis and number of diverticula
- NSAIDs use may increase the risk of bleeding

Genetics

No known genetic pattern

GENERAL PREVENTION

High-fiber diet (>30 g/d of fiber), or add nonabsorbable fiber (psyllium)

PATHOPHYSIOLOGY

Diverticulae form at the site of penetration of the mucosa by the vasa recta. Structural changes result in decreased resistance to intraluminal pressure. Diverticulitis occurs when perforation of the diverticulum occurs.

ETIOLOGY

- Increased intraluminal pressure from dense, fiber-depleted stools and abnormal colonic motility
- Occurs at areas of weakness from junctures of penetrating arteries in the muscular wall
- Bleeding is caused by medial thinning of the vasa recta and weakening of the artery.
- Diverticulitis occurs when increased intraluminal pressure results in local inflammation and necrosis leading to micro- or macroperforation.
- Previous belief that obstructing fecaliths were the common cause of diverticulitis is not supported

COMMONLY ASSOCIATED CONDITIONS

Connective tissue diseases, colon cancer, and inflammatory bowel disease

DIAGNOSIS

HISTORY

- Diverticulosis:
  - 80–85% of patients remain asymptomatic. Of the 15–20% with symptoms, 1–2% will need hospitalization, and 0.5% will need surgery.
  - Pain: Dull, colicky, mostly in left lower quadrant, can be worse after eating, some relief following bowel movement or passage of flatus
  - Diarrhea or constipation
- Diverticulitis: Uncomplicated (75%) and complicated (25%):
  - Pain: Acute onset, mostly localized in left lower quadrant; prominently associated with tenderness in same region
  - Fever with chills as severity increases
  - Anorexia, nausea (20–62%), or vomiting
  - Constipation (50%) or diarrhea (25–35%)
  - Dysuria, frequency if bladder involved
  - Pneumaturia, fecaluria if colovesical fistula develops
- Diverticular hemorrhage:
  - Melena, hematochezia
  - Painless rectal bleeding

PHYSICAL EXAM

- Diverticulosis:
  - May be completely normal
  - May have intermittent distension or tympany
  - No signs of peritoneal inflammation
- Diverticulitis:
  - Localized tenderness usually LLQ
  - Rebound tenderness, involuntary guarding, or rigidity
  - Palpable mass in LLQ (20%) that is tender, firm, or fixed
  - Abdominal distension and tympany
  - Bowel sounds hypoactive or could be high pitched and intermittent if obstruction ensues
  - Rectal exam may reveal tenderness, induration, or mass in the cul-de-sac.
  - Colovaginal, colovesical and perirectal fistulae may be the initial manifestation (rarely).
  - Important: If tenderness and guarding are generalized, have high suspicion for perforation

DIAGNOSTIC TESTS & INTERPRETATION

Lab

Initial lab tests

- WBC normal in diverticulosis; usually elevated with immature polymorphs in diverticulitis (normal in up to 45% of diverticulitis patients)
- Hemoglobin normal (unless bleeding)
- ESR elevated in diverticulitis
- UA may be abnormal with microscopic pyuria, hematuria, pneumaturia, or fecaluria (if fistula)
- Urine culture: Persistent infection in colovesical fistula
- Blood culture: Positive in diverticulitis with generalized peritonitis
- Malnutrition, steroids or immunosuppressive drugs may alter lab results

Imaging

Initial approach

- Diverticulosis:
  - Asymptomatic diverticulosis is commonly an incidental finding on colonoscopy
- Diverticulitis:
  - Plain film abdomen supine and upright; useful for urgent assessment of megacolon or free air
  - If suspected diverticulitis: CT scan with IV, oral, and rectal contrast (1)[A].
  - CT helps determine degree of acute perforation and assists in surgical planning.
  - Ultrasound is effective in identifying diverticulitis in the acute setting (2)[B].
  - Barium enema: not recommended due to risk of extravasation into the peritoneum.
- Diverticular bleeding/hematochezia:
  - Endoscopy is the test of choice for the evaluation of lower GI bleeding (3).
  - Angiography is used if massive bleeding obscures endoscopy or when endoscopy cannot visualize a source (3).

Follow-Up & Special Considerations

- After resolution of an initial episode of acute diverticulitis: Colonoscopy to exclude any associated malignancies, strictures, or inflammatory bowel disease (1).
- After an episode of lower GI bleeding, colonoscopy should be performed to exclude neoplasia (2).

Diagnostic Procedures/Surgery

- For evaluation of hematochezia in suspected diverticular hemorrhage:
  - A nasogastric tube should be placed to exclude upper GI sources of bleeding (3).
  - 99mTc-pertechnetate–labeled RBC scans can be used before angiography to evaluate if angiography can be effective or not in revealing a source; (not studied in a comparison trial) (3).
- For diverticulitis, gallium- or indium-labeled leukocytes to localize abscess (rarely used)

Pathological Findings

- Most right-sided diverticula are true diverticula (all layers of the colonic wall).
- Most left-sided diverticula are actually pseudodiverticula (outpouchings of the mucosa and submucosa).
- Surgical and autopsy studies show mycosis, a constellation of thickened circular muscle (pseudohypertrophy due to increased elastin in the taeniae), short taeniae, and luminal narrowing.
- Diverticulitis: Inflammation with lymphocytic infiltrate, ulceration, mucin depletion necrosis, Paneth cell metaplasia, and cryptitis.

DIFFERENTIAL DIAGNOSIS

Irritable bowel syndrome, lactose intolerance, carcinoma, inflammatory bowel disease, fecal impaction, incarcerated hernia, gallbladder disease, angiodysplasia, colitis, acute appendicitis, ectopic pregnancy

Pregnancy Considerations

Rule out ectopic pregnancy.

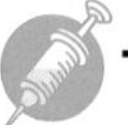

TREATMENT

MEDICATION

First Line

- Diverticulosis:
  - High fiber intake is recommended (preferably above 20–30 g/d).
- Symptomatic uncomplicated diverticular disease in the absence of a history of complicated disease can be treated with cyclical rifaximin or mesalamine continuously.
- Uncomplicated diverticulitis:
  - Oral antibiotics for outpatient treatment of mild disease: Cover for anaerobes and gram-negative rods with:
    - A quinolone (ciprofloxacin or levofloxacin) plus metronidazole (Flagyl) *(may use clindamycin if metronidazole intolerant) OR*
    - Bactrim plus metronidazole
    - Treat for 7–10 days
  - Inpatient: Use IV antibiotics:
    - Quinolone plus metronidazole
    - Mono therapy with a beta-lactam/beta-lactamase inhibitor: Zosyn or Unasyn or Ertapenem
    - Unresponsive or severe disease: Imipenem or Meropenem
  - Recurrences of acute diverticulitis may be decreased by using mesalamine ± rifaximin (4)[A] or probiotics
- Diverticular bleeding:
  - Consider Vasopressin 0.2–0.3 units/min through selective intra-arterial catheter
- Precautions:
  - Avoid morphine and other opiates that may increase intraluminal pressure or promote ileus.
  - Increased fiber intake is not recommended in the acute management of diverticulitis.

Second Line

- Outpatient: Augmentin or Moxifloxacin
- Severely ill inpatients: Ampicillin + metronidazole + a quinolone *OR* Ampicillin + metronidazole + an aminoglycoside

ADDITIONAL TREATMENT

General Measures

- Diverticulosis: Outpatient with fiber supplements to soften stools
- Outpatient diverticulitis: Pain, tenderness, leukocytosis, but no toxicity or peritoneal signs; use oral antibiotics. 1–2% of subjects require hospitalization for toxicity, septicemia, peritonitis, or failure of symptoms to be resolved in a few days. Up to 30% of patients may require surgery at first episode of diverticulitis. Up to 50% of patients with diverticulitis eventually may come to surgery.
- Toxic patients require hospitalization, bowel rest with clear liquids or nothing by mouth, and IV antibiotics at least until there is a positive response.
- Symptomatic improvement is expected within 2–3 days of initiating antibiotics, and antibiotics continued for 7–10 days (2).
- 80% of diverticular hemorrhages will resolve spontaneously (3).

Issues for Referral

Acutely suspected perforation, peritoneal signs, persistent bleeding requiring multiple transfusions

COMPLEMENTARY AND ALTERNATIVE MEDICINE

Probiotics may have benefit in symptomatic uncomplicated diverticular disease.

SURGERY/OTHER PROCEDURES

- Indication for emergent surgery: Peritonitis, uncontrolled sepsis, visceral perforation, colonic obstruction, or acute deterioration
- Surgery for nonemergent state controversial, sometimes even in complicated cases of diverticulitis
- Elective surgery after acute diverticulitis: Decision for elective resection should be made on a case-by-case basis (1)[B]:
  - After first episode, there is a 33% chance of recurrence; if it does recur, there is a 66% chance of a third bout.
  - Most complicated cases occur on the first presentation with subsequent presentations being uncomplicated.
  - Emergent surgery carries a 9-fold increase in mortality vs. elective (5).
  - Elective surgery recommendations should be based not on number of recurrences but on severity of complaints and complications (6).
  - Elective resection is typically advised after recovery from a complicated diverticulitis treated nonoperatively (1)[B].
  - Age: Younger patients more likely to have recurrence
  - Immunocompromised patients: More likely to present with acute complicated diverticulitis, fail medical management, and have complications from elective surgery.
- Large abscesses (>4 cm) are usually drained radiologically and many of these patients can be acutely managed nonoperatively (1).
- In diverticular hemorrhage, patients requiring more than 4 units of RBC transfused have a 60% chance of requiring surgical intervention to stop bleeding. Patients requiring <4 units typically do not need surgery (3).

IN-PATIENT CONSIDERATIONS

Initial Stabilization

IV fluids, analgesics, antibiotics, NG suction

Admission Criteria

~1–2% of subjects require hospitalization for toxicity, septicemia, peritonitis

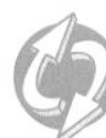

ONGOING CARE

DIET

- NPO during acute diverticulitis; progress to fluids, then high-fiber as bowel function returns
- Patients with known diverticulosis or a history of diverticulitis should eat a high-fiber diet (>30 g/d) to prevent recurrence (7).
- Nuts, corn, and popcorn do not increase risk for diverticulosis or diverticular complications (8).

PROGNOSIS

- Good with early detection and treatment of complications
- Recurrence risk increases with each bout.
- If diverticular bleeding, rebleeding occurs in up to 6%.

COMPLICATIONS

Hemorrhage, perforation, peritonitis, obstruction, abscess, or fistula

REFERENCES

1. Standards Committee of The American Society of Colon and Rectal Surgeons, Rafferty J, Shellito P, et al. Practice parameters for sigmoid diverticulitis. *Dis Colon Rectum*. 2006.
2. Stollman NH, Raskin JB. Diagnosis and management of diverticular disease of the colon in adults. Ad Hoc Practice Parameters Committee of the American College of Gastroenterology. *Am J Gastroenterol*. 1999;94:3110–21.
3. Zuccaro G. Management of the adult patient with acute lower gastrointestinal bleeding. American College of Gastroenterology. Practice Parameters Committee. *Am J Gastroenterol*. 1998;93:1202–8.
4. Gatta L, Vakil N, Vaira D, et al. Efficacy of 5-ASA in the treatment of colonic diverticular disease. *J Clin Gastroenterol*. 2010;44:113–9.
5. Novitsky YW, Sechrist C, Payton BL, et al. Do the risks of emergent colectomy justify nonoperative management strategies for recurrent diverticulitis? *Am J Surg*. 2008.
6. Klarenbeek BR, Samuels M, van der Wal MA, et al. Indications for elective sigmoid resection in diverticular disease. *Ann Surg*. 2010;251:670–4.
7. Ravikoff JE, Korzenik JR. Presentations the role of fiber in diverticular disease. *J Clin Gastroenterol*. 2011;45:S7–11.
8. Strate LL, Liu YL, Syngal S, et al. Nut, corn, and popcorn consumption and the incidence of diverticular disease. *JAMA*. 2008;300:907–14.

CODES

ICD9

- 562.10 Diverticulosis of colon (without mention of hemorrhage)
- 562.11 Diverticulitis of colon (without mention of hemorrhage)
- 562.12 Diverticulosis of colon with hemorrhage

CLINICAL PEARLS

- Diverticula occur in up to 20% of general population, but increases progressively with age, reaching up to 2/3 of people by the eighth decade.
- Patients with known diverticulosis should eat a high-fiber diet; nuts, corn, and popcorn do not increase risk for diverticular complications.
- WBC are not elevated in up to 45% of cases of diverticulitis

DOMESTIC VIOLENCE

Rhonda A. Faulkner, PhD
Meg Lekander, MD

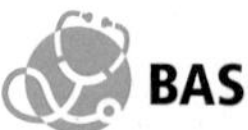

BASICS

DESCRIPTION

- Domestic violence (DV) is behavior in any relationship that is used to gain or maintain power and control over an intimate partner.
- May include physical, sexual, and/or emotional abuse, economic or psychological actions, or threats of actions that influence another person
- Although women are at greater risk of experiencing DV, it occurs among patients of any race, age, sexual orientation, religion, gender, socioeconomic background, and education level.
- Synonym(s): Intimate partner violence (IPV); Spousal abuse; Family violence

EPIDEMIOLOGY

Incidence

~8%; women are more likely to report partner violence than men (1)[B].

Prevalence

- DV occurs in 1 in 4 American families. In the US, 2–4 million women are abused by an intimate partner each year. Nearly 5.3 million incidents of DV occur each year among US women ≥18 years, and 3.2 million incidents among men.
- DV results in nearly 2 million injuries and 2,000–4,000 deaths nationwide each year.
- Reportedly, 30% of women and 22% of men have experienced physical, sexual, or psychological IPV during their lifetime in the US.
- 14–35% of adult female patients in emergency departments and 12–23% in family medicine offices report experiencing DV within the past year.
- Costs of DV are estimated to exceed $5.8 billion annually, of which $4.1 billion are for direct medical and mental health services.
- DV survivors have a 1.6–2.3-fold increase in health care use compared with nonabused population.

Geriatric Considerations

- ~4–6% of elderly are abused, with ~1–2 million elderly persons experiencing abuse and/or neglect each year. In 90% of cases, the perpetrator is a family member.
- Elder abuse is any form of mistreatment that results in harm or loss to an older person; may include physical, sexual, emotional, financial abuse, and/or neglect.

Pediatric Considerations

- >3 million children aged 3–17 years are at risk of witnessing acts of DV.
- ~1 million abused children are identified in the US each year.
- Children living in violent homes are at increased risk of physical, sexual, and/or emotional abuse; anxiety and depression; decreased self-esteem; emotional, behavioral, social, physical disturbances; and lifelong poor health.

Pregnancy Considerations

DV occurs during 7–20% of pregnancies. Women with unintended pregnancy are at 3 times greater risk of DV compared with those whose pregnancy was planned. 25% of abused women report exacerbation of abuse during pregnancy.

RISK FACTORS

- Patient/victim risk factors:
  - Substance abuse
  - Poverty/financial stressors/unemployment
  - Recent loss of social support
  - Family disruption and life cycle changes
  - History of abusive relationships or witness to abuse as child
  - Mental or physical disability in family
  - Social isolation
  - Pregnancy
- Abuser risk factors:
  - Substance abuse (e.g., heavy drinking)
  - Young age
  - Unemployment
  - Low academic achievement
  - Witnessing or experiencing violence as child
  - Depression
  - Personality disorders
- Relational risk factors:
  - Marital conflict
  - Marital instability
  - Economic stress
  - Traditional gender role norms
  - Poor family functioning

Geriatric Considerations

Factors associated with the abuse of older adults include increasing age, nonwhite race, low-income status, functional impairment, cognitive disability, substance use, poor emotional state, low self-esteem, cohabitation, and lack of social support.

Pediatric Considerations

Factors associated with child abuse or neglect include low-income status, low maternal education, nonwhite race, large family size, young maternal age, single-parent household, parental psychiatric disturbances, and presence of a stepfather.

DIAGNOSIS

- DV is often underdiagnosed, with only 10–12% of physicians conducting routine screening.
- Although prevalence of DV in primary care settings is 7–50%, <15% are screened.
- Pregnancy increases risk.
- 15–20% of women in US emergency departments are there related to DV.
- Barriers to screening: Time constraints, discomfort with the subject, fear of offending the patient, and lack of perceived skills and resources to manage DV.
- Abused patients may refuse to disclose abuse for many reasons:
  - Not feeling emotionally ready to admit the reality of the situation
  - Shame and self-blame
  - Feelings of failure if abuse is admitted
  - Fear of rejection by the physician
  - Fear of retribution from abuser
  - Belief that abuse will not happen again
  - Belief that no alternatives or available resources exist
- Physicians should introduce the subject of DV in a general way (i.e., "I routinely ask all patients about domestic violence. Have you ever been in a relationship where you were afraid?").
- How to screen:
  - Screen patient alone, without partner or others present.
  - Ask screening questions in patient's primary language; do not use children or other family members as interpreters.
- Partner Violence Screen (sensitivity 35–71%; specificity 80–94%):
  - "Have you ever been hit, kicked, punched, or otherwise hurt by someone within the past year? If so, by whom?"
  - "Do you feel safe in your current relationship?"
  - "Is there a partner from a previous relationship who is making you feel unsafe now?"
- CDC-recommended RADAR system:
  - R: Routinely screen every patient; make screening a part of everyday practice in prenatal, postnatal, routine gynecologic visits, and annual health screenings.
  - A: Ask questions directly, kindly, and be nonjudgmental.
  - D: Document findings in the patient's chart using the patient's own words, with details. Use body maps and photographs as necessary.
  - A: Assess the patient's safety and see if the patient has a safety plan.
  - R: Review options for dealing with DV with the patient and provide referrals.
- Additional DV screening tools:
  - SAFE Questions:
    - Stress/Safety: "Do you feel safe in your relationship?"
    - Afraid/Abused: "Have you ever been in a relationship where you were threatened, hurt, or afraid?"
    - Friends/Family: "Are your friends or family aware that you have been hurt? Could you tell them, and would they be able to give you support?"
    - Emergency Plan: "Do you have a safe place to go and the resources you need in an emergency?"
  - HITS Screening Tool (sensitivity 30–100%; specificity 86–99%):
  - Items scored as: 1, never; 2, rarely; 3, sometimes; 4, often; 5, frequently; score >10 is considered positive for abuse:
    - How often does your partner: Physically hurt you? Insult or talk down to you? Threaten you with harm? Scream or curse at you?

HISTORY

- Pregnancy difficulties such as poor/late prenatal care, low-birth-weight babies. and perinatal deaths
- Pelvic and abdominal pain, chronic without demonstrable pathology
- Headaches
- Back pain
- Gynecologic disorders
- Sexually transmitted infections including HIV/AIDS
- CNS disorders
- GI disorders
- Depression
- Suicidal ideation
- Anxiety
- Fatigue
- Substance abuse

- Eating disorders
- Overuse of health services/frequent emergency room visits
- Noncompliance

PHYSICAL EXAM

- Psychological signs and symptoms:
  - Signs of battered woman syndrome and/or PTSD (flat affect/avoidance of eye contact; evasiveness; heightened startle response; sleep disturbance; traumatic flashbacks)
  - Depression, anxiety, chronic fatigue, substance abuse
  - Suspicious partner accompaniment at appointment; overly solicitous partner and/or refusal to leave exam room
- Physical signs and symptoms:
  - Tympanic membrane rupture
  - Rectal or genital injury (centrally located injuries with bathing-suit pattern of distribution—concealable by clothing)
  - Head and neck injuries (site of 50% of abusive injuries)
  - Facial scrapes, loose or broken tooth, bruises, cuts, or fractures to face or body
  - Knife wounds, cigarette burns, bite marks, welts with outline of weapon (such as belt buckle)
  - Broken bones
  - Defensive posture injuries
  - Injuries inconsistent with the explanation given
  - Injuries in various stages of healing

DIAGNOSTIC TESTS & INTERPRETATION

- The US Preventive Services Task Force (USPSTF) found insufficient evidence to recommend for/against routine screening of parents or guardians for the physical abuse or neglect of children, of women for intimate partner violence, or of older adults or their caregivers for elder abuse.
- Other recommendations:
  - American College of Physicians recommends routine screening for DV in primary care settings and when women present for emergency care with traumatic injuries.
  - US Surgeon General and American Association of Family Practitioners recommend that physicians consider the possibility of DV as a cause of illness and injury.
  - The Partner Violence Screen is a 3-question screening tool with a high specificity.
  - There is no evidence of harm in screening for DV.

Pediatric Considerations

American Academy of Pediatrics (AAP) and American Medical Association (AMA) recommend that physicians remain alert for signs and symptoms of child physical and sexual abuse in the routine exam.

Pregnancy Considerations

ACOG and AMA guidelines on DV recommend that physicians routinely assess all pregnant women for DV.

Lab

Initial lab tests

LFTs, amylase, lipase if abdominal trauma is suspected

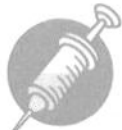

TREATMENT

- Treatment includes: Initial diagnosis; ongoing medical care; emotional support, counseling, and patient education regarding the DV cycle; referrals to community and supportive services as needed.
- Upon diagnosis, use the SOS-DoC intervention:
- S: Offer Support and assess Safety:
  - Support: "You are not to blame. I am sorry this is happening to you. There is no excuse for DV."
  - Remind patient of your commitment to confidential communication.
  - Safety: Listen and respond to safety issues for the patient: "Do you feel safe going home?"; "Are your children safe?"
- O: Discuss Options, including safety planning and follow-up:
  - Provide information about DV and help where needed. Make referrals to local resources:
    - "Do you need or want to access a safety shelter or DV service agency?"
    - "Do you want police intervention and if so, would you like me to call the police so they can make a report with you?"
    - Offer numbers to local resources and National DV Hotline: 1-800-799-SAFE (open 24/7; can provide physicians in every state with information on local resources).
- S: Validate patient's Strengths:
  - "It took courage for you to talk with me today. You have shown great strength in very difficult circumstances."
- Do: Document observations, assessment, and plans:
  - Use patient's own words regarding injury and abuse.
  - Legibly document injuries: Use a body map.
  - If possible, take instant photographs of patient's injuries if given patient consent.
  - Make patient safety plan. Prepare patient to get away in an emergency:
    - Encourage patient to keep the following items in a safe place: Keys (house and car); important papers (Social Security card, birth certificates, photo ID/driver's license, passport, green card); cash, food stamps, credit cards; medication for self and children; children's immunization records; important phone numbers/addresses (friends, family, local shelters); personal care items (e.g., extra glasses).
    - Encourage patient to arrange a signal with someone to let that person know when she or he needs help.
- C: Offer Continuity:
  - Offer a follow-up appointment and assess barriers to access.

ADDITIONAL TREATMENT

- National DV Hotline: 1-800-799-SAFE (7233)
- Post in all exam rooms posters in both English and Spanish; available at www.thehotline.org/resources/resource-download-center/

General Measures

- Reporting child and elder abuse to protective services is mandatory in most states. Several states have laws requiring mandatory reporting of IPV.
- Contact the local DV program to find out about laws and community resources before they are needed.
- Display resource materials (National DV Hotline: 1-800-799-SAFE) in the office, all exam rooms, and restrooms.

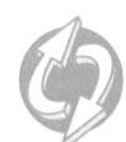

ONGOING CARE

FOLLOW-UP RECOMMENDATIONS

- Schedule prompt follow-up appointment.
- Inquire about what has happened since last visit.
- Review medical records and ask about past episodes to convey concern for the patient and a willingness to address this health issue openly.
- DV often requires multiple interventions over time before it is resolved.

PATIENT EDUCATION

- Counsel patients about nonviolent ways to resolve conflict.
- Educate patients about the cycle of violence.
- Counsel parents about developmentally appropriate ways to discipline their children.
- Educate parents about the negative consequences of arguments on children and each other.
- National Coalition Against Domestic Violence: www.ncadv.org
- CDC: www.cdc.gov/violenceprevention

PROGNOSIS

Most DV perpetrators do not voluntarily seek therapy unless pressured by partners or upon legal mandate. Current evidence is insufficient on effectiveness of therapy for perpetrators.

REFERENCE

1. Walton MA, Murray R, Cunningham RM, et al. Correlates of intimate partner violence among men and women in an inner city emergency department. *J Addict Dis*. 2009;28:366–81.

ADDITIONAL READING

- Cronholm PF, Fogarty CT, Ambuel B, et al. Intimate partner violence. *Am Fam Physician*. 2011;83:1165–72.
- Rhodes KV, Kothari CL, Ditcher M, et al. Intimate partner violence identification and response: Time for a change in strategy. *J Gen Intern Med*. 2011;15 March (Epub ahead of print).

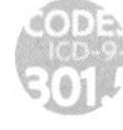

CODES

ICD9

- 995.80 Adult maltreatment, unspecified
- 995.81 Adult physical abuse
- 995.82 Adult emotional/psychological abuse

CLINICAL PEARLS

- Display resource materials in the office (e.g., posting abuse awareness posters/National DV Hotline, 1-800-799-SAFE, in both English and Spanish, in all exam rooms and restrooms).
- Despite lack of data, screen all women: "Have you ever been threatened, hit, kicked, or are you afraid of your partner?"
- For those who screen positive, offer resources, reassure confidentiality, and provide close follow-up.

DOWN SYNDROME

Michele Roberts, MD, PhD

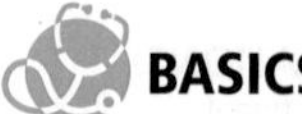

BASICS

DESCRIPTION
- Congenital condition associated with mental retardation and an increased risk of multisystem medical problems
- One of the most common identifiable causes of mental retardation
- System(s) affected: Neurologic (100%); Cardiac (40–50%); Gastrointestinal (GI) (8–12%)
- Etiology: The presence of all or part of an extra chromosome 21
- Synonym(s): Trisomy 21; DS

Pediatric Considerations
- Congenital heart disease is major cause of morbidity/mortality. Murmur may not be present at birth. Delay in recognition may lead to irreversible pulmonary hypertension.
- Early treatment of subclinical thyroid disease may improve growth and development (1)[B].

Geriatric Considerations
- Life expectancy has increased to 56 years in 2008 (2).
- Age-related health issues occur at earlier age than in general population.
- Communication difficulties may interfere with prompt recognition of:
  - Alzheimer disease, which is more prevalent and may occur at a younger age, and other psychiatric illness
  - Thyroid/autoimmune disorders
  - Cataracts/hearing loss

Pregnancy Considerations
- Most DS males are infertile:
- Females are subfertile but can conceive:
  - 36% of reported offspring have DS
  - Assess mental and physical fitness to carry pregnancy/care for child

EPIDEMIOLOGY

Incidence
In the US, 1 in 700 live births, 6,000 births/year in US

Prevalence
350,000 persons in the US

RISK FACTORS
- DS occurs in all races with equal frequency.
- Risk increases dramatically with mother's age:
  - Age 20, 1 in 1,445
  - Age 35, 1 in 270
  - Age 37, 1 in 100
  - Age 45, 1 in 25
- With prenatal screening of older mothers, relatively more DS infants are born to younger mothers.

Genetics
- Online Mendelian Inheritance in Man (OMIM) #190685
- Inheritance: Most commonly sporadic nondisjunction resulting in trisomy 21
- Chance of having another child with DS is:
  - 1% (or age risk, whichever is greater) after conceiving a pregnancy with nondisjunction trisomy 21
  - 10–15% for mothers and 3–5% for fathers who carry a balanced translocation
  - 100% if the parental translocation is 21:21(45,t [21:21])
- Unclear after child with mosaic DS, but ~1%
- Chromosome 21 has been sequenced; it is the smallest human chromosome.

GENERAL PREVENTION
- No prevention for nondisjunction
- The American College of Medical Genetics and the American College of Obstetrics and Gynecology recommend that all pregnant women be offered prenatal screening for DS.
- Preimplantation diagnosis with in vitro fertilization (IVF) or prenatal diagnosis and termination are current options.
- Maternal prenatal screening includes:
  - Pregnancy-associated plasma protein A (PAPP-A): First trimester
  - Quadruple test: Second trimester
  - Sequential/integrated screen combines both
  - Ultrasound (nuchal translucency or NT)
- Chorionic villi sampling or amniocentesis: If high a priori risk or positive screen

ETIOLOGY
- Trisomy 21: In 95% of patients, an extra chromosome 21 is found in all cells due to nondisjunction usually in maternal meiosis.
- Translocation DS: In 3% of patients, extra chromosome 21q material is translocated to another chromosome (usually 13, 14, or 21). For translocation trisomy 21, 2/3 are new, 1/3 have a parental carrier:
  - Translocation DS more likely if mother <30 years of age
- Mosaic trisomy 21: Found in 2% of patients with DS. Manifestations may be milder.

COMMONLY ASSOCIATED CONDITIONS
- Cardiac:
  - Congenital heart defects (40–50%):
  - Mostly endocardial cushion or ventricular septal defect (VSD)
- GI/Growth:
  - Structural defects (12%):
    - Duodenal or anal atresia/stenosis
    - Hirschsprung disease, annular pancreas
  - Gastroesophageal reflux
  - Constipation
  - Celiac disease
- Pulmonary:
  - Tracheal stenosis/tracheoesophageal fistula
  - Pulmonary hypertension
  - Obstructive apnea
- Genitourinary:
  - Cryptorchidism, hypospadias
  - Renal anomaly
- Hematologic/Neoplastic:
  - Macrocytosis (66%)
  - Transient leukemoid reaction (10%): Generally resolves spontaneously, but can be preleukemic (AMKL) in 20–30%
  - Leukemia (0.5–1%):
  - Acute lymphoblastic leukemia (ALL) risk: 10–20× that of ALL in non-DS
  - Decreased risk of most solid tumors; increased risk of germ cell tumors
- Endocrine:
  - Hypothyroidism: Congenital or acquired (20–40%)
  - Diabetes
  - Hypogonadism
- Skeletal:
  - Altered growth pattern
  - Atlantoaxial instability (15%); 2% symptomatic
  - Ligamentous laxity
  - Scoliosis (some cases have adult onset)
  - Hip problems (8%)
- Immune/Rheumatologic:
  - Abnormal immune function with increased rate of and mortality from infection, especially respiratory
  - Increased risk of autoimmune disorders including thyroid, celiac disease, lupus
- Neurologic:
  - Mental retardation ranging from near-normal to severe. Average is moderate retardation.
  - Seizures:
    - Infantile spasms (5–10%)
    - Increased risk child-/adult-onset seizures
  - Alzheimer disease: 100% develop neuropathologic changes, though not all develop symptoms
- Psychiatric:
  - Emotional/conduct disorders (25–33%)
  - Depression: Up to 10% of adults
- Sensory:
  - Hearing loss (60–90%): Mostly conductive due to high frequency of asymptomatic middle ear effusion
  - Visual impairment (60–70%): Mostly strabismus, nystagmus, cataracts
- Dermatologic, worsens with increasing age:
  - Palmoplantar hyperkeratosis (>75%), atopic or seborrheic dermatitis (50%), onychomycosis (50%), syringomas (30%), furunculosis/folliculitis (15%)

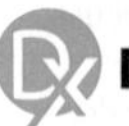

DIAGNOSIS
- The mother should be informed of the diagnosis promptly by a physician (preferably the obstetrician and pediatrician, or family physician), on the basis of clinical observations and before the karyotype is available, but with consideration of extenuating circumstances (e.g., mother's medical condition).
- The spouse/partner and infant should be present unless this would cause undue delay. The meeting should be private. Refer to the baby by name.
- The physician should be knowledgeable on the subject of DS, and should conduct a discussion with content that is current, respectful, balanced, informative, and realistic but not overly pessimistic, concentrating on what is relevant to the first year of life.
- A survey of mothers of children with prenatally diagnosed DS revealed a preference that the diagnosis be conveyed in person, that up-to-date printed materials on DS be provided, and that mothers be referred to local DS support groups (3).

HISTORY
85% of mothers of infants with DS learn of the diagnosis postnatally.

PHYSICAL EXAM
- DS-specific growth curves should be used.
- Infants and children:
  - Brachycephaly (100%)
  - Hypotonia (80%)
  - Small ears, often low set and simplified

- Upslanting palpebral fissure (90%)
- Epicanthic folds (90%)
- Brushfield spots
- Depressed nasal bridge
- Short neck, often with increased nuchal folds
- Abnormal dermatoglyphics, including single palmar crease, single flexion crease on fifth finger
- Increased space between toes 1 and 2; fifth finger clinodactyly; brachydactyly

- Adults: Features may become less obvious.

DIAGNOSTIC TESTS & INTERPRETATION

Lab

Initial lab tests

- A chromosome test is definitive and should always be done at the time of clinical suspicion.
- Parental chromosome study indicated only if translocation DS found in child.

Imaging

Initial approach

- Echocardiogram at the time of diagnosis. A ventricular septal defect (VSD)/endocardial cushion defect may not be apparent at birth.
- Radiographs of neck currently recommended for all children once between ages 3 and 5 years.

Follow-Up & Special Considerations

- Repeat neck films for minor trauma, neck pain, long-tract symptoms, or breathing problems.
- Cardiac follow-up as indicated

Pathological Findings

Upslanting palpebral fissures, epicanthic folds, fifth-finger clinodactyly, and single palmar crease individually may be a benign familial trait. Unilateral single palmar crease seen in 4% of general population; bilateral in 1%.

TREATMENT

ADDITIONAL TREATMENT

General Measures

- Genetic evaluation and counseling
- Now that many of the formerly life-threatening associated medical conditions may be treated successfully, increasing attention is paid to social issues, family impact, access to care, and unmet needs (4).

Issues for Referral

- Infant stimulation programs
- Physical/occupational/speech therapy
- Special needs educational support. Inclusion programs generally work well.

COMPLEMENTARY AND ALTERNATIVE MEDICINE

- Antioxidant therapy has theoretical basis for future benefits, although a 2008 randomized controlled trial provided no evidence to support the use of antioxidant or folinic acid supplements in children with DS (5).
- Vitamin E, selenium, and zinc may be beneficial (6)[C].
- Many unproven and dangerous procedures and therapies are offered to vulnerable parents:
  - Craniosacral manipulation is dangerous due to potential atlantoaxial instability.
  - Sicca is illegal in US, potentially dangerous, and without any evidence of benefit.
- Piracetam is much publicized, without scientific evidence of benefit.

SURGERY/OTHER PROCEDURES

Repair of congenital anomalies is appropriate. Plastic surgery for facial features generally not recommended.

IN-PATIENT CONSIDERATIONS

Discharge Criteria

If the social situation indicates adoption, there are families specifically seeking to adopt DS children.

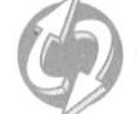

ONGOING CARE

FOLLOW-UP RECOMMENDATIONS

Patient Monitoring

Surveillance recommendations (7,8,9)[C] (repeat additionally for clinical suspicion):

- Vision: Assess for strabismus, cataracts, and nystagmus at birth and on each routine visit:
  - Should be seen by ophthalmologist by 6 months and every 2 years in early childhood, annually in later childhood and adulthood
- Hearing: Neonatal screen with ABR or OAE, then audiogram every 6 months until age 3 years, then annual hearing assessment
- Thyroid: Initial newborn screen. Repeat thyroid-stimulating hormone at 6 months, 12 months, and then annually.
- Screening for celiac disease is controversial, but does not appear to be cost effective.
- C-spine flexion/extension films once at 3–5 years of age and as indicated clinically.
- Echocardiogram for all newborns, regardless of murmur. Monitor clinically for later cardiac complications throughout life.

DIET

- No special diet, but caloric needs are lower in adolescents/adults with DS than in their peers
- Obesity is prevalent at all ages.
- No scientific evidence to support megavitamin therapy and dietary supplements that are widely discussed in the lay press

PATIENT EDUCATION

- National Down Syndrome Congress (800) 232-NDSC; http://www.ndsccenter.org
- National Down Syndrome Society (800) 221-4602; http://www.ndss.org
- The Down Syndrome Research Foundation provides information on the latest research and educational programs for people with DS: http://dsrf.org/index.cfm?fuseaction=publications.dsq

PROGNOSIS

- Associated congenital anomalies are the immediate concern during the newborn period.
- Adults can often work in protected situations; a few are largely independent.
- Earlier onset of age-related health issues, shortened life expectancy.
- Clinical Alzheimer disease in at least 1/3 of patients after age 35 years
- Children with DS, especially those of low socioeconomic status, may have more unmet medical needs and more negatively pronounced family impact, and may be less likely to have access to health care than do children with other special health care needs (4).

REFERENCES

1. van Trotsenburg AS, Vulsma T, van Rozenburg-Marres SL, et al. The effect of thyroxine treatment started in the neonatal period on development and growth of two-year-old Down syndrome children: A randomized clinical trial. *J Clin Endocrinol Metab*. 2005;90:3304–11.
2. http://www.ndss.org.
3. Skotko BG. Prenatally diagnosed Down syndrome: mothers who continued their pregnancies evaluate their health care providers. *Am J Obstet Gynecol*. 2005;192:670.
4. McGrath RJ, Stransky ML, Cooley WC, et al. National profile of children with Down syndrome: Disease burden, access to care, and family impact. *J Pediatr*. 2011.
5. Ellis JM, Tan HK, Gilbert RE, et al. Supplementation with antioxidants and folinic acid for children with Down's syndrome: Randomised controlled trial. *BMJ*. 2008;336:594–7.
6. Roizen NJ. Complementary and alternative therapies for Down syndrome. *MRDD Res Rev*. 2005;11:149–55.
7. American Academy of Pediatrics. Health supervision for children with Down syndrome *Pediatrics*. 2001;107:442–9.
8. Cohen WI. Current dilemmas in Down syndrome clinical care. *Am J Med Genet*. 2006;142C:141–8.
9. Smith DS. Health care management of adults with Down syndrome. *Am Fam Physician*. 2001;64: 1031–8.

ADDITIONAL READING

- Ranweiler R. Assessment and care of the newborn with Down syndrome. *Adv Neonatal Care*. 2009;9:17–24.
- Roizen NJ, Patterson D. Down's syndrome. *Lancet*. 2003;361:1281–9.
- Skotko BG, Capone GT, Kishnani PS, et al. Postnatal diagnosis of Down syndrome: Synthesis of the evidence on how best to deliver the news. *Pediatrics*. 2009;124:e751–8.

See Also (Topic, Algorithm, Electronic Media Element)

Algorithm: Mental Retardation

CODES

ICD9

- 318.0 Moderate intellectual disabilities
- 318.1 Severe intellectual disabilities
- 758.0 Down's syndrome

CLINICAL PEARLS

- DS can affect all systems, including neurologic, cardiac, GI, and endocrine.
- As life expectancy increases, regular health monitoring can improve outcomes.

DRUG ABUSE, PRESCRIPTION

Patricia Halligan, MD

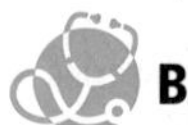

BASICS

DESCRIPTION

- Prescription drug abuse involves using a prescription medication for any reason beyond what it was prescribed for.
- Examples: Amphetamine use for weight loss, enhancing academic or sexual performance, euphoria or wakefulness; benzodiazepine use to boost an opiate high or ameliorate alcohol withdrawal; or opioid use to treat depression
- Diversion: Use of prescription drugs for recreational purposes; often person legally obtains Rx from provider and uses them inappropriately or sells them

EPIDEMIOLOGY

- Americans constitute only 4.6% of world's population and consume 80% of global opioid supply.
- Hydrocodone remains the #1 prescribed drug in US.
- In US, average sales of opioids/person have increased from 402% from 1997–2007. Among those who abused prescription drugs in past month, 56% received from a friend or family member, and 82% of those friends and relatives obtained prescription drug from just 1 doctor.
- Only 4% received the drug from a drug dealer and only 0.4% from the Internet.
- A 2010 study found 62% of college students diverted ADHD medicine and 35% diverted prescription analgesics. By 2008, emergency room visits for opioids increased by 614% over 13 years and 279% for benzodiazepines.
- Overdose deaths from prescription opioid analgesics have tripled from 1999–2006.

Incidence

- Predominant age opioid analgesics: 18–25 and over 50. Stimulants: 18–24.
- Predominant sex: Male > Female under 50. Older adult population: Female > Male.

Prevalence

- 6.2 million (2.5%) reported abusing prescription drugs in the past month.
- Pain relievers (1.7 million) are now the second most commonly abused illicit substance second to marijuana (4.2 million).
- Marijuana and pain relievers tied as most common drug used to initiate illicit drug use among first-time users (both 2.2 million).
- Lifetime prevalence of prescription drug abuse is highest for opioids, benzodiazepines, and stimulants.

RISK FACTORS

- Personal or family history of alcohol or drug abuse is the most strongly predictive factor.
- Male, single status, rural, major depressive episode in past year, axis 1 or 2 disorder diagnosis within past year
- Stimulant abusers: Full-time college students 18–24 years old
- Oxycodone abusers: White, male, younger (mean age 32), employed
- Patients with substance abuse and psychiatric history (past or current) are also at risk for abusing nonbenzo hypnotics (Ambien, Ambien CR, Lunesta, Sonata). Benzodiazepine dependence is seen in ~50% of those treated daily for more than 4 months.

GENERAL PREVENTION

- Avoid prescribing controlled substances to patients with personal or family history of substance abuse or with psychiatric disorders.
- Avoid prescribing controlled substances on the first visit. Take a thorough history, contact family members and past prescribers, perform observed urine drug screens. Stop prescribing opioid analgesics for chronic pain if they are not working, if patient is unable to take them as prescribed, or if there are problems. Look for and treat underlying substance abuse problems.

ETIOLOGY

- Increased quality measures around pain have left to a dramatic increase in the number of opioid prescriptions used to treat pain, despite any evidence of the efficacy for long-term opioid therapy for noncancer pain.
- Nonadherence to recommendations: Limit benzodiazepines to <2–4 weeks. American Psychiatric Association recommends against their use to treat generalized anxiety disorder or panic disorder, and long-term benzodiazepines do not aid sleep, etc.
- Prescriptions for controlled substances have increased faster than for noncontrolled pharmaceuticals (154.3% vs. 56.6%). Drug dealers are no longer the primary source of illicit drugs.
- There may be a genetic contribution to prescription drug abuse, as suggested by increased risk if a personal or family history of substance abuse.

COMMONLY ASSOCIATED CONDITIONS

- Benzodiazepines: Withdrawal syndromes/delirium, psychosis, sleep driving, blackout states, elderly with increased risk of falls/accidents, cognitive impairment, impaired driving, increased mortality
- Amphetamine: Hypertension, myocardial ischemia, dysrhythmias, seizures, hyperthermia, hallucinations, paranoia, anxiety, psychosis
- Opioids: Dysrhythmias (toursades de pointes), respiratory depression and death, low testosterone, sexual dysfunction, and fatigue
- Chronic opioid maintenance can produce hyperalgesia (increased pain perception); pain levels are reduced following successful detox. Sensorineural hearing loss can occur with hydrocodone. Chronic opioid use for low back pain is associated with longer disability, lower activity levels, worse pain, and more emergency room visits.

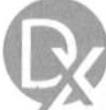

DIAGNOSIS

Screening: A single question: "How many times in the past year have you used an illegal drug or used a prescription medication for nonmedical reasons?": In primary care setting, resulted in sensitivity of 100% and specificity of ~75%.

HISTORY

A personal and family history of substance abuse, since this is the biggest predictor of prescription drug abuse. Talk to spouse/family members, past treaters, review medical records. Obtain prescription monitoring reports (PMRs) to detect doctor shopping, multiple pharmacy use, and early refills.

DIAGNOSTIC TESTS & INTERPRETATION

Urine drug screen (UDS): Order an expanded opiate panel to detect commonly used narcotics (ask specifically for hydrocodone, oxycodone, methadone, fentanyl, tramadol, buprenorphine, meperidine, propoxyphene). Also, clonazepam and lorazepam rarely show up as benzodiazepines in routine UDS and should be ordered specifically.

Lab

Interpretation: Positive if: A. It's positive for drugs that are not prescribed; B. Positive for illicit drugs (marijuana, cocaine); C. Is negative for prescribed drug (suspect diversion); and D. If patient refuses the test:

- OxyContin will only be positive for oxycodone, hydrocodone will be positive for hydrocodone and hydromorphone, codeine will be positive for codeine plus morphine, and heroin will be positive for morphine. Thus, if UDS is positive for morphine, it could mean that the patient took morphine, codeine, heroin, or hydrocodone. It's highly unlikely that a UDS is positive for marijuana based on second-hand smoke.

Diagnostic Procedures/Surgery

CAGE (Cut down, Anger at being questioned about use, Guilt about prior use, Eye-opener use early in day) or AUDIT to assess current alcohol use. DAST (drug abuse screening test) helps determine patient's involvement with drugs over the past year. Details: http://counsellingresource.com/lib/quizzes/drug-testing/drug-abuse/

Pathological Findings

Patient asks for dose escalations, early refills ("spilled the bottle, pharmacist shorted me, dog ate them, forgot the pills while on vacation"), has strong preference for 1 drug, targets appointments at end of day and after hours, shows hostile/threatening behavior, or can be overly flattering to doctor

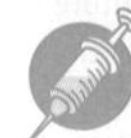

TREATMENT

- Whenever there is evidence of prescription drug abuse, the controlled substance should be stopped. Amphetamines may be stopped abruptly without risk of severe withdrawal or death.
- The opioid-abusing patient may be detoxed using clonidine, buprenorphine, or methadone. Buprenorphine has been shown to be more effective than clonidine in detox, and has demonstrated comparable effectiveness to methadone. However, buprenorphine has the advantage that withdrawal symptoms may resolve more quickly.

- Subutex (pure buprenorphine) lacks the naloxone component and should only be reserved for pregnant opioid-dependent patients; Subutex is prone to diversion and abuse, since patients can crush it and snort it, or shoot it and get high. This is not true of Suboxone. Methadone remains the gold standard of treatment for pregnant opiate-dependent women, although a 2008 study in Sweden showed less severity and less prolonged neonatal abstinence syndrome, higher-birth-weight babies, and shorter hospital stays in neonates born to mothers on Subutex compared to methadone (1)[B].
- Benzodiazepines cannot be stopped abruptly for risk of seizures and death. Cochrane Review supported a gradual withdrawal of benzodiazepines over a 10-week period. It did not find support for switching from short half-life to long half-life benzodiazepine before beginning the gradual taper, nor were any benefits discovered in using propranolol, buspirone, progesterone, hydroxyzine, or dothiepin.

MEDICATION

Use a chart demonstrating benzodiazepine equivalencies in order to convert the patient's benzodiazepine to diazepam to use for the duration of the taper. Sometimes, these charts tend to vary, but most North American conversion tables show that 10 mg of diazepam (Valium) is approximately equal to 1 mg of alprazolam (Xanax), 2 mg of lorazepam (Ativan), and 0.5 mg of clonazepam (Klonopin).

First Line

- Detox of opioid abuser: Clonidine 0.1–0.2 mg t.i.d. PRN autonomic hyperactivity (2)[A]. Buprenorphine 2–16 mg sublingual daily (3)[A]. Methadone 20–35 mg daily (4)(A).
- Maintenance opioid therapy in opioid-dependent patient:
  - Buprenorphine maintenance dose of 16–32 mg sublingual daily determined over a 3-day induction period (1)[B] equivalent to daily methadone doses of 60–100 mg in rates of treatment retention and opioid use.
  - Suboxone dose of 16 mg sublingual daily shown to be as effective as 90 mg methadone (1)[B]. Suboxone advantageous over methadone by not producing euphoria, not altering the person's consciousness/mood, not showing up in a urine drug screen at work, and low risk of respiratory depression and death. Another benefit of buprenorphine-based regimens is that withdrawal symptoms from cessation of long-term opioid maintenance therapy are often less with buprenorphine than with methadone.
  - Methadone starts very slowly at 10–30 mg daily, with very slow dose increases in the first few weeks, with daily recommended maintenance dose of 60–100 mg (1)[B].
- Benzodiazepine withdrawal: Convert to diazepam equivalent and taper slowly over ~10 weeks. The last half of the taper is the most difficult, so taper more slowly during the last few weeks. You may add carbamazepine 200–800 mg daily as adjunctive medication for benzodiazepine withdrawal symptoms, especially in patients who were dependent on 20 mg or more diazepam equivalents daily (5)[B].
- Stimulant withdrawal: Naltrexone 50 mg PO twice weekly has been shown to decrease amphetamine craving and reduce amphetamine use (6)[B].

Second Line

- Strattera may be helpful to manage ADHD symptoms at doses 40–100 mg daily in daily or b.i.d. dosing. Wellbutrin SR 150 mg b.i.d. can also be helpful in managing ADHD symptoms.
- Antidepressants may be helpful in reducing depression and anxiety commonly seen during benzodiazepine withdrawal, but randomized control trials are needed.

ADDITIONAL TREATMENT

General Measures

Self-help groups like Alcoholics Anonymous/Narcotics Anonymous may be helpful. Alanon/Alateen for family members. Cognitive behavior therapy aimed at anxiety reduction is helpful in benzodiazepine withdrawal.

Issues for Referral

Refer to chemical dependency groups/addiction specialists/pain management and psychiatry/psychology to treat underlying mood and anxiety disorders, PTSD, ADHD.

Additional Therapies

Behavioral sleep therapy may be helpful in managing insomnia.

COMPLEMENTARY AND ALTERNATIVE MEDICINE

Acupuncture, yoga, meditation, or martial arts may aid in anxiety management and stress reduction.

IN-PATIENT CONSIDERATIONS

Admission Criteria

Indications for inpatient detox are concomitant alcohol and benzodiazepine dependence (increased risk of seizures), mental confusion/delirium, history of seizures, psychosis, active suicidal ideation, serious comorbid medical issues, and absence of social support

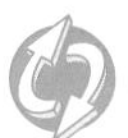

ONGOING CARE

PATIENT EDUCATION

- Advise patients receiving controlled medication to keep them hidden, inform them giving their medication to others may result in legal charges. When starting patients on controlled substances, warn them of potential addiction and withdrawal if the medication is stopped abruptly. Warn of the dangers of drug overdose causing respiratory depression and death with opioids and benzodiazepines (particularly if benzodiazepines are combined with alcohol or narcotics). Advise patients on controlled substances not to drink alcohol or use illicit drugs.
- Tell patient if he begins to need it in increasing amounts, uses it to feel high or overcome stress, or spends a lot of time craving it and thinking about his next dose to come to you and you will help him come up with a plan to comfortably stop the medication and try something new. Inform spouse/family members of this also.

REFERENCES

1. Maremmani I, Gerra G. Buprenorphine-based regimens and methadone for the medical management of opioid dependence: Selecting the appropriate drug for treatment. *Am J Addictions*. 2010;19:557–68.
2. Gowing L, Farrell M, Ali R, et al. Alpha 2-adrenergic agonists for the management of opioid withdrawal. *Cochrane Database Syst Rev*. 2009;CD002024.
3. Gowing L, Ali R, White JM, et al. Buprenorphine for the management of opioid withdrawal. *Cochrane Database Syst Rev*. 2009;CD002025.
4. Mattick RP, Breen C, Kimber J, et al. Methadone maintenance therapy versus no opioid replacement therapy for opioid dependence. *Cochrane Database Syst Rev*. 2009;CD002209.
5. Denis C, Fatseas M, Lavie E, et al. Pharmacological interventions for benzodiazepine monodependence management in outpatient settings. *Cochrane Database Syst Review*. 2008, issue 3.
6. Jayaram-Lindstrom N, Hammarberg A, Beck O, et al. Naltrexone for the treatment of amphetamine dependence: A randomized, placebo-controlled trial. *Am J Psychiatry*. 2008.

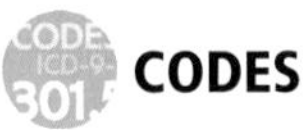

CODES

ICD9

- 305.40 Sedative, hypnotic or anxiolytic abuse, unspecified
- 305.50 Opioid abuse, unspecified
- 305.90 Other, mixed, or unspecified drug abuse, unspecified

CLINICAL PEARLS

- Screening: A single question: "How many times in the past year have you used an illegal drug or used a prescription medication for nonmedical reasons?"
- Avoid prescribing controlled substances and nonbenzodiazepine sleep aids (Ambien, Ambien CR) to patients at risk for substance abuse or axis 1 or axis 2 diagnoses.
- Discontinue prescription opioid analgesics if pain does not improve, if function does not improve, if there's evidence of prescription abuse or illicit drug abuse (i.e., positive UDS, DWI, accidental or intentional overdose, early refills).
- Try to limit benzodiazepine use to 2–4 weeks (i.e., when beginning an SSRI, but only until SSRI takes effect). Do not use benzos to treat depression, pain, or PTSD.
- Do frequent, observed urine drug screens.
- Addiction is a potentially fatal disease.

DUMPING SYNDROME

Hongyi Cui, MD, PhD
John J. Kelly, MD

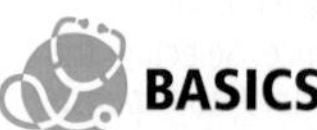

BASICS

DESCRIPTION

GI and vasomotor symptoms resulting from rapid gastric emptying and delivery of large amounts of hyperosmolar content into the small intestine. Usually occurs following gastric and esophageal surgery (gastrectomy, vagotomy, pyloroplasty, esophagectomy, Nissen fundoplication, or gastric bypass procedures).

EPIDEMIOLOGY

- Overall, about 10% of patients following gastric surgery and up to 50% of patients who undergo esophagectomy develop dumping symptoms.
- Predominant age: Middle age to elderly
- Predominant sex: Female > Male

Incidence

- In the US, 0.9% of proximal gastric vagotomy without any drainage procedure; 10–22% truncal vagotomy and drainage. After partial gastrectomy, 14–20% of patients develop symptoms of dumping.
- Prominent feature after bariatric surgery. Over 70% of gastric bypass patients experience varying degrees of dumping symptoms. Regarded as a beneficial feature of gastric bypass surgery, since patients learn to avoid calorie-rich foods and eat small meals.

RISK FACTORS

Accelerated gastric emptying resulting from gastric surgery is a main risk factor for dumping syndrome. In fact, the severity of dumping syndrome is proportional to the rate of gastric emptying. The common gastric surgical procedures associated with dumping syndrome are:

- Bariatric surgery (i.e., Roux-en-Y gastric bypass)
- Gastric drainage procedures (e.g., pyloroplasty)
- Partial gastrectomy
- Total gastrectomy: Those with pouch formation have significantly less dumping and heartburn (1)[A].
- Esophagectomy
- Antiulcer surgery (e.g., vagotomy)
- Antireflux surgery (e.g., Nissen fundoplication, especially in pediatric patients)

GENERAL PREVENTION

- Dietary modifications (i.e., eating frequent, small, dry meals that contain limited amount of refined carbohydrates; restrict fluids to between meals; avoid milk products and increase protein/fat intake and supplement dietary fibers, etc.)
- Postural changes (i.e., lying supine for 30 minutes after meals)
- New surgical techniques may reduce postoperative dumping syndrome in bariatric surgery (2)[B].

ETIOLOGY

The pathogenesis of dumping syndrome is multifactorial. It includes at least the following interplaying factors:

- Alterations in the storage function of the stomach and/or the pyloric emptying mechanism, leading to rapid delivery of hyperosmolar material into the intestine. This results in fluid shifts from the intravascular compartment into the bowel lumen, leading to rapid small-bowel distention and an increase in the frequency of bowel contractions (early dumping).
- Supraphysiologic release of various GI peptides/vasoactive mediators, leading to paradoxical vasodilation in a relatively volume-contracted state
- Reactive hypoglycemia secondary to hyperinsulinemia caused by high concentration of carbohydrates in the proximal small intestine and rapid absorption of glucose (late dumping)
- Pancreatic islet cell hyperplasia, rather than late dumping, is thought to be the underlying mechanism for hyperinsulinemic hypoglycemia with nesidioblastosis after gastric bypass. These patients do not respond to treatment for dumping syndrome, but the confirmation of such a rare condition is very cumbersome.

COMMONLY ASSOCIATED CONDITIONS

- Peptic ulcer disease
- Reactive hypoglycemia
- Gastrectomy/vagotomy/pyloroplasty
- Esophagectomy
- After Nissen fundoplication for reflux disease in pediatric population
- After gastric bypass procedure for morbid obesity

DIAGNOSIS

A suggestive symptom profile in a patient who has undergone gastric (including bariatric) or esophageal surgery warrants the investigation for dumping syndrome.

HISTORY

- History of gastric procedures
- GI symptoms (in early dumping):
  – Cramping abdominal pain
  – Diarrhea (postprandial)
  – Borborygmi
  – Bloating or epigastric fullness
  – Nausea/vomiting
- Systemic/vasomotor symptoms (both early and late dumping):
  – Palpitations
  – Diaphoresis
  – Faintness, fatigue, and headache
  – Flushing
  – Lightheadedness and desire to lie down
  – Confusion and syncope
  – Malnutrition and weight loss
- Early dumping symptoms include GI (abdominal pain, nausea, bloating, borborygmi and diarrhea, etc.) and vasomotor (perspiration and facial flushing, a desire to lie down, palpitations, weakness and syncope, etc.) symptoms; late dumping symptoms include perspiration, palpitations, hunger, weakness, confusion and syncope, etc.

PHYSICAL EXAM

- Diagnosis is mainly based on typical symptoms in patients with history of gastric procedures. A diagnostic scoring system has been developed by Sigstad based on various weighting factors allocated to the symptoms of dumping. A score index >7 is suggestive of dumping syndrome. The score index is very helpful in assessing a response to therapy.
- No physical signs are specific for dumping syndrome.

DIAGNOSTIC TESTS & INTERPRETATION

Lab

- Postprandial hypoglycemia
- Anemia
- Hypoalbuminemia
- Drugs that may alter lab results: Insulin
- Disorders that may alter lab results: Diabetes mellitus

Imaging

- Upper GI series: Barium rapidly emptying from stomach
- Nuclear medicine gastric emptying study
- Endoscopy (to define anatomy and exclude mechanical obstruction)

Diagnostic Procedures/Surgery

- Dumping syndrome is a clinical diagnosis based on typical symptoms in patients who have undergone gastric surgery.
- Oral glucose challenge test (i.e., oral intake of 50 g of glucose following 10-hour fasting) can elicit typical signs and symptoms in patients with dumping syndrome. A rise in heart rate by 10 beats per minute or more in the first hour is the best predictor for dumping syndrome.
- Hydrogen breath test after oral ingestion of glucose is also a sensitive test.

DIFFERENTIAL DIAGNOSIS

- Mechanical obstruction
- Gastroenteric fistula
- Celiac sprue
- Crohn disease
- Pancreatic exocrine insufficiency
- Neuroendocrine tumors (e.g., insulinoma and carcinoid)
- Irritable bowel syndrome
- Lactose intolerance

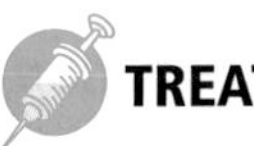

TREATMENT

Dietary modifications are the mainstay of treatment in patients with dumping syndrome. Medical therapy is effective in patients with incapacitating symptoms who fail dietary modifications. Remedial surgery is only considered in patients refractory to medical management.

MEDICATION

First Line

- Octreotide (Sandostatin, 100–500 μg SC b.i.d.) relieves dumping symptoms by delaying gastric emptying and inhibiting the release of GI hormones. Can be very expensive (3)[B]. Patients may have increased steatorrhea during octreotide treatment, and pancreatic enzyme supplement is effective in relieving this symptom. Gallstone formation is also associated with long-term use of octreotide.
- Late dumping symptoms can be ameliorated by the α-glucosidase inhibitor acarbose (100–200 mg PO t.i.d.), which lowers blood glucose by delaying GI absorption of carbohydrates. Patients on acarbose treatment often develop symptoms of bloating diarrhea due to bacterial fermentation of unabsorbed carbohydrate in the intestine.
- Pectin/guar gum (ingestion of up to 15 g with each meal) are effective by delaying glucose absorption and prolonging small-bowel transit time.

Second Line

Anticholinergics: Results generally are disappointing.

ADDITIONAL TREATMENT

General Measures

Most patients can be managed conservatively with dietary modification and medical treatment. Only a small percentage of patients ultimately require surgical intervention.

Additional Therapies

Continuous trophic enteral feeding via a jejunostomy has been reported to be an effective approach in patients refractory to all other treatment measures.

SURGERY/OTHER PROCEDURES

- Remedial surgery only if dietary and medical management unsuccessful and symptoms debilitating; the results are variable and unpredictable. A proper selection of the surgical intervention is very important. Most patients with dumping syndrome as a result of gastric bypass will find that the effects ameliorate with time (>2 years).
- Options of surgery include Roux-en-Y conversion (from Billroth I and II), pyloric reconstruction (for patients who have severe dumping following pyloroplasty), reversed jejunal segment (for patients who failed Roux-en-Y reconstruction), and conversion of Billroth II to Billroth I anastomosis.
- Patients with refractory dumping symptoms after loop gastrojejunostomy may benefit from simple takedown of the anastomosis; conversion to Roux-en-Y gastrojejunostomy is a reasonable option for patients with disabling dumping after distal gastrectomy. Other procedures have been attempted with limited success.
- The syndrome of hyperinsulinemic hypoglycemia with nesidioblastosis (a hyperplasia of islet cells) after Roux-en-Y gastric bypass (>1–2 year postop) can usually be managed with low-carbohydrate diet and alpha-glucosidase inhibitors. Subtotal or total pancreatectomy (as has been suggested in the literature) is usually unnecessary.

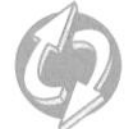

ONGOING CARE

FOLLOW-UP RECOMMENDATIONS

Lying supine for 30 minutes after eating or when symptoms occur may reduce the chance of syncope.

Patient Monitoring

Follow to be sure of adequate nutrition

DIET

- Low-carbohydrate, high-protein diet
- Add dietary fiber.
- Milk or milk products should be avoided.
- Frequent small meals with minimal liquid
- Avoid hyperosmolar liquids.

PATIENT EDUCATION

National Digestive Diseases Information Clearinghouse, Box NDDIC, Bethesda, MD 20892, (301) 468-6344, digestive.niddk.nih.gov

PROGNOSIS

Favorable

COMPLICATIONS

- Hypoglycemia
- Malnutrition and weight loss
- Electrolyte disturbances, including hypokalemia

REFERENCES

1. Gertler R, Rosenberg R, Feith M, et al. Pouch vs. no pouch following total gastrectomy: Meta-analysis and systematic review. *Am J Gastroenterol*. 2009; 104:2838–51.
2. Dikic S, Randjelovic T, Dragojevic S, et al. Early dumping syndrome and reflux esophagitis prevention with pouch reconstruction. *J Surg Res*. 2011.
3. Ukleja A. Dumping syndrome: Pathophysiology and treatment. *Nutr Clin Pract*. 2005;20:517–25.
4. Gonzalez-Sánchez JA, Corujo-Vázquez O, Sahai-Hernández M. Bariatric surgery patients: Reasons to visit emergency department after surgery. *Bol Asoc Med P R*. 2007;99:279–83.
5. Penning C, Vecht J, Masclee AA. Efficacy of depot long-acting release octreotide therapy in severe dumping syndrome. *Aliment Pharmacol Ther*. 2005;22:963–9.
6. Bouras EP, Scolapio JS. Gastric motility disorders: Management that optimizes nutritional status. *J Clin Gastroenterol*. 2004;38:549–57.

ADDITIONAL READING

Tack J, Arts J, Caenepeel P. Pathophysiology, diagnosis and management of postoperative dumping syndrome. *Nat Rev Gastroenterol Hepatol*. 2009;6:583–90.

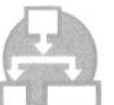

See Also (Topic, Algorithm, Electronic Media Element)

- Diarrhea, Chronic; Hypoglycemia, Nondiabetic; Peptic Ulcer Disease
- Algorithm: Diarrhea, Chronic

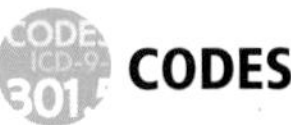

CODES

ICD9

564.2 Postgastric surgery syndromes

CLINICAL PEARLS

- Vagotomy affects gastric emptying through increased gastric tone and decreased receptive relaxation.
- Dumping syndrome is the most common cause for emergency room presentation after bariatric surgery (4)[B].
- An increase in heart rate of 10 BPM is noted after glucose challenge (50 g PO glucose) in patients with dumping syndrome.
- Depot octreotide has shown some promise as an alternative to standard SC octreotide (5)[B].
- Some side effects of octreotide are gallstones, steatorrhea, and diarrhea (6)[B].

DUPUYTREN CONTRACTURE

Jeffrey F. Minteer, MD

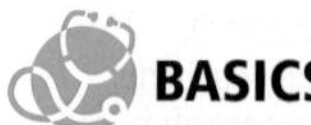

BASICS

DESCRIPTION

- Palmar fibromatosis; due to progressive fibrous proliferation and tightening of the fascia inside the palms, resulting in flexion deformities and loss of function
- Not the same as "trigger finger," which is caused by thickening of the distal flexor tendon
- Similar change may rarely occur in plantar fascia; it usually appears simultaneously.
- System(s) affected: Musculoskeletal

EPIDEMIOLOGY

Prevalence

- Unknown in US
- Norway: 9% males and 3% females

RISK FACTORS

- Smoking (mean 16 pack-years, odds ratio 2.8)
- Increasing age
- Male/Caucasian
- Workers exposed to vibration
- Diabetes mellitus (1/3 affected, increases with time, usually mild; middle and ring finger involved)
- Epilepsy
- Chronic illness (e.g., pulmonary tuberculosis, liver disease, HIV)
- Hypercholesterolemia
- Alcohol consumption

Genetics

- Autosomal-dominant with incomplete penetrance
- 68% of male relatives of affected patients develop disease at some time.

GENERAL PREVENTION

Avoid risk factors, especially with a strong family history.

ETIOLOGY

Unknown; possibly a T-cell–mediated autoimmune disorder

COMMONLY ASSOCIATED CONDITIONS

- Alcoholism
- Epilepsy
- Diabetes mellitus
- Chronic lung disease
- Occupational hand trauma (vibration white finger)
- Shoulder–hand syndrome
- Status postmyocardial infarction
- Hypercholesterolemia
- Carpal tunnel syndrome

DIAGNOSIS

HISTORY

- Caucasian male aged 50–60 years
- Family history
- Mild pain early
- Unilateral or bilateral (50%)
- Right hand more frequent
- Ring finger more frequent
- Ulnar digits more affected than radial digits

PHYSICAL EXAM

- Painless plaques or nodules in palmar fascia
- Extends into a cordlike band in the palmar fascia
- Skin adheres to fascia and becomes puckered.
- Nodules can be palpated under the skin.
- Digital fascia becomes involved as disease progresses.
- Reduced flexibility of metacarpophalangeal (MCP) and proximal interphalangeal (PIP) joints
- No sign of inflammation
- Web space contractures
- Dupuytren diathesis can involve plantar (Ledderhose—10%) and penile (Peyronie—2%) fascia
- Knuckle pads over PIP
- Disease stages:
  - Early: Skin pits (can also be seen in nevoid basal cell cancer and palmar keratosis)
  - Intermediate: Nodules and cords
  - Late: Contractures

DIAGNOSTIC TESTS & INTERPRETATION

Diagnostic Procedures/Surgery

MRI can assess cellularity of lesions that correlate with higher recurrence after surgery.

Pathological Findings

- Myofibroblasts
- First stage (proliferative): Increased myofibroblasts
- Second stage (residual): Dense fibroblast network
- Thrid stage (involutional): Myofibroblasts disappear

DIFFERENTIAL DIAGNOSIS

- Early for callosity
- Tendon abnormalities
- Camptodactyly: Early teens; tight fascial bands on ulnar side of small finger
- Diabetic cheiroarthropathy: All 4 fingers
- Volkmann ischemic contracture

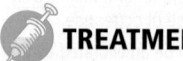

TREATMENT

MEDICATION

First Line

- Steroid injection for an acute tender nodule, painful knuckle pad
- Clostridial collagenase injections (FDA approved 2010):
  - Degrades collagen to allow manual rupture of diseased cord
  - Best for isolated cord of MCP joint
  - Recurrence rate at 8 years 67% in MCP joints, but less severe than initial contracture (1)[B]

Second Line
- Topical high-potency steroids: Case report of improvement with clobetasol 0.1% b.i.d. and at bedtime for 2–4 weeks
- Surgery for contracture >30%

ADDITIONAL TREATMENT
General Measures
- Physiotherapy alone is ineffective:
  - Intermittent splinting unlikely to be effective
  - Continuous splinting may be helpful in pre- and postoperative
- Isolated involvement of palmar fascia can be followed.
- MCP joint involvement can be followed if flexion contracture is <30°.

Issues for Referral
- Any involvement of PIP joints
- MCP joints contracted >30°
- Positive Hueston test

Additional Therapies
- Continuous elongation technique is useful to prepare a severely contracted PIP joint for surgery. The digit can frequently be completely extended; however, it will relapse if surgery is not performed.
- Prophylactic external beam radiation: 87% either no progression or improvement at 12 months; concern about local effects in a benign disease
- Intraoperative 5-fluorouracil ineffective
- Percutaneous and needle fasciotomy:
  - Best for MCP joint
  - Recurrence common
  - Not indicated in severe or recurrent disease

SURGERY/OTHER PROCEDURES
- Selective fascial ray release/partial fasciectomy (2)[B]
- Indications:
  - Any involvement of the PIP joints
  - MCP joints are contracted at least 30°.
  - Positive Hueston tabletop test: When the palm is placed on a flat surface, the digits cannot be simultaneously placed fully on the same surface as the palm because of flexion contractures.
- May require skin grafts for wound closure with severe cutaneous shrinkage. Reports of clinical regression with continuous passive skeletal traction in extension and under a skin graft.
- 80% have full range of movement if operated on early.
- Amputation of little finger if severe and deforming
- MCP joints respond better than PIP joints, especially if contracted >45°.

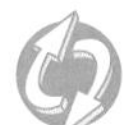

ONGOING CARE

FOLLOW-UP RECOMMENDATIONS
Patient Monitoring
Regular follow-up by physician every 6 months–1 year

PATIENT EDUCATION
- Avoid risk factors, especially with a strong family history.
- Mild disease: Passively stretch digits twice a day, and avoid recurrent gripping of tools.

PROGNOSIS
- Unpredictable, but usually slowly progressive
- 10% may regress spontaneously.
- Patients likely to have aggressive disease if 1 or more of the following are present: Age <40 years at onset, knuckle pads, positive family history, bilateral disease involving radial side of hand
- Recurrence rate after surgery is high; more with aggressive features
- Prognosis better for MCP joint vs. PIP joint after surgery and collagenase injection

COMPLICATIONS
- Postsurgery development of reflex sympathetic dystrophy
- Postoperative recurrence or extension in 46–80%
- Postoperative hand edema and skin necrosis
- Digital infarction

REFERENCES

1. Watt AJ, Curtin CM, Hentz VR, et al. Collagenase injection as nonsurgical treatment of dupuytren's disease: 8-year follow-up. *J Hand Surg Am*. 2010;35:534–9, 539.e1.
2. van Rijssen AL, Werker PM, et al. [Treatment of Dupuytren's contracture; an overview of options] *Ned Tijdschr Geneeskd*. 2009;153:A129.
3. Rayan GM. Clinical presentation and types of Dupuytren's disease. *Hand Clin*. 1999;15:87–96, vii.

ADDITIONAL READING

- Hunt TR. What is the appropriate treatment for Dupuytren contracture? *Cleve Clin J Med*. 2003;70:96–7.
- Hurst LC, Badalamente MA, Hentz VR, et al. Injectable collagenase clostridium histolyticum for Dupuytren's contracture. *N Engl J Med*. 2009;361: 968–79.
- Rayan GM. Duypuytren disease: Anatomy, pathology, presentation, and treatment. *J Bone Joint Surgery*. 2007;89(1):189–98.

CODES

ICD9
- 728.6 Contracture of palmar fascia
- 728.71 Plantar fascial fibromatosis

CLINICAL PEARLS
- 90% of cases are progressive.
- Refer those with any involvement of the PIP joints or MCP involvement >30°.
- Neither surgical nor enzymatic fasciotomy offers a cure; both have high rate of recurrence (3).

D

DYSFUNCTIONAL UTERINE BLEEDING

Pamela L. Grimaldi, DO
Kathryn Wilson, MD

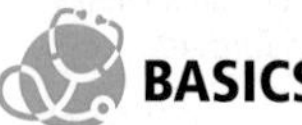

BASICS

DESCRIPTION

- Dysfunctional uterine bleeding (DUB) is irregular bleeding (usually heavy, prolonged, or frequent) that occurs in the absence of anatomic pathology.
- Associated with anovulatory menstrual cycles
- Typically is a diagnosis of exclusion: Need to exclude anatomic pathology and medical illnesses
- System(s) affected: Endocrine/metabolic, reproductive

EPIDEMIOLOGY

- Predominant age: 12–50 years
- Predominant gender: Women only
- Adolescents and perimenopausal women are affected most often.

Incidence

Accounts for 5–10% of outpatient gynecologic visits

Prevalence

Abnormal uterine bleeding occurs in:

- ~1 in 3 women of reproductive age
- ~1 in 10 postmenopausal women

RISK FACTORS

Risk factors for endometrial cancer (which can cause DUB):

- Age >40
- Obesity
- Diabetes mellitus
- Nulliparity
- Early menarche or late menopause (>55 years)
- Hypertension
- Chronic anovulation or infertility
- Unopposed estrogen therapy
- History of breast cancer or endometrial hyperplasia
- Tamoxifen use
- Family history: Gynecologic, breast, or colon cancer

Genetics

Unclear

PATHOPHYSIOLOGY

- Disruption of normal hormonal sequence of ovulatory menstrual cycle
- Anovulation accounts for 90% of DUB:
  - Loss of cyclic endometrial stimulation
  - Elevated estrogen levels stimulate endometrial growth.
  - Endometrium does not shed and eventually outgrows blood supply.
  - Tissue breaks down and sloughs from uterus.

ETIOLOGY

The diagnosis of DUB is made when pathologic causes of abnormal bleeding have been ruled out:

- Pregnancy:
  - Ectopic pregnancy, threatened or incomplete abortion, or hydatidiform mole
- Reproductive pathology and structural disorders:
  - Uterus: Leiomyomas, endometritis, hyperplasia, polyps, trauma
  - Adnexa: Salpingitis, functional ovarian cysts
  - Cervix: Cervicitis, polyps, STDs, trauma
  - Vagina: Trauma, foreign body
  - Vulva: Lichen sclerosis, STDs
- Malignancy of the vagina, cervix, uterus, and ovaries
- Systemic diseases:
  - Inflammatory bowel disease
  - Hematologic disorders (e.g., Von Willebrand disease, thrombocytopenia)
  - Advanced or fulminant liver disease
  - Chronic renal disease
- Diseases causing anovulation:
  - Hyperthyroidism/hypothyroidism
  - Adrenal disorders
  - Pituitary disease (prolactinoma)
  - Polycystic ovarian syndrome (PCOS)
  - Eating disorders
- Medications (iatrogenic causes):
  - Anticoagulants
  - Steroids
  - Tamoxifen
  - Hormonal medications: Intrauterine devices
  - SSRIs
  - Antipsychotic medications
- Other causes of abnormal uterine bleeding:
  - Excessive weight gain
  - Increased exercise
  - Stress

DIAGNOSIS

A thorough medical, surgical, social, and family history should be obtained.

HISTORY

- History of bleeding:
  - Onset, severity (quantified by pad/tampon use, presence and size of clots)
  - Association with other factors (e.g., coitus, contraception, weight loss/gain)
- Menstrual history:
  - Unpredictable or episodic, heavy or light bleeding
  - Menstrual symptoms typically do not precede bleeding
- Review of symptoms (exclude symptoms of pregnancy, symptoms of bleeding disorders, bleeding from other orifices, stress, exercise, recent weight change, visual changes, headaches, galactorrhea)
- Medication history (evaluate for use of aspirin, anticoagulants, hormones, herbal supplements)

ALERT

Postmenopausal bleeding is any bleeding that occurs >1 year after the last menstrual period; cancer must always be ruled out.

PHYSICAL EXAM

Discover anatomic or organic causes of DUB:

- Assess hemodynamic stability
- Evaluate for:
  - Obesity (body mass index)
  - Pallor
  - Visual field defects (pituitary lesion)
  - Hirsutism or acne (hyperandrogenism)
  - Goiter
  - Galactorrhea (hyperprolactinemia)
  - Purpura, ecchymosis (bleeding disorders)
- Pelvic exam:
  - Evaluate for uterine irregularities
  - Check for foreign bodies
  - Rule out rectal or urinary tract bleeding
  - Include Pap smear and tests for STDs

Pediatric Considerations

Premenarchal children with vaginal bleeding should be evaluated for foreign bodies, physical/sexual abuse, possible infections, and signs of precocious puberty.

DIAGNOSTIC TESTS & INTERPRETATION

Lab

Not always necessary

Initial lab tests

- Urine human chorionic gonadotropin (rule out pregnancy and/or hydatiform mole)
- CBC
- Thyroid-stimulating hormone (1)[B]
- Prolactin level
- Consider other tests based on differential diagnosis:
  - Follicle-stimulating hormone to evaluate for hypo- or hypergonadotropism
  - Coagulation studies and factors (2)[A]
  - Liver function tests
  - 17-hydroxyprogestrone
  - Androgenic hormones
  - *Neisseria gonorrhea*, *Chlamydia trachomatis* tests

Imaging

Initial approach

- Transvaginal US:
  - Indications: Postmenopausal patients, suspicion of pregnancy or anatomic abnormalities, PCOS
  - High sensitivity for endometrial carcinoma in postmenopausal women (3)[A]; if ≤4 mm, endometrial cancer is unlikely.
  - If endometrial thickness >5 mm, proceed to endometrial biopsy (EMB)
- Saline infusion sonohistogram: Often superior to TVUS in screening for anatomic abnormalities (4); can perform if TVUS is suspicious for lesion

Diagnostic Procedures/Surgery

- Pap smear to exclude cervical cancer
- EMB should be performed in women:
  - Women >35 years of age with DUB to rule out cancer or premalignancy
  - Women with endometrial thickness >5 mm
  - Women aged 18–35 with DUB and risk factors for endometrial cancer (see "Risk Factors")
  - Perform on or after day 18 of cycle if known; secretory endometrium confirms ovulation occurred
  - Does not diagnose leiomyosarcoma or fibroids because lesions are deep to endometrial lining
- Dilation and curettage:
  - Perform if bleeding is heavy, uncontrolled, and/or failed emergent medical management
  - Perform if unable to perform EMB in office
- Hysteroscopy if lesion suspected (diagnostic and therapeutic)

Pathological Findings

Pap smear could reveal carcinoma or inflammation indicative of cervicitis. Most EMBs show proliferative or dyssynchronous endometrium (suggesting anovulation).

DIFFERENTIAL DIAGNOSIS

See "Etiology."

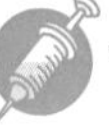

TREATMENT

Attempt to diagnose other causes of bleeding prior to instituting therapy.

MEDICATION

First Line

- Acute, emergent, nonovulatory bleeding (5):
  - Conjugated equine estrogen (Premarin): 25 mg IV q4h (maximum of 6 doses) or 2.5 mg PO q6h should control bleeding in 12–24 hours (6)[A]
  - Then change to OCP or progestin for cycle regulation
- Acute, nonemergent, nonovulatory:
  - Combination OCP with ≥30 μg estrogen given as a taper. An example of a tapered dose: 4 pills/d until bleeding stopped for 24 hours; 3 pills/d for 3 days; 2 pills/d for 3 days.
  - Then begin a once-a-day regimen (7)[B].
- Nonacute, nonovulatory:
  - OCPs: 20–35 μg estrogen plus progesterone (mono- or triphasic)
  - Progestins: Medroxyprogesterone acetate (Provera) 10 mg/d for 5–10 days each month. Daily progesterone for 21 days per cycle results in significantly less blood loss (8)[A].
  - Levonorgestrel intrauterine device (Mirena) is most effective (9)[A] and best suits most women long term (10)[A].
- Do not use estrogen if contraindications are present.
- Precautions:
  - Exclude endometrial hyperplasia and carcinoma before administering estrogen.
  - Consider deep vein thrombosis prophylaxis when treating with high-dose estrogens.
  - Failed medical treatment requires further workup.
  - Smokers >35 years of age should be counseled about the risk of thromboembolic disease when using OCPs.

Second Line

- GnRH agonists create a hypogonadotropic state, usually used as a bridge to definitive therapy.
- Danazol (Danocrine 200–400 mg/d) is more effective than NSAIDs but is limited by androgenic side effects and cost (11)[A]. It has been essentially replaced by GnRH agonists.
- Antifibrinolytics like tranexamic acid (Lysteda, 650 mg, 2 tablets t.i.d. (maximum of 5 days during menstruation) (12)[A].

ADDITIONAL TREATMENT

General Measures

NSAIDs (naproxen sodium 500 mg b.i.d., mefenamic acid 500 mg t.i.d., ibuprofen 600–1,200 mg/d):

- Decreases amount of blood loss compared with placebo (11)[A]
- Diminishes pain

Issues for Referral

- If an obvious cause for vaginal bleeding is not found in a pediatric patient, refer to a pediatric endocrinologist.
- Patients with persistent bleeding despite medical treatment require re-evaluation and referral to a gynecologist.

Additional Therapies

- Antiemetics if treating with high-dose estrogen
- Iron supplementation if anemia (usually iron deficiency) is identified

SURGERY/OTHER PROCEDURES

- Hysterectomy if there is endometrial cancer, if medical therapy fails, or if there is uterine pathology
- Endometrial ablation is less expensive than hysterectomy and has high satisfaction; medical treatment does not have to fail first (13)[A].

IN-PATIENT CONSIDERATIONS

Initial Stabilization

With acute bleeding, replace volume with crystalloid and blood as necessary.

Admission Criteria

Significant hemorrhage causing acute anemia with signs of hemodynamic instability

Nursing

Pad counts and clot size can be helpful to determine and monitor amount of bleeding.

Discharge Criteria

- Hemodynamic stability
- Control of vaginal bleeding

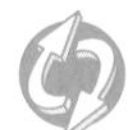

ONGOING CARE

FOLLOW-UP RECOMMENDATIONS

Routine follow-up with a primary care or OB/GYN provider

Patient Monitoring

Women treated with estrogen or OCPs should keep a menstrual diary to document bleeding patterns and their relation to therapy.

DIET

No restrictions

PATIENT EDUCATION

- Explain possible/likely etiologies
- Answer all questions, especially those related to cancer and fertility
- http://www.acog.org

PROGNOSIS

- Varies with pathophysiologic process
- Most anovulatory cycles can be treated with medical therapy and do not require surgical intervention.

COMPLICATIONS

- Iron-deficiency anemia
- Uterine cancer in cases of prolonged unopposed estrogen stimulation

REFERENCES

1. Albers J, et al. Abnormal uterine bleeding. *Am Fam Physician*. 2004;69:8.
2. Kouides PA, et al. Hemostasis and menstruation: Appropriate investigation for underlying disorders of hemostasis in women with extensive menstrual bleeding. *Fertil Steril*. 2005;84(5):1345–51.
3. Dijkhuizen FP, et al. The accuracy of transvaginal ultrasonography in the diagnosis of endometrial abnormalities. *Obstet Gynecol*. 1996;87(3): 345–9.
4. Maness DL, Reddy A, Harraway-Smith CL, et al. How best to manage dysfunctional uterine bleeding. *J Fam Pract*. 2010;59:449–58.
5. Casablanca Y. Management of dysfunctional uterine bleeding. *Obstet Gynecol Clin North Am*. 2008;35:219–34.
6. DeVore GR, et al. Use of intravenous Premarin in the treatment of dysfunctional uterine bleeding: A double-blind randomized control study. *Obstet Gynecol*. 1982;59(3):285–91.
7. Rimsza ME. Dysfunctional uterine bleeding. *Pediatr Rev*. 2002;23(7):227–33.
8. Lethaby A, et al. Cyclical progestogens for heavy menstrual bleeding. *Cochrane Database Syst Rev*. 2008;(1):CD001016.
9. Lethaby AE, Cooke I, Rees M, et al. Progesterone or progestogen-releasing intrauterine systems for heavy menstrual bleeding. *Cochrane Database Syst Rev*. 2005;CD002126.
10. Marjoribanks J, Lethaby A, Farquhar C, et al. Surgery versus medical therapy for heavy menstrual bleeding. *Cochrane Database Syst Rev*. 2006;CD003855.
11. Lethaby A, Augood C, Duckitt K, et al. Nonsteroidal anti-inflammatory drugs for heavy menstrual bleeding. *Cochrane Database Syst Rev*. 2007;CD000400.
12. Lethaby A, Farquhar C, Cooke I, et al. Antifibrinolytics for heavy menstrual bleeding. *Cochrane Database Syst Rev*. 2000;CD000249.
13. Lethaby A, Shepperd S, Cooke I, et al. Endometrial resection and ablation versus hysterectomy for heavy menstrual bleeding. *Cochrane Database Syst Rev*. 2000;CD000329.

ADDITIONAL READING

- Chen EC, Danis PG, Tweed E, et al. Clinical inquiries. Menstrual disturbances in perimenopausal women: What's best? *J Fam Pract*. 2009;58:E3.
- LaCour DE, Long DN, Perlman SE, et al. Dysfunctional uterine bleeding in adolescent females associated with endocrine causes and medical conditions. *J Pediatr Adolesc Gynecol*. 2010;23:62–70.
- Lethaby A, Irvine G, Cameron I, et al. Cyclical progestogens for heavy menstrual bleeding. *Cochrane Database Syst Rev*. 2008;CD001016.

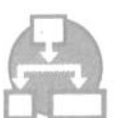

See Also (Topic, Algorithm, Electronic Media Element)

- Dysmenorrhea; Menorrhagia
- Algorithm: Menorrhagia

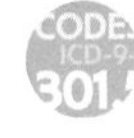

CODES

ICD9

- 626.7 Postcoital bleeding
- 626.8 Other disorders of menstruation and other abnormal bleeding from female genital tract
- 628.0 Infertility, female, associated with anovulation

CLINICAL PEARLS

- Uterine bleeding in premenarchal and postmenopausal women is always abnormal and should prompt immediate evaluation.
- DUB is irregular bleeding that occurs in the absence of pathology, making it a diagnosis of exclusion.
- Anovulation accounts for 90% of DUB.
- An EMB should be performed in all women >35 years of age with DUB to rule out cancer or premalignancy, and it should be considered in women aged 18–35 with DUB and risk factors for endometrial cancer.

D

DYSHIDROSIS

Rebecca A. Frye, DO
Scott Frye, MD

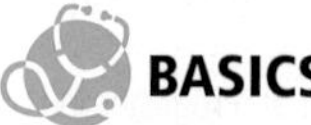

BASICS

DESCRIPTION

- A skin rash (dermatitis) of which there are several different classes within the family "dyshidrosis," and strict definitions are disputed
- Dyshidrotic eczema:
  - Common, chronic, or recurrent; nonerythematous; vesicular eruption primarily of the palms, soles, and interdigital areas
  - Associated with burning, itching, and pain
- Pompholyx (from Greek, "bubble"):
  - Rare condition characterized by abrupt onset of large bullae
  - Sometimes used interchangeably with dyshidrosis, although many believe them to be discrete entities
- Lamellar dyshidrosis:
  - Fine, spreading exfoliation of the superficial epidermis in the same distribution as described above
- System(s) affected: Dermatologic; Exocrine; Immunologic
- Synonym(s): Pompholyx; Cheiropompholyx; Keratolysis exfoliativa; Dyshidrotic eczema; Vesicular palmoplantar eczema; Desquamation of interdigital spaces; Palmar pompholyx reaction

EPIDEMIOLOGY

Incidence

- Incidence is 0.5%.
- Mean age of onset is <40 years.
- Male = Female
- Comprises 5–20% of hand eczema cases

Prevalence

20 cases per 100,000

RISK FACTORS

- Many risk factors are disputed in the literature, with none being consistently associated
- Atopy
- Other dermatologic conditions:
  - Atopic dermatitis (early in life)
  - Contact dermatitis (later in life)
  - Dermatophytosis
- Sensitivity to:
  - Foods
  - Drugs: Neomycin, quinolones, acetaminophen, and oral contraceptives
  - Nickel (seen in patients treated with disulfiram, which causes a high serum level of nickel)
  - Smoking in males

Genetics

- Atopy: 50% of patients with dyshidrotic eczema have atopic dermatitis.
- Rare autosomal dominant form of pompholyx found in Chinese population maps to chromosome 18q22.1–18q22.3 (1)

GENERAL PREVENTION

- Control emotional stress.
- Avoid excessive sweating.
- Avoid exposure to irritants.
- Avoid diet high in metal salts (chromium, cobalt, nickel).

PATHOPHYSIOLOGY

- Exact mechanism unknown; thought to be multifactorial
- On dermatopathology, vesicles are found in spongiotic dermatitis.

ETIOLOGY

- Exact cause not known
- Aggravating factors (debated):
  - Hyperhidrosis (in 40% of patients with the condition)
  - Climate: Hot or cold weather; humidity
  - Nickel sensitivity
  - Irritating compounds and solutions
  - Stress
  - Dermatophyte infection
  - Prolonged wear of occlusive gloves
  - IV immunoglobulin therapy
  - Smoking

COMMONLY ASSOCIATED CONDITIONS

- Atopic dermatitis
- Allergic contact dermatitis
- Parkinson disease

DIAGNOSIS

HISTORY

- Episodes of pruritic rash
- Recent emotional stress
- Familial or personal history of atopy
- Exposure to allergens or irritants (2):
  - Occupational, dietary, or household
  - Cosmetic and personal hygiene products
- Costume jewelry use
- IV immunoglobulin therapy
- HIV
- Smoking

PHYSICAL EXAM

- Symmetric distribution on the palms and soles; also may affect the dorsal aspects of hands and feet
- Early findings:
  - 1–2 mm, clear, nonerythematous, deep-seated vesicles
- Late findings:
  - Unroofed vesicles with inflamed bases
  - Desquamation
  - Peeling, rings of scale, or lichenification common

DIAGNOSTIC TESTS & INTERPRETATION

Lab

Follow-Up & Special Considerations

- Skin culture in suspected secondary infection (most commonly *Staphylococcus aureus*) (3)
- Consider antibiotics based on culture results and severity of symptoms.

Diagnostic Procedures/Surgery

- Diagnosis is based on clinical exam.
- KOH wet mount (if concerned about dermatophyte infection)
- Patch test (if suspect allergic cause)

Pathological Findings

- Fine 1–2-mm spongiotic vesicles intraepidermally with little to no inflammatory changes
- No eccrine glandular involvement
- Thickened stratum corneum

DIFFERENTIAL DIAGNOSIS

- Vesicular tinea pedis/manus
- Vesicular id reaction
- Contact dermatitis (allergic or irritant)
- Scabies
- Chronic vesicular hand dermatitis
- Drug reaction
- Dermatophytid
- Bullous disorders: Dyshidrosiform bullous pemphigoid, pemphigus, bullous impetigo, epidermolysis bullosa
- Pustular psoriasis
- Acrodermatitis continua
- Erythema multiforme
- Herpes infection
- Pityriasis rubra pilaris
- Vesicular mycosis fungoides

TREATMENT

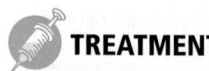

Identification and avoidance of aggravating factors

MEDICATION

First Line

- Mild cases: Topical steroids (high potency) (4)[B]:
  - Considered cornerstone of therapy, but limited published evidence
- Moderate-to-severe cases:
  - Ultrahigh-potency topical steroids with occlusion over treated area (3)[B]
  - Oral steroids 40–100 mg/d tapered after blister formation ceases (4)[B]
  - Psoralens plus ultraviolet (UV)-A therapy (PUVA), either oral *or* immersion in psoralens (5)[B]:
    - Oral 8-methoxypsoralen (8-MOP) dose: 0.6 mg/kg taken 1 hour prior to UVA irradiation
    - Immersion in 8-MOP: Solution of 5 mg/L of water × 15 minutes immediately preceding UVA irradiation
- Recurrent cases (3)[B]:
  - Systemic steroids at onset of itching prodrome
  - Prednisone 60 mg PO × 3–4 days

Second Line
- Topical calcineurin inhibitors (mitigate the long-term risks of topical steroid use):
  - Topical tacrolimus (6)[B]
  - Topical pimecrolimus (6)[B]
  - May not be as effective on plantar surface
- Other therapies (most likely to be limited to dermatologist use only):
  - Oral cyclosporine (3)[B]
  - Injections of botulinum toxin type A (BTXA) (6)[B]:
    - Newer topical forms of BTXA currently being developed and show promise
  - Systemic alitretinoin (6)[B]
  - Topical bexarotene (a retinoid X receptor agonist approved for use in cutaneous T-cell lymphoma) (6)[B]
  - Methotrexate (6)[C]

ADDITIONAL TREATMENT
- Radiation therapy (7)[C]
- UV-free phototherapy (6)[C]

General Measures
- Avoid possible causative factors: Stress, direct skin contact with irritants, nickel, occlusive gloves, smoking, sweating
- Moisturizers/emollients for symptomatic relief and to maintain effective skin barrier
- Skin care:
  - Wear shoes with leather rather than rubber soles (e.g., sneakers).
  - Wear socks and gloves made of cotton and change frequently.
  - Wash infrequently, carefully dry, then apply emollient.

Issues for Referral
- Allergist (if allergen testing required)
- Psychologist (if stress modification needed)

COMPLEMENTARY AND ALTERNATIVE MEDICINE
- Topical treatments to minimize pruritus (not curative) (3)[C]: Burrow solution (aluminum acetate) or vinegar compress
- Exposure to sunlight as maintenance therapy (8)[C]
- Dandelion juice (avoid in atopic patients) (6)[C]

ONGOING CARE

FOLLOW-UP RECOMMENDATIONS

Patient Monitoring
- Dyshidrotic Eczema Area and Severity Index (DASI)
- Parameters used in the DASI score:
  - Number of vesicles per square centimeter
  - Erythema
  - Desquamation
  - Severity of itching
  - Surface area affected
- Grading: Mild (0–15), moderate (16–30), severe (31–60)
- Monitor BP and glucose in patients receiving systemic corticosteroids.
- Monitor for adverse effects of medications.

DIET
- Consider diet low in metal salts if there is history of nickel sensitivity (3)[B].
- Updated recommendations for low-cobalt diet are available (9).

PATIENT EDUCATION
- Instructions on self-care, complications, and avoidance of triggers/aggravating factors
- Suggested Web site for patients: www.nlm.nih.gov

PROGNOSIS
- Condition is benign.
- Usually heals without scarring
- Lesions may spontaneously resolve.
- Recurrence is common.

COMPLICATIONS
- Secondary bacterial infections (*Staphylococcus aureus* most common)
- Dystrophic nail changes
- Fissures
- Skin tightening/discomfort
- Psychological distress

REFERENCES

1. Chen J, et al. The gene for a rare autosomal dominant form of pompholyx maps to chromosome 18q22.1–18q22.3. *J Invest Dermatol*. 2006;126: 300–4.
2. Guillet MH, Wierzbicka E, Guillet S, et al. A 3-year causative study of pompholyx in 120 patients. *Arch Dermatol*. 2007;143:1504–8.
3. Lofgren SM. Dyshidrosis: Epidemiology, clinical characteristics, and therapy. *Dermatitis*. 2006;17: 165–81.
4. Wollina U, et al. Pompholyx: A review of clinical features, differential diagnosis, and management. *Am J Clin Dermatol*. 2010;11:305–14.
5. Tzaneva S, Kittler H, Thallinger C, et al. Oral vs. bath PUVA using 8-methoxypsoralen for chronic palmoplantar eczema. *Photodermatol Photoimmunol Photomed*. 2009;25:101–5.
6. Wollina U. Pompholyx: What's new? *Expert Opin Investig Drugs*. 2008;17:897–904.
7. Sumila M, Notter M, Itin P, et al. Long-term results of radiotherapy in patients with chronic palmoplantar eczema or psoriasis. *Strahlentherapie und Onkologie*. 2008;184:218–23.
8. Leti M. Exposure to sunlight as adjuvant therapy for dyshidrotic eczema. *Med Hypotheses*. 2009.
9. Stuckert J, Nedorost S. Low-cobalt diet for dyshidrotic eczema patients. *Contact Dermatitis*. 2008;59:361–5.

ADDITIONAL READING

- Rashid RD, Salah W, Keuer EJ. Vexing vesicles. *J Med*. 2007;120:589–90.
- Thiers BH. What's new in dermatologic therapy. *Dermatol Ther*. 2008;21:142–9.
- Veien NK. Acute and recurrent vesicular hand dermatitis. *Dermatol Clin*. 2009;27:337–53.

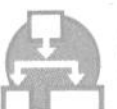

See Also (Topic, Algorithm, Electronic Media Element)

Algorithm: Rash, Focal

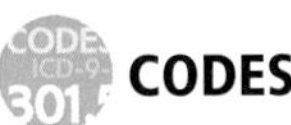

CODES

ICD9

705.81 Dyshidrosis

CLINICAL PEARLS
- Dyshidrosis is a transient, recurrent vesicular eruption most commonly of the palms, soles and interdigital areas.
- The etiology and pathophysiology are unknown, but are most likely related to a combination of genetic and environmental factors.
- The best prevention is limiting exposure to irritating agents and effective skin care.
- Treatments are based on severity of disease, and preferred treatments include topical steroids, oral steroid, and calcineurin inhibitors.
- The condition is benign and usually heals spontaneously and without scarring. Medical treatment decreases healing time and risk for progression to secondary bacterial infection.

DYSMENORRHEA

Pamela L. Grimaldi, DO, FAAFP
Kathryn Wilson, MD

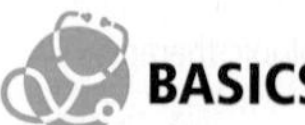

BASICS

DESCRIPTION
- Pelvic pain occurring at or around the time of menses; a leading cause of absenteeism for women <30 years
- Primary dysmenorrhea: Without pathologic physical findings
- Secondary dysmenorrhea: Often more severe than primary, having a secondary pathologic (structural) cause
- Classified by severity:
  - Mild: Pelvic discomfort, cramping, or heaviness on first day of bleeding with no associated symptoms
  - Moderate: Discomfort occurring during first 2–3 days of menses and accompanied by mild malaise, diarrhea, and headache
  - Severe: Intense, cramp-like pain lasting 2–7 days, often with nausea, diarrhea, back pain, thigh pain, and headache
- System(s) affected: Reproductive
- Synonym(s): Menstrual cramps

EPIDEMIOLOGY
- Predominant age:
  - Primary: Teens to early 20s
  - Secondary: 20s–30s
- Predominant sex: Women only

Prevalence
- >50% of adult women have menstrual pain.
- 10% are incapacitated for 1–3 days each cycle.

RISK FACTORS
- Primary:
  - Nulliparity
  - Obesity
  - Cigarette smoking
  - Positive family history
- Secondary:
  - Pelvic infection
  - Sexual transmitted diseases (STDs)
  - Endometriosis

Genetics
Not well studied

GENERAL PREVENTION
- Primary: Choose a diet low in animal fats, dairy products, and eggs. Increase vegetables, raw seeds, and nuts to increase production of beneficial prostaglandins. Consider supplementation with zinc 30 mg, taken 1–3 times daily for 1–4 days prior to the expected onset of menses.
- Secondary: Reduce risk of STDs

PATHOPHYSIOLOGY
See "Etiology."

ETIOLOGY
- Primary: Elevated production (2–7 times normal) of prostaglandins and other mediators in the uterus that produce uterine ischemia through:
  - Platelet aggregation
  - Vasoconstriction
  - Uterine contractions generating pressures higher than the systemic BP
- Secondary:
  - Congenital abnormalities of uterine or vaginal anatomy
  - Cervical stenosis
  - Pelvic infection
  - Adenomyosis
  - Endometriosis
  - Pelvic tumors, especially leiomyomata (fibroids)
  - Uterine polyps
  - Copper-containing intrauterine device (IUD)

Pediatric Considerations
Onset with first menses raises probability of genital tract anatomic abnormality, such as transverse vaginal septum, minimally perforated hymen, and uterine anomalies.

COMMONLY ASSOCIATED CONDITIONS
- Obesity
- Hyperestrogenic states
- Longer menstrual cycle length

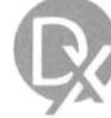

DIAGNOSIS

- Primary: History is characteristic.
- Based on characteristic history of cramping pain felt in suprapubic or low back
- Patients may have associated diarrhea, headache, or pain radiating into the inner thighs.

HISTORY
- Onset of symptoms
- Recurrence at or just before the onset of the menstrual flow:
  - Pelvic pain occurring between menstrual periods is not likely to be dysmenorrhea.
- Relief associated with:
  - Continued bleeding for the usual duration
  - Use of analgesics, especially NSAIDs
  - Orgasm
  - Local heat application
- Response to dietary supplements or NSAIDs helps confirm diagnosis.

PHYSICAL EXAM
- Primary: Physical exam typically is normal.
- Secondary: Exam may show evidence of uterine enlargement, tenderness, irregularity, or fixation.

DIAGNOSTIC TESTS & INTERPRETATION
Lab
- Pregnancy test to rule out ectopic pregnancy
- Cervical cultures to rule out infection
- Drugs that may alter lab results:
  - Antibiotics

Follow-Up & Special Considerations
Counsel regarding appropriate preventive measures for sexually transmitted infection and pregnancy.

Imaging
Initial approach
- Primary: Consider pelvic ultrasound to rule out secondary abnormalities if history is not characteristic.
- Secondary: Ultrasound or laparoscopy to define anatomy

Diagnostic Procedures/Surgery
Laparoscopy is rarely needed.

Pathological Findings
- Primary:
  - None
- Secondary:
  - Uterine enlargement
  - Leiomyomata
  - Ligamentous thickening
  - Fixation of pelvic structures
  - Endometritis
  - Salpingitis
  - Adenomyosis

DIFFERENTIAL DIAGNOSIS
- Primary:
  - History is characteristic
- Secondary:
  - Pelvic or genital infection
  - Complication of pregnancy
  - Missed or incomplete abortion
  - Ectopic pregnancy
  - Uterine or ovarian neoplasm
  - Endometriosis
  - UTI
  - Complication with IUD

Pregnancy Considerations
Consider ectopic pregnancy if there is a differential diagnosis of pelvic pain with vaginal bleeding.

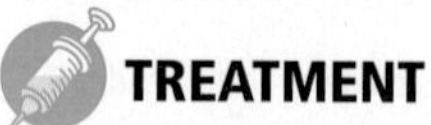

TREATMENT

- Reassure the patient that treatment success is very likely with adherence to recommendations.
- Relief may require the use of several treatment modalities at the same time.

MEDICATION
First Line
- NSAIDs (1): All NSAIDs studied have been found to be equally effective in the relief of dysmenorrhea. Because NSAIDs work by inhibiting prostaglandin synthesis, taking them at the very onset of menses (or whenever the cramping starts) provides the most relief.
  - Ibuprofen 400–600 mg q6h
  - Naproxen sodium 550 mg q12h
- Combination oral contraceptives (OCs) in monthly and especially in 3–5-month cycles may improve or eliminate dysmenorrhea, although they may be associated with increased breakthrough menstrual spotting (2)[B]:
  - Combination OCs containing $\leq$20 μg of ethinyl estradiol have not been found to be effective in reducing menstrual pain.
- Potential contraindications to NSAIDs and combination OC methods:
  - Platelet disorders
  - Gastric ulceration or gastritis
  - Thromboembolic disorders
  - Vascular disease
  - Other contraindications to OCs
- Precautions:
  - GI irritation
  - Lactation
  - Coagulation disorders
  - Impaired renal function
  - Congestive heart failure
  - Liver dysfunction

- Significant possible interactions:
  - Coumadin-type anticoagulants
  - Aspirin with other NSAIDs
  - Methotrexate
  - Furosemide
  - Lithium

Second Line

- Mefenamic acid 500 mg for 1 dose followed by 250 mg q6h may used if other NSAIDs are ineffective because it blocks production of prostaglandins as well as already-formed prostaglandins (1)[A].
- Progestin-containing IUD (Mirena) can help reduce bleeding and pain and even cause cessation of menses in suitable candidates.
- Behavioral interventions, such as relaxation exercises and meditation, have been shown to decrease pain during menstruation (3)[A].

ADDITIONAL TREATMENT

General Measures

- General physical conditioning: exercise raises endorphins and decreases pain
- High-frequency transcutaneous electrical nerve stimulation (TENS) was found to be effective for the treatment of dysmenorrhea, but with mild adverse events. No evidence for low-frequency TENS was found (4)[A].
- Secondary dysmenorrhea: Treatment of infections; suppression of endometrium if endometriosis suspected; remove copper IUD if suspected

COMPLEMENTARY AND ALTERNATIVE MEDICINE

- Osteopathic manipulation, including treatment of the sacrum and pelvis (5)[B]
- Aromatherapy with lavender, clary sage, rose oils, and abdominal massage decreases the intensity of pain (6)[B].
- Chinese herbal medicine shows promising evidence of decreasing pain, but more evidence is needed (7)[B].
- Acupuncture treatments have been shown to decrease pain in dysmenorrhea but further randomized, well-designed studies are needed (8)[B].

SURGERY/OTHER PROCEDURES

- Adenomyosis may require hysterectomy.
- Uterine artery embolization may be an alternative to hysterectomy for patients with leiomyomata (fibroid tumors) (9).

IN-PATIENT CONSIDERATIONS

Both primary and secondary dysmenorrhea usually are managed in the outpatient setting.

Initial Stabilization

- Primary: Outpatient care
- Secondary: Usually outpatient care

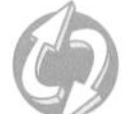

ONGOING CARE

FOLLOW-UP RECOMMENDATIONS

Normal

DIET

- Vitamin B_1 100 mg daily has been shown to be helpful in dysmenorrhea (10)[B].
- Magnesium has been shown to be useful, but the correct dosage has not been determined (10)[B].
- Insufficient evidence to show usefulness of fish oil, zinc, and vitamin E at this time (10)[B]
- Low-fat vegetarian diet can be helpful in some patients but difficult to adhere to

PATIENT EDUCATION

Reassure the patient that primary dysmenorrhea is treatable with use of dietary supplements and/or NSAIDs prior to menses and/or OCs, and that it will usually abate with age and parity.

PROGNOSIS

- Primary: Improves with age and parity
- Secondary: Likely to require therapy based on underlying cause

COMPLICATIONS

- Primary: Anxiety and/or depression
- Secondary: Infertility from underlying pathology

REFERENCES

1. Marjoribanks J, Proctor ML, Farquhar C, et al. Nonsteroidal anti-inflammatory drugs for primary dysmenorrhoea. *Cochrane Database Syst Rev.* 2003;CD001751.
2. Proctor ML, Roberts H, Farquhar CM, et al. Combined oral contraceptive pill (OCP) as treatment for primary dysmenorrhoea. *Cochrane Database Syst Rev.* 2001;CD002120.
3. Proctor ML, Murphy PA, Pattison HM, et al. Behavioural interventions for primary and secondary dysmenorrhoea. *Cochrane Database Syst Rev.* 2007;CD002248.
4. Proctor ML, Smith CA, Farquhar CM, et al. Transcutaneous electrical nerve stimulation and acupuncture for primary dysmenorrhoea. *Cochrane Database Syst Rev.* 2002;CD002123.
5. Chadwick K and Morgan A. The efficacy of osteopathic treatment for primary dysmenorrhea in young women. *The AAO Journal: A Publication of the American Academy of Osteopathy.* 1996 Fall;6(3):15–17, 29–31.
6. Han SH, Hur MH, Buckle J, et al. Effect of aromatherapy on symptoms of dysmenorrhea in college students: A randomized placebo-controlled clinical trial. *J Altern Complement Med.* 2006;12:535–41.
7. Zhu X, Proctor M, Bensoussan A, et al. Chinese herbal medicine for primary dysmenorrhoea. *Cochrane Database Syst Rev.* 2008;CD005288.
8. Smith CA, Zhu X, He L, et al. Acupuncture for primary dysmenorrhoea. *Cochrane Database Syst Rev.* 2011;CD007854.
9. Bradley LD, et al. Uterine fibroid embolization: A viable alternative to hysterectomy. *Am J Obstet Gynecol.* 2009;201:127–35.
10. Proctor ML, Murphy PA, et al. Herbal and dietary therapies for primary and secondary dysmenorrhoea. *Cochrane Database Syst Rev.* 2001;CD002124.

ADDITIONAL READING

- Cho SH, Hwang EW, et al. Acupuncture for primary dysmenorrhoea: A systematic review. *BJOG.* 2010;117:509–21.
- Eby G. Zinc treatment prevents dysmenorrhea. *Med Hypoth.* 2007;69.2:297–301.
- French L. Dysmenorrhea. *Am Fam Physician.* 2005;71:285–91.
- Giudice LC, et al. Clinical practice. Endometriosis. *N Engl J Med.* 2010;362:2389–98.
- Guerrera MP, Volpe SL, Mao JJ, et al. Therapeutic uses of magnesium. *Am Fam Physician.* 2009;80: 157–62.
- Harel Z, Biro FM, Kottenhahn RK, et al. Supplementation with omega-3 polyunsaturated fatty acids in the management of dysmenorrhea in adolescents. *Am J Ob Gyn.* 1996;174:1335–8.
- Milsom I, Hedner N, Mannheimer C. A comparative study of the effect of high-intensity transcutaneous nerve stimulation and oral naproxen on intrauterine pressure and menstrual pain in patients with primary dysmenorrhea. *Am J Obstet Gynecol.* 1994;170:123–9.
- Sanfilippo J, Erb T. Evaluation and management of dysmenorrhea in adolescents. *Clin Obstet Gynecol.* 2008;51:257–67.
- Stones RW, Mountfield J, et al. Interventions for treating chronic pelvic pain in women. *Cochrane Database Syst Rev.* 2000;CD000387.
- Transdermal nitroglycerine in the management of pain associated with primary dysmenorrhoea: a multinational pilot study. The Transdermal Nitroglycerine/Dysmenorrhoea Study Group. *J Int Med Res.* 1997;25:41–4.
- White AR. A review of controlled trials of acupuncture for women's reproductive health care. *J Fam Plan Reprod Health Care.* 2003;29:233–6.
- Yang H, Liu CZ, Chen X, et al. Systematic review of clinical trials of acupuncture-related therapies for primary dysmenorrhea. *Acta Obstet Gynecol Scand.* 2008:1–9.
- Zhao L, Li P. A survey of acupuncture treatment for primary dysmenorrhea. *J Tradit Chin Med.* 2009;29: 71–6.
- Ziaei S, Zakeri M, Kazemnejad A, et al. A randomised controlled trial of vitamin E in the treatment of primary dysmenorrhoea. *BJOG.* 2005;112:466–9.

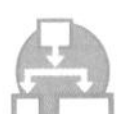

See Also (Topic, Algorithm, Electronic Media Element)

- Endometriosis
- Algorithm: Pelvic Girdle Pain

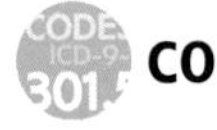

CODES

ICD9

625.3 Dysmenorrhea

CLINICAL PEARLS

- Dysmenorrhea is a leading cause of absenteeism for women <30 years old.
- Lifestyle and dietary supplement therapies are preferable for long-term treatment because they have equal or greater efficacy and pose fewer health risks than NSAIDs or hormonal contraceptives.
- All NSAIDs studied have been found to be equally effective in the relief of dysmenorrhea.

DYSPAREUNIA

Scott T. Henderson, MD

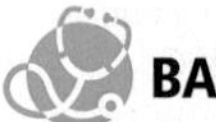

BASICS

DESCRIPTION

- Recurrent and persistent genital pain associated with sexual activity that is not exclusively due to lack of lubrication or vaginismus.
- May be the result of organic, emotional, or psychogenic causes:
  - Primary: Present throughout one's sexual history
  - Secondary: Arising from some specific event or condition (e.g., menopause, drugs)
  - Superficial: Pain at or near the introitus or vaginal barrel associated with penetration
  - Deep: Pain after penetration located at the cervix or lower abdominal area
  - Complete: Present under all circumstances
  - Situational: Occurring selectively with specific situations
- System(s) affected: Reproductive

EPIDEMIOLOGY

- Predominant age: All ages
- Predominant sex: Female > Male

Incidence

>50% of all sexually active women will report dyspareunia at some time.

Geriatric Considerations

Incidence increases dramatically in postmenopausal women primarily because of vaginal atrophy.

Prevalence

- Most sexually active women will experience dyspareunia at some time in their lives:
  - ~15% (4–40%) of adult women will have dyspareunia on a few occasions during a year.
  - ~1–2% of women will have painful intercourse on a more-than-occasional basis.
- Male prevalence is ~1%.

RISK FACTORS

- Fatigue
- Stress
- Depression
- Diabetes
- Estrogen deficiency:
  - Menopause
  - Lactation
- Previous pelvic inflammatory disease (PID)
- Vaginal surgery
- Alcohol/marijuana consumption
- Medication side effects (antihistamines, tamoxifen, bromocriptine, low-estrogen oral contraceptives, depo-medroxyprogesterone, desipramine)

Pregnancy Considerations

Pregnancy is a potent influence on sexuality; dyspareunia is common.

PATHOPHYSIOLOGY

See "Etiology" section.

ETIOLOGY

- Disorders of vaginal outlet:
  - Adhesions
  - Clitoral irritation
  - Episiotomy scars
  - Fissures
  - Hymeneal ring abnormalities
  - Inadequate lubrication
  - Infections
  - Lichen planus
  - Lichen sclerosus
  - Postmenopausal atrophy
  - Trauma
  - Vulvar papillomatosis
  - Vulvar vestibulitis/vulvodynia
- Disorders of vagina:
  - Abnormality of vault owing to surgery or radiation
  - Congenital malformations
  - Inadequate lubrication
  - Infections
  - Inflammatory or allergic response to foreign substance
  - Masses or tumors
  - Pelvic relaxation resulting in rectocele, uterine prolapse, or cystocele
- Disorders of pelvic structures:
  - Endometriosis
  - Levator ani myalgia
  - Malignant or benign tumors of the uterus
  - Ovarian pathology
  - Pelvic adhesions
  - Pelvic inflammatory disease
  - Pelvic venous congestion
  - Prior pelvic fracture
- Disorders of the GI tract:
  - Constipation
  - Crohn disease
  - Diverticular disease
  - Fistulas
  - Hemorrhoids
  - Inflammatory bowel disease
- Disorders of the urinary tract:
  - Interstitial cystitis
  - Ureteral or vesical lesions
- Chronic Disease
  - Behçet syndrome
  - Diabetes
  - Sjögren's syndrome
- Male:
  - Cancer of penis
  - Genital muscle spasm
  - Infection or irritation of penile skin
  - Infection of seminal vesicles
  - Lichen sclerosus
  - Musculoskeletal disorders of pelvis and lower back
  - Penile anatomy disorders
  - Phimosis
  - Prostate infections and enlargement
  - Testicular disease
  - Torsion of spermatic cord
  - Urethritis
- Psychological disorders:
  - Anxiety
  - Conversion reactions
  - Depression
  - Fear
  - Hostility toward partner
  - Phobic reactions
  - Psychological trauma

COMMONLY ASSOCIATED CONDITIONS

Vaginismus

Pregnancy Considerations

- Episiotomies do not have a protective effect (1)[A].
- Mediolateral episiotomy increases the risk of dyspareunia compared with no episiotomy (2)[B].

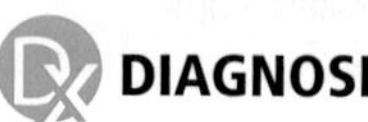

DIAGNOSIS

HISTORY

- Include menstrual, obstetric, reproductive, and sexual histories with medical and psychosocial history
- Identify pain characteristics:
  - Onset
  - Duration
  - Location: Entry vs. deep; single vs. multiple sites; positional
  - Intensity/quality: Varying degrees of pelvic/genital pressure, aching, tearing, and/or burning
  - Pattern (precipitating or aggravating factors): When pain occurs (at entry, during or after intercourse)
  - Relief measures: Avoid intercourse, change positions, have intercourse only at certain times of the month
- Question for history of domestic violence or history of rape.

PHYSICAL EXAM

- A complete exam, including a focused pelvic exam, to identify pathology and provide patient education
- Since exam often reproduces the pain, it must include inspection and palpation of vaginal area and urethral structures as well as palpation of the uterus.

DIAGNOSTIC TESTS & INTERPRETATION

Lab

Initial lab tests

Based on history and exam findings:

- Hormonal profile
- Wet mount
- Gonorrhea and chlamydia cultures
- Herpes culture
- Urinalysis and urine culture
- Pap smear

Imaging

Initial approach

Limited and based on history and exam findings

Follow-Up & Special Considerations

- Voiding cystourethrogram if urinary tract involvement
- GI contrast studies if GI symptoms
- Ultrasound and CT scan are of limited value; perform if clinically indicated

Diagnostic Procedures/Surgery

Based on history and exam findings:

- Colposcopy and biopsy if vaginal/vulvar lesions
- Laparoscopy if complex deep-penetration pain
- Cystoscopy if urinary tract involvement
- Endoscopy if GI involvement

Pathological Findings

Depends on etiology

DIFFERENTIAL DIAGNOSIS

Vaginismus

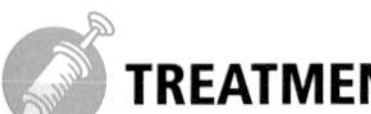

TREATMENT

- Primary dyspareunia might be related to vaginismus, low libido, and/or arousal disorders.
- Endocrine factors, such as primary amenorrhea, might reduce the biologic basis of sexual response.
- If pain prevents penetration, severe vaginismus may be present.

MEDICATION

First Line

Depends on the etiology:

- Antibiotics, antifungals, or antivirals as indicated for infection
- Estrogen for vaginal and vulvar atrophy
- Analgesics and topical anesthetics for pain
- Lubricants for dryness
- Vulvar vestibulitis/vulvodynia may respond to tricyclic antidepressants or gabapentin.

ADDITIONAL TREATMENT

General Measures

- Educate the patient and partner as to the nature of the problem. Reassure them that the problem can be solved.
- If an organic cause is identified during the initial evaluation, initiate specific treatment.
- Once organic causes are ruled out, treatment is a multidimensional and multidisciplinary approach (2)[C]:
  - Individual behavioral therapy: Indicated to help the patient deal with intrapersonal issues and assess the role of the partner.
  - Couple behavioral therapy:
    - Indicated to help resolve interpersonal problems
    - May involve short-term structured intervention or sexual counseling
    - Designed to systemically desensitize uncomfortable sexual responses and intercourse through a series of interventions over a period of weeks
    - Interventions range from muscle relaxation and mutual body massage to sexual fantasies and erotic massage.

Issues for Referral

Referral for long-term therapy may be necessary.

Additional Therapies

No benefit of therapeutic ultrasound (3)[A]

COMPLEMENTARY AND ALTERNATIVE MEDICINE

- Sitz baths may relieve painful inflammation.
- Perineal massage

SURGERY/OTHER PROCEDURES

- Laparoscopic excision of endometriotic lesions has shown benefit (4)[B].
- Surgical vestibulectomy can be considered if conservative measures fail with vulvar vestibulitis.

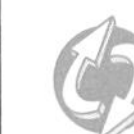

ONGOING CARE

FOLLOW-UP RECOMMENDATIONS

Patient Monitoring

- Outpatient follow-up depends on therapy.
- Every 6–12 months once resolved

DIET

A high-fiber diet may help if constipation is a contributing cause.

PATIENT EDUCATION

- Boston Women's Health Book Collective. *Our Bodies, Ourselves: A New Edition for a New Era*. New York: Simon & Schuster; 2005.
- Kegel exercise information
- Provide couples with information about sexual arousal techniques.

PROGNOSIS

Depends on underlying cause, but most patients will respond to treatment.

REFERENCES

1. Carroli G, Mignini L. Episiotomy for vaginal birth. *Cochrane Database Syst Rev*. 2009;CD000081.
2. Crowley T, Richardson D, Goldmeier D, et al. Recommendations for the management of vaginismus: BASHH Special Interest Group for Sexual Dysfunction. *Int J STD AIDS*. 2006;17:14–8.
3. Sartore A, De Seta F, Maso G, et al. The effects of mediolateral episiotomy on pelvic floor function after vaginal delivery. *Obstet Gynecol*. 2004;103: 669–73.
4. Ferrero S, Abbamonte LH, Giordano M, et al. Deep dyspareunia and sex life after laparoscopic excision of endometriosis. *Hum Reprod*. 2007;22(4): 1142–8.

ADDITIONAL READING

- Boardman LA, Stockdale CK, et al. Sexual pain. *Clin Obstet Gynecol*. 2009;52:682–90.
- Frank JE, Mistretta P, Will J. Diagnosis and treatment of female sexual dysfunction. *Am Fam Physician*. 2008;77:635–42.
- Steege JF, Zolnoun DA. Evaluation and treatment of dyspareunia. *Obstet Gynecol*. 2009;113:1124–36.

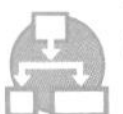

See Also (Topic, Algorithm, Electronic Media Element)

- Balanitis; Endometriosis; Pelvic Inflammatory Disease (PID); Sexual Dysfunction in Women; Vaginismus; Vulvovaginitis, Estrogen Deficient; Vulvovaginitis, Prepubescent
- Algorithms: Dyspareunia; Discharge, Vaginal

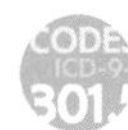

CODES

ICD9

- 302.76 Dyspareunia, psychogenic
- 625.0 Dyspareunia

CLINICAL PEARLS

- Careful history to determine if patient feels pain before, during, or after intercourse will help identify cause:
  - Pain before intercourse suggests a phobic attitude toward penetration and/or the presence of vestibulitis.
  - Pain during intercourse combined with the location of the pain is most predictive of the causes of pain.
  - Introital pain after intercourse suggests vestibulitis in women of childbearing age, hypertonic pelvic floor, or vulvovaginal dystrophia.
- Primary dyspareunia might be related to vaginismus, low libido, and/or arousal disorders.
- Episiotomy does not offer any benefit in the prevention of dyspareunia; a mediolateral episiotomy in fact may cause more future discomfort.

D

DYSPEPSIA, FUNCTIONAL

Marco Cornelio, MD
Macario C. Corpuz, Jr., MD, FAAFP

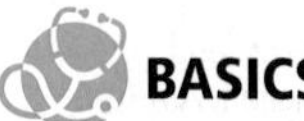

BASICS

DESCRIPTION

- A condition characterized by the presence of chronic intermittent symptoms for at least 3 months of epigastric pain, postprandial fullness, early satiety, or epigastric burning without mucosal lesions or other structural abnormalities of the GI tract (1)[A]
- Analogous to irritable bowel syndrome (IBS) of the upper GI tract
- System(s) affected: GI
- Synonym(s): Nonulcer dyspepsia; Moynihan dyspepsia; Pseudoulcer dyspepsia; Phantom ulcer; Nonorganic dyspepsia; Nervous dyspepsia

EPIDEMIOLOGY

Incidence

- 1–3% incidence of dyspepsia per year
- Accounts for 70% of patients with dyspepsia
- Accounts for ~5% of primary care visits

Prevalence

- 15–30% prevalence in developed countries
- Predominant age: Adults, but can be seen in children
- Predominant gender: Females > Males

RISK FACTORS

- Other functional disorders
- Anxiety
- Depression

Genetics

Possible link to G-protein β-3 subunit 825 CC genotype and serotonin transport genes

GENERAL PREVENTION

Avoid foods and habits known to exacerbate symptoms (see "Diet").

PATHOPHYSIOLOGY

- Not well understood
- Motility disorder
- Possible visceral hypersensitivity to gastric distention
- Psychosocial factors

ETIOLOGY

- Often unknown; may be of several different etiologies
- Evanescent ulcers (20–30% go on to develop ulcers)
- Gastric motility disorder (delayed or accelerated)
- Visceral hypersensitivity
- Impaired gastric accommodation
- Association with *Helicobacter pylori* infection
- Adverse drug effects (NSAIDs, bisphosphonate, corticosteroids)
- Carbohydrate malabsorption
- Food intolerance
- Psychosocial factors

COMMONLY ASSOCIATED CONDITIONS

Other functional bowel disorders

DIAGNOSIS

HISTORY

- Belching
- Aerophagia, gaseousness, abdominal distension
- Borborygmus
- Epigastric pain: Gnawing or burning; eating may improve or worsen symptoms
- Substernal pain: Gnawing or burning
- Early satiety
- Anorexia, nausea, or vomiting
- Change in bowel habits
- Abdominal tenderness
- Stress, anxiety, depression
- Exclude disorders in differential diagnosis (see below)

Pediatric Considerations

Look for family system dysfunction.

Pregnancy Considerations

Pregnancy may exacerbate condition.

Geriatric Considerations

Cancer risk is higher.

PHYSICAL EXAM

To rule out other disorders:

- Murphy sign for cholelithiasis
- Rebound and guarding for ulcer perforation

DIAGNOSTIC TESTS & INTERPRETATION

Lab

Initial lab tests

- CBC
- Chemistry panel
- *H. pylori* serology
- Stool for occult blood
- Liver function tests (if high suspicion of gallbladder disease present)

Imaging

Initial approach

- Usual:
  - Endoscopy (2)[A]:
    - For patients with alarm symptoms, patients who failed antisecretory medications, or patients who failed *H. pylori* test and treat strategy
- *Alarm symptoms*:
  - Onset of symptoms >45–55 years
  - Unexplained weight loss
  - Signs of a GI bleed
  - Family history of GI cancer
  - Progressive dysphagia
  - Persistent vomiting
- Sometimes:
  - Kidney, ureter, and bladder (KUB) x-ray for ulcer perforation
  - Right upper quadrant ultrasound for cholelithiasis

Diagnostic Procedures/Surgery

- Esophageal manometry (rarely needed)
- 24-hour intraesophageal pH monitoring (rarely needed unless dysphagia is present)

Pathological Findings

None (by definition)

DIFFERENTIAL DIAGNOSIS

- Gastroesophageal reflux disease (GERD)
- Cholecystitis
- Peptic ulcer disease
- Gastric cancer
- Esophageal spasm
- Malabsorption syndromes
- Pancreatic disease
- IBS
- Intestinal parasites
- Ischemic heart disease
- Diabetes mellitus
- Thyroid disease
- Connective tissue disorders
- Conversion disorder

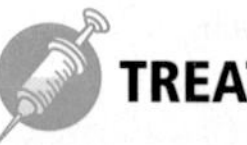

TREATMENT

MEDICATION

First Line

- 40% of patients improve with placebo.
- Acid reduction drugs:
  - H_2 antagonists: Ranitidine, famotidine (3)[A]
  - Over-the-counter omeprazole (4)[A]
  - *H. pylori* eradication (test and treat strategy)
- Significant possible interactions:
  - H_2 blockers interact with drugs metabolized by and affecting the liver.

Second Line

- Gastric motility drugs (3)[B]:
  - Metoclopramide (Reglan)
  - Erythromycin
- Amitriptyline: 50 mg at bedtime
- SSRIs
- Antacids
- Sucralfate
- Misoprostol
- Contraindications:
  - Avoid magnesium-containing antacids in patients with significant renal dysfunction.
- Precautions:
  - Calcium-containing antacids may precipitate the formation of kidney stones.
  - Metoclopramide can cause tardive dyskinesia and parkinsonian symptoms in older people.

ADDITIONAL TREATMENT

General Measures

- Appropriate health care: Outpatient
- Supportive measures:
  - Reassurance
  - Do not investigate excessively.
  - Dietary changes (see "Diet")
  - Elevate head of bed (where applicable).
  - Remain upright 30–60 minutes after eating.
  - Maintain ideal body weight.
  - Explore psychological issues.

Additional Therapies

- Stress reduction:
  - Relaxation techniques
  - Physical exercise
  - Reflux precautions where applicable
- Psychological therapy (1)[B]:
  - Cognitive-behavioral therapy
  - Hypnotherapy
  - Psychotherapy

COMPLEMENTARY AND ALTERNATIVE MEDICINE

- Peppermint oil
- Iberogast: Mixture of 9 plant extracts

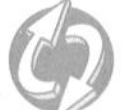

ONGOING CARE

FOLLOW-UP RECOMMENDATIONS

Patient Monitoring

- Usual duration of medication is 4 weeks, then 2 weeks intermittently for exacerbations. If chronic medication use is needed, endoscopy evaluation is indicated.
- Continue observation to provide support and reassurance.
- Minimize diagnostic studies unless disabling symptoms persist or new problems arise.

DIET

- Symptoms are frequently triggered or exacerbated by fatty foods.
- Eat frequent small meals.
- AVOID:
  - Foods known to exacerbate symptoms
  - Peppers, spices, citrus fruit
  - Regular and decaffeinated coffee
  - Tea, cocoa, and chocolate
  - Heavy alcohol use
  - Cigarette smoking
  - Aspirin-containing compounds and NSAIDs
  - Late evening meals

PATIENT EDUCATION

Prevention: Continue healthy habits listed under "Treatment" and "Diet" (i.e., avoid activities known to exacerbate problems, maintain healthy lifestyle, continue stress-reduction techniques).

PROGNOSIS

Long-term or chronic symptoms with symptom-free periods

COMPLICATIONS

Iatrogenic, from evaluation to rule out serious pathology

REFERENCES

1. Drossman DA. The functional gastrointestinal disorders and the Rome III process. *Gastroenterol.* 2006;130:1377–90.
2. Delaney B, Ford AC, Forman D, et al. Initial management strategies for dyspepsia. *Cochrane Database Syst Rev.* 2005:CD001961.
3. Loyd R, McClellan D. Update on the evaluation and management of functional dyspepsia. *Am Fam Phys.* 2011;83(5):547–52.
4. Lacy B, Cash B. A 32 year old woman with chronic abdominal pain. *JAMA.* 2008;299(5):555–65.

ADDITIONAL READING

- Choung RS, et al. Novel mechanisms in functional dyspepsia. *W J Gastroenterol.* 2006;12:673–7.
- Graham D, Rugge M. Clinical practice: Diagnosis & evaluation of dyspepsia. *J Clin Gastroenterol* 2010;44:167–72.
- Kandulski A, Venerito M, Malfertheiner P, et al. Therapeutic strategies for the treatment of dyspepsia. *Expert Opin Pharmacother.* 2010;11: 2517–25.
- Keohane J, et al. Functional dyspepsia and nonerosive reflux disease: Clinical interactions and their implications. *Med Gen Med.* 2007;9:31.
- Longstreth G. Functional dyspepsia—managing the conundrum. *N Engl J Med.* 2006;354:791–3.

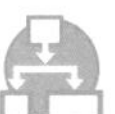

See Also (Topic, Algorithm, Electronic Media Element)

- Dyspepsia, Endoscopic-Negative Reflux Disease, Gastritis; Irritable Bowel Syndrome
- Algorithms: Dyspepsia; Epigastric Pain; Esophageal Regurgitation

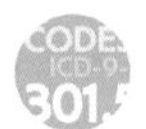

CODES

ICD9

536.8 Dyspepsia and other specified disorders of function of stomach

CLINICAL PEARLS

- When no organic cause for dyspepsia is found, it is considered functional or idiopathic.
- Extensive diagnostic testing is not recommended unless the patient presents with alarm symptoms (vomiting, early satiety, weight loss, or anemia).
- Consider empiric treatment with acid suppressants or *H. pylori* eradication if serology is positive.

DYSPHAGIA

Archit Sharma, MD
Mark D. Goodman, MD

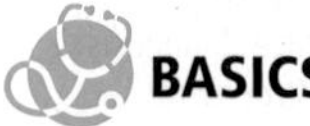

BASICS

Difficulty or discomfort during the progression of the alimentary bolus from the mouth to the stomach

DESCRIPTION

- Difficulty swallowing
- A disorder of transferring the food bolus from oropharynx to esophagus or of impairment in transport of the bolus through the esophagus
- Commonly divided based on:
  - Anatomic standpoint: Oropharyngeal or esophageal dysfunction
  - Pathophysiologic standpoint: Structure-related or functional causes
- Associated symptoms: *Odynophagia* (painful swallowing); *globus* (lump in throat)
- System(s) affected: GI; Nervous

EPIDEMIOLOGY

Incidence

- In US: 7% incidence during lifetime
- Predominant age: All ages; increasing prevalence with age
- Predominant sex: Male = Female

Prevalence

- 16–22% of people >50 years of age
- Up to 60% of nursing home residents
- 25% of hospitalized patients

RISK FACTORS

- Children: Hereditary and/or congenital malformations
- Adults: Age >50 years (esophageal cancer, neurologic disorders) more likely
- Smoking, excess alcohol intake, obesity
- Long history of GERD
- Medications (e.g., quinine, potassium chloride, vitamin C, tetracycline, Bactrim, clindamycin, NSAIDs)
- Neurologic events or diseases (CVA, neuromuscular disease, multiple sclerosis, Parkinson disease, ALS)
- Trauma or irradiation of head, neck, and chest

GENERAL PREVENTION

- Observe feeding of infants closely for aspiration; have suction available.
- Correct poorly fitting dentures in older patients.
- Avoid drinking alcohol with meals.
- Give consideration to positioning during meals and texture of foods being eaten.
- In infants/children: Discuss underlying problem and therapy for recurrent aspiration.
- Positioning and texture in older adults; dentures; supervision to prevent aspiration

ETIOLOGY

- Esophageal
  - Structural: Tumors (cancer or benign); strictures (peptic, chemical, trauma, radiation); lower esophageal rings (Schatzki rings); esophageal webs
  - Mechanical: Extrinsic compression from enlarged left atrium, aortic aneurysm, aberrant subclavian artery (termed *dysphagia lusoria*), substernal thyroid, cervical bony exostosis, and thoracic tumor
  - GERD
  - Neuromuscular: Achalasia, diffuse esophageal spasm, hypertensive lower esophageal sphincter, scleroderma, myasthenia gravis, nutcracker esophagus
- Oropharyngeal:
  - CVA
  - Parkinson disease
  - Neurodegenerative diseases (MS, ALS, Huntington disease, pseudobulbar palsy)
  - Zenker diverticulum
  - Myasthenia gravis
  - Polio
  - Cricopharyngeal achalasia
  - Cervical spondylosis (cervical osteophytes)
  - Obstructive lesions (tumors, inflammatory masses)

Pediatric Considerations

- Malformations: Congenital (esophageal atresia, cleft palate, choanal atresia, TE fistula, Zenker diverticulum)
- Malformations: Acquired (corrosive or herpetic esophagitis)
- Neuromuscular/neurologic: Delayed maturation, CP, MD, poliomyelitis
- GERD
- Tonsillar hypertrophy, large tongue, dental problems (overbite)

Geriatric Considerations

- Poor dentition and/or dentures
- Drug-induced

COMMONLY ASSOCIATED CONDITIONS

- Esophageal carcinoma
- GERD-induced peptic stricture
- Dysphagia lusoria (extrinsic compression)
- Achalasia
- Symptomatic diffuse esophageal spasm
- Eosinophilic esophagitis
- Foreign body
- Scleroderma
- Myasthenia gravis
- CVA

DIAGNOSIS

ALERT
Rapidly progressive symptoms and/or profound weight loss is indicative of malignant process; requires immediate attention; should undergo endoscopy with/without biopsy

HISTORY

- Is the dysphagia for solids, liquids, or both? Which started first?
- Does the food bolus feel stuck? If so, where?
- Are there symptoms of oropharyngeal dysfunction?
- Is there any cough while swallowing? Is it early in the swallowing or late?
- Is the dysphagia intermittent or progressive?
- Have you ever brought food back up or vomited?
- Is there a history of chronic heartburn?
- How much alcohol and/or tobacco do you use?
- Are there associated symptoms such as weight loss or chest pain?
- What medications are being taken?
- Is there odynophagia? (Does it hurt with just solid food or both solid and liquids?)
- Is there any halitosis?

PHYSICAL EXAM

- Oropharyngeal type:
  - Choking with swallowing
  - Coughing with swallowing
  - Nasal speech (wet voice)
  - Hoarseness of voice
  - Sialorrhea (drooling)
  - Frequent respiratory infections
  - Weight loss
  - Dysarthria
  - Nasopharyngeal regurgitation with swallowing
- Esophageal type:
  - Pressure sensation in midchest (localized below suprasternal notch highly likely to be esophageal disorder); narrow the diagnostic possibilities by asking if this occurs for solids, liquids, or both
  - Oral or pharyngeal regurgitation
  - Recurrent aspiration pneumonia
  - Weight loss
  - Symptoms of GERD
- Neck and oral cavity for lesions, masses, goiter
- Signs of collagen: Vascular disease
- Detailed neurologic exam, especially cranial nerves with gag reflex testing (CVA, neuromuscular disease, Parkinson)
- In infants:
  - Breastfeeding problems
  - Vomiting or spitting up during feeds
  - Lengthy feeding or eating times (>30 minutes)

DIAGNOSTIC TESTS & INTERPRETATION

- In infants/children:
  - Observe sucking/eating.
  - Attempt to pass NG tube to assess esophageal patency.
  - Radiography of neck and chest
  - Contrast radiography
  - Endoscopy
- In adults:
  - Barium swallow
  - Fiberoptic endoscopic examination of swallowing (FEES)
  - Gastroesophageal endoscopy
  - Barium cine/video esophagogram
  - Ambulatory 24-hour pH testing
  - Esophageal manometry
  - Videofluoroscopic swallowing study (VFSS)

Lab

As suggested by specific differential diagnosis under consideration

Initial lab tests

- CBC to screen for infectious and inflammatory condition
- Serum protein and albumin levels for nutritional assessment
- Thyroid function studies to detect dysphagia associated with hypothyroidism or hyperthyroidism

Imaging

- Barium swallow
- CT scan of chest
- MRI of brain and cervical spine
- VFSS

Diagnostic Procedures/Surgery
- Endoscopy with biopsy
- Esophageal manometry
- Esophageal pH monitoring

Pathological Findings
- Squamous cell or adenocarcinoma
- Barrett metaplasia
- Fibrous tissue of a ring, web, or stricture
- Loss of smooth muscle (scleroderma)
- Acute or chronic inflammatory changes
- Oropharyngeal lesions

DIFFERENTIAL DIAGNOSIS
- Cardiac chest pain
- Globus hystericus
- Functional heartburn or dysphagia

TREATMENT

MEDICATION

First Line
- **For spasms:** Calcium channel blockers: Nifedipine (Procardia) 10–30 mg t.i.d.; amitriptyline 0.5–2 mg/kg at bedtime; dicyclomine (Bentyl) 20 mg q.i.d.
- **For esophagitis:**
  - Antacids: Tums, Mylanta, Maalox
  - H_2 blockers: Cimetidine (Tagamet), ranitidine (Zantac), nizatidine (Axid), famotidine (Pepcid)
  - Proton pump inhibitors: Omeprazole (Prilosec), lansoprazole (Prevacid), rabeprazole (AcipHex), esomeprazole (Nexium), pantoprazole (Protonix)
  - Prokinetic agents: Metoclopramide (Reglan), erythromycin (Ery-Tab)
  - Contraindications:
    - Anticholinergics: Obstructive uropathy, glaucoma, myasthenia gravis, achalasia, dementia/delirium, advanced age
    - Nitrates: Early MI, severe anemia, increased ICP, HTN
  - Investigational: Cilostazol is under investigation for dysphagia in patients after a stroke; may improve swallowing and reduce risk of aspiration pneumonia; mechanism is not completely understood.
  - Precautions: May need to use liquid forms of medications because patients might have difficulty swallowing pills.

ADDITIONAL TREATMENT

General Measures
- Exclude cardiac disease.
- Ensure airway and pulmonary function.
- Assess nutritional status.
- Speech therapy evaluation is helpful.

Issues for Referral
- Need for endoscopy, refractory: Gastroenterology
- Failure of dilation or medications: Surgery for esophageal myotomy

Additional Therapies
Speech therapy for swallowing assessment, dietary and positioning recommendations, and muscle-strengthening exercise; no eating at bedtime; remaining upright after eating

SURGERY/OTHER PROCEDURES
- Esophageal dilatation (pneumatic or bougie)
- Esophageal stent; laser for cancer palliation
- Treatment for underlying problem (e.g., thyroid goiter, vascular ring, esophageal atresia)
- Nd:YAG laser incision of lower esophageal rings refractory to dilation
- Photodynamic therapy (cancer)
- Cricopharyngeal myotomy for oropharyngeal dysphagia
- Surgery for Zenker diverticulum, refractory strictures, or myotomy for achalasia
- Nissen fundoplication to prevent reflux

IN-PATIENT CONSIDERATIONS

Initial Stabilization
- Outpatient for conditions where patient is able to maintain nutrition and has little risk of complications
- Hospitalization may be required for either infants or adults when dysphagia is associated with total or near-total obstruction of esophageal lumen.
- Endoscopy and/or esophageal dilation may be needed for stenoses and strictures (often recur).
- Surgery may be required in either benign or malignant processes.

Admission Criteria
- Complete or partial esophageal obstruction with malnutrition or hypovolemia/dehydration
- Comorbid conditions complicating etiology of dysphagia
- Enteral feeding might be required in patients with:
  - Impaired level of consciousness
  - Massive aspiration or recurrent respiratory infections
  - Esophageal obstruction

IV Fluids
For dehydrated, hypovolemic patients and patients with impaired consciousness

Nursing
- Monitor for aspiration.
- Ensure correct posture of patient while feeding.
- Consider bedside screening tests using water swallowing and pulse oximetry to screen neurologic patients for dysphagia (1)[A].

Discharge Criteria
- Correction of dysphagia
- Tolerating adequate diet without nausea/pain
- Adequate nutritional intake
- Control of pain syndrome

ONGOING CARE

FOLLOW-UP RECOMMENDATIONS
- Sit upright for meals, stay upright afterward; appropriately fitting dentures
- Follow speech therapy/swallow therapy recommendations.
- Strengthening exercises and rehab after CVA

DIET
Depends on etiology and severity:
- Counsel the patient about avoiding irritating drugs.
- Counsel the patient about the importance of chewing food well.
- Speech therapy texture recommendations such as mechanical soft diet or pureed diet

PATIENT EDUCATION
Dietary modification, no eating at bedtime, remaining upright after eating, pharmacologic therapy, smoking cessation

PROGNOSIS
Course and prognosis vary with specific diagnosis (cancer, poor; esophageal peptic stricture, good).

COMPLICATIONS
- Aspiration/aspiration pneumonia
- Esophageal "asthma"
- Upper respiratory tract infections
- Malnutrition
- Esophagitis: Reflux based or pill induced
- Death

REFERENCE

1. Bours GJ, Speyer R, Lemmens J, et al. Bedside screening tests vs. videofluoroscopy or fibreoptic endoscopic evaluation of swallowing to detect dysphagia in patients with neurological disorders: Systematic review. *J Adv Nurs*. 2009;65:477–93.

ADDITIONAL READING

- Rofes L, Arreola V, Almirall J, et al. Diagnosis and management of oropharyngeal dysphagia and its nutritional and respiratory complications in the elderly. *Gastroenterol Res Pract*. 2011;2011.
- Speyer R, Baijens L, Heijnen M, et al. Effects of therapy in oropharyngeal dysphagia by speech and language therapists: A systematic review. *Dysphagia*. 2010;25:40–65.
- Verlaan JJ, Boswijk PF, de Ru JA, et al. Diffuse idiopathic skeletal hyperostosis of the cervical spine: An underestimated cause of dysphagia and airway obstruction. *Spine J*. 2011.

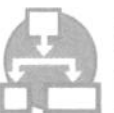

See Also (Topic, Algorithm, Electronic Media Element)

Gastroesophageal Reflux Disease

CODES

ICD9
- 530.3 Stricture and stenosis of esophagus
- 750.3 Congenital tracheoesophageal fistula, esophageal atresia and stenosis
- 787.20 Dysphagia, unspecified

CLINICAL PEARLS
- Taking a careful history of the types of food involved, progression, and associated symptoms will help to determine where the problem is.
- Alarming symptoms include weight loss, chest pain, rapid progression, and risk factors such as chronic GERD and alcohol or tobacco use.
- A barium study (esophagram) is the first step in evaluating patients with dysphagia if you suspect obstruction or achalasia, then endoscopy, or proceed directly to endoscopy if achalasia is less likely.
- An EGD with esophageal biopsies should be considered in patients with intermittent solid-food dysphagia to rule out eosinophilic esophagitis even if they have normal endoscopic findings.

ECTOPIC PREGNANCY

Janelle M. Evans, MD
Shaila V. Chauhan, MD

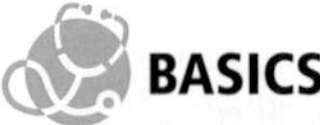

BASICS

DESCRIPTION

- Ectopic: Pregnancy occurs outside the confines of the uterine cavity.
- Tubal: Pregnancy implanted in any portion of the fallopian tube
- Abdominal: Pregnancy implanted intra-abdominally, most commonly in the posterior cul-de-sac.
- Heterotopic: Pregnancy implanted intrauterine and a separate pregnancy implanted outside uterine cavity.
- Ovarian: Implantation of pregnancy in ovarian tissue
- Cervical: Implantation in cervix (associated with large blood loss)
- Intraligamentary: Implantation of pregnancy within the broad ligament

EPIDEMIOLOGY

Incidence

- 108,800 cases in 1992 in the US according to Centers for Disease Control census (most recent data available). This is a 6-fold increase from 1970.
- 15.8 per 1,000 total reported pregnancies, or 9.5 per 10,000 women
- 28,000 hospitalizations reported in 2006 in the US for ectopic pregnancy
- Heterotopic pregnancy, although rare (1:30,000), occurs with greater frequency in women undergoing in vitro fertilization (IVF) (1–2/1,000)
- Leading cause of first-trimester maternal death and accounts for 9% of national pregnancy deaths

Prevalence

- Predominant age: >40% occur in women between ages 20 and 29
- 12–15% recurrence rate if prior ectopic pregnancy

RISK FACTORS

- History of tubal surgery (7:1,000 for tubal ligation)
- Previous ectopic pregnancy
- History of pelvic inflammatory disease (PID), endometritis, or current gonorrhea/chlamydia infection
- Pelvic adhesive disease (infection, prior surgery)
- Use of an intrauterine device: Reduction of the absolute risk of ectopic pregnancy overall, but increased likelihood of pregnancy being ectopic if pregnancy occurs
- Use of assisted reproductive technologies in up to 4% (e.g., IVF, embryo transfer)
- Diethylstilbestrol exposure in utero
- Cigarette smoking
- Some evidence that vaginal douching is a modifiable risk factor
- Patients with disorders that affect ciliary motility may be at increased risk.

GENERAL PREVENTION

- Reliable contraception or abstinence
- Screening and treatment of STDs (gonorrhea, chlamydia) that can cause PID and tubal scarring

PATHOPHYSIOLOGY

- 98% of ectopic pregnancies occur in the fallopian tube, 70% in the ampullary portion of the tube, 12% in the isthmus, 11% in the fimbria, and 2% in the cornua.
- Abdominal pregnancies account for 1.3% of all ectopics; ovarian and cervical sites account for 0.2% each.

ETIOLOGY

- For a tubal pregnancy:
  - Damage or compromise to the integrity of the fallopian tubes leads to dysfunction of the tubal cilia, which are required for proper movement of the fertilized ovum to the uterine cavity.
  - Scarring or narrowing of the tube damages tubal integrity.
- Other locations are rare and may occur from reimplantation of an aborted tubal pregnancy or uterine structural abnormalities (mainly cervical pregnancy).

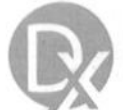

DIAGNOSIS

HISTORY

- In more than half of presenting cases, patients have sudden-onset abdominal pain coupled with cessation of/or irregular menses.
- Nausea and/or vomiting
- Abdominal pain or mass
- Referred shoulder pain (secondary to hemoperitoneum)

PHYSICAL EXAM

- Abdominal tenderness
- Vaginal bleeding
- Palpable mass on pelvic exam
- Cervical motion tenderness may also be appreciated.
- In cervical cases, an hourglass-shaped cervix might be noted.
- In cases of rupture and intraperitoneal bleeding, signs of shock such as pallor, tachycardia, and hypotension may be present.

DIAGNOSTIC TESTS & INTERPRETATION

Lab

Initial lab tests

- Human chorionic gonadotropin (HCG): Serial quantitative serum levels normally increase by ~66% every 48 hours:
  - Abnormal rise should prompt workup for gestational abnormalities.
- Serial hematocrit and abdominal exams to quantify blood loss only if not immediately going to the operating room
- Serum progesterone level (>20 mg/mL associated with lower risk of ectopic pregnancy)

Imaging

Initial approach

- Transvaginal ultrasound (TVUS) is the gold standard for diagnosis (1)[A]:
  - Doppler flowmetry is usually coupled with ultrasound for more accurate diagnosis.
- MRI is also useful, but costly, and rarely used if ultrasound is available.

Follow-Up & Special Considerations

Consider TVUS in the first trimester of future pregnancies.

Pathological Findings

- Tubal pregnancy: Chorionic villi within the tubal wall
- Ovarian pregnancy (Spiegelberg criteria):
  - Pregnancy found displacing or replacing the ovarian tissue
  - Possible utero-ovarian ligament attachment
  - Ovarian tissue identified as part of gestational sac
- Abdominal pregnancy—primary form:
  - Both ovaries and tubes appear normal.
  - No uteroperitoneal fistula is present.
  - Limited to peritoneal attachment of conceptus
- Cervical pregnancy: Villi seen in the cervical canal
- Intraligamentary pregnancy: The products of conception (POCs) are within the confines of the broad ligament.

DIFFERENTIAL DIAGNOSIS

- Missed or threatened abortion
- Appendicitis
- Salpingitis, PID
- Ruptured corpus luteum or hemorrhagic cyst
- Ovarian tumor, benign or malignant
- Ovarian torsion
- Endometrioma
- Cervical cancer
- Cervical phase of uterine abortion

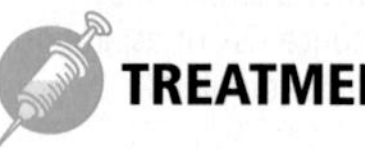

TREATMENT

MEDICATION

- Methotrexate: Primary treatment for unruptured tubal pregnancy or for remaining POCs after laparoscopic salpingotomy. It inhibits DNA synthesis via folic acid antagonism.
- Most effective when pregnancy is <3 cm diameter, HCG <5,000 mIU/mL, and no fetal heart rate is seen. Success rate is 85–90% with proper selection.
- Dosage:
  - Single: IM methotrexate: 50 mg/m^2 of body surface area; may repeat once (preferred method) if <15% decline in HCG by day 7
  - Multidose: Methotrexate 1 mg/kg IM/IV every other day, with leucovorin 0.1 mg/kg IM in between. Maximum 4 doses; course may be repeated 7 days after last dose if necessary.
- Contraindications:
  - Hemodynamic instability or any evidence of rupture
  - Fetal heart rate seen
  - Large gestational sac (>3 cm)
  - Noncompliance or limited access to hospital or transportation

- Precautions:
  - Immunologic, hematologic, renal, GI, hepatic, and pulmonary disease, or interacting medications
- Pretreatment testing: Serum HCG, CBC, liver and renal function tests, type and screen
- Patient counseling: During therapy, refrain from use of alcohol, aspirin, NSAIDs, and folate supplements (decreases efficacy of MTX); avoid excessive sun exposure

ADDITIONAL TREATMENT

- After evidence of repeat medical failure or rupture, surgery is necessary.
- Follow all patients treated medically to an HCG of 0 to prevent surgical intervention.
- Expectant management in asymptomatic patients with no evidence of rupture or hemodynamic instability coupled with an appropriately low BHCG, no evidence of fetal cardiac activity

Issues for Referral

- Refer to a gynecologist for medical treatment.
- Consult a gynecologist for surgical care.

COMPLEMENTARY AND ALTERNATIVE MEDICINE

Watchful waiting: If no clear adnexal mass and low HCG (usually 1,000–2,000), may follow with HCG/ultrasound. Rare cases of rupture have been described with low quants.

SURGERY/OTHER PROCEDURES

- Indications include ruptured ectopic, inability to comply with medical follow-up, previous tubal ligation, known tubal disease or current heterotopic pregnancy, desire for permanent sterilization at time of diagnosis.
- Laparoscopy is first-line surgical management.
- Salpingostomy preferred in patients who wish to maintain fertility:
  - Slightly higher recurrence rate than with salpingectomy
  - Slightly higher rate of persistent trophoblastic tissue with laparoscopy vs. open laparotomy (8% vs. 3.4%)
- Salpingectomy indicated for uncontrolled bleeding, recurrent ectopic pregnancy, severely damaged tube, gestational sac >4 cm, or patient desire for sterilization

IN-PATIENT CONSIDERATIONS

Initial Stabilization

Surgical emergency:

- 2 IV access lines should be placed immediately if suspicion of rupture; aggressive resuscitation as needed
- Blood product transfusion and fluids if necessary en route to operating room
- In cases of shock, pressors and cardiac support may be necessary.

Admission Criteria

Fails criteria for methotrexate management, suspicion of rupture, orthostatic, shock, and severe abdominal pain requiring IV narcotics

Nursing

Strict input/output, hourly vitals, orthostatics if mobile, frequent abdominal exams, serial hematocrit, pad counts if heavy vaginal bleeding

Discharge Criteria

Afebrile; abdominal pain resolving or resolved

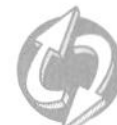

ONGOING CARE

FOLLOW-UP RECOMMENDATIONS

Patient Monitoring

- Serial serum quantitative HCG until level drops to negative
- Pelvic ultrasound for persistent or recurrent masses
- Pain control: Brief course of narcotics usually necessary
- Liver and renal function tests following methotrexate administration
- Delay of subsequent pregnancy for at least 3 months after treatment with methotrexate due to teratogenicity

DIET

- Avoid foods and vitamins high in folate due to interaction with methotrexate efficacy.
- Maintain excellent hydration.

PROGNOSIS

- Recurrence rate 12–15% for ectopic pregnancy
- Future fertility depends on fertility prior to ectopic, history of tubal compromise.
- Referral to reproductive endocrinologist appropriate if infertility persists beyond 12–18 months

COMPLICATIONS

- Hemorrhage and hypovolemic shock
- Persistent trophoblastic tissue after medical or surgical management
- Infection
- Infertility (more commonly with salpingectomy)
- Blood transfusions with associated infections/transfusion reaction
- Disseminated intravascular coagulation

REFERENCE

1. ACOG practice bulletin. Medical management of tubal pregnancy. Number 3, December 1998. Clinical management guidelines for obstetrician-gynecologists. American College of Obstetricians and Gynecologists. *Int J Gynaecol Obstet*. 1999;65:97–103.

ADDITIONAL READING

- Bisharah M, Tulandi T. Laparoscopic surgery in pregnancy. *Clin Obstet Gynecol*. 2003;46:92–7.
- Braude P, Rowell P. Assisted conception. III–problems with assisted conception. *BMJ*. 2003;327:920–3.
- Centers for Disease Control and Prevention. Sexually Transmitted Disease Surveillance 2007. Atlanta, GA: U.S. Department of Health and Human Services; December 2008.
- Elson J, et al. Expectant management of tubal ectopic pregnancy: Prediction of successful outcome using decision tree analysis. *Ultrasound Obstet Gynaecol*. 2004;23:552–6.
- Hajenius PJ, Mol F, Mol BW, et al. Interventions for tubal ectopic pregnancy. *Cochrane Database Syst Rev*. 2007;CD000324.
- Hoover KW, Tao G, Kent CK. Trends in the diagnosis and treatment of ectopic pregnancy in the United States. *Obstet Gynecol*. 2010;115(3):495–502.
- Lipscomb GH. Medical therapy for ectopic pregnancy. *Semin Reprod Med*. 2007;25:93–8.
- Mol F, Mol BW, Ankum WM, et al. Current evidence on surgery, systemic methotrexate and expectant management in the treatment of tubal ectopic pregnancy: A systematic review and meta-analysis. *Hum Reprod Update*. 2008;14:309–19.
- Murray H, et al. Diagnosis and treatment of ectopic pregnancy. *Can Med Assoc J*. 2005;173(8):905–12.
- Nama V, Manyonda I, et al. Tubal ectopic pregnancy: Diagnosis and management. *Arch Gynecol Obstet*. 2009;279:443–53.
- Ramakrishnan K, Scheid DC. Ectopic pregnancy: Expectant management of immediate surgery? *J Fam Pract*. 2006;55:517–22.
- Stein JC, Wang R, Adler N, et al. Emergency physician ultrasonography for evaluating patients at risk for ectopic pregnancy: A meta-analysis. *Ann Emerg Med*. 2010;56:674–83.
- Tay JI, Moore J, Walker JJ. Ectopic pregnancy. *BMJ*. 2000;320:916–9.

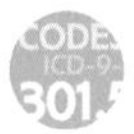

CODES

ICD9

- 633.00 Abdominal pregnancy without intrauterine pregnancy
- 633.10 Tubal pregnancy without intrauterine pregnancy
- 633.90 Unspecified ectopic pregnancy without intrauterine pregnancy

CLINICAL PEARLS

- Ectopic pregnancy is the leading cause of first-trimester maternal death and accounts for 9% of national pregnancy deaths.
- 98% of ectopic pregnancies occur in the fallopian tube.
- TVUS is the gold standard for diagnosis.
- When an ectopic pregnancy is <3 cm diameter, HCG <5,000 mIU/mL, and no fetal heart rate is seen, a single dose of methotrexate is the preferred medical treatment, with a success rate of 85–90%.
- Indications for surgery include ruptured ectopic, inability to comply with medical follow-up, previous tubal ligation, known tubal disease or current heterotopic pregnancy, or desire for permanent sterilization at time of diagnosis.

E

EJACULATORY DISORDERS

Andrew Leone, MD
Kyle D. Wood, MD

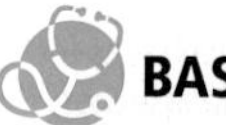

BASICS

DESCRIPTION

- Premature/rapid ejaculation: Inability to control the ejaculatory reflex is the most common type of sexual dysfunction affecting all age groups:
  - American Urological Association (AUA) 2003 Guidelines definition: Ejaculation that occurs sooner than desired, either before or shortly after penetration, causing distress to either one or both partners (1).
  - Natural biologic response is to ejaculate within 2–5 minutes after vaginal penetration.
  - Ejaculatory control is an acquired behavior that increases with experience.
- Delayed (retarded) ejaculation: Prolonged time to ejaculate despite desire, stimulation, and erection.
- Aspermia (lack of sperm in the ejaculate):
  - Anejaculation: Lack of emission or contractions of bulbospongiosus muscle
  - Retrograde ejaculation: Partial or complete ejaculation of semen into the bladder
  - Obstruction: Ejaculatory duct obstruction or urethral obstruction
- Painful ejaculation: Genital or perineal pain during or after ejaculation
- Ejaculatory anhedonia: Normal ejaculation lacking orgasm or pleasure
- Hematospermia: Presence of blood in the ejaculate
- Ejaculatory duct obstruction
- System(s) affected: Nervous; Reproductive
- Synonym(s): Premature ejaculation; Rapid ejaculation; Retarded ejaculation; Retrograde ejaculation; Anejaculation; Inhibited orgasm in males; Ejaculatory dysfunction

EPIDEMIOLOGY

- Premature ejaculation is common. Reported prevalence in US males ages 18–59: 21%
- Retarded ejaculation is reported in ~5–8% of men between 18 and 59, but <3% experience the problem for >6 months.
- Predominant age: All sexually mature age groups
- Predominant sex: Male only

Prevalence

20% of men affected

RISK FACTORS

See "Etiology."

PATHOPHYSIOLOGY

Male sexual response:

- Erection mediated by parasympathetic nervous system
- Ejaculation consists of 2 phases:
  - Emission phase: Semen is deposited into urethra by contraction of prostate, seminal vesicles, and vas deferens. Under autonomic sympathetic control.
  - Ejaculation phase: Semen is forcibly propelled out of urethra by rhythmic contractions of the bulbospongiosus and ischiocavernosus muscles. This is mediated by the somatic nervous system on the motor branches of the pudendal nerve.
- Bladder neck contracture occurs during the above process and is induced by alpha-adrenergic receptors to ensure anterograde ejaculation.
- Orgasm: The pleasurable sensation associated with ejaculation (cerebral cortex) (2)

ETIOLOGY

- Untreated erectile dysfunction is the most common treatable cause.
- Premature ejaculation (many potential causes but all without evidence base):
  - Penile hypersensitivity
  - 5-hydroxytryptamine (5-HT)-receptor sensitivity
  - Sexual inexperience
  - High level of sexual arousal and/or long interval since last ejaculation
  - Fear of sexual transmitted diseases (STDs)
  - Anxiety
  - Guilty feelings about sex
  - Lack of privacy
  - Interpersonal maladaptation (e.g., marital problems, unresponsiveness of partner)
- Retarded ejaculation:
  - Rarely may be caused by an underlying painful disorder (e.g., prostatitis, seminal vesiculitis)
  - May be psychogenic as part of erectile dysfunction
  - Sexual performance anxiety and other psychosocial factors
  - Some drugs may impair ejaculation (e.g., certain monoamine oxidase inhibitors [MAOIs], SSRIs, α- and β-blockers, thiazides, antipsychotics, tricyclic and quadricyclic antidepressants, NSAIDs, opiates, or alcohol).
- Never any ejaculate:
  - Congenital structural disorder (Müllerian duct cyst, Wolffian abnormality)
  - Acquired (radical prostatectomy, postinfectious, posttraumatic, T10–12 neuropathy)
- Anejaculation:
  - Medications (α- and β-blockers, benzodiazepines, SSRIs, MAOIs, TCAs, antipsychotics, aminocaproic acid)
  - Diabetes mellitus (DM) (neuropathy)
  - Retroperitoneal lymph node dissection
  - Sympathetic nerve injury (spinal cord injury, intraoperative injury)
  - Radical prostatectomy
- Retrograde ejaculation:
  - Transurethral resection of the prostate (25%) or other prostate resection procedures
  - Surgery on the neck of the bladder
  - Extensive pelvic surgery
  - Retroperitoneal lymph node dissection for testicular cancer (also may produce failure of emission)
  - Neurologic disorders (multiple sclerosis, DM)
  - Medications (α-blockers, in particular tamsulosin, ganglion blockers, antipsychotics)
  - Urethral stricture
  - Trauma
- Painful ejaculation:
  - Infection or inflammation (orchitis, epididymitis, prostatitis, urethritis)
  - Ejaculatory duct obstruction
  - Seminal vesicle calculi
  - Obstruction of the vas deferens
  - Psychological
- Ejaculatory anhedonia:
  - Medications
  - Psychological
  - Hormonal imbalances
  - Decreased libido
- Hematospermia:
  - Inflammation/infection
  - Calculi: Bladder, seminal vesicle, prostate, urethra
  - Trauma to genital area, i.e., cycling or constipation
  - Obstruction
  - Cyst
  - Tumor (prostate cancer [1–3% present with hematospermia])
  - Arteriovenous malformations
  - Iatrogenic
  - Hypertension
- Endocrinopathies can result in ejaculatory dysfunction

COMMONLY ASSOCIATED CONDITIONS

- Neurologic disorders (e.g., multiple sclerosis)
- Diabetes mellitus
- Prostatitis
- Ejaculatory duct obstruction
- Urethral stricture
- Psychologic disorders
- Endocrinopathies
- Relationship/interpersonal difficulties

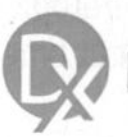

DIAGNOSIS

- Ejaculation occurs before individual wishes.
- Ejaculation does not occur following normal stimulation (including masturbation).

HISTORY

- Detailed sexual history, including:
  - Time frame of the problem
  - Evaluation of the quality of patient's sexual response
  - Sense of ejaculatory control and sexual distress
  - Overall assessment of the relationship
- Detailed history of recent and current medications
- History of past trauma or recent infections
- Past surgical history with particular attention to genitourinary (GU) surgeries
- Inquire about home remedies attempted.
- Many men do not distinguish initially between problems related to erection and ejaculation.
- Some men have unrealistic expectations of ejaculatory response and frequency.
- Include the sexual partner in the interview, especially if the patient expresses a belief that he is not meeting his partner's needs.
- In review of systems, elicit any evidence of testosterone deficiency or prolactin excess for diagnosis of anhedonia.

PHYSICAL EXAM

- Look for multiple sclerosis, spinal cord injury, and emotional disorders
- Thorough GU exam, including (3):
  - Size and texture of testes and epididymis
  - Verification of the presence of the vas deferens
  - Location and patency of urethral meatus
  - Digital rectal examination to evaluate prostate consistency and size and possible midline lesions

DIAGNOSTIC TESTS & INTERPRETATION

Lab

- Laboratory test results may be normal.
- Fasting blood sugar to rule out diabetes
- Postorgasmic urinalysis will confirm retrograde ejaculation. Sperm, fructose level, and viscosity can be measured.
- Anejaculation will have fructose negative, sperm negative, nonviscous postorgasmic urinalysis.
- In painful ejaculation, urinalysis and urine culture
- If prostate cancer is considered, check prostate-specific antigen (PSA).
- In anhedonia, consider checking testosterone, prolactin, and thyroid levels.

Imaging

- In hematospermia, painful ejaculation, or if ejaculatory duct obstruction is considered, transrectal ultrasound (TRUS) may be helpful.
- TRUS-guided seminal vesicle aspiration; if ejaculatory duct obstruction is present, then the aspirate will contain sperm.
- If suspicious of anatomic abnormality, can use ultrasound and/or MRI

TREATMENT

MEDICATION

- Premature ejaculation:
  - Treating underlying erectile dysfunction (if identified) may allow for a decrease in the rapidity.
  - Behavioral/sex therapy is important when appropriate.
  - Topical anesthetic gel applied (2.5% prilocaine + 2.5 % lidocaine [EMLA]) 2.5 g under a condom for 30 minutes prior to intercourse
  - Experimental PSD502 topical aerosol preparation of lidocaine/prilocaine effective in phase III trials (4)
  - Clomipramine 20–50 mg/d or sertraline 25–200 mg/d, fluoxetine 5–20 mg/d, or paroxetine 10–40 mg/d have been shown to delay ejaculation.
  - Clomipramine shown to be the most effective, but has higher rate of side effects
  - On-demand use of clomipramine 20–40 mg 4–24 hours before intercourse or sertraline 50 mg 4–8 hours before intercourse or paroxetine 20 mg 3–4 hours before intercourse
  - Switching antidepressants to bupropion, nefazodone, mirtazapine, or possibly trazodone may eliminate drug-induced ejaculatory disturbance.
- Delayed (retarded) ejaculation:
  - Retarded orgasm and ejaculation in patients who must continue SSRIs may respond to bupropion, buspirone, cyproheptadine, or yohimbine supplementation before intercourse.
  - Some evidence that cyproheptadine and amantadine may be helpful (5)
- Anejaculation/retrograde ejaculation:
  - α-agonists and antihistamines can be helpful but are not approved by the FDA:
    - Pseudoephedrine 60 mg PO every day to q.i.d.
    - Imipramine 25 mg PO b.i.d.
    - Ephedrine sulfate 50 mg PO q.i.d.
- Painful ejaculation:
  - Treat underlying infection/inflammatory process
  - α-blockers may have some benefit

ADDITIONAL TREATMENT

General Measures

- Identifying any medical cause (even if not reversible) helps patient accept condition.
- Improve partner communication.
- Psychological counseling may be beneficial for some patients.
- Reduce performance pressure through reassurance.
- Use of a variety of resources may be necessary (e.g., psychiatrist, psychologist, sex therapist, vascular surgeon, urologist, endocrinologist, neurologist).
- Premature ejaculation:
  - Use sensate focus therapy (gradual progression of nonsexual contact to sexual contact)
  - Quiet vagina: Female partner stops moving just prior to ejaculation
  - Techniques to learn ejaculatory control (e.g., coronal squeeze technique [squeezing the glans penis until ejaculatory urge ceases] or start-and-stop technique [cessation of penile stimulation when ejaculation approaches and resumption of stimulation when ejaculatory feeling ends])
- Delayed ejaculation:
  - Change medications to an antidepressant that is less likely to cause delayed ejaculation (citalopram, fluvoxamine, nefazodone).
  - If patient has diabetes, better control of diabetes may improve ejaculation.
  - Penile vibratory stimulation (not frequently used)
- Anejaculation/retrograde ejaculation:
  - Discontinue offending medication(s).
  - Diabetic control
  - If urethral obstruction present, refer to urology for management.
  - Retrograde ejaculation may be helped if intercourse occurs when bladder is full.
  - Consider penile vibratory stimulation (effective in spinal cord injuries >T10) or electroejaculation (place on monitor if lesions above T6 because autonomic dysreflexia may result) to collect sperm in anejaculation cases.
- Painful ejaculation:
  - Counseling may be beneficial.
  - If seminal vesicle stones possible, refer to urology.
- Hematospermia:
  - If persistent or high degree of suspicion for abnormality, refer to urologist for proper evaluation.

Issues for Referral

The following conditions, when suspected, should be referred to a urologist:

- Ejaculatory duct obstruction
- Seminal vesicle or prostatic stones
- Urethral obstruction
- Vas deferens obstruction
- Calculi
- Persistent or severe hematospermia

SURGERY/OTHER PROCEDURES

Surgical treatment of ejaculatory duct obstruction:

- Transurethral resection of the ejaculatory ducts

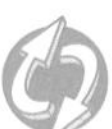

ONGOING CARE

PATIENT EDUCATION

See "General Measures."

PROGNOSIS

Often improves with therapy and counseling

COMPLICATIONS

Psychological impact on some males: Signs of severe inadequacy, self-doubt, additional anxiety, and guilt

REFERENCES

1. Montague DK, Jarow J, Broderick GA, et al. AUA guideline on the pharmacologic management of premature ejaculation. *J Urol*. 2004;172:290–4.
2. Master VA, Turek PJ. Ejaculatory physiology and dysfunction. *Urol Clin North Am*. 2001;28: 363–75, x.
3. Schuster TG, Ohl DA. Diagnosis and treatment of ejaculatory dysfunction. *Urol Clin North Am*. 2002;29:939–48.
4. Dinsmore WW, Wyllie MG. PSD502 improves ejaculatory latency, control and sexual satisfaction when applied topically 5 min before intercourse in men with premature ejaculation: Results of a phase III, multicentre, double-blind, placebo-controlled study. *BJU Int*. 2009.
5. McMahon CG, Abdo C, Incrocci L, et al. Disorders of orgasm and ejaculation in men. *J Sex Med*. 2004;1: 58–65.

ADDITIONAL READING

- Mercer CH, et al. Sexual function problems and health seeking behaviour in Britain: Probability sample survey. *Br Med J*. 2003;327:426–7.
- Richardson D, Goldmeier D, BASHH Special Interest Group for Sexual Dysfunction. Recommendations for the management of retarded ejaculation: BASHH Special Interest Group for Sexual Dysfunction. *Int J STD AIDS*. 2006;17:7–13.
- Waldinger MD. Premature ejaculation: Definition and drug treatment. *Drugs*. 2007;67:547–68.

CODES

ICD9

- 302.75 Premature ejaculation
- 608.87 Retrograde ejaculation
- 608.89 Other specified disorders of male genital organs

CLINICAL PEARLS

- If erectile dysfunction is contributing to ejaculatory difficulty, management of erectile dysfunction should precede attempted management of ejaculatory disorders.
- Medications should always be thoroughly reviewed, as they may be the primary cause of ejaculatory disorders.
- A multidisciplinary approach, including the primary care physician, urologists, psychologists, and other appropriate health care professionals, is essential to the proper treatment of ejaculatory disorders.

E

ELDER ABUSE

Thomas Price, MD

BASICS

DESCRIPTION

- Elder abuse, or elder mistreatment, is a condition in which the physical, psychological, or financial well-being of an older adult is infringed upon through intentional acts or lack of action, even if harm is not intended. 3 basic entities compose this problem:
  - Abuse: Includes physical, sexual, or psychological harm
  - Neglect: Withholding of necessary treatments or services
  - Exploitation: Use of an older adult's property counter to their needs or benefit
- Self-neglect is an additional subtype and may represent the most common form of elder mistreatment, though its exact prevalence is poorly understood (1).

EPIDEMIOLOGY

Incidence

10% of persons worldwide older than age 65 suffer abuse on an annual basis; as many as 1 new case every 8 hours (2,3)

Prevalence

Of persons older than age 60, in the past year:

- 5.2% encountered financial mistreatment by family members
- 5.1% suffered potential neglect
- 4.6% encountered emotional mistreatment, mostly by humiliation or verbal abuse
- 1.6% encountered physical mistreatment, mostly through battery
- 0.6% were sexually mistreated, mostly through forced intercourse (3)

RISK FACTORS

- Abuse victim risk factors (1,4):
  - Shared living situation with abuser
  - Dementia or other cognitive impairment
  - Social isolation or lower social network
  - Lower household income
  - Need for assistance with activities of daily living (ADLs)
  - Pre-existing poor relationship to abuser
  - Psychological distress or aggressive behaviors
- Abuse perpetrator risk factors (1):
  - Substance abuse (alcohol, narcotics, etc.)
  - Mental illness/alcohol abuse (abuser)
  - Financial/material dependence (abuser) on the victim
  - Unemployment
  - Family relationships

GENERAL PREVENTION

- Improve patient social contact and support
- Monitor patients for self-neglect and functional decline
- Recognition of caregiver stressors and burden
- Assist management of behavioral and functional changes that occur in dementia
- Though several screening tools exist, screening questionnaires are not helpful for use with patients with cognitive impairment (5). Common screening questions include:
  - Have you felt unsafe at home?
  - Has anyone hurt you, called you names, or taken things from you?
  - What happens when you disagree with [caregiver]?

ETIOLOGY

The most common scenario of abuse is a caregiver with poor family/social support who is providing care for an older person with a degree of disability. These caregivers are often relatives of the possible victim. Abuse can occur in any setting (home, assisted living, nursing home), and any older person with an impaired ability to defend or care for themself can be at risk.

COMMONLY ASSOCIATED CONDITIONS

- Patients diagnosed as suffering from elder abuse correlated with severity of cognitive impairment, presence of depression, delusions, pressure ulcers, actively resisting care, and conflict with family or friends (6)[B]:
  - Dementia manifesting with impaired decision making regarding finances may represent a higher risk pool (7).
- Older patients admitted with a geriatric syndrome of "failure to thrive" may be victims and should be screened for abuse.

DIAGNOSIS

Because neglect and exploitation are more common forms of elder mistreatment than abuse, the history is extremely important and will allow the practitioner to develop his or her own suspicion threshold for an individual case.

HISTORY

- Interviewing the patient separate from the suspected abuser is helpful. The patient may give vague explanations of the causes of injury or may refuse to answer questions.
- A history of dementia or functional decline can be associated with increased risk, as can an increase in physical and psychological aggression, which is often seen in dementia.
- Observe interaction between patient and caregiver. Suspicion is raised if the patient withdraws from the caregiver or the caregiver interrupts the patient and provides answers for him or her. Caregivers with anxiety, depression, and reduced social support are more likely to mistreat their care recipients (5)[C].

PHYSICAL EXAM

- Documentation of abnormal findings on physical exam may be used as evidence in court cases and should not include subjective or editorial comments or conclusions.
- Context of the physical condition of the patient is important. If they are examined in their own bed, look for bedding or mattress soiled by bodily fluids. If found on sheets, copious flakes of skin or shedded hair can point to restricted mobility and care:
  - Appearance of poor personal hygiene
  - Bruises and soft tissue injury:
    - Common areas include surfaces of the upper back, upper arms, and lower legs.
    - Lesions with shapes (such as buckles, snaps, or buttons) suggest prolonged immobility or blunt trauma.
  - Pressure ulcers can indicate neglect but are equivocal outside of context.
  - Poor dentition or evidence of oral sores, candidiasis, etc.
  - Findings of lice, scabies, or saprophytes
- Fearful or withdrawn affect
- A genital exam is indicated if sexual abuse is suspected, but should be performed with a documented chaperone of the patient's gender. The use of a rape kit if trained personnel is available may be appropriate.

DIAGNOSTIC TESTS & INTERPRETATION

Lab

The following workup is recommended:

- Urine and blood screen for narcotics, intoxicants, and other psychoactive agents (extended panels may be necessary depending on the laboratory)
- Nutritional assessment, including appropriate serology (albumin, prealbumin, iron), blood count, and extended blood chemistry
- Additional labs to consider in patients with cognitive impairment: Thyroid-stimulating hormone, syphilis serology, vitamin B_{12} level
- Assessment of infection (may include urinalysis and culture, chest radiograph, blood count, and cultures)
- If sexual abuse is suspected, culture and microscopy of any present exudate or residue and viral serology (rape kit lab package)

Imaging

- Radiographic imaging of areas below soft tissue injury is indicated if there is evidence of infection (osteomyelitis) at a pressure ulcer site or bruising of a limb (fracture).
- If physical abuse is suspected and cognitive impairment present, then cranial imaging to look for hemorrhage (e.g., subdural) is indicated.

Diagnostic Procedures/Surgery

- Pulse test: Check BP and pulse in presence and absence of suspected abuser. Elevation of either in the presence of the suspected abuser should raise suspicion. Useful in patients with dementia or other condition that makes history taking difficult.
- Documentation: Practitioners may make statements of "suspected mistreatment" but should avoid making definitive diagnosis of abuse in their initial assessment.

DIFFERENTIAL DIAGNOSIS

- Alzheimer disease alone can manifest with poor nutrition, withdrawal from society, and feelings of persecution.
- Delusions due to dementia, such as the Alzheimer type, may manifest early with accusations of theft and deception.
- Parkinson disease patients often fall and may exhibit fractures and bruises on a frequent basis that may mimic recurrent physical abuse.
- Coagulopathy such as that caused by use of antiplatelet or warfarin therapy can cause easy bruising of the forearms but usually spares the upper arm.
- Adenocarcinoma of the lung, prostate, and colon can present with weight loss, apathy, and pressure ulcers.
- Pancreatic adenocarcinoma may present with severe weight loss, depression, and a failure to thrive.
- Hypothyroidism can present with apathy, weight loss, and confusion that may be confused for neglect.
- Chronic lung disease can present as weight loss, reduced functional reserve, and withdrawal.
- Acute psychosis can be caused by infection, medications, or metabolic disturbances and may result in delusional accusations of harm and neglect.
- Impaired financial status often leads to a lack of access to appropriate food, clothing, shelter, and medical care.

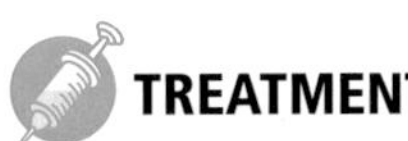

TREATMENT

In most states, the physician or allied health care worker is a mandated reporter of suspicion of elder abuse. This does not put a burden of charge on the physician.

IN-PATIENT CONSIDERATIONS

Initial Stabilization

Patient's living situation must be explored and determination of a safe alternative environment made. This is usually in conjunction with a social worker.

Admission Criteria

- Victims of elder abuse should be admitted to the hospital (observation status) if there are no safe discharge alternatives.
- Often, these victims will have acute or chronic medical illness that requires medical attention and possible conversion from observation to inpatient status.
- Cases of suspected abuse *must be reported* to the state's Adult Protective Services agency or a designated alternative (e.g., if patient resides in nursing home, then report to that state's regulatory entity). Social services may help. If physical harm has occurred, consider reporting to local law enforcement for investigation.
- Hospital security may need to be notified if restricted visitor access to a patient is required, and the patient's name may be hidden from the public hospital census.

Discharge Criteria

Victims should not be discharged to a potentially abusive environment without active investigation or protection (e.g., court order). Alternatives to discharge to the unsafe environment may include:

- Another friend or family member
- Nursing home
- Personal care home
- Assisted living facility
- Local victims' rescue or sheltering program if available

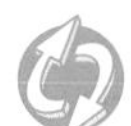

ONGOING CARE

FOLLOW-UP RECOMMENDATIONS

Victims of abuse should not be discharged without adequate follow-up, including:

- Primary care physician visit in 1 week
- Follow-up with Adult Protective Services or other agency
- Home Health Agency for assessment of safety (physical therapy)
- Follow-up with appropriate psychiatric or psychological care

Patient Monitoring

Frequent follow-up with appropriate state agency as discussed above

PATIENT EDUCATION

To locate the Elder Abuse Hotline in your state, go to: www.nccafv.org/state_elder_abuse_hotlines.htm

PROGNOSIS

Patients with corroborated elder abuse have a 3-fold increase in mortality over 10 years when compared with controls (8)[B].

COMPLICATIONS

Victims of elder abuse who are seen by an Adult Protective Services caseworkers are 4 times more likely to be admitted to a nursing home (9)[B].

REFERENCES

1. Mosqueda L, Dong X, et al. Elder abuse and self-neglect: "I don't care anything about going to the doctor, to be honest. . .". *JAMA*. 2011;306: 532–40.
2. National Center on Elder Abuse. *Elder Abuse Prevalence and Incidence*. Washinton, DC: American Public Human Services Association; 2005.
3. Acierno R, Hernandez MA, Amstadter AB, et al. Prevalence and correlates of emotional, physical, sexual, and financial abuse and potential neglect in the United States: The National Elder Mistreatment Study. *Am J Public Health*. 2010;100:292–7.
4. Lachs MS, Pillemer K, et al. Elder abuse. *Lancet*. 2004;364:1263–72.
5. Wiglesworth A, Mosqueda L, Mulnard R, et al. Screening for abuse and neglect of people with dementia. *J Am Geriatr Soc*. 2010;58:493–500.
6. Cooper C, Katona C, Finne-Soveri H, et al. Indicators of elder abuse: A crossnational comparison of psychiatric morbidity and other determinants in the Ad-HOC study. *Am J Geriatr Psychiatry*. 2006;14:489–97.
7. Widera E, Steenpass V, Marson D, et al. Finances in the older patient with cognitive impairment: "He didn't want me to take over." *JAMA*. 2011;305:698–706.
8. Lachs MS, Williams CS, O'Brien S, et al. The mortality of elder mistreatment. *JAMA*. 1998;280: 428–32.
9. Lachs MS, Williams CS, O'Brien S, et al. Adult protective service use and nursing home placement. *Gerontologist*. 2002;42:734–9.

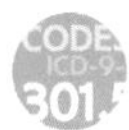

CODES

ICD9

- 995.82 Adult emotional/psychological abuse
- 995.83 Adult sexual abuse
- 995.84 Adult neglect (nutritional)

CLINICAL PEARLS

- Elder abuse, or elder mistreatment, is a condition in which the physical, psychological, or financial well-being of an older adult is infringed upon through intentional acts or lack of action, even if harm is not intended. 3 basic entities compose this problem:
  - Abuse: Includes physical, sexual, or psychological harm
  - Neglect: Withholding of necessary treatments or services
  - Exploitation: Use of an older adult's property counter to their needs or benefit
- Patients are diagnosed as suffering from elder abuse correlated with severity of cognitive impairment, presence of depression, delusions, pressure ulcers, actively resisting care, and conflict with family or friends.
- Patients with dementia or other psychiatric illness may accuse caregivers of physical harm or theft because of disease-induced delusions. Corroborating evidence may be needed to support suspicion of abuse, but these claims should not be summarily dismissed.

ENCEPHALITIS, VIRAL

Mary Cataletto, MD
Margaret McCormick, MS, RN

BASICS

DESCRIPTION

- Inflammatory process of the brain associated with clinical evidence of neurologic dysfunction
- System(s) affected: Nervous
- Synonym(s): Meningoencephalitis

EPIDEMIOLOGY

Incidence

3.5–7.4 per 100,000 persons per year

Prevalence

- Seasonal variation (e.g., arboviruses, enteroviruses, mumps, varicella)
- Nonseasonal: Most others (e.g., herpes simplex virus [HSV])

RISK FACTORS

- Age: Increased incidence among infants and elderly
- Contact with animals or insect vectors
- Impaired immune status
- Ingestions (e.g., raw meat)
- Occupation (e.g., lab or animal-care workers)
- Recreational activities (e.g., camping, hunting)
- Transfusion and transplantation
- Travel to endemic areas
- Recent vaccinations or unvaccinated status

GENERAL PREVENTION

- Appropriate clothing to protect against mosquitos
- Use of mosquito repellants (DEET, Picaridin)
- Avoidance and removal of ticks
- Elimination of mosquito breeding sources
- Vaccines, when available

PATHOPHYSIOLOGY

- Most common entry site is through the blood.
- Specific cell lines may be infected and are associated with specific symptom complexes:
  - Neurons: Associated with seizures
  - Oligodendroglia: May cause demyelination alone, cortical infection, or reactive parenchymal swelling; changes in state of consciousness
  - Brainstem neurons: Coma, respiratory failure
  - Microglia, macrophages: Neurologic dysfunction
- Pathologic changes seen with postinfectious and postvaccinal encephalomyelitis include perivascular infiltration of mononuclear inflammatory cells.

ETIOLOGY

- Vaccines have changed epidemiology in US.
- Despite extensive evaluations, the etiologic agent frequently is not identified (32–75%).
- Most commonly identified etiologies in US: HSV, West Nile, enteroviruses

COMMONLY ASSOCIATED CONDITIONS

- Seizures
- Hyperthermia
- Increased intracranial pressure (ICP)
- Inappropriate antidiuretic hormone (ADH) secretion

DIAGNOSIS

- Seek epidemiologic clues and assess risk factors in all patients with encephalitis.
- Consider acute disseminated encephalomyelitis (ADEM) with history of recent infectious illness or vaccination associated with clinical presentation of encephalitis (1)[B].
- Specific diagnostic studies should be done in the majority of patients (see "Diagnostic Tests & Interpretation" section) (1)[A].

HISTORY

The classic triad includes fever, headache, and altered mental status.

PHYSICAL EXAM

- General signs:
  - Rash
  - Mucus membrane lesions
  - Concurrent or prodromal upper respiratory findings
  - Parotitis
  - Erythema nodosum
  - Fever
- Neurologic findings:
  - Altered level of consciousness
  - Acute cognitive dysfunction
  - Behavioral changes
  - Neck stiffness
  - Focal neurologic signs
  - Motor weakness
- Other:
  - Loss of temperature or vasomotor control
  - Diabetes insipidus
  - Syndrome of inappropriate secretion of ADH

DIAGNOSTIC TESTS & INTERPRETATION

Lab

- Recommended general diagnostic studies (outside CNS) for all suspected encephalitis patients:
  - Blood cultures (1)[B]
  - Serum samples: At time of initial presentation and stored for future studies
- Additional studies based on risk factors and clinical findings:
  - Cultures of stool, nasopharynx, sputum (1)[B]
  - Skin scrapings of active vesicles (direct fluorescent antibody [DFA] testing to identify viral antigen)
  - Tissue biopsies with culture, antigen detection, nucleic acid amplification testing and histology (1)[A]
  - Serologic testing: IgM antibodies (1)[A], IgM and IgG capture ELISAs
  - Plaque reduction neutralization
  - Acute and convalescent phase serum to show seroconversion: Not helpful to initiate therapy but may be helpful for the retrospective diagnosis of a specific pathogen (1)[B]
  - Serum IgG antibodies should be considered in patients where the encephalitis may be the result of reactivation of a previously acquired infection.
  - Nucleic acid amplification tests (polymerase chain reaction [PCR]) (1)[B]

Initial lab tests

- Lumbar puncture is essential (unless specific contraindication) (1)[A]:
  - CSF shows pleocytosis (10–2,000 cells/mm^3). Mononuclear cells usually predominate. Finding of CSF eosinophils may suggest certain pathogens (e.g., highest with helminths but can also be seen with other pathogens).
  - CSF glucose normal or mildly depressed
  - CSF protein usually mild or moderately increased
  - Direct examination of CSF fluid with Gram stain for bacteria, acid–fast stain for *Mycobacteria*, by India ink for *Cryptococcus*, wet preparation for free-living amoeba, Giemsa stain for trypanosomes
  - CSF culture for bacteria, mycobacteria, fungi, amoeba, and viruses
  - CSF culture for viruses has limited value; not routinely recommended
  - CSF nucleic acid amplification tests (e.g., PCR) (1)[A]; herpes simplex PCR should be performed on all specimens (1)[A]; if negative, consider repeat in 3–7 days for those with compatible clinical syndrome or temporal lobe localization on neuroimaging (1)[B]
  - Viral-specific IgM (1)[A]
- In up to 10% of cases with viral encephalitis, CSF findings are normal.

Follow-Up & Special Considerations

- PCR may be negative early on; repeat in 48–72 hours; may be useful in detecting herpesvirus, enterovirus, seasonal and 2009 H1N1 influenza virus, and polyomavirus.
- Rapid influenza diagnostic tests (RIDTs) may be helpful in diagnosing seasonal and 2009 H1N1 in a clinically useful time frame. However, their sensitivity ranges from 10–70% and the currently available RIDTs cannot distinguish between the different influenza A subtypes (seasonal H1N1 vs. 2009 H1N1 vs. H3N2).

Imaging

Initial approach

- MRI: Most sensitive and most specific; however, in some cases, it may be normal either initially or during clinical course (2)[A]
- Diffusion-weighted imaging is superior to conventional MRI in encephalitis caused by herpes simplex virus, enterovirus, and West Nile virus.
- FLAIR (fluid attenuated inversion recovery) imaging may be helpful with enterovirus 71 encephalitis, flaviviruses, and eastern equine encephalitis.
- CT, with and without contrast enhancement, if MRI is not an option (1)[B]
- Fluorodeoxyglucose-positron emission tomography (FDG-PET) is not routinely recommended, but may be helpful as an adjunct diagnostic tool.

Follow-Up & Special Considerations

Imaging studies (e.g., CT, MRI, brain scan) may be normal early; later, nonspecific abnormalities may be seen (exception, herpes simplex encephalitis).

Diagnostic Procedures/Surgery

- Chest x-ray (CXR) may be helpful
- Electroencephalogram (EEG) is nondiagnostic but may be useful in early herpes simplex encephalitis and less commonly in other herpes viruses (VAV, EBV, HHV6):
  - Recommended for all patients with encephalitis (1)[A]
- Serologic testing
- Brain biopsy: *Rarely used and not routinely recommended*. Consider if unknown etiology and condition is deteriorating despite treatment with acyclovir (1)[B].

Pathological Findings

- Prominent inflammatory reaction in meninges and in a perivascular distribution
- Swelling and degenerative changes

DIFFERENTIAL DIAGNOSIS

- Vasculitis
- Paraneoplastic syndromes
- Postinfectious encephalitis
- Postimmunization encephalitis
- ADEM
- Secondary encephalopathy

TREATMENT

- Most will require intensive care.
- Initial empiric therapy includes prompt administration of IV acyclovir (unless there is a contraindication).
- When appropriate, combine with therapy for bacterial, rickettsial, or ehrlichial infection.
- Once an etiologic agent has been identified, therapeutic intervention should be re-evaluated, focusing on pathogen-specific therapy and discontinuing therapy if there is no available therapy against the specific etiologic agent.

MEDICATION

- No specific drug therapy is available for most types of viral encephalitis.
- Antiviral agents are available for encephalitides caused by herpes viruses, especially HSV, and for both seasonal and 2009 H1N1 influenza viruses.
- Acyclovir is recommended as immediate initial treatment for all patients with suspected encephalitis, pending results of diagnostic studies (3)[A].
- Appropriate antiviral therapy (i.e., Oseltamivir or Zanamivir) should be started as soon as possible for hospitalized patients with neurologic symptoms and suspected seasonal or 2009 H1N1 influenza infection (4)[C].
- Empiric antimicrobial therapy should be initiated if indicated by the clinical history or specific epidemiologic factors (1)[A].
- Doxycycline should be added to empiric regimen when clinical clues suggest rickettsial or ehrlichial infection (1)[A].
- Once etiology is determined, treat specifically.

ADDITIONAL TREATMENT

General Measures

- Supportive therapy
- Monitoring for drug-related toxicities

Issues for Referral

- Monitoring and management of ICP
- Evaluation and treatment of seizures
- Multidisciplinary teams often provide care.

Additional Therapies

Adjunctive agents: Limited data; consider risks and benefits, and consult infectious disease:

- Interferon (IFN) alpha: Tried with West Nile virus encephalitis; results inconclusive
- IFN alpha 2b (limited series): Reduce severity and duration of complications of St. Louis *encephalitis virus meningoencephalitis* (further studies needed)
- IV Ig containing high anti–West Nile virus antibody titers in patients with West Nile virus neuroinvasive disease (in trial)

SURGERY/OTHER PROCEDURES

The following procedures may be required during stabilization and care:

- ICP monitor
- Intubation and mechanical ventilation
- Central line for hemodynamic monitoring or total parenteral nutrition
- Arterial line
- Nasogastric tube placement
- Foley catheter placement

IN-PATIENT CONSIDERATIONS

- Admit suspected cases of encephalitis to hospital for evaluation, supportive care, and treatment. Most will require intensive care services.
- Although standard isolation precautions are appropriate for most viral encephalitides, droplet precautions are necessary for patients with confirmed or suspected seasonal or 2009 H1N1 influenza infection.

Initial Stabilization

- Protect airway when appropriate, and when indicated provide:
  - Supplemental oxygen
  - Intubation and mechanical ventilatory support
- Assessment and management of circulatory status, fluids, glucose, and electrolytes
- Precautions for seizure and altered mental status
- Consider isolation for immunosuppressed patients and those with exanthems.

Admission Criteria

- Suspicion of encephalitis
- Altered level of consciousness
- Need for intensive monitoring, airway protection, cardiopulmonary support

IV Fluids

- Monitor glucose, chemistries, and fluid balance
- Monitor for syndrome of inappropriate ADH hypersecretion
- Monitor for drug-specific toxicities

Nursing

- Isolation should be considered for immunosuppressed patients and those with exanthems.
- Precautions for seizure and altered mental status
- Comfort measures to reduce headache
- Injury prevention and safety
- Monitor level of consciousness, neurologic signs, cardiorespiratory parameters, and fluid balance.
- Establish and maintain open lines of communication with patient and family.
- Educate families about the importance of vaccines when available and postexposure prophylaxis for seasonal or 2009 H1N1 influenza virus.
- Skin care to prevent decubitus ulcers

Discharge Criteria

Resolution of acute symptoms:

- No longer need hospital-level care

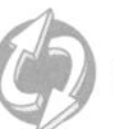

ONGOING CARE

Patients with suspected or proven encephalitis are best cared for, at least initially, in an intensive care unit.

FOLLOW-UP RECOMMENDATIONS

- Postencephalitis sequelae are primarily neurologic, and follow-up should be guided by patient's condition (e.g., anticonvulsants for seizures).
- Physical therapy may be necessary.

PATIENT EDUCATION

- DEET-containing mosquito repellants
- Avoidance of outdoor activities during periods of peak mosquito activity
- Use of protective clothing
- Adequate vector control and environmental sanitation
- Vaccines when available
- www.mayoclinic.com/health/encephalitis/DS00226

PROGNOSIS

Often difficult to predict; prognosis related to etiologic agent, age, and clinical course

COMPLICATIONS

Vary with age, etiologic agent, and clinical course

REFERENCES

1. Mandell G, et al. *Principles & Practice of Infectious Diseases*, 6th ed. New York: Elsevier; 2005: 1143–7.
2. Chaudhuri A, Kennedy PG. Diagnosis and treatment of viral encephalitis. *Postgrad Med J*. 2002;78:575–83.
3. Tunkel AR, Glaser CA, Bloch KC, et al. The management of encephalitis: Clinical practice guidelines by the Infectious Diseases Society of America. *Clin Infect Dis*. 2008;47:303–26.
4. CDC. Neurologic complications associated with novel influenza A (H1N1) virus infection in children—Dallas, Texas, May 2009. *MMWR*. 2009;58:773–8.

ADDITIONAL READING

Long SS. Encephalitis: Diagnosis and management in the real world. *Adv Exp Med Biol*. 2011;697: 153–73.

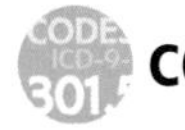

CODES

ICD9

049.9 Unspecified non-arthropod-borne viral diseases of central nervous system

CLINICAL PEARLS

- Neurologic signs are unlikely to distinguish etiologies, but location and type of skin lesions may be helpful.
- PCR may be negative early on; repeat in 48–72 hours.

ENCOPRESIS

Jay Gar-Yee Fong, MD
William T. Garrison, PhD

BASICS

DESCRIPTION

- The involuntary or intentional passage of feces into clothing or other inappropriate places by a child 4–18 years of age:
  - Age may be chronologic or developmental.
  - Absence of underlying organic process explaining these symptoms
  - At least 1 event per month for 3 months
  - Classified into functional constipation (retentive encopresis) and functional nonretentive fecal incontinence (FNRFI): Both cause fecal incontinence, but no constipation in FNRFI. *Functional constipation is more common.*
- System(s) affected: GI; Psychological
- Synonyms(s): Fecal incontinence, Soiling

EPIDEMIOLOGY

Incidence

Predominant sex: Male > Female (3:1). Constipation accounts for 3% of general pediatric referrals; up to 84% of constipated children have fecal incontinence at some point.

Prevalence

Occurs in 1–3% of children >4 years of age

RISK FACTORS

- Male gender
- Constipation
- Very low birth weight
- Painful defecation
- Difficulty with bowel training, including pressure related to early daycare placement
- Organic/anatomic causes
- Anxiety and depression

Genetics

None known, although incidence may be higher in children with family history of constipation

GENERAL PREVENTION

Family education regarding constipation: Avoid toilet training prior to readiness, optimal feeding, early detection of problems. Look for signs of relapse: Large-caliber stools, decrease in stool frequency, and soiling.

PATHOPHYSIOLOGY

- In 90% of cases, encopresis develops as a consequence of chronic constipation with resulting overflow incontinence, which typically is termed *retentive encopresis*. The other 10% are caused by specific organic etiologies.
- Chronic constipation due to irregular and incomplete evacuation results in progressive rectal distension and stretching of both the internal and external anal sphincters.
- As the child habituates to chronic rectal distension, he or she may no longer sense the normal urge to defecate. Eventually, soft or liquid stool begins to leak around the retained fecal mass, resulting in fecal soiling.
- Many children voluntarily withhold stool in response to the urge to defecate for fear of pain or due to a preoccupation with not interrupting social activities.

ETIOLOGY

- Psychological:
  - Stool withholding, fear, anxiety
  - Difficulty with toilet training, including unusual anxiety or conflict with parent
  - Resistance to using public toilet facilities, such as school bathrooms or outdoor toilets
  - Known association with sexual abuse in boys; likely similar association in girls as well
  - Developmental delay
- Anatomic:
  - Rectal distension and desensitization
  - Anal fissure or painful defecation
  - Muscle hypotonia
  - Slow intestinal motility
  - Hirschsprung disease
  - Cystic fibrosis
  - Spinal cord defects (e.g., spina bifida)
  - Congenital anorectal malformations
  - Anal stenosis
  - Anterior displacement of the anus
  - Postoperative stricture of anus or rectum
  - Pelvic mass
  - Neurofibromatosis
- Dietary or metabolic:
  - Lack of fiber
  - Excessive protein or milk intake
  - Inadequate water intake
  - Hypothyroidism
  - Hypercalcemia
  - Hypokalemia
  - DI or DM
  - Food allergy
  - Gluten enteropathy
- Medication side effects

COMMONLY ASSOCIATED CONDITIONS

- Common: Constipation, Hirschsprung disease
- Intermediate: Cerebral palsy, cystic fibrosis
- Less: Developmental and behavioral diagnoses, urinary incontinence

DIAGNOSIS

HISTORY

- Look for signs/symptoms of constipation:
  - Hard, large-caliber stools
  - <3 defecations/week
  - Pain or discomfort with stool passage, withholding of stool
  - Blood on stools
  - Decreased appetite
  - Abdominal pain improving with stool passage
  - Hiding while defecating before child is toilet trained; avoiding use of the toilet
  - Diet low in fiber or fluids, high in dairy
  - Passed stool within first 48 hours of life
  - Pasty stool found on underclothes
  - Recurrent UTIs
- Abrupt onset after age 5 years more likely to be associated with psychological trauma
- Overlap with ADD common in children >5 years of age
- Medications such as opiates, phenobarbital, and tricyclic antidepressants (TCAs)
- Family history of constipation

PHYSICAL EXAM

- Detailed history and physical exam usually make the diagnosis without need for lab testing.
- Neurologic exam of lower extremities and perineal area with attention to S1–S4 distribution, perineal sensation, cremasteric reflex, and anal sphincter tone
- Genital area
- Digital rectal exam: Assess for anal fissures, sphincter tone, rectal distension/impaction, presence of occult or visible blood
- Abdominal exam: Mild abdominal distension; palpable stool in left lower quadrant.

DIAGNOSTIC TESTS & INTERPRETATION

Lab

Most cases of fecal incontinence do not require extensive lab work.

Initial lab tests

Done to rule out organic causes when conventional treatment fails: UA/urine culture: UTI/glucosuria; thyroid function tests: hypothyroidism; electrolyte panel including calcium may show hypokalemia, hypercalcemia, or hyperglycemia

Follow-Up & Special Considerations

Failure to pass meconium within 48 hours of birth, failure to thrive, bloody diarrhea, or bilious vomiting in a neonate is almost always associated with aganglionic megacolon, and that history would warrant a barium enema and/or rectal biopsy. Constipation and diarrhea, rash, failure to thrive, or recurrent pneumonia should prompt evaluation for cystic fibrosis. Celiac disease should also be a consideration. Patients with abdominal distension or ileus should be evaluated for possible obstruction.

Imaging

Abdominal plain films may be useful if an impaction is suspected but not detected by abdominal or rectal exam.

Initial approach

Comprehensive history and physical exam. Management includes education, disimpaction if necessary, prevention, and follow-up.

Diagnostic Procedures/Surgery

Manometric studies may be useful in patients who have constipation that does not respond to treatment.

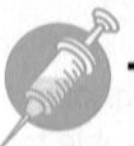

TREATMENT

A treatment approach that integrates both laxative treatment and behavioral therapy improves continence in children with fecal incontinence over laxative treatment alone (1).

MEDICATION

- Remove stool impaction, then start maintenance treatment program.
- No randomized, controlled studies have compared methods of disimpaction: Can use oral agents, enemas, and rectal suppositories; oral agents are least traumatic. Glycerin suppositories best option for infants.

First Line

- Disimpaction with PEG has been shown to be more effective than lactulose in 1 study (2)[B]:
  - Give 17 g (240 mL) water or juice: 1–1.5 g/kg/d × 3 days for disimpaction
  - 0.26–0.084 g/kg/d for maintenance
- Disimpaction with mineral oil for child >1 year also effective; give 15–30 mL/yr of age to maximum of 240 mL:
  - Maintenance: 1–3 mL/kg/d or divided b.i.d.
  - May mix with orange juice to make palatable; *avoid in infants to avoid aspiration and lipoid pneumonia*
- Other maintenance regimens include:
  - Milk of magnesia (MOM) 400 mg (5 mL): 103 mL/kg/d b.i.d. (3)[A]
  - Lactulose 10 g (15 mL): 1–3 mL/kg/d b.i.d.
  - Senna syrup 8.8 g sennoside (5 mL): Age 2–6 years: 2.5–7.5 mL/d b.i.d.; age 6–12 years: 5–15 mL/d b.i.d.
  - Bisacodyl suppository 10 mg: 0.5–1 suppository once or twice per day

Second Line

Another disimpaction protocol is as follows:

- Give 1 oz (28.4 g) of mineral oil the first day.
- On the next day, give 1–3 enemas until clear; this may be repeated over the next 1–2 days.
- Give an oil-retention enema.
- Follow the oil-retention enema with hypophosphate enemas (e.g., sodium phosphate [Fleet] 1 oz [28.4 g] per 20 lb [9.1 kg]) of body weight *or*
- Normal saline enemas: 2 tsp table salt/qt (946 mL) of warm water, and give 2 oz (60 mL)/yr of age to a maximum of 16 oz (480 mL)

ADDITIONAL TREATMENT

General Measures

- Anticipatory guidance relative to toilet training beginning at 18 months, with special attention to when children should reduce reliance on diapers or pull-ups during the daytime hours
- Eliminate impaction prior to maintenance Rx.
- Avoid frequent and repeated rectal exams, enemas, and suppositories, especially in infants.
- Once stools seem regular in frequency, child should sit on toilet b.i.d. at the same time each day for 10–15 minutes and for 10–15 minutes after meals. Incorporate positive reinforcement for successfully produced bowel movements.

Issues for Referral

If symptoms do not improve after 6 months of good compliance with a multifactorial treatment model, refer to pediatric GI for further evaluation.

Additional Therapies

Behavioral treatment and counseling

COMPLEMENTARY AND ALTERNATIVE MEDICINE

- Behavioral treatment is recommended as an adjunct to medical therapy in children with functional constipation.
- Children who receive behavioral treatment in addition to medications are more likely to have resolution of encopresis at 3 and 6 months than children who get medication alone.
- Biofeedback is not recommended because it does not improve outcomes when it is combined with medical therapy for functional constipation in children (1)[B].

SURGERY/OTHER PROCEDURES

If ongoing constipation refractory to a combination of medical and behavioral therapy, consider anorectal manometry to evaluate for internal anal sphincter achalasia (or ultrashort-segment Hirschsprung disease). If present, this condition can be treated successfully in the majority of patients with an internal sphincter myectomy.

IN-PATIENT CONSIDERATIONS

Initial Stabilization

Hospital admission and abdominal films may be necessary to ensure complete removal of impaction. This may include gastric administration of balanced electrolyte–polyethylene glycol solutions if the patient cannot tolerate the medication by mouth. Serial abdominal films as well as careful observation of the rectal effluent can help to determine when the patient is adequately treated.

Admission Criteria

Admission criteria should include:

- Continued soiling and recurrent impaction on outpatient medical therapy, whether from lack of medication efficacy or patient medication nonadherence
- Decreased PO intake for fluid and food
- Vomiting or obstructive-type symptoms

IV Fluids

IV fluids should be considered when the pediatric patient is heading toward dehydration while undergoing bowel cleanout.

Nursing

Nursing is essential to observing and documenting the stool consistency and clarity.

Discharge Criteria

- Stools becoming more loose in consistency and clear in appearance would signify a successful in patient endpoint.
- Abdominal radiograph showing much less fecal loading (compared with a pretreatment radiograph) plus improving serial abdominal exams

ONGOING CARE

FOLLOW-UP RECOMMENDATIONS

Patient Monitoring

- Continue the maintenance treatment program for at least 6 months, possibly 1–2 years.
- Visits every 4–10 weeks for support and to ensure compliance; more often with oppositional or anxious children
- Telephone availability to adjust doses and to provide continued encouragement to caregivers
- Treat redevelopment of impaction promptly.
- Chief target behaviors in a behavior plan for such children include compliance with medication, compliance with sits, and self-initiation of bathroom visits.
- Children who do not progress with a well-designed behavior plan should be referred for more in-depth mental health evaluation and counseling.

DIET

Hydration, high fiber, decrease or avoid cow's milk products if a trial shows this to be helpful. Avoid excessive bananas, rice, apples, and gelatin.

PATIENT EDUCATION

- Education and demystifying of the process
- Careful and full explanation of the treatment plan and dietary changes
- Avoid punishment for soiling.
- In children >4 years of age, explain to parents how overreliance on diapers and pull-ups, while convenient, can prolong the problem.
- Always attempt to use positive reinforcement first for successful toilet sits and medication compliance.
- If positive approach is unsuccessful, consider removing daily desired privileges (e.g., TV, video games, time with friends, etc.) for noncompliance with behavioral plan. Some children respond better to use of a token economy (chips or tickets to earn privileges the child desires).

PROGNOSIS

- Initial good response with a high relapse rate due to noncompliance by parents and/or child
- Depending on the study, anywhere from 30% to 50% of children still may have encopresis after 5 years of treatment.
- Children with psychosocial or emotional problems that preceded the encopresis are more recalcitrant to treatment.

COMPLICATIONS

- Colitis due to excessive enema/suppository
- Perianal dermatitis
- Anal fissure

REFERENCES

1. Brazzelli M. Behavioural and cognitive interventions with or without other treatments for the management of faecal incontinence in children. *Cochrane Database Syst Rev.* 2008;3:CD002240.
2. Loening-Baucke V, Pashankar DS. A randomized, prospective, comparison study of polyethylene glycol 3350 without electrolytes and milk of magnesia for children with constipation and fecal incontinence. *Pediatrics.* 2006;118:528–35.
3. Baker S. Evaluation and the treatment of constipation in infants and children: Recommendation of the North American Society for Pediatric Gastroenterology, Hepatology, and Nutrition. *J Pediatr Gastroenterol Nutr.* 2006; 43e1–13.

ADDITIONAL READING

Levitt M, Peña A. Update on pediatric faecal incontinence. *Eur J Pediatr Surg.* 2009;19(1):1–9.

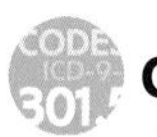

CODES

ICD9

- 307.7 Encopresis
- 787.60 Full incontinence of feces
- 787.62 Fecal smearing

CLINICAL PEARLS

- Most children (84%) with constipation have some fecal incontinence, but diagnosis of encopresis requires at least 1 event per month for 3 months.
- 90% of encopresis results from chronic constipation.
- Address toddler constipation early (decrease excessive milk intake, increase fruits/vegetables) to avoid future issues.

ENDOCARDITIS, INFECTIVE

William L. Marshall, MD
Wayra Salazar-Moreno, MD

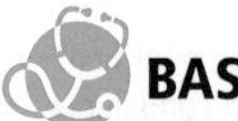

BASICS

DESCRIPTION

- An infection primarily of the valvular endocardium, and occasionally, the mural endocardium
- System(s) affected: Cardiovascular; Endocrine/Metabolic; Hematologic/Lymphatic; Immunologic; Pulmonary; Renal/Urologic; Skin/Exocrine; Neurologic
- Synonym(s): Bacterial endocarditis; Subacute bacterial endocarditis; Acute bacterial endocarditis

EPIDEMIOLOGY

Incidence

In the US: 1.5–6.2/100,000:

- Cumulative rate of endocarditis at 1 year after prosthetic valve replacement: 1.5–3.0%
- At 5 years: 3–6%
- Highest risk during 6-month period following valve replacement
- Incidence increased in the elderly

RISK FACTORS

- Injection drug use
- IV catheterization
- Certain malignancies (colon cancer)
- High-risk cardiac conditions:
  - Prosthetic cardiac valve
  - Previous infective endocarditis (IE)
  - Congenital heart disease (CHD):
    - Unrepaired cyanotic CHD, including palliative shunts and conduits
    - Repaired CHD with prosthetic device during the prior 6 months
    - Repaired CHD with residual defects at or near the site of prosthetic material
    - Cardiac transplantation recipients who develop valvulopathy (1)[B]

GENERAL PREVENTION

- Maintain good oral hygiene.
- Antibiotic prophylaxis is now only recommended for people with cardiac conditions predicting the highest risk of adverse outcome from IE (1).
- Procedures requiring prophylaxis:
  - Oral/upper respiratory tract: Manipulation of gingival tissue or periapical region of teeth or perforation of the oral mucosa (1)[C], invasive respiratory procedures involving incision, or biopsy of the respiratory mucosa:
    - Prophylaxis for dental/oral procedures (1)[C]
  - Amoxicillin: 2 g PO (if penicillin-allergic, clindamycin 600 mg PO) 30–60 minutes before procedure
  - Alternative: Ampicillin 2 g IV/IM (penicillin-allergic patients, clindamycin 600 mg IV), *or*
  - Cephalexin 2 g PO, *or*
  - Azithromycin/clarithromycin 500 mg PO, *or*
  - Cefazolin/ceftriaxone 1 g IV/IM 30 minutes before procedure
  - Pediatric doses: Amoxicillin 50 mg/kg PO; cephalexin 50 mg/kg PO; clindamycin 20 mg/kg PO; and ampicillin or ceftriaxone 50 mg/kg IM/IV
  - GI/GU: Only consider coverage for enterococcus (with penicillin, ampicillin, piperacillin, or vancomycin) for patients with an established infection undergoing procedures (1)[B].
  - Cardiac valvular surgery or placement of prosthetic intracardiac/intravascular materials (1)[B], perioperative prophylaxis with cefazolin 1–2 g IV 30 minutes preop, or vancomycin 15 mg/kg 60 minutes preop in the penicillin-allergic patient
  - Skin: Incision and drainage of infected tissue; use agents active against skin pathogens, e.g., cefazolin 1–2 g IV q8h or vancomycin 15 mg/kg q12h if penicillin-allergic or if MRSA suspected.

ETIOLOGY

- Acute endocarditis:
  - Gram-positive: *Staphylococcus aureus*; *Streptococcus* groups A, B, C, G; *Streptococcus pneumoniae*; *Staphylococcus lugdunensis*; *Enterococcus* spp.
  - Gram-negative: *Haemophilus influenzae* or *parainfluenzae*; *Neisseria gonorrhoeae*
- Subacute endocarditis:
  - Gram-positive: α-Hemolytic streptococci (Viridans group strep), *Streptococcus bovis*, *Enterococcus* spp., *S. aureus*, *Staphylococcus epidermidis*
  - HACEK organisms: ***H**aemophilus aphrophilus* or *paraphrophilus*, ***A**ctinobacillus (aggregatibacter) actinomycetemcomitans*, ***C**ardiobacterium hominis*, ***E**ikenella corrodens*, ***K**ingella kingae*
- Endocarditis in IV drug abusers (tricuspid valve):
  - Gram-positive: *S. aureus*, *Enterococcus* spp.
  - Gram-negative: *Pseudomonas aeruginosa*, *Burkholderia cepacia*, other bacilli
  - *Candida* spp.
- Early prosthetic-valve endocarditis (<60 days after valve implantation):
  - Gram-positive: *S. aureus*, *Staphylococcus epidermidis*
  - Gram-negative bacilli
  - Fungi: *Candida* spp., *Aspergillus* spp.
- Late prosthetic-valve endocarditis (>60 days after valve implantation):
  - Gram-positive: α-Hemolytic streptococci, *Enterococcus* spp., *S. epidermidis*
  - Fungi: *Candida* spp., *Aspergillus* spp.
- Culture-negative endocarditis:
  - *Bartonella quintana* (homeless people)
  - *Bartonella henselae* (cat owners)
  - Fastidious organism: *Brucella* spp., fungi, *Coxiella burnetii* (Q fever), *Chlamydia trachomatis*, *Chlamydia psittaci*, HACEK organisms
  - Use of antibiotics prior to blood cultures
  - Abiotrophia (formerly B_6-deficient streptococci)

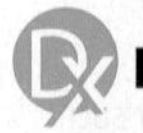

DIAGNOSIS

- Modified Duke Criteria for Diagnosis of IE (2)[B] (definite: 2 major criteria, or 1 major and 3 minor criteria, or 5 minor criteria; possible: 1 major and 1 minor criteria, or 3 minor criteria)
- Major clinical criteria:
  - Positive blood culture:
    - Typical microorganism for infective endocarditis (viridans strep., *S. aureus*, or community-acquired *Enterococcus*) from 2 separate blood cultures, *or*
    - Persistently positive blood culture
  - Single positive blood culture for *C. burnetii* or anti–phase-1 IgG antibody titer >1:800
  - Positive transesophageal echocardiogram recommended with prosthetic valves and "possible IE," or with complicated IE):
    - Oscillating mass on valve or supporting structures, in the path of regurgitant jets, on implanted material, *or*
    - Periannular abscess, *or*
    - New partial dehiscence of prosthetic valve
  - New valvular regurgitation (change in pre-existing murmur not sufficient)
- Minor criteria:
  - Predisposing heart condition or IV drug use
  - Fever ≥38.0°C (100.4°F)
  - Vascular phenomena: Major arterial emboli, septic pulmonary infarcts, mycotic aneurysm, intracranial hemorrhage, conjunctival hemorrhage, Janeway lesions
  - Immunologic phenomena: Glomerulonephritis, Osler nodes, Roth spots, rheumatoid factor
  - Microbiologic evidence: Positive blood culture, but not of major criterion (excluding single positive cultures for coagulase-negative staphylococci and organisms that do not cause endocarditis) or serologic evidence of infection with an organism likely to cause IE

HISTORY

- Fever (>38°C), chills; especially in subacute endocarditis: night sweats, weight loss, fatigue
- Predisposition to IE (e.g., injecting drug use); see "Risk Factors"
- Cough, dyspnea, orthopnea
- Symptoms of transient ischemic attacks, cerebrovascular accident (CVA), or myocardial infarction on presentation

PHYSICAL EXAM

- Heart murmur in most IE patients: Change in heart murmur is suggestive of IE, but rare; rales, edema
- Splinter hemorrhages in fingernail beds, Osler nodes on fleshy portions of extremities, "Roth Spot" retinal hemorrhages, Janeway lesions (cutaneous evidence of septic emboli), palatal or conjunctival petechiae
- Neurologic findings consistent with CVA, such as visual loss, motors weakness, and aphasia
- Splenomegaly, hematuria (due to emboli or glomerulonephritis)

DIAGNOSTIC TESTS & INTERPRETATION

Lab

- Positive blood cultures drawn >2 hours apart
- Leukocytosis in acute endocarditis
- Anemia in subacute endocarditis
- Elevated ESR, CRP
- Decreased C3, C4, CH50 in subacute endocarditis
- Hematuria, microscopic or macroscopic
- Rheumatoid factor in subacute endocarditis
- Consider serologies for *Chlamydia*, Q fever, and *Bartonella* in "culture-negative" endocarditis.

Imaging

- Transthoracic or transesophageal echocardiogram
- CT scan may be useful in locating abscesses (e.g., splenic abscess).

Pathological Findings

- Vegetations are composed of platelets, fibrin, and colonies of microorganisms. Destruction of valvular endocardium, perforation of valve leaflets, rupture

of chordae tendineae, abscesses of myocardium, rupture of sinus of Valsalva, and pericarditis may occur.
- Emboli, abscesses, and/or infarction may be found in any organ.
- Immune-complex glomerulonephritis

DIFFERENTIAL DIAGNOSIS
- Marantic endocarditis; connective tissue diseases; fever of unknown origin
- Intra-abdominal infections; rheumatic fever; salmonellosis; brucellosis
- Malignancy; tuberculosis; atrial myxoma; septic thrombophlebitis; infected central venous catheter

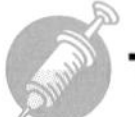

TREATMENT

MEDICATION
First Line
- PCN-susceptible Viridans group streptococci or *S. bovis*, native valve:
  - Pen G 12–18 million U/d IV either continuously or in 4–6 equally divided doses *or* ceftriaxone 2 g/d IV/IM in 1 dose, both for 4 weeks (2)[A].
  - For prosthetic valve infection, Pen G 24 million U/d IV either continuously or 4–6 equally divided doses for 6 weeks *or* ceftriaxone 2 g/d IV/IM in 1 dose ± gentamicin 3 mg/kg IV/IM q24h for 2 weeks (peak gentamicin level 3 μg/mL and trough <1 μg/mL).
- PCN-resistant Viridans group streptococci or *S. bovis,* native valve:
  - Pen G 24 million U/d IV either continuously or in 6 equally divided doses *or* ceftriaxone 2 g/d IV/IM in 1 dose for 4 weeks plus gentamicin 3 mg/kg IV/IM q24h for 2 weeks (peak gentamicin level 3 μg/mL and trough <1 μg/mL) (2)[B].
  - Regimen for prosthetic valve infection is equivalent, but length of therapy is 6 weeks for all antibiotics.
- *Staphylococcus* on native valve:
  - Oxacillin-sensitive: Oxacillin or nafcillin 2 g IV q4h for 4–6 weeks. Use of gentamicin 1 mg/kg q8h IV/IM for the first 3–5 days does not improve survival and increases the chance of nephrotoxicity.
  - Oxacillin-resistant: Vancomycin 15 mg/kg/d IV q12h for 6 weeks for goal trough of 15–20 μg/mL (2)[B].
- *Staphylococcus* of prosthetic valve:
  - Oxacillin-sensitive: Oxacillin or nafcillin 12 g/d IV in 6 equally divided doses plus rifampin 300 mg IV/PO q8h, for 6 weeks, plus gentamicin 1 mg/kg q8h IV/IM for the first 2 weeks (peak gentamicin level 3 μg/mL and trough <1 μg/mL) (2)[B].
  - Oxacillin-resistant: Vancomycin 15 mg/kg IV q12h, plus rifampin 300 mg IV/PO q8h, both for 6 weeks, plus gentamicin 3 mg/kg/d IV/IM in 2–3 doses for the first 2 weeks (peak gentamicin level 3 μg/mL and trough <1 μg/mL) (2)[B].
- Penicillin-sensitive *Enterococcus*, native or prosthetic valve: Ampicillin 2g IV q4h *or* Pen G 18–30 million U/d IV either continuously or in 6 equally divided doses, plus gentamicin 1 mg/kg IV q8h for 4–6 weeks (peak gentamicin level 3 μg/mL and trough <1 μg/mL) (2)[A]. Consider expert consultation for penicillin-resistant enterococci.
- HACEK organisms: Ceftriaxone 2 g IM or IV q24h for 4 weeks (2)[B] *or* ampicillin-sulbactam 2g IV q6h for 4 weeks (2)[B] *or* Ciprofloxacin 1 g/d PO or 800 mg/d IV in 2 equally divided doses for 4 weeks (2)[C].
- Precautions:
  - In patients with renal impairment, dosage adjustment should be made for penicillin G, gentamicin, cefazolin, ampicillin, ampicillin/sulbactam, ciprofloxacin, and vancomycin.
  - Rapid infusion of vancomycin <1 hour may cause "red-man syndrome" due to histamine release, not an allergic reaction. Treat with antihistamines and decrease infusion rate.
- Significant possible interactions:
  - Vancomycin plus gentamicin increases renal toxicity.
  - Rifampin increases the requirement for Coumadin and oral hypoglycemic agents.

Second Line
For patients allergic to penicillin:
- Penicillin-susceptible or resistant Viridans group streptococci or *S. bovis*: Vancomycin 30 mg/kg (not to exceed 2 g/d) IV for 4 weeks (6 weeks for prosthetic valve endocarditis) for goal trough of 10–15 μg/mL (2)[B].
- *Enterococcus*, native or prosthetic valve: Desensitization to penicillin should be considered. Vancomycin 15 mg/kg (usual dose, 1 g) IV q12h, plus gentamicin or streptomycin (peak gentamicin level 3 μg/mL and trough <1 μg/mL) for 4–6 weeks (6 weeks for prosthetic valve endocarditis) (2)[B].
- *Staphylococcus* of native valve: Cefazolin 2 g IV q8h (not to be used in patients with immediate-type hypersensitivity to penicillin) for 4–6 weeks (2)[B] *OR* vancomycin 30 mg/kg (usual dose, 1 g) IV q12h for a goal trough of 15–20 μg/mL, for 6 weeks (2)[B].

SURGERY/OTHER PROCEDURES
Surgical therapy (i.e., valve replacement) is required in 50% of IE cases. It should be considered for:
- CHF due to valve
- Embolic event in first 2 weeks of antibiotic therapy and stroke if hemorrhage has been excluded (2)[B]
- Persistent bacteremia after 1 week of antibiotic therapy or infection caused by resistant organisms (e.g., fungus, *Pseudomonas aeruginosa*, *S. marcescens*), *S. aureus* on a prosthetic valve, or most cases of relapsing IE (3)[B]
- Valve dehiscence, perforation, rupture or fistula, heart block, or large perivalvular abscess (2)[B]. Anterior mitral valve leaflet vegetation >10 mm in size, persistent vegetation after systemic embolization (2)[B], or increase in vegetation size despite antibiotic therapy (2)[C]
- Early prosthetic valve IE (3)[B]

ONGOING CARE

FOLLOW-UP RECOMMENDATIONS
Patient Monitoring
- Check gentamicin peak (~3 μg/mL) and trough (<1 μg/mL) levels if used for >5 days, and with renal dysfunction.
- Check vancomycin trough (15–20 μg/mL) levels in all patients (2)[B].
- Perform twice-weekly BUN and serum creatinine while on gentamicin.
- Consider audiometry baseline and follow-up during long-term aminoglycoside therapy.
- Baseline ECG, and monitor ECG for conduction disturbances/MI in initial weeks.
- TTE at the end of therapy
- Blood cultures q48h until negative

PROGNOSIS
In-hospital mortality is ~20%. Acute heart failure and cerebral embolism are the first 2 causes of death during IE (4).

COMPLICATIONS
- Arterial emboli and infarcts (e.g., myocardial infarction, mesenteric, splenic, cerebral infarct)
- Infectious emboli (e.g., abscesses of heart, lung, brain, meninges, bone, pericardium)
- Inflammatory/immune disorders (e.g., arthritis, myositis, glomerulonephritis)
- Other complications: CHF, ruptured valve cusp, sinus of Valsalva aneurysm, arrhythmia, and mycotic aneurysms

REFERENCES

1. Wilson W, et al. Prevention of infective endocarditis. Guidelines from the American Heart Association. A Guideline from the American Heart Association Rheumatic Fever, Endocarditis, and Kawasaki Disease Committee, Council on Cardiovascular Disease in the Young, and the Council on Cardiology, Council on Cardiovascular Surgery and Anesthesia, and the Quality of Care and Outcomes Research Interdisciplinary Working Group. *Circulation*. 2007;116:1736–54.
2. Baddour LM, Wilson WR, Bayer AS, et al. Infective endocarditis: Diagnosis, antimicrobial therapy, and management of complications: A statement for healthcare professionals from the Committee on Rheumatic Fever, Endocarditis, and Kawasaki Disease, Council on Cardiovascular Disease in the Young, and the Councils on Clinical Cardiology, Stroke, and Cardiovascular Surgery and Anesthesia, American Heart Association: Endorsed by the Infectious Diseases Society of America. *Circulation*. 2005;111:e394–434.
3. Head SJ, Mokhles MM, Osnabrugge RL, et al. Surgery in current therapy for infective endocarditis. *Vasc Health Risk Manag*. 2011;7:255–63.
4. Chu VH, Cabell CH, Benjamin DK, et al. Early predictors of in-hospital death in infective endocarditis. *Circulation*. 2004;109:1745–9.

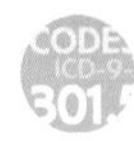

CODES

ICD9
- 041.10 Staphylococcus infection in conditions classified elsewhere and of unspecified site, staphylococcus, unspecified
- 421.0 Acute and subacute bacterial endocarditis

CLINICAL PEARLS
- Antibiotic prophylaxis is now only recommended for people with artificial heart valves, past history of IE, certain congenital heart diseases, and cardiac transplants with valvulopathy.
- Microbiologic, clinical, and echocardiographic findings lead to the diagnosis of IE. Treatment consists of prolonged courses of antibiotics, and often involves surgery.

ENDOMETRIAL CANCER AND UTERINE SARCOMA

Michael P. Hopkins, MD, MEd
Jonna M. Quinn, DO

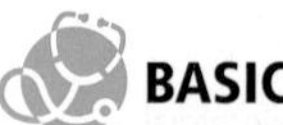

BASICS

DESCRIPTION

- Endometrial cancer: Malignancy of the endometrial lining of the uterus:
  - 2 types:
    - I: Estrogen dependent, lower grade, better prognosis
    - II: Estrogen independent, higher grade, more aggressive
- Cell types: Adenocarcinoma, adenosquamous (malignant squamous elements), clear cell, and papillary serous
- Sarcomas: Malignancy of the uterine mesenchyme and mixed tumors:
  - Mixed Müllerian sarcoma (carcinosarcoma): Heterologous sarcoma elements are not native to the Müllerian system (e.g., cartilage or bone); homologous sarcoma elements are native to the Müllerian system.
  - Endometrial stromal sarcoma develops from the stromal component of the endometrium.
  - Leiomyosarcoma develops in the myometrium or, rarely, in a myoma (fibroid).
  - Poorer prognosis
- Predominant age:
  - Endometrial cancer: The majority of patients are postmenopausal:
    - Median age: 66 years old
  - Sarcomas: Age 40–69 years old
- System(s) affected: Reproductive
- Synonym(s): Uterine cancer; Endometrial cancer; Corpus cancer

Pregnancy Considerations

This malignancy is not associated with pregnancy.

EPIDEMIOLOGY

Incidence

- Most common gynecologic malignancy, fourth most common cancer in women, eighth leading cause of cancer-related death in women
- ~40,000 new cases per year and 7,000 deaths per year

Prevalence

500,000 women in the US

RISK FACTORS

- Early menarche/late menopause
- Nulliparity
- Personal or family history of colon or reproductive system cancer
- Obesity
- Diabetes mellitus
- Hypertension
- Polycystic ovarian syndrome
- Menstrual irregularities
- Endometrial hyperplasia
- Unopposed estrogens
- Tamoxifen
- Age
- Prior pelvic irradiation (sarcoma)

Genetics

- Endometrial: Lynch syndrome (hereditary nonpolyposis colorectal cancer)
- Sarcoma: African American

GENERAL PREVENTION

- In young women who are obese or anovulatory, the risk of endometrial cancer can be reduced by taking oral contraceptive pills, permanently losing weight, or taking cyclic progesterone to prevent unopposed estrogens effects on the uterus.
- Estrogen replacement therapy should always include progesterone unless the woman has undergone a hysterectomy.
- Cigarette smoking has been associated with a lower risk of endometrial cancer; however, it is not recommended secondary to its many health risks.

PATHOPHYSIOLOGY

Continuous estrogen stimulation unopposed by progesterone

ETIOLOGY

- Endometrial: Unopposed estrogen:
  - Estrogen replacement therapy without concomitant progesterone increases the risk. Addition of progesterone decreases risk to that of general population.
- Sarcomas: Etiology unknown

COMMONLY ASSOCIATED CONDITIONS

- Endometrial hyperplasia: 1–25% will progress to endometria adenocarcinoma:
  - Simple without atypia
  - Complex without atypia
  - Simple with atypia
  - Complex with atypia:
    - 43% with complex hyperplasia with atypia have concurrent endometrial cancer
- Endometrial cancer patients should be screened regularly for breast and colon cancer because of an increased risk of these cancers.
- Patients who have breast or colon cancer are at increased risk for endometrial cancer.
- Granulosa cell tumors of the ovary produce estrogen; these patients will have an increased risk of endometrial cancer.

DIAGNOSIS

HISTORY

- Endometrial cancer:
  - Postmenopausal bleeding is the most frequent sign. Any spotting or abnormal discharge mandates evaluation.
- Sarcoma:
  - Mixed Müllerian sarcoma: Bleeding and prolapsing tissue, pain
  - Leiomyosarcoma: Increasing size of presumed uterine myomas, pain

PHYSICAL EXAM

Pelvic exam: Enlarged uterus

DIAGNOSTIC TESTS & INTERPRETATION

Lab

Initial lab tests

Liver and renal function tests

Follow-Up & Special Considerations

- A biopsy of a pregnant uterus can produce tissue that looks hyperplastic or premalignant.
- Pap smear is rarely positive.

Imaging

Initial approach

- Transvaginal ultrasound usually shows increased endometrial thickness.
- Levels of cancer antigen 125 (CA-125) may be elevated when intra-abdominal disease is present.
- Chest x-ray (CXR): Most common site of metastases is the lungs.
- Mammogram and colonoscopy: Endometrial cancer is associated with breast and colon cancer.

Follow-Up & Special Considerations

- CT scan, bone scan, liver spleen scan: Not part of the routine evaluation, but may be needed if metastasis is suspected.
- MRI has been reported to show the depth of myometrial penetration accurately but is not always cost effective.

Diagnostic Procedures/Surgery

- Office endometrial biopsy (90% accurate): If this is negative with high suspicion for cancer, a dilation and curettage is necessary. Endometrial stromal sarcoma and leiomyosarcoma rarely are diagnosed preoperatively.
- Fractional dilation and curettage is 99% accurate except in cases of sarcoma.
- Hysteroscopy may be associated with higher risk of positive washings/cytology; is controversial

Pathological Findings

- Stage I (confined to corpus uteri):
  - A. No or $<1/2$ myometrial invasion
  - B. Invision $\geq 1/2$ the myometrium
- Stage II: Tumor invades cervical stroma but does not extend beyond the uterus
- Stage III: Local and/or regional spread:
  - A. Uterine serosal and or adnexal invasion
  - B. Vaginal and/or parametrial involvement
  - C. Metastases to pelvic and/or para-aortic lymph nodes:
    - IIIC1: +pelvic nodes
    - IIIC2: +para-aortic lymph nodes positive pelvic lymph nodes
  - Stage IV: Tumor invades bladder and/or bowel mucosa and/or distant metastases:
    - A. Tumor invades bladder and/or bowel mucosa
    - B. Distant metastases, including intra-abdominal metastases and/or inguinal lymph nodes
- Federation of Gynecology and Obstetrics Staging System: revised 2009 (1)

DIFFERENTIAL DIAGNOSIS

- Atypical complex hyperplasia: A premalignant lesion of the endometrium
- Cervical cancer
- Ovarian cancer invading the uterus
- Endometriosis
- Adenomyosis

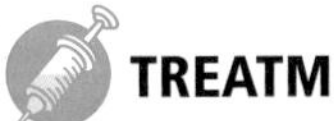

TREATMENT

MEDICATION

First Line

- Endometrial:
  - Chemotherapy for advanced or recurrent disease incurable with surgery and radiation (2,3)[A]:
    - Doxorubicin + Cisplatin + Paclitaxel
    - Paclitaxel + Carboplatin
  - Hormonal therapy:
    - Medroxyprogesterone acetate: For recurrence or metastases (2)[A]
    - Megestrol (Megace) 160 mg/d for 3 months for women with premalignant lesions, atypical complex hyperplasia, or well-differentiated endometrial cancer patients desiring fertility. Follow with dilation and curettage to determine cancer resolution.
    - Levonorgestrel-containing intrauterine device: As above for patients who desire future fertility
- Sarcoma:
  - Chemotherapy:
    - Doxorubicin as single agent or in combination (4)[A]
  - Hormonal:
    - Tamoxifen or aromatase inhibitors; not fully studied
    - Progesterones

Second Line

Ondansetron (Zofran), dronabinol (Marinol), metoclopramide (Reglan), and others to control nausea from chemotherapy

ADDITIONAL TREATMENT

General Measures

- Main treatment for uterine cancer is surgery.
- Radiation is used to prevent tumor recurrence at the vaginal cuff.

Additional Therapies

Radiation therapy:

- Nonoperative candidates: Radiation therapy alone (5)[A]
- Low risk: No adjuvant radiation therapy (5)[A]
- Intermediate risk: Consider adjuvant vaginal brachytherapy. Reduces local recurrences but has no effect on overall survival (5)[A].
- High risk: Chemotherapy and radiation therapy in some cases

SURGERY/OTHER PROCEDURES

Surgical staging:

- Extrafascial hysterectomy and bilateral salpingo-oophorectomy
- Cytologic washings
- Pelvic and para-aortic lymph node dissection
- Omental sampling as indicated
- Optimal tumor debulking

Geriatric Considerations

Older (and obese) patients may be at high risk for surgery. Alternative radiation therapy can be considered.

IN-PATIENT CONSIDERATIONS

Admission Criteria

- Excessive vaginal bleeding
- Preoperative stabilization

Nursing

Routine; ensure postoperative pain is controlled

Discharge Criteria

Postsurgical criteria: Pain controlled, tolerating diet, ambulating, and voiding

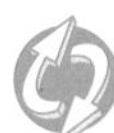

ONGOING CARE

FOLLOW-UP RECOMMENDATIONS

Speculum and rectovaginal exam every 3–4 months for 2–3 years, then every 6 months for 3 years, and then annually for life

Patient Monitoring

Annual CXR

DIET

As tolerated and according to comorbidities

PATIENT EDUCATION

After surgery:

- No intercourse for ~6 weeks
- No lifting >10–15 lbs
- No driving until pain free
- Do not expect resumption of full activity for 6 weeks.

PROGNOSIS

5-year survival rates:

- Uterine adenocarcinoma

Stage	Survival (%)
IA	88
IB	75
II	69
IIIA	58
IIIB	50
IIIC	47
IVA	17
IVB	15

- Uterine sarcoma

Stage	Survival (%)
I	70
II	45
III	30
IV	15

COMPLICATIONS

- Surgical: Excessive bleeding, wound infection, lymphedema, deep vein thrombosis (DVT), and damage to the urinary or intestinal systems
- Radiation: Diarrhea, ileus, bowel obstruction or fistula, radiation cystitis, proctitis, vaginal stenosis, DVT
- Chemotherapy: Per the drug given

REFERENCES

1. Creasman W. Revised FIGO staging for carcinoma of the endometrium. *Int J Gynaecol Obstet*. 2009;105(2):109.
2. Polyzos NP, Pavlidis N, Paraskevaidis E, et al. Randomized evidence on chemotherapy and hormonal therapy regimens for advanced endometrial cancer: An overview of survival data. *Eur J Cancer*. 2006;42:319–26.
3. Fleming GF, Brunetto VL, Cella D, et al. Phase III trial of doxorubicin plus cisplatin with or without paclitaxel plus filgrastim in advanced endometrial carcinoma: A Gynecologic Oncology Group Study. *J Clin Oncol*. 2004;22:2159–66.
4. Bramwell VH, Anderson D, Charette ML, et al. Doxorubicin-based chemotherapy for the palliative treatment of adult patients with locally advanced or metastatic soft tissue sarcoma. *Cochrane Database Syst Rev*. 2003:CD003293.
5. Einhorn N, Tropé C, Ridderheim M, et al. A systematic overview of radiation therapy effects in uterine cancer (corpus uteri). *Acta Oncol*. 2003;42:557–61.

ADDITIONAL READING

- American College of Obstetricians and Gynecologists. ACOG practice bulletin, clinical management guidelines for obstetrician-gynecologists, number 65, August 2005: Management of endometrial cancer. *Obstet Gynecol*. 2005;106:413–25.
- Gadducci A, Cosio S, Romanini A, et al. The management of patients with uterine sarcoma: A debated clinical challenge. *Crit Rev Oncol Hematol*. 2008;65:129–42.
- Humber C, et al. Chemotherapy for advanced, recurrent or metastatic endometrial carcinoma. *Cochrane Database Syst Rev*. 2005;(4):CD003915.

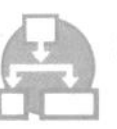

See Also (Topic, Algorithm, Electronic Media Element)

- Cervical Malignancy
- Algorithm: Pelvic Pain

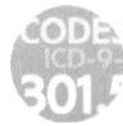

CODES

ICD9

- 179 Malignant neoplasm of uterus, part unspecified
- 182.0 Malignant neoplasm of corpus uteri, except isthmus

CLINICAL PEARLS

- Most common presenting symptom is abnormal uterine bleeding.
- Primary cause is unopposed estrogen.
- Endometrial thickness on transvaginal ultrasound of <5 mm makes endometrial cancer very unlikely.
- Primary treatment is with surgery with possible chemotherapy ± radiation.

ENDOMETRIOSIS

Pamela L. Grimaldi, DO, FAAFP
Kathryn Wilson, MD
Julie Scott Taylor, MD, MSc

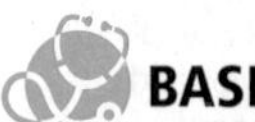

BASICS

DESCRIPTION

- Endometriosis is a common, recurring disease in women of reproductive age that may even persist into early menopause (1).
- Heterotopic islands of endometrial glands and stroma found outside the uterus:
  - Pelvic sites: Peritoneal surfaces (bladder, cul-de-sac, pelvic walls, ligaments, and fallopian tubes), vagina, cervix, lymph nodes, ovaries, bowel
  - Distant sites: Abdominal wall, spleen, gallbladder, stomach, nasal mucosa, spinal canal, lungs, breasts, diaphragm, pleura, pericardium
- Classified as peritoneal, ovarian, or deep endometriosis
- Staged according to the American Society for Reproductive Medicine surgical scoring system:
  - Based on disease severity: Extent and characteristics of endometrial implants and adhesions
  - Stage I (minimal) to IV (severe)
- System(s) affected: Reproductive
- Synonym(s): Endometriosis externa

ALERT
Staging is useful in therapeutic planning but does not correlate with severity of pain or predict response to treatment for symptoms or infertility.

EPIDEMIOLOGY

Incidence

- Affects 0.5–5% of fertile women
- Found in 30–50% of infertile women (2)
- Found in 50–60% of women and adolescent women with pelvic pain (3)

Pediatric Considerations

Endometriosis may begin with puberty, causing debilitating pelvic pain and severe dysmenorrhea associated with missed school, social, and family activities.

Pregnancy Considerations

Pelvic endometriosis generally is ameliorated with pregnancy, but infertility is significantly associated with the disease itself.

Geriatric Considerations

Although menopause often results in a resolution of symptoms, pelvic endometriosis may extend into menopause and is exacerbated by hormone replacement therapy (HRT).

Prevalence

- Predominant sex: Female only
- Affects 6–10% of reproductive-age women

RISK FACTORS

- Diethylstilbestrol exposure in utero
- Low birth weight
- Obstruction of menstrual flow (Müllerian anomalies)
- Prolonged exposure to endogenous estrogen:
  - Early menarche
  - Short menstrual cycles
  - Late menopause
  - Delayed childbearing
  - Obesity
- Hereditary/genetic predisposition
- Exposure to endocrine-disrupting chemicals
- Increased dietary intake of red meat and trans fats

Genetics

Genetic predisposition is common.

GENERAL PREVENTION

- Prevention is not possible, but some factors are considered protective:
  - Fruits, green vegetables, n-3 long-chain fatty acids
  - Multiple pregnancies
  - Prolonged lactation
- Early diagnosis and treatment might help prevent the possible sequelae.

PATHOPHYSIOLOGY

- Not fully understood; tendency for abnormal endometrial tissue to implant and proliferate, causing chronic peritoneal inflammation
- Endometrial-associated infertility is multifactorial:
  - Pelvic inflammation
  - Anatomic disruption of pelvic structures (involvement of the fallopian tube may cause isthmic tubal obstruction)
  - Proliferation and activation of peritoneal macrophages (may predispose to gamete phagocytosis)
  - Alteration in eutopic endometrium

ETIOLOGY

Not fully understood; theories include:

- Sampson theory: Retrograde menstruation results in peritoneal implantation and disease:
  - Affected women have an immune dysfunction that prevents clearing of implants
- Halban theory: Distant disease probably caused by hematogenous/lymphatic dissemination or metaplastic transformation
- Coelomic metaplasia: Coelomic epithelium undergoes metaplasia, forming functioning endometrium

COMMONLY ASSOCIATED CONDITIONS

Associated with increased risk of other autoimmune diseases (3); increased risk of ovarian, endometrioid, and clear-cell cancers as well as other cancers (e.g., non-Hodgkin lymphoma)

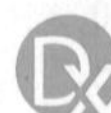

DIAGNOSIS

- Diagnosis can be challenging because symptoms overlap with many other gynecological and nongynecological conditions.
- A complete medical, surgical, social, and family history should be collected from patients.
- A complete physical exam, including a pelvic exam, should be performed.

HISTORY

- Dysmenorrhea (50–90% of cases)
- Dyspareunia
- Chronic pelvic pain ($\geq$6 months) that worsens with time and activity:
  - Intermittent or continuous
  - Dull, throbbing, or sharp
- Premenstrual spotting
- Dyschezia
- Cyclic nausea, abdominal distention, and early satiety
- Painful defecation
- Hematochezia
- Hematuria
- Infertility
- Spontaneous abortion (theoretical)
- History of pelvic pain, infertility, and hysterectomy in first- or second-degree relative

PHYSICAL EXAM

- Focal pain/tenderness on pelvic exam (associated with endometriosis in 66% of patients) (3)
- Pelvic mass
- Immobile pelvic organs (frozen pelvis)
- Rectovaginal exam revealing uterosacral nodules, beading, or tenderness

DIAGNOSTIC TESTS & INTERPRETATION

Lab

Initial lab tests

No special labs; CA-125 levels are not recommended (poor sensitivity and specificity) and may be falsely elevated due to peritoneal irritation.

Imaging

Initial approach

- Routine imaging is not recommended.
- If history and physical exam reveal adnexal pain or tenderness with/without fullness on pelvic exam:
  - Transvaginal US and MRI are equally effective in detecting ovarian endometriomas: Sensitivity 80–90% and specificity 60–98% for both (3)
  - US is preferred (less costly).
  - Both modalities are poor in detecting peritoneal implants and adhesions.

Diagnostic Procedures/Surgery

- Definitive diagnosis is made via visualization of lesions during surgery (laparoscopy or laparotomy).
- Hysterosalpingography for tubal occlusion (proximal or distal) and periadnexal adhesions

Pathological Findings

- Red and blue-black lesions, adhesions, and "chocolate cysts"
- Endometrial glands and stroma on histologic analysis of biopsied lesions

DIFFERENTIAL DIAGNOSIS

Differential diagnosis of pelvic pain includes all causes of acute abdomen and:

- Complications of intrauterine or ectopic pregnancy
- Pelvic adhesions
- Acute salpingitis/pelvic inflammatory disease
- Ruptured ovarian cyst
- Uterine leiomyomas
- Adenomyosis
- Irritable bowel syndrome
- Inflammatory bowel disease
- Intussusception
- UTI/cystitis
- Interstitial cystitis
- Malignancies
- Depression
- History of sexual abuse
- Myofascial pain

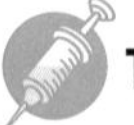

TREATMENT

MEDICATION

Medications may be helpful in treating symptoms of pain and dysmenorrhea, but symptoms frequently recur.

First Line

Empirical medical treatment is indicated for symptom management, but has not been shown to improve fertility (4):

- NSAIDs initiated at the beginning or just before menses
- Cyclic combined oral contraceptive pills (OCPs)

Second Line

- Continuous combined OCPs. Switch from cyclic to continuous OCPs for 3–6 months if symptoms persist or if there is chronic, noncyclic pelvic pain
- Progestogens:
  - Levonorgestrel IUD (Mirena), especially for symptomatic rectovaginal endometriosis (although not FDA approved) or instead of continuous OCPs in pain that persists despite first-line treatment
  - Medroxyprogesterone acetate 150 mg IM or 104 mg SC every 3 months
- GnRH agonists inhibit pituitary gonadotropin synthesis and induce a hypoestrogenic state (3)[A]:
  - Leuprolide acetate (Depo-Lupron) 3.75 mg IM each month or 11.25 mg IM every 3 months (gluteal)
  - Nafarelin (Synarel) intranasal spray 400 μg/d divided into 2 inhalations per day, 1 in each nostril (start between days 2 and 4 of menstrual cycle)
  - Goserelin (Zoladex) implant 3.6 mg SC in upper abdominal wall every 28 days for 6 months
- GnRH agonists should be given with estrogen-progestogen add-back therapy to minimize effects of hypoestrogenism (most importantly, reduced bone mineral density) (3)[A]:
  - Norethindrone acetate 5 mg PO once daily
  - Conjugated equine estrogen 0.635 mg PO once daily
- Danazol was an early treatment (now second or third line). Use is limited by androgenic side effects.

ADDITIONAL TREATMENT

General Measures

Calcium/vitamin D supplementation (1,000–1,500 mg/d) is recommended when using GnRH agonists to prevent calcium loss.

Issues for Referral

- Refer early to a board-certified reproductive endocrinologist or gynecologist with expertise in infertility if the patient has difficulty conceiving.
- Other indications for referral to a gynecologist include:
  - Need for definitive diagnosis (failure to respond to a conservative first-line therapy)
  - Chronic pelvic pain
  - Adolescent with severe dysmenorrhea/dyspareunia

Additional Therapies

Regular exercise and counseling for pain-management strategies (avoidance of narcotics is ideal)

COMPLEMENTARY AND ALTERNATIVE MEDICINE

- Physical therapy (3)[C]
- Acupuncture may be more effective than danazol to decrease pain, irregular menstruation, back pain, and perineal swelling (3)[C].
- Osteopathic manipulation (5)[B]

SURGERY/OTHER PROCEDURES

Surgery (laparoscopy or laparotomy) is both diagnostic and therapeutic (first line or when conservative measures fail):

- Peritoneal endometriosis: Laser ablation, excision, or fulguration
- Ovarian endometriosis (endometriomas) >3 cm: Ablation, excision, drainage

ALERT

Surgery for endometriomas may decrease ovarian reserve in advanced disease.

- Lysis of adhesions (LOA)
- Hysterectomy with bilateral salpingo-oophorectomy for debilitating symptoms refractory to other medical or surgical treatments (3)[C]:
  - Relieves pain in 80–90%, but pain recurs in 10% within 1–2 years after surgery
  - Postoperative HRT should include estrogen and progestogen (3)[C]
- Interruption of nerve pathways:
  - Laparoscopic ablations and presacral neurectomy improve dysmenorrhea (3)[A].
- Fertility procedures:
  - Ablation of lesions with LOA is recommended to treat infertility in stage I–II disease (3)[A]:
    - Spontaneous conception should be attempted for 1 year prior to assisted reproduction techniques
  - GnRH agonists 3–6 months before in vitro fertilization (IVF) increases live birth rates (3)[A]:
    - Disease does not endanger IVF pregnancies.

ONGOING CARE

FOLLOW-UP RECOMMENDATIONS

Routine gynecologic care

Patient Monitoring

- Symptomatic and asymptomatic pelvic masses <5 cm may be followed with serial US.
- Patients receiving GnRH agonist therapy should have serum estradiol levels monitored to assess degree of hypoestrogenemia and efficacy of add-back therapy: Estradiol between 30–45 pg/mL (109–164 pmol/L) prevents bone loss without stimulating disease.
- Endometriosis likely is an independent risk factor for the development of epithelial ovarian cancer.

DIET

No restrictions.

PATIENT EDUCATION

American Congress of Obstetrics and Gynecology at www.acog.org

PROGNOSIS

- Excellent, especially if diagnosis and treatment plans are initiated early in disease course
- Poor for recovery of fertility if the disease has progressed to stage III or IV

COMPLICATIONS

Possible sequelae include chronic pelvic pain, repetitive surgical intervention, costs, and infertility.

REFERENCES

1. Ozkan S, Murk W, Arici A. Endometriosis and infertility: Epidemiology and evidence-based treatments. *Ann N Y Acad Sci*. 2008;1127:92–100.
2. Härkki P, Tiitinen A, Ylikorkala O, et al. Endometriosis and assisted reproduction techniques. *Ann N Y Acad Sci*. 2010;1205:207–13.
3. Giudice LC, et al. Clinical practice. Endometriosis. *N Engl J Med*. 2010;362:2389–98.
4. Rodgers AK, et al. Treatment strategies for endometriosis. *Exp Opin Pharmacother*. 2008;9(2): 243–55.
5. Chadwick K, Morgan A. The efficacy of osteopathic treatment for primary dysmenorrhea in young women. *The AAO Journal: A Publication of the American Academy of Osteopathy*. 1996;6(3): 15–17, 29–31.

E

ADDITIONAL READING

- Brown J, Pan A, Hart RJ, et al. Gonadotrophin-releasing hormone analogues for pain associated with endometriosis. *Cochrane Database Syst Rev*. 2010;CD008475.
- Davis L, Kennedy SS, Moore J, et al. Modern combined oral contraceptives for pain associated with endometriosis. *Cochrane Database Syst Rev*. 2007:CD001019.
- de Ziegler D, Borghese B, Chapron C, et al. Endometriosis and infertility: Pathophysiology and management. *Lancet*. 2010;376:730–8.
- Ferrero S, Remorgida V, Venturini PL, et al. Current pharmacotherapy for endometriosis. *Expert Opin Pharmacother*. 2010;11:1123–34.
- Hughes E, Brown J, Collins JJ, et al. Ovulation suppression for endometriosis. *Cochrane Database Syst Rev*. 2007:CD000155.
- Jacobson TZ, Duffy JM, Barlow D, et al. Laparoscopic surgery for pelvic pain associated with endometriosis. *Cochrane Database Syst Rev*. 2009; CD001300.
- Vercellini P, Somigliana E, Viganò P, et al. Endometriosis: Current and future medical therapies. *Best Pract Res Clin Obstet Gynaecol*. 2008;22: 275–306.

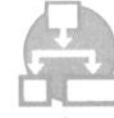

See Also (Topic, Algorithm, Electronic Media Element)

Algorithm: Pelvic Pain

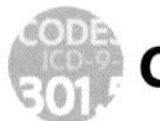

CODES

ICD9

- 617.0 Endometriosis of uterus
- 617.1 Endometriosis of ovary
- 617.9 Endometriosis, site unspecified

CLINICAL PEARLS

- Severe dysmenorrhea and dyspareunia are never normal. Failure to respond to NSAIDs and/or OCPs warrants further investigation.
- A rectovaginal exam can be useful in patients suspected of having endometriosis.

ENDOMETRITIS AND OTHER POSTPARTUM INFECTIONS

Justin P. Lavin, Jr., MD
Allison Kreiner, MD

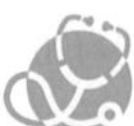

BASICS

DESCRIPTION

- Bacterial infection of the genital tract, usually within the first week after delivery, but can occur 1–6 weeks postpartum
- Endometritis (infection of the endometrium) is the *most common postpartum infection*.
- Less common are postpartum infections of the myometrium and parametrial tissues, vaginal and cervical infections, perineal cellulitis, pelvic cellulitis, septic pelvic vein thrombophlebitis, and parametrial phlegmon.
- System(s) affected: Reproductive
- Synonym(s): Postpartum infection; Endometritis; Endoparametritis; Endomyometritis; Myometritis; Endomyoparametritis; Metritis; Metritis with pelvic cellulitis

EPIDEMIOLOGY

Incidence

- Predominant age: Women of childbearing years
- Predominant sex: Female only

Prevalence

- Occurs in 1–3% of all births
- 10 times more likely with cesarean section:
  - 2–15% prior to labor
  - 30–35% after labor without prophylaxis
  - 2–15% after labor with prophylaxis
  - Accounts for 7% of maternal deaths
  - Fourth leading cause of maternal mortality

RISK FACTORS

- Cesarean delivery is the most important risk factor.
- Chorioamnionitis
- Bacterial vaginosis
- Group B streptococcal colonization of genital tract
- HIV infection
- Prolonged labor
- Prolonged rupture of membranes
- Multiple vaginal examinations
- Internal fetal monitoring during labor
- Operative vaginal delivery
- Manual extraction of the placenta
- Low socioeconomic status
- Obesity
- Anemia

GENERAL PREVENTION

- Avoid unnecessary vaginal examinations.
- Treat chorioamnionitis during labor.
- Spontaneous placental extraction
- Avoid retained placental fragments or membranes.
- Antibiotic prophylaxis for third- and fourth-degree laceration (1)[B]
- Use of aseptic technique during operative vaginal delivery
- No data to support antibiotic prophylaxis for operative vaginal delivery (2)[A]
- Administering prophylactic antibiotics before both emergency and scheduled cesarean reduces the prevalence of postpartum infection after cesarean (3)[A],(4)[B]:
  - Administering the antibiotics prior to skin incision in cesarean delivery (as opposed to the prior practice of waiting for cord clamping) is considered the standard of care.
  - Antibiotics should be administered within 1 hour of the surgery start time.
  - There is a 40% reduction in postpartum maternal infections without any increase in neonatal infectious outcomes or difficulty in evaluating the neonate (5)[B].
- Extending the spectrum of coverage to include not only a cephalosporin but also azithromycin decreases the incidence of infections (6)[A],(7)[B].
- Vaginal preparation with povidone-iodine solution immediately before cesarean delivery reduces the risk of postoperative endometritis (8)[A].

ETIOLOGY

- Endometritis commonly follows chorioamnionitis.
- Other infections follow trauma to the perineum, vagina, cervix, and uterus.
- Infection is nearly always polymicrobial and involves organisms that have ascended from the lower genital tract:
  - Aerobic isolates in 70%: *Streptococcus faecalis, S. agalactiae, S. viridans, Staphylococcus aureus, Escherichia coli*
  - Anaerobic isolates in 80%: *Peptococcus* sp., *Peptostreptococcus* sp., *Clostridium* sp., *Bacteroides bivius, B. fragilis, Fusobacterium* sp.
- Other genital mycoplasmata; very common (9)[B]

COMMONLY ASSOCIATED CONDITIONS

- Chorioamnionitis
- Wound infection

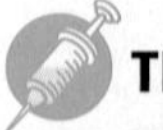

DIAGNOSIS

HISTORY

- Fever, chills, malaise, headache, anorexia
- Abdominal pain

PHYSICAL EXAM

- Oral temperature >38.7°C (101.6°F) in first 24 hours postpartum or >38°C (100.4°F) in 2 of first 10 days postpartum (excluding first 24 hours)
- Tachycardia
- Uterine tenderness on exam
- Other localized tenderness on exam
- Purulent or malodorous lochia
- Heavy vaginal bleeding
- Ileus
- Group A or B streptococcal bacteremia may have no localizing signs.

DIAGNOSTIC TESTS & INTERPRETATION

Lab

Initial lab tests

- CBC: Interpret with care, because *physiologic leukocytosis may be as high as 20,000 WBCs*.
- 2 sets of blood cultures (especially if sepsis is suspected)
- Note: Diagnosis is usually made clinically, but consider additional testing, including:
  - Genital tract cultures and rapid test for group B streptococci, which may be done while patient is in labor
  - Amniotic fluid Gram stain: Usually polymicrobial
  - Uterine tissue cultures: Prep the cervix with Betadine and use a shielded specimen collector or Pipelle. Difficult to obtain without contamination.

Imaging

Initial approach

If patient is not responsive to antibiotics in 24–48 hours:

- Ultrasound (US) for retained products of conception, pelvic abscess, or mass
- CT or MRI looking for pelvic vein thrombophlebitis, abscess, or deep-seated wound infection

Diagnostic Procedures/Surgery

Paracentesis or culdocentesis with culture rarely is necessary.

Pathological Findings

- Superficial layer of infected necrotic tissue in microscopic sections of uterine lining
- >5 neutrophils per HPF in superficial endometrium; ≥1 plasma cell in endometrial stroma
- Thrombosis of any of the pelvic veins, including the vena cava
- Phlegmon on leaves of the broad ligament
- Abscess

DIFFERENTIAL DIAGNOSIS

- UTI
- Viral syndrome
- Dehydration
- Pneumonia
- Wound infection
- Thrombophlebitis
- Thyroid storm
- Mastitis

TREATMENT

MEDICATION

First Line

- Clindamycin 900 mg IV q8h plus gentamicin 5 mg/kg IV q24h (10)[A]
- Potential side effects include nephrotoxicity, ototoxicity, pseudomembranous colitis, or diarrhea (in up to 6%).

Second Line

- Clindamycin 900 mg IV q8h plus aztreonam 1–2 g q8h (10)[A]
- Metronidazole 500 mg q12h plus penicillin 5 million units q6h, *OR*
- Ampicillin 2 g q6h plus gentamicin 5 mg/kg q24h (10)[A]
- Cefoxitin 2 g IV q6h. Add ampicillin 2 g IV q6h, if clinical failure after 48 hours (10)[A]
- Cefotetan 2 g IV q12h. Add ampicillin 2 g IV q6h, if clinical failure after 48 hours (10)[A].
- Note: Base therapy on cultures, sensitivities, and clinical response.
- Contraindications:
  - Drug allergy
  - Renal failure (aminoglycosides)
  - Avoid sulfa, tetracyclines, and fluoroquinolones before delivery and if breast-feeding. Metronidazole is relatively contraindicated if breast-feeding; however, clinical scenario should be considered.
- Precautions:
  - Clindamycin and other antibiotics occasionally cause pseudomembranous colitis.
- Significant possible interactions: Refer to the manufacturer's literature for each drug.
- Note: Consider adding a macrolide antibiotic (for chlamydia coverage) for infections occurring after 48 hours.
- Note: Heparin may be indicated for septic pelvic vein thrombophlebitis; requires 10 days of full anticoagulation.

SURGERY/OTHER PROCEDURES

- Curettage of retained products of conception
- Surgery to drain an abscess
- Surgery to decompress the bowel
- Surgical drainage of a phlegmon is not advised unless it is suppurative.

IN-PATIENT CONSIDERATIONS

Initial Stabilization

- Inpatient care for postpartum infections
- Most infections (94%) occur after hospital discharge.
- IV antibiotics and close observation for severe infections
- Open and drain infected wounds.
- Normalize fluid status.
- Note: Amnioinfusion during labor may decrease infections when membranes have been ruptured for >6 hours.

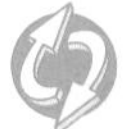

ONGOING CARE

FOLLOW-UP RECOMMENDATIONS

Patient Monitoring

- Individualize according to severity.
- IV antibiotics can be stopped when the patient is afebrile for 24–48 hours.
- Oral antibiotics on discharge are not necessary, except in cases of bacteremia; then continue oral antibiotics to complete a 7-day course.

DIET

As tolerated, although may be limited by ileus

PATIENT EDUCATION

- Advise patient to call her doctor if she has fever >38°C (100.4°F) postpartum, heavy vaginal bleeding, foul-smelling lochia, or other symptoms of infection.
- Information available at: www.healthline.com/yodocontent/pregnancy/infections-postpartum-endometritis.html

PROGNOSIS

- With supportive therapy and appropriate antibiotics, most patients improve within a few days.
- If no improvement occurs on antibiotics, consider retained placental fragments or membranes, abscess, wound infection, hematoma, cellulitis, phlegmon, or septic pelvic vein thrombosis.

COMPLICATIONS

- Resistant organisms
- Peritonitis
- Pelvic abscess
- Septic pelvic thrombophlebitis
- Ovarian vein thrombosis
- Sepsis
- Death

REFERENCES

1. Duggal N, Mercado C, Daniels K, et al. Antibiotic prophylaxis for prevention of postpartum perineal wound complications: A randomized controlled trial. *Obstet Gynecol*. 2008;111:1268–73.
2. Liabsuetrakul T, et al. Antibiotic prophylaxis for operative vaginal delivery. *Cochrane Databse Sys Rev*. 2009;1:CD004455.
3. Smaill FM, Gyte GM. Antibiotic prophylaxis versus no prophylaxis for preventing infection after cesarean section. *Cochrane Database of Sys Rev*. 2010;1:CD007482.
4. Dinsmoor MJ, Gilbert S, Landon MD, et al. Perioperative antibiotic prophylaxis for nonlaboring cesarean delivery. Eunice Kennedy Shriver National Institute of Child Health and Human Development Maternal-Fetal Medicine Units Network. *Obstet Gynecol*. 2009;114:752-6.
5. Owens SM, Brozanski BS, Meyn LA, et al. Antimicrobial prophylaxis for cesarean delivery before skin incision. *Obstet Gynecol*. 2009;114:573–9.
6. Costantine MM, Rahman M, Ghulmiyah L, et al. Timing of perioperative antibiotics for cesarean delivery: a metaanalysis. *Am J Obstet Gynecol*. 2008;199:301.e1–6.
7. Tita AT, Owen J, Stamm AM, et al. Impact of extended-spectrum antibiotic prophylaxis on incidence of postcesarean surgical wound infection. *Am J Obstet Gynecol*. 2008;199:303.e1–3.
8. Haas DM, Morgan AL, Darei S, et al. Vaginal preparation with antiseptic solution before cesarean section for preventing postoperative infections. *Cochrane Database of Sys Rev*. 2010;3:CD007892.
9. Roberts S, Maccato M, Faro S, et al. The microbiology of post cesarean wound morbidity. *Obstet Gynecol* 1993;81:383–6.
10. French LM, Smaill F. Antibiotic regimens for endometritis after delivery. *Cochrane Database Sys Rev*. 2009;1:CD001067.

ADDITIONAL READING

- American College of Obstetricians and Gynecologist. Use of Prophylactic Antibiotics in Labor. ACOG Practice Bulletin No. 120. *Obstet Gynecol*. 2011;117:1472–1483.
- Belfort MA, Clark SL, Saade GR, et al. Hospital readmission after delivery: Evidence for an increased incidence of nonurogenital infection in the immediate postpartum period. *Am J Obstet Gynecol*. 2010;202:35.e1–7.
- Maharaj D. Puerperal pyrexia: A review. Part I. *Obstet Gynecol Surv*. 2007;62:393–9.
- Maharaj D. Puerperal pyrexia: A review. Part II. *Obstet Gynecol Surv*. 2007;62:400–6.

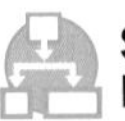

See Also (Topic, Algorithm, Electronic Media Element)

Algorithm: Pelvic Pain

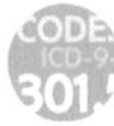

CODES

ICD9

- 658.40 Infection of amniotic cavity, unspecified as to episode of care or not applicable
- 670.00 Major puerperal infection, unspecified as to episode of care or not applicable
- 670.10 Puerperal endometritis, unspecified as to episode of care or not applicable

CLINICAL PEARLS

- Endometritis is a postpartum complication causing fever and uterine tenderness that occurs in 1–3% of all births.
- Infection is nearly always polymicrobial and involves organisms that have ascended from the lower genital tract.
- Evidence supports antibiotic prophylaxis prior to skin incision for all cesarean deliveries, but not for operative vaginal deliveries.
- Recommended treatment of endometritis is clindamycin 900 mg IV q8h and gentamicin 5 mg/kg q24h until the patient is afebrile for 24–48 hours.
- Antibiotics can be stopped completely when the patient has been afebrile for 24–48 hours, except in cases of documented bacteremia, which require a 7-day course of therapy.

ENURESIS

Melanie J.S. Malec, MD

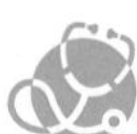

BASICS

DESCRIPTION

- Nocturnal enuresis (NE): Repeated spontaneous voiding of discrete amounts of urine during sleep after the anticipated age of bladder control (age 5)
- Daytime incontinence: Uncontrollable leakage of urine while awake
- Classification:
  - Primary NE: 1% of adult population; 80% of all cases; child/adult who has never established urinary continence on consecutive nights for a period of 6 months or more
  - Secondary NE: 20% of cases; resumption of enuresis after at least 6 months of urinary continence
- Also categorized as:
  - Monosymptomatic NE (uncomplicated): Bed wetting without lower urinary tract (LUT) symptoms other than nocturia and no history of bladder dysfunction
  - Nonmonosymptomatic NE: Bed wetting with LUT symptoms such as frequency, urgency, daytime wetting, hesitancy, straining, weak or intermittent stream, posturination dribbling, lower abdominal or genital discomfort, sensation of incomplete emptying
  - Daytime LUT condition: Bed wetting with LUT daytime symptoms
- Adult-onset NE with absent daytime incontinence is a serious symptom; complete urologic evaluation and therapy are warranted.
- System(s) affected: Nervous; Renal/Urologic
- Synonym(s): Bed wetting; Sleep enuresis; Nocturnal incontinence; Primary nocturnal enuresis

EPIDEMIOLOGY

Incidence

- Dependent upon family history
- Spontaneous resolution: 15% per year, 99% children are dry by age 15

Prevalence

- Very common. Affects 5–7 million children in the US
- 40% of 3-year-olds; 10% of 6-year-olds; 3% of 12-year-olds; 1% of adults
- Male > Female (3:1)
- Nocturnal > Day (3:1)

Geriatric Considerations

Infrequent; often associated with daytime incontinence (formerly referred to as diurnal enuresis)

RISK FACTORS

- Family history
- Stressors (emotional, environmental) common in secondary enuresis (e.g., divorce, death)
- Constipation and encopresis
- Organic disease: 1% of monosymptomatic NE (e.g., urologic and nonurologic causes)
- Psychological disorders:
  - Comorbid disorders are highest with secondary NE: Depression, anxiety, social phobias, conduct disorder, hyperkinetic syndrome, internalizing disorders
  - Association with attention deficit hyperactivity disorder (ADHD); more pronounced in ages 9–12 years
  - Abuse; 11% sexually abused girls
- Altered mental status or impaired mobility

Genetics

Most commonly, NE is an autosomal dominant inheritance pattern with high penetrance (90%):

- 1/3 of all cases are sporadic
- 75% of children with enuresis have a first-degree relative with the condition.
- Higher rates in monozygotic vs. dizygotic twins (68% vs. 36%)
- If both parents had NE, risk in child is 77%; 44% if 1 parent affected. Parental age of resolution often predicts when child's enuresis should resolve.

GENERAL PREVENTION

No known measures

PATHOPHYSIOLOGY

A disorder of sleep arousal, a low nocturnal bladder capacity, and nocturnal polyuria are the 3 factors that interrelate to cause nocturnal enuresis (1).

ETIOLOGY

- Both functional and organic causes; many theories, none absolutely confirmed
- Detrusor instability
- Deficiency of arginine vasopressin (AVP); owing to decreased inherent nocturnal AVP or decreased AVP stimulation secondary to an empty bladder (bladder distension stimulates AVP)
- Maturational delay of CNS
- Severe NE with some evidence of interaction between bladder overactivity and brain arousability: Association with children with severe NE and frequent cortical arousals in sleep
- Organic urologic causes in 1–4% of enuresis in children: UTI, occult spina bifida, ectopic ureter, lazy bladder syndrome, irritable bladder with wide bladder neck, posterior urethral valves
- Organic nonurologic causes: Epilepsy, diabetes mellitus, food allergies, obstructive sleep apnea, chronic renal failure, hyperthyroidism, pinworm infection, sickle-cell disease
- NE occurs in all stages of sleep.

COMMONLY ASSOCIATED CONDITIONS

- Obstructive sleep apnea syndrome; ↑ atrial natriuretic factor → inhibits renin-angiotensin-aldosterone pathway → ↑ diuresis
- Constipation (1/3 of NE patients)
- Behavioral problems (specifically ADHD)

DIAGNOSIS

HISTORY

- Age of onset, duration, severity
- LUT symptoms
- Constipation and encopresis (15% with comorbid encopresis)
- Daily intake patterns
- Voiding and elimination patterns (voiding diary)
- Psychosocial history
- Family history of enuresis
- Investigation and previous treatment history

PHYSICAL EXAM

- ENT: Evaluation for adenotonsillar hypertrophy
- Abdomen: Enlarged bladder, kidneys, fecal masses, or impaction
- Back: Look for dimpling or tufts of hair on sacrum
- Genital urinary exam:
  - Males: Meatal stenosis, hypospadias, epispadias, phimosis
  - Females: Vulvitis, vaginitis, labial adhesions, ureterocele at introitus; evidence of abuse.
- Rectal exam: Tone and constipation
- Neurologic exam, especially lower extremities

DIAGNOSTIC TESTS & INTERPRETATION

Lab

Initial lab tests

- Only obligatory test in children is urinalysis.
- Urinalysis and urine culture: UTI, pyuria, hematuria, proteinuria, glycosuria, and poor concentrating ability (low specific gravity) may suggest organic etiology, especially in adults.

Follow-Up & Special Considerations

Select tests for diagnosing causes of secondary enuresis: Serum glucose, BUN, creatinine, thyroid-stimulating hormone (TSH).

Imaging

Initial approach

- Urinary tract imaging is usually not necessary.
- If abnormal clinical findings or adult onset: Renal ultrasound (US) and bladder US.
- IV pyelogram, voiding cystourethrogram (VCUG), or retrograde pyelogram as indicated
- Spine radiographs for spina bifida occulta

Follow-Up & Special Considerations

In children, imaging and urodynamic studies are helpful for significant daytime symptoms, history of UTIs, suspected structural abnormalities, and refractory cases.

Diagnostic Procedures/Surgery

Urodynamic studies may be beneficial in adults and nonmonosymptomatic NE.

Pathological Findings

- Dysfunctional voiding
- Detrusor instability and/or reduced bladder capacity most common findings

DIFFERENTIAL DIAGNOSIS

- Primary NE:
  - Delayed physiologic urinary control
  - UTI (both)
  - Spina bifida occulta
  - Obstructive sleep apnea (both)
  - Idiopathic detrusor instability
  - Previously unrecognized myelopathy or neuropathy (e.g., multiple sclerosis, tethered cord, epilepsy)
  - Anatomic urinary tract abnormally (e.g., ectopic ureter)
- Secondary NE:
  - Bladder outlet obstruction
  - Neurologic disease, neurogenic bladder (e.g., spinal cord injury)

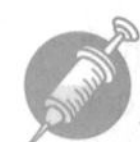

TREATMENT

- Prior to either alarm or pharmacologic treatment, supportive treatment measures should be attempted:
  - Counseling and information provision such as explanation of the 3 pathophysiologic factors

- Review of eating and drinking habits with emphasis on normal drinking patterns during daytime hours and reduction of intake in the hours prior to sleep.
- Positive reinforcement of the child should also be encouraged.

- If supportive measures have no success, combined therapy (e.g., enuresis alarm, bladder training, motivational therapy, and pelvic floor muscle training) is more effective than each component alone or than pharmacotherapy (2)[A].

MEDICATION

First Line

- Desmopressin (DDAVP): Synthetic analogue of vasopressin that decreases nocturnal urine output (3)[A]:
  - Adults only: 20 μg intranasally at bedtime
  - USFDA recommends against use in children due to reports of severe hyponatremia resulting in seizures and deaths in children using intranasal formulations of desmopressin
  - Oral DDAVP: Dose dependent: Begin at 0.2 mg tablet taken at bedtime on empty stomach; may titrate to 0.6 mg:
    - Maximally effective in 1 hour; cleared within 9 hour
    - Trial nightly for 6 months then stop for 2 weeks for test of dryness
    - Suspend dose in children who experience acute condition affecting fluid/electrolyte balances (fever, vomiting, diarrhea, vigorous exercise)
  - 10–70% success; safe even when used for >12 months; high relapse rate after discontinuation without a structured withdrawal program
- Anticholinergics:
  - Oxybutynin (Ditropan, Ditropan XL, Oxytrol patch): Anticholinergic; smooth muscle relaxant, antispasmodic; may increase functional bladder capacity and aids in timed voiding:
    - Ditropan: Adults and children >5 years of age: 5 mg PO t.i.d.–q.i.d.; children 1–5 years of age: 0.02 mg/kg/dose b.i.d.–q.i.d. (syrup 5 mg/5 mL)
    - Ditropan XL: Adults: 5 mg/d PO; increase to 30 mg/d PO (5-, 10-mg tabs)
    - Oxytrol patch: 1 patch every 3–4 days (3.9 mg/patch) (periodic trials off the medication, i.e., weekends or weeks at a time, will help determine efficacy and resolution of primary disturbance)
    - Ditropan 5–10 mg at night; 30–50% success; 50% relapse after stopped
  - Tolterodine (Detrol, Detrol LA): Anticholinergic; fewer side effects than Ditropan:
    - Detrol: 1–2 mg PO b.i.d.
    - Detrol LA: 2–4 mg/d

Pediatric Considerations

USFDA recommends against using intranasal formulations of desmopressin in children due to reports of severe hyponatremia resulting in seizures and deaths (4,5)[A].

Second Line

- Imipramine (Tofranil): Tricyclic antidepressant, anticholinergic effects; increases bladder capacity, antispasmodic properties:
  - Primarily in adults; use in children reserved for resistant cases
  - Dose: Adults, 25–75 mg and children >6 years, 10–25 mg PO at bedtime; increase by 10–25 mg at 1–2-week intervals; treat for 2–3 months; then taper
  - 25–30% success when used >3 months
  - Pretreatment ECG recommended to identify underlying rhythm disorders
- Precautions:
  - Oxybutynin: Glaucoma, myasthenia gravis, GI or genitourinary obstruction, ulcerative colitis, megacolon; use a decreased dose in the elderly.
  - Tolterodine: Urinary retention, gastric retention, or uncontrolled narrow-angle glaucoma; significant drug interactions with CYP2D6, CYP3A3/4 substrates
  - DDAVP: Avoid in patients at risk for electrolyte changes or fluid retention (congestive heart failure [CHF], renal insufficiency).
  - Imipramine: Do not use with monoamine oxidase inhibitors (MAOIs), hypotension, and arrhythmias; low toxic therapeutic ratio.
- Combination therapy with DDAVP and oxybutynin has better results than individual use.
- Prostaglandin inhibitors (e.g., indomethacin) have been studied; may increase bladder capacity.

ALERT

Imipramine: Cardiotoxicity and death with overdose have been described.

ADDITIONAL TREATMENT

General Measures

- Use nonpharmacologic approaches as first line before prescribing medications (6)[A].
- Simple behavioral interventions (e.g., scheduled wakening, positive reinforcement, bladder training, diet changes)
- Enuresis alarms (bells or buzzers):
  - 66–70% success rate; must be used nightly for 3–4 months; offers cure; significant parental involvement; disruption of sleep for entire family

Issues for Referral

- Primary NE: Persistent enuresis despite nonpharmacologic and pharmacologic therapies
- Diurnal incontinence or nonmonosymptomatic enuresis with voiding dysfunction or underlying medical condition

Additional Therapies

Individual psychotherapy, crisis intervention, and family therapy

COMPLEMENTARY AND ALTERNATIVE MEDICINE

Acupuncture and hypnosis are other treatments offered; few data support their use (7,8)[B].

SURGERY/OTHER PROCEDURES

Only for surgically correctable causes (e.g., tethered cord, ectopic ureter, benign prostatic hypertrophy, obstructive sleep apnea)

ONGOING CARE

FOLLOW-UP RECOMMENDATIONS

Patient Monitoring

Follow patient until condition resolved. Monitor therapy.

DIET

- Limit fluid and caffeine intake prior 2 hours to bedtime.
- Limit dairy products 4 hours prior to bedtime (decrease osmotic diuresis).

PATIENT EDUCATION

Web resources for alarms and supplies:

- www.bedwettingstore.com/index.htm
- www.pottypager.com/

PROGNOSIS

In children, NE is usually self-limiting; 1% will persist as adult; evaluate for organic causes.

COMPLICATIONS

UTI, perineal excoriation, psychological disturbance (especially in children)

REFERENCES

1. Robson WL. Current management of nocturnal enuresis. *Curr Opin Urol*. 2008;18:425–30.
2. Zaffanello M, Giacomello L, Brugnara M, et al. Therapeutic options in childhood nocturnal enuresis. *Minerva Urol Nefrol*. 2007;59:199–205.
3. Vande Walle J, Stockner M, Raes A, et al. Desmopressin 30 years in clinical use: A safety review. *Curr Drug Saf*. 2007;2:232–8.
4. Graham KM, Levy JB, et al. Enuresis. *Pediatr Rev*. 2009;30:165–72; quiz 173.
5. www.fda.gov/Drugs/DrugSafety/Postmarket DrugSafetyInformationforPatientsandProviders/ucm107924.htm.
6. Robson WL, et al. Clinical practice. Evaluation and management of enuresis. *N Engl J Med*. 2009;360:1429–36.
7. Neveus T, Eggert P, Evans J, et al. Evaluation of and treatment for monosymptomatic enuresis: A standardization document from the International Children's Continence Society. *J Urol*. 2010;183:441–7.
8. Libonate J, Evans S, Tsao JC, et al. Efficacy of acupuncture for health conditions in children: A review. *Sci World J*. 2008;8:670–82.

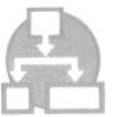

See Also (Topic, Algorithm, Electronic Media Element)

- Incontinence, Urinary Adult Female; Incontinence, Urinary Adult Male
- Algorithm: Enuresis

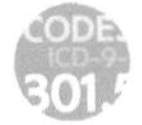

CODES

ICD9

- 307.6 Enuresis
- 788.30 Urinary incontinence, unspecified
- 788.36 Nocturnal enuresis

CLINICAL PEARLS

- Diagnosis is usually made based on history, physical examination, and urinalysis.
- If the condition is not distressing to child and caretakers, treatment is unnecessary.
- Dryness is possible for most children.

EOSINOPHILIC ESOPHAGITIS

Lauren Michal de Leon, MD
Edward Feller, MD

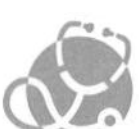

BASICS

Eosinophilic esophagitis (EE) is a disorder characterized by eosinophilic infiltration of esophageal mucosa commonly associated with chest pain, dysphagia, or food impaction.

DESCRIPTION

This entity is increasingly recognized as a cause of diverse symptoms, including gastroesophageal reflux disease (GERD) that is unresponsive to antireflux treatment.

EPIDEMIOLOGY

- All ages, most common in 20s–30s; male:female ratio = 3:1 in both children and adults
- Symptoms, most commonly dysphagia, have been present for a mean of 3–4 years prior to diagnosis.

Incidence

- Incidence in general population is 0.03% (1).
- Incidence in those with GERD/dysphagia symptoms: 2.8% (1)

Prevalence

Gradually increasing, perhaps due to better case finding, understanding of EE in multiple clinical guises; 4–6/100,000

RISK FACTORS

More than 50% with EE have personal history of allergic disorders, such as asthma, hay fever, or eczema (2)[A].

PATHOPHYSIOLOGY

Though not well understood, the pathophysiology of eosinophilic esophagitis is postulated to be due to increased recruitment and activation of eosinophils in the esophagus. Studies have been conducted to determine the chemoattractants responsible for recruitment. Thus far, eotaxin-3 and IL-5 activity have been implicated in this disease process.

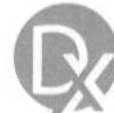

DIAGNOSIS

Definitive diagnosis can be established only by endoscopy and biopsy.

HISTORY

- Patients may complain of dysphagia and reflux-type symptoms. Often, the diagnosis is entertained after patients fail a trial of antireflux medications. Other common complaints include nausea or vomiting, regurgitation, chest pain, or decreased appetite.
- EE is a common cause of food impaction and should be considered in this clinical context.
- Patients may also have a history of food or environmental allergies as well as asthma or atopic conditions (e.g., dermatitis).

PHYSICAL EXAM

No specific physical exam findings are associated with the diagnosis. However, signs and symptoms of allergies or asthma with symptoms of ongoing dysphagia or GERD-like symptoms should raise suspicion; some patients will have signs indicating weight loss or malnutrition.

DIAGNOSTIC TESTS & INTERPRETATION

- GERD: Empiric trial of PPI symptoms if no warning "red flags"; if no improvement, consider EGD
- Dysphagia: EGD with biopsy is warranted if "red flags":
  - Dysphagia
  - Odynophagia
  - Weight loss
  - Early satiety or vomiting
  - Aspiration/wheezing or cough
  - GI bleeding
  - Unexplained iron-deficiency anemia
  - Male >45 years old with long-standing symptoms
- Consensus American Gastroenterologic Association guidelines for diagnosis include:
  - Clinical symptoms of esophageal dysfunction
  - >15 eosinophils in 1 high-power field on biopsy
  - Unresponsiveness to high-dose proton pump inhibitor (PPI) therapy
  - Normal pH monitoring of the distal esophagus

Lab

- Serum IgE levels can be elevated.
- Peripheral eosinophilia may be present in 10–50%, and in those instances, may be mild.

Diagnostic Procedures/Surgery

EGD should include multiple esophageal biopsies obtained along the full length of the esophagus. Biopsies of the stomach and duodenum should also be obtained to differentiate between eosinophilic esophagitis and eosinophilic gastroenteritis.

Pathological Findings

Criteria for diagnosis:

- Presence of >15 eosinophils per high-power field in 3 or more biopsies despite PPI treatment for 2 or more months
- Normal gastric and duodenal mucosal biopsies
- Exclusion of other causes of eosinophils in the esophagus and clinical symptoms

DIFFERENTIAL DIAGNOSIS

- GERD: Associated with esophageal eosinophilia; diseases may coexist in individual patients.
- Functional dyspepsia
- Congenital rings
- Connective tissue diseases
- Carcinoma
- Allergic vasculitis
- Esophageal motility disorder, such as achalasia

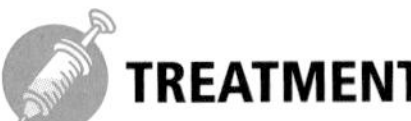

TREATMENT

Treatment regimens have not been formally established in large-scale randomized trials (3)[A].

MEDICATION

- Acid suppression: Diagnosis of eosinophilic esophagitis requires failure of acid therapy; many patients do have coexisting GERD. Acid suppression has been commonly used prior to diagnosis, but its impact on the natural history of eosinophilic esophagitis has not been shown to be beneficial.
- Esophageal dilatation: Reserved for patients with strictures or rings, but can result in perforation or tears. It does not impact the underlying inflammation.
- Elimination or elemental diets: Since there is an association with atopy, elimination diets have been studied in small cohorts. These small studies have shown clinical and histological improvement after initiating elimination diets based on food allergy testing. This testing and protocols have not been standardized, and have not been studied in adults (2).
- Systemic steroids: Patients showed clinical and histological improvements, but long-term toxicity limits use to brief treatment in patients with severe symptoms such as refractory dysphagia (2).
- Topical steroids (swallowed): Patients showed clinical and histological improvements with both topical fluticasone and suspension of budesonide, though an ideal dosage has not been established. Patients also relapsed after withdrawal of the medication; inhaled topical steroid trials are ongoing.
- Antihistamines: Case studies showed no benefit.
- Other options: Montelukast, mepolizumab, purine analogues, anti-TNF therapy. Varying results, not well studied.

First Line

- Given the strong circumstantial evidence of the role of food allergy, elimination diets established in conjunction with an allergist and nutritionist can be tried with children and adults (4):
  - In children, success rates of 77–98% have been reported for clinical and histologic remission using an elemental amino acid formula.
  - In adults, long-term restrictive diets are poorly tolerated and challenging.
- For a pharmacologic approach, swallowed fluticasone dose based on age should be tried for 6–8 weeks, with repeat for 4–6 weeks if patient fails the initial trial. Medication should be discontinued if patient develops side effects or other intolerances.

ADDITIONAL TREATMENT

Endoscopic dilation has been successful in patients with esophageal strictures, although reported complication rates are high.

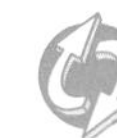

ONGOING CARE

DIET

A mainstay of treatment, especially in children

PROGNOSIS

Quality of life is affected to a minor degree in many; nutritional status can be maintained with appropriate care and diligence.

COMPLICATIONS

- Food impaction
- Esophageal stricture
- Nutritional deficits
- Subglottic stenosis or laryngeal edema is very rare.

REFERENCES

1. Sealock RJ, Rendon G, El-Serag HB, et al. Systematic review: The epidemiology of eosinophilic oesophagitis in adults. *Aliment Pharmacol Ther*. 2010;32:712–9.
2. Liacouras CA, Furuta GT, Hirano I, et al. Eosinophilic esophagitis: Updated consensus recommendations for children and adults. *J Allergy Clin Immunol*. 2011;128:3–20.e6.
3. Elliott EJ, Thomas D, Markowitz JE, et al. Non-surgical interventions for eosinophilic esophagitis. *Cochrane Database Syst Rev*. 2010;CD004065.
4. "American Gastroenterogical Association medical position statemnt: Guideline for the evaluation of food allergies." *Gatroenterology*. 2001;120(4): 1023–25.

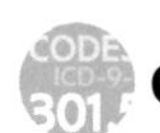

CODES

ICD9

530.13 Eosinophilic esophagitis

CLINICAL PEARLS

- EE commonly mimics more common disorders; hence, prolonged diagnostic delay is common.
- Consider EoE or functional dyspepsia if patient with GERD symptoms is unresponsive to PPI treatment.
- Remember "red flags" in patients with empiric GERD: Dysphagia, odynophagia, weight loss, early satiety or vomiting, aspiration/wheezing/cough, GI bleed, unexplained iron-deficiency anemia, age >50 years old

EPICONDYLITIS

Kevin Heaton, DO

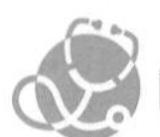

BASICS

DESCRIPTION

- Tendon injury characterized by pain and tenderness at the tendinous origins of the wrist flexors/ extensors on the epicondyles of the humerus
- May be acute (traumatic) or chronic (overuse)
- 2 types:
  - Medial epicondylitis or "golfer's elbow":
    - Involvement of the wrist flexors and pronators on the medial epicondyle
  - Lateral epicondylitis or "tennis elbow":
    - Involvement of the wrist extensors and supinators on the lateral epicondyle
- May be caused by many different athletic or occupational activities
- Common in carpenters, plumbers, gardeners, and politicians
- Usually occurs unilaterally on the epicondyles of the dominant arm
- Lateral epicondyle involvement is more common than medial.

EPIDEMIOLOGY

- Predominant age: >40
- Predominant sex: Male = Female

Incidence

- Very common site of overuse injury
- Lateral > Medial
- Estimated between 1% and 3%

Prevalence

- Lateral epicondylitis: 1.3%
- Medial epicondylitis: 0.4%

RISK FACTORS

- Repetitive wrist motions:
  - Flexion/pronation: Medial
  - Extension/supination: Lateral
- Smoking
- Obesity
- Upper extremity forceful activities

GENERAL PREVENTION

- Limit overuse of the wrist flexors, extensors, pronators, and supinators.
- Use proper techniques when working or playing racquet sports.
- Use lighter tools and smaller grips.

PATHOPHYSIOLOGY

- Acute (tendonitis):
  - Inflammatory response to injury
- Chronic (tendinosis):
  - Overuse injury
  - Tendon degeneration, fibroblast proliferation, microvascular proliferation, lack of inflammatory response

ETIOLOGY

- Repetitive wrist motions
- Tool/racquet gripping
- Shaking hands
- Sudden maximal muscle contraction
- Direct blow

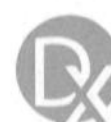

DIAGNOSIS

HISTORY

- Occupational activities
- Sport participation
- Direct trauma
- Duration of symptoms
- Treatments or medication use
- Pain with gripping
- Sensation of mild forearm weakness

PHYSICAL EXAM

- Localized pain just distal to the affected epicondyle
- Increased pain with wrist flexion/pronation (medial)
- Increased pain with wrist extension/supination (lateral)
- Medial epicondylitis:
  - Tenderness at origin of wrist flexor tendons
  - Increased pain with resisted wrist flexion and pronation
  - Normal elbow range of motion
  - Increased pain with gripping
- Lateral epicondylitis:
  - Tenderness at origin of wrist extensors
  - Increased pain with resisted wrist extension/ supination
  - Normal elbow range of motion
  - Increased pain with gripping

DIAGNOSTIC TESTS & INTERPRETATION

Imaging

Initial approach

No imaging is required for initial evaluation and treatment of a classic overuse injury.

Follow-Up & Special Considerations

- Anterior-posterior/lateral radiographs if decreased range of motion, trauma, or no improvement with initial conservative therapy. Assess for fractures or signs of arthritis.
- For recalcitrant cases:
  - Musculoskeletal ultrasound can show abnormal tendon appearance (e.g., tendon thickening, partial tear at tendon origin, calcifications) and neovascularity when color flow Doppler is used. It can also be used to guide steroid or other alternative injections.
  - MRI can show intermediate or high T2 signal intensity within the common flexor or extensor tendon or the presence of peritendinous soft tissue edema.

Diagnostic Procedures/Surgery

A local injection of anesthetic to document resolution of symptoms could be performed if the diagnosis is in doubt.

DIFFERENTIAL DIAGNOSIS

- Elbow osteoarthritis
- Fractures of the epicondyles
- Posterior interosseous nerve entrapment (lateral)
- Ulnar neuropathy (medial)
- Synovitis
- Medial collateral ligament injury
- Referred pain from shoulder or neck

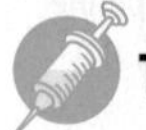

TREATMENT

MEDICATION

First Line

- Topical NSAIDs: Significantly more effective than placebo with respect to pain and participant satisfaction in the short term (≤6 weeks) with minimal adverse effects (1)[A]
- Oral NSAIDs: There is some evidence for short-term (≤6 weeks) benefit with respect to pain and function, but this benefit is not sustained. Associated with GI adverse effects (1)[A].

Second Line

Corticosteroid injections: Short-term (≤6 weeks) improvements in pain, global improvement, and grip strength compared to placebo, local anesthetic, and conservative treatments. No benefits found for intermediate or long-term outcomes (2)[A].

ADDITIONAL TREATMENT

General Measures

Initial treatment consists of activity modification, counterforce bracing, oral or topical NSAIDs, ice, and physical therapy:

- Observation: If left untreated, symptoms typically last between 6 months and 2 years. For patients with good function and minimal pain, conservative management with a "wait and see" policy may be considered.
- Activity modification, relative rest, and correction of faulty biomechanics
- Counterforce bracing with a forearm "tennis elbow" strap is easy to use and inexpensive. Systematic reviews have been unable to provide a solid conclusion about overall efficacy, but initial bracing may improve a patient's ability to perform daily activities in the first 6 weeks.
- Frequent ice application after activities
- Physical therapy:
  - Begin once acute pain resolved
  - Eccentric strength training regimen and stretching program
  - Ultrasound
  - Corticosteroid iontophoresis

Issues for Referral

Failure of conservative therapy

Additional Therapies

- Platelet-rich plasma injections (3)[B]:
  - Involves the injection of a concentrated portion of the patient's platelet-rich plasma. The localized injection leads to a local inflammatory response causing the platelets to degranulate, releasing growth factors, which then stimulates the physiologic healing cascade.
- Ultrasound-guided percutaneous needle tenotomy (4)[C]:
  - Involves the injection of a local anesthetic followed by ultrasound-guided tendon fenestration, calcification fragmentation and aspiration, and abrading the underlying bone. The procedure is thought to break apart scar tissue and stimulate an inflammatory and healing response.
- Prolotherapy (5)[B]:
  - Involves the injection of a dextrose solution into and around the tendon attachment. This stimulates a localized inflammatory response, leading to increased blood supply to the area, which increases the flow of nutrients and healing mediators to stimulate tendon healing.
- Glyceryl trinitrate (GTN) transdermal patch (6)[B]:
  - Nitric oxide (NO) is a small free radical generated by 3 isoenzymes called nitric oxide synthases. NO is expressed by fibroblasts and is postulated to aid in collagen synthesis. Topical application of glyceryl trinitrate theoretically improves healing by this mechanism. One-quarter of a 5-mg/24-hour GTN transdermal patch is applied once daily for up to 24 weeks.

COMPLEMENTARY AND ALTERNATIVE MEDICINE

Acupuncture (1)[A]:

- Effective for short-term pain relief for lateral epicondyle pain

SURGERY/OTHER PROCEDURES

- May be indicated in refractory cases
- Involves debridement and release of the involved tendons
- Can be performed open or arthroscopically

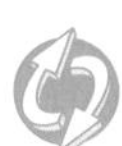

ONGOING CARE

PROGNOSIS

Good: Majority resolve with conservative care.

REFERENCES

1. Bisset L, Coombes B, Vicenzino B. Tennis elbow. *Clin Evid* (Online). 2011;2011.
2. Coombes BK, Bisset L, Vicenzino B. Efficacy and safety of corticosteroid injections and other injections for management of tendinopathy: A systematic review of randomised controlled trials. *Lancet*. 2010;376(9754):1751–67.
3. Taylor DW, Petrera M, Hendry M, et al. A systematic review of the use of platelet-rich plasma in sports medicine as a new treatment for tendon and ligament injuries. *Clin J Sport Med*. 2011.
4. McShane JM, Shah VN, Nazarian LN. Sonographically guided needle tenotomy for treatment of common extensor tendinosis in the elbow: Is a corticosteroid necessary? *J Ultrasound Med*. 2008;27(8):1137–44.
5. Rabago D, Best TM, Zgierska A, et al. A systematic review of four injection therapies for lateral epicondylosis: Prolotherapy, polidocanol, whole blood and platelet-rich plasma. *Br J Sports Med*. 2009;43;471–81.
6. Paoloni JA, Murrell GAC, Burch RM, et al. Randomised, double-blind, placebo-controlled clinical trial of a new topical glyceryl trinitrate patch for chronic lateral epicondylosis. *Br J Sports Med*. 2009;43:299–302.

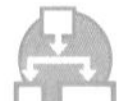

See Also (Topic, Algorithm, Electronic Media Element)

Algorithm: Pain in Upper Extremity

CODES

ICD9

- 726.31 Medial epicondylitis
- 726.32 Lateral epicondylitis

CLINICAL PEARLS

- Tendon injury characterized by pain and tenderness at the tendinous origins of the wrist flexors/extensors on the epicondyles of the humerus
- 2 types:
  - Medial epicondylitis or "golfer's elbow":
    - Involvement of the wrist flexors and pronators on the medial epicondyle
  - Lateral epicondylitis or "tennis elbow":
    - Involvement of the wrist extensors and supinators on the lateral epicondyle
- If left untreated, symptoms typically last between 6 months and 2 years.
- Majority of patients will improve with conservative treatment.
- NSAIDs first line; steroid injection second line
- Frequent ice application after activities
- Elbow straps during activity (counterforce bracing)
- Physical therapy as symptoms improve

EPIDIDYMITIS

Andrew Leone, MD
Kyle D. Wood, MD

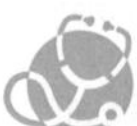

BASICS

- Acute epididymitis: Pain for <6 weeks
- Chronic epididymitis: Pain for >3 months

DESCRIPTION

Inflammation (infectious or noninfectious) of epididymis resulting in scrotal pain and swelling, induration of the posterior epididymis, and eventual scrotal wall edema, involvement of the adjacent testicle, and hydrocele formation:

- System(s) affected: Reproductive
- Synonym(s): Epididymo-orchitis
- Classification: Infectious (bacterial, viral, fungal, parasitic) versus sterile (chemical, traumatic, autoimmune, idiopathic, industrial, noninfectious, vasoepididymal reflux syndrome, vasal reflux syndrome); chronic versus acute

EPIDEMIOLOGY

- Predominant age: Usually younger, sexually active men or older men with UTIs; in older men usually secondary to bladder outlet obstruction
- Predominant sex: Male only

Pediatric Considerations

Occurs in prepubertal boys: Epididymitis is found to be the most common cause of acute scrotum, more common than testicular torsion.

Incidence

- Common (600,000 cases annually in the US)
- 1 in 1,000 males per year

Prevalence

Common

RISK FACTORS

- UTI, prostatitis
- Indwelling urethral catheter
- Urethral instrumentation or transurethral surgery
- Urethral or meatal stricture
- Transrectal prostate biopsy
- Prostate brachytherapy (seeds) for prostate cancer
- Anal intercourse
- High-risk sexual activity
- Strenuous physical activity
- Prolonged sedentary periods
- Bladder obstruction (benign prostatic hyperplasia, prostate cancer)
- HIV-immunosuppressed patient
- Severe Behçet disease
- Presence of foreskin (1)
- Constipation
- Sterile epididymitis:
  - Increased intra-abdominal pressure (occupation requiring frequent physical strain):
    - Military recruits, especially who begin physically unprepared
    - Laborers; restaurant kitchen workers
    - Full bladder during intense physical exertion

GENERAL PREVENTION

- Vasectomy or vasoligation during transurethral surgery
- Safer sexual practices
- Mumps vaccination
- Antibiotic prophylaxis for urethral manipulation
- Early treatment of prostatitis/benign prostatic hyperplasia (BPH)
- Avoid vigorous rectal exam with acute prostatitis.
- Sterile epididymitis:
  - Emptying the bladder prior to physical exertion
  - Physically conditioning the body prior to engaging in regular intense physical exertion (2)
  - Treating constipation

PATHOPHYSIOLOGY

- Infectious epididymitis:
  - Retrograde spread of urine or urinary bacteria from the prostate or urethra via the ejaculatory ducts and the vas deferens into the epididymis; rarely, hematogenous spread
  - Causative organism is identified in 80% of patients, and varies according to patient age.
- Sterile epididymitis:
  - Urine in full bladder when exposed to increased intra-abdominal pressure is pushed through internal urethral sphincter (located at proximal end of prostatic urethra).
  - Reflux of urine through orifice of ejaculatory ducts at verumontanum may occur with history of urethritis/prostatitis, as inflammation may produce rigidity in musculature surrounding orifice to ejaculatory ducts, holding them open.
  - Exposure of epididymis to foreign fluid may produce inflammatory reaction within 24 hours

ETIOLOGY

- <35 years and sexually active:
  - Usually *Chlamydia trachomatis* or *Neisseria gonorrhoeae*
  - Look for serous urethral discharge (chlamydia) or purulent discharge (gonorrhea).
  - With anal intercourse, likely *Escherichia coli* or *Haemophilus influenzae*
- >35 years:
  - Coliform bacteria usually, but sometimes *Staphylococcus aureus* or *S. epidermidis*
  - In elderly men, often with distal urinary tract obstruction, BPH, UTI, or catheterization
  - Tuberculosis, if sterile pyuria and nodularity of vas deferens (hematogenous spread)
  - Sterile urine reflux after transurethral prostatectomy
  - Granulomatous reaction following BCG intravesical therapy for bladder cancer
- Prepubertal boys:
  - Usually coliform bacteria
  - Evaluate for underlying congenital abnormalities, such as vesicoureteral reflux, ectopic ureter, or anorectal malformation (rectourethral fistula).
- Amiodarone may cause noninfectious epididymitis; resolves with decreasing drug dosage.
- Syphilis, blastomycosis, coccidioidomycosis, and cryptococcosis are rare causes, but brucellosis can be a common cause in endemic areas (3).

COMMONLY ASSOCIATED CONDITIONS

- Prostatitis/urethritis/orchitis
- Hemospermia
- Constipation
- UTI

DIAGNOSIS

- Scrotal pain, sometimes radiating to the groin region, may begin acutely over several hours.
- Urethral discharge or symptoms of UTI, such as frequency of urination, dysuria, cloudy urine, or hematuria (4)
- Initially, only the posterior-lying epididymis, usually the lowermost tail section, is very tender and indurated; will eventually progress to involvement of body and head of epididymis.
- Elevation of the testes/epididymis improves the discomfort (Prehn sign).
- Entire hemiscrotum becomes swollen and red, the testis becomes indistinguishable from the epididymis, the scrotal wall becomes thick and indurated, and reactive hydrocele may occur.
- Sterile epididymitis:
  - Unilateral scrotal pain and swelling preceded by intense physical exertion by several hours. Patient may recall full bladder prior to exertion.
  - No symptoms of infection

Pediatric Considerations

- In prepubertal patients, may be postinfectious inflammatory condition; treat with anti-inflammatories, analgesics, and usually no antibiotics (5)
- Bacteremia from *Haemophilus influenzae* infection may produce acute epididymitis.
- In adolescent males, particularly >13 years old, must rule out testicular torsion.
- History not helpful in distinguishing epididymitis from testicular torsion.

Geriatric Considerations

Diabetics with sensory neuropathy may have pain despite severe infection/abscess.

PHYSICAL EXAM

- The tail of the epididymis is larger in comparison to the contralateral side.
- Epididymis is markedly tender to palpation.
- Cremasteric reflex should be present in epididymitis; if absent, suspect testicular torsion.

DIAGNOSTIC TESTS & INTERPRETATION

Lab

Initial lab tests

- Urinalysis (pyuria and bacteruria suggestive of infectious origin)
- Urine culture (negative does not rule out)
- GC/chlamydia testing (urethral swab or urine testing)
- Gram stain urethral discharge
- WBC count may be elevated.
- Urinalysis clear and culture-negative suggest sterile epididymitis

Imaging

- If testicular torsion cannot be excluded (especially in pediatrics), Doppler ultrasound test of choice (6)
- In adult men, Doppler ultrasound: Sensitivity and specificity of 100% in evaluation of acute scrotum, but usually not needed (7)

Pediatric Considerations
Further radiographic imaging in children should be done to rule out anatomic abnormalities

Diagnostic Procedures/Surgery
This is a clinical diagnosis.

Pathological Findings
- Epididymis:
  - Surrounding tissue fibrosis and scarring
  - Interstitial nonspecific acute infiltration, edema, congestion, PMNs, and lymphocytes
  - Fine inflammatory adhesions
  - Can progress to abscess or necrosis (2)
- Vas deferens:
  - Possible fibrosis of this structure

DIFFERENTIAL DIAGNOSIS
- Epididymal congestion following vasectomy
- Testicular torsion
- Torsion of testicular appendages
- Orchitis
- Testicular malignancy
- Testicular trauma
- Epididymal cyst
- Inguinal hernia
- Urethritis
- Spermatocele
- Hydrocele
- Hematocele
- Varicocele
- Epididymal adenomatoid tumor
- Epididymal rhabdomyosarcoma
- Vasculitis (Henoch-Schönlein purpura)

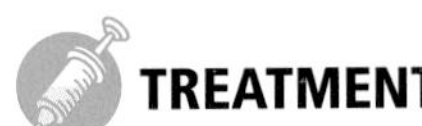

TREATMENT

- Bed rest or restriction on activity
- Athletic scrotal supporter
- Scrotal elevation
- Ice pack/warm compress
- If chemical epididymitis:
  - Cessation of strenuous physical activity for several weeks
  - Empty bladder prior to strenuous exercises.

MEDICATION
First Line
- <35 years, for chlamydia: Doxycycline 100 mg PO b.i.d. for 10 days PO ceftriaxone 250 mg IM × 1. Treat sexual partner(s) (8).
- If penicillin-allergic or participates in insertive anal intercourse: Ciprofloxacin (Cipro) 500 mg PO b.i.d. or ofloxacin (Floxin) 200 mg PO b.i.d. for 10 days
- Older men with bacteriuria:
  - Levofloxacin (Levaquin) 500 mg PO every day for 7–10 days (8)
  - Ofloxacin 300 mg PO b.i.d. for 10 days (8)
  - Ciprofloxacin (Cipro) 500 mg PO b.i.d. or ciprofloxacin (Cipro XL) 1,000 mg/d for 10–14 days
- Analgesia (infectious and chemical epididymitis):
  - NSAIDs (e.g., naproxen or ibuprofen) for mild to moderate pain
  - Consider corticosteroid if patient cannot tolerate NSAID.
  - Acetaminophen-codeine or acetaminophen-oxycodone for moderate-to-severe pain
- Septic or toxic patient:
  - Third-generation cephalosporin or aminoglycoside
- For Bechet, sarcoid, Henoch-Schönlein purpura:
  - Corticosteroids such as methylprednisolone 40 mg/d recommended

Second Line
- Trimethoprim-sulfamethoxazole (Bactrim, Septra) double-strength PO b.i.d. for 10–14 days; increasing bacterial resistance may limit effectiveness.
- Add rifampin (rifampicin) or vancomycin as required.

ADDITIONAL TREATMENT
General Measures
Spermatic cord block with local anesthesia in severe cases

Issues for Referral
- If suspicion is high for testicular torsion or cancer, consult a urologist.
- If failed medical management, should be referred to urologist to rule out anatomic abnormality or to diagnosis chemical epididymitis

SURGERY/OTHER PROCEDURES
- Vasostomy to drain infected material if severe or refractory case
- Scrotal exploration if unable to clinically distinguish between epididymitis or testicular torsion
- Drainage of abscesses, epididymectomy (acute suppurative), or epididymo-orchiectomy in severe cases refractory to antibiotics
- Surgery to correct underlying anatomic abnormality or obstruction

IN-PATIENT CONSIDERATIONS
Initial Stabilization
- The majority of cases can be managed with outpatient care.
- Inpatient care needed if septic or if surgery is scheduled

Admission Criteria
- Intractable pain
- Sepsis
- Abscess
- Persistent vomiting
- Purulent drainage

ONGOING CARE

FOLLOW-UP RECOMMENDATIONS
Patient Monitoring
- Office visits until all signs of infection have cleared
- In chemical epididymitis, follow-up in 4 weeks to assess efficacy of NSAIDs and lifestyle changes.

DIET
If constipation is contributing to chemical epididymitis, consider a high-fiber diet.

PATIENT EDUCATION
- Stress completing course of antibiotics, even when asymptomatic.
- Early recognition and treatment of UTI or prostatitis
- Safer sexual practices
- If chemical epididymitis, then educate on noninfectious etiology and proper lifestyle changes.

PROGNOSIS
- Pain improves within 1–3 days, but induration may take several weeks/months to completely resolve.
- If bilateral involvement, sterility may result
- In chemical epididymitis, symptoms usually resolve in <1 week.

COMPLICATIONS
- Recurrent epididymitis
- Infertility
- Oligospermia
- Testicular necrosis or atrophy
- Secondary abscess formation
- Fournier gangrene (necrotizing synergistic infection)

REFERENCES

1. Bennett RT, Gill B, Kogan SJ. Epididymitis in children: The circumcision factor? *J Urol*. 1998;160: 1842–4.
2. Wolin LH. On the etiology of epididymitis. *J Urol*. 1971;105:531–3.
3. Akinci E, Bodur H, Cevik MA, et al. A complication of brucellosis: epididymoorchitis. *Int J Infect Dis*. 2006;10:171–7.
4. Tracy CR, Steers WD, Costabile R. Diagnosis and management of epididymitis. *Urol Clin North Am*. 2008;35:101–8; vii.
5. Somekh E, Gorenstein A, Serour F. Acute epididymitis in boys: evidence of a post-infectious etiology. *J Urol*. 2004;171:391–4; discussion 394.
6. Trojian TH, Lishnak TS, Heiman D. Epididymitis and orchitis: An overview. *Am Fam Physician*. 2009;79: 583–7.
7. Süzer O, Ozcan H, Küpeli S, et al. Color Doppler imaging in the diagnosis of the acute scrotum. *Eur Urol*. 1997;32:457–61.
8. Drugs for sexually transmitted infections. *Treat Guidel Med Lett*. 2007;5:81–8.

CODES

ICD9
- 604.90 Orchitis and epididymitis, unspecified
- 604.91 Orchitis and epididymitis in diseases classified elsewhere
- 604.99 Other orchitis, epididymitis, and epididymo-orchitis, without mention of abscess

CLINICAL PEARLS

- With epididymitis, the pain is more gradual in onset, and the tenderness is mostly posterior to the testis. With testicular torsion, the symptoms are quite rapid in onset, the testis will be higher in the scrotum and may have a transverse lie, and the cremasteric reflex will be absent. The absence of leukocytes on urine analysis and decreased blood flow on scrotal ultrasound with Doppler will suggest torsion.
- Prostatic massage is contraindicated in epididymitis because the risk for worsening local infection and potential for sepsis is increased with acute prostatitis.
- Chemical epididymitis is a clinical diagnosis of exclusion, and infectious causes are much more common, but certain occupations, such as soldiers and laborers, must be considered.

EPIGLOTTITIS

Vassiliki P. Syriopoulou, MD

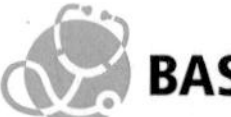

BASICS

DESCRIPTION

- An illness with acute onset characterized by inflammation and edema of the supraglottic structures, epiglottis, vallecula, arytenoepiglottic folds, and arytenoids
- System(s) affected: Pulmonary
- Synonym(s): Supraglottitis

EPIDEMIOLOGY

Incidence

- Has decreased dramatically since the introduction of the *Haemophilus influenzae* type b (Hib) vaccine in the mid-1980s (1,2)
- In adults: 1–3 per 100,000 per year
- In the pre-vaccine era, the most commonly affected group was children 2–4 years old.
- With use of Hib vaccine, the predominant age is shifting to older children (median age, 7 years) and adults (1,2).
- Predominant sex: Male > Female (1.8:1)

Prevalence

More prevalent in countries without universal immunization

RISK FACTORS

- Absence of immunization against Hib
- Immunocompromise

GENERAL PREVENTION

- *H. influenzae* type B vaccine is effective, although not 100% protective.
- Rifampin prophylaxis (20 mg/kg/d for 4 days, maximum daily dose 600 mg) for all household and daycare contacts of invasive Hib. Family and close contacts may be asymptomatic carriers of Hib.

Pediatric Considerations

Rare since introduction of Hib vaccine

Geriatric Considerations

Rare

PATHOPHYSIOLOGY

- In epiglottitis, usually a local invasion of the epiglottis occurs, followed by bacteremia.
- The epiglottis, aryepiglottic folds, false vocal cords, and supraglottic structures become inflamed and edematous, leading to narrowed airway and respiratory compromise.
- Inspiratory airway occlusion often occurs prior to total occlusion from supraglottic edema.

ETIOLOGY

- Bacterial:
  - Hib
  - *Streptococcus pyogenes*
  - *Streptococcus pneumoniae*
  - *Staphylococcus aureus*
  - Other bacteria (*P. multocida*, *N. meningitidis*, etc.)
- Fungal (*Candida spp.*)
- Viral
- Traumatic: Caustic ingestion
- Allergic reactions

DIAGNOSIS

HISTORY

- Sudden onset of severe symptoms and a fulminant course over a period of hours, unless airway control and medical management are initiated promptly.
- Fever is the first symptom, followed by stridor and labored breathing.
- Dysphagia, refusal to eat, drooling, and sore throat are common.
- Muffled voice/cry (vs. hoarseness in croup)
- Minimal cough (vs. barking cough in croup)
- Usually no history of prodromal upper respiratory infection (vs. positive history in croup)
- In adults, presentation is more indolent (sore throat and odynophagia are the predominant symptoms).

PHYSICAL EXAM

- Toxic appearance/shock (occasionally, due to associated septicemia)
- Marked restlessness, irritability, and anxiety are common.
- Airway obstruction resulting in respiratory distress
- Tripod position (sitting propped up on hands with head forward and tongue out)
- Stridor softer and less prominent than in croup
- Anterior neck exam may reveal tender adenopathy.
- Definitive diagnosis is established by visualizing a swollen and erythematous epiglottis during careful exam of the oropharynx, although this should not normally be attempted without specific training and equipment available to manage an obstructed airway, such as in an operating room (OR).
- Cyanosis indicates a poor prognosis.

DIAGNOSTIC TESTS & INTERPRETATION

Lab

Initial lab tests

- Blood culture (positive in >75–90% of children with Hib-acute epiglottitis). *Do not* visualize/swab epiglottis except in controlled environment (e.g., OR). Blood tests are also contraindicated until airway is secured.
- Epiglottic swab culture (positive in 70%)
- CBC: Leukocytosis with left shift
- Hib antigen test in serum/urine useful in children with previous antibiotic treatment
- Hypoxia usually not present until airway obstructed

Imaging

Initial approach

- Lateral neck radiographs typically show an enlarged edematous epiglottis (the thumbprint sign) (1,3); however, radiographs are contraindicated because of danger of sudden complete airway obstruction with delay of important airway intervention.
- If radiographs are obtained, ensure adequate staff in case complete airway obstruction occurs.
- Chest x-rays after intubation to check position of endotracheal tube and to rule out pneumonia, which may occur as a complication

Diagnostic Procedures/Surgery

- Visualization of epiglottis with tongue depressor is contraindicated because of danger of sudden complete airway obstruction.
- Controlled visualization of epiglottis at intubation in OR is diagnostic (cherry red, edematous epiglottis).
- Lumbar puncture is indicated if there is clinical suspicion of meningitis.
- In an adult, indirect laryngoscopy is generally safe.

DIFFERENTIAL DIAGNOSIS

- Viral croup (laryngotracheobronchitis)
- Acute angioneurotic edema (no fever)
- Aspirated foreign body (history, no fever)
- Bacterial tracheitis (pseudomembranous croup)
- Retropharyngeal or peritonsillar abscess
- Diphtheria in an unimmunized patient (often an adult)
- Sepsis from other cause

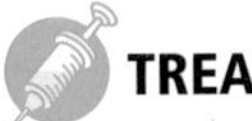

TREATMENT

There are 2 key aspects to the treatment of acute epiglottitis:

- Maintenance of an adequate airway should be the primary concern (1,2,3)[C].
- Administration of antimicrobial agents

MEDICATION

First Line

- Begin empiric antibiotic promptly after blood and epiglottic cultures are obtained. Use antibiotics guided by cultures thereafter. Duration of antimicrobial: 7–10 days (1,3)[C].
- Cefotaxime (Claforan) 100–200 mg/kg/d q8h IV (1,3)[C]
- Ceftriaxone (Rocephin) 50–100 mg/kg/d q12h IV (1,3)[C]

Second Line

- Other third- or fourth-generation cephalosporins IV or only ampicillin if Hib is sensitive (3)[C]
- Ampicillin-sulbactam (Unasyn) 150 mg/kg/d q6h, IV
- The role of steroids and racemic epinephrine remains controversial (1,3)[C].
- Antipyretics if necessary

ADDITIONAL TREATMENT

General Measures

- Each institution should have an emergency protocol involving a team of emergency room physicians, pediatricians, anesthesiologists, surgeons, pediatric intensivists, and pediatric intensive care unit (ICU) nurses (principles are similar for pediatric and adult patients).
- Call anesthesiologist to bedside.
- Have equipment for intubation and needle cricothyrotomy or percutaneous tracheostomy at bedside.
- Notify OR.
- Notify pediatric surgeon or ear/nose/throat (ENT) specialist for standby in OR in case tracheostomy becomes necessary.
- Keep patient quiet, calm, sitting up (in parent's arms).
- Avoid venipuncture, blood gases, oxygen masks, IV lines, injections, monitors, and radiographs.
- Judicious use of sedation that does not depress respirations may be appropriate.
- Racemic epinephrine is without benefit.
- Avoid examining the pharynx.
- Transport patient and parent together to OR in a wheelchair.
- Intubate all patients, preferably in OR under controlled circumstances by experienced anesthesiologist, with surgeon or ENT specialist on standby for emergency tracheostomy.
- Tracheostomy is not indicated unless intubation is unsuccessful (1,2,3)[C].
- Tape airway securely in place, and use a bite block if indicated.
- Splint elbows and restrain arms to avoid self-extubation.
- Use humidity and avoid T-piece (traction increases risk of accidental extubation).
- Continuous positive airway pressure, mechanical ventilation, and sedation are usually unnecessary.
- Pay attention to supervision and pulmonary suctioning to minimize risk of endotracheal tube plugs.

SURGERY/OTHER PROCEDURES

Emergency tracheotomy may be necessary (1,2,3)[C].

IN-PATIENT CONSIDERATIONS

Initial Stabilization

Acute epiglottitis is a medical emergency. During acute illness, hospitalize patient in ICU (1,2,3)[C].

Admission Criteria

Whenever the diagnosis of epiglottitis is suspected, immediate hospitalization is required.

IV Fluids

Initially, while intubated

Nursing

Expert respiratory nursing care is essential.

Discharge Criteria

Extubated patients afebrile in good clinical condition

ONGOING CARE

FOLLOW-UP RECOMMENDATIONS

Immunization

Patient Monitoring

- Rule out secondary foci of infection.
- Observe swallowing ability and presence of an air leak around endotracheal/nasotracheal tube.
- Follow-up with laryngoscopy prior to extubation (advocated by some).
- Observe in ICU for 24 hours following extubation.

DIET

IV fluid initially, then nasogastric feedings while intubated

PATIENT EDUCATION

Reassurance about treatment and outcome

PROGNOSIS

- Most patients can be extubated after 24–48 hours.
- Morbidity and mortality are low with appropriate intervention.

COMPLICATIONS

- Pneumonia, meningitis, septic arthritis, cervical adenitis, and cellulitis (rare)
- Progression of infection to deep neck tissue
- Epiglottic abscess
- Septic shock (~1%)
- Pneumothorax (rare)
- Death from asphyxia

REFERENCES

1. Mayo-Smith MF, Spinale JW, Donskey CJ, et al. Acute epiglottitis. An 18-year experience in Rhode Island. *Chest*. 1995;108:1640–7.
2. Guldfred LA, Lyhne D, Becker BC. Acute epiglottitis: Epidemiology, clinical presentation, management and outcome. *J Laryngol Otol*. 2008;122:818–23.
3. Glynn F, Fenton JE. Diagnosis and management of supraglottitis (epiglottitis). *Curr Infect Dis Rep*. 2008;10:200–4.

ADDITIONAL READING

- Cheung CS, Man SY, Graham CA, et al. Adult epiglottitis: 6 years experience in a university teaching hospital in Hong Kong. *Eur J Emerg Med*. 2009;16:221–6.
- Sobol SE, Zapata S, et al. Epiglottitis and croup. *Otolaryngol Clin North Am*. 2008;41:551–66, ix.
- Shah RK, Stocks C. Epiglottitis in the United States: National trends, variances, prognosis, and management. *Laryngoscope*. 2010;120:1256–62.
- Tibballs J, Watson T. Symptoms and signs differentiating croup and epiglottitis. *J Paediatr Child Health*. 2011;47:77-82.

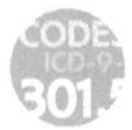

CODES

ICD9

- 464.30 Acute epiglottitis without mention of obstruction
- 464.31 Acute epiglottitis with obstruction
- 487.1 Influenza with other respiratory manifestations

CLINICAL PEARLS

- Acute epiglottitis is a medical emergency and requires immediate hospitalization. The airway must be secured before transport of all patients with suspected epiglottitis. Transport must be done by an experienced team.
- Evident respiratory distress, stridor, drooling, and shorter duration of symptoms are clinical features associated with a higher likelihood of airway obstruction in children with epiglottitis.
- Security of the airway is always of primary concern in acute epiglottitis; failure to intervene prior to loss of the airway associated with an increase in mortality. Avoid interventions that may upset the child, and proceed directly to operating room in parent's lap.
- Avoid use of tongue blade, which may worsen obstruction. Direct laryngoscopy should be done in OR.

EPISCLERITIS

Sindhu Kurian, MD
Peter J. Ziemkowski, MD

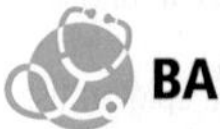

BASICS

- Episcleritis is inflammation of the vascular connective tissue located superficial to the sclera.
- It is usually a self-limited condition, typically lasting ~21 days (1).
- The majority of cases resolve without treatment.
- Recommended treatment is topical and is aimed at relieving symptoms.

DESCRIPTION

- Defined as edema and injection confined to the episcleral tissue
- 2 types: Simple or nodular

EPIDEMIOLOGY

Occurs equally in men and women

Incidence

- The condition is typically not seen in childhood.
- Men: Usually in their 30s and 60s, with peak incidence occurring in the 40s
- Women: Peak incidence in their 40s and 50s.
- Nodular episcleritis has a peak incidence in the fifth decade
- Simple episcleritis is more common in the fourth decade ($P \leq 0.05$) (2)

Prevalence

One study found all cases of rheumatoid-associated episcleritis in females, consistent with the higher incidence of rheumatoid arthritis in women (3).

PATHOPHYSIOLOGY

Pathogenesis can be either immune or nonimmune reactions:

- One example of a nonimmune mechanism is dry eye syndrome.
- Histologic examination of this syndrome reveals widespread vasodilation, edema, and lymphocytic infiltration (3).

COMMONLY ASSOCIATED CONDITIONS

- Rheumatoid arthritis
- Inflammatory bowel disease
- Gout
- Herpes zoster
- Hypersensitivity disorders:
  - Rosacea
  - Contact dermatitis
  - Penicillin sensitivity
  - Erythema multiforme

DIAGNOSIS

Episcleritis is a clinical diagnosis.

HISTORY

- A detailed history should be taken, including family history.
- Ask questions about any contact with chemical irritants/solvents, as well as if there is any history of rheumatic, connective tissue or skin disease, gout, venereal disease, tuberculosis or sarcoidosis (2).
- Discomfort occurs in 51% of patients and was equally common in simple and nodular types. The pain or discomfort was localized to the eye in 25% of patients with simple episcleritis and 33% of patients with nodular type (2).

PHYSICAL EXAM

- Check for visual acuity
- Simple episcleritis:
  - Diffuse edema of the episcleral tissue, sometimes infiltrated by greyish deposits appearing yellowish in red-free light.
  - The vessels retained their normal position and architecture.
  - Slit lamp examination shows how deep the edema is with the narrow beam.
  - Eyes were tender to touch in 33% of patients (2).
- Nodular episcleritis:
  - Edema and infiltration was localized to one part of the globe.
  - The nodules are usually single but can be multiple, reaching the size of a large pea.
  - Eyes were tender to touch in 40% of patients (2).
- It is important to exclude other complications such as glaucoma, uveitis, pars planitis, choroiditis, secondary retinal detachment, and optic neuritis.
- Complete physical exam (particularly the skin, joints, heart, and lung) should be done to assess for any associated conditions.

ALERT

Limitation of extraocular muscles and proptosis should lead to suspicion of involvement of posterior sclera.

DIAGNOSTIC TESTS & INTERPRETATION

- The majority of patients with episcleritis do not require any further lab work or diagnostic studies.
- Studies would be indicated in patients with persistent or recurrent episcleritis attacks.
- Evaluation can also be considered for patients whose history and physical exam suggest there is a systemic cause.

Lab

- CBC
- Rheumatoid arthritis latex agglutination test (typically used as the confirmatory test for rheumatoid factor)
- Serum uric acid
- ESR
- C-reactive protein (CRP)

DIFFERENTIAL DIAGNOSIS

- Scleritis which presents with intense pain, photophobia and a deep red or purplish scleral hue:
  - Slit-lamp examination is used to detect scleral edema and the involvement of the scleral vessels.
- Bacterial conjunctivitis
- Viral conjunctivitis
- Herpes keratitis

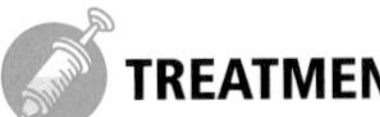

TREATMENT

MEDICATION

Treatment for episcleritis typically consists of symptomatic relief. The goal is to suppress the inflammation, which will in turn relieve the discomfort and prevent any destructive changes from occurring.

First Line

- Topical lubricants are typically used for initial management of episcleritis. Artificial tear preparations such as Refresh Plus or Bion Tears (3)[B].
- Topical NSAIDs (2)[C]
- Topical glucocorticoids such as prednisolone eye drops 0.5% hourly until 24 hours after inflammation has subsided. Then reduce to t.i.d. for 4 days (2)[B].
- Betamethasone (Betnesol) eye ointment 1% q.i.d. (2)[B]

ADDITIONAL TREATMENT

Only 16.7% of patients with episcleritis required more than topical corticosteroids for treatment and these patients required oral NSAIDs (4). Typically recommended is oral indomethacin and it is usually prescribed 25 mg PO t.i.d. (2)[C].

Issues for Referral

Rarely an episode of episcleritis at the initial presentation can progress to scleritis. At this time, an ophthalmology referral may be needed.

IN-PATIENT CONSIDERATIONS

Episcleritis rarely requires inpatient management.

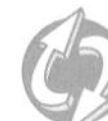

ONGOING CARE

FOLLOW-UP RECOMMENDATIONS

In one of the largest studies of episcleritis, it was found that episodes of episcleritis were usually self-limited and did not require any treatment.

PROGNOSIS

- Most of the patients have no ocular complications.
- Prognosis for episcleritis is excellent, with majority of patients making a full recovery.

COMPLICATIONS

Associated complications such as anterior uveitis, keratitis, glaucoma, or secondary cataract are uncommon and are never severe (4):

- Minimal corneal changes were seen in 15% of the patients with simple episcleritis and in 15% of patients with nodular disease, but none of these changes were severe.
- Keratitis was the most common complication in both simple and nodular disease (2).
- Low-grade anterior uveitis is seen with severe attacks of episcleritis: Onset of photophobia, pain, and decreased vision. This is best diagnosed by a slit lamp by an ophthalmologist (4).
- Anterior uveitis was present in 11% of patients with episcleritis and was mild. It is more commonly associated with scleritis (42%) than with episcleritis (11%) (5).

REFERENCES

1. Williams CP, Browning AC, Sleep TJ, et al. A randomised, double-blind trial of topical ketorolac vs artificial tears for the treatment of episcleritis. *Eye (Lond)*. 2005;19:739–42.
2. Watson PG, Hayreh SS, et al. Scleritis and episcleritis. *Br J Ophthalmol*. 1976;60:163–91.
3. McGavin DD, Williamson J, Forrester JV, et al. Episcleritis and scleritis. A study of their clinical manifestations and association with rheumatoid arthritis. *Br J Ophthalmol*. 1976;60:192–226.
4. Jabs DA, Mudun A, Dunn JP, et al. Episcleritis and scleritis: Clinical features and treatment results. *Am J Ophthalmol*. 2000;130:469–76.
5. Sainz de la Maza M, Jabbur NS, Foster CS, et al. Severity of scleritis and episcleritis. *Ophthalmology*. 1994;101:389–96.

CODES

ICD9

- 379.00 Scleritis, unspecified
- 379.02 Nodular episcleritis
- 379.09 Other scleritis and episcleritis

CLINICAL PEARLS

- Episcleritis typically is a benign disorder and the associated complications such as anterior uveitis, keratitis, secondary cataract and glaucoma are uncommon and never severe (5).
- It does not present with any decrease in visual acuity and rarely presents with pain.
- Treatment is aimed at symptomatic relief and attacks usually resolve quickly.
- Episcleritis can be an early presentation of scleritis, which is more severe. Accurate diagnosis of episcleritis is important.

EPISTAXIS

Julie Yeh, MD, MPH

BASICS

DESCRIPTION

- Hemorrhage from the nose involving either the anterior or posterior mucosal surfaces
- Synonym(s): Nosebleed

EPIDEMIOLOGY

Incidence

- In the US: Common
- Estimated lifetime incidence ~60%
- Bimodal, with peaks in children up to 15 and in adults >50
- Rare in children under age 2

RISK FACTORS

- Local irritation from multiple causes (see "Etiology")
- Medications/supplements, including aspirin and clopidogrel

GENERAL PREVENTION

- Humidification at night
- Cut fingernails to minimize picking.

PATHOPHYSIOLOGY

- Local vs. systemic disease. Large majority are due to local causes.
- Anterior: 90–95% of all cases (Kiesselbach plexus)
- Posterior: Usually branches of sphenopalatine arteries: May be asymptomatic or may present with other symptoms

ETIOLOGY

- Idiopathic
- Local inflammation/irritation:
  - Infection
  - Irritant inhalation
  - Topical steroid use
  - Septal deviation (more air movement on 1 side)
  - Low humidity
- Trauma:
  - Epistaxis digitorum (nose picking)
  - Foreign bodies
  - Septal perforation
  - Sinus fracture

COMMONLY ASSOCIATED CONDITIONS

- Vascular malformation/telangiectasia
- Neoplasm (rare, but consider in persistent unilateral cases)
- Systemic:
  - Coagulopathy, primary or iatrogenic
  - Thrombocytopenia
  - Cirrhosis
  - Renal failure
  - Alcoholism
- No proven association with hypertension (HTN), but may make control of bleeding more difficult.

DIAGNOSIS

HISTORY

- Initial presentation, including detail on where bleeding started (which side?)
- Trauma, including nose picking
- Previous episodes
- Comorbid conditions
- Current medications, including over-the-counter and supplements

PHYSICAL EXAM

- Blood loss through 1 or both nostrils in the majority of cases is due to anterior nasal septal bleeding and can often be directly visualized.
- Focus on localizing site of bleeding to anterior versus posterior nasal cavity.
- Patient seated, head forward, to avoid blood going down the posterior pharynx.

DIAGNOSTIC TESTS & INTERPRETATION

Indicated only in complicated cases

Lab

Lab testing is not indicated in the majority of uncomplicated cases in which bleeding is reasonably easily controlled and is not truly hemorrhagic.

Initial lab tests

- Mild cases, responsive to pressure: No labs
- For recurrent or intractable cases
- CBC, platelet count, prothrombin time (PT)
- PT/partial thromboplastin time (PTT) if on warfarin or other medications affecting coagulation
- Cross-match when appropriate
- Toxicology screen when nasal use of illicit drugs is suspected

Imaging

For most cases, imaging not indicated

Follow-Up & Special Considerations

If recurrent unilateral epistaxis, especially if not responding to treatment measures, consider evaluation for neoplasm.

Diagnostic Procedures/Surgery

Nasal endoscopy

DIFFERENTIAL DIAGNOSIS

- Diagnosis usually apparent; the differential for the etiology is key.
- Posterior bleeding must be included in the differential for any chronic blood loss.

Pediatric Considerations

More likely anterior, idiopathic, and recurrent

Geriatric Considerations

More likely to be posterior bleed

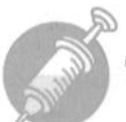

TREATMENT

- Most cases managed as outpatient
- Patient applies direct pressure by pinching the lower part of the nose for 5–20 minutes without a break. This will stop active bleeding in the majority of patients.
- An ice pack placed over the dorsum of the nose may help with hemostasis.
- Inspect the nasal septum for the bleeding site.

MEDICATION

First Line

If general measures fail, affected naris may be sprayed with topical vasoconstrictor such as phenylephrine or oxymetazoline.

Second Line

NosebleedQR: A nonprescription powder of hydrophilic polymer with potassium salt; induces formation of scab

ADDITIONAL TREATMENT

- Nasal packing: Either with ribbon gauze or preformed nasal tampons
- FloSeal: A biodegradable hemostatic sealant (a thrombin-type gel) in 1 study more effective and better tolerated than packing (1)[B]
- If an actively bleeding anterior septal site is visualized, this may be treated with gentle and specific silver nitrate cautery for ~10 seconds for definitive treatment.
- Limit cautery (silver nitrate) to 1 side of septum, or wait 4–6 weeks in between treatments to reduce risk of perforation.
- Posterior: Posterior packing or tamponade with balloon devices (Foley catheter has been used)
- Recurrent epistaxis: Cochrane Review of issue in children shows no difference in effectiveness between antiseptic nasal cream, petroleum jelly, silver nitrate cautery, or no treatment (2)[A]:
  - Silver nitrate cautery followed by 4 weeks of antiseptic cream may be better than antiseptic cream alone (3)[B].

General Measures

Resuscitation as indicated. Use universal "ABC" approach.

Issues for Referral

- Posterior bleeding, frequently requires an otolaryngology consultation
- Intractable bleeding. May require more specialized measures:
  - Endoscopic laser or electrocauterization
  - Angiography with arteriolar embolization

SURGERY/OTHER PROCEDURES

- Packing:
  - Layering of Vaseline ribbon gauze:
    - For gauze packing, be certain both ends of the ribbon gauze protrude from the nostril.
    - The packing is layered from the floor upward.
    - Secure packing with gauze across the outside of the nostril.
  - Nasal tampon may be used after lubricating the tip with KY Jelly or antibiotic cream or ointment.
  - Additional saline may be needed to expand the tampon if the bleeding has slowed.
  - Merocel and Rapid Rhino packs are easier to use than gauze packing and are usually well tolerated.
- Posterior bleed:
  - In the emergent setting, this may be attempted utilizing a Foley catheter or a specific posterior packing balloon.
  - With both methods, the tubing is introduced through the nose similar to the passage of a nasogastric tube. Once it reaches the posterior oral pharynx, the balloon is inflated and the tubing is pulled back outward to tamponade the posterior bleeding source:
    - If using a Foley catheter (10–14 French), the balloon can be inflated with 10 mL of saline.
    - Traction is maintained with an umbilical cord clamp with adequate padding between the clip and the nose to avoid injury.

IN-PATIENT CONSIDERATIONS

Consider hospitalization for elderly or for patients with posterior bleeding or coagulopathy. May also consider if significant comorbidities.

Initial Stabilization

Universal "Airway/Breathing/Circulation" (ABC) approach. Stop blood loss.

Admission Criteria

- Posterior bleed
- Hemodynamic changes
- Clotting dysfunction

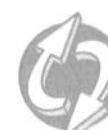

ONGOING CARE

FOLLOW-UP RECOMMENDATIONS

Patient Monitoring

- When significant blood loss, hemodynamic monitoring
- 24-hour minimum of packing in place; some authors recommend 3–5 days. The latter recommendation carries the risk of mucosal injury and toxic shock syndrome. The former has the risk of rebleed, which usually occurs between 24 and 48 hours.

PATIENT EDUCATION

- Demonstrate proper pinching pressure techniques.
- Avoidance of trauma or irritants is key.
- Management of systemic illness and proper use of medication

PROGNOSIS

- Most are self-limited.
- Good results with proper treatment

COMPLICATIONS

- Septal perforation
- Pressure-induced tissue necrosis of the nasal mucosa
- Toxic shock syndrome with packing
- Arrhythmias triggered by packing

REFERENCES

1. Mathiasen RA, Cruz RM. Prospective randomized, controlled clinical trial of a novel matrix hemostatic sealant in patients with acute anterior epistaxis. *Laryngoscope*. 2005;115:899–902.
2. Burton MJ, Dorée CJ. Interventions for recurrent idiopathic epistaxis (nosebleeds) in children. *Cochrane Database Syst Rev*. 2004:CD004461.
3. Calder N, Kang S, Fraser L, et al. A double-blind randomized controlled trial of management of recurrent nosebleeds in children. *Otolaryngol Head Neck Surg*. 2009;140:670–4.

ADDITIONAL READING

- Manes RP. Evaluating and managing the patient with nosebleeds. *Med Clin N Am*. 2010:903–912.
- Melia L, McGarry GW. Epistaxis: Update on management. *Curr Opin Otolaryngol Head Neck Surg*. 2011;19:30–35.
- Robertson S, Kubba H. Long-term effectiveness of antiseptic cream for recurrent epistaxis in childhood: Five-year follow up of a randomised, controlled trial. *J Laryngol Otol*. 2008:1–4.
- Schlosser RJ. Epistaxis. *N Engl J Med*. 2009:360: 784–9.

CODES

ICD9

784.7 Epistaxis

CLINICAL PEARLS

- Most episodes are anterior in etiology and respond to timed pressure over the anterior nares for 5–20 minutes.
- Most are idiopathic or as a result of nose picking.
- Posterior nosebleeds can be asymptomatic or present with nausea, hematemesis, or heme-positive stool.
- Consider evaluation for neoplasm if recurrent unilateral episodes.

EPSTEIN-BARR VIRUS INFECTIONS

Dennis E. Hughes, DO

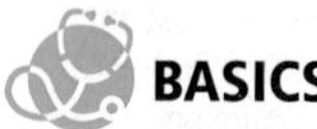

BASICS

DESCRIPTION

- Epstein-Barr virus (EBV) is a member of the herpes virus group.
- The primary infection occurs during childhood in vast majority of cases.
- System(s) affected: Hemic/Lymphatic/Immunologic
- May be a precursor to a spectrum of malignancies (potentially tumorigenic)

EPIDEMIOLOGY

Incidence

Worldwide, infects >90% of people (antibody-positive)

Prevalence

Primary Epstein-Barr viral infection:

- Military, college students, other cloistered, crowded populations have most active infection rate.
- Predominant age of primary infection is 10–19 years. (Manifests as infectious mononucleosis. Early childhood infections are usually asymptomatic.)
- Male = Female
- By ~20 years of age 60–90% of persons have a persistent (lifelong) anti-EBV antibody.

RISK FACTORS

- Age
- Sociohygienic level
- Geographic location
- Close, intimate contact

GENERAL PREVENTION

- Avoiding close physical contact with persons known to be currently symptomatic
- Good hand washing and hygiene
- EBV vaccine currently under development

PATHOPHYSIOLOGY

- A polyclonal B-cell proliferative response is characteristic of infectious mononucleosis. Relatively few circulating lymphocytes are infected by EBV and represent <0.1% of circulating mononuclear cells in the acute illness.
- After inoculation the virus replicates in the nasopharyngeal epithelium with resulting cell lysis and virion spread and viremia. The reticuloendothelia system is affected, resulting in a host response and the appearance of atypical lymphocytes in the peripheral blood.
- A persistent (asymptomatic) state ensues with the EBV genome maintained invisible to the immune system. Current thought is that a subsequent coinfection results in the development of a EBV-associated condition (malignancy as an example). Either by B-cell stimulation or diminished EBV-specific immune modulation, the previously latent EBV-infected B-cells replicate, allowing clinical manifestation of the EBV genome. The proteins produced may either modify host response to or contribute directly to the subsequent malignancy (1).

ETIOLOGY

- EBV, a member of the herpesvirus (DNA virus) group (human herpes virus 4)
- Humans are the only known reservoir.

COMMONLY ASSOCIATED CONDITIONS

- Infectious mononucleosis: The symptomatic primary EBV infection seen in otherwise healthy older children, adolescents, and young adults:
  - Clinical features vary in severity and duration: In children, generally mild; in adults, more severe and protracted
  - Incubation period is 30–50 days.
- X-linked lymphoproliferative syndrome (Duncan disease)
- Lymphoproliferative syndromes due to EBV infections in transplant patients
- Lymphomas (B-cell lymphoblastic, T-cell)
- Lymphocytic interstitial pneumonitis
- Hairy leukoplakia of the tongue, leiomyosarcoma, and CNS lymphomas in AIDS patients
- Burkitt lymphoma (most common childhood tumor in Africa and Papua New Guinea where malaria is endemic)
- Nasopharyngeal carcinoma (particularly in southeast China)
- Parotid carcinoma
- Hodgkin lymphoma (most common EBV-associated malignancy in US, EU)
- Postulated to be associated with multiple sclerosis (2–3 times incidence in EBV-positive individuals) (2)

DIAGNOSIS

HISTORY

- May begin abruptly or insidiously
- Syndrome of fatigue, malaise, and sore throat
- In adults, temperature may rise to 103°F (39.4°C) and gradually fall over a variable period of 7–10 days; in severe cases, temperature elevations of 104–105°F (40.0–40.6°C) may persist for 2 weeks.
- Children usually have a low-grade fever or may be afebrile.
- Diffuse hyperemia and hyperplasia of oropharyngeal lymphoid tissue
- Gelatinous, grayish white exudative tonsillitis persists for 7–10 days in 50%.
- Petechiae develop at border of hard and soft palates in 60%.
- Axillary, epitrochlear, popliteal, inguinal, mediastinal, and mesenteric nodes may also be affected (95% of patients) (3).
- Lymph node enlargement subsides over days or weeks.
- Chest pain (myocarditis and pericarditis)

PHYSICAL EXAM

- Fever, lymphadenopathy, pharyngitis in >50%, with palatal petechiae and hepatosplenomegaly ~10%
- Tender lymphadenopathy (cervical nodes are most commonly enlarged)
- Splenomegaly in 50%
- Skin manifestations (3–16%):
  - Erythematous macular or maculopapular rash
  - Petechial and purpuric exanthems have been reported.
  - Rash location: Trunk and upper arms; occasionally the face and forearms involved

DIAGNOSTIC TESTS & INTERPRETATION

Lab

Initial lab tests

- CBC with differential
- Lymphocytes and atypical lymphocytes:
  - Increased numbers of lymphocytes (especially atypical lymphocytes; may be up to 70% of leukocytes) in peripheral blood
  - In first week after onset, WBC count is normal or moderately decreased:
    - By the second week, lymphocytosis develops with >10% atypical lymphocytes.
  - During early illness, atypical lymphocytes are B-cells transformed by the EBV; later, atypical cells are primarily T-cells having an immunoregulatory function.
- Antibodies:
  - Heterophile antibodies in 80–90% of adults
  - Heterophile antibody is an IgM response, which appears during the first or second week of illness and persists for 3–6 months.
  - In general, agglutinin titer is higher in infectious mononucleosis than in other disorders; an unabsorbed heterophile titer >1:128 and 1:40 or higher after absorption is significant.
- Specific antibodies to EBV-associated antigens:
  - Develop regularly in infectious mononucleosis
  - Viral capsid-specific IgM and IgG are present early in illness.
  - Viral capsid-IgM responses disappear after several months, whereas viral capsid-IgG antibodies persist for life.
- Liver function studies; AST and ALT elevations and hyperbilirubinemia are common; frank jaundice is rare.
- Disorders that may alter lab results: Atypical lymphocytes are not specific for EBV infections and may be present in other clinical conditions, including rubella, infectious hepatitis, allergic rhinitis, asthma, and primary atypical pneumonia:
  - In infectious mononucleosis, increased numbers of atypical forms are present in peripheral blood; in other disorders, quantitative percentage is usually less.

Follow-Up & Special Considerations

Abnormal hepatic enzymes in 80% of patients for several weeks after onset; hepatomegaly in 15–20%

Imaging

Initial approach

- Abdominal ultrasound to monitor for splenic enlargement is not supported routinely (3).
- Consider for those wishing to return to strenuous activity or contact sports at day 21 of illness to evaluate for resolution of splenomegaly

Diagnostic Procedures/Surgery

Chest x-ray (CXR):

- Hilar adenopathy may be observed in infectious mononucleosis cases with extensive lymphoid hyperplasia.

Pathological Findings

- Mononuclear infiltrations involve lymph nodes, tonsils, spleen, lungs, liver, heart, kidneys, adrenal glands, skin, and CNS.
- Bone marrow hyperplasia develops regularly, and small granulomas may be present; these are nonspecific and have no prognostic significance.

DIFFERENTIAL DIAGNOSIS

- Streptococcal pharyngitis and tonsillitis
- Diphtheria
- Blood dyscrasias
- Rubella
- Measles
- Viral hepatitis
- Cytomegalovirus
- Toxoplasmosis

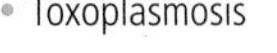

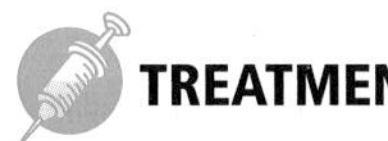

TREATMENT

MEDICATION

In primary infections:

- Antimicrobial agents (usually a penicillin) only if throat culture is positive for group A, beta-hemolytic streptococci
- Warm saline gargles for the pain of pharyngeal involvement and enlarged lymph nodes
- Corticosteroids:
  - Support unclear; may provide some symptomatic relief, but no improvement in resolution of illness
  - Consider in severe pharyngotonsillitis with oropharyngeal edema and airway encroachment. Dexamethasone (0.3 mg/kg/d) may be used for 1–3 days (3)[B].
  - Also for patients with marked toxicity or major complications (e.g., hemolytic anemia, thrombocytopenic purpura, neurologic sequelae, myocarditis, pericarditis)

ADDITIONAL TREATMENT

General Measures

- The treatment is chiefly supportive.
- NSAIDs
- During acute stage, limit activity for 4 weeks to reduce potential complications (splenic rupture, etc.) and aid in recovery.

Issues for Referral

- Development of clinical manifestations of expression of latent disease
- Not associated with a primary infection but in later years particularly in at-risk populations

SURGERY/OTHER PROCEDURES

With profound thrombocytopenia, refractory to corticosteroid therapy, splenectomy may be necessary.

IN-PATIENT CONSIDERATIONS

Admission Criteria

- Inability to eat food or drink fluids
- Splenic rupture

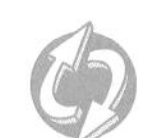

ONGOING CARE

FOLLOW-UP RECOMMENDATIONS

ALERT

Rupture of the spleen may be fatal if not recognized, and requires blood transfusions, treatment for shock, and splenectomy. Occurrence is estimated at 0.1% (3).

Patient Monitoring

- Avoid contact sports, heavy lifting, and excess exertion until spleen and liver have returned to normal size.
- Eliminate alcohol or exposure to other hepatotoxic drugs until liver function tests return to normal.
- Monitor patients closely during the first 2–3 weeks after the onset of symptoms. Thereafter, follow patients until their symptoms subside.
- Rarely, laboratory results resolve more slowly, and symptoms (malaise, fatigue, intermittent sore throat, lymphadenopathy) may persist for several months.

DIET

No restrictions. Hydration during acute phase is very important.

PATIENT EDUCATION

Mononucleosis on Familydoctor.org

PROGNOSIS

- Vast majority will be recovered by 4 weeks.
- Fatigue symptoms may persist for months (3).

COMPLICATIONS

- Neurologic (rare):
  - Aseptic meningitis
  - Bell palsy
  - Meningoencephalitis
  - Guillain-Barré syndrome
  - Transverse myelitis
  - Cerebellar ataxia
  - Acute psychosis
- Hematologic (rare):
  - Thrombocytopenia, slight to moderate, early in illness
  - Hemolytic anemia with marked neutropenia during early weeks
  - Aplastic anemia
  - Agammaglobulinemia
- Pneumonitis
- Splenic rupture:
  - Rare, but most often occurs in first 21 days of illness

REFERENCES

1. Klein G, Klein E, Kashuba E. Interaction of Epstein-Barr virus (EBV) with human B-lymphocytes. *Biochem Biophys Res Comm*. 2010;396(1):67–73.
2. Pohl D. Epstein-Barr virus and multiple sclerosis. *J Neurol Sci*. 2009.
3. Ebell MH. Epstein-Barr virus infectious mononucleosis. *Am Fam Physician*. 2006;70(7):1279–88.

ADDITIONAL READING

- Ascherio A, Munger KL. Epstein-Barr virus and multiple sclerosis: A review. *J. Neuroimmune Pharmacol*. 2010;5(3):271–7.
- Klutts JS, Ford BA, Perez NR, et al. Evidence-based approach for interpretation of Epstein-Barr virus serological patterns. *J Clin Microbiol*. 2009;47:3204–10.
- Munz C, Moorman A. Immune escape by Epstein-Barr virus associated maligancies. *Semin Cancer Biol*. 2008;18(6):381–7.

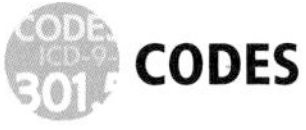

CODES

ICD9

075 Infectious mononucleosis

CLINICAL PEARLS

- False-negative monospot (heterophile antibody) in the first 10–14 days of illness
- 98% have fever, sore throat, cervical node enlargement, and tonsillar hypertrophy.
- Although splenic rupture is extremely rare, athletic activity should be curtailed for 3–4 weeks.
- Lab shows a lymphocytosis, not a monocytosis.

ERECTILE DYSFUNCTION

Chintan K. Patel, MD
Mark Sigman, MD

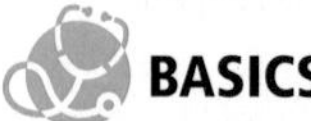

BASICS

DESCRIPTION

- Erectile dysfunction is defined as the consistent or recurrent inability to acquire or sustain an erection of sufficient rigidity and duration for sexual intercourse.
- In the past, erectile dysfunction was assumed to be a symptom of the aging process in men, but it can result from concurrent medical conditions of the patient or from medications that patients may be taking to treat those conditions.
- Sexual problems are frequent among older men and have a detrimental effect on their quality of life, but are infrequently discussed with their physicians (1).
- Synonym(s): Impotence

ALERT

When ED occurs in a younger man, it is associated with a significantly increased risk of future cardiac events, and thus should be a warning sign for all primary care providers (2).

EPIDEMIOLOGY

Incidence

It is estimated that over 600,000 new cases of erectile dysfunction will be diagnosed annually in the US, although this may be an underestimation of the true incidence, as erectile dysfunction is vastly underreported.

Prevalence

Overall prevalence for erectile dysfunction:

- 52% in men age 40–70 years
- Age-related increase ranging from 12.4% in men age 40–49 years up to 46.6% in men age 50–69 years

RISK FACTORS

- Advancing age
- Cardiovascular disease
- Diabetes mellitus
- Metabolic syndrome
- Cigarette smoking
- Urologic surgery, radiation, trauma/injury to pelvic area or spinal cord
- Medications that induce erectile dysfunction
- Central neurologic and endocrinologic conditions
- Substance abuse
- Psychological conditions: Stress, anxiety, or depression

Genetics

Rarely related to chromosomal disorders

GENERAL PREVENTION

The 2 best ways to prevent erectile dysfunction is by:

- Making healthy lifestyle choices by exercising regularly, eating well-balanced meals, and limiting alcohol and avoiding smoking
- Treating existing health problems and working with your patients to manage diabetes, heart disease, and other chronic problems

PATHOPHYSIOLOGY

- Erectile dysfunction is a neurovascular event:
  - With stimulation, there is release of nitrous oxide, which increases production of cGMP.
  - This leads to relaxation of cavernous smooth muscle, leading to increased blood flow to penis.
  - As cavernosal sinusoids distend with blood, there is passive compression of subtunical veins, which decreases venous outflow and this leads to an erection.
- Alterations in any of these events leads to erectile dysfunction.

ETIOLOGY

- Erectile dysfunction may result from problems with systems required for normal penile erection:
  - Vascular: Diseases that compromise blood flow:
    - Peripheral vascular disease, arteriosclerosis, essential hypertension
  - Neurologic: Diseases that impair nerve conduction to brain or penile vasculature:
    - Spinal cord injury, stroke, diabetes
  - Endocrine: Diseases associated with changes in testosterone, luteinizing hormone, prolactin levels
  - Psychological: Patients suffering from malaise, depression, performance anxiety
- Social habits such as smoking or excessive alcohol intake
- Medications may cause erectile dysfunction.
- Structural injury or trauma (bicycling accident)

Geriatric Considerations

Aging alone is not a cause.

COMMONLY ASSOCIATED CONDITIONS

- Cardiovascular disease:
  - Men with erectile dysfunction have a greater likelihood of having angina, myocardial infarction, stroke, transient ischemic attack, congestive heart failure, or cardiac arrhythmia compared to men without erectile dysfunction (3).
- Diabetes
- Psychiatric disorders

DIAGNOSIS

Inability to achieve or maintain erection satisfactory for intercourse

HISTORY

- Identify concurrent medical illnesses or surgical procedures, history of trauma, and a list of current medications
- Psychosocial history: Smoking, ethanol intake, recreational drug use, anxiety and depression, satisfaction with current relationship
- Detailed sexual history important to rule out premature ejaculation, as this is frequently confused with erectile dysfunction

PHYSICAL EXAM

- Signs and symptoms of hypogonadism: Gynecomastia, small testicles, decreased body hair
- Penile plaques (Peyronie disease)
- Detailed examination of the cardiovascular, neurologic, and genitourinary systems:
  - Check femoral and lower extremity pulses to assess vascular supply to genitals.
  - Check anal sphincter tone and genital reflexes, including cremasterics and bulbocavernosus.

DIAGNOSTIC TESTS & INTERPRETATION

Vascular and/or neurologic assessment, and monitoring of nocturnal erections may be indicated in select patients but not for routine workup (4)[C].

Lab

Initial lab tests

Diagnostic testing for erectile dysfunction should usually be limited to obtaining a fasting serum glucose level and lipid panel (most likely will be part of annual exams), thyroid-stimulating hormone level, and morning total testosterone level (3)[C].

Follow-Up & Special Considerations

Other hormonal tests, such as prolactin, should only be ordered when there is suspicion for a specific endocrinopathy.

Imaging

Initial approach

Doppler, angiogram, and cavernosogram are available radiologic modalities, but not recommended in routine practice for the diagnosis of erectile dysfunction (4)[C].

Follow-Up & Special Considerations

These tests may helpful when detailed information regarding vascular supply is needed.

Diagnostic Procedures/Surgery

Questionnaires can be offered to assess the severity of erectile dysfunction, including the International Index of Erectile Function (IEFF) and its validated and more easily administered abridged version, the Sexual Health Inventory for Men (SHIM) (4)[C].

DIFFERENTIAL DIAGNOSIS

- Premature ejaculation
- Decreased libido
- Anorgasmia

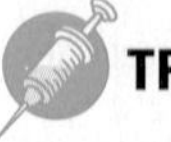

TREATMENT

Lifestyle modifications and managing medications contributing to erectile dysfunction is first-line therapy for ED (5)[C]. Use least invasive therapy first; reserve more invasive therapies for nonresponders.

MEDICATION

First Line

Phosphodiesterase type 5 (PDE-5) inhibitors are effective in the treatment of erectile dysfunction in many men, including those with diabetes mellitus and spinal cord injury, and sexual dysfunction associated with antidepressants (3)[A]. There is insufficient evidence to support the superiority of 1 agent over the others (5)[A]:

- Sildenafil (Viagra): Usual daily dose: 25–100 mg within at least 60 minutes of sexual intercourse on an empty stomach, at least 2 hours before meals. Duration up to 4 hours.
- Vardenafil (Levitra): Usual daily dose 5–20 mg within at least 60 minutes of sexual intercourse on an empty stomach, at least 2 hours before meals. Duration up to 4 hours.
- Tadalafil (Cialis): Usual daily dose 5–20 mg, at least 2 hours before intercourse. May take without regard to meals. Duration up to 36 hours:
  - Adverse effects of PDE-5 inhibitors: Headache, facial flushing, dyspepsia, nasal congestion, dizziness, hypotension, increased sensitivity to light (sildenafil and vardenafil), vision changes, lower back pain (tadalafil), and priapism (with excessive doses)

Geriatric Considerations

Use doses at the lower end of the dosing range for elderly patients:

- Sildenafil 25 mg daily
- Vardenafil 5 mg daily

Second Line

- Intraurethral and intracavernosal injectables are second-line therapies shown to be effective and should be administered based on patient preference (3)[B]. Intraurethral suppositories are a less invasive treatment option than intracavernosal injections; however, they are not as effective (5)[C]. Alprostadil, also known as prostaglandin E_1, causes smooth muscle relaxation of the arterial blood vessels and sinusoidal tissues in the corpora:
  - Intraurethral alprostadil (Muse):
    - Urethral suppository: 125-, 250-, 500-, and 1,000-mcg pellets. Administer 5–50 minutes before intercourse. No more than 2 doses in 24 hours are recommended.
  - Intracavernosal alprostadil (available in 2 formulations):
    - Alprostadil (Caverject): Usual dose: 10–20 mcg, with max dose of 60 mcg. Injection should be made at right angles into one of the lateral surfaces of the proximal third of the penis using a 0.5-inch 27- or 30-gauge needle. Do not use >3 times a week or > once in 24 hours.
    - Alprostadil may also be combined with papaverine (Bimix) plus phentolamine (Tri-Mix).

ALERT

- Initial trial dose should be administered under supervision of a specialist or primary care physician with expertise in these therapies.
- Patient should notify physician if erection lasts >4 hours for immediate attention.

- Vacuum pump devices are a noninvasive second-line option and are available over-the-counter. Do not use vacuum devices in men with sickle cell anemia or blood dyscrasias.
- Testosterone supplementation in men with hypogonadism improves erectile dysfunction and libido (3)[B]. Available formulations include injectable depots, transdermal patches and gels, SC pellets, and oral therapy.
- Contraindications:
  - Nitroglycerin (or other nitrates) and phosphodiesterase inhibitors: Potential for severe, potentially fatal hypotension
  - Precautions/side effects:
    - Testosterone: *Precautions*: Exogenous testosterone reduces sperm count and thus do not use in patients wishing to keep fertility; *side effects*: Acne, sodium retention
    - Intraurethral suppository: Local penile pain, urethral bleeding, dizziness, and dysuria
    - Intracavernosal injection: Penile pain, edema and hematoma, palpable nodules or plaques, and priapism
    - Sildenafil: Hypotension (caution for patients on nitrates)
    - PDE-5 inhibitors: Use caution with congenital prolonged QT syndrome, class Ia or II antiarrhythmics, nitroglycerin, α-blockers (e.g., terazosin, tamsulosin), retinal disease, unstable cardiac disease, liver and renal failure
    - Significant possible interactions:
      - PDE-5 inhibitor concentration is affected by CYP3A4 inhibitors (e.g., erythromycin, indinavir, ketoconazole, ritonavir, amiodarone, cimetidine, clarithromycin, delavirdine, diltiazem, fluoxetine, fluvoxamine, grapefruit juice, itraconazole, nefazodone, nevirapine, ritonavir, saquinavir, and verapamil). Serum concentrations and/or toxicity may be increased. Lower starting doses should be used in these patients.
      - PDE-5 inhibitor concentration may be reduced by rifampin and phenytoin.

ADDITIONAL TREATMENT

General Measures

- Psychotherapy alone or in combination with psychoactive drugs may be helpful in men whose erectile dysfunction is caused by depression or anxiety.
- Weight loss and increased physical activity for obese men with erectile dysfunction

Issues for Referral

Use of urologists, psychiatrists, psychologists, sex therapists, endocrinologists, or neurologists is often necessary for refractory cases.

Additional Therapies

Behavioral therapy: Couples therapy aimed at improving relationship difficulties found that men who received this therapy plus sildenafil had more successful intercourse than those who received only sildenafil (6)[A].

COMPLEMENTARY AND ALTERNATIVE MEDICINE

Yohimbine and herbal therapies are not recommended for the treatment of erectile dysfunction, as they have not proven to be efficacious (5)[C].

SURGERY/OTHER PROCEDURES

Penile prosthesis should be reserved for patients who have failed or are ineligible first- or second-line therapies (3)[B].

ONGOING CARE

FOLLOW-UP RECOMMENDATIONS

Patient Monitoring

Treatment should be assessed at baseline and after the patient has completed at least 1–3 weeks of a specific treatment: Monitor the quality and quantity of penile erections, and monitor the level of satisfaction patient achieves.

DIET

Diet and exercise recommended to achieve a normal body mass index; limit alcohol

PROGNOSIS

- All commercially available PDE-5 inhibitors are equally effective. In the presence of sexual stimulation, they are 55–80% effective (5)[A]:
  - Lower success rates with diabetes mellitus and radical prostatectomy patients who suffer from erectile dysfunction
- Overall effectiveness is 70–90% for intracavernosal alprostadil and 43–60% for intraurethral alprostadil (4)[B].
- Penile prostheses are associated with an 85–90% patient satisfaction rate (4)[C].

REFERENCES

1. Lindau ST, Schumm LP, Laumann EO, et al. A study of sexuality and health among older adults in the United States. *N Engl J Med*. 2007;357(8):762–74.
2. Inman BA, Sauver JL, Jacobson DJ, et al. A population-based, longitudinal study of erectile dysfunction and future coronary artery disease. *Mayo Clin Proc*. 2009;84(2):108–13.
3. Heidelbaugh JJ, et al. Management of erectile dysfunction. *Am Fam Physician*. 2010;81:305–12.
4. McVary KT. Clinical practice. Erectile dysfunction. *N Engl J Med*. 2007;357:2472–81.
5. The American Urological Association (AUA). Guideline on the management of erectile dysfunction: Diagnosis and treatment recommendations. Reviewed and Validitiy Confirmed in 2009.
6. Melnik T, Soares BGO, Nasselo AG. Psychosocial interventions for erectile dysfunction. *Cochrane Database Syst Rev*. 2007;(3):CD004825.

CODES

ICD9

- 302.72 Psychosexual dysfunction with inhibited sexual excitement
- 607.84 Impotence of organic origin

CLINICAL PEARLS

- Nitrates should be withheld for 24 hours after sildenafil or vardenafil administration and for 48 hours after use of tadalafil.
- Reserve surgical treatment for patients who do not respond to drug treatment.
- The use of PDE-5 inhibitors with alpha-adrenergic antagonists may increase the risk of hypotension. Tamsulosin is the least likely to cause orthostatic hypotension.
- Erectile dysfunction serves as a predictor for future cardiovascular events; thus, these patients should be followed vigilantly.

ERYSIPELAS

Khasha Touloei, DO
Mayha K. Patel, OMSIV
Alissa Craft, DO, MBA

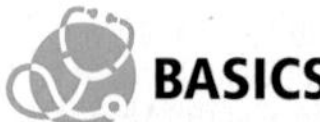

BASICS

DESCRIPTION
- Distinct form of cellulitis notable for acute, well-demarcated, superficial bacterial skin infection with lymphatic involvement almost always caused by *Streptococcus pyogenes*
- Usually acute, but a chronic recurrent form also exists (1)
- System(s) affected: Skin/Exocrine
- Synonym(s): Saint Anthony's fire

EPIDEMIOLOGY
- Predominant age: Infants, children, and adults >40 years
  – Greatest in elderly (>75 years)
- There is no gender or racial predilection

Incidence
- Erysipelas occurs in about 1/1,000 persons per year (2).
- Incidence on the rise since the 1980s (3)

Prevalence
Unknown

RISK FACTORS
- Disruption in the skin barrier (surgical incisions, insect bites, eczematous lesions, local trauma, abrasions, dermatophytic infections)
- Fissured skin (especially at the nose and ears)
- Toe-web intertrigo and lymphedema (2)
- Leg ulcers/stasis dermatitis
- Venous or lymphatic insufficiency (saphenectomy, varicose veins of leg, phlebitis, radiotherapy, mastectomy, lymphadenectomy)
- Chronic diseases (diabetes, malnutrition, nephrotic syndrome, heart failure)
- Morbid obesity
- Immunocompromised (HIV) or debilitated
- Alcohol abuse
- Recent streptococcal pharyngitis

GENERAL PREVENTION
- Good skin hygiene
- It is recommended that predisposing medical conditions such as tinea pedis and stasis dermatitis be appropriately managed first.
- Shaving within 5 days of facial erysipelas increases recurrence.
- Compression stockings should be encouraged for patients with lower extremity edema.
- Consider suppressive prophylactic antibiotic therapy such as penicillin in patients with >2 episodes in a 12-month period.

PATHOPHYSIOLOGY
- Group A streptococci induce inflammation and activation of the contact system: A proinflammatory pathway with antithrombotic activity; releasing proteinases and proinflammatory cytokines
- The generation of antibacterial peptides and the release of bradykinin, a proinflammatory peptide, increase vascular permeability and induce fever and pain.
- The M proteins from the group A streptococcal cell wall interact with neutrophils, leading to the secretion of heparin-binding protein, an inflammatory mediator that also induces vascular leakage.
- This cascade of reactions leads to the symptoms seen in erysipelas: Fever, pain, erythema, and edema.

ETIOLOGY
- Group A β-hemolytic streptococci primarily; occasionally other streptococcus groups C or G
- Rarely, group B streptococci or *Staphylococcus aureus* may be involved.

Pediatric Considerations
Group B streptococcus may be a cause of erysipelas in neonates/infants.

DIAGNOSIS

Prodromal symptoms before the skin eruption of erysipelas may include:
- Moderate- to high-grade fever
- Chills
- Headache
- Malaise
- Anorexia, usually in the first 48 hours
- Vomiting
- Arthralgias

ALERT
It is important to differentiate erysipelas from a MRSA infection, which usually presents with an indurated center, significant pain, and later evidence of abscess formation.

PHYSICAL EXAM
- Vital signs: Moderate- to high-grade fever with resultant tachycardia. Hypotension may occur.
- The presence of a fever in erysipelas can be considered a differentiating factor from other skin infections.
- Headache and vomiting may be prominent.
- Acute onset of erythematous plaque that is sharply demarcated, raised, fiery-red, tender, and spreads circumferentially over hours/days with marked swelling
- Peau d'orange appearance
- Vesicles and bullae may form, but are not uniformly present.
- Desquamation may occur later.
- Location:
  – Lower extremity 70–80% of cases
  – Face involvement is less common (5–20%), especially nose and ears
  – Chronic form usually recurs at site of the previous infection, and may recur years after initial episode.
- Patients on systemic steroids may be more difficult to diagnose because signs and symptoms of the infection may be masked by anti-inflammatory action of the steroids.
- Systemic toxicity resolves rapidly with treatment; skin lesions desquamate on days 5–10, but usually heal without scarring.
- In geriatric patients, facial involvement presents in a butterfly pattern. Pustules characteristically absent and regional lymphadenopathy with lymphangitic streaking is seen.

Pediatric Considerations
- Abdominal involvement more common in infants, especially around umbilical stump
- Face, scalp, and leg common in older children due to the excoriations of anterior rhinitis sicca allowing an easy port of entry

Geriatric Considerations
- Fever may not be as prominent.
- Face and lower extremity are the most common areas.
- High-output cardiac failure may occur in debilitated patients with underlying cardiac disease.
- More prone to complications

DIAGNOSTIC TESTS & INTERPRETATION
Lab
Reserve diagnostic tests for severely ill, toxic patients, or those who are immunosuppressed.

Initial lab tests
- Leukocytosis
- Blood culture (<5% positive)
- Elevated ESR and C-reactive protein (CRP)
- Streptococci may be cultured from exudate or noninvolved sites.

Pathological Findings
Biopsy is not needed. However, skin findings would show:
- Dermal and epidermal edema, extending into the SC tissues
- Peau d'orange appearance caused by edema in the superficial tissue surrounding the hair follicles
- Vasodilation and enlarged lymphatics
- Mixed interstitial infiltrate mainly consisting of neutrophils and mononuclear cells
- Endothelial cell swelling
- Gram-positive cocci in lymphatics and tissue with rare invasion of local blood vessels
- Fibrotic thickening of lymphatic vessel walls with possible luminal occlusion may be seen in recurrent erysipelas.

DIFFERENTIAL DIAGNOSIS
- Cellulitis (margins are less clear)
- Necrotizing fasciitis (systemic illness and more pain)
- Dermatophytes
- Impetigo (blistered or crusted appearance; superficial)
- Ecthyma (ulcerative impetigo)
- Herpes zoster (dermatomal distribution)
- Erythema annulare centrifugum (raised pink-red ring or bulls-eye marks)

- Contact dermatitis (no fever, pruritic)
- Giant cell urticaria (transient, wheal-appearance, severe itching)
- Angioneurotic edema (no fever)
- Scarlet fever (widespread rash with indistinct borders and without edema; rash is most common early in skin folds; develops generalized "sandpaper" feeling as it progresses)
- Toxic shock syndrome (diffuse erythema with evidence of multiorgan involvement)

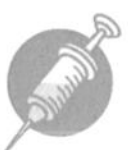

TREATMENT

MEDICATION

First Line

- Adults:
  - Extremities, nondiabetic:
    - Primary:
      - Penicillin G 1–2 million U IV q6h or (nafcillin or oxacillin 2 g IV q4h)
      - If not severe, dicloxacillin 500 mg PO q6h or cefazolin 1 g IV q8h
    - Alternative:
      - Erythromycin, Cefazolin, Azithromycin, Clarithromycin, Tigecycline (4)
      - Dapto 4 mg/kg/d IV (4)
      - Ceftobriprote (CFB) 500 mg IV q12h
  - Diabetics:
    - Early-mild:
      - TMP-SMX-DS 1–2 tabs PO b.i.d. and Penicillin VK 500 mg PO q.i.d. or cephalexin 500 mg PO q.i.d.
  - Severe disease:
    - IMP or MER or ERTA IV and linezolid 600 mg IV/PO b.i.d. or vancomycin IV or dapto 4 mg/kg IV q4h (4)
  - Facial:
    - Primary:
      - Vancomycin 1 g IV q12h
      - If the patient is over 100 kg, give 1.5 g IV q12h (4).
    - Alternative:
      - Dapto 4 mg/kg IV q24h or linezolid 600 mg IV q12h (4)
- Children:
  - Mild:
    - Penicillin VK:
      - <12 years: 25–50 mg/kg/d PO divided q6–8h max: 3 g/d
      - >12 years: Adult dose
    - Penicillin G procaine:
      - <30 kg: 300,000 U/d IM
      - >30 kg: Adult dose
  - Severe:
    - Nafcillin or oxacillin 2 g IV q4h or penicillin G parenterally is recommended for severe or complicated cases (1 million–2 million U q4–6h).
    - Ceftriaxone 50 mg/kg q12h or Cefazolin 100 mg/lg q8h
- In chronic recurrent infections, prophylactic treatment after the acute infection resolves:
  - Penicillin G benzathine 1.2 million U IM every month, or Penicillin VK 250 mg PO b.i.d.
- If staphylococcal infection is suspected or patient is acutely ill, a beta-lactamase-stable antibiotic should be considered.
- Consider community-acquired methicillin-resistant *Staphylococcus aureus* (MRSA) and, depending on regional sensitivity, may treat MRSA with trimethoprim-sulfamethoxazole, clindamycin, or tetracycline. If resistance is a concern or patient is clinically unstable, treat with vancomycin, daptomycin, or linezolid.

ADDITIONAL TREATMENT

Some patients may notice a deepening of erythema after initiating antimicrobial therapy. This may be due to the destruction of pathogens that release enzymes, increasing local inflammation. In this case, treatment with corticosteroids in addition to antimicrobials can mildly reduce healing time and antibiotic duration in patients with erysipelas. Consider prednisolone 30 mg/d with taper over 8 days (5)[B].

General Measures

- Symptomatic treatment of myalgias and fever
- Adequate fluid intake
- Local treatment with cold compresses
- Elevation of affected extremity
- Appropriate therapy for any underlying predisposing condition

Issues for Referral

Recurrent infection, treatment failure

IN-PATIENT CONSIDERATIONS

Initial Stabilization

Outpatient care

Admission Criteria

- Patient with systemic toxicity
- Patient with high-risk factors (e.g., elderly, lymphedema, postsplenectomy, diabetes)

IV Fluids

IV therapy if systemic toxicity or unable to tolerate PO

Discharge Criteria

No evidence of systemic toxicity with improvement of erythema and swelling

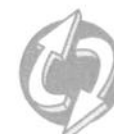

ONGOING CARE

FOLLOW-UP RECOMMENDATIONS

Bed rest with elevation of extremity during acute infection, then activity as tolerated

Patient Monitoring

Patients should be treated until all symptoms and skin manifestations have resolved.

PATIENT EDUCATION

Stress importance of completing prescribed medication regimen.

PROGNOSIS

- Patients should recover fully if adequately treated.
- Mortality <1% in patients receiving appropriate treatment.
- Bullae formation suggests longer disease course, and often indicates a concomitant *Staphylococcus aureus* infection that may require antibiotic coverage for MRSA.
- Chronic edema/scarring may result from chronic recurrent cases.
- Rarely, obstructive lymphadenitis may result from chronic recurrent cases.

COMPLICATIONS

- Recurrent infection
- Abscess (suggests staphylococcal infection)
- Necrotizing fasciitis
- Lymphedema
- Bacteremia (which may lead to sepsis or involvement of other organ systems)
- Sepsis
- Pneumonia (due to sepsis or toxin-producing organism)
- Meningitis (due to sepsis or toxin-producing organism)
- Embolism
- Gangrene
- Bursitis, septic arthritis, tendinitis, or osteitis

REFERENCES

1. Gabillot-Carré M, Roujeau JC. Acute bacterial skin infections and cellulitis. *Curr Opin Infect Dis*. 2007;20:118–23.
2. Bernard P. Management of common bacterial infections of the skin. *Curr Opin Infect Dis*. 2008; 21:122–8.
3. Celestin R, Brown J, Kihiczak G, et al. Erysipelas: A common potentially dangerous infection. *Acta Dermatovenerol Alp Panonica Adriat*. 2007;16: 123–7.
4. Gilbert D, Moellering R, Eliopoulos G, et al. The Sanford Guide to Antimicrobial Therapy 2010. Sperryville, VA: Sanford Guide; 2010.
5. Bergkvist PI, Sjöbeck K, et al. Antibiotic and prednisolone therapy of erysipelas: A randomized, double blind, placebo-controlled study. *Scand J Infect Dis*. 1997;29:377–82.

ADDITIONAL READING

- Breen JO. Skin and soft tissue infections in immunocompetent patients. *Am Fam Physician*. 2010;81:893–9.
- Stevens DL, et al. Practice guidelines for the diagnosis and management of skin and soft tissue infections. *Clin Infect Dis*. 2005;41:1973.

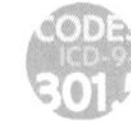

CODES

ICD9

035 Erysipelas

CLINICAL PEARLS

- Athlete's foot is the most common portal of entry for this superficial bacterial skin infection caused by *Streptococcus pyogenes*.
- Erysipelas is distinguished from cellulitis by its sharp, shiny, fiery-red, raised border.
- In recurrent cases, search for other possible source of streptococcal infection (e.g., tonsils, sinuses, intertrigo).
- Most erysipelas infections now occur on the legs, rather than the face.

ERYTHEMA MULTIFORME

Alina Markova, MD
Leslie Robinson-Bostom, MD

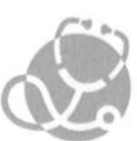

BASICS

- Erythema multiforme (EM) is an acute, self-limited hypersensitivity reaction:
  - Mostly triggered by infectious agents (more than 50% by herpes simplex virus [HSV]-1 or -2) or drugs (1,2)[B]
  - Involving the skin and the mucous membrane, most commonly the mouth (60–70% of all EM patients have oral lesions) (3)
  - Skin lesions include typical target or "iris" lesions, flat or raised atypical lesions, and macules with or without blisters.
- Currently, there are no universal diagnostic criteria for EM. It was previously considered to be a spectrum of disease, consisting of EM, EM major, Stevens-Johnson syndrome (SJS), and toxic epidermal necrolysis (TEN); however, it appears to be a growing consensus that EM is a distinct condition from SJS and TEN due to the differences in clinical presentation, histopathologic features, patient demographics, possible etiology and pathogenesis, and treatment plan (1,2,4,5)[C].

DESCRIPTION

- 2 subtypes, erythema multiforme minor (EMm) and erythema multiforme major (EMM), with the former involving none or 1 mucous membrane, and the latter involving at least 2 mucous sites (1)[C]
- Recurrent EM has a mean number of 6 attacks (range 2–24) per year and a mean duration of 9.5 years (range 2–36) (1)[B].
- System(s) affected: Skin/Exocrine
- Synonym(s): Erythema polymorphe

EPIDEMIOLOGY

Incidence

The annual incidence in the US has been estimated at between 0.01% and 1% (5)[C].

Prevalence

- Predominant age: Peak incidence in 20s and 40s; rare <age 3 and >age 50
- Predominant sex: Male > Female (3:2 to 2:1) (1,2)[C]

RISK FACTORS

Previous history of erythema multiforme

Genetics

Strong association with HLA-DQ3 in herpes-related cases; possible association in recurrent cases with HLA-B15, -B35, -A33, -DR53, DQB1*0301, and DQW3 (1)[C]

GENERAL PREVENTION

- Known or suspected etiologic agents should be avoided.
- Acyclovir or valacyclovir may help prevent herpes-related erythema multiforme (1,2)[B].

PATHOPHYSIOLOGY

- The exact pathophysiology of EM is unknown.
- Possible immunologically mediated lymphocytic reaction to an infectious agent or a drug at the dermal-epithelial junction
- HSV-triggered EM seems to involve CD4+ T-cell infiltration and associated IFN-γ activation.
- Drug-triggered EM involves CD8+ T-cells and associated TNF-α activation (5)[C].

ETIOLOGY

- Most cases appear to be due to a preceding infection.
- Viral infections, particularly herpes simplex (accounting for more than 50% of cases); also Epstein-Barr, coxsackie, echovirus, varicella, mumps, poliovirus, hepatitis C, cytomegalovirus, HIV, molluscum contagiosum virus
- Bacterial infections, particularly *Mycoplasma pneumoniae;* other occasional reported bacterial infections include *Treponema, Pallidum*, and *Gardnerella vaginalis*
- Fungal infection, including *Histoplasma capsulatum* and *Coccidioides immitis*
- Medications, including sulfonamides, penicillins, anticonvulsants (carbamazepine, phenytoin, phenylbutazone, phenothiazines, barbiturates), hydantoins, NSAIDs (including rofecoxib, valdecoxib), oral contraceptives, and statins. Other sparsely reported medications include cimetidine, salicylic acid, angiotensin receptor blockers (ARBs; candesartan cilexetil), metformin, bupropion, ciprofloxacin, sorafenib, gemfibrozil, risperidone, paclitaxel, metoprolol, tumor necrosis factor (TNF) inhibitors (adalimumab, etanercept, infliximab), and methotrexate (3)
- Vaccines: Tetanus/diphtheria, bacillus Calmette-Guérin, oral polio, hepatitis B, human papillomavirus, H1N1 influenza
- Occupational exposures: Herbicides (alachlor and butachlor), iodoacetonitrile
- Protozoan infections
- Radiation therapy
- Premenstrual hormone changes
- Sarcoidosis

COMMONLY ASSOCIATED CONDITIONS

Any of the infections or diseases listed under "Etiology"

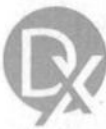

DIAGNOSIS

Diagnose clinically by careful review of the history and detailed physical examination; no specific labs are required for the diagnosis.

HISTORY

- Absent or mild prodromal symptoms
- Preceding HSV infection (over 50% of cases) 10–15 days before the skin eruptions (1,2)[B]
- Rash involving the skin and sometimes the mucous membrane, most commonly the mouth

PHYSICAL EXAM

- Skin pleomorphic eruption with a mixture of macules, papules of various sizes, and target lesions:
  - Typical target lesions: Raised and cyanotic center, edematous light intermediate ring and bright erythematous border (3 zones)
  - Flat or raised atypical target lesions: 2 zones only (center and intermediate ring) with poorly defined border
  - Symmetrically distributed eruption, mainly on the palms, soles, dorsum of the hands, and extensor surface of the extremities and the face
  - Lesions may coalesce and become generalized.
  - Body surface area with epidermal detachment <10% (1,2,4,5)[B]
- Mucosal involvement:
  - Minimal involvement in EM minor; if present, most commonly involves the mouth (usually cutaneous or mucosal lips (3)
  - At least 2 mucosal sites involved in EM major, including eyes (conjunctivitis, keratitis), mouth (stomatitis, cheilitis, characteristic blood-stained crusted erosions on lips) (3), and probable trachea, bronchi, GI tract, or genital tract (balanitis and valvulitis)
  - Multiple papules and vesicles, superficial irregular erosions, shallow painful ulcers with erythematous margin (1)[C]

DIAGNOSTIC TESTS & INTERPRETATION

Lab

- No specific lab test is indicated to make the diagnosis of EM (1,2,4,5)[B].
- Skin biopsy of lesional and perilesional tissue in equivocal conditions (1,2,4,5)[C]
- Direct and indirect immunofluorescence to differentiate EM from other vesiculobullous diseases (1)[C]. Direct immunofluorescence is detected on a biopsy of perilesional skin, and indirect immunofluorescence is detected from a blood sample.
- HSV tests in recurrent EM (serologic tests, swab culture, or tests using skin biopsy sample to check HSV antigens or DNA in keratinocytes by direct immunofluorescence [DFA] or polymerase chain reaction [PCR]) (5)[C]
- Antibody staining to IFN-γ and TNF-α to differentiate HSV-associated EM and drug-associated EM (5)[C]
- Elevated *M. pneumonia* antibody titer in *M. pneumonia* infection–associated EM (1)[C]

Imaging

Initial approach

No specific imaging studies are indicated in most cases.

Follow-Up & Special Considerations

Chest x-ray may be necessary if an underlying pulmonary infection (*M. pneumonia* infection) is suspected.

Pathological Findings

- Vacuolar interface dermatitis with CD4+ T lymphocytes and histocytes in papillary dermis and the epidermal-dermal junction
- Superficial perivascular lymphocytic inflammation
- Satellite cell necrosis
- Necrotic keratinocytes mainly in the basal layer
- Papillary dermal edema (1,2,5)[C]

DIFFERENTIAL DIAGNOSIS

- Stevens-Johnson syndrome (4)[C]:
  - Different pattern and location of the skin lesions
  - No typical target lesion
  - Atypical flat target lesions or macules, generalized or mainly in the trunk
  - Blisters and skin detachment <10% of the total body surface area
  - Usually with systemic complications (i.e., CNS, lung, GI system, kidney)
  - 1–5% mortality rate
- Toxic epidermal necrolysis (1,4)[C]:
  - Full-thickness skin necrosis and skin detachment >30% of the total body surface area
  - 10–30% mortality rate
- Urticaria
- Erythema annulare centrifugum
- Subacute cutaneous lupus erythematosus
- Necrotizing vasculitis
- Drug eruptions
- Contact dermatitis
- Pityriasis rosea
- Herpes simplex
- Secondary syphilis
- Tinea corporis
- Pemphigus vulgaris
- Pemphigoid
- Dermatitis herpetiformis
- Herpes gestationis
- Septicemia
- Serum sickness
- Viral exanthem
- Rocky Mountain spotted fever
- Mucocutaneous lymph node syndrome
- Meningococcemia
- Lichen planus
- Behçet syndrome
- Recurrent aphthous ulcers
- Herpetic gingivostomatitis
- Granuloma annulare

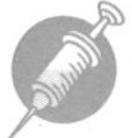

TREATMENT

MEDICATION

First Line

- Treatment of any underlying or causative disease (1,2)[B]
- Withdrawal of any drugs that might be the cause (1,2)[B]
- Symptomatic treatment with oral antihistamines and topical corticosteroids for mild cases (1,2)[B]
- Early treatment with acyclovir may lessen the number and duration of cutaneous lesions for patients with coexisting or recent HSV infection (2)[B]:
  - Acyclovir for adults: 200 mg, 5 times a day for 7–10 days in the onset of EM
  - For pediatric patients: 10 mg/kg or t.i.d. for 7–10 days
- Recurrent EM may be treated with oral acyclovir (400 mg b.i.d.), even if HSV infection has not been confirmed (2)[B].
- Valacyclovir (Valtrex, 500–1,000 mg/d) and famciclovir (Famvir, 125–250 mg/d) may be tried (2)[C]:
  - Reduce the dosage once the patient is recurrence-free for 4 months, and eventually discontinue the drug.

Second Line

- Recurrent EM cases nonresponsive to antiviral therapy could also try dapsone (100–150 mg/d), azathioprine (Imuran, 100–150 mg/d), thalidomide (100–200 mg per day), tacrolimus (0.1% ointment daily), mycophenolate mofetil (CellCept <2 g daily), hydroxychloroquine (<400 mg daily), colchicine (<1.2 mg daily) (2,6,7,8)[C].
- Cyclosporine given intermittently (4 mg/kg/d for a week) may also be used for recurrent EM (2)[C].
- Systemic steroid use is controversial, because it may decrease the patient's resistance to HSV and increase recurrent HSV infection and erythema multiforme eruptions (1,2)[C].
- Precautions: Refer to the manufacturer's profile of each drug.
- Significant possible interactions: Refer to the manufacturer's profile of each drug.

ADDITIONAL TREATMENT

General Measures

- Meticulous wound care and Burow solution or Domeboro solution dressings for severe cases with epidermal detachment followed by Vaseline gauze and curlex
- Mouth washes with warm saline or a solution of diphenhydramine, lidocaine (Xylocaine), and Kaopectate for oral lesions to provide symptomatic relief and oral hygiene, and to facilitate oral intake

IN-PATIENT CONSIDERATIONS

Admission Criteria

- Care at home
- Hospitalization needed for fluid, electrolyte management if patient with severe mucous membrane involvement, impaired oral intake and dehydration
- IV antibiotics if secondary infection develops

ONGOING CARE

FOLLOW-UP RECOMMENDATIONS

Patient Monitoring

- The disease is self-limiting.
- Complications are rare, with no mortality.

DIET

As tolerated with increased fluid intake

PATIENT EDUCATION

- The disease is self-limiting. However, the recurrence risk may be 30%.
- Antiviral therapy with acyclovir may reduce the duration and frequency of outbreaks.
- Avoid any identified etiological agents.

PROGNOSIS

- Rash evolves over 1–2 weeks and subsequently resolves within 2–6 weeks, generally without scarring or sequelae.
- Following resolution, there may be some postinflammatory hyper- or hypopigmentation.

COMPLICATIONS

Secondary infection

REFERENCES

1. Al-Johani KA, Fedele S, Porter SR. Erythema multiforme and related disorders. *Oral Surg Oral Med Oral Pathol Oral Radiol Endod*. 2007.
2. Lamoreux MR, Sternbach MR, Hsu WT. Erythema multiforme. *Am Fam Physician*. 2006;74:1883–8.
3. Sanchis JM, Bagán JV, Gavaldá C, et al. Erythema multiforme: Diagnosis, clinical manifestations and treatment in a retrospective study of 22 patients. *J Oral Pathol Med*. 2010;39:747–752.
4. Auquier-Dunant A, Mockenhaupt M, Naldi L, et al. Correlations between clinical patterns and causes of erythema multiforme majus, Stevens-Johnson syndrome, and toxic epidermal necrolysis: Results of an international prospective study. *Arch Dermatol*. 2002;138:1019–24.
5. Aurelian L, Ono F, Burnett J. Herpes simplex virus (HSV)-associated erythema multiforme (HAEM): A viral disease with an autoimmune component. *Dermatol Online J*. 2003;9:1.
6. Wetter DA, Davis MD, et al. Recurrent erythema multiforme: Clinical characteristics, etiologic associations, and treatment in a series of 48 patients at Mayo Clinic, 2000 to 2007. *J Am Acad Dermatol*. 2010;62:45–53.
7. Chen M, Doherty SD, Hsu S, et al. Innovative uses of thalidomide. *Dermatol Clin*. 2010;28:577–86.
8. Higgins E, Collins P. Recurrent bullous erythema multiforme treated with topical tacrolimus 0·1% ointment. *Br J Dermatol*. 2011;164(4):884–6.

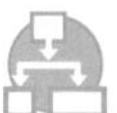

See Also (Topic, Algorithm, Electronic Media Element)

Cutaneous Drug Reactions; Dermatitis Herpetiformis; Herpes Gestationalis; Stevens-Johnson Syndrome; Toxic Epidermic Necrotisis; Urticaria

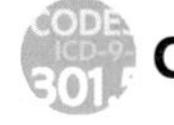

CODES

ICD9

- 695.10 Erythema multiforme, unspecified
- 695.13 Stevens-Johnson syndrome
- 695.14 Stevens-Johnson syndrome-toxic epidermal necrolysis overlap syndrome

CLINICAL PEARLS

- EM is diagnosed clinically by careful review of the history, through detailed physical examination, and by excluding other similar disorders. No lab tests are required for the diagnosis.
- Typical lesions are pleomorphic macules, papules, and characteristic target or "iris" lesions.
- Lesions are symmetrically distributed on palms, soles, dorsum of the hands, and extensor surfaces of extremities and face. The oral mucosa is the most affected mucosal region in EM.
- Management of EM involves determining the etiology when possible. The first step is to treat the suspected infection or discontinue the causative drug.
- Complications are rare. Most cases are self-limited. However, the recurrence risk may be as high as 30%.
- Recurrent cases often are secondary to herpes simplex infection. Antiviral therapy may be beneficial.

ERYTHEMA NODOSUM

Sophia L. Delano, MPP, MD
Nikki A. Levin, MD, PhD

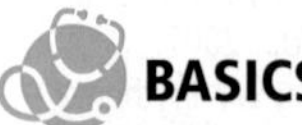

BASICS

DESCRIPTION

- A delayed-type hypersensitivity reaction to infectious agents, medications, or malignancies, or in the setting of autoimmune disorders, presenting as a SC panniculitis.
- Clinical pattern of multiple, bilateral, erythematous, tender SC nodules that undergo a characteristic pattern of color changes, similar to that seen in bruises. Unlike erythema induratum, the lesions of erythema nodosum do not typically ulcerate.
- Occurs most commonly on the shins, less commonly on the thighs and forearms
- May be accompanied by fever and arthralgias
- Often idiopathic but may be associated with a number of clinical entities
- Usually remits spontaneously in weeks to months without scarring or atrophy
- Synonym(s): Dermatitis contusiformis

Pregnancy Considerations

May have repeat outbreaks during pregnancy

EPIDEMIOLOGY

Incidence

- 1–5/100,000
- Predominant age: 20–30 years
- Predominant sex: Female > Male (3:1).

Prevalence

Varies geographically depending on the prevalence of disorders associated with erythema nodosum

RISK FACTORS

See "Etiology."

ETIOLOGY

- Idiopathic: 37–60%
- Bacterial: Streptococcal infections (most common cause in children), tuberculosis, leprosy, tularemia, gonorrhea, *Yersinia enterocolitica*, *Campylobacter*, *Salmonella*, *Shigella*
- Sarcoid
- Drugs: Sulfonamides, amoxicillin, oral contraceptives, bromides, azathioprine (1)
- Pregnancy
- Fungal: Dermatophytes, coccidioidomycosis, histoplasmosis, blastomycosis
- Viral/chlamydial: Infectious mononucleosis, lymphogranuloma venereum, paravaccinia, HIV (2)
- Enteropathies: Ulcerative colitis, Crohn disease, Behçet disease (3), celiac disease (4)
- Malignancies: Lymphoma/leukemia, sarcoma, myelodysplastic syndrome (5), after radiation therapy
- Sweet's syndrome (6)

COMMONLY ASSOCIATED CONDITIONS

See "Etiology."

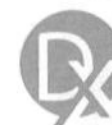

DIAGNOSIS

HISTORY

- Increasingly tender and aching nodules on the legs, usually over the shins.
- Fever, malaise, chills, fatigue
- Eruptions often preceded by symptoms of pharyngitis or upper respiratory infection
- Headache
- Arthralgias

PHYSICAL EXAM

- Initially warm, tender, brightly erythematous nodules, which may be raised, on anterior shins; lesions become bluish and fluctuant, gradually fading to yellowish, resembling a bruise.
- May occur on any area with SC fat
- Diameter usually 2–6 cm, but may rarely be larger

DIAGNOSTIC TESTS & INTERPRETATION

Diagnosis is usually clinical.

Lab

- ESR: May be elevated or normal
- CBC: Mild leukocytosis
- Antistreptolysin titers may be elevated.
- Throat culture (usually negative because the infection typically resolves before lesions appear)
- Stool culture and leukocytes, if indicated
- Skin testing for mycobacteria, if indicated
- Drugs that may alter lab results: Antecedent antibiotics may affect cultures.

Imaging

CXR for hilar adenopathy or infiltrates related to sarcoidosis or tuberculosis

Diagnostic Procedures/Surgery

Deep-incisional skin biopsy including SC fat; rarely necessary except in atypical cases with ulceration, duration >12 weeks

Pathological Findings

- Septal panniculitis without vasculitis
- Neutrophilic infiltrate in septa of fat tissue early in course
- Actinic radial (Miescher's) granulomas, consisting of collections of histocytes around a central stellate cleft, may be seen (7).
- Fibrosis, paraseptal granulation tissue, lymphocytes, and multinucleated giant cells predominate late in course.

DIFFERENTIAL DIAGNOSIS

- Nodular vasculitis or erythema induratum (warm ulcerating calf nodules)
- Superficial thrombophlebitis
- Cellulitis
- Septic emboli
- Weber-Christian disease (violaceous, scarring nodules)
- Lupus panniculitis
- Cutaneous polyarteritis nodosa
- Sarcoidal granulomas
- Cutaneous T-cell lymphoma
- Erythema nodosum leprosum (clinically similar to EN but shows vasculitis on histopathology)
- Vasculitis

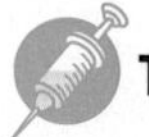

TREATMENT

- Medication usually more effective in acute than in chronic disease
- Condition often self-limited
- All medications listed as treatment for erythema nodosum are off-label uses of the medications. There are no FDA-approved medications for erythema nodosum.

MEDICATION

First Line

- NSAIDs:
  - Ibuprofen: 400 mg PO q4–6h (not to exceed 3,200 mg/d)
  - Indomethacin: 25–50 mg PO t.i.d.
  - Naproxen (Naprosyn): 250–500 mg PO b.i.d.
- Aspirin: 325 mg 1–2 tablets PO q4–6h (not to exceed 12 tablets a day); use enteric-coated tablets to decrease GI upset.
- Contraindications:
  - Active or recent peptic ulcer disease
  - History of hypersensitivity to NSAIDs

- Precautions:
  - GI upset/bleeding
  - Fluid retention
  - Dose reduction in elderly, especially those with renal disease, diabetes, or heart failure
  - May mask fever
  - NSAIDs may elevate liver function tests.
- Significant possible interactions:
  - May blunt antihypertensive effects of diuretics and β-blockers
  - NSAIDs can elevate plasma lithium levels.
  - Caution is advised with naproxen or any highly protein-bound drug because it may compete for albumin binding and elevate levels.
  - NSAIDs can cause significant elevation and prolongation of methotrexate levels.

Second Line

- Potassium iodide 400–900 mg/d divided 2–3×/day × 3–4 weeks (for persistent lesions). Need to monitor for hypothyroidism with prolonged use. Pregnancy class D.
- Corticosteroids for severe, refractory cases in which an infectious workup is negative. Prednisone 1 mg/kg/d for 1–2 weeks often helps resolve the lesions (8). Potential side effects include hyperglycemia, hypertension, weight gain, mood changes, bone loss, osteonecrosis, myopathy.
- Recent reports of improvement with colchicine 0.6–1.2 mg b.i.d.
- Hydroxychloroquine, thalidomide and cyclosporine may also be used.
- In a case of refractory erythema nodosum, minocycline 100 mg b.i.d. and tetracycline 500 mg b.i.d. were successfully used (9).

ADDITIONAL TREATMENT

General Measures

- Mild compression bandages and leg elevation may reduce pain. (Wet dressings, hot soaks, and topical medications are not useful.)
- Discontinue potentially causative drugs.
- Treat underlying disease

COMPLEMENTARY AND ALTERNATIVE MEDICINE

Vitamin B_{12} replacement. A single case report of resolution of lesions with B_{12} replacement in a patient who had B_{12} deficiency and erythema nodosum (10).

IN-PATIENT CONSIDERATIONS

Admission Criteria

Occasionally, admission may be needed for the antecedent illness (e.g., tuberculosis).

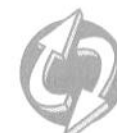

ONGOING CARE

FOLLOW-UP RECOMMENDATIONS

- Keep legs elevated.
- Elastic wraps or support stockings may be helpful when patients are ambulating.

Patient Monitoring

Monthly follow-up or as dictated by underlying disorder

DIET

No restrictions

PATIENT EDUCATION

- Lesions will resolve over a few weeks to months.
- No scarring is anticipated.
- Joint aches and pains may persist.
- <20% recur

PROGNOSIS

- Individual lesions resolve generally within 2 weeks.
- Total time course of 6–12 weeks but may vary with underlying disease.
- Joint aches and pains may persist for years.
- Lesions do not scar.
- Recurrences in 12–14% of patients: Occurs over variable periods, averaging several years; seen most often in sarcoid, streptococcal infection, pregnancy, and oral contraceptive use

COMPLICATIONS

- Vary according to underlying disease
- None expected from lesions of erythema nodosum

REFERENCES

1. de Fonclare AL, Khosrotehrani K, Aractingi S, et al. Erythema nodosum-like eruption as a manifestation of azathioprine hypersensitivity in patients with inflammatory bowel disease. *Arch Dermatol*. 2007;143:744–8.
2. Louthrenoo W, Lertprasertsuke N, Kasitanon N, et al. Erythema nodosum as a manifestation of HIV infection. *Asian Pac J Allergy Immunol*. 2002;20:175–8.
3. Psychos DN, Voulgari PV, Skopouli FN, et al. Erythema nodosum: The underlying conditions. *Clin Rheumatol*. 2000;19:212–6.
4. Bartyik K, Várkonyi A, Kirschner A, et al. Erythema nodosum in association with celiac disease. *Pediatr Dermatol*. 2004;21:227–30.
5. Then C, Langer A, Adam C, et al. Erythema nodosum associated with myelodysplastic syndrome: A case report. *Onkologie*. 2011;34:126–8.
6. Harris T, Henderson MC, et al. Concurrent Sweet's syndrome and erythema nodosum. *J Gen Intern Med*. 2011;26:214–5.
7. Schwartz RA, Nervi SJ, et al. Erythema nodosum: A sign of systemic disease. *Am Fam Physician*. 2007;75:695–700.
8. Requena L, Yus ES, et al. Erythema nodosum. *Dermatol Clin*. 2008;26:425–38, v.
9. Davis MD, et al. Response of recalcitrant erythema nodosum to tetracyclines. *J Am Acad Dermatol*. 2011;64:1211–2.
10. Volkov I, et al. Successful treatment of chronic erythema nodosum with vitamin B12. *J Am Board Fam Pract*. 2005;18:6.

E

ADDITIONAL READING

González-Gay MA, García-Porra C, Pujol RM, et al. Erythema nodosum: A clinical approach. *Clin Exp Rheumatol*. 2001;19:365–8.

CODES

ICD9

695.2 Erythema nodosum

CLINICAL PEARLS

- Lesions of erythema nodosum appear to be erythematous patches, but when palpated, their underlying nodularity is appreciated.
- Erythema nodosum in the setting of hilar adenopathy may be seen with multiple etiologies and does not exclusively indicate sarcoidosis.
- In patients with a history of Hodgkin's lymphoma, erythema nodosum may be a warning of impending recurrence.

ERYTHRASMA

Amena Hashmi, MD
Rahele Lameh, MD

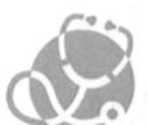

BASICS

Erythrasma is a bacterial infection of the skin folds, often misdiagnosed as a fungal infection, caused by *Corynebacterium minutissimum*.

DESCRIPTION

- *C. minutissimum* is a part of normal skin flora, but under moist, occluded conditions the diphtheroid bacteria will cause well-defined, reddish brown plaques in intertriginous areas such as the inguinal, intergluteal, interdigital, and inframammary folds.
- Also, ~30% of erythrasma infections may be concomitantly infected with a fungal infection, such as candida (1).
- In the immunocompetent patient, erythrasma may be a minor skin disorder; however, in the immunocompromised population, especially HIV patients, *C. minutissimum* can progress to severe cellulitis, abscess, or bacteremia (2).

EPIDEMIOLOGY

Incidence

Higher incidence in immunocompromised, predisposed, and elderly populations, but has been reported in all ages. Both sexes appear equally affected (3).

Prevalence

Erythrasma appears more in tropical areas, affecting ~4% of the population worldwide.

RISK FACTORS

- Obesity
- Diabetes
- Occlusive clothing/shoes
- Hyperhidrosis
- Immunocompromised state
- Advanced age

GENERAL PREVENTION

- Nonocclusive clothing and footwear
- Good hygiene
- Weight loss
- Good blood sugar control
- Avoiding constant skin friction

PATHOPHYSIOLOGY

C. minutissimum is a normal skin bacteria; however, under appropriate conditions, such as warmth, humidity, and occlusion, this bacteria invades the stratum corneum layer of epidermis causing it to thicken and scale. These diphtheroids produce porphyrin, which causes the fluorescence of the skin under Wood's light.

ETIOLOGY

Corynebacterium minutissimum

COMMONLY ASSOCIATED CONDITIONS

Coexisting fungal infections

DIAGNOSIS

HISTORY

- Normally, erythrasma is asymptomatic; however, it may present with pruritus (2).
- Reddish/brown discolored irregular patches
- Affects intertriginous areas, interdigital areas
- Consider when no improvement after antifungal therapy used for "fungal infection" (1)

PHYSICAL EXAM

Skin lesions present initially as red patches that are sharply demarcated, with irregular borders, that later may become brown/tan color. In toe webspaces, lesions can appear fissuring, macerated, and scaling (4). May be mistaken for tinea pedis.

DIAGNOSTIC TESTS & INTERPRETATION

Wood's lamp exam

Lab

- Gram stain may show gram-positive, rod-shaped organisms.
- Culture

Initial lab tests

Visualize skin lesions under Wood's lamp, though not always reliable (2)

Follow-Up & Special Considerations

Obtain skin scrapings if possible to view under microscope; consider KOH test to rule out dermatophytoses (2).

Pathological Findings

- Wood's lamp will show a coral red–colored fluorescence due to the presence of porphyrins.
- Under microscopic exam, rodlike bacteria are seen in the stratum corneum layer of skin (2).

DIFFERENTIAL DIAGNOSIS

- Psoriasis
- Familial pemphigus
- Dermatophytosis
- Acanthosis nigricans
- Intertriginous candidiasis
- Pitted keratolysis
- Tinea versicolor

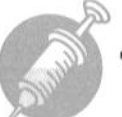

TREATMENT

- Erythromycin is treatment of choice, and a recent systematic review showed "convincing evidence" to recommend erythromycin; however, no evidence-based studies have clarified the best therapeutic options (2)[C],(5)[B].
- Red light photodynamic therapy may also be effective. One recent study showed ~23% of patients had complete recovery from lesions, while others had some reduction in extent of their lesions (6)[C].

MEDICATION

First Line

Erythromycin 250 mg q.i.d. for 14 days (1,2)[C]

Second Line

- Clarithromycin 1 g once (1)[C]
- Tetracycline 250 mg q.i.d. for 7–14 days (1)[C]
- Photodynamic therapy with red light (6)[C]

ADDITIONAL TREATMENT

- Topical erythromycin 2% b.i.d. 7–10 days (1)[C]
- Topical clindamycin 2% t.i.d. for 7 days (1)[C]

General Measures

- Athletes/military recruits should be treated for 48–72 hours prior to returning to contact situations (1)[C].
- Asymptomatic individuals, especially athletes, should be treated (1)[C].

Issues for Referral

In case of outpatient therapeutic failure or contraindication of systemic drugs, or immunocompromised, should be referred to specialists and may require inpatient therapy in the latter case due to possible complications.

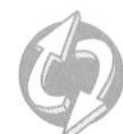

ONGOING CARE

PATIENT EDUCATION

Patients should be counseled to keep affected areas clean and dry and to avoid occlusive clothing and footwear.

PROGNOSIS

Good

COMPLICATIONS

Immunocompromised patients with erythrasma need to be cautious of septicemia, and patients with valvular heart disease or postsurgical wounds need to monitor for possible infective endocarditis and infection, respectively.

REFERENCES

1. Sedgwick PE, Dexter WW, Smith CT, et al. Bacterial dermatoses in sports. *Clin Sports Med*. 2007;26: 383–96.
2. Blaise G, Nikkels AF, Hermanns-Lê T, et al. Corynebacterium-associated skin infections. *Int J Dermatol*. 2008;47:884–90.
3. Husain Z, Cohen PJ, Schwartz RA, et al. Flexural and extensoral eruptions in dermatologic disease. *Clin Dermatol*. 2011;29:195–204.
4. Morales-Trujillo ML, Arenas R, Arroyo S, et al. [Interdigital erythrasma: Clinical, epidemiologic, and microbiologic findings]. *Actas Dermosifiliogr*. 2008;99:469–73.
5. Eekhof JA, Neven AK, Gransjean SP, et al. Minor derm ailments: How good is the evidence for common treatments? *J Fam Pract*. 2009;58:E2.
6. Darras-Vercambre S, Carpentier O, Vincent P, et al. Photodynamic action of red light for treatment of erythrasma: Preliminary results. *Photodermatol Photoimmunol Photomed*. 2006;22:153–6.

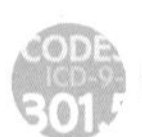

CODES

ICD9

039.0 Cutaneous actinomycotic infection

CLINICAL PEARLS

Erythrasma is a bacterial infection of the skin folds, often misdiagnosed as a fungal infection.

E

ESOPHAGEAL VARICES

Katherine Thompson, MD
Edward Feller, MD

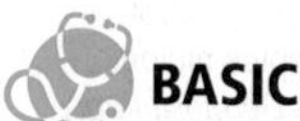

BASICS

DESCRIPTION

- Dilated veins in the distal esophagus that connect the portal and systemic circulations
- Result from resistance to portal blood flow
- Increased pressure and turbulent flow, as well as superficial location in the distal esophagus, make them prone to rupture, producing major GI bleeding with significant morbidity and mortality.

EPIDEMIOLOGY

Prevalence

- Esophageal varices in patients with cirrhosis (correlating with disease severity): 50%
- Patients with esophageal varices who bleed during their lifetime: 50%
- Bleeding from esophageal varices is associated with 15–20% mortality at 6 weeks.
- Predominant gender: Male > Female

RISK FACTORS

- Cirrhosis: Can result from alcohol abuse, viral hepatitis, autoimmune inflammation, hemochromatosis, Wilson disease, primary biliary cirrhosis, primary sclerosing cholangitis, nonalcoholic fatty liver disease, or medications
- In cirrhotics, thrombocytopenia (<68,000 platelets) and splenomegaly, correlated with portal hypertension, are independent predictors of esophageal varices (1).
- Noncirrhotic portal hypertension

Genetics

Rare hereditary causes of cirrhosis

GENERAL PREVENTION

- Prevention and treatment of causes of cirrhosis, including alcohol cessation, hepatitis B vaccine, clean needles, or detox in IVDU to avoid hepatitis C exposure; specific therapy for hepatitis B and C, hemochromatosis
- See "Treatment" section for prevention of first, second bleeds

PATHOPHYSIOLOGY

- Portal hypertension: Caused by elevated portal pressure due to splanchnic arteriolar vasodilatation and increased resistance to flow due to fibrous tissue and regenerative nodules
- Increased production of endothelin-1 (vasoconstrictor) and decreased production of nitrous oxide (vasodilator) causing intrahepatic vasoconstriction (2)

ETIOLOGY

- Portal hypertension: Defined as a pressure gradient >10 mm Hg between the portal vein and inferior vena cava. Collateral vessels (varices) form to decompress portal circulation.
- Cirrhotic portal hypertension:
  - >90% of cases (3)
  - Alcohol and hepatitis C are the most common etiologies.
  - Less common: Hemochromatosis, hepatitis B, nonalcoholic fatty liver disease
  - Uncommon: Biliary cirrhosis, autoimmune cirrhosis
- Noncirrhotic portal hypertension:
  - Extrahepatic portal or splenic vein thrombosis from umbilical vein infection, trauma, chronic pancreatitis, thrombotic conditions, and polycythemia
  - Malignant invasion of liver sinusoids or portal vein; in lymphoma, leukemia, hepatocellular, or other carcinomas
  - Metabolic disease altering liver sinusoids: Amyloidosis, Gaucher disease, Budd-Chiari syndrome, veno-occlusive disease (4)

COMMONLY ASSOCIATED CONDITIONS

- Portal hypertensive gastropathy, varices in stomach, duodenum, colon, rectum (causes massive bleeding, unlike hemorrhoids); rarely at umbilicus (caput medusa) or ostomy sites
- Hepatic encephalopathy, ascites, hepatorenal syndrome, spontaneous bacterial peritonitis
- Gastric varices: Isolated gastric varices also occur due to splenic vein thrombosis or stenosis from hypercoagulability or contiguous inflammation (most commonly, chronic pancreatitis). Tumors can compress or infiltrate the splenic vein leading to pressure increase in short gastric veins. Patients may show no clinical signs of portal hypertension.

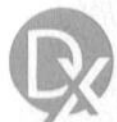

DIAGNOSIS

- First indication of varices can be GI bleeding: Painless hematemesis, hematochezia, and/or melena
- Occult bleeding with anemia: Uncommon
- Signs of cirrhosis or portal hypertension
- Endoscopic screening with known cirrhosis every 2–3 years (2)[C]; yearly in patients with decompensated cirrhosis (2)[C]

HISTORY

- Generally, a history of cirrhosis or liver disease
- Painless hematemesis, melena, or hematochezia
- Rapidly bleeding upper GI sites can present as rectal bleeding.

PHYSICAL EXAM

- Assess hemodynamic stability: Possible hypotension/tachycardia (if bleeding)
- Small, hard liver; hepatomegaly possible
- Splenomegaly, ascites
- Visible abdominal periumbilical collateral circulation (caput medusae)
- Spider angiomata on chest/back; palmar erythema
- Testicular atrophy; gynecomastia
- Anal varices (which collapse with digital pressure, whereas hemorrhoids do not)
- Hepatic encephalopathy
- Blood on rectal exam

DIAGNOSTIC TESTS & INTERPRETATION

Lab

Initial lab tests

- Anemia from blood loss; hemoglobin may be normal despite active bleed; may require 6–24 hours to equilibrate
- Platelet count <68,000: Most sensitive (71%) and specific (73%) lab parameter to indicate portal hypertension, large esophageal varices (1)
- Possibly abnormal AST, ALT, alkaline phosphatase, bilirubin, prolonged prothrombin time, or low albumin-reflecting cirrhosis
- BUN, creatinine to detect hepatorenal syndrome

Imaging

Initial approach

Esophagoscopy as part of esophagogastroduodenoscopy:

- Identify, treat nonbleeding varices appearing as protruding submucosal veins in the distal third of the esophagus (2)[C].
- Can identify actively bleeding varices as well as those with stigmata of recent hemorrhage
- Can treat actively bleeding vessels with esophageal band ligation (2)[A]; prevent rebleeding. Can also detect gastric varices, portal hypertensive gastropathy; diagnose alternative bleeding site, such as ulcer disease.

Diagnostic Procedures/Surgery

- Video capsule esophageal endoscopy, in early trials, has acceptable sensitivity and specificity for detecting but not treating varices; alternative for those unwilling to undergo screening UGI endoscopy
- Doppler sonography (second-line): Demonstrates patency, diameter, and flow in portal and splenic veins, and intra-abdominal collaterals; very sensitive for gastric varices and in surveillance to document patency after ligation or TIPS
- MRI (second-line, not routine): Demonstrates large vascular channels in abdomen, mediastinum:
  - Can demonstrate patency of intrahepatic portal vein and splenic vein. Venous-phase celiac arteriography: Demonstrates portal vein and collaterals; can diagnose hepatic vein occlusion.
  - Portal pressure measurement using retrograde catheter in hepatic vein

Pathological Findings

- Extensive collateral circulation in the mediastinum and abdomen in addition to large vessels in the esophageal submucosa
- When bleeding occurs, these large veins protrude into the submucosa of the esophagus and rupture into the lumen.

DIFFERENTIAL DIAGNOSIS

- Upper GI bleeding:
  - In patients with known varices, as many as 50% bleed from other, nonvariceal sources.
  - Peptic ulcer disease; gastritis
  - Gastric or esophageal malignancy
  - Congestive gastropathy of portal hypertension
  - Arteriovenous malformation (AVM)
  - Mallory-Weiss tears
  - Hemoptysis; nosebleed
- Lower GI bleeding:
  - Rectal varices
  - Hemorrhoids
  - Colonic neoplasia
  - Diverticulosis
  - Arteriovenous malformation
  - Rapidly bleeding upper GI site
- Continued or recurrent bleeding risk: Actively bleeding or large varix, high Childs-Pugh severity score, infection, renal failure

TREATMENT

MEDICATION

- ***Preventing varices from bleeding once present:***
  - Endoscope: Assesses variceal size, presence of red wale sign (varix with a weak wall), to determine risk stratification:
    - Endoscope every 2–3 years if cirrhosis but no varices, every 1–2 years if small varices and not receiving β-blockers
  - Nonselective β-blockers reduce portal pressure and decrease risk of first bleed from 25–15% in primary prophylaxis of bleeding (2). Used in cirrhosis plus small varices with increased hemorrhage risk (2)[C], as well as cirrhosis plus medium-to-large varices (2)[A]:
    - Propranolol: 40 mg b.i.d. increase until heart rate decreased by 25% from baseline
    - Nadolol 80 mg daily, increase as above
    - Contraindications: Severe asthma with β-blockers
  - *Nitrates should not be used in the primary prophylaxis of variceal bleed* (2)[A].
  - Obliteration of varices with esophageal banding for those intolerant of medication prophylaxis:
    - During ligation: Proton pump inhibitors such as lansoprazole 30 mg/d until varices obliterated
- ***Active bleeding:***
  - IV access; monitor intake and output.
  - Type and cross-match packed RBCs.
  - Appropriate resuscitation and maintenance of blood volume; transfuse to hemoglobin of 8 g/dL (2)[B]. Overtransfusion increases portal pressure and increases rebleeding risk.
  - Treat coagulopathy, if necessary. Be wary that fresh frozen plasma may increase blood volume and increase rebleeding risk.
  - Avoid sedation, monitor mental state, avoid nephrotoxic drugs
  - Inject thiamine as indicated, monitor blood glucose, delirium tremens
  - IV octreotide to lower portal venous pressure as adjuvant to endoscopic management (2)[A]. IV bolus of 50 mg followed by drip of 50 mg/h.
  - Urgent upper endoscopy for diagnosis and treatment (2)[A]:
    - Variceal band ligation or sclerotherapy for bleeding varices or nonbleeding medium-to-large varices to decrease bleeding risk
    - Variceal band ligation is preferred due to improved bleeding cessation, fewer complications (3).
  - Repeat ligation or sclerosant if bleeding recurs.
  - If endoscopic treatment fails to stop bleeding, may need Sengstaken Blakemore or Minnesota tube as emergency rescue therapy to stabilize patient for TIPS (5)[B].
  - During bleeding, consider antibiotic prophylaxis for spontaneous peritonitis, other infections with IV ciprofloxacin, or oral norfloxacin for 7–10 days (2,3)[A].
  - In active bleeding, avoid β-blockers, which decrease BP and blunt the physiologic increase in heart rate during acute hemorrhage.
- ***Preventing recurrence of bleeding:***
  - Vasoconstrictors: Terlipressin, octreotide (reduce portal pressure) (2)[A]
  - Endoscopic band ligation (EBL): If bleeding recurs or portal pressure measurement shows portal pressure remains >12 mm Hg
  - Endoscopic sclerotherapy: Second-line and uncommonly used (if EBL cannot be performed)
  - TIPS (2)[C]: Second-line therapy in those who fail above methods. TIPS decreases portal pressure by creating communication between hepatic vein and an intrahepatic portal vein branch.

ADDITIONAL TREATMENT

General Measures

- Treat comorbities, generally related to cirrhosis
- Refer for liver transplantation where appropriate.

Issues for Referral

Primarily those associated with liver transplantation

SURGERY/OTHER PROCEDURES

- Endoscopic variceal ligation: Preferred approach to those who cannot tolerate beta-blockers
- Transjugular intrahepatic portasystemic shunt (TIPS)
- Esophageal transection: In uncontrollable, exsanguinating bleeding
- Liver transplantation: Referral after diagnosis

IN-PATIENT CONSIDERATIONS

Admission Criteria

Inpatient for acute bleeding

Discharge Criteria

Cessation of bleeding, stability of other comorbidities, complications

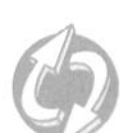

ONGOING CARE

FOLLOW-UP RECOMMENDATIONS

Patient Monitoring

- Close monitoring of vital signs if actively bleeding
- Endoscopic variceal ligation, repeated every 1–4 weeks until varices eradicated
- If TIPS, repeat endoscopy only if clinically bleeding
- If TIPS performed, follow-up recommended, usually Doppler sonogram every 6 months to assess shunt patency

PATIENT EDUCATION

National Digestive Information Clearinghouse, 2 Information Way, Bethesda, MD 20892 (digestive.niddk.nih.gov/) or American Liver Foundation, 1425 Pompton Way, Cedar Grove, NJ 07009 (www.liverfoundation.org)

PROGNOSIS

- Depends on prognosis of underlying condition
- With cirrhosis, 1-year survival for those who are alive 2 weeks after variceal bleed is 50%.
- Prognosis in noncirrhotic portal fibrosis is much better than that of cirrhotics.

COMPLICATIONS

- Bleeding
- Gastric, other uncommon varices may occur following eradication of esophageal varices
- Esophageal varices can recur after obliteration.
- Encephalopathy; renal dysfunction
- Infections after banding/ligation of varices

REFERENCES

1. Madhotra R, Mulcahy HE, Willner I, et al. Prediction of esophageal varices in patients with cirrhosis. *J Clin Gastroenterol*. 2002;34:81–5.
2. Garcia-Tsao G, Sanyal AJ, Grace ND, et al. Prevention and management of gastroesophageal varices and variceal hemorrhage in cirrhosis. *Hepatology*. 2007;46:922–38.
3. Cardenas A. Management of acute variceal bleeding: Emphasis on endoscopic therapy. *Clin Liver Dis*. 2010;14:251–262.
4. Sarin SK, Kumar A. Noncirrhotic portal hypertension. *Clin Liver Dis*. 2006;10:627–51.
5. Albillos A, Peñas B, Zamora J, et al. Role of endoscopy in primary prophylaxis for esophageal variceal bleeding. *Clin Liver Dis*. 2010;14:231–50.

ADDITIONAL READING

- Boyer TD, Haskal ZJ, American Association for the Study of Liver Diseases, et al. The role of transjugular intrahepatic portosystemic shunt (TIPS) in the management of portal hypertension: Update 2009. *Hepatology*. 2010;51:306.
- Cheung J, Zeman M, van Zanten SV, et al. Systematic review: Secondary prevention with band ligation, pharmacotherapy or combination therapy after bleeding from oesophageal varices. *Aliment Pharmacol Ther*. 2009;30:577–88.
- D'Amico G, Pagliaro L, Pietrosi G, et al. Emergency sclerotherapy versus vasoactive drugs for bleeding oesophageal varices in cirrhotic patients. *Cochrane Database Syst Rev*. 2010;CD002233.
- Groszmann RJ, Garcia-Tsao G, Bosch J, et al. Beta-blockers to prevent gastroesophageal varices in patients with cirrhosis. *N Engl J Med*. 2005;353:2254–61.

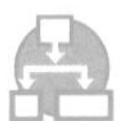

See Also (Topic, Algorithm, Electronic Media Element)

Cirrhosis of the Liver; Portal Hypertension

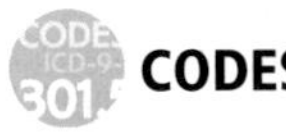

CODES

ICD9

- 456.0 Esophageal varices with bleeding
- 456.1 Esophageal varices without mention of bleeding
- 456.21 Esophageal varices in diseases classified elsewhere, without mention of bleeding

CLINICAL PEARLS

- Rapidly bleeding UGI sites can manifest as isolated rectal bleeding.
- In acute bleeding, avoid β-blockers, which decrease BP and blunt the physiologic increase in heart rate during acute hemorrhage.
- In acute bleeding, overtransfusion can elevate portal pressure, which increases bleeding risk.
- Thrombocytopenia: Sensitive marker of increased portal pressure, large esophageal varices
- During bleeding, consider antibiotic prophylaxis for spontaneous peritonitis and other infections with IV ciprofloxacin or oral norfloxacin for 7–10 days.

ESSENTIAL TREMOR SYNDROME

Jonathon M. Firnhaber, MD

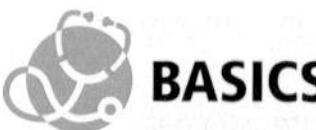

BASICS

DESCRIPTION

- A postural (occurring with voluntary maintenance of a position against gravity) or kinetic (occurring during voluntary movement) flexion–extension tremor that is slow and rhythmic and primarily affects the hands and forearms, head, and voice with a frequency of 4–12 Hz.
- Older patients tend to have lower-frequency tremors, while younger patients exhibit frequencies in the higher range.
- May be familial, sporadic, or associated with other movement disorders
- Can begin at any age, but the incidence and prevalence increase with age
- The tremor can be exacerbated by emotional or physical stresses, fatigue, and caffeine.
- System(s) affected: Neurologic; Musculoskeletal; Ear/Nose/Throat (ENT) (voice)

EPIDEMIOLOGY

Essential tremor is the most common pathological tremor in humans.

Incidence

- Can occur at any age, but bimodal peaks exist in the second and sixth decades
- Incidence rises significantly after age 49.

Prevalence

0.4–5% of the general population

RISK FACTORS

Genetics

- Positive family history in 50–70% of patients; autosomal dominant inheritance is demonstrated in many families, but twin studies suggest that environmental factors are also involved.
- There is a link to genetic loci on chromosomes 2p22–25, 3q13, and 6p23. In addition, a Ser9Gly variant in the dopamine D_3 receptor gene on 3q13 has been suggested as a risk factor.

PATHOPHYSIOLOGY

Suspected to originate from an abnormal oscillation within thalamocortical and cerebello-olivary loops, as lesions in these areas tend to reduce essential tremor. Essential tremor is not a homogenous disorder; many patients have other motor manifestations and nonmotor features, including cognitive and psychiatric symptoms.

COMMONLY ASSOCIATED CONDITIONS

Can be present in 10% of patients with Parkinson disease (PD); characteristics of PD that distinguish it from essential tremor include 3–5-Hz resting tremor; accompanying rigidity, bradykinesia, or postural instability; and no change from alcohol consumption.

DIAGNOSIS

HISTORY

- Core criteria for diagnosis:
  - Bilateral action (postural or kinetic) tremor of the hands and forearms (but not rest tremor)
  - Absence of other neurologic signs, with the exception of cogwheel phenomenon
  - May have isolated head tremor with no signs of dystonia
- Secondary criteria include long duration (>3 years), positive family history, and beneficial response to alcohol (1)[C].

PHYSICAL EXAM

- Tremor can affect upper limbs (~95% of patients).
- Less commonly, the tremor affects head (~34%), lower limbs (~30%), voice (~12%), tongue (~7%), face (~5%), and trunk (~5%).

DIAGNOSTIC TESTS & INTERPRETATION

Lab

Initial lab tests

- No specific biological marker or diagnostic test is available.
- Ceruloplasmin and serum copper to rule out Wilson disease
- Thyroid-stimulating hormone to rule out thyroid dysfunction
- Serum electrolytes, BUN, creatinine

Imaging

Initial approach

Brain MRI usually is not necessary or indicated unless Wilson disease is found or exam implies central lesion.

Diagnostic Procedures/Surgery

Electromyogram usually is not necessary.

Pathological Findings

Posture-related tremor

DIFFERENTIAL DIAGNOSIS

- Wilson disease
- Hyperthyroidism
- Multiple sclerosis
- Dystonic tremor
- Cerebellar tremor
- Asterixis
- Psychogenic tremor
- Orthostatic tremor
- Drug-induced or enhanced physiologic tremor (valproic acid, SSRIs, steroids, lithium, cyclosporine, β-adrenergic agonists, ephedrine, theophylline, tricyclic antidepressants [TCAs], antipsychotics)
- PD is manifested by a tremor at rest.

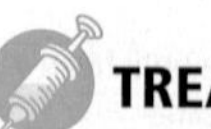

TREATMENT

MEDICATION

Pharmacologic treatment should be considered when tremor interferes with activities of daily living or causes psychological distress.

First Line

- Propranolol 60–320 mg/d in divided doses or in long-acting formulation reduces limb-tremor magnitude by ~50%, and almost 70% of patients experience improvement in clinical rating scales. There is insufficient evidence to recommend propranolol for vocal tremor. Single doses of propranolol, taken before social situations that are likely to exacerbate tremor, are useful for some patients.
- Primidone 25 mg at bedtime, gradually titrated to 150–300 mg at bedtime, improves tremor amplitude by 40–50%. Maximum dose is 750 mg/d, with doses >250 mg/d typically divided to b.i.d. or t.i.d. Low-dose therapy (<250 mg/d) is just as effective as high-dose (750 mg/d) therapy.
- Propranolol and primidone have similar efficacy when used as initial therapy for limb tremor; both carry a level A recommendation.

Second Line

- Topiramate at a mean dose of 292 mg/d demonstrated significantly greater reduction in tremor rating scale (TRS) compared with placebo (7.7 vs. 0.08; $p < .005$; baseline TRS = 37.0) in a small study combining results of 3 double-blind randomized controlled trials following a common protocol (2)[B]. Use is limited by dropout rates as high as 40% due to appetite suppression, weight loss, paresthesias, and concentration difficulties.
- Gabapentin up to 400 mg t.i.d.
- Sotalol, nadolol, and atenolol are alternative β-blockers; each has less evidence than propranolol to support use.
- Clonazepam and alprazolam should be used with caution because of abuse potential.
- Clozapine has shown efficacy at doses of 6–75 mg/d but is recommended only for refractory cases of limb tremor because of a 1% risk of agranulocytosis.
- Memantine, in a pilot study using doses up to 40 mg/d, showed significant benefit in a small subset of the study group. Adverse events at this dose included dizziness, somnolence, and poor energy (3).
- Other medications that have been used to treat essential tremor, with limited data to support their use, include acetazolamide, clonidine, flunarizine, levetiracetam, methazolamide, nimodipine, olanzapine, phenobarbital, pregabalin, quetiapine, sodium oxybate, and zonisamide.
- Alcohol may provide transient improvement in symptoms, but its brief duration of action, subsequent rebound, and associated risk of developing alcohol addiction make it an inappropriate treatment.
- Botulinum toxin A injections should be offered as a treatment option for cervical dystonia (Level A recommendation from American Association of Neurology), and may be offered for blepharospasm, focal upper extremity dystonia, adductor laryngeal dystonia, and upper extremity essential tremor (4)[B]. Limited data support its use for head and voice tremor (5).

ADDITIONAL TREATMENT

Issues for Referral

Referral to a neurologist can help to differentiate those with dystonia, neuropathic tremor, PD, or drug-induced tremor.

SURGERY/OTHER PROCEDURES

- Deep brain stimulation provides a magnitude of benefit that is superior to all available medications and may be used to treat medically refractory limb tremor and has fewer adverse effects than thalamotomy (6)[A].
- Bilateral thalamic stimulation is effective in reducing tremor and functional disability; however, dysarthria is a possible complication.
- Unilateral thalamotomy may be used to treat limb tremor that is refractory to medical management.
- Bilateral thalamotomy is not recommended because of adverse side effects.

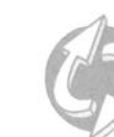

ONGOING CARE

DIET

Avoid caffeine.

PROGNOSIS

Tremor tends to worsen with age, increasing in amplitude.

REFERENCES

1. Bain P, Brin M, Deuschl G, et al. Criteria for the diagnosis of essential tremor. *Neurology*. 2000; 54:S7.
2. Connor GS, Edwards K, Tarsy D. Topiramate in essential tremor: Findings from double-blind, placebo-controlled, crossover trials. *Clin Neuropharmacol*. 2008;31:97–103.
3. Handforth A, Bordelon Y, Frucht SJ, et al. A pilot efficacy and tolerability trial of memantine for essential tremor. *Clin Neuropharm*. 2010;33: 223–6.
4. Simpson DM, et al. Therapeutics and Technology Assessment Subcommittee of the American Academy of Neurology. Assessment: Botulinum neurotoxin for the treatment of movement disorders (an evidence-based review): Report of the Therapeutics and Technology Assessment Subcommittee of the American Academy of Neurology. *Neurology*. 2008;70(19):1699–706.
5. Zesiewicz TA, et al. Practice parameter: Therapies for essential tremor: Report of the Quality Standards Subcommittee of the American Academy of Neurology. 2005;28;64(12):2008–20.
6. Flora ED, Perera CL, Cameron AL, et al. Deep brain stimulation for essential tremor: A systematic review. *Mov Disord*. 2010;25:1550–9.

ADDITIONAL READING

- Deuschl G, Raethjen J, Hellriegel H, et al. Treatment of patients with essential tremor. *Lancet Neurol*. 2011;10:148–61.
- Sullivan KL, Hauser RA, Zesiewicz TA. Essential tremor: Epidemiology, diagnosis, and treatment. *Neurologist*. 2004;10(5):250–8.

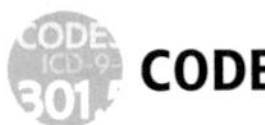

CODES

ICD9

333.1 Essential and other specified forms of tremor

CLINICAL PEARLS

- Core criteria for diagnosis of essential tremor include bilateral action (intention) tremor of the hands, forearm, and/or head without resting component.
- Beneficial response to alcohol and positive family history help to differentiate essential tremor from PD; PD is characterized by tremor at rest.
- 10% of patients with PD will have both resting tremors of PD and essential (intention) tremors.
- Wilson disease, thyroid disease, and medication effect should be ruled out.
- Brain MRI is usually not necessary or indicated.
- First-line treatments include propranolol and primidone.

E

EUSTACHIAN TUBE DYSFUNCTION

Teresa V. Chan, MD

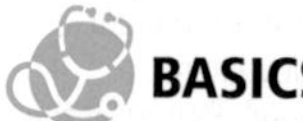

BASICS

DESCRIPTION
- Eustachian tube dysfunction (ETD) is classically described as a functional or structural obstruction of the eustachian tube due to not opening properly in response to atmospheric pressure changes and negative pressure in the middle ear.
- May occur in setting of pressure changes (e.g., scuba diving or plane travel) or acute upper airway inflammation (e.g., allergic or infectious rhinosinusitis)
- Chronic ETD may lead to a retracted tympanic membrane, recurrent serous effusions, recurrent otitis media, adhesive otitis media, chronic mastoiditis, or cholesteatoma.
- Patulous eustachian tube (PET) is a distinct entity in which the eustachian tube is excessively open. The patient may complain that his/her own voice, breathing, or heartbeat sounds like an echo or sounds excessively loud. This is autophony.
- System(s) affected: Auditory
- Synonym(s): Auditory tube dysfunction; Eustachian tube disorder; Blocked eustachian tube; Patulous eustachian tube

ALERT
- Sudden single-sided deafness (SSNHL) can be misdiagnosed as ETD.
- A simple 512-Hz tuning fork test lateralizes to the opposite ear in sudden sensorineural hearing loss and to the affected ear in ETD with conductive hearing loss.
- Any sudden sensorineural hearing loss is a medical emergency and should be referred to an otolaryngologist immediately.

EPIDEMIOLOGY
- Most common in children <5 years of age (1)
- Usually decreases with age

Incidence
70% of children by age 7 years have experienced ETD.

Prevalence
- Males > Females
- Highest prevalence amongst Native Americans, Inuits, Australian Aborigines, Hispanics, Africans

RISK FACTORS
- Adult and pediatric:
  - Allergic rhinitis, tobacco exposure, GERD, chronic sinusitis, adenoid hypertrophy or nasopharyngeal mass, neuromuscular disease, altered immunity
- Pediatric:
  - In addition to those listed above: prematurity and low birth weight, young age, daycare, exposure to many other children, crowded living conditions, low socioeconomic status, prone sleeping position, prolonged bottle use, craniofacial abnormalities (e.g., cleft palate, Down syndrome)

Pregnancy Considerations
ETD may be exacerbated by rhinitis of pregnancy; symptoms resolve postpartum.

Genetics
Twin studies show a genetic component (1). Specific genetic cause is still undefined.

GENERAL PREVENTION
- Control sources of upper airway inflammation: Allergies, infectious rhinosinusitis, GERD.
- Autoinsufflation of middle ear (i.e., blow gently against pinched nostril and closed mouth)
- Avoid atmospheric pressure changes (e.g., plane flight, scuba diving) in the setting of acute allergy exacerbation or URI.
- Avoid exposure to environmental irritants: Tobacco smoke, pollutants.

PATHOPHYSIOLOGY
- Under normal circumstances, the eustachian tube is closed, but it can open to let a small amount of air through to equalize pressure between the middle ear and the atmosphere.
- ETD is failure of the system at proximal end (ET, palate, nasal cavities, and nasopharynx) to regulate the middle ear and mastoid.
- Eustachian tube functions:
  - Ventilation/regulation of middle ear pressure
  - Protection from nasopharyngeal secretions
  - Drainage of middle ear fluid
  - ET is closed at rest and opens with yawning, swallowing, chewing.
- Cycle of dysfunction: Structural or functional obstruction of the ET compromises 3 functions of this system:
  - Negative pressure develops in middle ear.
  - Serous exudate is drawn from the middle ear mucosa by negative pressure or refluxed into the middle ear if the ET opens momentarily.
  - Infection of static fluid causes edema and release of inflammatory mediators, which exacerbates cycle of inflammation and obstruction.

ETIOLOGY
- In children, a horizontal and shorter ET predisposes to difficulties with ventilation and drainage (1).
- Adenoid hypertrophy can block the torus tubarius (proximal opening of the ET) (1).
- In adults, paradoxical closing with swallowing has been noted in a majority of patients (1).

COMMONLY ASSOCIATED CONDITIONS
- Hearing loss
- Middle ear effusion
- Recurrent otitis media
- Chronic mastoiditis
- Cholesteatoma
- Allergic rhinitis
- Chronic sinusitis
- URI
- Adenoid hypertrophy
- GERD
- Cleft palate
- Down syndrome
- Obesity
- Nasopharyngeal carcinoma or other tumor

DIAGNOSIS

HISTORY
- Fullness, pressure, clogged feeling in the ear is the most common complaint.
- Relief by "popping ears" (i.e., yawn or swallow tenses the tensor veli palatini, causing the ET to dilate)
- Subjective hearing loss may occur. Objective hearing loss may occur in setting of associated effusion or chronic ear disease.
- Determine unilateral or bilateral involvement. If an adult presents with persistent unilateral symptoms, workup for nasopharyngeal process such as tumor.
- Tinnitus (usually described as popping, fluttering, crackling instead of high-pitched ringing)
- Dizziness or lightheadedness is less common.
- History of previous ear infections, previous surgeries, including tympanostomy tubes
- Antecedent URI
- Rhinitis symptoms: Nasal congestion or rhinorrhea
- Head trauma (ears or nose)
- Voice change (hypo- or hypernasal voice, consider NP mass or palatal dysfunction)
- Recent flying or diving

PHYSICAL EXAM
- Pneumatic otoscopy: May see retracted tympanic membrane, effusion, decreased drum movement
- Toynbee maneuver: View changes of the drum while patient autoinsufflates against closed lips and pinched nostrils. May show various degrees of retraction:
  - Entire drum may be retracted and "lateralize" with insufflation.
  - Posterosuperior quadrant (pars flaccida) may form a retraction pocket. Early on, this can be "lateralized" with autoinsufflation. If long-standing or severe, this pocket is well established and even may be scarred down to the middle ear mucosa, ossicles, or filled with cholesteatoma.
- Tuning fork tests: 512-Hz fork placed on the forehead lateralizes to affected ear (Weber test) and the fork will be louder behind the ear on the mastoid than in front of the ear (bone conduction > air conduction, Rinne test) in a conductive hearing loss
- Nasopharyngoscopy: Adenoid hypertrophy or nasopharyngeal mass
- Anterior rhinoscopy: Deviated nasal septum, polyps, mucosal hypertrophy, turbinate hypertrophy

DIAGNOSTIC TESTS & INTERPRETATION

Lab
None

Imaging
- Radiologic studies are not performed routinely if clinical signs/symptoms suggest ETD.
- CT scan may show middle ear/mastoid opacification or other sequelae of chronic ETD and OM.

Diagnostic Procedures/Surgery
- Audiogram may show conductive hearing loss.
- Tympanometry: Type B or C tympanograms indicate fluid or retraction, respectively. Negative middle ear peak pressures seen even with normal (type A) tympanograms.

DIFFERENTIAL DIAGNOSIS
- SSNHL (a medical emergency)
- Tympanic membrane perforation
- Barotrauma
- TMJ disorder
- Ménière disease
- Superior semicircular canal dehiscence

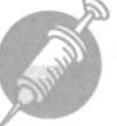

TREATMENT

- Reduce cycle of infection/inflammation.
- Tympanostomy tubes ± adenoidectomy when indicated for recurrent ear infections or severe progressive retractions

MEDICATION

- Few data exist to support pharmacologic treatments for ETD. Multiple retrospective Cochrane Reviews would argue against the use of decongestants, nasal steroids, or antihistamines for ETD (2)[A].
- Medication options below are provided for treatment of comorbid conditions; treat based on patient's symptoms and possible etiology.
- Decongestants, topical, oral (1)[C]:
  - Avoid prolonged use (>3 days) as can cause rhinitis medicamentosa
  - Decongestants are most useful for acute ETD related to a resolving URI.
  - Decongestants are not typically employed for relief of chronic ETD in children:
    - Phenylephrine (Dimetapp Cold Drops, PediaCare Children's Decongestant, Phenyl-T, Sudafed PE, Sudafed PE Congestion, Sudafed PE Quick Dissolve, Triaminic Thin Strips Cold) Adults and children >12 years: 1 (10 mg) tablet q4h PRN, children 6–11 years: 5 mg q4h PRN, children <4 years: 2.5 mg q4h PRN
    - Pseudoephedrine (Sudafed), Adults: 60 mg q4–6h PRN, children <12 years: 30 mg q4–6h PRN
    - Oxymetazoline (Afrin Nasal Spray), Adults and children >6 years: 1–2 sprays each nostril q12h PRN. Limit use to 3 days or less.
    - Phenylephrine (Neo-synephrine Nasal Spray) Adults: 1–2 sprays each nostril q4h PRN. Limit use to 3 days or less.
- Nasal steroids (may be beneficial for those with allergic rhinitis) (1)[B]:
  - Beclomethasone (Beconase, Vancenase), Adults and children >12 years: 1–2 sprays each nostril b.i.d., children 6-12 years: 1 spray each nostril b.i.d. Not recommended for children <6 years.
  - Budesonide (Rhinocort): Adults and children >6 years: 1 spray each nostril daily.
  - Ciclesonide (Omnaris) (a prodrug that is activated on nasal mucosa): Adults and children >6 years: 2 sprays each nostril daily.
  - Flunisolide (Nasarel, Nasalide): Adults and children >6 years: 2 sprays each nostril b.i.d.
  - Fluticasone furoate (Veramyst): Adults and children >12 years: 2 sprays each nostril daily, children 2–11 years: 1 spray each nostril daily.
  - Fluticasone propionate (Flonase): Adults 1–2 sprays each nostril daily, children >4 years: 1 spray each nostril daily.
  - Mometasone (Nasonex): Adults and children >12 years: 2 sprays each nostril daily, children 2–12 years: 1 spray each nostril daily. *Note: Only steroid nasal spray with indication for use in children ≥2 years.
  - Triamcinolone (Nasocort): Adults and children >6 years: 1–2 sprays each nostril daily, children 2–5 years: 1 spray each nostril daily
- Second-generation H_1 antihistamines (may be beneficial for those with ETD and chronic rhinitis) (1)[B]:
  - Cetirizine (Zyrtec) (tablets, chewable tablets or liquid available): Adults and children >6 years: 5–10 mg PO daily, children 6 months–5 years: 2.5–5 mg PO daily or divided b.i.d.
  - Desloratadine (Clarinex) (tablets, redi-tabs and liquid available): Adults and children >12 years: 5 mg PO daily, children 6–11 years: 2.5 mg PO daily, children 12 months-5 years: 1.25 mg PO daily, children 6–11 months: 1 mg PO daily
  - Fexofenadine (Allegra) (tablets, redi-tabs and liquid available): Adults and children >12 years: 60 mg PO b.i.d. or 180 mg PO daily, children 6–11 years: 30 mg PO b.i.d.
  - Levocetirizine (Xyzal) (tablets and liquid available): Adults and children >12 years: 2.5–5 mg PO every evening, children 6–11 years: 2.5 mg PO every evening, children 6 months–5 years: 1.25 mg PO every evening.
- Antihistamine nasal sprays (may be beneficial for those with ETD and chronic rhinitis):
  - Azelastine (Astepro or Astelin): Adults and children >12 years: 1–2 sprays each nostril b.i.d., children 6–11 years: 1 spray each nostril b.i.d.
  - Olopatadine (Patanase): Adults and children >12 years: 2 sprays each nostril b.i.d., children 6–11 years: 1 spray each nostril b.i.d.
- If ETD leads to OM associated with tympanic membrane perforation or if ventilation tube present, topical antibiotic drops are more efficacious than oral antibiotics (1)[A]:
  - Neomycin–polymyxin–hydrocortisone suspension (Cortisporin) 4 drops q.i.d. × 10 days
  - Ciprofloxacin–hydrocortisone suspension (Cipro HC) 5 drops b.i.d. × 7 days
  - Ofloxacin (Floxin): 5–10 drops b.i.d. × 10 days for acute otitis media
- Pain control, anti-inflammatory: Acetaminophen or other NSAIDs

SURGERY/OTHER PROCEDURES

- Myringotomy and pressure equalization tube placement to ventilate middle ear, relieve pressure, and prevent sequelae of chronically retracted drum (1)[A]
- Adenoidectomy if hypertrophied tissue is present:
  - In children, first set of tubes are typically placed alone. Adenoidectomy is performed in conjunction with second set of tubes if problems recur (1)[A].
  - Some advocate adenoidectomy even in absence of excess tissue; reduces frequency and number of subsequent tubes (3)[A].

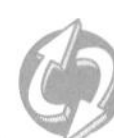

ONGOING CARE

FOLLOW-UP RECOMMENDATIONS

- Monitor pressure equalization tubes every 6–8 months in children and every 6–12 months in adults.
- Monitor tympanic membrane retraction pocket for progression every 6–12 months to allow for early intervention for progression in hearing loss, obvious ossicular erosion, or cholesteatoma.

DIET

- Generally no restrictions; avoid foods that would exacerbate reflux symptoms.
- In newborns, breast-feeding has been associated with a lower incidence of ETD and OM (1)[A].

PROGNOSIS

- May resolve with age in pediatric patients. If symptoms of ETD persist beyond age 7, patient is more likely to have long-term problems and require regular monitoring.
- For some, it is a chronic disorder; current treatments provide symptomatic relief; usually require prolonged use.

COMPLICATIONS

Morbidity related to hearing compromise or associated sequela of chronic ear infections

REFERENCES

1. Bluestone CD. Studies in otitis media: Children's Hospital of Pittsburgh-University of Pittsburgh progress report–2004. *Laryngoscope*. 2004;114: 1–26.
2. Simpson SA, Lewis R, van der Voort J, et al. Oral or topical nasal steroids for hearing loss associated with otitis media with effusion in children. *Cochrane Database Syst Rev*. 2011;5.
3. Bluestone CD, Hebda PA, Alper CM, et al. Recent advances in otitis media. 2. Eustachian tube, middle ear, and mastoid anatomy; physiology, pathophysiology, and pathogenesis. *Ann Otol Rhinol Laryngol Suppl*. 2005;194:16–30.

ADDITIONAL READING

Seibert JW, Danner CJ. Eustachian tube dfunction and the middle ear. *Otolaryngol Clin North Am*. 2006; 39(6):1221–35.

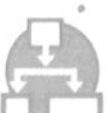

See Also (Topic, Algorithm, Electronic Media Element)

Algorithm: Ear Pain

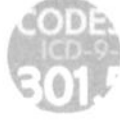

CODES

ICD9

- 381.60 Obstruction of Eustachian tube, unspecified
- 381.7 Patulous Eustachian tube
- 381.81 Dysfunction of Eustachian tube

CLINICAL PEARLS

- ETD can be an acute or chronic problem.
- Treatment is aimed at addressing potential contributing factors such as chronic rhinitis or GERD.
- SSNHL (medical emergency) can be misdiagnosed as ETD and should always be considered in the differential. A simple 512-Hz tuning fork test lateralizes to the opposite ear in sudden sensorineural hearing loss and to the affected ear in ETD with conductive hearing loss.

FACTITIOUS DISORDER/MÜNCHAUSEN SYNDROME

Irene C. Coletsos, MD
William G. Elder, Jr., PhD
Harold J. Bursztajn, MD

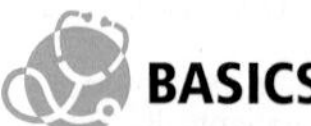

BASICS

DESCRIPTION

- Patients appear ill because they are feigning, exaggerating, or inducing symptoms.
- This is a mental disorder. These patients have an abnormal need for a sick role. They are *aware* that they are not ill, they are *aware* that their symptoms are not real, but will deny this.
- May come to light when there is a disease history stated in absence of symptoms, when symptom patterns are puzzling, or when there are nonhealing or unremitting symptoms despite repeated adequate and correct treatments.
- In factitious disorder by proxy, or Münchausen by proxy, an individual falsifies or induces illness in another person to vicariously accrue emotional payoffs, including sympathy, admiration, and/or feelings of power over care providers. Children are the usual victims and the mother is the usual perpetrator. The updated term for this activity is medical child abuse.
- Types of factitious disorder:
  - Factitious disorder with predominantly physical signs and symptoms:
    - Typically simulates one physical disease
  - Factitious disorder with predominantly psychological signs and symptoms:
    - These patients mimic the behavior of people with mental illnesses, claiming they are hearing voices or having visual hallucinations. In Ganser syndrome, patients may also give wrong answers to simple questions to support the image that they are mentally ill.
  - Münchausen syndrome is an extreme form usually with predominantly physical symptoms. Patients spend much of their lives seeking medical care from different providers and hospitals (changing hospitals when treatment is refused) and are willing to undergo painful procedures and surgeries to maintain their sick role. Named after an 18th-century nobleman who told tall tales.

EPIDEMIOLOGY

Incidence

Estimates vary on the incidence of medical child abuse. In the US, an estimated 200 new cases of serious abuse are expected to be uncovered yearly.

Prevalence

Factitious disorder with predominantly physical signs and symptoms: ~1–5% of people presenting with medical illness, according to some studies, but hard to estimate due to the secretive nature of the disorder. Identified as the probable cause of 3–9% of fevers of unknown origin in prospective studies.

RISK FACTORS

- Abuse/deprivation in childhood
- Childhood traumas, including hospitalizations
- Growing up with ill or emotionally unavailable caretakers
- Experience as health care professional
- Female gender 2:1 in factitious disorder
- Male gender 2:1 Münchausen syndrome
- Most by-proxy presentations involve a mother inducing symptoms in a child. Siblings of children known to have suffered this type of abuse are also at grave risk.

ETIOLOGY

- The psychological basis is thought to be an unresolved sense of deprivation from childhood that, in a time of stress in adulthood, leads to a false claim of medical illness in order to get care. In Münchausen, this behavior is chronic.
- Personality predisposition and shaping may be factors, evident in the high degree of deceitfulness, seeming lack of remorse, disregard for safety, inability to manage work and interpersonal situations, and unwillingness to conform to social norms.

COMMONLY ASSOCIATED CONDITIONS

- History of many medical procedures
- Substance abuse
- Suicide attempts
- Psychiatric comorbidities, including adjustment disorder, borderline personality disorder, depression, somatoform disorder, eating disorders
- In medical child abuse, the siblings of the currently affected child may have been improperly diagnosed with rare, intractable conditions or may even have died.
- Delusional disorder

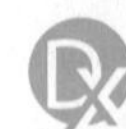

DIAGNOSIS

HISTORY

- A patient will relate a history of disease symptoms, often with "classic" textbook details, but has no signs of disease on examination. Or, if signs are noted, there may be evidence they were self-inflicted or are not medically caused.
- Careful elicitation of the developmental history may reveal early abuse or deprivations (1)[C].

PHYSICAL EXAM

- Normal, or evidence of self-inflicted wounds, such as scars
- Old wound with fresh bleeding (1)[C]
- Abscesses and rashes on body areas reachable by the patient. Areas not reachable by the patient are spared.
- Tenderness on palpation (while no tenderness noted by patient when the same areas are auscultated with pressure applied)

DIAGNOSTIC TESTS & INTERPRETATION

Lab

- Abnormal urine studies not reproducible if the patient is directly observed. (Patients may surreptitiously heat their thermometers or contaminate urine specimens.)
- Skin infection (abscesses, IV sites, Foley sites): Culture may show infection via *E. coli,* presumably a patient's own fecal material.
- Repeated blood cultures showing uncommon pathogens in a patient who is immunocompetent and has no history of IV drug use (2)[C]
- Lab results fail to show the expected disease markers suggested by the reported symptoms.
- Agents taken to mimic disease states (insulin, to produce hypoglycemia; thyroxine or Cytomel to produce hyperthyroidism; laxative or diuretics, to produce hypokalemia; self-injection of epinephrine or isoproterenol hydrochloride, to mimic Cushing disease; warfarin, to produce bleeding; quinidine, to produce purpura; alkylating agents, to produce pancytopenia)

Diagnostic Procedures/Surgery

- Patients often undergo many diagnostic or surgery procedures before the psychological nature of their illness is discovered. Procedures are often welcomed by the patient and, in the cases of medical child abuse, by the patient's caregiver. Avoid if possible.
- Psychological testing (3)[B]:
  - The Minnesota Multiphasic Personality Inventory, neuropsychological tests, and forensic tests are sensitive to faking and identify unusual profiles associated with factitious disorders.
- Cameras and other means of surveillance have frequently been used accidentally or purposely to detect patients (or parents) feigning (or inflicting) illnesses. Check with hospital attorney.

DIFFERENTIAL DIAGNOSIS

- Factious disorders are mental disorders where the patient has an abnormal need to maintain a sick role. Factitious disorders may be contrasted with other mental disorders where symptoms are beyond the patient's control, such as delusional disorders with bizarre somatic beliefs, and somatoform disorders where the patient has, and experiences, symptoms for psychological reasons:
  - In hypochondriasis the person believes or fears that they have a disorder. They are also anxious.
  - Somatization disorder involves recurrent physical symptoms where these symptoms cannot be explained fully by physical disorder. This often begins in late adolescence and worsens in times of stress.
  - Conversion disorder manifests in pseudoneurological symptoms classically originating from an unconscious psychological conflict.
- Shared paranoid disorder
- Factitious disorders may be contrasted with malingering, where secondary gain is sought (e.g., as a financial settlement, or to avoid responsibility). Malingering is the result of a conscious decision.
- Cultural differences in expressing pain and experiencing illness
- Occult medical illness (early stages of disease when blood tests may still show negative results)
- Unusual presentations of disease
- False-negative lab results
- For factitious disorder with predominantly psychological signs and symptoms, consider other medical etiologies:
  - Drug use, ingested as prescribed, or abused (e.g., benzodiazepines, cocaine, PCP, steroids), as well as drug withdrawal
  - Poisoning (alcohol, lead, mercury)
  - Stroke or traumatic brain injury
  - Also consider:
    - Infection (especially sepsis)
    - Postsurgical anesthesia
    - Pneumonia (especially in older patients)
    - UTI (especially in older patients)
    - Thiamine deficiency/Wernicke encephalopathy

ALERT

- Factitious disorder (or Münchausen syndrome) by proxy is a form of abuse.
- Parent may injure their child and then bring the child to care with a false history.
- Medical caregivers can help protect children by noting several warning signs, and being cautious about further testing and procedures for a child if: a child's disease is chronic, confusing, or unresponsive to treatment; a parent refuses to allow you to communicate with the child's other providers; a parent appears overly comfortable in the hospital setting, and not saddened or frightened by the child's illnesses. Always be aware of whether you are "treating" a parent's anxiety/demands vs. doing what is best for the child.
- A child in this situation may become quite ill, can have frequent hospitalizations, and may die from injuries.
- Older children who are victims of Münchausen by proxy may collude with the care provider who is victimizing them to maintain their relationship with the care provider (4)[C].
- Take steps to protect the child and siblings. Medical providers are legally required to report this and other types of abuse. Most experts recommend a multisystem approach that includes separating children from the abuser; therapy for the abuser, the abuser's significant other, and children; court monitoring to determine when/if the abuser can be reunited with children; medical monitoring to make sure future medical care for the child is warranted (and not part of an on-going abuse). Visits between the abuser and child can be therapeutic, but all must be carefully monitored to prevent the abuser from giving the child any food/drinks or medicine (5).

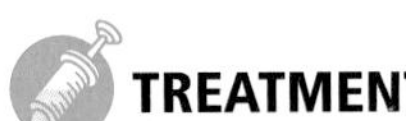

TREATMENT

ADDITIONAL TREATMENT

General Measures

- When possible, review medical and mental health records and mental health history. Mental disorders may be initially denied (3)[B].
- In cases of known or suspected factitious disorder, emergency department providers protect the patients (and protect themselves legally) by proceeding with the necessary treatment (e.g., if the patient has swallowed a foreign object, consult GI), putting the patient under observation during the hospital stay (to avoid having the patient inflict further self-injury), and consulting psychiatry as part of the treatment plan (6)[C].
- Management may be limited to clinician recognition of the disorder and making sure patients are not offered unnecessary drugs, risky procedures, or surgeries (7).
- Directly confronting patients ("You did this to yourself!") is usually met with angry denial. The patients often leave and try to get the treatment they had wanted from other providers and hospitals. Face-saving techniques that allow patients to give up their symptoms without being humiliated are thought to be more effective (8)[C].
- For example:
  - Patients with factitious disorder may accept a frank but empathetic assessment that their actions themselves constitute the disorder (6).
  - Use supportive measures such as regularly scheduled visits to help demonstrate that the patient's relationship with the provider does not have to be based on the conscious production of symptoms.
  - The Inexact Interpretation method may eventually help the patient begin to understand that the self-harm is part of a pattern of trying to cope with (usually) unresolved childhood stresses, without directly accusing them of the self-harm. This type of interaction has been found to advance the therapy and can help lessen the inclination to self-harm (8)[C].
  - A double-blind diagnostic explanation may assist remission (8)[C]. The clinician should perform a thorough physical examination and go through a rapport-building interview. The diagnosis is then delivered in 2 parts:
    - Part 1: "Sometimes people do things to make themselves ill. We call doing that factitious disorder."
    - Part 2: "Your problem is unusual and I believe it will respond to 1 more attempt to treat it. If that doesn't improve it, it is likely that you have a factitious disorder." The *medical* therapy should be a benign one, such as biofeedback, self-hypnosis, or, in the case of a "nonhealing" skin wound (due to a patient's persistent reinfecting of it), a skin graft and antibiotics.
- In treating perpetrators of by proxy/medical child abuse: They must be able to admit what they have done, have an appropriate emotional response, have strategies in place to treat their own emotional issues without abusing those they care for, and can demonstrate, over time (6–12 months), that they have put those strategies in place. The clinician advising the court on possible reunification of the abuser and child(ren) should be different from the one offering therapy. Despite therapy, relapse risk is high (9).
- Be aware of the possibility of countertransference. Remain aware of personal responses and feelings toward these patients. Anger at these patients hinders the therapeutic alliance, and could lead to missed diagnoses. On the other hand, overidentification with these patients (who are often health care providers themselves) interferes with the timely identification of this syndrome and treatment (6)[C]. In all cases, consider consulting with a psychiatrist or psychologist (7)[B].

IN-PATIENT CONSIDERATIONS

Initial Stabilization

- Form an alliance with the patient, identifying their suffering.
- Seek a detailed history of childhood events. Health history of parents and siblings may reveal early traumas to the patient (3)[B].

Admission Criteria

- Suicidality (10)[C]
- In by proxy/medical child abuse cases, children may have to be hospitalized for monitored detoxification from the unneeded medications they had been given.

Nursing

IV and other in-room equipment should be monitored for tampering.

ONGOING CARE

PROGNOSIS

- Fair to poor especially if etiology underlying the disorder cannot be addressed
- The long-term outcomes of patients with untreated factitious disorder have been judged to be worse than those with other severe mental disorders such as schizophrenic, bipolar, and delusional disorders.

COMPLICATIONS

Patient illness or death from self-harm and unnecessary medical interventions

REFERENCES

1. Peebles R, Sabella C, Franco K, et al. Factitious disorder and malingering in adolescent girls: Case series and literature review. *Clin Pediatr*. 2005; 44(3):237–43.
2. Galanos J, Perera S, Smith H, et al. Bacteremia due to three *Bacillus* species in a case of Munchausen's syndrome. *J Clin Microbiol*. 2003;41:2247–8.
3. Binder LM, Campbell KA. Medically unexplained symptoms and neuropsychological assessment. *J Clin Experiment Neuropsychol*. 2004;26(3): 369–92.
4. Awadallah N, Vaughan A, Franco K, et al. Munchausen by proxy: A case, chart series, and literature review of older victims. *Child Abuse Negl*. 2005;29:931–41.
5. Schreier H, et al. On the importance of motivation in Munchausen by Proxy: The case of Kathy Bush. *Child Abuse Negl*. 2002;26:537–49.
6. Jagoda P. Factitious disorder in the emergency department. *Primary Psychiatry*. 2009;16(1):61–6.
7. Krahn LE, Li H, O'Connor MK. Patients who strive to be ill: Factitious disorder with physical symptoms. *Am J Psychiatry*. 2003;160(6):1163–8.
8. Eisendrath SJ. Factitious physical disorders. *West J Med*. 1994;160:177–9.
9. Sanders MJ, Bursch B, et al. Forensic assessment of illness falsification, Munchausen by proxy, and factitious disorder, NOS. *Child Maltreat*. 2002;7: 112–24.
10. Johnson BR, Harrison JA. Suspected Munchausen's syndrome and civil commitment. *J Am Acad Psychiatry Law*. 2000;28:74–6.

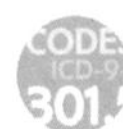

CODES

ICD9

- 300.16 Factitious disorder with predominantly psychological signs and symptoms
- 300.19 Other and unspecified factitious illness
- 301.51 Chronic factitious illness with physical symptoms

CLINICAL PEARLS

- Atypical emotional responses to illness are telling.
- Respond as you would to someone who cannot control self-harm rather than someone who wants to deceive you.
- In cases of by proxy disorders/medical child abuse, watch for children growing more ill after parental visits.

F

FACTOR V LEIDEN

Marc Jeffrey Kahn, MD, MBA
Rebecca Kruse-Jarres, MD, MPH

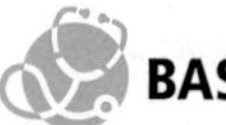

BASICS

DESCRIPTION

- Factor V Leiden is a genetic disease that is the most common hereditary cause of venous thrombosis. It leads to resistance to activated protein C.
- System(s) affected: Cardiovascular; Gastrointestinal; Hemic/Lymphatic/Immunologic; Nervous; Pulmonary; Reproductive
- Synonym(s): Factor V Leiden thrombophilia; Factor V Leiden mutation

Pediatric Considerations

Increased thrombosis risk in patients with factor V Leiden

Pregnancy Considerations

Heterozygous patients are not at increased risk for thromboembolism or fetal loss.

EPIDEMIOLOGY

- Predominant age: Thrombosis typically occurs after the second decade.
- Predominant sex: Male = Female

Prevalence

- ~3–12% of Caucasians are affected:
  - The mutation is rare in other ethnic groups, but has been reported in African and Native Americans.
- ~15–20% of patients who present with thrombosis have factor V Leiden.

RISK FACTORS

- Risk for venous embolism is 2.7-fold in heterozygous and 18-fold in homozygous factor V Leiden individuals, compared with individuals without the mutation.
- Oral contraceptives increase the risk of thrombosis:
  - In homozygotes, the risk increases 100-fold; in heterozygotes, 35-fold.
  - The increased risk is halved when the patient uses desogestrel-containing oral contraceptives.
- Hormone replacement therapy (HRT) and selective estrogen receptor modulators (SERMs) both increase the risk of thrombosis, and in patients with factor V Leiden, that risk is increased substantially.
- Pregnancy and homozygous factor V Leiden increase the risk of thrombosis 7–16-fold during pregnancy and the puerperium. Other complications of pregnancy may be increased in patients with factor V Leiden.
- Recurrence risk after an initial thrombosis is not increased in individuals who are heterozygous for factor V Leiden mutation. Data is conflicting in individuals who are homozygous, but it may not be increased (1).

Genetics

- Deep and superficial thrombosis of the venous system occurs with an odds ratio of 50–100 times greater for homozygotes.
- The odds ratio is closer to 2.5 times greater for heterozygotes.

GENERAL PREVENTION

Patients with factor V Leiden without thrombosis do not require prophylactic anticoagulation.

PATHOPHYSIOLOGY

- Point mutation causing substitution of arginine for glycine in residue 506 of factor V gene, rendering it less susceptible to inactivation by activated protein C
- Activated protein C is generated when protein C binds to its endothelial receptor, thrombomodulin.
- Activated protein C and its cofactor, protein S, lead to inactivation of factors V and VIII.
- Factor V Leiden is the most common cause of resistance to activated protein C.

ETIOLOGY

Genetic defect

COMMONLY ASSOCIATED CONDITIONS

Venous thrombosis

DIAGNOSIS

HISTORY

- Previous thrombosis
- Family history of thrombosis
- Family history of factor V Leiden mutation

PHYSICAL EXAM

- Arterial thrombosis is rare in adults with factor V Leiden.
- Thrombosis in unusual locations, such as the sagittal sinus, mesentery, and portal systems, is less common in patients with factor V Leiden than in patients with deficiency of protein C or S.
- Obstetric complications and venous thrombosis are increased in patients with factor V Leiden, and especially in those taking oral contraceptives.

DIAGNOSTIC TESTS & INTERPRETATION

Lab

Initial lab tests

- For evaluation of new clot in patient at risk: CBC with peripheral smear, PT/INR, aPTT, thrombin time, lupus anticoagulant, antiphospholipid antibodies, factor VIII, anticardiolipin antibody, anti-B2 glycoprotein I antibody, activated protein C resistance, protein S antigen and resistance, antithrombin III assay, fibrinogen, factor V Leiden, prothrombin G20210A, homocysteine
- Genetic test: DNA-based test for factor V mutation; is reliable while on anticoagulation
- Functional test: Plasma-based coagulation assay using factor V–deficient plasma to which patient plasma is added along with purified activated protein C. The relative prolongation of the activated partial thromboplastin time (aPTT) is used to assay for the defect. May be unreliable while taking heparin products (2).

Imaging

Initial approach

- Extremity ultrasound for deep vein thrombosis (DVT)
- V/Q scan of spiral CT for pulmonary embolism (PE)

Follow-Up & Special Considerations

- Ultrasound may not show DVT acutely; repeat in 1–2 days if strong suspicion.
- V/Q scan may be difficult to interpret in patients with other lung disease.

Diagnostic Procedures/Surgery

Magnetic resonance angiography (MRA), venography, or arteriography to detect thrombosis

Pathological Findings

Venous thrombus

DIFFERENTIAL DIAGNOSIS

- Protein C deficiency
- Protein S deficiency
- Antithrombin deficiency
- Other causes of activated protein C resistance (e.g., antiphospholipid antibodies)
- Dysfibrinogenemia
- Dysplasminogenemia
- Homocystinemia
- Prothrombin 20210 mutation
- Elevated factor VIII levels

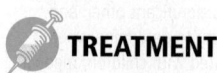

TREATMENT

Indicated for thrombosis

MEDICATION

First Line

- Low-molecular-weight heparin (LMWH) (2)[A]:
  - Enoxaparin (Lovenox): 1 mg/kg SC b.i.d., start warfarin simultaneously, continue Lovenox for at least 5 days and until international normalized ratio (INR) is >2, at which time it can be stopped
  - Fondaparinux (Arixtra): 7.5 mg SC daily
  - Tinzaparin (Innohep): 175 anti-Xa IU/kg SC daily for 6 days and patient is adequately anticoagulated with warfarin (INR of at least 2 for 2 consecutive days)
  - Dalteparin (Fragmin): 200 IU/kg SC daily
- Oral anticoagulant:
  - Warfarin (Coumadin) 5 mg daily PO initially and adjusted to an INR of 2–3
- Contraindications:
  - Active bleeding precludes anticoagulation (2)[A].
  - Risk of bleeding is a relative contraindication to long-term anticoagulation (2)[A].
  - Warfarin is contraindicated in patients with history of warfarin skin necrosis (2)[A].
  - Warfarin is contraindicated in pregnancy.

- Precautions:
  - Observe patient for signs of embolization, further thrombosis, or bleeding.
  - Avoid IM injections. Periodically check stool and urine for occult blood; monitor CBCs, including platelets.
  - Heparin: Thrombocytopenia and/or paradoxic thrombosis with thrombocytopenia
  - Warfarin: Necrotic skin lesions (typically breasts, thighs, or buttocks)
  - LMWH: Adjust dosage in renal insufficiency. May also need dose adjustment in pregnancy (check anti-Xa level).
- Significant possible interactions:
  - Agents that intensify the response to oral anticoagulants: Alcohol, allopurinol, amiodarone, anabolic steroids, androgens, many antimicrobials, cimetidine, chloral hydrate, disulfiram, all NSAIDs, sulfinpyrazone, tamoxifen, thyroid hormone, vitamin E, ranitidine, salicylates, acetaminophen
  - Agents that diminish the response to anticoagulants: Aminoglutethimide, antacids, barbiturates, carbamazepine, cholestyramine, diuretics, griseofulvin, rifampin, oral contraceptives

Second Line

- Heparin 80 mg/kg IV bolus followed by 18 g/kg/hr continuous infusion
- Adjust dose depending on aPTT.
- In patients requiring large daily doses of heparin, measure an anti-Xa level for dose guidance.
- Alternatively, unfractionated heparin can be given at 35,000 U/d SC, with subsequent dosing to maintain a therapeutic aPTT (3)[C].

ADDITIONAL TREATMENT

General Measures

- Patients with factor V Leiden and a first thrombosis should be anticoagulated initially with heparin or LMWH (4)[A].
- Treatment with LMWH is recommended over unfractionated heparin, unless the patient has severe renal failure (3)[B].
- Treat as outpatient, if possible (3)[B].
- Initiate warfarin with heparin on the first treatment day, and discontinue heparin after 5 days and when INR >2 (3)[A].
- Patients should be maintained on warfarin with an INR of 2–3 for at least 6 months (3)[A].
- Recurrent thrombosis requires indefinite anticoagulation (4)[B].
- Compression stockings for prevention

Issues for Referral

- Recurrent thrombosis on anticoagulation
- Difficulty anticoagulating
- Genetic counseling

SURGERY/OTHER PROCEDURES

- Anticoagulation must be held for surgical interventions.
- For most patients with deep vein thrombosis (DVT), recommendations are against routine use of vena cava filter in addition to anticoagulation (3)[A].
- Thrombectomy may be necessary in some cases.

IN-PATIENT CONSIDERATIONS

Initial Stabilization

Heparin

Admission Criteria

Complicated thrombosis, such as pulmonary embolus

Nursing

- Teach LMWH and warfarin use.
- See above for drug interactions.

Discharge Criteria

Stable on anticoagulation

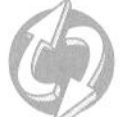

ONGOING CARE

FOLLOW-UP RECOMMENDATIONS

Patient Monitoring

Warfarin use requires periodic (~monthly after initial stabilization) INR measurements, with a goal of 2–3 (2)[A].

DIET

- No restrictions
- Large amounts of foods rich in vitamin K may interfere with anticoagulation with warfarin.

PATIENT EDUCATION

- Patients should be educated about:
  - Use of oral anticoagulant therapy
  - Avoidance of NSAIDs while on warfarin
- The role of family screening is unclear, as most patients with this mutation do not have thrombosis. In a patient with a family history of factor V Leiden, consider screening during pregnancy or if considering oral contraceptive use.

PROGNOSIS

- Most patients heterozygous for factor V Leiden do not have thrombosis.
- Homozygotes have about a 50% lifetime incidence of thrombosis.
- Recurrence rates after a first thrombosis are not clear, with some investigators finding rates as high as 5% and others finding rates similar to the general population.
- Despite the increased risk for thrombosis, factor V Leiden does not increase overall mortality.

COMPLICATIONS

- Recurrent thrombosis
- Bleeding on anticoagulation

REFERENCES

1. Lijfering WM, Middeldorp S, Veeger NJ, et al. Risk of recurrent venous thrombosis in homozygous carriers and double heterozygous carriers of factor V Leiden and prothrombin G20210A. *Circulation*. 2010;121:1706–12.
2. Moll S. Thrombophilias–practical implications and testing caveats. *J Thromb Thrombolysis*. 2006;21: 7–15.
3. Büller HR, Agnelli G, Hull RD, et al. Antithrombotic therapy for venous thromboembolic disease: The Seventh ACCP Conference on Antithrombotic and Thrombolytic Therapy. *Chest*. 2004;126:401S–28S.
4. Kim RJ, Becker RC. Association between factor V Leiden, prothrombin G20210A, and methylenetetrahydrofolate reductase C677T mutations and events of the arterial circulatory system: A meta-analysis of published studies. *Am Heart J*. 2003;146:948–57.

ADDITIONAL READING

Seligsohn U, Lubetsky A. Genetic susceptibility to venous thrombosis. *N Engl J Med*. 2001;344: 1222–31.

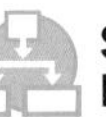

See Also (Topic, Algorithm, Electronic Media Element)

Deep Vein Thrombophlebitis (DVT)

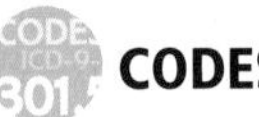

CODES

ICD9

289.81 Primary hypercoagulable state

CLINICAL PEARLS

- Extremely rare in Asian and African populations
- Asymptomatic patients with factor V Leiden do not need anticoagulation.

FAILURE TO THRIVE (FTT)

Keith Nokes, MD, MPH

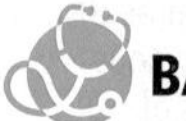

BASICS

DESCRIPTION

- Failure to thrive (FTT) is not a diagnosis but is a sign of inadequate nutrition in young children manifested by a failure of physical growth, usually affecting weight. In severe cases, decreased length and/or head circumference may develop.
- Various parameters are used to define FTT:
  - Weight for age less than fifth percentile on >1 occasion
  - Weight that drops 2 or more major percentile lines on standard growth charts
  - Weight <80% median weight for length
  - Weight <75% median weight for age
  - Weight for length less than fifth percentile
  - Height for age less than fifth percentile
- Weight for length may be the simplest method to identify FTT, but verify with other parameters.

Pediatric Considerations

- Children with genetic syndromes, intrauterine growth restriction (IUGR), or prematurity follow different growth curves.
- ~25% of children will decrease their weight or height crossing 2 or more major percentile lines in the first 2 years of life. These children are falling to their genetic potential or demonstrating constitutional growth delay (slow growth with a bone age < chronologic age). After shifting down, these infants grow at a normal rate along their new percentile and do not have FTT.

EPIDEMIOLOGY

Incidence

- Predominant age: 6–12 months; 80% <18 months
- Predominant sex: Male = Female

Prevalence

- As many as 10% of children seen in primary care have signs of growth failure.
- 1–5% of pediatric inpatient admissions are for FTT.

RISK FACTORS

- Psychosocial risks:
  - Poverty, parent(s) with mental health disorder or cognitive impairment, parent(s) with poor parenting skills or hypervigilant parents, families with unique health/nutritional beliefs, history of physical or emotional abuse, substance abuse, and social isolation
- Medical risks:
  - Intrauterine exposures, history of IUGR (symmetric or asymmetric), congenital abnormalities, oromotor dysfunction, premature or sick newborn, infant with physical deformity, acute or chronic medical conditions, developmental delay

Pregnancy Considerations

FTT is linked to intrauterine exposures, IUGR, and prematurity.

Genetics

Multiple genetic disorders can cause FTT.

GENERAL PREVENTION

- Educate parents on normal feeding and parenting skills
- Family support
- Access to supplemental feeding programs (WIC)

PATHOPHYSIOLOGY

- Mismatch between caloric intake and caloric expenditure
- Often grouped into 4 major categories:
  - Inadequate caloric intake (most frequent)
  - Inadequate caloric absorption
  - Excessive caloric expenditure
  - Defective utilization

ETIOLOGY

- Traditionally, FTT was classified as organic or nonorganic, but most cases are a combination of these factors.
- FTT often begins with a specific event, illness, or problem with transition. However, the caregivers and child may subsequently develop interaction difficulties that also need to be addressed.
- Causes of FTT can be grouped by pathophysiology (including examples):
  - Inadequate intake: Breast-feeding difficulty, incorrect formula preparation, poor transition to food (6–12 months), poor feeding habits (e.g., excessive juice, restrictive diets), mechanical problems (e.g., oromotor dysfunction, congenital anomalies, GERD, CNS or PNS anomalies), oral aversion, poverty, neglect, poor parent–child interaction
  - Inadequate absorption: Necrotizing enterocolitis, short gut syndrome, biliary atresia, liver disease, cystic fibrosis, celiac disease, milk protein allergy, vitamin/mineral deficiency
  - Increased expenditure: Hyperthyroidism, congenital/chronic cardiopulmonary disease, HIV, immunodeficiencies, malignancy, renal disease
  - Defective utilization: Metabolic disorders, congenital infections (TORCH)

DIAGNOSIS

HISTORY

- Prenatal and developmental history
- Past medical history: Acute/chronic disease affecting caloric intake, digestion, absorption, or causing increased energy need or defective utilization
- Medication history, including complementary and alternative medications
- Family history: Stature of parents and growth trajectories of siblings; chronic diseases; genetic disorders; developmental delay
- Diet history from birth: Breast or formula feeding; timing and introduction of solids; who feeds the child, when, and how often; placement of child during feeds; amounts consumed/caloric intake; beverages consumed; snacking; vomiting or stooling associated with feeds; oral aversions or unusual behaviors during feeding
- Social history: Family composition, socioeconomic status, child-rearing beliefs, stressors, parental depression, parental substance abuse, caretaker personal history of abuse/neglect
- Review of systems: Anorexia, activity level, mental status, fevers, dysphagia, vomiting, gastroesophageal reflux (GER), stooling pattern/consistency, dysuria, urinary frequency

PHYSICAL EXAM

- *Accurate* measurement of height, weight, and head circumference on National Center for Health Statistics (NCHS) growth charts (www.cdc.gov/growthcharts)
- The World Health Organization (WHO) growth charts may be more appropriate for breast-fed infants (www.who.int/childgrowth/standards/en/), and growth charts exist for many other syndromes/conditions such as Down syndrome, Turner syndrome, and premature infant.
- Exam should assess for the following:
  - Signs of dehydration or severe malnutrition:
    - Severity of malnutrition estimated via Gomez classification: Compare current weight for age with expected weight for age (50th percentile): Severe: <60% of expected; Moderate: 61–75%; Mild: 76–90%
  - Underlying medical disease
  - Dysmorphic features
  - Mental status (alert, responsive to stimuli)
  - Any signs of physical abuse and/or neglect
- Observe interaction with caregivers and feeding techniques, specifically bonding and social/psychological cues.

DIAGNOSTIC TESTS & INTERPRETATION

- Review newborn screening results in infants.
- Labs useful only in about 1% of cases, and usually those cases where underlying disease is suspected.
- A period of renutrition is preferable prior to extensive lab workup.

Lab

Labs should be ordered based on history and physical exam findings and the age of the patient.

Initial lab tests

- Tests often included in initial evaluation:
  - CBC
  - Electrolytes, BUN/creatinine, liver function tests
  - Urinalysis and urine culture
  - ESR
  - Lead level
- Other tests as dictated by the history and exam:
  - Thyroid-stimulating hormone (TSH), amylase/lipase, serum zinc level, iron studies, karyotype, genetic testing, sweat chloride test, stool for ova and parasite or fat/reducing substances, guaiac, alpha-1-antitrypsin and elastase, RAST testing for IgE food allergies, tissue transglutaminase and total IgA (celiac sprue), P-ANCA and ASCA (anti-*Saccharomyces cerevisiae* antibodies for IBD), TB test, HIV ELISA, hepatitis A, B, other infections

Follow-Up & Special Considerations

- Evaluation should include a home visit by the PCP or other clinician to observe infant feeding, interaction with caretakers, and home environment.
- Observe breast-feeding and/or formula preparation to ensure adequacy and offer instruction.
- Prospective 3-day food diary for accurate record of caloric intake should be obtained.
- Additional indicated evaluations may be performed by dietitians, occupational, physical and speech therapists, social workers, developmental specialists, psychiatrists, psychologists, visiting nurses, lactation consultants, and/or child protection services.

Imaging

Not routine. Performed only as indicated by specific history or physical exam findings.

Follow-Up & Special Considerations

Can consider:

- Skeletal survey if suspicion of physical abuse
- Bone age if possible endocrine disorder

- Swallowing studies, small bowel follow-through if possible oromotor dysfunction, GERD, structural abnormalities
- Brain imaging if microcephalic and/or neurologic findings on examination

DIFFERENTIAL DIAGNOSIS

Differentiate based on growth patterns:

- FTT classically presents as low weight for age, normal linear growth, normocephalic *or* low weight for age, followed by decreased linear growth *or* low weight for age, leading to decreased linear growth and decreased head circumference (without neurologic signs):
  - In this situation, consider the differential diagnosis as outlined in "Etiology" above.
- If low linear growth with normal weight for length *or* low linear growth and proportionately low weight and decreased head circumference:
  - Consider genetic potential (constitutional short stature or growth delay), genetic syndromes, teratogens, endocrine disorders
- If microcephaly with prominent neurologic signs with poor growth secondary to presumed neurologic disorder:
  - Consider TORCH infections, genetic syndromes, teratogens, brain injury (i.e., hypoxic/ischemic)

TREATMENT

MEDICATION

Use only for identified underlying conditions

ADDITIONAL TREATMENT

General Measures

- Treat underlying conditions.
- The goal is to improve nutrition to allow catch-up growth (weight gain 2–3 times > average for age).
- Calculate energy needs based on recommended energy intake for age, increased by 50%:
  - Recommended energy intake (use *expected*, not actual weight, to calculate needs):
    - 0–1 month: 120 kcal/kg/d
    - 1–2 months: 115 kcal/kg/d
    - 2–3 months: 105 kcal/kg/d
    - 3–6 months: 95 kcal/kg/d
    - 6 months to 3 years: 90 kcal/kg/d (1)[C]
- Alternatively, may calculate caloric requirements for infants to achieve catch-up growth:
  - kcal/kg/d required = [RDA for age (kcal/kg) × Ideal wt. for ht.] / Actual wt., where ideal wt. for ht. is the median wt. for the patient's ht.
- Try various strategies to increase caloric intake:
  - Optimize breast-feeding support, consider supplementation
  - Higher-calorie formulas
  - Addition of rice cereal or fats to current foods
  - Limit intake of milk to 24–32 oz/d.
  - Avoid juice and soda.
  - Vitamin and/or nutritional supplements
  - Assist with social and family problems (WIC, food stamps, and other transitional assistance).
- Rapid high-calorie intake can cause diarrhea, malabsorption, hypokalemia, hypophosphatemia. Therefore, increasing formulas above 24 kcal/oz is not recommended.
- The target energy intake should be slowly increased to goal over 5–7 days.
- Catch-up growth should be seen in 2–7 days.
- Accelerated growth should be continued for 4–9 months to restore weight and height.

Issues for Referral

- Refer as indicated for underlying conditions.
- Multidisciplinary care is beneficial (2)[B]. Specialized multidisciplinary clinics may be of benefit for children with complicated situations, failure to respond to initial treatment, or when the PCP does not have access to specialized services such as nutrition, psychology, PT/OT, speech therapy, etc.

Additional Therapies

In severe cases, nasogastric (NG) tube feedings or gastrostomy may be considered.

IN-PATIENT CONSIDERATIONS

Most cases of FTT can be managed as outpatients.

Initial Stabilization

- During catch-up growth, some children will develop nutritional recovery syndrome:
  - Symptoms include sweating, increased body temperature, hepatomegaly (increased glycogen deposits), widening of cranial sutures (brain growth > bone growth), increased periods of sleep, fidgetiness, and mild hyperactivity.
- There may also be an initial period of malabsorption with resultant diarrhea.

Admission Criteria

Hospitalization should be considered if:

- Outpatient management fails.
- There is evidence of severe dehydration or malnutrition.
- There are signs of abuse or neglect.
- There are concerns that the psychosocial situation presents harm to child.

Discharge Criteria

Catch-up growth should be seen in 2–7 days. If this is not seen, re-evaluation of causes is needed.

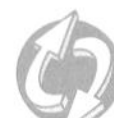

ONGOING CARE

FOLLOW-UP RECOMMENDATIONS

- If specific disease identified, follow-up as indicated.
- Close long-term follow-up with frequent visits is important to create and maintain a healthy, supportive environment.
- If the family fails to comply, child protection authorities must be notified.

DIET

Nutritional requirements for a "normal" child:

- Infant:
  - 120 kcal/kg/d, decreased to 95 kcal/kg/d at 6 months; if breast-fed, ensure appropriate frequency and duration of feeding.
  - Between 6 and 12 months, continue breast milk and/or formula, but pureed foods should be consumed several times a day during this period.
- Toddler:
  - 3 meals plus 2 nutritional snacks, 16–32 oz. milk/d, avoid juice and soda, and feed in a social environment.
  - Do not restrict fat and cholesterol in children <2 years old.
- Rate of weight gain expected for age:
  - 0–3 months: 26–31 g/d
  - 3–6 months: 17–18 g/d
  - 6–9 months: 12–13 g/d
  - 9–12 months: 9 g/d
  - 1–3 years: 7–9 g/d

PATIENT EDUCATION

- Families can be very anxious about poor infant growth. Counsel parents regarding the need to avoid "food battles," which worsen the problem.
- Educate parents regarding infant social and physiological cues, formula/food preparation, proper feeding techniques, and importance of relaxed and social mealtimes.
- When environmental deprivation is identified, educating in a nonpunitive way is essential.
- "Failure to Thrive: What This Means for Your Child," available from AAFP at: www.aafp.org/afp/2011/0401/p837.html
- The Women, Infants, and Children Program (WIC) provides grants to states for supplemental foods, health care referrals, and nutrition education for low-income pregnant, breast-feeding, and nonbreast-feeding postpartum women, and to infants and children up to age 5 at nutritional risk: www.fns.usda.gov/wic/

PROGNOSIS

- Many children with FTT show adequate improvement in dietary intake with intervention.
- Some studies looking at children with FTT have demonstrated an association with later problems with cognitive development, behavioral issues, and growth, but there is not a consensus on these long-term outcomes or their clinical significance (3).
- Children with FTT are at increased risk for future undernutrition, overnutrition, and eating disorders.

REFERENCES

1. Krugman SD, Dubowitz H. Failure to thrive. *Am Fam Physician*. 2003;68:879–84.
2. Cole SZ, Lanham JS. Failure to thrive: An update. *Am Fam Physician*. 2011;83(7):829–34.
3. Jaffe AC. Failure to thrive: Current clinical concepts. *Pediatr Rev*. 2011;32(3):100–7.

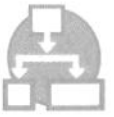

See Also (Topic, Algorithm, Electronic Media Element)

Down Syndrome; Irritable Bowel Syndrome; Turner Syndrome

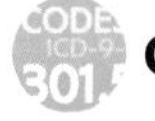

CODES

ICD9

- 783.41 Failure to thrive
- 783.7 Adult failure to thrive

CLINICAL PEARLS

- FTT is a sign of inadequate nutrition.
- Accurate and regularly measured weight, length, and head circumference are necessary to identify/evaluate FTT.
- Underlying medical issues are generally suggested by history and physical exam, and extensive laboratory or imaging tests are rarely needed.
- A multidisciplinary team approach to diagnosis and treatment is critical to help children with FTT and their families.

F

FATTY LIVER SYNDROME

Nilay Patel, MD
Edward Feller, MD

BASICS

Nonalcoholic fatty liver disease (NAFLD) describes a spectrum of fatty changes ranging from asymptomatic hepatic steatosis (fatty liver) to nonalcoholic steatohepatitis (NASH) and cirrhosis. NAFLD may be implicated in up to 90% of patients with asymptomatic, mild aminotransferase elevation not caused by alcohol, viral hepatitis, or medications. It may occur in 3–24% in the general population; increases to 58–74% of obese patients (1).

DESCRIPTION

- Fatty liver:
  - Reversible condition where large vacuoles of triglyceride fat accumulate in hepatocytes; liver biopsy diagnosis usually shows fatty deposits in >30% of liver cells; no necrosis, no fibrosis
  - ALT and AST enzymes usually normal, but may be elevated, rarely >3–4× the upper limit of normal
- NAFLD:
  - Fatty liver not due to excess alcohol consumption
  - Risk factors: Obesity, metabolic syndrome, dyslipidemia, insulin resistance, and type 2 diabetes
- NASH:
  - Progressive form of NAFLD; liver biopsy diagnosis of fatty deposits in >50% of liver cells associated with acute and chronic inflammation and fibrosis
  - Asymptomatic; ALT and AST elevated, generally <3–4× the upper limit of normal
  - Disease may progress to cirrhosis and/or hepatocellular cancer; incomplete data exist to assess natural history, although some evidence indicates that 30% with NASH have progression of fibrosis over 5 years.
- Both diseases usually identified in the fourth and fifth decade but may occur at any age
- Synonym(s): Steatosis; Steatonecrosis; Nonalcoholic fatty liver disease (NAFLD); Steatohepatitis; Nonalcoholic steatohepatitis (NASH)

Pregnancy Considerations

- A severe complication of third trimester is acute fatty liver of pregnancy. May be associated with signs of preeclampsia.
- Abrupt onset of confusion and restlessness with possible jaundice and right upper quadrant pain
- ALT, AST always elevated, usually <1,000 IU/L
- Emergency liver biopsy confirms diagnosis.
- Prompt delivery corrects the liver disease.
- Recurrence rare in subsequent pregnancies.

EPIDEMIOLOGY

NAFLD is the most common chronic liver disease globally, usually as benign, asymptomatic fatty liver (steatosis). NASH may be symptomatic with potential for progressive inflammation and fibrosis.

Incidence

- Present in up to 2/3 of obese (BMI >30) and in 90% of morbidly obese (BMI >39) persons
- Present in 5–10% type 2 DM patients
- Predominant age: 40s–50s; does occur in children
- Predominant sex: Male = Female

Prevalence

US prevalence is estimated at 6–24%

RISK FACTORS

- Obesity: BMI >30, DM, hypertension, hyperlipidemia (metabolic syndrome)
- Protein–calorie malnutrition
- TPN >6 weeks
- Severe acute weight loss, including starvation and bariatric surgery
- Organic solvent (e.g., chlorinated hydrocarbons, toluene) exposure; vinyl chloride; hypoglycin A
- Gene for hemochromatosis or other conditions with increased iron stores
- Drugs: Tetracycline, glucocorticoids, tamoxifen, methotrexate, valproic acid, fialuridine, most chemotherapy regimens, and nucleoside analogues

Pediatric Considerations

- Reye syndrome: Fatty liver with encephalopathy characterized by:
  - Vomiting with dehydration; usually postviral URI
  - Progressive CNS damage
  - Signs of hepatic injury: Liver morphologically shows extensive fatty vacuolization.
  - Hypoglycemia
- Etiology unknown; viral agents and drugs, especially salicylates, are implicated.
- Mortality rate 50%
- Tx: Mannitol, IV glucose, and FFP

Genetics

Largely unknown; carriers of hemochromatosis gene are more likely to be affected; possible genetic variants in the apolipoprotein C3 gene may play a role in fatty liver disease, insulin resistance, and hypertriglyceremia.

GENERAL PREVENTION

- Avoid excessive alcohol intake: >30 g/d for men, >20 g/d for women.
- Maintain or attain appropriate BMI.
- Avoid hepatotoxic medications.
- Obtain HAV and HBV vaccination if not immune.
- Obtain Pneumovax and yearly influenza vaccination.

PATHOPHYSIOLOGY

Primary derangement is *insulin resistance*, which leads to increased lipolysis, triglyceride synthesis, increased hepatic uptake of fatty acids.

ETIOLOGY

- NAFLD: Most commonly an impaired ability of the liver to remove fatty acids
- NASH: "2-hit" hypothesis involving macrovesicular steatosis due to increased hepatic lipid synthesis, reduced transfer of lipids from the liver, and increasing insulin resistance with increased hepatic oxidative stress (2). Mitochondrial damage leading to impaired restoration of ADT stores, lipid peroxidation, and increased iron stores each have been found in 25–40% of NASH patients.

COMMONLY ASSOCIATED CONDITIONS

Preeclampsia in pregnancy-related disease, central obesity, type 2 diabetes, insulin resistance, hyperlipidemia, hypertension

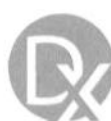

DIAGNOSIS

- Consider hepatic steatosis in any patient with asymptomatic aminotransferase elevation.
- Can occur with normal or fluctuating AST and ALT
- NASH has no distinguishing historical or laboratory features from other chronic liver disorders.
- Index of suspicion is higher with risk factors such as metabolic syndrome, insulin resistance, or obesity.
- Noninvasive biomarkers of steatosis or fibrosis are not sufficiently reliable. Liver biopsy is the definitive diagnostic test. Biopsy should be considered only when results are likely to change management.

HISTORY

Typically asymptomatic but some may experience fatigue and/or abdominal fullness.

PHYSICAL EXAM

Hepatomegaly: Incidentally observed enlarged liver or spleen on physical exam or imaging.

- Most common signs (each is infrequent):
  - Liver pain or tenderness
  - Mild to marked hepatomegaly
  - Splenomegaly
  - In advanced cases: Cutaneous stigmata of chronic liver disease or portal hypertension, variceal hemorrhage, ascites, hepatic encephalopathy, edema

DIAGNOSTIC TESTS & INTERPRETATION

Lab

- Both ALT and AST may be elevated:
  - Nonalcoholic, usually ALT:AST >1
  - If alcohol-induced, usually AST:ALT ≥2; serum alkaline phosphatase and direct bilirubin may be mildly elevated.
  - If advanced cirrhosis is present, marked, nonspecific enzyme abnormalities may exist.
- Level of enzyme elevation does not correlate with degree of fibrosis (3)[C].
- Severity in acute liver disease is marked by defects in ability to produce plasma proteins (serum albumin, prothrombin time), which are also clues to chronicity. Thrombocytopenia may indicate chronic liver disease and portal hypertension.
- Lipids almost always abnormal with elevated cholesterol, LDL, triglyceride, and decreased HDL
- Biomarkers of inflammation, increased oxidative stress or hepatocyte apoptosis such as leptin, adiponectin, CRP, serum caspase, and cytokeratin 18 remain investigational but may help differentiate NASH from NAFLD.

Initial lab tests

Serologic studies for viral hepatitis are vital: Serum ALT and AST, alkaline phosphatase, direct and total bilirubin, albumin and globulin, CBC, serum electrolytes, BUN, and creatinine.

Imaging

Initial approach

Fatty liver can be identified as hyperechoic liver on ultrasound, the first-line imaging modality for assessment of liver function abnormalities; MRI or CT may also be used.

Follow-Up & Special Considerations

- Imaging modalities such as Fibroscan, which detects tissue elasticity in cases of suspected hepatic fibrosis, and magnetic resonance spectroscopy are currently being evaluated (4)[B]. Newer contrast agents, particularly for MRI, are being evaluated to help characterize NAFLD (5).
- No imaging modality can distinguish between simple steatosis from steatohepatitis.

Diagnostic Procedures/Surgery

- Liver biopsy is the only reliable diagnostic method; however, it is not without risk, cost, and sampling error.
- Predictors associated with increased risk of fibrosis are BMI >30, age >50, insulin resistance or diabetes mellitus, and elevated serum ALT, AST.

Pathological Findings

- Liver biopsy is the gold standard to differentiate fatty liver with good prognosis from NASH (3)[B].
- In NASH, steatosis, ballooning, and lobular inflammation are minimal criteria for diagnosis; other common, but not necessary, findings include mild–moderate portal inflammation, acidophil bodies, perisinusoidal zone 3 fibrosis, megamitochondria, and Mallory hyaline in hepatocytes (6)[B].
- Staging is based largely on the extent of fibrosis.

DIFFERENTIAL DIAGNOSIS

- Viral hepatitis
- Alcoholic fatty liver (history of alcoholism may be difficult to document or exclude)
- Drug- or toxin-induced hepatitis
- Occupational exposure
- Metabolic liver disease
- Autoimmune hepatitis
- Celiac disease
- Muscle disease if nonhepatic cause of elevated enzymes are possible

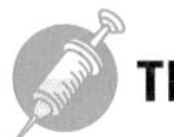

TREATMENT

Sustained weight loss has been the primary successful intervention in NASH. The most commonly cited recommendation is lifestyle modification through improved diet and regular exercise. Early promising results have been reported with weight loss pharmacotherapy and bariatric surgery. Studies assessing insulin-sensitizing and hepatoprotective agents are inconclusive; currently there is no proven medication treatment regimen.

MEDICATION

No specific therapy currently exists, but several promising agents are under investigation:

- There have been several studies that show drugs improving insulin resistance for patients with NAFLD may have a favorable role in decreasing aminotransferase levels and histologic evidence of disease, but they are not definitive. These include metformin and pioglitazone (7)[A].
- Vitamins E and C have shown mild improvement in hepatic steatosis and in inflammation, but results have not supported widespread utilization (8)[B]. New trials of vitamin E monotherapy and combination therapy are in progress (9).
- Several other drugs have been studied in small pilot trials and animal studies. These include fibrates, gemfibrozil, statins, omega-3 fatty acids, betaine, angiotensin-receptor blockers, and ursodeoxycholic acid. However, large randomized controlled studies have yet to be undertaken (8)[B].

ADDITIONAL TREATMENT

General Measures

- Aerobic exercise 3× weekly for 20–45 minutes or more
- DM should be tightly regulated.
- Components of metabolic syndrome (hypertension, dyslipidemia, and obesity) should be treated.
- Alcohol should be discontinued (3)[C].
- Avoid hepatotoxic medications.

Issues for Referral

Individuals with persistent liver enzyme elevation 2–3 times above the upper limit of normal or with fibrosis on biopsy benefit from hepatologist follow-up.

COMPLEMENTARY AND ALTERNATIVE MEDICINE

Be wary of potential hepatotoxicity of complementary medications, which may also contain impurities.

SURGERY/OTHER PROCEDURES

Bariatric procedures have been found to have a positive impact on NASH (3)[B]. Careful case selection assessing risk–benefit ratio is vital because natural history is generally uncomplicated. Bariatric surgery may be a more appropriate option with underlying morbid obesity (BMI >40) (9).

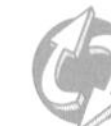

ONGOING CARE

FOLLOW-UP RECOMMENDATIONS

Patient Monitoring

- Repeat liver function tests yearly.
- Perform yearly US or CT scan to document diminution in fat.
- Changes toward normal provide major motivation to continue lifestyle changes.
- Routine liver biopsy is not recommended (3)[C].

DIET

Diet low in fat; low in simple carbohydrates; low in high fructose corn syrup; devoid of trans fats; replete with vitamins, minerals, and natural antioxidants; avoid alcohol

PATIENT EDUCATION

Planning for lifelong change in eating, exercise, and alcohol use is required.

PROGNOSIS

Within the spectrum of NALFD, only NASH has been convincingly shown to have a progressive course, potentially leading to cirrhosis, hepatocellular carcinoma, cholangiocarcinoma, or liver failure:

- Cirrhosis develops in up to 1/3 of patients with NASH within 10 years of follow-up, with liver failure from cirrhosis occurring in 1–5% (10).
- Transplantation is effective, but NASH may recur after transplantation (3)[C].

COMPLICATIONS

Progressive disease may be complicated by decompensated cirrhosis and portal hypertension, such as ascites, encephalopathy, bleeding varices, hepatorenal or hepatopulmonary syndromes.

REFERENCES

1. Foxx-Orenstein AE, et al. Gastrointestinal symptoms and diseases related to obesity: An overview. *Gastroenterol Clin North Am*. 2010;39: 23–37.
2. Edmison J, McCullough AJ, et al. Pathogenesis of non-alcoholic steatohepatitis: Human data. *Clin Liver Dis*. 2007;11:75–104, ix.
3. Ghali P, et al. The spectrum of nonalcoholic fatty liver disease. *J Clin Outcomes Managem*. 2005; 12:585–93.
4. Rafiq N, Younossi ZM, et al. Nonalcoholic fatty liver disease: A practical approach to evaluation and management. *Clin Liver Dis*. 2009;13: 249–66.
5. Browning JD, et al. New imaging techniques for non-alcoholic steatohepatitis. *Clin Liver Dis*. 2009; 13:607–19.
6. Brunt EM, et al. Nonalcoholic steatohepatitis. *Semin Liver Dis*. 2004;24:3–20.
7. Angelico F, Burattin M, Alessandri C, et al. Drugs improving insulin resistance for non-alcoholic fatty liver disease and/or nonalcoholic steatohepatitis. *Cochrane Database Syst Rev*. 2007;1:CD005166.
8. Torres D, Harrison S. Diagnosis and therapy of nonalcoholic steatohepatitis. *Gastroenterology*. 2008;134:1682–98.
9. Kadayifci A, Merriman RB, Bass NM, et al. Medical treatment of non-alcoholic steatohepatitis. *Clin Liver Dis*. 2007;11:119–40, ix.
10. Diehl AM, et al. Hepatic complications of obesity. *Gastroenterol Clin North Am*. 2005;34:45–61.
11. Schwimmer JB, Pardee PE, Lavine JE, et al. Cardiovascular risk factors and the metabolic syndrome in pediatric nonalcoholic fatty liver disease. *Circulation*. 2008;118:277–83.

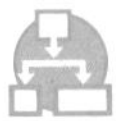

See Also (Topic, Algorithm, Electronic Media Element)

Alcohol Abuse and Dependence; Cirrhosis of the Liver; Diabetes Mellitus, Type 2; Metabolic Syndrome

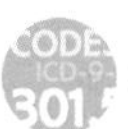

CODES

ICD9

- 571.0 Alcoholic fatty liver
- 571.8 Other chronic nonalcoholic liver disease

CLINICAL PEARLS

- NAFLD: Spectrum of liver damage ranging from simple steatosis to NASH, advanced fibrosis, and, rarely, progression to cirrhosis. It is increasingly recognized as a major cause of liver-related morbidity and mortality.
- NAFLD: Most common cause of liver disease in children. Overweight children with NAFLD are more likely to have metabolic syndrome and central obesity; elevated total cholesterol, LDL cholesterol, and triglycerides; low HDL cholesterol; elevated BP; and impaired fasting glucose (11)[B].
- NAFLD: A major cause of asymptomatic mild serum aminotransferase elevation.
- Benefit of statins in hypercholesterolemic patients generally outweighs risk of hepatoxicity. Continue statins and monitor hepatic enzymes.

FECAL IMPACTION

Robert A. Baldor, MD
Benjamin Hilliker, MD

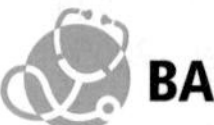

BASICS

DESCRIPTION

- Incomplete evacuation of feces, leading to formation of a large, firm, immovable mass of stool in the rectum (70%), sigmoid flexure (20%), or proximal colon (10%)
- System(s) affected: Gastrointestinal
- Synonym(s): Terminal reservoir syndrome

EPIDEMIOLOGY

Incidence

- General population: 1%
- Children: 1.5%
- Nursing home residents: 30%
- Constipation more common in women, nonwhites, low income, <12 years of education (1)[C]
- Predominant age: >60 years
- Predominant sex:
  - No sex preponderance in adults
  - Among children, 75% are boys.

Geriatric Considerations

- Much more likely to occur in patients >80 years of age
- Megarectum may be present in physically and mentally impaired elderly.
- Constipation appears to correlate with decreased caloric intake in the elderly.

RISK FACTORS

- Institutionalization
- Psychogenic illness
- Immobility, inactivity
- Pica
- Excessive seed consumption (common in Middle East cultures), leading to rectal seed bezoars
- Chronic renal failure; renal transplant recipients
- Urinary incontinence
- Cognitive decline, disability
- Constipation
- Heavy metal ingestion
- Poor toileting routines

Pediatric Considerations

- Habitual neglect of defecation urge, because of interference with play, may promote impaction.
- Fecal impaction has been reported to occur in >50% of all children with chronic constipation.

Genetics

Fecal impaction of the cecum may be seen in cystic fibrosis.

GENERAL PREVENTION

- Establish regular, consistent toilet time using gastrocolic reflex (2)[C].
- Maintain adequate hydration.
- Maintain high-fiber diet (2)[C].
- Regular exercise (2)[B]
- Install user-friendly commodes.
- Psyllium 7–24 g/d PO (1)[B]
- Use periodic enemas, if indicated.
- Periodic polyethylene glycol powder (MiraLax): 1 heaping tsp in 8 oz (240 mL) water daily × 2 weeks (1)[A]
- Lactulose 30–60 mL/d (1)[A]

PATHOPHYSIOLOGY

- The rectosigmoid colon dilates to accommodate mass, which, in turn, is not pliable enough to pass through the disproportionately small anal canal as a result of the patient's weak defecation effort.
- Impacted stool may exist as a single mass (stercolith) or as a composite of small, rounded fecal particles (scybalum).

ETIOLOGY

- Diet lacking in fiber and adequate fluids
- Drug side effects (2)[C]:
  - Stimulant laxatives
  - Opiates
  - Benzodiazepines
  - Tricyclic antidepressants
  - Phenothiazines
  - Antihypertensives (calcium channel blockers)
  - Aluminum (sucralfate, antacids)
  - Iron
  - Antispasmodics
  - Vinca alkaloids
  - 5HT3 antagonist
- Painful rectal conditions inhibiting voluntary defecation (e.g., anal fissure, hemorrhoids, fistulas)
- Neoplastic or inflammatory obstructing lesions (e.g., rectal bezoars)
- Neurogenic disorders:
  - Hirschsprung disease
  - Chagas disease
  - DM
  - Autonomic neuropathy
  - Multiple sclerosis
  - Spinal cord injury
  - Cauda equine
  - Parkinson disease
- Nonneurogenic:
  - Hypothyroidism
  - Hypokalemia
  - Hypercalcemia
  - Anorexia nervosa
  - Systemic sclerosis
  - Myotonic dystrophy
- Excess of GI inhibitory hormones (e.g., prolactin, endorphins, glucagon, secretin)
- Severe idiopathic chronic constipation
- Irritable bowel syndrome
- Pelvic floor dysfunction
- Pelvic floor dyssynergia
- Encopresis

COMMONLY ASSOCIATED CONDITIONS

- Pulmonary aspiration
- Urinary tract obstruction
- Recurrent UTIs
- Intestinal obstruction
- Spontaneous perforation of colon
- Stercoral ulceration
- Hernia
- Volvulus
- Megacolon or megarectum
- Rectal prolapse
- Pneumothorax
- Hypoxia
- Hypovolemic shock
- Iliac occlusion

Pregnancy Considerations

Impaction can produce dysfunctional labor, dystocia.

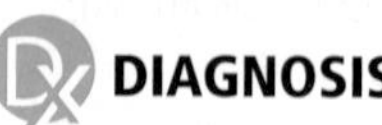

DIAGNOSIS

HISTORY

- Fecal incontinence, interpreted as diarrhea
- Postprandial abdominal pain
- Tenesmus
- Colic
- Nausea
- Vomiting
- Anorexia
- Weight loss
- Headache
- General malaise
- Agitation; confusion
- Urinary frequency
- Urinary incontinence

PHYSICAL EXAM

- Digital rectal exam (DRE):
  - Identify fissures or hemorrhoids.
  - Loss of sphincter tone: Neurologic disorders
  - Large mass of stool palpable in lower left quadrant and rectal vault
- The general physical exam may reveal secondary signs:
  - Weight loss
  - Dehydration
  - Agitation; confusion
  - Fever to 39.4°C (103°F)
  - Tachycardia
  - Tachypnea

DIAGNOSTIC TESTS & INTERPRETATION

Lab

Initial lab tests

Often normal

- Leukocytosis to 15,000 WBCs/mm^3
- Hyponatremia
- Hypokalemia
- Hypercalcemia
- TSH
- Stool may be positive for occult blood.
- Anemia, owing to chronic blood loss

Geriatric Considerations

Measure TSH, electrolyte activity, and BUN in elderly patients presenting with impaction.

Follow-Up & Special Considerations

Pediatrics:

- Antigliadin and antiendomysium antibodies
- Lead

Imaging

- Plain abdominal radiography may reveal stool or signs of obstruction if digital exam unrevealing.
- Stool retention is associated with megacolon.
- Barium enema can differentiate feces from tumor.

Diagnostic Procedures/Surgery

Sigmoidoscopy may be used to clarify the nature of a rectosigmoid mass.

DIFFERENTIAL DIAGNOSIS

- Irritable bowel syndrome
- Gastroenteritis, colitis
- Diverticulitis
- Appendicitis
- Carcinoma of the colon

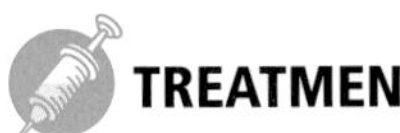

TREATMENT

MEDICATION

- A daily 1-L bolus of polyethylene glycol–electrolyte (GoLYTELY) solution given over 4–6 hours up to 3 days (2)[B]
- Polyethylene glycol-electrolyte (GoLYTELY) is better than lactulose in outcomes of frequency per week, form of stool, relief of abdominal pain, and the need for additional products (3)[A].
- Disimpaction in children; Consider combination:
  - Day 1: 1–2 phospho-soda enemas, 1 oz/10 kg; 4.5 oz maximum
  - Day 2: Bisacodyl suppository per rectum daily or b.i.d.
  - Day 3: Bisacodyl tablet PO daily or b.i.d.
  - Repeat 3-day cycle if needed once or twice.
- High-dose mineral oil: 15–30 mL PO per year of age per day to 8 oz maximum daily; b.i.d. for 3 days. Avoid if aspiration risk.
- Enemas: 1–2 oz/10 kg to 4.5 oz maximum, daily; b.i.d. for 1–2 days
- Children with constipation or fecal impaction who are treated with polyethylene glycol–electrolyte (GoLYTELY) have demonstrated consistently good outcomes. Dosages range from 0.3–0.7 g/kg/d (4)[A].
- Enemas and polyethylene glycol-electrolyte (GoLYTELY) were equally effective in treating fecal impaction in children. Polyethylene glycolelectrolyte (GoLYTELY) caused more fecal incontinence with comparable behavior scores (5)[B].
- Methylnaltrexone (Relistor) is approved for opioid-induced constipation by the FDA and can be considered in patients who do not have a reasonable response to a laxative regimen. Its use may be limited by cost (6)[B].
- Precautions:
  - Use magnesium citrate with caution in patients with renal insufficiency.
  - Be careful with lactulose; colonic distension can result from its bacterial fermentation.

ADDITIONAL TREATMENT

General Measures

- Manual fragmentation and extraction of fecal mass (after lubrication with lidocaine jelly) often required.
- Larger masses can be disimpacted with water jet directed through fiberoptic sigmoidoscope.
- Enemas containing 20% water-soluble contrast material (Hypaque) may help.
- If incomplete fragmentation: Suppositories or enemas with mineral oil, tap water, or sodium phosphate
- Ensure minimum fluid intake of 1.5–2 L/d.

Issues for Referral

In the pediatric population, consultation with a pediatric gastroenterologist should be considered if rectal medication is ineffective for disimpaction and in whom dietary changes and laxative therapy are ineffective.

COMPLEMENTARY AND ALTERNATIVE MEDICINE

Biofeedback improves constipation in patients with dyssynergic bowel function (7)[B].

SURGERY/OTHER PROCEDURES

- Laparotomy necessary only in extreme cases (2)[B]
- Electrohydraulic lithotripsy has been used to safely remove large, calcified fecaliths.

IN-PATIENT CONSIDERATIONS

Admission Criteria

- Disimpaction usually is performed in outpatient setting.
- Hospitalization is necessary if several attempts at outpatient management have failed.
- Presence of complications

ONGOING CARE

FOLLOW-UP RECOMMENDATIONS

Increased activity is important.

Patient Monitoring

<1 bowel movement every other day may lead to impaction.

DIET

- High fiber (25 g/d) with adequate fluid (minimum 2 L/d)
- Home remedy: Mix 2 cups bran, 2 cups applesauce, and 1 cup unsweetened prune juice; refrigerate; take 2–3 Tbs b.i.d.

PATIENT EDUCATION

- Comprehensive program, including use of laxatives, behavioral changes, dietary changes
- Effective education of the parents and child with regard to constipation is crucial in changing chronic behavior patterns.
- No hot water, soap, or hydrogen peroxide enemas. They may burn or irritate rectal mucosa, causing bleeding.
- "Obey the urge": Sit on toilet and attempt to defecate when the urge to move bowels is first sensed—usually after meal times. For children, have them sit on the toilet after meals.

PROGNOSIS

- Reimpaction is likely if program is not followed.
- Prognosis is poor for perforation with peritonitis.
- Mortality with impaction and obstruction is highest in the very young and the very old (up to 16%).

COMPLICATIONS

- Sepsis
- Hypotension
- Instrumental perforation
- Bleeding
- Postoperative obstruction

REFERENCES

1. Brandt LJ, Prather CM, Quigley EM, et al. Systematic review on the management of chronic constipation in North America. *Am J Gastroenterol*. 2005; 100(Suppl 1):S5–S21.
2. Hsieh C. Treatment of constipation in older adults. *Am Fam Physician*. 2005;72:2277–84.
3. Lee-Robichaud H, Thomas K, Morgan J, et al. Lactulose versus polyethylene glycol for chronic constipation. *Cochrane Database Syst Rev*. 2010;7:CD007570.
4. Candy D, Belsey J. Macrogol (polyethylene glycol) laxatives in children with functional constipation and faecal impaction: A systematic review. *Arch Dis Child*. 2009;94:156–60.
5. Bekkali N, van den Berg M, Dijkgraaf M, et al. Rectal fecal impaction treatment in childhood constipation: Enemas versus high doses oral PEG. *Pediatrics*. 2009;124;e1108–15.
6. Enck R. An overview of constipation and newer therapies. *Am J Hosp Palliat Care*. 2009;26(3): 157–8.
7. Rao SS, Seaton K, Miller M, et al. Randomized controlled trial of biofeedback, sham feedback, and standard therapy for dyssynergic defecation. *Clin Gastroenterol Hepatol*. 2007;5:331–8.

ADDITIONAL READING

- Constipation Guideline Committee of the North American Society for Pediatric Gastroenterology, Hepatology and Nutrition. Evaluation and treatment of constipation in infants and children: Recommendations of the North American Society for Pediatric Gastroenterology, Hepatology and Nutrition. *J Pediatr Gastroenterol Nutr*. 2006;43: e1–13.
- Tariq SH. Geriatric fecal incontinence. *Clin Geriatr Med*. 2004;20:571–87, ix.

See Also (Topic, Algorithm, Electronic Media Element)

Constipation; Diarrhea, Chronic; Encopresis

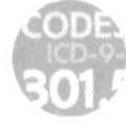

CODES

ICD9

- 560.32 Fecal impaction
- 564.00 Constipation, unspecified

CLINICAL PEARLS

- Any elderly person with a fever of uncertain cause should be assessed for fecal impaction with a DRE.
- When treating chronic pain patients with opioid preparations, be sure to supplement with stool softeners or osmotic laxatives.
- Hydrophilic colloid (fiber) is not that helpful in frail, end-of-life, or nonmobile patients.

FEMALE ATHLETE TRIAD

Christina Master, MD
Rahul Kapur, MD, BCSM

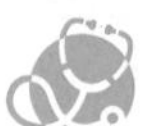

BASICS

Syndrome composed of 3 interrelated clinical entities: Low energy availability, menstrual dysfunction, low bone mineral density (BMD)

DESCRIPTION

- Female athlete triad terminology first used in 1992. Athletes may meet criteria for only 1 or 2 components of the triad.
- 2007 American College of Sports Medicine (ACSM) Position Stand:
  - Highlights that each component of the triad represents a continuous spectrum ranging from health to dysfunction
  - Underscores the importance of energy availability as fundamental to the propagation of the triad
  - Emphasizes that without correction of low energy availability, full recovery is not possible (1)[C]
- Energy availability:
  - Dietary energy intake minus exercise energy expenditure
  - Represents the amount of dietary energy remaining for bodily functions after exercise training
  - Low energy availability results in reducing mechanisms of cellular maintenance, thermoregulation, growth, and reproduction
  - Low energy availability occurs in the following settings: Increasing training disproportionately to energy intake; reducing energy intake by restricting, fasting, binging and purging, or by using diet pills, laxatives, diuretics, or enemas. Only some athletes will meet *Diagnostic and Statistical Manual* (DSM)-IV criteria for eating disorders, including anorexia nervosa and bulimia nervosa.
- Menstrual dysfunction:
  - Represents a spectrum ranging from eumenorrhea to amenorrhea, and includes athletes who have low estrogen levels, but still experience menstruation
  - Includes luteal suppression (shortened luteal phase, prolonged follicular phase, and decreased estradiol level), anovulation, oligomenorrhea (menstrual cycle >35 days), and primary and secondary hypothalamic amenorrhea
  - Primary amenorrhea, while less common, can occur in young athletes. Secondary amenorrhea is defined as the absence of menstrual cycles for >3 months after menarche has occurred.
  - Hypothalamic suppression is the most common cause of secondary amenorrhea in these athletes, although other causes must be ruled out prior to attributing the problem to low energy availability.
- Bone health:
  - Ranges from optimal bone health to osteoporosis, a skeletal disorder characterized by compromised bone strength predisposing a person to an increased fracture risk
  - Bone health refers to bone strength, or BMD, as well as bone quality. Current technology allows for the measurement of bone density but not quality, which helps to account for the fact that 2 athletes with the same BMD may have very different bone fracture histories:
    - Low bone density below the expected range for age for premenopausal women and low bone density for chronologic age for children describes athlete with a BMD Z-score that is 2 standard deviations (SD) below the mean.
    - Since most athletes have a higher BMD than nonathletes, ACSM recommends further workup for any athlete with a Z-score <−1, even in the absence of fracture (2)[C].
  - Endothelial dysfunction
  - Emerging evidence that the female athlete triad is associated with endothelial dysfunction. Athletic amenorrhea is associated with reduced brachial artery flow-mediated dilation. Abnormal brachial dilation has a 95% positive predictive value for coronary endothelial dysfunction. This additional association has sufficiently important implications for long-term women's health in addition to the triad above such that, in the future, this clinical syndrome may be best considered as a tetrad (3)[B].

EPIDEMIOLOGY

Unknown, as patients often avoid physicians and hide symptoms

Prevalence

- Overall prevalence: Difficult to ascertain for the complete triad; data suggests between 3.4% and 4.3%. 2 other triad studies found all 3 components of the triad in 2.7% of collegiate and 1.2% of high school athletes (4)[B]. 1 or 2 components of the triad may be found without the complete triad.
- Disordered eating: Prevalence of clinically diagnosed (DSM-IV) eating disorders in elite athletes 25–31% vs. 5.5–9% in the general population
- Menstrual dysfunction: Prevalence of secondary amenorrhea found to be as high as 69% in dancers and 65% in long-distance runners compared to 2–5% in the general population. Most patients exhibit a luteal deficiency or anovulatory cycle in 1 out of 3 menstrual cycles.
- Bone health: Using the World Health Organization (WHO) criteria for low BMD, prevalence of osteopenia (T-score between −1 and −2.5) ranges from 22–50% in female athletes, as compared to 12% in the normal population, and the prevalence of osteoporosis (T-score ≤−2.5) is as high as 13%, compared to 2.3% in the normal population.

RISK FACTORS

- Sports with an aesthetic component, e.g., ballet, figure skating, gymnastics, distance running, diving and swimming, or sports with weight classifications, e.g., martial arts and wrestling. Frequent weigh-ins, consequences for weight gain, domineering coaches or parents, and a win-at-all-cost attitude increase the risk of developing the triad.
- A lack of family or social support, either secondary to intense training hours causing social isolation or entering a new environment (boarding school or college). An athlete with comorbid psychological conditions, e.g., anxiety, depression, and/or obsessive–compulsive disorder, is more likely to develop the triad (4)[C].

GENERAL PREVENTION

- Education of athletes, coaches, trainers, parents, and physicians about the triad is crucial. Young athletes are extremely impressionable and may turn negative comments and unhealthy advice from adults into maladaptive eating and exercising habits. Primary care physicians should screen all adolescents for disordered eating, menstrual dysfunction, and injury history.
- Athletes presenting with "red flag" conditions such as fractures, weight changes, fatigue, amenorrhea, bradycardia, orthostatic hypotension, syncope, arrhythmia, electrolyte abnormalities, or depression should also be screened for the triad.

PATHOPHYSIOLOGY

- A baseline caloric deficit or low energy availability causes a disruption in the hypothalamic-pituitary-ovarian axis, decreasing the pulsatile release of gonadotropin-releasing hormone (GnRH).
- Low energy availability alters the levels of various metabolic hormones, some of which are thought to play a role in the regulation of GnRH secretion. Low GnRH levels subsequently decrease luteinizing hormone (LH) and follicle-stimulating hormone (FSH) levels causing a decrease in estrogen production, resulting in varying degrees of menstrual dysfunction.
- Estrogen deficiency also negatively affects bone density, and a chronic state of malnutrition reduces the rate of bone formation and increases the rate of bone resorption. This change in increased bone resorption and declined rate of bone formation begins within 5 days of a reduction in energy availability (5)[B].

COMMONLY ASSOCIATED CONDITIONS

- Anorexia nervosa or bulimia nervosa, and other psychological disorders, including low self-esteem, depression, and anxiety. In one study, 5.4% of athletes with eating disorders reported suicide attempts.
- Low BMD predisposes athletes to stress fractures and may not be fully reversible. This may lead to an even higher rate of fractures as these athletes reach postmenopausal status.

DIAGNOSIS

The female athlete triad is a clinical diagnosis based mainly on patient history. Screening for the female athlete triad should occur at annual sports physicals, routine exams, and acute visits for any concerning complaints or components of the triad (1)[C].

HISTORY

A 24-hour food recall diary may be helpful in this process. Athletes should be assessed for menstrual history (including oral contraceptive use), fracture history, and symptoms of depression (1)[C]. Special dietary practices, eating behaviors, and weight changes should also be collected. Body image; fear of weight gain; fluctuations in weight; history of disordered eating; and use of laxatives, diet pills, or enemas are crucial to understanding the extent of the disease.

PHYSICAL EXAM
- Height, weight, and vital signs
- Common findings in patients with disordered eating include bradycardia, orthostatic hypotension, hypothermia, cold or cyanotic extremities, lanugo, hypercarotenemia, parotid gland enlargement or tenderness, epigastric tenderness, eroded tooth enamel, and knuckle or hand calluses (Russell sign).
- Patients with primary amenorrhea should undergo a pelvic exam to determine the presence of a uterus. A pelvic exam in patients with secondary amenorrhea is warranted to rule out anomalies. Vaginal atrophy may be present in the hypoestrogen state (1)[C].

DIAGNOSTIC TESTS & INTERPRETATION
Lab
- Electrolytes and kidney function, CBC with differential, ESR, thyroid-stimulating hormone (TSH), 25-OH vitamin D, and urinalysis
- Primary evaluation for secondary amenorrhea includes a urine pregnancy test, FSH, LH, prolactin, and TSH (1)[B].

Imaging
- EKG to rule out a prolonged QT interval. The QT interval may be prolonged even in the absence of electrolyte abnormalities.
- Recommendation for BMD testing by dual-energy x-ray absorptiometry (DEXA) remains controversial. Current guidelines recommend DEXA studies for patients with disordered eating, eating disorders, amenorrhea, or oligomenorrhea for at least 6 months and/or patients with a history of stress fractures or fractures from minimal trauma. In patients with persistent components of the triad, re-evaluation by the same DEXA machine is recommended in 12 months from initial scan (1)[C].

DIFFERENTIAL DIAGNOSIS
The diagnosis of each component of the female athlete triad must be one of exclusion. Patients must be screened for anorexia nervosa and bulimia nervosa using the DSM-IV criteria. Similarly, before presuming a diagnosis of hypothalamic amenorrhea secondary to energy deficit, the following diagnoses must be ruled out:

- Pregnancy and endocrine abnormalities: Thyroid dysfunction, Cushing syndrome (4)[B]
- Hypothalamic dysfunction: Psychological stress-induced amenorrhea, medication-induced amenorrhea, Kallmann syndrome.
- Pituitary dysfunction: Prolactinoma or other pituitary neoplasm, Sheehan syndrome, sarcoidosis, empty-sella syndrome
- Ovarian dysfunction: Polycystic ovarian syndrome, premature ovarian failure, menopause, gonadal dysgenesis, Turner syndrome, ovarian neoplasm, autoimmune disease
- Uterine dysfunction: Asherman syndrome, absence of uterus

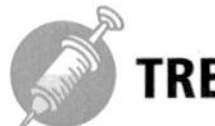

TREATMENT

- The treatment goal is to optimize nutritional status by establishing healthy eating behaviors and treating any associated maladaptive thought processes or psychological disorders.
- A multidisciplinary team, including a physician (or other health care provider), registered dietitian, and a mental health provider is crucial for treatment (1)[C]. Communication with team coaches, trainers, and family is also a critical intervention.
- Studies have shown a positive energy availability of more than 30 kcal/kg of fat-free muscle mass/day is sufficient to restore menstrual cycling, while an energy availability of more than 45 kcal/kg of fat-free muscle mass/day is likely needed for BMD improvement. Increases in body weight have been accompanied by improved BMD by up to 5% per year in previously amenorrheic athletes (1)[C].

MEDICATION
The use of oral contraceptive pills (OCPs), hormone replacement therapy (HRT), and/or bisphosphonates has not been clearly shown to increase BMD or aid in the restoration of normal menstrual cycling. OCPs can be considered to minimize further bone loss in patients over age 16, who, despite adequate nutrition and body weight gain, continue to have decreasing BMD and functional hypothalamic amenorrhea (1)[C].

IN-PATIENT CONSIDERATIONS
Patients with disordered eating or clinically diagnosable eating disorders must be evaluated for potentially life-threatening conditions requiring hospital admission, including bradycardia, severe orthostatic hypotension, significant electrolyte imbalances, hypothermia, arrhythmias, or prolonged QT interval on EKG (4)[C].

ONGOING CARE

- Patients with components of the triad should undergo frequent monitoring by all members of the multidisciplinary treatment team.
- In order to continue training and competing, athletes with disordered eating or clinically diagnosable eating disorders must agree to the following stipulations in the form of a behavior contract: To comply with all treatment strategies; to be closely monitored by health care providers; to place treatment goals over training goals; and to modify the type, duration, and intensity of training or competition if necessary.
- Athletes with disordered eating behaviors who do not comply with this agreement may need to be restricted from training (1)[C].

PATIENT EDUCATION
All young female patients should be counseled on the importance of proper nutrition, calcium, and vitamin D intake and the benefits of regular weightbearing exercise. Patients presenting with 1 or more components of the triad should be educated about the short-term and long-term effects of low BMD (6)[C].

PROGNOSIS
- The short- and long-term prognosis for patients with female athlete triad is dependent on time to diagnosis and response to treatment.
- Assuming early intervention with a multidisciplinary team, prognosis is very good. With adequate treatment and an increase in energy availability, patients will regain normal menstrual cycling and fertility and begin to increase BMD.
- Since the triad often occurs within the age window of optimal bone strengthening, patients with a prolonged disease course may suffer from complications of decreased BMD throughout their adolescent and adult life.
- In addition, patients with disordered eating behaviors may require long-term ongoing therapy to manage their disease (4)[C].
- The emerging association of the female athlete triad with endothelial dysfunction raises significant concerns for long-term cardiac endothelial implications in these athletes. It remains to be seen whether the endothelial dysfunction is reversible with intervention (3)[B].

REFERENCES

1. Nattiv A, Loucks AB, Manore MM, et al. American College of Sports Medicine position stand. The female athlete triad. *Med Sci Sports Exerc*. 2007; 39:1867–82.
2. International Society for Clinical Densitometry Writing Group for the ISCD Position Development Conference. Diagnosis of osteoporosis in men, women, and children. *J Clin Densitom*. 2004;7: 17–26.
3. Lanser EM, Zach KN, Hoch AZ, et al. The female athlete triad and endothelial dysfunction. *PM R*. 2011;3:458–65.
4. Hobart JA, Smucker DR. The female athlete triad. *Am Fam Physician*. 2000;61:3357–64, 3367.
5. The female athlete triad. *Med Sci Sports Exerc*. 2007;39:1867–82.
6. American Academy of Pediatrics. Committee on Sports Medicine and Fitness. Medical concerns in the female athlete. *Pediatrics*. 2000;106:610–3.

F

ADDITIONAL READING

Zach KN, Smith Machin AL, Hoch AZ, et al. Advances in management of the female athlete triad and eating disorders. *Clin Sports Med*. 2011;30:551–73.

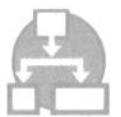

See Also (Topic, Algorithm, Electronic Media Element)

Algorithms: Amenorrhea, Primary (Absence of Menarche by Age 16); Amenorrhea, Secondary; Weight Loss

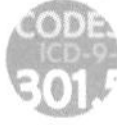

CODES

ICD9
- 307.50 Eating disorder, unspecified
- 626.0 Absence of menstruation
- 733.00 Osteoporosis, unspecified

CLINICAL PEARLS

- The female athlete triad consists of pathology in 3 clinical areas: Energy availability, menstrual function, and BMD. Athletes may exhibit varying degrees of dysfunction along each of the 3 spectra forming the triad. Endothelial dysfunction is emerging as a fourth component to be concerned about (1,3).
- Regular screening of adolescent and adult females at all routine and relevant acute visits is critical to early diagnosis and intervention.
- Immediate intervention by a multidisciplinary team, including physicians, registered dietitians, mental health professionals, coaches, trainers, and parents, is crucial to minimize further bone loss, recover BMD, and regain menstrual cycling.

FEVER OF UNKNOWN ORIGIN (FUO)

Scott T. Henderson, MD

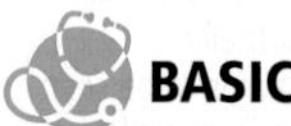

BASICS

DESCRIPTION

- Classic definition by Petersdorf and Beeson:
  - Fever over 38.3°C on several occasions
  - Fever duration at least 3 weeks
  - Uncertain diagnosis after 1 week of study in the hospital
- Modifications to the definition have been proposed, including eliminating the in-hospital evaluation and shortening the exam time.
- Some have suggested expansion of the definition to include nosocomial, neutropenic, and HIV-associated fevers that may not be prolonged.

EPIDEMIOLOGY

Incidence

No data on actual incidence

RISK FACTORS

- Recent travel
- Exposure to biologic or chemical agents
- HIV-infected patients with advanced disease
- Persons in AIDS risk group
- Elderly
- Drug abuse
- Immigrants
- Young female health care workers; consider factitious fever

ETIOLOGY

- >200 causes; each with prevalence ≤5%
- Most commonly an atypical presentation of a common condition
- Infection:
  - Abdominal abscesses
  - Amebic hepatitis
  - Catheter infections
  - Cytomegalovirus
  - Endocarditis/pericarditis
  - HIV (late stage)
  - Mycobacterial infection (often with advanced HIV)
  - Osteomyelitis
  - Renal
  - Sinusitis
  - Wound infections
  - Other miscellaneous infections
- Neoplasms:
  - Atrial myxoma
  - Colon cancer
  - Hepatoma
  - Lymphoma
  - Leukemia
  - Solid tumors (hypernephroma)
- Collagen vascular disease:
  - Giant cell arteritis
  - Polyarteritis nodosa
  - Polymyalgia rheumatica
  - Systemic lupus erythematosus
  - Rheumatic fever
  - Rheumatoid arthritis
- Other causes:
  - Alcoholic hepatitis
  - Cerebrovascular accident
  - Cirrhosis
  - Drug fever/medication induced:
    - Allopurinol, captopril, carbamazepine, cephalosporins, cimetidine, clofibrate, erythromycin, heparin, hydralazine, hydrochlorothiazide, isoniazid, meperidine, methyldopa, nifedipine, nitrofurantoin, penicillin, phenytoin, procainamide, quinidine, sulfonamides
  - Endocrinologic diseases
  - Factitious/fraudulent fever
  - Granulomatous diseases
  - Occupational causes
  - Periodic fever
  - Pulmonary emboli/deep vein thrombosis
  - Thermoregulatory disorders
- In up to 20% of cases, the cause of the fever will not be identified despite thorough workup.

Geriatric Considerations

Most common causes are acute leukemia, Hodgkin lymphoma, intra-abdominal infections, tuberculosis (TB), and temporal arteritis

- Infections account for over half of causes, with collagen-vascular diseases the second-most likely etiology.
- Inflammatory bowel disease is the common etiology in older children and adolescents.

DIAGNOSIS

HISTORY

- History should focus on relevant symptoms:
  - Constitutional symptoms almost always accompany a fever:
    - Chills, night sweats, myalgias, weight loss with an intact appetite (infectious)
    - Arthralgias, myalgias, fatigue (inflammatory)
    - Fatigue, night sweats, weight loss with loss of appetite (neoplasms)
- Past medical history should include information about previously treated chronic infections and any prior diagnosis of cancer.
- Past surgical history should include specific information about type of surgery performed, postoperative complications, and any indwelling foreign materials.
- Obtain a comprehensive list of all medications, including over-the-counter and herbal remedies.
- Family history to identify prior illnesses in family members that may have a genetic link, such as periodic fever syndromes, and recent illnesses in family members to which the patient may have been exposed

ALERT

Special attention should be paid to travel, occupational, sexual, and drug exposure.

Pediatric Considerations

About 50% of FUOs in published pediatric case series are ultimately shown to be due to infections; collagen vascular disease and malignancy also being common diagnoses (1)[A].

PHYSICAL EXAM

- Physical exam should focus on areas that have high diagnostic yield:
  - Funduscopic exam for choroid tubercles or Roth spots; temporal artery palpation; gums and oral cavity; auscultation for bruits and murmurs; abdominal palpation for organomegaly; rectal examination; testicular examination; palpate for adenopathy; skin and nail bed exam for clubbing, nodules, lesions, and rashes; focal neurologic signs; bony tenderness; and joint effusion
- Repeated exams are essential to determine cause.

DIAGNOSTIC TESTS & INTERPRETATION

Lab

Initial lab tests

- CBC
- Peripheral blood smear
- Liver function tests
- C-reactive protein
- ESR
- HIV antibody test
- Blood cultures (not to exceed 6 sets)
- Urinalysis and urine culture

Follow-Up & Special Considerations

- Rheumatoid factor and antinuclear antibody test
- Serologic tests: Epstein-Barr, hepatitis, syphilis, Lyme disease, Q fever, cytomegalovirus, amebiasis, coccidioidomycosis
- Serum ferritin
- Serum protein electrophoresis
- Sputum and urine cultures for TB
- Thyroid function tests
- Tuberculin skin test:
  - May not be helpful if anergic or acute infection
  - If test negative, repeat in 2 weeks

Imaging

Initial approach

- Chest x-ray (CXR)
- CT or MRI of abdomen and pelvis (plus directed biopsy, if indicated) (3)[C]

Follow-Up & Special Considerations

- Technetium-based scan if infectious process or tumor suspected (3)[B]
- Positron emission tomography (PET) scan using the radiolabeled glucose analogue ^{18}F-fluorodeoxyglucose if infectious process, inflammatory process, or tumor suspected; PET scans have a high negative predictive value (4)[B]
- Ultrasound of abdomen and pelvis (plus directed biopsy, if indicated) if mass lesions, renal obstruction, or gallbladder/biliary tree pathology suspected
- ECG if cardiac valve lesions (endocarditis), atrial myxomas, or pericardial effusion suspected (transthoracic vs. transesophageal)
- Leg Doppler if deep vein thrombosis/pulmonary embolism suspected
- CT scan of chest if pulmonary emboli suspected
- Indium-labeled leukocyte scanning if inflammatory process suspected
- Bone scan if osteomyelitis or metastatic disease suspected

Diagnostic Procedures/Surgery
- Liver biopsy if granulomatous disease suspected (3)[C]
- Temporal artery biopsy, particularly in the elderly (3)[B]
- Lymph node, muscle, or skin biopsy if clinically indicated
- Bone marrow biopsy if clinically indicated
- Spinal tap if clinically indicated

Pathological Findings
Depends on etiology

DIFFERENTIAL DIAGNOSIS
See "Etiology."

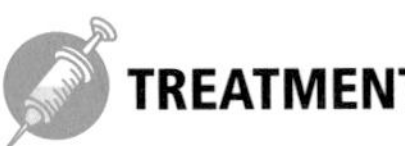

TREATMENT

MEDICATION
First Line
- First-line drugs are dependent on the diagnosis.
- Evidence does not support treatment of fever (4)[C].

Second Line
If the patient has symptoms with the fever or continues to decline, a therapeutic trial may be indicated:
- Antibiotic trial based on patient's history
- Antituberculous therapy if there is a high risk for granulomatous disease pending culture results
- Steroid trial based on patient's history (once occult malignancy is ruled out)

ALERT
If a steroid trial is initiated, patient may have a relapse after treatment or if certain conditions (such as TB) have been undiagnosed.

ADDITIONAL TREATMENT
General Measures
- Attempt to determine the etiology before initiating the therapy.
- Avoid therapeutic trials unless as a last resort and only if therapy is reasonably specific.
- "Shotgun" approaches are condemned, as they obscure the clinical picture, have untoward effects, and do not solve the problem (3)[C].

Additional Therapies
With temperature elevations, patients will have increased caloric and fluid demands.

SURGERY/OTHER PROCEDURES
Need for exploratory laparotomy has been largely eliminated with the advent of more sophisticated tests and imaging modalities.

IN-PATIENT CONSIDERATIONS
Admission Criteria
- Reserved for the ill and debilitated
- Consider if factitious fever has been ruled out or an invasive procedure is indicated

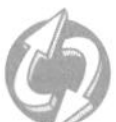

ONGOING CARE

FOLLOW-UP RECOMMENDATIONS
Patient Monitoring
If the etiology of the fever remains unknown, repeat the history and physical exam along with screening lab studies.

DIET
With temperature elevations, patients will have increased caloric and fluid demands.

PATIENT EDUCATION
Maintain an open line of communication between physician and patient/family as the workup progresses:
- The extended time required in establishing a diagnosis can be frustrating.

PROGNOSIS
- Depends on etiology and age:
  - Patients with HIV have the highest mortality.
- 1-year survival rates reflecting deaths due to all causes

Age	Survival
<35	91%
35–64	82%
>64	67%

COMPLICATIONS
Dependent on etiology

Pregnancy Considerations
Fever is known to increase the risk of neural tube defects and trigger preterm labor.

REFERENCES

1. Chow A, Robinson JL. Fever of unknown origin in children: A systematic review. *World J Pediatr*. 2011;7(1):5–10.
2. High KP, Bradley SF, Gravenstein S, et al. Clinical practice guideline for the evaluation of fever and infection in older adult residents of long-term care facilities: 2008 update by the Infectious Diseases Society of America. *J Am Geriatr Soc*. 2009;57:375–94.
3. Mourad O, Palda V, Detsky AS. A comprehensive evidence-based approach to fever of unknown origin. *Arch Intern Med*. 2003;163:545–51.
4. Keidar Z, Gurman-Balbir A, Gaitini D, et al. Fever of unknown origin: The role of 18F-FDG PET/CT. *J Nucl Med*. 2008;49:1980–5.
5. Plaisance KI, Mackowiak PA. Antipyretic therapy: Physiologic rationale, diagnostic implications, and clinical consequences. *Arch Intern Med*. 2000;160:449–56.

ADDITIONAL READING

- Cunha BA. Fever of unknown origin: Clinical overview of classic and current concepts. *Infect Dis Clin N Am*. 2007;21:867–915.
- Cunha BA. Fever of unknown origin: Focused diagnostic approach based on clinical clues from the history, physical examination, and laboratory tests. *Infect Dis Clin N Am*. 2007;21:1137–87.
- Varghese GM, Trowbridge P, Doherty T. Investigating and managing pyrexia of unknown origin in adults. *BMJ*. 2010;341:c5470.
- Williams J, Bellamy R, et al. Fever of unknown origin. *Clin Med*. 2008;8:526–30.

See Also (Topic, Algorithm, Electronic Media Element)

- Arthritis, Juvenile Idiopathic; Colorectal Cancer; Cytomegalovirus Inclusion Disease; Endocarditis, Infective; Hepatoma; HIV Infection and AIDS; Leukemia; Lupus Erythematosus, Discoid; Osteomyelitis; Polyarteritis Nodosa; Polymyalgia Rheumatica; Pulmonary Embolism; Rheumatic Fever; Sinusitis; Stroke, Acute; Temporal Arteritis
- Algorithms: Fever, Acute; Fever in the First 3 Months of Life; Fever of Unknown Origin

CODES

ICD9
780.60 Fever, unspecified

CLINICAL PEARLS

- The history, exam, diagnostic tests, and imaging should focus on the relevant causes of FUO:
  - A sequential approach leads to a rational sequential diagnosis or rules out causes of FUO.
- A "shotgun" approach to treatment should be avoided; empiric therapy should be used only in carefully defined circumstances.
- FUO cases that defy precise diagnosis after intensive investigation and prolonged observation generally carry a favorable prognosis.
- In many cases, FUO in older persons may represent atypical, nonclassic presentations of common infectious and noninfectious diseases.

FIBROCYSTIC CHANGES OF THE BREAST

Katherine M. Callaghan, MD
Dawn S. Tasillo, MD

BASICS

DESCRIPTION

- Fibrocystic changes (FCC) of the breast is a generalized term for a heterogeneous group of changes affecting the stromal and glandular tissues of the breast.
- It is the most common of all benign breast conditions.
- Commonly presents as mastalgia, engorgement, increased breast nodularity, and/or cysts:
  - Mastalgia (breast pain) is usually in upper outer quadrants of breast, bilateral, and may radiate to shoulders or upper arms.
  - Localized pain may occur with a rapidly enlarging cyst.
  - Nodules are usually small (2–10 mm), diffuse, and bilateral, with a rubbery consistency.
  - Cysts are more common in women in their 40s.
  - Larger cysts may have consistency of a water-filled balloon.
- Symptoms are most prominent in premenstrual (luteal) phase
- System(s) affected: Endocrine/Metabolic; Reproductive
- Synonym(s): Fibrocystic breast disease; Mammary dysplasia; Chronic cystic mastitis

EPIDEMIOLOGY

Most common in women of reproductive years; occasionally seen after menopause with hormone replacement

Incidence

Unknown but very frequent

Prevalence

50–60% of women without breast disease are found to have this pattern of fibrous change and cyst formation (1).

RISK FACTORS

- The effect of consumption of methylxanthine-containing substances (e.g., coffee, tea, cola, and chocolate) has not been found to be a contributing factor (2)[A].
- Diet high in fruits and vegetables and high parity independently decrease risk of FCC (3).
- Diet high in saturated fats may increase risk of FCC.

PATHOPHYSIOLOGY

May be the result of an exaggerated response of breast tissue to cycling hormones or a subtle imbalance in the ratio of estrogen to progesterone

ETIOLOGY

Estrogen likely a causative factor for many (4)[B]

COMMONLY ASSOCIATED CONDITIONS

Fibrocystic change found clinically confers no increased risk of breast cancer (1)

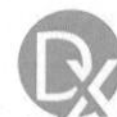

DIAGNOSIS

HISTORY

- May present in 3 overlapping, indistinct stages:
  - Mastoplasia (breast enlargement) and mastalgia, which may subside after menses; common in women in their 20s
  - Adenosis: Appearance of multiple small breast nodules; common in women in their 30s
  - Cystic phase: Tender cysts, usually small but up to 5 cm in diameter; common in women in their 40s
- Obtain personal history of breast biopsy and family history of breast disease (benign or malignant)

PHYSICAL EXAM

- With patient first upright, then supine turn rotated on to contralateral hip, evaluate all breast tissue from sternum to midaxillary line, from clavicle to mammary ridge.
- Using fingertip, proceed in a linear fashion from top of sternum past breast tissue using 3 different depths of pressure at each palpation. Continue superiorly again to clavicle in a "lawnmower" fashion.
- Quantitate size, consistency, mobility, location, and skin changes.
- Findings in FCC may include:
  - Smooth, tense, or fluctuant masses
  - Bilateral masses
  - Breast thickening
  - Nipple discharge
- Palpate for axillary lymph nodes.

DIAGNOSTIC TESTS & INTERPRETATION

- Evaluation should focus on excluding breast cancer.
- Testing may be conducted based on a level of clinical suspicion.

Imaging

Initial approach

- Ultrasound (US): Signs of malignancy include irregular mass, clustered masses, calcifications, architectural distortion, dilated duct; US is useful for differentiating cystic from solid lesions.
- Mammography may reveal mass or dense tissue ± calcifications.

Follow-Up & Special Considerations

- Mammogram may be normal in presence of malignancy and difficult to interpret in women <35 years of age due to dense breast tissue; US may be more helpful particularly in the presence of a palpable mass.
- MRI is indicated in patients with *BRCA1* or *BRCA2* mutation or in any woman with ≥25% lifetime risk for breast cancer (5).

Diagnostic Procedures/Surgery

- Fine-needle aspiration (FNA) and biopsy:
  - Allows differentiation of cystic and solid lesions
  - Aspirate may be straw-colored, dark brown, or green
  - Cells sent for cytology can reveal cancer with high accuracy
  - Low morbidity
- If mass disappears, no further evaluation is necessary (including cytologic evaluation of aspirated fluid).

Pathological Findings

- Certain histological changes in the setting of fibrocystic change confer an increased risk for breast cancer:
  - Atypia: Relative risk of 4.24
  - Proliferative changes without atypia: Relative risk of 1.88
  - Nonproliferative changes: Relative risk of 1.27 (6)

DIFFERENTIAL DIAGNOSIS

- Pain:
  - Mastitis
  - Costochondritis
  - Pectoralis muscle strain
  - Neuralgia
  - Breast cancer
  - Angina pectoris
  - Gastroesophageal reflux (GERD)
  - Superficial phlebitis of the thoracoepigastric vein (Mondor disease)
- Masses:
  - Breast cancer
  - Sebaceous cyst
  - Fibroadenoma
  - Lipoma
  - Fat necrosis
- Skin changes:
  - Breast cancer (peau d'orange: Thickened skin similar to peel of an orange)
  - Eczema

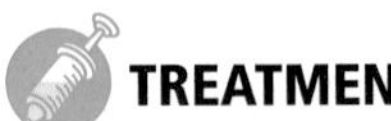

TREATMENT

- After ruling out malignancy by means of examination, and/or imaging and diagnostic procedures, FCC may not require treatment and often resolves with time.
- Cool compresses, avoiding trauma, and around-the-clock wearing of a well-fitting, supportive brassiere may be useful for symptom relief (7).

MEDICATION

First Line

For cyclic pain and swelling: NSAIDs:

- Ibuprofen 400 mg q.i.d./PRN
- Naproxen 500 mg b.i.d./PRN

Second Line

- Oral contraceptives may be useful in modulating symptoms or in preventing the development of new changes.
- For severe pain, consider (8):
  - Danazol (Danocrine) 100–400 mg/d divided in 2 doses × 4–6 months
  - Bromocriptine 2.5 mg b.i.d. × 3 months
  - Tamoxifen 10 mg/d × 3–6 months
  - These medications are not without serious side effects and thorough counseling is required. Consultation with a breast specialist may be considered.

ADDITIONAL TREATMENT

Issues for Referral

- If discrete palpable lesion in a woman ≤35 years, US then refer to a surgeon.
- If discrete palpable lesion in a woman >35 years, diagnostic mammography ± US then refer to surgeon.

COMPLEMENTARY AND ALTERNATIVE MEDICINE

Evidence supporting evening primrose oil, vitamin E, or pyridoxine as treatment for the discomforts of FCC is insufficient to draw conclusions about effectiveness (2).

SURGERY/OTHER PROCEDURES

Breast cyst aspiration can be both diagnostic and therapeutic.

ONGOING CARE

FOLLOW-UP RECOMMENDATIONS

Condition is benign, chronic, and recurrent.

Patient Monitoring

- The patient needs to be assessed with clinical examination, radiologic studies, and sometimes biopsy to be certain a lump is not malignant.
- Follow-up times are variable depending on the clinical situation.
- US is useful to differentiate cysts from solid lesions and in evaluating women <35 years of age for FCC but is not useful for screening.
- Screening mammograms should be obtained after age 40. Refer to the AAFP, ACOG, or ACS recommendations for screening schedules.
- Aspiration cytology is useful to differentiate cysts from solid lesions. The sensitivity and specificity of cyst aspirate cytology for cancer diagnosis depends on the skill of the clinician and cytopathologist and may be as high as 98%.
- When physical examination, mammography, and FNA are used in combination, detection rates for breast cancer range from 93–100%.

DIET

There is insufficient evidence that changes in diet (e.g., caffeine intake) effect symptoms from FCC. Individual patient response will vary.

PATIENT EDUCATION

- Patient info on fibrocystic breasts from the Mayo Foundation for Medical Education and Research: www.mayoclinic.com/health/fibrocystic-breasts/DS01070
- Info on breast cancer prevention from the National Cancer Institute: www.cancer.gov

REFERENCES

1. Santen RJ, Mansel R. Benign breast disorders. *N Engl J Med*. 2005;353:275–85.
2. Horner NK, Lampe JW. Potential mechanisms of diet therapy for fibrocystic breast conditions show inadequate evidence of effectiveness. *J Am Diet Assoc*. 2000;100:1368–80.
3. Wu C, Ray RM, Lin MG, et al. A case-control study of risk factors for fibrocystic breast conditions: Shanghai Nutrition and Breast Disease Study, China, 1995–2000. *Am J Epidemiol*. 2004;160: 945–60.
4. Meisner AL, Fekrazad MH, Royce ME. Breast disease: Benign and malignant. *Med Clin North Am*. 2008;92:1115–41, x.
5. Morris E. Diagnostic breast MR imaging: Current status and future directions. *Radio Clin N Am*. 2007;45(5).
6. Hartmann LC, Sellers TA, Frost MH, et al. Benign breast disease and the risk of breast cancer. *N Engl J Med*. 2005;353:229–37.
7. Giuliano AE, Hurvitz SA. Breast disorders. In: McPhee SJ, et al. *Current Medical Diagnosis & Treatment 2011*. New York: McGraw-Hill Medical; 2011.
8. Srivastava A, Mansel RE, Arvind N, et al. Evidence-based management of Mastalgia: A meta-analysis of randomised trials. *Breast*. 2007; 16:503–12.

ADDITIONAL READING

- Griffin JL, Pearlman MD, et al. Breast cancer screening in women at average risk and high risk. *Obstet Gynecol*. 2010;116:1410–21.
- Saslow D, et al. American Cancer Society guidelines for breast screening with MRI as an adjunct to mammography. *CA J Clin*. 2007;57(2):75–89.

F

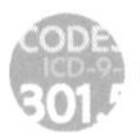

CODES

ICD9

- 610.0 Solitary cyst of breast
- 610.1 Diffuse cystic mastopathy
- 610.2 Fibroadenosis of breast

CLINICAL PEARLS

- Fibrocystic breast change is a common finding in reproductive aged women and generally does not confer an increased cancer risk.
- Symptoms can be managed expectantly, with NSAIDs, or oral contraceptives.
- Palpable breast lesions should be evaluated as clinically indicated.
- Immediate office aspiration of breast cysts is a relatively easy procedure and often provides pain relief.
- If a mass is still present after cyst aspiration, refer patient for further evaluation and diagnostic testing (biopsy).
- Certain histological subtypes of FCC found at time of biopsy are associated with breast cancer risk (see "Pathologic Findings").

FIBROMYALGIA

Alexander E. Davidovich, DO, MS
Tyler Cymet, DO

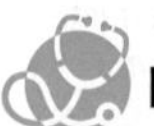

BASICS

DESCRIPTION

- Chronic widespread physically debilitating neurogenic pain syndrome:
  - Excessive generalized musculoskeletal tenderness at several defined anatomic sites on both sides of body and in axial skeleton
  - Pain exhibited as allodynia (nonpainful stimuli evoking pain), hyperpathia (painful stimuli evoking exaggerated and prolonged pain response), and hyperalgesia (extreme sensitivity to painful stimuli) (1)
  - Lasting ≥3 consecutive months
  - Commonly associated with symptoms such as:
    - Fatigue
    - Sleep disturbances
    - Cognitive dysfunction
    - Mood disorders
- Synonym(s): Fibrositis

EPIDEMIOLOGY

Incidence

- Predominant sex: Female > Male (~80% are females)
- Predominant age: 20–60 years

Prevalence

2–4% of adult US population

RISK FACTORS

- Female gender
- Poor functional status
- Negative/stressful life events

Genetics

- Genetics:
  - Inheritance is unknown but likely polygenic
  - High familial aggregation
  - Odds ratio may be as high as 8.5 for a first-degree relative of a familial proband
  - Commonly comorbid with mood or anxiety disorders in families
- Environmental:
  - Physical trauma or injury
  - Stressors (e.g., work, family, life events, and abuse)
  - Some studies report correlations to certain infections (e.g., Lyme disease and hepatitis C).

GENERAL PREVENTION

No specific prevention known

ETIOLOGY

- Combination of:
  - Abnormality in CNS pain processing
  - Genetic/familial/environmental factors
  - Mood or anxiety disorder
- Decrease in blood flow to the thalamus and caudate nucleus
- Afferent augmentation of peripheral nociceptive stimuli
- Alterations in neuroendocrine, neuromodulation, neurotransmitter, neurotransporter, biochemical, and neuroreceptor function/physiology (1)
- May be triggered or aggravated after a negative life event, physical injury, or illness

COMMONLY ASSOCIATED CONDITIONS

Arise in various parts of the body grouped as Somatic Syndromes, including (2):

- Irritable bowel syndrome, fatigue, rumination, muscle weakness, headache, abdominal pain, dizziness, insomnia, depression, constipation, nausea, nervousness, chest pain, blurred vision, fever, diarrhea, dry mouth, itching, wheezing, Raynaud phenomenon, hives, tinnitus, heartburn, oral ulcers, change in taste, seizures, dry eyes, dyspnea, loss of appetite, rash, sun sensitivity, hearing difficulties, easy bruising, hair loss, frequent urination, painful urination, and bladder spasms

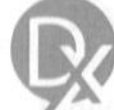

DIAGNOSIS

- Made clinically based on individual presentations; history and physical exam are paramount.
- Must consider psychosocial and emotional issues.
- Severity impacts the quality of life. Assess using the Revised Fibromyalgia Impact Questionnaire (FIQR) (1), as well as other scales.

HISTORY

- ≥3 months of symptoms centered at core triad including:
  - Chronic widespread, bilateral pain and in the axial skeleton
  - Generalized fatigue and sleep disturbances, with α-wave intrusions, causing deficient restorative sleep
  - Altered cognition/mood such as trouble concentrating, forgetfulness, disorganized thinking, and depression/anxiety
- Symptoms can wax and wane, vary in intensity from day to day, and by physical location.
- Associated somatic symptoms include nondermatomal paresthesias, temporomandibular joint dysfunction, morning stiffness, headache, urinary urgency, Raynaud phenomenon, visceral organ dysfunction (noncardiac chest pain, heartburn, and palpitations), interstitial cystitis, IBS (see list above).
- Impaired social/occupational functioning
- Absence of identifiable explanation for the pain
- Adverse effect of medication excluded (e.g., statins)

PHYSICAL EXAM

- Normal except for diffuse tenderness upon digital palpation of several body regions
- Multiple painful sites may be present; patient may have general hyperalgesia.
- Joints examined for swelling, tenderness, range of motion, crepitus, peripheral pain generators (e.g., RA, OA, tendonitis, adhesive capsulitis), and focal/objective weakness
- An absence of features in joints or skin of any inflammatory musculoskeletal disease
- Neurologic exam typically normal
- The American College of Rheumatology (ACR) 1990 diagnostic criteria used finding 11 of 18 specific anatomic tender point sites to diagnose fibromyalgia (sensitivity 88.4%, specificity 81.1%) (2).
- The ACR 2010 diagnostic criteria: (Sensitivity 96.6%, specificity 91.8% with Fibromyalgia Symptom scale (FS) score ≥13):
  - Diagnosed when the following 3 conditions met:
    - Widespread Pain Index (WPI) ≥7 and Symptom Severity (SS) scale score ≥5 or WPI 3–6 and SS score ≥9
    - Symptoms present at a similar level for at least 3 months
    - Absence of identifiable disorder to explain the pain
  - FS = WPI + SS (scale between 0 and 31)
  - WPI notes the number of areas in pain over past week (score between 0 and 19):
    - Above the waist:
      - Jaw, right and left
      - Neck
      - Shoulder girdle, right and left
      - Upper back
      - Upper arm, right and left
      - Lower arm, right and left
      - Chest
      - Abdomen
      - Lower back
    - Below the waist:
      - Hip (buttock, trochanter), right and left
      - Upper leg, right and left
      - Lower leg, right and left
  - The SS scale score is the sum of the severity of the 3 symptoms (fatigue, waking unrefreshed, cognitive symptoms) plus the extent (severity) of somatic symptoms in general during the previous 6 months. The final score is between 0 and 12:
    - The level of severity over the past week uses the following scale:
      - 0—No problem
      - 1—Slight or mild problems, generally mild or intermittent
      - 2—Moderate, considerable problems, often present and/or at a moderate level
      - 3—Severe: Pervasive, continuous, life-disturbing problems
    - Considering general somatic symptoms:
      - 0—No symptoms
      - 1—Few symptoms
      - 2—Moderate number of symptoms
      - 3—A great deal of symptoms

DIAGNOSTIC TESTS & INTERPRETATION

Lab

Initial lab tests

CBC with differential, ESR or CRP, CPK, TSH, comprehensive metabolic profile, BUN/creatinine, 25 OH vitamin D level, B12, RPR or VDRL

Imaging

Not indicated except to exclude other diagnoses

Diagnostic Procedures/Surgery

- Sleep studies to rule out obstructive sleep apnea or narcolepsy
- Neuropsychiatric evaluation for:
  - Depression
  - Anxiety
  - Cognitive disturbance
  - Memory

DIFFERENTIAL DIAGNOSIS

- Overlap syndromes:
  - Chronic fatigue syndrome
  - Myofascial pain (more anatomically localized than fibromyalgia)
- Common coexisting disorders:
  - Connective tissue diseases
  - Psychiatric illness
  - Sleep disorders
  - TMJ syndrome
- Medications: Statin-induced myopathy or opioid-induced hyperalgesia
- Hepatitides
- Hypothyroidism
- Inflammatory rheumatic diseases: Osteoarthritis, rheumatoid arthritis, systemic lupus erythematosus, polymyositis, polymyalgia rheumatica
- Spinal stenosis/neuropathies

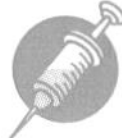

TREATMENT

- Mainstay of therapy includes combining medications with exercise, sleep hygiene, and psychotherapy (1).
- Daily aerobic and mixed-type exercises, and cognitive-behavioral therapy and operant behavioral therapy. Some data suggest benefit from hydrotherapy and water aerobics (3).

MEDICATION

- Pharmacotherapies should be selected to address individual patients' major complaints with the lowest effective therapeutic doses needed to improve daily functioning and quality of life (1).
- NSAIDs should be tried first but have limited efficacy.
- Caution if using opioids, hypnotics, anxiolytics, and certain skeletal-muscle due to the potential for abuse.
- The 3 FDA-approved drugs are: Pregabalin, Duloxetine, and Milnacipran (4); while others are used off-label.

First Line

- Amitriptyline: 25 mg PO at bedtime (5)[A], used for pain, fatigue, and sleep disturbances (6)
- Duloxetine: Initially 30 mg/d × 1 week, then increase to 60 mg/d (5)
- Milnacipran: Day 1: 12.5 mg/d; days 2–3: 12.5 mg b.i.d.; day 4–7: 25 mg b.i.d.; after day 7: 50 mg b.i.d.; max dose 100 mg PO b.i.d. (5)
- Pregabalin: Start with 150 mg/d, then advance to 300 mg/d within 1 week as needed. Max dose 450 mg/d
- Cyclobenzaprine 10–30 mg PO at bedtime (7)

Second Line

- Gabapentin 1,200–2,400 mg/d PO b.i.d.–t.i.d.; start with lower doses
- Tramadol 200–300 mg/d PO divided doses
- Fluoxetine 20–80 mg/d PO (higher doses may be needed)
- Clonazepam 0.5 mg PO at bedtime may help sleep.
- Acetaminophen 325–1,000 mg PO q.i.d. PRN
- Combinations of acetaminophen and tramadol effective for pain control
- Combinations of medicines such as amitriptyline and fluoxetine may be tried.

ADDITIONAL TREATMENT

General Measures

- Low-impact cardiovascular exercise and strength training mandatory (6).
- Cognitive-behavioral therapy (CBT) (7)
- Stress management
- Patient education; can consider group format (7)
- Sleep hygiene
- Psychosocial support
- Consider job/workplace modifications.

Issues for Referral

For nonresponders, may refer to rheumatology, psychiatry, and pain management centers.

COMPLEMENTARY AND ALTERNATIVE MEDICINE

- Physical therapy may be helpful as part of conditioning program/fitness.
- Moderate efficacy shown in some studies for:
  - Hydrotherapy (8), hypnotherapy, biofeedback
- Less evidence of efficacy:
  - Chiropractic, acupuncture, massage therapy, electrotherapy, ultrasonography

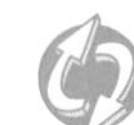

ONGOING CARE

FOLLOW-UP RECOMMENDATIONS

Patient Monitoring

For efficacy of therapy at 2–4 weeks

DIET

No restrictions; no proven efficacy of any specific diet

PROGNOSIS

- 50% with partial remission after 2–3 years of therapy
- Typically has fluctuating, chronic course
- Poorer outcome with:
  - Longer illness duration, more severe symptoms, depression, advanced age, lack of social support

REFERENCES

1. Smith HS, Barkin RL, et al. Fibromyalgia syndrome: A discussion of the syndrome and pharmacotherapy. *Dis Mon*. 2011;57:248–85.
2. Wolfe F, Clauw DJ, Fitzcharles MA, et al. The American College of Rheumatology preliminary diagnostic criteria for fibromyalgia and measurement of symptom severity. *Arthritis Care Res (Hoboken)*. 2010;62:600–10.
3. Smith HS, Bracken D, Smith JM, et al. Pharmacotherapy for fibromyalgia. *Front Pharmacol*. 2011;2:17.
4. Häuser W, Petzke F, Sommer C, et al. Comparative efficacy and harms of duloxetine, milnacipran, and pregabalin in fibromyalgia syndrome. *J Pain*. 2010;11:505–21.
5. Häuser W, Petzke F, Üçeyler N, et al. Comparative efficacy and acceptability of amitriptyline, duloxetine and milnacipran in fibromyalgia syndrome: A systematic review with meta-analysis. *Rheumatology (Oxford)*. 2011;50:532–43.
6. Hauser W, Bernandy K, Uceyler N, et al. Treatment of fibromyalgia syndrome with antidepressants: A meta-analysis. *JAMA*. 2009;301(2):198–209.
7. Hauser W, Bernhard M, Schiltenwolf M. Efficacy of multicomponent treatment in fibromyalgia syndrome: A meta-analysis of randomized controlled clinical trials. *Arth Rheum*. 2009; 61(2):216–24.
8. McVeigh JG, McGaughey H, Hall M, et al. The effectiveness of hydrotherapy in the management of fibromyalgia syndrome: A systematic review. *Rheumatol Int*. 2008;29(2):119–30.

ADDITIONAL READING

- American College of Rheumatology. Practice guidelines, patient education. Available at: www.rheumatology.org.
- National Fibromyalgia Association. Available at: www.fmaware.org.
- Wolfe F, Clauw DJ, Fitzcharles MA, et al. Fibromyalgia criteria and severity scales for clinical and epidemiological studies: A modification of the ACR Preliminary Diagnostic Criteria for Fibromyalgia. *J Rheumatol*. 2011;38:1113–22.

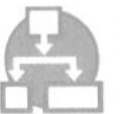

See Also (Topic, Algorithm, Electronic Media Element)

Algorithm: Fatigue

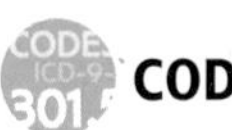

CODES

ICD9

729.1 Myalgia and myositis, unspecified

CLINICAL PEARLS

- Coexisting severe complaints of chronic pain, fatigue, multiple symptoms in the *absence* of laboratory or physical exam findings
- Biologic basis is still unclear, but the disease is considered a disorder of pain regulation termed *central sensitization*.
- Overlap with stress, depression, and anxiety must be recognized in treatment plan.
- Best outcomes occur in patients who understand their illness and are willing to engage in multimodal treatment, including exercise, medication, psychotherapy, and changing lifestyle habits.

F

FIBROSIS, PULMONARY

Amy Zhou, MD
Anna Rudnicki, MD

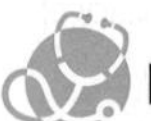

BASICS

DESCRIPTION

- Characterized by fibrosis of the lung parenchyma
- Chest CT shows reticular pattern and honeycombing with subpleural and lower lobe predominance.
- Lung biopsy shows "usual interstitial pneumonia" pattern.
- Classified based on etiology:
  - Idiopathic (IPF)
  - Nonidiopathic

EPIDEMIOLOGY

Incidence

- Incidence of IPF is 7–16 per 100,000 person-years.
- IPF is more common in men.
- Most patients with IPF are older than 60.
- Incidence of nonidiopathic pulmonary fibrosis is unknown.

Prevalence

- Prevalence of IPF is 2–39 cases per 100,000 people.
- Prevalence of nonidiopathic pulmonary fibrosis is unknown.

RISK FACTORS

- Family history of pulmonary fibrosis
- Gastroesophageal reflux
- Smoking
- Exposure to birds, livestock, dust from metals or wood, solvents

Genetics

- <5% of IPF is familial, and may involve mutations in surfactant protein A2 and C and/or abnormal telomere shortening.
- Most likely mode of transmission is autosomal-dominant with variable penetrance.

GENERAL PREVENTION

- No prevention for the idiopathic form.
- Avoid the risk factors mentioned above, such as smoking, certain occupational exposures, or drugs that induce pulmonary fibrosis.

PATHOPHYSIOLOGY

Postulated that microinjury to alveolar epithelial cells causes release of cytokines that activate fibroblasts

ETIOLOGY

Causes of the nonidiopathic form include:

- Occupational exposure
- Environmental exposure
- Drugs
- Systemic autoimmune diseases
- Granulomatous diseases

COMMONLY ASSOCIATED CONDITIONS

- Pulmonary hypertension: Occurs in 30–80% of patients with IPF, likely as a result of hypoxemic vasoconstriction
- GERD
- Nonidiopathic pulmonary fibrosis may be associated with collagen vascular diseases (such as rheumatoid arthritis and scleroderma).

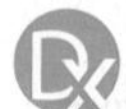

DIAGNOSIS

HISTORY

- Slowly progressive dyspnea
- Dry cough

PHYSICAL EXAM

- Tachypnea
- Fine inspiratory crackles
- Possible clubbing

DIAGNOSTIC TESTS & INTERPRETATION

Lab

Initial lab tests

- High-resolution chest CT (HRCT) is required to make diagnosis. Characteristic findings include a reticular pattern and honeycombing with a subpleural and lower lobe predominance (1).
- If the patient has characteristic findings of pulmonary fibrosis on chest CT and is of appropriate age for pulmonary fibrosis, then lung biopsy is not required (1).

Follow-Up & Special Considerations

- Surgical lung biopsy should be considered if clinical presentation and HRCT are not entirely characteristic with pulmonary fibrosis (1).
- Blood work to rule out associated collagen vascular disease (1)
- Bronchoscopy with BAL may help rule out other types of interstitial lung disease (1).

Imaging

Initial approach

Echocardiogram to evaluate for concomitant pulmonary hypertension

Diagnostic Procedures/Surgery

- Pulmonary function testing: Initially may see only decrease in diffusing capacity. Later in disease may develop decrease in lung volumes as well.
- Resting and exercise pulse oximetry to determine need for supplemental oxygen

Pathological Findings

Usual interstitial pneumonitis: Shows interstitial scarring, honeycombing, and fibroblastic foci

DIFFERENTIAL DIAGNOSIS

- Asbestosis
- Berylliosis
- Coal worker's pneumoconiosis
- Hypersensitivity pneumonitis
- Sarcoidosis
- Silicosis

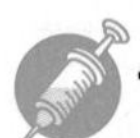

TREATMENT

MEDICATION

First Line

Supplemental oxygen if needed (1)[C]

Second Line

Combination therapy with prednisone, azathioprine, and N-acetylcysteine may be appropriate for a minority of patients, although evidence for benefit is weak and adverse effects of these drugs are considerable (1,2,3)[B].

ADDITIONAL TREATMENT

General Measures

- Pulmonary rehabilitation (1)[C]
- Consider treating for asymptomatic GERD (1)[B].
- Consider lung transplant.

Issues for Referral

- Patients should be evaluated and cared for longitudinally by a pulmonologist.
- If any uncertainty in diagnosis, then consider referral to thoracic surgery for lung biopsy.
- Depending on patient age, comorbidities, and preference, may consider referral for lung transplant.

Additional Therapies

- Limited studies have been done showing mixed evidence of benefit from interferon gamma 1-b, pirfenidone, and cyclosporine. These drugs are not currently approved for treating IPF in the US (4,5).
- Many other clinical trials are currently underway. Some of the targets being studied include TGF-β, connective tissue growth factor, IL-13, CCL2, CXCR4 and CXCL12, ACE, and angiotensin II (6).

COMPLEMENTARY AND ALTERNATIVE MEDICINE

None

SURGERY/OTHER PROCEDURES

Lung transplant carries a 5-year survival of 50–56% (1).

IN-PATIENT CONSIDERATIONS

Initial Stabilization

- Provide adequate supplemental oxygen.
- Work up other possible causes of respiratory decompensation.
- If no other cause found, then consider high-dose steroids.

Admission Criteria

Worsening shortness of breath and/or increased oxygen requirements

Nursing

Supplemental oxygen to keep saturations >90%

ONGOING CARE

FOLLOW-UP RECOMMENDATIONS

Patient should follow up with a pulmonologist.

Patient Monitoring

Disease progression can be monitored by periodic PFTs and HRCT.

DIET

No specific dietary requirements

PATIENT EDUCATION

- Patients should be counseled extensively regarding the prognosis of this diagnosis and given as much support as possible. Information about support groups in the local community and online may be helpful.
- Patients should be informed about the side effects of corticosteroid and/or cytotoxic therapy to decide whether to initiate pharmacologic treatment.
- American Lung Association: www.lungusa.org/lung-disease/pulmonary-fibrosis/
- Pulmonary Fibrosis Foundation: www.pulmonaryfibrosis.org/, which includes information about active pulmonary fibrosis clinical trials.

PROGNOSIS

- Median survival time was thought to be 2–3 years from time of diagnosis. However, recent data from clinical trials suggest that this may be an underestimate (1).
- Some patients may deteriorate quickly, while others can remain stable for an extended period of time. Acute exacerbations carry a high mortality, and ICU treatment (mechanical ventilation) is mostly unsuccessful.
- A higher extent of fibrosis increased the risk of death, while a higher percent-predicted DLCO reduced the risk of death.
- Biomarkers called pneumoproteins are currently being studied, and in the future may be able to provide individualized prognostic information for patients (7).

COMPLICATIONS

- Respiratory failure
- Infection
- Pulmonary hypertension
- Rib fractures secondary to prolonged coughing (especially in elderly patients with decreased bone density)

REFERENCES

1. Raghu G, Collard HR, Egan JJ, et al. An official ATS/ERS/JRS/ALAT statement: Idiopathic pulmonary fibrosis: Evidence-based guidelines for diagnosis and management. *Am J Respir Crit Care Med*. 2011;183:788–824.
2. Demedts M, Behr J, Buhl R, et al. High-dose acetylcysteine in idiopathic pulmonary fibrosis. *N Engl J Med*. 2005;353:2229–42.
3. Bradley B, Branley HM, Egan JJ, et al. Interstitial lung disease guideline: The British Thoracic Society in collaboration with the Thoracic Society of Australia and New Zealand and the Irish Thoracic Society. *Thorax*. 2008;63(Suppl 5):v1–58.
4. Hauber HP, Blaukovitsch M, et al. Current and future treatment options in idiopathic pulmonary fibrosis. *Inflamm Allergy Drug Targets*. 2010;9:158–72.
5. Azuma A, et al. Pirfenidone: Antifibrotic agent for idiopathic pulmonary fibrosis. *Expert Rev Respir Med*. 2010;4:301–10.
6. Datta A, Scotton CJ, Chambers RC, et al. Novel therapeutic approaches for pulmonary fibrosis. *Br J Pharmacol*. 2011;163:141–72.
7. Barlo NP, van Moorsel CH, van den Bosch JM, et al. Predicting prognosis in idiopathic pulmonary fibrosis. *Sarcoidosis Vasc Diffuse Lung Dis*. 2010; 27:85–95.

ADDITIONAL READING

- Castriotta RJ, Eldadah BA, Foster WM, et al. Workshop on idiopathic pulmonary fibrosis in older adults. *Chest*. 2010;138:693–703.
- Coward WR, Saini G, Jenkins G, et al. The pathogenesis of idiopathic pulmonary fibrosis. *Ther Adv Respir Dis*. 2010;4:367–88.
- Gogali A, Wells AU, et al. New pharmacological strategies for the treatment of pulmonary fibrosis. *Ther Adv Respir Dis*. 2010;4:353–66.
- Lynch DA, Godwin JD, Safrin S, et al. High-resolution computed tomography in idiopathic pulmonary fibrosis: Diagnosis and prognosis. *Am J Respir Crit Care Med*. 2005;172:488–93.
- Spagnolo P, Del Giovane C, Luppi F, et al. Non-steroid agents for idiopathic pulmonary fibrosis. *Cochrane Database Syst Rev*. 2010;CD003134.

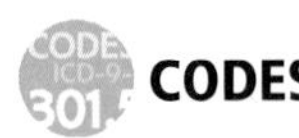

CODES

ICD9

- 501 Asbestosis
- 515 Postinflammatory pulmonary fibrosis
- 516.31 Idiopathic pulmonary fibrosis

CLINICAL PEARLS

- Pulmonary fibrosis can usually be diagnosed based on characteristic chest CT findings, which include a reticular pattern and honeycombing with a peripheral and basilar predominance.
- There are idiopathic and nonidiopathic forms of pulmonary fibrosis.
- Treatment options for pulmonary fibrosis are very limited and only serve to slow the progression of disease.

FLOPPY IRIS SYNDROME

Kunal K. Vyas, DO
Alissa Craft, DO, MBA

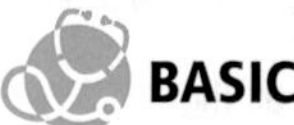

BASICS

DESCRIPTION

- Floppy iris syndrome (FIS) is a condition that involves a weakening of the iris dilating muscle that has been linked to alpha-1a antagonists, in particular tamsulosin.
- This condition becomes increasingly important in patients undergoing cataract surgery and trabeculectomy:
  - During surgery, the iris is dilated to help surgeons access the lens for removal. In patients with FIS, there may be poor pupil dilation, billowing of the iris, and progressive miosis during surgery. These responses increase the risk of surgical complications including:
    - Posterior capsule rupture with vitreous prolapse into the anterior chamber (1)
    - Iris trauma resulting in pupil deformity
    - Retinal detachment (2)

EPIDEMIOLOGY

Incidence

- There is a 2% occurrence of FIS in the general population undergoing cataract surgery.
- However, in a prospective study, there was a 90% occurrence of FIS in patients using alpha-1a antagonists and undergoing cataract surgery.

RISK FACTORS

Risk factors for this condition include the following medications:

- Alpha-1a antagonists:
  - Tamsulosin:
    - Tamsulosin has the highest affinity for alpha-1a receptors (3).
    - 85% of patients taking Tamsulosin experience FIS.
  - Terazosin
  - Doxazosin
  - Alfuzosin:
    - 15% of patients taking Alfuzosin experience FIS.
- Benzodiazepines
- Risperidone (4)
- Rivastigmine
- Donepezil

Genetics

There have been no studies that suggest a genetic predisposition for FIS.

GENERAL PREVENTION

- General prevention includes screening patients for cataracts before starting an alpha-1a antagonist.
- As the effect of alpha-1a antagonists may last for a prolonged period of time even after discontinuation, patients with cataracts should be considered for surgery prior to starting one of these agents.

PATHOPHYSIOLOGY

There have been 2 prominent theories proposed for the pathophysiology of FIS:

- The Theory of Anatomic Change:
  - This theory proposes that the parasympathomimetic effects of the alpha-1a blockers create an anatomic effect of pupil constriction.
  - This theory is predicated on clinical ophthalmologists experience with various topical and systemic parasympathomimetic drugs.
  - Ophthalmologists reported a 30–40% decrease in dilation on the day following the use of the drug (5).
  - This theory explains the inability of patients with FIS to experience normal pupil dilatation; however, does not explain the observation of the continued inability to experience pupil dilatation years after the alpha-blockers are stopped (6).
- The Theory of Iris Dilating Muscle Atrophy:
  - This theory hypothesizes that tamsulosin causes atrophy of the iris dilator muscle and in turn weakens it, resulting in the inability to dilate the pupil regardless of sympathetic stimulation (7).
  - These findings explain the inability of the iris to dilate in alpha-1a antagonist treated patients, and also address the lack of improvement years after discontinuation of the drug.
  - A recent case study has suggested that the iris muscle atrophy can be attributed to alpha-1a antagonistic activity on vasculature supplying the dilating muscle (8).

ETIOLOGY

- The primary cause of FIS has been shown to be alpha-1a antagonist drugs.
- In 86% of alpha-1a antagonist attributed FIS, tamsulosin has been the contributing agent.
- Other agents such as terazosin, alfuzosin, doxazosin, benzodiazepines, risperidone, rivastigmine, and donepezil can cause FIS.

COMMONLY ASSOCIATED CONDITIONS

None

DIAGNOSIS

- Although clues such as irregular pupil margins with history of alpha-1a antagonists use is enough for many ophthalmologists to take preventative measures during cataract surgery, the diagnosis of FIS can only be made intraoperatively.
- The FIS triad includes (1):
  - Progressive pupillary constriction during surgery
  - An iris that appears floppy or billows during normal irrigation and aspiration of the synthetic lens within the anterior chamber in the operated eye
  - A tendency of the iris to prolapse into the phacoemulsification and paracentesis incisions during cataract surgery

HISTORY

- Patient history is a very important part of anticipating who will develop intraoperative FIS.
- In male patients, it is important to have a high index of suspicion in those with benign prostatic hyperplasia (BPH), as alpha-1a antagonists are often used to control urinary retention symptoms in this disorder.
- In female patients, it is important to review medications in those receiving treatment for urinary retention.
- Other conditions that should prompt a review of medications in patients undergoing cataract surgery or trabeculectomy include:
  - Schizophrenia, due to the association with risperidone
  - Alzheimer disease, due to the association with rivastigmine and donepezil

PHYSICAL EXAM

During physical exam particular attention should be paid to pupillary reaction during illumination:

- Poor dilation does not always indicate FIS; however, in combination with a thorough medication history can help predict intraoperative FIS.

DIAGNOSTIC TESTS & INTERPRETATION

None. The diagnosis of FIS is made clinically.

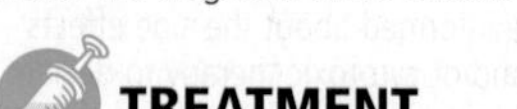

TREATMENT

- Treatment for FIS is directed at preventing pupillary constriction and facilitating pupillary dilatation during surgery:
  - Due to variability in the extent of iris billowing and prolapse, it is difficult to create definitive studies of treatment or prevention.
  - For this reason, any patient at risk of FIS who is undergoing cataract surgery should have placement of a malyugin ring, a device created to hold the iris open at 4 points (2).
  - This device can be inserted intraoperatively and has been demonstrated to reduce the complications associated with operating on a patient with FIS.

- Studies have also shown that discontinuing the alpha-1a blocker is not effective in preventing intraoperative FIS (6):
  - A potential preventative measure surrounds the use of finasteride, as opposed to alpha-1a antagonists in the treatment of urinary symptoms in patients with BPH.
  - Due to the finasteride mechanism of 5-alpha reductase inhibition, it has shown to not cause intraoperative FIS and may be equally efficacious in treating symptoms of BPH (9).

MEDICATION

Some sympathomimetic medications have been used to elicit pupil dilation, including atropine, phenylephrine, and epinephrine. However, ability to consistently cause uniform sustained pupil dilation through surgery is questionable.

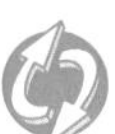

ONGOING CARE

FOLLOW-UP RECOMMENDATIONS

Recommendations for follow-up are based on the specific surgical complications and outcomes in patients with intraoperative FIS. All recommendations must be specific for that patient.

PATIENT EDUCATION

- Patients with even early cataract formation who may be surgical candidates in the future and who use are considering use of alpha-1a antagonists should be educated about the risk of intraoperative floppy iris syndrome.
- Physicians prescribing the alpha-1a antagonists should be aware of this risk as well and consider this when referring patients to ophthalmology for cataract procedures.

PROGNOSIS

Prognosis is based solely on the outcomes of potential surgical complications if a patient experiences FIS intraoperatively.

COMPLICATIONS

- Complications of this condition are primarily intraoperative and include:
  - Posterior capsule rupture with vitreous prolapse into the anterior chamber
  - Iris trauma resulting in pupil deformity
- Patients taking tamsulosin have a 2.3 times greater risk of postoperative complications as a result of cataract surgery. These complications may include loss of lens fragments and retinal detachment.

REFERENCES

1. Flach AJ, et al. Intraoperative floppy iris syndrome: Pathophysiology, prevention, and treatment. *Trans Am Ophthalmol Soc*. 2009;107:234–9.
2. Chang DF, Braga-mele R, Mamalis N, et al. Clinical experience with intraoperative floppy-iris syndrome. Results of the 2008 ASCRS member survey. *J Cataract Refract Surg*. 2008;34:1201–9.
3. Blouin M, Blouin J, Perreault S, et al. Intraoperative floppy iris syndrome associated with alpha-1 adrenoreceptors. Comparison of tamsulosin and alfuzosin. *J Cataract Refract Surg*. 2007;33: 1227–34.
4. Ford RL, Sallam A, Towler HMA. Intraoperative floppy iris syndrome associated with risperidone intake *Eur J Ophthalmol*. 2011;21(2):210–1.
5. Haddad NJ, Moyer NJ, Riley FC Jr. Mydriatic effect of phenylephrine hydrochloride. *Am J Ophthalmol*. 1970;70(5):729–33.
6. Chang DF, Campbell JR. Intraoperative floppy iris syndrome associated with tamsulosin (Flomax). *J Cataract Refract Surg*. 2005;31:664–73.
7. Santaella RM, Destafeno JJ, Stinnett SS, et al. The effect of alpha1-adrenergic receptor antagonist tamsulosin (Flomax) on iris dilator smooth muscle anatomy. *Ophthalmology*. 2010;117(9):1743–9.
8. Panagis L, Basile M, Friedman AH, et al. Intraoperative floppy iris syndrome: Report of a case and histopathologic analysis. *Arch Ophthalmol*. 2010;128(11):1437–41.
9. Lucia MS, Lambert JR. Growth factors in benign prostatic hyperplasia: Basic science implications. *Curr Urol Rep*. 2008;9(4):272–8.

ADDITIONAL READING

- Chadha V, Borooah S, Tey A, et al. Floppy iris behaviour during cataract surgery: Associations and variations. *Br J Ophthalmol*. 2007;91:40–2.
- Chang DF, Osher RH, Wang L, et al. A prospective multicenter evaluation of cataract surgery in patients taking tamsulosin (Flomax). *Ophthalmology*. 2007; 114:957–64.
- Nguyen DQ, Sebastian RT, Kyle G. Surgeon's experiences of the intraoperative floppy iris syndrome in the United Kingdom. *Eye*. 2007;21: 443–4.
- Oshika T, Ohashi Y, Inamura M, et al. Incidence of intraoperative floppy iris syndrome in patients on either systemic or topical alpha (1)-adrenoceptor antagonist. *Am J Ophthalmol*. 2007;143:150–1.
- Prata TS, Palmiero PM, Angelilli A, et al. Iris morphological changes related to alpha-1 adrenergic receptor antagonists: Implications for intraoperative floppy iris syndrome. *Ophthalmology*. 2009;116(5):877–81.

CODES

ICD9

364.81 Floppy iris syndrome

CLINICAL PEARLS

- FIS is diagnosed by the intraoperative triad of progressive pupillary constriction, an iris that appears floppy and billows during normal irrigation and aspiration of the synthetic lens, and a tendency of the iris to prolapse into the phacoemulsification and paracentesis incisions during cataract surgery.
- FIS is to be anticipated in patients who currently are using or have ever used alpha-1a antagonists.
- A malyugin ring holds the iris in its dilated position and has shown to remarkably improve postoperative results in patients at risk for FIS.
- In patients with cataracts and BPH, finasteride can be considered in place of alpha-1a antagonists, or cataract extraction before the start of alpha-1a antagonists should be considered.

FOLLICULITIS

Lara Stewart, DO, MPH

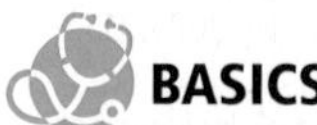

BASICS

DESCRIPTION

Inflammation of either superficial and/or deep hair follicle caused by infection, physical (traction) or chemical (tar/oils) irritation, or injury:

- Generally is an acute self-limiting disease that can occur anywhere on the body that hair is found
- Clusters of pink/red raised bumps that are often pruritic, occasionally painful, and frequently embarrassing/worrisome
- Most commonly associated with infection by *Staphylococcus aureus* or *Pseudomonas aeruginosa* (in the case of "hot tub folliculitis"), but also can be fungal or viral causality
- Noninfectious types include:
  - Eosinophilic pustular folliculitis (Ofuji disease in patients of Asian descent)
  - Eosinophilic folliculitis (seen in HIV-positive/immunocompromised)
  - Folliculitis decalvans
  - Pruritic folliculitis of pregnancy
- Pseudofolliculitis barbae is similar in appearance and historical causality, but a distinct disease process affecting the curly type hairs on the face/neck of primarily black males

EPIDEMIOLOGY

Incidence

- Folliculitis is a common disorder; a majority of people have been affected at some point in their lifetime.
- Affects persons of all ages, gender, and race

RISK FACTORS

- Hair removal (shaving/waxing)
- Other skin conditions: Eczema, acne
- Occlusive dressing/clothing
- Personal carrier of/or contact with methicillin-resistant *Staphylococcus aureus* (MRSA)-infected persons
- Obesity
- Immunosuppression (medications, chemotherapy, HIV)
- Use of hot tubs or saunas
- Diabetes mellitus

GENERAL PREVENTION

- Good hygiene practices:
  - Frequent hand washing
  - Antibacterial soaps
  - Frequent washing in hot water of towels/linens to avoid reinfection from contaminated clothing and washcloths, etc.
- Minimize friction from clothing.
- Good hair removal practices:
  - Exfoliate beforehand
  - Witch hazel, alcohol, or TendSkin afterward
  - Shave in direction of hair growth; use moisturizer/warm water; change razor frequently
  - Decrease frequency of shaving

PATHOPHYSIOLOGY

Predisposing factors to folliculitis:

- Nasal carriage of *S. aureus*
- Exposure to (poorly chlorinated) pools/hot tubs leading to folliculitis caused by *P. aeruginosa*
- Recent/prolonged antibiotic or corticosteroid use leading to *Candida* folliculitis

ETIOLOGY

- Bacteria:
  - Staphylococcal infection
  - MRSA due to increasing incidence of community-acquired infections
  - Pseudomonal folliculitis commonly erupts quickly after soaking in an infected spa or hot tub.
- Fungal:
  - Pityrosporum/Malassezia folliculitis may mimic acne, as it causes folliculitis of chest, back, shoulders, face, scalp
  - *Candida*
- Viral
  - Herpes simplex and Herpes zoster can cause folliculitis at the site/area of the herpes infection.
- Parasitic:
  - As a reaction to cutaneous larva migrans infestation
  - *Demodex* mite infection on the face and scalp
- Immunosuppression:
  - Transplant patients taking sirolimus are at risk for scalp folliculitis.
  - Eosinophilic folliculitis is uncommon in completely healthy adults, being more common in immunosuppressed (AIDS) patients, but in Japan it occurs as Ofuji disease.

COMMONLY ASSOCIATED CONDITIONS

- Conjunctivitis
- Impetigo
- Acne
- Eczema

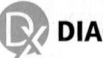

DIAGNOSIS

HISTORY

- Inquire as to exposures: Spa tubs, heat, topical agents, hair styling and shaving practices, recent antibiotics or steroids, HIV and cancer status
- Investigate MRSA exposures/carrier status, home and work environment (risk/exposure potential)
- Pityrosporum folliculitis occurs more often in warm, humid climates and more frequently in immunocompromised patients.
- Patient usually reports lesions have formed recently within the few days, or has been a recurrent issue of a periodic nature

PHYSICAL EXAM

- Characteristic lesions are multiple small papules and pustules, usually measuring $\leq$5 mm in diameter with erythematous base pierced by a central hair.
- Papular/pustular rash occurring on hair-bearing skin, especially the face (beard), proximal limbs, and scalp; often is pruritic
- Pseudomonal folliculitis appears as a widespread rash mainly on the trunk and limbs.
- In pseudofolliculitis barbae, the growing hair curls around and penetrates the skin, provoking a foreign-body reaction

DIAGNOSTIC TESTS & INTERPRETATION

Lab

Initial lab tests

- Diagnosis usually made clinically taking risk factors, history, and location of lesion into account
- Culture and Gram stain (gram-negative folliculitis occurs from long-term antibiotic therapy) for conclusive infectious identification and sensitivity profile
- Woods lamp fluorescence and potassium hydroxide preparation to look for budding yeast or hyphae

Follow-Up & Special Considerations

- If recurrent, consider HIV testing and A1C/fasting blood sugar testing to evaluate for diabetes.
- Punch biopsy

Pathological Findings

- Superficial/deep: Moderately intense infiltrate of inflammatory cells
- Pseudofolliculitis: Perifollicular inflammatory infiltrate
- Eosinophilic folliculitis: Collection of eosinophils within superficial follicle

DIFFERENTIAL DIAGNOSIS

- Acne vulgaris/acneiform eruptions
- Cutaneous candidiasis
- Contact dermatitis
- Rosacea folliculitis
- Milia
- Papular urticaria
- Insect bite

TREATMENT

MEDICATION

For most occurrences, antiseptic and supportive care is sufficient, and benefit of the use of systemic antibiotics is questionable.

First Line

- Staphylococcal folliculitis:
  - Mupirocin applied 2–5 times per day is preferred and most effective treatment
  - Cephalosporin (Cephalexin): 250 mg q.i.d. or 1,000 mg b.i.d. for 7–10 days
  - Dicloxacillin: 250 mg q.i.d. PO for 10–14 days
- For MRSA:
  - Bactrim DS 1–2 b.i.d. for 7–10 days
  - Clindamycin 300 mg PO q.i.d. for 7–10 days
  - Minocycline or doxycycline 100 mg PO b.i.d. for 10 days
- Pseudomonal folliculitis:
  - Usually self-limited; can be treated symptomatically; no antibiotic indicated
  - If severe or persistent, adults can use ciprofloxacin 500 mg b.i.d. PO for 10 days
  - Cephalexin 500 mg q6–8h for 7–10 days has been used in severe cases in children.
- Eosinophilic folliculitis/eosinophilic pustular folliculitis:
  - Good antiretroviral regimen of utmost importance (in HIV+ related cases)
  - Topical corticosteroids: e.g., fluocinonide 0.05% b.i.d.
  - NSAIDs: Systemic indomethacin
  - Itraconazole, metronidazole
  - Retinoids; e.g., topical isotretinoin
  - Some response seen in Ofuji disease with tacrolimus and UVB phototherapy
- Pityrosporum folliculitis:
  - Topical antifungals (e.g., ketoconazole 2% b.i.d.): Cream or shampoo
  - Systemic antifungals for relapses
- Herpetic folliculitis:
  - Valacyclovir 500 b.i.d. for 5 days
  - Famciclovir 125 mg b.i.d. for 5 days
  - Acyclovir 800 b.i.d. for 5 days

Second Line

- Recurrent disease:
  - Vitamin C (1 g/d × 4–6 weeks)
  - Mupirocin ointment (intranasally b.i.d. × 5 days)
  - Low-dose clindamycin (150 mg/d × 3 months)
- MRSA carrier status:
  - Nasal mupirocin ointment
  - Rifampin 600 mg/d PO × 10 days

ADDITIONAL TREATMENT

General Measures

- Supportive, local care to area of concern with warm compresses, topical antibiotics, and low-dose corticosteroids
- Intranasal mupirocin is mainstay of treatment for MRSA carriers and household/family members.
- Preventive measures are key to avoidance of recurrence:
  - Antibacterial soaps (Dial, chlorhexidine)
  - Good hand-washing techniques
  - Keep skin intact. Use moisturizers and avoid scratching.
  - Clean shaving instruments each day.
  - Change towels/washcloths and sheets daily.
  - Avoid contact with nasal secretions.
  - For obese individuals, weight reduction may be helpful.

Issues for Referral

Unusual or persistent cases should be biopsied if possible and then referred to dermatology.

Additional Therapies

Public Health Measures:

- Outbreaks of culture-positive pseudomonas hot tub folliculitis should be reported so that source identification can be determined and superchlorination (14 parts/million) can occur.

SURGERY/OTHER PROCEDURES

Incision and drainage is rarely necessary, and not preferred due to potential for scar formation.

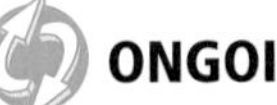

ONGOING CARE

FOLLOW-UP RECOMMENDATIONS

Patient Monitoring

- Resistant cases should be followed every 2 weeks until cleared.
- 1 return visit in 2 weeks if symptoms abate

DIET

For obese individuals, weight reduction may be helpful, as skin/skin friction will be lessened.

PATIENT EDUCATION

Avoid shaving in involved areas.

PROGNOSIS

- Usually resolves with treatment; however, *S. aureus* carriers may get recurrences.
- Mupirocin nasal treatment for carrier status and for family/household members may be required.
- Resistant or severe cases may warrant testing for diabetes mellitus or immunodeficiency (HIV).

COMPLICATIONS

- Primary complication of concern is recurrent folliculitis.
- Scarring/hyperpigmentation
- Progression to become furuncles or abscesses

ADDITIONAL READING

- Böer A, Herder N, Winter K, et al. Herpes folliculitis: Clinical, histopathological, and molecular pathologic observations. *Br J Dermatol*. 2006;154:743–6.
- Ellis E, et al. Eosinophilic pustular folliculitis: A comprehensive review of treatment options. *Am J Dermatol*. 2004;5(93):189–97.
- Fiorillo L, et al. The pseudomoneus hot foot syndrome. *N Eng J Med*. 2001;(345)335–8.
- Friedkin S, et al. MRSA disease in three communities. *N Eng J Med*. 2005;(352):1436–44.
- James D. Acne. *N Eng J Med*. 2005;(352):1463–72.
- Nervi SJ, Schwartz RA, Dmochowski M. Eosinophilic pustular folliculitis: A 40 year retrospect. *J Am Acad Dermatol*. 2006;55(2):285–9.

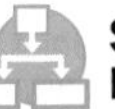

See Also (Topic, Algorithm, Electronic Media Element)

Algorithm: Rash, Focal

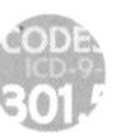

CODES

ICD9

704.8 Other specified diseases of hair and hair follicles

CLINICAL PEARLS

- The lesions of folliculitis measure ≤5 mm in size, are erythematous, pruritic, and usually cluster in groups. Considered a pyoderma of the hair follicle.
- MRSA is fast becoming the most common infectious cause, and should be considered in all difficult-to-treat cases:
  - Double-strength trimpterim-sulfamethoxazole (TMP-SMP) Bactrim/Septra 2 tablets b.i.d. plus rifampin in resistant/persistent infections complicated by abscess formation
- Patient education in proper skin care hygiene and preventive measures is vital to avoiding chronic or recurrent cases.
- Intranasal mupirocin treatment for chronic MRSA carrier state

F

FOOD ALLERGY

Stanley Fineman, MD

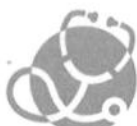

BASICS

DESCRIPTION
- Hypersensitivity reaction caused by certain foods
- System(s) affected: Gastrointestinal, Hemic/Lymphatic/Immunologic, Pulmonary, Skin/Exocrine
- Synonym(s): Allergic bowel disease; Dietary protein-sensitivity syndrome

EPIDEMIOLOGY
- Predominant age: All ages, but more common in infants and children
- Predominant sex: Male > Female (2:1)

Incidence
Prospective studies indicate ~2.5% of infants experience hypersensitivity reactions to cow's milk in their first year of life (1)[B].

Prevalence
- The prevalence of IgE-mediated food allergy is likely between 1% and 2% in the US (2,3)[A].
- In young children, the most common food allergies are cow's milk (2.5%), egg (1.3%), peanut (0.8%), and wheat (0.4%).
- Adults tend to have allergies to shellfish (2%), peanut (0.6%), tree nuts (0.5%), and fish (0.4%) (3)[B].
- In general, only 3–4% of children >4 years have persisting food allergy; therefore, it is frequently a transient phenomenon.
- 20% of children with peanut-protein allergy outgrow their sensitivity by school age (3,4)[B].

RISK FACTORS
- Persons with allergic or atopic predisposition have increased risk of hypersensitivity reaction to food.
- Family history of food hypersensitivity

Genetics
In family members with a history of food hypersensitivity, the probability of food allergy in subsequent siblings may be as high as 50%.

GENERAL PREVENTION
Avoidance of offending food

PATHOPHYSIOLOGY
Allergic response owing to immunologic mechanisms, such as the classic IgE-allergic response or nonimmunologic-mediated mechanisms

ETIOLOGY
- Any food or ingested substance can cause allergic reactions:
  - Most commonly implicated foods include cow's milk, egg whites, wheat, soy, peanuts, fish, tree nuts (walnut and pecan), shellfish, melons, sesame seeds, and sunflower seeds
- Several food dyes and additives can elicit allergic like reactions.

DIAGNOSIS

PHYSICAL EXAM
- GI (system usually affected):
  - More common: Nausea, vomiting, diarrhea, abdominal pain, occult bleeding, flatulence, and bloating
  - Less common: Malabsorption, protein-losing enteropathy, eosinophilic-enteritis, colitis
- Dermatologic:
  - More common: Urticaria/angioedema, atopic dermatitis, pallor, or flushing
  - Less common: Contact rashes
- Respiratory:
  - More common: Allergic rhinitis, asthma and bronchospasm, cough, serous otitis media
  - Less common: Pulmonary infiltrates (Heiner syndrome), pulmonary hemosiderosis
- Neurologic:
  - Less common: Migraine headaches
- Other symptoms:
  - Systemic anaphylaxis, vasculitis

DIAGNOSTIC TESTS & INTERPRETATION

Lab
- Eosinophilia in blood or tissue suggests atopy
- Epicutaneous (prick or puncture) allergy skin tests are used for documenting IgE-mediated immunologic hypersensitivity and can be done by commercially available extracts (variable sensitivities) or fresh-food skin testing.
- Skin testing using the suspect food is helpful. If positive on skin test, an oral challenge may aid in diagnosis. The overall correlation between commercially available allergy skin testing and oral food challenge is 60%, but increases to 90% when fresh-food skin testing is done. (i.e., a positive skin test correlates with a positive challenge to a particular food) (4)[A].
- Food-specific IgE assays can also detect specific IgE antibodies to offending foods
  - In certain laboratories, the ImmunoCap food-specific IgE was almost as accurate as a skin test in predicting positive oral challenges (5)[B].
- Periodic monitoring of the peanut-specific IgE levels every 2 years may be helpful. If the level of peanut-specific IgE falls below 0.5 kU/L, then a cautious oral challenge under the supervision of an allergist may be considered. A fresh-food skin test with peanut protein should be considered prior to the oral challenge.
- Patch tests for foods are useful for determining delayed-sensitivity immunologic reactions, in patients with eosinophilic esophagitis and atopic dermatitis, although the addition of these is considered of marginal benefit (6)[B].
- Widespread allergy skin testing or serum IgE tests are not recommended because of their poor predictive value without a clinical correlating history (7)[B].
- Leukocyte histamine release and assays for circulating immune complexes are predominantly research procedures and are of limited use in clinical practices:
  - Assays for IgG and IgG 4 subclass antibodies are commercially available.
  - No convincing data suggest that these tests are reliable for the diagnosis of food allergy.
- The provocative injection and sublingual provocative tests are highly controversial and have been proven to be useless for the diagnosis of food allergy.
- The leukocytotoxic assay is an unproven diagnostic procedure and is not useful for the diagnosis of allergy (6)[A].
- Other unproven diagnostic procedures that are not recommended include: Provocative neutralization, lymphocyte stimulation, hair analysis, and applied kinesiology (7)[B].

Diagnostic Procedures/Surgery
Elimination and challenge test is the best procedure for confirming food allergy:
- The suspected food is eliminated from the diet for 1–2 weeks.
- The patient's symptoms are monitored. If the patient's symptoms disappear or substantially improve, an oral challenge with the suspected food should be performed under medical supervision.
- Optimally, this challenge should be performed in a double-blind, placebo-controlled manner.
- Patients with history of anaphylaxis should not have an oral challenge unless lack of IgE sensitivity can be documented.
- Most allergic reactions will occur within 30 minutes to 2 hours after challenge, although late reactions have also been described, which may occur from 12–24 hours.

Pathological Findings
Pathologic findings are not common in food allergies; however, inflammatory changes can sometimes be seen in the GI tract. The diagnosis of eosinophilic esophagitis is defined by the finding of >15–20 eosinophils per high power field on esophageal biopsy (8)[B].

DIFFERENTIAL DIAGNOSIS
- A careful history is necessary to document a temporal relationship with the manifestations of suspected food hypersensitivity.
- The GI, dermatologic, respiratory, neurologic, or other systemic manifestations may mimic a variety of clinical entities.

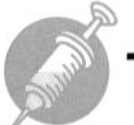

TREATMENT

MEDICATION

- Patients with significant type 1, IgE-mediated hypersensitivity should have epinephrine for autoinjection available in case of accidental ingestion and resulting severe anaphylactic reaction.
- After receiving epinephrine for a systemic anaphylactic reaction to a food, the patient should be monitored in a medical facility, since 15–20% of patients may require more than 1 dose of epinephrine.
- Symptomatic treatment for milder reactions (e.g., antihistamine)
- The use of cromolyn has been suggested but is not recommended for use in most patients with food allergy.

ADDITIONAL TREATMENT

General Measures

- Avoidance of the offending food is the most effective mode of treatment for patients with food allergies.
- Those patients with exquisite and severe allergy hypersensitivity to a food should be more cautious in their avoidance of that food. They should carry epinephrine for self-administration in the event that the offending food is ingested unknowingly and a subsequent immediate reaction develops.
- Immunotherapy or hyposensitization with food extracts by various routes, including SC immunotherapy or sublingual neutralization, are not recommended. Research studies are in progress, but immunotherapy is considered experimental.

COMPLEMENTARY AND ALTERNATIVE MEDICINE

There are reports of benefit using various Chinese herbal medicines in laboratory animals with induced food allergy. Benefits have not been reported in humans at this time.

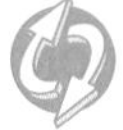

ONGOING CARE

FOLLOW-UP RECOMMENDATIONS

Patient Monitoring

As needed

DIET

- As determined by tests and clinical evaluation
- Strict avoidance of offending food

PATIENT EDUCATION

- Patients should be counseled by a dietitian to be sure that they maintain a nutritionally sound diet despite avoiding those foods to which the patient is sensitive.
- Patient support: Food Allergy and Anaphylaxis Network: 11781 Lee Jackson HWY, Suite 160, Fairfax, VA 22033-3309; 800.929.4040; Web site www.foodallergy.org
- Other information available at www.acaai.org and www.aaaai.org

PROGNOSIS

- Most infants will outgrow their food hypersensitivity by 2–4 years:
  - It may be possible to reintroduce the offending food cautiously into the diet (particularly helpful when the food is one that is difficult to avoid). It is critical that a specific IgE to the offending food is checked, optimally by fresh-food allergy skin test, and is negative prior to an oral challenge.
  - 20% of young children with peanut allergy experience resolution by the age of 5 years (9)[B].
  - 42% of children with egg allergy and 48% of children with milk allergy develop clinical tolerance and lose their sensitivity over time (7)[B].
- Adults with food hypersensitivity (particularly to milk, fish, shellfish, or nuts) tend to maintain their allergy for many years.

COMPLICATIONS

- Anaphylaxis
- Angioedema
- Bronchial asthma
- Enterocolitis
- Eosinophilic esophagitis
- Eczematoid lesions

REFERENCES

1. Høst A, Halken S. A prospective study of cow milk allergy in Danish infants during the first 3 years of life. Clinical course in relation to clinical and immunological type of hypersensitivity reaction. *Allergy*. 1990;45:587–96.
2. Chafen JJ, Newberry SJ, Riedl MA, et al. Diagnosing and managing common food allergies: A systematic review. *JAMA*. 2010;303:1848–56.
3. Sicherer SH, Sampson HA, et al. Food allergy. *J Allergy Clin Immunol*. 2010;125:S116–25.
4. Sampson HA. Utility of food-specific IgE concentrations in predicting symptomatic food allergy. *J Allergy Clin Immunol*. 2001;107:891–6.
5. Maloney JM, Rudengren M, Ahlstedt S, et al. The use of serum specific IgE measurements for the diagnosis of peanut, tree nut, and seed allergy. *J Allergy Clin Immunol*. 2008.
6. Spergel JM, Brown-Whitehorn T, Beausoleil JL, et al. Predictive values for skin prick test and atopy patch test for eosinophilic esophagitis. *J Allergy Clin Immunol*. 2007;119:509–11.
7. Boyce JA, Assa'ad A, Burks AW, et al. Guidelines for the diagnosis and management of food allergy in the United States: Report of the NIAID-Sponsored Expert Panel. *J Allergy Clin Immunol*. 2010;126:S1–58.
8. Furuta GT, Lacouras CA, et al. Eosinophilic esophagitis in children and adult: A systematic review and consensus recommendations for diagnosis and treatment. *Gastroenterology*. 2007;133:1342–63.
9. Sicherer SH, Sampson HA, et al. Peanut allergy: Emerging concepts and approaches for an apparent epidemic. *J Allergy Clin Immunol*. 2007;120.
10. Chapman JA, Bernstein IL. Food allergy: A practice parameter. *Ann Allergy Asthma Immunol*. 2006; 96:S1–68.
11. Greer FR, Sicherer SH, Burks AW, et al. Effects of early nutritional interventions on the development of atopic disease in infants and children: The role of maternal dietary restriction, breastfeeding, timing of introduction of complementary foods, and hydrolyzed formulas. *Pediatrics*. 2008; 121:183–91.

ADDITIONAL READING

Bernstein IL, Li JT, Bernstein DI, et al. Allergy diagnostic testing: An updated practice parameter. *Ann Allergy Asthma Immunol*. 2008;100:S1–148.

See Also (Topic, Algorithm, Electronic Media Element)

Anaphylaxis; Celiac Disease; Irritable Bowel Syndrome

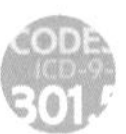

CODES

ICD9

- 708.0 Allergic urticaria
- 995.60 Anaphylactic shock due to unspecified food
- 995.7 Other adverse food reactions, not elsewhere classified

CLINICAL PEARLS

- Recent studies suggest that up to 20% of children with peanut allergy may outgrow their sensitivity:
  - Periodic monitoring of the peanut-specific IgE levels every 2 years may be helpful. If the level of peanut-specific IgE falls below 0.5 kU/L, then a cautious oral challenge under the supervision of an allergist may be considered. A fresh-food skin test with peanut protein should be considered prior to the oral challenge.
- Oral itching following ingestion of fresh fruit may be a warning of risk for anaphylaxis but may only represent oral allergy syndrome:
  - This syndrome is the result of cross-reacting proteins in pollens (example: Patients sensitive to birch tree pollen frequently have this cross-reactivity to fresh apples and pears. Cooked fruits are usually tolerated) (10)[B].
- Current evidence does not support a major role for maternal dietary restrictions during pregnancy or lactation in the prevention of atopic disease in infants. It is generally recommended to exclusively breast-feed for the first 6 months of life, particularly when there is a family history of atopy and food allergy. Although solid foods should not be introduced before 4–6 months of age, there is no convincing evidence that delaying their introduction beyond this period has a significant protective effect on the development of allergies (11)[B].

FOOD POISONING, BACTERIAL

Karl M. Schmitt, MD

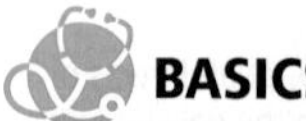

BASICS

DESCRIPTION

- Food poisoning, also called foodborne infection, is an illness resulting from the consumption of contaminated food.
- The illness may be produced by bacterial infection or by toxins produced by the bacteria.
- The most commonly recognized foodborne infections acquired in the US are those caused by the bacteria *Campylobacter*, *Salmonella*, and *C. perfringens*. Adding in traveler's diarrhea, *Escherichia coli* enters this group.
- *Vibrio* incidence rare, but increasing substantially in last 10 years (1)

EPIDEMIOLOGY

Incidence

In the US, it is estimated that there are more than 48 million cases of foodborne poisoning annually (the majority being viral in etiology), resulting in 128,000 hospitalizations and 3,000 deaths (1). ~1 in 6 Americans will have an episode.

RISK FACTORS

- Travel to developing countries
- Improper food storage or handling
- Cross-contamination during preparation of food
- Weakened immune system, pregnancy, elderly, and very young
- Underlying GI disorders
- Patients taking antacids, H2 blockers, and proton pump inhibitors

GENERAL PREVENTION

- When preparing food at home (1):
  - Clean:
    - Wash hands, cutting boards, and surfaces before food preparation and after preparing each food item.
    - Wash fresh produce thoroughly before eating.
  - Separate:
    - Keep raw meat, poultry, fish, and their juices away from other food.
    - Place cooked meat on clean platter.
  - Cook: Thoroughly cook meat to the following internal temperature (2):
    - Fresh beef, veal, pork, and lamb: 145°F
    - Ground meats and egg dishes: 160°F
    - Poultry: 165°F. Cook chicken eggs thoroughly until the yolk is firm.
  - Chill:
    - Refrigerate leftovers within 4 hours in clean, shallow, covered containers. If the temperature is >90°F, refrigerate within 1 hour.
- When traveling to underdeveloped countries (3):
  - Eat only foods that are freshly prepared.
  - Avoid beverages diluted with nonpotable water, such as ice and milk.
  - Avoid food washed in nonpotable water, like salads.
  - Other risky foods include raw or undercooked meat and seafood, unpeeled raw fruits and vegetables.
  - In developing nations, "Boil it, Cook it, Peel it, or Forget it."
  - Bottled, carbonated, and boiled beverages are generally safe to drink.
- Bismuth subsalicylate (Pepto-Bismol), two 262-mg tablets q.i.d. has been shown to protect travelers to developing countries ~60% of the time. However, it is not recommended for persons taking anticoagulants or other salicylates (4).

ETIOLOGY

- Short incubation period (1–6 hours): Likely preformed toxin-induced:
  - *Bacillus cereus*:
    - Food sources: Improperly cooked rice/fried rice and red meats
    - Causes sudden onset of severe nausea and vomiting. Diarrhea may be present.
  - *Staphylococcus aureus*:
    - Food sources: Unrefrigerated or improperly refrigerated meats, potato, and egg salads
    - Causes sudden onset of severe nausea and vomiting. Abdominal cramps and fever may be present.
- Medium incubation period (8–16 hours):
  - *Bacillus cereus* (toxin):
    - Food sources: Meat, stew gravy, vanilla sauce
    - Causes watery diarrhea, abdominal cramps, nausea
  - *Clostridium perfringens:*
    - Food sources: Dry or precooked meats and poultry
    - Causes watery diarrhea, nausea, abdominal cramps
- Long incubation period (>16 hours):
  - Toxin-producing organisms:
    - *Clostridium botulinum*: Food source is home-canned or improperly canned commercial foods. Causes vomiting, diarrhea, blurred vision, diplopia, dysphagia, and descending muscle weakness.
    - Enterohemorrhagic *E. coli* (e.g., 0157:H7): Food sources are undercooked beef, especially hamburger, unpasteurized milk, raw fruits and vegetables, and contaminated water. Causes severe diarrhea that often becomes bloody, abdominal pain, vomiting. More common in children <4 years of age.
    - Enterotoxigenic *E. coli*: Food sources are foods or water contaminated by human feces. Causes watery diarrhea, abdominal cramps, and vomiting.
    - *Vibrio cholerae*: Food sources are contaminated water, fish, and shellfish, especially food sold by street vendors. Causes profuse watery diarrhea and vomiting, which can lead to severe dehydration and death within hours.
  - Invasive organisms: Often bloody stool and fever:
    - *Campylobacter jejuni*: Food sources are raw and undercooked poultry, unpasteurized milk, contaminated meats. Causes diarrhea (may be bloody), cramps, vomiting, and fever.
    - *Salmonella*: Food sources are contaminated eggs, poultry, unpasteurized milk or juice, cheese, contaminated raw fruits and vegetables. Causes watery diarrhea, fever, abdominal cramps, vomiting.
    - *Shigella*: Food sources are food or water contaminated by human fecal material. Causes abdominal cramps, fever, diarrhea.
    - *Vibrio parahaemolyticus*: Food source is raw shellfish. Causes nausea, vomiting, diarrhea, and abdominal pain.
    - *Vibrio vulnificus:* Food source is undercooked and raw seafood; wounds exposed to sea water. Causes vomiting, diarrhea, abdominal pain, bacteremia, wound infections. Can be fatal in patients with liver disease or who are immunocompromised.
    - *Y. enterocolitica* and *Y. pseudotuberculosis*: Food sources are undercooked pork, unpasteurized milk, tofu, contaminated water. Causes appendicitislike symptoms: Abdominal pain, fever, diarrhea, and vomiting; occurs primarily in older children and younger adults.

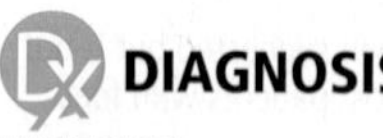

DIAGNOSIS

HISTORY

- Food poisoning most often presents as gastroenteritis (4).
- Most cases of gastroenteritis have a viral etiology. Suspect bacterial food poisoning when multiple persons have rapid onset after eating the same meal, have high fever, blood or mucus in stool, severe abdominal pain, or neurologic involvement.
- Suspect bacterial gastroenteritis if traveling in or recent travel to an underdeveloped country (4).
- Timing and presentation can aid in establishing an etiology.

PHYSICAL EXAM

- The physical exam should focus on signs of dehydration, including evaluating skin turgor and mucous membranes, and observing for hypotension or orthostatic changes.
- The abdominal exam should focus on abdominal distension with tenderness, suggestive of bowel obstruction. Auscultation may demonstrate increased bowel sound in obstruction or decreased bowel sounds with an ileus.
- Neurologic: Weakness, paresthesias, diplopia

DIAGNOSTIC TESTS & INTERPRETATION

Lab

Initial lab tests

- Culture of stool and sensitivity, fecal leukocytes, and Hemoccult testing; consider ova and parasites if history of foreign travel or symptoms lasting longer than 2 weeks
- May need to specify to lab if concerns for *Vibrio*, *E. coli* 0157:H7: Require special cultures
- BMP and WBC count if diarrhea is severe, temperature >101.5°F (38.5°C), persistently bloody stools, severe abdominal pain, or if patient is immunocompromised, elderly, or very young

Follow-Up & Special Considerations

Epidemiologic investigation may be warranted.

DIFFERENTIAL DIAGNOSIS

- Infectious gastroenteritis of any kind (i.e., viral)
- *C. difficile* colitis
- Inflammatory bowel disease
- Appendicitis and other acute abdominal surgical processes
- Hepatitis
- Malabsorption

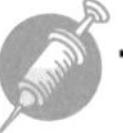

TREATMENT

- Most cases of food poisoning are self-limiting and do not require medication.
- A health care provider should be consulted for food poisoning if the following are present: High fever (≥101.5°F); blood in the stools; prolonged vomiting; signs of dehydration (decrease in urination, a dry mouth and throat, and feeling dizzy when standing up); diarrheal illness that lasts more than 3 days (3)[C]

MEDICATION

First Line

- Children, the elderly, and pregnant patients with signs of mild diarrhea should be started on oral rehydration solution to prevent dehydration (5)[B].
- Oral rehydration options can be purchased or mixed simply from common home ingredients. 6 tsp sugar, 1/2 tsp salt in 1 L of clean, potable water. May add 1/2 cup orange juice or mashed banana for taste and potassium.
- Travelers may consider empiric treatment for diarrhea with a single dose of ciprofloxacin 750 mg together with loperamide (see "Additional Treatment").

Second Line

For severe cases of food poisoning (up to 8% have bacteremia) or if the patient has a prosthetic valve, the following medications are recommended (6)[B]:

- *Bacillus cereus:*
  - Supportive care only
- *Campylobacter jejuni*:
  - Mild: Supportive care only
  - Severe: Children: Azithromycin 10 mg/kg/d for 3 days
  - Severe: Adults: Azithromycin 500 mg/d for 3 days
- *Clostridium botulinum*:
  - Supportive care. Antitoxin can be helpful if administered early in the course of the illness.
- *Clostridium perfringens:*
  - Supportive care only
- *Clostridium difficile:*
  - Metronidazole 500 mg t.i.d. for 10–14 days or vancomycin 125 mg PO q.i.d. for 10 days or rifaximin 400 mg q.i.d. for 10–14 days
- Enterohemorrhagic *E. coli* (e.g., 0157:H7):
  - Supportive care only. Closely monitor renal function, hemoglobin, and platelets. Infection associated with hemolytic uremic syndrome (HUS). Antibiotics may increase this risk.
- Enterotoxigenic *E. coli* (common cause of traveler's diarrhea):
  - Generally self-limited. Antibiotics shorten course of illness.
  - Children: Azithromycin 10 mg/kg/d for 3 days or ceftriaxone 50 mg/kg/d for 3 days
  - Adults: Ciprofloxacin 750 mg/d for 3 days or azithromycin 1 g × single dose. Rifaximin rising as an alternate.
- *Salmonella*:
  - Children: Ceftriaxone: 100 mg/kg/d divided b.i.d. for 7–10 days or azithromycin 20 mg/kg/d for 7 days
  - Adults: Levofloxacin 500 mg a day for 7–10 days or azithromycin 500 mg daily for 7 days. Either can be given for 14 days for immunosuppressed patients.
- *Shigella*:
  - Children: Azithromycin 10 mg/kg/d for 3 days or ceftriaxone 50 mg/kg/d for 3 days
  - Adults: Ciprofloxacin 750 mg/d for 3 days or azithromycin 500 mg/d for 3 days
- *S. aureus*:
  - Supportive care only
- *Vibrio cholerae*:
  - Children: Erythromycin 30 mg/kg/d given t.i.d. for 3 days or azithromycin 10 mg/kg/d for 3 days.
  - Adults: Doxycycline 300 mg 1-time dose or tetracycline 500 mg q.i.d. for 3 days or erythromycin 250 mg t.i.d. for 3 days or azithromycin 500 mg/d for 3 days
- *Vibrio parahaemolyticus*:
  - Supportive care only
  - May use doxycycline 300 mg 1 dose if severe
- *Vibrio vulnificus:*
  - Adults: Minocycline or doxycycline 100 mg b.i.d. plus either cefotaxime 2 g IV q8h or ceftriaxone 1 g IV daily with doses appropriately adjusted for underlying renal or hepatic disease
- *Yersinia*:
  - Usually supportive care only
  - Quinolones or third-generation cephalosporin if severe

ADDITIONAL TREATMENT

- Loperamide 4 mg initially, then 2 mg after each loose stool to a maximum of 16 mg in a 24-hour period may be used unless high fever, bloody diarrhea, and/or severe abdominal pain are present (signs of enteroinvasion). Among travelers with mild–moderate diarrhea and cramping, a single dose of ciprofloxacin 750 mg together with loperamide may eliminate the diarrhea. If symptoms persist after 24 hours, treat with antibiotics for an additional 1–2 days.
- Probiotics (i.e., *Lactobacillus* sp.) have shown decrease in duration of diarrhea by ~25 hours; more research is needed (7)[A]

ONGOING CARE

DIET

- Avoid food while nausea is present, but drink plenty of fluids in frequent sips.
- As the nausea subsides, drink adequate fluids, add in bland, low-fat meals and rest. Avoid alcohol, coffee, nicotine, spicy foods.
- Nursing infants should continue to be breast-fed on demand, and infants and older children should be offered their usual food (4).

PROGNOSIS

Most infections are self-limited and will resolve over the course of 4–5 days.

COMPLICATIONS

- Dehydration
- Hemolytic uremic syndrome (3–5% *E. coli* 0157:H7)
- Guillain-Barré syndrome after *Campylobacter* enteritis
- Reiter syndrome after *Salmonella* enteritis
- *Clostridium difficile* colitis after antibiotic use
- Postinfectious irritable bowel

REFERENCES

1. CDC. 2011 Estimates. www.cdc.gov/ncidod/dbmd/diseaseinfo/foodborneinfections_g.htm.
2. www.fsis.usda.gov/Is_It_Done_Yet/brochure_text.
3. www.cdc.gov/ncidod/dbmd/diseaseinfo/foodborneinfections_g.htm#howtreated.
4. Yates J. Traveler's diarrhea. *Am Fam Physician*. 2005;71:2095–100.
5. Ang JY, Mathur A. Traveler's diarrhea: Updates for pediatricians. *Pediatric Ann*. 2008;37:814–20.
6. Dupont HL. Bacterial diarrhea. *NEJM*. 2009;361:1560–9.
7. Probiotics for treating acute infectious diarrhea. *Cochrane Database Syst Rev*. 2010;11.

ADDITIONAL READING

- The Community Summary Report on Trends and Sources of Zoonoses and Zoonotic Agents in the European Union in 2007. *The European Food Safety Authority Journal*. 2009;223.
- Centers for Disease Control and Prevention. Trends in foodborne illness in the United States, 1996–2010. Available at: www.cdc.gov/foodborneburden/trends-infoodborne-illness.html.
- Diagnosis and management of foodborne illnesses: A primer for physicians. *MMWR Recomm Rep*. 2004;53(RR04):1–33.
- Reduced osmolarity oral rehydration solution. *Cochrane Database Syst Rev*. 2007;3.
- Rehydration Project. http://rehydrate.org/ors/made-at-home.
- Scorza K, Williams A, Phillips JD, et al. Evaluation of nausea and vomiting. *Am Fam Physician*. 2007;76:76–84.

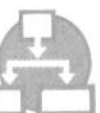

See Also (Topic, Algorithm, Electronic Media Element)

Appendicitis, Acute; Botulism; Brucellosis; Dehydration; Diarrhea, Acute; Guillain-Barré Syndrome; Hypokalemia; Intestinal Parasites; Salmonella Infection; Typhoid Fever

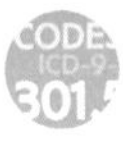

CODES

ICD9

- 003.9 Salmonella infection, unspecified
- 005.89 Other bacterial food poisoning
- 008.00 Intestinal infection due to e. coli, unspecified

CLINICAL PEARLS

- Consider bacterial food poisoning when multiple people present with symptoms after ingesting the same food and show fevers and blood or mucus in stool, or have recently returned from a developing nation.
- In developing nations, "Boil it, Cook it, Peel it, or Forget it."
- Consider culture and antibiotics in a prolonged febrile state with blood/mucus in stool, septicemic states, and traveler's diarrhea.
- Consider reporting to local/state health department for follow-up.
- Reintroduce food as soon as tolerated; use oral rehydration, limit high-fat foods and foods high in simple sugars. Lactose limitation is controversial.

F

FRAGILE X SYNDROME

Thomas J. Hansen, MD

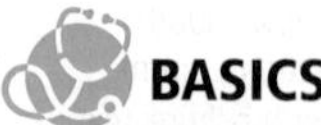

BASICS

DESCRIPTION

- Fragile X syndrome (FXS) is the most common inherited form of mental retardation (also referred to as mental impairment).
- Among the genetic causes of mental impairment, FXS is the second most common cause following Down syndrome.
- In addition to mental impairment, FXS is characterized by a group of symptoms that may include specific physical features, distinctive behavior patterns, defective speech and language, and cognitive deficits (1).
- Synonym(s): Marker X syndrome; Martin-Bell syndrome; Escalante's syndrome

EPIDEMIOLOGY

- Although this condition is seen in both sexes, males are usually more severely affected than females.
- Affected males almost always have mental impairment, mostly of moderate severity.
- Only 1/3–1/2 of the affected females have mental impairment, usually in the mild-to-moderate range (1).

Prevalence

- FXS with full mutation is seen in 1:4,000 males and 1:8,000 females (2).
- FXS with premutation is seen in 1:800 males and 1:200 females (1).

RISK FACTORS

Genetics

- This is an X-linked dominant disorder with variable penetrance.
- The syndrome is caused by an abnormal expansion of cytosine-guanine-guanine (CGG) on the fragile X mental retardation 1 (FMR1) gene. FMR1 normally synthesizes the fragile X protein (FMRP), but mutations in FMR1 lead to a lack of FMRP synthesis, which is important for normal brain development (3).
- The number of CGG repeats in the FMR1 gene are classified as:
  - Full mutation (>200 CGG repeats)
  - Premutation (~6–200 CGG repeats)
- Most males with full mutation have mental impairment in addition to some form of the physical and behavioral features.
- Males with premutation have normal intelligence but have an increased risk for tremor-ataxia syndrome between the ages of 50 and 60.
- Females with full mutation have an approximate 50% chance of having mental impairment in addition to some form of physical and behavioral features.
- Females with premutation have normal intelligence but have a 20% risk for premature ovarian failure.
- Since a male has only 1 X chromosome, it is never passed on to his son. He will pass the affected chromosome to all of his daughters.
- An affected female has a 50% chance of passing her affected chromosome to all of her children.

COMMONLY ASSOCIATED CONDITIONS

- Autistic spectrum disorder (2)
- Connective tissue manifestations, including flat feet and inguinal hernias (2)
- Mitral valve prolapse (develops during adolescence and adulthood) (2)
- Recurrent otitis media and sinusitis in childhood (2)
- Seizure disorder (15–20% for boys and 5% for girls) (3)
- Social phobias and other anxiety disorders (3)

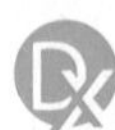

DIAGNOSIS

HISTORY

- Family history of mental impairment, particularly with multiple male relatives
- Family history of premature ovarian failure (POF) or fragile X-related tremor ataxia syndrome
- Delay of 1 or more developmental milestones, especially when there is mental impairment in the family (1)
- After the first year of life, delay in speech and language along with impaired fine motor skills

Pediatric Considerations

Average age at the time of diagnosis is 8 years, reflecting the subtlety of features in young children (1).

PHYSICAL EXAM

- Physical characteristics, which become more prominent with advancing age, include (2):
  - Large anterior fontanelle and macrosomia at birth
  - Macrocephaly
  - Prominent forehead
  - Pale blue iris
  - Long and thin face with a prominent jaw
  - Large ears
  - Midface hypoplasia
  - High arched palate
  - Dental overcrowding
  - Inability to touch the lips with the tongue
  - Soft stretchy skin
  - Plantar and hallucal crease
  - Single palmar crease
  - Double-jointed thumb
  - Hyperextensible metacarpophalangeal joints
  - Mitral valve prolapse
  - Pectus excavatum
  - Scoliosis
  - Pes planus
  - Macro-orchidism (usually seen after puberty)
- Cognitive deficits: Delayed language, math skills, problem-solving, abstract thinking, visuospatial abilities, short-term memory, adaptive behavior, and social skills (2)
- Behavioral characteristics include poor eye contact, tactile defensiveness, hand flapping, hand biting, perseverative speech (2), inattention, hypersensitivity to stimuli, overarousability, hyperactivity, and (mostly in men) explosive and aggressive behavior to others or self (3).

DIAGNOSTIC TESTS & INTERPRETATION

Diagnosis of FXS is made by DNA-based molecular tests, such as Southern blot test and PCR, to isolate the FMR1 gene mutation. Indications for testing include:

- Patients with a family history of mental impairment or FXS
- Any child with developmental delay of uncertain etiology or autism
- Individual with mental impairment of unknown etiology
- Women with premature ovarian failure of unknown cause
- Individuals with late-onset intentional tremor or ataxia, especially with a family history of movement disorders, FXS, or undiagnosed mental impairment
- Prenatal testing is offered only if maternal premutation or full mutation is present:
  - Chorionic villus sampling or amniocentesis is used for prenatal diagnosis.
  - Preimplantation genetic diagnosis may be another option for women with a premutation FXS; however, there are several limitations to this approach.

Imaging

Initial approach

Newborn screening for FXS is not routine at the present time (4)[B].

DIFFERENTIAL DIAGNOSIS

- Pervasive developmental disorder
- Learning disability
- Autism
- Attention deficit hyperactivity disorder (ADHD)
- Other causes of mental impairment

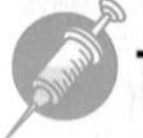

TREATMENT

- Treatment is usually supportive.
- Currently, there is no robust evidence to support recommendations on pharmacological treatments in patients with FXS in general, or in those with an additional diagnosis of ADHD or autism (5).

MEDICATION

Depending on the clinical presentation, pharmacotherapy may include (6)[B]:

- Atypical antipsychotics
- SSRIs
- Antiepileptics
- Methylphenidates
- Dextroamphetamines
- Clonidine
- Guanfacine

Second Line

Impossible to draw conclusions about the effect of folic acid on FXS patients due to the low quality of current evidence (7).

ADDITIONAL TREATMENT

Nonpharmacologic therapies are of tremendous value (8)[B] and include:

- Behavior therapy
- Speech and language therapy
- Psychotherapy and counseling
- Occupational and physical therapy
- Social skill training, support group
- Special education and preschool intervention programs (8)

Issues for Referral

- The proband and family should be referred for genetic counseling and tested for the FMR1 gene.
- Also see "Additional Treatment" section.

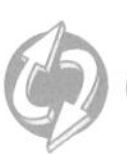

ONGOING CARE

PATIENT EDUCATION

- In young females with FXS who are planning for future pregnancies, one should review the reproductive options, such as egg donation, prenatal diagnosis, adoption, and preimplantation genetic diagnosis.
- Useful Web sites:
  - The National Fragile X Foundation (www.fragilex.org)
  - FRAXA Research Foundation (http://www.fraxa.org)
  - Gene Tests (www.genetests.org, www.geneclinics.org)
  - American College of Medical Genetics (www.acmg.net)
  - Dolan DNA Learning Center: Your Genes, Your Health (www.ygyh.org)
  - National Institute of Child Health and Human Development (www.nichd.nih.gov)

PROGNOSIS

- Patients with FXS have a normal lifespan.
- About 20–33% of women carrying a premutation for FXS are at increased risk for premature ovarian failure.
- 1/3 of males and, to a lesser extent, the females carrying the premutation are at increased risk for late-onset (>50 years of age) progressive neurodegenerative disorder. It is characterized by intentional tremor and ataxia, called fragile X-associated tremor/ataxia syndrome (FXTAS). Other associated findings include parkinsonism, autonomic dysfunction, peripheral neuropathy, and dementia.

REFERENCES

1. Wattendorf DJ, Muenke M. Diagnosis and management of fragile X syndrome. *Am Fam Physician*. 2005;72:111–3.
2. Visootsak J, Warren ST, Anido A, et al. Fragile X syndrome: An update and review for the primary pediatrician. *Clin Pediatr (Phila)*. 2005;44:371–81.
3. Tsiouris JA, Brown WT. Neuropsychiatric symptoms of fragile X syndrome: Pathophysiology and pharmacotherapy. *CNS Drugs*. 2004;18:687–703.
4. Bailey DB, Skinner D, Davis AM, et al. Ethical, legal, and social concerns about expanded newborn screening: Fragile X syndrome as a prototype for emerging issues. *Pediatrics*. 2008;121:e693–704.
5. Rueda JR, Ballesteros J, Tejada MI, et al. Systematic review of pharmacological treatments in fragile X syndrome. *BMC Neurol*. 2009;9:53.
6. Hagerman RJ, Berry-Kravis E, Kaufmann WE, et al. Advances in the treatment of fragile X syndrome. *Pediatrics*. 2009;123:378–90.
7. Rueda JR, Ballesteros J, Guillen V, et al. Folic acid for fragile X syndrome. *Cochrane Database Syst Rev*. 2011;CD008476.
8. Solomon M, Hessl D, Chiu S, et al. A genetic etiology of pervasive developmental disorder guides treatment. *Am J Psychiatry*. 2007;164:575–80.

ADDITIONAL READING

- American College of Obstetricians and Gynecologists Committee on Genetics. ACOG committee opinion. No. 338: Screening for fragile X syndrome. *Obstet Gynecol*. 2006;107:1483–5.
- Cornish KM, Gray KM, Rinehart NJ, et al. Fragile X syndrome and associated disorders. *Adv Child Dev Behav*. 2010;39:211–35.
- Garber KB, Visootsak J, Warren ST. Fragile X syndrome. *Eur J Hum Genet*. 2008.
- Hersh JH, Saul RA, Committee on Genetics, et al. Health supervision for children with fragile X syndrome. *Pediatrics*. 2011;127:994–1006.
- Huber K. Fragile X syndrome: Molecular mechanisms of cognitive dysfunction. *Am J Psychiatry*. 2007;164:556.
- McConkie-Rosell A, Finucane B, Cronister A, et al. Genetic counseling for fragile x syndrome: Updated recommendations of the national society of genetic counselors. *J Genet Couns*. 2005;14:249–70.
- Orr HT, Zoghbi HY. Trinucleotide repeat disorders. *Ann Rev Neurosci*. 2007;30:575–621.
- Penagarikano O, Mulle JG, Warren ST. The pathophysiology of fragile X syndrome. *Annu Rev Genomics Hum Genet*. 2007;8:109–29.
- Wiesner GL, Cassidy SB, Grimes SJ, et al. Clinical consult: Developmental delay/fragile X syndrome. *Prim Care*. 2004;31:621–5, x.

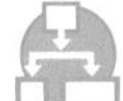

See Also (Topic, Algorithm, Electronic Media Element)

Algorithm: Mental Retardation

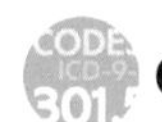

CODES

ICD9

759.83 Fragile X syndrome

CLINICAL PEARLS

- FXS is the most common inherited form of mental retardation.
- FXS is an X-linked dominant disorder with variable penetrance. Therefore, although this condition is seen in both sexes, males are usually more severely affected than females.
- Newborn screening for FXS is not routine.
- The average age at the time of diagnosis is 8 years old.

F

FROSTBITE

Alan M. Ehrlich, MD

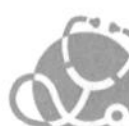

BASICS

DESCRIPTION
- A localized complication of exposure to cold, causing tissue to freeze, resulting in diminished blood flow to the affected part (especially hands, face, or feet)
- System(s) affected: Endocrine/Metabolic; Skin/Exocrine
- Synonym(s): Dermatitis congelationis; Frostnip; Environmental injuries

EPIDEMIOLOGY
- Predominant age: All ages
- Predominant sex: Male = Female

RISK FACTORS
- Previous cold-related injury
- Decreased caloric intake (<1,500 calories/d)
- Dehydration or hypovolemia
- Impaired cerebral function
- Under the effects of alcohol or drug abuse
- Underlying psychiatric disturbance
- Ambient temperature ≤−17.8°C (0°F)
- Smoker
- Elderly
- Lean body mass
- Low level of fitness
- Lack of proper clothing or shelter
- Raynaud phenomenon
- Peripheral vascular disease
- Diabetes mellitus
- Constriction from excessively tight clothing (including too many layers of socks)
- Vehicular failure leading to prolonged cold exposure

GENERAL PREVENTION
- Dress in layers with appropriate cold-weather gear.
- Avoid clothing that is too constricting.
- Cover exposed areas and extremities appropriately.
- Prepare properly for trips to cold climates.
- Minimize wind exposure.
- Stay dry.
- Avoid alcohol.
- Ensure adequate fluid and caloric intake.

PATHOPHYSIOLOGY
- Ice crystals form intracellularly.
- Vasoconstriction reduces blood flow and microclotting leads to ischemia.
- Dehydration, enzymatic destruction, and ultimately cell death occur.
- In severe cases, deep-tissue freezing may occur with damage to underlying blood vessels, muscles, and nerve tissue.

ETIOLOGY
- Prolonged exposure to cold
- Refreezing thawed extremities

COMMONLY ASSOCIATED CONDITIONS
Alcohol and/or drug abuse

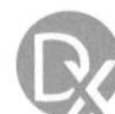

DIAGNOSIS

HISTORY
- Throbbing pain
- Paresthesia
- Excessive sweating
- Joint pain
- Determine duration and severity of cold exposure.

PHYSICAL EXAM
- Feet, hands, and face most commonly affected
- Injured area appears cold, hard, and white and is anesthetic to touch. It progresses to blotchy-red, swollen, and painful regions after rewarming.
- First degree: Redness and edema without blister formation
- Second degree: Redness, edema, and blister formation
- Third degree: Same as above with addition of hemorrhagic vesicles
- Fourth degree: Necrosis and gangrene
- Pallor
- Loss of cutaneous sensation
- Numbness
- Limited movement of affected joints
- SC edema
- Hyperemia
- Blistering
- Blue discoloration
- Skin necrosis
- Gangrene

DIAGNOSTIC TESTS & INTERPRETATION
ECG in hypothermia may show bradycardia, atrial fibrillation, atrial flutter, ventricular fibrillation, diffuse T-wave inversion, Osborn waves (upward-going "hump" following S wave in the RS–T segment).

Lab
- May show signs of hemoconcentration, such as elevated hemoglobin or high BUN/creatinine ratio
- Liver function tests for decreased hepatic function

Imaging
- Triple-phase bone scan can identify tissue viability at early stage and facilitate early debridement.
- Other imaging techniques sometimes used include MRI/MRA, infrared thermography, angiography, digital plethysmography, and laser Doppler studies.

Pathological Findings
- Ice crystallization in the intravascular extracellular space
- Atrophy
- Fibroblastic proliferation
- Skin necrosis

DIFFERENTIAL DIAGNOSIS
- Frostnip, a superficial cold injury that does not cause permanent damage
- Chilblains (pernio), an inflammatory reaction to short-term cold, wet exposure without tissue freezing
- Immersion syndrome (trench foot), inflammatory reaction to prolonged cold, wet exposure, typically socks or footwear

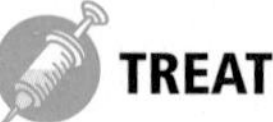

TREATMENT

Geriatric Considerations
- Associated disease states increase mortality.
- Periarticular osteoporosis complicates
- More prone to hypothermia

Pediatric Considerations
Loss of epithelial growth centers

ALERT
Acidosis

MEDICATION

First Line
- tPA administered within 24 hours of injury may prevent damage from thrombosis and may reduce amputation rate (1,2)[C].
- Aspirin 250 mg plus buflomedil 400 mg IV followed by 8 days of iloprost 0.5–2 ng/kg/min for 6 hours a day may prevent amputation in patients with frostbite extending to the proximal phalanx (3)[B].
- Tetanus toxoid
- Penicillin G 500,000 units q6h for 48–72 hours prophylactically (4)[B]
- Ibuprofen 400 mg q12h to inhibit prostaglandins (4)[C]
- NSAIDs for mild–moderate pain. For severe pain, narcotic analgesia.
- Precautions: tPA should not be used with history of recent bleeding, stroke, ulcer, etc.

Second Line
Pentoxifylline has been tried with some success (4)[C].

ADDITIONAL TREATMENT

General Measures
- If transport time will be short (1–2 hours at most), the risks posed by improper rewarming or refreezing outweigh the risks of delaying treatment for deep frostbite (5)[C].
- If transport will be prolonged (more than 1–2 hours), frostbite will often thaw spontaneously. It is more important to prevent hypothermia than to rewarm frostbite rapidly in warm water. This does not mean that a frostbitten extremity should be kept in the cold to prevent spontaneous rewarming. Anticipate that frostbitten areas will rewarm as a consequence of keeping the patient warm, and protect them from refreezing at all costs (5)[C].

- Rapid rewarming (6)[B]:
  - Immerse frozen body part in warm water (40–41°C [104–106°F]) whirlpool bath for at least 30 minutes and until thawing is complete.
  - Do not let affected part touch sides of whirlpool unit.
  - Continue rewarming until a red/purple color appears and the affected part becomes pliable.
  - It is critical not to allow refreezing after thawing has occurred.
  - Repeat treatment for 30 minutes b.i.d. until distinction of viable from nonviable tissue is clear or evidence of clear healing is present.
- After rewarming, injured parts should be covered with nonadhesive dressings, splinted, and elevated.
- Remove jewelry and clothing, if present, from the affected area.
- Application of topical aloe vera q6h
- Sterile cotton between fingers or toes, if applicable, to prevent maceration
- Keep the patient dry.
- If conscious, give the patient warm fluids with high sugar content.
- Prevent infection once treatment begins.
- Institute ongoing whirlpool therapy for cleansing and debridement.
- Prevent damage to other body parts.
- Prohibit use of nicotine-containing products (including cigarettes) or other vasoconstrictive agents.
- Maintenance: Gastric lavage, peritoneal dialysis, hemodialysis, and mediastinal lavage if needed (using warmed fluids)

Additional Therapies

- Heated oxygen
- Warm IV fluids via central venous pressure line

SURGERY/OTHER PROCEDURES

- Urgent surgery rarely needed except fasciotomy for compartment syndrome (suspect if tissue swollen and compartment pressures >37–40 mm Hg)
- Surgical debridement as needed to remove necrotic tissue
- Amputation should not be considered until it is definite that tissues are dead: May take ~3 weeks to know whether the tissue is permanently injured

IN-PATIENT CONSIDERATIONS

Initial Stabilization

- Institute emergency measures for hypothermic patient without pulse or respiration. Such measures may include CPR and internal warming with warm IV fluids and warm oxygen (see topic "Hypothermia").
- Prevent refreezing.
- It may be necessary to keep the frostbitten part frozen until the patient can be transported to a care facility. Prolonged freezing is preferable to warming and refreezing (7)[C].
- Remove nonadherent wet clothing.
- Treat for hypothermia.
- Treat for pain:
  - NSAIDs and/or narcotics if needed
- Do not rub areas to warm them; increased tissue damage may occur (1)[C].
- Do not allow patient with frostbitten feet to walk except when the life of the patient or rescuer is in danger (5)[C].

Admission Criteria

Hospitalization generally recommended (2)

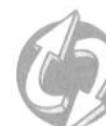

ONGOING CARE

FOLLOW-UP RECOMMENDATIONS

Outpatient or inpatient, depending on severity:

- As tolerated; protect injured body parts.
- Initiate physical therapy once healing progresses sufficiently.

Patient Monitoring

- Preferably electronic probe for temperature monitoring (rectal or vascular)
- Follow-up for physical therapy progress, infection, other complications

DIET

- As tolerated
- Warm oral fluids

PATIENT EDUCATION

- Refer to local library for information.
- Provide education on:
  - Exposure protection
  - Early signs and symptoms of frostbite

PROGNOSIS

- Anesthesia and bullae may occur.
- The affected areas will heal or mummify without surgery; the process may take 6–12 months for healing.
- Patient may be sensitive to cold and experience burning and tingling.
- Cyanotic nonblanching skin and blisters with dark fluid suggest worse prognosis (7)[C].

COMPLICATIONS

- Hyperglycemia
- Acidosis
- Refractory arrhythmias
- Tissue loss: Distal parts of an extremity may undergo spontaneous amputation.
- Gangrene
- Death

REFERENCES

1. Bruen KJ, Ballard JR, Morris SE, et al. Reduction of the incidence of amputation in frostbite injury with thrombolytic therapy. *Arch Surg*. 2007;142: 546–51; discussion 551–3.
2. Jurkovich GJ. Environmental cold-induced injury. *Surg Clin North Am*. 2007;87:247–67, viii.
3. Cauchy E, Cheguillaume B, Chetaille E, et al. A controlled trial of a prostacyclin and rt-PA in the treatment of severe frostbite. *N Engl J Med*. 2011;364:189–90.
4. Imray C, Grieve A, Dhillon S, et al. Cold damage to the extremities: Frostbite and non-freezing cold injuries. *Postgrad Med J*. 2009;85:481–8.
5. State of Alaska Cold Injury Guideline: Alaska Multi-level 2003 Version. www.chems.alaska.gov/EMS/documents/AKColdInj2005.pdf.
6. Hallam MJ, Cubison T, Dheansa B, et al. Managing frostbite. *BMJ*. 2010;341:c5864.
7. Biem J, Koehncke N, Classen D, et al. Out of the cold: management of hypothermia and frostbite. *CMAJ*. 2003;168:305–11.

ADDITIONAL READING

- Cappaert TA, Stone JA, Castellani JW, et al. National Athletic Trainers' Association position statement: Environmental cold injuries. *J Athl Train*. 2008; 43:640–58.
- Murphy JV, Banwell PE, Roberts AH, et al. Frostbite: Pathogenesis and treatment. *J Trauma*. 2000;48: 171–8.
- Twomey JA, Peltier GL, Zera RT. An open-label study to evaluate the safety and efficacy of tissue plasminogen activator in treatment of severe frostbite. *J Trauma*. 2005;59:1350–4; discussion 1354–5.

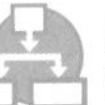

See Also (Topic, Algorithm, Electronic Media Element)

- Hypothermia
- Algorithm: Hypothermia

CODES

ICD9

- 991.0 Frostbite of face
- 991.1 Frostbite of hand
- 991.2 Frostbite of foot

CLINICAL PEARLS

- Frostbite is considered a tetanus-prone injury. Treat as any injury involving tissue destruction.
- Avoid rewarming en route to the hospital if there is a chance of refreezing. Avoid burns to affected areas, which may be numb and insensitive to heat.

FROZEN SHOULDER

Crystal L. Hnatko, DO

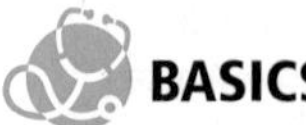

BASICS

DESCRIPTION
- A painful, gradual loss of both active and passive glenohumeral (GH) motion resulting from progressive fibrosis and ultimate contracture of the GH joint capsule in the absence of a known intrinsic shoulder disorder.
- Adhesive capsulitis (AC) is commonly categorized as primary (idiopathic) and secondary (underlying cause or associated condition).
- The clinical course is somewhat predictable (overlap and variability are present) and classically divided into 3 stages:
  - Stage 1, Freeze/Pain: The subacute onset of diffuse vague pain, 2–9 months
  - Stage 2, Frozen/Adhesive: The insidious onset of stiffness, 4–12 months
  - Stage 3, Thaw/Recovery: Protracted, often incomplete resolution, 5–24 months
- System(s) affected: Musculoskeletal
- Synonym(s): Adhesive capsulitis; Pericapsulitis; Scapulohumeral periarthritis

EPIDEMIOLOGY
- Predominant age: 40–60 years
- Predominant sex: Female > Male

ALERT
- The nondominant hand is more frequently affected.
- 20–30% of those affected will develop the condition in the opposite shoulder.

Prevalence
- General population: 2–5%
- Diabetics type I and type II: 10–20%

RISK FACTORS
- Sedentary vocation
- Age > 40 years
- Minor injury (20–30% of those with AC will report recent minor trauma to the shoulder)
- Systemic diseases: Endocrinopathies, autoimmune disorders, atherosclerotic disease (see "Commonly Associated Conditions")

Genetics
No known genetic predispositions

GENERAL PREVENTION
No current evidence regarding prevention

PATHOPHYSIOLOGY
Synovial inflammation and capsular fibrosis resulting in contracture of the rotator interval, coracohumeral ligament, and anterior shoulder capsule restricting movement of the shoulder (1)

ETIOLOGY
A poorly understood chronic inflammatory response with fibroblastic proliferation, which may be immunomodulated.

COMMONLY ASSOCIATED CONDITIONS
- Idiopathic AC is associated with:
  - History of AC in the contralateral shoulder
  - Dupuytren contractures
- Secondary AC is associated with: Diabetes type I and II (most common), thyroid disease (hypothyroidism, hyperthyroidism), autoimmune diseases, rotator cuff injury or minor shoulder trauma, surgery or immobilization of shoulder, prior cerebrovascular accident, or myocardial infarction

DIAGNOSIS

HISTORY
- Subacute onset of diffuse shoulder pain and the insidious, progressive loss of active and passive shoulder range of motion (ROM)
- Night pain often interrupts sleep.
- Pain is typically achy at rest and sharper with movement.
- Preceding injury, illness, or immobilization (secondary adhesive capsulitis)
- Loss of natural arm swing with gait
- Because of compensatory scapular elevation (to lift the arm), secondary muscle spasm and pain throughout neck, shoulder, and posterior thorax
- Muscle atrophy and weakness occur with time and disuse.
- Functional limitations: Inability to reach overhead or into a back pocket. Frequently unable to fasten the back of a garment.

PHYSICAL EXAM
- Diffuse shoulder tenderness with deep palpation
- Limited active and passive shoulder ROM in >1 plane (external rotation is usually the first to be restricted and the last to return)
- Normal 5/5 strength (if ROM permits testing and pain does not inhibit effort)
- Hawkins, Neer, Yergason, and Speed testing often positive (if ROM permits testing)
- No neurovascular deficits
- Early on, AC is almost indistinguishable from subacromial bursitis. The loss of passive external rotation (ER) may be the only finding on exam to differentiate early AC from the myriad of conditions that can cause subacromial bursitis. The only other condition that may cause loss of passive ER is GH arthritis.

DIAGNOSTIC TESTS & INTERPRETATION

Lab
Initial lab tests
No lab is diagnostic for primary (idiopathic) AC. If suspected, labs may be indicated to rule out any underlying systemic diseases associated with secondary AC.

Imaging
Initial approach
- Plain radiograph (anteroposterior [AP], axillary, supraspinatus outlet views) to rule out osteoarthritis, calcific tendinitis, avascular necrosis, osteomyelitis, fracture, dislocation, and tumor
- Radiographs should be normal but may demonstrate disuse osteopenia of the proximal humerus late in the course.
- Consider MRI to evaluate for thickening of the axillary pouch and to rule out other shoulder disorders. MRI with gadolinium may have some advantages to conventional MRI (2)[C].

Follow-Up & Special Considerations
Serial examination is advised in patients who present with nonspecific shoulder pain and normal radiographs eluding a specific diagnosis. At follow-up visits, the diagnosis is supported if restricted motion is demonstrated that may not have been present on initial presentation. Early in stage 1 pain is the predominant feature, and restriction of motion may be difficult to identify.

Diagnostic Procedures/Surgery
- Diagnostic subacromial injection of anesthetic may be used to differentiate AC from rotator cuff pathologies in some cases:
  - Resolution of pain and restored ROM after subacromial injection suggests rotator cuff pathology or other cause of impingement syndrome.
  - Intact muscle strength and persistent active and passive ROM deficits with a firm mechanical, tethered end point are consistent with AC.
- Joint aspiration if septic joint is suspected (rarely necessary)
- Arthroscopy to visualize fibrous bands in the joint space (rarely necessary)

Pathological Findings
If performed, surgical arthroscopy may demonstrate capsular thickening and synovial inflammation with adhesions to the humerus.

DIFFERENTIAL DIAGNOSIS
- Rotator cuff strain/tear/impingement syndrome
- Calcific tendinitis
- Septic or inflammatory arthropathy
- GH or acromioclavicular joint osteoarthritis (OA)
- Cervical strain/radiculopathy/OA
- Bony neoplasm/metastases
- Fracture/dislocation
- Avascular necrosis of humeral head
- Osteomyelitis
- Myofascial pain syndrome
- Thoracic outlet syndrome

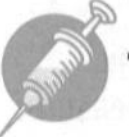

TREATMENT

- Optimizing treatment depends on recognition of the clinical stage at presentation in order to target the predominating process underlying the clinical symptoms with hopes of limiting the symptom severity (3)[C].
- Once the diagnosis is suspected, education and expectations should be discussed to include:
  - Protracted recovery (months to years) characterized by resolution of pain prior to the return of function
  - Full ROM may never be recovered; however, functional limitations are uncommon.
- There is no agreed-upon approach to treatment. Typical conservative therapy consists of any combination of physical therapy, oral medications, and joint or bursal injections.

- Other nonoperative therapies include hydrodilatation (capsular distention) and suprascapular nerve block (SSNB), both of which have demonstrated short-term improvements in pain and function.
- No therapy has definitively altered the long-term outcome, including surgical therapies such as capsular release and manipulation under anesthesia.
- Most sources suggest a minimum of 4–6 months of conservative therapies before more invasive surgical options are considered.

MEDICATION

First Line

- NSAIDs are widely used in the treatment of AC:
  - NSAIDs are of theoretical benefit in stage 1 for pain control.
  - NSAIDs are not without side effects and concomitant use with oral or injectable corticosteroids has no added benefit (4)[A].
  - If NSAIDs are contraindicated, it is reasonable to use acetaminophen or other opioid analgesics for pain control.
- Oral corticosteroids have demonstrated significant short-term improvement in pain and ROM (up to 6 weeks) (4,5)[A]. Like NSAIDs, oral steroids do not alter long-term outcomes and are not without side effects. Multiple different treatment regimens have been described and are likely most beneficial early in the course of the disease (stage 1 and early stage 2):
  - Prednisolone 30 mg daily for 3 weeks:
    - Alternatively 10 mg × 4 weeks, then 5 mg × 2 weeks
  - Triamcinolone 4 mg t.i.d. × 1 week, 4 mg b.i.d. × 1 week, 4 mg daily × 1 week
- Intra-articular corticosteroid injection has demonstrated significant short-term improvement in pain and ROM similar to that of oral corticosteroids. Improvements may persist up to 4 months if used in conjunction with physical therapy (3,4)[A].

Second Line

Tricyclic antidepressants (amitriptyline) have been used as neuromodulators. No evidence exists to support its use in AC.

ADDITIONAL TREATMENT

- Physical therapy: No known benefit to aggressive physical therapy vs. gentle stretching and active motion within the pain-free range. Despite common practice, there is no literature to support physical therapy alone in the treatment of AC (3)[A].
- Iontophoresis (electromotive drug administration) is generally not recommended in this condition.

General Measures

- Goal of all therapies: Control pain, preserve mobility, and allow for restful sleep.
- Heat and/or ice: May temporarily improve pain and secondary spasm
- Address underlying causes of secondary adhesive capsulitis (see "Associated Conditions").
- Patient education and reassurance must be ongoing.

Issues for Referral

- 7–12% of cases will not respond to nonoperative treatment (3).
- Indications for more invasive options remain highly subjective and need to be individualized to each patient.
- Orthopedic surgical referral should be considered if patient is considering a more invasive treatment option and the patient has not responded adequately to conservative treatment within 4–6 months.

Additional Therapies

- Capsular hydrodilatation (arthrography distention): Intra-articular injection of large volume normal saline, with or without corticosteroid, to distend and rupture capsular adhesions:
  - Improve pain and function in the short term (12 weeks) (6)[B]
- SSNB: Bupivacaine and corticosteroid injected into neurovascular bundle temporarily blocking afferent and efferent nerve signals:
  - Early evidence suggests short-term improvement in pain (3)[C].
- Low-power laser therapy: Superior to placebo (7)[C]

COMPLEMENTARY AND ALTERNATIVE MEDICINE

- Acupuncture: Unable to draw a conclusion on available evidence (7)
- Osteopathic manipulative technique: Evidence is lacking.

SURGERY/OTHER PROCEDURES

- Closed manipulation under anesthesia (MUA): Recent evidence questions the advantages of this procedure (6)[B]. Contraindicated in posttraumatic or postsurgical AC.
- Arthroscopic release: Most common surgical method for treating AC. Short-term benefits: Improved pain and function (3,6)[C]. Long-term benefits: Mixed findings (similar vs. superior to conservative therapy)

IN-PATIENT CONSIDERATIONS

Initial Stabilization

Outpatient care

ONGOING CARE

FOLLOW-UP RECOMMENDATIONS

Reinforce the natural course of the disease and discuss the various treatment options as the patient progresses through different stages of the disease. Many patients are more likely to request invasive procedures (injections, capsular distension, MUA, surgery) when the stiffness starts to affect activities of daily living (ADLs).

Patient Monitoring

Close monitoring and frequent encouragement are usually needed for successful recovery.

DIET

No restrictions

PATIENT EDUCATION

- Long-term course of treatment until resolution of symptoms. Stretching and ROM exercises daily during and after improvement.
- Codman pendulum exercises: Lean forward onto table or chair with unaffected arm bending at the waist; let the affected arm dangle. Now, swing the affected arm slowly by moving the torso. Try smaller and then bigger circles (clockwise and counterclockwise).
- Climbing the wall: Put the hand flat on a wall in front of you; use the fingers to "climb" the wall; pause 30 seconds every few inches. Repeat the exercise after turning 90° to wall (abduction).

PROGNOSIS

- Disorder is considered self-limiting
- Up to 50% have permanent restrictions of ROM (usually external rotation), which are rarely functionally significant

COMPLICATIONS

Surgical complications and complications due to MUA can be disabling, but are uncommon.

REFERENCES

1. Hand GC, Athanasou NA, Matthews T, et al. The pathology of frozen shoulder. *J Bone Joint Surg Br*. 2007;89(7):928–32.
2. Gokalp G, Algin O, et al. Adhesive capsulitis: Contrast-enhanced shoulder MRI findings. *J Med Imaging Radiat Oncol*. 2011;55(2):119–25.
3. Neviaser AS, Hannafin JA, et al. Adhesive capsulitis: A review of current treatment. *Am J Sports Med*. 2010;38:2346–56.
4. Favejee MM, Huisstede BM, et al. Frozen shoulder: The effectiveness of conservative and surgical interventions–systematic review. *Br J Sports Med*. 2011;45:49–56.
5. Buchbinder R, Green S, Youd JM, et al. Oral steroids for adhesive capsulitis. *Cochrane Database Syst Rev*. 2006.
6. Hsu J, Anakqenze O, Warrender W, et al. Current review of adhesive capsulitis. *J Shoulder Elbow Surg*. 2011;20:502–14.
7. Rookmoneea M, Dennis L, Brealey S, et al. The effectiveness of interventions in the management of patients with primary frozen shoulder. *J Bone Joint Surg Br*. 2010;92:1267–72.

ADDITIONAL READING

Blachard V, Barr S, Cerisola F. The effectiveness of corticosteroid injections compared with physiotherapeutic interventions for adhesive capsulitis: A systematic review. *Physiotherapy*. 2010;96(2): 95–107.

CODES

ICD9

726.0 Adhesive capsulitis of shoulder

CLINICAL PEARLS

- Early on in the course, AC is nearly indistinguishable from rotator cuff pathology, but restriction of external ROM is highly suggestive of adhesive capsulitis.
- Diagnostic subacromial bursa injection may assist in differentiating early AC from impingement syndrome. (In adhesive capsulitis, ROM deficits persist and strength is intact after injection.)
- Normal radiographs in the setting of progressive restriction of motion in more than 1 plane confirm the diagnosis.
- Treatment mainly consists of conservative measures: NSAIDs, oral or intra-articular corticosteroids, and physical therapy
- Invasive treatment options can be considered after 4–6 months: Capsular distention, MUA, and arthroscopy (about 10% of those affected)

FURUNCULOSIS

Zoltan Trizna, MD, PhD

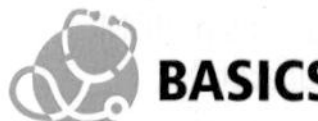

BASICS

DESCRIPTION
Acute bacterial abscess of a hair follicle (often *Staphylococcus aureus*):
- System(s) affected: Skin/Exocrine
- Synonym(s): Boils

EPIDEMIOLOGY
Incidence
- Predominant age:
  – Adolescents and young adults
  – Clusters have been reported in teenagers living in crowded quarters, within families, or in high school athletes.
- Predominant sex: Male = Female

Prevalence
Exact data are not available.

RISK FACTORS
- Carriage of pathogenic strain of *Staphylococcus* sp. in nares, skin, axilla, and perineum
- Rarely, polymorphonuclear leukocyte defect or hyperimmunoglobulin E–*Staphylococcus* sp. abscess syndrome
- Diabetes mellitus, malnutrition, alcoholism, obesity, atopic dermatitis
- Primary immunodeficiency disease and AIDS (common variable immunodeficiency, chronic granulomatous disease, Chediak-Higashi syndrome, C3 deficiency, C3 hypercatabolism, transient hypogammaglobulinemia of infancy, immunodeficiency with thymoma, Wiskott-Aldrich syndrome)
- Secondary immunodeficiency (e.g., leukemia, leukopenia, neutropenia, therapeutic immunosuppression)
- Medication impairing neutrophil function (e.g., omeprazole)
- The most important independent predictor of recurrence is a positive family history (1).

Genetics
Unknown

GENERAL PREVENTION
Patient education regarding self-care (see "General Measures"); treatment and prevention are interrelated.

PATHOPHYSIOLOGY
Infection spreads away from hair follicle into surrounding dermis.

ETIOLOGY
Pathogenic strain of *S. aureus* (usually); increasing incidence of community-acquired methicillin-resistant *S. aureus* (CA-MRSA)

COMMONLY ASSOCIATED CONDITIONS
- Usually normal immune system
- Diabetes mellitus
- Polymorphonuclear leukocyte defect (rare)
- Hyperimmunoglobulin E–*Staphylococcus* sp. abscess syndrome (rare)
- See "Risk Factors."

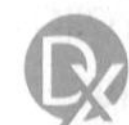

DIAGNOSIS

HISTORY
- Located on hair-bearing sites, especially areas prone to friction or repeated minor traumas (e.g., underneath belt, anterior aspects of thighs, nape, buttocks)
- No initial fever or systemic symptoms
- The folliculocentric nodule may enlarge, become painful, and develop into an abscess (frequently with spontaneous drainage).

PHYSICAL EXAM
- Painful erythematous papules/nodules (1–5 cm) with central pustules
- Tender, red, perifollicular swelling, terminating in discharge of pus and necrotic plug
- The lesions may be solitary or clustered.

DIAGNOSTIC TESTS & INTERPRETATION
Lab
Initial lab tests

Obtain culture if multiple abscesses, marked surrounding inflammation, cellulitis, systemic symptoms such as fever, or if immunocompromised.

Follow-Up & Special Considerations
- Immunoglobulin levels in rare (e.g., recurrent or otherwise inexplicable) cases
- If culture grows gram-negative bacteria or fungus, consider polymorphonuclear neutrophil leukocyte functional defect.

Pathological Findings
Histopathology (though a biopsy is rarely needed):
- Perifollicular necrosis containing fibrinoid material and neutrophils
- At deep end of necrotic plug, in SC tissue, is a large abscess with a Gram stain positive for small collections of *S. aureus*.

DIFFERENTIAL DIAGNOSIS
- Folliculitis
- Pseudofolliculitis
- Carbuncles
- Ruptured epidermal cyst
- Myiasis (larva of botfly/tumbafly)
- Hidradenitis suppurativa
- Atypical bacterial or fungal infections

TREATMENT

MEDICATION
First Line
- Systemic antibiotics usually unnecessary, unless extensive surrounding cellulitis or fever
- If suspect CA-MRSA, see "Second Line."
- If multiple abscesses, lesions with marked surrounding inflammation, cellulitis, systemic symptoms such as fever, or if immunocompromised: Place on antibiotics directed at *S. aureus* × 10–14 days:
  – Dicloxacillin (Dynapen, Pathocil) 500 mg PO q.i.d. *or* Cephalexin 250 mg PO q.i.d. *or* Clindamycin 150 mg q.i.d. if penicillin-allergic
- Suppression of pathogenic strain (if topical treatment fails):
  – Dicloxacillin/cloxacillin 500 mg b.i.d. × 10–14 days
  – Cephalexin or clindamycin (if penicillin-allergic)
  – If preceding fails, dicloxacillin/cloxacillin 500 mg plus rifampin 600 mg PO daily × 7–10 days *or* clindamycin 150 mg/d × 3 months (2)[C]
- Contraindications: Allergy to the particular drug selected
- Precautions: Cloxacillin and dicloxacillin: Anaphylactic reaction

Second Line

- Resistant strains of *S. aureus* (MRSA): Clindamycin 300 mg q6h or doxycycline 100 mg q12h or TMP-SMX DS 1 tab q8h or minocycline 100 mg q12h (3)[C]
- If known or suspected impaired neutrophil function (e.g., impaired chemotaxis, phagocytosis, superoxide generation), add vitamin C 1,000 mg/d × 4–6 weeks (prevents oxidation of neutrophils)
- If fail with antibiotic regimens:
  - May try oral pentoxifylline 400 mg t.i.d. × 2–6 months (4)[C]
  - Contraindications: Recent cerebral and/or retinal hemorrhage; intolerance to methylxanthines (e.g., caffeine, theophylline); allergy to the particular drug selected
  - Precautions: Prolonged prothrombin time (PT) and/or bleeding; if on warfarin, frequent monitoring of PT

ADDITIONAL TREATMENT

General Measures

- Moist, warm compresses (provide comfort, encourage localization/pointing/drainage) 30 minutes q.i.d.
- If pointing or large, incise and drain: Consider packing.
- Routine culture not necessary for localized abscess in nondiabetic patients with normal immune system
- Sanitary practices: Change towels, washcloths, and sheets daily; clean shaving instruments; avoid nose picking; change wound dressings frequently; do not share items of personal hygiene.

ONGOING CARE

FOLLOW-UP RECOMMENDATIONS

Patient Monitoring

Instruct patient to see physician if compresses unsuccessful.

DIET

Unrestricted

PROGNOSIS

- Self-limited: Usually drains pus spontaneously and will heal with or without scarring within several days
- Recurrent/chronic: May last for months or years
- If recurrent, usually related to chronic skin carriage of *Staphylococci* (nares or on skin). Treatment goals are to decrease or eliminate pathogenic strain *or* suppress pathogenic strain:
  - Culture nares, skin, axilla, and perineum (culture nares of family members).
  - Apply mupirocin ointment to anterior nares b.i.d. × 5 days (patient and family members/carriers).
  - Culture anterior nares every 3 months. If failure, retreat with mupirocin or consider oral antibiotics (5)[C].
  - See "Medications," "First Line," "Suppression of Pathogenic Strain."
- Especially in recurrent cases, wash entire body and fingernails (with nailbrush) daily for 1–3 weeks with povidone–iodine (Betadine), hexachlorophene (Hibiclens), or pHisoHex soap (all can cause dry skin).

COMPLICATIONS

- Scarring
- Bacteremia
- Seeding (e.g., septal/valve defect, arthritic joint)

REFERENCES

1. El-Gilany AH, Fathy H, et al. Risk factors of recurrent furunculosis. *Dermatol Online J*. 2009;15:16.
2. Klempner MS, Styrt B. Prevention of recurrent staphylococcal skin infections with low-dose oral clindamycin therapy. *JAMA*. 1988;260:2682–5.
3. *Up To Date 2007*. Impetigo, Folliculitis, Furunculosis, and Carbuncles.
4. Wahba-Yahav AV. Intractable chronic furunculosis: Prevention of recurrences with pentoxifylline. *Acta Derm Venereol*. 1992;72:461–2.
5. Doebbeling BN, et al. Long term efficacy of intranasal mupirocin, a prospective cohort study of *Staphylococcal aureus*. *Arch Int Med*. 1994;154:1505.
6. Winthropp KL, et al. An outbreak of mycobacterium furunculosis associated with footbaths at a nail salon. *N Engl J Med*. 2002;346(18):1366–71.

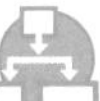

See Also (Topic, Algorithm, Electronic Media Element)

Folliculitis; Hidradenitis Suppurativa

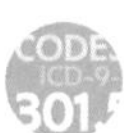

CODES

ICD9

- 680.0 Carbuncle and furuncle of face
- 680.3 Carbuncle and furuncle of upper arm and forearm
- 680.9 Carbuncle and furuncle of unspecified site

CLINICAL PEARLS

- The pathogens may be different in different localities. Keep up-to-date with the locality-specific epidemiology.
- If few, furuncles/furunculosis do not always need antibiotic treatment. If systemic symptoms (e.g., fever), cellulitis, or multiple lesions occur, oral antibiotic therapy is needed.
- Other treatments for MRSA include linezolid PO or IV and IV vancomycin.
- Folliculitis, furunculosis, and carbuncles are parts of a spectrum of pyodermas.
- Other causative organisms include anaerobic (e.g., *Escherichia coli, Pseudomonas aeruginosa,* and *Streptococcus faecalis*), anaerobic (e.g., *Bacteroides, Lactobacillus, Peptobacillius,* and *Peptostreptococcus*), and *Mycobacteria* (6).

F

GALACTORRHEA

Katherine M. Callaghan, MD
Dawn S. Tasillo, MD

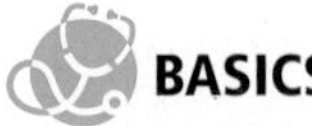

BASICS

DESCRIPTION

- Milky nipple discharge not associated with gestation or present more than 1 year after weaning. Galactorrhea does not include serous, purulent, or bloody nipple discharge.
- System(s) affected: Endocrine/Metabolic, Nervous, Reproductive
- Synonym(s): Disordered lactation; Nipple discharge

Pregnancy Considerations

Most cases of galactorrhea during pregnancy are physiologic.

EPIDEMIOLOGY

- Predominant age: 15–50 years (reproductive age)
- Predominant sex: Female > Male (rare, for example, in patients with MEN1 the most common anterior pituitary tumors are prolactinomas)

Incidence

Common

Prevalence

6.8% of women referred to physicians with a breast complaint have nipple discharge.

GENERAL PREVENTION

- Frequent nipple stimulation can cause galactorrhea.
- Keep medication causes in mind.

PATHOPHYSIOLOGY

Disorders of lactation are associated with elevated prolactin levels, either from overproduction or loss of inhibitory regulation by dopamine.

ETIOLOGY

- Nipple stimulation
- Pituitary gland overproduction:
  - Prolactinoma
- Loss of dopamine via hypothalamic dysregulation:
  - Craniopharyngiomas
  - Meningiomas or other tumors
  - Sarcoid
  - Irradiation
  - Vascular insult
  - Stalk disruption
  - Traumatic injury
- Medications that suppress dopamine:
  - Typical and atypical antipsychotics
  - SSRIs
  - Tricyclic antidepressants
  - Butyrophenones
  - Cimetidine
  - Ranitidine
  - Reserpine
  - Alpha-methyldopa
  - Verapamil
  - Estrogens
  - Isoniazid
  - Opioids
  - Stimulants
  - Neuroleptics
  - Metoclopramide
  - Domperidone
  - Protease inhibitors (1)
- Chest wall injury:
  - Zoster, surgical or other trauma
- Postoperative condition, especially oophorectomy
- Renal failure
- Other causes:
  - Primary hypothyroidism
  - Cirrhosis
  - Cushing disease
  - Ectopic prolactin secretion
  - Renal failure
  - Sarcoid
  - Lupus
  - Multiple sclerosis
  - Polycystic ovary syndrome
- Idiopathic:
  - Normal prolactin levels

COMMONLY ASSOCIATED CONDITIONS

See "Etiology."

DIAGNOSIS

- Findings vary with causes.
- Look for signs/symptoms of associated conditions:
  - Adrenal insufficiency
  - Acromegaly
  - Hypothyroidism
  - Chest wall conditions

HISTORY

- Usually bilateral milky nipple discharge, may be spontaneous or induced by stimulation
- Determine possibility of pregnancy, or recent discontinuation of lactation
- Signs of hypogonadism from hyperprolactinemia:
  - Oligomenorrhea, amenorrhea
  - Inadequate luteal phase, anovulation, infertility
  - Decreased libido (especially in affected males)
- Mass effects from pituitary enlargement:
  - Headache, cranial neuropathies
  - Bitemporal hemianopsia, amaurosis, scotomata

PHYSICAL EXAM

Breast examination should be performed with attention to the presence of spontaneous or induced nipple discharge.

DIAGNOSTIC TESTS & INTERPRETATION

Perform formal visual field testing if pituitary adenoma suspected.

Lab

Initial lab tests

- Prolactin level, thyroid-stimulating hormone, pregnancy test, liver, and renal functions
- Drugs that may alter lab results: Medications that can cause hyperprolactinemia
- Situations that may alter lab results:
  - Lab evaluation of prolactin may be falsely elevated by a recent breast examination
  - Vigorous exercise
  - Sexual activity
  - High-carbohydrate diet
  - Consider repeating the test under different circumstances if the value is borderline (30–40) elevated.
- Prolactin levels may fluctuate. Elevated prolactin levels should be confirmed with at least one additional level drawn in a fasting, nonexercised state, with no breast stimulation (2).
- Prolactin levels >250 ng/mL are highly suggestive of a pituitary adenoma (3).

Follow-Up & Special Considerations

- Consider follicle-stimulating hormone and leuteinizing hormone if amenorrheic
- Consider growth hormone levels if acromegaly suspected
- Check adrenal steroids if signs of Cushing disease

Imaging

- If a breast mass is palpated in the setting of nipple discharge, evaluation of that mass is indicated with mammogram and/or ultrasound
- Pituitary MRI with gadolinium enhancement if the serum prolactin level is significantly elevated (>200 ng/mL) or if a pituitary tumor is otherwise suspected

Diagnostic Procedures/Surgery

If diagnosis is in question, confirm by microscopic evaluation that nipple secretions are lipoid.

Pathological Findings

None unless pituitary resection required.

DIFFERENTIAL DIAGNOSIS

- Pregnancy-induced lactation or recent weaning
- Nonmilky nipple discharge:
  - Intraductal papilloma
  - Fibrocystic disease
- Purulent breast discharge:
  - Mastitis
  - Breast abscess
  - Impetigo
  - Eczema
- Bloody breast discharge: Consider malignancy (Paget disease, breast cancer)

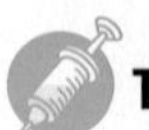

TREATMENT

- Avoid excess nipple stimulation.
- Idiopathic galactorrhea (normal prolactin levels) does not require treatment.
- Discontinue causative medications, if possible.
- Treat to manage symptoms, reduce patient anxiety, and restore fertility.

- Treat tumors >10 mm (even if asymptomatic) to reduce pituitary tumor size or prevent progression to avoid neurologic sequelae.
- If microadenoma, watchful waiting can be appropriate, as 95% do not enlarge.

MEDICATION

- Dopamine agonists work to reduce prolactin levels and shrink tumor size. Therapy is suppressive, not curative.
- Treatment is discontinued when tumor size has reduced or regressed completely or after pregnancy has been achieved.
- Bromocriptine:
  - Start at 1.25 mg/d PO with food and increase weekly by 1.25 mg/d until therapeutic response achieved. (Usually 2.5–15 mg/d, divided once daily/t.i.d.)
  - More expensive and more frequent dosing; however, most providers have experience with this effective drug.
  - Long-term treatment can cause woody fibrosis of the pituitary gland.
- Cabergoline (Dostinex):
  - Start at 0.25 mg PO weekly and increase by 0.25 mg monthly until prolactin levels normalize. Usual dose ranges from 0.25–1 mg PO once or twice weekly.
  - More effective and better tolerated than bromocriptine (3)
  - Convenient dosing
  - Although cabergoline has been associated with valvular heart disease in patients treated for Parkinson's disease, the lower doses used in treatment of prolactinomas have not been adequately studied (4).
- Contraindications are similar for all and include:
  - Uncontrolled hypertension
  - Sensitivity to ergot alkaloids
- Precautions:
  - Nausea, vomiting, and drowsiness are common.
  - Orthostasis, lightheadedness, or syncope
  - Hypertension, seizures, acute psychosis, and digital vasospasm are rare.
- Significant possible interactions:
  - Phenothiazines, butyrophenones, other drugs listed under "Etiology"

SURGERY/OTHER PROCEDURES

- Surgery:
  - Macroadenomas need surgery if medical management does not halt growth, if neurologic symptoms persist, if size >10 mm, or if patient cannot tolerate medications. Also considered in young patients with microadenomas in order to avoid long-term medical therapy (5).
  - Transsphenoidal pituitary resection
  - 50% recurrence after surgery
- Radiotherapy:
  - Radiation is an alternate tumor therapy for macroprolactinomas not responsive to other modes of treatment:
    - 20–30% success rate
    - 50% risk of panhypopituitarism after radiation
    - Risk of optic nerve damage, hypopituitarism, neurologic dysfunction, and increased risk for stroke and secondary brain tumors (5).

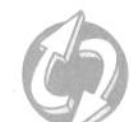

ONGOING CARE

FOLLOW-UP RECOMMENDATIONS

- Outpatient care unless pituitary resection required.
- Bromocriptine patients need adequate hydration.
- Dopamine agonist therapy should be discontinued in pregnancy (3).

Patient Monitoring

- Varies with cause; check prolactin levels every 6 weeks until normalized, then every 6–12 months.
- Monitor visual fields and/or MRI at least yearly until stable.

DIET

No restrictions

PATIENT EDUCATION

- Warn about symptoms of mass enlargement in pituitary
- Discuss treatment rationale and risks of treating and expectant management
- Patient education material available from American Family Physician: www.aafp.org/afp/20040801/553ph.html

PROGNOSIS

- Depends on underlying cause
- Symptoms can recur after discontinuation of dopamine agonist.
- Surgery can have 50% recurrence (6).
- Prolactinomas <10 mm can resolve spontaneously.

COMPLICATIONS

- If enlarging pituitary adenoma, risk of permanent visual field loss
- Panhypopituitarism can complicate radiation or surgical therapy.
- Osteoporosis if amenorrhea persists without estrogen replacement

REFERENCES

1. Molitch ME, et al. Drugs and prolactin. *Pituitary*. 2008;11:209–18.
2. Leung AK, Pacaud D. Diagnosis and management of galactorrhea. *Am Fam Physician*. 2004;70: 543–50.
3. Melmed S, Endocrine Society, et al. Diagnosis and treatment of hyperprolactinemia: An Endocrine Society clinical practice guideline. *J Clin Endocrinol Metab*. 2011;96(2):273–88.
4. Kars M, Pereira A, Bax, J et al. Cabergoline and cardiac valve disease in prolactinoma patients: Additional studies during long-term treatment are required. *Eur J Endocrinol*. 2008;159(4):363–7.
5. Mancini T, Casanueva FF, Giustina A. Hyperprolactinemia and prolactinomas. *Endocrinol Metab Clin North Am*. 2008;37:67–99.
6. Schlechte JA. Long-term management of prolactinomas. *J Clin Endocrinol Metab*. 2007;92: 2861–5.

ADDITIONAL READING

- Falkenberry S. Nipple Discharge. *OB GYN Clin*. 2002;29(1):21–9.
- Rodden AM, et al. Common breast concerns. *Prim Care*. 2009;36:103–13, viii.
- Santen R, Mansel R. Benign breast disorders. *NEJM*. 2005;353:275–85.

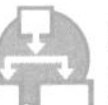

See Also (Topic, Algorithm, Electronic Media Element)

Hyperprolactinemia

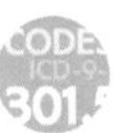

CODES

ICD9

- 611.6 Galactorrhea not associated with childbirth
- 676.60 Galactorrhea associated with childbirth, unspecified as to episode of care

CLINICAL PEARLS

- Galactorrhea is a common disorder, affecting up to 50% of reproductive-age women.
- Common causes include idiopathic, from excess nipple stimulation, dopamine-suppressing medications, or pituitary prolactinoma.
- Most cases may be adequately evaluated by thyroid-stimulating hormone, prolactin, and human chorionic gonadotropin measurement, with additional testing as suggested by the presence of other symptoms or signs.
- Lab evaluation of prolactin may be falsely elevated due to recent sexual activity, breast examination, exercise, or a high-carbohydrate diet. Repeat any borderline elevation before continuing evaluation or initiating treatment.
- Evaluate prolactin >200 ng/mL (or suspicion of pituitary macroadenoma) with a gadolinium-enhanced MRI.

G

GAMBLING ADDICTION

Amy Shah, MD
Christopher C. White, MD, JD, FCLM

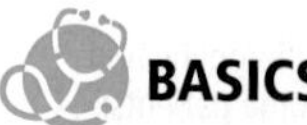

BASICS

DESCRIPTION

Gambling is the act of placing something of value at risk in the hopes of gaining something of greater value. Gambling addiction is an impulse-control disorder ranging in severity from problem gambling to the more severe pathologic gambling (PG). Disordered gambling is a dynamic behavior, and patients frequently move in both directions along the continuum of normal and PG behavior over relatively short time periods. Gambling addiction is further categorized into levels:

- Level 0: Nongamblers
- Level 1: Gambled without adverse consequences
- Level 2: Experienced negative consequences from gambling behavior but do not meet criteria for PG
- Level 3: Gambling meets *Diagnostic and Statistical Manual of Psychological Disorders*, 4th Edition (DSM-IV), criteria for PG: Persistent and recurrent maladaptive gambling behavior indicated by ≥5 DSM-IV criteria
- Level 4: Seeking help for gambling addiction regardless of degree of gambling addiction

EPIDEMIOLOGY

- Predominant sex: Male > Female
- The younger the person starts gambling, the more likely he or she is to become a pathologic gambler.
- A higher likelihood exists if parents have PG.
- Family history of substance abuse and mental disorders

Prevalence

- Lifetime pathologic gambling prevalence ranges from 0.4–4.0% in the US.
- 2.5% of the population of US and Canada meet criteria for problem gambling.

GENERAL PREVENTION

Focus on treatment, patient education, and awareness of risk factors, associated conditions, and warning signs of pathologic or problematic gambling behaviors.

RISK FACTORS

- Some types of gambling present a greater risk to cause PG than other types: Pull tabs, casino gambling, and bingo and cards outside a casino
- Being involved with several gaming modalities is related to PG and suggests that the gambler is very captivated with risking money for excitement as opposed to risking money for social pleasure or for an interest in sports.
- Alcohol abuse and dependence are correlated with problem gambling.
- Lower socioeconomic status positively correlates with increased gambling pathology because these persons have few financial resources and cannot recover as easily from losses. Persons even may believe that gambling is a way to ease their financial burden.

Genetics

SLC6A4 serotonin transporter gene has been associated with PG in males but not females.

PATHOPHYSIOLOGY

- The brains of pathologic gamblers may have some predisposition to illness. Functional MRI studies indicate that the ventromedial prefrontal cortex is less activated when gambling stimuli are presented to pathologic gamblers.
- Abnormalities in the neurotransmitters serotonin, norepinephrine, dopamine, and glutamate may be implicated in PG.
- Norepinephrine: Still unclear but plays a part in arousal or excitement
- Serotonin: Involved in impulse control
- Dopamine: May induce reversible PG in Parkinson patients who take dopamine agonists
- Gambling addiction can be classified as an addiction as well as an impulse control disorder, and medicine classes for each category have been used to treat it.

COMMONLY ASSOCIATED CONDITIONS

- Poor nutrition
- Stress-related medical conditions (e.g., peptic ulcer disease [PUD], hypertension, migraine)
- Suicidal ideation and attempts
- Substance abuse disorder
- Attention deficit hyperactivity disorder (ADHD)
- Bipolar disorder and other mood disorders
- Impulse-control disorders
- Personality disorders
- Incarceration
- Financial problems

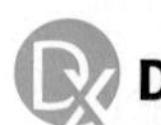

DIAGNOSIS

DSM-IV criteria for PG:

- Persistent and recurrent maladaptive gambling behavior, as indicated by 5 or more of the following:
  - Preoccupation with gambling
  - Need to gamble with increasing amounts of money to achieve the desired excitement
  - Repeated unsuccessful efforts to control, cut back, or stop gambling
  - Restless or irritable when attempting to cut down or stop gambling
  - Gambles as a way of escaping from problems or of relieving a dysphoric mood
  - After losing money gambling, often returns another day to get even
  - Lies to family members, therapist, or others to conceal the extent of involvement with gambling
  - Has committed illegal acts such as forgery, fraud, theft, or embezzlement to finance gambling
  - Has jeopardized or lost a significant relationship, job, or educational or career opportunity because of gambling
  - Relies on others to provide money to relieve a desperate financial situation caused by gambling
- The gambling behavior is not better accounted for by a manic episode.

HISTORY

- Preoccupation with gambling
- Preoccupation with money
- Unexplained new financial problems
- New participation in illegal or dishonest money-making endeavors or activities
- Disruptions in personal life or career
- Patient may ask his or her family and friends to pay off his or her debts ("bailing them out").

DIAGNOSTIC TESTS & INTERPRETATION

- Lie/bet method: Have you ever had to lie to people important to you about how much you gambled? Have you ever felt a need to bet more money?
  - A patient who answers at least 1 question with a "Yes" screens positively for PG.
  - This test has been shown to have >85% specificity and >95% sensitivity (1).
- South Oaks Gambling Screen (SOGS):
  - 20-question screen for PG
  - Score of 3–4 suggests problem gambling.
  - Score of 5 or more indicates probable PG.
  - Criticized as overestimating the number of pathologic gamblers and being too lengthy to administer (2)[B]
- Gamblers Anonymous 20 questions:
  - Easily obtainable from Gamblers Anonymous Web site
  - Scores of >7 are indicative of problem/PG.

Imaging

- Neuroimaging research indicates that the neural structures of the mesolimbic pathway are involved in PG, including the orbitofrontal cortex, amygdala, and ventral striatum/nucleus accumbens.
- Some data suggest the idea that because there is lower activity in the ventral striatum when receiving a reward in PG, these patients have decreased sensitivity to reward.

DIFFERENTIAL DIAGNOSIS

- Social gambling
- Professional gambling
- Bipolar disorder, manic episode
- Substance use disorder
- Personality disorder

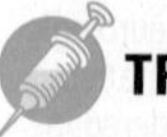

TREATMENT

In order to treat PG, treat the comorbidities first. The usual comorbid disorders are substance abuse, bipolar disorder, ADHD, and other impulse-control disorders (3,4). Nonpharmacologic therapies are more effective than pharmacologic therapies. There are some data suggesting that gambling abstinence is not necessary for treatment; patients still can exhibit controlled gambling.

MEDICATION

- There are no FDA-approved medicines for gambling addiction.
- SSRIs:
  - Beneficial for treating comorbid impulse-control disorders
  - Used to treat gambling addiction because of link with serotonergic dysfunction: Some studies show that low levels of serotonin cause a suppression of inhibitory responses.
  - Citalopram (Celexa) has shown significant improvement on all gambling measures, including number of days gambled, urge to gamble, and preoccupation with gambling. Celexa is also a low-cost medication with few drug interactions.
  - Fluvoxamine (Luvox) has been shown to be effective in a short-term acute trial as well.
  - Use of paroxetine (Paxil) in PG needs further studies.
- Modafinil helps pathologic gamblers with high impulsivity but increases gambling behavior in low-impulsivity pathologic gamblers. Modafinil shows decreases in motivation to gamble, risky decision making, and impulsivity in high-impulsivity pathologic gamblers (5)[B].
- Valproate and carbamazepine, as well as lithium carbonate, are effective treatments (5)[A].
- Opiate antagonists have the ability to decrease dopamine release in the dopamine reward pathway. Naltrexone and nalmefene are efficacious for PG and reduce urges to gamble. Positive family history of alcoholism predicted a positive response to opiate antagonist treatment (5).
- Selected antipsychotics have been shown to be ineffective in PG (i.e., olanzapine is not efficacious for the treatment of PG, and haloperidol may increase the desire to gamble in pathological gamblers) (5)[B].
- *N*-acetylcysteine (NAC), a glutamate-modulating agent, causes significant improvements in gambling thoughts and behaviors.
- Single case report indicated that disulfiram was helpful (6)[C]

ADDITIONAL TREATMENT

- Patients are often forced to come in for treatment after an ultimatum, such as threat of divorce or prosecution.
- Patients' personal characteristics (i.e., pride, denial, or impatience) can hinder therapy.
- Additionally, pathologic gamblers may leave when therapy does not work fast enough.
- Mental health workers must avoid negative transference.
- Because of increased suicide rates, patients may need to be hospitalized acutely for safety and to prevent gambling.
- Since patients are at increased risk from mental and physical illness, they benefit from relaxation exercises to reduce stress, identify triggers, substitute gambling with other activities, and a complete physical and lab work with nutrition evaluation.

General Measures

- Get a sense of the patient's readiness for change.
- Provide intervention/patient education. While there are no FDA-approved drug treatments for PG, make clinically based medication recommendations.
- Screen for and treat comorbid conditions.
- Provide referrals:
  - Addiction psychiatrist/counselor
  - Gamblers Anonymous
  - Consumer credit organizations
  - Bankruptcy lawyers
  - Gam-Anon for family members

Additional Therapies

- Cognitive-behavioral therapy (CBT) (7):
  - The main effective interventions for CBT are psychoeducation, cognitive restructuring, problem solving, social skills training, and relapse prevention. Studies indicated that CBT resulted in significant improvement for short-term therapy.
  - CBT may be done in several formats: Individual, group, brief group, and dual diagnosis. All these formats have been shown to be effective. Group therapy is favored because patients are often extroverted. Couple or family therapy also may be used.
- Gamblers Anonymous:
  - A 12-step program similar to Alcoholics Anonymous for a person suffering from a gambling addiction
  - Dropout rate is high if this is the only means of therapy (1)[B].
  - Patients may deny need to attend in the first place, and for that reason, Gamblers Anonymous may not be appropriate for patients who are in the precontemplation stage.
- Motivational enhancement therapy (MET):
  - Provides nonargumentative exploration of patient's stage of change
  - Patient receives positive reinforcement from clinician.
  - Motivational enhancement strategies support self-efficacy.
  - Improves patient rapport; aids in removing barriers to treatment
  - In one study, MET alone did not show any improvement, but MET and CBT together improved outcome measures (5)[B].

ONGOING CARE

FOLLOW-UP RECOMMENDATIONS

Patients seeking treatment for gambling addiction should be followed routinely to monitor the response to treatment, tolerance to medications, and possibility of relapse.

PATIENT EDUCATION

- Gamblers Anonymous:
  - www.gamblersanonymous.org
  - National hotline 1-888-GA-HELPS (888-424-3577)
- Gam-Anon: Support group for spouses, family, or close friends of compulsive gamblers: www.gam-anon.org
- Responsible Gambling Council: www.responsiblegambling.org
- Humphrey H. *This Must Be Hell: A Look at Pathological Gambling.* IUniverse; 2000.
- Lee B. *Born to Lose: Memoirs of a Compulsive Gambler.* Hazelden; 2005.

PROGNOSIS

- Patients with gambling addiction can be treated, but many relapse.
- 36–39% of patients did not experience any gambling-related problems according to one study, and only 7–12% sought formal treatment or Gamblers Anonymous meetings.
- Roughly 1/3 of patients who have a gambling addiction recover without any intervention.

REFERENCES

1. Potenza MN, Fiellin DA, Heninger GR, et al. Gambling: An addictive behavior with health and primary care implications. *J Gen Intern Med.* 2002;17:721–32.
2. Rossow I, Molde H. Chasing the criteria: Comparing SOGS-RA and the Lie/Bet screen to assess prevalence of problem gambling and "at-risk" gambling among adolescents. *Journal of Gambling Issues.* 2006;(18):57–71.
3. Potenza MN. Review. The neurobiology of pathological gambling and drug addiction: An overview and new findings. *Philos Trans R Soc Lond B Biol Sci.* 2008;363(1507):3181–9.
4. Chou K, Afifi TO. Disordered (pathologic or problem) gambling and axis I psychiatric disorders: Results from the national epidemiologic survey on alcohol and related conditions. *Am J Epidemiol.* 2011;173(11):1289–97.
5. Leung KS, Cottler LB. Treatment of pathological gambling. *Curr Opin Psychiatry.* 2009;22:69–74.
6. Mutschler J, Buhler M, Grosshans M, et al. Disulfiram, an option for treatment of pathological gambling? *Alcohol Alcohol.* 2010;45(2):214–6.
7. Okuda M, Balan I, Petry NM, et al. Cognitive-behavioral therapy for pathological gambling: Cultural considerations. *Am J Psych.* 2009;166(12):1325–30.

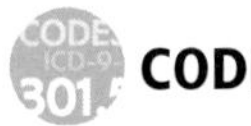

CODES

ICD9

- 312.31 Pathological gambling
- V69.3 Gambling and betting

CLINICAL PEARLS

- There are several brief screening strategies that can be used to identify PG, including the lie/bet method, the SOGS, and the Gamblers Anonymous 20 questions.
- To treat PG, first treat comorbidities such as substance abuse, bipolar disorder, ADHD, and other impulse-control disorders.
- Nonpharmacologic therapies are more effective than pharmacologic therapies. There is no FDA-approved therapy for PG.
- Patients seeking treatment for gambling addiction should be followed routinely by physicians and counselors to monitor the response to treatment, tolerance to medications, and possibility of relapse.

G

GANGLION CYST

Nathan P. Falk, MD
Cole Taylor, MD

BASICS

- Ganglions are common benign tumors that are not related to nerve tissue (as implied incorrectly by the name).
- Can be located throughout the body and usually located adjacent to or within joints and tendons, mostly on wrist, foot, and ankle
- Average size is 3 cm.
- Most are asymptomatic except for changing size, but local nerve compression can result in pain or activity limitation.

EPIDEMIOLOGY

- Can affect all age groups but unusual in children
- Most common in young adults and occur 3 times more commonly in women
- Mucous cysts are usually seen in older patients.
- Hand and wrist ganglions are commonly seen in dorsal wrist, radial wrist, and dorsum of the distal interphalangeal (DIP) joint (which is referred to as a mucous cyst).
- 60–70% of hand and wrist ganglions are in dorsal wrist, 15–20% are at the volar wrist.

Prevalence

- Prevalence of wrist ganglia in patients presenting with wrist pain has been reported as 19%.
- Prevalence of ganglia in patients with a palpable mass in the wrist has been reported as 27%.
- Prevalence of 5.6% in ankles has been reported.

RISK FACTORS

- More common in females
- Osteoarthritis for mucoid cysts
- No known occupational risk factors

Genetics

No specific genetic links have been found.

PATHOPHYSIOLOGY

Pathogenesis is unclear. Several theories:

- Mucoid degeneration of connective tissue results in formation of hyaluronic acid, leading to cystic space formation.
- Herniation of synovial lining creates a 1-way valve. This is supported by dye studies that show communication of fluid from the wrist joint into the cyst but not from the cyst to the joint. This is disputed by lack of epithelial lining of the cyst wall.
- A rent in the joint capsule or tendon sheath allows synovial fluid to leak into surrounding tissue. Local irritation leads to production of a pseudocapsule and ganglion. This would explain why no lining is seen on pathology.
- Recurrent stress and microtrauma at the synovial-capsular interface may stimulate mucin production by mesenchymal cells or fibroblasts.

ETIOLOGY

- Etiology is unknown.
- May be associated with trauma, but the majority of patients cannot recall specific trauma.

COMMONLY ASSOCIATED CONDITIONS

Mucous cysts are usually associated with some level of osteoarthritis of DIP joint.

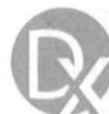

DIAGNOSIS

- Usually made on basis of history and physical examination
- Patients usually present when there is pain, increased size, interference with activities, or weakness.

HISTORY

- Patients usually present with asymptomatic mass present for months or years, decreasing and increasing in size.
- Mostly asymptomatic, but can be associated with pain and limitations in activity

PHYSICAL EXAM

- Mass is compressible, SC, transilluminating, and slightly mobile without overlying skin changes.
- Extension or flexion of wrist can cause pain through nerve compression.
- Small ganglions may only be palpable in full wrist flexion or extension.
- Occult ganglions are not palpable, but can be quite painful.

DIAGNOSTIC TESTS & INTERPRETATION

Unless diagnosis is unclear, most ganglions do not require imaging to confirm diagnosis.

Imaging

- Several options:
  - Ultrasound
  - MRI
  - Bone scintigraphy, arthroscopy
- Ultrasound and MRI have similar rates of sensitivity and specificity.
- Scintigraphy is less specific and not useful for this diagnosis.
- Ultrasound is less expensive than MRI but more operator-dependent.
- Arthroscopy is used for both diagnostic and therapeutic purposes and should be considered when initial workup is nondiagnostic, and conservative treatment is not effective.

Initial approach

Most are apparent clinically and do not need imaging.

Pathological Findings

- Gross pathologic evaluation shows that cysts are often multilobulated.
- Microscopic exam reveals outer wall with several layers of randomly oriented collagen fibers, relatively acellular with a few fibroblasts and mesenchymal cells in the collagen fibers.
- As pathology does not show an epithelial lining, it is therefore not a true cyst.
- Fluid contains glucosamine, albumin, globulin, and hyaluronic acid.
- Ganglions are histopathologically identical regardless of anatomic location.

DIFFERENTIAL DIAGNOSIS

- A mobile mass of extensor tendons of wrist may be a ganglion or tendon sheath, giant cell tumor, or tenosynovitis from infection or inflammation.
- Other tumors include lipoma, sarcoma, hamartoma, and interosseous neuroma.
- Firm mass may represent osteophyte.
- Overlying skin changes suggest an alternate diagnosis.

TREATMENT

4 primary treatment options (1):

- Reassurance and observation: Ganglia are not likely to be malignant or to cause damage:
  - 33% dorsal ganglions and 45% volar ganglions resolve spontaneously by 6 years; up to 80% of ganglion in children resolve.
- Closed rupture: Historically done by hitting cyst with a book:
  - Results in initial decreased clinical symptoms by 22–66%, but often leads to recurrence
- Aspiration: Can be done in an office under local anesthesia with 18-gauge or larger needle:
  - Studies demonstrate mixed results on aspirations of a ganglion; evidence supporting injecting steroids is weak, and splinting after the procedure may help cure rate, but recurrence may be as high as 80% after single aspiration. This can be reduced to 20% with multiple aspirations.

- Aspirations are more frequently being done with ultrasound guidance allowing direct visualization of the ganglion and perhaps more successful conservative treatment, although no studies to date have prospectively evaluated this (2).
- Volar ganglia should not be aspirated without ultrasound guidance due to risk of damage to neurovascular structures from blind aspiration attempts.
- Mucous cysts can be aspirated, but recurrence is >50% and pain may not resolve if it is due to underlying osteoarthritis.
- Surgical excision:
  - 1/3 of patients presenting with ganglion cyst elect for surgical intervention (3).

MEDICATION

Although evidence for steroid injection after aspiration is weak, this is still not an uncommon practice. No other medications have been shown to be effective.

SURGERY/OTHER PROCEDURES

- 6-year study comparing blind aspiration to surgery to watchful waiting found:
  - Recurrence rates: 58% after aspiration, 39% after surgery, and 58% in untreated patients
  - Satisfaction: 81% aspiration, 83% surgery, and 53% who were reassured, a significant difference
  - Persistent pain: 23% of patients who were satisfied vs. 45% who were unsatisfied
  - No significant difference seen in pain, weakness, or stiffness between groups.
  - Significant improvement in pain was seen in all groups.
  - Authors conclude that neither aspiration nor surgical excision provides a clear long-term benefit over the natural history of wrist ganglion, and the only benefit of surgery is early resolution of the appearance of the ganglia (4)[C].
- Bottom line:
  - Surgical excision yields less risk of recurrence but similar rates of pain, weakness, stiffness as aspiration or reassurance.
  - Patient satisfaction is higher with excision or aspiration; however, longer time out of work is seen with excision compared with aspiration and reassurance.
- 2 methods:
  - Arthroscopic compared to open excision: After 1 year, ~10% had recurrence; no significant difference in surgical approaches (5)[C].

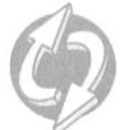

ONGOING CARE

May require supervised hand therapy after surgical repair to aid in pain reduction, improve stiffness and function

FOLLOW-UP RECOMMENDATIONS

- Hand therapy may be helpful if ganglion symptoms persist despite rest.
- Improved resolution rates with multiple aspirations
- Splinting is often used after surgical repair, and follow-up with orthopedics occurs for several weeks; hand therapy may be indicated for residual symptoms.

PROGNOSIS

- Very good
- Up to 50% will resolve with watchful waiting.
- Higher rate of resolution in children

COMPLICATIONS

- Risk of recurrence is present regardless of treatment; no specific recommendations to minimize this risk.
- Risks of surgical excision include:
  - Residual pain
  - Poor cosmesis
  - Neuropathy
  - Stiffness and instability of the wrist, especially scapholunate ligament instability; also may require open excision if arthroscopic fails to resolve symptoms

REFERENCES

1. Thommasen HV. Management of the occasional wrist ganglion. *Can J Rural Med*. 2006;11:51–3.
2. Jose J, Fourzali R, Lesniak B, et al. Ultrasound-guided aspiration of symptomatic intraneural ganglion cyst within the tibial nerve. *Skeletal Radiol*. 2011;40(11):1473–8.
3. Wong AS, Jebson PJ, Murray PM, et al. The use of routine wrist radiography is not useful in the evaluation of patients with a ganglion cyst of the wrist. *Hand*. 2007;2:117–9.
4. Dias JJ, Dhukaram V, Kumar P. The natural history of untreated dorsal wrist ganglia and patient reported outcome 6 years after intervention. *J Hand Surg Eur*. 2007;32:502–8.
5. Kang L, Akelman E, Weiss AP. Arthroscopic versus open dorsal ganglion excision: A prospective, randomized comparison of rates of recurrence and of residual pain. *J Hand Surg [Am]*. 2008;33:471–5.

ADDITIONAL READING

- Dias J, Buch K. Palmar wrist ganglion: does intervention improve outcome? A prospective study of the natural history and patient-reported treatment outcomes. *J Hand Surg [Br]*. 2003;28:172–6.
- Goldsmith S, Yang SS. Magnetic resonance imaging in the diagnosis of occult dorsal wrist ganglions. *J Hand Surg Eur Vol*. 2008;33:595–9.
- Lowden CM, Attiah M, Garvin G, et al. The prevalence of wrist ganglia in an asymptomatic population: Magnetic resonance evaluation. *J Hand Surg [Br]*. 2005;30:302–6.
- Lowden CM, et al. The prevalence of wrist ganglia in an asymptomatic population: Magnetic resonance evaluation. *J Hand Surg*. 2005;30B:3:302–6.
- Rizzo M, Berger RA, Steinmann SP, et al. Arthroscopic resection in the management of dorsal wrist ganglions: Results with a minimum 2-year follow-up period. *J Hand Surg [Am]*. 2004;29:59–62.
- Thornburg LE. Ganglions of the hand and wrist. *J Am Acad Orthop Surg*. 1999;7:231–8.

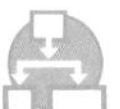

See Also (Topic, Algorithm, Electronic Media Element)

Algorithm: Pain in Upper Extremity

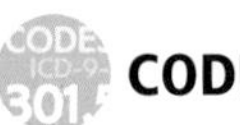

CODES

ICD9

- 727.41 Ganglion of joint
- 727.42 Ganglion of tendon sheath
- 727.43 Ganglion, unspecified

CLINICAL PEARLS

- Ganglia are the most common masses in the wrist and are not true cysts.
- Typical history and examination will make the diagnosis in most cases; plain films are expensive and not indicated.
- Can consider MRI or ultrasound if occult ganglion is suspected.
- Surgical excision may yield lower recurrence rates than aspiration.
- Volar wrist ganglia should not be aspirated without ultrasound guidance by an experienced provider due to the risk of damage to neurovascular structures from blind aspiration.

G

GASTRIC MALIGNANCY

Scott T. Henderson, MD

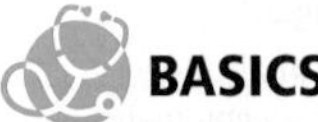

BASICS

DESCRIPTION
- May occur anywhere in the stomach
- Infiltration to lymph nodes, omentum, lungs, and liver is rapid.
- Uncommon in US natives
- Synonym(s): Linitis plastica

Pediatric Considerations
Rare

Pregnancy Considerations
- Rarely diagnosed during pregnancy
- Prognosis is poor if diagnosed.

EPIDEMIOLOGY
- Predominant age: >55 (2/3 >65)
- Predominant gender: Male > Female (1.7:1)
- Incidence is decreasing globally, but it remains the second-leading cause of cancer death.

Incidence
- 5.9/100,000 males (North America)
- 2.5/100,000 females (North America)
- 21,130 new cases per year (US)

RISK FACTORS
- *Helicobacter pylori* infection
- Achlorhydria
- Atrophic gastritis/intestinal metaplasia
- Pernicious anemia
- Prior gastric resection
- Polyps or dysplasia anywhere in alimentary canal
- Familial polyposis
- Barrett esophagus
- Smoking/tobacco abuse
- Patients in lower socioeconomic classes are at greater risk of developing gastric tumors.
- Diet rich in additives (e.g., smoked, pickled, or salted foods; highly spiced Asian foods)
- Low consumption of fruits and vegetables
- Overweight and obesity; strength of association increases with increasing body mass index (BMI) (1)[A]
- Ethnic background: Hispanic, Japanese, Chilean, Costa Rican:
  - Migrants from high-incidence areas (e.g., Iceland, Chile, or Japan) to low-incidence areas maintain an increased risk, whereas their offspring have an occurrence rate that corresponds to that of the new location.

Genetics
- More common in people with blood group A
- 2–4 times more common in first-degree relatives
- 1–3% of gastric cancers are associated with inherited gastric cancer predisposition syndromes, known as hereditary diffuse gastric cancer.

GENERAL PREVENTION
- A healthy lifestyle (not smoking, not consuming excess alcohol, avoiding obesity, and maintaining a good diet) is associated with reduced risk of gastric cancer:
  - Diets including 5–20 servings of both fruits and vegetables each week reduce the risk of gastric malignancy by ~1/2.
- Insufficient data to establish that screening would decrease mortality in US population
- Screening may be of benefit in high-prevalence areas.

ETIOLOGY
Unknown

COMMONLY ASSOCIATED CONDITIONS
- Giant hypertrophic gastritis (Ménétrier disease)
- Intestinal metaplasia of the stomach
- Atrophic gastritis
- *H. pylori* infection

DIAGNOSIS

HISTORY

ALERT
- Symptoms present late in the course.
- Anorexia/weight loss (70–80%)
- Cachexia
- Early satiety
- Nausea and vomiting
- Change in bowel habits
- Chronic noncolicky abdominal pain (especially in epigastrium):
  - Ranges from postprandial fullness to severe steady pain (70%)
  - Unrelieved by antacids
  - Exacerbated by food
  - Relieved by fasting
- Gross GI bleeding (10%)
- Dysphagia (rare)

PHYSICAL EXAM
- Abdominal palpation for masses and/or ascites
- Palpation for lymph nodes:
  - Left supraclavicular node (Virchow)
  - Sister Mary Joseph nodule at umbilicus
- Assess for jaundice

DIAGNOSTIC TESTS & INTERPRETATION

Lab

Initial lab tests
- CBC and platelet count:
  - Hemoglobin <12 g/dL (1.86 mmol/L)
  - Hematocrit <35 (0.35)
- Serum chemistry analysis:
  - Albumin 3 g/dL
- Coagulation studies
- *H. pylori* testing
- Stool guaiac

Follow-Up & Special Considerations
Pentagastrin test (stomach pH <6):
- Pernicious anemia may cause a false-positive pentagastrin test.

Imaging

Initial approach

CT scan of chest, abdomen, and pelvis with IV contrast and gastric distension with oral contrast or water should be performed routinely (2)[B].

Follow-Up & Special Considerations
In females, consider pelvic ultrasound.

Diagnostic Procedures/Surgery
- Upper endoscopy for direct visualization, cytology, and biopsy
- Endoscopic ultrasound is most accurate preoperative staging tool to identify proximal and distal extent of tumor (3)[B]
- Laparoscopy may be useful in select patients for staging (4)[C].

Pathological Findings
- Adenocarcinomas: 90% (Types: Intestinal [well-differentiated] and diffuse [undifferentiated/linitis plastica])
- Gastric lymphomas, sarcomas, and other rare types: 10%

DIFFERENTIAL DIAGNOSIS
- Angiodysplasia of the colon
- Carcinoma of body or tail of the pancreas
- Carcinoma of the colon
- Crohn disease
- Eosinophilic gastroenteritis
- Functional dyspepsia
- Gastric lymphoma
- Giant hypertrophic gastritis
- GI sarcoidosis
- Peptic ulcer with or without hemorrhage
- Small intestinal lymphoma

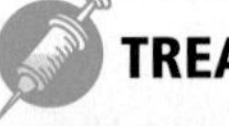

TREATMENT

MEDICATION

First Line
Combination chemotherapy improves survival compared to single-agent 5-FU (5)[A]:
- Among the combination chemotherapy regimens studied, best survival results are achieved with regimens containing 5-FU, anthracyclines, and cisplatin.
- In this category, epirubicin, cisplatin, and continuous-infusion 5-FU are tolerated best.

Second Line
- Ondansetron (Zofran), dronabinol (Marinol), metoclopramide (Reglan), and others for nausea control
- Pain control with opioids

ADDITIONAL TREATMENT

General Measures

- Multidisciplinary treatment is mandatory.
- Surgical excision of the tumor is only potentially curative option:
  - Extent of lymph nodes resection is controversial (6)[B].
  - Endoscopic mucosal resection for early gastric mucosal cancers (≤2 cm that are histologically differentiated and not ulcerated) and high-grade dysplasia may be curative (3)[B].
  - Even patients with incurable lesions should be offered an attempt at surgical reduction of the tumor:
    - Surgical reduction offers the best form of palliation and improves the likelihood of benefit if chemotherapy and/or radiation therapy is administered.
- Adjuvant chemotherapy may provide benefit compared to surgery alone (5)[A].
- Patients with inoperable, locally advanced disease should be offered chemotherapy and reassessed for surgery if response is favorable (3)[A].
- Patients with stage IV disease should be offered chemotherapy, which improves survival compared with the best supportive care (3)[A].
- Radiation therapy:
  - Used in combination with surgery and/or chemotherapy
  - Little benefit when used alone because of the radiation resistance of gastric tumors
  - Does have use in the palliation of pain, bleeding, and obstruction

Issues for Referral

Referral to a high-volume surgery center is usually indicated.

Additional Therapies

- The neoadjuvant use of radiotherapy is not recommended outside clinical trials.
- Role of treatment with anti-HER2 monoclonal antibodies being studied based on the evidence of HER2 overexpression in gastric cancer

COMPLEMENTARY AND ALTERNATIVE MEDICINE

Commonly used but with little supportive evidence

SURGERY/OTHER PROCEDURES

- Radical subtotal gastrectomy with gastrojejunostomy or gastroduodenostomy is the usual treatment of choice:
  - Large part of the stomach along with the greater and lesser omentum is removed en bloc.
  - Splenectomy or distal pancreatectomy is also sometimes performed.
  - Direct extensions also excised
- Total gastrectomy indicated only if necessary to remove the local lesion
- Local excision, endoscopic laser therapy, or electrocautery for palliation of incurable lesion by resection of bleeding area or area of obstruction

IN-PATIENT CONSIDERATIONS

Admission Criteria

- Inpatient care is common, but depends on stage at time of diagnosis.
- Most of the follow-up treatment is outpatient.

ONGOING CARE

FOLLOW-UP RECOMMENDATIONS

Symptom-driven follow-up visits to monitor disease state, assess treatments, monitor for recurrence/metastasis, and assess nutritional status (3)[B]

Patient Monitoring

Monitor vitamin B_{12} and iron levels following surgical resection; supplement if indicated.

DIET

- Patients at high nutritional risk should be considered for preoperative nutritional support.
- All patients undergoing surgery should be considered for early postoperative nutritional support:
  - Enteral route preferred
  - Consider placement of jejunostomy feeding tube.

PATIENT EDUCATION

- Contact local the American Cancer Society.
- Cancer Research Institute Helpbook: What to Do If Cancer Strikes. FDR Station, Box 5199, New York, NY 10150–5199.

PROGNOSIS

- Because most lesions do not produce symptoms until late in course, gastric carcinomas are usually advanced at the time of diagnosis.
- Overall 5-year relative survival rate is 24% (if local disease 61%, regional spread 24%, distant spread 3%).
- Early gastric cancers are usually detected as incidental findings or when screening endoscopy is performed in endemic areas.
- Primary gastric lymphoma is more treatable than gastric adenocarcinoma:
  - 5-year survival rate is 40–60% with subtotal gastrectomy followed by combination chemotherapy.

COMPLICATIONS

- Early lymphatic spread
- Aggressive metastatic disease (especially hepatic, cerebral, peritoneum, and pulmonary)
- Anemia (especially pernicious)
- Pyloric stenosis
- Dumping syndrome may occur following gastric surgery.

REFERENCES

1. Yang P, Zhou Y, Chen B, et al. Overweight, obesity and gastric cancer risk: Results from a meta-analysis of cohort studies. *Eur J Cancer*. 2009; 45(16):2867–73.
2. Scottish Intercollegiate Guidelines Network (SIGN). Management of oesophageal and gastric cancer. *A National Clinical Guideline*. Edinburgh (Scotland): Scottish Intercollegiate Guidelines Network (SIGN); 2006.
3. Okines A, Verheij M, Allum W, et al. Gastric cancer: ESMO Clinical Practice Guidelines for diagnosis, treatment and follow-up. *Ann Oncol*. 2010; 21(Suppl 5):v50–4.
4. Sarela AI, Lefkowitz R, Brennan MF, et al. Selection of patients with gastric adenocarcinoma for laparoscopic staging. *Am J Surg*. 2006;191:134–8.
5. Wagner AD, Unverzagt S, Grothe W, et al. Chemotherapy for advanced gastric cancer. *Cochrane Database Syst Rev*. 2010;3:CD004064.
6. McCulloch P, et al. Extended versus limited lymph nodes dissection technique for adenocarcinoma of the stomach (Cochrane Review). In: *The Cochrane Library*, Issue 4. Chichester, UK: John Wiley and Sons; 2005.

ADDITIONAL READING

- Clark CJ, Thirlby RC, Picozzi V, et al. Current problems in surgery: Gastric cancer. *Curr Probl Surg*. 2006;43:566–670.
- Khushalani N. Cancer of the esophagus and stomach. *Mayo Clin Proc*. 2008;83:712–22.
- Maconi G, Manes G, Porro GB. Role of symptoms in diagnosis and outcome of gastric cancer. *World J Gastroenterol*. 2008;14:1149–55.
- Wagner AD, et al. Chemotherapy for advanced gastric cancer (Cochrane Review). In: *The Cochrane Library*, Issue 4. Chichester, UK; 2005.
- Wagner AD, Moehler M. Gastric cancer: Development of targeted therapies in advanced disease. *Curr Opin Oncol*. 2009;21(4):381–5.

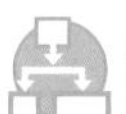

See Also (Topic, Algorithm, Electronic Media Element)

Multiple Endocrine Neoplasia (MEN)

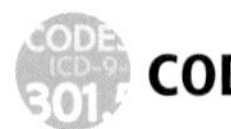

CODES

ICD9

- 151.0 Malignant neoplasm of cardia
- 151.1 Malignant neoplasm of pylorus
- 151.9 Malignant neoplasm of stomach, unspecified site

CLINICAL PEARLS

- Accurate preoperative staging is necessary to enhance survival.
- Endoscopic ultrasound is the most accurate preoperative staging tool.
- To enhance survival therapy with surgery, combination chemotherapy and radiation are necessary.

GASTRITIS

Michelle Whitehurst-Cook, MD

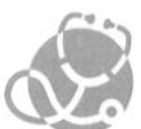

BASICS

DESCRIPTION

- Inflammatory reaction in the stomach: Typically involves the mucosa; seldom the full thickness of the stomach wall
- Patchy erythema of gastric mucosa: A common endoscopic finding; usually insignificant
- Erosive gastritis:
  - A reaction to mucosal injury by a noxious chemical agent (e.g., drugs especially NSAIDs or alcohol)
- Reflux gastritis:
  - A reaction to protracted reflux exposure to bile and pancreatic juice, usually associated with a defective pylorus
  - Typically limited to the prepyloric antrum
- Hemorrhagic gastritis (stress ulceration):
  - A reaction to hemodynamic disorder (e.g., hypovolemia or hypoxia [as in shock])
  - Also common in ICUs
  - Seen after severe burns
  - Seen after significant physical trauma
- Infectious gastritis:
  - Commonly associated with *Helicobacter pylori* (possibly causative, maybe opportunistic)
  - Viral infection, usually as a component of systemic infection, is common.
  - Significant infection by other specific microbes is rare.
- Atrophic gastritis:
  - Frequent, in varying degrees, in the elderly
  - Primarily from long-standing *H. pylori* infections (1)[A]
  - Major risk factor for onset of gastric cancer (1)[A]
  - Invariable in primary (pernicious) anemia
  - Autoimmune disease
  - Neutrophil cellular infiltration in acute gastritis
  - Patches of lymphoid follicles noted in chronic gastritis, along with plasma cells and macrophages; antibodies to parietal cells and intrinsic factor
  - >50% of humans are colonized with *H. pylori*.
- Synonym(s): Erosive gastritis; Reflux gastritis; Hemorrhagic gastritis; Acute gastritis

Geriatric Considerations

Persons >60 often harbor *H. pylori* infection.

Pediatric Considerations

Gastritis rarely occurs in infants or children.

EPIDEMIOLOGY

- Predominant age: All ages
- Predominant sex: Male = Female

RISK FACTORS

- Age >60
- Exposure to potentially noxious drugs or chemical agents, including alcohol or NSAIDS
- Hypovolemia, hypoxia (shock)
- Autoimmune diseases (thyroid and diabetes mellitus I)
- Family history of *H. pylori* and/or gastric cancer

Genetics

Unknown

GENERAL PREVENTION

- Patients should be warned of known or potentially injurious drugs or chemical agents.
- Patient with hypovolemia or hypoxia (especially patients confined to an intensive care ward) should receive prophylactic therapy with antacids.
- H_2 receptor antagonists, prostaglandins, or sucralfate used frequently in the ICU, burn and trauma victims
- Consider testing for *H. pylori* (and eradicating if present) in patients facing long-term NSAID therapy (2)[A].

PATHOPHYSIOLOGY

Noxious agents cause a breakdown in the gastric mucosal barrier leaving the epithelial cells unprotected.

ETIOLOGY

- Bacterial infection (e.g., *H. pylori*) most common cause
- Alcohol
- Aspirin and other NSAIDs
- Bile reflux
- Pancreatic enzyme reflux
- Stress (hypovolemia or hypoxia)
- Radiation
- *Staphylococcus aureus* exotoxins
- Viral infection
- Pernicious anemia
- Gastric mucosal atrophy
- Portal hypertensive (HTN) gastropathy
- Emotional stress

COMMONLY ASSOCIATED CONDITIONS

- Gastric or duodenal peptic ulcer
- Primary (pernicious) anemia
- Portal HTN
- Development of gastric lymphoma linked to the lymphoid follicles

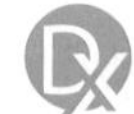

DIAGNOSIS

HISTORY

- Nondescript epigastric distress, often aggravated by eating, often severe, burning
- Anorexia
- Nausea, with or without vomiting
- Significant bleeding is unusual except in hemorrhagic gastritis.
- Hiccups
- Bloating or abdominal fullness

PHYSICAL EXAM

- Mild epigastric tenderness
- May have heme-positive stool
- Stool may be black in color.

DIAGNOSTIC TESTS & INTERPRETATION

- Nonendoscopic:
  - ^{13}C-urea breath test for *H. pylori* (not widely available)
  - Serologic test available for *H. pylori*, serum IgG (office and clinical laboratory):
    - Inexpensive
    - Cannot be used to assess eradication
  - Gastric acid analysis may be abnormal, but is not a reliable indicator of gastritis.
  - Stool analysis for *H. pylori* Ag
- Endoscopic:
  - Culture
  - PCR
  - Histology
  - Rapid urease testing

Lab

- Usually unremarkable, except when blood loss results in anemia
- Drugs that may alter lab results: Antibiotics or omeprazole may affect urea breath test for *H. pylori*.

Imaging

Nuclear scintigraphy is not done clinically.

Diagnostic Procedures/Surgery

Gastroscopy, usually with biopsy, is essential for a precise diagnosis. Recommended if there is a poor response to the initial treatment.

Pathological Findings

Acute or chronic inflammatory infiltrate in gastric mucosa, often with distortion or erosion of adjacent epithelium. Presence of *H. pylori* may be confirmed.

DIFFERENTIAL DIAGNOSIS
- Functional GI disorder
- Peptic ulcer disease
- Linitis plastica
- Viral gastroenteritis
- Pancreatic disease
- Gastric cancer (elderly)
- Cholecystitis
- Pancreatic disease (inflammation vs. tumor)

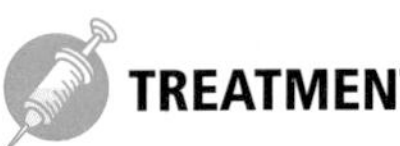

TREATMENT

MEDICATION
- Antacids: Best given in liquid form, 30 mL 1 hour after meals and at bedtime; useful mainly as an emollient
- H_2 receptor antagonists (e.g., cimetidine [Tagamet]): Oral cimetidine 300 mg q6h (or ranitidine [Zantac] or famotidine [Pepcid] or nizatidine [Axid]). Not shown to be clearly superior to antacids (3)[C]:
  - For severely ill patients: Priming dose of 300 mg IV, then a steady infusion of 37.5–75 mg/hr, dissolved in the running fluid
- Sucralfate (Carafate): 1 g q4–6h on an empty stomach; rationale uncertain, but empirically helpful
- Prostaglandins (e.g., misoprostol [Cytotec]): Can help allay gastric mucosal injury, suggested dosage of 100–200 mcg q.i.d.
- Proton pump inhibitors (PPIs) may be used if there is no response to antacids or H_2 receptor blockers
- To eradicate *H. pylori*:
  - Quadruple therapy is advised: PPI plus bismuth (Pepto-Bismol) 30 mL liquid or 2 tablets q.i.d. for 4 weeks plus metronidazole 250 mg q.i.d. for the first week, plus tetracycline 250 mg q.i.d. or amoxicillin 250 mg t.i.d. for 2–4 weeks has equal efficacy of triple therapy with PPI plus clarithromycin 500 mg b.i.d. for 2 weeks plus amoxicillin 250 mg t.i.d. for 2 weeks:
    - Quadruple therapy yields similar eradication rates to triple therapy (4)[A].
  - Dual therapy with omeprazole 20 mg b.i.d. plus amoxicillin 500 mg q.i.d. for 2 weeks
  - A short-course therapy with 1 week of metronidazole, omeprazole, and clarithromycin b.i.d. is 90% effective.
  - Consider newest recommendation of sequential antibiotic therapy with omeprazole 20 mg and amoxicillin 1 g b.i.d. for 5 days followed by clarithromycin 500 mg and tinidazole mg b.i.d. with omeprazole 20 mg for 5 days. Some studies show it works just as well as triple therapy (5)[B]
- Contraindications: Hypersensitivity to the drug(s)
- Precautions:
  - If bismuth is prescribed, warn the patient about the side effect of stool becoming black.
  - Refer to the manufacturer's profile of each drug.
- Significant possible interactions: Refer to the manufacturer's profile of each drug.

ADDITIONAL TREATMENT
General Measures
- Treatment of *H. pylori* is required to relieve symptoms, no specific therapy for the gastritis
- Parenteral fluid and electrolyte supplements required if vomiting prevents food intake
- Consider discontinuing NSAIDs or adding misoprostol.
- Encourage alcohol and smoking cessation.
- Endoscopy indicated for patients not responsive to treatment

IN-PATIENT CONSIDERATIONS
Gastritis may occur in ICU patients.

Initial Stabilization
Outpatient, except for severe hemorrhagic gastritis

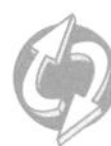

ONGOING CARE

FOLLOW-UP RECOMMENDATIONS
Usually no restrictions

Patient Monitoring
- Gastroscopy should be repeated after 6 weeks if gastritis has been severe or if symptomatic response to treatment has not been achieved.
- Patients with chronic gastritis are at increased risk for gastric carcinoma (lymphoma or adenocarcinoma).

DIET
Restrictions, if any, depend on the severity of the symptoms (e.g., bland, light, soft foods); it is wise to avoid caffeine and spicy foods, as well as alcohol.

PATIENT EDUCATION
- Explanation, reassurance
- Smoking cessation
- Dietary changes
- Relaxation therapy

PROGNOSIS
- Most cases clear spontaneously when the cause has been identified and treated.
- Recurrence of *H. pylori* infection may require a repeated course of treatment.

COMPLICATIONS
- Bleeding from extensive mucosal erosion or ulceration
- Clearing *H. pylori* before chronic gastritis develops may prevent development of gastric cancer.

REFERENCES

1. Rugge M, Pennelli G, Pilozzi E, et al. Gastritis: The histology report. *Dig Liver Dis*. 2011;43(Suppl 4): S373–84.
2. Lanza FL, Chan FK, Quigley EM, et al. Guidelines for prevention of NSAID-related ulcer complications. *Am J Gastroenterol*. 2009;104:728–38.
3. Nazareno J, Driman DK, Adams P. Is Helicobacter pylori being treated appropriately? A study of inpatients and outpatients in a tertiary care centre. *Can J Gastroenterol*. 2007;21:285–8.
4. Luther J, Higgins PD, Schoenfeld PS, et al. Empiric quadruple vs. triple therapy for primary treatment of *Helicobacter pylori* infection: Systematic review and meta-analysis of efficacy and tolerability. *Am J Gastroenterol*. 2010;105:65–73.
5. Graham Dy, Rimbara E. Understanding and appreciating sequential therapy for *Helicobacter pylori* eradication. *J Clin Gastroenterol*. 2011; 45(4):309–13.

ADDITIONAL READING

- Lahner E, Annibale B, Delle Gave G. Systemic review: *Heliocobacter pylori* infection and impaired drug absorption. *Aliment Pharmacol Ther*. 2009;(294): 379–86.
- McColl KE, et al. Clinical practice. *Helicobacter pylori* infection. *N Engl J Med*. 2010;362:1597–604.

CODES

ICD9
- 535.40 Other specified gastritis (without mention of hemorrhage)
- 535.50 Unspecified gastritis and gastroduodenitis (without mention of hemorrhage)
- 535.51 Unspecified gastritis and gastroduodenitis with hemorrhage

CLINICAL PEARLS
- Over half the population is colonized with *H. pylori*.
- *H. pylori* are the most common cause of gastritis.
- *H. pylori* antibodies decline in the year after treatment, but should not be used to determine eradication.
- *H. pylori* stool antigen tests can be used both before and after therapy.
- *H. pylori* antibody titers rise significantly with reinfection.

GASTROESOPHAGEAL REFLUX DISEASE

Ruben Peralta, MD

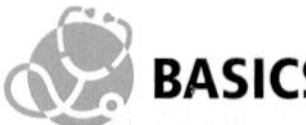

BASICS

DESCRIPTION

Reflux of gastroduodenal contents into the esophagus, larynx, or lungs, with or without resultant esophageal inflammation

Pediatric Considerations

Symptoms (vomiting, weight loss, failure to thrive) usually resolve by 18 months.

EPIDEMIOLOGY

Incidence

Children affected: 1/300–1,000

Prevalence

- Prevalence of gastroesophageal reflux disease (GERD): 10–20% in the US
- Prevalence of Barrett esophagus: 1.5%
- 65% adults have had heartburn; 15% have weekly symptoms
- In an European population-based study, reflux symptoms were found only in 40% of subjects with Barrett esophagus, and in 1/3 of patients with documented esophagitis.

RISK FACTORS

- Obesity
- Alcohol use
- Smoking
- Caffeine use
- Position of the acid pocket above the diaphragm in patients with hiatal hernia (see below) (1,2)

Genetics

Gene polymorphism identified

GENERAL PREVENTION

Positional treatment: Use infant seat for 2–3 hours after meals; thickened feedings:

- Avoid alcohol, nicotine, and caffeine.
- Avoid lying down immediately after a meal.
- Elevate head of bed.

ETIOLOGY

- Occurs with loss of the normal pressure gradient between the lower esophageal sphincter (LES) and the stomach
- Most commonly due to inappropriate relaxation of LES:
  - Foods (high fat, spicy, citrus, chocolate, peppermint, onions)
  - Medications (anticholinergic, smooth muscle relaxants, i.e., calcium channel blockers, nitrates)
- Other contributing factors include:
  - Pregnancy (progestational hormones decrease LES pressure)
  - Ineffective peristalsis
  - Scleroderma
  - Delayed gastric emptying
  - Positional: Recumbency, bending
- Obesity

COMMONLY ASSOCIATED CONDITIONS

- Reflux esophagitis: Due to exposure to acid, pepsin; classified as erosive (mucosal damage apparent, ulcers, friability) or nonerosive
- Extraesophageal reflux:
  - Aspiration
  - Chronic cough
  - Laryngitis, vocal cord granuloma
  - Sinusitis
  - Otitis media
- Halitosis
- Hiatal hernia: The position of the acid pocket (the zone of high acidity detected in the proximal stomach after a meal) above the diaphragm in patients with hiatal hernia is a major risk factor (1,2).
- Peptic stricture: In 10% with GERD
- Barrett esophagus
- Esophageal adenocarcinoma

DIAGNOSIS

- Heartburn (70–85%)
- Regurgitation of digested food (60%)
- Anginalike chest pain (33%)
- Abdominal pain (29%)
- Hoarseness (21%)
- Dysphagia (for solids; if solids and liquids, consider another cause) (20%)
- Bronchospasm (asthma) (15–20%)
- Aspiration (14%)
- Chronic cough
- Loss of dental enamel

HISTORY

- Heartburn: Retrosternal burning
- Regurgitation; sour or acid taste in mouth
- Symptoms with bending or recumbency
- Extraesophageal symptoms (e.g., cough)
- Diet, alcohol, smoking, and caffeine
- Diagnosis often made based on history alone, followed by a 1-week empiric trial with an antacid regimen

DIAGNOSTIC TESTS & INTERPRETATION

- Treated empirically if no red flags (dysphagia odynophagia, weight loss, early satiety, anemia, new onset, male >45 years) suggesting need to screen for more serious disease
- 24-hour pH monitoring: Gold standard for diagnosis; records number of reflux episodes and number that occur supine or upright; can be correlated with symptom diary
- Esophageal manometry records pressure of LES and effectiveness of peristalsis.

Lab

Check for anemia due to bleeding esophageal erosions or due to poor B_{12} absorption on proton pump inhibitor (PPI).

Imaging

Barium swallow:

- Presence of a sliding hiatal hernia appears to be a predictor of reflux esophagitis
- Mucosal irregularity due to inflammation and edema

Diagnostic Procedures/Surgery

- Endoscopy:
  - Not part of initial workup, unless anemia, unintentional weight loss, progressive dysphagia, GI bleeding, persistent vomiting, palpable epigastric mass, suspicion based on imaging study
  - Recommended for patients >55 who continue with symptoms after 4 weeks of treatment
  - Confirm mucosal injury; look for Barrett esophagus; biopsy for adenocarcinoma
  - ~50–70% of patients with heartburn have negative findings on endoscopy (nonerosive or endoscopy-negative reflux disease).
- Savary-Miller classification:
  - For grading esophagitis based on endoscopic findings:
    - Grade I: ≥1 nonconfluent reddish spots, with or without exudate
    - Grade II: Erosive and exudative lesions in the distal esophagus; may be confluent, but not circumferential
    - Grade III: Circumferential erosions in the distal esophagus
    - Grade IV: Chronic complications such as deep ulcers, stenosis, or scarring with Barrett metaplasia

Pathological Findings

- Acute inflammation (especially eosinophils)
- Hyperplasia of the basal zone of the epithelium seen in 85%
- Barrett epithelial change: Gastric columnar epithelium replaces squamous epithelium in distal esophagus.

DIFFERENTIAL DIAGNOSIS

- Infectious esophagitis (*Candida*, herpes, HIV, cytomegalovirus)
- Chemical esophagitis (lye ingestion)
- Pill-induced esophagitis
- Radiation injury
- Crohn disease
- Angina
- Stricture
- Esophageal carcinoma
- Achalasia
- Scleroderma
- Peptic ulcer disease

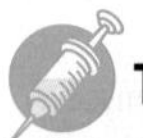

TREATMENT

MEDICATION

First Line

- Stepped therapy:
  - Phase I: Lifestyle and diet modifications, antacids plus H_2 blockers or PPIs
  - Phase II: Symptoms persist, consider endoscopic evaluation
  - Phase III: Surgery
- H_2 blockers in equipotent oral doses (e.g., cimetidine 800 mg b.i.d. or 400 mg q.i.d., or ranitidine 150 mg b.i.d., or famotidine 20 mg b.i.d., or nizatidine 150 mg b.i.d.)
- PPIs: Irreversibly bind proton pump, onset of effect 4 days. Include omeprazole 20 mg/d, lansoprazole 30 mg/d, pantoprazole 40 mg/d, rabeprazole 20 mg/d, esomeprazole 40 mg/d.
- Erosive esophagitis: PPI given for 8 weeks will be effective for healing in 90%:
  - PPI more effective than H_2 blocker for healing erosive esophagitis.

Pediatric Considerations

Antacids or liquid histamine type 2 blockers, omeprazole, metoclopramide

Second Line

- Antacids and agents like sucralfate may relieve breakthrough symptoms.
- Metoclopramide: 5–10 mg before meals
- Precautions:
  - Blood dyscrasias with PPIs and H_2 blockers
  - H_2 blockers must be renally dosed.
  - Metoclopramide is a dopamine blocker; risk of dystonia and tardive dyskinesia
  - On PPI, monitor B_{12}; B_{12} and iron absorption and calcium absorption compromised on PPI
- Significant possible interactions:
  - PPIs and H_2 blockers: Multiple cytochrome P450 drug interactions; examples include warfarin, phenytoin, antifungals

ADDITIONAL TREATMENT

General Measures

Lifestyle changes are first intervention:

- Elevate head of bed and avoid lying down soon after meals.
- Avoid stooping, bending, tight-fitting garments.
- Avoid medications that relax the LES (anticholinergic, calcium channel blockers).
- Lose weight.
- Stop smoking.
- Avoid alcohol.
- Decrease caffeine.

SURGERY/OTHER PROCEDURES

Open or laparoscopic Nissen fundoplication to increase pressure gradient between stomach and esophagus by wrapping gastric fundus around distal esophagus, often circumferential (360° fundoplication):

- Indications: Evidence of severe esophageal injury, incomplete response to medical treatment, medication treatment that has been or is expected to be prolonged
- Rule out esophageal dysmotility prior to surgery. If motility problems, consider a partial (270°, Toupet) wrap.
- Open and laparoscopic procedures both produce >90% response, equally effective for symptom reduction, quality of life, and decreased need for medications (3)[A].
- Cost analysis has indicated that if patient requires >10 years of PPI treatment, surgery may be more cost-effective.

Pediatric Considerations

Surgery for severe symptoms (apnea, choking, persistent vomiting)

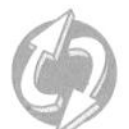

ONGOING CARE

FOLLOW-UP RECOMMENDATIONS

Patient Monitoring

- Follow symptomatically.
- Repeat endoscopy at 4–8 weeks for poor symptomatic response to medical therapy, especially in older patients.
- Current guideline is endoscopic surveillance every 2–5 years in patients with Barrett esophagus, assuming treatment if cancer is detected.

DIET

Avoid foods that make symptoms worse.

PATIENT EDUCATION

- Chocolate, peppermint, citrus, onions, spicy foods, and foods high in fat can make GERD symptoms worse.
- Eat small meals.
- Avoid lying down soon after meals.
- Elevate head of bed.
- Lifestyle changes, such as losing weight and smoking cessation and avoiding alcohol and caffeine, help.

PROGNOSIS

- Symptoms and esophageal inflammation often return promptly when treatment is withdrawn; to prevent relapse of symptoms, patients should be treated with continued antisecretory therapy:
  - PPI maintenance therapy may improve quality of life better than H_2 blocker maintenance.
  - Full-dose PPIs more effective than 1/2 dose for maintenance (3)[A]
  - In erosive esophagitis, daily maintenance therapy with a PPI has been proven to prevent relapse; intermittent PPI therapy has not been proven effective (4)[A].
- In terms of symptom reduction, medical and surgical therapy is equally effective (3)[A].
- Antireflux surgery:
  - 90–94% symptom response
  - 5% continued symptoms, should have anatomy evaluated by esophagram
  - Long-term follow-up shows some surgically treated patients may eventually require medical therapy.
- Regression of Barrett epithelium does not routinely occur despite aggressive medical or surgical therapy.

COMPLICATIONS

- Peptic stricture: 10–15%
- Barrett esophagus: 10%:
  - Adenocarcinoma from Barrett epithelium (rate of cancer development 0.5% annually)
- Extraesophageal symptoms: 5–10%, including hoarseness, aspiration, including aspiration pneumonia
- Bleeding due to mucosal injury
- Noncardiac chest pain

Geriatric Considerations

Complications more likely (e.g., aspiration pneumonia)

REFERENCES

1. Beaumont H, Bennink RJ, de Jong J, et al. The position of the acid pocket as a major risk factor for acidic reflux in healthy subjects and patients with GORD. *Gut*. 2010;59:441–51.
2. McColl KE, Clarke A, Seenan J, et al. Acid pocket, hiatus hernia and acid reflux. *Gut*. 2010;59:430–1.
3. Agency for Healthcare Research and Quality. Comparing effectiveness of management strategies for gastroesophageal reflux disease. An update to the 2005 report. Available at: http://effectivehealthcare.ahrq.gov. Accessed July 7, 2010.
4. Zacny J, Zamakhshary M, Sketris I, et al. Systematic review: The efficacy of intermittent and on-demand therapy with histamine H2-receptor antagonists or proton pump inhibitors for gastro-oesophageal reflux disease patients. *Aliment Pharmacol Ther*. 2005;21:1299–312.
5. Chang AB, Lasserson TJ, Kiljander TO, et al. Systematic review and meta-analysis of randomised controlled trials of gastro-oesophageal reflux interventions for chronic cough associated with gastrooesophageal reflux. *BMJ*. 2006;332:11–7.

ADDITIONAL READING

- Freedman ND, Murray LJ, Kamangar F, et al. Alcohol intake and risk of oesophageal adenocarcinoma: A pooled analysis from the BEACON Consortium. *Gut*. 2011;60:1029–37.
- Fuccio L, Zagari RM, Eusebi LH, et al. Meta-analysis: Can *Helicobacter pylori* eradication treatment reduce the risk for gastric cancer? *Ann Intern Med*. 2009;151:121–8.
- Lim LG, Tay H, Ho KY, et al. Curry induces acid reflux and symptoms in gastroesophageal reflux disease. *Dig Dis Sci*. 2011;56(12):3546–50.
- Reid BJ, Li X, Galipeau PC, Vaughan TL, et al. Barrett's oesophagus and oesophageal adenocarcinoma: Time for a new synthesis. *Nat Rev Cancer*. 2010;10:87–101.

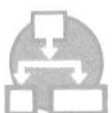

See Also (Topic, Algorithm, Electronic Media Element)

Algorithms: Dyspepsia; Epigastric Pain

CODES

ICD9

- 530.11 Reflux esophagitis
- 530.81 Esophageal reflux

CLINICAL PEARLS

- There is no evidence to support that treatment with PPI causes regression of Barrett esophagus or inhibits progression of esophageal dysplasia beyond benefits of symptomatic relief.
- GERD treatments are used to treat chronic cough. Meta-analysis of randomized clinical trials suggest PPIs help with cough resolution in some adults (5)[A].
- The role of *H. pylori* as an etiologic agent in GERD remains controversial.

GENERALIZED ANXIETY DISORDER

Michelle A. Tinitigan, MD

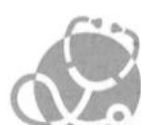

BASICS

DESCRIPTION

- Anxiety disorders are characterized by excessive worry that is difficult to control with at least 3 of the following symptoms: Restlessness, irritability, difficulty concentrating, muscle tension, sleep disturbances, and being easily fatigued. Symptoms must be distressing or impairing and not adequately explained by another related disorder (1).
- Occurs gradually, is recurrent, and remains chronic if not treated (1).

ALERT

Individuals with an anxiety disorder have a 15–20% lifetime risk of committing suicide.

Pediatric Considerations

Children and adolescents often present with worries concerning performance or competence.

EPIDEMIOLOGY

Prevalence

- Lifetime prevalence: 3–6%
- Primary-care setting prevalence: 5–8%
- Twice as common in women and commonly seen in middle age, with prevalence rates rising after age 35 in women and after age 45 in men (1)

RISK FACTORS

- Risk factors during childhood: Maternal internalizing symptoms (i.e., the mother's symptoms of anxiety and depression manifesting as insomnia, hopelessness, tension, somatic complaints), maltreatment, internalizing, conduct problems, and negative emotionality
- Family history
- History of other anxiety or mood disorders
- More common in ethnic minorities and in low socioeconomic status; some controversy over whether this results from more realistic worry about life situation

Genetics

Genetic factors play only a modest role in etiology of GAD. Heritability of female twin pairs was 30%.

PATHOPHYSIOLOGY

- Maladaptive response to stressful stimuli involving norepinephrine, serotonin, and γ-amino butyric acid
- Possible relationship between hypothalamic-pituitary-adrenal axis abnormalities and potential role of cholecystokinin

ETIOLOGY

GAD is likely a combination of genetic, developmental, and neurobiologic factors.

COMMONLY ASSOCIATED CONDITIONS

High rate of psychiatric comorbidity in patients with GAD, with 61% having multiple anxiety disorders, and 79% with >1 Axis I disorder (1); 35–50% of patients with major depression meet criteria for GAD.

DIAGNOSIS

- A 7-item anxiety questionnaire, GAD-7, has been developed in a primary care setting.
- Self-assessment screening tool; positive screen (score ≥8) should be followed by a clinician interview to establish a diagnosis.
- The first 2 items of GAD-7 (referred to as GAD-2), with a cutoff score of ≥3 warranting further evaluation; may be equally sensitive to GAD-7

HISTORY

- Initial interview: Unhurried and open-ended; when appropriate, family members should be involved.
- Medical history: Focused on contributing factors (e.g., medication side effects, substance abuse, or current medical condition)
- Psychosocial history: Screen for comorbid psychiatric disorders (major depression or agoraphobia), life stressors, family history, current social history, substance abuse history (including caffeine, nicotine, and alcohol), past sexual history, physical and emotional abuse, or emotional neglect.
- Diagnostic criteria from *DSM-IV* for GAD:
  - Excessive anxiety and worry about a number of events or activities, occurring more days than not for at least 6 months, that is out of proportion to the likelihood or impact of feared events, causing clinically significant social distress or functional impairment in social, occupational, or other important areas of functioning (2)
  - Anxiety is associated with at least 3 of the following somatic complaints: Restlessness, irritability, impaired concentration, muscle tension, fatigue, insomnia.
  - Affected patients have little insight into the connection between reported worries, current life stress, and their physical symptoms.
- Explore for causes of anxiety that may lead to other anxiety disorders:
  - Embarrassment in public (social phobia)
  - Having a panic attack (panic disorder)
  - Obsessions and rituals (OCD)
  - Separation from relatives (separation anxiety disorder)
  - Body image (anorexia nervosa)
- Assess for suicidality.
- Anxiety disorders have been shown to independently increase the risk of suicidality (panic disorder and social phobia more than GAD and OCD).

PHYSICAL EXAM

- Signs of common somatic symptoms include trembling, muscle tension, or muscle aches.
- Examine thyroid for signs of hyperthyroidism.
- Cardiac exam for tachycardia or atrial fibrillation

DIAGNOSTIC TESTS & INTERPRETATION

Lab

Initial lab tests

- CBC, comprehensive metabolic panel, TSH, urinalysis
- ECG (in patients >40 years of age with chest pain or palpitations)
- Serum or urine toxicology screen or drug levels if substance-induced anxiety suspected

DIFFERENTIAL DIAGNOSIS

- Other anxiety disorders: OCD, separation anxiety disorder, social phobia, posttraumatic stress disorder (PTSD), adjustment disorder with anxious mood, panic disorder, anorexia nervosa, hypochondriasis, somatization disorder
- Anxiety disorder owing to a general medical condition: Pheochromocytoma, hyperthyroidism, atrial fibrillation, stroke, parathyroid illness, vestibular nerve disease, mitral valve prolapse
- Anxiety associated with psychotic disorder or mood disorder; substance-induced anxiety disorder
- Dementia
- Medication-induced anxiety (e.g., steroids, thyroxine, theophylline, neuroleptics, SSRIs, tricyclic antidepressants, antihistamines, idiosyncratic reactions to other medications)

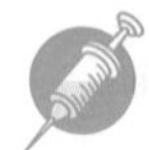

TREATMENT

MEDICATION

First Line

- SSRIs:
  - Paroxetine: 20 mg/d (number needed to treat [NNT] = 6.7)
    - May start at lower doses of 5–10 mg/d × 1 week to minimize adverse effect of restlessness and insomnia. Geriatric: 10 mg every morning; increase by 10 mg weekly to a maximum dose of 40 mg/d.
  - Escitalopram: Maintenance: 10–20 mg/d; geriatric: 10 mg/d; citalopram has shown efficacy in older patients (≥60 years old).
  - Sertraline: 25 mg/d; maintenance: 50–200 mg/d; may start at lower doses of 12.5–25 mg/d × 1 week
  - In children: Sertraline, fluoxetine, and fluvoxamine are effective in treating the symptoms of GAD in children and adolescents; should be reserved for individuals who have not responded to psychological therapies because of the risk of possible suicidal thoughts or behaviors.
  - Time of onset average 4 weeks; may co-administer a benzodiazepine to treat anxiety and agitation
  - Side effects: Sexual dysfunction, nausea, diarrhea, insomnia, withdrawal on discontinuation
- Serotonin norepinephrine reuptake inhibitors (SNRIs):
  - Venlafaxine: Initial: 37.5–75 mg/d; increase by 37.5-mg increments every 1–2 weeks until a dose of 150–300 mg is attained (NNT = 5.06).
  - Duloxetine: Initial: 30 mg/d PO × 1 week; then 60 mg/d PO
- It is recommended continuing therapy for at least 12 months rather than 6 months supported by previous research.

Second Line

- If monotherapy fails, try augmentation with a drug from another class, switch to drug with a different mechanism, or addition of psychotherapy. Second-line drugs include:
- Azapirones:
  - Buspirone (NNT = 4.4):
    - 15–30 mg b.i.d.; 30–60 mg/d given in 2 or 3 divided doses
    - Slow onset of action: Several weeks; variable intolerability

  - Appears to be useful in the treatment of GAD, especially for benzodiazepine-naïve patients, because it may be less addictive than benzodiazepines.
  - May alleviate decreased libido, diminished sexual arousal, or impaired orgasm associated with the use of antidepressants
- Tricyclic antidepressants (TCAs):
  - Imipramine 75 mg/d PO; increase to maximum of 200 mg/d (NNT = 4.07). May start at 10–20 mg at night, and titrate up to 75–300 mg at night. Usual maintenance: 50–150 mg/d. Geriatric: 25–75 mg at night; maximum of 200 mg/d
- Benzodiazepines (should be tapered as the antidepressant dose is titrated to therapeutic levels after 6–8 weeks):
  - Clonazepam: 0.25–0.5 mg PO b.i.d., titrated up to 1 mg b.i.d. or t.i.d.
  - Lorazepam: 0.5–1.0 mg PO t.i.d., titrated up to 1 mg PO t.i.d. or q.i.d.
  - Diazepam: 2–10 mg PO 2–4 times daily as needed; geriatric: 2–2.5 mg PO once or twice daily; increase gradually:
    - Have a rapid onset of action and are effective in GAD
    - Often recommended as adjunctive therapy to help patients in acute crisis or while waiting for a SSRI/SNRI to take effect.
    - Not recommended as monotherapy for depression, dysthymia, obsessive-compulsive disorder, and PTSD, which commonly occur with GAD.
    - Use for short-term treatment duration (up to 4 weeks) to avoid the risk of physical dependence and withdrawal (rebound anxiety).
    - Tapering usually takes months, with about 10% reduction per week.
    - If symptoms recur, it may be difficult to differentiate between benzodiazepine withdrawal or recurrence of GAD symptoms; symptoms that worsen within 2 weeks are most likely due to benzodiazepine withdrawal and suggest that the taper rate be decreased slightly.
    - Avoid in patients with polydrug or alcohol use, chronic pain disorders, and severe personality disorders, owing to high risk of dependence.
- Antihistamines:
  - Hydroxyzine: Associated side effects (in particular, sedation and anticholinergic effects), slow onset of action, and lack of efficacy for comorbid disorders (3)
- Pregabalin:
  - Approved in Europe for treatment of GAD (50–300 mg); has not been approved in the US4
  - Improves both psychic and somatic symptoms in adults with GAD, including the elderly
  - Discontinuation symptoms if abruptly stopped
- Atypical antipsychotic:
  - Quetiapine 50–150 mg/d:
    - Could be considered after other classes of drugs have proved ineffective or when certain types of symptoms are present (5)
    - Most trials used this for augmentation; however, more trials are needed to validate the efficacy of this class of drug

Pregnancy Considerations

- Paroxetine (Paxil): Association with congenital heart (septal) defects in first-trimester exposure and with persistent pulmonary hypertension in third-trimester exposure; Category D; fetal echocardiography should be considered for women who are exposed in early pregnancy.
- Venlafaxine (Effexor): Association with congenital heart defects in first-trimester exposure
- Benzodiazepines: First-trimester exposure is associated with craniofacial deformities. Maternal benzodiazepine use shortly before delivery is associated with floppy infant syndrome.

ADDITIONAL TREATMENT

Propranolol is not recommended for the treatment of GAD (no significant efficacy over placebo after 3 weeks in one randomized, controlled trial).

General Measures

Both psychological and medication therapies are effective and work well when used together.

Issues for Referral

Refer to a psychiatrist for comorbid depression, prolonged use of benzodiazepines, and for patients with suicidal ideation.

Additional Therapies

Cognitive-behavioral therapy can be an alternate first-line treatment or used in combination with medications. It has been shown to be superior to placebo in alleviating the symptoms of GAD.

COMPLEMENTARY AND ALTERNATIVE MEDICINE

- Kava, valerian root, and passion flower have been used to treat GAD; no adequate randomized trial of these medications (6).
- Kava has been temporarily taken off the market due to hepatotoxicity.
- Valerian is marketed principally for insomnia but also has been used as a mild sedative for anxiety disorders.
- Problems in methodology of randomized trials done on acupuncture limit conclusions on its effect on GAD.

IN-PATIENT CONSIDERATIONS

Initial Stabilization

Evaluate for suicidality, and begin pharmacologic treatment as soon as possible. Faster-acting medications (e.g., benzodiazepines) may be required for initial stabilization.

Admission Criteria

Inpatient admission is generally not necessary unless the patient expresses suicidal ideation.

Discharge Criteria

When suicidal ideation is no longer present and treatment has been started

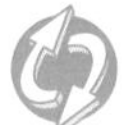

ONGOING CARE

FOLLOW-UP RECOMMENDATIONS

- Efficacy, medication tolerance, symptoms, and side effects should be assessed within 2 weeks of starting any new treatment.
- Once the patient has begun to experience relief from symptoms, follow-up should be every 4 weeks.

DIET

Discontinue or limit consumption of caffeine and other stimulant-type food/beverages.

PATIENT EDUCATION

- Patients should be presented with both medication and psychological treatment options.
- Patients treated with benzodiazepines should be made aware of the potential for dependence and the resulting short-term nature of this type of treatment.

PROGNOSIS

- GAD is a chronic disorder that rarely goes into remission, with long-term recovery achieved in only 1/3 of patients.
- Many patients will need chronic treatment with medication to prevent relapse; other patients may be treated with intermittent courses of acute treatment.
- Patients experience fluctuating levels of symptoms provoked by stressful life events. Augment treatment as needed.

REFERENCES

1. Davidson J, Feltner D, Dugar A. Management of generalized anxiety disorder in primary care: Identifying the challenges and unmet needs. *Prim Care Companion J Clin Psychiatry*. 2010;12(2): e1–e13.
2. American Psychiatric Association. *Diagnostic and Statistical Manual of Mental Disorders*, 4th ed, Primary Care Version (DSM-IV-PC). Washington, DC: American Psychiatric Association; 1995.
3. Bandelow B, Zohar J, Hollander E, et al. World Federation of Societies of Biological Psychiatry (WFSBP) guidelines for the pharmacological treatment of anxiety, obsessive-compulsive and post-traumatic stress disorders-first revision. *World J Biol Psychiatry*. 2008;9:248–312.
4. Lydiard RB, Rickels K, Herman B, et al. Comparative efficacy of pregabalin and benzodiazepines in treating the psychic and somatic symptoms of generalized anxiety disorder. *Int J Neuropsychopharmacol*. 2010;13:229–41.
5. Bandelow B, Chouinard G, Bobes J, et al. Extended-release quetiapine fumarate (quetiapine XR): A once-daily monotherapy effective in generalized anxiety disorder. Data from a randomized, double-blind, placebo- and active-controlled study. *Int J Neuropsychopharmacol*. 2010;13:305–20.
6. Lakhan SE, Vieira KF, et al. Nutritional and herbal supplements for anxiety and anxiety-related disorders: Systematic review. *Nutr J*. 2010;9:42.

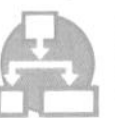

See Also (Topic, Algorithm, Electronic Media Element)

Depression

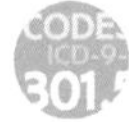

CODES

ICD9

- 300.00 Anxiety state, unspecified
- 300.02 Generalized anxiety disorder

CLINICAL PEARLS

- GAD is defined as excessive anxiety and worry more days than not for a period of 6 months or more, which the patient has a difficult time controlling and which causes significant impairment and distress.
- Patients should be evaluated for medical conditions that can cause hyperarousal, and other anxiety disorders.

G

GIARDIASIS

Kristyn Fagerberg, MD
Jill A. Grimes, MD

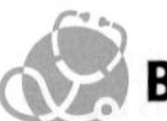

BASICS

DESCRIPTION

- Intestinal infection caused by the protozoan parasite *Giardia lamblia:*
  - *G. lamblia* is also called *G. duodenalis* and *G. intestinalis*.
- Infection results from ingestion of the cysts, which excyst into trophozoites:
  - Trophozoites colonize the small intestine and cause symptoms.
  - Cycle is continued when the trophozoites encyst in the small intestine and water, food, or hands are contaminated by feces of the infected person.
- Most infections result from fecal–oral transmission or ingestion of contaminated water (such as while swimming).
- Less commonly, giardiasis is the result of contaminated food.

EPIDEMIOLOGY

- Predominant age: All ages, but most common in early childhood ages 1–9 and adults 35–44 (1)[A]
- Predominant gender: Male > Female (slightly)

Pediatric Considerations

Common in early childhood

Prevalence

- 5% of patients with stools submitted for ova and parasite exams
- >19,000 cases/year in the US (although it is not reportable in Indiana, Kentucky, Mississippi, North Carolina, and Texas)

RISK FACTORS

- Daycare centers
- Anal intercourse
- Wilderness camping
- Travel to developing countries
- Children adopted from developing countries
- Public swimming pools

Genetics

No known genetic risk factors

GENERAL PREVENTION

- Good hand washing when caring for diapered children
- Water purification when camping and when traveling to developing countries
- Cooking all foods

PATHOPHYSIOLOGY

Giardia trophozoites colonize the surface of the proximal small intestine:

- The mechanism by which they cause diarrhea is unknown.

ETIOLOGY

Protozoan parasite (*G. lamblia*) infection acquired through fecal–oral transmission or ingestion of contaminated water, less commonly from contaminated food

COMMONLY ASSOCIATED CONDITIONS

Hypogammaglobulinemia and possibly IgA deficiency; diarrhea more severe and prolonged in these patients

DIAGNOSIS

HISTORY

- 25–50% of infected persons are symptomatic. Symptoms usually appear 1–2 weeks after an exposure.
- Chronic diarrhea (lasting >5–7 days and frequently weeks)
- Abdominal bloating
- Flatulence
- Loose, greasy, foul-smelling stools
- Weight loss
- Nausea
- Lactose intolerance

PHYSICAL EXAM

Nonspecific; abdominal bloating and afebrile

DIAGNOSTIC TESTS & INTERPRETATION

Lab

Initial lab tests

- Stool for ova and parasites:
  - Repeated 3 times if necessary
  - Cysts are seen in fixed or fresh stools and, occasionally, trophozoites are found in fresh diarrheal stools.
- Fluorescent antibody (FA) and ELISA tests of fecal specimens are available:
  - *A single FA or ELISA is at least as sensitive as 3 stools for ova and parasites.*
- Polymerase chain reaction (PCR) techniques have been found to be more sensitive than microscopy, but have not been widely adopted secondary to cost (2).

Follow-Up & Special Considerations

String test (Enterotest): A gelatin capsule on a string is swallowed and left in the duodenum for several hours or overnight. The end of the string is then visualized microscopically.

Diagnostic Procedures/Surgery

Esophagogastroduodenoscopy (EGD) with biopsy and sample of small intestinal fluid

Pathological Findings

Intestinal biopsy shows flattened, mild lymphocytic infiltration and trophozoites on the surface.

DIFFERENTIAL DIAGNOSIS

- Includes other etiologies of small intestinal diarrhea
- Infectious causes include cryptosporidiosis, isosporiasis, and cyclosporiasis.
- Other causes of malabsorption include celiac sprue, tropical sprue, bacterial overgrowth syndromes, and Crohn ileitis.
- Irritable bowel is suspected when diarrhea is not accompanied by weight loss.

TREATMENT

Outpatient for mild cases; inpatient if symptoms are severe enough to cause dehydration

MEDICATION

First Line

- Metronidazole (Flagyl): 250 mg t.i.d. for 5–7 days (3)[B]
- Tinidazole 2 g single dose (50 mg/kg up to 2 g for children) (3)[B]
- Albendazole 400 mg/d for 5 days:
  - Albendazole has comparable effectiveness to metronidazole with fewer side effects and low cost (4)[A].
- Precautions:
  - Theoretical risk of carcinogenesis with metronidazole
- Significant possible interactions: Occasional disulfiram reaction with metronidazole or tinidazole

Pregnancy Considerations

- Concern for potential teratogenicity of medications; consult infectious disease specialist or gastroenterologist for symptomatic disease
- Contraindications: Relatively contraindicated in pregnancy, especially first trimester

Second Line

- Furazolidone: 8 mg/kg/d t.i.d. for 10 days (slightly less effective, but commonly used in pediatrics because it is well tolerated)
- Paromomycin (Humatin): A nonabsorbable aminoglycoside that is probably less effective but commonly recommended in pregnancy because of theoretical risk of teratogenicity of other agents
- Quinacrine: 100 mg t.i.d. for 5–7 days; was the treatment of choice for giardiasis, but it has been withdrawn from the US market
- Nitazoxanide suspension was approved by the FDA in 2003 for treatment of giardiasis in children ages 1–11. Children ages 1–4 receive 100 mg b.i.d. and ages 5–11 receive 200 mg b.i.d. for 3 days (5)[B].

ADDITIONAL TREATMENT

- Lactose intolerance may follow *Giardia* infection and be a cause of persistent diarrhea post treatment.
- There have been anecdotal reports of herbal products containing *Mentha crispa* being effective in the treatment of Giardia. However, when studied, it was shown to be only 47.8% effective when compared to 84% for Secnidazole (a metronidazole analog) (6).

General Measures

- Medical therapy for all infected individuals
- Fluid replacement if dehydrated

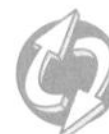

ONGOING CARE

FOLLOW-UP RECOMMENDATIONS

Patient Monitoring

Symptoms, weight, stool exams

DIET

Good nutrition, low lactose, low fat, monitor for dehydration

PATIENT EDUCATION

- Hand washing may be more important than water purification to prevent transmission in outdoor recreationalists (7)[A].
- CDC Facts about *Giardia* and Swimming Pools: www.cdc.gov/healthywater/pdf/swimming/resources/giardia-factsheet.pdf:
  - Don't swim when you have diarrhea.
  - Wash hands with soap after changing diapers before you return to the pool.
  - Do not put pool, lake, or river water in your mouth when you swim.

PROGNOSIS

- Untreated giardiasis lasts for weeks.
- Patients usually (90%) respond to treatment within a few days:
  - Most nonresponders or relapses respond to a second course with the same or a different agent.

COMPLICATIONS

Malabsorption and weight loss

REFERENCES

1. Yoder JS, Harral C, Beach MJ, et al. Giardiasis surveillance - United States, 2006–2008. *MMWR Surveill Summ*. 2010;59:15–25.
2. Haque R, Roy S, Siddique A, et al. Multiplex real-time PCR assay for detection of *Entamoeba histolytica, Giardia intestinalis,* and *Cryptosporidium* spp. *Am J Trop Med Hyg*. 2007;76:713–7.
3. Fallah M, Rabiee S, Moshtaghi AA. Comparison between efficacy of a single dose of tinidazole with a 7-day standard dose course of metronidazole in giardiasis. *Pak J Med Sci*. 2007;23(1):43–6.
4. Solaymani-Mohammadi S, Genkinger JM, Loffredo CA, et al. A meta-analysis of the effectiveness of albendazole compared with metronidazole as treatments for infections with *Giardia duodenalis*. *PLoS Negl Trop Dis*. 2010;4:e682.
5. Yoder JS, Beach MJ, Centers for Disease Control and Prevention (CDC). Giardiasis surveillance–United States, 2003–2005. *MMWR Surveill Summ*. 2007;56:11–8.
6. Teles NS, Fechine FV, Viana FA, et al. Evaluation of the therapeutic efficacy of *Mentha crispa* in the treatment of giardiasis. *Contemporary clinical trials*. 2011;32(6):809–13.
7. Welch TP, et al. Risk of giardiasis from consumption of wilderness water in North America: A systematic review of epidemiologic data. *Int J Infect Dis*. 2000;4:100–3.

ADDITIONAL READING

- Pawlowski SW, Warren CA, Guerrant R. Diagnosis and treatment of acute or persistent diarrhea. *Gastroenterology*. 2009;136(6):1874–86.
- Shields JM, Gleim ER, Beach MJ. Prevalence of *Cryptosporidium* spp. and *Giardia intestinalis* in swimming pools, Atlanta, Georgia. *Emerg Infect Dis*. 2008;14:948–50.

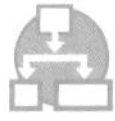

See Also (Topic, Algorithm, Electronic Media Element)

Algorithm: Diarrhea, Chronic

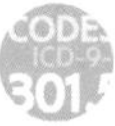

CODES

ICD9

007.1 Giardiasis

CLINICAL PEARLS

- Daycare facilities and public swimming pools are common sources of *Giardia* (don't assume camping or travel is required).
- Treatment with metronidazole is often poorly tolerated, but has higher cure rates.
- Most treatment failures respond to a second course of antibiotics (whether or not you switch drugs).

GILBERT DISEASE

Robert A. Marlow, MD, MA

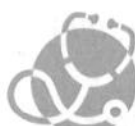

BASICS

DESCRIPTION

Mild chronic or intermittent unconjugated hyperbilirubinemia (not due to hemolysis) with otherwise normal liver function (1)

Pediatric Considerations

Rare for the disorder to be diagnosed before puberty

Pregnancy Considerations

The relative fasting that may occur with morning sickness can elevate the bilirubin level.

EPIDEMIOLOGY

- Predominant age: Present from birth, but most often presents in the second or third decade of life; heterozygous for single abnormal gene
- Predominant sex: Male > Female (2–7:1)

Prevalence

Prevalence in the US: ~7% of the population (2)

RISK FACTORS

Male gender

Genetics

A gene defect resulting in reduced bilirubin uridine diphosphate–glucuronosyltransferase-1 appears to be necessary but not sufficient for Gilbert syndrome (3).

ETIOLOGY

The hyperbilirubinemia results from impaired hepatic bilirubin clearance (~30% of normal). Hepatic bilirubin conjugation (glucuronidation) is reduced, although this is likely not the only defect.

COMMONLY ASSOCIATED CONDITIONS

Gilbert disease may be part of a spectrum of hereditary disorders that includes types I and II Crigler-Najjar syndrome.

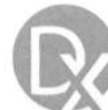

DIAGNOSIS

HISTORY

No significant symptoms, although a variety of nonspecific symptoms have been described.

PHYSICAL EXAM

No abnormal physical findings other than occasional mild jaundice

DIAGNOSTIC TESTS & INTERPRETATION

Lab

Initial lab tests

- Bilirubin: Elevated but <6 mg/dL (103 μmol/L) and usually <3 mg/dL (51 μmol/L), virtually all unconjugated (indirect)
- CBC with peripheral smear is normal.
- Reticulocyte count is normal.
- Liver function tests (aspartate aminotransferase [AST], alanine transaminase [ALT], alkaline phosphatase, and glutamyl transpeptidase [GGT]) are normal.
- Fasting and postprandial serum bile acids are normal.
- Up to 60% of patients have clinically insignificant mild hemolysis that frequently can only be detected with sophisticated red cell survival studies.
- Drugs that may alter lab results: Bilirubin level may be raised by nicotinic acid and lowered by phenobarbital.
- Disorders that may alter lab results: Bilirubin levels increase during fasting and may increase during a febrile illness.

Follow-Up & Special Considerations

If history, physical exam, and laboratory tests are normal, see the patient on 2–3 further occasions during the ensuing 12–18 months. If the patient develops no symptoms, reticulocytosis, or new liver function abnormalities, make the diagnosis of Gilbert disease.

Diagnostic Procedures/Surgery

- A liver biopsy is not usually needed to exclude other diagnoses (2).
- Some clinicians recommend confirming the diagnosis by reducing daily caloric intake to 400 kcal for 48 hours, which results in a 2–3-fold increase in unconjugated bilirubin.
- After 12 hours of fasting, an increase of total bilirubin to >1.9 mg/dL 2 hours after an oral dose of rifampin 900 mg distinguishes patients with Gilbert disease with a sensitivity of 100% and a specificity of 100% (4).

DIFFERENTIAL DIAGNOSIS

- Hemolysis
- Ineffective erythropoiesis (megaloblastic anemias, certain porphyrias, thalassemia major, sideroblastic anemia, severe lead poisoning, congenital dyserythropoietic anemias)
- Cirrhosis
- Chronic persistent hepatitis
- Pancreatitis
- Biliary tract disease

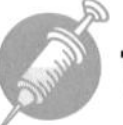

TREATMENT

Outpatient. The most important treatment is to make a positive diagnosis of Gilbert disease to reassure the patient and prevent further unnecessary procedures.

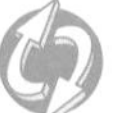

ONGOING CARE

FOLLOW-UP RECOMMENDATIONS

Patient Monitoring

If history, physical exam, and laboratory tests are normal, see the patient on 2–3 further occasions during the ensuing 12–18 months. If the patient develops no symptoms, reticulocytosis, or new liver function abnormalities, make the diagnosis of Gilbert disease.

PATIENT EDUCATION

Reassure the patient that the condition is benign with no known sequelae.

PROGNOSIS

The disorder is benign with an excellent prognosis. There is some preliminary evidence that patients with Gilbert disease may have a lower incidence of cardiovascular disease (5,6). Elevated levels of bilirubin may exert an antioxidation effect (6).

COMPLICATIONS

No known complications

REFERENCES

1. Bosma PJ. Inherited disorders of bilirubin metabolism. *J Hepatol*. 2003;38:107–17.
2. Radu P, Atsmon J. Gilbert's syndrome–clinical and pharmacological implications. *Isr Med Assoc J*. 2001;3:593–8.
3. Bosma PJ, Chowdhury JR, Bakker C, et al. The genetic basis of the reduced expression of bilirubin UDP-glucuronosyltransferase 1 in Gilbert's syndrome. *N Engl J Med*. 1995;333:1171–5.
4. Murthy GD, Byron D, Shoemaker D, et al. The utility of rifampin in diagnosing Gilbert's syndrome. *Am J Gastroenterol*. 2001;96:1150–4.
5. Inoguchi T, Sasaki S, Kobayashi K, et al. Relationship between Gilbert syndrome and prevalence of vascular complications in patients with diabetes. *JAMA*. 2007;298:1398–400.
6. Bulmer AC, Blanchfield JT, Toth I, et al. Improved resistance to serum oxidation in Gilbert's syndrome: A mechanism for cardiovascular protection. *Atherosclerosis*. 2008;199:390–6.

ADDITIONAL READING

- Claridge LC, Armstrong MJ, Booth C, et al. Gilbert's syndrome. *BMJ*. 2011;342:d2293.
- Strassburg CP. Pharmacogenetics of Gilbert's syndrome. *Pharmacogenomics*. 2008;9:703–15.

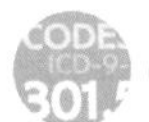

CODES

ICD9

277.4 Disorders of bilirubin excretion

CLINICAL PEARLS

- Gilbert disease: A mild chronic or intermittent unconjugated hyperbilirubinemia (not due to hemolysis) with otherwise normal liver function
- The hyperbilirubinemia results from impaired hepatic bilirubin clearance (~30% of normal). Hepatic bilirubin conjugation (glucuronidation) is reduced, although this is likely not the only defect.
- The most important reason to make the diagnosis of Gilbert disease is to reassure the patient that this is a benign condition with no known sequelae and to prevent unnecessary procedures.
- To diagnosis Gilbert disease: If history, physical exam, and laboratory tests (LFTs, reticulocytosis, etc.) are normal on visits every 6 months over 18 months
- A liver biopsy is not usually needed to rule out other liver diseases. The diagnosis can be confirmed by otherwise normal liver function tests, no evidence of hemolysis, and the response to fasting or a dose of rifampin.
- The etiology of Gilbert disease can result when the patient has a gene defect resulting in reduced conjugation of bilirubin. The gene defect is necessary but not sufficient to produce Gilbert disease.

G

GINGIVITIS

Hugh J. Silk, MD, MPH
Sheila O. Stille, DMD, MAGD
Stacy Temple, DMD

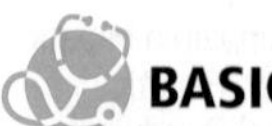

BASICS

DESCRIPTION

Gingivitis is a reversible form of inflammation of the gingiva. It is a mild form of periodontal disease. Classification includes:

- Plaque-induced
- Not plaque-induced (bacterial, viral, or fungal; e.g., acute necrotizing gingivitis, Vincent disease, denture-related)
- Modified by systemic factors (e.g., pregnancy, HIV, diabetes, leukemia)
- Modified by medications (antihypertensives, antipsychotics, antiepileptics, hormones)
- Modified by malnutrition (vitamin deficiencies)
- System(s) affected: Gastrointestinal
- Synonym(s): Mild periodontal disease; Gum disease

Geriatric Considerations

More frequent in this age group (due more to additive effects than to increased susceptibility)

Pediatric Considerations

Mild cases common in children (most common form of pediatric periodontal disease) and usually require no specific interventions

Pregnancy Considerations

- Very common in pregnant women; hormonal effect
- Hyperplasia
- Common; self-limited

EPIDEMIOLOGY

- Predominant age: >35 years old (but as young as 5)
- Predominant sex: Male = Female

Prevalence

- ~50% of children
- ~90% of adolescents and adult population
- ~30–75% of pregnant women

RISK FACTORS

- Poor dental hygiene/plaque formation
- Pregnancy
- Diabetes mellitus
- Malocclusion or dental crowding
- Smoking
- Mouth breathing
- Faulty dental restoration
- HIV-positive; AIDS
- Stress
- Vitamin C deficiency; coenzyme Q10 deficiency
- Dental appliances (dentures, braces)
- Eruption of primary or secondary teeth
- Necrotizing ulcerative gingivitis:
  - Stress
  - Lack of sleep
  - Malnutrition
  - Viral illness
  - Typically younger patients/teens and young adults
- Bronchial asthma (1)
- Rheumatoid arthritis (2)

Genetics

Possible genetic link (up to 30% of population). Rare condition called hereditary gingival fibromatosis associated with hirsutism.

GENERAL PREVENTION

- Good oral hygiene:
  - Adults:
    - Regular twice-daily brushing with fluoride toothpaste and increased benefit of using circular oscillating electric brush rather than regular brush (3)[A]
    - Daily high-quality flossing (many studies show that flossing does not help because it is often done incorrectly) (4)[A]
  - Pediatrics:
    - Regular twice-daily brushing with fluoride toothpaste under parental supervision until full manual dexterity (~8 years of age)
    - Regular flossing if no spaces between teeth
- Cleaning by a dentist or hygienist every 6 months or more frequently, if indicated
- Mouthrinse with essential oils (menthol, thymol, eucalyptol; e.g., Listerine) combined with brushing reduces gingivitis more than brushing alone (5). Caution: Long-term use of alcohol-based mouthrinse may be associated with an increase risk of oral cancer (6)[A].

PATHOPHYSIOLOGY

Inflammation of gingiva that may progress to deeper, destructive inflammation (see "Periodontitis")

ETIOLOGY

- Noncontagious
- Inadequate plaque removal
- Blood dyscrasias (pregnancy)
- Oral contraceptives
- Allergic reactions
- Nutritional deficiencies
- Vasoconstriction (nicotine)
- Endocrine/hormonal variations:
  - Pregnancy
  - Menses
  - Menarche
- Chronic debilitating disease
- Vincent disease:
  - Synergistic infection with fusiform bacillus (*Fusobacterium* spp.) and spirochete (*Borrelia vincentii*)

COMMONLY ASSOCIATED CONDITIONS

- Periodontitis
- Glossitis
- Pedunculated growths (pyogenic granulomata)

DIAGNOSIS

HISTORY

- Gum swelling and edema (usually painless)
- Gum erythema
- Bleeding of gums when brushing, flossing, or eating
- Inquire about HIV risk, pregnancy, nutritional deficiencies, diabetes, and other risk factors as indicated (see "Risk Factors").
- Smoking history
- Oral hygiene, dental visit history

PHYSICAL EXAM

- Normal gums should appear pink, firm, and shiny.
- Gum swelling and edema (usually painless)
- Erythema
- Bleeding with manipulation of gums
- Change of normal gum contours
- Plaque and calculus (not easily removed)
- Edema of interdental papillae
- HIV gingivitis:
  - Also called linear gingival erythema
  - Narrow band of bright red inflamed gum surrounding neck of tooth
  - Painful
  - Bleeds easily
  - Rapid destruction of tissue
- Vincent disease:
  - Ulcers
  - Fever
  - Malaise
  - Regional lymphadenopathy
  - Pain
  - Mouth odor

DIAGNOSTIC TESTS & INTERPRETATION

Lab

Initial lab tests

- Possible smear or culture to identify causative agent (HIV gingivitis includes gram-negative anaerobes, enteric strains, and candida)
- Labs for contributing conditions (HIV, pregnancy, diabetes, nutritional deficiencies)

Imaging

Initial approach

No tests usually needed

Pathological Findings

- Acute or chronic inflammation
- Hyperemic capillaries
- Polymorphonuclear infiltration
- Papillary projections in subepithelial tissue
- Fibroblasts

DIFFERENTIAL DIAGNOSIS

- Periodontitis (deeper inflammation, causing destruction to connective tissue, ligaments, and alveolar bone)
- Glossitis
- Desquamative gingivitis (painful, persistent, usually middle-aged women)
- Pericoronitis (gum flap traps food and plaque over partially erupted molar), common in adolescence
- Gingival ulcers (aphthous, herpetic, malignancy, TB, syphilis)
- Specific forms of gingivitis: See "Description" including acute necrotizing ulcerative gingivitis (Vincent disease) and HIV gingivitis (linear gingival erythema)

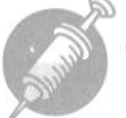

TREATMENT

MEDICATION

First Line

- Chlorhexidine rinses or varnishes may be used (7).
- Antibiotics indicated only for acute necrotizing ulcerative gingivitis (Vincent disease)
- Antibiotics:
  - Penicillin V: Pediatric dose, 25–50 mg/kg/d divided q6h; adult dose, 250–500 mg q6h, OR
  - Erythromycin: Pediatric dose 30–40 mg/kg/d divided q6h; adult dose, 250 mg q6h
- Topical corticosteroids:
  - Triamcinolone (0.147 mg/g) in Orabase (spray or ointment), applied locally t.i.d., q.i.d.
- Contraindications:
  - Allergy to specific medication
- Precautions:
  - Erythromycin frequently causes significant GI issues.

Second Line

- Acetaminophen or ibuprofen for any pain (rare)
- Other antibiotics or antifungal rinses or systemics according to culture or smear
- Decapinol oral rinse (surfactant that acts as a physical barrier, making it harder for bacteria to stick to tooth and mucosal surfaces) to reduce bacteria (not recommended for pregnant women or children under 12). Should be used in conjunction with other oral hygiene practices when those practices alone are not enough.

ADDITIONAL TREATMENT

General Measures

- Stop any contributing medications.
- Remove irritating factors (plaque, calculus, faulty dental restorations or dentures).
- Good oral hygiene (see "General Prevention")
- Regular dental checkups (for scaling and polishing if plaque and/or tartar are present)
- No smoking
- Warm saline rinses b.i.d.

Issues for Referral

- Dental referral for cleanings and further treatment as needed
- If gingivitis becomes periodontitis, deep root scaling and planing may be indicated.

COMPLEMENTARY AND ALTERNATIVE MEDICINE

- Bilberry: Potentially helpful in reducing inflammation and stabilizing collagen tissue
- Coenzyme Q10: Topically, to restore coenzyme Q10 deficiency
- Replace any other deficiencies (e.g., vitamin C).

SURGERY/OTHER PROCEDURES

- Debridement for acute necrotizing gingivitis
- Minor surgery may be necessary to correct tissue overgrowth for gingivitis caused by medicines.

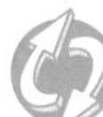

ONGOING CARE

FOLLOW-UP RECOMMENDATIONS

- Outpatient
- No restrictions

Patient Monitoring

Until clear; dental follow-up for continued cleanings and secondary prevention

DIET

- Well-balanced diet that includes fruits, vegetables, vitamin C; avoid sugary snacks and drinks, which contribute to plaque formation.
- Soft foods during flare, if significant inflammation/bleeding

PATIENT EDUCATION

- Good oral hygiene, including twice-daily brushing with fluoridated toothpaste and daily flossing; regular dental visits
- Printable and viewable patient information available under "periodontal diseases" from the American Dental Association at www.ada.org; and the American Academy of Periodontology at www.perio.org

PROGNOSIS

- Usual course: Acute, relapsing, intermittent, chronic
- Prognosis: Generally favorable, responds well to appropriate treatment
- Left untreated, may progress to periodontitis (controversial), which is a major cause of tooth loss

COMPLICATIONS

Severe periodontal disease (which is associated with heart disease, diabetes, and preterm birth)

REFERENCES

1. Mehta A, Sequeira PS, Sahoo RC, et al. Is bronchial asthma a risk factor for gingival diseases? A control study. *N Y State Dent J*. 2009;75:44–6.
2. Nilsson M, Kopp S. Gingivitis and periodontitis are related to repeated high levels of circulating tumor necrosis factor-alpha in patients with rheumatoid arthritis. *J Periodontol*. 2008;79:1689–96.
3. Deery C, Heanue M, Deacon S, et al. The effectiveness of manual versus powered toothbrushes for dental health: a systematic review. *J Dent*. 2004;32:197–211.
4. Berchier C E, Slot D E, Haps S, et al. The efficacy of dental floss in addition to a toothbrush on plaque and parameters of gingival inflammation: A systematic review. *Int J Dent Hygiene*. 2008;6(4):265–79.
5. Stoeken JE, Paraskevas S, van der Weijden GA. The long-term effect of a mouthrinse containing essential oils on dental plaque and gingivitis: A systematic review. *J Periodontol*. 2007;78(7):1218–28.
6. McCullough M, Farah CS. The role of alcohol in oral carcinogenesis with particular reference to alcohol-containing mouthwashes. *Aust Dent J*. 2008;53(4):302–305.
7. Puig-Silla M, Montiel-Company JM, Almerich-Silla JM. Use of chlorhexidine varnishes in preventing and treating periodontal disease. A review of the literature. *Med Oral Patol Oral Cir Bucal*. 2008;13:E257–60.

ADDITIONAL READING

- Armitage GC. Development of a classification system for periodontal diseases and conditions. *Ann Periodont*. 1999;4:1.
- Coventry J, Griffiths G, Scully C, et al. Periodontal disease: ABC of oral health. *Br Med J*. 2000;321:36–9.
- Loesche WJ, Grossman NS. Periodontal disease as a specific, albeit chronic, infection: Diagnosis and treatment. *Clin Microbiol Rev*. 2001;14:727–52.
- New Oral Rinse Helps Treat Gingivitis. *FDA Consumer* [serial on the Internet]. 2005, [cited July 22, 2008]; 39(4):5–6. Available from: Alt Health Watch.
- Oliver RC, Brown LJ, Loer H. Periodontal disease in the United States population. *J Periodontol*. 1998;69(2):269–78.

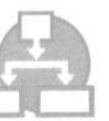

See Also (Topic, Algorithm, Electronic Media Element)

- Dental Infection; Glossitis
- Algorithm: Bleeding Gums

CODES

ICD9

- 523.00 Acute gingivitis, plaque induced
- 523.01 Acute gingivitis, non-plaque induced
- 523.10 Chronic gingivitis, plaque induced

CLINICAL PEARLS

- Gingivitis may be treated with regular dental cleanings, good oral hygiene, and use of chlorhexidine rinses.
- Untreated, gingivitis may progress to periodontitis, a possible contributor to systemic inflammation and its consequences (such as coronary artery disease and preterm labor).
- New-onset or difficult-to-treat gingivitis, consider differential of etiology: Pregnancy, HIV, diabetes, medications, vitamin deficiencies

GLAUCOMA, PRIMARY CLOSED-ANGLE

Michael C. Barros, PharmD, BCPS
J. Michael O'Connell, Jr., MD
Susan C. Kent, PharmD, CGP

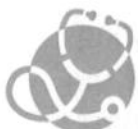

BASICS

DESCRIPTION

- Acute-angle closure (the term *glaucoma* is added when glaucomatous optic neuropathy is present):
  - At least 2 of the following symptoms: Ocular pain; nausea/vomiting; intermittent blurred vision with halos, *plus*
  - At least 3 of the following signs: Intraocular pressure (IOP) >21 mm Hg; conjunctival injection; corneal epithelial edema; middilated nonreactive pupil; shallower chamber in the presence of occlusion
- Primary-angle closure (the term *glaucoma* is added when glaucomatous optic neuropathy is present):
  - Occludable drainage angle *plus* signs that the peripheral iris has obstructed the trabecular meshwork (e.g., elevated IOP, lens opacities)
- Chronic angle-closure glaucoma: Refers to an eye with permanent closure of areas of the anterior chamber angle by peripheral anterior synechiae

Geriatric Considerations

Increased risk with age and prior history of cataract, hyperopia, and/or uveitis.

Pregnancy Considerations

Medications used may cross the placenta and be excreted into breast milk.

EPIDEMIOLOGY

- Leading cause of blindness due to glaucoma
- Age older than 40–50
- Female > Male
- Inuit and Asian > African and European
- Most common form of glaucoma worldwide, but only 10% of glaucoma in the US

Prevalence

Acute-angle closure glaucoma occurs in 1 in 1,000 Caucasians; 1 in 100 Asians; 2–4 in 100 Eskimos (lifetime)

RISK FACTORS

- Hyperopia
- Age >40–50 years old
- Shallow anterior chamber
- Female gender
- Family history of angle closure
- Asian or Inuit descent
- Pseudoexfoliation
- Short axial length
- Thick crystalline lens
- Medications that may induce angle-closure glaucoma:
  - ACE inhibitors (rare), adrenergic agonists (albuterol), anticholinergics, antihistamines, antidepressants including SSRIs and TCAs, cholinergic agents (pilocarpine), noncatecholamine adrenergic agonists, sulfa-based drugs, topiramate, warfarin (rare)

Genetics

Polygenic inheritance: First-degree relatives have a 2–5% lifetime risk.

GENERAL PREVENTION

- Routine eye exam with gonioscopy for high-risk populations
- US Preventive Services Task Force: Insufficient evidence to recommend for or against screening adults for glaucoma

PATHOPHYSIOLOGY

- Peripheral iris apposition to the trabecular meshwork obstructs the outflow of aqueous humor through the trabecular meshwork, which causes elevation in IOP.
- The underlying mechanism is anterior lens displacement or other anatomic abnormality, leading to pupillary block in which aqueous humor egress through the pupil is limited. This causes pressure to build posterior to the iris, leading to anterior iris displacement.

ETIOLOGY

Predisposing ocular anatomy

COMMONLY ASSOCIATED CONDITIONS

- Cataract
- Hyperopia
- Microphthalmos
- Systemic hypertension

DIAGNOSIS

HISTORY

- Patient's previous medical and ophthalmologic history
- Family history of glaucoma
- Obtain history of prescription and over-the-counter medications
- Precipitating factors (dim light, meds)
- Review of symptoms
- Acute:
  - Severe unilateral ocular pain
  - Blurred vision
  - Lacrimation
  - Photophobia
  - Halos around lights/objects
  - Frontal, ipsilateral, headache
  - Nausea and vomiting
- Chronic:
  - May have subacute symptoms (intermittent subacute attacks)
  - Compromised peripheral, then central vision
  - May be asymptomatic

PHYSICAL EXAM

- Includes, but is not limited to, the following in the undilated eye (1)[C]:
  - Visual acuity
  - Visual field testing and ocular motility
  - Pupil size and reactivity (middilated, minimally reactive)
  - External examination
  - Undilated fundus exam (congestion, cupping, atrophy of optic nerve)
  - Slit-lamp biomicroscopy (anterior segments)
  - Tonometry (determination of IOP)
  - Gonioscopy (visualization of the angle)
- Acute:
  - Elevated intraocular pressure (40–80 mm Hg)
  - Corneal microcystic edema (haze)
  - Lid edema, conjunctival hyperemia, and circumcorneal injection (ciliary flush)
  - Fixed middilated pupil (often oval) and firm globe
  - Shallow anterior chamber, often with inflammatory reaction (cell and flare)
  - Blepharospasm (severe cases)
  - Pain with eye movement
  - Closed angle by gonioscopy
- Chronic:
  - Multiple peripheral anterior synechiae
  - Normal or elevated intraocular pressure
  - Increased cup-to-disc ratio or excavation of disc
  - Glaucoma flecks (lens) and iris atrophy (previous acute attacks)

DIAGNOSTIC TESTS & INTERPRETATION

Imaging

Ultrasound biomicroscopy

Diagnostic Procedures/Surgery

Careful ophthalmic examination, including gonioscopy and tonometry (1,2,3)[C]

Pathological Findings

- Corneal stromal and epithelial edema
- Endothelial cell loss (guttata)
- Iris stromal necrosis
- Anterior subcapsular cataract (*glaukomflecken*)
- Optic disc congestion, cupping, excavation
- Optic nerve atrophy

DIFFERENTIAL DIAGNOSIS

- Acute orbital compartment syndrome
- Traumatic hyphema
- Conjunctivitis, episcleritis
- Corneal abrasion
- Glaucoma, malignant or neovascular
- Herpes zoster ophthalmicus
- Iritis and uveitis
- Orbital/periorbital infection
- Plateau iris syndrome
- Vitreous or subconjunctival hemorrhage
- Tight necktie, causing increased IOP
- Lens-induced angle closure

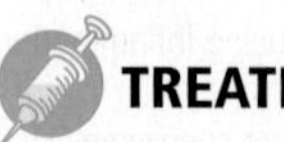

TREATMENT

Goals of treatment:

- Reverse or prevent angle-closure process
- Control IOP
- Prevent damage to the optic nerve

MEDICATION

- Practically speaking, acute angle glaucoma is managed with oral mannitol or glycerin for a rapid decrease in IOP, and then, after the cornea clears, a peripheral iridotomy is done.
- Initiate medical therapy first, using some or all of the following (1)[C],(4)[B]:
  - Topical/systemic carbonic anhydrase inhibitor:
    - Acetazolamide (Diamox) 500 mg IV, may repeat in 2–4 hours to a maximum of 1 g/d

- Dorzolamide (Trusopt) 2% eyedrops: Instill 1 drop in the affected eye(s) t.i.d.
- Brinzolamide (Azopt) 1% suspension: Instill 1 drop in the affected eye(s) t.i.d.:
  - Contraindications/precautions: Sulfa allergy (risk of cross-sensitivity), bitter taste, eyelid reactions
- β-blockers:
  - Timolol (Timoptic) 0.5% solution: Instill 1 drop in the affected eye(s) b.i.d.
  - Timolol (Istalol) 0.5% solution: Instill 1 drop once daily in the morning
  - Timolol (Timolol GFS, Timoptic-XE) 0.25–0.5% gel forming solution: Instill 1 drop once daily
  - Levobunolol (Betagan) 0.25–0.5% solution: Instill 1 drop in the affected eye(s) 1–2 times daily
  - Betaxolol (Betoptic) 0.5% solution: Instill 1–2 drops in the affected eye(s) b.i.d.
  - Carteolol (generic) 1% solution: Instill 1 drop in the affected eye(s) b.i.d.
  - Metipranolol (OptiPranolol) 0.3% solution: Instill 1 drop in the affected eye(s) b.i.d.:
    - Contraindications/precautions: Decompensated heart failure, sinus bradycardia $\geq$ second-degree, severe COPD/asthma; increased risk of bradycardia or heart block with digoxin, verapamil, diltiazem, or clonidine; effect on IOP may be lessened in patients taking oral β-blockers
- α_2-agonists:
  - Apraclonidine (Iopidine) 0.5% solution: Instill 1–2 drops in affected eye(s) t.i.d.
  - Brimonidine (Alphagan P) 0.15–0.2% solution: Instill 1 drop in affected eye(s) t.i.d.:
    - Contraindications/precautions: Use with current or within 14 days of MAO inhibitor therapy, CNS depression
- Prostaglandin analogs:
  - Latanoprost (Xalatan), travoprost (Travatan Z), bimatoprost (Lumigan): Instill 1 drop in the affected eye(s) every night:
    - Precautions: Irreversible changes to iris, eyelid and eyelash pigmentation, eyelash growth, itching, redness, edema
- Cholinergic agonists:
  - Pilocarpine (1%, 2%, 4% solution): Instill 1–2 drops up to 6 times daily); do not use unless directed by ophthalmologist
  - Carbachol 3% solution: Instill 1–2 drops up to t.i.d.
  - Echothiophate iodide (phospholine iodide) 0.125% solution; Instill 1 drop b.i.d.:
    - Precautions: May worsen the condition due to anterior rotation of the lens–iris diaphragm, impaired night vision,
- Combination products:
  - Timolol-dorzolamide (Cosopt) 0.5/2% solution: Instill 1 drop in the affected eye(s) b.i.d.
  - Timolol-brimonidine (Combigan) 0.5/0.2% solution: Instill 1 drop in the affected eye(s) b.i.d.

ADDITIONAL TREATMENT

General Measures

- For acute form:
  - Manage extraocular symptoms, such as nausea and pain.
  - Obtain an immediate ophthalmology consultation.
- Ocular goals of therapy through medical and surgical treatment:
  - Reduce IOP to <35 mm Hg or by >25% of presenting IOP (4)[B].
  - Prevent damage to the optic nerve.
  - Prevent central retinal artery occlusion.
  - Prevent or reverse angle closure.

Additional Therapies

- Initiate immediate emergency ophthalmologic treatment.
- Keep patient supine.

SURGERY/OTHER PROCEDURES

- Acute (1,5)[B]:
  - Laser peripheral iridotomy per ophthalmology (1,5)[B]
  - Perform surgical iridectomy if laser is not possible.
- Chronic:
  - Goniosynechialysis
  - Phacoemulsification

IN-PATIENT CONSIDERATIONS

Admission Criteria

- Patient requires metabolic $\pm$ electrolyte and volume status monitoring (with osmotic agents)
- Maintain ophthalmology follow-up.

IV Fluids

IV access

Nursing

Implement an emergency ophthalmic plan of care.

Discharge Criteria

Patient is stable for outpatient follow-up

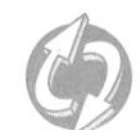

ONGOING CARE

FOLLOW-UP RECOMMENDATIONS

- Schedule an immediate ophthalmologic follow-up.
- Hospital admission if clinically warranted

Patient Monitoring

- Postsurgical follow-up
- Fellow eye evaluation
- Chronic monitoring post–acute attack per ophthalmology

DIET

Regular as tolerated

PATIENT EDUCATION

- Advise patient to seek emergency medical attention if experiencing a change in visual acuity, blurred vision, eye pain, or headache.
- New medication counseling
- If narrow angles but no peripheral iridotomy performed: Avoid decongestants, motion sickness medications, adrenergic agents, antipsychotics, antidepressants, and anticholinergic agents.
- Correct eyedrop administration technique
- Patients with significant visual impairment should be referred to vision rehab and social services.
- Patient education materials:
  - Glaucoma Research Foundation: www.glaucoma.org
  - National Eye Institute: www.nei.nih.gov
  - Glaucoma handout from American Academy of Family Physicians
  - Handout on using glaucoma eyedrops in *Am Fam Physician* 1999;59(7):1882

PROGNOSIS

- With timely treatment, most patients do not have permanent vision loss.
- Prognosis depends on ethnicity, underlying eye disease, and time-to-treatment.

COMPLICATIONS

- Chronic corneal edema
- Corneal fibrosis and vascularization
- Iris atrophy
- Cataract
- Optic atrophy
- Malignant glaucoma
- Central retinal artery/vein occlusion
- Permanent decrease in visual acuity
- Repeat episode
- Fellow eye attack

REFERENCES

1. American Academy of Ophthalmology. *Primary Angle Closure Preferred Practice Pattern*. San Francisco: American Academy of Ophthalmology; 2010. Available at: www.aao.org.
2. Asrani S, Sarunic M, Santiago C, et al. Detailed visualization of the anterior segment using fourier-domain optical coherence tomography. *Arch Ophthalmol*. 2008;126:765–71.
3. Barkana Y, Dorairaj SK, Gerber Y, et al. Agreement between gonioscopy and ultrasound biomicroscopy in detecting iridotrabecular apposition. *Arch Ophthalmol*. 2007;125:1331–5.
4. Choong YF, Irfan S, Menage MJ. Acute angle closure glaucoma: An evaluation of a protocol for acute treatment. *Eye*. 1999;13(Pt 5):613–6.
5. Saw SM, Gazzard G, Friedman DS. Interventions for angle-closure glaucoma: An evidence-based update. *Ophthalmology*. 2003;110:1869–78; quiz 1878–9, 1930.

ADDITIONAL READING

Tripathi RC, Tripathi BJ, Haggerty C. Drug-induced glaucomas: Mechanism and management. *Drug Saf*. 2003;26:749–67.

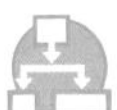

See Also (Topic, Algorithm, Electronic Media Element)

Glaucoma, Primary Open-Angle

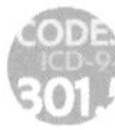

CODES

ICD9

- 365.20 Primary angle-closure glaucoma, unspecified
- 365.22 Acute angle-closure glaucoma
- 365.23 Chronic angle-closure glaucoma

CLINICAL PEARLS

- Examiner can determine if patient is hyperopic by observing the magnification of the patient's face through their glasses (myopic lenses minify).
- A careful history may reveal similar episodes of angle closure that resolved spontaneously.
- Miotics are ineffective in the setting of high IOP (due to iris sphincter ischemia) and potentially can worsen angle closure by causing anterior rotation of the lens–iris diaphragm.

GLAUCOMA, PRIMARY OPEN-ANGLE

Richard W. Allinson, MD

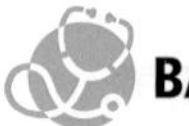

BASICS

DESCRIPTION

- Primary open-angle glaucoma (POAG) is an optic neuropathy resulting in visual field loss frequently associated with increased intraocular pressure (IOP).
- Normal IOP is 10–22 mm Hg. However, glaucomatous optic nerve damage also can occur with normal IOP and as a secondary manifestation of other disorders, such as corticosteroid-induced glaucoma.
- System(s) affected: Nervous
- Synonym(s): Chronic open-angle glaucoma

Pregnancy Considerations

Prostaglandins should be avoided during pregnancy in the treatment of POAG.

EPIDEMIOLOGY

Incidence

- Predominant age: Usually >40 years
- Increases with age
- Predominant gender: Male = Female

Prevalence

Prevalence of POAG in persons >40 years of age is ~1.8%.

Geriatric Considerations

Increasing prevalence with increasing age

RISK FACTORS

- Increased IOP
- Myopia
- Diabetes mellitus (DM)
- African American
- Elderly
- Hypothyroidism
- Positive family history
- Central corneal thickness <550 μm
- Larger vertical cup-to-disc ratio (C:D)
- Larger horizontal C:D
- Disc hemorrhage
- Prolonged use of topical, periocular, inhaled, or systemic corticosteroids

Genetics

A family history of glaucoma increases the risk for developing glaucoma.

GENERAL PREVENTION

Possible reduced risk of open-angle glaucoma with long-term use of oral statins

PATHOPHYSIOLOGY

- Abnormal aqueous outflow resulting in increased IOP
- Normally, aqueous is produced by the ciliary epithelium of the ciliary body and is secreted into the posterior chamber of the eye.
- Aqueous then flows through the pupil and enters the anterior chamber to be drained by the trabecular meshwork in the iridocorneal angle of the eye into the Schlemm canal and into the venous system of the episclera.
- 5–10% of the total aqueous outflow leaves via the uveoscleral pathway.

ETIOLOGY

- Impaired aqueous outflow through the trabecular meshwork
- Increased resistance within the aqueous drainage system

COMMONLY ASSOCIATED CONDITIONS

DM

DIAGNOSIS

HISTORY

Painless, slowly progressive visual loss; patients are generally unaware of the visual loss until late in the disease. Central visual acuity remains unaffected until late in the disease.

PHYSICAL EXAM

- Increased IOP
- C:D >0.5: Normal eyes show a characteristic configuration for disc rim thickness of inferior ≥ superior ≥ nasal ≥ temporal (ISNT rule).
- Earliest visual field defects are paracentral scotomas and peripheral nasal steps.

DIAGNOSTIC TESTS & INTERPRETATION

Imaging

Initial approach

- Optical coherence tomography can be useful in the detection of glaucoma by measuring the thickness of the retinal nerve fiber layer (RNFL).
- RNFL is thinner in patients with glaucoma.
- RNFL thickness is affected by age, ethnicity, axial length, and optic disc area. RNFL tends to be thinner with older age, Caucasians, greater axial length, and smaller optic disc area.
- Factors associated with variability in RNFL thickness measurements include signal-strength variability, low analysis confidence, and low RNFL thickness.

Diagnostic Procedures/Surgery

- Visual field testing: Perimetry
- Tonometry to measure IOP
- Ophthalmoscopy to assess optic nerve for glaucomatous damage

Pathological Findings

- Atrophy and cupping of optic nerve
- Loss of retinal ganglion cells and their axons produces defects in the retinal nerve fiber layer.

DIFFERENTIAL DIAGNOSIS

- Normal-tension glaucoma
- Optic nerve pits
- Anterior ischemic optic neuropathy
- Compressive lesions of the optic nerve or chiasm
- Posthemorrhagic (shock optic neuropathy)

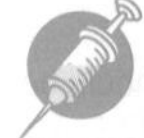

TREATMENT

MEDICATION

- >1 medication, with different mechanisms of action, may be needed.
- When ≥3 medications are required, compliance is difficult, and surgery may be needed. Ocular hypotensive agent categories:
  - β-adrenergic antagonists (nonselective and selective): Decrease aqueous formation: Timolol 0.5% 1 drop in affected eye q12h
  - Parasympathomimetics (miotic), including cholinergic (direct-acting) and anticholinesterase agents (indirect-acting parasympathomimetic): Increase aqueous outflow:
    - Pilocarpine 1–4% 1 drop in affected eye b.i.d.–q.i.d. (cholinergic)
    - Demecarium bromide 0.125% 1 drop in affected eye b.i.d. (anticholinesterase)
- Carbonic anhydrase inhibitors (oral, topical): Decrease aqueous formation:
  - Acetazolamide 250 mg PO q.i.d.
  - Dorzolamide 2% 1 drop t.i.d.
- Adrenergic agonists (nonselective and selective α_2-adrenergic agonists):
  - Epinephrine 0.5–2% 1 drop b.i.d. and dipivefrin 0.1% 1 drop b.i.d. (nonselective agents) increase aqueous outflow through the trabecular meshwork and increase uveoscleral outflow.
  - Brimonidine tartrate 0.1% 1 drop t.i.d. (α_2-adrenergic agonist) decreases aqueous formation and increases uveoscleral outflow.
- Prostaglandin analogues: Enhance uveoscleral outflow: Latanoprost 0.005% 1 drop at bedtime
- Hyperosmotic agents: Increase blood osmolality, drawing water from the vitreous cavity:
  - Mannitol 20% solution administered IV at 2 g/kg of body weight
  - Glycerin 50% solution administered orally; dosage is usually 4–7 oz
- Contraindications:
  - Nonselective β-adrenergic antagonists: Avoid in asthma, chronic obstructive pulmonary disease (COPD), second- and third-degree atrioventricular (A-V) block, and decompensated heart failure. Betaxolol is a selective β-adrenergic antagonist and is safer in pulmonary disease.
  - Parasympathomimetics (miotic): Indirect-acting parasympathomimetic agents increase risk of ocular and systemic side effects and are used rarely.
  - Carbonic anhydrase inhibitors:
    - Do not use with sulfa drug allergies.
    - Do not use with cirrhosis because of the risk of hepatic encephalopathy.
  - Adrenergic agonists: Caution recommended when using brimonidine and monoamine oxidase (MAO) inhibitor or tricyclic antidepressant (TCA) and in patients with vascular insufficiency. Brimonidine can cause excessive sleepiness and lethargy in children.
  - Prostaglandin analogues: Caution with uveitis and avoided during pregnancy
  - Hyperosmotic agents:
    - Glycerin can produce hyperglycemia or ketoacidosis in diabetic patients.
    - Can cause congestive heart failure
    - Do not use in patients with anuria.
- Precautions:
  - β-adrenergic antagonists: Caution with obstructive pulmonary disease, heart failure, and DM
  - Parasympathomimetics (miotic): Cause pupillary constriction and may cause decreased vision in patients with a cataract, and may cause an eye ache or myopia due to increased accommodation. All miotics break down the blood–aqueous barrier and may induce chronic iridocyclitis.

- Adrenergic agonists (e.g., brimonidine): Caution with vascular insufficiency
- Prostaglandin analogues may cause increased pigmentation of the iris and periorbital tissue (eyelid):
  - Increased pigmentation and growth of eyelashes
  - Should be used with caution in active intraocular inflammation (iritis/uveitis)
  - Caution is also advised in eyes with risk factors for herpes simplex, iritis, and cystoid macular edema.
  - Macular edema may be a complication associated with treatment.
- Hyperosmotic agents: Caution in diabetics; dehydrated patients; and those with cardiac, renal, and hepatic disease

- Significant possible interactions: β-adrenergic antagonists: Caution in patients taking calcium antagonists because of possible A-V conduction disturbances, left ventricular failure, or hypotension
- Parasympathomimetics (miotic): Indirect-acting parasympathomimetic agents, anticholinesterase eye drops, can reduce serum pseudocholinesterase levels. If succinylcholine is used for induction of general anesthesia, prolonged apnea may result.

ADDITIONAL TREATMENT

General Measures

- Early Manifest Glaucoma Trial:
  - Early treatment delays progression.
  - The magnitude of initial IOP reduction influences disease progression (1)[A].
- Ocular Hypertension Treatment Study:
  - Patients who only had increased IOP in the range of 24–32 mm Hg were treated with topical ocular hypotensive medication.
  - Treatment produced ~20% reduction in IOP.
  - At 5 years, treatment reduced the incidence of POAG by >50%: 9.5% in the observation group vs. 4.4% in the medication-treated group (2)[A].
- The Collaborative Normal-Tension Glaucoma Study Group:
  - Therapeutic intervention that resulted in a 30% decrease in IOP and helped to prevent progression of visual field loss (3)[A]
- The Advanced Glaucoma Intervention Study:
  - Eyes were randomized to laser trabeculoplasty or filtering surgery when medical therapy failed.
  - In follow-up, if the IOP was always <18 mm Hg, the visual fields tended to stabilize. When IOP was >17 mm Hg more than 1/2 of the time, patients tended to have worsening of their visual fields (4)[A].
  - Whites did better with trabeculectomy first, whereas African Americans did better with argon laser trabeculoplasty as the initial procedure.
- Collaborative Initial Glaucoma Treatment Study:
  - Both initial medical and surgical treatment achieved significant IOP reduction, and both had little visual field loss over time (5)[A].

SURGERY/OTHER PROCEDURES

- Argon laser trabeculoplasty (ALT):
  - Applied to 780° of the trabecular meshwork
  - Improves aqueous outflow
  - The Glaucoma Laser Trial Research Group showed in newly diagnosed, previously untreated patients with POAG that ALT was as effective as topical glaucoma medication within the first 2 years of follow-up.
  - Usually reserved for patients needing better IOP control while taking topical glaucoma drops
- Trabeculectomy (glaucoma filtering surgery):
  - Usually reserved for patients needing better IOP control after maximal medical therapy and who may have previously undergone an ALT
  - Mitomycin C can be applied at the time of surgery to increase the chances of a surgical success.
  - Subconjunctival bevacizumab may be a beneficial adjunctive therapy for reducing late surgical failure after trabeculectomy.
- Shunt (tube) surgery:
  - For example, Molteno and Ahmed devices
  - Generally reserved for difficult glaucoma cases in which conventional filtering surgery has failed or is likely to fail
- Tube Versus Trabeculectomy (TVT) Study:
  - After 3 years of follow-up, both procedures were associated with similar IOP reduction and the number of glaucoma medications needed (6)[A].
- Ciliary body ablation: Indicated to lower IOP in patients with poor visual potential or those who are poor candidates for filtering or shunt procedures
- Canaloplasty can control IOP in patients with POAG. Canaloplasty involves the placement of a microcatheter circumferentially through Schlemm canal, viscodilation of the canal, and placement of a nylon tensioning suture (7)[C].

ONGOING CARE

FOLLOW-UP RECOMMENDATIONS

Patient Monitoring

- Monitor vision and IOP every 3–6 months.
- Visual field testing every 6–18 months
- Optic nerve evaluation every 3–18 months depending on POAG control
- A worsening of the mean deviation by 2 dB on the Humphrey field analyzer and confirmed by a single test after 6 months had a 72% probability of progression.
- The IOP response to ocular hypotensive agents tends to be reduced in persons with thicker corneas.

PATIENT EDUCATION

POAG is a silent robber of vision, and patients may not appreciate the significance of their disease until much of their visual field is lost.

PROGNOSIS

- With standard glaucoma therapy, the rate of visual field loss in POAG is slow.
- Patients still may lose vision and develop blindness, even when treated appropriately.
- The rate of legal blindness from POAG over a follow-up of 22 years is 19%.
- The rate of progression of visual field loss increases with older age (8)[B].

COMPLICATIONS

Blindness

REFERENCES

1. Heijl A, Leske MC, Bengtsson B, et al. Reduction of intraocular pressure and glaucoma progression: Results from the Early Manifest Glaucoma Trial. *Arch Ophthalmol*. 2002;120:1268–79.
2. Kass MA, Heuer DK, Higginbotham EJ, et al. The Ocular Hypertension Treatment Study: A randomized trial determines that topical ocular hypotensive medication delays or prevents the onset of primary open-angle glaucoma. *Arch Ophthalmol*. 2002;120:701–13; discussion 829–30.
3. Comparison of glaucomatous progression between untreated patients with normal-tension glaucoma and patients with therapeutically reduced intraocular pressures. Collaborative Normal-Tension Glaucoma Study Group. *Am J Ophthalmol*. 1998;126:487–97.
4. The Advanced Glaucoma Intervention Study (AGIS): 7. The relationship between control of intraocular pressure and visual field deterioration.The AGIS Investigators. *Am J Ophthalmol*. 2000;130: 429–40.
5. Lichter PR, et al. CIGTS Study Group. Interim clinical outcomes in the Collaborative Initial Glaucoma Treatment Study comparing initial treatment randomized to medications or surgery. *Ophthalmol*. 2001;108:1943–53.
6. Gedde SJ, Schiffman JC, et al. Three-year follow-up of the tube versus trabeculectomy Study. *Am J Ophthalmol*. 2009;148:670–84.
7. Lewis RA, von Wolff K, et al. Canaloplasty: Three-year results of circumferential viscodilation and tensioning of Schlemm canal using a microcatheter to treat open-angle glaucoma. *J Cataract Refract Surg*. 2011;37:682–690.
8. Chauhan BC, Mikelberg FS, et al. Canadian glaucoma study: 3. Impact of risk factos and intraocular pressure reduction on the rates of visual field change. *Arch Ophthalmol*. 2010;128:1249–55.

ADDITIONAL READING

Lin HC, Kang JH, et al. Hypothyroidism and the risk of developing open-angle glaucoma: A five-year population-based follow-up study. *Ophthalmology*. 2010;117:1960–6.

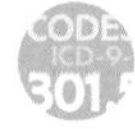

CODES

ICD9

365.11 Primary open angle glaucoma

CLINICAL PEARLS

- Topical or systemic steroids can cause the IOP to increase.
- Pain is not a frequent symptom of POAG.
- Painless, slowly progressive visual loss; patients generally are unaware of the visual loss until late in the disease. Central visual acuity remains unaffected until late in the disease.
- Patients still may lose vision and develop blindness, even when treated appropriately.

G

GLOMERULONEPHRITIS, ACUTE

Carla M. Nester, MD

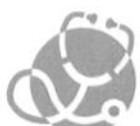

BASICS

DESCRIPTION

- Acute glomerulonephritis (GN) is an inflammatory process involving the glomerulus of the kidney, resulting in a clinical syndrome consisting of hematuria, proteinuria, hypertension, and renal insufficiency.
- Acute GN may be one of many primary diseases, or it may present as part of a systemic disease:
  - Postinfectious GN
  - IgA nephropathy–Henoch Schönlein purpura
  - Antiglomerular basement membrane disease (anti-GBM disease)
  - Antineutrophil cytoplasmic antibody (ANCA)-associated GN
  - Membranoproliferative GN (MPGN)
  - Lupus nephritis
  - Cryoglobulin-associated GN
- Clinical severity ranges from asymptomatic microscopic or gross hematuria to a rapid loss of kidney function (rapidly progressive GN: RPGN).

ALERT

Urgent investigation and treatment are required to avoid irreversible loss of kidney function.

EPIDEMIOLOGY

- Postinfectious GN:
  - Most commonly follows group A beta-hemolytic *Streptococcus* infection, but can occur as a result of other infections
  - Onset occurs 1–3 weeks after an infectious process (throat or skin).
  - Accounts for 80% of acute GN in children
- IgA nephropathy:
  - Most common form of primary acute GN
  - Occurs mainly in the second and third decades
  - Male:Female: 3:1
  - Incidence differs geographically: Asia > US
- Anti-GBM disease:
  - Also known as Goodpasture disease
  - A noted cause of the pulmonary–renal syndrome
  - Occurs most commonly in the second or third decade
  - Male:Female: 6:1
- ANCA-associated GN:
  - Uncommon: Often has a relapsing and remitting course
  - 3 disease presentations:
    - Wegener granulomatosis
    - Churg-Strauss disease
    - Microscopic polyangiitis
  - Older patients are more commonly affected, though this GN can affect any age group.
- MPGN:
  - May be primary or secondary
  - May present in the setting of a systemic viral or rheumatic illness
- Lupus nephritis:
  - 30–70% of systemic lupus patients will have renal involvement.
- Cryoglobulin-associated vasculitis:
  - 80% of cases are associated with hepatitis C infection.

RISK FACTORS

- Epidemics of nephritogenic strains of streptococci are triggers for postinfectious GN.
- Hepatic cirrhosis and celiac disease place patients at risk for IgA nephropathy.
- Anti-GBM disease has been associated with influenza A infection and inhaled hydrocarbon solvent exposure.
- ANCA-associated GN is increased in settings where there is increased silica exposure (i.e., earthquakes and farming).
- Infection with hepatitis B and/or C are known to be associated with MPGN.
- Infection with hepatitis C is a risk factor for developing cryoglobulinemic GN.
- Mutations in alternate complement pathway genes are associated with MPGN.

Genetics

Genetic factors are likely to play a role in susceptibility to many of the acute GNs, though these have not been sufficiently defined to be useful clinically.

GENERAL PREVENTION

Early detection is paramount.

ETIOLOGY

- In general, an immunologic mechanism triggers inflammation and proliferation of glomerular tissue.
- Postinfectious GN:
  - Host immune reaction to nephritogenic strains of streptococci are triggers.
- IgA nephropathy:
  - Relates to an abnormal glycosylation of IgA
- Anti-GBM disease:
  - Caused by autoantibodies that target type IV collagen of basement membranes
- ANCA-associated GN:
  - Autoantibodies against neutrophil granules are involved in the pathogenesis.
- MPGN:
  - An immune or genetic etiology is presumed, which triggers renal deposits and inflammation.
- Lupus nephritis:
  - An immune complex-mediated glomerular disease
- Cryoglobulin-associated GN:
  - An immune etiology is presumed, but not clearly defined.

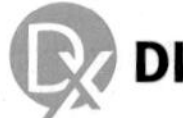

DIAGNOSIS

HISTORY

- Patients may complain of cola- or tea-colored urine and decreased urine volume.
- Edema occurs in many patients, typically face and lower extremities.
- Shortness of breath may occur with significant fluid overload.
- Generalized malaise
- Patients may also present with complaints more specific to the associated disease:
  - Joint pain or rash in lupus nephritis
  - Hemoptysis in anti-GBM disease
  - Sinusitis and pulmonary infiltrates in ANCA-associated GN
  - Abdominal or joint pain and purpura in IgA-Henoch Schönlein purpura
  - Purpura and skin vasculitis in cryoglobulinemia-associated GN

PHYSICAL EXAM

- A complete physical exam may discover clues to systemic disease as a potential cause.
- Sinus disease: ANCA-associated GN
- Pharyngitis or impetigo: Postinfectious GN
- Pulmonary abnormality: Anti-GBM disease or lupus nephritis
- Hepatomegaly or liver tenderness could point to cryoglobulinemia-associated GN or IgA nephropathy.
- Purpura may point to ANCA-associated GN or Henoch Schönlein purpura GN.

DIAGNOSTIC TESTS & INTERPRETATION

Lab

- Urinalysis with examination of sediment:
  - Dysmorphic RBCs or RBC casts on urine microscopy indicate glomerular hematuria and suggest the diagnosis of an acute GN.
- Electrolytes, BUN, creatinine, CBC
- Antistreptolysin O titer
- Streptozyme
- Complement levels (C3 and C4):
  - C3 complement levels are abnormal in postinfectious GN; C3 and C4 are abnormal in lupus nephritis and MPGN; C4 can be low in cryoglobulinemia.
- Proteinuria:
  - 24-hour collection or random urine protein/creatinine ratio
- Antinuclear antibody to rule out lupus nephritis
- ANCA antibody screen:
  - MPO and PR3 antibodies
- Anti-GBM antibody
- Hepatitis B antigen
- Hepatitis C antibody

Imaging
A chest x-ray may be useful to define the significance of hemoptysis or a suspected infiltrate on exam.

Pathological Findings
Renal biopsy:

- If clinical picture is consistent with postinfectious GN in a child, a biopsy may not be needed.
- If there is clinical suspicion for other causes of acute GN, renal biopsy should be done.
- Light microscopy:
  - Diffuse hypercellularity suggests a proliferative disease such as IgA nephropathy, lupus nephritis, or postinfectious GN.
- Immunofluorescence:
  - IgA staining is pathognomonic for IgA nephropathy, with the absence of staining suggesting ANCA-associated GN.
- Electron microscopy:
  - The location of immunoglobulin deposits is useful in pointing to a particular diagnosis.

DIFFERENTIAL DIAGNOSIS
- The differential for hematuria (without clear indication that it is from a glomerular origin) should include trauma, prostate diseases, urologic cancer, or renal stone disease.
- If the urine blood is felt to be of glomerular origin, the differential should include each of the glomerular diseases that can present as an acute GN.

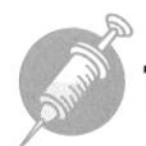

TREATMENT

Supportive in postinfectious

MEDICATION
First Line
- Hypertension:
  - Diuretics are useful, given that salt retention and edema are often present.
  - Calcium channel blockers
  - Avoid ACE inhibitors if significant renal dysfunction is present.
- Peripheral edema:
  - Loop diuretics are often required due to the degree of edema.
- Pulmonary edema:
  - Oxygen and diuretic
- Hyperkalemia:
  - Sodium polystyrene sulfonate (Kayexalate) resin: 15 g PO every day to q.i.d.
- Acidosis: Sodium bicarbonate 1–2 mEq/kg per dose (1–2 mmol/kg per dose) IV or PO

Second Line
- Each of the glomerular diseases often requires a specific treatment plan based on renal biopsy results; therefore, a nephrologist is often guiding care at this point.
- Pulse methylprednisolone has been reported to be useful in rapidly progressive forms of GN (1,2)[A].
- Crescents noted on renal biopsy are treated with the alkylating agent known as cyclophosphamide (1,2)[A].
- ANCA-associated renal disease, anti-GBM disease, and proliferative forms of lupus are treated with steroids, plus either cyclophosphamide or mycophenolate (1,2,3,4,5)[A].
- Plasmapheresis has been shown to be effective in cases of pulmonary hemorrhage and in some patients who present in renal failure (2)[A].
- Dialysis may be needed for uremia, hyperkalemia refractory to medical management, intractable acidosis, and diuretic-resistant pulmonary edema.

ADDITIONAL TREATMENT
Issues for Referral
Consultation with a nephrologist is often required in order to assist with renal biopsy to confirm diagnosis and to assist with management.

IN-PATIENT CONSIDERATIONS
Admission Criteria
Consider admission for patients with no urine output, significant hypertension, and suspicion of pulmonary hemorrhage or fluid overload that is compromising heart or respiratory function.

Discharge Criteria
Hemodynamically stable patients without complications may be managed as outpatients.

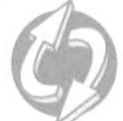

ONGOING CARE

FOLLOW-UP RECOMMENDATIONS
Patient Monitoring
Depends on type of GN:

- Regular BP checks and urinalysis to detect recurrence; assessment of renal function to detect acute or follow chronic renal disease as a result of the primary event; and regular clinical assessment to detect suspicious symptoms that may herald a recurrence (i.e., rash, joint complaint, hemoptysis)
- Periodic reassessment of serology tests to detect asymptomatic individuals

DIET
- No-added-salt diet and fluid restriction until edema and hypertension clear
- Avoid high-potassium foods if significant renal dysfunction is present.

PATIENT EDUCATION
- National Kidney Foundation, 30 E. 33rd Street, Suite 1100, New York, NY 10016; (212) 889-2210
- Web site: http://vsearch.nlm.nih.gov/vivisimo/cgi-bin/query-meta?v%3Aproject=medlineplus&query=glomerulonephritis&x=48&y=10 — then search under the individual disease

PROGNOSIS
- In general, the prognosis depends on the cause of the GN.
- The GN may be self-limited (i.e., postinfectious GN) or part of a chronic disease that makes the possibility of recurrence of acute disease likely with the potential for progressive loss of renal function over time.

COMPLICATIONS
- Hypertensive retinopathy and encephalopathy
- Rapidly progressive GN
- Microscopic hematuria may persist for years.
- Chronic kidney disease
- Nephrotic syndrome (~10%)

REFERENCES

1. Flanc RS, Roberts MA, Strippoli GF, et al. Treatment for lupus nephritis. *Cochrane Database Syst Rev.* 2004;CD002922.
2. Walters G, Willis NS, Craig JC. Interventions for renal vasculitis in adults. *Cochrane Database Syst Rev.* 2008;CD003232.
3. Hu W, Liu C, Xie H, et al. Mycophenolate mofetil versus cyclophosphamide for inducing remission of ANCA vasculitis with moderate renal involvement. *Nephrol Dial Transplant.* 2008;23(4):1307–12.
4. Walsh M, James M, Jayne D, et al. Mycophenolate mofetil for induction therapy of lupus nephritis: A systematic review and meta-analysis. *Clin J Am Soc Nephrol.* 2007;2(5):968–75.
5. Isenberg D, Appel GB, Contreras G, et al. Influence of race/ethnicity on response to lupus nephritis treatment: The ALMS study. *Rheumatology (Oxford).* 2010;49:128–40.

ADDITIONAL READING

Kaplan AA. The use of apheresis in immune renal disorders. *Ther Apher Dial.* 2003;7:165–72.

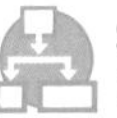

See Also (Topic, Algorithm, Electronic Media Element)

- Hyperkalemia; Hypertensive Emergencies; Renal Failure, Acute
- Algorithm: Hematuria

CODES

ICD9
580.9 Acute glomerulonephritis with unspecified pathological lesion in kidney

CLINICAL PEARLS

- Dysmorphic RBCs and RBC casts are a key component of the urinalysis in GN.
- Postinfectious GN in children is typically a self-limited disease.
- Searching for other organ involvement is useful in establishing a definitive diagnosis.
- With discovery of a GN, monitor the initial renal function labs frequently to identify a rapidly progressive GN.

GLOMERULONEPHRITIS, POSTSTREPTOCOCCAL

Alphonsus W. Kung, MD
Howard Alfred, MD

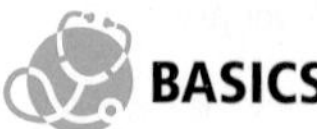

BASICS

DESCRIPTION

Poststreptococcal glomerulonephritis (PSGN) is caused by prior infection with certain strains of streptococcus, most commonly group A beta-hemolytic streptococcus (GAS). The clinical presentation varies from asymptomatic to the acute nephritic syndrome, characterized by gross hematuria, proteinuria, edema, hypertension, and acute kidney injury.

EPIDEMIOLOGY

97% in less developed countries with ~5,000 cases (1%) resulting in death

Incidence

- 9.5 to 28.5 per 100,000 individuals
- 470,000 cases per year worldwide

Prevalence

Unknown

RISK FACTORS

- Older patients (>60 years of age)
- Children 5–12 years of age (1)

GENERAL PREVENTION

- Early antibiotic treatment for streptococcal infections when indicated
- Prophylactic penicillin treatment to be used in closed communities and household contacts of index cases in areas where PSGN is prevalent

PATHOPHYSIOLOGY

- Glomerular immune complex disease induced by specific nephritogenic strains of streptococcus
- Proposed mechanisms for the glomerular injury (2):
  - Deposition of circulating immune complexes with streptococcal antigens (3)
  - In situ immune complex formation from deposition of streptococcal antigens within the glomerular basement membrane (GBM) and subsequent antibody binding
  - In situ glomerular immune complex formation promoted by antibodies to streptococcal antigens
  - Alteration of normal renal antigen that elicits autoimmune response

ETIOLOGY

- Glomerular immune complex causing complement activation and inflammation:
  - Nephritis-associated plasmin receptor (NAPlr)
  - Streptococcal pyrogenic exotoxin B (SPE B)
- Both activate the alternate complement pathway and enhance the expression of adhesion molecules. SPE B may also stimulate the production of chemotactic cytokines.

COMMONLY ASSOCIATED CONDITIONS

Streptococcal infection

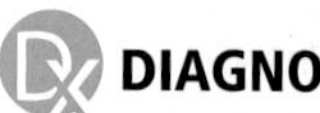

DIAGNOSIS

HISTORY

- Group A beta-hemolytic streptococcal (GAS) skin or throat infection
- The latent period between GAS infection and PSGN is dependent on the site of infection: 1–3 weeks following GAS pharyngitis and 3–6 weeks following GAS skin infection

PHYSICAL EXAM

- Edema: Present in about 2/3 of patients due to sodium and water retention
- Respiratory distress: Due to pulmonary edema
- Gross hematuria: Present in ~30–50% of patients
- Hypertension: Present in 50–90% of patients and varies from mild to severe secondary to fluid retention. Hypertensive encephalopathy is an uncommon but serious complication.
- Microscopic hematuria: Subclinical cases of PSGN

DIAGNOSTIC TESTS & INTERPRETATION

Lab

Initial lab tests

Urinalysis with hematuria. Can be with or without RBC casts and pyuria. Proteinuria present, but nephrotic range proteinuria is uncommon.

Follow-Up & Special Considerations

- Culture: PSGN usually presents weeks after a GAS infection, only ~25% of patients will have either a positive throat or skin culture.
- Complement: 90% of patients will have depressed C3 and CH50 levels in the first 2 weeks of the disease while C2 and C4 levels remain normal. C3 and CH50 levels return to normal within 4–8 weeks after presentation.
- Serology: Elevated titers of antibodies supports evidence of a recent GAS infection. Streptozyme test measuring antistreptolysin (ASO), antihyaluronidase (AHase), antistreptokinase (ASKase), anti–nicotinamide-adenine dinucleotidase (anti-NAD), and anti-DNAse B antibodies:
  - Positive in >95% of patients with PSGN due to pharyngitis and 80% with skin infections. In pharyngeal infection, ASO, anti-DNAse B, anti-NAD, and AHase titers elevated. In skin infection, only the anti-DNAse and AHase titers are typically elevated.

Diagnostic Procedures/Surgery

Renal biopsy only when diagnosis unsure

Pathological Findings

- Light microscopy: Diffuse proliferative glomerulonephritis with prominent endocapillary proliferation and numerous neutrophils with severity of involvement varies and correlates with the clinical findings. Crescent formation is uncommon and is associated with a poor prognosis.
- Immunofluorescence microscopy: Deposits of IgG and C3 distributed in a diffuse granular pattern
- Electron microscopy: Dome-shaped subepithelial electron-dense deposits that are referred to as humps. These deposits along with subendothelial deposits are immune complexes and correspond to the deposits of IgG and C3 found on immunofluorescence. Rate of clearance of these deposits affects recovery time.

- Renal biopsy: Usually not performed in most patients to confirm the diagnosis of PSGN as clinical history is highly suggestive and resolution of PSGN typically begins within 1 week of presentation. A biopsy is done when other glomerular disorders are being considered such as persistently low C3 levels beyond 6 weeks with possible diagnosis of membranoproliferative glomerulonephritis, recurrent episodes of hematuria suggestive of IgA nephropathy, or a progressive increase in serum creatinine not characteristic of PSGN.

DIFFERENTIAL DIAGNOSIS

The diagnosis of PSGN is generally by history once the diagnosis of acute nephritis is made, with documentation of a recent GAS infection, with nephritis beginning to resolve 1–2 weeks after presentation. However, if there is progressive disease beyond 2 weeks, persistent hematuria or hypertension beyond 4–6 weeks, or without adequate documentation of a GAS infection, the differential diagnosis of GN needs to be considered with renal biopsy in order:

- Membranoproliferative glomerulonephritis (MPGN): The presentation of MPGN may be indistinguishable initially with hematuria, hypertension, proteinuria, and hypocomplementemia after an upper respiratory infection. However, continues to have persistent nephritis and hypocomplementemia beyond 4–6 weeks and possibly a further elevation in serum creatinine. Patients with PSGN tend to have resolution of their disease and a return of normal C3 and CH50 levels within 2–4 weeks.
- Secondary causes of glomerulonephritis: Lupus nephritis and Henoch-Schönlein purpura nephritis have similar features to PSGN. Extrarenal manifestations and laboratory test of these underlying systemic diseases help differentiate them from PSGN. Hypocomplementemia is not characteristic of Henoch-Schönlein purpura and the hypocomplementemia that occurs in lupus nephritis is with reductions in both C3 and C4, while C4 levels are normal in PSGN. IgA nephropathy often presents after an upper respiratory infection. Distinguishing features from PSGN include a shorter time between the upper respiratory illness and hematuria as well as history of gross hematuria as PSGN recurrence is rare. IgA nephropathy is a chronic illness compared to PSGN with normal C3/C4.
- Both hepatitis B and endocarditis: Associated GN share common features with PSGN and also will present with reductions in C3 and C4.
- Postinfectious GN due to other microbial agents: Acute nephritis due to virus. Their clinical presentation is similar to PSGN except that there is no documentation of a GAS infection.

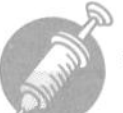

TREATMENT

MEDICATION

- There is no specific therapy for PSGN with no evidence that aggressive immunosuppressive therapy has a beneficial effect in patients with rapidly progressive crescentic disease. However, patients with more than 30% crescents on renal biopsy are often treated with steroids (4).
- Management is supportive with focus on treating the clinical manifestations of PSGN. These include hypertension and pulmonary edema:
  - General measures include sodium and water restriction and loop diuretics.
  - Infrequently, patients have hypertensive encephalopathy due to severe hypertension with use of calcium channel blocker to control hypertension and reverse the encephalopathy.
- Patients with evidence of persistent group A streptococcal infection should be given a course of antibiotic therapy.

SURGERY/OTHER PROCEDURES

In patients with severe acute renal failure, dialysis may be required.

ONGOING CARE

FOLLOW-UP RECOMMENDATIONS

Patient Monitoring

- Repeat urinalysis to check for clearance of hematuria and/or proteinuria.
- Consider other diagnosis if no improvement within 2 weeks.

DIET

Renal diet if requiring instances of dialysis

PROGNOSIS

- Most patients have an excellent outcome, even with renal failure and crescents on biopsy, with more than 90% of cases with recovery of renal function.
- Some patients, especially adults, develop hypertension, recurrent proteinuria, and renal insufficiency long after the initial illness.
- Hypertension is quite common in post-PSGN patients at 14%.
- Late renal complications associated with glomerulosclerosis on biopsy with possible irreversibly damaged glomeruli during acute episode followed by chronic compensatory hyperfiltration, leading to nonimmunologic glomerular injury with progressive renal dysfunction.

REFERENCES

1. Singh GR. Glomerulonephritis and managing the risks of chronic renal disease. *Pediatr Clin North Am*. 2009;56(6):1363–82.
2. Nadasdy T, Hebert LA. Infection-related glomerulonephritis: Understanding mechanisms. *Semin Nephrol*. 2011;31(4):369–75.
3. Uchida T, Oda T, Watanabe A, et al. Clinical and histologic resolution of poststreptococcal glomerulonephritis with large subendothelial deposits and kidney failure. *Am J Kidney Dis*. 2011;58(1):113–7.
4. Rodriguez-Iturbe B, Musser JM. The current state of poststreptococcal glomerulonephritis. *J Am Soc Nephrol*. 2008;19(10):1855–64.

ADDITIONAL READING

Ahn SY, Ingulli E. Acute poststreptococcal glomerulonephritis: An update. *Curr Opin Pediatr*. 2008;20(2):157–62.

CODES

ICD9

580.0 Acute glomerulonephritis with lesion of proliferative glomerulonephritis

CLINICAL PEARLS

- PSGN is caused by prior infection with certain strains of streptococcus, most commonly GAS.
- The clinical presentation varies from asymptomatic to the acute nephritic syndrome, characterized by gross hematuria, proteinuria, edema, hypertension, and acute kidney injury.
- Persistent nephritis and low C3 levels for more than 2 weeks should prompt evaluation for other causes of GN such as membranoproliferative glomerulonephritis or systemic lupus erythematosus nephritis.
- Management is supportive with focus on treating the clinical manifestations of PSGN, including hypertension and pulmonary edema.
- Proteinuria is associated with poor renal outcome.

GLOSSITIS

Karyn M. Sullivan, PharmD, MPH, RPh
George M. Abraham, MD, MPH

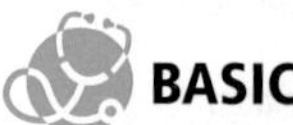

BASICS

DESCRIPTION

- An acute or chronic inflammation of the tongue, either as primary disease or a symptom of systemic disease
- Common forms:
  - Atrophic glossitis (AG) or smooth tongue
  - Benign migratory glossitis (BMG) or geographic tongue or erythema migrans
  - Median rhomboid glossitis (MRG)
  - Herpetic geometric glossitis (HGG)
- System(s) affected: Gastrointestinal

EPIDEMIOLOGY

- Predominant age: All ages; BMG more frequent in children
- Predominant gender:
  - Male > Female (3:1, MRG)
  - Female > Male (BMG)

Geriatric Considerations

Many patients with glossitis due to nutrition deficiencies are postmenopausal or elderly.

Prevalence

Varies; usual reported range: 1–14%

RISK FACTORS

- Poor nutrition
- Dentures
- Piercings
- Allergic background (e.g., asthma, eczema, hay fever)
- Smoking, smokeless tobacco
- Alcoholism
- Anxiety, stress
- Depression
- Hormonal disturbances
- Oral contraceptives
- Advancing age
- Immunocompromised state

Genetics

Familial history may be present with BMG.

GENERAL PREVENTION

- Evaluation of nutritional status, including B-vitamin deficiencies, anemias
- Cessation of tobacco use (including smokeless)
- Assess for irritation from teeth, dentures, or piercings.

PATHOPHYSIOLOGY

Tongue:

- AG: Atrophy of filiform papillae
- BMG: Erythematous, yellow-white lesions (dorsum)
- MRG: Atrophic filiform, plaquelike lesions (midline)
- HGG: Linear fissures (dorsum)

ETIOLOGY

- Systemic:
  - Nutritional deficiencies (e.g., B_{12}, folic acid)
  - Anemia (pernicious, iron deficiency)
  - HIV (opportunistic infections such as candidiasis, herpes simplex virus [HSV]; or HIV-associated changes such as loss of papillae)
  - Broad-spectrum antibiotics
  - Topical or inhaled corticosteroids
  - Various other medications (e.g., captopril, clarithromycin, enalapril, lansoprazole, lithium, metronidazole, NSAIDs)
- Local:
  - Infections (e.g., HSV, Epstein-Barr virus, candidiasis)
  - Trauma (ill-fitting dentures, piercings, burns, convulsive seizures)
  - Primary irritants (alcohol, tobacco, hot foods, spices, excessive peppermint, citrus)
  - Sensitization with chemical irritants (e.g., dyes, mouthwash, toothpaste, systemic drugs)
  - Malignancy (95% are squamous cell)

COMMONLY ASSOCIATED CONDITIONS

- Fissured tongue (BMG)
- HIV infection (rare)
- Reiter syndrome (rare)
- Down syndrome (rare)
- Crohn disease (rare)
- Celiac disease (possible correlation)

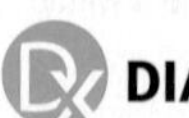

DIAGNOSIS

Some symptoms of glossitis have no organic cause. Treat symptoms and re-evaluate if no improvement.

HISTORY

- Many cases are asymptomatic.
- Oral discomfort
- Burning sensation on tongue (often associated with nutritional deficiency)
- Sensitivity to hot or spicy foods
- Sensation of foreign body in the mouth
- Paroxysmal ear pain
- Swollen or painful submandibular lymph nodes
- Symptoms tend to wax and wane (BMG).

PHYSICAL EXAM

- AG: Smooth, glossy, red or pink tongue (1,2)[B]
- BMG: Erythematous and white patches on the dorsum of tongue; lesions may lack papillae; irregular (maplike) and migratory lesions (3)[B]
- MRG: Erythematous, shiny, rhomboid-shaped plaque in middle of tongue; hypertrophic or atrophic surface changes (2,3)[B]
- HGG: Linear fissures on dorsal tongue; geometric pattern is common; herpetic lesions usually are absent on other mucosal surfaces (3)[B].

DIAGNOSTIC TESTS & INTERPRETATION

Lab

Serum B_{12}, folic acid, CBC with differential, ferritin, RPR, TSH

Initial lab tests

- AG: Test for B_{12}, folic acid, iron deficiency (1)[B]
- BMG: None (3,4)[B]
- MRG: Viral culture, fungal smear (3)[B]
- HGG: Viral culture, Tzanck smear (3)[B]

Diagnostic Procedures/Surgery

- Biopsy solitary lesions that do not respond to treatment (3,4)[B].
- Examine scrapings with 10% potassium hydroxide for suspected candidiasis (1).

Pathological Findings

Vary according to underlying causes

DIFFERENTIAL DIAGNOSIS

- Irritation fibroma
- Mucocele
- Granular cell tumor
- Tertiary syphilis
- Drug reaction
- Lichen planus
- Squamous cell carcinoma (rarely) (5)

Pediatric Considerations

Differential diagnosis includes local trauma and severe neutropenia (4).

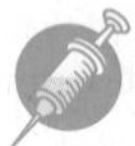

TREATMENT

MEDICATION

- AG:
  - Vitamin B_{12}, folic acid, iron (if deficient)
  - For candidiasis: Nystatin oral suspension 100,000 units/mL swish and spit 5 mL q.i.d. *OR* clotrimazole 1–2 troches 4–5 times a day (3)[B]
- BMG:
  - Usually no treatment
  - The following agents may be used to reduce tongue sensitivity or if lesions recur: Antihistamines, such as diphenhydramine liquid: Rinse with 5–10 mL, holding it over the tongue for a few minutes and then swallowing, 3–4 times a day (may also dilute in a 1:4 ratio with water) (2,6)[B] *or* Miracle Mouthwash: Swish and spit 5 mL, 3–4 times a day *OR* topical steroid gels, such as 0.1% triamcinolone oral dental paste (Oralone) (2)[B].

- MRG:
  - Usually no treatment
  - Topical antifungals (nystatin oral suspension or clotrimazole troches) may provide temporary improvement (3)[B].
- HGG:
  - Oral antivirals such as acyclovir 200 mg 5 times daily (3)[B],(7)[C]
- Contraindications:
  - Nystatin oral suspension: Hypersensitivity to nystatin products
  - Clotrimazole troche: Hypersensitivity to clotrimazole
  - Diphenhydramine:
    - Hypersensitivity to diphenhydramine
    - Newborns or premature infants
    - Nursing mothers
  - Acyclovir (oral): Hypersensitivity to acyclovir or valacyclovir
  - Triamcinolone (oral paste): Corticosteroid hypersensitivity
  - Precautions:
    - Clotrimazole troche: Hepatic impairment
    - Diphenhydramine:
      - May cause excitation in young children
      - Concurrent monoamine oxidase inhibitor (MAOI) therapy
      - Concurrent use of CNS depressants
      - Decreases mental alertness and psychomotor performance
      - Older adults are more susceptible to side effects.
      - Bladder neck obstruction
      - Symptomatic prostatic hypertrophy
      - Narrow-angle glaucoma
      - History of bronchial asthma, increased intraocular pressure, hyperthyroidism, cardiovascular disease, or hypertension
    - Acyclovir (oral):
      - Maintain adequate hydration
      - Geriatric patients (due to age-related decline in renal function)
      - Renal impairment
    - Triamcinolone (oral paste): Infections or sores in the mouth
  - Significant possible interactions:
    - Diphenhydramine: Alcohol (increased sedation)
    - Acyclovir (oral): Meperidine (increased risk of CNS stimulation and seizures)
  - Adverse effects:
    - Clotrimazole troche:
      - Nausea, vomiting, or diarrhea
      - Mild elevations in serum glutamic-oxaloacetic transaminase (SGOT) levels
    - Diphenhydramine:
      - Sedation
      - Dizziness
      - Urinary retention
    - Acyclovir (oral):
      - Nausea, vomiting, and diarrhea
      - Myalgia
      - Transient renal impairment
    - Triamcinolone (oral paste):
      - Burning
      - Itching
      - Irritation

Pediatric Considerations

- Diphenhydramine liquid: Rinse with 5–10 mL (depending on age and weight), holding it over the tongue for a few minutes and then swallowing, 3–4 times a day (6)[B].
- Topical antifungal/steroid agent: Triamcinolone acetonide 0.1% in nystatin suspension (8)[B]
- Alkaline saline mouth rinse (8)[B]
- Topical anesthetics/coating agents: 1:1 mixture of diphenhydramine liquid and Maalox (8)[B]

ADDITIONAL TREATMENT

General Measures

- Usually outpatient
- Avoid any possible sensitizing irritants or agents (such as acidic or spicy foods and drinks).
- Analgesics when needed
- Request dental evaluation.
- Scrupulous oral hygiene

IN-PATIENT CONSIDERATIONS

Initial Stabilization

If glossitis is secondary to a severe primary condition, attend to any acute needs of the primary problem.

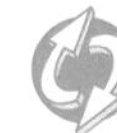

ONGOING CARE

FOLLOW-UP RECOMMENDATIONS

If lesions do not heal, biopsy is indicated.

Patient Monitoring

Revisit periodically when needed until healing occurs.

DIET

Bland or liquid diet

PATIENT EDUCATION

- Proper diet and nutrition
- Avoid irritants such as cigarette smoking and acidic or spicy foods.
- Maintain good oral hygiene.

PROGNOSIS

Prompt improvement when cause can be identified and treated

COMPLICATIONS

- Recurrence: Evaluate for systemic etiology.
- Chronicity: If not healing, biopsy is indicated.

REFERENCES

1. Terai H, Shimahara M. Atrophic tongue associated with *Candida*. *J Oral Pathol Med*. 2005;34:397–400.
2. Reamy BV, Derby R, Bunt CW. Common tongue conditions in primary care. *Am Fam Physician*. 2010;81:627–34.
3. Byrd JA, Bruce AJ, Rogers RS. Glossitis and other tongue disorders. *Dermatol Clin*. 2003;21:123–34.
4. Assimakopoulos D, Patrikakos G, Fotika C, et al. Benign migratory glossitis or geographic tongue: An enigmatic oral lesion. *Am J Med*. 2002;113:751–5.
5. Nelson BL, Thompson L. Median rhomboid glossitis. *Ear Nose Throat J*. 2007;86:600–1.
6. Sigal MJ, Mock D. Symptomatic benign migratory glossitis: Report of two cases and literature review. *Pediatr Dent*. 1992;14:392–6.
7. Grossman ME, Stevens AW, Cohen PR. Brief report: Herpetic geometric glossitis. *N Engl J Med*. 1993;329:1859–60.
8. Oh TJ, Eber R, Wang HL. Periodontal diseases in the child and adolescent. *J Clin Periodontol*. 2002;29:400–10.

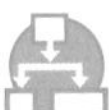

See Also (Topic, Algorithm, Electronic Media Element)

Candidiasis; HIV Infection and AIDS; Vitamin Deficiency

CODES

ICD9

529.0 Glossitis

CLINICAL PEARLS

- An acute or chronic inflammation of the tongue, either as primary disease or a symptom of systemic disease
- The most common forms are:
  - AG: Smooth, glossy, red or pink tongue
  - BMG or geographic tongue or erythema migrans: Erythematous and white patches on the dorsum of tongue; lesions may lack papillae; irregular (maplike) and migratory lesions
  - MRG: Erythematous, shiny, rhomboid-shaped plaque in middle of tongue; hypertrophic or atrophic surface changes
  - HGG: Linear fissures on dorsal tongue; geometric pattern is common; herpetic lesions usually are absent on other mucosal surfaces.
- Testing: Serum B_{12}, folic acid, CBC with differential, ferritin, RPR, TSH

GLUCOSE INTOLERANCE

Ramothea L. Webster, MD, PhD

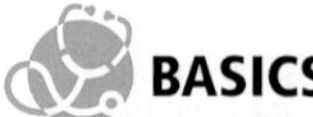

BASICS

DESCRIPTION

- Glucose intolerance is characterized by hyperglycemia resulting from defects in glucose and fat metabolism. Overt diabetes is classified as type 1 (T1DM), type 2 (T2DM), and gestational (GDM). Hyperglycemia not sufficient to meet the diagnostic criteria for diabetes is termed *prediabetes* and is categorized as either impaired fasting glucose (IFG) or impaired glucose tolerance (IGT).
- IFG and IGT are risk factors for developing diabetes and moderately increase the risk of cardiovascular disease (1)[A].

EPIDEMIOLOGY

- Diabetes affects almost 6% of the world's population
- ~97% of diabetic patients have T2DM
- ~79 million people in the US have prediabetes
- ~26 million people in the US (8.3%) have diabetes

Incidence

- Incidence of T1DM ranges from 7.61–25.7 per 100,000 per year in North America
- 1.9 million new cases of diagnosed diabetes in the US age ≥20 years in 2010

Prevalence

Prevalence of T2DM ranges from 6.69–28.2% in North America

RISK FACTORS

- T1DM:
  - First-degree relative with T1DM
  - Geography: increased incidence while traveling away from the equator
  - Possible risk factors:
    - Viral exposure (Epstein-Barr virus, cytomegalovirus, Coxsackie virus, mumps)
    - Low vitamin D levels
    - Being born with jaundice or experiencing respiratory infection just after birth
- Prediabetes and T2DM:
  - Body mass index [BMI] ≥25 kg/m
  - Hypertriglyceridemia, increased blood serum apolipoprotein A-1
  - Hypertension
  - Elevated liver enzymes (aspartate aminotransferase, alanine aminotransferase [ALT], γ-glutamyltransferase); note: ALT (gluconeogenic enzyme), gene expression suppressed by insulin
  - Physical inactivity:
    - Obesity increases the risk of developing T2DM 10-fold in women and 11.2-fold in men
  - First- or second-degree relative with T2DM
  - Race/ethnicity: Nonwhite race (African American, Latino, Native American, Asian American, Pacific Islander)
  - Many patients with T2DM also have the metabolic syndrome, which is characterized by central adiposity, insulin resistance, dyslipidemia, and hypertension.
- GDM:
  - Age >25 years
  - Delivery of a baby weighing >9 lb or unexplained stillbirth
  - Marked obesity, BMI >30
  - Family history of prediabetes/T2DM/GDM
  - Diagnosis of GDM with prior pregnancies
  - Nonwhite race

Genetics

- T1DM:
  - Multiple genetic predispositions and poorly defined environmental factors contribute to T1DM:
    - HLA-DR3 and HLA-DR4 associations exist with linkage to the *DQA* and *DQB* genes
- T2DM:
  - A stronger genetic predisposition than T1DM, contributed by multiple gene variations, strongest association is variation of *TCF7L2* gene

GENERAL PREVENTION

- A decrease in excess body fat provides the greatest risk reduction.
- Screening for prediabetes and diabetes should be performed at 3-year intervals beginning at age 45 (2)[A]:
  - Screen at younger ages or with increased frequency in those with additional risk factors or a BMI ≥25 kg/m^2 (2)[A]
- Patients with either IFG or IGT benefit from moderate weight loss (5–10%) and aerobic physical activity (150 min/wk) (1)[A]:
  - Metformin, acarbose, and orlistat effectively decrease the rate of progression to diabetes
- Patients with IFG or IGT should be monitored for diabetes every 1–2 years (2)[A].
- Patients with other cardiovascular risk factors (e.g., dyslipidemia, hypertension, obesity, tobacco use) should receive appropriate counseling to modify diet and exercise.

Pregnancy Considerations

- Screening for diabetes in pregnancy is based on risk factor analysis:
  - High risk: First prenatal visit
  - Average risk: 24–28 weeks' gestation
- Women with GDM should be screened for diabetes 6–12 weeks postpartum (2)[A].

ETIOLOGY

- T1DM:
  - Cellular-mediated autoimmune pathologic process leading to destruction of pancreatic islet β-cells and ultimately absolute insulin deficiency
- T2DM:
  - A multiorgan disease characterized by chronic and progressive insulin resistance and relative insulin deficiency:
    - Insulin resistance initially leads to an increase in functional β-cell mass, but this compensatory measure is often insufficient, and relative insulin deficiency, glucose intolerance, and hyperglycemia result.
  - Autoimmune destruction of β-cells does not occur.

COMMONLY ASSOCIATED CONDITIONS

- Hypertension
- Dyslipidemia
- Acanthosis nigricans
- Polycystic ovary syndrome
- Patients with T1DM are prone to other autoimmune disorders including celiac sprue, Grave disease, Hashimoto thyroiditis, Addison disease, vitiligo, myasthenia gravis, and pernicious anemia (2)[A].

DIAGNOSIS

HISTORY

- Characteristics of the onset of disease (e.g., diabetic ketoacidosis, routine lab evaluation)
- Diet and exercise history
- History of diabetes-related complications:
  - Microvascular: Eye, kidney, nerve
  - Macrovascular: Cardiac, cardiovascular disease, peripheral artery disease
  - Other: Sexual dysfunction, gastroparesis
- Tobacco and alcohol use
- Polyuria
- Polydipsia
- Unexplained weight loss (sometimes accompanied by polyphagia)
- Blurred vision

PHYSICAL EXAM

- BP, including orthostatics
- Dorsalis pedis and posterior tibialis pulses
- Funduscopic exam
- Thyroid palpation
- Skin exam (for acanthosis nigricans and insulin injection sites), trophic changes on toes
- Neurologic exam:
  - Patellar and Achilles reflexes
  - Proprioception, vibration, and monofilament sensation tests

DIAGNOSTIC TESTS & INTERPRETATION

Lab

Initial lab tests

- Prediabetes (2)[A]:
  - Categorized as IFG when diagnosed using glycosylated hemoglobin (HbA1c) or a fasting plasma glucose (FPG); IGT when diagnosed using the oral glucose tolerance test (OGTT):
    - IFG:
      - HbA1c between 5.7 and 6.4%
      - FPG ≥100 mg/dL and <126 mg/dL
    - IGT: A 2-hour plasma glucose between 140 mg/dL and 199 mg/dL after ingestion of a 75-g glucose load
  - Glucose tolerance test (GTT) is usually not necessary, except when diagnosing GDM.
  - HbA1c has advantages over FPG for diagnosis.
- Diabetes (2)[A]:
  - Diagnosed using any 1 of the following (on 2 or more occasions):
    - HbA1c ≥6.5% is diagnostic
    - Symptoms of diabetes plus:
      - Random plasma glucose (measured at any time of day, regardless of time since last meal) ≥200 mg/dL; or
      - FPG ≥126 mg/dL; or
      - A 2-hour plasma glucose ≥200 mg/dL following ingestion of a 75-g glucose load is diagnostic

Follow-Up & Special Considerations
- Fasting lipid profile
- Liver function tests
- Test for microalbuminuria
- Serum creatinine and calculated glomerular filtration rate
- Thyroid-stimulating hormones

DIFFERENTIAL DIAGNOSIS
Diabetes insipidus

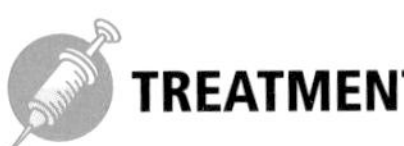

TREATMENT

Glycemic control and the preservation of β-cell function are central to the treatment of T1DM and T2DM.

MEDICATION
Noninsulin glucose-lowering agents:
- Sulfonylureas and meglitinides
- Metformin and acarbose: Reduce rates of glucose appearance in the circulation
- Thiazolidinediones: Modify fat-induced insulin resistance (2)[A]
- Incretins (exenatide and sitagliptin): targets pancreatic islet β-cell defects

First Line
- T1DM:
  - Insulin: Combination of intermediate- or long-acting basal insulin with premeal rapid or short-acting insulin (2)[A]
- T2DM:
  - Metformin combined with intensive, multidisciplinary lifestyle modification (7)[A]

Second Line
T2DM:
- Any of the following oral agents may be used in combination with metformin. Up to 3 oral agents may be used concurrently, but initiation of insulin therapy is preferred if treatment goals cannot be met using 2 oral agents (7)[A]:
  - Sulfonylurea
  - Glitazones
  - Acarbose

ALERT
- Metformin can cause lactic acidosis, a potentially fatal complication, in geriatric patients and patients with renal dysfunction and congestive heart failure (2)[A].
- Thiazolidinediones, including Avandia, Avandamet, and Avandaryl, may cause or exacerbate congestive heart failure in some patients. Initiation of these drugs in patients with established New York Heart Association class III or IV heart failure is contraindicated. After initiation of Avandia, Avandamet, or Avandaryl, and after dose increases, observe patients carefully for signs and symptoms of heart failure (including rapid weight gain, dyspnea, and/or edema) (4)[B].

ADDITIONAL TREATMENT
Weight loss of 5–10% improves glycemic control, increases insulin sensitivity, improves lipids, and lowers BP.

Issues for Referral
- Eye exam at time of initial diagnosis and annually thereafter
- Diabetes educator/registered dietician
- Exercise physiologist

IN-PATIENT CONSIDERATIONS
Initial Stabilization
- Monitor blood glucose levels, which should be considered an additional "vital sign."
- Critically ill and postsurgical diabetic patients usually require IV infusion of regular insulin:
  - Sliding-scale insulin regimens alone are ineffective and are not recommended (2)[A].
  - Prandial insulin doses should be given in relation to meals after correcting for premeal hyperglycemia.
- Monitor hospitalized patients closely for hypoglycemia.

Admission Criteria
- Diabetic ketoacidosis
- Nonketotic hyperosmolar syndrome

Discharge Criteria
Patient is no longer acidotic and is transitioned from IV insulin to either SC insulin or oral agents with appropriate glycemic control.

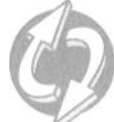

ONGOING CARE

FOLLOW-UP RECOMMENDATIONS
- At least 150 min/wk of moderate-intensity aerobic exercise and/or at least 90 min/wk of vigorous aerobic exercise (2)[A]
- Resistance exercise improves insulin sensitivity to the same extent as aerobic exercise; resistance training 3 times per week is recommended for those with T2DM (2)[A].

Patient Monitoring
- Self-monitoring of blood glucose
- The A1c should be measured at least twice a year in patients meeting treatment goals and quarterly in those whose therapy has changed or who are not meeting glycemic goals (2)[A]:
  - Therapeutic goal is to achieve an A1c (<7%) as close to normal as possible in the absence of hypoglycemia (2)[A].
- BP should be routinely measured.
- Annual testing for lipid abnormalities and microalbuminuria (for detection and therapy modification of incipient diabetic nephropathy)
- Annual dilated fundal exam
- Annual foot exam including monofilament testing for distal polyneuropathy

DIET
- Monitor carbohydrate intake: Match doses of insulin and insulin secretagogues to the carbohydrate content of meals (5)[B]
- Low-fat (<25%) intake (5)[B]:
  - Saturated fat intake should be <7% of total calories
  - Minimize *trans* fat intake
- Low-sodium intake (5)[B]
- High fiber (~50 g/d; 14 g/1,000 kcal) and whole-grain intake (5)[B]
- Maximize low-glycemic index foods
- Moderate alcohol intake

PROGNOSIS
- When appropriately treated, diabetes is not in itself a terminal disease.
- Most negative sequelae can be averted with consistent, longitudinal glycemic control.

COMPLICATIONS
- Cardiovascular disease
- Sexual dysfunction
- Gastroparesis
- Nephropathy and potential for renal failure
- Retinopathy and potential for loss of vision
- Peripheral and autonomic neuropathy

REFERENCES

1. Ford ES, Zhao G, Li C, et al. Pre-diabetes and the risk for cardiovascular disease: A systematic review of the evidence. *J Am Coll Cardiol*. 2010;55: 1310–7.
2. American Diabetes Association, et al. Standards of medical care in diabetes–2011. *Diabetes Care*. 2011;34 (Suppl 1):S11–61.
3. Saenz A, et al. Metformin monotherapy for type 2 diabetes mellitus. *Cochrane Database Sys Rev*. 2005;CD002966.
4. www.fda.gov/Drugs/DrugSafety/PostmarketDrugSafetyInformationforPatientsandProviders/ucm143349.htm.
5. American Diabetes Association, Bantle JP, Wylie-Rosett J, et al. Nutrition recommendations and interventions for diabetes: A position statement of the American Diabetes Association. *Diabetes Care*. 2008;31(Suppl 1):S61–78.

G

ADDITIONAL READING

- Adeghate E, Schattner P, Dunn E, et al. An update on the etiology and epidemiology of diabetes mellitus. *Ann N Y Acad Sci*. 2006;1084:1–29.
- Nyenwe EA, Dagogo-Jack SM, et al. Metabolic syndrome, prediabetes and the science of primary prevention. *Minerva Endocrinol*. 2011;36:129–45.

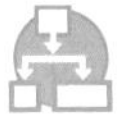

See Also (Topic, Algorithm, Electronic Media Element)

Algorithm: Hypoglycemia

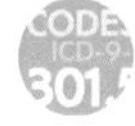

CODES

ICD9
- 790.21 Impaired fasting glucose
- 790.22 Impaired glucose tolerance test (oral)
- 790.29 Other abnormal glucose

CLINICAL PEARLS
- HbA1c ≥6.5% is diagnostic for diabetes and has advantages over FPG.
- GTT is usually not necessary, except when diagnosing GDM.

GONOCOCCAL INFECTIONS

Jill A. Grimes, MD

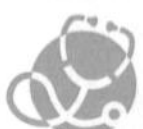

BASICS

DESCRIPTION

Gonorrhea is a sexually or vertically transmitted bacterial infection caused by *Neisseria gonorrhoeae*:

- *Neisseria gonorrhoeae* is a gram-negative intracellular diplococci.
- Commonly presents as urethritis, salpingitis, cervicitis, pelvic inflammatory disease (PID), epididymitis, or proctitis
- Hematogenous dissemination may also occur and lead to fever, skin lesions, arthralgias, purulent arthritis, tenosynovitis, endocarditis, or, rarely, meningitis.
- Asymptomatic carrier state can occur in both sexes.
- In newborns, gonococcal ophthalmia neonatorum, a purulent conjunctivitis, may occur after vaginal delivery by an infected mother and may lead to blindness if not treated promptly.
- System(s) affected: Cardiovascular; Musculoskeletal; Nervous; Reproductive; Skin/Exocrine
- Synonym(s): GC; Clap

EPIDEMIOLOGY

- Predominant age: 15–24 years
- Predominant sex: Prior to 1996, rates of gonorrhea among men were higher than rates among women:
  - 2009: Women 105.5/100,000 vs. Men 91.9/100,000

Incidence

- In 2009: 301,174 cases were reported to the CDC, resulting in rate of 99.1/100,000 US population.
- Highest rates are among black women aged 15–19 (2,613.8/100,000)
- Blacks (556.4/100,000) have 20.5 times greater rate than whites (27.2/100,000)
- The southern and midwest regions of the US have higher rates, with Mississippi having the highest rate by state (246.4/100,000)

Prevalence

As a treatable disease, incidence and prevalence of diagnosed disease are approximately equal. The asymptomatic nature of the disease (especially among women) suggests that the prevalence is higher than the reported incidence.

RISK FACTORS

- History of previous gonorrhea infection or other STIs
- Sexual exposure to an infected individual without barrier protection (condom)
- New or multiple sexual partners
- Inconsistent condom use
- Sex work or drug use
- Infants: Infected mother
- Children: Sexual abuse by infected individual
- Autoinoculation (finger to eye)
- For PID: Use of intrauterine devices

Genetics

Congenital deficiency of late components of complement cascade (C7,8,9) are prone to develop dissemination of local gonococcal infections.

GENERAL PREVENTION

- Condoms offer partial protection, but must be used for oral, anal, and vaginal intercourse to be effective.
- Treat sexual contacts; consider expedited partner therapy (EPT) (1)

PATHOPHYSIOLOGY

Infection requires 4 steps: (i) Mucosal attachment; (ii) Local penetration/invasion; (iii) Local proliferation; (iv) Inflammatory response or dissemination

ETIOLOGY

N. gonorrhoeae (gonococcus)

COMMONLY ASSOCIATED CONDITIONS

Other STIs:

- *Chlamydia*, syphilis, HIV, hepatitis B, herpes

DIAGNOSIS

HISTORY

- Sexual history:
  - Number of partners and age of onset of sexual activity; STI history
  - New/recent change in sexual partner
  - Contact with sex workers
  - Condom use
  - Menses, and possibility of pregnancy
- If symptoms: Onset, context, duration, timing, severity, associated symptoms, and modifying factors of symptoms:
  - Symptoms typically appear within 1–14 days after exposure (if present at all)
- 10% males and 20–40% of women are asymptomatic.
- Ocular symptoms: Discharge, itch, redness
- Pharyngeal symptoms: Asymptomatic infection (98%), sore throat
- GI symptoms: Acute diarrhea
- Urinary symptoms: Urinary frequency, urgency, dysuria
- Urethral symptoms: Copious urethral discharge:
  - Males: Scant to copious purulent urethral discharge (82%), dysuria (53%), testicular pain (1%), asymptomatic infection (10%), proctitis
  - Females: Asymptomatic cervical infection (20%), endocervical discharge (96%), vaginal discharge, Bartholin gland abscess, dysmenorrhea, menometrorrhagia, abdominal pain/tenderness, cervical motion tenderness, rebound, infertility, chronic pelvic pain
- Either sex, for receptive anal intercourse: Rectal discharge, tenesmus, rectal burning, asymptomatic
- Disseminated syndromes:
  - Fever, chills, malaise, dermatitis, polyarthralgia
  - Endocarditis: High fevers
  - Meningitis: Meningeal signs, headache, skin lesions, fever, altered mental status

PHYSICAL EXAM

- General: Fever, chills
- Ocular: Purulent discharge, conjunctivitis, chemosis, eyelid edema, corneal ulceration
- Pharyngeal infection: Exudative pharyngitis (<1%)
- GI: Acute diarrhea, hyperactive bowel sounds
- GU:
  - Males: Scant to copious purulent urethral discharge (82%), testicular tenderness (1%), asymptomatic infection (10%), proctitis
  - Females: Asymptomatic cervical infection (20%), endocervical discharge (96%), vaginal discharge, Bartholin gland abscess, abdominal pain/tenderness, cervical motion tenderness, rebound
- Either sex, for *receptive anal intercourse*: Rectal discharge; may appear normal
- Disseminated syndromes:
  - Fever, chills, malaise, tenosynovitis, dermatitis, polyarthralgia, purulent arthritis
  - Endocarditis: Rapid cardiac valve destruction, heart murmurs, high fevers
  - Meningitis: Meningeal signs, headache, skin lesions, fever, altered mental status

DIAGNOSTIC TESTS & INTERPRETATION

Lab

Initial lab tests

CDC recommends nucleic acid amplification as the most sensitive and specific test for *N. gonorrhoeae*. Other options include:

- Genital culture
- Add pharyngeal culture in adolescents (2)[A].
- Gram stain (recommended for urethritis)
- Urethral smear, sensitivity in symptomatic male: ≥95%. Sensitivity of endocervical smear in infected woman: 40–60%. Specificity: 100%
- DNA probes and PCR sensitivity: 92–99% dependent on population. Specificity: >97%; can replace culture
- Sensitivity of blood culture in disseminated disease: 50%. Sensitivity of joint fluid culture in septic arthritis: 50%
- Screen for additional STIs, especially chlamydia, syphilis, and HIV

Follow-Up & Special Considerations

- Test-of-cure testing is not generally recommended.
- Follow-up testing may be considered in cases of recurrent infection and/or in areas where significant antibiotic resistance exists.

Imaging

Initial approach

Imaging is not generally recommended.

Follow-Up & Special Considerations

Pelvic ultrasound or CT scan may demonstrate thick, dilated fallopian tubes or abscess formation.

Diagnostic Procedures/Surgery

Culdocentesis may demonstrate free purulent exudate and provide material for Gram staining and culture. Gram staining material from unroofed skin lesions may show typical organisms.

Pathological Findings

- Exudate of polymorphonuclear leukocytes is typical.
- Gram-negative intracellular *diplococci*
- Nonpathologic gram-negative *diplococci* may be found in extragenital locations. For this reason, Gram stain of pharyngeal or rectal swabs is not recommended.

DIFFERENTIAL DIAGNOSIS

Chlamydia trachomatis, UTIs, other vaginitis, or urethritis (bacterial, viral or parasitic)

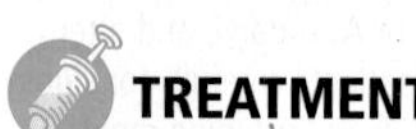

TREATMENT

MEDICATION

- *N. gonorrhoeae* antimicrobial resistance continues to increase.
- Quinolones not recommended since 2007; only cephalosporins now recommended

- *If treatment failure, check culture and sensitivities, and report to CDC through local health authorities.*
- Treat routinely with regimen that is also effective against uncomplicated genital chlamydial infection.

First Line

- Uncomplicated gonorrheal infection of the cervix, urethra, or rectum:
  - Ceftriaxone, 250 mg IM in a single dose (preferred) or Cefixime, 400 mg PO single dose
  - PLUS treatment for chlamydia (azithromycin 1 g PO single dose or doxycycline 100 mg PO b.i.d. for 7 days)
- Pharyngitis: Ceftriaxone, 250 mg IM once PLUS chlamydia treatment above
- Conjunctivitis: Ceftriaxone, 1 g IM
- PID: Parenteral and oral treatments are equivalent for mild- to moderate-severity PID. If using IV therapy, switch to PO within 24 hours of clinical improvement:
  - Cefotetan 2 g IV q12h OR Cefoxitin 2 g IV q6h PLUS Doxycycline 100 mg PO or IV q12h OR
  - Clindamycin 900 mg IV q8h PLUS Gentamicin loading dose IV or IM (2 mg/kg of body weight), followed by a maintenance dose (1.5 mg/kg) q8h (may substitute single daily dosing)
  - Preferred "oral" regimen includes:
    - Ceftriaxone, 250 mg IM once *plus* Doxycycline, 100 mg PO b.i.d. for 14 days
    - *With or without* Metronidazole, 500 mg PO b.i.d. for 14 days
- Disseminated infection in adults:
  - Ceftriaxone, 1 g IM or IV q24h until 24–48 hours after improvement begins, then switch to Cefixime 400 mg PO b.i.d. to complete at least 1 week of antibiotic treatment. *Also treat for chlamydial infection.*
- Meningitis and endocarditis:
  - Ceftriaxone, 1–2 g IV q12h 10–14 days for meningitis; 4 weeks for endocarditis
- *Contraindications: Doxycycline is contraindicated in pregnancy and young children.*

Pediatric Considerations

- Treatment of infants and children: <45 kg (patients >45 kg should receive full adult dose)
- Uncomplicated genital, pharyngeal, rectal, or conjunctival infection, and infants born to mothers with untreated gonorrhea:
  - Ceftriaxone, 125 mg IM in single dose
  - Disseminated infections: Ceftriaxone, 50 mg/kg IV or IM daily (max dose 1g) in single dose; bacteremia: 7 days; meningitis: 10–14 days; endocarditis: 4 weeks
- Ophthalmic neonatorum prophylaxis: Single application of Erythromycin (0.5%) ophthalmic ointment
- Neonatal conjunctivitis: Ceftriaxone 25–50 mg/kg IV or IM in a single dose (not to exceed 125 mg)
- Scalp abscesses (from scalp electrodes): Ceftriaxone 25–50 mg/kg/d IV or IM in a single daily dose for 7 days
- Asymptomatic infants born to mothers with untreated gonorrhea: Ceftriaxone 25–50 mg/kg IV or IM, not to exceed 125 mg, in a single dose

Second Line

- No second-line agent available in the US for gonococcal infections:
  - Recent gonococcal isolates within the US have demonstrated significant rates of resistance to both azithromycin and quinolones. Neither is currently recommended as a single agent for treatment (3)[A].
  - Progressive resistance to sulfonamides, penicillins, tetracyclines, fluoroquinolones and now developing resistance in Asia, Australia, and elsewhere to third-generation cephalosporins makes prevention critically important (4)[B].
- PID can be treated with clindamycin and gentamicin.
- For treatment options other than those listed in previous section, please see the CDC report on STD treatment guidelines at: www.cdc.gov/std/treatment/2010/gonococcal-infections.htm

ADDITIONAL TREATMENT

General Measures

- Counseling concerning risk reduction and condom use
- In children and adolescents, suspect sexual abuse.

IN-PATIENT CONSIDERATIONS

Admission Criteria

- Hematogenously disseminated infection
- Pneumonia or eye infection in infants
- PID: If unable to take oral medications, significant tubo-ovarian abscess, or patient is pregnant

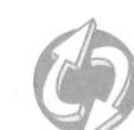

ONGOING CARE

FOLLOW-UP RECOMMENDATIONS

Patient Monitoring

US Preventive Services Task Force (USPSTF) recommends (5):

- Screen all sexually active women if they are at increased risk of infection (*simply having a new partner is considered "increased risk"*).
- Insufficient evidence to recommend screening men at increased risk of infection
- Strongly recommend prophylactic ocular topical medication for all newborns

PATIENT EDUCATION

- Counseling concerning risk reduction, condom use, future fertility, and full STI testing
- Encourage patient to notify partners; consider expedited partner therapy (1).
- **Gonorrhea is a reportable disease:**
  - *A provider must contact both the state health department and the CDC.*

PROGNOSIS

With adequate, early therapy, complete cure with return to normal function is the rule.

COMPLICATIONS

- Infertility
- Urethral stricture
- Corneal scarring
- Destruction of joint articular surfaces
- Cardiac valves

Pediatric Considerations

Vertical transmission to newborn infants is a significant risk among patients with gonococcal infection at the time of delivery.

REFERENCES

1. Gift TL, Kissinger P, Mohammed H, et al. The cost and cost-effectiveness of expedited partner therapy compared with standard partner referral for the treatment of chlamydia or gonorrhea. *Sex Transm Dis*. 2011;38:1067–73.
2. Giannini CM, Kim HK, Mortensen J, et al. Culture of non-genital sites increases the detection of gonorrhea in women. *J Pediatr Adolesc Gynecol*. 2010;23:246–52.
3. Update to CDC's sexually transmitted diseases treatment guidelines, 2006: Fluoroquinolones no longer recommended for treatment of gonococcal infections. *MMWR Morb Mortal Wkly Rep*. 2007;56(14):332–6.
4. Barry PM, Klausner JD. The use of cephalosporins for gonorrhea: The impending problem of resistance. *Expert Opin Pharmacother*. 2009;10: 555–77.
5. *Screening for Gonorrhea*, Topic Page. May 2005. U.S. Preventive Services Task Force. www.uspreventiveservicestaskforce.org/uspstf/uspsgono.htm Accessed 10/24/2011.

ADDITIONAL READING

- CDC. MMWR Cephalosporin susceptibility among *Neisseria gonorrhoeae* isolates–United States, 2000–2010; 2011;60(26):873–877.
- Ohnishi M, Golparian D, Shimuta K, et al. Is *Neisseria gonorrhoeae* initiating a future era of untreatable gonorrhea?: Detailed characterization of the first strain with high-level resistance to ceftriaxone. *Antimicrob. Agents Chemother*. 2011;55:3538–45.

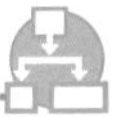

See Also (Topic, Algorithm, Electronic Media Element)

Chlamydial Sexually Transmitted Diseases; HIV Infection and AIDS; Pelvic Inflammatory Disease (PID); Syphilis

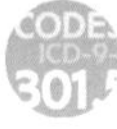

CODES

ICD9

- 098.0 Gonococcal infection (acute) of lower genitourinary tract
- 098.10 Gonococcal infection (acute) of upper genitourinary tract, site unspecified
- 098.11 Gonococcal cystitis (acute)

CLINICAL PEARLS

- Gonorrhea antibiotic resistance is a severe problem that continues to expand, and treatment recommendations have changed (see "Treatment").
- Patients testing positive for gonorrhea should also be considered for additional STI testing including chlamydia, syphilis, HIV, and hepatitis.
- Treat also for chlamydia, unless chlamydia infection ruled out.

G

GOUT

Wanda Cruz-Knight, MD

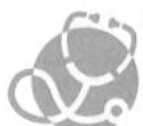

BASICS

DESCRIPTION

- Gout refers to a group of disorders related to hyperuricemia. Although hyperuricemia is necessary for the development of gout, it is not the only determining factor.
- Characterized by deposition of monosodium urate (MSU) crystals in tissue, resulting in acute and chronic arthritis, soft tissue masses called tophi, urate nephropathy, and uric acid nephrolithiasis
- Natural history involves 4 stages:
  - Asymptomatic hyperuricemia
  - Acute arthritis
  - Intercritical gout
  - Chronic tophaceous gout
- Acute gouty arthritis can affect ≥1 joints. The first metatarsophalangeal joint is most commonly involved at presentation (podagra).
- Other common sites include midtarsal, ankle, and knee joints.
- After an initial attack, patients can be attack-free for months or even years. Some patients will develop more frequent attacks or go on to develop chronic tophaceous gout.
- Management involves treating acute attacks and preventing recurrent disease by long-term reduction of serum uric acid levels through pharmacology and lifestyle adjustments.

Geriatric Considerations

- Presentation may lack acute pain, swelling, and inflammation
- More common in women >80
- Can present with tophi and finger joint pain
- Commonly triggered by diuretic use, especially in women

Pediatric Considerations

Often due to an inborn error of metabolism or other disease

EPIDEMIOLOGY

Incidence

Increases with age, especially in women

Prevalence

6 per 1,000 population for men; 1 per 1,000 population for women

RISK FACTORS

- Hyperuricemia
- Male gender (age <65)
- Increasing age
- Ethanol ingestion (beer and liquor > wine)
- Obesity (50%)
- Hypertension (50%)
- Diabetes
- Metabolic syndrome
- Medications: Diuretics induce 20% of secondary gout
- Diet: High-purine animal-origin foods (e.g., meats and seafood)
- Family history
- Keto- and lactic acidosis
- Surgery or trauma
- Renal impairment
- Hypothyroidism
- Parathyroid disease
- Hyperlipidemia types II, IV, V
- Paget disease
- Hyperproliferative skin disorders (psoriasis)
- Lymphoproliferative disorders, hemolytic anemia, hemoglobinopathies, pernicious anemia
- Glycogen storage diseases

Genetics

- Primary gout runs in families and follows multifactorial inheritance.
- Phosphoribosyl pyrophosphate (PRPP) deficiency and hypoxanthine-guanine-phosphoribosyltransferase (HGPRT) deficiency are inherited enzyme defects associated with a primary overproduction of uric acid.
- URAT1 (urate transporter) deficiency is also a hereditary enzyme defect resulting in primary underexcretion of uric acid.

GENERAL PREVENTION

- Treat underlying cardiovascular risk factors.
- Maintain weight at optimal BMI of <26.
- Regular exercise
- Diet modification
- Reduce alcohol consumption (beer and liquor).
- Maintain fluid intake and avoid dehydration.

PATHOPHYSIOLOGY

- Humans have a narrow window for urate to remain soluble before crystal precipitation due to lack of uricase enzyme.
- Precipitation of MSU crystals can occur in the synovium, joint cartilage, kidneys, and soft tissue.
- MSU crystals can initiate and sustain an inflammatory response, leading to an acute gout attack.
- Chronic and untreated hyperuricemia lead to tophi formation in and around the joint space.
- Tophi contribute to chronic synovitis, often resulting in joint damage.

ETIOLOGY

- Increased uric acid production
- renal under excretion of uric acid
- Enzyme defects
- Increased purine turnover
- Dehydration or starvation
- Malignancy

COMMONLY ASSOCIATED CONDITIONS

- Metabolic syndrome (obesity, hyperglycemia, hyperlipidemia, hypertension)
- Myeloproliferative disorders
- Lymphoproliferative disorders
- Alcoholism
- Endocrinopathies
- Lesch-Nyhan syndrome

DIAGNOSIS

HISTORY

- Rapid onset of severe pain, usually beginning in early morning with 1 or 2 joints (75% are monoarticular) ± fever
- Soft tissue redness, swelling, warmth
- Exquisite tenderness
- First metatarsophalangeal joint in 50% of initial attacks
- Acute untreated attacks last 2–21 days.
- Recurrent attacks last longer and occur more frequently with each recurrence.
- Between attacks, absence of inflammation (until the chronic or tophaceous phase occurs)
- Rarely polyarticular
- Migratory polyarthritis is a rare presentation.
- 50% untreated develop chronic arthritis
- SC or intraosseous nodules (20%), referred to as tophi, may affect ears (antihelix), extensor aspects of peripheral joints (e.g., olecranon), cornea, aorta, spine, even intracranial space (1).
- Pain with urination secondary to uric acid renal stones

PHYSICAL EXAM

- Examine suspected joint(s) for tenderness, swelling, and range of motion (ROM).
- Assess for presence of firm nodules known as tophi.

DIAGNOSTIC TESTS & INTERPRETATION

Lab

Initial lab tests

- Synovial fluid analysis: Urate crystals, (negatively birefringent under polarizing microscopy), cell count (WBC usually 5,000–50,000/mm^3; predominantly neutrophils); culture to rule out infection
- Blood studies: Elevated serum uric acid level, CBC (can show elevated WBC during acute attack)
- Urine studies: Urinalysis, 24-hour urine testing for uric acid and creatinine (urate excretion will likely not be accurate during an acute attack)

Imaging

Initial approach

- Radiograph is usually normal early in disease.
- Radiograph in chronic gout reveals "punched-out" erosions (lytic areas), often with periosteum overgrowing the erosion ("overhanging edge").
- Urate kidney stones are radiolucent, and thus invisible on radiograph.

Diagnostic Procedures/Surgery

- Arthrocentesis with polarizing optical examination
- Biopsy of synovial membrane or SC nodule, processing the specimen anhydrously (urate is water-soluble)

Pathological Findings

- Acute arthritis: Neutrophilic infiltrate throughout synovium
- Chronic arthritis: Intra-articular and periarticular tophi
- Tophi: Macrophages surround MSU crystals, forming a granuloma
- Gouty nephropathy: MSU crystals deposited in medullary interstitium

DIFFERENTIAL DIAGNOSIS

- Septic arthritis
- Pseudogout (calcium pyrophosphate deposition disease)
- Cellulitis
- Reactive arthritis
- Amyloidosis
- Osteoarthritis
- Hyperparathyroidism
- Spondyloarthropathy
- Rheumatoid arthritis (rarely)

TREATMENT

- Key component is lifestyle adjustment to avoid triggers and reduce risk
- Chronic treatment indicated if >2 attacks per year, tophi present, radiographic evidence of joint damage (2)[C]
- Goal for chronic treatment is serum uric acid <6 mg/dL (2)[B].

MEDICATION

First Line

Acute attack:

- NSAIDs (e.g., naproxen and indomethacin) at full dosage:
  - Taper a few days after symptoms resolve.
  - Use limited by GI side effects, including GI bleeding (1)[A]

Chronic treatment:

- Urate-lowering agents should not be prescribed until 2–3 weeks after acute attack has resolved, but should be continued if patient is taking them prior to attack.
  - Xanthine oxidase inhibitors:
    - Allopurinol start at 100 mg/d and adjust every 2–4 weeks until goal of serum uric acid is <6 mg/dL for 3–6 months (2)[B]:
      - Monitor for hypersensitivity reactions: Rash, hepatitis, interstitial nephritis, and toxic epidermal necrolysis.
      - Coprescribe with colchicine 0.5–1 mg/d OR low-dose NSAIDs daily on initiation of treatment to prevent rebound acute gout attacks (2)[B].
    - Febuxostat:
      - Approved by the FDA in 2009 for gout
      - Benefits include more selective xanthine oxidase inhibitor and no renal dose adjustment
      - Starting dose 40 mg/d; titrate to 80 mg/d to goal serum uric acid of <6 mg/dL (3,4)[B]

Second Line

- Acute attack:
  - Colchicine: Should be used within 12–24 hours of attack onset. 1 mg followed by 0.5 mg q2h until absence of symptoms or GI side effects occur (nausea, vomiting, diarrhea) (1)[A].
  - Systemic corticosteroids (5)[B]
  - Intra-articular long-acting corticosteroid is useful if 1 or a few joints involved (2)[B]
  - Adrenocorticotropic hormone (ACTH) 25 USP units SC for acute small-joint monoarticular gout. 40 USP units IM or IV for larger joints or polyarticular gout (2)[B].
- Chronic treatment:
  - Uricosuric agents
  - Use in patients refractory to allopurinol or in whom allopurinol is contraindicated. Ideal for patients <60 years with CrCl >80 mL/min, 24-hour urinary uric acid excretion ≤700 mg on normal diet, and without history of renal calculi:
    - Probenecid: Start at 250 mg PO b.i.d. and gradually increase to 500–2,000 mg (in 2 doses) until desired SUA in those with normal renal function (2)[B].
    - Sulfinpyrazone: Start at 50 mg PO b.i.d. and gradually increase to 100–400 mg/d (in 2 doses) until desired SUA in those with normal renal function (2)[B].
    - Initially coprescribe all uricosurics with either colchicine 0.5–1 mg/d for up to 6 months OR low-dose NSAIDs for up to 6 weeks.
  - Fenofibrate and losartan or amlodipine: Consider as alternative therapy for hyperlipidemia and HTN, respectively. Modest uricosuric effect (2,6)[B].
  - Ongoing studies: Puricase (PEG-uricase) for refractory chronic gout (7)[B]

ADDITIONAL TREATMENT

General Measures

Apply ice packs and rest affected joint.

SURGERY/OTHER PROCEDURES

Large tophi that are infected or interfering with joint motion may need to be surgically removed.

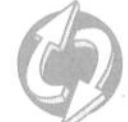

ONGOING CARE

FOLLOW-UP RECOMMENDATIONS

Patient Monitoring

Related to medicinal control of the acute attack and suppressing attacks:

- CBC, renal, liver function tests (LFTs), and urinalysis at 1 week, 6 weeks, and every 3 months

DIET

- Reduce ingestion of purine-rich foods of animal origin (meat and shellfish).
- Avoid alcoholic beverages, specifically beer and liquor.
- Increase low-fat dairy foods.
- Maintain adequate hydration.
- Consider additional vitamin C 500 mg/d (8).

PATIENT EDUCATION

Gout and Uric Acid Education Society: www.gouteducation.org

PROGNOSIS

- Gout can usually be successfully managed with proper treatment.
- Recurrent attacks may require long-term uric acid-lowering therapy.
- During the first 6–12 months of uricosuric or allopurinol therapy, acute gout attacks may occur.

COMPLICATIONS

- Increased susceptibility to infection
- Urate nephropathy
- Renal stones
- Nerve/spinal cord impingement

REFERENCES

1. Schlesinger N, Schumacher R, Catton M, et al. Colchicine for acute gout. *Cochrane Database Syst Rev*. 2006;CD006190.
2. Zhang W, Doherty M, Bardin T, et al. EULAR evidence based recommendations for gout. Part II: Management. Report of a task force of the EULAR Standing Committee for International Clinical Studies Including Therapeutics (ESCISIT). *Ann Rheum Dis*. 2006;65:1312–24.
3. Bruce SP. Febuxostat: A selective xanthine oxidase inhibitor for the treatment of hyperuricemia and gout. *Ann Pharmacother*. 2006;40:2187–94.
4. Schumacher HR, Becker MA, Wortmann RL, et al. Effects of febuxostat versus allopurinol and placebo in reducing serum urate in subjects with hyperuricemia and gout: A 28-week, phase III, randomized, double-blind, parallel-group trial. *Arthritis Rheum*. 2008;59:1540–8.
5. Janssens H, et al. Systemic corticosteroids for acute gout. *Cochrane Database Syst Rev*. 2008;16(2): CD005521.
6. Høieggen A, Alderman MH, Kjeldsen SE, et al. The impact of serum uric acid on cardiovascular outcomes in the LIFE study. *Kidney Int*. 2004;65: 1041–9.
7. Sundy JS, Ganson NJ, Kelly SJ, et al. Pharmacokinetics and pharmacodynamics of intravenous PEGylated recombinant mammalian urate oxidase in patients with refractory gout. *Arthritis Rheum*. 2007;56:1021–8.
8. Huang HY, Appel LJ, Choi MJ, et al. The effects of vitamin C supplementation on serum concentrations of uric acid: Results of a randomized controlled trial. *Arthritis Rheum*. 2005;52:1843–7.

ADDITIONAL READING

- Eggebeen AT. Gout: An update. *Am Fam Physician*. 2007;76:801–8.
- Keith MP, Gilliland WR. Updates in the management of gout. *Am J Med*. 2007;120:221–4.
- Liote F, et al. Gout: Update on some pathogenic and clinical aspects. *Rheum Dis Clin N Am*. 2006;32: 295–311.
- Terkeltaub RA. Clinical practice. Gout. *N Engl J Med*. 2003;349:1647–55.

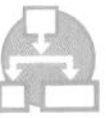

See Also (Topic, Algorithm, Electronic Media Element)

Alcohol Abuse and Dependence; Anemia, Sickle Cell

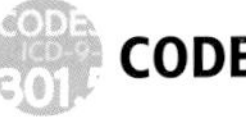

CODES

ICD9

- 274.00 Gouty arthropathy, unspecified
- 274.9 Gout, unspecified
- 274.10 Gouty nephropathy, unspecified

CLINICAL PEARLS

- Rapid onset of severe pain, usually beginning in early morning with 1 or 2 joints (75% are monoarticular)
- MSU crystals found in synovial fluid aspirate are pathognomonic for gout.
- Acute gout and sepsis can coexist.
- Asymptomatic hyperuricemia does not require treatment.
- Reducing serum uric acid level to <6 mg/dL to eliminate gout flare-ups and tophi.
- Insulin resistance and renal disease impair excretion of renal uric acid leading to gout.

GRANULOMA ANNULARE

Adam J. Tinklepaugh, MD
Alison Ehrlich, MD

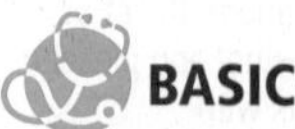

BASICS

DESCRIPTION

A benign skin condition characterized by grouped papules, which typically occur in an annular pattern. 5 variants have been described, the most common of which is localized granuloma annulare (GA). The other types are generalized, patch-type, SC (deep dermal), and perforating.

EPIDEMIOLOGY

Incidence

GA is not common, though its occurrence in the general population is unknown. It is seen more often in women, with a ratio of 2:1 over men. Most lesions resolve in 2–24 months, but may last up to 5–10 years. 2/3 of patients are <30 years old, and the age distribution varies by type, as follows:

- Localized: Children and adults <30 years old
- Generalized: Bimodal: Children <10 and adults 30–60 years old
- Patch-type: Adults >30 years old
- SC: Children 2–10 years old
- Perforating: Typically children, but also young adults

Prevalence

Among cases of GA, the approximate distribution is as follows:

- Localized: 75%
- Generalized: 10–15%
- Patch-type: <5%
- SC: <5%
- Perforating: <5% (perhaps higher in Hawaii)

RISK FACTORS

No definite risk factors have been identified. There is weak evidence for possible associations with diabetes mellitus, TB, HIV, EBV and other viral infections, interferon-alpha therapy, trauma, insect bites, and malignancies.

Genetics

There is some evidence for a possible hereditary component.

GENERAL PREVENTION

There are no established strategies for preventing GA.

ETIOLOGY

The cause of GA remains unknown.

COMMONLY ASSOCIATED CONDITIONS

See "Risk Factors." These noted associations are not common.

DIAGNOSIS

HISTORY

Cutaneous lesions of GA are generally asymptomatic. They may persist for months or years; longer duration is more often seen in the generalized subtype. They typically resolve spontaneously and they may recur.

PHYSICAL EXAM

- Localized: Small (1–2 mm) papules arranged in a ring, which may enlarge from 5 mm–5 cm. Color may range from skin colored to red. The most common locations are the dorsal aspects of the distal extremities.
- Generalized: Similar to localized, but a higher number of lesions, which are more diffuse distribution, often larger, and typically persist longer
- Patch-type: Erythematous, macules and patches distributed symmetrically on the extremities and trunk. The typical annular configuration may not be present.
- SC: Firm, nontender, SC nodule, which tends to grow rapidly. Usually solitary, but may occur in groups. Most common location is lower extremities, especially pretibial; other sites include upper extremities, scalp, buttocks.
- Perforating: Papules may be up to 4 mm and display umbilication, crusting, or scale. Lesions are often generalized and may occur anywhere.

DIAGNOSTIC TESTS & INTERPRETATION

Lab

Initial lab tests

Diagnosis is typically established by the history and physical, so lab investigations are rarely needed. Skin scraping/KOH test may be useful for excluding a fungal process.

Imaging

Initial approach

Rarely indicated, but may occasionally be useful in the workup of suspected SC subtype

Diagnostic Procedures/Surgery

Skin punch biopsy is useful to confirm the diagnosis and designate subtype. Immunohistochemical streptavidin-biotin-horseradish peroxidase (HRP) analysis for CD68/KP-1 is a sensitive histiocytic marker for confirming equivocal cases of GA.

Pathological Findings

Characterized by necrobiosis and palisading granulomas. Histologic variants include interstitial (histiocytic infiltrate between collagen fibers), classic (palisading dermal granulomas), and epithelioid (tuberculoid and sarcoidal granulomas).

DIFFERENTIAL DIAGNOSIS

- Localized: Tinea corporis, annular lichen planus, necrobiosis lipoidica, pityriasis rosea, erythema migrans of Lyme disease, leprosy
- Generalized: Sarcoidosis, lichen planus, cutaneous metastases
- Patch-type: Erythema migrans
- SC: Rheumatoid nodule
- Perforating: Molluscum contagiosum, sarcoidosis, insect bites

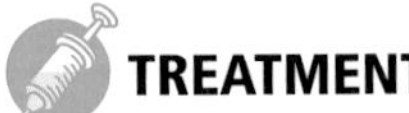

TREATMENT

MEDICATION

- There is no strong evidence supporting therapeutic intervention for GA. Reassurance with observation may be adequate treatment for localized, asymptomatic disease.
- The following therapies have been tried with variable success, and the possible benefit of treatment must be weighed against the significant toxicities of these treatments.

First Line

Corticosteroids:

- High-potency topical, with or without occlusion
- Intralesional triamcinolone 2.5–5 mg/mL (1)[B]

Second Line

Reported therapies (1)[B],(2)[B],(3)[B]:

- Methotrexate 15 mg IM weekly
- Rifampin 600 mg, ofloxacin 400 mg, minocycline 100 mg once-daily combination therapy
- Tacrolimus 0.1% ointment twice daily
- Pimecrolimus 1% cream twice daily
- Isotretinoin 0.5–0.75 mg/kg/d
- Dapsone 100 mg/d
- Chloroquine 3 mg/kg/d
- Hydroxychloroquine 6 mg/kg/d
- Cyclosporine 3–4 mg/kg/d
- Niacinamide 500 mg t.i.d.
- Infliximab 5 mg/kg IV

ADDITIONAL TREATMENT

General Measures

GA is a self-limited, asymptomatic condition that is likely to regress spontaneously (4)[C]. The clinician's primary role after diagnosis is to educate the patient regarding the anticipated natural history and to provide reassurance.

Additional Therapies

- Fractional thermolysis (Er:YAG fractionated laser) (5)[B]
- Psoralen ultraviolet A (PUVA) (6)[B]
- Cryotherapy
- Surgical excision for SC GA

ONGOING CARE

FOLLOW-UP RECOMMENDATIONS

Routine follow-up is not required unless treatment is initiated. Then follow-up may be important to monitor for possible adverse effects associated with treatment.

PATIENT EDUCATION

The patient should be educated that GA is a benign, self-limited condition that may persist a long time, resolve, and/or recur.

PROGNOSIS

Many cases resolve spontaneously, though recurrence—typically at the original site—is common.

COMPLICATIONS

Complications of treatment are much more likely than complications from GA.

REFERENCES

1. Cyr PR. Diagnosis and management of granuloma annulare. *Am Fam Physician*. 2006;74(10): 1729–34.
2. Marcus DV. Mahmoud BH. Hamzavi IH. Granuloma annulare treated with rifampin, ofloxacin, and minocycline combination therapy. *Arch Dermatol*. 2009;145(7):787–9.
3. Plotner AN, Mutasim DF. Successful treatment of disseminated granuloma annulare with methotrexate. *Br J Dermatol*. 2010;163(5):1123–4.
4. Misago N, Narisawa Y. Subcutaneous granuloma annulare with overlying localized granuloma annulare. *J Dermatol*. 2010;37(8):755–7.
5. Liu A, Hexsel CL, Moy RL. Granuloma annulare successfully treated using fractional photothermolysis with a 1,550-nm erbium-doped yttrium aluminum garnet fractionated laser. *Dermatol Surg*. 2011;37(5):712–5.
6. Browne F, Turner D, Goulden V. Psoralen and ultraviolet A in the treatment of granuloma annulare. *Photodermatol Photoimmuno Photomed*. 2011;27(2):81–4.

ADDITIONAL READING

- Duarte AF, Mota A, et al. Generalized granuloma annulare—response to doxycycline. *J Eur Acad Dermat and Vener*. 2009;23:84–5.
- Mazzatenta C, Ghilardi A, Grazzini M. Treatment of disseminated granuloma annulare with allopurinol: Case report. *Dermatologic Therapy*. 2010;23:S24–7.
- Shanmuga SC, Rai R, Laila A, et al. Generalized granuloma annulare with tuberculoid granulomas: A rare histiopathologic variant. *Indian J Dermatol Venereol Leprol*. 2010;76(1):73–5.

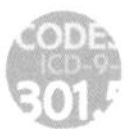

CODES

ICD9

695.89 Other specified erythematous conditions

CLINICAL PEARLS

This condition is benign. Most proposed treatments are not.

GRANULOMA, PYOGENIC

Albert Sohn, MD
Augustine J. Sohn, MD, MPH

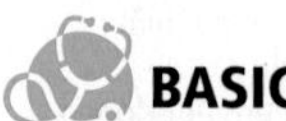

BASICS

DESCRIPTION

- Pyogenic granuloma are benign, acquired, solitary vascular proliferations that involve exposed areas of the skin such as the distal extremities (especially the hands) and face as well as oral cavity (most frequently the gingiva).
- Tendency to bleed easily due to the vascular nature of the lesion
- System(s) affected: Gastrointestinal; Skin (external ear canal)/Exocrine; Eye (i.e., eyelid, lacrimal sac)
- Synonym(s): Pregnancy tumor; Granuloma gravidum; Granuloma telangiectaticum; Lobular capillary hemangioma

EPIDEMIOLOGY

Mean age of patients with pyogenic granuloma is 40.5 years.

Incidence

- In children, pyogenic granuloma accounts for <1% of all skin nodules.
- 5% of pregnant women in the US are affected.

Prevalence

Relatively common condition

RISK FACTORS

- Pregnancy
- Trauma
- Intraoral trauma or surgery

GENERAL PREVENTION

Good oral hygiene

ETIOLOGY

- Thought to be an aberrant healing response to minor trauma in many cases
- May be related to hormonal changes in pregnancy
- Not caused by bacterial infection, but associated with capillary proliferation
- Not considered a hemangioma or neoplasm
- Associated with acute and chronic trauma, peripheral nerve injury, inflammatory systemic diseases, infection, drugs (systemic steroids, antiretroviral therapy, EGFR inhibitors) (1)

DIAGNOSIS

HISTORY

- Solitary lesion that develops rapidly from days to weeks after minor trauma
- Tends to bleed easily
- Grows early in pregnancy and partially regresses postpartum

PHYSICAL EXAM

- Most commonly located at head, neck, and upper extremities
- Among oral lesions, gingiva is the most common location
- Bright red, purple, yellow, or brown
- Moist and sometimes scaly-appearing surface
- Usually <1 cm, but ranges from a few millimeters to 2–3 cm in diameter
- Giant lesions may occur on areas such as the foot (rare)
- Soft; sessile or pedunculated
- Granular, smooth, or slightly nodular
- Solitary red papule, grows rapidly, forming a stalk, may bleed and ulcerate
- Red structureless areas surrounded by a white collarette intersected by white lines (2)[C]
- Erythematous, soft compressible papule with serosanguineous crusting and sharp demarcation

DIAGNOSTIC TESTS & INTERPRETATION

Lab

No labs are necessary for the diagnosis.

Diagnostic Procedures/Surgery

- Excisional biopsy
- Send for pathology

Pathological Findings

Microscopic examination reveals:

- Small, endothelial-lined vascular spaces
- Loose or dense connective tissue stroma
- Acute and chronic inflammatory cells
- No true granuloma formation
- Abundant mitotic activity
- Resembles granulation tissue in an edematous matrix, showing immature capillaries with interspersed tissue (3)[C]

DIFFERENTIAL DIAGNOSIS

- Peripheral ossifying granuloma
- Giant cell granuloma
- Odontogenic fibroma
- Kaposi sarcoma
- Malignant melanoma
- Angiolymphoid hyperplasia with eosinophilia
- Metastatic carcinoma
- Pilomatricoma
- In AIDS patients: Bacillary angiomatosis, deep mycoses
- Amelanotic/hypomelanotic melanoma (2)[C]

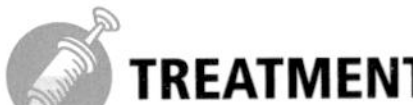

TREATMENT

MEDICATION

- Pyogenic granuloma that involve the nails may be treated with a 2–3-week course of a high-potency topical steroid under occlusion (e.g., clobetasol proprionate 0.05% ointment, betamethasone dipropionate 0.05% ointment, fluocinonide 0.1% cream) in the morning and topical antibiotic (2% mupirocin ointment) in the evening (4)[C].
- Small lesions can be cauterized without excision with topical silver nitrate; perform excisional biopsy if recurrent.

SURGERY/OTHER PROCEDURES

- Surgical excision with simple closure gives the best result with least recurrence (4)[C].
- Shave excision with cautery may be optimal treatment for a lesion on fingertips.
- Topical 5% imiquimod cream may be useful for children (5)[C].
- Electrosurgery (electrodesiccation and curettage)
- Topical 1.5% phenol solution may be used for periungual lesion (6)[C].
- CO_2-laser destruction
- Excision must be adequate to avoid recurrence. Even a small fragment of tissue left behind may lead to recurrence.
- Excisional biopsy should be tried in all situations if possible to ensure a proper diagnosis (i.e., not missing malignancies like amelanotic melanoma or basal cell carcinoma).

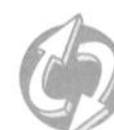

ONGOING CARE

PATIENT EDUCATION

Patient should avoid trauma to area following excision.

PROGNOSIS

- Some lesions spontaneously resolve on their own (usually within 6 months).
- Complete resolution is expected with adequate excision.

COMPLICATIONS

Recurrence: After removal or destruction of solitary lesion, multiple satellite lesions can form around original treatment site.

REFERENCES

1. Piraccini BM, Bellavista S, Misciali C, et al. Periungal and subungal pyogenic granuloma. *Br J Dermatol*. 2010;163(5):941–53.
2. Zalaudek I, Kreusch J, Giacomel J, et al. How to diagnose nonpigmented skin tumors: A review of vascular structures seen with dermoscopy: Part II. Nonmelanocytic skin tumors. *J Am Acad Dermatol*. 2010;63(3):377–86.
3. Greene AK, et al. Management of hemangiomas and other vascular tumors. *Clin Plast Surg*. 2011; 38:45–63.
4. Gilmore A, Kelsberg G, Safranek S, et al. Clinical inquiries. What's the best treatment for pyogenic granuloma? *J Fam Pract*. 2010;59:40–2.
5. Tritton SM, Smith S, Wong LC, et al. Pyogenic granuloma in ten children treated with topical imiquimod. *Pediatr Dermatol*. 2009;26(3):269–72.
6. Iglesias ME, DE Bengoa Vallejo RB, et al. Topical phenol as a conservative treatment for periungual pyogenic granuloma. *Dermatol Surg*. 2010;36(5): 675–8.

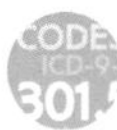

CODES

ICD9

- 522.6 Chronic apical periodontitis
- 528.9 Other and unspecified diseases of the oral soft tissues
- 686.1 Pyogenic granuloma of skin and subcutaneous tissue

CLINICAL PEARLS

- Benign, acquired, solitary vascular proliferation that involves exposed areas such as distal extremities and face as well as in the oral cavity
- Due mainly to aberrant healing response to minor trauma in many cases
- Excision must be adequate to avoid recurrence.
- Excisional biopsy recommended to ensure proper diagnosis (and to not miss a malignant lesion)
- Excision with primary closure or excision with cautery should be the first choice for treatment in most of the lesions.

GRAVES DISEASE

Katharine Barnard, MD

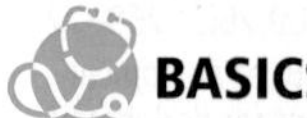

BASICS

DESCRIPTION

An autoimmune disease in which thyroid-stimulating antibodies cause increased thyroid function. The most common cause of hyperthyroidism. Classic findings are goiter and ophthalmopathy.

EPIDEMIOLOGY

Prevalence

- Overall prevalence of hyperthyroidism is estimated to be 2% for women and 0.2% for men.
- Graves disease accounts for 60–80% of all cases of hyperthyroidism.
- Predominant age: 30–40 years

RISK FACTORS

- Female sex (due to sex steroids)
- Postpartum period
- Stressful life events
- Medications: Iodine, amiodarone, lithium, highly active antiretroviral (HAART), rarely immune-modulating medications (i.e., interferon)
- Smoking (higher risk of developing ophthalmopathy)

Genetics

Higher risk with personal or family history of any autoimmune disease, especially Hashimoto thyroiditis

GENERAL PREVENTION

Screening thyroid-stimulating hormone (TSH) in asymptomatic patients is not recommended. No data conclusively show that treatment of subclinical thyroid dysfunction improves quality of life or clinical outcome measures (1).

PATHOPHYSIOLOGY

- Excessive production of TSH receptor antibodies from B cells primarily within the thyroid, likely due to genetic clonal lack of suppressor T cells
- Binding of these antibodies to TSH receptors in the thyroid causes increased production of thyroid hormone.
- Binding to similar antigen in retro-orbital connective tissue causes ocular symptoms.

COMMONLY ASSOCIATED CONDITIONS

- Mitral valve prolapse
- Hypokalemic periodic paralysis

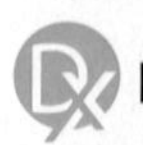

DIAGNOSIS

Thyroid hormone controls metabolic rate and affects many organ systems. Hyperthyroid patients appear hypermetabolic, with increased adrenergic tone.

HISTORY

- Tachycardia, palpitations
- Tremor, restlessness
- Anxiety, emotional lability, insomnia
- Sweating, heat intolerance
- Pruritus, skin changes
- Weight loss
- Fatigue, shortness of breath (due to muscle weakness)
- Oligo-/amenorrhea (women), erectile dysfunction (men), gynecomastia
- Loose, frequent stools
- Blurred vision or diplopia, lacrimation, photophobia, gritty sensation in eyes (ocular dryness), retro-orbital discomfort, painful eye movement, loss of color vision or visual acuity
- Worsening of chronic medical conditions (anxiety or bipolar disorder, glucose intolerance, heart failure or angina)

Geriatric Considerations

Elderly patients may not display classic symptoms; may present with atrial fibrillation or weight loss

PHYSICAL EXAM

- Thyroid: Enlarged, nontender, and without nodules; possible bruit (increased blood flow)
- Integumentary: Fine hair, warm skin, onycholysis of nails, palmar erythema, possible pretibial myxedema, possible hyperpigmented plaques (dermopathy)
- Cardiac: Resting tachycardia, hyperdynamic circulation, possible atrial fibrillation
- Ophthalmologic (present in 50% of cases): Lid lag, lid retraction, proptosis, corneal irritation, ophthalmoplegia; papilledema and loss of color vision may signify optic neuropathy
- Extremities: Tremor, hyperreflexia, proximal myopathy; rarely, soft tissue edema of extremities and clubbing of digits (acropachy)

DIAGNOSTIC TESTS & INTERPRETATION

Lab

Initial lab tests

- TSH is initial test. Very low or undetectable TSH confirms hyperthyroidism.
- Next, check T_4 level. T_4 will be high in Graves.

Pregnancy Considerations

TSH level at 36 weeks gestation is most predictive of neonatal hyperthyroidism. TSH and TRAb should be checked even in posttreatment pregnant patients taking thyroid hormone replacement. Infants of mothers with elevated TRAb in third trimester should be checked for hyperthyroidism after birth.

Imaging

Initial approach

After confirming suppressed TSH and high T_4, next step is radioactive iodine uptake (RAIU) and scan. Graves patients will have diffuse, elevated RAIU (vs. focal/nodular elevated uptake in adenoma and multinodular goiter, and decreased uptake in thyroiditis).

DIFFERENTIAL DIAGNOSIS

- Toxic multinodular goiter (multiple hormone-producing nodules)
- Toxic adenoma (single hormone-producing nodule)
- Thyroiditis (hormone leakage):
  - Subacute, usually postviral (thyroid will be tender)
  - Lymphocytic, including postpartum
  - Hashimoto thyroiditis (anti-TPO antibodies may stimulate TSH receptors)
- Iatrogenic (treatment-induced):
  - Iodine-induced (dietary, radiographic contrast, or medications)
  - Amiodarone
  - Thyroid hormone overreplacement (accidental or intentional)
- Tumor:
  - Pituitary adenoma producing TSH
  - Human chorionic gonadotropin (HCG)-producing tumors (stimulate TSH receptors)
  - Extraglandular thyroid hormone production (i.e., struma ovarii or metastatic thyroid cancer)

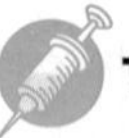

TREATMENT

MEDICATION

Goal of therapy is to correct the hypermetabolic state with the fewest side effects and lowest incidence of posttreatment hypothyroidism.

First Line

Radioactive iodine:

- Concentrates in the thyroid gland and destroys thyroid tissue
- Treatment of choice in the US for Graves disease
- High cure rate with single treatment, especially with high-dose regimen
- Risks: Side effects (neck soreness, flushing, decreased taste); worsening ophthalmopathy (15% incidence, higher in smokers); posttreatment hypothyroidism (80% incidence, not dosage-dependent); radiation thyroiditis (1% incidence); need to adhere to safety precautions until radiation is eliminated from the body.
- May worsen Graves orbitopathy (GO). Treatment for patients with moderate-to-severe GO is still guided by expert opinion pending further study (3).
- Pretreatment with antithyroid medication should be considered in patients with severe disease as symptom control and to reduce risk of posttreatment radiation thyroiditis. Pretreatment may, however, reduce cure rate with radioactive iodine, so is not uniformly recommended.
- May be repeated in as soon as 4 months if needed

Pregnancy Considerations

- Antithyroid drugs: Methimazole (MMI) and propylthiouracil (PTU):
  - Compete with the thyroid for iodine, thereby decreasing the synthesis of thyroid hormone; PTU also blocks peripheral conversion of T_4 to T_3
  - Treatment of choice for children and for adults who refuse radioactive iodine
  - May use as pretreatment (symptom control) for older or cardiac patients before radioactive iodine or surgery
  - MMI is usually first choice due to lower cost and once-daily dosing; additionally, the risk of hepatocellular inflammation (30%) and severe liver damage (0.1%) with PTU make it second-line to MMI for most patients (4).
  - No improvement in remission rates noted with higher-dose MMI; therefore, lowest effective dose should be used (5).

- Minor side effects (<5% incidence), which may be controlled by switching from one agent to another: Rash, fever, arthralgias, GI side effects
- Major side effects, which necessitate a change in treatment:
  - Polyarthritis (1–2%)
  - Agranulocytosis (<0.5%)
  - Cholestasis and jaundice (occurs rarely with MMI)
- Discontinue treatment after 1 year if patient is euthyroid and thyroid-stimulating antibody level is undetectable.
- 60% remission rate with 2 years of treatment (standard regimen); newer studies suggest no increased benefit to treatment beyond 18 months (6).
- Relapse rate of up to 50% in patients who respond initially; higher relapse rate if smoker, large goiter, or positive thyroid-stimulating antibodies at the end of treatment

- PTU is preferred in first trimester of pregnancy due to teratogenic effects of MMI. Switch to PTU in second and third trimester due to risk of hepatotoxicity (7).

Second Line

Plasmapheresis is under investigation as a treatment option (8), as is rituximab (immune modulator) for thyroid eye disease (9).

ADDITIONAL TREATMENT

Issues for Referral

- Endocrinologist for radioactive iodine therapy; if pregnant or breast-feeding patient
- Graves ophthalmopathy
- Surgery if failed drug therapy, or refusing RAI; obstruction or cosmesis

Additional Therapies

- Beta-blockers provide prompt control of adrenergic symptoms; start while workup is in progress. Long-acting propranolol is used most commonly and titrated to symptom control (40–320 mg daily). Calcium channel blockers are an alternative for heart rate control in patients who cannot take beta-blockers (8).
- Symptom control may be achieved with iodides, which block conversion of T_4 to T_3, and inhibit TSH release. Use for pregnant patients who do not tolerate antithyroid medication, or in conjunction with antithyroid medications. Should not be used long-term (may cause paradoxical increase in TSH release) or in combination with radioactive iodine.
- For corneal protection: Tinted glasses when outdoors, artificial tears, patching or taping the lids at night
- For orbitopathy: Moderate-to-severe cases should be treated with pulse-dose IV glucocorticoid, if patient does not have contraindication (10). Alternative is oral steroid (prednisone 60–80 mg daily for 2–4 weeks, then tapered off).
- For dermopathy, if local discomfort at site of plaques: Topical corticosteroid

SURGERY/OTHER PROCEDURES

Subtotal thyroidectomy preserves some thyroid function and only holds 25% postop incidence of hypothyroidism, but has less predictable outcome; therefore, total thyroidectomy is now standard of care (9).

IN-PATIENT CONSIDERATIONS

Indications for hospital admission:

- Thyroid storm (rare but life-threatening complication). Admit to intensive care unit (ICU) for symptom control and antithyroid medications.
- Ophthalmopathy with visual impairment. Admit with ophthalmology consult.
- Severe cardiac symptoms (congestive heart failure [CHF], rapid atrial fibrillation, angina). Admit for rate control and cardiology consult.

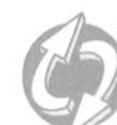

ONGOING CARE

FOLLOW-UP RECOMMENDATIONS

Patient Monitoring

- Monitoring is for resolution of hyperthyroidism and for development of hypothyroidism.
- Check TSH and T_4 levels every 1–2 months for first 6 months after treatment, then every 3 months for a year, then every 6–12 months thereafter. For patients on treatment with PTU and MMI, check anti-TSH receptor antibodies at 12 months of treatment to determine possibility of discontinuing medication.

Pregnancy Considerations

Postpartum exacerbation of hyperthyroidism is common for women not currently under treatment, so TSH and symptoms should be monitored.

DIET

Nutritional supplementation with L-carnitine may diminish hyperthyroid symptoms and may decrease bone demineralization (10).

PATIENT EDUCATION

Adherence to follow-up (surveillance) recommendations and medication regimens are the most important ways to achieve a good outcome and promote lifelong health.

PROGNOSIS

- Generally good with treatment
- May have irreversible ocular, cardiac, and psychiatric consequences
- Increased morbidity and mortality due to osteoporosis, atherosclerotic disease, insulin resistance and obesity, and endothelial cell dysfunction (thromboembolic risk) (8,11)

COMPLICATIONS

Hypothyroidism is most common consequence of treatment (25–80% depending on treatment modality). Patients should be monitored annually, even if asymptomatic.

REFERENCES

1. Helfand M, U.S. Preventive Services Task Force. Screening for subclinical thyroid dysfunction in nonpregnant adults: A summary of the evidence for the U.S. Preventive Services Task Force. *Ann Intern Med*. 2004;140:128–41.
2. Rivkees SA, Dinauer C. An optimal treatment for pediatric graves' disease is radioiodine. *J Clin Endocrinol Metab*. 2007;92:797–800.
3. Bartalena L. The dilemma of how to manage Graves' hyperthyroidism in patients with associated orbitopathy. *J Clin Endocrinol Metab*. 2011;96(3):592–9.
4. Cooper DS, Rivkees SA. Putting Propylthiouracil in perspective. *J Clin Endocrinol Metab*. 2009; 94(6):1881–2.
5. Benker G, Reinwein D. Is there a methimazole dose effect on remission rate in Graves disease? Results from a longterm prospective study. *Clin Endocrinol*. 2004;49(4).
6. Maugendre D, Gatel A. Antithyroid drugs and Graves disease—prospective randomized assessment of long-term treatment. *Clin Endocrinol*. 2004;50(1).
7. Lazarus JH, et al. Thyroid function in pregnancy. *Br Med Bull*. 2011;97:137–48.
8. Reid JR, Wheeler SF. Hyperthyroidism: Diagnosis and treatment. *Am Fam Physician*. 2005;72: 623–30.
9. Silkiss RZ, Reier A, Coleman M, et al. Rituximab for thyroid eye disease. *Ophthal Plast Reconstr Surg*. 2010;26(5):310–4.
10. Zang S, Ponto KA, Kahaly GJ. Clinical review: Intravenous glucocorticoids for Graves' orbitopathy: Efficacy and morbidity. *J Clin Endocrinol Metab*. 2011;96(2):320–2.
11. Barakate MS, Agarwal G. Total thyroidectomy is now the preferred option for the surgical management of Graves disease. *ANZ J Surg*. 2002;72(5).
12. Benvenga S, Ruggeri RM, Russo A, et al. Usefulness of L-carnitine, a naturally occurring peripheral antagonist of thyroid hormone action, in iatrogenic hyperthyroidism: A randomized, double-blind, placebo-controlled clinical trial. *J Clin Endocrinol Metab*. 2001;86:3579–94.
13. Burggraaf J, Lalezari S, Emeis JJ, et al. Endothelial function in patients with hyperthyroidism before and after treatment with propranolol and thiamazole. *Thyroid*. 2001;11:153–60.

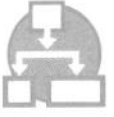

See Also (Topic, Algorithm, Electronic Media Element)

Algorithms: Anxiety; Cardiac Arrhythmias; Weight Loss

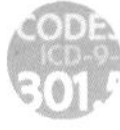

CODES

ICD9

- 242.00 Toxic diffuse goiter without mention of thyrotoxic crisis or storm
- 242.01 Toxic diffuse goiter with mention of thyrotoxic crisis or storm

CLINICAL PEARLS

Thyroid hormone controls metabolic rate and affects many organ systems. Hyperthyroid patients appear hypermetabolic, with symptoms and signs of increased adrenergic tone.

G

GROWTH HORMONE DEFICIENCY

Vibin Roy, MD
Manjula Julka, MD, FAAFP

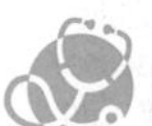

BASICS

DESCRIPTION

- Inadequate production of growth hormone (GH, also called *somatotropin*) in either adults or children.
- GH is a polypeptide hormone that stimulates growth and cell reproduction.
- Hypopituitarism is often used to describe growth hormone deficiency (GHD). However, hypopituitarism is actually defined as GHD plus a deficiency in at least one other anterior pituitary hormone.
- Panhypopituitarism is defined as a deficiency in all the hormones produced in the pituitary gland.
- System(s) affected: Endocrine; Musculoskeletal
- Synonym(s): Hypopituitarism

EPIDEMIOLOGY

Incidence

- Most common cause of GHD in children is idiopathic
- Most common cause of GHD in adults is a pituitary adenoma or treatment of the adenoma with surgery or radiotherapy:
  - 76% of patients with GHD had a pituitary tumor.
  - 13% had an extrapituitary tumor
  - 8% the cause was unknown
  - 1% had sarcoidosis
  - 0.5% had Sheehan syndrome

Prevalence

- In children, isolated GHD has been reported to affect 1 in 4,000.
- Adult-onset idiopathic GHD is extremely rare.

RISK FACTORS

Genetics

A variety of congenital genetic causes of GHD:

- Transcription factor defects (POU1F1/PIT-1, PROP-1, LHX3/4, HESX-1, and PITX-2)
- GHRH receptor gene defects
- GH secretagogue receptor gene defects
- GH gene defects
- GH receptor/postreceptor defects
- Prader-Willi syndrome
- Deletion and mutation of GH-1

PATHOPHYSIOLOGY

- GHD is caused by a complete lack of GH production or a decline in GH production. Causes can be genetic or acquired.
- Hypothalamus secretes GH-releasing hormone (GHRH), which stimulates the pituitary to secrete GH. Somatostatin is secreted by the hypothalamus to inhibit GH secretion. When GH pulses are secreted into the blood, then insulinlike growth factor (IGF)-1 is released. GHD may result from disruption of the GH axis at numerous places—in the higher brain, the hypothalamus, or the pituitary gland.

ETIOLOGY

- Congenital:
  - Genetic (see "Genetics")
  - Structural brain defects:
    - Agenesis of corpus callosum
    - Septo-optic dysplasia
    - Empty-sella syndrome
    - Encephalocele
    - Hydrocephalus
    - Arachnoid cyst
  - Associated midline facial defects:
    - Single central incisor
    - Cleft lip/palate
- Acquired:
  - Trauma:
    - Perinatal
    - Postnatal
  - CNS infection
  - Tumors of hypothalamus or pituitary:
    - Pituitary adenoma
    - Craniopharyngioma
    - Rathke cleft cyst
    - Glioma/astrocytoma
    - Germinoma
    - Metastatic
  - Cranial irradiation
  - Pituitary infarction
  - Surgery

COMMONLY ASSOCIATED CONDITIONS

- Macroadenoma
- Sarcoidosis
- Sheehan syndrome

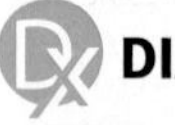

DIAGNOSIS

HISTORY

- Adults:
  - Fatigue
  - Muscle weakness
  - Depression
  - Social withdrawal
  - Poor memory
  - Loss of strength and/or stamina
  - Reduced physical performance
- Children:
  - Poor height velocity, slower muscular development and delayed gross motor milestones such as standing, walking, and jumping
  - Important questions to ask:
    - Birth weight and length
    - Previous growth points
    - Nutritional history
    - General health of child
    - Height of parents
    - Timing of puberty in parents

PHYSICAL EXAM

- Children with GHD:
  - Most common presentation is short stature and drop-off in height on the growth curve:
    - Strong suspicion if more than 2.5 SD below mean (corresponds to <0.5 percentile) for height (for chronological, age, sex, and background) and/or height velocity more than 2 SD below mean (corresponds to approximately less than third percentile) (1)
  - Newborns may present with hypoglycemia, prolonged jaundice, or micropenis.
  - Severe GHD children have maxillary hypoplasia and forehead prominence.
  - Accurately measure height and weight.
  - Assess pubertal status using Tanner staging system.
- Adults:
  - Decreased lean body mass
  - Poor bone density
  - Abnormal labs:
    - Altered lipid metabolism
    - Increased insulin resistance

DIAGNOSTIC TESTS & INTERPRETATION

Lab

Initial lab tests

- IGF-1, IGFBP-3
- Multiple GH levels
- Thyroid-stimulating hormone (TSH): Hypothyroidism should be excluded as a cause and thyroxine should be adequately replaced prior to testing for deficiency
- Serum electrolytes (low bicarbonate levels may indicate renal tubular acidosis)
- CBC and ESR
- Karyotype (in females to rule out Turner syndrome)

Follow-Up & Special Considerations

- Testing for GHD by random measurement of GH in a single blood sample is not beneficial, as GH is nearly undetectable for most of the day.
- In children, evaluate those who have significant discrepancy in growth curve (see "Physical Exam").
- Low levels of IGF-1 and IGF binding protein (IGFBP)-3
- Multiple blood-sample testing for GH levels
- GHD is effectively excluded in children with normal bone age and height velocity.

Imaging

Initial approach

Radiograph of hand and wrist to determine skeletal age in children

Follow-Up & Special Considerations

Brain MRI to evaluate for a tumor may be ordered.

Diagnostic Procedures/Surgery

Provocative tests should be done after abnormal levels of IGF-1 or IGFBP-3 are obtained and if they are not explicable by undernutrition:

- Give a dose of an agent that in a normal person causes a surge in the release of GH: Common agents used include arginine, clonidine, glucagons, insulin, levodopa, and propranolol (2)[C].
- After agent is given, GH serum levels are drawn every 15 minutes.
- GH levels are checked for over 60 minutes.
- Note the Insulin Tolerance Test is considered the gold standard in adults by American Association of Clinical Endocrinologists (AACE).

DIFFERENTIAL DIAGNOSIS

- Turner syndrome
- Renal failure
- Small size for gestational age in newborns
- Prader-Willi syndrome
- Idiopathic short stature
- Noonan syndrome
- Russell-Silver syndrome
- Down syndrome

TREATMENT

MEDICATION

- GHD is treated with GH replacement.
- Recombinant human growth hormone (rhGH) was first approved for childhood GHD in 1985.
- The recommended rhGH dose for children in the US is 0.175–0.35 mg/kg/wk with 0.3 mg/kg/wk being most commonly used. Stepwise increase during pubertal stages has been shown to improve growth velocity (3)[C].
- The rhGH therapy for GHD adults offers significant clinical benefits in body composition including skeletal integrity, lipids, quality of life, and exercise capacity. The dosing plans have evolved from weight-based to individualized dose-titration strategies based on age, gender, estrogen status, IGF-I levels, appropriate clinical response and avoidance of side effects (4)[C].
- Geref (sermorelin) has been removed from the market. It is a synthetic growth hormone-releasing hormone.
- Several growth hormone-releasing peptides (GHRPs) or nonpeptide analogs are to be evaluated in children and adults. It is too early to evaluate their long-term safety and efficacy.

ADDITIONAL TREATMENT

Issues for Referral

Patients with GHD would benefit from a referral to an endocrinologist.

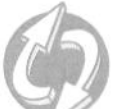

ONGOING CARE

FOLLOW-UP RECOMMENDATIONS

- Children: Regular follow-up with a pediatric endocrinologist
- Adults: Follow-up with an endocrinologist is recommended.

DIET

No restrictions

PROGNOSIS

- In children, the prognosis for GHD is good. GH therapy is effective.
- 5 independent predictors of pubertal growth:
  - Gender
  - Age at onset of puberty
  - Age at end of growth
  - Dose of growth hormone at onset of puberty
  - Deviation of target height from height at onset of puberty

COMPLICATIONS

- In children:
  - Slipped capital femoral epiphysis
  - Scoliosis
- In adults and children:
  - Metabolic effects
  - Antibodies to growth hormone
  - Cancer: Lymphoma, tumor recurrence
  - Fluid retention: Pseudotumor cerebri, carpal tunnel syndrome, pancreatitis, and edema

REFERENCES

1. Richmond EJ, Rogol AD, et al. Growth hormone deficiency in children. *Pituitary*. 2008;11:115–20.
2. Molich ME, et al. Clinical practice guideline: Evaluation and treatment of adult growth hormone deficiency. An endocrine society clinical practice guideline. *J Clin Endocrinol Metabol*. 2006;91: 1621–34.
3. Miller BS, et al. rhGH safety and efficacy update. *Adv Pediatr*. 2011;58:207–41.
4. Molitch ME, Clemmons DR, Malozowski S, et al. Evaluation and treatment of adult growth hormone deficiency: An Endocrine Society clinical practice guideline. *J Clin Endocrinol Metab*. 2011;96: 1587–609.

ADDITIONAL READING

- Cook D, et al. American Association of Clinical Endocrinologists Medical Guidelines for Clinical Practice for Growth Hormone Use in Growth Hormone-Deficient Adults and Transition Patients - 2009 Update. *AACE Guidelines*. 2009.
- Frohman LA, et al. Controversy about treatment of growth hormone-deficient adults: A commentary. *Ann Intern Med*. 2002;137:202–4.
- Hoffman AR, et al. Efficacy and tolerability of an individualized dosing regimen for adult growth hormone replacement therapy in comparison with fixed body weight-based dosing. *J Clin Endocrinol Metabol*. 2004;87:1974–9.

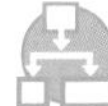

See Also (Topic, Algorithm, Electronic Media Element)

Pituitary Adenoma

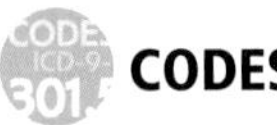

CODES

ICD9

- 253.2 Panhypopituitarism
- 253.3 Pituitary dwarfism

CLINICAL PEARLS

- Most common cause of GHD in children is idiopathic
- Most common cause of GHD in adults is pituitary adenoma
- Short stature and poor growth velocity are most common presentations of childhood GHD.
- Patients taking replacement GH therapy should have periodic monitoring for both adverse effects and physiologic benefits in addition to IGF-I levels.

G

GUILLAIN-BARRÉ SYNDROME

Amanda Westlake, MD
David Anthony, MD, MSc

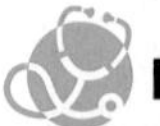

BASICS

DESCRIPTION

- A group of acquired autoimmune disorders causing acute peripheral neuropathy.
- Subtypes classified by pattern of neural injury:
  - Acute inflammatory demyelinating polyradiculoneuropathy (AIDP): Accounts for about 95% of cases in Europe and North America. Progressive limb weakness with areflexia.
  - Axonal injury: Accounts for about 5% of cases in Europe and North America, but 30–47% of cases in China, Japan, Central and South America:
    - *Acute motor axonal neuropathy (AMAN):* Pure motor neuropathy.
    - *Acute motor-sensory axonal neuropathy (AMSAN):* Combined motor-sensory neuropathy. Poor prognosis.
  - Miller Fisher Syndrome (MFS): Rare disorder. Ophthalmoplegia, ataxia, and areflexia.
- In Guillain-Barré Syndrome (GBS) symptoms progress for up to 4 weeks. This distinguishes it from subacute and chronic inflammatory demyelinating polyradiculoneuropathy (CIDP), in which the onset phase lasts 4–8 weeks or >8 weeks, respectively.
- Synonyms: GBS, Acute inflammatory demyelinating polyneuropathy; Landry-Guillain-Barré-Strohl syndrome; Acute inflammatory polyneuropathy; Idiopathic polyneuritis; Acute autoimmune neuropathy; Landry ascending paralysis

ALERT

25–30% of patients have respiratory paralysis. Rapidly progressive forms may cause quadriplegia and a need for mechanical ventilation within 48 hours.

ALERT

Absent reflexes are a red flag for GBS in patients with rapidly progressive limb weakness.

ALERT

A history of weakness preceded by respiratory or GI infection suggests GBS.

EPIDEMIOLOGY

Incidence

In the US: 1.8/100,000 (0.8/100,000 in children <18 years of age; 3.2/100,000 in adults >60 years of age)

Prevalence

- In the US: 3–10/100,000
- Male > Female (1.5:1)

PATHOPHYSIOLOGY

Autoimmune disorder targeted against myelin and/or axons causing destruction of peripheral nerves in susceptible individuals

ETIOLOGY

Leading hypothesis is that pathogenesis involves molecular mimicry (i.e., invoking an immune response to antigenic targets that are coincidentally shared by infectious organisms and peripheral nerve tissue).

COMMONLY ASSOCIATED CONDITIONS

- 2/3 of cases associated with antecedent bacterial or viral infection, usually of the respiratory or GI tract:
  - *Campylobacter jejuni:* The most common precipitant of GBS, seen in 21–32% of cases:
    - Associated with axonal degeneration, slower recovery, more severe residual disability
  - *Cytomegalovirus:* Primary CMV infection precedes 10–22% of cases
  - Also associated w/*Mycoplasma pneumoniae* (5%), influenza, Epstein-Barr virus, varicella zoster virus, and HIV infections
- Influenza vaccinations:
  - Risk of GBS following influenza infection 40–70 times greater than risk following seasonal influenza vaccine
  - Based on 1992–1994 data, inactivated seasonal flu vaccines are associated with a marginally significant, very small increase in the risk of GBS equivalent to about one case per million vaccines above background incidence. There was a steady decline in the number of cases of GBS associated with influenza vaccine in the US between 1993–94 (0.17 per 100,000 vaccinations) and 2002–03 (0.04 per 100,000).
  - *Of historical importance:* Increased incidence during 1976 US national immunization program against swine-origin influenza A H1N1 subtype A/NJ/76; vaccine attributable risk 8.8 per million recipients

DIAGNOSIS

HISTORY

- AIDP presents as an acute neuropathy, defined as progressive onset of limb weakness that reaches its worst within 4 weeks; 73% of patients reach a nadir of clinical function at 1 week.
- 2/3 of patients have had an antecedent infection, commonly a respiratory illness or gastroenteritis, within the previous 6 weeks (1)[C].
- Earliest symptoms are pain, numbness, paresthesias, or limb weakness. Numbness and paresthesias affect the extremities and spread proximally.
- Pain present in the majority, most commonly in the back and lower extremities; may be severe (2).
- A purely sensory syndrome, without weakness, excludes GBS.

PHYSICAL EXAM

- Diagnostic criteria for typical GBS (1)[C]:
  - Features required for diagnosis:
    - Progressive weakness of >1 limb
    - Areflexia
  - Features strongly supporting diagnosis:
    - Progression within 4 weeks
    - Relative symmetry
    - Mild sensory symptoms or signs
    - Cranial nerve involvement, especially bilateral weakness of facial muscles
    - Recovery beginning within 4 weeks after progression ceases
    - Autonomic dysfunction
    - Absence of fever at onset
    - Elevated CSF protein
    - CSF mononuclear leukocyte count $<10/\text{mm}^3$
    - Typical electrodiagnostic findings, including nerve conduction slowing or block

DIAGNOSTIC TESTS & INTERPRETATION

Lab

Initial lab tests

- Studies related to establishing the diagnosis:
  - CSF: Increase in CSF protein (>0.55 g/L) without pleocytosis (i.e., albuminocytologic dissociation). Elevated protein present in about 80% of patients but often normal within first 48 hours of symptom onset (1)[C]:
    - CSF should be analyzed before treatment with IVIg, which can cause aseptic meningitis.
  - Nerve conduction study: *The most useful confirmatory test;* conduction velocities abnormal in 85% of patients with demyelination, even early in the disease. If nondiagnostic, repeat after 1–2 weeks.
- Studies related to understanding causation:
  - Stool culture and serology for *C. jejuni*
  - Acute and convalescent serology for CMV, EBV, and *M. pneumoniae*
  - Stool culture for polio virus in pure motor syndromes
  - Anti-GQ1b antibodies in Miller Fisher variant

Follow-Up & Special Considerations

If indicated, labs targeted at specific differential diagnoses

Imaging

Initial approach

Imaging is not generally required as the diagnosis may be established based on clinical criteria, CSF analysis, and nerve conduction studies.

Diagnostic Procedures/Surgery

Sural nerve biopsy not indicated unless necessary to rule out vasculitis or amyloidosis.

DIFFERENTIAL DIAGNOSIS

Differential diagnosis of acute flaccid paralysis:

- Brain: Basilar artery stroke, brainstem encephalitis
- Spinal cord: Transverse myelitis, cord compression
- Motor neuron: Poliomyelitis
- Peripheral neuropathy other than GBS: Vasculitis, critical illness polyneuropathy, infectious (e.g., diphtheria, Lyme), CIDP, acute intermittent porphyria
- Neuromuscular junction: Myasthenia gravis, Eaton-Lambert, botulism, toxins (e.g., heavy metals, inhalant abuse, organophosphates)
- Muscle: Electrolyte disturbance (hypokalemia, hypophosphatemia), inflammatory myopathy, critical illness myopathy, acute rhabdomyolysis, trichonosis, periodic paralysis
- Psychological cause of weakness

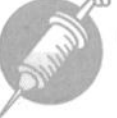

TREATMENT

MEDICATION

First Line

- Plasma exchange (PE):
  - Compared with supportive treatment, patients treated with plasma exchange fare significantly better in terms of time to recover walking, requirement for artificial ventilation, duration of artificial ventilation, full muscle strength recovery, and severe sequelae at 1 year (3)[A].
  - In mild GBS, 2 sessions of PE are superior to none. In moderate GBS, 4 sessions are superior to 2. In severe GBS, 6 sessions are not significantly better than 4 (3)[A].
  - More beneficial if started within 7 days of disease onset, but still beneficial at up to 30 days (3)[A].
  - Value of plasma exchange in children <12 is not known.
- IV immunoglobulin (IVIg) 0.4 g/kg/d for 5 days:
  - In severe disease, IVIg started within 2 weeks from onset hastens recovery as much as plasma exchange (4)[A].
  - In children, IVIg probably hastens recovery compared with supportive care alone (4)[B].
  - IVIg and plasma exchange are equally effective and associated with similar rates of adverse events. IVIg may be preferred due to convenience of administration (4)[A].
  - Treatment with IVIg after plasma exchange does not confer additional benefit compared with either treatment alone (4)[A].

Second Line

Corticosteroids given alone do not significantly hasten recovery from GBS or affect the long-term outcome (5)[A].

ADDITIONAL TREATMENT

General Measures

Pain: Both gabapentin and carbamazepine have been shown to decrease opiate requirements in patients with GBS. One study found gabapentin 300 mg t.i.d. superior to carbamazepine 100 mg t.i.d. in terms of pain control and need for supplementary analgesia. Opiates used with caution as risk of ileus already increased (2)[B].

IN-PATIENT CONSIDERATIONS

Initial Stabilization

- 25–30% of patients will require mechanical ventilation, yet classic signs of respiratory distress occur too late to serve as guidelines for management. Serial measurement of vital capacity (VC) and static inspiratory and expiratory pressures (PImax and PEmax) are the most useful parameters for evaluating respiratory compromise.
- Predictors of respiratory failure include rapid disease progression (≥3 days between onset of weakness and hospital admission), the presence of facial and/or bulbar weakness, VC <20 mL/kg, VC decrease >30% and Medical Research Council (MRC) sum score indicating muscle weakness (6)[B].
- Monitor closely for complications of autonomic dysfunction (e.g., hyper/hypotension, tachy/bradyarrhythmias, urinary retention, ileus).

Admission Criteria

- Admit any patient suspected of having GBS.
- Mildly affected patients who remain capable of walking unaided and are stable for more than 2 weeks are unlikely to progress and may be managed as outpatients.

Nursing

- Prevent complications of immobilization with graduated compression stockings and SC heparin.
- Respiratory care, aspiration precautions, and frequent turning
- Monitor bowel and bladder function for urinary retention and ileus.

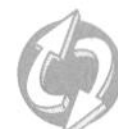

ONGOING CARE

FOLLOW-UP RECOMMENDATIONS

Patient Monitoring

- Pulmonary function testing (vital capacity, respiratory frequency) every 2–6 hours in the progressive phase and every 6–12 hours in the plateau phase (6)
- Monitor bulbar weakness and airway secretions.
- Telemetry in patients with severe disease

PATIENT EDUCATION

Important to emphasize expectation of full or significant recovery and explain phases of illness

PROGNOSIS

- If untreated, 3 phases of illness:
  - Initial progression phase up to 4 weeks; highest risk of death and complication during this phase
  - Variable plateau phase
  - Recovery phase (weeks–months): return of proximal followed by distal strength
- Mortality estimates range from 4–15% in all patients and up to 20% in those requiring mechanical ventilation. Major causes of death include sepsis, ARDS, pulmonary emboli, and arrhythmias.
- Around 80% achieve functional recovery within 6–12 months. Recovery is maximal at 18 months past onset.
- Up to 20% have residual disability at 1 year; neurologic sequelae include bilateral footdrop, intrinsic hand muscle wasting, sensory ataxia, and dysesthesia.
- Factors associated with poor functional outcome include age >60 years, rapid disease progression, severe disease indicated by GBS disability score or MRC sum score, preceding diarrhea, positive *C. jejuni* or CMV serology, axonal degeneration, and need for mechanical ventilation (6).

REFERENCES

1. Ropper AH, et al. The Guillain-Barré syndrome. *N Engl J Med*. 1992;326:1130–6.
2. Pandey CK, Raza M, Tripathi M, et al. The comparative evaluation of gabapentin and carbamazepine for pain management in Guillain-Barré syndrome patients in the intensive care unit. *Anesth Analg*. 2005;101:220–5, table of contents.
3. Raphael JC, Chevret S, Hughes RA, et al. Plasma exchange for Guillain-Barré syndrome. *Cochrane Database Syst Rev*. 2002;(2):CD001798.
4. Hughes RA, Swan AV, van Doorn PA. Intravenous immunoglobulin for Guillain-Barré syndrome. *Cochrane Database Syst Rev*. 2010;(6):CD002063.
5. Hughes RA, Swan AV, van Doorn PA. Corticosteroids for Guillain-Barré syndrome. *Cochrane Database Syst Rev*. 2010;(2):CD001446.
6. Walgaard C, Lingsma HF, Ruts L, et al. Prediction of respiratory insufficiency in Guillain-Barré syndrome. *Ann Neurol*. 2010;67(6):781–7.

ADDITIONAL READING

- Asbury AK, Cornblath DR, et al. Assessment of current diagnostic criteria for Guillain-Barré syndrome. *Ann Neurol*. 1990;27(Suppl):S21–4.
- Deeks SL, Lim GH, Simpson MA, et al. Estimating background rates of Guillain Barre Syndrome in Ontario in order to respond to safety concerns during pandemic H1N1/09 immunization campaign. *BMC Public Health*. 2011;11:329.
- Hughes RA, Cornblath DR, et al. Guillain-Barré syndrome. *Lancet*. 2005;366:1653–66.
- Lehmann HC, Hartung HP, Kieseier BC, et al. Guillain-Barré syndrome after exposure to influenza virus. *Lancet Infect Dis*. 2010;10:643–51.
- Newswanger DL, Warren CR, et al. Guillain-Barré syndrome. *Am Fam Physician*. 2004;69:2405–10.
- Orlikowski D, Prigent H, Sharshar T, et al. Respiratory dysfunction in Guillain-Barré syndrome. *Neurocrit Care*. 2004;1:415–22.
- Winer JB, et al. Guillain-Barre syndrome. *BMJ*. 2008;337:a671.

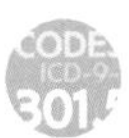

CODES

ICD9

- 357.0 Acute infective polyneuritis
- 357.82 Critical illness polyneuropathy

CLINICAL PEARLS

- The natural history of GBS is to resolve, and treatment with IVIg or plasma exchange speeds rate of recovery and reduces disability.
- The most useful diagnostic tests are lumbar puncture and nerve conduction studies.
- If GBS is suspected, initial evaluation must include measurement of vital capacity and inspiratory force to evaluate respiratory compromise.

GYNECOMASTIA

Timothy L. Black, MD

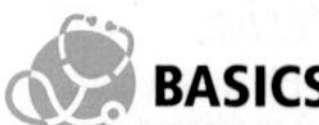

BASICS

DESCRIPTION
- Benign glandular enlargement of male breast that is generally bilateral (may be asymmetric or unilateral):
  - Type 1: Benign adolescent hypertrophy; physiologic discoid subacute mass
  - Type 2: Physiologic gynecomastia; generalized enlargement to greater degree
  - Type 3: Simulated by obesity
  - Type 4: Pectoral muscle hypertrophy
- System(s) affected: Endocrine/Metabolic; Skin/Exocrine
- Synonym(s): Male breast hypertrophy

EPIDEMIOLOGY
- Predominant age: Puberty; >65 years of age (especially with weight gain)
- Predominant sex: Male only

Pediatric Considerations
Transient gynecomastia is seen in neonatal boys.

Geriatric Considerations
Drug-induced form is more common in geriatric patients.

Prevalence
- 38–64% of pubertal males may have mild form. Usual onset is 11–12 years of age, with resolution by age 16–17 years.
- Nonpubertal forms are rare except when drug-induced.

RISK FACTORS
- Obesity
- Liver disease
- Renal disease
- Recovery from prolonged severe illness associated with malnutrition and weight loss (refeeding gynecomastia)
- Multiple therapeutic as well as nontherapeutic drugs (e.g., spironolactone, cimetidine, ranitidine, omeprazole, isoniazid, ketoconazole, amlodipine, captopril, diltiazem, enalapril, nifedipine, verapamil, diazepam, haloperidol, digitalis, statin drugs, anabolic steroids, androgens, estrogens, growth hormone, amphetamines, heroin, methadone, marijuana, and ethanol, among others) (1)
- Family history

Genetics
Some instances of familial gynecomastia may be inherited as male-limited autosomal trait

GENERAL PREVENTION
In men taking estrogen for prostate cancer: Low-dose radiation prior to institution of diethylstilbestrol

PATHOPHYSIOLOGY
The cause of pubertal gynecomastia is not clear (2)[C]:
- May be related to transient imbalance of androgens and estrogens
- May be related to higher leptin levels (may result in altered local estrogen levels)

ETIOLOGY
- Physiologic: Transient in neonatal boys and at puberty:
  - 60–90% of newborn males develop transient breast enlargement related to transplacental estrogen.
  - In pubertal boys, may require 1–3 years to regress or may not regress at all
  - Men age 60–90 years may develop gynecomastia related to declining levels of testosterone.
- Exposure to a high level of estrogen compared with testosterone concentration
- Identifiable syndrome/cause found in 12% of pubertal boys (3)[C]
- Tumors: Estrogen-secreting, gonadotropin-secreting, prolactin-secreting pituitary adenomas, hepatic fibrolamellar carcinoma
- Drugs (10–25% of gynecomastia) (1): Hormones, marijuana, digitalis, spironolactone, cimetidine, ketoconazole, phenytoin, furosemide, verapamil, cytotoxic drugs, antihypertensives, sedatives, antidepressants, amphetamines, heroin, methadone, anabolic steroids (2)[C]
- Systemic disorders: Cirrhosis, thyrotoxicosis, renal failure
- Androgen production deficiency
- Androgen-insensitivity syndromes
- Idiopathic (25% of gynecomastia)

COMMONLY ASSOCIATED CONDITIONS
- Peutz-Jeghers syndrome
- Male pseudohermaphroditism
- Hyperthyroidism
- Hypothyroidism
- Hepatic disease
- Prostate carcinoma
- Adrenal neoplasms (adenoma or carcinoma)
- Renal disease or dialysis
- True hermaphrodism
- Klinefelter syndrome
- Testicular failure (enzymatic defects of testosterone production, androgen insensitivity)
- Testicular neoplasms (germ cell, Leydig cell, Sertoli cell tumors)

DIAGNOSIS

HISTORY
- Determine onset and duration of symptoms.
- Investigate concurrent drug treatments.

PHYSICAL EXAM
- Careful breast exam to evaluate characteristics of breast:
  - May involve one or both breasts
  - Usually asymptomatic but may be tender if it has developed rapidly
  - Usually located concentrically beneath the nipple and areola
- Abdominal exam
- Testicular exam
- Rectal exam

DIAGNOSTIC TESTS & INTERPRETATION
- Most cases in teenage boys are self-limiting and require reassurance alone.
- Full endocrine investigations may be indicated if symptoms of other disease states are indicated:
  - Thyroid function studies, testosterone, estradiol, beta human chorionic gonadotropin, luteinizing hormone (LH), liver functions tests, GGT, prolactin, α-fetoprotein

Lab
Laboratory evaluation rarely indicated in teenage boys

Initial lab tests

If worsening symptoms or clinical suspicion of secondary cause, consider:
- Human chorionic gonadotropin (hGC) levels: High levels may indicate choriocarcinoma or other hCG-secreting tumor.
- Plasma testosterone and LH measurements: Help diagnose hypogonadism
- Serum estradiol (E_2)
- Serum prolactin
- Prostate-specific antigen (PSA)
- Liver function tests (LFTs)
- Others if clinically indicated (e.g., thyroid function, chromosomal analysis)

Follow-Up & Special Considerations

Disorders that may alter lab results:
- Cirrhosis
- Thyrotoxicosis
- Renal failure

Imaging
- CT scan of chest and abdomen if adrenal or extragonadal germ cell tumor is suspected
- Testicular ultrasound if there is a palpable mass or abnormality of one or both testicles (rarely indicated)
- MRI of pituitary fossa if prolactin levels are elevated (to exclude a prolactinoma)

Diagnostic Procedures/Surgery
Biopsy, if suspicious

Pathological Findings
- Dense, periductal, hyaline, collagenous connective tissue
- Hyperplastic ductal lining
- Plasma cell infiltrate

DIFFERENTIAL DIAGNOSIS
- Obesity with increase in adipose tissue
- Carcinoma of male breast
- Lipomas
- Neurofibromas
- Cystic hygroma

TREATMENT

- In teenage males, only reassurance and follow-up are usually indicated:
  - Spontaneous resolution in majority with the first 1–2 years
  - Persistent idiopathic gynecomastia in 7–8% of teenage boys at 3 years following diagnosis (2)[C]
- There is little evidence to recommend medical treatment of idiopathic gynecomastia in pediatric patients at this time (4).
- Consider medication or illicit drug use in adult males before initiating treatment.

MEDICATION

- Danazol (100 mg b.i.d. × 1 week followed by 100 mg t.i.d. × 2–6 weeks) (5)[B]:
  - Effective in 80% of patients
  - Especially effective in reducing tenderness
  - Dose can be repeated for responders.
  - Drug is licensed for treatment of gynecomastia in the UK.
- Tamoxifen (20–40 mg/d) has been used (5)[B]:
  - May be effective in 78–83% of men with gynecomastia
  - Less effective in breasts with a large amount of fatty tissue
  - May have high relapse rate
  - Short-term tamoxifen treatment also has been used successfully in the treatment of pubertal gynecomastia (6)[C].
- Anastrazole has been studied in pediatric patients with idiopathic gynecomastia and is not effective (4).
- Timing of treatment with medications may influence patient response:
  - Treatment early in the course of developing gynecomastia may be more beneficial (2)[C].
- Testosterone may be of some benefit but has not been well studied and is used infrequently.
- Clomiphene has been used infrequently.

ADDITIONAL TREATMENT

General Measures

- Correct underlying disorder.
- Withdraw causative drug (if feasible).
- Observe with reassurance that the problem is transient.

Issues for Referral

Refer to endocrinologist if abnormally elevated hormone levels are confirmed.

SURGERY/OTHER PROCEDURES

- Biopsy if suspicious for cancer:
  - Needle or excisional biopsy
  - Gynecomastia is felt to be a risk factor for the development of male breast cancer (7)
- SC mastectomy for severe, painful, or persistent cases or for patients with psychologic concerns (8)[C]:
  - Usually performed as outpatient surgery
  - General anesthesia required
  - Liposuction of the SC tissue may be required as well as skin removal if the breast is pendulous (9).

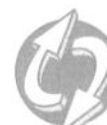

ONGOING CARE

FOLLOW-UP RECOMMENDATIONS

No restrictions

Patient Monitoring

- Every 3–6 months for physiologic gynecomastia
- Until well for nonphysiologic gynecomastia

DIET

- No special diet
- If obesity a problem, weight-loss diet

PATIENT EDUCATION

Surgical procedures for gynecomastia in pubertal boys are rarely covered by insurance because most insurance companies consider these procedures to be cosmetic.

PROGNOSIS

- Type 1: Resolves spontaneously
- Type 2: Clears without treatment (may take up to 2 years)
- Type 3: Little change without substantial weight loss
- Drug-induced: Drug withdrawal should result in resolution of gynecomastia in most cases.
- Other causes: Outcome depends on etiology.
- Good results with SC mastectomy

COMPLICATIONS

- Nipple inversion may occur following SC mastectomy.
- Asymmetry of breasts
- Postoperative fluid collection
- Withdrawal behavior related to drugs
- Depression
- Weight gain may be associated with danazol treatment.

REFERENCES

1. Eckman A, Dobs A. Drug-induced gynecomastia. *Expert Opin Drug Saf*. 2008;7:691–702.
2. Nordt CA, Divasta AD. Gynecomastia in adolescents. *Curr Opin Pediatr*. 2008;20:375–82.
3. Sher ES, et al. Evaluation of boys with marked breast development at puberty. *Clin Ped*. 1998;37:367–72.
4. Ma NS, Geffner ME. Gynecomastia in prepubertal and pubertal men. *Curr Opin Pediatr*. 2008;20:465–70.
5. Devalia HL, Layer GT, et al. Current concepts in gynaecomastia. *Surgeon*. 2009;7:114–9.
6. Derman O, Kanbur NO, Kutluk T. Tamoxifen treatment for pubertal gynecomastia. *Int J Adolesc Med Health*. 2003;15:359–63.
7. Brinton LA, Carreon JD, et al. Etiologic factors for male breast cancer in the U.S. Veterans Affairs medical care system database. *Breast Cancer Res Treat*. 2009. [epub ahead of print].
8. Gabra H, et al. Gynaecomastia in the adolescent: A surgically relevant condition. *Eur J Ped Surg*. 2004;14:3–6.
9. Cordova A, Moschella F. Algorithm for clinical evaluation and surgical treatment of gynaecomastia. *J Plast Reconstr Aesthet Surg*. 2007.

ADDITIONAL READING

Johnson RE, Murad MH, et al. Gynecomastia: Pathophysiology, evaluation, and management. *Mayo Clin Proc*. 2009;84:1010–5.

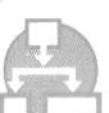

See Also (Topic, Algorithm, Electronic Media Element)

Algorithm: Gynecomastia

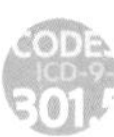

CODES

ICD9

611.1 Hypertrophy of breast

CLINICAL PEARLS

- The initial workup of gynecomastia is history, physical exam, and fasting labs including serum hCG, testosterone, LH, E_2, prolactin, PSA, and LFTs.
- Lab tests do not need to be done in boys with suspected pubertal gynecomastia, but they should be considered if the gynecomastia persists for >1 year.

G

HAMMER TOES

Janet Ricks, DO

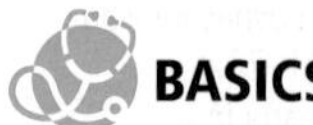

BASICS

Hammer toes are classified as a form of lesser toe (digits 2–5) deformities.

DESCRIPTION

- Plantar flexion deformity of the proximal interphalangeal (PIP) joint with varying degrees of hyperextension of the metatarsophalangeal (MTP) and distal interphalangeal (DIP) joints (1). Occurs primarily in sagittal plane.
- Can be flexible, semirigid, or fixed:
  - Flexible: Passively correctable to neutral position
  - Semirigid: Partially correctable to neutral position
  - Fixed: Not passively correctable to neutral position

EPIDEMIOLOGY

Most common deformity of lesser toes, typically affecting only 1 or 2 digits; second toe most commonly involved

Incidence

- Undefined with limited data
- Increases with age, duration of deformity (from flexible to rigid)

Prevalence

- More common in women than men (2): Female predominance from 2.5:1 to 9:1, depending on age group
- Can range from 1–20% of population studied
- Blacks more affected than whites (2)

RISK FACTORS

- Pes cavus and planus
- Hallux valgus
- Metatarsus adductus
- Ankle equinus
- Neuromuscular disease (rare)
- Trauma
- Improperly fitted shoes (e.g., with narrow toe box) and/or hosiery
- Abnormal metatarsal and/or digit length
- Inflammatory joint disease (e.g., rheumatoid arthritis)
- Connective tissue disease
- Diabetes mellitus

Genetics

- Specific genetic markers not identified
- Seen more frequently in families

GENERAL PREVENTION

- No documented means of prevention
- Modification of shoe wear using pressure dispersive devices reduces pain (1).
- Foot orthoses modulate biomechanical dysfunction and muscular imbalance, thereby preventing progression (2).
- Control of predisposing factors (e.g., inflammatory joint disease) may slow progression.

PATHOPHYSIOLOGY

- Any biomechanical dysfunction that results in loss of function of extensor digitorum longus (EDL) tendon at PIP joint and the flexor digitorum longus (FDL) tendon at the MTP joint. The intrinsic muscles sublux dorsally as the MTP hyperextends. This results in plantar flexion of the PIP joint and hyperextension of the MTP joint (2).
- Specific pathomechanics vary by etiology:
  - Toe length discrepancy or narrow toe box induces PIP joint flexion by forcing digit to accommodate shoe wear. May also lead to MTP joint synovitis secondary to overuse, with elongation of plantar plate and MTP joint hyperextension.
  - Rheumatoid arthritis causes MTP joint destruction and resultant subluxation

ETIOLOGY

- Congenital
- Acquired:
  - Any condition that compromises intra-articular and periarticular tissues, such as second ray longer than first, inflammatory joint disease, improper fitting shoes, and trauma (1). Damage to joint capsule, collateral ligaments, or synovia leads to unstable PIP joint or MTP joint.

COMMONLY ASSOCIATED CONDITIONS

- Hallux valgus
- Cavus foot
- Metatarsus adductus
- Dorsal callus

DIAGNOSIS

History and physical exam often sufficient for diagnosis of hammer toes. Additional testing available to exclude other conditions.

HISTORY

- Location, duration, severity, and rate of progression of foot deformity (3)[C]
- Type, location, duration of pain:
  - Patients often relate sensation of lump on plantar aspect of MTP joint.
- Degree of functional impairment
- Factors that improve and exacerbate the condition
- Type of footwear and hosiery worn
- Peripheral neurologic symptoms
- Any prior treatment rendered

PHYSICAL EXAM

- Note MTP joint hyperextension, PIP joint flexion, and DIP joint extension.
- Observe any adjacent toe deformities (e.g., hallux valgus, flexion contractures).
- Assess degree of flexibility and reducibility of deformity in both weight-bearing and non–weight-bearing positions (2)[C].
- Note any hyperkeratosis over the joint, ulcers, clavi (dorsal PIP joint, metatarsal head), adventitious bursa, erythema, or skin breakdown (2).
- Palpate for pain over dorsal aspect of PIP joint or MTP joint.
- Drawer test of MTP joint
- Palpate webspaces to exclude interdigital neuroma.
- Neurovascular evaluation (e.g., pulses, sensation, muscle bulk)

DIAGNOSTIC TESTS & INTERPRETATION

Lab

Initial lab tests

Not required unless clinically indicated to rule out suspected metabolic or inflammatory arthropathies (2)[C]. Rheumatoid factor, ANA, HLA-B27 serologies for inflammatory disease.

Imaging

Initial approach

Weight-bearing x-rays of affected foot in anterior–posterior (AP), lateral, and oblique views (2)[C]:

- AP view superior for assessing MTP subluxation or dislocation
- Lateral view best for evaluation of gross hammer toe deformity

Follow-Up & Special Considerations

MRI or bone scan if suspect osteomyelitis

Diagnostic Procedures/Surgery

- Nerve conduction studies or EMG if suspect neurologic disorder
- Doppler or plethysmography if impaired circulation and surgery is considered
- Computerized weight-bearing pressure testing indicated only in setting of neuromuscular deficiencies of toes

Pathological Findings

Histologic evaluation typically not necessary before treatment

DIFFERENTIAL DIAGNOSIS

Hammer toe: Hyperextension of the MTP and DIP joints and plantar flexion of the PIP joint

- Claw toe: Dorsiflexion of MTP joint and plantar flexion of the DIP joint
- Mallet toe: Fixed or flexible deformity of the DIP joint of the toe
- Overlapping fifth toe
- Interdigital neuroma
- Plantar plate rupture
- Nonspecific synovitis of MTP joint
- Exostosis
- Arthritis (e.g., rheumatoid, psoriatic)
- Fracture

TREATMENT

Goal of treatment is to reduce or relieve symptoms so that patients may return to their normal activity level. Management includes surgical and nonsurgical interventions. Mild cases, however, may not require treatment.

MEDICATION

Indicated if adequate pain relief achievable nonsurgically or patient is poor surgical candidate

First Line

NSAIDs may be helpful in managing symptoms of pain, as well as soft tissue and joint inflammation.

Second Line

Anti-inflammatory (cortisone) injectables if local inflammation or bursitis exists (1)[C]

ADDITIONAL TREATMENT

General Measures

Nonsurgical (conservative) treatment includes:

- Shoe modifications, such as wider and/or deeper toe box, may be used to accommodate the deformity and decrease the pressure over osseous prominences. Avoid high-heeled shoes (2)[C].
- Toe sleeve or orthodigital padding of the hammer toe prominence (4)[C]
- Hammer toe straightening orthotics or taping to reduce flexible deformities
- Debridement of hyperkeratotic lesions is effective in reducing symptoms. Topical keratolytics may be helpful (2)[C].
- Shoe orthotics may be used to control abnormal biomechanical influences.
- Physical therapy for stretching and strengthening of the toes may help to preserve flexibility.

Issues for Referral

If nonsurgical (conservative) treatment is unsuccessful and/or impractical or patient has combined deformity of MTP joint, PIP joint, and/or DIP joint, then patient may be referred to an orthopedic surgeon or surgical podiatrist for surgical interventions.

SURGERY/OTHER PROCEDURES

- Surgical procedures for the correction of hammer toes rely on the degree and flexibility of the contracture(s) and the related abnormalities that exist.
- Surgical interventions for *flexible* hammer toes include (1,4)[C]:
  - PIP joint arthroplasty (most common)
  - Flexor tendon lengthening/flexor tenotomy
  - Extensor tendon lengthening/tenotomy/MTP joint capsulotomy
  - Exostosectomy
  - Implant arthroplasty
- Surgical interventions for semirigid/rigid hammer toes include (1,4)[C]:
  - PIP joint resection arthroplasty or arthrodesis
  - Girdlestone-Taylor flexor-to-extensor transfer
  - Metatarsal shortening (Weil osteotomy)
  - Exostosectomy
  - Diaphysectomy of the proximal phalanx (less common)
  - Middle phalangectomy (less common)
  - Soft tissue releases/lengthening
- Procedures may be performed as isolated operations or in conjunction with other procedures.
- Contraindications for surgery: Active infection, inadequate vascular supply, and desire for cosmesis alone

ONGOING CARE

FOLLOW-UP RECOMMENDATIONS

- Radiographs should be taken immediately following surgery or at the first postoperative visit. Subsequent x-rays may be taken as needed.
- Full weight-bearing in a postoperative (surgical) shoe or other device is indicated based on the procedure(s) performed and on the individual patient.
- Elevate the foot above nose to minimize swelling, which can lead to pain and delay wound healing.
- Return to regular shoe wear depends on the postoperative course.
- Role and efficacy of postoperative physical therapy (3 times per week for 2–3 weeks) unclear

Patient Monitoring

In the absence of complications, the patient should be seen initially within the first week following the procedure(s). Frequency of subsequent visits is determined based on the procedure(s) performed and the postoperative course.

PATIENT EDUCATION

- Patients should be aware of mild-to-moderate swelling and plantar foot discomfort that may persist for many (1–6) months after surgery and may limit footwear options until resolved.
- MTP joint and PIP joint may remain stiff for extended period of time.
- "Molding" of the operative toe (assumes shape of adjacent toes)
- Encourage patients to wear shoes of adequate size with rounded or squared toe box in future.

PROGNOSIS

- Nonoperative (conservative) treatment usually alleviates pain; however, the deformity may progress despite diligent care.
- Surgical treatment of flexible hammer toe deformity reliably corrects the deformity and alleviates pain. Recurrence and progression are common, especially if the patient resumes wearing improperly fitted shoes.
- Surgical treatment of fixed hammer toe deformity provides reliable deformity correction and pain relief. Recurrence is uncommon.

COMPLICATIONS

- Common complications specific to digital surgery include, but are not limited to, the following:
  - Persistent edema
  - Recurrence of deformity
  - Residual pain
  - Excessive stiffness
  - Metatarsalgia
- Less common complications include the following:
  - Numbness (e.g., digital nerve palsy)
  - Flail toe
  - Symptomatic osseous regrowth
  - Malposition of toe
  - Malunion/nonunion
  - Infection
  - Vascular impairment (e.g., toe ischemia, gangrene)

REFERENCES

1. Academy of Ambulatory Foot and Ankle Surgery. *Hammertoe Syndrome*. Philadelphia: Academy of Ambulatory Foot and Ankle Surgery; 2003.
2. Clinical Practice Guideline Forefoot Disorders Panel of the American College of Foot and Ankle Surgeons. Diagnosis and treatment of forefoot disorders. Section 1: Digital deformities. *J Foot Ankle Surg*. 2009;48(2):230–8.
3. Schrier JC, Verheyen CC, Louwerens JW. Definitions of hammer toe and claw toe: An evaluation of the literature. *J Am Podiatr Med Assoc*. 2009;99: 194–7.
4. Smith BW, Coughlin MJ, et al. Disorders of the lesser toes. *Sports Med Arthrosc*. 2009;17:167–74.

ADDITIONAL READING

- Miller JM, Blacklidge DK, Ferdowsian V, et al. Chevron arthrodesis of the interphalangeal joint for hammertoe correction. *J Foot Ankle Surg*. 2010;49: 194–6.
- O'Kane C, Kilmartin T. Review of proximal interphalangeal joint excisional arthroplasty for the correction of second hammer toe deformity in 100 cases. *Foot Ankle Int*. 2005;26:320–5.
- Pietrzak WS, Lessek TP, Perns SV. A bioabsorbable fixation implant for use in proximal interphalangeal joint (hammer toe) arthrodesis: Biomechanical testing in a synthetic bone substrate. *J Foot Ankle Surg*. 2006;45:288–94.

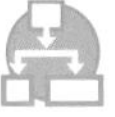

See Also (Topic, Algorithm, Electronic Media Element)

Algorithm: Foot Pain

CODES

ICD9

- 735.4 Other hammer toe (acquired)
- 754.71 Talipes cavus
- 755.66 Other anomalies of toes

CLINICAL PEARLS

- Hammer toe is plantar flexion deformity of PIP joint.
- Patients may complain of pain at the PIP joint or MTP joint.
- Perform a careful inspection and examination of foot, especially PIP joint and MTP joint.
- Initial management of hammer toe deformity consists of conservative therapy; however, if unsuccessful, surgical interventions are indicated.
- Well-fitting shoe wear is vital to minimizing recurrence after treatment.

H

HEADACHE, CLUSTER

Andrea Haas, MSIV
Ann Mitchell, MD

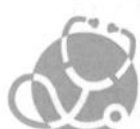

BASICS

DESCRIPTION
- Primary headache disease
- Multiple attacks of short-lived, excruciating, unilateral, sharp, searing, or piercing pain, typically localized in the periorbital area and temple accompanied by signs of ipsilateral autonomic dysfunction. *Severe* pain syndrome.
- Underdiagnosed and suboptimally treated
- Autonomic symptoms: Parasympathetic hyperactivity signs (ipsilateral lacrimation, eye redness, and nasal congestion) and sympathetic hypoactivity (ipsilateral ptosis and miosis)
- Attacks are without prodrome, rapidly escalating in intensity usually within 15 minutes, frequently have a circadian rhythmicity, and often wake patients 60–90 minutes after falling asleep. In contrast to other headache syndromes, the severe pain may cause patients to pace restlessly and occasionally exhibit agitated behavior.
- Individual attacks last 15–180 minutes if untreated and occur from once every other day to 8 times per day. 2 forms exist (ICHD-2 criteria):
  - Episodic: At least 2 cluster periods lasting 7 days–1 year, separated by a pain-free interval of >1 month (80–90% of cases)
  - Chronic: Cluster-free interval of <1 month in a 12-month period or greater

EPIDEMIOLOGY
Incidence
1-year incidence of 53 per 100,000

Prevalence
- Lifetime prevalence 56–326 per 100,000
- Predominant sex: Male > Female (4.3:1)
- Mean age of onset: Between 29.6 and 35.7 years
- Episodic cluster headaches (CH) > chronic CH

RISK FACTORS
- Male gender
- Age 30–60 years
- Cigarette smoking
- Family history of CH
- Alcohol induces attacks during a cluster, but not during remission.
- Small amounts of vasodilators (e.g., alcohol, nitroglycerin)
- Strong odors

Genetics
- Usually sporadic inheritance
- Autosomal-dominant inheritance in about 5% of cases, autosomal recessive or multifactorial pattern in other families
- Exact transmission pattern still debated
- First-degree relatives carry 5–18-fold; Second-degree 1–3-fold increased relative risk of disease.

PATHOPHYSIOLOGY
- Unknown
- Unlikely to arise from a single trigger zone
- Proposed mechanisms include:
  - Pain: Activation of trigeminal nerve
  - Autonomic symptoms: Activation of craniofacial parasympathetic nerve fibers secondary to pathological activation of trigemino-autonomic brainstem reflex. Trigger of trigeminofacial reflex might be in hypothalamus also explaining cyclical nature of cluster headache.

ETIOLOGY
Unknown

COMMONLY ASSOCIATED CONDITIONS
- Increased risk of suicide secondary to the extreme nature of the pain
- Medication-overuse headache
- History of migraine, frequently in female patients
- Sleep apnea
- Increased prevalence of cardiac right-to-left shunt and patent foramen ovale

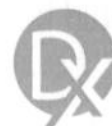

DIAGNOSIS

- Diagnosis is clinical.
- *International Classification of Headache Disorders* (2nd edition) criteria: At least 5 attacks of severe or very severe unilateral orbital, supraorbital, or temporal pain lasting 15–180 minutes if untreated
- At least 1 of the following:
  - Ipsilateral:
    - Conjunctival injection or lacrimation
    - Nasal congestion and/or rhinorrhea
    - Eyelid edema
    - Forehead and facial sweating
    - Miosis and/or ptosis
  - Sense of restlessness or agitation
- Attack frequency: 1 every other day to 8 per day
- Not attributed to another disorder
- Episodic CH: At least 2 cluster periods lasting 7 days–1 year, separated by a pain-free interval of >1 month (80–90% of cases)
- Chronic CH: Cluster-free interval of <1 month in a 12-month period or greater

HISTORY
- Excruciating, unilateral, sharp, searing, or piercing pain, typically localized in the periorbital area
- Nausea

PHYSICAL EXAM
- Acute distress, crying, screaming, restless, and/or agitated during attacks
- Ipsilateral lacrimation, injected conjunctivae, ptosis, and miosis
- Nasal stuffiness or rhinorrhea
- Bradycardia or tachycardia

DIAGNOSTIC TESTS & INTERPRETATION
- Diagnosis is primarily clinical; lab tests are not generally indicated.
- Consider neuroimaging (MRI/CT head and vascular imaging of brain):
  - Atypical CH presentation
  - Abnormal neurological exam
  - Suspect secondary CH (see "Differential Diagnosis")

DIFFERENTIAL DIAGNOSIS
- Other trigeminal autonomic cephalgias: Paroxysmal hemicrania, short-lasting unilateral neuralgiform headache attacks with conjunctival injection and tearing (SUNCT). Attacks last a few seconds only and respond to indomethacin.
- Hemicrania continua, hypnic headaches, trigeminal and other facial neuralgias, migraine, temporal arteritis, herpes zoster
- Secondary cluster headache:
  - Vertebral or carotid artery dissection
  - Brain arteriovenous malformations
  - Intracranial artery aneurysms
  - Pituitary adenomas
  - Nasopharyngeal carcinoma
  - Maxillary sinus foreign body/sinusitis
  - Cavernous hemangioma
  - Meningiomas/carcinomas/metastases

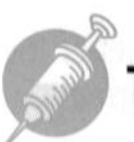

TREATMENT

Many of the medications discussed below are used off-label in the treatment of cluster headache.

MEDICATION
- Avoid pain therapy, especially narcotic analgesics, for acute attacks.
- Goal is abortion of acute attack and prophylaxis for expected duration of the cluster.
- Assess cardiovascular risk before instituting a vasoactive drug such as ergotamine or sumatriptan.

First Line
- For acute attacks:
  - Oxygen: 100% at 8–15 L/min for 15 minutes via nonrebreathing mask. Relief within 15 minutes. 70% obtain relief. Avoid in severe COPD as might affect hypoxic respiratory drive (1)[A].
  - Triptan medication: Sumatriptan (Imitrex): 6 mg SC, maximum 12 mg/24 hours with at least 1 hour between injections. Most effective medication for acute attacks: 74% of patients experience no further symptoms after 15 minutes. Adverse effects: Nonischemic chest pain, distal paresthesias, injection site reactions, nausea and vomiting, fatigue. Triptans contraindicated in ischemic cardiac disease, stroke, uncontrolled hypertension, Prinzmetal angina, basilar migraine, hemiplegic migraine, ischemic bowel disease, and peripheral vascular disease. Zolmitriptan nasal spray: 5- and 10-mg dosage both effective to relieve headaches at 30 minutes (2)[A]. Sumatriptan nasal spray: 20 mg effective within 30 minutes. Common adverse effect: Bitter taste (3)[B]. Zolmitriptan tablet: 5- and 10-mg tablets shown to be superior to placebo at 30 minutes with episodic CH, but not chronic CH (4)[B]. Oral administration is slower in onset and less efficacious than nonoral routes.
- Prophylaxis to shorten cluster period and severity and to prevent expected attacks. Prophylactic treatment does not prevent incitement of cluster period, but does prevent attacks within cluster period:
  - Verapamil: Starting dose should be 240–360 mg/d (120 mg t.i.d. or in SR formulation). Increase by 80 mg every 2 weeks with ECG control, until 720 mg dose is reached. Recommended clinical dose is 480 mg/d (5). If exceeded, informed consent has to be obtained. Doses up to 1,200 mg/d may be required. Has many drug-drug interactions, as it is a CYP3A4 inhibitor. Adverse effects include hypotension, arrhythmias, AV block, bradycardia, pr-prolongation, syncope, gum and ankle swelling, constipation, CHF.

- Lithium: One study compared lithium 800 mg/d to placebo in episodic CH. No difference in percentage of patients having cessation of attacks, although those on lithium felt subjectively better. Another study compared verapamil 360 mg/d to lithium 900 mg/d. 50% of verapamil group and 37% in lithium group improved. Seems more effective in chronic CH. Side effects: Confusion, dizziness, diabetes insipidus, polyuria, hypothyroidism, tremor, bradycardia, muscle hyperexcitability, headaches. Monitor levels, liver, renal, and thyroid function. Caution with nephrotoxic drugs, diuretics.
- *Though both verapamil and lithium are given a class C rating based on the trials done, extensive clinical experience as prophylaxis for cluster headaches is available. Verapamil is hence considered first-line prophylactic treatment.

Second Line

- Acute attack:
  - Lidocaine/Cocaine: 10 mg (1 mL) of lidocaine or 40–50 mg of 10% cocaine intranasal. Most common side effects are nasal congestion, unpleasant lidocaine taste.
  - Octreotide: SC 100 μg. Can be considered in patients when triptans are contraindicated. Main side effect is GI upset.
- Prophylaxis:
  - Civamide: 100 μL of 0.025% into each nostril daily. Only studied in episodic CH in one trial of 28 patients. Most common side effects were nasal burning, lacrimation, pharyngitis, rhinorrhea.
  - Melatonin: 9 mg at bedtime showed reduction in daily headache frequency vs. placebo. No side effects were reported.
  - Sodium valproate: Did not show any benefit vs. placebo. Not advised as preventive treatment.
  - Methylsergide: No studies available to confirm efficacy. Has serious adverse effects including pulmonary and retroperitoneal fibrosis. Cannot be given with triptans and ergots. Avoid use.

ADDITIONAL TREATMENT

Transitional preventive treatment:

- Used until longer-term preventive treatment becomes effective. Longer-term maintenance agents are started concurrently:
  - Steroids: Only 1 study using oral prednisone and it had serious limitations. In practice, a commonly used regimen is prednisone 60 mg/d for 3 days, then decreased by 10 mg every 3 days for a total of 18 days of treatment. Adverse effects for short-term use: Insomnia, psychosis, hyponatremia, edema, hyperglycemia, peptic ulcer.
  - Suboccipital steroid injection: One class I RCT showed benefit after 72 hours. 12.46 mg betamethasone dipropionate, 5.26 mg betamethasone disodium phosphate, and 0.5 mL 2% Xylocaine used.
  - Dihydroergotamine: 1 mg SC/IM b.i.d. for several days
  - Ergotamine tartrate: 1–2 mg/d or in divided doses; contraindicated with triptans
- Dihydroergotamine and ergotamine (no trials to prove efficacy)
- See "Acute and preventive pharmacologic treatment of cluster headache" by Francis et al. under "Additional Reading."

General Measures

- Avoid major changes in sleep habits.
- Stop smoking.
- Avoid use of alcohol during cluster period.
- Avoid prolonged physical exertion.
- Avoid extreme changes in altitude due to changes in oxygen levels.
- Avoid exposure to chemical agents/solvents.

Pregnancy Considerations

Collaboration between headache specialist, obstetrician, and pediatrician strongly encouraged. For abortive treatment, oxygen is most appropriate first-line therapy with nasal formulation of sumatriptan (pregnancy category B) or nasal lidocaine (pregnancy category B) as appropriate second-line therapies. As preventive therapy, verapamil (pregnancy category C) and steroids (pregnancy category C) remain the preferred options.

Issues for Referral

Consider a neurology or headache center referral for refractory or complicated patients.

SURGERY/OTHER PROCEDURES

- Various techniques focused on ablation of segments of trigeminal nerve root and sphenopalatine ganglion.
- Occipital nerve stimulation: 3 reports of occipital nerve stimulation found that ~60% of patients responded to treatment as defined by >50% reduction in headache severity or frequency. However, may not show improvement for weeks to 5 months (6).
- Deep brain stimulation (DBS):
  - Of the posterior inferior hypothalamus
  - Latest data showing that therapeutic effect of DBS might be related not to direct stimulation of hypothalamus but might modulate a local cluster headache generator in hypothalamus or mesencephalic gray matter or through nonspecific antinociceptive mechanisms (7).
- Surgery may be considered only for patients who are refractory to or have contraindications to medical therapy and whose cluster headaches occur on exclusively one side. Complications include facial analgesia. Hypothalamic or greater occipital nerve stimulation is now recommended over surgery due to avoidance of severing trigeminal nerve.

IN-PATIENT CONSIDERATIONS

Admission Criteria

Suicidal ideation, unwilling to contract for safety

ONGOING CARE

FOLLOW-UP RECOMMENDATIONS

Patient Monitoring

- Anticipate cluster bouts and initiate early prophylaxis.
- Watch for adverse medication response and side effects.
- Watch for unmasking of underlying cardiovascular disorder.
- Educate patient and family.

PROGNOSIS

- Unpredictable course. With aging, attack frequency often decreases.
- Poor prognosis associated with older age of onset, male gender, disease duration of >20 years for episodic form
- Possibility of transformation of episodic cluster to chronic cluster and occasionally chronic cluster to episodic cluster

COMPLICATIONS

- Side effects of medication, including unmasking of coronary heart disease
- Potential for drug abuse
- Problems with high-flow oxygen in patients with COPD or in those who smoke

REFERENCES

1. Cohen AS, Burns B, Goadsby PJ, et al. High-flow oxygen for treatment of cluster headache: A randomized trial. *JAMA*. 2009;302:2451–7.
2. Rapoport AM, Mathew NT, Silberstein SD, et al. Zolmitriptan nasal spray in the acute treatment of cluster headache: A double-blind study. *Neurology*. 2007;69:821–6.
3. van Vliet JA, Bahra A, Martin V, et al. Intranasal sumatriptan in cluster headache: Randomized placebo-controlled double-blind study. *Neurology*. 2003;60:630–3.
4. Bahra A, Gawel MJ, Hardebo JE, et al. Oral zolmitriptan is effective in the acute treatment of cluster headache. *Neurology*. 2000;54:1832–9.
5. Tfelt-Hansen P, Tfelt-Hansen J, et al. Verapamil for cluster headache. Clinical pharmacology and possible mode of action. *Headache*. 2009;49: 117–25.
6. Burns B, Watkins L, Goadsby PJ. Treatment of medically intractable cluster headache by occipital nerve stimulation: Long-term follow-up of eight patients. *Lancet*. 2007;369(9567):1099–106.
7. Fontaine D, Lanteri-Minet M, Ouchchane L, et al. Anatomical location of effective deep brain stimulation electrodes in chronic cluster headache. *Brain*. 2010;133:1214–23.

H

ADDITIONAL READING

Francis GJ, Becker WJ, Pringsheim TM, et al. Acute and preventive pharmacologic treatment of cluster headache. *Neurology*. 2010;75:463–73.

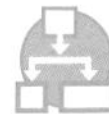

See Also (Topic, Algorithm, Electronic Media Element)

Algorithm: Headache, Chronic

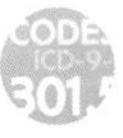

CODES

ICD9

- 339.00 Cluster headache syndrome, unspecified
- 339.01 Episodic cluster headache
- 339.02 Chronic cluster headache

CLINICAL PEARLS

- Patients are often agitated during the headache (vs. the quiet and withdrawn appearance of a migraine).
- Oxygen and triptans, not narcotics, are first-line therapy.

HEADACHE, MIGRAINE

Jay H. Levin, MD
Michelle L. Mellion, MD

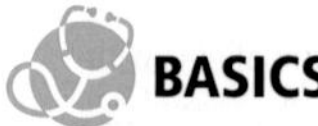

BASICS

DESCRIPTION

- Headache disorder with episodic manifestation characterized by recurrent painful paroxysms of moderate-to-severe, throbbing pain, typically unilateral, capable of altering daily function and lasting from 4–72 hours. Preheadache symptoms are nonspecific, may occur hours to days before headache. Most frequent subtypes are as follows:
  - Without aura (common migraine): Defining >80% of attacks, often associated with nausea, vomiting, photophobia, and/or phonophobia
  - With aura (classic migraine): Visual or other types of neurologic phenomenon lasting 5–60 minutes before the headache
- Other subtypes:
  - Chronic (Transformed) migraine: Chronic headache pattern evolving from episodic migraine. Migrainelike attacks are superimposed on a daily or near-daily headache pattern (e.g., tension headaches), >15 headache days per month for at least 3 months.
  - Medication overuse headache: Daily or near-daily use of acute medication perpetuating the headache pattern
  - Basilar-type migraine: Brainstem headache, with aura symptoms of dysarthria, vertigo, tinnitus, ataxia, and bilateral paresis or bilateral paresthesias
  - Hemiplegic migraine: Aura consisting of hemiplegia and/or hemiparesis
  - Ophthalmoplegic: Migrainelike neuralgia accompanied by palsy of an ocular cranial nerve during the headache phase
  - Retinal: Monocular symptoms of retinal vascular involvement during migraine
  - Menstrual-related (moliminal) migraine: Associated with onset of menstrual period
  - Childhood periodic syndromes (migraine equivalents): Recurrent, often cyclic, episodes of symptoms such as vomiting, intense nausea, and/or abdominal pain
  - Status migrainosus: Debilitating migraine that lasts longer than 72 hours
  - Migrainous infarction: Persistent or permanent neurologic deficits persisting beyond migraine attack, usually with neuroimaging changes

EPIDEMIOLOGY

Female > Male (3:1)

Prevalence

Affects over 28 million Americans:

- Adults: Women 18%; Men 6%

RISK FACTORS

- Sleep pattern disruption
- Diet: Skipped meals (40–56%), alcohol (29–35%), chocolate (19–22%), cheese (9–18%), caffeine overuse (14%), monosodium glutamate (MSG) (12%), and artificial sweeteners (e.g., aspartame, sucralose) (1)
- Menstrual cycle, excessive sleep, fatigue, emotional stress, letdown (relief of stress)
- Medications: Cyclic estrogen replacement, birth control pills, vasodilators
- Family history of migraine
- Female gender

Genetics

- >80% of patients have a positive family history.
- Familial hemiplegic migraine has been shown to be linked to both chromosomes 19 and 1.

GENERAL PREVENTION

- Avoid precipitants of attacks.
- Biofeedback, education, and psychological intervention
- Preventative therapy if attacks frequent, interfere with lifestyle, or are not controlled by acute interventions
- Lifestyle modifications may improve frequency and severity of headaches: Sleep hygiene, stress management, regular aerobic exercise (1)[C].

PATHOPHYSIOLOGY

Trigeminovascular hypothesis: Hyperexcitable trigeminal sensory neurons in brainstem stimulated and release neuropeptides such as substance P and calcitonin gene-related peptide (CGRP), leading to vasodilation and neurogenic inflammation (1,2).

ETIOLOGY

No longer believed to be primarily vascular in etiology; rather, cortical spreading depolarization/depression

COMMONLY ASSOCIATED CONDITIONS

- Depression, psychiatric disorders
- Sleep disturbance (e.g., sleep apnea)
- Cerebral vascular disease
- Peripheral vascular disease
- Seizure disorders
- Irritable bowel syndrome
- Obesity
- Patent foramen ovale (PFO)

DIAGNOSIS

A thorough history and neurologic examination is usually all that is necessary to make the diagnosis.

HISTORY

- Headache usually begins with mild pain that escalates into a unilateral (30–40% bilateral), throbbing (40% nonthrobbing) pain of 4–72 hours' duration.
- Intensified by movement and associated with systemic manifestations: Nausea (87%), vomiting (56%), diarrhea (16%), photophobia (82%), phonophobia (78%), muscle tenderness (65%), lightheadedness (72%), vertigo (33%)
- May be preceded by aura:
  - Visual disruptions are most common, including scotoma, hemianopsia, fortification spectra, geometric visual patterns, and occasionally hallucinations
  - Somatosensory disruption in face or arms
  - Speech difficulties
- Obtain adequate headache profile: Total number of headaches per month, number of days per month whereby headaches limit daily activities, frequency and amount of all headache medications used (3)
- Identify possible food triggers, nutritional history, and caffeine consumption (1).

PHYSICAL EXAM

Full neurologic exam to exclude other etiologies.

DIAGNOSTIC TESTS & INTERPRETATION

Testing indicated ONLY if abnormalities on exam or red flags in the history.

Imaging

Initial approach

Neuroimaging is ONLY appropriate with suspicious symptomatology and/or an abnormality on physical examination. Other red flags include:

- New onset in patient >50 years of age
- Change in established headache pattern
- Atypical pattern or unremitting/progressive neurologic symptoms
- Prolonged or bizarre aura

DIFFERENTIAL DIAGNOSIS

- Other primary headache syndromes
- If focal neurologic signs/symptoms present, consider transient ischemic attack, stroke
- Secondary headaches: Tumor, infection, vascular pathology, prescription or illicit drug use
- Drug-seeking patients
- Psychiatric disease
- Rarely, atypical forms of epilepsy

Pregnancy Considerations

- Migraine frequency may decrease in second and third trimesters.
- Nonpharamacologic methods are mainstay of treatment (see below).
- No treatment drug has FDA approval during pregnancy:
  - Acetaminophen, short-acting opioids, and antiemetics (e.g., prochlorperazine) can be considered for acute headaches during pregnancy.
  - Ergotamines are contraindicated.
  - Avoid herbal remedies (1)[C].
  - Early data for sumatriptan and naratriptan suggest no increase in birth defects.
  - Sumatriptan by injection is ideal for breast-feeding women with disabling migraines.
  - Propranolol is safe, effective for migraine prevention during pregnancy/lactation

TREATMENT

MEDICATION

First-Line Abortive Treatments

- Paracetamol (acetaminophen 1,000 mg) or aspirin (975 mg) plus the addition of a dopamine antagonist (e.g., metoclopramide 10 mg) may be as effective as oral sumatriptan 100 mg for acute migraine headache; NNT = 5.2 for 2-hour headache relief (5)[A].
- Aspirin 500 mg-acetaminophen 500 mg-caffeine 130 mg (AAC) combination (e.g., Excedrin Migraine) is an inexpensive, nonprescription, and FDA-approved treatment for acute migraine:
  - As early treatment for mild-to-moderate intensity migraines, AAC combination showed favorable results compared to oral sumatriptan 50 mg (4).

- Triptans are commonly used when OTC agents fail for moderate to severe attacks (2,4):
  - Oral sumatriptan 100 mg; NNT = 3.4 for 2-hour headache relief; expense varies, only some triptan generics available:
    - 44–77% of patients taking triptans report complete pain relief within 2 hours.
    - All triptans have similar effectiveness and tolerability, but some patients may respond better to one triptan over another (4).
    - Early intervention with triptans during the aura, prior to onset of pain, may prevent headache 89% of the time.
- Ergotamines (e.g., dihydroergotamine SC, IM, IV, or NS): Drug of choice in status migrainosus and nonpregnant patients with high degree disability
- NSAIDs such as ibuprofen, naproxen, and diclofenac are generally inexpensive and effective in up to 60% of cases (3,4)[A]:
  - Aspirin 1,000 mg plus the addition of a dopamine antagonist (e.g., metoclopramide 10 mg) may be as effective as oral sumatriptan 100 mg for acute migraine headache; NNT = 3.3 for 2-hour headache relief (3)[A].
- Antiemetics: Consider antinausea medications that antagonize dopamine receptors:
  - Metoclopramide, prochlorperazine
- IV dexamethasone: Use as adjunctive emergency therapy; 26% reduction of acute severe migraine recurrence, status migrainosus; NNT = 9 (4)[A].
- Contraindications to treatments:
  - Avoid 5-HT-1 agonists (triptans) and ergots in coronary heart disease, peripheral vascular disease, uncontrolled hypertension, complex migraine (e.g., basilar or hemiplegic migraine)
  - Triptans should not be used ergot derivative, MAOI, or other triptans.
  - Avoid narcotics or butalbital in addiction-prone patients and patients with frequent migraines.
- Precautions:
  - Frequent use of acute-treatment drugs may lead to increase in migraine patterns and medication overuse headache.

Second-Line Abortive Treatment

Opiates use is controversial:

- Some advocate the use of long-acting opioids in patients with refractory migraine.
- Opiates may contribute to medication overuse or chronic daily headache with use as few as 8 days per month (3)[C].

First-Line Preventative Treatment

- Consider starting preventative treatment when:
  - Quality of life is severely impaired (6)
  - 2 or more attacks occur per month
  - Migraine attacks do not respond to acute drug treatment
  - Frequent, very long, or uncomfortable auras occur
- For prevention of *episodic migraine*, FDA has approved propranolol, timolol, valproate, topiramate, and methysergide:
  - Topiramate 50–100 mg b.i.d. and (off-label) low-dose amitriptyline 25–75 mg daily are considered first-line migraine preventative treatments (6)[A].
  - Calcium channel blockers (e.g., verapamil) (off label) are effective for some patients. Other antihypertensives lack definitive data (6).
- For treatment of *chronic migraine*, FDA recently approved onabotulinumtoxinA (Botox) as it significantly reduced the frequency of headache days in chronic migraineurs (2).

ADDITIONAL TREATMENT

General Measures

- Most patients manage attacks with self-care.
- Cold compresses to area of pain
- Withdrawal from stressful surroundings
- Sleep is desirable.

Issues for Referral

- Obscure diagnosis, concomitant medical conditions, significant psychopathology
- Unresponsive to usual treatment
- Analgesic-dependent headache patterns

COMPLEMENTARY AND ALTERNATIVE MEDICINE

Oral supplements with evidence for effectiveness as preventives:

- Magnesium 400 mg daily (1)[A]
- Butterbur (Petasites hybridus; Petadolex) 75 mg b.i.d. × 1 month, then 50 mg b.i.d. (1)[A]
- Feverfew 100 mg daily (1)[B]
- CoQ10 300 mg daily (1)[B]
- Riboflavin (vitamin B_2) 400 mg daily (1)[B]

IN-PATIENT CONSIDERATIONS

Initial Stabilization

Monitor vital signs, patient comfort

Admission Criteria

Consider if diagnosis not clear; status migrainosus; may need to exclude intracranial bleeds, TIA, stroke.

IV Fluids

Fluids are a necessary part of inpatient management. Keeping patients hydrated and on antiemetics around the clock may be helpful.

Discharge Criteria

Judgment based on patient's overall clinical status, patient's ability to tolerate PO medications

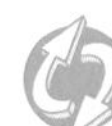

ONGOING CARE

FOLLOW-UP RECOMMENDATIONS

- Early intervention is key at the onset of an attack.
- Preventative treatment should aim to decrease frequency and severity of acute attacks, make acute treatments more efficacious, and minimize adverse drug reactions (6).

Patient Monitoring

- Monitor frequency of attacks, pain behaviors, and medication usage via headache diary.
- Encourage lifestyle modifications.

PATIENT EDUCATION

Educate patients about migraine triggers.

PROGNOSIS

- With increasing age, there may be a reduction in severity, frequency, and disability of attacks.
- Most attacks subside within 72 hours.

COMPLICATIONS

- Status migrainosus (>72 hours)
- Cerebral ischemic events (rare)
- Iatrogenic effects of treatment

REFERENCES

1. Sun-Edelstein C, Mauskop A. Food and supplements in the management of migraine headaches. *Clin J Pain*. 2009;25(5):446–52.
2. Marmura MJ, Silberstein SD, et al. Current understanding and treatment of headache disorders: Five new things. *Neurology*. 2011;76:S31–6.
3. Taylor FR, Kaniecki RG, et al. Symptomatic treatment of migraine: When to use NSAIDs, triptans, or opiates. *Curr Treat Options Neurol*. 2011;13:15–27.
4. Gilmore B, Michael M. Treatment of acute migraine headache. *Am Fam Physician*. 2011;83(3):271–80.
5. Derry S, Moore RA, McQuay HJ. Paracetamol (acetaminophen) with or without an antiemetic for acute migraine headaches in adults. *Cochrane Database Syst Rev*. 2010;(11):CD008040.
6. Fenstermacher N, Levin M, Ward T. Pharmacological prevention of migraine. *BMJ*. 2011;342:540–3.

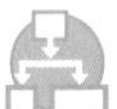

See Also (Topic, Algorithm, Electronic Media Element)

Algorithm: Headache, Chronic

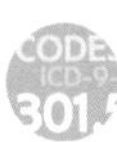

CODES

ICD9

- 346.00 Migraine with aura, without mention of intractable migraine without mention of status migrainosus
- 346.10 Migraine without aura, without mention of intractable migraine without mention of status migrainosus
- 346.90 Migraine, unspecified, without mention of intractable migraine without mention of status migrainosus

CLINICAL PEARLS

- Migraine is a chronic headache disorder of unclear etiology often characterized by unilateral, throbbing headaches that may be associated with additional neurologic symptoms.
- Accurate diagnosis of migraine is crucial.
- Consider nonspecific analgesics for milder attacks; migraine-specific treatments (triptans) for more severe attacks. Avoid opiates when possible. In frequent migraineurs, consider preventative treatments.

H

HEADACHE, TENSION

Kaelen C. Dunican, PharmD
Jill A. Grimes, MD

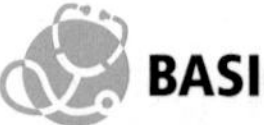

BASICS

DESCRIPTION

- Headache typically is characterized by bilateral mild to moderate pain and pressure, and it may be associated with pericranial tenderness at the base of the occiput.
- 2 types:
  - Episodic tension-type headache (ETTH) divided into:
    - Infrequent: <1 day per month
    - Frequent: ≥1 but <15 days per month
  - Chronic tension-type headache (CTTH): ≥15 days per month for >3 months
- Synonym(s): Muscle contraction headache; Stress headache

EPIDEMIOLOGY

Most common type of primary headache

Prevalence

- Lifetime prevalence is 79%.
- More prevalent among women
- Prevalence of CTTH is 3%.
- Prevalence of ETTH decreases with age, whereas the prevalence of CTTH increases with age.

RISK FACTORS

Associated with triggers/precipitating factors:

- Stress
- Change in sleep regimen
- Skipping meals
- Certain foods (caffeine, alcohol, chocolate)
- Physical exertion
- Environmental factors (sun glare, odors, smoke, noise, lighting)
- Poor or sustained posture
- Female hormonal changes
- Medications (e.g., nitrates, SSRIs, antihypertensives)
- Overuse of abortive headache medication

Genetics

An increased genetic risk has been suggested by studies, particularly for CTTH.

GENERAL PREVENTION

- Identification and avoidance of triggers/precipitating factors
- Minimize emotional stress.
- Encourage relaxation techniques:
  - Biofeedback, relaxation therapy, and physical therapy
  - Consider counseling/psychotherapy.

PATHOPHYSIOLOGY

- Debatable: Peripheral and/or central mechanisms
- Activation of peripheral nociceptors leads to muscle tenderness in ETTH.
- Central sensitization is associated with CTTH:
  - Nitric oxide may play an important role in central sensitization.
  - Debatable: Low platelet serotonin
- Peripheral: May provoke the central mechanism leading from ETTH to CTTH

ETIOLOGY

Stress is the most frequently reported precipitating factor.

COMMONLY ASSOCIATED CONDITIONS

- 83% of patients with migraine headaches also suffer from tension-type headaches.
- Debatable: Increased prevalence of comorbid anxiety and depression

DIAGNOSIS

Diagnosis is based on clinical symptoms:

- Diagnostic criteria provided by the International Headache Society (1):
  - Headache lasting 30 minutes to 7 days
  - At least 2 of the following:
    - Bilateral location
    - Pressing/tightening (nonpulsating) quality
    - Mild or moderate intensity
    - Not aggravated by routine physical activity
  - Not associated with nausea or vomiting (chronic type may be associated with nausea)
  - No more than 1 of the following: Photophobia or phonophobia
- Headache not due to another disorder
- Fronto-occipital or generalized pain (dull, pressing, or bandlike)
- Associated symptoms:
  - Fatigue
  - Irritability
  - Difficulty concentrating
  - Muscular tightness, tenderness, or stiffness in neck, occipital, and frontal regions

HISTORY

Obtain a thorough headache history to rule out other headache disorders, including severity, symptoms, onset, location and radiation of pain; quality of pain; concurrent medical conditions and medications; and recent trauma or other procedures:

- Onset of new headache in patients >40 years of age is cause for careful study, including imaging.

PHYSICAL EXAM

- General physical exam: Vital signs, funduscopic and cardiovascular assessment, palpation of the head and neck
- Neurologic exam: Mental status, pupillary responses, motor-strength testing, deep tendon reflexes, sensation, cerebellar function, gait testing, signs of meningeal irritation

DIAGNOSTIC TESTS & INTERPRETATION

Labs and neuroimaging (CT or MRI) *are only necessary when a secondary cause is suspected*:

- Atypical pattern of headache (does not fit specific category such as migraine, cluster, or tension) (2)[A]
- Focal neurologic findings
- New onset after age 40 years
- Sudden onset or worsening with exertion or Valsalva (2)[A]

Imaging

- CT scan, with and without contrast, is as sensitive as MRI and is the test of choice.
- Use MRI when lesions of the posterior fossa or aneurysm are suspected.

DIFFERENTIAL DIAGNOSIS

- Migraine headache
- Cluster headache
- Head trauma
- Subarachnoid hemorrhage
- Subdural hematoma
- Unruptured vascular malformation
- Ischemic cerebrovascular disease
- Temporal arteritis
- Arterial hypertension (HTN)
- Cerebral venous thrombosis
- Benign intracranial HTN
- Intracranial neoplasm, infection, or meningitis
- Low CSF pressure
- Medication (nonprescription analgesic dependency, nitrates)
- Caffeine dependency
- Metabolic disorders (hypoxia, hypercapnia, hypoglycemia)
- Toxic effects from drugs or fumes
- Temporomandibular joint syndrome
- Eyes: Glaucoma, refractive errors
- Sinusitis or middle-ear infection
- Cervical spondylosis
- Severe anemia or polycythemia
- Uremia and hepatic disorders
- Paget disease of bone

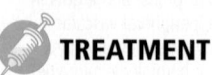

TREATMENT

- NSAIDs, acetaminophen (APAP), and aspirin (ASA) are effective for short-term pain relief of ETTH (3,4)[A].
- Tricyclic antidepressants (TCAs) are effective prophylaxis of CTTH (3,5)[A]. Amitriptyline should be considered first-line treatment for CTTH (4)[A].

MEDICATION

Choice of simple analgesic is based on patient-specific parameters:

- NSAIDs are most effective and should be considered first line in most patients for ETTH (3)[A]:
  - Ibuprofen and naproxen may be preferred due to better GI tolerability.
- APAP should be considered for patients taking warfarin, unable to tolerate NSAIDs, or allergic to ASA or NSAIDs.

First Line

- For acute attack (ETTH): NSAIDs, APAP, or ASA:
  - NSAIDs:
    - Ibuprofen (Motrin, Advil) 400–800 mg; may repeat q8h PRN (maximum 3.2 g/d)
    - Naproxen (Naprosyn) 375–500 mg or naproxen sodium (Aleve, Anaprox) 440–550 mg; may repeat q8–12h PRN (maximum 1,250 mg naproxen base/d)
    - Ketoprofen (Orudis) 12.5–50 mg; may repeat q6–8h PRN (maximum 300 mg/d)
    - Diclofenac (Voltaren, Cataflam) 50–100 mg; may repeat q8h PRN (maximum 150 mg/d)

- Contraindications:
  - ASA or NSAID allergy or bronchospasm, renal disease, bleeding disorders, increased risk of cardiovascular events (myocardial infarction [MI], stroke, new onset, or worsening of HTN)
- Drug interactions: Antihypertensives, anticoagulants, antiplatelet drugs, ASA, lithium, methotrexate
- Adverse effects:
  - Epigastric distress, peptic ulcer
- APAP (Tylenol) 1,000 mg; may repeat q6h PRN (maximum 4 g/d):
  - Adverse effects (rare): Rash, pancytopenia, liver damage
  - Precaution: Hepatic impairment, consumption of ≥3 alcoholic beverages per day
- Aspirin 500–1,000 mg; may repeat q6h PRN (maximum 4 g/d):
  - Contraindication: ASA or NSAID allergy or bronchospasm, bleeding disorders
  - Drug interactions: Anticoagulants, antiplatelet drugs, ACE inhibitors, β-blockers, corticosteroids, NSAIDs, sulfonylureas
  - Adverse effects: GI irritation/bleeding, thrombocytopenia
- Prophylaxis for CTTH: TCAs (amitriptyline [Elavil]), 10–75 mg/d:
  - Not FDA approved for CTTH.
  - Contraindications: Acute recovery phase of MI, use of monamine oxidase inhibitors (MAOIs) within 14 days
  - Drug interactions: Clonidine, MAOIs, quinolone antibiotics, SSRIs, sympathomimetics, azole antifungals, valproic acid
  - Adverse effects: Drowsiness, dry mouth, tachycardia, heart block, blurred vision, urinary retention, seizure

Second Line

- For acute attack (ETTH):
  - Caffeine combinations: 130 mg caffeine with 500 mg APAP and/or 500 mg ASA q6h PRN
  - Narcotic analgesics (rarely indicated; consider secondary causes of headache or secondary gain, such as drug-seeking behavior for personal use or diversion/sale)
  - Ketorolac: 60 mg IM, single dose
- For CTTH prophylaxis:
  - Mirtazapine 15–30 mg/d (not FDA approved for CTTH) (4)
  - Venlafaxine XR (Effexor XR): 37.5–300 mg/d (not FDA approved for CTTH) (4)
  - Alternative TCAs (not FDA approved for CTTH; although limited evidence of benefit, all are widely used for prophylaxis) (6):
    - Desipramine (Norpramin) 50–100 mg/d
    - Imipramine (Tofranil) 50–100 mg/d
    - Nortriptyline (Pamelor) 25–50 mg/d
    - Protriptyline (Vivactil) 25 mg/d

ALERT

Use of abortive agents >2 days per week may lead to *medication-overuse headaches*; must withdraw acute treatment to diagnose.

Pediatric Considerations

ASA and antidepressants are contraindicated.

ADDITIONAL TREATMENT

The combination of stress management therapy and a TCA (amitriptyline) may be most effective for CTTH.

General Measures

Relief measures: Relaxation routines; rest in quiet, dark room; hot bath or shower; massage of back of neck and temples

Additional Therapies

- Cognitive-behavioral interventions such as stress management programs may be helpful.
- Physical therapy, including positioning, ergonomic instruction, massage, transcutaneous electrical nerve simulation, and application of heat or cold may help
- Evidence regarding the usefulness of relaxation, biofeedback, and cognitive-behavioral therapies is conflicting.

COMPLEMENTARY AND ALTERNATIVE MEDICINE

- Topiramate 100 mg/d (limited clinical evidence for prevention of CTTH; not FDA approved for CTTH)
- Drugs with conflicting clinical evidence for CTTH (not FDA approved for CTTH):
  - Tizanidine 2–6 mg t.i.d.
  - Botulinum toxin type A 2–12 U injected into tender cranial muscles
  - Memantine 20–40 mg/d
- Alternative agents (not FDA approved for TTH):
  - Tiger Balm or peppermint oil applied topically to the forehead may be effective for ETTH.
  - Limited evidence: use of acupuncture (7)[A].

SURGERY/OTHER PROCEDURES

Chiropractic spinal manipulation cannot be recommended for the management of ETTH; recommendations cannot be made for CTTH (8)[A]

IN-PATIENT CONSIDERATIONS

Initial Stabilization

Outpatient treatment

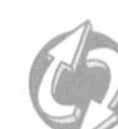

ONGOING CARE

FOLLOW-UP RECOMMENDATIONS

- Regulate sleep schedule.
- Regular exercise

DIET

- Identification and avoidance of dietary triggers
- Regulate meal schedule.

PATIENT EDUCATION

For additional information, contact:

- National Headache Foundation (888-643-5552, www.headaches.org)
- American Council for Headache Education (800-255-ACHE, www.achenet.org)

PROGNOSIS

- Usually follows a chronic course when life stressors are not changed
- Most cases are intermittent.

COMPLICATIONS

- Lost days of work and productivity (more with CTTH)
- Cost to health system
- Dependence/addiction to narcotic analgesics
- GI bleeding from NSAID use

REFERENCES

1. Headache Classification Subcommittee of the International Headache Society. The international classification of headache disorders: 2nd edition. *Cephalalgia*. 2004;24:1–151.
2. Detsky ME, McDonald DR, Baerlocher MO, et al. Does this patient with headache have a migraine or need neuroimaging? *JAMA*. 2006;296:1274–83.
3. Lenaerts ME. Pharmacotherapy of tension-type headache (TTH). *Expert Opin Pharmacother*. 2009;10:1261–71.
4. Bendtsen L, Evers S, Linde M, et al. EFNS guideline on the treatment of tension-type headache - report of an EFNS task force. *Eur J Neurol*. 2010;17: 1318–25.
5. Moja PL, Cusi C, Sterzi RR, et al. Selective serotonin re-uptake inhibitors (SSRIs) for preventing migraine and tension-type headaches. *Cochrane Database Syst Rev*. 2005:CD002919.
6. Verhagen AP, Damen L, Berger MY, et al. Lack of benefit for prophylactic drugs of tension-type headache in adults: A systematic review. *Fam Pract*. 2010;27:151–65.
7. Linde K, Allais G, Brinkhaus B, et al. Acupuncture for tension-type headache. *Cochrane Database Syst Rev*. 2009;CD007587.
8. Bryans R, Descarreaux M, Duranleau M, et al. Evidence-based guidelines for the chiropractic treatment of adults with headache. *J Manipulative Physiol Ther*. 2011;34:274–89.

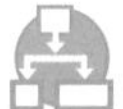

See Also (Topic, Algorithm, Electronic Media Element)

Algorithm: Headache, Chronic

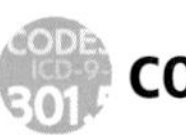

CODES

ICD9

307.81 Tension headache

CLINICAL PEARLS

- Tension-type headache may be difficult to distinguish from migraine without aura. A tension-type headache is typically described as bilateral, mild to moderate, dull pain, whereas a migraine is typically pulsating; unilateral; and associated with nausea, vomiting, and photophobia or phonophobia.
- Evidence suggests that NSAIDs may be more effective than APAP for ETTH. Consider APAP for patients who cannot tolerate or have a contraindication to NSAIDS. Initial dose of APAP should be 1,000 mg (500 mg may not be as effective).
- CTTH is difficult to treat, and these patients are more likely to develop medication-overuse headache. Clinical evidence supports the use of amitriptyline plus stress-management therapy for CTTH.
- Medication-overuse headaches must be avoided by limiting use of abortive agents to no more than 2 days per week.

H

HEARING LOSS

Teresa V. Chan, MD

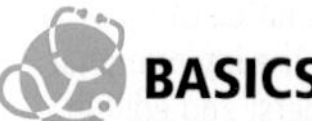

BASICS

DESCRIPTION

- Reduction in hearing manifested as decreased ability to detect or comprehend sound or speech
- May be conductive hearing loss (CHL or air–bone gap), sensorineural hearing loss (SNHL), or both
- System(s) affected: Auditory; External and middle ear (CHL), or inner ear (SNHL)

ALERT

- Any sudden SNHL (usually unilateral) is a medical emergency and should be referred to an otolaryngologist immediately.
- Treatment with high-dose steroids (1 mg/kg/d prednisone for 7–14 days, followed by taper) should begin ASAP, ideally within 1–2 weeks of onset.
- A simple 512-Hz tuning fork test lateralizes to unaffected ear in sudden SNHL (emergency) and lateralizes to the affected ear in CHL (not an emergency).

EPIDEMIOLOGY

- Predominant age: All ages affected; common in children (CHL) and elderly (SNHL)
- Predominant sex: Male = Female

Incidence

Hearing loss by age group:

- 3 in 10 people >60 years old
- 1 in 6 people ages 41–59 years old
- 1 in 14 people ages 29–40 years old
- At least 1.4 million children (18 or younger)

Prevalence

Hearing loss has doubled in the US during the past 30 years: 13.2 million people in 1971 to 28.2 million in 2000

Geriatric Considerations

- Age-related hearing loss is the most common cause in the US.
- ~50% of people >85 years have hearing loss.
- Hearing aids are underutilized.
- Loss of communication is a source of emotional stress and a physical risk for elderly.

Pediatric Considerations

Congenital hearing loss:

- 1–3/1,000 infants have hearing loss.
- Mandatory newborn screening (OAE and ABR testing is ideal)
- NICU screening before discharge
- Audiologic testing after major intracranial infection (meningitis)

Pregnancy Considerations

Otosclerosis (a CHL) can worsen during pregnancy.

RISK FACTORS

- Conductive:
  - Allergy
  - Chronic sinusitis
  - Cigarette smoking, second-hand smoke
  - Sleep apnea with CPAP use
  - Adenoid hypertrophy
  - Nasopharyngeal mass
  - Eustachian tube dysfunction
  - Head trauma
  - Neuromuscular disease
  - Family history/heredity
  - Altered immunity
  - Prematurity and low birth weight
  - Young age
  - Craniofacial abnormalities (e.g., cleft palate, Down syndrome)
  - Third mobile window (superior canal dehiscence or large vestibular aqueduct)
- Sensorineural:
  - Aging/older age
  - Loud noise/acoustic trauma
  - Dizziness/vertigo: Especially Ménière disease or history of labyrinthitis
  - Medications (aminoglycosides, loop diuretics, quinine, aspirin, chemotherapeutic agents)
  - Bacterial meningitis
  - Head trauma
  - Atherosclerosis
  - Vestibular schwannoma/skull base neoplasm
  - Previous ear surgery
- Sensorineural, pediatric-specific:
  - Postnatal asphyxia
  - NICU hospitalization
  - Mechanical ventilation lasting ≥5 days
  - In utero infections (TORCH)
  - Toxemia of pregnancy
  - Maternal diabetes
  - Rh incompatibility
  - Prematurity or birth weight <1,500 g
  - Hyperbilirubinemia; exchange transfusions
  - Anomalous temporal bone (Mondini or large vestibular aqueduct)
  - Infectious diseases: Chickenpox, measles, encephalitis, influenza, mumps

Genetics

- Connexin 26 (13q11–12): Most common cause of nonsyndromic genetic hearing loss
- Mitochondrial mutations or disorders:
  - May predispose to aminoglycoside ototoxicity
- Otosclerosis: Familial; no clear genetic cause
- Most common congenital syndromes:
  - Hemifacial microsomia
  - Stickler syndrome
  - Congenital cytomegalovirus
  - Usher syndrome
  - Branchio-oto-renal syndrome
  - Pendred syndrome
  - CHARGE association
  - Neurofibromatosis type II
  - Waardenburg syndrome

GENERAL PREVENTION

- Limit noise exposure; use hearing protection when exposure cannot be avoided.
- Avoid ear canal instrumentation (Q-tips, etc.).
- Limit ototoxic medications.

PATHOPHYSIOLOGY

- CHL:
  - Hearing loss can result from middle ear effusion, obstruction of canal (cerumen/foreign body, osteomas/exostoses, cholesteatoma, tumor), loss of continuity (ossicular discontinuity), stiffening of the components (myringosclerosis, tympanosclerosis, and otosclerosis), and loss of the pressure differential across the TM (perforation).
- SNHL:
  - Damage along the pathway from oval window, cochlea, auditory nerve, and brainstem. Examples include vascular/metabolic insult, mass effect, infection and inflammation, acoustic trauma (see below).
  - Noise-induced hearing loss is caused by acoustic insult that affects outer hair cells in organ of Corti causing them to be less stiff. Over time, severe damage occurs with fusion and loss of stereocilia. Eventually may progress to inner hair cells and auditory nerve as well.
- Large vestibular aqueduct or superior canal dehiscence: Third mobile window shunts acoustic energy away from cochlea.

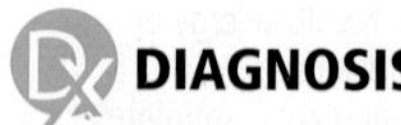

DIAGNOSIS

HISTORY

- Difficulty hearing:
  - Rapid vs. gradual decline: Rapid loss (<3 days) is a medical emergency. If suspicious of a sudden SNHL, refer to ENT ASAP.
  - Difficulty with discrimination
  - Difficulty hearing in crowds
  - Frequently having to ask speakers to repeat
  - Friends/family complain of hearing loss
  - TV, phone volume increasing
- Tinnitus, bilateral or unilateral
- Otalgia
- Otorrhea, clear or purulent
- Dizziness or vertigo
- Ear fullness
- Autophony (hearing own voice louder or echoing)
- Facial nerve twitching or asymmetry
- Depression
- Anxiety
- History of ear infections or ear surgeries
- History of trauma or noise exposure
- Family history of hearing loss
- History of recent viral infection
- Nasal obstruction
- Frequent epistaxis

PHYSICAL EXAM

- 512-Hz tuning fork tests:
  - Sensorineural loss:
    - Placed on the forehead: Lateralizes to nonaffected ear (Weber test)
    - Base of tuning fork placed on the mastoid and then fork end placed next to ear; heard louder next to ear (Rinne test)
  - Conductive loss:
    - Placed on the forehead or teeth lateralizes to affected or symptomatic ear
    - Placed on the mastoid and then next to ear; heard louder behind the ear on the side of conductive deficit
- Otoscopy: Assess for deformity, canal patency, and otorrhea; TM integrity/retraction/mobility with insufflation; canal; or middle ear mass.
- Facial symmetry
- Cranial nerve exam
- Nasopharyngoscopy: Adenoid hypertrophy or nasopharyngeal mass (mandatory in adult patient with new unilateral serous effusion)
- Pediatric: Survey for syndromic anomalies.

DIAGNOSTIC TESTS & INTERPRETATION

Lab

Often labs are not needed. If indicated:

- Pendred syndrome (goiter, mental retardation + SNHL): Perchlorate test, thyroid function tests
- Alport syndrome (nephritis + SNHL): Urinalysis, renal function tests
- Jervell and Lange-Nielsen syndrome (syncope, family history of sudden death + profound SNHL): EKG
- Any pediatric patient with SNHL: Consider genetic testing for connexin 26, mitochondrial studies
- TORCH screening test
- RPR or VDRL confirmed with FTA-ABS
- Lyme titer in endemic areas
- Antinuclear antibodies and sedimentation rate as a screen for autoimmune disease

Imaging

- Fine-cut CT temporal bones without contrast may help in the evaluation of CHL.
- MRI of brain and brainstem with gadolinium to evaluate SNHL in congenital hearing loss, early onset hearing loss, asymmetric hearing loss

Diagnostic Procedures/Surgery

- Audiometry: Pure tone (air and bone), speech testing, and impedance (middle ear pressure) testing
- Tympanometry: Type B or C tympanograms indicate fluid or retraction, respectively. Negative middle ear peak pressures seen even with normal (type A) tympanograms.
- Other tests:
  - Auditory brainstem response
  - Otoacoustic emissions: "Echo" of the cochlea
  - Behavioral (visual reinforcement) audiometry; used in children 6 months–5 years
- Myringotomy and tubes can be considered for persistent fluid with hearing loss.

Pathological Findings

Varies depending on etiology

DIFFERENTIAL DIAGNOSIS

- Conductive:
  - Cerumen impaction/foreign body
  - Perforation of tympanic membrane
  - Middle ear fluid (serous otitis media)
  - Acute otitis media
  - Adhesive otitis media
  - Cholesteatoma
  - Ossicular erosion (infection, cholesteatoma)
  - Myringosclerosis/tympanosclerosis
  - Temporal bone fracture
  - Otosclerosis
  - Congenital malleus fixation
  - Glomus tumor
  - Congenital aural atresia
  - Osteogenesis imperfecta
  - Superior canal dehiscence
- Sensorineural:
  - Presbycusis (hearing loss related to aging)
  - Noise-induced (recreational, occupational)
  - Ménière disease
  - Ototoxicity (aspirin, quinine, aminoglycosides)
  - Viral labyrinthitis
  - Cerebellopontine angle tumor
  - Large vestibular aqueduct syndrome
  - Syndromic hearing loss
  - Congenital cochlear malformation
  - Labyrinthine artery infarct
  - Idiopathic
  - Syphilis
  - CMV
  - Rubella
  - Temporal bone fracture
  - Metabolic (hyper-/hypothyroid)
  - Paget disease
  - Perilymphatic (inner ear) fistula
  - Autoimmune inner ear disease

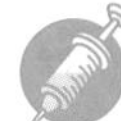

TREATMENT

- Early detection: If sudden single-sided deafness is suspected, refer ASAP to otolaryngologist for hearing testing and commencement of steroid therapy.
- Hearing rehabilitation:
  - Personal amplifiers, situation-specific amplification (e.g., amplified phone), or personal hearing aids can be considered for any individual who has significant communication difficulties due to hearing loss.
  - Cochlear implants for patients with bilateral severe-to-profound hearing loss who no longer derive benefit from hearing aids

MEDICATION

- Depends on cause. Hearing loss is a broad topic with many possible etiologies.
- Sudden SNHL: High-dose oral steroids: 1 mg/kg or 60–100 mg/d prednisone or 12–16 mg/d dexamethasone for 7–14 days, followed by a taper:
  - Some recent papers suggest simultaneous use of oral and intratympanic steroid use results in better outcomes. There is an ongoing multicenter trial comparing the efficacy of oral steroids and intratympanic steroids (1)[A],(2).
  - Evidence is conflicting regarding use of systemic steroids in sudden SNHL (2)[A].
- Vasodilators and vasoactive substances are being used to treat idiopathic SNHL, but evidence is conflicting (3)[A].

ADDITIONAL TREATMENT

Issues for Referral

- Audiology: If hearing loss is suspected, referral to audiology is warranted. Audiologists also provide hearing aid options and maintenance.
- Genetics: If congenital syndrome or familial hearing loss is suspected
- Speech therapist: If speech delay or speech impediment is present
- Endocrinology: Pendred syndrome, other associated endocrine disorder (hypo-/hyperthyroidism)
- Cardiology: Jervell and Lange-Nielsen syndrome
- Ophthalmology: Usher syndrome
- Neurotology and neurosurgery: CPA lesion, intracranial complication of middle ear disease

SURGERY/OTHER PROCEDURES

- CHL often has surgical options for repair:
  - Tympanostomy and tube placement
  - Tympanoplasty
  - Mastoidectomy
  - Ossicular chain reconstruction
  - Stapedectomy/stapedotomy
  - Canaloplasty
- Those with profound bilateral SNHL may qualify for cochlear implantation.

ONGOING CARE

FOLLOW-UP RECOMMENDATIONS

Patient Monitoring

Audiogram and clinical exam are primary means of monitoring patient.

DIET

Salt restriction to 2 g/d is helpful for Ménière disease patients.

PROGNOSIS

SNHL is usually permanent and may be progressive.

COMPLICATIONS

Acute middle ear problems may become chronic (perforations, cholesteatoma).

REFERENCES

1. Plontke SK, Löwenheim H, Mertens J, et al. Randomized, double blind, placebo controlled trial on the safety and efficacy of continuous intratympanic dexamethasone delivered via a round window catheter for severe to profound sudden idiopathic sensorineural hearing loss after failure of systemic therapy. *Laryngoscope*. 2009;119: 359–69.
2. Wei BP, Mubiru S, O'Leary S, et al. Steroids for idiopathic sudden sensorineural hearing loss. *Cochrane Database Syst Rev*. 2006;CD003998.
3. Agarwal L, Pothier DD, et al. Vasodilators and vasoactive substances for idiopathic sudden sensorineural hearing loss. *Cochrane Database Syst Rev*. 2009;CD003422.

ADDITIONAL READING

- Chau JK, Lin JR, Atashband S, et al. Systematic review of the evidence for the etiology of adult sudden sensorineural hearing loss. *Laryngoscope*. 2010;120:1011–21.
- For information on NIH-funded study. Available at: www.suddendeafness.org.
- National Institute on Deafness and Other Communication Disorders. Available at: www.nidcd.nih.gov/health/hearing/.

CODES

ICD9

- 389.00 Conductive hearing loss, unspecified
- 389.10 Sensorineural hearing loss, unspecified
- 389.9 Unspecified hearing loss

CLINICAL PEARLS

- In sudden hearing loss, if a 512-Hz tuning fork test (Weber test) lateralizes to the *unaffected ear*, suspect sensorineural causes (emergent evaluation needed), but if it lateralizes to the *affected* ear, the diagnosis is conductive hearing loss (not an emergency).
- ~50% of people >85 years have hearing loss, so encourage screening and treatment, especially in patients with early dementia (to maximize sensory input and sort out confusion vs. lack of hearing).

HEAT EXHAUSTION AND HEAT STROKE

Scott A. Fields, MD

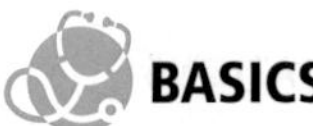

BASICS

DESCRIPTION

- A continuum of increasingly severe heat illnesses caused by dehydration, electrolyte losses, and failure of the body's thermoregulatory mechanisms:
  - Heat exhaustion is an acute heat injury with hyperthermia owing to dehydration.
  - Heat stroke is extreme hyperthermia with thermoregulatory failure and profound CNS dysfunction.
- System(s) affected: Endocrine/Metabolic; Nervous
- Synonym(s): Heat illness; Heat injury; Hyperthermia; Heat collapse; Heat prostration

Geriatric Considerations

Elderly persons are more susceptible.

Pediatric Considerations

Children are more susceptible.

Pregnancy Considerations

Pregnant women may be more prone to volume depletion with heat stress.

EPIDEMIOLOGY

- Predominant age: More likely in children or elderly
- Predominant sex: Male = Female

Incidence

Depends on intensity of heat; estimate of 20/100,000 persons per season

Prevalence

- Depends on predisposing conditions in combination with environmental factors
- Roughly 240 deaths per year in the US

RISK FACTORS

- Poor acclimatization to heat or poor physical conditioning
- Salt or water depletion
- Obesity
- Acute febrile or GI illnesses
- Chronic illnesses: Uncontrolled diabetes mellitus or hypertension, cardiac disease
- Alcohol and other substance abuse
- High heat and humidity, poor air circulation in environment
- Heavy, restrictive clothing
- Nutritional supplementation that includes ephedra

GENERAL PREVENTION

- The most important factor in preventing heat stress is adequate fluid replacement.
- Allow acclimatization to hot weather through proper conditioning and activity modification.
- Dress appropriately with loose-fitting, open-weave, light-colored clothing.

PATHOPHYSIOLOGY

Only those associated with major organ system failure

ETIOLOGY

Failure of heat-dissipating mechanisms or an overwhelming heat stress leading to a rise in core temperature, dehydration, and salt depletion

DIAGNOSIS

- Heat exhaustion: Symptoms are milder than in heat stroke, with no severe CNS derangements:
  - Fatigue and lethargy
  - Weakness
  - Dizziness
  - Nausea, vomiting
  - Myalgias
  - Headache
  - Profuse sweating
  - Tachycardia
  - Hypotension
  - Lack of coordination
  - Agitation
  - Intense thirst
  - Hyperventilation
  - Paresthesias
  - Core temperature elevated but <103°F (<39.4°C)
- Heat stroke: Divided into 2 categories: Classic and exertional:
  - Classic: Caused by environmental exposure, primarily in elderly or chronically ill patients, and may develop gradually over days
  - Exertional: Typically younger, very active patients; rapid onset:
    - Exhaustion
    - Confusion, disorientation
    - Delirium
    - Coma
    - Hot, flushed, and dry skin (sweating may continue in exertional heat stroke)
    - Core temperature >105°F (>40.5°C)

DIAGNOSTIC TESTS & INTERPRETATION

Lab

Used primarily to detect end-organ damage

Initial lab tests

- Electrolytes, urinalysis
- Creatinine, BUN
- Liver enzymes, muscle enzymes (creatine phosphokinase)
- CBC
- Increased urine specific gravity
- Results of these studies may indicate hypernatremia, hyperchloremia, and hemoconcentration.
- Drugs that may alter lab results: Diuretics

Diagnostic Procedures/Surgery

Rectal temperature monitoring

DIFFERENTIAL DIAGNOSIS

- Other causes of elevated temperature, dehydration, or circulatory collapse
- Febrile illnesses, sepsis
- Drug-induced fluid loss
- Cardiac arrhythmia or infarction
- Acute cocaine intoxication
- Neuroleptic malignant syndrome
- Malignant hyperthermia (an autosomally inherited disorder of skeletal and cardiac muscle in which patients have abnormal muscle metabolism on exposure to halothane or skeletal muscle reactants)

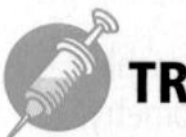

TREATMENT

MEDICATION

First Line

No medications are required in the initial management. Use isotonic saline solution to rehydrate (1,2)[C].

Second Line

- Consider immunomodulators such as corticosteroids (2)[C].
- Iced gastric, bladder, or peritoneal lavage (1,2)[C]
- Dantrolene 2–4 mg/kg for chemically assisted cooling (2)[C].
- In disseminated intravascular coagulopathy (DIC), consider appropriate replacement therapy.

ADDITIONAL TREATMENT

General Measures

- Fluid and electrolyte replacement with hypotonic oral fluids or IV 0.5–1 L normal saline initial bolus
- Consider central venous pressure (CVP) monitoring.
- Body immersion in ice water (1,2)[C]
- Evaporative cooling: Spraying water over the patient and facilitating evaporation and convection with the use of fans (1,2)[C]
- Immersing the hands and forearms in cold water (1,2)[C]
- Use of ice or cold packs on the neck, groin, and axillae (3)

IN-PATIENT CONSIDERATIONS

Initial Stabilization

- Emergency treatment; best in a hospital setting
- Rapid cooling: Remove clothing, wet patient down, and apply ice packs.

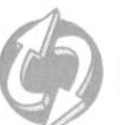

ONGOING CARE

FOLLOW-UP RECOMMENDATIONS

Rest with legs elevated (1,2)[C]

Patient Monitoring

- Rectal temperature monitoring: Cooling may be discontinued when the core temperature drops to 102°F (38.9°C) and stabilizes.
- Heat stroke patients may require airway management, hemodynamic monitoring, and careful fluid and electrolyte administration and monitoring.
- Consider CVP monitoring.

DIET

- Cool or cold clear liquids only (noncarbonated)
- Avoid caffeine.
- Unrestricted sodium

PATIENT EDUCATION

- The key to prevention is proper hydration.
- Stress the importance of proper conditioning and acclimatization.
- Instruct patients to recognize heat stress signs and symptoms.
- Maintain as much skin exposure as possible in hot, humid conditions while using proper sun-block protection.
- Avoid dehydration by consuming a proper amount of fluids during activity or exercise: 8 oz fluid intake for every 15 minutes of moderate exercise.
- Never leave children unattended in cars during hot weather.
- Try to gain access to air-conditioned environments during hot weather.

PROGNOSIS

- The prognosis is good when mental function is not altered and when serum enzymes are not elevated; recovery is within 24–48 hours in most cases.
- The mortality rate for heat stroke (10–80%) is directly related to the duration and intensity of hyperthermia, as well as to the speed and effectiveness of diagnosis and treatment.

COMPLICATIONS

- May involve failure of any major organ system
- Cardiac arrhythmias or infarction
- Pulmonary edema, acute respiratory distress syndrome
- Coma, seizures
- Acute renal failure
- Rhabdomyolysis
- DIC
- Hepatocellular necrosis

REFERENCES

1. Cleary M. Predisposing risk factors on susceptibility to exertional heat illness: Clinical decision-making considerations. *J Sport Rehabilitation*. 2007;16(3): 204–14.
2. Muldoon S. Identification of risk factors for exertional heat illness: A brief commentary on genetic testing. *J Sport Rehabilitation*. 2007;16(3): 222–6.
3. Gaffin SL, Gardner JW, Flinn SD. Cooling methods for heatstroke victims. *Ann Intern Med*. 2000;132: 678.

ADDITIONAL READING

- American College of Sports Medicine, Armstrong LE, Casa DJ, et al. American College of Sports Medicine position stand. Exertional heat illness during training and competition. *Med Sci Sports Exerc*. 2007;39: 556–72.
- Bouchama A, Dehbi M, Chaves-Carballo E. Cooling and hemodynamic management in heatstroke: Practical recommendations. *Crit Care*. 2007;11(3): R54.
- Bouchama A, Knochel JP. Heat stroke. *N Engl J Med*. 2002;346:1978–88.
- Charaton F. Ephedra supplement may have contributed to sportsman's death. *Br Med J*. 2003;326:464.
- Glazer JL. Management of heatstroke and heat exhaustion. *Am Fam Physician*. 2005;71(11): 2133–40.
- Smith JE. Cooling methods used in the treatment of exertional heat illness. *Br J Sports Med*. 2005;39: 503–7; discussion 507.
- Yeo TP. Heat stroke: A comprehensive review. *AACN Clin Issues*. 2004;15:280–93.

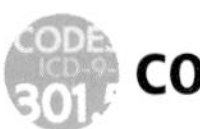

CODES

ICD9

- 992.0 Heat stroke and sunstroke
- 992.5 Heat exhaustion, unspecified

CLINICAL PEARLS

- The diagnosis of heat stroke relies on both hyperthermia and CNS dysfunction (e.g., irritability, ataxia, confusion, seizures, or coma).
- Start the cooling process immediately when heat exhaustion or heat stroke is recognized, beginning with wetting the skin with a cool mist and giving oral rehydration solutions containing saline, if the patient is alert and oriented.

HEMATURIA

Tracy O. Middleton, DO

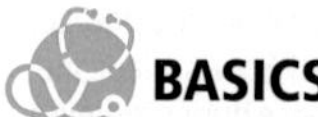

BASICS

DESCRIPTION

Blood or RBCs in the urine:

- Gross (visible) or microscopic (nonvisible)
- Symptomatic or asymptomatic

EPIDEMIOLOGY

Prevalence

- Microscopic hematuria in school-aged children: 0.5–2% (1)
- Microscopic hematuria in asymptomatic adults varies from 0.19–21%, depending on population studied (2,3).

RISK FACTORS

- Smoking
- Occupational exposures (dyes, rubber or tire manufacturing) (urothelial cancer)
- Analgesic abuse (e.g., phenacetin)
- Medications (e.g., cyclophosphamide)
- Pelvic irradiation
- Chronic infection, especially with calculi
- Recent upper respiratory tract infection
- Positive family history of renal diseases (stones, glomerulonephritis)
- Underlying primary renal disorder

ETIOLOGY

- Trauma:
  - Exercise-induced (resolves with rest)
  - Abdominal trauma and/or pelvic fracture with renal, bladder, or ureteral injury
  - Iatrogenic from abdominal or pelvic surgery; chronic indwelling catheters
  - Foreign body, physical/sexual abuse
- Neoplasms:
  - Malignancies: 30% of adult patients with painless, gross hematuria and ~10% with painless microscopic hematuria have a malignancy (2). Urothelial carcinoma of the bladder and renal tumors are of greatest concern in adults.
  - Benign tumors
  - Endometriosis of the urinary tract (suspect in females with cyclic hematuria)
- Inflammatory causes:
  - UTI: Most common cause of hematuria in adults
  - Renal diseases: Radiation nephritis, radiation cystitis, acute and chronic tubulointerstitial nephritis (due to drugs, infections, systemic disease)
  - Glomerular disease:
    - Goodpasture syndrome (antiglomerular basement membrane disease; autoimmune; associated pulmonary hemorrhage)
    - IGA nephropathy
    - Lupus nephritis
    - Henoch-Schönlein purpura
    - Membranoproliferative, poststreptococcal, or rapidly progressive glomerulonephritis
    - Wegener granulomatosis
  - Endocarditis/visceral abscesses
  - Other infections: Schistosomiasis, TB, syphilis
- Metabolic causes:
  - Calculus disease (85% of patients have hematuria):
    - Hypercalciuria: A common cause of both gross and microscopic hematuria in children (1)
    - Hyperuricosuria
- Congenital/Familial causes:
  - Cystic disease: Polycystic kidney disease, solitary renal cyst
  - Benign familial hematuria or thin basement membrane nephropathy (autosomal dominant)
  - Alport syndrome (X-linked in 85%; hematuria, proteinuria, hearing loss, corneal abnormalities) (4)
  - Fabry disease (X-linked recessive inborn error of metabolism; vascular kidney disease)
  - Nail-patella syndrome (autosomal dominant; nail and patella hypoplasia; hematuria in 33%)
  - Renal tubular acidosis type 1 (autosomal dominant or autoimmune)
- Hematologic causes:
  - Bleeding dyscrasias (e.g., hemophilia)
  - Sickle cell anemia/trait (renal papillary necrosis)
- Vascular causes:
  - Hemangioma
  - Arteriovenous malformations (rare)
  - Nutcracker syndrome: Compression of left renal vein and subsequent renal parenchymal congestion
  - Renal artery/vein thrombosis
  - Arterial emboli to kidney
- Chemical causes:
  - Nephrotoxins: Aminoglycosides, cyclosporine
  - Other drugs: Analgesics, oral contraceptives, Chinese herbs
- Obstruction:
  - Strictures or posterior urethral valves
  - Hydronephrosis, from any cause
  - Benign prostatic hyperplasia: Rule out other causes of hematuria.
- Other causes: Loin pain hematuria (most often in young women on oral contraceptives)

DIAGNOSIS

HISTORY

Considerations:

- Burning, urgency, frequency: UTI
- Dark cola-colored urine: Glomerular origin
- Arthritis/arthralgias/rash: Lupus, vasculitis, Henoch-Schönlein purpura
- Flank pain: Stones, infarction, pyelonephritis
- Recent upper respiratory infection (URI): Poststreptococcal GN, membranoproliferative GN; concurrent URI: IgA nephropathy
- Excessive vitamin use: Stones
- Marathon runner: Traumatic, rhabdomyolysis
- Travel: Schistosomiasis, tuberculosis
- Painless hematuria and/or weight loss: Malignancy
- Family history: Alport disease (hereditary nephritis), sickle cell, polycystic, IgA nephropathy, thin basement membrane disease

PHYSICAL EXAM

Considerations:

- Elevated BP, edema, and weight gain: Glomerular disease
- Fever: Infection
- Palpable kidney: Neoplasm, polycystic
- Genitalia: Look for meatal erosion, lesions

DIAGNOSTIC TESTS & INTERPRETATION

Pediatric Considerations

- Consider glomerulonephritis, Wilms tumor, child abuse
- Isolated asymptomatic microscopic hematuria may not need full workup; these pediatric patients rarely need cystoscopy, but must be observed for development of HTN, gross hematuria, or proteinuria (1,4)[B].
- Gross, or symptomatic, hematuria needs a full workup.
- If eumorphic RBCs, consider US (rule out stones, congenital abnormalities) and urinary Ca:Cr ratio (hypercalcemia) (4).
- If dysmorphic RBCs, consider renal consult.
- Renal ultrasound identifies most congenital and malignant conditions; CT reserved for cases of suspected trauma or stones (4)

Lab

Initial lab tests

- Urine dipstick (sensitivity 91–100%; specificity 65–99%):
  - False negatives are rare, but can be caused by high-dose vitamin C.
  - False positives: Oxidizers (povidone, bacterial peroxidases, bleach), myoglobin, alkaline urine (>9), semen, food coloring, food (beets, blackberries, rhubarb, paprika) (5)
  - Phenazopyridine may discolor the dipstick, making interpretation difficult.
- Microscopic urinalysis should always be done to confirm dipstick findings and quantify RBCs (6):
  - American Urological Association (AUA) defines clinically significant microscopic hematuria as ≥3 RBCs/hpf on microscopic evaluation of sediment from 2 of 3 properly collected (midstream, clean-catch) specimens (2,5,7)[C].
  - Exclude factitious or nonurinary causes, such as menstruation, mild trauma, exercise, poor collection technique, or chemical/drug causes, through cessation of activity/cause and a repeat urinalysis in 48 hours (1,2)[C].
- Differentiate intrinsic renal disease from other causes. Indicators of renal disease are significant (>500 mg/d) proteinuria, red cell casts (pathognomonic of glomerular disease), dysmorphic RBCs, and increased creatinine (7)[C].
- Urine culture if suspected infection/pyuria (4)
- In patients at high risk for lower tract cancer (e.g., former smokers, age >40, occupational exposures, etc.):
  - Urine cytology (sensitivity 66–79%; specificity 95–100%); preferably first void of morning on 3 consecutive days (AUA recommendation) (2); these patients will also require cystoscopy and upper urinary tract imaging (7)(C)
  - Cystoscopy for biopsy
  - Urinary tumor markers are available, but not currently recommended in the initial evaluation of hematuria.
- If persistent microscopic hematuria:
  - Renal function tests: BUN, creatinine, glomerular filtration rate
  - PT/INR for patients on warfarin or suspected of abusing warfarin
  - CBC:
    - Elevated WBCs with deeper infections
    - Anemia is unlikely from hematuria, although gross hematuria may produce significant blood loss.
  - Urine Ca:Cr ratio >0.2 mg/mg is suggestive of hypercalcuria in children >6 years (4).

Follow-Up & Special Considerations
Other tests depend on suspected etiology: STD testing, ANCA, C3, C4, ASO titer, hemoglobin electrophoresis (4)

Imaging

Initial approach

- For suspicion of stones, unenhanced helical CT; for upper tract disease, CT urography
- Multidetector CT urography (MDCTU); sensitivity 88–100%, specificity 93–100%:
  - The initial imaging of choice in nonpregnant adults with unexplained hematuria, especially if risk factors are present (5,8)[B]
  - Highly specific and relatively sensitive for the diagnosis of urinary tract neoplasms, especially when >1 cm (8)[B]
  - Higher radiation dose; weigh risk of disease vs. risk of radiation exposure (9)[B]
  - Does not obviate the need for cystoscopy, particularly in high-risk patients (8)[B]
  - Visualization of ureters is discontinuous.
  - Less cost-efficient
- CT:
  - Perform unenhanced helical CT as first test for suspected stone disease (2)[B].
- IV urography (IVU):
  - Limited sensitivity for small renal masses and for differentiating cystic from solid masses (7)[C]
  - Addition of ultrasound or CT often necessary to evaluate renal parenchyma (7)[C]
  - Potential reactions to IV iodine contrast media
- Renal US:
  - Best for differentiating cystic from solid masses
  - Sensitive for hydronephrosis
  - No radiation or iodinated contrast exposure, so a first choice for evaluating a patient with deteriorating renal function
  - Cost-efficient
  - Poor sensitivity for small renal masses (<3 cm) (7)[C]
  - Main disadvantage is inability to thoroughly evaluate the urothelium for transitional cell cancer
- MRI:
  - Similar to CT in sensitivity for renal masses
  - No radiation exposure
  - Least cost-efficient
  - Limited ability to reliably detect urinary tract calcifications (9)[B]

Pregnancy Considerations

Renal US is initial imaging choice for pregnant or pediatric patients (5)[C].

Follow-Up & Special Considerations
In the case of glomerulonephritis, consider CXR to rule out cardiac enlargement, effusions, or pulmonary bleeding (5)[C].

Diagnostic Procedures/Surgery

- Renal biopsy:
  - May be necessary to diagnose glomerulonephritis or in the face of increasing renal insufficiency
- Retrograde pyelogram:
  - Used to further evaluate filling defects detected on other modalities (9)[B]
  - Reserved for patients in which findings on MDCTU are equivocal or increased radiation is not justifiable (9)[B]
  - Sensitive for small lesions of supravesicular collecting system
  - Requires cystoscopy
- Flexible cystoscopy:
  - Best for evaluation of bladder pathology, especially small urothelial lesions; negative predictive value for bladder tumors is 99% (2)[B]
  - Fluorescence can be used to enhance detection of flat lesions (10)[C].
  - AUA recommends all patients with hematuria who are >40, younger with risk factors for bladder cancer, and/or those with abnormal cytology receive cystoscopy (2,7)[C].
- Ureteroscopy/pyeloscopy:
  - For visualization of suspected supravesical collecting system lesions
  - Biopsy, excision, fulguration, or extraction of lesions/stones possible
  - Requires anesthesia
  - Requires cystoscopy
  - Risk of injury to collecting system

Pathological Findings

Glomerulonephritis

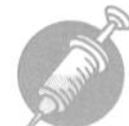

TREATMENT

MEDICATION

None indicated for undiagnosed hematuria

ADDITIONAL TREATMENT

Issues for Referral

Prompt nephrology referral for proteinuria, red cell casts, and elevated serum creatinine (2,7)[C]

SURGERY/OTHER PROCEDURES

Gross hematuria: Clots may require continuous bladder irrigation with a large-bore Foley catheter (2- or 3-way catheter may be helpful) to prevent clot retention.

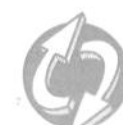

ONGOING CARE

FOLLOW-UP RECOMMENDATIONS

After initial workup, 35% of patients remain without a diagnosis.

Patient Monitoring

Although some experts still recommend periodic urinalysis and cytology, more recent literature suggests after thorough initial negative investigations (imaging, cystoscopy, cytology) no follow-up is indicated for the asymptomatic patient unless symptoms or frank hematuria develop (3)[B].

DIET

Not restricted, except in certain conditions (e.g., increased fluids for stones or clots; restricted animal proteins in stone disease)

PROGNOSIS

- Generally excellent for common causes of hematuria
- Poorer for malignant tumors and certain types of nephritis

REFERENCES

1. Bergstein J, Leiser J, Andreoli S. The clinical significance of asymptomatic gross and microscopic hematuria in children. *Arch Pediatr Adolesc Med*. 2005;159:353–5.
2. McDonald MM, Swagerty D, Wetzel L. Assessment of microscopic hematuria in adults. *Am Fam Physician*. 2006;73:1748–54.
3. Mishriki SF, Nabi G, Cohen NP. Diagnosis of urologic malignancies in patients with asymptomatic dipstick hematuria: Prospective study with 13 years' follow-up. *Urology*. 2008;71:13–6.
4. Massengill SF. Hematuria. *Pediatr Rev*. 2008;29: 342–8.
5. Choyke PL. Radiologic evaluation of hematuria: Guidelines from the American College of Radiology's appropriateness criteria. *Am Fam Physician*. 2008;78:347–52.
6. Rao PK, Gao T, Pohl M, et al. Dipstick pseudohematuria: Unnecessary consultation and evaluation. *J Urol*. 2010;183:560–4.
7. Grossfeld GD, Wolf JS, Litwan MS, et al. Asymptomatic microscopic hematuria in adults: Summary of the AUA best practice policy recommendations. *Am Fam Physician*. 2001;63: 1145–54.
8. Sudakoff GS, Dunn DP, Guralnick ML, et al. Multidetector computerized tomography urography as the primary imaging modality for detecting urinary tract neoplasms in patients with asymptomatic hematuria. *J Urol*. 2008;179: 862–7; discussion 867.
9. O'Connor OJ, McSweeney SE, Maher MM. Imaging of hematuria. *Radiol Clin North Am*. 2008;46:113–32, vii.
10. Sharma S, Ksheersagar P, Sharma P, et al. Diagnosis and treatment of bladder cancer. *Am Fam Physician*. 2009;80:717–23.

See Also (Topic, Algorithm, Electronic Media Element)

Algorithm: Hematuria

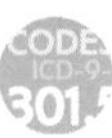

CODES

ICD9

- 599.70 Hematuria, unspecified
- 599.71 Gross hematuria
- 599.72 Microscopic hematuria

CLINICAL PEARLS

- Screening asymptomatic patients for microscopic hematuria is not recommended (2,4,10)[A].
- Asymptomatic hematuria and hematuria persisting after treatment of UTIs must be evaluated (2)[B].
- Patients with bladder cancer can have intermittent microscopic hematuria; a thorough evaluation in high-risk patients is needed after just 1 episode.
- Evaluation of upper and lower urinary tracts must be performed in all patients with gross hematuria and in high-risk patients with microscopic hematuria (7).
- After initial workup, 35% of patients remain without a diagnosis.
- Routine use of anticoagulants should not cause hematuria unless there is an underlying urologic abnormality (2)[B].

HEMOCHROMATOSIS

Robert A. Marlow, MD, MA

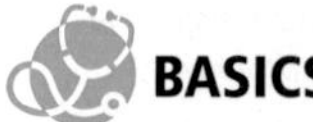

BASICS

DESCRIPTION

Hemochromatosis is a hereditary disorder in which the small intestine absorbs excessive iron (1,2):

- Early clinical features include arthralgia, fatigue, and decreased libido.
- Late effects include cirrhosis of the liver, diabetes, hypermelanotic pigmentation of the skin, and heart failure.
- Because there is no mechanism to excrete excess iron, the excess is stored in muscle and in organs, including the liver, pancreas, and heart, eventually resulting in severe damage to the affected organs.
- Liver damage ultimately may result in hepatocellular carcinoma.
- System(s) affected: Endocrine/Metabolic
- Synonym(s): Bronze diabetes; Troisier-Hanot-Chauffard syndrome

EPIDEMIOLOGY

Incidence

- Predominant age: Metabolic abnormality is congenital, but symptoms usually present in the fifth and sixth decades.
- Predominant sex: Gene frequency: Male = Female, although clinical signs are more frequent in men (8:1 male:female ratio) (3)

Prevalence

3/1,000 people (heterozygote frequency, 1/10) (4): The most common genetic abnormality in the US

Pediatric Considerations

Rarely, iron overload may occur as early as 2 years of age. The disorder can be diagnosed before iron overload is clinically apparent.

RISK FACTORS

- The disease is a genetic disorder.
- Affected individuals should not ingest iron supplements, eat raw shellfish, or eat large quantities of iron-rich food such as red meat.
- Alcohol increases the absorption of iron. (As many as 41% of patients with symptomatic disease are alcoholic.)
- Loss of blood, such as that which occurs during menstruation and pregnancy, delays the onset of symptoms.

Genetics

- Genetically heterogeneous disorder of iron overload; types 1, 2, and 3 are autosomal recessive; type 4 is autosomal dominant. Neonatal hemochromatosis is rare.
- Penetrance is incomplete; expressivity is variable.
- Factors contributing to variable expressivity include different mutations in the same gene, mitigating or exacerbating genes, and environmental factors.

GENERAL PREVENTION

- Family members of affected individuals should be screened.
- Screening of population is *not* recommended because the vast majority of those with homozygous hematomacrosis will remain asymptomatic and have a normal life span (7)[A].
- Pregnant women with the disorder should avoid iron supplements.

ETIOLOGY

- Type 1 hemochromatosis is caused by mutations in the *HFE* gene; type 2 by mutations in either the *HFE2* gene or *HAMP* gene; type 3 by mutations in the *TFR2* gene; and type 4 by mutations in the *SLC40A1* gene. The cause of neonatal hemochromatosis is unknown.
- The mechanism for increased iron absorption in the face of excessive iron stores is not clear. Iron metabolism appears normal in this disease except for a higher level of circulating iron.
- Iron overload may be caused by thalassemia, sideroblastic anemia, liver disease, excess iron intake, or chronic transfusion.

COMMONLY ASSOCIATED CONDITIONS

See "Complications."

DIAGNOSIS

HISTORY

- Weakness (83%)
- Abdominal pain (58%)
- Arthralgia (43%)
- Loss of libido or potency (38%)
- Amenorrhea (22%)
- Dyspnea on exertion (15%)
- Neurologic symptoms (6%)
- Symptoms of diabetes

PHYSICAL EXAM

- Hepatomegaly (83%)
- Increased skin pigmentation (75%)
- Loss of body hair (20%)
- Splenomegaly (13%)
- Peripheral edema (12%)
- Jaundice (10%)
- Gynecomastia (8%)
- Ascites (6%)
- Testicular atrophy
- Hepatic tenderness

DIAGNOSTIC TESTS & INTERPRETATION

After the diagnosis is established, consider having the patient take an oral glucose tolerance test to rule out diabetes and undergo an echocardiogram to rule out cardiomyopathy.

Lab

- Transferrin saturation (serum iron concentration ÷ total iron-binding capacity × 100): >70% is virtually diagnostic of iron overload; 45% or higher warrants further evaluation. Iron supplements and transfusions may elevate serum iron.
- Serum ferritin: >300 μg/L for men and postmenopausal women and 200 μg/L for premenopausal women (5); may be elevated by inflammatory reactions, other forms of liver disease, certain tumors (e.g., acute granulocytic leukemia), and rheumatoid arthritis
- Urinary iron
- Increased urine hemosiderin
- Hyperglycemia
- Decreased FSH
- Decreased LH
- Decreased testosterone
- Increased serum glutamic-oxaloacetic transaminase
- Hypoalbuminemia

Imaging

If the diagnosis is uncertain after laboratory testing, MRI may be helpful (1).

Diagnostic Procedures/Surgery

- Liver biopsy for stainable iron is the standard for diagnosis. Presence or absence of cirrhosis also can be ascertained. However, with the availability of genetic testing, liver biopsy is not frequently necessary to confirm the diagnosis (5)[C].
- DNA PCR testing for *HFE* gene mutations C282Y and H63D: Present in 85–90% of patients
- Homozygosity for the C282Y mutation with biochemical evidence for iron overload can confirm the diagnosis.

Pathological Findings

- Increased hepatic parenchymal iron stores
- Hepatic fibrosis and cirrhosis with hepatomegaly
- Pancreatic enlargement
- Excess hemosiderin in liver, pancreas, myocardium, thyroid, parathyroid, joints, skin
- Cardiomegaly
- Joint deposition of iron

DIFFERENTIAL DIAGNOSIS

- Repeated transfusions
- Hereditary anemias with ineffective erythropoiesis
- Alcoholic cirrhosis
- Porphyria cutanea tarda
- Atransferrinemia
- Excessive ingestion of iron (rare)

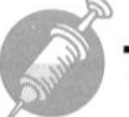

TREATMENT

MEDICATION

- None. Only when phlebotomy is not feasible or in the presence of severe heart disease should the iron-chelating agent deferoxamine (Desferal) be considered.
- Hepatitis A and hepatitis B immunizations should be done if there is no evidence of previous exposure (6).

ADDITIONAL TREATMENT

General Measures

- Remove excess iron by repeated phlebotomy once or twice weekly to establish and maintain a mild anemia (hematocrit of 35–39%) (5)[C].
- When the patient finally becomes iron deficient, a lifelong maintenance program of 2–6 phlebotomies a year to keep storage iron normal; maintain serum ferritin ≤50 μg/L

IN-PATIENT CONSIDERATIONS

Initial Stabilization

Outpatient treatment

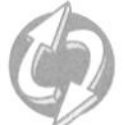

ONGOING CARE

FOLLOW-UP RECOMMENDATIONS

Full activity unless there is significant heart disease

Patient Monitoring

- Measure hematocrit before each phlebotomy; skip phlebotomy if hematocrit <36%.
- Schedule an additional phlebotomy when hematocrit >40%.
- When anemia becomes refractory, repeat transferrin saturation and serum ferritin to confirm depletion of iron stores.
- When iron stores are depleted, 2–6 phlebotomies a year should keep iron stores normal; maintain serum ferritin ≤50 μg/L.
- During maintenance therapy, measure transferrin saturation and serum ferritin yearly.

DIET

- An iron-poor diet is not of significant benefit.
- Avoid alcohol, iron-fortified foods, iron-containing supplements, and uncooked shellfish (increased susceptibility to *Vibrio* sp.).
- Restrict vitamin C to small doses between meals.
- Tea chelates iron and may be drunk with meals.

PATIENT EDUCATION

- Iron Overload Diseases Association, Inc., 525 Mayflower Rd, West Palm Beach, FL 33405
- American Hemochromatosis Society, Inc., 4044 W. Lake Mary Blvd., Unit 104, Lake Mary, FL 32746-2012

PROGNOSIS

- Patients diagnosed before cirrhosis develops and treated with phlebotomy have a normal life expectancy.
- Life expectancy is reduced in patients with cirrhosis and DM and those who require >18 months of phlebotomy therapy to return iron stores to normal.
- Patients with ferritin levels <1,000 μg/L are unlikely to have cirrhosis (2,3)

COMPLICATIONS

- Cirrhosis
- Hepatoma (only in patients with cirrhosis)
- Diabetes mellitus
- Cardiomyopathy
- Arthritis
- Hypogonadism

REFERENCES

1. van Bokhoven MA, van Deursen CT, Swinkels DW, et al. Diagnosis and management of hereditary haemochromatosis. *BMJ*. 2011;342:c7251.
2. Janssen MC, Swinkels DW, et al. Hereditary haemochromatosis. *Best Pract Res Clin Gastroenterol*. 2009;23:171–83.
3. Allen KJ, Gurrin LC, Constantine CC, et al. Iron-overload-related disease in HFE hereditary hemochromatosis. *N Engl J Med*. 2008;358: 221–30.
4. Brandhagen DJ, Fairbanks VF, Baldus W. Recognition and management of hereditary hemochromatosis. *Am Fam Phys*. 2002;65:853–60.
5. Qaseem A, Aronson M, Fitterman N, et al. Screening for hereditary hemochromatosis: A clinical practice guideline from the American College of Physicians. *Ann Intern Med*. 2005;143: 517–21.
6. Alexander J, Kowdley KV. Hereditary hemochromatosis: Genetics, pathogenesis, and clinical management. *Ann Hepatol*. 2005;4:240–7.
7. U.S. Preventive Services Task Force. Screening for hemochromatosis: Recommendation statement. *Ann Intern Med*. 2006;145:204–8.

ADDITIONAL READING

- Allen K, et al. Hereditary haemochromatosis—diagnosis and management. *Aust Fam Physician*. 2010;39:938–41.
- Pietrangelo A, et al. Hereditary hemochromatosis: Pathogenesis, diagnosis, and treatment. *Gastroenterology*. 2010;139:393–408.

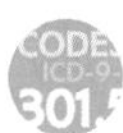

CODES

ICD9

- 275.01 Hereditary hemochromatosis
- 275.03 Other hemochromatosis

CLINICAL PEARLS

- The best laboratory tests available to screen a patient initially for hemochromatosis are serum ferritin and transferrin saturation. An elevated transferrin saturation is the earliest abnormality in hemochromatosis. Ferritin is a sensitive measure of iron overload but can be elevated in a variety of infectious and inflammatory conditions without iron overload being present.
- Liver biopsy need not be done to confirm the diagnosis or to check for cirrhosis if the patient is homozygous for C282Y or is heterozygous for C282Y/H63D. If the patient's serum ferritin is <1,000 μg/L, LFTs are normal, and hepatomegaly is not present, cirrhosis is very unlikely, so liver biopsy is not needed.
- Initially, a patient with hemochromatosis should have a phlebotomy weekly until the serum ferritin is <50 μg/L and the transferrin saturation falls to <30%. Then lifelong maintenance therapy of 2–6 phlebotomies a year is mandatory to keep the ferritin <50 μg/L and the transferrin saturation <50%.
- Most patients with hemochromatosis go undiagnosed. Because treatment with phlebotomy will prevent all complications when begun early, physicians should consider the diagnosis of hemochromatosis much more frequently. However, the US Preventive Services Task Force recommends against routine screening of asymptomatic average-risk populations.

H

HEMOPHILIA

Robyn D. Wing, MD
Patricia McQuilkin, MD

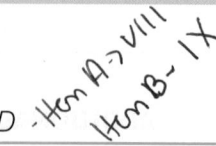

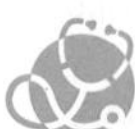

BASICS

DESCRIPTION

- Inherited bleeding disorders caused by a deficiency of coagulant factor VIII (hemophilia A) or factor IX (hemophilia B, also called Christmas disease). They are clinically indistinguishable but can be differentiated by assays that detect levels of factors VIII and IX.
- Disease severity is determined by the levels of the coagulant factor present:
  - Severe: <1%
  - Moderate: 1–5%
  - Mild: >5%
- Patients with >25% factor activity rarely bleed; however, bleeding after major surgery may occur in patients or carriers with factor VIII levels in the range of 25–35%.
- Synonym(s): Christmas disease (hemophilia B)

EPIDEMIOLOGY

- Congenital conditions: X-linked–recessive; therefore, they affect males almost exclusively.
- Females are generally asymptomatic carriers unless their factor level is <40%.

Incidence

Incidence of hemophilia A is 1:5,000 live male births; hemophilia B, 1:30,000 live male births.

Prevalence

Affect 500,000 worldwide; 2/3 undiagnosed

RISK FACTORS

Genetics

- Both hemophilia A and B are X-linked–recessive.
- 30% of cases are due to spontaneous mutation.

GENERAL PREVENTION

Consider testing family members for carrier status; may inform future reproductive decisions.

PATHOPHYSIOLOGY

- When blood vessel walls are damaged, exposure of subendothelial tissue initiates the primary hemostatic response, with plasma proteins and platelets interacting with this tissue to generate the platelet plug. Vascular injury also activates the coagulation pathway, which generates thrombin, an element essential to the creation of the fibrin net that stabilizes the platelet plug.
- Deficiencies in factor VIII or factor IX impair the coagulation pathway such that the platelet plug is inadequately stabilized, leading to excessive bleeding.

DIAGNOSIS

- Initial presentation:
  - May be known due to family history. All male infants born to known carriers should have factor level testing.
  - Intracranial bleeding, bleeding with circumcision, dental work, surgery, or injury
  - Excessive bruising, hematomas, hemarthroses
- Bleeding:
  - Depends on disease severity:
    - Severe: Spontaneous bleeding
    - Moderate: Bleeding with mild-to-moderate trauma
    - Mild: Bleeding with major trauma or surgery
  - Joints: Most common sites are ankle (children) and elbows, knees, and ankles (adolescents and adults). May present as irritability or decreased use of limb in an infant. In adults, prodromal stiffness and acute pain and swelling of joint:
    - Progressive arthropathy: Repeated bleeding into a joint damages cartilage and subchondral bone, causing fixed joints and resultant muscle wasting, which may significantly impair mobility.
  - Muscles: Hematoma formation most common in quadriceps, iliopsoas, and forearm
  - GI tract: Hematomas of bowel wall can cause obstruction or intussusception, as well as pain mimicking appendicitis.
  - CNS: Intracranial hemorrhage
  - Genitourinary (GU) tract: Hematuria
  - Posttraumatic: Delayed bleeding after injury or surgical procedures
- Compartment syndrome and ischemic nerve damage from large hematomas may occur, for example, femoral nerve neuropathy due to undetected retroperitoneal hemorrhage.
- Pseudotumor syndrome: Untreated hemorrhage causing a hematoma, which calcifies (named because it can be mistaken for cancer)

DIAGNOSTIC TESTS & INTERPRETATION

Lab

Initial lab tests

- Factor VIII, factor IX, aPTT, PT, platelet count, bleeding time, vWF antigen, and ristocetin cofactor activity
- Hemophilia A: Diagnostic test is low factor VIII.
- Hemophilia B: Diagnostic test is low factor IX.
- Activated partial thromboplastin time (PTT): Prolonged:
  - Corrected when mixed with normal plasma in absence of inhibitors
- Prothrombin time (PT): Normal
- Platelet count: Normal
- Bleeding time: Prolonged in 15–20% of patients with hemophilia A:
  - Recent aspirin use will increase bleeding time and can lead to confusion with Von Willebrand disease.

Follow-Up & Special Considerations

Inhibitors to factor VIII and IX (see "Complications"):

- Should be periodically measured with the Bethesda inhibitor assay, which quantifies the antibody titer
- Screen before invasive procedures and at regular intervals.

Diagnostic Procedures/Surgery

Prenatal diagnosis: Genetic testing of a sample of chorionic villus or fluid obtained at amniocentesis

Pathological Findings

In affected joints: Synovial hemosiderosis, articular cartilage degeneration, thickening of periarticular tissues, bony hypertrophy

DIFFERENTIAL DIAGNOSIS

- Von Willebrand disease
- Vitamin K deficiency (factor IX is vitamin K–dependent)
- Other factor deficiencies, afibrinogenemia, dysfibrinogenemia, fibrinolytic defects, platelet disorders
- Child abuse

TREATMENT

MEDICATION

First Line

- Primary prophylaxis:
  - Standard of care for patients with severe hemophilia
  - Regular and long-term treatment with deficient factor
  - Goal is to maintain the factor level above 1%, converting patient to moderate or mild hemophilia.
  - 3 times a week factor infusion for hemophilia A and twice-weekly infusions for hemophilia B have been demonstrated to reduce bleeding into joints, better prevent joint damage, and decrease frequency of hemorrhages when compared with patients treated on demand.
  - Optimal age to start treatment has not been established. Consensus is that it should be initiated before joint bleeds begin in order to most reduce the risk of subsequent arthropathy (usually within the first 2 years of life) (1)[B].
  - Questions remain about what dose of factor should be provided, when to escalate therapy, and how long prophylaxis should be given.
  - Barriers include cost and the need for frequent venous access. Stable venous access can be attained by CVLs or AV fistulae.
- On-demand therapy:
  - Hemophilia A:
    - Desmopressin (DDAVP): For mild hemophilia. Raises factor VIII levels by stimulating release of factor VIII from endothelial storage sites:
      - IV or SC: 0.3 mcg/kg infused 30 minutes prior to procedure; may repeat if needed
      - Intranasal: >50 kg = 150 mcg to each nostril (total = 300 mcg). <50 kg = 150 mcg to 1 nostril.
      - Adverse effect: Hyponatremic seizures, especially in children. Need to restrict fluids and watch sodium levels and urine output.
      - Children may have a lower therapeutic response, which may increase with age.
    - Purified factor VIII: Plasma-derived factor replacement is treated to inactivate viruses, an important innovation, because pooled plasma used previously carried high risk of HIV, hepatitis B, and hepatitis C transmission.
    - Recombinant factor VIII: Treatment of choice. Dosing: 1 U of factor VIII (the amount in 1 mL of plasma)/kg body weight will raise the plasma level of the recipient by 2%. Half-life of factor VIII is 8–12 hours. Therefore, b.i.d. or t.i.d. dosing is required with frequent factor-level checks.

- Hemophilia B:
  - Purified factor IX
  - Recombinant factor IX: Treatment of choice. Dosing: 1 U/kg will raise levels 1%. Half-life of factor IX is 16–17 hours.
- Amount and duration of factor replacement depends on location and severity of the bleed:
  - A target factor level of >30% is generally sufficient for mild bleeding episodes.
  - Major hemorrhages and large muscle bleeds require correction to levels between 50% and 100%.
  - Life-threatening bleeds require levels between 80% and 100%, which should be sustained with bolus dosing or continuous infusion.
- Both hemophilia A and B:
  - Antifibrinolytic agents: Enhance clot stabilization by inhibiting plasminogen activation. Effective in controlling mucosal bleeding, such as bleeding in oral cavity, epistaxis, and menorrhagia. Can also be used prophylactically, for example, prior to tooth extractions. Tranexamic acid (25 mg/kg PO q6–8h or 10 mg/kg IV q6–8h) and aminocaproic acid (Amicar) are also used.

Second Line

Patients with inhibitors:

- Low-titer (<5 BU/mL): Transient antibodies, which can be overcome with high amounts or longer duration of factor concentrate
- High-titer: Cannot be treated with deficient factor concentrates; must bypass the deficient factor in the clotting cascade:
  - Prothrombin complex concentrates and activated prothrombin complex concentrates (aPCC) may be used (both contain factors II, VII, IX, and X):
    - Risk of thrombus formation and disseminated intravascular coagulation (DIC) when used repeatedly or in higher doses
    - FEIBA VH dose: 50–100 U/kg q8–12h, but not to exceed 200 U/kg/d (2)[C]
  - Recombinant activated factor VII (rfVIIa): Avoids the risk associated with pooled donor plasma and does not cause a rise in antibody titer. However, it promotes coagulation only at the local level because it requires tissue factor to be active:
    - rfVIIa dose: 90–120 mcg/kg q2–3h or single dose of 270 mcg/kg for target joint bleeds (2)[B]
- Immune tolerance induction: Protocols to eliminate inhibitors. Regimens include frequent exposure to high-dose factor VIII therapy over 12–18 months, with or without immunosuppressive therapy (corticosteroids, cyclophosphamide, rituximab), until tolerance develops. Success rate shown to be 60–80% (3)[B].

ADDITIONAL TREATMENT

General Measures

- Avoid aspirin or other NSAIDs.
- Treat early; symptoms may occur before bleeding is clinically apparent.
- For surgical prophylaxis:
  - If major surgery is undertaken, factor levels should be maintained at >50% for at least 2–3 weeks after the procedure.
  - Dental extractions: Antifibrinolytics (Amicar, tranexamic acid) may be used.
  - Small procedures: May use DDAVP
- Hepatitis A and B vaccinations are recommended.
- Encourage physical activity. Patients should avoid high-impact contact sports.
- Female carriers: Majority of females are asymptomatic carriers, although an occasional carrier will bleed at time of surgery.

COMPLEMENTARY AND ALTERNATIVE MEDICINE

Gene therapy:

- Replacement of defective factor gene sequence with a corrected version, which would allow for increased factor production
- Animal studies have demonstrated safe, long-term expression of clotting factors using multiple gene-transfer strategies, but these findings have not been successful in patients (4)[B].
- Dramatic improvements seen with minimal increases in factor levels. For example, a patient may improve from a severe to a mild phenotype by increasing factor from <1% to >5%.

SURGERY/OTHER PROCEDURES

In patients with hemophilic arthropathy from recurrent hemarthrosis:

- Surgical or radionuclide synovectomy
- Total joint replacement

ONGOING CARE

FOLLOW-UP RECOMMENDATIONS

Restrict activities in proportion to the degree of factor deficiency.

Patient Monitoring

Regular evaluations every 6–12 months, including a musculoskeletal evaluation, an inhibitor screen, liver tests, and tests for antibodies to hepatitis viruses and HIV

PATIENT EDUCATION

- National Hemophilia Foundation at: www.hemophilia.org
- World Federation of Hemophilia at: www.wfh.org

PROGNOSIS

- Survival is normal for those with mild disease; mortality is increased 2–6-fold in those with moderate-to-severe disease.
- At one time, AIDS surpassed intracranial hemorrhage as the leading cause of death in hemophilia. Risk for HIV infection has declined significantly due to development of recombinant and virus-inactivated factor-replacement products.
- Hemophilic arthropathy is the main cause of morbidity in patients with severe hemophilia, as repeated hemarthroses result in eventual deformity and progressive disability.

COMPLICATIONS

- Hemophilic arthropathy: Symptoms include pain, limitation of motion, and contractures.
- Transmission of bloodborne infections, such as hepatitis A, B, C, D, and HIV. This risk has now been greatly reduced:
  - Hepatitis B and C increase risk for cirrhosis and hepatocellular cancer.
- Development of inhibitor autoantibodies: IgG antibodies that neutralize the deficient factor:
  - More common in hemophilia A (20–30% of patients compared to 5% in hemophilia B) (3)[B]
  - More common in patients with severe disease requiring multiple transfusions
  - Risk factors for inhibitor development include:
    - Specific genetic defect (family history); null mutations have higher inhibitor incidence
    - Very low or no circulating factor, therefore requiring multiple transfusions
    - Age of first exogenous factor exposure; previous studies report a higher incidence of developing antibodies in those exposed to exogenous factor at <6 months of age, but new studies show this may be due to severity of disease (5)[B].
    - Concurrent inflammation/infection when administering factor (2)[B] (e.g., surgical prophylaxis)
    - Duration of factor exposure (2)[B]
  - No increased risk of bleeding, but when bleeding occurs, it is more difficult to achieve hemostasis due to decreased response to factor replacement.

REFERENCES

1. Carcao M, Chambost H, Ljung R, et al. Devising a best practice approach to prophylaxis in boys with severe haemophilia: Evaluation of current treatment strategies. *Haemophilia*. 2010;16(Suppl 2):4–9.
2. Kempton CL, White GC, et al. How we treat a hemophilia A patient with a factor VIII inhibitor. *Blood*. 2009;113:11–7.
3. Carcao M, Lambert T, et al. Prophylaxis in haemophilia with inhibitors: Update from international experience. *Haemophilia*. 2010; 16(Suppl 2):16–23.
4. Murphy SL, High KA. Gene therapy for haemophilia. *Br J Haematol*. 2008;140:479–87.
5. Gouw SC, van der Bom JG, Marijke van den Berg H, et al. Treatment-related risk factors of inhibitor development in previously untreated patients with hemophilia A: The CANAL cohort study. *Blood*. 2007;109:4648–54.

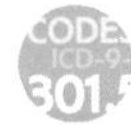

CODES

ICD9

- 286.0 Congenital factor viii disorder
- 286.1 Congenital factor ix disorder
- 286.2 Congenital factor xi deficiency

CLINICAL PEARLS

- Hemophilia A (factor VIII) and B (factor IX) are X-linked recessive conditions, affecting males almost exclusively.
- The severity of disease varies based on amount of factor present.
- Standard of care for treatment now includes primary prophylaxis with recombinant factor, as well as on-demand factor replacement with recombinant factor.
- Inhibitor formation should be suspected when treatment with deficient factor fails to correct coagulopathy.

HEMORRHOIDS

Juan Qiu, MD, PhD

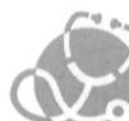

BASICS

DESCRIPTION

- Varicosities of the hemorrhoidal venous plexus
- External hemorrhoids are located below the dentate line and covered by squamous epithelium.
- Internal hemorrhoids are located above the dentate line.
- Both types of hemorrhoids often coexist.
- Classification of internal hemorrhoids:
  - First degree: Hemorrhoids do not prolapse.
  - Second degree: Prolapse through the anus on straining but reduce spontaneously
  - Third degree: Protrude and require digital reduction
  - Fourth degree: Cannot be reduced
- Hemorrhoids often progress from itching, bleeding stage to protrusion with easy reduction, then difficult reduction, and finally rectal prolapse. Thrombosis may occur at any protrusion stage.

Geriatric Considerations

Common in elderly along with rectal prolapse

Pediatric Considerations

- Uncommon in infants and children. Look for underlying cause (e.g., venacaval or mesenteric obstruction, cirrhosis, portal HTN).
- Occasionally, as in adults, hemorrhoids may result from chronic constipation, fecal impaction, and straining at stool. Surgery is rarely required in children.

Pregnancy Considerations

- Common in pregnancy
- Usually resolves after pregnancy
- No treatment required, unless extremely painful

EPIDEMIOLOGY

- Predominant age: Adults; peak between 45 and 65 years old
- Predominant sex: Male = Female

Incidence

Common

Prevalence

About 4–5% in general population in the US

RISK FACTORS

- Pregnancy
- Pelvic space-occupying lesions
- Liver disease
- Portal HTN
- Constipation
- Occupations that require prolonged sitting
- Loss of muscle tone in old age, rectal surgery, episiotomy, anal intercourse
- Obesity
- Chronic diarrhea

Genetics

No known genetic pattern

GENERAL PREVENTION

- Avoid constipation with high-fiber diet and hydration.
- Lose weight, if overweight.
- Avoid prolonged sitting on the toilet.

ETIOLOGY

- Dilated veins of hemorrhoidal plexus
- Tight internal anal sphincter
- Abnormal distention of the arteriovenous anastomosis
- Prolapse of the cushions and the surrounding connective tissues

COMMONLY ASSOCIATED CONDITIONS

- Liver disease
- Pregnancy
- Portal HTN
- Constipation

DIAGNOSIS

Diagnosis is usually made by history and inspection of the perineum, rectal exam, and anoscopy.

HISTORY

- All cases:
  - Classically, bright red blood per rectum; may be scant blood on toilet paper, or copious in the toilet bowl
  - Constipation or diarrhea
  - Straining with defecation
- Small or minimal external hemorrhoids: Episodic bleeding on stool or toilet paper, pruritus
- More extensive internal hemorrhoids: Feeling of incomplete evacuation

PHYSICAL EXAM

- Anorectal exam including anoscopy
- Inspection following straining at stool
- For protruding hemorrhoids: Mass, more prominent bleeding
- If not reducible, increased risk of strangulation and/or thrombosis with acute pain
- External hemorrhoids cause pain; internal hemorrhoids generally do not.
- Thrombosed hemorrhoids present as acute discomfort and the presence of a painful mass.

DIAGNOSTIC TESTS & INTERPRETATION

Diagnostic Procedures/Surgery

Sigmoidoscopy or colonoscopy depending on coexistent risk factors for malignancy in patients who present with bleeding.

DIFFERENTIAL DIAGNOSIS

- Rectal or anal neoplasia
- Condyloma
- Skin tag
- Inflammatory bowel disease (1)[B]
- Anal fistula, fissure, or abscess (2)[B]

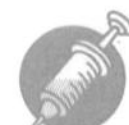

TREATMENT

All these treatments, except surgical, are outpatient with quick recovery time, usually <48 hours.

MEDICATION

- Prevention:
  - Fiber supplements
  - Stool softeners
- Pain:
  - Hydrocortisone ointment (0.5–1%)
  - Analgesic sprays or ointments—benzocaine, dibucaine (Nupercainal). Use sprays with caution as they may contain alcohol that can cause burning sensation when applied.
- Pruritus: Hydrocortisone (Anusol-HC, Cortifoam) ointment
- Bleeding:
  - Astringent suppositories (Preparation H)
  - Hydrocortisone (Anusol; Cortifoam) ointment
- Treatment for special cases:
  - Thrombosed external hemorrhoids: Fairly common complication of hemorrhoidal disease. With conservative treatment, the thrombus will be absorbed over the course of weeks and pain improves within 2–3 days (1)[B].
  - With severe acute pain, prompt excision should be performed under local anesthetic and the wound left open without packing. Sitz baths, topical anesthetics, and mild pain relievers for first 7–10 days after excision (1)[B].
  - Strangulated hemorrhoid: From irreducible third- or fourth-degree hemorrhoid. If untreated, can progress to ulceration and thrombosis. Treatment requires urgent or emergent hemorrhoidectomy.
  - Acute hemorrhoidal bleeding associated with portal HTN: Bleeding can be life threatening. Treatment should be suture of the bleeding site with incorporation of the mucosa, submucosa, and internal sphincter. Coagulopathy should be corrected.

ADDITIONAL TREATMENT

General Measures

- Hemorrhoids are a recurrent disease, even after surgical excision; measures for prevention should be taken.
- For mild symptoms or prevention:
  - Avoid prolonged sitting at stool.
  - Avoid straining.
  - Avoid constipation by eating a high-fiber diet or by taking fiber supplements; if necessary, take regular stool softeners.
  - Regular exercise
- For pain, sitz baths warm water or hypertonic Epsom salts (1 cup per 2 quarts of water)
- Mild and minimal hemorrhoids respond to changed diet, relief of constipation, and brief stooling.

- Pruritus or mild discomfort after stooling responds to hydrocortisone ointment, anesthetic ointments or sprays, and warm sitz bath.
- Constipation relief, anal hygiene, local ointments, and sitz baths are effective through the stage of easy reduction, but the more severe stages require rubber band ligation or rectal surgery.

COMPLEMENTARY AND ALTERNATIVE MEDICINE

Aloe vera cream on the surgical site after hemorrhoidectomy is effective in reducing postoperative pain, and decreasing both healing time and analgesic requirements (3)[B]

SURGERY/OTHER PROCEDURES

- Indications: Failure of medical and nonoperative therapy, symptomatic third- or fourth-degree symptoms in presence of a concomitant anorectal condition requiring surgery, or patient preference (2)[B],(4)
- Incision of thrombosed hemorrhoid: For severe pain
- Severe protruding hemorrhoids:
  - Rubber band ligation (internal hemorrhoids only)
  - Sclerotherapy: For symptomatic prolapsed stage I or II hemorrhoids; care must be (5) taken injecting near periprostatic parasympathetic nerves. Not for advanced disease or if evidence of infection, inflammation, ulceration is present (1)[B]:
    - Cryotherapy is no longer recommended due to high rate of complications (2)[B].
  - Prolapsed rectum:
    - Requires surgical correction
  - Surgical resection:
    - Gold standard: Conventional hemorrhoidectomy should be considered for grade III hemorrhoids not responding to banding (6)[A], mixed internal and external, grade IV hemorrhoids, or when complicated by fissures, fistula, or extensive skin tags.
- Newer technique:
  - Stapled hemorrhoidopexy; less painful than traditional surgery, but higher incidence of recurrences (7)[B]
  - Ligasure hemorrhoidectomy; reduces operating time, is superior in patient tolerance, and is equally effective as conventional hemorrhoidectomy in long-term symptom control

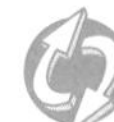

ONGOING CARE

FOLLOW-UP RECOMMENDATIONS

- Encourage physical fitness.
- Avoid prolonged sitting and straining on the toilet.

Patient Monitoring

As needed, depending on treatment

DIET

High-fiber (25–30 g of insoluble fiber/d), adequate fluids (6–8 glasses of water/d) and avoid excessive caffeine

PROGNOSIS

- Spontaneous resolution
- Recurrence

COMPLICATIONS

- Thrombosis
- Ulceration
- Anemia (rare)
- Incontinence
- Pelvic sepsis following hemorrhoidectomy (7)[B]

REFERENCES

1. Kaidar-Person O, Person B, Wexner SD. Hemorrhoidal disease: A comprehensive review. *J Am Coll Surg*. 2007;204:102–17.
2. Clinical Practice Committee, American Gastroenterological Association. American Gastroenterological Association medical position statement: Diagnosis and treatment of hemorrhoids. *Gastroenterology*. 2004;126:1461–2.
3. Eshghi F, Hosseinimehr SJ, Rahmani N, et al. Effects of Aloe vera cream on posthemorrhoidectomy pain and wound healing: Results of a randomized, blind, placebo-control study. *J Altern Complement Med*. 2010;16(6):647–50.
4. Castellvi J, Sueira A, Espinosa J, et al. Ligasure versus diathermy hemorrhoidectomy under spinal anesthesia or pudendal block with ropivacaine: A randomized prospective clinical study with 1-year follow-up. *Int J Colorectal Dis*. 2009;24(9):1011–8.
5. Nienhuiji S, de Hingh I. Conventional versus LigaSure hemorrhoidectomy for patients with symptomatic hemorrhoids (Review). *The Cochrane Library*. 2009:(2).
6. Shanmugam V, Hakeem A, Campbell KL, et al. Rubber band ligation versus excisional haemorrhoidectomy for haemorrhoids. *Cochrane Database Syst Rev*. 2005;1:CD005034. Updated 2011;3.
7. Nisar PJ, Acheson AG, Neal KR, et al. Stapled hemorrhoidopexy compared with conventional hemorrhoidectomy: Systematic review of randomized, controlled trials. *Dis Colon Rectum*. 2004;47:1837–45.

ADDITIONAL READING

- Giordano P, Gravante G, Sorge R, et al. Long-term Outcomes of stapled hemorrhoidopexy vs conventional hemorrhoidectomy. *Arch Surg*. 2009;144(3):266–72.
- Reese GE, von Roon AC, Tekkis PP, et al. Haemorrhoids. *Clin Evid (Online)*. 2009.

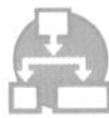

See Also (Topic, Algorithm, Electronic Media Element)

Colorectal Cancer; Portal Hypertension

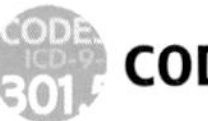

CODES

ICD9

- 455.0 Internal hemorrhoids without mention of complication
- 455.1 Internal thrombosed hemorrhoids
- 455.2 Internal hemorrhoids with other complication

CLINICAL PEARLS

- Hemorrhoids are uncommon in inflammatory bowel disease, and pain is most related to perianal inflammation, irritation, and swelling. Anal hygiene and symptomatic pain relief are the treatments of choice.
- No pain is associated with internal hemorrhoids. Pain occurs with external hemorrhoids only.

HENOCH-SCHÖNLEIN PURPURA

Kimberly A. Pesaturo, PharmD
Evan R. Horton, PharmD
Amy Pelletier, DO

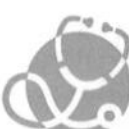

BASICS

DESCRIPTION

- Henoch-Schönlein purpura (HSP) is an immunologically mediated, nonthrombocytopenic, purpuric, systemic vasculitis involving small blood vessels (1).
- HSP is often self-limiting but can result in long-term renal damage (1).

EPIDEMIOLOGY

Incidence

- Up to 20.4/100,000 children <17 years of age per year, but incidence is variable (2)
- Predominant age: Highest incidence between 4 and 6 years of age (2)
- Most common in Caucasians, Japanese, and Native Americans (2)

Prevalence

- Year-round occurrence
- More common in late fall to early spring (3)

RISK FACTORS

Genetics

Possible genetic predisposition (1)

PATHOPHYSIOLOGY

- Immune-mediated disorder involving IgA complexes (specifically IgA1) that form and deposit in affected areas, triggering localized inflammation (1)
- Results in leukocytoclastic vasculitis and small blood vessel necrosis
- Proliferative glomerulonephritis with IgA deposition may be seen (4).

ETIOLOGY

- No single etiologic agent has been identified.
- Many cases are associated with preceding infections, usually involving group A β-hemolytic streptococci (3).
- Also reported following infections with (but not limited to): Parvovirus B19, adenovirus, hepatitis A and B viruses, Coxsackie virus, Epstein-Barr virus, varicella virus, *B. henselae*, *H. pylori*, and *M. pneumoniae* (3).
- Rare reports after drug ingestion, insect bites, and some vaccines

DIAGNOSIS

Palpable purpura with lower limb predominance with one or more of the following (4):

- Abdominal pain
- Biopsy with predominant IgA
- Arthralgia or arthritis
- Renal involvement (hematuria or proteinuria)

HISTORY

- Previous disease: Infections such as streptococcal infections, upper respiratory infections, and hepatitis (3)
- Rash: Initially may resemble urticaria prior to developing into palpable purpura (1)
- Headache
- Cough
- Vomiting
- Abdominal pain is the most common GI symptom (1).
- Transient arthritis of joints, most frequent in lower limbs (knees and ankles) (1)
- Edema of the periorbital region or ankles
- Hematuria
- Testicular pain or scrotal swelling (1)

PHYSICAL EXAM

- Rash is the hallmark of HSP (1). Rash may be petechial or purpuric in a pressure-dependent, symmetric distribution, usually predominating on lower limbs:
  - Rash may be briefly preceded by joint involvement or abdominal pain.
  - Skin lesions may spread to face and trunk; bullous lesions can develop.
- Abdomen often tender to palpation. Some form of bleeding may occur:
  - Abdominal symptoms may precede the rash by up to 2 weeks.
  - Intussusception is a possible complication.
- Hypertension may be present.
- Orchitis (less common) may occur and can mimic testicular torsion:
  - Swelling and bruising may be noted on the scrotum.
  - Testicular torsion also has been reported.
- Joints (mainly lower limb) should be examined for swelling and limited range of motion.
- CNS involvement may present with headaches, seizures, or behavioral changes (less common).
- Rare pulmonary involvement may be noted.

DIAGNOSTIC TESTS & INTERPRETATION

No definitive tests confirm the diagnosis of HSP.

Lab

The following labs may be useful in diagnosing HSP (1,3):

- CBC:
  - Normal platelet count differentiates from thrombocytopenic purpura.
  - Hemoglobin is usually normal; leukocytosis, eosinophilia especially, may be present.
  - Can detect anemia if there is GI blood loss.
- ESR:
  - Normal or elevated
- Prothrombin (PT) and partial thromboplastin time (PTT):
  - Normal
- IgA:
  - Often elevated in the acute phase of illness, with normal or increased IgG and IgM
- C3/C4:
  - Normal; sometimes decreased
- Antinuclear antibody:
  - Negative
- Throat culture for group A β-hemolytic streptococci:
  - May be positive
- Antistreptolysin O titer:
  - Determines preceding streptococcal infection
- Serum basic/comprehensive chemistries:
  - Elevated BUN and creatinine levels and decreased protein and albumin are seen with renal involvement.
- Urinalysis:
  - Gross hematuria and proteinuria are present in many patients. Microscopic blood, RBCs, WBCs, and casts suggest glomerulonephritis.
- Blood culture:
  - Evaluate for sepsis or bacteremia
- Stool guaiac

Imaging

The following imaging tests may be useful (1):

- Abdominal ultrasound for thickened bowel wall, intussusception
- Abdominal radiograph
- Renal tract ultrasound
- CXR
- Select neuroimaging

Diagnostic Procedures/Surgery

- Renal biopsy: Severe renal failure:
  - Epithelial crescent formation on renal biopsy suggests significant renal damage and inflammation.
- Skin biopsy of purpura: IgA deposition

DIFFERENTIAL DIAGNOSIS

- Petechial and purpuric rashes seen in thrombocytopenia from:
  - Idiopathic thrombocytopenic purpura
  - Sepsis/infection: Meningococcemia, Rocky Mountain spotted fever
  - Leukemia
  - Hemolytic-uremic syndrome
  - Coagulopathies
- Vasculitic rashes may result from primary and secondary vasculitides:
  - Polyarteritis nodosa
  - Wegener granulomatosis
  - Infection related
  - Connective tissue diseases (e.g., systemic lupus erythematosus) or Berger disease
  - Infantile acute hemorrhagic edema
  - Rheumatoid arthritis
  - Rheumatic fever
  - Kawasaki disease
- Other: Acute abdomen, bacterial endocarditis, abuse (3)

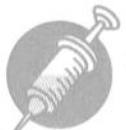

TREATMENT

MEDICATION

- HSP without nephritis usually resolves spontaneously without specific therapy.
- Early oral corticosteroids (1–2 mg/kg/d of prednisone for 2 weeks followed by taper) may reduce intensity of joint and abdominal pain (5)[B] and may be beneficial in reducing abdominal surgery (6)[C].
- Salicylates and other agents that affect platelet function should be avoided if GI tract bleeding is present. NSAIDs should be avoided in patients with renal disease (3).

ADDITIONAL TREATMENT

General Measures

- Treatment of hypertension may delay or prevent progression of renal disease in patients with glomerulonephritis.
- Rest and elevation of affected areas may limit purpura (3).

Issues for Referral

Pediatric nephrology and/or dermatology

IN-PATIENT CONSIDERATIONS

IV Fluids

Hospitalization is often unnecessary. Severe complications may require admission.

IV Fluids

Hydration should be maintained.

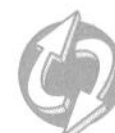

ONGOING CARE

FOLLOW-UP RECOMMENDATIONS

Patient Monitoring

- Patients should be seen weekly during the acute illness. Visits should include history and physical exam, along with BP measurement and urinalysis.
- All patients, even those who did not present with renal involvement, should have urine checked for blood weekly for 6 months and then monthly for 3 years because deterioration of renal function has been observed years after presentation in some patients.
- Women with a history of HSP should be monitored for proteinuria and HTN during pregnancy.

PATIENT EDUCATION

American Family Physician handout on HSP at www.aafp.org/afp/980800ap/980800b.html

PROGNOSIS

- Most patients are improved within 4 weeks of HSP onset.
- Younger age is associated with better prognosis.
- Recurrence within first 6 months in up to 33% (3)
- Extent of renal disease often dictates long-term prognosis (3).

COMPLICATIONS

- Hypertension
- End-stage renal disease
- Intussusception (most common GI tract complication, affecting 1–5% of patients)
- Protein-losing enteropathy
- Hemorrhagic pancreatitis
- Hydrops of the gallbladder
- Intestinal strictures
- Bowel perforations, ischemia, and infarctions, obstructions
- GI hemorrhage
- Pseudomembranous colitis
- Appendicitis
- Skin necrosis
- Subarachnoid, subdural, and cortical hemorrhage and infarction
- Peripheral mononeuropathies and polyneuropathies (Guillain-Barré syndrome)
- Pulmonary hemorrhage (uncommon but may result in death)
- Torsion of the testis and appendix testes and priapism
- Scrotal swelling and pain
- CNS complications
- Myocarditis

REFERENCES

1. McCarthy HJ, Tizard EJ. Diagnosis and management of Henoch-Schönlein purpura. *Eur J Pediatr*. 2010; 169:643–650.
2. Gardner-Medwin JM, Dolezalova P, Cummins C, et al. Incidence of Henoch-Schönlein purpura, Kawasaki disease, and rare vasculitides in children of different ethnic origins. *Lancet*. 2002;360: 1197–202.
3. Reamy BV, Williams PM, Lindsay TJ. Henoch-Schönlein purpura. *Am Fam Physician*. 2009;80(7): 697–704.
4. Ozen S, Pistorio A, Iusan SM, et al. EULAR/PRINTO/PRES criteria for Henoch-Schönlein purpura, childhood polyarteritis nodosa, childhood Wegener granulomatosis and childhood Takayasu arteritis: Ankara 2008. Part II: Final classification criteria. *Ann Rheum Dis*. 2010;69:798–806.
5. Weiss PF, Feinstein JA, Luan X, et al. Effects of corticosteroid on Henoch-Schönlein purpura: A systematic review. *Pediatrics*. 2007;120:1079–87.
6. Weiss PF, Klink AJ, Localio R, et al. Corticosteroids may improve clinical outcomes during hospitalization for Henoch-Schönlein purpura. *Pediatrics* 2010;126:674–81.

ADDITIONAL READING

- González LM, Janniger CK, Schwartz RA. Pediatric Henoch-Schönlein purpura. *Int J Dermatol*. 2009;48: 1157–65.
- Iqbal H, Evans A. Dapsone therapy for Henoch-Schönlein purpura: A case series. *Arch Dis Child*. 2005;90:985–6.
- Roberts PF, Waller TA, Brinker TM, et al. Henoch-Schönlein purpura: A review article. *South Med J*. 2007;100:821–4.

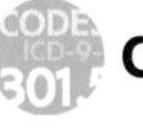

CODES

ICD9

- 287.0 Allergic purpura
- 287.8 Other specified hemorrhagic conditions

CLINICAL PEARLS

- HSP is a systemic vasculitis involving small blood vessels.
- Rash is the hallmark of HSP.
- HSP without renal involvement is often self-limiting.
- Early oral corticosteroid therapy may be beneficial.
- All patients, even those who did not present with renal involvement, should have urine checked for blood weekly for 6 months and then monthly for 3 years because deterioration of renal function has been observed years after presentation in some patients.

H

HEPARIN-INDUCED THROMBOCYTOPENIA

Adam B. Pesaturo, PharmD, BCPS
Patrick Mailloux, DO

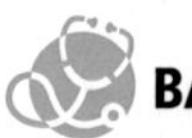

BASICS

DESCRIPTION

- Unexplained decrease in platelet count in a patient treated with heparin:
  - Minimum platelet count fall between 30% and 50% from baseline
- Antibody-mediated prothrombotic disorder initiated by heparin administration
- Idiosyncratic reaction
- 2 types: Nonimmune heparin-associated thrombocytopenia (previously called HIT type I) and HIT (immune induced; previously called HIT type II):
  - Nonimmune heparin-associated thrombocytopenia: More common, onset 1–4 days after starting heparin, mild thrombocytopenia (>100,000), few complications
  - HIT: Less common, onset 5–14 days after primary exposure to heparin, thrombocytopenia often <100,000 but usually >20,000, high risk of thrombosis:
    - Presentation of thrombocytopenia can be immediate if recent heparin exposure within past 100 days

EPIDEMIOLOGY

Incidence

- 10–15% of heparin-treated patients will experience decrease in platelet count.
- 0.3–3% will develop HIT.

RISK FACTORS

- Postsurgical > Medical > Obstetric:
  - Postcardiopulmonary bypass is the most significant risk factor
- Bovine unfractionated heparin (UFH) > porcine UFH > low-molecular-weight heparin (LMWH)
- Female > Male
- Heparin duration >4 days

GENERAL PREVENTION

- Inquire about recent heparin exposure and any history of HIT
- Proper documentation of past HIT reactions in patient's medical record
- No form of heparin should be administered once the diagnosis of HIT is confirmed.

PATHOPHYSIOLOGY

- Nonimmune heparin-associated thrombocytopenia: Potentially a result from direct platelet membrane binding with heparin
- HIT: Heparin can cause an increase in the blood concentration of platelet factor 4 (PF4), a chemokine. PF4 will form a complex with heparin.
- This heparin/PF4 complex can, in turn, stimulate the production of specific antiheparin/PF4 complex antibodies. These antibodies cause platelet activation and a prothrombotic state. Ultimately, this hypercoagulable state leads to thromboembolic complications in many patients.

COMMONLY ASSOCIATED CONDITIONS

- Venous thrombosis: Deep venous thrombosis (DVT), pulmonary embolism, adrenal vein thrombosis with hemorrhagic infarction
- Arterial thrombosis
- Skin lesions
- Acute systemic reactions

DIAGNOSIS

- Nonimmune heparin-associated thrombocytopenia: Asymptomatic drop in platelet count
- HIT: Thrombocytopenia or thrombosis with the presence of heparin-dependent antibodies:
  - A clinicopathologic syndrome, meaning the foundation for diagnosis is based on both clinical and serologic findings

HISTORY

- Duration of current heparin therapy
- Previous exposure to heparin, including heparin flushes and heparin-coated catheters
- In patients being treated with heparin for thrombosis in which thrombosis recurs during therapy, consider HIT as a potential cause.
- Pretest probability for HIT can be calculated using the "4 Ts" methodology (1):
  - Thrombocytopenia-new onset, timing of thrombocytopenia (5–10 days after exposure), thrombosis new onset and no other cause of thrombocytopenia
- The HIT Expert Probability score, though only validated once to date, may become an alternative pretest probability tool.

PHYSICAL EXAM

- Signs of venous or arterial thrombosis
- Skin necrosis (begins with erythema, progresses to ecchymosis and necrosis)
- Ischemic changes (signs of limb, renal, splenic, mesenteric ischemia)
- Bleeding (less common)

DIAGNOSTIC TESTS & INTERPRETATION

Lab

- Serial platelet counts in patients receiving heparin: Check platelets at baseline, after 24 hours, and then every other day for the first 14 days (2)[B].
- Confirmatory lab tests needed for a clinical diagnosis can use 1 of 3 serologic assays:
  - ELISA (antigenic assay): Up to 99% sensitive, poor specificity; thus, has an excellent negative predictive value for HIT
  - Heparin-induced platelet activation (platelet activation test): High specificity and low sensitivity
  - Serotonin release assay (platelet activation test): High specificity and moderate sensitivity
- Either a platelet activation assay or an antigenic assay alone may not be adequate for clinical diagnosis; their use in combination is usually recommended.
- The diagnostic interpretation of these laboratory tests must be made in the context of the clinical estimation of the pretest probability because HIT is a clinicopathologic syndrome. Patients may form heparin-dependent antibodies and still not develop HIT (3).

DIFFERENTIAL DIAGNOSIS

Other potential causes of thrombocytopenia include (list is not all-inclusive):

- Sepsis and other infections
- Drug reactions
- Autoimmune
- Transfusion reactions
- Physical destruction (i.e., during cardiopulmonary bypass)

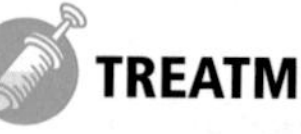

TREATMENT

Treatment is by prompt withdrawal of heparin and replacement with a suitable alternative anticoagulant.

MEDICATION

- Most patients will require anticoagulation either because of:
  - Pre-existing thrombosis *or*
  - Risk of thrombosis during 30 days after HIT diagnosis; consider anticoagulation for 30 days (4)[B]
- Dosing of anticoagulant will depend on indication (prophylaxis vs. treatment):
  - In cases where there is clinically a low suspicion/pretest probability of HIT and laboratory confirmation is pending, it may be appropriate to continue antithrombotic prophylaxis using nonheparin anticoagulants.
  - In cases with high suspicion/pretest probability of HIT and laboratory confirmation is pending, it is appropriate to begin anticoagulation treatment with a nonheparin product.
- Direct thrombin inhibitors (DTIs) (lepirudin, argatroban, and bivalirudin):
  - Reduce relative risk of thrombosis by 30%, on average (2)[B].
  - Can produce misleading elevation in international normalized ratio (INR) (most likely an in vitro reaction) (5):
    - Argatroban > Bivalirudin > Lepirudin
  - Lepirudin:
    - Initial dose, 0.1 mg/kg/hr; decrease dose with reduced renal function
    - Dose adjustments based on active partial thromboplastin time (aPTT) (goal: 1.5–2 times patient baseline); check aPTT q4h until steady state within goal aPTT range is achieved

- Argatroban:
  - Initial dose, 2 μg/kg/min; decrease dose with reduced hepatic function or with critical illness
  - Dose adjustments based on aPTT similar to lepirudin, except aPTT is initially checked q2h
- Bivalirudin:
  - Favorable pharmacologic profile; however, evidence for use is insufficient compared to lepirudin and argatroban
  - Initial dose is a 0.1 mg/kg bolus, followed by a continuous infusion rate of 0.2 mg/kg/hr, reduced dose with renal insufficiency (CrCl <30 mL/min)
  - Dose adjustments based on aPTT

- Factor Xa inhibitor (fondaparinux):
  - Reports of its use are theorized to be useful; however, there is minimal data supporting its efficacy for HIT, and an ideal dose has yet to be determined.
  - Association with the development of HIT has been reported (6)[C].
  - Optional agent for thromboembolic prophylaxis when practitioner wants to avoid heparin
  - Avoid in patients with renal dysfunction (CrCl <30 mL/min).
- Warfarin:
  - Must anticoagulate with an immediate-acting agent before starting warfarin
  - Use of warfarin without other anticoagulants should be avoided because it can cause thrombosis (2)[A].
  - Begin warfarin after platelet count >150,000 (2)[B].
  - Discontinue other anticoagulant and continue only warfarin after INR is therapeutic (2–3) for at least 5 days (2)[A]. This management differs from the normal heparin-to-warfarin transition in other conditions requiring anticoagulation.
- LMWH:
  - Although LMWH has a lower risk of initiating a HIT reaction, it should *not* be used when antibodies are already present. These antibodies can cross-react with LMWH and induce thrombosis and thrombocytopenia (2)[A].

ADDITIONAL TREATMENT

General Measures

- Discontinue all heparin products, including flushes and heparin-coated catheters.
- Nonimmune heparin-associated thrombocytopenia generally resolves when heparin is stopped:
  - Consider a nonheparin alternative such as fondaparinux if pharmacologic DVT prophylaxis is warranted.
- Avoid platelet transfusions (2)[C].
- Adverse reaction to heparin should be clearly documented in the medical record with instruction to avoid all heparin products.
- For patients with a documented history of HIT, under special circumstances only (such as the need for cardiopulmonary bypass), the use of heparin for a short duration may be acceptable if the absence of heparin/PF4 complex antibodies can be documented (7)[C].

IN-PATIENT CONSIDERATIONS

Nursing

- Avoid heparin flushes.
- Avoid platelet transfusion.
- Clearly document reaction in all medical records to avoid the future use of heparin.

ONGOING CARE

FOLLOW-UP RECOMMENDATIONS

- The transition period of anticoagulation with a DTI and warfarin in patients with HIT can be problematic.
- The INR while administering both a DTI and warfarin should be therapeutic (2–3) for at least 5 days before discontinuing the DTI.
- Warfarin therapy should not be commenced until the platelet count has stabilized within a normal range.
- DTIs can prolong INR; therefore, if INR is >4 while on both warfarin and a DTI, temporarily hold the DTI for 4–6 hours and recheck INR; this second INR will represent only the anticoagulant effect of warfarin.

Patient Monitoring

- Serial platelet counts
- Monitor PTT or INR as determined by the anticoagulation agent.

PATIENT EDUCATION

- Patient should inform all health care providers of any previous adverse reaction to heparin.
- HIT information available at: http://medlibrary.org/medwiki/Heparin-induced_thrombocytopenia

PROGNOSIS

- Thrombosis in HIT has 20–30% mortality, with additional morbidity from stroke and limb ischemia.
- Platelet counts normalize within weeks after stopping heparin.
- Risk of delayed thrombosis, especially in the first 30 days

REFERENCES

1. Lo GK, Juhl D, Warkentin TE, et al. Evaluation of pretest clinical score (4 T's) for the diagnosis of heparin-induced thrombocytopenia in two clinical settings. *J Thromb Haemost*. 2006;4:759–65.
2. Warkentin TE, Greinacher A, Koster A, et al. Treatment and prevention of heparin-induced thrombocytopenia: American College of Chest Physicians Evidence-Based Clinical Practice Guidelines (8th Edition). *Chest*. 2008;133: 340S–80S.
3. Shantsila E, Lip GY, Chong BH. Heparin-induced thrombocytopenia: A contemporary clinical approach to diagnosis and management. *Chest*. 2009;135:1651–64.
4. Dager WE, Dougherty JA, Nguyen PH, et al. Heparin-Induced Thrombocytopenia: Treatment Options and Special Considerations. *Pharmacotherapy*. 2007;27:564–87.
5. Warkentin TE, Greinacher A, Craven S, et al. Differences in the clinically effective molar concentrations of four direct thrombin inhibitors explain their variable prothrombin time prolongation. *Thromb Haemost*. 2005;94:958–64.
6. Warkentin TE, Maurer BT, Aster RH. Heparin-induced thrombocytopenia associated with fondaparinux. *N Engl J Med*. 2007;356:2653–5; discussion 2653–5.
7. Warkentin TE, Kelton JG, et al. Temporal aspects of heparin-induced thrombocytopenia. *N Engl J Med*. 2001;344:1286–92.

ADDITIONAL READING

- Cuker A, Arepally G, Crowther MA, et al. The HIT Expert Probability (HEP) Score: A novel pre-test probability model for heparin-induced thrombocytopenia based on broad expert opinion. *J Thromb Haemost*. 2010;8:2642–50.
- DocMD.com. Heparin induced thrombocytopenia [homepage]. www.heparininducedthrombocytopenia.com/.
- Martel N, Lee J, Wells PS. Risk for heparin-induced thrombocytopenia with unfractionated and low-molecular-weight heparin thromboprophylaxis: A meta-analysis. *Blood*. 2005;106:2710–5.

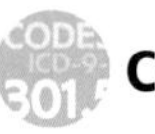

CODES

ICD9

289.84 Heparin-induced thrombocytopenia (HIT)

CLINICAL PEARLS

- Heparin exposure through virtually any preparation (including LMWH), any dose, or any route can cause HIT.
- LMWH is contraindicated in HIT; although LMWH is less likely to cause HIT, once HIT is present, the antibodies will cross-react and continue to cause a HIT reaction.
- If a patient is suspected of HIT (with or without confirmatory testing), immediately discontinue all forms of heparin.
- Patients will require anticoagulation either because of pre-existing thrombosis or the risk of thrombosis in first 30 days after HIT.
- A DTI should be used until a patient's INR is therapeutic (2–3) on warfarin for at least 5 days.
- The key to avoiding sequelae from HIT is awareness, vigilance, and a high degree of suspicion.

HEPATIC ENCEPHALOPATHY

Walter M. Kim, MD, PhD
Jyoti Ramakrishna, MD

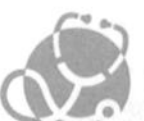

BASICS

DESCRIPTION

- Reversible altered mental and neuromotor functioning associated with acute or chronic liver disease and/or portal systemic shunting of blood
- The prominent features are confusion, impaired arousability, and a "flapping tremor" (asterixis).
- System(s) affected: Gastrointestinal; Nervous
- Synonym(s): HE; Portosystemic encephalopathy; Hepatic coma; Liver coma

EPIDEMIOLOGY

Predominant sex: Male = Female (reflecting underlying liver disease)

Prevalence

- Occurs in 1/3 of cirrhosis cases
- Occurs in all cases of fulminant hepatic failure
- Present in nearly 1/2 of patients who require transplantation
- Parallels the age predominance of fulminant liver disease: Peaks in the 40s; cirrhosis peaks in the late 50s; may occur at any age

RISK FACTORS

In patients with underlying liver disease, precipitating factors include:

- Infection (overt or occult, including spontaneous bacterial peritonitis)
- GI hemorrhage
- Use of sedative or opiate drugs
- Fluid or electrolyte disturbance ($Na+$, K^+, Mg^{2+}, or other electrolyte depletion)
- Transjugular intrahepatic portosystemic shunt (TIPS)

Genetics

- Unknown
- Conditions such as cystic fibrosis, α-1-antitrypsin deficiency, and Wilson disease can contribute to HE.

GENERAL PREVENTION

- Recognition of early signs and seeking of prompt treatment
- Avoidance of nonessential medications, particularly opiates and sedatives

PATHOPHYSIOLOGY

- Failure of liver to detoxify agents noxious to the CNS (e.g., ammonia, mercaptans, fatty acids)
- Increased aromatic and reduced branched-chain amino acids in blood
- These act as false neurotransmitters, possibly interacting with the gamma-aminobutyric acid (GABA) receptor.

ETIOLOGY

- Shunting of intestinal blood through the severely diseased liver without the intervention of viable liver cells
- Most common in long-standing cirrhosis of the liver with spontaneous shunting of intestinal blood through collateral vessels
- Shunting of such blood through collateral circulation or surgically constructed portacaval shunts
- TIPS, a widely used radiologically inserted shunt to lower portal pressure, produces HE.
- Acute onset of HE: Search for risk factors.

COMMONLY ASSOCIATED CONDITIONS

- Occurs rarely with portacaval shunt with normal liver function
- May occur as a complication of acute fatty liver of pregnancy

DIAGNOSIS

HISTORY

Pre-existing liver disease

PHYSICAL EXAM

- Ages 10–60 years:
  - Prominent signs of underlying liver disease (50%); jaundice most common, ascites second most common
  - GI hemorrhage with hematemesis or melena: 20%
  - Systemic infection, urinary tract or pulmonary: 20%
  - 4 stages of confusion and degree of obtundation described:
    - Stage 1: Forgetfulness, disturbance in nocturnal sleep, daytime drowsiness
    - Stage 2: Mild confusion, drowsy but arousable
    - Stage 3: Patient arousable, markedly confused, with limited orientation and inability to follow commands
    - Stage 4: Patient is unable to be aroused and exhibits extensive posturing.
  - Handwriting and hand coordination deteriorate in stages 1 and 2.
  - Asterixis prominent in stage 2
  - Reflexes symmetrically hyperactive in stage 3
  - Psychotic thoughts infrequent
  - Mental and neurologic signs change rapidly (over 6–12 hours).
- Age >60 years:
  - Signs of underlying liver disease diminish (25%).
  - Confusion more prominent
  - Precipitating GI hemorrhage or infection is less often identified.
  - Remains in stage 1 or 2 for many days
  - Progression slower
- Age <10 years:
  - Signs of underlying liver disease prominent; usually fulminant hepatic failure or extremely advanced cirrhosis
  - Progression through the stages is very rapid, often 6–12 hours.
  - Wilson disease can imitate HE.
- Vital signs:
  - Bradycardia
  - Increased BP suggestive of increased intracranial pressure
- Jaundice, ascites, and other correlates of liver disease
- CNS exam pertaining to stage of HE: Assess short-term memory and presence of asterixis.

DIAGNOSTIC TESTS & INTERPRETATION

- The clinical setting and findings are adequate to establish diagnosis in 80% of the cases.
- The treatment response often confirms the diagnosis.
- EEG: Shows symmetric slowing of basic (α) rhythm common with other forms of metabolic encephalopathy (1)[A]; useful to a limited extent
- Visual evoked potential: Specific in stages 2, 3, and 4
- Number connection test, line drawing test, clicker flicker frequency test, and other psychometric tests may be used to assess for minimal HE (2)[A].

Lab

Initial lab tests

- Liver tests, including aspartate aminotransferase (AST), alanine aminotransferase (ALT), and serum albumin to evaluate severity of underlying liver disease
- Prothrombin time (PT) elevated in liver failure
- Elevated ammonia often present (3)[A]; levels affected by infusion of amino acid solutions, opiate administration producing severe constipation, uremia, and rapid and severe tissue breakdown, massive burns, trauma, or infection
- Hematology to identify anemia and signs of infection
- Standard biochemistry profile to identify hypokalemia, bilirubinemia, altered calcium status, hypomagnesemia, and hypoglycemia
- BUN: creatinine ratio (BUN/Cr) >20 suggestive of GI bleeding or dehydration
- Blood, urine, and ascitic fluid cultures to identify infection, if clinically indicated
- Consider arterial blood gases.
- Toxicology screen for illicit drugs

Imaging

- Useful only to rule out other diagnoses
- CT scan of the head may be most useful (4)[A].
- MRI may demonstrate increased T1 signal in globus pallidus.

Diagnostic Procedures/Surgery

EEG has typical rhythm (see above).

Pathological Findings

- Brain edema in 100% of fatal cases
- Glial hypertrophy in chronic encephalopathy

DIFFERENTIAL DIAGNOSIS

- Metabolic encephalopathy related to anoxia, hypoglycemia, hypokalemia, hypo- or hypercalcemia, or uremia
- Head trauma, concussion, subdural hematoma
- Transient ischemic attack (TIA), ischemic stroke
- Alcohol withdrawal syndrome
- Alcohol intoxication
- Toxic confusion due to medication or drugs
- Meningitis
- Wilson disease
- Reye syndrome

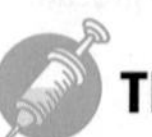

TREATMENT

MEDICATION

First Line

- Lactulose syrup (laxative action decreases colonic transit time, and bacterial digestion acidifies colon promoting excretion of ammonia): 30–60 mL of 50% solution PO q.i.d. Diminish to 15–30 mL b.i.d. when ≥3 bowel movements occur daily.

- Lactulose enema (for patients who cannot tolerate oral lactulose or have suspected ileus): 300 mL plus 700 mL tap water, retained for 1 hour
- If worsening occurs or no improvement in 2 days, add antibiotics:
  - Rifaximin: 400 mg PO t.i.d. (nonabsorbable antibiotic) (5)[A]; highly effective in reversing minimal HE (6)[A]
  - Neomycin: 1–2 g/d PO divided q6–8h, if renal status is good
  - Metronidazole and vancomycin are alternative antibiotics.
- Antacids as needed
- Contraindications:
  - Total ileus
  - Hypersensitivity reaction
- Precautions:
  - Hypokalemia
  - Electrolyte imbalance
  - Renal failure
- For significant possible interactions, refer to manufacturer's profile of each drug.

Second Line

Flumazenil

ADDITIONAL TREATMENT

General Measures

- Identify and vigorously treat precipitating causes: GI bleeding, infection, sedative drugs, and electrolyte imbalance are most common.
- Stage 2 or higher: Ensure adequate fluid intake and at least 1,000 kcal (4.19 megajoules) daily; avoid hypoglycemia.
- Give initial enema to all patients without diarrhea.
- If clumsiness and poor judgment are prominent, be sure the patient has the care needed to avoid falls, cuts on broken glass, smoking burns, and machinery/auto accidents.
- Avoid sedative or opiate medications. Benzodiazepine sedatives and opiate derivatives, such as diphenoxylate/atropine, have caused liver coma.
- Stage 4: Protect the airway, as aspiration is common (tracheal intubation is often used); feed intravenously or with jejunal feeding tube.

Issues for Referral

Refer early to a transplant center.

COMPLEMENTARY AND ALTERNATIVE MEDICINE

Probiotics and prebiotics have been associated with improvement of HE through modulation of gut flora (7)[C].

SURGERY/OTHER PROCEDURES

- Artificial liver perfusion devices have proven useful in fulminant hepatic failure to bridge the patient until a donor liver is available for transplantation.
- Stage 3 and 4 patients should be considered for liver transplantation.

IN-PATIENT CONSIDERATIONS

Initial Stabilization

- Monitor closely in stages 1 and 2 when diagnosis is clear, and watch for progression.
- Inpatient management for stages 3 and 4
- Stage 3 or 4 in fulminant hepatic failure is a strong indication for evaluation for liver transplantation; transfer to a transplant center should be considered.

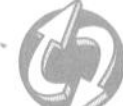

ONGOING CARE

FOLLOW-UP RECOMMENDATIONS

- Activity as tolerated
- Avoid driving or operating machinery.

Patient Monitoring

- To optimize treatment, a trail-making test should be followed (a pencil/paper connect-the-dots according to numbers). Apply to stage 1 and 2 patients to determine how much maintenance treatment is needed and what diet is appropriate. The test should be run daily at first and then at each visit when changes in drugs and diet are made.
- Patients with changed findings should be seen twice weekly.
- Stable patients should be seen monthly.
- Number connection test or line drawing test at each office visit
- In cirrhosis, evaluate for transplantation; death likely in 24 months

DIET

- Integrate with needs of underlying liver disease
- Lower total protein (0.8–1.2 g/kg/d); vegetable protein diets are better tolerated than animal protein diets; special IV/enteral formulations with increased branched-chain amino acids are available.
- Stage 3 and 4 patients need parenteral nutrition or jejunal feeds.
- As coma improves, increase dietary protein as tolerated.
- Have dietitian instruct patient in eating lower-protein diet.

PATIENT EDUCATION

Pamphlets suitable for patient and family are available from the American Association for the Study of Liver Diseases, 1729 King Street, Suite 200, Alexandria, Virginia 22314; (703) 299–9766; www.aasld.org

PROGNOSIS

- Acute or fulminant disease: With adequate aggressive treatment, disappears without residue or recurrence
- Chronic disease:
  - Coma returns
  - With each recurrence, becomes more and more difficult to treat
  - Plateau of maximum improvement shows a decrement over several years such that the degree of improvement with treatment is less and less; the mortality rate is 80%.

COMPLICATIONS

- Recurrence
- With many recurrences, permanent basal ganglion injury (non-Wilsonian hepatolenticular degeneration)
- Hepatorenal syndrome

REFERENCES

1. Saxena N, Bhatia M, Joshi YK, et al. Electrophysiological and neuropsychological tests for the diagnosis of subclinical hepatic encephalopathy and prediction of overt encephalopathy. *Liver*. 2002;22:190–7.
2. Weissenborn K, Ennen JC, Schomerus H, et al. Neuropsychological characterization of hepatic encephalopathy. *J Hepatol*. 2001;34:768–73.
3. Ong JP, Aggarwal A, Krieger D, et al. Correlation between ammonia levels and the severity of hepatic encephalopathy. *Am J Med*. 2003;114:188–93.
4. Quero Guillén JC, Herrerías Gutiérrez JM. Diagnostic methods in hepatic encephalopathy. *Clin Chim Acta*. 2006;365:1–8.
5. Bass NM, Mullen KD, Sanyal A, et al. Rifaximin treatment in hepatic encephalopathy. *N Engl J Med*. 2010;362:1071–81.
6. Sidhu SS, Goyal O, Mishra BP, et al. Rifaximin improves psychometric performance and health-related quality of life in patients with minimal hepatic encephalopathy (the RIME Trial). *Am J Gastroenterol*. 2011;106:307–16.
7. Liu Q, Duan ZP, Ha DK, et al. Synbiotic modulation of gut flora: Effect on minimal hepatic encephalopathy in patients with cirrhosis. *Hepatology*. 2004;39:1441–9.
8. Als-Nielsen B, et al. Non-absorbable disaccharides for hepatic encephalopathy: Systematic review of randomised trials. *Br Med J*. 2004;328:1046–511.

ADDITIONAL READING

- Blei AT, Córdoba J, Practice Parameters Committee of the American College of Gastroenterology. Hepatic encephalopathy. *Am J Gastroenterol*. 2001;96:1968–76.
- Ferenci P, Lockwood A, Mullen K, et al. Hepatic encephalopathy–definition, nomenclature, diagnosis, and quantification: Final report of the working party at the 11th World Congresses of Gastroenterology, Vienna, 1998. *Hepatology*. 2002;35:716–21.
- Kircheis G, Fleig WE, Görtelmeyer R, et al. Assessment of low-grade hepatic encephalopathy: A critical analysis. *J Hepatol*. 2007.

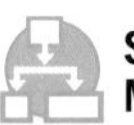

See Also (Topic, Algorithm, Electronic Media Element)

Algorithm: Delirium

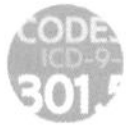

CODES

ICD9

572.2 Hepatic encephalopathy

CLINICAL PEARLS

- Closely monitor the mental status of your patient for confusion/drowsiness and through psychometric testing to determine if your patient with liver disease is developing HE.
- Although questions regarding the superiority of lactulose over antibiotics have been raised (8), at present, there is not sufficient evidence to change our current treatment recommendations.
- It is recommended that all patients with HE receive a liver transplantation evaluation.

H

HEPATITIS A

J. Scott Gaertner, MD

BASICS

DESCRIPTION

Infection with the hepatitis A virus (HAV) primarily involving the liver

EPIDEMIOLOGY

Pediatric Considerations

- Disease is often milder or asymptomatic in pediatric population.
- Infections are asymptomatic in 70% of children <6 years old.
- Hepatitis A infection severity increases with age.

Incidence

- In 2007, there were 2,979 HAV infections reported in the US.
- Prior to release of the HAV vaccine, there were 22,000–36,000 cases reported per year in the US (1)[B].
- Estimated cases: 25,000 HAV infections in 2007 (lowest ever recorded in US)
- Incidence in US: 1.1/100,000
- Predominant sex: Male = Female

Prevalence

Antibodies in 33% of US population

RISK FACTORS

- Foreign travel to developing countries accounts for over 50% of cases in North America and Europe.
- Employment in health care
- Household exposure
- Intimate exposure, especially men who have sex with men
- Institutionalized individuals
- Clotting factor disorders such as hemophilia
- Blood exposure/transfusion rare

Genetics

Autoimmune hepatitis is associated with human leukocyte antigen class II; DR3 and DR4 after active infection with HAV, although rare

GENERAL PREVENTION

- HAV vaccines: Havrix and Vaqta:
  - 0.5 mL IM for children >1 year; 1 mL IM for adults; second dose after 6–12 months.
  - Separate syringe site from immunoglobulin
  - Used for travelers, daycare staff/children, custodial facility employees, sewage workers, military, homosexual men, and food handlers
  - HIV-infected patients who are negative for HAV IgG should receive HAV vaccine series, preferably early in course of HIV infection:
    - If a patient's CD4 count is <200 cells/mm^3 or the patient has symptomatic HIV disease, it is preferable to defer vaccination until several months after initiation of antiretroviral (ARV) therapy in an attempt to maximize the antibody response to the vaccine (2)[A].
  - American Academy of Pediatrics recommends routine administration of HAV vaccine to all children 12–23 months of age in all states according to the CDC-approved immunization schedule:
    - Coadministration of the HAV vaccine with MMR and varicella vaccines did not impact the immunogenicity of any of the vaccines and was well tolerated (3)[B].
  - In 2007, self-reporting studies estimated vaccination coverage among adults aged 18–49 years at 12.1% (1)[B].
  - Seroprotection remain for at least 20 years after primary hepatitis A vaccine (4)[B]. *Booster vaccine is not recommended.*
  - HAV and hepatitis B virus: Twinrix
- Passive immunization: Immunoglobulin:
  - Immunoglobulin seems to be effective for both pre-exposure and postexposure prophylaxis of hepatitis A (5)[A]:
    - 0.02–0.06 mL/kg IM given within 2 weeks after exposure prevents illness in 80–90%
    - HAV vaccine has similar efficacy to immunoglobulin in postexposure prophylaxis if given within 2 weeks
    - Use immunoglobulin in cases where travelers need immediate protection, children <1 year of age, and pregnant females who will be traveling.
    - Use 0.06 mL/kg q5mo for long-term travelers if they are unable to receive the vaccine.
    - Do not give immunoglobulin with measles, mumps, rubella, or varicella vaccines.
- Good sanitation
- Good hygiene, including hand washing, especially for food handlers, healthcare, and daycare workers
- HAV is *not* killed by freezing.
- HAV is killed by heating to 185°F for 60 seconds, chlorine, and iodine.

PATHOPHYSIOLOGY

- Hepatitis A is a single-stranded linear RNA enterovirus and a member of the *Picornaviridae* family.
- Humans are the only natural host.

ETIOLOGY

- Incubation is 2–6 weeks (mean of 4 weeks)
- Greatest infectivity is during the 2 weeks before the onset of clinical illness.
- Infection occurs after eating or drinking food or water contaminated with HAV or direct contact with infected person who has poor personal hygiene.
- Food can become contaminated if handled by an infected individual with poor personal hygiene.
- Shellfish, such as clams and oysters, may be contaminated if harvested from waters contaminated with HAV.
- Bloodborne transmission occurs but is rare.
- No chronicity in HAV

COMMONLY ASSOCIATED CONDITIONS

- Arthritis
- Urticaria
- Anemia
- Immune complex nephritis

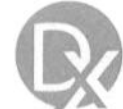

DIAGNOSIS

HISTORY

- Fever: 60%
- Malaise: 67%
- Nausea and vomiting
- Anorexia: 54%
- Dark urine: 84%
- Transient pale stools
- Right upper abdominal pain
- Fatigue
- Myalgias
- Symptom severity has direct correlation to age.
- Pediatric cases frequently asymptomatic

PHYSICAL EXAM

- Hepatomegaly
- Fever
- Jaundice
- Icterus
- Right upper abdominal tenderness

DIAGNOSTIC TESTS & INTERPRETATION

Lab

Initial lab tests

- Aspartate aminotransferase (AST) and alanine aminotransferase (ALT) elevated. May exceed 10,000. ALT usually >AST.
- Anti-HAV IgM: Positive at time of onset of symptoms
- Anti-HAV IgG: Appears soon after IgM and generally persists for years
- Alkaline phosphatase: Mildly elevated
- Bilirubin: Conjugated and unconjugated fractions usually increased. Usually follows rises in ALT and AST.
- Prothrombin time and partial thromboplastin time: Usually remains normal or near normal range:
  - Significant rises should raise concern.
- CBC: Mild leukocytosis; aplasia and pancytopenia are rare:
  - Initial thrombocytopenia may predict illness severity.
- Albumin, electrolytes, and glucose
- Urinalysis: Bilirubinuria

Follow-Up & Special Considerations

Illness usually resolves within 4 weeks from onset of symptoms.

Imaging

- Usually not needed
- Consider ultrasound to rule out differential diagnosis

Initial approach

Bed rest and appropriate nutrition/hydration

Follow-Up & Special Considerations

Usually can be managed outpatient

Diagnostic Procedures/Surgery

Liver biopsy usually not necessary

Pathological Findings

- Pronounced portal inflammation
- Immunofluorescent stains for HAV-antigen positive
- Positive serum markers in hepatitis A:
  - Acute disease: Anti-HAV IgM and IgG positive
  - Recent disease: Anti-HAV IgM and IgG positive
  - Previous disease: Anti-HAV IgM negative and IgG positive

DIFFERENTIAL DIAGNOSIS

- Hepatitis B, C, D, E
- Infectious mononucleosis
- Primary or secondary hepatic malignancy
- Ischemic hepatitis
- Drug-induced hepatitis
- Alcoholic hepatitis
- Autoimmune hepatitis
- Wilson disease

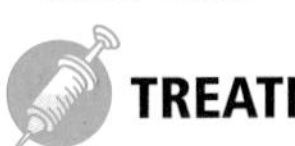

TREATMENT

MEDICATION

Postexposure prophylaxis to persons within 2 weeks of exposure to HAV:

- Administer hepatitis A vaccine to persons between the ages of 1 and 40.
- Administer immunoglobulin to persons <1 and >40 years of age.

First Line

- No antiviral medications indicated, as spontaneous resolution occurs in almost all patients.
- Steroids not indicated unless patient has autoimmune hepatitis

Second Line

- Antiemetics: Metoclopramide 5–20 mg IV/IM t.i.d.
- IV fluids
- Pruritus: Diphenhydramine 50 mg PO/IM q6h and cholestyramine 4 g b.i.d.
- If increased PT, give vitamin K 10–15 mg SC

ADDITIONAL TREATMENT

General Measures

- Monitor coagulation defects, fluid and electrolytes, acid–base imbalance, hypoglycemia, and impairment of renal function.
- Report acute cases to local public health department.

Issues for Referral

- Dictated by severity of illness
- Hepatic failure

COMPLEMENTARY AND ALTERNATIVE MEDICINE

Avoid botanicals with hepatotoxicity potential, including:

- Barberry, comfrey, golden ragwort, groundsel, huang qin, kava kava, pennyroyal, sassafras, senna, valerian, wall germander, wood sage

SURGERY/OTHER PROCEDURES

Liver transplant in fulminant hepatic failure

IN-PATIENT CONSIDERATIONS

Initial Stabilization

Treatment is usually outpatient

Admission Criteria

Dictated by severity of illness

IV Fluids

Treat dehydration and electrolyte imbalances.

Nursing

Routine

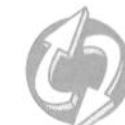

ONGOING CARE

FOLLOW-UP RECOMMENDATIONS

Return to work/school 10–14 days after onset of symptoms with diligence to hygiene

Patient Monitoring

- Monitor coagulation defects, fluid and electrolytes, acid–base imbalance, hypoglycemia, and impairment of renal function.
- Report acute cases to local public health department.
- Usually infectious 4 weeks from initial symptoms

DIET

- Adequate balanced nutrition
- Avoid alcohol.
- Avoid medications that may accumulate in the liver.

PATIENT EDUCATION

- Segregation of food handlers with HAV
- HAV immunity after infection

PROGNOSIS

- Excellent
- Mortality is 0.2%.

COMPLICATIONS

- Coagulopathy, encephalopathy, and renal failure
- Relapsing HAV: Usually milder than the initial case. Positive anti-HAV IgM. Total duration is usually <9 months.
- Prolonged cholestasis: Characterized by protracted periods of jaundice and pruritus (>3 months). Resolves without intervention.
- Autoimmune hepatitis: Good response to steroids
- Hepatic failure: Rare (1–2%)

REFERENCES

1. Lu PJ, Euler GL, Hennessey KA, et al. Hepatitis A vaccination coverage among adults aged 18–49 years in the United States. *Vaccine*. 2009;27(9):1301–5.
2. National Guideline Clearinghouse (NGC) Agency for Healthcare Research and Quality (AHRQ). Prevention of secondary disease: Preventive medicine. Viral hepatitis. 2011. www.guideline.gov.
3. Rinderknecht S, Michaels MG, Blatter M, et al. Immunogenicity and safety of an inactivated Hepatitis A vaccine when coadministered with measles-mumps-rubella and varicella vaccines in children less than 2 years of age. *Pediatric Infect Dis J*. 2011;30(10):e179–85.
4. Cornberg M, Manns MP, et al. [Prevention of virus hepatitis A to E]. *Internist (Berl)*. 2011;52:250–64.
5. Liu JP, Nikolova D, Fei Y. Immunoglobulins for preventing hepatitis A. *Cochrane Database Syst Rev*. 2009;(2):CD004181.

ADDITIONAL READING

- Garner-Spitzer E, Kundi M, Rendi-Wagner P. Correlation between humoral and cellular immune responses and the expression of the hepatitis A receptor HAVcr-1 on T cells after hepatitis A re-vaccination in high and low-responder vaccinees. *Vaccine*. 2009;27(2):197–204.
- Launay O, Grabar S, Gordien E. Immunological efficacy of a three-dose schedule of hepatitis A vaccine in HIV-infected adults: HEPAVAC study. *J Acquir Immune Defic Syndr*. 2008;49:272–5.
- Trofa AF, Klein NP, Paul IM, et al. Immunogenicity and safety of an inactivated hepatitis A vaccine when coadministered with diphtheria-tetanus-acellular pertussis and *Haemophilus influenzae* type B vaccines in children 15 months of age. *Pediatric Infect Dis J*. 2011;30(10):e179–85.

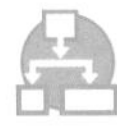

See Also (Topic, Algorithm, Electronic Media Element)

- Hepatitis B; Hepatitis C
- Algorithm: Hyperbilirubinemia

CODES

ICD9

070.1 Viral hepatitis a without mention of hepatic coma

CLINICAL PEARLS

- Hepatitis A vaccine is given in 2 doses 6–12 months apart.
- The vaccine is indicated for travelers, daycare staff/children, custodial facility employees, sewage workers, military, homosexual men, and food handlers.
- HAV disease severity directly correlates with age; children are often asymptomatic.

HEPATITIS B

Michael P. Curry, MD
Sanjiv Chopra, MBBS, MACP

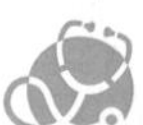

BASICS

DESCRIPTION

Systemic viral infection that may cause acute and chronic liver disease and hepatocellular carcinoma (HCC)

EPIDEMIOLOGY

Incidence

- Predominant age: All ages
- Predominant sex: Fulminant hepatitis B virus (HBV): Male > Female (2:1)
- In the US, 43,000 new infections in 2008, 70% due to IV drug use
- African Americans: Highest rate of acute HBV infection in US

Prevalence

- In the US, 800,000 to 1.4 million people have chronic HBV.
- Asia and the Pacific Islands have the largest populations at risk for HBV.
- Chronic HBV worldwide: 350–400 million persons:
  - Per year: 1,000,000 deaths:
    - 10th leading cause of death
    - Second most important carcinogen (behind tobacco)
    - Of chronic carriers, 25% die of cirrhosis or HCC.
    - Of chronic carriers, 75% are Asian.

RISK FACTORS

- Screen high-risk groups with HBsAg/sAb (1)[A]:
  - Persons born in endemic areas (45% of world)
  - Hemodialysis patients
  - IV drug users (IVDU), past or present
  - Men who have sex with men (MSM)
  - HIV- and HCV-positive patients
  - Household members of HBsAg carriers
  - Sexual contacts of HBsAg carriers
  - Inmates of correctional facilities
  - Patients with chronically elevated ALT/AST
- Vaccinate all above groups if negative.
- Additional risk factors:
  - Needle stick/occupational exposure
  - Recipients of blood/products; transplanted organ recipients
  - Intranasal drug users
  - Body piercing/tattoos

Genetics

Family history of HBV and/or HCC to determine exposure and future HCC risk

Pediatric Considerations

- Shorter acute course; fewer complications
- 90% of vertical/perinatal infections become chronic.

Pregnancy Considerations

- Screen all pregnant women for HBsAg (1)[A].
- High viral load at 28 weeks treated with oral meds from 32 weeks on reduces perinatal transmission.
- Infant of HBV-infected mother needs HB immune globulin (HBIg) (0.5 mL) plus HBV vaccine within 12 hours of birth and HBV series at 0, 1, and 6 months (1)[A].
- Breast-feeding is safe if HBIg and HBV vaccine are administered and nipples are without fissures.
- HIV coinfection significantly increases risk of vertical transmission.
- Continue medications if pregnancy occurs while on an oral antiviral therapy to prevent acute flare.

GENERAL PREVENTION

Most effective: HBV vaccination series (3 doses):

- Vaccinate:
  - All infants at birth
  - All at-risk patients (see "Risk Factors")
  - Health care and public safety workers
  - Sexual contacts of HBsAg carriers
  - Household contacts of HBsAg carriers
- Proper hygiene/sanitation by health care workers, IVDU, and tattoo/piercing artists:
  - Barrier precautions, safe handling of needles, sterilization of equipment, cover open cuts, clean blood spills with bleach
- Do not share personal items exposed to blood (e.g., nail clipper, razor, toothbrush).
- Safe sexual practices (condoms)
- HBsAg carriers cannot donate blood, tissue, or organs.
- Postexposure (e.g., needlestick): HBIg 0.06 mL/kg in <24 hours and vaccination

ETIOLOGY

HBV is a DNA virus of the family *Hepadnaviridae*.

COMMONLY ASSOCIATED CONDITIONS

Arthritis, polyarteritis nodosa, membranous glomerulopathy, anemia (including aplastic anemia), dermatitis, cardiomyopathy, hepatitis D virus infection, metabolic syndrome

DIAGNOSIS

HISTORY

- Exposure: Detailed family and social history
- Acute HBV:
  - Fever/malaise/fatigue/arthralgias/myalgias
  - Anorexia/nausea/vomiting
  - Jaundice/scleral icterus
  - Dark urine/pale stools
  - Right upper quadrant abdominal pain
- Chronic HBV: Typically asymptomatic

PHYSICAL EXAM

Acute: Ill; jaundice/scleral icterus; RUQ tenderness, hepatomegaly

DIAGNOSTIC TESTS & INTERPRETATION

Lab

Initial lab tests

- AST/ALT: Marked elevation in acute HBV, particularly of ALT, 400 to several thousand IU/mL (may be normal or mildly elevated in chronic HBV)
  - Elevated before bilirubin elevates
- Bilirubin: Normal to markedly elevated in acute HBV, conjugated/unconjugated
  - Last test to normalize as acute infection resolves
- Alkaline phosphatase: Mild elevation
- HBcAb IgM may be the only early finding ("window period," when HBsAg/sAb–).
- For acute hepatitis:
  - Monitor PT, albumin, electrolytes, glucose, CBC
  - If severe acute HBV, check for superinfection with hepatitis D (HDV Ag and HBDV Ab).
  - Hepatitis B serologic markers
- Hepatitis B e antigen (HBeAg+) indicates high replication/infectivity; confirmed with high HBV DNA ($\geq 10^5$ copies/mL); these patients benefit from medical therapy.
- HBV precore mutants have undetectable HBeAg despite active viral replication (confirm with HBV DNA level) as well as antibody to e antigen (HBeAb+).
- Screen for HIV, HCV, and immunity to HAV (HAV Ab total/IgG).

Follow-Up & Special Considerations

HBsAg+ persistence >6 months = chronic HBV:

- Measure HBV DNA level and ALT every 3–6 months.
- If age >40 and ALT borderline or mildly elevated, consider liver biopsy
- Measure baseline α-fetoprotein (AFP).
- Follow HBeAg for loss (every 6–12 months).
- Lifetime monitoring for progression, need for treatment, and screening for HCC

Imaging

- Ultrasound to demonstrate ascites, splenomegaly, portal hypertension, rule out obstruction, screen for HCC
- Contrast CT or MRI if abnormal ultrasound or elevated AFP

Diagnostic Procedures/Surgery

Liver biopsy or serum markers of fibrosis (Hepascore, Fibro test) determines extent of injury, excludes other liver disease, and guides therapy.

Pathological Findings

Liver biopsy in chronic HBV may show interface hepatitis and inflammation, necrosis, cholestasis, fibrosis, cirrhosis, or chronic active hepatitis.

DIFFERENTIAL DIAGNOSIS

- EBV; CMV; hepatitis A,C, or E
- Drug-induced, alcoholic, or autoimmune hepatitis
- Wilson disease or rheumatologic/immunologic disorders

Marker	Acute infection	Chronic infection	Inactive carrier	Resolved infection
HBsAg	+	+	+	–
HBsAb	–	–	–	+
HBcAb	+ IgM	– IgM; + total/IgG	+	+
HBeAg	+	±	–	–
HBeAb	–	±	+	±
HBV DNA	Present	Present	Low–negative	
Negative	ALT	Marked elevation	Transient mild elevation	Normal

TREATMENT

MEDICATION

First Line

- Acute HBV:
  - Supportive care; antiviral therapy not indicated; spontaneously resolves in 95% of immunocompetent adults. Treatment may be indicated in cases of severe acute HBV resulting in acute liver failure.
- Chronic HBV: Treatment based on HBeAg status:
  - FDA-approved drugs: Lamivudine 100 mg, adefovir 10 mg, entecavir 0.5–1 mg, telbivudine 600 mg, or tenofovir 300 mg, all given PO every day (dose based on renal function); pegylated interferon (peg-IFN) α2a SC weekly (1,2)[A]

ADDITIONAL TREATMENT

General Measures

- Monitor coagulation, electrolytes, glucose, renal function, phosphate, acid/base
- Report all HBsAg+ to public health department

Issues for Referral

- Refer all HBsAg+ patients for consideration of antiviral therapy.
- Refer to liver transplant program ASAP if fulminant acute hepatitis, end-stage liver disease, or HCC.

SURGERY/OTHER PROCEDURES

Liver transplantation, operative resection, radiofrequency ablation

IN-PATIENT CONSIDERATIONS

Admission Criteria

- Worsening course (marked increase in bilirubin, transaminases, or symptoms)
- Hepatic failure (high PT, low albumin)

Table 1 Chronic hepatitis B therapy (1)

HBeAg	HBV DNA Viral load	ALT*	Rec.
(+)	≥20,000 IU/mL	Elevated	Mono or combination therapy; biopsy or serum fibrosis marker prior to treatment
(−)	≥2,000 IU/mL	Elevated	Consider biopsy or serum fibrosis marker and treatment
(+)	≤20,000 IU/mL	Any	Monitor q6–12mo
(−)	≥2,000 IU/mL	Normal	Biopsy; treat if disease
(+)	≥20,000 IU/mL	Normal	Observe, consider treatment if ALT elevated. Biopsy if age >40 or ALT is high normal to mild elevation
(−)	≤2,000 IU/mL	Any	Monitor q6–12mo
Cirrhosis	Any	Any	Treat with mono or combination tx (3)
Decomp	Any	Any	Treat + refer for transplant

*ALT elevated if >2 × ULN; ULN for male = 30 IU/mL and for female = 19 IU/mL.

- Lamivudine no longer recommended first-line due to high rates of resistance
- Entecavir, tenofovir, peg-IFN are preferred first-line agents (1)[A]
- Oral agents given for extended period:
  - If HBeAg+, treat 6–12 months post loss of eAg/gain of eAb (1)[A]
  - If HBeAg–, treat indefinitely or until HBsAg clearance and HBsAb development (1)[A]
- Change/add drug based on development of resistance:
  - Confirm patient compliance with medications before assuming resistance.
  - Adherence to therapy or combination therapy lowers rate of resistance.
- Dose adjustment made for elevated creatinine
- Standard IFN (Intron A) no longer used in favor of peg-IFN:
  - Peg-IFN (Pegasys) injections given weekly for 48 weeks
  - Best efficacy in genotype A
  - Contraindicated if decompensated cirrhosis
- Goals of therapy: Undetectable HBV DNA, normal ALT, loss of HBeAg, + HBeAb; loss of HBsAg and + HBsAb.
- Precautions:
  - Oral drugs: Renal insufficiency, acute flare if discontinued, resistance/mutation development
  - Peg-IFN: Coagulopathy, myelosuppression, depression/suicidal ideation

Second Line

Emtricitabine effective; pending FDA approval

ONGOING CARE

Patient Monitoring

- Vaccinate for HAV if seronegative (1)[B].
- Monitor serial ALT and HBV DNA:
  - High ALT + low HBV DNA associated with favorable response to therapy
- Serologic markers: See chart
- Metabolic complications and renal function
- WBC/platelets with IFN therapy
- Monitor HBV DNA q3–6mo during therapy:
  - Undetectable DNA at week 24 of oral drug therapy associated with low resistance at year 2.
- Monitor for complications (ascites, encephalopathy, variceal bleed) in cirrhosis.

DIET

Avoid alcohol.

PATIENT EDUCATION

- Acute HBV:
  - Review transmission precautions (1)[A].
- Chronic HBV:
  - Alcohol/smoking increase progression of liver disease and should be avoided.
  - Strict compliance with oral medication is critical to prevent flare.
- Patient education materials in English and Spanish available at www.cdc.gov/hepatitis/B/PatientEduB.htm.

PROGNOSIS

- Acute infection: 95% of adults recover.
- Severity of encephalopathy predicts survival in fulminant hepatic failure.
- Acute HBV: Mortality 1%
- Acute HBV + HDV: Mortality 2–20%
- Chronic HBV:
  - Spontaneous resolution: 0.5% per year
  - Premature death from cirrhosis or HCC: 25%
  - Risk of HCC rises with rate of viral replication, even if no cirrhosis
  - US and AFP q6–12mo for screening (patient-specific guidelines) (1,3)[B]

COMPLICATIONS

- Acute or subacute hepatic necrosis; cirrhosis; hepatic failure
- Hepatocellular carcinoma (all chronic HBV patients are at risk)
- Severe flare of chronic HBV with corticosteroids:
  - Avoid if able; taper very slowly if used.
- Reactivation of resolved infection if immunosuppressed (e.g., chemotherapy): Prophylactic premedication recommended if HBsAg+ (1,3) or if HBcAb+ and received systemic chemotherapy.

REFERENCES

1. Lok AS, McMahon BJ, et al. Chronic hepatitis B: Update 2009. *Hepatology*. 2009;50:661–2.
2. Woo G, Tomlinson G, Nishikawa Y, et al. Tenofovir and entecavir are the most effective antiviral agents for chronic hepatitis B: A systematic review and Bayesian meta-analyses. *Gastroenterology*. 2010;139:1218–29.
3. Weinmaum C. Recommendations for identification and public health management of persons with chronic hepatitis B infection. *MMWR*. 2008;57:1–20.

See Also (Topic, Algorithm, Electronic Media Element)

- Cirrhosis of the Liver; Hepatitis A; Hepatitis C
- Algorithm: Hyperbilirubinemia

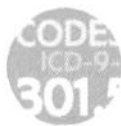

CODES

ICD9

- 070.30 Viral hepatitis b without mention of hepatic coma, acute or unspecified, without mention of hepatitis delta
- 070.32 Chronic viral hepatitis b without mention of hepatic coma without mention of hepatitis delta

CLINICAL PEARLS

- All patients born in endemic countries should be screened with HBsAg.
- Patients with chronic HBV need lifetime monitoring for progressive disease and HCC.

H

HEPATITIS C

Michael P. Curry, MD
Sanjiv Chopra, MBBS, MACP

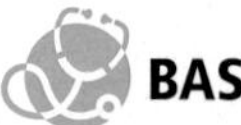

BASICS

DESCRIPTION

Acute or chronic systemic viral infection primarily involving liver

EPIDEMIOLOGY

- Predominant age: Highest incidence in ages 20–39; highest prevalence ages 30–49 years.
- Male = Female

Geriatric Considerations

Age >60 less likely to respond; treat earlier if able

Pediatric Considerations

- Prevalence: 0.3%
- Fewer symptoms or abnormal liver tests; more likely to clear spontaneously; slower rate of progression

Pregnancy Considerations

- Vertical transmission 1–5% if HIV negative
- Breast-feeding safe if no fissures (1)
- Ribavirin is teratogenic; contraindicated in pregnancy and in male partners of pregnant or impregnable women without contraception

Incidence

- In the US, 40,000 new cases of *chronic* hepatitis C virus (HCV) per year: Reports of *acute* infections rare (asymptomatic); 2/3 of people with chronic HCV are undiagnosed.
- Rate of new infections reduced since 1992 when effective donor blood screening began

Prevalence

- ~2.7–3.9 million in US (1.8%) HCV Ab+
- ~3 million have chronic HCV (HCV RNA+)
- ~12,000 deaths annually
- Most common cause of chronic liver disease and liver transplants in the US
- Genotype 1 predominant (75% of cases)

RISK FACTORS

- Screen patients with persistently elevated alanine aminotransferase (ALT) or known risk factors (1)[B]:
  - Hemodialysis
  - Blood ± product transfusion before 1992
  - Hemophilia treatment before 1987
  - IV drug use: 60–70% of new infections
    - *High transmission first use*; "once" is high risk
  - Sexually active homosexual male
  - HIV or hepatitis B infection
  - Household exposure to infected body fluids
  - Organ transplant recipients before 1992
  - Children of HCV+ mothers (test >18 months)
  - Current sexual partners of HCV+ persons
- Possible risk factors:
  - Inhaled cocaine use; shared works
  - Body piercing/tattoos
  - Unsterile medical equipment
  - Health occupational risks low unless needlestick
- Universal screening not recommended.

GENERAL PREVENTION

- No vaccine or postexposure prophylaxis available
- HCV Ab+ does not confer immunity to reinfection.
- Do not share razors/toothbrushes/nail clippers.
- Use and dispose of needles properly.
- Sexual transmission rare in long-term partners (1.5%) if monogamous (1)[C].

ETIOLOGY

Single-stranded RNA virus of family *Flaviviridae*

COMMONLY ASSOCIATED CONDITIONS

Diabetes, metabolic syndrome, iron overload, depression, substance abuse/recovery, autoimmune and hematologic disease, HIV and hepatitis B coinfections

DIAGNOSIS

HISTORY

- Determine exposure: *Complete* social history
- Chronic HCV: Vast majority mildly symptomatic (nonspecific fatigue) or asymptomatic elevated ALT/aspartate aminotransferase (AST)
- Acute HCV: *If* symptoms develop (rare):
  - Onset 2+ weeks postexposure and persist 2–12 weeks
  - Usually spontaneous clearance of fever; malaise/fatigue; arthralgias/myalgias; nausea/vomiting/anorexia; RUQ pain; jaundice/icterus/pruritus/dark urine/pale stools

PHYSICAL EXAM

- Typically normal unless advanced fibrosis/cirrhosis
- May have RUQ tenderness/hepatomegaly

DIAGNOSTIC TESTS & INTERPRETATION

Lab

Initial lab tests

- AST/ALT: Normal or transiently elevated in chronic HCV; ALT usually 1–2 × ULN; AST may be normal or elevated but < ALTAST/ALT ratio ≥1 associated with cirrhosis:
  - If ratio >2, rule out alcohol abuse
  - Marked elevation only in acute hepatitis (400 to several thousand U/L)
  - If acute, serial PT to monitor for liver failure (acute liver failure from HCV alone is exceedingly rare)
- Alkaline phosphatase and GGT: Usually normal; more likely abnormal if cirrhosis, alcohol/fatty liver, or biliary obstruction
- Bilirubin: Normal in chronic HCV unless end-stage disease; markedly elevated in acute HCV (both direct/indirect); occurs after ALT/AST increase, ≥6 weeks postexposure
- Albumin and PT normal until liver failure
- Anti-HCV negative until 8–9 weeks postexposure
- HCV RNA is positive 1–3 weeks postexposure
- Persistent HCV RNA >6 months = Chronic HCV
- False (+) antibody: Autoimmune disease; false (–): Immunosuppressed
- Screen for other liver disease (Differential DX):
  - Ferritin (moderately high levels typical in HCV), ceruloplasmin, ANA, α1-Antitrypsin phenotype, fasting glucose/lipid panel
- If chronic, baseline α-fetoprotein (AFP) serum markers in hepatitis C diagnosis

Follow-Up & Special Considerations

Vaccinate if seronegative for hepatitis A/B (1)[C].

Imaging

- Ultrasound: Hepatomegaly, fatty liver, rule out mass
- MRI with contrast if US or AFP abnormal; early cirrhosis not detectable by imaging

Diagnostic Procedures/Surgery

Liver biopsy or serum fibrosis marker (Hepascore, Fibro test) recommended in chronic HCV to determine extent of injury, exclude other disease, guide treatment, and determine prognosis (2)[C].

Pathological Findings

- Periportal lymphocytic inflammation
- Inflammation: Grade 0–4; fibrosis: Stage 0–4

DIFFERENTIAL DIAGNOSIS

Hepatitis A or B; EBV, CMV; alcoholic hepatitis; nonalcoholic steatohepatitis (NASH); hemochromatosis, Wilson disease, α1–Antitrypsin deficiency; ischemic, drug-induced, or autoimmune hepatitis

Table 1 Serum Markers in Hepatitis C Diagnosis

Result	Marker (Lab test)
(+)	Anti-HCV (antibody): • ELISA III • RIBA (distinguishes false-positive HCV Ab from spontaneous clearance)
(+)	HCV RNA (viral load): • Qualitative (TMA) • Quantitative, confirms (+) qualitative (PCR or bDNA)
1, 2, 3, 4, or 6 (rare) (also >50 subtypes)	Genotype (1)[A]: • Indeterminate if RNA too low, spontaneous clearance, or false-positive anti-HCV • 2a, 2b, 3a: Duration of therapy with pegylated interferon and ribavirin is 24 weeks • 1a, 1b: Duration of therapy is determined by response and includes pegylated interferon, ribavirin and a protease inhibitor such as telaprevir or boceprevir.

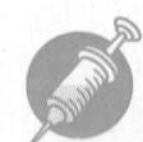

TREATMENT

MEDICATION

First Line

- Acute HCV: Antiviral therapy highly effective if given within 12 weeks of infection (2)[B]:
  - Pegylated interferon (IFN) alone or in combination with low-dose ribavirin, for 12–24 weeks
- Chronic HCV: Antiviral therapy variably effective Peg-IFN/ribavirin (1)[A]:
  - Peg-IFN/ribavirin/protease inhibitor combined therapy:
    - Peg-IFN α2b 1.5 μg/kg SC weekly *OR*
    - Peg-IFN α2a 180 mcg SC weekly *WITH*
    - Ribavirin 800–1,400 mg PO, divided b.i.d. (weight-based)
    - Telaprevir (Incivek) 375 mg, 2 tablets q8h with a snack containing fatty foods for 12 weeks *OR*
    - Boceprevir 200 mg, 4 tablets q8h with a snack starting on day 1 of week 5 of therapy

- Duration of therapy: 24–48 weeks based on genotype, cirrhosis and response guide therapy with assessment of HCV VL at weeks 4 and 12 for IFN/RBV and telaprevir and at weeks 8 and 24 for IFN/RBV and boceprevir.
- Treatment of HCV in the setting of HIV infection should be with IFN/RBV for 48 weeks regardless of HCV genotype.
- Telaprevir and boceprevir are not FDA approved for acute HCV infection, HIV and HCV infection, and nongenotype 1 HCV infection
- For genotype 2/3, 24 weeks sufficient if early viral response (EVR):
  - Cirrhosis lowers sustained viral response (SVR) by 50% in all genotypes.
  - Dose-reduced ribavirin/therapy interruption, especially before RNA negative, reduces SVR (3)[B]
- Contraindications: Mouse IG, egg, or neomycin allergy; pregnancy/breast-feeding; decompensated liver disease or renal failure; untreated psychiatric disease; corticosteroid use or uncontrolled autoimmune disease; DDI or D4T in HIV patients (substitute comparable agent)
- Precautions: Disorders of coagulation, anemia, or myelosuppression; seizures; depression/suicidal ideation (psychiatric clearance and monitoring recommended); retinopathy (diabetic/hypertensive) needs ophthalmology clearance/monitoring

ADDITIONAL TREATMENT

General Measures

- Report acute cases to the health department.
- Pretreatment patient counseling is critical.
- Control all other medical conditions prior to treatment.
- Side effects of IFN/ribavirin:
  - Fatigue, weight loss, insomnia, headache, depression/irritability, cognitive changes, nausea, rash, cough, thyroiditis, alopecia (temporary)
  - Premedicate injections with acetaminophen or NSAIDs if not contraindicated; early and prophylactic treatment of somatic and psychiatric side effects is key to adherence (4)
- Side effects of protease inhibitors:
  - Skin rash (mild to moderate in 50%, severe in 5%, Dress and Stevens Johnson syndrome seen in <1%), anemia, anorectal pain, dysgeusia
- Growth factors help maintain dose and tolerability (erythropoietin for ribavirin-induced anemia, G-CSF for IFN-induced neutropenia); however, not associated with improved SVR (3)[C]
- Team (PCP, GI/hepatologist/ID physician, counselor, help line/support group, insurance disease management program, family, 12-step sponsor) improves outcomes (4)

Issues for Referral

- Refer all patients to a specialist experienced with HCV therapy (2)[C] (clinical trial if uninsured)
- Refer to liver transplant program if fulminant acute hepatitis, at first complication of end-stage disease, or at diagnosis of HCC (2)[A].

Additional Therapies

Interferon-alfacon-1 (consensus IFN, Infergen) up to 37% cure rate in nonresponders/relapsers (5)[C].

COMPLEMENTARY AND ALTERNATIVE MEDICINE

- No medical evidence exists for using herbal or alternative therapy in HCV/cirrhosis/HCC (1)[C].
- Milk thistle (silymarin) generally safe and may reduce ALT but does not eradicate virus or improve outcomes; avoid while on IFN.
- Rate of HCC tripled in patients on herbal therapy compared to IFN therapy.

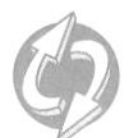

ONGOING CARE

FOLLOW-UP RECOMMENDATIONS

- If treatment is deferred, annual liver function tests; monitor for complications/associated conditions; and maintain sobriety/recovery.
- No need to monitor serial viral load unless on antiviral therapy; unrelated to disease severity or prognosis, and individual lab assays not well standardized.
- In cirrhosis, lifetime risk HCC 20%; screen with US/AFP every 6–12 months (2)[C].

Patient Monitoring

- Serial ALT/AST; serial fasting glucose
- Serial Hgb/Hct, WBCs, absolute neutrophil count, platelets
- Follow electrolytes, TSH, renal function, PT
- HCV qualitative RNA negativity at week 4 is rapid viral response (RVR); confers ~90% chance of SVR in all genotypes (1)
- HCV quantitative RNA negativity (or drop of ≥2 log) at week 12 is EVR; confers good chance SVR
- SVR also more likely in patients with (4) these factors: Age ≤40; female gender; Caucasian race; absence of bridging fibrosis/cirrhosis; HCV RNA <800,000 IU/mL; genotypes 2 and 3; BMI <30 kg/m^2; absence of insulin resistance and steatosis; absence of HIV; recent infection (e.g., needlestick)
- HCV RNA >1,000 IU/mL at week 4 or week 12 for patients on IFN/RBV and telaprevir requires discontinuation of therapy
- HVCV RNA >100 IU/mL at week 12 for patients on IFN/RBV and boceprevir requires discontinuation of therapy
- Monitor for decompensation (low albumin, ascites, encephalopathy, GI bleed) in cirrhotics.
- Goal of therapy is SVR: Eradication of HCV by negative qualitative RNA (TMA) 6 months posttreatment (relapse extremely rare after 6 months)

DIET

- Low-fat, high-fiber diet, and exercise to treat obesity/fatty liver
- Extra protein and fluids while on IFN therapy

PATIENT EDUCATION

- Avoid alcohol, tobacco, and drugs (including marijuana); refer to rehab/12-step program and monitor for relapse.
- Warn against claims of false cures.
- Recommend avoidance of herbs (may contain hepatotoxins and contaminants) and hepatotoxic medications and supplements.

PROGNOSIS

- Of acute infections, 70–80% become chronic.
- Of chronic infections, 30% will progress to cirrhosis at a rate of 1–3% per year over 10–30 years.
- Cirrhosis progresses to liver failure and/or cancer (HCC) in 30%; more rapid if older age when infected; male gender; alcohol/substance abuse; HIV or HBV coinfection; insulin resistance/diabetes (6)
- Chronic HCV is *curable* in ~70% of cases; in noncirrhotic genotype 2 or 3, cure rate ~90%

COMPLICATIONS

- Acute/subacute hepatic necrosis, liver failure, transplant and complications, death
- HCC: Risk factors include cirrhosis, age >55, male, obesity/diabetes/fatty liver, and ongoing alcohol/tobacco/marijuana/drug use.

REFERENCES

1. Ghany M, Strader D, et al. AASLD Practice Guidelines: Diagnosis, management, and treatment of Hepatitis C: An update. *Hepatology*. 2009;49: 1335–74.
2. Chronic Hepatitis C: Current Disease Management, NIH Pub. no. 07-4230 Nov. 2006. Available at: http://digestive.niddk.nih.gov/ddiseases/pubs/chronichepc/Accessed 5/15/10.
3. Shiffman ML. Optimizing the current therapy for chronic hepatitis C virus: Peginterferon and ribavirin dosing and the utility of growth factors. *Clin Liver Dis*. 2008;12:487–505, vii.
4. Agudelo E. Optimizing therapy in treatment-naïve genotype 1 patients. *Curr Hepatitis Rep*. 2008;7:64–71.
5. Leevy CB. Consensus interferon and ribavirin in patients with chronic hepatitis C who were nonresponders to pegylated interferon alfa-2b and ribavirin. *Dig Dis Sci*. 2008;53:1961–6.
6. Zein N. Steatosis and metabolic syndrome: An emerging enigma in the natural history of chronic hepatitis C. *Curr Hepatitis Rep*. 2008;7:61–3.

ADDITIONAL READING

Ghany MG, Nelson DR, Strader DB, et al. An update on treatment of genotype 1 chronic hepatitis C virus infection: 2011 practice guideline by the American Association for the Study of Liver Diseases. *Hepatology*. 2011;54:1433–44.

See Also (Topic, Algorithm, Electronic Media Element)

- Hepatitis A; Hepatitis B; Cirrhosis of the Liver
- Algorithm: Hyperbilirubinemia

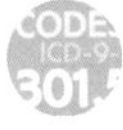

CODES

ICD9

- 070.54 Chronic hepatitis C without mention of hepatic coma
- 070.70 Unspecified viral hepatitis c without hepatic coma

CLINICAL PEARLS

- 1 in 10 patients with hepatitis C have no identifiable risk factors.
- Of infected persons, 15–25% spontaneously resolve infection without treatment.

H

HEPATITIS, AUTOIMMUNE

Michelle T. Martin, PharmD
Jamie Berkes, MD

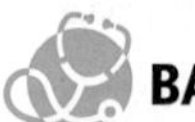

BASICS

DESCRIPTION

Autoimmune hepatitis (AIH) is a chronic inflammatory disorder of the liver, of unknown etiology, characterized by interface hepatitis, hypergammaglobulinemia, and autoantibodies:

- Clinical presentation can range from asymptomatic to acute, severe disease.
- AIH is diagnosed based on clinical, histologic, biochemical, and immunologic criteria.

EPIDEMIOLOGY

Incidence

0.1–1.9 per 100,000 per year in Caucasian populations. Lower incidence in Japan.

Prevalence

- 11.6–16.9 per 100,000 in Europe
- Females more affected than men for all types of AIH (3.6:1)
- Most common in Caucasians of northern European descent
- Bimodal age distribution for type I: Adolescents and adults in the fourth to sixth decades are most at risk.
- Type II is more often found in southern Europe vs. northern Europe, the US, or Japan. Primarily affects young females and children.

RISK FACTORS

- Female sex
- Triggers include: Medications, viruses (acute hepatitis A or B, Epstein-Barr)
- Associated autoimmune conditions

Genetics

- Associated with the complement allele C4AQO and with human leukocyte antigen (HLA) haplotypes B8, B14, DR3, DR4, and Dw3
- Studies show associations between microsatellite markers on chromosomes 11 and 18 (D11S902 and D18S464) and type I AIH (1).

PATHOPHYSIOLOGY

- Hepatic damage results from cell-mediated immunologic attack:
  - HLA facilitates presentation to antigen-processing cells, which encourage cytotoxic T-cell production.
  - Cytotoxic T-lymphocytes infiltrate hepatic tissue, release cytokines, and destroy hepatocytes.
  - Chronic inflammation of the liver leads to fibrosis and eventually cirrhosis in advanced cases.
- Acute fulminant inflammation can lead to acute liver failure in the absence of cirrhosis.
- Type I (80% of cases): Circulating antismooth muscle antibodies (SMA) and/or antinuclear antibodies (ANA)
- Type II: Antibodies to liver/kidney microsome type 1 (anti-LKM-1):
- Type III (least well-established type): Soluble liver antigen/liver pancreas antigen (SLA/LP); clinically identical to type I but with different antibody profile

ETIOLOGY

Idiopathic

COMMONLY ASSOCIATED CONDITIONS

- Type I diabetes mellitus
- Autoimmune thyroiditis
- Immune-mediated hemolytic anemia
- Idiopathic thrombocytopenic purpura
- Celiac sprue
- Ulcerative colitis
- Vitiligo
- Rheumatoid arthritis
- Primary biliary cirrhosis and primary sclerosing cholangitis occasionally overlap with AIH (1).

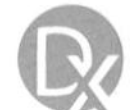

DIAGNOSIS

HISTORY

- 40% of cases are abrupt in onset; course is often fluctuating.
- Symptoms range from asymptomatic to vague nonspecific symptoms to acute fulminant hepatic failure:
  - Symptoms include: Right upper quadrant (RUQ) pain, nausea, jaundice, pruritus, fatigue, anorexia, arthralgias (usually of the small joints)
- Often history of other autoimmune disorders (15–34%), especially in type II AIH
- Obtain medication and alcohol use history.

PHYSICAL EXAM

Physical exam may be normal at the time of presentation, but may include:

- Hepatomegaly, splenomegaly, jaundice, stigmata of chronic liver disease

DIAGNOSTIC TESTS & INTERPRETATION

Simplified diagnostic criteria for AIH by the International Autoimmune Hepatitis Group, 2008 (2)[C] based on:

- Diagnosis:
  - $\geq$6 points: Probable AIH; $\geq$7 points: Definite AIH
- Autoantibodies (maximum of 2 points awarded for autoantibodies):
  - 1 point for ANA or SMA $\geq$1:40; 2 points for ANA or SMA $\geq$1:80
  - 2 points for anti-LKM or positive SLA
- IgG: 1 point for IgG > upper limit of normal (ULN); 2 points for IgG > 1.1 × ULN
- Histology: 1 point if compatible with AIH; 2 points if typical for AIH
- Exclusion of viral hepatitis: 2 points for negative viral hepatitis markers

Lab

Initial lab tests

- Aspartate aminotransferase (AST), alanine aminotransferase (ALT), alkaline phosphatase:
  - AST and ALT > 2–10 × ULN (3,4)[C]
  - Alk phos:AST (or ALT) ratio of <1.5 suggests AIH (3)[C]
- IgG > 1.5–2 × ULN suggests AIH (3,4)[C]
- Autoantibodies with titers >1:40–80 suggests AIH, including:
  - ANA, SMA (suggests type I AIH)
  - Anti-LKM-1, antiliver cytosol 1 antibodies (anti-LC1) (suggests type II AIH (3,4)[C]
  - Autoantibodies are suggestive but are not alone diagnostic of AIH.
- Presence of antimitochondrial antibodies (AMA) often indicates primary biliary cirrhosis (PBC).
- If patient negative for conventional autoantibodies but AIH is suspected, other serological markers, including at least anti-SLA and atypical perinuclear antineutrophil cytoplasmic antibody (pANCA), should be tested (5)[B]:
  - Soluble liver antigen/liver-pancreas autoantibodies (SLA/LP) in type III (6)[C]
- Viral hepatitis A, B, and C antibodies

Imaging

RUQ ultrasound and cholangiography can help distinguish obstructive from nonobstructive liver injury.

Diagnostic Procedures/Surgery

Liver biopsy

Pathological Findings

- Interface hepatitis; plasma cell infiltrate and rosettes also common (1)[C]
- Portal mononuclear cell infiltrate (4)[C]
- Eosinophils frequently present (4)[C]
- Biliary tree generally spared (4)[C]
- Fibrosis usually present with bridging in advanced cases (4)[C]

DIFFERENTIAL DIAGNOSIS

- AIH is a diagnosis of exclusion; hereditary, viral, and drug-induced causes must be ruled out.
- Primary biliary cirrhosis
- Primary sclerosing cholangitis
- Acute or chronic viral hepatitis
- Steatohepatitis (alcoholic or nonalcoholic)
- Systemic lupus erythematosus
- Wilson disease
- Hemochromatosis
- α1-antitrypsin deficiency
- Drug-induced hepatitis (e.g., minocycline, isoniazid, methyldopa, nitrofurantoin, atorvastatin); can case AIH-like syndrome with autoantibodies that usually disappear after medication discontinuation (3,4)

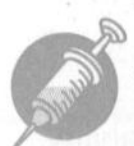

TREATMENT

MEDICATION

- Treatment generally indicated in the following conditions (5,6,7)[C]:
  - AST >10 × ULN
  - AST >5 × ULN with serum gamma globulin >2 × ULN (60% mortality at 6 months if left untreated)
  - Histologic features of bridging necrosis or multilobular necrosis (progress to cirrhosis in 82%, with 5-year mortality in 45% if left untreated)
- Treatment is indicated in pediatric patients with AIH diagnosis; disease is often more advanced.
- Treatment may be deferred in the following situations (6)[C]:
  - Asymptomatic interface hepatitis without necrosis
  - AST < 5 × ULN
  - Inactive cirrhosis
  - Decompensated inactive cirrhosis

First Line

- Prednisone (starting dose is 30–60 mg/d) with or without azathioprine (50–100 mg/d, or 1–2 mg/kg/d):
  - Combination therapy is preferred, especially for the following conditions (3,4,6,7)[B,C]:
    - Osteoporosis
    - Postmenopause
    - Diabetes
    - Hypertension (HTN)
    - Obesity
    - Acne
    - Depression
- Prednisone (20–60 mg) alone is preferred for the following conditions (3,4,6,7)[B,C]:
  - Thiopurine methyltransferase (TPMT) activity deficiency
  - Cytopenias (avoid azathioprine if WBC count $<2.5 \times 10^9$/L or platelet level $<50 \times 10^9$/L)
  - Pregnancy (azathioprine is Category D)
- To prevent bone disease, patients on corticosteroids should also take calcium with vitamin D and do weight-bearing exercise.

Second Line

- 6-mercaptopurine 1.5 mg/kg/d may be substituted for azathioprine (3,6)[C].
- Cyclosporine may be used in children who do not tolerate prednisone or who are steroid-resistant (1,3,6)[C].
- Cyclophosphamide, mycophenolate mofetil, deflazacort, and tacrolimus have shown some benefit in small trials (1,3)[C].

ADDITIONAL TREATMENT

General Measures

- Keep patient comfortable, with analgesics and antiemetics as necessary.
- Vaccinate against hepatitis A and B.

Geriatric Considerations

Use corticosteroids with caution in the elderly.

Pediatric Considerations

AIH is often more advanced in children, and treatment is generally advised.

Pregnancy Considerations

- AIH is associated with increased risk of low birth weight, prematurity, and fetal loss.
- Pregnancy is not a contraindication to treatment.
- Patients may require less immunosuppression during pregnancy; postpartum exacerbations can be anticipated, and steroid may be adjusted to prepregnancy dose 2 weeks prior to labor.
- β-blockers and short second stage of labor recommended if varices are present in second trimester.

SURGERY/OTHER PROCEDURES

Liver transplant for liver failure

IN-PATIENT CONSIDERATIONS

Admission Criteria

- No strict criteria; clinical judgment based on patient symptoms
- Severe cases should be admitted for monitoring of and to prevent fulminant hepatic failure.

IV Fluids

If significant nausea or vomiting occurs, replace fluid losses.

ONGOING CARE

FOLLOW-UP RECOMMENDATIONS

- Follow AST, ALT, total bilirubin, and IgG every 3–6 months during treatment.
- Continue treatment until levels normalize.
- Must continue treatment until liver histology is no longer inflammatory

Patient Monitoring

- Although clinical and laboratory findings can resolve within 2 weeks, treatment should be continued for at least 3–6 months after this because histologic improvement lags behind clinical improvement (4,6)[C].
- Liver biopsy should be obtained before discontinuing or reducing the maintenance immunosuppressive dose (6)[C].
- Liver biopsy may also be helpful for monitoring. Biopsy is suggested 1 year after normalization of laboratory values and/or 2 years after initial presentation (4)[C].
- Monitor AST, ALT, and autoantibodies regularly after discontinuing therapy. May decrease frequency of monitoring if no relapse occurs:
  - Treatment of relapse is the same as initial presentation of AIH.
- Long-term maintenance therapy is indicated for patients with multiple relapses.
- Consider screening for hepatocellular carcinoma in patients with cirrhosis every 6–12 months with ultrasound and α-fetoprotein measurements or yearly liver MRI.
- Eye examinations for cataracts and glaucoma for patients on prednisone
- CBC to monitor for cytopenias every 6 months while on azathioprine

DIET

As tolerated

PATIENT EDUCATION

- Diet to control weight and lipids is advised.
- Avoid hepatotoxic drugs such as alcohol and high doses of acetaminophen.

PROGNOSIS

- Untreated 5- and 10-year survival rates are 50% and 10%, respectively (1,3)[C].
- With treatment, survival >80% at 20 years (no statistical difference from general population) (4,6)[C]
- 80–90% will relapse following discontinuation of therapy (7)[C].
- 10% of patients will fail immunosuppressive therapy. These patients will ultimately need liver transplant (7)[C].
- Survival after liver transplant is 80–90% at 5 years and 75% at 10 years with recurrence of AIH up to 42% (4,7)[C].

COMPLICATIONS

- Fulminant hepatic failure requiring liver transplant
- Cirrhosis
- Hepatocellular carcinoma in patients who develop cirrhosis

REFERENCES

1. Teufel A, Galle PR, Kanzler S. Update on autoimmune hepatitis. *World J Gastroenterol.* 2009;15:1035–41.
2. Hennes EM, Zeniya M, Czaja AJ, et al. International Autoimmune Hepatitis Group. *Hepatology.* 2008;48(1):169–176.
3. Manns MP, Vogel A. Autoimmune hepatitis, from mechanisms to therapy. *Hepatology.* 2006;43:S132–44.
4. Krawitt EL. Autoimmune hepatitis. *N Engl J Med.* 2006;354:54–66.
5. Manns MP, Czaja AJ, Gorham JD, et al. Diagnosis and management of autoimmune hepatitis. *Hepatology.* 2010;51:2193–213.
6. Al-Khalidi JA, Czaja AJ. Current concepts in the diagnosis, pathogenesis, and treatment of autoimmune hepatitis. *Mayo Clin Proc.* 2001;76:1237–52.
7. Heathcote J. Treatment Strategies for Autoimmune Hepatitis. *Am J Gastroenterol.* 2006;101:S630–S632.

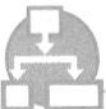

See Also (Topic, Algorithm, Electronic Media Element)

Algorithm: Hyperbilirubinemia

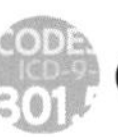

CODES

ICD9

571.42 Autoimmune hepatitis

CLINICAL PEARLS

- Treatment must continue for 3–6 months to allow for histologic changes, despite clinical and lab findings returning to normal within weeks.
- Alk phos: AST (or ALT) ratio of <1.5 suggests AIH.
- Children generally require treatment, but some adults may not progress enough to require medications.

HEPATOMA

E. James Kruse, DO, FACS
Angela L. Gucwa, MD

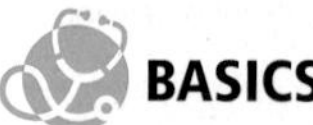

BASICS

DESCRIPTION

Also known as hepatocellular carcinoma (HCC), hepatoma is a primary malignant tumor of the liver arising from hepatic parenchymal cells (hepatocytes), excluding gallbladder and biliary ducts; 80% are associated with underlying liver disease, most commonly cirrhosis (exception: rare fibrolamellar type).

EPIDEMIOLOGY

Incidence

- Most common cause of cancer death worldwide
- Fifth most common malignancy worldwide, >1,000,000 new cases/year worldwide.
- 3–4 new cases/100,000 of the US population per year; 120 new cases/100,000 in Asia and Sub-Saharan Africa per year
- Among known cirrhotics, 2–5 cases/100 cirrhotics/year
- Incidence increasing since 1980s in the US (due to increase in hepatitis C infection)
- In 2010, the American Cancer Society estimates 24,120 new cases diagnosed and ~18,910 deaths.

Prevalence

- Asians > Native American > Hispanics > blacks > whites
- Predominant age: Median age 65 years in the West, fourth to fifth decades of life in Asia and Africa
- Predominant sex: Male > Female (3–4:1)

RISK FACTORS

- For HCC:
  - 80–90% of HCC associated with cirrhosis (1)[B]:
    - Cirrhosis can be from any etiology: Hepatitis B and C, alcoholism, hemochromatosis, nonalcoholic steatohepatitis, α_1–antitrypsin deficiency, biliary cirrhosis, autoimmune hepatitis, Wilson disease, glycogen storage disease
  - Fungal aflatoxins (contaminants of grain in Africa and Asia):
    - Synergistic effect with other causes of liver disease
  - Vinyl chloride
  - Thorium dioxide
  - Anabolic steroids
  - Arsenic
  - Nonalcoholic fatty liver disease/nonalcoholic steatohepatitis (2)[C]
- For fibrolamellar type: No identified risk factors
- For angiosarcoma: Vinyl chloride

Genetics

No known genetic pattern

GENERAL PREVENTION

- The major risk factor for HCC is cirrhosis. Prevention of cirrhosis and tumor surveillance in patients with or at risk for cirrhosis are key.
- Prevent hepatitis B virus (HBV) and hepatitis C virus (HCV) infection through safe sexual practices; avoidance of shared IV drug paraphernalia; and HBV vaccination.
- Treat chronic HBV and HCV with lamivudine, adefovir, entecavir, tenofovir, or ribavirin/pegylated interferon according to guidelines.
- Avoid excessive alcohol use.
- High-risk individuals:
  - Chronic hepatitis with HBV or HCV
  - Alcoholic cirrhosis
  - Genetic hemochromatosis
  - Exposure to vinyl chloride >10 years (screen every 6 months)
  - Primary biliary cirrhosis
- Screen high-risk patients by ultrasonography and alpha-fetoprotein every 6–12 months (3)[B].
- HCC progresses from dysplastic nodules to vascular invasion (after tumor is >2 cm in diameter).

ETIOLOGY

- Cirrhosis accounts for 80–90% of HCC. Alcoholic cirrhosis is most common in the western world. Reported risk in patients with alcoholic cirrhosis is 3–10% with micronodular pattern.
- HBV and HCV are independent and synergistic risk factors for HCC:
  - Associated with >70% of cases worldwide
  - Most important factor in Africa and Asia
- Chronic alcohol use
- Chronic smoking
- Mycotoxins (aflatoxins): Metabolite of the fungus *Aspergillus flavus* that contaminates foods
- Vinyl polymers associated with angiosarcoma and, less commonly, hepatocellular carcinoma

DIAGNOSIS

- In children:
  - Feminization, precocious puberty
  - Palpable liver mass, pain, asymmetrical hepatomegaly
- In adults:
  - Known cirrhosis or clinical signs of cirrhosis: 80%
  - Abdominal pain: 80%; right upper quadrant, dull ache to severe
  - Hepatomegaly: 80–90%; irregular, nodular, firm/hard, tender
  - Weight loss: 30%
  - Hepatic arterial bruit: 20%
  - Friction rub: Rare; more common in metastatic liver disease
  - Paraneoplastic syndromes: Hypertrophic osteoarthropathy, carcinoid syndrome, feminization, polycythemia
  - Unexplained deterioration of stable cirrhosis
  - Budd-Chiari syndrome (hepatic vein obstruction)
  - Portal vein thrombosis

DIAGNOSTIC TESTS & INTERPRETATION

Lab

Initial lab tests

Liver function tests, alkaline phosphatase, BUN and creatinine, CBC, calcium and α-fetoprotein (AFP).

Follow-Up & Special Considerations

- Liver function test abnormalities (aspartate aminotransferase, alanine aminotransferase, alkaline phosphatase)
- AFP:
  - Most important lab test for diagnosis of HCC
  - Not recommended as a sole screening test (60% sensitivity, 80% specificity) (1)[B].
  - Level of >400 ng/mL (>400 μg/L) is diagnostic. Level of >200 ng/mL is highly suspicious for HCC; level does not correlate with prognosis; level is useful in monitoring for recurrence.
  - Fibrolamellar carcinoma usually does not produce AFP:
- Some conditions may cause a slight elevation in AFP
  - Acute or chronic hepatitis
  - Germ cell tumors
  - Pregnancy
- Candidacy for specific treatments will be determined by the degree of liver impairment, commonly utilizing the Child-Pugh classification and/or Model for End-Stage Liver Disease score.
- Rare paraneoplastic syndrome: polycythemia, elevated calcium, low glucose

Imaging

- Ultrasound (US) (3)[B]:
  - Detects tumors >1 cm; performance dependent on examiner, technology, and amount of cirrhosis (decreases sensitivity)
  - More sensitive than AFP level
  - May be useful to follow patients with cirrhosis to help identify hepatocellular cancer at an early tumor stage
  - If US is positive, CT or MRI is performed to confirm (3)[B].
  - May be used as image guidance during percutaneous liver biopsy or other therapy (injection or ablation)
- Helical 3-phase CT scan:
  - Detects 1-cm tumors
  - Valuable in determining extrahepatic spread (most commonly to lung, periportal lymph nodes, bone, brain)
  - Delineates vascular anatomy to guide treatment (4)[A]
- Positron emission tomography (PET)/PET-CT improves CT detection rates.
- MRI:
  - More sensitive than helical CT scan for early detection of HCC
  - Helps differentiate benign from malignant tumors
  - Helpful in delineating the tumor and invasion of vessels
- Arteriography: Used rarely because of the accuracy of MRI and CT
- Imaging of a focal hepatic mass >2 cm with certain characteristic features can be sufficient for identification of HCC without tissue diagnosis (3)[B].

Diagnostic Procedures/Surgery

- Tissue diagnosis is used to confirm mass seen on imaging with atypical findings or in a noncirrhotic liver. Tissue confirmation is also useful to rule out liver metastases (3)[B].
- Liver biopsy: Performed using image guidance (US or CT) when nodules are not palpable. This is *not indicated* when a lesion has typical CT/MRI characteristics and an elevated AFP.
- Laparoscopy: To evaluate extent of cirrhosis and perform resection or ablation in skilled centers

- Preoperative workup: evaluation of extrahepatic metastases
- Unnecessary to biopsy a liver mass with typical radiographic features and elevated AFP. These findings are diagnostic.

Pathological Findings

- Nodular: 75%; usually in cirrhotic liver
- Massive: Common in children and noncirrhotic livers; are prone to rupture
- Diffuse: Rare; usually a large portion of liver is involved
- Hepatocellular: Most commonly multicentric and well differentiated; usually superimposed on underlying cirrhosis

DIFFERENTIAL DIAGNOSIS

- Small, asymptomatic tumors or underlying liver conditions:
  - Cirrhosis with regenerative nodules
  - Benign liver nodules
  - Hamartoma
  - Hemangioma
  - Metastatic adenocarcinoma
  - Cholangiocarcinoma
  - Adenomas
- Larger, symptomatic tumor with hepatomegaly:
  - Cirrhosis
  - Hepatic cyst
  - Adenoma
  - Hemangioma
  - Abscess
  - Metastatic malignancy of liver
  - Thrombosis of hepatic veins, portal vein, or inferior vena cava
  - Active viral hepatitis or alcoholic hepatitis
- Ruptured tumor: All causes of acute abdomen
- Traumatic hemoperitoneum

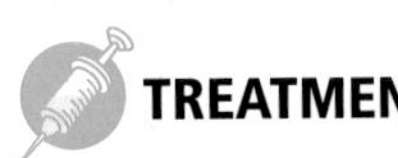

TREATMENT

MEDICATION

- Chemotherapy with sorafenib offers a small survival benefit in patients with disease that is not amenable to surgical intervention (5).
- Treatment of hepatoma in patients with active HCV with pegylated interferon-α and ribavirin prolongs survival and improves quality of life.

SURGERY/OTHER PROCEDURES

- Surgical resection and liver transplantation offer highest cure rate in HCC (1)[B]:
  - Resection should be considered in children and may include up to one lobe of the liver.
  - The resected specimen should contain 1-cm margins of normal liver tissue.
  - Intraoperative US should be performed to survey for additional lesions.
  - Resection is the preferred treatment in noncirrhotic patients with HCC if liver function is preserved and there is no evidence of portal hypertension (1)[B]:
    - Varies from segmental to trisegmental resection (up to 80% of the liver)
  - Transplantation is the preferred treatment for cirrhotic patients or unresectable tumors that meet transplantation criteria (1)[B].
  - Advanced liver disease, medical comorbidities, and extrahepatic metastases are common; therefore, only 15–30% of HCC patients are eligible for resection (1)[B].
  - The cure rate is high for both surgical options with the presence of ≤3 nodules, each <5 cm.
- Tumor ablation:
  - Ablation of tumors in patients not deemed candidates for resection or transplantation is often a safe alternative.
  - Ablation may be chemical with alcohol; cryotherapy with liquid nitrogen probes; or hyperthermic with radiofrequency, microwave, or laser.
  - Ablation may be performed surgically or percutaneously, depending on the location.
  - Radiofrequency ablation (RFA) is considered superior to alcohol injection for localized therapy (6)[B].
  - Recent trials show similar survival rates for RFA vs. surgical resection in small HCCs. There is insufficient evidence to change recommendations favoring surgery at this time (7)[B].
  - Irreversible electroporation is a newer technique that is undergoing clinical trials.
- Percutaneous treatments are best for unresectable disease, as a bridge to surgical resection or transplantation, and for early-stage tumors that are not amenable to surgery:
  - Regional transarterial therapy (delivers chemotherapy directly to the tumor via its immediate blood supply) or chemoembolization are used for intermediate-stage tumors; these modalities may provide palliation or down-stage the tumor, making surgery possible (8)[B]. These 2 approaches can be used together and may yield a better outcome than either treatment alone (8)[B].
- Fibrolamellar variant should be treated by surgical resection; this has shown excellent survival rates.

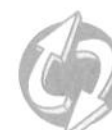

ONGOING CARE

FOLLOW-UP RECOMMENDATIONS

Patient Monitoring

Even after successful resection, there is a high risk of recurrence:

- AFP level every 3 months
- US every 4–6 months or contrast-enhanced CT/MRI scan depending on local expertise

DIET

Attention to nutrition: High-calorie diet

PATIENT EDUCATION

Emphasize preventive measures and HBV vaccine.

PROGNOSIS

- Dependent upon the amount of tumor replacing normal liver tissue and the degree of hepatic impairment
- Unresectable, symptomatic tumors: Grave; patients seldom live >6 months
- Resectable, asymptomatic tumors:
  - Surgery curative in >70% of children, 40% of adults
  - Surgery curative in >80% of cirrhotic adults with tumors <3 cm
- Transplantation: Similar to tumor-free patients with tumors <2 cm; 5-year survival rate of >70% with 1 tumor <5 cm or maximum of 3 lesions <3 cm (United Network of Organ Sharing criteria) (3)[B]

COMPLICATIONS

- Rupture
- Hemoperitoneum
- Liver failure
- Cachexia
- Metastases
- Thrombosis of portal, hepatic, renal veins:
  - Variceal bleeding

REFERENCES

1. Cha CH, Saif MW, Yamane BH, et al. Hepatocellular carcinoma: Current management. *Curr Probl Surg*. 2010;47:10–67.
2. Siegel AB, Zhu AX, et al. Metabolic syndrome and hepatocellular carcinoma: Two growing epidemics with a potential link. *Cancer*. 2009;115:5651–61.
3. El-Serag HB, Marrero JA, Rudolph L, et al. Diagnosis and treatment of hepatocellular carcinoma. *Gastroenterology*. 2008;134:1752–63.
4. Colli A, Fraquelli M, Casazza G, et al. Accuracy of ultrasonography, spiral CT, magnetic resonance, and alpha-fetoprotein in diagnosing hepatocellular carcinoma: A systematic review. *Am J Gastroenterol*. 2006;101:513–23.
5. NCCN Clinical Practice Guidelines Version 2.2011. Hepatocellular Cancers. www.nccn.org.
6. Cho YK, Kim JK, Kim MY, et al. Systematic review of randomized trials for hepatocellular carcinoma treated with percutaneous ablation therapies. *Hepatology*. 2009;49:453–9.
7. Delis S, Bakoyiannis A, Papailiou J, et al. Liver resection vs radio-frequency ablation in the treatment of small hepatocellular carcinoma. *Surg Oncol*. 2009.
8. Garrean S, Hering J, Helton WS, et al. A primer on transarterial, chemical, and thermal ablative therapies for hepatic tumors. *Am J Surg*. 2007;194: 79–88.

ADDITIONAL READING

Bruix J, Sherman M. Management of hepatocellular carcinoma: An update. *Hepatology*. 2011;53(3): 1020–1022.

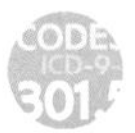

CODES

ICD9

155.0 Malignant neoplasm of liver, primary

CLINICAL PEARLS

- With benign liver tumors, most patients will have normal liver function tests; 97% with HCC will have >1 abnormal test.
- Hepatitis C is the biggest risk factor, especially if combined with alcohol abuse.
- Most common cause of cancer death worldwide; in the west, secondary to ethyl alcohol; in rest of world, secondary to hepatitis B and C

HEPATORENAL SYNDROME

Neil Crittenden, MD
Ashutosh Barve, MD, PhD

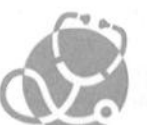

BASICS

Hepatorenal syndrome (HRS): Development of renal failure in patients with end-stage liver disease (ESLD) who have portal hypertension and ascites with poor prognosis.

DESCRIPTION

- HRS is a diagnosis of exclusion.
- Renal failure is a functional disorder because liver transplantation restores renal function.
- HRS classification:
  - Type 1: Rapid decline in serum creatinine >2.5 or a >50% drop in GFR in 2 weeks
  - Type 2: Slowly progressive (>2 weeks), usually associated with ascites resistant to diuretics
- Synonym(s): Renal failure of cirrhosis; Functional renal failure of cirrhosis; Hepatic nephropathy; Heyde syndrome; Oliguric renal failure of cirrhosis; Hemodynamic renal failure of cirrhosis

EPIDEMIOLOGY

- Up to 40% of patients with cirrhosis and ascites will develop HRS.
- Predominant age: Usually after fourth decade
- Predominant gender: Male > Female

Incidence

- Unclear; differentiation between HRS and acute tubular necrosis (ATN) or prerenal state not always made
- In a prospective study of 229 patients, the incidence of HRS in nonazotemic cirrhotic patients with ascites was reported as 18% at 1 year and 39% at 5 years.
- Estimate: 32–41 of 100 patients admitted to the hospital for cirrhosis with ascites develop HRS by 2 and 5 years.

Prevalence

In patients with cirrhosis and renal failure, the prevalence of type 1 HRS is 27–30% and of type 2 HRS is 15.8%.

RISK FACTORS

- Infections: Spontaneous bacterial peritonitis (SBP), bacteremia; HRS develops in 30% of patients with SBP.
- Any reduction of blood volume in cirrhosis:
  - Volume depletion (excessive diuretics, large-volume paracentesis, etc.)
  - Excessive diarrhea (lactulose induced) or vomiting
- Reduction in venous return with tense ascites
- GI bleeding (e.g., variceal bleeding)
- Protein-calorie malnutrition

Genetics

Only as risk for liver disease (e.g., Wilson Disease, hereditary hemochromatosis, alpha-1 antitrypsin deficiency)

GENERAL PREVENTION

- Avoid volume depletion in cirrhotic patients.
- Early diagnosis and aggressive treatment of infections in cirrhotic patients is essential.
- Careful management of patients with cirrhosis to prevent common precipitants (listed above).
- Recent trial of patients with cirrhosis and ascites showed pentoxifylline 400 mg PO t.i.d. reduced the incidence of HRS from 32% in the placebo group to 7% in the pentoxifylline group (1)[B].

PATHOPHYSIOLOGY

- Severe renal vasoconstriction from generalized vasodilation (especially in splanchnic circulation): Pooling of blood occurs in areas of vasodilation, causing reduction of effective arterial volume (EAV). Splanchnic vasodilation is mediated by vasodilator substances from high endothelial sheer stress from portal hypertension.
- Increased cardiac output initially maintains renal blood flow; later decreased EAV activates other compensatory mechanisms: renin-angiotensin, sympathetic nervous system, and ADH, causing vasoconstriction. HRS develops when increased cardiac output and renal intrinsic vasodilators can no longer counteract decreased EAV and renal vasoconstriction. AKI then develops from decreased renal blood flow.
- Renal vasoconstriction results in retention of sodium and water, aggravating ascites and edema. ADH release secondary to decreased EAV also results in water retention, which explains hyponatremia in HRS.
- Infections are a common precipitating factors of HRS in which vasoactive cytokines such as nitric oxide are produced, mediating splanchnic vasodilation. Reduction in EAV from hemorrhage, diarrhea, or vomiting large-volume paracentesis may also precipitate HRS. NSAIDs also cause HRS by inhibiting renal prostaglandin synthesis.

ETIOLOGY

HRS may develop in any patients with ESLD or acute fulminant hepatitis from any cause.

COMMONLY ASSOCIATED CONDITIONS

SBP, ESLD with ascites, alcoholic liver disease, hepatitis B and C, GI bleed, and other infections

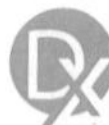

DIAGNOSIS

- Other causes of AKI must be excluded before diagnosing HRS. If no ascites, oligoria, and hyponatremia, then HRS is *unlikely*.
- Diagnostic criteria:
  - Presence of cirrhosis and ascites
  - Serum creatinine >1.5 mg/dL
  - No decrease of serum creatinine to <1.5 mg/dL after 48 hours of diuretic withdrawal and volume expansion with albumin at 1 g/kg/d up to 100 g/d
  - Absence of shock
  - Absence of parenchymal kidney disease

HISTORY

- Patient with advanced or severe acute liver failure presenting with declining renal function
- Renal failure progresses more rapidly in type 1 HRS, and patients are more severely ill as compared with patients with type 2 HRS.
- May have history of overdiuresis, infection, fever, abdominal pain, or bleeding
- Uremic encephalopathy on hepatic encephalopathy may cause severe deterioration of mental status.

PHYSICAL EXAM

- Oliguria (urine output <500 mL/d) with cirrhosis
- Jaundice
- Signs of portal hypertension: Ascites, encephalopathy, splenomegaly
- Signs of infection: Increased temperature, altered mental status
- Signs of SBP: Abdominal tenderness, increased temperature
- Tachycardia and bounding pulse

DIAGNOSTIC TESTS & INTERPRETATION

- The presence of proteinuria, hematuria, and sediment abnormalities in ESLD patient indicates a diagnosis other that HRS.
- Heavy proteinuria and RBC casts suggest glomerular disease.
- A diagnostic paracentesis with ascitic cell count, Gram stain, and culture should be preformed to rule out SBP. Ascitic neutrophils >250/mm^3 is diagnostic of SBP.

Lab

Initial lab tests

- Azotemia in the setting of cirrhosis with appropriate spot urine values (consistent with normal tubular function):
  - Urine sodium <10 mEq/L (10 mmol/L)
  - Fractional excretion of sodium <1%
  - No significant proteinuria
  - Urine/plasma creatinine >30:1
  - Osmolality: Mild to moderate reduction in ability to concentrate (400–600 mOsm/kg/H_2O)
  - All reversible causes should be ruled out (e.g., prerenal azotemia, obstruction).
- Urinalysis: Absence of ATN casts; <500 mg/dL protein, high specific gravity
- Minor criteria:
  - Urine volume <500 mL/d
  - Urine RBCs <50 per high-power field
  - Serum sodium <130 mEq/L
- Other:
  - Prolonged prothrombin time
  - Decreased serum albumin concentration
  - Elevated bilirubin

Follow-Up & Special Considerations

Follow BUN, creatinine, and electrolytes

Imaging

Initial approach

Renal US should be performed to rule out chronic kidney disease, hydronephrosis, or obstruction as the cause of AKI.

Follow-Up & Special Considerations

If ascites are not clinically apparent, an abdominal US can be done to evaluate for ascites.

Diagnostic Procedures/Surgery

Early nephrology and hepatology consultation should be considered.

Pathological Findings

- Liver: Cirrhosis or acute hepatitis
- Kidneys: Normal

DIFFERENTIAL DIAGNOSIS

For abrupt onset of oliguria in cirrhosis:

- Intravascular volume depletion
- GI fluid loss
- Cardiac failure (possibly alcoholic cardiomyopathy)
- Postrenal; obstruction
- Interstitial nephritis (drug induced)
- Intrinsic renal disease
- Renal artery or renal vein occlusion by thrombosis

TREATMENT

MEDICATION

- Reversal of HRS has been more successful using albumin combined with vasoconstrictors.
- Several meta-analyses showed a 40–60% reversal in HRS in patients with this combined treatment.
- Treatment is continued until serum creatinine <1.5 mg/dL with a mean time of reversal of 7 days.

First Line

- Albumin starts with priming dose of 1 g/kg body weight followed by 20–40 g/d.
- Vasoconstrictors: Availability differs by country. The most studied one, terlipressin, is presently unavailable in the US but is currently in a US clinical trial and may become available.
  - Terlipressin:
    - Dosage is started with 0.5 mg q4–6h
    - If serum creatinine does not decrease by more than 30% in 3 days the dose should be doubled (2)[A].
    - Maximum dose: 12 mg/d
    - Side effects are cardiovascular or ischemic complications in 12% of patients.
    - Research trials have used bolus dosing of terlipressin, but small trials recently have showed similar outcomes with continuous infusions equivalent to the same daily dose.
  - Combination therapy with midodrine and octreotide: Doses used are midodrine 7.5–12.5 mg PO t.i.d. and octreotide 100–200 mg SC t.i.d. titrated to an increase of mean arterial pressure (MAP) of at least 15 mm Hg (3)[B].
  - Norepinephrine:
    - Less studied than terlipressin, but 2 trials showed statistically similar results compared with terlipressin.
    - Dosage started at 0.5 mg/hr and is increased q4h by 0.5 mg/hr until an increase in the MAP of at least 10 mm Hg or an increase in 4-hour urine output to more than 200 mL (4)[B]
    - Maximum dose: 3 mg/hr

Second Line

- Pentoxifylline 400 mg PO t.i.d.
- N-Acetylcysteine 150 mg/kg IV over 2 hours followed by continuous infusion of 100 mg/kg daily for 5 days.
- Misoprostol 200–400 μg PO q.i.d.
- Low-dose dopamine once was thought to be beneficial; however, it failed in clinical studies.

ADDITIONAL TREATMENT

General Measures

- Discontinue diuretics.
- Avoid iatrogenic events that precipitate HRS, including excessive volume contraction.
- Avoid NSAIDs, aminoglycosides, or other nephrotoxins.
- Maximize left ventricular function, if possible.
- Relieve urinary obstruction when present.

Issues for Referral

A patient with HRS should follow up with a hepatologist 1 week after discharge and then every 3 months.

Additional Therapies

Dialysis is indicated only as ancillary support for patients awaiting liver transplant or in patients with acute, potentially reversible liver failure.

COMPLEMENTARY AND ALTERNATIVE MEDICINE

Patients must abstain from alcohol, and participation in treatment organizations has shown benefit.

SURGERY/OTHER PROCEDURES

- Definitive treatment is liver transplant with a survival rate of 65% in type 1 HRS.
- Transjugular intrahepatic portosystemic shunt (TIPS):
  - TIPS has been shown to improve renal function in several small trials (5)[B].
  - Use can be limited by high MELD scores in patients with HRS.
  - At least 2 studies have shown improved renal function following TIPS in patients with high MELD scores. Patients initially were treated with albumin and vasoconstrictor therapy to lower the creatinine, thus lowering the MELD score, and then proceeding with TIPS.

IN-PATIENT CONSIDERATIONS

Initial Stabilization

- Type 1 HRS will require hospitalization, whereas type 2 HRS may be managed in outpatient setting.
- Stop diuretics and provide volume with albumin.
- Evaluate for GI bleeding and SBP, and treat with antibiotics if either are present.

IV Fluids

Provide volume expansion with albumin (dose above). This is both therapeutic of volume depletion, as well as diagnostic. If the patient shows improvement, HRS is unlikely.

Nursing

- Monitor urine output and fluid balance.
- 2,000-mg sodium diet
- If the patient is not eating, place a Dobbhoff tube for tube feeds at target goal of 25 kcal/kg/d.
- If treating hepatic encephalopathy, titrate lactulose to 3–4 bowel movements a day
- Place a central venous catheter for central venous pressure monitoring if fluid status of the patient is unclear.

Discharge Criteria

- Persistent serum creatinine <1.5 mg/dL
- Following transplant

ONGOING CARE

FOLLOW-UP RECOMMENDATIONS

Patient Monitoring

- Monitor renal and hepatic function and serum electrolytes.
- Close follow-up with liver disease specialist as an outpatient

DIET

Sodium restriction to <88 mmol/d (<2,000 mg) to slow ascites accumulation

PATIENT EDUCATION

- Abstain from alcohol
- Low-sodium diet

PROGNOSIS

- Grave without liver transplant in patients with cirrhosis
- The time and degree of renal recovery after liver transplantation is variable, depending on the pretransplant renal function, but a substantial number of patients do show significant renal improvement.

COMPLICATIONS

- Death
- Dialysis dependency/end-stage renal disease
- Fluid overload with congestive heart failure or pulmonary edema
- Hepatic coma
- Secondary infections

REFERENCES

1. Tyagi P, Sharma P, Sharma BC, et al. Prevention of hepatorenal syndrome in patients with cirrhosis and ascites: A pilot randomized control trial between pentoxifylline and placebo. *Eur J Gastroenterol Hepatol*. 2011;23:210–7.
2. Gluud LL, Kjaer MS, Christensen E, et al. Terlipressin for hepatorenal syndrome. *Cochrane Database Syst Rev*. 2006;CD005162.
3. Skagen C, Einstein M, Lucey MR, et al. Combination treatment with octreotide, midodrine, and albumin improves survival in patients with type 1 and type 2 hepatorenal syndrome. *J Clin Gastroenterol*. 2009;43:680–5.
4. Sharma P, Kumar A, Shrama BC, et al. An open label, pilot, randomized controlled trial of noradrenaline versus terlipressin in the treatment of type 1 hepatorenal syndrome and predictors of response. *Am J Gastroenterol*. 2008;103:1689–97.
5. Runyon BA, AASLD Practice Guidelines Committee, et al. Management of adult patients with ascites due to cirrhosis: An update. *Hepatology*. 2009;49:2087–107.

ADDITIONAL READING

Guevara M, Arroyo V, et al. Hepatorenal syndrome. *Expert Opin Pharmacother*. 2011;12:1405–17.

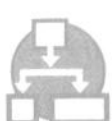

See Also (Topic, Algorithm, Electronic Media Element)

Acetaminophen Poisoning; Cirrhosis of the Liver; Hepatitis A; Hepatitis B; Hepatitis C; Renal Failure, Acute

CODES

ICD9

- 572.4 Hepatorenal syndrome
- 572.8 Other sequelae of chronic liver disease
- 586 Renal failure, unspecified

CLINICAL PEARLS

- HRS is a diagnosis of exclusion. Other causes of acute renal failure must be ruled out.
- HRS stems from hemodynamic changes associated with advanced liver disease, without intrinsic renal abnormalities.
- Treat correctable causes of azotemia. Initial therapy includes volume expansion with albumin.
- Liver transplantation is the treatment of choice.

HERNIA

Leah A. Burnett, MD
Harry W. Sell, Jr., MD, FACS

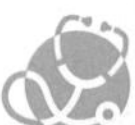

BASICS

DESCRIPTION

External hernias of groin and abdominal wall are an abnormal protrusion of the contents of the abdominal cavity through a fascial defect in the abdominal wall:

- Definitions:
  - Reducible: Extruded sac and its contents can be returned to original intra-abdominal position, either spontaneously or with gentle manual manipulation.
  - Irreducible/incarcerated: Extruded sac and its contents cannot be returned to original intra-abdominal position.
  - Strangulated: Compromise of blood supply to hernia sac contents
  - Richter: Partial circumference of bowel is incarcerated or strangulated. Partial wall damage may occur, increasing potential for bowel rupture and peritonitis.
  - Sliding: Wall of a viscus forms part of the wall of the inguinal hernia sac; i.e., R-cecum, L-sigmoid colon
- Types:
  - Groin: Inguinal and femoral
  - Inguinal:
    - Direct inguinal: Acquired; herniation through defect in transversalis fascia of abdominal wall medial to inferior epigastric vessels; increased frequency with age as fascia weakens
    - Indirect inguinal: Congenital; herniation lateral to the inferior epigastric vessels, through internal inguinal ring into inguinal canal. A "complete hernia" is one that descends into the scrotum, while an "incomplete hernia" remains within the inguinal canal.
  - Pantaloon: Combination of direct and indirect inguinal hernia with protrusion of abdominal wall on both sides of the epigastric vessels
  - Femoral: Descends through the femoral canal deep to the inguinal ligament. Because of the narrow neck of a femoral hernia, this type of hernia is especially prone to incarceration and strangulation.
  - Other: Obturator, sciatic, perineal
  - Incisional or ventral: Iatrogenic, herniation through a defect in the anterior abdominal wall at the site of a prior surgical incision; congenital, herniation through fascial defect in abdominal wall, secondary to collagen deficiency disease
  - Umbilical: Defect occurs at umbilical ring tissue.
  - Epigastric: Protrudes through the linea alba above the level of the umbilicus. These may develop at exit points of small paramidline nerves and vessels, or through an area of congenital weakness in the linea alba.
  - Interparietal (e.g., Spigelian hernia): Hernia sac insinuates itself between layers of the abdominal wall; strangulation common, often mistaken for tumor or abscess

Geriatric Considerations

Abdominal wall hernias increase with advancing age, with significant increase in risk during surgical repair.

Pregnancy Considerations

- Increased intra-abdominal pressure and hormone imbalances may contribute to increased risk of abdominal wall hernias.
- Umbilical hernias associated with multiple, prolonged deliveries

EPIDEMIOLOGY

Incidence

- 75–80% groin hernias: Inguinal and femoral
- 2–20% incisional/ventral, depending on whether a prior surgery was associated with infection or contamination
- 3–10% umbilical, considered congenital
- 1–3% other
- Groin:
  - 6–27% lifetime risk in adult men
  - 2-peak theory: Most inguinal hernias present before 1 year of age or after 55 years
  - ~50% of children under 2 will have a patent processus vaginalis, decreasing to 40% after age 2. Only between 25% and 50% will become clinically significant.
  - Inguinal hernia found in <5% of newborns, but M:F ratio is 10:1
  - Increased incidence in premature infants (1)[B]
  - Increased incidence in patients with abdominal aortic aneurysms
  - Femoral <10% of all groin hernias, 40% present as a surgical emergency
- Incisional/ventral: ~10–23% of abdominal surgeries complicated by an incisional hernia, most common in upper midline incisions. Incidence ratio M:F is 1:1.
- Umbilical: 10–20% of newborns (2). Most close by 5 years of age.

Prevalence

- Groin hernias more prevalent in men. Inguinal hernias more prevalent in men.
- Femoral and umbilical hernias more prevalent in women.
- Most inguinal hernias are indirect in both genders.
- Incisional/ventral hernias are more prevalent in obese or overweight men, as well as more prevalent among smokers. The opposite may be true for inguinal hernias (3)[C].

RISK FACTORS

Increased abdominal pressure, coughing, heavy lifting, constipation, pregnancy, ascites, prostatism, obesity, advancing age (loss of tissue turgor), smoking, steroid use, low birth weight, prematurity

Genetics

No known genetic pattern

PATHOPHYSIOLOGY

Loss of tissue strength and elasticity, especially with aging or congenital defect in abdominal fascia

ETIOLOGY

In general, a defect in the fascia of the abdominal wall. Most pediatric hernias are congenital defects (e.g., patent processus vaginalis), while most adult hernias are a result of acquired weakness in the tissues of the anterior abdominal wall.

COMMONLY ASSOCIATED CONDITIONS

Obesity, chronic obstructive pulmonary disease, multiple abdominal surgeries, pregnancy, advanced age, Ehlers-Danlos, Marfan, Hurler-Hunter, PKD, osteogenesis imperfecta, Beckwith-Wiedemann syndrome, Down syndrome, abdominal aortic aneurysm

DIAGNOSIS

HISTORY

- Many hernias are asymptomatic; symptoms may include pain, nausea, vomiting, bloating, and relief with reclining, necrosis of overlying skin.
- Hernia may be directly observed as protrusion through abdominal wall during maneuvers that increase intra-abdominal pressure.

PHYSICAL EXAM

- Examination should initially occur with patient standing and examiner placing finger in inguinal canal via the scrotum. Exam should also be performed with patient in supine position and with cough.
- Inguinal (superior to inguinal ligament):
  - Direct inguinal hernia: Finger in inguinal canal finds defect of the transversalis fascia as a deep (posterior to anterior) bulge palpated by pad of finger with increased intra-abdominal pressure.
  - Indirect inguinal hernia: Finger in inguinal canal finds a persistent process vaginalis as a bulge (lateral to medial) palpated by fingertip, and may extend down into scrotum.
- Femoral (inferior to inguinal ligament): Bulge in upper middle thigh; neck of the sac will protrude lateral to and below a finger placed on the pubic tubercle
- Umbilical: Palpable protrusion at umbilicus
- Incisional/ventral: Palpable protrusion at site of prior abdominal incision
- Epigastric: Majority occur just off midline, above umbilicus.

DIAGNOSTIC TESTS & INTERPRETATION

Imaging

Initial approach

Hernia evaluation rarely requires imaging; reserve for suspected abdominal hernia or unclear diagnosis. Plain radiographs are often used to look for evidence of obstructive signs, including dilated proximal bowel and bowel stacking:

- Ultrasonography can be used to assess inguinal hernias.
- CT or tangential radiography may also be used; best for incisional and abdominal wall hernias.
- Herniography is no longer recommended, but may be useful in interpreting obscure hernia symptoms in an atypical presentation (4)[A].
- CT imaging is frequently used to evaluate postsurgical patients with complaints of abdominal pain, and is considered the gold standard there.

Pediatric Considerations

There is insufficient evidence for contralateral exploration in pediatric patients, except using ultrasonography.

Follow-Up & Special Considerations

For occult hernias not well appreciated on exam or with imaging, diagnostic laparoscopy may be beneficial.

DIFFERENTIAL DIAGNOSIS

Lymphadenopathy, hydrocele, lipoma, varices, cryptorchidism, abscess, tumor, sports hernia (athletic pubalgia), pelvic fractures, adductor tears, omphalomesenteric duct, urachal cyst

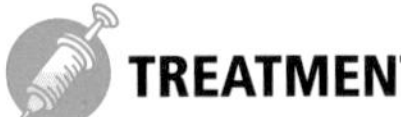

TREATMENT

- Elective setting:
  - Significantly lower morbidity and mortality when surgical repairs performed electively.
- Acute setting:
  - Pain medication recommended for symptomatic hernias
  - Strangulated hernias should be surgically repaired as early as possible to prevent complications such as necrosis and viscus perforation.
  - Manual reduction of incarcerated hernia improves outcomes by allowing for elective repair after improvement of acute swelling and inflammation (5).
  - Complication rate is near 20 times greater in emergent repair of pediatric inguinal hernias than elective procedures (6)[A].

MEDICATION

- Antibiotics: Antibiotic prophylaxis did not reduce wound infections after groin hernia repairs.
- Pain: Local anesthetic during surgical repair results in significant reduction of postoperative pain (6)[A]. Tension-free procedures such as Lichtenstein may be performed under local anesthesia.

ADDITIONAL TREATMENT

Geriatric Considerations

Use of a truss (external supportive device) for direct inguinal hernias common; no data exist on their long-term efficacy, and are often considered a temporizing measure

Issues for Referral

Warn patients symptoms or signs of incarceration or strangulation (acute abdominal pain, fever, bloody bowel movements) mandate immediate self-referral to emergency room.

SURGERY/OTHER PROCEDURES

All inguinal hernias should be surgically repaired, but watchful waiting in the asymptomatic patient is a safe option if significant comorbidities may compromise emergent repair (6)[A]:

- Incarceration and strangulation are absolute indications for hernia repair.
- Contraindications: Patients who are not surgical candidates based on cardiovascular risk factors:
  - Elective repair should be avoided in pregnant patients or those with active infections.
- Special considerations:
  - Umbilical hernias <0.5 cm usually obliterate and can be managed by observation (2).
  - Umbilical hernias in children age 2–4 years may be observed, as there is a high rate of spontaneous closure.
  - Semielective surgical repair can be safe during pregnancy if delayed until after second trimester.
  - Women had lower recurrence rates with laparoscopic methods than with Lichtenstein open method.
  - Ascites is not a strict contraindication for surgical repair. There is a greater risk of strangulation and complication without repair than the increased risks associated with repair in the presence of ascites.
  - The more emergent hernia operations can be performed using the same methods for nonacute situations. However, incarceration with strangulation my require laparotomy with partial bowel resection.
- Gold standard:
  - Inguinal hernia:
    - Open: Lichtenstein with mesh (37%) or mesh plug (34%): Decreased recurrence rates (6)[A]
    - Laparoscopic (14%) with mesh: Decreased hospital stay and postoperative pain (6)[A]:
      - Requires general anesthesia
      - Transabdominal preperitoneal (TAPP) vs. total extraperitoneal (TEP)
    - Pediatric: Recovery and outcome similar after open and laparoscopic repair. Laparoscopic hernia repair associated with increased operation/anesthesia time and postoperative pain.
  - Incisional/ventral:
    - Laparoscopic repair with mesh for simple, noncomplex hernias
    - Open repair with mesh for complex or recurrent hernias
  - Umbilical:
    - Pediatric: Open excision and closure with suture
    - Adult: Open repair with mesh or plug may reduce hernia recurrence.
- Newer techniques:
  - Prolene hernia system
  - Biologic wound closure system: Reduced recurrence in contaminated procedures
- Complications:
  - Recurrence
  - Postoperative pain, temporary or chronic: Improved in laparoscopic approach vs. open
  - Wound infection
  - Injury to cord structures in inguinal herniorrhaphy; with nerve injury, most symptoms will resolve

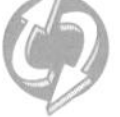

ONGOING CARE

PATIENT EDUCATION

- Cleveland Clinic: http://my.clevelandclinic.org/disorders/hernia/hic_hernia.aspx
- Groin hernias: University of Chicago Children's Hospital: www.uchicagokidshospital.org/specialties/general-surgery/patient-guides/inguinal-hernia.html
- Incisional/ventral: Society of American Gastrointestinal and Endoscopic Surgeons: http://sages.org/sagespublication.php?doc=PI10
- Umbilical hernias: Boston Children's Hospital: www.childrenshospital.org/az/Site1018/mainpageS1018P0.html

PROGNOSIS

- Groin (pediatric): Low recurrence rates (<3%) with surgical treatment; may spontaneously resolve in infants
- Groin (adult): ≥1%/year risk of bowel strangulation without surgical treatment; 0–10% postoperative recurrence rates, depending on surgeon experience level and method
- Incisional/ventral: 3–5% postoperative occurrence: 2–17% postrepair recurrence, increased to 20–46% in larger hernias
- Umbilical (pediatric):
  - High rate of spontaneous resolution
  - Hernia less likely to close further in older children and in children with larger defects
- Umbilical (adult): Up to 11% postoperative recurrence rate
- Epigastric: Most will ultimately become incarcerated and/or strangulated without surgical treatment. Recurrence is high due to frequency of missed defects during repair.

REFERENCES

1. Brandt ML. Pediatric hernias. *Surg Clin North Am*. 2008;88:27–43, vii–viii.
2. Snyder CL. Current management of umbilical abnormalities and related anomalies. *Semin Pediatr Surg*. 2007;16:41–9.
3. Rosemar A, Angerås U, Rosengren A. Body mass index and groin hernia: A 34-year follow-up study in Swedish men. *Ann Surg*. 2008;247:1064–8.
4. Ng TT, Hamlin JA, Kahn AM, et al. Herniography: Analysis of its role and limitations. *Hernia*. 2009;13:7–11.
5. Lau ST, Lee YH, Caty MG. Current management of hernias and hydroceles. *Semin Pediatr Surg*. 2007;16:50–7.
6. Matthews RD, Neumayer L. Inguinal hernia in the 21st century: An evidence-based review. *Curr Probl Surg*. 2008;45:261–312.

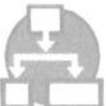

See Also (Topic, Algorithm, Electronic Media Element)

Algorithms: Abdominal Pain, Lower; Intestinal Obstruction; Pelvic Pain

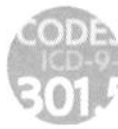

CODES

ICD9

- 550.10 Inguinal hernia, with obstruction, without mention of gangrene, unilateral or unspecified (not specified as recurrent)
- 550.90 Inguinal hernia, without mention of obstruction or gangrene, unilateral or unspecified (not specified as recurrent)
- 552.00 Unilateral or unspecified femoral hernia with obstruction

CLINICAL PEARLS

Types:

- Groin: Inguinal and femoral
- Inguinal:
  - Direct inguinal: Acquired; herniation through defect in transversalis fascia of abdominal wall medial to inferior epigastric vessels; increased frequency with age as fascia weakens
  - Indirect inguinal: Congenital; herniation lateral to the inferior epigastric vessels, through internal inguinal ring into inguinal canal. A "complete hernia" is one that descends into the scrotum, while an "incomplete hernia" remains within the inguinal canal.
- Pantaloon: Combination of direct and indirect inguinal hernia with protrusion of abdominal wall on both sides of the epigastric vessels
- Femoral: Descends through the femoral canal deep to the inguinal ligament. Because of the narrow neck of a femoral hernia, this type of hernia is especially prone to incarceration and strangulation.

HERPANGINA

Aamir Siddiqi, MD

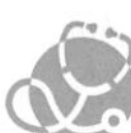

BASICS

DESCRIPTION
- Infectious disease caused by coxsackievirus group A
- Characteristics:
  - Fever of short duration
  - Typical vesicular or ulcerated lesions in the posterior pharynx or on the soft palate
  - Incubation period is 4 days.
- Usual course: Acute and self-limited
- System(s) affected: Endocrine/Metabolic; Gastrointestinal

EPIDEMIOLOGY
Incidence
- Year round in tropical climates
- Summer and autumn in temperate climates (1)[B]
- Predominant age: 3 months to 16 years
- Predominant sex: Male = Female

RISK FACTORS
Contact with infected person

GENERAL PREVENTION
- Avoid contact with infected individuals.
- The mode of transfer is fecal–oral, so general hygiene (hand washing) is suggested.
- Hand washing by preschool-aged children and their caregivers had a significant protective effect against herpangina from human enterovirus 71 infection (2).

ETIOLOGY
- Common:
  - Coxsackievirus A, types 1–10, 16, and 22 (3)[B]
- Infrequent:
  - Coxsackievirus B, types 1–5
  - Echovirus, types 6, 9, 11, 17, 22, and 25
  - Other enterovirus (4)[B]

DIAGNOSIS

HISTORY
The patient may have:
- Low- or high-grade fever
- General malaise
- Sore throat
- Characteristic oropharyngeal lesions
- Anorexia
- Irritability
- Listlessness

PHYSICAL EXAM
- Bilateral discrete vesicles, gray base
- Erythematous patches
- Vesicles may rupture to form ulcers.
- Posterior pharynx location:
  - Pharynx
  - Tonsils
  - Soft palate
- *Little involvement of anterior 2/3 of mouth*
- Oropharyngeal lesions in the form of vesicles with erythematous edges
- Drooling
- Fever
- Malaise
- Local pain
- Emesis
- Backache
- Headache
- Coryza
- Diarrhea

DIAGNOSTIC TESTS & INTERPRETATION
- This is a clinical diagnosis, so tests usually are not necessary.
- Complement fixation
- Hemagglutinin inhibition tests
- Serum antibodies to coxsackievirus:
  - Titers should show a 4-fold rise in serial samples.

Lab
- Generally no lab work is necessary.
- Slight leukocytosis
- Positive viral culture:
  - Mouth washings
  - Stool

DIFFERENTIAL DIAGNOSIS
- Herpes simplex:
  - Multiple ulcers on lips and anterior mouth
  - Diagnose with herpes culture.
- Drug reactions: Cutaneous lesions often present (urticaria, erythema multiforme)
- Recurrent aphthous stomatitis:
  - Buccal, labial, alveolar, mucosal ulcers
  - Recurrent crops
  - Few systemic symptoms
- Lichen planus: Painful ulcer, white lacy pattern on mucosa or may have cutaneous lesions that are purple and pruritic
- Hand, foot, and mouth disease: Classic distribution of vesicular rash on hands, buttocks, feet, and mouth

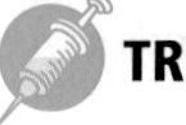

TREATMENT

Benign and self-limited course of the disease should be explained to the patient.

MEDICATION
First Line
- Analgesics:
  - Acetaminophen
  - NSAIDs:
    - Ibuprofen
    - Naproxen
- Topical anesthetics:
  - Viscous lidocaine 2% solution
- Mouthwash:
  - Aqueous solution of 1% dyclonine and 1% diphenhydramine (Benadryl) in 50% attapulgite (Kaopectate)
- Oral lozenges containing Dyclonine (Sucrets) may be used for soreness

ADDITIONAL TREATMENT

General Measures

- Self-limited
- Palliative and supportive
- Hydration

COMPLEMENTARY AND ALTERNATIVE MEDICINE

- Myrrh, an herbal antimicrobial, can improve the blister healing process and provide an analgesic effect, reducing the discomfort of topical ulcerations.
- Chewing licorice root has been found to be effective in soothing and curing mouth ulcers.

IN-PATIENT CONSIDERATIONS

Initial Stabilization

Outpatient

ONGOING CARE

FOLLOW-UP RECOMMENDATIONS

- No restrictions
- As tolerated, with no limitations

Patient Monitoring

Hydration

DIET

- Clear liquids
- Nonirritating foods such as milk products will be more palatable.

PROGNOSIS

Complete recovery

COMPLICATIONS

Complications are rare:

- Exanthem
- Aseptic meningitis
- Myocarditis
- Encephalitis

REFERENCES

1. Chen KT, Chang HL, Wang ST, et al. Epidemiologic features of hand-foot-mouth disease and herpangina caused by enterovirus 71 in Taiwan, 1998–2005. *Pediatrics*. 2007;120:e244–52.
2. Ruan F, Yang T, Ma H, et al. Risk factors for hand, foot, and mouth disease and herpangina and the preventive effect of hand-washing. *Pediatrics*. 2011;127:e898–904.
3. Melnick JL. Enteroviruses: Polioviruses, coxsackieviruses, echoviruses, and newer enteroviruses. In: Fields BN, Knipe DM, Howley PM, eds. *Field's Virology*. 1990:549–98.
4. Chang LY, Tsao KC, Hsia SH, et al. Transmission and clinical features of enterovirus 71 infections in household contacts in Taiwan. *JAMA*. 2004;291:222–7.
5. Frydenberg A, Starr M. Hand, foot and mouth disease. *Aust Fam Physician*. 2003;32:594–5.

ADDITIONAL READING

Wang SM, Liu CC, et al. Enterovirus 71: Epidemiology, pathogenesis and management. *Expert Rev Anti Infect Ther*. 2009;7:735–42.

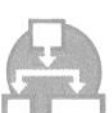

See Also (Topic, Algorithm, Electronic Media Element)

Herpes Simplex

CODES

ICD9

074.0 Herpangina

CLINICAL PEARLS

- Herpangina occurs commonly during the summer season.
- It is not practical to keep children out of school or child care because virus may be shed in feces for weeks (5)[B].
- Herpangina is caused most commonly by coxsackievirus A; less commonly it also may be caused by coxsackievirus B, enterovirus, and echovirus.
- Herpangina predominantly affects newborns and younger children.
- Herpangina is a clinical diagnosis; lab tests are not needed.

H

HERPES EYE INFECTIONS

Stephen Hendriksen, MD
Francesca L. Beaudoin, MS, MD

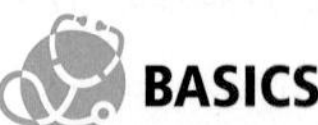

BASICS

DESCRIPTION

- Eye infection (blepharitis, conjunctivitis, keratitis, stromal keratitis, uveitis, retinitis, glaucoma, or optic neuritis) caused by herpes simplex virus (HSV) types 1 and 2 or varicella-zoster virus (VZV, or human herpes virus type 3)
- Categories: Neonatal, primary, and recurrent:
  - HSV keratitis more commonly HSV type I; VZV reactivation commonly called shingles or herpes zoster ophthalmicus (HZO) when there is involvement of the ophthalmic division of the fifth cranial nerve
  - Both HSV and HZO classically cause a dendritic keratitis best seen with fluorescein staining by slit-lamp examination
  - Reactivation of latent infection is most common for both
  - Primary HSV keratitis is more common in children
- System(s) affected: Eye; Skin; Central Nervous System (CNS) (neonatal)

EPIDEMIOLOGY

- Predominant age: HSV, any age; HZO, usually advancing age (>50 years old)
- Predominant sex: HSV, Male = Female; HZO Femal > Male

Incidence

- HSV ocular infection incidence estimated at 12–31 people per 100,000 annually; reoccurrence is more common
- Zoster: 2.2–3.4 per 1,000 people annually; lifetime risk is 20–30%:
  - HZO represents 10–20% of all cases of HZ

Prevalence

HSV ocular infection prevalence is around 150 per 100,000 population (1):

- HZO: 20–30% of the general population will develop HZ sometime in their lives with about a 1% chance of developing HZO

RISK FACTORS

- HSV: History or close contact with HSV-infected person:
  - General risk factors for reactivation: Stress, trauma, fever, UV light exposure, other viral infections
  - Risk factors for HSV keratitis: UV laser eye treatment, some topical ocular medications such as prostaglandin analogues, and primary/secondary immunosuppression
- HZO: History of varicella infection
  - Advancing age (>50), sex female > male, trauma, stress, immunosuppression

ALERT
Consider primary/secondary immunodeficiency disorders in all zoster patients <40 (e.g., AIDS, malignancy)

GENERAL PREVENTION

- Contact precautions with active lesions
- VZV can be spread to those who have not had chickenpox and are not immunized
- Antiviral prophylaxis while on topical steroids
- Varicella vaccination (Zostavax): Single 0.65 mL SC dose; no booster. No need to inquire about history of varicella or to perform testing for antibody. Can be given to those with prior zoster episode. Not used in treatment of acute zoster or postherpetic neuralgia (PHN).
- Acyclovir can be used prophylactically to prevent reoccurrence.

ALERT
Zoster vaccination is contraindicated if HIV-positive, other immunocompromised state, or active untreated tuberculosis (TB)

Pregnancy Considerations

- Pregnant women without history of chickenpox should avoid contact with persons with active zoster
- Pregnancy increases risk of recurrence.
- Live vaccine is contraindicated during pregnancy.

PATHOPHYSIOLOGY

- HSV and VZV are members of the *Herpesviridae* group (DNA viruses)
- Primary infection from contact with infected person leads to a latent state within trigeminal ganglia (HZO)
- Reactivation of the virus affecting the ophthalmic branch is common and can lead to direct ocular involvement.

ETIOLOGY

- Primary infections:
  - Neonatal is usually HSV-2
  - Primary ocular HSV is usually HSV-1
- Recurrent infections:
  - Reactivation from trigeminal ganglion
  - HSV-1, HSV-2, or VZV

COMMONLY ASSOCIATED CONDITIONS

Primary and secondary immunocompromised states

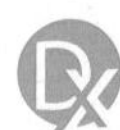

DIAGNOSIS

HISTORY

- Varies according to the virus and the ocular structures involved
- History of varicella or herpes simplex infection:
  - Recurrence of HSV keratitis is common and can lead to stromal infection
- Eye pain, headache, photophobia, tearing, ocular redness, discharge
- Decreased or blurry vision

PHYSICAL EXAM

- Varies according to the virus and the ocular structures involved (HSV most commonly affects the corneal epithelium; VZV most commonly affects corneal stroma and uvea)
- Typically unilateral in presentation:
  - HZO presents as early as 1–2 days after unilateral vesicular eruption in a dermatomal pattern
- HZO can present with a prodromal period of fever, malaise, headache, and eye pain before skin eruptions and visible eye lesions
- Decreased visual acuity
- Conjunctival injection
- Decreased corneal sensation
- Slit-lamp exam:
  - Fluorescein and rose bengal stain: Dendritic or geographic corneal epithelial staining pattern
  - Anterior chamber cells if uveitis present

ALERT
Unilateral dermatomal vesicular rash most commonly in ophthalmic branch (V_1) of trigeminal nerve (VZV):

- Hutchinson sign: Vesicular lesion on nose from VZV indicates an increased risk of HZO due to involvement of nasociliary branch of trigeminal nerve, which also innervates the eye

DIAGNOSTIC TESTS & INTERPRETATION

Lab

Initial lab tests

- Typically none needed, as diagnosis is primarily based on history and physical exam
- Other:
  - Corneal swab for HSV DNA by polymerase chain reaction (PCR) (PPV = 96%)
  - If vesicle present, can perform a Tzanck smear for VZV or HSV (multinucleated giant cells)
  - Antibody titers to assess exposure only; DFA (direct fluorescent antibody); tissue culture

ALERT
Urgent ophthalmology referral for slit-lamp exam, dilated fundus exam, and intraocular pressure measurement

DIFFERENTIAL DIAGNOSIS

- Any other cause of red, painful eye:
  - Bacterial, fungal, allergic, or other viral conjunctivitis
  - Acute angle closure glaucoma
- Corneal abrasion, recurrent corneal erosion, toxic conjunctivitis
- Temporal arteritis
- Trigeminal neuralgia

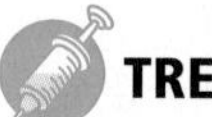

TREATMENT

MEDICATION

First Line

- HSV corneal epithelial disease:
  - Trifluorothymidine 1% (Trifluridine, Viroptic): Apply 1 drop q2h while awake to a max of 9 drops daily until re-epithelialization occurs, then 1 drop q4h for another 7 days (2)[A]
  - Ganciclovir 0.15% gel (Zirgan): Apply 1 drop in eye q3h while awake, around 5 times daily, until re-epithelialization occurs, then 1 drop q8h for 7 days (2)[A]
  - Vidarabine 3% ointment (Vira-A): Apply 0.5 inch into lower conjunctival sac 5 times daily q3h, until re-epithelialization occurs (2)[A]
  - Acyclovir: Ophthalmic ointment is available internationally but not approved in the US
  - Acyclovir: 400 mg PO 5 times per day was shown to be equivalent to topical acyclovir in one study (3)[B].
  - Epithelial debridement by an ophthalmologist: Removes virus quickly and may accelerate healing
  - Avoid topical steroids.
- HSV stromal keratitis or uveitis (without epithelial disease): Combination of antiviral and steroid treatment; requires ophthalmology evaluation:
  - Prednisolone acetate: 1% drops q.i.d. with slow taper

- Consider systemic steroids in severe uveitis.
- Trifluorothymidine: 1% drops q.i.d. for prophylaxis while on topical steroids
- Herpes zoster ophthalmicus (HZO):
  - Acyclovir: 800 mg PO 5 times a day for 7–10 days or valacyclovir (Valtrex) 1 g PO t.i.d. for 7–10 days or famciclovir (Famvir) 500 mg PO t.i.d. for 7–10 days (4,5)[A]
  - Topical antibiotic ophthalmic ointment to protect ocular surfaces (e.g., Bacitracin Polymyxin [Polysporin]): 0.5 inch ribbon 2–3 times a day for 7–10 days (5)[C]
  - If immunocompromised: Acyclovir 10–15 mg/kg IV q8h for 10 days (4,5)[A]
  - Prednisolone acetate: 1% drops q.i.d. with slow taper with an ophthalmologist (5)[B]
- Cycloplegic agent if anterior uveitis present; intraocular pressure-lowering agent if necessary

ALERT
- HZO: Antiviral therapy is most effective within the first 72 hours of rash onset but should still be initiated >72 hours after onset because of the possible complications of HZO
- Topical steroids:
  - Should only be prescribed by an ophthalmologist
  - Contraindicated with active corneal epithelial disease, which is best monitored with a slit lamp
  - Can increase intraocular pressure, cause corneal thinning, and, with long-term use, cause cataracts
- Topical antiviral agents:
  - Toxic to corneal epithelium
- Acyclovir:
  - Reduce dosage in renal insufficiency
- Prednisone:
  - Contraindicated in immunocompromised patients

Second Line
- HSV: Acyclovir 2 g/d PO in divided doses over 10 days in patients intolerant of topical antivirals (3)[B].
- Topical idoxuridine, acyclovir, brivudin while approved internationally are not approved for use in the US.
- Concomitant treatment with interferon may also improve outcomes but is not currently available.

ADDITIONAL TREATMENT
General Measures
- Avoid contact with nonimmune people.
- No contact lenses should be worn during treatment period
- Cool compresses
- Artificial tears
- Oral pain medications

Issues for Referral
Emergent or urgent ophthalmology referral, depending on severity of disease

Additional Therapies
- Recurrent HSV requires suppressive therapy:
  - Acyclovir 800 mg PO daily or valacyclovir 500 mg PO daily
- HZO leading to postherpetic neuralgia is very common and can be treated with gabapentin or pregabalin, TCAs, opioids, and lidocaine gel

SURGERY/OTHER PROCEDURES
Corneal transplantation for severe scarring or perforation

IN-PATIENT CONSIDERATIONS
Admission Criteria
- Severe systemic VZV disease
- Systemic HSV in children

Discharge Criteria
Resolution of systemic disease

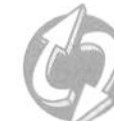

ONGOING CARE

FOLLOW-UP RECOMMENDATIONS
Patient Monitoring
- Monitor with slit-lamp exam every 1–2 days until improvement, then every 3–4 days until epithelial defect resolves
- Weekly after epithelial disease resolves until off topical antivirals

PATIENT EDUCATION
Educate patients about importance of early recognition of recurrent symptoms and need for prompt evaluation and treatment.

PROGNOSIS
- Many cases are self-limited but, depending on the ocular structure involved, can lead to permanent blindness, especially in the setting of recurrent disease.
- Recurrent ocular HSV:
  - HSV epithelial disease without treatment:
    - Without sequelae, 40% resolve
    - With treatment, 90–95% resolve without complication

Pediatric Considerations
- Neonatal primary HSV often disseminated with high mortality rate; 37% have vision worse than 20/200
- Pediatric cases more likely to be bilateral (26%); recurrent (48% in 15 months) and may cause amblyopia

COMPLICATIONS
- Recurrence
- Corneal neovascularization and scarring resulting in poor vision
- Neurotrophic ulcer with perforation
- Secondary bacterial or fungal infection
- Secondary glaucoma in 10%
- PHN in 20–40% with VZV, typically longer-lasting in older patients
- Vision loss from optic neuritis or chorioretinitis

REFERENCES

1. Liesegang TJ, Melton LJ, Daly PJ, et al. Epidemiology of ocular herpes simplex. Incidence in Rochester, Minn, 1950 through 1982. *Arch Ophthalmol.* 1989;107:1155–9.
2. Wilhelmus KR, et al. Antiviral treatment and other therapeutic interventions for herpes simplex virus epithelial keratitis. *Cochrane Database Syst Rev.* 2010;(12):CD002898.
3. Collum LM, McGettrick P, Akhtar J, et al. Oral acyclovir (Zovirax) in herpes simplex dendritic corneal ulceration. *Br J Ophthalmol.* 1986;70:435–8.
4. Carter WP, Germann CA, Baumann MR, et al. Ophthalmic diagnoses in the ED: Herpes zoster ophthalmicus. *Am J Emerg Med.* 2008;26:612–7.
5. Dworkin RH, Johnson RW, Breuer J, et al. Recommendations for the management of herpes zoster. *Clin Infect Dis.* 2007;44(Suppl 1):S1–26.

ADDITIONAL READING

- Ghaznawi N, Virdi A, Dayan A, et al. Herpes zoster ophthalmicus: Comparison of disease in patients 60 years and older versus younger than 60 years. *Ophthalmology.* 2011. [Epub ahead of print].
- Knickelbein JE, Hendricks RL, Charukamnoetkanok P, et al. Management of herpes simplex virus stromal keratitis: An evidence-based review. *Surv Ophthalmol.* 2009;54:226–34.
- Liesegang TJ, et al. Herpes zoster ophthalmicus natural history, risk factors, clinical presentation, and morbidity. *Ophthalmology.* 2008;115:S3–12.

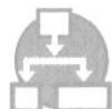

See Also (Topic, Algorithm, Electronic Media Element)

Algorithm: Eye Pain

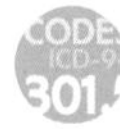

CODES

ICD9
- 053.20 Herpes zoster dermatitis of eyelid
- 053.21 Herpes zoster keratoconjunctivitis
- 053.22 Herpes zoster iridocyclitis

CLINICAL PEARLS

- HSV and VZV can lead to a wide array of ocular manifestations, ranging from self-limited disease to potentially vision-threatening disease and complications.
- A slit-lamp exam with fluorescein stain should be performed on all patients with possible HSV keratitis or HZO.
- Topical antiviral treatment is appropriate for HSV but systemic PO antiviral treatment is necessary for HZO.
- An ophthalmologist should be consulted before prescribing topical steroids.
- Hutchinson sign (vesicular lesion on nose from VZV) is a strong indicator of HZO.
- Zostavax is effective at preventing zoster and decreasing the duration of PHN.

HERPES SIMPLEX

Lara Stewart, DO, MPH

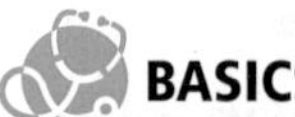

BASICS

DESCRIPTION

- Usually seen as an exanthem consisting of painful vesicles that occur often in clusters on skin, cornea, or mucous membranes
- Local skin lesions primarily located in oral and genital regions:
  - Herpes simplex virus (HSV)-1 associated with blisters on lips, in mouth, face, eyes
  - HSV-2 is primary source of genital herpes, although cross-reactivity is common with HSV-1 being a cause of genital sores as well due to oral–genital contact
- Viral disease with a wide range of sequelae. Complexity and variation of presentation dependent on if it is a disseminated infection, age and immune status of host, and whether the rash outbreak is primary or recurrence.
- Traditionally, HSV-1 is transmitted via infected saliva while HSV-2 is sexually transmitted.
- HSV can lead to meningitis/encephalitis and pneumonia among its systemic manifestations.
- Amount of viral shedding varies, but is greatest in the first/primary infection and lessens with subsequent infections.

EPIDEMIOLOGY

- Predominant age: Affects all ages; however, most HSV-1 is acquired in childhood, and most HSV-2 is acquired in young-middle adulthood
- Predominant sex: Male = Female

Incidence

- 29.2/100,000 office visits per year for herpes simplex-related codes
- HSV is never eliminated from the body, but stays dormant and can reactivate, causing symptoms.

Prevalence

- Widespread; 0.65–25% of adults may be excreting herpes simplex virus type 1 or 2 (HSV-1, HSV-2) at any given time, many of whom are unaware of this infection status.
- Prevalence of antibodies to HSV-1 is 90% by adulthood in the general population, and 30% of adults have antibodies to HSV-2.

RISK FACTORS

- Immunocompromised host, both acutely and chronic:
  - During presence of other illness or stress
  - Chemotherapy, malignancy/chronic disease states such as diabetes or AIDS, older age
- Atopic eczema, especially in children
- Prior HSV infection
- Sexual intercourse with infected person (condoms help minimize HSV transmission, but location of lesions outside condom-protected areas limit their effectiveness)
- Occupational exposure:
  - Dental professionals at higher risk for HSV-1 and resulting herpetic whitlow
- Neonatal herpes simplex: Primary perinatal infection is life threatening and usually acquired by vaginal birth via infected mother; fetal risk and neonatal risk are greater in mothers with primary genital herpes infection because shedding is more prolonged and the inoculum is greater; incubation from 5–7 days usually (rarely 4 weeks); cutaneous, mucous membrane, or ocular signs in only 70%

GENERAL PREVENTION

- Those with active disease should avoid direct contact with immunocompromised people, the elderly, and newborns.
- Wash hands often. Wash all linens with hot water immediately after lesions resolve.
- Kissing, sharing beverages from the same container, sharing food utensils or toothbrushes can transmit HSV
- Genital herpes: Avoid sexual contact while disease is active (recognizing herpes simplex is transmitted even when disease appears to be inactive), discuss condom benefits and limits, and reinforce benefits of mutually monogamous sexual relations.

ETIOLOGY

HSV, a DNA virus of 2 major types: HSV-1 and HSV-2. Most often, HSV-1 is associated with oral lesions, and HSV-2 with genital lesions, but reverse also occurs.

COMMONLY ASSOCIATED CONDITIONS

- Erythema multiforme: 50% of associated cases are caused by HSV I or II.
- All severe, unusual locations or treatment-resistant HSV cases should be screened for HIV.

DIAGNOSIS

HISTORY

- Most patients admit no known exposure to herpes, as transmission is often distant in time or via asymptomatic contacts.
- Report of a prodrome of fatigue, low-grade fever, itching, tingling, or hot skin area for a few days immediately prior to the rash outbreak
- In herpes labialis: Precipitating events may be sunlight, fever, trauma, menses, stress; prodrome of pain, burning, itching may last 6–48 hours before vesicles appear

PHYSICAL EXAM

- Vesicles: Usually cluster and open as painful ulcerated lesions, often with erythematous base
- Primary genital herpes: See "Herpes, Genital"
- Primary herpetic gingivostomatitis and pharyngitis: Usually in early childhood; incubation from 2–12 days, followed by fever, sore throat, pharyngeal edema, and erythema:
  - Small vesicles develop on pharyngeal and oral mucosa, rapidly ulcerate, and increase in number to involve soft palate, buccal mucosa, tongue, floor of mouth, and often lips and cheeks; tender gums may bleed; cervical adenopathy; fever, general toxicity, poor oral intake, and drooling contribute to dehydration; autoinoculation of other sites may occur; resolves in 10–14 days.
- Primary herpes keratoconjunctivitis: Unilateral conjunctivitis with regional adenopathy, as blepharitis with vesicles on lid margin, as keratitis with dendritic lesions, or with punctate opacities; lasts 2–3 weeks; systemic involvement prolongs process
- Eczema herpeticum: Diffuse poxlike eruption complicating atopic dermatitis; sudden appearance of lesions in typical atopic areas (upper trunk, neck, head); high fever, local edema, adenopathy
- Herpetic whitlow: Localized primary infection on a finger with intense itching and pain, followed by vesicles that may coalesce with swelling and erythema, and may mimic pyogenic paronychia; neuralgia and axillary adenopathy sometime occur; heals over 2–3 weeks without incision
- Congenital infection via prenatal transplacental virus transfer may present with jaundice, hepatosplenomegaly, disseminated intravascular coagulation (DIC), encephalitis, seizures, temperature instability, chorioretinitis, and/or conjunctivitis with or without skin vesicles
- Recurrent diseases from endogenous reactivation include:
  - Herpes labialis: Recurrent lesions on lips with HSV-1; usually <1 recurrence per 6 months, but 5–25% may have >1 attack per month; vesicles often at vermilion border, then ulcerate and crust within 48 hours; heals within 8–10 days generally; may have local adenopathy
  - Ocular herpes: May recur as keratitis, blepharitis, or keratoconjunctivitis; patients may have dendritic ulcers, decreased corneal sensation, less visual acuity; uveitis may cause permanent visual loss

DIAGNOSTIC TESTS & INTERPRETATION

Screen for other sexually transmitted infections (STIs) in patients with primary genital herpes. Viral: HIV, hepatitis B and C, human papillomavirus (HPV) have crossover; and bacterial: Gonorrhea, chlamydia should be screened for in new primary genital outbreaks.

Lab

- Tzanck smear shows multinucleated giant cells with 12–15 nuclei, often with eosinophilic intranuclear inclusions (scrape material from lesion onto slide, fix with ethanol or methanol, stain with Giemsa or Wright preparation); varicella (herpes zoster) has identical findings.
- HSV culture: On viral-specific media, swab and sample may need to be refrigerated; can take up to 6 days to be positive. Highly specific; hence, reliable if positive , but has 20% false-negative rate
- New type-specific Western blot blood-based antibody tests can reliably distinguish between HSV-1 and HSV-2 (now the gold standard). May take month or more for IgG to become positive, so better for subacute/recurrences.

Diagnostic Procedures/Surgery

Occasionally a biopsy is needed.

Pathological Findings

- See Tzanck prep above.
- Intraepithelial edema (ballooning degeneration) and intracellular edema
- A brain biopsy (in encephalitis) has hemorrhagic necrosis of gray and white matter with acute and chronic inflammation, thrombosis, and fibrinoid necrosis of parenchymal vessels, and intranuclear inclusions in astrocytes, oligodendroglia, and neurons.

DIFFERENTIAL DIAGNOSIS

- Impetigo: Straw-colored vesicles that crust
- Aphthous stomatitis: Grayish, shallow erosions with ring of hyperemia, usually only anterior in mouth and lips
- Herpes zoster: Unilateral dermatome distribution
- Syphilitic chancre: Usually painless ulcer
- Folliculitis: Herpes may mimic "shave bumps" in the genital area.

- Herpangina: Vesicles predominate on anterior tonsillar pillars, soft palate, uvula, and oropharynx but not more anteriorly on lips or gums (usually caused by group A coxsackievirus)
- Stevens-Johnson syndrome

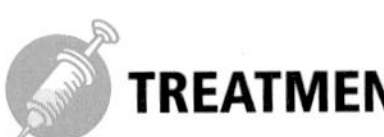

TREATMENT

MEDICATION

First Line

- In all cases, regardless of choice of agent, treatment should begin as early as possible, preferably in the prodromal phase even before lesions develop.
- Acyclovir (generic):
  - Mucocutaneous (or genital) HSV:
    - Primary/First infection: 400 mg t.i.d. × 7–10 days
    - If severe, start with IV q8h dosing for first few days, then complete 10-day course with oral route
    - Recurrence: 400 mg PO t.i.d. × 5 days or 800 mg b.i.d. × 5 days or 800 mg t.i.d. × 2 days
    - Suppression: 400 mg b.i.d. daily
  - Keratitis HSV: 400 mg PO 5 × per day; however, topical treatment is preferred first line
  - Pediatric dosing: Neonatal herpes simplex or encephalitis: 60 mg/kg/d IV divided q8h × 21 days:
    - Older (>3 months of age) immunocompetent is weight-based dosing (15 mg/kg/d divided q8h for 5–7 days)
  - Safe in pregnancy and lactation
- Penciclovir (Denavir): 10 mg/g cream. Apply to oral lesions q2h × 4 days
- Valacyclovir (Valtrex) (1):
- Primary genital herpes: 1 g PO b.i.d. for 7–10 days. Recurrent genital herpes: 500 mg PO b.i.d. for 3 days; suppression: 500–1,000 mg PO daily (depending on frequency of outbreaks). Labialis HSV (cold sores/oral lesions): 2,000 mg PO q12h × 1 day:
  - 500-mg daily dose if suppression is needed/desired
- Precautions:
  - Renal dosing required in all oral antivirals
  - Significant possible interactions: Probenecid with IV acyclovir and possibly probenecid with valacyclovir may reduce renal clearance and elevate antiviral drug levels.

Second Line

- Foscarnet:
  - Drug of choice for acyclovir resistance in immunocompromised persons with systemic HSV
  - 40 mg/kg IV q8h (assume valacyclovir and famciclovir resistance also if acyclovir resistance occurs)
- Other topicals:
  - Ophthalmic preparations for herpes keratoconjunctivitis; acyclovir, vidarabine (Vira-A), idoxuridine
  - Topical acyclovir and penciclovir improve healing times for recurrent herpes labialis by ~10% (2)[A].
  - Topical analgesics: Lidocaine 2% or 5% helps reduce the pain sequelae associated with vulvar and penile herpes outbreaks.
- Over-the-counter topical antivirals: Abreva

ADDITIONAL TREATMENT

General Measures

- Intermittent, cool, moist dressings with Domeboro or Burrow solution
- Painful urination and inability to void due to painful genital lesions is helped by pouring a cup of warm water over genitals while urinating or by sitting in a warm bath while urinating (Sitz baths)
- Children with gingivostomatitis who resist oral intake due to pain, or extensive skin disease (eczema herpeticum), may require IV hydration and volume replacement.

Issues for Referral

Recurrent cases of herpes keratoconjunctivitis should be referred to an ophthalmologist.

IN-PATIENT CONSIDERATIONS

Initial Stabilization

- Pregnancy considerations:
  - Caesarean section and/or acyclovir indicated if any active genital lesions (or prodrome) present the time of delivery; and should be considered if primary genital herpes occurred within the 4 weeks prior (3)[C]
  - Daily oral antivirals from 36 weeks onward in women with history of recurrent genital herpes to prevent outbreak near to/at time of delivery
  - Avoid fetal scalp electrodes if mother has history of genital HSV.
  - Risk of viral shedding at delivery from asymptomatic recurrent genital HSV is low (~1.6%); not predicted by monitoring cultures
- Pediatric considerations:
  - Neonates with likely exposure (high index of suspicion) to HSV at birth or with signs of infection should have culture of all bodily fluid sources and immediate treatment with IV acyclovir.

ONGOING CARE

FOLLOW-UP RECOMMENDATIONS

- For most typical cases, follow-up is not necessary. Lesions and symptoms resolve rapidly within 10 days. Extensive or primary cases should be rechecked in 1 week; monitor for secondary bacterial infections.
- Consider long-term suppression treatment.

DIET

If oral lesions present, avoid salty, acidic, or sharp foods (e.g., chips and orange juice)

PATIENT EDUCATION

- Explain the natural history of this viral illness, that timing of exposure is difficult to determine and that the virus will be in their system forever. Try to minimize the psychological impact of this diagnosis (reduce any stigma).
- Hygiene techniques to avoid self-spreading to other body areas (autoinoculation) or exposing others. Frequent hand washing; avoid scratching; and cover any active, wet lesions.

PROGNOSIS

- The usual course of the primary disease is 5 days to 2 weeks.
- Antiviral treatment can limit the length of disease state, reduce complicating sequelae, and nearly eliminate recurrences (if used daily).
- Viral shedding in recurrence is briefer than with the primary disease, and frequency of recurrence is extremely variable, dependent on individual patient factors.
- Newborns or immunocompromised individuals are at risk for major morbidity or mortality.
- HSV is never eliminated from the body but stays dormant and can reactivate, causing symptoms.

COMPLICATIONS

- Herpes encephalitis: A brain biopsy may be needed for diagnosis.
- Herpes pneumonia

REFERENCES

1. Cernik C, Gallina K, Brodell RT, et al. The treatment of herpes simplex infections: An evidence-based review. *Arch Intern Med*. 2008;168:1137–44.
2. Harmenberg J, Oberg B, Spruance S, et al. Prevention of ulcerative lesions by episodic treatment of recurrent herpes labialis: A literature review. *Acta Derm Venereol*. 2010;90:122–30.
3. Beauman JG. Genital herpes: A review. *Am Fam Physician*. 2005;72:1527–34,1541–42.

ADDITIONAL READING

- Chayavichitsilp P, Buckwalter JV, Krakowski AC, et al. Herpes simplex. *Pediatr Rev*. 2009;30(4): 119–29.
- Hollier LM, Straub H. Genital herpes. *Clin Evid (Online)*. 2011.
- Wilhelmus KR. Antiviral treatment and other therapeutic interventions for herpes simplex virus epithelial keratitis. *Cochrane Database Syst Rev*. 2010;(12):CD002898.

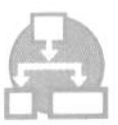

See Also (Topic, Algorithm, Electronic Media Element)

- Herpes, Genital
- Algorithm: Genital Ulcers

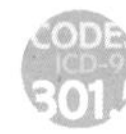

CODES

ICD9

- 054.3 Herpetic meningoencephalitis
- 054.6 Herpetic whitlow
- 054.9 Herpes simplex without mention of complication

CLINICAL PEARLS

- 25–30% of the US population has genital herpes, and more than 80% of the US population is seropositive for herpesvirus exposure/antibody evidence of infection.
- Most individuals are unaware that they have been infected and pass on the virus during asymptomatic periods.
- Chronic suppression for those with frequent recurrences is effective at preventing transmission and decrease outbreak frequency; recurrences naturally become less frequent over time, however.

HERPES ZOSTER

Robert J. Hyde, MD

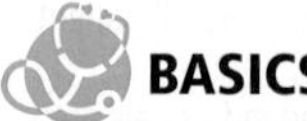

BASICS

DESCRIPTION

- Usually presents as a painful unilateral vesicular eruption within a dermatome
- Results from reactivation of varicella-zoster virus (human herpesvirus type 3)
- Postherpetic neuralgia (PHN) is usually defined as pain persisting at least 1 month after rash has healed. Because of variable definitions of PHN used in research, the term *zoster-associated pain* may be more clinically useful.
- System(s) affected: Nervous; Integumentary; Exocrine
- Synonym(s): Shingles

EPIDEMIOLOGY

Predominant sex: Male = Female

Incidence

- Incidence is increasing as population ages.
- Incidence increases with age: 2/3 of cases occur in adults ≥50 years old.
- Herpes zoster: 3.6 per 1,000 person-years (1).
- PHN: 18% in adult patients with herpes zoster; 33% ≥79 years old.

Prevalence

Nearly 1 million new herpes zoster cases yearly

Pregnancy Considerations

May occur during pregnancy.

Geriatric Considerations

- Increased incidence of zoster outbreaks
- Increased incidence of PHN

Pediatric Considerations

- Occurs less frequently in children.
- Has been reported in newborns primarily infected in utero.

RISK FACTORS

- The vast majority of persons affected have no underlying illness.
- Increasing age
- Reduced immunity associated with some malignancies (e.g., lymphoma)
- Treatment of malignancy (chemotherapy or radiotherapy)
- HIV infection
- Use of immunosuppressant drugs after organ transplant surgery or for disease management
- Spinal surgery

GENERAL PREVENTION

- Herpes zoster vaccination was licensed by the US FDA on May 25, 2006. Zostavax is available and ACIP recommended for patients ≥60 years of age (and in 2011, FDA approved for patients >50) (2):
  - Vaccine is proven to reduce cases of zoster, but no evidence yet to show decreased incidence of PHN beyond the direct effect of fewer cases of zoster (3).
- Zoster patients may transmit virus-causing varicella (chickenpox) to susceptible persons.

ETIOLOGY

Reactivation of varicella zoster virus (human herpesvirus type 3) from dorsal root or cranial nerve ganglia

COMMONLY ASSOCIATED CONDITIONS

Immunocompromised individuals, including HIV infection, posttransplantation, immunosuppressive drugs, and malignancy

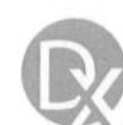

DIAGNOSIS

HISTORY

- Prodromal phase (sensations over involved dermatome prior to rash):
  - Tingling
  - Itching
  - Boring or knifelike pain
- Acute phase:
  - Constitutional symptoms variable (e.g., fatigue, malaise, headache, low-grade fever)
  - Dermatomal rash

PHYSICAL EXAM

- Acute phase:
  - Weakness (1% may have weakness in distribution of rash)
  - Initially erythematous and maculopapular; evolves rapidly to grouped vesicles
  - Vesicles become pustular and/or hemorrhagic in 3–4 days.
  - Resolution of rash, with crusts separating by 14–21 days
- Possible sine herpete (zoster without rash) and other chronic disorders associated with varicella-zoster virus without the typical rash
- Chronic phase:
  - PHN (15% overall; increases with age)
  - A small percentage (1–5%) may affect the motor nerves, causing weakness (called *zoster motorius*), facial nerve (e.g., Ramsay Hunt syndrome), spinal motor radiculopathies

DIAGNOSTIC TESTS & INTERPRETATION

Lab

- Rarely necessary because clinical appearance is usually sufficiently distinctive
- Viral culture
- Tzanck smear (does not distinguish from herpes simplex, and false-negative results occur)
- Polymerase chain reaction analysis
- Immunofluorescent antigen staining
- Varicella-zoster-specific IgM

Pathological Findings

- Multinucleated giant cells with intralesional inclusion
- Lymphatic infiltration of sensory ganglia with focal hemorrhage and nerve cell destruction

DIFFERENTIAL DIAGNOSIS

- Rash:
  - Herpes simplex virus
  - Coxsackievirus
  - Contact dermatitis
  - Superficial pyoderma
- Pain:
  - Cholecystitis
  - Appendicitis
  - Nephrolithiasis
  - Pleuritis
  - Myocardial infarction
  - Diabetic neuropathy

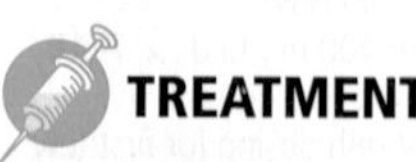

TREATMENT

MEDICATION

First Line

- Acute treatment:
  - Antiviral agents initiated within 72 hours of rash may relieve symptoms, speed resolution of rash, and prevent and/or ameliorate PHN (4)[A].
  - Valacyclovir: 1,000 mg t.i.d. × 7 days
  - Famciclovir: 500 mg t.i.d. × 7 days
  - Acyclovir: 800 mg q4h (5 doses daily) × 7 days
- Analgesics (acetaminophen, NSAIDs, opioids)
- Corticosteroids given acutely during zoster infection are ineffective in preventing PHN (5).
- Treatment of complications:
  - Secondary bacterial skin infections: Silver sulfadiazine topically and/or systemic antibiotics
- PHN and zoster-associated pain (4):
  - Tricyclic antidepressants (TCAs; amitriptyline 25 mg at bedtime and other low-dose TCAs) relieve pain acutely and may reduce pain duration.
  - Lidocaine patch 5% (Lidoderm) applied after skin rash closure over painful areas (limit 3 patches simultaneously or trim a single patch) for up to 12 hours has been reported to be effective in 1 limited trial.
  - Gabapentin: 100–600 mg t.i.d. for pain and other quality-of-life indicators; limited by adverse effects
  - Opioids, capsaicin cream, and other analgesics may be useful adjuncts.
  - Pregabalin: 50–100 mg t.i.d. reduces pain, but usefulness is limited by side effects.
- Prevention of PHN and zoster-associated pain: No treatment has been shown to prevent PHN completely, but treatment may shorten duration and/or reduce severity of symptoms (6):
  - Antiviral therapy with valacyclovir, famciclovir, or acyclovir given during acute skin eruption may be effective in limiting the duration of pain.
  - Low-dose amitriptyline in the same dosage as for treatment of PHN but started within 72 hours of rash onset and continued for 90 days may reduce PHN incidence or duration.
  - There is insufficient evidence that corticosteroids reduce incidence, severity, or duration of PHN (7).

- Contraindications: Refer to the manufacturer's profile of each drug.
- Precautions:
  - Assess renal function prior to using valacyclovir, famciclovir, or acyclovir.
  - Valacyclovir, famciclovir, and acyclovir are pregnancy category B.
  - Refer to the manufacturer's profile of each drug.
- Significant possible interactions: Refer to the manufacturer's profile of each drug.

Second Line

Numerous therapies have been advocated, but good supporting evidence is lacking.

ADDITIONAL TREATMENT

General Measures

- Treatment should be directed to control acute symptoms and prevent complications.
- Antiviral therapy decreases viral replication, lessens nerve damage and inflammation, and reduces the severity and duration of long-term pain syndromes (4)[A].
- Prompt analgesic control of pain may shorten the duration of zoster-associated pain.
- Lotions such as calamine and colloidal oatmeal may reduce itching and burning sensation.

IN-PATIENT CONSIDERATIONS

Initial Stabilization

Outpatient treatment, unless disseminated or occurring as complication of serious underlying disease requiring hospitalization

ONGOING CARE

FOLLOW-UP RECOMMENDATIONS

No restrictions

Patient Monitoring

Depends on symptoms

DIET

No special diet

PATIENT EDUCATION

- Inform patient that the duration of rash is 2–3 weeks.
- Encourage good hygiene and proper skin care.
- Warn of potential for dissemination (dissemination must be suspected with constitutional illness signs and/or spreading rash).
- Warn of potential PHN.
- Warn of potential risk of transmitting illness (chickenpox) to susceptible persons.

PROGNOSIS

- Immunocompetent individuals should experience spontaneous and complete recovery within a few weeks.
- Resolution of acute rash within 14–21 days
- PHN may occur in patients age ≥50 years despite treatment with antiviral medications.

COMPLICATIONS

- PHN
- Ophthalmic herpes zoster: 10–20%
- Superinfection of skin lesions:
  - Meningoencephalitis
  - Cutaneous dissemination
  - Hepatitis
  - Pneumonitis
  - Myelitis
  - Cranial and peripheral nerve palsies
  - Acute retinal necrosis

REFERENCES

1. Yawn BP, Saddier P, Wollan PC, et al. A Population-based study of the incidence and complication rates of herpes zoster before zoster vaccine introduction. *Mayo Clin Proc.* 2007;82(11): 1341–9.
2. FDA. Zostavax. www.fda.gov/biologics bloodvaccines/vaccines/approvedproducts/ ucm136941.htm Accessed 10/9/2011.
3. Chen N, Li Q, Zhang Y, et al. Vaccination for preventing postherpetic neuralgia. *Cochrane Database Syst Rev.* 2011;(3):CD007795.
4. Mounsey AL, Matthew LG, Slawson DC. Herpes zoster and postherpetic neuralgia: Prevention and management. *Am Fam Physician.* 2005;72: 1075–80.
5. Chen N, Yang M, He L, et al. Corticosteroids for preventing postherpetic neuralgia. *Cochrane Database Syst Rev.* 2010;(12):CD005582.
6. Weinberg JM, Vafaie J, Scheinfeld NS. Skin infections in the elderly. *Dermatol Clin.* 2004;22: 51–61.
7. Gnann JW, Whitley RJ. Clinical practice. Herpes zoster. *N Engl J Med.* 2002;347:340–6.

ADDITIONAL READING

- Harpaz R, Ortega-Sanchez IR, Seward JF, et al. Prevention of herpes zoster: Recommendations of the Advisory Committee on Immunization Practices (ACIP). *MMWR Recomm Rep.* 2008;57:1–30.
- Li Q, Chen N, Yang J, et al. Antiviral treatment for preventing postherpetic neuralgia. *Cochrane Database Syst Rev.* 2009;CD006866.
- Sampathkumar P, Drage LA, Martin DP. Herpes zoster (shingles) and postherpetic neuralgia. *Mayo Clin Proc.* 2009;84:274–80.

See Also (Topic, Algorithm, Electronic Media Element)

- Bell Palsy; Chickenpox (Varicella Zoster); Herpes Eye Infections; Herpes Simplex
- Algorithm: Genital Ulcers

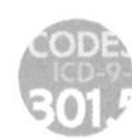

CODES

ICD9

- 053.9 Herpes zoster without mention of complication
- 053.19 Herpes zoster with other nervous system complications

CLINICAL PEARLS

- In herpes zoster ophthalmicus, Hutchinson sign is a vesicular rash at the nasal tip, indicating involvement of the external branch of cranial nerve V; associated with increased incidence of ocular zoster.
- Patients should be referred to an ophthalmologist for Hutchinson sign in the early phase of ophthalmic zoster or if they have visual complaints or an unexplained red eye (6).
- All patients should begin a course of antiviral therapy regardless of age. To be effective, therapy should be started within 72 hours of the onset of rash. After 72 hours, antiviral therapy is recommended for any immunocompromised patient who still has vesicles. However, no data examine the effect of antiviral medication after 72 hours.

HERPES, GENITAL

Terri Warren, MEd, BSN, MSN
Jill A. Grimes, MD

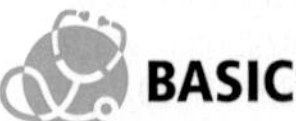

BASICS

DESCRIPTION

- Herpes simplex virus infection involving the genitals (anywhere within the waist to midthigh; innervation of the sacral ganglia)
- Primary, nonprimary first episode or recurrent
- Synonym(s): Herpes genitalis

EPIDEMIOLOGY

- Predominant age: 15–65 years, with increasing prevalence as ages increases (cumulative cases, no cure)
- Overall prevalence of HSV2 in the US: 16% of the population >14 and <50 years old
- Overall prevalence of HSV1 in the US: 57% of the population >14 and <50 years old
- Predominant sex: Female > Male; women are almost twice as likely as men to be infected due to receptive position with intercourse.
- African American 3× > Caucasian. ~50% of African Americans between the ages of 14 and 49 are infected with HSV2.

Incidence

300,000–1,500,000 cases. This makes genital herpes the third most incident STI in the US in 2011.

Prevalence

ALERT

45–50 million. HSV2 is the most prevalent STI in the US in 2011; *this number does not take into account cases of genital herpes that are caused by HSV1.*

RISK FACTORS

- Primary infection with HSV2:
  - Increasing age, lower socioeconomic status, black race, number of lifetime partners, and history of sexually transmitted diseases (STDs)
- Transmission of HSV2:
  - Incubation period: 1–10 days (mean, 5.8 days). *Most new cases are without symptoms.*
  - Annual risk: susceptible female acquiring disease from an infected male partner, ~10–30%; for susceptible male from infected female, ~5%. These risks include no condom use, no daily antiviral therapy, and sex with recognized symptoms.
  - Those with prior HSV1 infection are those least likely to display symptoms of HSV2 when it is acquired.
  - >70% new cases result from transmission during asymptomatic (clinically unrecognized) shedding.
  - Risk of HSV2 asymptomatic shedding: 13% of days; highest within 6 months of new infection (42% of days)
  - Daily antiviral therapy (e.g., valacyclovir 500 mg) reduces viral shedding and reduces transmission of HSV2 by 48%. Transmission studies have not been done on the other antiviral medicines (acyclovir and famciclovir) but they likely have similar results.
- Genital Transmission of HSV1:
  - Mostly due to receiving oral sex from someone who has oral HSV1 infection.
  - Can happen in the presence or absence of an active cold sore. Asymptomatic shedding occurs both orally and genitally.
  - Distinguishing between canker sores and cold sores is important when speaking with patients: Canker sores are *not* caused by herpes virus.
  - Daily antiviral therapy is also effective against HSV1 shedding, though very slightly less so than for HSV2.
- Recurrence triggers for genital herpes are unknown. Ultraviolet light is known trigger for oral herpes.

Pediatric Considerations

Neonatal infection occurs in 20–50/100,000 live births. 80% of infections result from asymptomatic maternal viral shedding.

GENERAL PREVENTION

- Oral, vaginal, and anal sexual abstinence is only option to provide complete protection.
- Condoms reduce transmission by about 30%.
- Reducing the frequency and number of partner changes likely reduces the risk of infection.
- Pregnant women who test antibody negative for HSV1 and HSV2 should avoid unprotected intercourse and receptive oral sex in late pregnancy.
- Screening with type-specific antibody in the general population and in pregnancy are not recommended by the USPSTF, though experts disagree about pregnancy:
  - Consider screening in asymptomatic patients with HIV infection and suppressive Rx if positive
  - Strongly consider HSV antibody testing as part of STD screening panel *or be certain patients know it is not included if it is not.*
  - Offer screening to discordant couples (one partner with known HSV, the other without)
  - Use antibody testing for patients whose genital symptoms cannot be definitely diagnosed as some other problem.
- Avoid sex if lesions or prodromal symptoms are present. Transmission is possible even when there are no symptoms present.
- Infants with possible HSV infection should be isolated in the nursery; maternal separation is not necessary; breast-feeding is allowed.

PATHOPHYSIOLOGY

HSV: A double-stranded DNA, *Alphaherpesvirinae* virus subfamily

ETIOLOGY

- HSV1: 10–50% (increasing incidence); now greater than HSV2 in some clinical settings. *~75% of new genital HSV among college students is HSV1.*
- HSV2: 60–90%; accounts for the significant majority of recurrent disease.

COMMONLY ASSOCIATED CONDITIONS

All STIs: Herpes labialis, syphilis, gonorrhea, nongonococcal urethritis/cervicitis, genital warts, HIV, and trichomonas

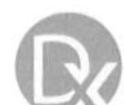

DIAGNOSIS

HISTORY

- 80% of patients with HSV2 are asymptomatic or do not recognize clinical manifestations of disease (1).
- Common presentations: Genital itching, pain, dysuria or visible blisters or sores; local symptoms can last 3–21 days.
- Constitutional symptoms are possible, mostly with first infection: Headache, photophobia, malaise, myalgia, fever

PHYSICAL EXAM

- Impossible to differentiate among primary, first-episode nonprimary, and recurrent disease on basis of symptoms and clinical findings
- Genital irritation, localized erythema, vulvar, penile, anal, perineal ulcers, sores, fissures, cracks, watery discharge from vagina or urethra, or pyuria without frequency and urgency:
  - Female: Pelvic examination of internal reproductive organs: External genitalia, vagina, cervix
  - Male: Penis and scrotum
  - Male and female: Rectum, thighs, buttocks, pubic hair area, mouth, inguinal lymph nodes
- Adenopathy, sacral paresthesias resulting in inability to urinate or defecate

Pediatric Considerations

Genital lesions in children suggest sexual abuse.

DIAGNOSTIC TESTS & INTERPRETATION

Lab

- Viral detection from lesion:
  - Swab lesions; PCR (2–3 × more sensitive than culture) preferred. Viral culture. Both should always include request for typing of virus.
  - Use Dacron or polyester-tipped swabs with plastic shafts, not cotton tips or wood shafts; both inhibit viral growth and/or replication.
- Type-specific serologic assays (TSST):
  - Western blot (gold standard), and type specific IgG antibody (glycoprotein G) ELISA to discriminate between HSV1 and HSV2
    - Seroconversion occurs 10 days to 4 months after infection. Use of daily herpes medicine may delay seroconversion. *Antibody testing is not necessary if a positive typed swab test has been obtained.*
    - Type specific antibody tests have a 4–6% false-positive rate. Anyone with a value of 1.1–3.5 on the type specific IgG HSV2 antibody test needs confirmation with another test, preferably herpes Western blot. If a low positive has been obtained early after possible infection, it is also acceptable to redo the ELISA when 3–4 months have passed in lieu of ordering a Western blot.
    - IgM antibody testing is never appropriate: Cannot distinguish with accuracy new from old infection, is often present with recurrent disease, and has many false positives.
- Commercially available ELISA tests include HerpesSelect-1 and 2 (ELISA), HerpesSelect 1/2 (immunoblot), Captia, and Biokit HSV-2 and SureVue HSV-2 (fingerstick, point-of-care) and herpes Western blot. Western blot is done only at the University of Washington in the US, but can be ordered through Quest Labs (test code 34534). A test kit can also be ordered directly from the University of Washington and sent to the health care provider for collection and return to the lab.

Pathological Findings

Histopathology–cytopathy is not a recommend method for diagnosing herpes because it cannot be typed and may be confused with other viruses in the herpes family.

DIFFERENTIAL DIAGNOSIS

- Primary syphilis
- Chancroid

- Lymphogranuloma venereum
- Herpes zoster
- Trauma
- Inflammatory bowel disease
- Behçet syndrome
- Stevens-Johnson syndrome
- Ulcerative balanitis
- Granuloma inguinale
- Neoplasia

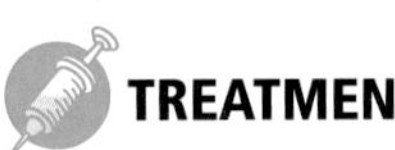

TREATMENT

MEDICATION

Antiviral medications should be started at the first sign or symptom of disease, preferably within 48 hours. People who are treating outbreaks episodically should have their prescription refill at home and be ready to take at the first sign of an outbreak.

First Line

- Acyclovir (Zovirax) (2)[A]:
  - First infection: 400 mg PO t.i.d. for 7–10 days or 200 mg PO 5 × a day for 7–10 days, longer if needed for incomplete healing.
  - Episodic therapy: 400 mg t.i.d. for 5 days or 800 mg b.i.d. for 5 days or 800 mg t.i.d. for 2 days. Shorter course, better compliance.
  - Daily suppression: 400 mg PO b.i.d.
  - Severe local or disseminated disease: 5–10 mg/kg IV q8h for 5–7 days
  - HIV infection: 400 mg PO 3–5 × a day until clinical resolution is attained
  - Precautions:
    - Pregnancy: Not approved by FDA for routine use (Category B). Studies have demonstrated safety of use.
    - Drug is excreted in breast milk
    - Modify dose in patients with renal insufficiency or who are taking nephrotoxic medicines.
    - Nephropathy and neuropathy are possible with high doses given IV
    - Rate of resistance in immunocompetent populations: 0.3%
- Valacyclovir (Valtrex) (2)[A], Pregnancy Category B, Pro-drug of acyclovir with better bioavailability, thus less frequent dosing possible:
  - First infection: 1 g PO b.i.d. for 7–10 days
  - Episodic therapy: 500 mg PO b.i.d. for 3–5 days or 1 g PO daily for 5 days
  - Daily suppression: 500 mg PO daily or 1,000 mg/d. If breaking through, attempt 500 mg b.i.d.
- Famciclovir (Famvir) (2)[A], Pregnancy Category B:
  - First infection: 250 mg PO t.i.d. for 7–10 days
  - Episodic therapy: 125 mg PO b.i.d. for 5 days or 1 g PO b.i.d. × 1 day
  - Daily suppression: 250 mg PO b.i.d.

Pregnancy Considerations

ACOG Clinical Management Guidelines (3,4)[A]:

- Primary HSV during pregnancy or lesions near/at term: Consider antiviral therapy (reduces duration/severity and viral shedding)
- Women with a history of genital herpes at or beyond 36 weeks should be offered suppression; may reduce C-section rate by 70%, clinical HSV, and HSV shedding; continue through delivery; acyclovir 400 mg t.i.d. or valacyclovir 500 mg b.i.d.

Second Line

- Foscarnet: 40 mg/kg IV q8h in severe disease with proven or suspected acyclovir-resistant strains
- Vidarabine: 10 mg/kg/d infused over 10 hours; benefits HIV patients with HSV1 infection failing acyclovir and foscarnet therapy
- Cidofovir (Vistide) topical: 0.1–0.3% gel for 5 days for progressive/resistant lesions
- Trifluridine (Viroptic) ophthalmic solution for mucocutaneous lesions resistant to acyclovir

Pediatric Considerations

- High-risk infant: Acyclovir, 30 mg/kg/d IV q9h for 10–14 days
- Low-risk infant, asymptomatic: Culture eyes, nose, and mouth at 24–36 hours and observe.

ADDITIONAL TREATMENT

General Measures

- Cool compresses of aluminum acetate (Burow solution) 4–6 times a day
- Ice packs to perineum, sitz baths, spray-on topical anesthetic
- Analgesics, NSAIDs

COMPLEMENTARY AND ALTERNATIVE MEDICINE

L-lysine is popular for those seeking a complementary alternative, but it has not been shown to be statistically beneficial in reducing outbreak duration or frequency.

ONGOING CARE

FOLLOW-UP RECOMMENDATIONS

- Avoid intercourse when symptomatic lesions are present.
- Make sex partners aware of herpes status prior to sexual activity.
- Use daily suppression therapy to reduce the risk of transmission by almost half.
- Have potential or current partners antibody tested prior to sexual activity; they may be infected and not know it.
- Concordant couples (i.e., both have the same type of herpes (HSV1 or HSV2) may have sex without worry about transmission or triggering outbreaks.

Patient Monitoring

- Latent infection: Check pregnant women at prenatal visits and onset of labor for presence of lesions. If yes, C-section recommended.
- Test for all other STDs in the setting of initial HSV infection.

DIET

No known benefits for any diet change, despite media-popular recommendations about increased intake of lysine and arginine avoidance.

PATIENT EDUCATION

- Herpes Resource Center: www.ashastd.org/herpes/herpes_overview.cfm.
- Warren T. *The Good News About the Bad News: Herpes: Everything you need to know*. Oakland, CA: New Harbinger Publications; 2009.

PROGNOSIS

- Resolution of signs/symptoms: 3–21 days.
- Latent infection: Recurrences in 80% of patients within 1 year of initial HSV2 infection; immunocompetent average 3–4 a year for genital HSV2; 1 a year for genital HSV1, 80% of people with HSV1 infection who do not experience a recurrence in the first year likely never will.
- HSV infection in immunocompromised (AIDS) patients: More severe, longer duration, more difficult to treat
- Treatment with antiviral agents does not eliminate virus from the body but significantly reduces transmission, shedding, and outbreaks.

Pediatric Considerations

Neonatal infection survival rates: Localized, >95%; CNS, 85%; systemic, 30%

COMPLICATIONS

- Urinary and bowel: Temporary nonfunction
- Transient aseptic meningitis
- Potential transmission to neonate, particularly in mothers with new infection during the third trimester, prolonged rupture of membranes, scalp electrodes, prematurity, and cervical lesions
- Increased risk for HIV infection (2–3 times) than in someone who does not have HSV2.
- Lowered self-esteem, guilt, anger, depression, fear of rejection, fear of transmission to partner

REFERENCES

1. Gupta R, Warren T, Wald A, et al. Genital herpes. *Lancet*. 2007;370:2127–37.
2. CDC. 2010 STD treatment guidelines. Atlanta, GA: Author. www.cdc.gov/std/treatment/2010/.
3. Money D, Steben M, Society of Obstetricians and Gynaecologists of Canada, et al. SOGC clinical practice guidelines: Guidelines for the management of herpes simplex virus in pregnancy. Number 208, June 2008. *Int J Gynaecol Obstet*. 2009;104: 167–71.
4. Sheffield JS, Hollier LM, Hill JB, et al. Acyclovir prophylaxis to prevent herpes simplex virus recurrence at delivery: A systematic review. *Obstet Gynecol*. 2003;102:1396–403.

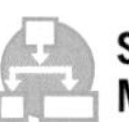

See Also (Topic, Algorithm, Electronic Media Element)

Algorithm: Genital Ulcers

CODES

ICD9

- 054.10 Genital herpes, unspecified
- 054.11 Herpetic vulvovaginitis
- 054.12 Herpetic ulceration of vulva

CLINICAL PEARLS

- Genital herpes infections are frequently contracted from oral sex.
- Condoms can decrease transmission by 30%.
- The majority of HSV genital infections are thought to be transmitted during asymptomatic shedding of the virus; make sure patients understand they are always potentially contagious, not just during outbreaks.

HERPETIC WHITLOW

Veena Kulchaiyawat, DO

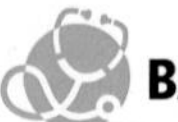

BASICS

DESCRIPTION

- Painful cutaneous viral infection of the finger(s), most commonly affecting the distal phalanx caused by direct inoculation by herpes simplex virus (HSV-1 or HSV-2)
- Highly contagious and easily spread via direct contact

EPIDEMIOLOGY

- Female-to-male ratio of 2.3:1 (1)
- Bimodal age distribution seen in children <10 years of age and adults 20–30 years of age (1,2)

Incidence

2.4 cases per 100,000 in 1 year (1)

RISK FACTORS

- Break in epidermis after minor trauma
- Direct contact between break in skin to secretions or lesions infected with herpes simplex virus:
  - Occupational risks that allow direct exposure of digits to oropharyngeal secretions (dentist, respiratory therapist, anesthesiologist, nurse, physician, or other health care personnel)
- Autoinoculation to self with existing herpes genitalis or gingivostomatitis:
  - Children with finger-sucking habits
  - Person with nail-biting habits

GENERAL PREVENTION

- Use universal fluid precautions (wash hands and wear protective gloves to prevent direct contact of digits to infected oropharyngeal or genital lesions).
- Avoid sharing toothbrush, washcloth, drinking glass, or utensils.
- Avoid wearing contact lenses to prevent transmission to the eyes.

PATHOPHYSIOLOGY

HSV enters epidermis through break in skin and infects the epithelial cells. Virus replication occurs and forms symptomatic vesicular lesions. Virus travels along the nerve root and remains dormant, but it can be reactivated to cause recurrent symptoms.

ETIOLOGY

- HSV-1 (oral mucosal membranes), most commonly in children
- HSV-1 or HSV-2 (genitalis), in adolescents and adults

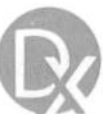

DIAGNOSIS

Diagnosis is based on the clinical history and physical exam (1,2,3,4,5)[C].

HISTORY

- Prodromal phase (3–7 days): Abrupt onset of digital pain described as burning, itching, and tingling after minor trauma to the digit
- Acute phase: 1 or more vesicle(s) will appear with surrounding erythema and swelling associated with severe constant throbbing pain of the digit(s).
- After acute phase has subsided (10–14 days), the pain will lessen and vesicles will dry and crust over or rupture, resulting in peeling of the skin with well-healed skin underneath.
- Systemic manifestations are not usually present, but occasionally can be associated with fever, malaise, chills, lymphadenopathy, or lymphangitis.
- Complete resolution within 18–28 days

PHYSICAL EXAM

There is a sequential pattern that is seen on physical exam:

- Erythema, edema, and vesicular lesions with clear fluid located at distal phalanx, most commonly occurring on the thumb or index finger
- Vesicles then coalesce to form honeycombed appearance.
- Satellite vesicular lesions may appear around the nail, and vesicular fluid may become more opaque or hemorrhagic in appearance.
- After vesicular spread has stopped, pain will improve and lesions will evolve, forming crusts and then peeling, which will subsequently leave well-healed epidermis.

DIAGNOSTIC TESTS & INTERPRETATION

History and physical will give you the diagnosis; however, further lab tests may be performed for confirmation if desired (2,3,4)[C].

Lab

- Viral culture from vesicular fluid can provide viral typing of HSV (1–4 days).
- Tzanck smear will reveal multinucleated giant cells on light microscopy:
  - Obtain scrapings from base of an unroofed vesicle or ulceration debrided of crust (avoid pulp space) and stain with Toluidine blue.
- Direct fluorescent or immunoperoxidase staining for HSV antigen from epithelial cells scraped from the vesicular base
- Blood serum HSV antibody titers:
  - Expect a rise in antibody titer from blood sampling at presentation and at 3 weeks.

Initial lab tests

None recommended unless confirmation is desired

Imaging

No imaging is indicated.

DIFFERENTIAL DIAGNOSIS

- Paronychia (vesicle with purulent fluid and positive Gram stain)
- Felon (abscess of distal pulp)
- Digital mucous cyst
- Drug eruption
- Blistering distal dactylitis

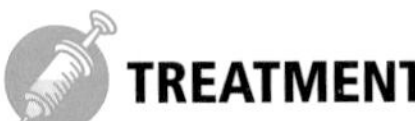

TREATMENT

Herpetic whitlow is a self-limited disease. Symptoms should improve after 10–14 days, and vesicular lesions should start to dry and crust over, resulting in well-healed skin, in 21–28 days (1,2,3)[C].

MEDICATION

Although there have been case reports of using topical, oral, and IV antivirals (acyclovir, famciclovir, valacyclovir) to help shorten the course of this condition and reduce viral shedding, further randomized controlled studies need to be performed to clearly define effective dosage and duration of antiviral medications (3)[C].

ADDITIONAL TREATMENT

General Measures

- Symptomatic treatment is the most important therapy (2,3,5)[C]:
  - Dry dressing to decrease possible viral spread
  - Analgesics, elevation, and immobilization to control pain
- Oral acyclovir may be considered to prevent recurrent symptoms; however, the dosage or duration of therapy has not been well studied with randomized controlled trials (2,3,6)[C].

SURGERY/OTHER PROCEDURES

- Consider decompression of the nail bed with partial removal of affected nail bed matrix to help relieve pain (5)[C].
- Simple perforation of nail over the involved matrix with segmental nail removal can also be performed to help improve discomfort (5)[C].

ALERT

Avoid incision and drainage of vesicular lesions that may seem to have purulent drainage, as this will delay resolution of this condition and lead to secondary bacterial infections.

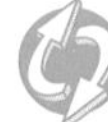

ONGOING CARE

COMPLICATIONS

- Recurrence of milder symptoms at same location can be triggered by physiological or psychological stressors (illness, fever, sun exposure, menstruation (1).
- Secondary bacterial infection
- Loss of work time
- Ocular infection
- Nail dystrophy or nail loss
- Localized hyperesthesia or hypoesthesia

REFERENCES

1. Gill MJ, Arlette J, Buchan KA. Herpes simplex virus infection of the hand. *J Am Acad Dermatol*. 1990;22:111–6.
2. Rubright JH, Shafritz AB. The herpetic whitlow. *J Hand Surg Am*. 2011;36:340–2.
3. Wu IB, Schwartz RA. Herpetic whitlow. *Cutis*. 2007;79:193–6.
4. Smith CA. Herpetic whitlow. *Clin Microbiol Newsletter*. 1985;7:1–3.
5. Polayes IM, Arons MS. The treatment of herpetic whitlow–a new surgical concept. *Plast Reconstr Surg*. 1980;65:811–7.
6. Laskin OL. Acyclovir and suppression of frequently recurring herpetic whitlow. *Ann Intern Med*. 1985;102:494–5.

ADDITIONAL READING

- Avitzur Y, Amir J. Herpetic whitlow infection in a general pediatrician—an occupational hazard. *Infection*. 2002;30:234–6.
- Clark DC. Common acute hand infections. *Am Fam Physician*. 2003;68:2167–76.
- Luxenberg EL, Silverman RA. Nail disorders in children. *Dermatol Nurs*. 2010;22:5–8.
- Schwandt NW, Mjos DP, Lubow RM, et al. Acyclovir and the treatment of herpetic whitlow. *Oral Surg Oral Med Oral Pathol*. 1987;64:255–8.
- Usatine RP, Tinitigan R. Nongenital herpes simplex virus. *Am Fam Physician*. 2010;82:1075–82.

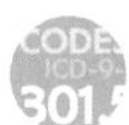

CODES

ICD9

054.6 Herpetic whitlow

CLINICAL PEARLS

- Incision and drainage of vesicular lesion is contraindicated, as this can cause secondary bacterial infection, delay resolution, and increase risk of systemic symptoms.
- Herpetic whitlow will not have a tense distal pulp on physical exam as compared to bacterial paronychia.
- Viral shedding of vesicle is active until the lesion crusts over.
- Recurrent infections can be triggered by fever, sun exposure, extreme temperatures, ultraviolet radiation, trauma, menstruation, or emotional stressors. Symptoms are usually milder and with a shorter duration.

H

HICCUPS

James H. Lewis, MD, FACP, FACG, AGAF

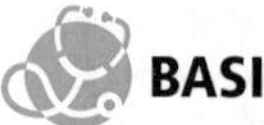

BASICS

DESCRIPTION

- Hiccups are caused by a sudden involuntary contraction of the inspiratory muscles (predominantly the diaphragm) terminated by abrupt closure of the glottis, stopping the inflow of air and producing the characteristic sound (1).
- System(s) affected: Nervous; Pulmonary
- Synonym(s): Hiccoughs; Singultus

Geriatric Considerations

Can be a serious problem among the elderly

Pregnancy Considerations

- Fetal hiccups are noted as rhythmic fetal movements (confirmed sonographically) that can be confused with contractions.
- Fetal hiccups often recur in subsequent pregnancies.

EPIDEMIOLOGY

- Predominant age: All ages (including fetus)
- Predominant sex: Male > Female (4:1)

Prevalence

Self-limited hiccups are extremely common, as are intra- and postoperative hiccups; intractable hiccups are rare.

RISK FACTORS

- General anesthesia; conscious sedation
- Postoperative state
- Genitourinary disorders
- Irritation of the vagus nerve branches
- Structural, vascular, infectious, neoplastic, or traumatic CNS lesions

GENERAL PREVENTION

- Identify and correct the underlying cause.
- Avoid gastric distention.
- Seek medical attention for frequent bouts or persistent hiccups.
- Acupuncture appears to be as or more efficacious than chronic drug therapy to control hiccups.

ETIOLOGY

- Pathophysiologic significance is unknown; may be a vestigial reflex; hiccups have been associated with >100 underlying disorders (1).
- Results from stimulation of $\geq$1 limbs of the hiccup reflux arc (vagus and phrenic nerves) with a "hiccup center" located in the upper spinal cord
- In men, >90% have an organic basis, whereas in women a psychogenic cause may be more likely.
- Specific underlying causes include:
  - Alcoholism
  - CNS lesions (brain-stem tumors, vascular lesions, Parkinson disease) (2)
  - Diaphragmatic irritation (tumors, pericarditis, eventration, splenomegaly, hepatomegaly, peritonitis)
  - Hair, insect, or foreign body irritating tympanic membrane
  - Pharyngitis, laryngitis
  - Mediastinal and other thoracic lesions (pneumonia, aortic aneurysm, tuberculosis [TB], myocardial infarction [MI], lung cancer, rib exostoses)
  - Esophageal lesions (reflux esophagitis, achalasia, *Candida* esophagitis, carcinoma, obstruction)
  - Gastric lesions (ulcer, distention, cancer)
  - Hepatic lesions (hepatitis, hepatoma)
  - Pancreatic lesions (pancreatitis, pseudocysts, cancer)
  - Inflammatory bowel disease
  - Cholelithiasis, cholecystitis
  - Prostatic disorders
  - Appendicitis
  - Postoperative, abdominal procedures (3)
  - Toxic metabolic causes (uremia, hyponatremia, gout, diabetes)
  - Drug-induced (dexamethasone, methylprednisolone, anabolic steroids, benzodiazepines, α-methyldopa)
  - Psychogenic causes (hysterical neurosis, grief, malingering)
  - Idiopathic

COMMONLY ASSOCIATED CONDITIONS

See "Etiology".

DIAGNOSIS

- Hiccup attacks usually occur at brief intervals and last only a few seconds or minutes. Bouts lasting >48 hours often imply an underlying physical or metabolic disorder.
- Intractable hiccups may occur continuously for months or years.
- Hiccups usually occur with a frequency of 4–60 per minute.

HISTORY

Recent surgery (especially genitourinary), general anesthesia (3); medications; alcoholism; GI, cardiac, or pulmonary disorders (see "Etiology") (1)

PHYSICAL EXAM

- See "Etiology" for specific findings to look for.
- Examine the ear canal for foreign bodies.

DIAGNOSTIC TESTS & INTERPRETATION

Lab

Consider CBC, metabolic panel as suggested by history

Imaging

Fluoroscopy is useful to determine whether 1 hemidiaphragm is dominant.

Diagnostic Procedures/Surgery

- Upper endoscopy, colonoscopy, CT scan (or other imaging) of brain, thorax, abdomen, and pelvis looking for etiological causes; exploratory laparoscopy or laparotomy for peritoneal lesions (carcinomatosis, etc.); GYN pathology, etc.
- The extent of the workup is often in proportion to the duration and severity of the hiccups.

DIFFERENTIAL DIAGNOSIS

See "Etiology"; burping (eructation) may be confused with hiccups (4).

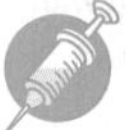

TREATMENT

- Outpatient (usually)
- Inpatient (if elderly, debilitated, or intractable hiccups)
- Nearly all hiccup treatments are anecdotal; those with recorded success are below (1).

MEDICATION

First Line

Possible drug remedies:

- Baclofen, a GABA analog, 5–10 mg t.i.d. (best choice) (5)[A]
- Chlorpromazine, 25–50 mg IV (1)[B]
- Haloperidol, 2–12 mg IM
- Phenytoin, 200 mg IV, then 100 mg q.i.d.
- Metoclopramide, 5–10 mg q.i.d. (1)[B].
- Nifedipine, 10–20 mg/d to t.i.d.
- Amitriptyline, 10 mg t.i.d.
- Lidocaine, 1.5 mg/kg IV infusion followed by 0.75 mg/kg on subsequent days
- Gabapentin (Neurontin), up to 1,800 mg/d in divided doses (6,7)[B]
- Contraindications: Refer to manufacturer's literature:
  - Baclofen is not recommended in patients with stroke or other cerebral lesions.

- Precautions: Refer to manufacturer's literature:
  - Abrupt withdrawal of baclofen should be avoided.
- Maintenance drug therapy (e.g., baclofen, 5–10 mg t.i.d.; phenytoin, 100 mg q.i.d.; valproic acid, 15 mg/kg undivided doses; nifedipine, 10–20 mg daily to t.i.d.; metoclopramide, 10 mg q.i.d.); gabapentin, up to 1,800 mg in divided doses

Second Line

- Amantadine, carbidopa-levodopa in Parkinson disease
- Steroid replacement in Addison disease
- Antifungal agent in *Candida* esophagitis
- Ondansetron in carcinomatosis with vomiting
- Nefopam (a nonopioid analgesic with antishivering properties related to antihistamines and antiparkinsonian drugs) is available outside the US in both IV and oral formulations (8)[B].

ADDITIONAL TREATMENT

General Measures

- Treat any specific underlying cause when identified (1):
  - Dilate esophageal stricture or obstruction.
  - Treat ulcers or reflux disease.
  - Remove hair or foreign body from ear canal.
  - Angostura bitters for alcohol-induced hiccups
  - Catheter stimulation of pharynx for operative and postoperative hiccups
  - Antifungal treatment for *Candida* esophagitis
  - Correct electrolyte imbalance.
- Medical measures:
  - Relief of gastric distention (gastric lavage, nasogastric aspiration, induced vomiting)
  - Counterirritation of the vagus nerve (supraorbital pressure, carotid sinus massage, digital rectal massage) to be used with caution
  - Respiratory center stimulants (breathing 5% CO_2)
  - Psychiatric (hypnosis, behavioral modification)
  - Phrenic nerve block or electrical stimulation (9) (or pacing) of the dominant hemidiaphragm
  - Miscellaneous (cardioversion)

Issues for Referral

For acupuncture or phrenic nerve crush, block, or electrostimulation (9,10)

COMPLEMENTARY AND ALTERNATIVE MEDICINE

- Acupuncture is increasingly being used to manage persistent hiccups (10)[B].
- Simple home remedies:
  - Swallowing a spoonful of sugar
  - Sucking on a hard candy or swallowing peanut butter
  - Holding breath and increasing pressure on diaphragm (Valsalva maneuver)
  - Tongue traction
  - Lifting the uvula with a cold spoon
  - Inducing fright
  - Smelling salts
  - Rebreathing into a paper (not plastic) bag
  - Sipping ice water
  - Rubbing a wet cotton-tipped applicator between hard and soft palate for 1 minute (11)[C]

SURGERY/OTHER PROCEDURES

- Phrenic nerve crush or transection of the dominant diaphragmatic leaflet
- Resection of rib exostoses

IN-PATIENT CONSIDERATIONS

Admission Criteria

Most patients can be managed as outpatients; those with severe intractable hiccups may require rehydration, pain control, IV medications, or surgery.

ONGOING CARE

FOLLOW-UP RECOMMENDATIONS

Patient Monitoring

Until hiccups cease

DIET

Avoid gastric distension from overeating, carbonated beverages, and aerophagia.

PATIENT EDUCATION

See "General Measures."

PROGNOSIS

- Hiccups often cease during sleep.
- Most acute benign hiccups resolve with home remedies or spontaneously.
- Intractable hiccups may last for years or decades.
- Hiccups have persisted despite bilateral phrenic nerve transection.

COMPLICATIONS

- Inability to eat
- Weight loss
- Exhaustion, debility
- Insomnia
- Cardiac arrhythmias
- Wound dehiscence
- Death (rare)

REFERENCES

1. Lewis JH. Hiccups and their cures. *Clin Perspect Gastroenterol*. 2000;3:277–83.
2. Miwa H, Kondo T. Hiccups in Parkinson's disease: An overlooked non-motor symptom? Parkinsonism Relat. *Disord*. 2010;16:249–51.
3. Kranke P, Eberhart LH, Morin AM. Treatment of hiccups during general anaesthesia or sedation: A qualitative systematic review. *Eur J Anaesthesiol*. 2003;20:239–44.
4. Hopman WP, van Kouwen MC, Smout AJ. Does (supra)gastric belching trigger recurrent hiccups? *World J Gastroenterol*. 2010;16:1795–9.
5. Ramírez FC, Graham DY. Treatment of intractable hiccup with baclofen: Results of a double-blind randomized, controlled, cross-over study. *Am J Gastroenterol*. 1992;87:1789–91.
6. Porzio G, Aielli F, Verna L, et al. Gabapentin in the treatment of hiccups in patients with advanced cancer: A 5-year experience. *Clin Neuropharmacol*. 2010;33(4):179–80.
7. Marinella MA. Diagnosis and management of hiccups in the patient with advanced cancer. *J Support Oncol*. 2009;7:122–7, 130.
8. Bilotta F, Rosa G. Nefopam for severe hiccups. *N Engl J Med*. 2000;343:1973–4.
9. Okuda Y, Kitajima T, Asai T. Use of a nerve stimulator for phrenic nerve block in treatment of hiccups. *Anesthesiology*. 1998;88:525–7.
10. Schiff E, River Y, Oliven A. Acupuncture therapy for persistent hiccups. *Am J Med Sci*. 2002;323:166–8.
11. Brostoff JM, Birns J, Benjamin E. The "cotton bud technique" as a cure for hiccups. *Eur Arch Otorhinolaryngol*. 2009;266(5):775–6.

ADDITIONAL READING

Cabane J, Bizec JL, Derenne JP, et al. [A diseased esophagus is frequently the cause of chronic hiccup. A prospective study of 184 cases.] *Presse Medicale*. Paris, France. 2010;39(6):e141–6.

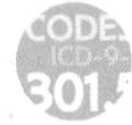

CODES

ICD9

- 306.1 Respiratory malfunction arising from mental factors
- 786.8 Hiccough

CLINICAL PEARLS

- An organic cause for persistent hiccups is more likely to be found in men.
- Rule out a foreign body in the ear canal as a trigger.
- Baclofen remains the only pharmacologic therapy proven effective in a clinical trial setting.
- Acupuncture is proving very effective in persistent hiccups refractory to other therapies.

HIDRADENITIS SUPPURATIVA

Francisco Aguirre, MD

BASICS

DESCRIPTION

- Acute, tender, cystlike abscesses in apocrine gland–bearing skin (axillae, anogenital area, pubis, areolae; also apocrine glands scattered around umbilicus, scalp, trunk, and face)
- Over time, fibrotic sinus tracts develop with intermittent drainage and periodic acute abscesses and may become chronic
- Common from late puberty through 40 years
- System(s) affected: Skin/Exocrine
- Synonym(s): Acne inversa; Apocrinitis; Hidradenitis axillaris

Geriatric Considerations

Rare after menopause

Pediatric Considerations

Rarely occurs before puberty

Pregnancy Considerations

No isotretinoin (Accutane) or tetracycline treatment during pregnancy. Disease may ease during pregnancy and rebound after parturition.

EPIDEMIOLOGY

- Predominant age: Peak onset age 11–30 years, commonly 30–40 years
- Predominant sex: 3:1 female-to-male ratio

Incidence

Peaks during second and third decades of life

Prevalence

0.3–4%

RISK FACTORS

- Obesity
- Acne
- Hyperandrogenism
- Hirsutism
- Smoking
- Lithium may trigger onset or exacerbate this condition.

Genetics

Unknown; possibly single gene transmission (autosomal dominant), possibly polygenic

GENERAL PREVENTION

- Weight loss if overweight or obese
- Avoid constrictive clothing/frictional trauma.
- Avoid heat exposure, sweating, shaving, depilation, and deodorants.
- Use antiseptic soaps, topical application of tea tree oil
- Smoking cessation

ETIOLOGY

- Traditionally considered a disorder of apocrine glands, but now believed to be primarily an inflammatory disorder of the hair follicle triggered by follicular plugging within apocrine gland–bearing skin
- Bacterial involvement is not a primary pathogenic event, but secondary.
- Sebum excretion is not an important factor.
- Smoking may be a major triggering factor.
- Considered part of follicular occlusive tetrad: Acne conglobata, dissecting cellulitis of scalp, hidradenitis suppurativa, and pilonidal sinus
- There may be a genetic predisposition component that is still being elucidated.

COMMONLY ASSOCIATED CONDITIONS

- Acne
- Perifolliculitis capitis abscedens et suffodiens (dissecting cellulitis of scalp)
- Arthritis
- Obesity with associated diabetes mellitus, atopy, acanthosis nigricans
- Crohn disease
- Pilonidal disease
- Smoking

DIAGNOSIS

HISTORY

- Multiple recurrences at the same site
- Recurrent deep boils >6 months in flexural sites
- Onset after puberty
- Poor response to conventional antibiotics
- Strong tendency toward relapse or recurrence
- Personal or family history of acne or pilonidal sinuses and premenstrual exacerbation of boils
- Early signs are pruritus, erythema, and local hyperhidrosis.
- Healing sites may be accompanied by scarring and sinus tracts.
- Associated arthritis and arthropathy, especially in the knees

PHYSICAL EXAM

- Tender nodules (dome-shaped) 0.5–3 cm in size are present:
  - Distribution is over the area of apocrine glands, with axillae and the groin being most common. Sites ordered by frequency of occurrence: Axillary, inguinal, perianal and perineal, mammary and inframammary, buttock, pubic region, chest, scalp, retroauricular, eyelid
  - Large lesions often are fluctuant.
  - Comedones may be present.
  - Possible malodorous discharge
- Staging: Most commonly done with the Hurley staging system, although it is likely that future studies will use the more detailed Sartorius staging system for clinical research:
  - Hurley staging system:
    - Stage I: Abscess formation (singular or multiple) without sinus tracts or scarring
    - Stage II: One or more widely separated, recurrent abscesses with tract formation and scars
    - Stage III: Multiple interconnected tracts and abscesses throughout an entire area

DIAGNOSTIC TESTS & INTERPRETATION

Lab

Initial lab tests

- Cultures of skin or aspirates of boils negative. When positive, often polymicrobial and have shown *Staphylococci aureus, Staphylococcus epidermidis, Streptococcus milleri, Streptococcus hominis, Bacteroides fragilis,* and *Bacteroides melaninogenicus*.
- Check sensitivities.
- May note increased ESR, leukocytosis, decreased serum iron, normocytic anemia, and changes in serum electrophoresis pattern, probably due to chronic inflammatory process
- Consider biopsy to differentiate from other diagnoses such as Crohn disease or squamous cell carcinoma, if appropriate.
- Consider these additional studies at baseline, depending on elected treatment:
  - CBC count with differential
  - Basic metabolic panel plus magnesium
  - Liver function tests
  - Glucose-6-phosphate dehydrogenase level
  - Fasting lipids
- Purified protein derivative

Follow-Up & Special Considerations

- There is a slightly increased risk of squamous cell carcinoma with chronic hidradenitis suppurativa; consider biopsy of concerning lesions.
- If patient is female with hirsutism, check:
  - Dehydroepiandrosterone sulfate
  - Testosterone: Total and free
  - Sex-hormone-binding globulin
  - Progesterone

Diagnostic Procedures/Surgery

- Incision and drainage of lesion(s) with culture and biopsy
- Mortimer clinical criteria for diagnosis: Recurrent boils in apocrine-gland-bearing skin for more than 3 months, presence of comedones in apocrine skin or retroauricular sites, and premenstrual exacerbation of disease (1)
- Ultrasound may be useful to assist in planning an entire excision to identify the full extent of sinus tracts.

Pathological Findings

- Histologically, chronic disease shows a dermis that contains inflammatory cells, giant cells, sinus tracts, SC abscesses, and, later, extensive fibrosis.
- Multiple comedones and follicular dilatation and possible occlusion by keratinized stratified squamous epithelium may be observed.

DIFFERENTIAL DIAGNOSIS

- Furunculosis/carbuncles: Differentiate by specific culture and by the response to specific antibiotics.
- Infected Bartholin or sebaceous cysts
- Hyperandrogenism
- Lymphadenopathy/lymphadenitis
- Cutaneous Langerhans cell histiocytosis
- Actinomycosis
- Granuloma inguinale
- Lymphogranuloma venereum
- Apocrine nevus
- Crohn with anogenital fistula (may coexist with hidradenitis suppurativa or be mistaken for it)
- Cutaneous tuberculosis
- Fox-Fordyce disease

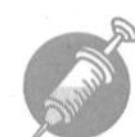

TREATMENT

- Conservative treatment includes all items under general prevention, plus use of warm compresses, sitz baths, and topical antiseptics for inflamed lesions and nonnarcotic analgesics (2)[C]. In addition, weight loss and smoking cessation have shown improvement (3).
- Medical treatment is often tried first because of extensive nature of surgical treatment.
- No medications are curative. Relapse is almost inevitable once medication is stopped. The strategy is to keep the disease contained with medications. If

a cure is sought and the disease is Hurley stage II–III, surgery should be considered.

MEDICATION

First Line

- Stage I disease: Consider either systemic or topical antibiotics:
  - Topical antibiotics: Select one of the following (clindamycin has the most evidence):
    - Clindamycin 1% solution b.i.d. (×12 weeks at a minimum) (2,4)
    - Benzoyl peroxide 5–10% solution b.i.d. (4)[C]
    - Chlorhexidine 4% solution b.i.d. (4)[C]
  - Systemic antibiotics: Select one of the following:
    - Tetracycline 500 mg b.i.d. (>12 weeks) (5)
    - Oral clindamycin 300 mg b.i.d. and rifampin 300 mg b.i.d. for 12 weeks (2,6)[B]
- Stage II–III disease:
  - Antibiotic therapy to address likely overlying bacterial infection, with a need to cover gram-negative, gram-positive, and anaerobic bacterial infections, with the antibiotic selection based on lesion location and characteristics. A range of regimens have been published with small studies of data available. One included a clindamycin/rifampin combination, another included rifampin/moxifloxacin/metronidazole.
  - Although antibiotic therapy is generally attempted, it is more likely that more aggressive approaches will be needed subsequently. This usually implies surgical treatment, but medical management may lead to progress once any infectious component has been addressed:
    - Immunosuppressive therapies with infliximab (2,7)[C]

Second Line

- Stage I:
  - Consider oral contraceptives for women if antibiotics fail. Low-dose progesterone birth control pills (e.g., Norinyl, Ortho-Novum) (2)[C].
  - Sulfamethoxazole/trimethoprim DS b.i.d. (4).
  - Oral amoxicillin 250–500 mg b.i.d., tetracycline, minocycline 50–100 mg b.i.d., doxycycline 50–100 mg b.i.d., or erythromycin (2)[C]
  - Limited lesions can be injected with corticosteroids, and flares can be addressed with short courses of oral or intralesional corticosteroids such as triamcinolone (2)[C].
  - Dapsone (2)[C]
  - Finasteride (consider only after menopause) (2,4)[C]
- Stage II–III disease or recalcitrant Stage I:
  - Systemic retinoids: Isotretinoin 40–80 mg PO every day for 4 months (2)[C]
  - Cyproterone acetate (if available) (2)[B]

ADDITIONAL TREATMENT

General Measures

- Symptomatic treatment for acute lesions
- Local cleansing (germicidal soap)
- Improve environmental factors that cause follicular blockage (see "General Prevention").
- Smoking cessation and weight loss if overweight.

Issues for Referral

- Lack of response to treatment or stage II–III disease is a reason to refer for surgical excision or radiation/laser treatment (stage II) or concern for malignancy such as squamous cell carcinoma.
- If significant psychosocial stress from diseases, referral for stress management and to a support group is recommended.

SURGERY/OTHER PROCEDURES

- Various surgical approaches have been used for stage II–III disease:
  - Incision and drainage is discouraged as it is rarely curative (2,8)[C].
  - Deroofing and marsupialization of the sinus tracts may be of benefit primarily for Hurley stage I–II disease, as healing time is reduced. Recurrences are sometimes seen but usually are smaller than the original lesions (2,8)[C].
  - Treatment for stage III or intractable cases: Wide full-thickness excision with healing by granulation or flap placement is the most definitive treatment and rarely has local recurrence if all sinus tracts are excised. Rates of local recurrence (within 3–72 months) are: axillary (3%), perianal (0%), inguinoperineal (37%), and submammary (50%) (9,10).
- CO_2 laser ablation with healing by secondary intention has recent data with good results (11).

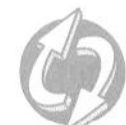

ONGOING CARE

FOLLOW-UP RECOMMENDATIONS

Follow up monthly or sooner to evaluate progress and assist with symptom management.

DIET

No limitations

PATIENT EDUCATION

- Severity can range from only 2 or 3 papules per year to extensive draining sinus tracts.
- Medications are temporizing measures and are rarely curative. Smoking cessation and weight loss can improve symptoms significantly.
- Attempts at local surgical "cures" do not affect recurrence at other sites.
- Hidradenitis suppurativa is considered a misnomer by many. *Acne inversa* is the more descriptive terminology.
- Hidradenitis Suppurativa Foundation: www.hs-foundation.org

PROGNOSIS

- Individual lesions (with or without drainage) heal slowly in 10–30 days.
- Recurrences may last for several years.
- Rare spontaneous resolution
- Relentlessly progressive scarring and sinus tracts are likely for chronic severe disease.
- Radical wide-area excision is the method that has shown the greatest likelihood for a lack of recurrence up to 5 years.

COMPLICATIONS

- Contracture formation at the sites of excisions in the case of surgery, possibly with restricted limb mobility
- Rarely, squamous cell carcinoma may develop in indolent sinus tracts (usually anogenital).
- Disseminated infection septicemia (unusual)
- Lymphedema
- Urethral/rectal fistula
- Anemia
- Asymmetrical pauciarticular to symmetrical polyarthritis/polyarthralgia in larger joints
- Amyloidosis and hypoproteinemia can lead to renal failure and even death.
- Interstitial keratitis
- Lumbosacral epidural abscess
- Sacral bacterial osteomyelitis

REFERENCES

1. Mortimer PS, Dawber RP, Gales MA, et al. Mediation of hidradenitis suppurativa by androgens. *Br Med J (Clin Res Ed)*. 1986;292: 245–8.
2. Lam J, Krakowski AC, Friedlander SF. Hidradenitis suppurativa (acne inversa): Management of a recalcitrant disease. *Pediatr Dermatol*. 2007;24: 465–73.
3. Sartorius K, Emtestam L, Jemec GB, et al. Objective scoring of hidradenitis suppurativa reflecting the role of tobacco smoking and obesity. *Br J Dermatol*. 2009;161(4):831–9.
4. Lee RA, Yoon A, Kist J. Hidradenitis suppurativa: An update. *Adv Dermatol*. 2007;23:289–306.
5. Jemec GB, Wendelboe P. Topical clindamycin versus systemic tetracycline in the treatment of hidradenitis suppurativa. *J Am Acad Dermatol*. 1998;39:971–4.
6. Mendonça CO, Griffiths CE. Clindamycin and rifampicin combination therapy for hidradenitis suppurativa. *Br J Dermatol*. 2006;154:977–8.
7. Grant A, Gonzalez T, Montgomery MO, et al. Infliximab therapy for patients with moderate to severe hidradenitis suppurativa: A randomized, double-blind, placebo-controlled crossover trial. *J Am Acad Dermatol*. 2010;62:205–17.
8. Slade DE, Powell BW, Mortimer PS. Hidradenitis suppurativa: Pathogenesis and management. *Br J Plast Surg*. 2003;56:451–61.
9. Kagan RJ, Yakuboff KP, Warner P, et al. Surgical treatment of hidradenitis suppurativa: A 10-year experience. *Surgery*. 2005;138:734–40; discussion 740–1.
10. Mandal A, Watson J. Experience with different treatment modules in hidradenitis suppurativa: A study of 106 cases. *Surgeon*. 2005;3:23–6.
11. Hazen PG, Hazen BP. Hidradenitis suppurativa: Successful treatment using carbon dioxide laser excision and marsupialization. *Dermatol Surg*. 2010;36:208–13.

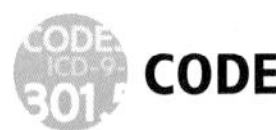

CODES

ICD9

705.83 Hidradenitis

CLINICAL PEARLS

- Hidradenitis suppurativa is an inflammatory disease of the apocrine skin areas that can be difficult to contain with behavior changes and medication.
- For those people with recalcitrant or severe disease, despite best-known medical treatments, surgery provides the only chance at a cure. Success rates depend on the location and extent of excision.

HIP FRACTURE

Kylee Eagles, DO
Lee A. Mancini, MD, CSCS, CSN

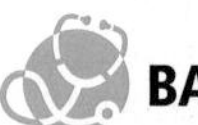

BASICS

DESCRIPTION

- Fracture of the femur head or neck, 90% of which are cause by a fall (1)
- Intracapsular:
  - Femoral neck, subcapital or transcervical
  - Intracapsular femoral neck fractures may disrupt the blood supply to the femoral head, resulting in avascular necrosis.
- Extracapsular:
  - Intertrochanteric
  - Subtrochanteric
- System(s) affected: Musculoskeletal, Neurological, Vascular
- Synonym(s): Subcapital fracture; Trochanteric fracture; Femoral neck fracture

Geriatric Considerations

Hip fractures are common in geriatric age group.

EPIDEMIOLOGY

- Predominant age: 80% occur in those >60 years old
- Predominant sex: Female > Male (3:1)

Incidence

- In the US, 250,000 patients per year >65 have fracture of hips (1).
- In the US, women >75 years: 1% incidence per year

Prevalence

- 77.2% hip fractures occur in women.
- ~794/100,000 women and ~369/100,000 men over age 65

RISK FACTORS

- Low bone-mineral density
- Metastatic cancer
- Neurologic disease with gait impairment
- Severe renal disease with secondary hyperparathyroidism
- Long-acting sedatives or hypnotics in the elderly (benzodiazepines, anticonvulsants)
- Age >65
- Propensity to fall
- History of previous fracture since age 50
- Weight loss
- Frailty
- Impaired vision, especially decreased depth perception
- Osteoarthritis
- Hyperthyroidism
- Deconditioning
- Cigarette smoking
- Alcohol use
- Diabetes mellitus
- Long-term proton pump inhibitor therapy (high doses)
- Sedentarism, especially if on feet <4 hours a day (2)

Genetics

No known genetic factor

GENERAL PREVENTION

- Prophylactic treatment for osteoporosis (2)[C]:
  - Calcium supplementation: 1,200 mg/d PO
  - Magnesium supplementation improves the bodies utilization of calcium
  - Vitamin D supplementation: >800 IU/d PO
  - Bisphosphonates
- Fall prevention:
  - Avoid long-acting sedatives and hypnotics in the elderly.
  - Use walking canes or walkers if patient has unsteady gait.
  - Use sturdy rails in showers, bathrooms, stairs, or ramps; avoid throw rugs and slippery surfaces.
  - Prescribe a structured exercise program (3)[C].
  - Ensure elderly patients have annual vision exams.
  - Minimize polypharmacy.
- Quantitative ultrasound and/or bone-mineral density measurements can be used to predict the likelihood of hip fracture in men and women.
- Treatment of osteoporosis to prevent hip fractures has been found successful with alendronate, but only when combined with weight-bearing exercise and aggressive vitamin D replacement. Data supporting other bisphosphonates to prevent hip fracture remains unclear.
- Bisphosphonates: Main adverse effect is esophageal irritation:
  - Alendronate (Fosamax), 35 (prevention)–70 mg (management) PO weekly
  - Risedronate (Actonel), 35 mg PO weekly
  - Ibandronate (Boniva), 150 mg PO monthly
  - Zoledronic acid (Reclast), 5 mg IV yearly:
    - Also approved as a fracture preventative after the occurrence of a hip fracture
  - Salmon calcitonin: Main adverse effect is nasal irritation and nausea:
    - Nasal spray (Miacalcin), 1 spray daily in alternate nostrils
    - Injectable (Calcimar), 100 IU/d SC or IM

ETIOLOGY

- Osteoporosis
- Direct blunt trauma
- Pathologic conditions (e.g., bone cancer)
- Stress fracture caused by overtraining
- Avascular necrosis

COMMONLY ASSOCIATED CONDITIONS

- Osteoporosis
- Metastatic malignancy

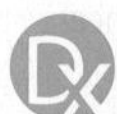

DIAGNOSIS

HISTORY

- Pain in hip: If severe, may indicate a displaced fracture. Mild pain usually occurs in nondisplaced fractures.
- Pain in knee: Pain is referred from hip and may occur in absence of hip pain.
- Inability to ambulate

PHYSICAL EXAM

- External rotation of leg
- Shortening of leg
- Pain with flexion abduction external rotation (FABER)
- Inability to straight leg raise or bear weight

DIAGNOSTIC TESTS & INTERPRETATION

Lab

Initial lab tests

Routine preoperative laboratory including CBC, chemical profile, electrolytes

Follow-Up & Special Considerations

Follow Hct postoperatively to evaluate for anemia.

Imaging

- Radiographs:
  - Anteroposterior and "frog leg" lateral of hip
  - Anteroposterior pelvis to rule out pelvic fracture
  - Remainder of femur to include knee
  - Any other tender or painful area, as other fractures are common and symptoms may be ignored in the face of severe pain of hip fracture.
- CT or MRI scans are not routinely indicated because the diagnosis is usually obvious from plain radiographs; however, MRI is 100% sensitive in delayed diagnosis of occult hip fracture.

Pathological Findings

Osteoporosis

DIFFERENTIAL DIAGNOSIS

Rule out primary or metastatic malignancy and pelvic fracture. If there was no direct trauma involved, investigate patient's history to rule out avascular necrosis or overtraining.

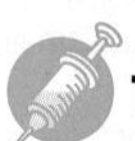

TREATMENT

- Treat urgently.
- Pain control

MEDICATION

- Analgesics:
  - Tylenol 1,000 mg PO q6h (max 3,000–4,000 mg/d).
  - If pain uncontrolled with Tylenol then use opioids such as Vicodin or Percocet. Avoid opioids in patients with a head injury or respiratory distress.
  - Transition to a long-acting opioid such as oxycodone. Dose based on usage of short-acting meds. Start low and increase slowly to achieve pain control.
  - NSAIDs are not recommended.
- Prophylactic anticoagulation with unfractionated low-dose heparin 5,000 U SC q8–12h or low-molecular-weight heparin (Lovenox) 40 mg SC q24h. Renally dose Lovenox if CrCl <30.
- Prophylactic antibiotics at induction of anesthesia: Cefazolin 1 g IV q8h × 3 doses. If penicillin allergic use clindamycin 600 mg IV q8h × 3 doses (1)[A].

First Line

If osteoporosis is present in a patient with a hip fracture, start bisphosphonates, calcium, and vitamin D as mentioned above in the general prevention section.

Second Line

Teriparatide (Forteo), 20 mEq/d SC for treatment of osteoporosis only:

- Avoid if patient has history of bone disease (i.e., osteosarcoma, Paget, malignancy).

ADDITIONAL TREATMENT

General Measures

- Oxygen therapy as needed per oximetry assessment
- Cyclical compression devices
- Situations where nonoperative treatment may be appropriate include:
  - End of life imminent
  - Nonambulatory, demented: Bed-bound, unable to transfer independently
- Compression-type fatigue fracture of the femoral neck:

- Occurs in normal bone exposed to excessive loads (e.g., young athlete)
- Patients must be compliant with 6–8 weeks of sharply restricted activity.

- Although patients with preoperative cognitive impairment require longer rehabilitation courses, they achieve short-term outcomes comparable to those who are cognitively unimpaired in the setting of a multidisciplinary hip fracture service. Cognitive impairment status should not be used as a determinant of which patients will benefit from surgery (4)[B].

SURGERY/OTHER PROCEDURES

- The majority of fractures are treated surgically with either internal fixation or arthroplasty.
- Surgery is recommended within 24–48 hours of presentation unless a patient has significant comorbidities that need to be addressed prior to surgery (2)[B]. Internal fixation is associated with a higher risk of implant failure than hemiarthroplasty (femoral head replacement).
- Undisplaced intracapsular fractures and extracapsular subtrochanteric fractures are most successfully repaired with hemiarthroplasty.
- Extracapsular intertrochanteric fractures are most often repaired with open reduction internal fixation (1).
- The choice of regional vs. general anesthesia has unknown effectiveness on morbidity or mortality outcomes (1)[B].

IN-PATIENT CONSIDERATIONS

Admission Criteria

- Virtually all patients should be admitted in anticipation of surgery.
- All patients should be on thromboprophylaxis (2)[A].
- Risk of DVT in patients with hip fracture is 50%.

IV Fluids

Used to maintain hydration while patient is NPO for surgery.

Nursing

- Assess for signs of delirium, which occurs in up to 62% of patients (1).
- Encourage PO intake because 20% of patients develop postop malnutrition (1).
- Use specialty mattress, frequent repositioning, and inspection of skin to avoid development of decubitus ulcers on the sacrum, heels, and malleoli (3)[A]
- Remove Foley within 24 hours of surgery to decrease incontinence and bladder infection (2)[B].

Discharge Criteria

- Patients should be ambulating with a walker or assistance (for toilet and prevention of deep vein thrombosis and decubiti) as soon as possible after surgery, usually the next day.
- In-patient evaluation by physical therapy and possibly occupational therapy/social services to determine discharge location and rehabilitation schedule. Begin rehab postoperative day 1 (2)[A].
- Prior to discharge assess for altered mental status, anemia, malnutrition, bladder and bowel function.

ONGOING CARE

FOLLOW-UP RECOMMENDATIONS

Patient Monitoring

- Radiographs of the hip are taken prior to discharge from the hospital and every 8–12 weeks thereafter until healed.
- Monitor postop physical therapy until full recovery. Rehab involves gait retraining, muscle stimulation, and a structured exercise program.

DIET

Nutritional supplementation with oral protein reduces postoperative complications and death (1)[B].

PROGNOSIS

- Hip fractures remain a serious injury in older people: 15–20% 3-month mortality in trochanteric fractures; 10% in neck fractures.
- 25% mortality in 1 year (3).
- Only 65% can be expected to return to their former state of health.
- 10% unable to return to former residence.
- A preop and postop interdisciplinary team approach results in better outcomes with fewer complications (1)[B].
- The overall risk of repeat hip fracture ranges from 2–10% and is greatest during the 12-month period following the first hip fracture.

COMPLICATIONS

- Mental deterioration:
  - Present in 90% of older patients for varying periods of time after surgery
  - Usually subsides, but may persist owing to pre-existing cognitive and mood disorders
- Infection:
  - More common in comminuted fractures and patients with diabetes
  - Surgical implants should be left in place and antibiotics given as indicated by culture and sensitivity.
  - May require incision and drainage
- Aseptic necrosis of femoral head:
  - Occurs in 25–30% of femoral neck fractures
  - Treatment requires a prosthetic replacement in older patients.
- Phlebitis:
  - Prophylaxis with warfarin (Coumadin) to keep INR 2–2.5 or prothrombin time 15–18 seconds, for at least 4 weeks, OR
  - Enoxaparin (Lovenox) 40 mg SC q24h beginning 12 hours after surgery and continuing until patient is mobile
- Nonunion:
  - In case of neck fractures, a prosthetic replacement is indicated.
  - In the intertrochanteric fracture, a bone graft, usually with replacement of the nail and plate, is indicated.

REFERENCES

1. Aaron-Gomez M, Miaota F. Medical management of hip fracture. *Clinics In Ger Med.* 2008;24(4).
2. Cherukuri M, Rao S. Management of hip fracture: The family physician's role. *Am Fam Physician.* 2006;73(12).
3. Jackman J, Watson T. Hip fracture in older men. *Clin Ger Med.* 2010;26(2).
4. Moncada LV, Andersen RE, Franckowiak SC, et al. The impact of cognitive impairment on short-term outcomes of hip fracture patients. *Arch Gerontol Geriatr.* 2006;43:45–52.

ADDITIONAL READING

- Frost SA. Risk factors for in-hospital post-hip fracture mortality. *Bone.* 2011;49(3):553–8.
- Ftouh S. Management of hip fracture in adults: Summary of NICE guidance. *BMJ* 2011;342:d3304.

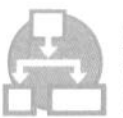

See Also (Topic, Algorithm, Electronic Media Element)

Osteoporosis

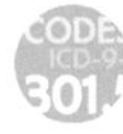

CODES

ICD9

- 820.01 Closed fracture of epiphysis (separation) (upper) of neck of femur
- 820.8 Closed fracture of unspecified part of neck of femur
- 820.9 Open fracture of unspecified part of neck of femur

CLINICAL PEARLS

- A structured exercise program has been shown to reduce falls and the fear of falling in frail older patients.
- Suspect a fracture in a patient with a shortened, externally rotated leg.

HIRSUTISM

Laura L. Novak, MD

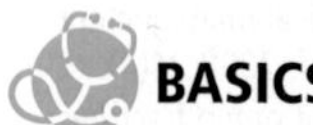

BASICS

DESCRIPTION
- Presence of excessive body and facial hair, in a male pattern, in women
- May be present in normal adults as an ethnic characteristic, or may develop as a result of androgen excess
- Often seen in association with polycystic ovarian syndrome (PCOS). May be accompanied by menstrual irregularities, insulin resistance, obesity, or acne.
- System(s) affected: Dermatologic; Endocrine/Metabolic; Reproductive
- Synonym(s): Excessive hair

Pregnancy Considerations
- May have related infertility. Offer intervention if desired.
- As hormone balance improves, fertility may increase; provide contraception as needed.
- Several medications used for treatment are contraindicated in pregnancy.

EPIDEMIOLOGY

Prevalence
8% of adult women

RISK FACTORS
- Family history
- Anovulation

Genetics
Multifactorial

GENERAL PREVENTION
- If there is associated insulin resistance or polycystic ovarian disease (PCOS), it can increase the risk of heart disease.
- Prolonged amenorrhea may, over time, put the patient at risk for endometrial hyperplasia or carcinoma.
- Women with late-onset congenital adrenal hyperplasia should be counseled that they may be carriers for the severe early-onset childhood disease.
- Avoid quackery and unlicensed electrolysis.

ETIOLOGY
Hirsutism is due to increased androgenic (male) hormones, either from increased peripheral binding (idiopathic) or increased production from the ovaries, adrenals, or fat. Exogenous medications can also be associated with hirsutism.

COMMONLY ASSOCIATED CONDITIONS
- PCOS: Most common cause of hirsutism, accompanied by menstrual irregularity or amenorrhea. Often associated with acne, obesity, and multicystic ovaries, but up to 50% of cases are atypical.
- Prolonged amenorrhea and anovulation
- Hypothyroidism or hyperprolactinemia
- Late-onset congenital adrenal hyperplasia: A genetic enzyme deficiency associated with more severe and earlier-onset hirsutism. Present in <2% of hirsute, amenorrheic patients.
- Tumor: Rare (<0.2%); ovarian or adrenal; especially if associated with virilization (rapid onset, clitoromegaly, balding, deepening voice)
- Cushing syndrome: Rare; characterized by central obesity, moon facies, striae, hypertension

DIAGNOSIS

HISTORY
- Age of onset (usually gradual), duration of symptoms
- Obtain a menstrual and fertility history: Irregular menses may indicate PCOS.
- Medication history: Look for use of valproic acid, testosterone, danazol, athletic performance drugs
- If galactorrhea is present, workup for hyperprolactinemia.

PHYSICAL EXAM
- The Ferriman-Gallwey scale (an instrument that rates hair growth in 9 areas on a scale of 0–4, with >8 being positive) may be used for diagnosis, but underrates localized hirsutism.
- Increased androgens may be associated with acne, obesity, insulin resistance, and hyperlipidemia.
- Increased hair growth on face, chest, and groin. May be hidden by plucking.
- Acanthosis nigricans: Velvety black skin in the axilla, neck, in insulin resistance
- Virilization: Deep voice, balding, clitoromegaly can indicate risk of tumor

DIAGNOSTIC TESTS & INTERPRETATION
- Diagnosis is clinical.
- Empiric treatment without lab workup is an acceptable option in mild–moderate hirsutism (1)[C].
- Lab testing is performed to rule out underlying tumor and pituitary diseases, which are rare.

Lab

Initial lab tests

Basic workup recommended by ACOG (2)[C]. Total testosterone, thyroid-stimulating hormone (TSH), and, if clinically suspicious, an insulin resistance workup:

- Testosterone: Random testosterone level is usually sufficient. A morning free testosterone is slightly more sensitive, but the difference isn't clinically relevant (3,2)[A]: Level >150 ng/dL may indicate ovarian tumor.
- TSH elevation indicates hypothyroidism.
- Insulin resistance testing: Results vary with age and ethnicity:
  - Fasting insulin level >20 or fasting glucose/insulin ratio <4.5 may indicate resistance.
  - ACOG recommends fasting and 2-hour glucose after 75-g glucose load in PCOS, but this may not be necessary.

Follow-Up & Special Considerations
- 17-hydroxyprogesterone (17-HP):
  - Elevations (>300) can indicate nonclassic congenital adrenal hyperplasia; rare (<2%)
  - Consider in patients with onset in early adolescence or high-risk group (Ashkenazi Jews)
  - Elevated levels require additional testing.
- Prolactin level if galactorrhea
- Dehydroepiandrosterone sulfate (DHEA-S) is no longer recommended routinely (4,5)[A]:
  - Levels >700 may indicate adrenal tumor.

Imaging
- If testosterone is >150, the patient may have a tumor. Testosterone is made by both the ovaries and adrenals, so both areas should be scanned. Ultrasound is best for the ovaries, and a CT is best for the adrenals.
- Ovarian ultrasound can help in the diagnosis of PCOS.

DIFFERENTIAL DIAGNOSIS
Hirsutism is associated with a number of different conditions (see "Etiology").

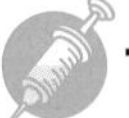

TREATMENT

MEDICATION

If idiopathic, no treatment is necessary, unless desired.

First Line

- Treatment goal is to decrease new hair growth and improve metabolic disorders.
- Oral contraceptives take 6 months to show effect; any brand is effective.
- Eflornithine (Vaniqa) HCl cream: Apply b.i.d.; reduces facial hair in 40% of women (with long-term use). Only FDA-approved hirsutism treatment.

Second Line

- Insulin sensitizers (metformin, thioglitazones) are mildly effective, but less so than oral contraceptives. May be used in diabetes or if oral contraceptives are contraindicated. Metformin is more effective than thioglitazones (6).
- Antiandrogenic drugs (used in combination with oral contraceptives to prevent menorrhagia and potential fetal toxicity) will further reduce hirsutism 15–25% (7,8). Usually begun after 6 months of first-line therapy if results are suboptimal. All should be avoided in pregnancy:
  - Spironolactone, 50–200 mg/d: Onset of action is slow; use with oral contraceptives to prevent menorrhagia. Watch for hyperkalemia, especially with drospirenone-containing OCP (Yasmin); contraindicated in pregnancy.
  - Finasteride: 5 mg/d decreases androgen binding; not approved by FDA. Use with contraception (pregnancy Category X).
  - Cyproterone, not available in the US: 12.5–100 mg/d day 5–15 of cycle combined with ethinyl estradiol 20–50 mcg day 5–25 of cycle
  - Flutamide: Nonsteroidal androgen receptor antagonist. Not recommended (1)[C].
- Steroids: Used in nonclassic congenital adrenal hyperplasia (NCCAH):
  - Dexamethasone 2 mg daily

ADDITIONAL TREATMENT

General Measures

- Treatment is slow and often lifelong.
- If patient desires pregnancy, induction of ovulation may be necessary.
- Provide contraception as needed.
- Encourage patient to maintain ideal weight.
- Treat accompanying acne.

COMPLEMENTARY AND ALTERNATIVE MEDICINE

- Saw palmetto (Serenoa repens): In small studies, decreases hair growth via blocking 5-α-reductase activity in the skin (3). Has similar peripheral action to finasteride (decreasing 5-α-reductase).
- Spearmint tea: 1 cup b.i.d.: In a study of 21 patients, 1 cup b.i.d. for 6 months led to decreased hirsutism (9).
- Licorice: In a small study, 9 women using 3.5 g daily for 2 cycles had benefit. Excess licorice can lead to hypokalemic hypertension (3).

ONGOING CARE

FOLLOW-UP RECOMMENDATIONS

No special activity

Patient Monitoring

Monitor for known side effects of medications.

DIET

No special diet

PATIENT EDUCATION

- Hormonal treatment stops further hair growth, but will not usually reverse present hair.
- Treatment takes 6 months to help and may be lifelong.
- Cosmetic measures include plucking, bleaching, shaving, electrolysis, laser hair removal, and cover-up cosmetics.
- If professional hair removal is chosen, laser/photoepilation is the preferred method, with the possible addition of eflornithine (Vaniqa) (1)[C].

PROGNOSIS

- Good (with long-term therapy) for halting further hair growth
- Moderate to poor for reversing current hair growth

COMPLICATIONS

- If PCOS is present, dysfunctional uterine bleeding and anemia
- If PCOS is present, anovulation may increase uterine cancer risk.
- Androgenic excess may adversely affect lipid status, cardiac risk, and bone density.
- Poor self-image/shame

REFERENCES

1. Martin, et al. 2008 Endocrinologic Society Guidelines. Evaluation and treatment of hirsutism in premenopausal women. *J Clin Endocrinol Metabol*. 2008;93(4):1105.
2. ACOG Clinical Practice Guideline No. 44. On the diagnosis and management of polycystic ovarian syndrome. Washington, DC: American College of Obstetrics and Gynecology; 2002.
3. Meletis C, Zabriskis N. Natural approaches for treating polycystic ovarian syndrome. *Altern Complement Ther*. 2006;12(4):157–64.
4. Azziz R. The evaluation and management of hirsutism. *Obstet Gynecol*. 2003;101:995–1007.
5. Rosenfeld RL. Hirsutism. *N Eng J Med*. 2005; 353(24):2578–88.
6. Harborne L, Fleming R, Lyall H, et al. Metformin or antiandrogen in the treatment of hirsutism in polycystic ovary syndrome. *J Clin Endocrinol Metab*. 2003;88:4116–23.
7. Farquhar C, Lee O, Toomath R, et al. Spironolactone versus placebo or in combination with steroids for hirsutism and/or acne. *Cochrane Database Syst Rev*. 2003;CD000194.
8. Swiglo BA, Cosma M, Flynn DN, et al. Clinical review: Antiandrogens for the treatment of hirsutism: A systematic review and metaanalyses of randomized controlled trials. *J Clin Endocrinol Metab*. 2008;93:1153–60.
9. Akdoan M, Tamer MN, Cüre E, et al. Effect of spearmint (Mentha spicata Labiatae) teas on androgen levels in women with hirsutism. *Phytother Res*. 2007;21(5):444–7.

ADDITIONAL READING

Radosh L, et al. Drug treatments for polycystic ovary syndrome. *Am Fam Physician*. 2009;79:671–6.

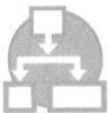

See Also (Topic, Algorithm, Electronic Media Element)

Acne Vulgaris; Infertility; Polycystic Ovarian Syndrome (PCOS)

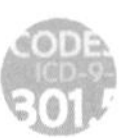

CODES

ICD9

- 256.4 Polycystic ovaries
- 704.1 Hirsutism

CLINICAL PEARLS

PCOS is the most common cause of hirsutism, accompanied by menstrual irregularity or amenorrhea. Often associated with acne, obesity, and multicystic ovaries, but up to 50% of cases are atypical.

HIV INFECTION AND AIDS

Adam Barta, MD

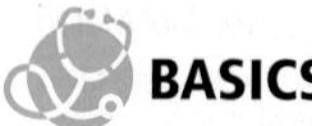

BASICS

DESCRIPTION

HIV is a retrovirus that integrates into CD4 T lymphocytes (a critical component of cell-mediated immunity), causing cell death and resulting in severe immunodeficiency, opportunistic infections, and malignancies:

- Because of treatment advances, HIV is now a chronic disease.
- The natural history of untreated HIV infection includes viral transmission, acute retroviral syndrome, recovery and seroconversion, asymptomatic chronic HIV infection, and symptomatic HIV infection or AIDS.
- Without antiretroviral treatment, the average patient develops AIDS ~10 years after transmission.
- All HIV-infected persons with CD4 <200 cells/mm^3 or having AIDS-defining illnesses are categorized as having AIDS.

EPIDEMIOLOGY

Incidence

- At end of 2008, 33.4 million people were estimated to be living with HIV/AIDS worldwide per UNAIDS and the World Health Organization. Yearly, 2.7 million new HIV infections and 2 million deaths are attributable to AIDS (1).
- US: 56,300 new cases; estimated 17,197 deaths of persons with AIDS in 2007 (2)

Prevalence

- Estimated 1.1 million persons in the US are living with HIV/AIDS; 25% of them are unaware of their status (1)
- HIV/AIDS cases are disproportionately high among racial/ethnic minority populations (1).
- Transmission of a drug-resistant virus is on the rise (1).
- Younger women and girls are particularly vulnerable (1).

RISK FACTORS

- Sexual activity (70% of world transmission): Viral load strongest predictor of heterosexual transmission with ulcerative urogenital lesions (3)[B].
- Male-to-male sexual contact accounted for 53% of newly diagnosed HIV/AIDS cases in 2007.
- Injection drug use
- Children of HIV-infected women:
  - Maternal HIV-1 RNA level is the best predictor of transmission risk.
  - HIV testing and use of antiretroviral drugs in pregnant women and their newborns has reduced the incidence of perinatal HIV transmission by >70% (from 25–29% without treatment to 8% with treatment) (4)[B].
  - Pregnant women should be treated until viral load is undetectable.
  - Can be transmitted through breast-feeding
- Recipients of blood products between 1975 and March 1985
- Occupational exposure

Genetics

People who lack CCR5, a cell-surface chemokine coreceptor used by HIV to infect cells, are highly resistant to HIV infection (5)[B].

GENERAL PREVENTION

Avoid unprotected sexual intercourse and injection drug abuse.

ETIOLOGY

HIV, a retrovirus

COMMONLY ASSOCIATED CONDITIONS

- Syphilis may be more aggressive in HIV-infected persons.
- Tuberculosis (TB) is coepidemic with HIV; test all persons with HIV for TB. Dually infected patients: 100× greater risk of developing active TB disease (compared with non-HIV) and higher rates of multidrug-resistant TB
- Patients coinfected with hepatitis C have a more rapid progression to cirrhosis.

DIAGNOSIS

- Acute retroviral syndrome: Precipitous decline in CD4 lymphocyte count and increased viremia ~1–4 weeks after transmission. Confirmed by demonstrating a high HIV RNA in the absence of HIV antibody.
- Mononucleosis-like syndrome, including:
  - Fever (97%)
  - Adenopathy
  - Pharyngitis (73%)
  - Rash (77%)
  - Myalgias/arthralgia (58%)
  - Less common: Headache, diarrhea, nausea, vomiting, hepatosplenomegaly, weight loss, thrush, and neurologic symptoms (12%)
  - Seroconversion: Development of a positive HIV antibody test usually occurs within 4 weeks of acute infection and invariably by 6 months.
  - Asymptomatic infection: Variable duration (average 8–10 years) and is accompanied by a gradual decline in CD4 cell counts and a relatively stable HIV RNA levels (the viral "set point"). Persistent lymphadenopathy: >1 cm in ≥2 extrainguinal sites; persists >3 months
- Symptomatic conditions:
  - Fever or diarrhea >1 month, bacillary angiomatosis, thrush, persistent candidal vulvovaginitis, cervical dysplasia or carcinoma in situ, oral hairy leukoplakia, herpes zoster, idiopathic thrombocytopenic purpura, pelvic inflammatory disease, peripheral neuropathy or myelopathy
- AIDS: defined by a CD4 cell count <200, a CD4 cell percentage of total lymphocytes <14% or one of several AIDS-related opportunistic infections: *Pneumocystis jiroveci (carinii)* pneumonia, cryptococcal meningitis, recurrent bacterial pneumonia, Candida esophagitis, CNS toxoplasmosis, tuberculosis and non-Hodgkin lymphoma (NHL), progressive multifocal encephalopathy, HIV nephropathy, Kaposi sarcoma, NHL, Hodgkin lymphoma, invasive cervical cancer.
- Advanced HIV disease: CD4 cell count <50. Most AIDS-related deaths occur at this time. Common late opportunistic infections: Cytomegalovirus (CMV) disease (retinitis, colitis) or disseminated *Mycobacterium avium* complex as well as HIV wasting syndrome (>10% wt loss) and HIV encephalopathy/dementia/minor cognitive-motor disorder.

HISTORY

- Medical history, including STDs and TB
- Review of systems: Fever, chills, night sweats, diarrhea, weight loss, fatigue, adenopathy, oral sores, odynophagia (esophageal candidiasis), cough, shortness of breath and dyspnea on exertion (early *Pneumocystis carinii* pneumonia), visual changes (CMV retinitis <200 CD4), skin rash, neurologic symptoms (CNS infection, malignancy, or dementia), sinusitis
- Social history, transmission risks, adherence
- Immunization review

PHYSICAL EXAM

Focus on weight, skin, retinal exam, oropharynx; lymph nodes; liver, spleen, mental status, sensation, genital and rectal examinations.

DIAGNOSTIC TESTS & INTERPRETATION

Lab

- Screening: ELISA reported as reactive or nonreactive; sensitivity and specificity >98%. Obtain HIV RNA if acute HIV infection is suspected:
  - New rapid and oral test available (home test kit, OraSure, OraQuickAdvanced Rapid HIV test).
- Confirmatory: Western blot:
  - Results positive, negative, or indeterminate
  - Per the CDC: Positive test is reaction with 2 of these 3 bands: P24, gp 41, and gp 120/160. If indeterminate, repeat test in 3–6 months.
- CD4 cell count and percentage (6)[A]
- HIV RNA viral load (6)[A]
- CBC with differential
- Serum chemistry
- Serologies: Hepatitis A, B, and C; syphilis.
- Urine screen for STIs (*Neisseria gonorrhoeae, Chlamydia trachomatis*)
- Cervical cytology
- PPD
- Glucose-6-phosphate levels
- Lipids at baseline and during highly active antiretroviral therapy (HAART)
- Genotypic tests for resistance to antiretrovirals for patients who have pretreatment HIV RNA >1,000 copies/m regardless of whether therapy will be initiated immediately (6)[A]

Imaging

Chest x-ray if pulmonary symptoms or positive PPD.

DIFFERENTIAL DIAGNOSIS

Order other tests/serologies if HIV RNA test is negative. Order throat cultures for bacterial/viral respiratory pathogens, Epstein-Barr virus VCA IgM/Igg, CMV IgM/IgG, human herpesvirus 6 IgM/IgG, and hepatitis serologies as appropriate to establish a diagnosis for patient's symptoms.

TREATMENT

- Antiretroviral therapy should be initiated in all patients with a history of an AIDS-defining illness or with a CD4 count <350 (6)[A]

- Antiretroviral therapy should be initiated regardless of CD4 count in patients with the following conditions: Pregnancy, HIV-associated nephropathy and HBV coinfections when treatment of hepatitis B virus is indicated (6)[A], rapidly declining CD4 counts (e.g., >100 cells/mm^3 decrease per year), higher viral load (e.g., >100,000 copies/mL) (6)[B]
- Antiretroviral therapy is recommended for all patients with CD4 count between 350 and 500 (6)[A].
- Consider for patients with CD4 count >500 (6)[B].

MEDICATION

- Nucleoside reverse transcriptase inhibitors (NRTIs):
  - Abacavir (ABC, Ziagen), didanosine (DDL, Videx), emtricitabine (FTC, Emtriva), lamivudine (3TC, Epivir), stavudine (d4T, Zerit), tenofovir (Viread), zalcitabine (ddC, Hivid), zidovudine (AZT, Retrovir), zidovudine + lamivudine (Combivir), zidovudine + lamivudine + abacavir (Trizivir), tenofovir + emtricitabine (Truvada)
- Nonnucleoside reverse transcriptase inhibitors (NNRTIs): Delavirdine (Rescriptor); efavirenz (Sustiva); nevirapine (Viramune); (Edurant); efavirenz, truvada (Atripla); rilpivirine, truvada (Complera)
- Protease inhibitors (PIs): Amprenavir (Agenerase), atazanavir (Reyataz), darunavir (Prezista), fosamprenavir (Lexiva), indinavir (Crixivan), lopinavir-ritonavir (Kaletra), nelfinavir (Viracept), ritonavir (Norvir), saquinavir (Fortovase, Invirase), tipranavir (Aptivus)
- Fusion inhibitors: Enfuvirtide (Fuzeon)
- Entry inhibitors: Maraviroc (Selzentry)
- Integrase inhibitors: Raltegravir (Isentress)
- Drug failure: Before selecting regimen, review clinical symptoms, history of HAART, and adherence. Perform resistance testing.
- Protease inhibitors can cause metabolic syndrome (lipodystrophy, decreased high-density lipoprotein, increased triglycerides, high BP, and hyperglycemia).
- HAART, especially the protease inhibitors, have potentially life-threatening interactions.

First Line

- NNRTI + 2 NNRTI (6)[A]
- PIs (preferably boosted with ritonavir) + 2 NRTI (6)[A]
- Integrase inhibitor + 2 NRTI (6)[A]

ADDITIONAL TREATMENT

General Measures

- Main goal of HAART: reduce the viral load, ideally to <50 HIV-1 RNA copies/mL), and delay immune suppression. Viral load is the most important indicator of response to HAART.
- An adequate CD4 response for most patients on therapy is defined as an increase in CD4 count in range of 50–150 cells/mm^3 per year with an accelerated response in the first 3 months (6).
- Prevent HIV-associated complications, short- and long-term adverse drug reactions, HIV transmission, HIV drug resistance, and preservation of HIV treatment options.
- Assess substance abuse, economic factors (e.g., unstable housing), social support, mental illness, comorbidities, high-risk behaviors, and other factors that are known to impair the ability to adhere to treatment and to promote HIV transmission.
- With prolonged use of HAART, virus may mutate; medication will be less effective, but resistant strains have more difficulty reproducing. (Medication is less effective than in a nonresistant patient.)
- Occupational exposure: Treatment after exposure in conjunction with expert consultation
- Prophylactic antimicrobial agents and vaccines:
  - *Pneumocystis jiroveci* (formerly *P. carinii*): TMP-SMX 1 DS daily or 1 SS daily indicated if CD4 <200/mm^3, prior PCP, thrush, or unexplained fever for >2 weeks
  - *Mycobacterium tuberculosis*: Treat if PPD >5 mm induration without prior prophylaxis or treatment, recent TB contact, or history of inadequately treated TB that healed. Confirmed by culture. Treatment is based on susceptibility.
  - *Toxoplasma gondii*: 33% per year risk of infection in untreated patients with CD4 <100/mm^3; prophylaxis: TMP-SMX DS daily.
  - *M. avium* complex: 20–40% risk with CD4 <50 and no HAART. Preferred prophylaxis is clarithromycin 500 mg PO b.i.d., or azithromycin 1,200 mg PO weekly.
  - Varicella: Seronegative and unexposed are at risk if exposed to chickenpox or shingles. Preferred regimen is VZIG 5 vials within 96 hours but preferably within 48 hours.
  - *Streptococcus pneumoniae*: 50–100 times increased risk of invasive infection compared with general population; Pneumovax every 5 years
  - Influenza vaccine each autumn
  - Hepatitis A and B vaccines for at-risk patients
  - Tetanus: dT vaccine in adults
  - Polio: Use *inactivated polio vaccine*, not oral polio vaccine, in children.

ONGOING CARE

FOLLOW-UP RECOMMENDATIONS

Patient Monitoring

- If HIV RNA is detectable at 2–8 weeks, repeat every 4–8 weeks until suppression to less than level of detection, then every 3–6 months (6)
- Monitor HIV RNA, CD4m and CBC every 3–4 months (6).
- Test fasting lipids and fasting glucose annually if normal. Basic chemistry, aspartate aminotransferase, alanine aminotransferase, T/D bilirubin every 6–12 months (6)
- HLA-B 5701 if considering abacavir (6)
- Pregnancy test if starting efavirenz (6)

DIET

- Encourage good nutrition and multivitamin use.
- Avoid raw eggs and unpasteurized milk. Severely immunocompromised patients should boil tap water to prevent *Cryptosporidium*.

PATIENT EDUCATION

- Provide nonjudgmental prevention counseling, reviewing routes and behaviors leading to transmission to others and acquisition of super infection with resistant strains.
- Counsel on importance of adherence to HAART and prevention of resistance.
- National AIDS Hotline: (800) 342-2437 [Spanish (800) 342-7432]
- National Institute of Health AIDS Clinical Trials Group: (800) 874-2572
- American Foundation for AIDS Research: (212) 719-0033 (new treatments and research)
- Information available at: www.aidsinfo.nih.gov

PROGNOSIS

- When untreated HIV infection leads to AIDS, the life expectancy is 3.7 years.
- AIDS-defining opportunistic infections usually do not develop until CD4 <200.
- In untreated HIV infection, CD4 counts decline at a rate of 50–80 per year, with more rapid decline as counts drop <200.
- Adherence failure—not drug resistance—is the most common cause of treatment failure (7)[B].

COMPLICATIONS

- Immunodeficiency
- Opportunistic infections
- Malignancy, including cervical or anal cancer

REFERENCES

1. Centers for Disease Control and Prevention (CDC). HIV prevalence estimates–United States, 2006. *MMWR Morb Mortal Wkly Rep*. 2008;57:1073–6.
2. Centers for Disease Control and Prevention: Diagnoses of HIV infection and AIDS in the United States and Dependent Areas, 2008 HIV Surveillance Report, Volume 2. Avialable at: www.cdc.gov/hiv/surveillance/resources/reports/2008report/ Page last updated: June 14, 2010.
3. Quinn TC, Wawer MJ, Sewankambo N, et al. Viral load and heterosexual transmission of human immunodeficiency virus type 1. Rakai Project Study Group. *N Engl J Med*. 2000;342:921–9.
4. US Public Health Service Task Force recommendations for use of antiretroviral drugs in pregnant HIV-1 infected women for maternal health interventions to reduce perinatal HIV-1 transmission in the US. *MMWR*. 2002;51:1–38.
5. Lama J, Planelles V. Host factors influencing susceptibility to HIV infection and AIDS progression. *Retrovirology*. 2007;4:52.
6. US Department of Health and Human Services. Guide for the Use of Antiretroviral Agents in HIV-1 Infected Adults and Adolescents. Available at: http://aidsinfo.nih.gov/guidelines/adult/AA_040705.
7. Simon V, Ho DD, Abdool Karim Q. HIV/AIDS epidemiology, pathogenesis, prevention, and treatment. *Lancet*. 2006;368:489–504.

CODES

ICD9

- 042 Human immunodeficiency virus (HIV) disease
- V08 Asymptomatic human immunodeficiency virus [HIV] infection status

CLINICAL PEARLS

- The symptoms of acute HIV infection include fever, sore throat, adenopathy, myalgias, and rash.
- Treatment guidelines are evolving to include earlier initiation of HAART in the course of the illness.
- The most common complications of HIV/AIDS are immunodeficiency, opportunistic infections, and malignancy.
- The prophylactic measures strongly recommended for HIV-infected patients are vaccination and prophylactic antibiotics based on history and CD4 count.

HODGKIN LYMPHOMA

Jennifer Gao, MD
Fred Schiffman, MD

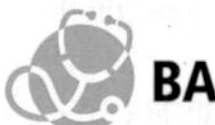

BASICS

DESCRIPTION

- Historical background:
  - Described in 1832 by Thomas Hodgkin in *On Some Morbid Appearance of the Absorbent Glands and Spleen*
  - First neoplasm to be: (i) Defined by cytological grounds based on presence of Reed-Sternberg cells, (ii) clinically staged neoplastic disease, and (iii) treated with chemotherapy and/or radiotherapy
- Neoplastic Reed-Sternberg (RS) cells of monoclonal lymphoid B-cell origin within inflammatory background of lymphocytes (T-helper type 2 and regulatory T-cells), eosinophils, histiocytes, and plasma cells (1)
- 2 subtypes: Classical Hodgkin's lymphoma (CHL, 95% of cases) and nodular lymphocyte predominant Hodgkin lymphoma (NLPHL, 5% of cases) (1):
  - NLPHL: B-cells, neoplastic LH cells with multilobulated nuclei, small nucleoli, and popcorn-like appearance
  - Classical Hodgkin lymphoma histologic subdivisions:
    - Nodular sclerosis (60%) Mixed cellularity (30%) Lymphocytic depletion (<10%) Lymphocytic rich (<10%)
- Frequency of lymph node involvement: Cervical > Mediastinal > Axillary > Para-aortic

EPIDEMIOLOGY

- 11.4% of all lymphomas in the US (2)
- Male > Female (1.4:1)
- Stage I/II at diagnosis: 50%
- Systemic symptoms: 25–40%
- Bone marrow involvement: 5%

Geriatric Considerations

- Poorer prognosis if present at ≥45 years (3):
  - Susceptibility to intensive therapy toxicities
  - Less likely to be included in clinical trials
  - Comorbidities affect toleration of standard treatment
- Benefit from doxorubicin in treatment regimen (3)

Pediatric Considerations

- Increased risk for males
- Young females (<30 years old) treated with thoracic radiation are at high risk for breast cancer (4):
  - Recommend early breast cancer screening

Pregnancy Considerations

- Abdominal ultrasonography to detect subdiaphragmatic disease (3)
- Treatment (3):
  - Delay until after delivery if asymptomatic and early-stage
  - ABVD safely used in second and third trimesters
  - Vinblastine monotherapy to control symptoms
  - First trimester: ABVD may or may not cause fetal malformations

Incidence

- 8,500 new cases in the US annually (5)
- Bimodal age distribution: Peak at 15–35 years and > 55 years (5)

RISK FACTORS

- Immunodeficiency (inherited or acquired)
- Autoimmune disorders
- EBV (6)
- Seasonal factors (6)

Genetics

- First-degree relative: 3–9× risk (6)
- Siblings of younger patients: 7× risk
- Weak correlation between familial HL and HLA class I regions containing HLA A1, B5, B8, B18 alleles (6)

ETIOLOGY

- Exact etiology unclear
- RS cells likely derived from germinal center B cells with mutations in immunoglobulin variable chain
- Seasonal features and higher frequencies with EBV suggest environmental factors (6)
- T-lymphocyte defects persist even after successful treatment

COMMONLY ASSOCIATED CONDITIONS

In HIV (3):

- AIDS-defining illness
- Predominantly mixed-cellularity or lymphocyte-depleted histologic subtypes
- At diagnosis: Widespread disease, extranodal involvement, systemic symptoms

DIAGNOSIS

HISTORY

- Asymptomatic lymphadenopathy (cervical or supraclavicular)
- Pel-Ebstein fever
- Night sweats
- Weight loss
- Fatigue
- Anorexia
- Alcohol-induced pain
- Pruritus
- Performance status

PHYSICAL EXAM

Palpate lymph nodes, spleen, and liver

DIAGNOSTIC TESTS & INTERPRETATION

Lab

Initial lab tests

- CBC
- Chemistry profile
- ESR
- Liver function tests
- Renal function tests
- HIV
- Hepatitis serology
- Pregnancy test (women of child-bearing age)
- Pulmonary function tests (diffusion capacity of the lung for carbon monoxide for ABVD or BEACOPP) (7)
- Drugs that may alter lab results: phenytoin may produce pseudolymphoma

Follow-Up & Special Considerations

- Fertility considerations (7):
  - Semen cryopreservation if chemotherapy or pelvic radiation therapy
  - In vitro fertilization or ovarian tissue/oocyte cryopreservation
- Radiation therapy (RT) considerations (7):
  - Splenic RT: pneumococcal, *H. flu*, meningococcal vaccines
  - Neck RT: Neck CT

Imaging

- Chest radiograph (7)
- Diagnostic CT scan of chest, abdomen, and pelvis (7)
- Positron emission tomography (PET) scan (for initial staging, midtreatment decision making, and end-of-treatment evaluation)
- Bone scan, gallium scan, abdominal US

Diagnostic Procedures/Surgery

- Excisional lymph node biopsy (7)
- Core needle biopsy (if diagnostic) (7)
- Immunohistochemistry (7)
- Bone marrow biopsy
- Liver biopsy (in selected cases)

Pathological Findings

Reed-Sternberg cell characteristics (7):

- Diameter: 20–50 micrometers
- Abundant acidophilic cytoplasm
- Bi- or polylobulated nucleus
- Acidophilic nucleoli
- CD30+, CD15+, CD45 negative, CD3 negative, CD20+ in 40% of cases
- RS cells necessary but not sufficient for diagnosis (need inflammatory background)

DIFFERENTIAL DIAGNOSIS

Non-Hodgkin's lymphoma, infectious lymphadenopathy, solid tumor metastases, sarcoidosis, autoimmune disease, AIDS/HIV, drug reaction

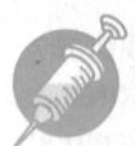

TREATMENT

- Ann Arbor staging with Cotswold modification: Needed to determine treatment modality (7):
  - Stage I: Single lymph node group - subscript E = extralymphatic organ or site involvement
  - Stage II: ≥2 node groups on the same side of the diaphragm - subscript E = extralymphatic organ or site involvement
  - Stage III: Node groups on both sides of the diaphragm - subscript E = extralymphatic organ or site involvement, subscript S = splenic involvement
  - Stage IV: Dissemination involving extranodal organs (except the spleen, which is considered lymphoid tissue)
  - Subclasses: A = no systemic symptoms; B = systemic symptoms (fever, night sweats, weight loss >10% body weight); X = bulky disease (widened mediastinum, >1/3 intrathoracic diameter, or >10-cm nodal mass)
  - Pathologic stage at given site denoted by superscript: M = bone marrow, H = liver, L = lung, O = bone, P = pleura, D = skin):
    - Splenectomy, liver biopsy, lymph node biopsy, bone marrow biopsy mandatory for pathological staging
- Treatment modalities: Radiation therapy and chemotherapy alone, or combined (5):
  - Early stages (favorable prognosis): Lower radiation doses and smaller fields, 2–4 chemotherapy cycles (8)[A]

- Early stages (unfavorable prognosis): Moderate chemotherapy (4–6 cycles) plus involved field radiation therapy (IFRT)
  - Advanced stages: Extensive chemotherapy (6–8 cycles) with or without RT
- Autologous bone marrow transplant: If fail conventional therapy
- Goal: Aim for cure
- All subsequent treatment and follow-up care recommendations based on National Comprehensive Caner Network (NCCN) consensus. Please refer to NCCN Practice Guidelines in Oncology for Hodgkin's Lymphoma (7).

MEDICATION

First Line

- ABVD chemotherapy: doxorubicin, bleomycin, vinblastine, dacarbazine (9):
  - Lower risk of secondary malignancy than with MOPP or MOPP/ABV
- Stanford V chemotherapy: doxorubicin, vinblastine, mechlorethamine, etoposide, vincristine, bleomycin, prednisone (9)

ALERT

- Must be monitored by experienced oncologist
- Contraindications: General for chemotherapy
- Precautions: Chemotherapy toxicity, bone marrow suppression:
  - Dacarbazine: Highly emetic, severe phlebitis
  - Bleomycin: Risk of pulmonary toxicity, death
  - Consider evaluating ejection fraction in doxorubicin regimens (7).

Second Line

- BEACOPP: Bleomycin, etoposide, doxorubicin, cyclophosphamide, vincristine, procarbazine, prednisone, G-CSF (5)
- Second-line chemotherapy: consider relapse pattern and previous regimens (7):
  - ICE: Ifosfamide, carboplatin, etoposide
  - C-MOPP: Cyclophosphamide, vincristine, procarbazine, prednisone
  - GVD: Gemcitabine, vinorelbine, pegylated liposomal doxorubicin
  - IGEV: Ifosfamide, gemcitabine, vinorelbine
- Stem cell transplant in progressive disease or relapse (7):
  - High-dose therapy and autologous stem cell transplant (HDT/ASCT): Improved event-free and progression-free survival compared with conventional chemotherapy
  - HDT/ASCT does not improve overall survival
- Rituximab: Excellent activity against lymphocyte-predominant variant due to CD20+ lymphocytes

ADDITIONAL TREATMENT

- Combined chemotherapy and radiation (7):
  - Bulky disease all stages: ABVD or Stanford V
  - Nonbulky disease stage I–II: ABVD or Stanford V
  - Nonbulky disease stage IB–IIB: BEACOPP
  - Bulky and Nonbulky disease stage III–IV: BEACOPP
- Radiation therapy alone: Uncommon except if lymphocyte-predominant (7):
  - Avoid high cervical regions and axillae (women only)

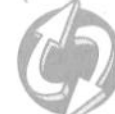

ONGOING CARE

FOLLOW-UP RECOMMENDATIONS

Patient Monitoring

- During therapy: CBC, nutrition, and hydration
- Restage with PET after 2–4 cycles of chemotherapy: Sensitive prognostic indicator (7)
- Posttreatment monitoring (7):
  - H&P: q2–4mo for first 2 years, then q3–6mo for next 3–5 years
  - Laboratory studies:
    - CBC, platelets, ESR, chemistry profile q2–4mo for 1–2 years, then q3–6mo for next 3–5 years
    - TSH annually if radiation to neck
  - Imaging:
    - Chest: Chest x-ray or CT q6–12mo during first 2–5 years
    - Abdominal/pelvic: CT q6–12mo during first 2–3 years
    - Annual breast mammogram or MRI beginning 8–10 years after therapy or at age of 40 years if chest or axillary irradiation
    - Surveillance PET should not be done routinely due to risk of false positives

PATIENT EDUCATION

- Reproductive impact
- Risks of secondary malignancy
- Oral and dental care during therapy
- Leukemia Society of America (www.lls.org)

PROGNOSIS

- Cure rate for classical Hodgkin lymphoma: 80% (2)
- Relapse or progression of disease rate: 5–20% (6)
- Overall survival rates (10):
  - 1-year survival: 92%
  - 5-year survival: 85%
  - 10-year survival: 81%
- International Prognostic Score for advanced disease (7):
  - Age ≥45 years
  - Male gender
  - Albumin <4 g/dL
  - Hemoglobin <10.5 g/dL
  - Lymphocytopenia: <600 lymphocyte cells/dL or lymphocytes <8% of WBC
  - WBC ≥15,000 cells/dL
  - Stage IV disease
- Main cause of death (10):
  - Initial 5 years: Hodgkin lymphoma
  - After 5–10 years: Leukemia, myelodysplastic syndrome
  - After 20 years: Second primary malignancy, cardiovascular disease (5)

COMPLICATIONS

- General: Chronic fatigue (10)
- Hematologic: Secondary malignancies, bone marrow suppression, anemia, ITP, TTP (10)
- Reproductive: Sterility, gonadal dysfunction, amenorrhea (10)
- Endocrine: Hypothyroidism (10)
- Infectious: Immunosuppressed infections including herpes zoster, overwhelming sepsis in asplenic patients
- Cardiac: Coronary artery disease, cardiomyopathy, valvular disease, pericardial disease (4)
- Pulmonary: Radiation pneumonitis, pulmonary fibrosis, chronic pleural effusion (5)
- Neurologic: Transient radiation myelopathy (Lhermitte sign)
- Oncologic: Cancers of the breast, cervix, colon, rectum, lung, bone and soft tissue, multiple myeloma, non-Hodgkin lymphoma, acute myelogenous leukemia (4,5)

REFERENCES

1. World Health Organization. *Cumulative Official Updates to ICD-10*. February 2010.
2. Jona A, Younes A. Novel treatment strategies for patients with relapsed classical Hodgkin lymphoma. *Blood Rev*. 2010;24:233–8.
3. Armitage JO. Early-stage Hodgkin's lymphoma. *N Engl J Med*. 2010;363:7.
4. Hodgson D, Grunfeld E, Gunraj N, et al. A population-based study of follow-up care for Hodgkin lymphoma survivors. *Cancer*. 2010: 3417–25.
5. Baxi SS, Matasar MJ. State-of-the-art issues in Hodgkin's lymphoma survivorship. *Curr Oncol Rep*. 2010;12:366–73.
6. Gascoyne Randy, Rosenwald A, Poppema S, et al. Prognostic markers in malignant lymphomas. *Leuk Lymphoma*. 2010; Early Online, 1–9.
7. NCCN Clinical Practice Guidelines in Oncology. *Hodgkin Lymphoma*. Version 2.2010. Available at: www.nccn.org.
8. Herbst C, Rehan FA, Skoetz N, et al. Chemotherapy alone versus chemotherapy plus radiotherapy for early stage Hodgkin lymphoma. *Cochrane Database Syst Rev*. 2011;CD007110.
9. Edwards-Bennett S, et al. Stanford V program for locally extensive and advanced Hodgkin lymphoma: The Memorial Sloan-Kettering Cancer Center experience. *Ann Oncol*. 2010;21: 574–81.
10. Czuczman M, Straus D, Gribben J, et al. Management options, survivorship, and emerging treatment strategies for follicular and Hodgkin lymphomas. *Leuk Lymphoma*. 2010;51(1):41–9.

CODES

ICD9

- 201.90 Hodgkin's disease, unspecified type, unspecified site
- 201.91 Hodgkin's disease, unspecified type, involving lymph nodes of head, face, and neck
- 201.92 Hodgkin's disease, unspecified type, involving intrathoracic lymph nodes

CLINICAL PEARLS

- Lymphoma with neoplastic Reed-Sternberg cells (monoclonal lymphoid B-cell) and inflammatory lymphocytes, eosinophils, histiocytes, and plasma cells
- Bimodal age distribution: Peak at 15–35 years and >55 years (prognosis worsens with age)
- Cure rate 80%, secondary malignancies common due to chemotherapy and radiation exposure

H

HOMELESSNESS

Dana Sprute, MD, MPH

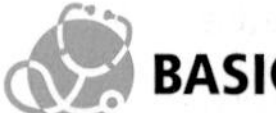

BASICS

DESCRIPTION

Federal definition: "Homeless" or "homeless individual or homeless person" includes: (i) An individual who lacks a fixed, regular, and adequate nighttime residence; and (ii) an individual who has a primary nighttime residence that is: (a) A supervised publicly or privately operated shelter designed to provide temporary living accommodations (including welfare hotels, congregate shelters, and transitional housing for the mentally ill); (b) an institution that provides a temporary residence for individuals intended to be institutionalized; (c) a public or private place not designed for, or ordinarily used as, a regular sleeping accommodation for human beings.

EPIDEMIOLOGY

Prevalence

3.5 million people in the US experience homelessness each year; 40% are homeless families (1):

- Since 2009, 1.2% increase in number of homeless families, 1.6% increase in homeless persons in a family, 1% decrease in number who are chronically homeless (1).

RISK FACTORS

- Social factors:
  - Poverty: Increase in US rates in the past 25 years:
    - 2011 federal poverty definition: $22,350 annual income for 4-person household (2)
    - 2 major contributors: Unemployment/eroding employment opportunities and decreasing availability of public assistance
    - In 2009, 14.3% of the US population fell below federal poverty definition; highest poverty rate since 1994. Children overrepresented in homeless population (children are 35.5% of people living in poverty, but only 24.5% of total population) (3).
  - Lack of affordable housing: Fall in federal support by 49% between 1980 and 2003
  - Increase in home foreclosures: 32% increase between April 2008 and April 2009 (4):
    - 10% become homeless as a result of foreclosure.
    - 49% report medical problems played role in foreclosure.
  - Unemployment: 9.2% official unemployment rate in the US, June 2011 (US Bureau of Labor Statistics, July 8, 2011)
  - Lack of affordable health care: 2009:
    - 50.7 million people in US without health insurance (3)
    - Source of insurance change: Private (63.9%) and employer (55.8%) based health insurance decreasing; rates of government insurance increasing (30.6%) (3)
- Domestic violence: 63% of homeless women experience domestic violence (2).
- Addiction disorders: 2/3 of homeless individuals report alcohol and/or drug use as a major factor contributing to homelessness; they face barriers to obtaining health care, including addiction treatment and support services (2).
- Psychiatric illness: 16% of single homeless adults suffer from persistent mental illness (2).
- At risk: Domestic violence; youth; veterans; rural; victims of violence
- Fundamental issues in homelessness and health care that require ongoing consideration:
  - Unstable housing; limited access to nutritious food and water; lack of transportation
  - Higher risk for abuse
  - Physical/cognitive impairments; behavioral health problems
  - Developmental discrepancies for children: Speech delay, chronic ear infection, insufficient opportunity to practice gross and fine motor skills
  - Higher risk for communicable disease
  - Lack of health insurance/resources; discontinuous/inaccessible health care; lack of a medical home; barriers to disability assistance
  - Cultural/linguistic barriers: Racial and ethnic groups overrepresented in homeless population
  - Limited education/literacy
  - Lack of social supports: Alienation from family and friends precipitates homelessness.
  - Criminalization of homelessness: Frequent arrests for loitering, sleeping in public places

GENERAL PREVENTION

- American Recovery and Reinvestment Act (ARRA), 2009: New/expanded programs to address homelessness and hunger. Provides support for: (i) Emergency Food and Shelter Program, (ii) Emergency Food Assistance Program, (iii) Neighborhood Stabilization Program, (iv) Homeless Prevention and Rapid Rehousing Program (5)
- Social Justice Policy Recommendations: Permanent affordable housing, foreclosure and homelessness prevention, increased funds for HUD McKinney-Vento programs (emergency, transitional, and permanent housing), rural homeless assistance, universal health care, universal livable income, employment/workforce services, prevention of hate crimes against the homeless, decriminalization of homelessness (6)

COMMONLY ASSOCIATED CONDITIONS

- Hunger: In 2009, 26% increase in demand for assistance (largest average increase since 1991) (5)
- Medical conditions:
  - Heart, lung, liver, renal disease, diabetes, HTN, cancer, pneumonia (2)
  - Infectious diseases:
    - Tuberculosis, HIV/AIDS, STIs (2)
    - Skin/nail infections (cellulitis, fungal infection) and infestation (lice and scabies)
    - Liver disease (e.g., hepatitis B or C, or alcohol-related)
  - Cognitive impairment: Traumatic brain injury, CVA, substance use
  - Dental problems (e.g., caries, periodontal disease)
  - Exposure-related conditions (frostbite, heatstroke) (2)
- Psychiatric illness (2)
- Traumatic injury: Increased risk of assault; victims of hate crimes (7)
- Criminalization of homelessness

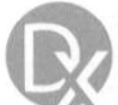

DIAGNOSIS

HISTORY

- Living conditions: Location, access to food, restrooms, place to store medicines, safety
- Prior homelessness: What precipitated it, first time, chronic
- Acute/chronic illness: Individual/family history of RAD, chronic otitis media, anemia, diabetes, CVD, TB, HIV/STIs, hospitalizations
- Family members, especially dependent children
- Medications: Current, psychiatric, contraception, OTC meds, dietary supplements, meds "borrowed" from others
- Prior providers: Oral health, primary care, current medical home
- Mental illness/cognitive deficit: Stress, anxiety, appetite, sleep, concentration, mood, speech, memory, thought process and content, suicidal/homicidal ideation, insight, judgment, impulse control, social interactions; symptoms of brain injury (headaches, seizures, memory loss, lability, irritability, dizziness, insomnia, poor organizational/decision making skills)
- Alcohol/nicotine/other drug use: Amount, frequency, duration; look for signs of substance abuse/dependence
- Sexual: Gender identity/orientation, behaviors, rape, pregnancies, hepatitis, HIV, other STIs
- Abuse: History or current abuse; emotional, physical, sexual; patient safety
- Legal problems/violence: Against persons/property, history of incarceration
- Regular/strenuous activities: Routines (treatment feasibility); level of strenuous activity
- Work history: Previous types of jobs, length held, veteran status, occupation injuries/toxic exposures; vocational skills, interest
- Education level/literacy: Highest level of education; ever in special education; assess ability to read/language skills/English fluency
- Nutrition/hydration: Diet, food resources, preparation skills, liquid intake
- Cultural heritage/affiliations: Family, friends, faith community, other sources of support
- Strengths: Coping skills, resourcefulness, abilities, interests

PHYSICAL EXAM

- Comprehensive exam: Height/weight, BMI, especially: Liver, dermatologic, oral, feet, neurologic, mental status
- Focused exams: For patients uncomfortable with full-body, unclothed exam at first visit
- Dental assessment: Age-appropriate teeth, obvious caries, dental/referred pain, diabetes

DIAGNOSTIC TESTS & INTERPRETATION

- Mental health: Patient Health Questionnaire (PHQ-9, PHQ-2), MHS-III, MDQ
- Cognitive assessment: Mini-Mental Status Exam (MMSE), Traumatic Brain Injury Questionnaire (TBIQ), Repeatable Battery for the Assessment of Neuro-Psychological Status (RBANS)

- Developmental assessment: Ages & Stages Questionnaires, Parents' Evaluation of Developmental Status (PEDS), Denver II or other standard screening tool
- Interpersonal violence: Domestic violence, rape, etc.
- Forensic evaluation: If strong evidence of abuse

Lab

- Baseline labs: EKG, lipid, electrolytes, BUN/creatinine levels, CBC, liver function tests, HIV, RPR
- PPD
- STI screening
- Substance abuse: SSI-AOD, urine drug screen

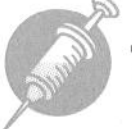

TREATMENT

- Establish rapport: Sensitivity to prior negative prior health care experiences
- Enlist resources: Mental health and substance abuse programs, free clinics, case management
- Health care maintenance: vaccinations (hepatitis A and B, pneumovax, TdaP, influenza) cancer and chronic disease screening for adults; EPSDT screening and vaccinations for children (8)
- Plan of care:
  - Basic needs: Food, clothing, housing may be higher priorities than health care.
  - Patient goals and priorities: Immediate/long-term health needs. Address patient wants first.
  - Action plan: Simple language, portable pocket card
  - After hours: Extended clinic hours
  - Safety plan: For violence and abuse suspected; mandatory reporting requirements
  - Emergency plan: Location of nearest ED, preparation for evacuation
  - Adherence plan: Use of interpreter, identification of potential barriers

MEDICATION

- Simple regimen: Low pill count, once-daily dosing if possible
- Dispensing: On site; small amounts at a time to promote follow-up, decrease risk of loss/theft/misuse. Determine resources for written prescriptions.
- Storage of medications: If no access to refrigeration, no prescription for meds requiring it
- Patient assistance: Free/low-cost drugs if readily available for continuous use
- Aids to adherence: Harm reduction, outreach/case management, directly observed therapy
- Side effects: Primary reason for nonadherence (diarrhea, polyuria, nausea, disorientation)
- Analgesia/symptomatic treatment: Contract, single provider for pain medication refills
- Dietary supplements: Multivitamins with minerals, nutritional supplements
- Managed care: Generics if possible, assistance getting prescription filled
- Lab monitoring: Monitor patients on antipsychotic medications for metabolic disorders.

ADDITIONAL TREATMENT

- Associated problems/complications:
  - No place to heal: Efficacy of medical respite/recuperative care, supportive housing
  - Fragmented care: Multiple providers. Use EMR; list prescribed meds on wallet-sized card.
  - Masked symptoms/misdiagnosis: e.g., weight loss, dementia, edema, lactic acidosis
  - Developmental discrepancies: Focus on immediate concerns, not possible future consequences.
  - Dual diagnoses: Integrated treatment for concurrent mental illness/substance use disorders
  - Loss of child custody: Support for parent of child abused by others and for abused parent
- Follow-up:
  - Contact info: Phone, reliable mail address, e-mail for patient/friend/family/case manager
  - Frequency: More frequent follow-up, incentives, nonjudgmental care regardless of adherence
  - Drop-in system: Anticipate/accommodate unscheduled clinic visits.
  - Transportation assistance: Provide car fare, tokens, help with transportation services.
  - Monitor school attendance: Address health/developmental problems with family/school.

IN-PATIENT CONSIDERATIONS

Admission Criteria

People who are homeless may be more likely to benefit from admission because:

- Living conditions are suboptimal.
- They have medical and psychiatric and/or substance use disorders.

Discharge Criteria

- Discharge treatment plans should be evaluated for feasibility.
- Bed rest, extended periods of elevation, rest, or icing are not feasible in most instances.
- Plans requiring multiple return visits are likely to fail if no support or return transportation.
- Attempt to assist patients who are amenable to treatment for drug, alcohol, nicotine abuse.
- Admission to inpatient rehabilitation if appropriate and possible

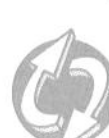

ONGOING CARE

FOLLOW-UP RECOMMENDATIONS

- Patients with a history of nonadherence need additional support (e.g., case manager, outreach) to succeed in ongoing care after hospital discharge.
- Limited access to telephones to schedule appointments, and may be unable to receive telephone messages with test results or rescheduled appointment times.
- Arrange appointments prior to discharge.
- Document the best way to contact the individual.
- Refer to a health care agency designed to address the needs of people who are homeless with integrated mental health, physical health, and substance use treatment.

PROGNOSIS

Mortality rates for chronically homeless adults are 4 times higher than the general population. Average life expectancy of homeless population is 42–52 years compared to 78 years for the general population (9).

REFERENCES

1. The 2010 Annual Homeless Assessment Report to Congress, U.S. Department of Housing and Urban Development, Office of Community Planning and Development.
2. www.nationalhomeless.org/factsheets/why.html, June 2009.
3. Income Poverty, and Health Insurance Coverage in the United States: 2009; issued September 2010. www.census.gov/prod/2010pubs/p60-238.pdf.
4. Foreclosure to Homelessness 2009: The Forgotten Victims of the Subprime Crisis, June 2009. www.nationalhomeless.org/advocacy/ForeclosuretoHomelessness0609.pdf.
5. The United States Conference of Mayors. Hungar and Homelessness Survey: A Status Report on Hunger and Homelessness in America's Cities, A 27-City Survey, December 2009. www. usmayors.org/pressreleases/uploads/USCMHungercompleteWEB2009.pdf.
6. Summary of Public Policy Recommendations, National Coalition for the Homeless, January 22, 2010. www.nationalhomeless.org.
7. Hate, Violence and Death on Main Street USA: A Report on Hate Crimes and Violence Against People Experiencing Homelessness in 2008. www.nationalhomeless.org/publications/hatecrimes/index.html.
8. Badiaga S, Raoult D, Brouqui P. Preventing and controlling emerging and reemerging transmissible diseases in the homeless. *Emerg Infect Dis*. 2008; 14:1353–9.
9. O'Connell JJ. *Premature Mortality in Homeless Populations: A Review of the Literature*. Nashville: National Health Care for Homeless Council, Inc.; 2005.

ADDITIONAL READING

Chronic Homelessness Policy Solutions, Chronic Homelessness Brief, March 2010. National Alliance to End Homelessness. www.endhomelessness.org.

CODES

ICD9

- V60.0 Lack of housing
- V60.1 Inadequate housing
- V60.89 Other specified housing or economic circumstances

CLINICAL PEARLS

- Stress related to difficulty meeting basic needs can interfere with engagement in health care.
- Assistance in gaining access to benefits or meeting basic needs may improve therapeutic relationship and allow individual to direct attention to physical health.
- Ending homelessness requires permanent housing with supportive services and implementing policies to prevent chronic homelessness. (www.endhomelessness.org/content/article/detail/1623). National Alliance to End Homelessness, January 2010.

H

HORDEOLUM (STYE)

Konstantinos E. Deligiannidis, MD, MPH
Alexandra A. Schultes, MD

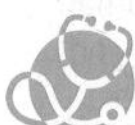

BASICS

DESCRIPTION
- An acute inflammation or infection of the eyelid margin involving the sebaceous gland of an eyelash (external hordeolum) or a meibomian gland (internal hordeolum)
- System(s) affected: Skin/Exocrine
- Synonym(s): Internal hordeolum; External hordeolum; Zeisian stye; Meibomian stye; Stye

EPIDEMIOLOGY
- Predominant age: None
- Predominant sex: Male = Female

Incidence
Unknown: Although external hordeolum is common, internal hordeolum is rare.

RISK FACTORS
- Poor eyelid hygiene
- Previous hordeolum
- Contact lens wearers
- Application of makeup
- Predisposing blepharitis (low-grade infections of the eyelid margin)
- Ocular rosacea

Genetics
No known genetic pattern

GENERAL PREVENTION
Eyelid hygiene

PATHOPHYSIOLOGY
- Bacterial infection of sebaceous or meibomian glands, causing an acute inflammatory reaction
- In an internal hordeolum, the meibomian gland may become obstructed, leading to a pustule on the conjunctival surface as opposed to the margin of the eyelid (1).

ETIOLOGY
- Most commonly caused by *Staphylococcus aureus* (~90–95% of all cases) or by *Staphylococcus epidermidis*.
- Seborrhea can predispose to infections of the eyelid.

COMMONLY ASSOCIATED CONDITIONS
- Acne
- Seborrhea
- An association may exist between hordeolum during childhood and developing rosacea in adulthood (2).

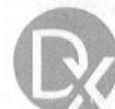

DIAGNOSIS

HISTORY
- Localized inflammation (vs. involvement of the entire eyelid or surrounding skin)
- Foreign body sensation in the eye
- Prior episodes are common.

PHYSICAL EXAM
- Localized inflammation of the eyelashes or a small pustule at the margin of the eyelid
- Localized swelling and tenderness on the internal or external aspect of the eyelid with an opening to either side
- To determine if an internal hordeolum is obstructed, the eyelid should be gently everted to examine for a pustule on the tarsal conjunctiva (1).
- Itching or scaling of the eyelids; collection of discharge, redness, and irritation leading to localized tenderness and pain

DIAGNOSTIC TESTS & INTERPRETATION

Lab
Culture of the eyelid margins usually is not necessary.

Diagnostic Procedures/Surgery
History and eye exam

Pathological Findings
Bacterial contamination and white cells in eyelid discharge

DIFFERENTIAL DIAGNOSIS
- Chalazion
- Blepharitis
- Eyelid neoplasms
- Periorbital cellulitis
- Dacryocystitis

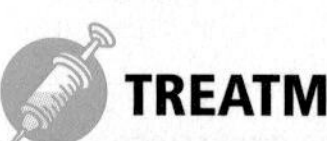

TREATMENT

MEDICATION

First Line
- Usually, a hordeolum spontaneously drains, aided by warm compresses to the area.
- Erythromycin ophthalmic 0.5% ointment, apply up to 6 times per day for 7–10 days
- Treat underlying dry eye with artificial tears.

Second Line
- Occasionally, the use of an aminoglycoside ophthalmic ointment, such as gentamicin or tobramycin, may be necessary if condition is refractory to simpler treatment.
- Oral dicloxacillin or cephalexin for 2 weeks if refractory to topical antibiotics

ADDITIONAL TREATMENT

General Measures
- The hordeolum should not be expressed.
- Warm compresses to the area of inflammation can help increase blood supply and encourage spontaneous drainage.
- Application of an antibiotic ointment (such as erythromycin) to the margin of the eyelid after proper cleansing (except in children <12 years old, in whom there is a risk of blurred vision and amblyopia) helps reduce bacterial proliferation.
- Good personal hygiene with attention to cleansing the eyelids on a daily basis to prevent recurrent infections

Issues for Referral
Consider referral if unresponsive to oral antibiotics.

COMPLEMENTARY AND ALTERNATIVE MEDICINE

Broncasma berna is a polyvalent antigen vaccine that may be useful in the treatment of recurrent hordeolum (3).

SURGERY/OTHER PROCEDURES

- If the infection becomes localized to a single gland, incision, drainage, or curettage sometimes is necessary. This is an in-office procedure with a local anesthetic:
  - Exercise caution because ocular perforation has been reported with the injection of an anesthetic to an infected lid (4)[C].
- The use of combined antibiotic ointment (neomycin sulfate, polymyxin B sulfate, and gramicidin) after surgery was not shown to have any statistically significant difference to artificial tears (5)[B].

IN-PATIENT CONSIDERATIONS

Initial Stabilization

Outpatient

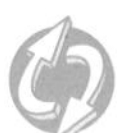

ONGOING CARE

FOLLOW-UP RECOMMENDATIONS

No restrictions

Patient Monitoring

The patient should be seen within several weeks to assess the effectiveness of therapy or should at least call the physician's office with a progress report.

DIET

No special diet

PATIENT EDUCATION

- The patient should be instructed in proper cleansing of the eyelids using a solution of tap water and baby shampoo or a commercially prepared hypoallergenic cleanser.
- The stye should not be squeezed or incised.

PROGNOSIS

- Usually responds well to good hygiene and warm compresses
- The inflammation usually improves within a week.
- Hordeolum tends to recur in some patients.

COMPLICATIONS

An internal hordeolum, if untreated, may lead to infections of adjacent glands and generalized cellulitis of the lid.

REFERENCES

1. Wald ER. Periorbital and orbital infections. *Infect Dis Clin North Am*. 2007;21:393–408, vi.
2. Bamford JT, Gessert CE, Renier CM, et al. Childhood stye and adult rosacea. *J Am Acad Dermatol*. 2006;55:951–5.
3. Nakatani M. Treatment of recurrent hordeolum with Broncasma Berna. *Eye*. 1999;13(Pt 5):692.
4. Kim JH, Yang SM, Kim HM, et al. Inadvertent ocular perforation during lid anesthesia for hordeolum removal. *Korean J Opththalmol*. 2006;20(3): 199–200.
5. Hirunwiwatkul P, Wachirasereechai K. Effectiveness of combined antibiotic ophthalmic solution in the treatment of hordeolum after incision and curettage: A randomized, placebo-controlled trial: a pilot study. *J Med Assoc Thai*. 2005;88:647–50.

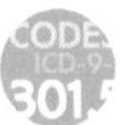

CODES

ICD9

- 373.11 Hordeolum externum
- 373.12 Hordeolum internum
- 373.13 Abscess of eyelid

CLINICAL PEARLS

- The hordeolum should not be expressed.
- Warm compresses to the area of inflammation can encourage spontaneous drainage.
- Application of an antibiotic ointment (such as erythromycin) to the margin of the eyelid after proper cleansing (except in children <12 years old, in whom there is a risk of blurred vision and amblyopia) helps reduce bacterial proliferation.
- Good personal hygiene with attention to cleansing the eyelids on a daily basis can prevent recurrent infections.

H

HORNER SYNDROME

Sana Syed, MD
Martina Vendrame, MD, PhD

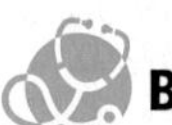

BASICS

DESCRIPTION

- Horner syndrome is caused by the interruption of sympathetic nerve supply to the eye, resulting in a classic triad of miosis, eyelid ptosis, and/or absence or decrease of sweating of the ipsilateral face and neck (hypohidrosis), with heterochromia in the pediatric population:
  – Central or preganglionic lesion (complete syndrome): First- or second-order neuron
  – Peripheral postganglionic lesion (incomplete syndrome, no anhydrosis): Third-order neuron
- System(s) affected: Nervous; Skin/Exocrine
- Synonym(s): Bernard-Horner syndrome; Bernard syndrome; Cervical sympathetic syndrome; oculosympathetic syndrome; Oculosympathetic paralysis; Oculosympathetic deficiency

EPIDEMIOLOGY

- Predominant age: None
- Predominant sex: Male = Female

Incidence

Unknown

Prevalence

Unknown

RISK FACTORS

- Most common: Apical bronchogenic carcinoma (Pancoast tumor) in smokers
- Aneurysm of the carotid or subclavian artery
- Injuries to the carotid artery high in the neck
- Dissection of the carotid arteries
- Carotid artery occlusion:
  – ~15% of patients with carotid artery occlusion develop ipsilateral Horner syndrome.
  – May occur without evidence of cerebral ischemia, neck injuries, or operative procedures
- Cluster headaches:
  – ~20% have an ipsilateral Horner syndrome

Genetics

Rare autosomal-dominant inheritance

PATHOPHYSIOLOGY

- Constellation of signs produced when sympathetic innervation to the eye is interrupted somewhere along the 3-neuron arc:
  – Absence of innervation of iris dilator and Müeller muscles leads to miosis and slight ptosis, respectively.
  – Sympathetic innervation also controls sweat glands; interruption causes anhydrosis.
- Sympathetic nerve fibers originate in the hypothalamus and travel down the lateral part of the brainstem to exit in the thoracic area. These fibers synapse in the cervical sympathetic ganglia (C8-T2, also called ciliospinal center of budge), and the postganglionic fibers travel to the eye along the wall of the carotid and ophthalmic arteries.
- Sympathetic fibers innervating sweat glands and vasodilatory muscles branch off before the cervical sympathetic ganglion traveling along the external carotid artery, so distal lesions will not result in anhydrosis.
- Lesions anywhere along this pathway will lead to ipsilateral Horner syndrome.

ETIOLOGY

- Idiopathic (40%), congenital, or acquired
- Best classified by which order neuron is affected and by age (pediatric vs. adult)
- First-order neuron (13%): Hypothalamus to cervical spinal cord (C8–T2):
  – Arnold-Chiari malformation
  – Basal meningitis (e.g., syphilis)
  – Basal skull tumors:
    ○ Cerebral vascular accident
    ○ Lateral medullary (Wallenberg) syndrome
  – Demyelinating disease (multiple sclerosis)
  – Intrapontine hemorrhage
  – Neck trauma
  – Pituitary tumor
  – Syringomyelia
- Second-order neuron (44%): Ascends with sympathetic trunk through brachial plexus over apex of lung to superior cervical ganglion (near common carotid artery bifurcation):
  – Pancoast tumor or infection of lung apex
  – Cervical rib
  – Aneurysm/dissection of aorta
  – Subclavian or common carotid artery
  – Central venous catheterization
  – Trauma/surgical injury
  – Chest tubes
  – Lymphadenopathy (Hodgkin, leukemia, tuberculosis, mediastinal tumors, sarcoid)
  – Mandibular tooth abscess
  – Lesions of the middle ear (acute otitis media)
- Third-order neuron lesions (43%): Ascends along adventitia of internal carotid artery through cavernous sinus close to the cranial nerve [CN] VI and then joins CN V_1 to innervate the iris dilator muscle and Müeller muscle in the eye:
  – Internal carotid artery dissection
  – Raeder syndrome (paratrigeminal syndrome)
  – Carotid cavernous fistula or other pathology
  – Cluster/migraine headaches
  – Herpes zoster
- Drugs: Acetophenazine, alseroxylon, bupivacaine, butaperazine, carphenazine, chloroprocaine, deserpidine, diacetylmorphine, diethazine, ethopropazine, etidocaine, guanethidine, influenza virus vaccine, levodopa, lidocaine, mepivacaine, mesoridazine, methdilazine, methotrimeprazine, oral contraceptives, perazine, prilocaine, procaine, prochlorperazine, promazine, propoxycaine, reserpine, thioproperazine, thioridazine, trifluoperazine

Pediatric Considerations

Most common etiology: Birth trauma to brachial plexus, chest surgery, neuroblastoma (paraspinal), and vascular anomalies of the carotid arteries

COMMONLY ASSOCIATED CONDITIONS

- Wallenberg syndrome
- Pancoast tumor
- C8 radiculopathy

DIAGNOSIS

HISTORY

- Ptosis (typically mild; 1–2 mm)
- Miosis (with an associated dilation lag)
- Anhydrosis or hypohidrosis (often not appreciated by patients or clinicians):
  – Ipsilateral side of the body: Central (first-order neuron)
  – Ipsilateral face: Preganglionic (second-order neuron)
  – Medial portion of forehead and side of nose: Postganglionic (third-order neuron after vasomotor and sudomotor fiber have branched off)

Pediatric Considerations

- In infants and children, loss of facial flushing is appreciated more than anhydrosis (Harlequin sign).
- First-order neuron may be associated with dysarthria, dysphagia, ataxia, vertigo, and nystagmus.
- Second-order neuron: History of previous trauma; neck, axillary, shoulder or arm pain; cough; hemoptysis; history of thoracic or neck surgery; history of chest tube or central venous catheter or neck swelling
- Third-order neuron: Diplopia (CN VI lesion), numbness in the distribution of the first and second division of the trigeminal nerve

ALERT

Horner syndrome in the presence of pain merits special consideration:

- Axial, shoulder, scapula, arm, or hand pain may be related to Pancoast tumor.
- Acute-onset, ipsilateral facial or neck pain: Consider carotid artery dissection until proven otherwise.
- Paratrigeminal syndromes:
  – Raeder paratrigeminal syndrome type I: Orbital pain, miosis, ptosis, with associated ipsilateral lesions of CN IIII; suspect middle cranial fossa mass lesion
  – Raeder paratrigeminal syndrome type II: Episodic retrobulbar or orbital pain, miosis, ptosis with no CN lesions; suspect migraine variant, syphilis, herpes zoster, hypertension.

PHYSICAL EXAM

- Complete neurological and chest examination are necessary to find associated physical findings.
- Measurement of pupillary diameter in dim and bright light and their reactivity to light and accommodative response:
  – Anisocoria greatest in dark, with affected pupil failing to dilate
  – Redilation (after light is removed) may lag 15–20 seconds on the affected side.
- Examine the upper lids for ptosis (<2 mm).

- Examination of the lower lids for "upside-down ptosis": Elevation of lower lid due to Müeller muscle weakness:
  - Illusion of enophthalmos secondary to narrowing of palpebral fissure
- Ipsilateral impaired flushing may be found.
- Loss of ciliospinal reflex. Pinching the skin of the back of the neck normally produces ipsilateral pupil dilation (unreliable).
- Biomicroscopic examination of the papillary margin and iris structure and color:
  - In congenital Horner syndrome, long-standing Horner syndrome, or Horner syndrome that occurs in children <2 years: Iris shows reduced pigmentation, blue-gray, mottling of the affected eye (heterochromia iridis) because formation of iris pigment early in life is under sympathetic control.
- Observation for the presence of nystagmus, facial swelling, lymphadenopathy, or vesicular eruptions
- Ophthalmoparesis, especially of CN VI

DIAGNOSTIC TESTS & INTERPRETATION

Lab

Initial lab tests

CBC, fluorescent treponemal antibody absorption test, venereal disease research laboratory, purified protein derivative, vanillylmandelic acid, homovanillic acid to rule out neuroblastoma in pediatric patients

Imaging

Initial approach

- Chest x-ray if patient is a smoker (apical bronchogenic carcinoma)
- CT/MRI/MRA of the brain, chest, and spinal cord:
  - If painful, order MRI/MRA to evaluate for carotid artery dissection emergently.
  - If acquired Horner syndrome in a child, suspect neuroblastoma and order MRI of sympathetic chain from abdomen to neck.

Diagnostic Procedures/Surgery

- Documentation of Horner syndrome:
  - 4–10% topical cocaine (2 drops):
    - A normal pupil will dilate. The miotic pupil in Horner syndrome will not dilate or will dilate poorly after 30 minutes because of the absence of norepinephrine at the nerve endings of the third-order neuron.
    - Positive test is anisocoria of 1 mm or more
    - Cocaine blocks the reuptake of norepinephrine by the neuron.
    - If the diagnosis is clear clinically, this test is not required.
    - Alternate test: Topical 0.5% apraclonidine
- Distinguishing a third-order neuron disorder from a first- or second neuron disorder:
  - Topical 1% hydroxyamphetamine:
    - If there is a first or second neuron lesion, dilation will take place 1 hour later.
    - Failure of the pupil to dilate, or poor dilation, indicates a third-order neuron lesion (positive when anisocoria increases by 1 mm or more).
    - No test exists to differentiate a first- or second-order neuron lesion.
    - Hydroxyamphetamine causes release of endogenous norepinephrine stored in the neuron.
    - Alternative test: 1% topical pholedrine
- Must wait >24 hours between the cocaine and hydroxyamphetamine tests

Pediatric Considerations

Due to transsynaptic degeneration in children, the hydroxyamphetamine test is not reliable.

Pathological Findings

- Brainstem lesion
- Massive hemisphere lesion
- Cervical cord lesion
- Root lesion
- Sympathetic chain lesion

DIFFERENTIAL DIAGNOSIS

- Neurological diseases
- Third nerve palsy
- Unilateral use of miotics
- Unilateral use of mydriatics
- Adie tonic pupil
- Iris sphincter muscle damage

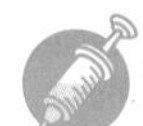

TREATMENT

MEDICATION

- Carotid artery dissection: Warfarin for 6 minutes (1)
- Antiplatelet therapy for stroke

ADDITIONAL TREATMENT

General Measures

- Horner syndrome in itself does not produce any disability or necessarily require treatment.
- Treat the underlying etiology.
- Search for a tumor or other compressive lesion.

Issues for Referral

- Neurologic, neuro-ophthalmic, oculoplastic
- Neurologic or vascular surgery: Interventional in cases of suspected carotid artery dissection or aneurysm
- Neurosurgery, surgical oncology, oncology, or radiotherapy consultation is dependent upon the particular etiology.

SURGERY/OTHER PROCEDURES

- Surgical care is dependent upon etiology.
- Consider ptosis repair surgery (oculoplastics).

ONGOING CARE

PROGNOSIS

- Postganglionic: Usually benign
- Central and preganglionic: Poorer prognosis

COMPLICATIONS

- Chronic pupillary constriction
- Cosmesis

REFERENCES

1. Nautiyal A, Singh S, DiSalle M, et al. Painful Horner syndrome as a harbinger of silent carotid dissection. *PLoS Med*. 2005;2(1):e19.
2. Aydin GB, Kutluk MT, Buyukpamukcu M, et al. Neurological complications of neuroblastic tumors: Experience of a single center. *Childs Nerv Syst*. 2010;26:359–65.
3. Bazari F, Hind M, Ong YE, et al. Horner's syndrome—not to be sneezed at. *Lancet*. 2010;375:776.
4. Freedman KA, Brown SM. Topical apraclonidine in the diagnosis of suspected Horner syndrome. *J Neuroophthalmo*. 2005;25(2):83–5.
5. Lee JH, Lee HK, Lee DH, et al. Neuroimaging strategies for three types of Horner syndrome with emphasis on anatomic location. *Am J Roentgenol*. 2007;188(1):W74–W81.

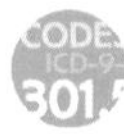

CODES

ICD9

- 337.09 Other idiopathic peripheral autonomic neuropathy
- 337.9 Unspecified disorder of autonomic nervous system
- 379.42 Miosis (persistent), not due to miotics

CLINICAL PEARLS

- Horner syndrome triad: Miosis, ptosis, and anhydrosis caused by a lesion in the sympathetic innervation to the neck, head, and eye
- Ptosis is mild, usually <2 mm.
- Red flags: Association with pain; central or preganglionic lesion suspected
- Confirm the diagnosis clinically with 2 drops of topical cocaine to the affected eye.
- Use hydroxyamphetamine to differentiate which order neuron is affected.
- Order imaging studies based on history and physical and hydroxyamphetamine testing.

H

HYDROCELE

Timothy L. Black, MD
James P. Miller, MD

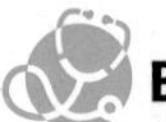

BASICS

DESCRIPTION

A collection of fluid within the scrotum:

- Communicating hydrocele:
  - Associated with a patent processus vaginalis
  - Has associated indirect inguinal hernia
- Noncommunicating hydrocele (the processus vaginalis is not patent):
  - Infantile type: Often spontaneous resolution
  - Adult type: Infrequent resolution
- Hydrocele of the cord: Distal portion of processus vaginalis has closed, midportion patent and fluid filled, proximal portion open or closed
- Acute hydrocele: Fluid collection resulting from an acute process within the tunica vaginalis
- System(s) affected: Reproductive

Pediatric Considerations

In communicating hydrocele, consider contralateral inguinal exploration.

EPIDEMIOLOGY

Predominant age: Childhood

Prevalence

- 1,000 per 100,000
- Estimated at 1% of adult men

RISK FACTORS

- Ventriculoperitoneal shunt
- Exstrophy of the bladder
- Cloacal exstrophy
- Ehlers-Danlos syndrome
- Peritoneal dialysis

ETIOLOGY

- Closure of processus vaginalis, trapping peritoneal fluid (noncommunicating)
- Closure of distal processus, trapping fluid in midportion of processus vaginalis (hydrocele of cord)
- Failure of closure of processus vaginalis (communicating hydrocele)
- Infection
- Tumors
- Trauma
- Ipsilateral renal transplantation

COMMONLY ASSOCIATED CONDITIONS

- Testicular tumors
- Trauma
- Ventriculoperitoneal shunt
- Nephrotic syndrome
- Renal failure with peritoneal dialysis

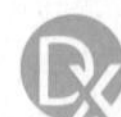

DIAGNOSIS

HISTORY

- Acute or subacute onset of scrotal swelling
- Frequent changes in size of the hydrocele (indicative of a communication)
- Swelling in scrotum or inguinal canal
- Usually not painful
- Sensation of heaviness in scrotum
- Pain radiating to back (occasionally)

PHYSICAL EXAM

- Swelling in scrotum or inguinal canal
- Demonstrated fluctuation in size (communicating hydrocele)
- Fluid collection in scrotum that transilluminates
- Scrotal mass, usually fluctuant

DIAGNOSTIC TESTS & INTERPRETATION

Lab

Lab studies usually are not helpful.

Imaging

- Abdominal radiograph: May be useful to distinguish incarcerated hernias from hydroceles (rarely needed)
- Inguinoscrotal ultrasound: Can demonstrate the presence of bowel (e.g., distinguish incarcerated hernia from a hydrocele of the cord) as well as presence of testicular torsion (1)
- Testicular nuclear scan or Doppler ultrasound: To distinguish testicular torsion

Diagnostic Procedures/Surgery

Aspiration of hydrocele for diagnosis should be discouraged.

Pathological Findings

Patent processus vaginalis in communicating hydroceles

DIFFERENTIAL DIAGNOSIS

- Indirect inguinal hernia
- Orchitis
- Epididymitis
- Traumatic injury to testicle
- Torsion of testicle or torsion of appendix testes

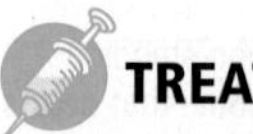

TREATMENT

ADDITIONAL TREATMENT

Issues for Referral

Recovery should be rapid and complete.

SURGERY/OTHER PROCEDURES

- In adults, no therapy is needed unless the hydrocele causes discomfort or unless there is a significant underlying cause such as tumor (2).
- Inguinal approach with ligation of processus vaginalis and excision, or distal splitting, or drainage of hydrocele sac in children (in hydrocele of cord, sac can be completely removed) (3)[B]
- Patients less <12 years old should undergo an inguinal approach, whereas scrotal approach can be considered in children >12 years old (4)[C].
- Scrotal approach with internal drainage of hydrocele in adults (highest recurrence rate) (5)[C]
- Scrotal approach with resection of hydrocele sac (highest complication rate, lowest recurrence rate) (5)[C]
- Jaboulay-Winkelmann procedure (for thick hydrocele sac): Hydrocele sac wrapped posteriorly around cord structures (5)[C],(6)[A]
- Lord procedure (for thin hydrocele sac): Radial sutures used to gather hydrocele sac posterior to testis and epididymis (5)[C],(6)[A]
- Aspiration of the hydrocele with instillation of sclerosing agent (talc is best) has been successfully used in adults (7)[B]:
  - Aspiration with instillation of sodium tetradecyl sulphate was compared prospectively with Jaboulay procedure (30 patients each group) (8)[B]:
    - Aspiration instillation group had fewer complications and was much less expensive, but had recurrence rate of 34% and high rate of patient dissatisfaction

IN-PATIENT CONSIDERATIONS

Initial Stabilization

- Outpatient surgery
- Observation in early infancy until definite communication demonstrated or until 1 year old

ONGOING CARE

FOLLOW-UP RECOMMENDATIONS

Full activity after surgery

Patient Monitoring

- Follow at 3–6-month intervals until decision for/against surgery is made.
- Postoperative follow-up at 2–4 weeks and then at intervals of 2–3 months until resolution of any postoperative (traumatic) hydrocele

COMPLICATIONS

- Complication rate for scrotal approach may reach 30% (9)[C].
- Preoperative antibiotics may be beneficial in reducing postoperative infections (9)[C].
- Postoperative traumatic hydrocele is common and usually resolves spontaneously.
- Injury to vas deferens or spermatic vessels
- Suture granuloma
- Hematoma
- Wound infection
- Recurrence of hydrocele
- Tense infantile abdominoscrotal hydrocele may have high complication rate (10)[C]:
  - May have significant rate of testicular dysmorphism (including hypoplasia)

REFERENCES

1. Clarke S, et al. Pediatric inguinal hernia and hydrocele: An evidence-based review in the era of minimal access surgery. *J Laparoendosc Adv Surg Tech A*. 2010;20:305–9.
2. de Castilla-Ramírez B, López-Flores SY, del Rocío Rábago-Rodríguez M, et al. [A clinical guideline for diagnosis and treatment of hydrocele in childhood]. *Rev Med Inst Mex Seguro Soc*. 2011;49:101–8.
3. Gahukamble DB, Khamage AS. Prospective randomized controlled study of excision vs. distal splitting of hernial sac and processus vaginalis in the repair of inguinal hernias and communicating hydroceles. *J Ped Surg*. 1995;30:624–5.
4. Wilson JM, Aaronson DS, Schrader R, et al. Hydrocele in the pediatric patient: Inguinal or scrotal approach? *J Urol*. 2008;180:1724–7; discussion 1727–8.
5. Ku JH, Kim ME, Lee NK, et al. The excisional placation and internal drainage techniques: A comparison of the results for idiopathic hydrocele. *BJU*. 2001;87:82–4.
6. Miroglu C, Tokuc R, Saporta L. Comparison of an extrusion procedure and eversion procedures in the treatment of hydrocele. *Int Urol Nephrol*. 1994;26:673–9.
7. Yilmaz U, Ekmekcioglu O, Tatlisen A, et al. Does pleurodesis for pleural effusions give bright ideas about the agents for hydrocele sclerotherapy? *Int Urol Nephrology*. 2000;32:89–92.
8. Khaniya S, Agrawal CS, Koirala R, et al. Comparison of aspiration-sclerotherapy with hydrocelectomy in the management of hydrocele: A prospective randomized study. *Int J Surg (London)*. 2009;7:392–5.
9. Swartz MA, Morgan TM, Krieger JN. Complications of scrotal surgery for benign conditions. *Urology*. 2007;69:616–9.
10. Cozzi DA, Mele E, Ceccanti S, et al. Infantile abdominoscrotal hydrocele: A not so benign condition. *J Urol*. 2008;180:2611–5; discussion 2615.

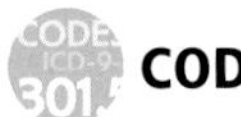

CODES

ICD9

603.9 Hydrocele, unspecified

CLINICAL PEARLS

- A diagnosis of hydrocele can virtually always be made by physical exam alone. Occasionally, scrotal ultrasound is needed, especially if there is concern about an underlying process.
- Aspirating a hydrocele as primary treatment is not recommended. If a hydrocele is confused with an incarcerated inguinal hernia, aspiration could result in significant complications. Otherwise, hydroceles simply recur following aspiration unless a sclerosing agent is injected as well.

H

HYDROCEPHALUS, NORMAL PRESSURE

Dennis E. Hughes, DO

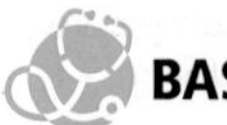

BASICS

DESCRIPTION

- Normal pressure hydrocephalus (NPH) is a clinical triad of gait instability, incontinence, and dementia (mnemonic: *wet, wobbly, wacky*). Originally described by Hakim and Adams in 1965, it occurs rarely, but is potentially treatable.
- Idiopathic
- Secondary to subarachnoid hemorrhage, head injury, or infection
- Absence of papilledema on clinical exam and normal CSF pressures at lumbar puncture

Geriatric Considerations

Idiopathic NPH primarily affects persons >60 years.

EPIDEMIOLOGY

Incidence

- No formal epidemiologic data exist regarding NPH because of the lack of consensus-derived diagnostic criteria. The natural history of untreated NPH has not been studied (1).
- Idiopathic form primarily affects elderly; at least >40 years of age.
- Secondary form can occur at any age.
- Affects both genders equally

Prevalence

Estimated to be the cause of dementia in ≤5% of affected individuals

RISK FACTORS

- Idiopathic risk is unknown.
- Secondary form is due to head trauma, subarachnoid hemorrhage, meningitis, or encephalitis.

PATHOPHYSIOLOGY

- This is a communicating hydrocephalus, a disorder of decreased CSF absorption. The subarachnoid granulations fail to maintain their baseline removal of CSF as a result of scarring or fibrosis.
- The result is a pressure gradient between the subarachnoid space and the ventricular system.
- CSF production decreases in the face of an increased pressure set-point (but still in excess of the amount of CSF absorbed).
- Elevated pressure distends ventricles and compresses the brain parenchyma.
- As a result of compression, ischemic changes occur in the parenchymal vasculature.

ETIOLOGY

- Some believe that the idiopathic form is a result of persistently insufficient removal of CSF by immature subarachnoid granulations from childhood.
- Secondary NPH may result from:
  - Subarachnoid hemorrhage
  - Head trauma
  - Resolved acute meningitis
  - Chronic meningitis (tuberculosis, syphilis)
  - Paget disease of the skull

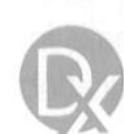

DIAGNOSIS

HISTORY

- Insidious and usually progressive; gait instability usually manifests initially, followed by changes in mentation, and eventually, urinary incontinence.
- Difficulty with initiation of movement: Feet appear "glued to the floor." Gait is wide-based, shuffling, and turning appears "en bloc."
- Inattention, forgetfulness, and lack of spontaneity often are seen with the subcortical dementia of NPH.
- Urinary urgency initially, followed by lack of inhibition and then frank incontinence
- Behavioral changes have been reported: Depression, mania, and psychotic features (1)
- A minimum duration of at least 3–6 months of symptoms and progression over time
- A remote trauma or infection suggests secondary vs. the idiopathic form.
- A lack of psychiatric, neurologic, or other medical conditions to explain the symptoms
- Because memory impairment may be present, it is important to include a knowledgeable informant who is familiar with the patient's premorbid state.
- The frontal lobe function is affected disproportionately to the memory impairment (objective testing may lead to an early diagnosis).

PHYSICAL EXAM

- Decreased step height and length
- Reduced speed of walking (cadence)
- Widened standing base
- Swaying of trunk during walking
- Decreased fine motor speed and accuracy
- Recall impaired for recent events
- Impaired ability to do multistep tasks or interpret abstractions

DIAGNOSTIC TESTS & INTERPRETATION

Lab

Initial lab tests

- Thyroid-stimulating hormone (TSH)
- Syphilis serology
- CBC
- Serum B_{12}, folate
- Metabolic profile
- Blood alcohol, analysis for drugs of abuse
- Urinalysis
- CSF analysis, including opening and closing pressures on lumbar puncture

Imaging

Initial approach

Imaging is essential:

- Either CT or MRI shows the ventriculomegaly with preservation of the cerebral parenchyma (as opposed to ventricular enlargement seen in other forms of dementia where brain atrophy is present).
- MRI can allow detection of other features such as signs of altered brain water content and callosal angles. However, these supportive findings are not independently diagnostic of NPH (1):
  - Enlargement of temporal horns of lateral ventricles colossal angle >40 degrees evidence of altered brain water content flow void on MRI

Diagnostic Procedures/Surgery

- Positron emission tomography (PET) scanning
- Nuclear cisternography
- CSF flow velocity (2)

DIFFERENTIAL DIAGNOSIS

- Alzheimer disease (may be a comorbid condition in as many as 75%)
- Parkinson disease
- Chronic alcoholism
- Intracranial infection
- Multi-infarct dementia
- Subdural hematoma
- Carcinomatous meningitis
- Collagen vascular disorders
- Depression
- Syphilis
- B_{12} deficiency
- Urologic disorders
- Other hydrocephalus disorders

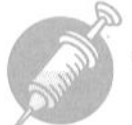

TREATMENT

MEDICATION

- No medication is significantly helpful.
- Use of carbonic anhydrase inhibitors (acetazolamide) with repeat lumbar punctures has provided mild and transient relief.
- Use of levodopa to rule out Parkinson disease may be helpful (NPH will display little, if any, significant improvement to dopamine agonist).

ADDITIONAL TREATMENT

Issues for Referral

- Neurology or neurosurgical consultation is helpful in suspected cases when other reversible medical conditions are ruled out.
- Recent cohort studies have demonstrated clinical improvement after surgical shunts. Perimeters of urinary continence, gait stability, and cognitive scores all improved at 1 year post shunt (3).

Additional Therapies

Gait training and use of ambulation assist devices as indicated

SURGERY/OTHER PROCEDURES

- Current therapy is limited to placement of ventriculoperitoneal or ventriculoatrial shunt from a lateral ventricle tunneled SC and drained into the peritoneal cavity (or right atrium).
- Success depends on appropriate patient selection. No specific test accurately identifies who will benefit from the CSF diversion.
- Patients whose symptoms have been present for a shorter period (<2 years) have a greater chance of improvement with shunting. Also, patients with a known cause of NPH tend to respond more favorably. However, improvement has been seen in patients with symptoms present for a long time (1).

IN-PATIENT CONSIDERATIONS

Admission Criteria

Usually only for planned surgical treatment

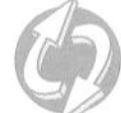

ONGOING CARE

FOLLOW-UP RECOMMENDATIONS

- Assessment and modification of environment for fall risks
- Evaluation for ability to operate a motor vehicle safely (if driving)

Patient Monitoring

- Repeat neuropsychological testing to evaluate the status of the dementia after treatment.
- Improvement in the incontinence and walking speed can also be objectively measured.

PATIENT EDUCATION

Information at: www.emedicinehealth.com/normal_pressure_hydrocephalus/article_em.htm

PROGNOSIS

The natural history is progressive deterioration. Patient's axial skeletal stability worsens with inability to walk, stand, sit, or turn over in bed.

COMPLICATIONS

- In patients treated surgically, cerebral infarcts, hemorrhage, infection, and seizures (in addition to the usual surgical risks): All usual age-related illnesses (as NPH is a condition affecting >65 years of age)
- Shunt malfunction (especially when symptoms recur after successful shunt placement)
- Falls due to gait instability
- UTIs
- Skin breakdown, pressure ulcers, infections as movement dysfunction progresses

REFERENCES

1. Relkin N, et al. Diagnosing idiopathic normal-pressure hydrocephalus. *Neurosurgery.* 2005; 57(3 Suppl):4–16.
2. Gallia GL, Rigamonti D, Williams MA. The diagnosis and treatment of idiopathic normal pressure hydrocephalus. *Nat Clin Pract Neurol.* 2006;2:375–81.
3. Hashimoto M, Ishikawa M, Mori E, et al. Diagnosis of idiopathic normal pressure hydrocephalus is supported by MRI-based scheme: A prospective cohort study. *Cerebralspinal Fluid Res.* 2010;7:18.

ADDITIONAL READING

- Ishikawa M, Hashimoto M, Kuwana N, et al. Guidelines for management of idiopathic normal pressure hydrocephalus. *Neurol Med Chir (Tokyo).* 2008;48(Suppl):S1–23.
- Pujari S, Kharkar S, Metellus P, et al. Normal pressure hydrocepalus long-term outcome after shunt surgery. *J Neuro Neurosurg Psychiatry.* 2008;79(11):1282–6.
- Razay G, Vreughenhil A, Liddell J. A prospective study of venriculo-peritoneal shunting for idiopathic normal pressure hydrocephalus. *J Clin Neurosci.* 2009;16(9):1180–3.
- Tarnaris A, Kitchen ND, Watkins LD. Noninvasive biomarkers in normal pressure hydrocephalus: Evidence for the role of neuroimaging. *J Neurosurg.* 2009;110(5):837–51.

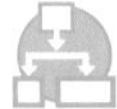

See Also (Topic, Algorithm, Electronic Media Element)

Algorithm: Ataxia

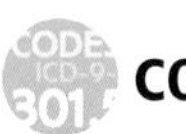

CODES

ICD9

331.5 Idiopathic normal pressure hydrocephalus (INPH)

CLINICAL PEARLS

- Consider in unexplained dementia
- Poor prognosis despite therapy

HYDRONEPHROSIS

Di Zhao, MD, PhD
Pang-Yen Fan, MD

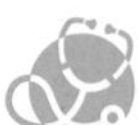

BASICS

DESCRIPTION

- Hydronephrosis refers to a structural finding—dilatation of the calyces and renal pelvis:
  - May occur with urinary tract obstruction, vesicoureteric reflux (VUR), high urine output, or physiologic changes in pregnancy
  - Sometimes accompanied with hydroureter
  - Presentation varies from incidental finding to UTI to severe pain.
- Hydronephrosis should not be used interchangeably with obstructive uropathy, which refers to the damage to renal parenchyma resulting from urinary tract obstruction.

EPIDEMIOLOGY

- Hydronephrosis is found in 3% of autopsy specimens.
- Acute unilateral obstruction is more common than bilateral.

PATHOPHYSIOLOGY

- Hydronephrosis develops with increased pressure in the urinary collecting system.
- Increased pressure within the renal collecting system can cause calyceal fornix rupture and urinary extravasation.
- Over time, pressures return to normal, but kidney function declines from intense renal vasoconstriction (1).
- With concomitant urinary infection, bacteria can enter the renal vasculature, resulting in sepsis.

ETIOLOGY

- Urinary tract obstruction: May be acute/chronic, partial/complete, uni-/bilateral:
  - Intraluminal obstruction: Calculi, sloughed renal papillae, blood clot
  - Intrinsic abnormality of the urinary collecting system: Transitional cell carcinomas, benign prostatic hypertrophy, prostate cancer, congenital ureteropelvic junction (UPJ) obstruction, ureterocele, neurogenic bladder (functional obstruction), urethral stricture or TB (can cause ureteral narrowing)
  - Extrinsic compression of the urinary collecting system: Extraurinary malignancy (lymphoma, colon, cervix), aortic/iliac aneurysm, retroperitoneal fibrosis, uterine prolapse (15% affected), endometriosis
- Vesicoureteric reflux (VUR) resulting in varying degrees of hydroureteronephrosis
- Physiologic hydronephrosis of pregnancy
- Hydronephrosis due to high urine output (e.g., diabetes insipidus, psychogenic polydipsia)
- Hydronephrosis of infection: Due to bacterial toxins inhibiting smooth muscle contraction of the renal pelvis and ureter

Pediatric Considerations

- Antenatal hydronephrosis is diagnosed in 1–5% of pregnancies, usually by ultrasound, as early as the 12th to 14th week of gestation.
- Children with antenatal hydronephrosis are at greater risk of postnatal pathology.
- Postnatal evaluation begins with ultrasound exam; further studies such as voiding cystourethrogram (VCUG) based on the severity of postnatal hydronephrosis
- In neonates, it is the most common cause of abdominal mass.
- The common etiologies in children are VUR, congenital UPJ obstruction, neurogenic bladder, and posterior urethral valves.
- Pediatric diagnostic algorithm differs from adult due to different differential diagnosis necessitating age-appropriate testing.

Pregnancy Considerations

- Physiologic hydronephrosis in pregnancy is more prominent on the right than left and can be seen up to 80% of pregnant women.
- Dilatation is caused by hormonal effects, external compression from expanding uterus, and intrinsic changes in the ureteral wall.
- Despite high incidence, most cases are asymptomatic.
- If symptomatic and refractory to medical management, ureteric calculus should be considered and urinary infection must be excluded.

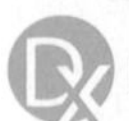

DIAGNOSIS

Symptoms vary according to cause, chronicity, location, and degree of obstruction.

HISTORY

- While often asymptomatic, hydronephrosis can be associated with pain ranging from vague intermittent discomfort to severe renal colic.
- Nausea, vomiting, chills may be associated with severe pain or infection.
- Fever with coexisting infection
- Polyuria may occur due to impaired urinary concentration in partial obstruction.
- Anuria if complete bilateral obstruction or complete obstruction of a solitary kidney
- Symptoms of chronic kidney disease: Anorexia, malaise, weight gain, edema, shortness of breath, mental state changes, tremors, GI bleeding
- Dietl crisis: Sudden attack of flank pain due to distension of renal pelvis caused by rapid ingestion of large amount of liquid or kinking of a ureter producing temporary occlusion of urine flow
- Symptoms of bladder outlet obstruction: Weak urine stream, nocturia, straining to void, overflow incontinence, urgency and frequency
- General medical and surgical history: Malignancy (extrinsic compression), radiotherapy (ureteric stricture/fibrosis), surgery (iatrogenic obstruction), trauma (hematoma or fibrosis), gynecologic disease (endometriosis, ovarian masses, uterine prolapse), smoking (urothelial cancer), drugs (methysergide-induced retroperitoneal fibrosis)

PHYSICAL EXAM

- General signs:
  - Volume overload (edema, rales, HTN)
  - Diaphoresis, tachycardia, tachypnea with pain
  - High-grade fever if infection
- Abdominal exam: CVA tenderness, palpable bladder, rarely palpable abdominal mass (may be visible, particularly in thin children)
- Pelvic exam: Pelvic mass, uterine prolapse, palpable enlarged prostate (cancer or benign), urethral meatal stenosis, phimosis

DIAGNOSTIC TESTS & INTERPRETATION

Lab

- Dipstick urinalysis: Hematuria, proteinuria, crystalluria, pyuria
- Midstream urine microscopy, culture, and sensitivity: Exclude infection or hematuria
- Creatinine, urea, and electrolytes: May demonstrate rising creatinine and urea if patient developing obstructive uropathy. Potassium may be elevated and bicarbonate decreased if patient is developing hyperkalemic metabolic acidosis.
- CBC: Anemia of chronic kidney disease (CKD), leukocytosis if infection; check platelet count prior to considering intervention
- PSA in adult males >50 or with abnormal digital rectal exam, or outlet obstruction signs or symptoms
- Urine cytology for malignant cells
- Note: CA 19-9 is elevated in benign hydronephrosis and not a useful marker for malignancy in these patients.

Imaging

- Ultrasound and noncontrast CT scanning are effective in diagnosing presence and cause of obstruction in most of the cases; radionuclide scanning only if indicated
- Ultrasound (US): Test of choice to rule out hydronephrosis:
  - Poor sensitivity for detecting cause and level of obstruction
  - Detection of renal parenchymal disease (decreased renal size, increased cortical echogenicity, cortical thinning, cysts)
  - Safe in pregnancy, contrast allergy, or renal dysfunction
  - Degree of hydronephrosis does not correlate with the duration or severity of the obstruction.
  - False positives (for urinary tract obstruction): Normal extrarenal pelvis, parapelvic cysts, VUR, excessive diuresis
  - False negatives: Dehydration; renal cortical cysts actually representing intrarenal calyceal dilatation; at immediate onset of acute obstruction before dilatation has occurred; retroperitoneal fibrosis
- CT without contrast (2)[A]:
  - Noncontrast helical CT of the abdomen and pelvis is the investigation of choice for suspected nephrolithiasis:
    - Stone is most commonly found at levels of ureteric luminal narrowing: UPJ, pelvic brim, and the vesico-ureteric junction.

  - If the obstruction is acute, proximal ureter and renal pelvis are dilated to the level of obstruction and perinephric stranding is seen as well as renal swelling.
  - If chronic, renal atrophy may be noted.
- Radionuclide renal scan (diuretic renal scintigraphy):
  - Useful in determining presence of true obstruction as well as total and separate (R vs. L) renal function
  - Advantages: Safe in contrast-allergic patients, no risk of contrast-induced acute kidney injury
  - Most common agents are DTPA and MAG-3.
  - Furosemide is given at 20 minutes after the agent was given; the t1/2 for the clearance of tracer from the system is measured.
  - T1/2 $<$10 minutes is unobstructed, $>$20 minutes is obstructed, and 10–20 minutes is equivocal; some experts consider $<$15 minutes normal.
  - False positives occur in patients with reduced creatinine clearance due to delayed excretion and in massive dilatation, causing a water-reservoir effect of delayed excretion without obstruction.
  - False negatives occur in dehydrated patients or inadequate diuretic challenges.
- Multiphase contrast-enhanced CT:
  - Nonenhanced phase detects stones and swelling
  - Parenchymal phase demonstrates decreased enhancement of renal parenchyma with acute obstruction; can identify extraurinary causes of obstruction and determine the relative GFR of each kidney with accuracy equal to diuretic renography.
  - Delayed phase allows visualization of the collecting system and soft tissue filling defects (e.g., urothelial cancer).
- If contrast is contraindicated (creatinine $>$2 mg/dL), magnetic resonance urography (MRU) is superior to noncontrast CT in diagnosing soft-tissue causes including strictures:
  - MRU disadvantages: Insensitive for stone detection (only 70%); increased expense; less availability; increased acquisition time compared to CT (35 minutes vs. 5 minutes)
  - MRU is also used in pregnancy.
- Voiding cystourethrogram to assess for the presence and severity of VUR when indicated.

Diagnostic Procedures/Surgery

Cystoscopy, retrograde pyelogram $\pm$ ureteroscopy and biopsy are occasionally used to determine the cause of obstruction (e.g., small urothelial cancer missed on imaging) or to confirm a normal distal ureter prior to pyeloplasty. In addition, such procedures are often needed to establish a definitive pathologic diagnosis for mass lesions.

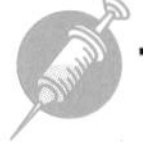

TREATMENT

ADDITIONAL TREATMENT

General Measures

- Treatment depends on cause and associated complications.
- Obstruction:
  - Bladder outlet obstruction: Urethral or suprapubic catheter
  - Ureteric obstruction: Retrograde (cystoscopic) or antegrade (percutaneous) stenting
- Correction of fluid and electrolyte abnormalities
- Analgesia
- Antibiotics as an adjunct to drainage if infection present
- VUR is often managed conservatively with antibiotics; surgical management required in severe cases in children or women of child-bearing age.

SURGERY/OTHER PROCEDURES

- Hydronephrosis due to obstruction:
  - Congenital UPJ obstruction: Pyeloplasty (open or laparoscopic), minimally invasive stricture incision (laser, Acucise cutting balloon catheter endopyelotomy)
  - Nephrolithiasis: ESWL (3), laser lithotripsy, ureteroscopy, percutaneous nephrostomy, ureteral stenting
  - Transitional cell cancer: Nephroureterectomy
  - Idiopathic retroperitoneal fibrosis: Ureterolysis (frees ureters from inflammatory mass)
  - Prostate disorders: Various treatment modalities including TURP and radical prostatectomy
- Nonobstructed hydronephrosis:
  - VUR: Ureteric reimplantation, endoscopic suburethral injection

IN-PATIENT CONSIDERATIONS

Initial Stabilization

Obstruction coexisting with infection (pyonephrosis) is a true urologic emergency requiring urgent drainage. Typically, this requires placement of percutaneous nephrostomy tube(s) as cystoscopic cannulation of the ureters is often difficult.

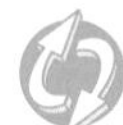

ONGOING CARE

FOLLOW-UP RECOMMENDATIONS

- Serial monitoring of kidney function (electrolytes, BUN, and creatinine) and BP until renal function stabilizes. Frequency of monitoring dependent on severity of renal dysfunction.
- Follow-up ultrasonography after stabilization of renal function to assess for resolution of hydronephrosis. If hydronephrosis persists, consider diuretic radionuclide study to rule out persistent obstruction.

PROGNOSIS

- Recovery of renal function depends on severity, acuity, and duration of obstruction.
- Significant recovery can occur despite days of complete obstruction, though some irreversible injury may develop within 24 hours.
- Course difficult to predict as diagnostic testing is of little value
- Course of incomplete obstruction highly unpredictable.

COMPLICATIONS

- Urine stasis: Increased risk of infection and calculus formation
- Obstruction causes progressive atrophy of kidney with irreversible loss of function:
  - Tubules lose ability to concentrate urine, conserve sodium, or excrete H^+.
- Spontaneous rupture of a calyx may occur with urine extravasation in the perinephric space.
- Postobstructive diuresis: Marked polyuria after relief of obstruction:
  - Caused mostly by fluid and solute overload, but may be exacerbated by impaired renal tubular concentrating ability
  - Urine output may exceed 500 mL/h.
  - Replace urine losses with hypotonic fluid (as the urine is often dilute) and only enough to avoid volume depletion. Replacement of urine output with equal amounts of saline will perpetuate the diuresis.

REFERENCES

1. Khalaf IM, Shokeir AA, El-Gyoushi FI, et al. Recoverability of renal function after treatment of adult patients with unilateral obstructive uropathy and normal contralateral kidney: A prospective study. *Urology*. 2004;64:664–8.
2. Worster A, Preyra I, Weaver B, et al. The accuracy of noncontrast helical computed tomography versus intravenous pyelography in the diagnosis of suspected acute urolithiasis: A meta-analysis. *Ann Emerg Med*. 2002;40:280–6.
3. El-Assmy A, El-Nahas AR, Sheir KZ. Is pre-shock wave lithotripsy stenting necessary for ureteral stones with moderate or severe hydronephrosis? *J Urol*. 2006;176:2059–62; discussion 2062.

ADDITIONAL READING

- Cerwinka WH, Qian J, Easley KA, et al. Appearance of dextranomer/hyaluronic acid copolymer implants on computerized tomography after endoscopic treatment of vesicoureteral reflux in children. *J Urol*. 2009.
- el-Nahas AR, Shoma AM, Eraky I, et al. Prospective, randomized comparison of ureteroscopic endopyelotomy using holmium:YAG laser and balloon catheter. *J Urol*. 2006;175:614–8; discussion 618.
- Grattan-Smith JD. MR urography: Anatomy and physiology. *Pediatr Radiol*. 2008;38(Suppl 2): S275–80.
- Lee RS, Cendron M, Kinnamon DD, et al. Antenatal hydronephrosis as a predictor of postnatal outcome: A meta-analysis. *Pediatrics*. 2006;118:586–93.

CODES

ICD9

- 591 Hydronephrosis
- 753.29 Other obstructive defects of renal pelvis and ureter

HYPERCALCEMIA ASSOCIATED WITH MALIGNANCY

Jenny Frazier, MD

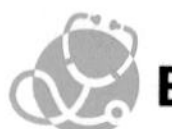

BASICS

DESCRIPTION

- Hypercalcemia associated with malignancy is the most common cause of severe hypercalcemia diagnosed in a hospital setting.
- Often a very poor prognostic sign
- Occurs with both solid tumors and hematologic malignancies; most commonly associated with multiple myeloma and breast and lung cancer; also associated with metastases to bone

EPIDEMIOLOGY

Incidence

Hypercalcemia is diagnosed in 20–30% of all cancer patients during the course of illness (1).

RISK FACTORS

- Dehydration
- Immobilization

GENERAL PREVENTION

Encourage adequate hydration and activity, especially in patients with multiple myeloma.

PATHOPHYSIOLOGY

- Increased bone resorption is involved in most cases, caused by either extensive local bone destruction or humoral factors.
- Humoral factors can interfere with the normal regulation of calcium by parathyroid hormone, calcitriol, and calcitonin.
- The humoral factors most commonly associated with cancer are parathyroid hormone (PTH)–related protein (rP) and 1,25-dihydroxyvitamin D (calcitriol); however, other bone-resorbing factors, including prostaglandins, transforming growth factors, tumor necrosis factor (TNF), colony-stimulating factors, and interleukins, may be involved in different types of malignancy.
- PTH-rP increases expression of receptor activator of nuclear factor κB ligand (RANKL) in bone. RANKL binds to RANK on the surfaces of osteoclast precursors, resulting in differentiation into osteoclasts and leading to bone resorption and the development of hypercalcemia.

ETIOLOGY

- Main mechanisms of hypercalcemia in malignancy:
  - Osteolytic metastases: Most commonly with breast cancer, multiple myeloma, lymphoma, and leukemia; accounts for about 20% of cases of hypercalcemia associated with malignancy
  - Humoral hypercalcemia: Ectopic production of PTH-rP; PTH-rP increases bone resorption by osteoclasts.
  - Associated with:
    - Non–small cell lung carcinoma
    - Breast cancer
    - Renal cell carcinoma
    - Prostate cancer
    - Melanoma
  - Ectopic PTH secretion: Very rare; has been seen with ovarian carcinoma, neuroectodermal tumor, thyroid papillary carcinoma, lung cancer, rhabdomyosarcoma, and pancreatic cancer
  - Calcitriol production: Lymphoma (non-Hodgkin, Hodgkin, and lymphomatosis/granulomatosis) and ovarian dysgerminomas
- In multiple myeloma, the elevated serum calcium may be due to the binding of the monoclonal protein with calcium. Multiple myeloma also may cause impaired renal function that decreases calcium excretion.

DIAGNOSIS

- The severity of symptoms depends on calcium level, rapidity of onset of hypercalcemia, state of hydration, and underlying malignancy.
- Early nonspecific symptoms often include nausea, vomiting, anorexia, depression, abdominal pain, constipation, and dizziness (1).
- Polyuria and polydipsia are more specific early symptoms (1).
- Cardiovascular:
  - Arrhythmias
  - QT-interval shortening
  - Calcium increases vascular tone.
- Genitourinary:
  - Nephrolithiasis, especially in the elderly
  - Polyuria because of impaired concentrating ability
- GI:
  - Peptic ulcers
  - Pancreatitis
  - Constipation
  - Anorexia
  - Nausea, vomiting
- Musculoskeletal:
  - Weakness, hypotonia
  - Hyporeflexia
  - Osteopenia, fractures
- Neuropsychiatric:
  - Depression, lethargy
  - Obtundation, coma
  - Memory impairment, confusion
  - Hallucinations
  - Headache
  - Seizures

DIAGNOSTIC TESTS & INTERPRETATION

Lab

- Serum calcium: Either ionized ("gold standard") or also must check albumin and correct: Ca(adj) = Ca(tot) + [0.8 × (4.5 – [alb])].
- Electrolytes including magnesium and phosphate (if hypercalcemia owing to PTH-rP, expect low phosphate, hyperchloremia, and mild alkalosis)
- Renal function: Urine calcium will be elevated.
- PTH: Levels of intact PTH should be measured routinely. Although ectopic PTH secretion is rare with malignancy, concomitant primary hyperparathyroidism is common (there is a higher incidence of cancer in patients with primary hyperparathyroidism and a higher incidence of primary hyperparathyroidism in patients with cancer).
- PTH-rP: In addition to helping with diagnosis, it is also a poor prognostic indicator and can be used to predict the response to treatment and is most commonly elevated in breast and lung cancer.
- Calcitriol: Should be measured when sarcoidosis, other granulomatous disorders, or the calcitriol lymphoma syndrome is in the differential diagnosis.
- If underlying malignancy is unknown, commence workup, for example, serum and urine electrophoresis for multiple myeloma.

ALERT

Lithium, thiazide diuretics, and vitamin D preparations all can increase serum calcium.

Imaging

None indicated for the immediate management of hypercalcemia, but studies such as a bone scan may be helpful for workup of underlying condition.

DIFFERENTIAL DIAGNOSIS

- Hyperparathyroidism
- Immobilization
- Calcium administration
- Renal causes:
  - Chronic or acute renal failure
  - Postrenal transplantation
- Hypocalciuric hypercalcemias:
  - Familial
  - Hypothyroidism
  - Adrenal insufficiency
  - Bartter syndrome
- Granulomatous disease:
  - Sarcoidosis
  - Histoplasmosis
  - Coccidioidomycosis
  - Tuberculosis
- Hyperthyroidism
- AIDS
- Hypophosphatemia
- Pheochromocytoma
- Acromegaly
- Drugs:
  - Calcium
  - Lithium
  - Theophylline
  - Thiazides
- Vitamin A or D toxicity

TREATMENT

MEDICATION

- Hydration:
  - The initial therapy of choice because many symptoms are caused by dehydration.
  - Vomiting and renal losses can cause profound dehydration.
  - Volume expansion with IV normal saline
- Loop diuretics (e.g., furosemide): Increase renal calcium excretion but only after adequate hydration. Recent literature review suggests that loop diuretics should not be used except in fluid overloaded patients because hydration with saline, particularly when combined with other agents such as bisphosphonates, is more effective and safer than hydration plus diuretic (2)[B].
- Bisphosphonates: Considered first-line medications; by inhibiting osteoclasts they reduce calcium release from bone, thereby counteracting the main mechanism of hypercalcemia of malignancy, which is bone reabsorption. They also decrease bone pain in patients with bone metastases (3)[B].
  - Zoledronic acid (Zometa):
    - Duration of action is 30 days.
    - Nephrotoxic potential, especially in myeloma patients receiving thalidomide
  - Pamidronate (Aredia): Normalizes calcium in up to 3 weeks
- Calcitonin: Also requires adequate rehydration; inhibits calcium reabsorption in the distal tubule:
  - Rapid onset of action (within 6–24 hours)
  - Side effects include nausea, vomiting, abdominal cramps, rash, flushing, diarrhea, and tachyphylaxis.
  - For life-threatening hypercalcemia, consider calcitonin injections every 12 hours (1)[B].
- Plicamycin (previously mithramycin):
  - May work via direct toxic effect on osteoclasts; reserved for patients who do not respond to bisphosphonates; can induce normocalcemia in 80% of those who receive it.
  - Side effects limit its use (e.g., nausea, vomiting, cellulitis at infusion site, cytopenias, hepatic toxicity, nephrotoxicity, and platelet inhibition); can have rapid rebound hypercalcemia
  - Onset of action within 12 hours, with maximal effect seen in 24–48 hours
- Gallium nitrate:
  - Works through multiple mechanisms, including inhibition of osteoclast-mediated bone resorption, alteration in bone structure, and stimulation of bone formation
  - Rarely used, except in cases of more severe hypercalcemia that has been unresponsive to initial therapy, because treatment requires 5-day continuous IV infusion
  - Onset of action 48–72 hours
  - Side effects: Nausea, vomiting, nephrotoxicity, hypophosphatemia, anemia, hypotension
- Inorganic phosphates:
  - Potentially lethal side effects limit use to patients with life-threatening hypercalcemia; IV use is no longer supported.
  - Side effects: Precipitation of calcium into tissues of the lung, heart, kidneys, and blood vessels can lead to organ damage, hypotension, and death.
  - Oral and rectal routes safer than IV
- Glucocorticoids:
  - Direct effects in treating hypercalcemia of malignancy are unclear.
  - Has direct tumoricidal effects on hematologic cancers such as multiple myeloma, lymphoma, and leukemias

ADDITIONAL TREATMENT

In cases where saline diuresis and medications fail, hemodialysis is an option. Hemodialysis is the treatment for patients with renal failure and life-threatening hypercalcemia (1)[B].

General Measures

- Treatment of underlying malignancy
- Monitor for hypophosphatemia, which is common in and can worsen hypercalcemia (3)[B]. Replace phosphorus PO or by nasogastric tube (3)[B].
- Discontinue use of oral calcium supplements and remove calcium from parenteral feeding solutions.
- Discontinue medications that can independently cause hypercalcemia (e.g., thiazides).
- Promote weight-bearing ambulation.

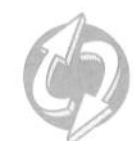

ONGOING CARE

FOLLOW-UP RECOMMENDATIONS

Avoid bed rest or immobilization as much as possible.

Patient Monitoring

Frequent serum calcium and electrolyte determinations; expect relapse

PROGNOSIS

- Median survival after diagnosis of tumoral hypercalcemia depends on type and extent of the malignancy but usually indicates a poor prognosis.
- >50% of patients die within 50 days of diagnosis of hypercalcemia (3).

REFERENCES

1. Zojer N, Ludwig H. Hematological emergencies. *Ann Oncol*. 2007;18(Suppl 1):i45–i48.
2. LeGrand SB, Leskuski D, Zama I. Narrative review: furosemide for hypercalcemia: An unproven yet common practice. *Ann Intern Med*. 2008;149: 259–63.
3. Higdon ML, et al. Treatment of oncologic emergencies. *AFP*. 2006;74:1874–80.
4. Deftos LJ. Hypercalcemia in malignancy and inflammatory diseases. *Endocrinol Metab Clin N Am*. 2002;31:141–58.
5. Stewart AF. Clinical practice. Hypercalcemia associated with cancer. *N Engl J Med*. 2005;352: 373–9.

ADDITIONAL READING

- Horwitz MJ, Stewart AF. Hypercalcemia associated with malignancy. In: Primer on the Metabolic Bone Diseases and Disorders of Mineral Metabolism. *American Society of Bone and Mineral Research*. 2006;31:195.
- Lipton A. Management of metastatic bone disease and hypercalcemia of malignancy. *Am J Cancer*. 2003;2(6):427–38.

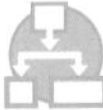

See Also (Topic, Algorithm, Electronic Media Element)

- Addison Disease; HIV Infection and AIDS; Hyperparathyroidism; Hyperthyroidism; Milk-Alkali Syndrome; Rhabdomyolysis; Sarcoidosis; Tuberculosis
- Algorithm: Hypercalcemia

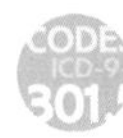

CODES

ICD9

- 198.5 Secondary malignant neoplasm of bone and bone marrow
- 275.42 Hypercalcemia

CLINICAL PEARLS

- Hypercalcemia of malignancy carries with it a very poor prognosis. The median survival after diagnosis is 6 weeks (3).
- Diagnosis may be difficult unless the patient has a known malignancy. Even with a known malignancy, other causes of hypercalcemia should be ruled out (4).
- The mnemonic for remembering the effects of hypercalcemia: Stones (kidney stones), bones (bone pain), moans (psychosis), groans (abdominal discomfort, constipation), and psychiatric overtones (including depression and confusion).
- Patients with hypercalcemia of malignancy do not need a low-calcium diet. Hypercalcemia decreases the absorption of calcium in the intestine (5).
- For severe hypercalcemia of malignancy, the initial treatment of choice is IV hydration. Volume depletion is the cause of many of the symptoms and the pathophysiology of hypercalcemia.

HYPERCHOLESTEROLEMIA

Sebastian T.C. Tong, MD, MPH
Joanne E. Wilkinson, MD, MSc

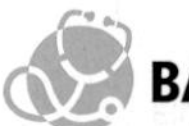

BASICS

DESCRIPTION

- Serum cholesterol >200 mg/dL (5.18 mmol/L):
  - Mainly caused by lifestyle habits in developed countries; however, rule out genetic and secondary causes
- Lipoprotein subtypes:
  - Low-density lipoproteins (LDL): Primary target of therapy, atherogenic
  - High-density lipoproteins (HDL): Atheroprotective
  - Triglycerides
- High cholesterol is a significant risk factor for cardiovascular disease.
- Categorized by Fredrikson Classification: Limited diagnostic/treatment implications except for specific genetic disorders
- System(s) affected: Cardiovascular; Endocrine/Metabolic

EPIDEMIOLOGY

Age: Increases with age (female onset delayed by 10–15 years compared with male)

Prevalence

- 54.9% of men and 46.5% of women in US with cholesterol >200 mg/dL (borderline high)
- 23.9% of men and 17.3% of women in US with cholesterol >240 mg/dL (high)

RISK FACTORS

Diet rich in saturated fat and cholesterol, obesity (BMI >30 kg/m^2), physical inactivity, heredity

Genetics

- Type 2 familial hypercholesterolemia (FH):
  - Most severe familial form
  - Autosomal dominant inheritance
  - Prevalence = 1/500 in US
  - High cholesterol levels from birth; atherosclerotic disease in early adulthood and high CHD risk in 40s–50s
  - Tendon xanthomas on Achilles and extensor tendons of hands common
  - Early lipid-lowering drug therapy shown to reduce CHD risk
- Other types: Mutation in apolipoprotein B-100 gene (APO-B) or proprotein convertase subtilisin/kexin type 9 gene (PCSK9)
- Early cholesterol testing of family members beneficial

GENERAL PREVENTION

- Reduced intakes of saturated fat and cholesterol
- Regular physical activity
- Weight control (see "Ongoing Care" section)

PATHOPHYSIOLOGY

- Deposition of cholesterol in vascular walls creating fatty streaks that become fibrous plaques
- Inflammation causes plaque instability leading to plaque rupture.

ETIOLOGY

- Primary: Diet, lack of physical activity, obesity
- Secondary: Hypothyroidism, diabetes, nephrotic syndrome, obstructive liver disease, chronic renal failure, medications (thiazide diuretics, carbamazepine, cyclosporine, progestins, anabolic steroids, corticosteroids, protease inhibitors).

COMMONLY ASSOCIATED CONDITIONS

Hypertension, diabetes mellitus, obesity

DIAGNOSIS

Screening recommendations:

- National Cholesterol Education Program (NCEP) Adult Treatment Panel (ATP) III: Fasting lipoprotein profile (total cholesterol, LDL-C, HDL-C, TG) (1)[A]:
  - All adults aged 20 yrs or older every 5 years
- US Preventive Services Task Force (USPSTF): Total cholesterol and HDL-C every 5 years:
  - All men aged 35 and older (2)[A]
  - Women aged 45 and older if at increased risk for coronary heart disease (2)[A]
  - Men aged 20–35 and women aged 20–45 if at increased risk for coronary heart disease (2)[B]
- American Diabetic Association: Yearly dyslipidemia screening for diabetics

HISTORY

- Emphasize possible secondary causes of hypercholesterolemia.
- Review medications that may change lipid levels.
- Assess other CHD risk factors.

PHYSICAL EXAM

Generally nonspecific findings and not important in diagnosis

DIAGNOSTIC TESTS & INTERPRETATION

Lab

Initial lab tests

- Fasting lipoprotein panel: Total cholesterol, LDL-C, HDL-C, triglycerides (1)[A]:
  - LDL-C is usually calculated value and is accurate if TG <350 mg/dL
- Nonfasting: Only cholesterol and HDL cholesterol usable (if TC >200 mg/d or HDL M40 mg/dL, follow-up lipoprotein profile needed), although LDL can be measured directly for nonfasting patients (2)[A]
- If elevated LDL-C or other form of hyperlipidemia, clinical/laboratory assessment to rule out secondary dyslipidemia before initiating lipid-lowering therapy: TSH, glucose, creatinine, liver enzymes, uric acid
- Consider genetic etiology in very high LDL (>190 mg/dL).

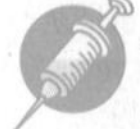

TREATMENT

Primary target in hypercholesterolemia therapy is lowering LDL-C (1)[A]:

Risk factors	LDL Goal
0–1	<160
2+	<130
CHD or CHD risk equivalent	<100

- Clinical evidence suggests optimal goal of LDL <70 for very high-risk patients although number needed to treat >100 people/yr
- Major risk factors that affect CHD risk:
  - Cigarette smoking
  - Hypertension (BP >140/90 mm Hg)
  - Low HDL cholesterol (<40 mg/dL) (if HDL >60 mg/dL, subtract 1 risk factor)
  - Family history of premature CHD (CHD in male first-degree relative <55 years; CHD in female first-degree relative <65 years)
  - Age (men >45, women >55)
- CHD risk equivalents:
  - Atherosclerotic disease: Peripheral arterial disease, abdominal aortic aneurysm, symptomatic carotid artery disease
  - Diabetes
  - Multiple risk factors that confer a 10-year risk for CHD >20%

MEDICATION

- Therapeutic lifestyle changes should be attempted first before drug therapy (diet and regular exercise; see "Ongoing Care").
- Start meds when >30 mg/dL over LDL goal.
- Check fasting lipoprotein profile (and LFTs if on a statin) 6 weeks after starting drug therapy to evaluate response
- Once goal reached: Monitor every 4–6 months
- Many more patients treated and medications used in US than elsewhere in the world without substantial evidence for improved outcomes.

ALERT

Elevated serum triglycerides:

- If >500, TG lowering becomes primary target until TG <500 to prevent acute pancreatitis
  - First line: Fibrate + therapeutic life changes; second line: nicotininc acid

First Line

HMG-CoA reductase inhibitors (statins):

- Types: Atorvastatin (Lipitor): 10–80 mg/d; fluvastatin (Lescol): 20–80 mg/d; lovastatin (Mevacor): 20–80 mg/d; pravastatin (Pravachol): 20–80 mg/d; rosuvastatin (Crestor): 5–20 mg/d; simvastatin (Zocor): 20–40 mg/d

ALERT

FDA alert: Simvastatin should no longer be prescribed at 80 mg/d doses due to increased risk of myopathy. Patients who have been at this drug dosage for >1 year can continue if no signs of myopathy.

- To be taken in the evening or at bedtime for best effect except atorvastatin and rosuvastatin (due to longer half-life)
- Effect: LDL-C ↓18–55%; TG ↓ 7–30%; HDL-C ↑ 5–15%; shown to decrease both CHD incidence and all-cause mortality
- Contraindications: Pregnancy, lactation, or active liver disease
- Possible interactions: Cyclosporine, macrolide antibiotics, various antifungal agents, cytochrome p-450 inhibitors, fibrates/nicotinic acid (to be used with caution)

- Adverse reactions:
  - Liver transaminase elevations (up to 3% of patients): ALT/AST before therapy to establish baseline, at 6 or 12 weeks and then every year:
    - Progression to severe hepatotoxicity rare
    - If LFTs 1–3× normal, can continue statin with frequent monitoring
    - If LFTs >3× normal, discontinue statin
    - Rechallenge of drug not contraindicated after LFTs return to normal
  - Myopathies (rare: ~0.1% of patients):
    - Regular creatine kinase (CK) monitoring not indicated
    - More likely in patients with multiple comorbidities or taking concurrent medications that increase statin concentrations
    - Instruct patients to report immediately if any muscle pain, muscle weakness, or brown urine
    - If myopathy or rhabdomyolysis suspected, discontinue statin use and draw serum CK
    - Can rechallenge statin at lower dose after resolution of symptoms
- Statins reduce major coronary events, CHD deaths, need for coronary procedures, and stroke although number needed to treat to prevent a single event varies widely and may be in 300–500 range/yr for primary prevention (less for secondary prevention) (1)[A]

Pregnancy Considerations

Statins contraindicated during pregnancy: Class XLactation: Possibly unsafe

ALERT

- Avoid grapefruit juice.
- New evidence suggests high-dose statins may be associated with increased risk of new-onset diabetes (3)[A].

Second Line

- Ezetimibe:
  - Can be taken by itself or in combination with a statin: Monotherapy (Zetia 10 mg/d) or ezetimibe/simvastatin (10/10, 10/20, 10/40, 10/80 mg/d)
  - Effect: In monotherapy, LDL ↓17%; in combo with a statin, an additional LDL ↓14% compared to only statin. No studies to date have shown CV benefit or decreased mortality rates: IMPROVE-IT trial studying CV benefit still ongoing.
  - Adverse reactions: Generally well tolerated; concern of increased cancer risk from ezetimibe therapy not well substantiated to date
- Fibric acid derivatives:
  - Types: Gemfibrozil (Lopid) 600 mg b.i.d., fenofibrate (Antara, Lofibra, Tricor, Triglide) 200 mg daily, clofibrate 1,000 mg b.i.d.
  - Effect: Most effective in lowering TG ↓20–50%; moderate effect in lowering LDL-C ↓5–20% and increasing HDL ↑10–35%. May increase LDL in those with high TG. Should not be used solely for HDL-raising effect.
  - Contraindications: Severe hepatic or renal insufficiency
  - Possible interactions: Potentiates effects of warfarin and oral hypoglycemic agents. Technically should be avoided with statins due to increased risk of rhabdomyolysis.
  - Adverse reactions: GI complaints; increased likelihood of cholesterol gallstones
- Nicotinic acid:
  - Types: Crystalline 1.5–4.5 g/d b.i.d. or t.i.d.; extended-release (Niaspan) 1–2 g at bedtime
  - Effect: Most effective lipid-lowering agent for raising HDL levels ↑15–35%; LDL-C ↓5–25%; TG↓20–50%, but little evidence for improved outcomes
  - Contraindications: Chronic liver disease, severe gout, hyperuricemia, high doses in type II diabetes
  - Adverse reactions: Cutaneous flushing, hyperglycemia, hyperuricemia/gout, upper GI distress, hepatotoxicity
- Bile acid sequestrant:
  - Types: Cholestyramine (Questran) 4–16 g/d; colestipol (Colestid) 5–30 g/d; colesevelam (Welchol) 2.6–3.6 g/d
  - Effect: LDL-C ↓15–30%; TG no effect; HDL-C ↑3–5%
  - Contraindications: Familial dysbetalipoproteinemia; TG >200 mg/dL (relative); TG >400 mg/dL (absolute); complete biliary obstruction; bowel obstruction
  - Possible interactions: Can decrease absorption of other drugs (take other drugs 1 hour before or 4 hours after administration of bile acid sequestrant); can decrease absorption of vitamins A, D, E, K
  - Adverse reactions: Upper and lower GI complaints common; no systemic adverse reactions because not absorbed from GI tract
- Nonstatin therapy lowers LDL-C but controversial as to whether it actually lowers CV outcomes and mortality (4)[C]

COMPLEMENTARY AND ALTERNATIVE MEDICINE

- Omega-3 fatty acids and fish oil intake:
  - Sources: Fish oil (salmon), plant sources (flaxseed, canola oil, soybean oil, nuts)
  - Mainly lowers triglyceride level, but has some benefit in lowering LDL and raising HDL although overall CV benefit and mortality reduction uncertain
  - AHA recommendation:
    - No history of CHD: Eat variety of oily fish twice a week
    - History of CHD: 1 g of combined EPA (eicosapentaenoic acid) and DHA (docosahexaenoic acid) daily; preferably from natural oily fish but can consider supplements with physician guidance
- Beta-sitosterols and red yeast rice (contains natural lovastatin-analogue) can reduce total cholesterol and LDL
- Garlic: Appears to have some lipid-lowering effect but more studies needed; effective dose not established but generally 1–2 cloves of raw garlic/d, 300 mg dried garlic powder tablet b.i.d. or t.i.d. or 7.2 g of aged garlic extract/d

ONGOING CARE

FOLLOW-UP RECOMMENDATIONS

Exercise:

- Sustained exercise for 30 minutes, 3–4 times per week: Increases HDL, lowers total cholesterol, and helps control weight

Patient Monitoring

Initially, lipid panel every 6 weeks until target goals reached, then every 4–6 months to promote compliance and monitor continued response. If taking a statin, check LFTs at baseline, at 6 or 12 weeks after therapy initiation, and then every year.

DIET

NCEP Therapeutic Lifestyle Changes Diet: Dietary fats: 25–35% of total calories. Saturated: <7% of total calories. Polyunsaturated: <10% of total calories. Monounsaturated: <20% of total calories. Carbohydrates: 50–60% of total calories from whole grains, fruits, vegetables. Fiber: 20–30 g/d. Cholesterol: <200 mg/d. Protein: ~15% of total calories.

PROGNOSIS

1% reduction in CV events for every 1.6 mg/dL reduction in LDL-C level

COMPLICATIONS

Atherosclerotic disease and generalized arteriosclerosis

REFERENCES

1. National Cholesterol Education Program (NCEP) Expert Panel on Detection, Evaluation, and Treatment of High Blood Cholesterol in Adults (Adult Treatment Panel III), et al. Third Report of the National Cholesterol Education Program (NCEP) Expert Panel on Detection, Evaluation, and Treatment of High Blood Cholesterol in Adults (Adult Treatment Panel III) final report. *Circulation*. 2002;106:3143–421.
2. U.S. Preventive Services Task Force. Screening for Lipid Disorders in Adults. Recommendation Statement. June 2008. http://uspreventiveservicestaskforce.org/uspstf08/lipid/lipidrs.htm.
3. Preiss D, Seshasai SRK, Welsh P, et al. Risk of incident diabetes with intensive-dose compared with moderate-dose statin therapy: A meta-analysis. *JAMA*. 2011;305:2556–64.
4. Murrow JR, et al. The role of nonstatin therapy in managing hyperlipidemia. *Am Fam Physician*. 2010;82:1056–7.

ADDITIONAL READING

Gillett RC, Norrell A, et al. Considerations for safe use of statins: Liver enzyme abnormalities and muscle toxicitiy. *Am Fam Physician*. 2011;83:711–6.

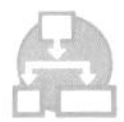

See Also (Topic, Algorithm, Electronic Media Element)

- Atherosclerosis; Hypothyroidism, Adult
- Algorithm: Hypercholesterolemia

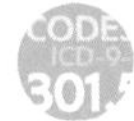

CODES

ICD9

272.0 Pure hypercholesterolemia

CLINICAL PEARLS

- Hypercholesterolemia is a significant risk factor for CHD. Primary target of therapy: lowering LDL-C.
- Diet and exercise should be tried before pharmaceutical interventions.
- Statins are considered first-line medications for hypercholesterolemia.
- Second-line therapy less well supported by evidence includes ezetimibe, fibric acid derivatives, niacin, and bile acid sequestrants.

H

HYPEREMESIS GRAVIDARUM

Scott A. Fields, MD

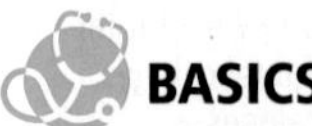

BASICS

DESCRIPTION

- Hyperemesis gravidarum is persistent vomiting in a pregnant woman that interferes with fluid and electrolyte balance as well as nutrition:
  - Usually associated with the first 8–20 weeks of pregnancy
  - Believed to have biomedical and behavioral aspects
  - Associated with high estrogen levels
  - Symptoms usually begin ~2 weeks after first missed period.
- System(s) affected: Endocrine/Metabolic; Gastrointestinal; Reproductive
- Synonym(s): Morning sickness

Pregnancy Considerations

Common condition during pregnancy, typically in the first and second trimesters but may persist into the third trimester.

EPIDEMIOLOGY

Incidence

Hyperemesis gravidarum occurs in 1–2% of pregnancies.

Prevalence

Hyperemesis gravidarum is the most common cause of hospitalization in the first half of pregnancy and the second most common cause of hospitalization of pregnant women.

RISK FACTORS

- Obesity
- Nulliparity
- Multiple gestations
- Gestational trophoblastic disease
- Gonadotropin production stimulated
- Altered GI function
- Hyperthyroidism
- Hyperparathyroidism
- Liver dysfunction

GENERAL PREVENTION

Anticipatory guidance in first and second trimesters regarding dietary habits in hopes of avoiding dehydration and nutritional depletion

Pregnancy Considerations

- 2% of pregnancies have electrolyte disturbances.
- 50% of pregnancies have at least some GI disturbance.

ETIOLOGY

- Unknown
- Possible psychologic factors
- Hyperthyroidism
- Hyperparathyroidism
- Gestational hormones
- Liver dysfunction
- Autonomic nervous system dysfunction

COMMONLY ASSOCIATED CONDITIONS

Hyperthyroidism

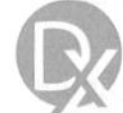

DIAGNOSIS

HISTORY

- Hypersensitivity to smell
- Alteration in taste
- Poor appetite
- Nausea
- Vomiting with retching
- Decreased urine output
- Fatigue
- Dizziness with standing

DIAGNOSTIC TESTS & INTERPRETATION

Lab

Initial lab tests

- Urinalysis: Glucosuria, albuminuria, granular casts, and hematuria (rare); ketosis more common
- Thyroid-stimulating hormone (TSH), T4
- Electrolytes, BUN, creatinine:
  - Electrolyte abnormalities due to nausea and vomiting and subsequent dehydration
  - Acidosis
- Calcium
- Increased uric acid
- Hypoalbuminemia

Follow-Up & Special Considerations

- If hypercalcemia, consider checking parathyroid hormone (PTH) for hyperparathyroidism.
- Drugs unlikely to alter lab results.

Imaging

No imaging is indicated for the diagnosis of hyperemesis gravidarum.

Diagnostic Procedures/Surgery

Indicated only if it is necessary to rule out other diagnoses as listed below

DIFFERENTIAL DIAGNOSIS

Other common causes of vomiting must be considered:

- Gastroenteritis
- Gastritis
- Reflux esophagitis
- Peptic ulcer disease
- Cholelithiasis
- Cholecystitis
- Pyelonephritis
- Anxiety
- Hyperparathyroidism

TREATMENT

Pyridoxine and metoclopramide (pregnancy Category A) are first-line treatments for hyperemesis gravidarum, followed by prochlorperazine (pregnancy Category C), prednisolone (pregnancy Category A), promethazine (pregnancy Category C), and ondansetron (pregnancy Category B1) (1,2).

MEDICATION

- Pyridoxine (vitamin B_6) 10–30 mg PO or IV daily
- Antihistamines (e.g., diphenhydramine [25–50 mg q4–6h] or doxylamine [12.5 mg PO b.i.d.])
- Phenothiazines (e.g., promethazine or prochlorperazine):
  - Precautions: Phenothiazines are associated with prolonged jaundice, extrapyramidal effects, hyper- or hyporeflexia in newborns
- Meclizine 25 mg PO q6h
- Methylprednisolone 16 mg PO × daily for 3 days, then taper over 2 weeks (3)
- Ondansetron 4–8 mg PO q8h

Pregnancy Considerations

All medications taken during pregnancy should balance the risks and benefits both to the mother and the fetus.

ADDITIONAL TREATMENT

General Measures

- Patient reassurance
- Bed rest
- If dehydrated, IV fluids. Repeat if there is a recurrence of symptoms following initial improvement.

COMPLEMENTARY AND ALTERNATIVE MEDICINE
- Ginger 350 mg PO t.i.d. may help (4).
- Motion sickness wristbands are another nonpharmacological intervention that may improve symptoms.
- Evidence is mixed regarding the impact of acupressure and acupuncture in treating hyperemesis gravidarum (1).
- Medical hypnosis may be a powerful adjunct to the typical medical treatment regimen (5)[B].

IN-PATIENT CONSIDERATIONS
Initial Stabilization
- Typically outpatient therapy
- In some severe cases, parenteral therapy in the hospital or at home may be required.
- Enteral volume and nutrition repletion may be indicated.

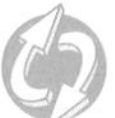

ONGOING CARE

FOLLOW-UP RECOMMENDATIONS
Activity as tolerated after improvement (4,6)[C]

Patient Monitoring
- In severe cases, follow up on a daily basis for weight monitoring.
- Special attention should be given to monitoring for ketosis, hypokalemia, or acid-base disturbances due to hyperemesis.

DIET
- NPO for first 24 hours if patient is ill enough to require hospitalization
- For outpatient: A diet rich in carbohydrates and protein, such as fruit, cheese, cottage cheese, eggs, beef, poultry, vegetables, toast, crackers, rice. Limit intake of butter. Patients should avoid spicy meals and high-fat foods.

PATIENT EDUCATION
- Attention should be given to psychosocial issues, such as possible ambivalence about the pregnancy.
- Patients should be instructed to take small amounts of fluid frequently to avoid volume depletion.
- Avoidance of individual foods known to be irritating to the patient
- Wet-to-dry nutrients (sherbet, broth, gelatin to dry crackers, toast)

PROGNOSIS
- Self-limited illness with good prognosis if patient's weight is maintained at >95% of prepregnancy weight
- With complication of hemorrhagic retinitis, mortality rate of pregnant patient is 50%.

COMPLICATIONS
- Patients with >5% weight loss are associated with intrauterine growth retardation and fetal anomalies.
- Hemorrhagic retinitis
- Liver damage
- CNS deterioration, sometimes to coma

REFERENCES

1. Sheehan P. Hyperemesis gravidarum—Assessment and management. *Aust Fam Physician*. 2007;36: 698–701.
2. Tan PC, Omar SZ. Contemporary approaches to hyperemesis during pregnancy. *Curr Opin Obstet Gynecol*. 2011;23(2):87–93.
3. Yost NP, McIntire DD, Wians FH, et al. A randomized, placebo-controlled trial of corticosteroids for hyperemesis due to pregnancy. *Obstet Gynecol*. 2003;102:1250–4.
4. Borrelli F, Capasso R, Aviello G. Effectiveness and safety of ginger in the treatment of pregnancy-induced nausea and vomiting. *Obstet Gynecol*. 2005;105:849–56.
5. Simon EP, Schwartz J. Medical hypnosis for hyperemesis gravidarum. *Birth*. 1999;26:248–54.
6. Cedergren M, Brynhildsen J, Josefsson A. Hyperemesis gravidarum that requires hospitalization and the use of antiemetic drugs in relation to maternal body composition. *Am J Obstet Gynecol*. 2008;198(4):412.e1–5.

ADDITIONAL READING

- Jewell D, Young G. Interventions for nausea and vomiting in early pregnancy. Cochrane Pregnancy and Childbirth Group. *Cochrane Database Syst Rev*. 2006;1.
- Poursharif B, Korst LM, Fejzo MS. The psychosocial burden of hyperemesis gravidarum. *J Perinatology*. 2008;28(3):176–81.
- Trogstad LI, Stoltenberg C, Magnus P, et al. Recurrence risk in hyperemesis gravidarum. *BJOG*. 2005;112(12):1641–5.
- Verberg MF, Gillott DJ, Al-Fardan N, et al. Hyperemesis gravidarum, a literature review. *Hum Reprod Update*. 2005;11:527–39.

CODES

ICD9
- 643.03 Mild hyperemesis gravidarum, antepartum
- 643.10 Hyperemesis gravidarum with metabolic disturbance, unspecified as to episode of care or not applicable
- 643.13 Hyperemesis gravidarum with metabolic disturbance, antepartum

CLINICAL PEARLS
- Do not allow patients to become volume depleted. Once this occurs, it is more difficult to interrupt the process.
- Do not be hesitant to use medications to assist the patient, as this may help avoid the volume depletion.

HYPEREOSINOPHILIC SYNDROME

Andrew M. Brunner, MD
Armando Bedoya, MD
Fred Schiffman, MD

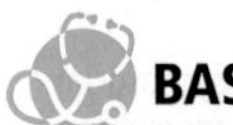

BASICS

DESCRIPTION

Hypereosinophilic syndrome (HES): A heterogeneous group of chronically high eosinophil states characterized by:

- A persistently elevated eosinophil count >1,500 cells/μL for at least 6 months
- Eosinophil-induced end-organ damage
- Exclusion of other causes of eosinophilia (e.g., parasitic infection, allergy, malignancy, collagen-vascular disease)
- There are several patient subsets within HES:
  - *FIP1L1/PDGFRα*-associated (F/P+) HES: Myeloproliferative HES, chronic eosinophilic leukemia (CEL)
  - F/P–HES:
    - Lymphocytic HES (L-HES): CD3–/CD4+ T-lymphocytes produce IL-5
    - Organ-restricted disease, e.g., eosinophilic esophagitis
  - Idiopathic HES
- System(s) affected: Hematologic; Cardiac; Cutaneous; Pulmonary; Neurologic; Gastrointestinal; Rheumatologic; Ocular
- Synonym(s): Disseminated eosinophilic collagen disease; Löeffler fibroplastic endocarditis with eosinophilia (not currently used)

EPIDEMIOLOGY

A rare condition, typically seen between 20 and 50 years of age

Incidence

- Peak incidence in fourth decade of life
- Uncommon in children
- Incidence decreases in elderly
- Predominant sex: Male > Female (9:1)
- Male predominance in F/P+ HES; other types more equally distributed

RISK FACTORS

Male gender (F/P+ HES)

Genetics

- F/P+ HES: Microdeletion at 4q12 causing gene fusion creates constitutively active tyrosine kinase.
- F/P– HES:
  - L-HES: Clonal T-cell expansion; mutations such as 16q breakage, partial 6q or 10p deletions, trisomy 7
  - Familial eosinophilia: Autosomal dominant, at 5q31–q33; eosinophilia at birth, often asymptomatic
  - Cardiac disease more in males, carriers of HLA-Bw44

GENERAL PREVENTION

No documented measures

PATHOPHYSIOLOGY

- Organ damage is similar among HES subsets and results from high eosinophil levels.
- Cytokines IL-3, IL-5, and GM-CSF stimulate bone marrow eosinophil production; IL-5 is most specific.
- Blood levels, organ migration regulated by chemokines, especially IL-5 and eotaxins
- HES: Eosinophils infiltrate organs and release toxic granules containing major basic protein, eosinophil peroxidase, eosinophil cationic protein (ECP), eosinophil-derived neurotoxin (EDN), Charcot Leyden crystal, VIP, and substance P. Neurotoxic, cytotoxic, and prothrombotic; creates oxidative burst, reactive oxygen species
- Cytokine release (IL-1, IL-3, IL-5, TNF-α) incites damage and activates inflammatory pathways.
- EDN and ECP activate fibroblasts: Fibrosis and organ dysfunction

ETIOLOGY

Variable, depends on patient subset:

- F/P+ HES: Clonal proliferation of myeloid cells with constitutively active tyrosine kinase (1)
- F/P– HES:
  - Clonal expansion of IL-5-producing CD3–/CD4+ T-lymphocytes (L-HES)
  - Enhanced activity of eosinophilogenic cytokines
  - Failure to normally regulate/suppress eosinophil activity

DIAGNOSIS

- Exclude secondary causes of eosinophilia.
- Highly variable presentation; depends on organ systems affected for any etiology; often indolent illness/incidental finding; occasionally acute onset, e.g., cardiac failure, thrombotic event

HISTORY

- Left upper quadrant pain (from splenomegaly)
- Most common sign and symptoms are weakness, fatigue, and anemia
- Cardiac manifestations (50–60%) may cause heart failure symptoms and chest pain.
- Neurologic manifestations (50%) may result from thromboembolic disease: Behavioral changes, memory loss, confusion.
- Cutaneous manifestations (69%) may cause pruritus.
- Pulmonary manifestations (40–60%) may cause dyspnea and nonproductive cough.
- GI manifestations (38%): Gastritis/enteritis: Diarrhea, vomiting, abdominal pain (embolic bowel infarction); hepatic manifestations of hepatitis, Budd-Chiari syndrome
- Ocular manifestations (20%): Blurry vision/blindness from microemboli
- Other: Myalgias, arthralgias

PHYSICAL EXAM

Various; depends on organ involvement

- Hematologic: Splenomegaly
- Cardiac:
  - Murmur
  - Signs of CHF
  - Microemboli, splinter hemorrhages
- Neurologic:
  - Signs of stroke/TIA
  - Sensory/motor deficits, usually symmetric
- Cutaneous: Angioedema, urticarial lesions, erythematous papules or nodules, mucosal ulcers, dermatographism
- Pulmonary: Crackles
- GI: Hepatomegaly (hepatitis, Budd-Chiari syndrome)
- Rheumatologic: Joint effusions

DIAGNOSTIC TESTS & INTERPRETATION

- May be discovered incidentally on routine laboratory testing
- Hematologic manifestations (100%):
  - Eosinophilia, leukocytosis
  - Thrombocytosis or thrombocytopenia
  - Hypercoagulable state (↑ tissue factor expression/altered thrombomodulin)

Lab

With the following, perform extensive workup to rule out secondary causes of eosinophilia:

- CBC:
  - ↓ Hematocrit (anemia of chronic disease, hypersplenism)
  - WBCs: eosinophils $\geq$1,500 cells/μL; leukocytosis of 10,000–30,000 (>90,000 carries poor prognosis)
  - Thrombocytosis; thrombocytopenia (hypersplenism)
- Genetics:
  - FISH analysis or RT-PCR: Assess *FIP1L1/PDGFRα* translocation/other TK mutations
  - RT-PCR or Southern blot: Assess IL-5-producing CD3–/CD4+ T-lymphocytes
- Chemistries:
  - ↑ Ig-E
  - ↑ Serum tryptase (F/P+ HES)
  - ↑ B_{12} levels
  - L-HES: ↑ IL-5, IgG, IgM, TARC levels
- ECG: T-wave inversion, restrictive cardiomyopathy

Initial lab tests

- Rule out other causes: Parasite serologies, stool ova and parasites × 3, HIV, ESR, CRP, rheumatoid factor, adrenal insufficiency
- CBC with differential, smear (eosinophil morphology is unreliable indicator); serum tryptase, B_{12}, immunoglobulins; ECG, troponin, CPK, LFTs, creatinine, BUN, PFTs (end-organ function)
- Peripheral blood screening for *FIP1L1-PDGFRA* first. If negative, then bone marrow biopsy and cytogenetics for *FIP1L1/PDGFRα, BCR/ABL, KIT* translocations; peripheral T-lymphocyte phenotyping with flow cytometry and TCR analysis (2)
- If all negative, consider idiopathic HES.

Imaging

- Echocardiogram
- Abdominal/chest CT: Assess splenomegaly, end-organ involvement

Diagnostic Procedures/Surgery

Tissue biopsy (organ-restricted disease)

Pathological Findings

Organ infiltration with eosinophils and lymphocytes, tissue necrosis, eosinophil degranulation, and microabscesses

DIFFERENTIAL DIAGNOSIS

- Extensive; first rule out secondary causes of eosinophilia: Parasitic infection, allergy, malignancy, drug hypersensitivity, connective-tissue disorders:
  - CEL: Clonality like F/P+ HES but differs by having 2–20% blasts peripherally or 5–20% blasts in the marrow
  - Acute eosinophilic leukemia: A form of AML with 50–80% eosinophils; may cause bronchospasm, heart failure

- Other conditions with high eosinophil levels: Hodgkin lymphoma, mastocytosis, chronic myelomonocytic leukemia (eosinophil variant), cutaneous T-cell lymphoma, Churg-Strauss syndrome/other vasculitides, toxicity (the eosinophilia–myalgia syndrome), HIV, HTLV, bronchopulmonary aspergillosis

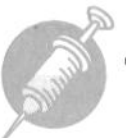

TREATMENT

- Treatment goal: Control and reduce end-organ damage.
- Some damage, such as cardiac fibrosis, may not be reversible.
- One must consider F/P transcript status.

MEDICATION

- F/P+ HES:
  - Tyrosine kinase inhibitors (TKIs) in all patients with or without symptoms
  - Danger of heart failure with therapy initiation (rapid release of killed eosinophil contents): Obtain troponin, monitor carefully, treat with corticosteroids 1–2 mg/kg/d concurrently or prior to initiation of therapy if complications arise, cardiac enzymes elevated, abnormal echocardiogram.
  - TKIs shown to induce complete molecular response (no F/P transcript); not yet known to be curative
- F/P– HES:
  - Corticosteroids are the mainstay of treatment.
  - A corticosteroid-sparing agent (interferon-α, anti-CD52 agents in L-HES, IL-5 inhibitors, chemotherapeutic agents) may be introduced if steroids poorly tolerated or fail to manage disease.
  - May respond to TKI, suggesting non-F/P tyrosine kinase activity

First Line

- F/P+ HES: Imatinib mesylate (Gleevec) started at 400 mg/d (3)[A]:
  - Generally, lower doses needed to induce/maintain remission than with CML. Therapy continued indefinitely
  - Side effects: Thrombocytopenia, anemia, nausea, diarrhea, ↑ LFTs
  - Resistance: T674I point mutation, similar to CML
- F/P– HES: Prednisone: Initial challenge of 60 mg once to determine responsiveness, followed by 1 mg/kg/d × 1–2 weeks. A taper should be initiated based on disease severity, persistent eosinophilia (4)[C]:
  - Side effects: Many; intolerance should prompt decreasing dose, adding second agent.
  - Once stable, may add corticosteroid-sparing agent

Second Line

- F/P + HES: Patients rarely have shown resistance to imatinib; initiate trial of other TKI such as nilotinib, sorafenib, or dasatinib (4)[C].
- F/P– HES:
- Interferon-α:
  - Effective dose 1–8 million U 3–7 times a week; start low, increase as tolerated.
  - Side effects: Flulike symptoms, cytopenias, depression, elevated LFTs, GI disturbances
- Hydroxyurea:
  - Start at 500–1,000 mg/d, increase to 2,000 mg/d.
  - Side effects: Cytopenias, nausea, rash, alopecia, diffuse pulmonary infiltrates, elevated LFTs, teratogen
- Mepolizumab (in clinical trials) (5):
  - Anti-IL5 (expressed on eosinophils) antibody; administered 750 mg IV every 4 weeks. Decreases steroid use
  - Side effects: Currently not well defined
- Alemtuzumab (L-HES use under evaluation) (6):
  - Anti-CD52 antibody, IV administration
  - Side effects: Hypotension, fever, fatigue, lymphopenia, neutropenia, fatal infection

ADDITIONAL TREATMENT

Issues for Referral

- Refer to a hematologist.
- Refer to appropriate specialist for organ dysfunction, e.g., cardiologist.

SURGERY/OTHER PROCEDURES

- Allogeneic stem cell transplant:
  - Patients failing other treatment modalities and/or aggressive disease
  - Patients with L-HES progressing to T-cell lymphoma
  - Role has not been well established
- Cardiac surgery for complications of HES has been efficacious. If valve replacement is necessary, use porcine valve because of underlying hypercoagulable state.

IN-PATIENT CONSIDERATIONS

Initial Stabilization

- Emergency treatment for eosinophilia >100,000 includes high-dose corticosteroids (prednisone 1 mg/kg).
- If levels fail to decrease significantly in 24 hours: Vincristine 1–2 mg/m^2, imatinib 400 mg, or plasmapheresis

Admission Criteria

Heart failure, splenic rupture, organ failure; admission also may be necessary for reduction of very high eosinophilia.

Discharge Criteria

Abatement of acute symptoms

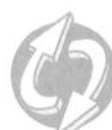

ONGOING CARE

FOLLOW-UP RECOMMENDATIONS

Frequency depends on etiology of disease, response to treatment, and severity of end-organ damage.

Patient Monitoring

- Weekly CBC on initiating treatment; longer intervals once stable
- L-HES: Increased risk of T-cell lymphoma; CBC every 3 months; flow cytometry biannually to monitor abnormal lymphocytosis (3)
- Patients on imatinib: LFTs and CBC monthly; RT-PCR for the F/P transcript; echocardiogram every 3 months
- Screen all patients for organ involvement every 6 months: Cardiac enzymes, PFTs, LFTs, renal function tests, ECG, echocardiogram.
- Anticoagulation unnecessary without thrombi

PROGNOSIS

- Better prognosis:
  - Absence heart disease
  - Presentation with angioedema
  - Corticosteroid responsive
  - Absent indicators of myeloproliferative disease (elevated B$_{12}$ or tryptase, splenomegaly, abnormal lymphocytes, cytogenetic abnormalities)
- Worse prognosis
  - Concurrent myeloproliferative disorder
  - Male sex
  - Peripheral blood blasts
  - WBC count >100,000

REFERENCES

1. Cools J, DeAngelo DJ, Gotlib J, et al. A tyrosine kinase created by fusion of the PDGFRA and FIP1L1 genes as a therapeutic target of imatinib in idiopathic hypereosinophilic syndrome. *N Engl J Med*. 2003;348:1201–14.
2. Tefferi A, Gotlib J, Pardanani A, et al. Hypereosinophilic syndrome and clonal eosinophilia: Point-of-care diagnostic algorithm and treatment update. *Mayo Clin Proc*. 2010;85: 158–64.
3. Baccarani M, Cilloni D, Rondoni M, et al. The efficacy of imatinib mesylate in patients with FIP1l1-PDGFRalpha-positive hypereosinophilic syndrome. Results of a multicenter prospective study. *Haematologica*. 2007;92(9):1173–9.
4. Fletcher S, Bain B. Diagnosis and treatment of hypereosinophilic syndromes. *Curr Opin Hematol*. 2007;14:37–42.
5. Rothenberg ME, Klion AD, Roufosse FE, et al. Treatment of patients with the hypereosinophilic syndrome with mepolizumab. *N Engl J Med*. 2008;358:1215–28.
6. Verstovsek S, Tefferi A, Kantarjian H, et al. Alemtuzumab therapy for hypereosinophilic syndrome and chronic eosinophilic leukemia. *Clin Cancer Res*. 2009;15:368–73.

ADDITIONAL READING

- Gotlib J, et al. World Health Organization-defined eosinophilic disorders: 2011 update on diagnosis, risk stratification, and management. *Am J Hematol*. 2011;86:677–88.
- Roufosse FE, Goldman M, Cogan E, et al. Hypereosinophilic syndromes. *Orphanet J Rare Dis*. 2007;2:37.
- Sheikh J, Weller PF. Clinical overview of hypereosinophilic syndromes. *Immunol Allergy Clin North Am*. 2007;27:333–55.

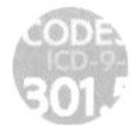

CODES

ICD9

288.3 Eosinophilia

CLINICAL PEARLS

- HS encompasses a group of diseases with eosinophils >1,500/μL and end-organ damage without an identifiable secondary cause.
- F/P+ transcript should be determined early in the course of treatment.
- Cardiac disease is a dangerous complication of this condition and may not be reversible.

H

HYPERKALEMIA

Ruben Peralta, MD, FACS
Mushreq Alani, MD

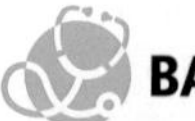

BASICS

DESCRIPTION

- Hyperkalemia is a common electrolyte disorder with a plasma potassium (K) concentration >5.5 mEq/L (>5 mmol/L).
- Hyperkalemia depresses cardiac conduction and can lead to fatal arrhythmias.
- Normal K regulation:
  - Ingested K enters portal circulation; pancreas releases insulin in response. Insulin facilitates K entry into cells.
  - K in renal circulation causes renin release from juxtaglomerular cells, leading to activation of angiotensin I, which is converted to angiotensin II in lungs. Angiotensin II acts in adrenal zona glomerulosa to stimulate aldosterone secretion. Aldosterone, at the renal collecting ducts, causes K to be excreted and sodium (Na) to be retained.
- 4 major causes:
  - Increased load: Either endogenous from tissue release or exogenous from a high intake, which is usually in association with impaired excretion
  - Decreased excretion: Due to decreased glomerular filtration rate
  - Cellular redistribution: Shifting of intracellular space (which is the major store of K) to extracellular space
  - Pseudohyperkalemia: Related to improper collection or transport of blood sample

Geriatric Considerations

Increased risk for hyperkalemia because of decreases in renin and aldosterone as well as increased number of comorbid conditions

EPIDEMIOLOGY

Prevalence

- 1–10% of hospitalized patients
- Predominant sex: Male = Female
- No age-related predilection

RISK FACTORS

- Impaired renal excretion of K
- Acidemia
- Massive cell breakdown (rhabdomyolysis, burns, trauma)
- Use of K-sparing diuretics
- Excess K supplementation

Genetics

Associated with some inherited diseases and conditions:

- Familial hyperkalemic periodic paralysis
- Congenital adrenal hyperplasia

GENERAL PREVENTION

Diet and oral supplement compliance

ETIOLOGY

- Pseudohyperkalemia:
  - Hemolysis of red cells in phlebotomy tube (spurious result is most common)
  - Thrombolysis
  - Leukocytosis
  - Thrombocytosis
  - Hereditary spherocytosis
  - Infectious mononucleosis
- Traumatic venipuncture or fist clenching during phlebotomy (spurious result)
- Transcellular shift (redistribution):
  - Metabolic acidosis
  - Insulin deficiency
  - Hyperglycemia
  - Tissue damage (rhabdomyolysis, burns, trauma) (1)
  - Tumor lysis syndrome
  - Cocaine abuse
  - Exercise with heavy sweating
  - Mannitol
- Impaired K excretion:
  - Renal insufficiency/failure
  - Addison disease
  - Mineralocorticoid deficiency
  - Primary hyporeninemia, primary hypoaldosteronism
  - Type IV renal tubular acidosis
- Medication-induced:
  - Excess K supplementation
  - ACE inhibitors (2)
  - Angiotensin receptor blockers
  - β-blockers
  - Cyclosporine
  - Digoxin toxicity
  - Ethinyl estradiol/drospirenone
  - Heparin
  - NSAIDs
  - Penicillin G potassium
  - Pentamidine
  - Spironolactone
  - Succinylcholine
  - Tacrolimus
  - Trimethoprim (2,3)

DIAGNOSIS

HISTORY

- Neuromuscular cramps
- Diarrhea
- Abdominal pain
- Myalgias
- Numbness
- Weakness

PHYSICAL EXAM

- Decreased deep tendon reflexes
- Flaccid paralysis of extremities

DIAGNOSTIC TESTS & INTERPRETATION

Lab

- Serum electrolytes
- Renal function: BUN, creatinine
- Urinalysis: K, creatinine, osmoles (to calculate fractional excretion of K and transtubular K gradient; both assess renal handling of K)
- Disorders that may alter lab results:
  - Acidemia: K shifts from the intracellular to extracellular space in an effort to buffer the acid load.
  - Insulin deficiency
  - Hemolysis of sample
- Cortisol and aldosterone levels to check for mineralocorticoid deficiency when other causes are ruled out

Diagnostic Procedures/Surgery

EKG:

- Peaked T wave in precordial leads (most common, usually earliest EKG change) (4).
- Loss of P wave
- Widened QRS
- Sine wave at very high K

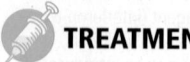

TREATMENT

MEDICATION

- After initial stabilization (see above), institute measures to decrease total body K:
  - Sodium polystyrene sulfonate (Kayexalate): 30–60 g PO or rectally
  - This is effective in 1–4 hours and is a definitive treatment. This may be repeated q6h, if necessary.
  - Enema form more quickly effective
- Diuretics (loop and thiazides)
- Consider the use of recombinant urate oxidase (Rasburicase) in patients with tumor lysis syndrome.
- Hemodialysis is the definitive therapy when other measures are not effective. Conditions such as digitalis toxicity or rhabdomyolysis exist in patients with end-stage renal disease, severe chronic kidney disease, acute kidney injury, or comorbidity.

ALERT

- Kayexalate provides a sodium load that may exacerbate fluid overload in cardiac or renal failure patients.
- Rapid administration of calcium in patients with suspected digitalis toxicity may result in a fatal dysrhythmia. Calcium should be administered slowly over 20–30 minutes in 5% dextrose with extreme caution.
- Calcium and dextrose/insulin are only temporizing measures and do not actually lower total body K levels.
- Sodium bicarbonate is no longer recommended to lower K, although it may be appropriate in patients with severe metabolic acidosis.

IN-PATIENT CONSIDERATIONS

Initial Stabilization

- If hyperkalemia is severe, treat first, then do diagnostic investigations.
- IV calcium to stabilize myocardium (caution in setting of digoxin toxicity, when calcium may worsen effects of toxicity)
- Insulin (usually 10 units IV, given with 50 mL of 50% glucose to avoid hypoglycemia); consider repeating if elevation persists
- Inhaled β_2-agonist (nebulized albuterol)
- Insulin and β_2-agonist facilitate K entry into cells and do not decrease total body K.
- Discontinue any medications that may increase K (e.g., K-sparing diuretics, exogenous K).

Admission Criteria

Admit for cardiac monitoring if EKG changes are present or if K is >6 mEq/L (6 mmol/L).

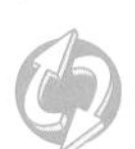

ONGOING CARE

FOLLOW-UP RECOMMENDATIONS

Patient Monitoring

- Reduction of plasma K should begin within the first hour of initiation of treatment.
- Serum K levels should be rechecked every 2–4 hours until the patient has stabilized and recurrent hyperkalemia is no longer a threat.
- Identification and elimination of possible causes and risk factors for hyperkalemia are essential.

DIET

≤80 mEq (≤80 mmol) of K per 24 hours

PATIENT EDUCATION

Consult with a dietitian about a low-K diet.

PROGNOSIS

- Associated with poor prognosis in heart failure patients
- Associated with poor prognosis in disaster medicine, trauma (1)
- Associated with poor prognosis in hemodialysis patients with higher dietary K^+ intake (5)

COMPLICATIONS

- Life-threatening cardiac arrhythmias
- Hypokalemia
- Potential complications of the use of ion-exchange resins for the treatment of hyperkalemia include volume overload and intestinal necrosis (6).

REFERENCES

1. Bosch X, Poch E, Grau JM. Rhabdomyolysis and acute kidney injury. *N Engl J Med*. 2009;361: 62–72.
2. Antoniou T, Gomes T, Juurlink DN, et al. Trimethoprim-sulfamethoxazole-induced hyperkalemia in patients receiving inhibitors of the renin-angiotensin system: A population-based study. *Arch Intern Med*. 2010;170:1045–9.
3. Weir MA, Juurlink DN, Gomes T, et al. Beta-blockers, trimethoprim-sulfamethoxazole, and the risk of hyperkalemia requiring hospitalization in the elderly: A nested case-control study. *Clin J Am Soc Nephrol*. 2010;5:1544–51.
4. Wong R, Banker R, Aronowitz P, et al. Electrocardiographic changes of severe hyperkalemia. *J Hosp Med*. 2011;6(4):240.
5. Noori N, Kalantar-Zadeh K, Kovesdy CP, et al. Dietary Potassium Intake and Mortality in Long-term Hemodialysis Patients. *Am J Kidney Dis*. 2010;56(2):338–47.
6. Sterns RH, Rojas M, Bernstein P, et al. Ion-exchange resins for the treatment of hyperkalemia: Are they safe and effective? *J Am Soc Nephrol*. 2010;21:733–5.

ADDITIONAL READING

- Cross NB, Webster AC, Masson P et al. Antihypertensives for kidney transplant recipients: systematic review and meta-analysis of randomized controlled trials. *Transplantation*. 2009;88:7–18.
- Hall AB, Salazar M, Larison DJ. The sequencing of medication administration in the management of hyperkalemia. *J Emerg Nurs*. 2009;35:339–42.
- Hollander-Rodriguez JC, Calvert JF. Hyperkalemia. *Am Fam Physician*. 2006;73:283–90.
- Kim HJ, Han SW. Therapeutic approach to hyperkalemia. *Nephron*. 2002;92(Suppl 1):33–40.
- Putcha N, Allon M, et al. Management of hyperkalemia in dialysis patients. *Semin Dial*. 2007;20:431–9.
- Stevens MS, Dunlay RW. Hyperkalemia in hospitalized patients. *Int Urol Nephrol*. 2000;32: 177–80.

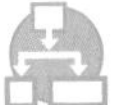

See Also (Topic, Algorithm, Electronic Media Element)

- Addison Disease; Hypokalemia
- Algorithm: Hyperkalemia

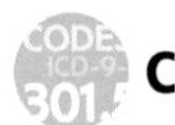

CODES

ICD9

276.7 Hyperpotassemia

CLINICAL PEARLS

- Emergency and urgent management of hyperkalemia takes precedent to a thorough diagnostic workup. Urgent treatment includes stabilization of the myocardium to protect against arrhythmias and mobilizing potassium from the extracellular (vascular) space into the cells.
- Multiple herbal medications can also increase K levels, including alfalfa, dandelion, horsetail nettle, milkweed, hawthorne berries, toad skin, oleander, foxglove, and ginseng.
- Many foods contain K. Those that are particularly high in K (>6.4 mEq per serving) include bananas, orange juice, other citrus fruits and their juices, tomatoes, tomato juice, cantaloupe, honeydew melon, peaches, potatoes, salt substitutes, and many herbal medications.
- To lower a patient's risk of developing hyperkalemia, have the patient follow a low-K diet, use selective β_1-blockers such as metoprolol or atenolol instead of nonselective β-blockers like carvedilol. Avoid NSAIDs. Concomitant use of kaliuretic loop diuretics may be useful.

HYPERNATREMIA

Fae G. Wooding, PharmD
Joshua M.V. Mammen, MD, PhD

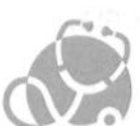

BASICS

DESCRIPTION

- Serum sodium (Na) concentration level >145 mEq/L often represents a state of hyperosmolality.
- Hypernatremia results from primary Na+ gain or water deficit.
- Hypernatremia may exist with hypo-, hyper-, or euvolemia.
- Hypovolemic hypernatremia: Most common type; occurs with a decrease in total body water (TBW) and a proportionately smaller decrease in total body Na.
- Euvolemic hypernatremia: No change in TBW with a proportionate increase in total body Na
- Hypervolemic hypernatremia: Increase in TBW and a proportionately greater increase in total body Na

Geriatric Considerations

- More common in the hospitalized patient; is an independent risk factor for mortality
- Hypernatremia may be caused by dehydration due to administration of loop diuretics.
- Increased risk because of impaired renal function and decline in thirst mechanism
- Chronically ill patients are at higher risk due to consumption of high-solute formulas.

Pediatric Considerations

- May occur in low-birth-weight newborns
- May result from improper preparation of infant formula or high concentration of Na in breast milk

EPIDEMIOLOGY

Incidence

- More common in elderly and young (1):
  - Occurs in 1% of hospitalized elderly patients (2)
- Gastroenteritis with diarrhea is the most common cause of hypernatremia in infants.

Prevalence

Females are at an increased risk due to decreased TBW.

RISK FACTORS

- Infants/children
- Old age
- Patients who are intubated or have altered mental status
- Diabetes mellitus
- Prior brain injury
- Surgery
- Diuretic therapy

Genetics

Some diabetes insipidus may be hereditary.

GENERAL PREVENTION

- Treatment or prevention of underlying cause
- Properly prepare infant formula and never add salt to any commercial infant formula.
- Keep patients well hydrated.

ETIOLOGY

- Excess Na (increase in total body Na) resulting from (3):
  - Incorrect infant formula preparation
  - Salt administered as punishment or prank
  - Sea water ingestion
  - Excessive use of $NaHCO_3$ antacid
  - IV NaCl or $NaHCO_3$ during cardiopulmonary resuscitation, metabolic acidosis, or hyperkalemia
  - Intrauterine NaCl for abortion
  - Excessive Na in dialysate solutions
  - Disorders of the adrenal axis (Cushing syndrome, Conn syndrome, congenital adrenal hyperplasia)
- Water deficit (total body Na normal) resulting from:
  - Adipsia (e.g., impaired thirst regulation, decreased access to water)
  - Nephrogenic diabetes insipidus (due to progressive renal dysfunction, hypercalcemia, hypokalemia, or medication-related)
  - Cranial diabetes insipidus (due to head trauma, stroke, or meningitis)
  - Increased insensible water loss (e.g., fever, hyperventilation, hypermetabolic state, sweat, severe burns, heat exposure, newborns under radiant warmers)
- Hypotonic fluid loss (total body Na decreased) resulting from:
  - Loss of fluid containing Na without adequate water replacement
- Urinary loss:
  - Osmotic diuretics
  - Diabetes mellitus (particularly new presentation or decompensated)
  - Diuresis from acute tubular necrosis or from relief of acute urinary obstruction
- GI loss:
  - Diarrhea, especially in children

COMMONLY ASSOCIATED CONDITIONS

- Gastroenteritis
- Altered mental status
- Burns
- Hypermetabolic conditions
- Head injury
- Renal dysfunction

DIAGNOSIS

HISTORY

- Obtain list of current and recent medications.
- Review recent illnesses and activities (1).

PHYSICAL EXAM

- Sinus tachycardia, hypotension, orthostatic hypotension, dyspnea
- Dry mucous membranes, cool or grey skin
- Excessive thirst, nausea, vomiting, diarrhea, oliguria, polyuria
- Fever, myalgia, muscle weakness
- Altered mental status, seizure, lethargy, irritability, coma, anophthalmus (1,3)[C]

DIAGNOSTIC TESTS & INTERPRETATION

Lab

Initial lab tests

- Serum Na, potassium, urea, creatinine, calcium, and osmolality (serum lithium if appropriate) (4)[C]
- Urine Na and osmolality
- Urinalysis
- Serum glucose
- Special tests:
  - Water deprivation (with diabetes insipidus, urine osmolality does not increase when hypernatremic)
  - Antidiuretic hormone stimulation (with nephrogenic diabetes insipidus, urine osmolality does not increase after ADH or DDAVP)
- Serum Na >150–170 mEq/L (>150–170 mmol/L) and BUN/creatine >20: Usually dehydration/ hypovolemia
- Serum Na >170 mEq/L (>170 mmol/L) and decreased urine Na: Usually diabetes insipidus
- Serum Na >190 mEq/L (>190 mmol/L): Usually chronic salt ingestion
- Diabetes insipidus:
  - Urine osmolality less than serum osmolality
  - Urine Na usually low
  - Polyuria
  - Neurogenic versus nephrogenic diabetes insipidus
- Hyperosmolar coma:
  - Blood sugar elevated
  - Decreased urine output
  - Increased urine osmolality
- Salt ingestion:
  - Increased urine Na
  - Increased urine osmolality
- Hypertonic dehydration:
  - Decreased urine Na
  - Increased urine osmolality

ALERT

A variety of medications may raise or lower Na levels.

Imaging

Initial approach

CT or MRI in diabetes insipidus to rule out craniopharyngioma, tumor, or median cleft syndrome (3,4)[C]

Diagnostic Procedures/Surgery

History, physical, laboratory studies, family history for neurogenic diabetes insipidus

DIFFERENTIAL DIAGNOSIS

- Diabetes insipidus
- Hyperosmotic coma
- Salt ingestion
- Hypertonic dehydration
- Hypothyroidism
- Cushing syndrome

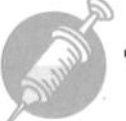

TREATMENT

MEDICATION

First Line

- Hypovolemia (usually Na 150–170) (4,5)[C]:
  - Isotonic saline (normal saline or Ringer lactate): 10–20 mL/kg IV over 1–2 hours. May repeat if ≥10% dehydration (4)[A].
  - Isotonic fluids: 5% dextrose with half-normal saline until urine output established (4)[B]
- Hypernatremia (usually due to chronic salt ingestion; Na >190):
  - Hypotonic fluids (NaCl or dextrose 5% in water) (4)[B]
  - Decrease serum Na by 0.5 mEq/L/hr (0.5 mmol/L/hr) or by no more than 20 mEq/L/d (20 mmol/L/d); allows idiogenic osmoles to resolve (mostly taurine in brain cell water).
  - Hypocalcemia may occur during correction of hypernatremia. Add calcium (50 mg/kg 10% calcium gluconate) to IV fluids.
  - Acidosis often is present in severely dehydrated patients. Add sodium bicarbonate, 50 mEq/L, to IV fluids. If both acidosis and hypocalcemia are present, correct the calcium deficit first.
  - Potassium and phosphate, if needed
  - Furosemide for hypervolemia. Dose varies depending on desired urine output.
- Neurogenic diabetes insipidus:
  - Desmopressin (DDAVP) acetate: Use parenteral form for acute symptomatic patients, and use intranasal or oral form for chronic therapy. Adults 10–40 μg intranasally in 1–3 divided doses; children 5–30 μg in a single evening dose or in 2 divided doses.
  - May use 2.5% dextrose in water if giving large volumes of water in diabetes insipidus or neurogenic diabetes insipidus to avoid glycosuria
  - May consider sulfonylureas or thiazide diuretics
- Nephrogenic diabetes insipidus:
  - Use of thiazide diuretic or indomethacin may be beneficial but should be used cautiously due to negative renal effects.
  - Lithium-induced nephrogenic diabetes insipidus: Hydrochlorothiazide 50 mg PO b.i.d. or indomethacin 50 mg PO t.i.d., or amiloride hydrochloride 5–10 mg PO b.i.d.
- Contraindications: Refer to manufacturer's literature.
- Precautions:
  - Rapid correction of hypernatremia can cause cerebral or pulmonary edema, seizures, or death. Hypocalcemia often occurs during correction.
  - Diabetes insipidus: High rates of dextrose 5% in water can cause hyperglycemia and glucose-induced diuresis.
- Significant possible interactions: Refer to manufacturer's literature.

Second Line

Consider NSAIDs in nephrogenic diabetes insipidus (3)[C].

ADDITIONAL TREATMENT

General Measures

- Appropriate health care: Inpatient (many patients are already hospitalized, and hypernatremia develops after admission)
- Treat hypovolemia first, then hypernatremia.
- Replace water orally if patient is conscious.
- Restore intravascular volume with IV fluids to normalize serum Na levels.
- Calculated water deficit (liters) = $[(0.6 \times \text{wt}) \times (\text{Na} - 140)] \div 140$:
  - Note: wt = weight in kilograms; Na = current serum Na
- Dialysis: Especially with serum Na >200 mEq/L (200 mmol/L)
- Speed of correction depends on severity of symptoms or rate of development of hypernatremia.

Issues for Referral

Underlying renal involvement associated with hypernatremia would benefit from a nephrology referral.

IN-PATIENT CONSIDERATIONS

Admission Criteria

Symptomatic patient with serum Na >155 mEq/L requires IV fluid therapy.

IV Fluids

Refer to "Medication" section.

Nursing

Bed rest until stable or underlying condition resolved or controlled

Discharge Criteria

Stabilization of serum Na level and symptoms are minimal

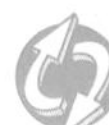

ONGOING CARE

FOLLOW-UP RECOMMENDATIONS

Patient Monitoring

- Frequent re-examinations in an acute setting
- Frequent electrolytes
- Urine osmolality and urine output in diabetes insipidus
- Ensure adequate ingestion of calories because patients may ingest so much water that they feel full and do not eat.
- Daily weights

DIET

- Ensure proper nutrition during acute phase.
- After resolution of acute phase, may want to consider Na-restricted diet for patient.
- Severe salt restriction in nephrogenic diabetes insipidus

PATIENT EDUCATION

Patients with nephrogenic diabetes insipidus must avoid salt and drink large amounts of water.

PROGNOSIS

Most recover, but neurologic impairment can sometimes be seen.

COMPLICATIONS

- CNS thrombosis or hemorrhage
- Seizures
- Mental retardation
- Hyperactivity
- Chronic hypernatremia: >2 days' duration has higher mortality
- Serum Na >180 mEq/L (>180 mmol/L): Often results in residual CNS damage

REFERENCES

1. Adrogue HJ, Madias NE. Hypernatremia. *N Engl J Med*. 2000;342:1493–9.
2. Bagshaw SM, Townsend DR, McDermid RC. Disorders of sodium and water balance in hospitalized patients. *Can J Anaesth*. 2009;56:151–67.
3. Kang SK, Kim W, Oh MS. Pathogenesis and treatment of hypernatremia. *Nephron*. 2002;92(Suppl 1):14–7.
4. Kraft MD, Btaichel F, Sachs GS, et al. Treatment of electrolyte disorders in adult patients in the intensive care unit. *Am J Health-System Pharm*. 2005;62:166382.
5. Weiss-Gullet E, Takala J, Jakob JM. Diagnosis and management of electrolyte emergencies. *Best Pract Res Clin Endocrinol Metab*. 2003;17(4):623–51.

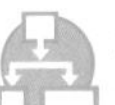

See Also (Topic, Algorithm, Electronic Media Element)

- Diabetes Insipidus
- Algorithm: Hypernatremia

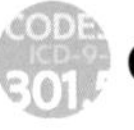

CODES

ICD9

276.0 Hyperosmolality and/or hypernatremia

CLINICAL PEARLS

- Determine if the patient has hypervolemic, euvolemic, or hypovolemic hypernatremia to determine differential diagnosis of etiology.
- Serum Na >150–170 mEq/L (>150–170 mmol/L) and BUN/creatine >20: Usually dehydration/hypovolemia
- Serum Na >170 mEq/L (>170 mmol/L) and decreased urine Na: Usually diabetes insipidus
- Serum Na >190 mEq/L (>190 mmol/L): Usually chronic salt ingestion
- Water replacement orally if patient is conscious (the preferred route)
- Speed of correction depends on severity of symptoms or rate of development of hypernatremia.

HYPERPARATHYROIDISM

Kyle D. Wood, MD
John Paul Lock, MD

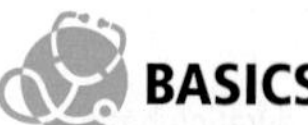

BASICS

DESCRIPTION

An acute or chronic dysfunction of the body's normal regulatory feedback mechanisms for parathyroid hormone (PTH):

- Primary: Intrinsic gland dysfunction and abnormal regulation of PTH secretion by calcium causing excessive PTH secretion
- Secondary: Gland hyperactivity that is a response to hypocalcemia, vitamin D deficiency, or renal failure
- Tertiary: Autonomous hyperfunction in the setting of long-standing secondary hyperparathyroidism (HPT)

EPIDEMIOLOGY

Incidence

Predominant sex: Female > Male (3:1)

Prevalence

Primary: ~1/750 adults

RISK FACTORS

Renal failure, age, poor nutrition, and/or family history

Genetics

Familial forms are rare, but include:

- Multiple endocrine neoplasia (MEN) types 1 and 2a: Patients with multiple gland hyperplasia in the absence of renal disease should be screened for MEN-1 gene mutation.
- Neonatal severe primary HPT
- HPT–jaw tumor syndrome
- Familial hypocalciuric hypercalcemia (FHH): Autosomal dominant
- Familial isolated HPT

GENERAL PREVENTION

Adequate intake of calcium and vitamin D may help prevent secondary HPT.

PATHOPHYSIOLOGY

- PTH is made in 4 parathyroid glands located behind the 4 poles of the thyroid gland (locations can vary).
- PTH releases calcium from bone by osteoclastic stimulation (bone resorption).
- PTH increases reabsorption of calcium in the distal tubules of the kidneys.
- PTH stimulates conversion of active vitamin D to increase calcium absorption from the GI tract.

ETIOLOGY

- Primary HPT: Unregulated increase of PTH production and release, causing increase in serum calcium:
  - Solitary adenoma (89%)
  - Double adenomas (5%)
  - Diffuse hyperplasia (6%) caused by multiple adenomas, MEN types 1 and 2a, familial hypocalciuric hypercalcemia
  - Parathyroid carcinoma (<2%)
- Secondary HPT: Adaptive parathyroid gland hyperplasia and hyperfunction:
  - Dietary: Vitamin D or calcium deficiency
  - Chronic renal disease resulting in:
    - Renal parenchymal loss causing hyperphosphatemia
    - Impaired calcitriol production causing hypocalcemia
    - General skeletal and renal resistance to PTH
- Tertiary HPT: Gland hyperplasia from prolonged hypocalcemia resulting in autonomous PTH oversecretion

COMMONLY ASSOCIATED CONDITIONS

- MEN syndromes type 1 and 2a
- Chronic renal failure

DIAGNOSIS

HISTORY

- Up to 75% are asymptomatic.
- Classic complaints of hypercalcemia include painful bones, renal stones, abdominal groans, and psychic moans.
- MEN is associated with pancreatic cancer, pituitary adenomas, medullary thyroid cancer, or pheochromocytoma.
- History of radiation to neck
- Medications: Thiazides or lithium

PHYSICAL EXAM

- Renal: Nephrolithiasis, nephrocalcinosis, reduced glomerular filtration rate, thirst, polydipsia, polyuria
- GI: Abdominal distress, gastroduodenal ulcer, pancreatitis, pancreatic calcification, constipation, vomiting, anorexia, weight loss
- Skeletal: Bone pain, cystic bone lesions, skeletal demineralization, spontaneous fracture, vertebral collapse, osteoporosis
- Mental: Fatigue, apathy, anxiety, depression, psychosis
- Neurologic: Somnolence, coma, diffuse EEG changes
- Neuromuscular: Muscle fatigue, weakness, hypotonia
- Cardiovascular: Hypertension, short QT interval, left ventricular hypertrophy
- Articular/periarticular: Arthralgia, gout, pseudogout, periarticular calcification
- Ocular: Band keratopathy, conjunctivitis, conjunctival calcium deposits

DIAGNOSTIC TESTS & INTERPRETATION

Lab

Initial lab tests

- Elevated serum calcium level (fasting): Simultaneous albumin to calculate a corrected serum calcium level or ionized calcium level; corrected calcium (mg/dL = measured calcium (mg/dL) = 0.8(4 – measured albumin)
- If hypercalcemia is confirmed, follow with intact PTH level:
  - High PTH suggests primary HPT.
  - Low PTH suggests non-PTH–mediated hypercalcemia.
- If elevated calcium is inconsistent, elevated ionized serum calcium in the setting of high PTH confirms diagnosis. Other findings may include low serum phosphate, elevated serum chloride, decreased serum CO_2, increased urinary cAMP, and abnormal 24-hour urine calcium excretion.
- In secondary HPT, an elevated phosphorus means chronic renal failure; a low phosphorus suggests another cause of vitamin D deficiency.

Follow-Up & Special Considerations

- A 24-hour urine calcium concentration to creatinine clearance ratio >0.02 suggests primary HPT; a ratio <0.01 may be normal or indicate FHH; important because FHH does not require surgery.
- Measure 25OH vitamin D—replete if ≤20 ng/mL. Hold off on management decisions (1).
- Consider serum protein electrophoresis.

Imaging

Initial approach

Imaging is not required in initial stages:

- In recent years, minimally invasive parathyroidectomy (MIP) has become more common, and imaging is required for surgical planning.
- Localization of a single adenoma allows a focused approach:
  - Technetium-99m sestamibi scan with single-photon-emission CT scan (2)[B]
  - Ultrasonography
- Imaging is indicated to localize hyperplasia or an ectopic parathyroid gland in repeat surgery.

Follow-Up & Special Considerations

- Obtain bone mineral density (DEXA) on patients with elevated PTH (3)[C].
- A baseline scan for occult nephrolithiasis is recommended (4)[C].
- Intraoperative measurement of intact PTH and/or gamma probe localization of abnormal glands with technetium-99m sestamibi scan has aided focused resections for patients with single-gland etiology (4)[C].

Diagnostic Procedures/Surgery

Consider EKG to assess for short QT interval.

Pathological Findings

See "Etiology."

- Positive inhalation challenge testing: A. Re-exposure to the environment. B. Inhalation challenge to the suspected antigen in a hospital setting.
- Histopathology showing compatible changes: Poorly formed, or noncaseating granulomas OR mononuclear infiltrate.
- Definitive HP:
  - Criteria 1, 2, and 3: Histopathological confirmation is not needed.
  - Criteria 1, 2, and 4A: BAL or histopathological confirmation is not needed.
  - Criteria 1, 2A, 3, and 5: Case cluster.
  - Criteria 2, 3, and 5: Diagnosis suspected after BAL or transbronchial lung biopsy.
- BAL (1):
  - Most sensitive tool to detect alveolitis in patients suspected of having HP.
  - A marked BAL lymphocytosis (>20% and often exceeding 50%) may be seen. The HP BAL CD4=/CD8+ ratio is usually decreased to <1 and the typical lymphocyte phenotype in BAL is CD3+/CD8+/CD56+/CD57+/CD10- in alveolitis HP.
- Other tests: Inhalation challenge to suspected environments lack standardization and can cause serious reactions (not recommended) (1)

Imaging

- CXR:
  - Acute: A micronodular, interstitial pattern in the lower and middle lung fields. Often normal.
  - Subacute: Same as acute, but the abnormalities are most predominant in the upper and middle lung fields.
  - Chronic: Upper lobe fibrosis, nodular or ground glass opacities, volume loss, emphysematous changes.
- CT scan of chest:
  - Acute: Often normal but may show the presence of ground glass opacities
  - Subacute: Ground glass opacities, poorly defined centrilobular nodules, mosaic attenuation on inspiratory images and air trapping on expiratory images.
  - Chronic: Fibrosis, irregular opacities, bronchiectasis, loss of lung volume, honeycombing, emphysematous changes
- HRCT appearance is a mid-to-upper zone predominance of centrilobular ground glass or nodular opacities with signs of air trapping (3).

Initial approach

Usually start with CXR; may progress to CT based on findings

Diagnostic Procedures/Surgery

- Pulmonary function tests (PFTs) (1):
  - Acute: Restrictive pattern, low diffusing capacity of the lung for carbon monoxide
  - Subacute: Restrictive pattern in some cases; may also have mixed restrictive and obstructive pattern; reduced DLCO.
  - Chronic: Moderate to severe restrictive pattern, may develop obstructive pattern due to emphysematous changes. The DLCO is invariably reduced and there is hypoxemia.
- Lung biopsy:
  - Transbronchial: Reveal small poorly formed noncaseating granulomas near respiratory or terminal bronchioles, large foam cells, peribronchial fibrosis.
  - Open lung biopsy: Highest yield in advanced disease. Reveals varying patterns of organizing pneumonia, centrilobular and perilobular fibrosis, multinucleated giant cells with clefts.

Pathological Findings

- Acute: Alveolar lymphocytosis is a major characteristic; poorly formed noncaseating granulomas; prominent giant cells
- Chronic: Noncaseating granulomas; constrictive bronchiolitis with or without organizing pneumonia; fibrosis develops as disease progresses (may resemble usual interstitial pneumonitis) (4)

DIFFERENTIAL DIAGNOSIS

- Acute: Acute infectious pneumonia: Influenza (or other viral pneumonia), mycoplasma, *Pneumocystis jiroveci* pneumonia, asthma
- Chronic: Sarcoidosis, chronic bronchitis, chronic obstructive pulmonary disease, tuberculosis, collagen vascular disease, idiopathic pulmonary fibrosis, lymphoma, fungal infections, *P. jiroveci* pneumonia

ALERT

HP in farmers must be distinguished from febrile, toxic reactions to inhaled dusts (organic dust toxic syndrome [ODTS]). Nonimmunologic reactions occur 30–50% more commonly than HP in farmers. ODTS is associated with intense exposure occurring on a single day.

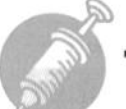

TREATMENT

MEDICATION

First Line

- Avoidance of offending antigen is primary therapy and results in regression of the disease (5)
- Corticosteroids (1): Usually prescribed for subacute or chronic forms, or for persistent symptoms
  - Prednisone: 0.5 go 1 mg/kg/d, max 60 mg PO daily.
  - For severe symptomatic patients, initial course of 1–2 weeks with taper 1
  - Maintenance therapy is rarely required.
- For hypersensitivity pneumonitis related to *Aspergillus*, antifungal therapy is not recommended (6)[C].

Second Line

- Bronchodilators and inhaled corticosteroids may symptomatically improve patients with wheeze and chest tightness (1)[B].
- Oxygen may be needed in advanced cases.
- Lung transplantation may be the last resort in severe cases unresponsive to therapy.

ADDITIONAL TREATMENT

General Measures

Outpatient except for acute pneumonitis cases and admission for workup (BAL, lung biopsy)

Issues for Referral

Referral to pulmonologist/immunologist

IN-PATIENT CONSIDERATIONS

Initial Stabilization

Supportive management as needed to maintain oxygenation and ventilation

Admission Criteria

- Unstable ventilation, oxygen requirement, mental status changes
- Need for invasive evaluation (lung biopsy)

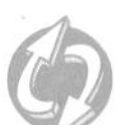

ONGOING CARE

FOLLOW-UP RECOMMENDATIONS

Patient Monitoring

- Initial follow-up should be weekly–monthly, depending on severity and course.
- Follow treatments with serial CXR, PFTs, circulating antibody levels.

DIET

No dietary restrictions

PATIENT EDUCATION

Note that chronic exposure may lead to a loss of acute symptoms with exposure (i.e., the patient may lose awareness of exposure–symptom relationship).

PROGNOSIS

- Acute: Good prognosis with reversal of pathologic findings if elimination of offending antigen early in disease.
- Chronic: Corticosteroids have been found to improve lung function acutely but offer no significant difference in long-term outcome (1)[C].

COMPLICATIONS

- Progressive interstitial fibrosis with eventual respiratory failure
- Cor pulmonale and right-heart failure

REFERENCES

1. Girard M, Lacasse Y, Cormier Y. Hypersensitivity pneumonitis. *Allergy*. 2009;64(3):322–34.
2. Navarro C, Mejía M, Gaxiola M, et al. Hypersensitivity pneumonitis: A broader perspective. *Treat Respir Med*. 2006;5(3):162.
3. Hanak V, Golbin J. High-resolution CT findings of parenchymal fibrosis correlates with prognosis in hypersensitivity pneumonitis. *Chest*. 2008;134(1):133.
4. Isabela C, et al. Hypersensitivity pneumonitis: Spectrum of high-resolution CT and pathologic findings. *AJR*. 2007;188(2):334–44.
5. Paul L, Lehrman S, et al. Hypersensitivity pneumonitis: Evaluation and management. *Compr Ther*. 2009;35(3-40):177.
6. Limper A, et al. An official American Thoracic Society statement: Treatment of fungal infections in adult pulmonary and critical care patients. *Am J Respir Crit Care Med*. 2011;183(1):96–128.

ADDITIONAL READING

Madison JM. Hypersensitivity pneumonitis: Clinical perspectives. *Arch Pathol Lab Med*. 2008;132:195–8.

CODES

ICD9

495.9 Unspecified allergic alveolitis and pneumonitis

CLINICAL PEARLS

- Skin testing is not useful for the diagnosis of HP.
- Once the disease is established, smoking does not appear to attenuate its severity, and it may predispose to more chronic and severe course.

H

HYPERSPLENISM

Nathan T. Connell, MD
Fred Schiffman, MD

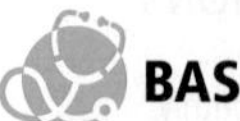

BASICS

DESCRIPTION

- Hypersplenism consists of the triad of:
  - Splenomegaly
  - Cytopenias with respective bone marrow hyperplasia of precursors
  - Resolution of the cytopenias with splenectomy (1)
- Commonly, hypersplenism is diagnosed without splenectomy. It is important to know that splenomegaly is not synonymous with hypersplenism. Some authors believe an overactive spleen without enlargement may be considered hypersplenism, such as is seen in immune thrombocytopenic purpura and autoimmune hemolytic anemia.

EPIDEMIOLOGY

May be as common as 30–70% in patients with cirrhosis and portal hypertension

PATHOPHYSIOLOGY

- Initial hypotheses stated that splenomegaly resulted in direct inhibition of bone marrow precursors, while others felt that hypersplenism was a result of sequestration of formed elements in the enlarged spleen.
- Increased numbers of splenic macrophages have been demonstrated in patients with portal hypertension, with concomitant increase in macrophage phagocytic activity (2).

ETIOLOGY

Many of the common etiologies are listed below. Almost any process involving the spleen or the hematologic system can result in hypersplenism:

- Infectious:
  - Tuberculosis
  - Malaria
  - Leishmaniasis
  - Candidiasis
  - Viral
  - Syphilis
  - Schistosomiasis
- Hematologic:
  - Myeloproliferative disorders
  - Polycythemia vera
  - Primary hypersplenism
  - Immune thrombocytopenic purpura
  - Autoimmune hemolytic anemia
- Neoplastic:
  - Hematologic malignancies
  - Melanoma
  - Various carcinomas
- Storage diseases:
  - Gaucher disease
  - Niemann-Pick disease
  - Amyloidosis
  - Glycogen storage disease
- Inflammatory:
  - Sarcoidosis
  - Systemic lupus erythematosus
  - Felty syndrome
- Congestive

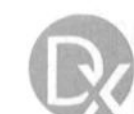

DIAGNOSIS

HISTORY

- Patients may complain of abdominal fullness or protrusion of the spleen through the abdominal wall. They may complain of early satiety if the spleen is compressing the stomach.
- Depending on etiology, patients may complain of tenderness in the left upper quadrant, especially in viral etiologies. In lymphoproliferative disorders, the spleen may be enlarged but asymptomatic unless there is splenic infarction. Given the location of the spleen next to the diaphragm, the sense of fullness may be referred through the phrenic nerve to the C3–5 dermatomes in the left shoulder.

PHYSICAL EXAM

- Jaundice: If hemolytic anemia is present
- Splenomegaly:
  - The normal spleen is usually not palpable. Physical examination demonstrating a palpable spleen may indicate pathology such as splenomegaly—and in turn hypersplenism in the appropriate clinical context—or it may indicate a wandering spleen.
  - Begin by percussing Traube semilunar space, which is demarcated by left anterior axillary line, the left costal margin, and the left sixth rib. This space is usually hollow. Splenic enlargement may cause dullness to percussion in this area. Other processes that may cause dullness include pleural or pericardial effusions. Additionally, if the patient recently ate a large meal, this area may be dull to percussion.
  - With the patient supine, allow your hand to gently rest on the abdomen. This will prevent sudden tensing of the abdominal musculature, which may obscure palpation. As the spleen enlarges, it moves caudally and medially. Start by palpating in the right lower quadrant and moving toward the umbilicus toward the left upper quadrant. If there is doubt about whether the spleen has moved beyond the costal margin, the patient may be asked to take a large breath, which will push the diaphragm, and in turn the spleen, toward the examiner's hands.

DIAGNOSTIC TESTS & INTERPRETATION

Lab

On CBC, any and all cell lines may be decreased, resulting in:

- Anemia
- Leukopenia
- Thrombocytopenia

Initial lab tests

- CBC
- Reticulocyte count if anemia
- If there is hemolysis, the reticulocyte count should be elevated along with evidence of hyperbilirubinemia.

Follow-Up & Special Considerations

Based on other historical and exam findings, testing for specific infectious etiologies may be warranted:

- Blood parasite smear for malaria
- EBV serologies
- HIV ELISA with Western blot
- JAK2 mutation in polycythemia vera
- PPD for tuberculosis

Imaging

- Ultrasound
- CT
- Tc-99m sulfur colloid scintigraphy
- PET
- MRI

Diagnostic Procedures/Surgery

Bone marrow biopsy

Pathological Findings

Hyperplasia of bone marrow precursors, especially those correlating with the patient's individual cytopenias

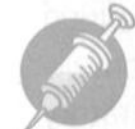

TREATMENT

MEDICATION

- No specific medication can be recommended for patients with hypersplenism. The most important item is to treat the underlying disorder.
- If ITP is the cause, the patient may benefit from:
  - Prednisone or methylprednisolone
  - IVIg
  - Rituximab
- If an infectious cause is discovered, treatment with appropriate antibiotic therapy may help the cytopenias improve.

SURGERY/OTHER PROCEDURES

- Many patients undergo splenectomy in order to alleviate severe cytopenias resulting from hypersplenism. These patients should ideally receive immunization to pneumococcus, meningococcus, *Haemophilus influenzae*, and influenza at least 14 days prior to splenectomy (3). If this cannot be done (i.e., in cases of emergent splenectomy), wait at least 14 days post splenectomy to immunize (4)[B].
- Pneumococcal vaccine:
  - Pneumococcal polyvalent-23 vaccine (PPSV23) for use in adults and fully immunized children 2 years of age or older
  - Pneumococcal polyvalent-13 vaccine (PCV13) for infants and young children 2 months of age or older
  - *Haemophilus influenzae* vaccine
  - Meningococcal vaccine:
    - Meningococcal conjugate vaccine (MCV4) for use in patients between 2 and 55 years of age
    - Meningococcal polysaccharide vaccine (MPSV4) for use in patients >55 years of age
  - Influenza vaccine should be administered yearly based on prevalent circulating strains. While patients are not at higher risk due to influenza itself, infection with influenza may place patients at higher risk for secondary bacterial infections.
- Radiofrequency ablation is becoming more available and can be successful at preventing recurrence of hypersplenism. It is not currently known whether there are differences between RFA and splenectomy in terms of postprocedure infectious risks (5).

IN-PATIENT CONSIDERATIONS

Admission Criteria

For patients with hypersplenism in general, admission is based on other factors, such as the underlying disorder and concurrent vital signs. For some patients, the large spleen compresses the stomach and prevents adequate oral intake.

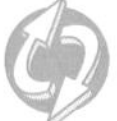

ONGOING CARE

- Adult patients who are splenectomized should also carry antibiotics with them to start treatment immediately should they develop fever. This may be the first sign of bacteremia, and early antibiotics reduce the mortality from overwhelming postsplenectomy sepsis.
- Controlled trials have not been performed, but some regimens include:
  - Amoxicillin-clavulanate 875 mg PO
  - Cefuroxime axetil 500 mg PO
- Patients allergic to beta-lactam antibiotics can be given an extended-spectrum fluoroquinolone such as levofloxacin 750 mg PO or moxifloxacin 400 mg PO
- In children with splenectomy, daily antibiotic prophylaxis for overwhelming postsplenectomy sepsis with penicillin VK or amoxicillin is recommended until age 5 or at least 3 years after splenectomy (6)[C]:
  - Age 2 months to 5 years: 125 mg PO b.i.d.
  - >5 years old: 250 mg PO b.i.d.

PATIENT EDUCATION

Patients who are splenectomized should be counseled extensively about the risk of overwhelming postsplenectomy sepsis and infection.

REFERENCES

1. Jandl JH, Aster RH, Forkner CE, et al. Splenic pooling and the pathophysiology of hypersplenism. *Trans Am Clin Climatol Assoc.* 1967;78:9–27.
2. Yongxiang W, Zongfang L, Guowei L, et al. Effects of splenomegaly and splenic macrophage activity in hypersplenism due to cirrhosis. *Am J Med.* 2002; 113:428–31.
3. Kroger AT, Atkinson WL, Marcuse EK, et al. General recommendations on immunization: Recommendations of the Advisory Committee on Immunization Practices (ACIP). *MMWR Recomm Rep.* 2006;55:1–48.
4. Shatz DV, Schinsky MF, Pais LB, et al. Immune responses of splenectomized trauma patients to the 23-valent pneumococcal polysaccharide vaccine at 1 versus 7 versus 14 days after splenectomy. *J Trauma.* 1998;44:(5):760–5; discussion 765–6.
5. Feng K, Ma K, Liu Q, et al. Randomized clinical trial of splenic radiofrequency ablation versus splenectomy for severe hypersplenism. *Br J Surg.* 2011; 98:354–61.
6. American Academy of Pediatrics. Children with asplenia or functional asplenia. In: Pickering LK, Baker CI, Kimberlin DW, et al., eds. *Red Book: 2009 Report of the Committee on Infectious Diseases*, 28th ed. Elk Grove Village, IL: American Academy of Pediatrics; 2009:72.

ADDITIONAL READING

- Abdella HM, Abd-El-Moez AT, Abu El-Maaty ME, et al. Role of partial splenic arterial embolization for hypersplenism in patients with liver cirrhosis and thrombocytopenia. *Indian J Gastroenterol.* 2010; 29:59–61.
- Iriyama N, Horikoshi A, Hatta Y, et al. Localized, splenic, diffuse large B-cell lymphoma presenting with hypersplenism: Risk and benefit of splenectomy. *Intern. Med.* 2010;49:1027–30.
- Peck-Radosavljevic M, et al. Hypersplenism. *Eur J Gastroenterol Hepatol.* 2001;13:317–23.
- Watanabe Y, Horiuchi A, Yoshida M, et al. Significance of laparoscopic splenectomy in patients with hypersplenism. *World J Surg.* 2007;31:549–55.

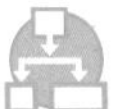

See Also (Topic, Algorithm, Electronic Media Element)

Anemia, Autoimmune Hemolytic; Immune Thrombocytopenic Purpura; Malaria; Polycythemia Vera; Tuberculosis

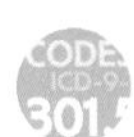

CODES

ICD9

289.4 Hypersplenism

CLINICAL PEARLS

- Splenectomy is often unnecessary to make the diagnosis.
- Avoid splenectomy in patients unless absolutely necessary. Splenectomized patients are at lifelong risk for overwhelming postsplenectomy infection and sepsis.
- If splenectomy is to be performed, give immunization for pneumococcus, meningococcus, *Haemophilus*, and influenza at least 14 days prior to surgery. Otherwise, wait until the 14th postoperative day to immunize.

H

HYPERTENSION, ESSENTIAL

David E. Burtner, MD

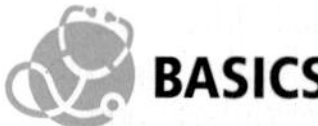

BASICS

DESCRIPTION

- Hypertension (HTN) is defined as 2 or more elevated BPs (systolic BP ≥140 mm Hg and/or diastolic BP ≥90 mm Hg) at ≥2 visits; operationally, any BP at which drug treatment results in a net benefit.
- HTN is a strong risk factor for cardiovascular disease.
- Pre-HTN: Systolic BP = 120–139 mm Hg or diastolic BP = 80–89 mm Hg
- Synonym(s): Benign, Chronic, Idiopathic, Familial, or Genetic HTN; High BP

Geriatric Considerations

- Isolated systolic HTN is common.
- Therapy has been shown to be effective and beneficial at preventing stroke, although target systolic BP is higher than in younger patients (around 150 mm Hg systolic), and adverse reactions to medications are more frequent. The benefit of therapy has been conclusively demonstrated in older patients (1).

Pediatric Considerations

Measure BP during routine exams.

Pregnancy Considerations

- Elevated BP during pregnancy may be either chronic HTN or pregnancy-induced preeclampsia. ACE inhibitors and angiotensin II receptor blockers (ARBs) are contraindicated.
- Maternal and fetal mortality benefit from treatment (see topic "Preeclampsia").

EPIDEMIOLOGY

Incidence

- Lifetime risk for men and women aged 55–65 years by age 80–85 is >90%.
- Predominant age: Essential (primary, benign, idiopathic) onset usually in the 20s–30s.
- Predominant sex: Male > Female; males tend to run higher than females and have a significantly higher risk of cardiovascular disease at any given pressure.

Prevalence

50 million (1988–1991 NHANES III); 20% of the US population

RISK FACTORS

Family history, obesity, alcohol use, excess dietary sodium, stress, and physical inactivity

Genetics

BP levels are strongly familial, but no clear genetic pattern exists. Familial risk for cardiovascular diseases should be considered.

ETIOLOGY

- >90% of HTN has no identified cause.
- Secondary causes of HTN: see topic "Hypertension, Secondary and Resistant":
  - Renal parenchymal: Glomerulonephritis, pyelonephritis, polycystic kidneys
  - Endocrine: Primary hyperaldosteronism, pheochromocytoma, hyperthyroidism, Cushing syndrome
  - Vascular: Coarctation of the aorta, renal artery stenosis
  - Chemical: Oral contraceptives, NSAIDs, decongestants, antidepressants, sympathomimetics, many industrial chemicals, corticosteroids, ergotamine alkaloids, lithium, cyclosporine, lead
  - Sleep apnea

DIAGNOSIS

HISTORY

- HTN is asymptomatic except in extreme cases or after related cardiovascular complications develop.
- Headache can be seen with higher BP, often present on awakening and occipital in nature.

PHYSICAL EXAM

- Retinopathy: Narrowed arteries, arteriovenous (AV) nicking, copper or silver wiring of retinal arterioles
- Increased A_2 heart sound
- Synchronous radial and femoral pulse can help to rule out coarctation of the aorta.

DIAGNOSTIC TESTS & INTERPRETATION

ECG to evaluate possible presence of left ventricular hypertrophy (LVH) or rhythm abnormalities affecting therapy

Lab

Initial lab tests

- Hemoglobin and hematocrit or CBC
- Complete urinalysis (may reveal proteinuria)
- Potassium, calcium, and creatinine
- Cholesterol (total and high-density lipoprotein [HDL])
- Fasting blood glucose, glycohemoglobin A1c
- Uric acid

Follow-Up & Special Considerations

- Special tests (only if history, physical, or lab indicates); see topic "Hypertension, Secondary and Resistant"
- Ambulatory (24-hour) BP monitoring if "white coat" hypertension is suspected
- Home BP monitoring is effective; elevated home BPs correlate with adverse outcomes, and normal readings are reassuring.

Imaging

Only if history or physical indicate (see topic "Hypertension, Secondary and Resistant")

Diagnostic Procedures/Surgery

- A presumptive diagnosis of HTN can be made if the average of at least 2 BP measurements exceeds either 140 mm Hg systolic or 90 mm Hg diastolic, assuming proper resting conditions, cuff size, and application are maintained.
- The Joint National Committee (JNC) (2) recommends emphasis on:
  - Family or personal history of HTN, cardiovascular, cerebrovascular, renal disease, and diabetes
  - Previous elevated BPs
  - Previous treatments
  - History of weight gain, exercise activities, sodium intake, fat intake, and alcohol use
  - Symptoms suggesting secondary HTN
  - Psychosocial and environmental factors affecting BP and risk for cardiovascular disease
  - Other cardiovascular risk factors, such as obesity, smoking, hyperlipidemia, and diabetes
  - Funduscopic exam for arteriolar narrowing, AV compression, hemorrhages, exudates, and papilledema
  - Body mass index (BMI)
  - Waist circumference
  - BP in both arms
  - Complete cardiac and peripheral pulse exam: Compare radial and femoral pulse for differences in volume and timing, auscultation for carotid and femoral bruits.
  - Abdominal exam for masses and bruits: Listen high in the flanks over the kidneys.
  - Neurologic assessment

DIFFERENTIAL DIAGNOSIS

Secondary HTN: Because of the low incidence of reversible secondary HTN, special tests should be considered only if the history, physical exam, or basic laboratory evaluation indicate the possibility. (See topic "Hypertension, Secondary and Resistant.")

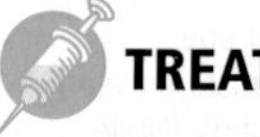

TREATMENT

MEDICATION

- The amount of BP reduction is probably more important than the choice of antihypertensive.
- Multiple drugs at submaximal dose may achieve target BP with fewer side effects.
- Thiazide diuretics have the most proven benefits (cost, compliance, and effectiveness). Chlorthalidone may be superior to more commonly used HCTZ due to longer half-life and more evidence to support (3,4)[A].
- Initial selection is based primarily on concomitant conditions (5).
- Sequential monotherapy attempts might be tried with different classes because individual responses vary.
- Majority of patients will require multiple meds.
- Benazepril combined with amlodipine has been shown to be superior to combination with HCTZ in high-risk patients (6)[A]. Some suggest that ACE/ARB plus dihydropyridine calcium channel blocker is first choice after monotherapy.
- β-blockers had been strongly recommended until recent meta-analyses. Atenolol may be particularly *ineffective* in reducing adverse outcomes of hypertension.
- ACE inhibitors should be used in patients with diabetes, proteinuria, atrial fibrillation, or congestive heart failure (CHF), but not in pregnancy.
- α-adrenergics are not the first choice for monotherapy (3)[A]. Might benefit males with benign prostatic hypertrophy (BPH).
- β-blockers might benefit patients with ischemic heart disease, CHF, or migraine.
- Calcium channel blockers could be considered in patients with isolated systolic hypertension, atherosclerosis, migraine, or asthma; well documented to reduce risk of stroke (3).

First Line

- Thiazide diuretics:
  - Hydrochlorothiazide: 6.25–50 mg daily
  - Chlorthalidone: 12.5–50 mg daily
  - Indapamide: 1.25–5 mg daily

- ACE inhibitors:
  - Captopril: 25–450 mg b.i.d.
  - Enalapril: 2.5–40 mg daily
  - Lisinopril: 5–40 mg daily
  - Ramipril: 2.5–20 mg daily
  - Quinapril: 10–80 mg daily
  - Benazepril: 10–40 mg daily
- ARBs:
  - Losartan: 25–100 mg in 1 or 2 doses; has unique but modest uricosuric effect
  - Valsartan: 80–320 mg daily
  - Irbesartan: 75–300 mg daily
  - Candesartan: 4–32 mg daily
  - Telmisartan: 40–80 mg daily
  - Olmesartan: 20-40 mg daily
- Renin inhibitor: Aliskiren 150–300 mg daily
- Calcium channel blockers:
  - Diltiazem CD: 180–360 mg daily
  - Felodipine: 5–20 mg daily
  - Nifedipine (sustained release): 30–90 mg daily
  - Verapamil (sustained release): 120–480 mg daily
  - Amlodipine: 2.5–10 mg daily
- β-blockers:
  - Atenolol: 25–100 mg daily; *no longer first-line*
  - Carvedilol: 6.25–25 mg b.i.d.
  - Labetalol: 100–900 mg b.i.d. (combined alpha-beta blocker)
  - Metoprolol tartrate: 50–200 mg b.i.d. or succinate ER daily
  - Pindolol: 5–30 mg b.i.d.; may be helpful if bradycardia on other β-blockers
  - Propranolol: 20–120 mg b.i.d.
  - Bisoprolol: 2.5–20 mg daily
- Contraindications:
  - Diuretics may worsen gout.
  - β-blockers (relatively) in reactive airway disease, heart block, diabetes, and peripheral vascular disease; probably should be avoided in patients with metabolic syndrome or insulin-requiring diabetes
  - Diltiazem or verapamil: Caution with systolic dysfunction heart failure or heart block
  - ACE inhibitors can worsen bilateral renovascular disease and are pregnancy Category D.

Second Line

- Many may be combined.
- Centrally acting adrenergic inhibitors:
  - Clonidine: 0.1–1.2 mg b.i.d. or weekly patch 0.1–0.3 mg daily
  - Guanfacine: 1–3 mg daily
  - Methyldopa: 250–2,000 mg b.i.d.
- α-adrenergic agents:
  - Prazosin: 1–10 mg b.i.d.
  - Terazosin: 1–20 mg daily
  - Doxazosin: 1–16 mg daily
- Peripherally acting adrenergic inhibitors: Rarely used:
  - Reserpine: 0.1–0.25 mg daily
- Vasodilators:
  - Hydralazine: 25–150 mg b.i.d.; risk of tachycardia, so generally combined with β-blocker; also drug-induced systemic lupus erythematosus (SLE)
  - Minoxidil: Rarely used due to adverse effects
- Loop diuretics (for volume overload):
  - Furosemide: 20–320 mg daily
  - Bumetanide: 0.5–2 mg daily
- K^+-sparing diuretics in patients with hypokalemia while taking thiazides, or suspected aldosteronism:
  - Amiloride: 5–10 mg daily
  - Spironolactone: 25–100 mg daily
  - Triamterene: 50–150 mg daily

ADDITIONAL TREATMENT

General Measures

- Treating patients to lower-than-standard BP targets, $\leq$140/90 mm Hg, does not further reduce mortality or morbidity (7)[A]. Individualize goal pressures based on risk factors; best target may be systolic BP near 150 mm Hg in patients $>$75–80 years of age.
- Primary focus is achieving systolic BP goal.
- Aerobic exercise
- Weight reduction for obese patients
- Smoking cessation
- Risk stratification affects the treatment:
  - Pre-HTN (120–139/80–89 mm Hg): Drug therapy for chronic renal disease or diabetes. Action to Control Cardiovascular Risk in Diabetes (ACCORD) trial did not support for noninsulin-dependent diabetes mellitus (NIDDM) patients (8).
  - Stage 1 HTN (140–159/90–99 mm Hg): Begin thiazide diuretics for most patients.
  - Stage 2 HTN ($>$160/$>$100 mm Hg): Consider starting 2 drugs.

COMPLEMENTARY AND ALTERNATIVE MEDICINE

Biofeedback and relaxation exercise

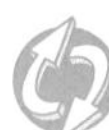

ONGOING CARE

FOLLOW-UP RECOMMENDATIONS

Patient Monitoring

- Re-evaluate patients every 3–6 months.
- Review compliance, effectiveness, and adverse reactions. Poor medication adherence is a leading cause of apparent medication failure.
- Quality-of-life issues, including sexual function, should be considered.
- Annual (at least) evaluation of urinalysis, creatinine, and potassium as part of a screening laboratory panel

DIET

- $\sim$20% of patients will respond to reduced-salt diet ($<$100 mmol daily; $<$6 g NaCl or $<$2.4 g Na).
- Consider Dietary Approaches to Stop Hypertension (DASH) diet: www.nhlbi.nih.gov/health/public/heart/hbp/dash/new_dash.pdf.
- Limit alcohol consumption to $<$1 oz daily.

PATIENT EDUCATION

- Emphasize the asymptomatic nature of HTN and importance of lifetime treatment.
- Review cardiovascular risk factors.
- Printed aids for high BP education available at www.nhlbi.nih.gov/health/public/heart/index.htm#hbp

COMPLICATIONS

Heart failure, renal failure, LVH, myocardial infarction, retinal hemorrhage, stroke, hypertensive heart disease, drug side effects

REFERENCES

1. Beckett NS, Peters R, Fletcher AE, et al. Treatment of hypertension in patients 80 years of age or older. *N Engl J Med*. 2008;358:1887–98.
2. Chobanian AV, Bakris GL, Black HR, et al. The Seventh Report of the Joint National Committee on Prevention, Detection, Evaluation, and Treatment of High Blood Pressure: The JNC 7 report. *JAMA*. 2003;289:2560–72.
3. ALLHAT Officers and Coordinators for the ALLHAT Collaborative Research Group. The Antihypertensive and Lipid-Lowering Treatment to Prevent Heart Attack Trial. Major outcomes in high-risk hypertensive patients randomized to angiotensin-converting enzyme inhibitor or calcium channel blocker vs diuretic: The Antihypertensive and Lipid-Lowering Treatment to Prevent Heart Attack Trial (ALLHAT). *JAMA*. 2002;288:2981–97.
4. Dorsch MP, Gillespie BW, Erickson SR, et al. Chlorthalidone reduces cardiovascular events compared with hydrochlorothiazide. *Hypertension*. 2011;57:689–94.
5. Mancia G, De Backer G, Dominiczak A, et al. Guidelines for the management of arterial Hypertension: The Task Force for the Management of Arterial Hypertension of the European Society of Hypertension (ESH) and of the European Society of Cardiology (ESC). *J Hypertens*. 2007;25:1105–87.
6. Chobanian AV. Does it matter how hypertension is controlled? *N Engl J Med*. 2008;359:2485–8.
7. Arguedas JA, Perez MI, Wright JM. Treatment blood pressure targets for hypertension. *Cochrane Database Syst Rev*. 2009:CD004349.
8. The ACCORD Study Group. Effects of intensive blood-pressure control in type 2 diabetes mellitus. *N Engl J Med*. 2010 Mar 14. PubMed PMID: 20228401.

ADDITIONAL READING

- Lindholm LH, Carlberg B, Samuelsson O. Should beta blockers remain first choice in the treatment of primary hypertension? A meta-analysis. *Lancet*. 2005;366:1545–53.
- NICE/BHS HTN Guideline Review, 28 June 2006. Available at: http://guidance.nice.org.uk/CG34/guidance/pdf/English.

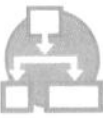

See Also (Topic, Algorithm, Electronic Media Element)

Hypertension, Secondary and Resistant; Hypertensive Emergencies; Polycystic Kidney Disease

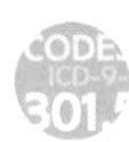

CODES

ICD9

- 401.0 Malignant essential hypertension
- 401.1 Benign essential hypertension
- 401.9 Unspecified essential hypertension

CLINICAL PEARLS

- Treatment of HTN reduces risk of many serious medical conditions with numbers needed to treat to prevent 1 serious event (such as stroke or MI) ranging from $\sim$20 patients per year for severe HTN to more than several hundred per year for mild HTN.
- Multiple submaximal doses are likely to have fewer side effects and more effectiveness than fewer maximum-dosed drugs.
- Patients presenting with symptoms should be made strongly aware that resolution of these symptoms does not mean BP elevation has resolved.

HYPERTENSION, SECONDARY AND RESISTANT

George Maxted, MD

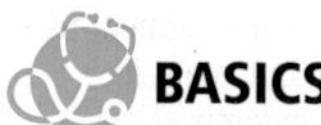

BASICS

DESCRIPTION

Uncontrolled hypertension comprises the following entities:

- Resistant hypertension: Defined by the Joint National Committee 7 as "failure to achieve goal BP (<140/90 mm Hg for the overall population and <130/80 mm Hg for those with diabetes or chronic kidney disease) when a patient adheres to maximum tolerated doses of 3 antihypertensive drugs including a diuretic" (1,2)
- Secondary hypertension: Elevated BP that results from an identifiable underlying mechanism (1,2)

Geriatric Considerations

- Onset of hypertension (HTN) in adults >60 years of age is a strong indicator of secondary HTN.
- In patients over 80 years of age, consider a higher target SBP of 150 or less (3).
- Elderly may be particularly responsive to diuretics and dihydropyridine calcium channel blockers (3).
- Systolic HTN is particularly problematic in the elderly.
- Secondary causes more common in the elderly include sleep apnea, renal disease, renal artery stenosis, and primary aldosteronism (2).

ALERT

Pseudoresistance:

- Inaccurate measurement of BP:
  - Cuff too small
  - Patient not at rest; sitting quietly for 5 minutes
- Poor adherence
  - In primary care settings, this has been estimated to occur in 40–60% of hypertensive patients (2).
- White-coat effect: prevalence 20–40%. Do not make clinical decisions about hypertension based solely on measurement in the clinic setting. Home BP monitoring and/or ambulatory BP monitoring are more reliable (4,5)
- Inadequate treatment (2)

EPIDEMIOLOGY

- Predominant age: In general, HTN has its onset between ages 30 and 50.
- Depending on etiology, age of onset can vary. Age of onset <20 years or >50 years increases likelihood that there is a secondary cause for HTN.
- The strongest predictors for resistant HTN are age (>75), presence of left ventricular hypertrophy (LVH), obesity (body mass index [BMI] >30), and high baseline systolic BP. Other predictors include chronic kidney disease, diabetes, living in the Southeastern US, African American race (especially women), excessive salt intake (2).
- In the ACCOMPLISH, INVEST, CONVINCE, ALLHAT, and LIFE studies, percent of patients reaching JNC-7 BP goals ranged from 45–82% (1).

Prevalence

The prevalence of resistant HTN is unknown. NHANES analysis indicates only 53% of adults are controlled to a BP of <140/90:

- Obstructive sleep apnea (OSA): 1 study diagnosed OSA in 83% of treatment-resistant hypertensives (2).
- Primary hyperaldosteronism (17–22% of resistant HTN cases) (2,6)
- Chronic renal disease (2–5% of hypertensives)
- Renovascular disease (0.2–0.7%, up to 35% of elderly, 20% of patients undergoing cardiac catheterization) (2)
- Cushing syndrome (0.1–0.6%)
- Pheochromocytoma (0.04–0.1% of hypertensives)

RISK FACTORS

Factors predictive of resistant or secondary hypertension: Female sex, African-American race, obesity, diabetes, worsening of control in previously stable hypertensive patient, onset in patients of age <20 or >50 years, lack of family history of hypertension, significant target end-organ damage, stage 2 HTN (systolic BP >160 mm Hg or diastolic BP >100 mm Hg), renal disease, alcohol or drug use

Genetics

In some patients, there is a possible relationship to ENaC gene variants (Liddle syndrome) and a CYP3A5 allele (cortisol metabolism, especially African Americans) (2).

GENERAL PREVENTION

The prevention of resistant and secondary hypertension is thought to be the same as for primary or essential hypertension. Adopting a DASH (Dietary Approaches to Stop Hypertension) diet, a low-sodium diet, weight loss in obese patients, exercise, limitation of alcohol intake, and smoking cessation may all be of benefit. Relaxation techniques may be of help, but data are limited.

PATHOPHYSIOLOGY

Depends on underlying etiology

ETIOLOGY

- Other rare causes: Hyperthyroidism, Hyperparathyroidism, Aortic coarctation, Intracranial tumor
- Drug-related causes:
  - Medications, especially NSAIDs (may also blunt effectiveness of ACE-inhibitors), decongestants, stimulants (e.g., amphetamines, attention deficient hyperactivity disorder [ADHD] medications), anorectic agents (e.g., modafinil, ephedra, guarana, ma huang, bitter orange), erythropoietin, natural licorice (in some chewing tobacco), yohimbine, glucocorticoids.
  - Oral contraceptives: Unclear association; mainly epidemiologic and with higher estrogen pills
  - Cocaine, amphetamines, other illicit drugs; drug and alcohol withdrawal syndromes
- Lifestyle factors:
  - Obesity, dietary salt may negate the beneficial effect of diuretics. Excessive alcohol, physical inactivity also contributors.

DIAGNOSIS

HISTORY

- Ask or review at every visit: "The Big Four" SANS mnemonic: 1. **S**alt intake, 2. **A**lcohol intake, 3. **N**SAID use, 4. **S**leep (author's suggestion, based on reference listed).
- Review home BP readings; consider ambulatory BP monitoring:
- History will vary with etiology of HTN:
  - Pheochromocytoma: Episodes of headache, palpitations, sweating
  - Cushing syndrome: Weight gain, fatigue, weakness, easy bruising, amenorrhea
  - Obstructive sleep apnea: Loud snoring while asleep, daytime somnolence
  - Increased intravascular volume: Swelling

PHYSICAL EXAM

- Ensure that the BP is measured correctly. The patient should be sitting quietly with back supported for 5 minutes prior to measurement. Proper cuff size: Bladder encircling at least 80% of the arm. Support arm at heart level. Minimum of 2 readings at least 1 minute apart. Check BP in both arms. Also check standing BP for orthostasis.
- Attention to findings related to possible etiologies: Renovascular HTN: Systolic/diastolic abdominal bruit. Pheochromocytoma: Diaphoresis, tachycardia. Cushing syndrome: Hirsutism, moon facies, dorsal hump, purple striae, truncal obesity. Thyroid disease: Enlarged thyroid, tremor, exophthalmos, tachycardia. Coarctation of the aorta: Upper limb HTN with decreased or delayed femoral pulses.
- Funduscopic exam

DIAGNOSTIC TESTS & INTERPRETATION

- ECG performed as part of the initial workup; LVH is an important marker of resistant HTN.
- Sleep study if history and physical indicate. Overnight oximetry is a good screen for nocturnal hypoxia. If positive, formal polysomnography may be indicated.

Lab

Initial lab tests

Initial limited diagnostic testing should include (2,6)[A]: Urinalysis, CBC, potassium, sodium, glucose, creatinine, lipids, TSH, calcium. 50% of patients with hyperaldosteronism may have normal potassium levels (1,2)

Follow-Up & Special Considerations

Further testing for primary aldosteronism (PA) may be considered:

- Empiric treatment with an aldosterone inhibitor may be preferable, and more clinically relevant: Spironolactone or eplerenone. Amiloride may be more effective in blacks
- Plasma aldosterone/renin ratio (ARR) is the preferred lab test *but* the test is difficult to properly perform and interpret. Consult your reference lab and interpret results with caution:
  - Further testing for pheochromocytoma: Plasma metanephrine screening test of choice: Confirmed by a 24-hour urinary metanephrine-to-creatinine ratio
  - Other tests to consider for resistant or secondary hypertension: 24-hour urine for free cortisol, calcium, parathyroid hormone (PTH), overnight 1-mg dexamethasone suppression test, urine toxicology screen

Imaging

- Imaging tests listed are necessary only if history, physical, or lab data indicate.
- Abdominal ultrasound: If renal disease is suspected
- MRA of renal vasculature: Preferred test for renovascular hypertension. Sensitive but low specificity. Conventional angiography or CT angiography second line after MRA to look at distal renal artery. Renal arteriography remains gold standard for renovascular disease

- Adrenal "incidentaloma" frequently arises in this era of multiple CT studies. If present in the setting of resistant hypertension, consider hyperaldosterone or hyperadrenalcorticoid states.
- Doppler or CT imaging of aorta along with chest x-ray looking for notched ribs (sign of coarctation)

Diagnostic Procedures/Surgery

Consider 24-hour ambulatory BP monitoring, especially if white-coat effect is suspected. Home BP monitor results predict mortality, stroke, and other target organ damage better than office BP (4,5). Optimal protocol involves 2 paired measurements morning and evening (4 measurements) over 4–7 days (7):

- Oscillometric, electronic, upper arm, fully automatic device with memory. Average multiple readings over several days.
- See www.dableducational.org for validated monitors.

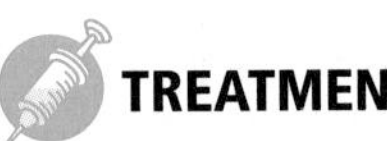

TREATMENT

- Treatment modality depends on etiology of HTN. Please see each etiology listed for information on proper treatment.
- Emphasize: Adherence to interventions according to JNC-7 recommendations. Lack of, or underuse of, diuretic therapy is often found. Nonpharmacologic measures include weight loss, dietary salt restriction, moderation of alcohol intake, increased physical activity:
  - Obese patients, blacks, elderly may be particularly responsive to diuretics (8).
  - Tolerance to diuretics may occur: Long-term adaptation to thiazides or the "braking effect." Consider increasing the dose of thiazide, or adding an aldosterone inhibitor (8).
- Treatment specific to certain secondary etiologies:
  - Primary aldosteronism: Aldosterone receptor antagonist: Spironolactone or eplerenone
  - Cushing syndrome: Aldosterone receptor antagonist
  - Obstructive sleep apnea: Continuous positive airway pressure (CPAP) $\pm$ oxygen, surgery, weight loss
  - Nocturnal hypoxia: Oxygen supplementation

MEDICATION

- Diuretics, especially chlorthalidone, are first line (8). Additional benefit has been demonstrated with ACE inhibitors, angiotensin II receptor blocker (ARB) agents, calcium channel blockers (2)[C].
- β-blockers are considered first line only for patients with ischemic heart disease or CHF. Combined a-β antagonists (e.g., labetalol) may be more effective for hypertension.
- Aldosterone antagonists may offer significant benefit (1)[C],(2,9).
- Central-acting agents (e.g., clonidine) are effective at reducing BP, but outcomes data are lacking.

ALERT

- Agents specific for treatment of hypertensive emergencies should be initiated under a situation in which immediate BP reduction will prevent or limit end-organ damage (see topic "Hypertensive Emergencies").
- Renovascular HTN: Angioplasty is the treatment of choice for fibromuscular dysplasia of a renal artery. Endovascular treatment of atherosclerotic disease is controversial, with no clear benefit over medical management. Cardiovascular Outcomes in Renal Atherosclerotic Lesions (CORAL) study is pending and may help determine risk/benefit (2).
- Referral to an HTN specialist or clinic: Retrospective studies indicate improved control rates for patients with resistant HTN referred to special HTN clinics (2)[C].

IN-PATIENT CONSIDERATIONS

Initial Stabilization

Hospitalization may be necessary for hypertensive urgency or emergency general measures.

ONGOING CARE

FOLLOW-UP RECOMMENDATIONS

Encourage aerobic activity of 30 min/d depending on patient condition.

DIET

- Reduced salt may lower BP.
- The Mediterranean Diet or DASH is recommended.

PATIENT EDUCATION

Home BP monitoring is recommended.

REFERENCES

1. Sarafidis PA, Bakris GL. Resistant hypertension: An overview of evaluation and treatment. *J Am Coll Cardiol*. 2008;52:1749–57.
2. Calhoun DA, et al. Resistant hypertention: Diagnosis, evaluation, and treatment. A scientific statement from the American Heart Association Professional Education Committee of the Council for High Blood Pressure Research. *Hypertension*. 2008;51(6):1403–19.
3. Aronow WS, Fleg JL, Pepine CJ, et al. ACCF/AHA 2011 expert consensus document on hypertension in the elderly: A report of the American College of Cardiology Foundation Task Force on Clinical Expert Consensus documents developed in collaboration with the American Academy of Neurology, American Geriatrics Society, American Society for Preventive Cardiology, American Society of Hypertension, American Society of Nephrology, Association of Black Cardiologists, and European Society of Hypertension. *J Am Coll Cardiol*. 2011;57:2037–114.
4. Powers BJ, Olsen MK, Smith VA, et al. Measuring blood pressure for decision making and quality reporting: Where and how many measures? *Ann Intern Med*. 2011;154:781–8.
5. Agarwal R, Bills JE, Hecht TJ, et al. Role of home blood pressure monitoring in overcoming therapeutic inertia and improving hypertension control: A systematic review and meta-analysis. *Hypertension*. 2011;57:29–38.
6. Gaddam KK, Nishizaka MK, Pratt-Ubunama MN, et al. Characterization of resistant hypertension: Association between resistant hypertension, aldosterone, and persistent intravascular volume expansion. *Arch Intern Med*. 2008;168:1159–64.
7. Johansson JK, Niiranen TJ, Puukka PJ, et al. Optimal schedule for home blood pressure monitoring based on a clinical approach. *J Hypertens*. 2010;28:259–64.
8. Ernst ME, Moser M. Use of diuretics in patients with hypertension. *N Engl J Med* 2009;361:2153–64.
9. Calhoun DA. Low-dose aldosterone blockade as a new treatment paradigm for controlling resistant hypertension. *J Clin Hypertens*. 2007;91(Suppl 1): 19–24.

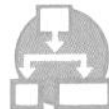

See Also (Topic, Algorithm, Electronic Media Element)

Aldosteronism, Primary; Coarctation of the Aorta; Cushing Disease and Cushing Syndrome; Hyperparathyroidism; Hypertension, Essential; Hyperthyroidism; Pheochromocytoma

CODES

ICD9

- 405.01 Malignant renovascular hypertension
- 405.09 Other malignant secondary hypertension
- 405.99 Other unspecified secondary hypertension

CLINICAL PEARLS

- Onset of HTN in adults >60 years of age is a strong indicator of secondary HTN.
- Common causes of resistant hypertension: Obstructive sleep apnea, excessive salt intake, medication nonadherence.
- Common secondary causes include sleep apnea, renal disease, renal artery stenosis, and primary aldosteronism.
- Home BP monitoring predicts outcomes better than office monitoring of BP.

H

HYPERTENSIVE EMERGENCIES

John A. Guisto, MD
Arthur B. Sanders, MD, MHA

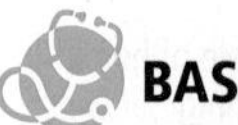

BASICS

DESCRIPTION

- Numerous terms can be used in the literature and often overlap (see "Synonyms"). Some definitions include a specific diastolic or systolic BP reading, whereas others emphasize an acute change in the BP or the presence of specific clinical syndromes.
- Severe HTN is defined as a diastolic BP of ≥115 mm Hg (15.3 kPa).
- A hypertensive emergency occurs only when an acute elevation of BP causes rapid and progressive end-organ damage, particularly in the cardiovascular, renal, and CNS.
- System(s) affected: Cardiovascular; Nervous; Pulmonary; Renal
- Synonym(s): Hypertensive crisis; Severe HTN; Malignant HTN; Accelerated HTN; Hypertensive emergency

EPIDEMIOLOGY

Incidence

Incidence of hypertensive emergency: 1% of patients with hypertension annually in the US

Prevalence

- Overall prevalence of HTN in the US: 29.3% based on 2003–2004 survey data
- Predominant age: Elderly

RISK FACTORS

- History of poorly controlled HTN
- Drug abuse
- Noncompliance with medications; abruptly stopping antihypertensive medication without supervision

Genetics

- Genetics: Risk of hypertensive emergency is higher in African Americans.
- Predominant sex: Male > Female

GENERAL PREVENTION

- Treat HTN.
- Counsel the patient about the importance of compliance with antihypertensive treatment and the dangers of stopping the medications abruptly.

PATHOPHYSIOLOGY

- Increased sympathetic tone leads to increased BP.
- Angiotensin II has multiple effects contributing to HTN and end-organ damage:
  - Stimulates sympathetic tone, aldosterone release, and antidiuretic hormone release
  - Chronic HTN induces vascular thickening and sclerosis.
  - Central effects include enhanced resorption of salt and water.
  - Chronic HTN shifts autoregulation of BP and cerebral blood flow.

ETIOLOGY

- Renal disease
- Abrupt withdrawal from antihypertensives, especially clonidine (Catapres)
- Withdrawal from CNS depressants
- Medications: SSRIs, decongestants, appetite suppressants, steroids (including oral contraceptives), MAOI interaction with certain foods or drugs, and drugs of abuse such as cocaine or amphetamine.
- Eclampsia/preeclampsia
- Thrombotic thrombocytopenic purpura
- Pheochromocytoma
- Severe burns
- Postoperative HTN

COMMONLY ASSOCIATED CONDITIONS

- Chronic renal failure
- Renovascular HTN
- Acute glomerulonephritis
- Renal vasculitis

Geriatric Considerations

Elderly patients may experience isolated systolic HTN due to decreased baroreceptor sensitivity.

Pediatric Considerations

- Usually associated with renal disease
- May present with abdominal pain
- Preferred agents for children include labetalol, nicardipine, and nitroprusside.

Pregnancy Considerations

- Hydralazine is drug of choice because nitroprusside decreases placental blood flow and cyanide metabolite crosses the placenta; may result in fetal toxicity with prolonged exposure.
- Treat preeclampsia.

DIAGNOSIS

Clinical presentation will vary depending on the organ system affected.

HISTORY

- Headache
- Altered mental status
- Nausea, vomiting
- Neurologic disturbance
- Shortness of breath, dyspnea, orthopnea
- Chest pain
- Abdominal pain
- Epistaxis

PHYSICAL EXAM

- HTN
- Focal neurologic deficits, stupor, coma
- Retinopathy: Funduscopic exam may reveal papilledema, exudates, or hemorrhages.
- Pulmonary edema
- Hemorrhage, thrombosis, embolus
- Renal or abdominal bruit
- Unequal BP or pulses in the extremities

DIAGNOSTIC TESTS & INTERPRETATION

Lab

Initial lab tests

- Urinalysis and renal function tests (red cell casts, hematuria, proteinuria are all common)
- Urine drug screen in selected patients
- Blood count and smear may indicate microangiopathic hemolytic anemia or thrombocytopenia.
- Serum electrolytes, which may indicate hypokalemic alkalosis
- Creatinine clearance
- Calcium, glucose

Follow-Up & Special Considerations

Subsequent workup pheochromocytoma in selected patients

Imaging

Initial approach

- Chest radiograph:
  - May show pulmonary edema and cardiomegaly due to CHF
  - Mediastinal widening and blunting of the aortic knob consistent with aortic aneurysm (potential rupture)
- If CNS symptoms, get CT scan or MRI of the head.
- If chest, abdominal, or back pain, consider contrast CT or MRI for suspected aortic dissection.

Follow-Up & Special Considerations

Subsequent workup for aldosteronism and for renal artery stenosis may be indicated in selected patients, especially young patients who may have fibromuscular dysplasia.

Diagnostic Procedures/Surgery

- ECG may reveal ischemia or left ventricular hypertrophy.
- The BP should be measured with an appropriately sized cuff, with ≥2 readings from both arms; then average readings.

Pathological Findings

Extreme BP elevations can overwhelm the autoregulatory mechanisms for organ blood flow, resulting in damage to the arteriolar and capillary beds. This process produces organ hemorrhages and edema.

DIFFERENTIAL DIAGNOSIS

- Myocardial infarction or angina pectoris
- Aortic dissection
- CHF
- Stroke
- Other CNS pathology (e.g., encephalopathy)
- Acute pulmonary edema
- Renal failure

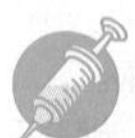

TREATMENT

MEDICATION

A 2008 Cochrane Review (1) noted that there are no randomized clinical trials showing a reduction in mortality from the recommended treatments and, similarly, no clear randomized trial basis for recommending one medication over another. However, the recommended medications have been shown to reduce BP in these circumstances, and the evidence levels reflect their effectiveness in this regard.

First Line

- IV unless otherwise indicated:
  - Nitroprusside (Nipride, Nitropress): Infusion 0.5–10 μg/kg/min; contraindicated in pregnancy (2,3)[A]
  - Fenoldopam (Corlopam): 0.1 μg/kg/min IV initial dose. Increase by 0.1 μg/kg/min q15min to desired effect. Maximum dose, 1.6 μg/kg/min (4)[A].
  - Hydralazine: Bolus 5–15 mg; preferred in pregnancy (2,3,5)[A]
  - Labetalol (Normodyne, Trandate): Bolus 20–80 mg q10–15min infusion 0.5–2 mg/min (2,3)[A]
  - Nitroglycerin (NTG): Infusion 5–100 μg/min (2,3,5)[A]
  - NTG: 0.4 mg SL tablet. Repeat q5min if needed. Consider IV infusion after 3 doses (2)[B].

– Phentolamine (Regitine): Bolus 5–10 mg q5–15min (2,3)[A]
– Esmolol: 0.05–0.3 mg/kg/min (2,3,5)[A]
– Enalapril: 0.625–1.25 mg (2,3)[B]
– Nicardipine: 4–15 mg/h (2,3,6)[B]

- The drug(s) used depends on the end organs affected and the patient's clinical status:
  – Hypertensive encephalopathy: Nicardipine, labetalol, esmolol, or enalaprilat (3)[A]
  – CNS events: Nicardipine, labetalol. In ischemic stroke, withhold treatment unless systolic >220 mm Hg or diastolic >120 mm Hg, except when needed for treating concomitant cardiovascular disease or pulmonary edema (2,3,5)[A]. In patients with intracerebral hemorrhage and systolic BP 150–220 mm Hg, acutely lowering to a systolic of 140 mm Hg is probably safe and may decrease additional bleeding (7)[B].
  – Subarachnoid hemorrhage: Nicardipine, labetalol, or esmolol (3,5)[A]
  – Myocardial ischemia: Nitroglycerin infusion, or labetalol, or esmolol (2,3,5)[A]
  – CHF: Nitroprusside infusion, or nitroglycerin infusion, or enalaprilat or nicardipine (2,3)[A]
  – Aortic dissection: Nitroprusside and β-blocker, esmolol or nitroglycerin infusion (2,3,5)[A]
  – Renal failure: Nitroprusside, labetalol, or nicardipine; consider dialysis (2,5)[A].
  – Pheochromocytoma: Phentolamine, or labetalol, or nitroprusside infusion (2)[A]
  – Antihypertensive withdrawal: Labetalol or phentolamine (2)[A]
  – Interactions between MAOIs and foods or drugs: Phentolamine or labetalol (2)[B]
  – Eclampsia/preeclampsia: Hydralazine, labetalol, or oral nifedipine (2,3,5)[A]

Second Line

- Oral clonidine: Oral loading dose of 0.2 mg followed by 0.1 mg/h until BP has been lowered or a total dose of 0.8 mg has been administered (2,5)[B]
- Trimethaphan (Arfonad): Infusion 0.5–5 mg/min (2)[B]
- Clevidipine: Start 1–2 mg/h, double q90sec until near goal, then smaller increases q5–10min. May be a good alternate choice for patients with signs/symptoms of acute heart failure
- Diazoxide in eclampsia/preeclampsia: 15 mg bolus q3min to maximum dose of 300 mg (8)[B]

ADDITIONAL TREATMENT

General Measures

- The general goal is to lower the mean arterial pressure (MAP) by ~20% or reduce the diastolic pressure to 100–110 mm Hg (13.3–14.6 kPa) over 1 hour.
- MAP is ~1/3 of the sum of twice the diastolic pressure plus the systolic pressure.
- If ongoing end-organ damage is thought to be secondary to the hypertensive state, prompt treatment with IV medication is indicated. Monitor patient closely so that a rapid fall in BP can be avoided.

COMPLEMENTARY AND ALTERNATIVE MEDICINE

Comfortable environment, which may lower the BP

SURGERY/OTHER PROCEDURES

- An arterial catheter may be used to monitor BP.
- Advantage over noninvasive monitoring not clearly proven (5)[C]

IN-PATIENT CONSIDERATIONS

Initial Stabilization

In general, lower the BP no more than 20% in the first hour; then, if stable, lower to 160/100–110 in the next 2–6 hours.

Admission Criteria

- All patients with true hypertensive emergencies should be hospitalized.
- Associated end-organ effects may require specific treatment (e.g., acute myocardial infarction).

IV Fluids

Fluid restriction may be appropriate for associated pathology such as pulmonary edema.

Nursing

Bed rest

Discharge Criteria

Patient should be stabilized on oral antihypertensives as appropriate (6)[A].

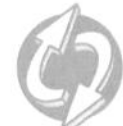

ONGOING CARE

FOLLOW-UP RECOMMENDATIONS

Close outpatient follow-up with primary care physician is recommended to ensure ongoing control of HTN.

Patient Monitoring

- Follow BP closely to avoid a rapid drop.
- Begin oral therapy as soon as possible after BP control has been achieved with IV medications.
- Ongoing BP control plus monitoring of affected organ system(s) (e.g., renal function) for evidence of continued morbidity

DIET

Low-sodium diet

PATIENT EDUCATION

- Avoid abrupt discontinuation of antihypertensive medicines.
- Stress importance of compliance.
- Emphasize the lack of symptoms with HTN until organ damage occurs.

PROGNOSIS

- BP should return to acceptable levels within 24 hours.
- Long-term prognosis depends upon extent of secondary end-organ damage in addition to ongoing BP control.

COMPLICATIONS

- Complications depend upon the organ system(s) that are secondarily affected.
- Abrupt or excessive lowering of BP may result in inadequate cerebral or cardiac blood flow, leading to stroke or myocardial ischemia.
- The benefits of aggressive treatment may outweigh the risks in patients with severe HTN but no end-organ damage. No studies have proven that aggressive treatment reduces the risk of long-term morbidity or mortality from hypertensive urgencies.

REFERENCES

1. Perez MI, Musini VM. Pharmacological interventions for hypertensive emergencies. *Cochrane Database Syst Rev*. 2008:CD003653.
2. Flanigan JS, Vitberg D. Hypertensive emergency and severe hypertension: What to treat, who to treat, and how to treat. *Med Clin North Am*. 2006;90:439–51.
3. Shayne PH, Pitts SR. Severely increased blood pressure in the emergency department. *Ann Emerg Med*. 2003;41:513–29.
4. Tumlin JA, Dunbar LM, Oparil S, et al. Fenoldopam, a dopamine agonist, for hypertensive emergency: A multicenter randomized trial. Fenoldopam Study Group. *Acad Emerg Med*. 2000;7:653–62.
5. Management of hypertension and hypertensive emergencies in the emergency department: The EMREG-International Consensus Panel Recommendations. *Ann Emerg Med*. 2008;51(3): S1–S38.
6. Chobanian AV, Bakris GL, Black HR, et al. The Seventh Report of the Joint National Committee on Prevention, Detection, Evaluation, and Treatment of High Blood Pressure: The JNC 7 report. *JAMA*. 2003;289:2560–72.
7. Morgenstern LB, et al. Guidelines for the management of spontaneous intracerebral hemorrhage: A guideline for healthcare professionals from the American Heart Association. *Stroke*. 2010;41:2108–29.
8. Hennessy A, Thornton CE, Makris A, et al. A randomised comparison of hydralazine and mini-bolus diazoxide for hypertensive emergencies in pregnancy: The PIVOT trial. *Aust N Z J Obstet Gynaecol*. 2007;47:279–85.

ADDITIONAL READING

- Baumann BM, Cline DM, Pimenta E. Treatment of hypertension in the emergency department. *J Am Soc Hypertension*. 2011;5(5)366–77.
- Marik PE, Varon J. Hypertensive crises: Challenges and management. *Chest*. 2007;131:1949–62.

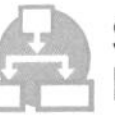

See Also (Topic, Algorithm, Electronic Media Element)

Aortic Dissection; Hypertension, Essential; Pheochromocytoma; Preeclampsia and Eclampsia (Toxemia of Pregnancy)

CODES

ICD9

401.9 Unspecified essential hypertension

CLINICAL PEARLS

- Treatment of severe HTN (hypertensive urgency) without evidence of acute end-organ damage is controversial. No emergent treatment is recommended in the emergency department. Initiation of oral medication may be indicated, with close follow-up.
- Avoid rapid prehospital lowering of BP.
- Treatment depends upon the organ systems affected.
- Esmolol and ACE inhibitors are contraindicated in pregnancy.

HYPERTHYROIDISM

Anup K. Sabharwal, MD, FACE
Atil Kargi, MD

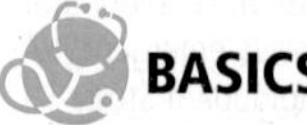

BASICS

Hyperthyroidism or thyrotoxicosis comprises a spectrum of clinical findings consistent with thyroid hormone excess. The former describes excess from the thyroid gland, whereas the latter can be produced from any other source or not identified.

DESCRIPTION

- Graves disease (GD): The most common form; diffuse goiter and thyrotoxicosis are common characteristics. Infiltrative orbitopathy is seen in 50% of patients. Infiltrative dermopathy is rare. Autoantibodies are directed at the thyrotropin-stimulating hormone (TSH) receptors.
- Toxic multinodular goiter (TMNG): Second most common; a TSH receptor mutation has been found in 60% of patients; patients older than age 40, insidious onset, frequent in iodine-deficient areas.
- Toxic adenoma: Younger patients, autonomously functioning nodules
- Iodine-induced hyperthyroidism
- Thyroiditis: Transient autoimmune process:
  - Subacute thyroiditis/De Quervain: Granulomatous giant cell thyroiditis, benign course; viral infections have been involved.
  - Postpartum thyroiditis
  - Drug-induced thyroiditis: Amiodarone, interferon alpha, interleukin 2, lithium
  - Miscellaneous: Thyrotoxicosis factitia, TSH-secreting pituitary tumors, and functioning trophoblastic tumors
- Subclinical hyperthyroidism: Suppressed TSH with normal thyroxine (T_4); may be associated with osteoporosis and atrial fibrillation (1)
- Thyroid storm: Rare hyperthyroidism; fever, tachycardia, systolic hypertension, CNS dysfunction (e.g., coma); up to 50% mortality

Geriatric Considerations

- Characteristic symptoms and signs may be absent.
- Atrial fibrillation is common when TSH <0.1 mU/L.

Pediatric Considerations

- Neonates and children are treated with antithyroids for 12–24 months.
- Radioactive iodine is controversial in patients under the ages of 15–18 years.

Pregnancy Considerations

Propylthiouracil (PTU) is currently the drug of choice during pregnancy. Treat with lowest effective dose. Avoid treatment-induced hypothyroidism. Radioiodine therapy is contraindicated.

EPIDEMIOLOGY

- 1.3% of population
- Predominant sex: Female > Male (7–10:1).
- Predominant age: Autoimmune thyroid disease in second and third decades. TMNG presents in patients older than age 40. GD is seen between 40 and 60 years of age.

Incidence

- Female 1:1,000
- Male: 1:3,000

RISK FACTORS

- Positive family history, especially in maternal relatives
- Female
- Other autoimmune disorders
- Iodide repletion after iodide deprivation, especially in TMNG

Genetics

The concordance rate for GD among monozygotic twins is 35%.

ETIOLOGY

- GD: Autoimmune disease
- TMNG: 60% TSH receptor gene abnormality; 40% unknown
- Toxic adenoma: Point mutation in TSH receptor gene with increased hormone production
- Thyroiditis:
  - Hashitoxicosis: Autoimmune destruction of the thyroid; antimicrosomal antibodies present
  - Subacute/De Quervain thyroiditis: Granulomatous reaction; genetic predisposition in specific human leukocyte antigens (HLAs); viruses such as coxsackievirus, adenovirus, echovirus, and influenza virus have been implicated; self-limited course, 6–12 months
  - Suppurative: Infectious
  - Drug-induced thyroiditis: Amiodarone produces an autoimmune reaction and a destructive process. Lithium, interferon-alpha, and interleukin 2 cause an autoimmune thyroiditis.
  - Postpartum thyroiditis: Autoimmune thyroiditis that lasts up to 8 weeks, and in 60% of patients, hypothyroidism manifests in the future.

COMMONLY ASSOCIATED CONDITIONS

- Autoimmune diseases
- Down syndrome
- Iodine deficiency

DIAGNOSIS

HISTORY

- Thyrotoxicosis is a hypermetabolic state where energy production exceeds needs, causing increased heat production, diaphoresis, and even fever.
- Thyrotoxicosis affects several different systems:
  - Constitutional: Fatigue, weakness, increased appetite, weight loss
  - Neuropsychiatric: Agitation, anxiety, emotional lability, psychosis, coma, and poor concentration and memory
  - GI: Increased appetite, hyperdefecation
  - Gynecologic: Oligomenorrhea, amenorrhea
  - Cardiovascular: Tachycardia (most common) and chest discomfort that mimics angina

Geriatric Considerations

Apathetic hyperthyroidism in the elderly

PHYSICAL EXAM

- Adults:
  - Skin: Warm, moist, pretibial myxedema (GD only)
  - Head, eye, ear, nose, throat (HEENT): Exophthalmos, lid lag
  - Endocrine: Hyperhidrosis, heat intolerance, goiter, gynecomastia, low libido, and spider angiomata (males)
  - Cardiovascular: Tachycardia, atrial fibrillation, cardiomegaly
  - Musculoskeletal: Skeletal demineralization, osteopenia, osteoporosis, fractures
  - Neurologic: Tremor, proximal muscle weakness, anxiety and lability, brisk deep tendon reflexes
  - Rarely: Thyroid acropathy (clubbing), localized dermopathy
- Children:
  - Linear growth acceleration
  - Ophthalmic abnormalities more common

DIAGNOSTIC TESTS & INTERPRETATION

Lab

- 95% have suppressed TSH and elevated free T_4. Total T_4 and triiodothyronine (T_3) represent the bound hormone and can be affected by pregnancy and hepatitis.
- T_3: Elevated especially in T_3 toxicosis or amiodarone-induced thyrotoxicosis
- T_4: Elevated; TSH autoantibodies rarely needed
- Free thyroxine index (FTI): Calculated from T_4 and thyroid hormone–binding ratio; corrects for misleading results caused by pregnancy and estrogens
- Inappropriately normal or elevated TSH with high T_4 suspicious for pituitary tumor or thyroid hormone resistance
- Drugs may alter lab results: Estrogens, heparin, iodine-containing compounds (including amiodarone and contrast agents), phenytoin, salicylates, steroids (e.g., androgens, corticosteroids)
- Drug precautions: Amiodarone and lithium may induce hyperthyroidism; MMI may cause warfarin resistance.
- Other findings that can occur: Anemia, granulocytosis, lymphocytosis, hypercalcemia, transaminase, and alkaline phosphate elevations.

Initial lab tests

- TSH, free T_4, T_4, T_3, TSI
- TSH-receptor (-R) antibodies (Abs): The routine assay is the TSH-binding inhibitor immunoglobulin assay (TBII). TSH-R Abs are useful in the prediction of postpartum Graves thyrotoxicosis and neonatal thyrotoxicosis.
- Thyroxine/triiodothyronine ratio: The T_4:T_3 ratio may be a useful tool when the iodine uptake testing is not available/contraindicated. ~2% of thyrotoxic patients have "T_3 toxicosis."

Follow-Up & Special Considerations

In severe cases, such as thyroid storm, hospitalize until stable, especially if >60 years of age, because of the risk of atrial fibrillation.

Imaging

- Nuclear medicine scanning (^{123}I or ^{131}I): The reference-range values for 24-hour radioiodine uptake is between 5% and 25%.
- Increased thyroid iodine uptake is seen with TMNG, toxic solitary nodule, and GD.
- GD shows a diffuse uptake and can have a paradoxical finding of high uptake at 4–6 hour but normal uptake at 24 hour because of the rapid clearance (2).
- TMNG will show a heterogeneous uptake, whereas solitary toxic nodule will show a warm or "hot" nodule.
- In iodine-deficient areas, an increased uptake is associated with low urine iodine levels.

- Hashimoto's thyroiditis can have an increased uptake at an early stage but no increased thyroid hormone production.
- Causes of thyrotoxicosis with low iodine uptake:
  - Acute thyroiditis, thyrotoxicosis factitia, and iodine intoxication with amiodarone or contrast material can cause low-uptake transient thyrotoxicosis. After thyroiditis resolves, the patient can become euthyroid or hypothyroid.
  - Iodine loading can cause iodine trapping and decreased iodine uptake (Wolff-Chaikoff effect).
  - Thyrotoxicosis factitia: Thyroglobulin levels are low in exogenous intake and high in endogenous production.
  - Other extrathyroidal causes include struma ovarii and metastatic thyroid carcinoma.
  - Technetium-99m scintigraphy: Controversial because it has a 33% discordance rate with radioactive iodine scanning.

Diagnostic Procedures/Surgery

Neck ultrasound will show increased diffuse vascularity in GD.

Pathological Findings

- GD: Hyperplasia
- Toxic nodule: Nodule formation

DIFFERENTIAL DIAGNOSIS

- Anxiety
- Malignancy
- Diabetes mellitus
- Pregnancy
- Menopause
- Pheochromocytoma
- Depression
- Carcinoid syndrome

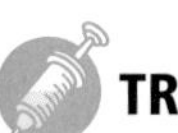

TREATMENT

- Radioactive iodine therapy (RAIT): Most common definitive treatment used in the US for GD and TMNG
- Pretreatment with antithyroid drugs is preferred to avoid worsening thyrotoxicosis. MMI is preferred over PTU as pretreatment because of decreased relapse, but it is held 3–5 days before therapy.
- There is concern for a slightly higher risk of lymphoma and leukemia in patients treated with RAIT.
- Usually patients become hypothyroid 2–3 months after therapy; therefore, antithyroid medications are continued after ablation.
- Glucocorticoids: Reduce the conversion of active T_4 to the more active T_3. In Graves ophthalmopathy, the use of prednisone before and after RAIT improves outcome.
- After RAIT, the release of antigens can worsen the inflammatory reaction and the ophthalmopathy.
- Smoking in GD patients is a risk factor for ophthalmopathy when treated with RAIT.
- For TMNG, the treatment of choice is RAIT. Medical therapy with antithyroid medications has shown a high recurrence rate. Surgery is considered only in special cases.
- Treatment for subacute thyroiditis is supportive with NSAIDs and beta blockers. Steroids can be used for 2–3 weeks.
- For amiodarone-induced thyrotoxicosis (AIT) type I, the treatment is antithyroid drugs and beta blockers. Potassium perchlorate also can be used as an iodine uptake inhibitor. Thyroidectomy is the last option. AIT type II is self-limited.
- Graves dermopathy: Difficult to treat in the chronic phase. Topical steroids with occlusive dressing may help in acute phase.

MEDICATION

First Line

- Antithyroid drugs: MMI and PTU are thionamides that inhibit iodine oxidation, organification, and iodotyrosine coupling. PTU can block peripheral conversion of T_4 to active T_3. Both can be used as primary treatment for GD and prior to RAIT or surgery (3)[A].
- Duration of treatment: 6 months to 2 years; 50–60% relapse after stopping; treatment beyond 18 months did not show any further benefit. The most serious side effects are hepatitis (0.1–0.2%), vasculitis, and agranulocytosis:
  - MMI: Adults: 10–15 mg q12h; children aged 6–10 years: 0.4 mg/kg/d PO once daily
  - PTU: Adults (preferred in thyroid storm and pregnant and lactating women): 100–150 mg PO q8h, not to exceed 200 mg/d during pregnancy
- β-adrenergic blocker: Propranolol in high doses (>160 mg/d) inhibits T_3 activation by up to 30%. Atenolol, metoprolol, and nadolol can be used.
- Glucocorticoids: Reduce the conversion of active T_4 to the more active T_3
- Cholestyramine: Anion exchange resin that decreases thyroid hormone reabsorption in the enterohepatic circulation; dose: 20–30 g/d
- Other agents:
  - Lithium: Inhibits thyroid hormone secretion and iodotyrosine coupling; can be dosed at 300 mg q8h with close monitoring of levels to avoid toxicity
  - Lugol solution: Saturated solution of potassium iodide (SSKI); blocks release of hormone from the gland but should be administered at least 1 hour after thionamide was given; acts as a substrate for hormone production (Jod-Basedow effect)
  - Potassium perchlorate: Especially for amiodarone-induced thyrotoxicosis
  - RAIT: See "Treatment" section.

Second Line

Ipodate sodium (Oragrafin): 0.5 g PO q.i.d. most effectively prevents conversion of T_4 to T_3 and thyroid hormone release; also useful in thyroid storm.

ADDITIONAL TREATMENT

Issues for Referral

Patients with Graves ophthalmopathy should be referred to an experienced ophthalmologist.

SURGERY/OTHER PROCEDURES

Thyroidectomy for compressive symptoms, masses, and thyroid malignancy may be performed in the second trimester of pregnancy only.

ONGOING CARE

FOLLOW-UP RECOMMENDATIONS

Patient Monitoring

- Repeat thyroid tests once a year, CBC and LFTs on thionamide therapy; continue therapy with thionamides for 12–18 months (3).
- After RAIT, thyroid function tests at 6 weeks, 12 weeks, 6 months, and annually thereafter if euthyroid; TSH may remain undetectable for months if patient is euthyroid; follow T_3 and T_4.

DIET

Sufficient calories to prevent weight loss

PROGNOSIS

Good (with early diagnosis and treatment)

COMPLICATIONS

- Surgery: Hypoparathyroidism, recurrent laryngeal nerve damage, and hypothyroidism
- RAIT: Postablation hypothyroidism
- GD: High relapse rate with antithyroid drug as primary therapy
- Graves ophthalmopathy, worsening heart failure if cardiac condition, atrial fibrillation, muscle wasting, proximal muscle weakness, increased risk of cerebrovascular accident (CVA) and cardiovascular mortality

REFERENCES

1. Cappola AR, Fried LP, Arnold AM, et al. Thyroid status, cardiovascular risk, and mortality in older adults. *JAMA*. 2006;295:1033–41.
2. Nayak B, Hodak SP. Hyperthyroidism. *Endocrinol Metab Clin North Am*. 2007;36:617–56.
3. Abraham P, Avenell A, Watson WA, et al. A systematic review of drug therapy for Graves' hyperthyroidism. *Cochrane Database Sys Rev*. 2005;153(4):489–98.

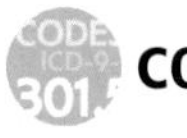

CODES

ICD9

- 242.00 Toxic diffuse goiter without mention of thyrotoxic crisis or storm
- 242.10 Toxic uninodular goiter without mention of thyrotoxic crisis or storm
- 242.20 Toxic multinodular goiter without mention of thyrotoxic crisis or storm

CLINICAL PEARLS

- Not all thyrotoxicoses are secondary to hyperthyroidism.
- GD presents with hyperthyroidism, ophthalmopathy, and goiter.
- Medical treatment for GD has a high relapse rate after stopping medications.
- Thyroid storm is a medical emergency that needs hospitalization and aggressive treatment.

H

HYPOGLYCEMIA, DIABETIC

Joseph A. Florence, MD

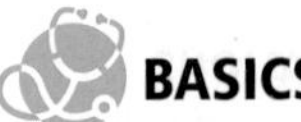

BASICS

DESCRIPTION

- Abnormally low concentration of glucose in circulating blood of diabetic; often referred to as an *insulin reaction*
- Classification includes:
  - Severe hypoglycemia: An event requiring assistance of another person to actively administer treatment
  - Documented symptomatic hypoglycemia: An event during which typical symptoms are accompanied by a measured plasma glucose of ≤70 mg/dL (3.9 mmol/L)
  - Asymptomatic hypoglycemia: An event not accompanied by symptoms, but a measured glucose of ≤70 mg/dL (3.9 mmol/L)
  - Probable symptomatic hypoglycemia: Event with symptoms, but glucose not tested
  - Relative hypoglycemia: An event with typical symptoms, but glucose >70 mg/dL (3.9 mmol/L)
- Hypoglycemia is the leading limiting factor in the glycemic management of type 1 and type 2 diabetes. Severe or frequent hypoglycemia requires modification of treatment regiments, including higher treatment goals (1).
- System(s) affected: Endocrine/Metabolic

ALERT

Hypoglycemic unawareness:

- Major risk factor for severe hypoglycemic reactions
- Most commonly found in patients with long-standing type 1 diabetes and children <7 years

EPIDEMIOLOGY

Incidence

From the Accord Study, the annual incidence of hypoglycemia was:

- 3.14% in the intensive treatment group
- 1.03% in the standard group
- Increased risk among women, African Americans, those with less than a high school education, aged participants, and those who used insulin at trial entry
- From the RECAP-DM study: Hypoglycemia was reported in 38% of type 2 patients who added a sulphonylurea or a thiazolinedione to metformin therapy during the past year.

RISK FACTORS

- Nearly 3/4 of severe hypoglycemic episodes occur during sleep.
- Autonomic neuropathy
- Illness, stress, and unplanned life events
- Duration of diabetes >5 years, advanced age, renal/liver disease, CHF, hypothyroidism, hypoadrenalism, gastroenteritis, gastroparesis (unpredictable CHO delivery)
- Starvation or prolonged fasting
- Alcoholism: Evening consumption of alcohol is associated with an increased risk of nocturnal and fasting hypoglycemia, especially in type 1 patients.
- Current smokers with type 1 diabetes
- Oral hypoglycemics with long duration and high potency have greater hypoglycemic risks.
- Insulin secretagogues: Sulfonylureas (Glipizide, Glibenclamide, Glibornuride, Gliclazide, Chlorpropamide, Glimepiride); glinide derivatives (Repaglinide, Nateglinide) stimulate insulin secretion and can cause hypoglycemia. Hypoglycemia is rare in diabetics not treated with insulin or insulin secretagogues (1).
- In patients 80 years or older, severe hypoglycemia is associated with comorbid conditions and in users of a long-acting sulphonylurea.
- Intensive insulin therapy (further lowering A1C from 7% to 6%) is associated with higher rate of hypoglycemia (2).

GENERAL PREVENTION

- Maintain routine schedule of diet, medication, and exercise.
- Stabilize daily carbohydrate intake.
- Regular blood glucose testing if taking insulin or insulin secretagogue:
  - ≥3 times daily testing if multiple injections of insulin, insulin pump therapy, or pregnant diabetic; frequency and timing dictated by needs and treatment goals
  - Particularly helpful for asymptomatic hypoglycemia
- Diabetes treatment and teaching programs (DTTPs) especially for high-risk type 1 patients, which teach flexible insulin therapy to enable dietary freedom
- Use of rapid-acting and long-acting insulin analogs is associated with less hypoglycemia (3).
- Hypoglycemia rates are reduced by up to 70% using continuous SC insulin infusion pumps compared with multiple daily injections (4)[C].
- Continuous glucose monitoring may supplement self-glucose monitoring and is especially useful with hypoglycemic unawareness and/or frequent hypoglycemic episodes (1).
- If pre-exercise glucose is <100 mg/dL and taking insulin or secretagogue, then carbohydrate consumption or reduction in medication may prevent hypoglycemia.

ETIOLOGY

- Loss of hormonal counter-regulatory mechanism in glucose metabolism
- Diet: Too little food (skipping meal), decreased carbohydrate intake
- Medication: Too much insulin or oral hypoglycemic agent (improper dose or timing)
- Erratic absorption of insulin or oral hypoglycemics
- Adverse reaction from other medications
- Exercise/physical activity: Unplanned or excessive
- Alcohol consumption
- Vomiting or diarrhea
- Gastroparesis

COMMONLY ASSOCIATED CONDITIONS

- Autonomic dysfunction
- Neuropathies
- Cardiomyopathies
- Older type 2 diabetics with severe hypoglycemia have a higher risk of dementia (5).

DIAGNOSIS

HISTORY

- Symptoms are idiosyncratic and vary considerably between individuals.
- Adrenergic hypoglycemia symptoms:
  - Hunger, trembling, pallor
  - Sweating, shaking, pounding heart, anxiety
- Neuroglycopenic hypoglycemia symptoms:
  - Dizziness, poor concentration, drowsiness, weakness, confusion, lightheadedness, slurred speech, blurred vision, double vision, unsteadiness, poor coordination
- Behavioral hypoglycemia symptoms:
  - Tearfulness, confusion, fatigue, irritability, aggressiveness

- Patients' reports of hypoglycemic symptoms are associated with a significantly lower treatment satisfaction and with barriers to adherence (6)[A].

PHYSICAL EXAM

- General: Confusion, lethargy
- HEENT: Diplopia
- Cor: Tachycardia
- Neuro: Tremulousness, weakness, paresthesias, stupor, seizure, or coma
- Mental status: Irritability, inability to concentrate, or short-term memory loss
- Skin: Pale, diaphoresis
- End-organ damage: Microvascular, macrovascular, ophthalmologic, neurologic, renal

DIAGNOSTIC TESTS & INTERPRETATION

Lab

- Plasma, serum or whole-blood glucose <70 mg/dL
- A hypoglycemic reading from a continuous glucose monitoring sensor should be verified by alternative glucose testing method prior to treatment.
- Suspect hypoglycemic unawareness in type 1 asymptomatic diabetes with low/normal HgbA1c.
- Chronic hypoglycemia is indicated by low glycohemoglobin level.
- Disorders that may alter lab results:
  - Hemoglobinopathies may alter HgbA1c results.

DIFFERENTIAL DIAGNOSIS

- Hypoglycemia seen in chronic alcoholics and binge drinkers.
- GI dysfunction causing postprandial hypoglycemia or alimentary reactive hypoglycemia
- Hormonal deficiency states (hormonal reactive hypoglycemia)
- Hypoglycemia of sepsis
- Islet cell tumors
- Factitious hypoglycemia from surreptitious injection of insulin
- Hypoglycemia may be found in early pregnancy, prolonged fasting, long periods of strenuous exercise, heart failure, malignancy, and renal or liver disease.

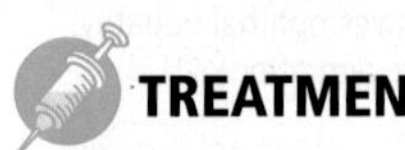

TREATMENT

MEDICATION

- Conscious patients:
  - Oral administration of small-molecule sugars (saccharose/glucose); glucose preferred; liquid preferred; any form of CHO that contains glucose may be used (7).
  - "Rule of 15": 15–20 g glucose (~60 calories simple carbohydrate) repeated q15min until blood sugar is ≥100 mg/dL (5.55 mmol/L)
  - Takes ~15 minutes for carbohydrates to be digested and enter bloodstream as glucose
  - Once sugar has normalized, then a meal or snack should be consumed to prevent recurrence of hypoglycemia (1)[C].

- Loss of consciousness at home:
  - Administer glucagon
  - IM or SC in the deltoid or anterior thigh:
    - <5 years old: 0.25–0.50 mg
    - 5–10 years old: 0.50–1 mg
    - >10 years old: 1 mg
- In unconscious, if emergency medical personnel are present or patient hospitalized:
  - Give 1/2 ampule 50% dextrose every 5–10 minutes until patient awakens.
  - Then feed orally and/or administer 5% dextrose IV at level that will maintain blood glucose >100 mg/dL.
  - Patients with hypoglycemia secondary to oral hypoglycemics should be monitored for 24–48 hours, because hypoglycemia may recur after apparent clinical recovery.
- Significant possible interactions:
  - Treatment may cause hyperglycemia (Somogyi phenomenon).
  - Clearance of certain oral hypoglycemics from plasma may be prolonged in persons with liver disease.

ADDITIONAL TREATMENT

General Measures

- Glucose: Preferred treatment; however, any form of carbohydrate that contains glucose should be effective (1)[C].
- Any sugar-containing food or beverage that can be rapidly absorbed: Juice (4–6 oz), candy (5–6 pieces of hard candy), or nondiet soda
- OTC glucose tablets or gels
- Glucagon: People in close contact with people with diabetes should be instructed in using an emergency glucagon kit (1)[C].
- Glucagon should be prescribed to patients at significant risk of severe hypoglycemia (1)[C].
- If a patient using acarbose suffers from a bout of hypoglycemia, the patient should eat something containing monosaccharides, such as glucose tablets. Since acarbose will prevent the digestion of complex carbohydrates, starchy foods will not effectively reverse a hypoglycemic episode in a patient taking it.
- Severe hypoglycemia combined with hypoglycemic unawareness should raise glycemic targets to avoid hypoglycemia.

Issues for Referral

- Frequent, recurring, or episodes that do not readily respond to treatment
- Consultant pharmacists can play a critical role in preventing hypoglycemia in long-term care facilities.

Additional Therapies

Use of a continuous glucose monitoring system in the management of severe hypoglycemia decreases the number of hypoglycemic values (8)[B]

IN-PATIENT CONSIDERATIONS

Admission Criteria

- Any doubt of cause
- Expectation of prolonged hypoglycemia (e.g., caused by sulfonylurea drug)
- Inability of patient to drink
- Treatment has not resulted in prompt recovery of sensorium.
- Seizures, coma, or altered behavior (e.g., ataxia, disorientation, unstable motor coordination, dysphasia) secondary to documented or suspected hypoglycemia

Discharge Criteria

Patient has normoglycemia and risk of severe hypoglycemia is negligible.

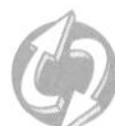

ONGOING CARE

FOLLOW-UP RECOMMENDATIONS

Rest until glucose is normal.

Patient Monitoring

Self-monitoring of blood glucose

DIET

- If alcohol consumed, combine with food to reduce risk of hypoglycemia.
- Protein does not slow absorption of carbohydrates.
- Fats may slow absorption of carbohydrates and may retard and then prolong the acute glycemic response (9)[C].

PATIENT EDUCATION

- Always have access to quick-acting carbohydrate.
- For planned exercise, consider a reduced insulin dosage; additional carbohydrates needed for unplanned exercise.
- For patients with hypoglycemia unawareness or 1 or more episodes of severe hypoglycemia, glycemic targets should be raised to avoid further hypoglycemia for at least several weeks.
- Educate patients and their relatives, close friends, teachers, and supervisors to be aware of diabetes diagnosis and signs/symptoms of hypoglycemia and treatment.
- Teach self-monitoring of blood glucose and self-adjustment for insulin therapy, diet control, and exercise regimen.
- Patient should wear medical alert identification bracelet or necklace.

PROGNOSIS

Full recovery usually depends on rapidity of diagnosis and treatment.

COMPLICATIONS

- Coma, seizure, MI, stroke (especially in elderly)
- Prolonged or severe hypoglycemia may cause permanent neurologic damage and/or cognitive impairment.

ALERT

In the ACCORD trial of adults with type 2 diabetes at especially high risk for heart attack and stroke, the medical strategy to intensively lower blood glucose (sugar) below current recommendations increased the risk of death compared with a less-intensive standard treatment strategy (10)[B].

REFERENCES

1. American Diabetes Association, et al. Standards of medical care in diabetes–2011. *Diabetes Care*. 2011;34(Suppl 1):S11–61.
2. Action to Control Cardiovascular Risk in Diabetes Study Group, Gerstein HC, Miller ME, et al. Effects of intensive glucose lowering in type 2 diabetes. *N Engl J Med*. 2008;358:2545–59.
3. Rosenstock J, Dailey G, Massi-Benedetti M, et al. Reduced hypoglycemia risk with insulin glargine: A meta-analysis comparing insulin glargine with human NPH insulin in type 2 diabetes. *Diabetes Care*. 2005;28:950–5.
4. Cohen ND, et al. Diabetes: Advances in treatment. *Internal Med J*. 2007;37:383–8.
5. Whitmer RA, Karter AJ, Yaffe K, et al. Hypoglycemic episodes and risk of dementia in older patients with type 2 diabetes mellitus. *JAMA*. 2009;301:1565–72.
6. Alvarez Guisasola F, Tofé Povedano S, Krishnarajah G, et al. Hypoglycaemic symptoms, treatment satisfaction, adherence and their associations with glycaemic goal in patients with type 2 diabetes mellitus: Findings from the Real-Life Effectiveness and Care Patterns of Diabetes Management (RECAP-DM) Study. *Diabetes Obes Metab*. 2008;10(Suppl 1):25–32.
7. American Diabetes Association, et al. Executive summary: Standards of medical care in diabetes–2011. *Diabetes Care*. 2011;34(Suppl 1):S4–10.
8. Ryan EA, Germsheid J, et al. Use of continuous glucose monitoring system in the management of severe hypoglycemia. *Diabetes Technol Ther*. 2009;11:635–9.
9. Franz MJ, Powers MA, Leontos C, et al. The evidence for medical nutrition therapy for type 1 and type 2 diabetes in adults. *J Am Diet Assoc*. 2010;110:1852–89.
10. National Institutes of Health. For safety, NHLBI changes intensive blood sugar treatment in clinical trial of diabetes and cardiovascular fitness. Accessed March 24, 2008 at: http://public.nhlbi.nih.gov/newsroom/home/GetPressRelease.aspx?id=2551.

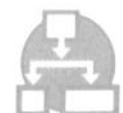

See Also (Topic, Algorithm, Electronic Media Element)

- Diabetes Mellitus, Type 1
- Algorithm: Hypoglycemia

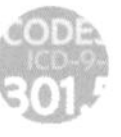

CODES

ICD9

- 250.80 Diabetes mellitus with other specified manifestations, type ii or unspecified type, not stated as uncontrolled
- 250.81 Diabetes mellitus with other specified manifestations, type I (juvenile type) not stated as uncontrolled

CLINICAL PEARLS

- Hypoglycemic unawareness is most common with tightly controlled, long-standing type 1 diabetes and children <7 years.
- Any form of carbohydrate that contains glucose should be effective for management, such as sugar-containing food or beverage that can be rapidly absorbed:
  - 6 oz juice; 6 pieces of hard candy; nondiet soda; OTC glucose tablets or gels

H

HYPOGLYCEMIA, NONDIABETIC

Matthew A. Silva, PharmD, RPh, BCPS
Pablo I. Hernandez Itriago, MD

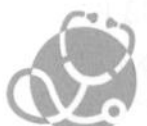

BASICS

DESCRIPTION
- Hypoglycemia defined by Whipple triad:
  - Low plasma glucose level (≤60 mg/dL)
  - Hypoglycemic symptoms that are relieved when glucose level is corrected
  - Occurs commonly in patients with diabetes receiving sulfonylurea or insulins; less commonly in patients without diabetes
- Reactive hypoglycemia:
  - Occurs in response to a meal, drugs, herbal substances, or nutrients
  - May occur 2–3 hours postprandially or later
  - Symptoms generally observed with serum glucose ≤60 mg/dL, lower in patients with hypoglycemic unawareness
  - Also seen after GI surgery (in association with dumping syndrome in some patients)
- Spontaneous (fasting) hypoglycemia:
  - May be associated with a primary condition, including hypopituitarism, Addison disease, myxedema, or in disorders related to hepatic dysfunction or renal failure
  - If hypoglycemia presents as a primary disorder, consider hyperinsulinism and extrapancreatic tumors.

EPIDEMIOLOGY
Incidence
- True incidence is unknown.
- 8.6% of hospitalized inpatients ≥65 years old:
  - Asymptomatic in 25% of cases

Prevalence
True prevalence is unknown:
- Predominant age: Older adult
- Predominant sex: Female > Male

RISK FACTORS
Refer to "Etiology."

Genetics
Some aspects may involve genetics (e.g., hereditary fructose intolerance).

GENERAL PREVENTION
- Follow dietary and exercise guidelines.
- Patient recognition of early symptoms and knowledge of corrective action

ETIOLOGY
- Reactive, postprandial:
  - Alimentary hyperinsulinism
  - Meals high in refined carbohydrate
  - Certain nutrients, including fructose, galactose, leucine
  - Glucose intolerance (prediabetes)
  - GI surgery
  - Idiopathic (unknown cause)
- Spontaneous:
  - Fasting
  - Alcohol or prescription medication (insulin, sulfonylureas, thiazolidinediones, incretin-mimetics, DPP-IV inhibitors, beta-blockers, salicylates, quinine, hydroxychloroquine, fluoroquinones, doxycycline, sertraline, disopyramide, pentamidine)
  - Nonprescription over-the-counter (OTC) agents, including performance-enhancing agents. Adulterated versions of phosphodiesterase inhibitors and performance-enhancing agents are routinely imported and may contain sulfonylureas and other hypoglycemic agents.
  - Consider medication errors as a source of unexplained hypoglycemia even in patients without diabetes.
  - Surreptitious drug use (self-injection of insulin or ingestion of oral hypoglycemic medications in patients with diabetes
  - Natural medicines or herbs (bitter melon, caffeine, cassia cinnamon, chromium, fenugreek, ginseng, guarana, mate, Stevia, vanadium)
  - Postsurgical (e.g., gastrectomy, Roux-en-Y) hypoglycemia/dumping syndrome
  - Islet cell hyperplasia or tumor (insulinoma)
  - Extrapancreatic insulin secreting tumor
  - Hepatic disease
  - Glucagon deficiency
  - Adrenal insufficiency
  - Catecholamine deficiency
  - Hypopituitarism
  - Hypothyroidism
  - Eating disorders
  - Exercise
  - Fever
  - Pregnancy
  - Renal glycosuria
  - Large tumors
  - Ketotic hypoglycemia of childhood
  - Enzyme deficiencies or defects
  - Severe malnutrition
  - Sepsis
  - Total parenteral nutrition therapy
  - Hemodialysis

Pediatric Considerations
- Usually divided into 2 syndromes
- Transient neonatal hypoglycemia
- Hypoglycemia of infancy and childhood
- Screening infants for hypoglycemia is appropriate when pregnancy was complicated by maternal diabetes.

Geriatric Considerations
- More likely to have underlying disorders or be causative medications
- Iatrogenic hypoglycemia is common in the hospitalized elderly with renal insufficiency.

COMMONLY ASSOCIATED CONDITIONS
- Severe liver disease; alcoholism
- Addison disease; adrenocortical insufficiency
- Myxedema
- Malnutrition (patients with renal failure)
- GI surgery
- Panhypopituitarism
- Insulinoma

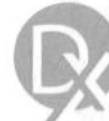

DIAGNOSIS

HISTORY
- CNS (neuroglycopenic) symptoms predominate with gradual glucose reduction:
  - Headache
  - Confusion
  - Lightheadedness
  - Fatigue and weakness
  - Visual disturbances
  - Changes in personality
- Adrenergic symptoms: More prominent in acute drop in glucose:
  - Anxiety
  - Tremulousness
  - Dizziness
  - Diaphoresis
  - Warmth/flushing
  - Heart palpitations
- GI symptoms:
  - Hunger
  - Nausea
  - Belching

PHYSICAL EXAM
- CNS (neuroglycopenic) symptoms predominate with gradual glucose reduction:
  - Convulsions
  - Coma
  - Hypotension
- Adrenergic symptoms: More prominent in acute drop in glucose:
  - Tremulousness
  - Diaphoresis
  - Warmth/flushing
  - Heart palpitations

DIAGNOSTIC TESTS & INTERPRETATION
Lab
Initial lab tests

Blood glucose ≤45 mg/dL (≤2.5 mmol/L) when symptomatic followed by symptom resolution with feeding (1,2)[C]:
- Plasma glucose overnight fasting: ≤60 mg/dL (≤3.33 mmol/L); confirm on 2 or more occasions (2)[C]

- Plasma glucose 72-hour fasting: ≤45 mg/dL (≤2.5 mmol/L) for females; ≤55 mg/dL (≤3.05 mmol/L) for males; fast may be ended when Whipple triad is achieved or hypoglycemia is demonstrated (2)[C]

Follow-Up & Special Considerations

- Oral glucose tolerance: ≤50 mg/dL (≤2.78 mmol/L) (1,2)[C]
- Misinterpretation of glucose tolerance tests may lead to misdiagnosis of hypoglycemia; ≥1/3 of normal patients have hypoglycemia, with or without symptoms, during the 4-hour glucose tolerance test. These patients may be at future risk for type 2 diabetes.
- C-peptide measurement (2)[C]
- Check liver studies, serum insulin, adrenocorticotrophic hormone (ACTH), and cortisol. Serum insulin should be suppressed when glucose is <60 mg/dL (2)[C].
- Serum b-hydroxybutyrate
- Insulin radioimmunoassay: Elevated insulin levels suggest islet cell hyperplasia or tumor (2)[C].
- Drugs may alter lab results: Many drugs can affect glucose levels; refer to drug or laboratory reference (2)[C].

Imaging

Initial approach

Abdominal CT to rule out abdominal tumor

Diagnostic Procedures/Surgery

- For definitive diagnosis, patient should have (2)[C]:
  - Documented low glucose levels
  - Symptoms when glucose levels are low
  - Evidence that symptoms are relieved specifically by ingestion of sugar or other food
  - Identification of the specific type of hypoglycemia
- Serum b-hydroxybutyrate <2.7 mg/dL in the presence of high serum insulin, C-peptide, and low serum glucose suggests excessive insulin production.

DIFFERENTIAL DIAGNOSIS

CNS disorders:

- Psychogenic
- Pseudohypoglycemia: Symptoms of hypoglycemia or self-diagnosis in patients in whom low blood glucose may not be detectable and who may be impossible to convince that they do not suffer from hypoglycemia after all tests are found to be normal

TREATMENT

MEDICATION

- Once diagnosis is established, begin therapy appropriate to underlying disorder.
- If unable to swallow: Glucagon 1 mg (1 unit) IM or SC. If no response, give IV bolus of 25–50 g of 50% glucose solution followed by continuous infusion until patient able to take by mouth (1)[C].
- Postsurgical gastrectomy patients unresponsive to dietary changes may benefit from propantheline, psyllium, fiber, or oat bran, which delays gastric emptying (1)[C].
- Insulinoma: See separate topic.

ADDITIONAL TREATMENT

General Measures

- Outpatient except for severe cases; may also be inpatient for testing
- Oral carbohydrate for alert patient without drug overdose (2–3 Tbs of sugar in glass of water or fruit juice, 1–2 cups of milk, piece of fruit, or several soda crackers) (1)[C]
- If unable to swallow: Use glucagon IM or SC (1)[C].
- If caused by medication or nutrients: Avoid or control causative agents (1)[C].
- If triggered by meals: Try high-protein diet with carbohydrate restriction (1)[C].
- Nonhypoglycemic hypoglycemia or pseudohypoglycemia:
  - Many patients (often females, aged 20–45) present with diagnosis of reactive hypoglycemia (self-diagnosed or misinterpretation of tests)
  - Symptoms may pertain to chronic fatigue and somatic complaints (stress often playing a role in these symptoms).
  - Management difficult; listening is important. Try 120-g carbohydrate diet (1)[C].
  - Counseling may be useful for stress and other problems.

SURGERY/OTHER PROCEDURES

If islet cell tumor (insulinoma) or other insulin-secreting tumor, surgery is treatment of choice. If inoperable, diazoxide may relieve symptoms.

IN-PATIENT CONSIDERATIONS

Admission Criteria

Hypoglycemia unresponsive to oral intake

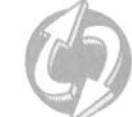

ONGOING CARE

FOLLOW-UP RECOMMENDATIONS

- Exercise routine or daily activity may need to be re-evaluated.
- Patients with recurrent hypoglycemia should have glucose source at hand for immediate ingestion during symptoms.

Patient Monitoring

- Depends on type and severity of symptoms and treatment of underlying cause
- Hypoglycemia from sulfonylureas can last for hours to days depending on half-life and renal function.

DIET

- High protein, low carbohydrate
- Frequent small feedings (6 daily)
- Avoid fasting.

PATIENT EDUCATION

- Dietary instruction
- Counseling for stress, if appropriate
- Recognition of early symptoms of hypoglycemia and how to take corrective action

PROGNOSIS

Favorable, with appropriate treatment

COMPLICATIONS

- Insulinoma: If tumor identified and removed, some surgical risk is involved.
- Organic brain syndrome: May occur with extensive, prolonged hypoglycemia

REFERENCES

1. Carroll MF, Burge MR, Schade DS. Severe hypoglycemia in adults. *Rev Endocr Meta Dis.* 2003;4(2):149–57.
2. Service FJ. Classification of hypoglycemic disorders. *Endocrinol Metab Clin North Am.* 1999;28: 501–17, vi.

ADDITIONAL READING

- Bharmal SV, Moyes V, Ahmed S, et al. Hypoglycaemia: Possible mediation by chromium salt medication. *Hormones (Athens).* 2010;9:181–3.
- Cansu DU, Korkmaz C. Hypoglycaemia induced by hydroxychloroquine in a non-diabetic patient treated for RA. *Rheumatology (Oxford).* 2008;47:378–9.
- Chan TY, et al. Outbreaks of severe hypoglycaemia due to illegal sexual enhancement products containing undeclared glibenclamide. *Pharmacoepidemiol Drug Saf.* 2009;18:1250–1.
- Chaubey SK, Sangla KS, Suthaharan EN, et al. Severe hypoglycaemia associated with ingesting counterfeit medication. *Med J Aust.* 2010;192:716–7.
- Lawrence KR, Adra M, Keir C. Hypoglycemia-induced anoxic brain injury possibly associated with levofloxacin. *J Infect.* 2006;52:e177–80.
- Pollak PT, Mukherjee SD, Fraser AD. Sertraline-induced hypoglycemia. *Ann Pharmacother.* 2001;35:1371–4.
- Singh M, Jacob JJ, Kapoor R, et al. Fatal hypoglycemia with levofloxacin use in an elderly patient in the post-operative period. *Langenbecks Arch Surg.* 2008;393:235–8.
- Yamada C, Nagashima K, Takahashi A, et al. Gatifloxacin acutely stimulates insulin secretion and chronically suppresses insulin biosynthesis. *Eur J Pharmacol.* 2006;553:67–72.

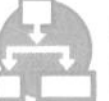

See Also (Topic, Algorithm, Electronic Media Element)

- Hypoglycemia, Diabetic; Insulinoma
- Algorithm: Hypoglycemia

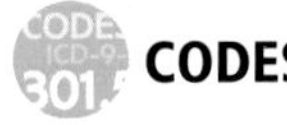

CODES

ICD9

251.2 Hypoglycemia, unspecified

CLINICAL PEARLS

- Symptoms coincide with low blood glucose levels.
- Symptoms resolve with PO/IV glucose or glucagon.
- Avoid known agents/nutrients that trigger hypoglycemia.
- Treat underlying cause.

H

HYPOKALEMIA

Ruben Peralta, MD, FACS
Mushreq Alani, MD

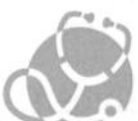

BASICS

DESCRIPTION

Hypokalemia is defined as a serum potassium concentration <3.5 mEq/L (normal range, 3.5–5 mEq/L).

EPIDEMIOLOGY

Predominant sex: Male = Female

Incidence

- Electrolyte abnormality is commonly encountered in clinical practice (1).
- Found in >20% of hospitalized patients (when defined as potassium <3.6 mEq/L).
- Higher incidence (5–20%) in individuals with eating disorders
- >10% of inpatients with alcoholism
- Higher incidence in patients with AIDS
- Associated risk after bariatric surgery

RISK FACTORS

Genetics

Some rare, familial disorders cause hypokalemia:

- Familial hypokalemic periodic paralysis: Hypokalemia after a high-carbohydrate or high-sodium meal or after exercise
- Congenital adrenogenital syndromes
- Liddle syndrome: Increases K+ secretion
- Familial interstitial nephritis

GENERAL PREVENTION

When initiating a diuretic, especially loop and thiazide diuretics, patients should be advised to increase their dietary potassium intake (see "Diet").

ETIOLOGY

Most common causes:

- Decreased intake: Deficient diet in alcoholics and elderly; anorexia nervosa
- GI loss: Vomiting, diarrhea, nasogastric tubes, laxative abuse, fistulas, villous adenoma, ureterosigmoidostomy, malabsorption, chemotherapy, radiation enteropathy, bulimia
- Intracellular shift of potassium: Metabolic alkalosis, insulin excess, β-adrenergic catecholamine excess (acute stress, B_2 agonists [2]), hypokalemic periodic paralysis, intoxications (theophylline, caffeine, barium, toluene)
- Renal potassium loss:
  - Drugs: Diuretics (especially loop and thiazides), amphotericin B, aminoglycosides (3,4,5)
  - Mineralocorticoid-excess states: Primary hyperaldosteronism; secondary hyperaldosteronism (congestive heart failure [CHF], cirrhosis, nephrotic syndrome, malignant hypertension, renin-producing tumors); renovascular hypertension; Bartter syndrome; Gitelman syndrome; congenital adrenogenital syndromes; exogenous mineralocorticoids (glycyrrhizic acid in licorice, carbenoxolone, steroids in nasal sprays); Liddle syndrome; vasculitis
- Glucocorticoid-excess states: Cushing syndrome, exogenous steroids, ectopic adrenocorticotrophic hormone (ACTH) production, II B hydroxysteroid dehydrogenase deficiency.
- Renal tubular acidosis (type I and II):
  - Leukemia
  - Magnesium depletion
  - Thyrotoxic hypokalemic paralysis
- Osmotic diuresis (e.g., poorly controlled diabetes)

COMMONLY ASSOCIATED CONDITIONS

Acute GI illnesses with severe vomiting or diarrhea

DIAGNOSIS

- Patients with hypokalemia often have no symptoms, especially if the hypokalemia is mild (serum potassium 3–3.5 mEq/L).
- Neuromuscular (most prominent manifestations):
  - Skeletal muscle weakness (proximal > distal muscles, lower limbs > upper limbs) may range from mild weakness to total paralysis, including respiratory muscles; it may lead to rhabdomyolysis and/or respiratory arrest in severe cases.
  - Smooth-muscle involvement may lead to GI hypomotility, producing ileus and constipation.
- Cardiovascular:
  - Ventricular arrhythmias; higher risk if underlying CHF, left ventricular failure (LVF), cardiac ischemia
  - Hypotension
  - Cardiac arrest
- Renal: Polyuria, polydipsia, nocturia owing to impaired ability to concentrate, myoglobinuria
- Metabolic: Hyperglycemia

HISTORY

Muscle weakness, hypotension, vomiting, diarrhea, polyuria, polydypsia, dyspnea on exertion

PHYSICAL EXAM

Skin turgor, hypotension, orthostasis, pulmonary congestion/rales, peripheral edema

DIAGNOSTIC TESTS & INTERPRETATION

Lab

- Serum potassium <3.5 mEq/L (<3.5 mmol/L)
- Disorders that may alter lab results: Leukemia and other conditions with high WBCs

Initial lab tests

- If not believed to be secondary to medications or GI losses: Serum electrolytes, urinary potassium, ECG.
- Calculate plasma anion gap normal (anion gap = Na – [Cl + HCO_3]); normal values, 12 ± 4 mEq/L. Must correct calculated anion gap for hypoalbuminemia. Increase calculated anion gap by 2.5 mEq/L for each 1 g/dL decrease in albumin below 4 g/dL.

Follow-Up & Special Considerations

- Excessive renal potassium loss: Urinary potassium is >20 mEq/d in the presence of hypokalemia:
  - In patients with excessive renal potassium loss and hypertension, plasma renin and aldosterone levels should be determined to differentiate adrenal from nonadrenal causes of hyperaldosteronism.
- If hypertension is absent and the patient is acidotic, renal tubular acidosis should be considered.
- If hypertension is absent and serum pH is normal to alkalotic, high urine chloride (>10 mEq/d [>10 mmol/d]) suggests hypokalemia secondary to diuretics or Bartter syndrome; low urine chloride (<10 mEq/d [<10 mmol/d]) suggests vomiting as a probable cause.
- ECG:
  - Hypokalemia increases the myocyte resting potential, which increases the refractory period; this can lead to arrhythmias.
  - Flattening or inversion of T waves
  - Increased prominence of U waves (small positive deflection after T wave, best seen in V2 and V3)
  - Depression of ST segment
  - Ventricular ectopia

Imaging

CT scan of adrenal glands if there is evidence of mineralocorticoid excess

Pathological Findings

In severe hypokalemia, necrosis of cardiac and skeletal muscle

DIFFERENTIAL DIAGNOSIS

- Spurious hypokalemia: Occurs when blood with high WBC count (>100,000/mm^3) is allowed to stand at room temperature (WBCs extract potassium from plasma)
- Thyrotoxicosis

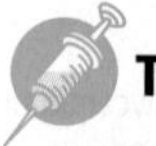

TREATMENT

MEDICATION

- Nonemergent conditions (serum potassium >2.5 mEq/L [>2.5 mmol/L], no cardiac manifestations):
  - Oral therapy preferred: 40–120 mEq/d (40–120 mmol/d) in divided doses usually is adequate
  - IV potassium should be given only when oral administration is not feasible (e.g., vomiting, postoperative state). Rate should not exceed 10 mEq/h, and concentration should not exceed 40 mEq/L. Up to 40 mEq in 100 mL over 1 hour can be given safely through a central venous line. The patient's cardiac rhythm should be closely monitored.
  - Potassium chloride is suitable for all forms of hypokalemia.

– Other potassium salts may be indicated if a coexisting disorder is present: Potassium bicarbonate or bicarbonate precursor (gluconate, acetate, or citrate) in metabolic acidosis or phosphate in phosphate deficiency
- Emergent situations (serum potassium <2.5 mEq/L [<2.5 mmol/L], arrhythmias), IV replacement:
  – Rate of administration should not exceed 20 mEq/h (20 mmol/h); maximum recommended concentration, 60 mEq/L (60 mmol/L) of saline for peripheral administration. Administration through central venous lines may allow for greater concentrations.
- Check serum magnesium and replace if needed; cannot adequately replace potassium in a setting of low magnesium.
- Precautions:
  – Any form of potassium replacement carries the risk of hyperkalemia.
  – Serum potassium should be checked more frequently in groups at higher risk: The elderly, diabetic patients, and patients with renal insufficiency.
  – Patients receiving digitalis and patients with diabetic ketoacidosis in whom intracellular shift in potassium is expected after insulin therapy is initiated must have more aggressive replacement.
- Significant possible interactions: Concomitant administration of potassium-sparing diuretics (spironolactone, triamterene, amiloride, ACE inhibitors) magnifies risk of hyperkalemia.

ADDITIONAL TREATMENT

General Measures

- For asymptomatic patients treated with oral replacement, outpatient follow-up is sufficient.
- Patients with cardiac manifestations require IV replacement with cardiac monitoring in an intensive care setting.

Geriatric Considerations

May need to correct magnesium depletion

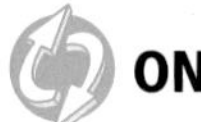

ONGOING CARE

FOLLOW-UP RECOMMENDATIONS

Patient Monitoring

- Patients receiving IV therapy should have cardiac monitoring and serum potassium level checked frequently (every 4–6 hours).
- Patients requiring potassium supplements should have serum potassium studied at intervals dictated by clinical judgment and patient compliance.

DIET

In patients with mild hypokalemia (potassium, 3–3.5 mEq/L [3–3.5 mmol/L]) not caused by GI losses, dietary supplementation may be sufficient; potassium-rich foods include oranges, bananas, cantaloupes, prunes, raisins, dried beans, dried apricots, and squash.

PATIENT EDUCATION

- Instructions for appropriate diet
- If potassium supplementation is necessary, stress the need for compliance.

PROGNOSIS

- Associated with higher morbidity and mortality because of cardiac arrhythmias
- Ease of correction of hypokalemia and need for prolonged treatment rest on the primary cause; if it can be eliminated (e.g., resolution of diarrhea, discontinuation of diuretics, removal of adrenal tumor), hypokalemia can be expected to resolve and no further treatment is indicated.

COMPLICATIONS

- Hyperkalemia can occur during the course of treatment (1).
- Increased risk of digoxin toxicity

REFERENCES

1. Crop MJ, Hoorn EJ, Lindemans J, et al. Hypokalaemia and subsequent hyperkalaemia in hospitalized patients. *Nephrol Dial Transplant*. 2007;22:3471–7.
2. Tran CT, Kjeldsen K, et al. Protection against β adrenoceptor agonist reduction of plasma potassium in severe but not in moderate hypokalemia. *Fundam Clin Pharmacol*. 2011;25: 452–61.
3. Ben Salem C, Hmouda H, Bouraoui K. Drug-induced hypokalaemia. *Curr Drug Saf*. 2009;4:55–61.
4. Ernst ME, Moser M, et al. Use of diuretics in patients with hypertension. *N Engl J Med*. 2009; 361:2153–64.
5. Cowtan T, et al. Thiazide diuretics. *N Engl J Med*. 2010;362:659; author reply 660.
6. Unwin RJ, Luft FC, Shirley DG, et al. Pathophysiology and management of hypokalemia: A clinical perspective. *Nat Rev Nephrol*. 2011;7:75–84.

ADDITIONAL READING

- Chan KE, Lazarus JM, Hakim RM, et al. Digoxin associates with mortality in ESRD. *J Am Soc Nephrol*. 2010;21:1550–9.
- Facchini M, Sala L, Malfatto G, et al. Low-K+ dependent QT prolongation and risk for ventricular arrhythmia in anorexia nervosa. *Int J Cardiol*. 2006; 106:170–6.
- Jones E. Hypokalemia. *N Engl J Med*. 2004;350: 1156.
- Osadchii OE, et al. Mechanisms of hypokalemia-induced ventricular arrhythmogenicity. *Fundam Clin Pharmacol*. 2010;24:547–59.
- Palmer BF, et al. A physiologic-based approach to the evaluation of a patient with hypokalemia. *Am J Kidney Dis*. 2010;56:1184–90.
- Zietse R, Zoutendijk R, Hoorn EJ. Fluid, electrolyte and acid-base disorders associated with antibiotic therapy. *Nat Rev Nephrol*. 2009;5:193–202.

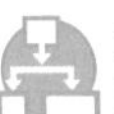

See Also (Topic, Algorithm, Electronic Media Element)

- Hyperkalemia
- Algorithm: Hypokalemia

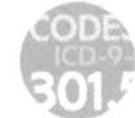

CODES

ICD9

276.8 Hypopotassemia

CLINICAL PEARLS

- In patients without heart disease, a low potassium level will rarely cause cardiac disturbances. In an otherwise healthy patient, gentle repletion using oral potassium or an increase in potassium-rich foods should be adequate.
- In patients with cardiac ischemia, heart failure, or left ventricular hypertrophy, even mild to moderate hypokalemia can cause arrhythmias. These patients should receive potassium repletion as well as cardiac monitoring.
- The safest way to safely prevent hypokalemia in diabetic and renal insufficiency patients is to ensure adequate dietary potassium intake with foods rich in potassium, including spinach, tomatoes, broccoli, squash, potatoes, bananas, cantaloupe, and oranges. Avoid potassium-sparing diuretics, if possible.
- Uncorrected hypomagnesemia can hinder the correction of hypokalemia. Check magnesium levels and replete as necessary (6).

HYPOKALEMIC PERIODIC PARALYSIS

Kinga K. Tomczak, MD, PhD
Rinat Jonas, MD

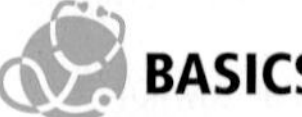

BASICS

DESCRIPTION
- Hypokalemic periodic paralysis (HPP) is a channelopathy characterized by episodic skeletal muscle weakness in the setting of a transient decrease in serum potassium (K) level. There are 2 forms:
  - Familial hypokalemic periodic paralysis (FHPP), classified as type 1 or type 2 (see "Etiology")
  - Hypokalemic periodic paralysis with thyrotoxicosis (thyrotoxic hypokalemic periodic paralysis [THPP])
- System(s) affected: Endocrine/Metabolic; Neuromuscular
- Synonym(s): Paroxysmal myoplegia

EPIDEMIOLOGY
- Predominant age: Onset of disease in late childhood or adolescence (FHPP), early adulthood (THPP). Onset >35 years of age is extremely rare.
- Age of onset depends on type of genetic mutation; earlier for type 1 FHPP by an average of 6 years (1)
- Predominant sex: FHPP, Male > Female (3:1); THPPs, Male > Female (20:1)
- THPP typically affects Asian males; rare in Caucasians (2,3)

Prevalence
- ~1/100,000 FHPP (estimated) (2)
- 4.3–13% of thyrotoxic Asian males develop THPP (3).

RISK FACTORS
- Male gender
- Age <35
- Family history (FHPP)
- Asian race (THPP)

Genetics
- FHPP: Autosomal dominant; incomplete penetrance in females (see "Etiology")
- THPP: Identifiable mutation in 1/3 of cases in 1 series, sporadic (4)

GENERAL PREVENTION
- See "Medication" (prevention of attacks) and "Diet."
- FHPP: Genetic counseling; 50% risk of transmitting abnormal gene to offspring and 50% chance of affected siblings
- National Institute of Neurological Disorders and Stroke (NINDS) Familial Periodic Paralyses Information Page: www.ninds.nih.gov/disorders/periodic_paralysis/periodic_paralysis.htm

PATHOPHYSIOLOGY
- Microelectrode studies show abnormal depolarization of skeletal muscle membrane (−50–60 mV instead of normal −90 mV) in presence of hypokalemia.
- Depolarization inactivates voltage-gated Na channels, preventing action potential propagation.
- New research suggests that "gating pore current" combined with a reduction in K_{ir} is sufficient to explain the pathologic muscle membrane depolarization observed in paralytic attacks of HPP (5,6).
- Cardiac and smooth muscles are not directly affected.
- Contractile apparatus is normal.
- Hypokalemia is caused by intracellular K shift; total body K is normal (i.e., hypokalemia not a result of K loss).

ETIOLOGY
- FHPP type 1 is caused by mutations in skeletal muscle voltage-gated *calcium channel genes*. FHPP type 2 is caused by mutations in *sodium channel* genes (1,7).
- The most common mutations identified in about 60–70% of patients with FHPP are in the calcium channel gene (CACNA1S); 10–15% are in the sodium channel gene (*SCN4A*).
- THPP is associated with a mutation in a voltage-gated *potassium channel* gene (*Kir2.6*) in 1/3 of cases (4).

COMMONLY ASSOCIATED CONDITIONS
THPP: Hyperthyroidism (2)

DIAGNOSIS

Signs and symptoms are mostly neuromuscular (paresis), but on rare occasions can also include cardiac (arrhythmias) and endocrine (hyperthyroidism in THPP only).

HISTORY
- Episodic attacks of focal or generalized muscle weakness lasting from a few hours to several days
- Typical attacks occur upon waking up from sleep or in the early morning.
- Attacks are usually provoked by strenuous exercise or high-carbohydrate meals, often several hours later or the next morning.
- Cold, stress, upper respiratory infections, high Na intake, alcohol, glucocorticoids, diuretics, insulin, or epinephrine may also exacerbate attacks
- Attacks are more common in summer and fall (THPP).
- Prodrome of stiff muscles, diffuse aching, and fatigue is common (3).
- Myalgias may be present.

PHYSICAL EXAM
- Limb muscle weakness: Lower extremity muscles are affected more than upper; proximal muscles are affected more than distal.
- Muscle weakness is usually symmetric.
- Muscles of the eyes, face, tongue, pharynx, larynx, diaphragm, and sphincters are rarely involved.
- Deep tendon reflexes may be hypoactive.
- Sensation is preserved.
- Strength between attacks is usually near normal.
- After years of attacks, persistent proximal weakness may be present.
- Patients with THPP may manifest signs of hyperthyroidism (especially systolic hypertension and tachycardia).

DIAGNOSTIC TESTS & INTERPRETATION
- Mild hypokalemia: ECG may show S-T depression, flattened T waves, or presence of U waves.
- Severe hypokalemia: ECG may show peaked P waves, prolonged P-R interval, or widened QRS.
- Electromyography (EMG) done during attack usually shows low postexercise compound motor action potential; pattern may help diagnose type 1 vs. type 2 FHPP.
- EMG is usually normal between attacks.
- Genetic testing (DNA sequencing) helps to differentiate type 1 from type 2 FHPP (Ca-channel vs. Na-channel mutations).

Lab
- Low serum potassium (as low as 1 mEq/L [1 mmol/L]) is a hallmark.
- Urine potassium is usually low as well.
- Serum phosphorous may be low.
- Serum creatine kinase level is normal or slightly increased.
- Acid–base balance is normal.
- Urine K/creatinine ratio is low (<2).
- T_3, T_4, free thyroid index are elevated, and thyroid-stimulating hormone (TSH) is decreased in THPP; may be only mildly abnormal (3).
- Hypercalciuria and hypophosphaturia are characteristic features of THPP.

Imaging
Thyroid scans using radioiodine (THPP only)

Diagnostic Procedures/Surgery
- During an acute attack, serum potassium level needs to be checked, both for diagnosis and to guide treatment.
- When high clinical suspicion but negative genetic testing, provocative testing can be done with 2 g/kg (50–100 g) PO glucose and/or 10 units SC regular or fast-acting insulin.
- Monitor closely for insulin-precipitated hypoglycemia.
- Patient should have cardiac monitoring during testing.
- Provocative testing with glucose and insulin can be risky. Safer alternative for diagnosis is monitoring for weakness and hypokalemia after exercise (30 minutes on a treadmill) or ACTH administration (80–100 IU IM).
- EMG may help confirm the diagnosis or discriminate between types of periodic paralysis.
- Negative tests do not exclude the diagnosis.

Pathological Findings
- Muscle biopsy may show atrophy, vacuoles, or tubular aggregates (vacuolar myopathy) (7)[C].
- Vacuolar myopathy is more likely in proximal muscles and is more common in FHPP than THPP.

DIFFERENTIAL DIAGNOSIS
- Andersen-Tawil syndrome (triad of periodic paralysis, ventricular dysthymias, and dysmorphic features)
- Hyperkalemic or normokalemic periodic paralysis (adynamia episodica)
- Secondary hypokalemia (laxative or diuretic use, diarrhea, vomiting, renal or adrenal disease, clay ingestion, barium poisoning)
- Myasthenia gravis
- Guillain-Barré syndrome
- Tick paralysis
- Akinetic epilepsy
- Cataplexy
- Drop attacks
- Episodic ataxia
- Hyperventilation
- Myotonia congenita
- Paramyotonia congenita
- Presyncope
- Sleep paralysis

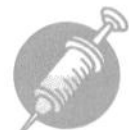

TREATMENT

Support by stabilizing airway, breathing, circulation (ABCs) if necessary. Hypokalemia must be confirmed prior to treatment.

MEDICATION
First Line
Acute attack:
- Goal is normalization of serum potassium
- Oral potassium chloride (KCl): 0.2–0.4 mEq/kg (up to 30 mEq), repeated q30min depending on response of ECG, serum K+, muscle strength (1)[C]
- In life-threatening situations can give 10–20 mEq/h IV KCL (not in dextrose solution); frequent ECG and potassium monitoring is necessary
- PO or IV propranolol (THPP only); PO dose is 3 mg/kg (2)[C]

Second Line
- Prevention of attacks in FHPP:
  - Acetazolamide: Usual dose 250 mg b.i.d. (type 1 FHPP or Ca-channel mutation only) (1,7)[B]. Acetazolamide can be cautiously tried in patients with type 2 FHPP or Na-channel mutation but it may precipitate attack (7)[C]
  - Dichlorphenamide: 50 mg b.i.d. is an alternative to acetazolamide
  - Spironolactone: 100 mg daily as a supplement to carbonic anhydrase inhibitor, or as an alternative
- Prevention of attacks in thyrotoxic hypokalemic periodic paralysis (2)[C]:
  - Antithyroid medications (propylthiouracil or methimazole), radioactive ablation of thyroid (2)[C]
  - Treat underlying thyrotoxicosis with nonselective β-adrenergic blocking agent (propranolol and others). Symptoms do not occur if patient is euthyroid.
- Contraindications:
  - Acetazolamide: Marked hepatic or renal dysfunction, hypersensitivity, adrenal failure, hyperchloremic acidosis, low serum Na, THPP
  - Propranolol: Cardiogenic shock, sinus bradycardia, second- or third-degree heart block, congestive heart failure, bronchial asthma, hypersensitivity
- Precautions and adverse reactions:
  - Infusion of IV or PO KCl must be monitored to avoid potentially fatal hyperkalemia (2)[B].
  - Rebound hyperkalemia may occur in patients who receive >90 mEq KCl in 24 hours and in patients with THPP who receive KCl and propranolol (2)[B].
  - Acetazolamide may cause fatigue, malaise, metallic taste, diarrhea, and may precipitate or worsen paralysis in patients with type 2 FHPP (2)[C].
  - Propranolol: Use with caution if impaired hepatic or renal function, Raynaud's, diabetes mellitus, second- or third-trimester pregnancy
- Possible drug interactions:
  - Acetazolamide: High-dose aspirin, amphetamines, methenamine
  - Propranolol: Phenothiazines, calcium channel blocker

ADDITIONAL TREATMENT
General Measures
- Mild hypokalemia or weakness: Outpatient K correction with close follow-up
- Severe hypokalemia or weakness: Inpatient K correction with cardiac monitoring

Issues for Referral
THPP: May need thyroid ablation

IN-PATIENT CONSIDERATIONS
Paralysis is often precipitated by surgery; therefore, close monitoring is warranted.

Initial Stabilization
May need respiratory support (rarely) and/or cardiac monitoring (usually done)

Admission Criteria
Severe weakness, hypokalemia with ECG findings, arrhythmias, respiratory compromise, need for IV KCl or propranolol

Discharge Criteria
Resolution of symptoms

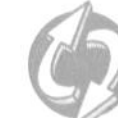

ONGOING CARE

FOLLOW-UP RECOMMENDATIONS
As tolerated, mild exercise may help.

Patient Monitoring
- Follow serum K and electrolytes (if on acetazolamide).
- Follow thyroid function tests (if on propranolol or antithyroid drugs).

DIET
Avoid high-carbohydrate, high-Na foods (7)[C].

PATIENT EDUCATION
- Strenuous exercise in combination with high-carbohydrate or high-Na meals may provoke attack.
- Attacks are also provoked by cold, stress, and alcohol.

PROGNOSIS
- Attack frequency usually lessens with age.
- Up to 2/3 of patients develop persistent proximal weakness (1)[C].
- Thyroid ablation resolves attacks (THPP only).

COMPLICATIONS
- Cardiac arrhythmias
- Respiratory collapse

REFERENCES

1. Venance SL, Cannon SC, Fialho D, et al. The primary periodic paralyses: Diagnosis, pathogenesis and treatment. *Brain*. 2006;129:8–17.
2. Lin SH. Thyrotoxic periodic paralysis. *Mayo Clin Proc*. 2005;80:99–105.
3. Kung AW. Clinical review; Thyrotoxic periodic paralysis: A diagnostic challenge. *J Clin Endocrinol Metab*. 2006;91(7):2490–5.
4. Ryan DP, da Silva MR, Soong TW, et al. Mutations in potassium channel Kir2.6 cause susceptibility to thyrotoxic hypokalemic periodic paralysis. *Cell*. 2010;140:88–98.
5. Francis DG, Rybalchenko V, Struyk A, et al. Leaky sodium channels from voltage sensor mutations in periodic paralysis, but not paramyotonia. *Neurology*. 2011;76(19):1635–41.
6. Tricarico D, Camerino DC. Recent advances in the pathogenesis and drug action in periodic paralyses and related channelopathies. *Front Pharmacol*. 2011;2:8.
7. Fontaine B, Fournier E, Sternberg D, et al. Hypokalemic periodic paralysis: A model for a clinical and research approach to a rare disorder. *Neurotherapeutics*. 2007;4:225–32.

ADDITIONAL READING

- Lin SH, Chu P, Cheng CJ, et al. Early diagnosis of thyrotoxic periodic paralysis: Spot urine calcium to phosphate ratio. *Crit Care Med*. 2006;34(12):2984–9.
- Sansone V, Meola G, Links TP, et al. Treatment for periodic paralysis. *Cochrane Database Syst Rev*. 2008:CD005045.

H

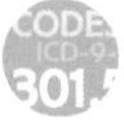

CODES

ICD9
359.3 Periodic paralysis

CLINICAL PEARLS

- Hypokalemic periodic paralysis should be suspected when a young, otherwise healthy male presents complaining of weakness on awakening, especially after exercising or eating a high-carbohydrate meal, and serum K is low, but he has no vomiting or diarrhea.
- Serum K, ECG, and TSH tests should be done immediately.
- The usual immediate therapy is to cautiously administer oral KCL 10–30 mEq, q30min, with cardiac monitoring and frequent serum K. If TSH is low, add propranolol, 3 mg/kg.

HYPONATREMIA

Ruben Peralta, MD, FACS
Rahma Salim, MD

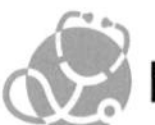

BASICS

DESCRIPTION

- Hyponatremia is a plasma sodium concentration of <135 mEq/L.
- System(s) affected: Endocrine/Metabolic

EPIDEMIOLOGY

Incidence

- Most common electrolyte disorder seen in the general hospital population (1).
- Predominant age: All ages
- Predominant sex: Male = Female

Prevalence

2.5% of hospitalized patients (1)

RISK FACTORS

Genetics

- Polymorphisms have been demonstrated.
- Mutations have been associated with nephrogenic syndrome of inappropriate antidiuresis (NSIAD).

GENERAL PREVENTION

Depends on underlying condition

PATHOPHYSIOLOGY

- Hypovolemic hyponatremia: Decrease in total body water and greater decrease in total body sodium; decreased extracellular fluid volume; orthostatic hypotension and other changes consistent with hypovolemia are present
- Euvolemic hyponatremia: Increase in total body water with normal total body sodium; extracellular fluid volume is minimally to moderately increased but with no edema
- Hypervolemic hyponatremia: Increase in total body sodium and greater increase in total body water; extracellular fluid increased markedly; edema present.
- Redistributive hyponatremia: Shift of water from intracellular compartment to extracellular compartment with resulting dilution of sodium; total body water and total body sodium unchanged; occurs with hyperglycemia
- Pseudohyponatremia: Dilution of aqueous phase by excessive proteins, glucose, or lipids; total body water and total body sodium unchanged; occurs in hypertriglyceridemia or multiple myeloma
- Low sodium creates an osmotic gradient between plasma and cells, and fluid shifts into cells, causing edema and increased intracranial pressure.

ETIOLOGY

- Hypovolemic hyponatremia: Extrarenal loss of sodium (<30 mmol/L in urine):
  - GI loss: Vomiting, diarrhea
  - Third spacing: Peritonitis, pancreatitis, burns, rhabdomyolysis
  - Skin loss: Burns, sweating, cystic fibrosis
  - Heat-related illnesses
- Hypovolemic hyponatremia: Renal loss of sodium (>30 mmol/L in urine):
  - Cerebral salt wasting syndrome
  - Adrenal pathology (e.g., Addison disease, hemorrhage, tuberculosis)
  - Diuretics
  - Osmotic diuresis
- Euvolemic hyponatremia (>30 mmol/L in urine):
  - Hypothyroidism
  - Hypopituitarism or other cause of glucocorticoid deficiency
  - Medications (e.g., carbamazepine, clofibrate, cyclosporine, levetiracetam, opiates, oxcarbazepine, phenothiazines, tricyclic antidepressants, vincristine) (2).
  - Primary polydipsia
  - Syndrome of inappropriate antidiuretic hormone secretion (SIADH)
  - Iatrogenic (e.g., excess hypotonic IV fluids)
- Hypervolemic hyponatremia (<30 mEq/L in urine, except chronic renal failure):
  - Nephrotic syndrome
  - Cirrhosis
  - Congestive heart failure (CHF)
  - Chronic renal failure
- Redistributive hyponatremia:
  - Hyperglycemia
  - Mannitol infusion
  - Hypertriglyceridemia
- Multiple myeloma

COMMONLY ASSOCIATED CONDITIONS

- Hypothyroidism
- Hypopituitarism
- Adrenocortical hormone deficiency
- HIV patients
- SIADH associated with cancers, pneumonia, tuberculosis, encephalitis, meningitis, head trauma, cerebrovascular accident, HIV infection (3).
- Acute neurological patients, brain injury
- Marathon runners in hot environments

DIAGNOSIS

- Symptoms related to the rate of fall in serum sodium and the degree of hyponatremia (3)
- Mild (130–135 mEq/L): Usually asymptomatic
- Moderate (120–130 mEq/L): Nausea, vomiting, malaise
- Severe: (115–120 mEq/L): Headache, lethargy, restlessness, disorientation
- Severe/rapid decreases can cause seizure, coma, and respiratory arrest and may be fatal.
- Other signs and symptoms: Weakness, muscle cramps, anorexia, hiccups, depressed deep tendon reflexes, hypothermia, positive Babinski responses, cranial nerve palsies, orthostatic hypotension

PHYSICAL EXAM

- Volume status: Skin turgor, jugular venous pressure, heart rate, orthostatic BP
- Exam for underlying illness: Signs of CHF, cirrhosis, hypothyroidism

DIAGNOSTIC TESTS & INTERPRETATION

Lab

Initial lab tests

- Comprehensive metabolic profile (BUN, creatinine, glucose, electrolytes, liver function studies, etc.)
- Thyroid-stimulating hormone (TSH)
- Lipid panel
- Serum osmolality
- Urine sodium and osmolality

Follow-Up & Special Considerations

- Serum sodium <135 mmol/L
- Plasma osmolality
- Urine sodium and osmolality
- Hypovolemic hyponatremia:
  - Plasma osmolality low
  - BUN: creatinine ratio >20:1
  - Urine sodium >20 mEq/L (>20 mmol/L): Renal loss
  - Urine sodium <10 mEq/L (<10 mmol/L): Extrarenal loss
  - Serum potassium >5 mEq/L (>5 mmol/L): Consider mineralocorticoid deficiency.
- Euvolemic hyponatremia:
  - Plasma osmolality low
  - BUN: creatinine ratio <20:1
  - Urine sodium >20 mEq/L (>20 mmol/L)
  - TSH test to rule out hypothyroidism
  - 1-hour cosyntropin-stimulation test to rule out adrenal insufficiency
- Hypervolemic hyponatremia:
  - Plasma osmolality low
  - Urine sodium <10 mEq/L (<10 mmol/L) in nephrotic syndrome, CHF, cirrhosis
  - Urine sodium >20 mEq/L (>20 mmol/L) in acute and chronic renal failure
- Redistributive hyponatremia:
  - Plasma osmolality normal or high
  - Glucose or mannitol levels elevated
- Pseudohyponatremia:
  - Plasma osmolality normal
  - Triglyceride, glucose, or protein levels elevated

Imaging

- CT scan of head if pituitary problem suspected or if SIADH from CNS problem suspected
- Chest x-ray to rule out pulmonary pathology if SIADH diagnosed

DIFFERENTIAL DIAGNOSIS

See "Etiology."

TREATMENT

MEDICATION

- Treatment tailored to clinical situation: Degree and rate of hyponatremia and whether or not the patient is symptomatic; some general principles apply (3)
- Formula to determine correction at: www.mdcalc.com/sodium-correction-rate-inhyponatremia and www.medcalc.com/sodium.html
- Asymptomatic, euvolemic patients can be treated with fluid restriction; the underlying cause also must be addressed.
- For severely hyponatremic/symptomatic patients, it is generally considered safe to increase the serum sodium by 0.6–2 mEq/L each hour, not to exceed 8 mEq/24 h.
- Treatment of underlying condition: Heart failure, cirrhosis, etc.

- In patients with euvolemic or hypervolemic hyponatremia, consider the use of new FDA-approved aquaretics (vaptans), such as tolvaptan, an oral vasopressin V_2-receptor antagonist, effective in increasing serum sodium concentrations (4).
- Rapid correction of severe symptomatic hyponatremia has been associated with central pontine myelinolysis, a neurologic disorder that induces loss of myelin and supportive structures in pons and occasionally in other areas of the brain. This results in irreversible injury. Symptoms are apparent 2–6 days after injury and include seizure, coma, spastic paraparesis, dysarthria, and dysphagia.
- Chronic hyponatremia owing to SIADH: Demeclocycline (inhibits ADH action at the collecting duct) if fluid restriction alone is not effective:
  - Contraindication: Can cause nephrotoxicity in patients with liver disease
  - In doses of 600–1,200 mg/d, the drug produces a nephrogenic diabetes insipidus.
  - Significant possible interactions: Oral anticoagulants, oral contraceptives, penicillin

ALERT

Caution: If severe, consider hypertonic saline (3% sodium chloride) with central line access; consult with a specialist before undertaking this treatment (5).

ADDITIONAL TREATMENT

General Measures

- Inpatient treatment is mandatory if acute hyponatremia or symptomatic; acute hyponatremia (developing over <48 hours) carries the risk of cerebral edema.
- Inpatient treatment is advised if asymptomatic and serum sodium <125 mEq/dL.
- Assess all medications patient is taking.
- Institute seizure precautions.

IN-PATIENT CONSIDERATIONS

Admission Criteria

- Admission is mandatory if the patient has acute hyponatremia or is symptomatic; acute hyponatremia (developing over <48 hours) carries the risk of cerebral edema.
- Admission is advised if patient is asymptomatic and has a serum sodium <125 mEq/dL.

ONGOING CARE

DIET

- Euvolemic hyponatremia: Restrict water to 1 L/d.
- Hypervolemic hyponatremia: Water and sodium restriction

PROGNOSIS

- In hospitalized patients, hyponatremia is associated with an elevated risk of adverse clinical outcomes and higher mortality (6).
- Recently, in community-dwelling, middle-aged and elderly adults, mild hyponatremia has been shown to be an independent predictor of death.
- Associated with poor prognosis in patients with acute pulmonary embolism
- Associated with poor prognosis in patients with liver cirrhosis and those waiting for liver transplant; it is associated with significant postoperative risk and short-term graft lost (6).

COMPLICATIONS

- Occult tumor may present with SIADH.
- Hypervolemia if saline used
- Osmotic demyelination (central pontine and extrapontine irreversible myelinolysis (5).
- Hyponatremia is the cause in 30% new-onset seizures in intensive care settings.
- Chronic hyponatremia is associated with increased odds of osteoporosis.

REFERENCES

1. Upadhyay A, Jaber BL, Madias NE. Epidemiology of hyponatremia. *Semin Nephrol*. 2009;29:227–38.
2. Meulendijks D, Mannesse CK, Jansen PA, et al. Antipsychotic-induced hyponatraemia: A systematic review of the published evidence. *Drug Saf*. 2010; 33:101–14.
3. Ellison DH, Berl T. Clinical practice. The syndrome of inappropriate antidiuresis. *N Engl J Med*. 2007;356: 2064–72.
4. Rozen-Zvi B, Yahav D, Gheorghiade M, et al. Vasopressin receptor antagonists for the treatment of hyponatremia: Systematic review and meta-analysis. *Am J Kidney Dis*. 2010;56:325–37.
5. Esposito P, Piotti G, Bianzina S, et al. The syndrome of inappropriate antidiuresis: Pathophysiology, clinical management and new therapeutic options. *Nephron. Clinical practice*. 2011;119:c62–c73.
6. Cárdenas A, Ginès P. Predicting mortality in cirrhosis–serum sodium helps. *N Engl J Med*. 2008;359:1060–2.

ADDITIONAL READING

- Callahan MA, Do HT, Caplan DW, et al. Economic impact of hyponatremia in hospitalized patients: A retrospective cohort study. *Postgrad Med*. 2009; 121:186–91.
- Cowtan T, et al. Thiazide diuretics. *N Engl J Med*. 2010;362:659–60.
- Ernst ME, Moser M, et al. Use of diuretics in patients with hypertension. *N Engl J Med*. 2009;361: 2153–64.
- Lim YJ, Park EK, Koh HC, et al. Syndrome of inappropriate secretion of antidiuretic hormone as a leading cause of hyponatremia in children who underwent chemotherapy or stem cell transplantation. *Pediatr Blood Cancer*. 2010;54: 734–7.

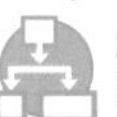

See Also (Topic, Algorithm, Electronic Media Element)

Algorithm: Hyponatremia

CODES

ICD9

276.1 Hyposmolality and/or hyponatremia

CLINICAL PEARLS

- Alcohol-dependent individuals with vitamin deficiencies, elderly women taking thiazide diuretics, and people with hypokalemia or burns are at increased risk of central pontine myelinolysis. A longer duration of hyponatremia is also a risk factor.
- The elderly have lower total body water, a decreased thirst mechanism, and decreased urinary concentrating ability; their kidneys are less responsive to ADH, and they show decreased renal mass, renal blood flow, and glomerular filtration rate.
- Bronchogenic carcinoma, pancreas, duodenal, prostate, thymoma, lymphoma, and mesothelioma are neoplastic diseases associated with SIADH.
- 3,4-Methylenedioxymethamphetamine (ecstasy) is an illicit drug that causes hyponatremia. The best approach is discontinuation of the drug.
- Mathematical formulas have been developed (Adrogue and Madias) for safe correction of hyponatremia and are available online (www.medcalc.com/sodium.html).
- Hyponatremia is seen frequently in patients with traumatic brain injury.
- For mild to moderate hyponatremia use isotonic saline solution (0.9%). For moderate to severe hyponatremia consider specialist consultation for use of hypertonic saline (3%) via central line access at a rate of 1–2 mL/kg body weight/h, increasing serum sodium levels by 0.5 mmol/L/h, and monitoring frequently the plasma sodium level (every 2–4 hours).
- In patients with severe hyponatremia (euvolemic and hypervolemic state), who do not respond to the above-mentioned approach, consider the use of newly FDA-approved aquaretics (vaptans), such as tolvaptan, an oral vasopressin V_2-receptor antagonist, or conivaptan for IV treatment of moderate to severe euvolemic and hypervolemic hyponatremia.

H

HYPOPARATHYROIDISM

Felix B. Chang, MD

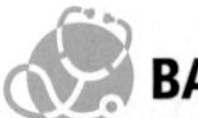

BASICS

DESCRIPTION

- Deficient secretion of parathyroid hormone. Often asymptomatic.
- Acute hypoparathyroidism with associated hypocalcemia results in tetany, with muscle cramps, carpopedal spasm, irritability, altered mental status, convulsion, stridor and tingling of the circumoral area, hands and feet
- Chronic: Lethargy, personality changes, anxiety, blurring of vision, parkinsonism, mental retardation
- Acquired hypoparathyroidism:
  - Surgical: Removal or damage to parathyroid glands or their blood supply. Thyroid, parathyroid or radical neck surgery for head and neck cancers.
  - Autoimmune: Isolated or combined with other endocrine deficiencies in polyglandular autoimmunity (PGA)
  - Deposition of heavy metals in gland: Copper (Wilson disease) or iron, radiation-induced destruction, and metastatic infiltration.
  - Functional hypoparathyroidism: Associated with hypomagnesemia. Hypermagnesemia.
- Congenital:
  - Calcium-sensing receptors (CaSR) abnormalities. Hypocalcemia with hypercalciuria.
  - HDR or Barakat syndrome: Deafness, renal dysplasia
  - Familial: Mutations of the TBCE gene. Abnormal PTH secretions.
- System(s) affected: Endocrine/Metabolic, Musculoskeletal, Nervous

Pediatric Considerations

- May occur in premature infants. Neonates born to hypercalcemic mothers may experience suppression of developing parathyroid glands. Congenital absence of parathyroids
- May appear later in childhood as autoimmune or APS-1

Geriatric Considerations

Hypocalcemia is fairly common in the elderly; however, it is rarely secondary to hypoparathyroidism.

Pregnancy Considerations

Use of magnesium as a tocolytic may induce functional hypoparathyroidism.

EPIDEMIOLOGY

Thyroid and parathyroid disease conditions resulting in surgical intervention are more common in women. Affects individuals of all ages.

Incidence

Rare, but most common cause of hypocalcemia. Most common after surgical procedure of the anterior neck. Transient hypoparathyroidism occurs in up to 20% of patients after surgery for thyroid cancer and permanent hypoparathyroidism occurs in 0.8–3% of patients after total thyroidectomy.

Prevalence

Wide variation. ADHH: 1 in 70,000 typically in infancy with hypocalcemic seizures.

RISK FACTORS

Neck surgery, especially thyroid, neck trauma, head and neck malignancies, family history of hypocalcemia, autoimmune polyglandular deficiency syndromes

Genetics

- Genetic defects may result in X-linked or in autosomal-recessive hypoparathyroidism due to abnormal parathyroid gland development. Associated with mutations in the transcription factor glial-cell missing B (BCMB).
- Mutations in transcription factors or regulators of parathyroid gland development:
  - Hypoparathyroidism may present as a component of a larger genetic syndrome (APS-1 or DiGeorge syndrome) or in isolation (X-linked hypoparathyroidism)
  - May be autosomal dominant (DiGeorge), autosomal recessive (APS-1), or X-linked recessive (X-linked hypoparathyroidism)
  - Congenital syndromes
    - 22q11.2 deletion syndrome, familial hypomagnesemia, hypoparathyroidism with lymphedema (1)
    - Hypoparathyroidism with sensorineural deafness
  - Autosomal dominant hypocalcemia with hypercalciuria (ADHH): Mutations gain-of-function of the CaSR gene suppressing the parathyroid gland, without elevation of the PTH.
  - PGA type 1: Childhood: Candidiasis, hypoparathyroidism, or Addison disease (2 criteria). Cataracts, uveitis, alopecia, vitiligo, or autoimmune thyroid disease. Fat malabsorption 20% and may present with weight loss, diarrhea, or malabsorption of vitamin D.

GENERAL PREVENTION

Intraoperative identification and preservation of parathyroid tissue

PATHOPHYSIOLOGY

- PTH is involved in the control of serum ionized calcium levels:
  - Mobilizes calcium and phosphorus from bone stores
  - Stimulates formation of 1,25-dihydroxy-vitamin D
  - Stimulates reabsorption of calcium in the distal nephron and phosphate excretion
- Loss of PTH action results in hypocalcemia, hyperphosphatemia, and hypercalciuria
- Magnesium is crucial for PTH secretion and activation of the PTH receptor; hypo- or hypermagnesemia may result in functional hypoparathyroidism.

ETIOLOGY

- Postsurgical: Transient, intermittent or permanent irradiation. Most common cause is surgical removal (any anterior neck procedure).
- Autoimmune: Genetic gain-of-function mutation in calcium-sensing receptor
- Infiltrative: Metastatic carcinoma, hemochromatosis, Wilson's disease, granulomas
- Hypo- (alcoholics) or hypermagnesemia: Chronic iron overloads

COMMONLY ASSOCIATED CONDITIONS

- DiGeorge syndrome
- Polyglandular autoimmune syndrome type I (APS-1)
- Multiple endocrine deficiency autoimmune candidiasis (MEDAC) syndrome
- Juvenile familial endocrinopathy
- Hypoparathyroidism
- Addison disease
- Moniliasis (HAM) syndrome a polyglandular deficiency syndrome, possibly genetic characterized by hypoparathyroidism
- Addison disease and chronic yeast infections

DIAGNOSIS

HISTORY

- Asymptomatic (2)
- Fatigue, circumoral or distal extremity paresthesias, muscle cramps, neuropsychiatric symptoms, seizures, previous neck trauma or surgery, head and neck irradiation, family history of hypocalcemia, presence of other autoimmune endocrinopathies

PHYSICAL EXAM

- Surgical scar on neck
- Chvostek sign: Positive sign is ipsilateral twitching of the upper lip upon tapping the facial nerve on the cheek.
- Trousseau sign: Positive sign is painful carpal spasm after 3-minute occlusion of brachial artery with BP cuff. BP cuff inflated to greater than systolic BP for 3 minutes leads to carpal spasm (flexion of metacarpophalangeal [MCP] joints, extension of interphalangeal [IP] joints, adduction of fingers and thumb)
- Tetany, laryngeo- or bronchospasm, cataracts, cardiac arrhythmias or failure. Dry hair, brittle nails

DIAGNOSTIC TESTS & INTERPRETATION

Lab

Initial lab tests

- Calcium: Total and ionized (low) (correct serum calcium level for albumin):
  - Corrected serum calcium = Total serum calcium + 0.8 (4 – serum albumin)
- Phosphorus (high)
- Intact PTH (low or inappropriately normal)
- Magnesium (low or high may cause hypoparathyroidism; may also be normal)
- BUN, creatinine, 25 OH vitamin D level (especially in elderly)
- Urinary calcium (normal or high)
- Calcium should be monitor after thyroid or parathyroid surgery

Follow-Up & Special Considerations

- EKG: Prolongation of ST and QTc intervals nonspecific repolarization changes dysrhythmias
- Urine calcium/creatinine ratio (normal 0.1–0.2) may be low before treatment but should be monitored to prevent stones due to hypercalciuria.
- Gene sequencing: Evaluation of other hormone levels may be required to diagnose APS-1.
- Hungry bone syndrome (transient hypoparathyroidism after parathyroid surgery):
  - Hypocalcemia due to hungry bone syndrome may persist despite recovery of PTH secretion from the remaining normal glands. Thus, serum PTH concentrations may be low, normal, or even elevated
- Infiltrative: Osteoblastic metastasis of prostate, breast or lung cancer

- Metabolic/nutritional: Renal failure neonatal hypocalcemia hypoalbuminemia malabsorption calcium (Ca++) chelators hypomagnesemia
- Familial hypocalcemia acute hyperphosphatemia (rare) vitamin D deficiency

Imaging

Radiographs may show absent tooth roots, calcification of cerebellum, choroid plexus, or cerebral basal ganglia. X-ray painful bones to rule out pathologic fractures.

Pathological Findings

Parathyroid gland parenchymal tissue completely or almost completely replaced by fat

DIFFERENTIAL DIAGNOSIS

- Vitamin D deficiency/resistance
- Pseudohypoparathyroidism, which presents in childhood, refers to a group of heterogeneous disorders defined by target organ (kidney and bone) unresponsiveness to PTH. It is characterized by hypocalcemia, hyperphosphatemia, and, in contrast to hypoparathyroidism, elevated rather than reduced PTH concentrations:
  - Hypoalbuminemia, renal failure, malabsorption, familial hypocalcemia, hypomagnesemia

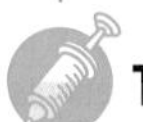

TREATMENT

MEDICATION

First Line

- Hypoparathyroid tetany, severe symptoms (tetany, seizures, cardiac failure, laryngospasm, bronchospasm):
  - IV calcium gluconate: 1 or 2 g, each infused over a period of 10 minutes. Central venous catheter preferred because calcium-containing solutions can irritate surrounding tissues. Follow with infusion 10 g calcium gluconate in 1 L 5% dextrose water at a rate of 1–3 mg calcium gluconate/kg of body weight/hr
- Maintenance:
  - Oral calcium: Calcium salts: 1–3 g PO daily.
  - Calcitriol: (Vitamin D 1,25-dihydroxycholecalciferol): 0.25 mcg daily. Doses 0.5–2 mcg/d are usually required.
- Hypomagnesemia: Acutely: 1–2 g IV q6h. Long-term magnesium oxide tablets (600 mg), once or twice per day.

Second Line

Cholecalciferol 10,000–50,000 units duration of action 4–8 weeks

ADDITIONAL TREATMENT

General Measures

- Monitor EKG during calcium repletion
- Maintenance therapy: May require lifelong treatment with calcium and calcitriol:
  - Maintain serum calcium in low normal range: 8–8.5 mg/dL (2–2.12 mmol/L)
- If hypercalcemia occurs, hold therapy until calcium returns to normal. Treat magnesium deficiency if present.
- Phosphate binders required if high calcium-phosphate product
- Thiazide diuretics combined with a low-salt diet may be used to prevent hypercalciuria, nephrocalcinosis, and nephrolithiasis.
- Oral calcium administration and vitamin D supplementation postthyroidectomy may reduce the risk for symptomatic hypocalcemia after surgery.

Issues for Referral

Endocrinologist, Nephrologist, Ophthalmologist

Additional Therapies

Parathyroid hormone 1–34 (SC) (3)[C],(4):

- May be as effective as calcitriol for maintaining growth and serum calcium levels in children with chronic hypoparathyroidism. Unproven method of treatment at this juncture; further study required

SURGERY/OTHER PROCEDURES

Transplantation of cryopreserved parathyroid tissue removed during prior surgery: Restore normocalcemia in 23% of cases

IN-PATIENT CONSIDERATIONS

Admission Criteria

Laryngospasm, seizures, tetany, QT prolongation

Discharge Criteria

Resolution of hypocalcemic symptoms, patient educated on hypoparathyroidism and treatment. Schedule follow-up.

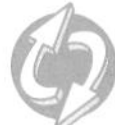

ONGOING CARE

FOLLOW-UP RECOMMENDATIONS

Patient Monitoring

- Goal of treatment is to reach a total corrected serum calcium level in low normal range (8–8.5 mg/dL or 2–2.12 mmol/L), 24-hour urine calcium below 300 mg and calcium-phosphate product below 55.
- Outpatient measurement of serum calcium, phosphorus, and creatinine weekly to monthly during initial management. Calcium, phosphate, and creatinine twice yearly when stable.
- Measurement of urine calcium and creatinine twice yearly
- Annual slit-lamp and ophthalmologic evaluation are recommended. Dexa scan.

DIET

Low phosphate diet in patients with hyperphosphatemia

PATIENT EDUCATION

- Provide careful and detailed instructions about maintenance therapy.
- Explain importance of periodic blood chemistry evaluations. Instruct patient to watch for signs and symptoms of over- and undertreatment.
- Educate patient to avoid hyperventilation (alkalosis increases calcium binding to albumin)

PROGNOSIS

Hypoparathyroidism following neck surgery is often transient. Length of required treatment may vary depending on origin. Symptoms and serum calcium can be well controlled with treatment.

COMPLICATIONS

- Neuromuscular symptoms: Paresthesias (circumoral, fingers, toes), hypercalciuria, nephrocalcinosis, nephrolithiasis; cataracts, basal ganglia calcifications with Parkinsonian symptoms
- If condition starts early in childhood: Stunting of growth, malformation of teeth (enamel defects), mental retardation. Atrophy, brittleness, and ridging of nails.
- Tetanus, seizures, pseudotumor cerebri has been described. Heart failure.

REFERENCES

1. Veerapandiyan A, Abdul-Rahman OA, Adam MP, et al. Chromosome 22q11.2 deletion syndrome in African-American patients: A diagnostic challenge. *Am J Med Genet A*. 2011;155A(9):2186–95.
2. Bilezikian J, Khan A, Potts J, et al. Hypoparathyroidism in the adult: Epidemiology, diagnosis, pathophysiology, target organ involvement, treatment, and challenges for future research. *J Bone Miner Res*. 2011;26(10):2317–37.
3. Winer KK, Sinaii N, Reynolds J, et al. Long-term treatment of 12 children with chronic hypoparathyroidism: A randomized trial comparing synthetic human parathyroid hormone 1–34 versus calcitriol and calcium. *J Clin Endocrinol Metabol*. 2010;95(6):2680–8.
4. Sikjaer T, Rejnmark L, Rolighed L, et al. The effect of adding PTH (1-84) to conventional treatment of hypoparathyroidism - A randomized, placebo controlled study. *J Bone Miner Res*. 2011;26(10): 2358–70.

ADDITIONAL READING

Krysiak R, Kobielusz-Gembala I, Okopien B, et al. Hypoparathyroidism in pregnancy. *Gynecol Endocrinol*. 2011;27:1–4.

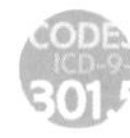

CODES

ICD9

252.1 Hypoparathyroidism

CLINICAL PEARLS

- Often asymptomatic, unless significant hypocalcemia is present
- Hypocalcemia, hyperphosphatemia and low parathyroid hormone levels are consistent with hypoparathyroidism
- Any dental changes, cataracts, and brain calcifications are permanent.
- Phenothiazine drugs should be administered with caution, since they may precipitate extrapyramidal symptoms in hypocalcemic patients. Furosemide should be avoided, since it may worsen hypocalcemia.

HYPOTENSION, ORTHOSTATIC

Martin A. Espinosa Ginic, MD
Bryan K. Moffett, MD

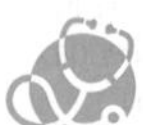

BASICS

Postural or orthostatic hypotension (OH) represents the failure of cardiovascular reflexes to maintain adequate BP on standing from a supine or sitting position.

DESCRIPTION

- OH is defined as a sustained and persistent drop in systolic BP (SBP) ≥20 mm Hg or diastolic BP (DBP) ≥10 mm Hg within 3 minutes of achieving a standing position, or head-up tilt to at least 60° on tilt table. Delayed OH can infrequently occur with a slow decline in SBP beyond 3 minutes of standing, and may be revealed by extending the period of orthostatic stress (1).
- Characteristic symptoms of OH are recurrent dizziness, lightheadedness, presyncope or syncope with assumption of an upright posture, typically relieved by achieving a recumbent position, and can be incapacitating. In the elderly, OH may be asymptomatic or present with nonspecific complaints of weakness.

EPIDEMIOLOGY

Asymptomatic OH is far more common than symptomatic OH, and is an independent risk factor for mortality and cardiovascular disease. OH is also a manifestation of many underlying diseases and may be the initial sign of autonomic failure in many neurologic disorders. The prevalence increases with age, hypertension, diabetes, and use of antihypertensive medication (2).

Incidence

80,095 orthostatic-related hospitalizations occurred in the US in 2004; OH was the primary diagnosis in 35%.

Prevalence

- ~6% of middle-aged persons, and 18% of individuals ≥65 years of age
- More common in those living in long-term care facilities (45% vs. 6% living in the community) (2)
- In those with hypertension, 13.4–32.1% (2)

RISK FACTORS

- Elderly, particularly in long-term care facilities
- Multiple comorbidities including HTN, diabetes, neurodegenerative disorders, and neuropathy
- Polypharmacy

GENERAL PREVENTION

- Avoid polypharmacy and monitor drug interactions.
- Adequate fluid balance

PATHOPHYSIOLOGY

- During standing, 500–1,000 mL of blood pools in the lower extremities and the splanchnic vasculature. This reduces cardiac preload but is opposed by an increase in sympathetic tone and vasopressin release that maintains cerebral perfusion pressure, by increasing peripheral vascular resistance. Impairment of these compensatory mechanisms by autonomic dysfunction, or nonneurogenic causes such as medications, hypovolemia, or cardiac pump failure leads to an inability to maintain effective cerebral perfusion pressure. Autonomic dysfunction also impairs norepinephrine-mediated proximal tubule renal sodium reabsorption, which contributes to OH through urinary sodium wasting and a consequent reduction in circulating plasma volume. In older people vascular stiffening and decreased baroreceptor sensitivity predispose to OH.
- Supine hypertension (SH), due to baroreflex dysfunction and fluid redistribution upon assuming a horizontal position, is common in patients with OH. Increased renal perfusion pressure in the recumbent position also leads to nocturnal natriuresis, which decreases circulating intravascular volume, worsening orthostatic tolerance in the morning.

ETIOLOGY

- Medications (iatrogenic causes):
  - Anticholinergics: Benztropine, orphenadrine, oxybutynin, trihexyphenidyl
  - Antidepressants: TCA, MAOIs, SSRIs, and SNRIs
  - Antihypertensives: Beta-blockers, calcium channel blockers, ACE-inhibitors, clonidine, vasodilators (alpha-blockers, hydralazine, nitrates)
  - Diuretics
  - Dopamine agonists: Levodopa, bromocriptine, ropinirole, pramipexole
  - Ethanol
  - Insulin (may exacerbate OH in the setting of diabetic neuropathy)
  - Narcotics/sedatives: Morphine, benzodiazepines, barbiturates, promethazine
  - Neuroleptics: Chlorpromazine, quetiapine
  - Neurotoxic drugs: Amiodarone, vincristine, cisplatin
- Neurogenic causes:
  - Idiopathic OH (1/3 of cases of OH)
  - Central autonomic nervous system diseases:
    - Familial dysautonomia (rare, childhood)
    - Lewy body dementia
    - Multisystem atrophy (uncommon)
    - Parkinson disease: 40% of patients with PD have OH.
    - Pure autonomic failure (rare)
  - Peripheral autonomic nervous system diseases:
    - Acute autonomic neuropathy and Guillain-Barré syndrome (acute onset, frequently preceded by viral syndrome)
    - Alcoholic polyneuropathy
    - Amyloidosis
    - Autoimmune autonomic ganglionopathy (rare)
    - Chronic renal failure: Uremic or beta-2 microglobulin neuropathy (dialysis)
    - Diabetes: Diabetic autonomic neuropathy (very common)
    - Exposure to neurotoxins
    - Hereditary sensory and autonomic neuropathies: Dopamine-beta-hydroxylase deficiency (rare)
    - HIV neuropathy
    - Paraneoplastic autonomic neuropathy: SCLC, NSCLC, GI neoplasias, prostate, breast, bladder, kidney, testicle, and ovary
    - Spinal cord pathologies: Trauma, myelitis, tumors, tabes dorsalis, multiple sclerosis, syringomyelia, infarction
    - Vitamin B_{12} deficiency
- Nonneurogenic causes:
  - Cardiac pump failure: Heart failure, arrhythmias, pericardial disease, severe aortic stenosis
  - Deconditioning
  - Intravascular volume depletion: Bleeding, diarrhea, diabetes insipidus, diuretics, poor oral intake, vomiting
  - Metabolic: Adrenal insufficiency, hypoaldosteronism, pheochromocytoma, carcinoid syndrome, hypokalemia (severe), hypothyroidism
  - Sepsis
  - Systemic mastocytosis
  - Venous pooling: Heat or vigorous exercise, postprandial splanchnic dilation, prolonged recumbency or standing

COMMONLY ASSOCIATED CONDITIONS

Diabetes mellitus with neuropathy, uncontrolled hypertension and antihypertensive treatment, Parkinson disease

DIAGNOSIS

Initial approach: Detailed history and physical examination with a focus on neurodegenerative disorders and neuropathy; thorough medication review; screening for reversible causes: 12-lead ECG, CBC, and BMP

HISTORY

- Postural symptoms: Dizziness, lightheadedness, palpitations, syncope or presyncope: Elderly patients may have vague complaints even before frank syncope: Generalized weakness, fatigue, nausea, difficulty with concentration or cognition, leg buckling, pure vertigo, visual blurring, headache or "coat-hanger" pattern neck-shoulder pain, orthostatic dyspnea, or angina.
- Aggravating factors: Warm environments, exertion, prolonged standing, ingestions of large or carbohydrate rich meals, alcohol intake (vasodilation)
- Volume depletion: Vomiting, diarrhea, poor PO intake, polyuria
- Cardiac pump failure: Orthopnea, edema, paroxysmal nocturnal dyspnea, angina
- Peripheral neuropathy: Numbness, pain, paresthesia, imbalance, or falls
- Associated diseases: Diabetes, Parkinson disease, dementia
- Autonomic symptoms: Altered sweating (hyper- or hypohydrosis), GI dysfunction (bloating, nausea, vomiting, constipation), impotence, bladder dysfunction, sicca symptoms
- Review all medications and herbal therapies.

PHYSICAL EXAM

- Measure BP while supine and standing: Patient should be supine for 5 minutes, then after standing, check the BP at 3 minutes. Use sitting measurements only if the patient is too dizzy or weak to stand. Use fall precautions: Do not check for OH in patients with supine SBP <90 mm Hg (shock) as it adds no useful information. Tachycardic response to standing may be a sign of hypovolemia or cardiac pump failure, while minimal or no change in heart rate may suggest a neurogenic cause. Orthostatic tachycardia without a significant drop in BP does not meet criteria for OH and may suggest postural orthostatic tachycardia syndrome (POTS).
- Cardiac exam: Jugular venous distention, pulse irregularity, edema, murmurs, S3
- Neurologic exam: Hypomimia, gait, tremor, cogwheel rigidity, motor strength, fine-touch, pain sensation, proprioception, Romberg maneuver, cerebellar signs, and myoclonus

DIAGNOSTIC TESTS & INTERPRETATION

Lab

Initial lab tests

- CBC: Anemia (hemorrhage) or leukocytosis (sepsis)
- BMP: Hypokalemia, alkalosis, and renal insufficiency suggesting volume depletion
- TSH

Follow-Up & Special Considerations

- If neuropathy is found on examination consider: Vitamin B_{12} levels, serum and urine protein electrophoresis (amyloidosis). Nerve conduction studies and electromyography: For suspected neuropathy.
- Adrenal insufficiency and pheochromocytoma evaluation is warranted in OH of uncertain cause: 8 a.m. cortisol level: If $<18\ \mu$g/dL, consider cosyntropin testing. 24-hour urinary or plasma fractionated metanephrines: Consider further testing depending on results.
- Antibodies to the neuronal nicotinic receptor (nAChR) in cases of suspected autoimmune autonomic ganglionopathy

Imaging

ECG: To rule out arrhythmias and detect structural heart disease. Echocardiogram: For abnormal ECG, new murmurs, or suspected heart failure. MRI: For suspected neurodegenerative disorders or spinal disease

Diagnostic Procedures/Surgery

- Tilt table testing: Indicated if orthostatic symptoms are persistent, significant, and characteristic despite a nondiagnostic clinical examination. Provocation with nitroglycerin or IV isoproterenol is not recommended, as it may cause false-positive results (3).
- Autonomic testing: Useful in cases where neurally mediated syncope vs. orthostatic syncope is unclear, and to diagnose subclinical cases. Includes HR and BP variability with deep inspiration and Valsalva maneuver, sudomotor evaluation, orthostatic vascular resistance, plasma norepinephrine response to orthostasis, and pharmacologic challenges (4,5).

DIFFERENTIAL DIAGNOSIS

Neurally mediated (reflex) syncope: Vasovagal syncope, situational syncope (cough, micturition, defecation, swallowing), carotid sinus hypersensitivity. Falls related to a neurologic disorder. Postprandial hypotension. Postural tachycardia syndrome (POTS). Shock (must have a normal lying BP before testing)

TREATMENT

- Abdominal binder or compression stockings (not TED hose), preferably waist high with 20 mm Hg of pressure (worn before rising) (3,4,6)[B]
- Perform gradual staged movements with postural changes: Arise slowly from supine to seated and rest before standing (3,4,6)[C]. Also, physical countermaneuvers (to increase vascular resistance and preload): Isometric contraction of leg muscles for 30 seconds at a time, repeated feet dorsiflexion, leg crossing and contraction, squatting, bending at the waist, leg elevation, and respiratory maneuvers like inspiration through pursed lips and inspiratory sniffing (3,4,6)[B]
- Moderate exercise (supine or sitting isotonic exercise if symptoms are severe): Improves orthostatic tolerance and reduces venous pooling (3,4,6)[B]
- Increase water and sodium intake: 2–2.5 L of fluid a day, and up to 10 g of sodium per day (if needed, salt tablets starting at 500 mg PO t.i.d. may be used). Encourage drinking water with meals and before exercise. Rapid ingestion of two 8-oz glasses of water (500 mL) over 3–4 minutes elicits a market pressor response lasting for up to 1 hour (3,4,6)[B].
- Elevate the head of the bed 20 degrees (4–6 inches) to reduce supine hypertension and nocturnal diuresis (3,4,6)[B].
- Avoid: Prolonged recumbency, increased intrathoracic pressure (straining, coughing), large meals especially if high in carbohydrates, and alcohol (3,4,6)[C]

MEDICATION

First identify and discontinue all potentially aggravating medications. Medication is indicated only when nonpharmacologic measures are insufficient to control symptoms. Goal of therapy is to improve functional capacity and quality of life without causing excessive supine hypertension, rather than to eliminate orthostatic drops in BP.

First Line

- Fludrocortisone: Synthetic mineralocorticoid that increases sodium and fluid retention and increases peripheral vascular resistance. Starting at 0.1 mg/d, titrate for symptoms every week up to 0.5 mg/d. Contraindicated in patients with HF and chronic renal insufficiency due to volume expansion (3,4,6)[B].
- Midodrine: Selective peripheral alpha-agonist that increases vascular resistance. Only drug currently FDA approved to treat OH. Start at 2.5 mg PO t.i.d. and titrate for symptoms up to 10 mg t.i.d. Avoid within 4 hours of bedtime to prevent worsening supine hypertension, and use with caution in patients with coronary artery disease (3,4,6)[A].

Second Line

- Pyridostigmine: Acetylcholinesterase inhibitor, increases sympathetic ganglionic neurotransmission. Dosage 30–60 mg PO t.i.d. (4,6)[B]
- Caffeine: Methylxanthine with pressor effect due to blockade of adenosine receptors. 100–250 mg PO t.i.d., as tablets or caffeinated beverages [B].
- Erythropoietin: Increases RBC mass. Consider only when significant anemia coexists. Dosage 25–75 U/kg SQ 3 times a week (maintenance dose may be lower). Iron studies and supplementation usually required (3,4)[B]
- Ephedrine: Mixed alpha and beta agonist. Dosage 25–50 mg PO t.i.d. (avoid within 4 hours before bedtime to prevent worsening supine hypertension) (3,4)[C]
- Pseudoephedrine: Mixed alpha and beta agonist. Dosage 30–60 mg PO t.i.d. (avoid within 4 hours before bedtime) (4)[C]
- Desmopressin: Vasopressin analogue. Dosage 5–40 μg/d nasal spray, or 100–800 μg/d PO (3,4)[C]
- L-dihydroxyphenylserine (Droxidopa): Prodrug that is converted to noradrenaline by dopadecarboxylase enzyme. Dosage 200–400 mg/d PO (3,5)[A]

ADDITIONAL TREATMENT

Consider bedtime nitrates or nifedipine to treat severe, sustained supine hypertension. May increase the risk of syncope and falls (4)[C]

Issues for Referral

Consider cardiology referral if there is significant heart disease or tilt table testing will be required. Consider neurology referral for confirmed or suspected primary neurologic pathologies.

ONGOING CARE

FOLLOW-UP RECOMMENDATIONS

Monitor for significant supine hypertension, fluid overload, electrolyte abnormalities, and heart failure in patients under medical treatment. In patients without an apparent cause of OH, follow-up is essential because OH alone may be the initial presentation of neurologic disorders.

PATIENT EDUCATION

Recognize symptoms and avoid aggravating factors. Educate on nonpharmacologic measures and goals of therapy.

COMPLICATIONS

Syncope, falls (hip fracture, head trauma), and rarely stroke

REFERENCES

1. Freeman R, et al. Consensus statement on the definition of orthostatic hypotension, neurally mediated syncope and the postural tachycardia syndrome. *Auton Neurosci*. 2011;161:46–8.
2. Benvenuto LJ, Krakoff LR, et al. Morbidity and mortality of orthostatic hypotension: Implications for management of cardiovascular disease. *Am J Hypertens*. 2011;24:135–44.
3. Lahrmann H, Cortelli P, Hilz M, et al. EFNS guidelines on the diagnosis and management of orthostatic hypotension. *Eur J Neurol*. 2006;13: 930–6.
4. Freeman R, et al. Clinical practice. Neurogenic orthostatic hypotension. *N Engl J Med*. 2008;358: 615–24.
5. Goldstein DS, Sharabi Y, et al. Neurogenic orthostatic hypotension: A pathophysiological approach. *Circulation*. 2009;119:139–46.
6. Figueroa JJ, Basford JR, Low PA, et al. Preventing and treating orthostatic hypotension: As easy as A, B, C. *Cleve Clin J Med*. 2010;77:298–306.

CODES

ICD9

458.0 Orthostatic hypotension

CLINICAL PEARLS

- OH is a clinical finding, not a disease. Treatment should be guided by symptoms rather than by absolute BP drop.
- Always check the medication list and volume status. Drug-related OH may be a sign of underlying autonomic dysfunction.
- Pharmacologic treatment is indicated only when nonpharmacologic measures are insufficient to control symptoms.

HYPOTHERMIA

Scott T. Henderson, MD

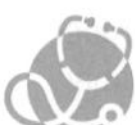

BASICS

DESCRIPTION

- A core temperature of <35°C (95°F)
- May take several hours to days to develop
- Patients with cold water immersion can appear to be dead but can still be resuscitated.
- System(s) affected: All body systems
- Synonym(s): Accidental hypothermia

EPIDEMIOLOGY

- Predominant age: Very young and the elderly
- Predominant sex: Male > Female

Geriatric Considerations

More common due to lower metabolic rate, impaired ability to maintain normal body temperature, and impaired ability to detect temperature changes

Prevalence

Estimates vary widely due to lack of pathologic evidence, and it is usually considered a secondary cause in diagnosing disorders.

RISK FACTORS

- Alcohol consumption
- Bronchopneumonia
- Cardiovascular disease
- Cold water immersion
- Dermal dysfunction (burns, erythrodermas)
- Drug intoxication
- Endocrinopathies (myxedema, severe hypoglycemia)
- Excessive fluid loss
- Hepatic failure
- Hypothalamic and CNS dysfunction
- Malnutrition
- Mental illness; Alzheimer disease
- Prolonged environmental exposure
- Renal failure
- Sepsis
- Trauma (especially head)
- Uremia

GENERAL PREVENTION

- Appropriate clothing with particular attention to head, feet, and hands
- For outdoor activities, carry survival bags with space blankets for use if stranded or injured.
- Avoid alcohol.
- Alertness to early symptoms and initiating preventive steps (e.g., drinking warm fluids)
- Identify medications that may predispose to hypothermia (e.g., neuroleptics, sedatives, hypnotics, tranquilizers).

ETIOLOGY

- Overwhelming environmental cold stress
- Decreased heat production
- Increased heat loss
- Impaired thermoregulation

COMMONLY ASSOCIATED CONDITIONS

- Addison disease
- CNS dysfunction
- Congestive heart failure
- Diabetes
- Hypopituitarism
- Hypothyroidism
- Ketoacidosis
- Pulmonary infection
- Sepsis
- Uremia

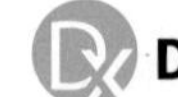

DIAGNOSIS

HISTORY

Presentation varies with the temperature of the patient at the time of presentation.

ALERT

History of prolonged exposure to cold may make the diagnosis obvious, but hypothermia may be overlooked, especially in comatose patients.

PHYSICAL EXAM

Exam findings vary with the temperature of the patient at the time of presentation:

- Mild (32–35°C):
  - Lethargy and mild confusion
  - Shivering
  - Tachypnea
  - Tachycardia
  - Loss of fine motor coordination
  - Increased BP
  - Peripheral vasoconstriction
- Moderate (28–32°C):
  - Delirium
  - Bradycardia
  - Hypotension
  - Hypoventilation
  - Cyanosis
  - Arrhythmias (prolonged PR interval; AV junctional rhythm; idioventricular rhythm; prolonged QT interval; altered T waves)
  - Semicoma and coma
  - Muscular rigidity
  - Generalized edema
  - Slowed reflexes
- Severe (<28°C):
  - Very cold skin
  - Rigidity
  - Apnea
  - Bradycardia
  - No pulse: Ventricular fibrillation or asystole
  - Areflexia
  - Unresponsive
  - Fixed pupils

ALERT

Use specially designed thermometers that can record low temperatures and measure core temperatures.

Pediatric Considerations

- Infants may present with bright red, cold skin and very low energy.
- A child's body temperature drops faster than an adult's when immersed in cold water.

DIAGNOSTIC TESTS & INTERPRETATION

Lab

Initial lab tests

- Arterial blood gases (corrected for temperature)
- CBC and platelet counts
- Serum electrolytes
- Urinalysis
- Coagulation studies
- Fibrinogen levels
- Blood culture
- BUN/creatinine
- Glucose
- Amylase
- Liver function studies
- Cardiac enzymes
- Calcium
- Magnesium
- Alcohol level

Follow-Up & Special Considerations

- Toxicology screen if mental status changes are more extreme than expected for temperature decrease
- Serum cortisol, if indicated
- Thyroid function tests, if indicated

Imaging

Initial approach

Cervical spine, chest, abdomen, if appropriate

Diagnostic Procedures/Surgery

EKG

Pathological Findings

- Moderate dilation of right heart
- Pulmonary edema

DIFFERENTIAL DIAGNOSIS

- Cerebrovascular accidents
- Intoxication
- Drug overdose
- Complications of diabetes, hypothyroidism, hypopituitarism

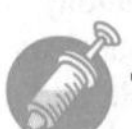

TREATMENT

MEDICATION

- For sepsis or bacterial infections: Antibiotics based on site and etiology
- For hypoglycemia, D50W at a dose of 1 mg/kg
- Thiamine, 100 mg, if alcoholic or cachectic
- Naloxone, 2 mg
- Levothyroxine 150–500 μg for myxedema
- For severe acidosis: Sodium bicarbonate
- Contraindications:
  - Medications, including epinephrine, lidocaine, and procainamide, can accumulate to toxic levels if used repeatedly.
  - Routine use of steroids or antibiotics has not been shown to increase survival or decrease postresuscitative damage.
- Precautions:
  - Medications should be avoided until core temperature is >30°C:
    - When temperature reaches >30°C, IV medications are indicated, but at longer than the standard intervals.
  - Avoid vasopressors due to arrhythmogenic potential and delayed metabolism.
- Significant possible interactions:
  - Use all drugs cautiously due to impaired metabolism and renal elimination.
- Once rewarming has occurred, there is mobilization of depot stores.

ADDITIONAL TREATMENT

General Measures

- Prehospital (1)[C]:
  - ABCs of basic life support
  - Remove wet garments.
  - Protect against heat loss and wind chill.
  - If far from definitive care, begin active rewarming but do not delay transport.
  - Give warm humidified oxygen if available.
- See "Initial Stabilization."

IN-PATIENT CONSIDERATIONS

Initial Stabilization

Rewarming dependent on severity of hypothermia and presence of cardiac arrest:

- If no cardiac arrest, consider active external rewarming (2)[B].
- If cardiac arrest present, consider active internal rewarming (2)[B].
- Warm center of body first.
- The rate of rewarming is determined by whether a perfusing cardiac output is present:
  - If a perfusing cardiac output is present, 1–2°C per hour is appropriate.
  - If not, then a faster rate of >2°C per hour should be used.
- Monitor core temperature; use a consistent method.
- Monitor BP and cardiac rhythm.
- Correct metabolic acidosis.
- Evaluate for frostbite and other trauma.
- Mild hypothermia:
  - Passive rewarming
  - Administration of heated IV solutions (D5NS)
  - Warm fluids may be given if fully alert.
- Moderate hypothermia:
  - Active external rewarming with forced warm air systems (3)[B]
- Severe hypothermia (active internal [core] rewarming):
  - Minimally invasive
  - Heated IV fluids
  - Heated humidified oxygen
  - Body cavity lavage:
    - Thoracic cavity lavage (43°C)
    - GI, colonic, or bladder lavage with warm fluids (43°C)
    - Peritoneal dialysis
  - Extracorporeal blood rewarming (3)[B]:
    - Cardiopulmonary bypass
    - Extracorporeal membrane oxygenation
    - Continuous arteriovenous rewarming
    - Hemodialysis and hemofiltration
- Cardiac arrhythmias:
  - Atrial fibrillation and sinus bradycardia are common, but patients usually convert to normal sinus rhythm with rewarming.
  - If ventricular fibrillation is present, it should be treated with 1 shock. If patient does not respond, further attempts should be deferred until the patient is rewarmed.
  - Do not treat transient ventricular arrhythmias.
  - If cardiac pacing required, preferable to use external noninvasive pacemaker

Admission Criteria

Patients with underlying disease, physiologic abnormalities, or core temperature 32°C should be admitted, preferably to the ICU.

IV Fluids

IVs should be heated to 40–42°C when possible, but should be no colder than the patient's core temperature.

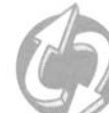

ALERT

- Avoid fluid overload.
- Avoid lactated Ringer solution because of decreased lactate metabolism.

Nursing

Because of the cold, heart is irritable and susceptible to arrhythmias; take special care in moving and transporting.

Discharge Criteria

Discharge from emergency department once normothermic, if mild hypothermia and no predisposing conditions or complications, and has suitable place to go.

ONGOING CARE

FOLLOW-UP RECOMMENDATIONS

Patient Monitoring

- During acute episode:
  - Monitor cardiac rhythm.
  - Monitor electrolytes and glucose frequently.
  - Monitor urinary output.
  - Follow blood gases.
- Following acute episode:
  - Continued therapy for any underlying disorder

DIET

Warm fluids only, if alert and able to swallow

PATIENT EDUCATION

- Alcohol intake increases risk of becoming hypothermic in cold conditions.
- Encourage persons with cardiovascular disease to avoid outdoor exercise in cold weather.
- If appropriate, referral to social service agency for help with adequate housing, heat, or clothing.

PROGNOSIS

- Mortality rates are decreasing due to increased recognition and advanced therapy.
- Mortality usually dependent on the severity of underlying cause of hypothermia
- In previously healthy individuals, recovery is usually complete.
- Mortality rate in healthy patients is <5%.
- Mortality rate in patients with coexisting illness is >50%.

Geriatric Considerations

Mortality rates increase with increasing age.

COMPLICATIONS

- Cardiac arrhythmias
- Hypotension
- Hyperkalemia
- Hypoglycemia
- Rhabdomyolysis
- Sepsis
- Pneumonia (aspiration and broncho)
- Pulmonary edema
- Acute respiratory distress syndrome
- Pancreatitis
- Peritonitis
- GI bleeding
- Acute tubular necrosis
- Bladder atony
- Intravascular thromboses/disseminated intravascular coagulation
- Metabolic acidosis
- Gangrene of extremities
- Compartment syndromes
- Seizures
- Cerebral ischemia
- Delirium

REFERENCES

1. American Heart Association. Part 10.4: Hypothermia. *Circulation*. 2005;112: IV-136–IV-138.
2. Kempainen RR, Brunette DD. The evaluation and management of accidental hypothermia. *Respir Care*. 2004;49:192–205.
3. McCullough L, Arora S. Diagnosis and treatment of hypothermia. *Am Fam Physician*. 2004;70: 2325–32.

ADDITIONAL READING

- Headdon WG, Wilson PM, Dalton HR, et al. The management of accidental hypothermia. *BMJ*. 2009;338:b2085.
- Schweitzer KS. Cold but not dead. *Air Med J*. 2008;27:94–8.
- van der Ploeg GJ, Goslings JC, Walpoth BH, et al. Accidental hypothermia: Rewarming treatments, complications and outcomes from one university medical centre. *Resuscitation*. 2010;81(11):1550–5.

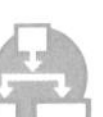

See Also (Topic, Algorithm, Electronic Media Element)

- Frostbite; Near Drowning
- Algorithm: Hypothermia

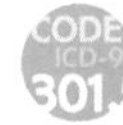

CODES

ICD9

991.6 Hypothermia

CLINICAL PEARLS

- Most common cause of hypothermia in the US is cold exposure due to alcohol intoxication.
- As long as core temperature is severely decreased, one should assume that resuscitation is possible unless there are obvious lethal injuries ("not dead until warm and dead").
- EKG changes are associated with hypothermia: Slowing of sinus rate with T-wave inversion, QT-interval prolongation, hypothermic J waves (Osborn waves) characterized by a notching of the QRS complex and ST segment

HYPOTHYROIDISM, ADULT

Barbara A. Majeroni, MD

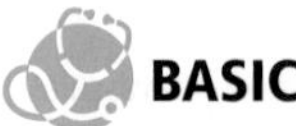

BASICS

DESCRIPTION
- Clinical state resulting from decreased circulating levels of free thyroid hormone or from resistance to hormone action
- Subclinical hypothyroidism: Elevated thyroid-stimulating hormone (TSH) (>4.5) with normal free T4
- System(s) affected: Endocrine/Metabolic
- Synonym(s): Myxedema

EPIDEMIOLOGY
Incidence
- Predominant age: >40 years
- Predominant gender: Female > Male, 5–10:1

Prevalence
- 3.7% in general population
- Common in elderly
- >65 years of age, increases to 6–10% of women, 2–3% of men
- Up to 20% of patients with major depressive disorder
- Subclinical hypothyroidism: 4–20%, depending on age and gender studied

RISK FACTORS
- Increasing age
- Personal or family history of autoimmune diseases, including type 1 diabetes mellitus (DM), Addison disease
- Previous postpartum thyroiditis
- Previous head or neck irradiation
- History of Graves disease
- Treatment with lithium, immune modulators such as IFN-α, or the iodine-containing antiarrhythmic amiodarone

Genetics
- No known genetic pattern for idiopathic primary hypothyroidism
- May be associated with type 2 autoimmune polyglandular syndrome, which is associated with HLA-DR3 and -DR4
- Secondary hypothyroidism frequently results from treatment for Graves disease, which may be familial.

ETIOLOGY
- Postablative: Follows radioactive iodine therapy or thyroid surgery; delayed hypothyroidism may develop in patients treated with thioamide drugs (e.g., propylthiouracil or methimazole) 4–25 years later
- Primary: May develop as result of autoimmune thyroiditis or be idiopathic
- With goiter: Most commonly a result of autoimmune disease, such as Hashimoto thyroiditis
- Other causes: Heritable biosynthetic defects, iodine deficiency (rare in US), or drugs (iodides, lithium, phenylbutazone, acetylsalicylic acid (ASA), amiodarone, aminoglutethimide, and IFN-α)
- Central or secondary: May be due to deficiency of thyrotropin-releasing hormone (TRH) from hypothalamus or TSH from pituitary
- Transient: May result from silent thyroiditis (most common in postpartum period) and subacute granulomatous thyroiditis

COMMONLY ASSOCIATED CONDITIONS
- Hyponatremia
- Anemia
- Idiopathic adrenocorticoid deficiency
- DM
- Hypoparathyroidism
- Myasthenia gravis
- Vitiligo
- Hypercholesterolemia
- Mitral valve prolapse
- Depression
- Rapid-cycling bipolar disorder
- Ischemic heart disease
- Metabolic syndrome
- Down syndrome

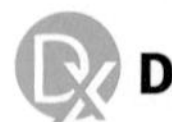

DIAGNOSIS

HISTORY
- Onset may be insidious, subtle
- Weakness, fatigue, lethargy
- Cold intolerance
- Decreased memory, concentration
- Hearing impairment
- Constipation
- Muscle cramps
- Arthralgias
- Paresthesias
- Modest weight gain (10 lb [4.5 kg])
- Decreased sweating
- Menorrhagia
- Depression
- Hoarseness
- Carpal tunnel syndrome

PHYSICAL EXAM
- Dry, coarse skin
- Dull facial expression
- Coarsening or huskiness of voice
- Periorbital puffiness
- Swelling of hands and feet (nonpitting)
- Bradycardia
- Hypothermia
- Reduced systolic BP
- Increased diastolic BP
- Reduced body and scalp hair
- Delayed relaxation of deep-tendon reflexes
- Macroglossia

Geriatric Considerations
- Characteristic signs and symptoms frequently changed or absent
- Diagnosis based on laboratory criteria

DIAGNOSTIC TESTS & INTERPRETATION
Lab
Initial lab tests
- Primary hypothyroidism (1)[C]:
  - TSH elevated
  - Serum free T4 decreased
- Central hypothyroidism:
  - TSH low
  - Serum free T4 decreased
  - Impaired TSH response to TRH
- Severe hypothyroidism:
  - Anemia
  - Elevated cholesterol
  - Elevated creatine phosphokinase, lactate dehydrogenase, aspartate aminotransferase
  - Hyponatremia
- Subclinical hypothyroidism:
  - TSH elevated (>4.5 mIU/L)
  - Serum free T4 normal

Follow-Up & Special Considerations
- Drugs that may alter lab results:
  - Thyroid supplement
  - Cortisone
  - Dopamine
  - Phenytoin
  - Estrogen or androgen therapy in excess of replacement
  - Amiodarone
  - Salicylates
- Disorders that may alter lab results:
  - Any severe illness
  - Pregnancy
  - Chronic protein malnutrition
  - Hepatic failure
  - Nephrotic syndrome

Imaging
Initial approach
- None necessary unless signs of cardiac involvement
- Chest radiograph may show enlarged heart (often due to pericardial effusion).

Pathological Findings
Thyroid may be small, atrophic, or enlarged.

DIFFERENTIAL DIAGNOSIS
- Nephrotic syndrome
- Chronic nephritis
- Neurasthenia
- Depression
- Euthyroid sick syndrome
- Congestive heart failure
- Primary amyloidosis
- Dementia from other causes

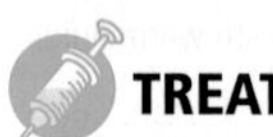

TREATMENT

MEDICATION
First Line
- Levothyroxine (Synthroid, Levothroid):
  - 1.6 mcg/kg/d; increase by 25 mcg/d every 4–6 weeks until TSH in normal range (2)[A]
  - Dosage requirements may vary with age, gender, residual secretory capacity of thyroid gland, other drugs being taken by patient, and intestinal function.
  - Elderly patients may require 2/3 of dose used in young adults because clearance is decreased.
  - Levothyroxine should be taken on an empty stomach. Administering at bedtime may result in higher levels than administering in the morning (3)[B].
- Contraindications:
  - Thyrotoxic heart disease
  - Uncorrected adrenocorticoid insufficiency

- Precautions:
  - Start with lower doses, such as 25 mcg, in elderly and in patients with heart disease.
  - Diabetic patients may need readjustment of hypoglycemic agents with institution of thyroxine.
  - Dosage of oral anticoagulants may need adjustment; monitor prothrombin time while initiating treatment.
- Significant possible interactions:
  - Oral anticoagulants
  - Insulin
  - Oral hypoglycemics
  - Estrogen
  - Oral contraceptives
  - Cholestyramine
  - Proton pump inhibitors
  - Ferrous sulfate, calcium carbonate, antacids, laxatives, colestipol, sucralfate, ciprofloxacin, and cholestyramine may decrease absorption.
- Controversy exists whether subclinical hypothyroidism should be treated if asymptomatic. Cochrane Review found no improvement in survival, cardiovascular morbidity, or health-related quality of life. Some evidence indicates improvement in lipid profiles and left ventricular function (4)[A]. Subclinical hypothyroidism should be treated in patients with iron deficiency anemia (5)[A], and in patients with TSH >10. Treatment may be indicated for patients with TSH between 4.5 and 10 if they are symptomatic.

Pregnancy Considerations

- Replacement therapy may need adjustment.
- TSH levels should be monitored monthly during first trimester (6)[C].
- Postpartum: Check TSH levels at 6 weeks.
- Painless subacute thyroiditis may occur in postpartum period, leading to transient hypothyroidism lasting 3 months. Treatment with replacement therapy may be warranted. Up to 30% of these individuals develop permanent hypothyroidism.

Second Line

No benefit to adding triiodothyronine (T_3) to thyroxine

ADDITIONAL TREATMENT

General Measures

- Outpatient, except for complicating emergencies (e.g., coma, hypothermia)
- Treatment goals: Restore and maintain euthyroid state.

Issues for Referral

- Central hypothyroidism, with low TSH and low free T4, would benefit from an endocrinology referral.
- Hypothyroidism unresponsive to treatment
- Serum TSH remains elevated despite full-dose treatment with levothyroxine

IN-PATIENT CONSIDERATIONS

Admission Criteria

Myxedema coma, hypothermia

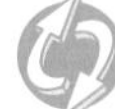

ONGOING CARE

FOLLOW-UP RECOMMENDATIONS

Monitor TSH.

Patient Monitoring

- Monitor TSH every 8–12 weeks until stabilized, then annually.
- Follow cardiac status closely in older patients.
- Check TSH more frequently in pregnancy, initiation of estrogen supplementation, or after large changes in body weight.
- In central hypothyroidism, TSH unreliable; must monitor free T4, T3

DIET

High-bulk diet may help avoid constipation.

PATIENT EDUCATION

- Stress importance of compliance with thyroid replacement therapy.
- Explain need for lifelong treatment.
- Instruct to report to physician any signs of infection or heart problems.
- Describe signs of thyrotoxicity.

PROGNOSIS

- Return to normal state is the rule.
- Relapses will occur if treatment is interrupted.
- If untreated, may progress to myxedema coma.

COMPLICATIONS

- Hypothyroid patients (mild to moderate) tolerate surgery with mortality and complications similar to euthyroid patients.
- If surgery is elective, render patient euthyroid prior to procedure.
- If surgery is urgent, proceed with procedure with individualized replacement therapy preoperatively and postoperatively.
- Treatment-induced congestive heart failure in people with coronary artery disease
- Myxedema coma: Life-threatening
- Increased susceptibility to infection
- Megacolon
- Organic psychosis with paranoia
- Adrenal crisis with vigorous treatment of hypothyroidism, especially in patients with undiagnosed polyendocrine syndromes
- Infertility
- Hypersensitivity to opiates
- Treatment over long periods can lead to bone demineralization.
- Subclinical hypothyroidism is associated with increased ischemic heart disease and increased all-cause mortality in men but not in women.

REFERENCES

1. Miller GD, Rogers JC, DeGroote SL. Which lab tests are best when you suspect hypothyroidism? *J Fam Pract*. 2008;57:613–9.
2. Roos A, et al. The starting dose of levothyroxine in primary hypothyroidism treatment: A prospective, randomized, double-blind trial. *Arch Int Med*. 2005;165:1714–20.
3. Nienke B, Visser TJ, Nijman J, et al. Effects of Evening vs morning levothyroxine intake, a randomized, double blind crossover trial. *Arch Int Mad*. 2010 170 (22):1996–2003.
4. Villar HCCE, Saconato H, Valente O, et al. Thyroid hormone replacement for subclinical hypothyroidism (Cochrane Review). In: *The Cochrane Library*, Issue 2. Chichester, UK: John Wiley and Sons, Ltd; 2008.
5. Cinemre H, Bilir C, Gokosmanoglu F, et al. Hematologic effects of levothyroxine in iron deficient subclinical hypothyroid patients: A randomized, double blind, controlled study. *J Clin Endocrinol Metabol*. 2009;94(1):151–6.
6. Alexander EK, Marqusee E, Lawrence J, et al. Timing and magnitude of increases in levothyroxine requirements during pregnancy in women with hypothyroidism. *N Engl J Med*. 2004;351:241–9.

ADDITIONAL READING

- Devdhar M, et al. Hypothyroidism. *Endocrinol Clin N Am*. 2007;36:595–615.
- Feldt-Rasmussen U. Treatment of hypothyroidism in elderly patients and in patients with cardiac disease. *Thyroid*. 2007;17:619–24.
- Razvi S, Weaver JU, Pearce SHS. Subclinical thyroid disorders: Significance and clinical impact. *J Clin Pathol*. 2010;63:379–86.
- Vaidya B, Pearce SHS. Management of hypothyroidism in adults. *BMJ*. 2008:337:284–9.

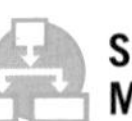

See Also (Topic, Algorithm, Electronic Media Element)

Hyperthyroidism; Thyroiditis

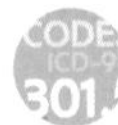

CODES

ICD9

- 244.0 Postsurgical hypothyroidism
- 244.1 Other postablative hypothyroidism
- 244.9 Unspecified acquired hypothyroidism

CLINICAL PEARLS

- Start low and go slow when starting thyroxine in an elderly patient or if known cardiovascular disease.
- Once a patient has attained the euthyroid state, maintain on the same brand of thyroxine. There can be up to 12.5% difference in brands considered bioequivalent.
- Monitor TSH every 8–12 weeks until stabilized, then annually.
- The symptoms of hypothyroidism may be vague and diffuse. Maintain a high index of suspicion, especially in women >50 years of age.

H

ID REACTION

Stanley Sagov, MD
Robert A. Baldor, MD

BASICS

DESCRIPTION

A generalized skin reaction associated with various infectious and inflammatory cutaneous conditions distant from the main rash of the disease:

- Id is a word termination often combined with a root reflecting the causative factor (i.e., bacterid, syphilid, and tuberculid). The dermatophytid is the most frequently referenced id reaction in dermatology. A dermatophytid is an autosensitization reaction in which a secondary cutaneous reaction occurs at a site distant to a primary fungal infection. The eruption begins typically within 1–2 weeks of the onset of the main lesion or following exacerbation of the main lesion.
- System(s) affected: Skin/Exocrine
- Synonym(s): Dermatophytid, Trichophytid, Autoeczematization

EPIDEMIOLOGY

- Predominant age: All ages
- Predominant sex: Male = Female

Incidence

Unknown; no good data source

Prevalence

Common

RISK FACTORS

- Fungal infection of the skin
- Stasis dermatitis

GENERAL PREVENTION

- Minimize factors for developing fungal infections.
- Promptly treat any developing fungal infection.

ETIOLOGY

Precise pathophysiology is uncertain. Circulating antigens may react with antibodies at sensitized areas of the skin, or abnormal immune recognition of autologous skin antigens may occur.

COMMONLY ASSOCIATED CONDITIONS

- Primary fungal infection
- Stasis dermatitis

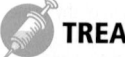

DIAGNOSIS

HISTORY

Itchy rash: Assess for the primary fungal or bacterial lesions that would have preceded the onset of the id reaction by days to weeks.

PHYSICAL EXAM

- Common:
  - Symmetric, pruritic vesicles on the hands
  - Tinea infection on the feet; contact or other eczematous dermatosis; or bacterial, fungal, or viral infection of the skin
  - Generalized reactions can occur.
- Less common:
  - Papules
  - Lichenoid eruption
- Eczematoid eruption

DIAGNOSTIC TESTS & INTERPRETATION

Lab

- Fungal infection at the primary site proven by potassium hydroxide (KOH) or fungal culture
- No fungal elements demonstrable at the site of the presumed id reaction
- Special tests: Skin shows a positive trichophyton reaction.

Follow-Up & Special Considerations

The id reaction resolves with successful eradication of the primary skin condition.

Pathological Findings

- Vesicles in the upper dermis
- Superficial perivascular lymphohistiocytic infiltrate
- Small numbers of eosinophils
- Moderate acanthosis
- Increased granular cell layer
- No infectious agents present in biopsy specimen

DIFFERENTIAL DIAGNOSIS

- Pompholyx (dyshidrotic eczema)
- Contact dermatitis
- Drug eruptions
- Pustular psoriasis
- Folliculitis
- Scabies

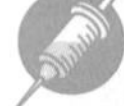

TREATMENT

MEDICATION

First Line

- Oral antihistamines for pruritus:
  - Chlorpheniramine 4 mg (peds: 0.35 mg/kg/24 hr div. q4–6h PRN; 2–6 years max 4 mg/24 hr; 6–12 years max 12 mg/24 hr) PO q4–6h PRN; max 24 mg/24 hr
  - Diphenhydramine 25–50 mg (peds: 5 mg/kg/24 hr divided q6h PRN; 2–5 years max 37.5 mg/24 hr; 6–11 years max 150 mg/24 hr; >12 years max 400 mg/24 hr) PO q4–6h PRN; max 400 mg/24 hr
  - Hydroxyzine 25–100 mg (peds: 2 mg/kg/24 hr divided q6h PRN) PO q6–8h PRN; max 600 mg/24 hr
- Topical treatments for pruritus:
  - Triamcinolone 0.1% ointment TID
  - Hydrocortisone 0.5%, 1%, 2.5%: Up to q.i.d.
  - Capsaicin 0.025%, 0.075% cream: Apply t.i.d. to q.i.d. PRN
  - Doxepin 5% cream: Apply q.i.d. for up to 8 days (to max of 10% of the body)
  - EMLA (2.5% lidocaine + 2.5% prilocaine): Apply prior to capsaicin
  - Permethrin 5% cream (for scabies):
    - Apply from neck down after bath.
    - Wash off thoroughly with water in 8–12 hours.
    - May repeat in 7 days.
  - Permethrin 1% cream rinse (for lice):
    - Shampoo, rinse, towel dry, saturate hair and scalp (or other affected area), leave on 10 min, then rinse.
    - May repeat in 7 days.
  - White petroleum emollients: Apply after short bath/shower in warm (not hot) water.
- Systemic steroids only if reaction is severe or generalized (e.g., Prednisone 20 mg)

Second Line

- Topical and/or systemic antifungals for identified associated fungal infection (common)
  - Tinea cruris/corporis:
    - Topical azole antifungal compounds (1)[C]
      - Econazole (Spectazole), ketoconazole (Nizoral): Usually applied b.i.d. × 2–3 weeks
      - Terbinafine (Lamisil): Over-the-counter (OTC) compound; can be applied once or b.i.d. × 1–2 weeks
      - Butenafine (Mentax): Applied once daily × 2 weeks; also very effective

– Tinea capitis:
  - Oral griseofulvin (2)[A] for *Trichophyton* and *Microsporum* sp.; microsized preparation available; dosage 125 mg/d in patients weighing 10–20 kg; 250 mg/d if weight is 20–40 kg; 500 mg/d if weight is >40 kg; taken b.i.d. or as a single dose daily × 6–12 weeks
  - Oral terbinafine (2)[A] can be used for *Trichophyton* sp. at 62.5 mg/d in patients weighing 10–20 kg; 125 mg/d if weight 20–40 kg; 250 mg/d if weight >40 kg; use for 4–6 weeks
  - Oral itraconazole (2)[A] can be used for *Microsporum* sp. and matches griseofulvin's efficacy while being better tolerated. Dosage of 3–5 mg/kg/d, but most studies have used 100 mg/d × 6 weeks in children >2 years of age.
- Topical or systemic antibiotics for any secondary bacterial infection

ADDITIONAL TREATMENT

General Measures

- Appropriate health care: Outpatient
- Treatment of the underlying infection or eczematous dermatitis
- Symptomatic treatment of pruritus with antihistamines and/or topical steroids if needed (may require class 1 or 2 steroid)
- Treatment for secondary bacterial infection

ONGOING CARE

PATIENT EDUCATION

Avoid hot, humid conditions that promote fungal growth. Aerate susceptible body areas (e.g., wear sandals or open footwear). If possible, wear boxer shorts or loose-fitting clothing, dry off wet skin after bathing, and use powders and antiperspirants to make the environment less conducive to fungal growth. Treat primary dermatitis promptly.

PROGNOSIS

After appropriate treatment, complete resolution in a few days to 2 weeks

COMPLICATIONS

Secondary bacterial infection (cellulitis)

REFERENCES

1. Bonifaz A, et al. Comparative study between terbinafine 1% emulsion-gel versus ketoconazole 2% cream in tinea cruris and corporis. *Eur J Derm*. 2000;10:107.
2. Gupta AK, Adam P, Dlova N, et al. Therapeutic options for the treatment of tinea capitis caused by *Trichophyton* species: Griseofulvin versus the new oral antifungal agents, terbinafine, itraconazole, and fluconazole. *Pediatr Dermatol*. 2001;18: 433–8.

ADDITIONAL READING

- Fuller LC, Smith CH, Cerio R, et al. A randomized comparison of 4 weeks of terbinafine vs. 8 weeks of griseofulvin for the treatment of tinea capitis. *Br J Dermatol*. 2001;144:321–7.
- Greaves MW, et al. Recent advances in pathophysiology and current management of itch. *Ann Acad Med Singap*. 2007;36:788–92.

CODES

ICD9

- 110.9 Dermatophytosis of unspecified site
- 692.89 Contact dermatitis and other eczema due to other specified agents

CLINICAL PEARLS

- When assessing an itchy rash, assess for the primary fungal or bacterial lesions that would have preceded the onset of the id reaction by days to weeks
- This is a diagnosis in the category of "If you don't think of it, you won't think of it," so when you see one skin lesion follow another, think of the id reaction.

I

IDIOPATHIC HYPERTROPHIC SUBAORTIC STENOSIS (IHSS)

Arka Chatterjee, MD
Ziad Alnabki, MD
Ihab Hamzeh, MD

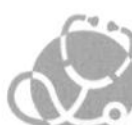

BASICS

DESCRIPTION

- IHSS (more commonly known as hypertrophic cardiomyopathy) is a form of primary myocardial hypertrophy, with or without presence of left ventricular outflow tract (LVOT) obstruction, and is characterized by 4 cardinal features:
  - Idiopathic left ventricular hypertrophy (LVH) in absence of other cardiac or systemic disease causing hypertrophy of such magnitude
  - Cardiac myocyte and myofibrillar disarray
  - Familial occurrence
  - Associated sudden cardiac death
- System(s) affected: Cardiovascular
- Synonym(s): Hypertrophic cardiomyopathy (HCM) (most accepted); Hypertrophic obstructive cardiomyopathy (HOCM); Muscular subaortic stenosis (MSS)

EPIDEMIOLOGY

- The disorder may present at any age.
- It is seen in equal frequency in both sexes, although it is often underrecognized in females and African Americans.
- Apical HCM is a variant seen more often in China and Japan (Yamaguchi apical variant).

Incidence

~1% of patients with HCM die annually, but this is no different from the overall population.

Prevalence

- Prevalence of phenotypically expressed IHSS in the adult general population is 1:500 (0.2%).
- Around 500,000 people are affected with IHSS in the US.
- It is the most common genetic cardiovascular disease.

RISK FACTORS

Risk factors for sudden cardiac death (SCD) include (1):

- A prior history of cardiac arrest or spontaneous sustained ventricular tachycardia (VT)
- Family history of premature SCD (especially in close relative or multiple)
- Unexplained syncope
- Extreme LVH measuring >30 mm
- Hypotensive response to exercise
- Nonsustained VT during Holter monitoring
- Other factors that may indicate risk are LVOT obstruction, high-risk mutation, atrial fibrillation, delayed enhancement on cardiac MRI, intense physical exertion, etc.

Genetics

- It is inherited as a mendelian autosomal dominant trait with >50% penetrance.
- 11 sarcomeric gene mutations are known, including, among others, beta myosin heavy chain, myosin binding protein C, and troponin I and T.

GENERAL PREVENTION

- Avoid strenuous exercise (particularly involving burst exertion) and heavy lifting (induces Valsalva maneuver).
- Maintain hydration to avoid volume depletion.
- Avoid alcohol.
- Certain drugs, such as nitrates, digoxin, beta agonists, vasodilators, and diuretics, are best avoided, particularly in presence of increased LVOT gradient.
- Implantable cardioverter defibrillator (ICD) is recommended for patients at high risk for sudden cardiac death (1,2)[C].

PATHOPHYSIOLOGY

- Left ventricular hypertrophy:
  - 1 or more regions of LV wall are thickened: Classically at the basal anterior septum, but may involve posterior septum or LV free wall and apex
  - Hypertrophy develops usually in adolescence, with an average 100% increase in LV mass.
- Systolic anterior motion (SAM) of the mitral valve:
  - Mitral valve abnormalities are primary manifestations of HCM: 1/both leaflets may be elongated.
  - SAM is the abrupt motion of the MV leaflet toward the septum, which creates dynamic LVOT obstruction on contact with the septum.
  - SAM is caused by drag effect of the high-velocity jet caused by ejection through a narrowed LVOT and/or a Venturi phenomenon.
- Disorganized myocardial architecture:
  - Myocytes and myofilaments are laid down in disorganized pattern, with increased matrix components causing myocyte disarray.
  - Microvascular disease leads to ischemia and replacement fibrosis.
- Diastolic dysfunction:
  - Result of reduced ventricular compliance; contributes predominantly to the symptoms of heart failure, like dyspnea

DIAGNOSIS

HISTORY

- Symptoms of heart failure: Dyspnea, paroxysmal nocturnal dyspnea, fatigue
- Angina pectoris
- Palpitations
- Exertional syncope or presyncope
- Symptoms may be worsened by anemia, hot and humid weather, a large meal, alcohol, or fever.
- Clinical symptoms correlate poorly with the severity of LVOT obstruction.
- 50% of these patients have positive family history for IHSS (and 50% are sporadic).

PHYSICAL EXAM

- A systolic crescendo/decrescendo murmur from LVOT obstruction is best heard at left lower sternal border.
- Intensity of murmur is dynamic and changes with maneuvers that affect the degree of obstruction.
- Maneuvers that decrease venous return (e.g., Valsalva, standing position, amyl nitrite) increase intensity of the murmur.
- Maneuvers that increase left ventricular afterload (e.g., handgrip) will soften the murmur.
- Bisferiens pulse
- Double or triple apical impulse
- Prominent S4
- Holosystolic murmur of mitral regurgitation may be heard at the apex.

DIAGNOSTIC TESTS & INTERPRETATION

- EKG: Common findings (50–90%):
  - Nonspecific ST-T wave abnormalities
  - LVH
- EKG: Less common findings (<50%):
  - Prominent and abnormal Q waves in anterior precordial and lateral limbs lead
  - Left atrial enlargement
  - Diffuse, marked, symmetric giant negative T waves in lateral precordial leads seen in patients with apical HCM
- Holter findings may include supraventricular tachycardia (SVT), ventricular premature contractions (PVC), nonsustained ventricular tachycardia (VT), and atrial fibrillation
- DNA analysis for known mutant genes is the definitive method for establishing the diagnosis of IHSS.

Imaging

- Chest x-ray may show cardiomegaly and left atrial enlargement.
- Echocardiogram helps establish the diagnosis most easily and reliably. Typical echo findings:
  - Asymmetric septal hypertrophy with septal-to-free-wall ratio >1.3:1 classically
  - Left ventricular hypertrophy (especially LV wall thickness in diastole >15 mm)
  - Small left ventricular chamber
  - In patients with apical IHSS, left ventricular cavity looks like a spade.
  - Abnormal systolic anterior motion of mitral valve leaflet
  - Continuous-wave Doppler best measures significant dynamic outflow obstruction.
  - Evidence of diastolic dysfunction
  - Provocative measures such as inhalation of amyl nitrate/Valsalva/dobutamine/exercise may be necessary to elicit significant LVOT gradients during echocardiography.
- 24-/48-hour Holter monitoring is recommended (3).
- Stress testing may be used to assess BP response with exercise (3).
- MRI of LV is useful if echo images are suboptimal or LV segmental hypertrophy is seen in an unusual location; delayed gadolinium enhancement can be used as a minor risk factor for SCD; mitral valve morphology can be better defined and may have a novel role in assessment.

DIFFERENTIAL DIAGNOSIS

- Valvular aortic stenosis
- Hypertensive heart disease, especially in elderly
- Athlete's heart: Differentiated by normal/enlarged LV cavity, regression of LVH on deconditioning
- Cardiac amyloidosis
- Noonan syndrome, mitochondrial myopathy, and metabolic storage disorders (e.g., Anderson Fabry disease and Friedrich ataxia)

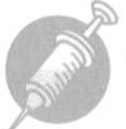

TREATMENT

- These patients must be counseled against competitive athletics irrespective of LVOT obstruction and associated symptoms.
- Adequate hydration should be maintained.
- Not a high-risk condition for endocarditis prophylaxis
- Genetic counseling may be appropriate.
- Only symptomatic patients will benefit from drug therapy.

MEDICATION

First Line

- β-blockers:
  - First-line drugs for patients with provocable gradient
  - 1/3–2/3 of patients experience symptomatic improvement.
- Disopyramide: Used as an adjunct with β-blockers or calcium channel blockers only, as it may accelerate AV conduction (2,4)[B]
- Verapamil: Ideally not used together with β-blockers and not first-line treatment, given the profound systemic vasodilatory effects of this agent

Second Line

- Atrial fibrillation is common and should be controlled.
- Maintenance of sinus rhythm should be aggressively pursued because of association of atrial fibrillation (AF) with heart failure symptoms and embolic phenomena (5)[C].
- Amiodarone is most effective for sinus rhythm maintenance in IHSS-associated atrial fibrillation.

ADDITIONAL TREATMENT

Pregnant patients with IHSS:

- IHSS patients who wish to become pregnant should be counseled prenatally regarding its autosomal dominant inheritance.
- Pregnancy is usually uneventful with increased plasma volume counteracting vasodilatation.
- Should be monitored closely in a tertiary care center during labor, as peripheral vasodilatation, fluid shift, and epidural analgesia pose a theoretical risk in presence of LVOT obstruction
- Spinal analgesia is contraindicated. Careful administration of epidural analgesia is controversial.

SURGERY/OTHER PROCEDURES

- Ventricular septal myotomy-myectomy (Morrow procedure):
  - The gold standard for drug-refractory symptomatic patients with obstructive IHSS (2,6)[B], and for relief of obstruction with outflow gradient >50 mm Hg at rest/with provocation
  - 5–10 gm of tissue is removed from the proximal septum.
  - Most (about 70%) patients achieve subjective improvement in symptoms lasting $\geq$5 years following their surgery.
  - Postoperative complications may include left bundle branch block (LBBB), ventricular septal defect (VSD), and aortic regurgitation.
- Heart transplant is advocated for nonobstructive IHSS patients with refractory severe symptoms due to restrictive physiology not responding to conventional treatment, including those with end-stage congestive heart failure.
- Percutaneous alcohol septal ablation:
  - Controlled alcohol-induced septal myocardial infarction resulting in an akinetic septal segment with instantaneous obliteration of the outflow obstruction and gradient
  - Preferred in patients at high risk from septal myectomy, those that refuse surgical therapy, and those who have failed surgical myectomy
- Implantable cardiac defibrillators for prevention of SCD in patient at high risk (1)[C]

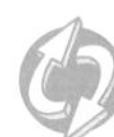

ONGOING CARE

FOLLOW-UP RECOMMENDATIONS

- Annual follow-up is recommended for stable patients.
- Among the first-degree relatives, screening with EKG and echocardiogram is recommended every 12–24 months between the ages of 12 and 21 years and every 5 years in adults, particularly if adverse IHSS-related events have occurred in the family.

PATIENT EDUCATION

- Patients with characteristic phenotype of IHSS (LVH) are excluded from all competitive sports except those with low static and dynamic intensity (e.g., golf).
- Gene carriers without the phenotype are not excluded from competitive sports.

PROGNOSIS

- Annual mortality of 1% is no different from the general US population
- Although it may be associated with important symptoms and premature SCD more frequently, these patients have no or relatively mild disability and normal life expectancy.

COMPLICATIONS

- Sudden death (1% per year)
- Ventricular arrhythmia
- Atrial fibrillation
- Infective mitral endocarditis
- Progressive heart failure

REFERENCES

1. Maron BJ, et al. Contemporary insights and strategies for risk stratification and prevention of sudden death in hypertrophic cardiomyopathy. *Circulation*. 2010;121:445–56.
2. Maron BJ, McKenna WJ, Danielson GK, et al. American College of Cardiology/European Society of Cardiology clinical expert consensus document on hypertrophic cardiomyopathy. A report of the American College of Cardiology Foundation Task Force on Clinical Expert Consensus Documents and the European Society of Cardiology Committee for Practice Guidelines. *J Am Coll Cardiol*. 2003;42: 1687–713.
3. Nishimura RA, Holmes DR, et al. Clinical practice. Hypertrophic obstructive cardiomyopathy. *N Engl J Med*. 2004;350:1320–7.
4. Sherrid MV, Barac I, McKenna WJ, et al. Multicenter study of the efficacy and safety of disopyramide in obstructive hypertrophic cardiomyopathy. *J Am Coll Cardiol*. 2005;45:1251–8.
5. Maron BJ, Olivotto I, Bellone P, et al. Clinical profile of stroke in 900 patients with hypertrophic cardiomyopathy. *J Am Coll Cardiol*. 2002;39: 301–7.
6. Maron BJ. Hypertrophic cardiomyopathy: A systematic review. *JAMA*. 2002;287:1308–20.

ADDITIONAL READING

- Fernandes VL, Nielsen C, Nagueh SF, et al. Follow-up of alcohol septal ablation for symptomatic hypertrophic obstructive cardiomyopathy the Baylor and Medical University of South Carolina experience 1996 to 2007. *JACC Cardiovasc Interv*. 2008;1: 561–70.
- Pelliccia A, Zipes DP, Maron BJ, et al. Bethesda Conference #36 and the European Society of Cardiology Consensus Recommendations revisited a comparison of U.S. and European criteria for eligibility and disqualification of competitive athletes with cardiovascular abnormalities. *J Am Coll Cardiol*. 2008;52:1990–6.

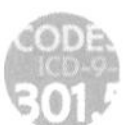

CODES

ICD9

425.1 Hypertrophic obstructive cardiomyopathy

CLINICAL PEARLS

ALERT

- IHSS should be considered in all patients with a history of unexplained sudden cardiac death.
- IHSS is the most common cause of sudden cardiac death in young athletes in the US.
- 75% patients do not have a sizeable resting gradient.
- Delayed de novo onset of left ventricular hypertrophy may occur in midlife.
- No antiarrhythmic therapy in asymptomatic HCM with high risk of SCD
- Intense competitive sports, strenuous exercise, and heavy lifting should be restricted because of high risk of SCD.

IDIOPATHIC THROMBOCYTOPENIC PURPURA (ITP)

Saurabh Sharma, MD

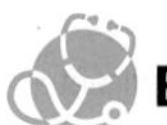

BASICS

DESCRIPTION

- Decrease in circulating number of platelets (<100,000) in absence of toxic exposure or disease associated with low platelet count
- Occurs as secondary effect of peripheral platelet destruction as well as decreased platelet production
- Diagnosis of exclusion
- Acute idiopathic thrombocytopenic purpura (ITP): Relatively common disease of childhood that often follows acute infection and has spontaneous resolution within 2 months; platelet counts <20,000
- Chronic ITP: Persists after 12 months without a specific cause; usually seen in adults and persists for months to years; platelet count typically 30,000–80,000. Spontaneous remission is rare in adults (9% in 1 series) (1).
- System(s) affected: Heme, Lymphatic, Immunologic
- Synonym(s): Postinfectious thrombocytopenia; Immune thrombocytopenic purpura; Werlhof disease

EPIDEMIOLOGY

- Predominant age:
  - Acute ITP (primarily a childhood disease): 2–6 years
  - Chronic ITP: >50 years
  - Uncommon in geriatric population; look for other cause of low platelet count
- Predominant gender:
  - Acute ITP: Male = Female
  - Chronic ITP: Female > Male (2:1)

Incidence

- Total incidence is >22 cases per million population per year
- Estimates from recent meta-analysis are 1.9–6.4 per 100,000 children/year and 3.3 per 100,000 adults/year (2)

Prevalence

- Due to its chronic nature, prevalence exceeds incidence
- Prevalence estimate in the US ~100 cases per million population

RISK FACTORS

- Acute infection
- Age (see "Epidemiology")
- Cardiopulmonary bypass
- Hypersplenism
- Antiphospholipid antibody syndrome
- Preeclampsia
- HIV infection

Genetics

No known genetic pattern

GENERAL PREVENTION

The patient should avoid medications (when feasible) that inhibit platelet function (such as aspirin) or those that suppress bone marrow.

PATHOPHYSIOLOGY

- IgG autoantibodies on platelet surface cause platelet uptake and destruction by reticuloendothelial phagocytes.
- There is also believed to be inhibition of megakaryocyte platelet production by specific IgG autoantibodies.

COMMONLY ASSOCIATED CONDITIONS

- Acute ITP:
  - Varicella, other viral infections (Epstein-Barr virus, cytomegalovirus)
- Chronic ITP:
  - HIV, *Helicobacter pylori*, hepatitis C
  - Graves disease, Hashimoto thyroiditis
  - Sarcoidosis
  - Systemic lupus erythematosus
- Autoimmune hemolytic anemia (Evans syndrome)

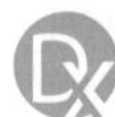

DIAGNOSIS

Diagnosis of exclusion; rule out other causes (infection, drugs, malignancy)

HISTORY

- Post-traumatic bleeding at 40,000–60,000 platelet count
- Bruising tendency, gingival bleeding, recurrent epistaxis
- GI bleeding
- Menometrorrhagia, menorrhagia
- Neurologic symptoms secondary to intracerebral bleeding
- Spontaneous bleeding may occur with platelet count <20,000.
- No constitutional symptoms (e.g., night sweats, bone pain, significant weight loss)

PHYSICAL EXAM

- Petechial hemorrhages, purpura
- Mucocutaneous hemorrhages
- No hepatosplenomegaly, lymphadenopathy, or stigmata of congenital disease (absence of splenomegaly is essential diagnostic criterion)

DIAGNOSTIC TESTS & INTERPRETATION

Lab

Initial lab tests

- CBC with differential, peripheral smear, bleeding time, PT, aPTT
- Decreased platelet count: Typical range of 5,000–75,000
- Relative lymphocytosis and slight eosinophilia
- Prolonged bleeding time (not useful in presence of thrombocytopenia)
- Prothrombin time/partial thromboplastin time normal

Follow-Up & Special Considerations

Platelet-associated antibody (PA-IgG): Bound test is superior: Sn 55%, Sp 83%:

- False-negative and false-positive results limit utility
- Not necessary for treatment decisions

Diagnostic Procedures/Surgery

- Bone marrow aspiration/biopsy (consider in refractory cases):
  - With classic ITP, marrow cellularity is normal; may see increase in megakaryocytes
  - Does not need to be done before giving γ-globulin
  - Not needed in patients <60 years who have typical clinical and lab presentation
- Consider in patients >60 years to rule out myelodysplasia
- Rarely indicated in children

Pathological Findings

- Peripheral smear:
  - Normal red and white cells with large platelets but diminished in number
  - Helps rule out pseudothrombocytopenia
- Marrow reveals abundant megakaryocytes with normal erythroid and myeloid precursors.

DIFFERENTIAL DIAGNOSIS

- Drug-induced immune thrombocytopenia: >150 drugs have been implicated
- Infections
- Acute leukemia
- Thrombotic thrombocytopenia purpura
- Hemolytic uremic syndrome
- Factitious: Platelet clumping on the peripheral smear
- Thrombocytopenia secondary to sepsis
- Myelodysplastic syndrome, particularly in older patients
- Decreased production in marrow: Malignancy, drugs, viruses, megaloblastic anemia
- Posttransfusion
- Gestational thrombocytopenia
- Isoimmune neonatal purpura
- Congenital thrombocytopenias
- Disseminated intravascular coagulation
- Alcohol-induced thrombocytopenic purpura

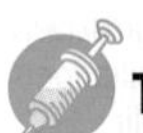

TREATMENT

MEDICATION

First Line

- Acute ITP: Oral prednisone 1–2 mg/kg/d for 2–4 weeks, then taper
- Chronic ITP (3):
  - Oral prednisone 1–2 mg/kg/d with tapers over 4–6 weeks; most responses occur within first week of treatment (4)[B]
  - Optimal duration of therapy unknown, but increased risk of complications if >2 months
  - Therapy does not appear to modify the natural history.
  - For patients who do not respond, consider IVIg 0.4 g/kg/d for 5 days, or anti-D, 50–75 μg/kg once (repeat as necessary), or dexamethasone 20–40 mg/d for 4 days; 3–4 cycles 2 weeks apart (4)[C]. Anti-D can only be used if patient is Rh+ and have not had splenectomy. It has FDA warning for severe hemolysis. Don't give in patients with bleeding causing decline in Hb or with evidence of autoimmune hemolysis.
  - If no response to these therapies, consider rituximab or splenectomy.
  - Also limited data supporting screening for and eradication of *H. pylori*
- Emergency treatment of patients with internal or mucocutaneous bleeding or who need emergent surgery treatment should include:
  - IVIg 1 g/kg/d for 2 days; can be repeated on day 3 for nonresponders
  - IV methylprednisolone 1 g/d for 3 days
  - Platelet transfusions (5 U q4–6h or 2 U/hr)
- Contraindications: Do not administer γ-globulin if patient has IgA deficiency.
- Other adverse events with IVIg include fever and renal failure.
- Possible interactions: Anaphylaxis in patients with IgA deficiency who have IgA autoantibodies

Second Line

- Acute ITP: IVIg (γ-globulin):
  - Single dose (1–2 g/kg) or 400 mg/kg/d for 5 days
  - Minor adverse reactions: Chills, nausea, headache, and joint pain may occur in 2–7% of the patients. If so, slow the rate of infusion.
  - γ-globulin may be effective alone or as pretreatment to facilitate platelet transfusion. This treatment may delay the need for a splenectomy.
- Chronic ITP: High doses of IV γ-globulin in emergencies (studies used platelet counts as surrogate marker and not bleeding outcomes)
- Anti-Rho(D) immunoglobulin 250 IU (50–75 μg/kg) as single dose or in 2 divided doses given over 2 days; indications for use:
  - Children with acute or chronic ITP
  - Adults with chronic ITP who are not antiglobulin (Coombs) test positive (otherwise are at risk for intravascular hemolysis)
  - ITP secondary to HIV infection
- Azathioprine: 1–4 mg/kg/d modified according to white blood cells
- Cyclophosphamide: 1–2 mg/kg/d
- Vincristine or vinblastine 2 mg IV/weekly
- Danazol: 400–800 mg/d
- Cyclosporin A: 3 mg/kg/d
- Rituximab 375 mg/m^2 weekly for 4 weeks (4)
- Mycophenolate mofetil
- Thrombopoietin receptor (C MPL)-agonists (stimulate thrombopoiesis): Both are FDA-approved for refractory ITP in adults. Studies are ongoing, but there are no published data to guide the use of these agents in children:
  - Eltrombopag (50 mg PO daily)
  - Romiplostim (1 mcg/kg SC weekly) (4,5)

ADDITIONAL TREATMENT

General Measures

- Outpatient management unless patient at risk for bleeding (platelet count <20,000)
- Admit patients with active bleeding.
- For children:
  - No treatment required if platelet count >30,000 and asymptomatic or for minor purpura
  - A single dose of IVIg (0.8–1 g/kg) or short course of corticosteroids should be used as first-line treatment. There is no evidence for longer course.
  - IVIg should be used instead of corticosteroids if rapid increase of platelet count is needed.
  - Anti-D may be considered for first-line therapy in Rh+ nonsplenectomized children with recognition of risks outlined above.
- For adults:
  - Consider treatment for patients with platelet count <30,000
  - Consider treatment for platelet count <50,000 with symptoms or risks for bleeding, such as hypertension or peptic ulcers
  - Longer courses of corticosteroids preferred over shorter courses.
  - IVIg may be used in conjunction with corticosteroids if rapid increase in platelet count is required.
- Specific treatment usually not necessary unless count <100,000; possibly <30,000 with chronic ITP
- Platelet transfusions for significant bleeding

Issues for Referral

Hematology consultation recommended for acute bleeding or who fail to respond to first-line therapies

SURGERY/OTHER PROCEDURES

Splenectomy:

- Reserved only for patients who fail medical therapy
- Patients should receive 23-valent pneumococcal vaccine and *Haemophilus influenza b (HIB)* at least 2 weeks prior to splenectomy; also should receive meningococcal group C conjugate vaccine if not previously immunized.
- Consider lifelong prophylactic antibiotics with penicillin or erythromycin.
- Criteria and timing of surgery remain poorly defined; decision based on severity, response to treatment, and patient preference regarding risks–benefits of surgery.
- Splenectomy considered if after 3–6 months patient needs >10–20 mg/d prednisone to keep platelets above 30,000/mm^3
- Should raise the platelet count to at least 20,000/mm^3 prior to surgery
- Reported 5–10-year efficacy is ~65% for all patients (4)
- Laparoscopic removal is becoming preferred technique

Pregnancy Considerations

- Dx if <50,000 platelet count: May consider caesarean section
- A patient in labor should receive IV γ-globulin due to the risk to the infant.
- Platelet autoantibodies cross the placenta and may cause neonatal thrombocytopenia. Consider prednisone 10–20 mg/d for 10–14 days prior to delivery.
- Preeclampsia or gestational thrombocytopenia may cause thrombocytopenia unrelated to ITP.

ONGOING CARE

FOLLOW-UP RECOMMENDATIONS

Patient Monitoring

Platelet counts weekly for patients on prednisone, monthly for stable patients

PATIENT EDUCATION

- Minimal activity to prevent injury or bruising, avoid contact sports.
- Avoid ASA and other platelet-inhibiting drugs.

PROGNOSIS

- Acute ITP:
  - ~80–85% of the patients completely recover within 2 months.
  - 15% proceed to chronic ITP
- Chronic ITP:
  - ~10–20% of the patients recover spontaneously.
  - Remainder with diminished platelets for months to years
  - May see spontaneous remissions (5%) and relapses
- ~10% are refractory (fail medical therapy and splenectomy)
- Chronic refractory ITP: Thrombocytopenia present for >3 months, failure to respond to splenectomy, platelet count of <50,000

COMPLICATIONS

- 1% mortality due to intracranial hemorrhage
- Severe blood loss
- Corticosteroid adverse effects
- Pneumococcal sepsis (if patient undergoes splenectomy)
- Better prognosis in children than adults

REFERENCES

1. Fogarty PF, et al. Chronic immune thrombocytopenia in adults: Epidemiology and clinical presentation. *Hematol Oncol Clin North Am*. 2009;23:1213–21.
2. Terrell DR, Beebe LA, Vesely SK, et al. The incidence of immune thrombocytopenic purpura in children and adults: A critical review of published reports. *Am J Hematol*. 2010;85:174–80.
3. Neunert C, Lim W, Crowtha M, et al. The American Society of Hematology 2011 evidence-based practice guideline for immune thrombocytopenia. *Blood*. 2011;117(16):4190–207.
4. Bussel JB, et al. Traditional and new approaches to the management of immune thrombocytopenia: Issues of when and who to treat. *Hematol Oncol Clin North Am*. 2009;23:1329–41.
5. Tarantino MD. The treatment of immune thrombocytopenic purpura in children. *Curr Hematol Rep*. 2006;5:89–94.

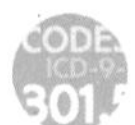

CODES

ICD9

287.31 Immune thrombocytopenic purpura

CLINICAL PEARLS

- Acute ITP: Relatively common disease of childhood that often follows acute infection and has spontaneous resolution within 2 months; platelet counts <20,000
- Chronic ITP: Persists after 12 months without a specific cause; usually seen in adults and persists for months to years; platelet count typically 30,000–80,000. Spontaneous remission is rare in adults.
- For acute ITP: Oral prednisone 1–2 mg/kg/d for 2–4 weeks, then taper
- For chronic ITP: Oral prednisone 1–2 mg/kg/d with tapers over 4–6 weeks

IgA NEPHROPATHY

Matthew R. Lawler, MD
Jahan Montague, MD

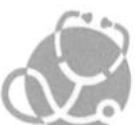

BASICS

DESCRIPTION

- First reported by Dr. J. Berger in 1968 as Berger disease
- Most common form of glomerulonephritis in the world
- Renal parenchymal damage and dysfunction are defined by predominant deposition of IgA in glomerular mesangium.
- Significant contributor to the incidence of end-stage renal disease (ESRD) in parts of Asia

EPIDEMIOLOGY

Incidence

In patients undergoing renal biopsy, the following incidence rates are reported: 30–40% in Asia, 15–20% in Europe, and 5–10% in North America.

Prevalence

- Highest prevalence in Pacific Rim, particularly Japan and Korea
- More common in Asians, whites, and American Indians vs. blacks in the US and Africa

RISK FACTORS

- Cirrhosis or advanced liver disease: Impaired removal of IgA by Kupffer cells in the liver predisposes individuals to IgA deposition in the kidney.
- Celiac disease: Ingestion of gliadin results in the formation of IgA antigliadin antibodies and deposition of immune complexes in the kidney.

Genetics

- Familial forms of IgA nephropathy (IgAN) exist
- No gene identified to date

PATHOPHYSIOLOGY

- Dimeric and polymeric forms of circulating IgA1 molecules deposit within the mesangium of the glomerulus.
- IgA deposition leads to an inflammatory reaction with neutrophilic infiltration, mesangial hypercellularity, and expansion.
- In proliferative forms of IgAN, diffuse endocapillary proliferation, fibrinoid necrosis, and epithelial cell crescents can be seen.
- The mechanisms of subsequent renal injury are similar to those seen in other forms of chronic glomerulonephritis.

ETIOLOGY

- Autoimmune in nature
- Aberrant O-glycosylation of IgA1 molecules has been implicated widely.
- Elevated levels of secretory IgA have also been studied, but a definitive link has not been established.

COMMONLY ASSOCIATED CONDITIONS

- Henoch-Schönlein purpura
- Hepatic failure
- Celiac disease
- Rheumatoid arthritis
- Ankylosing spondylitis
- Reiter syndrome
- HIV
- CMV

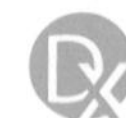

DIAGNOSIS

HISTORY

- Painless recurrent episodes of macroscopic hematuria concurrent to or immediately after viral pharyngitis (so called "synpharyngitic hematuria"); gastroenteritis is the presenting feature in 40–50% of cases
- Occasionally low-grade fever and flank pain accompanies hematuria.

PHYSICAL EXAM

- Hypertension
- Edema is common in patients with nephrotic syndrome.
- Rash seen in patients with Henoch-Schönlein purpura.
- Classically presents with palpable purpura in the lower extremity.

DIAGNOSTIC TESTS & INTERPRETATION

Lab

Initial lab tests

- Serum BUN and creatinine to evaluate for acute renal failure (<5% of cases)
- Complement levels should be normal
- Urinalysis for proteinuria and hematuria
- Urine microscopy to evaluate for dysmorphic RBCs and RBC casts
- Spot urine protein: Creatinine ratio or 24-hour urine protein

Imaging

Initial approach

- CT scan: To rule out nephrolithiasis or other possible causes of obstruction in a patient with painful hematuria or acute renal failure
- CT scan and cystoscopy: Useful in a setting of hematuria in middle-aged and elderly patients to rule out urologic malignancy
- Imaging is low yield for the workup of recurrent painless macroscopic hematuria in adolescent or young adult patients.

Follow-Up & Special Considerations

Imaging studies should be used during the initial approach if clinical concern for obstruction or malignancy exists.

Diagnostic Procedures/Surgery

Renal biopsy is the gold standard and currently is the only definitive method for the diagnosis IgAN.

Pathological Findings

- Light microscopy: Variable, nonspecific findings ranging from mesangial cell proliferation and expansion to crescentic or chronic sclerosing glomerulonephritis patterns
- Immunofluorescence microscopy: Pathognomonic finding of dominant or codominant IgA deposits in a diffuse pattern within the mesangium, often with paramesangial and subendothelial infiltration; IgG, IgM, C3, k, or l light chains may be codeposited.
- Electron microscopy: Electron-dense deposits are present in the mesangium.

DIFFERENTIAL DIAGNOSIS

- Thin basement membrane disease
- Alport syndrome
- Lupus nephritis
- Postinfectious glomerulonephritis
- Nephrolithiasis
- Urinary tract malignancy

TREATMENT

MEDICATION

First Line

- Use ACE inhibitor or angiotensin receptor blocker (ARB) to achieve BP target of 125/75 mm Hg and decrease proteinuria to <0.5 g/d (1)[A].
- In patients who continue to have sustained proteinuria >1 g/d despite maximal renin-angiotensin system (RAS) blockade and optimal BP control and have minor to moderate histologic lesions on biopsy, pulse or oral corticosteroid treatment should be considered in addition to continued RAS blockade (2,3)[B].
- Cyclophosphamide in combination with steroids has been shown to improve renal survival in patients with crescentic forms of IgAN on renal biopsy (4)[B].
- Oral prednisone (1 mg/kg/d for 30 days, tapered by 10 mg per month; all patients to be on 10 mg/d by 6 months); cyclophosphamide (monthly IV 0.5 mg/kg for 6 months)

Second Line

- Omega-3 fatty acids in large doses (12 g/d) may be beneficial in preserving renal function (5)[B].
- Tonsillectomy may be beneficial in patients whose IgA nephropathy symptoms are secondary to recurrent tonsillitis (6)[C].

ADDITIONAL TREATMENT

Issues for Referral

Persistent hematuria, persistent proteinuria, clinical features of nephrotic syndrome, and laboratory evidence of acute or chronic renal failure should prompt a referral to a nephrologist for diagnosis and management.

Additional Therapies

Lipid lowering therapies: All patients with chronic kidney disease (CKD) and dyslipidemia should be managed with a statin for cardiovascular risk reduction. This therapy also has been shown to slow the progression of renal disease.

SURGERY/OTHER PROCEDURES

In patients with advanced CKD requiring renal replacement, dialysis access placement and renal transplant may be scheduled.

IN-PATIENT CONSIDERATIONS

Admission Criteria

Acute kidney injury or complications related to CKD may prompt hospital admission for optimization of fluid status and management of metabolic derangements.

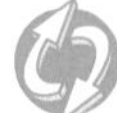

ONGOING CARE

FOLLOW-UP RECOMMENDATIONS

- Patients with mild proteinuria (<500 mg/d), normal renal function, and normal BP may be treated conservatively with regular follow-up at 6-month intervals.
- Patients with more aggressive disease characterized by persistent hematuria, high-grade proteinuria, difficult-to-control hypertension, or advanced CKD will require closer monitoring.

Patient Monitoring

- Pressure
- Serum electrolytes
- Serum creatinine
- Urine microscopic to evaluate disease activity
- Quantification of urine protein
- Repeat renal biopsy for histologic monitoring in patients with signs of progressive disease

DIET

In patients with advanced CKD, a renal diet consisting of fluid restriction, low protein, low potassium, low sodium, and low phosphorus should be followed.

PATIENT EDUCATION

In patients approaching ESRD, a nephrologist or nurse should educate the patient regarding options for dialysis and renal transplant.

PROGNOSIS

- Hypertension, proteinuria >1 g/d, male gender, elevated serum creatinine at diagnosis, and persistent microscopic hematuria (>6 months) are risk factors for progressive disease.
- Histologic findings including tubular dropout, interstitial fibrosis, and fibrous or cellular crescents are associated with a worse prognosis.
- <10% of all patients with IgAN have complete resolution of urinary abnormalities.
- 25–30% of patients will require renal replacement therapy (RRT; dialysis, transplant, etc.) within 20–25 years of presentation; 1.5% of patients with IgAN are calculated to reach ESRD per year (7)

COMPLICATIONS

- Progressive IgAN may lead to ESRD and necessitate RRT
- 5 years after renal transplant there is a 5% risk of graft failure secondary to a reoccurrence of IgAN (7).

REFERENCES

1. Cheng J, et al. ACEI/ARB therapy for IgA nephropathy: A meta analysis of randomized controlled trials. *Int J Clin Pract*. 2009;63(6): 880–8.
2. Cheng J, et al. Efficacy and safety of glucocorticoids therapy for IgA nephropathy: A meta-analysis of randomized controlled trials. *Am J Nephrol*. 2009; 30:315–22.
3. Manno C, et al. Randomized controlled clinical trial of corticosteroids plus ACE-inhibitors with long-term follow-up in proteinuric IgA nephropathy. *Nephrol Dial Transplant*. 2009;24:3694–701.
4. Tumlin J, et al. Crescentic, proliferative IgA nephropathy: Clinical and histological response to methylprednisolone and intravenous cyclophosphamide. *Nephrol Dial Transplant*. 2003;18:1321–9.
5. Donadio J, et al. A controlled trial of fish oil in IgA nephropathy. *NEJM*. 1994;331:1194–9.
6. Xie Y, et al. Relationship between tonsils and IgA nephropathy as well as indications of tonsillectomy. *Kidney International* 2004;65:1135–44.
7. Barratt J, Feehally J. IgA nephropathy. *J Am Soc Nephrol*. 2005;16:2088–97.

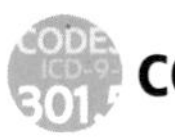

CODES

ICD9

583.89 Nephritis and nephropathy, not specified as acute or chronic, with other specified pathological lesion in kidney

CLINICAL PEARLS

- IgAN is a generally benign glomerulonephritis and is the most common cause of glomerulonephritis in the world; displays slow progression to ESRD.
- Persistent microscopic hematuria, moderate to severe proteinuria, and high-grade lesions on renal biopsy are risk factors for progressive disease.
- Renal biopsy is the only method of definitive diagnosis.
- Control of proteinuria and hypertension via RAS blockade with ACE inhibitors and/or ARBs are the mainstays of first-line therapy.

IMMUNODEFICIENCY DISEASES

Weily Soong, MD

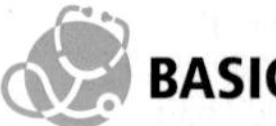

BASICS

DESCRIPTION

- Disorders caused by abnormal immune system function, resulting in increased susceptibility to infection
- Primary: An intrinsic defect in the immune mechanism:
  - Humoral (B-cell) immunodeficiencies:
    - Defects in antibody production
    - Agammaglobulinemia: X-linked (absent immunoglobulins; mutation in Bruton tyrosine kinase gene) and autosomal recessive (absent immunoglobulins [Ig]; defect in B-cell development)
    - IgA deficiency: Most common primary immunodeficiency; very low or absent IgA; defect unknown
    - Common variable immunodeficiency: Decreased levels of IgG, IgA, and/or IgM and poor responses to vaccinations; usually adult onset; genetic defects are known in a small percentage of cases
    - IgG subclass deficiency: Decrease in IgG subclasses; defect and clinical significance are unknown
    - Specific antibody deficiency: Poor antibody response to specific antigens; defect unknown
    - Transient hypogammaglobulinemia of infancy: Temporary decrease in IgG and IgA due to delayed maturation of the humoral system; unknown cause
    - Others: Includes Ig κ chain defects; Ig heavy chain gene deletions; defects in UNG and ICOS genes; NEMO
  - Combined immunodeficiencies:
    - Defects in the cellular effector (T- and B-lymphocytes and natural killer [NK] cells) and humoral mechanisms
    - Severe combined immunodeficiency (SCID): All forms have absent T cells, and depending on the genetic mutation, may or may not have B cells and NK-cells; X-linked or autosomal recessive; includes mutations in adenosine deaminase deficiency gene, common interleukin γ chain, *Jak3*, *CD45*, *RAG1*, and *RAG2* genes
    - Hyper-IgM syndrome: Normal to high IgM with low IgG and IgA; X-linked; defect in CD40 ligand and has features of a combined immunodeficiency; autosomal recessive; defect in *AID* gene and has features of a humoral immunodeficiency
    - Wiskott-Aldrich syndrome (WAS): X-linked; eczema, thrombocytopenia, repeated infections, decrease in T cells
    - Ataxia telangiectasia (A-T): Cerebellar ataxia, oculocutaneous telangiectasia, and cellular and humoral immunodeficiency; autosomal recessive
    - Omenn syndrome: Erythroderma, eosinophilia, hepatosplenomegaly, increased IgE; autosomal recessive
    - Purine nucleoside phosphorylase (PNP) deficiency: Severe lymphopenia, especially T cells; hemolytic anemia; neurologic abnormalities; autosomal recessive
    - Others: Includes ZAP70 and CD40 defects
  - Phagocytic immunodeficiencies:
    - Chronic granulomatous disease: Mutations in the oxidative burst mechanism of neutrophils; X-linked and autosomal-recessive variants
    - Chediak-Higashi syndrome: Mutations in lysosomal transport protein; albinism and neurologic symptoms; autosomal recessive
    - Leukocyte adhesion deficiency: Defects in leukocyte endothelial adherence and chemotaxis; autosomal recessive
    - Other: Cyclic neutropenia, glucose-6-phosphate dehydrogenase (G-6PD) deficiency, myeloperoxidase deficiency
  - Complement deficiencies; usually autosomal recessive:
    - Early complement (C1q, C1r, C2, C4); cause autoimmune diseases, such as lupus
    - Late complement (C5–C9); susceptible to recurrent neisserial infections and autoimmune diseases
    - C3 and mannose-binding lectin deficiency; susceptible to recurrent pyogenic infections
  - Pure cellular deficiencies and other well-defined syndromes:
    - DiGeorge syndrome: Thymic hypoplasia; decrease in T cells; associated with 22q11.2 chromosome deletions; de novo mutation or autosomal dominant
    - X-linked lymphoproliferative syndrome: Causes fatal infectious mononucleosis
    - Chronic mucocutaneous candidiasis or autoimmune polyglandular syndrome type 1: Mutations in the autoimmune regulator *AIRE* gene; causes autoimmune responses to endocrine tissues; autosomal recessive
    - Hyper-IgE syndrome (Job syndrome): Hgh IgE, chronic dermatitis, and recurrent infections; caused by gene mutation in stat3
    - Autoinflammatory disorders: Recurrent fevers (familial Mediterranean fever, Muckle-Wells, familial cold urticaria; autosomal recessive or dominant)
    - WHIM syndrome: Associated with warts, hypogammaglobulinemia, infection, myelokathexis (retention of leukocytes in the bone marrow); autosomal dominant
    - Autoimmune lymphoproliferative syndrome (ALPS): Defects in apoptosis; adenopathy, autoimmune cytopenias; autosomal recessive
- Secondary: A result of a secondary process, like another illness, age, injury, or treatment:
  - Premature and newborn
  - Hereditary and metabolic diseases:
    - Chromosomal abnormalities (Down syndrome) and sickle cell disease
    - Diabetes mellitus
    - Uremia and nephrotic syndrome
    - Malnutrition, vitamin, and mineral deficiencies; protein-losing enteropathies (1)
  - Medications: Immunosuppressive drugs, such as corticosteroids, immune modulators, radiation, chemotherapy; phenytoin
  - Infections: Includes HIV and mononucleosis
  - Infiltrative and hematological diseases: Includes sarcoidosis, leukemias, lymphomas, myeloma, aplastic anemia
  - Surgery and trauma: Burns, splenectomy
  - Other: Lupus and other autoimmune diseases, chronic hepatitis, cirrhosis, aging, thymoma, chronic stress

EPIDEMIOLOGY

Incidence

- Secondary immunodeficiencies are more common than primary.
- Children are most likely to present with primary immunodeficiencies.
- Primary immunodeficiencies occur in 1 in 10,000 births to 1 in 2,000 births:
  - 65% humoral deficiencies, 15% combined deficiencies, 10% phagocytic deficiencies, 5% cellular deficiencies, 5% complement deficiencies
- Infectious complications: In primary humoral disorders, they usually appear after 6 months of age. In cellular or combined disorders, they may appear shortly after birth.
- IgA deficiency is the most common primary immunodeficiency (~1 of every 500 people):
  - Patients may have poor response to antipneumococcal vaccines and a higher incidence of respiratory infections.
- Common variable immunodeficiency affects 1 in 30,000–50,000 people and usually appears during early adulthood.

RISK FACTORS

For secondary deficiencies: Depends on the etiology

Genetics

Primary: Inherited genetic defect (see "Description")

GENERAL PREVENTION

- For primary deficiencies: Goal is to avert infection by identification of at-risk newborns using genetic screening/counseling and prenatal diagnostic tests.
- For secondary deficiencies: Depends on the etiology

DIAGNOSIS

HISTORY

- A thorough personal history and family history will direct the proper search for a differential diagnosis.
- 10 warning signs suggestive of possible primary immunodeficiency (according to the Modell Foundation):
  - ≥8 new ear infections within 1 year
  - ≥2 serious sinus infections within 1 year
  - ≥2 months on antibiotics with little effect
  - ≥2 pneumonias within 1 year
  - Failure of an infant to gain weight or grow normally
  - Recurrent, deep skin or organ abscesses
  - Persistent thrush in mouth or elsewhere on skin after age 1 year
  - Need for IV antibiotics to clear infections
  - ≥2 deep-seated infections
  - A family history of primary immunodeficiency
- Unusual susceptibility to infection; type of infection might help to determine the type of immunodeficiency:
  - Humoral deficiencies:
    - Associated with bacterial and protozoan infections (e.g., chronic sinusitis, recurrent respiratory infection, chronic diarrheal disease)
    - Infections include *Streptococcus pneumoniae*, *Haemophilus influenzae*, *Staphylococcus aureus*, *Pseudomonas aeruginosa*, mycoplasma, enteroviruses, *Giardia*

- Combined deficiencies:
  - Associated with severe fungal, bacterial, protozoal, and viral infections
  - Infections include all viral infections; bacterial infections found in humoral deficiencies plus *Listeria* and *Salmonella*, enteric flora; mycobacteria; *Candida*; *Pneumocystis*; *Toxoplasma*; *Cryptococcus*
- Cellular deficiencies:
  - Associated with severe viral, mycobacterial, and fungal infections
  - Infections include *Salmonella*, *Mycobacteria*, and *Candida*
- Phagocytic defects:
  - Infections include *S. aureus*, enteric flora, *Serratia*, *Nocardia*, *P. aeruginosa*, *Salmonella typhi*, *Aspergillus fumigatus*, *Candida albicans*, *Pneumocystis*; *Mycobacteria*
- Complement deficiencies:
  - Infections include bacterial infections found in humoral deficiencies, especially *Neisseria meningitidis*

- Also associated with autoimmune disorders and malignancies, especially lymphoreticular

PHYSICAL EXAM
Physical exam may provide clues to correct diagnosis by allowing detection of subtle dysmorphology and site and type of infection.

DIAGNOSTIC TESTS & INTERPRETATION
Lab
Initial lab tests

High percentage of immunodeficiencies will be discovered by:

- CBC with differential smear. Normal total lymphocyte count in infants is higher than adults. Thus, a lymphocyte count of $<3{,}000/mm^3$ should be evaluated for an immunodeficiency (2).
- Serum protein electrophoresis for immunoglobulin levels, including IgG, IgA, IgM, and IgE; may include IgG subclasses. (Levels must be adjusted for age. Adults have higher levels than children.)
- Antibody responses to previous vaccines (tetanus, *Pneumococcus*, *H. influenzae*, diphtheria, varicella, pertussis)
- Infection evaluation, such as ESR, C-reactive protein, microbiology cultures
- Classical complement pathway test: CH50

Follow-Up & Special Considerations

These labs might be drawn depending on the history and initial labs:

- Flow cytometry to examine lymphocyte subsets (CD4, CD8, CD3, CD19, CD20)
- Lymphocyte proliferation responses to mitogens and antigens
- Specific complement levels
- Delayed hypersensitivity skin tests (anergy panel to mumps, *Candida*, tetanus, *Trichophyton*)
- Phagocyte function: Nitroblue-tetrazolium (NBT) test, dihydrorhodamine reductase test
- Specific cytokine function tests
- Genetic analysis

Imaging
Initial approach

Chest x-ray (CXR) of a newborn infant to look for an absence of a thymic shadow in SCID or DiGeorge

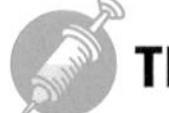

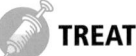

TREATMENT

MEDICATION
First Line
- Antibiotics with appropriate spectra for infecting organism(s):
  - May be used acutely, chronically, or prophylactically
- Antiviral therapy for HIV, varicella, herpes, influenza, and respiratory syncytial virus (RSV)
- Antifungal agents for specific fungal infections
- IV or SC Ig:
  - For diseases deficient in IgG, such as agammaglobulinemias, common variable, hyper-IgM, WAS, and A-T (3)[A]
  - Should *not* be used for IgG subclass deficiency
  - Periodic problems with the supply of the drug due to high demand
  - Enzyme replacement therapy for adenosine deaminase deficiency
  - For secondary immunodeficiencies, treatment depends on the specific etiology.

ADDITIONAL TREATMENT
General Measures
- If newborn has been identified as being at risk, consider cord blood storage for stem cell transplants, appropriate labs and genetic tests, and potential for isolation in sterile environment.
- If patient with cellular or combined defects must be transfused, must use irradiated and CMV-negative blood products.
- Avoid all live attenuated viral vaccines in patients with severe cellular or antibody immunodeficiencies (varicella, oral polio, measles, mumps, rubella, smallpox, Bacille Calmette-Guérin [BCG]).
- Bone marrow, stem cell, or thymic transplants for certain immunodeficiencies (e.g., SCID and DiGeorge) are best done at referral research centers.

Issues for Referral
Primary immunodeficiency patients should be referred to a physician specializing in allergy and clinical immunology for workup and management of immunodeficiency diseases.

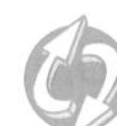

ONGOING CARE

FOLLOW-UP RECOMMENDATIONS
Patient Monitoring
- Monitor for infections and their complications.
- Infection control precautions: Depends on the situation and includes frequent hand washing, gloves, gowns, masks, safe water supply
- Monitor and maintain IgG levels in common variable hypogammaglobulinemia.

PATIENT EDUCATION
- Immune Deficiency Foundation, 25 West Chesapeake Ave. Room 206, Towson, MD 21204. Tel: 800-296-4433. www.primaryimmune.org.
- Jeffrey Modell Foundation, 747 3rd Avenue, New York, NY 10017. Tel: 212-819-0200. www.info4pi.org and www.jmfworld.com.

PROGNOSIS
- Short-term prognosis is related closely to the severity of the infectious complication.
- Long-term prognosis is related to the nature of the immune defect and the type and degree of immunodeficiency.

COMPLICATIONS
- Autoimmune disorders
- Reactions to immunoglobulin treatment
- Malignancies, especially lymphoreticular
- Overwhelming infection
- Fatal graft-versus-host disease following blood transfusions in patients with SCID

REFERENCES

1. Chinen J, Shearer WT, et al. Secondary immunodeficiencies, including HIV infection. *J Allergy Clin Immunol*. 2010;125:S195–203.
2. Oliveira JB, Fleisher TA, et al. Laboratory evaluation of primary immunodeficiencies. *J Allergy Clin Immunol*. 2010;125:S297–305.
3. Ballow M. Primary immunodeficiency disorders: Antibody deficiency. *J Allergy Clin Immunol*. 2002;109:581–91.

ADDITIONAL READING

- Carr TF, Koterba AP, Chandra R, et al. Characterization of specific antibody deficiency in adults with medically refractory chronic rhinosinusitis. *Am J Rhinol Allergy*. 2011;25:241–4.
- Jorgensen GH, Arnlaugsson S, Theodors A, et al. Immunoglobulin A deficiency and oral health status: A case-control study. *J Clin Periodontol*. 2010;37:1–8.
- Notarangelo LD, et al. Primary immunodeficiencies. *J Allergy Clin Immunol*. 2010;125:S182–94.

CODES

ICD9
- 279.00 Hypogammaglobulinemia, unspecified
- 279.01 Selective IgA immunodeficiency
- 279.3 Unspecified immunity deficiency

CLINICAL PEARLS
- Secondary causes of immunodeficiencies are more common than primary immunodeficiencies.
- If there is a history of any recurrent or unresolved infections, check IgG level. It is easy and inexpensive, and it probably is more useful than repeating other labs, such as a CBC.
- Consult a clinical immunologist if an immunodeficiency is suspected.

IMPETIGO

Elisabeth L. Backer, MD

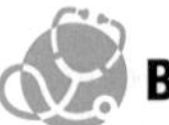

BASICS

DESCRIPTION

- A contagious, superficial, intraepidermal infection occurring prominently on exposed areas of the face and extremities.
- Infected patients usually have multiple lesions.
- Cultures positive in >80% cases for *Staphylococcus aureus* either alone or combined with group A β-hemolytic streptococci; *S. aureus* more common pathogen since 1990s
- Nonbullous impetigo: Most common form of impetigo. Formation of vesiculopustules that rupture, leading to crusting with a characteristic golden appearance; local lymphadenopathy may occur.
- Bullous impetigo: Staphylococcal impetigo that progresses rapidly to small-to-large flaccid bullae (newborns/young children) caused by epidermolytic toxin release; less lymphadenopathy; <30% of patients
- Folliculitis: Considered by some to be *S. aureus* impetigo of hair follicles
- Ecthyma: A deeper, ulcerated impetigo infection often with lymphadenitis
- System(s) affected: Skin/Exocrine
- Synonym(s): Pyoderma; Impetigo contagiosa; Impetigo vulgaris; Fox impetigo

EPIDEMIOLOGY

Incidence

- Predominant sex: Male = Female
- Predominant age: Children ages 2–5 years

Prevalence

In the US: Unreported

Pediatric Considerations

- Poststreptococcal glomerulonephritis may follow impetigo (in young children).
- Impetigo neonatorum may occur due to nursery contamination.

RISK FACTORS

- Warm, humid environment
- Tropical or subtropical climate
- Summer or fall season
- Minor trauma, insect bites
- Poor hygiene, poverty, crowding, epidemics, wartime
- Familial spread
- Poor health with anemia and malnutrition
- Complication of pediculosis, scabies, chickenpox, eczema/atopic dermatitis
- Contact dermatitis (Rhus)
- Burns
- Contact sports
- Children in daycare
- Possibly tobacco exposure
- Carriage of group A *Streptococcus* and *S. aureus*

GENERAL PREVENTION

- Close attention to family hygiene, particularly hand washing among children
- Covering of wounds
- Avoidance of crowding and sharing of personal items
- Treatment of atopic dermatitis

ETIOLOGY

- Coagulase-positive staphylococci: Pure culture ~50–90%; more contagious via contact
- β-hemolytic streptococci: Pure culture only ~10% of the time
- Mixed infections of streptococci and staphylococci common; data suggest increasing importance of staphylococci over past 20 years (1)[C]
- Direct contact or insect vector
- Can result from contamination at trauma site
- Regional lymphadenopathy

COMMONLY ASSOCIATED CONDITIONS

- Malnutrition and anemia
- Crowded living conditions
- Poor hygiene
- Neglected minor trauma
- Any chronic/underlying dermatitis

DIAGNOSIS

HISTORY

- Lesions are often described as painful (or pruritic).
- May be slow and indolent or rapidly spreading
- Most frequent on face around mouth and nose or at site of trauma

PHYSICAL EXAM

- Tender red macule or papule as early lesion
- Thin-roofed vesicle to bullae: Usually nontender
- Pustules
- Weeping, shallow, red ulcer
- Honey-colored crusts
- Satellite lesions
- Often multiple sites
- Bullae on buttocks, trunk, face

DIAGNOSTIC TESTS & INTERPRETATION

Lab

Initial lab tests

- None usually done; however, rarely consider the following:
  - Culture: Taken from the base of lesion after removal of crust will grow both staphylococci and group A streptococci
  - Antistreptolysin-O (ASO) titer: Can be weak positive for streptococci
  - Antideoxyribonuclease B (anti-Dnase B) and antihyaluronidase (AHT) response more reliable than ASO response
  - Streptozyme: Positive for streptococci
- Disorders that may alter lab results: Streptococcal pharyngitis will alter streptococcal enzyme tests.

Follow-Up & Special Considerations

Monitor for spread of disease and systemic manifestations.

Pathological Findings

Acute purulent infection of the skin due to *S. aureus*, group A β-hemolytic streptococci, or mixed bacteria

DIFFERENTIAL DIAGNOSIS

- Nonbullous:
  - Chickenpox
  - Herpes
  - Folliculitis
  - Erysipelas
  - Insect bites
  - Severe eczematous dermatitis
  - Scabies
  - Tinea corporis
- Bullous:
  - Burns
  - Pemphigus vulgaris
  - Bullous pemphigoid
- Stevens-Johnson syndrome

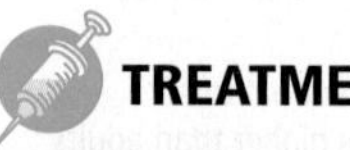

TREATMENT

MEDICATION

- In 2005, the Infectious Disease Society of America (IDSA) recommended topical treatment for limited lesions and oral medication when the disease is more severe/extensive (2)[C].
- Optimal treatment is unclear due to limited quality of evidence (3,4)[A].
- Penicillin and macrolide therapy is no longer recommended. Fluoroquinolones are not indicated due to resistance patterns.
- Dicloxacillin, cephalexin, clindamycin, topical mupirocin, and fusidic acid are effective unless local staphylococcal strains are resistant. (For methicillin-resistant *S. aureus* [MRSA] infections, treatment options include clindamycin and linezolid.)
- Consult the local hospital or health department for microbial resistance information.

- Nonbullous (minor spread, treat 7 days; widespread, treat 10 days); bullous (treat 10 days):
  - Retapamulin 1% ointment to be applied b.i.d. ×5 days (5)[B]
  - Mupirocin (Bactroban) topical ointment applied t.i.d. ×7–10 days (nonbullous only); not as effective on scalp as around mouth
  - Dicloxacillin: Adult 250 mg PO q.i.d.; pediatric 12–25 mg/kg/d divided q6h
- Contraindications: Drug allergy
- Precautions: Refer to manufacturer's profile for each drug.
- Significant possible interactions: Refer to manufacturer's profile for each drug.
- Oral doses
- First-generation cephalosporins: Children:
  - Cephalexin: 25–50 mg/kg/d divided q6h
  - Cefaclor: 20–40 mg/kg/d divided q8h
  - Cephradine: 25–50 mg/kg/d divided q6h–q12h
  - Cefadroxil: 30 mg/kg/d divided b.i.d.
- First-generation cephalosporins: Adults:
  - Cephalexin: 250 mg q.i.d.
  - Cefaclor: 250 mg t.i.d.
  - Cephradine: 500 mg b.i.d.
  - Cefadroxil: 1 g/d in divided doses
- Clindamycin
- Severe bullous disease may require IV therapy such as nafcillin or cefazolin.

ADDITIONAL TREATMENT

General Measures

- Prevention with mupirocin or triple antibiotic ointment t.i.d. to sites of minor skin trauma
- Removal of crusts, cleanliness with gentle washing 2–3× daily; clean with antibacterial soap, chlorhexidine, or Betadine.
- Washing of entire body may prevent recurrence at distant sites.

Issues for Referral

If resistant or extensive infections occur, especially in immunocompromised patients

Additional Therapies

Monitor for microbial resistance patterns.

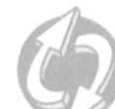

ONGOING CARE

FOLLOW-UP RECOMMENDATIONS

- Athletes restricted from contact sports
- School and daycare contagious restrictions

Patient Monitoring

If not clear within 7–10 days, culture the lesions.

PATIENT EDUCATION

Avoidance of infection spread is key; hand washing is vital.

PROGNOSIS

- Complete resolution in 7–10 days with treatment
- Antibiotic treatment will not prevent or halt glomerulonephritis, as it will rheumatic fever.
- If not clear within 7–10 days, culture is necessary to find resistant organism.
- Recurrent impetigo: Evaluate for carriage of *S. aureus* in nares (also perineum, axillae, toe web). Apply mupirocin ointment to nares b.i.d. × 5 days for clearance/decolonization.

COMPLICATIONS

- Ecthyma
- Erysipelas
- Poststreptococcal acute glomerulonephritis
- Cellulitis
- Bacteremia
- Osteomyelitis
- Septic arthritis
- Pneumonia
- Lymphadenitis

REFERENCES

1. Britton JW, Fajardo JE, Krafte-Jacobs B. Comparison of mupirocin and erythromycin in the treatment of impetigo. *J Pediatr*. 1990;117:827–9.
2. Stevens DL, Bisno AL, Chambers HF, et al. Practice guidelines for the diagnosis and management of skin and soft-tissue infections. *Clin Infect Dis*. 2005;41:1373–406.
3. Koning S, Verhagen AP, van Suijlekom-Smit LW, et al. Interventions for impetigo. *Cochrane Database Syst Rev*. 2004:CD003261.
4. George A, Rubin G. A systematic review and meta-analysis of treatments for impetigo. *Br J Gen Pract*. 2003;53:480–7.
5. Parish LC, Jorizzo JL, Breton JJ, et al. Topical retapamulin ointment (1%, wt/wt) twice daily for 5 days versus oral cephalexin twice daily for 10 days in the treatment of secondarily infected dermatitis: Results of a randomized controlled trial. *J Am Acad Dermatol*. 2006;55:1003–13.

ADDITIONAL READING

- Del Giudice P, Hubiche P. Community-associated methicillin-resistant *Staphylococcus aureus* and impetigo. *Br J Dermatol*. 2010;162:905.
- Kowalski TJ, Berbari EF, Osmon DR. Epidemiology treatment, and prevention of community-acquired methicillin-resistant *Staphylococcus aureus* infections. *Mayo Clin Proc*. 2005;80:1201–7; quiz 1208.

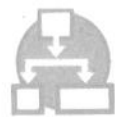

See Also (Topic, Algorithm, Electronic Media Element)

Algorithm: Rash, Focal

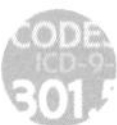

CODES

ICD9

684 Impetigo

CLINICAL PEARLS

- Superficial, intraepidermal infection
- Predominantly staphylococcal in origin
- Microbial resistance patterns need to be monitored.
- Topical treatment recommended for limited lesions and oral medication only when the disease is more severe/extensive.

I

INCONTINENCE, FECAL

Anita Krishnarao, MD, MPH
Samir A. Shah, MD
Adam Klipfel, MD

BASICS

Continuous or recurrent uncontrolled passage of fecal material (>10 mL) for >1 month

DESCRIPTION

- Involuntary passage of fecal material through the anal canal for >1 month in an individual >3 years old
- Major incontinence is the involuntary excretion of feces. Minor incontinence includes incontinence to flatus and occasional seepage of liquid stool.
- Fecal incontinence was the second-leading cause of nursing home placement:
  - Recurrent, involuntary loss of solid or liquid stools
  - Careful rectal exam to assess for rectal tone, voluntary squeeze, and overflow incontinence from fecal impaction
  - Endorectal ultrasound (EUS) is the simplest, most reliable, and least invasive test to find anatomic defects in the anal sphincters.
  - The goal of treatment should be to restore continence and improve quality of life.

Geriatric Considerations

- The prevalence of fecal incontinence increases with age.
- Idiopathic fecal incontinence: No identified cause; more common in middle-aged or elderly women.

EPIDEMIOLOGY

Incidence

Patients underreport fecal incontinence unless prompted. Studies may underestimate the number of patients affected.

Prevalence

- In younger persons, Women > Men
- 8% of adults overall
- 15% of adults >70 years old
- 56–66% of hospitalized older patients and over 50% in nursing home residents
- 50–70% of patients who have urinary incontinence also suffer from fecal incontinence.

Pregnancy Considerations

Obstetrical injury to the pelvic floor, during pregnancy or delivery, may result in initial temporary incontinence, which usually improves but many years later can result in subsequent incontinence.

Geriatric Considerations

- Fecal impaction and overflow diarrhea leading to fecal incontinence is a common scenario in older patients.
- Surgical history:
  - Anal surgery, including hemorrhoidectomy, anal fissure repair (sphincterotomy), anal dilatation, may predispose to fecal incontinence as a short-term or long-term complication.

RISK FACTORS

- Physical status:
  - Older age, female sex, obesity, limited physical activity
- Positive family history
- Neuropsychiatric conditions:
  - Multiple sclerosis, spinal cord injury, dementia, depression, stroke, diabetic neuropathy
- Trauma:
  - Prostatectomy, radiation
  - Risk factors at the time of delivery include the use of forceps and the need for an episiotomy.
  - Forceps delivery, occipitoposterior position, and prolonged second stage of labor
- Other:
  - Diarrhea, inflammatory bowel disease, irritable bowel syndrome, menopause, smoking, constipation
  - Potential association with child abuse and sexual abuse
  - Congenital abnormalities such as imperforate anus or rectal prolapse
  - Fecal impaction is a common cause of fecal incontinence in the elderly.

GENERAL PREVENTION

- Behavioral and lifestyle changes (obesity, limited physical activity or exercise, poor diet, and smoking are modifiable risk factors).
- Postmeal bowel regimen
- Avoid episiotomy when possible.
- Pelvic floor muscle training during pregnancy

PATHOPHYSIOLOGY

- Continence is dependent on the complex relationships involving temporal coordination of a variety of muscles, nerves, and reflex arcs.
- Important factors in maintaining continence include stool consistency, stool volume, colonic transit time, anorectal sensation, rectal compliance, anorectal reflexes, external and internal muscle sphincter tone, puborectalis muscle function, and the mental capacity.
- Disease processes or structural defects that alter any of these aspects can contribute to fecal incontinence.
- Diabetes is the most common metabolic disorder that may lead to fecal incontinence secondary to neuropathy of pudendal nerve.

ETIOLOGY

- Congenital: Spina bifida and myelomeningocele with spinal cord damage
- Trauma: Anal sphincter damage from vaginal delivery and surgical procedures
- Medical: Diabetes, stroke, spinal cord trauma, degenerative disorders of the nervous system, inflammatory conditions, rectal neoplasia

COMMONLY ASSOCIATED CONDITIONS

- Age >70 years
- Urinary incontinence or pelvic organ prolapse
- Chronic medical conditions such as diabetes, dementia, cerebrovascular accidents, cord compression, dementia, depression, immobility, chronic obstructive pulmonary disease, irritable bowel syndrome, urinary incontinence, or colectomy
- Obstetric injury at young age
- Surgeries in the anorectal area
- Stroke
- History of pelvic/rectal irradiation

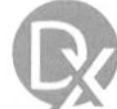

DIAGNOSIS

Diagnosis of fecal incontinence is primarily based on clinical history and physical findings

HISTORY

- Patients seldom volunteer information about fecal incontinence, so direct questioning is important.
- Determine by history:
  - Severity (soiling by liquid stools only or gross incontinence of solid stools)
  - Onset and duration (recent onset vs. chronic)
  - Frequency, presence of constipation or diarrhea
  - Review of medications
  - Assess diet, medical and obstetrical history, lifestyle, and mobility.
- Evaluate cognition with Mini-Mental Status Exam.
- Possible overlapping history of social withdrawal and depression

PHYSICAL EXAM

- The perianal area should be inspected.
- Inspect the perineum for chemical dermatitis, hemorrhoids, fistula, surgical scars, skin tags, rectal prolapse, soiling, and ballooning of the perineum (sarcopenia of pelvic musculature).
- A gaping anal orifice may indicate myopathy or neurologic disorder.
- Evaluate the external sphincter in response to perineal skin stimulation (anal wink). Absence is suggestive of neuropathic component.
- Ask the patient to bear down, preferably in standing position, to look for subclinical rectal prolapse.
- Digital rectal examination to estimate anal canal pressure while resting and during voluntary squeeze, rectal bleeding, hemorrhoids, neoplasm, fecal consistency, and clues to diarrhea or distal fecal impaction.
- Neurologic examination, including perianal sensation

DIAGNOSTIC TESTS & INTERPRETATION

History and physical exam will usually be enough for diagnosis. In selected patients, consider:

- EUS: Currently the simplest, most reliable, and least invasive test for defining anatomic defects in the external and internal anal sphincters, rectal wall, and the puborectalis muscle. Can be used to predict the therapeutic response to sphincteroplasty.
- Plain abdominal x-ray (impaction, constipation)
- Sigmoidoscopy/anoscopy/colonoscopy
- Defecography can measure the anorectal angle, evaluate pelvic descent, and detect occult or overt rectal prolapse.
- MRI defecography (dynamic MRI imaging) to further define pelvic floor anatomy
- Anorectal manometry: Measure parameters such as maximal resting anal pressure, amplitude and duration of squeeze pressure, the rectoanal inhibitory reflex, threshold of conscious rectal sensation, rectal compliance, and rectal and anal pressure during straining.
- Pudendal nerve terminal motor latency (PNTML): This technique is operator-dependent and has poor correlation with clinical symptoms and histologic findings.

- Electromyography: Sometimes helpful in evaluating neurogenic or myopathic damage in patients with fecal incontinence

Lab

Initial lab tests

- If history of travel, antibiotics, tube feedings, or have signs and symptoms of sepsis, the following stool studies may be indicated:
  - Culture and sensitivity
  - Ova and parasites
  - *Clostridium difficile* toxin assay
- Measure thyroid-stimulating hormone (TSH), electrolytes, and BUN in elderly patients with impaction.

Follow-Up & Special Considerations

Anorectal physiology laboratory

Imaging

- EUS may demonstrate anal sphincters, rectal wall, and the puborectalis muscle structural abnormalities (1).
- EUS can detect a sphincter injury in up to 35% of women who delivered vaginally.

Initial approach

The approach to the problem of fecal incontinence in older patients should be individualized, minimally invasive, convenient, and practically feasible.

DIFFERENTIAL DIAGNOSIS

- Anorectal disorders:
  - Inflammatory or infectious disorders
  - Neoplasms, radiation, ischemia, fistulas
  - Prolapsing internal hemorrhoids or rectal prolapse
  - Trauma: Obstetric, surgical, radiation, accidental
- Neurologic disorders:
  - Stroke, dementia, neoplasms, spinal cord injury, and/or diseases of altered level of consciousness
  - Pudendal neuropathy, neurosyphilis, multiple sclerosis, diabetes mellitus
- Miscellaneous causes:
  - Infectious diarrhea, fecal impaction and overflow, irritable bowel syndrome (IBS), laxative abuse, inflammatory bowel disease, short bowel syndrome, muscle diseases, senescence and frailty, collagen vascular disease, psychological and behavioral problems, radiotherapy

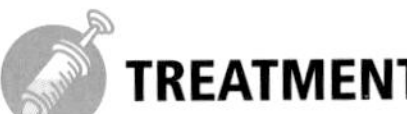

TREATMENT

MEDICATION

No specific medication has been proven to be of benefit for fecal incontinence (2)[A].

First Line

Specific treatment of underlying cause of diarrhea (such as infectious diarrhea or inflammatory bowel disease) may improve fecal continence.

Second Line

- Increase dietary fiber in milder forms of fecal incontinence are recommended to improve symptoms. Stool bulking agents include high-fiber diet, psyllium products, or methylcellulose (3)[B].
- Antidiarrheal agents, such as adsorbents or opium derivatives, may reduce fecal incontinence (3)[C].
- Patients with a fecal impaction and overflow incontinence should be disimpacted and treated with a bowel regimen to prevent recurrence.

ADDITIONAL TREATMENT

General Measures

- If ambulatory, prompted and scheduled defection (effective particularly in patients who have overflow incontinence)
- If bed-bound, schedule osmotic laxatives, or stimulant laxatives if constipated.
- Enemas, laxatives, and suppositories may help to promote more complete bowel emptying in appropriate patients and minimize further postdefecation leakage.
- Scheduled toileting and use of stool deodorants (Periwash, Derfil, Devrom).

Additional Therapies

- Biofeedback: Training involves teaching patient to recognize small volumes of rectal distension and to contract the external anal sphincter while simultaneously keeping intra-abdominal pressure low (4)[A]. Diabetics in particular may benefit.
- Patients with systemic neurologic disease, anal deformity, or frequent episodes of incontinence respond poorly.

SURGERY/OTHER PROCEDURES

- Surgery should be considered only when the nonsurgical approaches have failed.
- Sphincter repair should be offered for highly symptomatic patients with a defined defect of external anal sphincter (3)[B].
- Injectable therapy (tissue-bulking agent injected proximal to anus) seems to be safe and effective for patients with internal anal sphincter dysfunction (3)[B].
- Artificial anal sphincter implantation or dynamic graciloplasty (where gracilis muscle transposed into anus as modified sphincter) may be considered in patients with severe fecal incontinence with irreparable sphincter damage (3)[B].
- Stoma (colostomy or ileostomy) creation may be appropriate in patients with disabling fecal incontinence when other available therapeutic options have failed or when preferred by patient (3)[B].
- Sacral nerve stimulation (neuromodulation) via the implantation of SC electrodes that deliver low-amplitude electrical stimulation to sphincter muscles to improve overall rectal tone (5)[B]

IN-PATIENT CONSIDERATIONS

Initial Stabilization

If secondary to fecal impaction, manual fragmentation and extraction of fecal mass (after lubrication with lidocaine jelly)

Nursing

- Avoid catharsis.
- No hot water, soap, or hydrogen peroxide enemas.

Discharge Criteria

Outpatient care

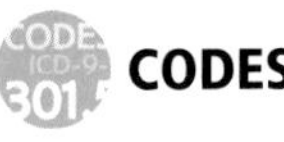

ONGOING CARE

FOLLOW-UP RECOMMENDATIONS

Periodic rectal exam

Patient Monitoring

Fewer than 1 bowel movement every other day with fecal incontinence might suggest impaction.

DIET

- High fiber (25 g/d) and at least 1.5 L fluid daily
- Avoid foods known to worsen symptoms (caffeine).

PATIENT EDUCATION

Kegel/sphincter training exercises alone do not work for fecal incontinence, but may supplement.

PROGNOSIS

- Reimpaction likely if bowel program not followed
- 50% failure rate over 5 years following overlapping sphincteroplasty

COMPLICATIONS

- Depression and social isolation
- Skin ulcerations
- Artificial bowel sphincter: 30% infection rate

REFERENCES

1. Woodfield CA, Krishnamoorthy S, Hampton BS, et al. Imaging pelvic floor disorders: Trend toward comprehensive MRI. *AJR Am J Roentgenol*. 2010;194:1640–9.
2. Cheetham MJ, Brazzelli M, Norton C, et al. Drug treatment for Faecal incontinence in adults. *Cochrane Database Syst Rev*. 2008;16(3): CD002116.
3. Tjandra JJ, Dykes SL, Kumar RR, et al. Practice parameters for the treatment of fecal incontinence. *Dis. Colon Rectum*. 2007;50:1497–507.
4. Norton C, Cody J, et al. biofeedback and or sphincter exercises for the treatment of faecal incontinence in adults. *Cochrane Library*. 2006;3:CD002111.
5. Wexner SD, et al. Sacral nerve stimulation: Time for critical appraisal. *Ann Surg*. 2011;254:175–6.

ADDITIONAL READING

Maeda Y, Laurberg S, Norton C, et al. Perianal injectable bulking agents as treatment for faecal incontinence in adults. *Cochrane Database Syst Rev*. 2010;5:CD007959.

I

CODES

ICD9

- 787.60 Full incontinence of feces
- 787.61 Incomplete defecation
- 787.62 Fecal smearing

CLINICAL PEARLS

- New onset of fecal incontinence may indicate spinal cord compression when observed with other neurologic symptoms.
- True incontinence must be differentiated from frequency and urgency without loss of bowel contents.

INCONTINENCE, URINARY ADULT FEMALE

Brent Matsuda, MD
Sheldon Riklon, MD

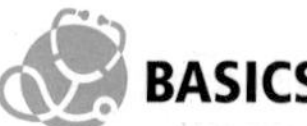

BASICS

DESCRIPTION

- Urinary incontinence is the involuntary loss of urine that is objectively demonstrable and is of medical, financial, social, and hygienic concern.
- Stress incontinence: Associated with increased intra-abdominal pressure, such as coughing, laughing, sneezing, or exertion
- Urge incontinence: Sudden uncontrollable urgency, leading to leakage of urine (also known as overactive bladder or detrusor overactivity)
- Mixed incontinence: Loss of urine from a combination of stress and urge incontinence
- Overflow incontinence: High residual or chronic urinary retention leads to urinary spillage from an overdistended bladder
- Functional incontinence: Loss of urine due to deficits of cognition and mobility
- Total incontinence: Continuous leakage of urine; leakage without awareness

EPIDEMIOLOGY

- Affects 25–45% of adult women (who experienced urine leakage at least once in the past year) (1,2,3)
- Affects 60–78% of women in nursing homes (3)
- Women 19–64 years of age have predominantly stress incontinence (20–25%), followed by mixed (15–20%), and urge (4–9%).
- In women 65–80 years of age, mixed is the most common (18%), followed by stress (16%), and urge (13%).
- In women over 80 years of age, mixed is the most common (28%), followed by urge (11%), and stress (8%) (4).

RISK FACTORS

Advanced age, obesity, menopause, pregnancy, vaginal childbirth, pelvic surgery or radiation, urethral diverticula, genital prolapse, smoking, chronic obstructive pulmonary disease (COPD), cognitive impairment, constipation, and pelvic floor dysfunction

GENERAL PREVENTION

Weight loss, pelvic floor exercises, smoking cessation, avoidance of bladder-irritant foods, increased fiber intake to reduce constipation, bladder retraining, and timed fluid intake

PATHOPHYSIOLOGY

- Stress incontinence: Occurs with increased intra-abdominal pressure without uninhibited detrusor contraction. 2 types:
  - Anatomic: Due to urethral hypermobility from lack of pelvic support
  - Intrinsic sphincter deficiency (ISD): Impairment of various intrinsic factors is responsible for the normal coaptation and closure of the urethra. Urethral mucosal seal and inherent closure from collagen, fibroelastic tissue, smooth and striated muscles, etc., may be lost secondary to surgical scarring, radiation, or hormonal and senile changes.
- Urge incontinence: May be due to detrusor overactivity, or may be idiopathic
- Overflow incontinence: Urinary retention (usually from lower motor paralytic neurogenic bladder)
- Total incontinence: Constant loss of urine in epispadias-exstrophy complex due to absence of bladder neck and urethra. Ectopic ureters in females usually open in the urethra distal to the sphincter or in the vagina, causing continuous leakage. Also may occur with fistulous connections between bladder, ureters, or urethra and vagina or uterus.

COMMONLY ASSOCIATED CONDITIONS

Pelvic organ prolapse, UTI, COPD, diabetes mellitus, neurological disease, obesity, chronic constipation, and any disease that results in chronic cough

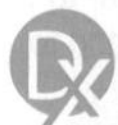

DIAGNOSIS

HISTORY

- Age: Stress incontinence is more common in women aged 19–64, whereas mixed incontinence is more common in women over 65. Incontinence dating from childhood indicates congenital causes (e.g., ectopic ureter, epispadias) or unresolved bedwetting issues.
- Childbirth: Weakness of the pelvic floor is more likely in multiparous women.
- Amount and nature of leakage: Severity of leakage should be graded by the number of pads used in 24 hours.
- Stress incontinence: Occurs in small spurts. Patients typically remain dry at night in bed.
- Urge incontinence: Sudden urge followed by leakage of large amounts, usually associated with frequency and nocturia
- Continuous slow leakage in between regular voiding indicates ectopic ureter, urinary fistula, etc.
- Pain: Suprapubic pain with dysuria implies urinary infection, dyspareunia, interstitial cystitis, etc.
- Medical history:
  - Neurologic conditions: cerebrovascular accident, parkinsonism, multiple sclerosis, myelodysplasia, diabetes, spinal cord injury
  - Radiation to pelvic and vaginal areas: Causes ISD, overactive bladder, fibrotic changes of pelvic floor musculature, and low bladder compliance
  - A history of smoking and chronic obstructive pulmonary disease with a chronic cough can aggravate incontinence.
  - A history of constipation can aggravate incontinence.
  - History of obesity
  - Hormonal status
  - Obstetrical history
- Medications:
  - Sympatholytic alpha-blockers (terazosin, prazosin, doxazosin, tamsulosin, alfuzosin, silodosin) can cause or worsen incontinence.
  - Sympathomimetic and tricyclic antidepressants (e.g., ephedrine, imipramine, amitriptyline, duloxetine) can cause retention with overflow incontinence.
  - Anticholinergic agents (e.g., tolterodine, oxybutynin, darifenacin, trospium chloride, solifenacin)
- Surgical history: Previous pelvic surgery, including gynecologic and bowel surgery, can injure the pelvic floor support and musculature, and affect the neurologic function.

PHYSICAL EXAM

- General status:
  - Obesity (BMI)
- General neurologic examination:
  - Mental status, speech, intellectual performance
  - Motor status: Gait, generalized or focal weakness, rigidity, tremor
  - Sensory status: Impairment of perineal-sacral area sensation helps localize the level of neurologic deficit.
  - Reflex: A bulbocavernous reflex implies contraction of the anal sphincter in response to squeezing the clitoris. This reflex tests the integrity of sacral 2, 3, 4 spinal cord segments.
- Urologic examination:
  - Abdomen: Masses, visible exstrophy-epispadias, incisional scars of previous surgeries
  - Suprapubic tenderness: May indicate cystitis
  - Palpable, distended bladder: Chronic urinary retention
- Pelvic examination:
  - Examination of the perineum and external genitalia including tissue quality and sensation.
  - Vaginal (half-speculum) examination for prolapse
  - Bimanual pelvic and anorectal examination for pelvic masses, pelvic floor function, etc.
    - Urethral hypermobility: Gauged by palpation of the descent of the proximal urethra on straining
    - Assessment of pelvic floor resting tone and function (ability to isolate and contract pelvic floor musculature)
  - Stress test for urinary incontinence: The patient is asked to cough or strain to reproduce incontinence.
  - Cystocele: If evident, is staged (grade 0–4)
  - Rectocele: If evident, is staged
  - Enterocele: If evident, is stage

DIAGNOSTIC TESTS & INTERPRETATION

Lab

- Urinalysis and urine culture
- Atypical urinary infections including ureaplasma and mycoplasma
- Renal function assessment: Recommended in patients with incontinence and a probability of renal impairment

Imaging

- Bladder scan to evaluate postvoid residual
- Upper tract imaging if upper tract involvement is suspected: CT scan, IV pyelogram, or renal sonography

Initial approach

- The ICIQ (International Consultation of Incontinence Modulator Questionnaire) is highly recommended for assessment of patient's perspective of symptoms of incontinence and their impact on quality of life.
- Bladder diary to evaluate oral intake, timing of leakage, and patient habits.

Diagnostic Procedures/Surgery

Urodynamic studies:

- Cystometric study of detrusor function: Determines bladder compliance, sensations, and detrusor responses to filling
- Uroflow with electromyography: Evaluates for any obstructive concerns
- Valsalva leak point pressure: Determines the intra-abdominal pressure at which leakage is observed

- Videourodynamic studies: Sophisticated combination of fluorocystourethrography and urodynamic studies

DIFFERENTIAL DIAGNOSIS

- Stress incontinence: Due to urethral hypermobility or ISD, though in the majority it is mixed or due to both
- Urge incontinence: Detrusor overactivity, conditions that irritate the bladder lining, but is often idiopathic
- Nocturnal enuresis: Idiopathic, detrusor overactivity, neurogenic, cardiogenic, or sleep apnea
- Continuous leakage: Ectopic ureter, urinary fistulas, exstrophy-epispadias complex
- Postvoid dribbling: Urethral diverticulum, idiopathic, iatrogenic, surgical

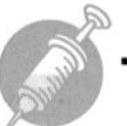

TREATMENT

Lifestyle changes and behavioral modification are first-line interventions and when properly trained, as effective as medications at reducing incontinence episode frequency. Should be maintained for 8–12 weeks prior to reassessment:

- Lifestyle changes: Weight loss is critical if obese, avoidance of certain foods that may make matters worse (e.g., caffeine, acidic foods).
- Behavioral modification: Supervised bladder training and Kegel exercises (training by professional improves outcomes); scheduled voiding

MEDICATION

First Line

- Urge incontinence: Anticholinergic agents:
  - Tolterodine (Detrol LA) 2–8 mg/d PO
  - Oxybutynin (Ditropan XL) 5–15 mg/d PO
  - Solifenacin (Vesicare) 5–10 mg/d PO
  - Darifenacin (Enablex) 7.5–15 mg/d PO
  - Trospium chloride (Sanctura XR) 60 mg/d PO
  - Transdermal oxybutynin (Gelnique) 10% applied daily
  - Fesoterodine (Toviaz) 4–8 mg/d PO
  - Imipramine (Tofranil) 10–60 mg PO at bedtime
  - Amitriptyline (Elavil) 10–100 mg PO at bedtime
- Stress incontinence:
  - Pelvic floor rehabilitation
  - Anticholinergics may be successful in mixed incontinence.

Second Line

Nonsurgical management: Helps about 50–65% of patients with milder symptom:

- Biofeedback and electrostimulation
- Occlusive and supportive devices (e.g., cones)
- Acupuncture (in selected cases)

ADDITIONAL TREATMENT

General Measures

- Treat correctable causes (e.g., UTI).
- Encourage weight loss in obese patients.
- Aggressive correction of constipation

SURGERY/OTHER PROCEDURES

- Surgical management for stress incontinence:
  - Periurethral injection of bulking agents: Collagen, carbon beads, hyaluronic acid, calcium hydroxylapatite
  - Slings (minimally invasive):
    - Tension-free vaginal tape procedures
    - Transobturator tape procedures
    - Single-incision sling (Mini-arc, Solyx)
  - Vaginal needle suspension: Raz, Stamey (not used commonly today)
  - Abdominal approaches: Marshall-Marchetti-Krantz cystourethropexy, Burch colposuspension, laparoscopic colposuspension
  - Artificial urinary sphincter placement (not approved by FDA in women)
- Of note: Up to 1/3 of women who have surgery undergo a second procedure during their lifetime.
- Surgical management for urge incontinence:
  - Sacral neuromodulation: Efficacy in 70–80% of patients who have failed other treatments
  - Percutaneous tibial nerve stimulation: Office-based therapy for urge, frequency, and urge incontinence
  - Botulinum toxin (intravesical injection) has a role with some patients (not FDA approved)
  - Bladder augmentation

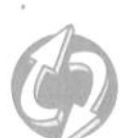

ONGOING CARE

FOLLOW-UP RECOMMENDATIONS

Patient Monitoring

- Postoperative assessment: Rule out UTI, check postvoid residual, check suture lines
- Periodic long-term follow-up with outcome-based questionnaire surveys

PROGNOSIS

Significant improvements are usually obtained with most patients.

COMPLICATIONS

- Prolonged exposure to urine causes skin breakdown and dermatitis, which may lead to ulceration and secondary infection.
- Inability for self-care is the precipitating factor for many nursing home admissions.
- Social isolation
- Weight gain (due to self-limiting exercise from fear of leakage)
- Avoidance of sexual activity

REFERENCES

1. Hunskaar S, Burgio K, Clark A, et al. Epidemiology of urinary and fecal incontinence and pelvic organ prolapse. In: *Incontinence, 3rd International Consultation on Incontinence*, vol. 1. Paris: Basic Evaluation; 2005:255.
2. Hunskaar S, Burgio K, Diokno A, et al. Epidemiology and natural history of urinary incontinence in women. *Urology*. 2003;62:16–23.
3. Landefeld CS, Bowers BJ, Feld AD, et al. National Institutes of Health State-of-the-Science Conference Statement: Prevention of fecal and urinary incontinence in adults. *Ann Intern Med*. 2008;148(6):449–58.
4. Shamliyan T, et al. Evidence Report/Technology Assessment, Number 161: Prevention of Urinary and Fecal Incontinence in Adults prepared for Agency for Healthcare Research and Quality, U.S. Department of Health and Human Services. AHRQ Publication No. 08-E003; 2007.

ADDITIONAL READING

- Abrams P, Andersson KE, Birder L, et al. Fourth International Consultation on Incontinence Recommendations of the International Scientific Committee: Evaluation and treatment of urinary incontinence, pelvic organ prolapse, and fecal incontinence. *Neurourol Urodyn*. 2010;29:213–40.
- Atiemo HO, Vasavada AS. Evaluation and management of refractory overactive bladder. *Curr Urol Rep*. 2006;7:370–5.
- Serati M, Salvatore S, Uccella S, et al. The impact of the mid-urethral slings for the treatment of stress urinary incontinence on female sexuality. *J Sex Med*. 2009;6(6):1534–42.

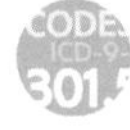

CODES

ICD9

- 788.30 Urinary incontinence, unspecified
- 788.31 Urge incontinence
- 788.33 Mixed incontinence (male) (female)

CLINICAL PEARLS

- Urinary incontinence is the involuntary loss of urine that is objectively demonstrable and is of medical, financial, social, and hygienic concern.
- Stress incontinence: Associated with increased intra-abdominal pressure, such as coughing, laughing, sneezing, or exertion
- Urge incontinence: Sudden uncontrollable urgency, leading to leakage of urine (also known as overactive bladder or detrusor overactivity)
- Rule out UTI by culture.
- Assume that a great percentage of women can be significantly helped by treatment.
- Physical therapy/pelvic floor rehabilitation by select physical therapists can be highly effective.
- Rule out STI and atypical urinary infections.
- Aggressively treat constipation.

INCONTINENCE, URINARY ADULT MALE

Elizabeth E. Houser, MD

BASICS

DESCRIPTION

- Urinary incontinence refers to the involuntary loss of urine that presents a medical, financial, social, or hygienic problem. 2 main types of incontinence exist: Stress incontinence and urge incontinence.
- Stress incontinence: Involuntary urine leaks secondary to increased intra-abdominal pressure being greater than the sphincter can control; may be precipitated by sneezing, laughing, coughing, exertion, etc.
- Urge incontinence: Involuntary leakage of urine associated with urgency; is believed to be secondary to uncontrolled contraction of the urinary bladder. It is also called detrusor overactivity.
- Mixed incontinence: Involuntary leakage of urine with urgency and with sneezing, laughing, coughing, exertion, etc.

EPIDEMIOLOGY

- Stress incontinence in men is rare, unless it is attributable to prostate surgery, neurologic disease, or trauma.
- Reported rates of incontinence range from 1% after transurethral resection to 2–57% after radical prostatectomy.

Prevalence

- Large studies have indicated that there is a 17% overall prevalence rate of incontinence among the male population (1).
- Prevalence of urinary incontinence in men increases sharply with age; only 5% younger than the age of 45 experience urinary incontinence, whereas 21% of those age ≥65 experience symptoms (2).
- Black men have the highest incidence of urinary incontinence (21%) among the male population (1).
- 31% of men ≥85 years of age experience incontinence (1).
- Incontinence in men of all ages is approximately half as prevalent as it is in women.

RISK FACTORS

- Age
- Neurologic disease
- Prostate surgery
- Pelvic trauma

GENERAL PREVENTION

Proper management of conditions, such as symptomatic bladder outlet obstruction caused by benign prostatic hyperplasia (BPH), early in the course may prevent continence problems later in life.

PATHOPHYSIOLOGY

- Incontinence secondary to bladder abnormalities:
  - Detrusor overactivity results in urge incontinence.
  - Detrusor overactivity commonly is associated with bladder outlet obstruction from BPH.
- Incontinence secondary to outlet abnormalities:
  - Sphincteric damage secondary to pelvic surgery or radiation
  - Sphincteric dysfunction secondary to neurologic disease
- Mixed incontinence is caused by abnormalities of both the bladder and the outlet overflow or caused by enlarged prostate or bladder neck contracture from prostate surgery.

COMMONLY ASSOCIATED CONDITIONS

- Neurologic disease (cerebrovascular accident, parkinsonism, multiple sclerosis, myelodysplasia, spinal cord injury)
- Pelvic radiation
- Pelvic trauma
- BPH
- Prostate surgery

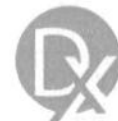

DIAGNOSIS

HISTORY

- Voiding symptoms:
  - Duration and characteristics of incontinence
  - Stress, urge, total
  - Precipitants and associated symptoms
  - Use of pads, briefs, diapers
  - Fluid intake
  - Alteration in bowel habits
  - Previous treatments and effect on incontinence
  - BPH symptoms
- Diabetes mellitus
- Associated conditions such as neurologic disease
- Medication use: Diuretics, drugs for BPH
- Alcohol and drug use, including caffeine
- Radical pelvic surgery or radiation:
  - Abdominoperineal resection
  - Prostatectomy: Radical or for benign disease

PHYSICAL EXAM

- Abdominal examination:
  - Suprapubic mass suggests retention.
  - Suprapubic tenderness suggests UTI.
  - Surgical scars suggesting pelvic surgery
  - Skin lesions associated with neurologic disease (such as neurofibromatosis and café au lait spots)
- External genitalia
- Prostate
- Spine/back
- Skeletal deformities
- Scars from previous spinal surgery
- Sacral abnormalities may be associated with neurogenic bladder dysfunction:
  - Cutaneous signs of spinal dysraphism:
    - SC lipoma
    - Vascular malformation, tuft of hair, or skin dimple on lower back
  - Cutaneous signs of sacral agenesis:
    - Low, short gluteal cleft
    - Flattened buttocks
    - Coccyx is not palpable
- Focal neurologic exam:
  - Motor function:
    - Inspect muscle bulk for atrophy.
    - Tibialis anterior (L4–S1): Dorsiflexion of foot
    - Gastrocnemius (L5–S2): Plantarflexion of foot
    - Toe extensors (L5–S2): Toe extension
- Sensory function
- Reflexes:
  - Anal reflex (S2–S5):
    - Gently stroke mucocutaneous junction of circumanal skin.
    - Absent visible contraction (wink) suggests peripheral nerve or sacral (conus medullaris) abnormality
  - Bulbocavernosus reflex (BCR) (S2–S4):
    - Elicited by squeezing glans to cause reflex contraction of anal sphincter
    - Absence of BCR suggests sacral nerve damage.

DIAGNOSTIC TESTS & INTERPRETATION

Lab

- Creatinine if significant retention suspected
- Urinalysis and urine culture to check for glucosuria, infection
- Prostate-specific antigen (PSA)

Imaging

- IV pyelogram, renal ultrasound, or CT of abdomen confirms normality of upper tracts.
- Voiding cystogram in select cases

Diagnostic Procedures/Surgery

- Urodynamics is useful for confirming bladder outlet obstruction as a possible cause of detrusor overactivity.
- Prostate ultrasound and biopsy if indicated by physical exam or PSA

DIFFERENTIAL DIAGNOSIS

- Urge incontinence
- Stress incontinence
- Mixed incontinence
- Overflow incontinence
- Intrinsic sphincter deficiency

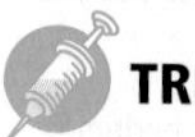

TREATMENT

- Best managed by combining lifestyle modification and medication
- Lifestyle changes: Weight loss (especially if overweight), limit fluids, toilet on a scheduled basis, eliminate certain foods that may make symptoms worse (e.g., caffeine, acidic foods)
- Bladder relaxation techniques (when trained by expert); unclear if pelvic floor exercises (Kegel) are effective for men; biofeedback

MEDICATION

First Line

- Urge incontinence (all equally efficacious; selection based upon side effect tolerance):
  - Oxybutynin (Ditropan XL) 5–15 mg PO every day
  - Tolterodine (Detrol LA) 2–4 mg PO every day
  - Darifenacin (Enablex) 7.5–15 mg PO every day
  - Solifenacin (Vesicare) 5–10 mg PO every day
  - Trospium chloride (Sanctura XR) 60 mg PO every day
  - Transdermal oxybutynin (Gelnique) 10% apply daily
  - Fesoterodine (Toviaz) 4–8 mg PO every day
- Stress incontinence:
  - No generally accepted drug therapy
  - Tricyclics sometimes used: Imipramine 10–25 mg PO b.i.d./t.i.d.

Second Line

- Urge incontinence
- Tricyclic antidepressants:
  - Imipramine 10–25 mg PO b.i.d./t.i.d.
- DDAVP for nocturnal symptoms:
  - 0.1–0.5 mg PO or intranasal at beditme
- Intradetrusor botulinum toxin injections (not FDA approved)

Geriatric Considerations

- Anticholinergics and tricyclics may result in significant cognitive impairment in elderly patients.
- DDAVP should be avoided in patients with known or potential cardiac disease.

ADDITIONAL TREATMENT

General Measures

- Bladder diaries are invaluable in helping patients understand patterns of incontinence.
- Time voiding to avoid significant bladder distention.

Additional Therapies

- Pelvic floor rehabilitation (Kegel exercises) may significantly improve both stress and urge incontinence in male patients.
- Timed voiding is a useful therapy for patients with urge incontinence.
- Overflow incontinence is usually caused by poor bladder contractility with urinary retention:
  - Indwelling catheter
  - Intermittent catheterization
  - Evaluate for outlet obstruction.

COMPLEMENTARY AND ALTERNATIVE MEDICINE

- Acupuncture in selected cases
- Physical therapy in selected cases

SURGERY/OTHER PROCEDURES

- Urge incontinence:
  - Sacral neuromodulation
  - Augmentation cystoplasty
- Stress incontinence:
  - Urethral bulking agents
  - Male sling procedures: Promising short-term results, but no long-term studies (3)[B]
  - Artificial urinary sphincter implant has excellent long-term continence rates (4)[A]

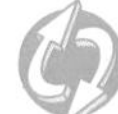

ONGOING CARE

FOLLOW-UP RECOMMENDATIONS

Patient Monitoring

Must monitor residual volume after voiding in patients taking anticholinergic medications

PROGNOSIS

Continence can be improved in almost all patients.

COMPLICATIONS

- Dermatitis
- Candidiasis
- Skin breakdown
- Social isolation
- Avoidance of sex
- Weight gain

REFERENCES

1. Anger JT, Saigal CS, Stothers L, et al. The prevalence of urinary incontinence among community dwelling men: Results from the National Health and Nutrition Examination survey. *J Urol*. 2006;176:2103–8; discussion 2108.
2. Giberti C, Gallo F, Schenone M, et al. The bone anchor suburethral synthetic sling for iatrogenic male incontinence: Critical evaluation at a mean 3-year followup. *J Urol*. 2009;181:2204–8.
3. Comiter CV. The male sling for stress urinary incontinence: A prospective study. *J Urol*. 2002; 167:597–601.
4. Elliott DS, Barrett DM. Mayo Clinic long-term analysis of the functional durability of the AMS 800 artificial urinary sphincter: A review of 323 cases. *J Urol*. 1998;159:1206–8.

ADDITIONAL READING

- Landefeld CS, Bowers BJ, Feld AD, et al. National Institutes of Health State-of-the-Science Conference Statement: Prevention of fecal and urinary incontinence in adults. *Ann Intern Med*. 2008; 148(6):449–58.
- Stewart WF, Van Rooyen JB, Cundiff GW, et al. Prevalence and burden of overactive bladder in the United States. *World J Urol*. 2003;20:327–36.

CODES

ICD9

- 788.30 Urinary incontinence, unspecified
- 788.31 Urge incontinence
- 788.32 Stress incontinence, male

CLINICAL PEARLS

- Always check postvoid residual to rule out overflow incontinence.
- Have patient complete a International Prostate Symptom Score and do uroflow.
- Check PSA.
- Urodynamics can be very helpful.
- Pelvic floor rehabilitation may have a significant effect for male patients.

I

INFERTILITY

Erika Mello, MD
Shaila V. Chauhan, MD

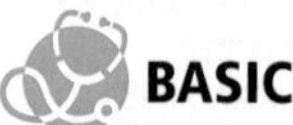

BASICS

DESCRIPTION

- Failure to conceive after 1 year of well-timed intercourse
- Evaluation after 6 months for women 35–39 years old and immediately if >39 years old

EPIDEMIOLOGY

Incidence

85% of couples conceive within 1 year, with 20% of women becoming pregnant during any one menstrual cycle.

Prevalence

- ~15% of all couples aged 35–40 years and >25% for women >40 years
- May be increasing as more women delay child-bearing; 20% of women in the US have their first child after age 35.
- 7.3 million women aged 15–44 years have impaired fecundity (1)[A].

RISK FACTORS

- Obesity, history of STD, endometriosis, irregular cycles, pelvic surgery or pathology, varicocele
- Medications, substance abuse, caffeine, smoking

Genetics

- Higher incidence of genetic abnormalities among infertile population (2), including Klinefelter syndrome (47XXY), Turner syndrome (45X or mosaic), and fragile X syndrome
- Balanced translocation may be present in phenotypically normal individuals, especially with a history of recurrent spontaneous abortion.
- Polycystic ovary syndrome (PCOS): Genetics are poorly understood but it is probably polygenetic.

GENERAL PREVENTION

- Encourage reproduction by 30–35 years.
- Maintain normal weight: 7 exercise level

PATHOPHYSIOLOGY

Complex and often multifactorial

ETIOLOGY

- Most couples have more than one factor (3).
- Tubal and ovulatory factors found in ~30% of couples:
  - *Chlamydia* infection is the most common cause of infertility in the US (owing to scarring and other effects on tubal function).
- Peritoneal (including endometriosis), uterine, cervical, general (i.e., psychogenic, nutritional, metabolic issues), and immunologic factors are less common: <10% each.
- Factors related to male partner are found in 30% of couples.
- Unexplained infertility is found in ~20% of couples.

COMMONLY ASSOCIATED CONDITIONS

- Risky sexual behavior
- Pelvic or lower abdominal pathology
- Endocrine dysfunction (thyroid, glucose metabolism, menstrual)
- Anovulation is commonly associated with hyperandrogenism and PCOS (4)[A]:
  - Obesity, hirsutism, and acne are common in women with PCOS (~80%).
  - Increased risk of endometrial hyperplasia
  - Metabolic problems with insulin resistance and lipid abnormalities are common.

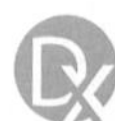

DIAGNOSIS

HISTORY

- Complete reproductive history:
  - Age at menarche, regularity of cycles, physical development
  - Primary or secondary infertility; infertility with previous partner
  - History of induced abortion, history of bilateral tubal ligation, vasectomy, other pelvic or abdominal surgery
- Abdominal pain or other abdominal symptoms
- STIs, especially pelvic inflammatory disease in women
- History of endocrine abnormalities (e.g., thyroid)
- History of malignancy: What kind? How was it treated?
- Chronic illness(es), including diabetes, HIV/AIDS, cystic fibrosis
- Family history:
  - Close relatives with congenital abnormalities or mental retardation
  - Infertility or early menopause in close relatives of female partner
- Medications, including alternative medicine
- Drug abuse, including tobacco, alcohol, street drugs
- Frequency of intercourse

PHYSICAL EXAM

- Evaluate for stigmata of polycystic ovary, Turner syndrome or thyroid disease, obesity or underweight, varicocele (men)
- Reproductive system evaluation: Hair patterns and pubertal development, including breasts

DIAGNOSTIC TESTS & INTERPRETATION

Lab

Initial lab tests

Evaluation is directed by history.

- Assessment of ovulation:
  - Luteal-phase progesterone at least 5 ng/mL on cycle days (CDs) 21–25 confirms ovulation.
  - Luteinizing hormone (LH) testing kit also can confirm ovulation.
  - Basal body temperature: ~1° increase during ovulation on morning evaluations, maintained over luteal phase, is indicative of ovulation.
  - Regular cycles with moliminal symptoms (i.e., breast tenderness, dysmenorrhea, and bloating) is 95% predictive of ovulation.
- Assessment of ovarian reserve:
  - CD 3 follicle-stimulating hormone (FSH) levels of <15 mIU/mL: Project possible reproductive potential (<10 suggests good ovarian reserve).
  - Clomiphene citrate challenge test: 100 mg/d on CDs 5–9 with measurement of FSH level on CD 3 and CD 10; FSH level of >15 on either CD 3 or CD 10 are associated with low reproductive potential, infertility, and higher rate of miscarriage.
- Semen analysis:
  - Normal: Volume >1.5 mL, count >20 million, motility >50%, and morphology >30% (or at least 14% by strict criteria)
  - If abnormal results, then do male evaluation as indicated clinically or consider referral.
  - Congenital bilateral absence of the vas deferens warrants cystic fibrosis screening.
- Additional labs:
  - CD 3 estradiol levels (related to follicular development), 25–75; abnormally high levels may represent diminished ovarian reserve.
  - CD 3 prolactin level, <24 ng/mL; increased levels interfere with ovulation and warrant further imaging for possible pituitary tumor.
  - Thyroid-stimulating hormone

Follow-Up & Special Considerations

Any abnormal value would warrant re-evaluation or possible referral if needed.

Imaging

Initial approach

- Transvaginal ultrasound to assess for anatomic abnormality (fibroid, polycystic ovaries, Müllerian anomalies)
- Sonohysterography detailed evaluation of the cavity.
- Hysterosalpingogram will evaluate patency of tubes and contour of the cavity; may be both diagnostic and therapeutic (4)[A].
- Semen analysis
- MRI of pelvis rarely needed

Follow-Up & Special Considerations

Abnormalities of imaging may require surgical evaluation, including referral if needed.

Diagnostic Procedures/Surgery

Laparoscopy is reserved for those at risk for endometriosis or for abnormal imaging findings.

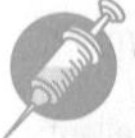

TREATMENT

MEDICATION

First Line

- Male factor: Intercourse, insemination, or in vitro fertilization (IVF). Consider lifestyle changes: Decrease heat to scrotum/testes, diet, exercise, eliminate substance abuse issues, and consider vitamin supplementation. Significant abnormalities warrant referral.
- Intrauterine insemination (IUI) or artificial insemination: This is performed easily in an office setting but requires specific sperm preparation for the procedure. It can be timed with natural cycles or stimulated cycles with LH kit assessment or ultrasound evaluation, leading to human chorionic gonadotropin injection to trigger ovulation. It can be performed with frozen sperm obtained from banks for severe male factor or for women lacking a male partner.
- Anovulation: Consider ovulation induction, most effectively with ~10% body weight loss if obese, but most commonly with clomiphene citrate (Clomid), typically 50 mg/d for 5 days; can start on CD 3, 4, or 5. If no ovulation, then increase dose by 50 mg/d in subsequent cycles; maximum, 150 mg/yr. Some will increase dose with ovulation but no pregnancy (4)[A].

- Anatomic issues: May need surgery, but if tubes are blocked, then referral for IVF is appropriate immediately.
- Unexplained infertility: Minor improvements with clomiphene or insemination alone; greater improvement with both together (5)[A].
- Coital or cervical problems: IUI (6)[C]
- Endometriosis: Either direct fertility treatments or surgery; medical therapy for endometriosis does not increase pregnancy rates after the therapy.
- Endocrine abnormalities may require treatment prior to pregnancy:
  - Stabilize thyroid disease or diabetes.
  - Consider bromocriptine or cabergoline for hyperprolactinemia.
  - Consider metformin or insulin sensitizer (e.g., glitazones) for insulin resistance.

Second Line

- If clomiphene fails to induce ovulation, can consider adding metformin (given initially as a low dose, but treatment dosing ultimately is ~1,500 mg/d; test renal function first), low-dose dexamethasone, oral contraceptives (OCPs) for 2 or more cycles, and then retry the clomiphene again immediately after stopping the OCPs (7)[A].
- Generally in subspecialty care: Gonadotropin therapies (injectable FSH or FSH plus LH) are effective, but riskier, treatments for infertility. They are effective for hypothalamic dysfunction, which clomiphene generally is not.
- Ultimately, IVF is a treatment option for all infertility patients when other therapies fail (4)[B].
- Surgery: For endometriosis and for anatomic issues

ADDITIONAL TREATMENT

General Measures

- Be aware of insurance coverage issues and requirements for each patient.
- Treatments increase estradiol levels, and the timing of the periovulatory mucus pattern may change to earlier in the cycle.
- Progesterone is responsible for the temperature changes in the cycle, and the premenstrual moliminal symptoms.
- Infertility and its treatment involve very emotional issues. Many patients may benefit from counseling and support measures.
- All female fertility patients should be taking folate supplementation of at least 400 μg/d.

Issues for Referral

Reproductive endocrinology and/or urology:

- Specialized lab prep is needed for IUI.
- Complications can be serious for these therapies.
- FSH plus LH therapies and IVF warrant referral in most cases.
- Consider reproductive/reconstructive surgery.

Additional Therapies

Increased age or with poor ovarian reserve, consideration of donor-egg IVF is warranted

COMPLEMENTARY AND ALTERNATIVE MEDICINE

Multiple types have been advocated for, but few have been fully evaluated.

SURGERY/OTHER PROCEDURES

- IVF clearly is the most effective infertility treatment available to patients.
- Male and female surgical issues should be addressed by experienced practitioners.

IN-PATIENT CONSIDERATIONS

Initial Stabilization

Rarely is hospitalization needed for infertility issues; however, it may be needed occasionally for issues related to problems in early pregnancy and ovarian hyperstimulation syndrome. If this occurs, recommend subspecialty consultation.

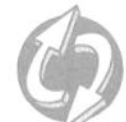

ONGOING CARE

FOLLOW-UP RECOMMENDATIONS

Patients often will need to consider more aggressive options as they progress through this process. From 3–6 cycles of oral ovulation induction would be an adequate trial prior to referral.

Patient Monitoring

- Cycle monitoring may be able to help mitigate some of the risks.
- Ultrasound monitoring can show the number of follicles developing during the cycle and may help to predict ovarian hyperstimulation and risk of multiple gestations.

DIET

- Healthy diet with minimization of fat, control of calories, and vitamin supplementation
- If obese, then diet modification is needed as above; low-fat, lower-calorie, high-fiber diet is most recommended.

PATIENT EDUCATION

Seek out patient education materials on the specific diagnoses involved. Good sources include:

- American Society for Reproductive Medicine (www.asrm.org)
- American College of Obstetricians and Gynecologists (www.acog.org)
- Resolve: National patient advocacy group revolving around infertility (www.resolve.org)

PROGNOSIS

- Generally excellent; most couples will achieve a pregnancy.
- Without therapy, ~50% of those couples not yet pregnant will conceive during both the second and third years of trying.

COMPLICATIONS

- Stress levels are high during treatment.
- Multiple pregnancy rates (even high-order ones) increase with all therapies involving ovulation induction with medications. Multiple rates are ~10% with oral medications, ~30% with injectable ones.
- Ovarian cysts are common during infertility treatments and can cause various problems.
- Ovarian hyperstimulation: Very rare with oral meds but more common with FSH treatments; can be life threatening
- Couples with infertility may have a slightly increased risk of congenital abnormalities in offspring in general, but no specific abnormalities.

REFERENCES

1. Centers for Disease Contol and Prevention. Reproductive health. Infertility FAQs. www.cdc.gov/reproductivehealth/Infertility/index.htm.
2. Clementini E, Palka C, Iezzi I, et al. Prevalence of chromosomal abnormalities in 2078 infertile couples referred for assisted reproductive techniques. *Human Reprod*. 2005;20:437–42.
3. Mayo Clinic. Infertility. www.mayoclinic.org/infertility/.
4. Thessaloniki ESHRE/ASRM-Sponsored PCOS Consensus Workshop Group. Consensus on infertility treatment related to polycystic ovary syndrome. *Fertil Steril*. 2008;89:505–22.
5. Hughes E, Collins J, Vandekerckhove P. Clomiphene citrate for unexplained subfertility in women. *Cochrane Database Syst Rev*. 2000:CD000057.
6. ASRM Publication. Infertility: An Overview. *A Guide for Patients*. 2003.
7. Palomba S, Oppedisano R, Tolino A, et al. Outlook: Metformin use in infertile patients with polycystic ovary syndrome: An evidence-based overview. *Reprod Biomed Online*. 2008;16:327–35.

ADDITIONAL READING

- Pavone ME, Hirshfeld-Cytron JE, Kazer RR, et al. The progressive simplification of the infertility evaluation. *Obstet Gynecol Surv*. 2011;66:31–41.
- Practice Committee of the American Society for Reproductive Medicine, supplement published in Fertility and Sterility in 2006, volume 86(Suppl 5) has multiple infertility-related articles.

See Also (Topic, Algorithm, Electronic Media Element)

- Endometriosis; Amenorrhea; Infertility; Metabolic Syndrome; Polycystic Ovarian Syndrome
- Algorithm: Infertility

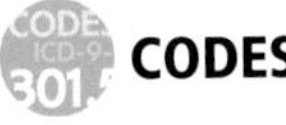

CODES

ICD9

- 628.0 Infertility, female, associated with anovulation
- 628.1 Infertility, female, of pituitary-hypothalamic origin
- 628.9 Infertility, female, of unspecified origin

CLINICAL PEARLS

- Infertility is a complex, multifactorial problem.
- Women <35 years of age should be evaluated for infertility after 1 year of unprotected intercourse; those ≥35 years should receive evaluation after 6 months, and those ≥40 years should receive assistance immediately.
- *Chlamydia* infection is the most common cause of infertility in the US.
- Clomiphene citrate is a selective estrogen receptor modulator that acts via estrogen antagonism at the hypothalamus, thus indirectly increasing FSH and LH production.
- Medical therapy for endometriosis does not increase pregnancy rates after the therapy. However, surgical treatment of endometriosis does improve pregnancy rates with subsequent infertility treatment.
- If a couple is able to do IVF, it is always their best chance of success for attaining a pregnancy.

INFLUENZA

Richard Kent Zimmerman, MD, MPH

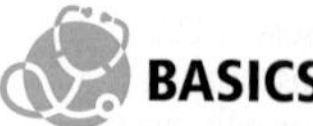

BASICS

DESCRIPTION

- Acute, usually self-limited, febrile infection caused by influenza virus types A and B
- Marked by inflammation of nasal mucosa, pharynx, conjunctiva, and respiratory tract
- Outbreaks occur almost every winter with varying degrees of severity.
- Influenza virus rarely displays antigenic shift (variation). This leads to strains of virus to which little immunologic resistance exists in a population, and it may result in pandemics. Displays minor antigenic variation called drift.
- Swine H1N1 also affects the GI system.
- System(s) affected: Head/Eyes/Ears/Nose/Throat; Pulmonary; with complications: Cardiac and CNS
- Synonym(s): Flu; Grippe; Acute catarrhal fever

EPIDEMIOLOGY

- Predominant age: Young and school-aged children (3 months–16 years old) and young adults:
  - Morbidity: Seasonal morbidity highest in elderly (>75 years) and those with concurrent medical illnesses, such as lung disease. Also higher in young preschool-aged children.
  - Hospitalization rates also higher in infants, elderly, and persons with chronic medical illnesses
- Predominant sex: Male = Female
- Pandemic novel H1N1 has increased morbidity and mortality in persons <65 years and those with concurrent medical illnesses and marked obesity.

Incidence

- Seasonal influenza in preuniversal vaccination: 95 million cases per year, typically fall/winter
- Attack rates in healthy children: 10–40% each year, prior to routine influenza vaccination

RISK FACTORS

- For contracting disease:
  - Semiclosed environments such as nursing homes, schools, and prisons
  - Crowded, close environments during epidemics
- For complications:
  - Neonates, infants, elderly
  - Pregnancy, especially in third trimester
  - Chronic pulmonary diseases
  - Cardiovascular diseases, including valvular problems and congestive heart failure (CHF)
  - Metabolic diseases
  - Hemoglobinopathies
  - Malignancies
  - Immunosuppression
  - Neuromuscular diseases that limit respiratory function and secretion handling
- Pandemic influenza causes morbidity in those <65 years.

GENERAL PREVENTION

- Incubation is 1–4 days; infected persons are most contagious during peak symptoms.
- Vaccination options include trivalent influenza vaccine (TIV) given IM or ID, high-dose trivalent influenza vaccine (TIV HD), or live attenuated influenza vaccine (LAIV), depending on indications and availability.
- Since fall 2010, influenza vaccine recommended universally for those aged ≥6 months
- TIV recommended annually for:
  - All persons aged ≥6 months
  - High-risk individuals, including pregnancy
  - Vaccine should be administered in the fall prior to influenza season.
  - Protection occurs 1–2 weeks after immunization.
  - Typically mild side effects include low-grade fever and local reaction at vaccination site
  - Inactivated IM dose: ≤3 years old: 0.5 mL; children 6–35 months old: 0.25 mL
  - Intradermal formulation for 18–64-year-olds uses a short 30-gauge needle in a single-use prefilled syringe with 0.1 mL vaccine; somewhat higher local reactions given ID
  - Single dose every year except for children <9 years old, who should receive 2 doses (4 weeks apart) the first year they receive influenza vaccine; if 1 or more doses given in 2010–2011 then only 1 dose needed in 2011–2012 season
  - Vaccine contraindication: Severe allergy such as anaphylaxis to eggs or other TIV components; guidelines have changed, as hives from eggs no longer considered a contraindication to TIV due to very low ovalbumin dose in current TIV and good safety information; observe egg-allergic patients for 30 minutes after vaccination; no skin testing with influenza vaccine needed in egg-allergic patients. Egg allergy is a contraindication to LAIV.
  - Precaution: Guillain-Barré syndrome within 6 weeks after a previous dose of influenza vaccine
- LAIV recommended annually for:
  - Healthy persons 2–49 years old
  - Includes health care providers, home care providers, staff and residents of nursing homes and other chronic care facilities, homeless, public safety workers, and close contacts of high-risk individuals, unless in contact with severely immunocompromised on reverse isolation
  - Vaccine contraindications: Anaphylaxis to eggs or other vaccine components, immunocompromising conditions, pregnancy, high-risk conditions including asthma or other chronic cardiopulmonary conditions, history of Guillain-Barré syndrome, chronic aspirin therapy in children
  - Single dose every year except for children <9 years old, who should receive 2 doses (4 weeks apart) the first year they receive influenza vaccine; if 1 or more doses given in 2010–2011 then only 1 dose needed in 2011–2012 season
- TIV-HD: High-dose trivalent inactivated influenza vaccine:
  - Contains 4 times the antigen concentration of TIV
  - Licensed for persons ≥65 years of age
  - Results in higher antibody levels but somewhat higher rates of local reactions
  - Effectiveness being studied
  - Advisory Committee on Immunization Practices does not express a preference for or against TIV-HD
- Antiviral prophylaxis depends on current resistance patterns each year; see www.cdc.gov/flu for the current patterns or check with local health department: Take for duration of outbreak if no vaccine given; discontinue after 14 days if used in addition to vaccine; may be used prophylactically:
  - In high-risk groups that have not been vaccinated or need additional control measures during epidemics. NOT a substitute for vaccination unless vaccine contraindicated (1)[B].
  - During influenza season for those with contraindications to vaccine
  - For staff and residents in nursing home outbreaks
  - For immune-deficient persons who are expected not to respond to vaccination
- For pandemic vaccine and antiviral recommendations, see www.cdc.gov/h1n1flu.

Pediatric Considerations

- Vaccinate children 6–23 months old with inactivated vaccine.
- Either TIV or LAIV in healthy children 2–18 years
- For prophylaxis, oseltamivir dosage varies by weight; zanamivir is approved for prophylaxis for children ≤5 years old at a dosage of 2 inhalations per day. For prophylaxis, the dosage of amantadine and of rimantadine is 5 mg/kg body weight/day up to 150 mg in 2 divided doses.

Pregnancy Considerations

- The CDC recommends vaccinating all women who will be pregnant during influenza season.
- Women at risk for influenza complications should receive inactivated influenza vaccine regardless of trimester.
- Recent evidence of excess morbidity during seasonal influenza supports vaccinating healthy pregnant women in the second or third trimester and those with comorbidities in any trimester (2)[B].
- Recent evidence of excess mortality in 2 previous influenza pandemics supports vaccinating women in any trimester during a pandemic. Oseltamivir, zanamivir, rimantadine, and amantadine are pregnancy Category C.

ETIOLOGY

Orthomyxovirus (influenza types A and B)

COMMONLY ASSOCIATED CONDITIONS

Bacterial pneumonia

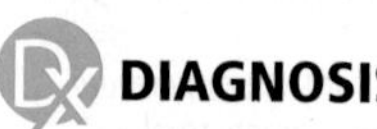

DIAGNOSIS

Sudden onset of:

- High fever
- Chills, malaise, myalgia
- Headache
- Rhinorrhea, nasal congestion
- Sore throat/pharyngitis/sinusitis
- Nonproductive cough

HISTORY

Close attention to local epidemiology (e.g., current outbreak in the community). Contact www.cdc.gov/flu/weekly/fluactivity.htm or state health department to determine type or perform testing.

DIAGNOSTIC TESTS & INTERPRETATION

Lab

- Leukopenia
- Leukocytosis may signal complications.
- Polymerase chain reaction from nasopharyngeal swab or aspirate is the gold standard: Accurate and timely (results in 24 hours)
- Rapid ELISA antigen test. Some rapid tests diagnose influenza A; others diagnose influenza A and B. Sensitivity and specificity vary by manufacturer, influenza strain, and patient age. False negatives are fairly common.

- Tissue culture of nasopharyngeal swab or aspirate: Takes time for results but allows subtyping for epidemiologic studies
- Pulse oximetry

Imaging

Chest x-ray:

- Usually normal unless secondary infection
- Basilar streaking

Pathological Findings

Inflammation of respiratory tract

DIFFERENTIAL DIAGNOSIS

- Respiratory viral infections, including respiratory syncytial virus, parainfluenza, adenovirus, enterovirus
- Infectious mononucleosis
- Coxsackievirus infections
- Viral or streptococcal tonsillitis
- Atypical *Mycoplasma* pneumonia
- Chlamydia pneumoniae
- Q fever

TREATMENT

MEDICATION

First Line

- Antiviral treatment depends on current resistance patterns each year; www.cdc.gov/flu or local health department for current patterns. Antivirals are most effective if administered within first 48 hours and in those with laboratory-confirmed or highly suspected influenza illness.
- Antivirals include amantadine, rimantadine, oseltamivir, zanamivir, and investigational peramivir.
- Antivirals considered for persons not at increased risk of complications from influenza whose onset of symptoms is within the last 48 hours and who wish to shorten the duration of illness and further reduce their relatively low risk of complications
- Symptomatic treatment for those patients *without risk factors* and *without* signs of lower respiratory tract infection (3)
- Antivirals within 48 hours of symptom onset recommended if at risk of complications (4)[B]
- Antivirals recommended for hospitalized patients (1)[B]
- Effect is reduction of symptoms by 24 hours and a reduction in complication rates:
  - Zanamivir dose: 2 inhalations b.i.d. for 5 days (age ≤7 years)
  - Rimantadine dose: 100 mg b.i.d. for ages 13–64 years; 100 mg daily for >65 years
  - Amantadine dose: 100 mg b.i.d. for ages 13–64 years; <100 mg daily for >65 years
  - Oseltamivir dose: 75 mg PO b.i.d. for 5 days (age ≤13 years)
  - If severe renal impairment, 75 mg PO once per day
  - Oseltamivir for children ≥1 year:
    - <15 kg, 30 mg b.i.d.
    - >15–23 kg, 45 mg b.i.d.
    - >23–40 kg, 60 mg b.i.d.
    - >40 kg, 75 mg b.i.d.
  - Oseltamivir for children <1 year: 3 mg/kg/dose b.i.d.
- Antipyretics:
  - Acetaminophen: In children
  - Contraindications: Allergy to a product
- Precautions:
  - Zanamivir may cause bronchospasm if the patient has chronic obstructive pulmonary disease (COPD) or asthma; the patient should have a bronchodilator available.
  - Amantadine: Has anticholinergic properties and should be used with caution in those with psychiatric, addiction, or neurologic disorders, as it may increase risk for suicide attempts or increase neurologic symptoms
  - Rimantadine may increase the risk of seizures in those with an underlying seizure disorder.
  - Oseltamivir:
    - May cause nausea and vomiting; may be less severe if taken with food
- Decrease dose of certain antivirals if creatinine clearance <30 mL/min.

Second Line

- Ibuprofen or other NSAIDs for symptomatic relief
- Aspirin: Should not be used in children <16 years due to risk of Reye syndrome, a rare and severe complication of aspirin use

ADDITIONAL TREATMENT

General Measures

- Symptomatic treatment (saline nasal spray, analgesic gargle)
- Cool-mist or ultrasonic humidifier to increase moisture of inspired air
- Modified respiratory isolation techniques. See www.cdc.gov/h1n1flu for pandemic isolation recommendations.
- Hospitalized patients may require oxygen or ventilatory support.
- Avoid smoking.

IN-PATIENT CONSIDERATIONS

Initial Stabilization

Outpatient except for treatment of severe complications or treatment of those in high-risk groups

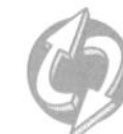

ONGOING CARE

FOLLOW-UP RECOMMENDATIONS

Patient Monitoring

- Mild cases: Usually no follow-up required
- Moderate or severe cases: Follow until symptoms resolve and any complications are treated effectively.

DIET

Increase fluid intake.

PATIENT EDUCATION

CDC: www.cdc.gov/flu

PROGNOSIS

Favorable

COMPLICATIONS

- Otitis media
- Acute sinusitis
- Croup
- Bronchitis
- Pneumonia
- Apnea in neonates
- Reye syndrome
- Rhabdomyolysis
- Postinfluenza asthenia
- COPD or CHF exacerbation
- Encephalopathy
- Death

Geriatric Considerations

Complications more likely in elderly

REFERENCES

1. Harper SA, Bradley JS, Englund JA, et al. Seasonal influenza in adults and children-diagnosis, treatment, chemoprophylaxis, and institutional outbreak management: Clinical practice guidelines of the Infectious Diseases Society of America. *Clin Infect Dis*. 2009;48(8):1003–32.
2. Mak TK, Mangtani P, Leese J, et al. Influenza vaccination in pregnancy: Current evidence and selected national policies. *Lancet Infect Dis*. 2008;8:44–52.
3. CDC. http://cdc.gov/H1N1flu/recommendations.htm#e.
4. Lalezari J, Campion K, Keene O, et al. Zanamivir for the treatment of influenza A and B infection in high-risk patients: A pooled analysis of randomized controlled trials. *Arch Int Med*. 2001;161(2):212–17.
5. Grayson ML, Melvani S, Druce J, et al. Efficacy of soap and water and alcohol-based hand-rub preparations against live H1N1 influenza virus on the hands of human volunteers. *Clin Infect Dis*. 2009;48(3):285–91.

ADDITIONAL READING

- American Academy of Pediatrics. Red Book Online Influenza Resource Page: Influenza Information for Health Care Professionals from the American Academy of Pediatrics. http://aapredbook.aappublications.org/flu
- CDC. Seasonal flue. www.cdc.gov/flu.
- Infectious Diseases Society of America. www.idsociety.org/Content.aspx?id=14220#seasonal

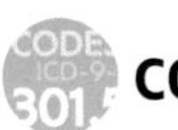

CODES

ICD9

- 487.0 Influenza with pneumonia
- 487.1 Influenza with other respiratory manifestations
- 487.8 Influenza with other manifestations

CLINICAL PEARLS

- Influenza is an acute, usually self-limited, febrile infection caused by influenza virus types A and B.
- Preventative measures are key, including vaccinations.
- Infection can cause significant morbidity and even mortality in the very young, very old, and those with pre-existing comorbidities.
- Hand hygiene either with soap and water (slightly superior) or with alcohol-based hand rubs are proven to reduce human influenza virus A on human hands (5)[C].

I

INGROWN TOENAIL

Steven E. Roskos, MD

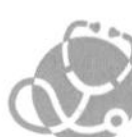

BASICS

DESCRIPTION

- In ingrown toenail, the distal margin of the nail plate grows into the lateral nail fold, causing irritation, inflammation, and sometimes bacterial or fungal infection:
  - Stage 1 (inflammation): Erythema, slight edema, tenderness of lateral nail fold
  - Stage 2 (abscess): Increased pain, erythema, and edema, as well as drainage (purulent or serous)
  - Stage 3 (granulation): Further increased erythema, edema, and pain, with granulation tissue growing over the nail plate
- Can be recurrent
- Synonym(s): Onychocryptosis

EPIDEMIOLOGY

- Great toenail is almost exclusively affected.
- Lateral edge of nail is more commonly affected than the medial edge.
- Most common in males ages 16–25 years
- More common in elderly females than in elderly males
- More common in those with lower incomes

Prevalence

- 24.5/1,000 overall
- 50/1,000 ≥65 years

RISK FACTORS

- Genetic factors:
  - Increased nail fold width
  - Decreased nail thickness
  - Medial rotation of the toe
- Many others proposed; none proven, including:
  - Distorted, thickened nail (onychogryphosis)
  - Fungal infection (onychomycosis)
  - Hyperhidrosis
  - Improper trimming of the lateral nail plate
  - Poorly fitting shoes
  - Trauma to nail or nail fold

GENERAL PREVENTION

- Properly fitting shoes
- Proper nail trimming

PATHOPHYSIOLOGY

- Nail plate penetrates the nail fold.
- This causes a foreign body reaction (inflammation).
- Bacteria or fungi may enter through the opening in the nail fold, causing infection and abscess formation.
- The inflamed and infected tissue hypertrophies, further covering the nail plate.

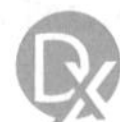

DIAGNOSIS

HISTORY

- Pain
- Redness
- Swelling
- Drainage

PHYSICAL EXAM

- Tenderness of lateral nail fold
- Erythema
- Edema
- Drainage (serous or purulent)
- Granulation tissue
- Hypertrophy of lateral nail fold

DIAGNOSTIC TESTS & INTERPRETATION

Lab

Initial lab tests

None needed unless patient appears septic: Then consider CBC and blood cultures

Imaging

- Consider MRI, x-ray, or bone scan if osteomyelitis is suspected.
- Consider x-ray if subungual exostosis is suspected.

DIFFERENTIAL DIAGNOSIS

- Cellulitis
- Felon (deep abscess on plantar aspect of toe)
- Onychogryphosis (gross thickening and hardening of the nail)
- Onycholysis (separation of nail from nail bed)
- Onychomycosis (fungal infection of the nail)
- Osteomyelitis
- Paronychia
- Subungual exostosis (osteochondroma beneath the nail)

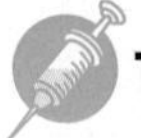

TREATMENT

- Simple nail avulsion (either partial or total) combined with the use of phenol is more effective than surgical excision of the nail bed at preventing symptomatic recurrence of ingrown toenails (1,2)[A].
- Flexible gutter splint is an option for effective treatment of stage 2 or 3 ingrown nails (3,4)[B].
- Oral or topical antibiotics are not helpful as an adjunct to surgical treatment of ingrown toenails (2,5)[B].

MEDICATION

- Some experts recommend oral or topical antibiotics for conservative management.
- Neither oral nor topical antibiotics are useful as an adjunct to surgical treatment (2,5)[B].
- NSAIDs are usually adequate for analgesia.
- Some experts use topical corticosteroids on the hypertrophic lateral nail fold, but this is not commonly practiced.

ADDITIONAL TREATMENT

General Measures

For stage 1:

- Warm water soaks twice a day
- Proper nail trimming
- Properly fitted shoes

Additional Therapies

- For stage 1 ingrown nails, several treatments are available:
  - Cotton wool:
    - Bluntly insert a wisp of cotton under the ingrown portion of the nail.
    - Instruct the patient to reinsert new cotton if the other comes out until the nail grows beyond the nail fold.
    - Consider adding silver nitrate cautery of the nail fold, which the patient then repeats at home.
  - Dental floss:
    - Bluntly insert some dental floss to lift the nail away from the lateral nail fold.
    - Instruct the patient to replace the floss as necessary if it comes out or gets dirty.
    - Keep floss in place until the nail grows beyond the nail fold.
  - Taping:
    - Apply surgical tape to both sides of toe.
    - Use another piece of tape from 1 side to the other to pull the lateral nail fold away from the nail plate.
    - Instruct the patient to keep taping until the nail grows beyond the fold.
  - Cryotherapy of the lateral nail fold
- For stage 2 ingrown nails, consider attempting conservative treatment, as above, especially cotton wool or cryotherapy.

SURGERY/OTHER PROCEDURES

- For stage 2 ingrown nails where conservative treatment has failed, stage 3 ingrown nails, or recurrent ingrown nails, consider either.
- Partial avulsion of the nail with phenol nail matrix ablation (1,2)[A]:
  - Achieve local anesthesia as described below.
  - Place a tourniquet.
  - Incise the nail longitudinally with scissors or a nail splitter a few millimeters from the ingrown border, starting at the distal edge and proceeding to the matrix.

– Elevate the ingrown part of the nail from the nail bed with a periosteal (Freer) elevator or hemostat.
– Pull this portion gently out with a hemostat.
– Dip a urethral swab in 80–88% phenol solution.
– Apply the phenol for 1 minute to the nail matrix under the proximal nail fold. Use multiple swabs if necessary.
– Wash the area with isopropyl (rubbing) alcohol to neutralize phenol.

- Flexible gutter splint (3,4)[B]:
  – Cut a 1–2-cm-long piece of sterilized plastic tube, such as IV tubing, 2–3 mm in diameter (alternatively, you may use a cap from a 29-gauge needle).
  – Make a slit in the tubing lengthwise, and cut the end off at an angle.
  – Apply local anesthesia.
  – Release the ingrown edge of the nail from the nail fold with a hemostat.
  – Slide the tube, angled end first, along the ingrown edge of the nail.
  – Consider fixing the tube in place with self-curing formable acrylic resin (used for dentures and sculptured nails), tape, or a single suture though the nail plate.
  – Leave the tube in place until nail has grown beyond the nail fold.
- Other options for nail matrix ablation include:
  – Electrocautery with a special flattened tip coated with Teflon on one side to protect the proximal nail fold
  – Curettage
  – Surgical excision
- Local anesthesia can be achieved with either:
  – Distal wing block: Infuse 1% lidocaine without epinephrine near the junction of the proximal and lateral nail folds. Continue infusing until the nail folds and the tip of the digit under the distal nail are white from the pressure of the anesthetic.
  – Digital ring block: Infuse 1% lidocaine without epinephrine on the medial and lateral surfaces of the involved digit to anesthetize the plantar and dorsal digital nerves. Lidocaine with epinephrine may be used in selected patients (no peripheral vascular disease, diabetes, cardiac problems, or any evidence of digital infection, gangrene, or bone fracture) (6).

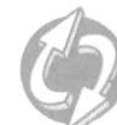

ONGOING CARE

FOLLOW-UP RECOMMENDATIONS

- Dress with antibiotic ointment or sterile petroleum jelly; cover with sterile gauze and tube gauze.
- Postoperative instructions should include:
  – Rest and elevate the foot for 12–24 hours.
  – Take NSAIDs for discomfort.
  – Change dressing and wash with soap and water daily.
  – Expect a sterile exudate for 2–6 weeks.
  – Avulsed nails may take 6–12 months to grow completely out (if no matrix ablation).
  – Call for increasing pain, redness, or swelling.
  – Average time to return to normal activities is 2 weeks.
- Patients treated conservatively should be followed up in the office every 7–10 days until marked improvement is noted.

PATIENT EDUCATION

- Trim nails straight across (do not round corners) and not too short.
- Wear properly fitting, comfortable shoes.

COMPLICATIONS

- Cellulitis after surgical procedure (uncommon)
- Damage to fascia or periosteum from overly aggressive matrix ablation
- Damage to nail bed
- Distal toe ischemia due to prolonged use of a tourniquet during surgery (rare)
- Nail plate deformity (due to damage to nail matrix)
- Osteomyelitis (rare)
- Permanent narrowing of nail (if matrix ablation is performed)
- Postoperative wound drainage
- Recurrence (40–80% with avulsion alone, 0.6–14% with matrix ablation, 6–13% with gutter splint)

REFERENCES

1. Rounding C, Bloomfield S. Surgical treatments for ingrowing toenails. *Cochrane Database Syst Rev*. 2003;1:CD001541.
2. Bos AM, van Tilburg MW, van Sorge AA, et al. Randomized clinical trial of surgical technique and local antibiotics for ingrowing toenail. *Br J Surg*. 2007;94:292–6.
3. Arai H, Arai T, Nakajima H, et al. Formable acrylic treatment for ingrowing nail with gutter splint and sculptured nail. *Int J Dermatol*. 2004;43:759–65.
4. Nazari S. A simple and practical method in treatment of ingrown nails: Splinting by flexible tube. *J Eur Acad Dermatol Venereol*. 2006; 20:1302–6.
5. Reyzelman AM, Trombello KA, Vayser DJ, et al. Are antibiotics necessary in the treatment of locally infected ingrown toenails? *Arch Fam Med*. 2000;9:930–2.
6. Altinyazar HC, Demirel CB, Koca R, Hosnuter M. Digital block with and without epinephrine during chemical matricectomy with phenol. *Dermatol Surg*. 2010;36(10):1568–71.

ADDITIONAL READING

- Chapeskie H. Ingrown toenail or overgrown toe skin?: Alternative treatment for onychocryptosis. *Can Fam Physician*. 2008;54:1561–2.
- Richert B. Basic nail surgery. *Dermatol Clin*. 2006;24:313–22.
- Woo SH, Kim IH. Surgical pearl: Nail edge separation with dental floss for ingrown toenails. *J Am Acad Dermatol*. 2004;50:939–40.

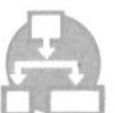

See Also (Topic, Algorithm, Electronic Media Element)

For a video of this procedure, go to: http://5minuteconsult.com/procedure/1508006 or http://emedicine.medscape.com/article/149627-overview#a01

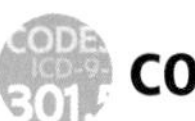

CODES

ICD9

703.0 Ingrowing nail

CLINICAL PEARLS

- The best treatment for a stage 1 ingrown toenail is to insert a wisp of cotton or dental floss between the nail plate and lateral nail fold.
- The best treatment for a stage 3 ingrown toenail is either partial nail avulsion with phenol matrix ablation or application of a flexible gutter splint.
- A patient can prevent ingrown toenails by trimming nails properly and wearing properly fitting shoes.
- Antibiotics are not useful in the treatment of ingrown nails in conjunction with surgical treatment; they may be useful for conservative treatment.

I

INJURY AND VIOLENCE

Monica Kaitz, MD
Edward Feller, MD

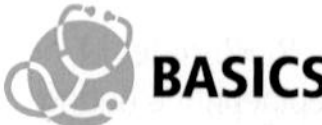

BASICS

EPIDEMIOLOGY

- Injury is the primary source of lost years of productive life for individuals <44 years of age.
- In industrialized countries, injury is the fifth leading cause of death overall and the leading cause of death for persons 1–14 years, accounting for 40% of all child death, 75% of youth death.
- Injury, intentional or not, is both predictable and preventable, with elderly and children most susceptible (1). Yearly, 1 in 3 adults aged >65 have falls. In women from 2004–2007, 54% of injuries occurred at home compared to 41% in men. Men acquired injuries more frequently in recreational (17%) and occupational settings (13%).

Incidence

- 63% unintentional, 34% intentional injury deaths in the US each year (1)
- Most common injuries:
  - During 2004–2007, 33.5 million reported injuries/year. Falls were leading cause of injury, ~40%, twice any other cause. The injury rate for falls was 17% higher among females (2)[A].
  - Falling is the most common injury in the young (43% of injuries) and elderly (64%).
  - Blunt trauma (20%) and overexertion (13%) are most common injuries in adolescents and adults, respectively. Bites/stings (4.8%), bicycle accidents (4.7%), and poisonings (1.8%) are uniquely common to children, while MVA are frequent in adolescents and adults (10%; third most common) as well as elderly (5%; fourth most common). Penetrating injury (8.1%) and blunt trauma/assault (4.9%) peak in adults, although absolute numbers have decreased since 2006 (3)[A].
- Most common fatal injuries:
  - MVA causes most deaths in children, adolescents, and adults, a close second in infants and the elderly superseded by unintentional suffocation and falls, respectively.
  - Children mostly die of unintentional injuries; in order: MVA, drowning, fire/burn, and suffocation.
  - Aside from MVA, most deaths in adolescents result from firearms, both homicide (second, fourth in adults) and suicide (third, third in adults). Suicide by suffocation is also pervasive in both adolescence (fourth) and adulthood (fifth).
  - Poisoning is particularly deadly in adults, with both unintentional (second) and suicidal (sixth) combined causing more deaths than MVA.
  - Homicide from firearm is fourth in children, second in adolescents, fourth in adults, while suicide by firearm is third in adolescents and adults, fourth in the elderly. It should be noted: Watch for homicide in infants (third) and adverse drug effects in the elderly.
  - Most firearm deaths are homicides in children and adolescents, suicides in adults and the elderly. Other common methods of suicide are suffocation, poisoning. Other common forms of homicide in adolescence (fourth) and adults (fifth) are penetrating injuries (3)[A].

Prevalence

- Firearms:
  - In 2001, 35% of adults reported living in a home with at least 1 firearm.
  - Gun violence costs $100 billion/yr of which $15 billion are from firearm injuries to children (1)[C].
- Child violence (1):
  - Homicide rate for children highest in US vs. other industrialized nations
  - 33% of rapes occur prior to 12 years of age; 50% by 18 years.
- Adolescent violence (4)[B]:
  - 33% of students are involved in fights annually; 13% of students participated in 1 or more fights at school in the last year.
  - 17% of students have carried a weapon in the last 30 days; 6.1% of students have carried a weapon to school. 9% of students have been injured by a weapon at school.
  - 16–19-year-olds at highest risk for motor vehicle crashes, boys twice that of girls (1)[C].
  - Dating violence: Prevalence has been reported to range from 9–46% (5)[C].
- Homicide (5)[C]:
  - Second leading cause of death for children 1–19 years of age
  - Leading cause of death among black 15–24-year-olds
- Bullying (5)[C]:
  - Prevalence 30% for children either bullying and/or being bullied in 6th–10th-graders
  - Bullying associated with low self-esteem, social isolation, and depression
  - 1 in 9 middle school students report being cyberbullied (via the Internet). ~50% of victims don't know perpetrator's identity.
- Interpersonal violence (IPV) (6):
  - 1 in 4 women and 1 in 7 men report a lifetime threatened or completed physical or sexual IPV. 1.4% of women and 0.7% of men reported IPV within the past year.
  - 40–70% of female homicides killed by boyfriends or husbands.
- Injury:
  - Youth are affected disproportionately, accounting for ~30% of potential life years lost before age 65 (more than cancer and heart disease combined) (1)[C].
  - 37.3% of all ED visits are injury-related (1)[C].
- Motor vehicle crashes (4)[C]:
  - 3 in 10 people are involved in an alcohol-related motor vehicle crash in their lifetime. 1 in 4 teens killed in a motor vehicle crash (2008) had a blood alcohol level >0.08 g/dL.
  - 18% of high school students do not wear seatbelts. 86% of youth under the age of 14 wear seatbelts; yet, 65% of these wear restraints that are inappropriate for their age or weight.
  - Mortality rate for male MVA 3 times greater than females. 50% of road traffic injuries are cyclists, pedestrians, and motorcycle riders (6).
- Poisonings:
  - Second leading cause of injury death overall, first for ages 35–54, incidence tripling from 4,000 in 1999 to 13,800 in 2006, 90% involving drugs, 40% involving opioid analgesics, in particular methadone. Risk varies with: Gender (males account for 75% of 2006 deaths), age, non-Hispanic white persons, and state.
- Drowning:
  - 86% were not wearing personal flotation devices (1).

RISK FACTORS

- Injuries and risk factors that contribute vary at different stages of life and development (4):
  - Infants, toddlers, and children (ages 0–9):
    - MVA: Unrestrained or improperly restrained. Only 37% are restrained in age-appropriate devices; of children killed in MVA, 68% are killed while riding with a driver under the influence of alcohol.
    - Bicycle: Collision with MV, self-reported speed >15 mph, age <6 or >39 years; less likely to wear helmet based on: Race, ethnicity, child age, household income, household education, helmet law
    - Suffocation (children <1 year old): Loose bedding, wedging, cosleeping, entrapment, hanging, sleeping in environments not intended for infants (couches, adult bed)
    - Drowning: Males, inadequate supervision, residential swimming pools
    - Falls: Walkers, open windows, open stairways, inadequate supervision, hazardous playground equipment
    - Homicides: Lack of access to social capital, community organization, and economic resources, familial instability, community and family violence, access to firearms
  - Adolescents (ages 10–24):
    - MVA: Male driver, inexperience, nighttime driving, speeding, tailgating, driving with other teenagers, cell phones, unrestrained occupants, alcohol and drug use
    - Homicide and suicide: Access to firearms, mental health, alcohol and drug use, exposure to suicidal behavior, history of aggressive behavior, cognitive deficits, poor supervision, exposure to violence, parental drug and alcohol use, poor peer-to-peer interaction, academic failure, poverty, lower socioeconomic class
    - Sports-related injuries
  - Adults (ages 25–64):
    - MVA: Alcohol and drug use, speeding, distractions (e.g., other passengers, cell phones)
    - Prescription drug overdose is a leading cause of accidental death in adults.
    - IPV: Female, young, history of IPV or sexual assault or child abuse, drugs, unemployment, depression, minority status, income or educational disparity, poverty, weak legal sanctions
  - Older adults (≥65):
    - MVA: Poor vision, medical condition, and comorbidities
    - Falls: Poor vision, medications, weakness, gait imbalance, environmental risk factors (loose rugs, poor lighting, lack of stair railings)
- In addition, individuals from low-income and racial and ethnic minority groups are at a greater risk for injury.

ETIOLOGY

Multifactorial

DIAGNOSIS

HISTORY

- Mechanism, timing, and location of injury:
  - Blunt vs. penetrating; intentional vs. unintentional; others injured vs. isolated injury; circumstances (weather, substance use, restrained vs. unrestrained)
  - Does history correlate with level of injury (i.e., level of suspicion for abuse [elderly, child, or partner])?
- IPV: Neurologic deficits, seizures, chronic pain, GI, STDs, pregnancy, psychiatric. Insufficient evidence per USPTF to recommend for or against routine screening of women for IPV.

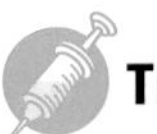

TREATMENT

- Prevention: Experts agree that most injuries are preventable. Prevention efforts have been framed as "the 5 E's": Enhanced education, engineering strategies, economic incentives, and enforcement/enactment of laws.
- Prevention by level of intervention: Primary (i.e., prevent crash—listed below by etiology), secondary (i.e., prevent injury upon crash), and tertiary (i.e., prevent poor outcomes upon injury)
- Motor vehicle injuries (4)[C]:
  - Infants, toddlers, and children: Age-appropriate child safety seats and passenger restraints with distribution programs, education programs for parents and caregivers, safety seat checkpoints, harsh penalties for drivers transporting children under the influence of drugs and/or alcohol, legislation regarding restraint of motor vehicle occupants
  - Adolescents and adults: Graduated driver licensing programs, blood alcohol concentration laws, minimum drinking age laws, sobriety checkpoints, programs for alcohol servers, zero alcohol tolerance laws for young drivers, school-based education programs on drinking and driving. Emergency medical services (EMS) response times, engineering cars for rapid extraction, organized trauma systems; collapsible automobile steering columns have been shown to decrease injury mortality and morbidity. Avoid alcohol: Effects on motorcycle riding skills observed at blood level as low as 0.05 g/dL. Motorcycle helmet decreases risk of death by 42%, head injury by 69% (1,6).
  - Older adults: Alternative transportation programs, screening for high-risk drivers, gradual curtailment of driving privileges, more frequent license renewal process
  - Bicycle helmets can reduce risk of head injury by 63–88%. Canadian helmet legislation decreased mortality by 52% (6).
  - Pedestrian injury: Reflective clothing
- Falls (4,6)[C]:
  - Infants/toddlers: Home safety assessments, window guards, elimination of walker use
  - Older adults: Home safety assessments, installation of handrails and grab bars, removal of tripping hazards, nonslip mats, exercise programs (improve strength and balance), night lights
  - Reduces rate of falls: Exercise 17%, vitamin D dosed 700–1,000 IU/d 19%, expedited first eye cataract surgery 34%, gradual withdrawal from psychotropic medications
- Drowning (4,6)[C]:
  - Improved supervision of young children (especially with epileptics and in bathtubs); current recommendations: Swimming lessons in those over 4; trained lifeguard supervision; fencing (1.2 m high, inclining toward climbers in ANEC study), locked gates, and pool alarms; personal flotation devices and boating safety awareness; parental certification in CPR
- Fire and burns:
  - Reducing temperature of hot water heaters to <54.4°C (130.1°F)
  - Smoke and carbon monoxide detectors; fire exit planning
  - Educational campaigns for those at highest risk for home fires (homes with children <4, adults >65, lower socioeconomic class, rural communities)
- Violence (homicide, suicide, assaults):
  - Most effective strategies focus on younger age groups' positive sense of self; emotional and behavioral regulation; decision-making skills; moral system of belief; and a positive connection with family and community.
  - Limited access to firearms and/or firearm safety training
  - Suicide: Access to mental health services, improved family and community support, development of healthy coping and problem-solving skills
  - IPV: Proven reduced by: Alcoholism treatment, intense interventions of >12 hours
  - Dating violence: 1 randomized trial of a school program was shown to be effective in decreasing self-reported dating violence 4 years out from the intervention (5).
- Sports-related injuries (4)[C]:
  - Proper equipment. Helmets can prevent 85% of bicyclist head injuries. States without helmet laws have doubled fatality rate from head injuries (1).
  - Plan of action for dealing with injuries such as concussion in young athletes, with guidelines regarding if or when it is safe to return to play.
- Musculoskeletal workplace injuries:
  - Back injuries: NIOSH review of literature shows insufficient evidence to substantiate backbelts as effective. Recommends employer implement comprehensive ergonomics program. Due to mechanical patient lifting devices, Bureau of Labor Statistics reported 35% decline in low back injuries in nurses 2003–2009 (7)[A].
  - Follow guidelines: Annual cost of farm-associated injuries among youth has been estimated at $1 billion annually. Guidelines established for parents match chores with their child's development, with follow-up unpublished data showing a 56% decline in youth farm injury rates from 1998–2009 (7). CDC prevention guidelines are available at: http://wonder.cdc.gov/wonder/prevguid/topics.html.
- Poisoning (1)[C]:
  - High rates in children: Call poison center hotline immediately after ingestion of toxin (90% occur at home).

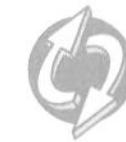

ONGOING CARE

COMPLICATIONS

- Injury-related medical expenditures are roughly 10% of US health care spending; $224–406 billion annually (1)
- Social burden of injury: Loss of productivity, emotional loss, nonmedical expenditures, reduced quality of life, litigation, rehabilitation, mental health costs, altered family and peer relationships, chronic pain, substance use and abuse, changes in lifestyle (3)

REFERENCES

1. Betz M, Li G. Injury prevention and control. *Emerg Med Clin N Am*. 2007;25:901–14.
2. Chen LH, Warner M, Fingerhut L, et al. Injury episodes and circumstances: National Health Interview Survey, 1997–2007. *Vital Health Stat* 2009;10(241). Available at www.cdc.gov/nchs/data/series/sr_10/sr10_241.pdf.
3. Centers for Disease Control and Prevention. National Center for Injury Prevention and Control. Web-based Injury Statistics Query and Reporting System (WISQARS). Available at: www.cdc.gov/ncipc/wisqars.
4. Centers for Disease Control and Prevention. National Center for Injury Prevention and Control. *CDC Injury Fact Book*. Atlanta: Author, 2006.
5. Committee on Injury, Violence, and Poison Prevention, et al. Policy statement–Role of the pediatrician in youth violence prevention. *Pediatrics*. 2009;124:393–402.
6. Curry P, Ramaiah R, Vavilala MS. Current trends and update on injury prevention. *Int J Crit Illn Inj Sci*. 2011;1:57–65.
7. Ten Great Public Health Achievements, United States 2001–2010. *MMWR*. 2011;60(19):619–23.

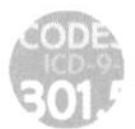

CODES

ICD9

- 959.8 Other specified sites, including multiple injury
- 959.9 Unspecified site injury

CLINICAL PEARLS

- Injury is the primary source of lost years of productive life for individuals <44 years of age.
- MVA causes most deaths in children and adolescents.
- Children die of unintentional injuries; in order: MVA, drowning, fire/burn, and suffocation.
- Homicide from firearm is fourth in children, second in adolescents, fourth in adults, while suicide by firearm is third in adolescents and adults, fourth in the elderly
- 1 in 4 women and 1 in 7 men report a lifetime threatened or completed physical or sexual intimate partner violence.

I

INTERSTITIAL CYSTITIS

Montiel T. Rosenthal, MD

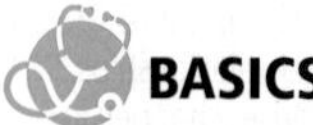

BASICS

DESCRIPTION

- A disease of unknown cause, probably representing a final common pathway from several etiologies
- Likely pathogenesis is disruption of urothelium, impaired lower urinary track defenses, and loss of bladder muscular wall elasticity. The symptoms in many patients are insidious and the disease progresses for years before the diagnosis is established.
- Mild: Normal bladder capacity under anesthesia. Ulceration, cracking, or glomerulation of mucosa (or not) with bladder distention under anesthesia. No incontinence. Symptoms wax and wane and may not progress. Interstitial cystitis is a bladder sensory problem.
- Severe: Progressive bladder fibrosis. Small true bladder capacity under anesthesia. Poor bladder wall compliance. Often, ulcers present at cystoscopy. May have overflow incontinence and/or chronic bacteriuria that is unresponsive to antibiotics.
- System(s) affected: Renal/urologic
- Synonym(s): Urgency frequency syndrome; Painful bladder syndrome

Pregnancy Considerations

Unpredictable symptom improvement or exacerbation during pregnancy. No known fetal effects from interstitial cystitis. Usual problems of unknown effect on fetus with medications taken during pregnancy

EPIDEMIOLOGY

- Occurs predominantly among whites
- Predominant sex: Female > Male (10:1)
- Predominant age:
  - Mild: 20–40 years
  - Severe: 20–70 years
- Pediatric considerations:
  - <10 years old and again at 13–17 years
  - Daytime enuresis, dysuria without infection

Prevalence

In the US:

- Up to 1,000,000 affected, but many cases likely are unreported
- 0.052%, but may be higher, up to 10% (1)[C]

RISK FACTORS

Unknown

ETIOLOGY

- Unknown, but is not primarily psychosomatic
- Possible causes:
  - Subclinical urinary infection
  - Damage to glycosaminoglycan mucus layer increasing bladder wall permeability to irritants such as urea
  - Autoimmune
  - Mast cell histamine release
- Neurologic upregulation/stimulation

COMMONLY ASSOCIATED CONDITIONS

- Fibromyalgia
- Allergies
- Chronic fatigue syndrome
- Depression
- Chronic prostatitis
- Chronic pelvic pain
- Irritable bowel syndrome
- Anal/rectal disease

DIAGNOSIS

- Frequent, urgent, relentless urination day and night; >8 voids in 24 hours
- Pain with full bladder that resolves with bladder emptying (except if bacteriuria is present).
- Urge urinary incontinence if bladder capacity is small.
- Sleep disturbance
- Dyspareunia, especially with full bladder
- Secondary symptoms from chronic pain and sleeplessness, especially depression

HISTORY

- Pelvic Pain and Urgency/Frequency Symptom Scale (2)[B]: Self-reporting questionnaire for screening potential interstitial cystitis patients
- Frequent UTIs, vaginitis, or symptoms during the week before menses

PHYSICAL EXAM

- Perineal/prostatic pain in men
- Anterior vaginal wall pain in women

DIAGNOSTIC TESTS & INTERPRETATION

Lab

- Urinalysis: Normal except with chronic bacteriuria (rare)
- Urine culture from catheterized specimen: Normal except with chronic bacteriuria (rare) or partial antibiotic treatment
- Urine cytology:
  - Normal: Reserve for men >40 years old and women with hematuria

Diagnostic Procedures/Surgery

- Cystoscopy (especially in men >40 years old or women with hematuria):
  - Bladder wall visualization
  - Hydraulic distention: No improved diagnostic certainty over history and physical alone
- No role for urodynamic testing
- K+ sensitivity test (2)[B]:
  - Insert catheter, empty bladder, instill 40 mL H_2O over 2–3 minutes, rank urgency on scale of 0–5 in intensity, rank pain on scale of 0–5 in intensity, drain bladder, instill 40 mL KCl 0.4 mol/L solution:
    - If immediate pain, flush bladder with 60 mL H_2O and treat with bladder instillations
    - If no immediate pain, wait 5 minutes and rate urgency and pain
  - If urgency or pain >2, treat as above
- Pain or urgency >2 is considered a positive test and strongly correlates with interstitial cystitis if no radiation cystitis or acute bacterial cystitis is present.

Pathological Findings

- Nonspecific chronic inflammation on bladder biopsies
- Urine cytology negative for dysplasia and neoplasia
- Possible mast cell proliferation in mucosa

DIFFERENTIAL DIAGNOSIS

- Uninhibited bladder (urgency, frequency, urge incontinence, less pain, symptoms usually decrease when asleep)
- Urinary infection: Cystitis, prostatitis
- Bladder neoplasm
- Bladder stone
- Neurologic bladder disease
- Nonurinary pelvic disease (STIs, endometriosis, pelvic relaxation)

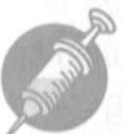

TREATMENT

MEDICATION

Randomized controlled trials of most medications for interstitial cystitis demonstrate limited benefit over placebo; there are no clear predictors of what will benefit an individual. Prepare the patient that treatment may involve trial and error.

First Line

- Pentosan polysulfate (Elmiron) 100 mg t.i.d. May take several months to become effective; rated as modestly beneficial in systematic drug review (3)[A] (only FDA-approved treatment for interstitial cystitis).
- Tolterodine 1–2 mg b.i.d.
- Triple drug therapy: 6 months of pentosan, hydroxyzine, doxepin
- Behavioral therapy combined with oral agents found improved outcomes compared to medications alone.
- Antibacterials for bacteriuria
- Hydroxyzine
- Amitriptyline ≥50 mg/d (4)[C]
- Oxybutynin, hyoscyamine, and other anticholinergic medications decrease frequency.
- Prednisone (only for ulcerative lesions)
- Montelukast
- Doxepin decreases frequency.
- NSAIDs for pain and any inflammatory component
- Bladder instillations:
  - Lidocaine, sodium bicarbonate, and heparin or pentosan polysulfate sodium
  - Dimethyl sulfoxide (DMSO) every 1–2 weeks for 3–6 weeks, then as needed
  - Heparin sometimes added to DMSO
  - Other agents: Steroids, silver nitrate, oxychlorosene (Clorpactin)
- Contraindications:
  - No anticholinergics for patients with closed-angle glaucoma
- Significant possible interactions:
  - Refer to manufacturer's profile of each drug.

Second Line

Phenazopyridine, a local bladder mucosal anesthetic, usually is not very effective.

ADDITIONAL TREATMENT

General Measures

- Appropriate health care: Outpatient
- Eliminate foods and liquids that exacerbate symptoms on individual basis.
- Biofeedback bladder retraining

Additional Therapies

Myofascial physical therapy (targeted pelvic, hip girdle, abdominal trigger point massage) (5)[C]

COMPLEMENTARY AND ALTERNATIVE MEDICINE

Guided imagery

SURGERY/OTHER PROCEDURES

- Hydraulic distention of bladder under anesthesia: Symptomatic but transient relief
- Cauterization of bladder ulcer
- Augmentation cystoplasty to increase bladder capacity and decrease pressure, with or without partial cystectomy. Expected results in severe cases: Much improved, 75%; with residual discomfort, 20%; unchanged, 5%
- Urinary diversion with total cystectomy only if disease completely refractory to medical therapy

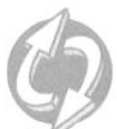

ONGOING CARE

FOLLOW-UP RECOMMENDATIONS

Patient Monitoring

Not specifically needed unless symptoms are unresponsive to treatment

DIET

- Variable effects from person to person
- Common irritants include caffeine, chocolate, citrus, tomatoes, carbonated beverages, K^+-rich foods, spicy foods, acidic foods, and alcohol.

PATIENT EDUCATION

Interstitial Cystitis Association, 110 Washington St. Suite 340, Rockville, MD 20850; 1(800) HELPICA; www.ichelp.org

PROGNOSIS

- Mild: Exacerbations and remissions of symptoms; may not be progressive; does not predispose to other diseases
- Severe: Progressive problems that usually require surgery to control symptoms

COMPLICATIONS

Severe with long-term, continuous high bladder pressure could be associated with renal damage.

REFERENCES

1. Parsons CL, Tatsis V. Prevalence if interstitial cystitis in young women. *Urology.* 2004;64:866.
2. Parsons CL, Dell J, et al. Increased prevalence of interstitial cystitis; previously unrecognized urologic and gynecological cases identified using a new symptom questionnaire and intravesical potassium sensitivity. *Urology.* 2002;60:573–8.
3. Dimitrakov J, Kroenke K, Steers WD, et al. Pharmacologic management of painful bladder syndrome/interstitial cystitis: A systematic review. *Arch Intern Med.* 2007;167:1922–9.
4. Foster HE, Hanno PM, Nickel JC, et al. Effect of amitryptylline on symptoms in treatment naive patients with interstitial cystitis/painful bladder syndrome. *J Urol.* 2010;183:1853–8.
5. Fitzgerald MP, Anderson RU, Potts J, et al. Randomized multicenter feasibility trial of myofascial physical therapy for treatement of urologic chronic pelvic pain syndrome. *J Urol.* 2009;182:570–80.

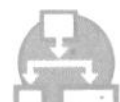

See Also (Topic, Algorithm, Electronic Media Element)

- Urinary Tract Infection (UTI) in Females
- Algorithm: Pelvic Girdle Pain (Pregnancy or Postpartum Anterior Pelvic Pain)

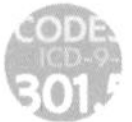

CODES

ICD9

595.1 Chronic interstitial cystitis

CLINICAL PEARLS

- The potassium sensitivity test has been the most useful in confirming an initial diagnosis of interstitial cystitis.
- K+ sensitivity test (2):
  - Insert catheter, empty bladder, instill 40 mL H_2O over 2–3 minutes, rank urgency on scale of 0–5 in intensity, rank pain on scale of 0–5 in intensity, drain bladder, instill 40 mL KCl 0.4 mol/L solution
- Submucosal petechial hemorrhages and/or ulceration at the time of bladder distention and cystoscopy further support the diagnosis.
- At present, there is no definitive treatment for interstitial cystitis.
- Most patients with severe disease receive multiple treatment approaches. Regular multidisciplinary follow-up, pharmacological therapy, avoidance of symptom triggers, psychological and supportive therapy are all important because this disease tends to wax and wane. Monitor patients for comorbid depression.
- Empowering patients to be managers of their symptoms, to communicate regularly with their physicians, and to learn as much as they are able about this disease can help them to optimize their outcome.

INTERSTITIAL NEPHRITIS

Fozia A. Ali, MD

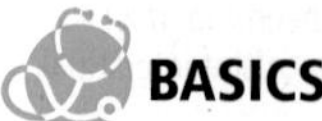

BASICS

DESCRIPTION

- Acute interstitial nephritis (AIN) is an inflammatory response of the kidney involving interstitial edema and, at times, tubular cell damage. It may be an acute reaction or a result of long-term damage.
- System(s) affected: Renal/Urologic, Endocrine/Metabolic, Immunologic
- Synonym(s): Tubulointerstitial nephritis (TIN), Acute interstitial allergic nephritis

EPIDEMIOLOGY

Pediatric Considerations

Children exposed to lead poisoning are more likely to develop nephritis as a young adult:

- TIN with uveitis presents in adolescent females
- Atherosclerotic or ischemic nephritis is more common in the elderly.

Incidence

- Interstitial nephritis accounts for 10–15% of kidney disease in the US.
- Analgesic-induced nephritis is 5–6× more common in women.
- Peak incidence in women 60–70 years of age

Geriatric Considerations

The elderly have more severe disease and increased risk of permanent damage.

GENERAL PREVENTION

- Early recognition and prompt discontinuation of offending agents
- Remove all sources of heavy metals, including ceramics.
- Avoid further nephrotoxicity.

PATHOPHYSIOLOGY

- AIN:
  - Delayed hypersensitivity reaction, usually owing to drugs
  - May cause acute renal insufficiency
  - Regardless of the severity of the damage to the tubular epithelium, the renal dysfunction generally is reversible, possibly reflecting the regenerative capacity of tubules with preserved basement membrane.
- Chronic interstitial nephritis (CIN):
  - Follows long-term exposure to offending agents
  - Often found on routine labs or evaluation for hypertension (HTN)
  - Characterized by interstitial scarring, fibrosis, and tubule atrophy, resulting in progressive chronic renal insufficiency
- TIN is sometimes associated with uveitis.

ETIOLOGY

- AIN:
  - Hypersensitivity to drugs (70%):
    - Antibiotics: Penicillin, cephalosporins, sulfonamides, rifampin
    - NSAIDs/analgesics (more common in elderly people because of the higher incidence of arthritic disorders in this population)
    - Sulfa-containing diuretics
    - Phenytoin
    - Allopurinol
  - Infectious
  - AIN is associated with primary renal infections such as acute bacterial pyelonephritis, renal tuberculosis, and fungal nephritis.
  - Acute transplant rejection
  - Immunologic: Systemic lupus erythematosus (SLE), Sjögren's syndrome, sarcoidosis, Wegener's granulomatosis, cryoglobulinemia
  - Idiopathic (isolated or with uveitis)
- CIN:
  - Drugs: Analgesics, lithium, antineoplastics, antibiotics, anticonvulsants, antihypertensives, immunosuppressants, diuretics, Chinese herbal medicines
  - Heavy metals: Lead, cadmium
  - Obstruction: Stones, neoplasm, prostatic hypertrophy
  - Metabolic: Hypercalcemia, hyperoxaluria, chronic hypokalemia, cystinosis
  - Vascular changes: Cholesterol emboli, HTN, sickle hemoglobinopathy, radiation
  - Toxins: Snakebite venom (hemotoxic or myotoxic)
  - Other: Balkan-endemic nephropathy, Epstein-Barr virus

COMMONLY ASSOCIATED CONDITIONS

- Alport syndrome
- Medullary cystic disease
- Inflammatory bowel disease
- Multiple myeloma
- Primary biliary cirrhosis

DIAGNOSIS

- AIN:
  - Fever: 80%
  - Transient maculopapular rash: 25–50%
  - Acute renal insufficiency:
    - Decreased urine output: 50%
    - Signs of fluid overload or depletion
    - Altered mental status
    - Nausea, vomiting
- CIN:
  - HTN
  - Decreased urine output or polyuria
  - Inability to concentrate urine
  - Polydipsia
  - Acidosis
  - Anemia
  - Fanconi syndrome

HISTORY

- Medications
- Alcohol and illicit drug use
- Exposure to heavy metals
- Tobacco use
- Dyslipidemia/atherosclerosis
- Cancer
- HTN

PHYSICAL EXAM

- Increased BP
- Altered mental status
- Rash accompanying renal findings in acute AIN
- Pericardial rub if uremic pericarditis
- Lung crackles if fluid overload
- Extremity swelling
- Weight gain from fluid retention

DIAGNOSTIC TESTS & INTERPRETATION

Lab

- CBC:
  - Eosinophilia (80%): Not seen in NSAID-induced AIN
  - Anemia
- Chemistry:
  - Acidosis
  - Hypokalemia/hyperkalemia
  - Elevated BUN and creatinine
- Urinalysis with urine lytes:
  - Hematuria (95%)
  - Mild proteinuria (present to variable degrees, usually <1 g/24 h, except in AIN associated with NSAIDs)
  - Specific gravity
  - Pyuria, WBC casts
  - Eosinophiluria
- Serologic testing for immunologic disease: Sarcoidosis, Sjögren syndrome, Wegener granulomatosis, Behçet syndrome
- Lead level:
  - Not useful in chronic lead exposure
  - >90% of lead resides in bone
  - If chronic lead exposure is suspected, consider EDTA lead mobilization test.
- Liver function tests: Elevated serum transaminase levels (in patients with associated drug-induced liver injury)

Imaging

- Kidneys, ureters, and bladder (KUB)
- Gallium scan (a negative gallium scan does not preclude the diagnosis because false-negative results can be seen)
- Renal ultrasonography may demonstrate kidneys that are normal to enlarged in size with increased cortical echogenicity, but there are no ultrasonographic findings that will reliably confirm or exclude AIN versus other causes of acute renal failure.
- The role of IV pyelography (IVP) remains in question (in many instances, similar information can be obtained by ultrasound without exposing the patient to potentially nephrotoxic contrast dye).

Follow-Up & Special Considerations

Patients who do not recover renal function and those with chronic TIN should receive long-term follow-up care to protect kidneys from further potentially nephrotoxic therapies.

Diagnostic Procedures/Surgery

- Renal biopsy is the gold standard and definitive method of establishing diagnosis of AIN. However, it is not needed in all patients.
- Indications for renal biopsy: Patients who do not improve following withdrawal of likely precipitating medications, who have no contraindications to renal biopsy and do not refuse the procedure, and who are being considered for steroid therapy are good candidates for renal biopsy.
- Contraindications: Renal biopsy is contraindicated in bleeding diathesis, solitary kidney, end-stage renal disease with small kidneys, severe uncontrolled HTN and sepsis, or renal parenchymal infection.

Pathological Findings
- Acute:
  - Cellular infiltration with eosinophilia
  - In cholesterol microembolism in the kidney, the finding of a characteristic needle-shaped cleft in medium- or small-sized renal arterioles is diagnostic.
- Chronic: Chronic TIN is characterized by tubular atrophy, fibrosis, and cellular infiltration with mononuclear cells.

DIFFERENTIAL DIAGNOSIS
- Acute renal failure
- Urinary tract obstruction

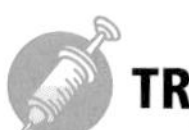

TREATMENT

For AIN, data on corticosteroids' efficacy has been limited (1)[B].

MEDICATION
- Mainstay of treatment is supportive therapy.
- Offending drugs should be discontinued.
- If patient is taking multiple offending drugs, a reasonable clinical approach should include whether any suspected drug can be substituted easily with another medication.
- If renal failure persists after removing agent, attempt medication therapy.

First Line
- Prednisone 0.5–2 mg/kg/d PO or equivalent IV dose × 1–2 weeks, followed by a gradual taper over 3–4 weeks
- In patients who do not respond to corticosteroids within 2–3 weeks, treatment with cyclophosphamide (Cytoxan) can be considered.
- Studies support steroid use in chronic, not acute, interstitial nephritis (1)[B],(2),(3)[C],(4)[A].
- Continue corticosteroids for 6 months in patients with sarcoidosis (2)[C].

Second Line
- Lead toxicity: Repeated chelation therapy may improve renal function (5)[A]:
  - Succimer 10 mg/kg PO q8h × 5 days, then q12h × 14 days, *or*
  - EDTA 2 g IV/IM; if IM, use with 2% lidocaine.
- SLE nephritis: Steroids plus cyclophosphamide or azathioprine (4)[A]
- Urate nephropathy:
  - Allopurinol to decrease urate level (2)[C]
  - Use with caution because allopurinol is nephrotoxic.
- Lithium-induced nephritis: Use amiloride as adjunct (2)[C].
- Cidofovir-induced nephritis: Use probenecid as adjunct (2)[C].

ADDITIONAL TREATMENT
General Measures
- Discontinue offending agent.
- Reduce exposure to other nephrotoxic agents.
- Supportive measures
- Maintain adequate hydration.
- Symptomatic relief for fever, rash, and systemic symptoms
- Control of BP and anemia.
- Correct electrolyte imbalances.
- Dialysis if criteria is met

Issues for Referral
Most patients presenting with renal insufficiency, proteinuria, and/or acid–base electrolyte disorders require consultation with a nephrologist.

IN-PATIENT CONSIDERATIONS
Patients with acute renal failure or with serious electrolyte or acid–base disorders may require inpatient care until stabilization or resolution.

Initial Stabilization
- Arterial blood gases
- ECG

Admission Criteria
- Oliguria or anuria persists
- Severe electrolyte abnormalities
- ECG changes

Discharge Criteria
- Stable vitals, labs, and ECG
- Normal urine production

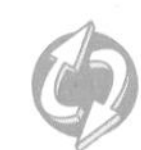

ONGOING CARE

FOLLOW-UP RECOMMENDATIONS
Patient Monitoring
If patients must remain on nephrotoxic medications, measure renal function, electrolytes, and phosphorus frequently.

DIET
- Low fat/low cholesterol
- Low protein (6)[A]
- Low sodium
- Low potassium

PATIENT EDUCATION
Printed materials for patients are available at the National Kidney Disease Education Program, (866) 4-KIDNEY, www.nkdep.nih.gov.

PROGNOSIS
- If the associated AIN is detected early (within 1 week of the rise in serum creatinine) and the drug is discontinued promptly, the long-term outcome is favorable for a return to baseline serum creatinine.
- Renal biopsy reveals extent of damage.
- AIN:
  - Recovery within weeks to months
  - Acute dialysis is needed for 1/3 of patients before resolution.
  - Rarely progresses to end-stage renal disease (ESRD)
- CIN: Can progress to ESRD
- TIN with uveitis:
  - Renal disease remits in 1 year if untreated.
  - Uveitis has relapsing course, requiring systemic corticosteroids
- Untreated acute renal failure has a 45–70% mortality.

COMPLICATIONS
- Papillary necrosis
- Chronic tubulointerstitial disease may progress to ESRD requiring dialysis or transplantation.
- Analgesics increase the risk of transitional cell cancers of the uroepithelium.

REFERENCES

1. Clarkson MR, et al. Acute interstitial nephritis: Clinical features and response to corticosteroid therapy. *Nephrol Dialysis Transplant*. 2004;19:2778–83.
2. Braden GL, O'Shea MH, Mulhern JG. Tubulointerstitial diseases. *Am J Kidney Dis*. 2005;46:560–72.
3. Markowitz GS, Perazella MA. Drug-induced renal failure: A focus on tubulointerstitial disease. *Clinica Chimica Acta*. 2005;351:31–47.
4. Flanc RS, et al. Treatment for lupus nephritis. *Cochrane Database Sys Rev*. 2004;1:CD002922.
5. Lin JL, Lin-Tan DT, Hsu KH, et al. Environmental lead exposure and progression of chronic renal diseases in patients without diabetes. *N Engl J Med*. 2003;348:277–86.
6. Fougue D, Laville M. Low-protein diets for chronic kidney disease in nondiabetic adults. *Cochrane Database Sys Rev*. 2009;(3):CD001892.

ADDITIONAL READING

- http://emedicine.medscape.com/article/243597-followup
- http://jasn.asnjournals.org/cgi/reprint/9/3/506
- www.aafp.org/afp/20030615/2527.html

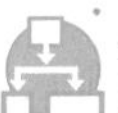

See Also (Topic, Algorithm, Electronic Media Element)

Algorithm: Hematuria

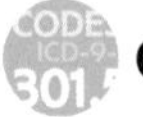

CODES

ICD9
- 580.89 Acute glomerulonephritis with other specified pathological lesion in kidney
- 582.89 Chronic glomerulonephritis with other specified pathological lesion in kidney
- 583.89 Other nephritis and nephropathy, not specified as acute or chronic, with specified pathological lesion in kidney

CLINICAL PEARLS

- The symptoms of AIN are more dramatic and sudden (days to weeks) than those of CIN, which is slower and progressive.
- The best treatment is to first remove the offending agent.
- Hypercalcemia is both a cause and an effect of CIN. Treating hypercalcemia slows the progression of CIN.
- Finding eosinophilia on the CBC rules out NSAID-induced AIN.
- The gold standard in diagnosing interstitial nephritis is a renal biopsy.

INTESTINAL OBSTRUCTION

Anita Krishnarao, MD, MPH
Samir A. Shah, MD
Adam Klipfel, MD

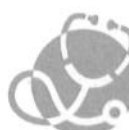

BASICS

DESCRIPTION

- Intestinal obstruction exists when there is an impairment of the normal transit of intestinal contents.
- This can be partial or complete and may be mechanical or functional.
- Obstruction should be considered in the context of abdominal pain, distention, emesis, and obstipation.
- System(s) affected: Gastrointestinal (GI)

Geriatric Considerations

If patient is elderly, must consider:

- Colonic neoplasm
- Chronic constipation/fecal impaction
- Pseudo-obstruction (Ogilvie syndrome)
- Volvulus

Pediatric Considerations

If patient is in early infancy, must consider:

- Pyloric stenosis: Infant 3–6 weeks old with postprandial, nonbilious, projectile vomiting
- Intestinal malrotation/volvulus: Sudden-onset, bilious vomiting with acute abdomen symptoms
- Hirschsprung disease: Failure to pass stool in first days of life, explosive expulsion of gas and stool after digital rectal exam

EPIDEMIOLOGY

Predominant sex: Male = Female

Prevalence

In US: Accounts for ~20% of all admissions for acute abdominal conditions

RISK FACTORS

- Previous abdominal and/or pelvic surgery
- Hernia
- Chronic constipation
- Cholelithiasis
- Inflammatory bowel disease
- Ingested foreign bodies: Pica, enteric potassium tablets, etc.
- Diverticular disease

Genetics

Unknown

GENERAL PREVENTION

Prevention depends on the cause. Treatment of conditions (such as tumors and hernias) that are related to obstruction may reduce your risk.

PATHOPHYSIOLOGY

Mechanical obstruction of bowel causes bowel distention and accumulation of fluid and gas in bowel lumen. Increased intraluminal pressure and peristaltic contractions increase capillary and venous pressure of bowel wall and decrease absorption and lymphatic drainage, which may lead to bowel ischemia and necrosis if obstruction is prolonged.

ETIOLOGY

- Luminal lesions:
  - Impactions
  - Gallstones
  - Meconium in newborns
  - Intussusception
- Intrinsic lesions:
  - Congenital (e.g., atresia and stenosis, imperforate anus, duplications, Meckel diverticulum)
  - Trauma
  - Inflammatory (e.g., Crohn disease, diverticulitis, ulcerative colitis, radiation, toxic [ingestions])
  - Neoplastic (most common cause of colon obstruction in adults)
  - Miscellaneous (e.g., endometriosis)
  - Pseudomyxoma peritonei is an appendiceal tumor.
- Extrinsic lesions:
  - Adhesions (most common cause of small bowel obstruction)
  - Hernia and wound dehiscence
  - Masses (e.g., annular pancreas, anomalous vasculature, abscess and hematoma, neoplasms)
  - Volvulus
  - Neuromuscular defect (e.g., megacolon, neuro-/myopathic motility disorders)

DIAGNOSIS

HISTORY

- Abdominal pain: Diffuse, poorly localized abdominal cramping at intervals of 5–15 minutes
- Abdominal distention: More commonly seen in distal obstruction
- Emesis: Usually occurs immediately after obstruction of bowel:
  - More frequent in proximal obstruction; unusual in colon obstruction until small bowel distension occurs
- Obstipation: Common symptom; may pass contents distal to obstruction within first 24 hours of obstruction, especially in proximal intestinal obstruction; pain followed by explosive diarrhea is seen often in partial obstruction.

PHYSICAL EXAM

- Inspection: Distension (a late finding) less likely in proximal obstructions
- Auscultation: High-pitched bowel sounds, peristaltic rushes
- Palpation: Tenderness, mass, presence of peritoneal signs (these suggest strangulation or perforation)
- Rectal examination: May reveal fecal impaction; occult blood may suggest colon malignancy.

DIAGNOSTIC TESTS & INTERPRETATION

Lab

Initial lab tests

Laboratory studies are not particularly helpful in diagnosing intestinal obstruction, but may help in the evaluation of associated dehydration and complications of intestinal obstruction:

- WBC count: Slight increase (15,000/mm^3); significant increases and leftward shift with strangulation, ischemic bowel
- Hematocrit: Moderate rise associated with extracellular fluid loss
- Renal: Urine specific gravity 1.025–1.030 and increase in BUN and creatinine reflect degree of extracellular volume loss
- Serum lactate elevated in bowel strangulation and mesenteric ischemia
- Arterial blood gas:
  - Metabolic alkalosis often a result of frequent emesis
  - Metabolic acidosis can result from bowel ischemia directly related to obstruction or from associated severe dehydration.

Imaging

Initial approach

The diagnosis of intestinal obstruction is primarily made based upon clinical and radiographic findings:

- Abdominal and chest radiographs:
  - Primary radiographic study to confirm diagnosis of intestinal obstruction:
    - *Most patients will not require further radiologic tests.*
  - Distension of small bowel or colon
  - Air–fluid levels (may be seen in ileus, gastroenteritis, constipation)
  - Lack of colon gas
  - Free intraperitoneal air (strangulation with perforation)
  - "Coffee bean sign" or "bent inner tube" appearance for colonic volvulus
  - Foreign-body visualization
- CT:
  - Adjunctive study of choice to help determine presence, location, cause, and severity of obstruction
  - Closed-loop obstruction: Distended, fluid-filled, C-shaped or U-shaped loop of bowel with prominent mesenteric vasculature converging on point of torsion/incarceration
  - Bowel ischemia: Intestinal pneumatosis and mesenteric changes (may not be detected in mild ischemia)

Follow-Up & Special Considerations

- Contrast studies:
  - Water-soluble (Gastrografin) enema is useful for the diagnosis of colonic obstruction, and may be therapeutic in intussusception.
  - Gastrografin (preferred over barium) orally may differentiate obstruction from ileus.
  - Enteroclysis may identify the site of small bowel obstruction (rarely used).
- Ultrasound may be used for pregnant patients or as a bedside test for the critically ill, although it is not as helpful as CT.

Diagnostic Procedures/Surgery

- Rigid proctoscopy: May be therapeutic in sigmoid volvulus
- Flexible sigmoidoscopy/colonoscopy

Pathological Findings

- Edema of mucosa
- Hypersecretion
- Necrosis

DIFFERENTIAL DIAGNOSIS

- Adynamic ileus
- Colonic pseudo-obstruction (Ogilvie syndrome)

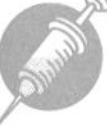

TREATMENT

- Inpatient management is generally recommended.
- Clinically stable patients may be treated conservatively with bowel rest, nasogastric suction, and IV fluid resuscitation.
- Surgery is warranted if obstruction does not resolve within 48–72 hours of initiation of conservative therapy (1)[B].
- Immediate surgical exploration is warranted if any of the following are present:
  - Severe leukocytosis or acidosis concerning for sepsis
  - Peritonitis
  - Intestinal ischemia/bowel necrosis
  - Perforation
  - Irreducible or strangulated hernia
- Consider use of intraperitoneal prophylactic agents for preventing intra-abdominal adhesions (2)[A]—a major risk factor for the development of intestinal obstruction.
- Continuous IV lidocaine during and after abdominal surgery may reduce postoperative ileus, improve patient rehabilitation, and shorten hospital stay (3,4)[A].

MEDICATION

Antibiotic use is controversial in the absence of sepsis, but prophylactic broad-spectrum antibiotics (gram-negative, gram-positive, and anaerobic coverage) are appropriate before the surgery.

ADDITIONAL TREATMENT

General Measures

- IV fluids
- Nasogastric suction
- Foley catheter

Issues for Referral

Early surgical evaluation should be part of the initial management for a suspected intestinal obstruction.

SURGERY/OTHER PROCEDURES

- Timing of operative intervention is critical; must correct electrolytes and volume quickly before surgery.
- Surgical procedures:
  - Closed bowel procedures: Lysis of adhesions, reduction of intussusception, reduction of volvulus, reduction of incarcerated hernia
  - Enterotomy for the removal of bezoars, foreign bodies, gallstones
  - Resection of bowel for obstructing lesions, strangulated bowel
  - Bypass of intestine around obstruction
  - Colostomy or cecostomy, with or without mucous fistula, proximal to obstruction

IN-PATIENT CONSIDERATIONS

IV Fluids

Normal saline or Lactated Ringer's solution with potassium supplementation as necessary

Nursing

Careful attention to input/output and volume status

ONGOING CARE

FOLLOW-UP RECOMMENDATIONS

Patient Monitoring

- Daily monitoring in hospital
- Follow outpatient postoperatively in 1–2 weeks.

DIET

NPO until obstruction resolved

PROGNOSIS

Prognosis depends on the underlying etiology and patient's general medical condition. In general, mortality from intestinal obstruction ranges from <1% to >20% depending on etiology, bowel viability, and comorbidities.

COMPLICATIONS

- Slow return of bowel function
- Higher risk of subsequent obstruction
- Sepsis
- Bowel ischemia and necrosis

REFERENCES

1. Jackson P, Raiji M. Evaluation and management of intestinal obstruction. *Am Fam Physician.* 2011;83.2.
2. Kumar S, Wong PF, Leaper DJ. Intra-peritoneal prophylactic agents for preventing adhesions and adhesive intestinal obstruction after nongynaecological abdominal surgery. *Cochrane Database Syst Rev.* 2009;CD005080.
3. Marret E, Rolin M, Beaussier M, et al. Meta-analysis of intravenous lidocaine and postoperative recovery after abdominal surgery. *Br J Surg.* 2008;95: 1331–8.
4. McCarthy GC, Megalla SA, Habib AS, et al. Impact of intravenous lidocaine infusion on postoperative analgesia and recovery from surgery: A systematic review of randomized controlled trials. *Drugs.* 2010;70:1149–63.

ADDITIONAL READING

- ASGE Standards of Practice Committee, Harrison ME, Anderson MA, et al. The role of endoscopy in the management of patients with known and suspected colonic obstruction and pseudo-obstruction. *Gastrointest Endosc.* 2010;71:669–79.
- Blanch AJ, Perel SB, Acworth JP. Paediatric intussusception: Epidemiology and outcome. *Emerg Med Australas.* 2007;19(1):45–50.
- Diaz JJ, Bokhari F, Mowery NT, et al. Guidelines for management of small bowel obstruction. *J Trauma.* 2008;64:1651–64.
- Harvey KP, Adair JD, Isho M, et al. Can intravenous lidocaine decrease postsurgical ileus and shorten hospital stay in elective bowel surgery? A pilot study and literature review. *Am J Surg.* 2009;198:231–6.
- Rathore MA, Andrabi SI, Mansha M. Adult intussusception—a surgical dilemma. *J Ayub Med Coll Abbottabad.* 2006;18(3):3–6.

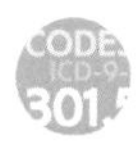

CODES

ICD9

- 560.39 Other impaction of intestine
- 560.9 Unspecified intestinal obstruction
- 751.1 Congenital atresia and stenosis of small intestine

CLINICAL PEARLS

- 15–20% of patients with colorectal cancer present with colonic obstruction.
- Initial management in most cases of suspected intestinal obstruction should be conservative and include early surgical consultation, IV fluid resuscitation, nasogastric decompression, and Foley catheter placement to monitor fluid status.
- Most patients do not require imaging beyond x-rays to establish diagnosis.

INTESTINAL PARASITES

Douglas W. MacPherson, MD, MSc(CTM), FRCPC

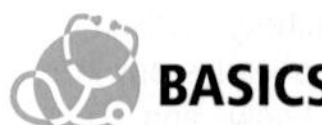

BASICS

DESCRIPTION

- Parasites are divided into 2 groups:
  - Protozoa: Single-cell organisms; typically multiply within the host; intestinal protozoa: Transmission by direct fecal–oral route; do not cause eosinophilia
  - Helminths (worms): Multicellular organisms; rarely multiply within the host (exceptions *Strongyloides stercoralis, Hymenolepis nana*); infection may cause a degree of eosinophilia. Level of eosinophilia is associated with the degree of tissue invasiveness. Worms have a limited life span, and without reinfection, most eventually die on their own.
- Some are invasive, and some do not release their infective forms into the bowel. This latter group (e.g., *Toxoplasma gondii, Echinococcus* sp., *Trichinella spiralis*) is not reviewed here.
- Most worms require incubation outside the host before being infectious or need a vector for transmission. *Enterobius vermicularis* (pinworm) eggs are infectious shortly after being passed; autoinfection occurs readily.
- Person-to-person transmission of worms is uncommon, except for pinworm.
- System(s) affected: Gastrointestinal (GI)

Pediatric Considerations

Most common age group affected

Pregnancy Considerations

Many of the treatments are contraindicated.

EPIDEMIOLOGY

Acquisition involves personal, food, and/or water sanitation and migration from higher-prevalence areas.

Incidence

- Predominant sex: Male = Female
- Predominant age: Pediatric

Prevalence

- US laboratory statistics: 5–30% of general population. Random testing finds at least 1 GI parasite in 5–10% of all people.
- From daycare surveys: Asymptomatic 20–30%; symptomatic 50–80%
- Intestinal protozoa account for most parasite findings in North America. Helminths account for <10% of GI parasites.
- *Blastocystis hominis* is a commensal enteric fungus of no clinical significance found in 20–30% of stools.

RISK FACTORS

- Age (children)
- Low socioeconomic status and poor sanitation: Personal, food, water; crowding: Day care centers, institutional care
- International travel or migration
- Multiple medical conditions, pregnancy, gastric hypoacidity, immunosuppression (AIDS)

GENERAL PREVENTION

- Intestinal parasites are usually acquired by direct fecal–oral contact via ingested contaminated food or water. Rarely, infected arthropod vectors are involved in transmission. Person-to-person transmission may occur through this mechanism.
- Safe food and water precautions ("Wash it, cook it, peel it, or forget it"); enteric and hand hygiene is the means of preventing infections. Infrastructure systems for safe food and water processing contribute to the low prevalence of intestinal parasites.

PATHOPHYSIOLOGY

- The pathophysiology of GI parasitic infections is host–parasite-specific.
- Most intestinal parasitic infections are eventually self-limiting. Most worms have a defined life expectancy in the host. Autoreinfection does occur in some worm infections (e.g., strongyloidiasis, pinworm).

ETIOLOGY

- Protozoan pathogens:
  - *Giardia lamblia:* Common
  - *Entamoeba histolytica, Cryptosporidium* sp., *Isospora belli, Balantidium coli, Cyclospora cayetanensis, Microsporida*
- Possible protozoan pathogens: *Dientamoeba fragilis*
- Probable nonpathogenic protozoa:
  - Amoebas: All other *Entamoeba* sp., *Endolimax nana*
  - All other intestinal flagellates
- Helminthic pathogens: Nematodes (roundworms): *Enterobius vermicularis, Trichuris trichiura, Ascaris lumbricoides*, hookworm (*Necator americanus, Ancylostoma duodenale*), *Strongyloides stercoralis, Capillaria philippinensis, Trichostrongylus* sp.
- Helminthic pathogens: Trematodes (flukes): *Fasciolopsis buski, Clonorchis sinensis, Opisthorchis viverrini, Heterophyes, Fasciola hepatica, Paragonimus westermani, Schistosoma mansoni, S. japonicum, S. hematobium, S. mekongi*
- Helminthic pathogens: Cestodes (tapeworms): *Taenia saginata, T. solium, Diphyllobothrium latum, Hymenolepis nana, H. diminuta, Dipylidium caninum*

COMMONLY ASSOCIATED CONDITIONS

- GI parasitic infections and diseases may be associated with HIV infection or AIDS, steroid use, immune deficiencies, and blood type.
- Intestinal parasite infection appears to protect against allergic sensitization (1)[A].

DIAGNOSIS

HISTORY

Historical or physical features alone cannot separate intestinal parasites from other GI infections or the noninfectious enteric diseases except the actual finding of a typical worm (i.e., a tapeworm segment or roundworm: Ascarid, whipworm, or pinworm):

- Acute bacterial or viral GI syndromes tend to be sudden onset and short duration.
- Fever is uncommon with GI parasites unless there is tissue invasion (e.g., amoebiasis, strongyloidiasis).
- Chronic bloating, excessive gas, and intermittent/unpredictable diarrhea without blood is typical of giardiasis.
- Extraintestinal symptoms and signs are uncommon with GI parasites, except invasive strongyloidiasis.
- A water, food, or fecal contamination exposure history (e.g., international travel, migration, high-risk environments [day care centers, camping]) may suggest a particular parasitic agent.
- A family or personal history of inflammatory or irritable bowel syndromes does not exclude GI parasites.

PHYSICAL EXAM

- Will generally appear well even if distressed with GI complaints; usually afebrile
- Diffuse, migratory rash (cutaneous larva currens) with invasive strongyloidiasis; this is a medical emergency.
- Weight loss and anorexia may be present (e.g., chronic giardiasis, invasive amoebiasis, chronic helminths).
- Anemia may be present with heavy hookworm infections.
- Excessive gas: Bloating, eructation, flatulence, borborygmi
- Nausea or vomiting: Intermittent, recurrent
- Abdominal pain/tenderness
- May have bowel tenderness, but liver and spleen are usually normal
- Diarrhea: Persistent and recurrent, chronic but dysentery (i.e., frank GI bleeding) is rare, except with *E. histolytica, B. coli*
- Pruritus ani: *E. vermicularis, T. trichiura, S. stercoralis*, tapeworms. Perirectal or vulvar rash.
- Passing a roundworm or tapeworm or a worm segment

DIAGNOSTIC TESTS & INTERPRETATION

- Stool specimens that are properly collected, preserved, and transported for examination in a qualified and proficient laboratory by a dedicated parasitology technologist team have the highest diagnostic yield for GI parasites.
- Special diagnostics for *Cryptosporidium, I. belli, Cyclospora, Microsporidia*, and *Strongyloides*: Give specific laboratory notice.
- Pinworm paddles provide a greater diagnostic yield for *E. vermicularis*. Multiple tests (2) may be needed to exclude pinworms.
- Parasite culture is possible for *G. lamblia, E. histolytica*, and *S. stercoralis* but is rarely indicated; only done in reference laboratories
- Rarely, a biopsy and histology will demonstrate the presence of an invasive helminth on tissue section.
- Tissue biopsies of intestine, liver, or bladder may show granulomatous reactions of schistosome eggs.

Lab

- A single stool specimen collected into a preservative (i.e., sodium acetate formalin [SAF]), well mixed to fix and preserve all elements, yields an accurate diagnosis in 90%. Additional specimens improve diagnostic accuracy (3)[A].
- Newer lab techniques for stool specimens currently provide little diagnostic advantage. Exception: *Giardia* antigen—fluorescent antibody (FA) and ELISA tests: A single FA or ELISA may be at least as sensitive as 3 stools for ova and parasites.
- Serology: Useful if parasite is not found in stool samples normally or if low numbers of parasites; available only through reference centers, that is, *Strongyloides*, amebiasis, schistosomiasis
- Drugs that may alter lab results: Use of antibiotics; oil-based laxatives, and barium in the stool interfere with microscopy.

Initial lab tests

Screening blood eosinophilia is not recommended.

Follow-Up & Special Considerations

- A single negative stool examination does not rule out intestinal parasitic infection, but when performed under best conditions is highly accurate. Repeat testing may be indicated for primary diagnosis.
- Population-based intestinal parasite screening in North America (e.g., daycare attendees, personal-care providers, food handlers, immigrants) has low diagnostic utility and is not recommended.

Imaging

Diagnostic radiology is rarely needed. Exception: Invasive disease due to amebiasis for colitis, amebomas, and liver abscesses.

Diagnostic Procedures/Surgery

- Invasive diagnostic procedures are rarely needed or indicated.
- Egg granulomata of schistosomiasis may be demonstrated in affected tissues.
- With hemorrhagic colitis due to invasive amebiasis, sigmoidoscopy is diagnostic.
- Upper intestinal endoscopy can yield fluid to be examined for *G. lamblia* trophozoites and *S. stercoralis* larvae.

Pathological Findings

- Most intestinal parasites are not invasive and produce nonspecific or no changes in bowel histology.
- Invasive amebiasis produces a classic endoscopic and histologic picture of ulceration and inflammation in the colon.
- Protozoa or helminths may be seen in bowel biopsy histology.

DIFFERENTIAL DIAGNOSIS

- Other nonparasitic intestinal infections
- Food poisoning
- Malabsorption: Commonly lactose, gluten enteropathy; rarely celiac disease, tropical or nontropical sprue
- Inflammatory and irritable bowel diseases
- Hemorrhoid or rectal fissures

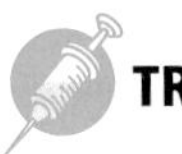

TREATMENT

Specific antiparasitic treatment should be selected on patient needs, parasite biology, and epidemiology.

MEDICATION

- Protozoa (4)[A]:
  - *E. histolytica:* Asymptomatic infection needs individual assessment.
  - *E. histolytica* symptomatic intestinal: Iodoquinol or diloxanide furoate
  - *E. histolytica* invasive disease: Iodoquinol or diloxanide furoate plus metronidazole alone or metronidazole alone or emetine plus chloroquine phosphate
  - *G. lamblia:* Metronidazole or tinidazole or furazolidone or quinacrine. *Note:* Albendazole, available in the US only from manufacturer, may have activity against *G. lamblia*.
- *Cryptosporidium:* None proven effective
- *I. belli* protozoa: Trimethoprim–sulfamethoxazole
- *B. coli*: Tetracycline or iodoquinol or metronidazole
- *Cyclospora:* Sulfamethoxazole-trimethoprim
- *Microsporidia*: Albendazole (some species)
- Helminths:
  - Nematodes (except *Strongyloides* and *Trichostrongylus*): Mebendazole or pyrantel pamoate or piperazine citrate or albendazole (available in US only from manufacturer)
  - *Strongyloides* and *Trichostrongylus:* Thiabendazole or albendazole (available in US only from manufacturer)
  - Cestodes: Praziquantel or niclosamide
  - Trematodes: Niclosamide or praziquantel

Pediatric Considerations

Nitazoxanide 7.5 mg/kg PO b.i.d. × 3 days or single-dose tinidazole 50 mg/kg (not available in the US) may be used.

ADDITIONAL TREATMENT

General Measures

- Not all patients need to be treated with drugs.
- Symptomatic treatment is indicated for patient comfort once specific therapy has been initiated.
- Drugs inhibiting intestinal motility are relatively contraindicated in patients with diarrhea caused by invasive organisms.

Issues for Referral

Treatment failures, complex patients (including drug intolerances or allergies), multiple parasitic infections, and complicated medical (e.g., HIV/AIDS, diabetes, chronic steroid use, etc.) or surgical conditions: Specialist in tropical medicine or infectious diseases

COMPLEMENTARY AND ALTERNATIVE MEDICINE

- Many complementary and alternative therapies exist, but none are effective for primary treatment.
- Consequences of intestinal parasitic infections include lactose intolerance, irritable bowel syndrome, or nutritional deficiencies of calorie–protein deficiencies, dehydration, vitamin B_{12} deficiency.

SURGERY/OTHER PROCEDURES

- Surgical procedures play little role except for amebic liver abscesses, which may need to be drained, especially left lobe abscesses.
- Surgery possible for bowel or organ obstruction, *A. lumbricoides* migration, or for complicated amebic colitis.

IN-PATIENT CONSIDERATIONS

Nosocomial intestinal parasitic infections are rare, as are hospital-based parasitic GI outbreaks. Invasive strongyloidiasis may occur in hospitals for other reasons (e.g., surgery, use of high-dose steroids, etc.).

Admission Criteria

Admission is rarely required except for intestinal obstruction, dysentery, or systemic invasion.

ONGOING CARE

FOLLOW-UP RECOMMENDATIONS

Patient Monitoring

For the majority of intestinal parasitic infections, testing for clearance is not indicated. Repeat stool examination for clearance should be timed taking into account the life cycle of the parasite and the risk of reinfection.

DIET

Many patients experience symptoms of irritable bowel syndrome and/or lactose intolerance during and following bowel infections, especially when infected with *G. lamblia*.

PATIENT EDUCATION

Important to reduce the risk of reinfection or transmission

COMPLICATIONS

Complications are rare and include chronic persistent diarrhea, irritable bowel syndrome, and chronic malabsorption.

REFERENCES

1. Feary J, Britton J, Leonardi-Bee J. Atopy and current intestinal parasite infection: A systematic review and meta-analysis. *Allergy*. 2011;66(4):569–78.
2. Strand EA, Robertson LJ, Hanevik K, et al. Sensitivity of a *Giardia* antigen test in persistent giardiasis following an extensive outbreak. *Clin Microbiol Infect*. 2008;14:1069–71.
3. Senay H, MacPherson DW. Parasitology: Diagnostic yield of stool examination. *Can Med Assoc J*. 1989;140:1329–31.
4. Abramowicz M, ed. Drugs for parasitic infections. In: *The Medical Letter*. New York: The Medical Letter; September 2007, pg 1–15.

ADDITIONAL READING

- CDC. Parasites and Health. Parasites of the intestinal tract. Available at: www.dpd.cdc.gov/dpdx/html/para_health.htm.
- Escobedo AA, Alvarez G, González ME, et al. The treatment of giardiasis in children: Single-dose tinidazole compared with 3 days of nitazoxanide. *Ann Trop Med Parasitol*. 2008;102:199–207.
- Leonardi-Bee J, Pritchard D, Britton J. Asthma and Current intestinal parasite infection: Systematic review and meta-analysis. *Am J Respir Crit Care Med*. 2006.

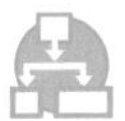

See Also (Topic, Algorithm, Electronic Media Element)

Algorithm: Hematemesis (Bleeding, Upper GI)

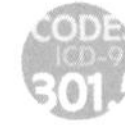

CODES

ICD9

- 127.4 Enterobiasis
- 127.9 Intestinal helminthiasis, unspecified
- 129 Intestinal parasitism, unspecified

CLINICAL PEARLS

- Consider GI parasites when dealing with a history of travel, recent immigration, children, or other vulnerable populations, or a story of chronic or persistent diarrhea or seeing worms in the stool.
- Stools correctly collected in the proper preservative will detect most intestinal parasites. Exceptions: *S. stercoralis*, *E. vermicularis*, *Cryptosporidium*, *Cyclospora*, and *Microspora* sp.
- Checking for eosinophilia is not a reliable screening method.

I

INTUSSUSCEPTION

Timothy L. Black, MD
James P. Miller, MD

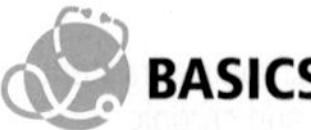

BASICS

DESCRIPTION

- Invagination of a portion of intestine into itself:
  - May involve any part of small intestine or ileocolic (95%) or colocolic segment
- System(s) affected: Gastrointestinal

Geriatric Considerations

- Adult intussusception represents 5% of all intussusceptions and fewer than 5% of intestinal obstruction cases in adults (1)[B].
- 90% have pathologic lead point (site of initiation of event) (1)[B].

Pediatric Considerations

- Usually no identified lead point; only present in 2–12%
- Represents the most common abdominal emergency in infancy (2)[C]
- Postoperative intussusception (1–24 days postoperatively) is virtually always in small bowel and only rarely can be reduced hydrostatically.

EPIDEMIOLOGY

- Predominant age:
  - 5–10 months (65% are <1 year of age)
  - Only 10–25% of cases occur at >1 year of age.
  - Adults represent about 5% of all intussusceptions.
- Predominant sex: Male > Female (3:2). Male preponderance is more obvious in older infants.

Incidence

In the US:

- 1.5–4/1,000 live births
- 0.5% after laparotomy

RISK FACTORS

- Henoch-Schönlein purpura
- Leukemia
- Lymphoma
- Cystic fibrosis
- Recent upper respiratory tract infection: 21%
- Recent operation (1–24 days previously)
- Recent viral GI illness
- Meckel diverticulum
- Recent rotavirus vaccine administration (3)[C]
- Small bowel carcinoma
- Polyps
- Stricture

ETIOLOGY

- Children:
  - Marked hypertrophy of Peyer patches: 92–98%
  - Lead point in 2–12%: Polyp, Meckel diverticulum, duplication cyst, ectopic pancreas, lymphoma, Henoch-Schönlein purpura, lipoma, carcinoma
  - Allergic reactions, diet changes, and changes in intestinal activity may be other causes.
  - Possible adenovirus or rotavirus infection
  - 1998 Rotashield vaccine showed that 1/10,000–1/32,000 vaccines developed intussusception (3)[C]:
    - Vaccine was administered 3–14 days before the onset of current symptoms.
    - Infants usually >3 months of age
  - 2006 and 2008 Rotavirus vaccines (RV5 and RV1) show no increase in cases of intussusception over placebo recipients (4)[A]. Since 2006, more than 14 million doses of RV5 have been administered, and the CDC Immunization Safety Office summary of postlicensure safety monitoring of RV5 does not indicate that immunization with RV5 is associated with intussusception. Monitoring of RV1 is ongoing.
  - Recent operative procedure
- Adults: Virtually always associated with lead point

COMMONLY ASSOCIATED CONDITIONS

- Henoch-Schönlein purpura
- Cystic fibrosis

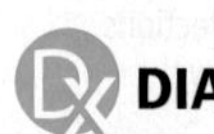

DIAGNOSIS

HISTORY

- History of intermittent colicky abdominal pain (almost all children), with episodes lasting 5–10 minutes, frequently with completely asymptomatic period separating the episodes
- Almost all have history of vomiting associated with at least some of the painful episodes.
- History of bloody stool
- Blood per rectum ("currant jelly" stools): 65–95%, highest percentage in infants
- Diarrhea: 7%

PHYSICAL EXAM

- Lethargy (more pronounced with longer duration of illness): 22%
- Palpable mass: 16–41%
- Prolapse of intussusceptum through anus: 3%
- Fever
- Extreme pallor in some
- In postoperative patients, usually presents as small bowel obstruction (5)[C]
- Abdominal distension sometimes marked, depending on the duration of symptoms
- Bowel sounds hyperactive initially; may be absent later

DIAGNOSTIC TESTS & INTERPRETATION

Lab

- Electrolytes
- CBC
- Urinalysis
- Stool guaiac

Imaging

- Ultrasound is diagnostic (2)[C],(6)[B].
- Transient small bowel intussusception is seen frequently in patients with gastroenteritis; these usually resolve spontaneously without additional treatment. (Most of these actually will resolve during the ultrasound observation period.)
- Plain film: Flat and upright abdominal films may suggest the diagnosis.
- CT scan may be helpful, especially in adults (7)[C].

Diagnostic Procedures/Surgery

- Contrast enema (barium, water-soluble contrast material, or air)
- Abdominal ultrasound
- Colonoscopy may be useful in evaluation of adult patients presenting with subacute or chronic colonic obstruction (1)[B].

Pathological Findings

- Hyperplasia of Peyer lymphatic patches of terminal ileum (92%), with or without mesenteric lymphadenopathy
- Recognizable lead point, 2–12% (see list in "Etiology")

DIFFERENTIAL DIAGNOSIS

- Adhesive-band small bowel obstruction
- Appendicitis
- Gastroenteritis
- Rectal prolapse (if intussuscepted bowel protrudes from anus)

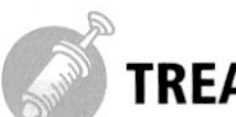

TREATMENT

ADDITIONAL TREATMENT

General Measures

- IV fluid resuscitation
- Foley catheter (if child is severely dehydrated)
- Nasogastric tube
- Antibiotics useful only if necrotic bowel present
- Nonoperative care (2)[C],(6)[B]:
  - Hydrostatic/pneumatic reduction of intussusception (50–80% success)
  - Barium column should be 40–42 inches high.
  - Enema is continued as long as progress is made. Contrast material may be drained and the enema repeated up to 3×.
  - Pneumatic reduction pressure should not exceed 120–140 mm Hg (16–18.6 kPa).

SURGERY/OTHER PROCEDURES

- Right lower quadrant incision
- Gentle manipulation by pushing intussusception (not pulling)
- If unable to reduce nonviable bowel, segmental resection with reanastomosis
- Enterotomy if lead point suspected
- Incidental appendectomy usually done
- Some centers are using laparoscopy or laparoscopically assisted reduction/resection.
- Postoperative intussusception usually requires laparotomy and operative reduction (5)[C].
- Many adults do not have preoperative diagnosis of intussusception (only 65% in one series) (7)[C].
- In adults, segmental bowel resection usually is required.
- In adults, ventral rectopexy has low recurrence rates and improves fecal incontinence (8)[A].

IN-PATIENT CONSIDERATIONS

Initial Stabilization

Inpatient until resolved

Admission Criteria

Infants are frequently admitted for overnight observation after nonoperative reduction owing to high incidence of recurrence in the first 24 hours.

Discharge Criteria

Normal bowel function, tolerating regular diet, no abdominal pain

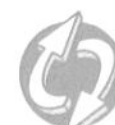

ONGOING CARE

FOLLOW-UP RECOMMENDATIONS

As tolerated after reduction

Patient Monitoring

Office visit 1–2 weeks after discharge

DIET

Liquids are started after abdominal distension resolves and bowel function returns.

PATIENT EDUCATION

- Instruct family on the possibility of recurrence (5–13%).
- Most recurrences occur in the first 24 hours after reduction.

PROGNOSIS

- Mortality should not exceed 1–2%.
- Possible recurrence after hydrostatic reduction: 5–13%
- Possible recurrence after operative reduction: 3%

COMPLICATIONS

- Bowel perforation during attempted reduction (in 0.16–2.8% of patients with pneumatic reduction)
- Prolonged ileus
- Adhesions with intestinal obstruction
- Incisional hernia
- Ischemic intestine requiring second operation
- Electrolyte abnormality
- Anemia
- Pleural effusion
- Sepsis
- Recurrence

REFERENCES

1. Marinis A, Yiallourou A, Samanides L, et al. Intussusception of the bowel in adults: A review. *World J Gastroenterol*. 2009;15:407–11.
2. Sorantin E, Lindbichler F. Management of intussusception. *Eur Radiol*. 2004;14(Suppl 4): L146–54.
3. Bines JE. Rotavirus vaccines and intussusception risk. *Curr Opin Gastroenterol*. 2005;21:20–5.
4. Committee on Infectious Diseases. Prevention of rotavirus disease: Updated guidelines for use of rotavirus vaccine. *Pediatrics*. 2009;123:1412–20.
5. Holcomb GW, Ross AJ, O'Neill JA. Postoperative intussusception: Increasing frequency or increasing awareness? *South Med J*. 1991;84:1334–9.
6. Applegate KE. Clinically suspected intussusception in children: Evidence-based review and self-assessment module. *AJR Am J Roentgenol*. 2005;185:S175–83.
7. Wang N, Cui X, et al. Adult intussusception: A retrospective review of 41 cases. *World J Gastroenterol* 2009;15:3303–8.
8. Samaranayake CB, Luo C, Plank AW, et al. Systematic review on ventral rectopexy for rectal prolapse and intussusception. *Colorectal Dis*. 2010; 12(6):504–12.

ADDITIONAL READING

- Applegate KE, et al. Intussusception in children: Evidence-based diagnosis and treatment. *Pediatr Radiol*. 2009;39(Suppl 2):S140–3.

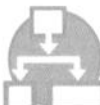

See Also (Topic, Algorithm, Electronic Media Element)

Cystic Fibrosis; Henoch-Schönlein Purpura; Intestinal Obstruction

CODES

ICD9

560.0 Intussusception

CLINICAL PEARLS

- Some patients may need a KUB if bowel obstruction is suspected, but diagnostic confirmation with ultrasound is the "gold standard." A contrast enema then serves both diagnostic and, hopefully, therapeutic purposes.
- A lead point is present in only 10% of children <1 year of age and is most commonly a Meckel diverticulum.

IRON TOXICITY, ACUTE

David C. Mackenzie, MD

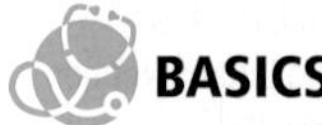

BASICS

DESCRIPTION

- Acute iron (Fe) overload from accidental or intentional ingestion
- Unintentional ingestion by children is common, because Fe-containing compounds are readily available, brightly colored, and sometimes sugar-coated.
- Acute symptoms are characterized by vomiting, diarrhea, and abdominal pain. More severe clinical findings include cyanosis, altered mental status, acidosis, hematemesis, shock, and coma.
- The most serious exposures involve prenatal vitamins and pure Fe preparations that contain ferrous sulfate. The toxic dose of Fe depends on the amount (mg/kg) of elemental Fe ingested.
- Clinically evident toxicity is more common with ingestions >40 mg/kg, typically as transient GI symptoms. Persistent vomiting, diarrhea, or abdominal pain are suggestive of a more significant ingestion.
- Metabolic acidosis is an indicator of Fe-induced toxicity. Death from Fe overdose has been reported from a wide range of exposures (60–300 mg/kg).
- Morbidity and mortality is greater among patients with intentional ingestion.
- System(s) affected: Cardiovascular; Gastrointestinal; Hematologic/Lymphatic/Immunologic
- Synonym(s): Iron poisoning; Iron overdose

Pediatric Considerations

For a 2-year-old, the average lethal dose of elemental Fe is 3 g. This is fewer than 50 iron sulfate 325-mg tablets.

EPIDEMIOLOGY

Incidence

>4,000 cases/year of elemental Fe overdose reported to Association of Poison Control Centers (AAPCC) (1)

Prevalence

- Fe ingestion is a common cause of morbidity in children, but mortality from Fe exposure is decreasing (2,3).
- In 2008, 4,479 elemental Fe and 19,707 vitamin-containing Fe exposures were reported to the AAPCC; no deaths were reported (1).

RISK FACTORS

- Access to Fe-containing products by children resulting in accidental ingestion
- A pregnant mother or the birth of a sibling within 6 months was identified as a risk factor for children <3 years old, likely due to the presence of prenatal vitamins or Fe supplements.

GENERAL PREVENTION

- Keep prescription and over-the-counter (OTC) Fe products/vitamins out of the reach of children.
- Unit-dose packaging of Fe supplements has resulted in a reduction of Fe poisoning in children and should be recommended as the preferred packaging to patients (4)[B].

PATHOPHYSIOLOGY

- Tissue damage from Fe is due to free-radical production and lipid peroxidation, leading to the following conditions:
  - Direct vasodilation
  - Increased capillary permeability
  - Necrosis of mucosal cells
  - Altered mitochondrial lipid membrane
  - Biochemical effects (i.e., uncoupling of oxidative phosphorylation and Krebs cycle enzymatic process inhibition)
  - Inhibition of serum proteases (e.g., thrombin)
- The following conditions can result:
  - Local: Fe-induced damage to the GI mucosa
  - Systemic toxicity: Injury to the cardiovascular system and liver

ETIOLOGY

- Excessive Fe ingestion: The average human lethal dose is 200–250 mg elemental Fe/kg of body weight. Ferrous sulfate contains ~60 mg of elemental iron/325-mg tablet.
- Serious toxicity or even death has been associated with >60 mg/kg of elemental Fe ingestion (~1 tablet/kg).

DIAGNOSIS

HISTORY

- Determine type and quantity of Fe ingested.
- Note times of ingestion and symptom onset.
- Was the ingestion intentional or accidental?
- Identify those who are severely ill or who have subtle features of a significant ingestion.
- Ask about possible coingested substances.
- For children: Other siblings at risk?

PHYSICAL EXAM

Classically, 5 phases occur after toxic ingestions (but do not occur in all patients, and often overlap; for example, in massive overdose, patients may present in shock):

- From 0.5–6 hours: GI symptoms predominate, including vomiting, hematemesis, abdominal pain, diarrhea, GI bleeding, lethargy, shock, and metabolic acidosis
- Latent: From 6–24 hours: Apparent recovery; observe patient closely for hypoperfusion and acidosis.
- From 6–72 hours: Profound cardiovascular toxicity, shock, severe acidosis, cyanosis, and fever; potential recurrence of GI bleeding and vomiting; coagulopathy (preceding liver dysfunction) can occur.
- From 12–96 hours: Hepatotoxicity and necrosis may occur, leading to coma, coagulopathy, and jaundice. Symptoms may recur and can include pulmonary edema, shock, acidosis, convulsions, anuria, hyperthermia, and death.
- From 2–8 weeks: Delayed GI scarring and bowel obstruction

DIAGNOSTIC TESTS & INTERPRETATION

Lab

Initial lab tests

- Obtain measurement of serum Fe 6 hours after ingestion:
  - Serum Fe >500 μg/dL correlated with moderate to severe toxicity
  - Serial measures may not be helpful.
  - Total iron-binding capacity (TIBC) cannot be used to manage Fe overdose (5); inaccurate in setting of Fe overload; affected by deferoxamine
- CBC with differential, chemistry panel, liver function tests (LFTs), prothrombin time (PT), partial thromboplastin time (PTT), type and cross-match. WBC count of 15,000/mm^3 correlates with Fe levels >300 μg/dL (100% specificity, 50% sensitivity) (5).
- Glucose level: Glucose of 1,150 mg/dL correlates with Fe level >300 μg/dL (same specificity and sensitivity as WBC count) (5).
- Amylase and lipase
- Arterial blood gases (ABGs) to detect anion-gap metabolic acidosis
- Drugs that may alter lab results: Deferoxamine can falsely lower serum Fe unless a reducing agent is added to the specimen; should obtain a free Fe concentration.

Follow-Up & Special Considerations

Tests to monitor for complications:

- Electrolytes, BUN and creatinine
- Coagulation tests: PT/PTT/INR
- Serum bicarbonate
- Liver function tests in severe overdose
- Amylase and lipase
- ABG/VBG to detect metabolic acidosis

Imaging

Initial approach

Abdominal radiograph to evaluate for tablets in the GI tract

Diagnostic Procedures/Surgery

Acute Fe poisoning is a clinical diagnosis (5).

Pathological Findings

- Hepatic, renal, and myocardial necrosis
- Irritation and ulceration of stomach and small intestine

DIFFERENTIAL DIAGNOSIS

- Conditions that present similarly to acute iron toxicity:
  - Gastritis
  - Small bowel obstruction
  - Drug intolerance/overdose
  - Alcohol toxicity
  - Viral illness
  - Diabetic ketoacidosis
  - Metabolic acidosis
- Other poisonings, including aspirin, NSAIDs, theophylline, organophosphates, carbamates, other metals and metalloids, paraquat, caustic agents, colchicines, nicotine, and mushrooms

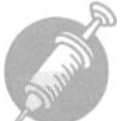

TREATMENT

MEDICATION

- Ensure adequate airway, breathing, and circulation.
- Begin fluid replacement for signs of volume depletion or shock: IV access followed by fluid bolus of 20 mL/kg
- GI decontamination:
  - Activated charcoal does not bind Fe; administration probably not helpful unless coingestions are present (3,5)[C]
  - Gastric lavage and syrup of ipecac not recommended by most toxicologists (3,5)
  - Case reports suggest whole-bowel irrigation may be useful (5)[C]:
    - Polyethylene glycol (Colyte, GoLYTELY) via nasogastric tube at 500 mL/h for children and up to 1.5–2 L/h for adults. End point: Clear rectal effluent; disappearance of radiopacities.
    - Consider endoscopic or surgical removal of Fe-containing bezoar if unresponsive to irrigation.
- IV deferoxamine:
  - Chelates free iron ions. May work best if initiated early, before Fe absorption from GI tract is complete.
  - Indications: Ingestion above levels associated with serious toxicity (>40 mg/kg Fe); clinical signs of severe toxicity (persistent vomiting or diarrhea, altered mental status, evidence of shock); metabolic acidosis; serum Fe level >500 μg/dL (5)[B]
  - Starting dose: 15 mg/kg/h
  - Maximum dose: 35 mg/kg/h
  - Contraindications: Relatively contraindicated in severe renal disease or anuria or primary hemochromatosis
  - Precautions: Discuss administration with poison control. Can cause histamine-mediated hypotension, urticaria, or flushing. Longer infusions (>24 hours) associated with ARDS.

Pregnancy Considerations

- Treatment same as that for nonpregnant women (5)
- Transplacental absorption limited
- Phase 3 toxicity associated with spontaneous abortion, preterm delivery, maternal death

ADDITIONAL TREATMENT

General Measures

Consult with a poison control center (1-800-222-1222).

Issues for Referral

Explore psychological issues if it was an intentional ingestion

Additional Therapies

Hemodialysis, peritoneal dialysis, and exchange transfusion have been used in lethal overdoses. Limited experimental data suggest hyperbaric oxygen may have benefit.

SURGERY/OTHER PROCEDURES

Fe pill bezoars can lead to perforation and may need removal by endoscopy or gastrostomy.

IN-PATIENT CONSIDERATIONS

Initial Stabilization

- Emergency room for acute ingestion
- In-patient for severe ingestion
- Supportive treatment

Admission Criteria

Ingestion with suspicion for intentional self-harm; ingestions of ≥60 mg/kg elemental Fe or severe or persistent symptoms requiring deferoxamine; consider admission or 6–12 hours ED observation for ingestions >40 mg/kg

IV Fluids

- Normal saline boluses of 20 mL/kg
- Keep hydrated while on deferoxamine.

Nursing

Supportive nursing care

Discharge Criteria

- Make sure that patient is not in phase 2 (latent) toxicity. Observe for 6–12 hours postingestion.
- Patients with ingestion of <40 mg/kg elemental Fe and no or mild symptoms may be observed at home (3)[C].
- Resolution of symptoms and education on possible complications after treatment for severe toxicity

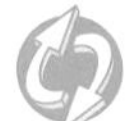

ONGOING CARE

PATIENT EDUCATION

- Undertake prevention counseling on proper storage of Fe products (out of the reach of children).
- Encourage purchase of Fe supplements in unit-dose packaging.
- Educational material from poison control centers may be available to use.

PROGNOSIS

Depends on amount ingested, time to presentation, and timing of therapy

COMPLICATIONS

At 2–4 weeks after severe ingestion, pyloric or antral stenosis, hepatic cirrhosis, and CNS damage may occur.

REFERENCES

1. Bronstein AC, Spyker DA, Cantilena LR, et al. 2008 annual report of the American Association of Poison Control Centers' National Poison Data System (NPDS): 26th Annual Report. *Clin Toxicol (Phila)*. 2009;47:911–1084.
2. Cheney K, Gumbiner C, Benson B. Survival after a severe iron poisoning treated with intermittent infusions of deferoxamine. *J Toxicol Clin Toxicol*. 1995;33:61–6.
3. Manoguerra A. Iron ingestion: An evidence-based consensus guideline for out-of-hospital management. *Clin Toxicol*. 2005;43:553–70.
4. Tenenbein M. Unit-dose packaging of iron supplements and reduction of iron poisoning in young children. *Arch Pediatr Adolesc Med*. 2005;159:557–60.
5. Madiwale T, Liebelt E. Iron: Not a benign therapeutic drug. *Curr Opin Pediatr*. 2006;18:174–9.

ADDITIONAL READING

- Consensus guideline for out-of-hospital management of Fe ingestion. American Association of Poison Control Centers. *National Guideline Clearinghouse*. 2005;19:8054.
- www.AAPCC.org.

CODES

ICD9

964.0 Poisoning by iron and its compounds

CLINICAL PEARLS

- Fe overdose has been a leading cause of fatalities from toxic agents in children <6 years of age.
- Serious toxicity or even death has been associated with >60 mg/kg of elemental Fe ingestion (~1 tablet/kg).
- Outpatient GI decontamination with ipecac syrup or other entities is not recommended.
- It is critical to differentiate if a patient is exhibiting mild GI symptoms with resolving toxicity or if the patient is simply in the latent phase and needs continued observation or treatment with deferoxamine.

IRRITABLE BOWEL SYNDROME

Kelly O'Callahan, MD

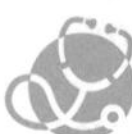

BASICS

DESCRIPTION

- A condition characterized by a chronic abdominal pain associated with alteration in bowel habits in the absence of organic pathology.
- May be characterized as diarrhea-predominant or constipation-predominant; or may alternate between diarrhea and constipation.
- Synonym(s): Spastic colon, irritable colon

EPIDEMIOLOGY

Irritable bowel syndrome (IBS) accounts for up to 50% of GI visits in some practices and is second to upper respiratory infection as cause for lost workdays.

Prevalence

- Estimated to be ~15% of the population of North America:
  - However, only 15% of these patients actually seek medical attention.
- Predominant age: Teens to late 20s:
  - If >age 50, consider other diagnoses
- Predominant sex: In the US, Female > Male (2:1)

RISK FACTORS

- Other family members with similar GI disorder
- History of childhood sexual abuse
- Sexual or domestic abuse in women
- Depression
- Can occur after an infectious colitis

Pregnancy Considerations

No risk to mother or fetus

Genetics

Unknown, but more common in families of IBS patients

GENERAL PREVENTION

See "Diet."

ETIOLOGY

- The etiology is unknown, but patients demonstrate intestinal motility abnormalities with enhanced sensitivity to visceral stimuli.
- The trigger may be luminal or environmental.

COMMONLY ASSOCIATED CONDITIONS

- Migraine
- Urinary frequency and urgency
- Fibromyalgia
- Dyspareunia
- Depression

DIAGNOSIS

- Rome II criteria: ≥12 weeks in last 12 months of abdominal pain or discomfort that has 2 of 3 features:
  - Relieved by defecation
  - Onset associated with change in frequency of stool
  - Onset associated with change in form of stool
- Symptoms can also include:
  - Mucus in stools
  - Constipation
  - Bloating
  - Diarrhea
  - Abdominal distention
  - Upper abdominal discomfort after eating
  - Straining for normal consistency stools
  - Urgency of defecation
  - Feelings of incomplete evacuation
  - Abnormal stool form
  - Nausea, vomiting (rarely)

HISTORY

- As above, but also may have history of abuse or depression
- Patient may note worsening of symptoms with stress or around menses.
- IBS is unlikely in patients with a history of weight loss, bleeding, nocturnal diarrhea, fever, or anemia.

PHYSICAL EXAM

Generally normal, but may have abdominal tenderness to palpation

DIAGNOSTIC TESTS & INTERPRETATION

- In the setting of a typical history and in the absence of warning signs such as anemia or weight loss, it is reasonable to obtain baseline labs as discussed below and begin treatment.
- In those who do not respond to treatment, further evaluation with imaging studies and endoscopy is warranted to exclude organic pathology.

Lab

As needed to rule out other pathology specific to the patient's symptoms:

- Diarrhea-predominant: ESR, CBC, tissue transglutaminase, TSH, and stool for ova and parasites
- Constipation-predominant: CBC, TSH, electrolytes, calcium
- Abdominal pain: LFTs and amylase

Follow-Up & Special Considerations

Consider lactulose breath test to assess for small bowel bacterial overgrowth associated with IBS (1)[C].

Imaging

- Abdominal CT scan or abdominal ultrasound to evaluate pain is generally normal.
- Small-bowel series or video capsule endoscopy to rule out Crohn disease of small intestine may be considered, and will also be normal.
- Sitz Marker study may be used to evaluate colon transit in patients with constipation.

Diagnostic Procedures/Surgery

Sigmoidoscopy/colonoscopy may be used to rule out inflammatory bowel disease or microscopic colitis.

ALERT

Colonoscopy should be performed in all persons >50 years of age for colorectal cancer screening

Pathological Findings

None

DIFFERENTIAL DIAGNOSIS

- Inflammatory bowel disease
- Lactose intolerance
- Infections (*Giardia lamblia, Entamoeba histolytica, Salmonella, Campylobacter, Yersinia, Clostridium difficile*)
- Celiac sprue
- Microscopic colitis
- Cathartic use
- Magnesium-containing antacids
- Hypo-/hyperthyroidism
- Pancreatic insufficiency
- Depression
- Small bowel bacterial overgrowth
- Somatization
- Villous adenoma
- Endocrine tumors
- Diabetes mellitus
- Radiation damage to colon or small bowel

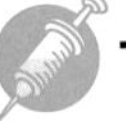

TREATMENT

MEDICATION

- Alternating diarrhea and constipation:
  - Fiber supplements, such as Metamucil or Citrucel, 1–2 Tbs/d can improve consistency of stool, but do not help abdominal pain (2)[B]
  - Synthetic agents such as Citrucel are less likely to cause bloating.
  - Peppermint oil may help with cramping.
- Constipation-predominant:
  - Fiber as above
  - GlycoLax (Miralax) 17 g/d
  - Lubiprostone (Amitiza) 8 mcg b.i.d. (3)[B]
- Diarrhea-predominant:
  - Fiber as above
  - Antispasmodics: Levsin .125 mg q.i.d.; dicyclomine (Bentyl) 10–20 mg b.i.d. or q.i.d.; chlordiazepoxide-clidinium (Librax) 1 or 2 before meals and every night at bedtime; phenobarbital-scopolamine-hyoscyamineatropine (Donnatal) 1 or 2 tablets before meals and at bedtime (4)[B]
  - Antidepressants: Tricyclic antidepressants such as Elavil 10–50 mg at bedtime are effective in decreasing neuropathic pain and may slow gut transit (5)[B].
  - Loperamide (Imodium), 4 mg initial dose, then 2 mg after each unformed stool, or diphenoxylate-atropine (Lomotil) 2.5–5 mg (1–2 tablets) after each unformed stool
  - SSRIs and other antidepressants may be of use if depression is a factor.
  - Cholestyramine (Questran) 1 pkt. every day-b.i.d. can be helpful in patients with IBS, particularly postcholecystectomy.
  - Probiotics have demonstrated modest benefit in patients with IBS, particularly those with bloating and diarrhea; however, the most beneficial strains have yet to be identified. Probiotics are available as oral supplements or additives to yogurt (6)[C].
  - Antiflatulents: Simethicone (Mylicon), 2–4 tablets after meals and at bedtime; Beano
  - Xifaxan (rifaximin) 550 mg PO t.i.d. for 2 weeks, may help bloating and diarrhea (7)[C]
- Lactose intolerance: Lactase (Lactaid) capsules or tablets; 1–2 tablets prior to ingesting dairy products

ADDITIONAL TREATMENT

General Measures

Outpatient evaluation as outlined above with focus on explaining mechanism of disease and reassurance. Biofeedback and stress reduction can help.

Issues for Referral

Possible psychiatric referral for those with depression

Additional Therapies

The evidence for the role of small intestine bacterial overgrowth (SIBO) in IBS and subsequent antibiotic therapy is conflicting; older age and female gender are predictors of SIBO within IBS (8)[C].

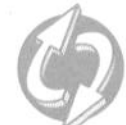

ONGOING CARE

FOLLOW-UP RECOMMENDATIONS

Patient Monitoring

As needed for symptoms

DIET

- Increase fiber slowly to avoid increased intestinal gas production.
- During initial evaluation may wish to try 2 weeks of lactose-free diet to rule out lactose intolerance as etiology of symptoms.
- Avoid large meals, fatty foods, and caffeine, which can often exacerbate symptoms.
- Some patients note improvement in all symptoms with a low-carbohydrate diet.

PATIENT EDUCATION

Patients should not be given the impression that this is a psychiatric illness.

PROGNOSIS

- No progression to cancer or inflammatory disease
- Expect recurrences, especially when under stress.

REFERENCES

1. Shah ED, Basseri RJ, Chong K, et al. Abnormal breath testing in IBS: A meta-analysis. *Digest Dis Sci*. 2010.
2. Ruepert L, Quartero AO, de Wit NJ, et al. Bulking agents, antispasmodics and antidepressants for the treatment of irritable bowel syndrome. *Cochrane Database Syst Rev*. 2011;CD003460.
3. Drossman DA, Chey WD, Johanson JF, et al. Clinical trial: lubiprostone in patients with constipation-associated irritable bowel syndrome - results of two randomized, placebo-controlled studies. *Aliment Pharmacol Ther*. 2008.
4. Poynard T, Regimbeau C, Benhamou Y. Meta-analysis of smooth muscle relaxants in the treatment of irritable bowel syndrome. *Aliment Pharmacol Ther*. 2001;15:355–61.
5. Jackson JL, O'Malley PG, Tomkins G, et al. Treatment of functional gastrointestinal disorders with antidepressant medications: A meta-analysis. *Am J Med*. 2000;108:65–72.
6. Hong KS, Kang HW, Im JP, et al. Effect of probiotics on symptoms in Korean adults with irritable bowel syndrome. *Gut Liver*. 2009;3:101–7.
7. Schey R, Rao SS, et al. The role of rifaximin therapy in patients with irritable bowel syndrome without constipation. *Expert Rev Gastroenterol Hepatol*. 2011;5:461–4.
8. Reddymasu SC, Sostarich S, McCallum RW, et al. Small intestinal bacterial overgrowth in irritable bowel syndrome: Are there any predictors? *BMC Gastroenterol*. 2010;10:23.
9. Rahimi R, Nikfar S, Rezaie A, et al. Efficacy of tricyclic antidepressants in irritable bowel syndrome: A meta-analysis. *World J Gastroenterol*. 2009;15:1548–53.

ADDITIONAL READING

- Hun L et al. Bacillus coagulans significantly improved abdominal pain and bloating in patients with IBS. *Postgrad Med*. 2009;121:119–24.
- Moayyedi P, Ford AC, Talley NJ, et al. The efficacy of probiotics in the therapy of irritable bowel syndrome: A systematic review. *Gut*. 2010;59(3):325–32.

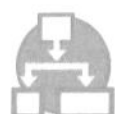

See Also (Topic, Algorithm, Electronic Media Element)

Algorithm: Diarrhea, Chronic

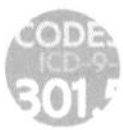

CODES

ICD9

564.1 Irritable bowel syndrome

CLINICAL PEARLS

- Aim treatment at predominant symptom (9)[A].
- Bulking agents or fiber is generally useful, but must be added slowly to not aggravate symptoms.

KAPOSI SARCOMA

Johra Nasreen, MD

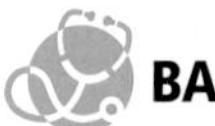

BASICS

Kaposi sarcoma (KS) was originally described in 1872 by a Hungarian dermatologist named Moritz Kaposi.

DESCRIPTION

- A low-grade vascular tumor associated with HHV-8
- Kaposi sarcoma–associated herpesvirus (KSHV), another name is human herpesvirus 8 (HHV-8), is the etiologic agent of all clinical forms of Kaposi sarcoma (KS) and several other malignancies.
- KSHV is also linked to other lymphoproliferative diseases, including primary effusion lymphoma (PEL) and multicentric Castleman disease (MCD).
- 4 major forms are seen:
  - AIDS-related (epidemic) KS: Have high levels of inflammation and oxidative stress as a result of host responses to HIV infection and chronic inflammation (1)[A]
  - Iatrogenic/immunosuppressive KS: Most commonly organ transplant–associated
  - African (endemic) KS: Seen in equatorial Africa, especially sub-Saharan
  - Indolent (classic) KS: Rare, mostly seen in elderly men in the Mediterranean and Eastern European regions, is ubiquitously associated with high level of inflammation and oxidative stress because of its close link with aging (1)
- Systems affected: Hemolytic/Lymphatic/Immunologic; Skin/Exocrine; Gastrointestinal; Pulmonary
- Synonym(s): Endotheliosarcoma; Multiple idiopathic hemorrhagic sarcoma

EPIDEMIOLOGY

- Predominant age: 16–70 years; African KS predominantly affects young; classic KS those older; AIDS-related KS most commonly in middle-aged adults
- Predominant sex: Male-to-female ratio for epidemic KS in the US is ~50:1, while male-to-female ratio is ~10:1 for classic and endemic KS.
- Among those with HIV, most common in homosexual or bisexual men

Incidence

- The US incidence of KS after transplantation is estimated to be <1% (2).
- Incidence of KS among HIV-seropositive individuals has decreased greatly with the advent of highly active antiretroviral therapy (HAART): 15.2/1,000 from 1992–1996 compared with 4.9/1,000 from 1997–1999 (2).
- ~2,500 cases of KS occur annually in the US.

Prevalence

- Before HAART became available, KS was >20,000 times more common in AIDS patients than in the general population and 300 times more common in an AIDS host than in other immunosuppressed hosts; with the advent of HAART, this ratio has decreased. AIDS-related KS in the US decreased 10% per year from 1990–1997 (2).
- The seroprevalence of KSHV in the US is 1–5%; in certain parts of Africa, rates are >70%.
- KS previously was the most common malignancy in HIV-infected patients; some new studies have demonstrated that non–AIDS-defining malignancies may be more common in HIV-infected patients on HAART (3).
- AIDS-related KS may occur at normal CD4 cell counts, though is more common at CD4 <2,003 cells/m.
- In eastern and southern Africa, KS represents nearly 20% of all pediatric cancers (2); in sub-Saharan Africa, KS is also the most frequent cancer among men and the third most frequent cancer among women (4).
- Fulminant lymphadenopathic disease is a subtype of endemic KS occurring in young children with a mean age of 3 years (2).

RISK FACTORS

- HIV infection
- Living in endemic areas (e.g., Zimbabwe, Uganda)
- Immunosuppression (e.g., immunosuppressant medications, transplantation, chemotherapy)
- High-risk sexual practices
- Maternal–fetal or maternal–child transmission
- Injection drug use
- Exposure to infectious saliva
- Contact with KS skin lesions
- Blood transfusions (may transmit HHV-8)
- HHV-8 viremia (detection of HHV-8 in peripheral blood associated with >10-fold increased risk of developing KS)
- High antibody titers to HHV-8 related to faster development of KS

Genetics

Genetic predisposition is suggested by the occurrence of classic KS in men of Mediterranean or Eastern European Ashkenazi descent (2).

GENERAL PREVENTION

Safe sex practices, antiviral prophylaxis medication, avoid needle sharing, and careful screening of transplant organs

PATHOPHYSIOLOGY

- Incompletely understood mechanisms involving HHV-8–induced viral oncogenesis, cytokine-induced growth, and angiogenesis in a setting of immunocompromise
- Ongoing debate about whether KS is a clonal malignancy vs. polyclonal inflammatory response that can progress to sarcoma given host characteristics (5)
- HIV infection may promote KS progression by inducing cytokines as well as indirectly by impairing host immunity.
- Certain HIV gene products may play a role in promoting tumorigenesis in KS; for instance, the TAT gene may be responsible for conversion of the KS cell into a malignant phenotype (5).

ETIOLOGY

- HHV-8 was identified as the etiologic agent in 1994; HHV-8 is necessary, but not sufficient to induce KS.
- HHV-8, immunocompromised status, and cytokine-induced growth represent preconditions for development of KS (5).
- HHV-8 can be transmitted through blood transfusions, solid-organ transplants, and possibly through saliva.
- Recent epidemiologic data suggest that sexual transmission is not a major source of HHV-8 infection in the general population.

COMMONLY ASSOCIATED CONDITIONS

HIV infection/AIDS; lymphoma

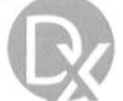

DIAGNOSIS

HISTORY

- Elicit prognostic factors: Age at onset of KS or AIDS, occurrence of tumor before/after onset of AIDS, comorbid conditions
- Commonly presents with cutaneous involvement
- May have tumor-associated lymphedema, with lower extremity and/or facial swelling
- GI involvement is usually asymptomatic, but may present as nausea/vomiting, abdominal pain, dysphagia, or bowel obstruction.
- Pulmonary involvement may be asymptomatic or present with symptoms such as cough, dyspnea, hemoptysis, or chest pain.

PHYSICAL EXAM

- Full physical exam, including dermatologic exam to evaluate for cutaneous involvement
- The skin lesions characterized by:
  - Macular, papular, nodular, or plaquelike appearance
  - Can be discrete or confluent, typically in symmetric distribution
  - Variable color (can be brown, pink, red, or violaceous) and can be difficult to assess in dark-skinned individuals
  - Size varies from millimeters to several centimeters in diameter
  - Nearly all palpable and nonpruritic
  - May be located anywhere on body, but typically found on lower extremities and head/neck region, with mucous membrane involvement common

DIAGNOSTIC TESTS & INTERPRETATION

Lab

- Serostatus can be determined with enzyme-linked immunoassay for antibody to KSHV (ELISA)
- Viral load of KSHV can be measured with quantitative PCR testing.
- CD4 lymphocyte count and HIV viral load determination should be performed in those with HIV infection.

Imaging

- CXR, CT scan, or MRI (chest, abdomen) to assess organ involvement
- Thallium or gallium scans may help to differentiate pulmonary KS from infection.

Diagnostic Procedures/Surgery

- Biopsy of skin or lymph node
- Bronchoscopy with biopsy of suspicious lung lesions
- Endoscopy

Pathological Findings

- Neovascularization with aberrant proliferation of small vessels
- Atypical spindle-shaped cell with leukocytic infiltration
- Angiogenesis
- Extravasated RBCs
- Hemosiderin-laden macrophages

DIFFERENTIAL DIAGNOSIS

- Bacillary angiomatosis
- Granuloma faciale
- Vascular proliferation
- Purpuric lesions
- Dermatofibrosarcoma protuberans

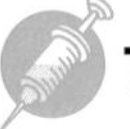

TREATMENT

The major goals of treatment are symptom palliation, prevention of disease progression, and shrinkage of tumor to alleviate edema, organ compromise, and psychological stress (6).

MEDICATION

First Line

- Highly active antiretroviral therapy (HAART) is recommended for virtually all patients with AIDS-related KS (7,8).
- The need for treatment beyond HAART and the choice among the various options depend upon the extent of disease, the rapidity of tumor growth, the HIV-1 viral load, the CD4 cell count, and the patient's overall medical condition (8).
- Localized therapy for limited, cutaneous disease: Radiation for individualized lesions, intralesional chemotherapy (e.g., with vinblastine), topical alitretinoin gel, cryotherapy, laser therapy, photodynamic therapy, surgical excision (2,9)[A]
- Cytotoxic chemotherapy for disseminated disease: Liposomal anthracyclines (e.g., pegylated liposomal doxorubicin (PLD), daunorubicin); liposomal formulations offer improved outcome with less toxicity (9)[A].
- Intralesional chemotherapy used to induce regression of injected tumors and is preferred for small lesions. Vinblastine is the most widely used, injected directly into a KS lesion as a 0.2–0.3 mg/mL solution with a volume of 0.1 mL per 0.5 cm^2 of lesion. Multiple injections may be necessary for larger lesions. A second series of injections is often necessary 3–4 weeks later. Treated lesions will fade and regress, although typically not resolve completely (10).

Second Line

- Cytotoxic chemotherapy: Paclitaxel (9)[A]
- Other chemotherapy agents (use limited by side effects): Vinca alkaloids, bleomycin

ADDITIONAL TREATMENT

General Measures

- In AIDS-related KS, optimize control of HIV replication with HAART; HAART increases KSHV-specific immune responses and reduces the risk of progression from KSHV to Kaposi sarcoma by 90% (4)[A].
- Recommendation is for viral suppression with continuous HAART rather than interrupted CD4 T-cell-guided HAART (3)[A].
- In immunosuppressant medication–related KS, reduce dosage or stop if possible.
- Treatment otherwise is determined by the extent and location of the disease.

Issues for Referral

- Consider referral to HIV specialist to maximize HAART.
- Oncologist, surgeon, and/or dermatologist as needed and provider's comfort with specific therapies

Additional Therapies

- Experimental therapies: Include recombinant interleukin-12, thalidomide, imatinib, temsirolimus, intralesional human chorionic gonadotropin (hCG), vitamin D analogues, and interferon-alfa
- Interferon-alfa is not used frequently due to poor tumor response and high toxicity compared with pegylated liposomal doxorubicin.
- Antiviral therapy against HHV-8: Some studies show treatment benefit with foscarnet and ganciclovir; acyclovir has no activity against HHV-8 and is not recommended.

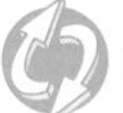

ONGOING CARE

FOLLOW-UP RECOMMENDATIONS

Patient Monitoring

- In HIV patients with KS, other opportunistic infections must be treated aggressively.
- Since non–AIDS-defining malignancies are becoming more common than KS in the HIV population, standard cancer preventative measures should be encouraged (3)[B].

DIET

No particular diet recommended

PATIENT EDUCATION

- HIV risk prevention
- Injection drug rehabilitation
- Promoting adherence to HAART for patients with AIDS-related KS

PROGNOSIS

- AIDS-related KS tends to have aggressive clinical course; however, improved HIV treatments have resulted in enhanced survival for patients with AIDS-related KS.
- Prognostic factors: Immunologic status as measured by CD4 count, age at onset, occurrence of tumor before/after onset of AIDS, comorbid conditions, organ involvement
- Pulmonary involvement is a poor prognostic factor; most common cause of mortality with KS is uncontrolled pulmonary hemorrhage.
- Indolent/classic KS: 10–15-year survival; rarely metastasizes; most deaths due to unrelated cause
- Endemic KS: Some subtypes can be rapidly fatal.
- AIDS-related KS: With appropriate HAART, course typically chronic; no cure, rarely fatal
- Iatrogenic/transplant KS: Course can be chronic or rapidly progressive, and spontaneous remission after discontinuation of immunosuppressive therapy is typical.

COMPLICATIONS

- Extensive pulmonary involvement may lead to hypoxemia.
- Extensive lymphatic involvement may lead to severe edema.
- Pediatric intussusception can be caused by AIDS-associated Kaposi sarcoma.
- KS may develop as an immune reconstitution inflammatory syndrome (IRIS) among HIV-seropositive individuals at the advent of HAART (11).

REFERENCES

1. Ye F, Gao SJ, et al. A novel role of hydrogen peroxide in Kaposi sarcoma-associated herpesvirus reactivation. *Cell Cycle (Georgetown, Tex.)*. 2011;10:3237–8.
2. Hengge UR, Ruzicka T, Tyring SK, et al. Update on Kaposi's sarcoma and other HHV8 associated diseases. Part 1: Epidemiology, environmental predispositions, clinical manifestations, and therapy. *Lancet Infect Dis*. 2002;2:281–92.
3. Silverberg MJ, Neuhaus J, Bower M, et al. Risk of cancers during interrupted antiretroviral therapy in the SMART study. *AIDS*. 2007;21:1957–63.
4. Sullivan SG, Hirsch HH, Franceschi S, et al. Kaposi sarcoma herpes virus antibody response and viremia following highly active antiretroviral therapy in the Swiss HIV Cohort study. *AIDS*. 2010;24(14):2245–52.
5. Hengge UR, Ruzicka T, Tyring SK, et al. Update on Kaposi's sarcoma and other HHV8 associated diseases. Part 2: Pathogenesis, Castleman's disease, and pleural effusion lymphoma. *Lancet Infect Dis*. 2002;2:344–52.
6. Dezube BJ, Pantanowitz L, Aboulafia DM. Management of AIDS-related Kaposi sarcoma: Advances in target discovery and treatment. *AIDS Read*. 2004;14:236.
7. Bower M, Collins S, Cottrill C et al. British HIV Association guidelines for HIV-associated malignancies 2008. *HIV Med*. 2008;9:336.
8. Stebbing J, Sanitt A, Nelson M, et al. A prognostic index for AIDS-associated Kaposi's sarcoma in the era of highly active antiretroviral therapy. *Lancet*. 2006;367:1495.
9. Di Lorenzo G, Konstantinopoulos PA, Pantanowitz L, et al. Management of AIDS-related Kaposi's sarcoma. *Lancet Oncol*. 2007;8:167–76.
10. Ramírez-Amador V, Esquivel-Pedraza L, Lozada-Nur F, et al. Intralesional vinblastine vs. 3% sodium tetradecyl sulfate for the treatment of oral Kaposi's sarcoma. A double blind, randomized clinical trial. *Oral Oncol*. 2002;38: 460.
11. Feller L, Lemmer J. Insights into pathogenic events of HIV-associated Kaposi sarcoma and immune reconstitution syndrome related Kaposi sarcoma. *Infect Agent Cancer*. 2008;3:1.

CODES

ICD9

- 176.0 Kaposi's sarcoma, skin
- 176.1 Kaposi's sarcoma, soft tissue
- 176.9 Kaposi's sarcoma, unspecified site

CLINICAL PEARLS

- HHV-8 (also known as KSHV) is the etiologic agent for KS.
- HHV-8, immunocompromise, and cytokine-induced growth represent preconditions for the development of KS.
- AIDS-related KS can occur at normal CD4 counts.
- Staging for KS is usually based on the system of the AIDS Clinical Trial Group (ACTG), consisting of extent of tumor (T), immune status (I), and severity of systemic illness (S).
- Cytotoxic chemotherapy is the gold standard for treatment of disseminated disease.

KAWASAKI SYNDROME

Kelly B. Han, MD
Richard A. Moriarty, MD

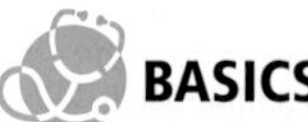

BASICS

DESCRIPTION

Kawasaki syndrome is an acute, self-limited, systemic inflammatory process that causes a febrile, exanthematous, vasculitic disease in young children, notable for its cardiac sequelae:

- Vasculitis affecting the coronary arteries can result in aneurysms or ectasia, further leading to MI/ischemia or sudden death.
- System(s) affected: Cardiovascular; Gastrointestinal; Hematologic/Lymphatic/Immunologic; Musculoskeletal; Nervous; Pulmonary; Renal/Urologic; Skin/Exocrine
- Synonym(s): Mucocutaneous lymph node syndrome (MCLS), Infantile polyarteritis, Kawasaki syndrome

ALERT

Kawasaki syndrome should be considered in any child with extended high fever unresponsive to antibiotics or antipyretics, rash, and nonexudative conjunctivitis.

EPIDEMIOLOGY

Incidence

- Worldwide: Affects all races, but most prevalent in Asia, especially Japan where annual incidence rate approaches 200/100,000 in children <5 years old
- In the US, the annual incidence rate among children <5 years of age is 33/100,000 for Americans of Asian and Pacific Islander descent, 17/100,000 for non-Hispanic blacks, 11/100,00 for Hispanics, and 9/100,000 for whites. Highest incidence in Hawaii.
- Leading cause of acquired heart disease in children in developed countries:
  - Predominant age: 1–5 years
  - 85% cases are children <5 years of age and 50% <2 years of age

Prevalence

- Highest to lowest prevalence: Asians > Blacks > Hispanics > Whites
- Seasonal variation: Increased in winter and early spring in temperate places, summer in Asia, and outbreaks at 2–3-year intervals

RISK FACTORS

Genetics

- The risk of occurrence in twins is ~13%.
- Siblings of patients in Japan have a 10-fold relative risk. Increased occurrence of KD in children whose parents also had illness in childhood (1).

GENERAL PREVENTION

No preventive measures available

PATHOPHYSIOLOGY

- Acute Kawasaki syndrome causes inflammation in the smooth muscle layer of medium arteries, especially the coronary arteries.
- Inflammatory cells in the media secrete cytokines, interleukins, and matrix metalloproteases that cause fragmentation of the internal elastic lamina.
- Necrosis may develop and result in aneurysmal dilation of these arteries.
- A prominence of IgA plasma cells and IgA deposits are characteristic features of KS. Similar IgA plasma cells are found in the respiratory tract of patients with KS (2).
- During the period of greatest vascular damage, there is a progressive increase in the platelet count.
- As the process resolves over weeks to months, active inflammatory cells are replaced by fibroblasts and monocytes; tissue repair and remodeling and may cause vascular fibrosis and stenosis.

ETIOLOGY

- Unknown. However, an infectious cause is favored owing to the acute, self-limited nature, community-wide outbreaks, seasonality, and laboratory features indicating respiratory route of entry (2).
- Working hypothesis: KD is caused by a childhood transmissible infectious agent that causes clinical symptoms in genetically susceptible individuals.

DIAGNOSIS

- ≥5 days of fever and ≥4 of following 5 principal clinical features; or <4 features and presence of coronary artery disease on 2D echocardiography:
  - Nonpurulent conjunctival injection with limbic sparing
  - Erythematous mouth and pharynx, tongue, and lips
  - A polymorphous, generalized, erythematous rash
  - Changes in the skin of the peripheral extremities
  - Cervical lymphadenopathy

ALERT

Prolonged fever without rash and treated with antibiotics may cause clinicians to believe that later rash development is due to a drug reaction.

- Incomplete Kawasaki syndrome:
  - ≥5 days of fever, ≥2 principle clinical features, labs indicating systemic inflammation, and exclusion of other diseases
  - Incomplete cases that exhibit <4 clinical criteria often occur in infants ≤6 months old or older children/adolescents. The frequency of coronary artery aneurysms (CAAs) is often higher in patients with missed diagnosis or delayed treatment. For this reason, in infants with prolonged fever and few or no clinical features, echocardiography and labs for inflammation should be considered.

HISTORY

- Fever is the first sign during the acute phase.
- Symptoms may not occur all at once but usually occur in close proximity.

PHYSICAL EXAM

- High-spiking and remittent fever for ≥5 days:
  - Fever is high (103–105°F [39.4–40.5°C]) and unresponsive to antibiotics.
  - May be prolonged (3–4 weeks, with mean duration of 11 days)
  - Extreme irritability is a very common feature.
- Bilateral painless nonpurulent conjunctival injection without corneal ulceration, or edema. Limbic sparing usually seen.
- Changes in lips and oral cavity:
  - Redness and swelling of lips in the acute stage; cracking, fissuring, bleeding in subacute phase
  - Strawberry or erythematous tongue
- Extensive erythematous polymorphous rash: Within 5 days of fever
  - Morbilliform is most common. May be maculopapular, scarlatiniform; can resemble erythema multiforme, erythroderma, urticarial exanthem; rarely micropustular.
  - Perineal desquamation especially in skin folds
- Extremity changes:
  - Reddened palms and soles on days 3–5.
  - Edema of hands and feet on days 4–7; painful induration
  - Desquamation of fingers and toes that begins in periungual area at 2–3 weeks
- Acute, unilateral cervical lymphadenopathy (least common symptom):
  - ≥1 lymph nodes >1.5 cm, firm and nonfluctuant. Usually none to slight tenderness.
  - Generalized lymphadenopathy usually absent
- Cardiac exam: Tachycardia, gallop rhythms, hyperdynamic precordium, innocent flow murmurs, depressed contractility
- Other organ system involvement:
  - Cardiovascular: Myocarditis; pericarditis (often subclinical), CAA, and other medium-sized arterial aneurysms
  - GI: Anorexia, abdominal pain, vomiting or diarrhea, acute gallbladder hydrops, hepatic enlargement, jaundice
  - Renal: Nephritis, urethritis
  - Respiratory: Pneumonitis, atelectasis or pleural effusion, cough
  - Joints: Polyarthritis of small joints in acute phase; weight-bearing joints affected after 10th day from onset of fever
  - Neurologic: Irritability, aseptic meningitis, peripheral neuropathy (unilateral facial palsy), transient high-frequency hearing loss

DIAGNOSTIC TESTS & INTERPRETATION

Lab

- Initial workup should include appropriate testing to rule out sepsis: CBC with differential, urine analysis and culture, blood culture; lumbar puncture if <4 months of age or if signs or symptoms of meningitis:
  - Leukocytosis (12K–40K cells/mm^3) with immature and mature granulocytes
  - Anemia: Normochromic, normocytic
  - Thrombocytosis (500,000 to >1,000,000/mm^3) in second and third weeks. Thrombopenia during acute phase is associated with CAA and MI.
- Elevated CRP (>35 mg/L in 80% cases), ESR (>60 mm/hr in 60% cases), and α_1-antitrypsin

ALERT

ESR can be artificially high after immunoglobulin IV (IVIG) therapy. CRP is a better test.

- Hyponatremia
- Moderately elevated AST, ALT, GGT, and bilirubin
- Decreased albumin
- Abnormal plasma lipids: Low cholesterol, high-density lipoprotein (HDL), and apo-AI
- CSF pleocytosis may be seen (lymphocytic with normal protein and glucose)
- Sterile pyuria but not seen in suprapubic collection
- Nasal swab to rule out adenovirus

Imaging

- Once Kawasaki syndrome is suspected, all patients need a cardiac evaluation, including ECG and echocardiogram:

– ECG may show arrhythmias, prolonged PR interval, and ST/T-wave changes.
– Echocardiography has a high sensitivity and specificity for detection of abnormalities of proximal LMCA and RCA (3)[C]; may show perivascular brightening, ectasia, decreased left ventricular contractility, pericardial effusion, or aneurysms.
– Cardiac stress test if CAA seen on echo

- Baseline CXR: May show pleural effusion, atelectasis, and congestive heart failure (CHF)
- Hydrops of the gallbladder may be associated with abdominal pain or may be asymptomatic

Diagnostic Procedures/Surgery

- No laboratory study proves diagnosis; the diagnosis rests on constellation of clinical features and exclusion of other illnesses in differential diagnosis.
- Patients with complex coronary artery lesions may benefit from coronary angiography after the acute inflammatory process has resolved; generally recommended in 6–12 months (3)[C]

DIFFERENTIAL DIAGNOSIS

- Bacterial: Staphylococcal scalded-skin syndrome, toxic shock syndrome, scarlet fever, bacterial cervical lymphadenitis, *Mycoplasma* infection, leptospirosis, Lyme disease, Rocky Mountain spotted fever
- Viral: Measles, adenovirus, Epstein-Barr virus infections
- Toxoplasmosis
- Reiter syndrome
- Hypersensitivity drug reactions (erythema multiforme minor, Stevens-Johnson syndrome)
- Juvenile rheumatoid arthritis
- Acrodynia (mercury poisoning)
- Other vasculitides

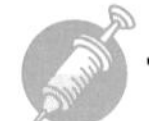

TREATMENT

Inpatient care with IV access and cardiac monitoring until stable is warranted.

MEDICATION

- Optimal therapy is IVIG 2 g/kg IV over 10 hours with high-dose aspirin preferably within 7–10 days of fever, followed by low-dose aspirin until follow-up echocardiograms indicate a lack of coronary abnormalities (4)[A].
  – IVIG lowers the risk of CAA and may shorten the duration of fever.
  – The extreme irritability often resolves very quickly after IVIG is given.
- Retreatment with IVIG if clinical response is incomplete or fever persists/returns 48 hours after start of IVIG treatment (3)[C]:
  – ≥10% of patients do not respond to initial IVIG treatment. 2/3 of nonresponders respond to the second dose of IVIG.
  – Nonresponders tend to have ↑ bands, ↓ albumin, and an abnormal echo.
- Aspirin, 80–100 mg/kg/d in 4 doses beginning with IVIG administration (3)[A]. Switch to low-dose aspirin (3–5 mg/kg/d) when afebrile for 48–72 hours. Maintain low dose for 6–8 weeks until follow-up echocardiogram is normal (3)[C]. Continue salicylate regimen in children with coronary abnormalities long term or until documented regression of aneurysm (3)[B].
- Contraindications:
  – IVIG: Documented hypersensitivity, IgA deficiency, anti-IgE/IgG antibodies, severe thrombocytopenia, coagulation disorders.
  – Aspirin: Vitamin K deficiency, bleeding disorders, liver damage, documented hypersensitivity, hypoprothrombinemia
- Precautions:
  – No statistically significant difference noted between different preparations of IVIG (4)[A]
  – High-dose aspirin therapy can result in tinnitus, decrease of renal function, and increased transaminases.
  – Do not use ibuprofen in children with coronary artery aneurysms who are taking aspirin for antiplatelet effects.
  – Significant possible interactions: Aspirin therapy has been associated with Reye syndrome in children who develop viral infections, especially influenza B and varicella. Yearly influenza vaccination thus is recommended for children requiring long-term treatment with aspirin (3)[C]. Delay any live vaccines, especially varicella and measles, for 11 months after IVIG treatment.

Second Line

Corticosteroids should be used only if ≥2 IVIG treatments have failed. The addition of corticosteroids to IVIG and aspirin during initial treatment has not showed clear benefits (no reduction of CAA).

ADDITIONAL TREATMENT

General Measures

Antibiotics are given until bacterial etiologies are excluded (e.g., sepsis or meningitis).

Issues for Referral

Referral to pediatric cardiologist if coronary abnormalities suspected on echo or if extensive stenosis/pathology is suspected

Additional Therapies

- In patients with coronary disease, treatment and prevention of thrombosis are crucial.
- Antiplatelet agents (clopidogrel, dipyridamole), heparin, low-molecular-weight heparin, or warfarin are sometimes added to the low-dose aspirin regimen depending on severity of coronary involvement (3)[C].

SURGERY/OTHER PROCEDURES

- Very unlikely to be needed. Coronary artery bypass grafting (CABG) for severe obstruction or after recurrent myocardial infarction (3)[C]. Younger patients have a higher mortality rate.
- Coronary revascularization via percutaneous coronary intervention for patients with evidence of ischemia on stress testing (3)[C]

IN-PATIENT CONSIDERATIONS

Admission Criteria

All children with suspected Kawasaki syndrome

IV Fluids

Normal saline (NS) for rehydration and 1/2 NS for maintenance

Discharge Criteria

Children are usually discharged after 24–48 hours of remaining afebrile after IVIG treatment.

ONGOING CARE

FOLLOW-UP RECOMMENDATIONS

With giant or multiple aneurysms, contact and high-risk sports should be avoided.

Patient Monitoring

- Repeat ECG and echo at 6–8 weeks. If abnormal, repeat at 6–12 months.
- Patients with complex coronary artery lesions may benefit from coronary angiography; generally recommended in 6–12 months (3)[C].

PROGNOSIS

- Usually self-limited
- Moderate-sized aneurysms usually regress in 1–2 years, resolving in 50–66% of cases.
- Recurrence (3% in Japan, <1% in the US)
- Sudden death in early adulthood (rare)

COMPLICATIONS

- 15–25% of untreated patients develop coronary artery aneurysms in convalescent phase.
- 2–7% of treated patients develop aneurysms. 1% develop giant aneurysms.
- Risk factors for aneurysm:
  – Male, age <1 year old, high ESR >4 weeks, fever >2 weeks in treated patients, fever >48 hours after IVIG treatment
- Mortality of 0.08–0.17% is due to cardiac disease.

REFERENCES

1. Takahashi K, Oharaseki T, Yokouchi Y, et al. Pathogenesis of Kawasaki disease. *Clin Exp Immunol*. 2011;164 (Suppl 1):20–2.
2. Rowley AH, Shulman ST, et al. Pathogenesis and management of Kawasaki disease. *Expert Rev Anti Infect Ther*. 2010;8:197–203.
3. Newburger JW, Takahashi M, Gerber MA, et al. Diagnosis, treatment, and long-term management of Kawasaki disease: A statement for health professionals from the Committee on Rheumatic Fever, Endocarditis, and Kawasaki Disease, Council on Cardiovascular Disease in the Young, American Heart Association. *Pediatrics*. 2004;114:1708–33.
4. Oates-Whitehead RM, Baumer JH, Haines L, et al. Intravenous immunoglobulin for the treatment of Kawasaki disease in children. *Cochrane Database Syst Rev*. 2003;(4):CD004000.

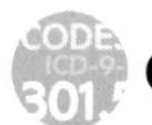

CODES

ICD9

446.1 Acute febrile mucocutaneous lymph node syndrome (MCLS)

CLINICAL PEARLS

- The diagnosis of Kawasaki syndrome rests on a constellation of clinical features.
- Once Kawasaki syndrome is suspected, all patients need an inpatient cardiac evaluation, including ECG and echocardiogram.
- Optimal therapy is IVIG 2 g/kg IV over 10 hours with high-dose aspirin 80–100 mg/kg/d in 4 doses.

KELOIDS

Patrick W. Joyner, MD, MS
Kristyn Fagerberg, MD

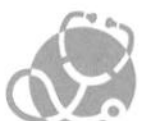

BASICS

DESCRIPTION

- Abnormally large overgrowths of fibrous tissue (scar) occurring as a result of trauma or irritation that do not subside with time
- System(s) affected: Skin/Exocrine

EPIDEMIOLOGY

Incidence

- Predominant age: 10–30 years
- Higher incidence during puberty and pregnancy
- Predominant sex: Female > Male
- However, mean age between the 2 sexes is almost identical, with females getting first keloid at 22.3 years of age and males developing first keloid at 22.8 years.

Prevalence

- 4–16% of the black and Hispanic populations
- Also a higher incidence in the Asian population
- Data from the UK demonstrated that <1% of Caucasians had keloids.

RISK FACTORS

- Family history of keloids
- Dark skin pigment
- Certain locations on the body (e.g., deltoids, chest, neck, earlobes)
- Pregnancy
- Adolescence

Genetics

- More common in blacks and Asians (5–15×) than in whites; in all races, more darkly pigmented individuals are at higher risk.
- Both autosomal dominant and autosomal-recessive familial inheritance have been reported.

GENERAL PREVENTION

- Primary prevention: Avoid elective surgery, body piercing, and tattooing in high-risk patients.
- Wounds should be kept clean to prevent infection.
- When feasible, laparoscopic approaches are preferred in keloid formers.
- Compressive pressure dressings may be useful in high-risk (e.g., burn) patients. Local steroid injection postoperatively in high-risk patients is also effective.
- Physicians should be alert to delays in wound healing, persistent erythema, or pruritus as impending symptoms of possible keloid formation and make all reasonable attempts to reduce inflammation and tension on the skin with appropriate methods.

ETIOLOGY

- Wounds: Traumatic, surgical, body piercing (foreign-body reaction)
- Wound infection
- Burn injury
- Other injuries:
  - Insect bite
  - Folliculitis barbae and nuchae
  - Acne
  - Chickenpox
- Vaccination (especially bacille Calmette-Guérin)
- Rarely occur in places on body lacking sebaceous glands; thus, sebaceous glands, and the body's reaction to this sebum, are hypothesized to be an etiologic factor in keloid development. Moreover, humans are the only mammals with sebaceous glands and the only mammals affected by keloids.
- Increased ratio of type I to type III collagen
- Increased density and proliferation rate of fibroblasts

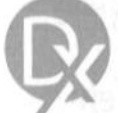

DIAGNOSIS

HISTORY

- Pain
- Tenderness
- Hyperesthesia
- Pruritus (occasional)
- May be asymptomatic
- Grow beyond the border of the original wound

PHYSICAL EXAM

- Firm, smooth, elevated scar with sharply demarcated borders
- Initially may be pale or mildly erythematous
- Older lesion hypopigmented or hyperpigmented
- Scar extends beyond margins of the initial wound.
- Over period of years, keloids may continue to grow and may develop clawlike projections.
- Keloids occur more frequently on the chest, shoulders, upper back, back of the neck, and earlobes.

DIAGNOSTIC TESTS & INTERPRETATION

Biopsy only if unable to differentiate from carcinoma or infectious disease because a biopsy may increase the keloid's size. Use a 2-mm punch biopsy to minimize trauma.

Pathological Findings

Histology shows whorl-like arrangements of hyalinized collagen bundles, with pressure thinning of papillary dermis and minimal elastic tissue.

DIFFERENTIAL DIAGNOSIS

- Hypertrophic scar (usually regresses spontaneously, does not cross wound margins, and rarely more than 1 cm in thickness and width)
- Dermatofibroma
- Infiltrating basal cell carcinoma
- Sclerosing metastatic malignancies
- Desmoplastic melanoma
- Sarcoidosis
- Leprosy (nodular LL type)
- Other fibronodular skin diseases (e.g., neurofibromatosis, post–kala-azar dermal leishmaniasis)

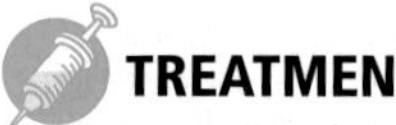

TREATMENT

- Given the high recurrence rates and significant expense associated with treatment, prevention of keloids should take priority. Avoidance of known risk factors such as piercings, tattoos, and elective surgery is highly recommended in people with either a family or personal history of keloids.
- A recent meta-analysis of 70 studies has shown that all the currently accepted treatment options have fairly comparable efficacy, with a mean improvement of 60% (1). Also of note is that keloids do not regress spontaneously.
- Treatment options should be based on the type of keloid. Characteristics to take into consideration: (i) Presence/absence of scar contractures; (ii) size; and (iii) number of keloids:
  - Small, single keloids can be treated more aggressively.
  - Large or multiple keloids are typically more complicated to treat and should be evaluated on an individual basis (2).

MEDICATION

First Line

- Triamcinolone (Kenalog) suspension 10 mg/mL (3)[A]:
  - Most commonly used treatment option. Likely more effective if combined with cryotherapy, pulsed dye laser, or 5-fluorouricil. No difference when combined with excision versus monotherapy (2).
  - 72% showed symptomatic improvement in 1 trial (3).
  - Use 27–30-gauge needle and a TB syringe (total dose 20–30 mg triamcinolone); may inject 3 lesions at a time using 10 mg/lesion.
  - Advance the needle while injecting to distribute medication evenly.
  - Early keloids are more responsive to this therapy than are older lesions.
  - Reinject every 4 weeks until keloid shrinks to near skin surface.
  - If no response to 10 mg/mL triamcinolone suspension, may try 40 mg/mL suspension
  - May mix dilute triamcinolone (5–10 mg/mL) with local anesthetic for excision of keloids; postoperative steroid injections at 2–4 weeks and then monthly for 6 months help to prevent recurrences
  - Contraindications: Active skin infection at injection site
  - Precautions:
    - Systemic absorption with reversible adrenal suppression, hyperglycemia
    - Local effects: Skin atrophy, ulceration, depigmentation, telangiectasias
    - Both types of side effects are more common with 40 mg/mL triamcinolone suspension.
  - Significant possible interactions: Rare interactions (only with very large doses of corticosteroids and systemic absorption)

- Silica gel sheeting: First-line prophylaxis after surgical procedure or keloid excision (3)[A],(4)[C]:
  - Patient compliance limits effectiveness.
  - Sheets are cut to fit and must be worn for at least 12 hours and, optimally, 24 hours a day.
  - Unclear whether benefit is from silicone or occlusive effect
  - Adverse effects are generally from irritation: Pruritus, rash, erosion, and maceration. There is complete resolution within a few days of removal.

Second Line

- Cryotherapy is likely to be more useful in early, smaller lesions. It is not recommended for larger areas owing to pain and decreased skin pigmentation (2).
- Verapamil locally may be helpful as an adjuvant following excision and topical silicone (3)[C].
- Interferon-α2b may be helpful after excision (3)[C].
- Topical imiquimod (Aldara) may be helpful after excision.
- Intralesional 5-fluorouracil (3)[C]: One study showed a 92% reduction in lesion size when combined with triamcinolone and excision (5).
- Intralesional bleomycin (3)[C]
- Radiation therapy has greater success rates when used in combination with surgical excision. There are some concerns about precipitating malignant lesions with radiation; however, a direct correlation has not been made (2).

Pregnancy Considerations

Radiation therapy, 5-fluorouracil, and bleomycin are unsafe in pregnancy.

ADDITIONAL TREATMENT

General Measures

- Appropriate health care: Outpatient
- Intralesional corticosteroid injection causes atrophy, telangiectasia, and pigment changes in half of patients but is the most successful therapy (3)[A].
- Pressure bandages must maintain 24 mm Hg and should be worn for 6–12 months (3)[C]. Bandages should not be removed for >30 min/d.
- Pressure clips (Zimmer splints) are useful for earlobes (6)[C]. Designer splints look like fashion earrings.
- Cryotherapy may be useful for small keloids (e.g., acne scars) (3)[C].
- Use 10–30-second freeze–thaw cycles every month; may cause permanent hypopigmentation.
- Topical agents: No evidence to support efficacy of retinoic acid, vitamin E, allantoin, or onion extract (3); some evidence for imiquimod. Generally, retinoids are tolerated in patients with pigmented skin; however, the treating physician must be cognizant of the development of retinoid dermatitis, which can induce postinflammatory hyperpigmentation. Regimen reduction/modification and possibly cessation of the drug is the treatment.

Issues for Referral

When intralesional steroids fail, referral to dermatologist or plastic surgeon may be indicated.

Additional Therapies

- Local radiotherapy may be effective after excision but carries a small risk of carcinogenesis (7)[B].
- Physical therapy useful if contractures associated

COMPLEMENTARY AND ALTERNATIVE MEDICINE

None proven (3)

SURGERY/OTHER PROCEDURES

- Surgery: High recurrence rate (45–100%) if used alone; therefore, is used only for the debulking of large keloids or if a lesion is unresponsive to steroid injections or other therapy; combine with preoperative steroid injection and possibly other modalities (3). Debulking just enough for symptomatic improvement is recommended (2).
- Pulsed-dye laser surgery: No definitive evidence of efficacy or advantage over other methods; therefore, use only if other methods fail, and then use in conjunction with them (3)[C]; some promise is seen in combination with triamcinolone and 5-fluorouracil (4)[C].

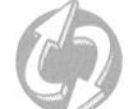

ONGOING CARE

FOLLOW-UP RECOMMENDATIONS

Patient Monitoring

Monthly visits for up to 1 year for evaluation and possible steroid reinjections

DIET

No special diet

PATIENT EDUCATION

- Stress the possibility of recurrence despite appropriate treatment.
- May require many months of treatment with combined modalities
- Prevention: In those with risk factors or previous keloids, caution against activities or procedures that may entail dermal disruption, and suggest early treatment of any such events.

PROGNOSIS

When treatment is successful, lesions gradually diminish over 6–18 months with therapy, leaving a flat, shiny scar. While keloids can improve with treatment, cure is unlikely.

COMPLICATIONS

Skin atrophy, ulceration, depigmentation, and telangiectasias can occur as a result of local steroid injections.

REFERENCES

1. Leventhal D, Furr M, Reiter D. Treatment of keloids and hypertrophic scars: A meta-analysis and review of the literature. *Arch Facial Plast Surg*. 2006;8: 362–8.
2. Ogawa R, et al. The most current algorithms for the treatment and prevention of hypertrophic scars and keloids. *Plast Reconstr Surg*. 2010;125:557–68.
3. Mustoe TA, Cooter RD, Gold MH, et al. International clinical recommendations on scar management. *Plast Reconstr Surg*. 2002;110: 560–71.
4. Asilian A, Darougheh A, Shariati F. New combination of triamcinolone, 5-Fluorouracil, and pulsed-dye laser for treatment of keloid and hypertrophic scars. *Dermatol Surg*. 2006;32: 907–15.
5. Davison SP, Dayan JH, Clemens MW, et al. Efficacy of intralesional 5-fluorouracil and triamcinolone in the treatment of keloids. *Aesthet Surg J*. 2009; 29(1):40–6.
6. Russell R, Horlock N, Gault D. Zimmer splintage: A simple effective treatment for keloids following ear-piercing. *Br J Plast Surg*. 2001;54:509–10.
7. Ogawa R, Mitsuhashi K, Hyakusoku H, et al. Postoperative electron-beam irradiation therapy for keloids and hypertrophic scars: Retrospective study of 147 cases followed for more than 18 months. *Plast Reconstr Surg*. 2003;111:547–53; discussion 554–5.

ADDITIONAL READING

- Geria AN, Lawson CN, Halder RM, et al. Topical retinoids for pigmented skin. *J Drugs Dermatol*. 2011;10:483–9.
- Seifert O, Mrowietz U, et al. Keloid scarring: Bench and bedside. *Arch Dermatol Res*. 2009;301:259–72.
- Viera MH, Caperton CV, Berman B, et al. Advances in the treatment of keloids. *J Drugs Dermatol*. 2011;10:468–80.

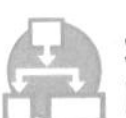

See Also (Topic, Algorithm, Electronic Media Element)

Bites; Burns; Leprosy; Warts

CODES

ICD9

701.4 Keloid scar

CLINICAL PEARLS

- The most successful treatment of hypertrophic scar or keloid is achieved while the scar is still immature, but the overlying epithelium is intact, although this is not as yet confirmed in the literature.
- Keloids extend beyond the margins of the original wound and do not regress with time; this is a way of differentiating from hypertrophic scars. Treatment is similar, but keloids are much more likely to recur.
- Closing wounds with a minimum of suture tension, avoiding midsternal incisions and crossing joint lines, and injecting steroids into the incision postoperatively reduce the chance of keloids forming following unavoidable surgery.

KERATOACANTHOMA

Wesley Wu, MD
Leslie Robinson-Bostom, MD
Raymond G. Dufresne, Jr., MD

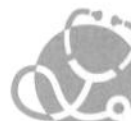

BASICS

DESCRIPTION

- Atypical squamous epithelial neoplasm, most frequently classified as a benign variant of a well-differentiated squamous cell carcinoma (SCC)
- Rapidly proliferating, firm, skin-colored, dome-shaped papule or nodule in early stages with subsequent development of a smooth central crater filled with a keratin plug
- May spontaneously resolve and become an atrophic scar within months to a year
- Management is primarily surgical excision.
- Clinical and histologic differentiation from SCC can be difficult and is not always predictive.
- System(s) affected: Skin

EPIDEMIOLOGY

- Greatest incidence during seventh decade of life with few cases below 20 years of age
- Presentation increased during summer and early fall seasons
- More frequent in males to females, 2:1
- More common in Caucasians

RISK FACTORS

- Sunlight exposure and fair skin
- Chemical carcinogens, including pitch, tar, and smoking
- Trauma with development after 1 month
- Tattoos
- Immunocompromised state
- Discoid lupus erythematosus

Genetics

- Multiple gene mutations, including p53
- Ferguson-Smith (AD)
- Gzybowski (sporadic)
- Witten-Zak (AD)
- Muir-Torre (AD)
- Incontinentia pigmenti (XLD)
- Xeroderma pigmentosum (AR)

GENERAL PREVENTION

Sun protection

PATHOPHYSIOLOGY

- Hair follicle histogenesis and keratinocyte proliferation, with or without inflammation
- Regression may be due to immune cytotoxicity or terminal differentiation of keratinocytes.

ETIOLOGY

Unclear, but multiple etiologies have been suggested, including trauma, UV damage, chemical carcinogen exposure, viral infections such as HPV or Merkel cell polyomavirus, immunosuppression, and a genetic predisposition.

COMMONLY ASSOCIATED CONDITIONS

- Commonly associated with lesions induced by sun damage, including solar lentigines, solar elastosis, actinic keratoses, and other skin cancers
- Less commonly with nevus sebaceous and inflammatory disorders
- If part of Muir-Torre syndrome, may see sebaceous neoplasms and malignancy involving the genitourinary and GI systems

DIAGNOSIS

HISTORY

- Asymptomatic with occasional tenderness
- Classic solitary lesion grows rapidly, up to 2.5 cm within several weeks.
- Remains stable in its mature state for several weeks, and may regress. However, may also behave as an aggressive SCC.
- If multiple lesions are present, family history is important to elicit.

PHYSICAL EXAM

- Firm, pink or skin-colored, dome-shaped papule or nodule with smooth, shiny surface and a central crater keratin plug and telangiectasia may be present at borders (1)
- Most commonly occurs as a solitary lesion but can also occur in multiples, with or without eruptive characteristics, or may enlarge up to 30 cm as a keratoacanthoma centrifugum marginatum
- Frequently distributed on sun-exposed areas, such as the face, neck, dorsum of upper extremities, and the posterior legs
- Less frequently on buttocks, thighs, penis, ears, scalp, mucosal surfaces, and subungually
- Subungual lesions are usually on the first 3 digits, are painful, and can be associated with incontinentia pigmenti.

DIAGNOSTIC TESTS & INTERPRETATION

- Shave biopsy may be insufficiently deep to distinguish keratoacanthomas (KA) from a more malignant form of SCC.
- Excisional biopsy is necessary to confirm diagnosis, although many believe that it is not possible to completely and reliably differentiate SCC from KA.

Imaging

- Not necessary, but radiograph of digit in subungual keratoacanthoma usually shows crescent-shaped radiolucent defect due to osteolysis
- Aggressive tumors may need CT with contrast for evaluation of lymph nodes and MRI if there is concern over perineural invasion.

Pathological Findings

- Well-differentiated squamous epithelium with glassy eosinophilic cytoplasm surrounding a well-demarcated central core of keratin (2)
- Entrapped elastic fibers within the squamous epithelium are common.
- May see lymphocytes, eosinophils, and intratumoral neutrophilic abscesses
- Differentiated from SCCs by epithelial lip and well-demarcated tumor and stroma outline without the presence of ulceration, mitosis, and pleomorphism
- Resolving keratoacanthoma shows flattening and fibrosis at base of lesion.

DIFFERENTIAL DIAGNOSIS

- SCC
- Cutaneous horn
- Merkel cell carcinoma
- Metastasis to the skin
- Molluscum contagiosum
- Prurigo nodularis
- Verruca vulgaris
- Verrucous carcinoma
- Hypertrophic actinic keratosis
- Sebaceous adenoma
- Hypertrophic lichen planus
- Hypertrophic lupus erythematosus
- Deep fungal infection
- Atypical mycobacterial infection

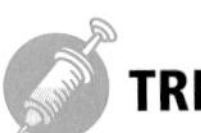

TREATMENT

Medical treatment should be attempted for up to 4 weeks and stopped if lesions show no signs of involution (3).

MEDICATION

- Only used for cases in which surgical intervention is not feasible or desirable, such as those with lesions not amenable to surgery due to number, size, location, or patient's cormorbidites
- Limited data are available for the best initial medical treatment and are listed below in no particular order:
  - Intralesional methotrexate 0.4–1.5 mg (12.5 or 25 mg/mL) $\times 2$ injections
  - Imiquimod cream 5% every 2 days
  - Topical 5-fluorouracil cream 5% daily
  - Intralesional 5-fluorouracil 0.2–0.5 of 50 mg/mL 2–5 doses weekly in proliferative growth phase
  - IFNα2b for actinic or HPV-related lesions
- If lesions are recurrent or multiple, consider isotretinoin 1.5 mg/kg daily.

ADDITIONAL TREATMENT

Radiotherapy, primary or adjuvant: These tumors may regress with low doses of radiation and may require doses up to 40–50 GY in 10–20 fractions in treating for possible SCC.

Issues for Referral

Refer to a dermatologist if suspected lesions are >2 cm, numerous, mucosal, or subungual.

SURGERY/OTHER PROCEDURES

Keratoacanthoma has been highly debated as a squamous cell variant, which despite spontaneous regression, requires treatment as an SCC. Treatment is primarily surgical for a solitary keratoacanthoma, creating 3–5-mm margins:

- Excision is the standard. If small (<2 cm) and at a low-risk site (e.g., trunk, extremities), curettage with or without electrodessication
- Cryosurgery for small solitary or multiple lesions when surgery is less practical
- Mohs micrographic surgery if >2 cm, recurrent, perineural, or persistent in areas of high recurrence or requiring tissue conservation such as the face, digits, or genitalia

ONGOING CARE

FOLLOW-UP RECOMMENDATIONS

1-month follow-up to assess resolution, with follow-up every 6 months after

Patient Monitoring

Self skin exams with detailed instructions by:

- The Skin Cancer Foundation: www.skincancer.org/Self-Examination>
- The American Academy of Dermatology: www.aad.org/skin-conditions/skin-cancer-detection/about-skin-self-exams

PATIENT EDUCATION

- Sun protection measures ,including sun block with SPF >15, wide-brimmed hats, long sleeves, dark clothing, while avoiding tanning salons
- Trauma can induce KA, and patient should avoid procedures such as body peels, carbon dioxide laser resurfacing, megavoltage radiation therapy, and cryotherapy.
- Avoid tar, pitch, and smoking.

PROGNOSIS

- Atrophic scarring may occur with intervention, but is significantly reduced.
- Very few cases of invasion and metastasis
- 4–8% recurrence
- Mucosal and subungual lesions do not regress.
- If multiple KAs present in patient or family members, evaluate for Muir-Torre syndrome and obtain a colonoscopy beginning at age 25, as well as testing for genitourinary cancer.

REFERENCES

1. Cribier B, Asch PH, Grosshans E. Differentiating squamous cell carcinoma from keratoacanthoma using histopathological criteria: Is it possible? A study of 296 cases. *Dermatology.* 1999;199: 208–12.
2. Schwartz RA. Keratoacanthoma: A clinico-pathologic enigma. *Dermatol Surg.* 2004;30: 326–33.
3. Ko CJ. Keratoacanthoma: Facts and controversies. *Clin Dermatol.* 2010;28:254–61.

ADDITIONAL READING

Schwartz RA. Keratoacanthoma. *J Am Acad Dermatol.* 1994;30:1–19.

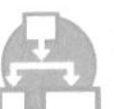

See Also (Topic, Algorithm, Electronic Media Element)

Cutaneous Squamous Cell Carcinoma

CODES

ICD9

238.2 Neoplasm of uncertain behavior of skin

CLINICAL PEARLS

- Suspect KA if there is a rapidly growing nodular lesion with a hyperkeratotic core.
- Excision of suspected lesion is necessary to differentiate from SCC and treatment in most cases.
- Consider KA in subungual lesions if it is painful and does not regress.
- May behave aggressively and cannot be reliably separated from SCC

KERATOSIS, ACTINIC

Zoltan Trizna, MD, PhD

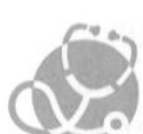

BASICS

DESCRIPTION

- Common, usually multiple, premalignant lesions of sun-exposed areas of the skin
- Common consequence of excessive cumulative ultraviolet (UV) light exposure
- Synonym(s): Solar keratosis

Geriatric Considerations

Frequent problem

Pediatric Considerations

Rare (if child, look for freckling and other stigmata of xeroderma pigmentosum)

EPIDEMIOLOGY

Incidence

- Incidence: Between 12.6% and 43.4% per year
- Rates vary with age group and exposure to sun.
- Predominant age: ≥40 years; progressively increases with age
- Predominant sex: Male > Female
- Common in those with blonde and red hair; rare in darker skin types

Prevalence

- Age-adjusted prevalence rate for actinic keratoses (AKs) in US Caucasians is 6.5%.
- For 65–74-year-old males with high sun exposure: It is 55.4%, and for those with low sun exposure, it is 18.5%.

RISK FACTORS

- Exposure to UV light (especially long-term and/or repeated exposure due to outdoor occupation or recreational activities, indoor or outdoor tanning)
- Skin type: Burns easily, does not tan
- Immunosuppression, especially organ transplantation

Genetics

The *p53* chromosomal mutation has been shown consistently in both AKs and squamous cell carcinomas (SCCs). Many new genes have been shown recently to have similar expression profiles in AKs and SCCs.

GENERAL PREVENTION

Sun avoidance and protective techniques are helpful.

PATHOPHYSIOLOGY

The epidermal lesions are characterized by atypical keratinocytes at the basal layer with occasional extension upward. Mitoses are present. The histopathologic features resemble those of SCC in situ or SCC, and the distinction depends on the extent of epidermal involvement.

ETIOLOGY

Cumulative UV exposure

COMMONLY ASSOCIATED CONDITIONS

- SCC
- Other features of chronic solar damage: Lentigines, elastosis, and telangiectasias

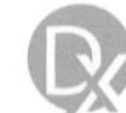

DIAGNOSIS

HISTORY

- The lesions are frequently asymptomatic; symptoms may include pruritus, burning, and mild hyperesthesia.
- Lesions may enlarge, thicken, or become more scaly. They also may regress or remain unchanged.
- Most lesions occur on the sun-exposed areas (head and neck, hands, forearms).

PHYSICAL EXAM

- Usually small (<1 cm), often multiple red, pink, or brown macules, papules, or plaques that are rough to palpation
- Yellow or brown adherent scale is often present on top of the lesion.
- Several clinical variants exist:
  - Atrophic: Dry, scaly macules with indistinct borders and an erythematous base
  - Hypertrophic: Overlying hyperkeratosis (in an extreme form: Cutaneous horn) may be impossible to differentiate from SCC clinically.
  - Pigmented: Smooth tan/brown plaque, spreading centrifugally
  - Bowenoid: Red scaly plaques with distinct borders
  - Actinic cheilitis: Inflammatory lesion involving usually the lower lip

DIAGNOSTIC TESTS & INTERPRETATION

Diagnostic Procedures/Surgery

- The diagnosis is usually made clinically, except where there is a suspicion of carcinoma.
- Skin biopsy is especially recommended if large, ulcerated, indurated, or bleeding; or if the lesions are nonresponsive to treatment.

Pathological Findings

- Dysplastic keratinocytes in lower levels of epidermis with a dermal lymphocytic infiltrate
- Neoplastic cells, mostly found in the lower epidermal layers, are cytologically identical to those of SCCs.
- If neoplastic cells extend throughout entire epidermis or into the dermis, the lesions will qualify as an SCC in situ or invasive SCC, respectively.
- Malignant cells are sparse except in the bowenoid variety.
- Hypertrophic, atrophic, bowenoid, acantholytic, and pigmented varieties show the corresponding epidermal findings.

DIFFERENTIAL DIAGNOSIS

- SCC (hypertrophic type)
- Keratoacanthoma
- Bowen disease
- Basal cell carcinoma
- Verruca vulgaris
- Less likely: Verrucous nevi, warty dyskeratoma, lichenoid keratoses, seborrheic keratoses, porokeratoses, seborrheic dermatitis or psoriasis (near hairline), lentigo maligna, solar lentigo, discoid lupus erythematosus

TREATMENT

First-line treatment is cryotherapy (technically, this is considered surgery, especially by insurance companies) (1,2)[A].

MEDICATION

First Line

- Topical treatments target both visible and subclinical lesions.

- Topical fluorouracil (Efudex, Carac, Fluoroplex cream, Fluoroplex solution):
  - Every day–b.i.d. for 3–6 weeks, depending on the brand, concentration, and formulation
  - Can be very irritating
- Topical imiquimod (Aldara) 5% cream:
  - Apply every day, 2 days per week, for up to 4 months to an area not larger than the forehead or 1 cheek.
  - Can be irritating
- Topical imiquimod (Zyclara) 3.75% cream:
  - Apply once a day for 2 weeks, followed by no treatment for the next 2 weeks; then apply once a day for another 2 weeks.
  - Can be irritating
- 3% diclofenac (Solaraze) gel:
  - b.i.d. for up to 3 months

Second Line

- Topical tretinoin (Retin-A) or tazarotene (Tazorac): May be used to enhance the efficacy of topical fluorouracil
- Systemic retinoids: Used infrequently

ADDITIONAL TREATMENT

General Measures

- Sun-protective techniques
- Sunscreens and physical sun protection recommended

Additional Therapies

Close monitoring with no treatment is an appropriate option for mild lesions.

SURGERY/OTHER PROCEDURES

- Cryosurgery ("freezing," liquid nitrogen):
  - Most common method
  - Cure rate: 75–98.8%
  - May leave scars
  - May be superior to photodynamic therapy for thicker lesions
- Photodynamic therapy with a photosensitizer (e.g., aminolevulinic acid) and "blue light":
  - May clear >90% of AKs
  - Less scarring than cryotherapy
  - May be superior to cryotherapy, especially in the case of more extensive skin involvement
- Curettage and electrocautery (ED&C, "scraping and burning")
- Medium-depth peels, especially for the treatment of extensive areas
- CO_2 laser therapy
- Dermabrasion
- Surgical excision (excisional biopsy)

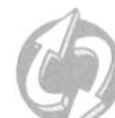

ONGOING CARE

FOLLOW-UP RECOMMENDATIONS

Patient Monitoring

Depends on associated malignancy and frequency with which new AKs appear

PATIENT EDUCATION

- Teach sun-protective techniques:
  - Limit outdoor activities between 10 a.m. and 4 p.m.
  - Wear protective clothing and wide-brimmed hat.
  - Proper use (including reapplication) of sunscreens with SPF >30, preferably a preparation with broad-spectrum (UV-A and UV-B) protection
- Teach self-examination of skin (melanoma, squamous cell, basal cell).
- Patient education materials:
  - http://dermnetnz.org/lesions/solar-keratoses.html
  - www.skincarephysicians.com/actinickeratosesnet/index.html
  - www.skincancer.org/Actinic-Keratosis-and-Other-Precancers.htm

PROGNOSIS

Very good. A significant proportion of the lesions may resolve spontaneously (3).

COMPLICATIONS

- AKs are premalignant lesions that may progress to SCCs. The rate of malignant transformation is unclear; the reported percentages vary (3).
- Patients with AKs are at increased risk for other cutaneous malignancies.

REFERENCES

1. Helfand M, Gorman AK, Mahon S, et al. AHRQ evidence report from OHSU Evidence-Based Practice Center. 2001.
2. de Berker D, McGregor JM, Hughes BR, et al. Guidelines for the management of actinic keratoses. *Br J Dermatol*. 2007;156:222–30.
3. Criscione VD, Weinstock MA, Naylor MF, et al. Actinic keratoses: Natural history and risk of malignant transformation in the Veterans Affairs Topical Tretinoin Chemoprevention Trial. *Cancer*. 2009;115:2523–30.

ADDITIONAL READING

- Kanellou P, Zaravinos A, Zioga M, et al. Genomic instability, mutations and expression analysis of the tumour suppressor genes p14(ARF), p15(INK4b), p16(INK4a) and p53 in actinic keratosis. *Cancer Lett*. 2008;264:145–61.
- Rossi R, Mori M, Lotti T. Actinic keratosis. *Int J Dermatol*. 2007;46:895–904.

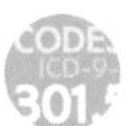

CODES

ICD9

702.0 Actinic keratosis

CLINICAL PEARLS

- AKs are premalignant lesions.
- Often more easily felt than seen
- Therapy-resistant lesions should be biopsied, especially on the face.

KERATOSIS, PILARIS

Zoltan Trizna, MD, PhD

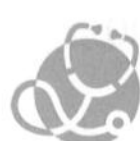

BASICS

- Keratosis pilaris (KP) is a benign skin disorder resulting in a process of hyperkeratinization of the hair follicles.
- Generally asymptomatic, often improving with age

DESCRIPTION

Small (1–2 mm) keratotic papules are localized to hair follicles, most frequently on the lateral aspects of the arms and thighs. Often described as chicken skin or goose bumps.

EPIDEMIOLOGY

There is a slight female predominance.

Prevalence

KP affects up to 80% of adolescents, often worsening during puberty, and up to 40% of adults.

RISK FACTORS

Genetics

Autosomal dominant inheritance with variable penetrance has been described, and many (30–50%) will report a positive family history of the disorder.

GENERAL PREVENTION

Moisturize to prevent excessive drying of the skin. Use only mild soaps (cleansers). Avoid hot showers.

PATHOPHYSIOLOGY

The abrasive ("sandpaper-like", "chicken-skin," or "goosebump-like") texture of the skin is caused by excess buildup of keratin. An underlying hair may be found in some of the papules. In the inflammatory variant, mild perifollicular erythema is present.

ETIOLOGY

Autosomal-dominant inheritance with variable penetrance

COMMONLY ASSOCIATED CONDITIONS

Ichthyosis, xerosis, atopic dermatitis

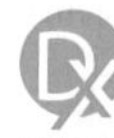

DIAGNOSIS

HISTORY

- Patients often complain about a "rough" skin, sometimes with pruritus (which indicates inflammation).
- Most patients are asymptomatic, but they worry about their cosmetic appearance.
- Family history is positive in up to 50% of cases.

PHYSICAL EXAM

- Firm, minimally rough, 1–2-mm, follicle-based papules, some with perilesional erythema. The distribution is frequently symmetrical.
- Most common on the lateral-proximal aspects of the arms and thighs; less common on the cheeks and gluteal areas

DIAGNOSTIC TESTS & INTERPRETATION
The diagnosis is visual.

Diagnostic Procedures/Surgery
Skin biopsy if diagnosis in doubt

Pathological Findings
Hyperkeratosis, hypergranulosis, and follicular plugging are typical. A mild superficial perivascular inflammatory infiltrate may be noted.

DIFFERENTIAL DIAGNOSIS
- Acne
- Folliculitis
- Rare dermatologic conditions (e.g., keratosis follicularis, lichen spinulosus, lichen nitidus, perforating folliculitis)

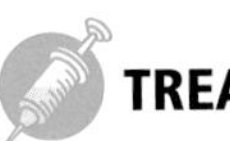

TREATMENT

Daily measures to prevent dry skin, such as using mild cleansers, along with moisturizers, are the mainstay of treatment.

MEDICATION
First Line
- Lactic acid 12% creams or lotions (e.g., ammonium lactate: AmLactin, LacHydrin)
- Urea (in 40–50% topical preparations).

Second Line
Emollient-based topical steroids (e.g., Cloderm, Locoid Lipocream)

ADDITIONAL TREATMENT
General Measures
Moisturize. Use emollients.

Additional Therapies
- Topical retinoids: Tretinoin (Retin-A), adapalene (Differin), tazarotene (Tazorac)
- Tacrolimus (Protopic) ointment

SURGERY/OTHER PROCEDURES
Microdermabrasion, laser (Nd:YAG, pulsed dye)

ONGOING CARE

PROGNOSIS
Most cases improve with age.

COMPLICATIONS
Hair loss is rare. If the lateral eyebrows are involved, consider the diagnosis of KP atrophicans faciei (ulerythema ophryogenes).

ADDITIONAL READING

Hwang S, Schwartz RA, et al. Keratosis pilaris: A common follicular hyperkeratosis. *Cutis*. 2008;82: 177–80.

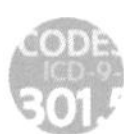

CODES

ICD9
701.1 Keratoderma, acquired

CLINICAL PEARLS

- KP is frequently mistaken for acne.
- Patients often self-manage with over-the-counter acne treatment products or medications originally prescribed for their facial acne.
- Daily measures to prevent dry skin, such as using mild cleansers, along with moisturizers, are the mainstay of treatment.

K

KLINEFELTER SYNDROME

Kimberly Bombaci, MD
Robert A. Baldor, MD

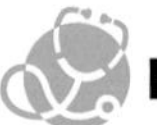

BASICS

DESCRIPTION

- A common genetic abnormality that presents in males who have ≥1 additional X chromosomes (47,XXY). Presentation is highly variable; many patients do not have the "textbook" features.
- A common cause of primary hypogonadism and infertility in males.
- Usually undiagnosed before puberty and many present in adulthood with infertility.
- Klinefelter syndrome has been associated with both increased morbidity and mortality believed to be related to genetic, hormonal, and socioeconomic factors (1).

EPIDEMIOLOGY

Prevalence

- ~1 in 600 males
- Significantly underdiagnosed:
  - Only 25% diagnosed in their lifetime
  - Only 4–10% diagnosed before puberty
  - Accounts for 3% of male infertility

RISK FACTORS

Risk increases with maternal age.

Genetics

- Mutations are spontaneous and patients have no family history.
- It is usually a result of maternal meiotic nondisjunction.

PATHOPHYSIOLOGY

- Primary hypogonadism with variable Leydig cell function
- Low or low-normal testosterone
- High or high-normal gonadotropins (LH and FSH)
- Unclear whether many aspects of syndrome are caused by hormonal abnormalities or extra X chromosome

ETIOLOGY

- ~90% have the XXY karyotype, which is caused by meiotic nondisjunction of the X chromosome during gametogenesis.
- ~10% have a mosaic karyotype, caused by nondisjunction of the X chromosome during early mitosis of the zygote.

Pregnancy Considerations

- Prenatal diagnosis is possible by karyotyping cells obtained from amniocentesis.
- Parents should be counseled about the highly variable phenotypic range of Klinefelter syndrome and the risks associated with amniocentesis.

COMMONLY ASSOCIATED CONDITIONS

- Azoospermia and infertility (>99%)
- Gynecomastia
- Developmental abnormalities:
  - Learning difficulties, especially with language development
  - Gross motor delay
  - Autism spectrum behavior
- Psychiatric illness:
  - ADHD
  - Problems with regulation of emotion and behavior
  - Psychotic disorder
- Cardiovascular disorders:
  - Thromboembolic disease
  - Recurrent leg ulcers owing to venous insufficiency and postthrombotic syndrome
  - Mitral and aortic valve disease
- Metabolic disorders:
  - Osteoporosis
  - Metabolic syndrome and diabetes
- Essential tremor
- Taurodontism (enlargement of the pulp and thinning of the surface of the teeth)
- Autoimmune diseases (uncommon)
- Malignancies (rare):
  - Breast cancer
  - Mediastinal germ cell tumors

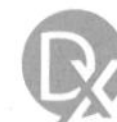

DIAGNOSIS

HISTORY

- Fertility history (infertility nearly universal)
- Learning disabilities, poor school performance
- Psychosocial problems and psychiatric illness
- Cardiovascular disease and risk factors
- Reproductive goals

PHYSICAL EXAM

- Small, firm testes (3–8 mL) (95%)
- Sparse facial and body hair (88%), female pubic hair distribution (53%)
- Gynecomastia (27%)
- Tall, long legs, narrow shoulders, broad arm span, and abdominal adiposity
- Poor muscle tone (76%) and increased fat:muscle ratio
- Specific mild dysmorphic features (2):
  - Clinodactyly (74%)
  - Hypertelorism (69%)
  - Mild elbow dysplasia (36%)
  - High arched palate (37%)

Pediatric Considerations

- Infants:
  - No pathognomonic features
  - Increased incidence of congenital abnormalities of all types, undescended testes, and micropenis
- Children:
  - Tall
  - Increased BMI (on average) (2) and increased fat:muscle ratio
  - Poor muscle tone
  - Small penis and testicles
  - Specific mild dysmorphic features (see above)

DIAGNOSTIC TESTS & INTERPRETATION

Lab

Initial lab tests

- Chromosomal analysis:
  - Gold standard: Cytogenetic analysis (karyotype)
  - Alternative: Barr body analysis (if diagnosis suspected, PPV = 0.86, NPV = 0.94) (3)
  - Rapid polymerase chain reaction technique looking at the copy number of the androgen receptor (AR) gene (located to Xq11.2–q12) has been described as a screen for Klinefelter syndrome and other X-chromosome aneuploidies (4).
- Hormonal testing (neither sensitive nor specific; become more pronounced at puberty):
  - Blood testosterone levels are low.
  - Blood FSH and LH levels are elevated.
  - Urinary gonadotropin levels are increased.

Follow-Up & Special Considerations

- Semen analysis (if indicated): Azoospermia
- Consider diabetes evaluation.
- Consider hypercoagulability screening.

Imaging

Follow-Up & Special Considerations

- Consider bone density screening.
- Consider echocardiogram to evaluate for valve disease.
- Consider dental radiographs for diagnosis of taurodontism.

Pathological Findings

- XXY karyotype (or variation)
- Testicular biopsy in an adult demonstrates hyalinization of the seminiferous tubules and hyperplasia of Leydig cells.

DIFFERENTIAL DIAGNOSIS

- Secondary hypogonadism (low FSH and LH)
- Acquired primary hypogonadism (exposure to toxins, specific medications, radiation, mumps, or chronic disease)
- XYY karyotype (normal testicles and hormone levels, usually fertile)
- 46,XY/XO karyotype (features of Turner syndrome)
- Congenital anorchia (severe hypogonadism)
- Myotonic dystrophy (muscle weakness and pain, family history)
- Idiopathic hypogonadism

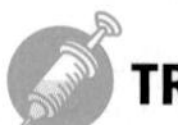

TREATMENT

MEDICATION

First Line

Testosterone therapy:

- Benefits:
  - Increases body hair and penis length and improves libido
  - Improves bone density (5)[C]
  - May reduce gynecomastia and abdominal adiposity and increase muscle mass (5)[C] (not replicated in all studies)
  - May improve mood, energy level, cognition, and social functioning and decrease aggression (5)[B]
  - May lower serum total cholesterol (5) and improve metabolic syndrome (6)[C]
  - May possibly reduce hypercoagulability (7), improve autoimmune disease (8)[C]

- Risks and side effects:
  - Erythrocytosis
  - Acne
  - Lowering of HDL
  - Worsening of aggression
  - Peliosis hepatitis, hepatic adenomas, and hepatocellular carcinoma
  - Worsening of subclinical prostate cancer
  - May accelerate infertility in adolescents and young men; cryopreservation of existing sperm should be considered before starting therapy.
- Contraindications:
  - Prostate cancer
  - Liver disease
- Dosage and administration:
  - Oral: Initial: 60–80 mg b.i.d.; maintenance: 20–60 mg b.i.d. (not available in the US)
  - Buccal: 30 mg b.i.d.
  - Transdermal patch: 2.5–7.5 mg/d
  - Transdermal gel: 5 g/d
  - IM injection: 50–400 mg every 2–4 weeks
  - SC pellets: 150–450 mg every 3–6 months
  - Titrate to symptoms and to maintain testosterone levels in middle of normal range. Normalization of gonadotropins may not be possible.
- Monitoring:
  - Monthly during initial therapy, less frequently when dosage stabilized: CBC, liver enzymes, testosterone, FSH, LH, PSA (if appropriate)
  - Serial prostate exams in older men
  - Consider annual or semiannual lipid panel.
  - Aggression and irritability levels

Pediatric Considerations

- Testosterone therapy, beginning at age 11–13, recommended by experts (9)[C]; consider semen cryopreservation before starting therapy.
- In addition to parameters listed above, monitor bone age.
- Micropenis in infants and children has been treated with topical or IM testosterone (9)[C].
- Consider pediatric endocrinology consultation.

ADDITIONAL TREATMENT

General Measures

- Preventive dental care
- Calcium and vitamin D supplementation
- Breast self-exams

Issues for Referral

- Adolescents and young men wishing to preserve fertility should be referred for cryopreservation of existing sperm if sperm are present on semen analysis.
- Fertility treatment may be offered using testicular fine-needle aspiration (TEFNA) or testicular sperm extraction (TESE) followed by in vitro fertilization. Embryos are at a modestly increased risk of cytogenetic abnormalities, but most of the resulting pregnancies are healthy.

Additional Therapies

Individual or family counseling, if indicated

Pediatric Considerations

- Infertility progresses rapidly during adolescence and early adulthood; therefore, adolescents should be referred for cryopreservation of sperm.
- Consider referrals for speech therapy, occupational therapy, physical therapy, and educational support.

SURGERY/OTHER PROCEDURES

Mastectomy can be performed to correct gynecomastia, which can be a cause of psychological strain and increase the risk of breast cancer.

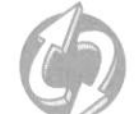

ONGOING CARE

FOLLOW-UP RECOMMENDATIONS

If patient is treated with testosterone, consider semiannual visits when the dosage is stabilized: Review interval history, symptoms, side effects, and therapy risks–benefits.

Patient Monitoring

- Annual diabetes screening
- Annual clinical breast exam
- Periodic bone density testing

PATIENT EDUCATION

- Presentation is variable, with most patients appearing physically normal.
- Patients are likely infertile, but there are options for reproductive therapy.
- There is high incidence of learning disabilities and psychiatric illness. Appropriate therapy should be utilized.
- Risk of diabetes and importance of regular screening and maintaining a healthy weight
- Risk of osteoporosis and importance of calcium, vitamin D, and weight-bearing exercise
- Regular dental care
- American Association for Klinefelter Syndrome Information and Support, www.aaksis.org
- Klinefelter Syndrome Support Group, http://klinefeltersyndrome.org

PROGNOSIS

- Infertility is nearly universal.
- Physical findings are generally subtle.
- Behavioral characteristics are highly variable.
- On average, adults have modestly reduced intelligence, verbal reasoning, language skills, and motor dexterity.
- Increased number of X chromosomes is correlated with increased phenotypic severity.

Pediatric Considerations

- Developmental and behavioral problems are common:
  - 77% of children have difficulty learning to read.
  - 42% of children have delayed speech.
  - Motor delay
  - Difficulty with social interaction (autism-like behavior)
  - Sensory avoidance, gaze avoidance, and a passive demeanor
- Children are at risk of poor school performance and school failure.
- Children are more likely to require psychiatric care.

REFERENCES

1. Bojesen A, Gravholt CH, et al. Morbidity and mortality in Klinefelter syndrome (47,XXY). *Acta Paediatr*. 2011;100:807–13.
2. Zeger MP, Zinn AR, Lahlou N, et al. Effect of ascertainment and genetic features on the phenotype of Klinefelter syndrome. *J Pediatr*. 2008;152:716–22.
3. Kamischke A, Baumgardt A, Horst J, et al. Clinical and diagnostic features of patients with suspected Klinefelter syndrome. *J Androl*. 2003;24:41–8.
4. Ottesen AM, Garn ID, Aksglaede L, et al. A simple screening method for detection of Klinefelter syndrome and other X-chromosome aneuploidies based on copy number of the androgen receptor gene. *Mol Hum Reprod*. 2007;13:745–50.
5. Wang C, et al. Long-term testosterone gel (AndroGel) treatment maintains beneficial effects on sexual function and mood, lean and fat mass, and bone mineral density in hypogonadal men. *J Clin Endo Metab*. 2004;85(9):2085–98.
6. Spark RF. Testosterone, diabetes mellitus, and the metabolic syndrome. *Curr Urol Rep*. 2007;8: 467–71.
7. Zitzmann M, Junker R, Kamischke A, et al. Contraceptive steroids influence the hemostatic activation state in healthy men. *J Androl*. 2002;23: 503–11.
8. Koçar IH, Yesilova Z, Ozata M, et al. The effect of testosterone replacement treatment on immunological features of patients with Klinefelter's syndrome. *Clin Exp Immunol*. 2000;121:448–52.
9. Bojesen A, et al. Klinefelter syndrome in clinical practice. *Nat Clin Prac*. 2007;4(4):192–201.

ADDITIONAL READING

- Bruining H, Swaab H, Kas M, et al. Psychiatric characteristics in a self-selected sample of boys with Klinefelter syndrome. *Pediatrics*. 2009;123: e865–70.
- Wattendorf DJ, Muenke M. Klinefelter syndrome. *Am Fam Physician*. 2005;72:2259–62.

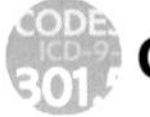

CODES

ICD9

758.7 Klinefelter's syndrome

CLINICAL PEARLS

- Klinefelter syndrome males have ≥1 additional X chromosome (XXY karyotype).
- Most men do not have the "textbook" features.
- Accounts for 3% of male infertility
- Frequently undiagnosed until adulthood
- Testosterone therapy, beginning in adolescence, has many benefits.

K

KNEE PAIN

Jennifer Schwartz, MD
J. Herbert Stevenson, MD

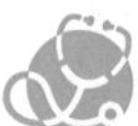

BASICS

DESCRIPTION

Knee pain is a common complaint in the outpatient setting. Onset may be acute or chronic, or it may present as an acute exacerbation of a chronic condition. Trauma, overuse, and degenerative conditions are frequent causes. Acuity of onset, patient age, pain location, associated symptoms, and mechanism of injury can help narrow the differential diagnosis.

EPIDEMIOLOGY

Incidence

- Knee pain accounts for 1.9 million primary care visits annually.
- The incidence of knee osteoarthritis is 240 cases per 100,000 person years (1).

Prevalence

- The knee is the most common site of lower extremity injury among runners (2). Patellofemoral syndrome is one of the most common diagnoses.
- Osteoarthritis is one of the leading causes of disability in the US.

RISK FACTORS

- Obesity
- Malalignment
- Poor flexibility, muscle imbalance or weakness
- Rapid increases in training volume and intensity
- Improper footwear, training surfaces, technique
- Activities involving cutting, jumping, deceleration
- Previous injuries

GENERAL PREVENTION

- Maintain normal body mass index; weight loss if obese.
- Use sound exercise training principles.
- Correct strength and flexibility imbalances.

ETIOLOGY

- Trauma (ligament or meniscal injury, fracture, dislocation)
- Overuse (tendinopathy, apophysitis)
- Age related (arthritis, degenerative conditions)
- Rheumatologic (rheumatoid arthritis [RA], gout, pseudogout)
- Infectious (bacterial, postviral, Lyme)
- Referred pain (hip, back)

COMMONLY ASSOCIATED CONDITIONS

- Fracture, contusion
- Effusion, hemarthrosis
- Patellar dislocation/subluxation
- Meniscal injury
- Ligamentous injury
- Tendinopathy
- Bursitis
- Osteochondral injury
- Arthritis
- Septic joint
- Muscle strain

DIAGNOSIS

HISTORY

- Pain:
  - Diffuse pain: Osteoarthritis, patellofemoral pain syndrome/chondromalacia
  - Pain ascending/descending stairs: Meniscal injury, patellofemoral pain syndrome/chondromalacia
  - Pain with prolonged sitting, standing from sitting: Patellofemoral pain syndrome/chondromalacia
- Mechanism of injury:
  - Hyperextension, deceleration, cutting: Anterior cruciate ligament (ACL) injury
  - Hyperflexion, fall on flexed knee, "dashboard injury": Posterior cruciate ligament (PCL) injury
  - Lateral force (valgus load): Medial collateral injury
  - Twisting on planted foot: Meniscal injury
- Effusion:
  - Rapid onset (2 hours): ACL tear, patellar subluxation, tibial plateau fracture. Hemarthrosis is common.
  - Slower onset (24–36 hours), smaller: Meniscal injury, ligament sprain
  - Swelling behind the knee: Popliteal cyst; prepatellar: Bursitis

PHYSICAL EXAM

- Observe for antalgic gait, patellar tracking abnormalities.
- Inspect for malalignment, atrophy, swelling.
- Palpate for effusion, warmth, tenderness.
- Evaluate active/passive range of motion (ROM) and flexibility.
- Evaluate strength, muscle tone.
- Pay attention to: Joint instability, locking, catching

DIAGNOSTIC TESTS & INTERPRETATION

- Patellar apprehension test: Patellar instability. Patellar grind test: Patellar dysfunction.
- Lachman, anterior drawer test: ACL integrity. Lachman is more sensitive and specific.
- Posterior drawer, posterior sag sign: PCL integrity
- Valgus/varus stress test: Medial/lateral collateral ligament (MCL/LCL) integrity
- McMurray test: Meniscal injury
- Ober test: Iliotibial band (ITB) tightness

Lab

- Suspected septic joint, gout, pseudogout:
  - Arthrocentesis with cell count, Gram stain, culture, protein/glucose, synovial fluid analysis
- Suspected rheumatoid arthritis:
  - CBC, ESR, rheumatoid factor. Consider Lyme titer.

Imaging

- Radiographs may be needed to rule out fracture in patients with acute knee trauma per the Ottawa rules:
  - Age >55 years *or*
  - Tenderness at the patella or fibular head *or*
  - Inability to bear weight 4 steps *or*
  - Inability to flex knee to 90°
- Radiographs may help in diagnosing osteoarthritis, osteochondral lesions, patellofemoral pain syndrome:
  - Upright anteroposterior, lateral, merchant/sunrise, notch/tunnel, weightbearing views
- CT scan may be required if occult fracture is suspected.
- MRI is "gold standard" for imaging muscle, ligamentous, and intra-articular structures.

Diagnostic Procedures/Surgery

Arthroscopy may be beneficial in the diagnosis of certain conditions, including meniscal and ligamentous injuries.

DIFFERENTIAL DIAGNOSIS

- *Acute onset*: Fracture, contusion, cruciate or collateral ligament tear, patellar dislocation/subluxation. If systemic symptoms: Osteomyelitis, septic arthritis, gout, pseudogout, Lyme.
- *Insidious onset*: Patellofemoral pain syndrome/chondromalacia, iliotibial band syndrome, osteoarthritis, rheumatoid arthritis, bursitis, tumor, tendinopathy, loose body, bipartite patella, degenerative meniscal tear
- *Anterior pain*: Patellofemoral pain syndrome/chondromalacia, patellar injury, patellar tendinopathy, pre- or suprapatellar bursitis, tibial apophysitis, fat pad impingement, quadriceps tendinopathy, osteoarthritis
- *Posterior pain*: PCL injury, posterior horn meniscal injury, popliteal cyst/aneurysm, hamstring or gastrocnemius injury
- *Medial pain*: MCL injury, medial meniscal injury, pes anserine bursitis, medial plica syndrome, osteoarthritis
- *Lateral pain*: LCL injury, lateral meniscal injury, ITB syndrome, osteoarthritis

Geriatric Considerations

OA, degenerative meniscal tears, and gout are more common.

Pediatric Considerations

- 3 million pediatric sports injuries occur annually.
- Must be concerned about physeal/apophyseal and joint surface injuries in skeletally immature:
  - Acute: Patellar subluxation, avulsion fractures, ACL tear
  - Overuse: Patellofemoral pain syndrome, apophysitis, osteochondritis dissecans, patellar tendonitis, stress fracture
  - Other:
    - Neoplasm, juvenile rheumatoid arthritis, infection, referred pain from slipped capital femoral epiphysis

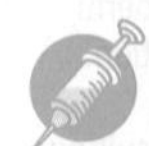

TREATMENT

MEDICATION

- Oral medications:
  - Acetaminophen: Up to 3–4 g/d. Safe and effective in osteoarthritis (1)[A].
  - NSAIDs:
    - Ibuprofen: 200–800 mg t.i.d.
    - Naproxen: 250–500 mg b.i.d.:
      - Useful for acute ligament sprains, muscle strains (3)[C]
      - Useful for short-term pain reduction in osteoarthritis. Long-term use not recommended due to side effects (1)[A].

- Not recommended for fracture, stress fracture, chronic muscle injury: May be associated with delayed healing; low dose and brief course only if necessary (3)[C].
  - Tramadol/narcotics: Not recommended as first-line treatment (1). Can be used with acute injuries.
- Topical medications:
  - Topical NSAIDs may provide pain relief in osteoarthritis and are more tolerable than orals (4)[C].
  - Topical capsaicin may be an adjunct for pain management in osteoarthritis (4)[C].
- Injections:
  - Intra-articular corticosteroid injection may provide short-term benefit in knee osteoarthritis (1,5)[A].
  - Viscosupplementation may improve pain and function in patients with osteoarthritis after other methods have been exhausted (1,6)[A].

ADDITIONAL TREATMENT

General Measures

Acute injury: PRICEMM therapy (*p*rotection, *r*elative rest, *i*ce, *c*ompression, *e*levation, *m*edications, *m*odalities)

Issues for Referral

- Acute trauma, young athletic patient
- Joint instability
- Lack of improvement with conservative measures
- Salter-Harris physeal fractures

Additional Therapies

- Physical therapy is recommended as initial treatment for patellofemoral pain syndrome (7)[A].
- Exercise, muscle strengthening improves outcome in osteoarthritis (1)[A].

COMPLEMENTARY AND ALTERNATIVE MEDICINE

May reduce pain and improve function in OA:

- Glucosamine sulfate (500 mg t.i.d.) (1,8)[B]
- Chondroitin (400 mg t.i.d.) (8)[B].
- S-adenosylmethionine (SAMe), ginger extract, methylsulfonylmethane: Less reliable improvement and evidence

SURGERY/OTHER PROCEDURES

- Surgery may be required for ligamentous and cartilaginous injuries.
- Chronic conditions refractory to conservative therapy may require surgical intervention.

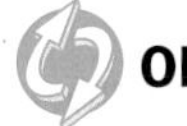

ONGOING CARE

FOLLOW-UP RECOMMENDATIONS

- Activity modification in overuse conditions
- Rehabilitative exercise in OA:
  - Low-impact exercise: Walking, swimming, cycling
  - Strength, ROM, and proprioceptive training

Patient Monitoring

- After initial treatment in acute injury, consider rehabilitation.
- In chronic and overuse conditions, assess functional status, rehabilitative exercise compliance, and pain control at follow-up visit.

DIET

Weight reduction for overweight patient with osteoarthritis

PATIENT EDUCATION

- Review activity modifications.
- Encourage the patient to play an active role in the rehabilitative process.
- Review risks and benefits of pharmaceutical interventions.

PROGNOSIS

Varies with diagnosis, severity of injury, chronicity of condition, patient motivation to participate in rehabilitative exercises, and whether surgical intervention is required.

COMPLICATIONS

- Disability
- Arthritis
- Chronic joint instability
- Deconditioning

REFERENCES

1. Bijlsma JW, Berenbaum F, Lafeber FP. Osteoarthritis: An update with relevance to clinical practice. *Lancet*. 2011;377(9783):2115–26.
2. van Gent RN, et al. Incidence and determinents of lower extremity running injuries in long distance runners: A systematic review. *Br J Sports Med*. 2007;41:469–80.
3. Ziltener JL, Leal S, Fournier PE. Non-steroidal anti-inflammatory drugs for athletes: An update. *Ann Phys Rehabil Med*. 2010;53(4):278–82.
4. Altman RD, Barthel HR. Topical therapies for osteoarthritis. *Drugs*. 2011;71(10):1259–79.
5. Bellamy N, Campbell J, Welch V, et al. Intraarticular corticosteroids for treatment of osteoarthritis of the knee. *Cochrane Database System Review*. 2011: CD005328.
6. Bellamy N, Campbell J, Welch V, et al. Viscosupplementation for the treatment of osteoarthritis of the knee. *Cochrane Database Sys Rev*. 2011;CD005321.
7. Bolgla LA, Boling MC. An update for the conservative management of patellofemoral pain syndrome: A systematic review. *Int J Sports Phys Ther*. 2011;6(2):112–25.
8. Vangsness CT Jr, Spiker W, Erickson J. A review of evidence based medicine for glucosamine and chondroitin sulfate use in knee osteoarthritis. *Arthroscopy*. 2009;25(1):86–94.

ADDITIONAL READING

- Caine D, DiFiori J, Maffulli N. Physeal injuries in children's and youth sports: Reasons for concern? *Br J Sports Med*. 2006;40:749–60.
- Calmbach WL, Hutchens M. Evaluation of patients presenting with knee pain: Part 1. *Am Fam Physician*. 2003;68(5):907–12.
- Debbi EM, Agar G, Fichman G, et al. Efficacy of a methylsulfonylmethane supplement on osteoarthritis of the knee- a randomized control trial. *BMC Complement Altern Med*. 2011;11(1):50.
- Fransen M, McConnell S. Exercise for osteoarthritis. *Cochrane Datatbase Syst Rev*. 2008:CD004376.
- Jackson JL, O'Malley PG, Kroenke K. Evaluation of acute knee pain in primary care. *Ann Intern Med*. 2003;129:575–88.
- Jalili M, Gharebaghi H. Validation of the Ottawa Knee Rules in Iran: A prospective study. *Emerg Med J*. 2010;27(11):849–51.
- Ringdahl E, Pandit S. Treatment of knee osteoarthritis. *Am Fam Physician*. 2011;83(11): 1287–92.
- Rutjes AWS, Neusch E, et al. S-adenosylmethionine for osteoarthritis of the knee or hip. *Cochrane Database Syst Rev*. 2010:CD007321.

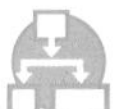

See Also (Topic, Algorithm, Electronic Media Element)

Algorithms: Knee Pain; Popliteal Mass

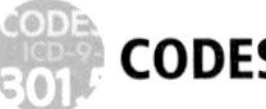

CODES

ICD9

- 715.36 Osteoarthrosis, localized, not specified whether primary or secondary, lower leg
- 715.96 Osteoarthrosis, unspecified whether generalized or localized, involving lower leg
- 719.46 Pain in joint, lower leg

CLINICAL PEARLS

- Knee pain is a common presentation for both acute and chronic injuries.
- Presence of an effusion in a patient younger than 30 years of age signifies a significant knee injury needing accurate/prompt diagnosis.
- Acute mechanism: Consider ligamentous injury, meniscal tear, fracture.
- Overuse mechanism: Consider osteoarthritis, patellofemoral pain syndrome, tendinopathy, bursitis, and stress fracture.
- Pediatric patient with knee pain: Consider possible physeal, apophyseal, or articular cartilage injuries. Don't forget referred pain from the hip/knee/back!

LABYRINTHITIS

Teresa V. Chan, MD

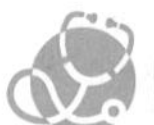

BASICS

DESCRIPTION

- Acute inflammation of the labyrinth (the organs of hearing and balance that comprise the bony inner ear). Infection (viral or bacterial) and subsequent inflammation of the inner ear is felt to be the most common etiology (see "Differential Diagnosis"). This typically presents with persistent room-spinning vertigo lasting for hours or days AND often sudden hearing loss in 1 ear.
- System(s) affected: Nervous; Special sensory (auditory and vestibular)
- Synonym(s): Acute peripheral vestibulopathy; vestibular neuronitis (vertigo/dizziness only); vestibular neuritis (vertigo/dizziness only)

ALERT

- "Vertigo" and "dizziness" are commonly used terms. Symptoms should be clarified with patients by giving them options of alternative descriptions such as lightheadedness, dysequilibrium, room-spinning vertigo, or imbalance.
- Vertigo is not a diagnosis; it is a symptom.
- Benign positional vertigo (BPPV) is the most common cause of room-spinning vertigo. Unlike labyrinthitis, BPPV is episodic and typically occurs when extending the neck with the head turned to one side (e.g., when lying down or turning in bed). The associated room-spinning vertigo is often severe and lasts <1 minute each time. Rarely, some may report a sense of dysequilibrium lasting for hours after the initial event.

Geriatric Considerations

- Acute infectious labyrinthitis is often associated with vestibular hypofunction of the involved ear. Peripheral vertigo improves over time with central compensation.
- Elderly patients are less likely to fully compensate and they may report symptoms of dizziness and dysequilibrium lasting weeks after resolution of the acute vertigo. Vestibular physical therapy in elderly patients is often warranted after an acute episode of labyrinthitis.
- Avoid excessive use of scopolamine, meclizine, and other vestibular suppressants following the initial event, especially in the elderly, as this will delay central compensation. These medications should be used only on an as-needed basis for severe symptoms.

Pediatric Considerations

Unusual in this age group, except meningogenic suppurative labyrinthitis, which more commonly affects children <2 years.

EPIDEMIOLOGY

- Predominant age: Rare in children; most common in middle age (30–60 years old)
- Predominant sex: Male = Female

Incidence

- Viral labyrinthitis is the most common etiology.
- Suppurative or serous labyrinthitis secondary to otitis media is increasingly rare in the postantibiotic era; exact incidence is unknown:
  - Estimated 0.5–3% of intratemporal complications of otitis media in recent studies
  - Higher rates in cases with cholesteatoma

Prevalence

In the US, second most common cause of dizziness due to persistent peripheral vestibular hypofunction (9%); benign positional vertigo (16%) is most common

RISK FACTORS

- Viral upper respiratory infection
- Herpes zoster infection
- Head trauma
- Otitis media
- Cholesteatoma
- Meningitis
- Vestibulotoxic/ototoxic medications
- Otosyphilis (congenital or acquired)
- Cerebrovascular disease
- Autoimmune disease

Genetics

No known genetic pattern

GENERAL PREVENTION

- Scheduled immunizations (see "Common Viral Pathogens" under "Risk Factors")
- Prevent maternal transmission of pathogens, including syphilis, HIV

PATHOPHYSIOLOGY

Acute inflammation or damage to the inner ear, involving the peripheral special sensory organs of hearing and balance:

- Viruses may pass hematogenously into the labyrinth or directly from the middle ear to labyrinth via the round window or oval window.
- Bacterial toxins and host inflammatory mediators (e.g., cytokines) from a middle ear infection may reach the inner ear. In serous labyrinthitis, bacteria are not present in the inner ear.
- In suppurative labyrinthitis, the infecting organism obtains direct access into the inner ear:
  - Otogenic: Usually unilateral. Enters via round window or oval window to the labyrinth. May also enter via dehiscent horizontal semicircular canal if there is associated cholesteatoma.
  - Meningogenic: Can be bilateral. Enters by way of CSF via internal auditory canal or cochlear aqueduct.
- Ischemia: Ischemic or thromboembolic events involving the labyrinthine artery can cause symptoms that mimic acute labyrinthitis. May have other associated neurologic symptoms.
- Autoimmune: Local or systemic inflammatory processes may affect the inner ear directly via autoantibodies or indirectly via a vasculitis of the labyrinthine artery.

ETIOLOGY

- Infections:
  - Common viral: Cytomegalovirus, mumps virus, varicella zoster virus, rubeola virus, influenza virus, parainfluenza virus, herpes simplex virus, adenovirus, coxsackievirus, respiratory syncytial virus, HIV
  - Common bacterial: *Streptococcus pneumoniae*, *Haemophilus influenzae*, *Moraxella catarrhalis*, *Neisseria meningitidis*, *Streptococcus* sp., *Staphylococcus* species, *Borrelia burgdorferi*
  - Treponemal: *Treponema pallidum*
- Autoimmune:
  - Autoimmune inner ear disease
  - Wegener granulomatosis
  - Cogan syndrome
  - Systemic lupus erythematous
  - Polyarteritis nodosa
  - Behçet disease
  - Others
- Ischemia/infarction
- Ototoxic drugs (e.g., aminoglycosides, cisplatin)

COMMONLY ASSOCIATED CONDITIONS

- Viral upper respiratory infection
- Otitis media
- Cholesteatoma
- Head injury

DIAGNOSIS

HISTORY

- Vertigo AND (often) hearing loss in 1 ear
- Vertigo is acute in onset and lasts days to weeks.
- Nausea and vomiting are common.
- Fullness of affected ear
- Tinnitus of affected ear (roaring, ringing)
- Upper respiratory tract infection symptoms (preceding or concurrent)
- Otorrhea (not common with viral causes)
- Otalgia (not common with viral causes)
- Severe headache, fever, and nuchal rigidity in the setting of meningitis.
- Recurrent or progressive symptoms should raise suspicion for autoimmune causes.
- Profound imbalance or associated focal neurologic signs (motor or sensory weakness) are not typical and should prompt imaging (1) (see "Diagnostic Tests and Interpretation")

PHYSICAL EXAM

- Nystagmus:
  - Fast-beating nystagmus toward affected ear (acutely)
  - Fast-beating nystagmus away from affected ear (chronically)
- Symptoms improve in supine position and with eyes closed
- Otologic exam may be unremarkable in the setting of viral labyrinthitis
- Serous or purulent effusion in the middle ear may be present.
- Retraction of the tympanic membrane and keratinaceous debris may be present in the setting of cholesteatoma.

DIAGNOSTIC TESTS & INTERPRETATION

Lab

- Routine laboratory studies are not helpful in making the diagnosis unless an autoimmune cause is highly suspected.
- Consider culture of otorrhea or middle ear fluid to direct antibiotic choice.
- Consider lumbar puncture if associated meningitis is suspected.
- RPR or VDRL to screen for syphilis when clinically indicated by risk factors/history. Positive tests should be followed by FTA-Abs.

Imaging

- Imaging is not required for the diagnosis of acute labyrinthitis; however, if associated neurologic symptoms are present (e.g., motor/sensory weakness), an MRI and MRA of brain and brain stem would be indicated.

- An MRI of the brain with and without contrast is the study of choice for suspected lesions involving the eighth cranial nerve.

Follow-Up & Special Considerations

Labyrinthitis ossificans is fibrosis of the internal auditory canal following bacterial meningitis and is thought to occur due to a suppurative labyrinthitis. This can occur rapidly, especially after *S. pneumoniae* meningitis. Severity and progression of hearing loss will determine urgency for cochlear implant consideration. MRI of brain/brain stem may show loss of T2 signal in the internal auditory canal and MRI ± CT should be performed prior to cochlear implantation in these patients.

Diagnostic Procedures/Surgery

- Audiogram should be obtained for every patient with suspected labyrinthitis
- Vestibular tests are not typically indicated in the acute setting. However, if vertigo and dizziness persist after expected resolution of symptoms, the following tests should be utilized: Electronystagmography (ENG). This may include a battery of tests, depending on the resources of the audiologist. At the very least, bithermal caloric testing should be performed.

Pathological Findings

- Audiogram may show hearing loss of varying degrees and loss in discrimination to varying degrees.
- Caloric testing may show relative weakness of the horizontal semicircular canal of the affected side.

DIFFERENTIAL DIAGNOSIS

- Vestibular neuritis/neuronitis
- Benign paroxysmal positional vertigo (BPPV): Episodic, vertigo lasting seconds/minutes, worse when lying down or looking up
- Ménière disease: Episodic vertigo lasting minutes to hours, associated with ear fullness, tinnitus, and hearing loss
- Idiopathic sudden single-sided deafness
- Autoimmune inner ear disease
- Postconcussive syndrome
- Acute otitis media
- Ototoxicity
- CVA/brain-stem infarct
- Cerebellopontine-angle tumors (e.g., vestibular schwannoma)
- Vestibular migraine
- Multiple sclerosis
- Parainfectious encephalomyelitis
- Parainfectious cranial polyneuritis
- Ramsay Hunt syndrome
- Cerebral or systemic vasculitis
- Temporal lobe epilepsy
- HIV infection
- Perilymphatic fistula
- Superior canal dehiscence
- Syphilis

TREATMENT

- Close follow-up.
- Vestibular suppressants as needed (see "Medication"). Optimally used for severe acute attacks of vertigo only. Patients should be advised NOT to use these medications as a scheduled medication or for prophylaxis without symptoms.
- Persistent dizziness following acute labyrinthitis should be managed with vestibular physical therapy through a licensed physical therapist.
- Sudden single-sided hearing loss (onset within 2 weeks) should be managed with high-dose oral steroids ASAP. There are ongoing studies to test the efficacy of oral vs. intratympanic steroids for sudden sensorineural hearing loss.
- For suppurative labyrinthitis, appropriate antibiotics to eradicate infection, supportive care, prevention of spread of infection: Can be associated with labyrinthitis ossificans; decisions regarding cochlear implantation may need to be made early if both ears develop severe to profound hearing loss.

MEDICATION

- Use of the following drugs should be on an as-needed basis. No patient should take vestibular suppressants as chronic medication. Benzodiazepines are better vestibular suppressants and are preferred over antihistamine/anticholinergics such as meclizine. Sublingual benzodiazepines are very effective for vertigo and should be considered first-line therapy.
- Vestibular suppressants:
  - Lorazepam (Ativan): 0.5–2 mg SL/PO b.i.d. PRN or Diazepam (Valium) 2–5 mg q.i.d. PO PRN
  - Meclizine (Antivert, Bonine, Zentrip [dissolvable]) 12.5–25 mg PO b.i.d.–t.i.d. PRN
  - Dimenhydrinate (Dramamine) 25–50 mg PO q4h PRN
- Antiemetics:
  - Odansetron (Zofran) 4–8 mg PO t.i.d. PRN or Granisetron (Kytril) 1 mg PO t.i.d. PRN
  - Meclizine (Antivert, Bonine) 12.5–25 mg PO q4h PRN
  - Promethazine (Phenergan) 12.5–25 mg PO/PR qid prn or Prochlorperazine (Compazine) 25 mg PR q.i.d. PRN
  - Metoclopramide (Reglan) 10 mg PO t.i.d. PRN
  - Scopolamine (Transderm Scop Patch) 1 transdermal q3days PRN (avoid in the elderly)
- Antivirals:
  - Acyclovir 800 mg PO 5 times per day for 7 days is used in labyrinthitis associated with herpes zoster but is otherwise not indicated.
- Steroids:
  - Prednisone 1 mg/kg PO daily × 1 week and then taper over 1–2 weeks
  - Given early in the setting of bacterial meningitis, may decrease the otologic sequelae, specifically labyrinthitis ossificans
  - Used in treatment of labyrinthitis for associated sudden sensorineural hearing loss
  - Other immunosuppressants such as etanercept (Enbrel) have been studied in the treatment of AIED and are beyond the scope of this topic.

Pregnancy Considerations

Of the vestibular suppressants and antiemetics listed above, dimenhydrinate, diphenhydramine, odansetron, granisetron, and metoclopramide are Pregnancy Class B.

ADDITIONAL TREATMENT

General Measures

- Treat underlying disorder when possible.
- Symptomatic treatment and reassurance during acute period
- Minimize vestibular suppressants after acute period of vertigo to promote central compensation.
- Visual–vestibular exercises for prolonged symptoms and unilateral vestibular loss

Issues for Referral

- Consider neuro-otology referral for other peripheral causes of vertigo or unremitting vertigo.
- Consider neurology referral for suspected central causes of vertigo or dizziness.
- Consider otolaryngology referral for progressive bilateral hearing loss and vertigo after preliminary laboratory workup excluding rheumatologic causes.

Additional Therapies

For labyrinthitis, use of vestibular rehabilitation exercises is effective in decreasing symptoms (2).

IN-PATIENT CONSIDERATIONS

Initial Stabilization

Usually outpatient management

Admission Criteria

Systemic infection, young age, intractable vertigo with nausea and vomiting (e.g., unable to tolerate oral diet or function independently)

ONGOING CARE

FOLLOW-UP RECOMMENDATIONS

Patient Monitoring

Follow hearing loss weekly with audiograms until hearing stabilizes.

DIET

Avoid alcohol as this may exacerbate symptoms.

PATIENT EDUCATION

Lie still with eyes closed in a darkened room during acute attacks. Otherwise, encourage activity as tolerated. Minimize rapid head movement until symptoms resolve. Vestibular physical therapy important after acute symptoms to manage unilateral vestibular loss.

PROGNOSIS

Depends on cause

COMPLICATIONS

Permanent hearing loss and chronic impairment of balance

REFERENCES

1. Baloh RW, et al. Differentiating between peripheral and central causes of vertigo. *Otolaryngol Head Neck Surg*. 1998;119:55–9.
2. Hillier SL, Hollohan V. Vestibular rehabilitation for unilateral peripheral vestibular dysfunction. *Cochrane Database Syst Rev*. 2007;CD005397.

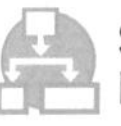

See Also (Topic, Algorithm, Electronic Media Element)

Ménière Disease; Postconcussive Syndrome; Tinnitus

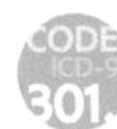

CODES

ICD9

- 386.30 Labyrinthitis, unspecified
- 386.31 Serous labyrinthitis
- 386.32 Circumscribed labyrinthitis

L

LACRIMAL DISORDERS

Asma Ashraf, MBBS, BSC
Manjula Julka, MD, FAAFP

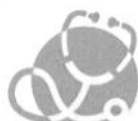

BASICS

DESCRIPTION
- Diseases and abnormalities of tear production and maintenance of tear film
- The most common lacrimal disorder is dry eye syndrome, which is often referred to as dysfunctional tear syndrome (1).
- Lacrimal duct disorders usually result in overflow tearing.
- System(s) affected: Skin/Exocrine

EPIDEMIOLOGY
Prevalence
Very common throughout the US, more often seen in arid climates:
- Predominant gender: Female $>$ Male
- Predominant age: Dry eye symptoms increase with age and are most often seen in the elderly.

RISK FACTORS
- Exposure to dry environments (e.g., high altitudes) (2)
- History of collagen vascular disease, such as rheumatoid arthritis, Sjögren syndrome, thyroid disease, rosacea, Bell palsy, eyelid abnormalities
- Medications including oral contraceptives, diuretics, β-blockers, antihistamines, and antidepressants (3)
- Posttraumatic stress disorder (4)
- Smoking (5)
- Vitamin A deficiency
- Eye surgery (6): Blepharoplasty, cataract (7), laser vision correction (8)

GENERAL PREVENTION
- Prevent exposure to eye irritants from pollution, cigarette smoke, and sun exposure.
- Ensure adequate vitamin A intake through diet or as a supplement.
- Patients with prior laser vision correction should wait at least 6 months before undergoing blepharoplasty because of the effects on corneal sensation, tear production, and tear film alteration (8).
- Increasing awareness of this condition among people residing in dry environments

PATHOPHYSIOLOGY
Tear film is composed of 3 layers:
- Mucin layer: Allows spread of aqueous tears
- Thick aqueous layer: Produced by lacrimal gland
- Lipid layer: Controls tear evaporation

ETIOLOGY
- Results from poor tear production, rapid tear evaporation, and/or an abnormal concentration of mucin or lipid in tear film
- Most common cause of dry eye symptoms is aqueous tear deficiency
- Decreased androgens are thought to contribute to a decrease in tear production.

COMMONLY ASSOCIATED CONDITIONS
Sjögren syndrome, rheumatoid arthritis, thyroid disease, rosacea, pregnancy, menopause, malnutrition

DIAGNOSIS

HISTORY
- Dry sensation in eyes
- Foreign-body sensation
- Blurry vision
- Itching
- Ocular pain
- Photophobia
- Burning
- Occasional tearing due to excessive reflex tearing:
  - Patient's symptoms usually worsen in dry, smoky environments, while reading, driving, or using a computer for extended periods

Pediatric Considerations
Lacrimal duct obstruction should be suspected in an infant presenting with excessive tearing (epiphora).

PHYSICAL EXAM
Slit-lamp exam reveals decreased tear film and may reveal punctate epithelial defects on cornea.

DIAGNOSTIC TESTS & INTERPRETATION
Lab
Initial lab tests

Tear production can be measured using a Schirmer filter strip after instillation of topical anesthetic. Wetting of $<$10 mm of the slip after 5 minutes is indicative of insufficient tear production.

Diagnostic Procedures/Surgery
- Staining of the ocular surface with fluorescein will show areas of abnormal uptake and patches of drying. It allows the tear break-up time (TBUT) to be calculated. A TBUT of $<$10 seconds is abnormal.
- Rose bengal will be taken up by dead or dying epithelial cells, and it may be a more sensitive test.

Pathological Findings
In Sjögren syndrome, infiltration of the lacrimal gland with inflammatory cells may be evident.

DIFFERENTIAL DIAGNOSIS
- Ocular: Allergy, conjunctivitis, contact lens complication, exposure keratopathy
- Other: Ocular rosacea, thyroid ophthalmopathy, ocular manifestation of HIV, Bell palsy, vitamin A deficiency

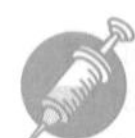

TREATMENT

MEDICATION
First Line
- Preservative-free artificial tears: 1 drop in each eye several times a day to prevent discomfort (9)[A]
- Ophthalmic lubricating ointment may be used in each eye at bedtime (10)[B].

Second Line
- Dry eye has been identified as having an inflammatory component that responds in refractory cases to topical immunosuppressives, such as cyclosporine (Restasis) 0.05%, 1 drop to each eye b.i.d. (11,12)[A].
- Emerging therapies include topical androgens, secretagogues (e.g., oral pilocarpine), cytokine-blocking agents, and a P2Y2 receptor agonist (Diquafosol).

ADDITIONAL TREATMENT
General Measures
- Those with systemic illnesses predisposed to dry eye should be informed and instructed in the appropriate use of artificial tear supplements.
- Symptoms of dry eye may decrease with an increase in home humidification and hydration.

Issues for Referral
Rheumatology referral if systemic collagen vascular disease is suspected

Additional Therapies

- Fatty acid (omega-3), linoleic acid, and gamma-linoleic acid supplements (13)[B]
- Lid massage and warm compresses several times a day

Pediatric Considerations

The vast majority of babies born with nasolacrimal duct obstructions will clear spontaneously during the first year of life. On occasion, surgical probing is necessary.

SURGERY/OTHER PROCEDURES

Punctal occlusion, with either punctal plugs or laser, is used in moderate to severe dry eye if medical therapy fails.

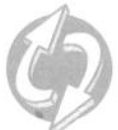

ONGOING CARE

FOLLOW-UP RECOMMENDATIONS

Patient Monitoring

- Monitor early to assess efficacy of treatment.
- The viscosity of artificial tears and frequency of use can be increased for symptom relief.

DIET

- Diet rich in omega-3 fatty acids and/or linoleic acids may benefit some patients
- Adequate vitamin A intake

PATIENT EDUCATION

All individuals with systemic illnesses predisposed to dry eye, postmenopausal women, and those residing in arid climates, or >60 years should be instructed in the use of artificial tear supplements to combat dry eye symptoms.

PROGNOSIS

- Lacrimal disorders can be adequately managed with artificial tear supplements.
- Blocked tear ducts can be managed with probing and punctal dilation and/or dacryocystorhinostomy procedures in more severe cases.

COMPLICATIONS

Severe dry eye may lead to the following:

- Corneal breakdown
- Secondary invasion by bacteria
- Eye infections

REFERENCES

1. Behrens A, Doyle JJ, Stern L, et al. Dysfunctional tear syndrome: A Delphi approach to treatment recommendations. *Cornea*. 2006;25:900–7.
2. Gupta N, Prasad I, Himashree G, et al. Prevalence of dry eye at high altitude: A case controlled comparative study. *High Alt Med Biol*. 2008; 9:327–34.
3. Schaumberg DA, Dana R, Buring JE, et al. Prevalence of dry eye disease among US men: Estimates from the Physicians' Health Studies. *Arch Ophthalmol*. 2009;127:763–8.
4. Galor A, Feuer W, Lee DJ, et al. Prevalence and risk factors of dry eye syndrome in a United States veterans affairs population. *Am J Ophthalmol*. 2011;152(3):377–84.
5. Sahai A, Malik P, et al. Dry eye: Prevalence and attributable risk factors in a hospital-based population. *Indian J Ophthalmol*. 2005;53: 87–91.
6. Pacella SJ, Codner MA, et al. Minor complications after blepharoplasty: Dry eyes, chemosis, granulomas, ptosis, and scleral show. *Plast Reconstr Surg*. 2010;125:709–18.
7. Cho YK, Kim MS, et al. Dry eye after cataract surgery and associated intraoperative risk factors. *Korean J Ophthalmol*. 2009;23:65–73.
8. Lee WB, McCord CD, Somia N, et al. Optimizing blepharoplasty outcomes in patients with previous laser vision correction. *Plast Reconstr Surg*. 2008;122:587–94.
9. Ousler GW, Michaelson C, Christensen MT. An evaluation of tear film breakup time extension and ocular protection index scores among three marketed lubricant eye drops. *Cornea*. 2007;26: 949–52.
10. Tauber J. Efficacy, tolerability and comfort of a 0.3% hypromellose gel ophthalmic lubricant in the treatment of patients with moderate to severe dry eye syndrome. *Curr Med Res Opin*. 2007;23:2629–36.
11. Hardten DR, Brown MJ, Pham-Vang S. Evaluation of an isotonic tear in combination with topical cyclosporine for the treatment of ocular surface disease. *Curr Med Res Opin*. 2007;23:2083–91.
12. Roberts CW, Carniglia PE, Brazzo BG. Comparison of topical cyclosporine, punctal occlusion, and a combination for the treatment of dry eye. *Cornea*. 2007;26:805–9.
13. Barabino S, Rolando M, Camicione P. Systemic linoleic and gamma-linoleic acid therapy in dry eye syndrome with an inflammatory component. *Cornea*. 2003;22:97–101.

ADDITIONAL READING

- Barabino S, Rolando M, Camicione P, et al. Systemic linoleic and gamma-linolenic acid therapy in dry eye syndrome with an inflammatory component. *Cornea*. 2003;22:97–101.
- Dogru M, Tsubota K. New insights into the diagnosis and treatment of dry eye. *Ocul Surf*. 2004;2:59–75.
- Karadayi K, Ciftci F, Akin T. Increase in central corneal thickness in dry and normal eyes with application of artificial tears: A new diagnostic and follow-up criterion for dry eye. *Ophthalmic Physiol Opt*. 2005;25:485–91.
- Perry HD, Donnenfeld ED. Dry eye diagnosis and management in 2004. *Curr Opin Ophthalmol*. 2004;15:299–304.
- Stern ME, Gao J, Siemasko KF. The role of the lacrimal functional unit in the pathophysiology of dry eye. *Exp Eye Res*. 2004;78:409–16.

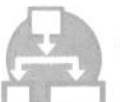

See Also (Topic, Algorithm, Electronic Media Element)

Sjögren Syndrome

CODES

ICD9

- 375.9 Unspecified disorder of lacrimal system
- 375.15 Tear film insufficiency, unspecified

CLINICAL PEARLS

- Dry eye syndrome is common in the US, affecting postmenopausal women more than any other population.
- Symptoms are usually adequately managed with preservative-free artificial tears and humidified environments.
- Dry eye symptoms that are refractory to medical treatment and/or punctal plugs should raise the suspicion of an underlying systemic condition, and a rheumatology consult should be considered.

L

LACTOSE INTOLERANCE

Mohammad Ansar Mughal, MD
Fozia A. Ali, MD

BASICS

DESCRIPTION

- Inability to digest lactose (the primary sugar in milk) into its constituents, glucose and galactose, because of low levels of the lactase enzyme in the brush border of the duodenum:
  - *Congenital lactose intolerance*: Very rare
  - *Primary lactose intolerance*: Common in adults in whom a low level of lactase has developed after childhood
  - *Secondary lactose intolerance:* The inability to digest lactose caused by any condition injuring the intestinal mucosa (e.g., diarrhea) or a reduction of available mucosal surface (e.g., resection):
    - Typically transient, with the duration of the intolerance determined by the nature and course of the primary condition
  - Symptoms are experienced after consumption of milk and milk-containing products.
  - Intolerance varies with amount of lactose consumed and rate of gastric emptying (faster emptying times being associated with greater symptoms).
  - Infants with induced acute or chronic diarrhea may develop lactose intolerance, especially with rotavirus disease.
  - *Lactose malabsorption* is defined as the inability to absorb lactose. This does not necessarily parallel lactose intolerance.
- System(s) affected: Endocrine/Metabolic; Gastrointestinal
- Synonym(s): Lactase deficiency

Pediatric Considerations

- Primary lactose intolerance usually begins in late childhood.
- No consensus exists on whether young children (<5 years of age) should avoid lactose following diarrheal illness.
- Lactose-free formulas are available.
- Exclude a milk protein allergy.

EPIDEMIOLOGY

Incidence

- Primary lactose intolerance varies according to race:
  - Up to 15% of northern European descendants
  - 80% of blacks and Latinos
  - 100% of Native American and Asians (1)
- Secondary lactose intolerance:
  - ≥50% of infants with acute or chronic diarrheal disease have lactose intolerance, especially with rotavirus disease.
  - Lactose intolerance also is fairly common with giardiasis and ascariasis, irritable bowel syndrome (IBS), tropical and nontropical sprue, and the AIDS malabsorptive syndrome.

Prevalence

- Predominant age:
  - Primary: Teenage and adult
  - Secondary: Depends on underlying condition
- Predominant sex: Male = Female

RISK FACTORS

- Race: Adult-onset lactase deficiency varies widely among countries.
- Age:
  - Signs and symptoms usually do not become apparent until after age 6–7 years, and recent studies actually have shown that hypolactasia may begin even after age 20.
  - Symptoms may not be apparent until adulthood depending on dietary lactose intake and rate of decline of intestinal lactase activity.
  - Lactase enzyme activity is highly correlated with age, regardless of symptoms.

Genetics

- The gene responsible for lactase has been identified (2)[A]. The wild-type presentation is associated with the decline of lactase activity.
- Genetic polymorphisms associated with lactase persistence are concentrated predominantly in northern Europeans.

GENERAL PREVENTION

Avoidance of lactose in large quantities will relieve symptoms. Patients can learn what level of lactose is tolerable in their diet.

ETIOLOGY

- Primary lactose intolerance: Normal decline in the lactase activity in the intestinal mucosa after weaning is genetically controlled and permanent.
- Secondary lactose intolerance: Associated with gastroenteritis in children
- Secondary lactose intolerance is also associated with nontropical and tropical sprue, regional enteritis, abetalipoproteinemia, cystic fibrosis, ulcerative colitis, and immunoglobulin deficiencies in both adults and children.

COMMONLY ASSOCIATED CONDITIONS

- Tropical or nontropical sprue
- Giardiasis
- Immunoglobulin deficiencies
- Crohn disease
- Cystic fibrosis

DIAGNOSIS

Evaluation of lactose intolerance includes a careful medical history, review of symptoms, and physical examination.

HISTORY

- Symptoms may arise 30 minutes to 2 hours after consumption of products containing lactose and may be distinguished from IBS with a trial of a lactose-free diet.
- Symptoms include bloating, cramping, abdominal discomfort, diarrhea or loose stools, and flatulence.
- The abdominal pain may be crampy in nature and often is localized to the periumbilical area or lower quadrant.
- The stools usually are bulky, frothy, and watery.
- Only 1/3–1/5 of the people with lactose malabsorption will develop symptoms.
- The degree of symptoms varies with the lactose load and with other food consumed at the same time.

PHYSICAL EXAM

Borborygmi may be audible on physical examination and to the patient.

DIAGNOSTIC TESTS & INTERPRETATION

Lab

Initial lab tests

- Lactose breath hydrogen test (especially in children): The test is begun by giving oral lactose in the fasting state, at a usual dose of 2 g/kg (maximum dose 25 g). Breath hydrogen is sampled at baseline and at 30-minute intervals after the ingestion of lactose for 3 hours. The postlactose and baseline values are compared. We generally consider a breath hydrogen value of 10 ppm as normal. Values between 10 and 20 ppm may be indeterminate unless accompanied by symptoms, whereas values over 20 ppm are considered diagnostic of lactose malabsorption.
- Lactose absorption test: Alternative to lactose breath hydrogen test in adults (more invasive and equivalent in sensitivity and specificity to breath test). Following oral administration of a 50-g test dose in adults (or 2 g/kg in children), blood glucose levels are monitored at 0, 60, and 120 minutes. An increase in blood glucose by <20 mg/dL (1.1 mmol/L) plus the development of symptoms is diagnostic. False-negative results may occur in patients with diabetes or bacterial overgrowth.
- Low fecal pH and reducing substances are only valid when stools are collected fresh and assayed immediately. Test is fairly insensitive.

Diagnostic Procedures/Surgery

Small bowel biopsy for assay of lactase activity: May be normal if deficiency is focal or patchy (not readily available and usually not necessary)

Pathological Findings

Lactase deficiency in intestinal mucosa may be patchy or focal.

DIFFERENTIAL DIAGNOSIS

- Sucrase deficiency
- Diarrhea
- IBS
- Protein intolerance
- Malabsorption syndromes

TREATMENT

The treatment of lactose malabsorption in the absence of a correctable underlying disease includes 4 general principles:

- Reduced dietary lactose intake
- Substitution of alternative nutrient sources to maintain energy and protein intake
- Administration of a commercially available enzyme substitute
- Maintenance of calcium and vitamin D intake

MEDICATION

Lactase (Lactaid, Lactrase) tablets (1)[A]:

- Commercially available "lactase" preparations are actually bacterial or yeast β-galactosidases.
- Take 1–2 capsules or tablets prior to ingesting milk products.
- These vary in effectiveness at preventing symptoms.
- Can add tablets or contents of capsules to milk before drinking; also available in milk in some areas
- Not effective for all people with lactose intolerance

COMPLEMENTARY AND ALTERNATIVE MEDICINE

Certain probiotic formulations taken with meals may alleviate some of the symptoms of lactose intolerance in select patients (3)[B].

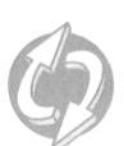

ONGOING CARE

DIET

- Reduce or restrict dietary lactose to control symptoms.
- Yogurt and fermented products, such as hard cheese, are better tolerated than milk.
- Supplement calcium in the form of calcium carbonate.
- Prehydrolyzed milk (Lactaid) is available and effective.

PATIENT EDUCATION

- Patients must read labels on commercial products, because milk sugar is used in many products and may cause symptoms.
- Lactose-intolerant patients may tolerate whole milk or chocolate milk better than skim milk due to slower rate of gastric emptying.
- Lactose consumed with other food products is better tolerated than when it is consumed alone.
- Primary lactase deficiency is permanent; secondary lactose intolerance usually is temporary, although it may persist for several months after the inciting disease has been cured.
- 20% of prescription drugs and 6% of over-the-counter (OTC) medicines use lactose as a base.
- Most patients still can tolerate 12–15 g of lactose despite their lactose intolerance or malabsorption (4)[A].

PROGNOSIS

- Normal life expectancy
- Symptoms can be controlled through diet alone if lactase tablets are ineffective.

COMPLICATIONS

Calcium deficiency: Avoidance of milk and other dairy products can lead to reduced calcium intake, which may increase the risk for osteoporosis and fracture.

REFERENCES

1. Levri KM, Ketvertis K, Deramo M, et al. Do probiotics reduce adult lactose intolerance? A systematic review. *J Fam Pact*. 2005;54:613.
2. Waud JP, Matthews SB, Campbell AK. Measurement of breath hydrogen and methane, together with lactase genotype, defines the current best practice for investigation of lactose sensitivity. *Ann Clin Biochem*. 2008;45:50–8.
3. Sanders SW, Tolman KG, Reitberg DP. Effect of a single dose of lactase on symptoms and expired hydrogen after lactose challenge in lactose-intolerant subjects. *Clin Pharm*. 1992;11:533–8.
4. Shaukat A, Levitt MD, Taylor BC, et al. Systematic review: Effective management strategies for lactose intolerance. *Ann Intern Med*. 2010;152:797–803.

ADDITIONAL READING

- Brannon PM, Carpenter TO, Fernandez JR, et al. NIH Consensus Development Conference Statement: Lactose intolerance and health. *NIH Consensus and State-of-the-Science Statements*. 2010;27.
- Swagerty DL, Walling AD, Klein RM. Lactose intolerance. *Am Fam Physician*. 2002;65:1845–50.

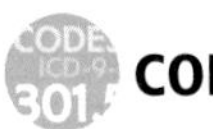

CODES

ICD9

271.3 Intestinal disaccharidase deficiencies and disaccharide malabsorption

CLINICAL PEARLS

- Keeping a food diary with symptomatic episodes documented can help to identify food sources that may be problematic.
- Patients should read ingredient labels to look for milk or lactose, but also for ingredients such as whey and curd, which indicate the presence of lactose.
- Lactose-intolerant patients may tolerate whole milk or chocolate milk better than skim milk due to a slower rate of gastric emptying.
- Many patients with lactose intolerance avoid dairy products to an unnecessary degree, causing inadequate intake of of calcium and vitamin D, which may predispose them to osteoporosis.

LARYNGEAL CANCER

Hugh J. Silk, MD, MPH
Sheila O. Stille, DMD, MAGD

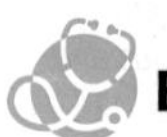

BASICS

DESCRIPTION

- A friable, granular tumor of the larynx that leads to hoarseness, hemoptysis, and cough
- Of all malignant lesions, <1%; squamous cell carcinomas constitute 95–98% of all malignant neoplasms of the larynx.
- Laryngeal cancer accounts for <2% of all carcinomas.
- At the time of diagnosis, 62% will have local disease, 26% regional disease, and 8% distant disease in the lungs, liver, and/or bone.
- No racial predilection
- System(s) affected: Pulmonary; ENT
- Synonym(s): Cancer of the larynx; Throat cancer; Cancer of the voice box

EPIDEMIOLOGY

Incidence

- Per year, 5/100,000 (12,250 new cases per year in the US). These are usually squamous cell carcinomas that arise from the glottis.
- Predominant age:
  - Median age of occurrence in sixth and seventh decades
  - <1% of laryngeal cancers arise in patients <30 years of age.
- Predominant sex: Male > Female (4:1); increasing incidence in women who smoke; synergistic with alcohol abuse

Prevalence

- About 3,700 deaths from disease in the US yearly
- Second most common site for head and neck cancer (26% of all cases)
- 11th most common cancer in males

RISK FACTORS

See "Etiology."

Genetics

Unknown

GENERAL PREVENTION

- Avoidance or cessation of smoking and/or alcohol abuse (85% attributed to smoking or alcohol abuse)
- Wearing proper respiratory masks/respirators if chronic exposure to certain chemicals, gases, and wood dust
- Treating chronic laryngopharyngeal reflux
- Indirect laryngoscopy for at-risk patients with persistent hoarseness lasting beyond 1–2 weeks

ETIOLOGY

- Smoking (dose dependent) (1)
- Heavy alcohol use (1)
- Smoking plus moderate alcohol use (1)
- Possibly chronic laryngopharyngeal reflux (small studies)
- Occupational hazards (asbestos, pesticides, polycyclic aromatic hydrocarbons, woodworkers)
- HPV (less than oropharyngeal 35% vs. 24%) (2)[A]

COMMONLY ASSOCIATED CONDITIONS

Up to 10% of patients may have a synchronous squamous cell carcinoma in the lower or upper aerodigestive tract, most notably in the esophagus or lungs.

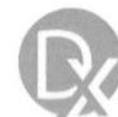

DIAGNOSIS

Early laryngeal cancer generally has a good prognosis, with a 5-year disease specific survival rate of more than 90% for T1 tumors.

HISTORY

- Persistent hoarseness in an elderly or middle-aged cigarette smoker (3)
- Dyspnea and/or stridor
- Ipsilateral otalgia
- Dysphagia
- Odynophagia
- Chronic cough
- Hemoptysis
- Weight loss due to poor nutrition
- Halitosis due to tumor necrosis
- Chronic exposure to known risk factors (see "Etiology")

PHYSICAL EXAM

- Visualization of larynx initially by mirror and then a full nasolaryngoscopic exam
- Physical observation of vocal cord mobility, airway patency, and any regional spread
- Cervical lymph node exam
- Mass in the neck from metastatic lymph node
- Laryngeal tenderness secondary to tumor necrosis or suppuration
- Broadening of the larynx on palpation with loss of crepitation
- Fullness of the cricothyroid membrane

DIAGNOSTIC TESTS & INTERPRETATION

Imaging

- CT scan or MRI if chest, liver, or brain metastasis suspected
- Bone scan if bone metastasis suspected

Diagnostic Procedures/Surgery

Indirect and/or direct laryngoscopy and biopsy to determine stage of disease as well as histologic confirmation

Pathological Findings

- Laryngoscopy: Fungating, friable tumor with heaped-up edges and granular appearance, with multiple areas of central necrosis and exudate surrounding areas of hyperemia
- Squamous cell carcinoma in 95% of cases

DIFFERENTIAL DIAGNOSIS

- Acute or chronic laryngitis secondary to allergies, voice overuse, chemical exposures
- Benign vocal cord lesions such as polyps, nodules, and papillomas
- Tuberculosis or fungal infection (candidiasis) of the larynx (4)

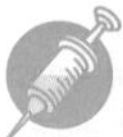

TREATMENT

- Radiotherapy tends to be the treatment of choice in northern Europe, Australasia, and Canada, whereas surgery tends to be the treatment of choice in southern Europe and many centers in the US.
- Increased use of transoral endoscopic laser microsurgery, improved delivery of radiotherapy and concomitant chemoradiotherapy have been used over the past 10 plus years with promising results (5)

MEDICATION

- Narcotics may be necessary for pain control during treatment for mucositis (of the mouth) secondary to radiation therapy. Viscous lidocaine can be helpful as well.
- Nystatin mouth rinses for oral thrush

ADDITIONAL TREATMENT

General Measures

- Tracheotomy care, when applicable
- If patient is diagnosed during pregnancy: Natural history of disease and treatment side effects have to be weighed against the possibilities of continuing on to delivery.

Issues for Referral

- ENT for direct visualization of larynx; biopsy and surgery
- Depending on patient's management plan, nutritional and dental consults may be needed.
- Treatment may result in need for voice rehabilitation and be the cause of social isolation, job loss, and depression; therefore, refer to psychology, social work, and/or support groups as indicated (5).

Additional Therapies

Radiotherapy:

- There is increased focus on radiation therapy (RT), combined chemotherapy and RT, and function-preserving laryngectomy surgery due to patient fear of voice loss (5).
- Early disease may be treatable by either RT or laser cordectomy on an outpatient basis. No randomized, controlled trial has proven superiority of either when last reviewed by Cochrane in 2007. 90% cure rates are the rule (6)[A].
- BCCIP protein (BRCA2 and CDKN1A [p21(Waf1/Cip1)] interacting protein) can be a prognostic marker for RT, with loss of the protein indicating a worse prognosis (7).

SURGERY/OTHER PROCEDURES

- Tracheotomy may be necessary if a tumor is large enough to cause upper airway obstruction.
- More advanced disease needs inpatient care, necessitating partial or total laryngectomy and postoperative RT 4–5 weeks after surgery depending on the stage of disease.

IN-PATIENT CONSIDERATIONS

Initial Stabilization

Primarily outpatient care

Admission Criteria

- More advanced disease, surgical intervention, and complication management
- Nutritional or airway issues/complications

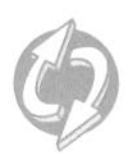

ONGOING CARE

FOLLOW-UP RECOMMENDATIONS

Patient may remain fully active unless debilitated from more advanced disease and/or greater degree of surgery.

Patient Monitoring

- Repeat indirect laryngoscopy and complete head and neck exams periodically for at least 5 years after treatment to detect early recurrence or second primary
- Yearly chest x-rays (and liver function text monitoring) for metastatic disease
- Patients with dysphagia should undergo barium swallow and/or esophageal endoscopy to rule out second synchronous tumor in the esophagus.
- Patients with unexplained pain should have appropriate radiologic or nuclear medicine bone scans.
- Mental status change warrants CT scan of the brain to rule out brain metastases.

DIET

- Nasogastric or gastrostomy feeding may be necessary if tumor involves esophageal inlet.
- No special diet otherwise

PATIENT EDUCATION

Material is available from local cancer society.

PROGNOSIS

- Early disease is expected to have >90% cure rate with laryngeal and voice preservation.
- If lesion enlarges or metastasizes to regional cervical lymph nodes, the cure rate usually drops by 50%.
- Most recurrences occur within the first 2 years of initial treatment.

COMPLICATIONS

- Temporary odynophagia or dysphagia secondary to mucositis and/or thrush during RT
- Persistent hoarseness despite adequate treatment, necessitating further adjunctive procedures and/or speech therapy
- Tracheostoma stenosis requiring stenting with laryngectomy tubes or further surgery
- Dysphagia secondary to upper esophageal stricture after total laryngectomy, necessitating dilation
- Aspiration after partial laryngectomy, necessitating complete laryngectomy or tracheotomy
- Inability to decannulate after partial laryngectomy because of laryngeal stenosis and/or aspiration
- Radiation-induced chondronecrosis, which mimics tumor recurrence
- Radiation edema, necessitating emergent tracheotomy
- Hypothyroidism secondary to laryngectomy and RT (8)

REFERENCES

1. La Vecchia C, Zhang ZF, Altieri A. Alcohol and laryngeal cancer: An update. *Eur J Cancer Prev*. 2008;17(2):116–24.
2. Kreimer AR, Clifford GM, Boyle P, et al. Human papillomavirus types in head and neck squamous cell carcinomas worldwide: A systematic review. *Cancer Epidemiol Biomarkers Prev*. 2005;14(2): 467–75.
3. Chu EA, Kim YJ. Laryngeal cancer: Diagnosis and preoperative work-up. *Otolaryngol Clin N Am*. 2008;41:673–95.
4. Nunes FP, Bishop T, Prasad ML. Laryngeal candidiasis mimicking malignancy. *Laryngoscope*. 2008;118:1957–9.
5. American Society of Clinical Oncology, Pfister DG, Laurie SA. American Society of Clinical Oncology clinical practice guideline for the use of larynx-preservation strategies in the treatment of laryngeal cancer. *J Clin Oncol*. 2006;24:3693–704.
6. Dey P. Radiotherapy vs. open surgery vs. endolaryngeal surgery (with or without laser) for early laryngeal squamous cell cancer. *Cochrane Database Syst Rev*. 2002;2:CD002027.
7. Rewari A, Lu H, Parikh R. BCCIP as a prognostic marker for radiotherapy of laryngeal cancer. *Radiother Oncol*. 2009;90(2):183–8.
8. Alkan S, Baylancicek S, Ciftçic M. Thyroid dysfunction after combined therapy for laryngeal cancer: A prospective study. *Otolaryngol Head Neck Surg*. 2008;139:787–91.

ADDITIONAL READING

- Ferlito A, Bradley PJ, Rinaldo A. What is the treatment of choice for TI squamous cell carcinoma of the larynx? *J Laryngol Otol*. 2004;118:747–9.
- Huang SH, Lockwood G, Irish J. Truths and myths about radiotherapy for verrucous carcinoma of larynx. *Int J Radiat Oncol Biol Phys*. 2008.
- Silver CE, Beitler JJ, Shaha AR, et al. Current trends in initial management of laryngeal cancer: The declining use of open surgery. *Eur Arch Otorhinolaryngol*. 2009;266:1333–52.
- Stewart SL, Cardinez CJ, Richardson LC, et al. Surveillance for cancers associated with tobacco use—1999 to 2004. *MMWR*. 2008;57(SS08):1–33.

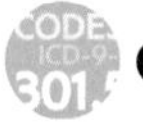

CODES

ICD9

- 161.0 Malignant neoplasm of glottis
- 161.1 Malignant neoplasm of supraglottis
- 161.2 Malignant neoplasm of subglottis

CLINICAL PEARLS

- Persistent hoarseness in an at-risk older person should prompt investigation with indirect and/or direct laryngoscopy.
- RT and multimodal therapies have reduced the need for laryngectomy except in advanced cases. ENT and radiation oncology consultations are recommended.
- Counsel all patients about primary prevention (no smoking, limit alcohol use) and counsel patients with cancer on secondary prevention.

LARYNGITIS

Hugh J. Silk, MD, MPH
Sheila O. Stille, DMD, MAGD

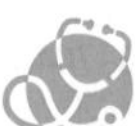

BASICS

DESCRIPTION

- Laryngitis is inflammation, erythema, and edema of the mucosa of the larynx and/or vocal cords. Characterized by hoarseness, loss of voice, or coughing.
- There is a range of severity, but most cases are acute and are associated with viral upper respiratory infection, irritation, or acute vocal strain
- System(s) affected: Pulmonary; ENT
- Synonym(s): Laryngotracheitis; Acute laryngitis; Chronic laryngitis; Croup (in children)

EPIDEMIOLOGY

- Predominant age: Affects all ages
- Children more susceptible than adults due to increased risk of symptomatic inflammation from smaller airways
- Predominant gender: Male = Female

Incidence

Common

Prevalence

Common

RISK FACTORS

- Acute:
  - Upper respiratory tract infection
  - Voice overuse
  - Pneumonia
  - Influenza
  - Lack of immunization for pertussis or diphtheria
  - Immunocompromised
- Chronic:
  - Allergy
  - Chronic rhinitis/sinusitis
  - Voice abuse
  - Gastroesophageal reflux disease (GERD)/ laryngopharyngeal reflux disease (LPRD) (rare) (1)[A]
  - Smoking: Primary or secondhand
  - Excessive alcohol use
  - Constant exposure to dust or other irritants; environmental pollution
  - Previous endotracheal intubation
  - Medications: Inhaled steroids, anticholinergics, and antihistamines

Geriatric Considerations

May be more ill, slower to heal

Pediatric Considerations

- Common in this age group
- Consider congenital causes.

GENERAL PREVENTION

- Avoid overuse of voice (voice training helpful for vocal musicians/public speakers)
- Influenza virus vaccine is suggested for high-risk individuals.
- Quit smoking and avoid secondhand smoke.
- Limit or avoid alcohol/caffeine/acidic foods.
- Maintain proper hydration status.
- Avoid allergens.
- Good hand washing (infection prevention)

ETIOLOGY

- Misuse or abuse of voice
- Virus infections: Influenza A, B; parainfluenza; adenovirus; coronavirus; rhinovirus; human papillomavirus; cytomegalovirus; varicella-zoster virus; herpes simplex virus; respiratory syncytial virus; coxsackievirus
- Bacterial infections (uncommon): β-hemolytic streptococcus, *Streptococcus pneumoniae*, *H. influenzae*, tuberculosis (TB), leprosy, *Moraxella catarrhalis*, *Mycoplasma pneumoniae*, *Chlamydophila pneumoniae*
- Fungal infections (rare): Histoplasmosis, blastomycosis, coccidioides, cryptococcus, and candida
- Secondary syphilis left untreated
- Leprosy (in 30–55% of those with leprosy, larynx is affected; tropical and warm countries)
- Laryngeal TB
- Inhaling irritating substances (e.g., air pollution, cigarette smoke)
- Aspiration of caustic chemicals
- Aging changes: Muscle atrophy, loss of moisture in larynx, and bowing of vocal cords
- GERD/LPRD
- Excessively dry environment
- Allergic
- Idiopathic
- Iatrogenic: Inhaled steroids such as those used to treat asthma, surgical injury, or compression of recurrent laryngeal nerve
- Vocal cord nodules/polyps ("singer's nodes")
- Bowing of vocal cords with age
- Retropharyngeal abscess
- Cancer
- Neuromuscular disorder (e.g., myasthenia gravis); stroke
- Rheumatoid arthritis
- Trauma (e.g., endotracheal intubation, blunt or penetrating trauma to neck)

COMMONLY ASSOCIATED CONDITIONS

- Viral pharyngitis
- Diphtheria (rare): Membrane can descend into larynx
- Pertussis: Larynx involved as part of the respiratory system
- Bronchitis
- Pneumonitis

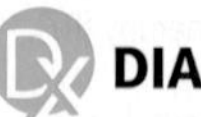

DIAGNOSIS

HISTORY

- Hoarseness, throat tickling, rawness, and cough
- Abnormal-sounding voice
- Constant urge to clear the throat
- Possible fever
- Malaise
- Dysphagia/odynophagia
- Regional lymphadenopathy
- Stridor or possible airway obstruction in children (2)
- Hemoptysis
- Laryngospasm or sense of choking
- Allergic rhinitis/rhinorrhea/postnasal drip (PND)
- Occupation or other reasons for voice overuse
- Smoking history
- Blunt or penetrating trauma to neck
- GERD/LPRD

PHYSICAL EXAM

- Head and neck exam including cervical nodes; cranial nerve exam
- ENT referral for persistent symptoms (>2–3 weeks) or fear of foreign body

DIAGNOSTIC TESTS & INTERPRETATION

Lab

- Rarely needed
- WBCs elevated in bacterial laryngitis
- Viral culture (seldom necessary)

Imaging

Barium swallow, only if needed for differential diagnosis

Diagnostic Procedures/Surgery

- Fiber-optic or indirect laryngoscopy: Looking for red, inflamed, and occasionally hemorrhagic vocal cords; rounded edges and exudate (Reinke edema)
- Consider otolaryngologic evaluation and biopsy: Laryngitis lasting more than 2 weeks in adults with history of smoking or alcohol abuse to rule out malignancy.

- pH probe (24-hour): No difference in incidence of pharyngeal reflux as measured by pH probe between patients with chronic reflux laryngitis and healthy adults (3)
- Strobovideo laryngoscopy for diagnosis of subtle lesions

DIFFERENTIAL DIAGNOSIS

- Diphtheria
- Vocal nodules or polyps
- Laryngeal malignancy
- Thyroid malignancy
- Upper airway malignancy
- Epiglottitis
- Pertussis
- Laryngeal nerve trauma/injury

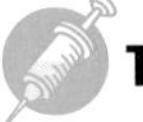

TREATMENT

- Evidence is limited, but good, that treatment beyond supportive care is ineffective.
- Antibiotics usually not indicated because it is viral. The bacterial form is rare.
- Corticosteroids in severe cases of laryngitis to reduce inflammation, such as croup
- May need voice training, if voice overuse

MEDICATION

Usually none

First Line

- Analgesics
- Antipyretics (rare)
- Cough suppressants
- Throat lozenges
- Plenty of fluids

Second Line

- Inhaled corticosteroids (consider if allergy-induced)
- Oral corticosteroids: Only if urgent need (presenter, singer, actor); evidence of benefit has been studied with single-dose dexamethasone in children ages 6 months to 5 years for moderate severity croup (for croup)
- Standard of care is to prescribe proton pump inhibitors for chronic laryngitis if GERD or LPRD is suspected; however, evidence suggests only a modest benefit, if any (4).
- Treat nonviral infectious underlying causes
- Candidal laryngitis:
  - Mild cases: Oral antifungal (fluconazole)
  - Amphotericin B or an echinocandin can be given in life-threatening cases.

ADDITIONAL TREATMENT

General Measures

- Acute:
  - Usually a self-limited illness lasting <3 weeks and not severe
  - Antibiotics of no value (5)[A]
  - Avoid excessive voice use, including whispering
  - Steam inhalations or cool-mist humidifier
  - Increase fluid intake, especially in cases associated with excessive dryness
  - Avoid smoking (or secondhand exposure)
  - Saltwater gargles
- Chronic:
  - Symptomatic treatment as above
  - Voice therapy (for patients with intermittent dysphagia and vocal abuse)
  - Stop smoking
  - Reduce or stop alcohol intake
  - Occupational change or modification, if exposure
  - Consider discontinuing inhaled corticosteroids
- Reflux laryngitis: Elevate head of bed, other antireflux management; proton pump inhibitors

Issues for Referral

- Consider otolaryngologic evaluation and biopsy for laryngitis lasting more than 2 weeks in adults with history of smoking or alcohol abuse to rule out malignancy.
- Consider GI consult to rule out GERD/LPRD.

COMPLEMENTARY AND ALTERNATIVE MEDICINE

The following, although not well studied, have been recommended by some experts:

- Barberry, blackcurrant, echinacea, eucalyptus, German chamomile, goldenrod, goldenseal, hot lemon and honey, licorice, marshmallow, peppermint, saw palmetto, slippery elm, vitamin C, zinc

SURGERY/OTHER PROCEDURES

- Vocal cord biopsy of hyperplastic mucosa and areas of leukoplakia if cancer or TB is suspected
- Removal of nodules or polyps if voice therapy fails

ONGOING CARE

PATIENT EDUCATION

- Educate on the importance of voice rest, including whispering
- Provide assistance with smoking cessation
- Help the patient with modification of other predisposing habits or occupational hazards

PROGNOSIS

Complete clearing of the inflammation without sequelae

COMPLICATIONS

Chronic hoarseness

REFERENCES

1. Joniau S. Reflux and laryngitis: A systemic review. *Otolarygol Head Neck Surg*. 2007;136:686–92.
2. Gallivan GJ, Gallivan KH, Gallivan HK. Inhaled corticosteroids: Hazardous effects on voice—an update. *J Voice*. 2007;21:101–11.
3. Johnson DA. Medical therapy of reflux pharyngitis. *J Clin Gastroenterol*. 2008;42(5):589–93.
4. Tulunay OE. Laryngitis—Diagnosis and management. *Otolaryngol Clin N Am*. 2008;41: 437–52.
5. Reveiz L, Cardona AF, Ospina EG. Antibiotics for acute laryngitis in adults. *Cochrane Database Syst Rev*. 2007;CD004783.

ADDITIONAL READING

- Banfield G, Tandon P, Solomons N. Hoarse voice: An early symptom of many conditions. *Practitioner*. 2000;244:267–71.
- Gilbert CR, Vipul K, Baram M. Novel H1N1 influenza A viral infection complicated by alveolar hemorrhage. *Respir Care*. 2010;55:623–5.
- Moore JM, Vaezi MF. Extraesophageal manifestations of gastroesophageal reflux disease: Real or imagined? *Curr Opin Gastroenterol*. 2010;26:389–94.
- Reveiz L, Cardona AF, Ospina EG. Antibiotics for acute laryngitis in adults. *Cochrane Database Syst Rev*. 2007;CD004783.
- Rosen CA, Anderson D, Murry T. Evaluating hoarseness: Keeping your patient's voice healthy. *Am Fam Physician*. 1998;57:2775–82.
- Wheeler DS, Dauplaise DJ, Giuliano JS. An infant with fever and stridor. *Pediatr Emerg Care*. 2008;24:46–9.

CODES

ICD9

- 464.00 Acute laryngitis without mention of obstruction
- 476.0 Chronic laryngitis

CLINICAL PEARLS

- Laryngitis is usually self-limited and needs only comfort care.
- Refer to ENT for direct visualization of vocal cords for prolonged laryngitis.
- Standard treatment is voice rest.

L

LAXATIVE ABUSE

Lauren Michal de Leon, MD
Edward Feller, MD

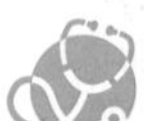

BASICS

DESCRIPTION
- Laxative abuse may be intentional or unintentional, and manifests commonly as watery diarrhea caused by self-medication or as apparent diarrhea caused by adding various fluids to stool:
  - Common cause of chronic diarrhea
- System(s) affected: Gastrointestinal; Nervous; Psychiatric
- Synonym(s): Factitious diarrhea; Cathartic colon; Münchausen syndrome (self or by proxy)—most dramatic form

EPIDEMIOLOGY
- Predominant age: 18–40 years with bulimia or anorexia nervosa; 40–60 years without eating disorders
- Common in the elderly (*unintentional*)
- Predominant sex (*intentional abuse*): Female (90%) > Male
- Children may be given excess laxation by caregivers (especially mothers), an example of Münchausen syndrome by proxy.
- May coexist with diverse manifestations of factitious illness (endocrine, skin, neurologic)

Prevalence
Laxative abuse in different groups (1):
- As many as 15% undergoing evaluation for chronic diarrhea
- Unexplained chronic diarrhea after routine investigations: 3.5–7%
- Patients with binging/purging anorexia and bulimia nervosa: As many as 70%
- Referrals to tertiary-care centers for evaluation of chronic diarrhea: As high as 15%
- Chronic use of constipating medications such as opioids

Geriatric Considerations
Elderly in nursing homes at increased risk for laxative overuse (usually inadvertent)

RISK FACTORS
In patients with eating disorders (2):
- Longer duration of illness
- Comorbid psychiatric diagnoses (e.g., major depression, obsessive–compulsive disorder, posttraumatic stress disorder, anxiety, borderline personality disorder)
- Early age of appearance of eating disorder symptoms

GENERAL PREVENTION
- Educate patients about normal bowel function, potential adverse effects of excessive laxation, and use of additional medications (e.g., magnesium-containing antacids) that can cause diarrhea.
- Ask patients specifically about laxative use. Inadvertent overuse is common.

ETIOLOGY
- Chronic ingestion of any laxative agent:
  - Osmotic diarrhea: Magnesium sulfate, nonabsorbable sugars, sodium phosphate
  - Secretory diarrhea: Dihydroxy bile salts, castor oil, docusate sodium
- Psychologic factors:
  - Bulimia or anorexia nervosa
  - Secondary gain of attention: Disability claims or need for concern, caring from others
  - Hysterical behavior
  - Inappropriate perceptions of "normal" bowel habits
  - Chronic constipation, especially in the elderly

COMMONLY ASSOCIATED CONDITIONS
- Anorexia nervosa; bulimia nervosa
- Use of constipating medications (opioids, iron supplements)
- Any chronic disorder associated with constipation
- Depression and anxiety
- Borderline personality
- Self-injurious behaviors/suicidal ideation
- Impulsive behavior
- Münchausen syndrome/Münchausen syndrome by proxy; may have associated factitious symptoms involving diverse organ systems

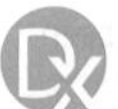

DIAGNOSIS

Chronic diarrhea can be characterized into 4 types: Secretory, osmotic, inflammatory, and fatty diarrhea. Be certain to rule out other causes of chronic diarrhea, even if laxative abuse is a high probability on the differential diagnosis list.

HISTORY
- Suspicion in patients with undiagnosed chronic diarrhea, especially when refractory; some patients may not be aware of the association of some over-the-counter medications with chronic diarrhea (3).
- Signs and symptoms: Increasing frequency of bowel movements; large volume, watery diarrhea; nocturnal bowel movements that are typically absent in osmotic diarrhea or in irritable bowel syndrome
- Additional symptoms: Abdominal pain, rectal pain, nausea, vomiting, weight loss, malaise, muscle weakness; be wary of chronic constipation with long-term laxative abuse.
- Additional signs: Hypokalemia, hyperphosphatemia, hypernatremia, skin pigmentation, finger clubbing, cyclic edema, kidney stones, melanosis coli, cardiac arrhythmias with severe hypokalemia
- Monitor "doctor hopping."

PHYSICAL EXAM
- No specific findings, but may include cachexia, evidence of dehydration, abdominal pain or distension, and edema; fever may be due to self-infected wounds or thermometer manipulation
- Bulimics or anorexics who purge may have Reynold sign (excoriation of fingers from repeated self-induced retching)
- Rarely, severe cases may be associated with renal failure, cardiac arrhythmias, skeletal muscle paralysis, signs of anemia from blood-letting or self-induced skin wounds.

DIAGNOSTIC TESTS & INTERPRETATION
Lab
- Serum chemistries: Hypokalemia, metabolic alkalosis (4)[C]
- Urinalysis: Bisacodyl, senna, cascara, magnesium, and phosphate titers
- Urine volume and electrolytes (help assess volume status and need for hospitalization)
- Stool sodium, potassium (see algorithm below); stool osmolality (some patients may exaggerate stool volume or add water or hypotonic urine)
- Stool pH (alkalinization suggests presence of phenolphthalein)
- Stool for laxative titers (bisacodyl, senna, cascara, magnesium, phosphate, castor oil, mineral oil)

Initial lab tests
- Serum electrolytes will show hypokalemia secondary to increased intestinal fluid loss:
  - Acute diarrhea: Metabolic acidosis due to hypovolemia
  - Chronic diarrhea: Metabolic alkalosis secondary to hypokalemia-induced inhibition of chloride uptake in the intestine, thereby inhibiting bicarbonate secretion
- CBC and stool cultures: Rule out infectious cause if history is suspicious.

Follow-Up & Special Considerations
If history and initial lab tests are suspicious for laxative abuse, the following algorithm can be used to confirm diagnosis and determine what type of laxative is being used (5):
- Collect 24-hour stool: If solid, workup is over.
- Calculate stool osmolality, stool electrolytes, and osmolal gap (= 290 – 2($Na^+ + K^+$), where Na^+ and K^+ are the concentrations from the stool sample):
  - If osmolality >400 mOsm/kg, rule out urine contamination of stool. Measure urea and creatinine of sample.
  - If osmolality <250–400 mOsm/kg, rule out water added to stool (colon cannot dilute stool to osmolality plasma).
  - If osmolality = 250–400 mOsm/kg, measure osmolal gap:
    - Gap >50: Unmeasured solute; check fecal fat and stool magnesium levels.
    - Gap <50: Rule out use of secretory laxative; urinalysis and stool analysis for laxative titers. Do not obtain serum laxative titers, as they peak 1–2 hours after ingestion. Urine titers can be 10 × as high as plasma titers.
- Thin-layer chromatography may produce false-positive tests for bisacodyl and false-negative tests for senna.
- Confirm diagnosis with multiple stool analyses before confronting patient with intentional use.

Imaging
- Not usually necessary for diagnosis of laxative abuse; colonoscopy, small-bowel endoscopy, or imaging studies may be needed to evaluate other causes of chronic diarrhea.
- Be cautious about perpetuating Münchausen syndrome through extensive workup.
- Melanosis coli on sigmoidoscopy may document overuse of anthracene laxatives.

Pathological Findings

- Melanosis coli: Dark-brown discoloration of colon with lymph patches visible through mucosa; also can be diagnosed by demonstrating pigment-containing macrophages in lamina propria; only occurs with abuse of anthraquinone-containing laxatives, such as senna or cascara.
- Cathartic colon: Refers to dilatation and ahaustral appearance of the atonic colon on barium enema or plain film; result of severe and prolonged laxative abuse

DIFFERENTIAL DIAGNOSIS

Any etiology of chronic diarrhea, especially in high-risk groups

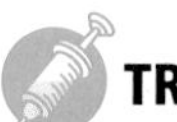

TREATMENT

MEDICATION

- Replace needed vitamins, electrolytes, and minerals (6).
- Nonstimulant laxatives if needed to treat constipation:
  - Senna best during pregnancy and lactation
  - Lactulose
  - High-fiber diet
- Avoid danthron due to hepatotoxicity.
- Precautions: Patients may be manipulative in attempts to deny problem; may hide laxatives in hospital rooms.
- Significant possible interactions:
  - Increased rate of intestinal motility may affect rate of absorption of medications (e.g., antibiotics, hormones).
  - Docusate sodium may potentiate hepatotoxicity of other drugs.

ADDITIONAL TREATMENT

General Measures

- Psychological support is essential.
- Confront the patient gently with support and understanding. Have a detailed plan for intervention and ongoing treatment.
- Wean patient off laxatives, and substitute high-fiber diet and bulk preparations or short-term saline enemas.
- Treat constipation.
- Treat metabolic abnormalities with potassium supplements, etc. (oral preferred).

Issues for Referral

In cases of Münchausen syndrome by proxy, legal proceedings must be considered, especially because most victims are children.

SURGERY/OTHER PROCEDURES

Avoid exploratory surgery and repetitive evaluations with invasive procedures.

IN-PATIENT CONSIDERATIONS

Admission Criteria

- Persistent diarrhea with evidence of hemodynamic instability
- Electrolyte/metabolic complications, including lactic acidosis
- Cardiac arrhythmias
- Inability to contract for safety

IV Fluids

Resuscitate based on clinical presentation. If patient is hemodynamically stable and without significant abnormalities in serum sodium, can give normal saline boluses or oral replacement to correct metabolic alkalosis (chronic) or acidosis (acute) as needed. If patient is hemodynamically unstable, treat volume status as in hypovolemic shock, while monitoring serum electrolytes closely (especially sodium, potassium, and bicarbonate).

Nursing

- If stable, patient does not need continuous telemetry. Depending on psychiatric history, patient may need constant observation. Special care must be taken to ensure adequate nutrition, discard laxatives. If patient is unstable, telemetry and appropriate vital-signs monitoring may be necessary.
- If surreptitious laxative ingestion is suspected, do not perform unauthorized room searches due to legal constraints.

Discharge Criteria

- Psychological support
- Diet and bowel programs

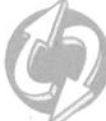

ONGOING CARE

FOLLOW-UP RECOMMENDATIONS

Patient Monitoring

- Careful psychological counseling
- Careful medical support; show concern by frequent visits as needed.
- Assess serum electrolytes.

DIET

Ensure good nutritional habits:

- Increase fiber intake.
- Adequate calories, especially with bulimia

PROGNOSIS

- Natural history is unclear, dependent on underlying cause.
- Prognosis related to psychological response in intentional abuse
- Prognosis poor with anorexia nervosa; very poor in Münchausen syndrome
- Cathartic colon commonly refractory to treatment

COMPLICATIONS

- Risk of multiple tests, procedures, and surgeries (intentional use)
- Malnutrition
- Electrolyte imbalances (hypokalemia)
- Renal failure
- Fatalities, especially in children given laxatives by parents; eating disorders
- Renal calculi
- Cathartic colon with constipation as a consequence of prolonged irritant laxative use. No diarrhea, fever, or blood loss.
- Fecal impaction in elderly
- Recurrences are common for factitious abuse, even after confrontation.

REFERENCES

1. Roerig JL, Steffen KJ, Mitchell JE, et al. Laxative abuse: Epidemiology, diagnosis and management. *Drugs*. 2010;70:1487–503.
2. Sim LA, McAlpine DE, Grothe KB, et al. Identification and management of eating disorders in the primary care setting. *Mayo Clin Proc*. 2010;85:746–51.
3. Toney RC, Agrawal RM. Medication induced constipation and diarrhea. *Pract Gastroenterol*. 2008;34:12–28.
4. Thomas PD, Forbes A, Green J, et al. Guidelines for the investigation of chronic diarrhoea, 2nd ed. *Gut*. 2003;52(Suppl 5):v1–15.
5. Shelton JH, Santa Ana CA, Thompson DR. Factitious diarrhea induced by stimulant laxatives: Accuracy of diagnosis by a clinical reference laboratory using thin layer chromatography. *Clin Chem*. 2007;53:85.
6. Kent AJ, Banks MR. Pharmacologic management of diarrhea. *Gastroenterol Clin N Am*. 2010;39: 495–507.

ADDITIONAL READING

- Kovacs D, Palmer RL. The associations between laxative abuse and other symptoms among adults with anorexia nervosa. *Int J Eat Disord*. 2004;36:224–8.
- Xing JH, Soffer EE. Adverse effects of laxatives. *Dis Colon Rectum*. 2001;44:1201–9.

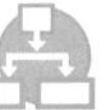

See Also (Topic, Algorithm, Electronic Media Element)

Algorithm: Diarrhea, Chronic

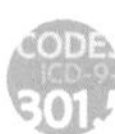

CODES

ICD9

- 305.90 Other, mixed, or unspecified drug abuse, unspecified use
- 307.51 Bulimia nervosa
- 564.89 Other functional disorders of intestine

CLINICAL PEARLS

- Laxative abuse may be intentional or unintentional; it is a common feature of eating disorders and has a female predilection.
- As many as 15% of patients referred to tertiary-care centers for unexplained chronic diarrhea abuse laxatives.
- Presentation is diverse and nonspecific, including weight loss, weakness, and hypotension without acknowledgment of diarrhea, when intentional.
- Consider the diagnosis in patients with watery diarrhea, especially when unexplained or refractory.

L

LEAD POISONING

Jason Chao, MD, MS

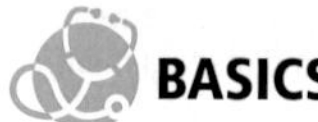

BASICS

DESCRIPTION

- Consequence of a high body burden of lead (Pb), an element with no known physiologic value
- Synonym(s): Lead poisoning, Inorganic

EPIDEMIOLOGY

- Predominant age: 1–5 years; adult workers
- Predominant sex: Male > Female (1:1 in childhood)

Prevalence

- Incidence of elevated lead levels declined steadily from 7.5% in 1997 to under 2% in 2006.
- 1999–2002: Centers for Disease Control (CDC) estimated that 1.6% of US children aged 1–5 years had blood Pb levels >10 μg/dL, but levels are variable among communities and populations.
- Sporadic cases in adults

RISK FACTORS

- Children with pica or with iron-deficiency anemia
- Residence in or frequent visitor to deteriorating pre-1960 housing with lead-painted surfaces
- Soil/dust near Pb industries or urban roads
- Sibling or playmate with Pb poisoning
- Dust from clothing of Pb worker
- Pb dissolved in water from Pb or Pb-soldered plumbing
- Pb-glazed ceramics, especially with acidic food or drink
- Recent refugee
- Folk remedies and cosmetics:
  - Mexico: Azarcon, greta
  - Dominican Republic: Litargirio, a topical agent
  - Asia and Middle East: Chuifong tokuwan, pay-loo-ah, ghasard, bali goli, kandu, ayurvedic herbal medicine from South Asia, kohl (alkohl, ceruse), surma, saoott, cebagin
- Hobbies: Glazed pottery making, target shooting, Pb soldering, preparing Pb shot or fishing sinkers, stained-glass making, car or boat repair, home remodeling
- Occupational exposure: Plumbers, pipe fitters, Pb miners, auto repairers, glass manufacturers, shipbuilders, printers, plastics manufacturers, Pb smelters and refiners, steel welders or cutters, construction workers, rubber product manufacturers, battery manufacturers, bridge reconstruction workers
- Dietary: Zinc or calcium deficiency
- Imported toys with Pb

Pediatric Considerations

- Children are at increased risk because of incomplete development of the blood–brain barrier at <3 years of age, allowing more Pb into the CNS; ingested Pb has 40% bioavailability in children compared with 10% in adults.
- Common childhood behaviors such as frequent hand-to-mouth activity and pica (repeated ingestion of nonfood products) greatly increase the risk of ingesting Pb.

GENERAL PREVENTION

- Family should receive counseling on potential sources of Pb and methods to decrease Pb exposure. Children at high risk should receive blood Pb screening (1)[C].
- Warn parents about the dangers posed by unsafe renovation methods and to be cognizant of the possibility of new and re-emerging sources of lead in children's environments.
- Wet mopping and dusting with a high-phosphate solution (e.g., powdered automatic dishwasher detergent with 1/4 cup/gal of water) will help to control Pb-bearing dust. But high-phosphate detergent is no longer available in some states.
- Pregnant women with community-specific or any individual risk factor for Pb poisoning should be screened for Pb toxicity (2)[C].

PATHOPHYSIOLOGY

Pb replaces calcium in bones. Pb interferes with heme synthesis; causes interstitial nephritis; and interferes with neurotransmitters, especially glutamine; high levels affect blood–brain barrier and lead to encephalopathy, seizures, and coma.

ETIOLOGY

Inhalation of Pb dust or fumes or ingestion of Pb

COMMONLY ASSOCIATED CONDITIONS

Iron-deficiency anemia

DIAGNOSIS

HISTORY

- Often asymptomatic
- Mild-to-moderate toxicity:
  - May cause myalgia or paresthesia, fatigue, irritability, lethargy
  - Abdominal discomfort, arthralgia, difficulty concentrating, headache, tremor, vomiting, weight loss, muscular exhaustibility
- Severe toxicity: 3 major clinical syndromes:
  - Alimentary type: Anorexia, metallic taste, constipation, severe abdominal cramps due to intestinal spasm and sometimes associated with abdominal wall rigidity
  - Neuromuscular type (characteristic of adult plumbism): Peripheral neuritis, usually painless and limited to extensor muscles
  - Cerebral type or Pb encephalopathy (more common in children): Seizures; coma; and long-term sequelae, including neurologic defects, retarded mental development, and chronic hyperactivity
- Chronic exposure may cause renal failure.

PHYSICAL EXAM

Often normal; abdominal tenderness may be severe. Neurologic exam may reveal neuropathy or encephalopathy.

DIAGNOSTIC TESTS & INTERPRETATION

Lab

- Blood Pb >10 μg/dL (0.48 μmol/L), collected with Pb-free container
- Use a laboratory that can achieve routine performance within 2 μg/dL.
- CDC Lead Poisoning Classification

Class	Lead (μg/dL)
I	<10
II	10–19
III	20–44
IV	45–69
V	>70

- Screening capillary Pb levels >10 μg/dL (0.48 μmol/L) should be confirmed with a venous sample.
- Hemoglobin and hematocrit slightly low; eosinophilia or basophilic stippling on peripheral smear may be seen but is not diagnostic of Pb toxicity.
- Renal function is decreased in late stages.

Imaging

- Abdominal radiograph for Pb particles in gut if recent ingestion is suspected
- Radiograph of long bones may show lines of increased density in the metaphyseal plate resulting from growth arrest, but does not usually alter management and is not routinely recommended.
- X-ray fluorescence for the total body burden of Pb is experimental.

DIFFERENTIAL DIAGNOSIS

- Alimentary type may be confused with acute abdomen.
- Neuromuscular type may be confused with other polyneuropathies.
- Cerebral type may be confused with ADD, mental retardation, autism, dementia, and other causes of seizures.
- Elevated erythrocyte protoporphyrin may be caused by iron-deficiency anemia or, less commonly, hemolytic anemia.
- Erythropoietic protoporphyria produces a very high erythrocyte protoporphyrin level.

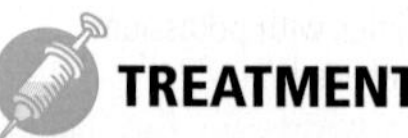

TREATMENT

- Class I: If Pb level is between 5 and 10 μg/dL, more frequent Pb screening (every 6 months) might be appropriate. Educate family on sources of Pb (3)[C].
- Class II: Repeat Pb testing in 1–3 months. Treat as class III if levels remain elevated (4)[C]. Educate family on sources of Pb.
- Classes III–V: Case report to local health department; complete inspection of home or workplace to determine source of Pb. Screen all family members. Consider chelation for class III; treat classes IV and V (4)[C].

MEDICATION

- Consider oral chelation for class IV; chelation (preferably parenteral) for class V or symptomatic class III or IV (4)[C].
- Do not begin chelation until Pb particles present in gut are cleared (4)[C].

First Line

- Oral chelation: Succimer (Chemet), dimercaptosuccinic acid (DMSA) 10 mg/kg q8h × 5 days; then 10 mg/kg q12h × 2 weeks. This may be repeated after 2 weeks off if Pb levels are not stabilized below 15 μg/dL (<0.72 μmol/L) (4)[C].
- Parenteral chelation (begin after establishment of adequate urine output):
  - Class V or symptomatic: Dimercaprol (British anti-Lewisite [BAL]) 75 mg/m^2 given deep IM; then BAL 450 mg/m^2/d divided q4h × 5 days plus Ca edetate calcium disodium (EDTA) 1,500 mg/m^2/d continuous IV infusion × 5 days. If rebound Pb level ≥45 μg/dL (≥2.17 μmol/L), chelation may be repeated after 2-day interval if symptomatic, after 5-day interval if asymptomatic.
  - Class IV asymptomatic: Ca EDTA 1,000 mg/m^2/d × 5 days; may be repeated after 5–7 days
- Diazepam for initial control of seizures; further control maintained with paraldehyde
- Contraindications: BAL should not be given to patients allergic to peanuts (the drug solution contains peanut oil).
- Precautions:
  - Succimer: GI upset, rash, nasal congestion, muscle pains, elevated liver function tests
  - Ca EDTA: Renal failure, increased excretion of zinc, copper, and iron
  - BAL: Nausea, vomiting, fever, headache, transient hypertension, hepatocellular damage
- Significant possible interactions:
  - Vitamins should not be given concurrently with oral chelation.
  - BAL may precipitate hemolytic crisis in a patient with glucose-6-phosphate dehydrogenase deficiency.

Second Line

Oral chelation with penicillamine (d-penicillamine, Depen, Cuprimine) (4)[C]:

- Penicillin-allergic patient should not receive penicillamine (cross-sensitivity is common).
- 10–15 mg/kg/d given b.i.d. mixed in apple juice/sauce on empty stomach (*not* approved by the FDA)
- Penicillamine may cause GI upset, renal failure, granulocytopenia, liver dysfunction, iron deficiency, and drug-induced lupuslike syndrome.

ADDITIONAL TREATMENT

Remove patient from potential source of Pb for class IV or V until complete home inspection is performed (5)[C].

Issues for Referral

Consider consultation if parenteral chelation is required.

IN-PATIENT CONSIDERATIONS

Initial Stabilization

Outpatient care unless parenteral chelation is required or immediate removal from contaminated environment

Admission Criteria

- Blood Pb level >70 μg/dL
- If symptomatic, blood Pb level >35 μg/dL

Discharge Criteria

If Pb source is in the home, the patient must reside elsewhere until the abatement process is completed.

ONGOING CARE

FOLLOW-UP RECOMMENDATIONS

Avoid visit to any site of potential contamination.

Patient Monitoring

- After chelation, check for rebound Pb level in 7–10 days. Follow with regular monitoring, initially biweekly or monthly.
- Correct iron deficiency or any other nutritional deficiencies present.
- For class II or higher, repeat testing every 3 months until class I level is achieved.

DIET

- If symptomatic, avoidance of excessive fluids
- Avoidance of pica
- Adequate calcium, iron, zinc, and vitamin C to reduce absorption and retention of Pb (6)[B]

PATIENT EDUCATION

- Needleman HL, Landrigan PJ. *Raising Children Toxic Free: How to Keep Your Child Safe from Lead, Asbestos, Pesticides, and Other Environmental Hazards*. New York: Avon Books; 1995.
- National Lead Information Center, 422 South Clinton Avenue, Rochester, NY 14620; (800) 424-5323; www.epa.gov/lead/
- National Safety Council, 1121 Spring Lake Drive, Itasca, IL 60143-3201; (800) 621-7615; www.nsc.org/news_resources/Resources/Documents/Lead_Poisoning.pdf

PROGNOSIS

- Symptomatic Pb poisoning without encephalopathy generally improves with chelation, but subtle CNS toxicity may be long-lasting or permanent.
- If encephalopathy occurs, permanent sequelae (e.g., mental retardation, seizure disorder, blindness, and hemiparesis) occurs in 25–50%.

COMPLICATIONS

- CNS toxicity may be long-lasting or permanent.
- Long-term Pb exposure may cause chronic renal failure (Fanconi-like syndrome), gout, or Pb line (blue–black) on gingival tissue.
- Pb exposure in pregnancy is associated with reduced birth weight and premature birth.
- Pb is an animal teratogen.

REFERENCES

1. Centers for Disease Control and Prevention. Recommendations for blood lead screening of Medicaid-eligible children aged 1–5 years: An updated approach to targeting a group at high risk. *MMWR*. 2009;58(No. RR-9):1–11.
2. Centers for Disease Control and Prevention. *Guidelines for the Identification and Management of Lead Exposure in Pregnant and Lactating Women*. U.S. Department of Health and Human Services. Atlanta, GA; November 2010.
3. Binns HJ, Campbell C, Brown MJ, et al. Interpreting and managing blood lead levels of less than 10 microg/dL in children and reducing childhood exposure to lead: Recommendations of the Centers for Disease Control and Prevention Advisory Committee on Childhood Lead Poisoning Prevention. *Pediatrics*. 2007;120:e1285–98.
4. American Academy of Pediatrics Committee on Drugs. Treatment Guidelines for Lead Exposure in Children. *Pediatrics*. 1995;96:155–60.
5. Centers for Disease Control and Prevention. *Managing Elevated Blood Lead Levels among Young Children: Recommendations from the Advisory Committee on Childhood Lead Poisoning Prevention*. Atlanta, GA: Centers for Disease Control and Prevention; 2002.
6. Woolf AD, Goldman R, Bellinger DC. Update on the clinical management of childhood lead poisoning. *Pediatr Clin North Am*. 2007;54:271–94, viii.

ADDITIONAL READING

- American Academy of Pediatrics Committee on Environmental Health. Lead exposure in children: Prevention, detection, and management. *Pediatrics*. 2005;116:1036–46.
- Chandramouli K, Steer CD, Ellis M, et al. Effects of early childhood lead exposure on academic performance and behaviour of school age children. *Arch Dis Child*. 2009;94:844–8.

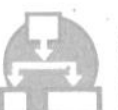

See Also (Topic, Algorithm, Electronic Media Element)

Anemia, Iron Deficiency

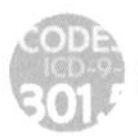

CODES

ICD9

- 984.0 Toxic effect of inorganic lead compounds
- 984.9 Toxic effect of unspecified lead compound

CLINICAL PEARLS

- The following children should have Pb screening:
  - 6–11 months of age with 1 or more risk factors:
    - Live in or visit a house built before 1960 with peeling paint or recent renovation
    - Sibling/playmate with elevated Pb
    - Live with adult with job or hobby involving Pb
    - Live near industry likely to release Pb
  - Children living in high-risk communities (>12% elevated Pb) should be tested yearly from ages 1–5.
  - Newly arrived refugees
  - Children in low-risk areas should be screened by a questionnaire.
- There is no clear safe Pb level. A level <10 μg/dL is used to define "normal," but there is increasing evidence that levels <10 μg/dL are detrimental to neural development in young children. Many experts are treating Pb levels >4 μg/dL as elevated.
- There are no studies that show benefit of chelation at asymptomatic class III. Removal of sources of Pb is paramount.

L

LEGG-CALVE-PERTHES DISEASE

Bryan G. Beutel, MD

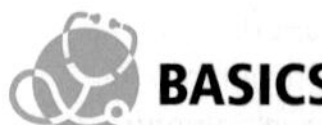

BASICS

DESCRIPTION

- Legg-Calve-Perthes disease (LCPD) defined as idiopathic ischemic osteonecrosis of the femoral head
- Leads to impaired growth of epiphysis and deformity of femoral head
- Occurs in pediatric patients
- Majority of cases are unilateral. 10% of cases are bilateral, but generally do not occur simultaneously.
- System(s) affected: Musculoskeletal

EPIDEMIOLOGY

- Predominant age: Susceptible age is 2–12 years. However, ~80% occur between the ages of 4 and 9 years.
- Predominant sex: Males > Females (4:1)
- In bilateral cases, males predominate (7:1). However, females seem to have more severe involvement.

Incidence

Annual international incidence of ~1:1,200

Prevalence

~5:100,000

RISK FACTORS

Increased risk in children with:

- Low birth weight
- Factors predisposing to thrombophilia (e.g., Factor V Leiden deficiency, protein C or S deficiency, etc.)
- Lower socioeconomic status
- ADD
- Exposure to secondhand smoke
- Caucasian or Asian ethnicity

Genetics

No specific gene locus has been identified for LCPD. Avascular necrosis of femoral head (unrelated to LCPD) may develop sporadically or as autosomal-dominant disorder with type II collagen mutation.

GENERAL PREVENTION

Since etiology is not clearly understood, prevention is challenging.

ETIOLOGY

- Generally idiopathic, but may be due to trauma, sickle-cell crisis, congenital dislocation of the hip, toxic synovitis
- It is hypothesized that the interruption of the blood supply to the femoral epiphysis is an important factor causing femoral head osteonecrosis in the early stages of LCPD. Other sources, in addition to the epiphyseal vasculature, supply the proximal femoral growth plate (1)[B].
- Deformity may result from growth arrest of the capital femoral epiphysis and physis, asymmetric repair, iatrogenic causes, or devitalized articular cartilage and weakening mechanical properties of bone leading to trabecular collapse (2)[B].

COMMONLY ASSOCIATED CONDITIONS

- Short stature
- Delayed bone age (observed in 89% of LCPD patients)
- Possible association with hypercoagulable states (see "Risk Factors")

DIAGNOSIS

HISTORY

- Typically, there is an insidious onset with no known trauma or injury. A traumatic event, however, may exacerbate or unveil symptomatology.
- Pain primarily localized to the hip or groin, although referred pain to the medial portion of the ipsilateral knee and lateral thigh is not uncommon.
- May report symptoms in 1 or both hips. Bilateral cases usually do not become symptomatic at the same time.

PHYSICAL EXAM

- Commonly presents with a limp/antalgic gait
- Short, thin stature is common.
- Leg-length discrepancy secondary to collapse of the femoral head or adduction contracture
- Limited range of motion (ROM), especially in internal rotation and abduction
- Possible hip flexion contracture (10–20°)
- Atrophy of thigh, gluteus, calf musculature may be present secondary to disuse due to pain

DIAGNOSTIC TESTS & INTERPRETATION

Lab

- CBC with differential to rule out infection, if suspected
- ESR to rule out infection, if suspected

Imaging

- Serial radiographs (anteroposterior [AP] and frog-leg lateral) of the pelvis are essential for determining extent of involvement and progression of healing. Catterall, Salter-Thompson, and Herring (Lateral Pillar) are the 3 most commonly used radiographic classification systems for LCPD. The Lateral Pillar classification may be the most reliable and easiest to implement (3)[B]:
  - Catterall: 4-group classification, based upon radiographic signs and degree of capital femoral epiphysis involvement
  - Salter-Thompson: 2-group system, based upon degree of subchondral fracture/resorption
  - Herring (Lateral Pillar): 3-group classification, based upon femoral head shape and degree of lateral pillar involvement
- Radiographs demonstrate progression of disease: Arrest of femoral epiphyseal growth, subchondral fracture, resorption, reossification, then healed state
- Full extent of involvement may not be evident for several months because radiographic findings lag symptoms.
- MRI is most sensitive test; facilitates early diagnosis of necrosis and visualization of articular surface (4)[B]:
  - Does not, generally, accurately depict healing process
- Dynamic arthrography is used to assess congruency of femoral head; may demonstrate flattening of femoral head and hinge abduction
- Radionuclide (technetium[99]) bone scan may be helpful in delineating the extent of avascular changes.

Diagnostic Procedures/Surgery

Hip joint aspiration to rule out septic arthritis if clinical suspicion of infection exists

Pathological Findings

- Early (necrosis, resorption) stage:
  - Inflammation leads to widening of distance between acetabulum and femoral head.
  - Necrosis of bone with subchondral bone fracture and subsequent collapse
- Late (healing) stage: Revascularization by creeping substitution of necrotic bone and reconstitution of femoral head

DIFFERENTIAL DIAGNOSIS

- Unilateral:
  - Septic arthritis
  - Osteomyelitis
  - Juvenile rheumatoid arthritis
  - Toxic synovitis
  - Slipped capital femoral epiphysis
  - Neoplasm
  - Abscess of psoas muscle
- Bilateral:
  - Spondyloepiphyseal dysplasia
  - Metaphyseal dysplasia
- Other: Hypothyroidism

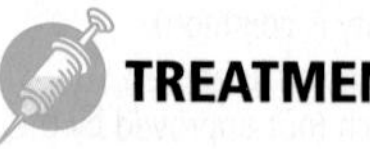

TREATMENT

- Depending upon the severity of the disease, the treatment options range from observation and frequent follow-up to reconstructive hip surgery (5)[B].
- The evidence that supports conservative treatment for children with LCPD is not of high quality. However, there is no scientific evidence that conservative treatments modify the natural history of LCPD (6)[B].

MEDICATION

First Line

Ibuprofen 10 mg/kg PO t.i.d.–q.i.d. to reduce inflammation and pain symptomatology:

- Contraindications: Allergy to ibuprofen
- Precautions: GI irritation or bleeding

Second Line

Acetaminophen as needed for pain relief

ADDITIONAL TREATMENT

General Measures

Primary goals of treatment:

- Relieve weightbearing across affected hip, thereby reducing irritability of the hip.
- Obtain and maintain hip range of motion (7)[B].
- Maximize regeneration and spherical development of the femoral head by containing the femoral epiphysis within the acetabulum (7)[B].

Issues for Referral

Baseline pediatric orthopedic surgery referral is recommended.

Additional Therapies

- Physical therapy may be prescribed by pediatric orthopedist to maintain hip motion.
- Bed rest and traction for short period if severe pain
- Maintain internal rotation and abduction of hip to keep femoral head reduced in acetabulum:
  - Orthotic devices and braces achieve this containment.

SURGERY/OTHER PROCEDURES

- Surgical outcome depends on age at presentation and severity of disease at the time of surgery (8)[A]:
  - Children over 8 years of age at time of onset of LCPD with over 50% of lateral pillar height maintained have superior outcomes with surgical than nonsurgical interventions (9)[B].
- Adductor tenotomy may be used to help restore ROM secondary to adductor contracture (10)[B].
- Femoral and/or pelvic osteotomy may be used to help contain femoral epiphysis within the confines of the acetabulum (in older children or in cases of hip subluxation) (10)[B]:
  - Varus osteotomy of proximal femur most common
  - Pelvic osteotomies include: Shelf operation, acetabular rotational osteotomy, medial displacement/Chiari osteotomy
  - Triple pelvic osteotomy is effective option for patients with >50% lateral pillar height maintained or younger patients with <50% maintained (11)[C]
- Percutaneous innominate pelvic osteotomy without the use of bone graft may be a less aggressive alternative (12)[C].
- Arthrodiastasis (procedure for distracting joint surface while preserving mobility) effective in patients <8 years of age (13)[C]

IN-PATIENT CONSIDERATIONS

Initial Stabilization

- Pediatric orthopedic consultation
- Ambulatory treatment is typical; however, some patients may require inpatient traction or surgical procedures.

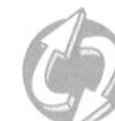

ONGOING CARE

FOLLOW-UP RECOMMENDATIONS

- Ambulatory status dependent upon extent/stage of disease
- Limit weightbearing in cases of hip irritation.

Patient Monitoring

- Initially, close pediatric orthopedic follow-up, including radiographic evaluation, is needed to determine extent of necrosis.
- Once healing phase is entered, follow-up can be incremental (every 6 months).
- Long-term follow-up is necessary to determine final outcome.

DIET

Avoid obesity, as the hip is a weightbearing joint.

PROGNOSIS

- Most patients have a favorable outcome.
- Outcome depends on patient's age at the time of diagnosis (the younger, the better).
- Prognosis also is related to the degree of involvement of the femoral head (as determined by radiography).
- The 4 main prognostic factors are:
  - Patient's age at the onset of the disease
  - Degree of limitation of range of motion
  - Extent of involvement of the femoral epiphysis
  - Any additional radiographic "head-at-risk" signs (e.g., calcification lateral to epiphysis, horizontal physis, radiolucency in lateral epiphysis/ metaphysis, etc.) (5)

COMPLICATIONS

- Permanent distortion of the femoral head
- Distorted joint prone to early degenerative joint disease (osteoarthritis):
  - Most notably due to irregularly contoured femoral head, flattening of acetabular wall
- Limb-length discrepancy leading to chronic limp

REFERENCES

1. Kim HK, Stephenson N, Garces A, et al. Effects of disruption of epiphyseal vasculature on the proximal femoral growth plate. *J Bone Joint Surg Am*. 2009;91(5):1149–58.
2. Koob TJ, Pringle D, Gedbaw E, et al. Biomechanical properties of bone and cartilage in growing femoral head following ischemic osteonecrosis. *J Orthop Res*. 2007;25:750–7.
3. Mahadeva D, Chong M, Langton DJ, et al. Reliability and reproducibility of classification systems for Legg-Calvé-Perthes disease: A systematic review of the literature. *Acta Orthop Belg*. 2010;76:48–57.
4. Dillman JR, Hernandez RJ, et al. MRI of Legg-Calve-Perthes disease. *AJR Am J Roentgenol*. 2009;193:1394–407.
5. Nelitz M, Lippacher S, Krauspe R, et al. Perthes disease: Current principles of diagnosis and treatment. *Dtsch Arztebl Int*. 2009;106: 517–23.
6. Sinigaglia R, Bundy A, Okoro T, et al. Is conservative treatment really effective for Legg-Calvé-Perthes disease? A critical review of the literature. *Chir Narzadow Ruchu Ortop Pol*. 2007;72:439–43.
7. Thompson GH, Price CT, Roy D, et al. Legg-Calvé-Perthes disease: Current concepts. *Instr Course Lect*. 2002;51:367–84.
8. Grzegorzewski A, Kozlowski P, Szymczak W, et al. Leg length discrepancy in Legg-Calve-Perthes disease. *J Pediatr Orthop*. 2005;2005:206–9.
9. Herring JA, Kim HT, Browne R. Legg-Calve-Perthes disease. Part II: Prospective multicenter study of the effect of treatment on outcome. *J Bone Joint Surg Am*. 2004;86-A(10): 2121–34.
10. Herring JA. The treatment of Legg-Calve-Perthes disease. A critical review of the literature. *J Bone Joint Surg Am*. 1998;73A:448–458.
11. Wenger DR, Pring ME, Hosalkar HS, et al. Advanced containment methods for Legg-Calve-Perthes disease: Results of triple pelvic osteotomy. *J Pediatr Orthop*. 2010;30(8): 749–57.
12. Sanchez Mesa PA, Yamhure FH, et al. Percutaneous innominate pelvic osteotomy without the use of bone graft for femoral head coverage in children 2–8 years of age. *J Pediatr Orthop B*. 2010;19:256–63.
13. Aly TA, Amin OA, et al. Arthrodiastasis for the treatment of Perthes' disease. *Orthopedics*. 2009;32:817.

ADDITIONAL READING

Lee MC, Eberson CP, et al. Growth and development of the child's hip. *Orthop Clin North Am*. 2006;37: 119–32, v.

CODES

ICD9

732.1 Juvenile osteochondrosis of hip and pelvis

CLINICAL PEARLS

- LCPD is a common cause of hip pain in children.
- In the setting of a pediatric patient presenting with knee pain, always examine the hip joint.
- Serial radiographs (with application of an appropriate classification scheme) necessary for diagnosis and monitoring of disease course
- Obtain pediatric orthopedic surgery consultation.
- Surgical outcome depends on age at presentation and severity of disease at the time of surgery.

L

LEGIONNAIRES' DISEASE

Kristen Koenig, MD, CPT, MC
Major Dena George, MD

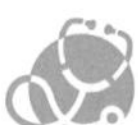

BASICS

DESCRIPTION

- The term *Legionnaires' disease* was coined for an epidemic of lower respiratory tract disease occurring among people attending an American Legion convention in Philadelphia in 1976. Until this outbreak, the causative bacteria was unknown. It was isolated, identified, and named *Legionella pneumophila*, due to its ability to cause pneumonia and flulike illnesses. The bacteria inhabit manmade water system in hotels, hospitals, and air conditioning cooling towers:
  - Ranks among the 3 most common pneumonias in the clinical setting
  - Most common atypical pneumonia
- System(s) affected: Gastrointestinal; Pulmonary
- Synonym(s): Legionella pneumonia; Legionellosis

EPIDEMIOLOGY

- Predominant age: 15 months–84 years old; increased >50 years old
- Predominant gender: Male > Female

Incidence

- Reported cases increased from 1,310 in 2002, to 2,223 in 2003, with >2,000 cases per year from 2003–2005
- Outbreaks occur most often at the end of the summer and early fall.

RISK FACTORS

- Impaired cellular immunity (*Legionella* are intracellular pathogens)
- Smoking
- Alcohol abuse
- Immunosuppression/HIV
- Chronic cardiopulmonary disease
- Surgery
- Advanced age
- Transplant recipients

GENERAL PREVENTION

- *Not transmitted person to person* (isolation is unnecessary)
- Superheat and flush water systems: Water is heated to 70°C, and distal outlets are flushed with hot water for 30 minutes.
- Ultraviolet light or copper-silver ionization are bactericidal.
- Monochloramine disinfection of municipal water supplies is associated with decreased risk for *Legionella* infection (1)[B].

ETIOLOGY

- *Legionella pneumophila*, a weak gram-negative aerobic organism, is a saprophytic freshwater bacterium, widely distributed in soil and water. Bacteria are motile by bipolar flagella. Optimum temperature for growth is 40–45°C.
- Exists as an intracellular parasite of protozoa, colonizes surfaces and grows in biofilms, which persist in nematodes
- Serogroups 1–6 account for cases of disease.
- In the lung, *Legionella* infects alveolar macrophages.
- Mode of transmission:
  - Aspiration
  - Direct transmission into the lungs by equipment, such as respiratory equipment
  - Most important mode: Aerosolization and airborne dissemination of contaminated water, such as inhaling organisms while showering
- Recently, community outbreaks have been associated with whirlpools, spas, and fountains.
- Not spread between humans

COMMONLY ASSOCIATED CONDITIONS

Pontiac fever: Self-limited flulike illness without pneumonia caused by *Legionella* species

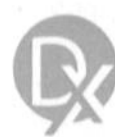

DIAGNOSIS

- Range of illness from asymptomatic seroconversion, mild febrile illness, to severe pneumonia
- Wound infections with *Legionella* have been reported.
- Incubation period of 2–10 days

HISTORY

- Signs and symptoms (percentage that can be affected):
  - Dry cough (92%), which may become productive
  - Fever/chills (90%)
  - Dyspnea (62%)
  - Pleuritic chest pain (35%)
  - Headache (48%)
  - Myalgia/arthralgia (40%)
  - Watery diarrhea (50%)
  - Nausea and vomiting (49%)
  - Neuropsychiatric symptoms of confusion, disorientation, obtundation, depression, hallucinations, insomnia, seizure
- History:
  - Identify immunosuppression risk factors.

PHYSICAL EXAM

- Fever
- Relative bradycardia
- Rales on lung auscultation with signs of consolidation

DIAGNOSTIC TESTS & INTERPRETATION

Lab

Initial lab tests

- Diagnosis:
  - Gold standard is sputum culture for *Legionella*. Alert lab about possible diagnosis (sample needs buffered charcoal yeast extract agar) (2)[C]. This method has variable sensitivity (10–80%) (3), and is time consuming (up to 7 days for results). Another difficulty is that <50% of patients produce sputum.
  - Serology has a sensitivity of 41–94% (3):
    - Its primary limitation is that an increase in antibody titer cannot be detected prior to 3–4 weeks, and is not useful in early stages of the disease.
  - Urinary antigen detects serogroup 1, which causes most human disease (2,3)[A]. Urinary antigen tests are highly specific (99%) but variably sensitive (3,4)[A]. *Legionella* antigenuria can be detected within 1–2 days after onset of disease and persists for days to weeks. It is limited by the fact that it only detects serogroup 1, and it is estimated that it may miss up to 40% of cases.
  - The combination of respiratory specimen cultures and urine *Legionella* antigen testing are optimal for diagnosis.
  - Silver and Gimenez stains are used for lung tissue/specimens.
  - Disorders that may alter lab results: Direct immunofluorescence can cross-react with *Pseudomonas* and *Bacteroides* sp., *E. coli*, and *Haemophilus*.
- Other lab abnormalities, notable because these are not seen with other forms of pneumonia:
  - Hyponatremia
  - Hypophosphatemia
  - Mildly elevated serum transaminases
  - Elevated creatinine kinase
  - Microscopic hematuria
  - Highly elevated CRP
  - Highly elevated ferritin

Imaging

Initial approach

Chest radiograph (5)[B]:

- Not specific for *Legionella*
- Commonly shows lower lobe patchy alveolar infiltrate with consolidation, usually unilateral
- Cavitation or abscess formation, more common in immunocompromised
- Pleural effusion in up to 50%
- May take from 1–4 months for the radiograph to return to normal. Progression of infiltrate on x-ray can be seen despite antibiotic therapy.

Diagnostic Procedures/Surgery

Transtracheal aspiration or bronchoscopy for sputum/lung samples may be needed.

Pathological Findings

- Multifocal pneumonia with alveolitis and bronchiolitis, with fibrinous pleuritis; may have serous or serosanguineous pleural effusion
- Abscess formation occurs in up to 20% of patients.
- Progression of infiltrates, despite appropriate therapy, may be suggestive of Legionnaires' disease. Also, improvement on radiograph may not correlate with clinical findings (longer lag times on radiographic findings).

DIFFERENTIAL DIAGNOSIS

- Other bacterial pneumonias, especially atypical pneumonias such as *Mycoplasma pneumonia*, Q fever (*Coxiella burnetii*), *Chlamydophila pneumoniae*, *C. psittaci*, *Francisella tularensis*
- Viral pneumonias, especially adenovirus, influenza, CMV

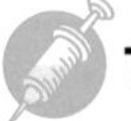

TREATMENT

MEDICATION

First Line

- Antibiotics that achieve high intracellular concentrations are most effective. first-line treatment is levofloxacin (6,7,8)[B]; however, there are no prospective randomized controlled trials comparing fluoroquinolones to macrolides for the treatment of *Legionella*. In retrospective and observational studies, levofloxacin has been shown to result in more rapid defervescence, result in fewer complications, and decrease hospital stay compared to macrolide antibiotics. Antibiotics should be initiated via the parenteral route due to the GI symptoms associated with *Legionella*:
  - Levofloxacin is the preferred agent (6,7,8)[B]:
    - Levofloxacin 750 mg/d IV (switch to PO when patient is afebrile/tolerating PO) for 10–14 days
  - Azithromycin may also be used first line (6,7)[B]. It requires a shorter duration of treatment than levofloxacin due to a longer half-life:
    - Azithromycin 500 mg/d IV (switch to PO when afebrile/tolerating PO) for 7–10 days
- Contraindications: Hypersensitivity reactions
- Precautions: Liver disease
- Significant possible interactions:
  - Can increase theophylline, carbamazepine, and digoxin levels; can increase activity of oral anticoagulants
  - May decrease the effectiveness of oral anticoagulants, steroids, digoxin, quinidine, oral contraceptives, and hypoglycemic agents
- Longer courses of treatment (up to 21 days) may be needed in immunocompromised patients.

Second Line

- Doxycycline 200 mg IV/PO q12h for 72 hours, then 100 mg IV/PO q12h for total 14 days
- Doxycycline cannot be used in pregnant patients and is not approved for children under 8 years of age.

ADDITIONAL TREATMENT

General Measures

- The severity of the illness and the support available in the outpatient setting will dictate the appropriate site for care.
- Supportive care:
  - Oxygenation, hydration, and electrolyte balance with antibiotic therapy
- Extrapulmonary complications and higher mortality rate occur with AIDS patients.

IN-PATIENT CONSIDERATIONS

Admission Criteria

- Inability to tolerate oral antibiotics
- Hypoxemia

Discharge Criteria

- Afebrile
- Able to tolerate oral antibiotics
- Normal oxygen saturation

ONGOING CARE

FOLLOW-UP RECOMMENDATIONS

Patient Monitoring

- Respiratory status, hydration, and electrolyte status should be monitored closely.
- A chest radiograph is not useful to monitor the clinical response.

PATIENT EDUCATION

- Educate patients regarding prevention/avoidance measures, risk reduction, the expected disease progression, and the lack of person-to-person transmission.
- Disease prevention: Elimination of the pathogens from water supplies

PROGNOSIS

- Recovery is variable; some patients experience rapid improvement with defervescence in 3–5 days and recovery is complete in 6–10 days, whereas others may have a much more protracted course despite treatment.
- Mortality rate can approach 50% with nosocomial infections.

COMPLICATIONS

- Dehydration
- Hyponatremia
- Respiratory insufficiency requiring ventilator support
- Bacteremia or abscess formation in immunocompromised patients
- Extrapulmonary disease can occur in the form of:
  - Encephalitis
  - Cellulitis
  - Sinusitis
  - Pancreatitis
  - Pyelonephritis
  - Endocarditis (most common extrapulmonary site)
  - Pericarditis
  - Perirectal abscess
- Renal failure
- Disseminated intravascular coagulation
- Multiple organ dysfunction syndrome (MODS)
- Coma
- Death occurs in 10% of treated immunocompetent patients, and in up to 80% of untreated immunocompromised patients.

REFERENCES

1. Flannery B, Gelling LB, Vugia DJ, et al. Reducing Legionella colonization in water systems with monochloramine. *Emerg Infect Dis*. 2006;12: 588–96.
2. Yzerman EP, den Boer JW, Lettinga KD, et al. Sensitivity of three urinary antigen tests associated with clinical severity in a large outbreak of Legionnaires' disease in The Netherlands. *J Clin Microbiol*. 2002;40:3232–6.
3. Tronel H, Hartemann P. Overview of diagnostic and detection methods for legionellosis and *Legionella* spp. *Lett Appl Microbiol*. 2009;48(6):653–6.
4. Shimada T, Noguchi Y, Jackson JL, et al. Systemic review and metaanalysis: Urinary antigen tests for legionellosis. *Chest*. 2009.
5. Tan MJ, Tan JS, Hamor RH, et al. The radiologic manifestations of Legionnaire's disease. The Ohio Community-Based Pneumonia Incidence Study Group. *Chest*. 2000;117:398–403.
6. Blázquez Garrido RM, Espinosa Parra FJ, et al. Antimicrobial chemotherapy for Legionnaires disease: Levofloxacin versus macrolides. *Clin Infect Dis*. 2005;40:800–6.
7. Mykietiuk A, Carratala J, Fernandez-Sabe N, et al. Clinical Outcomes for hospitalized patients with *Legionella* pneumonia in the antigenuria era: The influence of levoflaxacin therapy. *CID*. 2005(40): 794–9.
8. Sabria M, Pedro-Botet ML, Gomez J, et al. Fluoroquinolones vs macrolides in the treatment of Legionnaires disease. *Chest*. 2005;(128):1401–5.

ADDITIONAL READING

- *Committee on Infectious Diseases of American Academy of Pediatrics*. *Red Book*. Elk Grove Village: American Academy of Pediatrics; 2009.
- Cunha BA. Legionnaire's disease: Clinical differentiation from typical and other atypical pneumonias. *Infect Dis Clin N Am*. 2010;24:73–105.
- Hilbi H, Jarraud S, Hartland E, Buchrieser C. Update on Legionnaires' disease: pathogenosis, epidemiology, detection and control. *Molecular Microbiology*. 2010;76(1):1–11.
- Mandell LA, Wunderink RG, Anzueto A, et al. Infectious Diseases Society of America/American Thoracic Society Consensus Guidelines on the Management of Community-Acquired Pneumonia in Adults. *Clin Inf Dis*. 2007;44:S27–72.

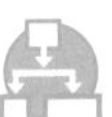

See Also (Topic, Algorithm, Electronic Media Element)

Pneumonia, Bacterial

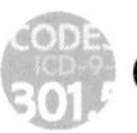

CODES

ICD9

482.84 Pneumonia due to Legionnaires' disease

CLINICAL PEARLS

- Consider Legionnaires disease in pneumonia in presence of GI symptoms, especially diarrhea; neurologic findings, especially confusion; fever >39°C; Gram stain of respiratory secretions with many neutrophils but few organisms; hyponatremia.
- Consider Legionnaires' disease in nosocomial pneumonia.
- Because an increase in *Legionella* antibody titers cannot be detected prior to 3–4 weeks, serology is not useful in early stages of the disease.
- The combination of respiratory specimen cultures and urine *Legionella* antigen testing are optimal for diagnosis.

The views expressed in this chapter are those of the author and do not reflect the official policy or position of the Department of the Army, Department of Defense, or the US government. Opinions, interpretations, conclusions, and recommendations herein are those of the author and are not necessarily endorsed by the US Army.

LEUKEMIA, ACUTE LYMPHOBLASTIC IN ADULTS (ALL)

Richard A. Larson, MD

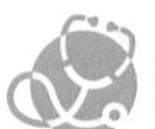

BASICS

DESCRIPTION
- ALL in adults is a malignant proliferation and accumulation of immature lymphocytes.
- System(s) affected: Hemic/Lymphatic/Immunologic
- Synonym(s): Acute lymphocytic leukemia

Pregnancy Considerations
Many chemotherapy drugs are teratogenic.

EPIDEMIOLOGY
- Predominant age: Median age, 35–40 years; incidence increases with age.
- Predominant sex: Male > Female (slightly)

Incidence
In the US: 1,000 adult cases per year

RISK FACTORS
- Age >60 years
- Incidence seems to increase after exposure to chemical agents, such as benzene, or to radiation, but acute myeloid leukemia (AML) is more common.
- May follow aplastic anemia

Genetics
- Increased incidence in children with Down syndrome or in rare familial diseases such as ataxia-telangiectasia, Bloom syndrome, Fanconi anemia, Klinefelter syndrome, and neurofibromatosis
- Can rarely occur in adult identical twins

ETIOLOGY
- Unknown
- Epstein-Barr virus is implicated in Burkitt leukemia/lymphoma.

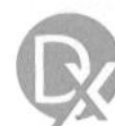

DIAGNOSIS

HISTORY
- Anemia: Fatigue, shortness of breath, lightheadedness, angina, headache
- Thrombocytopenia: Easy bruising
- Neutrocytopenia: Fever, infection
- Lymphocytosis: Bone pain
- CNS: Confusion

PHYSICAL EXAM
- Thrombocytopenia: Petechiae, ecchymoses, epistaxis, retinal hemorrhages
- Anemia: Pallor
- Neutrocytopenia: Fever, infection
- Lymphocytosis: Lymphadenopathy, splenomegaly; less often, hepatomegaly
- CNS: Cranial nerve palsies, confusion

DIAGNOSTIC TESTS & INTERPRETATION

Lab

Initial lab tests

CBC with differential, liver function tests, uric acid, ESR, or C-reactive protein:
- Anemia: Normochromic, normocytic
- Thrombocytopenia
- Peripheral blood lymphoblasts
- Elevated lactate dehydrogenase
- Elevated uric acid

Follow-Up & Special Considerations

Special tests:
- Immunophenotyping of marrow/blood lymphoblasts: B-lineage (CD19, CD20, CD24); T-lineage (CD2, CD5, CD7); common ALL antigen (CD10); human leukocyte antigen (HLA)-DR; terminal deoxynucleotidyl transferase (TdT); aberrant myeloid antigens (CD13, CD33); stem cell antigen (CD34)
- Cytochemical stains: Myeloperoxidase, negative; Sudan black B, usually negative; TdT, positive; periodic acid Schiff, ± is variable, depending on subtype:
  - Cytogenetics: Specific recurring chromosomal abnormalities have independent diagnostic and prognostic significance (hyperdiploidy >50 chromosomes or t(14q11q13) are favorable; the Philadelphia chromosome, t[9;22], t[4;11], −7 and +8 are unfavorable). A translocation t(8;14) or t(2;8) or t(8;22) identifies Burkitt-type leukemia that requires specific therapy.
  - Reverse transcription polymerase chain reaction for rapid diagnosis of BCR/ABL + ALL
  - HLA typing of patient and siblings for hematopoietic cell transplantation

Imaging
- Chest radiograph to evaluate for mediastinal mass or hilar adenopathy and for pulmonary infiltrates suggestive of infection
- Ultrasound exam to assess splenomegaly or renal enlargement suggestive of leukemic infiltration

Diagnostic Procedures/Surgery
- Bone marrow examination with aspiration, biopsy, immunophenotyping, cytochemistry, and cytogenetics
- Lymph node biopsy is rarely necessary but can be diagnostic.
- Lumbar puncture is typically done both for diagnosis of CNS involvement and for intrathecal treatment. It should be done if neurological symptoms or signs are present. Repeat lumbar puncture after bone marrow remission is achieved to evaluate occult CNS involvement, and continue prophylactic CNS treatment.

Pathological Findings
Diffuse replacement of marrow and lymph node architecture by sheets of malignant lymphoblasts

DIFFERENTIAL DIAGNOSIS
- Malignant disorders: Other leukemias, especially AML; chronic myeloid leukemia in lymphoid blast phase; prolymphocytic leukemia; malignant lymphomas; multiple myeloma; bone marrow metastases from solid tumors (breast, prostate, lung, renal); myelodysplastic syndromes (1)[A]
- Nonmalignant disorders: Aplastic anemia; myelofibrosis; autoimmune diseases (Felty syndrome, lupus); infectious mononucleosis; pertussis; autoimmune thrombocytopenic purpura; leukemoid reaction to infection

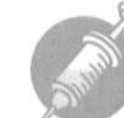

TREATMENT

MEDICATION

First Line
Optimal therapy is not yet known (1,2)[A]. ALL should be treated at a comprehensive oncology center. All treatment regimens are still investigational, but clearly effective for some fraction of patients. Cancer and Leukemia Group B protocol 9111 is an example of therapy (3)[A]:
- Remission induction:
  - Cyclophosphamide: 1,200 mg/m^2 IV on day 1 (800 mg/m^2 if >60 years old)
  - Daunorubicin: 45 mg/m^2 IV on days 1, 2, and 3 (30 mg/m^2 if >60 years old)
  - Vincristine: 2 mg IV on days 1, 8, 15, and 22
  - Asparaginase (L-asparaginase): 6,000 units/m^2 SC or IM on days 5, 8, 11, 15, 18, and 22
  - Prednisone: 60 mg/m^2 on days 1–21 (days 1–7 if >60 years old)
  - Filgrastim, G-CSF: 5 μg/kg/d SC starting on day 4 has been shown to shorten the duration of neutropenia and improve the complete remission rate, especially in older patients.
  - Imatinib mesylate: 600–800 mg/d is effective alone and in combination with chemotherapy for Philadelphia chromosome–positive ALL (4)[B].
- Consolidation (repeat twice in 8 weeks):
  - Cyclophosphamide: 1,000 mg/m^2 IV on day 1
  - Intrathecal (IT) methotrexate: 15 mg with hydrocortisone 50 mg on day 1
  - Mercaptopurine (6-mercaptopurine): 60 mg/m^2 on days 1–14
  - Cytarabine: 75 mg/m^2 SC on days 1–4 and 8–11
  - Vincristine: 2 mg IV on days 15 and 22
  - Asparaginase: 6,000 U/m^2 SC or IM on days 15, 18, 22, and 25
- CNS prophylaxis and interim maintenance—2,400 cGy cranial irradiation:
  - IT-methotrexate: 15 mg with hydrocortisone 50 mg on days 1, 8, 15, 22, and 29
  - Mercaptopurine (6-mercaptopurine): 60 mg/m^2 on days 1–70, taken in the evening
  - Oral methotrexate: 20 mg/m^2 on days 36, 43, 50, 57, and 64
- Late intensification:
  - Doxorubicin: 30 mg/m^2 IV on days 1, 8, and 15
  - Vincristine: 2 mg IV on days 1, 8, and 15
  - Dexamethasone: 10 mg/m^2 on days 1–14
  - Cyclophosphamide: 1,000 mg/m^2 IV on day 29
  - Thioguanine (6-thioguanine): 60 mg/m^2 on days 29–42
  - Cytarabine: 75 mg/m^2 SC on days 29–32 and 36–39
- Prolonged maintenance:
  - Vincristine: 2 mg/mo IV for 16 months
  - Prednisone: 60 mg/m^2 for 5 days with the vincristine
  - Mercaptopurine (6-mercaptopurine): 60 mg/m^2/d for 16 months, taken in the evening
  - Oral methotrexate: 20 mg/m^2/wk for 16 months

- Philadelphia chromosome–positive ALL:
  - Imatinib mesylate (400–800 mg/d) is effective alone and in combination with chemotherapy (4)[B].
- Contraindications: Doses and schedule may need to be altered for older patients and for concurrent infection and organ toxicity (2)[B].
- Precautions:
  - Tumor lysis syndrome (elevated uric acid, potassium, and phosphate with decreased calcium, leading to renal failure, disseminated intravascular coagulation, and cardiac arrhythmias) may be prevented by administering allopurinol 300 mg/d. Begin 2 days before chemotherapy begins. Reduce doses if used with mercaptopurine or azathioprine. Give increased fluids; IV urate oxidase (rasburicase) can be used to treat hyperuricemia rapidly.
  - Oral sulfamethoxazole-trimethoprim or aerosolized pentamidine is given for *Pneumocystis carinii* prophylaxis.
  - Profound immunosuppression: Take appropriate precautions when patient is neutropenic.
  - High-dose cyclophosphamide causes severe nausea and vomiting. Use appropriate antiemetic regimen to prevent.
  - Neurotoxicity, ileus with vincristine
  - Asparaginase may cause severe allergic reactions as well as impaired pancreatic and liver function. Monitor serum glucose concentrations frequently and carefully. Pancreatitis or thrombosis may occur. Peg-asparaginase has been approved and can be used IV or IM in place of native *Escherichia coli* asparaginase.
  - Rituximab (anti-CD20 monoclonal antibody) appears to improve the outcome of patients with ALL if CD20 is expressed on more than 20% of their blast cells.
  - Also note: Burkitt leukemia/lymphoma (ALL-L3):
    - The outcome is clearly better if high-dose methotrexate and alkylating agents are used for initial therapy.
    - Only 18 weeks of treatment are required.
    - Rituximab (anti-CD20 monoclonal antibody) improves the outcome of patients with Burkitt leukemia when added to chemotherapy.

Second Line

Clofarabine has been approved for relapsed childhood ALL. Pegylated asparaginase (IV or IM) has been used in place of *E. coli*–derived L-asparaginase. Other anthracyclines, investigational chemotherapy agents and monoclonal antibodies (e.g., rituximab; alemtuzumab). Allogeneic hematopoietic stem cell transplantation is recommended for any patient with relapsed ALL (5,6)[A].

ADDITIONAL TREATMENT

General Measures

- Appropriate health care:
  - Inpatient care during remission induction chemotherapy
  - Postremission therapy is usually outpatient.
- Protective isolation from infection
- Adequate calcium and vitamin D supplementation may reduce bone injury from corticosteroids and avascular necrosis of large joints.

Issues for Referral

ALERT

ALL can become a fatal disorder quickly. As soon as the diagnosis is suspected, patients should be referred quickly to an appropriate oncology center.

COMPLEMENTARY AND ALTERNATIVE MEDICINE

Unproven and may result in dangerous drug interactions with chemotherapy

SURGERY/OTHER PROCEDURES

Surgical placement of a percutaneous, silastic, double-lumen central venous catheter

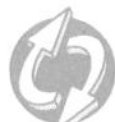

ONGOING CARE

FOLLOW-UP RECOMMENDATIONS

Ambulatory as tolerated

Patient Monitoring

- Daily during induction chemotherapy for metabolic and infectious complications
- Weekly during remission consolidation chemotherapy
- Monthly during maintenance therapy
- Every 3 months thereafter

DIET

- Nutritional support, including IV hyperalimentation, if necessary
- Avoid alcohol.
- Calcium and vitamin D

PATIENT EDUCATION

- Risks of infection, transfusion, chemotherapy
- Stop smoking.

PROGNOSIS

- ~80–95% of patients <60 years old will achieve a complete remission, and 35–60% will remain free of disease at 5 years (3,6,7,8,9)[A].
- Older patients (>60 years) do less well, but 80% may achieve a complete remission (2)[B].
- Patients with unfavorable cytogenetic subtypes [especially t(9;22) and t(4:11)] should undergo allogeneic stem cell transplantation in first remission if an HLA-identical donor were available (1,4,5,6)[A]

COMPLICATIONS

- Infections (*P. carinii* pneumonia, bacterial pneumonia or sepsis, fungal pneumonia)
- Bleeding
- Coagulopathy (deep vein thrombosis) from asparaginase therapy
- Need for transfusions
- Sterility from treatment
- Arachnoiditis and CNS effects from intrathecal chemotherapy and irradiation
- Pancreatitis and liver dysfunction from chemotherapy
- Osteonecrosis of joints (avascular necrosis) related to corticosteroids
- Relapse of ALL in marrow or extramedullary sites (CNS, testis)

REFERENCES

1. Faderl S, O'Brien S, Pui CH, et al. Adult acute lymphoblastic leukemia: Concepts and strategies. *Cancer*. 2010;116:1165–76.
2. Larson RA. Management of acute lymphoblastic leukemia in older patients. *Semin Hematol*. 2006;43:126–33.
3. Larson RA, Dodge RK, Linker CA, et al. A randomized controlled trial of filgrastim during remission induction and consolidation chemotherapy for adults with acute lymphoblastic leukemia: CALGB study 9111. *Blood*. 1998;92: 1556–64.
4. Stock W, et al. Current treatment options for adult patients with Philadelphia chromosome-positive acute lymphoblastic leukemia. *Leuk Lymphoma*. 2010;51:188–98.
5. Oliansky DM, Larson RA, Weisdorf D, et al. The role of cytotoxic therapy with hematopoietic stem cell transplantation in the treatment of adult acute lymphoblastic leukemia: Update of the 2006 evidence-based review. *Biol Blood Marrow Transplant*. 2011.
6. Mattison RJ, Larson RA, et al. Role of allogeneic hematopoietic cell transplantation in adults with acute lymphoblastic leukemia. *Curr Opin Oncol*. 2009;21:601–8.
7. Kantajian H, Hoelzer D, Larson RA, eds. Advances in the treatment of adult acute lymphocytic leukemia: Parts I and II. *Hematol Oncol Clin North Am*. 2000.
8. Pieters R, Carroll WL, et al. Biology and treatment of acute lymphoblastic leukemia. *Hematol Oncol Clin North Am*. 2010;24:1–18.
9. Campana D, et al. Role of minimal residual disease monitoring in adult and pediatric acute lymphoblastic leukemia. *Hematol Oncol Clin North Am*. 2009;23:1083–98, vii.

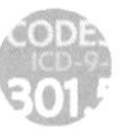

CODES

ICD9

- 204.00 Lymphoid leukemia, acute, without mention of having achieved remission
- 204.01 Lymphoid leukemia, acute, in remission
- 204.02 Acute lymphoid leukemia, in relapse

CLINICAL PEARLS

- ALL can become fatal quickly; as soon as diagnosis is suspected, refer patient to an oncology center.
- Optimal therapy is not yet known (1,2)[A]. ALL should be treated at a comprehensive oncology center. All treatment regimens are still investigational, but clearly are effective for some fraction of patients.

LEUKEMIA, ACUTE MYELOID

Jan Cerny, MD, PhD

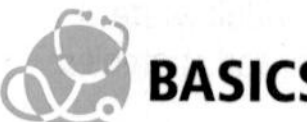

BASICS

DESCRIPTION

- Acute myeloid leukemia (AML) is characterized by proliferation and accumulation of abnormal immature myeloid progenitors (blasts) with reduced capacity to differentiate into more mature cellular elements. This leads to bone marrow failure and results in a variety of systemic symptoms.
- The former French–American–British (FAB) classification system divided AML based on the cell morphology with the addition of cytogenetics (subtypes M0–M7).
- The World Health Organization (WHO) classification attempts to provide more meaningful prognostic information:
  - AML with characteristic genetic abnormalities: Translocation t(8;21), t(15;17) and inversion in chromosome 16 inv(16)
  - AML with multilineage dysplasia: Presence of a prior myelodysplastic syndrome (MDS) or myeloproliferative disease (MPD) that transformed into AML
  - AML and MDS, therapy-related
  - AML not otherwise categorized
  - Acute leukemias of ambiguous lineage (*biphenotypic acute leukemia*)

EPIDEMIOLOGY

- ~13,500 cases diagnosed in 2007; second most common type of leukemia in adults
- Predominant sex: Male ≥ Female

Incidence

The incidence of AML increases with age and median age is more than 70 years.

RISK FACTORS

- Genetic predisposition (e.g., Down syndrome); other familial disorders are Bloom syndrome (~25% develop AML), Fanconi anemia (52%), neurofibromatosis, Li-Fraumeni syndrome, Wiskott-Aldrich syndrome, Kostmann syndrome, and Diamond-Blackfan anemia
- Radiation exposure
- Immunodeficiency states
- Chemical and drug exposure (nitrogen mustard and alkylating agents; benzene)
- Myelodysplastic syndrome (preleukemia)
- Cigarette smoking

Genetics

- Unknown; some are familial
- Cytogenetics and genetics play a very important role in diagnosis and prognosis of AML and have implications for therapy.
- 3 risk groups:
  - Good risk: inv(16), t(8;21), t(15;17)
  - Standard risk: Normal karyotype
  - Poor risk: Monosomy 5 and 7 (typically secondary AML), deletion 5q, abnormalities of 11q23 or complex karyotype
- FLT3 gene mutations, especially internal transmembrane duplications (FLT3-ITD), have been associated with poor survival in AML. These and other (onco)gene (e.g., WT1, NPM1 and P53) mutations are studied to further risk-stratify patients (1).

GENERAL PREVENTION

None currently identified, but treatment of high-risk myelodysplastic syndrome with demethylating agents (Vidaza, 5-azacytidine) has been shown to prolong time to transformation from MDS into AML (2).

ETIOLOGY

Precise causes unknown, but some risk factors have been identified (see also "Risk Factors")

COMMONLY ASSOCIATED CONDITIONS

The following are oncologic emergencies:

- Disseminated intravascular coagulopathy (DIC) usually in acute promyelocytic leukemia (APL), but may be seen in any AML
- Leukostasis (high blast number and increased adhesive ability of blasts)
- Tumor lysis syndrome (TLS): Spontaneous or in response to chemotherapy

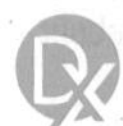

DIAGNOSIS

HISTORY

Fatigue (anemia or tumor burden). Bleeding (low platelets or DIC). Difficulty clearing infections (neutropenia or immune dysregulation).

PHYSICAL EXAM

- Mostly nonspecific and related to marrow or tissue infiltration:
  - Fever
  - Bleeding
  - Pallor
  - Splenomegaly
  - Hepatosplenomegaly
  - Lymphadenopathy (usually reactive)
- If CNS is involved, symptoms of increased intracranial pressure can be present.
- Occasionally patients will present with prominent extramedullary sites of leukemia (e.g., skin infiltration or ultimately as a granulocytic sarcoma).

DIAGNOSTIC TESTS & INTERPRETATION

Lab

- CBC shows subnormal RBCs, neutrophils, and platelets
- Bone marrow for histology, flow cytometry, and cytogenetics to establish diagnosis and prognosis
- ESR
- Lactate dehydrogenase (LDH) and uric acid can be elevated (e.g., TLS).
- Coagulation profile can be normal or prolonged (e.g., DIC).
- Drugs that may alter lab results: Chemotherapy agents, corticosteroids
- Other special tests: Spinal tap may reveal fluid with leukemic cells.

Imaging

Ultrasonography or CT scan of the abdomen may discover organomegaly.

Diagnostic Procedures/Surgery

Bone-marrow studies are necessary to make the diagnosis:

- Aspirates: For cell morphology, cytochemistries, immunophenotyping (can confirm differentiation stage of AML); cytogenetics: Chromosomal aberration (prognostic value; see "Genetics")
- Biopsies provide valuable information for cellularity, architecture, etc.

Pathological Findings

- The marrow will be hypercellular and the normal architecture effaced; leukemic blasts is >20%.
- The liver and spleen may be infiltrated with leukemic cells.

DIFFERENTIAL DIAGNOSIS

- Virus-induced cytopenia, lymphadenopathy, and organomegaly
- Immune cytopenias (including systemic lupus erythematosus [SLE])
- Drug-induced cytopenias
- Other marrow failure and infiltrative diseases (e.g., aplastic anemia, paroxysmal nocturnal hemoglobinuria, myelodysplastic syndromes, Gaucher disease)

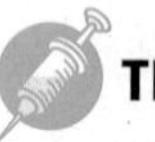

TREATMENT

- Chemotherapy is the backbone of AML therapy and consists of induction and consolidation phase ± maintenance (APL).
- Bone marrow transplantation (BMT) for high-risk AML
- Only modest improvements have been made in AML induction chemotherapy. Supportive care has improved significantly.

Geriatric Considerations

- Older patients (>60 or 65 years) remain a therapeutic challenge, as they do not tolerate intensive therapies. These patients are offered so-called reduced-intensity or nonmyeloablative bone marrow transplantation.
- Adding growth factors (granulocyte-colony stimulating factor [G-CSF]) may reduce toxicity in older patients (however not generally accepted).
- 5-azacitidine significantly prolongs survival in older adults with low marrow blast count (<30%) (3).

Pediatric Considerations

Tolerate intense treatments better

Pregnancy Considerations

Chemotherapy is a viable option in the second and third trimesters.

MEDICATION

First Line

- Acute promyelocytic leukemia [APL, AML with t(15;17)]:
  - All-trans retinoic acid (ATRA) and arsenic trioxide both promote maturation to granulocytes.
  - Idarubicin can be added to induction therapy.
- Treatment of AML in younger adults: AML (other than APL)
- Induction (daunorubicin or idarubicin [anthracycline and cytarabine]): the generally accepted combination is 3 + 7 (anthracycline is given for 3 and cytarabine for 7 days)
- Remission is typically consolidated in younger patients by:
  - In good-risk AML, 3–4 cycles of high-dose cytarabine (HiDAC) and bone marrow transplant (BMT) is reserved for time of recurrence.
  - In poor-risk patients, 1–2 cycles of HiDAC (until donor is identified) are followed by allogeneic BMT.

- Intermediate-risk AML should be treated based on individual patient's features, donor availability, and access to clinical trials. Recent meta-analysis showed that even intermediate-risk patients benefit from allogeneic BMT (4).
- Treatment of AML in older adults (e.g., >65 years) remains a challenge. These patients have poor performance status, more likely secondary AML, higher incidence of unfavorable cytogenetics, comorbidities, shorter remissions, and overall survival:
  - Intensive chemotherapy only for selected patients; alternative regimens with e.g., mitoxantrone, fludarabine, and clofarabine. New drugs (demethylating agents as above (3), FLT3 inhibitors, monoclonal antibodies, etc.) are being studied in clinical trials.
- Contraindications: Comorbidities; therapy has to be individualized.
- Precautions:
  - If organ failure, some drugs may be avoided or dose-reduced (e.g., no anthracyclines in patients with pre-existing cardiac problems).
  - Patients will be immunosuppressed during treatment. Avoid live vaccines. Administer varicella-zoster or measles immunoglobulin as soon as exposure of patient occurs.
- Significant possible interactions: Allopurinol accentuates the toxicity of 6-mercaptopurine.

Second Line

Healthy, younger patients usually are offered reinduction chemotherapy and allogeneic BMT.

ADDITIONAL TREATMENT

General Measures

- Ongoing assessment of bone marrow, liver, heart, and kidney functions during therapy
- Close monitoring of coagulation parameters (risk for DIC)
- Supportive therapy with:
  - Good hydration
  - Transfusions of packed RBCs and platelets based on patient's needs (threshold as for platelets as low as 5,000); use leukoreduced, irradiated blood products in BMT candidates
  - Avoid antiplatelet agents (e.g., aspirin products).
  - Follow febrile neutropenic guidelines in neutropenic patient who becomes febrile (even low-grade fever).

Issues for Referral

- AML should be managed by specialized team led by a hematologist/oncologist.
- Refer patient to a transplant center early because a search for a donor may be necessary.

SURGERY/OTHER PROCEDURES

Bone marrow transplant: Decision between myeloablative and nonmyeloablative approach should be based on patient's performance status, comorbidities, and AML risk factors:

- Allogeneic BMT is acceptable in first remission in poor-risk AML or in second remission in all other AML patients. Matched related donor used to be preferred over matched unrelated donor (lower risk of graft-versus-host disease), recent data suggest equal outcomes as allogeneic transplant regimens and post-transplant care have improved significantly.
- Cord blood may be used as alternative source of hematopoietic stem cells even for adults
- Autologous BMT may be acceptable in specific situations (e.g., no donor is available).

IN-PATIENT CONSIDERATIONS

Admission Criteria

Induction treatment for AML requires inpatient care, usually on a specialized ward. Episodes of febrile neutropenia typically require admission and IV antibiotics.

IV Fluids

Appropriate hydration to prevent TLS

Nursing

IV may lead to chemical burns in the event of extravasation.

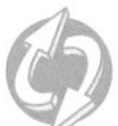

ONGOING CARE

FOLLOW-UP RECOMMENDATIONS

Ambulatory as tolerated; no intense or contact sports; no aspirin due to risk of bleeding

Patient Monitoring

- Repeat bone-marrow studies to document remission and also if a relapse is suspected.
- Follow CBC with differential, coagulation studies, uric acid level, and other chemistries related to TLS (creatinine, potassium, phosphate, calcium); monitor urinary function at least daily during induction phase and less frequently later.
- Physical evaluation, including weight and BP, should be done frequently during treatment.

DIET

Ensure adequately balanced calorie/vitamin intake. TPN if case of severe mucositis

PATIENT EDUCATION

- Leukemia Society of America 600 Third Avenue, New York, NY 10016, 212-573-8484
- National Cancer Institute, Bethesda, MD, has pamphlets and telephone education.
- *You and Leukemia: A Day at a Time*, by Dr. Lynn S. Baker (Saunders).

PROGNOSIS

AML remission rate is 60–80%, with only 20–40% long-term survival. The wide variable prognosis is due to prognostic group (age, cytogenetics, and genetics).

COMPLICATIONS

- Acute side effects of chemotherapy, including febrile neutropenia
- TLS
- DIC
- Late-onset cardiomyopathy in patients treated with anthracyclines
- Chronic side effects of chemotherapy (secondary malignancies)
- Graft-versus-host disease in patient who received allogeneic BMT

REFERENCES

1. Döhner H, Estey EH, Amadori S, et al. Diagnosis and management of acute myeloid leukemia in adults: Recommendations from an international expert panel, on behalf of the European Leukemia. *Net Blood*. 2010;115:453–74.
2. Fenaux P, Mufti GJ, Hellstrom-Lindberg E, et al. Efficacy of azacitidine compared with that of conventional care regimens in the treatment of higher-risk myelodysplastic syndromes: A randomised, open-label, phase III study. *Lancet Oncol*. 2009;10:223–32.
3. Fenaux P, Mufti GJ, Hellström-Lindberg E, et al. Azacitidine prolongs overall survival compared with conventional care regimens in elderly patients with low bone marrow blast count acute myeloid leukemia. *J Clin Oncol*. 2010;28:562–9.
4. Koreth J, Schlenk R, Kopecky KJ, et al. Allogeneic stem cell transplantation for acute myeloid leukemia in first complete remission: Systematic review and meta-analysis of prospective clinical trials. *JAMA*. 2009;301:2349–61.

ADDITIONAL READING

- Devita VT Jr, Rosenberg SA, Lawrence TS, eds. *DeVita, Hellman, and Rosenberg's Cancer: Principles & Practice of Oncology*, 8th ed. Philadelphia: Lippincott Williams & Wilkins; 2008.
- O'Donnell MR, Appelbaum FR, Coutre SE, et al. Acute myeloid leukemia. *J Natl Compr Canc Netw*. 2008;6:962–93.

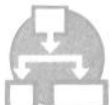

See Also (Topic, Algorithm, Electronic Media Element)

Disseminated Intravascular Coagulopathy (DIC); Leukemia Acute Lymphoblastic in Adults (ALL); Leukemia, Chronic Myelogenous (CML); Myelodysplastic Syndromes (MDS); Myeloproliferative Neoplasms

CODES

ICD9

- 205.00 Myeloid leukemia, acute, without mention of having achieved remission
- 208.00 Leukemia of unspecified cell type, acute, without mention of having achieved remission

CLINICAL PEARLS

- Prognosis of leukemia depends on the cytogenetic and molecular profile of the disease.
- Allogeneic transplant remains the only therapy with curative potential for patients with intermediate- and high-risk AML.

L

LEUKEMIA, CHRONIC LYMPHOCYTIC

Jan Cerny, MD, PhD
Deepa Jagadeesh, MD, MPH

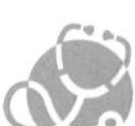

BASICS

DESCRIPTION

- Chronic lymphocytic leukemia (CLL) is a monoclonal disorder characterized by a progressive accumulation of mature but functionally incompetent lymphocytes.
- CLL can be distinguished from prolymphocytic leukemia (PLL). Based on percentage of prolymphocytes, the disease may be regarded as CLL (<10% prolymphocytes), PLL (>55% prolymphocytes), or CLL/PLL (>10% and <55% prolymphocytes).
- Small lymphocytic lymphoma is a lymphoma variant of CLL.
- System(s) affected: Hematologic/Lymphatic/Immunologic

EPIDEMIOLOGY

Incidence

- With 15,000–17,000 new cases reported every year, CLL represents the most common form of leukemia in adults in the US.
- Predominant age: CLL primarily affects elderly individuals, median age of diagnosis being 70 years. The incidence continues to rise in those >55 years.
- Predominant sex: Male > Female (1.7:1)
- The incidence is higher among whites than among African Americans.

RISK FACTORS

- As in the case of most malignancies, the exact cause of CLL is uncertain.
- Possible chronic immune stimulation is suspected, but is still being elucidated.
- Monoclonal B-cell lymphocytosis: 1% risk progression to CLL

Genetics

CLL is an acquired disorder, and reports of truly familial cases are exceedingly rare.

GENERAL PREVENTION

Unknown

PATHOPHYSIOLOGY

- The cell of origin in CLL is a clonal B cell arrested in the B-cell differentiation pathway, intermediate between pre-B cells and mature B cells. In the peripheral blood, these cells resemble mature lymphocytes and typically show B-cell surface antigens: CD19, CD20, CD21, and CD23. In addition, they express CD5 (usually found on T cells).
- The *bcl2* proto-oncogene is overexpressed in B-CLL. *Bcl2* is a known suppressor of apoptosis (programmed cell death), resulting in extremely long life of the affected lymphocytes.

ETIOLOGY

Unknown, but genetic mutations leading to disrupted function and prolonged survival of affected lymphocytes are suspected.

COMMONLY ASSOCIATED CONDITIONS

- Immune system dysregulation is common.
- Autoimmune hemolytic anemia (AIHA) may accompany CLL.
- Immune thrombocytopenic purpura (ITP) may accompany CLL.

DIAGNOSIS

HISTORY

- Insidious onset; it is not unusual for CLL to be discovered incidentally. Up to 40% of patients are asymptomatic at the time of diagnosis.
- Others may have:
  - Repetitive infections (pneumonia, but also mucocutaneous herpetic infections, etc.)
  - Enlarged lymph nodes
  - Early satiety and/or abdominal discomfort related to an enlarged spleen
  - Mucocutaneous bleeding and/or petechiae due to thrombocytopenia
  - Fatigue-related and/or other symptoms of anemia
  - Fevers, night sweats, >10% weight loss (B symptoms)

PHYSICAL EXAM

- Localized or generalized lymphadenopathy
- Splenomegaly (30–40%)
- Hepatomegaly (20%)
- Mucocutaneous bleeding (thrombocytopenia)
- Skin petechiae (thrombocytopenia)
- Pallor

DIAGNOSTIC TESTS & INTERPRETATION

Lab

Initial lab tests

- CBC with differential shows absolute lymphocytosis with >5,000 lymphocytes/μL. The blood smear also shows ruptured lymphocytes ("smudge" cells).
- Exam of the blood smear is important in diagnosis of CLL.
- The diagnosis can be confirmed by immunophenotyping: CLL cells are positive for CD19, CD20, and CD24, as well as CD5. They have low levels of surface membrane IgM or IgD. The monoclonality is proven by the presence of a single immunoglobulin light chain (κ or λ). FMC-7 is absent.
- CBC shows anemia and/or thrombocytopenia.
- Plasma β_2–microglobulin may be elevated.
- Serum protein electrophoresis (some patients may have monoclonal gammopathy)
- Lactate dehydrogenase (LDH) may be elevated (due to disease activity or to AIHA).
- Hypogammaglobulinemia
- In case associated with AIHA, labs consistent with hemolysis may be present (elevated LDH, total bilirubin; reticulocyte count does not have to be elevated due to bone marrow infiltration).

Follow-Up & Special Considerations

Frequency and type of follow-up depend on severity of symptoms as well as risk factors (see "Prognosis").

Imaging

Initial approach

- Liver/spleen ultrasound may demonstrate organomegaly.
- CT scan of chest/abdomen/pelvis typically is not necessary for staging. However, it may help to identify compression of organs or internal structures from enlarged lymph nodes.

Diagnostic Procedures/Surgery

- Although bone marrow biopsy has its prognostic value (diffuse infiltration is a risk factor), it is not done routinely.
- Consider a lymph node biopsy if lymph node(s) begin to enlarge rapidly in a patient with known CLL to assess the possibility of transformation to a high-grade lymphoma (Richter syndrome), especially when accompanied by fever, weight loss, and pain.

Pathological Findings

A bone marrow aspirate usually shows >30% lymphocytes.

DIFFERENTIAL DIAGNOSIS

- Infectious causes:
  - Bacterial (tuberculosis)
  - Viral (mononucleosis)
- Malignant causes:
  - Leukemic phase of non-Hodgkin lymphomas
  - Hairy cell leukemia
  - Waldenstrom macroglobulinemia
  - Large granular lymphocytic leukemia

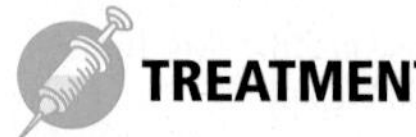

TREATMENT

MEDICATION

First Line

- Most patients are asymptomatic and do not need active treatment unless they have generalized (so-called B) symptoms, progressive marrow failure, AIHA or thrombocytopenia, progressive splenomegaly, massive lymphadenopathy, or progressive lymphocytosis (increase >50% in 2 months or a doubling time of <6 months).
- Low-risk disease, Rai stage 0, and Binet stage A require only periodic follow-up.
- Intermediate-risk group, Rai stage I and II, and Binet stage B could be observed until there is evidence of disease progression or development of symptoms.
- Treatment should be initiated in high-risk patients, Rai stage III and IV, and Binet stage C.
- Early treatment in low-risk group is not recommended.
- 3 main groups of drugs used are alkylating agents (chlorambucil, and recently bendamustine), purine analogs (fludarabine and pentostatin), and monoclonal antibodies (rituximab and alemtuzumab)

- Single-agent (fludarabine, bendamustine, or chlorambucil) or combination regimens commonly used
- Fludarabine-based regimens are FC (in combination with cyclophosphamide) FR (fludarabine + rituximab), and FCR (fludarabine + cyclophosphamide + rituximab).
- FCR is the widely used regimen of choice if patient can tolerate it.
- PCR (pentostatin + cyclophosphamide + rituximab) is another regimen that is effective.
- Steroids (prednisone) are useful in patients with autoimmune manifestations of CLL (e.g., AIHA, ITP).

Second Line

- Combinations of chemotherapeutic agents that patient did not fail yet. Occasionally, some patients can be retreated with a drug used previously.
- Alemtuzumab (anti-CD52) has shown activity in relapsed and refractory disease.
- Newer agents like ofatumumab (novel anti-CD20), lenalidomide, and others have shown promising activity.
- Consider splenectomy (surgery or radiation) if massive splenomegaly causes significant anemia and thrombocytopenia.
- Allogenic and autologous stem cell transplant can be considered in high-risk and younger patients (limited data available).

ADDITIONAL TREATMENT

General Measures

Patients with frequent infections associated with hypogammaglobulinemia are likely to benefit from monthly infusions of IVIG.

Issues for Referral

- Surgical consultation for splenectomy in selected patients
- Bone marrow transplant in young patients with refractory disease (however, still considered experimental therapy)

Additional Therapies

Patients requiring therapy who are high risk for tumor lysis syndrome should be given allopurinol to prevent uric acid nephropathy.

SURGERY/OTHER PROCEDURES

Splenectomy in selected patients

IN-PATIENT CONSIDERATIONS

Admission Criteria

No specific criteria, but due to complications of disease (e.g., AIHA) or complications of therapy (e.g., febrile neutropenia) or significant tumor lysis syndrome after initiation of chemotherapy

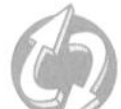

ONGOING CARE

FOLLOW-UP RECOMMENDATIONS

- Low-risk CLL: Physical exam and CBC with differential every 3 months
- Patients in remission after treatment should also be followed every 3–6 months.

Patient Monitoring

- CBC with differential (lymphocytosis) every 3 months, LDH, β_2-microglobulin, IgG level
- Physical exam (lymphadenopathy, splenomegaly)

DIET

- Ensure adequately balanced calorie/vitamin intake.
- Follow weight.

PATIENT EDUCATION

Leukemia and Lymphoma Society has educational pamphlets: www.webmd.com/cancer/tc/leukemia-topic-overview.

PROGNOSIS

- 2 staging systems are used: The Rai in the US and the Binet in Europe. Neither is completely satisfactory.
- The Rai staging system:
  - Stage 0: Lymphocytosis only; median survival of 120 months
  - Stage I: Lymphocytosis and adenopathy; median survival of 95 months
  - Stage II: Lymphocytosis and splenomegaly and/or hepatomegaly; median survival of 72 months
  - Stage III: Lymphocytosis and anemia (hemoglobin <10 g/dL); median survival of 30 months
  - Stage IV: Lymphocytosis and thrombocytopenia (platelets $<100 \times 10^9$/L); median survival of 30 months
- The Binet staging system:
  - Stage A: Hemoglobin ≥10 g/dL, platelets $\geq 100 \times 10^9$, and <3 lymph node areas involved (Rai stages 0, I, and II); survival >120 months
  - Stage B: Hemoglobin and platelet levels as in stage A and 3 or more lymph node areas involved (Rai stages I and II); survival is 61 months
  - Stage C: Hemoglobin <100 g/L, platelets $<100 \times 10^9$, or both (Rai stages III and IV); survival is 32 months
- Adverse risk factors:
  - Advanced Rai or Binet stage
  - Peripheral lymphocyte doubling time <12 months
  - Diffuse marrow infiltration
  - Increased number of prolymphocytes or cleaved cells
  - Poor response to chemotherapy
  - High β_2-microglobulin and thymidine kinase levels and low microRNAs (miRNAs)
  - Abnormal karyotyping: Deletion of 17p- and 11q-
  - New IgVH unmutated status (expression of ZAP-70 >20% or CD38 >30% evaluated by immunophenotyping are surrogate markers)
  - *P53* mutation or deletion

COMPLICATIONS

- Acute or long-term effects of chemotherapy
- Richter syndrome (above)
- AIHA (in some cases may be related to the use of fludarabine)

ADDITIONAL READING

- Chiorazzi N, Rai KR, Ferrarini M. Chronic lymphocytic leukemia. *N Engl J Med*. 2005;352:804–15.
- National Comprehensive Cancer Network guidelines at www.nccn.org
- Shanafelt TD, Kay NE. Comprehensive management of the CLL patient: A holistic approach. *Hematology Am Soc Hematol Educ Program*. 2007:324–31.

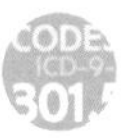

CODES

ICD9

- 204.10 Lymphoid leukemia, chronic, without mention of having achieved remission
- 204.11 Chronic lymphoid leukemia, in remission

CLINICAL PEARLS

- CLL represents the most common form of leukemia in adults in the US.
- Predominant age: CLL primarily affects elderly individuals, median age of diagnosis being 70 years. The incidence continues to rise in those >55 years.
- Clinical monitoring of asymptomatic and low-risk patients is a reasonable approach ("watch and wait").
- High-risk patients, bulky disease, or patients who fail fludarabine and rituximab-based therapies have typically poor prognosis and may require intensive therapies, including allogeneic transplantation.
- Median survival is 3–10 years, depending on stage.

L

LEUKEMIA, CHRONIC MYELOGENOUS

Jan Cerny, MD, PhD

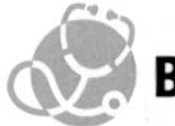

BASICS

DESCRIPTION

- Chronic myelogenous leukemia (CML) is a myeloproliferative disorder characterized by clonal proliferation of myeloid precursors in the bone marrow with continuing differentiation into mature granulocytes.
- Hallmark of CML is Philadelphia chromosome [translocation t(9;22)]
- Natural history of the disease evolves in 3 clinical phases: A chronic phase, an accelerated phase, and blast phase or crisis (transformation to acute leukemia)

EPIDEMIOLOGY

Incidence

- Per year, 1.6 cases/100,000 persons
- Predominant age: 50–60 years
- Predominant sex: Male > Female (1.3:1)

Prevalence

Accounts for 15–20% of adult leukemias

RISK FACTORS

Ionizing radiation exposure (uncommon)

Genetics

Acquired genomic changes

GENERAL PREVENTION

None currently identified

PATHOPHYSIOLOGY

Philadelphia chromosome is a balanced translocation between *BCR* (on chromosome 22) and *ABL* (on chromosome 9) genes t(9;22)(q34;q11). This fusion gene, *BCR-ABL,* codes for an abnormal constitutively active tyrosine kinase that affects numerous signal transduction pathways, resulting in uncontrolled cell proliferation and reduced apoptosis.

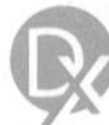

DIAGNOSIS

85–90% of patients present in the chronic phase and the disease can be found accidentally during routine screening.

HISTORY

- Chronic phase: Fatigue, weight loss, night sweats, abdominal fullness owing to enlarged spleen, early satiety, dyspnea, bleeding; rare: bruising, left upper quadrant abdominal pain, sternal pain (owing to expanding bone marrow), and gouty arthritis; up to 30% of patients are asymptomatic.
- Accelerated phase: Progressive splenomegaly and left upper quadrant abdominal pain occasionally referred to the left shoulder (owing to splenic infarction or rupture), progressive weight loss and sweats, unexplained fever or bone pain, chloromas (extramedullary tumors)
- Blast phase: Bleeding, bruising, infections, prominent constitutional symptoms

PHYSICAL EXAM

- Splenomegaly (50–90%), hepatomegaly (up to 50%)
- Less common: Splenic friction rub, lymphadenopathy

DIAGNOSTIC TESTS & INTERPRETATION

Lab

- CBC:
  - Hematocrit: May be normal, slightly increased, or decreased
  - WBC count: Markedly increased (50,000–100,000/μL) with granulocytes in all stages of development, including occasional blasts <10% in chronic phase, basophilia, eosinophilia
  - Platelets: Normal, elevated (34%), or occasionally low
  - In accelerated phase: Anemia, 10–19% blood or marrow blasts, basophils plus eosinophils >20%, thrombocytopenia
  - Blast phase: Blood or marrow blasts >20%
- Genetics:
  - Demonstration of the Philadelphia chromosome, t(9,22), by cytogenetic techniques, FISH, or reverse-transcription-polymerase chain reaction (RT-PCR)
  - Additional cytogenetic abnormalities occur in the accelerated and blast phases [monosomy 7, t(3,21), trisomy 8 and 19, Philadelphia chromosome duplication, abnormalities of chromosome 17 such as monosomy, trisomy, and isochromosome mutations]. These may contribute to resistance to tyrosine kinase inhibitors (TKIs; e.g., imatinib). Further molecular testing (mutations within *BCR-ABL*) is suggested in case of loss of response to therapy.
- Others:
  - Low or absent leukocyte alkaline phosphatase in neutrophils
  - High lactate dehydrogenase (LDH)
  - Elevated uric acid

Initial lab tests

CBC, LDH, uric acid, bone marrow biopsy and aspirate, cytogenetics on bone marrow and FISH for *BCR-ABL*, RT-PCR, liver function tests

Follow-Up & Special Considerations

- Mutation analysis of tyrosine kinase domain of *ABL* kinase, as they may cause resistance to therapy with TKIs.
- HLA-A*02 positive is associated with CML and a protective effect is seen with the HLA-B*35 allele (pooled odds ratio 0.64, 95% confidence interval 0.48–0.86 (1)[A].

Imaging

Abdominal ultrasound or CT scan shows splenomegaly; not mandatory

Diagnostic Procedures/Surgery

Bone marrow aspiration and biopsy

Pathological Findings

Myeloid hyperplasia with elevated myeloid: Erythroid ratio, normal maturation, marrow basophilia, and increased reticulin fibrosis

DIFFERENTIAL DIAGNOSIS

- Chronic myelomonocytic leukemia, chronic neutrophilic leukemia, chronic eosinophilic leukemia, juvenile myelomonocytic leukemia, infectious mononucleosis, leukemoid reaction, polycythemia vera, and treatment with granulocyte-stimulating factors
- Acute myelogenous leukemia resembles blast crisis with myeloid blasts, and acute lymphoblastic leukemia resembles blast crisis with lymphoid blasts.
- Atypical CML is a chronic myeloproliferative disorder with a clinical hematologic picture similar to CML, but it lacks Philadelphia chromosome and *BCR-ABL* rearrangement.

TREATMENT

MEDICATION

- TKIs (tyrosine kinase inhibitors (e.g., imatinib) provide durable, long-term control of disease.
- The response to TKIs is assessed at specific time points from the beginning of treatment and is categorized as follows:
  - Complete hematologic response (CHR): Normalization of peripheral counts, no disease symptoms, no immature cells
  - Minor/partial/complete cytogenetic response (CCR): 35–90%, 1–34%, no Philadelphia-positive metaphases
  - Major molecular response (MMR): Decreased level of *BCR-ABL* transcript by PCR 3-log
  - Complete molecular response (CMR): *BCR-ABL* transcript is undetectable by PCR.

First Line

- Gleevec (imatinib mesylate), an oral TKI, 400 mg/d PO
- Side effects: Thrombocytopenia, anemia, elevated liver enzymes, edema, GI disturbances, rash
- International Randomized Study of Interferon Versus STI571 (IRIS) established imatinib as first-line therapy (2).
- Imatinib dose can be increased to 600 and 800 mg/d if only partial cytogenetic response to 400 mg/d is achieved at 6 months of treatment.
- Second-generation TKIs have shown higher efficacy and less side effects and are approved for first-line therapy of chronic phase CML: Nilotinib (Tasigna) and dasatinib (Sprycel) (3,4,5,6).

Second Line

- Dasatinib (Sprycel), second-generation TKI, active against most of *BRC-ABL* mutants, not active in T315I mutation:
  - 100 mg/d in patients resistant or intolerant to imatinib and 70 mg twice a day for patients in accelerated or blastic phase
  - Side effects: Pleural effusions, cytopenias
- Nilotinib (Tasigna), also second-generation TKI, highly selective and more potent *BCR-ABL* TKI, active against most *BRC-ABL* mutants, not active in T315I mutation:
  - 400 mg PO bid in patients resistant or intolerant to imatinib in chronic or accelerated phase
  - Side effects: Cytopenias, QTc prolongation, pancreatitis

ADDITIONAL TREATMENT

Issues for Referral

All patients with CML should be referred to a hematologist.

SURGERY/OTHER PROCEDURES

Allogenic bone marrow transplant (BMT):

- It is the only known cure; however, 71% of patients who achieve complete cytogenetic response with imatinib maintain that response for 7 years, and no patient progressed on the trial between years 5 and 6 of treatment (2)
- Most effective in patients <50 years of age who are in the chronic phase
- Initial mortality is higher (related to the use of myeloablative regimens) than medical management but provided higher rates of survival in pre-imatinib era. Matched related donors used to have a better prognosis than matched unrelated donors for allogeneic donation (less graft-versus-host disease).
- Significant improvement in transplant techniques leading to better outcomes, such as alternative sources of stem cells; nonmyeloablative regimes have shown improvements in transplant-related mortality.
- Transplant option should be thoroughly discussed with young patients in chronic phase and considered an alternative to imatinib, dasatinib, or nilotinib, especially if the patient does not tolerate TKIs or disease is not responding.
- Can be considered in patients who fail to achieve complete hematologic response by 3 months, have no cytogenetic response or cytogenetic relapse, or have T315I mutation

IN-PATIENT CONSIDERATIONS

Initial Stabilization

- Hydroxyurea to rapidly reduce the WBC count
- Allopurinol to prevent tumor lysis syndrome in patients with very high counts; to be administered before chemotherapy is instituted; probably not necessary when imatinib is used

Admission Criteria

Acute abdominal symptoms (infarcted or ruptured spleen); tumor lysis syndrome owing to initial therapy; complications of BMT

Discharge Criteria

Abatement of acute symptoms

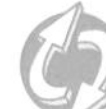

ONGOING CARE

FOLLOW-UP RECOMMENDATIONS

- Frequency depends on stage at presentation and response to first-line therapy.
- While splenomegaly persists, avoid contact sports or trauma to abdomen.

Patient Monitoring

- CBC with differential: Weekly until blood counts stable, then every 2–4 weeks during complete hematologic response, once in CCR and stable, patient can be followed less frequently (3-month intervals)
- Bone marrow cytogenetics (evaluation for clonal evolution) every 6 months while in CHR, every 12–18 months while in complete cytogenic response, MMR, CMR
- Quantitative RT-PCR every 3 months (peripheral blood)
- Liver function tests monthly on imatinib

PROGNOSIS

- With treatment, 5-year survival >50%
- Without treatment: CML invariably will progress to accelerated phase within 2–5 years and blast phase within several months of the accelerated phase.
- Poor prognosis: Patients presenting in accelerated or acute leukemia, or presenting with very large spleen size, platelets >700,000/μL, and patients resistant to current therapies (T315I mutation)

COMPLICATIONS

- Splenic infarct or rupture
- Progression to accelerated or blast phase
- Thrombotic events owing to elevated platelets
- Bleeding owing to low or dysfunctional platelets
- Sequelae of anemia

REFERENCES

1. Naugler C, Liwski R, et al. Human leukocyte antigen class I alleles and the risk of chronic myelogenous leukemia: A meta-analysis. *Leuk Lymphoma*. 2010; 51:1288–92.
2. O'Brien SG, Guilhot F, Goldman JM, et al. International randomized study of interferon versus STI571 (IRIS) 7-year follow-up: Sustained survival, low rate of transformation and increased rate of major molecular response (MMR) in patients (pts) with newly diagnosed chronic myeloid leukemia in chronic phase (CMLCP) treated with imatinib (IM). *ASH Ann Meeting Abstracts*. 2008;112:186.
3. Kantarjian HM, Baccarani M, Jabbour E, et al. Second-generation tyrosine kinase inhibitors: The future of frontline CML therapy. *Clin Cancer Res*. 2011;17:1674–83.
4. Cortes J, O'Brien S, Borthakur G, et al. Efficacy of dasatinib in patients (pts) with previously untreated chronic myelogenous leukemia (CML) in early chronic phase (CML-CP). *ASH Ann Meeting Abstracts*. 2008;112:182.
5. Rosti G, Palandri F, Castagnetti F, et al. Nilotinib for the frontline treatment of Ph+ chronic myeloid leukemia. *Blood*. 2009;114:4933–8.
6. Saglio G, Kim DW, Issaragrisil S, et al. Nilotinib versus imatinib for newly diagnosed chronic myeloid leukemia. *N Engl J Med*. 2010;362: 2251–9.

ADDITIONAL READING

- Goldman JM, Marin D. Management decisions in chronic myeloid leukemia. *Semin Hematol*. 2003;40: 97–103.
- Kantarjian H, Pasquini R, Hamerschlak N. Dasatinib or high-dose imatinib for chronic-phase chronic myeloid leukemia after failure of first-line imatinib: A randomized phase 2 trial. *Blood*. 2007;109: 5143–50.

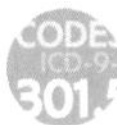

CODES

ICD9

- 205.10 Myeloid leukemia, chronic, without mention of having achieved remission
- 205.11 Myeloid leukemia, chronic, in remission

CLINICAL PEARLS

- CML belongs to the myeloproliferative disorders group.
- The gold standard for diagnosis of CML is detection of the Philadelphia chromosome or its products, *BCR-ABL* mRNA, and fusion protein.
- Tyrosine kinase inhibitors provide durable, long-term control of the disease and have dramatically altered treatment.
- Atypical CML is a form of clinically typical CML but without the presence of the typical *BCR-ABL* translocation.
- Blast crisis is a form of acute leukemia that is a possible complication of CML.

L

LEUKOPLAKIA, ORAL

Christine K. Jacobs, MD

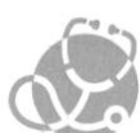

BASICS

DESCRIPTION

- *Oral leukoplakia* is a nonspecific clinical term used to describe a white patch on the oral mucosa that remains despite attempts to rub or scrape it off.
  - It has no pathologic or microscopic correlation with any specific disease and may be related to a variety of lesions, from benign hyperkeratosis to squamous cell carcinoma.
- System(s) affected: Gastrointestinal

EPIDEMIOLOGY

- Develops most often before age 40
- Predominant sex: Male > Female
- Some studies show no gender difference.

Prevalence

- 1–3% of the adult population is affected.
- Mean age of onset is 40 years.

Geriatric Considerations

Malignant transformation to carcinoma is more common in older patients.

RISK FACTORS

- Tobacco, particularly smokeless tobacco
- Alcohol use
- Repeated or chronic mechanical trauma from dental appliances or cheek biting
- Chemical irritation to oral regions
- Diabetes

Genetics

P53 overexpression correlates with leukoplakia and particularly squamous cell carcinoma (1).

GENERAL PREVENTION

- Avoid tobacco of any kind, alcohol, habitual cheek biting, tongue chewing.
- Use well-fitting dental prosthesis.
- Regular dental check-ups to avoid bad restorations
- Diet rich in fresh fruits and vegetables may help to prevent cancer.

PATHOPHYSIOLOGY

Hyperkeratosis or dyskeratosis of the oral squamous epithelium

ETIOLOGY

- Tobacco use in any form
- Alcohol consumption/alcoholism
- Oral infections
- *Candida albicans* infection may induce dysplasia and increase malignant transformation (2).
- Human papillomavirus, types 11 and 15
- Sunlight
- Vitamin deficiency
- Syphilis
- Dental restorations
- Prosthetic dental appliances
- Estrogen therapy
- Chronic trauma or irritation
- Epstein-Barr virus (oral hairy leukoplakia)
- Areca nut/betel (Asian populations)
- Mouthwash preparations and toothpaste containing the herbal root extract sanguinaria

COMMONLY ASSOCIATED CONDITIONS

- Leukokeratosis nicotina palati is rarely malignant.
- HIV infection is closely associated with hairy leukoplakia.
- Erythroplakia in association with leukoplakia, "speckled leukoplakia," or erythroleukoplakia is a marker for underlying dysplasia.
- Proliferative verrucous leukoplakia may develop into either squamous cell carcinoma or verrucous hyperplasia.

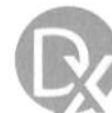

DIAGNOSIS

Leukoplakia is an asymptomatic white patch on the oral mucosa.

HISTORY

- Usually asymptomatic
- History of tobacco or alcohol use or oral exposure to irritants

PHYSICAL EXAM

- Location:
  - 50% on tongue, mandibular alveolar ridge, and buccal mucosa
  - Also seen on maxillary alveolar ridge, palate, and lower lip
  - Infrequently seen on floor of the mouth and retromolar areas
  - Floor of mouth, ventrolateral tongue, and soft palate complex are more likely to have dysplastic lesions.
- Appearance:
  - Clinical appearance of lesion does not necessarily correspond to malignant potential.
  - Varies from homogeneous, nonpalpable, faintly translucent white areas to thick, fissured, papillomatous, indurated plaques
  - May feel rough or leathery
  - Lesions can become exophytic or verruciform.
  - Color may be white, gray, yellowish white, or brownish gray, although mixed white and red lesions ("speckled leukoplakia") are more likely to be dysplastic or malignant.
  - Cannot be wiped or scraped off
  - Macular or plaquelike
  - Nodular and verrucous variants are more likely to be malignant.

DIAGNOSTIC TESTS & INTERPRETATION

Biopsy may assess the degree of dysplasia but does not correlate with the risk of subsequent malignant transformation (3).

Lab

Initial lab tests

Laboratory tests generally are not indicated:

- Consider saliva culture if *C. albicans* infection is suspected.

Follow-Up & Special Considerations

If no clear diagnosis, consider CBC, RPR, and biopsy.

Imaging

No imaging is indicated.

Diagnostic Procedures/Surgery

- Biopsy is necessary to rule out carcinoma if lesion is persistent, changing, or unexplained.
- Noninvasive brush biopsy and analysis of cells with DNA–image cytometry constitute a sensitive and specific screening method.
- Patients with dysplastic or malignant cells on brush biopsy should undergo more formal excisional biopsy.

Pathological Findings

- Biopsy specimens range from hyperkeratosis to invasive carcinoma.
- At initial biopsy, 6% are invasive carcinoma.
- 0.13–6% subsequently undergo malignant transformation.
- Location is important: 60% on floor of mouth or lateral border of tongue are cancerous; buccal mucosal lesions are generally not malignant but require biopsy if not resolving.

DIFFERENTIAL DIAGNOSIS

- White oral lesions that can be wiped away: Acute pseudomembranous candidiasis (4)
- White oral lesions that cannot be rubbed off (5):
  - Chronic hyperplastic candidiasis
  - Traumatic or frictional keratosis (e.g., linea alba)
  - Leukoedema (benign milky opaque lesions that disappear with stretching)
  - Aspirin burn (from holding aspirin in cheek)
  - Lichen planus (bilateral fairly symmetric lesions, reticular pattern of slightly raised gray-white lines)
  - Verrucous carcinoma
  - Lupus
  - Squamous cell carcinoma
  - Oral hairy leukoplakia, commonly on the lateral border of the tongue with a bilateral distribution (in HIV patients with Epstein-Barr virus infection)
  - Smoker's palate (leukokeratosis nicotina palati)
  - White sponge nevus (congenital benign spongy lesions)
  - Syphilitic oral lesion
  - Dyskeratosis congenita (a rare inherited multisystem disorder)

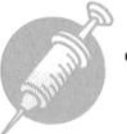

TREATMENT

- Treatment may include:
  - Surgical removal of the lesion
  - Topical or systemic medical treatment
  - Removal of predisposing habits (alcohol and tobacco)
  - Other treatment such as photodynamic therapy
- Treatment does not prevent malignant transformation.

MEDICATION

- Vitamin A, retinoids, beta-carotene, and lycopene may heal the oral leukoplakia (6)[A].
- No treatment has been shown to prevent relapse or malignant transformation (6)[A].
- Leukoplakia:
  - Isotretinoin (Accutane), 1–2 mg/kg/d PO may lead to temporary remission, but side effects are poorly tolerated.
  - Systemic administration of lycopene may have some efficacy in patients, similar to a subcontinental Indian population, for the short-term resolution of oral epithelial dysplasia (7)[B].
- Hairy leukoplakia:
  - Acyclovir, 2–4 g/d PO systemically is effective, but the lesions recur when the treatment is stopped.
  - Topical retinoids
  - Topical podophyllin 25% resin applied twice, 1 week between applications; however, the bad taste is poorly tolerated.

ADDITIONAL TREATMENT

General Measures

- Eliminate habitual lip biting.
- Correct ill-fitting dental appliances, bad restorations, or sharp teeth.
- Stop smoking and using alcohol.
- If dysplasia is evident, remove lesion. Consider otolaryngologist or oral surgery referral.
- Some small lesions may respond to cryosurgery.
- Beta-carotene, lycopene, retinoids, and cyclooxygenase 2 (COX-2) inhibitors may cause partial regression (experimental).
- For hairy tongue: Tongue brushing

SURGERY/OTHER PROCEDURES

- Complete excision is standard treatment for dysplasia or malignancy.
- Scalpel excision, laser ablation, electrocautery, or cryoablation
- Photodynamic therapy resolves lesions in 80% of patients with oral leukoplakia or erythroplakia (8).

IN-PATIENT CONSIDERATIONS

Initial Stabilization

- Eliminate etiologic factors.
- Re-evaluate in 7–14 days.
- Biopsy if lesion is persistent.

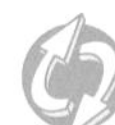

ONGOING CARE

FOLLOW-UP RECOMMENDATIONS

Patient Monitoring

- Regular, close follow-up, even after successful treatment
- Biopsy as needed.

DIET

Regular

PATIENT EDUCATION

- If biopsy is negative, stress importance of periodic and careful follow-up.
- Initiate a dental referral to eliminate dental factors.
- Stress importance of stopping tobacco and alcohol use.
- Encourage participation in smoking-cessation program.

PROGNOSIS

- Most leukoplakia is benign.
- Cancer is curable if detected early.
- 0.13–6% of initially benign lesions subsequently develop into cancer.
- More likely to be cancerous if on floor of mouth or lateral border of tongue

COMPLICATIONS

- New lesions may develop after treatment.
- Without surgical intervention, 4% develop carcinoma after 6.6 years (9).
- Larger lesions and nonhomogeneous leukoplakia are associated with higher rates of malignant transformation.

REFERENCES

1. Duarte EC, Ribeiro DC, Gomez MV, et al. Genetic polymorphisms of carcinogen metabolizing enzymes are associated with oral leukoplakia development and p53 overexpression. *Anticancer Res*. 2008;28:1101–6.
2. Cao J, Liu HW, Jin JQ, et al. [The effect of oral candida to development of oral leukoplakia into cancer.] *Zhonghua Yu Fang Yi Xue Za Zhi*. 2007; 41(Suppl):90–3.
3. Holmstrup P, Vedtofte P, Reibel J, et al. Oral premalignant lesions: Is a biopsy reliable? *J Oral Pathol Med*. 2007;36:262–6.
4. Akpan A, Morgan R, et al. Oral candidiasis. *Postgrad Med J*. 2002;78:455–9.
5. Canaan TJ, Meehan SC. Variations of structure and appearance of the oral mucosa. *Dent Clin North Am*. 2005;49:1–14, vii.
6. Lodi G, Sardella A, Bez C, et al. Interventions for treating oral leukoplakia. *Cochrane Database Syst Rev*. 2006;CD001829.
7. Brennan M, Migliorati CA, Lockhart PB, et al. Management of oral epithelial dysplasia: A review. *Oral Surg Oral Med Oral Pathol Oral Radiol Endod*. 2007.
8. Jerjes W, Upile T, Hamdoon Z, et al. Photodynamic therapy outcome for oral dysplasia. *Lasers Surg Med*. 2011;43:192–9.
9. Holmstrup P, Vedtofte P, Reibel J, et al. Long-term treatment outcome of oral premalignant lesions. *Oral Oncol*. 2006;42:461–74.

ADDITIONAL READING

- Greer RO. Pathology of malignant and premalignant oral epithelial lesions. *Otolaryngol Clin North Am*. 2006;39:249–75, v.
- Hardy ML. Dietary supplement use in cancer care: Help or harm. *Hematol Oncol Clin North Am*. 2008;22:581–617, vii.
- Maraki D, Becker J, Boecking A. Cytologic and DNA-cytometric very early diagnosis of oral cancer. *J Oral Pathol Med*. 2004;33:398–404.
- Reamy BV, Derby R, Bunt CW, et al. Common tongue conditions in primary care. *Am Fam Physician*. 2010;81:627–34.
- Warnakulasuriya S, Dietrich T, Bornstein MM, et al. Oral health risks of tobacco use and effects of cessation. *Int Dent J*. 2010;60:7–30.

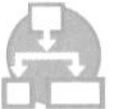

See Also (Topic, Algorithm, Electronic Media Element)

Epstein-Barr Virus Infections; HIV Infection and AIDS

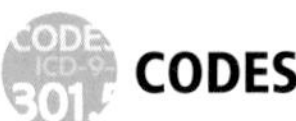

CODES

ICD9

528.6 Leukoplakia of oral mucosa, including tongue

CLINICAL PEARLS

- Linea alba: A white line on the buccal mucosa along the occlusal plane
- Low but significant rate of malignant transformation is not prevented with medical or surgical treatment; thus, long-term surveillance is essential.
- To lessen risk of malignant transformation, tobacco and alcohol cessation, and consider *C. albicans* eradication

LICHEN PLANUS

Herbert P. Goodheart, MD

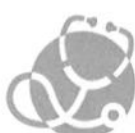

BASICS

Lichen planus (LP) is an idiopathic eruption with characteristic shiny, flat-topped papules (Latin: planus, "flat") purple (violaceous) papules on the skin, often accompanied by characteristic mucous membrane lesions (Wickham striae). Itching may be severe.

DESCRIPTION

- Classic (typical) LP is a relatively uncommon cutaneous inflammatory disorder of the skin and mucous membranes; hair and nails may also be affected:
  – Small, flat, angular, red-to-violaceous, shiny, pruritic papules on the skin; fine, white, lacy patches or erosions on oral mucosa
  – Most commonly seen on the flexor surfaces of the upper extremities, extensor surfaces of the lower extremities, the genitalia, and on the mucous membranes
  – Course is unpredictable; onset is abrupt or gradual. May resolve spontaneously, recur intermittently, or persist for many years.
- Drug-induced LP:
  – Clinical and histopathologic findings may mimic those of classic LP. Lesions usually lack Wickham striae (see below).
  – There is generally a latent period of months from drug introduction before lesions appear.
  – Lesions resolve when the inciting agent is discontinued, often after a prolonged period.
- LP variants:
  – Follicular: On scalp (lichen planopilaris) and skin
  – Annular: Appear on glans penis and oral mucosa
  – Linear: May be an isolated finding
  – Atrophic: Rare, most often the result of resolved lesions
  – Lichen planus pemphigoides: A combination of LP and bullous pemphigoid
- System(s) affected: Skin/Exocrine
- Synonym(s): Lichenoid eruptions

EPIDEMIOLOGY

- Predominant age: 30–60 years old; rare in children and the geriatric population
- Predominant sex: Female > Male

Prevalence

In the US, 450/100,000

RISK FACTORS

Exposure to certain drugs or chemicals:

- Thiazides, furosemide, beta-blockers, sulfonylureas, antimalarials, penicillamine, gold salts, and ACE inhibitors
- Rarely: Photo-developing chemicals, dental materials, tattoo pigments

ETIOLOGY

LP is considered to be a cell-mediated immune response of unknown origin.

COMMONLY ASSOCIATED CONDITIONS

- An association has been noted between lichen planus and hepatitis C virus infection (more common in Japan and Italy), chronic active hepatitis, lichen nitidus, and primary biliary cirrhosis. Hepatitis should be considered in patients with widespread presentations of LP.
- Lichen planus has also infrequently been reported to be found in association with other diseases of altered immunity than would be expected by chance:
  – Bullous pemphigoid
  – Alopecia areata
  – Myasthenia gravis
  – Vitiligo
  – Ulcerative colitis
  – Graft versus host reaction
  – Lupus erythematosus (lupus erythematosus–lichen planus overlap syndrome)
  – Morphea and lichen sclerosis et atrophicus

DIAGNOSIS

LP is most commonly diagnosed by its appearance, despite its range of clinical presentations. A skin biopsy should be performed if the diagnosis is in doubt.

HISTORY

A minority of patients have a family history of LP. Affected families have an increased frequency of human leukocyte antigen B7 (HLA-B7).

PHYSICAL EXAM

- Skin (often severe pruritus):
  – Papules: 1–10 mm, shiny, flat-topped (planar) lesions that occur in crops; lesions may have a fine scale
  – Evidence of scratching (i.e., crusts and excoriations) is usually absent.
  – Color: Violaceous, with white lacelike pattern (Wickham striae) on surface of papules. Wickham striae are best seen after topical application of mineral oil, and if present, are virtually pathognomonic for lichen planus.
  – Shape: Polygonal or oval. Annular lesions may appear on trunk and mucous membranes. Various shapes and sizes may be noted (polymorphic).
  – Arrangement: May be grouped, linear, or scattered individual lesions
  – Koebner phenomenon (isomorphic response): New lesions may be noted at sites of minor injuries, such as scratches or burns.
  – Distribution: Ventral surface of wrists and forearms, dorsa hands, glans penis, dorsa feet, groin, sacrum, shins, and scalp. Hypertrophic (verrucous) lesions may occur on lower legs and may be generalized.
  – Postinflammatory hyperpigmentation: Lesions typically heal, leaving darkly pigmented macules in their wake.
- Mucous membranes (40–60% of patients with skin lesions; 20% have mucous membrane lesions without skin involvement):
  – Most commonly asymptomatic, nonerosive, milky-white lines with an elegant, lacy, netlike streaked pattern
  – Usually seen on buccal mucosa, but may appear on tongue, gingiva, palate, or lips
  – May be erosive, rarely bullous
  – Painful, especially if ulcers present
  – Lesions may develop into squamous cell carcinoma (1–3%).
  – Glans penis, labia minora, vaginal vault, and perianal areas may be involved (1,2).
- Hair and nails:
  – Scalp: Atrophic scalp skin and destruction of hair follicles. May result in permanent patchy, scarring alopecia (lichen planopilaris).
- Nails (10%): Involvement of nail matrix may cause proximal-to-distal linear grooves and partial or complete destruction of nail bed with pterygium formation.

DIAGNOSTIC TESTS & INTERPRETATION

Lab

If suggested by history:

- Serology for hepatitis B and C
- Liver function tests

Diagnostic Procedures/Surgery

- Skin biopsy
- Direct immunofluorescence helps to distinguish lichen planus from discoid lupus erythematosus.

Pathological Findings

- Vacuolar degeneration of the basal layer
- Hyperkeratosis and irregular acanthosis, increased granular layer
- Basement membrane thinning with "saw-toothing"
- Degenerative keratinocytes, known as colloid or Civatte bodies, are found in the lower epidermis.
- Dense, bandlike (lichenoid) lymphocytic infiltrate of the upper dermis
- Melanin pigment in macrophages

DIFFERENTIAL DIAGNOSIS

- Skin:
  – Lichen simplex chronicus
  – Eczematous dermatitis
  – Psoriasis
  – Discoid lupus erythematosus
  – Other lichenoid eruptions (those that resemble lichen planus)
  – Pityriasis rosea
  – Lichen nitidus
- Oral mucous membranes:
  – Leukoplakia
  – Oral hairy leukoplakia
  – Candidiasis
  – Squamous cell carcinoma (particularly in ulcerative lesions)
  – Aphthous ulcers
  – Herpetic stomatitis
  – Secondary syphilis
- Genital mucous membranes:
  – Psoriasis (penis and labia)
  – Nonspecific balanitis, Zoon balanitis
  – Fixed drug eruption (penis)
  – Candidiasis (penis and labia)
  – Pemphigus vulgaris, bullous pemphigoid, and Behçet disease (all rare)
- Hair and scalp:
  – Scarring alopecia (pseudopelade)

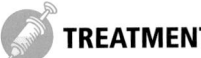

TREATMENT

Although LP can resolve spontaneously, treatment is usually demanded by patients who may be severely symptomatic or troubled by its cosmetic appearance.

MEDICATION

First Line

Pediatric Considerations

Children may absorb a proportionally larger amount of topical steroid because of larger skin surface-to-weight ratio:

- Skin: Superpotent topical steroids (e.g., 0.05% clobetasol propionate) b.i.d. for 2 weeks:
  - Potent topical steroids such as triamcinolone acetonide 0.1% or fluocinonide 0.05% under occlusion
  - Intralesional corticosteroids (e.g., triamcinolone [Kenalog] 5–10 mg/mL) for recalcitrant and hypertrophic lesions
  - Antihistamines (e.g., hydroxyzine, 25 mg PO q6h) have limited benefit for itching, but may be helpful for sedation at bedtime.
  - "Soak and smear" technique: Can lead to a rapid improvement of symptoms in even a day or 2 and may obviate the need for systemic steroids. Soaking allows water to hydrate the stratum corneum. Soaking also allows the anti-inflammatory steroid in the ointment to penetrate more deeply into the skin. Smearing of the ointment traps the water in the skin because water cannot move out through greasy materials:
    - Soaking is done in a bathtub using lukewarm plain water for 20 minutes at night, then, without drying the skin, affected skin is immediately smeared with a thin film of the steroid ointment containing clobetasol or another superpotent topical steroid. A topical steroid cream is applied thereafter during the daytime hours, if necessary.
    - The soaking and smearing may be done for 4–5 days or longer, if necessary. The treatments are best done at night because the greasy ointment applied to the skin gets on pajamas (instead of on daytime clothes) and the ointment is on the skin during sleep.
- Mucous membranes for erosive, painful lichen planus:
  - Topical corticosteroids (0.1% triamcinolone [Kenalog] in Orabase) or 0.05% clobetasol propionate ointment b.i.d.
  - Intralesional corticosteroids
  - Topical 0.1% tacrolimus (Protopic Ointment) b.i.d. (3,4)[A]
  - Topical 1% pimecrolimus (Elidel) cream b.i.d. (5)[A]
  - Topical retinoids (e.g., 0.05% tretinoin [retinoic acid] in Orabase)

Second Line

Skin and mucous membranes:

- Intralesional corticosteroids
- Topical 0.1% tacrolimus (Protopic Ointment) b.i.d. (4,5)
- Topical 1% pimecrolimus (Elidel) cream b.i.d. (6)
- Oral prednisone: Used only for a short course (e.g., 30–60 mg/d for 2–4 weeks) or IM triamcinolone (Kenalog) 40–80 mg every 6–8 weeks:
  - Precautions with systemic steroids
  - Systemic absorption of steroids may result in hypothalamic-pituitary-adrenal axis suppression, Cushing syndrome, hyperglycemia, or glucosuria.
  - Increased risk with high-potency topical steroids (i.e., use over large surface area, prolonged use, occlusive dressings)
  - In pregnancy: Usually safe, but benefits must outweigh the risks
- Oral retinoids: Isotretinoin in doses of 10 mg PO for 2 months and acitretin 30 mg have resulted in improvement in some refractory cases.
- Oral metronidazole 500 mg b.i.d. for 20–60 days can be given as a safer alternative to systemic corticosteroids.
- Cyclosporine may be used in severe cases, but cost and potential toxicity limit its use. Topical use for severe oral involvement refractory to other treatments (3).
- Thalidomide
- Psoralen ultraviolet-A (PUVA), broad-band or narrow-band ultraviolet-B (UVB) (6)
- Griseofulvin
- Azathioprine
- Mycophenolate mofetil

ALERT

Avoid oral and topical retinoids during pregnancy.

ADDITIONAL TREATMENT

General Measures

- Goal is to relieve itching and resolve lesions
- Asymptomatic oral lesions require no treatment.

IN-PATIENT CONSIDERATIONS

Initial Stabilization

Outpatient care

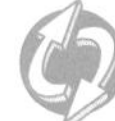

ONGOING CARE

FOLLOW-UP RECOMMENDATIONS

Patient Monitoring

Serial oral examinations for erosive/ulcerative lesions

PATIENT EDUCATION

- Oral, erosive, or ulcerative lichen planus: Annual follow-up to screen for malignancy (7)
- Avoid spicy foods, cigarettes, and excessive alcohol.
- Avoid crispy foods such as corn chips, pretzels, and toast.

PROGNOSIS

- Spontaneous resolution in weeks is possible, but disease may persist for years, especially oral lesions and hypertrophic lesions on the shins.
- There is a tendency toward relapse.
- Recurrence in 12–20%, especially in those with generalized involvement

COMPLICATIONS

- Alopecia
- Nail destruction
- Squamous cell carcinoma of the mouth or genitals

REFERENCES

1. Belfiore P, Di Fede O, Cabibi D, et al. Prevalence of vulval lichen planus in a cohort of women with oral lichen planus: An interdisciplinary study. *Br J Dermatol*. 2006;155(5):994–8.
2. Di Fede O, Belfiore P, Cabibi D, et al. Unexpectedly high frequency of genital involvement in women with clinical and histological features of oral lichen planus. *Acta Derm Venereol*. 2006;86:433–8.
3. Conrotto D, Carbone M, Carrozzo M, et al. Ciclosporin vs. clobetasol in the topical management of atrophic and erosive oral lichen planus: A double-blind, randomized controlled trial. *Br J Dermatol*. 2006;154:139–45.
4. Morrison L, Kratochvil FJ, Gorman A. An open trial of topical tacrolimus for erosive oral lichen planus. *J Am Acad Dermatol*. 2002;47:617–20.
5. Passeron T, Lacour JP, Fontas E, et al. Treatment of oral erosive lichen planus with 1% pimecrolimus cream: A double-blind, randomized, prospective trial with measurement of pimecrolimus levels in the blood. *Arch Dermatol*. 2007;143:472–6.
6. Ultraviolet-B treatment for cutaneous lichen planus: Our experience with 50 patients. Pavlotsky F, Nathansohn N, et al. *Photodermatol Photoimmunol Photmed*. 2008:83–6.
7. Gonzalez-Moles MA, Scully C, Gil-Montoya JA. Oral lichen planus: Controversies surrounding malignant transformation. *Oral Dis*. 2008;14(3):229–43.

CODES

ICD9

697.0 Lichen planus

CLINICAL PEARLS

- Remember the 7 Ps of lichen planus: *P*urple, *p*lanar, *p*olygonal, *p*olymorphic, *p*ruritic (not always), *p*apules that heal with *p*ostinflammatory hyperpigmentation.
- Serial oral or genital examinations are indicated for erosive/ulcerative LP lesions to monitor for the development of squamous cell carcinoma.
- An association has been noted between LP and hepatitis C virus infection, chronic active hepatitis, and primary biliary cirrhosis.
- The "soak and smear" technique can lead to a rapid improvement of symptoms in even a day or 2 and may obviate the need for systemic steroids.

LICHEN SIMPLEX CHRONICUS

Jennifer Crombie, MD
Dori Goldberg, MD

BASICS

DESCRIPTION

- A chronic dermatitis resulting from continued, repeated rubbing, or scratching of the skin
- System(s) affected: Skin/Exocrine
- Synonym(s): Lichen simplex; neurodermatitis; neurodermatitis circumscripta

EPIDEMIOLOGY

Geriatric Considerations

Common in those >60 years

Pediatric Considerations

Rare in preadolescents

Incidence

- Common
- Peak incidence 35–50 years of age
- Females > Males (F:M = 2:1)

Prevalence

Common

RISK FACTORS

Any pre-existing pruritic dermatosis can result in the development of secondary lichen simplex chronicus.

Genetics

Polymorphisms of the serotonin transporter gene (5-HTT) have been implicated.

GENERAL PREVENTION

Avoid common triggers such as psychological distress, environmental factors such as heat and excessive dryness, skin irritation, and the development of pruritic dermatoses.

PATHOPHYSIOLOGY

- Scratching may be secondary to habit or a conditioned response to anxiety.
- Repeated scratching or rubbing causes inflammation and pruritus.
- Pruritus results in continued scratching.
- The formation of a itch–scratch cycle leads to a chronic dermatosis.

ETIOLOGY

- Primary lichen simplex chronicus occurs de novo in tissue with previously normal appearance.
- This is idiopathic in many instances.
- Secondary forms begin as a pruritic skin disease that evolves into neurodermatitis after resolution of the primary dermatitis.
- Precursor dermatoses include atopic dermatitis, contact dermatitis, lichen planus, lichen sclerosis, stasis dermatitis, psoriasis, fungal infections, and insect bites.
- There is a possible relation between disease development and underlying neuropathy, particularly radiculopathy or nerve-root compression.
- Pruritus-specific C neurons are temperature sensitive, which may explain itching that occurs in warm environments.
- Anxiety and emotional stress appear to play a role.

COMMONLY ASSOCIATED CONDITIONS

- Prurigo nodularis is a nodular variety of the same disease process.
- Atopic dermatitis
- Anxiety, depression, and obsessive–compulsive disorders

DIAGNOSIS

HISTORY

- Gradual onset
- Begins as a localized area of pruritus
- Most patients acknowledge that they respond with vigorous rubbing, itching, or scratching, which brings temporary satisfaction.
- Pruritus is typically paroxysmal, worse at night, and may lead to scratching during sleep.
- Most commonly involves easily accessible areas, including nape of neck, ankles, extensor surfaces of forearms, scalp, and anogenital region

PHYSICAL EXAM

- Erythematous, scaling, lichenified plaques with varying amounts of overlying excoriation
- Accentuation of normal skin lines
- In cases of long-standing duration, hyperpigmentation and hypopigmentation can be seen.
- Scarring may result following ulcer formation or secondary infection.

DIAGNOSTIC TESTS & INTERPRETATION

Lab

Initial lab tests

- None are diagnostic
- Microscopy and culture preparation may be helpful in identifying a superimposed fungal infection.

Diagnostic Procedures/Surgery

A skin biopsy to identify characteristic changes on pathology can be beneficial if the diagnosis is in question.

Pathological Findings

- Hyperkeratosis
- Acanthosis
- Lengthening of rete ridges
- Hyperplasia of all components of epidermis
- Chronic inflammatory infiltrate of dermis with perivascular infiltrates of lymphocytes and occasional macrophages

DIFFERENTIAL DIAGNOSIS

- Atopic dermatitis
- Contact dermatitis
- Fungal infection
- Lichenified psoriasis
- Lichen planus
- Mycosis fungoides
- Lichen amyloidosis
- Stasis dermatitis

TREATMENT

MEDICATION

First Line

- Reducing inflammation:
  - Topical steroids are first-line agents.
  - High-potency steroids alone, such as 0.05% betamethasone dipropionate cream or 0.05% clobetasol propionate cream, can be used initially but not on the face, anogenital region, or intertriginous areas. They should be used on small areas only for no longer than 2 weeks except under the close supervision of a physician (1)[C].
  - Switch to intermediate- or low-potency steroids as response allows.
  - An intermediate-potency steroid, such as 0.1% triamcinolone cream, may be used for initial treatment of the face and intertriginous areas, and for maintenance treatment of other areas.
  - A low-potency steroid, such as 1% hydrocortisone cream, should be used for maintenance treatment of the face and intertriginous areas.
  - Steroid tape, flurandrenolide, has optimized penetration and provides a barrier to continued scratching.
  - Intralesional steroids, such as triamcinolone acetate, are also safe and effective (2)[C].
  - Contraindications:
    - High-potency topical steroids should not be used on the face or intertriginous areas.
  - Precautions:
    - Topical steroid therapy can cause epidermal and dermal atrophy as well as hypopigmentation.
- Preventing the itch–scratch cycle:
  - Antipruritic agents such as 1% menthol preparations and pramoxine
  - Oral antihistamines such as diphenhydramine and hydroxyzine for antipruritic and sedative effects
  - Sedating tricyclics, such as doxepin and amitriptyline, for nighttime itching

Second Line

- Topical aspirin has been shown to be helpful in treating neurodermatitis (3)[C].
- Topical doxepin cream 5% has significant antipuritic activity (4)[C].
- Topical capsaicin cream can be helpful for treatment of early disease manifestations (5)[C].
- A case report showed that topical 0.1% tacrolimus was effective in treating lichen simplex chronicus of the face (6)[C].
- Topical pimecrolimus may decrease the symptoms of vulvar lichen simplex chronicus (7)[C].
- Gabapentin was found to decrease symptoms in patients who are nonresponsive to steroids (8)[C].
- Botulinum toxin injected intradermally has been reported to improve symptoms in patients with recalcitrant pruritus (9)[C].
- Transcutaneous electrical nerve stimulation may relieve pruritus in patients for whom topical steroids were not effective (10,11)[C].
- SSRIs may be effective in controlling compulsive scratching.

ADDITIONAL TREATMENT

General Measures

- Patient education
- Treat pruritus to interrupt the scratch–itch cycle
- Treat underlying pruritic skin conditions

Issues for Referral

- No response to treatment
- Presence of signs and symptoms suggestive of a systemic cause of pruritus
- Consultation with a psychiatrist for patients with severe stress, anxiety, or compulsive scratching
- Consultation with an allergist for patients with multisystemic atopic symptoms

Additional Therapies

- Cooling of the skin with ice or cold compresses
- Soaks and lubricants to improve barrier layer function
- Provide barrier protection with bandages or Unna boots
- Nail trimming

COMPLEMENTARY AND ALTERNATIVE MEDICINE

- Cognitive-behavioral therapy may improve awareness and help to identify coping strategies (12)[C].
- Hypnosis may be beneficial in decreasing pruritus and preventing scratching (12)[C].
- Homeopathic remedies (i.e., thuja and graphites) may provide resolution of symptoms (13)[C].

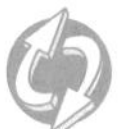

ONGOING CARE

FOLLOW-UP RECOMMENDATIONS

Patient Monitoring

Patients should be followed closely and regularly for response to therapy, complications from therapy, and secondary infections.

DIET

Regular balanced diet

PATIENT EDUCATION

- Patients should understand the cause of this disease and their role in its resolution.
- Stress reduction techniques can be useful for patients for whom stress plays role.
- Emphasize that scratching and rubbing must stop for lesions to heal.
- Avoid exposure to known triggers.

PROGNOSIS

- Often chronic and recurrent
- Good prognosis if the itch–scratch cycle can be broken
- After healing, the skin should have a normal appearance unless a severe secondary infection or ulcer formation has occurred.
- Postinflammatory pigmentary changes may be slow to resolve.

COMPLICATIONS

- Secondary infection
- Scarring is rare.
- Complications related to therapy, as mentioned in medication precautions
- Squamous cell carcinoma within affected regions is rare.

REFERENCES

1. Datz B, Yawalkar S. A double-blind, multicenter trial of 0.05% halobetasol propionate ointment and 0.05% clobetasol 17-propionate ointment in the treatment of patients with chronic, localized atopic dermatitis or lichen simplex chronicus. *J Am Acad Dermatol*. 1991;25:1157–60.
2. Richards RN. Update on intralesional steroid: Focus of dermatoses. *J Cutan Med Surg*. 2010; 14(1):19–23.
3. Yosipovitch G, Sugeng MW, Chan YH. The effect of topically applied aspirin on localized circumscribed neurodermatitis. *J Am Acad Dermatol*. 2001;45:910–3.
4. Drake L, Millikan E, the Doxepin Study Group. The antipuritis effect of 5% doxepin cream in patients with eczematous dermatitis. *Arch Dermatol*. 1995;131:1403–8.
5. Kantor GR, Resnik KS. Treatment of lichen simplex chronicus with topical capsaicin cream. *Acta Derm Venereol*. 1996;76:161.
6. Aschoff R, Wozel G. Topical tacrolimus for the treatment of lichen simplex chronicus. *J Dermatolog Treat*. 2007;18(2):115–7.
7. Goldstein AT, Parneix-Spake A. Pimecrolimus cream 1% for treatment of vulvar lichen simplex chronicus: An open label trial. *Obstet Gynecol*. 2006;107(4 Suppl):54S–5S.
8. Gencoglan G, Inanir I, Gunduz K. Therapeutic hotline: Treatment of prurigo nodularis and lichen simplex chronicus with gabapentin. *Dermatol Ther*. 2010;23(3):194–8.
9. Heckmann M, Heyer G, Brunner B. Botulinum toxin type A injection in the treatment of lichen simplex: An open pilot study. *J Am Acad Dermatol*. 2002;46:617–9.
10. Engin B, Tufekci O, Yazici A. The effect of transcutaneous electrical nerve stimulation in the treatment of lichen simplex: A prospective study. *Clin Exp Dermatol*. 2009;34:324–8.
11. Yuksek J, Sezer E, Aksu M, et al. Transcutaneous electrical nerve stimulation for reduction of pruritis in macular amyloidosis and lichen simplex. *J Dermatol*. 2011;38(6):546–52.
12. Shenefelt PD. Biofeedback, cognitive-behavioral methods, and hypnosis in dermatology: Is it all in your mind? *Dermatol Ther*. 2003;16:114–22.
13. Gupta R, Manchanda RK, et al. Homoeopathy for the treatment of lichen simplex chronicus: A case series. *Homeopathy*. 2006;95:245–7.

ADDITIONAL READING

- Hercogová J, et al. Topical anti-itch therapy. *Dermatol Ther*. 2005;18:341–3.
- Kirtak N, Inaloz H, Akcali C, et al. Association of serotonin transporter gene-linked polymorphic region and variable number of tandem repeat polymorphism of the serotonin transporter gene in lichen simplex chronicus patients with psychiatric status. *Int J Dermatol*. 2008;47:1069–72.
- Konuk N, Koca R, Atik L, et al. Psychopathology, depression and dissociative experiences in patients with lichen simplex chronicus. *Gen Hosp Psychiatry*. 2007;29:232–5.
- Lotti T, Buggiani G, Prignano F. Prurigo nodularis and lichen simplex chronicus. *Dermatol Ther*. 2008;21:42–6.
- Lynch P. Lichen simplex chronicus (atopic/neurodermatitis) of the anogenital region. *Dermatol Ther*. 2004;17:8–19.
- Rajalakshmi R, Thappa DM, Jaisanker TJ, et al. Lichen simplex chronicus of the anogenital region: A clinico-etiological study. *Indian Venereol Leprol*. 2011;77(1):28–36.
- Solak O, Kulac M, Yama M, et al. Simplex chronicus as a symptom of neuropathy. *Clin Exper Dermatol*. 2008;34:476–80.
- Wu M, Wang Y, Bu W, et al. Squamous cell carcinoma arising in lichen simplex chronicus. *Eur J Dermatol*. 2010;20(6):858–9.

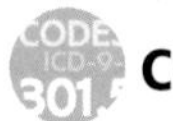

CODES

ICD9

698.3 Lichenification and lichen simplex chronicus

CLINICAL PEARLS

- Primary lichen simplex chronicus originates de novo while secondary lichen simplex chronicus occurs in the setting of a pruritic dermatologic condition.
- This is a chronic inflammatory condition that results from repeated scratching and rubbing.
- The diagnosis is made clinically based on history and skin examination.
- If the diagnosis is unclear, consider empiric treatment with close monitoring or skin biopsy.
- Stopping the itch–scratch cycle through patient education, skin lubrication, and topical antipruritic medications is key.

LIPOMA

Manjula Cherukuri, MD
Lisa O. Jolly, MD

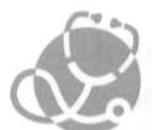

BASICS

DESCRIPTION

- Lipomas are the most common benign SC tumors.
- They are composed of mature fat cells, enveloped by a thin, fibrous capsule.
- Slow growing, often asymptomatic, and usually have a soft doughy feel on palpation
- Some lipomas are believed to have developed following blunt trauma.
- Lipomas rarely, if ever, become malignant, but must be differentiated from liposarcomas and other tumors.

EPIDEMIOLOGY

- They can occur at any age, but are most common in middle-aged adults, peaking in the 40–60-year age group.
- They are rare in children.

Incidence

The incidence of lipomas is 1 per 1,000 individuals annually.

Prevalence

Occur in about 1% of population

RISK FACTORS

- Soft tissue trauma frequently has been cited as a cause, especially if the patient develops a posttraumatic hematoma.
- Alcohol consumption may be a predisposing factor for Madelung disease, or benign symmetric lipomatosis, with lipomas on the head, neck, shoulders, and proximal upper extremities. This may present with the characteristic "horse collar" cervical appearance, resulting in swallowing or respiratory problems and sudden death.

Genetics

- May appear as a hereditary syndrome in patients with hereditary multiple lipomatosis, an autosomal dominant condition. This is found most frequently in men, characterized by extensive, symmetric, sometimes giant lipomas mostly on extremities and trunk.
- Congenital lipomas have been observed in children.

PATHOPHYSIOLOGY

- The pathogenetic link between soft tissue trauma and the formation of posttraumatic lipomas is still controversial.
- There are 2 potential explanations to correlate soft tissue trauma and adipose tissue tumor growth:
  - The first is the formation of so-called posttraumatic pseudolipomas by prolapsing adipose tissue through fascia resulting from direct impact.
  - A second possibility points toward lipoma formation as a result of preadipocyte differentiation and proliferation mediated by cytokine release following soft tissue trauma and hematoma formation.

ETIOLOGY

They are reported to occur after trauma, but most are idiopathic.

COMMONLY ASSOCIATED CONDITIONS

- Admixture of other tissue types leads to fibrolipomas, angiolipomas, and myolipomas.
- Unusual presentations of lipoma can occur, like giant lipomas in hereditary multiple lipomatosis, adiposis dolorosa (multiple tender, diffuse lesions), Gardner syndrome with intestinal polyposis, and Madelung disease (numerous symmetrically distributed lipomas of the upper trunk).
- Liposarcomas rarely develop from benign lipomas. They can occur anywhere in the body, mostly in deep structures.

DIAGNOSIS

HISTORY

- Useful questions on history gathering are duration, associated symptoms, tenderness, recurrence, progression, similar lesions, and weight loss.
- Generally slow growing; may take years before being noticed
- If fast growing, may indicate a liposarcoma
- Individuals can have single lesions or a few. In ~5% of cases, patients have multiple lesions.
- Lipomas are usually SC and often found in the upper trunk, especially the shoulders, back, neck, and head, but can be anywhere in or on the body.
- Lipomas have been reported in anatomic locations as varied as cardiac, intrathoracic, endobronchial, retroperitoneal, breast, intermuscular, calf, thigh, scapular, intraosseous, fingers, palmar, toe, epidural, spinal, intra-articular (knee), parapharyngeal, nasopharyngeal, adrenal, inguinal, bladder, scrotal, ovarian, intracranial, intraneural, and GI tract (most often in the ileum).
- Usually asymptomatic
- Infrequently may cause pain; seen with angiolipoma, a highly vascular lipoma
- Depending on location, lipomas can cause respiratory distress due to bronchial obstruction if in major airways or can cause cord compression if in dural/medullary components of the spinal cord.
- Neuropathic symptoms from compression may develop (mass effect from lipoma) in locations such as the forearm or ankle.
- In the GI tract, lipomas can present as submucosal fatty tumors. The most common locations include the esophagus, stomach, and small intestine. Symptoms may occur from luminal obstruction or bleeding.
- Most often patients show them to physicians for explanation and reassurance.
- They may be first noted by physicians on a physical exam.

PHYSICAL EXAM

- Lipomas are usually soft, homogeneous, oval, and nontender, and the overlying skin is mobile over them.
- They are commonly from 1–5 cm in diameter. If larger, this raises suspicion for liposarcoma.
- Rubbery or doughy consistency; if harder, suspect liposarcoma, sebaceous (epidermoid) cyst, or abscess.
- Overlying skin is normal; if erythematous, might indicate an abscess.
- The tumor will be felt to slip out from under your fingers ("slippage sign") as opposed to a sebaceous cyst or an abscess, which is tethered by surrounding induration.

DIAGNOSTIC TESTS & INTERPRETATION

Most SC lipomas can be diagnosed based on history and physical, and no imaging studies are required.

Imaging

- MRI and CT scan are used mostly for atypical locations and as a preoperative measure.
- Because of differences in treatment, prognosis, and long-term follow-up, it is important to preoperatively distinguish simple lipomas from well-differentiated liposarcomas.
- MRI is extremely sensitive in the detection of well-differentiated liposarcomas and very specific in the diagnosis of simple lipomas. When an extremity or body wall lesion is considered suspicious for well-differentiated liposarcoma, it is more likely (64%) to represent one of many benign lipoma variants (1).
- Reported MRI findings suggestive of liposarcoma include a partially ill-defined margin, neurovascular involvement, enhancing thick/nodular septum, and a partially bright signal intensity on T1-weighted images. A thick/nodular septum was identified as the most statistically significant predictor of liposarcoma (2).
- If liposarcoma is suspected, fine- and core-needle aspirations have been proposed along with imaging. A core-needle biopsy has been proposed as the preferred biopsy method; it can provide accurate diagnosis and assessment of malignant potential and grade if examined by an experienced pathologist (3).

Diagnostic Procedures/Surgery

If diagnosis is uncertain, excisional biopsy is a preferred assessment tool.

Pathological Findings

- Lipomas are composed of adipose tissue, with varying amounts of a network of connective tissue.
- Lipomas are surrounded by a fibrous, well-defined capsule that is separate from the surrounding tissue.
- Lipomas differ from normal fat with increased levels of lipoprotein lipase and a larger number of precursor cells.

DIFFERENTIAL DIAGNOSIS

- Differential diagnosis includes epidermoid cyst (sebaceous cyst), hematoma, vasculitis, panniculitis, rheumatic nodules, metastatic disease, or infections.
- Sebaceous (epidermoid) cysts are also rounded and SC. They can be differentiated from lipomas by their characteristic central punctum and surrounding induration.
- Abscess typically has pain along with overlying induration and erythema.
- Benign lipomas must be differentiated from liposarcomas. Rapid growth and hard consistency should prompt consideration of malignancy.

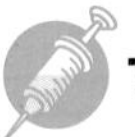

TREATMENT

- Most lipomas can be observed without treatment (4)[C].
- They need treatment if there is diagnostic uncertainty, hard consistency on palpation, rapid growth, associated pain, compression of nerves/vital organs, or cosmetic concern.
- Treatment of lipoma varies from nonsurgical treatments like steroid injection or liposuction, which can be cosmetically useful in certain locations (such as facial), or surgical treatments like excision or enucleation by "squeeze technique" (4)[C].
- A successful trial of lipomas treated with SC deoxycholate injections has been reported suggesting that low-concentration deoxycholate may be a relatively safe and effective treatment for small collections of fat. However, controlled clinical trials will be necessary to substantiate these observations (5)[C].
- Spinal lipomas should be operated on as soon as possible on a prophylactic basis, and careful and constant follow-up should be carried out to permit prompt reintervention in cases with deterioration (6)[C].

SURGERY/OTHER PROCEDURES

- Plan the incision to follow skin lines, if possible, to minimize scarring. Use a surgical marker to draw out the palpable margins of the lipoma and the planned incision. The incision should be about 60% of the lipoma width. Be prepared to extend the incision if needed.
- After anesthetizing the skin with a local anesthetic, a linear incision is carried out down to the level of the capsule using a number 11 or 15 blade.
- Blunt dissection (curved hemostat) and sharp dissection (iris scissor) are used to separate the fibrous capsule from the surrounding soft tissue. Care must be taken not to invade the capsule to maintain proper aesthetics.
- As the lobule is lifted, the dissection is continued to free up the entire tumor.
- Apply pressure to the outside of the lipoma to express it through the skin opening (7)[C]. In many cases, the lipoma will just pop out. If not, more dissection may be needed, or the incision may be lengthened.
- After the lipoma is out, pressure with gauze is usually all that is needed to obtain good hemostasis. If bleeding persists, use electrocoagulation before closing the incision.
- The dead space may be closed with deep absorbable sutures, but often this is not necessary.
- The skin may be closed with nonabsorbable simple interrupted sutures. For small lipomas, closure may be performed with wound-closure strips or the linear incision left open.
- If excessive skin remains, the linear incision can be turned into an ellipse to avoid redundant skin.

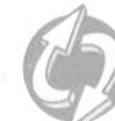

ONGOING CARE

FOLLOW-UP RECOMMENDATIONS

Usual surgical follow-up is needed to monitor for any complications such as hematoma formation or infection.

PATIENT EDUCATION

Handout: "What Are Lipomas?" *American Family Physician*. March 1, 2002. www.aafp.org/afp/20020301/905ph.html

PROGNOSIS

Most lipomas grow very slowly and are benign, asymptomatic, and remain stable. Recurrence after excision is rare unless excision was incomplete.

COMPLICATIONS

- Hematoma and seroma formation or infection is rare but possible.
- Occasionally, a bilobar lipoma may be missed, resulting in "recurrence." The local recurrence rate of simple lipomas involving SC tissues is ~1–2%.
- Lipomas that grow rapidly or become painful or nodular must be evaluated for liposarcoma.

REFERENCES

1. Gaskin CM, Helms CA. Lipomas, lipoma variants, and well-differentiated liposarcomas (atypical lipomas): Results of MRI evaluations of 126 consecutive fatty masses. *AJR Am J Roentgenol*. 2004;182:733–9.
2. Jaovisidha S, Suvikapakornkul Y, Woratanarat P, et al. MR imaging of fat-containing tumours: The distinction between lipoma and liposarcoma. *Singapore Med J*. 2010;51:418–23.
3. Strauss DC, Qureshi YA, Hayes AJ, et al. The role of core needle biopsy in the diagnosis of suspected soft tissue tumours. *J Surg Oncol*. 2010;102(5):523–9.
4. Bancroft LW, Kransdorf MJ, Peterson JJ, et al. Benign fatty tumors: Classification, clinical course, imaging appearance, and treatment. *Skeletal Radiol*. 2006;35:719–33.
5. Rotunda AM, Ablon G, Kolodney MS. Lipomas treated with subcutaneous deoxycholate injections. *J Am Acad Dermatol*. 2005;53:973–8.
6. Jindal A, Mahapatra AK, et al. Spinal lipomatous malformations. *Indian J Pediatr*. 2000;67:342–6.
7. Salam GA, et al. Lipoma excision. *Am Fam Physician*. 2002;65:901–4.

ADDITIONAL READING

- Aust MC, Spies M, Kall S, et al. Posttraumatic lipoma: Fact or fiction? *Skinmed*. 2007;6:266–70.
- Blount JP, Elton S. Spinal lipomas. *Neurosurg Foc*. 2001;10(1):e3.
- Pandya KA, Radke F, et al. Benign skin lesions: Lipomas, epidermal inclusion cysts, muscle and nerve biopsies. *Surg Clin North Am*. 2009;89:677–87.
- Salam GA. Lipoma excision. *Am Fam Physician*. 2002;65:901–4.

CODES

ICD9

- 214.0 Lipoma of skin and subcutaneous tissue of face
- 214.1 Lipoma of other skin and subcutaneous tissue
- 214.9 Lipoma, unspecified site

CLINICAL PEARLS

- Slow growing, often asymptomatic, and usually diagnosed by palpation
- Asymptomatic SC lipomas can be followed clinically and only need treatment if they cause pain, are growing rapidly, or causing compression of vital organs/nerves.
- Most symptomatic lipomas are removed surgically, but for small ones, liposuction or steroid injection has been reported to be successful.
- In the SC location, the primary differential diagnosis is a sebaceous (epidermoid) cyst or an abscess.
- Consider referral to subspecialty if a lipoma in a delicate anatomic location needs removal or if there is concern that the lesion might be malignant.

L

LUMBAR (INTERVERTEBRAL) DISK DISORDERS

Captain Michael R. Brackman, DO
Major Dena George, MD

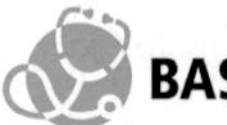

BASICS

DESCRIPTION

- Many patients with low back pain have lumbar disk disease.
- Lumbar disk disease may progress to disk degeneration, disk herniation, spinal narrowing, and arthritic proliferation of the facet joint.
- Disk degeneration/herniation may involve the surrounding spinal ligaments, muscles, joints, and skeleton.
- Management is based on symptoms and disability.
- Distinguishing between the normal aging of the spine and pathologic findings is difficult.
- Nonradicular low back pain (acute and chronic) remains near the waist and is caused by soft tissue or disk injury.
- Radicular low back pain (acute and chronic) radiates in a dermatomal pattern into the buttocks, hips, or legs rather than the back.
- Signs of weakness, numbness, or loss of reflexes may or may not be present.
- In younger patients, the source of the pain is likely to be mechanical compression or chemical irritation due inflammation of a nerve root.
- Spinal stenosis is more likely to be the cause of radicular pain in patients >55 years.
- System(s) affected: Musculoskeletal, Nervous
- Synonym(s): Degenerative disk disease, Intervertebral disk dislocation, Herniated disk, Herniated nucleus pulposus

EPIDEMIOLOGY

Incidence

- Nonspecific mechanical back low back pain is the fifth most common reason for all physician visits (1).
- Accounts for 2.3% of all physician visits, with an annual incidence rate of 5–8%.
- Among patients with acute back pain, only 4% have nerve root symptoms due to a herniated disk.
- $50 billion is spent annually on low back pain in the US (2).

Prevalence

- 1-year prevalence of 22–65%.
- Lifetime prevalence of low back pain is 11–84%.

Geriatric Considerations

Usually multifactorial, sources to consider: Lesions of spine, degenerative spondylolisthesis, spinal stenosis with neurogenic claudication; disk disease, and osteoporotic compression fractures also possible

Pregnancy Considerations

Increased incidence of low back pain (sacroiliac dysfunction) and/or sciatica; conservative treatment

RISK FACTORS

- Normal aging process after age 20
- Cigarette smoking
- Obesity
- Occupations with prolonged standing, heavy lifting, and vibrating tools
- Anxiety, depression
- Pregnancy

GENERAL PREVENTION

- Modification of job to reduce exposure to known risk factors
- Avoid smoking (persisting pain more common in smokers).
- Maintain a normal body weight.
- Routine exercise
- Back classes for prevention of recurrent back pain

PATHOPHYSIOLOGY

- Nerve roots exiting the spinal canal through the spinal neural foramen are susceptible to injury and irritation.
- The neural foramen may be compromised by a bulging disk, herniated nucleus pulposus, degenerative changes of the spine, masses, or fractures.
- Inflammation leads to chemical irritation of the nerve roots.

ETIOLOGY

- Trauma, major or minor
- Frequent lifting of heavy objects, especially bending at the waist and twisting movements
- Vibration (e.g., driving motor vehicles)
- Degenerative changes

COMMONLY ASSOCIATED CONDITIONS

- Poor physical conditioning or posture
- Obesity
- Osteoarthritis
- Osteoporosis
- Depression or other psychiatric disorders

DIAGNOSIS

HISTORY

- Assess location, onset, aggravating/relieving factors, and associated symptoms.
- Red flag conditions that may indicate a more serious etiology include:
  - Fracture: Major/minor trauma, strenuous lifting, steroid use
  - Cancer: Age over 50 or under 20, history of non–skin cancer, weight loss, severe nighttime pain
  - Infection: IV drug use, skin infection, UTI, immunosuppression
  - Cauda equina syndrome: Saddle anesthesia, bladder dysfunction, neurologic deficits in lower extremities
- Yellow flag conditions that may indicate risk for development of prolonged pain:
  - Depression
  - Impaired global functioning
  - Job dissatisfaction
  - Disputed compensation claims (1)

PHYSICAL EXAM

- Assess ROM
- Palpate the spine for bony tenderness.
- Assess motor strength in lower extremities:
  - Brief screening tests include raising heels off ground and walking on toes, and raising toes off ground and walking on heels.
- Assess reflexes in the Achilles and patellar tendons.
- Straight leg raise (SLR) test: In supine position, elevation of affected leg between 30° and 60° elicits pain radiating into the leg (sensitivity = 0.91, specificity = 0.26)
- Crossed SLR test: In supine position, elevation of the leg opposite the side of pain between 30° and 60° elicits pain (sensitivity = 0.29, specificity = 0.88)

DIAGNOSTIC TESTS & INTERPRETATION

Lab

Follow-Up & Special Considerations

- Labs only indicated if red flags are present. CBC, ESR, or C-reactive protein (elevation may signify infection, autoimmune arthropathy, or cancer).
- Urinalysis if suspecting urinary system etiology

Imaging

Follow-Up & Special Considerations

- Imaging indicated for red-flag symptoms or findings
- Lumbosacral plain films: Rarely indicated, may identify tumor, vertebral compression fracture, osteoarthritis, spondylolisthesis
- MRI preferred over CT scan and myelogram. However, in asymptomatic adults getting MRI of the lumbar spine, disk herniation is found in about 1/3 of the patients, and disk bulging is found in >1/2 of these patients.

Diagnostic Procedures/Surgery

- Myelograms are not common (used for surgical candidate evaluation or to help rule out more serious etiology such as tumor, infection, fracture)
- Electromyography useful to distinguish peripheral neuropathy from cord or nerve root impairment, and may confirm level of lesion

Pathological Findings

Difficult to distinguish the normal aging process of disk degeneration from specific lesions causing low back pain and sciatica

DIFFERENTIAL DIAGNOSIS

- Acute or chronic lumbosacral strain
- Facet joint disease
- Piriformis syndrome
- Spondylosis
- Spondylolisthesis
- Spinal arthritis
- Sciatica
- Fibromyalgia
- Compression fracture
- Metastatic and primary tumors
- Vertebral infection
- Pain referred from hip, retroperitoneum, aneurysms, or pelvis, neurogenic claudication
- Cauda equina syndrome

TREATMENT

MEDICATION

First Line

- Analgesia with NSAIDs or acetaminophen
- Consider muscle relaxants
- Precautions: Elderly, HTN, prior peptic ulcer disease or bleeding, renal disease, liver disease, cardiac dysfunction, addiction

- Opioids, even short term, increase odds of patient developing chronic back pain. Use with caution and discuss with patients the potential for physical dependence.

Second Line

- Injections: Epidural steroid injections may benefit some patients in the short term, but the evidence is not strong for long-term relief (5)[A].
- Tricyclic antidepressants or gabapentin/pregabalin may benefit patients with radiculopathy.
- Opioids: No more effective in relieving low back symptoms than safer analgesics such as acetaminophen, aspirin, or other NSAIDS.

ADDITIONAL TREATMENT

General Measures

- Initial conservative therapy:
  - Self-care: Avoid bed rest for more than a few days, daily activities as tolerated, local heat
  - Analgesics, muscle relaxants
  - Physical therapy, spinal manipulation
- Conservative treatment is recommended for the first 4–6 weeks. >80% of herniated disks improve with time. For persistent or severe pain and neurologic deficits, consider evaluating the patient for surgery.
- Emergent surgical referral for cauda equina syndrome (6)[A]

Issues for Referral

- Progressive or severe neurologic deficit
- Cauda equina syndrome
- Persistent sciatica for at least 1 month with corresponding clinical and imaging findings
- Persistent neurologic deficit despite 4–6 weeks of conservative therapy

COMPLEMENTARY AND ALTERNATIVE MEDICINE

- For chronic nonradicular pain: Improve physical fitness with low-impact aerobic exercise.
- Manipulation and physical therapy have been shown to be beneficial (3).
- Acupuncture: Short-term benefit for chronic low back pain (3).
- Transcutaneous electrical nerve stimulation (TENS)
- Massage, acupressure
- Exercise, yoga

SURGERY/OTHER PROCEDURES

- Surgical discectomy: Techniques include open and microsurgical discectomy, percutaneous laser, percutaneous suction, and arthroscopic discectomies.
- Absolute indications for discectomy:
  - Cauda equina syndrome
  - Progressive neurologic deficit despite conservative treatment
- Relative indications for discectomy:
  - Intolerable pain
  - Multiple episodes of radiculopathy
  - Persistent dysfunctional pain: These patients have been reported to improve more rapidly postoperatively, but long-term results show little difference from nonoperative treatment.
  - Static neurologic deficit: No reported difference between operative or nonoperative treatment for the improvement in weakness or sensory disturbance
  - Spinal fusion (arthrodesis): Indicated for spinal instability.
  - Disc prothesis versus rehabilitation in patients with low back pain and degenerative disc disease (4):
    - Study does not apply to patients with nerve root compression from herniated discs or spinal stenosis.
    - No difference in return to work, life satisfaction, fear avoidance beliefs, drug use, or scores on a back performance scale at 2 years follow-up.

IN-PATIENT CONSIDERATIONS

Initial Stabilization

- Inpatient admission uncommon
- Evaluate for more serious causes of back pain.
- Consider pain-management consultation.

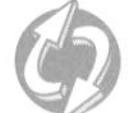

ONGOING CARE

FOLLOW-UP RECOMMENDATIONS

- Follow-up if pain or neurologic deficit is increasing
- Return visit ~10 days to 2 weeks following initial visit; pain may take 2 weeks to begin to improve
- Thereafter, monitor every 2–4 weeks until fully functional.

Patient Monitoring

- Follow pain history and neurologic status.
- Monitor exercise program

PATIENT EDUCATION

Maintain good posture, proper body mechanics, and physical fitness.

PROGNOSIS

- Acute low back pain (90%) and/or radiculopathy (75–90%) can be expected to recover spontaneously with conservative therapy.
- Chronic nonradicular low back pain: Most patients respond to conservative management such as manipulation, fitness, weight reduction, and education regarding back care.
- Chronic radicular pain: Careful selection of surgical candidates leads to satisfactory results (85% in long-term studies).

COMPLICATIONS

- Foot drop with weakness of anterior tibial, posterior tibial, and peroneal muscles
- Loss of ankle jerk
- Bladder and rectal sphincter weakness with retention or incontinence
- Limitation of movement and restricted activity
- Narcotic addiction

REFERENCES

1. Chou R, Qaseem A, Snow V, et al. Diagnosis and treatment of low back pain: A joint clinical practice guideline from the American College of Physicians and the American Pain Society. *Ann Intern Med*. 2007;147:478–91.
2. National Institute of Neurological Disorders and Stroke. *Low Back Pain Fact Sheet*. June 15, 2011. August 20, 2011. www.ninds.nih.gov/disorders/backpain/detail'backpain.htm.
3. Chou R, Loeser J, Owens D. Interventional therapies, surgery, and interdisciplinary rehabilitation for low back pain: An evidence-based clinical practice guideline from the American Pain Society. *Spine*. 2009;34(10):1066–77.
4. Hellum C, et al. Surgery with disc prosthesis versus rehabilitation in patients with low back pain and degenerative disc: Two year follow-up of randomised study. *BMJ*. 2011;342:d2786.
5. Abdi S, Datta S, Trescot AM, et al. Epidural steroids in the management of chronic spinal pain: A systematic review. *Pain Physician*. 2007;10:185–212.
6. van Tulder MW, Koes B, Seitsalo S, et al. Outcome of invasive treatment modalities on back pain and sciatica: An evidence-based review. *Eur Spine J*. 2006;15(Suppl 1):S82–92.

ADDITIONAL READING

- Atlas SJ, Keller RB, Wu YA, et al. Long-term outcomes of surgical and nonsurgical management of sciatica secondary to a lumbar disc herniation: 10 year results from the maine lumbar spine study. *Spine*. 2005;30:927–35.
- Jarvik JG, Deyo RA. Diagnostic evaluation of low back pain with emphasis on imaging. *Ann Intern Med*. 2002;137:586–97.
- Smeal WL, Tyburski M, Alleva J, et al. Conservative management of low back pain, part I. Discogenic/radicular pain. *Dis Mon*. 2004;50:636–69.
- Weinstein JN, Lurie JD, Tosteson TD, et al. Surgical vs nonoperative treatment for lumbar disk herniation: The Spine Patient Outcomes Research Trial (SPORT) observational cohort. *JAMA*. 2006;296:2451–9.

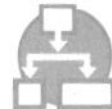

See Also (Topic, Algorithm, Electronic Media Element)

- Low Back Pain
- Algorithm: Low Back Pain, Acute

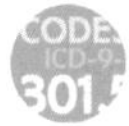

CODES

ICD9

- 722.52 Degeneration of lumbar or lumbosacral intervertebral disc
- 722.73 Intervertebral disc disorder with myelopathy, lumbar region
- 722.93 Other and unspecified disc disorder, lumbar region

CLINICAL PEARLS

- Initial imaging is rarely required, except in the presence of red flags.
- Features that predict best surgical outcome:
  - Definable neurologic deficit
  - Pathology in imaging that correlates with deficit
  - Positive nerve root tension signs
  - Leg pain >back pain
  - No response to nonsurgical therapy for 4–6 weeks
- Adverse psychosocial factors to resolving back pain:
  - Pending litigation or compensation
  - Depressed or hostile patient
  - Prolonged use of narcotics or alcohol

The views expressed in this chapter are those of the author and do not reflect the official policy or position of the Department of the Army, Department of Defense, or the US Government. Opinions, interpretations, conclusions, and recommendations herein are those of the author and are not necessarily endorsed by the US Army.

LUNG ABSCESS

Ruben Peralta, MD, FACS

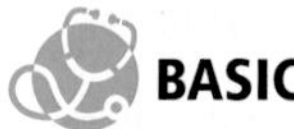

BASICS

DESCRIPTION

- A localized collection cavity of necrotic lung tissue and pus resulting from pyogenic bacteria:
  - Presentation may be acute or chronic (symptoms for >4 weeks).
  - Usual course is subacute progression of symptoms.
- Synonym(s): Pulmonary abscess

EPIDEMIOLOGY

Incidence

- Predominant age: Mainly fourth to sixth decades
- Predominant sex: Male > Female (4:1)

Prevalence

Unknown; relatively rare since advent of antibiotics

Pediatric Considerations

Staphylococcus most common organism in children

RISK FACTORS

- Periodontal disease (gingivitis), dental abscess, dental surgery
- Risk for aspiration:
  - Alcohol intoxication (loss of consciousness) is most common cause of aspiration.
  - Epilepsy
  - Cerebrovascular accident (CVA) with oropharyngeal dysfunction
  - Sinusitis
  - General anesthesia with surgery
  - Dysphagia
  - Tracheal/nasogastric tube
  - Severe gastroesophageal reflux disease (GERD)
  - Cerebral palsy
- Large bacterial burden:
  - Necrotizing pneumonia
  - Bacteremia (especially *Staphylococcus*)
  - Septic embolism (especially in endocarditis)
  - Disseminated septic phlebitis
- Airway obstruction:
  - Bronchial stenosis
  - Pulmonary embolism
  - Cavitary infarction
  - Lung neoplasia
  - Enlarged lymph node
  - Foreign body: Stent-associated respiratory tract infection (SARTI)
- Immunocompromise:
  - Diabetes mellitus
  - HIV infection
  - Chronic steroid use
- Amebic lung abscess: Most often from direct extension from liver abscess through the diaphragm to the right lower lobe

Genetics

- No known genetic pattern
- Immunodeficiency associated with *FCN3* mutation and ficolin-3 deficiency may predispose patients to lung infections (1).

GENERAL PREVENTION

- Treatment of predisposing diseases
- Aspiration precautions
- Treatment of periodontal diseases

ETIOLOGY

- May be due to aspiration of anaerobic oral flora (most common); 24–48 hours after aspiration, lung abscess forms.
- Less commonly, septic emboli from endocarditis and others (1,2,3)
- Usually mixed flora with predominance of anaerobes
- Oral flora anaerobes (60–75% of cases):
  - *Peptostreptococcus*
  - *Prevotella*
  - *Fusobacterium*
  - *Bacteroides* sp.
- Aerobes (10–20%):
  - *Staphylococcus aureus*
  - *Streptococcus pyogenes*
  - *Klebsiella* sp.
  - *Pseudomonas aeruginosa*
  - *Streptococcus milleri*
- Atypical aerobes:
  - *Legionella*
  - *Nocardia*
- *Actinomyces*

COMMONLY ASSOCIATED CONDITIONS

- Periodontal disease
- Pneumonia
- Alcoholism
- Empyema (if necrosis of the abscess wall allows entry into pleural space)
- Tuberculosis
- Immunocompetent patient

DIAGNOSIS

HISTORY

- Fever
- Malaise
- Diaphoresis
- Night sweats
- Anorexia
- Weight loss
- Dyspnea
- Chest pain/pleurisy
- Cough with purulent, foul-smelling, putrid, sour-tasting sputum
- Hemoptysis

PHYSICAL EXAM

- Vital signs: Tachypnea, tachycardia
- Lung exam:
  - Decreased breath sounds
  - Cavernous breath sounds
  - Crackles
  - Wheezing
  - Dullness to percussion
  - Consolidation by auscultation
- Clubbing of digits

ALERT

The posterior segment of the right upper lobe is the most common location for a lung abscess.

DIAGNOSTIC TESTS & INTERPRETATION

Lab

- CBC shows leukocytosis and anemia.
- Hypoalbuminemia
- Sputum smear: Neutrophils, mixed bacteria
- Sputum culture: Often grows normal respiratory flora; may help in atypical presentations
- Blood culture: Often negative in anaerobic abscess
- Drugs that may alter lab results: Prior antibiotics

Imaging

- CXR:
  - Lung cavity with air–fluid level
  - Consolidation with radiolucency, infiltrates, pleural effusion, mediastinal adenopathy
- Ultrasound:
  - Color Doppler ultrasound: Great sensitivity, specificity, positive predictive value, and negative predictive value when identification of vessel signals in a pericavitary consolidation is achieved.
- CT scan:
  - Defines location and extent (typical location depends on segments such as posterior segments of upper lobes or superior segments of lower lobes)
  - May detect obstructing lesion
  - May demonstrate cavitary opacities
  - May show multiple thrombus of neck vessels (infectious thrombophlebitis) (4)

Diagnostic Procedures/Surgery

- Bronchoscopy if obstruction is suspected
- Bronchoscopic brushing
- Bronchoalveolar lavage
- Transthoracic needle aspiration (rarely done)
- Percutaneous catheter-guided drainage (5)

Pathological Findings

- Solitary abscess
- Multiple abscesses
- Cavitation with necrosis
- Effusion/empyema

DIFFERENTIAL DIAGNOSIS

- Bronchogenic carcinoma
- Bronchiectasis
- Empyema with bronchopulmonary fistula
- Tuberculosis
- Mycotic lung infections
- Vasculitis
- Parasitic lung infections
- Infected pulmonary bulla
- Wegener granulomatosis
- Pulmonary sequestration
- Subphrenic or hepatic abscess with perforation into a bronchus
- Bronchogenic or parenchymal cyst
- Aspirated foreign body

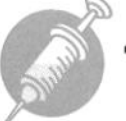

TREATMENT

MEDICATION

First Line

Antibiotics according to culture and sensitivity results; for presumed anaerobes, clindamycin 600 mg q6h IV followed by 300 mg q6h PO × 4 weeks

Second Line

- Historically, standard therapy had been penicillin G 1 million–2 million units IV q4h until improvement, followed by 1.2 million units (750 mg) PO q6h × 3–4 weeks; now many relevant pathogens produce β-lactamase.
- Cefoxitin 2 g IV q8h
- Piperacillin-tazobactam 3.375 g IV q6h
- Ticarcillin-clavulanate 3.1 g IV q6h
- Metronidazole has not proven as effective as clindamycin but often is recommended for use as an adjunctive therapy (500 mg IV q6h).
- Full course of therapy may be needed for 8 weeks.

ADDITIONAL TREATMENT

General Measures

- Postural drainage
- Nasotracheal suctioning if needed
- Prolonged course of antibiotics
- Pulmonary physiotherapy
- Bronchoscopy with selective therapeutic lavage (rarely done)
- In general, 10% require surgical intervention, such as drainage of abscess or empyema.

SURGERY/OTHER PROCEDURES

- Antibiotic treatment is successful in most patients; surgical options are considered when medical therapy fails.
- Endoscopy drainage
- Tube thoracostomy with medical failure or prohibitive operative risk
- Thoracoscopy drainage (6)
- Percutaneous catheter-guided drainage (5)
- Pulmonary resection only if complications occur or if patient fails therapy (mortality 11–16%)

IN-PATIENT CONSIDERATIONS

Initial Stabilization

Inpatient care for monitoring and treatment

ONGOING CARE

FOLLOW-UP RECOMMENDATIONS

Activity reduced until radiographic evidence of clearing

Patient Monitoring

Serial radiographs until resolution of cavity

DIET

No restrictions

PATIENT EDUCATION

- Pulmonary physiotherapy techniques
- American Academy of Family Physicians at www.aafp.org
- American Lung Association: Possible Complications of Pneumonia: www.lungusa.org/lung-disease/pneumonia/understanding-pneumonia.html

PROGNOSIS

- Clinical improvement with decrease in fever expected 3–4 days after starting antibiotics
- Defervescence expected in 7–10 days
- Prognosis depends on the underlying disease or immunosuppression.
- Patients with primary abscess (otherwise healthy, typical aspiration) have cure rates of 90–95%.
- Certain factors tend to have worse prognosis:
  - Large abscess (>6 cm)
  - Anatomic obstruction
  - Right lower lobe location
  - Certain bacteriologic species: *S. aureus*, *Klebsiella*, *Pseudomonas*
- Overall mortality 15–20%
- Patients with secondary abscess (underlying neoplasm, obstruction, HIV) have 75% mortality.

Geriatric Considerations

Mortality higher in the elderly

COMPLICATIONS

- Extension
- Empyema
- Massive hemoptysis
- Pneumothorax
- Brain abscess

REFERENCES

1. Munthe-Fog L, Hummelshøj T, Honoré C, et al. Immunodeficiency associated with FCN3 mutation and ficolin-3 deficiency. *N Engl J Med*. 2009;360:2637–44.
2. Chirinos JA, Garcia J, Alcaide ML, et al. Septic thrombophlebitis: Diagnosis and management. *Am J Cardiovasc Drugs*. 2006;6:9–14.
3. Mawdsley JE, Maleki N, Benjamin E, et al. Oesophageal perforation with asymptomatic lung abscess formation. *Lancet*. 2006;368:2104.
4. Velagapudi P, Turagam M, Are C, et al. "A forgotten disease": A case of lemierre syndrome. *Sci World J*. 2009;9:331–2.
5. Chen CH, Chen W, Chen HJ, et al. Transthoracic ultrasonography in predicting the outcome of small-bore catheter drainage in empyemas or complicated parapneumonic effusions. *Ultrasound Med Biol*. 2009.
6. Nagasawa KK, Johnson SM, et al. Thoracoscopic treatment of pediatric lung abscesses. *J Pediatr Surg*. 2010;45:574–8.

ADDITIONAL READING

- Huang CT, Chen CY, Ho CC, et al. A rare constellation of empyema, lung abscess, and mediastinal abscess as a complication of endobronchial ultrasound-guided transbronchial needle aspiration. *Eur J Cardiothorac Surg*. 2011;40:264–5.
- Medford AR, Bennett JA, Free CM, et al. Endobronchial ultrasound-guided transbronchial needle aspiration (EBUS-TBNA): Applications in chest disease. *Respirology*. 2010;15:71–9.

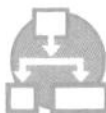

See Also (Topic, Algorithm, Electronic Media Element)

Pneumonia, Bacterial

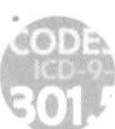

CODES

ICD9

- 513.0 Abscess of lung
- 513.1 Abscess of mediastinum

CLINICAL PEARLS

- Bacteria are carried to the dependent portions of the lung, with the posterior segment of the right upper lobe being the most common location for abscess.
- Percutaneous drainage and surgical resection could be considered treatment options when medical therapy fails. Endoscopic drainage techniques show promise as an alternative.
- Lemierre syndrome is a complication of *Fusobacterium necrophorum* oropharyngeal infection (usually pharyngitis). The infection extends to the internal jugular vein, causing thrombophlebitis. The thrombophlebitis, in turn, produces septic emboli, including emboli that produce lung abscess or pneumonia (2).

L

LUNG, PRIMARY MALIGNANCIES

Maryann R. Cooper, PharmD
Gerald Gehr, MD

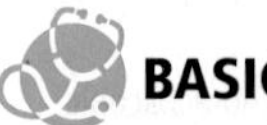

BASICS

DESCRIPTION

- Leading cause of cancer-related death in the US (estimated 157,300 deaths in 2010, 28% of all cancer-related deaths) (1)
- Divided into 2 broad categories:
  - Non–small cell lung cancer (NSCLC) (>85% of all lung cancers):
    - Adenocarcinoma (~40% of NSCLC): Most common type in the US, most common type in nonsmokers, metastasizes earlier than squamous cell, poor prognosis, bronchoalveolar, a subtype of adenocarcinoma has better prognosis
    - Squamous cell carcinoma (<25% of NSCLC): Dose-related effect with smoking, slower growing than adenocarcinoma
    - Large cell (~10% of NSCLC): Prognosis similar to adenocarcinoma
  - Small cell lung cancer (SCLC) (16% of all lung cancers): Centrally located, early metastases, aggressive
- Other: Mesothelioma, carcinoid tumor, and sarcoma
- Staging:
  - NSCLC: Staged from 0–IV based on: Primary tumor (T), lymph node status (N), and presence of metastasis (M)
  - SCLC: Staged based on disease location: Limited to ipsilateral hemithorax (stages I–IIIB); extensive if metastatic beyond hemithorax (stages IIIB and IV)
- Tumor locations: Upper: 60%, lower: 30%, middle: 5%, overlapping and main stem: 5%
- May spread by local extension to involve chest wall, diaphragm, pulmonary vessels, vena cava, phrenic nerve, esophagus, or pericardium
- Most commonly metastasize to lymph nodes (pulmonary, mediastinal), then liver, adrenal, bone (osteolytic), kidney, brain

EPIDEMIOLOGY

Incidence

- Estimated 222,520 new cases in the US in 2010 (1)
- Predominant age: >40 years; peak at 70 years
- Predominant sex: Male > Female

Prevalence

- Most common cancer worldwide
- Lifetime probability (1):
  - Men: 1 in 13
  - Women: 1 in 16

RISK FACTORS

- Smoking (relative risk [RR] 10–30)
- Second-hand smoke exposure
- Radon
- Environmental and occupational exposures:
  - Asbestos exposure (synergistic increase in risk for smokers)
  - Air pollution
  - Ionizing radiation
  - Mutagenic gases (halogen ethers, mustard gas, aromatic hydrocarbons)
  - Metals (inorganic arsenic, chromium, nickel)
- Lung scarring from tuberculosis
- Radiation therapy to the breast or chest

Genetics

NSCLC

- Oncogenes: Ras family (H-ras, K-ras, N-ras)
- Tumor suppressor genes: Retinoblastoma, *p-53*

GENERAL PREVENTION

- No cost-effective screening measure
- Prevention via aggressive smoking-cessation counseling and therapy; a 20–30% risk reduction occurs within 5 years of cessation
- Avoid supplemental β-carotene and vitamin E in smokers
- Avoid hormone replacement therapy in postmenopausal smokers or former smokers (increased risk of death from NSCLC)

ETIOLOGY

Multifactorial; see "Risk Factors."

COMMONLY ASSOCIATED CONDITIONS

- Paraneoplastic syndromes: Hypertrophic pulmonary osteoarthropathy, Lambert-Eaton syndrome, Cushing syndrome, hypercalcemia from ectopic parathyroid hormone releasing hormone, syndrome of inappropriate antidiuretic hormone (SIADH)
- Hypercoagulable state
- Pancoast syndrome
- Superior vena cava syndrome
- Pleural effusion
- Chronic obstructive pulmonary disease (COPD), other sequelae of cigarette smoking

DIAGNOSIS

HISTORY

- May be asymptomatic for most of course
- Pulmonary:
  - Cough (new or change in chronic cough)
  - Wheezing and stridor
  - Dyspnea
  - Hemoptysis
  - Pneumonitis (fever and productive cough)
- Constitutional:
  - Malaise
  - Bone pain (metastatic disease)
  - Fatigue
  - Weight loss, anorexia
  - Fever
  - Anemia
  - Clubbing of digits
- Other presentations:
  - Chest pain (dull, pleuritic)
  - Shoulder/arm pain (Pancoast tumors)
  - Dysphagia
  - Plethora (redness of face or neck)
  - Hoarseness (involvement of recurrent laryngeal nerve)
  - Horner syndrome
  - Neurologic abnormalities (e.g., headaches, syncope, weakness, cognitive impairment)
  - Pericardial tamponade (pericardial invasion)

PHYSICAL EXAM

- General: Pain, performance status, weight loss
- Head, eye, ear, nose, throat (HEENT): Horner syndrome, dysphonia, stridor, scleral icterus
- Neck: Supraclavicular/cervical lymph nodes, mass
- Lungs: Effusion, wheezing, airway obstruction, pleural effusion
- Abdomen/groin: Hepatomegaly or lymphadenopathy
- Extremities: Signs of hypertrophic pulmonary osteoarthropathy, DVT
- Neurologic: Rule out cognitive and focal motor defects

DIAGNOSTIC TESTS & INTERPRETATION

Lab

Initial lab tests

- CBC
- BUN, serum creatinine
- Liver function tests (LFTs), LDH
- Electrolytes:
  - Hypercalcemia (Paraneoplastic syndrome)
  - Hyponatremia (SIADH)
- Sputum cytology

Follow-Up & Special Considerations

CBC, BUN, serum creatinine, LFTs prior to each cycle of chemotherapy

Imaging

- Chest x-ray (CXR) (compare with old films):
  - Nodule or mass, especially if calcified
  - Persistent infiltrate
  - Atelectasis
  - Mediastinal widening
  - Hilar enlargement
  - Pleural effusion
- CT scan of chest (with IV contrast material):
  - Nodule or mass (central or peripheral)
  - Lymphadenopathy
- Evaluation for metastatic disease:
  - Brain MRI: Lesions may be necrotic, bleeding.
  - Abdomen: Hepatic, adrenal, renal masses
- Positron emission tomography (PET) scan: To evaluate metastasis
- Bone scan: Advanced disease or bone pain

Diagnostic Procedures/Surgery

- Biopsy with pathology review to determine NSCLC versus SCLC
- Pulmonary function tests
- Enlarged mediastinal lymph nodes necessitate staging by mediastinoscopy, video-assisted thoracoscopy, or fine-needle aspiration
- Transbronchial biopsy (Wang needle)
- Bronchoscopy for surgical planning
- Bone marrow aspirate (small cell)
- Cervical mediastinoscopy (the upper, middle peritracheal, and subcarinal lymph nodes)
- Anterior mediastinotomy (the posterior mediastinum and peritracheal, subazygous, hilar, and aortopulmonary window nodal regions)
- Video-assisted thoracoscopy (associated pleural disease and suspected mediastinal nodal spread)

Pathological Findings

Pathologic changes from smoking are progressive: Basal cell proliferation, development of atypical nuclei, stratification, metaplasia of squamous cells, carcinoma in situ, and then invasive disease

DIFFERENTIAL DIAGNOSIS

- COPD (may coexist)
- Granulomatous (tuberculosis, sarcoidosis)
- Cardiomyopathy
- Congestive heart failure (CHF)

TREATMENT

MEDICATION

- Chemotherapy is the mainstay of treatment for SCLC and advanced NSCLC.
- Adjuvant chemotherapy following surgery improves survival in patients with fully resected stage II–III NSCLC (2)[A].
- Palliative measures: Analgesics
- Dyspnea: Oxygen, morphine

First Line

- NSCLC:
  - Stages II–III: adjuvant chemotherapy:
    - Cisplatin-based doublets (combination with etoposide, vinorelbine, docetaxel, and others)
    - Carboplatin plus paclitaxel is an alternative to cisplatin-based regimens in patients that are unlikely to tolerate cisplatin
    - Cisplatin plus pemetrexed (non–squamous cell)
  - Stage IV:
    - Cisplatin-based doublets with or without bevacizumab (non–squamous cell) or cetuximab
    - Erlotinib is an alternative in patients with tumors that express EGFR
- SCLC:
  - Cisplatin or carboplatin plus etoposide

Second Line

- NSCLC:
  - Cisplatin-based doublets with or without bevacizumab (non–squamous cell) or cetuximab
  - Docetaxel or pemetrexed (non–squamous cell only) or erlotinib (EGFR-positive tumors)
- SCLC:
  - Topotecan or CAV (cyclophosphamide, doxorubicin, vincristine), gemcitabine, docetaxel, paclitaxel

ADDITIONAL TREATMENT

General Measures

- NSCLC (3)[C]:
  - Stage I, stage II, and selected stage III tumors are surgically resectable. Neoadjuvant or adjuvant therapy is recommended for many patients with stage II and III NSCLC. Patients with resectable disease who have medical contraindications to surgery are candidates for curative radiation therapy.
  - Patients with unresectable or N_2, N_3 disease are treated with radiation therapy in combination with chemotherapy. Selected patients with T_3 or N_2 disease can be treated effectively with surgical resection and either preoperative or postoperative chemotherapy or chemoradiation therapy.
  - Patients with distant metastases (M_1) can be treated with radiation therapy or chemotherapy for palliation or best supportive care alone.
- SCLC (4)[C]:
  - Limited stage: Concurrent chemotherapy and radiation
  - Extensive stage: Combination chemotherapy
  - Consider prophylactic cranial irradiation (PCI) in patients achieving a complete response (5)[B]
- Quality-of-life assessments: Karnofsky Performance Scale (KPS), Eastern Cooperative Oncology Group (ECOG)
- Discussions with patient and family about end-of-life care

Additional Therapies

- Smoking cessation counseling
- Consider bisphosphonates or denosumab in patients with bone metastases to reduce skeletal related events.

SURGERY/OTHER PROCEDURES

- Resection for NSCLC, for stages I, II, and IIIa, if medically fit to undergo surgery
- Resection of isolated, distant metastases has been achieved and may improve survival.
- Resection involves lobectomy in 71%, wedge in 16%, and complete pneumonectomy in 18%
- Resection should be accompanied by lymph node dissection for pathologic staging.

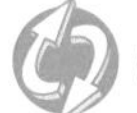

ONGOING CARE

FOLLOW-UP RECOMMENDATIONS

Patient Monitoring

- Depends on clinical history, but in general, postoperative visits every 3–6 months in the year after surgery with physical and CXR
- Follow-up CT scans as indicated

PATIENT EDUCATION

- www.cancer.gov/cancertopics
- www.smokefree.gov/

PROGNOSIS

- For combined, all types and stages, 5-year survival rate is 16% (NSCLC: 17%; SCLC 6%) (1)
- NSCLC (3):
  - Localized disease (stages I and II): 49%
  - Regional disease: 16%
  - Distant metastatic disease: 2%
- SCLC (4):
  - Without treatment: Median survival from diagnosis of only 2–4 months
  - Limited-stage disease: Median survival of 16–24 months; 5-year survival rate: 14%
  - Extensive-stage disease: Median survival of 6–12 months; long-term disease-free survival is rare

COMPLICATIONS

- Development of metastatic disease, especially to brain, bones, adrenals, and liver
- Local recurrence of disease
- Postoperative complications
- Side effects of chemotherapy or radiation

REFERENCES

1. American Cancer Society: *Cancer Facts and Figures 2010*. Atlanta, GA: American Cancer Society, 2010.
2. Pignon JP, Tribodet H, Scagliotti GV, et al. Lung adjuvant cisplatin evaluation: A pooled analysis by the LACE Collaborative Group. *J Clin Oncol*. 2008; 26:3552–9.
3. www.cancer.gov/cancertopics/pdq/treatment/non-small-cell-lung/healthprofessional.
4. www.cancer.gov/cancertopics/pdq/treatment/small-cell-lung/healthprofessional.
5. Slotman B, Faivre-Finn C, Kramer G, et al. Prophylactic cranial irradiation in extensive smallcell lung cancer. *N Engl J Med*. 2007;357:664–72.

ADDITIONAL READING

- Arriagada R, Bergman B, Dunant A, et al. Cisplatin-based adjuvant chemotherapy in patients with completely resected non-small-cell lung cancer. *N Engl J Med*. 2004;350:351–60.
- Collins LG, Haines C, Perkel R, et al. Lung cancer: Diagnosis and management. *Am Fam Physician*. 2007;75:56–63.
- Hanna N, Shepherd FA, Fossella FV, et al. Randomized phase III trial of pemetrexed versus docetaxel in patients with non-small-cell lung cancer previously treated with chemotherapy. *J Clin Oncol*. 2004;22:1589–97.
- Pirker R, Pereira JR, Szczesna A, et al. Cetuximab plus chemotherapy in patients with advanced non-small-cell lung cancer (FLEX): An open-label randomised phase III trial. *Lancet*. 2009;373: 1525–31.
- Sandler A, Gray R, Perry MC, et al. Paclitaxel-carboplatin alone or with bevacizumab for non-small-cell lung cancer. *N Engl J Med*. 2006;355: 2542–50.
- Shepherd FA, Rodrigues Pereira J, Ciuleanu T, et al. Erlotinib in previously treated non-small-cell lung cancer. *N Engl J Med*. 2005;353:123–32.
- Sundstrøm S, Bremnes RM, Kaasa S, et al. Cisplatin and etoposide regimen is superior to cyclophosphamide, epirubicin, and vincristine regimen in small-cell lung cancer: Results from a randomized phase III trial with 5 years' follow-up. *J Clin Oncol*. 2002;20:4665–72.
- von Pawel J, Schiller JH, Shepherd FA, et al. Topotecan versus cyclophosphamide, doxorubicin, and vincristine for the treatment of recurrent small-cell lung cancer. *J Clin Oncol*. 1999;17: 658–67.

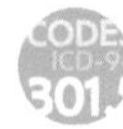

CODES

ICD9

- 162.3 Malignant neoplasm of upper lobe, bronchus or lung
- 162.4 Malignant neoplasm of middle lobe, bronchus or lung
- 162.9 Malignant neoplasm of bronchus and lung, unspecified

CLINICAL PEARLS

- Prognosis and treatment of lung cancer differs greatly between small cell and non–small cell histologies.
- Adjuvant cisplatin based chemotherapy improves survival in patients with completely resected stage II-III NSCLC.
- Chemotherapy with or without radiation can be offered to patients with advanced NSCLC or SCLC.
- There is little role for surgery in the treatment of SCLC.

LUPUS ERYTHEMATOSUS, DISCOID

Johra Nasreen, MD

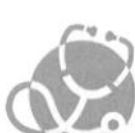

BASICS

DESCRIPTION

- Discoid lupus erythematosus (DLE) is the most common form of cutaneous LE. It is a chronic, disfiguring, inflammatory skin disease that typically manifests as erythematous, indurated, scaly plaques that have the potential to cause permanent scarring and dyspigmentation.
- Synonym(s): Chronic cutaneous LE; subacute cutaneous LE

Pediatric Considerations

Neonatal LE is a syndrome of cutaneous lupus occasionally with systemic manifestations, infrequently including congenital heart block. It is caused by transplacental passage of any of several maternal antibodies.

Pregnancy Considerations

Be aware if systemic retinoids are used in treatment (pregnancy Category X).

EPIDEMIOLOGY

Up to 28% of discoid LE patients are susceptible to developing systemic LE (1).

Incidence

DLE occurs at all ages and among all ethnic groups; it occurs more frequently in women than in men. All forms of cutaneous LE are most common among women of childbearing age:

- Predominant age: 25–45 years
- Predominant sex:
  - Localized DLE: Female > Male (3:1)
  - Generalized DLE: Female > Male (9:1)

Prevalence

- White women: 3 of 100,000
- African American women: 8 of 100,000

RISK FACTORS

DLE most commonly afflicts young adult women, especially African American and Hispanics, though it may occur at any age and it occurs worldwide.

Genetics

- DLE probably occurs in genetically predisposed individuals.
- A haplotype of cytotoxic T-lymphocyte-associated protein 4 (CTLA4) showed association with DLE.

GENERAL PREVENTION

- Avoid sunlight exposure. Excessive heat, excessive cold, and trauma to the affected regions may make the condition worse.
- Sunscreens with ultraviolet (UV) B and UVA blockers are recommended.
- Protective clothing (dark colors and closely woven fabrics) and hats are effective sun blockers.

PATHOPHYSIOLOGY

The pathophysiology of DLE is not well understood. It has been suggested that a heat shock protein is induced in the keratinocyte after UV light exposure or stress, and this protein may act as a target for gamma (delta) T-cell–mediated epidermal cell cytotoxicity.

COMMONLY ASSOCIATED CONDITIONS

- Systemic lupus erythematosus (SLE)
- Mixed connective tissue disease
- Antiphospholipid syndrome

DIAGNOSIS

The diagnosis of discoid lupus is generally made based on clinical features. Histology may be required to confirm the diagnosis.

HISTORY

- The disease predominantly affects *sun-exposed sites* such as the face, especially the malar areas, bridge of nose, lower lip, lower eyelids, and ears; the dorsal hands; and the scalp, although it can be disseminated.
- DLE starts as an erythematous papule or plaque, usually on the head or neck, with an adherent scale (2).
- Lesions occasionally are lightly pruritic or stinging
- Photosensitivity
- Koebner response (precipitation by cutaneous trauma)

PHYSICAL EXAM

- 2 forms are prevalent:
  - Localized DLE: Occurs on sun-exposed areas of the face, particularly the bridge of the nose, lower eyelids, lower lip, and ears. Antibodies against double-stranded DNA are almost always absent.
  - Generalized or widespread DLE: Occurs when other areas are affected. Lesions are seen on upper extremities and thorax most often, along with usual sites for localized DLE.
- "Carpet-tack" appearance of skin when scale removed
- Oral ulceration in 15% of the patients
- The lesion tends to spread centrifugally and as it progresses there is follicular plugging and pigmentary changes, generally hyperpigmentation at the periphery, and hypopigmentation with atrophy, scarring, and telangiectasia at the center of the lesion (2).
- Involvement of the scalp commonly produces a scarring alopecia. Scarring alopecia presents in patients with DLE and mainly is associated with a prolonged disease course (2).

DIAGNOSTIC TESTS & INTERPRETATION

Lab

- Due to the risk of SLE development in DLE patients, complete skin exams, joint assessments, and laboratory tests including antinuclear antibody (ANA), ESR, and CBC should be performed regularly for DLE patients (1).
- Localized DLE: Positive ANAs in low titer (30%)
- Generalized DLE: May find increased sedimentation rate, positive ANAs (60–80%), positive SS-A (80%) and positive SS-B (40%) autoantibodies, positive double-stranded DNA (dsDNA; <5%), leukopenia, hematuria, and albuminuria if concomitant SLE
- Immunofluorescent staining of skin biopsies (lupus band test)
- Disorders that may alter lab results: Concomitant SLE

Diagnostic Procedures/Surgery

Skin biopsy

Pathological Findings

- Hyperkeratosis and parakeratosis
- Focal epidermal atrophy
- Hydropic degeneration of basal cell layer
- Edema, mucin, and inflammation of dermis
- Follicular plugging
- Mononuclear cell infiltration at the dermal–epidermal junction and in the dermis around blood vessels
- Basement zone thickened with strong periodic acid–Schiff reaction staining
- Dermal mucinosis
- Immunofluorescence reveals a granular pattern of immunoglobulin and complement deposition at the dermal–epidermal border in involved skin.

DIFFERENTIAL DIAGNOSIS

- Actinic keratoses
- Granuloma annulare
- Sarcoidosis
- Psoriasis, plaque
- Rosacea
- Eczema
- Polymorphous light eruption
- Drug eruptions
- Cutaneous leishmaniasis
- Lupus vulgaris
- Seborrheic dermatitis
- Lichen planus
- Pemphigus erythematosus
- Keratoacanthoma
- Granuloma faciale
- Dermatomyositis
- Squamous cell carcinoma

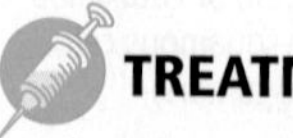

TREATMENT

- The cornerstone of therapy includes topical and intralesional glucocorticoids, and broad-spectrum sunscreens are recommended for all patients. Antimalarial agents, such as hydroxychloroquine, chloroquine, and quinacrine, are indicated when topical or intralesional therapy fails to control skin disease.
- DLE can cause permanent scarring, which can be prevented by early treatment.

MEDICATION

First Line

- Localized DLE:
  - Current study showed fluocinonide 0.05% cream (a potent topical corticosteroid) to be better than hydrocortisone 1% cream (a mild corticosteroid) (3)[A]
  - Topical corticosteroids:
    - The mainstay of treatment of DLE. Patients usually start with a potent topical steroid (fluocinonide 0.05% cream) applied b.i.d., then switch as soon as possible to a lower-potency steroid (e.g., triamcinolone 0.1%) applied b.i.d. The minimal use of steroids reduces recognized side effects such as atrophy, telengiaectasia, striae, and purpura (2)[A].
  - Intralesional steroids:
    - For example, triamcinolone 2.5–5 mg/mL for the face or 5–10 mg/mL elsewhere; are particularly useful to treat chronic lesions, hyperkeratotic lesions, and those that do not respond adequately to topical steroids:
      - Lesions at particular sites (e.g., the scalp) may also benefit.

- Recognized side effects of intralesional steroids include cutaneous atrophy and dyspigmentation, which are not significant risks in experienced hands.
  - Oral steroids may be required for the control of systemic lupus but are not generally beneficial in DLE:
    - Patients with progressive or disseminated disease, or those with localized disease that does not respond to topical measures, may require the addition of systemic agents.
- Generalized DLE:
  - Antimalarials (2)[A]:
    - Treatment with antimalarial drugs constitutes first-line systemic therapy for DLE. Therapy with antimalarials, either used singly or in combination, is usually effective.
    - 2 commonly used preparations are chloroquine and hydroxychloroquine (4).
    - Hydroxychloroquine: 200 mg/d for an adult
    - It may take between 4 and 8 weeks for any clinical improvement; if there are no untoward GI or other side effects, to increase the dose to b.i.d.
    - No more than 6.5 mg/kg/d should be administered.
    - In some patients who do not respond to hydroxychloroquine, chloroquine 250 mg/d may be more effective.
    - In general, hydroxychloroquine is a safe, well-tolerated drug and adverse effects are relatively few, the most widely recognized of which is retinal toxicity.
    - Chloroquine causes macular pigmentation that progresses to a typical bull's eye lesion and then to widespread retinal pigment epithelial atrophy, resembling retinitis pigmentosa.
    - Other adverse effects of antimalarials include GI symptoms (e.g., nausea and vomiting) and cutaneous side effects, including pruritus, lichenoid drug reactions, annular erythema, hyperpigmentation, and hematological disturbances such as leukopenia and thrombocytopenia.

Second Line

- Localized DLE:
  - Intralesional triamcinolone: 2.5 mg/mL injected at monthly intervals
  - Prednisone: 15 mg b.i.d., then tapered after response
- Generalized DLE:
  - Quinacrine: 100 mg/d
  - Dapsone: 100 mg/d
  - Azathioprine: 100 mg/d
  - Systemic retinoid (e.g., etretinate 1 mg/kg)
  - Thalidomide 50–300 mg/d also is effective (5)[C].
  - Dapsone is useful in patients who also have vasculitis. It is the treatment of choice for patients with bullous lupus.
- Recent case reports have shown successful treatments with IVIG, the monoclonal antibody efalizumab, and the immunomodulatory drug tacrolimus.
- Both tacrolimus and pimecrolimus show efficacy in localized DLE (6)[A].

ADDITIONAL TREATMENT

R-salbutamol sulphate, a well-known molecule with anti-inflammatory effects

General Measures

Avoid sun exposure, excessive heat, cold, or trauma.

Issues for Referral

Given the scarring nature of this illness, dermatology referral is frequently indicated. Also, the treatment consists of medications less commonly used by primary care providers.

SURGERY/OTHER PROCEDURES

- Excision of burned-out scarred lesions is possible; however, reactivation of inactive lesions has been reported in some patients.
- Laser therapy may be useful for lesions with prominent telangiectases. Reactivation also is a consideration with this form of therapy.

ONGOING CARE

FOLLOW-UP RECOMMENDATIONS

Follow patients with DLE at regular intervals. Response to therapy varies from several weeks to several months. At each visit, question the patient about new symptoms that may reflect systemic disease.

Patient Monitoring

- Initially recheck patients once or twice per month, then annually in otherwise asymptomatic patients.
- Perform routine laboratory studies for assessment, including CBC, renal function tests, and urinalysis, at regular intervals.
- Ophthalmology follow-up at 6-month intervals, if patient is taking antimalarials
- If lesions subside, reduce dosage of antimalarials over 2–3 months and then discontinue.

PATIENT EDUCATION

- Teach patients proper use of sunscreens and other measures to prevent sun exposure (e.g., wide-brimmed hats, long sleeves).
- Advise patients about symptoms of SLE for which they should watch.

PROGNOSIS

- 40% of patients may have complete remission; 1–5% may develop systemic lupus (these patients usually have generalized DLE).
- Cutaneous lupus has the tendency to change over time. Some patients may progress through several different subsets of cutaneous lupus and ultimately evolve into systemic lupus.
- Not life threatening unless it turns into systemic type

COMPLICATIONS

- Cicatricial alopecia
- Lupoid rash
- Lupus mastitis (7)
- Squamous cell carcinoma

REFERENCES

1. Chong BF, Song J, Olsen NJ, et al. Determining risk factors for developing systemic lupus erythematosus in discoid lupus erythematosus patients. *The British journal of dermatology*. Epub 2011 Dec 5.doi: 10.1111/j.1365–2133. 2011. 10610.x.
2. Panjwani S. Early diagnosis and treatment of discoid lupus erythematosus. *J Am Board Fam Med*. 2009;22(2):206–13.
3. Jessop S, Whitelaw DA, Delamere FM. Drugs for discoid lupus erythematosus. *Cochrane Database Syst Rev*. 2009;4:CD002954.
4. Abarientos C, Sperber K, Shapiro DL, et al. Hydroxychloroquine in systemic lupus erythematosus and rheumatoid arthritis and its safety in pregnancy. *Expert Opin Drug Saf*. 2011;10:705–14.
5. James WD, et al. *Andrews' Diseases of the Skin*, 10th ed. Philadelphia: WB Saunders; 2006:157–65.
6. Tzellos TG, Kouvelas D. Topical tacrolimus and pimecrolimus in the treatment of cutaneous lupus erythematosus: An evidence-based evaluation. *Eur J Clin Pharmacol*. 2008;64:337–41.
7. Kinonen C, Gattuso P, Reddy VB, et al. Lupus mastitis: An uncommon complication of systemic or discoid lupus. *Am J Surg Pathol*. 2010;34:901–6.

ADDITIONAL READING

- Järvinen TM, Hellquist A, Koskenmies S, et al. Tyrosine kinase 2 and interferon regulatory factor 5 polymorphisms are associated with discoid and subacute cutaneous lupus erythematosus. *Exp Dermatol*. 2010;19:123–31.
- Lin JH, Dutz JP, Sontheimer RD, et al. Pathophysiology of cutaneous lupus erythematosus. *Clin Rev Allergy Immunol*. 2007;33:85–106.

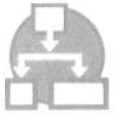

See Also (Topic, Algorithm, Electronic Media Element)

Systemic Lupus Erythematosus (SLE)

CODES

ICD9

695.4 Lupus erythematosus

CLINICAL PEARLS

- Patients with cutaneous DLE have a small chance of developing SLE over a span of months to years.
- Screening patients with cutaneous disease for systemic symptoms such as oral ulcers, arthritis, etc., is a good first step.
- If patient has any systemic symptoms, laboratory testing of blood for ANAs is indicated.
- Systemic steroids are rarely indicated in DLE.

L

LUPUS NEPHRITIS

Weizhen Tan, MD
Neena Gupta, MD

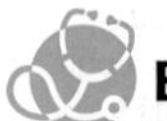

BASICS

DESCRIPTION

- Lupus nephritis (LN) is the renal manifestation of systemic lupus erythematosus (SLE).
- Per American College of Rheumatology (ACR) criteria for diagnosis of SLE, renal involvement is defined as persistent proteinuria >500 mg/d (3+ on dipstick) or presence of cellular casts.
- Clinical manifestations primarily due to immune complex–mediated glomerular disease, but tubulointerstitial and vascular involvement often seen. Diagnosis by clinical, urinary abnormalities, autoantibodies, and requires renal biopsy.
- Treatment and prognosis depend on ISN/RPS 2003 histologic class—risk of end-stage renal disease (ESRD) highest in class IV.
- Delay in diagnosis/treatment increases risk of ESRD.
- For proliferative LN (class III, IV, V + III/IV features): Induction of remission by steroids + IV cyclophosphamide or mycophenolate mofetil (MMF) and maintenance of remission by low-dose steroids and Azathioprine (AZA) or MMF.

EPIDEMIOLOGY

- Peak incidence of SLE is 15–45 years, with female-to-male ratio of 10:1.
- Once SLE develops, LN affects both genders equally, is more severe in children and men, and less so in older adults.

Incidence

- SLE: 1.4–21.9/100,000 (1)
- Up to 60% of patients with SLE develop LN over time, and 25–50% present initially with renal involvement.

Pediatric Considerations

LN is more common and severe in children. 60–80% have LN at or soon after SLE onset.

Prevalence

SLE: 7.4–159.4/100,000 (1)

RISK FACTORS

Risk factors for LN include younger age, African American or Hispanic race, more ACR criteria met for diagnosis of SLE, longer duration of the disease, hypertension, lower socioeconomic status, family history of SLE, anti-dsDNA antibodies.

Genetics

No clear pattern but multigenic inheritance supported by racial differences, clustering in families, ~25% concordance in identical twins.

PATHOPHYSIOLOGY

- Immune complex–mediated inflammatory response injures glomeruli, tubules, interstitium, and vasculature.
- Glomeruli: Varying degrees of mesangial proliferation, crescent formation (see "Pathological Findings"), fibrinoid necrosis causing reduced GFR
- Persistence of inflammation (chronicity) leads to sclerosis and loss of glomeruli.
- Tubulointerstitial injury (seen as edema, inflammatory cell infiltrate acutely, and tubular atrophy in chronic phase) with or without tubular basement membrane immune complex deposition contributes to reduced renal function.
- Vascular lesions: Immune complex deposition and noninflammatory necrosis in arterioles

ETIOLOGY

- SLE is a multifactorial disease with a multigenic inheritance, but exact etiology is still elusive.
- Defective T-cell autoregulation and polyclonal hyperactivity of B cells
- Dysregulated apoptosis and impaired clearance of apoptic cells causes breakdown of self-tolerance to nuclear antigens.
- Development of anti-DNA, anti-C1q, anti-α-actin, and other nuclear component autoantibodies
- Deposition of circulating immune complexes or formation of complexes by these antibodies attaching to local nuclear antigens leads to complement activation; plays a key role in tissue injury and inflammation.
- Interaction of genetic hormonal and environmental factors leads to great variability in LN severity.

COMMONLY ASSOCIATED CONDITIONS

Other organ systems such as skin, hematologic, cerebral, pulmonary, GI, and cardiac are often involved as part of SLE.

DIAGNOSIS

HISTORY

- LN can present with proteinuria, hematuria, active urine sediment, edema, hypertension, increased creatinine. Other symptoms related to acute kidney injury or reduced renal function
- Symptoms related to other organ involvement
- Renal involvement is relatively uncommon in drug-induced lupus.

PHYSICAL EXAM

- Detailed exam for signs of active SLE
- High BP, peripheral edema

DIAGNOSTIC TESTS & INTERPRETATION

Lab

- Active urine sediment suggests nephritis.
- Autoantibodies, low complement levels
- Renal biopsy is gold standard for diagnosis, treatment, and prognostication.

Initial lab tests

- Urinalysis may show hematuria, proteinuria (protein/creatinine ratio >0.2), or nephrotic range proteinuria (>3.5 g/24 hr) and active urine sediment (RBC casts and granular casts) (2)[C].
- Serum-Lytes, BUN, creatinine, albumin, routine serological markers of SLE like ANA, anti-dsDNA, anti-Ro, anti-La, anti-RNP, anti-Sm, antiphospholipid antibody, C3,C4, CH50, CBC with differential and CRP (2)[C]

Follow-Up & Special Considerations

- Monitor every 3 months for disease activity (2)[C]: Urinalysis for hematuria, proteinuria; blood for C3, C4, anti-dsDNA, serum albumin, and creatinine
- Patients with eGFR <60 mL: Follow National Kidney Foundation Guidelines for chronic kidney disease.
- Drug level monitoring if on immunosuppressants

Pregnancy Considerations

- Pregnancy leads to worsening of renal function in LN. Risk factors include renal impairment at baseline, active disease, hypertension, and proteinuria.
- Risk factors for fetal loss include elevated serum creatinine, heavy proteinuria, hypertension, and anticardiolipin antibodies.

Imaging

Initial approach

Renal ultrasound (2)[C]

Diagnostic Procedures/Surgery

Renal biopsy is the gold standard for diagnosing and classifying LN.

Pathological Findings

- Adequate renal biopsy (at least 10 glomeruli for light microscopy or total 20–25 glomeruli) is essential. Light, immunofluorescence, and electron microscopy needed for accurate classification.
- On immunofluorescence microscopy: Immune complex deposits consisting of IGG, IGA, IGM, C1q, and C3 (full house) highly suggestive of LN.
- Revised ISN/RPS 2003 histologic classification guides therapeutic decisions.
- LN is classified as purely mesangial (class I, II), focal proliferative: <50% glomeruli (class III), diffuse proliferative: ≥50% (class IV), membranous (class V), and advanced sclerosis (class VI). Subdivisions for activity (A) and chronicity (C) in class III/IV and for segmental (S) or global (G) glomerular involvement in class IV [Class III A, C, A/C and class IV S(A), G(A), S(A/C), S(C), G(C)].
- Lesions may change to another class over time or with therapy.
- Focal and diffuse proliferative LN (classes III and IV) are common forms of LN and are the ones most likely to progress to ESRD.

DIFFERENTIAL DIAGNOSIS

- LN has to be differentiated from other primary glomerular disease, secondary renal involvement in other systemic disorders such as ANCA associated vasculitis, HSP, antiglomerular basement membrane disease, and viral infections.
- Mixed connective tissue disorder may have glomerulonephritis indistinguishable from LN.
- Clinical data have to be combined with serologic and renal biopsy patterns to differentiate LN from other processes

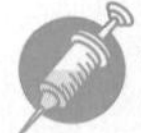

TREATMENT

MEDICATION

First Line

Class I + II LN: No specific therapy needed, as long-term renal prognosis is good. Renin–angiotensin system blockade for BP and proteinuria.

Proliferative LN (Class III,IV,V+III/IV): Treatment involves induction and maintenance phase. Principles of treatment:

- Avoid delay in treatment.
- Inducing response/remission in a short time period (3–6 months)
- Maintaining response and avoiding iatrogenic morbidity (5–10 years)

INDUCTION: Steroids + immunosuppressive agent (for mild class III, high-dose steroids alone may be enough):

- Glucocorticoids: Methylprednisolone pulse 0.5–1 g/d for 3 days followed by oral prednisone 0.5–1 mg/kg/d PO (max 60 mg/d, taper after 4–8 weeks) (3,4)[A] *AND*
- Cyclophosphamide: IV cyclophosphamide (high dose = 0.75–1 g/m^2 monthly × 6 doses—NIH regimen; low dose = 0.5 g q2wk × 6 doses—EuroLupus regimen) or daily oral cyclophosphamide (1.5 mg/kg/d) for no longer than 6 months (to prevent premature ovarian failure) (5)[A] *OR*
- MMF: 1–3 g/d PO divided b.i.d. (target 3 g/d as tolerated) for 6 months (6)[A]

MAINTENANCE:

- Glucocorticoids: Oral prednisone tapered to low doses (generally <10 mg/d by 6 months) **AND**
- MMF **OR** AZA (azathioprine): MMF 1–2 g/d divided b.i.d. PO or AZA 1–2.5 mg/kg/d (3,4)[A]
- Cyclophosphamide IV quarterly for 1–2 year after renal remission; not used now due availability of less toxic regimen.

Class V LN: Good prognosis in general, treatment not standardized

- For subnephrotic patients, no specific treatment except renin–angiotensin system blockade.
- Options for nephrotic patients include steroids with either calcineurin inhibitors, IV cyclophosphamide, AZA, or MMF (4)[B].
- Class V LN with presence of class III or class IV biopsy findings need aggressive combination regimen as for class III/IV.

Second Line

- Rituximab, an anti-CD20 chimeric monoclonal antibody: Rescue treatment in proliferative LN.
- Biologics/new agents: Ocrelizumab (humanized anti-CD-20), epratuzumab (anti-CD-22 monoclonal antibody), Abatacept (T-cell costimulation modulator), and Belimumab (anti–B-cell stimulator antibody) are all currently being studied (4)[C].
- Other treatments used in selected patients: Plasma exchange, IVIG

ADDITIONAL TREATMENT

General Measures

- Monitor bone density, optimize vitamin D and calcium intake in patients on glucocorticoids.
- Low-salt diet for hypertension, edema
- Avoid sun or ultraviolet light exposure.

Issues for Referral

- Patients should be referred to a nephrologist for initial management: Renal biopsy, induction therapy.
- Refer also for relapse of LN (e.g., new onset HTN, proteinuria, nephrotic syndrome).

Additional Therapies

- BP control
- Dyslipidemia treatment, management of other modifiable cardiovascular risk factors
- Anticoagulation for symptomatic antiphospholipid antibody syndrome

SURGERY/OTHER PROCEDURES

- Renal transplant for ESRD when clinical and serologic inactivity for a year
- Patient and graft survival rates are similar to non-SLE patients (1)[C].
- Risk of recurrent LN in renal transplant recipients usually low but range between 0% and 30% in different studies; graft loss due to recurrence is rare.

IN-PATIENT CONSIDERATIONS

Initial Stabilization

- Control hypertension and proteinuria if present.
- Labs to help confirm SLE/LN, renal ultrasound
- Consult nephrologist for further management and renal biopsy.

Admission Criteria

- Uncontrolled hypertension, acute kidney injury
- Severe extrarenal manifestation

IV Fluids

Patients who have nephrotic syndrome or acute kidney injury should be fluid restricted.

Discharge Criteria

Once the patient is stabilized and renal biopsy is performed, management may be as an outpatient.

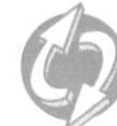

ONGOING CARE

FOLLOW-UP RECOMMENDATIONS

Patient Monitoring

- Monitor urine protein/creatinine ratio, urine microscopy, serum albumin and creatinine, antibody titers (especially anti-dsDNA), C3, C4, BP at least every 3 months for first 2–3 years (2)[C].
- Once stable on maintenance therapy with no active disease, follow-up can be spaced every 6–12 months (2)[C].

DIET

Low-salt diet

PATIENT EDUCATION

Teach the patient the importance of medication adherence to control disease and self-monitoring for relapse of symptoms.

PROGNOSIS

- LN has negative impact on survival in SLE patients: 10-year survival 88% and 94% in patients with and without renal involvement (7)
- LN patients suffer relapse at a rate of ~35%, and between 10% and 20% of patients progress to ESRD within 10 years (5) depending on population studied, histologic class, activity and chronicity index, response to treatment, and many other factors.
- Prognosis of patients with proliferative LN has improved greatly. 5-year renal survival of class IV LN was <30% before 1970 and is >80% in last 2 decades (1).
- Early and complete remission with treatment is the best prognostic factor. Predictors of remission include low baseline proteinuria, normal creatinine, Caucasian race, and treatment initiation within 3 months of clinical diagnosis.
- Indicators of poorer prognosis include diffuse proliferative LN, esp. crescentic, higher activity/chronicity index on biopsy, African American race, lower socioeconomic status, poor response to treatment, high creatinine at baseline, uncontrolled hypertension, and relapse.

COMPLICATIONS

- Risks from immunosuppression: Infections, malignancy
- Treatment side effects: Cyclophosphamide causes primary amenorrhea and is thus recommended for induction phase only.
- MMF may cause GI upset, nausea, and is a teratogen. (Azathioprine recommended for women who desire pregnancy)
- Risk of vascular thromboses (hypercoagulable state from antiphospholipid antibodies)
- About 10–20% of patients will eventually develop ESRD from progressive disease refractory to treatment and require dialysis/kidney transplantation (7).

REFERENCES

1. Ortega LM, Schultz DR, Lenz O, et al. Review: Lupus nephritis: Pathologic features, epidemiology and a guide to therapeutic decisions. *Lupus*. 2010;19:557–74.
2. Mosca M, et al. EULAR recommendations for monitoring patients with SLE in clinical practice and in observational studies. *Ann Rheum Dis*. 2010:69: 1269–74.
3. Ponticelli C, Glassock RJ, Moroni G, et al. Induction and maintenance therapy in proliferative lupus nephritis. *J Nephrol*. 2010;23:9–16.
4. Bomback AS, Appel GB, et al. Updates on the treatment of lupus nephritis. *J Am Soc Nephrol*. 2010;21:2028–35.
5. Houssiau FA, Ginzler EM, et al. Current treatment of lupus nephritis. *Lupus*. 2008;17:426–30.
6. Appel GB, Contreras G, Dooley MA, et al. Mycophenolate mofetil versus cyclophosphamide for induction treatment of lupus nephritis. *J Am Soc Nephrol*. 2009;20:1103–12.
7. Houssiau FA, et al. Management of lupus nephritis: An update. *J Am Soc Nephrol*. 2004;15:2694–704.

ADDITIONAL READING

Weening JJ, D'Agati VD, Schwartz MM, et al. The classification of glomerulonephritis in systemic lupus erythematosus revisited. *J Am Soc Nephrol*. 2004;15: 241–50.

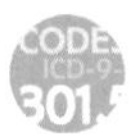

CODES

ICD9

- 581.81 Nephrotic syndrome in diseases classified elsewhere
- 710.0 Systemic lupus erythematosus

CLINICAL PEARLS

- Early diagnosis, classification via biopsy, and treatment are imperative for improved renal survival in patients with LN.
- Treatment of proliferative/progressive LN is based on the principle of short induction course followed by longer maintenance course with glucocorticoids and immunosuppressants.

L

LYME DISEASE

Barbara A. Majeroni, MD

BASICS

DESCRIPTION

- A multisystem infection caused by the spirochetes of *Borrelia* strains, which is transmitted primarily by ixodid ticks, *I. scapularis* (deer ticks) in the New England and Great Lakes areas, and *I. pacificus* in the West, also known as black-legged ticks and Western black-legged ticks
- Early localized Lyme disease includes a characteristic expanding skin rash (erythema migrans) (70%) and constitutional flulike symptoms.
- Disseminated Lyme disease may present with involvement of ≥1 organ systems. Neurologic, cardiac, and pauciarticular arthritis are most common.
- Post-Lyme disease syndrome involves arthritis (50%) and chronic neurologic syndromes.
- System(s) affected: Hemic/Lymphatic/Immunologic; Musculoskeletal; Skin/Exocrine; Cardiac; Neurologic
- Synonym(s): Lyme arthritis; Lyme borreliosis

EPIDEMIOLOGY

Incidence

- Most cases of Lyme disease in the US occur in southern New England; southeastern New York; New Jersey; eastern Pennsylvania; eastern Maryland; and parts of Minnesota, Wisconsin, and Michigan.
- In states where Lyme disease is endemic, the incidence is 0.5 per 1,000, but can be substantially higher in local areas (1)[B]. Cases have been reported from 46 states and the District of Columbia.

Prevalence

- The most common tickborne infection in the US and Europe
- Annually Europe: 65,500; North America: 16,500; Asia: 3,500; North Africa: 10 (2)
- Predominant age: Can occur in all ages, but most common in children ages 5–14 and in the 55–70-year age group
- Predominant sex: Male > Female in the US

RISK FACTORS

- Exposure in tick-infested area; most common April–November
- Those who reside or are employed in areas where ticks are found are at increased risk.
- Ixodid ticks are commonly found on deer. Hunters may be at an increased risk.

Genetics

Human leukocyte antigen: Haplotype DR4 or DR2 may be more susceptible to prolonged arthritis.

GENERAL PREVENTION

- Prevention of the infection is possible by careful exam of skin for ticks after outdoor activities.
- The prompt removal of ticks may limit transmission.
- Clothing that covers the ankles should be worn in endemic areas, and the use of insect repellants containing DEET is recommended.
- No vaccine is currently available.
- Prophylactic treatment with 1 dose of 200 mg of doxycycline within 72 hours of a tick bite in highly endemic areas has been suggested. (This is contraindicated in pregnancy and children; no prophylactic agent is approved for these groups.) (3)[A]

ETIOLOGY

- Infection with spirochete *B. burgdorferi* in the US, or *B. afzelii* or *B. garinii* in Europe, transmitted by the bite of ixodid ticks
- Primary animal reservoir is the white-footed mouse

COMMONLY ASSOCIATED CONDITIONS

Southern tick–associated rash illness may be mistaken for Lyme disease. It is seen in the southeastern and south central US, and is associated with the bite of the Lone Star tick, *Amblyomma americanum*.

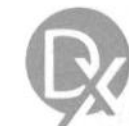

DIAGNOSIS

HISTORY

- History of a tick bite followed by illness with erythema migrans is the key to diagnosis (4)[C].
- Early Lyme disease:
  - Some patients may be asymptomatic.
  - Fever
  - Headache
  - Myalgias
  - Arthralgias
- Disseminated Lyme disease:
  - Facial palsies or other cranial neuropathies
  - Joint pain (usually large joint monoarthritis)
  - Iritis, conjunctivitis
- Late untreated Lyme disease:
  - Recurrent synovitis
  - Recurrent tendonitis and bursitis
  - Encephalopathic symptoms:
    - Headaches
    - Decreased memory
    - Difficulty concentrating
    - Confusion
    - Fatigue
  - Symptoms mimicking other CNS diseases:
    - Multiple sclerosislike symptoms
    - Strokelike symptoms
    - Transverse myelitis
  - Peripheral neuropathic symptoms; motor, sensory, or autonomic neuropathies
  - Meningitis

PHYSICAL EXAM

- Early Lyme disease:
  - Erythema migrans
- Disseminated Lyme disease:
  - Multiple erythema migrans
  - Facial palsies or other cranial neuropathies
  - Heart block
  - Pericarditis
  - Arthritis
  - Other neurologic signs

ALERT

- *Transmission does not occur if tick attachment is <48 hours*, and only 25% transmission occurs for attachments of >72 hours.
- Infection is preceded by a tick bite, although patient may be unaware of tick attachment.

DIAGNOSTIC TESTS & INTERPRETATION

Lab

Initial lab tests

- Testing and treatment not indicated if tick attachment is <48 hours
- Diagnosis is based mainly on clinical findings in endemic areas.
- ELISA for IgM and IgG *B. burgdorferi* antibodies, followed by a Western blot test if positive or equivocal (4)[A]
- Culture of CSF for *B. burgdorferi*
- Use of plasma polymerase chain reaction (PCR) is of little value, but PCR of synovial fluid may be helpful.

Follow-Up & Special Considerations

- Late-stage disease with negative serology may be seen in patients who received early antibiotic treatment.
- Disorders that may alter lab results: False-positive response has been seen with Rocky Mountain spotted fever, syphilis, systemic lupus erythematosus, and rheumatoid arthritis.
- PCR for Lyme disease in synovial fluid is both sensitive and specific for diagnosing Lyme arthritis.
- PCR of CSF has a very low sensitivity for Lyme meningitis, which is likely in the setting of CSF pleocytosis with erythema migrans, papilledema, and cranial neuropathies.
- There are CDC warnings against using nonvalidated testing methods, including urine antigen test, immunofluorescent staining for cell wall-deficient forms of *B. burgdorferi*, and lymphocyte transformation tests to aid in the diagnosis of Lyme disease (4).
- After an infection, antibodies may persist for months to years. *Serologic tests do not distinguish active from past infection.*
- Antibodies are not protective.

Imaging

Initial approach

No imaging indicated

Diagnostic Procedures/Surgery

Lumbar puncture when neurologic findings are present, with ELISA of CSF for *B. burgdorferi* antibodies

Pathological Findings

Culture of *B. burgdorferi* from blood or skin biopsy has a very low yield.

DIFFERENTIAL DIAGNOSIS

- Juvenile rheumatoid arthritis
- Viral syndromes
- Later stages may mimic many other diseases.
- Coinfection with babesiosis has been reported. Suggested by high fever.

TREATMENT

Antibiotic prophylaxis is recommended for the prevention of Lyme disease in endemic areas following an *Ixodes* tick bite (3)[A].

MEDICATION

First Line

- Erythema migrans:
  - Doxycycline (Vibramycin): 100 mg PO b.i.d. for 10 days (10–21) (do not use in children <8 or in pregnancy); OR
  - Amoxicillin: 500 mg PO t.i.d. for 14 days (14–21) (pediatric dose 50 mg/kg/d); OR
  - Cefuroxime axetil 500 mg PO b.i.d. for 14 days (14–21):
    - 1 randomized, controlled trial of patients with erythema migrans found 10 days of treatment as effective as 20 days.
- Neurologic disease:
  - Normal CSF, treat for 14–21 days: Doxycycline 100 mg PO b.i.d. or amoxicillin 500 mg PO t.i.d.
  - With abnormal CSF, treat for 4 weeks: Ceftriaxone (Rocephin) 2 g/d IV, cefotaxime 2g q8h, or penicillin G 5 million U q6h.
  - Cardiac disease:
    - Mild (first-degree AV block, PR <300 msec): Doxycycline 100 mg PO b.i.d. or amoxicillin 500 mg PO t.i.d. for 14 days (14–21)
    - More serious: Ceftriaxone 2 g q24h IV for 30 days
- Arthritis without neurologic disease:
  - Oral treatment for 28 days with doxycycline 100 mg b.i.d. or amoxicillin 500 mg t.i.d.
  - If oral treatment fails, begin an IV treatment for 2–4 weeks with ceftriaxone 2 g/d.
- Contraindications:
  - Allergy to agent
  - Doxycycline is contraindicated in children and in women who are pregnant or breastfeeding.
- Precautions: Refer to the manufacturer's profile of each drug:
  - In ~15% of patients treated with IV therapy, a Jarish-Herxheimer-type reaction develops within 24 hours of initiation of therapy.
- Significant possible interactions:
  - If the patient is taking oral anticoagulants, it may be necessary to reduce the dose.
  - Oral contraceptives may be less effective.

Pediatric Considerations

- The drug of choice in pediatrics is amoxicillin.
- Tetracyclines are contraindicated.

Pregnancy Considerations

- Because *B. burgdorferi* can cross the placenta, pregnant patients with active disease should receive parenteral antibiotics.
- Doxycycline should not be used in pregnancy.

Second Line

Azithromycin, 500 mg PO daily for 7 days, can be used for those allergic to beta-lactams and unable to take tetracyclines, but is less effective.

ADDITIONAL TREATMENT

General Measures

- Early and disseminated Lyme disease can usually be treated as an outpatient except in the case of complications, such as carditis or meningitis, requiring parenteral antibiotics.
- For post-Lyme disease syndrome in a patient who has received adequate treatment, evidence suggests that further courses of antibiotics offer no benefit (5)[A].

IN-PATIENT CONSIDERATIONS

Admission Criteria

- Admission and monitoring are recommended for patients with Lyme carditis and symptoms of chest pain, syncope, or dyspnea, and for those with second- or third-degree heart block or first-degree heart block of ≥300 msec.
- Also for symptoms of meningitis

ONGOING CARE

FOLLOW-UP RECOMMENDATIONS

Patient Monitoring

Based on the severity of symptoms, patients with Lyme carditis, neurologic syndromes, or arthritis may require monitoring for months to years.

DIET

No restrictions

PATIENT EDUCATION

In endemic areas, patients should be advised to protect themselves against tick exposure.

PROGNOSIS

- Early treatment with antibiotics can shorten the duration of the symptoms and prevent later disease.
- Response of late-stage disease is vàriable and may take several weeks after beginning treatment.

COMPLICATIONS

- Recurrent synovitis, tendonitis, bursitis
- Chronic neurologic symptoms
- Peripheral neuropathies

REFERENCES

1. Murray TS, Shapiro ED. Lyme Disease. *Clin Lab Med*. 2010;30(1).
2. Hubalek Z. Epidemiology of Lyme *Borrelliosis*. *Curr Probl Dermatol*. 2009:31–50.
3. Warshafsky S, Lee DH, Francois LK, et al. Efficacy of antibiotic prophylaxis for the prevention of Lyme disease: An updated systematic review and meta-analysis. *J Antimicrob Chemother*. 2010;65: 1137–44.
4. Centers for Disease Control and Prevention. Notice to readers: Caution regarding testing for Lyme disease. *MMWR*. 2005;54:125.
5. Lantos PM, Charini WA, Medoff G, et al. Final report of the Lyme disease review panel of the Infectious Disease Society of America. *Clin Infect Dis*. 2010;51(1):1–5.

ADDITIONAL READING

- American Lyme Disease Foundation: www.aldf.com
- Bratton RL, Whiteside JW, Hovan MJ, et al. Diagnosis and treatment of Lyme disease. *Mayo Clin Proc*. 2008;83:566–71.
- Hoppa E, Bachur R. Lyme disease update. *Curr Opin Pediatr*. 2007;19:275–80.
- Treatment of Lyme disease. *Med Lett Drugs Ther*. 2007;49:49–51.
- www.nih.gov
- www.cdc.gov

CODES

ICD9

- 088.81 Lyme disease
- 320.7 Meningitis in other bacterial diseases classified elsewhere
- 711.80 Arthropathy associated with other infectious and parasitic diseases, site unspecified

CLINICAL PEARLS

- The presence of erythema migrans following a tick bite in an area endemic for Lyme disease warrants empiric treatment.
- Doxycycline is the drug of choice, but it is contraindicated in women who may be or may become pregnant and in children <8 years old. Amoxicillin or cefuroxime axetil can be used.
- Transmission does not occur if tick attachment is <48 hours, and only 25% transmission occurs in >72 hours, so daily skin exam and removal of ticks can prevent Lyme disease.

L

LYMPHANGITIS

Kinjal Amin, PharmD
Paul Beninger, MD

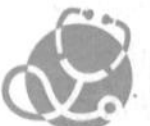

BASICS

DESCRIPTION

- Local inflammation of lymphatic vessels:
  - Acute or chronic
- Usually due to trauma and/or infection of the nearby skin

RISK FACTORS

- Diabetes mellitus
- Chronic steroid use
- Prolonged time with a peripheral venous catheter in place
- Varicella infection
- Immunocompromise
- Human, animal, or insect bites
- Fungal skin infections
- Any trauma to the skin
- IV drug abuse

GENERAL PREVENTION

Proper wound care (1)[A]

ETIOLOGY

- Acute or chronic infection of the skin causing inflammation of lymphatic channels
- Acute infection:
  - Usually caused by group A beta-hemolytic *Streptococcus*
  - Less commonly caused by:
    - *Staphylococcus aureus*
    - *Pasteurella multocida*
    - *Spirillum minus* (rat-bite disease)
    - *Pseudomonas*
    - Other *Streptococcus* sp.
- Chronic infection:
  - Caused by parasites (filariasis) or fungi (sporotrichosis)
  - Immunocompromised patients can be infected with gram-negative rods, gram-negative bacilli, or fungi.
  - In fresh water, think *Aeromonas hydrophila*.
  - Filariasis (most common worldwide causative agent is *Wuchereria bancrofti*) (2)

COMMONLY ASSOCIATED CONDITIONS

- Lymphedema
- Lymph node dissection
- Athlete's foot
- Sporotrichosis
- Cellulitis (may coexist)
- Erysipelas (often coexists)
- Filarial infection (*Wuchereria bancrofti*)

DIAGNOSIS

HISTORY

- History of trauma to skin, cut, abrasion, or fungal infection (e.g., athlete's foot)
- Systemic symptoms:
  - Malaise
  - Fever and chills
  - Loss of appetite
  - Headache
  - Muscle aches
- Travel to a tropical region

PHYSICAL EXAM

- Look for abscess
- May have lymph node tenderness
- Local signs:
  - Red macular linear streaks from site of infection toward the regional draining lymph node
  - Tenderness and warmth over affected skin
  - May have lymph node involvement
  - May have blistering of affected skin

DIAGNOSTIC TESTS & INTERPRETATION

Lab

- CBC may show leukocytosis or filarial infection
- Blood cultures

Imaging

Plain radiology unnecessary

Diagnostic Procedures/Surgery

- Aspirate and culture any pus.
- Use sensitivity to guide antibiotic treatment.

DIFFERENTIAL DIAGNOSIS

- Septic thrombophlebitis (1)[C]
- Superficial thrombophlebitis (1)[C]: Feel for induration over the vein.
- Contact dermatitis (1)[C]
- Allergic reaction (1)[C]: Less likely to be allergic if >24 hours after exposure (e.g., insect bite)

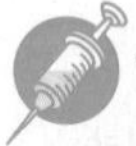

TREATMENT

MEDICATION

- If nontoxic and >3 years of age, treat as an outpatient with oral antibiotics.
- If no improvement after 48 hours of oral antibiotics, change to IV antibiotics.
- If systemic involvement, start IV antibiotics immediately.
- If group A hemolytic *Streptococcus* is suspected, treat aggressively.

First Line

- Antibiotics for suspicion of bacterial infection:
  - Amoxicillin:
    - Dosing:
      - Adults:
        - Mild to moderate: 500 mg PO q12h or 250 mg PO q8h
        - Severe: 875 mg PO q12h or 500 mg PO q8h
      - Children <3 months: 30 mg/kg/d PO divided q12h
      - Children ≥3 months, ≤40 kg:
        - Mild to moderate: 25 mg/kg/d PO divided q12h or 20 mg/kg/d divided q8h
        - Severe: 45 mg/kg/d PO divided q12h or 40 mg/kg/d divided q8h
      - Children ≥3 months, ≥40 kg:
        - Refer to adult dosing
    - Common adverse effects:
      - Diarrhea
    - Serious adverse effects:
      - Anaphylaxis, Stevens-Johnson syndrome (SJS), toxic epidermal necrolysis (TENS)
    - Drug interactions:
      - Methotrexate, venlafaxine, warfarin, hormonal contraceptives
    - Contraindications:
      - Hypersensitivity to penicillins
  - Ampicillin/Sulbactam:
    - Dosing:
      - Adults: 1.5–3 g (ampicillin plus sulbactam component) IV/IM q6h; MAX 4 g sulbactam/d
      - Children <40 kg: 300 mg/kg/d IV infusion, in divided doses q6h; MAX 4 g sulbactam/d
      - Children ≥40 kg: Refer to adult dosing
    - Common adverse effects:
      - Diarrhea, rash, and injection site reactions
    - Serious adverse effects:
      - Clostridium difficile diarrhea, pseudomembranous enterocolitis, dysuria
    - Drug interactions:
      - Hormonal contraceptives
    - Contraindications:
      - Hypersensitivity to penicillins
  - Ceftriaxone:
    - Dosing:
      - Adults: 1–2 g IV/IM q24h or in divided doses b.i.d.; maximum 4 g/d
      - Children: 50–75 mg/kg/d IV/IM once daily or in divided doses q12h; maximum 2 g/d
    - Common adverse effects:
      - Injection site reactions, diarrhea, thrombocytosis, eosinophilia
    - Serious adverse effects:
      - SJS, TENS, erythema multiforme, renal failure, pseudomembranous enterocolitis, hemolytic anemia anaphylaxis

- Drug interactions:
  - Contraindicated with the use of calcium containing products (e.g., calcium chloride, calcium gluconate, lactated ringers solution)
- Contraindications:
  - Hypersensitivity to cephalosporins
  - Concurrent use of calcium containing IV fluids
  - Use in neonates; increased risk of kernicterus

– Cephalexin:
- Dosing:
  - Adults: 500 mg PO q12h
  - Children: 25–50 mg/kg/d divided q12h
- Common adverse effects:
  - Diarrhea
- Serious adverse effects:
  - SJS, TENS, interstitial nephritis, renal failure, pseudomembranous enterocolitis, anaphylaxis
- Drug interactions:
  - Cholestyramine, metformin
- Contraindications:
  - Hypersensitivity to cephalosporins

– Azithromycin (if penicillin or cephalosporin allergy):
- Dosing:
  - Adults: 500 mg PO on day 1 followed by 250 mg/d PO on days 2–5
  - Children ≥2 years: 12 mg/kg/d PO (maximum dose: 500 mg/d) once daily for 5 days
- Common adverse effects:
  - Abdominal pain, nausea, vomiting, diarrhea, increased liver enzymes, headache
- Serious adverse effects:
  - Prolonged QT interval, torsades de pointes, liver failure, Lambert-Eaton syndrome, myasthenia gravis, corneal erosion, anaphylaxis
- Drug interactions:
  - Contraindicated with the use of ergot derivatives, pimozide and dronedarone
  - Disopyramide, class III antiarrhythmics, propafenone, ziprasidone, warfarin, digoxin, fentanyl, simvastatin
- Contraindications:
  - Hepatic dysfunction or cholestatic jaundice with prior treatment
  - Hypersensitivity to macrolide or ketolide (azithromycin, erythromycin, clarithromycin)

- Diethylcarbamazine, ivermectin, albendazole, and doxycycline are used for treatment of filarial infection
- Acetaminophen or ibuprofen for pain and fever

ADDITIONAL TREATMENT

General Measures

- Hot, moist compresses to affected area
- If lymphedema is involved, compression garments and weight loss may help.

SURGERY/OTHER PROCEDURES

Incision and drainage of abscessed areas

IN-PATIENT CONSIDERATIONS

Initial Stabilization

- ABCs
- Fluids if in hypotensive shock

Admission Criteria

- If patient requires IV antibiotic therapy
- If symptoms are severe (3)[C]:
  - High fever
  - Rigor
  - Systemic toxicity
  - Shock
- Altered mental status

Discharge Criteria

Patient can be discharged on oral antibiotics after systemic symptoms resolve.

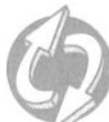

ONGOING CARE

FOLLOW-UP RECOMMENDATIONS

- Elevate affected area when at rest, if possible (4)[C].
- 48-hour follow-up to ensure proper antibiotic coverage (if outpatient)

Patient Monitoring

Close follow-up to ensure decreasing inflammation

PATIENT EDUCATION

Instruct patients on proper wound care (and foot care, if applicable).

PROGNOSIS

- Good prognosis for uncomplicated lymphangitis
- Antimicrobial therapy is effective in 90% of patients.
- Untreated, can spread rapidly, especially group A *Streptococcus*

COMPLICATIONS

- Sepsis
- Bacteremia
- Cellulitis extending from vessels

REFERENCES

1. Falagas ME, Bliziotis IA, Kapaskelis AM. Red streaks on the leg. *Am Fam Phys*. 2006;73(6):1061–2.
2. Taylor MJ, Hoerauf A, Bockarie M, et al. Lymphatic filariasis and onchocerciasis. *Lancet*. 2010;376: 1175–85.
3. Edlich RF, Winters KL, Britt LD. *BJ Long-Term Effects Med Implants*. 2005;15(5):499–510.
4. Bonnetblanc JM, Bédane C. Erysipelas: Recognition and management. *Am J Clin Dermatol*. 2003;4:157–63.

ADDITIONAL READING

- Badger C, Seers K, Preston N, et al. Antibiotics/anti-inflammatories for reducing acute inflammatory episodes in lymphoedema of the limbs. *Cochrane Database Syst Rev*. 2004;CD003143.
- Del Giudice P, et al. Cutaneous complications of intravenous drug abuse. *Br J Dermatol*. 2004;150: 1–10.
- Haddad FG, Waked CH, Zein EF. Peripheral venous catheter-related inflammation. A randomized prospective trial. *J Med Liban*. 2006;54:139–45.
- Pereira de Godoy JM, Azoubel LM, Guerreiro Godoy Mde F. Erysipelas and lymphangitis in patients undergoing lymphedema treatment after breast-cancer therapy. *Acta Dermatovenerol Alp Panonica Adriat*. 2009;18:63–5.

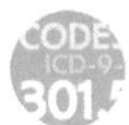

CODES

ICD9

457.2 Lymphangitis

CLINICAL PEARLS

- The classic presentation of lymphangitis is red, linear streaks along the skin from an infected site (e.g., bite, cut, abrasion) to the draining lymph node for that region.
- Patients who have lymph node dissection as part of their breast cancer treatment may have difficulty draining lymphatic fluid properly, leading to lymphedema and an increased predisposition to infection and lymphangitis.
- A patient with severe systemic symptoms (e.g., high fever, rigors, shock, septic, altered mental status) should be admitted and treated with IV antibiotics. A patient with moderate systemic symptoms (e.g., fever, chills, muscle aches) should be monitored closely for worsening but could be treated as an outpatient.
- Patients can take ibuprofen or acetaminophen for the pain and/or fever associated with lymphangitis. Ibuprofen also helps with inflammation at high doses.
- Usually parasitic or fungal infections cause chronic lymphangitis.

LYMPHEDEMA

Kim House, MD

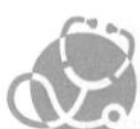

BASICS

DESCRIPTION

- Swelling of a body part due to an abnormality in regional lymphatic drainage
- Results in increased interstitial volume secondary to the accumulation of tissue (lymphatic) fluid
- Most common in the lower limb (80%), but also can occur in the arms, face, trunk, and external genitalia

EPIDEMIOLOGY

Incidence

- Predominant sex: Female > Male
- Predominant age: Any age
- 13% of breast cancer patients treated with surgery; 42% of those treated with surgery and radiation therapy
- Estimated to be between 1/6,000 and 1/300 live births; Milroy disease presents at birth.
- Meige disease develops during puberty.

Prevalence

- 120 million people worldwide are affected with filariasis.
- 3 million–5 million people are affected by secondary lymphedema in the US.

RISK FACTORS

- Filariasis: Most common cause worldwide
- Mastectomy
- Prior trauma
- Infection of affected limb
- History of prior surgical or radiation therapy for malignancy
- Long history of venous insufficiency
- Obesity

Genetics

- Milroy disease: Autosomal dominant; diagnosed either at birth or the first year of life
- Lymphedema praecox has onset between the ages of 1 and 35 years.
- Lymphedema tarda occurs >35 years

GENERAL PREVENTION

Treatment of congestive heart failure (CHF), venous insufficiency

PATHOPHYSIOLOGY

- Postoperative: Gradual failure of distal lymphatics, which have to "pump" lymph at a greater pressure through damaged proximal ducts
- Risk is higher with postoperative radiation because radiation reduces regrowth of ducts due to fibrous scarring.

ETIOLOGY

Secondary lymphedema:

- Trauma; recurrent infection; malignancy, including metastatic disease
- Developing countries: Most common cause is filariasis (*Wucheria bancrofti*).

COMMONLY ASSOCIATED CONDITIONS

Venous disease

DIAGNOSIS

HISTORY

Recent surgery: Vein stripping can significantly exacerbate mild lymphedema (1)[B]:

- First symptom: Painless swelling
- Feeling of heaviness in the limb, especially at the end of the day and in hot weather

PHYSICAL EXAM

- Initial: Pitting edema, can spread proximally
- Later: Nonpitting; after first year, does not spread proximally/distally but spreads radially
- Hyperkeratosis (thicker skin)
- Papillomatosis (rough skin)
- Increase in skin turgor
- Positive Stemmer sign (inability to pinch the skin of the dorsum of the second toe between the thumb and forefinger): Exclude heart failure.

DIAGNOSTIC TESTS & INTERPRETATION

- Lack of response to elevation or diuretic therapy may indicate a lymphatic insufficiency (2)[B].
- Diuretics increase excretion of salt and water, thereby decreasing plasma volume, venous capillary pressure, and filtration. Diuretics improve filtration edema, but don't improve lymph drainage over the long term.

Lab

Initial lab tests

- Comprehensive chemistry panel: Evaluate for hepatic or renal impairment.
- Urinalysis: Protein-losing nephropathy

Imaging

Initial approach

- Ultrasound: Evaluate for acute/chronic deep vein thrombosis (DVT). Gives information about soft tissue changes but does not tell about truncal anatomy of the lymphatics (1)[B].
- Duplex ultrasound: Lymphedema causes gradual impedance of venous return that aggravates the edema; 82% of patients with unexplained limb edema were diagnosed using a combination of duplex ultrasound and lymphoscintigram (3)[A].

Follow-Up & Special Considerations

- Lymphangiogram: Direct cannulation of lymphatics through the skin; risk for infection, local inflammation; not used commonly (3)[C]
- Lymphoscintigram: Radiolabeled protein technetium-99m-labeled colloid:
  - Measures lymphatic function, lymph movement, lymph drainage, and response to treatment
  - Sensitivity 73–97%; specificity 100%
  - Best to use 1-hour and delayed images together (3)[A]
- CT scan: Calf skin thickening, thickening of the SC compartment, increased fat density, thickened perimuscular aponeurosis; typical honeycomb appearance (3)[B]
- MRI: Circumferential edema, increased volume of SC tissue, honeycomb pattern above the fascia between the muscle and subcutis; cannot differentiate primary from secondary lymphedema (3)[B]

DIFFERENTIAL DIAGNOSIS

- CHF
- Renal failure
- Hypoalbuminemia
- Protein-losing nephropathy
- Lipidemia
- DVT
- Chronic venous disease
- Postoperative complications following ipsilateral surgery
- Cellulitis
- Baker cyst
- Idiopathic edema

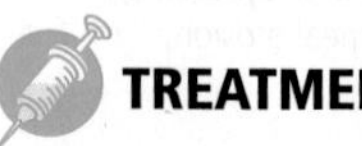

TREATMENT

MEDICATION

- Micronized purified flavonoid fraction (Daflon 500 mg) is effective in decreasing venous stasis and idiopathic cyclic edema, chronic venous insufficiency, and postmastectomy lymphedema. It also reduces capillary permeability and the inflammatory component (4)[C].
- Benzopyrenes (coumarin): Reduces edema fluid by increasing the number of macrophages and enhancing proteolysis, resulting in the removal of protein, increasing softness in the limbs, and decreasing elevated skin temperature:
  - Decreases symptoms and signs and decreases instances of secondary infection
  - Some reports of hepatotoxicity (4)[C]

ADDITIONAL TREATMENT

General Measures

- Elevation of affected limb: May be difficult for some patients to comply
- Prevent disease progression.
- Achieve mechanical reduction and maintenance of limb size.
- Alleviate symptoms.
- Prevent skin infection.

Issues for Referral

- Refer to physical therapist with lymphedema training for manual decongestive therapy.
- Provide education for patient/family for self-administration of therapy in future.
- Education for family about bandaging
- Fitting for compression garments

Additional Therapies

- Exercise: Lymph flow occurs as a result of inspiratory reduction in the intrathoracic pressure associated with inspiration. Best results are achieved with combination of flexibility, strength, and aerobic training (3)[B].
- Compression with custom-made elastic stocking (minimum pressure is 40 mm Hg):
  - Protection against external incidental trauma
  - Decreases the intrinsic trauma on the skin due to chronically increased interstitial pressures, which cause stretch of the skin and SC tissues
  - No data on preference of custom-made versus prefabricated
  - Replace every 3–6 months or when starting to lose elasticity (1)[B].
- Multilayer bandaging: Inner layer of tubular stockinette followed by foam and padding to protect the joint flexures and to even out the contours of the limb so that pressure is distributed evenly; outer layer of at least 2 short-stretch extensible bandages; more effective than hosiery alone (1)[B]
- Pneumatic pumps: Development of high pressure up to 150 mm Hg; can reduce limb girth by 37–68.6%; wear a compression stocking when not using pump; high risk of genital edema; no metastasis in limb due to risk of spread (1)[B]

COMPLEMENTARY AND ALTERNATIVE MEDICINE

Heat therapy: Hot water immersion, microwave, and electromagnetic irradiation may be helpful (1)[C].

SURGERY/OTHER PROCEDURES

- Debulking procedures (Charles procedure): Radical excision of SC tissue with primary or staged skin grafting:
  - Men had less improvement than women.
  - Main risk is infection and necrosis of the skin graft.
- Bypass procedures: Creation of lymphatic–venous anastomosis: Reserved for highly refractory cases only

IN-PATIENT CONSIDERATIONS

Initial Stabilization

- May admit to specialized rehabilitation unit for combination treatment in patients with heart failure or severe pulmonary disease
- IV antibiotics for infection

Admission Criteria

Systemic signs of infection

Nursing

- Leg elevation
- Encourage patient mobilization/exercise.
- Patient education for bandaging/wound care

Discharge Criteria

- Resolution of signs/symptoms of infection (e.g., elevated WBC count, fever, abnormal vital signs)
- Clinical improvement in wound appearance

ONGOING CARE

FOLLOW-UP RECOMMENDATIONS

Lymphedema will return in several days if patient stops wearing compression garments during the day and bandaging at night.

Patient Monitoring

- Daily visit to therapist for acute treatment
- Monthly visits for maintenance care

DIET

Low sodium

PATIENT EDUCATION

- Use compression garments, especially when exercising.
- Avoid affected limb(s) being dependant for long period of time: Patient should perform daily skin examination.

PROGNOSIS

Good with daily care

COMPLICATIONS

- Infection (local versus systemic): Common
- Risk of wound formation (venous wounds/abrasions) that are difficult to heal: Common
- Lymphangiosarcoma: Found in lymphedematous arms of patients following radical mastectomy; also in patients with Milroy disease; treatment is radiotherapy with surgery, reserved for patients with discrete nonmetastatic disease

REFERENCES

1. Warren A, et al. Lymphedema: A comprehensive review. *Ann Plastic Surg.* 2007;59(4):464–72.
2. Mortimer P. Implications of the lymphatic system in CVI-associated edema. *Angiology.* 2000;51(1):3–7.
3. Brennan MJ, Miller LT. Overview of treatment options and review of the current role and use of compression garments, intermittent pumps, and exercise in the management of lymphedema. *Cancer.* 1998;83:2821–7.
4. Tiwari A, Cheng KS, Button M, et al. Differential diagnosis, investigation, and current treatment of lower limb lymphedema. *Arch Surg.* 2003;138: 152–61.

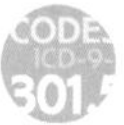

CODES

ICD9

- 125.9 Unspecified filariasis
- 457.0 Postmastectomy lymphedema syndrome
- 457.1 Other lymphedema

CLINICAL PEARLS

- Use short-stretch bandages for wrapping (not ACE wraps).
- Heat/whirlpool typically makes the wounds/lymphedema worse, not better.
- Patients with lymphedema are at much higher risk for infection than patients with only venous insufficiency.

L

LYMPHOGRANULOMA VENEREUM

Larissa Calka, MD
Marie Ellen Caggiano, MD, MPH

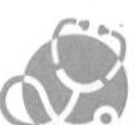

BASICS

Lymphogranuloma venereum (LGV) is a rare systemic STD caused by virulent strains of *Chlamydia trachomatis*. The incidence of LGV has been increasing in the US among men who have sex with men (MSM).

DESCRIPTION

- LGV may initially present as a painless vesicular or ulcerative lesions on the external genitalia. These self-limited lesions are seen in early disease and are followed by tender inguinal/femoral lymphadenopathy, usually unilateral. If untreated, proctocolitis can occur causing severe anogenital inflammation and scarring.
- Historically thought of as a disease of the tropics, more recently, outbreaks have been reported in Europe, North America, and Australia.
- System(s) affected: Gastrointestinal; Hemic/Lymphatic/Immunologic; Reproductive
- Synonym(s): Tropical bubo; Climatic bubo; Strumous bubo; Poradenitis inguinalis; Durand-Nicolas-Favre disease; Lymphogranuloma inguinale; fourth, fifth, or sixth venereal disease

EPIDEMIOLOGY

- Predominant age: Third decade; corresponding with average age of peak sexual activity
- Predominant sex: Male > Female (5:1)

Incidence

In the US, about 300 cases reported each year.

Prevalence

In the US, incidence is increasing among MSM.

Pregnancy Considerations

LGV may be acquired passing through infected birth canal; congenital transmission is not known to occur.

RISK FACTORS

- Unprotected intercourse
- Anal intercourse
- Residing in tropical or developing countries
- Prostitution
- MSM
- HIV (+)

GENERAL PREVENTION

- Treat sexual contact(s).
- Condoms may provide protection against genital–anogenital transmission, but they have no impact on transmission between other sites.

PATHOPHYSIOLOGY

Tissue damage from lymphatic inflammation and obstruction

ETIOLOGY

3 of 15 known strains of *C. trachomatis*, described as serovars L1, L2, and L3, are responsible for LGV. The strains of *C. trachomatis* that cause urethritis appear to infect only squamocolumnar cells; LGV strains are more invasive, capable of replication in macrophages, and can spread to lymphatic tissue at the site of infection, leading to systemic illness.

COMMONLY ASSOCIATED CONDITIONS

Screening for comorbid STIs should include testing for gonorrhea, hepatitis B, hepatitis C, herpes, HIV, and syphilis.

DIAGNOSIS

LGV is a rare disease, predominantly diagnosed by clinical suspicion based on history, physical examination, and exclusion of other diagnoses. Where available, serologic testing can be helpful. Calling a reference lab is often helpful for determining the best available test. Swabs obtained from infected lesions or aspirates of affected lymphatic tissue may be examined by culture, direct immunofluorescence, or nucleic acid amplification (NAAT).

HISTORY

Recent unprotected intercourse with a prostitute or MSM, especially anal intercourse, attendance at sex parties, use of sex toys, or intercourse with a person recently visiting from the tropics such as Africa, the Caribbean, South America, East Asia, or Indonesia

PHYSICAL EXAM

3 stages:

- Primary: Superficial painless lesions such as papules, vesicles, ulcers, or erosions appear on the external genitalia, in the area of inoculation, 3–30 days after exposure. These disappear in a few days, leaving no scar.
- Secondary: The inguinal syndrome (bubonic stage) or hemorrhagic proctitis (following rectal intercourse). Femoral lymphics can also be involved, often unilaterally:
  - Fever, chills, headache, myalgias, malaise
  - Inguinal syndrome: Regional lymphadenopathy, usually unilateral, develops 2–6 weeks after the primary stage. Buboes begin as firm, tender, enlarged, matted lymph nodes, and eventually involve the overlying skin causing erythema, adhesions, and severe groin pain. Within 1–2 weeks, the buboes may become fluctuant and rupture, relieving the pain but leaving fistulas to drain or involute and form firm inguinal masses (1)[C]. Drainage patterns in women can affect deep pelvic lymph nodes causing pelvic, abdominal, and lower back pain (2)[C].
  - Proctitis: Anal pruritus and mucoid rectal discharge, multiple discrete superficial ulcerations with irregular borders, rectal pain, and tenesmus (3)[C]. Discharge and lesions may be seen on anoscopy or endoscopy.
- Tertiary: Anogenital stage:
  - Lymphatic obstruction and scarring
  - Severe inflammation of genitalia or anorectal canal
  - Occurs predominantly among women and MSM
  - Lymphatic obstruction may produce perianal growths or lymphoid tissue resembling hemorrhoids.
  - Perirectal abscesses, ischiorectal and rectovaginal fistulas, anal fistulas, and rectal strictures or stenosis may occur.

DIAGNOSTIC TESTS & INTERPRETATION

Lab

- Specimens may be obtained from urine, the urethra, endocervix, or rectum (if proctitis is present) and tested for *C. trachomatis*. Lymph node specimens (aspirate or biopsy) and tissue obtained from rectal biopsy can also be evaluated for organism (4)[C].
- Cultures obtained from primary lesions may be used to isolate organism. Polymerase chain reaction (PCR)–based genotyping can be used to differentiate LGV from other chlamydial strains.
- Dry swabs should be stored and shipped frozen. Swabs stored in chlamydia transport medium should be kept frozen at −80°C if culture will be done or −20°C if culture will not be done. Check with the laboratory for specific protocols.
- Serologic tests are more useful after LGV has become invasive (i.e., secondary or tertiary LGV), although serovar specific tests are not widely available.

Initial lab tests

- NAAT will identify all *C. trachomatis* serovars, including those associated with LGV. NAAT is licensed for genital samples but not FDA approved for rectal samples. However, some data exist supporting validity of testing rectal samples, and certain laboratories may be able to process samples (4)[C]. Positive NAAT samples can be sent for LGV genotyping.
- Confirmation by genotyping for LGV via DNA sequencing or restriction fragment length polymorphism (RFLP) is definitive (i.e., differentiates LGV from other chlamydial strains) (4)[B].
- Cultures from a primary lesion may grow chlamydia, but genotyping is necessary to differentiate LGV from other *C. trachomatis* strains (2)[C].
- Urine can be tested with NAAT and positives sent for LGV genotyping; samples should be stored and shipped frozen.
- Serum Igm microimmunofluorescence (MIF-IgG) testing is more readily available but not definitive of LGV. It is important that the L serovar be included as an antigen for testing (4)[C].
- Serum antibody levels to L1, L2, and L3 serovars of *C. trachomatis* also measured using complement fixation, although cross-reactivity with other chlamydial organisms is possible.
- A 4-fold rise in MIF titer to LGV antigen (>1:256) or a complement fixation titer >1:64, with the proper clinical scenario, is strongly suggestive of LGV (4)[C].

Follow-Up & Special Considerations

- CBC and differential may reveal lymphocytosis or monocytosis.
- ESR may be elevated.
- Consider syphilis, gonorrhea, hepatitis B and hepatitis C, herpes simplex virus (HSV), HIV testing.

Imaging

Imaging is only necessary to clarify or define complications or to exclude other diagnoses.

Initial approach

- CT scan for retroperitoneal adenitis
- Barium enema may reveal the characteristic elongated stricture of rectal LGV.

Diagnostic Procedures/Surgery

- Buboes may require infiltration of 2–5 mL of sterile saline prior to aspiration.
- Endoscopy may visualize characteristic rectal pathology.

DIFFERENTIAL DIAGNOSIS

- Painful genital ulcer, often with adenitis (in order of frequency): Genital herpes, chancroid, LGV. Patients should also be evaluated for syphilis and HIV. Not all ulcers are infectious in etiology; on the other hand, polymicrobial infections may occur.
- Painless genital ulcer: Syphilis, granuloma inguinale (donovanosis), LGV. Patients should also be evaluated for herpes and HIV.
- Inguinal adenitis:
  - Genital herpes, syphilis, chancroid, granuloma inguinale (donovanosis)
  - Other considerations for inguinal adenitis include cat scratch disease, local skin infection, lymphoma, HIV, and reactive adenopathy.
  - Less common: Lymphoproliferative buboes
- Buboes or suppurative adenitis: Chancroid, donovanosis, plague, tularemia, sporotrichosis, actinomycosis, or tuberculosis
- Retroperitoneal adenitis: Malignancy
- Proctitis: Gonococcal and non-LGV chlamydial proctitis, inflammatory bowel disease
- Lymphatic obstruction: Schistosomiasis or malignancy

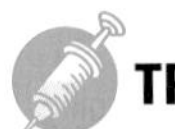

TREATMENT

Oral antibiotics administered in the ambulatory setting are effective in most uncomplicated cases.

MEDICATION

Consider treating empirically for LGV if specific LGV diagnostic testing is not available for patients with a compatible clinical syndrome (e.g., proctocolitis, genital ulcer disease with lymphadenopathy) (3)[C].

First Line

- For acute cases: Doxycycline 100 mg PO b.i.d. for 21 days (5)[B]
- For chronic or relapsing cases: Consider longer course of therapy and alternating antibiotics (4)[C].

Second Line

- Erythromycin base 500 mg PO q.i.d. for 21 days (4)[C]
- Azithromycin 1 g PO once weekly for 3 weeks (4)[C]
- Trimethoprim-sulfamethoxazole 80 mg/400 mg PO b.i.d. for 21 days (4)[C]
- Tetracycline hydrochloride 500 mg PO q.i.d. for 21 days (4)[C] or minocycline 300 mg loading dose, followed by 200 mg b.i.d. for 21 days (4)[C]

Pregnancy Considerations

Treat pregnant and lactating women with erythromycin (3)[C]. There is no current evidence supporting the efficacy of azithromycin in pregnant women; however, it may prove to be a useful treatment. Doxycycline is contraindicated in pregnancy.

ADDITIONAL TREATMENT

General Measures

Any person having sexual contact with an individual diagnosed with LGV within 60 days of symptoms onset should be examined, tested, and treated for chlamydial infection (3)[C]. The current recommendation for treatment of exposed partners is azithromycin 1 g PO single dose or doxycycline 100 mg PO b.i.d. for 7 days (3)[C]. Some sources recommend doxycycline 100 mg PO b.i.d. for full 21-day course (2)[C].

Issues for Referral

Surgical intervention for complications associated with LGV should be delayed until antibiotic therapy has been administered for at least a few days and fever has resolved.

SURGERY/OTHER PROCEDURES

In the bubonic stage, nodes should be aspirated through intact skin for diagnostic purposes, and this may also improve symptoms. Nodes may also be incised and drained (I&D) for diagnostic purposes and to possibly prevent inguinal or femoral ulcerations. There is controversy as to whether I&D or excision of nodes improves symptoms as opposed to delaying healing.

IN-PATIENT CONSIDERATIONS

Inpatient treatment is rarely necessary.

Admission Criteria

Unable to tolerate oral antibiotics, ambulate, or perform self-care due to pain or other complications, or patients preparing to undergo a surgical intervention for extensive disease.

Nursing

Public health nurses can help track and treat sexual contacts.

Discharge Criteria

When stable and able to perform self-care

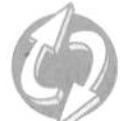

ONGOING CARE

FOLLOW-UP RECOMMENDATIONS

Patients should be observed until signs and symptoms resolve and routine chlamydial tests are negative. Test of microbiological cure is recommended 3–5 weeks after treatment (4)[C]. Serology should not be used to monitor treatment response, as the duration of antibody response has not been defined.

Patient Monitoring

- Fever and buboes usually abate within 1–2 days after starting antibiotics. For persistent fever or malaise, monitor closely for complications such as an abscess or superinfection.
- Treatment has no effect on existing scar tissue; therefore, monitor for surgical complications.
- Dual infections with other STDs are common; appropriate monitoring should be performed, especially for gonorrhea, hepatitis B, hepatitis C, HIV, and syphilis.

DIET

Tetracyclines should be taken on an empty stomach except for doxycycline, which can be taken with food.

PATIENT EDUCATION

LGV is an STD. The patient should be counseled about other STDs and safer sex practices. Patients should abstain from intercourse or other sexual contact until treatment is complete.

PROGNOSIS

- Improved by early treatment
- Complete resolution of symptoms is expected if treatment is undertaken before scarring.
- Reinfection and/or inadequate treatment may result in relapse.

COMPLICATIONS

- Scarring, including possible ureteral or bowel obstruction, persistent rectovaginal fistula, or gross destruction of the anal canal, anal sphincter, or perineum may occur. Repair of such complications, as well as relief of lymphatic obstruction, such as genital elephantiasis, are the more common surgical indications. Surgery should be performed only after antibiotic treatment has been initiated.
- Mild rectal strictures can occasionally be dilated on an outpatient basis.
- Squamous cell carcinoma has been associated with LGV.

REFERENCES

1. Martin-Iguacel R, Llibre JM, Nielsen H, et al. Lymphogranuloma venereum proctocolitis: A silent endemic disease in men who have sex with men in industrialized countries. *Eur J Microbiol Infect Dis*. 2010;29:917–25.
2. Lymphogranuloma venereum (LGV). In: HIV Clinical Resource: Office of the Medical Director, New York State Department of Health AIDS Institution in collaboration with the Johns Hopkins University Division of Infectious Disease; 2007:1–10.
3. Workowski KA, Berman SM. Sexually transmitted disease treatment guidelines, 2010. *MMWR Recomm Rep.*. 2010;59:1–26.
4. Herring A, Richens J. Lymphogranuloma venereum (LGV). In: *Sexually Transmitted Infections: UK National screening and testing guidelines*. London (UK): British Association for Sexual Health and HIV (BASHH); 2006:57–62.
5. McLean CA, Stoner BP, Workowski KA. Treatment of lymphogranuloma venereum. *Clin Infect Dis*. 2007;44(Suppl 3):S147–52.

ADDITIONAL READING

- Herring A, Richens J. Lymphogranuloma venereum. *Sex Transm Infect*. 2006;82(Suppl 4):iv23–5.
- MacDonald N, Wong T. Canadian guidelines on sexually transmitted infections, 2006. *CMAJ*. 2007; 176:175–6.

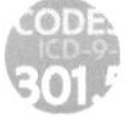

CODES

ICD9

099.1 Lymphogranuloma venereum

CLINICAL PEARLS

- In MSM presenting with colorectal symptoms (mucopurulent or bloody discharge, rectal pain, tenesmus, abdominal pain, constipation), clinicians should place LGV proctocolitis in their differential diagnosis. It can occasionally be misdiagnosed as Crohn disease.
- Once the diagnosis of LGV is made, it is very important to test for other associated STDs, especially hepatitis C and HIV.

LYMPHOMA, BURKITT

Jennifer J. Greene Welch, MD

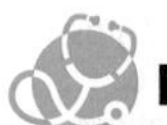

BASICS

DESCRIPTION

- Mature B-cell neoplasm that arises in lymph node germinal centers
- Highly aggressive, rapidly growing malignancy
- Can present as lymphoma or leukemia
- 3 distinct forms, differing in epidemiology, clinical presentation, and genetics:
  - Endemic, or African
  - Sporadic
  - Immunodeficiency-related:
    - HIV/AIDS-related
    - Post solid organ transplant
    - Congenital immunodeficiency
- Associated with Epstein-Barr virus (EBV):
  - Almost 100% of endemic cases
  - Up to 30% of sporadic cases
- Specific chromosome translocation [t(8;14)]
- Similar disease characteristics to diffuse large B-cell lymphoma (DLBCL)
- System(s) affected: Hematologic, Lymphatic
- Synonym(s): Mature B-cell high-grade lymphoma, mature B-cell acute lymphoblastic leukemia, L3 type (FAB classification), Burkitt cell leukemia

Pediatric Considerations

Common age group (30% of cases in the US)

Geriatric Considerations

Unusual in this age group. Toxicity with chemotherapy may be increased in the elderly.

Pregnancy Considerations

With aggressive treatment, good maternal and fetal outcome

EPIDEMIOLOGY

- Varies by disease form
- Endemic:
  - One of most common tumors of childhood in Africa, most frequently occurring in children 4–7 years old
  - Rare in adults
- Sporadic (1):
  - In the US, trimodal peaks of age incidence around ages 10, 40, and 75
  - More common in Caucasians
  - Male > Female (3:1 or 4:1)

Incidence

Rare in the US, incidence 0.27 per 100,000 person-years; 50 times more common in endemic regions of Africa

Prevalence

Comprises <1% of adult non-Hodgkin's lymphoma (NHL); accounts for 30–40% of NHL in children in the US and western Europe

RISK FACTORS

Endemic: Children with early acquisition of EBV infection are at increased risk. Coinfection with malaria and EBV 100-fold increase in incidence.

GENERAL PREVENTION

No known methods to prevent Burkitt lymphoma

ETIOLOGY

- Activation and overexpression of *c-myc* oncogene
- Monoclonal proliferation of B lymphocytes resulting from dysregulation of *c-myc*:
  - Translocation of *c-myc* to immunoglobulin coding regions results in constitutive expression of gene product.
  - EBV-infected cells in germinal-center reactions may increase the risk of translocation.
- Poorly regulated proliferation of genetically unstable B cells increases chance of translocations:
  - Immunodeficiency patients with persistent generalized lymphadenopathy and polyclonal B-cell activation

COMMONLY ASSOCIATED CONDITIONS

- EBV infection
- Immunodeficiency, especially AIDS

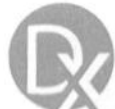

DIAGNOSIS

HISTORY

- Rapidly progressive bulky adenopathy or extranodal mass
- Symptoms of bone marrow involvement:
  - Fatigue, exercise intolerance, bruising, epistaxis, other bleeding, fever
- Abdominal presentation:
  - Abdominal pain, nausea, vomiting, bowel obstruction, GI bleeding, symptoms mimicking acute appendicitis or intussusception
- Endemic (African): Jaw or facial bone tumor, with mouth pain, loose teeth, or jaw mass
- Nonendemic: Extranodal disease, abdominal presentation typical
- Can present as acute leukemia (L3-ALL) with predominant bone marrow involvement and no mass lesions
- Renal function impairment and significant metabolic derangement may quickly manifest due to the rapid progression and spread of the tumor.

PHYSICAL EXAM

- Endemic: Mass on jaw or facial bone, pallor, petechiae, hepatosplenomegaly
- Sporadic: Lymphadenopathy, any mass lesion, abdominal tenderness, pallor, petechiae, hepatosplenomegaly
- Immunodeficiency-associated: Lymphadenopathy. pallor, petechiae, hepatosplenomegaly

DIAGNOSTIC TESTS & INTERPRETATION

Lab

Initial lab tests

- Biopsy of mass lesion: Diagnosis by cellular morphology on histologic examination
- CBC with differential: Anemia, neutropenia, and/or thrombocytopenia
- Order electrolytes, BUN, creatinine, calcium, magnesium, phosphorus, serum lactate dehydrogenase (LDH), uric acid: Hypokalemia, hypophosphatemia, hypercalcemia, hyperuricemia, renal insufficiency, elevated LDH
- Hepatitis B virus serologies prior to rituximab

Follow-Up & Special Considerations

- Diagnosis requires immunophenotypic and cytogenetic data.
- Immunophenotype studies:
  - Cells express surface IgM and B-associated antigens (CD19, CD20, CD22, CD79a), as well as CD10, HLA-DR, and CD43
  - Cells also show nuclear staining for BCL-6 protein
- Cytogenic studies to visualize chromosomal translocation:
  - Reciprocal chromosome translocation involving *c-myc* and immunoglobulin heavy chain (IgH) gene [t(8;14)] (80%)
  - Reciprocal chromosome translocation involving *c-myc* and immunoglobulin light chain (IgL) genes [t(2;8) or t (8;22)]
  - Fluorescence in situ hybridization (FISH) or long-segment polymerase chain reaction (PCR) may be necessary to identify translocation
- EBV testing in lesional cells
- Gene expression profiling can help distinguish Burkitt lymphoma from DLBCL.

Imaging

Initial approach

- Chest x-ray
- CT scan of chest, abdomen, pelvis
- Whole body positron emission tomography (PET) to identify active disease
- Dedicated imaging of any site suspected to be involved by tumor

Diagnostic Procedures/Surgery

- Bone marrow aspiration and biopsy for morphology and flow cytometry
- Lumbar puncture for CSF cell count, differential, and cytology
- Lymph node biopsy: Most suggestive lymph nodes should be selected for excisional biopsy:
  - Frozen sections and needle biopsies discouraged as lymph node architecture helpful for diagnosis.
- Diagnostic laparotomy with resection of localized disease

Pathological Findings

- Monotonous diffuse infiltrate of medium-size round cells, with round or oval nuclei, several nucleoli, and coarse chromatin. Cytoplasm is intensely basophilic and moderately abundant.
- Mitotic rate is high; close to 100% of viable cells will be actively engaged in cell cycle
- Classic starry-sky histologic appearance:
  - Results from the presence of scattered macrophages with phagocytic cell debris
  - Characteristic of, although not pathognomonic, for Burkitt's lymphoma

DIFFERENTIAL DIAGNOSIS

- Other non-Hodgkin's lymphomas:
  - Burkitt-like lymphoma: Intermediate immunophenotype and molecular characteristics between classic Burkitt's lymphoma and DLBCL
  - DLBCL: Large, irregular cells, often with BCL rearrangement
  - Precursor B-lymphoblastic lymphoma
  - Precursor T-lymphoblastic lymphoma
  - Mantle cell lymphoma, blastoid variant
- Hodgkin lymphoma
- Acute lymphoblastic leukemia
- Other causes of lymphadenopathy
  - Infection (e.g., bacterial lymphadenitis, mononucleosis, tuberculosis, atypical mycobacterium, cat-scratch disease)
  - Reactive lymphoid hyperplasia
  - Histiocytosis
- Other primary malignancies of childhood (e.g., Wilms tumor, neuroblastoma, peripheral neuroectodermal tumor)
- Other metastatic malignancies

TREATMENT

If available, all patients should be offered participation in an appropriate clinical trial.

MEDICATION

- Intensive, short-term, multiagent chemotherapy administered in cycles (2,3,4)[A]:
  - Chemotherapeutic agents include cyclophosphamide, methotrexate, vincristine, prednisone, high-dose methotrexate, high-dose cytarabine, etoposide, isophosphamide, and doxorubicin.
  - Type and extent of therapy depend on stage of disease
- Rituximab in combination with chemotherapy may improve outcome (3)[B].
- Nonintensive chemotherapy protocols utilized in developing countries can be effective (5)[B]:
  - Cyclophosphamide, methotrexate
  - Areas with limited financial and medical resources
- CNS prophylaxis for most patients:
  - Not necessary for limited disease far from CNS
  - Intrathecal methotrexate, with or without IV methotrexate and cytarabine, may be used for CNS prophylaxis
  - Prophylactic irradiation does not improve outcome
- Chemotherapy cycles should be initiated as soon as hematologic recovery permits:
  - Delay of chemotherapy may result in regrowth of resistant tumor between cycles.
- Management of tumor lysis syndrome with initial cycle of chemotherapy

Second Line

- Rituximab may be effective if not used previously.
- Hematopoietic stem cell transplantation in combination with high-dose chemotherapy (6)

ADDITIONAL TREATMENT

Issues for Referral

All patients should be managed by a pediatric or adult hematologist/oncologist.

COMPLEMENTARY AND ALTERNATIVE MEDICINE

Many possible complementary and alternative therapies exist to assist in management of side effects of chemotherapy. These should be considered individually with the patient.

SURGERY/OTHER PROCEDURES

- Biopsy and staging:
  - All patients require a biopsy to establish the diagnosis pathologically
- Surgical resection:
  - Treatment for small, completely resectable abdominal tumors (in addition to chemotherapy)
  - For patients with intestinal obstruction who cannot begin chemotherapy immediately
- Most patients require placement of a central venous line for administration of chemotherapy.

IN-PATIENT CONSIDERATIONS

Initial Stabilization

- Burkitt's lymphomas have high-growth fractions and short doubling times:
  - Rapid initiation of definitive chemotherapy is essential.
- Management of tumor lysis syndrome with initial cycle of chemotherapy:
  - Aggressive hydration without potassium
  - Close monitoring of electrolytes, renal function, and uric acid initially q6–8h.
  - Rasburicase (0.2 mg/kg IV once daily for up to 5 days depending on response to therapy) to break down uric acid
  - Allopurinol (10 mg/kg PO divided 2–3 times per day) if rasburicase not available:
    - Consider alkalization of urine with bicarbonate-containing IV fluids (goal urine pH 7–8) with allopurinol use
  - Use of phosphate binder if serum phosphorus becomes elevated
  - Medical management of hyperkalemia

IV Fluids

Aggressive IV hydration with first cycle of chemotherapy:

- Typically D5/0.5 NS at 125 cc/m^2/hr (twice the maintenance rate)
- No potassium in IV fluids.

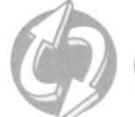

ONGOING CARE

FOLLOW-UP RECOMMENDATIONS

Patient Monitoring

- Close monitoring of serum chemistries is critical due to high risk of tumor lysis syndrome and uric acid nephropathy.
- CBC, liver function tests, and renal function should also be closely monitored throughout chemotherapy.
- Surveillance physical exam and imaging for detection of recurrence
- All patients, particularly children, should be followed indefinitely for long-term effects of chemotherapy.

PATIENT EDUCATION

Educational materials are available online from:

- Leukemia and Lymphoma Society (www.leukemia-lymphoma.org)
- Curesearch (www.curesearch.org)

PROGNOSIS

- Localized disease, 5-year disease-free survival >90%
- Aggressive treatment of advanced disease yields >80% 5-year disease-free survival.
- Recurrent disease tends to be more resistant to therapy.
- Mortality for endemic form remains high where access to health care is limited.

COMPLICATIONS

- Complications of extensive abdominal disease include obstructive jaundice and pancreatitis, bowel obstruction, and intestinal perforation.
- Tumor lysis syndrome with renal failure (uric acid nephropathy) secondary to high tumor burden and rapid cell turnover may occur prior to and especially following the start of chemotherapy.
- Rituximab has been associated with reactivation of hepatitis B virus resulting in fulminant liver failure.
- Other short- and long-term complications of chemotherapy include alopecia, myelosuppression, life-threatening infection, nausea, mucositis, infusion reactions, peripheral neuropathy, seizures, infertility, congestive heart failure, and secondary malignancy.

REFERENCES

1. Mbulaiteye SM, Anderson WF, Bhatia K, et al. Trimodal age-specific incidence patterns for Burkitt lymphoma in the United States, 1973–2005. *Int J Cancer*. 2010;126:1732–9.
2. Pillon M, Arico M, Basso G, et al. NHL-Committee of the Italian Associaiation of Pediatric Hematology, Oncology. Long-term results of AIEOP-8805 protocol for acute B-cell lymphoblastic leukemia of childhood. *Pediatr Blood Cancer*. 2011;56(4): 544–50.
3. Mohamedbhai SG, Sibson K, Marafioti T, et al. Rituximab in combination with CODOC-M/IVAC: A retrospective analysis of 23 cases of non-HIV related B-cell non-Hodgkin lymphoma with proliferation index >95%. *Br J Haematol*. 2011; 152(2)175–81.
4. Okebe JU, Lasserson TJ, Meremikwu MM, et al. Therapeutic interventions for Burkitt's lymphoma in children. *Cochrane Database Syst Rev*. 2006; CD005198.
5. Beogo R, Nacro B, Ouedraogo D, et al. Endemic Burkitt lymphoma of maxillofacial region: Results of induction treatment with cyclophosphamide plus methotrexate in West Africa. *Pediatr Blood Cancer*. 2011;56(7):1068–70.
6. Gross TG, Hale GA, He W, et al. Hematopoietic stem cell transplantation for refractory or recurrent non-Hodgkin lymphoma in children and adolescents. *Biol Blood Marrow Transplant*. 2010; 16:223–30.

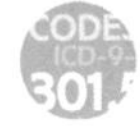

CODES

ICD9

- 200.20 Burkitt's tumor or lymphoma, unspecified site
- 200.21 Burkitt's tumor or lymphoma involving lymph nodes of head, face, and neck
- 200.22 Burkitt's tumor or lymphoma involving intrathoracic lymph nodes

CLINICAL PEARLS

- Burkitt's lymphoma is an aggressive mature B-cell malignancy most commonly diagnosed in childhood.
- Burkitt's lymphoma is strongly associated with t(8;14) and EBV infection.
- Burkitt's lymphoma is highly treatable with intense multiagent systemic and intrathecal chemotherapy.

L

MACULAR DEGENERATION, AGE-RELATED (ARMD)

Richard W. Allinson, MD

BASICS

DESCRIPTION

- Pigmentary changes in the macula or typical drusen associated with visual loss to the 20/30 level or worse, not caused by cataract or other eye disease, in individuals >50 years old
- Some definitions exclude age or visual acuity criteria.
- Leading cause of irreversible, severe visual loss in persons >65 years old
- Stages:
  - Atrophic/nonexudative
  - Neovascular/exudative
- System(s) affected: Nervous
- Synonym(s): Senile macular degeneration; Subretinal neovascularization; Age-related macular degeneration (ARMD)

EPIDEMIOLOGY

- Neovascular/exudative form is rare in blacks and more common in whites.
- Predominant gender: Female

Incidence

- In the Framingham Eye Study (FES), drusen were noted in 25% of all participants who were ≥52 years old. ARMD-associated visual loss was noted in 5.7%.
- Atrophic/nonexudative stage accounts for 20% of cases of severe visual loss.
- Neovascular/exudative stage accounts for 80% of cases of severe visual loss.

Prevalence

Per FES study:

- People 65–74 years old: 11%
- People ≥75 years old: 27.9%

RISK FACTORS

- Obesity (increased body mass index [BMI])
- Ethnicity: Non-Hispanic whites
- Cigarette smoking
- *Chlamydia pneumoniae* infection
- Family history
- Excess sunlight exposure
- Blue or light iris color
- Hyperopia
- History of cardiovascular disease (hypertension [HTN], circulatory problems)
- Short stature

Genetics

- Genetic susceptibility may be a factor in ARMD. ~25% genetically determined.
- Complement factor H is an important susceptibility gene for ARMD.

GENERAL PREVENTION

- Ultraviolet (UV) protection for eyes
- Routine ophthalmologic visits:
  - Every 2–4 years for patients 40–64 years
  - Every 1–2 years after age 65
- Patients who take statin drugs, which modify lipid profiles, may have a reduced risk.

PATHOPHYSIOLOGY

- Breaks in Bruch membrane allow choroidal neovascular membranes (CNVMs) to invade the retinal pigment epithelium (RPE) and grow into the subretinal space.
- Atrophic/nonexudative: Drusen and/or pigmentary changes in the macula
- Neovascular/exudative: Growth of blood vessels underneath the retina

ETIOLOGY

- Visible light can result in the formation and accumulation of metabolic byproducts in the RPE, a pigment layer underneath the retina that normally helps remove metabolic byproducts from the retina. Excess accumulation of these metabolic byproducts interferes with the normal metabolic activity of the RPE and can lead to the formation of drusen.
- Neovascular stage generally arises from the atrophic stage.
- Most do not progress beyond the atrophic/nonexudative stage; however, those who do are at a greater risk of severe visual loss.

COMMONLY ASSOCIATED CONDITIONS

- Presumed ocular histoplasmosis syndrome
- Exudative retinal detachment
- Vitreous hemorrhage
- Other causes of CNVMs

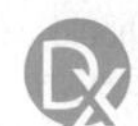

DIAGNOSIS

HISTORY

- Patients frequently notice distortion of central vision.
- Patients may notice straight lines appear crooked (e.g., telephone poles).

PHYSICAL EXAM

Retinal exam:

- Atrophic/nonexudative stage:
  - Drusen:
    - ○ Small yellowish white lesions
    - ○ Can be subdivided into types such as hard drusen and soft drusen
  - Atrophy of the RPE
- Neovascular/exudative stage:
  - Blood vessels growing underneath the retina from the choroid are called CNVMs or subretinal neovascularization (SRN). The choroid is the vascular layer underneath the RPE.
  - Subretinal fluid
  - Exudates
  - Subretinal hemorrhage
  - On Amsler grid testing, the horizontal or vertical lines may become broken, distorted, or missing.
- Disciform scar: An advanced stage resulting in a fibrovascular scar

DIAGNOSTIC TESTS & INTERPRETATION

Diagnostic Procedures/Surgery

- Amsler grid testing
- Fluorescein angiography:
  - Detection of CNVMs
  - Differentiate between atrophic and neovascular ARMD.
- Indocyanine green videoangiography: May identify occult or hidden CNVMs
- Optical coherence tomography (OCT) may be useful in identifying CNVMs, subretinal fluid, and retinal thickening.

Pathological Findings

Drusen: Deposits of hyaline material between the RPE and Bruch membrane (the limiting membrane between the RPE and the choroid)

DIFFERENTIAL DIAGNOSIS

- Idiopathic SRN
- Presumed ocular histoplasmosis syndrome
- Diabetic retinopathy
- Hypertensive retinopathy

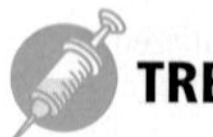

TREATMENT

MEDICATION

- Atrophic/nonexudative macular degeneration:
  - Free radical formation in the retina, induced by visible light, may play a role in cellular damage that results in ARMD.
- Age-Related Eye Disease Study (AREDS) found that a high-dose regimen of antioxidant vitamins and mineral supplements reduces progression of ARMD in some cases:
  - Recommended daily doses: Vitamin C 500 mg, vitamin E 400 IU, β-carotene 15 mg, zinc oxide 80 mg, and cupric oxide 2 mg (1)[A]
  - Exercise caution with β-carotene use in smokers due to potential link to lung cancer.
- Laser photocoagulation to treat drusen is not recommended.

First Line

Ranibizumab (Lucentis):

- Antibody fragment that inhibits all active forms of vascular endothelial growth factor (VEGF)
- Approved for neovascular (wet) age-related macular degeneration
- Injected intravitreally, at a dose of 0.5 mg, every 4 weeks
- 1 year after treatment, up to 40% of patients treated with ranibizumab gained at least 3 lines of vision, and ~95% maintained vision (2)[A].
- Ranibizumab is superior to verteporfin in the treatment of predominately classic CNVMs (3)[A].
- The PrONTO Study demonstrated OCT-guided, variable-dosing regimen with ranibizumab resulted in similar results to the MARINA and ANCHOR studies with monthly injections (4)[A].
- When comparing ranibizumab and bevacizumab in a multicenter study, both treatments were effective in stabilizing visual loss, and no difference was found in the visual outcome between the 2 treatment groups. There was a slightly higher rate of serious systemic adverse events noted in the bevacizumab group (5)[A].

Second Line

- Pegaptanib sodium (Macugen) is a compound that binds to and neutralizes VEGF. The usual dose is 0.3 mg injected intravitreally every 6 weeks as needed for the treatment of neovascular ARMD. Pegaptanib preserves vision rather than improving it. 70% of treated patients lost fewer than 15 letters of visual acuity at 1 year.
- Bevacizumab (Avastin) is a full-length antibody to VEGF, administered intravitreally at a dose of 1.25 mg, and is being evaluated in the treatment of neovascular ARMD. Widely used off-label because of its lower cost.
- VEGF Trap is being investigated in the treatment of neovascular ARMD. VEGF Trap has a higher binding affinity for all VEGF-A isoforms than does ranibizumab (6)[C].

ADDITIONAL TREATMENT

General Measures

Low-vision aids may be helpful.

SURGERY/OTHER PROCEDURES

- Neovascular/exudative macular degeneration:
  - The Macular Photocoagulation Study (MPS) demonstrated a treatment benefit for laser treatment of CNVMs that were ≥200 microns (200 microns = 0.2 mm) from the center of the macula.
- Treatment of CNVMs 1–199 microns from the center of the macula has been studied by the Age-Related Macular Degeneration Study-Krypton Laser (ARMDS-K). The benefit of laser treatment was greatest among patients without evidence of HTN. No benefit was observed among patients who had highly elevated BP and/or used antihypertensive medication.
- Vitrectomy has been used to remove CNVMs, but this is generally not recommended.
- CNVMs can bleed spontaneously, leaving blood underneath the retina. Vitrectomy to remove subretinal blood may be of benefit and should be performed within 7 days of the bleed. Tissue plasminogen activator (tPA) instilled into the eye may help remove a subretinal hemorrhage. In some cases, intravitreal gas with or without tPA may displace submacular blood:
  - Intravitreal bevacizumab may be helpful in the treatment of neovascular age-related macular degeneration associated with a large submacular hemorrhage (7)[C].
- Macular translocation involves intentionally creating a retinal detachment and attempting to shift the macula away from the CNVM. Laser is then applied to the CNVM after the retina is translocated. This procedure is associated with potentially serious surgical risks.
- Photodynamic therapy (PDT) with verteporfin reduces vision loss in patients with >50% "classic" subfoveal CNVMs. Verteporfin is administered IV, and a diode laser at 689 nm is applied to the CNVM:
  - After 24 months of follow-up in patients who underwent PDT to treat predominately classic subfoveal CNVM, 59% of the verteporfin-treated eyes vs. 31% of the placebo-treated eyes lost fewer than 15 letters from baseline.
  - In occult subfoveal CNVMs with no classic component, PDT significantly reduced the risk of moderate and severe vision loss.
  - PDT treatment benefit may not only depend on lesion type, but also on lesion size and presenting visual acuity. The treatment benefit may be related to smaller lesion size and worse presenting visual acuity.
  - Patients should be informed of a ~4% risk of acute, severe vision loss after PDT.
  - Intravitreal triamcinolone combined with PDT may result in improved visual acuity for patients with CNVMs.
- Combination therapy combining intravitreal ranibizumab with PDT and/or intravitreal triamcinolone is being evaluated.

ONGOING CARE

FOLLOW-UP RECOMMENDATIONS

Patient Monitoring

- Laser-treated patients should be re-examined promptly if new visual symptoms occur.
- Amsler grid can aid in discovering visual disturbances.
- Patients with soft drusen or pigmentary changes in the macula are at an increased risk of visual loss. They should monitor their vision, such as by daily Amsler grid testing and subjective measures of visual acuity, such as reading ability. If there are no new symptoms, follow-up examination in 6–12 months.

DIET

- Eating dark green, leafy vegetables (spinach or collard greens), which are rich in carotenoids, may decrease the risk of developing the neovascular/exudative stage.
- Fish consumption with omega-3 fatty acid intake reduces the risk of ARMD.

PATIENT EDUCATION

Instruct visually impaired patients to check with the local low-vision center for aids.

PROGNOSIS

- Patients with bilateral soft drusen and pigmentary changes in the macula but no evidence of exudation have an increased likelihood of developing CNVMs and subsequent visual loss.
- Patients with bilateral drusen carry a cumulative risk of 14.7% over 5 years of suffering significant visual loss in 1 eye from the neovascular stage of ARMD.
- Patients with neovascular stage in 1 eye and drusen in the opposite eye are at an annual risk of 5–14% of developing the neovascular stage in the opposite eye with drusen.
- High incidence of recurrence after thermal laser treatment for CNVMs.
- After 2 years of monthly ranibizumab injections, visual loss is commonly associated with impaired function of the photoreceptors and RPE and not from active leakage from CNVMs (8)[A].

COMPLICATIONS

Blindness

REFERENCES

1. Age Related Eye Disease Study Research Group. A randomized, placebo-controlled, clinical trial of high-dose supplementation with vitamins C and E, beta carotene, and zinc for age-related macular degeneration and vision loss: AREDS report no. 8. *Arch Ophthalmol*. 2001;119:1417–36.
2. Rosenfeld PJ, Brown DM, Heier JS, et al. Ranibizumab for neovascular age-related macular degeneration. *N Engl J Med*. 2006;355:1419–31.
3. Brown DM, Michels M, Kaiser PK, et al. Ranibizumab versus verteporfin photodynamic therapy for neovascular age-related macular degeneration: Two-year results of the ANCHOR study. *Ophthalmology*. 2009;116:57–65.e5.
4. Fung AE, Lalwani GA, Rosenfeld PJ, et al. An optical coherence tomography-guided, variable dosing regimen with intravitreal ranibizumab (Lucentis) for neovascular age-related macular degeneration. *Am J Ophthalmol*. 2007;143:566–83.
5. CATT Research Group, Martin DF, Maguire MG, et al. Ranibizumab and bevacizumab for neovascular age-related macular degeneration. *N Engl J Med*. 2011;364:1897–908.
6. Nguyen QD, Shah SM, Browning DJ, et al. A phase I study of intravitreal vascular endothelial growth factor trap-eye in patients with neovascular age-related macular degeneration. *Ophthalmology*. 2009;116:2141–8.e1.
7. Stifter E, Michels S, Prager F, et al. Intravitreal bevacizumab therapy for neovascular age-related macular degeneration with large submacular hemorrhage. *Am J Ophthalmol*. 2007;144:886–92.
8. Rosenfeld PJ, Shapiro H, Tuomi L, et al. Characteristics of patients losing vision after 2 years of monthly dosing in the phase III ranibizumab clinical trials. *Ophthalmology*. 2011;118:523–30.

ADDITIONAL READING

Gupta OP, Shienbaum G, Patel AH, et al. A treat and extend regimen using ranibizumab for neovascular age-related macular degeneration: Clinical and economic impact. *Ophthalmology*. 2010;117:2134–40.

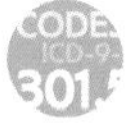

CODES

ICD9

- 362.50 Macular degeneration (senile) of retina, unspecified
- 362.51 Nonexudative senile macular degeneration of retina
- 362.52 Exudative senile macular degeneration of retina

CLINICAL PEARLS

- Patients frequently notice distortion of central vision.
- Patients may notice straight lines appear crooked (e.g., telephone poles).
- Hyperopia is a risk factor for ARMD.
- AREDS found that a high-dose regimen of antioxidant vitamins and mineral supplements reduces progression of ARMD in some cases.

MALARIA

Paul Arguin, MD

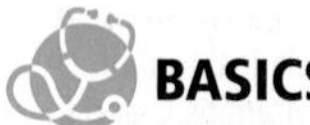

BASICS

DESCRIPTION

- Acute or chronic infection transmitted to humans by *Anopheles* spp. mosquitoes
- Most morbidity and mortality caused by *P. falciparum*; it is responsible for >1 million deaths annually, the majority of which occur in children <5 years in sub-Saharan Africa.
- Nonimmune individuals are most susceptible to rapid progression to severe disease.
- System(s) affected: Lymphatic; Immunologic; Vascular; Hematologic; Renal; Cerebral

EPIDEMIOLOGY

Incidence

- Most US cases (>99%) are imported. Very rare cases reported from local transmission after introduction, transfusion transmission, and congenital transmission.
- 1,000–1,500 cases and 5 deaths per year in the US
- Cases imported to the US: 40% *P. falciparum*; 16% *P. vivax*; 2% *P. malariae*; 2% *P. ovale*; 40% unknown

Prevalence

- Predominant age: All ages
- Predominant gender: Male = Female

RISK FACTORS

- Traveling and/or migration from an area where malaria is endemic (most from sub-Saharan Africa)
- Rarely, blood transfusion, mother-to-fetus transmission, and autochthonous transmission

Genetics

Unknown genetic predilection, but inherited conditions may affect disease severity and susceptibility (glucose-6-phosphate deficiency, sickle cell disease or trait, and hereditary elliptocytosis)

GENERAL PREVENTION

- Mosquito avoidance measures: Insect repellent, clothing that covers most of the body, mosquito nets treated with permethrin, air conditioning, and avoiding outdoor activity dusk to dawn (1)[A]
- Malarial chemoprophylaxis when in endemic area
- Mefloquine: Begin at least 2 weeks before arrival and continue for 4 weeks after leaving area. Adults, 250 mg (1 tablet) weekly; children ≤9 kg, 5 mg/kg; children >9–19 kg, 1/4 tablet weekly; children >19–30 kg, 1/2 tablet weekly; children >30–45 kg, 3/4 tablet weekly; children >45 kg as adult:
  - Caution: Mefloquine-resistant areas
- Atovaquone/proguanil: Begin 1–2 days before arrival and continue for 1 week after leaving area. Adults, 1 adult tablet daily; children 5–8 kg, 1/2 pediatric tablet daily; children >8–10 kg, 3/4 pediatric tablet daily; children >10–20 kg, 1 pediatric tablet daily; children >20–30 kg, 2 pediatric tablets daily; children >30–40 kg, 3 pediatric tablets daily; children >40 kg, 1 adult tablet daily
- Doxycycline: Begin 1–2 days before arrival and continue for 4 weeks after leaving area. Adults, 100 mg daily; children, 2 mg/kg up to 100 mg daily (not for children <8 years old)
- Chloroquine: Begin 1–2 weeks before arrival and continue for 4 weeks after leaving area. Adults, 300 mg base (500 mg salt) weekly; children, 5 mg base/kg weekly up to 300 mg:
  - Caution: Chloroquine-resistant areas
- Primaquine: Begin 1–2 days before arrival and continue for 1 week after leaving area; adults 30 mg/d; children, 0.5 mg/kg/d up to adult dose

PATHOPHYSIOLOGY

- Malarial parasites digest red cell proteins and make the RBC membrane less deformable, causing hemolysis, increased splenic clearance, and anemia.
- Red cell lysis stimulates release of cytokines and TNF-α.
- *P. falciparum* induces human RBCs to secrete a protein that makes RBCs stick to the intravascular surface of small blood vessels, causing obstruction and end-organ ischemia.

ETIOLOGY

P. falciparum, *P. malariae*, *P. vivax*, *P. ovale*, and *P. knowlesi* in parts of Southeast Asia

COMMONLY ASSOCIATED CONDITIONS

Bacterial coinfections

DIAGNOSIS

HISTORY

- First symptoms of malaria are nonspecific. Suspect in anyone ill returning from endemic area:
  - Fever, malaise, myalgias, chills, headache, nausea, splenomegaly (with chronic infection), hypotension, anemia (with chronic or severe disease), thrombocytopenia, jaundice, vomiting and diarrhea resembling gastroenteritis
- *P. falciparum*:
  - Incubation usually 12–14 days, symptoms within 2 months of infection in most individuals (partially immune individuals such as immigrants may become ill up to 1 year after last exposure)
  - Severe disease and complications: Vascular collapse, CNS impairment, renal failure, and acute respiratory distress syndrome
- *P. vivax* and *P. ovale:*
  - Incubation period 12–18 days for primary infection and up to 12 months (and longer) for relapses; generally presents with fevers
  - Dormant parasites may remain in liver and reactivate years after initial infection.
  - Can be severe
- *P. malariae* (benign quartan malaria):
  - Incubation period ~35 days
  - May become chronic; untreated can persist asymptomatically in human host for years
- *P. knowlesi*:
  - Incubation period ~12 days
  - Possibly severe

PHYSICAL EXAM

- Often not specific
- General: Elevated temperature, fatigue, tachycardia, tachypnea
- Chronic: Pallor, splenomegaly (hyperactive malarial splenomegaly syndrome)

DIAGNOSTIC TESTS & INTERPRETATION

Lab

- Malarial smear thick and thin preparations:
  - Microscopy to evaluate for presence of parasite forms, determine species, and quantify the percentage of RBCs that are infected (2)[A]
  - Test should be performed on site right away with results available within hours.
  - Rapid antigen capture enzyme: Can detect the presence of malaria parasites within minutes. Cannot determine species or quantify parasitemia. Positive and negative results must always be confirmed by microscopy.
  - Other tests: Species-specific PCR (confirms species)
- General laboratory findings (nonspecific):
  - In uncomplicated infection:
    - Elevated liver function tests and lactate dehydrogenase
    - Thrombocytopenia, anemia, and leukopenia
- Note: A low to low-normal platelet count or a slightly high bilirubin is typical and should alert the clinician of the diagnosis after exposure in an endemic setting.
- Note: Antimalarial agents may reduce parasitemia.

Initial lab tests

- CBC with differential and platelets
- Basic chemistry panel including bilirubin
- Malaria thick and thin blood films (if negative, repeat every 12–24 hours for at least 3 sets)

Follow-Up & Special Considerations

Nonimmune individuals with suspected or confirmed *P. falciparum* should be hospitalized.

Imaging

Use only for respiratory disease (chest x-ray) or cerebral malaria (scan prior to spinal tap)

Pathological Findings

Malaria causes hemolysis.

DIFFERENTIAL DIAGNOSIS

- Infections (disseminated or localized): Abscess, viral, gastroenteritis, typhoid/paratyphoid, other bacteremias, rickettsial disease, mycobacteria
- Collagen vascular disease (SLE, vasculitides)
- Neoplasms (lymphoma, leukemia, other blood dyscrasias, other tropical causes of splenomegaly)
- Severe malaria infection may mimic hepatitis, pneumonia, stroke, or sepsis.

TREATMENT

MEDICATION

First Line

- For uncomplicated chloroquine-resistant *P. falciparum* (most *P. falciparum*), chloroquine-resistant *P. vivax*, or when species is unknown, the following regimens are recommended:
  - Atovaquone-proguanil (Malarone): Adult tablet: 250 mg atovaquone and 100 mg proguanil. Pediatric tablet: 62.5 mg atovaquone and 25 mg proguanil. Adults: 4 adult tablets once per day for 3 days. Children 5–8 kg: 2 pediatric tablets once per day for 3 days; children 9–10 kg: 3 pediatric tablets once per day for 3 days; children 1–20 kg: 1 adult tablet once per day for 3 days; children 21–30 kg: 2 adult tablets once per day for 3 days; children 31–40 kg: 3 adult tablets once per day for 3 days; children >40 kg: 4 adult tablets once per day for 3 days (1)[A]

- Artemether-lumefantrine (Coartem): Tablet contains 20 mg artemether and 120 mg lumefantrine. Persons 5–<15 kg: 1 tablet b.i.d. for 3 days; persons 15–<25 kg: 2 tablets b.i.d. for 3 days; persons 25–<35 kg: 3 tablets b.i.d. for 3 days; persons ≥35 kg: 4 tablets b.i.d. for 3 days (1)[A]
- Quinine sulfate plus doxycycline or clindamycin: Adults: Quinine sulfate 650 mg (salt) t.i.d. for 3 days (should be extended to 7 days for infections acquired in southeast Asia). Doxycycline 100 mg b.i.d. for 7 days. Clindamycin 20 mg (base)/kg/d divided t.i.d. for 7 days. Children: Quinine sulfate 10 mg (salt)/kg t.i.d. for 3 days (should be extended to 7 days for infections acquires in SE Asia) plus clindamycin dosed as above.
- Mefloquine: Adults: 750 mg followed by 500 mg 8 hours later. Children: 15 mg/kg followed by 10 mg/kg 8 hours later (not to exceed adult dose)

- Oral therapy for *P. ovale, P. malariae*, chloroquine-sensitive *P. falciparum* (rare), and chloroquine-sensitive *P. vivax* (New Guinea has highest rates of CQ resistant *P. vivax*):
  - Chloroquine phosphate: Adults: 600-mg base followed by 300 mg at 6, 24, and 48 hours. Children: 10 mg base/kg (max 600 mg), then 5 mg/kg at 6, 24, and 48 hours
  - Primaquine phosphate (should be added to chloroquine therapy for cure of dormant forms of *P. vivax* and *P. ovale*): Adults: 30-mg base (52.6 mg) daily for 2 weeks or 45-mg base (79 mg) weekly for 8 weeks. Children: 0.6-mg base/kg/d for 2 weeks (3)[A]. See "Precautions."
- Therapy for severe *P. falciparum:*
  - Clinical features defining severe malaria:
    - Impaired level of consciousness (LOC)
    - Respiratory distress, jaundice
    - Repeated convulsions, shock
  - Laboratory features:
    - Hypoglycemia (glucose <40 mg/dL)
    - Elevated bilirubin (total >2.5 mg/dL)
    - Acidosis (plasma bicarbonate <15 mmol/L)
    - Lactic acidosis (serum lactate >45 mg/dL)
    - Elevated aminotransferase (>3 times)
    - Serum creatinine >3 mg/dL
- Parenteral therapy:
  - Quinidine gluconate 10 mg/kg in normal saline over 1–2 hours followed by 0.02 mg/kg/min continuous infusion, or repeat
  - Intensive care monitoring is necessary, especially when initiating quinidine therapy.
- In severe malaria, CDC should be contacted for assistance; CDC Malaria Branch: 770-488-7100; www.cdc.gov/Malaria/.
- In 2007, CDC made artesunate available in the US for severe malaria and in special circumstances under an investigational protocol. Contact the CDC for assistance as noted above.
- Oral therapy for chloroquine-resistant *P. vivax*:
  - Atovaquone/Proguanil or quinine sulfate plus doxycycline or mefloquine: Dosages above. Should follow with primaquine for liver-dormant forms (3)[B]
  - Mefloquine:
    - Adults: 1,250 mg once (usually divided as 750 mg, then 500 mg 8 hours later)
    - Children: 15 mg/kg, then 10 mg/kg 8 hours later (high GI adverse event profile) (1)[B]. Should follow with primaquine for liver-dormant forms

ADDITIONAL TREATMENT

Issues for Referral

Infectious disease or tropical medicine expert for most cases

Additional Therapies

Exchange transfusions may be necessary in severe disease or with very high parasitemia; discuss with expert or CDC.

Pediatric Considerations

- Children are particularly susceptible to severe disease.
- All children, even infants, should receive chemoprophylaxis if traveling to an endemic area.
- Malaria commonly resembles acute gastroenteritis in children.
- Children with severe disease are particularly prone to hypoglycemia. IV fluids with glucose should be used for maintenance and frequent blood glucose measurements taken.

Pregnancy Considerations

- Chloroquine is safe in the doses recommended for prevention and treatment of malaria; FDA Category C.
- Mefloquine is safe in the doses recommended for prevention and treatment of malaria; FDA Category B.
- Atovaquone-proguanil (Malarone) has not been studied in pregnant women; it has not been shown to cause birth defects or other problems in animal studies; FDA Category C.
- No primaquine (FDA class undetermined) or tetracyclines (FDA class D) in pregnancy.
- Quinine/quinidine (FDA class X/C, respectively) should be used during pregnancy or breast-feeding when benefit outweighs risk.

COMPLEMENTARY AND ALTERNATIVE MEDICINE

None. Many deaths have resulted from using unapproved alternatives to medications.

SURGERY/OTHER PROCEDURES

Rarely, splenectomy must be performed in patients with HSM and medically unresponsive hematologic disorders.

IN-PATIENT CONSIDERATIONS

Initial Stabilization

- Inpatient care for all cases of *P. falciparum* malaria in nonimmune patients or any patient, despite the species, with signs of severe illness; outpatient care for others (1)[C]
- Nonimmune with *P. falciparum* may progress from mild symptoms to death within 12 hours. All patients treated on outpatient basis should have follow-up within 24 hours.

Admission Criteria

- All nonimmune patients with confirmed or suspected *P. falciparum*
- All patients with signs of severe disease (see "Treatment")

IV Fluids

Maintenance IV fluids with glucose, because of risk of hypoglycemia, is recommended if unable to tolerate fluids by mouth. Excess fluids may result in iatrogenically induced pulmonary edema.

Nursing

Observe for fluid excess, renal insufficiency (urine output), and hypoglycemia.

Discharge Criteria

Clinical improvement, ability to tolerate oral medications and fluids, with documented decreasing parasitemia levels

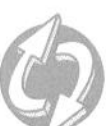

ONGOING CARE

PATIENT EDUCATION

- Malarial chemoprophylaxis prior to travel
- Travel information may be obtained at the CDC travel Web site: www.cdc.gov/travel

PROGNOSIS

- Only *P. falciparum* infection carries a poor prognosis, with high mortality if untreated. However, if diagnosed early and treated appropriately, the prognosis is excellent.
- *P. vivax* and other nonfalciparum may be severe, particularly with comorbidities.

COMPLICATIONS

- *P. falciparum*: If not treated early, may cause cerebral malaria, acute renal failure, acute gastroenteritis, pulmonary edema, and massive hemolysis. Chronic malaria: Splenomegaly or splenic rupture. Death from malaria is virtually limited to *P. falciparum* infection or infection with other species in a patient with other underlying illness.
- *P. malariae*: Nephrotic syndrome may develop in patients with chronic infection.
- Other complications: Seizures, anuria, delirium, coma, dysentery, algid malaria, blackwater fever, hyperpyrexia

REFERENCES

1. Centers for Disease Control and Prevention. Treatment of Malaria (Guidelines for clinicians). Updated 9/23/11 at www.cdc.gov/malaria/pdf/treatmenttable.pdf.
2. Chen LH, Keystone JS. New strategies for the prevention of malaria in travelers. *Infect Dis Clin North Am*. 2005;19:185–210.
3. Griffith KS, Lewis LS, Mali S, et al. Treatment of malaria in the United States: A systematic review. *JAMA*. 2007;297:2264–77.

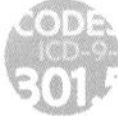

CODES

ICD9

- 084.0 Falciparum malaria [malignant tertian]
- 084.1 Vivax malaria [benign tertian]
- 084.6 Malaria, unspecified

CLINICAL PEARLS

- Rapid malaria tests are useful in the acute setting for determining if a patient has *P. falciparum* malaria (high negative predictive value). However, blood smears should also be performed on all suspected cases.
- Children with malaria frequently clinically appear to have gastroenteritis or nonspecific viral infections.
- Nonimmune persons with suspected or confirmed *P. falciparum* malaria are at high risk and must be managed aggressively (i.e., hospitalized).

M

MARFAN SYNDROME

Michele Roberts, MD, PhD

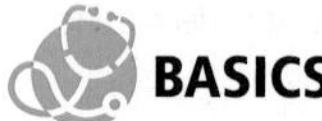

BASICS

DESCRIPTION

- Marfan syndrome (MFS) is an inherited disorder of connective tissue.
- Because many features of MFS appear in the general population, specific diagnostic criteria (Ghent nosology) were established, recognizing a constellation of features, with major and minor criteria for establishing the diagnosis (1).
- The nosology was revised (2,3) because the previous criteria were not sufficiently validated, were not consistently applicable in children, or necessitated expensive and specialized tests.
- System(s) affected: Musculoskeletal; Cardiovascular; Ocular; Pulmonary; Skin/Integument; Connective tissue (dura)

Pediatric Considerations

Early surgical intervention may reduce the degree of scoliosis.

Pregnancy Considerations

- Manage pregnancy in MFS as high risk, preferably with a cardiologist. Prepregnancy evaluation should include a screening transthoracic echocardiogram for aortic root dilation.
- Beta-blockers should be considered in all pregnancies to minimize the risk of aortic dilation throughout the pregnancy.
- 1% complication rate if aortic root diameter <40 mm; 10% if >40 mm. Consider elective surgery before pregnancy if >47 mm.

EPIDEMIOLOGY

- Congenital. Although clinical manifestations may be apparent in infancy, affected individuals may not present until adolescence or young adulthood.
- No gender, ethnic, or racial predilection. With advanced paternal age, a slightly increased risk of de novo mutation resulting in MFS in offspring.

Prevalence

1/3,000–1/5,000

RISK FACTORS

Genetics

- Mutations of the *fibrillin-1 (FBN1)* gene on chromosome 15q21.1 are responsible for Marfan syndrome, OMIM #154700.
- MFS is an autosomal-dominant condition with complete penetrance and variable expressivity. Apparent nonpenetrance may be due to lack of recognition of MFS in a mildly affected individual.
- Each child of an affected parent has a 50% chance of inheriting the disorder, and may be more or less severely affected. 25% of cases result from de novo mutation.

GENERAL PREVENTION

- Prenatal diagnosis is possible in families with a known mutation.
- Antibiotic prophylaxis against endocarditis for dental and other procedures is no longer routinely recommended by the ADA/AHA.
- Athletes who are especially tall should be screened for aortic root dilation.

ETIOLOGY

Genetic abnormality; mutations of the *FBN1* (fibrillin) gene. Fibrillin is an extracellular matrix protein widely distributed in elastic and nonelastic connective tissue.

COMMONLY ASSOCIATED CONDITIONS

- High prevalence of obstructive sleep apnea in MFS; may be a risk factor for aortic root dilatation (4)
- Increased prevalence of migraine in MFS

DIAGNOSIS

- In the revised Ghent nosology:
  - CV manifestations (aortic root aneurysm/dissection) and ectopia lentis have more weight.
  - Molecular genetic testing for *FBN1* plays a more prominent diagnostic role, but is not required.
  - Less specific manifestations were removed or made less influential, thus avoiding obligate thresholds that were not evidence based. Careful follow-up diminishes risk of missed diagnosis.
  - New criteria explicitly allow for alternative diagnoses, where additional features warrant: Shprintzen-Goldberg syndrome (SGS), Loeys-Dietz syndrome (LDS), or vascular-type Ehlers-Danlos syndrome (vEDS).
  - Z-score calculator for aortic root enlargement: www.marfan.org
- In the absence of a family history of MFS:
  - Aortic root dilatation or dissection ($Z \geq 2$) (Ao) *and* ectopia lentis (EL): Unequivocal diagnosis of MFS, irrespective of systemic features, except where they are diagnostic of SGS, LDS, or vEDS
  - Ao *and* a *bona fide FBN1* mutation: Diagnostic of MFS, even in the absence of EL
  - Where Ao is present but EL is absent and the *FBN1* status is negative (or unknown), diagnosis of MFS requires systemic findings score ≥7 points using a new scoring system (see below) and exclusion of SGS, LDS, and vEDS.
  - With EL but without Ao, *FBN1* mutation previously associated with Ao is required for diagnosis of MFS.
- Systemic features, scoring system (see "Physical Examination"):
  - Wrist *and* thumb sign +3; wrist *or* thumb sign +1
  - Pectus carinatum deformity +2; pectus excavatum or chest asymmetry +1
  - Hindfoot deformity +2; pes planus +1
  - Pneumothorax +2
  - Dural ectasia +2
  - Protrusio acetabuli +2 by x-ray, CT, or MRI
  - Reduced upper-to-lower segment ratio (US/LS) *and* increased arm/height *and* no severe scoliosis +1
  - Scoliosis or thoracolumbar kyphosis +1
  - Reduced elbow extension +1
  - Facial features (3/5) +1
  - Skin striae +1
  - Myopia >3 diopters +1
  - Mitral valve prolapse (all types) +1
- Maximum: 20 points; score ≥7 indicates systemic involvement
- Positive family history requires a family member independently diagnosed using above criteria.
- With a positive family history, MFS can be diagnosed with ectopia lentis, *or* systemic score ≥7, *or* aortic root dilatation with $Z \geq 2$ in persons >20 years old, *or* $Z \geq 3$ in persons <20 years old.
- In persons <20 years old who have negative family history and suggestive findings but who do not meet Ghent criteria, "nonspecific connective tissue disorder" is diagnosed, and close clinical follow-up is recommended.
- In the presence of a relevant *FBN1* mutation, "potential MFS" is diagnosed, and close follow-up is recommended.
- In adults who have suggestive findings but who do not meet Ghent criteria, consider alternative diagnoses: Ectopia lentis syndrome (ELS), mitral valve prolapse syndrome (MVPS), MASS phenotype.

PHYSICAL EXAM

- Facial features: Dolichocephaly, enophthalmos, downslanting palpebral fissures, malar hypoplasia, retrognathia
- Thumb sign: Distal phalanx of thumb protrudes from clenched fist. Wrist sign: Thumb and fifth digit overlap when circling wrist.
- Pectus carinatum deformity: Pectus excavatum or chest asymmetry beyond normal variation
- Hindfoot valgus with forefoot abduction and lowering of the midfoot; should be distinguished from pes planus
- Reduced US/LS: 0.93 in unaffected individuals vs. ≤0.85 in affected white adults, ≤0.78 in affected black adults. US is measured from the top of the head to the top of the midpubic bone; LS is measured from the top of the pubic bone to the sole of the foot. In children, abnormal US/LS: US/LS <1, age 0–5 years; US/LS <0.95, 6–7 years; US/LS <0.9, 8–9 years; <0.85, age ≥10 years.
- Increased arm span to height ratio >1.05
- Scoliosis or thoracolumbar kyphosis is diagnosed if, upon bending forward, there is a vertical difference ≥1.5 cm between the ribs of the left and right hemithorax.
- Reduced elbow extension if angle between upper and lower arm measures ≤170 on full extension
- Skin: Striae atrophicae are significant if not associated with significant weight changes (or pregnancy) and if located on midback, lumbar region, upper arm, axilla, or thigh.
- Because of lack of specificity, the following criteria were removed from the current nosology: Joint hypermobility, high arched palate, and recurrent or incisional herniae (2).

DIAGNOSTIC TESTS & INTERPRETATION

Lab

- Other than *FBN1* mutation, no specific laboratory abnormalities are associated with MFS.
- Specific criteria have been established (2) for *FBN1* mutations causative of MFS, including those found in families with MFS. *FBN1* mutation is a valuable marker for risk or aortic dissection (5). In a small subset of patients with unequivocal MFS, no known *FBN1* mutation is found.
- In patients whose physical examination is suggestive of MFS, urinary homocystine should be measured to rule out homocystinuria, an inborn error of methionine metabolism.

Imaging

- Anteroposterior (AP) radiograph: Diagnosis of protrusio acetabuli. Results from deepening of hip sockets during growth; does not cause problems during childhood
- Scoliosis: Cobb angle ≥20 on radiographs. Imaging for MFS diagnosis, or as per clinical exam.
- Hindfoot valgus with forefoot abduction and lowering of the midfoot: Anterior and posterior views if clinically indicated

- Echocardiography: Measure aortic root at the level of sinuses of Valsalva; check for mitral valve prolapse.
- MRI or CT to evaluate for dural ectasia for diagnosis, and if symptomatic, symptoms highly variable, nonspecific, and include lower back pain

Diagnostic Procedures/Surgery
- Ectopia lentis is diagnosed on slit-lamp examination after maximal dilatation of the pupil. Lens dislocation is most often upward and temporal.
- Myopia: Common in the general population; myopia $>$3 diopters contributes to MFS systemic score

Pathological Findings
- Cystic medial necrosis of the aorta
- Myxomatous degeneration of cardiac valves

DIFFERENTIAL DIAGNOSIS
Several conditions present clinical manifestations overlapping with MFS in cardiovascular, ocular, and skeletal systems:
- Ectopia lentis syndrome—no aortic root dilatation
- Mitral valve prolapse syndrome—MVP, limited systemic features may include pectus excavatum, scoliosis, mild arachnodactyly; aortic enlargement and ectopia lentis preclude this diagnosis.
- MASS phenotype—(*M*itral valve prolapse; myopia; borderline, nonprogressive *A*ortic enlargement (Z $<$2); and nonspecific *S*keletal and *S*kin involvement). Aortic involvement in MASS is usually nonprogressive; some risk for more severe vascular involvement.
- Shprintzen-Goldberg syndrome; Loeys-Dietz syndrome; Ehlers-Danlos syndrome
- Homocystinuria—Marfanoid habitus, thrombosis, mental retardation; urine amino acid analysis is diagnostic; lens dislocates downward.
- Familial thoracic aortic aneurysm
- Stickler syndrome; congenital contractural arachnodactyly; Weill-Marchesani syndrome; multiple endocrine neoplasia, type 2B

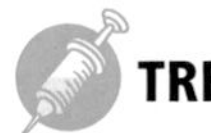

TREATMENT

MEDICATION
- Prevention of aortic complications: Labetalol or other β-adrenergic blockers. Dosage adjusted to target heart rate (resting rate 60 beats/min, increase to $\leq$110 beats/min after moderate exertion; or $<$100 beats/min after submaximal exercise) (2)[C].
- Other agents used if β-blockers contraindicated. Calcium channel blockers, ACE inhibitors, and angiotensin receptor blockers also retard aortic dilation in children and adolescents (6)[B].

ADDITIONAL TREATMENT
Issues for Referral
Genetics, Cardiology, Orthopedics, Ophthalmology

SURGERY/OTHER PROCEDURES
- When cardiac symptoms develop or aortic root diameter is $\geq$5 cm, consider surgical intervention (7). Many MFS patients will ultimately require reconstructive cardiovascular surgery:
  - Dissection of ascending aorta (type A) is a surgical emergency. Consider prophylactic surgery when diameter of sinus of Valsalva approaches 5 cm (2). Other considerations include family history, rate of change, other cardiac pathology, pregnancy.
  - Dissection of descending thoracic aorta (type B) surgical indications include intractable pain, limb or organ ischemia, aortic diameter $>$5.5 cm (or rapidly increasing) (2)
- Mitral valve repair: For severe mitral valve regurgitation or progressive LV dilatation or dysfunction, or in patients undergoing valve-sparing root replacement (2)
- Lens subluxation: Incidence of glaucoma is high, so surgery is performed only if the condition cannot be treated with corrective lenses. Surgical removal of lens in lens opacity, impending complete luxation, lens-induced glaucoma or uveitis, or anisometropia or refractive error not amenable to optical correction (2).
- Severe pectus excavatum may require surgery.
- Scoliosis: Bracing for curves 20–40 until growth is complete, or surgery if $>$40
- Surgery only for most severe cases of dural ectasia
- Hip replacement in middle age or later if protrusio acetabulae has led to severe arthritic change

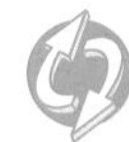

ONGOING CARE

FOLLOW-UP RECOMMENDATIONS
- Avoid sports that can increase aortic root enlargement or pneumothorax, including weightlifting and acceleration/deceleration sports. Low-risk sports include bowling, golf, skating (but not ice hockey), snorkeling, brisk walking, treadmill walking or stationary biking, modest hiking (8)[C].
- Exercise restrictions based on individual circumstances (8). Recommendation from the National Marfan Foundation (www.marfan.org) and guidelines from the American Heart Association/ American College of Cardiology task forces. In general, avoid contact sports, Valsalva, and exhaustion.

Patient Monitoring
Frequent examinations (at least twice per year) while patient is still growing, with particular attention to cardiovascular system and to scoliosis:
- Yearly echocardiograms (initially), more frequent if aortic diameter is increasing rapidly ($\geq$5 cm/yr) or is approaching the surgical threshold ($\geq$4.5 cm in adults)
- Aortic root dilatation in MFS is usually progressive, warrants vigilance even when not seen on initial examination. Age $<$20, yearly echocardiogram. Adults with repeatedly normal aortic root measurements, echocardiogram every 2–3 years (2).
- Regular imaging after surgical repair of aorta
- Scoliosis or pectus deformity: Standard orthopedic management. Clinical evaluation for scoliosis earlier than in general population. Plain radiographs of spine during growth years to detect and measure scoliosis.
- Annual ophthalmologic evaluation for detection of ectopia lentis, myopia, cataract, glaucoma, and retinal detachment. Myopia is very common in MFS and may have early onset, rapid progression, and high degree of severity. Early monitoring, aggressive refraction to prevent amblyopia (2).

PATIENT EDUCATION
- National Marfan Foundation, 382 Main St., Port Washington, NY 11959; 800-8MARFAN, www.marfan.org
- American Heart Association at www.americanheart.org

PROGNOSIS
Life-threatening complications involve cardiovascular dysfunction. In 1972, life span was 32 years. Currently, life span is nearly normal.

COMPLICATIONS
Bacterial endocarditis, aortic dissection, aortic or mitral valve insufficiency, dilated cardiomyopathy, retinal detachment, glaucoma, pneumothorax

REFERENCES

1. De Paepe A, Devereux RB, Dietz HC, et al. Revised diagnostic criteria for the Marfan syndrome. *Am J Med Genet*. 1996;62:417–26.
2. Loeys BL, Dietz HC, Braverman AC, et al. The revised Ghent nosology for the Marfan syndrome. *J Med Genet*. 2010;47:476–85.
3. Faivre L, Collod-Beroud G, Callewaert B, et al. Pathogenic FBN1 mutations in 146 adults not meeting clinical diagnostic criteria for Marfan syndrome: Further delineation of type 1 fibrillinopathies and focus on patients with an isolated major criterion. *Am J Med Genet A*. 2009;149A:854–60.
4. Kohler M, Blair E, Risby P, et al. The prevalence of obstructive sleep apnoea and its association with aortic dilatation in Marfan's syndrome. *Thorax*. 2009;64(2):162–6.
5. Faivre L, Collod-Beroud G, Child A, et al. Contribution of molecular analyses in diagnosing Marfan syndrome and type I fibrillinopathies: An international study of 1009 probands. *J Med Genet*. 2008;45:384–90.
6. Williams A, Davies S, Stuart AG, et al. Medical treatment of Marfan syndrome: A time for change. *Heart*. 2008;94:414–21.
7. Benedetto U, Melina G, Takkenberg JJ, et al. Surgical management of aortic root disease in Marfan syndrome: A systematic review and meta-analysis. *Heart*. 2011;97:955–8.
8. Maron BJ, Chaitman BR, Ackerman MJ, et al. Recommendations for physical activity and recreational sports participation for young patients with genetic cardiovascular diseases. *Circulation*. 2004;109:2807–16.

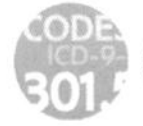

CODES

ICD9
759.82 Marfan syndrome

CLINICAL PEARLS
- Because many features of MFS appear in the general population, diagnostic criteria have been established. Molecular diagnostic testing for *FBN1* mutations will play an increasing role.
- Early diagnosis of homocystinuria is important, because clinical complications, which include a high risk of vascular thrombosis, can be minimized with appropriate diet and medication.

MARIJUANA ABUSE

Riabianca Garcia, MD
David Anthony, MD

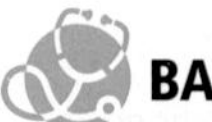

BASICS

DESCRIPTION

Marijuana or cannabis abuse is classified in DSM-IV as a disorder that involves:

- Periodic use and intoxication, which may interfere with an individual's performance at school or work and even be physically hazardous in a multitude of situations, such as driving a car or heavy machinery
- Legal problems and negative consequences, such as arrest for possession
- Arguments with spouses or parents because of the possession in the home or its presence around others
- May also lead to significant levels of tolerance along with psychological and physical problems associated with compulsive use, at which time a diagnosis of marijuana dependence should be considered rather than marijuana abuse

EPIDEMIOLOGY

- The US is ranked first among 17 European and North American countries by the World Health Organization for prevalence of marijuana use.
- About 42% of teens will have tried marijuana by the time they graduate from high school (1).
- An estimated 2.2 million Americans used marijuana for the first time in 2008; >50% were under age 18 (1).
- In the US, 10% of those who ever use marijuana become daily users, and 20–30% become weekly users.

RISK FACTORS

- Age (highest use among those 18–25 years)
- Male sex
- Comorbid psychiatric disorders (i.e., bipolar disorder, PTSD)
- Other substance use (i.e., alcohol, cocaine)
- Lower educational achievement (rates of dependence lowest among college graduates)

PATHOPHYSIOLOGY

- Main active ingredient in marijuana: Delta-9-tetrahydrocannibinol (THC)
- When marijuana is smoked, THC rapidly passes from the lungs into the blood and to the brain, where it binds to cannabinoid receptors (CBRs).
- CBRs are responsible for memory, thinking, concentration, sensory and time perception, pleasure, movement, and coordination.
- THC artificially stimulates the CBRs, disrupting the function of endogenous cannabinoids. A marijuana "high" results from overstimulation of these receptors.
- Over time, overstimulation alters the function of CBRs, which can lead to addiction and to withdrawal symptoms when drug use stops.
- Effects of smoked marijuana can last 1–3 hours.
- Effects from marijuana consumed in foods or beverages appear later, usually in 30 minutes to 1 hour, but can last up to 4 hours.
- Smoking marijuana delivers significantly more THC into the bloodstream than eating or drinking the drug.

DIAGNOSIS

- Screen for marijuana use along with other lifestyle questions like tobacco and alcohol use.
- Ask for frequency and amount used (e.g., "How long does a nickle bag last you?").
- Unexplained deterioration in school or work performance may be a red flag for abuse (2)[C].
- Problems with or changes in social relationships (such as spending more time alone or with persons suspected of using drugs) and recreational activities (such as giving up activities that were once pleasurable) may indicate abuse.
- If available, information from concerned parents or spouses should be obtained (2)[C].
- DSM-IV-TR criteria for cannabis dependence: A maladaptive pattern of cannabis use resulting in clinically significant impairment or distress, as indicated by 3 or more of the following at any time during the same 12-month period:
  - Tolerance, defined by using increased amounts of cannabis to achieve the desired effect or intoxication or diminished effect with continued use of the same amount of cannabis
  - Cannabis is often taken in larger amounts or over a longer period than was intended.
  - There is a persistent desire or there are unsuccessful efforts to cut down or control cannabis use.
  - A great deal of time is spent obtaining cannabis, using it, or recovering from its effects.
  - Important social, occupational, or recreational activities are neglected because of cannabis use.
  - Persistent cannabis use despite knowledge of having a recurrent or ongoing physical or psychological problem that is probably caused or exacerbated by cannabis, such as a chronic cough related to smoking or a decrease in goal-related activities

HISTORY

- Clinical presentation of acute intoxication:
  - Euphoria, elation, laughter, heightened sensory perception, altered perception of time, increased appetite
  - Poor short-term memory, concentration
  - Fatigue, depression
  - Occasionally, distrust, fear, anxiety, panic
  - With large doses, acute psychosis: Delusions, hallucinations, loss of sense of personal identity
- Withdrawal symptoms include:
  - Nausea
  - Weight loss
  - Decreased appetite
  - Insomnia
  - Depressed mood

PHYSICAL EXAM

- Evaluate for:
  - Conjunctival injection
  - Xerostomia
  - Nystagmus
  - Increased heart rate
  - Altered pulmonary status
  - Altered body temperature
  - Reduced muscle strength
  - Decreased coordination
- Withdrawal findings include:
  - Restlessness/agitation
  - Irritability
  - Tremor
  - Diaphoresis
  - Increased body temperature

DIAGNOSTIC TESTS & INTERPRETATION

Positive urine drug screen. Cannabinoids can be detected in urine weeks to months after marijuana use.

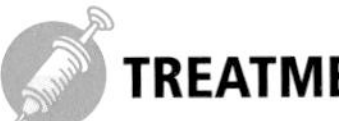

TREATMENT

- 4 methods of behavioral-based interventions:
  - Cognitive-behavioral therapy
  - Motivational interviewing
  - Motivational enhancement therapy
  - Contingency management
- No intervention to date has proved consistently effective for marijuana abuse (3)[C].
- Despite this, trials on cognitive-behavioral therapy and contingency management have shown better outcomes in reduction in marijuana use and maintaining abstinence (4)[A].
- For younger persons, family-based interventions may be more effective (3)[C].
- With marijuana abuse most prevalent among patients suffering from other psychiatric disorders, studies indicate that treating the mental health disorder may help reduce marijuana use, particularly among heavy users and those with more chronic mental disorders (1)[C].
- Advice to give to patients for management of withdrawal (3)[C]:
  - Gradually reduce amount of marijuana used before cessation.
  - Delay first use of marijuana until later in the day.
  - Consider use of nicotine replacement therapy if planning to stop separate tobacco use at the same time.
  - Relaxation, distraction
  - Avoid cues and triggers associated with cannabis use.
- Prescribe short-term analgesia and sedation for withdrawal symptoms if required (3)[C].
- If irritability and restlessness are marked, consider prescribing very-low-dose diazepam for 3–4 days (3)[C].
- Provide user and family members with information regarding marijuana abuse and withdrawal to increase understanding of the abuse and reduce likelihood of relapse.
- Withdrawal symptoms peak on day 2 or 3, and most are over by day 7. Sleep and vivid dreams can continue for 2–3 weeks.

MEDICATION

- No effective medication for the treatment of marijuana abuse as of yet
- One study suggested that oral THC could be used to abate marijuana withdrawal in individuals who are trying to quit (5)[C].
- Another study concluded that medications used to treat other drug use disorders, such as buspirone, lithium, and fluoxetine, may have therapeutic benefit (6)[C].

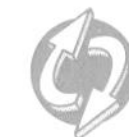

ONGOING CARE

FOLLOW-UP RECOMMENDATIONS

- Monitor cessation of marijuana use with urine tests over several weeks for the inactive metabolite of cannabis (carboxy-tetrahydrocannabinol).
- Heavy smokers may continue to be positive for marijuana for up to 6 weeks.

PATIENT EDUCATION

To learn more about marijuana abuse, visit the National Institute on Drug Abuse (NIDA) Web site at www.drugabuse.gov. Other NIDA Web sites include:

- http://backtoschool.drugabuse.gov/
- http://marijuana-info.org
- http://teens.drugabuse.gov

COMPLICATIONS

- Acute adverse effects:
  - Anxiety and panic, especially in naive users
  - Psychotic symptoms at high doses
  - Motor vehicle accidents if a person drives while intoxicated
- Chronic adverse effects:
  - Subtle cognitive impairment
  - Poor educational outcomes, lower income, greater welfare dependence, and unemployment
  - Chronic bronchitis and impaired respiratory function in regular smokers
  - Psychotic symptoms and disorders in heavy users, especially those with a history of psychotic symptoms or a family history of these disorders

REFERENCES

1. National Institute on Drug Abuse. *Research Report Series: Marijuana Abuse*, 2010.
2. Hubbard J, Franco S, Onaivi E. Marijuana: Medical Implications. *Am Fam Physician*. 1999;60: 2583–93.
3. Winstock A, Ford C, Witton J. Assessment and management of cannabis use disorders in primary care. *BMJ*. 2010;340:800–804.
4. Denis C, Lavie E, Fatseas M, et al. Psychotherapeutic interventions for cannabis abuse and/or dependence in outpatient settings. *Cochrane Database Syst Rev*. 2008;3:CD005336.
5. Budney A, Vandrey R, Hughes J, et al. Oral delta-9-tetrahydrocannabinol suppreses cannabis withdrawal symptoms. *Drug Alcohol Depend*. 2007;86:22–29.
6. Vandrey R, Haney M. Pharmacotherapy for cannabis dependence: How close are we? *CNS Drugs*. 2009;23:543–53.

ADDITIONAL READING

- Fergusson D, Boden J. Cannabis use and later life outcomes. *Addiction*. 2008;103:969–76.
- Hall W, Degenhardt L. Adverse health effects of non-medical cannabis use. *Lancet*. 2009;374: 1383–91.

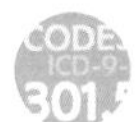

CODES

ICD9

- 305.20 Cannabis abuse, unspecified
- 305.21 Cannabis abuse, continuous
- 305.22 Cannabis abuse, episodic

CLINICAL PEARLS

- Marijuana abuse may result in poor performance in school or work, legal problems, and arguments with family.
- Patients should be screened for marijuana use. Questions asked may include frequency and amount.
- Effects of smoked marijuana can last 1–3 hours. Effects from foods or beverages appear later, usually in 30 minutes to 1 hour, but can last up to 4 hours.
- Smoking marijuana delivers significantly more THC into the bloodstream than eating or drinking the drug.
- Acute marijuana intoxication is manifested by: Conjunctival injection, increased heart rate, euphoria, heightened sensory perception, altered perception of time, increased appetite, poor short-term memory and concentration, fatigue. Large doses may result in acute psychosis: Delusions, hallucinations.
- Withdrawal symptoms include nausea, weight loss, decreased appetite, insomnia, depressed mood. Peaks on day 2 or 3, and most are over by day 7.
- Cognitive-behavioral therapy, motivational interviewing, motivational enhancement therapy, and contingency management are 4 methods of behavioral-based interventions used in the treatment of marijuana abuse.

MASTALGIA

Eduardo Lara-Torre, MD
Amanda Murchison, MD
Patrice Weiss, MD

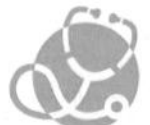

BASICS

DESCRIPTION

- Painful breast tissue, often bilateral, that can be cyclic or noncyclic:
  - 2/3 of breast pain is cyclic and is usually associated with hormonal changes related to menses, external hormones, pregnancy, or menopause.
  - 1/3 is noncyclic and often is related to a breast or chest wall lesion.
- Synonym(s): Mastodynia; Breast pain

EPIDEMIOLOGY

Incidence

- Predominant sex: Most common in women but occurs occasionally in men
- Predominant age: Generally seen from adolescence through menopause
- Frequency of breast cancer with those reporting breast pain ranges from 1.2–6.7% (1).
- Up to 70% of women report some degree of breast pain at some point in their lives (2).
- Most describe mild pain, but 11% describe pain as moderate to severe.

RISK FACTORS

- Diet high in saturated fats
- Cigarette smoking
- Recent weight gain
- Pregnancy
- Large, pendulous breasts (caused by stretching of Cooper ligament)
- Exogenous hormones
- Caffeine has *not* been shown to be a risk factor (3)[B].

Genetics

Familial tendency

GENERAL PREVENTION

- Avoid exposure to risk factors.
- Properly fitted bra support

PATHOPHYSIOLOGY

- Causative pathophysiology remains unclear but is thought to be related to hormonal or nutritional factors.
- When fibrocystic disease is the source, growth and distension of the cyst with hormonal fluctuation can cause pain.
- Hormonal factors (e.g., hormone-replacement therapy, oral contraceptives, pregnancy, menses, puberty, and menopause) may influence the diverse conditions that cause mastalgia or may themselves cause breast tenderness and pain.

ETIOLOGY

- Benign breast disorders (e.g., fibrocystic changes)
- Trauma (including sexual abuse/assault)
- Diet and lifestyle
- Lactation problems (e.g., engorgement, mastitis, breast abscess)
- Breast masses, including breast cancer
- Hidradenitis suppurativa
- Costochondritis (Tietze syndrome)
- Postthoracotomy syndrome
- Spinal and paraspinal disorders
- Potential side effects of medications
- Postradiation effects
- Referred pain (e.g., pulmonary, cardiac, or gallbladder disease)
- Ductal ectasia

DIAGNOSIS

HISTORY

- Location, duration, frequency, severity, associated symptoms, related activities (e.g., trauma), and aggravating and ameliorating factors
- Complete medical history with focus on gynecologic/obstetric history
- Complete systematic review of systems
- Diet/smoking history
- Detailed family history for risk assessment for breast cancer

PHYSICAL EXAM

- Examine breasts systematically in both standing and sitting positions.
- Assess for skin changes, breast symmetry and contour, dimpling, localized tenderness, bruising, masses, nipple discharge, and lymphadenopathy. Look for signs that are suggestive of breast malignancy.

DIAGNOSTIC TESTS & INTERPRETATION

Lab

Initial lab tests

- If galactorrhea is found, check a fasting prolactin level.
- Possibly thyroid-stimulating hormone

Imaging

- Consider an ultrasound in women with focal, persistent breast pain.
- Mammogram ± ultrasound in women aged 30–35 years of age or older

Pediatric Considerations

Ultrasound is the imaging test of choice for children and adolescents. A mammogram is not useful.

Diagnostic Procedures/Surgery

- Cysts may need to be aspirated to relieve symptoms or verify diagnosis.
- Biopsies may be indicated based on the results of examination, ultrasound, or mammography.

Pediatric Considerations

In children and adolescents, do not perform biopsies unless there is suspicion for cancer. Refer to a specialist in pediatric breast disease.

Pathological Findings

- Normal breast tissue
- Benign: Fibrocystic changes, duct ectasia, solitary papillomas, simple fibroadenomas
- Small increased risk of breast cancer: Ductal hyperplasia without atypia, sclerosing adenosis, diffuse papillomatosis, complex fibroadenomas
- Moderate increased risk: Atypical ductal hyperplasia, atypical lobular hyperplasia
- Breast cancer

DIFFERENTIAL DIAGNOSIS

- The major alternate disease to consider is breast cancer, particularly if pain is localized.
- Manipulation or trauma also can worsen symptoms.
- Chest wall pain or referred pain resulting from splenomegaly also must be differentiated from mastalgia.
- Sometimes cyclic pain is concurrent with premenstrual syndrome.
- Ductal ectasia of the breast

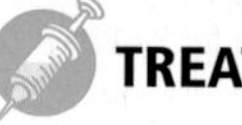

TREATMENT

MEDICATION

First Line

Acetaminophen, NSAIDs either oral or topical (such as diclofenac sodium or piroxicam) (4)[A]

Second Line

- Oral contraceptives may help some patients prevent fibrocystic disease but may worsen pain in some sensitive patients.
- If the patient is on an oral contraceptive, switch to one that has a lower estrogen component.
- In some patients with mastalgia only during their menses, menstrual suppression with continuous oral contraceptives may be of benefit.
- Oral progesterone: 10 mg PO daily
- Other possibilities for patients with refractory symptoms, used infrequently because of potential side effects, include these:
  - Danazol: 100 mg b.i.d. (possibly lower doses) may be the most effective; major adverse effects include menstrual irregularities, weight gain, acne, hirsutism, and voice change; *may be used during luteal phase only;* approved by the FDA for this indication
  - Toremifene: 30 mg PO daily (5)[A]
  - Bromocriptine: 5 mg PO daily and cabergoline 0.5 mg PO weekly both during the second half of the menstrual cycle are equally effective, but cabergoline has fewer side effects (6)[A].

ADDITIONAL TREATMENT

If the patient is breast-feeding, correct any breast-feeding difficulties; treat underlying mastitis or breast abscess.

General Measures

- Stop or modify the current hormonal therapy.
- A repeat examination may help to establish any cyclic nodularity pattern.
- Wear a properly fitted support bra (may be fitted by a professional).
- Reassurance (sufficient for most patients)
- Weight loss for obese patients
- Smoking cessation
- Relaxation training

Pediatric Considerations

Children and adolescents may require referrals to a specialist.

COMPLEMENTARY AND ALTERNATIVE MEDICINE

- Vitamin E and evening primrose oil have not been found to be of benefit for chronic mastalgia (1,7)[B].
- Flaxseed oil is not effective for the treatment of mastalgia (8)[C].

SURGERY/OTHER PROCEDURES

Some patients may need surgical breast reduction.

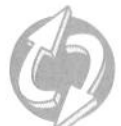

ONGOING CARE

FOLLOW-UP RECOMMENDATIONS

As needed

Patient Monitoring

- As needed for patients not receiving pharmacotherapy
- Time of follow-up will vary by type of pharmacotherapy and patient's particular problems

DIET

- Decrease fat intake to 20% of total calories.
- There is no strong evidence that reduction in caffeine intake may help to decrease the severity or incidence of the disease (9)[C].

PATIENT EDUCATION

Avoid or adjust risk factors.

PROGNOSIS

- Premenstrual mastalgia increases with age and then generally stops at menopause unless the patient is receiving hormone therapy (HT).
- Most patients can control symptoms without receiving HT.
- Several months of HT may provide several more months of relief, but mastalgia may recur.
- Cyclic mastalgia responds better than noncyclic mastalgia to treatment.
- Effects of long-term HT are unknown.

REFERENCES

1. Smith RL. Evaluation and management of breast pain. *Mayo Clinic Proc.* 2004;79:353.
2. Ader DN, Shriver CD. Cyclical mastalgia: Prevalence and impact in an outpatient breast clinic sample. *J Am Coll Surg.* 1997;185:466–70.
3. Levinson W, Dunn PM. Nonassociation of caffeine and fibrocystic breast disease. *Arch Intern Med.* 1986;146:1773–5.
4. Ahmadinejad M, Delfan B, Haghdani S, et al. Comparing the effect of diclofenac gel and piroxicam gel on mastalgia. *Breast J.* 2010;16: 213–4.
5. Gong C, Song E, Jia W. A double-blind randomized controlled trial of toremifene therapy for mastalgia. *Arch Surg.* 2006;141:43–7.
6. Aydin Y, Atis A, Kaleli S, et al. Cabergoline versus bromocriptine for symptomatic treatment of premenstrual mastalgia: A randomised, open-label study. *Eur J Obstet Gynecol Reprod Biol.* 2010;150(2):203–6.
7. Pruthi S, Wahner-Roedler DL, Torkelson CJ, et al. Vitamin E and evening primrose oil for management of cyclical mastalgia: A randomized pilot study. *Altern Med Rev.* 2010;15:59–67.
8. Basch E, Bent S, Collins J. Flax and flaxseed oil (linum usitatissimum): A review by the Natural Standard Research Collaboration. *J Soc Integr Oncol.* 2007;5:92–105.
9. Gumm R, Cunnick GH, Mokbel K. Evidence for the management of mastalgia. *Curr Med Res Opin.* 2004;20:681–4.

ADDITIONAL READING

- Blommers J, de Lange-De Klerk ES, Kuik DJ. Evening primrose oil and fish oil for severe chronic mastalgia: A randomized, double-blind, controlled trial. *Am J Obstet Gynecol.* 2002;187:1389–94.
- Brennan M, Houssami N, French J. Management of benign breast conditions. Part 1–Painful breasts. *Aust Fam Physician.* 2005;34:143–4.
- Campagnoli C, Ambroggio S, Lotano MR, et al. Progestogen use in women approaching the menopause and breast cancer risk. *Maturitas.* 2009;62:338–42.
- Colak T, Ipek T, Kanik A. Efficacy of topical nonsteroidal antiinflammatory drugs in mastalgia treatment. *J Am Coll Surg.* 2003;196:525–30.
- McFadyen IJ, Chetty U, Setchell KD. A randomized double blind-cross over trial of soya protein for the treatment of cyclical breast pain. *Breast.* 2000;9:271–6.
- Miltenburg DM, Speights VO. Benign breast disease. *Obstet Gynecol Clin North Am.* 2008;35:285–300, ix.
- Olawaiye A, Withiam-Leitch M, Danakas G. Mastalgia: A review of management. *J Reprod Med.* 2005;50:933–9.
- Qureshi S, Sultan N. Topical nonsteroidal anti-inflammatory drugs versus oil of evening primrose in the treatment of mastalgia. *Surgeon.* 2005;3:7–10.

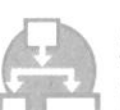

See Also (Topic, Algorithm, Electronic Media Element)

- Premenstrual Syndrome (PMS) and Premenstrual Dysphoric Disorder
- Algorithms: Breast Discharge; Breast Pain

CODES

ICD9

611.71 Mastodynia

CLINICAL PEARLS

- When evaluating a patient with breast pain, always rule out cancer first.
- In the adolescent population, do not biopsy; instead, refer to a pediatric specialist.
- Premenstrual mastalgia increases with age and then generally stops at menopause unless the patient is receiving HT.

M

MASTITIS

Montiel T. Rosenthal, MD

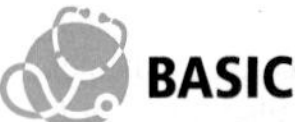

BASICS

DESCRIPTION

- Inflammation of the breast parenchyma, and possibly associated tissues (areola, nipple, SC fat)
- Usually associated with bacterial infection (and milk stasis in the postpartum mother)
- Usually an acute condition, but can become chronic cystic mastitis

EPIDEMIOLOGY

- Predominantly affects females
- Mostly in the puerperium
- Neonatal form
- Posttraumatic:
  - Ornamental nipple piercing increases risk of transmission of bacteria to deeper breast structures:
    - *S. aureus* is the predominant organism.
    - Epidemic form rare in the age of reduced hospital stays for mothers and newborns

Incidence

- 2.5% of breast-feeding mothers develop nonepidemic mastitis.
- Greatest incidence among breast-feeding mothers 2–3 weeks postpartum
- Neonatal form:
  - 1–5 weeks of age with equal gender risk and unilateral presentation
- Pediatric form:
  - Around or after puberty
  - 82% of cases in girls

RISK FACTORS

- Breast-feeding
- Milk stasis:
  - Inadequate emptying of breast
    - Scarring of breast due to prior mastitis
    - Scarring due to previous breast surgery
  - Breast engorgement:
    - Interruption of breast-feeding
- Ornamental nipple piercing increases risk of transmission of bacteria to deeper breast structures:
  - *S. aureus* predominant organism
- Neonatal colonization with epidemic *Staphylococcus*
- Neonatal:
  - Bottle-fed babies
  - Manual expression of "witch's milk"
  - Can predispose to lethal necrotizing fasciitis
- Maternal diabetes
- Maternal HIV
- Maternal vitamin A deficiency (in animal models) (1)

GENERAL PREVENTION

Regular emptying of both breasts and nipple care to prevent fissures when breast-feeding (2)

PATHOPHYSIOLOGY

- Micro-abscesses along milk ducts and surrounding tissues
- Inflammatory cell infiltration of breast parenchyma and surrounding tissues
- Nonpuerperal (infectious):
  - *S. aureus*, *Bacteroides* sp., Peptostreptococcus, Staphylococcus (coagulase neg.), *Enterococcus faecalis*
  - *Histoplasma capsulatum*
- Puerperal (infectious):
  - *S. aureus*, *Streptococcus pyogenes* (group A or B), *Corynebacterium* sp., *Bacteroides* sp., Staphylococcus (coagulase neg.), *E. coli*, *Salmonella* sp.
  - MRSA (3)[C]
- Rare secondary site for tuberculosis in endemic areas (1% of mastitis cases in these areas):
  - Single breast nodule with mastalgia
- *Corynebacterium* sp. associated with greater risk for development of chronic cystic mastitis
- Granulomatous mastitis:
  - Idiopathic:
    - Predilection for Asian and Hispanic women
    - Association with alpha-1-antitrypsin deficiency, hyperprolactinemia with galactorrhea, oral contraceptive use, and breast trauma
    - Most women with history of lactation in previous 5 years
  - Lupus; autoimmune

ETIOLOGY

- Puerperal:
  - Retrograde migration of surface bacteria up milk ducts
  - Bacterial migration from nipple fissures up breast lymphatics
  - Secondary monilial infection in the face of recurrent mastitis and/or diabetes
  - Seeding from mother to neonate in cyclical fashion
- Nonpuerperal:
  - Ductal ectasia
  - Breast carcinoma
  - Inflammatory cysts
  - Chronic recurring SC or subareolar infections
  - Parasitic infections: *Echinococcus*; filariasis; Guinea worm in endemic areas
  - Herpes simplex (4)[C]
  - Cat-scratch disease
- Lupus

COMMONLY ASSOCIATED CONDITIONS

Breast abscess

DIAGNOSIS

- Fever and malaise
- Nausea ± vomiting
- Localized breast tenderness, heat, and redness
- Possible breast mass

HISTORY

- Breast pain
- "Hot cords burning in chest wall"

PHYSICAL EXAM

- Breast tenderness
- Localized breast induration, redness, and warmth
- Peau d'orange appearance to overlying skin

DIAGNOSTIC TESTS & INTERPRETATION

Lab

Initial lab tests

Mastitis is typically a clinical diagnosis. Labs rarely needed except for patients ill enough to be hospitalized:

- CBC
- Blood culture
- In epidemic puerperal mastitis:
  - Milk leukocyte count
  - Milk culture
  - Neonatal nasal culture

Follow-Up & Special Considerations

Lactating mothers produce salty milk from affected side (higher Na and Cl concentrations) as compared with unaffected side.

Imaging

- No imaging required for postpartum mastitis in a breast-feeding mother that responds to antibiotic therapy
- Mammography for women with nonpuerperal mastitis
- Breast ultrasound to rule out abscess formation in women:
  - Special consideration for this in women with breast implants who have mastitis

Diagnostic Procedures/Surgery

Options if further progression to abscess formation:

- Needle aspiration
- I&D
- Excisional biopsy

DIFFERENTIAL DIAGNOSIS

- Abscess (bacterial, idiopathic granulomatous mastitis, fungal, tuberculosis)
- Tumor:
  - Idiopathic granulomatous mastitis
  - Inflammatory breast cancer
  - Wegener granulomatosis
  - Sarcoidosis
  - Foreign-body granuloma
- Ductal cyst (ductal ectasia)
- Consider monilial infection in lactating mom, especially if mastitis is recurrent.

TREATMENT

A recent Cochrane Review found that there is insufficient evidence to confirm or refute the effectiveness of antibiotic therapy for the treatment of lactational mastitis (5)[A].

MEDICATION

- Prioritized on the basis of likelihood of MRSA as etiologic factor and clinical severity of condition
- Treat for 10–14 days (6)[B].
- For idiopathic granulomatous mastitis, prednisone in 1 mg/kg prolonged taper (± methotrexate or azathioprine) (7)[C]

First Line

- Outpatient:
  - Dicloxacillin 500 mg q.i.d.
  - Cephalexin 500 mg q.i.d.
  - TMP/SMX; DS b.i.d. (MRSA possible)
- Inpatient:
  - Nafcillin 2 g q4h
  - Oxacillin 2 g q4h
  - Vancomycin 1 g q12h (MRSA possible)
- Breast-feeding beyond 1 month:
  - PCN, ampicillin, or erythromycin (5)[A]

Pediatric Considerations

- TMP/SMZ given to breast-feeding mothers with mastitis can potentiate jaundice for neonates.
- Clindamycin IM, IV, or PO with dosing based on age and weight

Second Line
- If mastitis is odoriferous and localized under areola, add metronidazole 500 mg t.i.d. IV or PO.
- If yeast is suspected in recurrent mastitis, add topical, oral, and neonatal nystatin.

ADDITIONAL TREATMENT
Issues for Referral
- Abscess formation
- Need for breast biopsy

Additional Therapies
- Warm packs (or ice packs) to affected breast for comfort
- The use of a breast pump may aid in breast emptying, especially if the infant is unable to assist in doing this.
- Wear supporting bra that is not too tight

SURGERY/OTHER PROCEDURES
In cases of biopsy-proven idiopathic granulomatous mastitis, surgical removal can result in a 5–50% chance of recurrence, fistula formation, and poor wound healing.

IN-PATIENT CONSIDERATIONS
If a new mother is admitted to the hospital for treatment of her mastitis, rooming-in of the infant with the mother is mandatory so that breast-feeding can continue. In some hospitals, rooming-in may require hospital admission of the infant (8).

Initial Stabilization
- Oral antibiotics
- Frequent emptying of breasts if breast-feeding
- Analgesics for pain:
  - Acetaminophen
- NSAIDs

Admission Criteria
- Failure of outpatient/oral therapy:
  - Patient unable to tolerate oral therapy
  - Patient noncompliant with oral therapy
  - Severe illness without adequate supportive care at home
- Neonatal mastitis

Nursing
- Breast-feeding/pumping of breasts encouraged
- Start infant with feedings on affected side.
- Abscess drainage is not a contraindication for breast-feeding.

Discharge Criteria
- Afebrile
- Tolerating oral antibiotics well

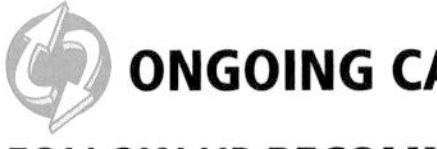

ONGOING CARE

FOLLOW-UP RECOMMENDATIONS
Rest for lactating mothers, up to bathroom

DIET
- Encourage oral fluids
- Multivitamin including vitamin A

PATIENT EDUCATION
- Encourage oral fluids
- Rest essential
- Regular emptying of both breasts with breast-feeding
- Nipple care to prevent fissures

PROGNOSIS
- Puerperal:
  - Good with prompt (within 24 hours of symptom onset) antibiotic treatment and breast emptying; 96% success rate
  - 11% risk of abscess if left untreated with antibiotics
  - Antibodies develop in breast glands within first few days of infection, which may provide protection against infection or reinfection.
- Rare risk of abscess formation beyond 6 weeks postpartum if no recurrent mastitis

COMPLICATIONS
- Breast abscess
- Recurrent mastitis with resumption of breast-feeding or with breast-feeding after next pregnancy
- Bacteremia
- Sepsis

REFERENCES

1. Chew BP, Zamora CS, Luedecke LO, et al. Effect of vitamin A deficiency on mammary gland development and susceptibility to mastitis through intramammary infusion with *Staphylococcus aureus* in mice. *Am J Vet Res*. 1985;46:287–93.
2. Crepinsek MA, Crowe L, Michener K, et al. Interventions for preventing mastitis after childbirth. *Cochrane Database Syst Rev*. 2010; CD007239.
3. Gastelum DT, Dassey D, Mascola L, et al. Transmission of community-associated methicillin-resistant *Staphylococcus aureus* from breast milk in the neonatal intensive care unit. *Pediatr Infect Dis J*. 2005;24:1122–4.
4. Soo MS, Ghate S. Herpes simplex virus mastitis: Clinical and imaging findings. *AJR Am J Roentgenol*. 2000;174:1087–8.
5. Jahanfar S, Ng CJ, Teng CL, et al. Antibiotics for mastitis in breastfeeding women. *Cochrane Database Syst Rev*. 2009;CD005458.
6. Gilbert DN, Moellering RC, et al. *The Sanford Guide to Antimicrobial Therapy 2010,* 40th ed.
7. Patel RA, Strickland P, Sankara IR, et al. Idiopathic granulomatous mastitis: Case reports and review of the literature. *J Gen Intern Med*. 2009;25:270–3.
8. Academy of Breastfeeding Medicine Protocol Committee. ABM clinical protocol #4: Mastitis. Revision, May 2008. *Breastfeed Med*. 2008;3: 177–80.

ADDITIONAL READING

Spencer JP, et al. Management of mastitis in breastfeeding women. *Am Fam Physician*. 2008;78:727–31.

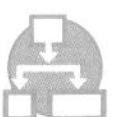

See Also (Topic, Algorithm, Electronic Media Element)

Algorithms: Breast Discharge; Breast Pain

CODES

ICD9
- Puerperal:
  - 611.0 Inflammatory disease of breast
  - 675.20 Nonpurulent mastitis associated with childbirth, unspecified as to episode of care or not applicable
  - 675.23 Nonpurulent mastitis associated with childbirth, antepartum condition or complication
- NonPuerperal:
  - 675.24 Nonpurulent mastitis associated with childbirth, postpartum condition or complication
  - 675.21 Nonpurulent mastitis associated with childbirth, delivered, with or without mention of antepartum condition
- 675.22 Nonpurulent mastitis associated with childbirth, delivered, with mention of postpartum complication

CLINICAL PEARLS

- Complete emptying of the breasts on a regular schedule, avoiding constrictive clothing or bras that might obstruct breast ducts, meticulous attention to nipple care, "adequate rest," and a liberal intake of oral fluids for the mother can all reduce the risk of a breast-feeding mother's developing mastitis.
- The first-line treatment for puerperal mastitis is Dicloxacillin 500 mg PO q.i.d. × 10–14 days. Most mastitis can be treated with oral therapy.
- Among breast-feeding mothers, if the symptoms of mastitis fail to resolve within several days of appropriate management including antibiotics, further investigations may be required to confirm resistant bacteria, abscess formation, an underlying mass, or inflammatory or ductal carcinoma.
- More than 2 recurrences of mastitis in the same location or with associated axillary lymphadenopathy warrant evaluation with ultrasound and/or mammography to rule out an underlying mass.

MASTOIDITIS

Jaime Wagner, MD
Francesca L. Beaudoin, MS, MD

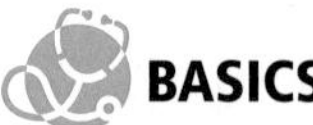

BASICS

Suppurative complication of acute otitis media (AOM) affecting the mastoid air cells or posterior process of the temporal bone

DESCRIPTION

- Inflammatory process of the mastoid bone
- Acute mastoiditis is a suppurative infection that typically presents after acute otitis media. Symptoms are present for <1 month. Subdivided into 2 stages:
  – Acute mastoiditis with periosteitis: Involvement of the periosteum of the mastoid bone, purulence within the mastoid air cells
  – Acute mastoid osteitis (coalescent mastoiditis): Destruction of the bony septae that separate air cells; leads to an empyema and involvement of more serious head and neck complications
- Subacute mastoiditis (masked mastoiditis): Indolent process, may occur with recurrent AOM that was not sufficiently treated
- Chronic mastoiditis: Due to chronic suppurative otitis media that has failed treatment; usually associated with cholesteatoma; symptoms lasting months to years

EPIDEMIOLOGY

- Children > Adults
- Most common in children <2 years old
- In pediatrics: Males > Females
- Incidence down since introduction of antibiotics; controversial whether incidence is now rising due to antibiotic-resistant *Staphylococcus pneumoniae*

Incidence

1–4 cases per 100,000 person year (1)

Prevalence

Unknown

RISK FACTORS

- Cholesteatoma
- Recurrent acute otitis media or chronic suppurative otitis media
- Immunocompromised patient

Genetics

No known genetic pattern

GENERAL PREVENTION

- Adequate antibiotic treatment for acute otitis media
- Prevention of recurrent acute otitis media
- Early referral to ENT for chronic otitis media
- Treatment of chronic eustachian tube dysfunction (i.e., pressure equalization tubes)
- Early identification of cholesteatoma
- Pneumococcal conjugate vaccine

PATHOPHYSIOLOGY

- Subclinical stage begins with acute otitis media causing inflammation of mastoid air cells (likely present in all cases of AOM)
- Obstruction of the aditus ad antrum (the connection between the tympanic cavity and the mastoid) during severe cases of AOM:
  – Blocks outflow tract of mastoid air cells
  – Accumulation of edema and purulent material with penetration of mucosa and periosteum (acute mastoiditis with periosteitis)
- Increased pressure from fluid within the air cells leads to destruction of bony septae (acute mastoid osteitis or acute coalescent mastoiditis)
- Acute mastoid osteitis can then lead to pus dissecting to adjacent areas in head and neck and subsequent abscess formation:
  – Subperiosteal abscess (most common complication), Bezold abscess, suppurative labyrinthitis, suppurative CNS complications

ETIOLOGY

- AOM: *Haemophilus influenzae, Streptococcus pneumoniae*
- Acute mastoiditis: *Streptococcus pneumoniae* (most common organism), *Streptococcus pyogenes, Haemophilus influenzae, Staphylococcus aureus* (including MRSA):
  – Introduction of the 7-valent pneumococcal conjugate vaccine in 2000 has led to increase in multidrug-resistant *Streptococcus pneumoniae* serotype 19A (2)
- Chronic mastoiditis: *Pseudomonas aeruginosa, Staphylococcus aureus,* Enterobacteriaceae, anaerobic bacteria

DIAGNOSIS

HISTORY

- At time of admission (1)[A]:
  – 42% of children had previous history of otologic disease.
  – 54% were on antibiotic therapy.
  – Average duration of symptoms 9.8 days
- Most common symptoms (1)[A]:
  – Lethargy/malaise or irritability
  – Fever
  – Poor feeding/decreased appetite
- Otalgia/possible otorrhea
- Hearing loss
- Headache
- Pain/redness/swelling noted over mastoid

PHYSICAL EXAM

- Postauricular changes: Erythema, tenderness, edema, and/or fluctuance (81–85%) (1)[A]
- Bulging, erythematous, or dull tympanic membrane (60–71%)
- Protrusion of auricle (79%)
- Fever (76%)
- Possible otorrhea if tympanic membrane is perforated
- Narrowing of external auditory canal
- Subperiosteal abscess
- Tympanic membrane can be normal in 10% of patients: Suspicious for mastoiditis when symptoms of acute otitis media persist >2 weeks

DIAGNOSTIC TESTS & INTERPRETATION

Lab

Initial lab tests

- CBC with differential: Increased leukocyte count (3)[C]
- Elevated ESR and CRP (3)
- Blood cultures
- Myringotomy/tympanocentesis: Send for cultures, Gram stain, acid-fast stain (1)[B]

Follow-Up & Special Considerations

Interpret normal WBC with caution in immunocompromised patient with symptoms.

Imaging

- Mastoiditis is often a clinical diagnosis, but CT imaging is often pursued to confirm the diagnosis and look for complications.
- If obvious physical exam and/or historical findings are absent, temporal bone imaging is recommended for patients with cervical or postauricular findings (4).

Initial approach

- Plain radiographs of mastoid area (low diagnostic yield):
  – Distortion of mastoid outline or clouding of mastoid air cells (not diagnostic, also seen in AOM)
  – Coalescence of air cells; diagnostic but rare
- CT scan findings (97% sensitivity, 94% predictive value) (5):
  – Clouding or opacification of air cells (a finding also present in AOM)
  – Mastoid air cell coalescence
  – Cortical bone erosion
  – Rim-enhancing fluid collections
- CT of temporal bone with contrast (4)[C]:
  – Useful for identifying suppurative extension or asymptomatic complications
- Technetium-99m bone scan: More sensitive to osteolytic changes than CT
- Indications for CT scan in pediatrics (5)[C]:
  – Neurologic signs
  – Vomiting/lethargy
  – Suspected cholesteatoma
  – Fever after 48–72 hours of therapy
  – Local progression of disease
- MRI is being used with increasing frequency; may see increased fluid signal of mastoid air cells on T2-weighted MRI:
  – Not an effective screening tool, often an incidental finding in the absence of clinical signs

Diagnostic Procedures/Surgery

- Tympanocentesis should be performed to obtain middle ear fluid for culture and sensitivity (1)[B].
- Myringotomy with culture (also therapeutic)
- Audiography if suspected hearing loss
- Obtain CSF if suspect intracranial extension.
- Biopsy if tissue protruding through TM or tympanostomy tube

Pathological Findings

- Inflammatory tissue in air cell system
- Granulation tissue
- Osteitis

DIFFERENTIAL DIAGNOSIS

- Postauricular inflammatory adenopathy
- Severe external otitis
- Postauricular cellulitis
- Benign neoplasm: Aneurysmal bone cyst, fibrous dysplasia
- Malignant neoplasm: Rhabdomyosarcoma, neuroblastoma
- Deep neck space infections
- Furuncle of meatus of ear
- Parotitis
- Local trauma to auricula

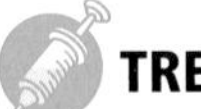

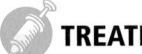

TREATMENT

IV antibiotics and myringotomy (± tympanostomy tubes) is now the mainstay of therapy for uncomplicated acute mastoiditis, reflecting a shift away from surgical treatment (6)[C].

MEDICATION

First Line

- Empiric antibiotics directed against most common organisms: *S. pneumoniae* (including multiple resistant strains), *S. pyogenes*, *S. aureus* (including MRSA), *P. aeruginosa*
- Use third-generation cephalosporin with additional coverage for resistant strain (4)[C].
- Ceftriaxone 1–2 g IV q24h:
  - Pediatric dosing: 50–75 mg/kg/d IV divided q12–24h
  - Precaution: Adjust dose with renal impairment.
- New recommendation of adding clindamycin to ceftriaxone for coverage of ceftriaxone-resistant *S. pneumoniae* in pediatric patients (4)[C]:
  - Clindamycin pediatric dosing: 20–40 mg/kg/d IV divided q6–8h
- Cefotaxime 1–2 g IV q4–8h depending on severity:
  - Pediatric dosing: 100–200 mg/kg/d divided q6–8 hours
- Add vancomycin 30–60 mg/kg/d divided q8–12 hours if concerned for MRSA:
  - Pediatric dosing: 15 mg/kg/dose q6–8h
  - Precaution: Adjust dose with renal impairment.
- For chronic mastoiditis, treat with piperacillin/tazobactam 3.375 g IV q6h:
  - Pediatric dosing: 300 mg/kg/d based on piperacillin component divided q6–8h
- For other significant contraindications, precautions, or interactions, please refer to the manufacturer's literature.

Second Line

- Oral antibiotics are given after 7–10 days of IV antibiotics and once myringotomy/blood cultures narrow pathogen and sensitivities, typically:
  - Amoxicillin-clavulanate (Augmentin) or clindamycin PLUS third-generation cephalosporin for 3 weeks or total treatment duration of 4 weeks
- For chronic mastoiditis: Use topical drops, ofloxacin otic solution (0.3%), neomycin, polymyxin B, and hydrocortisone 3 drops, 3–4 times per day

ADDITIONAL TREATMENT

General Measures

- Inpatient care during acute phase for IV antibiotics
- Keep affected ear dry.

Issues for Referral

All cases of mastoiditis should be referred to ENT specialists for both adult and pediatric patients.

SURGERY/OTHER PROCEDURES

- Tympanocentesis should be performed to obtain cultures and guide antibiotic choice (1)[B].
- Myringotomy to allow drainage of the middle ear is performed in most patients (6)[C] with or with placement of tympanostomy tubes:
  - Tympanostomy tubes allow for prolonged drainage.
- Treatment of subperiosteal abscess is becoming controversial (6):
  - Trial of conservative therapy with IV antibiotics, tympanostomy tubes, and retroauricular puncture; if conservative treatment fails or neurologic symptoms are present, consider incision and drainage or mastoidectomy (5)[C].
- Mastoidectomy is reserved for those patients whose condition fails to improve or progresses within 24–48 hours despite IV antibiotics and myringotomy, or those with meningeal or intracranial complications (5)[C].
- Frequent cleaning of ear canal under microscope to ensure pressure-equalization tube patency and adequate drainage of middle ear
- Topical antibiotic drops are also usually used after insertion of pressure-equalization tubes.

IN-PATIENT CONSIDERATIONS

Initial Stabilization

- Hospitalize any patient with acute mastoiditis; start IV antibiotics.
- ENT referral (for tympanostomy or surgery if complications suspected)

Admission Criteria

Clinical or imaging evidence of acute mastoiditis

Nursing

Caution patient about getting affected ear wet.

Discharge Criteria

- Afebrile for 48 hours before IV antibiotics are discontinued
- Clinical improvement
- Able to take oral antibiotics

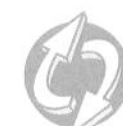

ONGOING CARE

FOLLOW-UP RECOMMENDATIONS

- Oral antibiotics for 3 weeks following satisfactory course of IV antibiotics (total duration of antibiotics is 4 weeks)
- For chronic mastoiditis, consider antimicrobial prophylaxis with amoxicillin for several months.

Patient Monitoring

- Postoperative: Audiogram after acute flare-up has subsided to assess for hearing loss
- Follow up with ENT as outpatient, with closer follow-up for patients who had intracranial complications or hearing loss.

DIET

No special diet

PATIENT EDUCATION

- Precaution about getting affected ear wet
- Follow-up with ENT as outpatient.

PROGNOSIS

- Depends on severity and stage of disease
- Conductive hearing loss may require reconstructive surgery.
- Most cases of mastoiditis recover fully when early treatment is initiated.

COMPLICATIONS

- Total estimated complication rate 17.9% (3)
- Subperiosteal abscess (most common complication)
- Gradenigo syndrome (palsy of the sixth cranial nerve, draining ear, and retro-orbital pain)
- Bezold abscess (abscess of sternocleidomastoid muscle)
- Sigmoid sinus thrombosis
- Meningitis
- Intracranial abscess epidural/subdural/intraparenchymal
- Periosteitis
- Osteomyelitis of the temporal bone
- Central venous sinus thrombosis
- Suppurative labyrinthitis (resulting in deafness)
- Citelli abscess (osteomyelitis of the calvaria)
- Facial nerve paralysis

REFERENCES

1. van den Aardweg MT, Rovers MM, de Ru JA, et al. A systematic review of diagnostic criteria for acute mastoiditis in children. *Otol Neurotol*. 2008;29:751–7.
2. Ongkasuwan J, Valdez TA, Hulten KG, et al. Pneumococcal mastoiditis in children and the emergence of multidrug-resistant serotype 19A isolates. *Pediatrics*. 2008;122:34–9.
3. Bilavsky E, Yarden-Bilavsky H, Samra Z, et al. Clinical, laboratory, and microbiological differences between children with simple or complicated mastoiditis. *Int J Pediatr Otorhinolaryngol*. 2009;73:1270–3.
4. Lin HW, Shargorodsky J, Gopen Q, et al. Clinical strategies for the management of acute mastoiditis in the pediatric population. *Clin Pediatr (Phila)*. 2010;49:110–5.
5. Bakhos D, Trijolet JP, Morinière S, et al. Conservative management of acute mastoiditis in children. *Arch. Otolaryngol Head Neck Surg*. 2011;137:346–50.
6. Tamir S, Shwartz Y, Peleg U, et al. Shifting trends: Mastoiditis from a surgical to a medical disease. *Am J Otolaryngol*. 2010;31:467–71.

ADDITIONAL READING

- Roddy MG, Glazier SS, Agrawal D. Pediatric mastoiditis in the pneumococcal conjugate vaccine era: Symptom duration guides empiric antimicrobial therapy. *Pediatr Emerg Care*. 2007;23:779–84.
- Smith J, et al. Complications of chronic otitis media and cholesteatoma. *Otolaryngol Clin N Am*. 2006;39(6):1237–55.

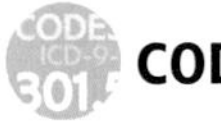

CODES

ICD9

- 383.00 Acute mastoiditis without complications
- 383.01 Subperiosteal abscess of mastoid
- 383.9 Unspecified mastoiditis

CLINICAL PEARLS

- Tympanic membrane can be normal in 10% of patients: Suspect mastoiditis when symptoms of acute otitis media persist >2 weeks with a normal TM.
- Hospitalize all patients with acute mastoiditis.
- Start with broad-spectrum IV antibiotics, and collect middle ear fluid cultures to further guide treatment.
- Early involvement of ENT consultation for possible surgical intervention

MEASLES (RUBEOLA)

Herbert L. Muncie, Jr., MD
Marin Dawson-Caswell, DO

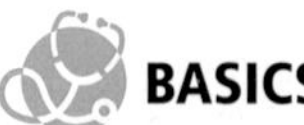

BASICS

DESCRIPTION

- A highly communicable, acute viral illness characterized by a maculopapular rash; begins at the head, spreads inferiorly to trunk and extremities
- Rash is preceded by fever and the classic triad: Cough, coryza, and conjunctivitis, and pathognomonic Koplik spots
- Major public health problem in the developing world, with significant morbidity and mortality
- System(s) affected: Primarily Hematologic/Lymphatic/Immunologic; Pulmonary; Skin; all systems may be affected by measles virus and/or its complications.
- Synonym(s): Rubeola

EPIDEMIOLOGY

- Transmission: Direct contact with infectious droplets or airborne spread (less common):
  - Droplets can remain in the air for hours.
  - In 2000, ongoing transmission declared eliminated in the US as a result of high rates of vaccination.
- Infectivity: Highly infectious; 75–90% of susceptible contacts will develop the disease:
  - Infectivity: Greatest during the prodromal phase
  - Patients are considered contagious from 5 days before symptoms until 4 days after rash appears.
  - Immunocompromised patients are considered contagious for entire duration of disease.
- Incubation period: Averages 12.5 days from exposure to onset of prodromal symptoms (1)
- Predominant age: Varies based on local vaccine practices and disease incidence. In developing countries; most cases occur in children <2 years of age.

Incidence

- In the US: No longer considered an endemic disease by the CDC (2); isolated outbreaks still occur, with most cases imported to those who are unvaccinated
- First 5 months of 2011, more cases of measles were reported in the US than during any period since 1996. 118 cases were reported:
  - Of these, 89% were unvaccinated.
  - Young children aged 6–23 months traveling abroad are at increased risk if unvaccinated (3).
- Worldwide: An estimated 20 million measles cases occur each year, with 242,000 measles deaths in 2006. Over 95% of measles deaths occur in countries with per capita gross national income of <US$1,000 and weak health infrastructures.

RISK FACTORS

- For developing measles:
  - Not being immunized or failure to receive 2 doses of vaccine
  - Travel to countries where measles is endemic
  - Contact with exposed individuals, travelers, or immigrants
- For severe measles or measles complications:
  - Immunodeficiency
  - Malnutrition
  - Pregnancy
  - Vitamin A deficiency
  - Age <5 years or >20 years

GENERAL PREVENTION

- Totally preventable disease with vaccination and positive externalities due to herd immunity (4)
- Measles vaccine (active immunization):
  - Live further-attenuated vaccine available as monovalent vaccine, but usually given in combination with mumps and rubella (MMR); varicella now has been added
  - Primary vaccination of general population requires 2 doses (0.05 mL SC):
    - First dose given at 12–15 months; 95% develop immunity.
    - Second dose given at time of school entry (or any time >4 weeks after first measles vaccine); almost always initial nonresponders develop immunity.
    - HIV-infected children should be vaccinated while asymptomatic or before CD4+ cell count drops below 500/mm^3.
  - Common adverse reactions:
    - Fever and rarely febrile seizures 6–12 days after vaccination (5–15%)
    - Transient, mild, measleslike rash 7–10 days after vaccination (5%, with decreasing incidence during second vaccination)
    - Mild allergic reaction
    - If hypersensitivity reaction occurs, test for immunity; if immune, second dose is not needed.
    - Epidemiologic evidence has not substantiated any link between MMR vaccine and autism (5)[A].
  - Contraindications:
    - Pregnancy: Live vaccine is contraindicated in pregnant women (theoretical risk of fetal infection).
    - Anaphylactic reaction to gelatin or neomycin; consult allergist before vaccination.
    - Egg anaphylaxis is not considered a contraindication.

PATHOPHYSIOLOGY

Measles virus enters respiratory mucosa and replicates locally, then spreads to regional lymphatic tissues, then on to other reticuloendothelial sites via the bloodstream.

ETIOLOGY

- Measles virus, an RNA virus of genus *Morbillivirus*, family *Paramyxoviridae*
- Humans are the only natural host.

COMMONLY ASSOCIATED CONDITIONS

- Immunosuppression
- Malnutrition

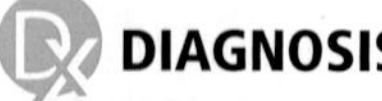

DIAGNOSIS

HISTORY

- Prodromal period: Usually 2–3 days before rash, but may be up to 8 days:
  - Fever:
    - Begins 8–12 days after exposure; persists until 2–3 days after onset of rash
    - High temperatures seen (39–40.5°C); can precipitate febrile seizures
    - Fever more than 3 days after rash suggests complication
  - Classic triad of "croupy" cough, coryza, and conjunctivitis
  - Cough may persist for up to 2 weeks.
  - Prodromal symptoms typically intensify over 2–4 days and peak on first day of rash before subsiding.
- Loose stools, malaise, irritability, photophobia (from iridocyclitis), sore throat, headache, and abdominal pain

PHYSICAL EXAM

- Koplik spots:
  - Pathognomonic of prodromal measles
  - 2–3-mm, gray–white, raised lesions on erythematous base that appear on buccal mucosa
  - Occur ~48 hours before measles exanthem
- Rash (not pathognomonic):
  - Maculopapular, blanches
  - Begins at ears and hairline and spreads head to toe, reaching hips by day 2
  - Discrete erythematous patches become confluent over time, with greater confluence on upper body than lower body.
  - Clinical improvement usually occurs within 48 hours of appearance of rash.
  - 3–4 days after rash appears, it fades and changes to brown color, followed by fine desquamation.
- Lymphadenopathy and pharyngitis may be seen during exanthem period.

DIAGNOSTIC TESTS & INTERPRETATION

Lab

Initial lab tests

- Measles IgM assay from serum or saliva is gold standard of World Health Organization (WHO):
  - Simplest diagnostic method
  - In countries with low measles prevalence, this approach may lead to false-positive results, so in low-prevalence countries, the use of paired acute and convalescent sera for antimeasles IgM and IgG is suggested.
  - IgM may be undetectable on first day of exanthem; usually detectable 3 days after exanthem:
    - At least a 4-fold increase is indicative of infection.
    - Sensitivity: 77% within 72 hours of rash onset; 100% 4–11 days after rash onset; if negative but rash lasts >72 hours, repeat
- Measles IgG is undetectable up to 7 days after exanthem; peaks about 14 days after exanthem:
  - An IgG concentration with 4-fold increase at least 7 days after rash onset vs. 14 days later by standard serologic assay is confirmatory.
- Culturing measles virus is difficult; not commonly performed.
- Mild neutropenia is common.
- Liver transaminases and pancreatic amylase may be elevated, particularly in adults.

ALERT

Suspected measles cases in the US must be reported to the local or state health department.

Imaging

CXR is appropriate when suspicion exists of secondary pneumonia.

DIFFERENTIAL DIAGNOSIS
- Drug eruptions
- Rubella
- *Mycoplasma pneumoniae*
- Infectious mononucleosis
- Parvovirus B19 infection
- Roseola
- Enteroviruses
- Rocky Mountain spotted fever
- Dengue
- Toxic shock syndrome
- Meningococcemia
- Kawasaki disease

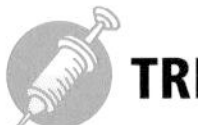

TREATMENT

MEDICATION
- No approved antiviral therapy is available. Immunosuppressed children with severe measles have been treated with IV or aerosolized ribavirin, but no controlled data exist, and this use is not approved by the FDA.
- Antibiotics:
  - Reserved for patients with clinical signs of bacterial superinfection
  - Although a 2006 Cochrane Review reported insufficient evidence to justify prophylactic antibiotics for prevention of measles-associated pneumonia, a small 2006 randomized, double-blinded trial resulted in an 80% (number needed to treat [NNT] = 7) decrease in measles-associated pneumonia with use of prophylactic antibiotics; authors suggest the use of prophylactic antibiotics in patients with a high risk of complications (6)[B].
- Vitamin A:
  - Children 6–12 months of age receive 100,000 IU as 1 dose.
  - Children >12 months of age receive 200,000 IU as 1 dose:
    - American Academy of Pediatrics recommends only in limited circumstances: Hospitalized children aged 6–12 months; children >6 months of age with other risk factors for complications
    - Limited evidence exists to generalize efficacy to developed countries.
- Outbreak control:
  - The CDC defines an outbreak of measles as a single case.
  - Prompt immunization (within 72 hours) of people at risk of exposure or already exposed who cannot provide documentation of measles immunity:
    - Monovalent vaccine may be given to infants 6 months–1 year of age, but 2 further doses of vaccine after 12 months must be given for appropriate immunization.
    - Monovalent or combination vaccine may be given to all measles-exposed susceptible individuals where not contraindicated.
    - Individuals who have not been immunized within 72 hours of exposure should be excluded from school, child care, and health care settings until 2 weeks after onset of rash in last case of measles.
  - Immunoglobulin (passive immunity) may be necessary for certain high-risk individuals exposed to measles where vaccine is inappropriate:
    - IM immunoglobulin should be given within 6 days of exposure to measles; CDC recommends 0.25 mL/kg to maximum of 15 mL; immunocompromised individuals receive 0.5 mL/kg to a maximum of 15 mL.
    - Children <1 year old
    - Pregnant women
    - Individuals with severe immunosuppression

ADDITIONAL TREATMENT

General Measures
- Supportive therapy (i.e., antipyretics, antitussives, humidification, increased consumption of oral fluids)
- Control:
  - All patients with measles should be placed in respiratory isolation until 4 days after onset of rash; immunocompromised patients should be isolated for duration of illness.
  - Notify public health officials of suspected cases.

IN-PATIENT CONSIDERATIONS
Outpatient care is appropriate, except where complications develop (e.g., encephalitis, pneumonia).

ONGOING CARE

FOLLOW-UP RECOMMENDATIONS
Patients are advised to call their doctor if they develop any:
- Difficulty breathing or noisy breathing
- Changes in vision
- Changes in behavior, confusion
- Chest or abdominal pain

PATIENT EDUCATION
- Avoid exposure to other individuals, particularly unimmunized children and adults, pregnant women, and immunocompromised persons, until 4 days after rash onset.
- Avoid contact with potential sources of secondary bacterial pathogens until respiratory symptoms resolve.

PROGNOSIS
- Typically self-limited; prognosis good
- High fatality rates may be seen among malnourished or immunocompromised children, particularly in developing countries.
- Complications occur in up to 40% of cases.

COMPLICATIONS
- Otitis media (occurs in 5–15%)
- Respiratory complications:
  - Bronchopneumonia (occurs in 5–10%):
    - Accounts for most measles-related deaths
    - May be viral or bacterial
  - Interstitial pneumonitis: In immunocompromised patients
  - Laryngotracheobronchitis ("measles croup"): Occurs in younger age group (<2 years of age)
- GI complications: Diarrhea (may lead to dehydration)
- Neurologic complications:
  - Febrile seizures
  - Acute disseminated encephalomyelitis with seizures and variety of neurologic abnormalities (occurs in 1/1,000 cases): Presents soon after measles resolves
  - Subacute sclerosing panencephalitis (SSPE):
    - Rare degenerative CNS disease resulting from persistent measles infection following natural disease
    - Presents 5–15 years after infection
    - Disappearing as a result of mass vaccination
- Ocular complications: Keratitis:
  - Can lead to permanent scarring, blindness
  - Vitamin A deficiency predisposes to more severe keratitis and its complications.
- Other secondary bacterial infections
- Death: Results from complications, mainly pneumonia, rather than the virus itself

REFERENCES

1. Lessler J, Reich NG, Brookmeyer R, et al. Incubation periods of acute respiratory viral infections: A systematic review. *Lancet Infect Dis*. 2009;9: 291–300.
2. Orenstein WA, Papania MJ, Wharton ME. Measles elimination in the United States. *J Infect Dis*. 2004;189(Suppl 1):S1–3.
3. Centers for Disease Control and Prevention (CDC), et al. Measles imported by returning U.S. travelers aged 6-23 months, 2001-2011. *MMWR Morb Mortal Wkly Rep*. 2011;60:397–400.
4. Althouse BM, Bergstrom TC, Bergstrom CT, et al. Evolution in health and medicine Sackler colloquium: A public choice framework for controlling transmissible and evolving diseases. *Proc Natl Acad Sci USA*. 2010;107(Suppl 1): 1696–701.
5. Demicheli V, Jefferson T, Rivetti A, et al. Vaccines for measles, mumps and rubella in children. *Cochrane Database Syst Rev*. 2005;CD004407.
6. Garly ML, Balé C, Martins CL, et al. Prophylactic antibiotics to prevent pneumonia and other complications after measles: Community based randomised double blind placebo controlled trial in Guinea-Bissau. *BMJ*. 2006;333:1245.

CODES

ICD9
- 055.1 Postmeasles pneumonia
- 055.79 Measles with other specified complications
- 055.9 Measles without mention of complication

CLINICAL PEARLS
- Measles is a highly communicable viral disease whose natural transmission has been halted in the US by mass immunization.
- Immunization of the general public requires 2 doses: 1 at 12–15 months of age and 1 at school age (4–6 years of age).
- Presentation includes a prodrome of fever, cough, coryza, and conjunctivitis, followed by a descending maculopapular rash.
- Suspected measles cases must be reported to state or local health departments, and measures taken to contain outbreak.
- Measles-associated pneumonia is the most common cause of mortality.

MEASLES, GERMAN (RUBELLA)

Jennifer P. Herbert, MD

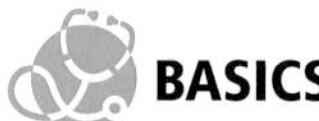

BASICS

DESCRIPTION

- Rubella is a mild viral exanthematous infection of children and adults, generally self-limiting, with rare complications. Nonimmune women who become infected with rubella while pregnant may have devastating fetal effects. Up to 50% of infections may be asymptomatic (1).
- Systems affected: Hematologic; Nervous; Pulmonary; Exocrine; Ophthalmologic; Skeletal
- Synonyms: German measles; 3-day measles

Pregnancy Considerations

- Pregnancy-associated rubella infection may lead to congenital rubella syndrome (CRS) with potentially devastating fetal outcomes.
- CRS is present in 90% of fetuses exposed during the first 11 weeks of gestation and 20% of fetuses exposed by 20 weeks of gestation (2).
- Most effective prevention of CRS is screening pregnant women for rubella immunity and immunizing nonimmune women postpartum (2)[B].
- Women vaccinated against rubella are advised not to become pregnant for 28 days: The vaccine-type virus can cross the placenta. No case of CRS has occurred after inadvertent vaccination, but a risk of 0.5–1.3% cannot be ruled out (2)[C].
- PCR–based method (87–100% sensitive) of detecting viral RNA in amniotic fluid allows rapid diagnosis of fetal infection if performed after 15 weeks gestation; however, recent studies have indicated that fetal blood sampling at the same gestation yielded rubella-specific RNA where amniotic fluid failed (3)[B].

EPIDEMIOLOGY

- A 50–70 nm RNA togavirus of the genus *Rubivirus* (1)
- 13 genotypes have been identified (4).
- Live attenuated vaccine made first available in the US in 1969
- Since 2004, not endemic in the US. All cases are of imported origin: Travelers with inadequate immunity (1).
- Average incubation: 14 days; range of 12–23 days
- Infectious period between 7 days before and 5–7 days after rash onset
- Transmitted by respiratory droplets
- Temporal association: Late winter and early spring
- Only natural host is the human (1)

Incidence

- US incidence <10/100,000 since 2001
- 5 cases were reported in the US in 2010.
- Still occurs worldwide in developing countries: 100,000 cases of CRS reported annually.

RISK FACTORS

Inadequate immunization or immunity after prior vaccination, immunodeficiency states, immunosuppressive therapy, crowded living/working conditions, international travel (1)[C]

Genetics

Children with CRS and children with type I DM share a high frequency of HLA-DR3 histocompatibility Ag and a high prevalence of islet cell Ab.

GENERAL PREVENTION

- Vaccination most effective preventive strategy
- Available combined with measles and mumps (MMR), combined MMR and varicella (MMRV), or as monovalent rubella vaccine
- Rubella vaccine (strain RA 27/3):
  - A 2-dose schedule combined MMR vaccine recommended for those born after 1957. The first dose recommended at ages 12–15 months; second dose recommended either at 4–6 or at 11–12 years of age. Children with HIV should receive MMR vaccine at 12 months of age if no contraindications exist. If an outbreak occurs, immediate vaccination for infants 6–11 months old is recommended (2).
  - Recommended for nonimmune people in the following groups: Prepubertal boys and girls, premarital or postpartum women, college students, daycare personnel, health care workers, and military personnel
- Contraindicated: Pregnancy, immunodeficiency (except HIV infection), within 3 months of IVIG or blood administration, severe febrile illness, or hypersensitivity to vaccine components. Patients who receive rubella vaccine do not transmit rubella to others, although the virus can be isolated from the pharynx (1).
- During outbreaks, serologic screening before vaccination is NOT recommended because rapid mass vaccination is necessary to stop the spread of the disease (2)[A].
- Debate about safety of MMR vaccine: Continued studies conducted prove the dissociation of the MMR vaccine with autism (5). Cochrane systematic review stated that it is unlikely to be associated with Crohn disease or ulcerative colitis. It is likely to be associated with benign thrombocytopenic purpura, parotitis, joint and limb complaints, febrile seizures, and aseptic meningitis (mumps).
- Children who receive the MMRV vaccine experience a 2-fold increase in incidence of febrile seizures than those who receive MMR and varicella vaccines separately (5).
- Because the US has adequate vaccination capabilities, antibody screening in prenatal care is recommended by the CDC and the ACOG, and should be reinforced (6)[B].

PATHOPHYSIOLOGY

- The virus invades the respiratory epithelium, spreads hematogenously to the lymphatics, where it starts replicating. Once infected, the patient starts shedding the virus from the nasopharynx 3–8 days after inoculation, lasting up to 14 days after the rash starts.
- Progression from prodromal stage (1–5 days), to lymphadenopathy (5–10 days), and finally to a light pink, pruritic, maculopapular rash: Starts on the face and spreads inferiorly to the trunk and extremities, sparing the palms and soles (14–17 days after onset of initial symptoms)
- 90% of fetuses exposed to rubella in the first 11 weeks of gestation (organogenesis) will develop CRS. 20% chance of developing CRS if exposed 12–20 weeks of gestation, and after 20 weeks gestation the risk drops to 2% (2).

ETIOLOGY

- German measles first described by German authors in the mid-18th century; thought to be a variant form of either measles or scarlet fever
- In 1815, described in the English literature by Manton; felt to be a separate entity from measles or scarlet fever
- Given the name rubella in 1866 by Veale
- 1962–1965: Global pandemic resulting in an estimated 12.5 million cases in the US with a devastating 2,000 cases of encephalitis, 11,250 cases of therapeutic or spontaneous abortions, 2,100 neonatal deaths, and 20,000 infants born with CRS (1)
- LAV licensed in the US in 1969 for the purpose of preventing CRS

DIAGNOSIS

Counsel of State and Territorial Epidemiologists (CSTE) Case Definition Classifications of Rubella (1):

- Clinical Case Definition:
  - Acute onset of generalized maculopapular rash
  - Temperature >99°F (37.2°C), if measured
  - Arthralgia or arthritis, lymphadenopathy or conjunctivitis
- Laboratory criteria for diagnosis:
  - Isolation of virus from: Throat or nasal swabs, serum, CSF, urine, or cataracts if removed from infected infant
  - 4-fold rise in acute- and convalescent-phase titers of serum IgG Ab
  - Positive serologic test for IgM Ab
  - PCR positive for virus

HISTORY

- Most cases of postnatal rubella are due to inadequately immunized travelers returning from endemic areas.
- Rubella can spread quickly among persons residing in close quarters.
- Postnatal rubella: Low-grade fever, sore throat, nausea, anorexia, arthritis, arthralgia, malaise. 50% may be asymptomatic.
- CRS: Parental concerns about hearing or vision impairment, jaundice, or developmental delay
- Deafness could be the only manifestation and not be noticed until second year of life (2).

PHYSICAL EXAM

- Postnatal rubella: Low-grade fever, lymphadenopathy (postauricular, occipital, posterior cervical), exanthem (mild, pink, discrete 1–4 mm maculopapular), soft palate petechiae (Forchheimer sign) (20%)
- CRS: Microcephaly, large anterior fontanelle, sensorineural hearing loss (58%), cataracts, glaucoma, microphthalmia, pigmentary retinopathy, purpuric ("blueberry muffin") skin lesions, murmur (50%) consistent with PDA or PPAS, hepatosplenomegaly with jaundice, cryptorchidism, inguinal hernia, radiolucent bone disease

DIAGNOSTIC TESTS & INTERPRETATION

Lab

- Because 50% of cases are subclinical, laboratory testing is the only way to confirm the diagnosis (1).
- Detection of wild-type virus is considered the gold standard (1).

- Enzyme immunoassay (EIA): Preferred testing for IgM antibodies, which may not be detectable before 5 days after the onset of rash (1)
- Hemagglutination inhibition (HAI) test: Was once the standard. A 4-fold increase of IgG Ab levels from acute to convalescent phase is diagnostic for recent infection (1).
- Latex agglutination (LA) test: Appears to be sensitive and specific, but dependent on experienced lab personnel (1)
- Immunofluorescent antibody (IFA) assay: Used for detection of IgG and IgM Ab to the virus (1)
- Avidity test: Not routine and should be performed in reference labs. Purpose: Distinguish between recent and past infections (1).
- Serum collection should be performed within 7–10 days after the onset of the illness. When testing for IgM, repeat collection may be necessary if the sample was taken before day 5. When testing for seroconversion, a second sample for IgG testing should be collected 2–3 weeks after the first specimen (acute to convalescent phase). In most cases, IgG is detectable 8 days after rash onset (1).
- The virus may be isolated from 1 week prior to 2 weeks after the rash onset. Maximal viral shedding occurs up to day 4 after rash onset. Best results yielded from throat swabs (1).
- Viral genotyping by RT-PCR is performed to help determine the country of origin for epidemiology. For typing, throat swabs should be collected 4 days after the rash onset and sent directly to the CDC (1).
- In general, viral cultures of CSF are only reserved for suspected cases of CRS or rubella encephalitis (1).
- If a pregnant female is exposed, amniotic fluid for PCR or fetal blood may be obtained at 15 weeks gestation for viral detection. Placental biopsy may be done at 12 weeks, but is performed less often. If positive, the parents should be offered genetic counseling (1).
- As the incidence of rubella decreases, the PPV of IgM results decreases. False positives can occur in patients with parvovirus B19, mononucleosis, and positive rheumatoid factor (1).
- After re-exposure, a person with a low level of Ab from past infection or vaccination may experience an acute, small rise in Ab levels. This is not associated with a high incidence of contagion to others or of fetal risk (1).

Follow-Up & Special Considerations

- Reporting: State dependent. Samples should be sent to the CDC for genotyping. Cases of CRS, report to the National Congenital Rubella Syndrome Registry (1,2).
- Infants with CRS may shed virus up to 1 year. Place on contact isolation during all admissions until their first birthday, unless they have 2 negative throat cultures and urine specimens a month apart once they are 3 months old (2).

Pathological Findings

- Pink, discrete, maculopapular rash that begins on the face and spreads down
- Congenital cataracts
- Purpuric lesions in the neonate ("blueberry muffin" baby)
- Congenital hearing loss

DIFFERENTIAL DIAGNOSIS

- Postnatal rubella:
  - Measles virus (rubeola)
  - Scarlet fever
  - Infectious mononucleosis
  - Erythema infectiosum (parvo B19/ Fifth disease)
  - Roseola infantum (i.e., exanthem subitum)
  - Toxoplasmosis
  - Drug eruptions
  - Other exanthematous enteroviral infections
- Congenital rubella:
  - Measles
  - Parvo B19
  - Human herpesvirus 6
  - Other exanthematous entero- or arboviruses

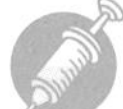

TREATMENT

- Supportive for mild cases
- Isolate patients for 5–7 days after the rash onset.
- Postnatal rubella: Mild and self-limited; treat for symptomatic relief. Hospitalize for complications: ITP or encephalitis, which may be associated with the vaccine.
- CRS: Supportive care unless neurologic or hemorrhagic complications develop; phototherapy may be indicated for jaundice; multidisciplinary management of long-term complications

MEDICATION

- No specific therapy available for mild cases
- Age- and dose-appropriate antipyretics
- NSAIDs can be used for arthritis and arthralgias in adults and infants older than 6 months.
- IVIG can be given in severe thrombocytopenia, but most cases are auto-limited.

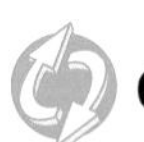

ONGOING CARE

FOLLOW-UP RECOMMENDATIONS

Patient Monitoring

- People immune to rubella via natural infection or vaccine may be reinfected when re-exposed; such infection is usually asymptomatic and detectable only by serology. Those who have received the vaccine have lower measurable IgG levels than those who had the natural disease.
- In CRS, it is extremely important to detect auditory and visual impairment early so that adequate education and counseling can begin (2).
- 2/3 of internationally adopted children have no written record of immunizations (4).

PATIENT EDUCATION

- Make every effort to avoid exposing infected patient to pregnant women.
- JAMA Patient Page on Rubella located at www.jama.com; go to Patient Page Index; click on "Previous Topics, Rubella (1/23–30/2002)."
- www.cdc.gov/rubella/
- www.nlm.nih.gov/medlineplus/ency/article/001574.htm

PROGNOSIS

- Postnatal rubella: Complete and full recovery without sequelae is the rule.
- CRS:
  - Varied and unpredictable spectrum ranging from stillbirth to completely normal infancy and childhood
  - Infants may remain contagious for up to 1 year after birth (2).
  - Detectable levels of IgG persist for years and then may decline (does not drop at the expected 2-fold dilution/month). By age 5, 20% have no detectable antibody (2).
  - IgM may not be detectable until 1 month after birth and may persist for 6–12 months (2).
  - Overall mortality 10%; greatest during first 6 months
  - 70% of encephalitis cases develop residual neuro defects, including autistic syndrome.
  - Prognosis is excellent when only minor congenital defects are present.

COMPLICATIONS

- Postinfectious encephalitis (1/5,000 cases)
- Thrombocytopenic purpura (1/3,000 cases)
- CRS: Incidence dependent on trimester exposed
- Rubella vaccine may rarely cause encephalitis or idiopathic thrombocytopenic purpura (ITP):
  - ITP is self-limited and is not a contraindication to the vaccine.

REFERENCES

1. Centers for Disease Control and Prevention. Manual for the surveillance of vaccine-preventable diseases, 4th ed; Chapter 14-Rubella. 2008 [cited 2011 July]; Available at: www.cdc.gov/vaccines/pubs/surv-manual/chpt14-rubella.html.
2. Centers for Disease Control and Prevention. Manual for surveillance of vaccine-preventable diseases 4th ed; Chapter 15-Congenitial Rubella Syndrome. 2008 [cited 2011 July]; Available at: www.cdc.gov/vaccines/pubs/surv-manual/chpt15-crs.html.
3. Tang J, Aarons E, Hesketh L, et al. Prenatal diagnosis of congenital rubella infection in the second trimester of pregnancy. *Prenat Diagn*. 2003:23(6):509–12.
4. Abernathy E, Hubschen J, Muller C, et al. Status of global virologic surveillance for rubella viruses. *JID*. 2011;204:524–32.
5. Lai J, Fay K, Bocchini J. Update on childhood and adolescent immunizations: Selected review of US recommendations and literature: Part 2. *Curr Opin Pediatr*. 2011;23:470–81.
6. Centers for Disease Control and Prevention. Recommendations of the Advisory Committee on Immunization Practices. *MMWR*. 2011:(2).

ADDITIONAL READING

- Morbidity and Mortality Weekly Report for case tracking
- Walling A. Measles, mumps, and rubella in pregnant women. *Am Fam Physician*. 2006;73(5):907–8.

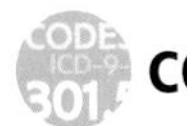

CODES

ICD9

- 056.00 Rubella with unspecified neurological complication
- 056.9 Rubella without mention of complication
- 771.0 Congenital rubella

CLINICAL PEARLS

The only vaccine designed to protect someone other than the vaccine recipient

M

MELANOMA

Richard F. DeSouza, MD

BASICS

DESCRIPTION

- Tumor arising from malignant degeneration of cells from the melanocytic system:
  - Most arise in the skin but also may present as a primary lesion in any tissue. Ocular, GI, genitourinary, lymph node, and leptomeninges are the primary extracutaneous sites.
  - Metastatic spread to any region in the body
- There are 4 main subtypes of malignant melanoma based on pathology: Superficial spreading melanoma, nodular, acral lentiginous, and lentigo maligna. The superficial spreading variant is the most common. The lentigo maligna variant is the slowest growing with the least tendency to metastasize.
- System(s) affected: Skin/Exocrine

Geriatric Considerations

Lentigo maligna is seen most commonly in elderly patients who have had a slowly enlarging pigmented lesion. This type is usually found on the face, beginning as a circumscribed macular patch of mottled pigmentation showing shades of dark brown, tan, or black.

Pediatric Considerations

Congenital large nevi (>5 cm) are risk factors and have a >2% lifetime risk of malignant conversion. Blistering sunburns in childhood significantly increase adult risk.

Pregnancy Considerations

- Because melanocyte-stimulating hormone (MSH) levels are markedly increased during pregnancy and melanoma is one of the few carcinomas that can spread to the placenta, there has been concern that pregnancy exacerbates melanoma. Data now suggest that there is no increased risk of melanoma with pregnancy (1)[B].
- It has been suggested to wait 1–2 years if further pregnancy is desired for patients with recent melanomas.

EPIDEMIOLOGY

Incidence

- In 2010, an estimated 68,130 invasive melanomas were diagnosed in the US.
- 1 in 63 Americans will develop melanoma (1) in their lifetime.
- Sixth most common cancer overall in the US (1), being the fifth most common in men and seventh most common in women
- Highest annual incidence rate of any cancer in whites between the ages of 25 and 29 years and in white males between 35 and 39 years of age
- Predominant age: Median age = 55 years; >50% of all individuals with melanoma are between 20 and 40 years of age.
- Predominant sex: Male > Female (1.5×)
- Incidence among whites is 10–20× greater than that among blacks or Hispanics.

Prevalence

- >29/100,000 white males and >19/100,000 white females
- ~2% of all cancer deaths
- In women, the most common location is the legs, and in men, the trunk.

RISK FACTORS

- Heavy ultraviolet A (UVA) and ultraviolet B (UVB) exposure
- Previous pigmented lesions (especially dysplastic or melanocytic nevi)
- Fair complexion, freckling, blue eyes, and blond or red hair
- Those with increased numbers of nevi (>100), highest predictor of risk
- Family history of melanoma
- Tanning bed use before age 30 years (controversial)
- Changing nevus
- Large (>5 cm) congenital nevi
- Other skin cancers
- Immunosuppression
- Blistering sunburns in childhood
- Occupational exposure to ionizing radiation
- Does not appear to be affected by pregnancy, oral contraceptives, or hormone replacement

Genetics

- In individuals with dysplastic nevi, a family history of dysplastic nevus syndrome with melanoma conveys a nearly 100% lifetime risk of development of melanoma. Close surveillance is indicated.
- An estimated 8–12% of patients with melanoma have a family history of the disease.
- Changes in oncogenes, suppressor gene growth factors, and receptors have been suggested as genetic effects from these chromosomal associations. Certain genes, such as CDKN2A and CDK4, have been suggested to play a role in some cases of melanoma.

GENERAL PREVENTION

- Avoidance of sunburn, especially in childhood, is important. Up to 2/3 of melanoma may be attributed to excessive sunlight exposure.
- While data on the effectiveness of sunscreen is limited, it is recommended that if one is going to be exposed to sunlight, it is best to generously apply sunscreen to all exposed skin using a product with a sun protection factor (SPF) of at least 15, reapplying every 2 hours.
- Avoid tanning beds.
- Primary prevention by large-scale screening has failed.
- Screening of high-risk individuals is likely to be successful.

PATHOPHYSIOLOGY

Under investigation, but clearly associated with exposure to UVA and UVB

COMMONLY ASSOCIATED CONDITIONS

- Dysplastic nevus syndrome
- Heavy mole formers are individuals on whom >50 nevi are found. These patients may have a higher lifetime risk of melanoma than the general population because 50–75% of all melanomas arise in pre-existing nevi.
- Giant congenital nevus syndrome is associated with an approximate 6% lifetime incidence of melanoma.
- Xeroderma pigmentosum is a rare condition associated with an extremely high risk of skin cancers, including melanoma.

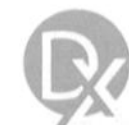

DIAGNOSIS

HISTORY

Change in a pigmented lesion: Hypo- or hyperpigmentation, bleeding, scaling, size change, texture change

PHYSICAL EXAM

- Use the ABCDE mnemonic: *A*symmetry; *B*order irregularity; *C*olor variegation (especially red, white, black, and blue hues); *D*iameter >6 mm; or *E*levation above skin surface
- Any new and/or changing nevus, bleeding or ulcerated
- Location on whites is primarily the back and lower leg, and on blacks is the hands, feet, and nails.
- Individuals at high risk for melanoma should have a careful ocular exam to assess for presence of melanoma in the iris, retina, or other pigmented eye cells (2)[C].

DIAGNOSTIC TESTS & INTERPRETATION

Lab

With metastatic disease, lactate dehydrogenase (LDH) determination may be helpful.

Imaging

Initial approach

Imaging studies are of benefit only in detecting metastatic disease, which is usually to the brain, lymph nodes, and lungs.

Diagnostic Procedures/Surgery

- Surgical biopsy is the only appropriate diagnostic procedure. Any suspicious nevus or pigmented lesion should be excised. A full-thickness biopsy with a cuff of fat should be sent for pathologic evaluation (3). Lesions never should be curetted, electrodesiccated, or shaved (known or strongly suspected melanoma), although low-likelihood lesions are sometimes removed by deep shave technique. Any irregularly pigmented lesion >2 cm in a preadolescent individual should be considered for excision.
- Frozen sections are also not indicated.
- Once diagnosed, see below for surgical management.

Pathological Findings

- Gross pathologic features include 4 clinical types:
  - Superficial spreading melanoma: 70–75%
  - Nodular: 15%
  - Acral lentiginous: 2–8%
  - Lentigo maligna: 4–10% (a small percentage are amelanotic)
- Nodular melanoma is primarily vertical growth, whereas the other 3 types are horizontal.
- Importance of number of mitoses and presence of ulceration increasing (3)
- Immunohistochemical testing on melanoma cells increases sensitivity of lymph node biopsies, but clinical application is still being investigated (1,4).

DIFFERENTIAL DIAGNOSIS
- Dysplastic and blue nevi
- Vascular skin tumor
- Actinic keratosis
- Traumatic hematoma
- Lentigo
- Pigmented squamous cell and basal cell carcinomas, seborrheic keratoses, other changing nevi

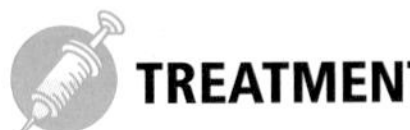

TREATMENT

MEDICATION
- While at the early stage surgical excision is curative in most cases; in most patients with stage IV disease systemic treatment with chemotherapy is required.
- Single-agent cytotoxic chemotherapy, most commonly with agents such as dacarbazine or temozolomide, can cause partial remissions, though the effect appears transient and there is no increase in survival.
- Combination chemotherapy also has not shown an increase in survival and does not appear to have any advantage over a single-agent regimen.
- High-dose interleukin-2 (IL-2) immunotherapy is associated with prolonged survival in a certain select group of patients, and may actually result in cure. Due to its associated toxicity, not all patients will be able to tolerate or be candidates for this treatment.
- Ipilimumab, a monoclonal antibody targeting CTLA-4, has been shown to increase overall survival in patients with advanced melanoma who have failed previous systemic therapy, and is recommended for those who are not candidates for high-dose IL-2 therapy.
- Interferon-alfa-2b has not shown increased benefit in disease-free time and overall survival (4,5)[B].

ADDITIONAL TREATMENT

General Measures
Fully excise lesion with a 2-mm rim of normal skin is the primary treatment for melanoma.

Issues for Referral
- Consultation with oncology is highly recommended for consideration of chemotherapeutic options.
- Referral to a regional melanoma center is often done.
- Cosmetic surgery is often needed once final excision is done.
- Isolated metastases may be treated surgically.
- Localized metastases (i.e., extremity) may be treated with regional chemotherapy (3).

Additional Therapies
- Molecular targeted therapies are under investigation, for example the use of inhibitors of *BRAF* in those patients who have the characteristic mutations in the *BRAF* gene.
- Early benefit with vaccines has not stood the test of time (4,5)[B].

COMPLEMENTARY AND ALTERNATIVE MEDICINE
Many have been tried with no lasting benefits.

SURGERY/OTHER PROCEDURES
- Appropriate treatment for melanoma is surgical excision.
- Extent of excision margins is becoming standardized. Generally, achieve margins of 1 cm if the lesion is <1 mm thick. If 1–2 mm, extend margins to 1–2 cm (4,6)[B].
- Sentinel lymph node biopsy for lesions of 1–4 mm deep has become standard of care in many locations. However, increased survival has not been demonstrated.
- Elective lymph node dissection is no longer an option (4,6)[B].

IN-PATIENT CONSIDERATIONS

Initial Stabilization
Most surgeries are done as outpatients with no stabilization needed.

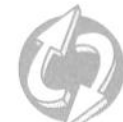

ONGOING CARE

FOLLOW-UP RECOMMENDATIONS
Once diagnosed, close follow-up and avoidance of UVA and UVB are highly advised.

Patient Monitoring
- Skin exams every 3–6 months in patients with history of melanoma
- Those with 1 melanoma diagnosed are at much greater risk for subsequent new primary melanomas.
- Thorough skin self-exams weekly

DIET
No data suggesting the benefit or risk of dietary manipulations

PATIENT EDUCATION
- Teach patients who are at risk or have had melanoma the principles of ABCDE examinations.
- Patients with a history of melanoma or dysplastic nevus syndrome must have frequent total-body examinations for any abnormal-appearing or changing nevi.
- Educational materials are available at the National Cancer Institute, Department of Health and Human Services, Public Inquiries Section, Office of Cancer Communications, Building 31, Room 101-18, 9000 Rockville Pike, Bethesda, MD 20892; (301) 496-5583.

PROGNOSIS
Prognosis is based on staging of the initial lesion:
- Staging (falls into 3 categories):
  - Breslow: 70% 5-year survival of patients without local or distant lymphatic spread
  - Clark staging depends on depth of invasion by skin layer. The best prognosis is for lesions that are <0.85 mm (especially if restricted to the stratum granulosum or higher), which carry 95–100% 5-year survival. Spread to lymphatics or regional lymph nodes carries a $<5\%$ 5-year survival.
  - American Joint Committee on Cancer (AJCC): Stage 0 in situ and lentigo maligna, stages I and II localized to skin, stage III regional lymph node or satellite lesions, stage IV distant metastases
- Women have a better prognosis than men.
- Truncal lesions have a poorer prognosis.
- With distant metastases, disease is uniformly lethal.
- Lesions with ulceration at the time of presentation have a significantly poorer prognosis.

COMPLICATIONS
- Metastatic spread
- Unsatisfactory cosmetic results following the primary surgery

REFERENCES

1. Markovic SN, Erickson LA, Rao RD, et al. Malignant melanoma in the 21st century, part 1: Epidemiology, risk factors, screening, prevention, and diagnosis. *Mayo Clin Proc.* 2007;82:364–80.
2. Bataille V, deVries E. Melanoma-Part 1: Epidemiology, risk factors and prevention. *BMJ.* 2008:337:a2249, 1287–91.
3. Thurwell C, Nathan P, Melanoma-Part 2: Management. *BMJ.* 2008:337:a2488, 1345–8.
4. Lane JE, Dalton RR, Sanguqza OP. Cutaneous melanoma. *J Fam Prac.* 2007;56(1):18–28.
5. Gogas HJ, Kirkwood JM, Sondak VK. Chemotherapy for metastatic melanoma: Time for a change? *Cancer.* 2007;109:455–64.
6. Markovic SN, Erickson LA, Rao RD, et al. Malignant melanoma in the 21st century, part 2: Staging, prognosis, and treatment. *Mayo Clin Proc.* 2007; 82:490–513.

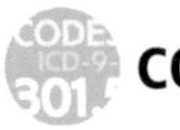

CODES

ICD9
- 172.0 Malignant melanoma of skin of lip
- 172.1 Malignant melanoma of skin of eyelid, including canthus
- 172.9 Melanoma of skin, site unspecified

CLINICAL PEARLS
- Up to 5% of new melanomas are from an unknown primary. Always consider melanoma if a lymph node is enlarged and nontender.
- Don't forget that amelanotic melanomas exist; the physician should biopsy new sites of no pigment or loss of pigment.
- 80% of cutaneous melanomas arise in existing nevi. Any changing nevi should be considered for full-thickness biopsy.

MÉNIÈRE DISEASE

Shanin Gross, DO

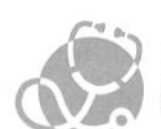

BASICS

DESCRIPTION

- An inner ear (labyrinthine) disorder characterized by recurrent attacks of hearing loss, tinnitus, vertigo, and sensations of aural fullness. Generally believed to be caused by, or related to, an increase in the volume and pressure of the inner ear endolymph fluid (endolymphatic hydrops).
- Often unilateral initially, but it is estimated that nearly half become bilateral over time.
- Severity and frequency of vertigo may diminish over time, but hearing loss is often progressive and/or fluctuating.
- Usually idiopathic (Ménière disease), but may be secondary to another condition causing endolymphatic hydrops (Ménière syndrome)
- System(s) affected: Nervous
- Synonym(s): Ménière syndrome; Endolymphatic hydrops

EPIDEMIOLOGY

- Predominant age of onset: 40–60 years
- Predominant gender: Female > Male (1.3:1)
- Race/ethnicity: White, northern European > blacks

Incidence

Estimates 1–150/100,000/year

Prevalence

Varies from ~7.5 to >200/100,000

RISK FACTORS

Not well understood, but *may* include:

- Stress
- Allergy
- Increased salt intake
- Caffeine, alcohol, or nicotine intake
- Chronic exposure to loud noise
- Family history of Ménière
- Certain vascular abnormalities (patients may also have history of migraines)
- Certain viral exposures (especially herpes simplex virus [HSV])

Genetics

Some families show increased incidence, but genetic vs. environmental influences are not well understood.

GENERAL PREVENTION

Reduce risk factors: Stress; salt, alcohol, and caffeine intake; smoking; noise exposure; ototoxic drugs (aspirin, quinine, aminoglycosides, etc.)

PATHOPHYSIOLOGY

Not fully understood; theories include increased pressure of the endolymph fluid due to increased fluid production or decreased resorption. This may be caused by endolymphatic sac pathology, abnormal development of the vestibular aqueduct, or inflammation caused by circulating immune complexes. Increased endolymph pressure may cause rupture of membranes and changes in endolymphatic ionic gradient.

ETIOLOGY

Idiopathic (Ménière *disease)*, but Ménière *syndrome* may be secondary to injury or other disorder (e.g., reduced middle ear pressure, allergy, endocrine disease, lipid disorders, vascular, viral, syphilis, autoimmune). Any disorder that could cause endolymph hydrops could be implicated in Ménière *syndrome*.

COMMONLY ASSOCIATED CONDITIONS

- Endolymphatic hydrops
- Anxiety (secondary to the disabling symptoms)
- Migraines
- Theorized: Hypothyroidism
- Hyperprolactinemia

DIAGNOSIS

Diagnosis is clinical. Tests rule out other conditions (1)[B].

HISTORY

Attacks are typically spontaneous, but may be preceded by an aura of increasing fullness in the ear and tinnitus. These may occur in clusters with long intervening symptom-free remissions. Signs and symptoms to look for include:

- Formal criteria for diagnosis from AAO-HNS:
  - At least 2 episodes of rotational-horizontal vertigo >20 minutes in duration
  - Tinnitus or aural fullness
  - Hearing loss: Low frequency (sensorineural) confirmed by audiometric testing
  - Other causes (acoustic neuroma, etc.) excluded
  - During severe attacks: Pallor, sweating, nausea, vomiting, falling, prostration
  - Symptoms are exacerbated by motion.
  - Between attacks, affected patients may experience motion-related imbalance without vertigo.
  - Caution: Many conditions may produce auditory and vestibular findings identical to those associated with Ménière disease.

PHYSICAL EXAM

- Physical exam rules out other conditions; no finding is unique to Ménière disease.
- Horizontal nystagmus may be seen during attacks.
- Otoscopy is typically normal.
- Triggering of attacks in the office with Dix-Hallpike maneuver suggests diagnosis of benign paroxysmal positional vertigo, not Ménière.

DIAGNOSTIC TESTS & INTERPRETATION

Testing done to rule out other conditions, and does not necessarily confirm or exclude Ménière disease

Lab

Initial lab tests

- Consider serologic tests specific for *Treponema pallidum* in at-risk populations: Microhemagglutination (MHA), fluorescent treponemal antibody (FTA), *Treponema* immobilization test (TPI) (1)[C]
- Thyroid, fasting blood sugar, and lipid studies

Imaging

MRI to rule out acoustic neuroma or other CNS pathology, including tumor, aneurysm, and multiple sclerosis (MS).

Initial approach

- Detailed history and physical exam
- Labs, audiometry, consider MRI

Diagnostic Procedures/Surgery

- Auditory:
  - Audiometry using pure tone and speech to show low-frequency sensorineural (nerve) loss and impaired speech discrimination. Usually shows low-frequency sensorineural hearing loss.
  - Tuning fork tests (i.e., Weber and Rinne) will confirm validity of audiometry.
  - Auditory brainstem response audiometry (ABR) to rule out acoustic neuroma
  - Electrocochleography (ECOG) may be useful to confirm etiology (1).
- Vestibular:
  - Caloric testing: Electronystagmography (ENG) may show reduced caloric response. Can obtain reasonably comparable information with use of 0.8 mL of ice water caloric testing. Reduced activity on either side is consistent with Ménière diagnosis, but is not itself diagnostic.
  - Drugs that may alter lab results: Any sedating medication may affect and invalidate vestibular testing.

Pathological Findings

Histologic temporal bone analysis (at autopsy). Dilation of inner ear fluid system may be seen.

DIFFERENTIAL DIAGNOSIS

- Acoustic neuroma or other CNS tumor
- Syphilis
- Perilymphatic fistula
- Viral labyrinthitis
- Transient ischemic attack (TIA), migraine
- Vertebrobasilar disease
- Other labyrinthine disorders that produce similar symptoms (e.g., Cogan syndrome, benign positional vertigo, temporal bone trauma)
- Diabetes or thyroid dysfunction
- Vestibular neuronitis
- Medication side effects
- Otitis media

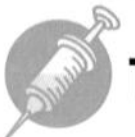

TREATMENT

- Can usually be managed in outpatient setting
- A paucity of evidence-based guidelines exist regarding treatment for Ménière disease; therefore, there is no "gold standard" treatment.
- Medications are given primarily for symptomatic relief of vertigo and nausea, not to change disease progression.
- During attacks, bed rest with eyes closed and protection from falling. Attacks rarely last >4 hours.

MEDICATION

First Line

- Acute attack: Initial goal is immediate stabilization and symptom relief. For severe episodes, choose 1 (2)[C]:
  - Benzodiazepines (such as diazepam): Decrease vertigo and anxiety
  - Antihistamines (meclizine/dimenhydrinate): Decrease vertigo and nausea
  - Anticholinergics (transdermal scopolamine): Prevents nausea and emesis associated with "motion sickness"
  - Antidopaminergic (metoclopramide, promethazine): Decreases nausea, anxiety
  - Rehydration therapy and electrolyte replacement
  - Steroid taper for acute hearing loss
- Maintenance (goal is to prevent/reduce attacks)
- Lifestyle changes (low-salt diet, etc.) are needed.

- Diuretics are frequently used, and may help reduce attacks by decreasing the pressure and volume of endolymphatic fluid; however, there is insufficient evidence at this time (2)[C],(3)[A]:
  - Hydrochlorothiazide/Triamterene (Dyazide, Maxzide)
  - Acetazolamide (Diamox)
- Contraindications:
  - Atropine: Cardiac disease, especially SVT and other arrhythmias, prostatic enlargement
  - Scopolamine: Children and elderly, prostatic enlargement
  - Diuretics: Electrolyte abnormalities, renal disease
- Precautions:
  - Sedating drugs should be used with caution, particularly in the elderly. Patients should be cautioned not to operate motor vehicles or machinery. Atropine and scopolamine should be used with particular caution.
  - Diuretics: Monitor electrolytes. Use with caution in patients with sulfa allergy.
- Significant possible interactions: Transdermal scopolamine: Anticholinergics, belladonna products, antihistamines, tricyclic antidepressants, other

Second Line

- Steroids have been used, both intratympanic and systemically (PO or IV) for longer treatment of hearing loss:
  - Intratympanic administration results in higher steroid levels in the inner ear and may be more effective and safer than systemic (2)[C].
  - Addition of prednisone 30 mg/d to diuretic treatment reduced severity and frequency of tinnitus and vertigo in one pilot study.
- In Europe, one of the preferred drugs is betahistine, a histamine agonist (unavailable in the US). Insufficient evidence to state effectiveness: Other vasodilators, such as isosorbide dinitrate, niacin and histamine, have also been used, but evidence of their effectiveness is sparse (2)[C].
- Famvir has also been studied for the treatment of vertigo and stabilization of hearing. Evidence is lacking, but indicates more improvement in hearing than balance [B].
- Inner ear perfusion with gentamicin and steroids have helped control and stabilize vertigo and hearing loss in Ménière disease (4)[A].

ADDITIONAL TREATMENT

Issues for Referral

- Consider ear, nose, throat (ENT)/neurology referral for confirmation, further testing.
- All patients need formal audiometry to confirm hearing loss.

Additional Therapies

- Application of intermittent pressures via a myringotomy using a Meniett device has been found in some studies to relieve dizziness:
  - Safe; requires a long-term tympanostomy tube
- Vestibular rehabilitation may be beneficial for patients with persistent vestibular symptoms (5)[A]:
  - Safe and effective treatment for unilateral vestibular dysfunction
  - When attacks are disabling, the patient should be encouraged to slowly resume activity as soon as able.

COMPLEMENTARY AND ALTERNATIVE MEDICINE

Insufficient evidence to support effectiveness, but many integrative (CAM) techniques have been tried, including (2)[C]:

- Acupuncture (6)[A], acupressure, tai chi
- Niacin, bioflavonoids, lipoflavonoids, ginger, ginkgo biloba, and other herbal supplements

SURGERY/OTHER PROCEDURES

- Interventions that preserve hearing (7)[B]:
  - Endolymphatic sac surgery, either decompression or drainage of endolymph into mastoid or subarachnoid space:
    - Less invasive; may decrease vertigo, may influence hearing or tinnitus
    - There is insufficient evidence of the beneficial effect of endolymphatic sac surgery in Ménière disease (8)[A].
  - Vestibular nerve section (intracranial procedure):
    - More invasive due to intracranial location
    - Decreases vertigo and preserves hearing
  - Tympanostomy tube: May decrease symptoms by decreasing the middle ear pressure
- Interventions for patients with no serviceable hearing (7)[C]:
  - Labyrinthectomy: Very effective at controlling vertigo, but causes deafness
  - Vestibular neurectomy
  - Many patients may be candidates for cochlear implantation if they have lost serviceable hearing.

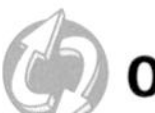

ONGOING CARE

FOLLOW-UP RECOMMENDATIONS

Patient Monitoring

Due to the possibility of progressive hearing loss despite eventual decrease in vertiginous attacks, it is important to have close follow-up to monitor changes in hearing, and continue surveillance for more serious underlying causes (acoustic neuroma, etc.).

DIET

- Diet is usually not a factor, unless attacks are brought on by certain foods.
- Some physicians restrict salt, but this is not supported by randomized controlled trials (1)[C].

PATIENT EDUCATION

- Limit activity during attacks.
- Between attacks, patient may be fully active, but is often limited due to fear or lingering symptoms. This can be severely disabling.
- Patient information, including support group contacts, is available from the Vestibular Disorders Association (www.vestibular.org) and the American Academy of Otolaryngology-Head and Neck Surgery (www.entnet.org/HealthInformation/menieresDisease.cfm).

PROGNOSIS

- Alternating attacks and remission
- 1/2 of cases resolve spontaneously within 2–3 years, but can last >20 years. Severity and frequency of attacks diminish, but hearing loss is often progressive.
- 90% of patients can be managed successfully with medication. 5–10% of patients require surgery for incapacitating vertigo.
- Clinicians must not overlook possibility of acoustic tumor, which produces an identical clinical picture.

COMPLICATIONS

Loss of hearing; injury during attack; inability to work

REFERENCES

1. Sajjadi H, Paparella MM. Meniere's disease. *Lancet*. 2008;372:406–14.
2. Coelho DH, Lalwani AK. Medical management of Ménière's disease. *Laryngoscope*. 2008;118(6): 1099–108.
3. Thirlwall AS, Kundu S. Diuretics for Ménière's disease or syndrome. *Cochrane Database Syst Rev*. 2006;3:CD003599.
4. Hamid M, et al. Medical management of common peripheral vestibular diseases. *Curr Opin Otolaryngol Head Neck Surg*. 2010;18:407–12.
5. Hillier SL, Hollohan V. Vestibular rehabilitation for unilateral peripheral vestibular dysfunction. *Cochrane Database Syst Rev*. 2007;CD005397.
6. Long AF, Xing M, Morgan K, et al. Exploring the evidence base for acupuncture in the treatment of Meniere's syndrome–A systematic review. *Evid Based Complement Alternat Med*. 2009. Epub ahead of print.
7. van Benthem PP, Giard JL, Verschuur HP. Surgery for Ménière's disease (Protocol). *Cochrane Database Syst Rev*. 2005;3:CD005395.
8. Pullens B, Giard JL, Verschuur HP, van Benthem PP, et al. Surgery for Ménière's disease. *Cochrane Database Syst Rev*. 2010;CD005395.

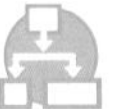

See Also (Topic, Algorithm, Electronic Media Element)

- Hearing Loss; Labyrinthitis; Tinnitus
- Algorithm: Vertigo

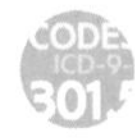

CODES

ICD9

- 386.00 Meniere's disease, unspecified
- 386.01 Active Ménière's disease, cochleovestibular
- 386.02 Active Ménière's disease, cochlear

CLINICAL PEARLS

- Diagnosis of Ménière disease is clinical, based on repeated episodes of vertigo, hearing loss, and tinnitus or aural fullness.
- Multiple medical, surgical, and rehabilitative treatments are available to decrease the severity and frequency of attacks. Some of these may preserve hearing, while some destroy it.
- A patient is likely to have progressive hearing loss despite a natural progression toward fewer vertigo attacks.
- When considering Ménière disease in a patient with vertigo and hearing loss, acoustic neuromas must also be considered.
- Take symptoms seriously, as they may be disabling.

M

MENINGITIS, BACTERIAL

Paul R. Gordon, MD, MPH

BASICS

DESCRIPTION

- Bacterial meningitis is an inflammation of the pia-arachnoid and its fluid and the fluid of the ventricles:
  - Always cerebrospinal
- System(s) affected: Nervous

ALERT

Bacterial meningitis is a medical, neurological, and sometimes neurosurgical emergency. Community-acquired meningitis caused by *Streptococcus pneumoniae* has case fatality rates from 19–37% in adults.

Geriatric Considerations

Signs and symptoms may be less evident and less specific in elderly patients with other disorders, such as congestive heart failure and pneumonia.

EPIDEMIOLOGY

- Predominant age: Neonates, infants, and elderly
- Predominant sex: Male = Female

Incidence

3–10/100,000 population

RISK FACTORS

- Immunocompromised host
- Alcoholism, diabetes
- Neurosurgical procedure or head injury
- Abdominal surgery at risk for gram-negative infection

Genetics

Individuals of Navajo Indian or American Eskimo descent may have genetic or acquired vulnerability to invasive disease.

GENERAL PREVENTION

- Prompt medical treatment for infections
- Strict aseptic techniques when treating patients with head wounds or skull fractures
- Look for evidence of CSF fistula in patients with recurrent meningitis.
- Meningitis caused by *Haemophilus influenzae* has been nearly eliminated due to routine vaccination.
- Conjugate vaccines against *S. pneumoniae* may reduce the burden of disease in childhood and may produce herd immunity among adults.
- Persons with close contact to patients with meningococcal meningitis must receive chemoprophylaxis to eradicate carriage.

PATHOPHYSIOLOGY

Bacterial infection causes inflammation of the pia-arachnoid and its fluid and the fluid of the ventricles.

ETIOLOGY

Bacteria are divided into age groups to guide empiric therapy (percentages indicate relative incidence). Any organism can cause meningitis in any age group; therapy should be guided by culture whenever possible:

- Neonates:
  - Group B *Streptococcus*: 50% of cases
  - *Escherichia coli*: 25%
  - Other gram-negative rods: 8%
  - *Listeria monocytogenes*: 6%
  - *S. pneumoniae*: 5%
  - Group A *Streptococcus*: 4%
  - *H. influenzae*: 3%
- In adults up to age 60:
  - *S. pneumoniae*: 60%
  - *Neisseria meningitidis*: 20%
  - *H. influenzae*: 10%
  - *L. monocytogenes*: 6%
  - Group B *Streptococcus*: 4%
- In adults ≥60 years old:
  - *S. pneumoniae*: 70%
  - *L. monocytogenes*: 20%
  - *N. meningitidis*: 3–4%
  - Group B *Streptococcus*: 3–4%
  - *H. influenzae*: 3–4%

COMMONLY ASSOCIATED CONDITIONS

The following conditions are associated with a worse prognosis:

- Coma
- Seizures
- Alcoholism
- Old age
- Infancy
- Diabetes mellitus
- Multiple myeloma
- Head trauma

DIAGNOSIS

HISTORY

- Antecedent upper respiratory infection
- Fever
- Headache
- Vomiting
- Photophobia
- Seizures
- Nausea
- Rigors
- Profuse sweats
- Weakness
- Elderly: Subtle findings, commonly including confusion

PHYSICAL EXAM

The triad of fever, neck stiffness, and altered mental status has low sensitivity (44%). However, almost all patients present with at least 2 out of 4 symptoms: Headache, fever, neck stiffness, and altered mental status:

- Meningismus
- Signs of cerebral dysfunction
- Altered mental status
- Focal neurologic deficits
- Meningococcal rash: Macular and erythematous at first, then petechial or purpuric

DIAGNOSTIC TESTS & INTERPRETATION

Lab

Initial lab tests

- CSF analysis: Turbid:
  - Neonates:
    - ○ >10 WBCs in CSF
    - ○ CSF Blood glucose ratio <0.6
    - ○ CSF protein >150 mg/dL
  - Infants/children:
    - ○ >5 WBCs in CSF
    - ○ CSF:Blood glucose ratio <0.6
    - ○ CSF protein >50 mg/dL
  - Adults:
    - ○ 1,000–100,000 WBCs in CSF
    - ○ CSF: Blood glucose ratio <0.4
    - ○ CSF protein >45 mg/dL (usually 150–400 mg/dL)
    - ○ Suspect ruptured brain abscess when WBC count is unusually high (>100,000).
  - In all age groups:
    - ○ CSF opening pressure >180 mm H_2O (1.77 kPa) (kilopascal)
    - ○ CSF gram positive in 75% of untreated patients
    - ○ CSF culture positive: 70–80% of cases
    - ○ Bacterial testing using polymerase chain reaction (PCR) (particularly in those with negative cultures) (*not yet routinely recommended*)
- Serum WBCs: Rarely useful in differentiating bacterial from viral illness
- Serum blood cultures:
  - Blood culture positive: 40–60% of cases
- Serum electrolytes
- Evaluation of clotting function if petechiae or purpuric lesions are noted

Imaging

- CT scan of head if concern for increased intracranial pressure or warning signs of space-occupying lesion (new-onset seizure, evolving signs of brain tissue shift, or papilledema)
- Chest radiograph may reveal silent area of pneumonitis or abscess.
- Sinus/skull radiographs may reveal cranial osteomyelitis, paranasal sinusitis, or skull fracture, but rarely indicated.
- Later in course, head CT scan, if hydrocephalus, brain abscess, subdural effusions, and subdural empyema are considered or in those patients who have not responded clinically after 48 hours of appropriate antibiotics.

Diagnostic Procedures/Surgery

Lumbar puncture

Pathological Findings

- Pleocytosis in CSF
- Bacterial antigen tests should be reserved for cases in which the initial CSF Gram stain is negative and CSF culture is negative at 48 hours of incubation.
- PCR of CSF and blood is most helpful for documenting meningococcal disease in the patient with negative cultures.

DIFFERENTIAL DIAGNOSIS

- Bacteremia
- Sepsis
- Brain abscess
- Seizures
- Other nonbacterial meningitides

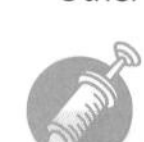

TREATMENT

- If diagnosis is suspected, lumbar puncture should be done in office with antimicrobial therapy begun before transfer to hospital; if not possible, administer antibiotics promptly.
- Inpatient care: ICU often required

MEDICATION

Empiric IV therapy until culture results available:

- Consider local patterns of bacterial sensitivity.
- See "Etiology" for age definitions and likely organisms.

First Line

The following regimens are somewhat simplified but will adequately treat patients pending culture results. Additional subgroupings may simplify treatment in some patients. Penicillin-allergic patients present a special challenge not covered here; seek infectious disease consultation:

- Neonates (give both) (1)[B]:
  - Ampicillin: 100–400 mg/kg/d divided q6–12h
  - Tobramycin: 7.5 mg/kg/d q6–8h (premature or <1 week of age, 2.5 mg/kg q12h)
- Infants >4 weeks of age:
  - Ampicillin: 300–400 mg/kg/d divided q4–6h (maximum, 2 g q3–4h) AND
  - Chloramphenicol: 75–100 mg/kg/d divided q6h OR
  - Ceftriaxone: 100 mg/kg/d divided q12–24h (maximum, 2 g q12h) or cefotaxime 200 mg/kg/d divided q4–6h AND
  - Vancomycin: 10–15 mg/kg q12h (maximum, 1,500 mg q12h)
- Adults (2,3)[A]:
  - Vancomycin: 1 g IV q12h AND
  - Ceftriaxone: 1–2 g IV q12–24h (maximum, 2 g q12h) *OR* cefotaxime 2 g IV q4–6h
- Precaution: Ototoxicity from aminoglycoside
- Contraindications: Allergies to specific antibiotics
- Treatment duration:
  - *N. meningitidis*, *H. influenzae*: 7–10 days
  - *S. pneumoniae*: 10–14 days
  - Group B *Streptococcus* organisms, *E. coli*, *L. monocytogenes*: 14–21 days
  - Neonates: 12–21 days or at least 14 days after a repeated culture is sterile
- Corticosteroids (4)[A]:
  - Early treatment with dexamethasone decreases mortality and morbidity for pediatric patients >1 month old and in adults with acute bacterial meningitis, and does not increase the risk of GI bleeding. However, data support this practice only in high-income countries (5).
  - Dexamethasone: 0.15 mg/kg q6h (10 mg for adults), started 15–20 minutes before or with the antibiotic for 4 days

Second Line

- Antipseudomonal penicillins
- Aztreonam
- Quinolones (e.g., ciprofloxacin)
- Meropenem

ADDITIONAL TREATMENT

General Measures

- Appropriate empiric antibiotic therapy, initiated promptly
- Vigorous supportive care with constant nursing to ensure prompt recognition of seizures and prevention of aspiration
- Therapy for coexisting conditions
- Measures to prevent hypothermia and dehydration

Issues for Referral

Consultation from ICU specialist

IN-PATIENT CONSIDERATIONS

Admission Criteria

Bacterial meningitis requires hospitalization.

IV Fluids

There is no evidence to support other than maintenance fluid therapy (2,6)[A].

Nursing

- ICU monitoring may be needed to recognize changes in the patient's consciousness and the development of new neurologic signs, subtle seizures, and to treat severe agitation effectively.
- Patients with suspected meningococcal infection require respiratory isolation for 24 hours.

Discharge Criteria

May consider home therapy for the completion of IV antibiotic course once patient is clinically stable and culture and sensitivity results are known

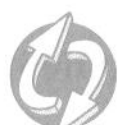

ONGOING CARE

FOLLOW-UP RECOMMENDATIONS

Patient Monitoring

Brainstem auditory evoked response test should be performed on infants before hospital discharge:

- Further follow-up will depend on its results and course of meningitis while in hospital.

DIET

Regular as tolerated, except when syndrome of inappropriate secretion of antidiuretic hormone complicates course

PATIENT EDUCATION

Available at the American Academy of Pediatrics, 141 Northwest Point Blvd., P.O. Box 927, Elk Grove Village, IL 60009-0927; (800) 433-9016; www.aap.org/

PROGNOSIS

Overall case fatality 14%:

- *H. influenzae*: 5%
- *N. meningitidis*: 10%
- *S. pneumoniae*: 19–37%

COMPLICATIONS

- Seizures: 20–30%
- Focal neurologic deficit
- Cranial nerve palsies (III, VI, VII, VIII):
  - Comprises 10–20% of the cases
  - Usually disappear within a few weeks
- Sensorineural hearing loss: 10% in children
- Neurodevelopmental sequelae: 30% subtle learning deficits
- Obstructive hydrocephalus
- Subdural effusions
- Decline in consciousness that may be due to meningoencephalitis

REFERENCES

1. Chávez-Bueno S, McCracken GH. Bacterial meningitis in children. *Pediatr Clin North Am.* 2005;52:795–810, vii.
2. Prasad K, Singhal T, Jain N, Gupta PK. Third generation cephalosporins versus conventional antibiotics for treating acute bacterial meningitis. *Cochrane Library, Cochrane Collaboration.* 2005 Volume 4.
3. Schut ES, de Gans J, van de Beek D, et al. Community-acquired bacterial meningitis in adults. *Pract Neurol.* 2008;8:8–23.
4. Assiri AM, Alasmari FA, Zimmerman VA, et al. Corticosteroid administration and outcome of adolescents and adults with acute bacterial meningitis: A meta-analysis. *Mayo Clin Proc.* 2009;84:403–9.
5. Brouwer MC, McIntyre P, de Gans J, et al. Corticosteroids for acute bacterial meningitis. *Cochrane Database Syst Rev.* 2007;(1):CD004405.
6. Maconochie I, Baumer H, Stewart ME. Fluid therapy for acute bacterial meningitis. *Cochrane Database Syst Rev.* 2008;CD004786.

ADDITIONAL READING

Thigpen MC, Whitney CG, Messonnier NE, et. al. Bacterial meningitis in the United States, 1998-2007. *N Engl J Med.* 2011;364:2016–25.

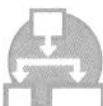

See Also (Topic, Algorithm, Electronic Media Element)

- Meningitis, Viral; Meningococcemia
- Algorithm: Delirium

CODES

ICD9

- 320.0 Hemophilus meningitis
- 320.1 Pneumococcal meningitis
- 320.9 Meningitis due to unspecified bacterium

CLINICAL PEARLS

- Suspected bacterial meningitis is a medical emergency, and immediate diagnostic steps must be taken to establish the specific cause. Antibiotic therapy should be initiated immediately after the lumbar puncture is performed if the clinical suspicion for meningitis is high.
- Neuroimaging is indicated in infants and children with signs or symptoms of complications and/or recurrent meningitis.
- Neurologic sequelae, including deafness, mental retardation, spasticity and/or paresis, and seizures, occur in 15–25% of infants and children.
- *Streptococcus pneumoniae* and *Neisseria meningitidis* are the most common causes of bacterial meningitis in infants and children >1 month of age.
- Neonatal meningitis should be suspected in any infant <1 month of age who presents with clinical findings of sepsis or meningitis. The most commonly reported signs are fever (rectal temperature >38°C), hypothermia (rectal temperature ≤36°C), irritability, and poor feeding or feeding intolerance. Bulging fontanelle and nuchal rigidity are observed in a minority of infants.

MENINGITIS, VIRAL

Luis K. Abrishamian, MD
Andrew D. Goldberg, MD

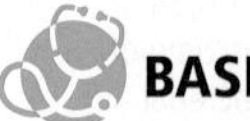

BASICS

DESCRIPTION

- System(s) affected: Nervous
- Synonym(s): Abacterial meningitis, Aseptic meningitis:
  - Aseptic meningitis is a clinical syndrome characterized by acute meningeal inflammation without an identifiable bacterial pathogen in the CSF.

EPIDEMIOLOGY

Incidence

- Estimated 26,000–42,000 hospitalizations each year in the US for viral meningitis (VM)
- In 2006, there were 72,000 meningitis-related hospitalizations, with 58% of those having meningitis as the primary reason for hospitalization. Of all 72,000 hospitalizations, 56.4% were determined to be viral cases (1)[A]
- More common than bacterial meningitis:
  - The annual incidence of viral meningitis is higher than total number cases of meningitis caused by all other etiologies combined
- Peaks in late summer to early fall:
  - Enteroviruses and arthropod-borne viruses predominate in warm months
  - Mumps usually occurs in the winter and spring, often in epidemics
- Occurs in both outbreak and sporadic forms

RISK FACTORS

- Close contact with known cases of VM
- Immunocompromised hosts may be more susceptible to cytomegalovirus (CMV), herpes simplex virus (HSV), and adenovirus
- Lymphocytic choriomeningitis virus (LCMV) is commonly transmitted via exposure to rodent feces, bodily fluids, or nesting materials:
  - Rodent bites and vertical transmission as mechanisms of infection are possible but unconfirmed

Geriatric Considerations

Cases of VM in the elderly are rare but documented. Consider alternative diagnoses (e.g., carcinomatous meningitis, NSAID- or medication-induced meningitis, etc.) in the elderly population.

Genetics

No genetic predispositions have been established relating to increased susceptibility to VM.

GENERAL PREVENTION

Limit exposure to known hosts, hand washing, and general hygiene.

PATHOPHYSIOLOGY

- First described by Wallgren in 1925
- In immunocompetent hosts, VM is generally caused by a systemic viral infection with predilection to neurologic involvement.
- Less commonly, direct neural transmission occurs from a self-limited infection such as HSV already present in the immunocompetent host.

ETIOLOGY

- >90% of cases caused by enterovirus family, which includes coxsackievirus A and B, echovirus, poliovirus, and E# variants: E9 and E30 strains specifically implicated in eastern and western hemispheres, respectively
- Less common causes include HSV-1 and HSV-2, varicella-zoster virus, adenovirus, LCMV, CMV, Epstein-Barr virus (EBV), HIV, and mumps
- Recurrent (Mollaret's) meningitis shows 80% association with HSV-2
- Arthropod-borne viruses: West Nile virus, St. Louis encephalitis virus, and California encephalitis virus
- Parvovirus B19 is found in the CSF of 4.3% of undiagnosed meningoencephalitis patients (2)[B]

COMMONLY ASSOCIATED CONDITIONS

- Encephalitis
- Neurologic deficits
- Myopericarditis
- Neonatal enteroviral sepsis

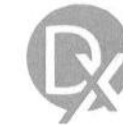

DIAGNOSIS

Predominant symptoms include:

- Fever
- Headache
- Photophobia
- Myalgias
- Nausea
- Vomiting
- Malaise

HISTORY

- Travel and exposure history
- Sexual activity (e.g., HSV, HIV, etc.)
- Outdoor exposure (Lyme disease)
- Rodent feces and/or urine exposure (LCMV)
- Solid-organ transplant (LCMV, CMV)

PHYSICAL EXAM

- Nuchal rigidity
- Altered mental status
- Fever (>100.4°F/38°C)
- Meningeal signs should not be used exclusively to diagnose or rule out meningitis (1)[C]; these include:
  - Nuchal rigidity
  - Brudzinski sign: Neck flexion elicits involuntary knee flexion in supine patient
  - Kernig sign: Resistance to knee extension following flexion of hips and knees by physician
- In the presence of erythema chronicum migrans or cranial neuropathy, consider Lyme meningitis given correlation with exposure and endemic area
- Be aware of mucocutaneous findings such as dermatologic manifestations (e.g., vesicular rash in hand, foot, and mouth disease), herpangina, and generalized maculopapular rash:
  - Zoster rash usually occurs after meningeal infection with VZV meningitis

DIAGNOSTIC TESTS & INTERPRETATION

Lab

Initial lab tests

- Lumbar puncture (LP) is standard of care in patients with high clinical suspicion:
  - Indications for LP include fever, sudden abrupt mental status change, headache, and/or lethargy.
  - Clinical judgment is to be used in all cases.
  - In patients with high suspicion of bacterial meningitis, antibiotic treatment should be started immediately.
- CSF analysis: Glucose, protein, WBC count with differential, RBC count, Gram stain, culture
- Typical CSF findings in viral meningitis:
  - Elevated WBC count: 10–1,000/mm^3, classically with a lymphocyte predominance
  - Initial phase of illness (first 24–48 hours) may show neutrophil predominance.
  - Protein normal to slightly elevated (<150 mg/dL):
    - One 3-year retrospective study found elevated CSF protein levels in patients with meningitis secondary to HSV-2 or VZV infection compared to enteroviruses
  - Negative Gram stain and bacterial culture
  - Elevated opening pressure:
    - Culture CSF for enteroviruses, HSV, and mumps. However, viral culture may yield no additional benefit when nucleic acid amplification has been employed (3)[C]:
      - In diagnosing enteroviral infections (EVs), nucleic acid tests are more sensitive than cultures.
    - Polymerase chain reaction (PCR) has a sensitivity of 95–100% for HSV-1 and -2, EBV, and enterovirus, allowing for earlier hospital discharge and less intervention.
    - Reverse-transcriptase PCR test is approved by the FDA for enteroviral meningitis: Results are available within 2.5 hours.
- Peripheral PMN count of >16 × 10(9)/L, serum C-reactive protein of >100 mg/L and hemorrhagic rash are shown to strongly and independently correlate with the diagnosis of bacterial meningitis and meningococcal septicemia.
- EEG in some cases, especially if encephalitis is a consideration
- CBC: Normal or mildly elevated WBCs
- Serum procalcitonin and CSF lactate concentrations appear to be highly discriminative parameters for the differential diagnosis of BM and VM, respectively.
- Viral cultures and/or antibody titers
- Serum procalcitonin (>0.5 ng/mL) and CSF protein (>0.5 g/L) have high correlation with pediatric bacterial vs. aseptic meningitis.
- Serum and stool specimens can assist in diagnosing enteroviral infections in children.

Follow-Up & Special Considerations

- Exercise clinical judgment regarding contraindications to LP. They include:
  - Increased intracranial pressure owing to mass lesion
  - Ventricular obstruction

- Local infection at potential LP site or suspected epidural abscess
- Anticoagulation or coagulopathy:
  - Level of coagulopathy that increases risk is unclear
- Possibility of cardiorespiratory compromise secondary to patient positioning during procedure

- Disorders that may alter lab results:
  - Diabetes: Consider blood sugar level to correlate with CSF glucose level
  - Pre-existing neurologic diseases (e.g., intracranial neoplasm, demyelinating disease)

Imaging

Initial approach

- Indication for imaging rests with consideration of alternative diagnoses; may be performed prior to LP in the presence of papilledema, spinal cord trauma, altered mental status, or focal neurologic findings. Prior to performing LP, CT scan may not be clinically necessary in the absence of risk factors.
- Standard techniques include noncontrast brain CT scan or MRI

DIFFERENTIAL DIAGNOSIS

- Bacterial meningitis
- Encephalitis
- Epidural abscess
- Other infectious agents:
  - Tuberculosis
  - Syphilis
  - Leptospirosis
  - Lyme disease
- Parameningeal infections (e.g., subdural empyema)
- Postinfectious encephalomyelitis
- Viral syndrome (e.g., influenza)
- Leukemia and carcinomatous meningitis
- Migraine headache
- Acute metabolic encephalopathy
- Chemical meningitis
- Brain abscess

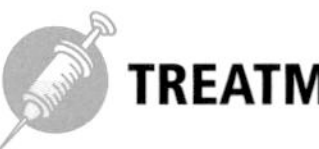

TREATMENT

MEDICATION

- Analgesics (adult doses):
  - Morphine: 0.05–0.1 mg/kg IV, titrated to pain relief
  - Hydromorphone (Dilaudid): 1–2 mg IV, titrated to pain relief
  - Hydrocodone (Vicodin): 5/500 mg 1–2 tablets PO q6h *or* oxycodone (Percocet) 5/325 mg 1–2 tablets PO q4–6h
- Antiemetics:
  - Prochlorperazine (Compazine): 10 mg IM/IV q4h
  - Ondansetron (Zofran): 4–8 mg IV q8h
  - Metoclopramide (Reglan): 10–20 mg IV/IM q4–6h
- Antipyretics: Acetaminophen (Tylenol): 650 mg PO or rectal suppository q4h
- Antiviral agents: Initiate empiric acyclovir at 10 mg/kg IV q8h for patients with CSF pleocytosis, negative Gram stain, and suspicion for HSV while awaiting results of definitive (e.g., HSV PCR) testing (4)[A]
- Antibiotics:
  - Not indicated for treatment of viral meningitis
  - If unclear etiology, treat symptomatically, and follow the patient closely in the hospital setting
  - If in doubt, initiate an IV or IM broad-spectrum antibiotic with good CSF penetration.
- Precautions: Aspirin should be avoided in children and adolescents owing to a possible association with Reye syndrome.

ADDITIONAL TREATMENT

General Measures

- Management is largely supportive.
- IV fluids if oral intake is poor or vomiting is present
- Pain management

IN-PATIENT CONSIDERATIONS

Admission Criteria

Generally, VM is treated on an outpatient basis, in contrast to the bacterial form; those with VM plus complicating factors may be hospitalized.

IV Fluids

May use normal saline bolus or continuous infusion, based on clinical judgment.

Nursing

- Neurologic monitoring for changes in mental status, fever, etc. to assess disease progression or alternate diagnosis
- Contact precautions until bacterial meningitis is ruled out
- Private room indicated with sterile precautions
- Encourage hand washing.

Discharge Criteria

Symptomatic relief

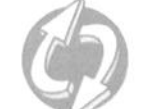

ONGOING CARE

FOLLOW-UP RECOMMENDATIONS

Follow-up with primary care physician

Patient Monitoring

- Monitor for relapse or exacerbation of symptoms after treatment course.
- Observe for potential neurological and neuroendocrine complications:
  - Seizures
  - Cerebral edema
  - Syndrome of inappropriate antidiuretic hormone (SIADH) secretion

DIET

- Determined by symptoms
- May need to order NPO owing to nausea or vomiting with advancement to clear fluids and regular diet as tolerated

PATIENT EDUCATION

- Discuss possibility, but low probability, of transmission to contacts.
- Expected duration of illness (5–10 days)
- For patient education materials, refer patients to the online EBSCO Health Library article Viral Meningitis (http://healthlibrary.epnet.com/GetContent.aspx?token=38405ca3-6cab-4817-9cba-dc64dc5c69f1&chunkiid=11469).

PROGNOSIS

- Complete recovery generally within 5–7 days
- Headaches and other uncomfortable symptoms may persist intermittently for 1–2 weeks.
- Only 0.6% of hospitalizations for VM resulted in death in a recent study.
- European studies have shown some residual postmeningeal cognitive impairment.

COMPLICATIONS

- Post-LP headache:
  - 36.5% of patients within 48 hours
- Fatigue
- Irritability
- Muscle weakness
- Seizures (rare)

REFERENCES

1. Thomas KE, et al. The diagnostic accuracy of Kernig's sign, Brudzinski's sign, and nuchal rigidity in adults with suspected meningitis. *Clin Infect Dis*. 2002;35(1):46–52.
2. Barah F, et al. Association of human parvovirus B19 infection with acute meningoencephalitis. *Lancet*. 2001;358(9299):2168.
3. Polage CR, Petti CA. Assessment of the utility of viral culture of cerebrospinal fluid. *Clin Infect Dis*. 2006;43:1578–9.
4. Swadron SP, et al. Pitfalls in the management of headache in the emergency department. *Emerg Med Clin North Am*. 2010;28:127–47.

ADDITIONAL READING

Logan SA, MacMahon E. Viral meningitis. *BMJ*. 2008;336:36–40.

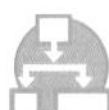

See Also (Topic, Algorithm, Electronic Media Element)

Algorithm: Delirium

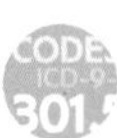

CODES

ICD9

- 047.0 Meningitis due to coxsackie virus
- 047.1 Meningitis due to echo virus
- 047.8 Other specified viral meningitis

CLINICAL PEARLS

- Viral vs. bacterial meningitis cannot be distinguished clinically; refer all suspected meningitis cases to hospital for diagnosis and management.
- Viral meningitis is more common than bacterial meningitis in the pediatric population. As age increases, the likelihood of a bacterial cause also increases.
- Antibiotic administration hours or days prior to CSF analysis may result in "partially treated" bacterial meningitis that mimics viral meningitis.
- IV acyclovir should be administered if there is a high clinical suspicion for VM
- If bacterial meningitis is in the differential diagnosis, broad-spectrum antibiotics with effective CSF penetration should be given:
  - Antibiotics should be continued until the diagnosis of bacterial meningitis is ruled out.
- Morbidity with VM is low, but increases with associated encephalitis.
- There is no evidence to support meningitis prophylaxis in basilar skull fracture with or without CSF leakage.

MENINGOCOCCEMIA

Glenn Skow, MD, MPH

BASICS

DESCRIPTION

- Caused by *Neisseria meningitidis* in the blood, which results in a broad spectrum of clinical manifestations
- Bacteremia without sepsis: Meningococcal bacteremia rarely occurs without sepsis.
- Bacteremia without meningitis: Patient is acutely ill and may have skin manifestations (rashes, petechiae, and ecchymosis) and hypotension.
- Bacteremia with meningitis:
  - Predominant clinical picture of meningitis: Sudden onset of fever, nausea, vomiting, headache, decreased ability to concentrate, and myalgias
  - Disease progression is usually quite rapid with a transition from health to severe disease in a matter of hours.
  - Skin manifestations and hypotension may also be present:
    - A petechial rash appears as discrete lesions 1–2 mm in diameter, most frequently on the trunk and lower portions of the body and will be seen in more than 50% of patients on presentation
    - Purpura fulminans is a severe complication of meningococcal disease and occurs in up to 25% of cases. It is characterized by the acute onset of cutaneous hemorrhage and necrosis due to vascular thrombosis and disseminated intravascular coagulopathy.

EPIDEMIOLOGY

Incidence

- The US mortality rate is 0.5–1.1/100,000, or ~13%:
  - 11–19% of survivors suffer serious sequelae, including deafness, neurologic deficit, or limb loss.
- Disease is seasonal, with cases peaking in December and January.
- Annually, about 1,000 cases of invasive meningococcal disease occur in the US (1):
  - Among adolescents and young adults, ages 14–24, the occurrence is 20%.
  - Among infants under 1 year of age, the occurrence is 16%.

RISK FACTORS

- Age: 3 months–1 year
- Late complement component deficiency (C5, C6, C7, C8, or C9)
- Asplenia (1)
- Close contacts (e.g., household, nurseries, day care, dormitories, military barracks)
- Exposure to active and passive tobacco smoke (1).

Genetics

Late complement component deficiency has an autosomal-recessive inheritance.

GENERAL PREVENTION

- 2 vaccines are currently licensed for use in the US. Each contains antigens to serogroups A, C, Y, and W-135. Neither vaccine provides immunity against serotype B, which is responsible for 1/3 of cases in the US (2):
  - Meningococcal Polysaccharide Vaccine (MPSV4): Recommended for patients 55 years of age or older with elevated risk (1):
    - Duration of protection is short. 1–3 years for patients under 5 years of age and 3–5 years for adolescents and adults (2)
    - Reasonable for patients requiring short protection such as those traveling to endemic areas; for college freshmen; and for those who are experiencing community outbreaks (2)
  - Meningococcal Conjugate Vaccine (MCV4): Recommended for patients ages 2 through 55 (1)
- Protective levels of antibody are achieved in ~7–10 days after primary immunization (2)
- Vaccine is recommended for all persons 11–18 and persons 19–55 at increased risk for the disease:
  - Guillain-Barré syndrome has been associated with the MCV4 vaccine, so a personal history of Guillain-Barré is a relative contraindication for receiving this vaccine.
- CDC International Travel Advisory:
  - Vaccine is required by the Government of Saudi Arabia for Hajj pilgrims above age 2.
  - The vaccine should be given to travelers to sub-Saharan Africa ("meningitis belt") during dry season.

ETIOLOGY

- *Neisseria meningitidis*, a gram-negative diplococcus with at least 13 serotypes
- Major serogroups in the US: B, C, Y, and W-135:
  - Serogroup B is the predominant cause of meningococcemia in children <1 year of age.
  - Serogroup C is the most common cause of cases in the US.
  - Serogroup Y is the predominant cause of meningococcemia in the elderly (2).
- Major serogroups worldwide are A, B, C, Y, and W-135:
  - W-135 is the major cause of disease in the "meningitis belt" of sub-Saharan Africa.

DIAGNOSIS

HISTORY

- Symptoms:
  - Sudden onset of fever, nausea, vomiting, headache, myalgias, chills, rigor, and/or sore throat (nonsuppurative):
    - Pharyngitis may be mistaken for streptococcal pharyngitis.
    - Myalgia may be mistaken for severe "flu" with a peak incidence coinciding in winter months.
  - Changes in mental status, decreased ability to concentrate, stiff neck, convulsions
- Be sure to ask about possible exposures.

PHYSICAL EXAM

- Neurological: Nuchal rigidity, focal neurologic findings, coma, seizure:
  - Focal neurologic findings and seizures are more commonly seen with *H. influenzae* or *Streptococcus pneumoniae*.
- Cardiovascular: Hypotension, tachycardia, shock, heart failure with pulmonary edema
- Dermatologic: Maculopapular rash, petechiae, ecchymosis, purpura
- Median time of onset of specific meningitis symptoms (e.g., neck stiffness, photophobia, bulging fontanelle) was ~12–15 hours after onset of illness (3).
- Late signs of meningitis (e.g., unconsciousness, delirium, or seizures) occurred at a median of 15 hours in infants under 1 year of age and at a median of 24 hours in older children (3).

DIAGNOSTIC TESTS & INTERPRETATION

ALERT

- The gold standard for the diagnosis of systemic meningococcal infection is the isolation of *N. meningitidis* from a usually sterile body fluid such as blood or CSF.
- Antibiotic administration may render blood and/or CSF culture negative within 2 hours, so begin treatment and then test.

Lab

Initial lab tests

- CBC with differential:
  - Leukocytosis or leukopenia
  - Left shift of leukocytes, toxic granulation
  - Thrombocytopenia
- Lactic acid:
  - Lactic acidosis
- Coagulation studies:
  - Prolonged PT/PTT
  - Low fibrinogen
  - Elevated fibrin degradation products
- Blood culture:
  - Blood culture growing *N. meningitis*
  - Positive in 50–60% of cases
- CSF:
  - Cloudy
  - Increased WBCs with polymorphonuclear cells predominant
  - Gram stain showing gram-negative diplococci
  - Glucose-to-blood glucose ratio <0.4
  - Protein >45 mg/dL
  - Positive for *N. meningitidis* antigen (MAT or PCR)
  - Culture positive for *N. meningitidis*:
    - Positive in 80–90% of cases

Imaging

Initial approach

CT scan of head if there is concern for space-occupying lesions

Diagnostic Procedures/Surgery

- Blood culture
- Lumbar puncture:
  - After a brief history and physical exam have suggested meningitis, initiate antibiotics within 30 minutes and then proceed with a lumbar puncture.

Pathological Findings

- Disseminated intravascular coagulation
- Exudates on meninges
- Polymorphonuclear infiltration of meninges
- Hemorrhage of adrenal glands

DIFFERENTIAL DIAGNOSIS

- Septicemia due to other microorganisms
- Meningitis due to other pyogenic bacteria
- Gonococcemia
- Acute bacterial endocarditis
- Rocky Mountain spotted fever
- Hemolytic uremic syndrome
- Gonococcal arthritis dermatitis syndrome
- Influenza

TREATMENT

MEDICATION

First Line

- Dexamethasone:
  - Indications:
    - Known or suspected pneumococcal meningitis in selected adults
    - Children with *H. influenzae* type b meningitis
  - Dexamethasone is often given initially in adults and children with bacterial meningitis while awaiting microbiologic data.
  - Dexamethasone has not been shown to be of benefit in meningococcal meningitis and should be discontinued once this diagnosis is established.
  - Dosage:
    - Infants and children >6 weeks: IV 0.15 mg/kg/dose q6h for the first 2–4 days of antibiotic treatment
    - Start 10–20 minutes before or with the first dose of antibiotic.
- Antibiotics:
  - Treatment for suspected meningococcal meningitis must begin as soon as possible; coverage for other possible causes of meningitis must be given until a definitive diagnosis is made.
  - Age influences the etiologic organism:
    - Preterm to <1 month: Ampicillin plus cefotaxime or Ampicillin plus Gentamicin:
      - Cefotaxime:
        - 0–7 days: 50 mg/kg q12h
        - 8–28 days: 50 mg/kg q8h
      - Ampicillin:
        - >2,000 g:
          - 0–7 days: 50 mg/kg q8h
          - 8–28 days: 50 mg/kg q6h
        - <2,000 g:
          - 0–7 days: 50 mg/kg q12h
          - 8–28 days: 50 mg/kg q8h
    - 1 month to 50 years: Cefotaxime or Ceftriaxone plus Vancomycin:
      - If severe penicillin allergy: Chloramphenicol plus TMP-SMX plus Vancomycin
    - >50 years of age or patients with alcoholism, debilitating disease, or impaired immunity: Ampicillin plus Ceftriaxone plus Vancomycin:
      - Ampicillin: 2 g IV q4h
      - Ceftriaxone: 2 g IV q12h
      - Vancomycin: 500–750 mg IV q6h
      - If severe penicillin allergy: TMP-SMX plus Vancomycin
  - Penicillin G:
    - Meningococcal meningitis is well treated with Penicillin G if the isolate is proven to be penicillin-susceptible.
    - Penicillin can be used if the isolate has a penicillin minimum inhibitory concentration (MIC) of <0.1 mcg/mL.
    - For isolates with a penicillin MIC of 0.1–1 mcg/mL, treatment with high-dose penicillin is effective, but a third-generation cephalosporin is preferred (4).
    - Penicillin G: 4 million units IV q4h (pediatric dose: 0.25 mU/kg IV q4–6h) or ampicillin: 2 g IV q4h (pediatric dose: 200–300 mg/kg IV q6h)
- Duration of treatment: 7 days (4)
- Chemoprophylaxis:
  - Indications:
    - Close contacts: Those who have had prolonged (>8 hours) contact while in close proximity (<3 ft) to the patient, or who have been directly exposed to the patient's oral secretions between 1 week before the onset of the patient's symptoms until 24 hours after initiation of appropriate antibiotic therapy (2):
      - Examples: Household members and personnel in nurseries, daycare centers, nursing homes, dormitories, and other closed institutions
    - No chemoprophylaxis is indicated for casual contacts, including most health care workers, unless there is exposure to respiratory secretion.
  - Timing:
    - Ideally <24 hours after identification of the index patient
    - Chemoprophylaxis administered >14 days is not recommended by the CDC
  - Regimens:
    - Rifampin, Ciprofloxacin, and Ceftriaxone:
      - Ceftriaxone:
        - Recommended for pregnant women
        - Adults: 250 mg IM as a single dose
      - Rifampin (meningococcal meningitis prophylaxis):
        - Adult: 600 mg IV or PO q12h for 2 days
        - Pediatric:
          - <1 mo: 10 mg/kg/d in divided doses q12h for 2 days
          - Infants and children: 20 mg/kg/d in divided doses q12h for 2 days (max: 600 mg/dose)
      - Ciprofloxacin:
        - Adults: 750 mg PO as a single dose (5)[B]
      - Vaccination:
        - For household contacts (if the case is from a vaccine-preventable serogroup)
- Precautions:
  - Adjust the dosage of both medications in patients with severe renal dysfunction.

Second Line

- For meningitis:
  - Chloramphenicol: 1 g IV q6h (pediatric dose: 75–100 mg/kg q6h) or ceftriaxone 2 g IV q12h (pediatric dose: 80–100 mg/kg q12–24h)
  - In large outbreaks, a single dose of long-acting chloramphenicol has been used. Single-dose ceftriaxone shows equal efficacy in one RCT.
- Precautions:
  - Ceftriaxone should not be used in patients with a history of anaphylactic reactions to penicillin (e.g., hypotension, laryngeal edema, wheezing, hives).
  - Chloramphenicol may cause aplastic anemia.

ADDITIONAL TREATMENT

General Measures

- Appropriate antibiotic
- Supportive care
- Close monitoring (e.g., seizure activity)

Issues for Referral

Potential complications:

- Disseminated intravascular coagulation (DIC)
- Acute respiratory distress syndrome
- Renal failure
- Adrenal failure

IN-PATIENT CONSIDERATIONS

Initial Stabilization

- If meningitis is suspected, initiate antibiotics and then proceed to an immediate lumbar puncture.
- Droplet isolation for 24 hours from the beginning of antibiotic therapy

IV Fluids

- Replace volume as needed.
- Patient may present with septic shock and will require resuscitation with large volumes of crystalloid.

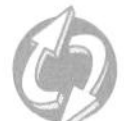

ONGOING CARE

FOLLOW-UP RECOMMENDATIONS

- Patients should have close follow-ups with their physicians upon discharge from the hospital.
- In patients with neurologic deficits, follow-up with a neurologist may be needed.

PATIENT EDUCATION

- Educate family and close contacts regarding the risk of contracting meningococcal infections.
- Educate health care personnel who are not at risk of contracting meningococcal infections.

PROGNOSIS

Overall mortality is 13%.

COMPLICATIONS

- DIC
- Acute tubular necrosis
- Neurologic: Sensorineural hearing loss, cranial nerve palsy, seizures
- Obstructive hydrocephalus
- Subdural effusions
- Acute adrenal hemorrhage
- Waterhouse-Friderichsen syndrome

REFERENCES

1. Centers for Disease Control and Prevention. Factsheet: Meningococcal Disease and Meningococcal Vaccine. Available at: www.cdc.gov/vaccines/vpd-vac/mening/vac-mening-fs.htm.
2. Gardner P. Prevention of meningococcal disease. *N Engl J Med*. 2006;355:1466–73.
3. Thompson MJ, Ninis N. Clinical recognition of meningococcal disease in children and adolescents. *Lancet*. 2006;367(9508):397.
4. Tunkel AR, et al. Practice guidelines for the management of bacterial meningitis. *Clin Infect Dis*. 2004;39(9):1267.
5. Fraser A, Gafter-Gvili A, Paul M. Antibiotics for preventing meningococcal infections. *Cochrane Database Syst Rev*. 2005;CD004785.

CODES

ICD9

- 036.0 Meningococcal meningitis
- 036.2 Meningococcemia

CLINICAL PEARLS

- Chemoprophylaxis is needed for close contacts.
- Prevention with vaccinations is key.
- Treatment should never be delayed for diagnostic tests.

MENISCAL INJURY

Bryan G. Beutel, MD

BASICS

DESCRIPTION

- The menisci are 2 (medial, lateral) semilunar fibrocartilaginous structures located between the femoral condyles and tibial plateau of the knee.
- Each meniscus comprises 3 segments: Body, anterior horn, and posterior horn.
- The menisci serve as crucial parts of the knee joint for stabilization, energy absorption, joint lubrication, and load distribution (30–55%) across the knee. Menisci also aid in preventing the anterior displacement of the tibia.
- After the age of 10 years, the meniscus begins to devascularize, and by adulthood, only the peripheral 10–30% of the medial, and 10–25% of the lateral menisci are vascular.
- Injuries to the menisci can be *acute* or *degenerative*. The injury is more likely to be degenerative in people older than 40 years (particularly men). The medial meniscus is more likely to be injured than the lateral meniscus because of its reduced mobility and role as the primary weight-bearing surface.

Geriatric Considerations

Meniscal tears in geriatric patients are more likely due to *chronic degeneration* of the meniscus that can result in a tear with minimal acute trauma.

Pediatric Considerations

- *Discoid meniscus* is an anatomic variant (incidence of 3.5–5%) that can cause an atraumatic snapping or popping sensation in the child's or adolescent's knee.
- It is rare to sustain a meniscal injury under the age of 10 years, but it can be associated with a discoid meniscus.
- Most discoid meniscal tears are lateral.

EPIDEMIOLOGY

- Predominant age: Males aged 31–40 years; females aged 11–20 years
- Predominant gender: Male:Female ratio varies from 2.5:1 to 4:1

Incidence

- Observed in various sports, including football, soccer, basketball, skiing, and baseball
- Between 80% and 90% of meniscal injuries in children and adolescents occur during athletics. True overall incidence in individuals <18 years of age, however, remains unknown.

Prevalence

Estimated to be 60–70 cases per 100,000 people

RISK FACTORS

- Increased age:
  - Highest risk if >40 years old.
- Obesity and smoking are risk factors for degenerative meniscal tears.
- High degree of physical activity (especially contact sports)
- Tibiofemoral arthritis
- Anterior cruciate ligament (ACL) insufficiency
- Posterior cruciate ligament (PCL) insufficiency

Genetics

A congenital abnormality leading to discoid meniscus increases the risk of meniscal tear among children. No specific gene locus has been identified.

GENERAL PREVENTION

- Strengthening of quadriceps and hamstring muscles
- Conditioning while participating in sports
- Treatment and rehabilitation of previous knee injuries, particularly ACL injuries
- Improving core proprioception may prevent knee injuries in female athletes.

ETIOLOGY

- Acute tears typically occur due to a twisting motion of the knee while the foot is planted.
- Sports injuries occur while cutting, decelerating, hyperflexing, or landing from a jump.
- Degenerative tears occur secondary to minimal trauma.

COMMONLY ASSOCIATED CONDITIONS

- ACL is concomitantly torn in 1/3 of cases:
  - The patient may feel or hear a "pop."
  - More common in children and adolescents
- Medial collateral (MCL) and lateral collateral (LCL) ligament tears
- Tibial plateau fractures
- Femoral shaft fractures
- Tibiofemoral joint dislocation (seen occasionally)

DIAGNOSIS

HISTORY

- Obtain description of the mechanism of injury.
- Inquire about previous knee injuries.
- Pain associated with activities requiring flexion of the knee, such as climbing stairs or squatting
- Swelling for days after the injury:
  - Swelling is often delayed; immediate swelling is associated with an ACL tear.
- Locking, catching, popping, crunching (at the time of injury), or buckling
- The patient may have a limp or be unable to bear weight.
- Pain on side of knee where meniscal tear is present

PHYSICAL EXAM

- Overall, positive predictive value of physical exam is as high as 91.5%; accuracy as high as 94.5%.
- Compare with noninjured knee.
- Examine for effusion. May indicate peripheral meniscal tear or synovitis. If effusion is too large, re-evaluate knee in 1 week.
- Assess for joint line tenderness (sensitivity: 79%; specificity: 15%; and positive predictive value: 50%) (1)[B].
- Decreased active and passive range of motion ("locked" knee)
- Pain with full flexion (posterior horn tears) or extension (anterior horn tears) of the knee
- McMurray test (sensitivity: 53%; specificity: 59%) (1)[B]
- The Apley grind test for meniscal tear is neither specific nor sensitive, and it rarely should be used.
- Assess for coexisting ligament injury by applying varus, valgus, anterior, and posterior stresses across the knee.

DIAGNOSTIC TESTS & INTERPRETATION

Lab

Laboratory evaluation is generally not indicated unless there are signs of septic joint, which would warrant arthrocentesis with synovial fluid analysis, ESR, C-reactive protein (CRP), WBC count, etc.

Imaging

Initial approach

Plain radiographs should be obtained to detect fractures, loose bodies, or arthritic changes.

Follow-Up & Special Considerations

- MRI is the optimal study for intra-articular pathology; however, it should only be performed if the diagnosis is unclear or if an MRI will change the management. Overall, positive predictive value of an MRI is 91.5% and accuracy is 95.5% for a meniscal tear. Sensitivity and specificity for lateral tears are 79% and 96%, respectively, and 93% and 88% for medial tears, respectively (2)[B].
- The sagittally oriented short echo time (TE) sequence is best for identifying meniscal tears.
- Abnormal MRI changes may be due to degenerative disease rather than an acute tear.
- 61% of adult patients without knee symptoms were found to have incidental meniscal tears with an MRI (3)[B].

Diagnostic Procedures/Surgery

Arthroscopy may be needed for diagnostic purposes if the MRI is indeterminate.

DIFFERENTIAL DIAGNOSIS

- ACL or collateral ligament tear
- Contusion
- Discoid meniscus
- Pathologic plica
- Osteochondritis dissecans
- Loose body or fracture
- Osteoarthritis (OA)
- Patellofemoral syndrome
- Gout, pseudogout
- Rheumatoid arthritis

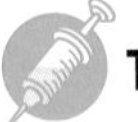

TREATMENT

MEDICATION

- NSAIDs
- Narcotic analgesics if needed for severe pain

ADDITIONAL TREATMENT

General Measures

- RICE: Rest, Ice, Compression, Elevation
- Meniscal preservation should be the goal of treatment in order to decrease any future complication of OA.
- The treatment depends on the type, location, and extent of the tear as well as the age and activity of the patient.
- Small, nondisplaced peripheral tears (because this region is vascular), especially in the lateral meniscus, may heal on their own or become asymptomatic and, therefore, do not require surgery.
- Aggressive physical therapy/rehabilitation should be provided as the initial form of treatment in most patients, as a majority of them will become symptom-free from strengthening alone:
  - Patients >30 years who do not have a "locked" knee should undergo 6–12 weeks of rehabilitation. If they are symptomatic after rehabilitation, surgery should be considered.
- A "locked" knee requires immediate surgery.
- In patients >40 years with OA and meniscal injury, surgery should be offered after a failure of 3–6 months of rehabilitation.
- If the patient is <30 years and very active in sports or at work, surgery may be required.
- Activity should be restricted to weight-bearing as tolerated. Crutches may be needed the patient is unable to bear weight.

Issues for Referral

Surgical consult for injuries that may require surgery

Additional Therapies

- Rehabilitation is required for surgical and nonsurgical patients. Strengthening and increasing the range of motion (ROM) is the primary goal of rehabilitation.

SURGERY/OTHER PROCEDURES

- Most surgeries can be performed arthroscopically.
- Meniscal repairs have a better functional outcome and decrease the risk of OA compared with (partial) meniscectomy (4)[B]. Whereas repairs reapproximate the meniscus with sutures or other fixation techniques, meniscectomy resects the injured portion of meniscus.
- Surgically implanted collagen meniscal implants do not improve postoperative function in patients with acute meniscal injury when compared to meniscectomy alone.
- Meniscal allograft transplantation improves function in patients with prior meniscectomy (5)[B].

ONGOING CARE

FOLLOW-UP RECOMMENDATIONS

- After meniscal repair, patients can weight-bear in 4–6 weeks and return to full activity in 4–6 months if they are symptom-free, have a full ROM, sufficient strength, and a normal physical exam.
- After a meniscectomy, patients can weight-bear in 1–2 days and return to full activity in 2–4 weeks.
- Combined ACL and meniscal repair requires 6 months of postoperative rehabilitation before the patient can return to sports.

PATIENT EDUCATION

- Educate the patient on how to ambulate on crutches, if needed.
- Teach the patient about the risks and benefits of surgery vs. conservative treatment.

PROGNOSIS

- The prognosis is more favorable if surgery is done within 8 weeks, the tear is in the periphery, the tear is <2.5 cm, the tear is in the lateral meniscus, and/or the patient is <30 years of age.
- The strongest predictors of *poor* functional outcome after an arthroscopic partial meniscectomy are greater articular cartilage degeneration observed during surgery, greater size of meniscal resection, greater laxity of the ACL, and prior surgery of the knee (6)[B].
- Young athletes generally recover faster than older patients.

COMPLICATIONS

- Meniscectomies may eventually lead to OA. Consequently, meniscal repair should be performed over meniscectomy when appropriate:
  - At 10–20 years after the injury, about 50% of patients will have OA, with associated pain and functional impairment.
  - Risk factors for greater radiographic evidence of OA after an arthroscopic partial meniscectomy are a greater size of meniscal resection and female gender (6)[B].
- Surgery may cause injury to neurovascular structures.

REFERENCES

1. Strayer RJ, Lang ES. Evidence-based emergency medicine/systematic review abstract. Does this patient have a torn meniscus or ligament of the knee? *Ann Emerg Med*. 2006;47:499–501.
2. Rosas HG, De Smet AA, et al. Magnetic resonance imaging of the meniscus. *Top Magn Reson Imaging*. 2009;20:151–73.
3. Englund M, Guermazi A, Gale D. Incidental meniscal findings on knee MRI in middle-aged and elderly persons. *N Engl J Med*. 2008;359:1108–15.
4. Stein T, Mehling AP, Welsch F, et al. Long-term outcome after arthroscopic meniscal repair versus arthroscopic partial meniscectomy for traumatic meniscal tears. *Am J Sports Med*. 2010;38(8): 1542–8.
5. LaPrade RF, Wills NJ, Spiridonov SI, et al. A prospective outcomes study of meniscal allograft transplantation. *Am J Sports Med*. 2010;38(9): 1804–12.
6. Meredith DS. Factors predicting functional and radiographic outcomes after arthroscopic partial meniscectomy: A review of the literature. *Arthroscopy*. 2005;21(2):211–23.

ADDITIONAL READING

- Konan S, Rayan F, Haddad FS, et al. Do physical diagnostic tests accurately detect meniscal tears? *Knee Surg Sports Traumatol Arthrosc*. 2009;17: 806–11.
- Osti L, Papalia R, Del Buono A, et al. Good results five years after surgical management of anterior cruciate ligament tears, and meniscal and cartilage injuries. *Knee Surg Sports Traumatol Arthrosc*. 2010;18:1385–90.

See Also (Topic, Algorithm, Electronic Media Element)

Algorithm: Knee Pain

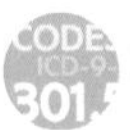

CODES

ICD9

- 836.0 Tear of medial cartilage or meniscus of knee, current
- 836.1 Tear of lateral cartilage or meniscus of knee, current
- 836.2 Other tear of cartilage or meniscus of knee, current

CLINICAL PEARLS

- Increasing core proprioception may prevent knee injuries in female athletes.
- The MRI is the preferred imaging modality to identify meniscal pathology.
- Nonsurgical and surgical candidates require rehabilitation.
- Meniscal preservation should be the goal of treatment to prevent OA.
- Meniscal repairs (suturing the meniscus) have a better functional outcome and decrease the risk of OA compared with meniscectomy.

MENOPAUSE

Rebecca Blumhofer, MD, MPH
Stacy E. Potts, MD, MEd

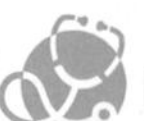

BASICS

DESCRIPTION

- Natural menopause: Permanent cessation of menstrual periods for at least 12 consecutive months in a nonpregnant woman ≥45 years old:
  - Resulting from ovarian follicular depletion
  - Not associated with a pathologic etiology
- Perimenopause: From the onset of menstrual changes through the first year of menopause (average length of perimenopause is 4–5 years)
- Postmenopause: Usually accounts for >1/3 of a woman's life
- Premature menopause: Menopause occurring before age 40; may be associated with sex chromosome abnormalities

EPIDEMIOLOGY

- Average age of perimenopause onset is 47.5 years.
- Mean age of menopause onset is 51–52 years.
- Earlier menopause in Hispanic women as compared to Caucasian

Incidence

In the US, 1.3 million women reach menopause annually.

RISK FACTORS

- Aging
- Oophorectomy
- Sex chromosome abnormalities (e.g., Turner syndrome)
- Age of maternal menopause
- Reproductive history: Nulliparous, short cycles during adolescence

GENERAL PREVENTION

Goal is not to prevent menopause but to retard development of osteoporosis related to menopause:

- Weight-bearing exercise
- Avoid smoking.
- Avoid excessive alcohol and caffeine intake.
- Maintain healthy weight.
- Calcium intake 1,200–1,500 mg/d beginning in adolescence
- Adequate vitamin D (800–1,200 IU daily)

PATHOPHYSIOLOGY

Normal physiologic process

ETIOLOGY

- As women age, the number of ovarian follicles decreases: Ovarian production of estrogen and inhibin decreases, and luteinizing (LH) and follicle-stimulating (FSH) hormone production increases:
  - Without estrogen, failure of endometrial development occurs and menstrual cycles become irregular, then cease.
  - Symptoms directly or indirectly due to decrease in estrogen
- Surgical: Removal of functioning ovaries due to disease or incidental to hysterectomy
- Other:
  - Treatment of endometriosis
  - Treatment of breast cancer with antiestrogens (which is reversible)
  - May occur after cancer chemotherapy (permanent or reversible)

DIAGNOSIS

HISTORY

- Cessation of menses:
  - Generally preceded by a period of irregular cycles as well as heavy or diminished bleeding
- Vasomotor symptoms: Hot flashes and sweating, often at night (30–80%):
  - First and most common manifestation of menopause
  - Prevalence of symptoms varies across cultures
  - Last ~3–4 minutes, occur at unpredictable intervals
  - Frequency usually declines with time
- Mood changes (8–38%), anxiety, depression
  - More common in women with less education attainment and/or personal history of depression
- Sleep disorders (35–60%):
  - Lengthening of latent phase
  - Less time spent asleep
- Urogenital atrophy:
  - Atrophic vaginitis causes vaginal dryness (17–30%), itch, dyspareunia, and possible sexual dysfunction.
  - Urethral atrophy causes urgency, frequency, dysuria, and stress incontinence.
  - Atrophy of paravaginal tissues that support bladder and rectum can lead to urocele, rectocele, and uterine prolapse.
  - Increased pH and atrophy increase risk of vaginal infections and UTIs.
- Osteopenia and osteoporosis
- Change in intensity and severity of migraines
- Skin thinning, hair loss, hirsutism, brittle nails
- Breast pain

Geriatric Considerations

Vaginal bleeding in postmenopausal women is abnormal; endometrial cancer must be ruled out.

PHYSICAL EXAM

- Decrease in breast size and change in breast texture
- External, speculum, and bimanual pelvic exams: Atrophic vaginal mucosa (urogenital atrophy)

DIAGNOSTIC TESTS & INTERPRETATION

Lab

Initial lab tests

- Generally none required; the patient's age and symptoms establish the diagnosis
- If laboratory confirmation is desired:
  - Elevated serum FSH level >30 mIU/mL indicates ovarian failure.
  - Symptoms may precede changes in lab parameters.
- Drugs that may alter lab results: Estrogens, androgens, oral contraceptive pills (OCPs)
- LH has no role in diagnosing menopause.

Imaging

Initial approach

Annual mammography is recommended for menopausal women (upper age limit for discontinuation remains uncertain)

Follow-Up & Special Considerations

- Brain MRI if pituitary tumor suspected
- Abnormal vaginal bleeding in a postmenopausal patient should be evaluated by transvaginal ultrasound (TVUS) and/or endometrial biopsy:
  - If endometrial stripe is <5 mm on TVUS, endometrial carcinoma is unlikely.
- Bone mineral density (BMD) testing with dual energy x-ray absorptiometry (DEXA) scan in postmenopausal women <65 years with additional risk factors (not otherwise indicated at onset of menopause):
  - Previous history of fractures, low body weight, cigarette smoking, family history of fractures should be tested if osteoporosis is a concern (not usually indicated at onset of menopause).

Pathological Findings

- Abnormal BMD and DEXA scan results:
  - T-score on DEXA of 1–2.5 = Osteopenia
  - T-score >2.5 = Osteoporosis
  - Defer to femoral neck T-score value over spine T-score
- Z-score measures age-matched mean bone density (not clinically useful)

DIFFERENTIAL DIAGNOSIS

Pregnancy, polycystic ovarian syndrome, pituitary adenoma, anorexia nervosa causing amenorrhea, hypothalamic dysfunction, Asherman syndrome, obstruction of uterine outflow tract, Sheehan syndrome, thyroid disease

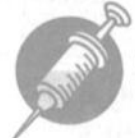

TREATMENT

Treatment choice depends on the severity of symptoms.

MEDICATION

First Line

Hormone therapy (HT) (1):

- The primary indication for HT is the treatment of moderate to severe vasomotor symptoms. Combination estrogen–progestin therapy is effective treatment for these symptoms, and other menopausal symptoms (sleep disorders, urogenital atrophy). It is also useful for preventing osteoporotic fractures and colorectal cancer and may help with mood symptoms (2,3)[A].
- Current recommendations for HT suggest use for a limited duration (i.e., few years) in treating menopausal symptoms in women near menopause and do not have a history of and are not at high risk for coronary artery disease (CAD), stroke, breast cancer, or thromboembolism. If these risk factors are present, or if the woman is asymptomatic, consider alternative treatments to prevent bone loss.
- If HT is selected, estrogen should be given in combination with progestin for women with an intact uterus. Depending on duration of use, unopposed estrogen carries a 2–6.7-fold higher risk of endometrial cancer. Most data available are for continuous treatment (as opposed to cyclical) with combined conjugated equine estrogen (CEE) 0.625 mg and medroxyprogesterone acetate 2.5 mg. However, considerable evidence supports the use of low-dose HT, which is associated with 50% lower rates of irregular bleeding. Low dose = 0.3 or 0.45 mg/d of CEE (4)[A].

- Precautions:
  - The Women's Health Initiative (WHI) study, in 2002, done in women without established coronary heart disease (CHD), found those treated with combination estrogen–progestin therapy had an increased relative risk of invasive breast cancer, CHD, stroke, and pulmonary embolism at 5 years of use (3)[A]. This risk of breast cancer was found to be independent of mammography screening frequency (1)[B]. Put another way, for every 100 women treated with HT for 5 years, 1 will have a serious adverse event.
  - The Heart and Estrogen/Progestin Replacement study (HERS), done in women with established CHD, demonstrated improvements in the lipid profiles of women on HT, but the overall risk of vascular mortality did not decline.
  - There is an increased risk of ovarian cancer in women who take HT. One out of every 8,300 women who take hormone replacement therapy each year has been shown to suffer from ovarian cancer (5)[B].
  - Higher doses of estrogen can cause hypercoagulability, breast tenderness, gallbladder disease, and hypertension (HTN).
  - Contraindications to HT:
    - Estrogen-dependent malignancies
    - Unexplained uterine bleeding
    - History of thromboembolism or stroke
    - CAD
    - Active liver disease
- For osteoporosis:
  - Women with a history of hip or vertebral fracture or personal history of osteoporosis should be treated.
  - Bisphosphonates inhibit osteoclast action and resorption of bone:
    - Alendronate (Fosamax): Treatment dose: 70 mg/wk or 10 mg/d. Prevention dose: 35 mg/wk or 5 mg/d.
    - Risedronate (Actonel): 35 mg once a week or 5 mg/d. Same dose for prevention and treatment.
    - Zoledronic acid (Reclast or Zometa): 5 mg IV annually. Same dose for prevention and treatment.
    - Ibandronate (Boniva): 2.5 mg/d or 150 mg/mo. Same dose for prevention and treatment:
      - The BONE trial demonstrated that ibandronate decreased the risk of vertebral fracture, but it failed to demonstrate a decrease in the risk of extravertebral fractures.
  - Selective estrogen receptor modulators (SERMs) selectively inhibit or stimulate estrogenlike action in various tissues. The SERM used for the treatment of osteoporosis is the following:
    - Raloxifene (Evista): 60 mg/d for prevention and treatment; because raloxifene is a less potent antiresorptive drug than alendronate, risedronate, or estrogen, it is best suited for the prevention or treatment of mild osteoporosis (7)[A].
    - Raloxifene should be used in postmenopausal women who cannot tolerate bisphosphonates and/or those who are at risk for invasive breast cancer.
    - Raloxifene should be used primarily in postmenopausal women with predominantly spinal osteoporosis (7,8)[A].
    - The EFFECT trial demonstrated that raloxifene decreased the risk of vertebral fracture but failed to demonstrate a decrease in the risk of extravertebral fractures.
    - Calcium: 1,200–1,500 mg elemental calcium PO daily
    - Vitamin D: 800–1,200 IU PO daily
- For atrophic vaginitis:
  - Topical estrogen therapy (ET): Conjugated estrogens (Premarin cream); best for local therapy of atrophic vaginitis. ET applied to vaginal mucosa as needed reverses vaginal atrophy, enhances blood flow, reduces pH and UTIs. Data are insufficient to recommend annual endometrial surveillance in women using ET with no vaginal bleeding. ET should be continued as long as distressing symptoms remain. Women with a history of hormone-dependent cancer should consult with an oncologist before using (9)[B].

Second Line

Nonhormonal treatments may be helpful to treat vasomotor symptoms in women who wish to or need to avoid HT (e.g., breast CA):

- Antidepressants venlafaxine (37.5–75 mg/d), paroxetine (10–20 mg/d), or fluoxetine (20 mg/d) are options that have been shown to result in 1 fewer hot flash a day.
- Gabapentin (300–900 mg/d) has been shown to have some effect in reducing vasomotor symptoms by up to 2 hot flashes per day (10)[A].
- Clonidine may be used to treat mild hot flashes, although it is less effective than antidepressants or gabapentin. Initial oral dose is 0.05 mg b.i.d.; some women may require 0.1 mg b.i.d.
- All trials of second-line therapies have been of short duration (i.e., a few months) (8,10)[A].

COMPLEMENTARY AND ALTERNATIVE MEDICINE

Trials of nonprescribed therapies are difficult to interpret due to variability of components and doses:

- Soy isoflavone showed a mixed effect in placebo-controlled trials in reduction of hot flashes.
- Red clover, black cohosh, reflexology, aerobics, and magnet therapy showed no impact on hot flashes when compared to placebo.
- Small clinical trials of evening primrose, dong quai, ginseng, and wild yam do not support their use for relief of hot flashes.

ONGOING CARE

FOLLOW-UP RECOMMENDATIONS

Patient Monitoring

A DEXA scan is indicated at age 65 for all women and at age 60 for women at risk for osteoporotic fractures (6)[B].

DIET

Calcium and vitamin D supplements as above

PATIENT EDUCATION

Encourage lifestyle modifications:

- Smoking cessation
- Weight-bearing exercise
- Avoid excess alcohol and caffeine.
- Address cardiovascular risk factor modification.

PROGNOSIS

If untreated:

- Ultimate disappearance of vasomotor symptoms; usually takes several years
- Osteoporosis: Possible fractures of the hip, vertebrae, and wrists

COMPLICATIONS

- Osteoporosis: At menopause, women have accelerated bone loss up to 3–5% per year for 5–7 years.
- Increased risk of CAD

REFERENCES

1. Chlebowski RT, Kuller LH, Prentice RL, et al. Breast cancer after use of estrogen plus progestin in postmenopausal women. *N Engl J Med*. 2009;360:573–87.
2. Nelson HD. Commonly used types of postmenopausal estrogen for treatment of hot flashes: Scientific review. *JAMA*. 2004;291: 1610–20.
3. Rossouw JE, Anderson GL, Prentice RL, et al. Risks and benefits of estrogen plus progestin in healthy postmenopausal women: Principal results From the Women's Health Initiative randomized controlled trial. *JAMA*. 2002;288:321–33.
4. Lobo RA, et al. Should symptomatic menopausal women be offered hormone therapy? *Med Gen Med*. 2006;8(3):40–58.
5. Mørch LS, Løkkegaard E, Andreasen AH, et al. Hormone therapy and ovarian cancer. *JAMA*. 2009;302:298–305.
6. Sambrook PN, Geusens P, Ribot C, et al. Alendronate produces greater effects than raloxifene on bone density and bone turnover in postmenopausal women with low bone density: Results of EFFECT (Efficacy of FOSAMAX versus EVISTA Comparison Trial) International. *J Intern Med*. 2004;255:503–11.
7. Riggs BL, Hartmann LC. Selective estrogen-receptor modulators – mechanisms of action and application to clinical practice. *N Engl J Med*. 2003;348:618–29.
8. North American Menopause Society. The role of local vaginal estrogen for treatment of vaginal atrophy in postmenopausal women. *Menopause*. 2007;14(3):357–69.
9. National Guideline Clearinghouse. Menopause. www.guideline.gov.
10. USPSTF. www.ahrq.gov/clinic/epcsums/osteoporosis.pdf.

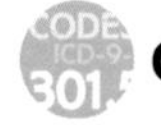

CODES

ICD9

- 256.31 Premature menopause
- 627.2 Symptomatic menopausal or female climacteric states

CLINICAL PEARLS

- Menopause is usually diagnosed by history alone.
- HT can be used short term for relief of moderate to severe vasomotor symptoms but not in the longer term for prevention of cardiovascular disease.

MENORRHAGIA

Donald A.F. Nelson, MD

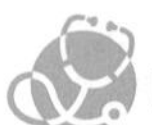

BASICS

DESCRIPTION

- Excessive amount or duration of menstrual flow, at more or less regular intervals. Flow ≥80 mL per cycle, compared to normal average 30–40 mL (1,2).
- Distinguishable from but may overlap with the following:
  - Metrorrhagia: Irregular or frequent flow, noncyclic
  - Menometrorrhagia: Frequent, excessive, irregular flow (menorrhagia plus metrorrhagia)
  - Polymenorrhea: Frequent flow, cycles of 21 days or fewer
  - Intermenstrual bleeding: Bleeding between regular menses
  - Dysfunctional uterine bleeding (DUB): Abnormal endometrial bleeding of hormonal cause and related to anovulation
- System(s) affected: Reproductive

EPIDEMIOLOGY

Prevalence

- The prevalence of abnormal uterine bleeding (AUB) is estimated at 11–13% in the general population and increases with age, reaching 24% in those aged 36–40 years (3).
- ~30% of women complain of excessive bleeding at some point (1).
- Predominant sex: Female only
- Predominant age:
  - Menarche to menopause; ~50% of cases occur in patients >40 years old
  - Dysfunctional bleeding is fairly common in adolescence and near menopause.
  - In adolescence, irregular bleeding due to anovulation and immaturity of the hypothalamic-pituitary-ovarian axis is common.

Pediatric Considerations

Genital bleeding before puberty can result from trauma, foreign bodies, vaginal infection, or exogenous hormone administration.

Pregnancy Considerations

Bleeding in pregnancy is not menorrhagia. Complications of pregnancy or cervical/vaginal lesions should be considered.

Geriatric Considerations

True menorrhagia cannot occur after menopause. However, genital atrophy as well as uterine and ovarian cancers may be associated with vaginal bleeding in the elderly.

RISK FACTORS

- Obesity
- Anovulation
- Estrogen administration (± progestin)
- Prior treatment with progestational agents or oral contraceptives increases risk of endometrial atrophy, but it decreases the risk of endometrial hyperplasia or neoplasia.

GENERAL PREVENTION

Periodic Pap smears and pelvic examinations at appropriate intervals based on age and risk factors

ETIOLOGY

- Hypothyroidism
- Endometrial proliferation/excess/hyperplasia:
  - Anovulation, oligo-ovulation
  - Ovarian tumor
  - Prolonged estrogen, progestin, or oral contraceptive administration
  - Polycystic ovarian syndrome
- Local factors:
  - Endometrial atrophy, postmenopause
  - Abnormal endometrial prostaglandin levels
  - Endometrial polyps
  - Endometrial neoplasia
  - Adenomyosis/endometriosis
  - Uterine myomata (fibroids)
  - Intrauterine device (IUD)
  - Uterine sarcoma
- Coagulation disorders:
  - Thrombocytopenia, platelet disorders
  - Von Willebrand disease, factor deficiencies
  - Leukemia
  - Ingestion of aspirin/acetylsalicylic acid or anticoagulants
  - Renal failure/dialysis

COMMONLY ASSOCIATED CONDITIONS

Metrorrhagia, menometrorrhagia, androgenic disorders

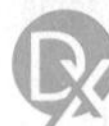

DIAGNOSIS

HISTORY

- Excessive menstrual flow is defined subjectively and varies greatly from woman to woman.
- Useful features:
  - Bleeding substantially heavier than usual flow (or >80 mL per cycle if quantified)
  - Bleeding lasting >7 days
  - Flow associated with significant clots
  - Anemia
- Symptoms that suggest cycles are ovulatory:
  - Regular menstrual interval
  - Midcycle pain (mittelschmerz)
  - Dysmenorrhea
  - Premenstrual symptoms: Breast soreness/tenderness, mood changes
- Abdominal pain or cramps at other times of the cycle may be associated with structural causes:
  - Myomas
  - Polyps
  - Ovarian tumors

PHYSICAL EXAM

- Hirsutism, acne, or obesity may accompany chronic anovulation.
- Pelvic/rectal examination to detect/exclude other causes of bleeding:
  - Cervical or vaginal bleeding
  - Pelvic or adnexal masses
  - Signs of pelvic infection

DIAGNOSTIC TESTS & INTERPRETATION

Lab

Initial lab tests

- Pregnancy test: Exclude pregnancy first.
- CBC to assess severity of blood loss and to rule out thrombocytopenia and leukemia (2)
- In selected cases:
  - TSH test
  - Coagulation screen, with follow-up testing if screen is abnormal
  - Creatinine, BUN
  - Serum progesterone: 5–20 ng/mL (15.9–63.6 nmol/L) in luteal phase, <1 ng/mL (<3.18 nmol/L) in follicular phase or anovulatory cycle

Imaging

Initial approach

- Transvaginal ultrasonography can help distinguish bleeding due to atrophy from bleeding caused by hyperplasia, polyps, or myomas.
- Ultrasonography to evaluate adnexal masses or myomas suspected from pelvic exam.
- A CT is used to investigate potentially malignant pelvic masses.
- An MRI is not recommended as a first-line procedure (3).

Diagnostic Procedures/Surgery

- Endometrial biopsy detects hyperplasia, dysplasia, or atrophy. If done before expected menses, it may also help confirm the diagnosis of anovulation or luteal phase defect.
- After age 35–40, endometrial carcinoma is a significant cause of bleeding. Obtain endometrial sampling before attempting hormonal treatment (4)[C].

Pathological Findings

- Vary with etiology. In ~50% of cases, no uterine pathology is found (1).
- Progestins used before endometrial biopsy may cause decidualization and obscure correct diagnosis.

DIFFERENTIAL DIAGNOSIS

- Pregnancy complications:
  - Threatened abortion
  - Incomplete abortion
  - Ectopic pregnancy
- Nonuterine bleeding:
  - Cervical ectropion/erosion
  - Cervical neoplasia/polyp
  - Cervical or vaginal trauma/foreign body
  - Condylomata
  - Atrophic vaginitis
- Pelvic inflammatory disease:
  - Endometritis
  - Tuberculosis

TREATMENT

MEDICATION

First Line

- For acute control of severe bleeding:
  - Estrogen, conjugated (Premarin): 25 mg IV q4h up to 6 doses or 10–20 mg/d PO in 4 divided doses until bleeding abates (4)[C]
- For less severe bleeding (usual case) or after control of acute bleeding has been achieved:
  - Medroxyprogesterone acetate (Provera): 10–30 mg/d for 5–10 days
  - Any combination oral contraceptive (i.e., usually a high-dose oral contraceptive) 1 tablet q.i.d. for 5–7 days
- To prevent heavy bleeding in subsequent cycles:
  - Medroxyprogesterone acetate: 5–30 mg/d for 10 days per month
  - Usual cyclic dose of a combination oral contraceptive (4)[C]

Second Line

- Nonsteroidal prostaglandin-synthetase inhibitors (e.g., naproxen, mefenamic acid, ibuprofen) can reduce blood loss ~25% with ovulatory cycles and reduce dysmenorrhea (5)[B].
- Tranexamic acid (Cyklokapron), a plasminogen activation inhibitor, 2 g/d PO is equally or more effective than medroxyprogesterone 10 mg b.i.d. (6)[B].
- Norethindrone acetate (Aygestin): 2.5–10 mg/d for 10–21 days per month
- Levonorgestrel intrauterine system (Mirena IUD) can reduce blood loss >90% (5)[B].
- Danazol and GnRH agonists are also effective therapies but are more likely to have adverse side effects. Mifepristone (RU-486) has been used experimentally (1).

ADDITIONAL TREATMENT

Additional Therapies

Nausea and vomiting are common from IV estrogen; antiemetics are helpful.

SURGERY/OTHER PROCEDURES

- Endometrial ablation by laser, electrosurgical, microwave, or thermal means is a conservative alternative to hysterectomy and usually successful, although some patients require additional therapy in the long term (1,7)[A].
- Hysterectomy when indicated to treat coexisting conditions (myomas, endometrial dysplasia) or for bleeding unresponsive to other measures (1,8).

IN-PATIENT CONSIDERATIONS

Initial Stabilization

- Most cases can be managed as outpatient in an office or emergency department.
- Rule out pregnancy complications and nonuterine bleeding.
- Treat severe or life-threatening bleeding acutely:
  - Circulatory support, transfusion if necessary
  - IV estrogen
  - Curettage if necessary
  - Hysterectomy in extreme cases

Admission Criteria

- Bleeding leading to orthostatic hypotension
- Hematocrit <25%

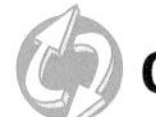

ONGOING CARE

FOLLOW-UP RECOMMENDATIONS

Proceed to identify the underlying cause of bleeding and treat to prevent recurrence:

- Hormonal therapy
- Dilatation and curettage for cases that fail to respond to hormone therapy
- Consider endometrial ablation or hysterectomy in persistent cases in which fertility is not a concern.
- Specific treatment for neoplasia, polyps, systemic disease
- Patients in whom fertility is a consideration may also need appropriate treatment for anovulation, endometriosis, and myomas.

Patient Monitoring

- Varies with cause of bleeding
- Medical treatment of hyperplastic/dysplastic endometrium should be followed by a repeat biopsy to confirm that histologic structure has returned to normal.

DIET

Iron supplementation may help correct for increased blood loss.

PATIENT EDUCATION

Information about side effects of medications should be provided.

PROGNOSIS

- Varies with cause of bleeding
- Most patients whose condition results from hormonal causes will respond to hormonal manipulation.

COMPLICATIONS

- Anemia
- Estrogen may precipitate acute intermittent porphyria or cholestatic jaundice in susceptible patients.

REFERENCES

1. Oehler MK, Rees MC. Menorrhagia: An update. *Acta Obstet Gynecol Scand*. 2003;82:405–22.
2. Siegel JE. Abnormalities of hemostasis and abnormal uterine bleeding. *Clin Obstet Gynecol*. 2005;48:284–94.
3. Marret H, Fauconnier A, Chabbert-Buffet N, et al. Clinical practice guidelines on menorrhagia: Management of abnormal uterine bleeding before menopause. *Eur J Obstet Gynecol Reprod Biol*. 2010;152:133–7.
4. Management of anovulatory bleeding. *ACOG Practice Bulletin 14, March 2000, reaffirmed* 2009.
5. Reid PC, Virtanen-Kari S. Randomised comparative trial of levonorgestrel intrauterine system and mefenamic acid for the treatment of idiopathic menorrhagia. *BJOG*. 2005;112:1121–5.
6. Kriplani A, Kulshrestha V, Agarwal N. Role of tranexamic acid in management of dysfunctional uterine bleeding in comparison with medroxyprogesterone acetate. *J Obstet Gynaecol*. 2006;26:673–8.
7. Practice Committee of American Society for Reproductive Medicine, et al. Indications and options for endometrial ablation. *Fertil Steril*. 2008; 90:S236–40.
8. Showstack J, Lin F, Learman LA. Randomized trial of medical treatment versus hysterectomy for abnormal uterine bleeding: Resource use in the Medicine or Surgery (Ms) trial. *Am J Obstet Gynecol*. 2006;194:332–8.

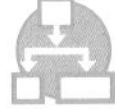

See Also (Topic, Algorithm, Electronic Media Element)

- Abnormal Pap and Cervical Dysplasia; Amenorrhea; Cervical Malignancy; Cervical Polyps; Cervicitis, Ectropion, and True Erosion; Dysfunctional Uterine Bleeding; Dysmenorrhea; Menopause; Polycystic Ovarian Syndrome (PCOS); Uterine Myomas
- Algorithm: Menorrhagia (Excessive Bleeding)

CODES

ICD9

- 626.2 Excessive or frequent menstruation
- 626.3 Puberty bleeding
- 626.6 Metrorrhagia

CLINICAL PEARLS

- Menorrhagia is defined as an excessive amount or duration of menstrual flow at more or less regular intervals and has a wide variety of potential causes.
- Pregnancy should be ruled out as part of the initial evaluation.
- Because endometrial carcinoma is a significant cause of bleeding in women over age 35, an endometrial biopsy to rule out endometrial carcinoma is recommended before using any hormonal treatments.
- Iron supplementation will help correct for increased blood loss while the underlying etiology is being identified and treated.

MENTAL RETARDATION

Jennifer L. Ayres, PhD

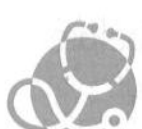

BASICS

- Mental retardation (MR) is a global deficit in cognitive functioning evidenced by a significant difference between one's mental and chronological ages (also known as *intelligence quotient* [IQ]) and significantly impaired adaptive functioning (1).
- Although these cognitive issues typically have a pervasive impact, patients with MR will display highly variable levels of functioning and subsequent service needs.
- Patients must be evaluated individually. Treatment plans must be tailored to specific needs.
- The current *Diagnostic Statistical Manual of Mental Disorders, 4th edition, Text Revision*, diagnosis is "Mental Retardation." However, because that term has been deemed to be pejorative and culturally insensitive, the term "intellectual disability" should be used instead.

DESCRIPTION

- MR is defined as an IQ ≤70 and a significant impairment in an area of adaptive functioning such as communication, self-care, activities of daily living, socialization, use of community and resources, or health/safety (1).
- These issues are present prior to the age of 18 years.
- Currently, MR is subgrouped according to IQ level: mild, IQ ~55–69; moderate, ~40–54; severe, ~25–39; and profound, ~0–24. A diagnosis of "Mental Retardation, Severity Unspecified" may be used for individuals who are unable to undergo formal assessment.
- The 3 most common causes of MR are Down syndrome, Fragile X syndrome, and fetal alcohol syndrome (FAS).
- Synonym(s): Intellectual disability; Cognitive disability

ALERT

For some causes of MR, prenatal testing is available.

EPIDEMIOLOGY

Incidence

- 1 in 63 to 1 in 83 (found in 2 surveillance studies in Atlanta, GA, in 1996 and 2000) (2)
- By definition, MR begins in childhood and must be diagnosed prior to the age of 18 years.
- Predominant sex: Male > Female: 2:1 for mild MR, 1.5:1 for severe MR

Prevalence

In the US, 1–2.5% of the population

RISK FACTORS

- Maternal substance abuse during pregnancy
- Maternal infection during pregnancy
- For some causes, family history
- Mild MR is more common in children of women who did not complete high school; is likely related to genetic and socioeconomic factors (e.g., nutritional deficiencies, poverty).

Genetics

A number of genetic and epigenetic causes are known, and more are under investigation (3).

GENERAL PREVENTION

- Public health efforts to reduce alcohol and drug use by pregnant women
- Prenatal folic acid supplementation

ETIOLOGY

- The cause of mild MR is identified in <50% of cases. The cause of severe MR is identified in >75% of cases.
- Causes:
  - Maternal substance abuse (e.g., alcohol); FAS is a leading environmental cause of MR.
  - Maternal infections: TORCH viruses (*T*oxoplasma, *o*ther infections, *r*ubella, *c*ytomegalovirus, and *h*erpes simplex)
  - Down syndrome
  - Sex chromosome abnormalities: Fragile X, Turner syndrome, Klinefelter syndrome
  - Autosomal-dominant conditions: Neurocutaneous syndromes (e.g., neurofibromatosis, tuberous sclerosis)
  - Autosomal-recessive conditions:
    - Amino acid metabolism (e.g., phenylketonuria, maple-syrup urine disease)
    - Carbohydrate metabolism (e.g., galactosemia, fructosuria)
    - Lipid metabolism
    - Tay-Sachs disease
    - Gaucher disease
    - Niemann-Pick disease (e.g., mucopolysaccharidosis)
    - Purine metabolism (e.g., Lesch-Nyhan disease)
    - Other (e.g., Wilson disease)
- Maternal use of prescription medications (e.g., Accutane, Dilantin)
- Perinatal factors:
  - Prematurity
  - Birth injuries
  - Perinatal anoxia
- Postnatal factors:
  - Childhood diseases (e.g., meningitis, encephalitis, hypothyroidism)
  - Trauma (e.g., accidents, physical abuse)
  - Severe deprivation
  - Poisoning (e.g., lead, carbon monoxide, household products)

COMMONLY ASSOCIATED CONDITIONS

- Seizures
- Mood disorders
- Behavioral disorders

DIAGNOSIS

A diagnosis of MR/intellectual disability should be made only through a psychodiagnostic assessment conducted by a mental health provider who is trained and licensed to conduct formal psychological testing.

HISTORY

- 3-generation family history
- Children with profound or severe MR typically are diagnosed at birth or during the newborn period and are more likely to have dysmorphic features.
- Children with MR often are identified because they fail to meet motor or language milestones.

PHYSICAL EXAM

Careful examination by a physician trained in the assessment of morphologic features suggestive of a specific etiology for MR (e.g., microcephaly) (4)

DIAGNOSTIC TESTS & INTERPRETATION

- Visual and hearing tests to rule out these etiologies as a cause of impairment and provide an assessment of visual and auditory functioning, which often are impaired in children and adults with MR
- Formal testing of intellectual and adaptive functioning:
  - A child's communication skills must be considered in test selection. For example, a patient with auditory processing issues or limited expressive or receptive language skills may need to be assessed using a nonverbal IQ test, such as the Leiter-R, Test of Nonverbal Intelligence, or other nonverbal measures.
  - Commonly used intelligence tests (e.g., Bayley Scales of Infant Development, Stanford-Binet Intelligence Scale, Wechsler Intelligence Scales) are determined by age/developmental level of the child.
  - Common tests of adaptive functioning include the Vineland Adaptive Behavior Scales, 2nd edition, and Adaptive Behavior Assessment System, 2nd ed. These tests assess areas of functioning, such as age-appropriate communication, social skills, activities of daily living, and motor skills.

Lab

- Metabolic screening is not routine unless evidence in history and physical or no newborn screening records (5)[B]
- Lead as per current targeted guidelines (5)[B]
- Thyroid-stimulating hormone if systemic features present or no newborn screening (5)[B]
- Routine cytogenetic testing (karyotype) (5)[B]:
  - Fragile X screening (*FMR1* gene), particularly if there is family history of intellectual disability (5)[B]
  - Rett syndrome (*MECP2* gene) in women with unexplained moderate-to-severe intellectual disability (5)[B]
- Molecular screening such as array comparative genomic hybridization is used increasingly and may yield a diagnosis in 10% undiagnosed cases (4)[B].

Imaging

- Neuroimaging (MRI more sensitive than CT) is routinely recommended. The presence of physical findings (microcephaly, focal motor deficit) will increase the yield of a specific diagnosis (5)[B].
- MRI may show mild cerebral abnormalities but is unlikely to establish etiology of MR (4).

Follow-Up & Special Considerations

Electroencephalogram is not routine unless epilepsy or a specific epileptiform syndrome is present (5)[C].

DIFFERENTIAL DIAGNOSIS

- Brain tumors
- Auditory, visual, and/or speech/language impairment
- Autistic disorder (language and social skills are more affected than other cognitive abilities); however, 75% of individuals with an autistic disorder may meet criteria for a comorbid diagnosis of MR.
- Expressive or receptive language disorders
- Cerebral palsy
- Emotional or behavioral disturbance
- Learning disorders (reading, math, written expression)
- Auditory or sensory processing difficulties
- Lack of environmental opportunities for appropriate development

TREATMENT

- Early intervention services tailored to the individual's specific needs
- Caregiver support, including:
  - Training caregiver(s) to address behavioral issues and support socialization development
  - Encouraging caregivers to create a structured home environment that is based on the child's developmental level and specific needs rather than age-appropriate expectations
  - Providing caregiver(s) with an opportunity to address their reactions to the diagnosis and their child's special needs
  - Informing caregivers about advocacy groups and available community, state, and national resources (6,7)
- Individualized education plans and, depending on the level of impairment, social skills and behavioral plans/training
- Refer to job training programs and independent living opportunities if appropriate.
- Take notice of all changes in behavior, which may be indicative of pain or illness, particularly in individuals with limited communication skills.
- Assess for abuse and neglect.

MEDICATION

Medication may be appropriate for comorbid conditions (e.g., anxiety, ADHD, depression).

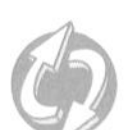

ONGOING CARE

The physician should match his or her communication of exam procedures, test results, and treatment recommendations to the patient's level of cognitive functioning and receptive language skills:

- The vast majority of patients with MR will fall within the mild range and are fully capable of understanding information if it is provided at the appropriate level.
- Provide oral and written explanations directly to the patient instead of solely to his or her caregivers. The dignity of the patient must be respected at all times. This includes providing honest information, responding to patient's questions with respect, and not infantilizing the patient due to his or her intellectual disability.

FOLLOW-UP RECOMMENDATIONS

- Many adults and children with MR exhibit poor physical fitness. Preliminary studies suggest that structured exercise programs are effective to engage this population in healthy activities (8)[A].
- Linkage to community-based resources for job training, independent living, caregiver support, school-based services

Patient Monitoring

- Primary care with attention to associated medical conditions
- Vision testing at least once before age 40 (age 30 in Down syndrome) and every 2 years thereafter (9)[B]
- Hearing evaluations every 5 years after age 45 (every 3 years throughout life in Down syndrome) (9)[B]
- Screen for sexual activity and offer contraception and testing for STIs (9)[B].
- Abuse and neglect of people with MR are common. Screen at least annually and assess for abuse if behavior change is noted. Report abuse or neglect to appropriate protective agencies (9)[B].
- Dysphagia and aspiration are common; consider speech pathology evaluation and swallowing study (10)[B].
- Monitor for and treat constipation (10)[B].
- Osteoporosis: Common; low threshold to order imaging studies after traumatic injury (10)[B]

DIET

No restrictions, except in cases of metabolic and storage disorders (e.g., phenylketonuria). Ensure that the patient has access to appropriate information regarding healthy eating and nutrition.

PATIENT EDUCATION

- Families should be referred to the local Association for Retarded Citizens: www.thearc.org
- American Association of Intellectual and Developmental Disabilities: www.aaidd.org
- Refer to local family support group (e.g., Parent To Parent, local Down Syndrome Association, local Autism Association)
- Special Olympics: www.specialolympics.org

PROGNOSIS

Although MR is a lifelong diagnosis, individuals with MR are capable of living a fulfilling, purposeful life that includes having a career, living independently, marrying/participating in a committed relationship, and becoming a parent.

REFERENCES

1. American Psychiatric Association. *Diagnostic and Statistical Manual of Mental Disorders,* 4th ed, text revision. Arlington, VA: American Psychiatric Association; 2000.
2. www.cdc.gov/ncbddd/dd/.
3. Grant ME. The epigenetic origins of mental retardation. *Clin Genet*. 2008;73:528–30.
4. van Karnebeek CDM, Jansweijer MCE, Offringa M. Diagnostic investigations in individuals with mental retardation: A systematic literature review of their usefulness. *Eur J Human Genet*. 2005;13:6–25.
5. Shevell M, Ashwal S, Donley D, et al. Practice parameter: Evaluation of the child with global developmental delay: Report of the Quality Standards Subcommittee of the American Academy of Neurology and The Practice Committee of the Child Neurology Society. *Neurology*. 2003;60:367–80.
6. Shogren KA, Bradley VJ, Gomez SC, et al. Public policy and the enhancement of desired outcomes for persons with intellectual disability. *Intellect Dev Disabil*. 2009;47:307–19.
7. Rizzolo MC, Hemp R, Braddock D, et al. Family support services for persons with intellectual and developmental disabilities: Recent national trends. *Intellect Dev Disabil*. 2009;47:152–5.
8. Heller T, Hsieh K, Rimmer JH. Attitudinal and psychosocial outcomes of a fitness and health education program on adults with down syndrome. *Am J Ment Retard*. 2004;109:175–85.
9. Sullivan WF, Heng J, Cameron D, et al. Consensus guidelines for primary health care of adults with developmental disabilities. *Can Fam Physician*. 2006;52:1410–8.
10. Prater CD, Zylstra RG. Medical care of adults with mental retardation. *Am Fam Physician*. 2006;73:2175–83.

ADDITIONAL READING

Moeschler JB, Shevell M, American Academy of Pediatrics Committee on Genetics. Clinical genetic evaluation of the child with mental retardation or developmental delays. *Pediatrics*. 2006;117:2304–16.

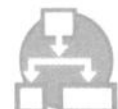

See Also (Topic, Algorithm, Electronic Media Element)

- Attention Deficit/Hyperactivity Disorder; Cerebral Palsy; Down Syndrome; Fragile X Syndrome; Lead Poisoning
- Algorithm: Mental Retardation

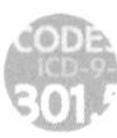

CODES

ICD9

- 317 Mild intellectual disabilities
- 318.0 Moderate intellectual disabilities
- 319 Unspecified mental retardation

CLINICAL PEARLS

- The term *mental retardation* may be interpreted as culturally insensitive and disrespectful to patients and their caregivers. *Intellectual disability* is the preferred term.
- Overall functioning with MR is highly variable and influenced by multiple factors, including appropriateness of school placement/special education services, exposure to early intervention, behavioral therapy, parent training, self-esteem, and social skills.
- Previous stereotypes of people with MR (e.g., always happy, poor prognosis, unable to function independently) have been refuted. People with MR are showing a level of functioning variability that parallels what is found in the non-MR population.
- Be aware of the unique parenting needs that caregivers may face. Link families to community resources that can provide practical and emotional support when appropriate.
- Because children with developmental disabilities are at higher risk of being abused than their peers without developmental disabilities, discuss with caregivers how to educate children about safety precautions in a developmentally appropriate manner.

MESENTERIC ADENITIS

Karen Buch, MD
Daniel J. Kowal, MD

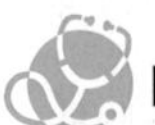

BASICS

Mesenteric adenitis is inflammation of the mesenteric lymph nodes, typically a self-limited disease.

DESCRIPTION

Both acute and chronic episodes of mesenteric adenitis have been described:

- May clinically mimic acute appendicitis

EPIDEMIOLOGY

- It is a commonly misdiagnosed condition, making definite incidence unknown.
- Estimated at around 20% in patients presenting for appendectomy (1)

Prevalence

- Mesenteric adenitis generally affects males and females equally:
  - However, adenitis secondary to *Yersinia* infection is more prevalent in boys than girls (2).
- The prevalence of etiological agent *Yersinia enterocolitica* is most common in North America, Eastern Europe, and Australia (2).

RISK FACTORS

- Typically preceded by upper respiratory infection or pharyngitis (3)
- History of ingesting undercooked pork (2)

Genetics

Mesenteric adenitis can occur in adults, but it is more common in children and adolescents younger than 15 years. This condition during childhood or adolescence is linked to a significantly reduced risk of ulcerative colitis in adulthood (3).

GENERAL PREVENTION

Minimize risk by eating fully cooked foods, especially meat (2).

PATHOPHYSIOLOGY

- On gross inspection, lymph nodes are enlarged and soft.
- Adjoining mesentery may be edematous and may or may not present with exudates (3).
- In instances of infectious etiologies, pathogens are ingested, translocate intestinal epithelium and gain access to lymph nodes via intestinal lymphatics via Peyer's patches (3).

ETIOLOGY

Underlying infectious process or intra-abdominal inflammatory process:

- Infectious agents include (3,4):
  - *Y. enterocolitica*
  - Beta-hemolytic *Streptococcus* species
  - *Staphylococcus* species
  - *Streptococcus viridans*
  - *Escherichia coli*
  - *Mycobacterium tuberculosis*
  - *Giardia lamblia*
  - EBV
  - Acute HIV infection
  - Coxsackie viruses
  - Rubeola virus
  - Cat-scratch disease
  - Adenovirus species

COMMONLY ASSOCIATED CONDITIONS

- Appendicitis (4,5)
- Crohn disease (1,5)
- Ulcerative colitis (1,5)

DIAGNOSIS

HISTORY

The onset of symptoms is variable, and usually nausea or abdominal pain are the first presenting symptoms. Generally, symptoms are nonspecific:

- Nausea and vomiting (which may precede abdominal pain)
- Abdominal pain: Nonspecific and diffuse tenderness
- Malaise or fatigue
- Diarrhea
- Fevers
- Anorexia
- Recent history of upper respiratory tract infection

PHYSICAL EXAM

- Fevers
- Right lower quadrant tenderness, may or may not exhibit rebound tenderness
- Peripheral/generalized lymphadenopathy
- Toxic appearance
- Rectal tenderness
- Rhinorrhea
- Hyperemic pharynx

DIAGNOSTIC TESTS & INTERPRETATION

Lab

Initial lab tests

- CBC: Leukocytosis
- Basic metabolic panel: May show contraction alkalosis and azotemia
- Stool cultures for diarrhea
- Serologic testing of etiologic agents
- Blood cultures: Patients with septicemia

Imaging

Initial approach

- CT scan: Enlarged mesenteric lymph nodes that tend to be increased in size, number, and distribution compared to that seen in appendicitis:
  - A specific CT appearance is described as a minimum of 5 clustered lymph nodes measuring at least 3 mm in the short axis diameter (6)[B],(7)[B].
  - May or may not have evidence of ileal or ileocecal wall thickening
  - Appendix appears normal
- Ultrasound: Used for exclusion of other potential differential diagnoses:
  - Preferred imaging modality in children
  - May elicit focal tenderness with transducer pressure (7)[B]

Diagnostic Procedures/Surgery

- Lymph node biopsy: Applicable only for those patients already subjected to laparotomy to isolate the causative organism.
- Surgery is usually indicated in cases of suppuration and/or abscess formation, with signs of peritonitis, or if acute appendicitis cannot be excluded with certainty.

Pathological Findings

- Microscopically, lymph nodes display nonspecific hyperplasia. If a suppurative infection is present, lymph nodes may contain necrotic material with pus formation (1[B],4[C]).
- Lymphatic sinuses may be enlarged.
- Immune cell infiltration may be observed.
- In cases of *Y. entercolitica* infection, lymph node capsules may be thickened with surrounding edema present. There may be hyperplasia with infiltration from immune-mediated cells and plasma cells (4[C]).

DIFFERENTIAL DIAGNOSIS

- Appendicitis, pyelonephritis, cholecystitis, inflammatory bowel disease, benign neoplasm of small bowel
- UTI, salpingitis, chronic mesenteric ischemia, ectopic pregnancy
- Intestinal duplication, regional enteritis, intussusception, intestinal lymphoma, cecal tumor
- Vasoocclusive crises, porphyria, familial Mediterranean fever

TREATMENT

MEDICATION

First Line

- Supportive and symptomatic treatment for uncomplicated cases
- IV fluid resuscitation for patients with clinical evidence of hypovolemia
- Correction of any underlying electrolyte aberrations

Second Line

- Empiric broad-spectrum antibiotic administration for moderately to severely ill patients with adjustment for subsequently isolated pathogens
- Treatment duration is variable based on the cause and severity of illness. For uncomplicated cases, antibiotic treatment is not necessary.

SURGERY/OTHER PROCEDURES

- Surgery is usually indicated in cases of suppuration and/or abscess formation, with signs of peritonitis, or if acute appendicitis cannot be excluded with certainty.
- At laparotomy, the diagnosis is generally clear. An appendectomy should be performed in view of the tendency for recurrence and the difficulty in differentiating adenitis from appendicitis.

IN-PATIENT CONSIDERATIONS

Initial Stabilization

Volume resuscitation as needed and correction of any underlying electrolyte abnormalities

Admission Criteria

Indicated for patients with complications and hemodynamic instability

IV Fluids

- IV fluid hydration may be indicated for patients who cannot tolerate PO intake secondary to nausea or vomiting.
- Aggressive fluid hydration is indicated for patients who show evidence of sepsis.

Discharge Criteria

Hemodynamic stability, able to tolerate a PO diet

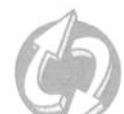

ONGOING CARE

FOLLOW-UP RECOMMENDATIONS

Patient Monitoring

Close outpatient monitoring is needed to ensure total resolution of symptoms.

DIET

There are no specific dietary recommendations. Oral intake can be temporarily held until nausea and vomiting resolve.

PATIENT EDUCATION

In cases of *Yersinia* infection, patients should avoid unpasteurized milk, raw pork, and contaminated water.

PROGNOSIS

- Generally self-limiting and benign condition
- Increased morbidity/mortality for patients presenting with concomitant sepsis

COMPLICATIONS

- Increased GI losses leading to hypovolemia and electrolyte imbalance
- Abscess formation
- Peritonitis
- Sepsis
- Latent extraintestinal manifestations, including arthralgias, truncal and extremity rashes, erythema nodosum in instances of *Y. enterocolitica* infection
- Postinfectious chronic complications of *Yersinia* infection including reactive arthritis, conjunctivitis, and urethritis

REFERENCES

1. Frisch M, Pedersen BV, Andersson RE. Appendicitis, mesenteric lymphadenitis, and subsequent risk of ulcerative colitis: Cohort studies in Sweden and Denmark. *BMJ*. 2009;338:b716.
2. Currie B. *Yersinia enterocolitica*. *Pediatr Rev*. 1998;19(7):250; discussion 251.
3. Blattner RJ. Acute mesenteric lymphadenitis. *J Pediatr*. 1969:479–81.
4. Kelly CS, Kelly RE Jr. Lymphadenopathy in children. *Pediatr Clin North Am*. 1998;45:875–88.
5. Zganjer M, Roic G, Cizmic A. Infectious ileocecitis—appendicitis mimicking syndrome. *Bratisl Lek Listy*. 2005;106:201–2.
6. Rao PM, Rhea JT, Novelline RA. CT diagnosis of mesenteric adenitis. *Radiology*. 1997;202:145–9.
7. Sivit CJ. Imaging children with acute right lower quadrant pain. *Pediatr Clin North Am*. 1997;44: 575–89.

ADDITIONAL READING

Bhandarkar DS, Shah RS, Katara AN, et al. Laparoscopic biopsy in patients with abdominal lymphadenopathy. *J Minim Access Surg*. 2007;3(1): 14–8.

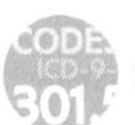

CODES

ICD9

289.2 Nonspecific mesenteric lymphadenitis

CLINICAL PEARLS

- This is a self-limited inflammatory process involving the mesenteric lymph nodes that may mimic appendicitis.
- It is more common in children, rather than adults, and may follow an upper respiratory tract infection.
- Treatment is mainly supportive.

M

METABOLIC SYNDROME

Deepali Tukaye, MD, PhD
Nancy Kubiak, MD

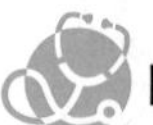

BASICS

DESCRIPTION

- A common disorder that is a risk factor for type 2 diabetes mellitus, cardiovascular disease, stroke, fatty liver and certain cancers
- Involves a cluster of metabolic abnormalities:
  – Intra-abdominal obesity
  – Dyslipidemia
  – Hypertension
  – Insulin resistance with or without impaired glucose tolerance
  – Proinflammatory state
  – Prothrombotic state

EPIDEMIOLOGY

- Predominant age: >60 years old (~50% of cases)
- Predominant sex: Male = Female
- Ethnicity: Mexican Americans (highest risk)

Prevalence

- Affects 34% of US adults >20 years old; increasing with the aging population and the prevalence of obesity
- Data vary among populations depending on the criteria used, but available literature suggests that metabolic syndrome is a rapidly growing epidemic worldwide.

Pediatric Considerations

- Obese children and adolescents are at high risk for the metabolic syndrome (prevalence of 6.4% in the US). Risk factors of metabolic syndrome in children and adolescents include heredity, low birth weight, childhood weight gain and obesity, endocrine abnormalities, hostility, maternal gestational diabetes, and poor health habits.
- International Diabetes Federation consensus report (1) defined criteria in 3 age groups (6 to <10 years; 10 to <16 years; 16+ years, adult criteria applicable). Obesity defined by waist circumference ≥90th percentile; rest of the diagnostic criteria (triglycerides [TGs], high-density lipoprotein-cholesterol [HDL-C], hypertension [HTN], and fasting blood sugar/type 2 diabetes mellitus [DM]) are largely the same as in adults for children ≥10 years, with some exceptions, and warrant treatment. Clinical significance of metabolic syndrome in pediatric population is not well established. Focus on established risk factors rather than diagnosis.

RISK FACTORS

- Obesity/intra-abdominal obesity
- Insulin resistance
- Older age
- Ethnicity
- Family history
- Physical inactivity
- High-carbohydrate diet
- Smoking
- Postmenopausal status
- Low socioeconomic status
- Alteration of gut flora

Genetics

Genetic factors contribute significantly to causation. Most identified genes are transcription factors or regulators of transcription and translation. It is a multifactorial disease with evidence of complex interactions between genetics and environment.

GENERAL PREVENTION

- Effective weight loss and maintenance of normal body weight long term
- Regular and sustained physical activity
- Diet low in saturated fats and simple sugars

PATHOPHYSIOLOGY

- Adipose tissue dysfunction and insulin resistance.
- Decreased levels of adiponectin, an adipocytokine, known to protect against type 2 DM, HTN, atherosclerosis, and inflammation.
- Increase in intra-abdominal and visceral adipose tissue.
- Abnormal fatty acid metabolism, endothelial dysfunction, systemic inflammation, oxidative stress, elevated renin-angiotensin system activation, and a prothrombotic state (increased tissue plasminogen activator inhibitor-1) are also associated.

ETIOLOGY

The main etiological factors are:

- Obesity (particularly abdominal)/excess adipose tissue
- Insulin resistance
- Other contributing factors:
  – Advancing age
  – Proinflammatory state
  – Genetics
- Endocrine (e.g., postmenopausal state)

COMMONLY ASSOCIATED CONDITIONS

- Polycystic ovary syndrome
- Fatty liver disease (nonalcoholic steatohepatitis)
- Chronic renal disease
- Obstructive sleep apnea
- Gallstones (cholesterol)
- Erectile dysfunction (in men)
- Hyperuricemia and gout

DIAGNOSIS

HISTORY

- Family history of metabolic syndrome, type 2 DM, and cardiovascular disease
- Symptoms indicating cardiovascular disease or diabetes
- Comprehensive lifestyle history:
  – Diet, including intake of carbohydrates and fats
  – Weight history, including onset of obesity and previous weight loss attempts
  – Exercise regimen
  – Alcohol intake
- Cigarette smoking
- Assess cardiovascular risk with Framingham risk assessment tool

PHYSICAL EXAM

Various criteria-based definitions have been proposed, including those by the World Health Organization, the International Diabetes Federation, and the National Cholesterol Education Program's Adult Treatment Panel III (ATP III). According to ATP III, a diagnosis of metabolic syndrome can be made when ≥3 of the following 5 characteristics are present (2):

- Abdominal obesity: Men >102 cm, women >88 cm (ATP III recommends lowering threshold in population prone to insulin resistance, especially Asian Americans)
- BP ≥130/85 mm Hg
- TGs ≥150 mg/dL
- HDL: Men <40 mg/dL, women <50 mg/dL
- Fasting glucose ≥100 mg/dL

DIAGNOSTIC TESTS & INTERPRETATION

Lab

Initial lab tests

- Fasting lipids (particularly TGs and HDL)
- Fasting glucose

Follow-Up & Special Considerations

- Formal 75-mg oral glucose tolerance test for diagnosis of impaired fasting glucose/impaired glucose tolerance (IGT)
- Serum-free testosterone, sex hormone-binding globulin
- Liver function tests
- Measurement of insulin levels is controversial

Imaging

None necessary to diagnose metabolic syndrome

Diagnostic Procedures/Surgery

- May require 24-hour BP monitoring (rules out white coat hypertension)
- ECG, stress test, coronary angiography may be used for diagnosis of cardiovascular disease arising as a complication of the syndrome

Pathological Findings

- Microalbuminuria
- Increased WBC count
- Increased C-reactive protein
- Increased fibrinogen
- Increased proinflammatory cytokines (e.g., tumor necrosis factor alpha)
- Increased uric acid
- Increased homocysteine
- Type 2 DM
- Fatty liver (complicated by end-stage liver disease and hepatocellular carcinoma)
- Hypertensive and/or diabetic eye disease
- Renal impairment/failure
- Peripheral vascular disease
- Coronary artery disease
- Cerebrovascular disease

DIFFERENTIAL DIAGNOSIS

Individual components of the syndrome may be present without fulfilling all the ATP III diagnostic criteria

TREATMENT

The primary therapeutic goal is to prevent or reduce obesity. Aggressive lifestyle modification (diet and exercise) is considered first-line therapy.

MEDICATION

- Daily treatment with aspirin is recommended for patients with cardiovascular disease or those at high risk.
- Consult clinical guidelines for treatment of dyslipidemia, hypertension, IGT, and diabetes
- Multiple medications usually are required to achieve adequate BP control.
- The diagnosis and treatment of insulin resistance is controversial.

First Line

Lifestyle modification alone as initial strategy is applicable to individuals with low 10-year Framingham risk for coronary artery disease (CAD). In individuals with higher 10-year risk, more aggressive risk factor based approach is recommended in addition to lifestyle modifications (3):

- Obesity: Lifestyle changes are the cornerstone of treatment. Aim for a gradual ~5–10% weight reduction. Any amount of weight loss is associated with significant benefits.
- Physical activity: 30–60 minutes of moderate-intensity aerobic activities like brisk walking 5–7 d/wk; increase in daily lifestyle activities and resistance training 1–2 d/wk. In patients with established CAD, assess detailed history of physical activity and exercise tolerance to guide activity prescription. Advise medically supervised programs for high-risk population (recent acute coronary syndrome [ACS], congestive heart failure, recent revascularization). Cumulative exercise time over the day contributes to health benefit.
- Dyslipidemia: Drug therapy can be commenced after 6 weeks of lifestyle modification. Target of therapy depends of patient's level of cardiovascular risk:
  - Statin if predominantly high low-density lipoprotein (LDL)
  - Fibrate with fish oils if predominantly high TGs and/or low HDL
  - Target LDL-cholesterol based on Framingham risk: high risk, <100 mg/dL; moderate risk, <130 mg/dL; low risk, <160 mg/dL.
  - If TGs are >200 mg/dL after achieving goal LDL-cholesterol, consider additional therapies for non–HDL-C (the goal is 30 mg/dL higher than LDL-cholesterol goal for each risk group).
  - If HDL-C remains low after non–HDL-C goal is achieved, intensify lifestyle modification or add drug therapy depending on patients risk category.
- HTN: Aim for similar targets to patients with diabetes (<130/80 mm Hg).
  - ACE inhibitor or angiotensin receptor blocker (e.g., losartan 50 mg/d if ACE inhibitor intolerance) is usually prescribed for patients with diabetes.
- Impaired glucose tolerance:
  - Current guidelines emphasize that treatment should be with diet and exercise. The role of oral hypoglycemic agents to prevent diabetes in patients with the metabolic syndrome is unclear. Metformin, 500 mg to 1 g, 1–3 times daily, may be considered (4).
- Prothrombotic state: Low-dose aspirin for patients with 10-year risk for CAD ≥10% or known atherosclerotic CAD or type 2 DM or others in high-risk category. Use clopidogrel if aspirin is contraindicated in these groups.
- If CAD or type 2 DM is already evident, treat as per guidelines.

ADDITIONAL TREATMENT

General Measures

- Aggressive treatment of individual risk factors
- Avoid or stop smoking.
- Avoid excess alcohol intake.

Issues for Referral

- Nutrition
- Exercise program
- Smoking cessation

COMPLEMENTARY AND ALTERNATIVE MEDICINE

Fish oils and plant sterol esters for cardioprotective effects

SURGERY/OTHER PROCEDURES

- Surgery to treat obesity in severely obese patients who have failed trials of lifestyle modification and pharmacotherapy (4); surgery recommended if body mass index [BMI] >40 or BMI >35 with obesity-related comorbidities.
- Liposuction of abdominal adipose tissue does not reduce insulin resistance or cardiovascular risk factors.

IN-PATIENT CONSIDERATIONS

Management usually does not require admission.

Admission Criteria

Serious complications (e.g., ACS, hypertensive crisis, diabetic coma)

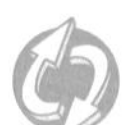

ONGOING CARE

FOLLOW-UP RECOMMENDATIONS

- Regular 30-minute exercise will improve all components of the metabolic syndrome. Cumulative small periods of exercise over the day provide significant health benefits.
- Encourage changing sedentary activity choices (e.g., driving car, taking elevator, and the like) to more active ones (e.g., walking, cycling).
- Regular monitoring of weight, abdominal circumference measurements, BP, fasting lipids, and sugar levels

Patient Monitoring

- Regular monitoring of weight, abdominal circumference measurements, BP, fasting lipids, and sugar levels
- Fasting lipids, fasting sugar, and/or oral glucose tolerance test should be checked annually.

DIET

- Weight reduction to correct abdominal obesity is a primary goal achieved by reduction of energy intake and increased physical activity (5)[A]. Reduction by 500 calories per day will usually achieve a weight loss of 0.5 kg/wk.
- Current recommendations include: Saturated fats <7% total calories; reduction in transfats; dietary cholesterol <200 mg/d; total fat 25–35% of total calories. Diet composed of unsaturated fat with limitation of simple sugars. Encourage salt restriction, increased consumption of fresh fruits and vegetables, alcohol moderation, increased fiber and whole grains.

PROGNOSIS

Increased risk of type 2 DM (~5-fold), CAD (~1.5–3-fold), acute myocardial infarction (~2.5-fold), and all-cause mortality (~1.5-fold) (6).

COMPLICATIONS

Long-term complications are primarily CAD and type 2 DM. Recent evidence demonstrates an increased risk of nonalcoholic fatty liver disease, stroke, and an increased risk of developing certain cancers, especially breast cancer in postmenopausal women.

REFERENCES

1. Zimmet P, Alberti KG, Kaufman F, et al. The metabolic syndrome in children and adolescents - an IDF consensus report. *Pediatr Diabetes*. 2007;8: 299–306.
2. National Cholesterol Education Program (NCEP) Expert Panel on Detection, Evaluation, and Treatment of High Blood Cholesterol in Adults (Adult Treatment Panel III), et al. Third Report of the National Cholesterol Education Program (NCEP) Expert Panel on Detection, Evaluation, and Treatment of High Blood Cholesterol in Adults (Adult Treatment Panel III) final report. *Circulation*. 2002;106:3143–421.
3. Grundy SM, Cleeman JI, Daniels SR, et al. Diagnosis and management of the metabolic syndrome: An American Heart Association/National Heart, Lung, and Blood Institute scientific statement: Executive Summary. *Crit Pathw Cardiol*. 2005;4:198–203.
4. Clinical Guidelines on the Identification, Evaluation, and Treatment of Overweight and Obesity in Adults: The Evidence Report. National Institutes of Health. *Obes Res*. 1998;6(Suppl 2):51S–209S.
5. Slentz CA, Duscha BD, Johnson JL, et al. Effects of the amount of exercise on body weight, body composition, and measures of central obesity: STRRIDE–a randomized controlled study. *Arch Intern Med*. 2004;164:31–9.
6. Kassi E, Pervanidou P, Kaltsas G, et al. Metabolic syndrome: Definitions and controversies. *BMC Med*. 2011;9:48.

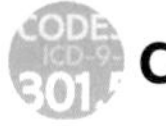

CODES

ICD9

- 272.8 Other disorders of lipoid metabolism
- 277.7 Dysmetabolic syndrome x
- 278.00 Obesity, unspecified

CLINICAL PEARLS

- Abdominal circumference should be measured as part of a cardiovascular risk assessment.
- Prevention or reduction of obesity is the cornerstone of management of metabolic syndrome. Cumulative physical activity over the day significantly adds to the benefit of regular 30–60-minute exercise regimen.
- Aggressive lifestyle modification is first-line lifelong treatment for all patients.

M

METATARSALGIA

Kenneth M. Bielak, MD
Eric J. Kujawski, DO

BASICS

DESCRIPTION
- Defined as pain in the metatarsal region of the foot, but more commonly refers to pain of the plantar surface of the forefoot in the metatarsal head region
- System(s) affected: Musculoskeletal

EPIDEMIOLOGY
Incidence
Especially common in athletes with high-impact sports involving the lower extremities (running, jumping, dancing, etc.)

Prevalence
Common

RISK FACTORS
- Obesity
- High heels or narrow shoes
- Competitive athletes for weight-bearing sports (e.g., ballet, basketball, running, soccer, baseball, football)
- Foot deformities (e.g., pes planus, pes cavus, tight Achilles tendon, tarsal tunnel syndrome, hallux valgus, prominent metatarsal heads, excessive pronation, hammer toe deformity, tight toe extensors)

Geriatric Considerations
- Arthritis should be ruled out early.
- More frequent in older athletes
- Symptoms are more pronounced in older people.
- Age-related atrophy of the metatarsal fat pad may increase the risk for metatarsalgia.

Pediatric Considerations
- Muscle imbalance disorders (e.g., Duchenne muscular dystrophy) are a cause of foot deformities in children.
- In adolescent girls, consider Freiberg infraction (i.e., aseptic necrosis of the metatarsal head usually due to trauma in adolescents who jump or sprint).
- Salter I injuries may affect subsequent growth and healing of the epiphysis.

Pregnancy Considerations
- Forefoot pain during pregnancy usually results from change in gait, increased weight, and joint laxity.
- Properly fitted low-heeled shoes are especially important in this group of patients.

GENERAL PREVENTION
- Wear properly fitted shoes with good padding.
- Start weight-bearing exercise programs gradually.

PATHOPHYSIOLOGY
- General:
  - Excessive or repetitive stress: Wearers of high heels, ballet dancers, competitive athletes
  - Soft tissue dysfunction: Intrinsic muscle weakness, laxity in the Lisfranc ligament
  - Abnormal foot posture: Forefoot varus or valgus, cavus or equinus deformities, loss of the metatarsal arch, splay foot, pronated foot
  - Dermatologic: Warts, calluses
- Great toe:
  - Hallux valgus (bunion), either varus or rigidus
- Lesser metatarsals:
  - Freiberg infraction (i.e., aseptic necrosis of the metatarsal head usually due to trauma in adolescents who jump or sprint)
  - Hammer toe or claw toe
  - Morton syndrome (i.e., long second metatarsal)

ETIOLOGY
Abnormal pressure distribution plantar to the metatarsal heads

COMMONLY ASSOCIATED CONDITIONS
See "Etiology."

DIAGNOSIS

HISTORY
- Gradual chronic onset is more common than acute presentation.
- Predisposition with pes cavus deformity and hyperpronation
- Acute, chronic, or recurrent symptoms located in the region of the metatarsal heads usually on the plantar surface
- Pain: Often described as seeming like walking with a pebble in the shoe; aggravated during midstance or propulsion phases of walking or running

PHYSICAL EXAM
- Point tenderness over plantar metatarsal heads
- Pain in the interdigital space or a positive metatarsal squeeze test suggests Morton neuroma.
- Plantar keratosis (callus formation) often noted
- Swelling
- Tenderness of the metatarsal head(s) with pressure applied by the examiner's finger and thumb
- Erythema (occasionally)

DIAGNOSTIC TESTS & INTERPRETATION
Lab
Initial lab tests
- Only if diagnosis is in question: ESR, rheumatoid factor, human leukocyte antigen (HLA), rapid plasma reagin (RPR), uric acid, glucose, CBC with differential
- Disorders that may alter lab results: Acute infections

Imaging
Initial approach
- Weight-bearing radiographs: Anteroposterior, lateral, and oblique views. Occasionally metatarsal or sesamoid axial films (to rule out sesamoid fracture) or skyline view of the metatarsal heads to assess the plantar declination of the metatarsal heads: Obtained with the metatarsophalangeal joints in dorsiflexion (to evaluate alignment).
- Increasing use of sonography and MRI, but still no benefit over clinical assessment
- MR arthrography of the MTP joint can delineate capsular tears, typically of the distal lateral border of the plantar plate, an often underrecognized cause of metatarsalgia (1)[C].
- Bone scan if high index of suspicion of stress fracture exists

Diagnostic Procedures/Surgery
Plantar pressure distribution analysis: Although still early in its development, this modality may be helpful to distinguish patterns of pressure distribution due to malalignment.

Pathological Findings
Because of its 2 sesamoid bones, the first metatarsal head usually carries about 30% of the weight when walking. A normal metatarsal arch also ensures this balance. The first metatarsal head has adequate padding to accommodate it. A pronated splayfoot disturbs this balance, causing equal weight-bearing on all metatarsal heads. Any foot deformity also changes distribution of weight to areas of the foot that do not have sufficient padding. Reactive tissue can build up a callus around the metatarsal head, which compounds the pain.

DIFFERENTIAL DIAGNOSIS
- Stress fracture (most commonly second metatarsal)
- Morton neuroma (i.e., interdigital neuroma)
- Sesamoiditis or sesamoid fracture
- Salter I fracture in pediatric population
- Arthritis (e.g., gouty, rheumatoid, inflammatory, osteoarthritis, septic, calcium pyrophosphate, dihydrate crystal deposit disease [CPPD]
- Lis Franc injury
- Avascular necrosis of the metatarsal head
- Infection (e.g., cellulitis, diabetic foot, Lyme disease, leprosy)
- Bone tumors (rare)
- Ganglion cyst
- Foreign body
- Vasculitis (diabetes)
- Cavovarus foot

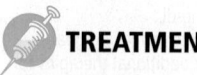

TREATMENT

MEDICATION
- NSAIDs (ibuprofen 800 mg t.i.d. 7–14 days or naproxen 500 mg b.i.d. 7–14 days)
- Contraindications: GI bleeding or ulcer
- Precautions in patients with:
  - Renal disease
  - Hepatic disease
  - Coagulation disorders

- Significant possible interactions:
  - Anticoagulants
  - Digoxin
  - Lithium
  - Methotrexate
  - Cyclosporin

ADDITIONAL TREATMENT

Issues for Referral

Athletes may warrant early podiatric or orthopedic evaluation.

Additional Therapies

- Low-heeled (<2 cm height) wide-toe-box shoes
- Metatarsal pads and arch supports
- Orthotics/rocker bar (prescriptive orthotics have been shown to be effective treatment)
- Thick-soled shoes
- Shaving the callus may provide temporary relief, but should not be excised.
- Improve flexibility and strength of the muscles of the foot with:
  - Exercises (e.g., towel grasps, pencil curls)
  - Physical therapy to maintain range of motion (ROM) and restore normal biomechanics

COMPLEMENTARY AND ALTERNATIVE MEDICINE

Magnetic insoles not effective for chronic nonspecific foot pain

SURGERY/OTHER PROCEDURES

- If no improvement with conservative therapy for 3 months, referral to foot/ankle orthopedic or surgical podiatrist may be necessary.
- If a correctable anatomic abnormality exists: Bunionectomy, partial osteotomy, or surgical fusion (2)[C]. Success rates vary depending on procedure. The Weil osteotomy is a safe and effective treatment for metatarsalgia (3)[C]. The most commonly reported complication of the Weil osteotomy was floating toe with an overall occurrence of 36%. Recurrence was reported in 15% of the cases. Transfer metatarsalgia was reported in 7% of the cases, whereas delayed union, nonunion, and malunion were collectively reported in 3% of the cases (4)[C].
- Morton neurectomy for the treatment of metatarsalgia reported 82% excellent or good results (5)[C].
- Surgery only as a last resort if no anatomic abnormality is present (6)[C]

IN-PATIENT CONSIDERATIONS

Initial Stabilization

- Relieve pain
- Ice initially
- Rest: Temporary alteration of weight-bearing activity; use of cane or crutch. For more physically active patients, suggest an alternative exercise or cross-training:
  - Moist heat later
  - Taping or gel cast
  - Stiff-soled shoes will act as a splint.
- Relieve the pressure beneath the area of maximal pain by redistributing the pressure load of the foot, which can be achieved by weight loss.

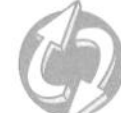

ONGOING CARE

FOLLOW-UP RECOMMENDATIONS

Patient Monitoring

If stress fracture has been ruled out and patient's condition has not improved >3 months of conservative treatment, consider surgical evaluation.

PATIENT EDUCATION

- Instruct about wearing proper sort of shoes and gradual return to activity.
- Cross-training until symptoms subside
- Patient teaching: Prevention
- Biomechanical evaluation is advised by appropriately skilled clinician

PROGNOSIS

Outcome depends on the severity of the problem and whether surgery is required to correct it.

COMPLICATIONS

- Back, knee, and hip pain due to change in gait
- Transfer metatarsalgia following surgical intervention, which subsequently transfers stress to other areas

REFERENCES

1. Kier R, Abrahamian H, Caminear D, et al. MR arthrography of the second and third metatarsophalangeal joints for the detection of tears of the plantar plate and joint capsule. *AJR Am J Roentgenol*. 2010;194:1079–81.
2. Thomson CE, Gibson JN, Martin D. Interventions for the treatment of Morton's neuroma. *Cochrane Database Systematic Review*. 2004;(3):CD003118.
3. Khurana A, Kadamabande S, James S, et al. Weil osteotomy: Assessment of medium term results and predictive factors in recurrent metatarsalgia. *Foot Ankle Surg*. 2011;17:150–7.
4. Highlander P, Vonherbulis E, Gonzalez A, et al. Complications of the weil osteotomy. *Foot Ankle Spec*. 2011;4:165–70.
5. Pace A, Scammell B, Dhar S, et al. The outcome of Morton's neurectomy in the treatment of metatarsalgia. *Int Orthop*. 2010;34:511–5.
6. Espinosa N, Brodsky JW, Maceira E, et al. Metatarsalgia. *J Am Acad Orthop Surg*. 2010;18:474–85.

ADDITIONAL READING

- Adams WR, et al. Morton's neuroma. *Clin Podiatr Med Surg*. 2010;27:535–45.
- Birbilis T, Theodoropoulou E, Koulalis D. Forefoot complaints–the morton's metatarsalgia. The role of MR imaging. *Acta Medica (Hradec Kralove)*. 2007;50:221–2.
- Burns J, Landorf KB, Ryan MM, et al. Interventions for the prevention and treatment of pes cavus. *Cochrane Database Syst Rev*. 2007;(4):CD006154.
- Espinosa N, Maceira E, Myerson MS. Current concept review: Metatarsalgia. *Foot Ankle Int*. 2008;29:871–9.
- Gregg J, Marks P. Metatarsalgia: An ultrasound perspective. *Australas Radiol*. 2007;51:493–9.
- Gregg JM, Schneider T, Marks P. MR imaging and ultrasound of metatarsalgia-the lesser metatarsals. *Radiol Clin North Am*. 2008;46:1061–78.
- Hockenbury RT. Forefoot problems in athletes. *Med Sci Sport ecerc*. 1999;31(suppl 7):S448–58.
- Iagnocco A, Coari G, Palombi G, et al. Sonography in the study of metatarsalgia. *J Rheumatol*. 2001;28:1338–40.
- Janisse DJ, Janisse E. Shoe modification and the use of orthoses in the treatment of foot and ankle pathology. *J Am Acad Orthop Surg*. 2008;16(3):152–8.
- Kanatli U. Pressure distribution patterns under the metatarsal heads in healthy individuals. *Acta Orthop Traumatol Turc*. 2008;42(1):26–30.
- Ko PH, Hsiao TY, Kang JH, et al. Relationship between plantar pressure and soft tissue strain under metatarsal heads with different heel heights. *Foot Ankle Int*. 2009;30:1111–6.
- Sharp RJ, et al. The role of MRI and ultrasound imaging in Morton's neuroma and the effect of size of lesion on symptoms. *J Bone Joint Surg*. 2003;85(7):999–1005.
- van Wyngarden TM. The painful foot, Part I: Common forefoot deformities. *Am Fam Physician*. 1997;55:1866–76.
- Wu KK. Morton neuroma and metatarsalgia. *Curr Opin Rheumatol*. 2000;12:131–42.

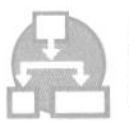

See Also (Topic, Algorithm, Electronic Media Element)

Morton Neuroma (Interdigital Neuroma)

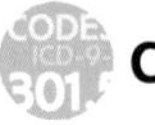

CODES

ICD9

- 359.1 Hereditary progressive muscular dystrophy
- 726.70 Enthesopathy of ankle and tarsus, unspecified
- 732.5 Juvenile osteochondrosis of foot

CLINICAL PEARLS

- Pain of the plantar surface of the forefoot in the metatarsal head region
- Common especially in athletes with high-impact sports involving the lower extremities (running, jumping, dancing, etc.)
- Point tenderness over plantar metatarsal heads
- Athletes may warrant early podiatric or orthopedic evaluation.

METHANOL POISONING

Ernest Pedapati, MD

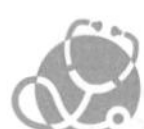

BASICS

DESCRIPTION

- Methanol (wood alcohol) is a clear, colorless solvent found in antifreeze, cleaning solutions, copy machine fluid, gasoline additives, paint, paint thinner, and liquid fuel (1).
- Methanol is less expensive than ethanol and may be used by chronic alcoholics as a substitute.
- Intoxication also can be secondary to methanol-contaminated grain alcohol (moonshine), accidental ingestion, or a suicide attempt.
- Methanol produces inebriation, and its metabolic products may cause metabolic acidosis, blindness, and death.

Pregnancy Considerations

Avoid ethanol therapy as a treatment for methanol poisoning during the first trimester of pregnancy; you may substitute fomepizole, which is a pregnancy category C drug.

EPIDEMIOLOGY

Incidence

- Predominant age: Most >18 years of age, followed by <6 years of age
- Predominant sex: Male > Female

Prevalence

In the US, 683 methanol exposures were reported in 2007. 68 cases resulted in moderate to severe outcomes, and there were 9 fatalities.

RISK FACTORS

- Alcoholism
- Epidemics may occur in institutionalized settings where ethyl alcohol is unavailable (e.g., prisons).
- Inappropriate storage, leading to access by children

GENERAL PREVENTION

- Substance education for those at risk
- Proper storage of methanol-containing products

PATHOPHYSIOLOGY

- Methanol metabolism in brief has the following characteristics (1,2):
  - Methanol is readily absorbed and quickly distributed.
  - The liver slowly metabolizes methanol into formaldehyde via alcohol dehydrogenase.
  - Formaldehyde is rapidly converted into formic acid via aldehyde dehydrogenase.
  - Formic acid is slowly converted to carbon dioxide and water through a folate-dependent process.
  - A limited amount of methanol is also eliminated essentially unchanged through exhalation (12%) and through the urine (3%).
- Methanol is minimally toxic, but formic acid causes anion-gap metabolic acidosis and ocular toxicity. Increased lactate owing to systemic toxicity contributes to the acidosis (1).
- A fatal dose is 15–240 mL, depending on concentration.
- Peak blood levels occur 30–60 minutes after ingestion (1).

COMMONLY ASSOCIATED CONDITIONS

Alcoholism

DIAGNOSIS

- The classic clinical picture includes nausea, vomiting, abdominal pain, visual disturbances, and metabolic acidosis. There is a latent period after ingestion of 6–24 hours before onset of symptoms; this may be delayed further with concomitant ethanol ingestion (2).
- Overt clinical signs are expected with severe exposure, but at low doses (i.e., occupational exposure), elevated methanol levels may be the only sign.

HISTORY

- Initial CNS depression or inebriation (1)
- Headache, vertigo, lethargy, confusion; severely intoxicated patients can present with coma and convulsions.
- Visual disturbances, ranging from mild blurring to complete blindness "like standing in a snowfield" (3)
- GI symptoms may include nausea, vomiting, and marked abdominal pain.
- Dyspnea

PHYSICAL EXAM

Key physical findings (1,2):

- Initially, inebriation and gastritis
- Heart rate abnormalities, including bradycardia in late stages
- Tachypnea with onset of metabolic acidosis
- Visual field defects, blurred or double vision; loss of visual acuity or pupillary reaction
- A funduscopic exam may reveal retinal edema, hyperemia, or loss of disc cupping.
- Abdominal tenderness
- Stupor, confusion, seizure, or coma may be present.
- Parkinson-type symptoms have been reported in severe acute and low-level chronic methanol poisoning (4).

DIAGNOSTIC TESTS & INTERPRETATION

Lab

- Serum methanol may be elevated acutely.
- After a latent period, serum formate is a better measure of toxicity.
- Elevated osmolar gap and anion gap; include lactate and ethanol levels to help identify acid contributing to elevated anion gap
- Urinalysis may show myoglobinuria.
- Other useful labs:
  - Arterial blood gas
  - Electrolytes, BUN, creatinine, calcium, liver function tests, amylase, lipase, creatinine phosphate
  - Toxicologic screens if coingestants are suspected

Imaging

A CT scan or MRI of the brain if indicated by neurologic exam. Brain imaging may reveal optic pathway damage, hypodensities in the putamen or caudate nucleus, cerebral edema, cerebral hemorrhage, or cerebral infarct (1).

DIFFERENTIAL DIAGNOSIS

- Ingestion of other alcohols, including ethyl alcohol, ethylene glycol, benzyl alcohol, and isopropyl alcohol
- Other toxic ingestions, including paraldehyde and formaldehyde
- Increased anion-gap metabolic acidosis caused by renal failure, diabetic ketoacidosis, or lactic acidosis

TREATMENT

MEDICATION

- Ethanol and fomepizole saturated aldehyde dehydrogenase prevent the formation of formic acid.
- Metabolism of formic acid is a folate-dependent pathway.
- Criteria for initiation of therapy in patients with known or suspected methanol poisoning (1)[C]:
  - Plasma methanol >20 mg/dL *or*
  - Recent history of ingestion of toxic amounts of methanol and an osmolar gap >10 mOsm/L *or*
  - Suspected methanol ingestion with at least 2 of the following:
    - Arterial pH <7.3
    - Serum bicarbonate <20 mmol/L
    - Osmolar gap >10 mOsm/L

First Line

Fomepizole:

- First 48 hours: IV load with 15 mg/kg, then dosed 10 mg/kg q12h for 4 doses (1)[C]
- After 48 hours: Induces P-450 enzymes, so increase to 15 mg/kg until serum methanol <20 mg/dL (1)[C].
- Increase dosing to every 4 hours for hemodialysis. No adjustments in dosing are needed for renal or hepatic disease.
- Side effects: Mildly increased levels of alanine aminotransferase and aspartate aminotransferase that resolve without consequence (5)

Second Line

- Folinic acid (Leucovorin): May enhance formic acid metabolism (5)[C]:
  - 1 mg/kg (up to 50 mg) initially
  - Folic acid can be given q6h at the same dose until metabolic acidosis resolves.
- Ethanol:
  - IV loading dose, then maintenance dosing based on hourly serum ethanol levels; target therapeutic ethanol level is 100–150 mg/dL. Treat until serum methanol is <20 mg/dL (1)[C].
  - Side effects include inebriation, hypoglycemia, phlebitis, and volume overload.
  - Avoid ethanol therapy with CNS depressants, and watch for disulfiram reactions.

ADDITIONAL TREATMENT

General Measures

- Prioritize management on timing and amount of exposure; if patient is intoxicated, history may be unreliable.
- A low or nondetectable methanol level does not rule out ingestion.
- Initial stabilization: IV access and isotonic fluids to maintain adequate urine output and prevent renal failure
- Initial management: Focused on preventing metabolic acidosis and ophthalmic complications
- Consider gastric decontamination with induced emesis, charcoal, or gastric lavage only if concomitant ingestion is known (1)[C].
- Sodium bicarbonate can be considered if serum pH <7.2.
- Hemodialysis (see "In-Patient Considerations")

Issues for Referral

- For patients with substance abuse, referral to detox, rehabilitation, and/or AA/NA
- Ophthalmology follow-up for patients with visual disturbances

IN-PATIENT CONSIDERATIONS

Consider urgent hemodialysis with the following (1,6):

- Significant acidosis (pH <7.2) unresponsive to therapy
- Deteriorating vital signs despite intensive support
- Renal failure
- Severe electrolyte imbalance
- Visual or funduscopic abnormalities
- Serum methanol concentration >50 mg/dL or >30 g ingested

IV Fluids

Isotonic IV fluid to maintain urine output

ONGOING CARE

FOLLOW-UP RECOMMENDATIONS

- Restricted activity if patient is inebriated, has altered level of consciousness, or has visual impairments
- Referral to psychiatry for suicidal patients

DIET

Thiamine supplementation for patients with long-term alcoholism

PATIENT EDUCATION

- Anticipatory guidance for parents regarding storage of hazardous chemicals
- Motivational interviewing for those with substance dependence and referral for additional treatment
- American Academy of Clinical Toxicology: www.clintox.org

PROGNOSIS

- The outcome varies, depending on time to presentation and the quantity of methanol ingested.
- The outcome is related to the degree of acidosis, coma, or seizures at time of presentation.
- Diagnostic and treatment delays are correlated with a poor outcome (3)[C].

COMPLICATIONS

- Blindness and other visual disturbances
- Myoglobinuric renal failure
- Pancreatitis
- Parkinson syndrome

REFERENCES

1. Barceloux DG. American Academy of Clinical Toxicology practice guidelines on the treatment of methanol poisoning. *Clin Toxicol*. 2002;40:415–46.
2. Kraut JA, Kurtz I. Toxic alcohol ingestions: Clinical features, diagnosis, and management. *Clin J Am Soc Nephrol*. 2008;3(1):208–25.
3. Hovda KE. Methanol outbreak in Norway 2002–2004. *J Int Med*. 2005;258:181–90.
4. Airas L, Paavilainen T, Marttila RJ. Methanol intoxication-induced nigrostriatal dysfunction detected using 6-[18F]fluoro-l-dopa PET. *Neurotoxicology*. 2008;29(4):671–4.
5. Brent J. Fomepizole for ethylene glycol and methanol poisoning. *N Engl J Med*. 2009;360:2216–23.
6. Mégarbane B, Borron SW, Baud FJ. Current recommendations for treatment of severe toxic alcohol poisonings. *Intensive Care Med*. 2005;31:189–95.

ADDITIONAL READING

- Comolu S, Ozen B, Ozbakir S. Methanol intoxication with bilateral basal ganglia infarct. *Australas Radiol*. 2001;45:357–8.
- Litovitz TL, Klein-Schwartz W, White S. 2000 Annual report of the American Association of Poison Control Centers Toxic Exposure Surveillance System. *Am J Emerg Med*. 2001;19:337–95.

CODES

ICD9

980.1 Toxic effect of methyl alcohol

CLINICAL PEARLS

- Formic acid, the toxic agent in methanol poisoning, causes anion-gap metabolic acidosis, optic disc edema, and myelin breakdown by direct toxic effects (1)[C].
- Ethanol has the longest history of use, is inexpensive, and is widely available. Fomepizole is preferred because dosing is simpler, it does not require hourly blood draws, and it is not a CNS depressant. No direct comparison of the 2 treatments is available.
- Common indications for hemodialysis in a methanol overdose include severe acidosis, visual symptoms, unstable vital signs, refractory electrolyte disturbances, and methanol level >50 mg/dL (1)[C].
- Recent literature has suggested that, in the absence of neurologic impairment, ocular symptoms, and severe metabolic acidosis, fomepizole may obviate the need for hemodialysis (5,6)[B].

M

MILD COGNITIVE IMPAIRMENT

Birju B. Patel, MD, FACP
N. Wilson Holland, MD, FACP

BASICS

DESCRIPTION

- Mild cognitive impairment (MCI) is defined as significant cognitive impairment in the absence of dementia, as measured by standard memory tests:
  - Report of memory problems, preferably corroborated by another person
  - Ability to perform activities of daily living (ADLs) is maintained.
  - Normal general thinking and reasoning skills
  - Other terms used in the literature relating to MCI: Isolated memory impairment; cognitive impairment not dementia (CIND); predementia; mild cognitive disorder; age-associated memory impairment; age-related cognitive decline; benign senescent forgetfulness. Some of these conditions are not felt to progress to dementia (i.e., benign senescent forgetfulness, age-associated memory impairment, age-related cognitive decline).
- Annual rates of conversion of MCI to dementia are 2–15% in the elderly.

EPIDEMIOLOGY

Incidence

- Predominant sex: Male > Female (1)
- Predominant age:
  - Higher in older persons or those with less education
  - 12–15/1,000 person-years in those aged ≥65 years
  - 54/1,000 person-years in those aged ≥75 years

Prevalence

- MCI is more prevalent than dementia in the US.
- 3–5% for those aged ≥60 years
- 15% for those aged ≥75 years

RISK FACTORS

- Age
- Diabetes
- Hypertension
- Dyslipidemia
- Sleep apnea
- Apolipoprotein (APO) E4 genotype

Genetics

APO E4 genotype: Various pathways exist leading to amyloid accumulation and deposition thought to be associated with dementia.

PATHOPHYSIOLOGY

- Subtypes of MCI:
  - Single-domain amnestic
  - Multiple-domain amnestic
  - Nonamnestic single-domain
  - Nonamnestic multiple-domain
- The amnestic subtype is higher risk for progression to Alzheimer disease.

ETIOLOGY

Vascular, degenerative, traumatic, metabolic, psychiatric, or combination

COMMONLY ASSOCIATED CONDITIONS

See "Risk Factors."

DIAGNOSIS

HISTORY

- Focus on cognitive deficits and impairment.
- Review all medications that may affect cognition. Particular emphasis should be given to anticholinergic medications (patients on these may be mistakenly classified as having MCI).
- Rule out depression.
- Assess function (ADLs, instrumental ADLs) and subtle changes in daily function (such as in their workplace).
- Impact on interpersonal relationships and caregiver stress

PHYSICAL EXAM

- A general exam focusing on clinical clues to identifying vascular disease (e.g., bruits, abnormal BP)
- Neurologic exam to rule out reversible CNS causes of cognitive impairment or other causes of cognitive impairment (e.g., Parkinson disease)
- Office measure of cognitive function

DIAGNOSTIC TESTS & INTERPRETATION

Lab

Initial lab tests

- CBC
- Comprehensive metabolic profile
- Thyroid-stimulating hormone
- Vitamin B_{12}
- Lipids
- Also consider HIV testing in the appropriate risk setting.

Follow-Up & Special Considerations

Consider referral to a memory evaluation center for more comprehensive evaluation of MCI looking for specific cognitive domains involved.

Imaging

- CT scan can detect structural CNS conditions leading to cognitive impairment:
  - Subdural hematoma
  - Normal-pressure hydrocephalus
  - Metastatic disease
- MRI further evaluates vascular, infectious, neoplastic, and inflammatory conditions.

Initial approach

- Rule out reversible causes of cognitive impairment.
- Cognitive testing is important (e.g., Montreal Cognitive Assessment [MOCA], Mini Mental Status Exam [MMSE], Saint Louis University Mental Status [SLUMS]); MOCA may be more sensitive for detecting MCI.
- Neuropsychological testing for complex and atypical presentations
- Vascular risk factor reduction and treatment

Follow-Up & Special Considerations

- Document progression of functional impairment, cognitive decline, concurrent depression, and comorbidities.
- Advanced planning while patient is competent
- Early education of caregivers on safety, maintaining structure, managing stress, and future planning

Pathological Findings

- Little is known about MCI pathology due to a lack of longitudinal studies.
- Alzheimer dementia pathophysiology:
  - Neurofibrillary tangles in hippocampus
  - Senile plaques (amyloid deposition)
  - Neuronal degeneration
- Those with MCI have intermediate amounts of pathologic findings of Alzheimer's disease with amyloid deposition and neurofibrillary tangles in the mesial temporal lobes compared with those with dementia.
- Amnestic MCI is associated with white-matter hyperintensity volume on MRI, whereas nonamnestic MCI is associated with infarcts (2).

DIFFERENTIAL DIAGNOSIS

- Delirium
- Dementia
- Depression
- "Reversible" cognitive impairment:
  - Medications (anticholinergics and medications with anticholinergic properties)
  - Hypothyroidism
  - Vitamin B_{12} deficiency
- Reversible CNS conditions
- Give consideration to sleep conditions, especially sleep apnea, that can contribute to cognitive deficits.

TREATMENT

MEDICATION

- The use of cholinesterase inhibitors (ChEIs) in MCI is not associated with any delay in the onset of Alzheimer disease or dementia. Moreover, the safety profile showed that the risks associated with ChEIs are not negligible (3). Therefore, ChEIs are not recommended routinely (4).
- Consider symptomatic treatment with ChEIs only if memory complaints appear to be affecting quality of life in individual patients or in patients with an amnestic subtype of MCI.

ADDITIONAL TREATMENT

General Measures

Atherosclerotic risk factors should be treated aggressively.

Issues for Referral

Consider referral to a memory specialist (i.e., geriatrician, neurologist, geropsychiatrist) to evaluate and differentiate subtypes of MCI and specific cognitive deficits.

COMPLEMENTARY AND ALTERNATIVE MEDICINE

There is no evidence of the efficacy of vitamin E in the prevention or treatment of people with MCI. More research is needed to identify the role of vitamin E, if any, in the management of cognitive impairment.

IN-PATIENT CONSIDERATIONS

- Delirium is more common in patients hospitalized with all forms of cognitive impairment.
- Avoid medications that may worsen or precipitate cognitive decline (e.g., anticholinergics, antihistamines, etc.).
- Patients may be extremely sensitive to the hospital environment:
  - Moderate level of stimulation is best.
  - Avoid sensory deprivation. Make sure that patients have access to hearing aids and eyeglasses.

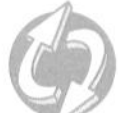

ONGOING CARE

FOLLOW-UP RECOMMENDATIONS

Patients should be re-evaluated every 6–12 months to determine if symptoms are progressing.

Patient Monitoring

Appropriate cognitive and functional testing should be used to evaluate progression, along with clinical history and exam. If a medication is started, patients need to be followed more frequently to evaluate for efficacy, side effects, dose titration, etc. Declining executive function may be an early marker to progression of MCI to dementia, and clinicians should monitor and advise patients and families proactively to look for this (5).

DIET

Diets that are promoted by the American Heart Association to minimize atherosclerotic risk factors should be emphasized.

PATIENT EDUCATION

- Encourage lifestyle changes:
  - Physical activity such as walking 30 minutes daily on most days of the week
  - Mental activity that stimulates language skills and psychomotor coordination should be encouraged. Computer activities, reading books, crafts, crossword puzzles, and games may be linked to decreased risk of development of MCI.
- Cognitive rehabilitation strategies may be beneficial in helping with daily activities relating to memory tasks in MCI (6).

PROGNOSIS

- Conversion rates from MCI to dementia range from 5–15% annually.
- Amnestic subtypes of MCI are most likely to progress to dementia.

REFERENCES

1. Petersen RC, Roberts RO, Knopman DS, et al. Prevalence of mild cognitive impairment is higher in men. The Mayo Clinic Study of Aging. *Neurology.* 2010;75(10):889–97.
2. Luchsinger JA, Brickman AM, Reitz C, et al. Subclinical cerebrovascular disease in mild cognitive impairment. *Neurology.* 2009;73:450–6.
3. Patel BP, Holland NW. *Adverse Effects of Acetylcholinesterase Inhibitors Clinical Geriatrics.* 2011:19(1):27–30.
4. Larner AJ, et al. Cholinesterase inhibitors: Beyond Alzheimer's disease. *Expert Rev Neurother.* 2010; 10:1699–705.
5. Marshall GA, Rentz DM, Frey MT, et al. Executive function and instrumental activities of daily living in mild cognitive impairment and Alzheimer's disease. *Alzheimers Dement.* 2011;7(3):300–8.
6. Kinsella GJ, Mullaly E, Rand E, et al. Early intervention for mild cognitive impairment: A randomised controlled trial. *J Neurol Neurosurg Psychiatr.* 2009;80:730–6.

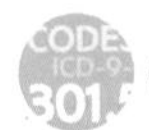

CODES

ICD9

331.83 Mild cognitive impairment, so stated

CLINICAL PEARLS

- Amnestic MCI affects primarily memory and is more likely to progress to Alzheimer dementia.
- Screen for reversible factors, particularly anticholinergic medications, depression, and sleep disorders.
- Look closely at vascular risk factors, and modify them as best as possible.
- ChEIs should not be used routinely unless memory complaints are affecting quality of life in patients. Potential side effects of these medications should be thoroughly discussed with patients and their families. A baseline EKG should be done prior to initiation of ChEIs due to risk of bradycardia and syncope.
- Encourage both physical and mental exercises.

MITRAL REGURGITATION

Yongkasem Vorasettakarnkij, MD, MSc
Peerawut Deeprasertkul, MD

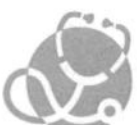

BASICS

DESCRIPTION

- Disorder of mitral valve (MV) closure, either organic or functional, resulting in a backflow of the left ventricular (LV) stroke volume into the left atrium (LA); uncompensated, this leads to LV and LA enlargement, elevated pulmonary pressures, atrial fibrillation, heart failure, and sudden cardiac death.
- Types of mitral regurgitation (MR):
  - Acute vs. chronic
  - Organic vs. functional:
    - Functional: No valvular abnormalities are found, and the disease results from valve deformation, caused by LV remodeling or dilatation
    - MV structures include not only the mitral annulus, MV leaflets, chordae tendineae, and papillary muscles but also posterior LA wall and LV wall.
- System(s) affected: Cardiac; Pulmonary

EPIDEMIOLOGY

Moderate to severe MR affects 2.5 million people in the US (2000 data). It is the most common valvular disease, and its prevalence is expected to double by 2030 (1).

Prevalence

- By severity on echocardiography:
  - Mild MR: 19% (up to 40% if trivial jets included)
  - Moderate MR: 1.9%
  - Severe MR: 0.2%
- By category (1):
  - Degenerative (myxomatous disease, annular calcification): 60–70%
  - Ischemic: 20%
  - Endocarditis: 2–5%
  - Rheumatic: 2–5%

RISK FACTORS

Age, hypertension, rheumatic heart disease, endocarditis, anorectic drugs

GENERAL PREVENTION

- Risk factor modification for coronary artery disease (CAD)
- Antibiotic prophylaxis for poststreptococcal rheumatic heart disease
- Endocarditis prophylaxis for MR is no longer recommended

PATHOPHYSIOLOGY

- Acute MR: Acute damage to MV leads to sudden LA and LV volume overload. Sudden rise in LV volume load without compensatory LV remodeling results in impaired forward cardiac output and possible cardiogenic shock.
- Chronic MR: LV eccentric hypertrophy compensates for increased regurgitant volume to maintain forward cardiac output and alleviate pulmonary congestion. However, ongoing LV remodeling can result in LV dysfunction. Simultaneously, LA compensatory dilatation for the larger regurgitant volume predisposes patients to develop atrial fibrillation (AF).
- Ischemic MR: Papillary muscle rupture, ischemia during acute MI, and incomplete coaptation of valve leaflets or restricted valve movement resulting from ischemia

ETIOLOGY

- Acute MR:
  - Flail leaflet: Myxomatous disease, infective endocarditis, or trauma
  - Ruptured chordae tendineae: Trauma, spontaneous rupture, infective endocarditis, or rheumatic fever
  - Ruptured or displaced papillary muscle: Acute myocardial infarction (MI), severe myocardial ischemia, or trauma
- Chronic MR:
  - Structural:
    - Degenerative: Mitral annular calcification, mitral valve prolapse (MVP)
    - Infective endocarditis
    - Rheumatic heart disease (RHD)
    - Inflammatory diseases: Lupus, eosinophilic endocardial disease
    - Anorectic drugs
    - Congenital (cleft leaflet)
  - Functional:
    - Ischemic: CAD/MI
    - Nonischemic: Cardiomyopathy, LV dysfunction from any cause
    - Hypertrophic cardiomyopathy

COMMONLY ASSOCIATED CONDITIONS

MVP with MR common in Marfan syndrome

DIAGNOSIS

HISTORY

- Associated conditions: RHD, prior MI, connective tissue disorder
- Acute MR:
  - Sudden onset of dyspnea
  - Orthopnea, paroxysmal nocturnal dyspnea
  - Chronic MR:
    - Exertional dyspnea
    - Fatigue
    - Palpitation: Paroxysmal or persistent AF

PHYSICAL EXAM

- Acute MR:
  - Rapid and thready pulses
  - Sign of poor tissue perfusion with peripheral vasoconstriction
  - Hyperdynamic precordium without apical displacement
  - S_3 and S_4 (if in sinus rhythm)
  - Systolic murmur at left sternal border and base:
    - Early, middle, or holosystolic murmur
    - Often soft, low-pitched, decrescendo murmur
  - Rales
- Chronic MR:
  - Brisk upstroke of arterial pulse
  - Leftward displaced LV apical impulse
  - Systolic thrill at the apex (suggests severe MR)
  - Soft S_1 and widely split S_2
  - Loud P_2 (if pulmonary hypertension)
  - S_3 gallop
  - Holosystolic murmur at apex that radiates to axilla
  - Ankle edema, jugular venous distension, and ascites, if development of right-sided heart failure

DIAGNOSTIC TESTS & INTERPRETATION

Lab

- Chest x-ray (CXR):
  - Acute MR: Pulmonary edema, normal heart size
  - Chronic MR: LA and LV enlargement
- ECG:
  - Acute MR:
    - Varies depending on etiologies (e.g., acute MI)
  - Chronic MR:
    - P mitrale from LA enlargement
    - LV hypertrophy
    - Q waves from prior MI
    - AF

Initial lab tests

- Cardiac enzymes and brain natriuretic peptide (BNP), if appropriate
- See workup for MI, CAD, and congestive heart failure (CHF)

Imaging

Initial approach

Transthoracic echocardiogram (TTE):

- Indications for TTE (2):
  - Baseline evaluation of LV function, right ventricular and LA size, pulmonary artery pressure, and severity of MR
  - Delineation of mechanism of MR
  - Surveillance of asymptomatic moderate–severe LV function (ejection fraction [EF] and end-systolic dimension [ESD])
  - Evaluate MV apparatus and LV size and function after a change in signs or symptoms in a patient with MR.
  - Evaluate after MV repair or replacement.
- Findings in acute MR:
  - Evidence of etiology: Flail leaflet or infective vegetations
  - Normal LA and LV size
- Findings in chronic MR:
  - Evidence of degenerative, rheumatic, ischemic, congenital, and other causes
  - Enlarged LA and LV

Follow-Up & Special Considerations

- Intervals for follow-up TTE: See "Follow-Up" below.
- Transesophageal echocardiogram (TEE):
  - Intraoperatively to define severity/cause of MR and/or LV function
  - Nondiagnostic TTE
  - Evaluation of prosthetic heart valves
- Exercise Doppler echo:
  - Assess exercise tolerance and the effects of exercise on pulmonary artery pressure in asymptomatic patients with severe MR (2)[C].
- Cardiovascular magnetic resonance: When regurgitant severity is indeterminant on echocardiography, especially in patients with LV dysfunction

Diagnostic Procedures/Surgery

- Cardiac catheterization (2):
  - Hemodynamic measurements: Pulmonary pressure is discordant to the severity of MR as assessed by noninvasive testing.

- Left ventriculography and hemodynamic measurement:
  - Noninvasive tests are inconclusive regarding severity of MR
  - Regurgitant severity is discordant between clinical and noninvasive findings
- Coronary angiography: Prior to MV surgery in patients at risk for CAD

Pathological Findings

Quantification of severe MR requires integration of:

- Structural parameters:
  - LA size: Dilated, unless acute
  - LV size: Dilated, unless acute
  - Leaflets: Abnormal
- Doppler parameters
- Quantitative parameter

DIFFERENTIAL DIAGNOSIS

- Aortic stenosis (AS): Usually midsystolic but can be long, difficult to distinguish from holosystolic, at apical area, and radiating to the carotid arteries (unlike MR)
- Tricuspid regurgitation: Holosystolic but at left lower sternal border, does not radiate to axilla or increase in intensity with inspiration (unlike MR)
- Ventricular septal defect (VSD): Harsh holosystolic murmur at lower left sternal border but radiates to right sternal border (not axilla)

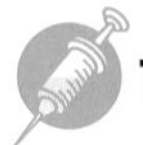

TREATMENT

Acute, severe MR (2):

- Medical therapy has a limited role and is aimed primarily to stabilize hemodynamics preoperatively.
- Urgent surgical consultation

MEDICATION

Chronic MR:

- Structural:
  - Asymptomatic: No proven long-term medical therapy
  - Symptomatic: Diuretics and vasodilators
- Functional: LV dysfunction or symptomatic: ACEIs, β-blockers (particularly carvedilol and long-acting metoprolol)

SURGERY/OTHER PROCEDURES

- Isolated MV surgery is not indicated for patients with mild to moderate MR (2)[C].
- Acute, severe MR secondary to acute MI:
  - Acute rupture of papillary muscle: Emergency MV repair or replacement
  - Papillary muscle displacement:
    - Aggressive medical stabilization, and intra-aortic balloon pump
    - Valve surgery usually required in addition to revascularization
- Chronic severe MR:
  - MV repair in an experienced center is recommended over MV replacement in most circumstances (3):
    - Survival rate: Early and overall mortality were lower after MV repair than after MV replacement
    - 10-year rate of stroke: 10% (repair) vs. 12% (bioprosthetic-valve replacement) vs. 23% (mechanical-valve replacement)
    - Risk of endocarditis: 1.5% at 15 years vs. 0.3–1.2% per year
    - Overall rates of reoperation are similar.
  - Indications for MV surgery in chronic severe degenerative MR (2):
    - Symptomatic (NYHA functional class II–IV):
      - Absence of severe LV dysfunction (EF ≥30% and ESD ≤55 mm)
      - Severe LV dysfunction (EF <30% and/or ESD >55 mm). Only if repair is highly likely to be successful.
    - Asymptomatic:
      - Mild to moderate LV dysfunction (EF 30–60% and/or ESD ≥40 mm)
      - Preserved LV function (EF >60% and ESD <40 mm): MV repair in experienced surgical centers is reasonable if chance of successful repair without residual MR is >90%
      - Preserved LV function with new onset atrial fibrillation or with pulmonary hypertension (PASP >50 mm Hg at rest or PASP >60 mm Hg with exercise)
  - Indications for surgery in chronic ischemic MR (4)[C]:
    - Severe MR: LVEF >30% undergoing CABG
    - Moderate MR: Undergoing CABG if repair is feasible
    - Symptomatic, severe MR: LVEF <30%, and option for CABG
    - Severe MR, LVEF >30%: no option for revascularization, refractory to medical therapy, and low comorbidity
  - Percutaneous repair with mitral valve clip may be considered: Less effective at reducing MR but superior safety (5)
- Nonischemic functional, severe MR: In selected patients, consider the following:
  - Cardiac resynchronization therapy
  - Percutaneous mitral annuloplasty
  - Percutaneous repair with mitral valve clip

Geriatric Considerations

- Medical therapy alone for patients >75 years of age with MR is preferred owing to increased operative mortality and decreased survival (compared with those with AS), especially with preexisting CAD or need for MV replacement.
- MV repair is preferable to MV replacement.

IN-PATIENT CONSIDERATIONS

Initial Stabilization

Acute MR:

- Stabilize ABCs. Initiate IV, O_2, and monitoring
- Nitroprusside (+ dobutamine and/or aortic balloon counterpulsation if hypotensive) (3)[C]
- Treat underlying causes (e.g., MI).
- Treat acute pulmonary edema with furosemide, morphine
- Urgent surgical consultation

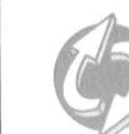

ONGOING CARE

FOLLOW-UP RECOMMENDATIONS

Chronic MR: Asymptomatic:

- Mild MR with normal LV size and function and no pulmonary hypertension: Annual clinical evaluation to assess symptom progression
- Moderate MR: Annual clinical evaluation and echocardiography to assess LV function
- Severe MR: Clinical evaluation and echocardiography every 6–12 months
- Consider serial CXRs and ECGs, and consider stress test if exercise capacity is doubtful

PATIENT EDUCATION

- Exercise after MV repair: Avoid sports with risk for bodily contact or trauma. Low-intensity competitive sports are allowed.
- Competitive athletes with MR:
  - Asymptomatic with normal LV size and function, normal pulmonary artery pressures, and sinus rhythm: No restrictions
  - Mildly symptomatic and those with LV dilatation: Activities with low to moderate dynamic and static cardiac demand allowed
- AF and anticoagulation: No contact sports

PROGNOSIS

- Acute, severe MR: Mortality risk with surgery, 50%; mortality risk with medical therapy alone, 75% in first 24 hours; 95% at 2 weeks
- Chronic MR:
  - Asymptomatic severe MR with normal LVEF: 10% yearly rate of progression to symptoms and subnormal resting LVEF
  - Symptomatic severe MR: 8-year survival rate, 33% without surgery; mortality rate, 5% yearly

Pregnancy Considerations

MR with NYHA functional class III–IV at high risk for maternal and/or fetal risk

COMPLICATIONS

Acute pulmonary edema, CHF, atrial fibrillation, bleeding risk with anticoagulation, endocarditis, sudden cardiac death

REFERENCES

1. Enriquez-Sarano M, Akins CW, Vahanian A. Mitral regurgitation. *Lancet*. 2009;373:1382–94.
2. Bonow RO, et al. Focused update incorporated into the ACC/AHA 2006 guidelines for the management of patients with valvular heart disease. *Circulation*. 2008;118:e523–661.
3. Foster E. Clinical practice. Mitral regurgitation due to degenerative mitral-valve disease. *N Engl J Med*. 2010;363:156–65.
4. Vahanian A, Task Force on the Management of Valvular Heart Disease of the European Society of Cardiology, ESC Committee for Practice Guidelines, et al. Guidelines on the management of valvular heart disease: The Task Force on the Management of Valvular Heart Disease of the European Society of Cardiology. *Eur Heart J*. 2007;28:230–68.
5. Feldman T, Foster E, Glower DG, et al. Percutaneous repair or surgery for mitral regurgitation. *N Engl J Med*. 2011;364:1395–406.

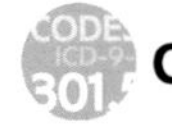

CODES

ICD9

- 394.1 Rheumatic mitral insufficiency
- 424.0 Mitral valve disorders
- 746.6 Congenital mitral insufficiency

CLINICAL PEARLS

- Follow-up for mild to moderate MR: Serial exam and/or echo unless LV structural changes
- Severe MR is usually managed with mitral valve repair.
- Endocarditis prophylaxis is not recommended.

M

MITRAL STENOSIS

Viola Chu, MD, MS
Jill SM Omori, MD

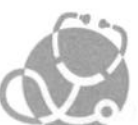

BASICS

DESCRIPTION

- Resistance to diastolic filling of the left ventricle due to narrowing of mitral valve orifice
- Normal valve orifice 4–6 cm^2; symptoms typically seen when orifice is <2.5 cm^2
- Hemodynamic consequences are due to passive transmission of left atrial pressure to the pulmonary circulation.

EPIDEMIOLOGY

- Most common acquired valvular disease secondary to rheumatic heart disease (60% of cases)
- Predominant age: Symptoms primarily occur in fourth to seventh decade
- Predominant sex: Female > Male (2:1)

Incidence

Decreased incidence of mitral stenosis seen in the US because of decreased incidence of rheumatic heart disease (better detected) and treatment of group A streptococcal infection, as well as a shift in prevalence away from rheumatogenic strains. However, global burden remains significant (1).

RISK FACTORS

- Rheumatic fever is the greatest risk factor:
  - 30–40% of rheumatic fever patients eventually develop mitral stenosis, presenting an average of 20 years after dx of rheumatic fever.
  - Acute rheumatic fever occurs 2–3 weeks after episode of untreated group A streptococcal pharyngitis caused by rheumatogenic organism.
  - Low socioeconomic status (i.e., crowded conditions) favor the spread of streptococcal infection.
- Aging (increasing valvular calcification)
- Chest irradiation (increasing tissue fibrosis)

GENERAL PREVENTION

- Prompt recognition and treatment of group A streptococcal infection; recognition of cardinal signs and symptoms of acute rheumatic fever via Jones criteria
- Jones criteria: Diagnosis requires evidence of streptococcal infection plus 2 major criteria or 1 major plus 2 minor criteria.

Evidence of Strep Infection	ASO titer or positive throat culture
Major criteria	Carditis, polyarthritis, Sydenham chorea, erythema marginatum, SC nodules
Minor criteria	Migratory arthralgias, fever, acute phase reactants (elevated ESR, leukocytosis), prolonged PR interval on EKG

PATHOPHYSIOLOGY

- Obstruction between LA and LV impairs LV filling during diastole leads to increased LA pressure
- Increased LA pressure is transmitted passively ("back pressure") to the pulmonary circulation; over time, pulmonary HTN results.
- Over time, LA pressure overload can dilate the chamber and interrupt the cardiac conduction system, resulting in atrial fibrillation.
- Pulmonary hypertension also can cause increased collateralization between pulmonary and bronchial circulation, resulting in intraparenchymal hemorrhage with hemoptysis.

ETIOLOGY

- Rheumatic fever: Most common (see "Risk Factors")
- Aging (extension of mitral annular calcification)
- Rare causes:
  - Congenital (associated with mucopolysaccharidoses)
  - Autoimmune: SLE, rheumatoid arthritis
  - Malignant carcinoid
  - Other acquired: Left atrial myxoma, left atrial thrombus

COMMONLY ASSOCIATED CONDITIONS

- Atrial fibrillation (30–40% of symptomatic patients) and thromboembolic complications
- Associated valve lesions due to chronic inflammation (aortic stenosis, aortic insufficiency)
- Pulmonary congestion and pulmonary hypertension
- Pulmonary embolism (10%)
- Systemic congestion
- Systemic embolism
- Infection (1–5%)

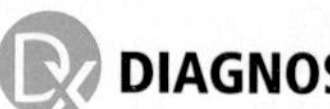

DIAGNOSIS

HISTORY

- History of rheumatic fever
- Severity of presentation depends on valve area; most early cases will be asymptomatic.
- Presenting features usually due to pulmonary vascular congestion:
  - Palpitations
  - Dyspnea on exertion
  - Fatigue
  - Pulmonary edema
  - Paroxysmal nocturnal dyspnea
- Atrial fibrillation
- Embolic event
- In advanced disease, symptoms of pulmonary hypertension and right heart failure predominate: Jugular venous distention, hepatomegaly, ascites, and peripheral edema
- Rare presentations: Hemoptysis, hoarseness (compression of recurrent laryngeal nerve by enlarged pulmonary artery or LA), dysphagia (compression)

PHYSICAL EXAM

- Auscultation:
  - Classic Murmur: Accentuated S1, opening snap, apical early decrescendo diastolic rumble with presystolic accentuation
  - Murmur variability seen in severe stenosis:
    - With mobile, noncalcified valve, murmur persists throughout diastole and S1 and the opening snap remains loud.
    - With a heavily calcified valve, murmur often is difficult to hear. S1 and the opening snap may be soft to absent.
- Prominent *a* wave in jugular venous pulse
- If pulmonary hypertension is present: Right ventricular lift, increased P2, high-pitched decrescendo diastolic murmur of pulmonic insufficiency (Graham Steell murmur)
- May also find associated aortic or, less commonly, tricuspid murmurs due to aortic or tricuspid valve involvement from rheumatic heart disease

DIAGNOSTIC TESTS & INTERPRETATION

Imaging

Initial approach

- EKG (2):
  - LA enlargement (manifested by broad, notched P waves in lead II [P mitrale] with a negative terminal deflection of the P wave in lead V1)
  - Atrial fibrillation common
  - RVH, RAD, and a large R wave in V1 possible
- Chest radiograph:
  - LA enlargement, straightening of the left heart border, a "double density" and elevation of the left mainstem bronchus
  - Prominent pulmonary arteries at the hilum with rapid tapering
  - RVH
  - Pulmonary edema pattern with Kerley B lines (late presentation)
- Echocardiogram indications:
  - Class I:
    - Diagnosis of mitral stenosis
    - Assess severity
    - Reassess after change in symptoms
    - Exercise Doppler for discrepancies between symptoms and echo findings
    - TEE to evaluate possible LA thrombus
    - TEE when transthoracic echo nondiagnostic
  - Class II:
    - Reassess asymptomatic patients
    - Severe MS: Yearly
    - Moderate MS: Every 1–2 years
    - Mild MS: Every 3–5 years
  - Class III:
    - Satisfactory result of transthoracic echo
- Echocardiogram findings (3):
  - MV anterior leaflet doming
  - Immobility of the posterior leaflet
  - Echo can demonstrate alternative causes of MS if not rheumatic.
  - Mitral valve area defined:
    - Normal: 4–6 cm^2
    - Mild MS: <2 cm^2
    - Moderate MS: 1–1.5 cm^2
    - Severe MS: <1 cm^2
- Cardiac catheterization indications:
  - Class I recommendations:
    - When echo is nonconclusive
    - Discrepancy between echo and symptoms
    - Discrepancy between echo and valve area
  - Class II recommendations:
    - To assess response of LA and pulmonary artery pressures to exercise when symptoms and echo findings do not match
    - Assess cause of severe pulmonary hypertension out of proportion to echo results
  - Class III recommendations:
    - Satisfactory result of echo

Follow-Up & Special Considerations
- If valve area >1.5 cm^2 and pressure gradient <5 mm Hg, then no further initial workup is needed.
- If valve area is <1.5 cm^2, then do further workup prior to surgical correction.

Diagnostic Procedures/Surgery
Exercise or Dobutamine stress test:
- When symptoms are severe but echo findings are mild
- To determine if surgery is needed

Pathological Findings
Rheumatic fever–induced pathologic changes:
- Leaflet thickening
- Leaflet calcification
- Commissural fusion
- Chordal shortening

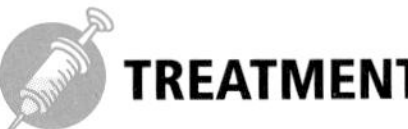

TREATMENT

MEDICATION

First Line
- Antibiotic prophylaxis against rheumatic fever and/or carditis is recommended for patients with history of rheumatic fever
  - Penicillin V (PO) or G (IM): IM is more effective than PO (4)
  - Sulfadiazine
  - Erythromycin
  - Take antibiotic continuously to prevent recurrence of rheumatic fever or carditis.
  - Duration of rheumatic fever prophylaxis:
    - Rheumatic fever without carditis: Take for 5 years or until age 21, whichever is longer
    - Rheumatic fever with carditis but no residual heart disease: Take for 10 years or well into adulthood, whichever is longer.
    - Rheumatic fever with carditis plus residual heart disease: Take for 10 years or until 40 years old, whichever is longer.
- Antibiotic prophylaxis against infective endocarditis is not routinely recommended (5).
- β-blockers for tachycardia or exertional symptoms
- Calcium channel blockers for tachycardia or exertional symptoms
- Diuretics for symptoms of pulmonary congestion
- Digitalis for atrial fibrillation if LV or right ventricle dysfunction
- Anticoagulation:
  - Class I recommendations:
    - MS and atrial fibrillation or history of atrial fibrillation
    - MS and prior embolic event
    - MS and left atrial thrombus
  - Class IIb recommendations
    - Asymptomatic MS but with severe MS and LA dimension >54 mm by echo
    - Severe MS, enlarged LA and spontaneous contrast on echo
- Warfarin (international normalized ratio) range 2–3
- Heparin in the acute atrial fibrillation setting

Second Line
Amiodarone for rate control if β-blockers or calcium channel blockers cannot be used

ADDITIONAL TREATMENT

General Measures
- Exercise:
  - Mild MS patients are usually asymptomatic even with strenuous exercise.
  - Usually recommend low-level aerobic exercise, limited by symptoms of dyspnea.
- Counsel patients that MS usually is slowly progressive but can have sudden onset of atrial fibrillation, which could become rapidly fatal. Call 911 for marked worsening of symptoms.
- Atrial fibrillation accompanying MS impairs left ventricular filling, especially with a rapid ventricular response:
  - Rate control with beta or calcium channel blockers or amiodarone.
  - Cardioversion for medical failure or if patient is unstable
  - If the atrial fibrillation has been present for longer than 24–48 hours, then:
    - Anticoagulate for 3 weeks then cardiovert
    - Heparinize, perform TEE, and if no atrial thrombus then cardiovert
  - After cardioversion, patient needs long-term anticoagulation.
  - These patients can critically decompensate due to loss of atrial contractility causing an inability to fill the LV.

SURGERY/OTHER PROCEDURES
- Balloon valvotomy:
  - Symptomatic patients with NYHA Class II, III, or IV symptoms with valves that look favorable and with favorable comorbidities
- Mitral valve surgery (6):
  - When MS is severe and balloon valvotomy is contraindicated due to unfavorable anatomy

Pregnancy Considerations
Volume expansion during pregnancy can exacerbate heart failure symptoms. For this reason, MS often presents during the intrapartum period. For patients with known severe MS, intervention should be pursued prior to pregnancy. Pregnancy in a patient with severe MS has a high rate of both maternal and fetal complications, including death. Percutaneous balloon valvotomy can be performed in symptomatic pregnant patients.

ONGOING CARE

FOLLOW-UP RECOMMENDATIONS
- Ascertain the valve gradient and pulmonary arterial pressure with echocardiogram.
- Follow-up will depend on the severity of the mitral stenosis and the patient's symptoms:
  - Asymptomatic patients: Annual history and examination; other tests can be deferred.
  - Symptomatic patients are reviewed according to individual therapy, symptoms, and signs; echocardiogram to evaluate for changes

DIET
Salt restriction for pulmonary congestion

PROGNOSIS
Natural history:
- Asymptomatic latent period after rheumatic fever for 10–30 years. 10-year survival for asymptomatic or minimally symptomatic patients is 80%. 10-year survival after onset of symptoms is 50–60%.
- Symptoms typically become debilitating 10 years after onset of symptoms.
- 10-year survival after onset of debilitating symptoms is only 0–15%.
- Mean survival with significant pulmonary hypertension is <3 years.
- The severity of MS progresses over time in almost all patients. There are no known medical therapies, apart from prevention of recurrent rheumatic fever, that alter this natural history. When symptoms develop, balloon valvotomy, open mitral commissurotomy, or closed mitral commissurotomy provides effective means of reducing stenosis but is not curative. Restenosis sometimes occurs and can be early (<5 years) or late (>20 years).
- Appropriate medical treatment can delay necessity for surgery, and surgical treatment substantially prolongs survival in patients with severe MS.

COMPLICATIONS
Left and right heart failure, atrial fibrillation and systemic embolization, pulmonary hypertension, bacterial endocarditis

REFERENCES

1. Ray S. Changing epidemiology and natural history of valvular heart disease. *Clin Med*. 2010;10(2): 168–71.
2. Chandrasekhar Y. Mitral stenosis. *Lancet*. 2009; 374(9697):1271–83.
3. Maganti K, et al. Valvular heart disease: Diagnosis and management. *Mayo Clin Proc*. 2010;85(5): 483–500.
4. Manyemba J, Mayosi BM. Penicillin for secondary prevention of rheumatic fever. *Cochrane Database Syst Rev*. 2002;(3).
5. Nishimura RA, et al. ACC/AHA 2008 guideline update on valvular heart disease: Focused update on infective endocarditis: A report of the American College of Cardiology/American Heart Association Task Force on Practice Guidelines endorsed by the Society of Cardiovascular Anesthesiologists, Society for Cardiovascular Angiography and Interventions, and Society of Thoracic Surgeons. *Catheter Cardiovasc Interv*. 2008;72(3):E1–12.
6. Zakkar M, et al. Rheumatic mitral valve disease: Current surgical status. *Prog Cardiovasc Dis*. 2009;51(6):478–81.

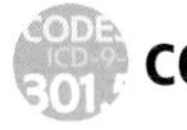

CODES

ICD9
- 394.0 Mitral stenosis
- 394.1 Rheumatic mitral insufficiency
- 394.2 Mitral stenosis with insufficiency

CLINICAL PEARLS
- Asymptomatic patients may be followed clinically with yearly exams for development of symptoms, with periodic echocardiography to evaluate valve area.
- Once symptoms of MS develop, initiate appropriate medical therapy but advise patient that, for most patients, surgical therapy will be needed to prolong survival. Almost all cases of mitral valve stenosis progress in severity over time.

MITRAL VALVE PROLAPSE

Peerawut Deeprasertkul, MD
Yongkasem Vorasettakarnkij, MD, MSc

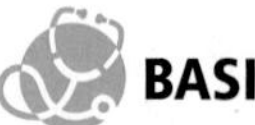

BASICS

DESCRIPTION

- Generally, mitral valve prolapse (MVP) is a systolic billowing of one or both mitral leaflets into the left atrium during systole ± mitral regurgitation (MR).
- More specifically, MVP is a single or bileaflet prolapse of at least 2 mm superior displacement into left atrium during systole on the parasternal long-axis annular plane of the valve on echocardiogram ± leaflet thickening:
  - Classic: Prolapse with >5 mm of leaflet thickening
  - Nonclassic: Prolapse with <5 mm of leaflet thickening (1)
- Synonym(s): Systolic click-murmur syndrome; Billowing mitral cusp syndrome; Myxomatous mitral valve; Floppy valve syndrome; Redundant cusp syndrome; Barlow syndrome

EPIDEMIOLOGY

Incidence

- Predominant age: MVP has been described in all age groups.
- Initial descriptions based on clinical examinations suggested a 2:1 female predominance. Using modern echocardiogram criteria, men and women are affected equally (2).
- The most serious consequences of hemodynamically significant MR occur in men older than 50 years.

Prevalence

MVP is the most common valvular abnormality, affecting 1–2.5% of the general population (2,3) depending on the precise definition.

RISK FACTORS

- MVP is a primary cardiovascular disorder.
- MVP is more likely to occur in patients with connective tissue disorders (see "Commonly Associated Conditions").
- Physical characteristics associated with MVP:
  - Straight thoracic spine
  - Pectus excavatum
  - Asthenic body hiatus
  - Low BMI
  - Scoliosis or kyphosis
  - Hypermobility of the joints
  - Arm span > height
  - Narrow anteroposterior (AP) diameter of the chest

Genetics

- Familial MVP is inherited as an autosomal-dominant trait but with variable expressivity and incomplete penetrance.
- 2 genetic loci identified:
  - *MMVP1* on chromosome 16p11.2-p12.1
  - *MMVP2* on chromosome 11p15.4 (1)

PATHOPHYSIOLOGY

- The pathology causing MVP is multifactorial and includes the following:
  - Abnormal valve tissue:
    - Myxomatous degeneration: Redundant layers of leaflet "hooding" the cords, chordal elongation, and annular dilatation
    - Myxoid leaflets are more elastic and less stiff than normal valves.
    - Chordal rupture is more common.
  - Disparity in size between the mitral valve and the left ventricle
  - Connective tissue disorders (1)
- MVP is often associated with variable degrees of MR.
- Frequently there is enlargement of the left atrium (LA) and left ventricle (LV).
- Mitral annulus is often dilated.
- Involvement of other valves may occur (tricuspid valve prolapse 40%, pulmonic prolapse and aortic prolapse 2–10%)
- Possible increased vagal tone
- Possible increased urine epinephrine and norepinephrine
- MVP patients often have orthostatic hypotension and tachycardia.

ETIOLOGY

- Genetics cause proliferation of the spongiosa layer of the leaflets (3).
- Fibrosis on surface of leaflets (3)
- Thinning and elongation of chordae tendineae
- The mitral valve differentiates during days 35–42 of fetal development, the same time as differentiation of the vertebrae and ribs.

COMMONLY ASSOCIATED CONDITIONS

- Marfan syndrome (91% of Marfan syndrome patients have mitral valve prolapse) (1)
- Ehlers-Danlos syndrome
- Hypertrophic cardiomyopathy
- Pseudoxanthoma elasticum
- Osteogenesis imperfecta
- Von Willebrand disease (3)
- Primary hypomastia

DIAGNOSIS

Physical exam and echocardiography

HISTORY

- Most patients are asymptomatic.
- The most frequent symptom is palpitations.
- Symptoms related to autonomic dysfunction:
  - Anxiety and panic attacks
  - Arrhythmias
  - Exercise intolerance
  - Palpitations and atypical chest pains
  - Fatigue
  - Orthostasis, syncope, or presyncope
  - Neuropsychiatric symptoms
- Symptoms related to progression of mitral regurgitation:
  - Fatigue
  - Dyspnea
  - Exercise intolerance
  - Orthopnea
  - Paroxysmal nocturnal dyspnea
  - Congestive heart failure (CHF)
- Symptoms occur as a result of an associated complication (stroke, arrhythmia).

PHYSICAL EXAM

- Auscultatory examination:
  - Mid-to-late systolic click:
    - May vary in timing and intensity based on ventricular beat-to-beat volume variations
    - At low ventricular volumes, the valve may prolapse earlier during systole and further into the LA than during volume overload.
    - It may or may not be followed by a high-pitched, mid-to-late systolic murmur at the cardiac apex.
  - Murmur: A mid-to-late crescendo systolic murmur best heard at apex, middle- to high-pitched, occasionally musical or honking in quality
  - Occasionally, only the ejection click is present.
  - The duration of the murmur corresponds with the severity of MR.
- Dynamic auscultation:
  - Maneuvers that move the click and murmur toward S_1:
    - Arterial vasodilation
    - Amyl nitrate
    - Valsalva
    - Augmented contractility
    - Decreased venous return (which can be induced by standing up)
  - Maneuvers that move the click and murmur toward S_2:
    - Squatting
    - Leg raise
    - Isometric exercise

DIAGNOSTIC TESTS & INTERPRETATION

Imaging

Initial approach

- Echocardiogram:
  - Indicated for the diagnosis of MVP and assessment of MR, leaflet morphology, and left ventricular systolic function in asymptomatic patients with physical signs of MVP
  - Routine repetition of echocardiography is not indicated for the asymptomatic patient who has MVP and no MR, or MVP and mild MR with no changes in clinical signs and symptoms.
  - Most useful and definitive imaging study
  - Parasternal long-axis view most specific for diagnosis
  - Valve prolapse of ≥2 mm above the mitral annulus is most highly associated with MVP ± leaflet thickening.
  - Other findings may include the following:
    - Anterior leaflet billowing
    - Leaflet thickening of ≥5 mm
    - Leaflet redundancy
    - Mitral regurgitation
    - Posterior leaflet displacement
  - Nondiagnostic transthoracic echocardiogram: ≤10%
  - Transesophageal echocardiography is helpful to visualize the leaflet anatomy, especially if a valve repair operation is being considered and/or if there is a flail leaflet.
- Angiography indicated in patients with severe and symptomatic MR for whom cardiac surgical referral is being contemplated:
  - Impaired LV systolic function to evaluate for mitral valve surgery
  - Rarely used for diagnostic purposes
- ECG is usually normal:
  - May be nonspecific ST-T wave changes
  - T-wave inversions
  - Prominent Q waves
  - QT prolongation

- A chest x-ray (CXR) is not necessary for diagnosis:
  - Typically, the CXR is normal.
  - Other findings:
    - Possible pulmonary edema: Pulmonary edema may be asymmetric with acute chordal rupture and flail leaflet.
    - Possible calcification of the mitral annulus
- Holter monitoring is optional if patient has palpitations. Order Holter monitoring as usual for syncope or dizziness.

Follow-Up & Special Considerations

Patients with a first-degree relative who has myxomatous mitral valve prolapse should be screened with echocardiography (1).

Pathological Findings

- Myxomatous proliferation of the middle layer (spongiosa) of the valve, resulting in increased mucopolysaccharide deposition and myxomatous degeneration
- By electron microscopy, the collagen fibers in the valve leaflets are disorganized and fragmented.
- With increased stroma deposition, the valve leaflets enlarge and become redundant.
- The endothelium is usually noncontiguous and a frequent site for thrombus or infective vegetation.

DIFFERENTIAL DIAGNOSIS

- Mitral regurgitation
- Tricuspid regurgitation
- Tricuspid valve prolapse
- Papillary muscle dysfunction
- Hypertrophic cardiomyopathy
- Ejection clicks (don't change timing with systole)

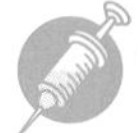

TREATMENT

MEDICATION

- Asymptomatic MVP is treated with reassurance; normal lifestyle and regular exercise is encouraged (3).
- MVP and transient ischemic attacks (TIA) are treated with aspirin 75–325 mg daily (Class I recommendation) (3)[C].
- MVP with history of cryptogenic stroke, or atrial fibrillation with $CHADS_2$ score <2, is generally treated with aspirin 75–325 mg daily (3)[C].
- MVP with atrial fibrillation with $CHADS_2$ score ≥ 2 is treated with warfarin (3)[C].
- MVP with history of stroke plus atrial fibrillation or left atrial appendage thrombus is treated with warfarin (3)[C]
- MVP with palpitations is treated with β-blockers and/or recommendation to discontinue alcohol, cigarettes, and caffeine. Continuous ambulatory ECG monitoring may be useful to detect significant arrhythmias (3).

ADDITIONAL TREATMENT

General Measures

Treat MVP with orthostatic symptoms by liberalizing fluid and salt intake. If severe, mineralocorticoids or clonidine may rarely be used. Support stockings may also be beneficial.

Additional Therapies

- Endocarditis prophylaxis is not recommended for MVP (3)[B].
- Patients with prior endocarditis undergoing dental, respiratory tract, infected skin, or musculoskeletal should receive prophylaxis for endocarditis with amoxicillin 30–60 minutes prior to procedure (3)[B]. Ampicillin, cefazolin, or ceftriaxone IM or IV may be used if unable to tolerate oral medications.

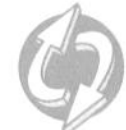

SURGERY/OTHER PROCEDURES

- Referral for surgery is recommended for patients with severe MR with impaired LV systolic function or flail leaflet owing to ruptured chordae tendineae (3).
- Minimally invasive mitral valve repair may have less pain or shorter postoperative hospital stay compared to conventional median sternotomy open repair for patients with bileaflet prolapse and severe mitral regurgitation (4).
- Surgical repair of mitral regurgitation due to isolated posterior leaflet prolapse is associated with a low reoperation rate (5).

ONGOING CARE

FOLLOW-UP RECOMMENDATIONS

- Asymptomatic MVP patients with no significant MR can be followed clinically every 3–5 years.
- Patients who are symptomatic or have high-risk features on initial echocardiogram, including moderate to severe MR, may need serial echocardiograms and should be followed clinically once per year.
- Patients with MVP and severe MR may require coronary angiography and transesophageal echocardiography if cardiac surgical referral is planned.

PATIENT EDUCATION

Patient education on avoidance of alcohol, caffeine, stimulants, and nicotine may be sufficient to control symptoms in some instances:

- No contraindication to pregnancy
- Restriction from competitive sports if patient has MVP with one of the following features (6):
  - A history of syncope associated with document arrhythmia
  - A family history of MVP-related SCD
  - Sustained or repetitive and nonsustained supraventricular tachycardia or frequent and/or complex ventricular tachyarrhythmias on ambulatory Holter monitoring
  - Severe MR
  - A prior embolic event
  - Left ventricular systolic dysfunction
- Explain the hereditary nature of familial MVP.

PROGNOSIS

- Excellent prognosis for asymptomatic patients
- For patients with severe MR or reduced ejection fraction, the prognosis is similar to that for nonischemic MR.

COMPLICATIONS

- Sudden cardiac death (yearly rate of 1.9/10,000 per year) is twice the rate in the general population; risk is 50–100 times greater (0.9–1.9% per year) if significant MR is present.
- Chordae rupture with acute mitral insufficiency (higher risk of cardiac death; up to 2% per year)
- Endocarditis
- Cerebrovascular ischemic event
- Fibrin emboli
- Heart failure with progressive MR
- Arrhythmia:
  - Atrial premature beats, 35–90%
  - Supraventricular tachycardia, 3–32%
  - Ventricular premature beats, 58–89%
  - Complex ventricular ectopy, 30–56%
- Pulmonary hypertension
- CHF
- Progressive MR

REFERENCES

1. Hayek E, Gring CN, Griffin BP. Mitral valve prolapse. *Lancet*. 2005;365:507–18.
2. Freed LA, Levy D, Levine RA, et al. Prevalence and clinical outcome of mitral-valve prolapse. *N Engl J Med*. 1999;341:1–7.
3. Bonow RO, Carabello BA, Chatterjee K. 2008 focused update incorporated into the ACC/AHA 2006 guidelines for the management of patients with valvular heart disease: A report of the American College of Cardiology/American Heart Association Task Force on Practice Guidelines (Writing Committee to revise the 1998 guidelines for the management of patients with valvular heart disease). Endorsed by the Society of Cardiovascular Anesthesiologists, Society for Cardiovascular Angiography and Interventions, and Society of Thoracic Surgeons. *J Am Coll Cardiol*. 2008;52: e1–142.
4. Speziale G, Nasso G, Esposito G, et al. Results of mitral valve repair for Barlow disease (bileaflet prolapse) via right minithoracotomy versus conventional median sternotomy: A randomized trial. *J Thorac Cardiovasc Surg*. 2011;142:77–83.
5. Johnston DR, Gillinov AM, Blackstone EH, et al. Surgical repair of posterior mitral valve prolapse: Implications for guidelines and percutaneous repair. *Ann Thorac Surg*. 2010;89:1385–94.
6. Maron BJ, Ackerman MJ, Nishimura RA. Task Force 4: HCM and other cardiomyopathies, mitral valve prolapse, myocarditis, and Marfan syndrome. *J Am Coll Cardiol*. 2005;45:1340–5.

CODES

ICD9

424.0 Mitral valve disorders

CLINICAL PEARLS

- MVP patients often have orthostatic hypotension and tachycardia.
- Asymptomatic MVP patients with no significant MR can be followed clinically every 3–5 years.
- Patients who are symptomatic or have high-risk features on initial echocardiogram, including moderate to severe MR, may need serial echocardiograms and should be followed clinically once per year.

M

MOLLUSCUM CONTAGIOSUM

Gillian S. Stephens, MD, MSc

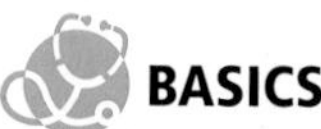

BASICS

DESCRIPTION

- Common, benign, viral (*Poxviridae*) skin infection
- 1–5 mm, "pearly" white or flesh-colored
- Dome-shaped papules; central umbilication (difficult to see in young children)
- Highly contagious; autoinoculation, skin-to-skin contact, sexual contact, shared clothing, towels, bathing water
- Self-limited in immunocompetent
- Difficult to treat/disfiguring in immunocompromised

EPIDEMIOLOGY

Incidence

- Up to 20% children in tropics
- 30% in AIDS patients

Prevalence

- Children 2–15 years
- Sexually active young adults
- 5–18% HIV population

RISK FACTORS

- Skin-to-skin contact with infected person
- Contact sports
- Sexual activity with infected partner
- Immunocompromised: HIV, chemotherapy, corticosteroid therapy, transplant patients

GENERAL PREVENTION

- Avoid skin-to-skin contact with host (e.g., contact sports, sexual activity).
- Avoid sharing clothing, towels, bathing water.

PATHOPHYSIOLOGY

- Virions invade and replicate in cytoplasm of epithelial cells.
- Cause abnormal cell proliferation
- Genome encodes proteins to evade host immune system
- Incubation period: 1–7 weeks
- Not associated with malignancy

ETIOLOGY

- DNA virus; *Poxviridae* family
- 4 major types, clinically indistinguishable
- No cross-hybridization or reactivation by other poxviruses

COMMONLY ASSOCIATED CONDITIONS

- Atopic dermatitis
- HIV/AIDS
- Immunosuppression: Corticosteroids, chemotherapy

DIAGNOSIS

HISTORY

- Contact with known infected person
- Participation in contact sports
- Sexual activity

PHYSICAL EXAM

- Discrete, firm papules with a central umbilication
- Umbilication not obvious in small children
- White curdlike core under umbilicated center
- Lesions are flesh, pearl, or red in color
- May have surrounding erythema or dermatitis
- Immunocompetent hosts: Average of 11–20 lesions, 2–5 mm diameter (range: 1–10 mm)
- Hosts with HIV/AIDS: Hundreds of widespread lesions
- Children: Trunk, extremities, face, anogenital region
- Sexually active: Inner thighs, anogenital area
- Perform thorough skin exam including conjunctiva and anogenital area.

Pediatric Considerations

- Infants <3 months, consider vertical transmission (1)
- Children: Fever, >50 lesions, limited response to therapy, consider immunodeficiency (2)
- Children: Anogenital lesions, consider autoinoculation/possible sexual abuse (2)

DIAGNOSTIC TESTS & INTERPRETATION

Lab

Initial lab tests

- Virus cannot be cultured.
- Scrape lesion; Tzanck preparation; molluscum cytoplasmic inclusion bodies (2)
- Culture lesion if concern is secondary infection.
- Sexual transmission: Test for other STIs, including HIV.

Imaging

Initial approach

Microscopy

Diagnostic Procedures/Surgery

Clinical; using magnifying lens

Pathological Findings

Molluscum cytoplasmic inclusion bodies within keratinocytes

DIFFERENTIAL DIAGNOSIS

- AIDS patients: Cryptococcus, penicilliosis, histoplasmosis, coccidiomycosis
- Basal cell carcinoma
- Benign appendageal tumors: Syringomas, hydrocystomas, ectopic sebaceous glands
- Condyloma acuminatum
- Dermatofibroma
- Eyelid: Abscess, chalazion, foreign body granuloma
- Folliculitis/furunculosis
- Keratoacanthoma
- Oral squamous cell carcinoma
- Trichoepithelioma
- Verruca vulgaris
- Warty dyskeratoma

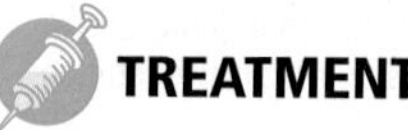

TREATMENT

MEDICATION

First Line

- Cantharidin solution 0.7–0.9%: Apply sparingly to lesions, cover with occlusion dressing, wash off in 2–6 hours or sooner if blistering. Repeat treatment every 1–4 weeks until lesions resolve (in-office treatment) (2,3)[C]:
  - Adverse effects: Blistering, erythema, pain, pruritus
  - Precautions: Do not use on face or on genital mucosa
- Cimetidine 40 mg/kg/d divided t.i.d. for 2 months. Maximum dose 800 mg t.i.d. (2,4)[C]:
  - Adverse effects: Headache, diarrhea, gynecomastia
  - Precautions: Pregnancy Category B. Not recommended for use while nursing.
- Imiquimod cream 5%: Optimal dosing regimen unknown. Genital area: Apply to lesions 1 time daily 3 times per week until lesions resolve, up to 16 weeks (2,3)[C]:
  - Adverse effects: Erythema, edema, pruritus, postinflammatory pigment changes
  - Contraindications: Pregnancy

Second Line

- Limit treatment to small areas 4–10 cm^2:
  - Podofilox cream 0.5%: Apply to lesions b.i.d. for 3 days, none for 4 days; may repeat this cycle 4–6 times (3)[C]:
    - Adverse effects: Erythema, edema, pain
    - Contraindications: Pregnancy
  - Podophyllin 10–25% solution: Apply sparingly to lesions 1 time weekly for 4–6 weeks (in-office treatment) (3)[C]:
    - Adverse effects: Erythema, edema, pain
    - Contraindications: Pregnancy, infants, children, oral mucosa
- For HIV/AIDS patients with refractory lesions, consider:
  - Starting or maximizing HAART therapy (2)[C]
  - IV or topical cidofovir (2,3)

ADDITIONAL TREATMENT

General Measures

- Natural resolution
- No single intervention has been shown to be convincingly effective in treating molluscum contagiosum (5).

COMPLEMENTARY AND ALTERNATIVE MEDICINE

Australian lemon myrtle oil: Apply 10% solution once daily for 21 days (6)[C].

SURGERY/OTHER PROCEDURES

- Cryotherapy: 5–10 seconds with 1–2 mm margins. Repeat every 3–4 weeks as needed until lesions disappear (2,3)[C]:
  - Adverse effects: Erythema, edema, pain, blistering
  - Contraindications: Cryoglobulinemia, Raynaud disease
- Curettage (± electrodessication) under local or topical anesthesia (2,3)[C]:
  - Adverse effects: Pain, scarring
- Incision and expression of central particle (2):
  - Adverse effects: High rate of scarring
- CO_2 (3) or pulsed dye (2,3)[C] lasers (for recalcitrant lesions, usually in HIV/AIDS patients):
  - Adverse effects: Pain, edema, scarring, postinflammatory pigment changes
- Photodynamic therapy (ALA/MAL-PDT) (7)[C]

Pediatric Considerations

- Surgical interventions: Second-line in small children; pain associated
- Pain control: Pretreat with topical lidocaine or EMLA before surgical treatment.
- Note: Adverse effect:
  - Lidocaine or EMLA over large body surface area: Methemoglobinemia and CNS toxicity. Refer to manufacturer's recommendations on dosing and use in children.

Pregnancy Considerations

- Safe in pregnancy: Curettage, cryotherapy, incision, and expression
- Contraindicated: Podophyllin, podofilox, or imiquimod; teratogenic

ONGOING CARE

FOLLOW-UP RECOMMENDATIONS

Patient Monitoring

Depends on type of treatment

DIET

Regular

PATIENT EDUCATION

- Cover lesions to prevent spread.
- Avoid scratching.
- Avoid contact sports.
- Avoid sharing towels, baths.
- Avoid sexual activity.
- Avoid swimming pools.

PROGNOSIS

- Immunocompetent: Self-limited, resolves in 3–12 months (range: 2 months–4 years)
- Immunocompromised: Lesions difficult to treat, may persist for years

COMPLICATIONS

- Secondary infection
- Scarring, hyper-/hypopigmentation

REFERENCES

1. Connell CO, Oranje A, Van Gysel D, et al. Congenital molluscum contagiosum: Report of four cases and review of the literature. *Pediatr Dermatol*. 2008;25:553–6.
2. Brown J, Janniger CK, Schwartz RA, et al. Childhood molluscum contagiosum. *Int J Dermatol*. 2006;45:93–9.
3. Ting PT, Dytoc MT. Therapy of external anogenital warts and molluscum contagiosum: A literature review. *Dermatol Ther*. 2004;17:68–101.
4. Jones S, Kress D. Treatment of molluscum contagiosum and herpes simplex virus cutaneous infections. *Cutis*. 2007;79(suppl 4):11–17.
5. van der Wouden JC, Menke J, Gajadin S, et al. Inteventions for cutaneous molluscum contagiosum. *Cochrane Database Syst Rev*. 2009;(4):CD004767.
6. Burke BE, Baillie JE, Olson RD. Essential oil of Australian lemon myrtle *(Backhousia citriodora)* in the treatment of molluscum contagiosum in children. *Biomed Pharmacother*. 2004;58:245–7.
7. Rossi R, Bruscino N, Ricceri F, et al. Photodynamic treatment for viral infections of the skin. *G Ital Dermatol Venereol*. 2009;144:79–83.

ADDITIONAL READING

Dohil MA, Lin P, Lee J, et al. The epidemiology of molluscum contagiosum in children. *J Am Acad Dermatol*. 2006;54:47–54.

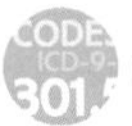

CODES

ICD9

078.0 Molluscum contagiosum

CLINICAL PEARLS

- Natural resolution is preferred treatment in healthy patients (5)[A].
- Reassure parents that lesions will heal naturally and generally resolve without scarring (5)[A].
- No one specific treatment has been identified as superior to any other (5)[A].
- Consider topical corticosteroids or antihistamines for pruritus or associated dermatitis (2)[C].

M

MONONUCLEOSIS

Renata Gazzi, MD

BASICS

DESCRIPTION

Infectious mononucleosis (IM) is an acute illness resulting from Epstein-Barr virus (EBV) infection that occurs mainly in adolescents and young adults.

EPIDEMIOLOGY

Incidence

- Not a reportable disease, but by age 5 years, ~50% of all Americans have been infected; 90% by age 25 years.
- IM accounts for fewer than 2% of pharyngitis cases in adults:
  - The vast majority of adults are not susceptible to infection because of prior exposure.
- The incidence is ~30× higher in whites than in blacks in the US.
- No seasonal peak

Prevalence

~50% of people who are infected with the virus will develop symptoms; others can carry the virus, not knowing they have it.

RISK FACTORS

- Age between 10 and 30 years
- Populations with many young adults, such as active-duty military personnel, high school and college students

Genetics

Unknown

GENERAL PREVENTION

- No blood donation for at least 6 months
- Avoid saliva of infected person.
- Vaccine is under research.

PATHOPHYSIOLOGY

- EBV replicates primarily in B-lymphocytes but also replicates in the epithelial cells of the pharynx and parotid duct.
- EBV is spread by saliva (i.e., coughing, sneezing, kissing, and sharing drinks and utensils).
- The incubation period is 4–8 weeks.
- EBV also has been isolated in both cervical epithelial cells and in male seminal fluid, suggesting that transmission also may occur sexually.

ETIOLOGY

EBV is a double-stranded DNA herpesvirus.

COMMONLY ASSOCIATED CONDITIONS

- Streptococcal pharyngitis may be associated in 30% of patients.
- A history of infectious mononucleosis significantly increases the risk of multiple sclerosis (1)[A].

DIAGNOSIS

HISTORY

- Individuals between 10 and 30 years of age with a history of sore throat and significant fatigue
- The syndrome is often heralded by malaise, headache, and low-grade fever.
- Prodrome typically evolves into the classic triad:
  - Fever
  - Tonsillar pharyngitis
  - Lymphadenopathy

PHYSICAL EXAM

- Lymphadenopathy (100%):
  - Typically symmetric
  - More commonly involves the posterior cervical chain, but it also may become more generalized
  - Peaks in the first week and then subsides gradually over 2–3 weeks
- Fever (98%)
- Pharyngitis (85%)
- Splenomegaly (50–60%)

DIAGNOSTIC TESTS & INTERPRETATION

Lab

Initial lab tests

- CBC: An increase in total lymphocyte >35% and atypical lymphocytes of at least 10%
- Elevated aminotransferases: Seen in the vast majority of patients but typically self-limited
- Heterophile antibodies (monospot test):
  - In 40% of patients, positive in first week
  - 90% of patients in third week
  - May remain positive for 2 years for up to 20% of infected individuals
- EBV-specific antibodies:
  - Viral capsid antigen (VCA):
    - IgG and IgM peak at 3–4 weeks.
    - IgG then declines but persists for life.
    - IgM declines rapidly and is undetectable by 3 months.
  - EB nuclear antigen (EBNA):
    - Develops after 2 months and persists indefinitely
    - Presence early in the course of illness excludes acute EBV infection.
  - Early antigen (EA):
    - IgG to EA is present at the onset of clinical illness and persists for 2–3 months.

Follow-Up & Special Considerations

- In a patient with compatible syndrome and a negative heterophile antibody, the monospot test can be repeated because this test can be negative during the first week of clinical illness.
- EBV-specific antibodies should be determined if the patient has a repeatedly negative monospot test.

Imaging

Initial approach

Imaging not indicated initially

Follow-Up & Special Considerations

- Ultrasound if clinically important to diagnose or follow splenomegaly
- CT scan of abdomen is preferred to rule out splenic rupture.

DIFFERENTIAL DIAGNOSIS

- Cytomegalovirus
- Toxoplasmosis
- Rubella
- Adenovirus
- Herpesviruses
- Drug adverse effects
- Streptococcal pharyngitis
- Viral tonsillitis
- Diphtheria
- Viral hepatitis
- Lymphoma or leukemia
- Human herpesvirus 6
- Roseola
- Mumps
- Primary HIV infection

Pregnancy Considerations

Differentiating between IM caused by EBV and a similar syndrome owing to cytomegalovirus (CMV) or HIV infection often is not possible clinically, and it is particularly important if the patient is pregnant because CMV, HIV, and *Toxoplasma* infections can have significant adverse effects on pregnancy outcomes.

Pediatric Considerations

EBV acquired during childhood years is often subclinical.

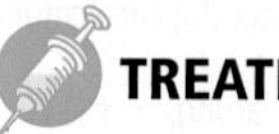

TREATMENT

MEDICATION

First Line

- Acetaminophen
- NSAIDs
- Lozenges
- Gargling with 2% lidocaine (Xylocaine) solution

Second Line

- Acyclovir (Zovirax): Not recommended; no clinical benefit
- Corticosteroids: Recommended in patients with significant pharyngeal edema that threatens respiratory compromise

- Steroids are not recommended for routine treatment but do improve fever and hematologic abnormalities and may shorten length of infirmary stay (2)[B].

ADDITIONAL TREATMENT

General Measures

Symptomatic treatment, the mainstay of care, includes adequate hydration, analgesics, antipyretics, and adequate rest. Complete bed rest is unnecessary.

Issues for Referral

- Emergent ENT consultation for an impending airway obstruction
- Surgery consultation if suspicious of splenic rupture; the typical manifestations are abdominal pain and/or a falling hematocrit.

Additional Therapies

The preferred treatment for splenic rupture is nonoperative with intensive supportive care and splenic preservation, but some require splenectomy.

SURGERY/OTHER PROCEDURES

- Splenectomy
- Tonsillectomy

IN-PATIENT CONSIDERATIONS

Initial Stabilization

Outpatient usually; 95% of patients recover uneventfully without specific complication.

Admission Criteria

Suspicion of splenic rupture or airway obstruction

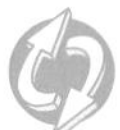

ONGOING CARE

FOLLOW-UP RECOMMENDATIONS

A generalized maculopapular, urticarial, or petechial rash is seen occasionally. Rash is more common following the administration of ampicillin or amoxicillin.

DIET

Soft diet followed by gradually advanced diet if severe sore throat

PATIENT EDUCATION

- For athletes planning to resume noncontact sports, training can be restarted gradually 3 weeks from symptom onset. For strenuous contact sports or activities associated with increased intraabdominal pressure, patient should wait a minimum of 4 weeks after illness onset (3)[B].
- There is no set time to go back to school or work. Individuals with IM tend to be most contagious during the incubation period, the 4–6 weeks before they get sick, and during the acute phases of their illness. Some people even may shed EBV when they are no longer sick.
- Because the EBV resides in the body for life, it can reactivate, but in most cases it won't cause symptoms unless the immune system becomes severely compromised.

PROGNOSIS

Fatigue, myalgias, and need for sleep may persist for several months after the acute infection has resolved.

COMPLICATIONS

- Chronic EBV infections (i.e., chronic fatigue syndrome, the diagnosis of which remains highly controversial)
- Splenic rupture (rare, 0.1–0.5% of patients with proven IM)
- Hemolytic anemia (mild)
- Thrombocytopenia
- Hemolytic-uremic syndrome
- Seizures and other neurologic abnormalities
- Nerve palsies
- Meningoencephalitis
- Reye syndrome
- Myocarditis/ECG changes
- Airway obstruction
- Acute interstitial nephritis

REFERENCES

1. Handel AE, Williamson AJ, Disanto G, et al. An updated meta-analysis of risk of multiple sclerosis following infectious mononucleosis. *PLoS ONE*. 2010;5.
2. Dickens KP, Nye AM, Gilchrist V, et al. Clinical inquiries. Should you use steroids to treat infectious mononucleosis? *J Fam Pract*. 2008;57:754–5.
3. Eichner ER. Sports medicine pearls and pitfalls–defending the spleen: Return to play after infectious mononucleosis. *Curr Sports Med Rep*. 2007;6:68–9.

ADDITIONAL READING

- Candy B, Hotopf M, et al. Steroids for symptom control in infectious mononucleosis. *Cochrane Database Syst Rev*. 2006;3:CD004402.
- Ebell MH. Epstein-Barr infectious mononucleosis. *Am Fam Phys*. 2004;70:1279–87.
- Putukian M, O'Connor FG, Stricker P, et al. Mononucleosis and athletic participation: An evidence-based subject review. *Clin J Sport Med*. 2008;18:309–15.

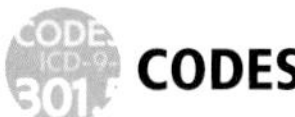

CODES

ICD9

075 Infectious mononucleosis

CLINICAL PEARLS

- IM should be suspected in patients 10–30 years of age who present with sore throat and significant fatigue, palatal petechiae, posterior cervical or auricular adenopathy, marked axillary adenopathy, or inguinal adenopathy.
- Patients with suspected IM, based on history and physical exam, should have a CBC with differential and a heterophile antibody test. In addition, patients also should have a diagnostic evaluation for streptococcal infection by culture or antigen test.
- In a patient with a compatible syndrome and a negative heterophile antibody test, the monospot test can be repeated because this test can be negative during the first week of clinical illness. EBV-specific antibodies (e.g., VCA IgM and IgG and EBNA) should be determined if the patient has repeatedly negative monospot tests.
- The presence of IgG EBNA or the absence of IgG and IgM VCA excludes primary EBV infection and should prompt consideration of alternative etiologies of a mononucleosislike illness.
- An increase in monocytes does not suggest mononucleosis; an increase in total lymphocytes >35% and atypical lymphocytes >10% does suggest mononucleosis.

MORTON NEUROMA (INTERDIGITAL NEUROMA)

Jake D. Veigel, MD
Anastasia Grivoyannis, MD
J. Herbert Stevenson, MD

BASICS

DESCRIPTION

- Perineural fibrosis of the common digital nerve as it passes between metatarsals; the most common site is the interspace between the third and fourth metatarsals; the interspace between the third and second metatarsals is the second most common site.
- System(s) affected: Musculoskeletal; Nervous
- Synonym(s): Plantar digital neuritis

EPIDEMIOLOGY

Prevalence

- Unknown
- Mean age: 45–50 years
- Predominant sex: Female > Male (8:1)

RISK FACTORS

- High-heeled shoes: Cause more weight to be transferred to the front of the foot
- Tight-toed shoes (tight toe boxes): Cause lateral compression
- Pes planus (flat feet): Causes nerve to be pulled more medially, which increases irritation
- Obesity
- Ballet dancing, basketball, aerobics, tennis, running, and similar activities

GENERAL PREVENTION

- Wear properly fitting shoes.
- Avoid high heels and shoes with narrow toe boxes.

PATHOPHYSIOLOGY

- Lateral plantar nerve combines with part of medial plantar nerve; the 2 nerves combine, creating a nerve with larger diameter than nerves going to other digits.
- Nerve lies in SC tissue, deep to the fat pad of foot, just superficial to the digital artery and vein.
- Overlying the nerve is the strong, deep transverse metatarsal ligament that holds the metatarsal bones together.
- With each step the patient takes, the inflamed nerve becomes compressed between the ground and the deep transverse metatarsal ligament.

ETIOLOGY

- Excessive stress of the forefoot
- Repetitive trauma
- Congenitally enlarged plantar digital nerve

DIAGNOSIS

HISTORY

- Most common complaint is pain localized to interspace between third and fourth toes.
- Pain is less severe when not bearing weight.
- Pain, cramping, or numbness of the forefoot during weight bearing or immediately after strenuous foot exertion
- Radiation of pain to the toes
- Pain is relieved by removing the shoe and massaging the foot.
- Patients often state: "It feels like I am walking on a marble."
- A burning pain in the ball of the foot that may radiate into the toes
- Tingling or numbness in the toes
- Aggravated by wearing tight or narrow shoes

PHYSICAL EXAM

- A palpable nodule in the metatarsal interspace is an occasional finding.
- Positive Mulder sign: See "Diagnostic Procedures."
- Intense pain on pressure between metatarsal heads
- Assess midfoot motion and digital motion to determine if arthritis or synovitis.
- Palpate along metatarsal shafts to assess for metatarsalgia or stress fractures.

DIAGNOSTIC TESTS & INTERPRETATION

Imaging

Initial approach

- Radiographs may help to rule out osseous pathology if diagnosis is in question, but films usually are normal in patients with a Morton neuroma.
- Ultrasound shows a hypoechoic nodule between the metatarsal interspace. Ultrasound had a 65% specificity and a 98% sensitivity for Morton neuromas, but it is not good at assessing the size of the lesion (1)[C].
- MRI is used to ensure that compression is not caused by a malignant tumor in the foot. MRI is helpful in determining how much of the nerve to resect surgically, and it has a sensitivity of 83% and a specificity of 99% (1)[C].

Diagnostic Procedures/Surgery

- Mulder sign: A "click" and pain produced by squeezing the metatarsal heads together and simultaneously compressing the neuroma between the thumb and index finger of the other hand
- Corticosteroid injection can significantly reduce symptoms. Inject 1–2 mL lidocaine and 0.5–1 mL dexamethasone just proximal to the metatarsal heads. More than 1 injection is often needed, usually once a week for 3 weeks (2,3).

Pathological Findings

Chronic fibrosis and thickening of the digital nerve

DIFFERENTIAL DIAGNOSIS

- Stress fracture
- Hammer toe
- Metatarsophalangeal synovitis
- Metatarsalgia
- Arthritis
- Bursitis
- Foreign body

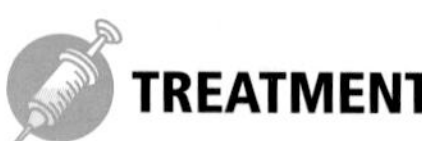

TREATMENT

MEDICATION

First Line

Injectable steroids (e.g., betamethasone phosphate/acetate or methylprednisolone): Use if general measures fail (2,3)[C]

Second Line

NSAIDs for temporary symptom relief (1,2)[C]

ADDITIONAL TREATMENT

General Measures

- Wear flat shoes with a roomy toe box (4)[A].
- Metatarsal pads placed immediately proximal to the 2 involved metatarsal heads (4)[A]
- Corticosteroid injection into the dorsal part of the foot with medium- or long-acting steroid (e.g., betamethasone, methylprednisolone) mixed with local anesthetic (e.g., lidocaine) (4)[A]
- If patient has pes planus, use an arch support (4)[A].
- Literature suggests wide variability in success rate (50–98%) (4)[A].

Issues for Referral

Continued pain despite conservative treatments and injections

Additional Therapies

Serial alcohol injection therapy into the neuroma to sclerose the nerve has been successful (5)[C].

SURGERY/OTHER PROCEDURES

Surgical removal of the neuroma, release of the transverse metatarsal ligament, or both in refractory cases

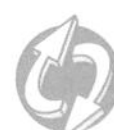

ONGOING CARE

FOLLOW-UP RECOMMENDATIONS

If no improvement after 3 months of conservative treatment, consider corticosteroid injection. Repeat injection if no improvement after 2–4 weeks.

PATIENT EDUCATION

Wearing of properly fitted, comfortable shoes

PROGNOSIS

- 40–50% improve after 3 months of conservative treatment.
- 45–50% improve after steroid injection.
- 96% improve after surgery.

COMPLICATIONS

Hip and knee pain related to gait changes

REFERENCES

1. Sharp RJ, et al. The role of MRI and ultrasound imaging in Morton's neuroma and the effect of size of lesion on symptoms. *Br J Bone Joint Surg*. 2003;85:999–1005.
2. Tallia AF, Cardone DA. Diagnostic and therapeutic injection of the ankle and foot. *Am Fam Physician*. 2003;68:1356–62.
3. Schreiber K, Khodaee M, Poddar S, et al. Clinical Inquiry. What is the best way to treat Morton's neuroma? *J Fam Pract*. 2011;60:157–8, 168.
4. Thomson CE, Gibson JN, Martin D, et al. Interventions for the treatment of Morton's neuroma. *Cochrane Database Syst Rev*. 2004; CD003118.
5. Hughes RJ, Ali K, Jones H, et al. Treatment of Morton's neuroma with alcohol injection under sonographic guidance: Follow-up of 101 cases. *Am J Roentgenol*. 2007;188:1535–9.

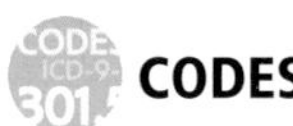

CODES

ICD9

355.6 Lesion of plantar nerve

CLINICAL PEARLS

- Diagnosis of Morton neuroma usually is made clinically.
- Footwear modification, metatarsal pads, and shoe inserts are mainstays of treatment.
- Corticosteroid injection into the neuroma may be helpful.

M

MOTION SICKNESS

Courtney I. Jarvis, PharmD
Allison Hargreaves, MD

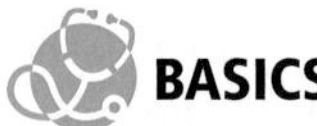

BASICS

DESCRIPTION

- Not a true sickness, but a normal response to a situation in which sensory conflict about body motion exists among visual receptors, vestibular receptors, and body proprioceptors
- Also can be induced when patterns of motion differ from those previously experienced
- System(s) affected: Nervous
- Synonym(s): Car sickness; Sea sickness; Air sickness; Space sickness; Physiologic vertigo

EPIDEMIOLOGY

Incidence

Predominant sex: Female > Male

RISK FACTORS

- Motion (auto, plane, boat, amusement rides)
- Travel
- Visual stimuli (e.g., moving horizon)
- Poor ventilation (fumes, smoke, carbon monoxide)
- Emotions (fear, anxiety)
- Zero gravity
- Pregnancy, menstruation, oral contraceptive use
- History of migraine headaches
- Other illness or poor health

GENERAL PREVENTION

See "General Measures."

Pediatric Considerations

- Rare in children <2 years of age
- Incidence peaks between the ages of 3 and 12 years.
- Antihistamines may cause excitation in children.

Geriatric Considerations

- Age confers some resistance to motion sickness.
- Elderly at increased risk of anticholinergic side effects from treatment

Pregnancy Considerations

- Pregnant patients more likely to experience motion sickness
- Treat with medications thought to be safe during morning sickness (e.g., meclizine, dimenhydrinate).

ETIOLOGY

- Precise etiology unknown; thought to be due to a mismatch of vestibular and visual sensations
- Nausea and vomiting occur as a result of increased levels of dopamine and acetylcholine, which stimulate chemoreceptor trigger zone and vomiting center in CNS.

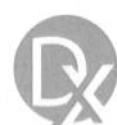

DIAGNOSIS

HISTORY

Presence of the following signs and symptoms in the context of a typical stimulus:

- Nausea
- Vomiting
- Diaphoresis
- Pallor
- Hypersalivation
- Yawning
- Hyperventilation
- Anxiety
- Panic
- Malaise
- Fatigue
- Weakness
- Confusion
- Dizziness

DIFFERENTIAL DIAGNOSIS

- Mountain sickness
- Vestibular disease
- Gastroenteritis
- Metabolic disorders
- Toxin exposure

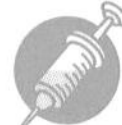

TREATMENT

- Follow guidelines under "General Measures" section to prevent motion sickness (1)[C].
- Premedicate before travel with antidopaminergic, anticholinergic, or antihistamine agents (1)[A]:
  - For extended travel, consider treatment with scopolamine transdermal patch (2)[A].
  - Second-generation (nonsedating) antihistamines are not effective at preventing motion sickness (3)[B].
  - Serotonin (5-HT3) antagonists (e.g., ondansetron) do not appear effective in preventing motion sickness (4)[B].
- Conflicting data exist on the efficacy of acupressure for nausea and vomiting associated with motion sickness (5)[B].
- Benzodiazepines suppress vestibular nuclei but would not be considered first line due to sedation and addiction potential (6)[C].

MEDICATION

First Line

- Scopolamine transdermal patch: Apply 2.5 cm^2 (4-mg) patch behind ear at least 4 hours (preferably 6–12 hours) before travel, and replace every 3 days (2)[A]:
  - Scopolamine may also be given in tablets, capsules, or oral solution; all are more effective than placebo (2)[A].
- Dimenhydrinate (Dramamine): Take 30–60 minutes before travel:
  - Adults and adolescents: 50–100 mg q4–6h, maximum 400 mg/d
  - Children 6–12 years of age: 25–50 mg q6–8h, maximum 150 mg/d
  - Children 2–6 years of age: 12.5–25 mg q6–8h, maximum 75 mg/d
- Meclizine (Antivert): Take 30–60 minutes before travel. Adults and adolescents >12 years of age: 12.5–25 mg q12–24h

- Cyclizine (Marezine): Take 30–60 minutes before travel:
  – Adults and adolescents: 50 mg q4–6h, maximum 200 mg/d
  – Children 6–12 years of age: 25 mg up to t.i.d.
- Promethazine (Phenergan): Take 30–60 minutes before travel:
  – Adults and adolescents: 25 mg q12h; 25–50 mg IM if already developed severe motion sickness
  – Children 2–12 years of age: 0.5 mg/kg q12h, maximum 25 mg b.i.d. *Caution:* Increased risk of dystonic reaction in this age group
- Contraindications: Patients at risk for acute-angle closure glaucoma
- Precautions:
  – Young children
  – Elderly
  – Pregnancy
  – Urinary obstruction
  – Pyloric-duodenal obstruction
- Adverse reactions:
  – Drowsiness
  – Dry mouth
  – Blurred vision
  – Confusion
  – Headache
  – Urinary retention
- Significant possible interactions:
  – Sedatives (antihistamines, alcohol, antidepressants)
  – Anticholinergics (belladonna alkaloids)

Second Line

- Benzodiazepines: Take 1–2 hours before travel:
  – Diazepam 2–10 mg PO q6–12h
  – Lorazepam1–2 mg PO q8h
- Contraindications:
  – Severe respiratory dysfunction
  – Severe liver dysfunction
- Precautions:
  – Alcohol/drug abuse
  – Elderly
  – Sedation
  – Addiction is possible.

ADDITIONAL TREATMENT

General Measures

- Minimize exposure (sit in middle of plane or boat).
- Improve ventilation; avoid noxious stimuli.
- Semirecumbent seating
- Fix vision on horizon, avoid fixation on moving objects, keep eyes fixed on still, distant objects.
- Avoid reading while actively traveling.
- Minimize food intake before travel; avoid alcohol.
- Increase airflow around face.
- Acupressure on point PC6 has been shown to reduce feelings of nausea but not the incidence of vomiting during pregnancy, after surgery, and in cancer chemotherapy. However, conflicting evidence of efficacy has been found for motion sickness. Point PC6 (Neiguan on pericardium meridian): 2 cm proximal of transverse crease of palmar side of wrist between tendons of the palmaris longus and the flexor carpi radialis.

COMPLEMENTARY AND ALTERNATIVE MEDICINE

Ginger: 940 mg or 1 g; take 4 hours before travel (evidence controversial)

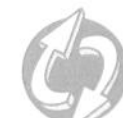

ONGOING CARE

FOLLOW-UP RECOMMENDATIONS

- Semirecumbent seating
- Avoid reading while actively traveling.

DIET

- Decrease oral intake or take frequent small feedings.
- Avoid alcohol.

PROGNOSIS

- Symptoms should resolve when motion exposure ends.
- Resistance to motion sickness seems to increase with age.

COMPLICATIONS

- Hypotension
- Dehydration
- Depression
- Panic
- Syncope

REFERENCES

1. Committee to advise on tropical medicine and travel. Statement on motion sickness. *CCDR*. 2003; 29:1–12.
2. Spinks A, Wasiak J, Bernath V. Scopolamine (hyoscine) for preventing and treating motion sickness. *Cochrane Database Syst Rev*. 2011;6: CD002851.
3. Cheung BS, Heskin R, Hofer KD. Failure of cetirizine and fexofenadine to prevent motion sickness. *Ann Pharmacother*. 2003;37:173–7.
4. Hershkovitz D, Asna N, Shupak A, et al. Ondansetron for the prevention of seasickness in susceptible sailors: An evaluation at sea. *Aviat Space Environ Med*. 2009;80:643–6.
5. Streitberger K, Ezzo J, Schneider A. Acupuncture for nausea and vomiting: An update of clinical and experimental studies. *Auton Neuro*. 2006;129: 107–17.
6. Zajonc TP, Roland PS. Vertigo and motion sickness. Part II: Pharmacologic treatment. *Ear Nose Throat J*. 2006;85:25–35.

ADDITIONAL READING

Carroll ID, Williams DC. Pre-travel vaccination and medical prophylaxis in the pregnant traveler. *Travel Med Infect Dis*. 2008;6:259–75.

See Also (Topic, Algorithm, Electronic Media Element)

Algorithm: Vertigo

CODES

ICD9

994.6 Motion sickness

CLINICAL PEARLS

- The scopolamine patch should be applied at least 4 hours before travel, although it may be more effective if placed 6–12 hours before departure.
- Oral medications should be administered 30–60 minutes before departure.
- Although acupressure wristbands have been found to be effective by systematic reviews in postoperative and chemotherapy-induced nausea and vomiting, conflicting data exist for motion sickness.

M

MRSA SKIN INFECTIONS

Stephen A. Martin, MD, EdM
Paul Belliveau, PharmD, RPh

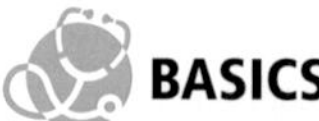

BASICS

DESCRIPTION

- Community-acquired methicillin-resistant *Staphylococcus aureus* (CA-MRSA) has properties that allow it to create skin and soft tissue infections (SSTIs) in otherwise healthy hosts:
  - CA-MRSA has a different virulence and disease pattern than hospital-acquired MRSA (HA-MRSA).
- MRSA infections acquired by persons who have not been recently (<1 year) hospitalized or had a medical procedure (e.g., dialysis, surgery, catheters) are known as CA-MRSA infections:
  - This definition is evolving, given the increasing intersection of HA- and CA-MRSA.
- *The prevalence of CA-MRSA is rapidly increasing in the US.*
- CA-MRSA typically causes mild-to-moderate SSTIs, particularly abscesses, furuncles, and carbuncles:
  - Severe disease from CA-MRSA is less frequent, but can include:
    - Necrotizing pneumonia with abscesses
    - Necrotizing fasciitis
    - Septic thrombophlebitis
    - Sepsis
  - In 1 review, 77% of CA-MRSA infections were SSTIs; only 6% of infections were invasive (e.g., bacteremia, osteomyelitis).
- Although less frequent, HA-MRSA can still cause SSTIs in the community, and clinicians should be alert to this possibility. 1 study showed no significant difference in hospitalization rates among CA-MRSA, HA-MRSA, and methicillin-sensitive *Staphylococcus aureus* (MSSA).
- System(s) affected: Skin; Soft tissue

EPIDEMIOLOGY

- Predominant age: All ages, generally younger
- Predominant sex: Female > Male

Incidence

- 316/100,000/year (2004–2005)
- 25/100,000/year pediatric MRSA SSTI hospitalizations (2006)

Prevalence

- Still significantly affected by local epidemiology
- 25–30% of US population is colonized with *S. aureus*; up to 7% is colonized with MRSA.
- CA-MRSA was isolated in 59% of skin and soft tissue infections presenting to 11 emergency departments (range 15–74%). In 1993, 1.5 million SSTIs were seen in US emergency rooms (ERs). In 2005, this had increased to 3.4 million. Hospital admission data indicate a 29% increase in SSTIs from 2000–2004.
- CA-MRSA accounts for up to 75% of all community staphylococcal infections in children.

RISK FACTORS

- Although several factors are associated with CA-MRSA, their presence or absence cannot reliably predict CA-MRSA itself; in 1 study, almost 1/2 the patients with CA-MRSA had no established risk factor. Physician suspicion for MRSA has been found to be a poor predictor.
- Any antibiotic use in past month
- Presence of an abscess
- Reported "spider bite"
- History of MRSA infection
- Close contact with a similar infection
- Children, particularly in daycare centers
- Competitive athletes
- Incarceration
- High prevalence in the community
- Hospitalization in the past 12 months (although *S. aureus* can colonize for years)

GENERAL PREVENTION

- Prior research has established colonization (particularly of the anterior nares) as a risk factor for subsequent *S. aureus* infection. It is not yet clear whether this is also the case for CA-MRSA. Recent work has indicated that rectal colonization may be more significant.
- CA-MRSA may be transmitted much more through the environment, including households, than via nares colonization.
- Health care workers have been found to be a major vector of MRSA for hospitalized patients, reinforcing the need for aggressive cleaning of hands and common equipment.
- Research for a vaccine is underway.

ETIOLOGY

- First noted in 1980, CA-MRSA's current US epidemic began in 1999. The USA 300 clone is predominant.
- CA-MRSA is currently distinguished from HA-MRSA by:
  - Lack of a multidrug-resistant phenotype
  - Presence of exotoxin virulence factors
  - Type IV staphylococcus cassette cartridge (contains the methicillin-resistance gene *mecA*)

COMMONLY ASSOCIATED CONDITIONS

Many patients are otherwise healthy.

DIAGNOSIS

HISTORY

- Potential risk factors
- Complaint of "spider bite"
- Prior MRSA skin infection
- Risk factors alone cannot rule in or rule out a CA-MRSA infection (1)[B].

PHYSICAL EXAM

- Exam consistent with a furuncle/carbuncle (boils) or abscess, sometimes with a surrounding cellulitis. A nonsuppurative cellulitis is also possible, although it is a less common presentation of CA-MRSA.
- Erythema
- Increased warmth
- Tenderness
- Swelling
- Fluctuance
- Infected wound
- Folliculitis, pustular lesions
- Appearance like an insect or spider bite
- Tissue necrosis

DIAGNOSTIC TESTS & INTERPRETATION

Lab

Initial lab tests

- Wound cultures are essential for diagnosis.
- Susceptibility testing; many labs use oxacillin instead of methicillin.
- A "D-zone disk-diffusion test" evaluates for inducible clindamycin resistance in CA-MRSA resistant to erythromycin (2)[C].

Imaging

Initial approach

- In unclear cases, ultrasound may help delineate an abscess.
- Although CT or MRI may show fascial plane edema in necrotizing fasciitis, it should not delay intervention.

Diagnostic Procedures/Surgery

Purulent lesions should be incised and drained (I&D), cultured, and tested for susceptibilities.

DIFFERENTIAL DIAGNOSIS

Skin and soft tissue infections due to another cause

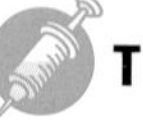

TREATMENT

- Evidence for the treatment of CA-MRSA SSTIs, including oral antibiotics, are generally based on results of small case series, anecdotal reports, and anticipated susceptibility profiles. Randomized controlled trials are beginning to accumulate and generally show no additional benefit to antibiotic treatment over I&D alone.
- A recent guideline recommends antibiotics with certain conditions, such as: Severe, systemic infection; immunosuppression; extremes of age; location difficult to drain; drainage failure (3)[C]
- Systematic review does not recommend agents to eliminate MRSA colonization for patients with infection or their close contacts (4)[C].
- Most CA-MRSA infections are localized SSTIs and do not require hospitalization or vancomycin therapy (4)[C].
- Initial empirical antibiotic coverage should be based on local CA-MRSA prevalence and individual patient risk factors. In 1 pediatric model, cephalexin was the optimal antibiotic for an SSTI only when CA-MRSA prevalence was <10%.

MEDICATION

ALERT

- For purulent infections, basic principles include surgical drainage and debulking, wound culture, and narrow-spectrum antimicrobials:
  - *Successful I&D may have more of an effect than antibiotics in mild cases for both adults and children*, and is important in general.
  - Moist heat may work for small furuncles.
  - Patients with an abscess are frequently cured by drainage alone.
- CA-MRSA is resistant to β-lactams (including oral cephalosporins and antistaphylococcal penicillins) and often macrolides, azalides, and quinolones.
- Although most CA-MRSA isolates are susceptible to rifampin, this drug should *never* be used as a single agent because of concerns for rapid emergence of resistance. The role of combination therapy with rifampin in CA-MRSA SSTIs is still not clearly defined.
- There has been increasing resistance to clindamycin, both initial (~33%) and induced.

- Although CA-MRSA isolates are susceptible to vancomycin, oral vancomycin cannot be used for CA-MRSA SSTIs due to limited GI absorption.

First Line

CA-MRSA SSTIs: Treat with a 7–14-day course of one of the following agents (duration of therapy depends on severity and clinical response):

- Trimethoprim/sulfamethoxazole: DS (160 mg TMP and 800 mg of SMX) 1–2 tablet(s) PO b.i.d. daily (8–12 mg/kg/d of trimethoprim component in 2 divided doses for children)
- Doxycycline or minocycline: 100 mg PO b.i.d. (children >8 years and <45 kg; 2–5 mg/kg/d PO in 1–2 divided doses, not to exceed 200 mg/d; children >8 years and >45 kg: Use adult dosing), taken with a full glass of water
- Clindamycin: 300–600 mg PO t.i.d. (10–20 mg/kg/d PO in 3 divided doses for children), taken with full glass of water. Check D-zone test in erythromycin-resistant, clindamycin-susceptible *S. aureus* isolates (test is positive with induced resistance).

Second Line

The above medication options are not sufficient for treatment of severe CA-MRSA SSTIs requiring hospitalization or for HA-MRSA SSTIs. For such infections, consider one of the following (3)[A]:

- Vancomycin: Generally 1 g IV q12h (30 mg/kg/d IV in 2 divided doses; in children: 40 mg/kg/d IV in 4 divided doses)
- Linezolid: 600 mg IV/PO b.i.d. (Uncomplicated: Children <5 years of age, 30 mg/kg/d in 3 divided doses; 20 mg/kg/d IV/PO in 2 divided doses for children 5–11 years of age; children >11 years, use adult dosing. Complicated: Birth–11 years, 30 mg/kg/d IV/PO in 3 divided doses; older, use adult dosing).
- Clindamycin: 600 mg IV t.i.d.; in children, 10–13 mg/kg/dose q6–8h up to 40 mg/kg/d
- Daptomycin: 4 mg/kg/d IV (safety/efficacy not established in patients <18 years of age) if no pulmonary involvement
- Tigecycline: 100 mg IV once, then 50 mg IV q12h (for adults). An increase in all-cause mortality was observed in early studies involving tigecycline-treated patients.
- Telavancin: 10 mg/kg/d IV once a day (for adults)

Pediatric Considerations

- Tetracyclines not recommended <8 years
- TMP-SMX not recommended <2 months

Pregnancy Considerations

- Tetracyclines are contraindicated.
- TMP-SMX not recommended in third trimester

Geriatric Considerations

A recent review notes no prospective trials in this age and recommends use of general adult guidelines.

ADDITIONAL TREATMENT

General Measures

- Modify therapy as necessary based on culture and susceptibility testing.
- Determine if household or other close contacts have SSTI or other infections, and facilitate evaluation.
- Treat underlying condition (e.g., tinea pedis).
- Restrict contact if wound cannot be covered.
- Elevate affected area.

Issues for Referral

In addition to inpatient concerns, consider consultation with an infectious disease specialist in cases of:

- Refractory CA-MRSA infection
- Plan to attempt decolonization

SURGERY/OTHER PROCEDURES

Progression to serious SSTIs, including necrotizing fasciitis, is possible and mandates prompt surgical evaluation.

IN-PATIENT CONSIDERATIONS

Initial Stabilization

Depends on severity of SSTI, presence of SSTI complications (sepsis, necrotizing fasciitis), and comorbidities

Admission Criteria

Consider admission in patients either:

- Systemically ill (e.g., febrile) with stable comorbidities, or
- Systemically well with comorbidities that may delay or complicate resolution of their SSTI

Nursing

Contact precautions

Discharge Criteria

If admitted for IV therapy:

- Afebrile for 24 hours
- Clinically improved
- Able to take oral medication
- Has adequate social support and available for outpatient follow-up

ONGOING CARE

FOLLOW-UP RECOMMENDATIONS

Patient Monitoring

For outpatients:

- Return promptly if patient develops systemic symptoms, worsening local symptoms, or does not improve within 48 hours.
- Consider a follow-up within 48 hours of initial visit to assess response and review culture.

PATIENT EDUCATION

- Keep wounds that are draining covered with clean, dry bandages.
- Clean hands regularly with soap and water or alcohol-based gel. Hot shower daily with soap.
- Do not share items that may be contaminated (including razors or towels).
- Clean clothes, towels, and bed linens.

PROGNOSIS

- In outpatients, improvement should occur within 48 hours.
- Data are limited as to risk of recurrence.

COMPLICATIONS

- Necrotizing pneumonia or empyema (after an influenzalike illness)
- Necrotizing fasciitis
- Sepsis syndrome
- Pyomyositis and osteomyelitis
- Purpura fulminans
- Disseminated septic emboli
- Endocarditis

REFERENCES

1. Daum RS. Clinical practice. Skin and soft-tissue infections caused by methicillin-resistant *Staphylococcus aureus*. *N Engl J Med*. 2007;357:380–90.
2. Moellering RC. A 39-year-old man with a skin infection. *JAMA*. 2008;299:79–87.
3. Liu C, Bayer A, Cosgrove SE, et al. Clinical practice guidelines by the infectious diseases society of america for the treatment of methicillin-resistant *Staphylococcus aureus* infections in adults and children. *Clin Infect Dis*. 2011;52:e18–55.
4. Stryjewski ME, Chambers HF. Skin and soft-tissue infections caused by community-acquired methicillin-resistant *Staphylococcus aureus*. *Clin Infect Dis*. 2008;46(Suppl 5):S368–77.
5. Chuck EA, Frazee BW, Lambert L, et al. The benefit of empiric treatment for methicillin-resistant *Staphylococcus aureus*. *J Emerg Med*. 2010;38:567–71.

ADDITIONAL READING

- Breen JO, et al. Skin and soft tissue infections in immunocompetent patients. *Am Fam Physician*. 2010;81:893–9.
- The CDC has gathered information for health care professionals, including clinical guides, via the National MRSA Education Initiative (accessed 7/30/2011) at www.cdc.gov/mrsa/. These include a treatment appraoch: www.cdc.gov/mrsa/treatment/outpatient-management.html.
- David MZ, Daum RS, et al. Community-associated methicillin-resistant *Staphylococcus aureus*: Epidemiology and clinical consequences of an emerging epidemic. *Clin Microbiol Rev*. 2010;23:616–87.
- Dryden MS, et al. Complicated skin and soft tissue infection. *J Antimicrob Chemother*. 2010;65(Suppl 3):iii35–44.

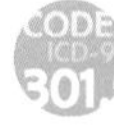

CODES

ICD9

- 041.12 Methicillin resistant Staphylococcus aureus in conditions classified elsewhere and of unspecified site
- V02.54 Carrier or suspected carrier of Methicillin resistant Staphylococcus aureus
- V09.0 Infection with microorganisms resistant to penicillins

CLINICAL PEARLS

- Incise and drain purulent lesions and send for wound culture.
- Know the prevalence and susceptibilities of CA-MRSA in your location. Consider use of an algorithm to help guide clinical decisions (5)[B].
- Use 1/4 cup household bleach diluted in 1 gallon of water to clean surfaces; no evidence that widespread cleaning (with sprays/foggers) works any better than focused cleaning of frequently touched areas.

MULTIPLE MYELOMA

Deepa Jagadeesh, MD, MPH
William V. Walsh, MD

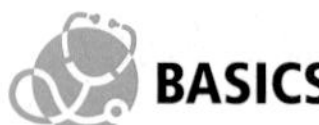

BASICS

DESCRIPTION

- Multiple myeloma (MM) is a clonal proliferation of malignant plasma cells.
- It accounts for 10–13% of all hematological malignancy and 1% of all cancers.
- MM characterized by monoclonal protein in the blood and urine and evidence of end organ damage ("CRAB": Hypercalcemia, renal insufficiency, anemia, and bone lesions)
- Monoclonal gammopathy of undetermined significance (MGUS) is a common disorder with limited monoclonal plasma cell proliferation that progresses to MM; risk of progression is about 1%/yr.
- MGUS progresses to smouldering or asymptomatic MM and eventually to symptomatic MM.
- Synonym(s): Plasma cell myeloma; Plasma cell leukemia

EPIDEMIOLOGY

- Median age of diagnosis is 70 years old, 37% diagnosed at age ≥75 years (1)
- Male > Female (slightly) blacks are almost twice more commonly affected than whites

Incidence

5.56 new cases/100,000 annually (2)

Prevalence

In 2007, there were 61,642 cases in the US (2).

RISK FACTORS

- Most cases have no known risks associated.
- Known risk factors include age, sex, and race.
- Chemicals like dioxin, herbicides, insecticides, petroleum, heavy metals, plastics, and ionizing radiation increase the risk of MM.
- MGUS: Median time to progression to MM is 4.8 years; probability of progression increases with time.

Genetics

Rare family clusters

GENERAL PREVENTION

None known

PATHOPHYSIOLOGY

- Clonal proliferation of plasma cells derived from postgerminal center B cells (3)
- Plasma cells undergo multiple chromosomal mutations to progress to MM.
- Genetic damage in developing B-lymphocytes at time of isotype switching, transforming normal plasma cells into malignant cells, arising from single clone
- Earliest chromosomal translocations involve immunoglobulin heavy chains on chromosome 14q32 and partner genes c-MAF (16q23), FGFR3/MMSET (4p16.3), cyclin D1 (11q13), and cyclin D3 (6p21).
- Activation of K-RAS, and N-RAS, mutations in TP53, and changes in c-myc are associated with disease progression (1).
- Malignant cells multiply in bone marrow, suppressing normal bone marrow cells and producing large quantities of monoclonal immunoglobulin (M) protein.
- Malignant cells stimulate osteoclasts that cause bone resorption and inhibit osteoblasts that form new bone, causing lytic bone lesions.

ETIOLOGY

Unknown

COMMONLY ASSOCIATED CONDITIONS

Secondary amyloidosis commonly due to MM

DIAGNOSIS

HISTORY

- 34% of patients are asymptomatic at the time of presentation.
- Hypercalcemia (28%): Anorexia, nausea, somnolence, and polydipsia
- Renal failure (20–50%)
- Anemia (73%)
- Bony lesions (80%): Lytic lesions causing bone pain (58%) (1), osteoporosis or pathologic fracture (26–34%)
- Other symptoms: Fatigue, peripheral neuropathy, weight loss, recurrent infections, hyperviscosity syndrome, and cord compression

PHYSICAL EXAM

- Dehydration
- Skin findings of amyloidosis: Waxy papules, nodules, or plaques that may be evident in the eyelids, retroauricular region, neck, or inguinal and anogenital regions; petechiae and ecchymosis; "pinch purpura"
- Hyperviscosity syndrome in 7%: Retinal hemorrhages, prolonged bleeding, neurologic changes
- Tender bones and masses

DIAGNOSTIC TESTS & INTERPRETATION

Lab

Criteria for diagnosis: The diagnosis of MM requires all of the following:

- Bone marrow (BM) involvement with ≥10% of plasma cells (PC) or the presence of a plasmacytoma
- Monoclonal protein (M-spike) in the blood and urine
- Presence of "CRAB" (hypercalcemia, renal insufficiency, anemia, and bone lesions)

Initial lab tests

- CBC with differential to evaluate anemia, other cytopenias
- BUN, creatinine
- Serum electrolytes, serum albumin, serum calcium
- Serum lactate dehydrogenase (LDH), β_2-microglobulin
- Serum protein electrophoresis (SPEP), serum immunofixation electrophoresis (SIFE): M protein level elevated; 2% localized band on serum protein electrophoresis, 93% monoclonal protein on immunoelectrophoresis
- Quantitative serum immunoglobulin levels: IgG, IgA, and IgM
- Quantitative serum free light chain (FLC) levels: Kappa and lambda chains
- Elevated ESR
- Urine analysis: 24-hour urine for protein, urine protein electrophoresis (UPEP), urine immunofixation electrophoresis (UIFE); 20% positive urine protein (3)
- Bone marrow aspirate and biopsy for histology, immunohistochemistry, flow cytometry, cytogenetics, and fluorescence in situ hybridization (FISH)

Follow-Up & Special Considerations

- Bone marrow aspirate and biopsy to monitor response to treatment
- SPEP with SIFE: M protein helps to track progression of myeloma and response to treatment.
- Serum immunoglobulins and free light chains can be used to monitor response or relapse.
- Plasma cell labeling index may be helpful to identify the fraction of the myeloma cell population that is proliferating (3).

Imaging

Initial approach

- Skeletal survey: For lytic bone lesions, osteopenia, osteoporosis, or compression fractures
- MRI for any back pain or earliest signs/symptoms of spinal cord compression

Follow-Up & Special Considerations

- CT scan: If high suspicion for bone lesions despite normal skeletal survey; can differentiate malignant from benign vertebral compression fractures in patients who are not MRI candidates
- Positron-emission tomographic (PET) scans: Used if suspected bone issue is suspected despite a normal skeletal survey, MRI, and CT
- Baseline bone densitometry may be indicated (3).

Diagnostic Procedures/Surgery

Staging:

- Durie Salmon stage:
  - Stage I: Hemoglobulin >10 g/L, serum calcium normal (<12 mg/dL), normal bone or solitary plasmacytoma, IgG <5 g/dL, IgA <3 g/dL, urine Bence Jones (BJ) protein <4 gm/24 hr
  - Stage II: Neither stage I nor stage III
  - Stage III: Hemoglobulin <8.5 g/L, serum calcium >12 mg/dL, bone lesions, IgG >7 g/dL, IgA >5 g/dL, urine BJ protein >12 g/24 h
- International staging system (ISS):
  - Stage I: Albumin ≤3.5 g/dL and β_2-microglobulin <3.5 μg/mL
  - Stage II: Neither stage I nor stage III
  - Stage III: β_2-microglobulin ≥5.5 μg/mL
- Mayo clinic risk stratification:
  - Standard risk: t(11:14), t((6:14), and hyperdiploidy
  - High risk: t(4:14), t(14:16), del 17 p, del 13q by cytogenetics, hypodiploidy, and plasma cell labeling index (PCLI) >3%

Pathological Findings

Bone marrow involvement with plasma cells ≥10%; Russell bodies

DIFFERENTIAL DIAGNOSIS

- MGUS: Monoclonal protein <3 g/dL, BM plasma cells <10%, and absence of "CRAB" symptoms:
  - Prevalence 5.3% if >70 years of age
  - Progress to MM 1%/yr
  - Increased risk of progression if IgA or IgM, higher percentage of marrow plasma cells
- Smouldering MM: Monoclonal protein ≥3 g/dL, BM plasma cells ≥10%, and absence of "CRAB" symptoms:
  - Higher risk of progression to MM; 10%/yr in the first 5 years

- Increased risk of progression if higher percentage of marrow PC, greater M-spike, and significantly abnormal FLC ratio
- Metastatic cancer to bone
- Waldenström macroglobulinemia: IgM monoclonal gammopathy with >10% marrow lymphoplasmacytic infiltrate
- Systemic AL amyloidosis: Amyloid-related syndrome with positive amyloid stain plus monoclonal plasma cell disorder
- POEMS syndrome: *P*olyneuropathy, *o*rganomegaly, *e*ndocrinopathy, *m*onoclonal gammopathy, *s*kin changes

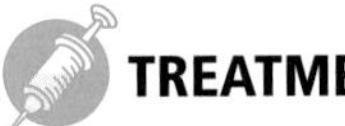

TREATMENT

- Treatment varies depending on how active disease is and the stage of MM.
- Treatment for smoldering MM is close monitoring at 3-month intervals. Clinical trials are ongoing to determine whether newer agents would delay progression.
- Key determinant factor in choosing chemotherapy regimen is to establish if the patient is a transplant candidate or not.
- Autologous stem cell transplant (ASCT) following induction chemotherapy is standard of care for patients with symptomatic disease <65 years of age or those >65 years of age and able to undergo procedure. Although not curative, ASCT has shown to improve complete response rates, progression free survival (PFS), and overall survival (OS) in randomized trial (4).

MEDICATION

- Induction chemotherapy for SCT eligible patients:
  - VTD (Velcade [bortezomib]/thalidomide/dexamethasone); RVD (Revlimid [lenalidomide]/Velcade (bortezomib)/dexamethasone); TD (thalidomide/dexamethasone); Rd (lenalidomide/low-dose dexamethasone); Vd (bortezomib/dexamethasone); CyBorD (cyclophosphamide/bortezomib/dexamethasone)
- ASCT can be used either as consolidation therapy in patients with good response to induction chemo or at the time of relapse.
- Maintenance lenalidomide or thalidomide after ASCT has shown to improve PFS.
- Induction chemotherapy for SCT-ineligible patients:
  - MPT (melphalan/prednisone/thalidomide); VMP (bortezomib/melphalan/prednisone); MPR-R (melphalan/prednisone/lenalidomide and lenalidomide maintenance); Rd or Vd

First Line

- Proteasome inhibitors:
  - Bortezomib (Velcade):
    - Inhibits the ubiquitin-proteasome catalytic pathway in cells by binding to the 20S proteasome complex
    - Toxicity: Peripheral neuropathy, cytopenias, nausea
    - Consider herpes simplex virus (HSV) prophylaxis.
- Cyclophosphamide:
  - Nitrogen mustard–derivative alkylating agent
  - Often used in combination with prednisone or thalidomide in cases of relapsed disease
  - Toxicity: Cytopenias, anaphylaxis, interstitial pulmonary fibrosis, secondary malignancy, impaired fertility
- Immunomodulators:
  - Thalidomide and lenalidomide (Revlimid):
    - Works by antiangiogenesis inhibition, immunomodulation, and inhibition of tumor necrosis factor
    - Toxicity: Birth defects, deep vein thrombosis (DVT), neuropathy, rash, nausea, bradycardia
    - DVT prophylaxis, usually with aspirin
- Dexamethasone:
  - Low doses (40 mg/wk) superior to higher doses
  - Increases risk of DVT
- Bisphosphonates (5)[A]:
  - No effect on mortality but decrease pain, pathological vertebral fractures, and fractures of other bones
  - No bisphosphonate is superior to others.
  - Dose-adjust/monitor renal function.
  - Monitor for osteonecrosis of jaw.

Second Line

- If recurred more than 1 year after treatment then initial chemo can be used again.
- Thal/dex, Rd, or VD can be used to treat relapsed or refractory MM.

ADDITIONAL TREATMENT

- Local radiation therapy for bone pain:
  - Should be limited for patients with disabling pain who have not responded to analgesics and/or chemotherapy
  - Avoid extensive radiation therapy.
- Allogenic stem cell transplant:
  - Theoretical advantages over autologous stem cell transplant include lack of graft contamination with tumor cells and lack of graft vs. MM effect.
  - Its role in treatment of MM is controversial and investigational.

General Measures

Maintain adequate hydration to prevent renal insufficiency.

Issues for Referral

For spinal or other bone pathology refer to orthopedics for support.

Additional Therapies

- Effective pain management:
  - Avoid NSAIDS due to nephrotoxicity.
- Kyphoplasty/vertebroplasty: Consider for symptomatic vertebral compressions.
- Plasmapheresis: For hyperviscosity syndrome (a rare complication)
- Erythropoietin: For selected patients with anemia
- Patients should receive vaccines for pneumococcus and influenza.
- Do not administer zoster vaccine and other live-virus vaccines.

IN-PATIENT CONSIDERATIONS

Initial Stabilization

- Avoid IV radiographic contrast materials due to risk for contrast-induced nephropathy.
- Adequate hydration
- Avoid NSAIDs to decrease chance of renal insufficiency.
- Manage hypercalcemia and control hyperuricemia.

Admission Criteria

Indications: Pain, infections, cytopenias, renal failure, bone complications, spinal cord compression

ONGOING CARE

PATIENT EDUCATION

www.myeloma.org

PROGNOSIS

- Median survival overall is 3 years.
- Median survival by ISS stage:
  - Stage I: 62 months
  - Stage II: 44 months
  - Stage III: 29 months
- Median survival in patients with high-risk multiple myeloma (see "staging" for definition) is <2–3 years, even after autologous stem cell transplant; however, with more modern therapies, survivals of 10 years or more are being seen.

COMPLICATIONS

Many, including infection, pain, lytic bone lesions, hypercalcemia, hyperuricemia, spinal cord compression, anemia, hyperviscosity syndrome, renal insufficiency

REFERENCES

1. Palumbo A, Anderson K. Multiple myeloma. *N Engl J Med* 2011;364:1046–60.
2. National Cancer Institute, SEER cancer statistics review, 1975–2007. http://seer.cancer.gov/csr/1975_2007/results_merged/sect_18_myeloma.pdf.
3. The NCCN Multiple Myeloma Clinical Practice Guidelines in Oncology (Version 2.2008). © 2008 National Comprehensive Cancer Network, Inc. Available at: www.nccn.org. Accessed April 29, 2010.
4. Attal M, Harousseau JL, Stoppa AM, et al. Intergroupe Francais Myelome. A prospective, randomized trial of autologous bone marrow transplantation and chemotherapy in multiple myeloma. *N Engl J Med*. 1996;335:91–7.
5. Mhaskar R, Redzepovic J, Wheatley K, et al. Bisphosphonates in multiple myeloma. *Cochrane Database Syst Rev*. 2010;3:CD003188.

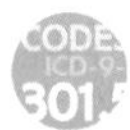

CODES

ICD9

- 203.00 Multiple myeloma, without mention of having achieved remission
- 203.01 Multiple myeloma, in remission
- 203.02 Multiple myeloma, in relapse

CLINICAL PEARLS

- MM is a plasma cell malignancy that causes end-organ damage.
- Suspect MM if high total protein:albumin ratio.
- High index of suspicion for spinal cord compression
- Avoid nephrotoxins (radiographic contrast material, NSAIDs, dehydration).
- Patients with MM are immunocompromised.

MULTIPLE SCLEROSIS

Yolanda Backus, MD
James J. Arnold, DO

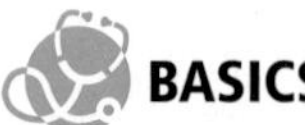

BASICS

DESCRIPTION

- A chronic disease involving inflammation and degeneration leading to demyelinization of the white matter of the brain and spinal cord with axonal damage.
- 4 internationally recognized forms (1):
  - Relapsing/remitting multiple sclerosis (RRMS): (85%) Periods of relapse during which time new symptoms can appear and old ones worsen followed by periods of remission. Can result in residual deficits or full recovery between symptomatic periods.
  - Secondary progressive MS (SPMS): Steady progression of clinical neurologic damage with or without relapses and minor remissions. 50% of patients with RRMS will develop SPMS; patients may have experienced RRMS for 2–40 years or more. Relapses and remissions will decrease over time.
  - Primary progressive MS (PPMS): Gradual progression of the disease from onset with no relapses or remissions.
  - Progressive relapsing MS (PRMS) (least common): Steady, cumulative progression of clinical neurologic damage with superimposed relapses and remissions.
- Clinically isolated syndromes (CIS): Initial clinical manifestation of demyelination; most commonly consisting of optic neuritis, transverse myelitis, and brainstem syndromes (1)

Pregnancy Considerations

- Relapses are less frequent during pregnancy, especially in the third trimester, as well as in the postpartum period.
- Pregnancy does not alter the overall course of MS.
- Relapse rate is unaffected by breast-feeding

EPIDEMIOLOGY

- Predominant age: 20–40 years old. Exception: PRMS is typically diagnosed in patients >40 years old.
- Predominant sex: Female > Male. Males experience a more malignant course than females.

Incidence

3.6 cases per 100,000 person years worldwide (2)

Prevalence

In the US, 400,000 people have MS; 2.5 million cases worldwide

RISK FACTORS

- 0.1% (1 out of 1,000) risk of developing the disease in the general population (3)
- Northern European descent
- Family history of the disease; 1–3% risk of MS among first-degree relatives
- Temperate climate: However, the latitude gradient (the higher the latitude, the higher the incidence) present in older incidences studies of MS is decreasing (2). Ethnic groups along the equator have the lowest incidence of disease (4).

Genetics

- Strong genetic component in determining susceptibility to the disease. HLA-DRB1 has been particularly associated.
- Patients with MS are more likely to have other autoimmune disorders.

GENERAL PREVENTION

No known preventive measures. Avoid factors that may precipitate an exacerbation, such as stressful life events.

PATHOPHYSIOLOGY

- Neurodegeneration within plaques leads to disability; disease is radiologically active during periods of apparent clinical stability.
- Disease occurs in genetically susceptible people with breaches in the blood–brain barrier (BBB); invasion of autoreactive T cells (primarily Th-1) and intrathecal B cells damage the CNS
- Histological findings: Perivascular infiltration of leukocytes, parenchymal edema, loss of myelin and oligodendrocytes, widespread axonal damage, plasma cells, myelin-filled macrophages, hypertrophic astrocytes (5)

ETIOLOGY

Unknown but various theories:

- Autoimmune theory supported by human leukocyte antigen (HLA) linkage, hereditary pattern, immunocytes in plaques, changes in peripheral blood immunocytes
- Low vitamin D levels and limited sun exposure
- Combined theory: Autoimmune disorder triggered in genetically susceptible individuals as an infrequent response to environmental factors

COMMONLY ASSOCIATED CONDITIONS

- Optic neuritis: Unilateral eye pain, worse with movements: Scotoma (loss of mainly central vision); color desaturation; Marcus Gunn pupil (afferent pupillary defect)
- Internuclear ophthalmoplegia (INO): Horizontal nystagmus of abducting eye: Lost/delayed adduction
- Lhermitte phenomenon: Shocklike sensation with head and/or neck movement

DIAGNOSIS

Primarily clinical diagnosis of 2 or more distinct episodes of CNS dysfunction separated by both time (at least 3 months) and space (2 distinct neurologic deficits) with eventual partial resolution of CNS symptoms: Some patients may experience a prodrome. Minimum duration for relapse is 24 hours.

HISTORY

- Fatigue
- Painful loss of vision in 1 eye
- Urinary urgency or retention
- Hyperesthesia/paresthesias, radicular pain
- Clumsiness/incoordination/tremor, vertigo
- Blurred or double vision
- Constipation
- Emotional lability
- Sexual dysfunction
- Seizure

PHYSICAL EXAM

- Ocular paralysis (INO)
- Hemiparesis or monoparesis
- Hyperactive deep tendon reflexes or clonus
- Genital anesthesia
- Loss of position/vibration sense
- Ataxia
- Spasticity: Lower extremity > upper extremity

DIAGNOSTIC TESTS & INTERPRETATION

Lab

- CSF shows oligoclonal bands, abnormal colloidal gold curve, elevated gamma-globulin IgG, mild mononuclear pleocytosis with lymphocytic predominance (<40 cells/mL), myelin debris, and normal or slightly elevated protein.
- Tests to exclude other disorders: Serology for syphilis (serum and CSF), ESR, B_{12}, thyroid-stimulating hormone, antinuclear antibody, Lyme titer

Imaging

MRI of head/spine (more sensitive than CT):

- T2 image: Hyperintense lesions: Enhancement is due to breach in BBB.
- T1 image: Hypointense lesions: Black holes, gray holes: Negative prognostic indicators
- Lesions can disappear with serial imaging due to resolution of edema and remyelination.
- Affected areas (need 1 lesion in 2/4 areas per McDonald criteria (6):
  - Periventricular white matter (pathognomonic finding)
  - Juxtacortical
  - Infratentorial
  - Spinal cord

Diagnostic Procedures/Surgery

Electrophysiological testing: Sensory evoked potential testing (visual, brainstem auditory, and somatosensory): Helpful in identifying neurolesions not evident on MRI

DIFFERENTIAL DIAGNOSIS

- Tumors (brainstem, cerebellar, spinal cord)
- CNS infections
- Syphilis, HIV
- Trigeminal neuralgia
- Epilepsy
- Transverse myelitis
- Ataxias (Friedreich ataxia, hereditary ataxia)
- Amyotrophic lateral sclerosis
- Progressive multifocal leukoencephalopathy
- Syringomyelia, Chiari malformation
- Ruptured intervertebral disc, disc herniation
- Small cerebral infarcts
- Vasculitides (giant cell arteritis)
- Behçet disease
- Systemic lupus erythematosus
- Sarcoidosis
- Pernicious anemia

TREATMENT

Treatment is preventive and disease mitigating, not curative or restorative. Early treatment can slow progression to clinically definite MS during CIS. The frequency of relapses early in the course of MS has predictive value for future disability (1,2)[B].

MEDICATION

- Relapses: Methylprednisolone: 500–1,000 mg/d IV for 3–5 days; no oral taper (1)[A]; Prednisone: 300 mg b.i.d. for 3 days; no oral taper (1)[B]
- Disease modifying therapy: Interferon-β (IFN-β): Betaseron (IFN-β-1b) 250 μg SC every other day, Avonex (IFN-β-1a) [30 μg IM weekly], Rebif (IFN-β-1a) 22 or 44 μg SC 3×/wk (1)[B]:
  - Monitor CBC and liver function tests before starting therapy and every 6 months.
  - Can prophylactically treat with NSAIDs to reduce side effects, including flulike symptoms and injection-site reactions; titrating IFN-β therapy can decrease liver dysfunction
  - Glatiramer acetate (Copaxone): 20 mg/d SC (1)[A]:
    - Improved side-effect profile when compared with interferon-β
    - >50% of patients will have injection-site reaction; alternate injection sites
  - Natalizumab (Tysabri): 300 mg IV every 4 weeks (2)[A]: Second-line therapy due to previous safety concerns in combination therapy; FDA approved as monotherapy in 2006
  - Fingolimod (Gilenya): 0.5 mg PO daily FDA approved in 2010:
    - Side effects: Bradycardia and AV block within first 6 hours of first dose, macular edema, basal cell carcinoma with higher doses
    - Monitor liver function and observe for at least 6 hours after first dose
  - Mitoxantrone (Novantrone): 12 mg/m^2 short IV infusion q3mo (2)[C]:
    - Not indicated in treatment of PPMS
    - Serious cardiotoxicity side effects; regular monitoring of left ventricular ejection fraction is recommended
- Symptomatic therapies: (2)[C],(4):
  - Spasticity: Baclofen, diazepam, gabapentin
  - Pain: NSAIDs, carbamazepine, gabapentin, lamotrigine, topiramate, tricyclic antidepressants
  - Bladder dysfunction: [Urgency] oxybutynin, tolterodine tartrate; [retention] intermittent self-catheterization
  - Constipation: High-fiber diet, stool softeners, bulk-producing agents, laxatives, suppositories
  - Sexual dysfunction: Alprostadil, sildenafil, vardenafil
  - Fatigue: Amantadine, modafinil, stimulants (pemoline, methylphenidate, 4-aminopyridine)
  - Tremors: Clonazepam, β-blockers, primidone
  - Depression: SSRIs, cognitive-behavioral therapy
  - Paranoia/mania: Haloperidol, lithium, atypical antipsychotics

ADDITIONAL TREATMENT

Shepherd MS relapse protocol (1,2)[C]:

- Rule out possible precipitating events (heat exposure, overexertion, UTI, upper respiratory infection).
- If any infection is suspected, screen and treat accordingly. Hold steroids.
- If there are no clear-cut precipitating events, determine the severity of the symptoms and any impact on activities of daily living.
- If the symptoms are not significantly affecting activities of daily living, observe.
- If activities of daily living are affected, consider steroid therapy. Review medical history for any relative contraindications (diabetes mellitus type 2, hypertension, pregnancy, poorly controlled psychiatric disease, past history of poor tolerance for steroids).
- If there are no contraindications, proceed with steroids: IVMP 1 g/d for 3 days. No oral taper. Oral prednisone 300 mg b.i.d. for 3 days. No oral taper. (May consider taper in patients who report general malaise after 3 days of IV or oral steroids.)
- Consider lorazepam 1 mg PO q8h for patients with a history of anxiety while on steroids or 1 mg PO at bedtime for insomnia.
- Practice varies on whether to prescribe antacids or H2 blockers during steroids; generally not recommended.
- For patients intolerant to steroids or pregnant women, consider IVIG 0.4 g/kg/d for 5 days; some patients do seem to respond to IVIG for relapses.
- For patients with tightly controlled diabetes mellitus, steroids can be used with caution by using sliding-scale insulin. May consider IVIG as above for these patients as well.

General Measures

Rehabilitation including physical and occupational therapy. Psychotherapy and support. Yoga, Pilates, and water therapies can all be helpful. Sunlight can increase levels of vitamin D, which may improve relapse frequency and duration (7).

ONGOING CARE

FOLLOW-UP RECOMMENDATIONS

Treat relapses with corticosteroids to minimize disease progression and duration of relapse. Maintain regular activity but avoid overwork and fatigue. Rest during periods of acute relapse.

Patient Monitoring

Progression of disease is measured by the Kurtzke disability status scale (KDSS). 1 is the least disabling and 10 is death. Kurtzke disability status scale:

- No disability and minimal neurologic signs
- Minimal disability (e.g., slight weakness or stiffness, mild gait or visual disturbance)
- Moderate disability (e.g., monoparesis, mild hemiparesis, moderate ataxia, disturbing sensory loss, prominent urinary or eye symptom, or combination of lesser dysfunction)
- Relatively severe disability but fully ambulatory without aid, self-sufficient and able to be up around 12 hr/d, does not prevent the ability to work or carry on normal living activities, excluding sexual dysfunction
- Disability is severe enough to preclude working, maximal motor function involves walking unaided up to 500 m
- Needs assistance with walking (e.g., cane, crutches, or braces)
- Restricted to a wheelchair but able to wheel oneself and enter and leave chair without assistance
- Restricted to bed or chair, retains many self-care functions and has effective use of arms
- Helpless and bedridden
- Death due to MS (from respiratory paralysis, coma, following repeated or prolonged epileptic seizures)

DIET

High fluid intake and a high-fiber diet to prevent or treat constipation (2)[C]. Vitamin D: 50,000 IU/wk; ergocalciferol for 8 weeks; recheck vitamin D levels (goal of >40 ng/mL): Maintenance with vitamin D_3 at 1,000–2,000 IU/d once deficiency/insufficience has been corrected (1,7)[B]

PATIENT EDUCATION

- National Multiple Sclerosis Society, 205E 42nd St., New York, NY 10017; (800) 624-8236. At: www.nationalmssociety.org/index.aspx
- National Institute of Neurological Disorders and Stroke: www.ninds.nih.gov/disorders/multiple_sclerosis/multiple_sclerosis.htm

PROGNOSIS

- ~70% of patients lead active, productive lives with prolonged remissions. 30% relapse in 1 year, 20% in 5–9 years, and 10% in 10–30 years
- 50% of patients are using a cane (KDSS 6), 15% are wheelchair dependent (KDSS 7) within 10 years
- Variable course; can cause early death or disability if disease is rapidly progressive or relapses frequent
- Life expectancy of patients with MS is nearly the same as that of the unaffected population

COMPLICATIONS

Emotional lability, chronic pain (55–65%), nystagmus or optic nerve atrophy, sexual dysfunction, infections such as UTIs, paraplegia, delirium or coma

REFERENCES

1. Thrower BW, et al. Relapse management in multiple sclerosis. *Neurologist*. 2009;15:1–5.
2. Alonso A, Hernan MA. Temporal trends in the incidence of multiple sclerosis-a systematic review. *Neurology*. 2008;71:1329–135.
3. Courtney AM, Treadaway K, Remington G, et al. Multiple sclerosis. *Med Clin North Am*. 2009;93.
4. Rejdak K, Jackson S, Giovannoni G, et al. Multiple sclerosis: A practical overview for clinicians. *Br Med Bull*. 2010;95:79–104.
5. Frohman EM, Racke MK, Raine CS. Multiple sclerosis–The plaque and its pathogenesis. *NEJM*. 2006;354:942–55.
6. Polman CH, et al. Diagnostic criteria for multiple sclerosis: 2010 revisions to the McDonald criteria. *Ann Neurol*. 2011;69:292–302.
7. Solomon AJ, Whitham RH, et al. Multiple sclerosis and vitamin D: A review and recommendations. *Curr Neurol Neurosci Rep*. 2010;10(5):389–96.

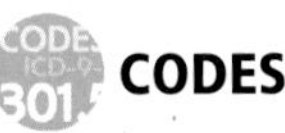

CODES

ICD9

340 Multiple sclerosis

CLINICAL PEARLS

- MS is an inflammatory and neurodegenerative disorder affecting the CNS.
- Treat relapses with steroids; ongoing disease modification is the mainstay of therapy, as there is no cure.
- MS is a clinical diagnosis and can only be appropriately diagnosed over time.

MUMPS

Frances Y. Wu, MD

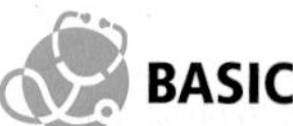

BASICS

Acute, generalized paramyxovirus infection usually presenting with unilateral or bilateral parotitis

DESCRIPTION

- Painful parotitis occurs in 95% of *symptomatic* mumps, but 1/3 of mumps cases may be asymptomatic.
- Epidemics in late winter and spring with transmission by respiratory secretions
- Incubation ~14–24 days
- System(s) affected: Hematologic/Lymphatic/Immunologic; Reproductive; Skin/Exocrine
- Synonym(s): Epidemic parotitis; Infectious parotitis

EPIDEMIOLOGY

- Predominant age: 85% occur before age 15:
  - Adult cases typically more severe
- Predominant sex: Male = Female
- Geriatric population: Most are immune.
- Acute epidemic mumps:
  - Most cases occur in children aged 5–15 years.
  - Recent (2006) US epidemic in vaccinated college students aged 18–24 years with 5,700 US cases:
    - Another US epidemic 2009–2010 in NY/NJ, over 1,500 cases (1)
  - Unusual in children <2 years of age
  - Most infants <1 year are immune.
  - Urban epidemics among nonvaccinated populations
  - Communicable period 24 hours before to 72 hours after parotitis onset
  - Incubation period 18 days

Incidence

- 0.09/100,000 persons in the US
- Occasional epidemic outbreaks in a given region

Prevalence

- 0.0064/100,000 persons
- 90% of adults are seropositive even without history.

RISK FACTORS

- Foreign travel/exposure: 43% of other nations do not vaccinate for mumps.
- Crowded environments such as dormitories
- Waning immunity after single-dose vaccination; even after 2 doses immunity drops from 95–86% in 9 years (2)[C].

GENERAL PREVENTION

- Vaccination:
  - 2 doses of live mumps vaccine or measles-mumps-rubella (MMR) vaccine recommended, first at 12–15 months and second at 4–6 years of age
  - 95% effective in studies, but field trials show 75–95% efficacy, which may be below level needed for herd immunity to prevent epidemic spread (3)[C]. Successful prevention (Finland) may require 95% first-dose plus >80% second-dose compliance (4).
  - Adverse effects: Most common proven effect is ITP, with incidence of 3.3/100,000 doses.
  - No relationship between MMR vaccine and autism
- Immunoglobulin not effective in prevention
- Postexposure vaccination does not protect from recent exposure.
- Isolate hospitalized patients until 5 days past onset (5)[C]; exclude nonimmune individuals for 26 days after last case onset.

Pregnancy Considerations

- There are no proven complications of vaccine, but theoretically should not vaccinate in pregnancy.
- Immunization of family may protect against later exposures but not the present one.

PATHOPHYSIOLOGY

Mumps virus replicates in glandular epithelium of parotids, pancreas, and testes:

- Leads to interstitial edema and inflammation
- Interstitial glandular hemorrhage may occur.
- Pressure caused by edema of the testes against the tunica albuginea can lead to necrosis.

ETIOLOGY

- Mumps paramyxovirus
- Other viruses, such as coxsackievirus (rare)

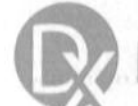

DIAGNOSIS

HISTORY

- Initial parotid swelling just behind jaw
- Swelling peaks in 1–3 days, lasts 3–7 days.
- Sour foods cause pain in parotid gland region.
- Moderate fever, usually not above 104°F (40°C):
  - High fever frequently associated with complications

PHYSICAL EXAM

- Parotid pain and swelling in one or both glands
- Rare prodrome of fever, neck muscle ache, and malaise
- Meningeal signs in 15%, encephalitis in 0.5%
- Rarely arthritis, orchitis, thyroiditis, mastitis, pancreatitis, oophoritis, and myocarditis
- Rare maculopapular, erythematous rash
- Up to 50% of cases may be very mild.
- Obscures angle of mandible
- Elevates earlobe
- Redness at opening of Stensen duct but no pus
- Swelling in sternal area; rare, but pathognomonic of mumps

DIAGNOSTIC TESTS & INTERPRETATION

Lab

- The following 3 special tests to confirm an outbreak should be ordered and reported to health department:
  - IgM titer (positive by day 5 in 100% of nonimmunized patients)
  - Swab of parotid duct or other affected salivary ducts for viral isolation
  - Rise in IgG titer samples; test should be ordered if patient previously immunized, first sample within 5 days of onset, second 2 weeks later.
- Other potential findings: Serum amylase may be elevated; CSF leukocytosis and leukopenia may be present.

Imaging

Testicular ultrasound may be useful to differentiate mumps orchitis from testicular torsion.

Initial approach

Clinical diagnosis (swelling of one or both parotid glands):

- Lasting 2 or more days
- No other apparent cause
- Rare presentation of meningitis without parotitis (1–10%)

Diagnostic Procedures/Surgery

If meningitis is present, lumbar puncture may be required to prove aseptic meningitis.

Pathological Findings

Periductal edema and lymphocytic infiltration in affected glands

DIFFERENTIAL DIAGNOSIS

- If not epidemic, other viruses are more common: Parainfluenza parotitis, Epstein-Barr virus, coxsackievirus, adenovirus, parvovirus B19
- Suppurative parotitis: Often associated with *Staphylococcus aureus* (presence of Wharton duct pus on massaging parotid gland nearly excludes diagnosis of mumps)
- Recurrent allergic parotitis
- Salivary calculus with intermittent swelling
- Lymphadenitis from any cause, even HIV infection
- Cytomegalovirus parotitis in immunocompromised patients
- Mikulicz syndrome: Chronic, painless parotid and lacrimal gland swelling of unknown cause that occurs in tuberculosis, sarcoidosis, lupus, leukemia, lymphosarcoma, and malignant or benign salivary gland tumors
- Sjögren syndrome, diabetes mellitus, uremia, malnutrition
- Drug-related parotid enlargement (iodides, guanethidine, phenothiazine)

- Other causes of the complications of mumps (meningoencephalitis, orchitis, oophoritis, pancreatitis, polyarthritis, nephritis, myocarditis, prostatitis)
- Mumps orchitis must be differentiated from testicular torsion and from chlamydial or bacterial orchitis. (Testicular sonogram can be useful.)

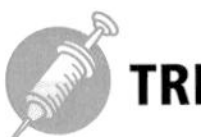

TREATMENT

- No specific antiviral therapy
- Analgesics to relieve pain
- Avoid corticosteroids for mumps orchitis because they can reduce testosterone concentrations and increase testicular atrophy.
- IVIG only successful for certain autoimmune-based sequelae: Postinfectious encephalitis, Guillain-Barré syndrome, or ITP
- Interferon-α2b improved severe bilateral orchitis and decreased testicular atrophy in small studies.

MEDICATION

First Line

- Corticosteroids or a NSAID may diminish pain and swelling in acute orchitis and arthritis mumps, but usually are not necessary.
- May use acetaminophen for fever and/or pain.
- Contraindications: Refer to manufacturer's profile for each drug.
- Precautions: Avoid aspirin for pain in children. Aspirin use in children with viral infections has been associated with Reye syndrome.
- Significant possible interactions: Refer to manufacturer's profile for each drug.

Second Line

- Mumps arthritis may improve with corticosteroids or an NSAID.
- Interferon-α2b $\times$ 7 days has been used experimentally in small studies (2)[C] for severe bilateral orchitis to prevent infertility.

ADDITIONAL TREATMENT

General Measures

- High fever and testicular pain: May hospitalize for steroids or interferon
- Orchitis:
  - Ice packs to scrotum can help to relieve pain.
  - Scrotal support with adhesive bridge while recumbent and/or athletic supporter while ambulatory

IN-PATIENT CONSIDERATIONS

Initial Stabilization

Outpatient supportive care if no complications

Admission Criteria

Hospitalize only if CNS symptoms occur.

IV Fluids

If severe nausea or vomiting accompanies pancreatitis

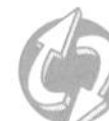

ONGOING CARE

FOLLOW-UP RECOMMENDATIONS

Mumps orchitis:

- Bed rest and local supportive clothing (e.g., 2 pairs of briefs) or adhesive-tape bridge
- Must be out of school until no longer contagious: About 9 days after onset of pain

Patient Monitoring

Most cases will be mild. Monitor hydration status.

DIET

Liquid diet if cannot chew

PATIENT EDUCATION

Orchitis is common in older children but rarely results in sterility, even after bilateral orchitis.

PROGNOSIS

- Complete recovery is usual; immunity is lifelong.
- Transient sensorineural hearing loss occurs in 4% of adults.
- Rare recurrence after 2 weeks may be recurrent nonepidemic parotitis.

COMPLICATIONS

- May precede, accompany, or follow salivary gland involvement and may occur (rarely) without primary involvement of the parotid gland
- Orchitis is common (30%) in postpubertal boys:
  - It starts within 8 days after parotitis.
  - Fever, swollen testis of 4 days' duration
  - Impaired fertility in 13%, but absolute sterility is rare.
- Meningitis (1–10%) or encephalitis (0.1%) may present 5–10 days after first symptoms of illness. Aseptic meningitis typically is mild, but meningoencephalitis may lead to seizures, paralysis, hydrocephalus, or in 2% of encephalitis patients, death.
- Acute cerebellar ataxia has been reported after mumps infections; self-resolving in 2–3 weeks.
- CSF pleocytosis, usually lymphocytes, found in 65% of patients with parotitis
- Oophoritis in 7% of postpubertal females; no decreased fertility
- Pancreatitis, usually mild
- Nephritis, thyroiditis, and arthralgias are rare.
- Myocarditis: Usually mild, but may depress ST segment, may be linked to endocardial fibroelastosis
- Deafness: 1/15,000 unilateral nerve deafness; may not be permanent
- Inflammation about the eye (keratouveitis) rarely
- Dacryoadenitis, optic neuritis

Pediatric Considerations

- Orchitis is more common in adolescents.
- Young children are less likely to develop complications.
- Most complications occur in postpubertal group.
- Avoid aspirin use in children with viral symptoms.

Pregnancy Considerations

Disease may increase the rate of spontaneous abortion in first trimester; however, perinatal mumps has been reported to take a benign course.

REFERENCES

1. Centers for Disease Control and Prevention (CDC). Update: Mumps outbreak–New York and New Jersey, June 2008–Jan 2010. *Morb Mortal Wkly Rep*. 2010;59(05):125–9.
2. Hviid A, Rubin S, Mühlemann K. Mumps. *Lancet*. 2008;371:932–44.
3. Hindiyeh MY, Aboudy Y, Wohoush M, et al. Characterization of large mumps outbreak in vaccinated Palestinian refugees. *J Clin Microbiol*. 2009.
4. MacDonald N, Hatchette T, Elkout L, et al. Mumps is back: Why is mumps eradication not working? *Adv Exp Med Biol*. 2011;697:197–220.
5. Centers for Disease Control and Prevention (CDC). Updated recommendations for isolation of persons with mumps. *Morb Mortal Wkly Rep*. 2008;57: 1103–5.

ADDITIONAL READING

- Centers for Disease Control and Prevention (CDC). Brief report: Update: Mumps activity–United States, January 1–October 7, 2006. *Morb Mortal Wkly Rep*. 2006;55:1152–3.
- Gemmill IM. Mumps vaccine: Is it time to re-evaluate our approach? *CMAJ*. 2006;175:491–2.
- Kancherla VS, Hanson IC. Mumps resurgence in the United States. *J Allergy Clin Immunol*. 2006;118: 938–41.

CODES

ICD9

- 072.0 Mumps orchitis
- 072.8 Mumps with unspecified complication
- 072.9 Mumps without mention of complication

CLINICAL PEARLS

- Mumps is a clinical diagnosis, including swelling of one or more parotid glands for 2 or more days without other obvious cause, but confirmatory tests must be done for epidemics.
- Ultrasound is useful to distinguish testicular torsion from testicular pain related to mumps orchitis.
- MMR vaccine is only 75–95% effective in field trials; therefore, expect some cases of mumps despite completed vaccinations.

MUSCULAR DYSTROPHY

Austin Larson, MD
Brian Alverson, MD

BASICS

- Primary inherited myopathies caused by dysfunctional proteins of muscle fibers
- Distribution of weakness, other associated symptoms, and disease prognosis depend on the specific mutated gene and the severity of the mutation.

DESCRIPTION

- Duchenne muscular dystrophy (DMD):
  - Highest-incidence muscular dystrophy, X-linked inheritance, early onset, rapidly progressive
  - Patients are wheelchair-dependent prior to age 13
- Becker muscular dystrophy (BMD):
  - Less severe phenotype than Duchenne, also caused by mutation in DMD gene (dystrophin protein)
  - Distinction from DMD is clinical: Patients are wheelchair-dependent after age 16.
- Myotonic muscular dystrophy (MMD):
  - Myotonia (slow relaxation after muscle contraction), distal and facial weakness
- Limb-girdle muscular dystrophy (LGMD):
  - Proximal weakness and atrophy, variable prognosis with 19 different identified mutations
- Fascioscapulohumeral muscular dystrophy (FSHMD):
  - Pattern of weakness with primarily facial and shoulder muscles affected
- Emery-Dreifuss muscular dystrophy (EDMD):
  - Characterized by early development of joint contractures and cardiac involvement
- Congenital muscular dystrophies (CMD):
  - Heterogeneous group of myopathic diseases presenting in infancy with generally poor prognosis
  - Includes Fukuyama CMD, Ullrich CMD, Walker Warburg syndrome, and other conditions
- Oculopharyngeal muscular dystrophy (OPMD):
  - Adult onset, affects extraocular and pharyngeal muscles
- System(s) affected: Musculoskeletal; Cardiac; Nervous

EPIDEMIOLOGY

Incidence

- DMD: 30/100,000 male births
- BMD: 3/100,000 male births
- MMD: 10/100,000 births
- FSHMD: 5/100,000 births

RISK FACTORS

Genetics

- Autosomal dominant:
  - Generally later onset and less severe than diseases with recessive or X-linked inheritance
  - FSHMD, OPMD, some forms of LGMD and EDMD (some types)
  - MMD:
    - Trinucleotide repeat expansion with earlier onset of symptoms in subsequent generations due to accumulation of repeats
- Autosomal recessive:
  - LGMD (some subtypes), CMD
- X-linked:
  - DMD/BMD:
    - 30% of affected males have a de novo mutation (mother is not a carrier).
    - 20% of female carriers have some manifestation of the mutation (usually mild muscle weakness).
    - 50% of female carriers have serum CK greater than twice the upper limit of normal.
    - Female phenotype is dependent on the pattern of X chromosome inactivation.

GENERAL PREVENTION

Genetic counseling for known carriers

PATHOPHYSIOLOGY

Mutations affect proteins connecting cytoskeleton to cell membrane and extracellular matrix:

- Phenotype is also seen with some nuclear membrane and Golgi-associated protein mutations.
- Muscle fibers become fragile and easily damaged by contraction.
- Satellite cells replace dead muscle fibers:
  - Population of satellite cells is exhausted, resulting in decreasing numbers of muscle fibers and progressive weakness and atrophy.

ETIOLOGY

- DMD/BMD:
  - Defective protein is dystrophin; translated from the largest known human gene (DMD), making up 1.5% of the X chromosome.
  - DMD phenotype results from mutations that cause profound loss of dystrophin function; 90% of mutations in DMD are frameshift mutations, resulting in undetectable levels of functional dystrophin protein.
  - BMD phenotype results from less severe mutations to DMD gene; patients have low but detectable levels of functional dystrophin.
- MMD: Results from trinucleotide repeat expansion in the untranslated region of the gene DMPK on chromosome 19; encodes myotonin protein kinase
- LGMD: Results from mutations to genes encoding proteins associated with dystrophin; calpain-, dysferlin-, and fukutin-related proteins are affected most commonly
- EDMD: Mutated proteins are associated with the nuclear membrane in muscle fibers; emerin in X-linked form, lamin A and C in autosomal forms
- OPMD: Trinucleotide repeat expansion on chromosome 14 results in defective polyadenylate binding protein; results in accumulation of protein in the cell nucleus
- FSHMD: Deletion in untranslated region of chromosome 4

COMMONLY ASSOCIATED CONDITIONS

- Decreased IQ: On average, 1 SD below the mean in DMD
- Dilated cardiomyopathy and conduction abnormalities:
  - Can be severe in EDMD
  - Can affect otherwise asymptomatic female carriers of DMD

DIAGNOSIS

HISTORY

- DMD: Normal attainment of early motor milestones with subsequent abnormal gait and slowing gross motor development; clumsiness, weakness in toddlers and young children
- BMD: Progressive difficulty with ambulation and frequent falls in adolescence
- MMD: Slurred speech, muscle wasting, difficulty with ambulation
- LGMD: Back pain, lordosis/inability to rise from a chair, climb stairs, and use arms overhead
- FSHMD: Facial weakness, inability to close eyes completely
- EDMD: Contractures of elbows and ankles, difficulty with ambulation in teens
- OPMD: Ptosis and dysphagia in middle age, often with family history

PHYSICAL EXAM

- DMD/BMD:
  - Muscle weakness, proximal more affected than distal
  - Gower sign: Use of arms to push upper body into standing posture from lying prone
  - Trendelenburg gait (hip waddling)
  - Winged scapulae and lordosis
  - Pseudohypertrophy of the calf (caused by proliferation of fat and connective tissue)
  - Contractures of lower extremity joints and elbows
- MMD:
  - Characteristic facial appearance: Narrow face, open triangular mouth, high arched palate, concave temples, drooping eyelids, frontal balding in males
  - Slit-lamp eye exam: Cataracts
  - Myotonia: Inability to relax muscles after contraction
  - Distal muscle weakness and wasting
- FSHMD:
  - Winged scapulae, pronounced weakness with arms above head
  - Protruding lips, unable to whistle
- CMD:
  - Arthrogryposis at birth (multiple joint contractures)
  - Diffuse hypotonia and muscle wasting with thin appearance

DIAGNOSTIC TESTS & INTERPRETATION

Lab

Initial lab tests

- Creatine kinase (CK): Initial screening test if muscular dystrophy is suspected (1)
- Elevated in DMD (10–100×); elevated at birth, peaks at time of presentation, and falls through course of illness. Other MD may result in normal or only mildly elevated CK.
- Genetic testing:
  - For definitive diagnosis in patient with characteristic presentation and elevated CK
  - Deletion and duplication analysis by polymerase chain reaction will identify the majority of patients
  - If not diagnostic, then may proceed to full sequencing of DMD gene for point mutations
  - Specific genetic testing is available for most non-DMD muscular dystrophies and may be chosen based on age, family history, pattern of affected muscles, and other symptoms.

Diagnostic Procedures/Surgery

- Muscle biopsy: Second-line diagnostic instrument if DNA analysis is nondiagnostic; can have prognostic value if interpreted by experienced neuromuscular pathologist
- Dystrophin protein assay: Severe reduction or complete absence of dystrophin is diagnostic of DMD.
- Immunohistochemical staining for other known protein defects in muscular dystrophies
- Electromyography and nerve conduction studies are not necessary unless considering alternative diagnoses.
- ECG: Abnormalities found in >90% of males and up to 10% of female carriers of DMD. Q waves in anterolateral leads, tall R waves in V1, shortened PR interval, arrhythmias (2).

Pregnancy Considerations

Prenatal diagnosis (optional):

- Amniocentesis, chorionic villus sampling, or fetal muscle biopsy for affected families
- Genetic diagnosis at 10–13 weeks' gestation

Pathological Findings

- Heterogeneic muscle fibers: Atrophy and hypertrophy of fibers with proliferation of connective tissue in muscle
- Immunohistochemical staining for dystrophin protein:
  - DMD: No detectable dystrophin in most fibers; occasional revertant fibers with normal dystrophin
  - BMD: Highly variable staining for dystrophin throughout muscle

DIFFERENTIAL DIAGNOSIS

- Glycogen storage diseases and other metabolic myopathies
- Mitochondrial myopathies: MELAS, MERRF
- Inflammatory myopathies: Polymyositis, dermatomyositis, inclusion-body myositis
- Neuromuscular junction diseases: Myasthenia gravis, Lambert-Eaton
- Motor neuron diseases: Amyotrophic lateral sclerosis, spinal muscular atrophy
- Charcot-Marie-Tooth disease
- Friedreich ataxia
- Viral myositis
- Malnutrition
- Hypothyroid or hyperthyroid myopathy
- Cushing syndrome

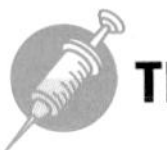

TREATMENT

Trials of agents that affect dystrophin gene expression as well as gene therapy with viral vectors are an active area of research; however, steroid treatment is the only clinically available regimen at this time.

MEDICATION

Prednisone 0.75 mg/kg/d (1,3,4):

- Slows the decline in muscle function, progression to scoliosis, and degradation of pulmonary function; prolongs functional ambulation; possible reduction in cardiac morbidity
- Initiate therapy when motor function ceases to improve, prior to decline in function.
- Monitor adverse effects and intervene to mitigate harm:
  - Some use bisphosphonates for preventing loss of bone density.
  - Annual exam for development of cataracts
  - Avoid NSAID use due to risk of peptic ulcers
  - Stress-dose steroids during surgeries and illnesses.
  - Monitor and treat hypertension.
  - Patients should be aware of immune suppression and notify emergency providers.
  - Controversial: 10-day-on/10-day-off schedule of prednisone may reduce side effects.

ADDITIONAL TREATMENT

General Measures

Goal of management: Lessen impairments, reduce functional limitations:

- Ambulation prolonged by use of knee-ankle-foot orthoses
- Serial casting to treat contractures
- Diagnose sleep apnea with polysomnography; treat with noninvasive ventilation.
- Adaptive devices to improve function
- Avoid overexertion and strenuous exercise (5).

Issues for Referral

- Refer to neuromuscular diseases specialist for definitive diagnosis and treatment
- Coordinated multidisciplinary clinic specific to these illnesses (6)
- Cardiology for management of cardiomyopathy
- Pulmonology for monitoring of pulmonary function and clearance regimen

SURGERY/OTHER PROCEDURES

- Spinal surgery for scoliosis
- Scapular fixation for scapular winging can be beneficial.
- May consider surgical treatment of ankle or knee contractures

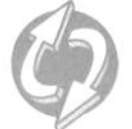

ONGOING CARE

- Individualized education plan and developmental evaluation for school accommodations
- Maintenance of current influenza and pneumococcal vaccination status

FOLLOW-UP RECOMMENDATIONS

Patient Monitoring

- ECG, echocardiogram, and consultation with a cardiologist at diagnosis and annually after age 10
- Annual spinal radiography for scoliosis
- DEXA scanning and serum marker testing for osteoporosis
- Pulmonary function testing twice yearly if no longer ambulatory

DIET

- Obesity is common due to steroid treatment and wheelchair confinement.
- Weight control can improve quality of life.
- Diet may be limited by dysphagia; swallow evaluation can determine appropriate foods.
- Calcium and vitamin D supplementation is indicated for patients on steroids.

PATIENT EDUCATION

Muscular Dystrophy Association: www.mda.org

PROGNOSIS

- DMD/BMD:
  - Progressive weakness, contractures, inability to walk
  - Kyphoscoliosis and progressive decline in respiratory vital capacity
  - Significantly shortened lifespan (DMD: 16 ± 4 years; BMD: 42 ± 16 years)
- Other types: Slow progression and near-normal life span with functional limitations

COMPLICATIONS

- Cardiac arrhythmia, cardiomyopathy
- Dysphagia, GERD, constipation
- Scoliosis, joint contractures
- Obstructive sleep apnea
- Malignant hyperthermialike reaction to anesthesia
- Respiratory failure and early death

REFERENCES

1. Bushby K, Finkel R, Birnkrant DJ, et al. Diagnosis and management of Duchenne muscular dystrophy, part 1: Diagnosis, and pharmacological and psychosocial management. *Lancet Neurol*. 2010;9: 77–93.
2. Takami Y, Takeshima Y, Awano H, et al. High incidence of electrocardiogram abnormalities in young patients with Duchenne muscular dystrophy. *Pediatr Neurol*. 2008;39:399–403.
3. Manzur AY, Kuntzer T, Pike M, et al. Glucocorticoid corticosteroids for Duchenne muscular dystrophy. *Cochrane Database Syst Rev*. 2008;CD003725.
4. Cossu G, Sampaolesi M, et al. New therapies for Duchenne muscular dystrophy: Challenges, prospects and clinical trials. *Trends Mol Med*. 2007;13:520–6.
5. van der Kooi EL, Lindeman E, Riphagen I. Strength training and aerobic exercise training for muscle disease. *Cochrane Database Syst Rev*. 2005; CD003907.
6. Bushby K, Finkel R, Birnkrant DJ, et al. Diagnosis and management of Duchenne muscular dystrophy, part 2: Implementation of multidisciplinary care. *Lancet Neurol*. 2010;9:177–89.

CODES

ICD9

- 359.0 Congenital hereditary muscular dystrophy
- 359.1 Hereditary progressive muscular dystrophy
- 359.21 Myotonic muscular dystrophy

CLINICAL PEARLS

- Pediatricians should have a low threshold to obtain serum CK as a screening test in the face of gross motor delay or muscular weakness, especially in boys.
- Steroids should be initiated in DMD patients when gross motor function ceases to progress.
- High-quality care of patients with muscular dystrophy requires a medical home; a multidisciplinary team of physicians, therapists, and other providers; and extensive patient and family support.

MYASTHENIA GRAVIS

Shaylin Cersosimo, MD, MPH
Macario C. Corpuz, Jr., MD, FAAFP

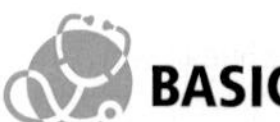

BASICS

DESCRIPTION

Primary disorder of neuromuscular transmission characterized by fluctuating muscle weakness:

- Ocular myasthenia gravis (MG) (15%): Weakness limited to eyelids and extraocular muscles
- Generalized MG (85%): Commonly affects ocular as well as a variable combination of bulbar, proximal limb, and respiratory muscles
- 50% of patients who present with ocular symptoms develop generalized MG within 2 years.
- Onset may be sudden and severe, but it is typically mild and intermittent over many years.
- System(s) affected: Neurologic; Hematologic, Lymphatic, Immunologic; Musculoskeletal

EPIDEMIOLOGY

Occurs at any age, but a bimodal distribution to the age of onset:

- Female predominance: 20–40
- Male predominance: 60–80

Incidence

Estimated annual incidence 2–4 cases per 1,000,000

Prevalence

In the US, 100–200 per million; increasing over the past 5 decades

Pediatric Considerations

A transient form of neonatal MG seen in 10–20% of infants born to MG mothers. It occurs as a result of the transplacental passage of maternal antibodies that interfere with function of the neuromuscular junction. Resolves in weeks to months.

RISK FACTORS

- Familial MG
- D-Penicillamine (drug-induced MG)
- Other autoimmune diseases

Genetics

- Congenital MG syndrome describes a collection of rare hereditary disorders. This condition is not immune-mediated but instead results from the mutation of a component of the neuromuscular junction (autosomal recessive).
- Familial predisposition seen in 5% of cases.

PATHOPHYSIOLOGY

- Reduction in the acetylcholine receptors (AChR) at muscle endplates, resulting in insufficient neuromuscular transmission
- Seropositive MG: 80–85% of all MG patients:
  - Anti-acetylcholine receptor (anti-AChR): A humoral, antibody-mediated, T-cell–dependent attack of the AChRs or receptor-associated proteins at the postsynaptic membrane of the neuromuscular junction.
  - Patients without anti-AChR antibodies may have antibodies against muscle-specific kinase (MuSK) (1)[C]. Females tend to be anti-MuSK positive, and respiratory and bulbar muscles are frequently involved.
  - Seronegative MG (SNMG): 6–12% (2)[C].

ETIOLOGY

- Poliovirus has been found in macrophages inside thymic tissue, suggesting a possible viral component (3).
- Also documented immediately after viral infections (measles, EBV, HIV, and HTLV)

COMMONLY ASSOCIATED CONDITIONS

- Thymic hyperplasia (60–70% of MG patients)
- Thymoma (10–15% of MG patients)
- Autoimmune thyroid disease (3–8%)

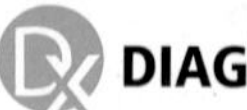

DIAGNOSIS

Myasthenia Gravis Foundation of America Clinical Classification (4)[A]:

- Class I: Any eye muscle weakness, possible ptosis, no other evidence of muscle weakness elsewhere
- Class II: Eye muscle weakness of any severity, mild weakness of other muscles
  - Class IIa: Predominantly limb or axial muscles
  - Class IIb: Predominantly bulbar and/or respiratory muscles
- Class III: Eye muscle weakness of any severity, moderate weakness of other muscles:
  - Class IIIa: Predominantly limb or axial muscles
  - Class IIIb: Predominantly bulbar and/or respiratory muscles
- Class IV: Eye muscle weakness of any severity, severe weakness of other muscles:
  - Class IVa: Predominantly limb or axial muscles
  - Class IVb: Predominantly bulbar and/or respiratory muscles (can also include feeding tube without intubation)
- Class V: Intubation needed to maintain airway

HISTORY

The hallmark of MG is fatigability:

- Fluctuating weakness that worsens during the day and after prolonged use of affected muscles, may improve with rest
- Early symptoms are transient with asymptomatic periods lasting days or weeks.
- With progression, asymptomatic periods shorten and symptoms fluctuate from mild to severe.
- More than 50% of patients present with ocular symptoms (ptosis and/or diplopia). Eventually 90% of patients with MG develop ocular symptoms.
- Ptosis might be unilateral, bilateral, or shifting from eye to eye.
- 15% present with bulbar symptoms.
- <5% present with proximal limb weakness alone.

ALERT

Myasthenic crisis: Respiratory muscle weakness producing respiratory insufficiency and pending respiratory failure

PHYSICAL EXAM

- Ptosis may worsen with propping of opposite eyelid (curtain sign) or sustained upward gaze.
- "Myasthenic sneer," in which the midlip rises, but corners of mouth do not move
- Muscle weakness is usually proximal and symmetric.

DIAGNOSTIC TESTS & INTERPRETATION

Lab

Initial lab tests

- Antiacetylcholine receptor (anti-AChR) antibody (74–85% are seropositive):
  - Generalized myasthenia: 75–85%
  - Ocular myasthenia: 50%
  - MG and thymoma: 98–100%
  - Poor correlation between antibody titer and disease severity (5)[C]
  - False-positive results in thymoma without MG, Lambert-Eaton myasthenic syndrome, small cell lung cancer, and rheumatoid arthritis treated with penicillamine
- Antimuscle-specific tyrosine kinase (anti-MuSK) antibody:
  - Used if MG suspected, patient seronegative
  - Present in 40–50% of seronegative patients with generalized MG; absent in ocular MG (1,5)[C]
  - These patients are less likely to respond to acetylcholine esterase inhibitors, which may actually worsen symptoms, but they are more likely to respond to plasmapheresis and selected immunotherapy (5)[C]
- Antistriated muscle (anti-SM) antibody:
  - Present in 84% of patients with thymoma who are <40 years old
  - Anti-SM AB can be present without thymoma in patients >40 years old.

Imaging

- Chest radiographs or CT scans may identify a thymoma.
- MRI of brain and orbits to rule out other causes of cranial nerve deficit.

Diagnostic Procedures/Surgery

- Tensilon (Edrophonium) test:
  - Initial 2-mg IV dose, followed by another 2 mg every 60 seconds up to a maximum dose of 10 mg.
  - A positive test shows improvement of strength within 30 seconds of administration.
  - Sensitivity 80–90% (5)[C]
  - Cardiac disease and bronchial asthma are relative contraindications, especially in elderly.
  - Atropine: 0.4–0.6 mg IV may rarely be required as antidote; must be available.
- Ice pack test:
  - For patients with ptosis in whom Tensilon test is contraindicated
  - Ice pack applied to closed eyelid for 60 seconds, then removed; extent of ptosis immediately assessed
  - Ice will decrease the ptosis induced by MG.
  - Sensitivity 80% in patients with prominent ptosis
- Electrophysiology testing:
  - Repetitive nerve stimulation (RNS):
    - Widely available, most frequently used
    - Moderately sensitive for both generalized MG (75%) and ocular MG (50%) (5)[C]
  - Single-fiber EMG (SFEMG):
    - Assesses temporal variability between 2 muscle fibers within same motor unit (jitter).
    - Sensitive (90–95%) but less specific (5)[C].
    - Technically difficult to perform; limited availability

Pathological Findings

- Lymphofollicular hyperplasia of thymic medulla occurs in 65% of patients with MG, thymoma in 15%
- Immunofluorescence: IgG antibodies and complement on receptor membranes

DIFFERENTIAL DIAGNOSIS

- Thyroid ophthalmopathy
- Oculopharyngeal muscular dystrophy

- Myotonic dystrophy
- Kearns-Sayre syndrome
- Chronic progressive external ophthalmoplegia
- Brain-stem and motor cranial nerve lesions
- Botulism
- Motor neuron disease (e.g., ALS)
- Lambert-Eaton myasthenic syndrome
- Drug-induced myasthenia
- Congenital myasthenic syndrome
- Depression
- Dermatomyositis/Polymyositis
- Sarcoidosis and neuropathy
- Tolosa-Hunt syndrome

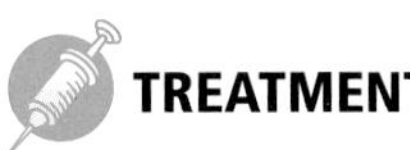

TREATMENT

MEDICATION

First Line

Symptomatic treatments (anticholinesterase agents):

- Pyridostigmine bromide (Mestinon):
  - Most commonly prescribed since available in oral tablet
  - Starting dose of 30 mg PO t.i.d.
  - Maximum dose: 120 mg q3–4h
- Neostigmine methylsulfate (Prostigmin):
  - Starting dose of 0.5 mg SC or IM q3h
  - Titrate dosage to clinical need.
- Ambenonium (Mytelase):
  - Longer duration of action than neostigmine, which leads to longer effect at night and upon waking (6)[C]
  - Use with caution in patients with asthma and Parkinson disease
  - Starting dose of 5 mg PO t.i.d. or q.i.d.
  - Maintenance dose of 15–100 mg/d, usual 40 mg/d
  - Maximum dose: 50–75 mg PO t.i.d. or q.i.d.

Second Line

- Immunosuppressants (7)[B]: Oral corticosteroids are first choice of drugs when immunosuppression is necessary:
  - Prednisone: Start as in-patient with a 60 mg/d PO; taper the dosage every 3 days; switch to alternate day regimen within 2 weeks. Taper very slowly to establish the minimum dosage necessary to maintain remission.
  - Cyclophosphamide: Adults: 1–5 mg/kg/d PO; Children: 2–8 mg/kg/d PO
  - Cyclosporine: Adults: 5 mg/kg/d PO (nephrotoxicity and drug interactions)
  - Mycophenolate: 1 g PO or IV b.i.d.
  - Azathioprine: 100–200 mg/d PO:
    - Most frequently used for long-term immunomodulation
    - Benefit may not be apparent for up to 18 months after initiation of therapy
    - Prednisolone plus azathioprine may be effective when used as a corticosteroid-sparing agent
- Acute immunomodulating treatments:
  - Plasmapheresis: Bulk removal of 2–3 L of plasma 3 times per week, repeated until rate of improvement plateaus (6)[B]:
    - Improves weakness in nearly all and can last up to 3 months
  - Immunoglobulin: 2 g/kg IV over 2–5 days (7)[B]
  - Plasmapheresis and immunoglobulin have comparable efficacy in treating moderate to severe MG (8)
  - Rapid onset of effect but short duration of action
  - Used for acute worsening of MG to improve strength prior to surgery, prevent acute exacerbations induced by corticosteroids and as a chronic intermittent treatment to provide relief in refractory MG
- Other immunosuppressant therapies:
  - Tacrolimus: Effective in MG (9)
  - Rituximab: Monoclonal antibody directed against antigens on B cells shows benefit in MG (10):
    - Seronegative MuSK-antibody positive MG patients may have better response to Rituximab than conventional therapies.

ALERT

Avoid aminoglycosides and other drugs with the potential for neuromuscular blockade, which may precipitate weakness.

ADDITIONAL TREATMENT

General Measures

- Treatment based on age, gender, severity of disease, and disease progression.
- 3 basic approaches: Symptomatic, immunosuppressive, and supportive. Few should receive a single therapeutic modality.

SURGERY/OTHER PROCEDURES

- Thymectomy recommended for most patients
- No clear clinical benefit if onset at ≥60 years unless thymoma present

Pediatric Considerations

- Infants with severe weakness from transient neonatal myasthenia may be treated with oral pyridostigmine; general support is necessary until the condition clears.
- Corticosteroids limited only to severe disease

IN-PATIENT CONSIDERATIONS

Initial Stabilization

- Plasmapheresis
- IV gamma-globulin

Admission Criteria

- Management of pulmonary infections
- Myasthenic or cholinergic crises

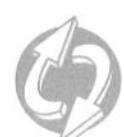

ONGOING CARE

PATIENT EDUCATION

MG Foundation of America (MGFA): www.myasthenia.org

PROGNOSIS

- Overall good, but highly variable
- Myasthenic crisis associated with substantial morbidity and 4% mortality
- Seronegative patients are more likely to have purely ocular disease, and those with generalized SNMG have a better outcome after treatment (11)[C].

COMPLICATIONS

Acute respiratory arrest; chronic respiratory insufficiency

REFERENCES

1. McConville J, Farrugia ME, Beeson D. Detection and characterization of MuSK antibodies in seronegative myasthenia gravis. *Ann Neurol*. 2004;55:580–4.
2. Chan KH, Lachance DH, Harper CM. Frequency of seronegativity in adult-acquired generalized myasthenia gravis. *Muscle Nerve*. 2007;36:651–8.
3. Cavalcante P, Barberis M, et al. Detection of poliovirus-infected macrophages in thymus of patients with myasthenia gravis. *Neurology*. 2010;74:1118–26.
4. Jaretzki A, Barohn RJ, Ernstoff RM. Myasthenia gravis: Recommendations for clinical research standards. Task Force of the Medical Scientific Advisory Board of the Myasthenia Gravis Foundation of America. *Neurology*. 2000;55:16–23.
5. Meriggioli MN, Sanders DB. Myasthenia gravis: Diagnosis. *Semin Neurol*. 2004;24:31–9.
6. Angelini C. Diagnosis and management of autoimmune myasthenia gravis. *Clin Drug Investig*. 2011;31:1.
7. Hart IK, Sathasivam S, Sarshar T. Immunosuppressive agents for myasthenia gravis. *Cochrane Database Syst Rev*. 2007;17:CD005224.
8. Barth D, Nabavi Nouri M, et al. Comparison of IVIg and PLEX in patients with myasthenia gravis. *Neurology*. 2011;76:2017–23.
9. Evoli A, Di Schino C, Marsili F, et al. Successful treatment of myasthenia gravis with tacrolimus. *Muscle Nerve*. 2002;25:111–4.
10. Zebardast N, Patwa HS, Novella SP, et al. Rituximab in the management of refractory myasthenia gravis. *Muscle Nerve*. 2010;41:375–8.
11. Deymeer F, Gungor-Tuncer O, Yilmaz V. Clinical comparison of anti-MuSK- vs anti-AChR-positive and seronegative myasthenia gravis. *Neurology*. 2007;68:609–11.

ADDITIONAL READING

Cavalcante P, Le Panse R, et al. The thymus in myasthenia gravis: Site of "innate autoimmunity"? *Muscle Nerve*. 2011;44:467–84.

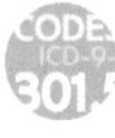

CODES

ICD9

- 358.00 Myasthenia gravis without (acute) exacerbation
- 358.01 Myasthenia gravis with (acute) exacerbation
- 775.2 Neonatal myasthenia gravis

CLINICAL PEARLS

- An autoimmune disease, marked by abnormal fatigability and weakness of selected muscles (often ocular), which is relieved by rest, and medications.
- Anticholinesterase medication and a thymectomy lessen the severity of the symptoms.
- Steroid therapy, plasma exchange, or immunoglobulin can be used in severely affected patients.

MYELODYSPLASTIC SYNDROMES

Richard A. Larson, MD

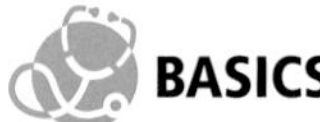

BASICS

DESCRIPTION

Myelodysplastic syndromes (MDSs) constitute a heterogeneous group of acquired hematopoietic stem-cell disorders characterized by cytologic dysplasia in the bone marrow and blood and by various combinations of anemia, neutropenia, and thrombocytopenia:

- The natural progression of disease evolves as cellular maturation becomes more arrested and blast cells accumulate. There is a great deal of overlap between arbitrary diagnostic subgroups.
- World Health Organization classification (1):
  - Refractory cytopenia with unilineage dysplasia:
    - Refractory anemia (RA); refractory neutropenia; refractory thrombocytopenia
    - <5% blasts and <15% ring sideroblasts in marrow; <1% blasts in blood
  - Refractory anemia with ring sideroblasts (RARS):
    - <5% blasts in marrow; ≥15% of erythroid precursors are ring sideroblasts; no blasts in blood
    - Also known as acquired idiopathic sideroblastic anemia
  - Refractory cytopenia with multilineage dysplasia:
    - Marked trilineage dysplasia but without excess blasts in marrow; no Auer rods; <1% blasts in blood
  - Refractory cytopenia with multilineage dysplasia and ring sideroblasts
  - Refractory anemia with excess blasts-1 (RAEB-1):
    - 5–9% blasts in marrow; no Auer rods; <5% blasts in blood; <1,000 monocytes/mm^3
  - RAEB-2:
    - 10–19% blasts in marrow; 5–19% blasts in blood; ± Auer rods; <1,000 monocytes/mm^3
  - MDS associated with isolated del(5q) (2):
    - RA with erythroid hyperplasia, increased megakaryocytes with hypolobated nuclei, and normal or increased platelets; <5% blasts in marrow; <1% blasts in blood
  - Acute MDS with sclerosis:
    - RAEB with marked myelosclerosis
  - Chronic myelomonocytic leukemia (CMMoL or CMML) is now grouped with myelodysplastic/myeloproliferative disorders:
    - <20% blasts and promonocytes in marrow and blood with >1,000 monocytes/mm^3
  - RAEB in transformation is now considered acute myeloid leukemia (AML):
    - 20–30% blasts in marrow; >20% blasts in blood
    - Incidence: 2:1 (female > male)
  - Therapy-related MDS (t-MDS) (3,4):
    - Seen 3–7 years after treatment with alkylating agents and/or radiotherapy
    - Evolves to AML over ~6 months
    - Classified by the World Health Organization as therapy-related myeloid neoplasm
- System(s) affected: Hematologic; Lymphatic; Immunologic
- Synonym(s): Dysmyelopoietic syndrome; Hemopoietic dysplasia; Preleukemia; Smoldering or subacute myeloid leukemia

Pediatric Considerations

Pediatric presentations of MDS:

- Monosomy 7 syndrome
- Juvenile chronic myelogenous leukemia

EPIDEMIOLOGY

- Predominant age: Median age, >65 years; uncommon in children and young adults
- Predominant sex: Male = Female

Incidence

Apparent increased incidence (1–2 per 100,000 per year) in recent years may be due to improved diagnosis; incidence increases markedly with older age.

RISK FACTORS

- Primary MDS is associated with older age, occupational exposure to petroleum solvents (benzene, gasoline), and smoking.
- Secondary (therapy-related) MDS is associated with prior treatment with alkylating agents or radiotherapy.

Genetics

- Most are clonal neoplasms by cytogenetics, G6PD isoenzyme analysis, or restriction fragment length polymorphism analysis.
- Mutations in RAS oncogene
- Mutations in *RPS14* gene on chromosome 5q

COMMONLY ASSOCIATED CONDITIONS

- Anemia
- Neutropenia
- Thrombocytopenia
- Pancytopenia
- Opportunistic infections
- Bleeding, bruising
- Sweet syndrome (neutrophilic dermatosis)

DIAGNOSIS

HISTORY

- Fatigue
- Fever
- Easy bruising

PHYSICAL EXAM

- Anemia:
  - Fatigue
  - Shortness of breath
  - Lightheadedness
  - Angina
- Leukopenia:
  - Fever
  - Infection
- Thrombocytopenia:
  - Ecchymoses
  - Petechiae
  - Epistaxis
  - Purpura
- Splenomegaly (uncommon):
  - Mild to moderate enlargement may be encountered, particularly in CMMoL.
- Skin infiltrates:
  - Sweet syndrome

DIAGNOSTIC TESTS & INTERPRETATION

- Cytogenetics (5,6)[A]:
  - At least 50% of patients with primary MDS and nearly all with t-MDS have clonal chromosomal abnormalities: +8,–7,–5, del(5q), del(7q), del(20q), iso(17), and complex karyotypes
  - Detection of clonal abnormality establishes a diagnosis of neoplasm and rules out a nutritional, toxic, or autoimmune disorder.
  - Cytogenetic analysis of metaphase cells from a bone marrow aspirate provides more information than fluorescence in situ hybridization analysis on blood cells.
- Granulocyte function tests: Abnormal in 50% (decreased myeloperoxidase activity, phagocytosis, chemotaxis, and adhesion)
- Platelet function tests: Impaired aggregation
- Marrow colony assays in vitro:
  - Results are variable and correlate poorly with clinical course.
  - Poor clonal growth may suggest more rapid evolution to AML.
- Immunophenotyping:
  - Nonspecific myeloid markers are present.
  - Occasionally, evidence can be found for concomitant lymphoproliferative disorder.
  - Loss of CD59 expression suggests paroxysmal nocturnal hemoglobinuria (PNH).

Lab

Initial lab tests

- CBC
- Review of the peripheral blood smear for the presence of dysplasia

Follow-Up & Special Considerations

- Anemia: Often macrocytic; occasional poikilocytosis, anisocytosis; variable reticulocytosis
- Granulocytopenia: Hypogranular or agranular neutrophils with poorly condensed chromatin; Pelger-Huet anomaly with hyposegmented nuclei
- Thrombocytopenia: Occasionally giant platelets or hypogranular platelets
- Fetal hemoglobin may be elevated.
- Flow cytometry to detect loss of CD59 on RBCs, CD16 on granulocytes, and CD14 on monocytes; typical of PNH.
- Direct antiglobulin (Coombs) test
- Paraprotein: Present in some
- Erythropoietin: Usually normally elevated for the degree of anemia unless renal failure is present
- Increased serum and tissue iron (ferritin), especially if anemia has been long-standing
- Serum copper level

Imaging

Liver/spleen scan or CT, although rarely necessary, may disclose occult splenomegaly or lymphadenopathy.

Diagnostic Procedures/Surgery

- Review peripheral blood smear.
- Bone marrow aspiration, biopsy, and cytogenetics

Pathological Findings

- Ineffective hematopoiesis with dysplasia in 1 or more cell lineages dominates the bone marrow picture in MDS (1).
- Marrow cellularity usually is normal or increased for the patient's age, but may be hypoplastic in ~10%.
- Reticulin fibrosis usually is minimal except in t-MDS and acute MDS with sclerosis.

- Myeloblasts may be clustered in the intertrabecular spaces with abnormal localization of immature precursors.

DIFFERENTIAL DIAGNOSIS

- Other malignant disorders:
  - Evolving AML or erythroleukemia
  - Chronic myeloproliferative disorders
  - Polycythemia vera
  - Myeloid metaplasia with myelofibrosis
  - Malignant lymphoma
  - Metastatic carcinoma
- Nonmalignant disorders:
  - Aplastic anemia
  - Autoimmune disorders (Felty syndrome, lupus, hemolytic anemia)
  - Nutritional deficiencies (vitamin B_{12}, pyridoxine, copper, protein malnutrition)
  - Heavy metal intoxication
  - Alcoholism
  - Chronic liver disease
  - Hypersplenism
  - Chronic inflammation
  - Recent cytotoxic therapy or irradiation
  - HIV infection
  - Paroxysmal nocturnal hemoglobinuria

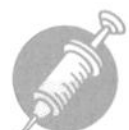

TREATMENT

MEDICATION

First Line

- Epoetin alfa or darbepoetin can increase hemoglobin levels in MDS patients who have low serum erythropoietin levels at baseline.
- Only azacitidine, decitabine, and lenalidomide have been approved by the FDA for MDS (7,8)[B].
- Azacitidine and decitabine have been proven in randomized controlled trials to be more effective for these heterogeneous disorders than supportive care with antibiotics and transfusions as needed (9,10)[A].
- Vitamins, iron, corticosteroids, androgens, or thyroid hormone are rarely helpful, unless evidence of a specific deficiency exists.
- Clinical trials show azacitidine, 75 mg/m^2 SC for 7 days and repeated every 28 days, decreases RBC transfusion requirements, yields longer times to AML or death, and improves quality of life (9)[A].
- Decitabine was approved with a continuous IV schedule that usually requires hospitalization (10)[A]. More commonly, it is given at 20 mg/m^2/d IV over 1 hour as an outpatient, repeated every 4 weeks.
- Lenalidomide, 10 mg PO daily for 21 days every 4 weeks has yielded complete remission in patients with MDS and del(5q) (2)[A]. It is less effective in patients with MDS without del(5q).
- Intensive chemotherapy:
  - Younger patients with MDS may benefit from AML chemotherapy, especially if Auer rods are present, but toxicity may be severe for older patients.
  - Remission durations are variable (median, ~1 year).
- Allogeneic hematopoietic stem cell transplantation:
  - Recommended for younger patients with human leukocyte antigen–matched donors to eradicate the malignant clone and resupply normal hematopoietic stem cells
- Aminocaproic acid (epsilon-aminocaproic acid) or tranexamic acid may benefit patients with chronic, severe thrombocytopenia and bleeding.
- Contraindications: Cytotoxicity of chemotherapy may increase the risk of bleeding and infection and the need for transfusion support.
- Precautions: Aspirin, salicylates, and NSAIDs should be avoided.

Second Line

- Danazol or prednisone may benefit concomitant autoimmune thrombocytopenia.
- Investigational agents:
  - Low doses of cytarabine, tretinoin (all-trans retinoic acid), homoharringtonine, 13-cis retinoic acid, arsenic trioxide, histone/protein deacetylase inhibitors, interferon, cyclosporine, antithymocyte globulin, granulocyte macrophage colony-stimulating factor or granulocyte colony-stimulating factor, and interleukin-3
  - Agents such as thalidomide that inhibit the production of tumor necrosis factor in the marrow
- Amifostine may stimulate the proliferation of normal hematopoiesis.

ADDITIONAL TREATMENT

General Measures

- Immunize for pneumococcal pneumonia and influenza and hepatitis B.
- RBC transfusions to alleviate symptoms
- Platelet transfusions only for bleeding or before surgery to avoid alloimmunization
- Early use of antibiotics for fever, even while culture results are pending, due to quantitative and qualitative granulocyte disorder
- Iron chelation therapy to avoid iron overload from chronic transfusions

Issues for Referral

- Refer younger adults for allogeneic hematopoietic cell transplantation.
- Refer patients with symptoms or transfusion requirements for clinical trials.

ONGOING CARE

FOLLOW-UP RECOMMENDATIONS

Usually outpatient except when necessary to hospitalize for the treatment of infection, blood transfusions, or intensive chemotherapy

Patient Monitoring

- At least monthly during supportive care
- More frequently if receiving treatment

DIET

Reduce alcohol use and iron intake (unless patient is iron deficient).

PATIENT EDUCATION

- Stop smoking.
- Seek early medical attention for fever, bleeding, or symptoms of anemia.
- Advise about the risks of chronic transfusion therapy.

PROGNOSIS

- Median survival for RA and RARS is 5 years, but it may extend much longer.
- RA with del(5q) syndrome is quite favorable (2).
- Median survival for RAEB, RCMD, and CMMoL is ~1 year; 50% of patients evolve to AML and the other 50% die of infection or bleeding.

COMPLICATIONS

- Infection
- Bleeding
- Complications of anemia and transfusions

REFERENCES

1. Swerdlow SH, Campo E, Harris NL, et al., eds. *WHO Classification of Tumours of Haematopoietic and Lymphoid Tissues*. Lyon, France: IARC Press; 2008.
2. List A, Dewald G, Bennett J, et al. Lenalidomide in the myelodysplastic syndrome with chromosome 5q deletion. *N Engl J Med*. 2006;355:1456–65.
3. Singh ZN, Huo D, Anastasi J, et al. Therapyrelated myelodysplastic syndrome: Morphologic subclassification may not be clinically relevant. *Am J Clin Pathol*. 2007;127:197–205.
4. Larson RA, Le Beau MM. Therapy-related myeloid leukaemia: A model for leukemogenesis in humans. *Chem Biol Interact*. 2005;153–54: 187–95.
5. Greenberg P, Cox C, LeBeau MM, et al. International scoring system for evaluating prognosis in myelodysplastic syndromes. *Blood*. 1997;89:2079–88.
6. Cheson BD, Greenberg PL, Bennett JM, et al. Clinical application and proposal for modification of the International Working Group (IWG) response criteria in myelodysplasia. *Blood*. 2006; 108:419–25.
7. Larson RA. Myelodysplasia: When to treat and how. *Best Pract Res Clin Haematol*. 2006;19: 293–300.
8. Greenberg PL, Attar E, Battiwalla M, et al. Myelodysplastic syndromes. *J Natl Compr Canc Netw*. 2008;6:902–26.
9. Silverman LR, Demakos EP, Peterson BL, et al. Randomized controlled trial of azacitidine in patients with the myelodysplastic syndrome: A study of the cancer and leukemia group B. *J Clin Oncol*. 2002;20:2429–40.
10. Kantarjian H, Issa JP, Rosenfeld CS, et al. Decitabine improves patient outcomes in myelodysplastic syndromes: Results of a phase III randomized study. *Cancer*. 2006;106:1794–803.

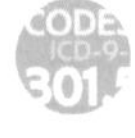

CODES

ICD9

- 238.72 Low grade myelodysplastic syndrome lesions
- 238.75 Myelodysplastic syndrome, unspecified
- 285.0 Sideroblastic anemia

CLINICAL PEARLS

- MDSs constitute a heterogeneous group of acquired, hematopoietic stem-cell disorders characterized by cytologic dysplasia in the bone marrow and blood and by various combinations of anemia, neutropenia, and thrombocytopenia.
- The natural progression of disease evolves as cellular maturation becomes more arrested and blast cells accumulate.
- Initial lab: CBC with differential and review of peripheral smear for dysplasia

MYELOPROLIFERATIVE NEOPLASMS

Daniel J. Shaheen, PharmD
Gerald Gehr, MD

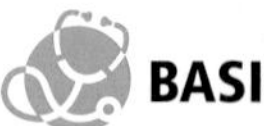

BASICS

DESCRIPTION

- Over 60 years ago William Dameshek recognized similarities in clinical features and bone marrow morphology between a group of disorders he termed myeloproliferative disorders (MPD).
- In 2008, the World Health Organization (WHO) revised the classification of myeloproliferative disorders to myeloproliferative neoplasms (MPNs) (1).
- This includes the "classic" MPNs: Chronic myelogenous leukemia ([CML], positive for *BCR-ABL1* [Philadelphia (Ph) chromosome]); polycythemia vera (PV); essential thrombocythemia (ET); and primary myelofibrosis (PMF). Also the classification now includes the "nonclassic" conditions of chronic neutrophilic leukemia (CNL), chronic eosinophilic leukemia not otherwise specified (CEL-NOS), systemic mastocytosis (SM), and myeloproliferative neoplasm unclassifiable (MPN-u).
- With each disorder, the proliferation of a particular cell line tends to dominate. These disorders can mimic one another; CML is the only one that is readily distinguished by the Ph chromosome.
- CML: Characterized by splenomegaly, hepatomegaly, night sweats, and increased granulocytes; runs a generally mild course (*chronic phase*) until it transforms to a frankly leukemic phase (*accelerated phase → blast crisis*); predilection for the elderly
- PV: Characterized by erythrocytosis, though patients may exhibit increased splenomegaly and bone marrow fibrosis consistent with myelofibrosis
- PMF: Usually has a severe course, and unlike PV and ET, survival is usually reduced
- ET: Dominated by markedly elevated platelets; may transform into AML
- CNL: Marked by neutrophilic leukocytosis; predilection for the elderly; and absence of *BCR-ABL* (Ph chromosome).
- CEL-NOS: Characterized by the abnormal proliferation of eosinophil precursors with 5–19% myeloblasts in the bone marrow or >2% in blood
- SM: Almost always involves bone marrow; characterized by aggregates of abnormal mast cells; serum elevations of tryptase can be a useful marker; the *KIT* D816V mutation is usually present
- System(s) affected: Hematologic/Immunologic

EPIDEMIOLOGY

Incidence

Overall, the classic MPNs have a cumulative incidence of ~4–5/100,000 per year (2010):

- CML: 1.6/100,000 per year; median age at diagnosis 65 years; male > female (1.6:1)
- PMF: 0.5–1.5/100,000 per year; median age at diagnosis 60 years; male = female
- ET: 0.8/100,000 per year; median age at diagnosis 60 years, though second peak of ET in younger patients at ~30 years; female > male (1.4:1)
- PV: 1/100,000 per year; male > female (1.3:1)

RISK FACTORS

- Family history of MPNs or *JAK2* V617F gene mutation
- CML: Exposure to ionizing radiation

Genetics

Cytogenetics (2,3):

- CML is defined by the *BCR-ABL1* gene (99%). This is the result of fusion between genes *BCR and ABL1*. The fusion is most often caused by the translocation of chromosomes 9 and 22, and results in an abnormal chromosome 22 (Ph chromosome).
- The other classic MPNs are collectively known as BCR-ABL1-negative MPNs; a single mutation in the Janus kinase 2 (*JAK2* V617F) gene is the most prevalent mutation found in this group (96% in PV, 65% in PMF, and 55% in ET).
- A somatic mutation in the myeloproliferative leukemia virus (*MPL*) gene has been described in 10% of PMF patients and in 3% of ET patients.
  - Some patients may have multiple *MPL* mutations or even co-occurrence with *JAK2* V617F.
- Patients with SM may have mutations of *KIT* and/or *PDGFRA*; rates have not been characterized yet.
- TET oncogene family member 2 (*TET2*) mutations have been described in classic as well as in nonclassic MPNs, though with limited prognostic utility.

PATHOPHYSIOLOGY

- MPNs are characterized by increasing amounts of myeloid lineage cells without dyserythropoiesis, monocytosis, or granulocytic dysplasia.
- More recently, mutant tyrosine kinases, specifically *JAK2* V617F, as well as mutations in *KIT, MPL,PDGFRA, and TET2,* were identified for the MPNs. These mutations induce unregulated tyrosine kinase activity, which can result in massive cell proliferation and the inhibition of apoptosis.

ETIOLOGY

Unknown; familial component described in PV, ET, and PMF; if *JAK2* and *MPL* mutations, consider familial testing

COMMONLY ASSOCIATED CONDITIONS

- Clonal evolution into acute myeloid leukemia; most common with CML
- Thrombosis/bleeding
- Immunologic abnormalities reported with PMF, including antinuclear antibodies, elevated rheumatoid factor titers, and Coombs positivity

DIAGNOSIS

HISTORY

- A history of abdominal pain or fullness, bruising, bleeding, thrombosis, bone/joint pain, fevers, jaundice, and/or ascites
- Thromboses in the venous system may occur, including deep venous thrombosis or mesenteric thrombosis. Portal vein thrombosis may cause Budd-Chiari syndrome.
- Most thrombotic events occur about 2 years before diagnosis.

PHYSICAL EXAM

- General: Hypermetabolic state (fever, sweating), acute gouty arthritis, fatigue, splenomegaly, skin findings (e.g., petechiae, jaundice)
- CML: Splenomegaly (>75% of patients), hepatomegaly, abdominal pain
- PV: Pruritus, headache, weakness, erythromelalgia
- PMF: Severe fatigue, splenomegaly in virtually all patients, hepatomegaly in ~50%, lymph node enlargement, jaundice, edema, and ascites
- ET: May have no symptoms or findings in >50% patients; for other patients, easy bruising, transient ischemic attacks, or even frank strokes may occur, as well as a higher incidence of cardiovascular events

DIAGNOSTIC TESTS & INTERPRETATION

Lab

- Genotyping for *JAK2* V617F mutation. Positive results make PV, ET, or PMF very likely. If negative, PV is unlikely, but ET or PMF are still possible, so testing for the *MPL* mutation is recommended.
- CML: The presence of *BCR-ABL1* is diagnostic. Marked leukocytosis. CML is characterized by 3 phases: Chronic, acute, and blast crisis with peripheral blood and bone marrow blast cell levels of <10%, 10–19%, and >20%, respectively. Elevated serum vitamin B_{12} level. Elevated lactate dehydrogenase. Hyperuricemia. Markedly decreased leukocyte alkaline phosphatase (LAP) (absent in 5–10%). Platelet count may be normal or elevated.
- PMF (1,2) (WHO criteria): Diagnosis requires meeting all 3 major criteria and 2 minor criteria:
  - *Major criteria:* 1. Megakaryocyte proliferation and atypia accompanied by either reticulin or collagen fibrosis; 2. Not meeting WHO criteria for CML, PV, MDS, or other myeloid neoplasm; 3. Demonstration of *JAK2* V617F or other clonal marker or absence of marker with no evidence of secondary marrow fibrosis
  - *Minor criteria:* 1. Leukoerythroblastosis; 2. Increased serum LDH level; 3. Anemia; 4. Palpable splenomegaly
- ET (1,2) (WHO criteria): Diagnosis requires meeting all 4 major criteria:
  - *Major criteria:* 1. Thrombocytosis with persistent level ≥450,000 platelets/L; 2. Megakaryocyte proliferation with large and mature morphology; 3. Not meeting WHO criteria for CML, PV, PMF, MDS, or other myeloid neoplasm; 4. Demonstration of *JAK2* V617F or other clonal marker or absence of clonal marker with no evidence of reactive thrombocytosis
  - Bone marrow biopsy showing increased numbers of enlarged, mature megakaryocytes
  - ~60–70% will have *MPL* or *JAK2* V617F mutation; absence of the Ph chromosome
- PV (1,2) (WHO criteria): Diagnosis requires either both major criteria and 1 minor criterion or the first major criterion and 2 of the minor criteria:
  - *Major criteria:* 1. Hemoglobin>18.5 g/dL in men, >16.5 g/dL in women or other evidence of increased red cell volume; 2. Presence of *JAK2* V617F or other functionally similar mutation (e.g., *JAK2* exon 12 mutation)
  - *Minor criteria:* 1. Bone marrow biopsy showing hypercellularity for age with trilineage myeloproliferation; 2. Subnormal serum erythropoietin (Epo) level; 3. Endogenous erythroid colony formation

Initial lab tests
For clinical suspicion, obtain a peripheral blood smear; if positive, consider a bone marrow test.

Imaging
- PMF: Radiographic osteosclerosis in 25–66% of patients
- ET: Imaging may be necessary for confirmation of venous thromboses (usually mesenteric, lower extremity, or hepatic).

Diagnostic Procedures/Surgery
Cytogenetic and molecular studies: RT-PCR to detect *BCR-ABL1*, *MPL*, or *JAK2* V617F mutations

Pathological Findings
- PMF: Bone marrow megakaryocytic hyperplasia and atypia, reticulin and/or collagen fibrosis, osteosclerosis (new bone formation); foci of extramedullary hematopoiesis may be seen at multiple sites (e.g., spleen, liver, kidneys, lymph nodes, lungs, and spinal column); leukoerythroblastosis; anemia
- ET: Bone marrow proliferation of megakaryocytic lineage

DIFFERENTIAL DIAGNOSIS
- CML: Leukemoid reaction (low or absent LAP, which is also seen in paroxysmal nocturnal hemoglobinuria); chronic myelomonocytic leukemia (CMML)
- PMF: Spent PV (late stage of PV), CML-secondary myelofibrosis
- ET: Secondary thrombocytosis (inflammation, iron deficiency, and neoplasia), PV, CML
- PV: Other neoplasias known to cause erythrocytosis; hypoxemia secondary to other causes

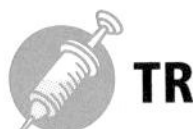

TREATMENT

MEDICATION
First Line
- CML (4,5) (see "Leukemia, Chronic Myelogenous"):
  - Imatinib mesylate (Gleevec): 400 mg daily, a potent inhibitor of the ABL tyrosine kinase
  - Allogeneic stem cell transplant
- PV and ET (6,7): The goal of therapy is to prevent thrombohemorrhagic complications, not to cure:
  - Evidence supports the antithrombotic benefit of low-dose aspirin in PV, while its use in ET is generally accepted provided an absence of contraindications.
  - Hydroxyurea is typically used to control thrombocytosis in high-risk ET/PV patients. Thrombosis risk is reduced by controlling the WBC count within the low normal range.
  - IFN-α or busulfan is considered for those who have resistance or an intolerance to hydroxyurea. IFN-α can also be used for pregnant patients.
- PMF (7,8): Therapy is indicated for the treatment of anemia and symptomatic splenomegaly:
  - Anemia is often treated with androgenic steroids: fluoxymesterone, 10 mg t.i.d.; testosterone enanthate, 400–600 mg IM weekly; prednisone, (0.5–1 mg/kg/d).
  - Hydroxyurea is useful for controlling splenomegaly and thrombocytosis.
  - Allogeneic bone marrow transplantation is the only intervention known to prolong survival for patients with PMF.
- Promising therapies for classic MPNs involve molecular targeting of *JAK2*.

Second Line
- CML (5): Tyrosine kinase inhibitors; Nilotinib, 300 mg b.i.d.; or Dasatinib, 100 mg daily
- PMF: Androgens and glucocorticoids may improve anemia. Corticosteroids can be used if autoimmune hemolysis is present.

ADDITIONAL TREATMENT
General Measures
- Splenectomy has no impact on mortality but is occasionally carried out for symptomatic relief. Extreme thrombocytosis and progressive and massive liver enlargement may ensue.
- CML: Molecularly targeted therapy (with imatinib); chemotherapy (for advanced disease). Bone marrow transplantation is the only known curative option.
- PMF: No standard therapy; rule out other treatable causes for anemia. Radiotherapy for symptomatic tumors or symptomatic splenomegaly. Successful bone marrow transplantation can lead to the reversal of established fibrosis.
- ET: Young, asymptomatic patients with platelet counts of $<1,500,000/\mu L$ usually are not treated. Lower the platelet count in those >60 years of age with a history of cardiovascular risk factors or if the platelet count >1,500,000/L.

Issues for Referral
Usually comanaged with the guidance of a hematologist/oncologist; surgical oncology, radiation oncology, and palliative care

Additional Therapies
Massive splenomegaly or foci of extramedullary hematopoiesis may require palliative radiation.

SURGERY/OTHER PROCEDURES
No role unless for splenectomy or relief of organ compression by foci of hematopoiesis in PMF

IN-PATIENT CONSIDERATIONS
Initial Stabilization
Treatment to relieve symptoms and prevent infections

Admission Criteria
Severe cachexia; extramedullary hematopoiesis and sequelae, including renal failure and hepatomegaly; severe splenomegaly necessitating treatment; severe bleeding; petechiae; anemia

IV Fluids
Hydration status should be kept optimized during hospitalization to prevent tumor lysis syndrome.

Nursing
Comfort measures such as pain control

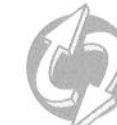

ONGOING CARE

FOLLOW-UP RECOMMENDATIONS
Restrictions depend on the symptoms.

PROGNOSIS
- CML: Median survival is >5 years from the time of diagnosis; 85% will die in blast crisis. Pregnancy does not affect the course of the disease; >95% of mothers survive to delivery.
- PMF: Progressive splenomegaly, anemia. Median survival is 5 years from the time of diagnosis, and about 30% lower than in matched controls. Patients usually die from hemorrhagic or thrombotic complications and infections.
- ET/PV: Near-normal life expectancy

COMPLICATIONS
- Transformation to acute leukemia, gout, or nephropathy owing to hyperuricemia
- PMF: Portal hypertension, splenic infarcts, Budd-Chiari syndrome, pulmonary hypertension
- ET: Thrombohemorrhagic complications in 1/3 of patients; erythromelalgia (a vasoocclusive syndrome with localized pain of distal extremities); first-trimester abortion; medication-related side effects

REFERENCES

1. Wadleigh M, Tefferi A. Classification and diagnosis of myeloproliferative neoplasms according to the 2008 World Health Organization criteria. *Int J Hematol*. 2010;91:174–9.
2. Tefferi A, Vainchenker W, et al. Myeloproliferative neoplasms: Molecular pathophysiology, essential clinical understanding, and treatment strategies. *J Clin Oncol*. 2011;29:573–82.
3. Tefferi A, et al. Novel mutations and their functional and clinical relevance in myeloproliferative neoplasms: JAK2, MPL, TET2, ASXL1, CBL, IDH and IKZF1. *Leukemia*. 2010;24:1128–38.
4. Levine RL, Gilliland DG. Myeloproliferative disorders. *Blood*. 2008;112:2190–8.
5. NCCN clinical practice guidelines in oncology: *Chronic Myelogenous Leukemia*. Fort Washington, PA: National Comprehensive Cancer Network, 2011. (Accessed August 11, 2011 at www.nccn.org/professionals/physician_gls/pdf/cml.pdf).
6. Squizzato A, Romualdi E, Middeldorp S, et al. Antiplatelet drugs for polycythaemia vera and essential thrombocythaemia. *Cochrane Database Syst Rev*. 2008;CD006503.
7. Tefferi A, et al. Essential thrombocythemia, polycythemia vera, and myelofibrosis: Current management and the prospect of targeted therapy. *Am J Hematol*. 2008;83:491–7.
8. Mesa RA. New drugs for the treatment of myelofibrosis. *Curr Hematol Malig Rep*. 2010;5:15–21.

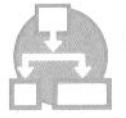

See Also (Topic, Algorithm, Electronic Media Element)

Leukemia, Chronic Myelogenous; Polycythemia Vera

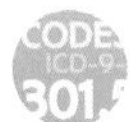

CODES

ICD9
- 205.10 Myeloid leukemia, chronic, without mention of having achieved remission
- 238.4 Polycythemia vera
- 238.79 Neoplasm of uncertain behavior of other lymphatic and hematopoietic tissues

CLINICAL PEARLS
- CML, characterized by splenomegaly and increased granulocytes, runs a generally mild course until it transforms to a frankly leukemic phase and is positive for BCR-ABL, the Ph chromosome.
- Splenectomy has no impact on mortality but is occasionally carried out for symptomatic relief. Extreme thrombocytosis and progressive and massive liver enlargement may ensue.

MYOCARDIAL INFARCTION, NON–ST-SEGMENT ELEVATION (NSTEMI)

Samuel Joffe, MD
Matthew McGuiness, MD

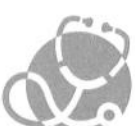

BASICS

DESCRIPTION
- Non–ST-segment elevation myocardial infarction (NSTEMI) is an acute coronary syndrome (ACS) defined by the presence of elevated cardiac biomarkers, typically Troponin or MB fraction of creatinine kinase (CKMB), together with the absence of ST-segment elevations on ECG.
- NSTEMI typically presents with anginal symptoms as well as ST-segment depressions and/or T-wave inversions on ECG.
- Elevated cardiac biomarkers may not be detectable for several hours following the onset of symptoms.

EPIDEMIOLOGY
- Incidence increases with age (1).
- Men > Women. Presentation in women is on average 10 years later.

Incidence
- Of 1.57 million annual ACS admissions in the US, ~570,000 have a discharge diagnosis of NSTEMI.
- Incidence ~190 per 100,000 per year

Prevalence
- ~7.5 million people in the US are affected by MI.
- Prevalence 2,500 per 100,000 (2.5%)

RISK FACTORS
- Age
- Hypertension
- Tobacco use
- Diabetes mellitus
- Dyslipidemia
- Family history of early coronary artery disease (CAD)
- Sedentary lifestyle
- Overweight/obesity

GENERAL PREVENTION
- Smoking cessation, healthy diet, weight control, physical activity
- If risk factors are present: BP control, lipid-lowering therapy, daily aspirin (in select patients)

PATHOPHYSIOLOGY
NSTEMI is usually caused by acute rupture of an atherosclerotic plaque, causing thrombosis and partial or total occlusion of a coronary artery.

ETIOLOGY
- Platelet-rich thrombus on a disrupted plaque is the most common cause.
- Coronary vasospasm, often caused by cocaine or methamphetamine abuse
- Dynamic obstruction (coronary spasm, vasoconstriction, muscle bridge)
- Progressive mechanical limitation of coronary flow
- Coronary arterial inflammation
- Coronary dissection/rupture and thrombogenesis
- Myocardial oxygen demand exceeds supply

COMMONLY ASSOCIATED CONDITIONS
- Abdominal aortic aneurysm
- Carotid disease
- Peripheral vascular disease

DIAGNOSIS

HISTORY
- Chest heaviness/tightness, with or without exertion
- Pain or discomfort radiating to the neck, jaw, interscapular area, upper extremities, or epigastrium
- Associated symptoms of dyspnea, nausea, diaphoresis, light-headedness, dysphoria
- History of myocardial ischemia (stable or unstable angina, MI, coronary bypass surgery, or percutaneous coronary intervention [PCI])
- Family history of CAD or MI
- Risk factors for CAD and bleeding
- Use of phosphodiesterase-5 inhibitors and concomitant nitrates
- Use of cocaine or amphetamines
- Medications and recent medication changes

PHYSICAL EXAM
- General: Abnormal vital signs including tachycardia or bradycardia, hypertension or hypotension, widened pulse pressure, tachypnea, fever
- Neuro: Dizziness, syncope, fatigue, weakness, altered mental status
- Cardiovascular: Dysrhythmia, jugular venous distention (JVD), new murmur, rub or gallop
- Respiratory: Tachypnea, increased work of breathing, crackles
- Musculoskeletal: Sharp pain reproducible with movement or palpation is unlikely to be cardiac
- Skin: Cool skin, pallor, diaphoresis

Geriatric Considerations
Elderly patients as well as women and those with diabetes may have an atypical presentation without classic anginal symptoms.

DIAGNOSTIC TESTS & INTERPRETATION

Lab

Initial lab tests
- 12-lead ECG (2)[A]:
  - ST-segment depression and/or T-wave inversion:
    - ≥1-mm ST depression in ≥2 contiguous leads
    - T-wave inversions, other changes
    - ST depression and/or tall R-wave in V1/V2 with upright T waves may indicate transmural STEMI of posterior wall.
    - If initial ECG nondiagnostic but symptoms persist with suspicion for ACS, perform serial ECGs at 15–30-minute intervals (2).
- Serum biomarkers:
  - NSTEMI is strictly defined as elevated serum biomarkers (usually Troponin) exceeding the 99th percentile of a normal reference population in the absence of evidence of STEMI.
  - Troponin concentration rises 3–6 hours after onset of ischemic symptoms.
  - CK-MB increases 3–4 hours after onset of myocardial injury.
  - Myoglobin: Early marker for myocardial necrosis. Increases 2 hours after onset of myocardial necrosis.
  - Patients with negative biomarkers within 6 hours of the onset of symptoms should have biomarkers remeasured 8–12 hours from onset of symptoms (2)[B].

Follow-Up & Special Considerations
- Fasting lipid profile
- CBC, basic metabolic panel, activated partial thromboplastin time (aPTT)
- Other laboratory tests:
  - Lactate dehydrogenase: Increases within 24 hours, peaks 3–6 days, baseline 8–12 days (not routinely ordered)
  - Leukocytes: Increase within several hours after MI, peak in 2–4 days
  - Brain natriuretic peptide (BNP): Increases with MI, may not indicate heart failure

Pregnancy Considerations
Findings mimicking NSTEMI in pregnancy: ST depression after anesthesia, increase in CK-MB after delivery, and mild increase in troponin in preeclampsia and gestational hypertension. Spontaneous coronary dissection is a rare cause of ST elevation in pregnancy.

Imaging

Initial approach
- Chest x-ray
- Consider transthoracic echocardiography if not recently performed (2)[B].

Diagnostic Procedures/Surgery
- Coronary angiography (discussed below under "Treatment")
- If serial cardiac enzymes are negative and symptoms have resolved, consider stress testing including either standard exercise treadmill test (ETT), stress echocardiography, or stress nuclear study (2)[B].
- Transesophageal echocardiography, contrast chest CT scan, or MRI generally reserved for differentiating STEMI and other causes of chest pain from aortic dissection.

Pathological Findings
- Subendocardial myocardial necrosis may be present.
- Atherosclerosis

DIFFERENTIAL DIAGNOSIS
- Unstable angina (presentation similar to NSTEMI but with negative biomarkers)
- Aortic dissection
- Pulmonary embolism
- Pleuropericarditis
- Perforating ulcer
- Gastroesophageal reflux disease (GERD) and spasm
- Biliary or pancreatic pain
- Dysrhythmia

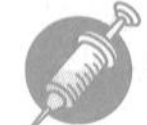

TREATMENT

MEDICATION

First Line
- Aspirin, nonenteric-coated, initial dose of 162–325 mg PO or chewed (2)[A]
- For ASA-intolerant patients as well as patients planned for PCI who are not at high risk for complex disease requiring coronary artery bypass graft (CABG) surgery, administer clopidogrel loading dose 300–600 mg followed by 75 mg daily (2)[A], or prasugrel loading dose 60 mg followed by 10 mg daily (2)[B].

- Nitroglycerin sublingual 0.4 mg q5min for total of 3 doses, then assess need for IV NTG (2)[C]
- Supplemental oxygen 2–4 L/min, maintaining arterial oxygen saturation >90% (2)[B]
- Morphine sulfate 2–4 mg IV (with increments of 2–8 mg IV repeated at 5–15-minute intervals (2)[A]
- Oral beta-blocker (cardioselective agent such as metoprolol or atenolol preferred) if no contraindication (2)[B]
- Risk stratify using the TIMI or GRACE score to select use of early invasive approach (within 12–24 hours of admission) vs. medical therapy.
- Risks and benefits of the early invasive approach:
  - 33% relative risk reduction for both the endpoints of refractory angina and rehospitalization at 6–12 months (3)[A]
  - 27% and 22% relative risk reduction in rates of MI at 6–12 months and 3–5 years, respectively (3)[A]
  - Doubled risk of procedure-related MI and increased risk of minor periprocedural bleeding (2)[A].
- Invasive management: Benefits more pronounced in higher-risk patients, such as those with ECG changes or diabetes (3)[A]. (Subsequent recommendations all (2): For patients with elevated risk for clinical events or refractory angina or hemodynamic or electrical instability, initiate anticoagulant: Enoxaparin or unfractionated heparin (UFH) or bivalirudin. Prior to angiography, add GP IIb/IIIa inhibitor (eptifibatide or tirofiban) or thienopyridine (clopidogrel or prasugrel). Use both agents in patients for whom PCI is planned or who are at high risk for recurrent ischemia or delayed angiography.
- Medical management: For low-risk or selected intermediate-risk patients; based on patient or physician preference; or in chronic renal insufficiency stage IV: Initiate anticoagulant therapy: Enoxaparin or UFH or fondaparinux; enoxaparin or fondaparinux preferable. Initiate clopidogrel or prasugrel.
- Contraindications: Prasugrel is contraindicated in patients over 75 or those with history of CVA/TIA or increased bleeding risk. Enoxaparin is contraindicated in patients with renal insufficiency.

Second Line

- ACE inhibitor in patients with pulmonary congestion or left ventricular ejection fraction (EF) ≤40%. Substitute angiotensin receptor blocker (ARB) for ACE-intolerant patients (2)[A].
- Nondihydropyridine calcium channel blocker (CCB) (verapamil or diltiazem) to reduce myocardial oxygen demand when beta-blockers are contraindicated if normal EF (2)[B]. Use oral long-acting CCB only after beta-blockers and nitrates have been fully used (2)[C].
- Long-term nitrate therapy for recurrent angina/ischemia or heart failure (2)[C]
- Sublingual NTG at discharge (2)[C]
- Lipid-lowering therapy: High-dose statin (preferred due to nonlipid benefit on vascular function) (2)[A], niacin, or fibrate (2)[C]

ADDITIONAL TREATMENT

General Measures

- Bed/chair rest with continuous ECG monitoring
- Antiarrhythmics as needed
- Anxiolytics as needed
- Deep vein thrombosis prophylaxis
- Continuation of aspirin, clopidogrel or prasugrel, beta-blockers, ACE inhibitors (or ARBs if ACE-intolerant), lipid-lowering therapy
- Tight BP control
- Treatment for depression PRN (common post-MI)
- Cardiac rehabilitation and increased physical activity
- Smoking cessation
- Annual influenza vaccine

Issues for Referral

Cardiology consultation usually appropriate

SURGERY/OTHER PROCEDURES

- Coronary reperfusion:
  - PCI with stent placement
  - Coronary artery bypass graft (CABG) surgery
- Intra-aortic balloon pump for severe ischemia, hypotension, refractory pain

IN-PATIENT CONSIDERATIONS

Initial Stabilization

Bed rest with continuous ECG monitoring, assess for reperfusion therapy, relieve ischemic pain, treat life-threatening complications, admit to coronary care unit.

Admission Criteria

All patients with definite or suspected acute MI, ongoing pain, positive cardiac markers, ST deviations, hemodynamic abnormalities, probable or definite acute coronary syndrome (ACS)

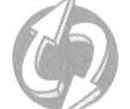

ONGOING CARE

FOLLOW-UP RECOMMENDATIONS

- Follow-up within 2–6 weeks (low risk) and 14 days (high risk).
- Refer to cardiac rehabilitation.

DIET

- Diet low in saturated fat, cholesterol, and sodium
- Request dietary consult

PATIENT EDUCATION

- Education on new medications, diet, exercise, smoking cessation, lifestyle modification
- Resume exercise, sexual activity after outpatient re-evaluation

PROGNOSIS

NSTEMI patients have a lower inhospital mortality than those with STEMI, but a similar or worse long-term outcome.

COMPLICATIONS

- Cardiogenic shock
- Heart failure
- Myocardial rupture
- Ventricular aneurysm
- Dysrhythmia
- Acute pulmonary embolism
- Acute thromboembolic stroke
- Pericarditis/Dressler syndrome
- Depression (increases mortality risk)
- Hyperglycemia

REFERENCES

1. *Heart Disease and Stroke Statistics 2008 Update*. Dallas, TX: American Heart Association, 2008.
2. Anderson JL, Adams CD, Antman EM, et al. 2011 ACCF/AHA Focused Update Incorporated Into the ACC/AHA 2007 Guidelines for the Management of Patients With Unstable Angina/Non-ST-Elevation Myocardial Infarction: A report of the American College of Cardiology Foundation/American Heart Association Task Force on Practice Guidelines. *Circulation*. 2011;123:e426–579.
3. Hoenig MR, Aroney CN, Scott IA. Early invasive versus conservative strategies for unstable angina and non-ST elevation myocardial infarction in the stent era (review). *Cochrane Database Syst Rev*. 2010;3.

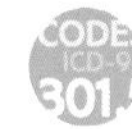

CODES

ICD9

- 410.70 Subendocardial infarction, episode of care unspecified
- 410.71 Subendocardial infarction, initial episode of care
- 410.72 Subendocardial infarction, subsequent episode of care

CLINICAL PEARLS

- Discontinue NSAIDs, nonselective or selective cyclooxygenase (COX)-2 agents, except for ASA, due to increased risks of mortality, reinfarction, hypertension, heart failure, and myocardial rupture.
- Discontinue clopidogrel or prasugrel 5–7 days before elective CABG.
- Do not use nitrate products in patients who recently used a phosphodiesterase-5 inhibitor (24 hours of sildenafil or 48 hours of tadalafil).
- Duration of antithrombotic therapy after NSTEMI is dependent on type of stent received and medications administered.
- In right ventricular infarctions, avoid nitrates and other BP-lowering medications, administer IV fluids aggressively for hypotension, consider the possibility of bradycardia and need for atropine and temporary pacing.
- Avoid beta-blockers in cocaine users.

MYOCARDIAL INFARCTION, ST-SEGMENT ELEVATION (STEMI)

Fae G. Wooding, PharmD
Ivan A. Arenas, MD, PhD
Juyong Lee, MD, PhD

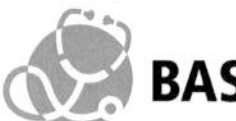

BASICS

DESCRIPTION

Acute myocardial infarction (AMI) is the rapid development of myocardial necrosis resulting from a sustained and complete absence of blood flow to a portion of the myocardium. ST-segment elevation myocardial infarction (STEMI) occurs when coronary blood flow ceases following thrombotic occlusion of a coronary artery (usually) affected by atherosclerosis, causing transmural ischemia. This is accompanied by release of serum cardiac biomarkers and ST elevation (and likely a Q wave when infarction occurs) on an ECG.

EPIDEMIOLOGY

Incidence

In the US, estimated annual incidence of MI is 600,000 new and 320,000 recurrent attacks.

Prevalence

- Leading cause of morbidity and mortality in the US
- ~7.5 million people in the US are affected by MI.
- Prevalence increases with age and is higher in men (5.5%) than women (2.9%).

RISK FACTORS

Advancing age, hypertension, tobacco use, diabetes mellitus, dyslipidemia, family history of premature onset of coronary artery disease (CAD), sedentary lifestyle

GENERAL PREVENTION

Smoking cessation, consume healthy diet, weight control, regular physical activity, maintain goal BP

PATHOPHYSIOLOGY

Atherosclerotic lesions may be smooth and concentric or rough, eccentric, and fissured. Plaques that are rough and eccentric are more unstable, thrombogenic, and prone to rupture.

ETIOLOGY

- Atherosclerotic coronary artery disease
- Nonatherosclerotic:
  - Emboli: For example, thrombi from left ventricle or atrium
  - Mechanical obstruction: Chest trauma, dissection of aorta or coronary arteries
  - Increased vasomotor tone, variant angina
  - Arteritis, others: Hematologic (DIC), aortic stenosis, cocaine, IV drug use, severe burns, prolonged hypotension

COMMONLY ASSOCIATED CONDITIONS

Abdominal aortic aneurysm, extracranial cerebrovascular disease, atherosclerotic peripheral vascular disease

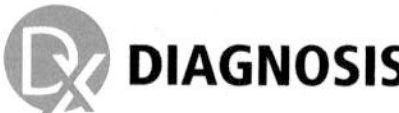

DIAGNOSIS

HISTORY

- Classically, sudden-onset chest heaviness/tightness, with or without exertion, lasting at least minutes
- Pain or discomfort radiating to neck, jaw, interscapular area, upper extremities, and epigastrium
- Previous history of myocardial ischemia (stable or unstable angina, MI, coronary bypass surgery, or percutaneous coronary intervention [PCI])
- Assess risk factors for CAD, history of bleeding, noncardiac surgery, family history of premature CAD
- Medications: Phosphodiesterase-5 inhibitors (if recent use, avoid concomitant nitrates)
- Alcohol and drug abuse (especially cocaine)

PHYSICAL EXAM

- General: Restless, agitated, hypothermia, fever
- Neuro: Dizziness, syncope, fatigue, asthenia, disorientation (especially in the elderly)
- Cerebrovascular (CV): Dysrhythmia, hypotension, widened pulse pressure, S3 and S4, jugular venous distention (JVD)
- Respiratory: Dyspnea, tachypnea, crackles
- GI: Abdominal pain, nausea, vomiting
- Musculoskeletal: Pain in neck, back, shoulder, or upper limbs
- Skin: Cool skin, pallor, diaphoresis

Geriatric Considerations

Elderly patients may have an atypical presentation, including silent or unrecognized MI, often with complaints of syncope, weakness, shortness of breath, unexplained nausea, epigastric pain, altered mental status, or dementia. Patients with diabetes mellitus may have fewer and less dramatic chest symptoms.

DIAGNOSTIC TESTS & INTERPRETATION

Lab

Initial lab tests

- Coronary angiography
- 12-lead ECG: ST-segment elevation in a regional pattern $\geq$1 mm ST elevation, with or without abnormal Q waves. ST depression $\pm$ tall R wave in V1/V2 may be STEMI of posterior wall. Absence of Q waves represent partial or transient occlusion or early infarction. New ST- or T-wave changes indicative of myocardial ischemia or injury. Consider right-sided and posterior chest leads if inferior MI pattern (V3R, V4R, V7-V9).

Follow-Up & Special Considerations

- Serum biomarkers:
  - Troponin I and T (cTnI, cTnT) rise 3–6 hours after onset of ischemic symptoms. Elevations in cTnI persist for 7–10 days, while those in cTnT persist for 10–14 days after MI.
  - Myoglobin fraction of creatine kinase (CK-MB): Rises 3–4 hours after onset of myocardial injury; peaks at 12–24 hours and remains elevated for 2–3 days. CK-MB adds little diagnostic value in assessment of possible ACS to troponin testing.
  - Myoglobin: Early marker for myocardial necrosis. Rises 2 hours after onset of myocardial necrosis, reaches peak at 1–4 hours, and remains elevated for 24 hours. Myoglobin adds little diagnostic value in assessment of possible ACS to troponin testing.
- Fasting lipid profile, CBC with platelets, electrolytes, magnesium, BUN, serum creatinine, and glucose. International normalized ratio (INR) if anticoagulation contemplated. Brain natriuretic peptide (BNP) is elevated in acute MI; may or may not indicate heart failure.

Pregnancy Considerations

Findings mimicking acute MI in pregnancy: ST-segment depression after anesthesia, increase in CK-MB after delivery, and mild increase in troponin I levels in preeclampsia and gestational hypertension

Imaging

Initial approach

ECG with continuous monitoring:

- 2-D and M-mode echocardiography is useful in evaluating regional wall motion in MI and left ventricular function.
- Portable echo can clarify diagnosis of STEMI if concomitant left bundle branch block (LBBB).
- Useful in assessing mechanical complications and mural thrombus

Diagnostic Procedures/Surgery

High-quality portable chest x-ray. Transthoracic and/or transesophageal echocardiography, contrast chest CT scan, or MRI may occasionally be of value acutely. Coronary angiography is definitive test.

ALERT

Isosmolar contrast medium or low-molecular-weight contrast medium other than ioxaglate or iohexol is indicated in patients with chronic kidney disease undergoing angiography who are not undergoing chronic dialysis.

Pathological Findings

Myocardial necrosis and atherosclerosis, if etiologic

DIFFERENTIAL DIAGNOSIS

Unstable angina, aortic dissection, pulmonary embolism (PE), perforating ulcer, pericarditis, dysrhythmias, gastroesophageal reflux disease (GERD) and spasm, biliary or pancreatic pain, hyperventilation syndrome

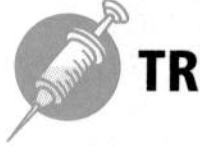

TREATMENT

MEDICATION

Medication recommendations based upon 2009 ACC/AHA focused guideline updates (1)

First Line

- Supplemental oxygen 2–4 L/min, maintaining arterial oxygen saturation >90%
- Nitroglycerin (NTG) sublingual 0.4 mg q5min for total of 3 doses, followed by nitroglycerin IV if ongoing pain and/or hypertension and/or management of pulmonary congestion
- Morphine sulfate 2–4 mg IV (with increments of 2–8 mg IV repeated at 5–15-minute intervals to relieve pain or pulmonary congestion
- Antiplatelet agents:
  - Aspirin (ASA), nonenteric-coated, initial dose 162–325 mg chewed
  - A loading dose of a thienopyridine is recommended for STEMI patients for whom PCI is planned:
    - At least 300–600 mg of clopidogrel should be given as early as possible before or at the time of primary or nonprimary PCI or

    - Prasugrel 60 mg should be given as soon as possible for primary PCI. Do not use in patients likely to undergo CABG or with active bleeding, history of TIA or stroke, or additional risk factors for bleeding (body weight <60 kg or concomitant use of medications that increase risk of bleeding). Generally not recommended for patients age ≥75 years of age.
    - Duration of therapy with a thienopyridine varies. 12 months for patients receiving drug-eluting stent (DES) during PCI for ACS. Consider earlier discontinuation if risk of morbidity due to bleeding outweighs the benefits of therapy. May continue clopidogrel or prasugrel for longer than 15 months in patients undergoing DES placement. Discontinue clopidogrel for at least 5 days or prasugrel at least 7 days prior to planned CABG.
  - For STEMI patients undergoing nonprimary PCI:
    - Continue clopidogrel in a patient who has received fibrinolytic therapy and has been given clopidogrel.
    - Administer loading dose of clopidogrel 300–600 mg if patient received a fibrinolytic without a thienopyridine, or, once the coronary anatomy is known and PCI is planned, administer a loading dose of prasugrel as soon as possible, but no later than 1 hour after PCI. Administer loading dose of clopidogrel 300 mg in patients <75 years of age who received fibrinolytic therapy or who do not receive reperfusion therapy.
    - Clopidogrel 75 mg should be given with aspirin in patients with STEMI regardless of reperfusion therapy.
- Beta-blocker (BB) within 24 hours, if no contraindications exist
- Glycoprotein IIb/IIIa receptor antagonists at time of primary PCI in selected patients: Abciximab, eptifibatide, or tirofiban
- ACE inhibitors should be initiated orally within the first 24 hours of STEMI in patients with anterior infarction or LVEF <0.40 in the absence of contraindications. Initiate ACE inhibitors within 24 hours of STEMI in all patients if no contraindications exist.
- Coronary reperfusion therapy:
  - Primary PCI:
    - If patient presents within 12 hours of symptom onset and "door-to-balloon inflation" within 90 minutes of presentation at a facility with PCI capability
    - If substantial risk for intracranial hemorrhage (ICH)
    - Age <75 with STEMI or LBBB who develop shock within 36 hours of acute MI (AMI)
    - Severe congestive heart failure and/or pulmonary edema (Killip class III)
    - Not eligible to receive fibrinolytic therapy within 12 hours of onset of symptoms
    - Patients with onset of symptoms within the prior 12–24 hours and 1 or more of the following: Severe CHF, hemodynamics or electrical instability, or persistent ischemic symptoms
- Fibrinolysis:
  - If presenting at a hospital without PCI capability and cannot be transferred to a PCI-capable facility to undergo PCI within 90 minutes of first medical contact, administer fibrinolytic therapy, "door-to-needle," within 30 minutes of presentation.
  - If no contraindications, administer within 12 hours, but not beyond 24 hours, of onset of symptoms to patients with STEMI in ≥2 contiguous leads and new or presumably new LBBB:
    - Alteplase (rt-PA): 15-mg IV bolus, followed by 0.75 mg/kg (up to 50 mg) IV over 30 minutes, then 0.5 mg/kg (up to 35 mg) over 60 minutes; max 100 mg over 90 minutes
    - Reteplase (r-PA): 10 units IV bolus over 2 minutes, give second bolus 30 minutes later
    - Tenecteplase (TNK-tPA): 30–50 mg (based on weight) IV bolus over 5–10 seconds
  - Combination reperfusion with abciximab and half-dose r-PA or TNK-tPA
  - Use anticoagulants (unfractionated heparin [UFH], enoxaparin, or fondaparinux) as ancillary therapy to reperfusion therapy for minimum 48 hours and duration of admission (up to 8 days). Avoid UFH if >48 hours of anticoagulant required: Recommend supportive anticoagulant regimens in patients proceeding to primary PCI who have been treated with ASA and thienopyridine. Administer additional boluses of UFH as needed to maintain therapeutic clotting time levels in patients who received prior treatment with UFH. Bivalirudin recommended as a supportive measure for primary PCI in patients with or without prior treatment with UFH.

Second Line

- Long-acting nondihydropyridine calcium channel blocker (CCB) when BB is ineffective or contraindicated if ejection fraction (EF) is normal
- Aldosterone receptor antagonist if already receiving therapeutic doses of an ACE inhibitor and BB. Avoid use in patients with decreased renal function.
- Lipid-lowering therapy: Statin (preferred because of additional nonlipid effects on vascular function), niacin, or fibrate

ADDITIONAL TREATMENT

General Measures

- Admit to telemetry/coronary care unit with continuous ECG monitoring and bed rest. Anxiolytics if needed. Stool softeners.
- Antiarrhythmics as needed for unstable dysrhythmia. Deep vein thrombosis (DVT) prophylaxis.
- Continuation of aspirin, clopidogrel, BB, ACE inhibitors (or ARB if ACE-intolerant), lipid-lowering therapy, tight BP control, progressively increased physical activity, smoking cessation, annual influenza vaccine
- Elicit symptoms or signs of depression and treat with an SSRI or psychotherapy if present.

Issues for Referral

Cardiac rehabilitation, neurology/neurosurgery if intracranial hemorrhage

SURGERY/OTHER PROCEDURES

Intra-aortic balloon pump for cardiogenic shock. PCI of the left main coronary artery with stents as an alternative to CABG in patients with favorable anatomy and comorbidities that may increase risk of adverse surgical outcomes if CABG chosen. Coronary artery bypass graft (CABG).

IN-PATIENT CONSIDERATIONS

Initial Stabilization

All patients with STEMI should be admitted to a CCU for evaluation and treatment. Transfer high-risk patients who receive fibrinolytic therapy as primary reperfusion therapy at a non–PCI-capable facility to a PCI-capable facility as soon as possible.

Admission Criteria

Definitive or suspected acute MI, ongoing pain, positive cardiac markers, ST deviations, hemodynamic abnormalities

IV Fluids

Right ventricular infarction may need fluid resuscitation for hypotension.

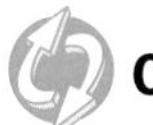

ONGOING CARE

FOLLOW-UP RECOMMENDATIONS

F/U in 3–6 weeks of d/c. Identify high-risk patients for implantable cardioverter defibrillator (ICD) placement (especially those with EF <30%).

DIET

NPO for first 4–12 hours due to risk of emesis or aspiration; request dietary consult if lipid, weight, or glucose issues

PATIENT EDUCATION

May resume sexual activity within 10 days, consistent with current exercise capacity. Driving can resume 1 week after discharge. Low-fat diet.

COMPLICATIONS

Heart failure, myocardial rupture/left ventricular aneurysm, pericarditis, dysrhythmias, acute mitral regurgitation, severe depression (common)

REFERENCE

1. Kushner FG, et al. 2009 focused updates: ACC/AHA guidelines for the management of patients with ST-elevation myocardial infarction and ACC/AHA/SCAI guidelines on percutaneous coronary intervention. *J Am Coll Cardiol*. 2009;54: 2205–41.

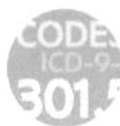

CODES

ICD9

- 410.90 Acute myocardial infarction of unspecified site, episode of care unspecified
- 410.91 Acute myocardial infarction of unspecified site, initial episode of care
- 410.92 Acute myocardial infarction of unspecified site, subsequent episode of care

CLINICAL PEARLS

Discontinue clopidogrel at least 5–7 days before elective CABG. Do not administer nitrates to patients who have recently used PDE-5 inhibitors.

MYOCARDITIS

Francesca L. Beaudoin, MS, MD
Ron Van Ness-Otunnu, MD

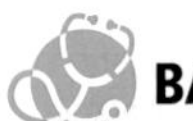

BASICS

DESCRIPTION

- Inflammatory disease of myocardium, most commonly from viral infection. Etiologies include infectious pathogens, autoimmune disease, drug-induced hypersensitivity reactions, systemic eosinophilic syndromes, and toxins.
- Clinical presentation varies widely from mild chest discomfort or dyspnea, to shock, heart failure, and sudden cardiac death.
- The range of treatment is broad and dependent upon the cause and severity of the disease, from basic pharmacologic therapy for left ventricular dysfunction, to vasopressor and inotropic support for hemodynamic compromise, to ventricular assist devices, extracorporeal membrane oxygenation, or heart transplants for severely compromised patients.
- While more often there is a resolution of disease with supportive or directed care, unresolved disease may lead to chronic dilated cardiomyopathy with a high risk of increased morbidity and mortality.

EPIDEMIOLOGY

- Male > Female
- Infant mortality as high as 75%
- Child mortality as high as 25% (1)

Incidence

Unknown

Prevalence

- Large prospective study implicated myocarditis as the cause of dilated cardiomyopathy in 9% of cases (2)
- Based on prospective postmortem data, myocarditis is associated with sudden cardiac death in young adults at rates between 8.6% and 12% (2)
- In HIV-related deaths, myocarditis is the most common cardiac finding on autopsy (50% prevalence)
- Most common cause of new heart failure in previously healthy children (3)

RISK FACTORS

- Community viral endemic or other infection
- Hypersensitivity reaction
- Autoimmune disease
- Drug or toxin exposure
- Travel to area endemic to specific pathogens
- Eosinophilic syndromes

PATHOPHYSIOLOGY

3-phase progression:

- Acute direct or indirect myocyte injury from pathogen or toxin and initiation of innate immune response
- Acquired immune system activation with immune dysregulation: T-cell response, B-cell activation, possible antibody cross-reaction with endogenous myocardial epitopes (molecular mimicry) leads to myocytolysis or worsening inflammatory response
- Progression to persistent cardiomyopathy and either chronic infection or eventual recovery

ETIOLOGY

- Viral:
  - Enteroviruses (coxsackie B particularly) are the most common cause of myocarditis overall (and found in 32% of viral-mediated myocarditis)
- Bacterial:
  - *Staphylococcus*, *Streptococcus*, Mycobacterial
- Fungal:
  - *Aspergillus*, *Candida*, Coccidioides, *Cryptococcus*
- Protozoal:
  - *Trypanosoma cruzi*, Entamoeba
- Parasitic:
  - Schistosoma, *Larva migrans*, *Trichinella*
- Spirochetal:
  - Borrelia burgdorferi
- Immunologic:
  - Giant cell, sarcoidosis, Kawasaki disease, systemic lupus erythematosus (SLE)
- Drug-induced hypersensitivity reactions:
  - Antibiotics, anticonvulsants, antipsychotics
- Systemic hypereosinophilic syndromes
- Toxins:
  - Cocaine, sulphonamides, chemotherapeutics

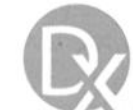

DIAGNOSIS

The diagnosis of myocarditis is based upon a combination of clinical, laboratory, and imaging findings (see "Diagnostic Tests & Interpretation"):

- Fulminant myocarditis: Severe hemodynamic compromise, distinct viral prodrome, abrupt onset. Echocardiography: Nondilated wall thickening, hypocontractile left ventricle. Best long-term prognosis among those patients presenting with heart failure (4)
- Subacute myocarditis: Less severe presentation, but worse long-term prognosis due to increased likelihood of chronic dilated cardiomyopathy

HISTORY

- Viral prodrome (fever, malaise, myalgias, upper respiratory and/or GI symptoms) within previous 2 weeks. Reported viral prodrome incidence highly variable (2)
- Exertional dyspnea (72%)
- Chest pain or discomfort (32%)
- Decreased exercise tolerance
- Palpitations
- Syncope (predictor of increased mortality)
- Wide range of clinical presentations, from asymptomatic with EKG abnormalities to cardiogenic shock or sudden death
- Most patients presenting with acute dilated cardiomyopathy have mild disease (4).
- Children have a more fulminant presentation and are frequently initially misdiagnosed with asthma, pneumonia, or sepsis (1).
- Important to distinguish:
  - Acute lymphocytic: Unclear onset, rare hemodynamic compromise, frequently requires cardiac transplant; increased mortality
  - Fulminant lymphocytic: Abrupt onset (<3 days) with 2-week viral prodrome, hemodynamic compromise, good prognosis with supportive care
- High-risk presentations (4):
  - Heart failure with eosinophilia
  - Giant cell myocarditis (high risk of death or cardiac transplant)
  - Heart failure + dilated left ventricle + new ventricular arrhythmia, heart block, or poor response to treatment over 2 weeks
- Coexistence with cardiac amyloidosis or hypertrophic cardiomyopathy can worsen prognosis
- Clinical suspicion for high morbidity/mortality presentation should prompt endomyocardial biopsy

PHYSICAL EXAM

- Arrhythmias (18%)
- Friction rub (concurrent pericarditis), gallop
- Increased jugular venous pressure
- Hypotension
- Decreased pulse pressure
- Hemodynamic collapse/cardiogenic shock
- Pulmonary hypertension, bundle branch block, EF <40% predict increased mortality
- In children, the most common findings are tachycardia, tachypnea, intercostal retractions, and grunting.

DIAGNOSTIC TESTS & INTERPRETATION

- Lab tests, EKG, and echocardiography are insensitive and frequently nonspecific, but they may in combination yield important diagnostic information.
- EKG findings (4)[C]:
  - Sinus tachycardia
  - Ventricular arrhythmia
  - Atrioventricular conduction block
  - Diffuse ST elevation and PR depression
  - Signs of acute myocardial infarction (ST-segment elevations in ≥2 leads, T-wave inversions, ST segment depressions, pathologic Q waves)
- Echocardiography to rule out causes of heart failure; identifies global or focal left ventricular abnormality, dilated cardiomyopathy
- Cardiac catheterization for alternative diagnoses
- Chest x-ray may reveal cardiac enlargement and/or pulmonary congestion
- Endomyocardial biopsy (EMB) is infrequently indicated (<5% of cases warrant biopsy). Higher yield if within <4 weeks of symptom onset (4)[B]
- The EMB may be useful when a particular cause is suspected and confirmation will alter the treatment plan. The risk of a serious complication from biopsy is <1% in centers experienced with the technique.
- Biopsy is recommended if common causes of dilated cardiomyopathy are excluded and there is one of the following (2)[C]:
  - Ventricular arrhythmias or progressive conduction disease
  - Heart failure with rash, fever, or eosinophilia
  - History of collagen vascular disease
  - Amyloidosis, sarcoidosis, hemochromatosis
  - Suspected giant cell myocarditis (poor prognosis: Median survival of 5.5 months from onset)
  - Rapidly progressive cardiomyopathy
- Amyloidosis is a negative prognostic factor for a heart transplant.
- Due to rapid deterioration, identification of giant cell disease prompts mechanical circulatory support or a heart transplant.

Lab

Initial lab tests

- Cardiac enzymes:
  - Creatine kinase: Low predictive value
  - Troponin I or T: 30–50% sensitive, 90% specific, 80–90% positive predictive value (2) for myocardial injury

- Myocyte-specific major histocompatibility complex antigens: 80–85% sensitive and specific (2)
- ESR not recommended: Poor sensitivity and specificity

Imaging

Noninvasive imaging (2,5):

- Cardiac MRI:
  - May be a viable alternative to biopsy, identifies patients that may benefit from biopsy, guides biopsy, evaluates disease progression
  - Gadolinium late enhancement and T2-weighted
- Echocardiography:
  - Segmental wall abnormalities and nondilated wall thickening
  - Gadolinium enhanced spin-echo, segmented inversion recovery gradient-echo pulse sequence
  - Ultrasonic tissue characterization ≥90% specific
- Nuclear imaging with antimyosin antibodies:
  - $Gallium^{67}$ uptake for myocyte inflammation highly specific, but not sensitive
  - $Indium^{11}$ for myocyte necrosis
  - $Technetium^{99m}$ highly sensitive

Diagnostic Procedures/Surgery

- Cardiac catheterization if symptoms or EKG findings suggest acute myocardial infarction
- Immunohistochemistry: Immunoperoxidase staining of human leukocyte antigens
- Viral PCR

Pathological Findings

Dallas Criteria (histopathologic definition of myocarditis):

- Inflammatory cellular infiltrate with myocyte necrosis
- No longer the gold standard due to (2): Sampling error (>17 samples required to diagnose 80% cases), intraobserver variability, diagnostic in only 10–20% cases of hypersensitivity myocarditis

DIFFERENTIAL DIAGNOSIS

- Aortic dissection
- Pericarditis
- Acute myocardial infarction
- Pulmonary embolus
- Congestive heart failure
- Sepsis
- Cardiomyopathies (dilated, restrictive, hypertrophic, transient stress [Takotsubo disease])
- Pericardial effusion
- Pneumonia

TREATMENT

- The treatment of myocarditis is largely supportive with specific treatment aimed at heart failure and underlying etiologies.
- Hemodynamic and cardiovascular supportive care; pacing for complete heart block; additional management based on presentation or suspected underlying cause (4)
- In suspected acute viral myocarditis, advise the patient to limit physical activity because it may increase viral replication and worsen condition (5)[C].
- Follow the latest American College of Cardiology/American Heart Association recommendations for the treatment of left ventricular systolic dysfunction: Diuretics, β-adrenergic blockers, ACE inhibitors, and angiotensin II receptor blockers as indicated (2)[B].
- Avoid NSAIDs: These are associated with increased mortality (4)[C].
- Drug-induced hypersensitivity: Withdraw agent
- Systemic hypereosinophilic syndrome: Treat underlying disorder
- Cardiac sarcoidosis: Use corticosteroids regardless of cardiac dysfunction severity
- Kawasaki disease: IVIG
- Hepatitis C: May respond to interferon (4)[C]
- Systemic autoimmune (SLE, scleroderma, polymyositis, giant cell myocarditis): Immunosuppressants may be beneficial (2)[C]
- Consider an intra-aortic balloon pump or left ventricular assist device for severe myocarditis as a temporizing measure or bridge to heart transplantation (rescue therapy) (4)[C].

MEDICATION

See "Congestive Heart Failure" for management of heart failure aspects.

ADDITIONAL TREATMENT

Limit physical activity in the acute setting. Exercise training may improve clinical status for patients with current or prior symptoms of heart failure and reduced left ventricular ejection fraction (6)[B].

Issues for Referral

All myocarditis patients should be referred to a cardiologist.

SURGERY/OTHER PROCEDURES

- Intra-aortic balloon pump
- Implantable cardioverter-defibrillator

IN-PATIENT CONSIDERATIONS

Initial Stabilization

- Cardiopulmonary monitoring and support
- Vasopressors or inotropes if indicated
- EKG, echocardiogram, cardiac catheterization
- Intra-aortic balloon pump, ventricular assist device

Admission Criteria

- Admit all patients with suspected myocarditis for supportive care, etiology-specific treatment as appropriate, and cardiologic evaluation.
- Particularly concerning presentations:
  - Hemodynamic compromise
  - Arrhythmia
  - Uncorrected high BP
  - Acute myocardial ischemia
  - Severe infection
  - Syncope

Discharge Criteria

- Hemodynamically stable
- Medical workup completed
- Outpatient medication plan and follow-up arranged

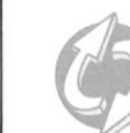

ONGOING CARE

FOLLOW-UP RECOMMENDATIONS

Regular follow-up for at least 3 years due to possible recurrence

DIET

Salt restriction with heart failure

PATIENT EDUCATION

- Most cases are expected to resolve without severe morbidity or mortality.
- Follow-up for as long as 3 years may be required.
- Patients must adhere to medication and diet plans to avoid worsening of heart failure.

PROGNOSIS

- Spontaneous improvement in 50–57%
- 3–5-year survival of 56–83%
- Acute fulminant: 93% survival at 11 years
- Acute nonfulminant: 45% survival at 11 years (5)

COMPLICATIONS

- If previous history of myocarditis or idiopathic cardiomyopathy, may have chronic myocardial persistence of virus, leading to progressive left ventricular deterioration
- Up to 50% develop dilated cardiomyopathy

REFERENCES

1. Freedman SB, Haladyn JK, Floh A, et al. Pediatric myocarditis: Emergency department clinical findings and diagnostic evaluation. *Pediatrics*. 2007;120:1278–85.
2. Magnani JW, Dec GW. Myocarditis: Current trends in diagnosis and treatment. *Circulation*. 2006;113: 876–90.
3. Durani Y, Giordano K, Goudie BW. Myocarditis and pericarditis in children. *Pediatr Clin N Am*. 2010;57: 1281–303.
4. Cooper LT. Myocarditis. *N Engl J Med*. 2009;360: 1526–38.
5. Dennert R, Crijns HJ, Heymans S. Acute viral myocarditis. *Eur Heart J*. 2008;29(17):2073–82.
6. Hunt SA, Abraham WT, Chin MH, et al. American College of Cardiology/American Heart Association 2005 Guideline Update for the Diagnosis and Management of Chronic Heart Failure in the Adult. *Circulation*. 2005;112:e154–235.

ADDITIONAL READING

- Japanese Circulation Society. Guidelines for diagnosis and treatment of myocarditis. *Circ J*. 2011;75:734–43.
- Jessup M, Abraham WT, Casey DE, et al. 2009 focused update: ACCF/AHA Guidelines for the Diagnosis and Management of Heart Failure in Adults. *Circulation*. 2009;119:1977–2016.

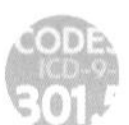

CODES

ICD9

- 422.90 Acute myocarditis, unspecified
- 422.91 Idiopathic myocarditis
- 429.0 Myocarditis, unspecified

CLINICAL PEARLS

- Most patients recover with only supportive care. However, unresolved disease may lead to chronic dilated cardiomyopathy with a high risk of increased morbidity and mortality.
- An endomyocardial biopsy should be reserved for high-risk presentations and/or where it is suspected the information may change the management plan.
- General heart failure treatment guidelines are applicable to patients with heart failure due to myocarditis.

NARCOLEPSY

Jeffrey F. Minteer, MD

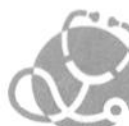

BASICS

DESCRIPTION

- Disorder of unknown etiology characterized by excessive daytime sleepiness typically associated with cataplexy (sudden bilateral weakness of skeletal muscles) and other REM sleep phenomena, such as sleep paralysis and hypnagogic hallucinations
- Commonly misconceived as representing low intelligence and/or poor motivation
- Frequently overlooked disorder with an average of 15 years of symptoms prior to diagnosis
- System(s) affected: Nervous

EPIDEMIOLOGY

Incidence

- Onset usually in teenage years
- Bimodal distribution peak at 15 and 36 years of age
- Predominant sex: Male = Female
- Occurrence: 0.74/100,000 persons

Pediatric Considerations

Uncommon in childhood

Prevalence

25–50 cases/100,000 people.

RISK FACTORS

- Head trauma
- CNS infectious disease
- Anesthesia
- Psychological stress
- Pregnancy
- Family history
- High body mass index (BMI)

Genetics

- Increased incidence in families with positive history: 1–2% in first-degree relative of index case (10–40 times the general population)
- Twin concordance is 25–31% (suggests environmental contribution)
- Most are sporadic.
- 85–95% of patients with narcolepsy and cataplexy have biologic HLA DQB1*0602; 40% of patients with narcolepsy without cataplexy express this antigen. (HLA) DQB1*0602 is present in 24% of the general population.
- Autosomal-recessive inheritance pattern
- 12% of Asians, 25% of whites, and 38% of African Americans are gene carriers.

ETIOLOGY

- Unknown
- Neurodegenerative disorder resulting from selective loss of neurons containing hypocretin in the hypothalamus
- 85% of patients with narcolepsy and cataplexy have low hypocretin in CSF.
- Possible involvement of immune system and environmental influences

COMMONLY ASSOCIATED CONDITIONS

Obstructive sleep apnea, obesity, anxiety

DIAGNOSIS

HISTORY

- Classic tetrad of excessive daytime sleepiness, cataplexy, sleep paralysis, and hypnagogic hallucinations (4 most common symptoms): Only 10–20% of patients have all 4 symptoms.
- 3 general forms:
  - Narcolepsy without cataplexy: 40%
  - Narcolepsy with cataplexy: 60%
  - Narcolepsy due to a medical condition: Unknown
- Excessive daytime sleepiness and sleep attacks:
  - Primary symptom and required for diagnosis
  - Instantaneous, irresistible REM sleep
  - First and most disabling symptom
  - Tendency to take naps lasting 5–10 minutes
  - Episodes last minutes to hours
  - 1–8 naps a day but 24-hour duration of sleep is normal
  - Associated with dreaming
  - Nap restores wakefulness for several hours
  - More likely to happen in a monotonous, warm environment; after a large meal; or with strong emotions
- Cataplexy: Auxiliary symptom (60%):
  - Pathognomonic if present
  - Sudden bilateral weakness of skeletal muscles
  - Provocation by sudden strong wave of emotion
  - Consciousness and memory are not impaired.
  - Short duration (less than a few minutes)
  - Can be limited to a particular muscle group (e.g., jaw droop with inability to speak; arm, neck, or leg weakness)
- Sleep paralysis: Auxiliary symptom (50%):
  - When falling asleep or on awakening, the patient wants to but cannot move, but this can end abruptly when the patient is touched or spoken to.
  - Brain wakes from sleep while body remains paralyzed in REM sleep.
  - Lasts seconds to minutes
  - Patients are aware of events around them but cannot open eyes or move.
  - Can be preceded by hallucinatory phenomena
  - 50% of the normal population have ≥1 episodes (so this symptom is nonspecific).
- Hypnagogic hallucinations: Auxiliary symptom (60%):
  - Vivid, frightening visual or auditory illusions or hallucinations at onset of sleep
  - Dreamlike experiences that occur during wakefulness or suddenly at sleep onset
  - Characteristic hallucinations include seeing human or animal faces or feeling that someone else is in the room.
  - Hallucinations also can be auditory.
- Disturbed nocturnal sleep (66%):
  - Normal total sleep with decreased sleep efficiency
  - More frequent transitions from wakefulness to sleep
  - Retrograde amnesic and automatic behavior lasting minutes to hours
  - Increased periodic leg movements (50%)
  - Depression (18–37%)
  - Automatic behavior: Activity without memory of the event

PHYSICAL EXAM

- A complete exam is useful to rule out other causes of hypersomnia.
- If cataplexy is witnessed, examiner will be unable to elicit deep tendon reflexes.

DIAGNOSTIC TESTS & INTERPRETATION

Lab

Follow-Up & Special Considerations

- HLA typing for DQB1 in ambiguous cases
- Low CSF hypocretin-1 level: 99% specificity, 87% sensitivity in patients with cataplexy; useful in children unable to do a multiple sleep latency test (MSLT, described below)

Imaging

Initial approach

- Nighttime polysomnography (PSG): Monitoring of patients in a sleep laboratory will usually document fragmented sleep with a normal amount of REM sleep but a pattern of sleep-onset REM. The PSG is useful to rule out other causes of excessive daytime sleepiness, including sleep apnea syndromes and nocturnal myoclonus.
- MSLT: Begins ≥90 minutes after nighttime test:
  - The patient is monitored during 4–5 naps taken at 2-hour intervals; rapidity of sleep onset and type of sleep pattern are documented. The supportive test includes mean sleep latency (time to fall asleep) of ≤5 minutes and 1 or more sleep-onset REM periods.
  - Sensitivity 77%; specificity 97%; positive predictive value 73%

Diagnostic Procedures/Surgery

- Diagnostic criteria according to the International Classification of Sleep Disorders
- Minimal criteria are B + C or A + D + E + G:
  - A. Excessive sleepiness—required
  - B. Recurrent lapses into sleep daily for ≥3 months
  - C. Cataplexy
  - D. Associated features: Sleep paralysis, hypnagogic hallucinations, disrupted sleep
  - E. MSLT abnormalities (as described above)
  - F. Biologic markers (see "Genetics")
  - G. Absence of medical or psychiatric disorder
  - H. Low CSF hypocretin-1 level

DIFFERENTIAL DIAGNOSIS

Excessive daytime sleepiness is present in 4% of the general population, although most individuals are not narcoleptic. Possible etiologies include:

- Sleep apnea syndromes (40–50% of those with excessive somnolence)
- Epileptic seizures and syncope
- Idiopathic CNS hypersomnolence (5–10% of those with excessive somnolence)
- Nocturnal myoclonus
- Psychomotor seizures
- Recurrent hypersomnia that lasts days to weeks and recurs months later
- Hypersomnia related to a medical condition such as Parkinson disease

TREATMENT

MEDICATION

First Line

- Excessive daytime sleepiness:
  - Modafinil (Provigil):
    - Structurally distinct from amphetamines
    - 200–400 mg/d; start with 100 mg/d and increase over 3–4 days (1)[A].
    - First-line treatment: 60% effective and 20% partially effective
    - Half-life of 14 hours, so can dose daily
    - No decrease in cataplexy
  - Armodafinil (Nuvigil):
    - Enantiomeric form of modafinil with slightly longer half-life of 15 hours
    - 150–250 mg every morning
  - Sodium oxybate (Xyrem):
    - 2.5–9 mg; may take 3 months to achieve full response
    - Preferred treatment for narcolepsy with cataplexy and disturbed nocturnal sleep
    - Give 1/2 dose at bedtime and 1/2 dose 4 hours later; date rape drug with abuse potential (1)[A]
    - Can use with modafinil in severe cases
    - May worsen sleep-disordered breathing in patients with obstructive sleep apnea
- Cataplexy:
  - Sodium oxybate: See above
  - Serotonin-norepinephrine reuptake inhibitors:
    - Venlafaxine: 75–375 mg daily
  - Tricyclic antidepressants:
    - High side-effect profile
    - Abrupt withdrawal causes rebound cataplexy
    - Protriptyline: 2.5–10 mg/d
  - Amphetamines:
    - Methylphenidate (Ritalin): Initial dose 30 mg/d divided b.i.d. or t.i.d.; maximum dose 100 mg/d (1)[B], short-acting
    - Dextroamphetamine: Initial dose 15 mg/d divided b.i.d. or t.i.d.; maximum dose 100 mg/d (1)[B]
    - Combination regimen of long- and short-acting medicines: Pemoline plus single or multiple doses of methylphenidate
- Auxiliary symptoms (e.g., cataplexy [2][C], hypnagogic hallucination, sleep paralysis [2][C]):
  - Antidepressants suppress REM sleep:
    - Imipramine: 75–150 mg/d
    - Protriptyline: 10–40 mg/d
    - Clomipramine: 150–250 mg/d
    - Fluoxetine: 20–60 mg/d
    - Venlafaxine: 75–150 mg b.i.d.
  - Although often used, quality evidence is lacking to demonstrate improvement in cataplexy symptoms from antidepressants (2)[A].
- Contraindications: Stimulants in hypertensive patients
- Precautions:
  - Amphetamines:
    - If the patient develops a tolerance to stimulants, switch drugs rather than to increase dose; there is little cross-tolerance.
    - Headaches, irritability, hypertension (HTN), psychosis, anorexia, habituation, rebound hypersomnia
    - Pemoline: Fewer cardiovascular side effects, longer acting, liver toxicity, little abuse potential
  - Other:
    - Imipramine: Dry mouth, sedation, urinary retention, impotence
    - Modafinil: Less rebound hypersomnia; may become drug of choice; does not affect BP; tolerance limited; best if initial treatment; does not treat cataplexy; main side effect is headache; increased metabolism of oral contraceptives (so use 50-μg pill)
    - The patient may develop a tolerance to the anticataplectic effect of tricyclic antidepressants (TCAs) and can get a rebound of cataplexy when a drug is withdrawn.
- Significant possible interactions: Combination of TCAs and stimulants can lead to significant HTN.

Second Line

- Excessive daytime sleepiness:
  - Amphetamines:
    - Methylphenidate (Ritalin): Initial dose 30 mg/d divided b.i.d. or t.i.d.; maximum dose 100 mg/d (1)[B], short acting, most potent amphetamine available
    - Dextroamphetamine: Initial dose 15 mg/d divided b.i.d. or t.i.d.; maximum dose 100 mg/d (1)[B]
  - Selegiline: Selective MAO-B inhibitor; anticataplectic effective for excessive daytime sleepiness; 20–40 mg/d divided morning and noon (1)[B]
- Contraindications: Stimulants in hypertensive patients
- Precautions:
  - Amphetamines:
    - If the patient develops a tolerance to stimulants, switch drugs rather than to increase dose; there is little cross-tolerance.
    - Headaches, irritability, HTN, psychosis, anorexia, habituation, rebound hypersomnia
  - Other: Selegiline: Doses >20 mg require a low-tyramine diet because the drug begins to lose selectivity.
  - The patient may develop a tolerance to the anticataplectic effect of antidepressants and can get a rebound of cataplexy when a drug is withdrawn.

ADDITIONAL TREATMENT

General Measures

- None of the currently available medications enable people with narcolepsy to consistently maintain a fully normal state of alertness.
- Drug therapy should be supplemented by various behavioral strategies.
- Well-timed 20-minute naps may be helpful.
- Avoid sedative drugs.
- Use safety precautions, particularly when driving. People with untreated narcoleptic symptoms are involved in automobile accidents roughly 10× more frequently than the general population. However, accident rates are at normal levels among patients who have received appropriate medication therapy.

Issues for Referral

- Unresponsive to primary medications
- Patient support groups can be very beneficial.

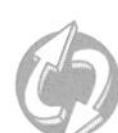

ONGOING CARE

FOLLOW-UP RECOMMENDATIONS

Patient Monitoring

Frequent BP checks and regular follow-ups (approximately every 6 months) are recommended.

DIET

Selegiline: Doses >20 mg require a low-tyramine diet because the drug begins to lose selectivity.

PATIENT EDUCATION

- Narcolepsy information from the National Institute of Neurological Disorders and Stroke at www.ninds.nih.gov/disorders/narcolepsy/narcolepsy.htm
- Narcolepsy Network, Inc., 79 Main Street, North Kingstown, RI 02852; e-mail: narnet@narcolepsynetwork.org; Web site: www.narcolepsynetwork.org

PROGNOSIS

Narcolepsy is a lifelong disease. Symptoms can worsen with aging. In women, symptoms can improve after menopause.

REFERENCES

1. Mohsenin V. Narcolepsy–master of disguise: Evidence-based recommendations for management. *Postgrad Med.* 2009;121:99–104.
2. Vignatelli L, D'Alessandro R, Candelise L. Antidepressant drugs for narcolepsy. *Cochrane Database Syst Rev.* 2008;CD003724.

ADDITIONAL READING

- Dauvilliers Y, Arnulf I, Mignot E. Narcolepsy with cataplexy. *Lancet.* 2007;369:499–511.
- Zaharna M, Dimitriu A, Guilleminault C. Expert opinion on pharmacotherapy of narcolepsy. *Expert Opin Pharmacother.* 2010;11(10):1633–45.

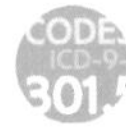

CODES

ICD9

- 347.00 Narcolepsy without cataplexy
- 347.01 Narcolepsy with cataplexy

CLINICAL PEARLS

- Narcolepsy is a frequently missed disorder with an average of 15 years of symptoms before a definitive diagnosis is made (1)[A].
- The classic tetrad of symptoms includes excessive daytime sleepiness, cataplexy, sleep paralysis, and hypnagogic hallucinations.
- The International Classification of Sleep Disorders has specific diagnostic criteria for narcolepsy.
- Medications are helpful but not curative.

N

NEAR DROWNING

Mia D. Sorcinelli, MD

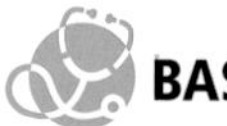

BASICS

DESCRIPTION

- Multisystem, potentially fatal disease resulting from near suffocation secondary to submersion of a person's face or head in a liquid
- A form of acute respiratory distress syndrome (ARDS) with neurologic complications
- System(s) affected: Cardiovascular; Nervous; Pulmonary; Renal

EPIDEMIOLOGY

Incidence

- In 2007, there were 3,237 deaths in the US; about 10 per day, 2 of whom are under age 14.
- 54 infants accidentally drowned in the US in 2007.
- In 2007, there were 4,321 near drownings in the US; the actual number is likely much higher due to underreporting.
- Second leading cause of injury-related death (after automobile crashes) for US children, 1–12 years of age, in 2006
- Predominant age: Teenagers and toddlers
- Predominant sex: Male > Female

Prevalence

- Drowning was the sixth leading cause of accidental death for all ages in the US in 2006.
- For every child under age 15 who dies from drowning, 5 more children are seen in the emergency room for nonfatal submersion injuries.

ALERT

Proper water safety techniques may help to avoid this problem.

RISK FACTORS

- Alcohol ingestion
- Seizure disorder
- Inability to swim
- Hyperventilation prior to underwater swimming
- Improper pool fencing
- Inadequate adult supervision of children
- Cardiac arrhythmias: Familial long QT and familial polymorphic ventricular tachycardia (VT)
- Residence within sunbelt states
- Adolescents: May be intoxicated or using drugs
- Adults: Most near drownings are associated with boating accidents ± alcohol

GENERAL PREVENTION

- Proper adult supervision of children
- Knowledge of water safety guidelines
- Mandatory pool fencing and pool alarms
- Fences higher than 54 in. (137 cm.) for home pools
- Avoidance of alcohol or recreational drugs around water
- Swimming instruction at an early age
- Cardiopulmonary resuscitation (CPR) instruction for pool owners, parents
- Boating safety knowledge
- Personal flotation device (such as a preserver, if necessary)

Pediatric Considerations

Children should never be left alone near water. Young children can drown in very small amounts of water such as in bathtubs, buckets, and toilets.

PATHOPHYSIOLOGY

Hypoxemia and acidosis cause most of the physiologic problems.

ETIOLOGY

- Swimming accidents: Head trauma while swimming; hyperventilation before underwater swimming
- Bathtub and bucket drowning in children <1 year of age
- Pool drowning in children 1–4 years of age
- Drug or alcohol overdose
- Boating mishaps, water sports, scuba diving
- Motor vehicle accidents (e.g., automobile submerged in water)
- Suicide

COMMONLY ASSOCIATED CONDITIONS

- Cardiopulmonary arrest before submersion
- Trauma, especially to the head, causing altered mental status
- Seizure disorder
- Alcohol or drug overdose
- Hypothermia

DIAGNOSIS

HISTORY

- Victim found in or near water
- Water temperature may be important, although no conclusive evidence exists.
- Look for signs of trauma.

PHYSICAL EXAM

- Level of consciousness: Altered or comatose
- Absent or weak pulse
- Tachypnea or agonal respirations, cough
- Cyanosis
- Wheezing
- Abdominal distension
- Hypothermia
- Poorly reactive, dilated, and fixed pupils
- Poor peripheral perfusion
- Rectal temperature

DIAGNOSTIC TESTS & INTERPRETATION

Lab

Initial lab tests

- Arterial blood gases (ABGs): Hypoxia, hypercarbia
- Electrolytes: Hypokalemia, hyponatremia (especially freshwater), hypernatremia (especially saltwater)
- Blood glucose: Increased levels may impair neurologic recovery after ischemic brain injury.
- Urea, creatinine, total creatinine kinase
- Urinalysis: Rare oliguria, albuminuria
- Coagulation studies
- CBC with differential
- Blood cultures for critically ill patients
- Tracheal aspirate cultures recommended by some sources for patients with pneumonia or intubated patients.
- Toxicology for drug overdoses
- Any underlying condition that may alter normal fluid and electrolyte balance can affect lab results (e.g., congestive heart failure [CHF]) or alter normal pulmonary function (e.g., emphysema).

Follow-Up & Special Considerations

Serum electrolyte monitoring

Imaging

Initial approach

A chest x-ray (CXR) may show pulmonary edema, consolidation from aspiration, atelectasis, or pneumothorax.

Follow-Up & Special Considerations

A repeat CXR may raise suspicion for pneumonia.

Diagnostic Procedures/Surgery

- Central venous pressure (CVP) monitoring
- ECG
- EEG if question of seizure as cause

Pathological Findings

- "Dry lungs": ~10% of victims drown without aspiration; may be due to prolonged laryngospasm, but some controversy exists
- "Wet drowning": 80–90% of victims show aspiration of water, sand, and mud into the lungs.
- Loss of normal pulmonary architecture occurs with both fresh- and saltwater aspiration.
- Loss of surfactant, with alveolar consolidation, atelectasis, hyaline membrane formation, development of intrapulmonary right-to-left shunting
- Increased lung weight and intra-alveolar hemorrhages; decreased lung compliance
- Pneumonia, abscess, and ARDS in those who survive only a few hours or days
- Cardiac: Low cardiac index, elevated right- and left-sided heart-filling pressures, elevated systemic and pulmonary vascular resistance
- Renal: Acute tubular necrosis from hypoxemia, shock, hemoglobinuria, myoglobinuria
- Neurologic: Hypoxia followed by ischemia, infarctions in "watershed" areas, damage especially to the hippocampus, insular cortex, and basal ganglia

DIFFERENTIAL DIAGNOSIS

Head trauma, arrhythmia, seizure, alcohol or other substance overdose

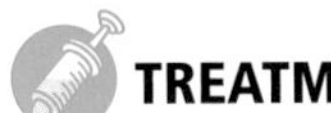

TREATMENT

Immediate reversal of hypoxemia should form the foundation of any treatment plan. Anticipate the need for critical care and a tertiary medical center in advance, and plan accordingly.

MEDICATION

First Line

- For bronchospasm: Aerosolized bronchodilator (1)[C]: Albuterol (Proventil, Ventolin), 3 mL of 0.083% solution *or* 0.5 mL of 0.5% solution diluted in 3 mL of saline
- Patients who develop pneumonia: Appropriate antibiotic based on sputum or endotracheal lavage culture (2)[A]
- Prophylactic antibiotics and steroids are not helpful (2)[B].

Second Line

Pressors as needed for resulting sepsis

ADDITIONAL TREATMENT

General Measures

- Never approach a struggling victim alone.
- Start with the basics: Airway, breathing, circulation (ABCs).
- Initiate rescue breathing while still in water if possible (1).
- Remove from water quickly and place in a normal CPR position (1).
- Avoid abdominal thrusting unless an obvious foreign body is present (1).
- Use cricoid pressure to limit aspiration (2)[B].
- Routine cervical collar use is not needed unless there is high suspicion for trauma (2).
- Supplemental oxygen, early intubation as needed (2)[A]
- If patient is breathing on his or her own, place in the right lateral decubitus position to prevent aspiration of vomit or gastric contents (1).
- Rough handling of victims of cold-water drowning may increase risk of ventricular fibrillation during resuscitation.

Issues for Referral

Refer severe cases to an intensivist or a trauma specialist.

Additional Therapies

- Oxygen for all patients
- Hypothermia may respond well to immediate rewarming on transport, as well as to cardiopulmonary bypass if the patient is severely hypothermic and asystolic (3)[C].
- More research is needed regarding intentional hypothermia in the initial days of treatment for patients, especially children, who underwent hypothermic near drowning. Ongoing studies eventually may lead to mild therapeutic hypothermia as a cornerstone of therapy in the pediatric population following cardiac arrest of many etiologies (4).
- Some small case studies suggest that in adults and children, particularly after hypothermic near-drowning, combinations of ECMO and extended therapeutic hypothermia (for up to 7 days) can dramatically improve neurologic and pulmonary outcomes (5).

COMPLEMENTARY AND ALTERNATIVE MEDICINE

Core warming with gastric or bladder lavage and/or providing warmed air through a ventilator may be necessary (2)[C].

SURGERY/OTHER PROCEDURES

ICU procedures as warranted for advanced life support

IN-PATIENT CONSIDERATIONS

Initial Stabilization

ABCs

Admission Criteria

- Hospitalize all patients initially.
- Monitor patients in an ICU setting, except for those few who present to the emergency department in an alert condition without evidence of respiratory compromise.

IV Fluids

To maintain adequate intravascular volume (1)[C]

Nursing

- Bed rest for at least the initial 24 hours
- Careful monitoring of neurologic status
- Continuous pulse oximetry monitoring

Discharge Criteria

Patients with Glasgow Coma Scale $\geq$13, a normal CXR, lack of clinical evidence of respiratory distress, and normal oxygen saturation on room air can be discharged after 8 hours of observation (2).

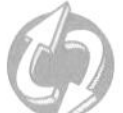

ONGOING CARE

FOLLOW-UP RECOMMENDATIONS

Appropriate follow-up with orthopedic, neurologic, cardiac, etc., specialists as warranted

Patient Monitoring

- Frequent check of O_2 saturation
- ABG monitoring (2)
- A pulmonary artery catheter may be needed for hemodynamic monitoring in unstable patients (1)[C].
- Intracranial pressure monitoring in selected patients (1)[C]
- Serum electrolyte determinations (2)

DIET

NPO until mental status normalizes

PATIENT EDUCATION

Re-emphasize preventive measures on discharge from hospital. Educate parents, and recommend pool safety, etc.

PROGNOSIS

- Patients who are alert or mildly obtunded at the time they present to the hospital have an excellent chance for a full recovery.
- Patients who are comatose or receiving CPR at the time of presentation, or who have dilated and fixed pupils and no spontaneous respiratory activity have a more guarded and often poor prognosis.
- Secondary drowning from neurogenic pulmonary edema may occur within 48 hours of initial presentation.

COMPLICATIONS

- Early:
  - Bronchospasm
  - Vomiting/aspiration
  - Hypoglycemia
  - Hypothermia
  - Seizure
  - Hypovolemia
  - Electrolyte abnormalities
  - Arrhythmia from hypoxia or hypothermia (rarely from electrolyte imbalance)
  - Hypotension
- Late:
  - ARDS
  - Anoxic encephalopathy
  - Pneumonia
  - Lung abscess/empyema
  - Renal failure
  - Coagulopathy
  - Sepsis
  - Barotrauma
  - Seizure

REFERENCES

1. Orlowski JP, Szpilman D. Drowning. Rescue, resuscitation, and reanimation. *Pediatr Clin North Am*. 2001;48:627–46.
2. Salomez F, Vincent JL. Drowning: A review of epidemiology, pathophysiology, treatment and prevention. *Resuscitation*. 2004;63:261–8.
3. Giesbrecht GG, Hayward JS. Problems and complications with cold-water rescue. *Wilderness Environ Med*. 2006;17:26–30.
4. Kochanek PM, Fink EL, Bell MJ, et al. Therapeutic hypothermia: Applications in pediatric cardiac arrest. *J Neurotrauma*. 2009;26(3)421–7.
5. Guenther U, Varelmann D, Putensen C, et al. Extended therapeutic hypothermia for several days during extracorporeal membrane-oxygenation after drowning and cardiac arrest: Two cases of survival with no neurological sequelae. *Resuscitation*. 2009;80:379–81.

ADDITIONAL READING

- American Heart Association Guidelines for Cardiopulmonary Resuscitation and Emergency Cardiovascular Care. Part 10.3: Drowning. *Circulation*. 2005;112(24S):133–5.
- Committee on Injury, Violence, and Poison Prevention, et al. Policy statement—prevention of drowning. *Pediatrics*. 2010;126(1):178–85.

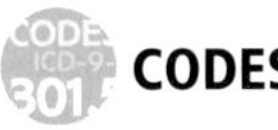

CODES

ICD9

994.1 Drowning and nonfatal submersion

CLINICAL PEARLS

- The single most important treatment for near-drowning victims is prompt reversal of the hypoxic state. This should form the cornerstone for all other treatment modalities. Without oxygenation, other treatment is futile.
- Family physicians and pediatricians should review water safety tips and guidelines with parents and children at yearly visits. Encourage pool owners and parents with young children to become CPR certified. Prevention of drowning can save many lives each year.
- Despite successful resuscitation, patients are at risk for ARDS due to delayed pulmonary edema that may start hours after their submersion incident. For this reason, careful monitoring of every resuscitated patient is essential.

NEPHROPATHY, URATE

Jaspreet Singh, DO

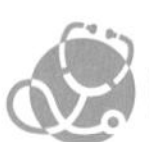

BASICS

- The water-insoluble nature of uric acid presents a unique problem in the acidic environment of the distal nephron of the kidney. Due to the lack of the enzyme uricase, which converts uric acid into a more soluble compound, allantoin, the human kidney is more susceptible to the side effects of uric acid crystal deposition.
- There are 3 different types of renal diseases induced by uric acid or urate crystal deposition:
  - Acute uric acid nephropathy (UAN)
  - Chronic urate nephropathy
  - Uric acid nephrolithiasis

DESCRIPTION

- Renal parenchymal damage and dysfunction associated with disordered uric acid metabolism
- Affects the renal/urologic system; several syndromes may present:
  - Acute UAN: Precipitated by renal tubular obstruction resulting from acute massive elevation of serum uric acid, often due to cell lysis during induction chemotherapy or radiation; furthermore, crystallization of uric acid or calcium phosphate in renal tubules affects renal function.
  - Uric acid nephrolithiasis: Seen most commonly in patients with underlying hyperuricemia or gout who have abnormally low urine pH due to low ammonia excretion:
    - Frequency of stone formation increases with increasing serum uric acid levels and urinary uric acid excretion rates.
    - ~20% of patients with gout will form uric acid stones.
  - Hyperuricemia of chronic renal failure: An early result of chronic renal failure due to retention of uric acid resulting from decreased tubular secretion or altered postsecretory reabsorption or both; secondary gout occurs in <1% of all patients
- Chronic urate nephropathy: Renal insufficiency attributed to parenchymal damage secondary to medullary urate deposition; effect of hyperuricemia on development and progression of chronic renal disease in humans is largely unknown. Studies in animals have shown an association between hyperuricemia and intrarenal vascular disease (1).

EPIDEMIOLOGY

Incidence

- 1 in every 114 patients newly diagnosed with gout develops uric acid stones per year. Uric acid stones are more common in patients with gout, and the chance of stone formation increases with increasing serum urate levels and urine excretion rates. Uric acid nephrolithiasis has a peak incidence in the fifth decade of life.
- Predominant age: Adults
- Predominant sex: Male > Female (4:1). In the US, the prevalence rate is 4–9% in men and 1.7–4.1% in women.

Prevalence

- Gout 1%, hyperuricemia 5–10%, uric acid nephrolithiasis 0.1% in the US
- Uric acid calculi account for 5–10% of all stones in the US.
- The overall prevalence of uric acid calculi in persons with primary gout is estimated to be 22%.

RISK FACTORS

- Hyperuricemic acute renal failure (2):
  - Chemotherapy of neoplastic disorders
  - Sudden increase in uric acid load
  - Volume depletion
  - Pre-existing acute or chronic renal insufficiency
  - Large tumor burden
  - Lactate dehydrogenase (LDH) >1,500 IU
  - Extensive bone marrow involvement
  - Elevated tumor sensitivity to chemotherapeutic agents
- Uric acid nephrolithiasis (3):
  - Decreased urine pH
  - Diminished urinary volume
  - Excessive urinary uric acid
  - Acute diarrheal states and inflammatory bowel disease
  - Diabetes mellitus
  - Metabolic syndrome
  - Probenecid and aspirin use

GENERAL PREVENTION

- Appropriate pretreatment prior to chemotherapy for leukemia or lymphoma
- Avoidance of factors that can cause abrupt or persistent increases in serum uric acid or urinary uric acid excretion

ETIOLOGY

- Hyperuricemic acute renal failure:
  - Endogenous uric acid overproduction: Rapid cell turnover/destruction due to malignancy or rhabdomyolysis, enzymatic/metabolic abnormalities, inappropriate high dose of uricosuric agent in hyperuricemic individual
  - Exogenous uric acid overproduction: Excessive dietary purine ingestion
- Uric acid nephrolithiasis:
  - Idiopathic: Sporadic
  - Familial (primary hyperuricemia):
    - Congenital gout, hypertension (HTN), and hyperuricemia (autosomal dominant)
    - Congenital hypoxanthine–guanine phosphoribosyltransferase deficiency (Lesch-Nyhan syndrome, X-linked recessive)
    - Congenital phosphoribosyl pyrophosphate overactivity (X-linked recessive)
    - Congenital glycogen storage disease type I
  - Secondary hyperuricemia:
    - Lead intoxication
    - Diuretics
    - Cytotoxic chemotherapy or radiation in leukemia or lymphoma
    - Heat stress and exercise
    - Diabetic ketoacidosis
    - Starvation ketosis
    - Chronic myeloproliferative disease
    - Psoriasis
  - Secondary hyperuricosuria: Primary gout, excessive purine intake, tubular reabsorptive defect, uricosuric drugs (e.g., cyclosporine, ethambutol, probenecid, phenylbutazone, pyrazinamide, salicylates, vitamin A, tacrolimus, radiocontrast materials)
  - Dehydration: GI or skin loss

Pediatric Considerations

- Gout and uric acid nephrolithiasis may have onset in infancy or childhood with familial causes of hyperuricemia, such as Lesch-Nyhan syndrome.
- It may occur more often in pediatric patients because of the increased incidence of acute lymphoblastic leukemia and Burkitt lymphoma in this population.

COMMONLY ASSOCIATED CONDITIONS

- Treatment of neoplastic disorders
- Gout (4)
- HTN (1)
- Myocardial infarction (1)
- Stroke (1)
- IgA nephropathy: Worse prognosis with elevated uric acid levels (1)

DIAGNOSIS

- Hyperuricemic acute renal failure (2):
  - Precipitated by chemotherapy for leukemia or lymphoma or some solid-tumor malignancies
  - Hyperkalemia: Weakness, paresthesias, muscle cramps, nausea, vomiting, diarrhea, anorexia
  - Hyperphosphatemia: Acute nephrocalcinosis
  - Hypocalcemia: Muscle cramps, tetany, cardiac arrhythmia, seizures
  - Oliguria
  - Anuria
  - Anorexia, nausea, vomiting, encephalopathy, and other manifestations of uremia
  - HTN
  - Dehydration
- Uric acid nephrolithiasis:
  - Flank pain
  - Groin pain
  - Microscopic or gross hematuria
  - Anorexia
  - Nausea, vomiting
  - Ureteral obstruction
  - UTI
  - Dehydration
- Hyperuricemia of chronic renal failure:
  - Established chronic renal failure with glomerular filtration rate (GFR) <15–20 mL/min
  - Serum uric acid 7–10 mg/dL chronically
  - Acute onset of uremic symptoms

HISTORY

Nonspecific, but includes nausea, vomiting, and fatigue; predisposing causes help to direct clinical suspicion

DIAGNOSTIC TESTS & INTERPRETATION

Lab

- Hyperuricemic acute renal failure:
  - Serum uric acid >15–20 mg/dL (0.88–1.18 mmol/L)
  - Rising BUN and creatinine
  - Urinary uric acid/creatinine ratio >1; ratio of 0.6–0.75 suggests another cause of renal failure (2)[C]
  - Uric acid crystals in urine
- Uric acid nephrolithiasis:
  - Urine pH <6 (Nitrazine paper) (3)[A].
  - Uric acid crystals in urine; urate crystals tend to be needle-shaped or flat, square plates; both are strongly birefringent
  - 24-hour urinalysis: Urinary uric acid often >4,800 μmol/d in men and >4,400 μmol/d in women or uric acid/creatinine ratio >530 μmol/mmol (hyperuricosuria) (5)[A]

– Measure serum uric acid, calcium, and creatinine: Serum uric acid is often normal, especially with low urine pH <6.2 (3)[A]
– Hematuria
– Stone analysis: Uric acid or mixed uric acid with calcium oxalate or calcium phosphate
- Hyperuricemia of chronic renal failure:
  – Serum uric acid is usually 7–10 mg/dL and is rarely >10 mg/dL due to compensatory increase in GI secretion of uric acid (1)[A].
  – Serum uric acid remains normal until GFR <20 mL/min (6)[C].

Imaging

- IV pyelography: Filling defects (3)
- Nonenhanced CT scan: Lower density than calcium stones (3)[A]; CT attenuation values between 300 and 400 HU (7)

Diagnostic Procedures/Surgery

- Cystoscopy and retrograde pyelography (3)
- Renal biopsy

Pathological Findings

- Hyperuricemic acute renal failure: Uric acid crystals in collecting ducts, eventually obstructing nephrons (2)
- Uric acid nephrolithiasis: Radiolucent, often orange or red stones that can occlude ureters or entire renal collecting system (3)
- Chronic urate nephropathy: Birefringent, needlelike crystals in the tubular lumen or in the interstitium with surrounding inflammatory cells and fibrosis (5)

DIFFERENTIAL DIAGNOSIS

- Hyperuricemic acute renal failure: Prerenal failure, contrast nephropathy, acute tubular necrosis, tumor infiltration of kidneys, obstruction
- Uric acid nephrolithiasis: Calcium oxalate, calcium phosphate, struvite, cystine stones; 20% of patients with calcium nephrolithiasis have hyperuricemia (3)
- Chronic urate nephropathy: Other causes of chronic renal failure, including diabetes, atherosclerotic disease, HTN, and glomerular disease, are more likely. Environmental lead poisoning is another consideration in a patient with hypertension, gout, hyperuricemia, and chronic kidney disease (8).

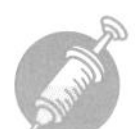

TREATMENT

MEDICATION

- Hyperuricemic acute renal failure: Prevent by pretreating with allopurinol or rasburicase and hydrating patient prior to administration of chemotherapeutic agents for leukemia or lymphoma (2,9)[A]:
  – Begin hydration 2 days prior to and continue for 2 days after induction chemotherapy (2)[A].
  – Allopurinol 200–600 mg/d (adults) (2)[A] and 10 mg/kg q8h (children) (10)[A]
  – Rasburicase 0.2 mg/kg/d IV during initial chemotherapy for pediatric patients with advanced-stage lymphoma or high-tumor-burden leukemia (9,10)[B]
  – Promptly correct metabolic abnormalities (2)[A].
  – Dialyze when renal failure fails to resolve with conservative management or when life-threatening electrolyte or volume-overload disorders are present (2)[A].
- Uric acid nephrolithiasis:
  – Encourage hydration to obtain urine output 1.5–2 L (5,7)[A].
  – Alkali to maintain urine pH at 6–7; give potassium alkali 20–30 mEq b.i.d. to t.i.d. (3,5)[A]
  – If hyperuricosuric and urinary alkalinization is unsuccessful, give allopurinol starting at 100–300 mg/d (5)[B].
- Hyperuricemia of chronic renal failure: Consider allopurinol only in patients with prior history of gout or nephrolithiasis (6)[C].
- Asymptomatic hyperuricemia: There is insufficient evidence to indicate treatment of asymptomatic hyperuricemia (1)[A].
- Precautions:
  – In patients with renal impairment, dosing for allopurinol, which is cleared renally, must be adjusted (2)[A].
  – Avoid abrupt decreases or increases in serum uric acid, which may precipitate acute gouty arthritis.
- Significant possible interactions of allopurinol:
  – Inhibits metabolism of mercaptopurine and azathioprine
  – Ethanol decreases its effects.
  – Increases likelihood of skin rash when used with amoxicillin or ampicillin
  – Risk of nephrolithiasis with excess vitamin C

ADDITIONAL TREATMENT

General Measures

- Hyperuricemic acute renal failure:
  – IV hydration
  – Hemodialysis in severe cases
- Uric acid nephrolithiasis:
  – Hydration to increase urine output
  – Normalize renal uric acid excretion.
  – Normalize urine pH.
  – Antibiotic treatment of UTI

SURGERY/OTHER PROCEDURES

Uric acid nephrolithiasis resistant to conservative management: Lithotripsy, cystoscopic stenting, percutaneous nephrostomy (3)[A]

IN-PATIENT CONSIDERATIONS

Initial Stabilization

Outpatient treatment except for complicated nephrolithiasis and hyperuricemic acute renal failure

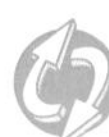

ONGOING CARE

DIET

- Moderation of purine intake (5)[C]
- For nephrolithiasis, ensure that fluid intake is adequate to produce urine output of at least 2 L/d unless urine output is limited by acute or chronic renal failure (5)[A].
- In renal failure, restrict sodium for HTN and potassium for hyperkalemia.

PROGNOSIS

- With effective drug therapy and general management, prognosis is excellent in patients with hyperuricemic acute renal failure (2) and nephrolithiasis (3).
- Development of progressive renal insufficiency in patients with gout or hyperuricemia is unlikely to occur unless caused by underlying renal disease or associated medical conditions with adverse renal effects (4).

COMPLICATIONS

- Gout and asymptomatic hyperuricemia: No renal complications proven in humans (1)
- Hyperuricemic acute renal failure (2):
  – Irreversible renal failure (end-stage renal disease)
  – Residual renal insufficiency
  – Persistent renal tubular functional defects
- Uric acid nephrolithiasis (4):
  – Urinary obstruction
  – UTI, pyelonephritis
  – Renal insufficiency
- Hyperuricemia of chronic renal failure: Progression to end-stage renal failure

Geriatric Considerations

Renal insufficiency is more likely because of age and associated medical conditions.

REFERENCES

1. Kanellis J, Feig DI, Johnson RJ. Does asymptomatic hyperuricaemia contribute to the development of renal and cardiovascular disease? An old controversy renewed. *Nephrology (Carlton)*. 2004;9:394–9.
2. Davidson MB, et al. Pathophysiology, clinical consequences, and treatment of tumor lysis syndrome. *Am J Med*. 2004;1116(8):546–54.
3. Coe FL, Evan A, Worcester E. Kidney stone disease. *J Clin Invest*. 2005;115:2598–608.
4. Nakagawa T, Mazzali M, Kang DH, et al. Uric acid–a uremic toxin? *Blood Purif*. 2006;24:67–70.
5. Reynolds TM. ACP Best Practice No 181: Chemical pathology clinical investigation and management of nephrolithiasis. *J Clin Pathol*. 2005;58:134–40.
6. Snaith ML. ABC of rheumatology: Gout, hyperuricemia, and crystal arthritis. *Br Med J*. 1995;310:521–4.
7. Becker G. Uric acid stones. *Nephrology (Carlton)*. 2007;12(Suppl 1):S21–5.
8. Lin JL, Yu CC, Lin-Tan DT, et al. Lead chelation therapy and urate excretion in patients with chronic renal diseases and gout. *Kidney Int*. 2001;60:266–71.
9. Coiffier B, Altman A, Pui CH, et al. Guidelines for the management of pediatric and adult tumor lysis syndrome: An evidence-based review. *J Clin Oncol*. 2008;26:2767–78.
10. Goldman SC, Holcenberg JS, Finklestein JZ, et al. A randomized comparison between rasburicase and allopurinol in children with lymphoma or leukemia at high risk for tumor lysis. *Blood*. 2001;97:2998–3003.

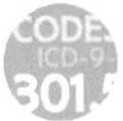

CODES

ICD9

- 274.10 Gouty nephropathy, unspecified
- 274.11 Uric acid nephrolithiasis

CLINICAL PEARLS

- Uric acid is water-insoluble in the acidic environment of the distal nephron of the kidney.
- Due to the lack of the enzyme uricase, which converts uric acid into a more soluble compound, allantoin, the human kidney is more susceptible to the side effects of uric acid crystal deposition

N

NEPHROTIC SYNDROME

Carla M. Nester, MD

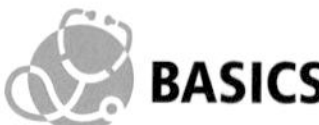

BASICS

DESCRIPTION

- A clinical syndrome of heavy proteinuria (>3.5 g/1.73 m^2/24 hours), hypoalbuminemia, hyperlipidemia, and edema
- Includes both primary and secondary forms
- Associated with many types of kidney disease

EPIDEMIOLOGY

Based on definitive diagnosis:

- Diabetic nephropathy:
  - Most common cause of secondary nephrotic syndrome
- Minimal change disease (MCD):
  - Most common nephrotic syndrome in children, peaks at 2–8 years
  - Associated with drugs or lymphoma in adults
- Amyloidosis:
  - Rare
- Lupus nephropathy (LN):
  - Adult women are affected about 10× more often than men.
- Focal segmental glomerulosclerosis (FSGS):
  - 25% of nephrotic syndrome in adults
  - Most common primary nephrotic syndrome in African Americans
  - Has both primary and secondary forms
- Membranous nephropathy:
  - Most common primary nephrotic syndrome in Caucasians
  - Associated with malignancy and infection
- Membranoproliferative glomerulonephritis (MGN):
  - May be primary or secondary
  - May present in the setting of a systemic viral or rheumatic illness

RISK FACTORS

- Drug addiction (e.g., heroin [FSGS])
- Hepatitis B and C, HIV, other infections
- Immunosuppression
- Nephrotoxic drugs
- Vesicoureteral reflux (FSGS)
- Cancer (usually MGN, may be MCD)
- Chronic analgesic use/abuse
- Preeclampsia
- Diabetes mellitus

Genetics

Genetic factors are likely to play a role in susceptibility to the various nephrotic syndromes, though these have not been sufficiently defined to be useful clinically.

GENERAL PREVENTION

In general, there are few preventive measures, except avoidance of known causative medications.

PATHOPHYSIOLOGY

- Increased glomerular permeability to protein molecules, especially albumin
- Edema results primarily from renal salt retention, with arterial underfilling from decreased plasma oncotic pressure playing an additional role.
- Hyperlipidemia is thought to be a consequence of increased hepatic synthesis resulting from low oncotic pressure and urinary loss of regulatory proteins.
- The hypercoagulable state that can occur in some nephrotic states is likely due to loss of antithrombin III in urine.

ETIOLOGY

- Primary renal disease:
  - Minimal change disease
  - FSGS
  - MGN
  - IgA nephropathy
  - Membranoproliferative glomerulonephritis
- Secondary renal disease (associated primary renal disease shown in parentheses):
  - Diabetic nephropathy
  - Amyloidosis
  - LN
  - FSGS
  - Infections (MGN)
  - Cancer (MCD or MGN)
  - Drugs (MCD or MGN)

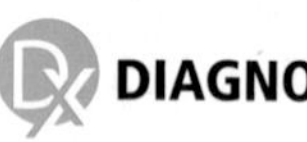

DIAGNOSIS

HISTORY

- Look for signs or symptoms of systemic disease:
  - Joint complaint, rash, edema, infectious complaint, fevers, anorexia, oliguria, foamy urine, acute flank pain, hematuria, etc.
- Look for a recent drug history that may be causative, especially NSAIDs.
- Assess for risk factors.

PHYSICAL EXAM

A complete physical exam may discover clues to systemic disease as a potential cause and/or may suggest the severity of disease:

- Fluid retention: Abdominal distention, abdominal fluid shift, extremity edema, puffy eyelids, scrotal swelling, weight gain, shortness of breath:
  - Pericardial rub and decreased breath sounds with pleural effusions may develop.
- Hypertension
- Orthostatic hypotension

ALERT

The potential for thromboembolic disease leading to pulmonary embolism is one of the most life-threatening aspects of a patient who is actively nephrotic.

DIAGNOSTIC TESTS & INTERPRETATION

Lab

Initial lab tests

- Confirm proteinuria is present:
  - By urine dipstick initially, and then quantitate by 24-hour urine or urine protein to creatinine ratio
- Rule out urine infection with urine culture.
- Full blood count and coagulation screen
- Renal function tests:
  - BUN, creatinine with estimated glomerular filtration rate
- Glucose to rule out overt diabetes
- Blood cultures to rule out a postinfectious process
- Lipid panel to judge the relative effect of loss of protein into the urine
- Liver function tests to exclude liver disease or infection
- Look for autoimmune disease:
  - Antinuclear antibody and/or antidouble-stranded DNA (dsDNA) positivity would suggest lupus.
  - Complement levels: A low C3 may suggest a postinfectious or membranoproliferative process, whereas both low C3 and C4 point to lupus.
- Serum protein electrophoresis/urine immune electrophoresis to rule in a paraproteinemia
- Hepatitis B and C screen
- HIV and rapid plasma reagent:
  - Urinalysis to evaluate for the presence of cellular casts

Imaging

- Renal ultrasound to verify the presence of 2 kidneys of normal shape and size
- Chest x-ray to detect presence of pleural effusion or infection
- If thrombosis suspected:
  - Doppler ultrasound of the legs
  - MRI or venography for renal vein thrombosis
  - Ventilation/perfusion nuclear medicine lung scan and/or CT may be required to rule out pulmonary embolism.

Diagnostic Procedures/Surgery

Renal biopsy:

- Rarely done in children with first episode of nephrotic syndrome, as minimal-change disease is common and empiric steroid therapy is the standard of care.
- Often required to confirm the clinical diagnosis in adults and assist with making a treatment plan

Pathological Findings

- Light microscopy:
  - May see nothing (e.g., MCD)
  - Sclerosis (e.g., FSGS or diabetic nodules in diabetes)
  - Diffuse hypercellularity suggests a proliferative disease such as IgA nephropathy, LN, or postinfectious GN.
- Immunofluorescence:
  - Mesangial IgA suggests IgA nephropathy, Henoch-Schönlein; other staining patterns are specific for other disease processes.
- Electron microscopy:
  - The location of immunoglobulin deposits is useful in pointing to a particular diagnosis.

DIFFERENTIAL DIAGNOSIS

- Edema and proteinuria:
  - See "Etiology."
- Edema alone:
  - Other diseases to rule out in patients who have edema without proteinuria include:
    - Congestive heart failure, cirrhosis, hypothyroidism, nutritional hypoalbuminemia, protein-losing enteropathy

TREATMENT

MEDICATION

First Line

- Edema: Salt restriction and salt-wasting diuretics (loop and thiazide diuretics):
  - Salt restriction to <6 g of sodium chloride (<2.4 g sodium/d)
  - Restrict fluid intake to <1.5 L/d if hyponatremic.
  - Target weight loss of 0.5–1 kg/d (1–2 lbs/d)
- Statins have been shown to improve endothelial function (1)[A] and decrease proteinuria (2)[A].
- ACE inhibitors or angiotensin II receptor blockers thought to reduce proteinuria, hyperlipidemia, thrombotic tendencies, progression of renal failure (1,3)[A] and to control hypertension if present.
- For steroid-responsive disease (MCD and FGS), steroids dosed in consultation with nephrologist

Second Line

- Many of the nephrotic diseases will require escalation in therapy above steroids. These include rapidly relapsing forms as well as MGN, LN, and IgA nephropathy:
  - Bolus steroids and other immunosuppressives are required in this circumstance (cyclophosphamide, mycophenolate mofetil, chlorambucil, cyclosporine).
- Randomized controlled data have been insufficient to determine which patients require prophylactic anticoagulation (4)[A]. One practice is to anticoagulate with heparin and then warfarin in patients who have persistent nephrotic-range proteinuria. This decision is made based on patient's history of edema, hypoalbuminemia, history of thromboembolism, or immobility.
- Hypocalcemia from vitamin D loss should be treated with oral vitamin D (dihydrotachysterol) 0.2 mg/d.

ADDITIONAL TREATMENT

Ambulation or range-of-motion exercises to lower risk of deep vein thrombosis (DVT)

Issues for Referral

Consultation with a nephrologist is often required in order to assist with renal biopsy to confirm diagnosis and to assist with management of edema. Cytotoxic medications may be called for, depending on the disease process, and this may best be handled by the nephrologists.

IN-PATIENT CONSIDERATIONS

Admission Criteria

Respiratory distress, sepsis/severe infection, thromboses, renal failure, hypertension, or other complications

Discharge Criteria

Hemodynamically stable patients without complications may be managed as outpatients.

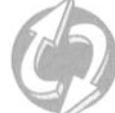

ONGOING CARE

FOLLOW-UP RECOMMENDATIONS

Patient Monitoring

- Frequent monitoring is required for relapse, disease progression, and for detecting signs of toxicity of medical management.
- Re-evaluate for azotemia, urine protein, hypertension, edema, loss of renal function, cholesterol, and weight.

DIET

- Normal protein (1 g/kg/d)
- Low fat (cholesterol)
- Reduced sodium
- Supplemental multivitamins and minerals, especially vitamin D and iron
- Fluid restriction if hyponatremic

PATIENT EDUCATION

- Printed material for patients: National Kidney Foundation, 30 E. 33rd Street, Suite 1100, New York, NY 10016; (800) 622-9010:
  - Childhood Nephrotic Syndrome
  - Diabetes and Kidney Disease
  - Focal Glomerulosclerosis
- Web site: National Institutes of Health: Nephrotic syndrome

PROGNOSIS

The nephrotic syndrome in children (MCD) is typically self-limited and carries a good prognosis. In the adult, the prognosis is variable. Complete remission is expected if the basic disease is treatable (infection, malignancy, drug induced); otherwise, a relapsing and remitting course is possible, with progression to dialysis seen in more aggressive forms (diabetic glomerulosclerosis).

COMPLICATIONS

- Thromboembolism:
  - DVT and/or renal vein thrombosis may occur.
  - The risk appears to be greater the lower the serum albumin.
  - Pulmonary embolism is a known complication.
- Pleural effusion
- Ascites
- Hyperlipidemia, cardiovascular disease
- Acute renal failure, progressive renal failure
- Protein malnutrition/muscle wasting
- Infection secondary to low serum IgG concentrations, reduced complement activity, and depressed T-cell function:
  - Peritonitis, pneumonia, or cellulitis
- Loss of vitamin D (vitamin D–binding protein loss in urine) leading to bone disease

REFERENCES

1. Randomized placebo-controlled trial of effect of ramipril on decline in glomerular filtration rate and risk of terminal renal failure in proteinuric, non-diabetic nephropathy. *The GISEN Group (Gruppo Italiano di Studi Epidemiologici in Nefrologia) Lancet*. 1997;349:1857–63.
2. Fried LF, Orchard TJ, Kasiske BL. Effect of lipid reduction on the progression of renal disease: A meta-analysis. *Kidney Int*. 2001;59:260–9.
3. Kunz R, Friedrich C, Wolbers M, et al. Meta-analysis: Effect of monotherapy and combination therapy with inhibitors of the renin angiotensin system on proteinuria in renal disease. *Ann Intern Med*. 2008;148:30–48.
4. Kulshrestha S, Grieff M, Navananeethan SD. Interventions for preventing thrombosis in adults and children with nephrotic syndrome (protocol). *Cochrane Database Syst Rev*. 2006;(2):CD006024.

ADDITIONAL READING

- Madaio MP, Harrington JT. The diagnosis of glomerular diseases: Acute glomerulonephritis and the nephrotic syndrome. *Arch Intern Med*. 2001;161:25–34.
- Meyrier A. An update on the treatment options for focal segmental glomerulosclerosis. *Expert Opin Pharmacother*. 2009;10:615–28.
- Schwarz A. New aspects of the treatment of nephrotic syndrome. *J Am Soc Nephrol*. 2001; 12(Suppl 17):S44–7.

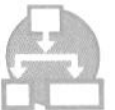

See Also (Topic, Algorithm, Electronic Media Element)

Amyloidosis; Diabetes Mellitus, Type 1; Diabetes Mellitus, Type 2; Glomerulonephritis, Acute; HIV Infection and AIDS; Lupus Erythematosus, Discoid; Multiple Myeloma; Renal Failure, Acute

CODES

ICD9

- 581.1 Nephrotic syndrome with lesion of membranous glomerulonephritis
- 581.3 Nephrotic syndrome with lesion of minimal change glomerulonephritis
- 581.9 Nephrotic syndrome with unspecified pathological lesion in kidney

CLINICAL PEARLS

- A clinical syndrome of heavy proteinuria, hypoalbuminemia, hyperlipidemia, and edema often associated with diabetes and NSAIDs
- Pediatric nephrotic syndrome typically carries a good prognosis and is easily treated with steroids. Recurrences are common.
- Nondiabetic adults with nephrotic syndrome will require a renal biopsy to determine cause.
- Have a high index of suspicion for symptoms that may represent an embolic event

NEUROFIBROMATOSIS TYPE 1

Tracey Samko, MD
Michele Roberts, MD, PhD

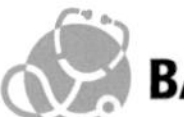

BASICS

DESCRIPTION

- Neurofibromatosis type 1 (NF1) and 2 (NF2) are neurocutaneous syndromes (phakomatoses). Although they share a name and are both autosomal-dominant disorders, they are distinct and unrelated conditions with genes on different chromosomes. NF2 is a rare condition that causes bilateral vestibular schwannomas.
- NF1 is a multisystem disorder that may affect any organ. It is the most common of the phakomatoses.
- System(s) affected: Musculoskeletal; Nervous; Skin/Exocrine; Cardiovascular; Neuro-ophthalmologic
- Synonym(s): von Recklinghausen disease, formerly *peripheral NF*

EPIDEMIOLOGY

Incidence

- Predominant sex for NF1: Male = Female
- Birth incidence NF1: 1 in 2,500–3,000

Prevalence

1 in 3,000 to 1 in 4,000

RISK FACTORS

- Having an affected first-degree relative is a diagnostic criterion for NF1, although relatives may be unaware of their condition.
- Affected individuals with a positive family history, as well as those with a new mutation, have a 50% risk of transmitting NF1 to each of their offspring; 1 in 12 will be severely affected.
- Individuals with segmental NF1 may have gonadal mosaicism and may be at risk for transmission of the mutated gene.

Genetics

- Online Mendelian Inheritance in Man #162200
- Caused by a mutation in the *NF1* gene on chromosome 17q11.2; autosomal-dominant inheritance; protein product is called *neurofibromin*
- 50% of cases are attributed to new mutations. Prenatal diagnosis is possible with a positive family history.
- Penetrance is nearly 100%; expressivity is highly variable.
- *NF1* is a large gene with a variety of mutations causing neurofibromatosis. Molecular technology can detect 95% of clinically important *NF1* mutations, but it is usually not indicated because clinical diagnosis frequently can be established in childhood.
- ~5% of individuals with NF1 have a large deletion of the entire *NF1* gene (or nearly so). These individuals usually have a more severe phenotype.
- A variant of NF1, known as *segmental NF*, is limited to a single body region and may be explained by mosaicism for the *NF1* mutation.

PATHOPHYSIOLOGY

- Neurofibromin belongs to a family of guanosine triphosphatase–activating proteins and acts as a tumor suppressor by down-regulating a cellular proto-oncogene, *p21-ras,* that enhances cell growth and proliferation.
- Neurofibromata are benign tumors composed of Schwann cells, fibroblasts, mast cells, and vascular components that develop along nerves.
- The 2-hit hypothesis has been invoked to explain malignant transformation in *NF1*.

COMMONLY ASSOCIATED CONDITIONS

Cardiovascular disease: Congenital heart disease, pulmonary stenosis, hypertension, renal artery stenosis

DIAGNOSIS

- NF1 can be diagnosed by routine exam by ages 6–8 years, with attention to skin stigmata; diagnostic criteria for include ≥2 of the following (1):
  - ≥6 café-au-lait (light brown) macules, ≥5 mm in prepubertal individuals or ≥15 mm in adults
  - ≥2 neurofibromata of any type or 1 plexiform (noncircumscribed) neurofibroma
  - Axillary or inguinal freckling
  - ≥2 Lisch nodules (benign iris hamartomas, asymptomatic)
  - Optic glioma by MRI
  - Characteristic osseous lesions: Sphenoid dysplasia, long-bone cortical thinning, ribbon ribs, angular scoliosis
  - First-degree relative with NF1 according to above criteria
- Prenatal diagnosis is possible when there is a known mutation or with linkage testing when there is a positive family history, although it is not predictive of the clinical course. Molecular genetic testing of the *NF1* gene is available in several laboratories (www.genetests.org), although often it is not necessary for diagnosis.

HISTORY

- Family history of a first-degree relative with NF1
- Manifestations generally are not visible at birth, although plexiform neurofibromata usually are congenital and tibial bowing is congenital.
- In addition to cutaneous lesions, NF1 may present with painful neurofibromata, pathologic fractures, or headaches secondary to hypertension caused by pheochromocytomas.

PHYSICAL EXAM

- Skin:
  - Café-au-lait macules develop during the first 3 years of childhood and are usually the presenting feature of NF1. Evenly pigmented, irregularly shaped (coast-of-California borders), light brown macules present in 97% of patients with NF1; many unaffected individuals have 1–3 such macules.
  - Neurofibromata: Can be cutaneous, SC, or plexiform and may be soft or firm; buttonhole invagination is pathognomonic. Cutaneous neurofibromata usually begin to appear during late childhood or adolescence.
  - Plexiform neurofibromata are present in up to 50% of individuals with NF1:
    - Usually congenital but may be subtle during infancy.
    - Freckling or hypertrichosis may be present over plexiform neurofibromata; may affect underlying structures or cause focal hyperplasia.
    - Many are internal and are not obvious during a physical exam.
  - Evaluate for new lesions and progression of pre-existing ones. Rapidly growing cutaneous lesions should be evaluated thoroughly.
  - Axillary freckling (Crowe sign) or inguinal freckling (91%)
- Ophthalmologic: 30% have Lisch nodules
- Skeletal:
  - Scoliosis and vertebral angulation
  - Localized bone hypertrophy, especially of the face
  - Limb abnormalities:
    - Pseudoarthrosis of the tibia
    - Tibial dysplasia (anterolateral bowing of the tibia) is congenital, if present.
    - Nonossifying fibromas of the long bones in adolescents and adults are uncommon but can increase risk of fracture.
- Pay particular attention to neurologic examination or new focal pain.
- Measure BP yearly. Hypertension is more common in patients with NF1 and could be secondary to renal artery stenosis, aortic stenosis, or pheochromocytoma.
- Evaluate neurodevelopmental progress in children.

Geriatric Considerations

In NF1, cutaneous lesions and tumors increase in size and number with age.

Pediatric Considerations

Children who have inherited the *NF1* gene of an affected parent usually are identified by age 1, but external stigmata may be subtle. If there are no stigmata by age 2, NF is unlikely but the child should be re-examined at age 5. Definite diagnosis can be made by age 8 using National Institute of Health (NIH) criteria (1).

DIAGNOSTIC TESTS & INTERPRETATION

Lab

- Clinical diagnosis: DNA sequence and deletion/duplication analysis of the *NF1* gene can identify mutations in ~96% of those with a clinical diagnosis.
- Diagnostic laboratory information is available at www.genetests.org.

Imaging

- Characteristic radiographic findings in NF1 include sphenoid dysplasia, long-bone cortical thinning, ribbon ribs, and angular scoliosis. Screening radiographs of the knees in adolescents is controversial. CT scan can demonstrate bony changes.
- MRI may demonstrate findings of the orbits, brain, or spine (86%). The value of performing routine head MRI scanning in asymptomatic individuals with NF1 is controversial. Optic gliomata (seen on MRI, 11–15%) may lead to blindness. Although areas of increased T_2 signal intensity (unidentified bright objects) are commonly identified on brain MRI, they are not diagnostic of NF1 and are of no clinical significance.
- The NIH Consensus Development Conference does not recommend routine neuroimaging as a means of establishing a diagnosis (1,2).

Diagnostic Procedures/Surgery
- Ophthalmologic evaluation, including slit-lamp examination of the irides
- Neuropsychological testing: Intelligence usually is normal, although significant deficits in language, visuospatial skills, and neuromotor skills may be present.

DIFFERENTIAL DIAGNOSIS
Familial café-au-lait spots (autosomal dominant, no other NF1 features); Watson syndrome; LEOPARD syndrome; McCune-Albright syndrome; neurocutaneous melanosis; proteus syndrome; lipomatosis

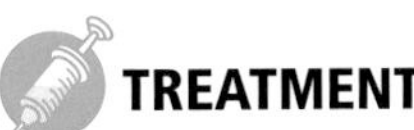

TREATMENT

MEDICATION
First Line
Anticonvulsants for seizure control, medications for ADHD, etc.

Second Line
Multiple clinical trials for NF1 are recruiting patients (see www.clinicaltrials.gov).

ADDITIONAL TREATMENT
Issues for Referral
- Patients with more than minimal manifestations of NF1 should be referred to a multidisciplinary NF clinic.
- Referral for psychosocial issues of family and affected individuals
- Educational intervention for children with learning disabilities or ADHD (40%)
- Early referral to orthopedics for congenital tibial bowing

Additional Therapies
- Occupational therapy for children with NF1 who present with fine motor difficulties
- There is no evidence supporting laser therapy for café-au-lait spots.
- The Children's Tumor Foundation (CTF) has established the NF Clinical Trials Consortium and the CTF NF Clinic Network to facilitate future clinical trials and help identify best practices (3).

SURGERY/OTHER PROCEDURES
Surgical treatment for severe scoliosis, plexiform neurofibromata, or malignancy

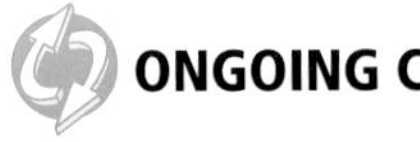

ONGOING CARE

FOLLOW-UP RECOMMENDATIONS
NF1 health supervision 2008 guidelines (4):
- Infancy to 1 year:
  - Growth and development: Mild short stature, macrocephaly due to increased brain volume; also aqueductal stenosis/obstructive hydrocephalus, hydrocephalus
  - Check for focal neurologic signs or asymmetric neurologic exam.
  - Skeletal abnormalities, especially of spine and legs
  - Neurodevelopmental progress
- 1–5 years:
  - Café-au-lait spots and axillary freckling have no clinical significance.
  - Annual ophthalmologic exam
  - Order brain MRI for visual changes, persistent headaches, seizures, marked increase in head size, plexiform neurofibroma of the head.
  - Assess speech and language: Hypernasal speech due to velopharyngeal insufficiency and delayed expressive language development
  - Developmental evaluation of learning and motor abilities; may benefit from preschool services, speech/language and/or motor therapy, and special education
  - Monitor BP annually.
- 5–13 years:
  - Evaluate for skin tumors causing disfigurement and obtain consultation if surgery is desired to improve appearance or function.
  - Evaluate for premature or delayed puberty. If sexual precocity is noted, evaluate for an optic glioma or hypothalamic lesion. Review the effects of puberty on NF.
  - Evaluate for learning disabilities and ADHD.
  - Evaluate social adjustment, development, and school placement.
  - Monitor ophthalmologic status yearly until age 8; complete eye examination every 2 years.
  - Monitor BP annually.
  - Refer patient to a clinical psychologist or child psychiatrist for problems with self-esteem if indicated.
  - Discuss growth of neurofibromata during adolescence and pregnancy.
  - Counsel parents about discussing diagnosis with child.
- 13–21 years:
  - Examine the adolescent for abnormal pubertal development.
  - Perform a thorough skin examination for plexiform neurofibromata and a complete neurologic exam for findings suggestive of deep plexiform neurofibromata. Obtain surgical consultation if there are signs of pressure on deep structures.
  - Continue to monitor BP yearly.
  - Continue ophthalmologic examination every 2 years until age 18.
  - Discuss genetics of NF1 or refer for genetic counseling.
  - Discuss sexuality, contraception, and reproductive options.
  - Discuss effects of pregnancy on NF1, if appropriate. Neurofibromata may enlarge and new tumors may develop during pregnancy.
  - Review prenatal diagnosis or refer the patient to a geneticist.

PATIENT EDUCATION
- Genetic counseling and patient education regarding future complications about family planning
- The CTF: www.CTF.org. Support groups are important.

PROGNOSIS
Variable; most patients have a mild expression of NF1 and lead normal lives.

COMPLICATIONS
- Disfigurement: Skin neurofibromata develop primarily on exposed areas. The number tends to increase with puberty or pregnancy.
- Scoliosis: 10–30%, but most cases are mild; bowing of long bones, 2%
- A large head is common but rarely associated with hydrocephalus.
- Increased risk of malignancy: Malignant peripheral nerve sheath tumor (MPNST) occurs in 5–10% of individuals with NF1, usually in adults (1). Typically, MPNST arises from a plexiform neurofibroma. Slightly increased risk for other malignancies, e.g., pheochromocytoma, rhabdomyosarcoma, leukemia, Wilms tumor. Optic glioma or other CNS tumors arise, usually during childhood (5–15%).
- Learning disability: ~50%; may be associated with ADHD; mental retardation 4–8%
- GI neurofibromata may cause a range of GI disturbances.
- Seizures 6–7%
- Hypertension is a frequent finding in adults and may occur during childhood.
- Disorders of puberty

Pregnancy Considerations
Increased risk of perinatal complications, stillbirth, intrauterine growth constriction; risk of cord compression and outlet obstruction by pelvic neurofibromata.

REFERENCES

1. DeBella K, Szudek J, Friedman JM. Use of the national institutes of health criteria for diagnosis of neurofibromatosis 1 in children. *Pediatrics*. 2000; 105:608–14.
2. National Institutes of Health Consensus Development Conference Statement: neurofibromatosis. Bethesda, MD; July 13–15, 1987. *Neurofibromatosis*. 1988;1:172–8.
3. Williams VC, Lucas J, Babcock MA, et al. Neurofibromatosis type 1 revisited. *Pediatrics*. 2009;123:124–33.
4. Hersh JH. and Committee on Genetics. Health supervision for children with neurofibromatosis. *Pediatrics*. 2008;121:3:633–42.

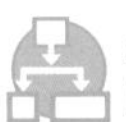

See Also (Topic, Algorithm, Electronic Media Element)

Tuberous Sclerosis Complex; von Hippel–Lindau Disease

CODES

ICD9
- 237.71 Neurofibromatosis, type 1, von Recklinghausen's disease
- 252.01 Primary hyperparathyroidism

CLINICAL PEARLS
- NF1 and NF2 are 2 distinct genetic disorders.
- NF1 has marked clinical variability. Even minimal findings necessitate monitoring. External stigmata may be subtle or absent in young children. Minimally affected children may become severely affected adults.
- A single café-au-lait spot is of no concern in a child, but having ≥6 is 1 of the diagnostic criteria for NF1.

N

NEUROPATHIC PAIN

Christian D. Gonzalez, MD

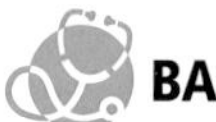

BASICS

DESCRIPTION

- Neuropathic pain is defined as pain in association with primary injury or dysfunction of the nervous system, with or without ongoing tissue damage.
- Divided into 2 groups based on the location of the suspected lesion: Central vs. peripheral:
  - Newer data suggest a possibility that most neuropathic syndromes have a component of both central and peripheral mechanisms.
- An important consideration with a patient with neuropathic pain is the absence of any deficit or injury. Socially, the patient appears "normal," yet suffers from a chronic painful condition. This can lead to psychosocial distress, as the patient is labeled "drug seeking."
- May be triggered by numerous insults, including direct nerve injury, infection, metabolic dysfunction, autoimmune disease, neoplasm, drugs, radiation, and neurovascular disorders
- May reflect the pathologic operation of a dysfunctional nervous system rather than a manifestation of any underlying pathology itself (i.e., phantom limb pain, complex regional pain syndrome [CRPS]):
  - Patients may paradoxically experience pain and hypersensitivity in an area of denervation.
- System(s) affected: Nervous; Musculoskeletal

EPIDEMIOLOGY

Incidence

Epidemiologic data are limited. It will also be varied, depending on the inclusion criteria: Radiculopathies, peripheral neuropathy, etc.:

- >3 million Americans suffer from painful diabetic neuropathy (PDN).
- 1 million Americans suffer from postherpetic neuralgia (PHN).

Prevalence

Estimated at 1.5% of the population, although recent studies in England, Germany, and France place it around 6–8% of the population.

RISK FACTORS

- Radiculopathy
- Polyneuropathy (diabetes mellitus, alcohol induced, postchemotherapy, heritable neuropathies)
- Trauma (nerve entrapment, postsurgical, nerve injury)
- Infection (HIV, herpes zoster)
- Central mechanisms (stroke, multiple sclerosis [MS], spinal cord injury, limb amputation)
- Nutritional deficiencies (B_{12}, folate)
- Medications (AIDS medications DDC and DDI, antibiotics metronidazole and isoniazid, some chemotherapeutics, amiodarone, hydralazine, phenytoin, nitrofurantoin)

PATHOPHYSIOLOGY

- Positive symptoms due to changes in peripheral nerves, loss of inhibitory mechanisms in CNS, and central sensitization
- Negative symptoms likely due to axonal or neuronal loss

ETIOLOGY

- Associated with a predisposing factor
- In addition to possible etiologies listed as risk factors above, others include:
  - Demyelinating disorders (MS, Guillain-Barré)
  - Neoplasm (primary or metastatic)
  - Neurovascular (central post-stroke syndrome, trigeminal neuralgia)
  - Autoimmune disease (Sjögren syndrome, polyarteritis nodosa)
  - Structural disease (herniated disc disease)

COMMONLY ASSOCIATED CONDITIONS

- Depression
- Anxiety
- Sleep disturbance
- Fibromyalgia

DIAGNOSIS

HISTORY

- May have history of nerve trauma; however, absence does not exclude the diagnosis of neuropathic pain
- Clinical manifestation can include both negative and positive sensory symptoms and signs. Motor dysfunction is rare.
- Pain is often described as burning, shocklike, tingling, numbing, or intensely hot or cold.

PHYSICAL EXAM

- Positive signs and symptoms:
  - Hyperalgesia: An exaggerated pain response to a noxious stimulus
  - Allodynia: The perception of pain due to a nonnoxious stimuli; for instance, gentle mechanical pressure, light pinprick, hot or cold stimuli, and vibration cause pain.
- Negative signs and symptoms: Reduced sensation to touch, pinprick, temperature, or vibration
- Motor signs and symptoms: Signs may include hypotonia, tremor, dystonia, ataxia, hypo-/hyperreflexia, or motor neglect. Motor symptoms include weakness, fatigability, decreased range of motion, joint stiffness, and spontaneous muscle spasm.

DIAGNOSTIC TESTS & INTERPRETATION

Lab

Initial lab tests

None specifically for neuropathic pain, but tests to rule out other causes should be considered:

- Serum B_{12}
- 25 hydroxy vitamin D
- Thyroid-stimulating hormone (TSH)
- Rapid plasma reagin (RPR) or venereal disease reaction level (VDRL)
- Fasting glucose, creatinine
- Lyme serology

Follow-Up & Special Considerations

Studies may include nerve conduction, electromyography, evoked potentials, quantitative sensory testing, thermography, radiologic imaging

Imaging

Initial approach

- Used to rule out other causes for pain
- Consider imaging based on affected area. MRI shows greatest anatomic detail for spine.
- Positron emission tomography (PET) and single-photon emission computed tomography (SPECT) scans, standard MRI, and functional MRI all have been used to map synaptic activity in the thalamus and somatosensory cortex. Initial studies using these imaging techniques have suggested maladaptive reorganization of the thalamus and somatosensory cortex.

Diagnostic Procedures/Surgery

- Sympathetic nerve blocks
- Epidural steroids
- Peripheral nerve blocks
- Dorsal column stimulator and peripheral nerve stimulator

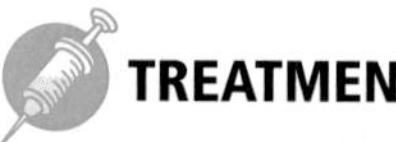

TREATMENT

MEDICATION

First Line

- All first-line agents are those that have been studied the most. However, the more we understand about chronic opioid therapy, the more we recommend *not* starting an opioid until other neuropathic agents have failed. In general, moving from 1 anticonvulsant or tricyclic antidepressant (TCA) to the other should be considered the first step of action.
- Gabapentin:
  - An anticonvulsant that has the broadest evidence for efficacy against neuropathic pain, FDA approved for its treatment (1)[A]
  - Evidence supports efficacy in PDN, PHN, phantom limb pain, Guillain-Barré syndrome, acute and chronic pain from spinal cord injury, and CRPS type 1 (2)[A]
  - Start 300 mg daily, increase gradually; dosing up to 600 mg t.i.d. is suggested; max dose of 3,600 mg/d in divided doses; adjust dose in renal insufficiency
  - Adequate trial of 3–8 weeks of therapy at full dose before considering it a failure
  - Interactions: No major drug–drug interactions
  - Adverse effects: Dizziness, somnolence, GI symptoms, peripheral edema
- Tricyclic antidepressants:
  - This class has the most evidence supporting a role in neuropathic pain (3)[A].
  - Dosing: Start at 10–25 mg at bedtime, then titrate up to antidepressant drug levels.
  - Secondary amines (nortriptyline, desipramine) are safer than amitriptyline and imipramine.
  - Precautions: Small therapeutic-to-toxic window; use caution in prescribing to those with cardiac risk factors, glaucoma, urinary retention; suicide susceptibility
  - Should obtain a pretreatment ECG for documentation and monitoring any arrhythmias

- Absolute contraindication with monamine oxidase inhibitors (MAOIs)
- Interactions: Numerous possible drug–drug interactions (type 1C antiarrhythmics, SSRIs, anticholinergics, sympathomimetics, CNS depressants)
- Adverse effects: QT interval abnormalities, arrhythmias, sedation, dry mouth, constipation, sexual dysfunction, weight gain, postural hypotension

- Tramadol (4)[A]:
  - Norepinephrine and serotonin inhibitor with a major metabolite that acts as an opioid (mu receptor) agonist
  - Dosage: 250 mg/d divided doses, max 400 mg/d
  - Precautions: Avoid in those with seizure history
  - Interactions: Increased seizure risk in those taking SSRIs, TCAs, MAOIs, neuroleptics concomitantly; increased risk of serotonergic symptoms if used with SSRIs, MAOIs; adjust dose for renal insufficiency, hepatic disease
  - Adverse effects: Dizziness, nausea, constipation, somnolence, orthostatic hypotension
- Pregabalin:
  - FDA approved for treatment of neuropathic pain secondary to PHN and diabetic polyneuropathy. Also approved for fibromyalgia (5)[A].
  - Dosage: Start at 75 mg b.i.d., maximum dose 300 mg b.i.d.
  - Interactions: No major drug–drug interactions
- Opioids (2)[A]:
  - According to the World Health Organization, should be used in "ladder" fashion, added to nonopioid agents if they are insufficient. However, this is usually for palliative cancer patients. Chronic opioid therapy can be detrimental to psychosocial environment of the patient.
  - Evidence for increased efficacy when used in conjunction with gabapentin
  - Controlled-release opioids recommended (controlled-release oxycodone, morphine, transdermal fentanyl, methadone)
  - Dosage: Start with short-acting analgesic equivalent to oral morphine sulfate 5–15 mg q4h; after 1–2 weeks of treatment, calculate equivalent dose of long-acting agent and use short-acting opioids for breakthrough.
  - No clear maximum dosage, but trials do not show benefits at doses higher than 180 mg/d of morphine.
  - Precaution: Avoid in those with history of substance abuse, use with caution in the elderly, may cause respiratory depression
  - Interactions: Additive effects with CNS depressants, increased risk of serotonin syndrome with serotonergic agents
  - Adverse effects: Constipation, sedation, nausea, lightheadedness
  - Adjuvant therapies with opioids should be used to treat nausea/vomiting, constipation, sedation, pruritus, etc.

Second Line

- Some evidence suggests use of other medications:
  - Antidepressants: Paroxetine, venlafaxine, duloxetine, bupropion, citalopram (2)
  - Duloxetine has comparable efficacy and tolerability to gabapentin and pregabalin in treatment of diabetic peripheral neuropathic pain (6)[A].
  - Anticonvulsants: Topiramate, Zonegran, lamotrigine, carbamazepine, oxcarbazepine
  - Antiarrhythmics: Mexiletine
  - NMDA receptor antagonists: Ketamine, dextromethorphan (5)
  - Other agents: Baclofen, clonidine, capsaicin
- Topical lidocaine; 5% lidocaine patch:
  - FDA approved for treatment of PHN, but has been used for other focal neuropathic pain syndromes
  - Dosage: Up to 3 patches for 12 hours daily
  - Interactions: No significant drug–drug interactions
  - Adverse effects: Mild skin reactions
  - Cochrane Review in 2007 showed insufficient evidence to recommend as first line.

ADDITIONAL TREATMENT

Issues for Referral

Referral to pain clinic or neurosurgery is appropriate if refractory to initial treatment.

Additional Therapies

- Transcutaneous electrical nerve stimulation (TENS) may be helpful; optimal dosing is yet to be established (7)[B].
- Spinal cord stimulation may be effective for chronic pain, especially if back surgery failed (8)[B].

COMPLEMENTARY AND ALTERNATIVE MEDICINE

See "Additional Therapies."

SURGERY/OTHER PROCEDURES

Nerve destructive procedures:

- Should be used with caution, as a refractory to treatment to different pain can ensue. If nononcological nerve damage, most neurolytic procedures are not recommended.
- Sympathetectomy: More studies needed for effectiveness and safety
- Dorsal root entry zone lesion (dorsal rhizotomy)
- Lateral cordotomy
- Trigeminal nerve ganglion ablation

ONGOING CARE

FOLLOW-UP RECOMMENDATIONS

- Multidisciplinary team improves care.
- Opioid contracts to prevent abuses

Patient Monitoring

Random urinalysis for specific prescribed drug and all drugs of abuse for patients receiving opioid therapy

PROGNOSIS

Chronic course of pain symptoms often requires management with numerous medications and adjunctive therapies.

COMPLICATIONS

Long-term disability is a possibility. Drug addiction is possible.

REFERENCES

1. Wiffen PJ, et al. Gabapentin for acute and chronic pain. *Cochrane Database Syst Rev*. 2007;4: CD005452.
2. Schmader KE. Epidemiology and impact on quality of life of postherpetic neuralgia and painful diabetic neuropathy. *Clin J Pain*. 2002;18:350–4.
3. Saarto T, Wiffen PJ. Antidepressants for neuropathic pain. *Cochrane Database Syst Rev*. 2007;4:CD005454.
4. Hollingshead J, et al. Tramadol for neuropathic pain. *Cochrane Database Syst Rev*. 2007;2:CD003726.
5. Galluzzi KE. Managing neuropathic pain. *J Am Osteopath Assoc*. 2007;107:ES39–48.
6. Quilici S, Chancellor J, Lothgren M, et al. Meta-analysis of duloxetine vs. pregabalin and gabapentin in the treatment of diabetic peripheral neuropathic pain. *BMC Neurol*. 2009;9:6.
7. Carrol D, et al. TENS for chronic pain. *Cochrane Database Syst Rev*. 2007;4:2007.
8. Mailis-Gagnon A, et al. Spinal cord stimulation for chronic pain. *Cochrane Database Syst Rev*. 2007; 4:CD003783.

ADDITIONAL READING

- Eisenberg E, McNicol E, Carr DB. Opioids for neuropathic pain. *Cochrane Database Syst Rev*. 2006;3:CD006146.
- Kroenke K, Krebs EE, Bair MJ. Pharmacotherapy of chronic pain: A synthesis of recommendations from systematic reviews. *Gen Hosp Psychiatry*. 2009;31:206–19.
- Raja SN, Haythornthwaite JA. Combination therapy for neuropathic pain–which drugs, which combination, which patients? *N Engl J Med*. 2005;352:1373–5.
- Torrance N, Smith BH, Benett MI, et al. The epidemiology of chronic pain of predominantly neuropathic origin. Results from a general population survey. *J Pain*. 2006;7(4):281–9.
- Wiffen PJ, McQuay HJ, Moore RA. Carbamazepine for acute and chronic pain. *Cochrane Database Syst Rev*. 2005;CD005451.

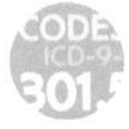

CODES

ICD9

- 349.9 Unspecified disorders of nervous system
- 356.9 Unspecified idiopathic peripheral neuropathy
- 729.2 Neuralgia, neuritis, and radiculitis, unspecified

CLINICAL PEARLS

- Multidisciplinary approach to pain management is suggested.
- Gabapentin is first-line for neuropathic pain, followed by other anticonvulsants, TCAs and SNRIs.
- A trial of interventional nerve blockage should be recommended prior to committing to chronic analgesic therapy.
- Opioids are used after 2 or 3 other attempts at treatment, in combination with other first-line agents. Opioids are generally considered weak neuropathic agents. Thus, high dosages are required to be effective in dealing with chronic pain. This presents a problem with potential for side effects, misuse, and addiction.

NEURORETINITIS

Michael Smit, OD, OMS IV
Melicien Tettambel, DO

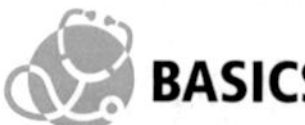

BASICS

DESCRIPTION

- Neuroretinitis (NR) is an acute inflammatory condition of the retina defined by optic disc edema and stellate maculopathy:
  - A characteristic pattern of macular exudates surrounds the fovea.
  - Vitreous cells are common.
- While many cases remain idiopathic, a broad list of infectious and autoimmune conditions has been associated.
- Various forms of neuroretinitis include the following:
  - Leber's idiopathic stellate neuroretinitis
  - Diffuse unilateral subacute neuroretinitis
  - Idiopathic retinitis
  - Vasculitis
  - Idiopathic retinal vasculitis, aneurysms, and neuroretinitis (IRVAN)
  - Recurrent neuroretinitis

EPIDEMIOLOGY

- There is no gender predilection (1).
- Ages have been reported from 8–55, with an average of 28 years old.
- Epidemiological data are limited for neuroretinitis.

Incidence

Unknown

Prevalence

Unknown

RISK FACTORS

Varies by underlying etiology

Genetics

No known genetic component

GENERAL PREVENTION

See prevention of underlying etiologies

PATHOPHYSIOLOGY

- The underlying pathophysiology involves increased permeability of disc vasculature, but the exact etiology is not fully defined:
  - Autoimmune
  - Infectious
- Optic disc edema is thought to be from the leakage of vessels within the optic nerve as demonstrated by fluorescein angiography.
- Juxtapapillary leakage may contribute to focal detachment and exudates.
- Exudates within the outer plexiform layer form the characteristic stellate pattern. These exudates get reabsorbed by macrophages (2).

ETIOLOGY

- Idiopathic (up to 50% of cases)
- Various bacterial, viral, protozoal, and parasitic causes have been described or suspected:
  - More commonly described are *Bartonella henselae*, *Rickettsia typhi*, Mycobacterium tuberculosis, *Borrelia burgdorferi*, *Treponema pallidum*, *Leptospira* spp., *Toxoplasmosis gondii*, HIV, HSV, HZV, EBV, hepatitis B, hepatitis C, mumps, Coxsackie B, *Toxocara canis*, Histoplasmosis Capsulatum, *Brucella* spp.
- Autoimmune conditions include antiphospholipid syndrome and sarcoidosis.

COMMONLY ASSOCIATED CONDITIONS

- See the broad list of underlying etiologies.
- Variations include Leber's idiopathic stellate neuroretinitis, diffuse unilateral subacute neuroretinitis (associated with nematode infection), idiopathic retinitis, vasculitis, IRVAN, and recurrent neuroretinitis.

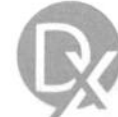

DIAGNOSIS

HISTORY

- Painless decrease in vision:
  - Typically unilateral
  - Less commonly bilateral
- Viral prodrome common
- Comprehensive social history including:
  - Travel and exposure history
  - Animal contacts
  - Foods
  - Sexual history

PHYSICAL EXAM

- Complete physical exam for suspected underlying association
- Neurological evaluation
- Complete eye exam with dilated funduscopy:
  - Decreased visual acuity, typically unilateral
  - Color vision changes
  - Desaturation of vision in the affected eye
  - Relative afferent pupillary defect
  - Optic disc edema
  - Retinal edema, exudates, stellate maculopathy
  - Deep, pale yellow–white retinal lesions

DIAGNOSTIC TESTS & INTERPRETATION

Lab

Directed to suspected underlying etiology

Initial lab tests

Evaluation might include:

- CBC
- ACE
- ANA
- Antidouble-stranded DNA
- C3
- ESR
- FTA-ABS
- Serologies for viral, fungal, and bacterial etiologies
- ELISA for *Toxocara canis*
- Tuberculin skin test

Follow-Up & Special Considerations

- The stellate macular appearance may develop subsequently to the optic nerve involvement and should be monitored in the first weeks after initial presentation.
- Rarely, a CSF evaluation may be indicated.

Imaging

Initial approach

MRI of the head and orbits

Diagnostic Procedures/Surgery

- Visual field testing may show a central scotoma affecting vision in the central field or a cecocentral scotoma, which includes the blind spot and extends into the area of central fixation due to involvement of the papillomacular bundle.
- Color vision testing
- Fluorescein angiography
- Optical coherence tomography (OCT)
- Diagnostic vitrectomy when appropriate

DIFFERENTIAL DIAGNOSIS

- Optic neuritis
- Hypertensive retinopathy
- Diabetic papillitis
- Anterior ischemic optic neuropathy

ALERT

If a bilateral presentation is found, the differential diagnosis should expand to include increased intracranial pressure or mass effect.

TREATMENT

- The treatment is directed at the underlying etiology:
  - High-dose oral steroids are commonly used in idiopathic and recurrent neuroretinitis with occasional high-dose IV steroids used in recurrent neuroretinitis (3)[C].
  - Steroids do not appear to alter visual outcomes (1).
- Consider antibiotics for cat-scratch disease (CSD) while serologies are pending:
  - Adults: Ciprofloxacin or azithromycin
  - Children: Azithromycin or sulfamethoxazole-trimethoprim (3)

MEDICATION

Direct to underlying etiology

ADDITIONAL TREATMENT

Laser treatment has been utilized for *Toxocara canis* (4).

Issues for Referral

Refer for neurological and ophthalmological consultation upon initial suspicion.

COMPLEMENTARY AND ALTERNATIVE MEDICINE

N/A

SURGERY/OTHER PROCEDURES

Laser treatment can be directed at the invading organism in helminthic infections (4).

IN-PATIENT CONSIDERATIONS

As necessary for underlying systemic or neurologic complications

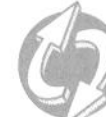

ONGOING CARE

FOLLOW-UP RECOMMENDATIONS

- Systemic monitoring will depend on the symptoms and underlying etiology.
- Ophthalmologic monitoring may be weekly initially to monitor for development of macular star and depending on underlying etiology and severity, followed by less frequent monitoring until a resolution of optic nerve involvement and macular involvement.
- Macular involvement may take longer to subside (5).

Patient Monitoring

Directed to underlying etiology

DIET

No specific diet

PROGNOSIS

- Generally favorable outlook with typical reported recovery of vision to 20/40 or better within 2 months (6)
- The optic disc edema resolves over 8–12 weeks (2).

COMPLICATIONS

- Permanent vision loss
- Retinal detachment
- Optic atrophy
- Retinal pigment epithelial defects

REFERENCES

1. Dreyer RF, Hopen G, Gass JD, et al. Leber's idiopathic stellate neuroretinitis. *Arch Ophthalmol.* 1984;102:1140–5.
2. Ray S, Gragoudas E, et al. Neuroretinitis. *Int Ophthalmol Clin.* 2001;41:83–102.
3. Purvin V, Sundaram S, Kawasaki A, et al. Neuroretinitis: Review of the literature and new observations. *J Neuroophthalmol.* 2011;31:58–68.
4. Narayan SK, Kaliaperumal S, Srinivasan R, et al. Neuroretinitis, a great mimicker. *Ann Indian Acad Neurol.* 2008;11:109–13.
5. Maitland CG, Miller NR, et al. Neuroretinitis. *Arch Ophthalmol.* 1984;102:1146–50.
6. Casson RJ, O'Day J, Crompton JL. Leber's stellate neuroretinitis: Differential diagnosis and approach to management. *Aust N Z J Ophthalmol.* 1999 Feb;27(1):65–9.

ADDITIONAL READING

Spencer BR, Digre KB, et al. Treatments for neuro-ophthalmologic conditions. *Neurol Clin.* 2010;28:1005–35.

CODES

ICD9

363.05 Focal retinitis and retinochoroiditis, juxtapapillary

CLINICAL PEARLS

- For a patient with painless unilateral vision loss after a viral-like prodrome, consider neuroretinitis and refer immediately to an ophthalmologist for further evaluation including a complete eye exam with dilated funduscopy.
- Many of the underlying etiologies can present with various eye manifestations in addition to neuroretinitis, including anterior uveitis, retinitis, chorioretinitis, posterior uveitis, optic neuritis, and endophthalmitis.

NEUTROPENIA, CYCLIC

Eyad Akrad, MD
Timothy J. Barreiro, DO, FCCP, FACOI

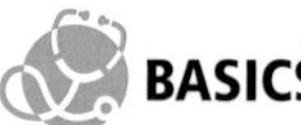

BASICS

DESCRIPTION

- A rare hematological disorder characterized by recurrent fevers, mouth ulcers, and infections attributable to regularly recurring severe neutropenia
- Although inherited in an autosomal-dominant pattern, mutations in the gene for neutrophil elastase (ELA-2), sporadic mutations can occur.
- Exhibits oscillations of neutrophils with 21-day periodicity, but cycle length may vary from 14–40 days
- During the neutropenic period, blood neutrophil levels fall to $<0.2 \times 10^9$/L for 3–5 days, before increasing to near the lower limit of normal, about 2×10^9/L.

EPIDEMIOLOGY

- Most patients present before the age of 5:
  - 32% are <1 year
  - 27% are between ages 1–5
- Occurs equally in both sexes

Incidence

1 in a million persons in the general population

RISK FACTORS

Family history is predictive, although patients proven to have the (ELA) mutation will lack positive family history due to subclinical presentation among family members, new mutation, or variability in expression

Genetics

- Inherited as an autosomal-dominant disorder with full penetrance but varying severity of clinical manifestations (expression)
- Most commonly sporadic
- Due to mutations in the gene for neutrophil elastase (ELA-2 or ELANE) on chromosome 19p13.3

GENERAL PREVENTION

Genetic counseling

PATHOPHYSIOLOGY

- Bone marrow during neutropenia demonstrates "maturation arrest" at the promyelocyte and myelocyte stage of development
- At least 80% of cases of cyclic neutropenia are attributable to the mutations for neutrophil elastase (ELA-2/ELANE). The effect of these mutations shortens survival of neutrophil progenitors through accelerated apoptosis, making neutrophil production inefficient. It is not known if any other mutations can cause this disease.

ETIOLOGY

The cause of acquired cyclic neutropenia is unknown.

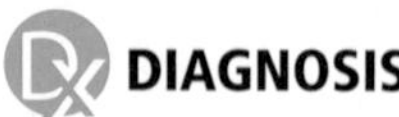

DIAGNOSIS

HISTORY

- Usually an infant (age <1 year)
- Recurrent clinical syndrome and infections correlating with cyclic neutropenia
- May be asymptomatic during neutropenic periods
- Patients are usually asymptomatic, with normal exam between neutropenic periods
- The clinical syndrome (1)[C]:
  - Phase 1:
    - 1–3 days
    - Patient feels listless and irritable
    - Dullness to the eyes
    - Swelling of lips
    - Pallor
    - Low-grade fever
  - Phase 2:
    - 1–3 days
    - Aphthous ulcers
    - Tender cervical lymphadenopathy
    - Temperature peaks
  - Phase 3:
    - Fever resolves
    - Return of well-being
    - Healing of oral aphthae
- Additional manifestations:
  - Most common:
    - Gingivitis
    - Furunculosis
    - Cellulitis
    - Infection of cuts or abrasions
    - Pharyngitis
    - Sinusitis
    - Otitis
  - Less common:
    - Pneumonia
    - Perianal abscesses
    - Necrotic bowels and spontaneous perforation
    - Bacteremia (*Clostridium septicum*)

PHYSICAL EXAM

Evaluate for bowel perforation (rare); with signs of peritonitis in presence of abdominal pain

DIAGNOSTIC TESTS & INTERPRETATION

Lab

- Diagnostic:
  - Serial blood counts are necessary to make the diagnosis (2)[C]:
    - Obtained at least 3 days a week for 6 weeks or longer
    - Should show at least 2 neutrophil counts (nadirs) $<0.2 \times 10^9$/L
    - Cycle length should be about 21 days
    - Neutrophilic troughs are synchronous with mouth ulcers and other inflammatory features.
  - Genetic testing (3)[A]:
    - Sequencing of *ELA-2* gene is helpful in diagnosis.
    - Not yet established as the primary method to establish the diagnosis
    - Some patients with severe congenital neutropenia have mutations in the same region of *ELA-2* gene.
  - Bone marrow examination is only necessary to rule out other diagnoses.
- Nondiagnostic lab findings:
  - Neutropenic episodes are usually associated with normal or near normal total leukocyte counts.
  - Oscillations in monocyte, reticulocyte, and platelet counts are frequently observed (cyclic hematopoiesis).
  - The cyclic oscillation of monocytes and reticulocytes is reciprocal to that of neutrophils; whereas, platelet oscillation is similar.
  - Typically, there is a monocytosis throughout most of the cycle.
  - Despite cycling of blood elements, hemoglobin concentration and platelet counts remain in the normal range.

Follow-Up & Special Considerations

25 OH vitamin D level

Imaging

Bone mineral density scan once diagnosis is made

DIFFERENTIAL DIAGNOSIS

- Kostmann agranulocytosis (severe congenital neutropenia)
- Neutropenia due to myelopoiesis and lymphopoiesis:
  - Reticular dysgenesis (congenital aleukia)
- Neutropenia with associated B- or T-lymphocyte abnormalities:
  - X-linked agammaglobulinemia (Bruton disease)
  - Dysgammaglobulinemia
- Neutropenia with associated inherited metabolic diseases:
  - Disorders of propionate and methylmalonate
  - Branched chain organic aciduria
  - Type 1B glycogen storage disease
- Neutropenia with associated phenotypic abnormalities:
  - Shwachman syndrome
  - Cartilage-hair hypoplasia
  - Dyskeratosis congenita
- Neutropenia with associated neutrophil morphologic abnormalities:
  - Myelokathexis
- Drug-induced neutropenia:
  - Antibiotics: Penicillins, chloramphenicol, sulfonamides
  - Antithyroid medication
  - NSAIDs
- Autoimmune neutropenia (chronic benign neutropenia)
- Neutropenia as part of aplastic anemia
- Neutropenia due to marrow infiltration by cancer cells
- Neutropenia due to sepsis

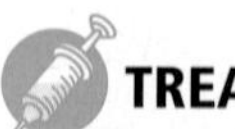

TREATMENT

MEDICATION

First Line

- Patients respond well to treatment with granulocyte colony-stimulating factor (G-CSF) (4,5,6)[A].
- SC G-CSF on a daily or alternate-day basis is usually well tolerated by patients of all ages (7)[A].
- Initial dose is 1–2 mg/kg/d; most patients can be managed on <3 mg/kg/d.

- The required response is:
  - To shorten the duration of neutropenia, usually reflected by resolution of mouth ulcers, fever, and other inflammatory symptoms
  - To elevate the neutrophil counts at all other phases of the cycle
  - To shorten the cycle length
- Avoidance of very high counts by constant low-dose treatment may prevent side effects:
  - Bone pain and osteoporosis
  - Myalgia and arthralgia
  - Headaches
- Some patients with confirmed diagnosis and typical mutation are relatively asymptomatic and do not require G-CSF treatment.

Second Line

There is ***no other clearly beneficial therapy:***

- Granulocyte-macrophage colony-stimulating factor (GM-CSF) has side effects and is less potent.
- Corticosteroids, lithium, and androgens are ineffective.
- Cyclic neutropenia can be cured by hematopoietic cell transplantation in an animal model, and has been transferred from an affected human donor to a recipient following bone marrow transplantation. However, stem cell transplantation has not been used because of G-CSF effectiveness.

ADDITIONAL TREATMENT

There are no absolute guidelines regarding the use of antibiotics. Experienced clinicians suggest (8)[C]:

- Antibiotics are not required for every neutropenic period.
- Clinical judgement is more important than superficial microbial cultures.
- After infancy, mouth, throat, and skin ulcers and inflammation during neutropenic periods can generally be managed without antibiotics.
- Antibiotics are recommended in the case of otitis, sinusitis, or lower respiratory tract infection.
- Neutropenic ileocolitis requires parenteral antibiotics if suspected [4].

General Measures

- Genetic counseling
- Regular and aggressive dental care
- Antibacterial mouthwash Peridex is useful in decreasing gingivitis (8)[A].
- Bone density screening is recommended; osteoporosis can develop during prolonged G-CSF treatment (5)[C].
- Maintaining adequate levels of vitamin D is recommended.

IN-PATIENT CONSIDERATIONS

Admission Criteria

- Routine hospitalization for episodes of febrile neutropenia is usually not required, as the patients have active monocytosis during neutropenia and lymphocyte-mediated immunity is not impaired.
- Hospitalization is recommended in the case of severe abdominal symptoms (neutropenic ileocolitis) to prevent bowel necrosis and spontaneous perforation, with the following measurements (8)[C]:
  - Bowel rest
  - IV hydration
  - Parenteral antibiotics to cover enteric organisms, especially clostridial species

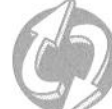

ONGOING CARE

FOLLOW-UP RECOMMENDATIONS

Patient Monitoring

Once the diagnosis is established and G-CSF treatment has started (2)[C]:

- Blood counts should be obtained periodically to avoid overtreatment or undertreatment.
- On reaching a stable dose of G-CSF, blood counts can be monitored every few months.

DIET

No specific diet is generally recommended.

PATIENT EDUCATION

- Because of the great regularity of cycles, patients can learn to organize their lives around the disease.
- Patients can predict the neutropenic periods and avoid activities that might cause minor injuries.
- Dental work and surgery can be planned to avoid neutropenic periods.
- Patients can be reassured that incidental infections should respond uniformly and readily to antimicrobials.
- Patients should be counseled to seek medical attention if abdominal pain is persistent or associated with significant abdominal tenderness.

PROGNOSIS

- Cyclic neutropenia is a benign disease; patients grow and develop normally.
- Sepsis and death from bacteremias are uncommon, but they are a source of fear and concern for patients and their parents.
- Evolution to myeloid leukemia is not a recognized complication with or without treatment with G-CSF.
- Evolution to myelodysplasia is not reported.
- Symptoms and the oscillations in the blood count abate as the patient gets older.

COMPLICATIONS

- Chronic gingivitis
- Increased dental caries
- Premature tooth mobility and loss
- Septic shock due to perforating colonic ulcers and infections of clostridial species and gram-negative organisms
- Increased rate of spontaneous abortions in women

REFERENCES

1. Wright DG, Dale DC, Fauci AS, et al. Human cyclic neutropenia: Clinical review and long-term follow-up of patients. *Medicine (Baltimore)*. 1981;60:1–13.
2. Dale DC, Welte K, et al. Cyclic and chronic neutropenia. *Cancer Treat Res*. 2011;157:97–108.
3. Aprikyan AA, Dale DC, et al. Mutations in the neutrophil elastase gene in cyclic and congenital neutropenia. *Curr Opin Immunol*. 2001;13:535–8.
4. Dale DC, Bonilla MA, Davis MW, et al. A randomized controlled phase III trial of recombinant human granulocyte colony-stimulating factor (filgrastim) for treatment of severe chronic neutropenia. *Blood*. 1993;81:2496–502.
5. Dale DC, Cottle TE, Fier CJ, et al. Severe chronic neutropenia: Treatment and follow-up of patients in the Severe Chronic Neutropenia International Registry. *Am J Hematol*. 2003;72:82–93.
6. Heussner P, Haase D, Kanz L, et al. G-CSF in the long-term treatment of cyclic neutropenia and chronic idiopathic neutropenia in adult patients. *Int J Hematol*. 1995;62:225–34.
7. Jayabose S, Tugal O, Sandoval C, et al. Recombinant human granulocyte colony stimulating factor in cyclic neutropenia: Use of a new 3-day-a-week regimen. *Am J Pediatr Hematol Oncol*. 1994;16:338–40.
8. Dale DC, Hammond WP, et al. Cyclic neutropenia: A clinical review. *Blood Rev*. 1988;2:178–85.

ADDITIONAL READING

- Dale DC, Bolyard AA, Aprikyan A, et al. Cyclic neutropenia. *Semin Hematol*. 2002;39:89–94.
- Dale DC, Bolyard AA, Hammond WP, et al. Cyclic neutropenia: Natural history and effects of long-term treatment with recombinant human granulocyte colony-stimulating factor. *Cancer Invest*. 1993;11:219–23.
- Haurie C, Dale DC, Mackey MC, et al. Cyclical neutropenia and other periodic hematological disorders: A review of mechanisms and mathematical models. *Blood*. 1998;92:2629–40.
- Wright DG, Kenney RF, Oette DH, et al. Contrasting effects of recombinant human granulocyte-macrophage colony-stimulating factor (CSF) and granulocyte CSF treatment on the cycling of blood elements in childhood-onset cyclic neutropenia. *Blood*. 1994;84:1257–67.

CODES

ICD9

288.02 Cyclic neutropenia

CLINICAL PEARLS

- Cyclic neutropenia is a benign disease; bowel necrosis and perforation are rare, but may be associated with mortality.
- While establishing the diagnosis requires obtaining 3 blood counts a week for 6 weeks to demonstrate the specific findings mentioned above, genetic testing can confirm the diagnosis.
- The mainstay of treatment is SC recombinant G-CSF, which is effective and well tolerated.

NICOTINE ADDICTION

Brett White, MD

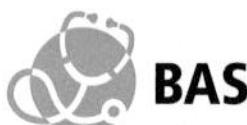

BASICS

DESCRIPTION

Nicotine addiction is characterized by signs of dependence (compulsive use of a substance despite knowledge of its adverse effects).

EPIDEMIOLOGY

Incidence

20–25% of the US population smokes.

Prevalence

70 million Americans ≥12 years of age reported current use of tobacco (58.7 million were cigarette smokers, 13.3 million smoked cigars, 8.6 million used smokeless tobacco, 2.1 million smoked pipes) (1)[B].

Pediatric Considerations

7.1% of 8th graders, 13.6% of 10th graders, and 19.2% of 12th graders have used cigarettes in the past 30 days (1).

RISK FACTORS

- Mental illness (depression, posttraumatic stress disorder, bipolar disorder, and schizophrenia)
- Low socioeconomic status
- Low educational status
- Early firsthand nicotine experience increases risk for chronic abuse.
- Environmental factors are critical for smoking initiation; genetic factors contribute to smoking persistence and difficulty quitting.

Genetics

- Mutation in the b1$_4$ subunit of nicotinic acetylcholine receptors (nAChRs) expressed by neurons was found to lower the threshold for the induction of nicotine dependence.
- Specific genes have been isolated that are associated with nicotine dependence, including *CHRNB3,* the b2$_3$ nicotine receptor subunit gene.
- T-variant gene associated with decreased activity of CYP2B6 (enzyme that breaks down nicotine in the brain); may lead to increased craving during smoking cessation. These patients are also 1.5 times more likely to resume smoking during treatment.

GENERAL PREVENTION

- Physician advice:
  - The USPSTF strongly recommends clinicians screen all adults for tobacco use and provide tobacco cessation interventions for those who use tobacco products. Rating: A Recommendation.
  - The USPSTF strongly recommends clinicians screen all pregnant women for tobacco use and provide augmented pregnancy-tailored counseling to those who smoke. Rating: A Recommendation.
  - The USPSTF concludes the evidence is insufficient to recommend for or against routine screening for tobacco use or interventions to prevent and treat tobacco use and dependence among children or adolescents. Rating: I Recommendation.
- School-based smoking-prevention education

PATHOPHYSIOLOGY

- Mechanism by which nicotine binds to nAChR and how this leads to dependence is still poorly understood, though likely involves activation of the mesocorticolimbic system with resulting dopamine release.
- Nicotine has both stimulating and depressing effects within the CNS; relaxing and euphoric effects may contribute to psychological dependence.

Pregnancy Considerations

- Carbon monoxide and nicotine may interfere with oxygen supply to the fetus, resulting in fetal growth restriction and decreased birth weight.
- Smoking may increase the incidence of spontaneous abortion and SIDS, as well as learning or behavioral problems and an increased risk of obesity in children (1).

ETIOLOGY

Polymorphisms in neuronal nAChR genes could be associated with increased susceptibility to tobacco dependence.

COMMONLY ASSOCIATED CONDITIONS

- COPD (emphysema and chronic bronchitis)
- Cancers (lung, oral/pharyngeal, kidney, bladder, cervical, anal)
- Coronary artery disease
- Periodontal disease

DIAGNOSIS

DIAGNOSTIC TESTS & INTERPRETATION

Spirometry: Decreased FEV$_1$ (may be present in COPD)

Diagnostic Procedures/Surgery

Using spirometry to determine "lung age" (approximation of age of patient's lungs based on the faster decline in FEV1 than is expected with normal aging)

DIFFERENTIAL DIAGNOSIS

- Depression
- COPD
- b1$_1$-antitrypsin deficiency
- Asthma
- CHF
- Respiratory infections
- Lung cancer
- Cystic fibrosis

TREATMENT

Counseling:

- Advice from doctors helps people who smoke to quit.
- Providing brief, simple advice about quitting smoking increases likelihood that someone who smokes will successfully quit and remain a nonsmoker 12 months later. More intensive advice (i.e., motivational interviewing, etc.) may result in higher rates of quitting. Providing follow-up support after offering the advice may increase the quit rates slightly (2)[A].
- The USPSTF strongly recommends screening all adults for tobacco use and providing tobacco cessation interventions for those who use tobacco products. Rating: A recommendation.

MEDICATION

First Line

- Varenicline (Chantix) is a nicotinic acetylcholine partial agonist for the treatment of nicotine addiction. Trials have suggested this agent may be more efficacious than bupropion (3)[A]. Longer-term therapy (up to 24 weeks) may delay or prevent relapse:
  - Starter package includes 0.5 mg/d for 3 days, then 0.5 mg b.i.d. for 4 days, then 1 mg/d starting on day 7.
  - Maintenance package includes 1 mg b.i.d. (continue for 12 weeks total).
- Nicotine replacement therapy (NRT). All forms of NRT increase the chance of stopping smoking by 50–70%. There is no overall difference in effectiveness of different forms of NRT nor a benefit for using patches beyond 8 weeks. Heavier smokers may need higher doses. Starting NRT before planned quit date may increase the chance of success (4)[A]:
  - Nicotine gum (Nicorette): For >25 cigarettes/d habit, 4-mg gum q1–2h for 6 weeks; for <25 cigarettes/d habit, 2-mg gum q1–2h for 6 weeks; decrease dosing by q1–2h for 3 weeks; chew, then tuck between cheek and gingiva
  - Nicotine transdermal (NicoDerm CQ): For >10 cigarettes/d habit, 21-mg patch/d for 6 weeks, then 14-mg patch/d for 2 weeks, then 7-mg patch/d for 2 weeks; for <10 cigarettes/d habit, 14-mg patch/d for 6 weeks, then 7-mg patch/d for 2 weeks
  - Nicotine lozenge (Commit): For patients who have first cigarette within 30 minutes of waking, 4-mg lozenge PO q1–2h for 6 weeks; first cigarette >30 minutes after waking, 2-mg lozenge PO q1–2h for 6 weeks; decrease dosing by q1–2h for 3 weeks.
  - Nicotine nasal (Nicotrol NS): 1–2 sprays (0.5 mg/spray) each nostril q1h for 8 weeks, then taper; maximum 10 sprays/h and 80 sprays/d
  - Nicotine inhaler (Nicotrol inhaler): 6–16 cartridges inhaled (4 mg/cartridge) per day for 6–12 weeks, then taper
- Medications:
  - Bupropion (Zyban): An antidepressant; start 150 mg/d PO for 3 days, then 150 mg PO b.i.d.; stop smoking 5–7 days after starting treatment; continue 7–12 weeks

ALERT

Varenicline (Chantix) has not been studied when used in patients with serious psychiatric illness. It should be used with extreme caution in patients with serious psychiatric disorders (bipolar disorder, depression, or schizophrenia), as use may exacerbate these conditions.

Second Line

- Nortriptyline: Tricyclic antidepressant; start 25 mg/d, gradually increase to target dose of 75–100 mg/d; stop smoking 2–4 weeks after starting treatment; continue for 12 weeks:
  - Contraindications: Narrow-angle glaucoma or heart disease (AMI, AV, or bundle-branch block, QT prolongation)
  - Caution: Pregnancy Category D

- Clonidine: 0.1-mg patch per week, increase dose as needed; continue for 3–10 weeks:
  - Caution: Must monitor BP closely and taper when discontinuing.
- Benzodiazepines: Although this class of drug has not improved rates of abstinence from smoking, patients with a high level of anxiety possibly could benefit from anxiolytics as a smoking-cessation intervention.

ADDITIONAL TREATMENT

Pregnancy Considerations

- The USPSTF strongly recommends clinicians screen all pregnant women for tobacco use and provide augmented pregnancy-tailored counseling to those who smoke. Rating: A recommendation.
- Other interventions:
  - Smokers who get support from partners and other people are more likely to quit.
  - Group programs double cessation rates more than being given self-help materials without face-to-face instruction and group support. It is unclear whether groups are better than individual counseling or other advice, but they are more effective than no treatment. Not all smokers making a quit attempt want to attend group meetings, but for those who do, they are likely to be helpful.
- Smokers should be given a choice of quitting methods, either reducing smoking before quitting or abruptly quitting, as neither has demonstrated superior quit rates.

Pregnancy Considerations

Interventions were effective in helping women to stop smoking during pregnancy (overall by ~6%). The most effective intervention appeared to be providing incentives, which helped around 24% of women to quit smoking during pregnancy. The smoking cessation interventions reduced the number of babies with low birth weight and preterm births, confirming that smoking cessation can reduce the adverse effects of smoking on newborn infants.

General Measures

- Brief strategies to help the patient willing to quit tobacco use—the "5 A's":
  - *Ask* the patient if he or she uses tobacco.
  - *Advise* him or her to quit.
  - *Assess* willingness to make a quit attempt.
  - *Assist* those who are willing to make a quit attempt.
  - *Arrange* for follow-up contact to prevent relapse (5).
- Enhancing motivation to quit tobacco—the "5 R's":
  - *Relevance*—Encourage the patient to indicate why quitting is personally relevant.
  - *Risks*—Ask the patient to identify potential negative consequences of tobacco use.
  - *Rewards*—Ask the patient to identify potential benefits of stopping tobacco use.
  - *Roadblocks*—Ask the patient to identify barriers or impediments to quitting, and provide treatment (e.g., problem-solving counseling or medication) that could address barriers.
  - *Repetition*—The motivational intervention should be repeated every time an unmotivated patient visits the clinic setting (6)[A].

COMPLEMENTARY AND ALTERNATIVE MEDICINE

- Acupuncture: No consistent evidence acupuncture is effective for smoking cessation
- Hypnotherapy: No good evidence to show whether or not hypnotherapy can help people trying to quit smoking

IN-PATIENT CONSIDERATIONS

- Programs to stop smoking that begin during a hospital stay and include follow-up support for at least 1 month after discharge are effective. Programs are effective when administered to all hospitalized smokers, regardless of admitting diagnosis.
- Consider NRT to all inpatients who smoke to decrease withdrawal symptoms.

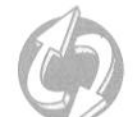

ONGOING CARE

FOLLOW-UP RECOMMENDATIONS

- Patients motivated to quit smoking and who have initiated therapy should follow up routinely with the physician to monitor response and observe for any medication side effects.
- Encourage routine exercise as a component of smoking-cessation treatment.

DIET

Weight gain (4–5 kg over 10 years) possible after smoking cessation

PATIENT EDUCATION

- www.smokefree.gov
- www.nicotine-anonymous.org
- http://quitnet.com

PROGNOSIS

More than 85% of those who try to quit on their own relapse, most within a week (1).

REFERENCES

1. National Institute on Drug Abuse. *Tobacco Addiction*. National Institute of Health; 2009 June. NIH Publication Number 09-4342.
2. Stead LF, Bergson G, Lancaster T. Physician advice for smoking cessation. *Cochrane Database Syst Rev*. 2008;2:CD000165.
3. Cahill K, Stead LF, Lancaster T. Nicotine receptor partial agonists for smoking cessation. *Cochrane Database Syst Rev*. 2008;3:CD006103.
4. Stead LF, Perera R, Bullen C, et al. Nicotine replacement therapy for smoking cessation. *Cochrane Database Syst Rev*. 2008;1:CD000146.
5. Dixon LB, Medoff D, Goldberg R, et al. Is implementation of the 5 A's of smoking cessation at community mental health centers effective for reduction of smoking by patients with serious mental illness? *Am J Addict*. 2009;18:386–92.
6. The Clinical Practice Guideline Treating Tobacco Use and Dependence 2008 Update Panel, Liaisons, and Staff. A Clinical Practice Guideline for Treating Tobacco Use and Dependence: 2008 Update A U.S. Public Health Service Report. *Am J Prev Med*. 2008; 35:158–76.

ADDITIONAL READING

The Agency for Health Care Policy and Research Smoking Cessation Clinical Practice Guideline. *JAMA*. 1996;275:1270–80.

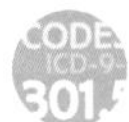

CODES

ICD9

- V15.82 Personal history of tobacco use
- 305.1 Tobacco use disorder
- 649.00 Tobacco use disorder complicating pregnancy

CLINICAL PEARLS

- Smoking cessation should be encouraged to all patients who smoke.
- There is no one type of NRT that is best; they are equally effective. Choice, therefore, should be based on patient preference.
- Consider NRT to all inpatients who smoke to decrease withdrawal symptoms.

NOSOCOMIAL INFECTIONS

Cheryl Durand, PharmD, RPh
Edward L. Yourtee, MD

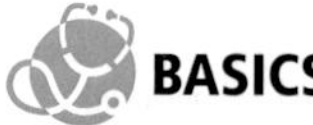

BASICS

DESCRIPTION

- Also known as *health care–associated infections* (HAIs)
- Infection must not have been present or incubating on admission to health care facility
- CDC categories:
  - Catheter-associated urinary tract infection (CAUTI)
  - Surgical site infection (SSI)
  - Ventilator-associated pneumonia (VAP)
  - Central line-associated bloodstream infection (CLABSI)
  - *Clostridium difficile* infection (*C. diff, C. difficile*, CDAD, CDI)
- The National Healthcare Safety Network (NHSN) at www.cdc.gov/nhsn monitors the epidemiology of emerging HAI pathogens and their mechanisms of resistance and evaluates alternative surveillance and prevention strategies .
- *Medicare and Medicaid will not provide payment for the treatment of certain hospital-acquired conditions (HAC), including catheter-associated UTIs, central line–associated bloodstream infections, and some surgical site infections.*

EPIDEMIOLOGY

- General:
  - 13/1,000 patient-days in the ICU (1)
  - 6.9/1,000 patient-days in high-risk nurseries (2)
  - 2.6/1,000 patient-days in nurseries (1)
  - Estimated cost of HAIs is $20 billion per year (3).
- Infection-specific:
  - Catheter-associated UTI:
    - Hospital stay increased by 1–3 days
    - Cost up to $600 per infection
  - Ventilator-associated pneumonia:
    - Hospital stay increased by 6 days
    - Cost up to $5,000 per infection
  - Central line–associated bloodstream infection:
    - Hospital stay increased by 7–20 days
    - Cost up to $56,000 per infection (4)
  - Surgical-site infection:
    - Hospital stay increased 7.3 days
    - Cost >$3,000 per infection
    - May not be apparent until 1 month after surgery
  - *Clostridium difficile* infection (see topic "*Clostridium Difficile* Infection")

Incidence

- 1.7 million HAIs in 2002 (1)
- 5–10% of hospital stays are complicated by HAIs (3).
- The majority of patients affected have a single-site infection.
- UTI: 36% of HAIs (1):
  - 424,060 cases in 2002 in the US (1)
  - 2.39/100 admissions
- Pneumonia: 11% of HAIs (1):
  - 129,519 cases in 2002 in the US (1)
  - 0.60/100 admissions
- Bloodstream infection: 11% of HAIs (1):
  - 133,368 cases in 2002 in the US (1)
  - 0.27/100 admissions
- Surgical-site infection: 20% of HAIs (1):
  - 244,385 cases in 2002 in the US (1)
  - 3% of all surgeries (2)
  - 20% of emergency abdominal surgeries (2)
- Others: 22% of HAIs (1): 263,810 cases in 2002 in the US (1)
- Resistance rates are increasing among several problematic gram-negative pathogens that are often responsible for serious nosocomial infections, including carbapenemase-producing *Klebsiella* and *Acinetobacter* (5).
- In 2008, 70% of nosocomial infections were resistant to at least 1 antimicrobial drug that was effective previously (6).

RISK FACTORS

- Extremes of age
- Chronic disease (including diabetes, renal failure, and malignancy)
- Immunodeficiency
- Malnutrition
- Medications such as antibiotics, antacids, and sedatives
- Colonization with pathogenic strains of flora
- Breakdown of mucosal or cutaneous barriers, including trauma and battle wounds
- Anesthesia

GENERAL PREVENTION

- Prevention efforts should address both patient-specific and facility-related risk factors.
- Hand hygiene:
  - Before direct patient contact (7)[B]
  - After contact with blood, excretions, body fluids, wound dressings, nonintact skin, mucous membranes (7)[A]
  - After contact with intact skin (7)[B]
  - When hands will be moving from contaminated to clean body site (7)[C]
  - Alcohol-based product: When hands are not visibly soiled (7)[A]
  - Soap and water:
    - When visibly soiled (7)[A]
    - When in contact with spores (7)[C]
- Antibiotic stewardship: The use of narrow-spectrum antibiotics reduces the risk of multidrug resistant organisms and the occurrence of *C. difficile*.
- Hospital-based surveillance programs
- Infection control programs with specially trained employees (7)[B]
- Employee education on HAIs (7)[B]
- Minimize invasive procedures.
- Isolation of known pathogen carriers (7)[A]:
  - Contact precautions:
    - Pathogens spread by direct contact.
    - Gloves when entering room (7)[B]
    - Gown if clothing will touch patient or environment (7)[B]
    - Includes methicillin-resistant *Staphylococcus aureus* (MRSA), vancomycin-resistant *Enterococcus*, *C. difficile*, extended-spectrum β-lactamase-producing gram-negative rods
  - Droplet precautions:
    - Infectious particles measure $>5\ \mu m$
    - Mask when entering room (7)[B]
    - Shed via talking, coughing, sneezing, mucosal shedding, airway suctioning, bronchoscopy
    - Includes *Neisseria meningitis*, influenza, *Haemophilus influenzae*, diphtheria, *Bordetella pertussis*
  - Airborne precautions:
    - Infectious particles measure $<5\ \mu m$
    - Fit-tested National Institute of Occupational Safety and Health (NIOSH)–approved N-95 or higher respirator on entering room (7)[B]
    - Shed via coughing
    - Includes tuberculosis, varicella-zoster virus, measles
- Infection-specific measures:
  - Catheter-associated UTI:
    - Employee education on urinary catheters (e.g., indications, placement, maintenance) (8)[C]
    - Sterile catheter placement technique (8)[C]
    - Closed urine collection system (8)[C]
    - Use of catheter only as necessary (8)[B]
    - Removal of catheter as early as possible (8)[B]
  - Ventilator-associated pneumonia:
    - Intubation only as necessary (9)[C]
    - Perform oral decontamination with an antiseptic agent (10)[A].
    - Avoidance of nasotracheal intubation (9)[B]
    - Inline suctioning (9)[C]
    - Head elevation of 30–45° (9)[C]
  - Central line–associated bloodstream infection:
    - Employee education on IV catheters (e.g., indications, placement, maintenance) (11)[A]
    - Sterile catheter placement technique (including chlorhexidine prep, maximal barrier precautions) (11)[A]
    - Prompt removal of catheter (11)[A]
    - Hand hygiene in addition to glove use (11)[A]
    - Regular monitoring of catheter site (11)[B]
  - Surgical-site infection:
    - Proper surgical hand hygiene (3)[B]
    - Prophylactic antibiotic therapy when indicated (3)[A]
    - Elimination of underlying infections before surgery (3)[A]
    - Hair removal with electric clippers or depilatory agent (3)[B]
    - Postoperative blood sugar control
  - *Clostridium difficile* infection:
    - Hand hygiene with soap and water (spores are resistant to alcohol-based products) (3)
    - Restrict use of cephalosporins and clindamycin when possible (3).
    - The use of probiotics has not shown to reduce the incidence of antibiotic-related *C. difficile* infections (3).

PATHOPHYSIOLOGY

- Endogenous spread: Patient's own normal flora causes invasive disease (majority of cases).
- Exogenous route: Flora acquired from within health care facility causes invasive disease.

ETIOLOGY

- UTI: *Escherichia coli*, *Klebsiella* spp., *Serratia* spp., *Enterobacter*, *Pseudomonas aeruginosa*, *Enterococcus* spp., *Candida albicans*
- Pneumonia: Aerobic gram-negative bacilli, *S. aureus*, *P. aeruginosa*
- Bloodstream infection: *Staphylococcus* spp.
- Surgical-site infection: *S. aureus*, gram-negative bacilli

DIAGNOSIS

Consistent with nature of infection

HISTORY

- Exposure to health care facility
- Recent surgery or open wounds
- History of invasive procedure:
  - Urinary catheter placement
  - Indwelling vascular catheter
- Recent intubation/mechanical ventilation
- Past infections (e.g., MRSA)

PHYSICAL EXAM

Consistent with nature of infection

DIAGNOSTIC TESTS & INTERPRETATION

As appropriate for suspected infection

Pathological Findings

Consistent with underlying infection

DIFFERENTIAL DIAGNOSIS

- Community-acquired infection
- Noninfectious process

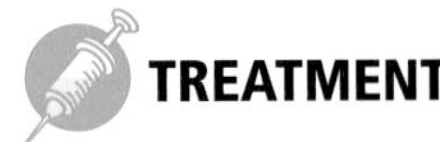

TREATMENT

MEDICATION

- As appropriate for specific nature of infection
- Several agents have been approved recently for the treatment of antibiotic-resistant gram-positive infections:
  - Linezolid
  - Daptomycin
  - Telavancin
  - Tigecycline
  - Ceftaroline
- *Some emerging resistant gram-negative infections have been found to be resistant to nearly all antibiotics and require expert consultation for management.*

ADDITIONAL TREATMENT

General Measures

- Treat the underlying infection as indicated.
- Specific measures as appropriate for type of infection:
  - UTI: Remove urinary catheters.
  - CLABSI: Remove IV catheter.
  - *Clostridium difficile*: Stop all antibiotics not being used to treat *C. difficile*.

Issues for Referral

As appropriate

SURGERY/OTHER PROCEDURES

- As appropriate for specific nature of infection
- Screening for nasal carriage of MRSA and isolation have been shown to reduce the nosocomial spread of MRSA.
- Treating proven nasal carriers of *Staphylococcus* or MRSA with mupirocin prevents *S. aureus* nosocomial infections after surgery. This screen-and-treat approach is cost-saving as long as the prevalence of mupirocin resistance is low (12)[B].

IN-PATIENT CONSIDERATIONS

IV Fluids

As needed

Nursing

- Hand washing should be performed upon entering and exiting the patient room even if there is no direct contact with the patient.
- Isolation precautions as indicated

Discharge Criteria

When infection has resolved or patient is stable

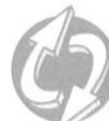

ONGOING CARE

FOLLOW-UP RECOMMENDATIONS

Patient Monitoring

As appropriate for specific type of infection

PROGNOSIS

- 99,000 deaths in 2002 in the US (1)
- Bloodstream infection mortality: 27% (13)
- Pneumonia mortality: 33–50% (14)
- Surgical-site infection mortality: 11% (1)

COMPLICATIONS

Related to specific nature of infection

REFERENCES

1. Klevens RM, Edwards JR, Richards CL, et al. Estimating health care-associated infections and deaths in U.S. hospitals, 2002. *Public Health Rep*. 2007;122:160–6.
2. Barie PS, Eachempati SR. Surgical site infections. *Surg Clin North Am*. 2005;85:1115–35, viii–ix.
3. Society for Healthcare Epidemiology of America; Infectious Diseases Society of America. A compendium of strategies to prevent healthcare-associated infections in acute care hospitals. *Infect Control Hosp Epidemiol*. 2008;29(suppl 1):S1–S92.
4. O'Grady NP, et al. Guidelines for the prevention of intravascular catheter-related infections. *MMRW*. 2002;51:1–32.
5. Slama TG. Gram-negative antibiotic resistance: There is a price to pay. *Crit Care*. 2008;12(Suppl 4):S4.
6. Carmeli Y. Strategies for managing today's infections. *Clin Microbiol Infect*. 2008;14(Suppl 3):22–31.
7. Siegel JD, Rhinehart E, Jackson M, et al. 2007 Guideline for isolation precautions: Preventing transmission of infectious agents in health care settings. *Am J Infect Control*. 2007;35:S65–164.
8. Hooton TM, Bradley SF, Cardenas DD, et al. Diagnosis, prevention, and treatment of catheter-associated urinary tract infection in adults: 2009 international clinical practice guidelines from the Infectious Disease Society of America. *Clin Infect Dis*. 2010;50:625–63.
9. Tablan OC, et al. Guidelines for preventing health-care associated pneumonia, 2003: Recommendations of CDC and the healthcare infection control practices advisory committee. *MMWR*. 2004;53:1–40.
10. Chan EY, Ruest A, Meade MO, et al. Oral decontamination for prevention of pneumonia in mechanically ventilated adults: Systematic review and meta-analysis. *BMJ*. 2007;334:889.
11. O,Grady NP, Alexander M, Burns LA, et al. Guidelines for the Prevention of Intravascular Catheter-related Infections, 2011. Accessed June 28, 2011. www.cdc.gov/hicpac/BSI/01-BSI-guidelines-2011.html.
12. Van Rijen M, Bonten M, Wenzel R, et al. Mupirocin ointment for preventing *Staphylococcus aureus* infections in nasal carriers. *Cochrane Database Syst Rev*. 2009;1:CD006216.
13. Wisplinghoff H, Bischoff T, Tallent SM, et al. Nosocomial bloodstream infections in US hospitals: Analysis of 24,179 cases from a prospective nationwide surveillance study. *Clin Infect Dis*. 2004;39:309–17.
14. American Thoracic Society, Infectious Diseases Society of America. Guidelines for the management of adults with hospital-acquired, ventilator-associated, and healthcare-associated pneumonia. *Am J Respir Crit Care Med*. 2005; 171:388–416.

ADDITIONAL READING

Tacconelli E, et al. Screening and isolation for infection control. *J Hosp Infect*. 2009;73:371–7.

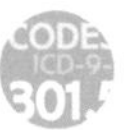

CODES

ICD9

- 486 Pneumonia, organism unspecified
- 599.0 Urinary tract infection, site not specified
- 998.59 Other postoperative infection

CLINICAL PEARLS

- Nosocomial infections are associated with increased mortality, length of stay, and admission cost.
- Prevention efforts should address both patient-specific and facility-related risk factors.
- Proper use of an alcohol-based hand product should be carried out before and after each patient encounter, even when gloves are used. Alcohol-based hand rubs are not effective for killing spores formed by *Clostridium difficile*. Hand washing with soap and water after exposure to spores is the appropriate alternative.
- Contact, droplet, or airborne precautions should be employed when appropriate to reduce the spread of infection.
- The risk of developing a resistant nosocomial infection can be reduced by emphasizing the use of narrow-spectrum antibiotics and frequent evaluation of necessity of continuing antibiotics in the health care setting.

NOVEL INFLUENZA A (2009 H1N1)

Sumanth Gandra, MD, MPH
Raul Davaro, MD

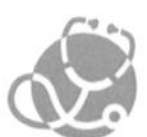

BASICS

Novel influenza (2009 H1N1):

- 2009 H1N1 virus is a novel influenza A virus originating from a reassortment of influenza viruses that circulated in North American and Eurasian pig herds.
- The 2009 H1N1 pandemic started in March 2009 in Mexico and then spread to many countries, including the US.
- The pandemic was declared to be over in August 2010 by the World Health Organization (WHO) (1).
- Although pandemic is over, 2009 H1N1 virus still exists and can cause disease.
- Generally self-limited and uncomplicated disease course
- Typically presented with influenzalike symptoms, but patients may be symptomatic with diarrhea and vomiting (2).
- Susceptible to neuraminidase inhibitors, but resistant to adamantine antiviral agents (3)

EPIDEMIOLOGY

- The CDC estimates that between 43 million and 89 million cases of 2009 H1N1 occurred between April 2009 and April 2010 in the US, including ~274,000 hospitalizations and 12,470 deaths (4).
- 90% of the reported cases were accounted for by patients under the age of 64 (4).

Incidence

- Predominant sex: Male = Female
- Affected mostly young people
- Older people are protected because they had pre-existing antibodies that cross-reacted with 2009 H1N1.

RISK FACTORS

- Similar to regular influenza transmission, with exposure to respiratory secretions accounting for the main avenue of infection
- Close contact (<6 ft) with confirmed case increased the possibility for large-droplet transmission (2)
- Risk factors for complications of or severe illness with 2009 H1N1 virus infection (5):
  - Age <5 years or >65 years
  - Pregnancy
  - Morbid obesity
  - Chronic medical conditions (diabetes, chronic cardiovascular conditions, cirrhosis, end-stage renal disease [ESRD] on hemodialysis [HD])
  - Chronic lung disorders (chronic obstructive pulmonary disease [COPD], asthma, cystic fibrosis)
  - Immunosuppression (associated with HIV infection, organ transplantation, receipt of chemotherapy or corticosteroids, or malnutrition)
  - Sickle cell disease

GENERAL PREVENTION

- 2009 H1N1 vaccination, monovalent or trivalent. The 2010–2011 seasonal influenza has 2009 H1N1 included.
- CDC recommends 2009 H1N1 vaccine for all persons 6 months or older.
- Observing hand hygiene and appropriate cough etiquette
- Health care personnel observed droplet precautions (surgical mask or N95 mask and protective goggles) in addition to contact precautions for patients presenting with symptoms of an influenzalike illness (fever with cough or sore throat).
- When leaving their rooms, patients were outfitted with a surgical mask to contain their respiratory secretions.

ETIOLOGY

- 2009 H1N1 influenza was a quadruple-reassortant strain with the individual gene segments of the virus originating from humans, birds, North American pigs, and Eurasian pigs.
- Reservoirs included infected human and pig populations.

DIAGNOSIS

HISTORY

- Incubation period: 1.5–3 days but may be as long as 7 days
- Clinical spectrum ranged from afebrile upper respiratory illness to fulminant viral pneumonia.
- Symptoms were similar to regular seasonal influenza, most patients presented with (5)[B]:
  - Fever
  - Sore throat
  - Cough
  - Myalgias
  - Nasal congestion
  - Rhinorrhea
- GI symptoms with nausea, vomiting, and diarrhea were more common than with seasonal influenza (5)[B].
- Close contact with a suspected or confirmed case

DIAGNOSTIC TESTS & INTERPRETATION

- Rapid flu tests (6)[B]:
  - The rapid antigen test and direct fluorescent antibody (DFA) had low sensitivities to detect 2009 H1N1 (17.8% and 46.7%, respectively)
- Viral culture and polymerase chain reaction (PCR) test were highly sensitive (88.9% vs. 97.8%) (6)[B].
- PCR (respiratory viral panel) was the test of choice .

Lab

Initial lab tests

- CBC with differential
- Basic metabolic panel
- Blood cultures
- Liver function tests (LFTs)

Imaging

Chest x-ray (CXR): Among those hospitalized for 2009 H1N1 infection, 50% had infiltrates on CXR (2).

Pathological Findings

Most consistent histopathologic findings were varying degrees of diffuse alveolar damage with hyaline membranes and septal edema, tracheitis, and necrotizing bronchiolitis.

DIFFERENTIAL DIAGNOSIS

- Seasonal influenza
- Respiratory viral infections from such agents as coronavirus, rhinovirus, and adenovirus
- Croup
- Pneumonia (typical and atypical)
- Infectious mononucleosis
- Pharyngitis (viral or streptococcal)
- HIV syndrome

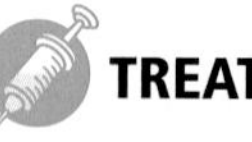

TREATMENT

- Most infections were self-limited and uncomplicated.
- Use of medications was guided by clinical judgment.
- Treatment was recommended to high-risk patients with suspected 2009 H1N1 infection, as well as to patients with symptoms severe enough to require hospitalization with suspected infection.
- High-risk patients (mentioned in "Risk Factors")
- Treatment with neuraminidase inhibitors was most effective when administered within 48 hours of symptom onset (7)[A].

MEDICATION

- 2009 H1N1 was found to be susceptible to the neuraminidase inhibitors oseltamivir (Tamiflu) and zanamivir (Relenza) (3)[B].
- Genetic sequencing indicated resistance to the adamantine antivirals (e.g., amantadine).

First Line

- Oseltamivir (7)[B]:
  - Adult dosage: 75 mg PO b.i.d. × 5 days
  - Pediatric dosage (safety and efficacy not established for children <1 year of age):
    - ≤15 kg: 30 mg PO b.i.d. × 5 days; 16–23 kg: 45 mg PO b.i.d. × 5 days; 24–40 kg: 60 mg PO b.i.d. × 5 days; >40 kg: 75 mg PO b.i.d. × 5 days
  - Pediatric dosage <1 year old: <3 months: 12 mg PO b.i.d. × 5 days; 3–5 months: 20 mg PO b.i.d. × 5 days; 6–11 months: 25 mg PO b.i.d. × 5 days
  - Chemoprophylaxis: Adult dosage: 75 mg PO daily × 10 days
  - Pediatric dosage (safety and efficacy not established for children <1 year of age):
    - ≤15 kg: 30 mg PO daily × 10 days
    - 16–23 kg: 45 mg PO daily × 10 days
    - 24–40 kg: 60 mg PO daily × 10 days
    - >40 kg: 75 mg PO daily × 10 days

- Postexposure prophylaxis was indicated for high-risk patients, health care personnel, public health workers, and first responders in close contact with suspected case of 2009 H1N1.
- Adverse effects: Most common symptoms include nausea and vomiting, occurring in 9–10% of patients. Neuropsychiatric events (e.g., hallucinations, delirium, and abnormal behavior) are rare symptoms. Other rare symptoms include anaphylaxis and severe skin reactions, such as Stevens-Johnson syndrome and toxic epidermal necrolysis.
- Other considerations: Metabolized by liver; pregnancy Class C medication

- Zanamivir (7)[B] (not recommended for patients with respiratory conditions such as COPD or asthma):
  - Adult dosage: 2 puffs of 5 mg INH b.i.d. × 5 days
  - Pediatric dosage: >7 years old: 2 puffs of 5 mg INH b.i.d. × 5 days
  - Chemoprophylaxis: Adult dosage: 2 puffs of 5 mg INH daily × 5 days; Pediatrics: >5 years old: 2 puffs of 5 mg INH daily × 5 days
  - Limited quantities of IV zanamivir were made available.
  - Adverse effects: Most notably may cause bronchospasm, especially in patients with pre-existing respiratory illnesses. Common adverse symptoms include headache, nausea, dizziness, and cough. Rare symptoms are similar to those of Tamiflu, including neuropsychiatric symptoms, anaphylaxis, and severe skin reactions.
  - Other considerations: Metabolized by liver; pregnancy Class C medication
  - Sporadic cases of neuraminidase inhibitors were recognized in the 2009 H1N1, typically in viruses with the H275Y mutation, but remained susceptible to zanamivir.
- Peramivir:
  - FDA issued emergency use authorization (EUA) for peramivir, an investigational neuraminidase inhibitor for treatment of severely ill cases of confirmed or suspected cases of 2009 H1N1.
  - Administered IV
  - EUA for peramivir expired in June 2010

ADDITIONAL TREATMENT

Additional Therapies

- Broad-spectrum antibiotics as needed for treatment of bacterial coinfections
- In patients with 2009 H1N1 who had acute respiratory distress syndrome (ARDS), extracorporeal membrane oxygenation was utilized.

REFERENCES

1. World Health Organization. In focus: H1N1 now in the post-pandemic period. August 10, 2010. www.who.int/csr/disease/swineflu/en/index.html.
2. Novel Swine-Origin Influenza A (H1N1) Virus Investigation Team. Emergence of a novel swine-origin influenza A (H1N1) virus in humans. *N Engl J Med*. 2009.
3. Centers for Disease Control and Prevention (CDC). Update: Drug susceptibility of swine-origin influenza A (H1N1) viruses, April 2009. *MMWR*. 2009;58:433–5.
4. Updated CDC Estimates of 2009 H1N1 Influenza Cases, Hospitalizations and Deaths in the United States, April 2009 – April 10, 2010. www.cdc.gov/h1n1flu/estimates_2009_h1n1.htm.
5. Writing Committee of the WHO Consultation on Clinical Aspects of Pandemic (H1N1) 2009 Influenza; Bautista E, Chotpitayasunondh T, et al. Clinical aspects of pandemic 2009 influenza A (H1N1) virus infection. *N Engl J Med*. 2010; 362:1708–19.
6. Ginocchio CC, Zhang F, Manji R, et al. Evaluation of multiple test methods for the detection of the novel 2009 influenza A (H1N1) during the New York City outbreak. *J Clin Virol*. 2009;45:191–95.
7. Harper SA, Bradley JS, Englund JA, et al. Seasonal influenza in adults and children-diagnosis, treatment, chemoprophylaxis, and institutional outbreak management: Clinical practice guidelines of the Infectious Diseases Society of America. *Clin Infect Dis*. 2009.

CODES

ICD9

- 488.11 Influenza due to identified novel H1N1 influenza virus with pneumonia
- 488.12 Influenza due to identified novel H1N1 influenza virus with other respiratory manifestations
- 488.19 Influenza due to identified novel H1N1 influenza virus with other manifestations

CLINICAL PEARLS

- 2009 H1N1 was *not* contracted from eating pork or pork products.
- 2009 H1N1 pandemic started in March 2009 and was declared to be over in August 2010.
- Affected mostly young people because older people had pre-existing antibodies that cross-reacted with 2009 H1N1
- Most cases are self-limited and uncomplicated.
- Up to 25% of patients reported vomiting and diarrhea in addition to fever, headache, sore throat, and cough.
- PCR (respiratory viral panel) was the test of choice.
- Susceptible to neuraminidase inhibitors (oseltamivir and zanamivir), but resistant to adamantine antiviral agents

OBESITY

Maya Leventer-Roberts, MD, MPH
Frank J. Domino, MD

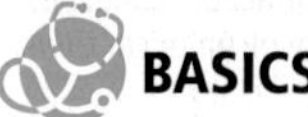

BASICS

DESCRIPTION

- Excess adipose tissue is often associated with negative health outcomes.
- Body mass index (BMI) can indicate status as underweight, normal weight, overweight, obese, and morbidly obese.
- Increased risk of morbidity and mortality is more closely related to abdominal obesity than it is to gluteal obesity.
- System(s) affected: Endocrine/Metabolic; Cardiac; Respiratory; Gastrointestinal; Musculoskeletal
- Synonym(s): Overweight; Adiposis; Adiposity

Geriatric Considerations

The BMI associated with the lowest risk of mortality increases as age increases.

EPIDEMIOLOGY

- Predominant age: All ages
- Predominant sex: Female > Male

Prevalence

- Mean prevalence of obesity is 32.2% in the US.
- Overweight: 40% of men and 25% of women
- Obese: 20% of men and 25% of women

Pediatric Considerations

- Obesity during adolescence and young adulthood predicts obesity in adulthood.
- The prevalence of obesity among the pediatric population is rising.
- Risk factors include decreased physical activity, increased consumption of sweetened beverages and potatoes, and increased television viewing.

RISK FACTORS

- Parental obesity
- Sedentary lifestyle
- High-calorie diet
- Pregnancy
- Low socioeconomic status
- >2 hours of television viewing per day

Genetics

- Rare genetic syndromes such as Prader-Willi and Bardet-Biedl
- Studies are inconclusive regarding specific genetic predictors of obesity.

GENERAL PREVENTION

- Encourage routine exercise, limited TV viewing, and moderation in diet.
- Avoid calorie-dense and nutrient-poor foods such as sweetened beverages and processed foods.
- Most obese patients underestimate the amount of ingested calories per day.

ETIOLOGY

- Obesity is caused by an imbalance between food intake and energy expenditure.
- Uncommon causes include insulinoma, hypothalamic disorders, hypothyroidism, and Cushing syndrome.
- Menopause and smoking cessation are associated with significant weight gain.
- Medications: corticosteroids, neuroleptics (particularly the "atypical" antipsychotics), and antidepressants

DIAGNOSIS

HISTORY

- Prior attempts at weight loss
- Reported readiness to change lifestyle
- Social support and resources
- Diet and exercise habits
- Associated risk factors: Diabetes mellitus type 2, hypertension, hyperlipidemia, sleep apnea
- History of incest
- Symptoms suggesting hypothyroidism, Cushing syndrome, genetic syndromes

PHYSICAL EXAM

Elevated BMI and excess adipose tissue:

- BMI = body weight (kg)/body height (m^2):
  - Overweight: BMI = 25–29.9 kg/m^2
  - Obese: BMI ≥30 kg/m^2
- Morbidly obese: ≥40 kg/m^2

Table 1 BMI obesity threshold by height

Height	BMI = 25 Weight (lb/kg)	BMI = 27 Weight (lb/kg)	BMI = 30 Weight (lb/kg)
5′0	128/58	138/63	153/70
5′2	136/61	147/67	164/74
5′4	145/66	157/71	174/79
5′6	155/70	167/76	186/84
5′8	164/74	177/81	197/89
5′10	174/79	188/85	209/95
6′0	184/83	199/90	221/100
6′2	194/88	210/95	233/106
6′4	205/92	221/101	246/112

- Fat distribution pattern:
  - Waist circumference is measured around the abdomen at the level of the umbilicus:
    - >40 in (102 cm) for men and >35 in (88 cm) for women is associated with increased risk for most obesity-related medical conditions (1)[C].

DIAGNOSTIC TESTS & INTERPRETATION

Lab

- Used to monitor associated risk factors and conditions
- Serum lipid panel and fasting glucose
- Hypothyroidism is uncommon cause of obesity, consider obtaining thyroid-stimulating hormone

Pathological Findings

- Hypertrophy and/or hyperplasia of adipocytes
- Cardiomegaly
- Hepatomegaly

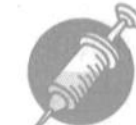

TREATMENT

MEDICATION

- National Institute of Health guidelines suggest nonpharmacologic treatment for at least 6 months.
- Medication treatment may be initiated for unsatisfactory weight loss in those with a BMI >30 or with a BMI >27 combined with associated risk factors (e.g., coronary heart disease, diabetes, sleep apnea, hypertension, hyperlipidemia).
- Diet, exercise, and behavior therapy *must* be included with pharmacologic treatment for those without comorbidities (1)[B].

First Line

- Medications produce modest weight loss (2)[A].
- The lipase inhibitor orlistat decreases the absorption of dietary fat. Dose: 120 mg PO t.i.d. with meals. Patients must avoid taking fat-soluble vitamin supplements within 2 hours of taking orlistat. The FDA has approved orlistat to be sold over the counter as a weight-loss aid.
- Contraindications:
  - Orlistat: Chronic malabsorption syndromes, cholestasis
- Precautions: Relapse after discontinuation of drug
- Significant possible interactions:
  - Pulse and BP elevations possible with sibutramine.
  - Concurrent use with general anesthetics may cause arrhythmias.
  - Serotonergic agents may cause "serotonin syndrome" in combination with sibutramine.

Second Line

- Appetite suppressants recommended for short-term treatment (≤6 months)
- Only beneficial in patients who exercise and eat reduced calorie diet

- Schedule IV drugs:
  – Diethylpropion: 25 mg before meals t.i.d.; discontinue if no response after 4 weeks
  – Phentermine: 15, 30, 37.5 mg PO every morning; discontinue if tolerance or no response after 4 weeks
- Pending FDA approval:
  – Combination of phentermine 15 mg + topiramate 92 mg/d; side effects include hypertension, arrhythmia
  – Combination of bupropion 360 mg + naltrexone 32 mg/d; side effects unclear
- Schedule III drugs: Benzphetamine, phendimetrazine

ADDITIONAL TREATMENT

General Measures

- The following assessments can determine the status and plan of action:
  – Degree of health risk from BMI and waist circumference (1)[C] (see "Diagnosis")
  – Motivation to lose weight (1)[C]
  – Patient-specific goals of therapy
  – Necessary counseling or referral to a dietitian for diet, exercise, and behavior modification (1)[B]
  – Long-term follow-up (1)[C]
- Goal for therapy is to achieve and sustain weight loss up to 10% of body weight for overweight and obese patients (1)[A].
- Behavior therapy and cognitive-behavioral methods can result in modest weight loss, but are most effective when combined with dietary and exercise treatments (3)[A].
- Use of commercial weight loss programs (e.g., Weight Watchers) more effective than "standard of care" counseling (4)[B]

Pregnancy Considerations

- Weight loss is not appropriate for most pregnant or lactating women (1)[C].
- During pregnancy, obese women should gain less than the 25 pounds recommended for nonobese women.

SURGERY/OTHER PROCEDURES

Patients meeting criteria (including severe obesity [BMI >40 kg/m^2]) can be considered for gastric bypass procedures:

- Malabsorptive surgery reduces the length of the small intestine.
- Restrictive surgery reduces the stomach's capacity.
- Gastric bypass requires complex presurgical evaluation, surgery, and follow-up in a skilled treatment center (1)[C].
- Lifelong medical surveillance is necessary after obesity surgery (1)[C].
- Surgical treatment is the most effective long-term weight-loss treatment available for morbidly obese patients (5)[B].
- Lap Band data is conflicting; but the most recent data is encouraging.

ONGOING CARE

FOLLOW-UP RECOMMENDATIONS

- Exercise is an integral part of any weight-loss program, yet exercise alone rarely results in significant weight loss (1)[A].
- Exercise regimens should last 30–90 minutes, 5–7 times per week.
- Combination of weight training and aerobic activity is preferred over aerobic activity alone.

Patient Monitoring

Long-term routine follow-up is crucial to prevent relapse after weight loss or further weight gain.

DIET

- Long-term studies suggest net calorie reduction of 500–1,000 kcal/d and ease of use are more important than diet composition for long-term results:
  – A reduction of 500 kcal/d intake can result in ~1 lb (0.45 kg) weight loss per week (1)[A].
  – Low-saturated-fat, high-complex-carbohydrate, and high-fiber diets are recommended most often (1)[A].
  – Portion-controlled servings are recommended.
- Low glycemic index diet: Primarily eating foods that result in slowed absorption of carbohydrates
- Very-low-calorie diet (400–800 kcal/d):
  – Can result in more rapid weight loss than higher-calorie diets but are less effective in the long term
  – Complications can include dehydration, orthostatic hypotension, fatigue, muscle cramps, constipation, headache, cold intolerance, and relapse after discontinuation.
  – Contraindications: Recent myocardial infarction or cerebrovascular accident, renal disease, cancer, pregnancy, insulin-dependent diabetes mellitus, and some psychiatric disturbances.

PATIENT EDUCATION

- Emphasize the value of a healthy BMI.
- Recommended Web sites:
  – www.shapeup.org for general information and specific resources
  – www.nal.usda.gov/fnic/foodcomp/search for the FDA nutritional content in common foods
  – Lose It! application for iTunes (http://itunes.apple.com/us/app/lose-it/id297368629?mt=8)
  – Low Glycemic Index Diet List: www.the-gi-diet.org/lowgifoods/

PROGNOSIS

- Lowest mortality associated with a BMI of 22
- Long-term maintenance of weight loss is extremely difficult.
- A motivated patient is most likely to achieve successful weight loss.
- There have been several controversial studies suggesting that a BMI in the mildly overweight range is associated with a decreased risk of mortality relative to a BMI in the underweight or obese range (6)[B].

COMPLICATIONS

- Cardiovascular disease
- Stroke (in men)
- Thromboembolism
- Heart failure
- Hypertension
- Hypoventilation and sleep apnea syndromes
- Higher death rates from cancer: Colon, breast, prostate, endometrial, gallbladder, liver, kidney
- Diabetes mellitus
- Skin changes
- Hyperlipidemia
- Gallbladder disease
- Osteoarthritis
- Gout
- Poor self-esteem
- Discrimination
- Increased sick leave

REFERENCES

1. National Institutes of Health Clinical guidelines on the identification, evaluation, and treatment of overweight and obesity in adults: The evidence report. NIH Publication No. 98-4083, 1998.
2. Padwal R, Li SK, Lau DCW. Long-term pharmacotherapy for obesity and overweight (Cochrane Review). *The Cochrane Library*. Issue 4. Chichester, UK: Wiley & Sons; 2005.
3. Shaw K, et al. Psychological interventions for overweight and obesity (Cochrane Review). *The Cochrane Library*. Issue 4. Chichester, UK: Wiley & Sons; 2005.
4. Jebb SA, Ahern AL, Olson AD, et al. Primary care referral to a commercial provider for weight loss treatment versus standard care: A randomised controlled trial. *Lancet*. 2011;378:1485–92.
5. Colquitt J, et al. Surgery for morbid obesity (Cochrane Review). *The Cochrane Library*. Issue 4. Chichester, UK: Wiley & Sons; 2005.
6. Flegal K, Graubard B, Williamson D, et al. Excess deaths associated with underweight, overweight, and obesity. *JAMA*. 2005;293(15):1861–7.

ADDITIONAL READING

Thomas DE, Elliott EJ, Baur L. Low glycaemic index or low glycaemic load diets for overweight and obesity. *Cochrane Database Syst Rev*. 2007:CD005105.

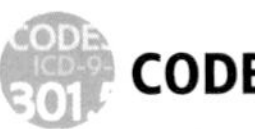

CODES

ICD9

- 278.00 Obesity, unspecified
- 278.01 Morbid obesity

CLINICAL PEARLS

- Drug treatment with a first-line medication may be indicated when nonpharmacologic treatment for 6 months has been ineffective and the patient has a BMI >30 or a BMI >27 with associated risk factors. Medications produce (at most) a modest long-term weight loss.
- Surgical treatment may be indicated in patients with a BMI >40 who have failed more conservative treatment, particularly when there are associated risk factors such as diabetes mellitus.
- There is no convincing evidence that any specific diet is more effective than any other diet of equivalent caloric content.

OBSESSIVE-COMPULSIVE DISORDER (OCD)

Anna K. Morin, PharmD, RPH
Robert A. Baldor, MD

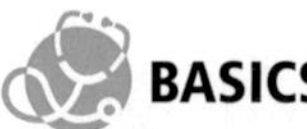

BASICS

DESCRIPTION

- A psychiatric condition classified as an anxiety disorder characterized by obsessions (recurrent intrusive thoughts, ideas, or images) and compulsions (repetitive, ritualistic behaviors or mental acts) causing significant patient distress
- Not to be confused with obsessive-compulsive personality disorder

EPIDEMIOLOGY

Incidence

- Predominant age: Mean age of onset 22–36 years:
  - Male = Female (males present at younger age)
  - Child/adolescent onset in 33% of cases
  - 1/3 of cases present by age 15 years.
  - 85% of cases present at <35 years of age.
  - Diagnosis rarely made at >50 years of age.
- Predominant gender: Male > Female (3:1)

Pediatric Considerations

Insidious onset; consider brain insult in acute presentation of childhood obsessive-compulsive disorder (OCD).

Geriatric Considerations

Consider neurologic disorders in new-onset OCD in the elderly.

Prevalence

- 2.3% lifetime in adults
- 1–2.3% prevalence in children/adolescents

RISK FACTORS

- Exact cause of OCD is not fully elucidated.
- Combination of biologic and environmental factors likely involved:
  - Link between low serotonin levels and development of OCD
  - Link between brain insult and development of OCD (i.e., encephalitis, pediatric streptococcal infection, or head injury)

Genetics

- Greater concordance in monozygotic twins
- Positive family history: Prevalence rates of 7–15% in first-degree relatives of children/adolescents with OCD

GENERAL PREVENTION

- OCD cannot be prevented.
- Early diagnosis and treatment can decrease patient's distress and impairment.

PATHOPHYSIOLOGY

- Exact pathophysiology unknown
- Dysregulation of serotonergic pathways
- Dysregulation of corticostriatal-thalamic-cortico (CSTC) pathways

ETIOLOGY

- Exact etiology unknown
- Genetic and environmental factors
- Pediatric autoimmune disorder associated with streptococcal infections

COMMONLY ASSOCIATED CONDITIONS

- Major depressive disorder
- Panic disorder
- Social phobia
- Phobia
- Tourette syndrome
- Substance abuse
- Eating disorder
- Body dysmorphic disorder

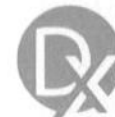

DIAGNOSIS

HISTORY

- Patient presents with either obsessions or compulsions, which cause marked distress, are time-consuming (>1 h/d), and cause significant occupational/social impairment.
- 4 criteria support diagnosis of obsessions:
  - Patients are aware that they are thinking the obsessive thoughts; thoughts are not imposed from outside (as in thought insertion).
  - Thoughts are not just excessive worrying about real-life problems.
  - Recurrent thoughts are persistent, intrusive, and inappropriate, causing significant anxiety and distress.
  - Attempts to suppress intrusive thoughts are made with some other thought or activity.
- 2 criteria support a diagnosis of compulsions:
  - The response to an obsession is to rigidly perform repetitive behaviors (e.g., hand washing) or mental acts (e.g., counting silently).
  - Although done to reduce stress, the responses are either not realistically connected with the obsession or they are excessive.
  - In children, check for precedent streptococcal infection.
- Common obsessive themes:
  - Harm (i.e., being responsible for an accident)
  - Doubt (i.e., whether doors or windows are locked or the iron is turned off)
  - Blasphemous thoughts (i.e., in a devoutly religious person)
  - Contamination, dirt, or disease
  - Symmetry or orderliness
- Common rituals or compulsions:
  - Hand washing, cleaning
  - Checking
  - Counting
  - Hoarding
  - Ordering, arranging
  - Repeating
- Neither obsessions nor compulsions are related to another mental disorder (i.e., thoughts of food and presence of eating disorder).
- 80–90% of patients with OCD have obsessions and compulsions.
- 10–19% of patients with OCD are pure obsessional.

PHYSICAL EXAM

- Dermatologic problems caused by excessive hand washing may be observed.
- Hair loss caused by compulsive pulling or twisting of the hair (trichotillomania) may be observed.

DIAGNOSTIC TESTS & INTERPRETATION

Lab

No diagnostic laboratory findings identified

Imaging

None indicated; consider brain MRI to rule out neurologic disorder.

Diagnostic Procedures/Surgery

- Yale-Brown Obsessive-Compulsive Scale (Y-BOCS) or CY-BOCS for children
- Maudsley Obsessive-Compulsive Inventory (MOCI)

Pathological Findings

- Compulsions are designed to relieve the anxiety of obsessions; they are not inherently enjoyable (ego-dynastic) and do not result in completion of a task.

DIFFERENTIAL DIAGNOSIS

- Obsessive-compulsive personality disorder:
  - In personality disorder, traits are ego-syntonic and include perfectionism and preoccupation with detail, trivia, or procedure and regulation. Patients tend to be rigid, moralistic, and stingy. These traits are often rewarded in the patient's job as desirable.
- Impulse-control disorders: Compulsive gambling, sex, or substance abuse: The compulsive behavior is not in response to obsessive thoughts, and the patient derives pleasure from the activity.
- Depression
- Brooding, but ideas not as senseless as in OCD
- Schizophrenia: Patient perceives thought to be true and coming from an external source.
- Generalized anxiety disorder, phobic disorders, separation anxiety: Similar response on heightened anxiety, but presence of obsessions and rituals signifies OCD diagnosis.
- Anxiety disorder due to a general medical condition: Obsessions or compulsions are assessed to be a direct physiologic consequence of a general medical condition.

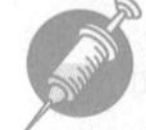

TREATMENT

MEDICATION

First Line

- Adequate trial at least 10–12 weeks
- Optimal doses may exceed typical doses for depression.
- Current evidence suggests SSRIs as first-line agents (1,2)[A]:

- Fluoxetine (Prozac):
  - Adults: 20 mg/d; increase by 10–20 mg every 4–6 weeks until response; range: 20–80 mg/d
  - Children (7–17 years of age): 10 mg/d; increase 4–6 weeks until response; range: 20–60 mg/d
- Sertraline (Zoloft):
  - Adults: 50 mg/d; increase by 50 mg every 4–7 days until response; range: 50–200 mg/d; may divide if above 100 mg/d
  - Children (6–17 years of age): 25 mg/d; increase by 25 mg every 7 days until response; range: 50–200 mg/d
- Paroxetine (Paxil):
  - Adults: 20 mg/d; increase by 10 mg every 4–7 days until response; range: 40–60 mg/d
  - Children: Safety and effectiveness in patients <18 years have not been established.
- Fluvoxamine (Luvox):
  - Adult: 100 mg/d; increase by 50 mg every 4–7 days until response; range: 200–300 mg/d
  - Children (8–17 years of age): 25 mg/d; increase by 25 mg every 4–7 days until response; range: 50–200 mg/d
- Absolute SSRI contraindications:
  - Hypersensitivity to SSRIs
  - Within 14 days of monoamine oxidase inhibitor (MAOI)
- Relative SSRI contraindications:
  - Severe liver impairment
  - Seizure disorders (lower seizure threshold)
- Precautions:
  - Watch for suicidal behavior or worsening depression during first few months of therapy or after dosage changes with antidepressants, particularly in children, adolescents, and young adults.
  - Long half-life of fluoxetine (>7 days) may be troublesome if patient has an adverse reaction.
  - May cause drowsiness and dizziness when therapy initiated; warn patients about driving and heavy-equipment hazards.

Pregnancy Considerations

All SSRIs are pregnancy Category C, except paroxetine, which is Category D.

Second Line

- Try switching to another SSRI.
- Tricyclic acid (TCA), clomipramine (Anafranil):
  - Adults: 25 mg/d; increase gradually over 2 weeks to 100 mg/d, then to 250 mg/d (maximum dose) over next several weeks, as tolerated.
  - Children (10–17 years of age): 25 mg/d; titrate as needed and tolerated up to 3 mg/kg or 200 mg/d (whichever is less).
  - Absolute clomipramine contraindications:
    - Within 6 months of an MI
    - Hypersensitivity to clomipramine or other TCA
    - Within 14 days of an MAOI
    - Third-degree atrioventricular (AV) block
  - Relative clomipramine contraindications:
    - Narrow-angle glaucoma (increased intraocular pressure)
    - Prostatic hypertrophy (urinary retention)
    - First- or second-degree AV block, bundle-branch block, and congestive heart failure (proarrhythmic effect)
    - Pregnancy Category C
  - Precautions:
    - Dangerous in overdose
    - Pretreatment ECG for patients >40 years of age
    - Watch for suicidal behavior or worsening depression during first few months of therapy or after dosage changes with antidepressants, particularly in children, adolescents, and young adults.
    - May cause drowsiness and dizziness when therapy is initiated; warn patients about driving and heavy-equipment hazards.

ADDITIONAL TREATMENT

General Measures

- Combined medications and cognitive-behavioral therapy (CBT) is most effective (1,2)[A].
- Family psychoeducation
- Parent behavior management training if patient is a child or adolescent

Issues for Referral

- Psychiatric referral for CBT (in vivo exposure and prevention of compulsions)
- Psychiatric evaluation if obsessions and compulsions significantly interfere with patient's functioning in social, occupational, or educational situations

Additional Therapies

Dopamine receptor antagonists (antipsychotic agents) alone are not effective in treatment of OCD. They can be used as augmentation to SSRI therapy for treatment-resistant OCD; they also can worsen OCD symptoms (2). Some evidence that addition of quetiapine or risperidone to antidepressants will increase efficacy; data with olanzapine too limited to draw conclusions (3):

- Pimozide (Orap): Initial dose: 0.5 mg/d; target dose: 1–6 mg/d
- Haloperidol (Haldol): Initial dose: 0.5 mg/d; target dose: 0.5–6 mg/d
- Risperidone (Risperdal): Initial dose: 0.5 mg/d; target dose: 0.5–2 mg/d
- Olanzapine (Zyprexa): Initial dose: 1.25 mg/d; target dose: 1.25–30 mg/d
- Quetiapine (Seroquel): Initial dose: 25 mg/d; target dose: 600 mg/d

ONGOING CARE

FOLLOW-UP RECOMMENDATIONS

Y-BCOS or MOCI surveys to track progress

Patient Monitoring

Monitor for decrease in obsessions and time spent performing compulsions.

DIET

No dietary modifications or restrictions are recommended.

PATIENT EDUCATION

- Importance of medication adherence
- Importance of psychotherapy (CBT)
- International OCD Foundation, PO Box 961029, Boston, MA 02196; 617-973-5801; www.ocfoundation.org
- Obsessive Compulsive Anonymous, PO Box 215, New Hyde Park, NY 11040; 516-739-0662; http://obsessivecompulsiveanonymous.org

PROGNOSIS

- Chronic waxing and waning course in majority of patients:
  - 24–33% fluctuating course
  - 11–14% phasic periods of remission
  - 54–61% chronic progressive course
- Early onset a poor predictor

COMPLICATIONS

- Depression in 1/3 of patients with OCD
- Avoidant behavior (phobic avoidance):
  - Children may drop out of education.
  - Adults may become home-bound.
- Anxiety and paniclike episodes associated with obsessions

REFERENCES

1. Gava I, et al. Psychological treatments versus treatment as usual for obsessive compulsive disorder (OCD). *Cochrane Database Sys Rev.* 2007;2:CD005333.
2. Stein DJ, et al. Obsessive-compulsive disorder: Diagnostic and treatment issues. *Psychiatr Clin N Am.* 2009;32:665–85.
3. Komossa K, Depping AM, Meyer M, et al. Second-generation antipsychotics for obsessive compulsive disorder. *Cochrane Database Sys Rev.* 2010;12:CD008141.

ADDITIONAL READING

- *Diagnostic and Statistical Manual of Mental Disorders DSM-IV (Text Revision)*, 4th ed. Washington, DC: American Psychiatric Association, 2000.
- Koran LM, et al. Practice guideline for the treatment of patients with obsessive-compulsive disorder. *Am J Psychiatry.* 2007;164:5–53.
- Kurlan R, Kaplan EL, et al. The pediatric autoimmune neuropsychiatric disorders associated with streptococcal infection (PANDAS) etiology for tics and obsessive-compulsive symptoms: Hypothesis or entity? Practical considerations for the clinician. *Pediatrics.* 2004;113:883–6.
- Nestadt G, et al. Genetics of obsessive compulsive disorder. *Psychiatr Clin N Am.* 2010;33:141–58.

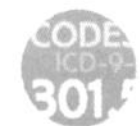

CODES

ICD9

300.3 Obsessive-compulsive disorders

CLINICAL PEARLS

- CBT is initial treatment of choice for mild OCD.
- CBT plus an SSRI or an SSRI alone is the treatment choice for more severe OCD.
- >65–70% of patients with OCD respond to first SSRI treatment.
- Improvement in symptoms is often incomplete and ranges from 25–60%.

OCULAR CHEMICAL BURNS

Vinod P. Mitta, MD
Chris Tang, MD

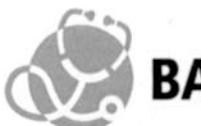

BASICS

DESCRIPTION

- Chemical exposure to the eye can result in rapid, devastating, and permanent damage, and is one of the true emergencies in ophthalmology.
- Separate alkaline from acid chemical exposure:
  - Alkaline burns: More severe—alkali compounds are lipophilic, penetrating rapidly into eye tissue; saponification of cells leads to necrosis and may produce injury to lids, conjunctiva, cornea, sclera, iris, and lens (cataracts)
  - Acid burns: Acid usually does not damage internal structures because protein denatures, creating a barrier to further acid penetration (hydrofluoric and, to a lesser extent, sulfurous acids are an exception to this rule). Injury is often limited to lids, conjunctiva, and cornea.
- System(s) affected: Nervous; Skin/Exocrine
- Synonym(s): Chemical ocular injuries

EPIDEMIOLOGY

- Predominant age: Can occur at any age, peak from 16–25 years of age
- Predominant sex: Male > Female

Incidence

- Estimated 300/100,000 per year
- Alkali burns twice as common as acid burns

RISK FACTORS

- Construction work (plaster, cement, whitewash)
- Use of cleaning agents (drain cleaners, ammonia)
- Automobile battery explosions (sulfuric acid)
- Industrial work (many possible agents)
- Alcoholism
- Any risk factor for assault (~10% of injuries due to deliberate assault)

GENERAL PREVENTION

Safety glasses to safeguard eyes

PATHOPHYSIOLOGY

- Hydration of glycosaminoglycans causes corneal opacification.
- Saponification of cell membranes causes cell death.
- Cation binding to collagen results in hydration, thickening, and shortening of collagen fibrils. This can mechanically elevate intraocular pressure through distortion of the trabecular meshwork.

ETIOLOGY

Sources of alkaline and acidic compounds

Alkali Compounds	Typical Sources
Calcium Hydroxide (Lime)	Cement, whitewash
Sodium Hydroxide (Lye)	Drain cleaner
Potassium Hydroxide (Lye)	Drain cleaner
Ammonia	Cleaning agents
Ammonium Hydroxide	Fertilizers
Acidic Compounds	**Typical Sources**
Sulfuric Acid	Car batteries
Sulfurous Acid	Bleach
Hydrochloric Acid	Chemistry laboratories
Acetic Acid	Vinegar
Hydrofluoric Acid	Glass polish

COMMONLY ASSOCIATED CONDITIONS

Facial cutaneous chemical or thermal burns

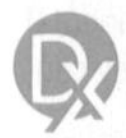

DIAGNOSIS

HISTORY

- In alkaline burns, can have initial pain that later diminishes
- Mild burns: Pain and blurred vision
- Moderate-to-severe burns: Severe pain and markedly reduced vision

PHYSICAL EXAM

- Mild burns:
  - Blurry vision
  - Eyelid skin erythema and edema
  - Corneal epithelial defects or superficial punctate keratitis
  - Conjunctival chemosis, hyperemia, and hemorrhages without perilimbal ischemia
  - Mild anterior chamber reaction
- Moderate-to-severe burns:
  - Reduced vision
  - Second- and third-degree burns of eyelid skin
  - Corneal edema and opacification
  - Corneal epithelial defects
  - Marked conjunctival chemosis and perilimbal blanching
  - Moderate anterior chamber reaction
  - Increased intraocular pressure
  - Local necrotic retinopathy

DIAGNOSTIC TESTS & INTERPRETATION

Imaging

Not necessary unless suspicion of intraocular or orbital foreign body is present

Diagnostic Procedures/Surgery

- Measure pH of tear film with litmus paper or electronic probe:
  - Irrigating fluid with nonneutral pH (e.g., normal saline has pH of 4.5) may alter results.
- Careful slit-lamp exam, fundus ophthalmoscopy, tonometry, and measurement of visual acuity
- Full extent of damage from alkaline burns may not be apparent until 48–72 hours after exposure.

Pathological Findings

- Corneal epithelial defects or superficial punctate keratitis, edema, opacification
- Conjunctival chemosis, hyperemia, and hemorrhages
- Perilimbal ischemia
- Anterior chamber reaction
- Increased intraocular pressure

DIFFERENTIAL DIAGNOSIS

- Thermal burns
- Ocular cicatricial pemphigoid
- Other causes of corneal opacification
- Ultraviolet radiation keratitis

TREATMENT

Copious irrigation and removal of corneal or conjunctival foreign bodies are always the initial treatment (1,2)[A]:

- Passively open patient's eyelid and have them look in all directions while irrigating.
- Be sure to remove all reservoirs of chemical from the eyes.
- Continue irrigation until the tear film and superior/inferior cul-de-sac is of neutral pH and pH is stable (2)[C]:
  - Severe burns should be irrigated for at least 15 minutes to as much as 2–4 hours; this irrigation should not be interrupted during transportation to hospital (2)[C].
  - It is impossible to overirrigate.
- Initial pH testing should be done on both eyes even if the patient claims to only have unilateral ocular pain/irritation so that a contralateral injury is not neglected.
- Use whatever nontoxic fluid is available for irrigation on scene. In hospital, sterile water, normal saline, normal saline with bicarbonate, balanced salt solution (BSS) or lactated Ringer's solution may be used:
  - No therapeutic difference in effectiveness has been noted between types of solutions (1)[C].
- A topical anesthetic can be used to provide for patient comfort (e.g., proparacaine, tetracaine).
- Sweep the conjunctival fornices every 12–24 hours to prevent adhesions (2)[C].
- Eye patching may relieve pain, but has not been shown to improve outcomes (3)[C].

MEDICATION

First Line

- Further treatment (depending on severity and associated conditions):
  - Topical prophylactic antibiotics: Any broad-spectrum agent (e.g., bacitracin–polymyxin B [Polysporin] ointment q2–4h, ciprofloxacin [Ciloxan] drops q2–4h, chloramphenicol [Chloroptic] ointment q2–4h) (1)[C]:
    - Some experts suggest that systemic tetracycline derivatives (especially doxycycline) may be beneficial because studies performed in animals have shown an additional anti-inflammatory effect (by inhibiting metalloproteinases) and improved corneal healing in alkali burns (4)[C].
  - Tear substitutes: Hydroxypropyl methylcellulose (HypoTears PF, Refresh Plus) drops q4h, carboxymethylcellulose (Refresh PM) ointment at bedtime (1)[C]:
    - Most beneficial in those with impaired tear production (elderly patients)
  - Cycloplegics for photophobia and/or uveitis: Cyclopentolate 1% t.i.d., or scopolamine 1/4% b.i.d. (1)[C]
  - Antiglaucoma for elevated intraocular pressure (IOP): Latanoprost (Xalatan) 0.005% q24h, or timolol (Timoptic) 0.5% b.i.d., or levobunolol (Betagan) 0.5% b.i.d., and/or acetazolamide (Diamox) 125–250 mg PO q6h, or methazolamide (Neptazane) 25–50 mg PO b.i.d., and/or IV mannitol 20% 1–2 g/kg as needed (1)[C]
  - Corticosteroids for intraocular inflammation: Prednisolone (Pred-Forte) 1% or equivalent q1–4h for 7–10 days; if severe, prednisone 20–60 mg PO daily for 5–7 days. Taper rapidly if epithelium is intact by this time (1)[C]:
    - Use of corticosteroids >10 days may do harm by inhibiting repair and cause corneoscleral melt (1,5)[C].
  - Consider vitamin C (ascorbic acid) 500 mg PO q.i.d. and/or acetylcysteine (Mucomyst) 10–20% topically q4h if corneal melting occurs (1)[C].
- Precautions:
  - Timolol and levobunolol: History of congestive heart failure (CHF) or chronic obstructive pulmonary disease (COPD)
  - Acetazolamide and methazolamide: History of nephrolithiasis or metabolic acidosis
  - Mannitol: History of CHF or renal failure
  - Scopolamine: History of urinary retention
  - Topical corticosteroids must be used with caution in the presence of damaged corneal epithelium because iatrogenic infection can occur. Daily follow-up or consultation with an ophthalmologist is recommended.

ADDITIONAL TREATMENT

Issues for Referral

See "Medication."

SURGERY/OTHER PROCEDURES

- Goal of subacute treatment is restoration of the normal ocular surface anatomy, control of glaucoma, and restoration of corneal clarity.
- Surgical options include:
  - Debridement of necrotic tissue (1)[C]
  - Conjunctival/tenon advancement (tenoplasty) to restore vascularity in severe burns (1)[C]
  - Tissue adhesive (e.g., isobutyl cyanoacrylate) for impending or actual corneal perforation of <1 mm (1)[C]:
    - Tectonic keratoplasty for acute perforation >1 mm (1)[C]
  - Limbal autograft transplantation for epithelial stem cell restoration (1)[C]
  - Conjunctival or mucosal membrane transplant to restore ocular surface in severe injury (1)[C]
  - Lamellar or penetrating keratoplasty for tectonic stabilization or visual rehabilitation (1)[C]

IN-PATIENT CONSIDERATIONS

Initial Stabilization

Usual for patient

Admission Criteria

Based on ophthalmic consultation and concomitant burn injuries

Discharge Criteria

Emergency department evaluation with inpatient admission and ophthalmology consultation, depending on severity

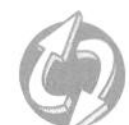

ONGOING CARE

FOLLOW-UP RECOMMENDATIONS

Patient Monitoring

- Depending on severity of ocular injury:
  - From daily to weekly visits initially
- May be inpatient
- If on mannitol or prednisone, consider frequent serum electrolytes.

DIET

Regular as tolerated

PATIENT EDUCATION

- Safety glasses
- Need for immediate ocular irrigation with any available water following chemical exposure to the eyes

PROGNOSIS

- Depends on severity of initial injury. Increasing amounts of limbal ischemia and corneal opacification correlate with poorer prognosis (Roper-Hall classification system)
- For mildly injured eyes, complete recovery is the norm.
- For severely injured eyes, permanent loss of vision is not uncommon.

COMPLICATIONS

- Persistent epitheliopathy
- Fibrovascular pannus
- Corneal ulcer/perforation
- Corneal scarring
- Progressive symblepharon and entropion
- Neurotrophic keratitis
- Lid malposition secondary to cicatricial changes
- Glaucoma
- Cataract
- Hypotony
- Phthisis bulbi
- Blindness

REFERENCES

1. Wagoner MD. Chemical injuries of the eye: Current concepts in pathophysiology and therapy. *Survey Ophthalmol*. 1997;41:275–313.
2. Kuckelkorn R, Schrage N, Keller G, et al. Emergency treatment of chemical and thermal eye burns. *Acta Ophthalmol Scand*. 2002;80:4–10.
3. Spector J, Fernandez WG, et al. Chemical, thermal, and biological ocular exposures. *Emerg Med Clin North Am*. 2008;26:125–36, vii.
4. Ralph RA, et al. Tetracyclines and the treatment of corneal stromal ulceration: A review. *Cornea*. 2000;19:274–7.
5. Fish R, Davidson RS, et al. Management of ocular thermal and chemical injuries, including amniotic membrane therapy. *Curr Opin Ophthalmol*. 2010; 21:317–21.

ADDITIONAL READING

Rodrigues Z, et al. Irrigation of the eye after alkaline and acidic burns. *Emerg Nurse*. 2009;17:26–9.

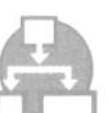

See Also (Topic, Algorithm, Electronic Media Element)

Burns

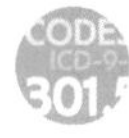

CODES

ICD9

- 940.0 Chemical burn of eyelids and periocular area
- 940.2 Alkaline chemical burn of cornea and conjunctival sac
- 940.3 Acid chemical burn of cornea and conjunctival sac

CLINICAL PEARLS

- Prompt irrigation of all chemical burns, even prior to arrival to the emergency room, is essential to ensure best outcomes.
- All patients with chemical injuries to their eyes should be urgently referred to ophthalmology staff for further assessment.

ONYCHOMYCOSIS

Natasha A. Travis, MD
Christiane Mbianda, MD

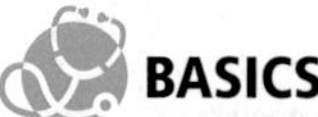

BASICS

DESCRIPTION

- Chronic fungal infection of fingernails or toenails
- Caused mostly by dermatophytes, also yeasts, molds
- Toenails more commonly affected than fingernails
- System(s) affected: Skin/Exocrine
- Synonym(s): Tinea unguium; Ringworm of the nail

EPIDEMIOLOGY

Prevalence

- Occurs in 2–8% in general population
- Predominant age: 14–28% in adults >60 years of age
- Rare before puberty

RISK FACTORS

- Older age
- Tinea pedis
- Cancer
- Diabetes
- Peripheral vascular disease
- Psoriasis
- Cohabitation with others with onychomycosis
- Immunodeficiency
- Swimming
- Smoking
- Peripheral vascular disease
- Children with Down's syndrome

ETIOLOGY

- Dermatophytes: *Trichophyton* (*T. rubrum* most common), *Epidermophyton*, *Microsporum*
- Yeasts: *C. albicans* (most common), *C. parapsilosis*, *C. tropicalis*, *C. krusei*
- Molds: *Scopulariopsis brevicaulis*, *Hendersonula toruloidea*, *Aspergillus* sp., *Alternaria tenuis*, *Cephalosporium*, *Scytalidium hyalinum*
- Dermatophytes cause 90% of toenail and most of fingernail onychomycoses.
- Fingernail onychomycosis is more often caused by yeasts than is the case for toenail onychomycosis.
- Dermatophytes invade normal keratin, whereas molds invade altered keratin.

COMMONLY ASSOCIATED CONDITIONS

- Immunodeficiency or chronic metabolic disease
- Tinea pedis or manuum

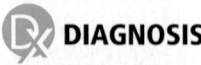

DIAGNOSIS

PHYSICAL EXAM

- Dermatophytes: Commonly preceded by dermatophyte infection at another site; 80% involve toenails, especially hallux; simultaneous infection of fingernails and toenails is rare. 4 clinical forms occur:
  - Distal or lateral subungual onychomycosis (most common): Spreads from distal or lateral margins to nail bed to nail plate; subungual hyperkeratosis; subungual paronychia; onycholysis; nail dystrophy; discoloration—yellow-brown; yellow streaking laterally; bois vermoulu ("worm-eaten wood"); onychomadesis
  - Proximal subungual onychomycosis (rare): Hands or feet; leukonychia—begins under posterior nail groove, appearing to occur from the proximal underside of the nail (or direct invasion of the nail plate from above); spreads to nail plate and lunula; seen with immunodeficiency
  - Superficial white onychomycosis (rare): Hallux preferentially affected; infection of outer surface of nail plate; opaque white spots on nail plate eventually merge to involve entire surface of the nail
- Candidal:
  - Hands, 70%, especially for the dominant hand
  - Middle finger most common
  - Pain mild, unless secondarily infected
  - Increases on prolonged contact with water
  - Primarily affects tissue surrounding nail
  - Begins with cuticle detachment
  - Dark yellowish to blackish brown to green zone along lateral border of nail
  - Secondary ungual changes: Convex, irregular, striated nail plate with dull, rough surface
  - Onycholysis, especially on hands
  - Distal subungual onychomycosis may occur.
  - Primary involvement of the nail plate is uncommon (thin, crumbly, opaque, brownish nail plate deformed by transverse grooves).
  - Periungual edema/erythema may occur (club-shaped, bulbous fingertips).
- Molds:
  - More common in those >60 years of age
  - More common in nails of hallux
  - Resembles distal and lateral onychomycosis

Pediatric Considerations

Candidal infection presents more commonly as superficial white onychomycosis.

DIAGNOSTIC TESTS & INTERPRETATION

- Accurate diagnosis requires both laboratory and clinical evidence.
- If onychomycosis is suspected clinically and initial diagnostic laboratory tests are negative, the tests should be repeated.

Lab

Initial lab tests

- Direct microscopy with potassium hydroxide (KOH) preparation:
  - Clip away diseased, discolored nail plate.
  - Collect debris from stratum corneum of most proximal area (beneath nail or crumbling nail itself) with 1-mm curette or scalpel.
  - Larger sample improves sensitivity.
  - KOH (5%) plus gentle heat.
  - High sensitivity if >2 preparations examined
- Cultures: False negative in 30% (secondary to loss of dermatophyte viability; improved by immediate culture on Sabouraud cell culture medium)
- Histologic examination of nail clippings; punch biopsy: Proximal lesions; stain both with periodic acid–Schiff (PAS) stain
- Discontinue all topical medication for some time before obtaining a sample.

Pathological Findings

Pathogens within the nail keratin

DIFFERENTIAL DIAGNOSIS

- Psoriasis (most common alternate diagnosis)
- Traumatic dystrophy
- Lichen planus
- Onychogryphosis
- Eczematous conditions
- Hypothyroidism
- Drugs and chemicals
- Yellow nail syndrome
- Neoplasms
- Only 50% of dystrophic nails are due to onychomycosis.

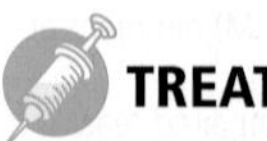

TREATMENT

MEDICATION

Pregnancy Considerations

Oral antifungals and ciclopirox are pregnancy Category B (terbinafine, ciclopirox) or C (itraconazole, fluconazole, and griseofulvin). Because treatment of onychomycosis usually can be postponed until after pregnancy, treatment should be avoided during pregnancy.

First Line

- Oral antifungals are preferred due to higher rates of cure, but they have systemic adverse effects and drug–drug interactions.
- Terbinafine: 250 mg/d PO × 6 weeks for fingernails and 3 months for toenails, most effective in cure and prevention of relapse, most cost-effective with higher patient satisfaction compared with itraconazole pulse. It has similar tolerance to terbinafine pulse (500 mg/d × 1 week per month for 3 months), and fewer drug–drug interactions (1)[C],(2)[A].
- Itraconazole pulse: 400 mg/d PO or 200 mg PO b.i.d. × 1 week, then 3 weeks off, repeat for 2 cycles for fingernails and 3–4 cycles for toenails (lower cost and lower pill burden than itraconazole continuous, more effective than terbinafine for *Candida* and molds, do not need to monitor liver function tests (1)[C],(2)[A]
- Itraconazole continuous: 200 mg/d PO × 6 weeks for fingernails and 3 months for toenails (may be more effective than itraconazole pulse, more effective than terbinafine for *Candida* and molds) (1)[C],(2)[A]

Second Line

- Fluconazole pulse: 150–300 mg PO weekly × 6 months (less frequent dosing but lower cure rate) (1)[C],(2)[A]
- Griseofulvin: 500–1,000 mg/d PO for up to 18 months (lower cure rate, needs to be continued until the diseased nail is completely replaced) (1)[C],(2)[A]
- Ciclopirox: 8% nail lacquer: Apply once daily to affected nails (if without lunula involvement) for up to 48 weeks, and every 7 days, remove lacquer with alcohol, then file away loose nail material and trim nails (low cure rate, avoids systemic adverse effects, less cost-effective). Application after PO treatment may reduce recurrences (3)[A].

- Contraindications for oral antifungals:
  - Hepatic disease
  - Pregnancy (see "Pregnancy Alert")
  - Current or history of congestive heart failure (CHF) (itraconazole)
  - Porphyria (griseofulvin)
- Precautions/adverse effects:
  - Oral antifungals:
    - Hepatotoxicity
    - Neutropenia
    - Hypersensitivity
    - Photosensitivity, lupuslike symptoms, proteinuria (griseofulvin)
    - Chronic kidney disease (avoid terbinafine for patients with CrCl <50 mL/min, decrease fluconazole dose)
    - CHF, peripheral edema, pulmonary edema (itraconazole)
  - Ciclopirox: Rash, nail disorders; avoid contact with skin other than skin immediately surrounding nail; use with caution on broken skin or in vascular compromise
- Significant drug–drug interactions:
  - Terbinafine (inhibits CYP2D6): β-Blockers, cimetidine, cyclosporine, dextromethorphan, monoamine oxidase inhibitors (MAOIs), rifampin, SSRIs, tricyclic antidepressants (TCAs), warfarin
  - Itraconazole, fluconazole (inhibit CYP3A4): Antiarrhythmics, benzodiazepines, cisapride, ergot alkaloids, HMG CoA reductase inhibitors, alfentanil, buspirone, calcium channel blockers, carbamazepine, cimetidine, corticosteroids, cyclosporine, haloperidol, hydrochlorothiazide, hypoglycemics, losartan, oral contraceptives, phenytoin, pimozide, protease inhibitors, rifamycins, sirolimus, tacrolimus, TCAs, theophylline, tolterodine, vinca alkaloids, warfarin, zidovudine, zolpidem
  - Griseofulvin: Barbiturates, cyclosporine, oral contraceptives, salicylates, warfarin

ADDITIONAL TREATMENT

General Measures

- Avoid factors that promote fungal growth (i.e., heat, moisture, occlusion).
- Treat underlying disease risk factors.
- Treat secondary infections.

COMPLEMENTARY AND ALTERNATIVE MEDICINE

Melaleuca alternifolia (tea tree) oil has a 10% mycologic cure.

SURGERY/OTHER PROCEDURES

- Nail debridement to remove infected keratin (efficacy not well studied):
  - Mechanical: Soften with occlusive dressing with 40% urea gel; detach from nail bed with tweezers or file with abrasive stone.
  - Chemical: Protect peripheral tissue with adhesive strips; apply ointment of 30% salicylic acid, 40% urea, or 50% potassium iodide under occlusive dressing.
  - Surgical avulsion: For involvement of a few nails; used by some for pain control
- Laser/light therapy may have potential in the treatment of onychomycosis (4).

ONGOING CARE

FOLLOW-UP RECOMMENDATIONS

- Formation of a new fingernail takes 4–6 months and a new toenail takes 12–18 months.
- Cure defined as (5)[C]:
  - 100% absence of clinical signs and/or
  - Negative mycology with $\geq$1 of the following clinical signs:
    - Distal subungual hyperkeratosis or onycholysis leaving <10% of the nail plate affected
    - Nail plate thickening that does not improve with treatment because of comorbid condition

Patient Monitoring

- Topical agents: Slow response expected; visits every 6–12 weeks
- Terbinafine, griseofulvin: Baseline and as needed liver function tests (LFTs) and CBC
- Itraconazole continuous: Baseline and as needed LFTs

PATIENT EDUCATION

- Advise patient to:
  - Keep affected area clean and dry.
  - Avoid rubber or other occlusive footwear.
  - Avoid tight or ill-fitting footwear.
  - Wear absorbent cotton socks; avoid synthetic fibers.
  - Change clothing and towels frequently, and launder them in hot water.
- Cure of all toenails may not be attainable.
- Nails may not appear normal after cure.

PROGNOSIS

- Complete clinical cure in 25–50% (higher mycologic cure rates)
- Recurrence is 10–50% (relapse or reinfection).
- Poor prognostic factors (5)[C]:
  - Areas of nail involvement >50%
  - Significant proximal or lateral disease
  - Subungual hyperkeratosis >2 mm
  - White/yellow or orange/brown streaks in the nail (includes dermatophytoma)
  - Total dystrophic onychomycosis (with matrix involvement)
  - Nonresponsive organisms (e.g., *Scytalidium* mold)
  - Patients with immunosuppression
  - Diminished peripheral circulation

COMPLICATIONS

- Secondary infections with progression to soft tissue infection or osteomyelitis
- Toenail discomfort or pain that can limit physical mobility or activity
- Anxiety, negative self-image

REFERENCES

1. Finch JJ, Warshaw EM. Toenail onychomycosis: Current and future treatment options. *Dermatol Ther*. 2007;20:31–46.
2. Hinojosa JR, Hitchcock K, Rodriguez JE. Clinical inquiries. Which oral antifungal is best for toenail onychomycosis? *J Fam Pract*. 2007;56:581–2.
3. Crawford F, Hollis S. Topical treatments for fungal infections of the skin and nails of the foot. *Cochrane Database Syst Rev*. 2007;(3):CD001434.
4. Landsman AS, Robbins AH, Angelini PF, et al. Treatment of mild, moderate, and severe onychomycosis using 870- and 930-nm light exposure. *J Am Podiatr Med Assoc*. 2010;100:166–77.
5. Scher RK, Tavakkol A, Sigurgeirsson B. Onychomycosis: Diagnosis and definition of cure. *J Am Acad Dermatol*. 2007;56:939–44.

ADDITIONAL READING

- de Berker D. Clinical practice. Fungal nail disease. *N Engl J Med*. 2009;360:2108–16.
- Welsh O, Vera-Cabrera L, Welsh E. Onychomycosis. *Clin Dermatol*. 2010;28:151–9.

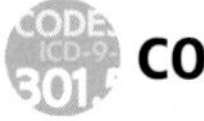

CODES

ICD9

- 110.1 Dermatophytosis of nail
- 112.3 Candidiasis of skin and nails

CLINICAL PEARLS

- Psoriasis and chronic nail trauma are commonly mistaken for fungal infection.
- Diagnosis should be based on both clinical and mycologic laboratory evidence.
- Oral antifungals generally are well tolerated and more effective than topical antifungals, with terbinafine being the most effective.
- LFT monitoring is necessary for most oral antifungal regimens.
- The patient should understand that treatment is long term, recurrence is common, and nails may not appear normal even after treatment.

OPTIC ATROPHY

Birgit Khandalavala, MD

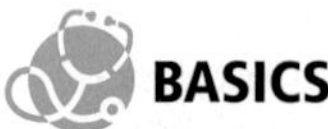

BASICS

DESCRIPTION

- Loss of the ganglion cell axons that form the optic nerve. Clinical sign not a diagnosis (1). Because this loss is irreversible, the term optic neuropathy may be preferable:
  - May be primary inherited optic atrophy, congenital nongenetic, or secondary to inherited or acquired disease
  - Optic nerve aplasia is an extremely rare congenital, nongenetic abnormality of unknown etiology associated with other ocular malformations.
  - Optic nerve hypoplasia is a more common congenital abnormality associated with:
    - Many genetic syndromes
    - Metabolic disorders
    - Chromosomal abnormalities
    - Developmental abnormalities
    - Maternal alcohol consumption, diabetes, illicit drugs
  - Acquired optic atrophy may be ischemic, inflammatory, infectious, traumatic, drug-induced, radiation-induced, toxic, nutritional, or related to compression, usually developing several months after the initial injury.
- System(s) affected: Nervous
- Synonym(s): Leber hereditary optic neuropathy; Optic neuropathy

Pediatric Considerations

Optic atrophy in small children may be difficult to recognize because disks normally have a pale appearance.

EPIDEMIOLOGY

- Predominant age: May be congenital:
  - Inherited forms occur from shortly after birth to the third decade.
  - Acquired forms tend to occur later in life.
- Predominant sex: Male > Female (inherited forms)
- Leber hereditary optic neuropathy: Predominately 20–30-year-old men (2)

RISK FACTORS

- Genetic
- Acquired:
  - Diabetes mellitus
  - Hypertension
  - Radiation exposure
  - Alcoholism
  - Renal failure
  - Arteriosclerosis

Genetics

- Inherited forms may be autosomal-recessive, autosomal-dominant, X-linked–recessive (3)[C], or mitochondrial (4)[C]:
  - Leber hereditary optic neuropathy (LHON):
    - Mitochondrial inheritance (maternal)
    - Complex I of mitochondrial respiratory chain
    - Bilateral subacute optic neuropathy
    - Degeneration of retinal ganglion cells and their axons
    - Primarily affecting young adult men
  - Autosomal-dominant optic atrophy, Kjer type:
    - Affects children in the first decade of life
    - Bilateral, slowly progressive loss of vision
    - OPA1 gene on chromosome 3q28
    - Autosomal gene affects mitochondrial function.
  - Autosomal-recessive optic atrophies (OPA6, rare)
- Optic atrophies associated with genetic metabolic conditions
- Disorders of amino acid metabolism:
  - Hyperhomocysteinemia is associated with ischemic optic neuropathy.
- Wolfram syndrome
- Mitochondrial disorders
- Peroxisomal disorders:
  - Refsum disease
  - Adrenoleukodystrophy
- Lysosomal storage diseases:
  - Tay-Sachs
  - Niemann-Pick
  - Mucopolysaccharidoses
- Other inherited neurodegenerative conditions:
  - Hereditary ataxia
  - Charcot-Marie-Tooth disease
  - Familial dysautonomia

GENERAL PREVENTION

Regular ophthalmologic exam in high-risk groups

ETIOLOGY

- Nongenetic optic neuropathy
- Compression of the optic nerve:
  - Glaucoma
  - Chronic papilledema
  - Tumor
  - Aneurysm
  - Hydrocephalus
- Inflammation:
  - Graves disease
  - Chronic optic neuritis
- Trauma
- Syphilis
- Ischemic optic neuropathy
- Central retinal artery or vein occlusion
- Retinal degeneration
- Congenital optic atrophy: Possibly due to lack of oxygen during pregnancy, labor, or early neonatal period
- Radiation neuropathy
- Drugs:
  - Amiodarone
  - Chloroquine
  - Ethambutol
  - Oral contraceptives
  - Streptomycin
  - Vincristine
- Nutritional deficiencies:
  - Vitamin B_{12}
  - Folic acid
  - Thiamine
- Demyelinating disorders (e.g., multiple sclerosis)
- Toxins/poisons:
  - Cyanide
  - Lead
  - Methanol
- Tobacco

COMMONLY ASSOCIATED CONDITIONS

- Multiple sclerosis
- Diabetes
- Cardiovascular disease

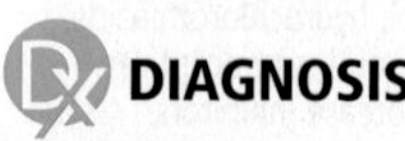

DIAGNOSIS

HISTORY

- Family history of visual loss
- Congenital disorders
- Painless loss of visual acuity:
  - Bilateral can be synchronous or metachronous
  - In primary optic atrophies, often the only clinical feature

PHYSICAL EXAM

- Funduscopic exam:
  - Small, pale optic disk is diagnostic.
  - Enlarged peripapillary atrophy if glaucoma is the cause
  - Unilateral disk swelling points toward nerve compression.
- Loss of pupillary reactions
- Visual-field defects
- Abnormalities in color vision and contrast sensitivity

DIAGNOSTIC TESTS & INTERPRETATION
- Automated visual-field test (e.g., Humphrey)
- Color vision testing
- Visual-evoked potentials
- Fluorescein angiography

Lab
- CBC
- Electrolytes
- Antinuclear antibody test
- ESR
- C-reactive protein
- Vitamin B_{12}, folate, and thiamine levels
- Fluorescent treponemal antibody absorption test
- Serologic test for syphilis
- Heavy-metal screen
- Genetic testing if indicated, especially for Leber hereditary optic neuropathy

Imaging
- CT or MRI of head may be indicated for unexplained or isolated optic atrophy.
- Optical coherence tomography is a new technique with potential to distinguish the thickness of the retinal nerve fiber without radiation.

Initial approach
- A complete ophthalmic examination, including a comprehensive history, will lead to an underlying diagnosis in 92% of cases.
- Ancillary testing is only indicated when the cause is not apparent by clinical evaluation.

Diagnostic Procedures/Surgery
- Complete neurologic exam for multiple sclerosis
- Complete ophthalmologic exam, including dilated evaluation of retina
- Carotid ultrasound (adult-acquired optic atrophy)

DIFFERENTIAL DIAGNOSIS
- Glaucomatous optic atrophy particularly in late-stage disease can be indistinguishable
- Myopia
- Postoperative cataract extraction (no natural yellow color from the human lens)

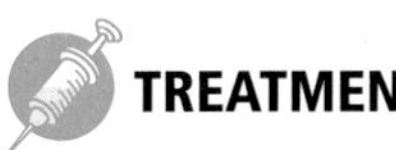

TREATMENT

MEDICATION
- Corticosteroids may briefly improve visual acuity when optic neuritis is present.
- Long-term benefits are unproven.

ADDITIONAL TREATMENT
Associated conditions may require specific treatment for nutritional deficiencies, coexistent inflammatory syndromes, or multiple sclerosis.

General Measures
- Optic nerve damage is usually permanent, so early detection is important (3)[C].
- Treat the underlying cause, if treatable.
- Correction of an underlying nutritional deficiency or discontinuation of the causative drug may halt progression.
- Optic nerve pressure may be relieved by neurosurgery.

Issues for Referral
- Genetic counselling
- Neurosurgical referral if secondary to compression
- Rheumatology referral if associated with systemic diseases
- Neurological referral for multiple sclerosis

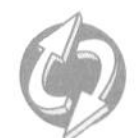

ONGOING CARE

FOLLOW-UP RECOMMENDATIONS
- Determined by the associated cause
- Progressive optic atrophy may require more frequent follow-up.

Patient Monitoring
- Annual evaluations if stable
- May be gradually discontinued if optic atrophy is unexplained and nonprogressive

DIET
No special diet

PATIENT EDUCATION
- Low-vision counseling
- Genetic counseling if inherited
- Glaucoma education
- For patient education materials favorably reviewed on this topic, contact the National Eye Institute, Information Officer, Department of Health and Human Services, 9000 Rockville Pike, Bethesda, MD 20892; (301) 496-5248
- American Council of the Blind: (800) 424-8666

PROGNOSIS
- Visual loss occurs over weeks to months.
- Correction of an underlying nutritional deficiency or discontinuation of the causative drug may halt progression.
- Optic neuropathy is usually not reversible.

REFERENCES

1. Golnik K, et al. Nonglaucomatous optic atrophy. *Neurol Clin*. 2010;28:631–40.
2. Teive HA, Troiano AR, Raskin S, et al. Leber's hereditary optic neuropathy–case report and literature review. *Sao Paulo Med J*. 2004;122: 276–9.
3. Huizing M, et al. Optic atrophies in metabolic disorders. *Mol Genet Metabol*. 2005;86:51–60.
4. Howell N. LHON and other optic nerve atrophies: The mitochondrial connection. *Dev Ophthalmol*. 2003;37:94–108.

ADDITIONAL READING

- Barboni P, Savini G, Valentino ML, et al. Retinal nerve fiber layer evaluation by optical coherence tomography in Leber's hereditary optic neuropathy. *Ophthalmology*. 2005;112:120–6.
- University of Michigan Kellogg Eye Center. Available at: www.kellogg.umich.edu.

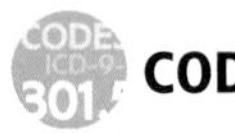

CODES

ICD9
- 377.10 Optic atrophy, unspecified
- 377.11 Primary optic atrophy
- 377.12 Postinflammatory optic atrophy

CLINICAL PEARLS
- The hallmark of optic atrophy, which is a sign not a diagnosis, is a small, pale optic disk on funduscopic exam.
- Optic atrophy with systemic symptoms typically leads to the diagnosis of a metabolic cause of optic atrophy.
- Optic atrophy is inherited by autosomal-dominant, autosomal-recessive, X-linked, or mitochondrial inheritance.
- The best treatment for optic atrophy is early diagnosis, which can assist in halting progression, but damage is usually irreversible.
- The types of visual loss involved with optic atrophy are blurred vision, abnormal peripheral vision, abnormal color vision, and decreased brightness. Bilateral loss is either synchronous or metachronous.

OPTIC NEURITIS

Olga M. Ceron, MD
Pablo I. Hernandez Itriago, MD

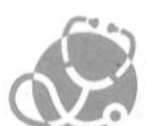

BASICS

DESCRIPTION

- Inflammation of the optic nerve (cranial nerve II)
- Most common form is acute demyelinating optic neuritis (ON), but other causes include infectious disease and systemic autoimmune disorders
- Optic disc may be either normal in appearance at onset (retrobulbar ON, 67%) or swollen (papillitis, 33%)
- Key features:
  - Abrupt visual loss
  - Periorbital pain especially with eye movement (90%)
  - Dyschromatopsia: Color vision deficits
  - Afferent pupillary defect
- Usually unilateral in adults; bilateral disease more common in children
- Presenting complaint in 25% of multiple sclerosis (MS) patients
- In children, headaches are common.
- System(s) affected: Nervous
- Synonym(s): Papillitis; Demyelinating optic neuropathy; Retrobulbar optic neuritis

EPIDEMIOLOGY

Incidence

- 5 cases per 100,000 seen annually
- More common in northern latitudes
- More common in whites than in other races
- Predominant age: Typically 18–45 years; mean age 30
- Predominant sex: Female > Male (3:1)

PATHOPHYSIOLOGY

- In both MS-associated and isolated monosymptomatic ON, the cause is presumed to be a demyelinating autoimmune reaction.
- Possible mechanisms of inflammation in immune-mediated ON are the cross-reaction of viral epitopes and host epitopes, and the persistence of a virus in CNS glial cells
- Neuromyelitis optica (NMO) IgG autoantibody, which targets the water channel aquaporin-4

ETIOLOGY

- Primarily idiopathic
- MS
- Viral infections: Measles, mumps, varicella-zoster, coxsackievirus, adenovirus, hepatitis A and B, HIV, herpes simplex virus, cytomegalovirus
- Nonviral infections: Syphilis, tuberculosis, meningococcus, cryptococcosis, cysticercosis, bacterial sinusitis, streptococcus B, *Bartonella*, Lyme disease, fungus
- Systemic inflammatory disease: Sarcoidosis, systemic lupus erythematosus, vasculitis
- Local inflammatory disease: Intraocular or contiguous with the orbit, sinus, or meninges
- Toxic: Lead, methanol, arsenic, radiation
- Vascular lesions affecting the optic nerve
- Posterior uveitis
- Tumors
- Medications: Ethambutol, chloroquine, isoniazid, chronic high-dose chloramphenicol, tumor necrosis factor α antagonist, infliximab (Remicade), adalimumab (Humira), etanercept (Enbrel)

COMMONLY ASSOCIATED CONDITIONS

- MS (common): ON is associated with an increased risk of MS.
- Other demyelinating diseases: Guillain-Barré syndrome, Devic neuromyelitis optica, multifocal demyelinating neuropathy, acute disseminated encephalomyelitis

DIAGNOSIS

HISTORY

- Decreased visual acuity, deteriorating in hours to days, usually reaching lowest level after 1 week
- Usually unilateral but can also be bilateral
- Brow ache, globe tenderness, deep orbital pain exacerbated by eye movement (92%)
- Retro-orbital pain may precede visual loss.
- Desaturation of color vision (dull or faded colors), especially red tones
- Apparent dimness of light intensities
- Impairment of depth perception (80%); worse with moving objects (Pulfrich phenomenon)
- Transient increase in visual symptoms with increased body temperature and exercise (Uhthoff phenomenon)
- May present with a recent flulike viral syndrome
- Detailed history and review of systems, looking for a history of demyelinating, infectious, or systemic inflammatory disease

PHYSICAL EXAM

Complete general exam, full neurologic exam, and ophthalmologic exam looking for the following:

- Decreased visual acuity and color perception
- Central, cecocentral, arcuate, or altitudinal visual field deficits
- Papillitis: Swollen disc $\pm$ peripapillary flame-shape hemorrhage or often normal disc exam
- Temporal disc pallor seen later at 4–6 weeks (1)[A]
- Relative afferent pupillary defect (Marcus-Gunn pupil): The pupil of the affected eye dilates with a swinging light test unless disease is bilateral.

DIAGNOSTIC TESTS & INTERPRETATION

Lab

Initial lab tests

- In typical presentations, ESR is standard, but other labs are unnecessary. Antinuclear antibodies (ANAs), angiotensin-converting enzyme level, fluorescent treponemal antibody absorption (FTA-ABS), and chest radiograph have been shown to have no value in typical cases (1)[A].
- In atypical presentations, including absence of pain, a very swollen optic nerve, >30 days without recovery, or retinal exudates, labs may be indicated to rule out underlying disorders:
  - CBC
  - ANA test
  - Rapid plasma reagin test
  - FTA-ABS test

Follow-Up & Special Considerations

- Visual field test (Humphrey 30–2); to evaluate for visual field loss: Diffuse and central visual loss more predominant in the affected eye at baseline (2)[A]
- A novel blood test called an *NMO-IgG* checks for antibodies for neuromyelitis optica.

Imaging

Initial approach

- MRI of brain and orbits: Thin cuts (2–3 mm) gadolinium enhanced and fat suppression images to look for Dawson fingers of MS (periventricular white matter lesions oriented perpendicular to the ventricles) and to also look for enhancement of the optic nerve
- CT scan of chest to rule out sarcoidosis if clinical suspicion is high

Diagnostic Procedures/Surgery

- In atypical cases including bilateral deficits, young age, or suspicion of infectious etiology, lumbar puncture (LP) with neurology consultation is indicated.
- LP for suspected MS is a physician-dependent decision. Some studies indicate that it may not add value to MRI for MS detection (1)[A], but there is no consensus on the subject.

DIFFERENTIAL DIAGNOSIS

- Demyelinating disease, especially MS
- Infectious/systemic inflammatory disease
- Neuroretinitis: Virus, toxoplasmosis, *Bartonella*
- Toxic or nutritional optic neuropathy
- Acute papilledema (bilateral disc edema)
- Compression:
  - Orbital tumor/abscess compressing the optic nerve
  - Intracranial tumor/abscess compressing the afferent visual pathway
  - Orbital pseudotumor
  - Carotid–ophthalmic artery aneurysm
- Temporal arteritis or other vasculitides
- Trauma or radiation
- Neuromyelitis optica (Devic disease)
- Anterior ischemic optic neuropathy
- Leber hereditary optic neuropathy
- Kjer-type autosomal-dominant optic atrophy
- Severe systemic hypertension
- Diabetic papillopathy

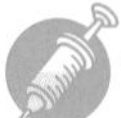

TREATMENT

Most persons with optic neuritis recover spontaneously.

MEDICATION

First Line

- IV methylprednisolone has been shown to speed up the rate of visual recovery but without significant long-term benefit; consider for patients who require fast recovery (i.e., monocular patients or those whose occupation requires high-level visual acuity). For significant vision loss, parenteral corticosteroids may be considered on an individualized basis:
  - Observation and corticosteroid treatment are both acceptable courses of action (3)[A].
  - High-dose IV methylprednisone (250 mg q6h × 3 days) followed by oral corticosteroids (1 mg/kg/d PO × 11 days, taper over 1–2 weeks) (3)[A]
- Others use IV Solu-Medrol infusion (1 g in 250 mL D_5 1/2 normal saline infused over 1 hour daily for 3–5 days).
  - No evidence of long-term benefit (1)[A],(4)[B]
  - May decrease recovery time (3)[A],(4)[B]
  - May decrease risk of MS at 2 but not 5 years (3)[A]
- Give antiulcer medications with steroids.

Second Line

- Disease-modifying agents such as interferon-β-1a (IFN-β-1a; Avonex, Rebif) and IFN-β-1b (Betaseron) are used to prevent or delay the development of MS in people with ON who have ≥2 brain lesions evident on MRI.
- These medications have been proposed for use in patients with one episode of ON (clinically isolated syndrome) at high risk of developing MS (1+ lesion on brain MRI).
- The Controlled High Risk Avonex Multiple Sclerosis Trial study has shown that IFN-β1–a reduces the conversion to clinically definite MS in high-risk patients by ~50%.
- Decisions should be made individually with neurology consultation.

ALERT

Never use oral prednisone alone as the primary treatment because this may increase the risk for recurrent ON and should be avoided (3)[A].

Pediatric Considerations

- No systematic study defining high-dose corticosteroids in childhood ON has been conducted. *Walsh & Hoyt's Clinical Neuro-ophthalmology* recommends methylprednisolone 1–2 mg/kg × 3–5 days, followed by a longer taper. Farris and Pickard used doses of methylprednisolone ranging from 0.25–6.26 mg/kg, with 50% the patients receiving doses of 125 or 250 mg q6h × 5 days, followed by a taper.
- Optic disc swelling and bilateral disease are more common in children, as is severe loss of visual acuity (20/200 or worse).
- Consider infectious and postinfectious causes of optic nerve impairment.

ADDITIONAL TREATMENT

General Measures

Referral to a neurologist and/or ophthalmologist

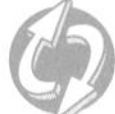

ONGOING CARE

FOLLOW-UP RECOMMENDATIONS

Patient Monitoring

Monthly follow-up to monitor visual changes and steroid side effects

PATIENT EDUCATION

- Provide reassurance about recovery of vision.
- If the disease is believed to be secondary to demyelinating disease, patient should be informed of the risk of developing MS.
- For patient education materials favorably reviewed on this topic, contact:
  - National Eye Institute, Information Officer, Department of Health and Human Services, 9000 Rockville Pike, Bethesda, MD 20892, 301-496-5248
  - North American Neuro-Ophthalmology Society (NANOS), 5841 Cedar Lake Road, Suite 204, Minneapolis, MN 55416, phone: 952-646-2037, fax: 952-545-6073, www.nanosweb.org

PROGNOSIS

- Orbital pain usually resolves within 1 week.
- Visual acuity:
  - Rapid spontaneous improvement at 2–3 weeks and continues for several months (may be faster with IV corticosteroids)
  - Often returns to normal or near-normal levels (20/40 or better) within 1 year (90–95%), even after near blindness
- Other visual disturbances (e.g., contrast sensitivity, stereopsis) often persist after acuity returns to normal.
- Recurrence risk of 35% within 10 years: 14% affected eye, 12% contralateral, 9% bilateral; recurrence is higher in MS patients (48%)
- ON is associated with increased risk of developing MS; 35% risk at 7 years, 58% at 15 years:
  - Brain MRI helps to predict risk:
    - 0 lesions: 16%
    - 1–2 lesions: 37%
    - 3+ lesions: 51% (5)
- Poor prognostic factors:
  - Absence of pain
  - Low initial visual acuity
  - Involvement of intracanalicular optic nerve
- Children with bilateral visual loss have a better prognosis than adults.

COMPLICATIONS

Permanent loss of vision (6)

REFERENCES

1. Vedula SS. Corticosteroids for treating optic neuritis. *Cochrane Database Syst Rev.* 2007;1: CD001430.
2. Keltner JL, Johnson CA, Cello KE, et al. Visual field profile of optic neuritis: A final follow-up report from the optic neuritis treatment trial from baseline through 15 years. *Arch Ophthalmol.* 2010;128:330–7.
3. Simsek I, Erdem H, Pay S. Optic neuritis occurring with anti-tumour necrosis factor alpha therapy. *Ann Rheum Dis.* 2007;66:1255–8.
4. Gleicher N, et al. *Principles and Practice of Medical Therapy in Pregnancy*, 3rd ed. Norwalk, CT: Appleton and Lange; 1998:1396–9.
5. Kaufman DI, Trobe JD, Eggenberger ER. Practice parameter: The role of corticosteroids in the management of acute monosymptomatic optic neuritis. Report of the Quality Standards Subcommittee of the American Academy of Neurology. *Neurology.* 2000;54:2039–44.
6. Carter J. e-Medicine, *Optic Neuritis* August 8, 2009.
7. Optic Neuritis Study Group. Visual function 15 years after optic neuritis: A final follow-up report from the Optic Neuritis Treatment Trial. *Ophthalmology.* 2008;115:1079–1082.e5.

ADDITIONAL READING

- Arnold AC. Evolving management of optic neuritis and multiple sclerosis. *Am J Ophthalmol.* 2005;139: 1101–8.
- Balcer LJ. Clinical practice. Optic neuritis. *N Engl J Med.* 2006;354:1273–80.
- Galetta SL. The controlled high risk Avonex multiple sclerosis trial (CHAMPS Study). *J Neuroophthalmol.* 2001;21:292–5.
- Rizzo JF, Andreoli CM, Rabinov JD. Use of magnetic resonance imaging to differentiate optic neuritis and nonarteritic anterior ischemic optic neuropathy. *Ophthalmology.* 2002;109:1679–84.

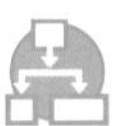

See Also (Topic, Algorithm, Electronic Media Element)

Multiple Sclerosis

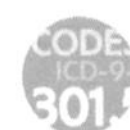

CODES

ICD9

- 377.30 Optic neuritis, unspecified
- 377.31 Optic papillitis
- 377.39 Other optic neuritis

CLINICAL PEARLS

- The MRI is the procedure of choice for determining relative risk and possible therapy for MS prevention.
- The ONTT showed that high-dose IV methylprednisolone followed by oral prednisone accelerated visual recovery but did not improve the 6-month or 1-year visual outcome compared with placebo, whereas treatment with oral prednisone alone did not improve the outcome and was associated with an increased rate of recurrence of ON.

ALERT

Results of 15-year Optic Neuritis Study Group:

- After the initial period of recovery after an acute episode of ON, visual acuity remained stable in most patients.
- Overall, 72% of affected eyes had visual acuity of 20/20 or better, with 2/3 of patients having 20/20 or better vision in both eyes.
- In most patients, there was little change in vision between the 10- and 15-year follow-up. examinations. 6 patients (2%) had visual acuity of 20/40 or worse in both eyes. Visual function was slightly better in patients without MS compared with those with MS (7).

ORAL REHYDRATION

William A. Primack, MD

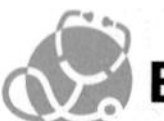

BASICS

Oral rehydration is a clinically useful, cost-effective, and safe technique to treat all but the most severe dehydration.

DESCRIPTION

- Dehydration and ongoing fluid losses from infectious gastroenteritis (GE) can be treated effectively with oral rehydration solution (ORS) except in the most severe cases, in which initial parenteral fluid resuscitation is required (1)[B],(2)[B],(3)[A].
- ORSs for rehydration should have a sodium (Na) content of ~75 mEq/L (75 mmol/L). Maintenance ORSs, with an Na content of 40–50 mEq/L (40–50 mmol/L), are useful for repair of mild dehydration and treatment of ongoing losses with relatively low Na content (e.g., rotavirus) (2)[A].
- High Na diarrheal losses (such as with cholera) may require higher Na content ORSs (WHO solution = 90 mEq/L [90 mml/L] Na). In 2002, the WHO reduced the Na content of its ORS from 90 mEq/L to 75 mEq/L, and in 2003, the CDC endorsed this approach.
- System(s) affected: Endocrine/Metabolic; Gastrointestinal

EPIDEMIOLOGY

Incidence

- Predominant age: Primarily infants and children, but effective for all ages
- Predominant sex: Male = Female

PATHOPHYSIOLOGY

This therapy takes advantage of the coupled transport of Na and glucose in the small intestine even during a course of GE. Water follows osmotically after Na entry. Potassium is passively absorbed via solvent drag. A glucose concentration of 2% allows most efficient Na absorption (5).

DIAGNOSIS

HISTORY

- Frequency and volume of urination
- Vomiting: Duration and amount
- Diarrhea: Duration and amount
- Fever
- Weight loss: Amount
- Travel
- Exposure to others with GE
- Recent antibiotic use

PHYSICAL EXAM

- Level of consciousness
- Capillary refill (abnormal if >2 seconds)
- Mucous membranes: Dry, cracked
- Tears: Decreased
- Heart rate (HR): Increased
- RR: Increased
- BP: Orthostasis
- Pulse: Faint
- Skin turgor: Decreased, tenting
- Eyes: Sunken
- Urine output: Decreased

DIAGNOSTIC TESTS & INTERPRETATION

Lab

Initial lab tests

- None usually necessary
- If moderate to severe, obtain Na, potassium, bicarbonate, chloride, glucose, BUN, creatinine.

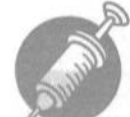

TREATMENT

MEDICATION

First Line

Many comparable generic formulations are available.

Comparison of oral rehydration products

Solution	Type*	Na^+	K^+	HCO_3
WHO (1975)	R	90	20	20
WHO (2002)	R	75	20	10
Pedialyte	M	45	20	25
Enfalyte**	M	50	25	34

*R = rehydration; M = maintenance; Na^+ = Na (mEq/L or mmol/L); K^+ = potassium (mmol/L); COH_3 = carbohydrate (g/L)
**Contains rice syrup solids.

Second Line

In areas where malnutrition is more likely, supplementation with 20 mg oral zinc daily shortens the course of diarrhea and lessens costs (6)[B]. Probiotics may also shorten course of diarrhea, but which probiotic is optimal is not yet clear (7)[B].

ADDITIONAL TREATMENT

General Measures

- In developed countries, most diarrheal losses are low Na; consequently, maintenance ORSs can be used for rehydration (2)[A].
- If patient is obtunded or has paralytic ileus, use IV hydration.
- ORS is not to be diluted.
- If vomiting occurs, small amounts of ORS given frequently are usually effective. Antiemetics (ondansetron or metoclopramide) may reduce vomiting but may increase diarrhea (8)[B]
- If the patient is not vomiting and is alert, thirst is an excellent indicator of fluid needs. Very important to replace any ongoing losses and add maintenance fluids.
- Estimate replacement at 60 mL/kg for mild dehydration and 80–100 mL/kg for moderate dehydration over the first 4–8 hours.
- Replace ongoing stool losses with an ORS. In an infant, estimate 5–10 mL/kg per stool, or weigh diapers.
- Maintenance oral rehydration therapy begins when the deficit is replaced and provides for ongoing losses. Maintenance ORS or a combination of ORS and water or other clear liquids can be used.
- Add maintenance requirements to replacement:
  - Estimate:
    - 0–10 kg: 4 mL/kg/hr
    - Plus 10–20 kg: 2 mL/kg/hr
    - Plus >20 kg: 1 mL/kg/hr
  - Use a maintenance ORS:
    - For example, an 18-kg child who has moderate dehydration would require ~56 mL/hr for maintenance [(10 kg × 4 mL/hr) + (8 kg × 2 mL/hr)]. Replacement fluid would be about 1,500–1,800 mL over 4–8 hours or about 300 mL/hr, giving a total rate of about 350 mL or 12 oz/hr. The child should receive additional ORSs for any ongoing losses.
  - Traditional clear fluids (e.g., fruit juice, soda) are inappropriate for oral rehydration therapy.
- If the patient has hypertonic dehydration, oral rehydration should be planned for 12–24 hours.

- Effective at all ages:
  - If child refuses because of taste, flavor with a commercial flavoring such as sugar-free grape-flavored Kool-Aid, and use ~1/4 tsp to 4 oz ORS.
  - Prepackaged ORS-flavored freeze pops (often well accepted)
- If necessary, rehydration by NG tube is appropriate.
- Begin feeding as soon as rehydration is achieved.
- Contraindications:
  - Conditions predisposing to risk of aspiration: Altered consciousness, seizure activity, severe hypotension, shock
  - Persistent vomiting (as in pyloric stenosis)
  - Absent bowel sounds
- Precautions:
  - The ingredients should be provided in premixed packets to avoid iatrogenic errors in mixing. In the US, Pedialyte premixed powder packets to be diluted in 8 oz (240 mL) of water.
  - If water safety is questionable, it should be boiled or treated for purification.
  - Discard the solution after 12 hours if held at room temperature or 24 hours if refrigerated.
  - After rehydration is complete, ORSs should not be used as the only fluid intake because the high Na content may lead to hypernatremia.

COMPLEMENTARY AND ALTERNATIVE MEDICINE

The probiotics may shorten the duration of diarrhea, especially in patients within developed countries (7)[B].

IN-PATIENT CONSIDERATIONS

Admission Criteria

Failure of oral therapy: Estimated failure rate is 4% (3)[A].

IV Fluids

To be used for initial resuscitation in severe cases or if failure of ORS.

Nursing

If vomiting occurs, small amounts of ORS given frequently are usually effective.

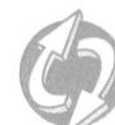

ONGOING CARE

FOLLOW-UP RECOMMENDATIONS

- Primarily outpatient
- Designed to be administered by family members

DIET

- For breast-feeding infants, the mother should continue nursing.
- For bottle-fed babies, there should be an early institution of formulas. Lactose-free formulas rarely are required.
- Age appropriate:
  - Complex carbohydrate-rich (e.g., rice, bread, potato, cereal), low-fat foods should be offered as soon as the dehydration deficit is replaced.
- Cow's milk can be added to diet after several days.

PATIENT EDUCATION

- Awareness and availability of ORSs markedly diminishes morbidity from GE.
- Travelers concerned with severe diarrhea should carry ORS packets on trips.

PROGNOSIS

- Rapid clinical improvement despite continuing diarrhea is the usual course.
- The overall complication rate for oral rehydration is similar to that for parenteral rehydration in cases of mild and moderate dehydration (1)[B],(3)[A].

COMPLICATIONS

Change to IV hydration if the patient has increasing weight loss (fluid deficit), clinical deterioration, or intractable vomiting.

REFERENCES

1. Spandorfer PR, Alessandrini EA, Joffe MD, et al. Oral versus intravenous rehydration of moderately dehydrated children: A randomized, controlled trial. *Pediatrics.* 2005;115:295–301.
2. Hahn S, Kim S, Garner P. Reduced osmolarity oral rehydration solution for treating dehydration caused by acute diarrhoea in children. *Cochrane Database Syst Rev.* 2002;CD002847.
3. Hartling L, Bellemare S, Wiebe N. Oral versus intravenous rehydration for treating dehydration due to gastroenteritis in children. *Cochrane Database Syst Rev.* 2006;3:CD004390.
4. Murphy CK, Hahn S, Volmink J. Reduced osmolarity oral rehydration solution for treating cholera. *Cochrane Database Syst Rev.* 2004;4:CD003754.
5. Duggan C, Fontaine O, Pierce NF. Scientific rationale for a change in the composition of oral rehydration solution. *JAMA.* 2004;291:2628–31.
6. Lazzerini M, Ronfani L. Oral zinc for treating diarrhoea in children. *Cochrane Database Syst Rev.* 2008;3:CD005436.
7. Canani RB, Cirillo P, Terrin G. Probiotics for treatment of acute diarrhoea in children: Randomised clinical trial of five different preparations. *BMJ.* 2007;335:340.
8. Alhashimi D, Al-Hashimi H, Fedorowicz Z. Antiemetics for reducing vomiting related to acute gastroenteritis in children and adolescents. *Cochrane Database Syst Rev.* 2009;2:CD005506.

ADDITIONAL READING

Fonseca BK, Holdgate A, Craig JC. Enteral vs intravenous rehydration therapy for children with gastroenteritis: A meta-analysis of randomized controlled trials. *Arch Pediatr Adolesc Med.* 2004;158:483–90.

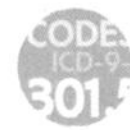

CODES

ICD9

- 009.0 Infectious colitis, enteritis, and gastroenteritis
- 276.51 Dehydration

CLINICAL PEARLS

- ORSs are more effective and less costly than IV hydration yet are underutilized in the developed world.
- In developed countries, most diarrheal losses are low Na; consequently, maintenance ORSs can be used for rehydration.
- ORSs should not be diluted.

OSGOOD-SCHLATTER DISEASE

David P. Sealy, MD

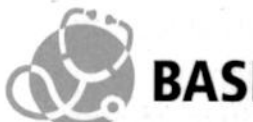

BASICS

DESCRIPTION

- A syndrome associated with traction apophysitis in adolescent boys and girls consisting of pain in the tibial tubercle with swelling
- System(s) affected: Musculoskeletal

EPIDEMIOLOGY

Prevalence

- Not known, but common (13% of athletes in 1 Finnish study)
- Incidence in girls increasing

RISK FACTORS

- Ages 11–18 years
- Girls 8–12, boys 10–16
- Male sex slightly more common
- Rapid skeletal growth
- Involvement in repetitive-jumping sports such as football, volleyball, basketball, hockey, soccer, skating, gymnastics, and ballet (2-fold risk compared to nonathletes)
- Sports involving heavy quadriceps activity

GENERAL PREVENTION

- Avoidance of sports involving heavy quadriceps loading
- Patients may compete if pain is minimal.
- Increase hamstring and quadriceps flexibility.

PATHOPHYSIOLOGY

Traction apophysitis of the tibial tubercle due to repetitive strain on the secondary ossification center of the tibial tuberosity (1)

ETIOLOGY

- Basic etiology unknown, but clearly exacerbated by exercise. Jumping and pivoting sports are the worst—repetitive trauma the most likely source.
- Possible association with tight hip flexors, quadriceps, and hamstring muscle groups

COMMONLY ASSOCIATED CONDITIONS

Shortened (tight) rectus femoris in 75% with OSD

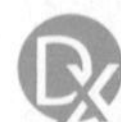

DIAGNOSIS

HISTORY

- Unilateral or bilateral (30%) tibial tuberosity pain
- Pain exacerbated by exercise, especially jumping and landing after jumping

PHYSICAL EXAM

- Knee pain with squatting or crouching
- Absence of effusion or condyle tenderness
- Tibial tuberosity swelling and tenderness
- Pain increased with knee extension against resistance or kneeling
- Erythema over tibial tuberosity

DIAGNOSTIC TESTS & INTERPRETATION

Lab

Initial lab tests

No blood tests are indicated unless other diagnostic considerations are entertained.

Imaging

Initial approach

Radiographic imaging of the proximal tibia and knee may show heterotopic calcification in the patellar tendon:

- X-rays are rarely diagnostic.
- Calcified thickening of the tibial tuberosity with irregular ossification at insertion of tendon to tibial tubercle

Diagnostic Procedures/Surgery

- Bone scan may show increased uptake in the area of the tibial tuberosity; will have increased uptake in apophysis in any child, but may be more than the opposite side.
- Ultrasound is becoming an excellent alternative, with characteristic findings and classification (2).
- MRI has characteristic findings of fragmentation of the tibial tubercle and bone edema.

Pathological Findings

Biopsy is not necessary but would show osteolysis and fragmentation of the tibial tubercle.

DIFFERENTIAL DIAGNOSIS

- Stress fracture of the proximal tibia
- Pes anserinus bursitis
- Quadriceps tendon avulsion
- Patellofemoral stress syndrome
- Chondromalacia patellae
- Proximal tibial neoplasm
- Osteomyelitis of the proximal tibia
- Tibial plateau fracture
- Sinding-Larsen-Johansson syndrome (patellar apophysitis)—pain over inferior patellar tendon
- Patellar fracture
- Infrapatellar bursitis
- Patellar tendinitis—pain over inferior patellar tendon and inferior pole of patella

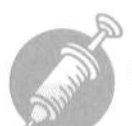

TREATMENT

MEDICATION

First Line

None in particular, but all analgesics may be considered. NSAIDs are of minimal benefit; however, narcotics are not recommended (3)[B].

Second Line

- More potent analgesics such as narcotics may be considered for short-term use or in extreme situations.
- Injectable corticosteroids universally not recommended due to reports of SC atrophy (3)[C]

ADDITIONAL TREATMENT

General Measures

- Frequent ice applications after exercise
- Rest
- Knee immobilization in extension (severe cases)
- In more severe cases, avoidance of activities that increase pain or swelling
- Consider physical therapy referral for quadriceps isometric strengthening, hip extensions, adductor strengthening, and hamstring and quadriceps stretching exercises.
- Open- and closed-chain eccentric quadriceps strengthening
- Patients with marked pronation may benefit from orthotics.

Issues for Referral

When conservative therapy is unsuccessful, consideration of surgery warrants referral.

SURGERY/OTHER PROCEDURES

- Débridement of a thickened, cosmetically unsatisfactory tibial tubercle (rare) or removal of heterotopic bone
- Surgical excision of a painful tibial tubercle rarely needed (<5%) (3)[C]
- 75% return to normal sport activity and 89% are not restricted from competition due to recurrent pain (4)[B].

ONGOING CARE

FOLLOW-UP RECOMMENDATIONS

- Athletes may return to play if tolerated.
- Presence of pain does not preclude competition.

Patient Monitoring

With worsening of symptoms only

PATIENT EDUCATION

- Consider avoidance of jumping sports. Assure family that symptoms and findings will diminish with time and rest.
- Can play sports with mild pain
- Quad stretching and strengthening important

PROGNOSIS

Except in rare complicated cases, this is a self-limiting illness that resolves within 2 years of full skeletal maturation. However, up to 60% of adults with prior Osgood-Schlatter disease (OSD) still report occasional symptoms and have pain with kneeling. Most persons with OSD will have residual "knobby" tibial tubercles that never completely resolve. They may decline in size but will remain throughout life to some extent.

COMPLICATIONS

Rarely, the heavily fragmented and inflamed tibial ossicle will avulse and require surgery.

REFERENCES

1. Gholve PA, Scher DM, et al. Osgood Schlatter Syndrome. *Curr Opin Pediatr*. 2007;19(1):44–50.
2. Zaid AA, et al. The immature athlete. *Clin Sports Med*. 2002;21:3.
3. Bloom OJ, Mackler L. What is the best treatment for Osgood Schlatter disease? *J Fam Prac*. 2004;53(2):153–6.
4. Pihlamajaki HK, Visuri TI. Longterm outcome after surgical treatment of unresolved Osgood Schlatter Disease in young men: Surgical technique. *J Bone Joint Surg Am*. 2010;(Suppl 1) Pt 2:258–64.

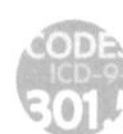

CODES

ICD9

732.4 Juvenile osteochondrosis of lower extremity, excluding foot

CLINICAL PEARLS

- Pain starting below the patella in an athlete during rapid growth spurt is OSD, patellar tendinosis, or Sindig-Larsen-Johansson syndrome.
- Only OSD hurts directly over the tibial tubercle.

OSTEITIS DEFORMANS (PAGET DISEASE OF BONE)

Bryan G. Beutel, MD

BASICS

DESCRIPTION

- Inflammatory focal disorder of hyperactive bone resorption followed by equally hyperactive and excessive bone formation (remodeling):
  - Stimulated by abnormal osteoclasts
- Results in enlarged, disorganized, weakened, and highly vascularized mosaic of bone
- Often painful, with easily deformed bone that is subject to fractures with minimal trauma
- Proclivity to affect axial skeleton and proximal long bones of lower extremities:
  - Less commonly affects the joints
- Cranial and vertebral involvement can also lead to neurologic deficits.
- Synonym(s): Paget's disease of bone

EPIDEMIOLOGY

- Predominant age: >50 years; occasionally seen in ages 20–50 years
- Predominant sex: Slightly more common in males than females (3:2)

Prevalence

- Prevalence generally increases with increasing age:
  - 2% among 55–59-year-old men, 20% among men >85 years of age
- More prevalent if ancestry is Caucasian, especially from United Kingdom, Northern Europe (excluding Scandinavia), Italy, Australia, and New Zealand:
  - 3% of Caucasians >50 years of age have at least 1 focus.
- Rare in African Americans and Asians
- Overall, prevalence is decreasing for unknown reasons.

Geriatric Considerations

Common

RISK FACTORS

- First-degree relative with osteitis deformans:
  - 15–30% of patients note a family history of osteitis deformans.
- Caucasian, European ethnicity
- See "Genetics" section.

Genetics

- Mutations in SQSTM1 gene, predominately ubiquitin-binding associated (UBA) domain and P392L, have been identified (1)[B]. Product of SQSTM1 affects osteoclast differentiation and activation.
- Recent data suggests an 18q locus is involved.

GENERAL PREVENTION

Avoid excessive mechanical stress on afflicted bones to reduce chance of fractures and other complications.

ETIOLOGY

Etiology generally unknown, although several theories have been proposed:

- Viral infection, especially paramyxovirus (controversial)
- Zoonotic infections
- Occupational exposure to toxins
- Childhood malnourishment resulting in vitamin D deficiency or low dietary calcium

COMMONLY ASSOCIATED CONDITIONS

- Hyperparathyroidism
- Gouty diathesis
- Secondary osteoarthritis
- Mottled retinal degeneration
- Peyronie disease
- Accelerated atherosclerosis
- Osteoporosis circumscripta
- Frontotemporal dementia (rare)
- Hereditary inclusion-body myopathy (rare)
- Bone sarcoma (rare)
- Angioid streaks (rare)

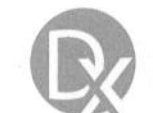

DIAGNOSIS

HISTORY

- Frequently asymptomatic (70–90% of patients); finding is often incidental
- Bone pain is most common complaint, notable at rest and night, likely stemming from periosteal distortion or hypervascularity.
- Secondary osteoarthritis
- Hearing loss (secondary to cranial nerve VIII compression)
- Headaches
- Head enlargement (e.g., patient may report an increase in hat size)
- Pathologic fractures
- Possible muscle weakness secondary to compression of nerve roots

PHYSICAL EXAM

- Neurologic examination for deficits:
  - Audiogram for sensorineural or conductive hearing loss (if skull involvement)
  - Visual field study for visual impairment (if skull involvement)
  - Peripheral neuropathies
- Skeletal deformities may be present, often asymmetric:
  - Skull involvement including enlarged maxilla or frontal bossing
  - Bowed leg
- Renal calculi (due to increased calcium, uric acid)
- Warmth and increased skin temperature over affected areas
- Carpal/tarsal tunnel syndromes may manifest as positive Tinel and Phalen tests
- Ophthalmic examination may reveal mottled retinal degeneration (rare).
- Cardiovascular effects resulting in valvular/endocardial calcification and high-output congestive heart failure (rare)

DIAGNOSTIC TESTS & INTERPRETATION

Lab

- Serum *calcium, phosphorus, parathyroid hormone* levels usually normal; rarely increased
- Serum *alkaline phosphatase* (total or bone-specific) typically elevated (95% of patients) (2)[B]
- Serum *gamma glutamyl transpeptidase* often normal
- Serum *osteocalcin* (binary ghost-pulse constraint) usually increased
- Urinary *pyridinoline collagen crosslinks* typically elevated
- Serum and urinary *N- and C-telopeptide* (collagen crosslinks) usually increased
- Drugs that may alter laboratory results:
  - Vitamin D and its metabolites
  - Hepatotoxic drugs
- Disorders that may alter lab results:
  - See "Differential Diagnosis."
  - Osteomalacia
  - Liver disorders
  - Traumatic fractures

Imaging

- X-rays may demonstrate various pagetic bone elements:
  - Resorptive fronts with osteolysis appear as radiolucencies.
  - "Framed vertebrae" (enlarged vertebral bodies, thickened cortices, vertical striations)
  - "Brim sign" (thickened iliopectineal line)
  - "Cotton wool" skull pattern
  - "Blade of grass" (V-shaped pattern demarcating pagetic from normal bone)
- Radionuclide bone scans more sensitive than radiographs:
  - Show intense uptake in focal pattern
- CT and MRI demonstrate extra-bony extension if sarcomatous degeneration occurs.

Diagnostic Procedures/Surgery

Bone biopsy needed only in confounding cases.

Pathological Findings

3 pathological phases have been identified:

- Lytic phase: Osteo*clasts* are large, contain 10–100 nuclei, and have abnormal configuration:
  - Electron photomicroscopy demonstrates that nuclei and cytoplasm contain myriad inclusion bodies resembling viral nucleocapsids.
  - Leads to increase in bone resorption
- Mixed phase: Excessive osteo*blastic* bone formation predominates from increase in number of osteoblasts; nonlinear collagen deposition results.
- Sclerotic phase: Sclerotic bone–containing cement lines forming a mosaic pattern (woven bone), infiltration of vasculature and fibrous connective tissue

DIFFERENTIAL DIAGNOSIS

- Osteoporosis
- Osteoarthritis
- Polyostotic fibrous dysplasia
- Primary bone neoplasms
- Osteitis fibrosis cystica (skeletal hyperparathyroidism)
- Osteolytic, osteoblastic metastases

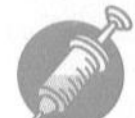

TREATMENT

MEDICATION

Medical treatment primarily implemented to relieve bone pain, as well as prevent progression of disease leading to skeletal deformities, neurologic issues, etc. (3)[B]. Bisphosphonates are the mainstay of medical treatment, as their structure mimics that of pyrophosphate and inhibits osteoclastic activity.

First Line

Add NSAIDs to the following drugs for secondary osteoarthritis. COX-2 inhibitors may be substituted:

- Synthetic injectable salmon calcitonin (Miacalcin): 50 IU SC/IM 3 times weekly to 100 IU SC/IM daily, courses 1.5–3 years; *or*
- Etidronate (Didronel), 5 mg/kg PO daily (~400 mg; taken on an empty stomach) for 6 months. Rarely, 20 mg/kg/d for 1 month. Courses may be repeated after a 3–6-month rest period; *or*
- Alendronate (Fosamax) 40 mg PO daily (taken on an empty stomach) for 6 months; *or*
- Risedronate (Actonel) 30 mg PO daily (taken on an empty stomach) for 2 months; *or*
- Pamidronate (Aredia) 60 mg/d by 4–6-hour infusions for 2–3 days. Alternately, 30 mg/d by 4–6-hour infusions once a week for 6 weeks. May be repeated several months later if effect wears off.
- Zoledronic acid (Reclast) 5-mg infusion over 15 minutes plus 1,500-mg elemental calcium (divided) and 1,000 IU vitamin D per day for minimal 2 weeks after infusion
- Contraindications:
  - History of allergy or hypersensitivity
  - For alendronate and risedronate, esophageal dysfunction, severe upper GI tract symptoms, gastroesophageal reflux disease, etc.
- Precautions:
  - Adverse side effects may require ameliorative measures or temporary dose reduction.
  - Salmon calcitonin: Nausea, vomiting, anorexia, flushing, rash, including urticaria (rare)
  - Etidronate disodium: Nausea, vomiting, diarrhea, increased bone pain
  - Alendronate and risedronate: Heartburn, epigastric pain, and musculoskeletal pain. Take on an empty stomach with copious water. No food, beverages, or other medications for 30–60 minutes. Remain upright for 1 hour.
  - Pamidronate disodium: Transient fever, leukopenia, hypocalcemia, headache, malaise, loss of appetite
- Significant possible interactions: None
- IV therapy has been shown to improve serum alkaline phosphatase levels more than oral administration of bisphosphonates (4)[B]. Studies have demonstrated, however, that intensive bisphosphonate treatment provides no significant difference in clinical manifestations of osteitis deformans when compared to symptomatic management (5)[B].

Second Line

NSAIDs or COX-2 inhibitors for mildly symptomatic disease in nonstrategic areas

ADDITIONAL TREATMENT

General Measures

- Rarely, splints for severely resorbed areas with high risk of fracture
- Shoe raises may be utilized to counteract limb shortening.
- Hearing aids for severe deafness: May be of some value in sensorineural deafness

COMPLEMENTARY AND ALTERNATIVE MEDICINE

Physiotherapy, hydrotherapy, or transcutaneous electrical nerve stimulation may be used to treat pain.

SURGERY/OTHER PROCEDURES

- Total joint replacement (hip, knee) may be indicated if joints affected: May restore mobility and ameliorate pain
- Osteotomy procedures for extreme deformity
- Decompression procedures (skull, spinal column) for acute neurologic deficits (rarely needed)
- Bone biopsy (rarely needed) to help confirm diagnosis if remains unclear
- Extirpative surgery for sarcomatous complications
- Open reduction and fixation of pathologic fractures

IN-PATIENT CONSIDERATIONS

- Osteitis deformans is generally treated on an outpatient basis, except when surgery or IV treatment is used.
- Bisphosphonates are indicated preoperatively to mitigate surgical blood loss and reduce risk of implant loosening in the setting of a total joint replacement (6)[B].

ONGOING CARE

FOLLOW-UP RECOMMENDATIONS

- Full activity to maintain function
- Avoid excessive mechanical stress on involved bones.

Patient Monitoring

- Follow-up visits every 2–4 months during drug therapy; yearly if drugs not being used:
  - Alkaline phosphatase level (total or bone-specific) before each visit
- Repeat x-rays and bone scan every 3–5 years or as needed.

DIET

Sufficient dietary intake of calcium and vitamin D is crucial, especially for those undergoing bisphosphonate treatment.

PATIENT EDUCATION

Paget Foundation, 120 Wall St., Suite 1602, New York, NY 10005; tel. (212) 509-5335; fax (212) 509-8492; www.paget.org

PROGNOSIS

- Depends on severity, often asymptomatic
- Slow progression if untreated
- Significant amelioration with treatment (≥85%)
- Poor prognosis if bone sarcoma develops (5-year survival of ~6%) (2)[B]

COMPLICATIONS

- Fractures
- Severe deformities
- Head enlargement
- Acetabular protrusion
- Neurologic deficits
- Deafness
- Visual impairment
- Nephrocalcinosis
- Peyronie syndrome
- Sarcomatous degeneration (<1% of cases)

REFERENCES

1. Seton M, et al. Paget's disease: Epidemiology and pathophysiology. *Curr Osteoporos Rep*. 2008;6: 125–9.
2. Ralston SH, Langston AL, Reid IR, et al. Pathogenesis and management of Paget's disease of bone. *Lancet*. 2008;372:155–63.
3. Rubin DJ, Levin RM. Neurologic complications of Paget disease of bone. *Endocr Pract*. 2009;15(2): 158–66.
4. Hosking D, et al. Pharmacological therapy of Paget's and other metabolic bone diseases. *Bone*. 2006;38:S3–7.
5. Langston AL, Campbell MK, Fraser WD, et al. Randomized trial of intensive bisphosphonate treatment versus symptomatic management in Paget's disease of bone. *J Bone Miner Res*. 2010;25:20–31.
6. Wegrzyn J, Pibarot V, Chapurlat R, et al. Cementless total hip arthroplasty in Paget's disease of bone: A retrospective review. *Int Orthop*. 2010; 34:1103–9.

ADDITIONAL READING

- Ankrom MA, Shapiro JR. Paget's disease of bone (osteitis deformans). *J Am Geriatr Soc*. 1998;46: 1025–33.
- Noor M, Shoback D. Paget's disease of bone: Diagnosis and treatment update. *Curr Rheumatol Rep*. 2000;2:67–73.
- Rothschild BM. Paget's disease of the elderly. *Compr Ther*. 2000;26:251–4.
- Siris ES. Paget's disease of bone. *J Bone Miner Res*. 1998;13:1061–5.
- Wallach S. Identifying and controlling Paget's disease. *J Musculoskel Med*. 1997;14:66–82.

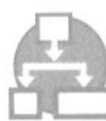

See Also (Topic, Algorithm, Electronic Media Element)

Arthritis, Osteo; Bone Tumor, Primary Malignant; Hyperparathyroidism

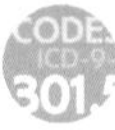

CODES

ICD9

- 731.0 Osteitis deformans without mention of bone tumor
- 731.1 Osteitis deformans in diseases classified elsewhere

CLINICAL PEARLS

- Most patients with osteitis deformans are asymptomatic.
- Bone pain is most common symptom.
- Radiographic signs of osteolysis and thickened cortices are seen in osteitis deformans.
- Bisphosphonates are the primary medical treatment.
- Follow-up for evidence of sarcomatous transformation.

OSTEOCHONDRITIS DISSECANS

John Spittler, MD, MS
Morteza Khodaee, MD, MPH

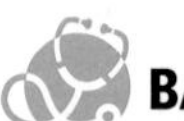

BASICS

DESCRIPTION

- Osteochondritis dissecans (OCD) is a lesion of the subchondral bone that may secondarily cause separation and instability of the overlying articular cartilage.
- The loose piece of bone and cartilage may migrate into joint, making the joint unstable or seeming to "lock up."
- Most common cause of intra-articular loose body in adolescents
- Knee is the most commonly affected joint; can occur in any diarthrodial joint, including, in decreasing order of frequency: Elbow (capitellum), ankle (talar dome or tibial plafond), tarsal navicular, hip (femoral capital epiphysis), shoulder (humeral head or glenoid), and wrist (scaphoid)
- System(s) affected: Musculoskeletal

EPIDEMIOLOGY

Incidence

- Unknown: Estimated 2–5/10,000 persons
- Predominant age: Young adults between 10 and 40 years of age
- Juvenile type (JOCD) in children and adolescents prior to physeal closure
- Predominant sex: Male > Female (5:3)

RISK FACTORS

- Trauma
- Being very active (children and adults)
- Participating in multiple sports, especially gymnastics and overhead sports
- Abnormal mechanical axis of the leg can be a risk factor (1)[C]:
  - Varus axis and medial condyle OCD
  - Valgus axis and lateral condyle OCD

Pediatric Considerations

Although still idiopathic, the mean age in JOCD is decreasing, and the prevalence in girls is increasing with changes in athletic participation by children (2)[C].

Genetics

No genetic pattern known, but bilateral lesions have been noted in up to 30% of patients.

GENERAL PREVENTION

There is no clear way to avoid the development of OCD.

PATHOPHYSIOLOGY

- Primary change happens in the bone and necrosis occurs in a focal area.
- Overlying cartilage changes are secondary to these bony changes.
- Loss of subchondral bone support leads to degenerative cartilage changes: Softening and fibromatous fissuring
- A fragment may detach and become a loose body within the affected joint.
- Cartilage itself is without a vascular supply, and healing occurs by vascular supply to underlying bone, which stimulates inflammation, repair, and remodeling.
- It is difficult to predict which lesions will go on to heal and remodel.

ETIOLOGY

- Controversial and unclear
- Theories include trauma or repetitive microtrauma, ischemia, familial predisposition, fragile blood supply of the physeal line, epiphyseal abnormalities, and endocrine imbalance (currently most credited theory is repetitive microtrauma with possible vascular insufficiency) (3)
- Most commonly affected joints are:
  - Knee: Overuse and with patellar dislocation and with injury to the anterior cruciate ligament; bilateral involvement noted in up to 30% of patients
  - Elbow: Overuse injury in overhead throwers and racket sports, as well as gymnasts
  - Ankle: Frequently associated with history of previous ankle sprain
- Relationship between adult and juvenile forms of OCD remains unclear

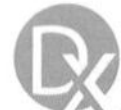

DIAGNOSIS

HISTORY

- Insidious (most common) or posttraumatic onset of pain, which improves with rest
- Pain usually described as a deep and vague ache
- Pain may be associated with clicking, swelling, locking (usually with a loose body), and stiffness.

PHYSICAL EXAM

- May be associated with secondary muscle atrophy, mild effusion, decreased range of motion (ROM), joint-line tenderness, or tenderness over the lesion
- The Wilson test may be positive (i.e., pain with knee extension and tibial internal rotation) in some patients with knee involvement.

DIAGNOSTIC TESTS & INTERPRETATION

Lab

Initial lab tests

No specific laboratory tests are helpful in the diagnosis of OCD.

Imaging

Initial approach

- The diagnosis is usually made by standard radiographs. Typical findings include small articular surface radiolucency or irregularity and bony fragmentation with partial or complete separation of the articular cartilage:
  - Knee: Anteroposterior (AP), lateral, sunrise, and tunnel views (most likely location for abnormality in the lateral portion of the medial condyle)
  - Elbow: Routine AP and lateral elbow series (common involvement of the humeral capitellum)
  - Ankle: AP, lateral, and mortise views (lesions most commonly involve the posteromedial or anterolateral talar dome)
- MRI can delineate the bony lesion, involvement of cartilage, and any fluid behind the fragment. It also allows for staging of the lesion:
  - Stage I: Thickening of the articular cartilage and low signal change (stable)
  - Stage II: Articular cartilage breached, low signal rim behind fragment indicating fibrous attachment (stable)
  - Stage III: Articular cartilage breached, high signal changes behind fragment and underlying subchondral bone (unstable)
  - Stage IV: Loose body (unstable)
- CT scan provides architectural description of the bony lesion; however, it provides less information than MRI.
- Bone scan may be useful in evaluation of healing potential, but this is controversial at present.

DIFFERENTIAL DIAGNOSIS

- In the knee:
  - Meniscal tear
  - Patellofemoral pain syndrome
- Stress fracture
- Tendinopathy
- Avascular necrosis
- Acute fracture
- Neoplasm

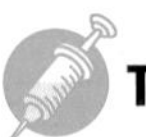

TREATMENT

MEDICATION

Acetaminophen, NSAIDs, or other pain medications for symptomatic relief

ADDITIONAL TREATMENT

General Measures

- Goals of treatment:
  - Maintain smooth, congruous joint surface.
  - Alleviate pain.
  - Prevent degenerative joint disease.
  - Promote revascularization of necrotic fragment and regeneration of affected cartilage.
- There are no randomized, controlled trials, but in JOCD initial nonsurgical treatment is the standard of care.
- Treatment options include periods of immobilization, activity modification, and non–weight-bearing. Type and duration of immobilization remain controversial.
- If non–weight-bearing immobilization is used, add intermittent maintenance of ROM.
- Physical therapy can often be helpful to establish an exercise plan.
- Follow closely for 12 weeks to ensure healing.
- Casting is often used for 6-week intervals, especially with JOCD, due to issues of compliance in this age group.

Issues for Referral

- Patients in whom surgery may be considered as an early treatment option (loose fragments, adults, or lesions >1 cm)
- Unstable lesions on MRI, including presence of an intra-articular loose body
- Failure of conservative, symptomatic treatment

SURGERY/OTHER PROCEDURES

- Surgical treatment is used when:
  - Conservative measures have failed
  - Physeal closure has occurred, which carries a worse prognosis for healing (adult form)
  - Unstable lesions are visualized on MRI, including presence of an intra-articular loose body
  - Lesion are large (>1 cm)
- Arthroscopic surgery is the preferred method. In addition, arthroscopy is a valuable tool to evaluate the stability of the lesion and visualize the overlying cartilage.
- Surgical treatment includes fragment excision, microfracture technique (drilling) to increase blood supply, screw fixation of the loose fragment, allograft insertion, autologous chondrocyte implantation. Fragment excision has fallen out of favor due to poor long-term results (3)[B],(4)[B].

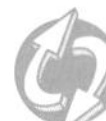

ONGOING CARE

FOLLOW-UP RECOMMENDATIONS

- Outpatient care usually utilized
- Inpatient treatment usually not indicated, unless postoperative

Patient Monitoring

- Initially should be followed every 6 weeks with serial radiographs to evaluate healing and monitor for possible displacement
- Healing is expected within 4–6 months.
- In JOCD, radiographs at 1 year may show no residual abnormality.
- If postoperative and remains symptomatic, the patient may be followed with MRI or SPECT/CT to evaluate healing (5)[C].

DIET

Vitamin D supplementation

PATIENT EDUCATION

The critical importance of compliance with the treatment plan should be stressed.

PROGNOSIS

- Factors associated with good prognosis:
  - Younger age
  - Open growth plate
  - Smaller lesions (<160 mm^2)
  - Stable lesions
  - Non–weight-bearing location of the lesion
- The absence of a sclerotic rim on x-rays at the time diagnosis can be an indication for conservative treatment for OCD of the knee, due to the resultant high probability for spontaneous recovery (6)[C].
- An incongruous joint surface may lead to degenerative changes in the future.
- Clinical improvement may proceed radiologic healing.

COMPLICATIONS

- Failure to revascularize and heal
- Displacement of a fragment becoming a loose body within a joint
- Predisposition for early osteoarthritis in the affected joint

REFERENCES

1. Jacobi M, Wahl P, Bouaicha S, et al. Association between mechanical axis of the leg and osteochondritis dissecans of the knee: Radiographic study on 103 knees. *Am J Sports Med*. 2010;38(7):1425–28.
2. Kocher MS, Tucker R, Ganley TJ, et al. Management of osteochondritis dissecans of the knee: Current concepts review. *Am J Sports Med*. 2006;34:1181–91.
3. Pape D, Filardo G, Kon E, et al. Disease-specific clinical problems associated with the subchondral bone. *Knee Surg Sports Traumatol Arthrosc*. 2010;18:448–62.
4. Vasiliadis HS, Danielson B, Ljungberg M, et al. Autologous chondrocyte implantation in cartilage lesions of the knee: Long-term evaluation with magnetic resonance imaging and delayed gadolinium-enhanced magnetic resonance imaging technique. *Am J Sports Med*. 2010;38:943–9.
5. Konala P, Iranpour F, Kerner A, et al. Clinical benefit of SPECT/CT for follow-up of surgical treatment of osteochondritis dissecans. *Ann Nuc Med*. 2010;24:621–4.
6. Ramirez A, Abril JC, Chaparro M, et al. Juvenile osteochondritis dissecans of the knee: Perifocal sclerotic rim as a prognostic factor of healing. *J Pediatr Orthop*. 2010;30:180–5.

ADDITIONAL READING

- Bruce EJ, Hamby T, Jones DG, et al. Sports-related osteochondral injuries: Clinical presentation, diagnosis, and treatment. *Prim Care*. 2005;32:253–76.
- Cahill BR, Ahten SM, et al. The three critical components in the conservative treatment of juvenile osteochondritis dissecans (JOCD). Physician, parent, and child. *Clin Sports Med*. 2001;20:287–98, vi.
- Crawford DC, Safran MR, et al. Osteochondritis dissecans of the knee. *J Am Acad Orthop Surg*. 2006;14:90–100.
- Wall EJ, Vourazeris J, Myer GD, et al. The healing potential of stable juvenile osteochondritis dissecans knee lesions. *J Bone Joint Surg Am*. 2008;90:2655–64.

CODES

ICD9

732.7 Osteochondritis dissecans

CLINICAL PEARLS

- OCD is a lesion of the subchondral bone that may secondarily cause separation and instability of the overlying articular cartilage; may sometimes become loose in joint, causing it to "lock up"; knee most commonly affected.
- Many lesions heal without surgical intervention with adherence to a conservative management plan.
- Compliance with immobilization and possibility of further trauma should be emphasized, especially with younger athletes.
- Frequent follow-up every 6 weeks is important to ensure healing.
- Patients in whom surgery may be considered as an early treatment option (loose fragments, adults, or lesions >1 cm)

OSTEOMALACIA AND RICKETS

Elizabeth Ann Nelson, MD
Lauren Ferrara, MD

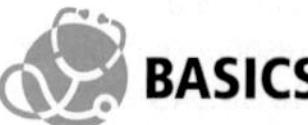

BASICS

DESCRIPTION

- A metabolic bone disorder due to decreased bone mineralization (calcification) and increased organic bone matrix that results in decreased bone density
- Referred to as *renal osteodystrophy* when secondary to renal disease
- System(s) affected: Musculoskeletal

EPIDEMIOLOGY

- Children: Median age of presentation is 15 months.
- Adults: Elderly

Incidence

In the US, occurs almost exclusively in breast-fed infants without vitamin D supplementation or sun exposure

RISK FACTORS

- Children:
  - Nutritional rickets:
    - Breast-feeding as a sole source of nutrition without vitamin D supplementation
    - Dark skin
    - Limited exposure to sunlight
    - Vegetarian diet without vitamin supplementation
    - Malabsorption syndromes
  - Prematurity
  - Maternal vitamin D deficiency
- Adults:
  - Poor diet
  - Poverty
  - Food faddism
  - Anorexia nervosa
  - Renal failure
  - Gastrectomy

Genetics

Rare causes of rickets in children include:

- Vitamin D–dependent rickets: An autosomal-recessive disorder caused by deficiency of renal 25-hydroxyvitamin D3 1-alpha-hydroxylase or altered calcitriol receptors
- Vitamin D–resistant rickets: An X-linked dominant or autosomal disorder caused by decreased proximal renal tubular reabsorption of phosphorus

GENERAL PREVENTION

- Adequate vitamin D intake: Encourage foods such as fatty fish, cod liver oil, egg yolks, and fortified foods:
  - Adults: Vitamin D, 400–800 U/d
- American Academy of Pediatrics recommends a minimum vitamin D intake of 400 U/d starting within the first few days of life (1):
  - Infants who consume >1 L/d of vitamin D–fortified formula or whole milk will receive the recommended vitamin D intake.
  - Supplementation is recommended for breast-fed infants and children consuming <1 L/d of vitamin D–fortified formula or milk.
- Sunlight exposure: 10–15 minutes on face, hands, and arms 2–3 days per week
- Adequate calcium intake: Encourage high-calcium foods or supplements.

PATHOPHYSIOLOGY

- Children: Defective mineralization of cartilage in the epiphyseal growth plates:
  - Failure of growing bone to mineralize due to inadequate substrate (low calcium or phosphate) or interference with mineralization (such as vitamin D deficiency or toxic exposure)
  - Lack of calcified osteoid and accumulation of unossified cartilage
- Adults: Disorder of mineralization of newly formed bone matrix

ETIOLOGY

- Hypophosphatemia from secondary hyperparathyroidism, due to vitamin D deficiency is the primary cause in adults
- Vitamin D metabolism abnormalities, including hepatic or renal disease
- Resistance to vitamin D
- Inadequate dietary calcium
- Impaired intestinal absorption of calcium or phosphorus due to celiac disease, cystic fibrosis, or postgastrectomy
- Inadequate dietary phosphorus
- Impaired renal phosphate absorption associated with proximal or distal renal tubular defects
- Causes that inhibit mineralization of the growth plate and osteoid:
  - Alkaline phosphatase deficiency
  - Aluminum toxicity
  - Fluoride toxicity
  - Primary hyperparathyroidism
- Drugs that may affect absorption or metabolism of calcium, phosphorus, or vitamin D:
  - Antacids
  - Antiepileptic drugs
  - Corticosteroids
  - Loop diuretics
- Drugs that inhibit mineralization: Bisphosphonates
- Oncogenic osteomalacia

COMMONLY ASSOCIATED CONDITIONS

- Children with vitamin D–deficiency rickets:
  - Secondary hyperparathyroidism
  - Dilated cardiomyopathy
  - Marrow fibrosis with pancytopenia or microcytic hypochromic anemia
  - Dysregulation of immune function and cellular differentiation and proliferation
- Adults with osteomalacia:
  - Chronic renal disease
  - Gastrectomy
  - Epilepsy
  - Malnutrition

DIAGNOSIS

HISTORY

- Common presentations in children:
  - Muscle weakness: May not be able to stand until age 3
  - Bowed legs
  - Diffuse limb pain
  - Hypocalcemic seizures
  - Carpopedal spasms
  - Signs and symptoms of hypocalcemia:
    - Muscle cramps
    - Numbness
    - Paresthesias
    - Tetany
    - Seizures
    - Diarrhea
- Common presentations in adults:
  - Dull, bony pain and tenderness typically in lower spine and pelvis that is aggravated by activity and weight bearing
  - Muscle weakness, especially the proximal lower extremity
  - Fractures may occur with little or no trauma

PHYSICAL EXAM

Perform a complete physical and dental examination in children:

- General:
  - Palpate entire skeletal system to search for tenderness and bony abnormalities.
  - Evaluate for growth abnormalities such as decreased height and spinal deformity.
- Head, ears, eyes, nose, and throat (HEENT):
  - Craniotabes (thinning and softening of occipital and parietal bones)
  - Late closing of fontanelles
  - Fontal bossing of skull
  - Tooth abnormalities
- Chest:
  - Rachitic rosary (enlarged costochondral joints felt lateral to nipple line)
  - Harrison groove (flaring of ribs at diaphragm level)
  - Pigeon breast (protrusion of the sternum)
- Back:
  - Lordosis/kyphosis
  - Scoliosis
- Extremities:
  - Bowing or widening of the physis
  - Genu valgum (leg bowing)
  - Flaring of the wrists
  - Fraying and cupping of metaphysis
  - Genu varum (knock knees)
- Neurologic:
  - Gait disturbances in an ambulatory child
  - Signs of hypocalcemia:
    - Hyperreflexia
    - Neuromuscular instability: Chvostek sign (tap cranial nerve VII), Trousseau sign (carpopedal spasm 2–3 minutes after BP cuff is inflated proximally)
    - Tetany, myopathy, seizures, spasm, muscle weakness
- In adults:
  - Proximal muscle weakness, possible muscle wasting, hypotonia, and discomfort with movement
  - Waddling gait
  - Bone pain and tenderness to palpation: Most pronounced in the lower spine, pelvis, and lower extremities

DIAGNOSTIC TESTS & INTERPRETATION

Lab

- In children with vitamin D–deficiency rickets (1):
  - Serum phosphorus: Decreased
  - Serum calcidiol (25-hydroxy vitamin D3): Decreased
    - Indicative of overall vitamin D status
  - Urinary calcium: Decreased
- In adults with vitamin D–deficiency osteomalacia (2):
  - Serum phosphorus: Decreased
  - Plasma calcium: Decreased/normal
  - Serum calcidiol: Decreased
  - Alkaline phosphatase: Increased
- In adults with phosphate-wasting osteomalacia (2):
  - Serum phosphorous: Decreased
  - Phosphate clearance: Increased
  - Serum calcium: Normal
  - Alkaline phosphatase: Normal

Initial lab tests

- Blood tests:
  - Serum calcium (total and ionized), phosphate, BUN, creatinine, electrolytes
  - Serum calcidiol
  - Alkaline phosphatase
  - Parathyroid hormone
- Urinalysis:
  - Calcium, phosphate, creatinine in spot urine sample
  - pH, protein, and glucose

Imaging

Initial approach

- Anteroposterior radiograph of rapidly growing skeletal areas including knees, wrists, and anterior rib ends
- Children: Radiographic changes in rapidly growing skeletal areas (knee, wrist), including widening of the distal epiphysis, fraying and widening of the metaphysis, and angular deformities of the arm and leg bones (1)
- Adults (3):
  - Most common: Reduced bone density with thinning of the cortex
  - Changes in vertebral bodies: Loss of radiologic distinctness and concavity of the vertebral body
  - Characteristic finding: Looser zones:
    - Pseudofractures, fissures, or narrow radiolucent lines, 2–5 mm in width with sclerotic borders
    - Usually located at the femoral neck, on the medial part of the femoral shaft, immediately under the lesser trochanter, or a few centimeters beneath the pubic and ischial rami

Diagnostic Procedures/Surgery

The most accurate diagnosis is made by bone biopsy using double tetracycline labeling. Tetracyclines are deposited as a band at the mineralization front and, because they are fluorescent, they are easily visualized under a fluorescence microscope. After 2 courses of the antibiotic, separated by a period of days, the growth rate of the skeleton can be estimated in iliac crest biopsies by measuring the distance between the bands of deposited tetracycline. In normal adults, this distance is ~1 micron/d:

- 2 changes occur in osteomalacia:
  - Distance between tetracycline bands is reduced
  - Unmineralized matrix appears as a widened osteoid seam (>15 microns), and the osteoid volume is >10%.
- Both features are necessary for the diagnosis because other disorders may show one of these findings (2).
- Bone biopsy is not usually done in adults because the diagnosis can be made from the history, physical examination, and a combination of laboratory and radiologic studies.

Pathological Findings

- Children (1):
  - Widening of distal physis
  - Fraying and widening of the metaphysis
  - Angular deformities of arm and leg bones

DIFFERENTIAL DIAGNOSIS

- Children:
  - Liver disease
  - Anticonvulsant drugs
  - Failure to thrive
  - Developmental delay
  - Orthopedic abnormalities
  - Congenital syphilis
  - Osteogenesis imperfecta
  - Child abuse
  - Alkaline phosphatase deficiency
  - Aluminum toxicity
  - Fluoride toxicity
  - Primary hyperparathyroidism (rare)
- Adults:
  - Osteoporosis
  - Hyperparathyroidism
  - Metastatic bone disease
  - Lymphoma or myeloma
  - Fibromyalgia

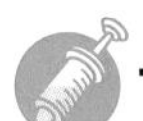

TREATMENT

A combination of calcium and vitamin D is recommended:

- A study in Nigerian children with nutritional rickets showed that treatment with calcium and vitamin D combined compared with treatment with vitamin D alone is more likely to produce radiographic evidence of nearly complete healing of rickets (58% vs. 19%) (4).

MEDICATION

First Line

- Children with vitamin D–deficiency rickets:
  - Ergocalciferol (calciferol) 150,000- or 300,000-U single dose:
    - Can be administered IM or PO in liquid or capsule form
    - Capsules can be softened in water and mixed with food
  - Calcium 1,000 mg/d PO
- Adults with vitamin D–deficiency osteomalacia:
  - Ergocalciferol (Calciferol) 50,000 U once or twice per week for 6–12 months
  - Followed by ergocalciferol 400 U/d
  - If the deficiency is due to malabsorption:
    - Ergocalciferol 10,000–50,000 U/d
    - Calcidiol 0.05–0.125 mg/d
  - Calcium 1,000 mg/d PO:
    - If the patient has malabsorption, 4 g of calcium per day

ADDITIONAL TREATMENT

Calcium and phosphorus supplementation if serum levels are low

SURGERY/OTHER PROCEDURES

Surgery may be necessary to repair severe bone abnormalities.

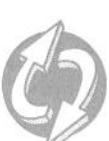

ONGOING CARE

FOLLOW-UP RECOMMENDATIONS

- For children, monitor:
  - Serum calcium, phosphorus, alkaline phosphatase, calcidiol:
    - Serum phosphorus should increase during the first week of treatment, followed by an increase in serum calcium.
  - Urinary calcium and phosphorus levels, spot urine calcium
- For adults taking calcium supplements, monitor:
  - Plasma concentration and urinary levels of calcium

PROGNOSIS

- Varies depending on the etiology
- Vitamin D deficiency causes of rickets:
  - Radiographic findings will normalize within 1 week of treatment.
  - Reversible physical findings will normalize within 6 months of treatment.

COMPLICATIONS

- Fractures: Typically involve the ribs, vertebrae, and long bones
- Osteomyelitis
- Renal failure
- Renal tubular acidosis
- Hypocalcemic seizures or muscle spasms
- Growth deformity and bowing of the long bones in children

REFERENCES

1. Wagner CL, Greer FR, American Academy of Pediatrics Section on Breastfeeding, et al. Prevention of rickets and vitamin D deficiency in infants, children, and adolescents. *Pediatrics*. 2008;122:1142–52.
2. Bingham CT, Fitzpatrick LA. Noninvasive testing in the diagnosis of osteomalacia. *Am J Med*. 1993;95:519.
3. Frame B, Parfitt AM. Osteomalacia: Current concepts. *Ann Intern Med*. 1978;89:966.
4. Thacher TD, Fischer PR, Pettifor JM, et al. A comparison of calcium, vitamin D or both for nutritional rickets in Nigerian children. *N Engl J Med*. 1999;341(8):563.

CODES

ICD9

- 268.0 Rickets, active
- 268.2 Osteomalacia, unspecified
- 268.9 Unspecified vitamin D deficiency

CLINICAL PEARLS

In the US, occurs almost exclusively in breast-fed infants without vitamin D supplementation or sun exposure. Ensure adequate vitamin D supplementation.

O

OSTEOMYELITIS

Colleen M. Prinzivalli, PharmD, BCPS
Michael C. Barros, PharmD, BCPS
J. Michael O'Connell, Jr., MD

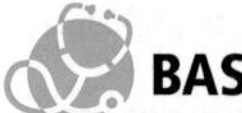

BASICS

DESCRIPTION

- An acute or chronic inflammation of the bone. Osteomyelitis can occur as a result of hematogenous seeding, contiguous spread of infection, or direct inoculation into intact bone (trauma or surgery).
- 2 major classification systems for osteomyelitis (1):
  - Waldvogel classification:
    - Classified according to the duration of the disease (acute or chronic), the mechanism of infection (hematogenous or contiguous), and the presence of vascular insufficiency
  - Cierny-Mader classification:
    - Based on the portion of bone affected, the physiologic status of the host, and other risk factors
- Special situations:
  - Vertebral osteomyelitis (2,3):
    - Acute, subacute, or chronic
    - May result from hematogenous seeding, direct inoculation, or contiguous spread
    - Back pain (most common initial symptom)
    - Lumbar spine (most commonly involved) followed by thoracic spine
    - Bone biopsy (open technique) has 93% pathogen recovery.
  - Infections of prosthetic joints:
    - Obtaining specific diagnosis and targeted therapy quicker (easy access)
    - X-ray of joint initially done, then 3-phase bone scan, since MRI/CT scans of limited use in this circumstance
    - Treat with combination of antibiotics, including rifampin, especially in prosthetic joint infections.
  - Posttraumatic infections:
    - Depends on type of fracture, level of contamination, and severity of tissue injury
    - Tibia most commonly involved
- System(s) affected: Musculoskeletal

EPIDEMIOLOGY

- Predominant age: Commonly seen in older adults
- Predominant sex: Male > Female
- Hematogenous osteomyelitis:
  - Adults (most patients >50 years old): Vertebral
  - Children: Long bones
- Contiguous osteomyelitis:
  - Predominantly found in patients with diabetes mellitus or vascular insufficiency

Incidence

- Incidence is low due to high resistance of normal bone to infection and occur in patients with risk factor.
- 25% lifetime risk of diabetics of developing foot complication

Prevalence

Up to 66% of diabetics with foot ulcers (1)

RISK FACTORS

- Diabetes mellitus
- Recent trauma/surgery
- Foreign body (e.g., prosthetic implant)
- Neuropathy and vascular insufficiency
- Immunosuppression
- Sickle-cell disease
- Injection drug use
- Previous osteomyelitis

GENERAL PREVENTION

- Antibiotic prophylaxis:
  - Clean bone surgery:
    - Antibiotics should be administered IV from 30 minutes before skin incision to no longer than 24 hours after the operation.
  - Closed fractures:
    - Antistaphylococcal penicillins or first- or second-generation cephalosporins
  - Open fractures:
    - In patients who can receive antibiotics within 6 hours of injury and who receive prompt operative treatment, give antistaphylococcal penicillins or first- or second-generation cephalosporins for 24 hours.
- All patients with diabetes mellitus should have a complete foot examination by a health care professional yearly (1).

PATHOPHYSIOLOGY

- Infection is caused by biofilm bacteria, which protects bacteria from antimicrobial agents and host immune responses (3).
- Acute: Suppurative infection of bone with edema and vascular compromise leading to sequestra
- Chronic: Presence of necrotic bone or sequestra or recurrence of previous infection

ETIOLOGY

- Hematogenous osteomyelitis (commonly a monomicrobial infection) (1):
  - *S. aureus* (most common) with high percentage of MRSA (50%) (3)
  - Coagulase-negative staphylococci and aerobic gram-negative bacteria
  - *Salmonella* sp. (sickle-cell patients)
  - *M. tuberculosis* and fungi (rare) in endemic areas or in immunocompromised hosts
- Contiguous focus osteomyelitis (commonly a polymicrobial infection):
  - Diabetes or vascular insufficiency:
    - Coagulase-positive and -negative staphylococci
    - Streptococci, gram-negative bacilli, anaerobes (*Peptostreptococcus* sp.)
  - Prosthetic device:
    - Coagulase-negative staphylococci and *S. aureus*

COMMONLY ASSOCIATED CONDITIONS

See "Risk Factors."

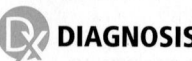

DIAGNOSIS

HISTORY

- Hematogenous osteomyelitis:
  - Conditions predisposing to bacteremia (diabetes, renal insufficiency, invasive procedures and IV drug use) (3)
  - Other sites of infection
- Contiguous osteomyelitis and vascular insufficiency–associated infection:
  - Recent trauma/surgery within 1–2 months
  - Presence of prosthetic device
  - History of diabetes
- Chronic osteomyelitis:
  - History of acute osteomyelitis

PHYSICAL EXAM

- Restriction of movement of the involved extremity or refusal to bear weight
- Pain or tenderness in the infected area
- Signs of localized inflammation
- Fever and/or chills
- Motor and sensory deficits (vertebral infection)
- Visible or palpable bone with a metal probe ("positive probe-to-bone test")
- Ulcer >2 cm wide and >3 mm deep increases likelihood in diabetic foot ulcers (1)[B].
- In patients with diabetes, classic signs and symptoms of infection may be masked due to vascular disease and neuropathy.

DIAGNOSTIC TESTS & INTERPRETATION

Lab

Initial lab tests

Labs (1)[C]:

- WBC is not a reliable indicator and can be normal even when infection is present (3).
- CRP is usually elevated but nonspecific.
- ESR is high in most cases:
  - ESR >70 mm/hr increases likelihood in diabetic lower extremity ulcer (4)[B].
- Drugs that may alter lab results: Antimicrobial agents given prior to culture
- Disorders that may alter lab results: Immunosuppression, chronic inflammatory disease, other/adjacent sites of infection

Follow-Up & Special Considerations

- A persistently elevated CRP but not ESR at 4–6 weeks can be associated with persistent osteomyelitis (1)[C].
- Patients receiving prolonged antimicrobial therapy should have the following tests to monitor for adverse reactions (1)[C]:
  - Weekly CBC
  - Liver and kidney function tests

Imaging

Initial approach

- Routine radiography standard first-line imaging (5)[C]: Classic triad for osteomyelitis is demineralization, periosteal reaction, and bone destruction:
  - Bone destruction is not apparent on plain films until after 10–21 days of infection.
  - Bone must undergo 30–50% destruction before it is evident on films.
- MRI:
  - For visualization of septic arthritis, spinal infection, and diabetic foot infections (5)[C]
  - T1-weighted image: Low signal intensity
  - T2-weighted image: High signal intensity
  - MI with gadolinium sensitivity and specificity range from 60–100% and 50–90%, respectively (3)[C]

- CT:
  - Better than standard radiography in fragments and sequestration, but inferior to MRI in soft tissue and bone marrow assessment
  - Useful to define surrounding soft tissues and identification of sequestra
  - Bone scan would typically be first test after plain x-ray in setting of joint prosthesis.

Follow-Up & Special Considerations

- Radionuclide scanning (e.g., technetium, indium, or gallium) is useful when diagnosis is ambiguous or extent of disease is in question, but is limited by reports of low sensitivity and specificity.
- MRI is not helpful in assessing the response to therapy due to persistence of bony edema (1)[C].

Diagnostic Procedures/Surgery

- Cultures:
  - Definitive diagnosis is made by blood culture (hematogenous) and by needle aspiration/bone biopsy with subsequent demonstration of the microorganism by culture and sensitivity or histology.
  - Appropriate pathogen isolated in blood culture combined with radiographic evidence may obviate need for bone culture.
  - Wound swabs and sinus tract cultures have utility for infection control and correlate well with the presence of *S. aureus* in deep cultures.
- Image-guided bone biopsy for vertebral osteomyelitis unless (+) blood culture and (+) radiographic evidence

Pathological Findings

Inflammatory process of bone with pyogenic bacteria, necrosis

DIFFERENTIAL DIAGNOSIS

- Systemic infection from other source
- Aseptic bone infarction
- Localized inflammation or infection of overlying skin and soft tissues (e.g., gout)
- Brodie abscess
- Neuropathic joint disease (Charcot foot)
- Fractures/trauma
- Tumor

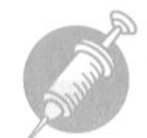

TREATMENT

MEDICATION

- Duration of therapy 4–6 weeks for acute osteomyelitis and generally >8 weeks for chronic osteomyelitis
- Determine therapy based on culture results.
- Fluoroquinolones may be used as an alternative to β-lactam antibiotics (use with caution to limit antibiotic resistance).
- Antibiotic dosing dependent upon creatinine clearance (utilizing Cockcroft-Gault equation)

First Line

- *Staphylococcus aureus* or coagulase-negative staphylococci (1)[C]:
  - Methicillin-sensitive (MSSA):
    - β-lactam at high dose (nafcillin or oxacillin 2 g IV q6h) or cefazolin 1–2 g IV q8h (2)
  - Methicillin-resistant (MRSA) (6):
    - Vancomycin 15 mg/kg IV q8–12h with target trough of 15–20 mcg/mL
- *Streptococcus* sp. (2,7):
  - Penicillin G 4 million units q4–6h
- *Enterobacter* sp. (2,7):
  - Fluoroquinolone (levofloxacin 750 mg IV/PO q24h) or ceftriaxone 2 g IV q24h
- *Pseudomonas aeruginosa* (2,7):
  - Cefepime or ceftazidime 2 g IV q8h (consider adding aminoglycoside)
- Anaerobes (2):
  - Clindamycin 600 mg IV q6–8h

Second Line

- *S. aureus* (1)[C],(2,7):
  - MSSA: Fluoroquinolone plus rifampin (levofloxacin 750 mg IV/PO q24h plus rifampin 300 mg PO q12h)
  - MRSA: Linezolid 600 mg PO/IV q12h or daptomycin 6 mg/kg IV q24h
- *Streptococcus* sp. (2,7):
  - Ceftriaxone 2 g IV q24h or cefazolin 1–2 g IV q8h
- *Enterobacter* sp. (quinolone-resistant, including extended-spectrum β-lactamase–producing *E. coli*) (2,7):
  - Carbapenem (imipenem/cilastatin 500 mg IV q6h)
- *Pseudomonas aeruginosa* (2,7):
  - Piperacillin/tazobactam 4.5 g IV q6h
- Anaerobes (2,7):
  - Metronidazole 500 mg IV/PO q6–8h

ADDITIONAL TREATMENT

General Measures

- Adequate nutrition
- Smoking-cessation counseling
- Control of diabetes

Additional Therapies

- Hyperbaric oxygen therapy may be useful as an adjunctive treatment, but data are limited.
- Negative pressure wound therapy is also a possible adjunctive treatment.

SURGERY/OTHER PROCEDURES

Surgical drainage, dead-space management, adequate soft tissue coverage, restoration of blood supply, and removal of necrotic tissues are of utmost importance to effect cure.

Pediatric Considerations

Medullary osteomyelitis (stage 1) in children may be treated without surgical intervention.

IN-PATIENT CONSIDERATIONS

Initial Stabilization

Correct electrolyte imbalances, hyperglycemia, azotemia, and acidosis; control pain

Nursing

Bed rest and immobilization of the involved bone and/or joint

Discharge Criteria

Clinical and laboratory evidence of resolving infection and appropriate outpatient therapy

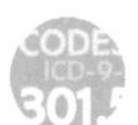

ONGOING CARE

FOLLOW-UP RECOMMENDATIONS

Patient Monitoring

Blood levels of antimicrobial agents, ESR, CRP, and repeat plain radiography

PATIENT EDUCATION

Diabetic glycemic control and foot care

PROGNOSIS

- Superficial and medullary osteomyelitis treated with antimicrobial and surgical therapy have a response rate of 90–100%.
- Morbidity and mortality are contingent on the underlying health of the host.
- Up to 36% recurrence in diabetics
- Increased mortality after amputation

COMPLICATIONS

- Abscess formation
- Bacteremia
- Fracture/nonunion
- Loosening of prosthetic implant
- Postoperative infection
- Sinus tract formation can be associated with neoplasms, especially in presence of long-standing infection

REFERENCES

1. Sia IG, Berbari EF. Osteomyelitis. *Best Prac Res Clin Rheum*. 2006;20(6):1065–81.
2. Zimmerli, Werner. Vertebral osteomyelitis. *N Engl J Med*. 2010;362:1022–9.
3. Bhavan KP, Marschall J, Olsen MA, et al. The epidemiology of hematogenous vertebral osteomyelitis: A cohort study in a tertiary care hospital. *BMC Infect Dis*. 2010;10:158.
4. Dinh MT, et al. Diagnostic accuracy of the physical examination and imaging tests for osteomyelitis underlying diabetic foot ulcers: Meta analysis. *Clin Inf Dis*. 2008;47:519–27.
5. Stumpe KD, Strobel K, et al. Osteomyelitis and arthritis. *Semin Nucl Med*. 2009;39:27–35.
6. Malloy KM, Davis GA. Summary of ASHP/IDSA/SIDP vancomycin monitoring recommendations: A focus on osteomyelitis. *Orthopedics*. 2009;32:499.
7. Lew D, Waldvogel. Osteomyelitis. *Lancet*. 2004; 364:369–79.

CODES

ICD9

- 730.00 Acute osteomyelitis, site unspecified
- 730.10 Chronic osteomyelitis, site unspecified
- 730.20 Unspecified osteomyelitis, site unspecified

CLINICAL PEARLS

- Hematogenous osteomyelitis is usually monomicrobial, whereas osteomyelitis due to contiguous spread or direct inoculation is usually polymicrobial.
- *S. aureus*, coagulase-negative staphylococci, and aerobic gram-negative bacilli are the most common organisms.
- Acute osteomyelitis typically presents with gradual onset of pain. Local findings (e.g., tenderness, warmth, erythema, and swelling) and systemic symptoms (e.g., fever and chills) also may be present.
- Treatment of osteomyelitis often requires both surgical débridement and antimicrobial therapy. At least 6 weeks of antimicrobial therapy is recommended.

OSTEONECROSIS

Joselyn Jedick, DO

BASICS

Definition: Cellular death ("necrosis") of the elements of bone ("osteo") due to interruption of the blood supply to that bone. Classified as traumatic (most common) vs. nontraumatic.

DESCRIPTION

- Primarily involves the epiphysis of long bones (most commonly femoral head, humeral head, and the femoral condyles) but small bones in the hand, foot, ankle, and face are also affected
- System(s) affected: Musculoskeletal
- Synonym(s): Idiopathic osteonecrosis; Avascular necrosis (AVN); Lunatomalacia/Kienböck disease (involving lunate); Subchondral fracture; Aseptic necrosis; Legg-Calve-Perthes syndrome (children with idiopathic necrosis of the femoral head)

EPIDEMIOLOGY

- Predominant age: Third–fifth decade
- Predominant sex: Male > Female ratio 4–8:1

Incidence

- There are 10,000–20,000 new cases reported in the US per year.
- Disease is bilateral in at least 50% of all nontraumatic cases and in 75–95% of cases associated with steroid use (1).

Prevalence

- Hip: Occurs in ~10% of undisplaced femoral neck fractures, 15–30% of displaced femoral neck fractures, and 10% of hip dislocations
- Jaw: Occurs in 3–12% of oncology patients taking high-dose IV bisphosphonates at 36 months of exposure and in <1% of nononcology patients with osteoporosis (2)
- Special population: Occurs in 21–25% of patients during early postoperative period following renal transplant

RISK FACTORS

- Top 3: Trauma, prolonged corticosteroid use, alcoholism
- Others: Bisphosphonate use, sickle cell disease, diabetes mellitus, type II or IV hyperlipemia, oral contraceptives, pregnancy, decompression sickness (aka "bends," "caisson disease," "divers disease"), chronic pancreatitis, Crohn disease, myeloproliferative disorders, radiation treatment, rheumatoid arthritis (RA), systemic lupus erythematosus (SLE), chronic renal failure and hemodialysis, Gaucher disease, organ transplant, trauma, tobacco use, HIV, hypercoagulable state, developmental hip dysplasia, idiopathic

GENERAL PREVENTION

- Limiting alcohol use: Dose-dependent relationship with RR of 3.3 for <400 mL/wk consumed compared to RR of 17.9 for >1,000 mL/wk consumed
- Smoking cessation: Smokers with RR of 3.9 vs. nonsmokers with no significance found to cumulative effect
- Limiting corticosteroid use: Cumulative dose is directly correlated to increased risk of osteonecrosis (3)[B]
- Screening: No definitive evidence but screening of asymptomatic patients at high risk for osteonecrosis may be of value if prophylactic treatment of asymptomatic osteonecrosis is proven useful (4)[B]

PATHOPHYSIOLOGY

- Pathophysiology is multifactorial and not fully understood, but the final common pathway is interruption of the blood flow to the bone.
- Lack of blood supply leads to hyperemia, demineralization, trabecular thinning, and subchondral plate fracture, which eventually leads to collapse of the necrotic segment (1)
- The collapse of the bone is irreversible, painful, often requires surgery for symptom relief, and is a risk factor for developing osteoarthritis (OA).

ETIOLOGY

- Traumatic: Disruption of blood supply due to physical disruption of a vessel due to fracture or dislocation
- Nontraumatic: Possible mechanisms include:
  - Impedance of blood flow due to vascular compression/vasospasm
  - Extraluminal obliteration from marrow edema
  - Intraluminal obstruction from thromboembolism, nitrogen bubbles, fat emboli, intravascular coagulation, or vascular stasis (1)

DIAGNOSIS

- Consider AVN in any individual with bone pain and history of trauma or other risk factors.
- Pain in the affected joint is typically the presenting symptom.

HISTORY

- Hip/femoral head: Dull, aching groin/hip pain that is progressive and worsened with weight bearing
- Knee: Dull, aching knee pain that is worsened with weight bearing, stair climbing, and at night
- Humeral head: Shoulder pain that is severe and poorly localized, worsened at night, and with activity
- Lunate (Kienböck disease): Pain and stiffness to dorsal wrist of dominant hand

PHYSICAL EXAM

- Hip/femoral head:
  - Decreased hip range of motion, especially in rotation and abduction
  - Antalgic or Trendelenburg gait
  - Synovitis = pain throughout range of motion
- Knee:
  - Pseudolocking secondary to pain, effusion, or muscle contracture
- Humeral head:
  - Active motion inhibited by pain
  - Passive motion and strength preserved
- Lunate (Kienböck disease):
  - Dorsal swelling with tenderness over radiocarpal joint
  - Restricted and painful dorsiflexion of wrist
  - Weakness of grip

DIAGNOSTIC TESTS & INTERPRETATION

- No specific physical findings or laboratory tests can reliably establish the diagnosis.
- Clinically suspected osteonecrosis can be confirmed only by diagnostic imaging or biopsy.
- Imaging options:
  - Plain films: First line:
    - Early stages: Unremarkable
    - Mild to moderate AVN: Sclerosis and changes in bone density
    - Advanced disease: Bony deformities such as flattening, subchondral radiolucent lines (crescent sign), and osseus collapse
    - Views to order based on location:
      - Hip/femoral head: Anteroposterior (AP) and frog lateral views of both hips
      - Knee: AP, lateral, and tunnel view of knee
      - Humeral head: AP, true AP, and axillary views of shoulder
      - Lunate: Standard wrist films
  - MRI: Gold standard for diagnosis with sensitivity and specificity >98% (5)[B]; obtain if x-ray findings are normal and clinical suspicion is high:
    - Early stages: Decreased signal intensity of the subchondral region on both T1- and T2-weighted images (water signal)
    - Mild to moderate AVN: High signal intensity line within 2 parallel rims of decreased signal intensity on T2-weighted scans (double line sign)
    - Advanced disease: Deformity and calcification of the articular surface
  - Bone scan: Alternative to MRI; when used with SPECT imaging is 85% sensitive and 100% specific:
    - Central area of decreased uptake surrounded by an area of increased uptake (doughnut sign)

Lab

Consider testing for sickle cell disease (Hb electrophoresis), hyperlipidemia (fasting lipid profile), and coagulopathies (protein C, protein S, factor V Leiden) with atraumatic etiology

Imaging

- Bone marrow edema on MRI should be considered a marker for potential progression to advanced osteonecrosis and collapse of the femoral head.
- Several different staging systems available for classifying osteonecrosis of the femoral head (6):
  - FICAT: Stages 0–4 based on symptoms, x-ray, and MRI findings
  - Steinberg: Stages 0–6 based on imaging and subdivided into categories based on percentage of the femoral head affected
  - ARCO (international classification of osteonecrosis of the femoral head): Stages 0–6 based on clinical symptoms and imaging findings with focus on status of the femoral head

DIFFERENTIAL DIAGNOSIS
- Hip/femoral head:
  - Osteoarthritis, femoral neck fracture, labral tear, osteomyelitis, muscle strain, groin injury, transient synovitis, bone marrow edema syndrome
- Knee:
  - Osteoarthritis, septic arthritis, meniscal tear, bone bruise, transient osteopenia of the knee, pes anserine bursitis, osteochondritis desiccans
- Humeral head:
  - Adhesive capsulitis, rotator cuff tear/tendonitis, osteomyelitis
- Lunate (Kienböck disease):
  - TFCC injury, tenosynovitis of extensor compartments, rheumatoid arthritis, degenerative joint disease, occult ganglion, other carpal bone injury

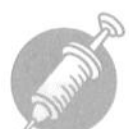

TREATMENT

- The treatment depends on the age, location, stage of the disease, and overall health of the patient.
- The goal of therapy is to preserve the native joint for as long as possible.
- Early diagnosis is important to maximize treatment options.

MEDICATION
- No medical treatment has been proven effective for arresting the disease process.
- NSAIDs and other analgesics should be given as needed for pain relief.
- Prophylactic alendronate at 70 mg/wk PO for 25 weeks found to prevent collapse of femoral head (NNT = 2) and need for total hip arthroplasty (NNT = 2) at 2 years in patients with Steinberg stage 2 or 3 nontraumatic AVN of femoral head with necrotic area >30% (7)[B]

ADDITIONAL TREATMENT
General Measures
- Usually managed as an outpatient but may be inpatient if surgery indicated
- Crutches or other assistive devices to avoid weight bearing in early disease if weight-bearing joint is affected.

Issues for Referral
Refer for an evaluation by orthopedic surgeon once a diagnosis is made to determine if surgery is appropriate.

COMPLEMENTARY AND ALTERNATIVE MEDICINE
Noninvasive modalities of electrical stimulation, shock wave therapy, and electromagnetic field therapy undergoing trials but currently no evidence to support these

SURGERY/OTHER PROCEDURES
- Surgical options are controversial and depend on severity and site of disease.
- Hip/femoral head:
  - Early stages (precollapse) treated surgically with bone decompression and possible bone graft
  - Later stages (postcollapse) treated with total hip arthroplasty
- Knee: Arthroscopy, osteochondral grafts, high tibial osteotomy, core decompression, unicompartmental knee arthroplasty, total knee arthroplasty
- Humeral head: Arthroscopy, core decompression, hemiarthroplasty, total shoulder arthroplasty
- Lunate (Kienböck disease): Lunate excision with or without replacement, joint-leveling procedures, intercarpal fusions, revascularization, salvage procedures

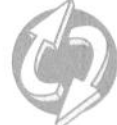

ONGOING CARE

- Physical therapy and occupational therapy as adjunctive treatments
- Sickle cell patients: No evidence that adding hip core decompression to physical therapy achieves clinical improvement in people with avascular necrosis of bone compared to physical therapy alone, per Cochrane Review

PATIENT EDUCATION
- Physicians prescribing bisphosphonates should counsel their patients about potential oral complications linked to using these medications and advise patients to notify their dentists that they are taking the drugs.
- Other high-risk patients should be educated about the risk of developing osteonecrosis and should be advised to report symptoms as soon as possible.

PROGNOSIS
- Poor prognostic factors include age >50, advanced disease at time of diagnosis, necrosis of >1/3 of the femoral head weight-bearing area, lateral femoral head involvement, and nonmodifiable risk factors.
- Progression of asymptomatic osteonecrosis of the femoral head proportional to lesion size with small lesions (<15% involvement) unlikely to progress and large lesions (>30% involvement) likely to progress
- >50% of patients with osteonecrosis require surgical treatment within 3 years of diagnosis.
- Osteonecrosis of the humeral head accounts for 10% of total joint replacement procedures performed annually in the US (5).

COMPLICATIONS
- Secondary to surgery-induced trauma, including nonunion, malunion, peroneal nerve palsy, deep venous thrombosis, intraoperative fracture, and postoperative dislocation (5)
- Progression of disease leads to OA of the involved joint to a varying degree.

REFERENCES

1. Lafforgue P. Pathophysiology and natural history of avascular necrosis of bone. *Joint Bone Spine*. 2006; 73(5):500–7.
2. Khan AA, Sándor GK, Dore E. Bisphosphonate associated osteonecrosis of the jaw. *J Rheumatol*. 2009;36:478–90.
3. Powell C, Chang C, Naguwa SM, et al. Steroid induced osteonecrosis: An analysis of steroid dosing risk. *Autoimmun Rev*. 2010;9:721–43.
4. American College of Radiology (ACR) Appropriateness Criteria for avascular necrosis of the hip. *National Guideline Clearinghouse*. 2010; 31:15734.
5. Assouline-Dayan Y, Chang C, Greenspan A. Pathogenesis and natural history of osteonecrosis. *Semin Arthritis Rheum*. 2002;32:94–124.
6. Steinberg ME, Steinberg DR. Classification systems for osteonecrosis: An overview. *Orthop Clin North Am*. 2004;35:273–83, vii–viii.
7. Lai K-A, Shen W-J, Yang C-Y, et al. The use of alendronate to prevent early collapse of the femoral head in patients with nontraumatic osteonecrosis. *J Bone and Joint Surg Am*. 2005;87:2155–59.

ADDITIONAL READING

- Matsuo K, Hirohata T, Sugioka Y, et al. Influence of alcohol intake, cigarette smoking and occupational status on idiopathic osteonecrosis of the femoral head. *Clin Orthop Relat Res*. 1998:115–23.
- National Institute of Arthritis and Musculoskeletal and Skin Diseases: Osteonecrosis. www.niams.nih.gov/health_info/osteonecrosis/.
- Tofferi J, Gilliland W. E-medicine rheumatology: Avascular necrosis. http://emedicine.medscape.com/article/333364-overview.

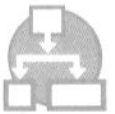

See Also (Topic, Algorithm, Electronic Media Element)

Arthritis, Osteo; Hip Avascular Necrosis; Legg-Calvé-Perthes Disease

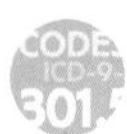

CODES

ICD9
- 733.40 Aseptic necrosis of bone, site unspecified
- 733.41 Aseptic necrosis of head of humerus
- 733.42 Aseptic necrosis of head and neck of femur

CLINICAL PEARLS

- Trauma, alcoholism, and prolonged glucocorticoid use are the most common risk factors for the development of osteonecrosis.
- When prescribing systemic corticosteroids, use the minimum effective dose and duration; warn patients of the risk for developing osteonecrosis (3).
- Identify at-risk patients and suspect osteonecrosis in this population if they present with bone or joint pain.
- Initiate a workup with appropriate radiographs, then proceed to an MRI if indicated (4)[A].

OSTEOPOROSIS

Karen L. Maughan, MD

BASICS

DESCRIPTION

A skeletal disease characterized by low bone mass, disruption of skeletal microarchitecture, and increased skeletal fragility, resulting in fractures occurring with a fall from standing height or less or with no trauma

EPIDEMIOLOGY

- Predominant age: Elderly >60 years of age
- Predominant sex: Female > Male (80%/20%)

Incidence

In 2000, there were 9 million osteoporotic fractures worldwide.

Prevalence

- 12 million Americans have osteoporosis.
- Women >50 years of age: 24%
- Men >50 years of age: 7.5%
- 50% of postmenopausal women will have an osteoporotic fracture during their lifetime.

RISK FACTORS

- Nonmodifiable:
  - Advanced age (>65 years)
  - Female gender
  - Caucasian or Asian
  - Family history of osteoporosis
  - History of atraumatic fracture
- Modifiable:
  - Low body weight (<58 kg or body mass index <20)
  - Calcium or vitamin D deficiency
  - Inadequate physical activity
  - Cigarette smoking
  - Excessive alcohol intake (>2 drinks/d)
  - Medications: Chronic corticosteroids, excessive thyroid hormone replacement, medroxyprogesterone acetate, heparin, proton pump inhibitors

Genetics

- Familial predisposition
- More common in Caucasians and Asians than in African Americans and Hispanics

GENERAL PREVENTION

The aim in the prevention and treatment of osteoporosis is to prevent fracture.

- Exercise (weight-bearing, aerobic, and strength training) increases bone mineral density (BMD), although it is unclear if it prevents fractures (1)[B].
- Calcium (1,200 mg) and vitamin D (800 IU) daily
- Avoid smoking.
- Limit alcohol use (<2 drinks/d).
- Screen all women ≥65 years of age and women ≥60 years of age who are at high risk for fracture (www.ahrq.gov/clinic/uspstf/uspsoste.htm).
- Consider screening elderly men who are at high risk for fracture (2)[C].
- Correct treatable medical conditions and other risk factors.

PATHOPHYSIOLOGY

- Imbalance between bone resorption and bone formation
- Trabecular bone (vertebral) more active than cortical (hip) bone

ETIOLOGY

- Aging
- Hypoestrogenemia

COMMONLY ASSOCIATED CONDITIONS

- Malabsorption syndromes: Gastrectomy, inflammatory bowel disease, celiac disease
- Hypoestrogenism: Menopause, hypogonadism, eating disorders, elite athletes
- Chronic liver disease, hemochromatosis
- Endocrinopathies: Hyperparathyroidism, hyperthyroidism
- Multiple myeloma, multiple sclerosis, osteomalacia, rheumatoid arthritis
- Medications (see "Medications" under "Risk Factors")

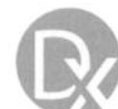

DIAGNOSIS

HISTORY

- Review risk factors.
- Online risk factor assessment tools are available, although external validation is lacking (e.g., FRAX [www.sheffield.ac.uk/FRAX/index.htm], Garvan [http://garvan.org.au/promotions/bone-fracture-risk/calculator/]).
- Often no clinical findings until fracture occurs

PHYSICAL EXAM

- Thoracic kyphosis
- Height loss >1.5 cm

DIAGNOSTIC TESTS & INTERPRETATION

Dual-energy x-ray absorptiometry (DEXA) of the lumbar spine/hip is the "gold standard" for the diagnosis of osteoporosis (see "Initial Approach" under "Imaging").

Lab

Initial lab tests

To elicit common causes of secondary osteoporosis:

- 25-hydroxyvitamin D, CBC, serum calcium, total protein, creatinine, alkaline phosphatase

Follow-Up & Special Considerations

Consider further lab work depending on initial evaluation, *Z*-score <–2, or young age.

- Parathyroid hormone (PTH), ionized calcium (hyperparathyroidism)
- Thyroid-stimulating hormone (hyperthyroidism)
- Testosterone (hypogonadism in men)
- Serum protein electrophoresis (multiple myeloma)
- Urinary-free cortisol (Cushing disease)
- Vitamin B_{12} level and intrinsic-factor antibody (pernicious anemia)
- IgA antiendomysial antibodies (celiac sprue)
- Serum and 24-hour urine calcium, serum phosphate (osteomalacia)
- Markers of bone resorption (urine *N*-telopeptides of type 1 collagen, serum C-telopeptides of type 1 collagen, serum N-terminal propeptide of type 1 procollagen): No prospective studies supporting use in osteoporosis diagnosis and management; potential role for identifying patients at high risk for fracture and monitoring response to therapy

Imaging

Initial approach

- DEXA of the lumbar spine/hip is the "gold standard" for measuring BMD and making a diagnosis of osteoporosis.
- BMD is expressed in terms of T-scores and *Z*-scores:
  - T-score is the number of standard deviations (SDs) a patient's BMD deviates from the mean for young normal (age 25–40 years) control individuals of the same sex.
  - The World Health Organization (WHO) defines normal BMD as a T-score ≥–1, osteopenia as a T-score between –1 and –2.5, and osteoporosis as a T-score ≤–2.5.
  - WHO thresholds can be used for postmenopausal women and men >50 years of age.
  - The Z-score is a comparison of the patient's BMD with an age-matched population.
  - A Z-score <–2 should prompt evaluation for causes of secondary osteoporosis.
- Ultrasound densitometry is used to measure BMD at the calcaneus (heel). It is lower in cost and involves no radiation exposure but is not as accurate as DEXA, and no studies support its use in determining therapy.
- Plain radiographs lack sensitivity to diagnose osteoporosis, but an abnormality (e.g., widened intervertebral spaces, rib fractures, vertebral compression fractures, etc.) should prompt evaluation of BMD.

Diagnostic Procedures/Surgery

Bone biopsy rarely is needed to rule out neoplasms and other metabolic bone diseases.

Pathological Findings

- Reduced skeletal mass, trabecular bone thinned or lost more so than cortical bone
- Osteoclast and osteoblast number variable
- No evidence of other metabolic bone diseases and no increase in unmineralized osteoid
- Marrow normal or atrophic

DIFFERENTIAL DIAGNOSIS

- Multiple myeloma or other neoplasms
- Osteomalacia
- Type I collagen mutations
- Osteogenesis imperfecta

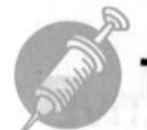

TREATMENT

Treat patients with a T-score ≤–2.5 with no risk factors, patients with a T-score ≤–2 and 1 or more risk factors, and patients with a prior history of osteoporotic fracture at the spine or hip.

MEDICATION

Calcium, 1,500 mg; vitamin D, 800 IU/d

First Line

- Bisphosphonates:
  - Alendronate, 10 mg PO daily or 70 mg PO weekly
  - Risedronate, 5 mg PO daily, 35 mg PO weekly, 75 mg PO twice monthly, or 150 mg PO monthly
  - Zoledronic acid, 5 mg IV yearly
- These drugs become incorporated into skeletal tissue, where they inhibit the resorption of bone by osteoclasts.
- Number needed to treat (NNT) to prevent vertebral fracture = 17

- NNT to prevent hip fracture = 100 (3)[A]
- Ibandronate increases bone density but does not appear to decrease fractures.

Second Line

- Raloxifene, 60 mg PO daily:
  - Selective estrogen receptor modulator with positive effects on BMD and fracture risk but no stimulatory action on breasts or uterus
  - NNT with 60 mg/d for 3 years to prevent 1 postmenopausal woman with osteoporosis from developing a vertebral fracture = 29.
  - Decreases vertebral but not hip fractures (4)[A]; increases risk of thromboembolism
- Teriparatide, 20 mg SC daily:
  - Recombinant formulation of PTH; when given daily, it promotes new bone formation.
  - Studies have shown a reduction in the incidence of vertebral fractures by 65% (5)[B].
  - No data exist on its safety and efficacy after >2 years of use.
  - Primarily indicated for those with worsening osteoporosis despite bisphosphonate therapy
- Estrogen, 0.625 mg PO daily (with progesterone if women has a uterus): Effective in prevention and treatment of osteoporosis (35% reduction in hip and vertebral fractures after 5 years of use), but the risks (e.g., increased rates of myocardial infarction, stroke, breast cancer, pulmonary embolus, and deep vein thrombosis) must be weighed against the benefits, and have decreased interest in this regiment (6)[B].
- Strontium, 2 g PO daily:
  - Appears to inhibit bone resorption and increase bone formation
  - Available for use in Europe
  - NNT to prevent vertebral fracture = 13
  - NNT to prevent hip fracture = 50 (7)[B]
- Denosumab:
  - Human monoclonal antibody RANKL receptor
  - Inhibits osteoclast formation
  - NNT to prevent vertebral fracture = 20 after 3 years
  - NNT to prevent hip fracture = 200 after 3 years (8)
- Calcitonin:
  - Acts by reducing the number of osteoclasts, therefore decreasing bone turnover
  - Has been shown to increase BMD, but no studies have shown conclusively a reduction in the occurrence of fractures.
  - May decrease acute vertebral compression-fracture pain (analgesic).

ADDITIONAL TREATMENT

- Exercise: Any weight-bearing exercise for 30 minutes 3 times per week (1)[B]
- Smoking cessation
- Decrease any fall risk.
- Evaluate and treat all patients presenting with fracture resulting from minimal trauma.

Issues for Referral

Endocrinology for recurrent bone loss/fracture despite treatment of osteoporosis and evaluation and treatment of possible secondary causes

Additional Therapies

Physical therapy to help with muscle strengthening to decrease fall risk

COMPLEMENTARY AND ALTERNATIVE MEDICINE

Isoflavones not better than placebo for bone density and fracture risk

SURGERY/OTHER PROCEDURES

Options for patients with painful vertebral compression fractures failing medical treatment:

- Vertebroplasty: Orthopedic cement is injected into the compressed vertebral body.
- Kyphoplasty: A balloon is expanded within the compressed vertebral body to reconstruct volume of vertebrae. Cement is injected into the space.

IN-PATIENT CONSIDERATIONS

Initial Stabilization

Inpatient care for pain control of acute back pain secondary to new vertebral fractures and for acute treatment of femoral and pelvic fractures

Discharge Criteria

- Pain controlled; fracture stabilized
- Rehabilitation, nursing home, or home care may be needed following peripheral fractures.

ONGOING CARE

FOLLOW-UP RECOMMENDATIONS

Patient Monitoring

- Weight-bearing exercises such as walking, jogging, stair climbing, and tai chi have been shown to decrease falls.
- All successful studies on the treatment of osteoporosis involve weight-bearing exercise.
- BMD should be tested no earlier than 2 years after starting bisphosphonate. It is uncertain whether repeat DEXA scanning is of value (9).
- For many women, 5 years of treatment with a bisphosphonate is as good as 10 years of treatment. Those at high risk for vertebral fracture or with very low BMD may benefit by continuing treatment beyond 5 years (10)

DIET

- Diet to maintain normal body weight
- Calcium, 1,500 mg; vitamin D, 800 IU daily

PATIENT EDUCATION

National Osteoporosis Foundation: www.nof.org

PROGNOSIS

- With treatment, 80% of patients stabilize skeletal manifestations, increase bone mass, increase mobility, and have reduced pain.
- 15% of vertebral and 20–40% of hip fractures may lead to chronic care and/or premature death.

COMPLICATIONS

- Severe, disabling pain
- Dorsal/lumbar neurologic deficits secondary to vertebral fracture (rare)

REFERENCES

1. Bonaiuti D, Shea B, Iovine R. Exercise for preventing and treating osteoporosis in postmenopausal women. *Cochrane Database Syst Rev.* 2002;CD000333.
2. Qaseem A, Snow V, Shekelle P. Screening for osteoporosis in men: A clinical practice guideline from the American College of Physicians. *Ann Intern Med.* 2008;148:680–4.
3. Wells GA, Cranney A, Peterson J, et al. Alendronate for the primary and secondary prevention of osteoporotic fractures in postmenopausal women. *Cochrane Database Syst Rev.* 2008;1:CD001155.
4. Ettinger B, Black DM, Mitlak BH. Reduction of vertebral fracture risk in postmenopausal women with osteoporosis treated with raloxifene: Results from a 3-year randomized clinical trial. Multiple Outcomes of Raloxifene Evaluation (MORE) Investigators. *JAMA.* 1999;282:637–45.
5. Neer RM, Arnaud CD, Zanchetta JR. Effect of parathyroid hormone (1-34) on fractures and bone mineral density in postmenopausal women with osteoporosis. *N Engl J Med.* 2001;344:1434–41.
6. Cauley JA, Robbins J, Chen Z. Effects of estrogen plus progestin on risk of fracture and bone mineral density: The Women's Health Initiative randomized trial. *JAMA.* 2003;290:1729–38.
7. O'Donnell S, Cranney A, Wells GA, et al. Strontium ranelate for preventing and treating postmenopausal osteoporosis. *Cochrane Database Sys Rev.* 2006;4.
8. Cummings SR, San Martin J, McClung MR, et al. Denosumab for prevention of fractures in postmenopausal women with osteoporosis. *N Engl J Med.* 2009;361:756–65.
9. Hillier TA, Stone KL, Bauer DC, et al. Evaluating the value of repeat bone mineral density measurement and prediction of fractures in older women: The study of osteoporotic fractures. *Arch Intern Med.* 2007;167:155–60.
10. Black DM, Schwartz AV, Ensrud KE, et al. Effects of continuing or stopping alendronate after 5 years of treatment: The Fracture Intervention Trial Long-term Extension (FLEX): A randomized trial. *JAMA.* 2006;296:2927–38.

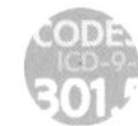

CODES

ICD9

- 733.00 Osteoporosis, unspecified
- 733.01 Senile osteoporosis
- 733.02 Idiopathic osteoporosis

CLINICAL PEARLS

- Screen all women ≥65 years of age with DEXA scans.
- Screen both men and women ≥60 years of age at increased risk for osteoporosis with DEXA scans.
- Premenopausal women with osteoporosis should be screened for secondary causes, such as malabsorption syndromes, hyperparathyroidism, hyperthyroidism, and medication sensitivity.
- Evaluate and treat all patients presenting with fractures from minimal trauma.
- If the patient is not responding to treatment, consider screening for a secondary, treatable cause of osteoporosis.

OTITIS EXTERNA

Douglas S. Parks, MD

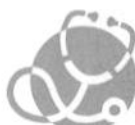

BASICS

DESCRIPTION

Inflammation of the external auditory canal:

- Acute diffuse otitis externa: The most common form; an infectious process, usually bacterial, occasionally fungal (10%)
- Acute circumscribed otitis externa: Synonymous with furuncle; associated with infection of the hair follicle, a superficial cellulitic form of otitis externa
- Chronic otitis externa: Same as acute diffuse but of longer duration (>6 weeks)
- Eczematous otitis externa: May accompany typical atopic eczema or other primary skin conditions
- Necrotizing malignant otitis externa: An infection that extends into the deeper tissues adjacent to the canal; may include osteomyelitis and cellulitis; rare in children
- System(s) affected: Skin/Exocrine
- Synonym(s): Swimmer's ear

EPIDEMIOLOGY

Incidence

- Unknown; higher in the summer months and warm, wet climates
- Predominant age: All ages
- Predominant sex: Male = Female

Prevalence

- Acute, chronic, and eczematous: Common
- Necrotizing: Uncommon

RISK FACTORS

- Acute and chronic otitis externa:
  - Traumatization of external canal
  - Swimming
  - Hot, humid weather
  - Hearing aid use
- Eczematous: Primary skin disorder
- Necrotizing otitis externa in adults:
  - Advanced age
  - Diabetes mellitus (DM)
  - Debilitating disease
  - AIDS
- Necrotizing otitis externa in children (rare):
  - Leukopenia
  - Malnutrition
  - DM
  - Diabetes insipidus

GENERAL PREVENTION

- Avoid prolonged exposure to moisture.
- Use preventive antiseptics (acidifying solutions with 2% acetic acid [white vinegar] diluted 50/50 with water or isopropyl alcohol, or 2% acetic acid with aluminum acetate [less irritating]) after swimming and bathing.
- Treat predisposing skin conditions.
- Eliminate self-inflicted trauma to canal with cotton swabs and other foreign objects.
- Diagnose and treat underlying systemic conditions.
- Use ear plugs when swimming.

ETIOLOGY

- Acute diffuse otitis externa:
  - Traumatized external canal (e.g., from use of cotton swab)
  - Bacterial infection (90%): *Pseudomonas* (67%), *Staphylococcus*, *Streptococcus*, gram-negative rods
  - Fungal infection (10%): *Aspergillus* (90%), *Candida*, *Phycomycetes*, *Rhizopus*, *Actinomyces*, *Penicillium*
- Chronic otitis externa: Bacterial infection: *Pseudomonas*
- Eczematous otitis externa (associated with primary skin disorder):
  - Eczema
  - Seborrhea
  - Psoriasis
  - Neurodermatitis
  - Contact dermatitis
  - Purulent otitis media
  - Sensitivity to topical medications
- Necrotizing otitis externa:
  - Invasive bacterial infection: *Pseudomonas*
  - Associated with immunosuppression

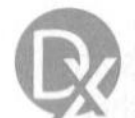

DIAGNOSIS

HISTORY

Variable-length history of itching, plugging of ear, ear pain, and discharge from ear

PHYSICAL EXAM

- Ear canal red, containing purulent discharge and debris
- Pain on manipulation of the pinnae
- Possible periauricular adenitis
- Possible eczema of pinna
- Cranial nerve (VII, IX–XII) involvement (extremely rare)

DIAGNOSTIC TESTS & INTERPRETATION

Lab

- Gram stain and culture of canal discharge (occasionally helpful)
- Antibiotic pretreatment may affect results.

Imaging

Radiologic evaluation of deep tissues in necrotizing otitis externa with high-resolution CT scan, MRI, gallium scan, and bone scan

Pathological Findings

- Acute and chronic otitis externa: Desquamation of superficial epithelium of external canal with infection
- Eczematous otitis externa: Pathologic findings consistent with primary skin disorder; secondary infection on occasion
- Necrotizing otitis externa: Vasculitis, thrombosis, and necrosis of involved tissues; osteomyelitis

DIFFERENTIAL DIAGNOSIS

- Idiopathic ear pain
- Otitis media with perforation
- Hearing loss
- Cranial nerve (VII, IX–XII) palsy with necrotizing otitis externa
- Wisdom tooth eruption
- Basal cell or squamous cell carcinoma

TREATMENT

Outpatient treatment, except for resistant cases and necrotizing otitis externa

MEDICATION

Resistance is an increasing problem. *Pseudomonas* is the most common bacteria and it is more susceptible to fluoroquinolones such as ciprofloxacin or ofloxacin, whereas *Staphylococcus* is equally susceptible to both fluoroquinolones and polymyxin B combinations. If a patient has recurring episodes or is not improved in 2 weeks, change the class of antibacterial and consider cultures and sensitivities.

First Line

- Acute bacterial and chronic otitis externa:
  - Neomycin/polymyxin B/hydrocortisone (Cortisporin): 5 drops q.i.d. If the tympanic membrane is ruptured, use the suspension; otherwise, the solution may be used; may be ototoxic and resistance-developing in *Staphylococcus* and *Streptococcus* sp. (2)[B]. Least expensive
  - Acetic acid 2% with hydrocortisone 1%: 3–5 drops q4–8h × 7 days; may cause minor local stinging. This is as effective as neomycin–polymyxin B (3)[B] but is expensive. It may take up to 2 days longer to achieve resolution of symptoms (1)[A].
  - A wick may be helpful in severe cases by keeping the canal open and keeping antibiotic solution in contact with infected skin (4)[C].
  - Oral antibiotics are indicated only if there is associated otitis media or cellulitis of the outer ear (red canal without discharge).
  - Analgesics as needed; narcotics may be necessary.

- Recurrent otitis externa may be prevented by applying equal parts white vinegar and isopropyl alcohol (OTC rubbing alcohol) to external auditory canals after bathing and swimming.
- Fungal otitis externa:
  - Topical therapy, antiyeast for *Candida* or yeast: 2% acetic acid 3–4 drops q.i.d.; clotrimazole 1% solution; itraconazole oral
  - Parenteral antifungal therapy: Amphotericin B
  - Patients with Ramsay-Hunt syndrome: Acyclovir IV
- Eczematous otitis externa: Topical therapy:
  - Acetic acid 2% in aluminum acetate
  - Aluminum acetate (5%; Burow solution)
  - Steroid cream, lotion, ointment (e.g., triamcinolone 0.1% solution)
  - Antibacterial, if superinfected
- Necrotizing otitis externa:
  - Parenteral antibiotics: Antistaphylococcal and antipseudomonal
  - 4–6 weeks of therapy
  - Quinolones PO × 2–4 weeks
- Contraindications:
  - Hypersensitivity to topical or parenteral therapy
  - Renal or hepatic failure when using amphotericin B
- Precautions:
  - Dosage adjustment for amphotericin B in patients with renal or hepatic dysfunction
  - Sensitivity to neomycin
- Significant possible interactions:
  - Hypokalemia associated with amphotericin B may lead to digitalis toxicity.
  - Concurrent administration of nonabsorbable anions, such as carbenicillin, may exacerbate hypokalemia.

Second Line

- Acute bacterial and chronic otitis externa:
  - Ciprofloxacin 0.3% and dexamethasone 0.1% suspension (Cipro dex): 3–4 drops b.i.d. × 7 days or ofloxacin (Floxin Otic): 0.3% solution 10 drops once a day × 7 days (1)[A]. Less ototoxicity and reported antibiotic resistance, but branded drugs are far more expensive.
  - Betamethasone 0.05% solution may be as effective as a polymyxin B combination without the risk of ototoxicity or antibiotic resistance. However, the data are not very robust and more study is needed (1)[A].
- Azole antifungals for fungal otitis externa

ADDITIONAL TREATMENT

General Measures

- Cleaning the external canal may facilitate recovery.
- Analgesics as appropriate for pain
- Antipruritic and antihistamines (eczematous form)
- Ear wick (Pope) for nearly occluded ear canal

Issues for Referral

Resistant cases or those requiring surgical intervention

COMPLEMENTARY AND ALTERNATIVE MEDICINE

- Over-the-counter white vinegar; 3 drops in affected ear for minor case
- Tea tree oil in various concentrations has been used as an antiseptic (5)[B]. Ototoxicity has been reported in animal studies at very high doses.
- Grapefruit seed extract in various concentrations has been described as useful in the lay literature.

SURGERY/OTHER PROCEDURES

For necrotizing otitis externa or furuncle

IN-PATIENT CONSIDERATIONS

Admission Criteria

Necrotizing otitis media requiring parenteral antipseudomonal antibiotics

Discharge Criteria

Resolution of infection

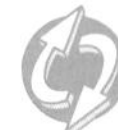

ONGOING CARE

FOLLOW-UP RECOMMENDATIONS

No restrictions

Patient Monitoring

- Acute otitis externa:
  - 48 hours after therapy instituted to assess improvement
  - At the end of treatment
- Chronic otitis externa:
  - Every 2–3 weeks for repeated cleansing of canal
  - May require alterations in topical medication, including antibiotics and steroids
- Necrotizing otitis externa:
  - Daily monitoring in hospital for extension of infection
  - Baseline auditory and vestibular testing at beginning and end of therapy

DIET

No restrictions

PROGNOSIS

- Acute otitis externa: Rapid response to therapy with total resolution
- Chronic otitis externa: With repeated cleansing and antibiotic therapy, most cases will resolve. Occasionally, surgical intervention is required for resistant cases.
- Eczematous otitis externa: Resolution will occur with control of the primary skin condition.
- Necrotizing otitis externa: Usually can be managed with debridement and antipseudomonal antibiotics; recurrence rate is 100% when treatment is inadequate. Surgical intervention may be necessary in resistant cases or if there is cranial nerve involvement. Mortality rate is significant, probably secondary to the underlying disease.

COMPLICATIONS

- Mainly a problem with necrotizing otitis externa; may spread to infect contiguous bone and CNS structures
- Acute otitis externa may spread to pinna, causing chondritis.

REFERENCES

1. Kaushik V, Malik T, Saeed SR, et al. Interventions for acute otitis externa. *Cochrane Database Syst Rev*. 2010;CD004740.
2. Cantrell HF, Lombardy EE, Duncanson FP. Declining susceptibility to neomycin and polymyxin B of pathogens recovered in otitis externa clinical trials. *South Med J*. 2004;97:465–71.
3. van Balen FA, Smit WM, Zuithoff NP. Clinical efficacy of three common treatments in acute otitis externa in primary care: Randomised controlled trial. *BMJ*. 2003;327:1201–5.
4. Block SL. Otitis externa: Providing relief while avoiding complications. *J Fam Pract*. 2005;54: 669–76.
5. Farnan TB, McCallum J, Awa A. Tea tree oil: In vitro efficacy in otitis externa. *J Laryngol Otol*. 2005;119: 198–201.

ADDITIONAL READING

Dohar JE, Roland P, Wall GM, et al. Differences in bacteriologic treatment failures in acute otitis externa between ciprofloxacin/dexamethasone and neomycin/polymyxin B/hydrocortisone: Results of a combined analysis. *Curr Med Res Opin*. 2009;25: 287–91.

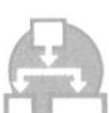

See Also (Topic, Algorithm, Electronic Media Element)

Algorithm: Ear Pain

CODES

ICD9

- 380.10 Infective otitis externa, unspecified
- 380.15 Chronic mycotic otitis externa
- 380.22 Other acute otitis externa

CLINICAL PEARLS

- Acute diffuse otitis externa is the most common form: Bacterial (90%), occasionally fungal (10%).
- Acute circumscribed otitis externa is associated with infection of the hair follicle.
- Chronic otitis externa is the same as acute diffuse but of longer duration (>6 weeks).
- Eczematous otitis externa may accompany typical atopic eczema or other primary skin conditions.
- Necrotizing malignant otitis externa is an infection that extends into the deeper tissues adjacent to the canal. It may include osteomyelitis and cellulitis; it is rare in children.

OTITIS MEDIA

David B. Gilchrist, MD
Hugh J. Silk, MD, MPH

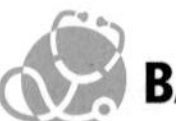

BASICS

DESCRIPTION

- Inflammation of the middle ear
- Acute otitis media (AOM): Inflammation of the middle ear often following or associated with a viral upper respiratory infection (URI). Rapid onset; cause may be infectious, either viral (AOM-v) or bacterial (AOM-b), but there is also a sterile etiology (AOM-s)
- Recurrent AOM: ≥3 episodes in 6 months or ≥4 episodes in 1 year
- Otitis media with effusion (OME): Persistent middle ear fluid that is associated with AOM but can arise without prior AOM
- Chronic otitis media with or without cholesteatoma
- System(s) affected: Nervous; ENT
- Synonym(s): Secretory or serous otitis media

EPIDEMIOLOGY

Incidence

- AOM:
  - Predominant age: 6–24 months; declines >7 years; rare in adults
  - Predominant sex: Male > Female
  - By age 7 years, 93% of children have had ≥1 episodes of AOM; 39% have had ≥6.
  - Placement of tympanostomy tubes is second only to circumcision as the most frequent surgical procedure in infants.
  - Increased incidence in the fall and winter
- OME:
  - ~90% of children aged 6 months to 4 years have at least 1 episode.

Prevalence

- Most common infection for which antibacterial agents are prescribed in the US
- Diagnosed 5 million times per year in the US

RISK FACTORS

- Premature birth
- Bottle-feeding while supine
- Routine daycare attendance
- Frequent pacifier use after 6 months of age
- Smoking in household
- Male gender
- Native American/Inuit ethnicity
- Low socioeconomic status
- Family history of recurrent otitis
- AOM before age 1 is a risk for recurrent AOM
- Presence of siblings in the household
- Underlying ear, nose, or throat (ENT) disease (e.g., cleft palate, Down syndrome, allergic rhinitis)

Genetics

- Strong genetic component in twin studies for recurrent and prolonged AOM
- May be influenced by skull configuration or immunologic defects

GENERAL PREVENTION

- PCV-7 immunization reduces the number of cases of AOM by about 6–28% (however, evidence shows that this is offset by an increase in AOM caused by other bacteria) (1)[C]. The effect of the introduction of the PCV-13 vaccine on the incidence of AOM has yet to be studied.
- Influenza vaccine reduces AOM by about 30% in children older than age 2 (by preventing influenza).
- Breast-feeding for ≥6 months is protective.
- Avoiding supine bottle-feeding, passive smoke, and pacifiers >6 months may be helpful.
- Secondary prevention: Adenoidectomy and adenotonsillectomy for recurrent AOM has limited short-term efficacy for children older than 3 years of age and is associated with its own adverse risks.

ETIOLOGY

- AOM-b (bacterial): Usually, a preceding viral URI produces eustachian tube dysfunction:
  - *S. pneumoniae*: 20–35%, *H. influenzae*: 20–30%, *M. (B.) catarrhalis*: 15%, Group A streptococci: 3%, *S. aureus*: 12% produce β-lactamases that hydrolyze amoxicillin and some cephalosporins.
- AOM-v (viral): 15–44% of AOM infections are caused primarily by viruses (e.g., respiratory syncytial virus, parainfluenza, influenza, enteroviruses, adenovirus, human metapneumovirus, and parechovirus).
- AOM-s (sterile/nonpathogens): 25–30%
- OME: Eustachian tube dysfunction; allergic causes are rarely substantiated.

COMMONLY ASSOCIATED CONDITIONS

URI

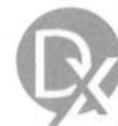

DIAGNOSIS

- AOM: Acute history, signs, and symptoms of middle ear inflammation and effusion:
  - Earache (LR = 3–7.3)
  - Preceding or accompanying URI symptoms
  - Decreased hearing
- Infectious AOM:
  - Fever (although it is debatable whether OM itself causes fever or fever is due to accompanying viral illness)
  - Decreased eardrum mobility (with pneumatic otoscopy) (LR = 51)
  - Eardrum bulging (LR = 51), cloudy (LR = 34), distinctly red (LR = 8.4). Presence of air–fluid level behind the tympanic membrane.
  - Redness alone is not a reliable sign.
  - Otorrhea if eardrum is perforated
- AOM in infants and toddlers:
  - May cause few symptoms in the first few months of life
  - Irritability may be the only symptom.
- OME:
  - Usually asymptomatic
  - Decreased hearing
  - Eardrum often dull but not bulging
  - Decreased eardrum mobility (pneumatic otoscopy)
  - Presence of air–fluid level
  - Weber test is positive to affected ear for an ear with effusion.

DIAGNOSTIC TESTS & INTERPRETATION

Lab

Initial lab tests

The WBC count may be higher in bacterial AOM than in sterile AOM, but this is almost never useful.

Diagnostic Procedures/Surgery

- To document the presence of middle ear fluid, pneumatic otoscopy can be supplemented with tympanometry and acoustic reflex measurement.
- Hearing testing is recommended when hearing loss persists for ≥3 months or at any time language delay, significant hearing loss, or learning problems are suspected.
- Language testing should be performed for children with hearing loss.
- Tympanocentesis for microbiologic diagnosis is recommended for treatment failures; may be followed by myringotomy.

DIFFERENTIAL DIAGNOSIS

- Tympanosclerosis
- Redness because of crying
- Trauma
- AOM vs. OME
- AOM-b vs. AOM-v vs. AOM-s
- Referred pain from the jaw, teeth, or throat
- Otitis externa
- Otitis-conjunctivitis syndrome

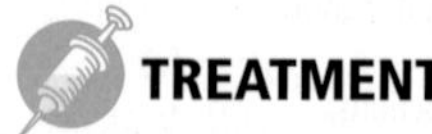

TREATMENT

MEDICATION

First Line

- AOM: The American Academy of Pediatrics (AAP)-AAFP Consensus Guideline recommends amoxicillin, 80–90 mg/kg/d; children >2 years old with no complications, 5–7-day course; 10-day course for children <2 years old. It is unclear if daily or b.i.d. dosing is as effective as t.i.d. or q.i.d. dosing (2)[A].
- If penicillin-allergic:
  - Non–type 1 hypersensitivity reaction: Cefdinir, 14 mg/kg/d; cefpodoxime, 10 mg/kg/d; or cefuroxime 30 mg/kg b.i.d.
  - Type 1 hypersensitivity to penicillin: Azithromycin (10 mg/kg/d [maximum dose 500 mg/d] as a single dose on day 1 and 5 mg/kg/d [maximum dose 250 mg/d] for days 2–5)
  - Other alternatives: Clarithromycin, 15 mg/kg/d (b.i.d. dose); erythromycin-sulfisoxazole, 50 mg/kg/d; or sulfamethoxazole–trimethoprim, 6–10 mg/kg/d based on trimethoprim
- A single dose of parenteral ceftriaxone (50 mg/kg) is as effective as a full course of antibiotics in uncomplicated AOM.
- A single dose of azithromycin has been approved by the FDA, but studies did not include otitis-prone children or have criteria for AOM diagnosis.
- Consider treatment of children between 6 months and 2 years old with antibiotics to reduce duration of symptoms (3)[A].
- OME: See "General Measures"; no benefit to treatment. Medications promote transitory resolution in 10–15%, but the effect is short-lived.

Second Line

- Alternative antibiotics are indicated for the following AOM patients:
  - Persistent symptoms after 48–72 hours of amoxicillin
  - AOM within 1 month of amoxicillin therapy
  - Severe earache
  - Age <6 months with high fever
  - Immunocompromised:
    - Amoxicillin-clavulanate, 90 mg/kg–6.4 mg/kg/d, divided b.i.d.
    - Ceftriaxone, 50 mg/kg IM or IV q24h for 3 consecutive days can be reserved for those who are too sick to take oral medications or who unsuccessfully took amoxicillin-clavulanate. Neither erythromycin-sulfisoxazole nor trimethoprim-sulfamethoxazole should be used as a second-line agent in treatment failures.
- Recurrent AOM: Antibiotic prophylaxis for recurrent AOM (>3 distinct, well-documented episodes in 6 months) with amoxicillin, 20 mg/kg/d for 3 months, resulted in a benefit of ~1 fewer episode per child per year. The possibility of increased resistance and side effects are not thought to be worth risking.

ADDITIONAL TREATMENT

General Measures

- Assess pain.
- Acetaminophen, ibuprofen, benzocaine drops (additional but brief benefit over acetaminophen)
- Significant disagreement exists about the usefulness of antibiotic treatment for this often self-resolving condition. Studies suggest that ~15 children need to be treated with antibiotics to prevent 1 case of persisting AOM pain at 1–2 weeks (NNT= ~15); the NNT to cause harm (primarily diarrhea) is 8–10.
- If antibiotics are not used, 81% of patients over 2 years of age are better in 1 week vs. 94% if antibiotics are used.
- The delay of antibiotics found a modest increase in mastoiditis from 2/100,000 to 4/100,000.
- The AAP/AAFP guidelines recommend the following for observation vs. antibacterial therapy, although these guidelines are not rigorously evidence-based:
  - <6 months of age: Antibacterial therapy should be administered to any child, regardless of the degree of diagnostic certainty.
  - Children >6 months: Antibacterial therapy is recommended when the diagnosis of AOM is certain and the illness is severe (i.e., moderate to severe otalgia or fever ≥39°C in the previous 24 hours).
  - Observation is an option when the diagnosis is certain, but illness is not severe, and in patients with an uncertain diagnosis.
- OME: Watchful waiting for 3 months per AAP/AFPP guidelines for those not at risk (see "Complications"). Of these cases, 25–90% will recover spontaneously over this period. There is no benefit of antihistamines or decongestants (4)[A] or antibiotics or systemic steroids.

COMPLEMENTARY AND ALTERNATIVE MEDICINE

- It is unclear whether alternative and homeopathic therapies are effective for AOM, including mixed evidence about the effectiveness of zinc supplementation of reducing AOM.
- Xylitol, probiotics, herbal ear drops, and homeopathic interventions may be beneficial in reducing pain duration, antibiotic use, and bacterial resistance.

SURGERY/OTHER PROCEDURES

- Recurrent AOM: Consider referral for surgery if ≥3 episodes of well-documented AOM within 6 months, ≥4 episodes within 12 months, or AOM episodes occur while on chemoprophylaxis.
- Tympanostomy tubes may be effective in selective patients.
- Adenoidectomy has limited or no effect.
- Adenotonsillectomy reduced the rate of AOM by 0.7 episode per child only in the first year after surgery and had a 15% complications rate.
- OME: Referral for surgery for tympanostomy should be individualized. It can be considered if >4–6 months of bilateral OME and/or >6 months of unilateral OME and/or hearing loss >25 dB or for high-risk individuals at any time.
- Tympanostomy tubes may reduce recurrence of AOM minimally, but it does not lower the risk of hearing loss (5)[A].
- Adenoidectomy is indicated in specific cases; tonsillectomy or myringotomy is never indicated (6)[A].

IN-PATIENT CONSIDERATIONS

Initial Stabilization

Outpatient treatment except when surgery is indicated or for AOM in febrile infants <2 months old or children requiring ceftriaxone who also require monitoring for 24 hours

ONGOING CARE

FOLLOW-UP RECOMMENDATIONS

Patients with otitis media who do not respond within 48–72 hours should be re-evaluated:

- If therapy was delayed and diagnosis is confirmed, start therapy with high-dose amoxicillin.
- If therapy was initiated, consider changing the antibiotic; options are limited because macrolides have limited benefit against *H. influenza* over amoxicillin, and most oral cephalosporins have no improved outcomes.

Patient Monitoring

- AOM: Up to 40% may have persistent middle ear effusion at 1 month, with 10–25% at 3 months.
- OME: Repeat otoscopic or tympanometric exams at 3 months as indicated, as long as OME persists or sooner if there are red flags (see above).

PROGNOSIS

- See "Treatment" under "General Measures."
- Recurrent AOM and OME: Usually subsides in school-age children; few have complications.

COMPLICATIONS

- AOM: Serious complications are rare: Tympanic membrane perforation/otorrhea, acute mastoiditis, facial nerve paralysis, otitic hydrocephalus, meningitis, hearing impairment
- OME: Speech and language disabilities may occur. Hearing loss is not caused by OME, but in children who are at risk for speech, language, or learning problems (e.g., autism spectrum, syndromes, craniofacial disorders, developmental delay, and children already with speech/language delay), it could lead to further problems because they are less tolerant of a hearing impairment.
- Recurrent AOM and OME: Atrophy and scarring of eardrum, chronic perforation and otorrhea, cholesteatoma, permanent hearing loss, chronic mastoiditis, other intracranial suppurative complications

REFERENCES

1. Eskola J, Kilpi T, Palmu A. Efficacy of a pneumococcal conjugate vaccine against acute otitis media. *N Engl J Med*. 2001;344:403–9.
2. Thanaviratananich S, Laopaiboon M, Vatanasapt P. Once or twice daily versus three times daily amoxicillin with or without clavulanate for the treatment of acute otitis media. *Cochrane Database Syst Rev*. 2008;CD004975.
3. Hoberman A, Paradise JL, Rockette HE, et al. Treatment of acute otitis media in children under 2 years of age. *N Engl J Med*. 2011;364:105–15.
4. Coleman C, Moore M. Decongestants and antihistamines for acute otitis media in children. *Cochrane Database Syst Rev*. 2008;CD001727.
5. Lous J, Burton MJ, Felding JU. Grommets (ventilation tubes) for hearing loss associated with otitis media with effusion in children. *Cochrane Database Syst Rev*. 2005;CD001801.
6. American Academy of Family Physicians, American Academy of Otolaryngology-Head and Neck Surgery, American Academy of Pediatrics Subcommittee on Otitis Media With Effusion. Otitis media with effusion. *Pediatrics*. 2004;113: 1412–29.

ADDITIONAL READING

- Gould JM, Matz PS. Otitis media. *Pediatr Rev*. 2010;31:102–16.
- Shaikh N, Hoberman A, Kaleida PH, et al. Videos in clinical medicine. Diagnosing otitis media—otoscopy and cerumen removal. *N Engl J Med*. 2010;362:e62.

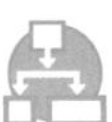

See Also (Topic, Algorithm, Electronic Media Element)

Algorithm: Ear Pain

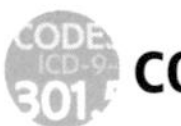

CODES

ICD9

- 381.00 Acute nonsuppurative otitis media, unspecified
- 381.3 Other and unspecified chronic nonsuppurative otitis media
- 381.10 Chronic serous otitis media, simple or unspecified

CLINICAL PEARLS

- Pneumatic otoscopy is the single most specific and clinically useful test for diagnosis.
- Consider a delay of antibiotics for 24–48 hours in uncomplicated children >2 years old who do not have severe illness.
- First-line treatment is amoxicillin, 80–90 mg/kg/d for 10 days for children <2 years old; consider a 5–7-day course in children >2 years old.
- Erythema and effusion can persist for weeks.
- Antibiotics, antihistamines, and steroids are not indicated for OME.

OTITIS MEDIA WITH EFFUSION

Leanne Zakrzewski, MD
Daniel T. Lee, MD

BASICS

DESCRIPTION

- Also called serous otitis media, secretory otitis media, or "glue ear"
- Otitis media with effusion (OME) is defined as the presence of a middle-ear effusion (MEE) in the absence of acute signs of infection.
- In children, OME most often arises following an acute otitis media (AOM). In adults, it often occurs in association with eustachian tube dysfunction.

EPIDEMIOLOGY

Incidence

- It is difficult to determine the incidence of OME because it is asymptomatic. In addition, many cases self-resolve quickly, making it challenging to diagnose OME.
- A 2-year prospective study of 2–6-year-old preschool children revealed MEE, as diagnosed via monthly otoscopy and tympanometry, occurred at least once in 53% of children in the first year and 61% of children in the second year (1).
- A second study followed 7-year-old children monthly for 1 year and found, using tympanometry, a 31% incidence of MEE in study children. In 25% of children with persistent MEE, spontaneous recovery was noted after an average of 2 months (2).
- Nearly all children have experienced 1 episode of OME by the age of 3 years.
- Predominant sex: Male = Female

Prevalence

The prevalence of OME varies with age and the time of year. It is more prevalent in the winter months than in the summer months.

RISK FACTORS

- Risk factors for children include a family history of OME, bottle-feeding, attending daycare, and exposure to tobacco smoke.
- In adults, eustachian tube dysfunction has been noted to be a predisposing factor.

GENERAL PREVENTION

OME is generally not preventable, although smoke exposure may reduce risk.

ETIOLOGY

- In children, it was thought that effusions of OME resulted from chronic inflammation, for example, after AOM, and that the effusions frequently were sterile; however, some recent studies have demonstrated that a biofilm forms by bacterial otopathogens. A bacterial pathogen is identified in ~1/3 of effusions from OME in children who undergo myringotomy and tube placement, most often in children younger than 2 years old. The common pathogens include nontypeable *H. influenzae*, *S. pneumoniae*, and *M. catarrhalis*.
- The contribution of allergies to OME in children is still controversial. One study of 209 children with OME in a UK allergic clinic found a history of allergic rhinitis, asthma, and eczema in 89%, 36%, and 24%, respectively (3).
- Gastroesophageal reflux has been hypothesized to be a cause of OME in children as well. However, studies measuring the concentration of pepsin and pepsinogen in middle-ear fluid have reported conflicting results.
- In adults, OME often occurs in association with eustachian tube dysfunction, but can also result from barotrauma or allergy.

DIAGNOSIS

HISTORY

- OME is often asymptomatic. It can be characterized by hearing loss or a sense of aural fullness. Older children and adults usually recognize the hearing impairment. An infant will not be able to express the hearing loss, but it may be apparent to the parent when observing and interacting with the child. Sleep disturbances are often reported by parents.
- OME is transient in most children and may not be diagnosed.
- Vertigo may occur, though it is not a common complaint. In the young child, vertigo can be recognized by imbalance, falling, stumbling, or clumsiness. The older child or adult with vertigo may describe a feeling of spinning or turning.
- In adults, there may be a history of recurrent episodes of AOM or a recent upper respiratory tract infection. There may also be an exacerbation in seasonal allergy symptoms or recent airplane travel.

PHYSICAL EXAM

- Clinical signs of acute illness or AOM are, by definition, absent in patients with OME, including bulging or erythema of the TM.
- Otoscopic findings of OME are fluid (often yellowish, but sometimes clear) visible behind a retracted tympanic membrane.

DIAGNOSTIC TESTS & INTERPRETATION

Diagnostic Procedures/Surgery

- A subcommittee comprised of members from the American Academy of Pediatrics, the American Academy of Family Physicians, and the American Academy of Otolaryngology-Head and Neck Surgery (AAP/AAFP/AAOHNS) developed a clinical practice guideline that delineates current diagnosis and management of children between 2 months and 12 years of age with OME (4).
- The gold standard to make the diagnosis is pneumatic otoscopy, which demonstrates reduced or absent mobility of the tympanic membrane secondary to fluid in the middle ear (4)[A].
- Tympanometry and acoustic reflectometry may also be used to support the diagnosis, especially when the presence of MEE is difficult to determine based upon routine physical exam and pneumatic otoscopy.

DIFFERENTIAL DIAGNOSIS

- Acute otitis media
- Bullous myringitis
- Tympanosclerosis (may cause decreased or absent motion of the tympanic membrane)
- Sensorineural hearing loss, including retrocochlear lesions

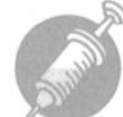

TREATMENT

- OME resolves without medical intervention in most patients.
- The goals of management are to eliminate the effusion, restore normal hearing, and prevent future episodes, if possible.
- Management options include watchful waiting, medications in limited situations, and surgery. Which strategy is chosen depends on many factors, including the risk of, or presence of, any associated speech, language, or learning delays and on the severity of any associated hearing loss.
- Many studies support the strategy of watchful waiting:
  - A 2005 Cochrane review was done on the use of tympanostomy tubes for hearing loss associated with OME in children. While children who received tympanostomy tubes spent less time with effusion during the first postoperative year, the gains seen in hearing diminished over time. In addition, no significant effects were seen on language development or cognition in otherwise healthy children.
  - Another longitudinal study evaluated children younger than 3 years old with persistent MEE and timing of tympanostomy tubes. Children were randomly assigned to prompt (<3 months) or delayed insertion of tubes, and development outcomes were assessed at periodic intervals from 3–11 years of age. No difference was noted between the 2 groups in literacy, attention, social skills, and academic achievement (5).

MEDICATION

- The AAP/AAFP/AAOHNS guideline recommends against routine use of antibiotics in treatment of OME (4)[A]:
  - Antibiotics have been found in a meta-analysis to improve clearance of the effusion within the first month after treatment, but relapses of an effusion were common, and no benefit was noted past the first month.
  - Amoxicillin is preferred for treatment of OME when antibiotics are used. Other antibiotics, including amoxicillin-clavulanate and ceftibuten, have been tested in clinical trials, but none has been clearly shown to have significant advantage over the others.
- Antihistamines and decongestants have little effect on OME in children and are not recommended (4)[A]. Multiple randomized, double-blind trials have shown that antihistamines plus decongestants fail to shorten the time to resolution of effusions.
- The AAP/AAFP/AAOHNS guideline recommends against administering oral or intranasal corticosteroids (4)[A].
- In adults, eustachian tube dysfunction secondary to allergic rhinitis or recent URI can be the cause of OME. As a result, most patients are treated with decongestants, antihistamines, and/or nasal steroids, despite a lack of data demonstrating a clear benefit. The majority of effusions will self-resolve over the course of 12 weeks, and most adult patients can be observed during this time.

ADDITIONAL TREATMENT

Issues for Referral

- The following are indications for referral to a surgeon for evaluation of tympanostomy tube placement:
  - Children with hearing loss ≥40 dB
  - Children who have structural damage to the tympanic membrane or middle ear (prompt referral is recommended)
  - Children who have OME of ≥4 months' duration with persistent hearing loss (≥21 dB) or other signs or symptoms related to the effusion (4)[B]
- It is also recommended that children with recurrent or persistent OME who are at risk of speech, language, or learning problems have early referral to a specialist, regardless of hearing status.

Additional Therapies

- Autoinflation, which refers to the process of opening the eustachian tube by raising intranasal pressure (e.g., by forced exhalation with closed mouth and nose or by mechanical device) has been evaluated, and it may be beneficial in the short term. A 2006 Cochrane review of 6 studies comparing any form of autoinflation to no autoinflation in children with OME found improvement in patients' tympanogram or audiometry results beyond 1 month.
- Studies of autoinflation have not been published in adults to date, but the maneuver is free, without significant adverse effects, and may be helpful for some patients.

SURGERY/OTHER PROCEDURES

- Adenoidectomy should not be performed in children with persistent OME alone unless there is a distinct indication for the procedure for another problem (e.g., chronic sinusitis or nasal obstruction) (4)[B]. Adenoidectomy (and concurrent tube placement) may be considered when repeat surgery for OME is necessary (e.g., when effusion recurs after tubes have fallen out or are removed) (4). In these cases, adenoidectomy has been shown to decrease the need for future procedures for OME.
- Tonsillectomy does not appear to improve the outcome for OME and is generally not advised (4)[B].
- In adults, myringotomy may be effective with few adverse effects; however, no randomized trials have been published to date evaluating myringotomy and tube placement in adults.

ONGOING CARE

FOLLOW-UP RECOMMENDATIONS

Patient Monitoring

- Children who are at risk for speech, language, or learning problems, and whose OME persists for ≥3 months should undergo hearing evaluation. The results of the hearing test can help determine the management strategy:
  - Children with hearing loss ≤20 dB and without speech, language, or developmental problems can be managed with watchful waiting.
  - Children with hearing loss 21–39 dB can be managed with watchful waiting or referred for surgery.
  - Children with hearing loss ≥40 dB should be referred for surgical evaluation (4)[B].
- Re-evaluation and repeat hearing tests should be performed every 3–6 months until the effusion has resolved or the child develops an indication for surgical referral. It is also reasonable to refer patients for surgical evaluation if the child has had bilateral OME for ≥3 months, unilateral OME ≥6 months, or cumulative duration of OME ≥12 months.
- For children with mild conductive hearing loss (21–39 dB) whose parents prefer the watchful waiting strategy, interventions in the home can help. These include speaking in close proximity to the child, facing the child and speaking clearly, and providing preferential seating in the classroom.

PROGNOSIS

Regular follow-up and evaluation are important to detect any hearing loss, speech, language, or learning delay. Surgical referral is important when indicated to prevent long-term sequelae. The prognosis for OME is otherwise good in low-risk children and adults.

COMPLICATIONS

- The most significant complication of OME is permanent conductive hearing loss, but pain, balance disturbance, and tinnitus may also occur.
- If the tympanic membrane becomes severely retracted, a cholesteatoma can occur. Another potential complication is tympanosclerosis, which is characterized by whitish plaques in the tympanic membrane.

REFERENCES

1. Casselbrant ML, Brostoff LM, Cantekin EI, et al. Otitis media with effusion in preschool children. *Laryngoscope*. 1985;95:428–36.
2. Lous J, Fiellau-Nikolajsen M, et al. Epidemiology and middle ear effusion and tubal dysfunction. A one-year prospective study comprising monthly tympanometry in 387 non-selected 7-year-old children. *Int J Pediatr Otorhinolaryngol*. 1981;3: 303–17.
3. Alles R, Parikh A, Hawk L, et al. The prevalence of atopic disorders in children with chronic otitis media with effusion. *Pediatr Allergy Immunol*. 2001;12:102–6.
4. American Academy of Family Physicians, American Academy of Otolaryngology-Head and Neck Surgery, American Academy of Pediatrics Subcommittee on Otitis Media With Effusion, et al. Otitis media with effusion. *Pediatrics*. 2004;113: 1412–29.
5. Paradise JL, Feldman HM, Campbell TF, et al. Effect of early or delayed insertion of tympanostomy tubes for persistent otitis media on developmental outcomes at the age of three years. *N Engl J Med*. 2001;344:1179.

ADDITIONAL READING

- Cantekin EI, Mandel EM, Bluestone CD, et al. Lack of efficacy of a decongestant-antihistamine combination for otitis media with effusion ("secretory" otitis media) in children. Results of a double-blind, randomized trial. *N Engl J Med*. 1983;308:297–301.
- Chan KH, Mandel EM, Rockette HE, et al. A comparative study of amoxicillin-clavulanate and amoxicillin. Treatment of otitis media with effusion. *Arch Otolaryngol Head Neck Surg*. 1988;114: 142–6.
- Gates GA, Avery CA, Prihoda TJ, Cooper JC, et al. Effectiveness of adenoidectomy and tympanostomy tubes in the treatment of chronic otitis media with effusion. *N Engl J Med*. 1987;317:1444–51.
- Hall-Stoodley L, Hu FZ, Gieseke A, et al. Direct detection of bacterial biofilms on the middle-ear mucosa of children with chronic otitis media. *JAMA* 2006;296:202.
- Lieu JE, Muthappan PG, Uppaluri R. Association of reflux with otitis media in children. *Otolaryngol Head Neck Surg*. 2005;133:357.
- Lous J, Burton MJ, Felding JU, et al. Grommets (ventilation tubes) for hearing loss associated with otitis media with effusion in children. *Cochrane Database Syst Rev*. 2005;1:CD001801.
- Mandel EM, Casselbrant ML, Kurs-Lasky M, et al. Efficacy of ceftibuten compared with amoxicillin for otitis media with effusion in infants and children. *Pediatr Infect Dis J*. 1996;15:409.
- Mandel EM, Rockette HE, Bluestone CD, et al. Efficacy of amoxicillin with and without decongestant-antihistamine for otitis media with effusion in children. Results of a double-blind, randomized trial. *N Engl J Med*. 1987;316:432–7.
- O'Reilly RC, He Z, Bloedon E, et al. The role of extraesophageal reflux in otitis media in infants and children. *Laryngoscope*. 2008;118:1.
- Paradise JL, Feldman HM, Campbell TF, et al. Tympanostomy tubes and developmental outcomes at 9 to 11 years of age. *N Engl J Med*. 2007;356: 248.
- Perera R, Haynes J, Glasziou P, et al. Autoinflation for hearing loss associated with otitis media with effusion. *Cochrane Database Syst Rev*. 2006;4: CD006285.
- Williams RL, Chalmers TC, Stange KC, et al. Use of antibiotics in preventing recurrent acute otitis media and in treating otitis media with effusion. A meta-analytic attempt to resolve the brouhaha. *JAMA*. 1993;270:1344.

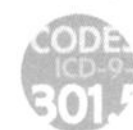

CODES

ICD9

381.20 Chronic mucoid otitis media, simple or unspecified

CLINICAL PEARLS

- OME is defined as the presence of an MEE in the absence of acute signs of infection.
- In children, OME most often arises following an AOM. In adults, it often occurs in association with eustachian tube dysfunction.
- The gold standard to make the diagnosis is pneumatic otoscopy.
- Avoid the use of antihistamines, decongestants, or corticosteroids (oral or intranasal) routinely for the management of OME in children, as they have not been shown to offer significant benefit.
- Management options include watchful waiting, medications in limited situations, and surgery. Which strategy is chosen depends upon many factors, including the risk of, or presence of, any associated speech, language, or learning delays and on the severity of any associated hearing loss.

OVARIAN CANCER

Elizabeth B. Pelkofski, MD
Lindsay Abcunas, MD
Susan L. Zwiezig, MD

BASICS

There are over 22,000 new cases of ovarian cancer annually, and >13,000 women will die of their disease, making this the most lethal of gynecologic cancers.

DESCRIPTION

Malignancy that arises from the epithelium (85–90%), stroma, or germ cells of the ovary; also, tumors metastatic to the ovary; histologic types include:

- Epithelial:
  - Serous (tubal epithelium)
  - Mucinous (cervical and GI mucinous epithelium)
  - Endometrioid (endometrial epithelium)
  - Clear cell (mesonephroid)
  - Brenner (transitional cell epithelium)
  - Carcinosarcoma
- Stromal:
  - Granulosa cell tumor
  - Theca cell tumor
  - Sertoli–Leydig cell tumors
  - Gynandroblastoma
  - Lipid cell tumor
- Germ cell:
  - Teratoma (immature)
  - Dysgerminoma
  - Embryonal carcinoma
  - Gonadoblastoma
  - Endodermal sinus tumor
  - Embryonal carcinoma
  - Choriocarcinoma
- Metastatic disease from:
  - Breast
  - Endometrium
  - Lymphoma
  - GI tract (Krukenberg tumor)
  - Primary peritoneal
- System(s) affected: Gastrointestinal; Reproductive; Endocrine; Metabolic

EPIDEMIOLOGY

Incidence

- 21,880 new cases/yr in the US; 13,850 deaths/yr
- Leading cause of gynecologic cancer death in women; mortality from ovarian cancer has decreased only slightly during the last 4 decades.
- 75% diagnosed at advanced stage
- Predominant age:
  - Epithelial: Mid-50s
  - Germ cell malignancies: Usually observed in patients <20 years of age

Prevalence

Lifetime risk for general population: 1 in 70 women develops ovarian cancer.

RISK FACTORS

- 90% of ovarian cancer is sporadic and not inherited, but family history is the most significant risk factor. One first-degree relative increases risk to 5%; 2 relatives, to 7%; individuals in families with familial cancer syndromes have 20–60% risk of developing ovarian cancer.
- Nulligravity (or infertility), early menarche, late menopause, endometriosis
- Environmental (talc, smoking, obesity)

Genetics

- Breast/ovarian cancer syndrome: Early-onset breast or ovarian cancer, autosomal-dominant transmission, usually associated with *BRCA-1* or *BRCA-2* mutation
- Lynch II syndrome: Autosomal-dominant inheritance; increased risk for colorectal, endometrial, stomach, small bowel, breast, pancreas, and ovarian cancers; defect in mismatch repair genes

GENERAL PREVENTION

For epithelial cancer, frequency of ovulation appears to be important. The following factors are protective:

- Use of oral contraceptives: 5 years of use decreases risk by 20%; 15 years, by 50%:
  - The progestin component of oral contraceptive preparations (OCPs) may protect against ovarian cancer by regulating apoptosis of the ovarian epithelium.
- Multiparity
- Breast-feeding
- Tubal ligation or hysterectomy
- Recent studies have shown that no clear association exists between ovarian cancer and use of ovulation-induction agents such as clomiphene, but more long-term studies are necessary.
- NSAID and acetaminophen use have been shown to reduce risk of ovarian cancer (1)[B].
- Recommendations for high-risk populations:
  - Women with a family history of a hereditary ovarian cancer syndrome should undergo pelvic examinations, CA-125 level measurement, and transvaginal ultrasonography every 6–12 months beginning at ages 25–35.
  - Women with family histories of ovarian cancer or premenopausal breast cancer should be referred for genetic counseling.
  - Prophylactic oophorectomy is advised for mutation carriers after child-bearing is completed or by age 35:
    - Risk of primary peritoneal carcinoma is 1% after prophylactic oophorectomy.
- Screening: No effective screening exists for ovarian cancer:
  - Routine use of CA-125 and transvaginal ultrasound for screening in women of average risk is discouraged. Annual pelvic examinations are recommended, particularly in postmenopausal women. An adnexal mass in a premenarchal female or a palpable adnexa in a postmenopausal female warrants further evaluation.

PATHOPHYSIOLOGY

- Malignant transformation of the ovarian epithelium from repeated minor trauma during ovulation may lead to this change.
- Most ovarian cancer (75%) presents as advanced disease. Metastatic disease may develop at the same time as the primary tumor.

COMMONLY ASSOCIATED CONDITIONS

- Ascites
- Pleural effusion
- Decrease of serum albumin
- Breast carcinoma
- Bowel obstruction
- Carcinomatosis

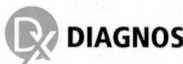

DIAGNOSIS

HISTORY

- Bloating
- Early satiety, anorexia, dyspepsia
- Sense of abdominal fullness, increased abdominal size
- Abdominopelvic pain or cramping
- Urinary frequency or urgency in absence of infection
- Fatigue
- Dyspareunia
- Weight loss
- Severe pain secondary to ovarian rupture or torsion most frequent in germ cell tumors
- Precocious puberty (choriocarcinoma, embryonal carcinoma)

PHYSICAL EXAM

- Ascites
- Cul-de-sac and/or pelvic nodularity
- Pelvic mass
- Pleural effusion
- Omental mass
- Cachexia
- Adenopathy
- Hirsutism in androgen-secreting germ cell tumors

DIAGNOSTIC TESTS & INTERPRETATION

Lab

Initial lab tests

- CA-125 (not specific for ovarian cancer)
- Liver function tests (LFTs) to rule out hepatic disease
- CBC
- Urinalysis
- Serum albumin
- Carcinoembryonic antigen (CEA) if GI primary suspected
- If nonepithelial tumor suspected: Chorionic gonadotropin (β-hCG [dysgerminoma, choriocarcinoma, embryonal carcinoma]), α-fetoprotein (endodermal sinus tumor, embryonal carcinoma), lactate dehydrogenase (LDH [dysgerminoma]), or inhibin (granulosa cell tumor)

Follow-Up & Special Considerations

Disorders that may alter lab results: CA-125 may be elevated from gynecologic causes (e.g., menses, pregnancy, endometriosis, peritonitis, myomas, pelvic inflammatory disease) and with ascites, pleural effusion, congestive heart failure (CHF), pancreatitis, systemic lupus erythematosus (SLE), or liver disease.

Imaging

Initial approach

- Pelvic ultrasound
- CXR
- Abdominopelvic CT scan with contrast material

Follow-Up & Special Considerations

- Patients with ovarian cancer need current mammography.
- Barium enema or colonoscopy if a colon primary is suspected

Diagnostic Procedures/Surgery

- Endometrial biopsy if abnormal bleeding present
- Surgery is necessary for definitive diagnosis.
- Paracentesis if patient with symptomatic ascites and not an operative candidate

Pathological Findings

Epithelial ovarian cancer commonly involves the peritoneal surfaces of the abdomen and pelvis, especially the cul-de-sac, paracolic gutters, and diaphragmatic surfaces.

DIFFERENTIAL DIAGNOSIS

- GI, fallopian, or endometrial malignancies
- Irritable bowel syndrome
- Colitis
- Hepatic failure with ascites
- Diverticulitis
- Pelvic kidney
- Tubo-ovarian abscess or hydrosalpinx
- Uterine fibroids
- Endometriomas
- Physiologic cysts
- Benign or borderline neoplasms

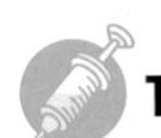

TREATMENT

MEDICATION

First Line

- After surgery, most patients will require chemotherapy. Stage 1a, grade 1 and most stage 1b, grade 1 tumors do not require adjuvant therapy. Patients with clear cell carcinomas, grade 3 tumors, or tumors staged 1c or worse require adjuvant therapy. Patients should be encouraged to participate in clinical trials whenever possible.
- Paclitaxel (Taxol) is recommended in combination with platinum-based therapy as the first-line treatment of epithelial ovarian cancer.
- Intraperitoneal (IP) chemotherapy in combination with IV chemotherapy improves survival in advanced ovarian cancer (2)[A]. IP chemotherapy is associated with more toxicity.
- Germ cell cancers: Bleomycin, etoposide, platinum agent (3)[A]
- Contraindications: Poor functional status, excessive toxicity, hypersensitivity
- Precautions: All regimens cause bone marrow suppression. Cisplatin is associated with ototoxicity, renal toxicity, and peripheral neuropathy. Taxol can cause neutropenia and neuropathy.
- Antiemetic: Ondansetron (Zofran), dronabinol (Marinol), metoclopramide (Reglan), prochlorperazine (Compazine), promethazine (Phenergan)

Second Line

- Liposomal doxorubicin
- Carboplatin/gemcitabine
- Topotecan
- Taxotere
- Etoposide
- Bevacizumab
- Cyclophosphamide
- Tamoxifen may be used in recurrent disease when chemotherapy is not appropriate (4)[B].

SURGERY/OTHER PROCEDURES

- Surgical exploration with staging and debulking is critical. Maximal cytoreduction of tumor burden enhances effectiveness of adjuvant therapy and is associated with longer survival.
- For epithelial malignancies, careful staging, tumor excision/debulking includes:
  - Cytologic evaluation of peritoneal fluid (or washings from peritoneal lavage)
  - Bilateral salpingo-oophorectomy with hysterectomy and tumor reductive surgery
  - Excision of omentum
  - Inspection and palpation of peritoneal surfaces
  - Cytologic smear of right hemidiaphragmatic surface
  - Biopsy of adhesions or any suspicious areas
  - Biopsy of paracolic recesses, pelvic sidewalls, posterior cul-de-sac, and bladder peritoneum
  - Pelvic and para-aortic lymph node biopsies
- Germ cell cancers (less likely to be bilateral): Salpingo-oophorectomy (unilateral if only 1 ovary involved) in young patient

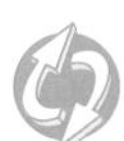

ONGOING CARE

FOLLOW-UP RECOMMENDATIONS

Patient Monitoring

- Physical exam every 3 months for the first 2 years after diagnosis; every 6 months until 5 years and then yearly thereafter (5)[C]
- If CA-125 elevated at diagnosis, can follow levels after treatment to detect recurrence (is often elevated 2–5 months before clinical detection of relapse) (5,6)[C]
- Germ cell/sex-cord stromal cancer: Physical exam and tumor markers every 3 months for the first 2 years after diagnosis:
  - Tumor markers for sex-cord stromal cancers should be checked every 6 months for 10 years, as recurrences can occur remote from initial diagnosis (5)[C].
- CT scan of chest, abdomen, and pelvis and/or PET scan when suspect recurrence
- Screening with CXR, MRI, CT, or PET not recommended, as insufficient data to support

PROGNOSIS

- Recurrence rates:
  - Early-stage disease: 25%
  - Advanced disease: >80%
- 5-year survival rates for ovarian cancer based on FIGO data:

Stage I	a 90%	b 86%	c 83%
Stage II	a 71%	b 66%	c 71%
Stage III	a 47%	b 42%	c 33%
Stage IV	19%		

COMPLICATIONS

- Pleural effusion
- Pseudomyxoma peritonei
- Ascites
- Toxicity of chemotherapy
- Bowel obstruction
- Malnutrition
- Electrolyte disturbances
- Fistula formation

REFERENCES

1. Collaborative Group on epidemiological Studies of Ovarian cancer: Beral V, Doll R, Hermon C, et al. Ovarian cancer and oral contraceptives: Collaborative reanalysis of data from 45 epidemiological studies including 23,257 women with ovarian cancer and 87,303 controls. *Lancet*. 2008;371:303–14.
2. Armstrong DK, Bundy B, Wenzel L, et al. Intraperitoneal cisplatin and paclitaxel in ovarian cancer. *N Engl J Med*. 2006;354:34–43.
3. Schumer ST, Cannistra SA. Granulosa cell tumor of the ovary. *J Clin Oncol*. 2003;21:1180–9.
4. Orlando M, Costanzo MV, Chacon RD. Randomized trial of combination chemotherapy versus monotherapy in relapsed ovarian carcinoma: A meta-analysis of published data. *J Clin Oncol*. 2007;25:280s.
5. Salani R, Backes F, Fung M, et al. Posttreatment surveillance and diagnosis of recurrence in women with gynecologic malignancies: Society of Gynecologic Oncologists recommendations. *Am J Obstet Gynecol*. 2011;204:466–76.
6. Gadducci A, Cosio S, Zola P, et al. Surveillance procedures for patients treated for epithelial ovarian cancer: A review of the literature. *Int J Gynecol Cancer*. 2007;17:21–31.

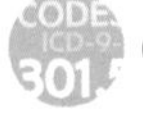

CODES

ICD9

183.0 Malignant neoplasm of ovary

CLINICAL PEARLS

- Family history of ovarian cancer or early-onset breast cancer is the most significant risk factor for the development of ovarian cancer, yet the vast majority of cases remain sporadic.
- The diagnosis of ovarian cancer should be suspected in women with persistent bloating, upper abdominal discomfort, or GI symptoms of unknown etiology.
- Surgery is the mainstay of treatment for ovarian cancer, though many patients benefit from adjuvant chemotherapy.
- The prognosis of ovarian cancer is poor and requires close follow-up by physical exam, tumor markers, and imaging when indicated.

OVARIAN CYST, RUPTURED

Leah Wilson, MD
Mark J. Manning, DO, MsMEL

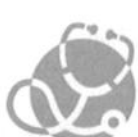

BASICS

- Ovarian cysts are very common. Women of reproductive age develop ovarian cysts with each ovulatory cycle.
- Ovarian cyst rupture and hemorrhage (of follicle or corpus luteum) are essentially physiologic events.
- A ruptured ovarian cyst is usually asymptomatic but sometimes causes pain ranging from mild to severe due to peritoneal irritation (blood and sebaceous material most irritating).
- Symptomatic ruptured ovarian cysts can usually be managed as an outpatient but occasionally require surgical intervention.

DESCRIPTION

Types of ovarian cysts that may rupture fall into 2 groups: Physiologic and pathologic (1)[C]:

- Physiologic or functional cysts form as a result of normal hormonal stimulation of the ovary. Most are asymptomatic and spontaneously resolve in 60–90 days:
  - Follicular cysts form when a growing follicle fails to rupture and release an egg:
    - Most common type of functional cyst
    - Unilateral and filled with serous fluid
  - Corpus luteum cysts occur when an egg is released and pregnancy does not occur. The residual structure does not regress and may hemorrhage internally (hemorrhagic cysts).
  - Theca-lutein cysts result from excessive stimulation of beta-human chorionic gonadotropin such as in infertility patients, molar pregnancies, or choriocarcinoma. These cysts are also susceptible to internal hemorrhage.
- Pathologic cysts are caused by a process other than normal hormonal stimulation. When followed, these cysts remain stable in size or may grow:
  - Endometriomas are cysts or collections of blood clot that form as a result of cycling endometrial tissue on the ovary. Also called "chocolate cysts" due to their appearance.
  - Mature cystic teratoma (dermoid) develop from totipotent germ cells:
    - Most commonly, they contain mucinous material and hair.
    - Up to 14% are bilateral and can grow very large.
    - <1% rupture spontaneously but may lead to shock, hemorrhage, and acute peritonitis.
  - Cystadenomas may have solid or mucinous areas and are usually benign but may have borderline malignant areas. They rarely rupture.
  - Other cystic-appearing adnexal structures include paratubal cysts, tubo-ovarian abscess, hydrosalpinx, ectopic pregnancy.

EPIDEMIOLOGY

- The exact incidence difficult to determine due to asymptomatic nature of most cysts and cyst rupture.
- Annual incidence of acute pelvic pain attributed to ovarian cysts in the US has been quoted at 65,000 (2)[B].
- 4% of women are admitted to hospital with an ovarian cyst by age 65 (3)[B].

RISK FACTORS

Increased risk of developing physiologic cysts associated with:

- Smoking
- Levonorgesterel IUD (4)[B]
- Tamoxifen (5)[B]

GENERAL PREVENTION

For patients with painful, recurrent ovarian cysts, oral contraceptive pills can be prescribed to suppress ovulation:

- This may help prevent the formation of new cysts but will not impact cysts that have already formed (6)[A].

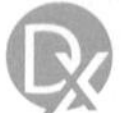

DIAGNOSIS

- A ruptured ovarian cyst may be asymptomatic or present as abdominal pain, varying from dull to acute.
- The broad range of presentations can prove to be a diagnostic dilemma for many physicians.

HISTORY

- A general past medical and surgical history should be reviewed.
- Risk factors for gynecologic pain should be elicited:
  - Possibility of pregnancy
  - Menstrual history with attention to symptoms suggestive of endometriosis or history of cysts
  - STD history
  - Levonorgestrel-containing intrauterine device (up to 12% of users experience ovarian cysts) (4)[B]
  - Infertility treatment
- Typical features of pain due to ruptured ovarian cyst include:
  - Pain often begins during strenuous activity (exercise or intercourse)
  - Sudden onset, unilateral pelvic pain that becomes more dull and generalized over time.
  - Pain is worse with movement
- Other causes of acute abdominal pain should also be considered, including GI and urologic etiologies.

ALERT

Patients with bleeding diathesis or undergoing anticoagulation therapy may experience significant bleeding from hemorrhagic cysts.

PHYSICAL EXAM

- Vital signs are typically normal. Low-grade fever may be present.
- If significant blood loss has occurred, may have signs of hypovolemic shock (uncommon).
- Tenderness in unilateral lower quadrant (right side more common)
- Peritoneal signs may be present depending on degree of peritoneal irritation.
- May have cervical motion tenderness

DIAGNOSTIC TESTS & INTERPRETATION

Lab

- Pregnancy test is an important first test for ruling out ectopic pregnancy as a cause of the pain.
- CBC is useful:
  - Hematocrit is best compared to a baseline hematocrit.
  - Elevated WBC count or left shift may indicate infectious etiology.
  - Low platelets can worsen bleeding.
- Cervical cultures if pelvic inflammatory disease is suspected
- Urinalysis to evaluate possibility of infection or stones
- Blood type and cross-matching if the patient is hemodynamically unstable and surgery is planned
- Tumor markers (i.e., CA-125): Not recommended for initial evaluation. May be elevated in a number of benign conditions including hemoperitoneum. Not likely to help in diagnosis or management

Imaging

- Transvaginal ultrasound is first-line imaging modality (1)[C],(7)[B]
- Findings may include:
  - Adnexal mass: Features may suggest type of cyst/tumor
  - Free fluid in pelvis: Usually small amount but large amount may indicate ongoing hemorrhage
- CT scan is second line and not typically helpful. Use if nongynecologic pathology suspected

DIFFERENTIAL DIAGNOSIS

Should include all causes of acute abdominal pain, both gynecologic and nongynecologic, such as:

- Ectopic pregnancy
- Ovarian torsion
- Pelvic inflammatory disease ± tubo-ovarian abscess
- Ovarian hyperstimulation syndrome (OHSS)
- Ovarian cancer with ascites
- Appendicitis
- Diverticulitis
- Nephrolithiasis
- Bowel obstruction or perforation

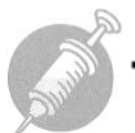

TREATMENT

MEDICATION

- For uncomplicated cyst ruptures (absence of hemodynamic instability, acute abdomen, enlarging hemoperitoneum, ultrasound evidence of malignancy), goal should be conservative therapy if possible.
- Pain due to an uncomplicated cyst rupture is usually self-limiting and can be managed on an outpatient basis with pain medication and rest (3)[B].

First Line

NSAIDs are the most effective at relieving pain due to peritoneal irritation.

Second Line

Narcotic pain medications may also be necessary acutely.

ADDITIONAL TREATMENT

Issues for Referral

- The vast majority of ruptured ovarian cysts are a result of functional cysts in reproductive-age women and the risk of malignancy is very low.
- Referral to a gynecologic oncologist should be made in any postmenopausal female with an adnexal mass that has concerning ultrasound findings, an elevated CA-125, ascites, a nodular, fixed pelvic mass and a family history of breast or ovarian cancer (1,7).

SURGERY/OTHER PROCEDURES

For complicated ovarian cyst rupture (hemodynamic instability, significant hemoperitoneum, concern for ovarian torsion) or if patient is deteriorating, surgical evaluation is recommended (3)[B]:

- Laparoscopy is typically preferred but approach should be based on surgeon's comfort and expertise, patient factors (clinical condition, body habitus, previous abdominal surgeries, etc) (1)[C],(7)[B].
- Surgery includes suction-evacuation of any fluid or blood found in the pelvis as well as achieving hemostasis, if needed, at the site of the cyst:
  - If a cyst wall is present, it should be removed.
- In the vast majority of cases, oophorectomy is not necessary.
- Laparoscopic excision of the cyst and capsule of endometriomas substantially decreases risk of recurrence (8)[A].

IN-PATIENT CONSIDERATIONS

Inpatient management may include IV hydration, monitoring of vital signs, serial hematocrits, and pain control.

ONGOING CARE

FOLLOW-UP RECOMMENDATIONS

- Patient should have follow up ultrasound in 6 weeks.
- Most functional cysts resolve spontaneously without treatment and "watchful waiting" with serial transvaginal ultrasounds for 2–3 cycles is appropriate.
- If cysts fail to resolve or develop concerning ultrasound findings (increasing size or complexity, nodules, septations, excrescences), they may be pathologic and surgical evaluation is recommended (6)[A].
- With an uncomplicated cyst rupture, fluid typically resorbs in 24 hours and symptoms resolve within 2–3 days

Pregnancy Considerations

Ovarian cysts in pregnancy:

- With the widespread use of ultrasonography during pregnancy, up to 4% of pregnant women are found to have adnexal masses, most of which are follicular cysts which spontaneously resolve by 16 weeks' gestation.
- <2% will spontaneously rupture or torse during pregnancy; however, this can lead to preterm labor and delivery, which may cause poor obstetric outcomes.
- If they are painful, large (>8 cm), or have ultrasound characteristics that are concerning for malignancy, elective surgical evaluation may be considered (1)[C],(7)[B].

PATIENT EDUCATION

Patient handout on pelvic pain at aafp.org

REFERENCES

1. Stany MP, Hamilton CA, et al. Benign disorders of the ovary. *Obstet Gynecol Clin North Am*. 2008;35: 271–84, ix.
2. Kruszka PS, Kruszka SJ. Evaluation of acute pelvic pain in women. *Am Fam Physician*. 2010;82(2): 141–47.
3. Bottomley C, Bourne T, et al. Diagnosis and management of ovarian cyst accidents. *Best Pract Res Clin Obstet Gynaecol*. 2009;23:711–24.
4. Mirena [package insert]. Wayne, NJ: Bayer HealthCare Pharmaceuticals Inc.; 2009.
5. Tamoxifen citrate [package insert]. Wilmington, DE: riston Meyers Squibb Pharmaceuticals Inc: 2003.
6. Grimes DA, Jones LB, et al. Oral contraceptives for functional ovarian cysts. *Cochrane Database Syst Rev*. 2009;2:CD006134.
7. Management of Adnexal Masses ACOG Practice Bulletin No. 83. *Obstet Gynecol*. 2007;110: 201–14.
8. Hart RJ, Hickey M, Maouris P, et al. Excisional surgery versus ablative surgery for ovarian endometriomata. *Cochrane Database Syst Rev*. 2008;2:CD004992.

ADDITIONAL READING

- Falcone T. Risk of complications from gynecological surgery is lower with laparoscopy than with laparotomy. *Evidence Based Obstet Gynecol*. 2004;4:185–6A.
- Hoo WL, Yazbek J, Holland T, et al. Expectant management of ultrasonically diagnosed ovarian dermoid cysts: Is it possible to predict outcome? *Ultrasound Obstet Gynecol*. 2010;36:235–40.
- Huchon C, Staraci S, Fauconnier A, et al. Adnexal torsion: A predictive score for pre-operative diagnosis. *Hum Reprod*. 2010;25:2276–80.
- Møller LM, et al. [Complications of gynaecological operations. A one-year analysis of a hospital database] *Ugeskr Laeg*. 2005;167:4654–9.
- Raziel A, Ron-El R, et al. Current management of ruptured corpus luteum. *Eur J Obstet Gynecol Reprod Biol*. 1993;50:77–81.
- Saunders BA, Podzielinski I, Ware RA, et al. Risk of malignancy in sonographically confirmed septated cystic ovarian tumors. *Gynecol Oncol*. 2010;118: 278–82.

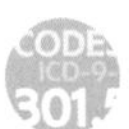

CODES

ICD9

620.2 Other and unspecified ovarian cyst

CLINICAL PEARLS

- Functional ovarian cysts are very common in reproductive-age women and usually resolve spontaneously in 60–90 days.
- If a cyst does rupture, the pain is usually self-limited and can be treated with oral pain medications on an outpatient basis.
- Surgery may be necessary if pain is extreme or if the patient is unstable. This usually involves laparoscopically evacuating irritating fluid and blood from the abdominal cavity, achieving hemostasis, and removing the cyst wall if possible.

OVARIAN HYPERSTIMULATION SYNDROME (OHSS)

Kimberly E. Liu, MD, FRCSC, MSI
Ellen Greenblatt, MD, FRCSC

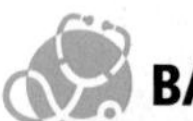

BASICS

DESCRIPTION

- Iatrogenic physiologic complication of controlled ovarian hyperstimulation (most often related to treatment for infertility)
- Results in ovarian enlargement, increased vascular permeability with resulting third-space loss and intravascular fluid depletion, electrolyte imbalance, hemoconcentration, and ascites
- Classification of OHSS is based on clinical symptoms and ultrasound findings:
  - Mild: Abdominal distension and discomfort
  - Moderate: Abdominal distension, enlarged ovaries (8–10 cm^3) and ascites on ultrasound (largest pocket <3 cm)
  - Severe: Clinical evidence of ascites and/or hydrothorax, hemoconcentration >45%
  - Critical: Hemoconcentration >55%, creatinine clearance <50 mL/min, renal failure, thromboembolism, ARDS
- Symptoms of OHSS may occur early (within 10 days of hCG administration) or late (more than 10 days after hCG administration). Late OHSS is usually associated with a pregnancy and may often be more severe.

EPIDEMIOLOGY

Incidence

- Predominant age: Women of reproductive age
- With controlled ovarian hyperstimulation (COH) and in vitro fertilization (IVF):
  - Mild OHSS: 20–33% of cycles
  - Moderate OHSS: 3–6% of cycles
  - Severe OHSS: 0.1–2% of cycles

RISK FACTORS

- Previous history of OHSS
- Young age
- Low body weight
- Polycystic ovary syndrome (PCOS) or polycystic ovaries on ultrasound
- Large number of resting follicles (>10 follicles between 2 and 8 mm) per ovary
- High doses of gonadotropins
- Large number of intermediate-sized follicles
- Number of oocytes retrieved
- Rapidly rising estradiol levels
- High estradiol levels >3,000/4,000 pg/mL
- Use of human chorionic gonadotropin (hCG) for luteal support
- Achievement of a pregnancy
- Multiple pregnancy

GENERAL PREVENTION

- Patients who have had OHSS are more at risk for OHSS in the future, and this should be taken into consideration in subsequent treatment cycles. Patients need to inform their health care providers of a history of OHSS when considering further assisted reproductive technology treatment.
- A general principle in the prevention of OHSS is to recognize patients at high risk based on the above listed risk factors and to use low doses of stimulation and frequent monitoring.
- If a patient develops risk factors during stimulation, consideration should be given to canceling the cycle by withholding the preovulatory injection of hCG, proceeding with a lower dose of hCG, the use of a GnRH agonist to trigger ovulation in GnRH antagonist cycles, "coasting" or withholding stimulatory drugs for several days to allow for estradiol levels to plateau or decrease, avoiding the use of hCG for luteal supporting, or freezing all viable embryos without proceeding with an embryo transfer (1)[B].
- Recent evidence suggests that the off-label use of dopamine agonists (cabergoline 0.5 mg) after hCG administration may decrease the incidence of OHSS (2)[A].

PATHOPHYSIOLOGY

- Ovarian hyperstimulation leads to increased capillary permeability and intravascular fluid shifts (3).
- Fluid shifts can lead to ascites and pleural effusions.
- Intravascular volume depletion can lead to hemoconcentration, decreased renal perfusion, and thrombosis.
- The ovarian renin–angiotensin system, cytokines, and other inflammatory mediators, such as vascular endothelial growth factor (VEGF), may play a role in the pathophysiology of OHSS.

ETIOLOGY

- OHSS is an iatrogenic syndrome that occurs during controlled ovarian hyperstimulation (COH) for infertility treatment.
- Generally, OHSS is associated with the use of exogenous gonadotropins, such as recombinant or purified follicle-stimulating hormone (FSH).
- OHSS rarely has been associated with types of ovarian stimulation, such as clomiphene citrate.

COMMONLY ASSOCIATED CONDITIONS

- Infertility
- PCOS
- Assisted reproductive technologies

DIAGNOSIS

OHSS is a clinical diagnosis based on history, physical exam, ultrasound findings, and laboratory results.

HISTORY

- Details of stimulation cycle:
  - Medications used
  - Date of oocyte retrieval and embryo transfer
- Symptoms of dehydration
- Abdominal pain and distension
- Nausea, vomiting, diarrhea
- Shortness of breath
- Loss of appetite
- Weight changes
- Fluid intake
- Lethargy
- Risks factors such as PCOS or previous OHSS

PHYSICAL EXAM

- Vital signs, including O_2 saturation if shortness of breath
- Weight (daily)
- Monitoring of ins and outs (daily or more often as needed)
- Chest and cardiovascular exam
- Abdominal circumference measured at the umbilicus (daily)
- Gentle abdominal exam to detect ascites

ALERT

Pelvic and bimanual examinations are contraindicated to avoid ovarian hemorrhage or rupture.

DIAGNOSTIC TESTS & INTERPRETATION

Lab

Initial lab tests

- CBC:
  - Hemoconcentration (hematocrit >45% indicates severe disease, >55% indicates critical disease)
  - WBC >15,000 indicates severe disease
- Electrolytes to look for hyponatremia and hyperkalemia
- Renal function tests
- Liver enzymes
- Coagulation profile
- β-hCG

Follow-Up & Special Considerations

For patients with mild or moderate OHSS being monitored as an outpatient, CBC and electrolytes should be performed every 1–2 days, until improvement in symptoms.

Imaging

Initial approach

- Abdominal/pelvic ultrasound to assess ovarian size, ovarian torsion or rupture, and abdominal ascites
- CXR to evaluate pleural effusion in presence of shortness of breath

Follow-Up & Special Considerations

Repeat abdominal/pelvic ultrasound as needed to assess ascites and guide management for paracentesis.

Pathological Findings

- Ovarian enlargement
- Decreased renal perfusion
- Thromboembolism
- Abdominal ascites
- Pleural effusions
- Pericardial effusions

DIFFERENTIAL DIAGNOSIS

- Hemorrhagic ovarian cyst
- Ovarian torsion
- Ectopic pregnancy
- Pelvic infection

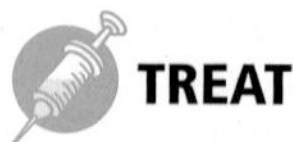

TREATMENT

MEDICATION

- Heparin 5,000 units SC q8–12h; all hospitalized patients should be on anticoagulation prophylaxis and graduated compression stockings to prevent thrombotic events (4)[C].
- Full anticoagulation therapy should be started if there is evidence of a thromboembolic event.

ADDITIONAL TREATMENT

General Measures

- Mild to moderate OHSS: Generally managed as outpatient:
  - Oral fluid intake of at least 1 L daily of a balanced electrolyte solution (sports drinks) (4)[C]
  - Monitor daily weight, abdominal circumference, and urine output (4)[C].
  - Avoid physical exertion or abdominal trauma.
  - Monitor for development of further symptoms.
  - Frequent follow-up is required.
  - For moderate OHSS, frequent assessments every 1–2 days including a physical examination and blood work, should occur.
  - Consider hospitalization with worsening signs or symptoms:
    - Severe abdominal pain
    - Severe oliguria or anuria
    - Tense ascites
    - Dyspnea or tachypnea
    - Hypotension, dizziness, or syncope
    - Severe electrolyte imbalance: Hyponatremia <135 mEq/L, hyperkalemia >5 mEq/L, hemocrit >45%
- Severe OHSS: Should be managed as an inpatient (5):
  - Daily weight and abdominal circumference
  - Frequent monitoring of vital signs every 2–8 hours
  - Strict monitoring of input and output to maintain urine output of 20–30 cc/hr
  - Bed rest or reduced activity; the enlarged ovaries are at risk of torsion and ovarian hemorrhage either spontaneously or from injury or trauma
  - With severe illness, oral fluids should be limited and rehydration provided with IV fluids until evidence of symptom resolution such as spontaneous diuresis (7)[A].
  - IV fluids should be administered to maintain urine output to 20–30 mL/hr. Normal saline with 5% dextrose is preferred to Ringer's lactate (4)[C].
  - Once third-space edema re-enters the intravascular space, hemoconcentration reverses and the patient begins to diurese spontaneously.
  - Monitor leukocyte count, hematocrit and hemoglobin, electrolytes, creatinine, and liver enzymes.
  - Thrombosis prophylaxis (4)[C]
  - Intensive monitoring may be required for pulmonary support in cases of acute respiratory distress syndrome, thromboembolic events, or for renal failure.

Issues for Referral

Consultation with a reproductive endocrinology specialist or a gynecologist with experience in the management of OHSS and its complications.

SURGERY/OTHER PROCEDURES

- Paracentesis/thoracentesis may be required for symptomatic control and for pulmonary and/or renal compromise. An ultrasound-guided approach for paracentesis is recommended to avoid the enlarged ovaries:
  - Indications for paracentesis include severe discomfort or pain, respiratory compromise, evidence of hydrothorax, or persistent oliguria/anuria despite adequate fluid replacement.
- Surgery should be avoided whenever possible in these patients.
- When ovarian hemorrhage is suspected, surgery may be necessary. The goal should be hemostasis, and the ovaries should be conserved when possible.
- In a situation of ovarian torsion, surgery may be performed to attempt to revascularize the ovary by unwinding the adnexa.

IN-PATIENT CONSIDERATIONS

Inpatients should have a CBC and electrolytes daily. Renal function, liver enzymes, and coagulation profile should be repeated as needed.

Initial Stabilization

Vital signs and O_2 saturation

Admission Criteria

- Abdominal pain suspicious of torsion or hemorrhage
- Intolerance of food or liquids
- Hypotension
- Significant ascites or plural effusions
- Hemoconcentration: Hematocrit >50%; WBC count >25,000
- Hyponatremia (Na <135 mEq/L)
- Hyperkalemia (K >5 mEq/L)

IV Fluids

- With severe illness, IV fluid rehydration should be used. After an initial bolus of 500–1,000 mL, fluid administration should continue to maintain a urine output of at least 20–30 mL/hr. D_5NS is preferred over Ringer's lactate because of the risk of hyponatremia.
- Albumin 25% (50–100 g) should be reserved for situations in which IV fluids are inadequate to maintain hemodynamic stability or urine output.
- Diuretics should be used cautiously and only after intravascular volume has been restored. Diuretics may aggravate hypovolemia and hemoconcentration.

Discharge Criteria

- Tolerating oral liquids and diet
- Resolution of hemoconcentration and electrolyte imbalances
- Adequate urine output

ONGOING CARE

FOLLOW-UP RECOMMENDATIONS

Patients discharged from the hospital should be followed with frequent health care provider contact until symptom resolution.

Patient Monitoring

Patients who have conceived should have an early ultrasound to confirm pregnancy and rule out multiple gestations and then routine antenatal care as indicated by their pregnancy.

DIET

Consume 1–1.5 L daily of a balanced salt solution, such as a sports drink, until resolution of symptoms.

PATIENT EDUCATION

- Monitor oral intake and urinary output.
- Reduce activity to avoid abdominal trauma or impact
- American Congress of Obstetricians and Gynecologists (ACOG) at www.acog.org

PROGNOSIS

OHSS is a self-limited disease that will run its course over 10–14 days in the absence of an ensuing pregnancy and may persist for weeks in a pregnant patient. Supportive treatment is initiated to prevent further deterioration of the patient's condition.

COMPLICATIONS

- Ovarian hemorrhage or torsion
- Arterial and venous thrombosis
- Acute respiratory distress syndrome (ARDS)
- Liver or renal failure

Pregnancy Considerations

- Patients who conceive a multiple gestation are at higher risk of OHSS.
- Studies have shown an increased risk of prematurity, low birth weight, pregnancy-induced hypertension, and gestational diabetes in women who had severe OHSS (6)[B].

REFERENCES

1. Vloeberghs V, Peeraer K, Pexsters A, et al. Ovarian hyperstimulation syndrome and complications of ART. *Best Pract Res Clin Obstet Gynaecol*. 2009; 23:691–709.
2. Youssef MA, van Wely M, Hassan MA, et al. Can dopamine agonists reduce the incidence and severity of OHSS in IVF/ICSI treatment cycles? A systematic review and meta-analysis. *Hum Reprod Update*. 2010.
3. Gómez R, Soares SR, Busso C, et al. Physiology and pathology of ovarian hyperstimulation syndrome. *Semin Reprod Med*. 2010;28:448–57.
4. Practice Committee of American Society for Reproductive Medicine. Ovarian hyperstimulation syndrome. *Fertil Steril*. 2008;90:S188–93.
5. Sansone P, Aurilio C, Pace MC, et al. Intensive care treatment of ovarian hyperstimulation syndrome (OHSS). *Ann N Y Acad Sci*. 2011;1221:109–18.
6. Raziel A, Schachter M, Friedler S, et al. Outcome of IVF pregnancies following severe OHSS. *Reprod Biomed Online*. 2009;19:61–5.
7. Youssef MA, Al-Inany HG, Evers JL, et al. Intra-venous fluids for the prevention of severe ovarian hyperstimulation syndrome. *Cochrane Database Syst Rev*. 2011;CD001302.

ADDITIONAL READING

- Aboulghar M, et al. Treatment of ovarian hyperstimulation syndrome. *Semin Reprod Med*. 2010;28:532–9.
- Genazzani AR, Monteleone P, Papini F, et al. Pharmacotherapy of ovarian hyperstimulation syndrome. *Expert Opin Pharmacother*. 2010;11: 2527–34.
- Humaidan P, Quartarolo J, Papanikolaou EG, et al. Preventing ovarian hyperstimulation syndrome: Guidance for the clinician. *Fertil Steril*. 2010;94: 389–400.

CODES

ICD9

256.1 Other ovarian hyperfunction

CLINICAL PEARLS

- Patients who have had OHSS are more at risk for OHSS in the future.
- Abdominal and pelvic exams are contraindicated in patients with OHSS.
- OHSS is a self-limited disease. Management is mainly supportive.

OVARIAN TUMOR (BENIGN)

Emily Von Bargen, MD
Mark J. Manning, DO, MsMEL

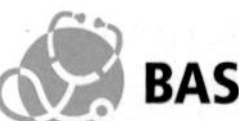

BASICS

DESCRIPTION

- The ovaries are a source of many tumor types (benign and malignant) because of the histologic variety of their constituent cells.
- Benign ovarian tumors create difficulties in differential diagnosis because of the need to identify malignancy and discriminate tumor from cysts, infectious lesions, ectopic pregnancy, and endometriomas.
- Tumors are often clinically silent until well developed; may be solid, cystic, or mixed; and they may be functional (producing sex steroids, as with arrhenoblastomas and gynandroblastomas) or nonfunctional.
- System(s) affected: Endocrine/Metabolic; Reproductive

Geriatric Considerations

Because incidence of malignancy increases with age, postmenopausal patients warrant comprehensive evaluation and follow-up.

Pediatric Considerations

Malignancy must be ruled out in premenarchal patients. Early neonatal cysts are rare.

EPIDEMIOLOGY

Incidence

- 30% of regularly cycling females
- 50% of women without regular cycles
- Predominant age: Premenarchal girls have a 6–11% risk of cancer in an ovarian tumor, and postmenopausal women have a 29–35% risk:
  - High percentage of ovarian tumors are malignant in girls younger than 15 years old.

RISK FACTORS

- As yet poorly characterized for benign tumors; cigarette smoking doubles the relative risk for developing functional ovarian cysts.
- Possible contributory factors are early menarche, obesity, infertility, and hypothyroidism.
- Tamoxifen increases risk of ovarian cyst formation (15–30%).
- Risks for ovarian cancer include age >60 years; early menarche; late menopause; nulliparity; infertility; endometriosis; family history of ovarian, breast, or colon cancer; a personal history of breast or colon cancer; or BRCA mutation.
- Risk for ovarian cancer is decreased in women who have used OCPs, been pregnant, or breast-fed.

GENERAL PREVENTION

- Although oral contraceptives do not appear to increase rates of cyst resolution, they do decrease risk for forming new ovarian cysts.
- A large British cohort of 5,479 women demonstrated that the resection of benign cysts has no impact on future risk for ovarian cancer (1).
- A case-control study of 299 women found no evidence that ovulation-induction treatment predisposes women to the development of borderline ovarian growths (2).

ETIOLOGY

- Endometriosis with localized, repeated ovarian hemorrhage
- Physiologic cysts
- Tumorigenesis, with genetics as yet poorly defined

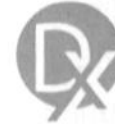

DIAGNOSIS

- A careful history is important.
- Usually asymptomatic
- Pain related to torsion, endometriosis, or rupture

HISTORY

- Early satiety
- Dyspepsia/bloating
- Increased abdominal girth
- Bowel pressure or bladder pressure sensations
- Menstrual irregularities
- Dyspareunia
- Hirsutism or sexual precocity
- Severe acne
- Deepening of the voice
- Virilization

PHYSICAL EXAM

- Examine lymph nodes for enlargement.
- Chest auscultation can reveal a pleural effusion.
- Abdominal exam may identify ascites, masses, or increased abdominal girth.
- Pelvic exam

DIAGNOSTIC TESTS & INTERPRETATION

Lab

Initial lab tests

- CBC for WBCs helpful if pelvic inflammatory disease (PID) suspected
- Serum B-HCG
- Urinalysis
- Serum estrogens and androgens if signs of androgen excess
- Serum tumor markers may be considered but often confuse rather than help to resolve diagnosis; choose carefully (3):
  - CA-125 should not be ordered in a premenopausal patient for screening purposes. If an ovarian tumor in a premenopausal patient is highly suspicious for cancer by ultrasound, a CA-125 level >200 u is concerning. In a postmenopausal patient, cancer must be ruled out and a CA-125 >35 u is concerning.
  - α-Fetoprotein and human chorionic gonadotropin (hCG) can be ordered for suspected germ cell tumor.
- Disorders that may alter lab results:
  - CA-125: Endometriosis, peritonitis, PID, Meigs syndrome, uterine fibroids, hepatitis, pancreatitis, SLE, diverticulitis
  - β-hCG: Pregnancy, hydatidiform mole
  - α-Fetoprotein: Hepatocellular carcinoma, hepatic cirrhosis, acute or chronic hepatitis
  - Human epididymis protein 4 (HE4) may offer superior specificity compared to CA-125 for the differentiation of benign and malignant adnexal masses in premenopausal women (4).

Imaging

- Transvaginal ultrasound is the best means to determine the architecture of an ovarian cyst or mass (5).
- Transvaginal ultrasonography may differentiate tumors from other pelvic lesions and identify features that place the patient at greater risk for malignancy (e.g., solid component, papillations, multiple septations, ascites, bilaterality, fixed and irregular, rapidly enlarging, accompanied by cul-de-sac nodules).
- Transabdominal ultrasonography can help identify ascites.
- Color-flow Doppler evaluation also may be helpful. Color flow to the solid component of the tumor is concerning for cancer. Gray scale may be an important method of differential diagnosis of ovarian growths (6).
- MRI with apparent diffusion coefficient mapping may be useful in the differential diagnosis of cystic masses. MRI can be helpful in better defining masses in women with low risk of ovarian cancer but who have an "indeterminant" mass on ultrasound (7).
- Cystoscopy if hematuria is present in the absence of infection or if IV pyelogram reveals intravesical surface irregularity
- Abdominopelvic CT scan with contrast material, if MRI unavailable (8)
- Barium enema, colonoscopy, or IV pyelogram, as indicated

Diagnostic Procedures/Surgery

Exploratory laparoscopy or laparotomy

Pathological Findings

- Follicular (fluid distension of atretic follicle) and corpus luteum cysts (corpus luteum hematoma). Follicular cysts are the most common ovarian cysts in the premenopausal nonpregnant female.
- Endometrioma
- Pregnancy luteoma (composed of hyperplastic stromal theca–lutein cells)
- Serous and mucinous cystadenomas and mixed serous/mucinous cystadenomas
- Granulosa cell tumors
- Benign connective tissue tumors (thecomas, fibromas, Brenner tumors)
- Cystic teratoma (dermoid cyst); teratomas are the most common benign neoplasms.
- Germinal inclusion cyst (regarded by some as the precursor for epithelial ovarian cancer)

Pregnancy Considerations

- Most cysts discovered during pregnancy are corpus luteum or follicular cysts.
- The 2 most commonly encountered tumors during pregnancy are cystadenomas (serous or mucinous) and dermoid cysts.

DIFFERENTIAL DIAGNOSIS

- Ovarian malignancies
- Endometrioma
- Uterine leiomyoma
- Appendicular cysts
- Diverticulitis or bowel abscess
- PID with tubo-ovarian abscess
- Distended urinary bladder
- Ectopic pregnancy
- Hydrosalpinx
- Functional cysts (follicular and corpus luteum cysts)
- Polycystic ovaries
- Ovarian lipoma

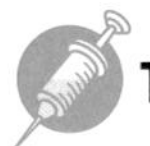

TREATMENT

MEDICATION

Oral contraceptives decrease risk for forming new ovarian cysts. They do not aid in resorption of current ovarian cysts (9).

First Line

NSAIDs or narcotics may be helpful for discomfort.

ADDITIONAL TREATMENT

General Measures

- In premenopausal patients with cystic lesions <10 cm in diameter, simple observation for 4–6 weeks is acceptable. No evidence suggests that use of a contraceptive pill is more effective than time alone in facilitating ovarian cyst resorption.
- If a large cyst remains unchanged after 4–6 weeks of observation, then surgical exploration is indicated.
- Unilocular ovarian cysts <5 cm in premenopausal patients were not considered suspicious.

SURGERY/OTHER PROCEDURES

- Cystectomy or wedge resection for cyst with benign features (10)
- Surgical removal of tumor to establish diagnosis when:
  - Premenopausal cysts >5 cm that persist >12 weeks
  - Mass is solid.
  - Mass is >10 cm.
  - Mass in a premenarchal or postmenopausal female
  - Suspicion of torsion or rupture
  - Postmenopausal cysts
  - Cysts with worrisome features on ultrasound (e.g., papillations)
  - For masses that are worrisome for cancer, consider referral to a GYN-oncologist for initial surgery (11).

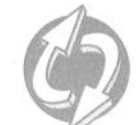

ONGOING CARE

FOLLOW-UP RECOMMENDATIONS

Patient Monitoring

- Most require only yearly exams.
- Varies by diagnosis

PATIENT EDUCATION

A variety of excellent patient education materials (e.g., "Ovarian Cyst") can be downloaded from the American Association of Family Physicians and American College of Obstetricians and Gynecologists Internet sites: www.aafp.org/afp and www.acog.com.

PROGNOSIS

Complete cure

COMPLICATIONS

Complications of untreated dermoid and mucinous cysts may include rupture and pseudomyxoma peritonei.

REFERENCES

1. Crayford TJ, Campbell S, Bourne TH, et al. Benign ovarian cysts and ovarian cancer: A cohort study with implications for screening. *Lancet*. 2000; 355:1060–3.
2. Cusidó M, Fábregas R, Pere BS, et al. Ovulation induction treatment and risk of borderline ovarian tumors. *Gynecol Endocrinol*. 2007;23:373–6.
3. Clarke-Pearson D. Screening for ovarian cancer. *NEJM*. 2009;361:170–7.
4. Holcomb K, Vucetic Z, Miller MC, et al. Human epididymis protein 4 offers superior specificity in the differentiation of benign and malignant adnexal masses in premenopausal women. *Am J Obstet Gynecol*. 2011;205(4):358.e1–6. Epub 2011 May 14.
5. Givens V, Mitchell G. Diagnosis and management of adnexal masses. *AAFP*. 2009;80(8):815–822.
6. Marchesiini AC, et al. A critical analysis of Doppler velocimetry in the differential of malignant and benign ovarian masses. *J Women Health*. 2008;17(10):97–102.
7. Nakayama T, et al. Diffusion-weighted echo-planar MR imaging and ADC mapping in the differential diagnosis ovarian cystic masses: Usefulness of detecting keratinoid substances in mature cystic teratomas. *J Magn Reson Imag*. 2005;22(2):271–8.
8. Iyer VR, Lee SI, et al. MRI, CT, and PET/CT for ovarian cancer detection and adnexal lesion characterization. *AJR Am J Roentgenol*. 2010; 194:311–21.
9. Holt VL, Cushing-Haugen KL, Daling JR. Oral contraceptives, tubal sterilization, and functional ovarian cyst risk. *Obstet Gynecol*. 2003;102: 252–8.
10. Labarge PY, et al. Short-term morbidity and long-term recurrence rate of ovarian dermoid cysts treated by laparoscopy vs. laparotomy. *J Obstet Gynecol Can*. 2006;28(9):789–93.
11. Borgfeldt C, Andolf E. Cancer risk after hospital discharge diagnosis of benign ovarian cysts and endometriosis. *Acta Obstet Gynecol Scand*. 2004;83:395–400.

ADDITIONAL READING

- Kirilovas D, Schedvins K, Naessén T, et al. Conversion of circulating estrone sulfate to 17beta-estradiol by ovarian tumor tissue: A possible mechanism behind elevated circulating concentrations of 17beta-estradiol in postmenopausal women with ovarian tumors. *Gynecol Endocrinol*. 2007;23:25–8.
- Zwiesler D, Lewis SR, Choo YC, et al. A case report of an ovarian lipoma. *South Med J*. 2008;101: 205–7.

CODES

ICD9

220 Benign neoplasm of ovary

CLINICAL PEARLS

- Cigarette smoking doubles the relative risk of developing a functional ovarian cyst.
- Transvaginal pelvic ultrasound is the imaging test of choice to initially determine the architecture of an ovarian cyst or mass.
- Malignancy must be ruled out in both premenarchal and postmenopausal patients.
- Do not order CA 125 on premenopausal patients with an ovarian mass unless it is highly suspicious for cancer.

O

PAGET DISEASE OF THE BREAST

Adam P. Vasconcellos, MD
Fred Schiffman, MD

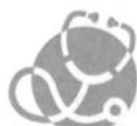

BASICS

DESCRIPTION

- An uncommon presentation of breast malignancy involving the nipple-areolar complex and characterized by eczematous changes, erythema, ulceration, bleeding, and/or itching (1,2)
- System(s) affected: Skin/Exocrine

EPIDEMIOLOGY

Incidence

In the US: 1,000–4,000 new cases each year:

- 1–3% of breast cancers (1)
- Peak incidence females ages 50–60 (1,2)

Prevalence

<1% of population

RISK FACTORS

Same risk factors apply as for noninherited breast cancers:

- Female gender
- Age >40
- Previous breast cancer
- First-degree relative with history of breast cancer
- Jewish/Caucasian
- Menarche <12 years of age
- Menopause >50 years of age
- Nulliparity or first child after age 34
- History of ionizing radiation exposure
- History of alcohol abuse

Genetics

No known genetic pattern, although studies suggest 80% or higher Her-2/Neu overexpression (3)

PATHOPHYSIOLOGY

- Epidermotropic theory:
  - Ductal carcinoma cells migrate from underlying mammary ducts to epidermis of the nipple to become Paget cells.
- Transformation theory (not favored):
  - Epidermal cells of nipple/areola transform into Paget cells (1).

ETIOLOGY

Cause is unknown, but risk factors for Paget disease appear similar to those of developing breast cancer in general (see above).

COMMONLY ASSOCIATED CONDITIONS

- Associated with underlying in situ or invasive breast cancer in 82–100% of patients (3)
- Multifocal/multicentric-associated underlying carcinomas in 32–41% of patients (1,2)

DIAGNOSIS

HISTORY

- Nipple itching, burning, bleeding
- Lesion usually located first on the nipple, then may spread to areola (1,2)
- Nipple/areolar skin changes that have not responded to conservative treatment

PHYSICAL EXAM

- Eczematous nipple changes
- Nipple erythema and scaling
- Nipple erosion or ulceration
- Bloody nipple discharge
- Nipple retraction
- Nipple fissures
- Palpable breast mass
- Thickening in breast tissue without nipple change (2)

DIAGNOSTIC TESTS & INTERPRETATION

Imaging

Initial approach

Mammography and breast ultrasound:

- Recommended for all patients with Paget disease on skin biopsy (3)

Follow-Up & Special Considerations

Breast MRI:

- Recommended if negative mammography and ultrasound (3)
- Recommended if considering breast-conserving surgery (4)
- Some recommend breast MRI for all patients with a new Paget disease diagnosis (4).
- More sensitive than mammography or breast ultrasound in detecting multifocal or multicentric breast cancer (1,3)
- Higher false-positive rate—patients should be made aware of this

Diagnostic Procedures/Surgery

Definitive diagnosis obtained by biopsy. Any chronic or nonhealing nipple lesions should be biopsied:

- If positive findings on clinical exam/imaging: Core biopsy and full-thickness skin biopsy of nipple–areola complex (5)

Pathological Findings

- Malignant cell invasion of the epidermis with large, pale cytoplasm, hyperchromatic nuclei with prominent nucleoli (1)
- Underlying ductal adenocarcinoma

DIFFERENTIAL DIAGNOSIS

- Eczema
- Contact dermatitis
- Psoriasis
- Skin tumors (e.g., Bowen disease)
- Squamous cell carcinoma
- Basal cell carcinoma

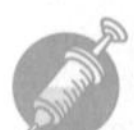

TREATMENT

MEDICATION

Following surgery:

- Chemotherapy per oncology study protocols
- Doxorubicin (Adriamycin)-based regimen
- Cyclophosphamide, methotrexate, 5-fluorouracil (CMF)
- Tamoxifen
- Paclitaxel (Taxol)

ADDITIONAL TREATMENT

Issues for Referral

- Surgery
- Medical oncology
- Radiation oncology

Additional Therapies

Possible breast reconstructive surgery with plastic surgery

SURGERY/OTHER PROCEDURES

- Mastectomy:
  - Due to high rate of false-negative findings on mammography and high incidence of multicentric or multifocal in situ or invasive carcinomas discovered in mastectomy specimens (3)
- Breast-conserving surgery:
  - If Paget disease found to be confined to nipple–areola complex without underlying neoplasm (2)
  - If disease limited to central segment of breast (6)
  - Approximate 5% risk of local recurrence at 5 years (3)
- Sentinel node biopsy:
  - For evaluation of axillary nodes
  - Recommended in patients diagnosed with invasive cancer
  - Recommended in patients undergoing mastectomy (3,6)

IN-PATIENT CONSIDERATIONS

Initial Stabilization

Dependent on cancer histology, size, and stage (see topic on "Breast Cancer"):

- Radiotherapy
- Chemotherapy
- Hormonal manipulation

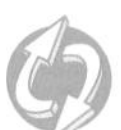

ONGOING CARE

FOLLOW-UP RECOMMENDATIONS

Oncology consultation

Patient Monitoring

Routine screening for women >40 years:

- Annual physician exams, with physician/patient conversation regarding frequency of imaging studies
- Per USPSTF guidelines, mammography at least biennially for women ages 50–74
- Monthly self-exams (although evidence does not support efficacy)

PATIENT EDUCATION

- National Cancer Institute, Department of Health and Human Services, Public Inquiries Section, Office of Cancer Communications, Building 31, Room 101-18, 9000 Rockville Pike, Bethesda, MD 20892; (301) 496-5583
- www.cancer.gov/cancertopics/factsheet/Sites-Types/pagets-breast

PROGNOSIS

Paget disease may correlate with higher-grade tumors, multifocal disease, and Her-2/Neu overexpression, all suggesting poorer prognosis:

- Prognosis by presence/absence of palpable mass prior to excision:
  - 92% 5-year survival, 82% 10-year survival postexcision if no palpable mass
  - 38% 5-year survival, 22% 10-year survival postexcision if palpable mass present
- Prognosis by stage of underlying breast carcinoma (see (7) for Breast Cancer staging descriptions):

Stage	5-yr relative survival
0	100%
I	100%
II	86%
III	57%
IV	20%

COMPLICATIONS

Risk factors for recurrence:

- Axillary lymph node metastases
- Underlying invasive cancer
- Palpable tumor in the breast (8)

REFERENCES

1. Caliskan M, Gatti G, Sosnovskikh I, et al. Paget's disease of the breast: The experience of the European Institute of Oncology and review of the literature. *Breast Cancer Res Treat*. 2008;112: 513–21.
2. Kim HS, Seok JH, Cha ES, et al. Significance of nipple enhancement of Paget's disease in contrast enhanced breast MRI. *Arch Gynecol Obstet*. 2010;282:157–62.
3. Siponen E, Hukkinen K, Heikkilä P, et al. Surgical treatment in Paget's disease of the breast. *Am J Surg*. 2010;200:241–6.
4. Zakhireh J, Gomez R, Esserman L, et al. Converting evidence to practice: A guide for the clinical application of MRI for the screening and management of breast cancer. *Eur J Cancer*. 2008;44:2742–52.
5. Carlson RW, Allred DC, Anderson BO, et al. Invasive breast cancer. *J Natl Compr Canc Netw*. 2011;9:136–222.
6. Morrogh M, Morris EA, Liberman L, et al. MRI identifies otherwise occult disease in select patients with Paget disease of the nipple. *J Am Coll Surg*. 2008;206:316–21.
7. www.cancer.org/Cancer/BreastCancer/DetailedGuide/breast-cancer-staging.
8. Dalberg K, Hellborg H, Wärnberg F, et al. Paget's disease of the nipple in a population based cohort. *Breast Cancer Res Treat*. 2008;111:313–9.

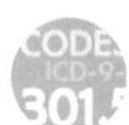

CODES

ICD9

- 174.0 Malignant neoplasm of nipple and areola of female breast
- 174.8 Malignant neoplasm of other specified sites of female breast
- 174.9 Malignant neoplasm of breast (female), unspecified

CLINICAL PEARLS

- Any chronic or nonhealing nipple or breast lesions should be biopsied to rule out malignancy.
- Paget disease is an uncommon presentation of breast malignancy involving the nipple–areolar complex and characterized by eczematous changes, erythema, ulceration, bleeding, and/or itching.

PALLIATIVE CARE

Felix B. Chang, MD

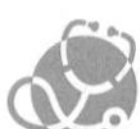

BASICS

Palliative care (from Latin *palliare*, to cloak): The active total care of patients whose disease is not responsive to curative treatment.

DESCRIPTION

- The goal of palliative care is preventing and relieving suffering, while supporting the best quality of life in people facing serious illness.
- Pain control includes the evaluation and management of its physical, emotional, social, economic, and spiritual components (1).
- Home-based comfort measures: Only 35% of patients want to die at home (2).
- Hospice care eligibility: Terminal illness and an estimated prognosis of 6 months or less.
- Palliative medicine skills: Communication, decision making, management of complications, psychosocial care of the patient and family, symptom control, care of the dying, coordination of care.

EPIDEMIOLOGY

- Estimate of patients receiving medical benefits for hospice and palliative care is >500,000.
- In 2003, more than 260,000 Medicare beneficiaries enrolled in hospice for terminal cancer.
- By 2008, only 31% had cancer and 69% died from chronic diseases.
- The most common reason to enter palliative care is advanced cancer. Other diseases include HIV/AIDS, CHF, COPD, RF, liver failure, dementia, and stroke.
- More than 80% of hospice beneficiaries are over age 65 years and a third are >85 years of age.

Incidence

Measuring the number of patients in palliative care is difficult.

GENERAL PREVENTION

Appropriate and aggressive use of advance directives:

- State-by-state laws and forms: www.aarp.org/relationships/caregiving/info-01-2011/caregiver_map.html
- More specific directive forms: www.coalitionccc.org/advance-health-planning.php

COMMONLY ASSOCIATED CONDITIONS

- Pain is the single most prevalent symptom: Headache, bone pain, ascites, chest pain
- 60% have shortness of breath commonly due to lung cancer and advanced CHF.
- 62% anorexia, nausea and vomiting, constipation, dysphagia. Anxiety, depression, and hopelessness are common with terminally ill cancer patients.
- Delirium between 40% and 85% in the last weeks of life

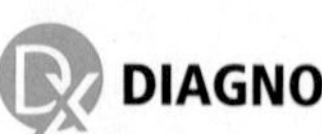

DIAGNOSIS

The **PEACE** tool evaluates:

- **P**hysical symptoms
- **E**motive and cognitive symptoms
- **A**utonomy and related issues
- **C**ommunication: Contribution to others, and closure of life affairs related issues
- **E**conomic burden and other practical issues, also transcendent and existential issues

HISTORY

- Personhood issues (spiritual/faith, cultural, family/community resource support) assume a co-equal place in assessing the palliative care patient.
- Evaluate possible barriers to timely consideration of a palliative approach to care:
  - The impression that palliation means "there is nothing more I can do for you"
  - Difficulty in recognizing when "aggressive" interventions have lost ability to prolong life
  - Not recognizing that quality-of-care therapies can be of value
  - Patients and decision-responsible caregivers equate palliative measures with "giving up."
- Assessment:
  - Emotive and cognitive symptoms (2): Sadness (grief), anxiety, depression, and delirium
  - Autonomy (3):
    - Do you feel in control of your care? Are we doing all and only the things you desire? Do you know the nature of your illness and what to expect on it?
    - Do you feel heard/listened to? Are we following your directions to your satisfaction? Are your treatment preferences in writing?
  - Closure of life affairs: Is there anyone whom you have not seen or need to talk to? Do you have regrets? What do you still want to accomplish in your life?
  - Economic burden: Are you worried about financial burden? Do you worry that you may become a burden to your family? Do you need help with insurance agencies?
- Transcendental and existential issues: Evaluate sense of peace, meaning, and hopes vs. torment or agony. Are you suffering? Would you like a chaplain/counselor to visit?

PHYSICAL EXAM

- Physical symptoms: Pain, anorexia, and other appetite or oral intake–related issues, incontinence and other genitourinary symptoms (constipation, vomiting, diarrhea), respiratory symptoms (dyspnea, cough), nausea and other GI symptoms (constipation, vomiting, diarrhea), ulcerations and other skin complaints, level of functioning, fatigue or asthenia, and side effect of common treatments.
- Vitals: Weight, midarm circumference
- General: Orientation, cognition. Assess ability to contribute meaningfully.
- Eyes, ears, nose, throat: Vision and hearing adequate for communication purposes
- Oral: Assess tongue whether it is moist, dry, or with thrush. Check for presence of ketone breath, gag reflex, dentures, gingivitis, tooth decay, and abscess. Assess risk for aspiration.
- Neck: Assess lymphadenopathy, thyromegaly, hepatojugular (H-J) reflux, stiff/supple neck, paracervical pain triggers (common cause of headaches in elderly), and kyphosis
- Cardiovascular: Murmurs/splits/gallops, PMI
- Lungs: Inspection, palpation, percussion, auscultation; BP (sitting and standing); pulse and respiration
- Abdomen/genitourinary: Distention, presence of artificial feeding device. Digital rectal exam for constipation/impaction and Hemoccult
- Musculoskeletal/neurologic: Pain sites, weakness, paresthesia, pathologic reflexes (Hoffman, Babinski), contractures, posture, range of motion
- Skin: Presence of rash, bed sores, wounds

DIAGNOSTIC TESTS & INTERPRETATION

Lab

Initial lab tests

Urinalysis, comprehensive metabolic panel, CBC

Follow-Up & Special Considerations

Interdisciplinary teamwork (IDTW): One key to effective care is adopting a model of interdisciplinary team care. Providing proficient care enlists most often the following team players: Physician, nurse, social worker, home health aide, pastor, administrator, pharmacist, medical supplier (beds, nebulizers, oxygen, commodes, wheelchairs), respite and home health agencies, community resources (Meals on Wheels, volunteers), allied health practitioners (e.g., aromatherapy, massage, OMM, acupuncture, meditation, ethicist)

Imaging

Should be reserved for the identification of conditions that will change treatment when present

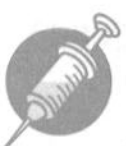

TREATMENT

MEDICATION

- Consider trimming medications that appear to offer little in the way of improving quality of life or meaningfully extending duration of life.
- Assure compliance by addressing patient/caregiver understanding and consensus, written record for them, and assurance that language/functional illiteracy are not issues.
- Pain:
  - Immediate-release morphine PO/IV treats dyspnea effectively and typically at doses lower than would be necessary for the relief of moderate pain.
  - Once pain is controlled, convert to a long-acting narcotic with short-acting agents made available as tolerance develops and/or patient develops breakthrough pain.
- Vomiting associated with a particular opioid may be relieved by substitution with an equianalgesic dose of another opioid or a sustained-release formulation. Dopamine-receptor antagonists are commonly used (metoclopramide, prochlorperazine, promethazine)
- Constipation: A prophylactic bowel regimen of stool softeners (docusate) and stimulants (bisacodyl or senna) should be started when opioid treatment is begun to avoid constipation. Polyethylene glycol started with initiation of narcotics may prevent onset, hydration (4)[A].
- Dyspnea: Oxygen, narcotics, and if CHF, diuretics and/or long-acting nitrates, benzodiazepines (5)
- Delirium: Lowest doses necessary of benzodiazepines or antipsychotics (Haldol, others)
- Brain metastases: Radiation, oral steroids (Decadron), etc.
- Patient safety and nonpharmacologic strategies to assist orientation (clocks, calendars, environment, and redirection). Some may be "pleasantly confused," and decision by family and clinician not to treat delirium may be justified. When cause of delirium cannot be identified/corrected rapidly, consider neuroleptics (haloperidol or risperidone)

ALERT

Bone pain: NSAIDs added to narcotics are more effective than narcotics alone.

ADDITIONAL TREATMENT

General Measures

Shift from biomedical problem list to a symptom-management care plan. Polypharmacy is common; research for adverse effects and drug interactions.

Issues for Referral

- Eligibility for hospice care: Determining prognosis and appropriateness of hospice referral:
  - (I) The patient's condition is life limiting, and the patient and/or family have been informed of this condition.
  - (II) The patient and/or family have elected treatments goals directed toward the relief of symptoms, rather than a cure of the underlying disease.
  - (III) The patient has either of the following: A. Documented clinical progression of disease, which may include: 1. Progression of the primary disease process as listed in disease-specific criteria; as documented by serial physician assessment, laboratory, radiologic, or other studies. 2. Multiple emergency department visit or inpatient hospitalizations over the prior 6 months. 3. For homebound patients receiving home health services, nursing assessment may be documented. For patients who do not qualify for 1, 2, or 3, a recent decline in functional status may be documented. B. Documented recent impaired nutritional status related to the terminal process. 1. Unintentional, progressive weight loss of >10% over the prior 6 month. 2. Serum albumin <2.5 g/dL may be helpful prognostic indicator, but should not be used in isolation from other factors in I–III
- Eligibility for Medicare hospice benefit: Eligibility for Medicare part A (hospital insurance), Medicare approved hospice. The patient signs a statement choosing hospice care instead of regular Medicare. The patient's personal physician and the hospice medical director both certify that the patient has a terminal illness and <6 months to live (6).

ONGOING CARE

PATIENT EDUCATION

Get palliative care: www.getpalliativecare.org/

PROGNOSIS

- For seriously ill patients with advanced COPD, heart failure, or end-stage liver disease, clinical prediction criteria are not effective in identifying a population with a survival prognosis of 6 months or less (7).
- Guidelines for determining prognosis in selected noncancer diseases:
  - Heart disease: For congestive heart failure symptoms at rest (optimize with diuretics, vasodilators, ACE inhibitors) Uncontrollable arrhythmias (control symptoms), history of cardiac arrest/resuscitation, cardiogenic brain embolism
  - Pulmonary disease:
    - Dyspnea at rest from decreased functional activity, exacerbated by fatigue, cough
    - Presence of cor pulmonale or right heart failure
    - Hypoxemia at rest on supplemental oxygen. Hypercapnia. Unintentional weight loss of >10% of body weight over 6 months; resting tachycardia (>100/min) in COPD
  - Dementia:
    - Functional assessment ≥ stage 7: Unable to ambulate, dress or bathe; urinary or fecal incontinence; unable to communicate meaningfully
    - Comorbid conditions: Aspiration pneumonia, pyelonephritis, or urinary infections; septicemia, decubitus ulcer; recurrent fever; difficulty swallowing or refusal to eat
  - HIV:
    - CD4+ count below 25 cells/mm^3
    - Viral load >100,000 copies/mL
    - Life-threatening concomitant conditions
    - Chronic persistent diarrhea for 1 year; persistent serum albumin <2.5 gm/dL; substance abuse; age >50; decision to forgo retroviral, chemotherapeutic prophylaxis drug therapy related specifically to HIV disease, congestive heart failure
  - Liver disease:
    - Laboratory indicators of severely impaired liver function: Prothrombin time prolonged >5 seconds over control; serum albumin <2.5 g/dL
    - Clinical indicators of end-stage liver disease: Ascites, refractory to sodium restriction and diuretics, or patient noncompliant, spontaneous bacterial peritonitis, hepatorenal syndrome, hepatic encephalopathy, refractory to protein restriction and lactulose or neomycin, or patient noncompliant; recurrent variceal bleeding
    - Worsening prognosis: Progressive malnutrition, muscle wasting with reduced strength and endurance; continued active alcoholism, >80 g ethanol per day, hepatocellular carcinoma, hepatitis B surface antigen positivity
  - Renal diseases:
    - Laboratory criteria for renal failure: Creatinine clearance of <10 cc/min (<15 cc/min for diabetes) and serum creatinine of <8 mg/dL (>6 mg/dL in diabetics).
    - End-stage renal disease discontinuing dialysis, or dialysis eligible and refusing, with renal failure: Uremia; oliguria; intractable hyperkalemia; uremic pericarditis; hepatorenal syndrome; intractable fluid overload
    - In hospitalized patients with acute renal failure, other comorbid conditions that predict early mortality: Mechanical ventilation; malignancy-other organ systems; chronic lung disease; advanced cardiac disease; sepsis; immunosuppression/AIDS; albumin <3.5 g/dL; cachexia; platelet count <25,000; age >75; disseminated intravascular congestion; GI bleeding
  - Stroke and coma: I. During the acute phase immediately following a hemorrhagic or ischemic stroke: A. Coma or persistent vegetative state beyond 3 days' duration. B. In postanoxic stroke, coma or severe obtundation, accompanied by severe myoclonus, persisting beyond 3 days past the anoxic event. C. Comatose patients with any 4 of the following on day 3 of coma: Abnormal brain stem response; absent verbal response; absent withdrawal response to pain; serum creatinine >1.5 mg/dL, age >70. D. Dysphagia severe enough to prevent the patient from receiving food and fluids necessary to sustain life. E. CT or MRI findings indicating decreased likelihood of survival. II. Once the patient has entered the chronic phase: A. Age >70. B. Poor functional status, as evidenced by Karnofsky score of <50%. C. Poststroke dementia, as evidenced by a FAST score >7. D. Poor nutritional status, whether on artificial or not: Aspiration pneumonia; upper UTI, sepsis; refractory stage 3–4 decubitus ulcer; fever recurrent after antibiotics

REFERENCES

1. Hall S, Kolliakou A. Improving palliative care for older people in care homes. *Cochrane Database Syst Rev*. 2011;3:CD007132.
2. Meuser T, Pietruck C, et al. Symptoms during cancer pain treatment following WHO-guidelines: A longitudinal follow-up study of symptoms prevalence, severity and etiology. *Pain*. 2001; 93:247.
3. Lo B, Quill T, et al. Discussing palliative care with patients. ACP-ASIM End-of-Life Care Consensus Panel. American College of Physicians-American Society of Internal Medicine. *Ann Intern Med*. 1999;130:744.
4. Phillip G, Cavenagh J. Medically assisted hydration for adult palliative care patients. *Cochrane Database Syst Rev*. 2008;2:CD006273.
5. Simon S, Higginson I. Benzodiazepines for the relief of breathlessness in a advanced malignant and nonmalignant diseases in adult. *Cochrane Database Syst Rev*. 2010;1:CD007354.
6. Medicare Hospice Benefits, Health care Financing Administration, Publication No. HCFA02154, Revised August 1999.
7. Fox E, Landrum NcNiff, et al. Evaluation of prognostic criteria for determining hospice eligibility in patients with advanced lung, heart, or liver disease. SUPPORT Investigators. Study to Understand Prognosis and Preferences for Outcomes and Risks of Treatments. *JAMA*. 1999;282:1638.

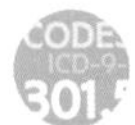

CODES

ICD9

V66.7 Encounter for palliative care

CLINICAL PEARLS

- Palliative medicine is not just for terminally ill patients.
- Under-treatment of cancer pain is as high as 40%.
- The treatment of pain at the end of life is the right of the patient and a moral duty, as well as a legal obligation.
- Benzodiazepines do not appear to reduce breathlessness in patient with advanced cancer or COPD.

PANCREATIC CANCER

Sarah Lee, MD
Edward Feller, MD

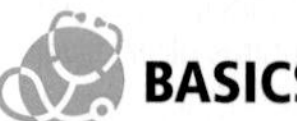

BASICS

DESCRIPTION

- Carcinoma of the exocrine pancreas is the fourth most common cause of cancer death in the US.
- Rarely curable: Overall 1-year and 5-year relative survival rates of 25% and 5%, respectively.
- 60–70% occur in the head, 15% in the body, 5% in the tail; 20% diffusely involve the gland.
- <20% are localized at diagnosis. For localized, small cancers (<2 cm) with no lymph node metastases and no extension beyond the capsule, surgical resection has 5-year survival rates of 18–24%.
- In apparently resectable disease, 20–40% have unresectable lesions at surgery.
- Ampullary, duodenal, or distal bile duct tumors may mimic pancreatic carcinoma and are more likely to be resectable and curable.
- For advanced or unresectable cancers, survival is <1% at 5 years; most patients die within 1 year.

EPIDEMIOLOGY

During 2003–2007, the median age at diagnosis for pancreatic cancer was 72 years. It is rare among those younger than age 45; after 45, occurrence rises sharply.

Incidence

- An estimated 42,470 people were diagnosed in 2009 (21,040 men and 21,420 women); there were 35,240 deaths.
- More common in black and white races, 16.7 and 10.3 in 100,000 men and 14.4 and 10.3 in 100,000 women, respectively. Among Hispanic and Asian/Pacific Islanders there is an incidence of 10.9 and 8.3 in 100,000 men and 10.1 and 8.3 in 100,000 women, respectively (1).

Prevalence

In 2008, in the US, ~34,657 men and women (16,811 men and 17,846 women) were alive who had a history of pancreatic cancer.

RISK FACTORS

- Smoking: Relative risk (RR) = 1.5; correlates with amount smoked
- Diabetes: RR = 2.1 (95% CI, 1.6–2.8); as many as 1 in 6 become diabetic within 6 months before diagnosis.
- Prior partial gastrectomy or cholecystectomy: 2–5-fold increased risk 15–20 years after gastrectomy
- Familial aggregation/genetic factors: 5–10% of patients have a first-degree relative with the disease.
- Hereditary chronic pancreatitis: Cumulative risk by ages 50 and 75 is 10% and 54%, respectively.
- Chronic pancreatitis: Tropical and nontropical
- High intake of dietary fat and obesity
- Coffee and alcohol consumption: Studies fail to demonstrate a convincing relationship.
- Aspirin and NSAID use: Large cohort studies have not found any link.

Genetics

- Multifactorial: Activation of oncogenes (e.g., *K-ras* mutation 90%); inactivation of tumor suppressor genes (e.g., p16/*CDKN2A* [95%], TP*53* [75–85%], SMAD4 [30%], and *BRCA2* genes [10%]); and defects in DNA mismatch repair genes (e.g., *hMLH1* and *hMSH2* [4% of pancreatic tumors])
- Hereditary pancreatitis: Cumulative risk of pancreatic cancer in affected family members by age 70 is estimated to be 40%.
- Inherited cancer syndromes:
  - Peutz-Jeghers syndrome: Related genes: *PRSS1* and *STK 11*; lifetime risk is as high as 36%.
  - Hereditary breast/ovarian cancer: 5% lifetime risk for pancreas cancer; related genes: *BRCA2* and *BRCA1*
  - Familial atypical multiple-mole melanoma syndrome: 19% lifetime risk; related gene: *CDKN2A*
  - Ataxia-telangiectasia: Related gene: *ATM*
  - Li-Fraumeni syndrome: Related gene: *p53*

GENERAL PREVENTION

Routine screening is not recommended. Even with a strong family history or predisposition syndromes, utility and cost-effectiveness of screening are unclear.

PATHOPHYSIOLOGY

Pancreatic intraepithelial neoplasia: Best characterized precursor lesion. Progression to more severe dysplasia is marked by expression of multiple oncogenes.

COMMONLY ASSOCIATED CONDITIONS

- See "Genetics."
- Chronic pancreatitis; diabetes mellitus; inherited cancer syndromes as noted above

DIAGNOSIS

HISTORY

- Dependent on tumor location; majority become symptomatic late in disease course.
- Weight loss 90%; pain 75% (progressive midepigastric dull ache that often radiates to the back); malnutrition 75%; jaundice 70%; anorexia 60%; pruritus 40%; diabetes mellitus 15%; weakness, fatigue, malaise 30–40%; acholic stools, dark urine, steatorrhea.
- Uncommon: Unexplained thrombophlebitis; acute pancreatitis from tumor obstruction of the pancreatic duct; new-onset diabetes mellitus.

PHYSICAL EXAM

- Muscle wasting and malnutrition are common; skin lesions are indicative of pruritus.
- Palpable abdominal mass or ascites in 20%
- Jaundice: 70% if tumor obstructs bile duct; 10% with body or tail carcinoma
- Courvoisier sign (painless jaundice with a palpable gallbladder): Uncommon; usually associated with pancreatic head tumors, periampullary carcinoma, and primary bile duct tumors; hepatomegaly in advanced disease
- Virchow node (left supraclavicular) and Sister Mary Joseph node (umbilical) in metastatic disease; palpable rectal shelf (nonspecific sign of carcinomatosis)
- Migratory thrombophlebitis (uncommon); associated with hypercoagulability in mucin-producing pancreatic cancer
- GI bleeding from tumor erosion into adjacent viscera (colon); portal hypertension-related bleeding (uncommon)
- Pancreatic panniculitis: SC areas of nodular fat necrosis

DIAGNOSTIC TESTS & INTERPRETATION

- Cross-sectional imaging commonly is used to evaluate symptoms or abnormal lab results.
- Endoscopic ultrasound-guided biopsy: Best modality for tissue diagnosis; sensitivity of ~75–90%, specificity near 100% for diagnosis of a pancreatic mass

Lab

Routine laboratory tests may reveal elevated serum bilirubin and alkaline phosphatase (cholestasis), anemia, or decreased serum albumin (malnutrition)

Initial lab tests

- Most patients do not require measurement of serum tumor markers for diagnosis or management.
- Elevated CA 19-9 antigen: 80% sensitivity, 90% specificity; individuals with Lewis-negative blood group antigen phenotype (5–10%) are unable to synthesize CA 19-9. Elevations can occur in benign pancreatic or biliary diseases and in nonpancreatic malignancy. Not recommended as a screening test.

Follow-Up & Special Considerations

During therapy, increase in CA 19-9 may identify progressive tumor growth. Normal CA 19-9 does not exclude recurrence.

Imaging

- Mass within the pancreas, which often obstructs the pancreatic duct or biliary tract
- Assesses presence of metastases and extrapancreatic extension, including vascular involvement (2)

Initial approach

- CT scan using thin section, multiphase multidetector helical CT is procedure of choice for diagnosis and staging: 85–90% sensitivity and 90–95% specificity; useful for evaluation of distant metastasis and prediction of resectability
- Abdominal ultrasound (US): Common initial test to assess jaundice and duct dilatation; less sensitive than CT for pancreatic masses.
- Endoscopic US (EUS) is accurate for tissue biopsy, local tumor and node staging, predicting vascular invasion (90% specificity, 73% sensitivity), and when no mass is identified on CT.
- Endoscopic retrograde cholangiopancreatography (ERCP): Invasive procedure with 90% sensitivity and 95% specificity for ductal cancer; useful in jaundice when endoscopic stent is indicated for biliary obstruction; generally confined to high probability for therapeutic intervention on biliary or pancreatic ductal systems.
- MRI: No advantage over contrast-enhanced CT.

- MR cholangiopancreatography: Noninvasive; 90% sensitivity and 95% specificity. Preferred in specific settings: Gastric outlet or duodenal stenosis or after surgical rearrangement (Billroth II) or ductal disruption; to detect bile duct obstruction, after attempted ERCP is either unsuccessful or provides incomplete information.

Diagnostic Procedures/Surgery

- Percutaneous fine-needle aspiration biopsy with US or CT guidance: 80–90% sensitivity and 98–100% specificity
- EUS–guided biopsy: 85–90% sensitivity and virtually 100% specificity for pancreatic mass
- Staging laparoscopy and US: 92% sensitivity, 88% specificity, and 89% accuracy
- Positive peritoneal cytology has a positive predictive value of 94%, specificity of 98%, and sensitivity of 25% for determining unresectability (3).
- Positron emission tomography scan: 90% sensitivity but 70% specificity; limited anatomic information
- Tumor staging:
  - Stage I: Tumors limited to the pancreas
  - Stage II: Regionally invasive; may involve lymph nodes, but without celiac or mesenteric artery involvement
  - Stage III: Direct involvement of celiac or superior mesenteric artery involvement
  - Stage IV: Distant metastases

Pathological Findings

- Duct cell carcinoma: 90%
- Others: Acinar, papillary mucinous, signet ring, adenosquamous, mucinous, giant or small cell, cystadenocarcinoma, undifferentiated, unclassified carcinoma

DIFFERENTIAL DIAGNOSIS

- Duodenal cancer, cholangiocarcinoma, lymphoma, islet cell tumor, sarcoma, cystic neoplasms, tumor metastatic to pancreas (rare)
- Nonmalignant conditions: Choledocholithiasis, acute pancreatitis, biliary tract stricture, adenoma; chronic mesenteric ischemia
- Tuberculosis or fungal abscess in AIDS.
- Patients may present with back pain mimicking musculoskeletal disease.

ALERT

Be wary of chronic pancreatitis, which can present with a similar pain pattern, weight loss, jaundice, and an inflammatory mass on imaging.

TREATMENT

- Surgical resection: Only chance of cure; no role for resection in metastatic disease. As few as 15–20% are candidates for resection.
- Criteria for unresectability: Extrapancreatic spread, encasement or occlusion of major vessels, distant metastases

MEDICATION

- Analgesics
- Stage I and II:
  - Radical pancreatic resection plus chemotherapy
  - ESPAC-3 trial after pancreatic resection: Compared with 5-fluororacil (FU) and folinic acid, gemcitabine did not improve overall survival (4)[A].
  - Currently, postoperative gemcitabine alone or in combination with 5-FU–based chemoradiation is the current standard of care; preoperative neoadjuvant treatment trials are in progress (5).
- Stage III:
  - Standard: Chemotherapy with gemcitabine-based regimens (6)[A]; chemoradiation is controversial
  - Palliation of biliary obstruction by endoscopic, surgical, or radiologic methods
  - Intraoperative radiation therapy and/or implantation of radioactive substances
- Stage IV:
  - Chemotherapy: Gemcitabine with erlotinib, a platinum agent, or a fluoropyrimidine may modestly prolonged survival compared to Gemcitabine alone (6)[A].
  - Pain-relieving procedures (celiac or intrapleural block) and supportive care; palliative decompression

ADDITIONAL TREATMENT

- For resected tumors: Postoperative radiation therapy with other chemotherapeutic agents
- Intraoperative radiation therapy and/or implantation of radioactive substances (ongoing trials)

Additional Therapies

- Biliary decompression with endoprostheses or transhepatic drainage
- Celiac axis and intrapleural nerve blocks can provide effective pain relief for some patients.
- Opiates may be needed for pain control.

SURGERY/OTHER PROCEDURES

- Standard treatment options:
  - Pancreaticoduodenectomy, Whipple procedure, en bloc resection of the head of the pancreas, distal common bile duct, duodenum, jejunum, and gastric antrum
  - Total pancreatectomy
  - Distal pancreatectomy for body and tail tumors
- Nonstandard surgeries:
  - Pylorus-preserving pancreaticoduodenectomy, regional pancreatectomy
  - Palliative bypass:
    - Biliary decompression; gastrojejunostomy for gastric outlet obstruction; duodenal endoprosthesis for obstruction

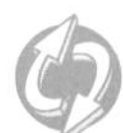

ONGOING CARE

DIET

- Frequently, malabsorption caused by exocrine insufficiency contributes to malnutrition; pancreatic enzyme replacement can help to alleviate symptoms.
- Fat-soluble vitamin deficiency may require replacement therapy.

PROGNOSIS

- Median survival: 10–20 months
- 5-year survival: ~30% if node-negative; 10% if node-positive
- Metastatic cancer: 1–2% 5-year survival
- For localized disease and small cancers (<2 cm) with no lymph node involvement and no extension beyond the capsule of the pancreas, complete surgical resection can yield a 5-year survival: 18–24%.

COMPLICATIONS

- Diabetes mellitus, malabsorption
- Surgical complications: Intra-abdominal abscess, postgastrectomy syndromes, pancreatico-jejunostomy, gastric and biliary anastomotic leaks; operative mortality varies

REFERENCES

1. Altekruse SF, et al. SEER Cancer Statistics Review, 1975–2007, National Cancer Institute Bethesda, MD, http://seer.cancer.gov/csr/1975_2007/, based on November 2009 SEER data submission, posted to the SEER Web site, 2010.
2. Kinney T. Evidence-based imaging of pancreatic malignancies. *Surg Clin N Am*. 2010;90:411–425.
3. Callery MP, Chang KJ, Fishman EK, et al. pretreatment assessment of resectable and borderline resectable pancreatic cancer; expert consensus statement. *Ann Surg Oncol*. 2009; 16: 1727-33.
4. Neoptolemos JP, Stocken DD, Ghaneh P, et al. Adjuvant chemotherapy with flurouracil plus folinic acid vs gemcitabine following pancreatic cancer resection. *JAMA*. 2010; 304:1073–81.
5. Hidalgo M. Pancreatic cancer. *N Engl J Med*. 2010; 362:1605–17.
6. Heinemann V, Boeck S, Hinke S, et al. Meta-analysis of randomized trials: Evaluation of benefits from gemcitabine-based combination chemotherapy applied to advanced pancreatic cancer. *BMC Cancer*. 2008;8:82.

ADDITIONAL READING

Verbesey JE, Munson JL. Pancreatic cystic neoplasms. *Surg Clin N Am*. 2010;90:411–25.

CODES

ICD9

- 157.0 Malignant neoplasm of head of pancreas
- 157.1 Malignant neoplasm of body of pancreas
- 157.2 Malignant neoplasm of tail of pancreas

CLINICAL PEARLS

- Sudden onset of diabetes mellitus in nonobese adults aged >40 years warrants consideration of pancreatic cancer.
- Cancer of the exocrine pancreas is rarely curable and has an overall 5-year survival rate of <4%. Fewer than 20% of cases are localized at diagnosis.
- Be wary of chronic pancreatitis, which can present with similar pain pattern, weight loss, jaundice and an inflammatory mass on imaging.

PANCREATITIS, ACUTE

Robert L. Frachtman, MD

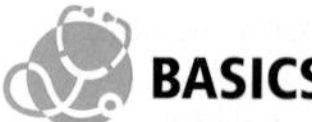

BASICS

DESCRIPTION

Acute inflammatory process of the pancreas with variable involvement of regional tissue or remote organ systems:

- Inflammatory episode with symptoms related to intrapancreatic activation of enzymes with pain, nausea, and vomiting and associated intestinal ileus
- Varies widely in severity (including death), complications, and prognosis
- Complete structural and functional recovery, provided no necrosis or pancreatic ductal disruption

EPIDEMIOLOGY

Incidence

- 1–5/10,000
- Predominant age: None
- Predominant sex: Male = Female

Prevalence

Acute: 19/10,000

RISK FACTORS

See "Etiology."

Genetics

Hereditary pancreatitis is a rare condition with an autosomal-dominant inheritance pattern.

GENERAL PREVENTION

- Avoidance of alcohol excess, especially over a prolonged period
- Avoidance of cigarette smoking
- Correction of underlying causes (hypertriglyceridemia or hypercalcemia)
- Discontinuation of medications associated with pancreatitis as soon as it is diagnosed
- Cholecystectomy if symptomatic cholelithiasis

PATHOPHYSIOLOGY

Autodigestion of the pancreas, interstitial edema with severe third spacing, hemorrhage, necrosis, release of vasoactive peptides, acute fluid collection (within 6 weeks), pseudocyst or postnecrotic collection (>6 weeks), pancreatic ductal disruption, injury to surrounding vascular structures such as the splenic vein (thrombosis) and splenic artery (pseudoaneurysm)

ETIOLOGY

- Alcohol
- Gallstones (including microlithiasis)
- Trauma/surgery
- Acute discontinuation of medications for diabetes or hyperlipidemia
- Following endoscopic retrograde cholangiopancreatography (ERCP)
- Medications (most common, but not exhaustive list):
  - ACE inhibitors
  - Angiotensin receptor blockers (ARBs)
  - Thiazide diuretics and furosemide
  - Antimetabolites (Purinethol and azathioprine) (1)[A]
  - Corticosteroids
  - Exenatide (Byetta) (2)[A]
  - Pentamidine
  - Statins, especially simvastatin (1)[A]
  - Mesalazine (1)[A]
  - Pancreatitis may occur only after several months' administration of some of the implicated medications.
  - When a patient presents with pancreatitis, all medications should be reviewed in the PDR and accessible literature and should be continued only if the benefit justifies the risk of continuing a potential cause of pancreatitis, especially if no other causes are identified.
- Metabolic causes:
  - Hypertriglyceridemia
  - Hypercalcemia
  - Acute renal failure
  - Hereditary causes (uncommon)
  - Systemic lupus erythematosus/polyarteritis
  - Infections (list not exhaustive):
    - Mumps, Coxsackie, cryptosporidiosis
- Penetrating peptic ulcer (rare)
- Cystic fibrosis and CFTR gene mutations
- Tumors (e.g., ampullary)
- Pancreas divisum
- Sphincter of Oddi dysfunction
- Scorpion venom
- Vascular disease
- Acute fatty liver of pregnancy
- Idiopathic

COMMONLY ASSOCIATED CONDITIONS

- Consider coexistent alcohol withdrawal, alcoholic hepatitis, and ascending cholangitis.
- Obesity or overweight adds a prognostic factor of severity, local complications, and mortality (3)[A].

DIAGNOSIS

Symptoms and objective evidence (imaging, amylase/lipase) do not always correlate.

HISTORY

- Fairly rapid onset of epigastric pain, which may radiate posteriorly, often with emesis
- Alcohol use
- History of gallstones
- Family history of gallstones
- Medication use
- Abdominal trauma
- Recent significant weight loss (via causing cholelithiasis)

PHYSICAL EXAM

- Abdominal findings: Epigastric tenderness, loss of bowel sounds
- Other findings: Fever, tachycardia, hypotension/shock, jaundice, rales/percussive dullness
- Rare (with hemorrhagic pancreatitis):
  - Flank discoloration (Grey–Turner sign) or umbilical discoloration (Cullen sign)

DIAGNOSTIC TESTS & INTERPRETATION

The laboratory and radiographic assessment of both acute and chronic pancreatitis must be used together, as there can be many false positives and false negatives.

Lab

- Elevated serum amylase >3× upper limit of normal (severity is not related to degree of elevation)
- Elevated serum lipase >3× upper limit of normal (may stay elevated longer than amylase in mild cases)
- Elevated total bilirubin to 3 mg/dL is not uncommon with pancreatitis, per se, but more elevated levels create consideration of common bile duct obstruction.
- Transaminases can quickly rise to near 1,000 U/L with acute bile duct obstruction, but should rapidly fall as the alkaline phosphatase rises; a 3-fold elevation in the ALT in the setting of acute pancreatitis has a 95% positive predictive value for gallstone pancreatitis.
- Triglyceride levels >1,000 mg/dL suggest hypertriglyceridemia as the cause.
- Glucose is increased in severe disease.
- Calcium is decreased in severe disease.
- WBCs can be 10,000–25,000/μL without active infection.
- Rising hemoglobin is a poor prognostic sign (severe third spacing). Rising BUN and creatinine imply volume depletion or acute renal failure.
- Disorders that may alter results for amylase or lipase:
  - Biliary tract disease, penetrating peptic ulcer, intestinal obstruction, intestinal ischemia/infarction, ruptured ectopic pregnancy, renal insufficiency, burns, macroamylasemia, or macrolipasemia

Initial lab tests

Admit labs should be supplemented by early and frequent follow-up labs to assess renal function, hydration, sepsis, biliary obstruction, and O_2 saturation.

Imaging

- Plain film of abdomen is useful to rule out mechanical small bowel obstruction, but ileus secondary to pancreatitis is common.
- CXR is useful to evaluate for early ARDS and pleural effusion; if upright, can rule out free subdiaphragmatic air.
- Ultrasound is useful to rule out cholelithiasis; choledocholithiasis can occasionally be seen.
- CT scan:
  - Will confirm the diagnosis, assess the severity, establish a baseline, and rule out other possibilities
  - IV contrast is not essential on the initial CT scan regarding evaluation for necrosis and should be avoided in volume-depleted patients.
  - A negative CT scan will not rule out noncalcified cholelithiasis.
  - If not contraindicated, a CT scan with IV contrast at day 3 can assess the degree of necrosis when necrotizing pancreatitis is suspected because of O_2 saturation <90%, systolic BP <90 mm Hg, etc.
- MRCP is useful (if it can be performed) to assess the likelihood of choledocholithiasis; as a bonus, one may find pancreas divisum, a dilated pancreatic duct, or chronic ductal changes.
- EGD may occasionally be necessary to rule out a penetrating duodenal ulcer or an obstructing ampullary neoplasm if suggested by laboratory or imaging studies.
- ERCP may be necessary for emergency common bile duct decompression due to an impacted stone.
- Endoscopic ultrasonography (EUS) may be useful when a patient with "idiopathic pancreatitis" has a second episode.

Initial approach

The ultrasound, followed quickly by the CT scan, has largely replaced the plain film of the abdomen.

Follow-Up & Special Considerations

If renal function is stable, a contrast-enhanced CT scan is very useful at day 3 to assess for necrosis, a major prognostic indicator. Later in the course, if a fluid or semisolid collection develops and there is a sudden worsening in the temperature curve, material can be aspirated via CT scan to assess for secondary infection.

DIFFERENTIAL DIAGNOSIS

- Penetrating peptic ulcer
- Acute cholecystitis
- Cholangitis
- Macroamylasemia, macrolipasemia
- Mesenteric vascular occlusion and/or infarction
- Perforation of a viscus
- Intestinal obstruction
- Aortic aneurysm (dissecting or rupturing)
- Inferior wall myocardial infarction
- Lymphoma

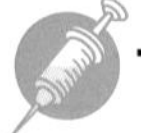

TREATMENT

MEDICATION

- Analgesia:
  - Hydromorphone (Dilaudid) 0.5–1 mg IV q1–2h PRN (morphine sulfate can increase sphincter of Oddi pressure, worsening the pancreatitis and increasing ductal pressure).
  - Demerol should be avoided due to the potential of accumulation of a toxic metabolite.
- Antibiotics:
  - Carbapenems can be considered for prophylaxis in necrotizing/severe pancreatitis if >30% necrosis on the CT scan (the usage of prophylactic antibiotics remains controversial, however, and seems to be losing favor)
  - Beta-lactam blockers with semisynthetic penicillin (e.g., Zosyn) or fluoroquinolones if cholangitis
  - Be vigilant for monilial superinfections when giving prophylactic antibiotics.

ADDITIONAL TREATMENT

General Measures

- Confirm diagnosis and rule out other possibilities, if needed (see above).
- Unless extremely mild, most cases require hospitalization.
- Fluid resuscitation:
  - If moderate or severe pancreatitis, there could easily be a 3-L deficit due to third spacing.
  - Infusion rates of 500 mL/hr for the first several hours, followed by 200–300 mL/hr for 48 hours, would not be unreasonable in those circumstances.
  - Urine output goal should be 0.5–1 mL/kg/hr.
- Eliminate all unnecessary medications, especially those that could potentially cause pancreatitis.
- Analgesia (see above)
- NG tube is needed if there is intractable emesis, which could be secondary to a generalized ileus or a gastric outlet obstruction secondary to extrinsic duodenal compression.
- Follow status regarding renal function, volume, calcium, and oxygenation.
- Imaging studies as needed (e.g., contrasted CT scan in 48–72 hours, if no contraindications, to evaluate for necrotizing pancreatitis, which increases the incidence of fluid collections)
- Intermittent pneumatic compression device
- Enteral nutrition at level of ligament of Treitz if oral feeding will not be possible within 5–7 days (preferable to TPN due to decreased infection rate), to be discontinued if there are increases in pain, amylase/lipase levels, or fluid collection volume
- TPN (without lipids if triglycerides are elevated) if oral or nasoenteric feedings are not tolerated

Issues for Referral

Refer to a tertiary center if pancreatitis is either already severe or actively evolving and when advanced imaging or endoscopic therapy is being considered.

SURGERY/OTHER PROCEDURES

- Necrosectomy for infected necrosis
- ERCP early if evidence of acute cholangitis or at 72 hours if evidence of ongoing biliary obstruction
- Resection or embolization for bleeding pseudoaneurysms
- Plasma exchange if necrotizing pancreatitis secondary to hypertriglyceridemia

IN-PATIENT CONSIDERATIONS

Discharge Criteria

- Pain control
- Diet tolerance
- Alcohol rehab and smoking cessation, if needed
- Low-grade fever and mild leukocytosis do not necessarily indicate infection and may take weeks to resolve. However, patients must be warned that infections may occur even after 10 days, due to secondary infection of necrotic material.

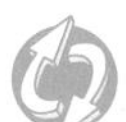

ONGOING CARE

FOLLOW-UP RECOMMENDATIONS

- Follow-up imaging studies may be required in several weeks, especially if the original CT scan showed a fluid collection or necrosis, or if the amylase or lipase continue to be elevated:
  - Pseudocyst or abscess (sudden onset of fever)
  - Splenic vein thrombosis (gastric variceal hemorrhage can occur rarely)
  - Pseudoaneurysm (splenic, gastroduodenal, intrapancreatic) hemorrhages (life threatening)
- Mild exocrine and endocrine dysfunction occur, but are usually subclinical.

DIET

- Begin diet after pain, tenderness, and ileus have resolved; small amounts of high-carbohydrate, low-fat, and low-protein foods; advance as tolerated; NPO or nasogastric tube if patient is vomiting
- TPN if oral is not tolerated (no lipids if triglycerides are increased) (4)[A]
- Enteral nutrition at level of ligament of Treitz is preferable to TPN if tolerated (less infection, decreased organ failure).

PROGNOSIS

85–90% resolve spontaneously; 3–5% mortality (17% in necrotizing pancreatitis). APACHE II scoring is most accurate but difficult to apply (5)[A]; Ranson criteria (see below) have a sensitivity of ~40%:

- On admission: Age >55 years, WBCs >16,000/mm, blood glucose >200 mg/dL (11.1 mmol/L), serum lactate dehydrogenase (LDH) >350 IU/L, AST >250 IU/L
- Within 48 hours: Hematocrit decreases >10%, serum calcium <8 mg/dL, BUN increase >8 mg/dL, arterial PO_2 <60 mm Hg, base deficit >4 mEq/L, fluid retention >6 L
- Ranson scoring:
  - Ranson score of 0–2: Minimal mortality
  - Ranson score of 3–5: 10–20% mortality
  - Ranson score of >5: >50% mortality

REFERENCES

1. Nitsche CJ, Jamieson N, Lerch MM, et al. Drug induced pancreatitis. *Best Pract Res Clin Gastroenterol*. 2010;24:143–55.
2. Anderson SL, Trujillo JM, et al. Association of pancreatitis with glucagon-like peptide-1 agonist use. *Ann Pharmacother*. 2010;44:904–9.
3. Wang SQ, Li SJ, Feng QX, et al. Overweight is an additional prognostic factor in acute pancreatitis: A meta-analysis. *Pancreatology*. 2011;11:92–8.
4. Oláh A, Romics L, et al. Evidence-based use of enteral nutrition in acute pancreatitis. *Langenbecks Arch Surg*. 2010;395:309–16.
5. Gravante G, Garcea G, Ong SL, et al. Prediction of mortality in acute pancreatitis: A systematic review of the published evidence. *Pancreatology*. 2009;9:601–14.

ADDITIONAL READING

- Eltookhy A, Pearson N. Drug-induced pancreatitis. *CPJ/RPC*. 2006;139:58–60.
- Wu BU, Conwell DL, et al. Acute pancreatitis part I: Approach to early management. *Clin Gastroenterol Hepatol*. 2010;8.410–6.
- Wu BU, Conwell DL, et al. Acute pancreatitis part II: Approach to follow-up. *Clin Gastroenterol Hepatol*. 2010;8:417–22.

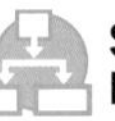

See Also (Topic, Algorithm, Electronic Media Element)

Choledocholithiasis; Peptic Ulcer Disease; Substance Use Disorders; Systemic Lupus Erythematosus (SLE)

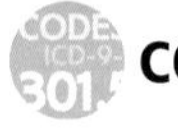

CODES

ICD9

577.0 Acute pancreatitis

CLINICAL PEARLS

- Review all medications upon admission and discontinue any that have been implicated as causing pancreatitis, especially ACE inhibitors (in this author's experience).
- Fluid resuscitation is critical early since inadequate resuscitation has been implicated in converting mild pancreatitis into necrotizing pancreatitis.
- Referral to tertiary center is needed if acute pancreatitis is severe or evolving/worsening.
- Outpatient follow-up, particularly reimaging, is very important.

PANCREATITIS, CHRONIC

Robert L. Frachtman, MD

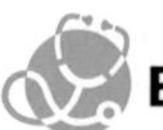

BASICS

DESCRIPTION

Irreversible:

- Progressive destruction of the pancreas
- May result in either or both exocrine and endocrine insufficiency
- Pain, malabsorption, diabetes mellitus, and increased risk of pancreatic cancer are the major features.

EPIDEMIOLOGY

Incidence

Predominant age:

- 35–45 years (usually related to alcohol)
- Predominant sex: Male = Female

Prevalence

8.3/10,000

RISK FACTORS

See "Etiology."

Genetics

Hereditary pancreatitis is a rare condition with an autosomal-dominant inheritance pattern.

PATHOPHYSIOLOGY

- Calcification
- Fibrosis/atrophy
- Pancreatic ductal strictures

ETIOLOGY

- Alcohol
- Familial
- Autoimmune

DIAGNOSIS

Symptoms and objective evidence (imaging, amylase/lipase) do not always correlate.

HISTORY

- Fairly rapid onset of epigastric pain, which may radiate posteriorly, often with emesis, with acute superimposed on chronic pancreatitis. Chronic vague abdominal pain occurs with classical chronic pancreatitis.
- Alcohol use
- Steatorrhea
- Weight loss
- Children:
  - Recurrent postprandial epigastric pain
  - Family history of chronic pancreatitis
  - Growth failure
  - Diabetes

PHYSICAL EXAM

- Acute superimposed on chronic pancreatitis:
  - See "Acute Pancreatitis" topic.
- Chronic pancreatitis:
  - Mild, diffuse tenderness
  - Ascites

DIAGNOSTIC TESTS & INTERPRETATION

The laboratory and radiographic assessment of both acute and chronic pancreatitis must be used together, as there can be many false positives and negatives.

Lab

- Features and considerations:
  - Amylase and lipase usually normal or near normal
  - Hyperglycemia
  - Steatorrhea (fecal fat >15 g/d on 100 g of fat per day diet), with other malabsorptive consequences such as low B_{12} level
  - Flare-ups may mimic acute pancreatitis.
  - Elevated alkaline phosphatase and bilirubin imply obstruction of the intrapancreatic common bile duct by extrinsic fibrosis or cancer.
  - Hereditary pancreatitis: Mutations in PRSSI gene and SPINKI gene
  - Autoimmune pancreatitis: Elevated serum IgG4, autoantibodies to lactoferrin and carbonic anhydrase
  - Decreased fecal elastase: Pancreatic insufficiency
- Disorders that may alter results for amylase or lipase:
  - Biliary tract disease, penetrating peptic ulcer, intestinal obstruction, intestinal ischemia/infarction, ruptured ectopic pregnancy, renal insufficiency, burns, macroamylasemia, or macrolipasemia

Imaging

- Plain film of abdomen: Might show pancreatic calcification if severe
- Ultrasound: Not terribly helpful for pancreas, but will assess the common bile duct diameter
- CT scan of abdomen: Pseudocysts, pancreatic duct dilation, and calcifications
- Magnetic resonance cholangiopancreatography (MRCP): Pancreatic ductal deformities/strictures (with or without pancreatic ductal stones), retained common bile duct stones
- Endoscopic ultrasound (EUS): Might help diagnose pancreatic cancer arising out of chronic pancreatitis

DIFFERENTIAL DIAGNOSIS

- Pancreatic cancer
- Lymphoma
- Other malabsorptive processes, such as bacterial overgrowth, celiac disease, etc.

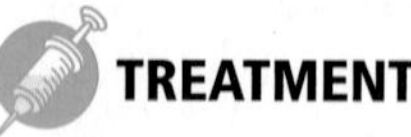

TREATMENT

MEDICATION

- Analgesics
- Pancreatic enzyme supplements, e.g., Pancrease or Creon MT (2 24,000 IU capsules at the beginning of each meal), are microencapsulated now and do not require acid inhibition for protection for most cases.
- Some experts believe that uncoated enzymes, not available in the US currently, are much more efficacious for pain control (when given with proton pump inhibitors [PPIs] to protect their integrity) than are coated enzymes (1)[C],(2)[B].
- Octreotide (Sandostatin) can be supplemental therapy for pancreatic ductal fistulae.

ADDITIONAL TREATMENT

General Measures

- Discontinue cigarette smoking, which can exacerbate chronic pancreatitis (3)[B].
- Analgesia: Consider pain management consultation regarding narcotic requirements.
- Exocrine and endocrine replacement therapy (enzymes and insulin, respectively)
- Consider more advanced therapy for pain: Celiac ganglion block, endoscopic or surgical decompression of partially obstructed pancreatic duct

SURGERY/OTHER PROCEDURES

- Pseudocyst drainage:
  - Conservative approach is recommended.
  - Endoscopic (via endoscopic ultrasound) or surgical approach if mature wall
  - Percutaneous approach if rapidly enlarging or if thin wall
- Pancreatic ascites with disruption of the main pancreatic duct:
  - Endoscopic placement of pancreatic ductal stent is preferred, if possible (4)[B].
  - Lateral pancreaticojejunostomy if endoscopic therapy is not possible
- Biliary obstruction (secondary to chronic pancreatitis, not choledocholithiasis):
  - Placement of retrievable metal stent or multiple plastic stents, if possible
  - Choledochojejunostomy if endoscopic therapy is not possible
- Pancreatic ductal obstruction by stone:
  - Endoscopic pancreatic sphincterotomy with stone extraction

IN-PATIENT CONSIDERATIONS

Discharge Criteria

- Pain control
- Resolution of problems secondary to ductal disruption, if present
- Alcohol rehab and smoking cessation, if needed

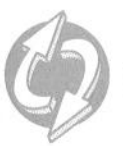

ONGOING CARE

FOLLOW-UP RECOMMENDATIONS

Depends on the source of the pain and whether or not a ductal disruption exists

DIET

- Small meals high in protein, ~20 g/d of fat; adjust if diabetes mellitus is present
- Pancreatic enzyme replacement therapy (preferably noncoated)

PROGNOSIS

- Patient may have recurrent episodes of acute pancreatitis.
- Slow progression
- May "burn out" with resolution of symptoms
- Narcotic addiction occurs frequently.
- Pancreatic exocrine and/or endocrine insufficiency may occur years later.

REFERENCES

1. Slaff J, et al. Protease-specific suppression of pancreatic exocrine secretion. *Gastroenterology.* 1984;87:44–52.
2. Puylaert M, Kapural L, Van Zundert J, et al. 26. Pain in chronic pancreatitis. *Pain Pract.* 2011;11(5): 492–505.
3. Yadav D, et al. Alcohol consumption, cigarette smoking, and the risk of recurrent acute and chronic pancreatitis. *Arch Intern Med.* 2009;169(11):1035.
4. Kozarek R, Ball T, Patterson D, et al. Endoscopic transpapillary therapy for disrupted pancreatic duct and peripancreatic fluid collections. *Gastroenterology.* 1991;100(5 Pt 1):1362.

ADDITIONAL READING

- Bornman PC, Botha JF, Ramos JM, et al. Guideline for the diagnosis and treatment of chronic pancreatitis. *S Afr Med J.* 2010;100(12 Pt 2): 845–60.
- Giuliano CA, Dehoorne-Smith ML, Kale-Pradhan PB. Pancreatic enzyme products: Digesting the changes. *Ann Pharmacother.* 2011;45(5):658–66.

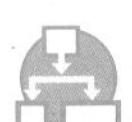

See Also (Topic, Algorithm, Electronic Media Element)

Choledocholithiasis; Peptic Ulcer Disease; Substance Use Disorders; Systemic Lupus Erythematosus (SLE)

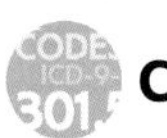

CODES

ICD9

577.1 Chronic pancreatitis

CLINICAL PEARLS

- Pancreatic enzyme replacement therapy is always the foundation of therapy.
- Pancreatic ductal injury must be considered and addressed.
- All patients with chronic pancreatitis do not yet necessarily have clinically significant pancreatic insufficiency.
- Fat malabsorption precedes carbohydrate and protein malabsorption.
- It may be very difficult to differentiate between chronic pancreatitis and pancreatic cancer arising from chronic pancreatitis.

PANIC DISORDER

Michael Golding, MD
Darpreet Kaur, MBBS, DGO

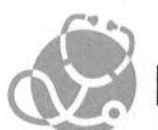

BASICS

DESCRIPTION

- The key feature of a panic attack is a brief period of sympathetic nervous system hyperarousal accompanied by psychological terror.
- In panic disorder there are multiple panic attacks: Some unexpected, over the course of at least 1 month, with worry about them.

EPIDEMIOLOGY

Incidence

- Predominant age: All ages; in school-age children, panic disorder can be confused with conduct disorder and school avoidance
- Peak age of onset is early to mid-20s
- Predominant sex: Female > Male (2:1)

Prevalence

- Lifetime prevalence: 1–3%
- ~8% of patients in a primary care practice population have panic disorder
- Of patients presenting with chest pain in the emergency room, 25% have panic disorder
- Chest pain is more likely due to panic if atypical, younger age, female, known problems with anxiety

RISK FACTORS

- Life stressors of any kind can precipitate attacks.
- History of sexual abuse and physical abuse, anxious and overprotective parents
- Substance abuse, bipolar disorder, major depression, obsessive–compulsive disorder, simple phobia

Genetics

Twin and family studies support a genetic predisposition.

PATHOPHYSIOLOGY

- Noradrenergic neurotransmission from the locus coeruleus causes increased sympathetic stimulation throughout the body.
- Current neurobiologic research is focusing on abnormal responses to anxiety-producing stimuli in the hippocampus, amygdala, and prefrontal cortex; e.g., there appears to be limbic kindling in which an original frightening experience dominates future responses even when subsequent exposures are not objectively threatening.
- Brain pH disturbances (e.g., excess lactic acid) from normal mentation in genetically vulnerable patients may activate the amygdala and generate unexpected fear responses.

ETIOLOGY

Unknown:

- Biologic theories focus on limbic system malfunction in dealing with anxiety-evoking stimuli.
- Psychological theories speak of deficits in managing strong affects such as fear and anger.
- Agoraphobia may be a learned response to panic attacks or a learned response to a cluster of subclinical panic symptoms; e.g., if a person has a panic attack in the grocery store, he may learn to fear the grocery store and other situations in which subclinical or clinical panic attacks occur.

COMMONLY ASSOCIATED CONDITIONS

- Of patients with panic disorder, >70% also have 1 or more other psychiatric diagnoses: PTSD (recalled trauma precedes panic attack), social phobia (fear of scrutiny precedes panic attack), simple phobia (fear of something specific precedes panic), major depression, bipolar disorder, substance abuse, obsessive–compulsive disorder, separation anxiety disorder
- Panic disorder is more common in patients with hypertension, mitral valve prolapse, reflux esophagitis, interstitial cystitis, irritable bowel syndrome, fibromyalgia, nicotine dependence

DIAGNOSIS

- Panic attack: A discrete period of intense fear, reaching a peak within 10 minutes in which 4 (or more) of the following symptoms develop abruptly: (i) palpitations, pounding heart, or accelerated heart rate; (ii) sweating; (iii) trembling or shaking; (iv) sensations of shortness of breath or feeling smothered; (v) a choking sensation; (vi) chest pain or discomfort; (vii) nausea or abdominal distress; (viii) feeling dizzy, unsteady, lightheaded, or faint; (ix) derealization (feelings of unreality) or depersonalization (feeling detached from oneself); (x) fear of losing control or going crazy; (xi) fear of dying; (xii) paresthesias; (xiii) chills or hot flushes
- Panic disorder: Recurrent unexpected panic attacks not better accounted for by another psychiatric condition (e.g., PTSD, OCD, separation anxiety disorder) AND not induced by drugs of abuse, medical conditions, or prescribed drugs AND with more than 1 month of at least one of the following: (a) worry about additional attacks; (b) worry about the implications of the attack (e.g., losing control, having a heart attack, "going crazy"); and/or (c) a significant change in behavior related to the attacks
- Specify "panic with agoraphobia" if anxiety about being in places or situations from which escape might be difficult (or embarrassing)

HISTORY

- Panic attacks are not subtle, but obtaining a clear history, especially with a new patient, is difficult for 2 reasons:
  - In the throes of a panic attack, many patients are convinced that the disorder is physically dangerous because of the frightening physical symptoms they are experiencing.
  - Patients are often deeply embarrassed by their problem, which they see as a personal failure.
- The best way to get a good history is through tactful, nonjudgmental questioning after the worst of the attack is over.
- A thorough medication and substance abuse history is important.

PHYSICAL EXAM

- During an attack, there will be tachycardia, hyperventilation, and sweating.
- Check the thyroid for fullness or nodules.
- Cardiac exam to check for a murmur or arrhythmias
- Lung exam to rule out asthma (limited airflow, wheezing)

DIAGNOSTIC TESTS & INTERPRETATION

Consider EKG and pulse oximetry to rule out certain serious causes of panic; consider Holter monitoring

Lab

No specific lab tests are indicated except to rule out conditions in the differential diagnosis. Consider these tests:

- Finger-stick blood sugar in acute setting in a diabetic patient
- Thyroid-stimulating hormone (TSH), electrolytes, CBC

Imaging

Initial approach

Consider ordering echocardiogram if you suspect mitral valve prolapse

Diagnostic Procedures/Surgery

If a medical cause of anxiety is strongly suspected, do the workup appropriate for that condition.

DIFFERENTIAL DIAGNOSIS

- Medication use may mimic panic disorder and create anxiety: Antidepressants to treat panic may paradoxically initially cause panic; antidepressants in bipolar patients can cause anxiety/mania/panic; short-acting benzodiazepines (alprazolam), beta blockers (propranolol), and narcotics can cause interdose rebound anxiety; benzodiazepine treatment causes panic when patients take too much and run out of these medicines early; bupropion, levodopa, amphetamines, steroids, albuterol, sympathomimetics, fluoroquinolones, and interferon can cause panic.
- Substances of abuse: Alcohol withdrawal, benzodiazepine withdrawal, narcotic withdrawal, caffeine, marijuana (panic with paranoia), amphetamine abuse, MDMA, hallucinogens (PCP, LSD), dextromethorphan abuse
- Medical illnesses: Hypo/hyperthyroidism, mitral valve prolapse, asthma/chronic obstructive pulmonary disease (COPD), reflux esophagitis with hyperventilation, tachyarrhythmias, premenstrual dysphoric disorder, menopause, pregnancy, hypoglycemia (in diabetes), hypoxia, inner ear disturbances (labyrinthitis), myocardial infarction, pulmonary embolus, TIAs, carcinoid syndrome, pre- and postictal states (e.g., in TLE), celiac disease and autoimmune disease, pheochromocytoma, Cushing syndrome, hyperaldosteronism, Wilson disease
- Psychiatric conditions that have overlapping symptomatology include mood, anxiety, and personality disorders such as major depression, bipolar disorder, posttraumatic stress disorder, borderline personality disorder, social phobia, obsessive–compulsive disorder, and generalized anxiety disorder. In PTSD, there is always a recollection or visual image that precedes the panic attack. In social phobia, fear of scrutiny precedes the panic attack. In bipolar disorder, major depression, borderline personality disorder, and substance abuse, the patient often complains first of panic and anxiety and minimizes other potentially relevant symptoms and behaviors.
- Somatization disorder is also an illness of multiple unexplained medical symptoms, but the presenting picture is usually one of chronic symptoms rather than the acute, dramatic onset of a panic attack. Somatization disorder and panic can be (and often are) diagnosed together.

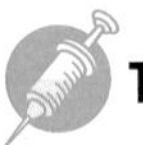

TREATMENT

Combined antidepressant therapy and psychotherapy is superior to either alone during active treatment. Cognitive-behavioral therapy (CBT) provides long-lasting treatment, often without subsequent need for medications (1)[A].

MEDICATION

- Medication management is indicated if psychotherapy is not successful or may be initiated together with psychotherapy.
- Patient preference plays a big part in this decision.
- Because patients typically are anxious about their treatment, the therapeutic alliance is critical for the chronic care of this disorder.
- If medications are started, they should be maintained for at least 6 months after symptom control.

First Line

- In nonbipolar patients start a low-dose antidepressant (e.g., 5 mg escitalopram, 25 mg sertraline, 10 mg paroxetine) and consider doubling the dose after 2 or 3 weeks; while waiting for the antidepressant to work, schedule frequent visits, give the patient reassurance, teach a relaxation technique, encourage the patient to do vigorous aerobic exercise (e.g., running in place) as soon as a panic attack begins (if medically appropriate and in an appropriate situation) (2)[B]; refer the patient to a competent therapist for CBT.
- In bipolar patients, treat the underlying bipolar disorder with a mood stabilizer rather than an antidepressant and panic symptoms often resolve.
- FDA-approved choices for the treatment of panic disorder include sertraline, paroxetine, fluoxetine, alprazolam, and clonazepam, but avoid giving benzodiazepines to those with a history of substance abuse or those who are currently abusing alcohol or benzodiazepines, unless utilizing a detoxification protocol.
- All antidepressants except bupropion can treat panic disorder, but fluoxetine and selegiline patch can cause more initial nervousness than other antidepressants.

Second Line

- Tricyclic antidepressants, particularly imipramine (start 25 mg/d in the evening and increase up to 25 mg every 3 days to a maximum of 200 mg/d). Slower titration and lower doses are often as effective. Imipramine is as efficacious as SSRIs in the treatment of panic. Tricyclic antidepressants are considered second line because of difficulty in dosing, more side effects, and greater risk associated with overdose compared with the SSRIs.
- Alprazolam (0.5–1 mg) and lorazepam (0.5–1 mg) can be given as a single dose to help with panic symptoms. If antidepressants are only partially effective, consider adding a longer acting benzodiazepine like clonazepam (0.5–1.5 mg b.i.d.).
- Benzodiazepines, particularly longer-acting benzodiazepines like clonazepam, can be considered as single agents to treat panic in patients with bipolar disorder and those with no mood symptoms or anxiety symptoms other than panic.

ADDITIONAL TREATMENT

General Measures

CBT, tailored for panic disorder, consists of several steps: Education, changing cognitions about the attack and the illness, relaxation and controlled breathing techniques, and, if appropriate, exposure to anxiety-provoking conditions coupled with in vivo relaxation exercises

Issues for Referral

Consider referral to a psychiatrist for panic disorder that is comorbid with bipolar disorder, borderline personality disorder, schizophrenia, suicidality, alcohol or substance abuse

Additional Therapies

Aerobic exercise reduces symptoms better than placebo (3)[B].

IN-PATIENT CONSIDERATIONS

Admission Criteria

- In an outpatient clinic or emergency room, if certain life-threatening mimics of panic disorder have not been ruled out, such as a myocardial infarction (MI) or pulmonary embolus (PE), inpatient hospitalization is needed to complete the evaluation.
- If a panic disorder patient is suicidal with intention to act on the idea, a psychiatric admission is indicated.

ONGOING CARE

PATIENT EDUCATION

- www.nlm.nih.gov/medlineplus/panicdisorder.html
- Patient information handouts in *American Family Physician* 2005;71:740 and 2006;74:1393.
- www.nimh.nih.gov/health/publications/when-fear-overwhelms-panic-disorder/index.shtml

PROGNOSIS

- Most patients recover with treatment.
- Though it can recur, panic can be successfully treated again.

COMPLICATIONS

- Iatrogenic benzodiazepine dependence
- Iatrogenic mania in bipolar patients treated for panic with unopposed antidepressants
- Misdiagnosis of more serious psychiatric conditions as panic disorder, or of panic disorder comorbid with more serious psychiatric conditions

REFERENCES

1. Furukawa TA, Watanabe N, Churchill R. Combined psychotherapy plus antidepressants for panic disorder with or without agoraphobia. *Cochrane Database Syst Rev.* 2007(1);CD004364.
2. Esquivel G, Díaz-Galvis J, Schruers K, et al. Acute exercise reduces the effects of a 35% CO_2 challenge in patients with panic disorder. *J Affect Disord.* 2008;107(1–3):217–20.
3. Broocks A, Bandelow B, Pekrun G, et al. Comparison of aerobic exercise, clomipramine, and placebo in the treatment of panic disorder. *Am J Psychiatry.* 1998;155:603–9.

ADDITIONAL READING

- Ham P, Waters DB, Oliver MN. Treatment of panic disorder. *Am Fam Physician.* 2005;71:733–9.
- McIntosh A. Clinical Guidelines for the Management of Anxiety. *Management of anxiety (panic disorder, with or without agoraphobia, and generalized anxiety disorder) in adults in primary, secondary and community care.* National Institute for Clinical Evidence NICE, 2004.
- Roy-Byrne PP, Craske MG, Stein MB. Panic disorder. *Lancet.* 2006;368:1023–32.
- Roy-Byrne PP, Wagner AW, Schraufnagel TJ. Understanding and treating panic disorder in the primary care setting. *J Clin Psychiatry.* 2005; 66(Suppl 4):16–22.
- Shedler J, Beck A, Bensen S. Practical mental health assessment in primary care. Validity and utility of the Quick PsychoDiagnostics Panel. *J Fam Pract.* 2000;49:614–21.
- Simon NM, Fischmann D. The implications of medical and psychiatric comorbidity with panic disorder. *J Clin Psychiatry.* 2005;66(Suppl 4):8–15.
- *Treatment of Patients with Panic Disorder*, 2nd ed. Arlington, VA: American Psychiatric Association; January 2009.

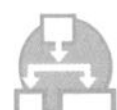

See Also (Topic, Algorithm, Electronic Media Element)

Algorithm: Anxiety

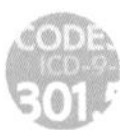

CODES

ICD9

- 300.01 Panic disorder
- 300.21 Agoraphobia with panic disorder

CLINICAL PEARLS

- Encouraging patients (who are medically able) to do 10 minutes of vigorous aerobic exercise the moment a panic attack seems to be starting is often a very effective way to help patients to feel safe during panic attacks. They often notice, and you can point out, that through exercise they can raise their heart rate beyond that which occurs in a panic attack. If a normal, healthy activity like exercise can do that, they conclude, panic attacks probably aren't endangering their hearts after all. In addition, such exercise often makes patients feel better in itself and can treat panic.
- Always check that a patient with panic is not suicidal: Patients with panic disorder are at increased risk.
- Once the panic attacks are eliminated, any agoraphobia often needs to be separately treated by gentle exposure to the feared environment, even though the physiological effects of panic are no longer present.

PARANOID PERSONALITY DISORDER

Margo Lauterbach, MD
Patrick Smallwood, MD

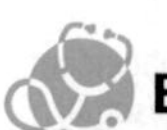

BASICS

DESCRIPTION

- Paranoid personality disorder is a maladaptive, persistent pattern of behavior characterized by suspiciousness, inappropriate mistrust of people, and hostility toward others who often are perceived as malicious. Consequently, patients avoid intimate relationships, bear grudges, and expect to be exploited by others.
- Paranoid personality disorder is one of the Cluster A personality disorders.

EPIDEMIOLOGY

Incidence

- Predominant age: First manifests during childhood or adolescence
- Predominant sex: Male > Female
- Increased in families with delusional disorder (persecutory type) and chronic schizophrenia

Prevalence

- 0.5–2.5% of the general population
- 2–10% of psychiatric outpatients
- 10–30% of psychiatric inpatients

RISK FACTORS

- Family history of paranoid personality disorder
- Childhood abuse/neglect

Genetics

Genetic predisposition may play a role (see "Incidence").

PATHOPHYSIOLOGY

Paranoid sense of mistrust can result from childhood abuse/neglect and/or genetic predisposition to paranoia.

ETIOLOGY

Specific causes are unknown.

COMMONLY ASSOCIATED CONDITIONS

- May develop major depressive disorder and may be at increased risk for obsessive–compulsive disorder and agoraphobia
- At risk for alcohol or other substance abuse or dependence

DIAGNOSIS

HISTORY

- Thorough psychiatric history and mental status examination
- Collateral history to establish pervasive pattern of behavior
- Diagnosis is based on fulfilling 4 of 7 *DSM-IV* criteria for the disorder (1,2)[C]:
  - Suspects exploitation, harm, or deceit by others
  - Unjustified doubt of others' loyalty or trustworthiness
  - Fears malicious retaliation if confides in others, and thus avoids doing so
  - Believes benign remarks or situations are threatening or demeaning
  - Unforgiving; hypersensitive to slights
  - Unjustifiably perceives attacks on character/reputation and may become hostile or counterattack
  - Suspects infidelity of spouse/sexual partner
- Associated features include:
  - Strong sense of autonomy
  - Stubborn
  - Litigious
  - Can be perceived as fanatic
  - May form closed groups or cults
  - Can foster fear in others

DIAGNOSTIC TESTS & INTERPRETATION

Psychological testing (e.g., Minnesota Multiphasic Personality Inventory)

Imaging

Brain imaging may rule out organic disease for those with emerging symptoms.

DIFFERENTIAL DIAGNOSIS

- Although brief psychotic states can result from significant stressors, primary psychotic disorders including paranoid schizophrenia, delusional disorder (paranoid type), and mood disorder with psychotic features must be ruled out.
- Schizoid personality disorder; avoidant personality disorder
- Medical disorders (e.g., temporal lobe epilepsy) with behavioral changes
- Culturally appropriate behavior, sometimes marked by defensiveness or guardedness, must not be mistaken for paranoia. Minorities, immigrants, and refugees also can present similarly but may be plagued by unfamiliarity.
- Paranoid traits can develop in the face of physical handicaps, such as hearing impairment.

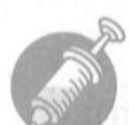

TREATMENT

MEDICATION

- Although little evidence suggests that the core personality features of paranoid personality disorder respond to psychopharmacologic treatment, psychotic paranoid ideation, acute hostility, anxiety, or psychosis can respond to low-dose antipsychotics and/or short-term benzodiazepines (3,4)[C].
- Short-term benzodiazepines, such as diazepam, can be useful in treating acute agitation, hostility, or anxiety.
- Acute psychotic states and delusional thinking can respond to low-dose antipsychotics, such as haloperidol.
- Taking medications can be interpreted by the patient as powerlessness and loss of autonomy.

ADDITIONAL TREATMENT

General Measures

- Treatment is difficult and often avoided by the patient (3,4)[C].
- Supportive psychotherapy, a form of therapy that is predictable, respectful, and straightforward, is preferred. Overly warm and empathetic styles can be regarded as intrusive (4)[A].
- Mistrust issues can undermine group therapy and behavioral therapy.
- Family therapy may be helpful.

Issues for Referral

The patient should be referred for individual psychotherapy and psychiatric follow-up if psychiatric medication(s) are indicated.

IN-PATIENT CONSIDERATIONS

Admission Criteria

Patients who become suicidal or homicidal may require psychiatric hospitalization for safety and stabilization. Patients with acute psychotic states also may require hospitalization if they are unable to care for themselves or pose a risk to others.

Discharge Criteria

A hospitalized patient usually is discharged after appropriate therapeutic interventions and discharge planning have taken place. Suicidal ideation, homicidal ideation, and/or acute psychotic states must be resolved.

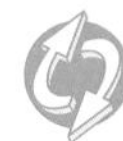

ONGOING CARE

PATIENT EDUCATION

National Institute of Mental Health at www.nimh.nih.gov

PROGNOSIS

- Good prognosis for those with good ego strength and strong support system
- Poor prognosis for those with poor insight, lack of primary support system, or comorbid Axis I psychiatric diagnosis

COMPLICATIONS

Significant impairment in work and interpersonal relationships

REFERENCES

1. American Psychiatric Association. *Diagnostic and Statistical Manual of Mental Disorders*, 4th ed. Washington, DC: American Psychiatric Press; 2000.
2. Svrakic DM, Cloninger CR. Paranoid personality disorder. In: Sadock BJ, Sadock VA, eds. *Kaplan & Sadock's Comprehensive Textbook of Psychiatry*, 8th ed. Philadelphia: Lippincott Williams & Wilkins; 2005:2081.
3. Bender DS, Dolan RT, Skodol AE, et al. Treatment utilization by patients with personality disorders. *Am J Psychiatry*. 2001;158:295–302.
4. Verheul R, Herbrink M. The efficacy of various modalities of psychotherapy for personality disorders: A systematic review of the evidence and clinical recommendations. *Int Rev Psychiatry*. 2007;19:25–38.

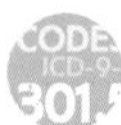

CODES

ICD9

301.0 Paranoid personality disorder

CLINICAL PEARLS

- Paranoid personality disorder is a maladaptive, persistent pattern of behavior characterized by suspiciousness, inappropriate mistrust of people, and hostility toward others.
- Although little evidence suggests that the core personality features of paranoid personality disorder respond to psychopharmacologic treatment, psychotic paranoid ideation, acute hostility, anxiety, or psychosis can respond to low-dose antipsychotics or short-term benzodiazepines.
- Poor prognosis for those with poor insight, lack of primary support system, or a comorbid Axis I psychiatric diagnosis

PARKINSON DISEASE

Alicia R. Desilets, PharmD
Mildred LaFontaine, MD

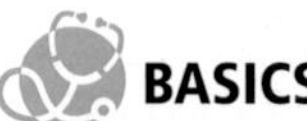

BASICS

DESCRIPTION

- Parkinson disease (PD) is a progressive neurodegenerative disorder caused by degeneration of dopaminergic neurons in the substantia nigra pars compacta.
- Cardinal symptoms include resting tremor, rigidity, bradykinesia, and gait dysfunction.
- Diagnosis is based primarily on history and examination.

EPIDEMIOLOGY

Incidence

- Average age of onset: ~60 years
- Slightly more common in men than women

Prevalence

- Second most common neurodegenerative disease after Alzheimer disease
- 0.3% of general population and 1–2% of those 60 years of age and older (prevalence increases with age)
- Affects 1 million people in the US

RISK FACTORS

- Age is the greatest risk factor.
- History of smoking may reduce risk.
- Weak association with exposure to toxins (herbicides and insecticides); however, relationship is not clear

Genetics

Mutations in multiple autosomal-dominant and automal-recessive genes have been linked to PD or parkinsonian syndrome. Genes investigated in PD include *LRRK-2*, *GBA*, and *alpha-synuclein*.

PATHOPHYSIOLOGY

- Pathologic hallmark: Selective loss of dopamine-containing neurons in the pars compacta of the substantia nigra
- Loss of neurons accompanied by presence of Lewy bodies, pale bodies (predecessor of the Lewy body), and Lewy neuritis

ETIOLOGY

Dopamine depletion in the substantia nigra and the nigrostriatal pathways results in almost all motor complications of PD.

COMMONLY ASSOCIATED CONDITIONS

Nonmotor-associated symptoms include cognitive abnormalities, autonomic dysfunction (e.g., constipation, urinary urgency), sleep disturbances, mental status changes (depression, psychosis, hallucinations, dementia), orthostatic hypotension, and pain.

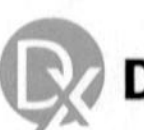

DIAGNOSIS

- Diagnosis during life is based on clinical impression.
- True gold standard for diagnosis is neuropathologic exam.
- Historically, 2 of the 3 cardinal manifestations must be present; tremor, bradykinesia, and rigidity have been shown to lead to misdiagnosis during autopsy.
- High level of probability if patient has resting tremor, prominent asymmetry, and good response to levodopa

HISTORY

Symptoms are often subtle and/or falsely attributed to aging:

- Gradual decreased emotion displayed in facial features
- General motor slowing and stiffness (1 or both arms do not swing with walk)
- Resting tremor (often initially 1 hand)
- Speech soft or mumbling
- Falls or difficulty with balance (tends to occur with disease progression)

PHYSICAL EXAM

- Tremor:
  - Resting tremor (4–6 Hz) in a limb that is often asymmetric
  - Disappears with voluntary movement
  - Frequently emerges in a hand while walking and may present as pill rolling
  - May also present in jaw, chin, lips, tongue
- Bradykinesia
- Rigidity:
  - Cogwheel (catching and releasing) or lead pipe (continuously rigid)
- Postural instability

DIAGNOSTIC TESTS & INTERPRETATION

Lab

Initial lab tests

- Thyroid testing
- Ceruloplasmin and copper in patients <50 years of age to rule out Wilson disease

Imaging

Initial approach

- Diagnosis mainly is clinical
- MRI of brain to rule out other disorders, particularly in patients thought to have PD but who are not responding to therapy
- Positron emission tomography and single-photon emission CT may be somewhat helpful with diagnosis, but often are not required

Pathological Findings

Lewy bodies

DIFFERENTIAL DIAGNOSIS

- Essential tremor: Bradykinesia is not present; often symmetric and occurs mostly during action or when holding hands outstretched
- Drug-induced parkinsonism: Reversible, although it may take weeks or months after offending medication is stopped:
  - Neuroleptics (most common cause)
  - Antiemetics (e.g., prochlorperazine and promethazine), metoclopramide
  - SSRIs
  - Calcium channel blockers (e.g., flunarizine and cinnarizine),
  - Amiodarone
  - Lithium
  - Cholinergics
  - Chemotherapeutics
  - Amphotericin B
  - Estrogens
  - Valproic acid
- Psychogenic parkinsonism
- Progressive supranuclear palsy: Impairment in vertical eye movements (particularly down gaze), hyperextension of neck, and early falling
- Multiple system atrophy: Presence of prominent orthostatic hypotension or concomitant cerebellar signs
- Dementia with Lewy bodies
- Other considerations: Huntington disease, Hallervorden-Spatz disease, Wilson disease, dopa-responsive dystonia

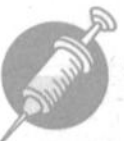

TREATMENT

MEDICATION

- PD treatment goal: Improve motor and nonmotor deficits
- Agents are chosen based on patient age and symptoms present
- First-line agents in early PD: Levodopa, dopamine agonists, monoamine oxidase (MAO)-B inhibitors (1)[A]:
  - Levodopa vs. dopamine agonist is controversial (2)[B]:
    - Most patients eventually will develop motor fluctuations with levodopa. Younger patients are more likely to develop motor fluctuations. Some recommend delaying initiation of levodopa to decrease drug-induced motor fluctuations early in the disease.
    - Older patients often are unable to tolerate the adverse events of dopamine agonists.
    - All patients eventually will require levodopa therapy.
  - MAO-B inhibitors (rasagiline) should be considered as initial monotherapy (2)[B]; also being investigated for potential neuroprotective effects
- Second-line agents in early PD: β-adrenergic antagonists (postural tremor), amantadine, anticholinergics (young patients with tremor) (1)[A]; there is lack of good evidence for symptom control.
- Treatment of levodopa-induced motor complications:
  - End of dose wearing off:
    - Entacapone (with each levodopa dose) or rasagiline preferred (3)[A]
    - May also consider dopamine agonist, apomorphine, selegiline (4)[B]
  - Dyskinesias:
    - Typically occur at peak dopamine level
    - Amantadine may be considered; however, its efficacy is questionable (1)[B].

First Line

- Carbidopa plus levodopa (carbidopa inhibits peripheral conversion of levodopa):
  - Immediate release (Sinemet):
    - Tablets (mg): 10/100, 25/100, 25/250
    - Usual initial maintenance dose: 25/100 mg PO t.i.d. Most patients will require 25 mg of carbidopa to inhibit peripheral conversion of levodopa.
    - Watch for nausea, orthostatic hypotension, sedation, vivid dreams, and vomiting.
  - Orally disintegrating (Parcopa):
    - Tablets (mg): 10/100, 25/100, 25/25
  - Sustained release (Sinemet CR):
    - Tablets (mg): 25/100, 50/200
    - Dose agents initially b.i.d.

- Carbidopa plus levodopa plus entacapone (Stalevo):
  - Tablets (mg): 12.5/50/200, 18.75/75/200, 25/100/200, 31.25/125/200, 37.5/150/200, 50/200/200
  - Addition of entacapone as a single agent should be initiated prior to use of this combination:
    - Once daily dose of carbidopa/levodopa has been identified, may convert to Stalevo
    - Dose of levodopa may need to be decreased with the addition of entacapone
  - Side effects are the same, plus diarrhea and brownish orange urine.
- Dopamine agonists (Nonergot): Side effects include nausea, vomiting, hypotension, sedation, lower extremity edema, vivid dreaming, compulsive behavior, confusion, lightheadedness, and hallucinations:
  - Pramipexole (Mirapex): Tablets (mg): 0.125, 0.25, 0.5, 1, 1.5
    - Start with 0.125 mg t.i.d., gradually increase every 5–7 days to 0.5–1.5 mg t.i.d.
    - CrCl 35–59 mL/min 0.125 mg PO b.i.d.
    - CrCl 15–34 mL/min 0.125 mg PO daily
  - Pramipexole ER (Mirapex ER): Tablets (mg): 0.375, 0.75, 1.5, 3, 4.5; start with 0.375 PO daily
  - Ropinirole (Requip): Tablets (mg): 0.25, 0.5, 1, 2, 3, 4, 5; start with 0.25 mg t.i.d., increase gradually to 3–8 mg t.i.d.
  - Requip XL: Tablets (mg): 2, 4, 6, 8, 12; start at a 2-mg dose once daily, increase in 1–2 weeks
- Dopamine agonists (ergot): Increased adverse event profile makes these agents nonpreferred to nonergot dopamine agonists
- Bromocriptine (Parlodel):
  - Tablets: 2.5 mg
  - Capsules: 5 mg
  - Start with 1.25 mg b.i.d., increase by 2.5 mg every 2–4 weeks up to effective dose (30–90 mg/d in 3 divided doses).
  - Same as nonergot and increases risk for pulmonary fibrosis (decreased efficacy compared with other agents)
- Selective MAO-B inhibitors: Side effects include insomnia, jitteriness, hallucinations; mostly found with selegiline; rasagiline shown to have similar adverse events as placebo in clinical trials. Rasagiline is metabolized via CYP 1A2; caution with other medications utilizing this enzyme system (e.g., ciprofloxacin):
  - Both agents contraindicated with meperidine and numerous other agents metabolized via CYP1A2
  - At therapeutic doses, unlikely to induce a "cheese reaction" (tyramine storm)
- Selegiline (Eldepryl):
  - Tablets (mg): 5 mg; initiate 5 mg PO b.i.d.
  - Orally disintegrating tablet (Zelapar): 1.25 mg; 1.25 mg PO daily for 6 weeks; increase as needed to maximum of 2.5 mg daily
  - Transdermal patch (Emsam): 6 mg/24 hr, 9 mg/24 hr, 12 mg/24 hr; start with 6 mg/24 hr and titrate up every 2 weeks as needed to a maximum of 12 mg/24 hr
- Rasagiline (Azilect): Tablets (mg): 0.5, 1; initiate 0.5–1 mg daily

Second Line

- Anticholinergic agents: Usually avoided due to lack of efficacy (only useful for tremor) and increased adverse event profile, including blurred vision, confusion, constipation, dry mouth, memory difficulty, sedation, and urinary retention:
  - Trihexyphenidyl:
    - Tablets (mg): 2, 5
    - Start with 1–2 mg daily, increase by 2 mg every 3–5 days until usual dose is 5–15 mg in 3–4 divided doses
  - Benztropine (Cogentin):
    - Tablets (mg): 0.5, 1, 2
    - Start with 0.5–6 mg in 1–2 divided doses; increase by 0.5 mg every 5–6 days
- N-methyl-D-aspartic acid antagonist: Exact mechanism is unknown and efficacy is questionable; however, it may be useful for dyskinesias. Side effects include confusion, dizziness, dry mouth, livedo reticularis, and hallucinations:
  - Amantadine (Symmetrel):
    - Tablets: 100 mg
    - Start with 100 mg b.i.d.; may increase to 300 mg daily in divided doses; must be renally adjusted
- Catechol-O-methyl transferase (COMT) inhibitors: Entacapone preferred due to hepatotoxicity associated with tolcapone. Adverse events include nausea and orthostatic hypotension:
  - Tolcapone (Tasmar):
    - Tablets (mg): 100, 200
    - Start 100 mg t.i.d.; maximum dose 600 mg/d; must be taken with carbidopa/levodopa
  - Entacapone (Comtan):
    - Tablets: 200 mg
    - 200 mg with each dose of carbidopa/levodopa; maximum dose, 1,600 mg/d
- Apomorphine (Apokyn): Nonergot-derived dopamine agonist given SC for off episodes. Adverse events include nausea, vomiting, dizziness, hallucinations, orthostatic hypotension, and somnolence:
  - Effective dose ranges from 2–6 mg per injection; most patients require 0.06 mg/kg
  - Monitor for orthostatic hypotension after initial dose; this is a potent emetic, so initiate an antiemetic (e.g., trimethobenzamide) 3 days prior to start and continue for 2 months. Avoid ondansetron (combination causes severe hypotension and syncope) and dopamine antagonists such as prochlorperazine and metoclopramide.
  - Indicated only for "off" episodes with levodopa therapy

ADDITIONAL TREATMENT

General Measures

- Multidisciplinary rehabilitation with standard physical and occupational therapy components to improve functional outcomes
- Physiotherapy to help with gait re-education, enhancement of aerobic capacity, improvement in movement initiation, improvement in functional independence, and help with home safety
- Emotional and psychological support of patient and family
- Speech and language therapy, dysphagia evaluation and therapy

Issues for Referral

All patients with suspected PD immediately should be referred to a specialist for an accurate diagnosis and management (1).

SURGERY/OTHER PROCEDURES

Deep brain stimulation (bilateral subthalamic nucleus or globus pallidus interna) for patients with motor complications refractory to best medical treatment who are healthy, have no significant active comorbidity, are responsive to levodopa, and do not have depression or dementia (1)

ONGOING CARE

DIET

- Increase dietary fluids and fiber, and increase activity for constipation
- For dysphagia, consider soft food, swallowing evaluation, and increased time for meals

PATIENT EDUCATION

- www.apdaparkinson.org
- www.parkinson.org
- http://guidance.nice.org.uk/CG35

PROGNOSIS

PD is a chronic progressive disease; prognosis varies based on patient-specific symptoms.

COMPLICATIONS

Psychosis can be caused by medication (most common); simplify medication regimen by discontinuing anticholinergics, dopamine agonists, amantadine, COMT inhibitors and selegiline; and a decrease in levodopa:

- Clozapine is useful but needs frequent monitoring due to agranulocytosis.
- Quetiapine (Seroquel) may be considered a better option.

REFERENCES

1. National Institute for Health and Clinical Excellence. *Parkinson's Disease: Diagnosis and Management in Primary and Secondary Care*. London: NICE; 2006.
2. Chen JJ, Swope DM. Pharmacotherapy for Parkinson's disease. *Pharmacotherapy*. 2007;27:161s–73s.
3. Pahwa R, Factor SA, Lyons KE, et al. Practice parameter: Treatment of Parkinson disease with motor fluctuations and dyskinesia (an evidence-based review): Report of the Quality Standards Subcommittee of the American Academy of Neurology. *Neurology*. 2006;66:983–95.
4. Diaz NL, Waters CH. Current strategies in the treatment of Parkinson's disease and a personalized approach to management. *Expert Rev. Neurother*. 2009;9(12):1781–9.

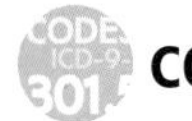

CODES

ICD9

332.0 Paralysis agitans

CLINICAL PEARLS

- Emphasize the importance of exercise and movement to help preserve function as long as possible.
- Pharmacotherapeutic regimens need to be individualized based on patient-specific symptoms and age.

PARONYCHIA

Robert A. Baldor, MD

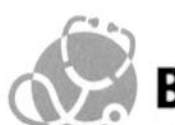

BASICS

DESCRIPTION

- Infectious or eczematous inflammation of the folds of skin surrounding the fingernail or toenail; may be acute or chronic:
  - Acutely, it often appears 2–5 days after trauma.
  - May be considered work-related among bartenders, waitresses, nurses, and others who often wet their hands
- System(s) affected: Skin/Exocrine
- Synonym(s): Eponychia; Perionychia

Pediatric Considerations

Thumb/finger-sucking is a risk factor (anaerobes and *Escherichia coli* may be present).

EPIDEMIOLOGY

Incidence

- Common in the US
- Predominant age: All ages
- Predominant sex: Female > Male (3:1)

RISK FACTORS

- Acute: Trauma to skin surrounding nail, ingrown nails, manicured/sculptured nails, diabetes mellitus (DM)
- Chronic: Frequent immersion of hands in water (e.g., cooks, chefs, bartenders, housekeepers, swimmers), DM, immunosuppression (reported association with antiretroviral therapy for HIV and with use of epidermal growth factor inhibitors)

GENERAL PREVENTION

- Chronic: Avoid allergens and frequent wetting of hands; wear rubber gloves with a cloth liner.
- Good diabetic control
- Expectant treatment for candidiasis
- Chronic: Keep fingers dry; avoid allergens.

PATHOPHYSIOLOGY

- A paronychial infection usually starts in the lateral nail fold.
- Occasionally, the infection includes the complete margin of skin around the nail plate, which results from mechanical separation of the nail plate from the perionychium.
- Early in the course of this disease process (<24 hours), cellulitis alone may be present. An abscess can form if the infection does not resolve quickly.
- Chronic infections most likely represent eczematous reaction with secondary infection and multifocal etiology.

ETIOLOGY

- Acute: *Staphylococcus aureus* and *Streptococcus pyogenes;* less frequently, *Pseudomonas pyocyanea* and *Proteus vulgaris*. In digits exposed to oral flora, also consider *Eikenella corrodens, Fusobacterium, and Peptostreptococcus*.
- Chronic: Eczematous reaction with secondary *Candida albicans* (~95%); less frequently, dermatophytes and, occasionally, molds (*Scytalidium, Fusarium*)

COMMONLY ASSOCIATED CONDITIONS

- DM
- If chronic, eczema or atrophic dermatitis
- Certain medications: Cetuximab, paclitaxel, antiretroviral therapy (especially protease inhibitors and lamivudine, with toes more commonly involved)
- If multiple, consider pemphigus vulgaris (rare)

DIAGNOSIS

HISTORY

- Localized pain and tenderness
- Previous trauma (bitten nails, ingrown nails, manicured nails)
- Contact with herpes infections
- Contact with allergens or irritants (frequent water immersion, latex)

PHYSICAL EXAM

- Acute: Red, hot, tender, tense nail fold ± abscess
- Chronic: Swollen, tender, boggy nail fold ± abscess
- Occasional elevation of nail bed
- Separation of nail fold from nail plate
- Red, painful swelling of skin around nail plate
- Purulent drainage
- Secondary changes of nail plate
- Green changes in nail (*Pseudomonas*)
- Positive digital pressure test (light pressure over the area causes digital blanching and demarcation of the abscess)
- Chronic; symptoms similar to acute with possible retraction of nail fold and absence of adjacent cuticle, thickening of nail plate, with prominent transverse ridges known as *Beau lines*

DIAGNOSTIC TESTS & INTERPRETATION

Lab

None required unless condition is severe; resistant to treatment or methicillin-resistant *S. aureus* (MRSA) is suspected; then:

- Gram stain
- Culture and sensitivity
- Potassium hydroxide wet mount plus fungal culture
- Drugs that may alter lab results: Use of over-the-counter antimicrobials or antifungals

Diagnostic Procedures/Surgery

- Scraping for wet mount and culture in chronic cases
- Incision and drainage for suppurative or cases not responding to conservative management
- Tzanck testing or viral culture in suspected viral cases

DIFFERENTIAL DIAGNOSIS

- Herpetic whitlow (similar in appearance, very painful, often associated with vesicles)
- Felon (abscess of fingertip pulp; urgent diagnosis required)
- Allergic contact dermatitis (latex, acrylic)
- Reiter disease
- Psoriasis
- Chronic; squamous cell carcinoma, malignant melanoma, metastases, eczema, psoriasis, Reiter syndrome

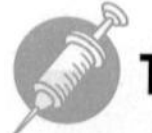

TREATMENT

MEDICATION

First Line

- Tetanus booster when appropriate
- No evidence that antibiotics are better or worse than incision and drainage, although if there is an obvious pus pocket, incision and drainage is recommended.
- Acute (mild cases):
  - Antibiotic cream alone or in combination with a topical steroid
  - Antibiotic cream applied t.i.d.–q.i.d. (e.g., mupirocin or gentamicin/neomycin/polymyxin B) for 5–10 days
  - If eczematous: Topical steroid applied b.i.d. (e.g., betamethasone 0.05% cream) for 7–14 days
- Acute (exposure to oral flora):
  - Clindamycin (Cleocin) 315–450 mg t.i.d.–q.i.d. for 7 days:
    - Pediatric: 10 mg/kg q8h
  - Amoxicillin–clavulanate potassium (Augmentin): 875 mg/125 mg q12h or 500 mg/125 mg t.i.d. for 7 days:
    - Pediatric: 45 mg/kg q12h (for <40 kg)

- Acute (no exposure to oral flora):
  - Dicloxacillin 250 mg t.i.d. for 7 days
  - Cephalexin (Keflex) 500 mg b.i.d.–t.i.d. for 7 days
- Acute (suspected MRSA):
  - Trimethoprim/sulfamethoxazole 160 mg/800 mg b.i.d. for 7 days
  - Doxycycline 100 mg b.i.d. for 7 days
- Chronic:
  - Topical steroids: e.g., betamethasone 0.05%; applied b.i.d. for 7–14 days with or without antifungal
  - Topical antifungal: e.g., econazole, clotrimazole, or nystatin; applied topically t.i.d. for up to 30 days
- Contraindications: Allergy to antibiotic, may consider erythromycin as alternative
- Precautions: Erythromycin may cause significant GI upset.
- Significant possible interactions:
  - Erythromycin affects levels of theophylline and effects of carbamazepine, digoxin, and corticosteroids. Cardiac toxicity with terfenadine or astemizole is possible.
  - Ketoconazole, astemizole, itraconazole, fluconazole: Terfenadine, statin drugs

Second Line

- Systemic antifungals (rarely needed):
  - Itraconazole (Sporanox) 200 mg/d for 90 days (may have longer action because it is incorporated in nail plate); pulse therapy may be useful (200 mg b.i.d. for 7 days, repeated monthly for 2 months)
  - Terbinafine (Lamisil) 250 mg/d for 6 weeks (fingernails) or 12 weeks (toenails)
  - Fluconazole (Diflucan) 150 mg/wk for 4–6 months
- Antipseudomonal drugs (e.g., third-generation cephalosporins, aminoglycosides)

ADDITIONAL TREATMENT

General Measures

- Acute: Water or vinegar/water (1:1) soaks (t.i.d.–q.i.d.), warm compresses, elevation
- Chronic: Keep fingers dry. Apply moisturizing lotion after hand washing; avoid exposure to irritants; improved diabetic control.

Issues for Referral

Chronic; treatment failure, consider biopsy and/or in cases of recalcitrant chronic paronychia referral for possible en bloc excision of the nail fold or eponychial marsupialization with or without nail removal

SURGERY/OTHER PROCEDURES

- Incision and drainage of abscess, if present
- A subungual abscess or ingrown nail requires partial or complete removal of nail.

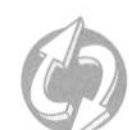

ONGOING CARE

FOLLOW-UP RECOMMENDATIONS

Chronic: Avoid frequent immersion, triggers, allergens, or nail biting and finger sucking.

DIET

If patient is diabetic, institute appropriate dietary changes for better control.

PATIENT EDUCATION

Avoid trimming cuticles; stress importance of good diabetic control; avoid contact irritants; use rubber gloves with cotton liners to avoid exposure to moisture

PROGNOSIS

- With adequate treatment and prevention, healing can be expected.
- If no response in chronic lesions, rarely benign or malignant neoplasm may be present, and referral should be considered.

COMPLICATIONS

- Acute: Subungual abscess
- Chronic: Secondary ridging, thickening, and discoloration of nail, nail loss

ADDITIONAL READING

- Rigopoulos D, Alevizos A. Acute and chronic paronychia. *Am Fam Physician*. 2008;177(3): 339–46.
- Rockwell PG. Acute and chronic paronychia. *Am Fam Physician*. 2001;63:1113–6.
- Shaw J, Body R. Best evidence topic report. Incision and drainage preferable to oral antibiotics in acute paronychial nail infection? *Emerg Med J*. 2005; 22:813–4.
- Tosti A, Piraccini BM, Ghetti E, et al. Topical steroids versus systemic antifungals in the treatment of chronic paronychia: An open, randomized double-blind and double dummy study. *J Am Acad Dermatol*. 2002;47:73–6.

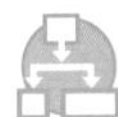

See Also (Topic, Algorithm, Electronic Media Element)

Onychomycosis

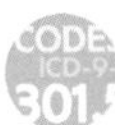

CODES

ICD9

- 681.02 Onychia and paronychia of finger
- 681.11 Onychia and paronychia of toe

CLINICAL PEARLS

- Tetanus booster when appropriate
- No evidence that antibiotics are better or worse than incision and drainage, although incision and drainage is recommended for an obvious pus pocket.

PARAROTITIS, ACUTE AND CHRONIC

Meera Shah, MD
Kathleen Ferrer, MD

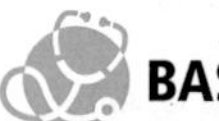

BASICS

DESCRIPTION

- Parotitis is inflammation of the parotid gland caused by infection (viral or bacterial), noninfectious systemic illnesses, mechanical obstruction, or medications.
- The parotid gland is the largest of the salivary glands, located lateral to the masseter muscle anteriorly and extending posteriorly over the sternocleidomastoid muscle behind the angle of the mandible.
- The parotid duct, also called the Stensen's duct, pierces the buccinator muscle to enter the buccal mucosa just opposite the second maxillary molar.
- The branches of the seventh cranial nerve divide the gland into lobes.
- The parotid gland contains lymph nodes.
- Parotitis can be unilateral or bilateral, acute or chronic.

EPIDEMIOLOGY

- Prior to widespread vaccination, parotitis was primarily caused by mumps virus:
  - ~150,000 cases of mumps parotitis occurred per year in the prevaccine era.
  - Now, ~1,600 cases/yr occur due to occasional sporadic outbreaks.
- Acute bacterial parotitis occurs more frequently in elderly patients, neonates (especially preterm infants), and postoperative patients.
- Chronic bilateral parotid enlargement is a common manifestation of HIV infection; for perinatally HIV-infected children, the average age of onset for parotid enlargement is 5 years of age .
- Juvenile recurrent parotitis is the most common inflammatory salivary gland disorder in the US; first onset of symptoms occurs between the ages of 3 and 6.

RISK FACTORS

- Acute viral parotitis: Lack of mumps, measles, rubella (MMR) vaccination
- Acute bacterial parotitis:
  - Conditions that predispose to salivary stasis, such as dehydration, debilitation, poor oral hygiene, Sjögren syndrome, cystic fibrosis, bulimia/anorexia, sialolithiasis (stones), ductal stenosis, trauma
  - Medications such as anticholinergics, antihistamines, diuretics, tricyclic antidepressants, thioridazine, iodine
  - Immunosuppression, HIV, chemotherapy, radiation, malnutrition, alcoholism
- Chronic parotitis:
  - Ductal stenosis, HIV, tuberculosis, Sjögren syndrome, and sarcoidosis

GENERAL PREVENTION

- MMR vaccination with the first dose between 12 and 15 months and second dose between 4 and 6 years of age; of note, mumps vaccination does not guarantee prevention, possibly due to waning immunity in adolescence
- Maintaining adequate hydration and good dental hygiene
- Sucking on hard or sour candies can stimulate salivary flow and prevent salivary stasis.
- Smoking cessation, abstinence from alcohol, and avoidance of chronic purging

PATHOPHYSIOLOGY

- Acute viral parotitis begins as a systemic infection that localizes to the parotid gland, resulting in inflammation and swelling of the gland:
  - Mumps, or paramyxovirus, has a predilection for the parotid gland and classically has been linked with parotitis.
- For bacterial parotitis, stasis of salivary flow allows retrograde introduction of bacterial pathogens into parotid gland, resulting in localized infection.
- Chronic parotitis in HIV-infected patients can be due to the presence of benign lymphoepithelial cysts, follicular hyperplasia of parotid lymph nodes, or diffuse infiltrative lymphocytosis syndrome (DILS) causing infiltration of the parotid gland by CD8 cells:
  - Parotitis may also be secondary to immune reconstitution after initiation of combination antiretroviral therapy in HIV-infected patients (1).

ETIOLOGY

- Acute parotitis due to infection:
  - Viral:
    - Paramyxovirus (mumps), parainfluenza virus types 1 and 3, influenza A, coxsackieviruses, Epstein-Barr virus (EBV)
    - Cytomegalovirus (CMV) and adenovirus have been seen in patients with HIV.
  - Bacterial:
    - *Staphylococcus aureus* and anaerobes (oral flora) are most commonly seen.
    - *Streptococcus pneumoniae*, *Escherichia coli*, and *Haemophilus influenza* (less common)
    - Gram-negative rods such as *E. coli*, *Klebsiella*, *Enterobacter*, and *Pseudomonas* can be seen in chronically ill or hospitalized patients.
  - Fungal:
    - *Candida* has been isolated in chronically ill or hospitalized patients.
    - Actinomyces can be found in patients with a history of trauma or dental caries.
- Acute, recurrent parotitis:
  - Juvenile recurrent parotitis may be secondary to chronic inflammation; etiology is unknown, but a genetic component has been described.
  - Mechanical: Sialolithiasis, ductal stenosis
  - Pneumoparotitis may occur when air is trapped in the ducts of the parotid gland; may be seen in wind instrument players, glass blowers, and SCUBA divers
  - Medications: Anticholinergics, antihistamines, tricyclic antidepressants, thioridazine, iodine
  - Other: Diabetes, alcoholism, bulimia
- Chronic parotitis:
  - HIV
  - Tuberculosis, syphilis (rare)
  - Autoimmune: Sjögren syndrome (parotid enlargement, xerostomia, and keratoconjunctivitis)
  - Inflammatory: Sarcoidosis:
    - Heerfordt syndrome (parotid enlargement, facial palsy, and uveitis) is rare manifestation of sarcoidosis

COMMONLY ASSOCIATED CONDITIONS

HIV, Sjögren syndrome, sarcoidosis, sialolithiasis

DIAGNOSIS

HISTORY

- Acute parotitis presents with sudden-onset pain and swelling of the cheek usually extending to and obscuring the angle of the mandible:
  - Viral parotitis is usually bilateral and accompanied by a prodrome of malaise, anorexia, headaches, myalgias, arthralgias, and fever; no pus is noted at Stensen's duct.
  - Bacterial parotitis is typically unilateral with induration, warmth, and erythema over the affected cheek; fever is often noted.
  - Juvenile recurrent parotitis is usually unilateral; pain and swelling usually resolve within 2 weeks and exacerbations occur until puberty; purulent exudate is not typical, but superinfection may occur .
  - Sialolithiasis is characterized by recurrent acute swelling and pain, exacerbated by eating; sialolithiasis affects the submandibular gland more frequently.
  - Other frequently reported symptoms include trismus (inability to open mouth), pain exacerbated by chewing or worsened by foods that stimulate production of saliva (i.e., sour candies), dry mouth with abnormal taste, difficulty with drinking/eating, anorexia, or dehydration.
- Chronic parotitis presents with recurrent or chronic nontender swelling of 1 or both parotid glands:
  - Sjögren syndrome, sarcoidosis, HIV, tuberculosis
  - Chronic parotitis may predispose to superinfection, which would present similarly to an acute parotitis.

PHYSICAL EXAM

- Characterized by swelling or enlargement of parotid gland, which overlies the masseter muscle; may obscure the angle of the mandible or cause the ear to protrude upward and outward:
  - Tender and bilateral suggests viral etiology; tender and unilateral suggests bacterial etiology
  - Nontender in HIV, tuberculosis, Sjögren, sarcoidosis
- Trismus can be noted.
- Pus from Stensen's duct is suggestive of bacterial parotitis or superinfection; duct may also be edematous and erythematous.
- In juvenile recurrent parotitis, Stensen's duct is often enlarged, dilated, erythematous, and swollen.
- Halitosis and dental decay are often associated with acute exacerbations.
- Facial nerve palsy can be seen in severe cases.

DIAGNOSTIC TESTS & INTERPRETATION

Lab

- Performing aerobic culture and Gram stain of purulent drainage from Stensen's duct or aerobic and anaerobic culture from needle aspiration of gland or abscess can be helpful to identify causative organism:
  - Anaerobic culture from Stensen's duct will likely contain oropharyngeal contamination; hence, it is recommended to perform anaerobic cultures only from needle aspirate fluid.
- Aerobic and anaerobic blood culture may also identify causative organism.
- Acute bacterial parotitis often demonstrates an elevated white cell count and amylase.
- For suspected mumps, obtain mumps IgM antibody or mumps reverse transcription-polymerase chain reaction (RT-PCR). Also, a 4-fold increase of mumps IgG antibody indicates infection.
- Consider sending EBV, respiratory virus PCR if viral parotitis suspected; CMV titers should be sent in immunocompromised patients
- For chronic, recurrent, or nontender parotitis, consider HIV test, PPD, SS-A SS-B antibodies, rheumatoid factor, antinuclear antibodies

Imaging

- Consider obtaining CT scan or ultrasound of parotid area to assess for abscess, cystic masses, parotid tumors, ductal stenosis, or sialolithiasis.
- Imaging studies can also identify features consistent with HIV or juvenile recurrent parotitis.

Diagnostic Procedures/Surgery

Consider performing a biopsy or fine-needle aspiration of gland if there is suspicion for tuberculosis, Sjögren syndrome, or sarcoidosis.

Pathological Findings

- Findings characteristic of HIV are described in in the "Pathophysiology" section.
- Noncaseating granulomas can be seen in sarcoidosis, and caseating granulomas may be found in tuberculosis.

DIFFERENTIAL DIAGNOSIS

Nonparotid swelling or erythema may sometimes appear similar to parotitis: Lymphoma, neoplasm, lymphangitis, cervical adenitis, external otitis media, dental abscess, cellulitis can be considered in the differential. Differentiating between nonparotid swelling and parotitis can sometimes be difficult:

- Parotid swelling or enlargement typically obscures the angle of the mandible (unlike cervical adenitis).
- Involvement of Stensen's duct is also unique to parotitis.

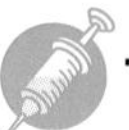

TREATMENT

- Usually a self-limiting course that requires primarily supportive treatment with rest, adequate hydration, analgesia, and antipyretics:
  - Can also stimulate glands to produce saliva by sucking on sugarless lemon drops or glycerin swabs
  - Local heat and gentle massage of gland can provide symptomatic relief.
  - For chronic presentations encourage good dental hygiene and treat underlying etiology of parotitis (HIV, tuberculosis).
- For suspected bacterial component, can empirically initiate antibiotics to cover *S. aureus*, anaerobes (oral flora), and *S. pneumoniae*
- Patients should be isolated; isolate up to 5 days after parotid swelling is noted.

MEDICATION

- Acute bacterial parotitis:
  - Outpatient management: Amoxicillin/clavulanate or clindamycin
  - Chronically ill or hospitalized: Ampicillin/sulbactam or clindamycin or nafcillin; if methicillin-resistance is probable, consider vancomycin or linezolid
- Pilocarpine and cevimeline can stimulate saliva production and provide symptomatic relief for patients with underlying Sjögren syndrome

SURGERY/OTHER PROCEDURES

- Consider needle aspiration for bacterial parotitis with abscess formation or clinical deterioration with increasing pain, erythema, and swelling, not responding to medication
- May perform serial drainage for symptomatic cysts
- Consider superficial parotidectomy for severe recurrent parotid infections in patients with underlying predisposing etiology (such as Sjögren syndrome)
- For sialolithiasis or ductal stenosis, consult otolaryngology for possible duct ligation, ductoplasty, or parotidectomy; interventional sialoscopy has been shown to be a therapeutic tool for strictures (2)[C].
- Sclerotherapy has been shown to be effective in the treatment of cysts in HIV parotitis (3)[C].

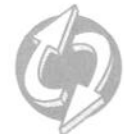

ONGOING CARE

FOLLOW-UP RECOMMENDATIONS

Antibiotic therapy initiated at diagnosis combined with adequate hydration should result in improvement within 48 hours. If not, patient should be re-evaluated.

DIET

- Ensure adequate fluid intake.
- Suggest hard or sour candies to stimulate salivary flow.

PROGNOSIS

- Viral infection in immunocompetent individuals often resolves with excellent prognosis.
- Parotid cysts found in HIV-infected patients are usually benign lymphoepithelial lesions with infrequent malignant transformation.
- Increased incidence of malignant lymphoma or lymphoepithelial carcinoma can be seen in patients with Sjögren syndrome.

COMPLICATIONS

- For mumps, potential complications include orchitis, pancreatitis, meningitis, or nephritis.
- Untreated bacterial parotitis can lead to local extension, abscess formation, and facial paralysis.

REFERENCES

1. Ortega KL, Ceballos-Salobreña A, Gaitán-Cepeda LA, et al. Oral manifestations after immune reconstitution in HIV patients on HAART. *Int J STD AIDS*. 2008;19:305–8.
2. Koch M, Iro H, Zenk J, et al. Role of sialoscopy in the treatment of Stensen's duct strictures. *Ann Otol Rhinol Laryngol*. 2008;117:271–8.
3. Berg EE, Moore CE, et al. Office-based sclerotherapy for benign parotid lymphoepithelial cysts in the HIV-positive patient. *Laryngoscope*. 2009;119:868–70.

ADDITIONAL READING

- Brook I, et al. Acute bacterial suppurative parotitis: Microbiology and management. *J Craniofac Surg*. 2003;14:37–40.
- Brook I, et al. The bacteriology of salivary gland infections. *Oral Maxillofac Surg Clin North Am*. 2009;21:269–74.
- Patel A, Karlis V, et al. Diagnosis and management of pediatric salivary gland infections. *Oral Maxillofac Surg Clin North Am*. 2009;21:345–52.

CODES

ICD9

- 072.9 Mumps without mention of complication
- 527.2 Sialoadenitis

CLINICAL PEARLS

- Physical exam is usually sufficient for diagnosis (parotid swelling and tenderness with or without purulent drainage from Stensen's duct)
- In recurrent or chronic cases, must consider other underlying etiologies, such as HIV.
- *S. aureus* and anaerobes (oral flora) are the most common organisms isolated in acute bacterial parotitis.
- Encouraging good oral hygiene and adequate hydration in chronically ill, debilitated, and hospitalized patients can reduce the occurrence of parotitis.

PARVOVIRUS B19 INFECTION

Luis T. Garcia, MD

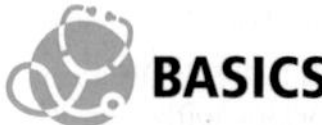

BASICS

DESCRIPTION

- Human parvovirus B19 is the primary cause of erythema infectiosum (EI, or fifth disease).
- Complications in susceptible individuals include transient aplastic crisis (TAC) in patients with increased RBC turnover (e.g., sickle-cell anemia), chronic anemia in immunodeficient individuals, and arthritis and arthralgias in normal hosts:
  - Pregnant women who are not immune are at risk of intrauterine infection, with potentially significant consequences to the fetus.
- System(s) affected: Mainly Hemic/Lymphatic/Immunologic; Musculoskeletal; Skin/Exocrine; possibly Central Nervous System (CNS); Cardiac; Renal

Pregnancy Considerations

Documentation of acute infection during pregnancy should prompt referral to maternal–fetal medicine specialist. Maternal B19 infection between 9 and 20 weeks' gestation may be associated with a significant risk for developing fetal anemia.

EPIDEMIOLOGY

- Infection is common in childhood.
- Predominant age: Peak age for EI is 4–12 years.
- 50% of children 15 years of age are parvovirus B19–seropositive.
- Predominant sex: Male = Female
- Epidemics occur in late spring every 2–4 years.

Prevalence

- Extremely common in the US; >50% of adults have evidence of prior infection. Most common as community epidemics in winter and spring in nontropical regions.
- Antibody IgG prevalence:
  - 1–5 years, 2–15%
  - 6–9 years, 20–40%
  - 11–19 years, 35–60%
  - >50 years, >75%

RISK FACTORS

- School-related epidemic and nonimmune household contacts have a secondary attack rate of 50%.
- Highest secondary attack rates are for daycare providers and school personnel in contact with affected children.
- Those with increased cell turnover (e.g., SS anemia, thalassemia) at risk for aplastic crisis
- Immunodeficiency may increase risk of chronic anemia.
- 40% of pregnant women are not immune, with 1.5% seroconversion/yr.

Genetics

Erythrocyte P antigen–negative individuals are resistant to infection.

GENERAL PREVENTION

- Standard hygienic practices with good hand washing can minimize spread.
- Because EI is so common, it is impossible to avoid exposure completely. Also, period of contagion is before clinical illness (rash) appears.
- Pregnant health care workers should avoid caring for patients with transient aplastic crises.
- Pregnant childcare workers are at some increased risk; however, exclusion from the workplace will not eliminate this risk and, therefore, is not recommended.

PATHOPHYSIOLOGY

- Natural host of B19 is human erythroid progenitor
- Infection of proerythroblasts causes cessation of RBC production.

ETIOLOGY

- Small (20–25 mm), nonenveloped, single-stranded DNA virus. Only known parvovirus to infect humans and belongs to the family *Parvoviridae*.
- Respiratory secretions and rarely blood products are sources of human spread of virus.
- Maternal viremia with transplacental passage is the source of fetal infection.
- In EI, the rash is thought to be autoimmune due to IgM complexes.

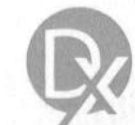

DIAGNOSIS

HISTORY

- Headache, pharyngitis, coryza, myalgia, arthralgias, arthritis, and GI disturbances are more frequent and severe in adults (nonspecific flulike illness).
- Pruritus (especially soles of feet) and mild arthralgia may occur.

PHYSICAL EXAM

- Onset of rash is first noted on the face ("slapped-cheek appearance").
- Second stage follows 1–4 days later with a lacy reticular rash on the trunk and limbs.
- A third stage of rash is characterized by marked evanescence and recrudescence, sometimes associated with bathing, exercise, sun exposure, or emotional stress.

DIAGNOSTIC TESTS & INTERPRETATION

Lab

Initial lab tests

- CBC shows anemia and reticulocytopenia.
- Usually no need for serology because diagnosis is made clinically
- B19-specific IgM (detected 10–14 days after infection) and IgG recommended for immunocompetent patient when needed
- B19-specific DNA detection for fetus, neonate, patients with TAC, and immunosuppressed patients
- To exclude congenital B19 in infants with negative B19 IgM, one must follow an infant's B19 IgG serology in the first year of life.
- Maternal serum α-fetoprotein may be increased in fetuses with hydrops fetalis.

Follow-Up & Special Considerations

- Joint disease:
  - In adults, 80% of patients may manifest arthritis and/or arthralgia (female > male).
  - In children, joint symptoms are less common.
  - Knees, hands, and ankles (frequently symmetric) are involved most commonly.
  - Joint symptoms usually subside within 3 weeks but may persist for months. No joint erosions on x-ray.
- TAC:
  - Seen in patients with increased RBC turnover, such as sickle-cell anemia, spherocytosis, thalassemia, and pyruvate kinase deficiency
  - Aplastic event is self-limited, with reticulocytes reappearing in 7–10 days and full recovery in 2–3 weeks.
  - In children with sickle cell hemoglobinopathies and heredity spherocytosis, fever is the most common symptom (73%), and rash is highly unlikely.
- Chronic anemia:
  - Seen in immunodeficient individuals with no IgM response
  - No manifestations of fever, rash, or joint symptoms usually.
- Fetal/neonatal infection:
  - Risk of transplacental spread of virus ~33% in infected mothers
  - A pregnant woman with a new rash or arthralgia should be tested for the virus.
  - Clinical manifestations range from asymptomatic seroconversion and normal pregnancy (most commonly), to variable degrees of fetal hydrops, to second- and third-trimester intrauterine fetal demise without hydrops.
  - B19 infection always should be suspected in cases of nonimmune hydrops.
  - The principal organ involved in the fetus is the bone marrow. RBC survival is shortened, and profound anemia can result from B19-induced erythroid bone marrow aplasia.
  - Over 95% of fetal complications (fetal hydrops and death) occur within 12 weeks of acute parvovirus B19 infection in pregnancy.
  - Risk of fetal loss in pregnancy is highest with B19 infections in the first trimester (9%).
  - Fetal anemia is the most common manifestation of later infection, but seroconversion after 21 weeks had no severe anemia (1).
  - In one study, 84% of B19-infected pregnant women who carried to term delivered normal infants.
  - Parvovirus B19 infection does not increase the risk of birth defects or mental retardation.
  - There are no known long-term developmental problems in infant survivors.
- Papular purpuric gloves and socks syndrome (PPGSS): Strong association with B19. Severe petechial and ecchymotic rash in hand–foot distribution with associated febrile tonsillopharyngitis and oral ulcerations (2).

Imaging

Initial approach

Documented acute maternal infection in the first trimester warrants weekly fetal ultrasound (US) for 8–12 weeks to access for hydrops development (3)[C].

Pathological Findings

- Skin biopsy usually normal but may show mild inflammation consisting of perivascular infiltrations of mononuclear cells
- In hydrops fetalis, may see intranuclear inclusions in nucleated RBCs
- In stillbirths related to maternal B19 infection, virus can be detected in all tissues.

DIFFERENTIAL DIAGNOSIS

- Rubella
- Enteroviral disease
- Systemic lupus erythematosus
- Drug reaction
- Lyme disease
- Rheumatoid arthritis

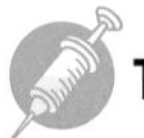

TREATMENT

MEDICATION

- No therapy is needed usually.
- Anti-inflammatory agents may alleviate arthritic symptoms.

ADDITIONAL TREATMENT

General Measures

- IVIG for B19-related refractory anemia, especially if patient is immunodeficient (4)[C]
- Cessation of immunosuppressive therapy has allowed some patients to clear chronic infections.
- RBC transfusions may be required for aplastic crisis.
- Intrauterine RBC transfusions have been shown to reduce mortality significantly in hydrops/anemia diagnosed by US or cordocentesis. There is a firm recommendation for intrauterine transfusion for parvovirus B19–induced hydrops (5)[A].

Issues for Referral

Documentation of acute infection during pregnancy should prompt referral to maternal–fetal medicine specialist.

IN-PATIENT CONSIDERATIONS

Initial Stabilization

- Outpatient management for EI
- Inpatient management for aplastic crisis, which may require RBC transfusions

ONGOING CARE

FOLLOW-UP RECOMMENDATIONS

Patient Monitoring

Periodic blood counts for anemic patients

PATIENT EDUCATION

- Parvovirus B19 (fifth disease): www.cdc.gov/ncidod/dvrd/revb/respiratory/parvo_b19.htm
- Parvovirus B19 infection and pregnancy: www.cdc.gov/ncidod/dvrd/revb/respiratory/B19&preg.htm
- Parvovirus B19: What you should know: www.aafp.org/afp/20070201/377ph.htm
- Physicians should counsel pregnant women with respect to prevention and management of maternal B19 infection (6)[C].
- Pregnant women should avoid exposure to patients with active or chronic infections. However, exclusion of pregnant women from the workplace where EI is occurring is not recommended.
- Children with symptoms are no longer infectious and may attend childcare or school.

PROGNOSIS

- Usually self-limited
- Joint symptoms subside in weeks (often by 2 weeks but may last months).
- ~20% of infections result in delayed virus elimination and viremia persisting for several months to years.
- Full recovery from aplastic crisis in 2–3 weeks

COMPLICATIONS

Conditions associated with B19 but not proven:

- Chronic fatigue syndrome
- Glomerulonephritis and other renal diseases have been reported in both immunocompromised and immunocompetent patients.
- Nephrotic syndrome/glomerulonephritis
- Hepatitis
- Neurologic manifestations/stroke/meningoencephalitis
- Henoch-Schönlein purpura or vasculitis
- Myocarditis
- Pericarditis

REFERENCES

1. Simms RA, Liebling RE, Patel RR, et al. Management and outcome of pregnancies with parvovirus B19 infection over seven years in a tertiary fetal medicine unit. *Fetal Diagn Ther*. 2009;25(4).
2. Fretzayas A, Douros K, Moustaki M, et al. Papular-purpuric gloves and socks syndrome in children and adolescents. *Pediatr Infect Dis J*. 2009;28(3):250–2.
3. Enders M, Weidner A, Rosenthal T, et al. Improved diagnosis of gestational parvovirus B19 infection at the time of nonimmune fetal hydrops. *J Infect Dis*. 2008;197:58.
4. Orange JS, Hossny EM, Weiler CR, et al. Use of intravenous immunoglobulin in human disease: A review of evidence by members of the Primary Immunodeficiency Committee of the American Academy of Allergy, Asthma and Immunology. *J Allergy Clin Immunol*. 2006;117:S525–53.
5. de Jong EP, de Haan TR, Kroes AC, et al. Parvovirus B19 infection in pregnancy. *J Clin Virol*. 2006;36: 1–7.
6. Beigi RH, Wiesenfeld HC, Landers DV, et al. High rate of severe fetal outcomes associated with maternal parvovirus B19 infection in pregnancy. *Infect Dis Obstet Gynecol*. 2008;2008:524–601.

ADDITIONAL READING

- March of Dimes Fifth Disease in Pregnancy: www.marchofdimes.com/professionals/14332_25586.asp.
- Ramirez MM, Mastrobattista JM. Diagnosis and management of human parvovirus B19 infection. *Clin Perinatol*. 2005;697–704.
- Tolfvenstam T, Broliden K, et al. Parvovirus B19 infection. *Semin Fetal Neonatal Med*. 2009;14: 218–21.

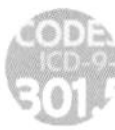

CODES

ICD9

- 057.0 Erythema infectiosum (fifth disease)
- 079.83 Parvovirus B19

CLINICAL PEARLS

- Parvovirus B19 infection is usually a benign, self-limited illness with no long-term effects.
- The rash of EI signifies that the patient is no longer infectious.
- Patients with increased RBC turnover (SS, thalassemia) are at risk for transient aplastic crisis.
- Immunocompromised patients may be at risk for chronic anemia.
- Documentation of acute infection before 20 weeks gestation warrants maternal–fetal consultation for serial monitoring of fetal well-being for 3 months via ultrasound.

PATELLOFEMORAL PAIN SYNDROME

Jake D. Veigel, MD
Anastasia Grivoyannis, MD
J. Herbert Stevenson, MD

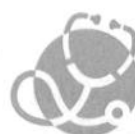

BASICS

DESCRIPTION

- Peri- or retropatellar pain resulting from biomechanical forces in the patellofemoral joint
- System(s) affected: Musculoskeletal

EPIDEMIOLOGY

Prevalence

- May affect 25% of athletes (1)
- Common among adolescents
- Difference between sexes is negligible (a 3% higher prevalence has been reported among female vs. male athletes).
- Higher incidence during the second and third decades of life. Incidence decreases with age in both men and women.

RISK FACTORS

- Increased Q angle (>20°) (2,3)[B]
- Weakness of the quadriceps and/or hip abductors (2,3)[B]
- Iliotibial (IT) band tightness (2)[B]
- Inflexibility of the hamstrings, quadriceps, or hip flexors (2)[B]
- Generalized ligamentous laxity (2)[B]
- Lateral retinacular tightness (2)[B]

Genetics

Unknown

GENERAL PREVENTION

- Injury prevention program for those with potential risk factors
- In runners, wearing properly fitting footwear
- Proper training programs with appropriate slow increases in mileage

PATHOPHYSIOLOGY

Repetitive contact of the undersurface of the patella against the trochlea of the femur with or without maltracking of the patella

ETIOLOGY

Precise cause unknown, likely multifactorial; can be categorized into 3 subsets:

- Anatomic (malalignment, abnormal patellar height, shallow trochlear groove, muscular dysfunction)
- Dynamic (muscle imbalance, overload, or overuse)
- Specific (chondral, plica, or neuroma)

COMMONLY ASSOCIATED CONDITIONS

- IT band friction syndrome
- Patellar tendinopathy

DIAGNOSIS

HISTORY

- An accurate history should differentiate pain from instability (e.g., pain quality, swelling, giving way, mechanical symptoms, and grinding, inciting events, overuse, and history of trauma)
- Most common symptom: Anterior knee pain exacerbated by physical activity or an increase in physical activity
- Pain often exacerbated when squatting
- Anterior knee pain when descending/ascending stairs, ambulating over uneven surfaces, or running
- Theater sign or movie-goer sign: Anterior knee pain upon arising after prolonged sitting
- Crepitus with knee range of motion
- Often can have pain after activity as well as during activity

PHYSICAL EXAM

- In some athletes, physical findings may be subtle or absent. Observe patella position in the knee at 90° and track for a J sign (3).
- Pain at the area of the patellofemoral articulation (e.g., patella facets, trochlea, and peripatellar area) (3).
- Apprehension sign: Compress the patella against the femur and ask the patient to contract quadriceps muscles; pain upon contraction is consistent with patellofemoral pain syndrome (3), although pain may be present in normal individuals as well.
- Reproduction of pain with compression of patella against the trochlea (3)
- Q angle is assessed by taking the angle of the intersection of 2 lines: 1 drawn from the anterior superior iliac spine to the midpatella and the other line drawn from the midpatella to the tibial tubercle. An angle of >20° is a potential risk factor.

DIAGNOSTIC TESTS & INTERPRETATION

Lab

None indicated

Imaging

In general, imaging is unnecessary and not helpful in diagnosing this condition. If imaging is indicated because of severity, atypical symptoms, or persistence of symptoms despite treatment, 4 views of the knee, including lateral, Merchant or sunrise, standing anteroposterior, and posteroanterior tunnel views are recommended to view patellar tilt and to rule out other potential etiologies of anterior knee pain. Radiographic findings may not correlate with symptoms.

Follow-Up & Special Considerations

Radiographic images may be normal until late stages, when the posterior patellar surface becomes irregular and cartilage erosion becomes radiographically detectable.

Pathological Findings

Should be absent, and any presence of pathology indicates other diagnosis.

DIFFERENTIAL DIAGNOSIS

- Patellofemoral joint osteoarthritis (2)
- Chondromalacia patella
- Patellar tendinopathy
- Articular cartilage injury
- Hoffa disease
- IT band syndrome
- Loose bodies
- Neuromas
- Osgood-Schlatter disease
- Osteochondritis dissecans
- Patellar instability/subluxation
- Patellar fracture
- Patellar stress fracture
- Pes anserine bursitis
- Plica synovialis
- Bone tumors
- Prepatellar bursitis
- Previous surgery
- Quadriceps tendinopathy
- Referred pain from lumbar spine or hip joint pathology
- Saphenous neuritis
- Sinding-Larsen-Johansson syndrome
- Symptomatic bipartite patella

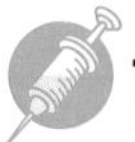

TREATMENT

Most important is abstaining from activity thought to induce the problem and training in a different manner.

MEDICATION

- There is limited evidence for the effectiveness of NSAIDs for short-term pain relief (4)[C].
- The evidence for glycosaminoglycan polysulphate is conflicting and merits further investigation (4).
- Nandrolone may be effective, but it is too controversial to recommend for treatment (4).

ADDITIONAL TREATMENT

Ice packs after activity have been found to improve clinical symptoms.

General Measures

- Physical therapy referral for exercises are effective (1,5)[A].
- Specific home exercises may be employed, but guidance from a physical therapist is preferred (1,5)[A], particularly for athletes.
- Knee braces and taping can be helpful at the initiation of physical therapy, but do not replace a well-designed exercise program (1,5)[A].
- Orthotic arch support may be helpful (5)[C].
- Rest from painful activity and substitute aggravating activities with crosstraining exercises (e.g., swimming) (5)[C].
- Applying ice for 10–15 minutes at a time may be helpful (5)[C].

Issues for Referral

Referral for surgery is a last resort after all conservative measures fail.

SURGERY/OTHER PROCEDURES

- Attempts to correct maltracking of the patellofemoral joint with a lateral retinacular release or tibial tubercle transposition have shown variable results.
- Rarely indicated

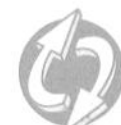

ONGOING CARE

PATIENT EDUCATION

Patient education and exercises: http://familydoctor.org/online/famdocen/home/healthy/physical/injuries/479.html

REFERENCES

1. Collado H, Fredericson M, et al. Patellofemoral pain syndrome. *Clin Sports Med*. 2010;29:379–98.
2. Waryasz GR, et al. Patellofemoral pain syndrome (PFPS): A systematic review of anatomy and potential risk factors. *Dynam Med*. 2008;7:1476–1459.
3. Fredericson M, Yoon K, et al. Physical examination and patellofemoral pain syndrome. *Am J Phys Med Rehabil*. 2006;85:234–43.
4. Heintjes E, Berger MY, Bierma-Zeinstra SM, et al. Pharmacotherapy for patellofemoral pain syndrome. *Cochrane Database Syst Rev*. 2004;(3):CD003470.
5. Dixit S, DiFiori JP, Burton M, et al. Management of patellofemoral pain syndrome. *Am Fam Physician*. 2007;75:194–202.

ADDITIONAL READING

Bizzini M, Childs JD, Piva SR, et al. Systematic review of the quality of randomized controlled trials for patellofemoral pain syndrome. *J Orthop Sports Phys Ther*. 2003;33(1):4–20.

See Also (Topic, Algorithm, Electronic Media Element)

Algorithm: Knee Pain

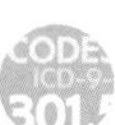

CODES

ICD9

719.46 Pain in joint involving lower leg

CLINICAL PEARLS

- Patellofemoral pain syndrome is the most common cause of anterior knee pain in active adults (age 20–39), affecting men and women almost equally.
- The clinical diagnosis is made by taking a history and the use of the apprehension sign (compress the patella against the femur and ask the patient to contract quadriceps muscles; pain with contraction is consistent with patellofemoral pain syndrome).
- Well-designed exercises geared at quadriceps strengthening, hamstring and IT band flexibility, and hip stabilizers are the most effective evidence-based treatment.

PATENT DUCTUS ARTERIOSUS

Cody Mead, DO, CPT, MC, USA
Vernon Wheeler, Jr., MD, FAAFP

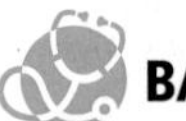

BASICS

DESCRIPTION

- Patent ductus arteriosus (PDA) is the failure of the ductus arteriosus, a vessel connecting the pulmonary artery and aorta, to close after birth. 75% of cases occur as an isolated defect:
  - Clinical presentation depends on the size of the ductus arteriosus and gestational age at delivery.
  - Predominant left-to-right shunt leads to vascular congestion of the lungs.
  - Premature infants present with apnea and/or respiratory distress.
  - PDA is considered pathological when it persists beyond 3 months of age or is associated with symptoms.
  - Spontaneous closure after 5 months is rare in the full-term infant.
  - Ibuprofen is considered the drug of choice for symptomatic PDA. Efficacy is the same as indomethacin, but ibuprofen reduces the risk of NEC and renal insufficiency. Long-term studies are lacking (1)[A].
- System(s) affected: Cardiovascular; Pulmonary
- Synonym(s): Aorticopulmonary shunt; Aorticopulmonary communication

Pediatric Considerations

Some infants with coexisting cardiac anomalies benefit temporarily from a PDA to provide shunting to the lungs (right heart obstructions) or periphery (coarctation of the aorta). Definitive treatment should proceed as soon as feasible.

Pregnancy Considerations

Women with small-to-moderate-sized ductus and left-to-right shunt can expect an uncomplicated pregnancy. High risk in those with high pulmonary resistance and right-to-left shunt.

EPIDEMIOLOGY

PDA is the fifth most common congenital cardiac defect in the US, representing 5–10% of all congenital heart diseases.

Incidence

- Predominant age: Infancy
- Predominant sex: Female > Male (2:1)
- 8 in 1,000 premature live births
- In term infants, the incidence is about 1 in 2,000–2,500 live births

RISK FACTORS

- Premature birth, high altitudes
- Maternal rubella in the first trimester
- Coexisting cardiac anomalies
- Any condition resulting in hypoxia (pulmonary, hematologic, etc.)
- Prenatal indomethacin exposure associated with increased incidence and severity of postnatal PDA

Genetics

- Siblings of patients with PDA have 2–4% increase in frequency of PDA
- Autosomal-dominant inheritance in some families

GENERAL PREVENTION

- Prophylactic IV indomethacin in preterm infants reduces symptomatic PDA, length of supplemental oxygen requirement, need for surgical ligation, and grade 3 or 4 intraventricular hemorrhage. Unfortunately, there was no effect on mortality or neurodevelopment, and there are no studies showing long-term outcomes (2,3)[A].
- Similarly, prophylactic ibuprofen decreased the incidence of symptomatic PDA, decreased the need for rescue treatment with cyclo-oxygenase inhibitors, and decreased the need for surgical closure. Again, this treatment is not recommended until long-term outcomes have been studied (4)[A].

PATHOPHYSIOLOGY

- The ductus arteriosus (DA) is normally open during fetal life. It is kept patent by low arterial oxygen levels and circulating prostaglandin E2. At birth, closure is triggered by a decrease in circulating prostaglandin E2 and increase in arterial oxygen tension.
- Closes by 24 hours in 50% of full-term neonates, by 48 hours in 90%, and by 72 hours in virtually all neonates. A PDA occurs when the DA fails to completely close postnatally.
- The main features of the natural history include spontaneous ductal closure, bacterial endocarditis, late congestive heart failure (CHF), and the development of pulmonary vascular obstructive disease.

ETIOLOGY

- Prematurity, congenital
- Hypoxia, prostaglandins

COMMONLY ASSOCIATED CONDITIONS

- Coarctation of the aorta
- Pulmonary valve stenosis or atresia
- Peripheral pulmonary stenosis (maternal rubella)
- Aortic stenosis, ventricular septal defect
- Necrotizing enterocolitis in preterms
- Bronchopulmonary dysplasia
- Club feet, cataracts, blindness, systemic arterial stenosis (associated with maternal rubella)

DIAGNOSIS

HISTORY

- Children:
  - Many are asymptomatic.
  - Failure to grow, easy fatigability
  - Recurrent respiratory infections
  - Dyspnea on exertion
- Adults:
  - Leg fatigue, fatigue, syncope
  - Shortness of breath, angina

PHYSICAL EXAM

- Signs (left-to-right shunt):
  - Rough systolic murmur
  - Continuous "machinery" murmur
  - Thrill at left upper sternal border
  - Bounding pulse with wide pulse pressure
  - Prominent, displaced apical impulse
  - Systolic ejection click
  - Diastolic flow murmur (across mitral valve)
  - Excessive sweating
  - Tachypnea, tachycardia, rales in failure
- Signs (right-to-left shunt):
  - Cyanosis, especially lower extremities
  - Clubbing
  - Diastolic Graham-Steell murmur (high-velocity pulmonic insufficiency secondary to pulmonary hypertension)
  - Right ventricular heave
- Signs of congestive heart failure: Tachycardia, hyperactive precordium, edema, decreased urine output

DIAGNOSTIC TESTS & INTERPRETATION

Lab

Initial lab tests

- Arterial blood gas
- ECG in children and adults may show left ventricular and left atrial hypertrophy.
- ECG in infants usually normal
- Brain natriuretic peptide (BNP) levels correlate with symptoms and magnitude of ductal shunt.

Imaging

Initial approach

- Chest radiograph usually normal in infants
- Chest radiograph in children and adults (shunt vascularity, calcifications, left ventricle and left atrial enlargement, dilated ascending aorta, dilated pulmonary arteries)
- Chest radiograph may show cardiomegaly, signs of heart failure.

Follow-Up & Special Considerations

- Echocardiography/Doppler
- Contrast echocardiography
- Radionuclide angiography
- MRI

Diagnostic Procedures/Surgery

- Doppler echocardiography: Preferred procedure in confirming the diagnosis and characterizing PDA
- Cardiac catheterization and angiography: Will demonstrate the shunt and determine the degree of shunting, pulmonary pressures, and other coexisting cardiac abnormalities

Pathological Findings

- Infolding of endothelial cells and migration of undifferentiated smooth muscle cells fail.
- Left ventricular and atrial enlargement
- Patent ductus may have abnormal intima (maternal rubella).

DIFFERENTIAL DIAGNOSIS

- Venous hum
- Total anomalous pulmonary venous return
- Ruptured sinus of Valsalva
- Arteriovenous communications
- Anomalous origin of left coronary artery from pulmonary artery
- Absence or atresia of pulmonary valve
- Aortic insufficiency with ventricular septal defect
- Peripheral pulmonary stenosis (maternal rubella)
- Truncus arteriosus
- Aortopulmonary fenestration
- Coronary artery fistula

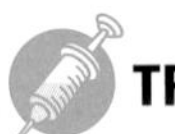

TREATMENT

MEDICATION

Pharmacologic therapy is used strictly in the premature infant, and prostaglandin inhibitors are the initial intervention.

First Line

- Ibuprofen lysine (IV preparation): Only for infants 500–1,500 g and ≤32 weeks' gestation: Dose is 10 mg/kg IV followed by 5 mg/kg 24 and 48 hours later
- Indomethacin 0.2 mg/kg per dose IV q12h for 3 doses. Decreased efficacy in term infants; not effective in children or adults (5)[A]
- Oxygen, diuretics
- Indomethacin contraindications:
  - Renal dysfunction, overt bleeding
  - Shock, necrotizing enterocolitis
  - Myocardial ischemia
- Precautions: With indomethacin treatment, oliguria, hyponatremia; can have significant adverse effects on renal, GI, and cerebrovascular blood flow

Second Line

- Ibuprofen and indomethacin appear to have similar efficacy in closing PDA; however, ibuprofen reduces risk of NEC and transient renal insufficiency (1)[A].
- Oral ibuprofen dosed at 10 mg/kg followed by 5 mg/kg at 24 and 48 hours is an option if the IV preparation is unavailable, but patients with borderline renal function should be evaluated and followed closely (6)[B].
- Alprostadil (prostaglandin E1) treatment to maintain patency of duct in ductal-dependent lesions
- Antibiotic prophylaxis to prevent infective endocarditis with dental, GI, GU, or respiratory tract procedures is no longer recommended unless the patient has unrepaired cyanotic congenital heart disease.

ADDITIONAL TREATMENT

General Measures

- Appropriate health care: Inpatient surgery
- Small, asymptomatic shunts may not need closure.

SURGERY/OTHER PROCEDURES

- Surgical transection and ligation for moderate/large shunts best option in premature infants when medical treatment has failed or is contraindicated (7)[A]
- Preterm infants with severe pulmonary dysfunction
- Persistent PDA on echocardiography despite 2 courses of pharmacologic treatment
- Complications on indomethacin, such as decreased renal output (<1 mL/kg/hr), intestinal bleeding, intestinal perforation
- Contraindications to pharmacologic (severe thrombocytopenia, evolving intracranial hemorrhage, bleeding diathesis)
- Transfemoral catheter technique to occlude PDA with coil embolization, wire mesh, or double umbrella for larger duct option for larger infants and children

IN-PATIENT CONSIDERATIONS

Initial Stabilization

- Pulmonary support, oxygen to correct hypoxia
- Sodium and fluid restriction

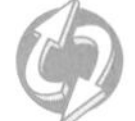

ONGOING CARE

FOLLOW-UP RECOMMENDATIONS

- No need for antibiotic prophylaxis after surgical repair
- Timely closure of a PDA is generally definitive treatment, and no special care or follow-up is necessary.
- In medically treated patients, echocardiography to confirm ductus closure after 3-day course of medication, with additional 3 days of pharmacologic treatment if luminal patency

Patient Monitoring

- Annual routine follow-up after closure
- Shunts that have not been closed should be followed more closely.

DIET

No specific diet

PATIENT EDUCATION

Discuss prematurity and explain different treatments of premature infants and full-term infants.

PROGNOSIS

- Before 3 months, closure in premature infants is 75%.
- Before 3 months, closure in term infants is 40%.
- Best postoperative results if closed before age 3 years.
- Increased pulmonary vascular resistance and pulmonary hypertension more common if closed after age 3 years
- No firm statistics, but decreased survival for large shunts
- In adults, the prognosis depends on the condition of pulmonary vasculature and the status of the myocardium if congestive cardiomyopathy was present prior to ductal closure.

COMPLICATIONS

- Left heart failure, pulmonary hypertension
- Right heart hypertrophy and failure
- Eisenmenger physiology
- Bacterial endocarditis, myocardial ischemia
- Necrotizing enterocolitis

REFERENCES

1. Ohlsson A, Walia S, et al. Ibuprofen for the treatment of patent ductus arterisousus in preterm and/or low birth weight infants. *Cochrane Database Syst Rev.* 2010;4.
2. Fowlie PW, Davis PG, McGuire W. Prophylactic intravenous indomethacin for preventing mortality and morbidity in preterm infants. *Cochrane Database Syst Rev.* 2010;7:CD000174.
3. Cooke L, Steer P, et al. Indomethacin for asymptomatic patent ductus arteriosus in preterm infants. *Cochrane Database Syst Rev.* 2008;3.
4. Ohlsson A, Shah SS. Ibuprofen for the prevention of patent ductus arteriosus in preterm and/or low birth weight infants. *Cochrane Database Syst Rev.* 2011;7.
5. Van Overmeire B, Smets K, Lecoutere D, et al. A comparison of ibuprofen and indomethacin for closure of patent ductus arteriosus. *N Engl J Med.* 2000;343:674–81.
6. Gokmen T, Erdeve O, Altug N, et al. Efficacy and safety of oral versus intravenous ibuprofen in very low birth weight preterm infants with patent ductus arteriosus. *Journal of Pediatrics.* 2011;158:549–54.
7. Malviya M, Ohlsson A, Shah S. Surgical versus medical treatment with cyclooxygenase inhibitors for symptomatic patent ductus arteriosus in preterm infants. *Cochrane Database Syst Rev.* 2006;1.

ADDITIONAL READING

- Pass R, et al. Multicenter USA Amplatzer PDA occlusion device trial: Initial and mid-term results. *Circulation.* 2002;106:II486.
- Tavera M, Bassereo P, Biddau R, et al. Role of echocardiography on the evaluation of patent ductus arteriosus in newborns. *J Matern Fetal Neonatal Med.* 2009;22(S3):10–3.

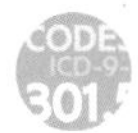

CODES

ICD9

747.0 Patent ductus arteriosus

CLINICAL PEARLS

- Ibuprofen is currently the treatment of choice in preterm infants with PDA and is preferred over indomethacin due to equal efficacy and reduced incidence of NEC and reduced renal impairment; surgical treatment is second line and used for symptomatic infants or those in whom the PDA does not close spontaneously or with pharmacologic treatment.
- PDA increases incidence of necrotizing enterocolitis in premature infants.
- Left untreated, patients develop Eisenmenger syndrome: Right-to-left shunting. At this point, pulmonary vascular disease is irreversible, and closure of PDA is contraindicated.

The views expressed in this chapter are those of the author and do not reflect the official policy or position of the Department of the Army, Department of Defense, or the US Government. Opinions, interpretations, conclusions, and recommendations herein are those of the author and are not necessarily endorsed by the US Army.

PEDICULOSIS (LICE)

Kaelen C. Dunican, PharmD
Julie Scott Taylor, MD, MSc

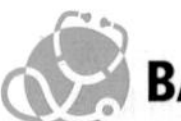

BASICS

DESCRIPTION

- A very contagious parasitic infection caused by lice (blood-sucking insects, obligate parasites)
- 2 species of lice infest humans:
  - *Pediculus humanus* has 2 subspecies: The head louse (var. *capitis*) and the body louse (var. *corporis*). Both species are 1–3-mm long, flat, and wingless and have 3 pairs of legs that attach closely behind the head.
  - *Phthirus pubis* (pubic or crab louse): Resembles a sea crab and has widespread claws on the second and third legs
- System(s) affected: Skin/Exocrine
- Synonym(s): Lice; Crabs

EPIDEMIOLOGY

Incidence

- In the US: 6–12 million new cases/yr
- Predominant age:
  - Head lice: Most common in children 3–12 years of age; more common in girls than boys
  - Pubic lice: Most common in adults

Prevalence

Head lice: 1–3% in industrialized countries

RISK FACTORS

- General: Overcrowding and close personal contact
- Head lice:
  - School-aged children, gender (girls)
  - Sharing combs, hats (including helmets), clothing, and bed linens
  - African Americans rarely have head lice; theories include twisted hair shaft and increased use of thick hair products
- Body lice: Poor hygiene, homelessness
- Pubic lice: Promiscuity (very high transmission rate)

GENERAL PREVENTION

- Environmental measures: Wash, dry-clean, or vacuum all items that may have come in contact with infected individuals.
- Screen and treat affected household contacts.
- Head lice: Follow-up by school nurses may help to prevent recurrence and spread.
- Pubic lice: Limit the number of sexual partners (note: condoms do not prevent transmission nor does shaving pubic hair).
- Body lice: Proper hygiene

PATHOPHYSIOLOGY

Itching is a hypersensitivity reaction to the saliva of the feeding louse.

ETIOLOGY

- Infestation by lice: *P. humanus* var. *capitis*, *P. humanus* var. *corporis*, or *P. pubis*
- Characteristics of lice:
  - The adult louse is dark grayish and moves quickly but does not jump or fly.
  - Eggs (sometimes referred to as nits) camouflage with the individuals' hair color and are cemented to the base of the hair shaft (within 4 mm of the scalp).
  - Nits (empty egg casings) appear white (opalescent) and remain cemented to the hair shaft.
  - Lice feed solely on human blood by piercing the skin, injecting saliva, and then sucking blood.
- Transmission: Direct human-to-human contact
  - Head lice: Direct head-to-head contact or contact with infested fomite (less common)
  - Body lice: Contact with contaminated clothing or bedding
  - Pubic lice: Typically transmitted sexually (fomite transmission is unlikely)

COMMONLY ASSOCIATED CONDITIONS

Up to 1/3 of patients with pubic lice have at least 1 concomitant STD.

DIAGNOSIS

HISTORY

- Pruritus is common, mostly at night.
- Investigate contacts of infected individuals.

PHYSICAL EXAM

- Diagnosis is confirmed clinically by visualization of live lice.
- *P. capitis* (head lice):
  - Found most often on the back of the head and neck and behind the ears (warmer areas of the hair)
  - Eyelashes may be involved.
  - Eggs, found cemented on the base of a hair shaft, are difficult to remove.
  - Pruritus may be accompanied by local erythema and small papules.
  - May see excoriations around hairline
  - Scratching can cause inflammation and secondary bacterial infection.
  - Pyoderma and lymphadenopathy in severe infestation
- *P. corporis* (body lice):
  - Poor hygiene
  - Adult lice and nits in the seams of clothing
  - Intense pruritus involving area covered by clothing (trunk, axillae, and groin)
  - Uninfected bites present as erythematous macules, papules, and wheals.
  - Pyoderma and excoriation may be seen.
- *P. pubis* (pubic louse):
  - Pubic hair is the most common site, but lice may spread to hair around anus, abdomen, axillae, chest, beard, eyebrows, and eyelashes.
  - Eggs are present at the base of hair shafts.
  - Anogenital pruritus
  - Blue macules may be seen in the surrounding skin.
  - Delay in treatment may lead to development of groin infection and regional adenopathy.

DIAGNOSTIC TESTS & INTERPRETATION

- Head lice: Comb hair thoroughly with a fine-toothed louse comb (0.2–0.3 mm between teeth) to identify live lice (1,2)[C]. Simple visual inspection is of similar sensitivity to wet combing but about 25% as effective as dry combing with a metal comb (3).
- Body lice: Examine the seams of clothing to locate lice and their eggs (2)[C].

Lab

- Carefully examine hair shafts under the microscope; lice and eggs can be seen easily under a microscope.
- In contrast to dandruff, eggs and nits cannot be removed easily from a hair shaft.

Follow-Up & Special Considerations

- Empty nits will remain on hair shafts for months after eradication of the live infestation. On Wood's lamp exam, live nits fluoresce white and empty nits fluoresce gray.
- Pubic lice: Patients should be evaluated for other STDs.

DIFFERENTIAL DIAGNOSIS

- Scabies and other mite species that can cause cutaneous reactions in humans
- Dandruff and other hair debris can sometimes look like head lice but do not stick to hair shafts like eggs and nits do.

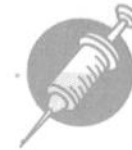

TREATMENT

Since the early 1990s, lice have acquired some degree of resistance to insecticides (3).

MEDICATION

Permethrin (over the counter [OTC]), synergized pyrethrin (OTC), spinosad (Rx), benzyl alcohol (Rx), and malathion (Rx) are effective for head lice (1,4,5)[A]. Permethrin, synergized pyrethrin, and malathion are effective for pubic lice (4)[A]:

- Permethrin may be preferred because it has residual activity for up to 3 weeks (2)[C]. However, newer shampoos may reduce the residual effect (1)[C].
- Malathion and spinosad are considered second line for head lice but may be more effective due to ovicidal activity (1,5)[B].

First Line

- Head and pubic lice:
  - Pyrethrum insecticides: Permethrin 1% cream rinse (Nix) or pyrethrins 0.33% with piperonyl butoxide 4% (synergized pyrethrins, Rid, Pronto): Apply for 10 minutes, then wash.
    - Reapplication in 7–10 days (day 9 is optimal) is always required with use of synergized pyrethrin and may be necessary with use of permethrin, especially if live lice are observed.
    - Side effects: Application-site erythema; ocular erythema, and application-site irritation
- Body lice: Best treated with synergized pyrethrin lotion applied once and left on for several hours.
- Eyelash infestation: Apply petroleum jelly b.i.d. × 10 days.
- Precautions:
  - Pyrethrins: Avoid in patients with ragweed allergy (may cause respiratory symptoms).
  - Pediculicides should never be used to treat eyelash infections.

Second Line

- Head lice and pubic lice:
  - Malathion 0.5% lotion (Ovide):
    - Apply for 8–12 hours, then wash off.
    - Excipients isopropyl alcohol (78%) and terpineol (12%) may contribute to its efficacy.
    - Flammable and has a bad odor
    - A second application may be necessary after 7–10 days (day 9 is optimal) if live lice are observed.
  - Dual therapy with 1% permethrin and oral trimethoprim/sulfamethoxazole (TMP/SMX) only for cases of multiple treatment failures or suspected cases of lice-related resistance to therapy (TMP/SMX is not approved by the FDA for lice)

- Lindane 1% shampoo: Apply for 4 minutes, then wash (should *not* be repeated).
  - Side effects: Neurotoxicity (seizures, muscle spasms), aplastic anemia
  - Contraindications: Uncontrolled seizure disorder, premature infants
  - Precautions: Do not use for excoriated skin, immunocompromised patients, conditions that increase seizure risk, or with medications that decrease seizure threshold
  - Possible interactions: Concomitant use with medications that lower the seizure threshold
- Head lice:
  - Spinosad 0.9% lotion (Natroba):
    - Apply to dry hair and scalp for 10 minutes, then rinse with warm water. Repeat in 7 days if live lice are observed.
    - Side effects: Application-site erythema, ocular erythema, and application-site irritation
  - Benzyl alcohol 5% lotion (Ulesfia):
    - Apply to dry hair by using a sufficient amount to saturate the scalp and hair (amount depends on hair length), rinse after 10 minutes, and repeat in 7 days.
    - Side effects: Pruritus, erythema, pyoderma, ocular irritation, application-site irritation
  - Mechanical removal of lice and nits by wetting hair and then systematically combing with a fine-toothed comb every 3–4 days × 2 weeks to remove all lice as they hatch

ALERT

Lindane: FDA black box warning of severe neurologic toxicity (use only when first-line agents have failed). The National Pediculosis Association strongly advises against using lindane at all.

Pediatric Considerations

- Avoid synergized pyrethrin and permethrin in infants <2 months of age, malathion in children <2 years of age, and benzyl alcohol and spinosad in children <6 months of age.
- Lindane: Not recommended in patients who weigh <50 kg, including infants

Pregnancy Considerations

Permethrin, synergized pyrethrin, malathion, spinosad, and benzyl alcohol are pregnancy category B. Lindane is category C.

ADDITIONAL TREATMENT

- Several classes of alternative physically acting (vs. physiologically acting) treatments are under investigation, the most promising of which are silicone mixtures that work by blocking the louse respiratory tract (3).
- For "difficult to treat" cases of head lice, oral ivermectin (400 mcg/kg), given twice at a 7-day interval, had superior efficacy when compared with topical 0.5% malathion lotion (6)[A].

General Measures

- Head lice: Wash all bedding, towels, clothes, headgear, combs, brushes, and hair accessories in hot water (60°C).
- Vacuum furniture and carpets.
- Any personal articles that cannot be washed in hot water, dry cleaned, or vacuumed should be sealed in a plastic bag and stored for at least 2 weeks.
- All household members and close contacts should be examined and treated concurrently if infested.
- Insecticide sprays are not necessary.
- Pubic lice: Avoid sexual activity until both partners are successfully treated. Shaving pubic hair does not improve treatment outcomes.
- Nit and egg removal:
  - It is particularly important to remove eggs that are within 1 cm of the scalp to prevent reinfestation.
  - After treatment with shampoo or lotion, eggs and nits remain in the scalp or pubic hair until mechanically removed.
  - Eggs and nits are best removed with a very fine nit comb.

COMPLEMENTARY AND ALTERNATIVE MEDICINE

- Ivermectin: 200 μg/kg repeated in 7–10 days
  - Should not be used in children weighing <15 kg; pregnancy Category C
  - Not approved by the FDA for lice
- Head lice:
  - Dry-on, suffocation-based pediculicide: Nuvo or Cetaphil lotion:
    - Apply thoroughly to hair, comb, dry with hairdryer, shampoo after 8 hours.
    - Repeat once a week until cured, up to a maximum of 3 applications.
    - Not approved by the FDA for lice
  - Dimethicone 4% lotion: Apply to hair for 8 hours; repeat in 1 week (not approved by the FDA for lice)
  - No home remedies (e.g., vinegar, isopropyl alcohol, olive oil, mayonnaise, melted butter, and petroleum jelly) to treat head lice infestations are effective.
  - Herbal shampoos and pomades have not been evaluated in clinical trials and are not approved by the FDA for lice.
  - Lavender oil and tea tree oil have been implicated in triggering prepubertal gynecomastia in boys, so they should not be used against lice (3).

ONGOING CARE

FOLLOW-UP RECOMMENDATIONS

Children may return to school after completing topical treatment, even if nits remain in place. No-nit policies are not necessary (1).

Patient Monitoring

Drug resistance should be suspected if live lice are still present 12–24 hours after treatment.

PATIENT EDUCATION

- National Pediculosis Association at www.headlice.org
- CDC at www.cdc.gov/ncidod/dpd/parasites/headlice/default.htm
- www.headliceinfo.com/faqs.htm

PROGNOSIS

- With appropriate treatment, >90% cure rate
- Recurrence common, mainly from reinfection or failure to comply with treatment

COMPLICATIONS

- Poor sleep due to pruritus
- Persistent itching may be caused by too frequent use of the pediculicide.
- Missed school; social stigma
- Secondary bacterial infections
- Body lice can transmit typhus and trench fever.

REFERENCES

1. Frankowski BL, Bocchini JA Jr. The Council on School Health and Committee on Infectious Disease. *Head lice. Pediatrics*. 2010;126:392–403.
2. Orion E, Marcos B, Davidovici B. Itch and scratch: Scabies and pediculosis. *Clin Dermatol*. 2006;24:168–75.
3. Burgess IF. Current treatments for pediculosis capitis. *Curr Opin Infect Dis*. 2009;22:131–6.
4. Flinders DC, De Schweinitz P. Pediculosis and scabies. *Am Fam Physician*. 2004;69:341–8.
5. Cole SW, Lundquist LM. Spinosad for treatment of head lice infestation. *Ann Pharmacother*. 2011;45:954–9.
6. Chosidow O, Giraudeau B, Cottrell J, et al. Oral ivermectin versus malathion lotion for difficult-to-treat head lice. *N Engl J Med*. 2010;362:896–905.

ADDITIONAL READING

- Diamantis SA, Morrell DS, Burkhart CN. Treatment of head lice. *Dermatol Ther*. 2009;22:273–8.
- Lebwohl M, Clark L, Levitt J. Therapy for head lice based on life cycle, resistance, and safety considerations. *Pediatrics*. 2007;119:965–74.

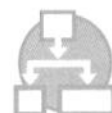

See Also (Topic, Algorithm, Electronic Media Element)

Arthropod Bites and Stings; Scabies

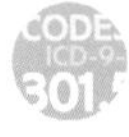

CODES

ICD9

- 132.1 Pediculus corporis (body louse)
- 132.2 Phthirus pubis (pubic louse)
- 132.9 Pediculosis, unspecified

CLINICAL PEARLS

- Proper product application is essential; improper product application should be considered when assessing treatment failure.
- The prevalence of resistant infestations is increasing, so if live lice are present 12–24 hours after proper treatment, resistance should be suspected and an alternative agent from another class should be used.
- Routine re-treatment on day 9 is recommended for nonovicidal products (permethrin and synergized pyrethrins).
- With all treatment options, patients' hair should be reinspected after 7–9 days and, if live lice are detected, treatment should be repeated on day 9.
- No-nit policies are not necessary because empty nits may remain on hair shafts for months after eradication.

PELVIC INFLAMMATORY DISEASE (PID)

Shannon Demas, MD
Marie Ellen Caggiano, MD, MPH

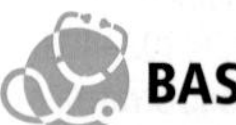

BASICS

DESCRIPTION

- An acute infection of the upper genital tract in women caused by the ascent of organisms, often sexually transmitted, from the vagina and endocervix to the uterus, fallopian tubes, ovaries, and contiguous structures
- *Pelvic inflammatory disease* (PID) is a broad term that encompasses a variety of upper genital tract infections, including endometritis, salpingitis, oophoritis, tubo-ovarian abscess, peritonitis, and perihepatitis.
- Accurate diagnosis is challenging and incorrect in up to 1/3 of women.
- System(s) affected: Reproductive
- Synonym(s): Salpingitis; Salpingo-oophoritis; Adnexitis; Pyosalpinx; Tubo-ovarian abscess; Pelvic peritonitis; Upper genital tract infection

EPIDEMIOLOGY

- Predominant age: 1/3 of patients are <20 years of age; 2/3 are <25 years of age.
- Predominant sex: Female only

Incidence

In the US, 1 million women are treated for PID each year.

Prevalence

100–200 per 100,000 women

RISK FACTORS

- Sexually active and age <25 years
- First sexual activity at young age
- New/multiple sexual partners
- Nonbarrier contraceptive methods (i.e., oral contraceptive pills)
- Previous history of PID; 20–25% will have a recurrence.
- History of *Chlamydia trachomatis*; 10–40% will develop PID.
- History of gonococcal cervicitis; 10–20% will develop PID.

GENERAL PREVENTION

- Educational programs about safer sex practices and STI prevention
- Barrier contraceptives, especially condoms and spermicidal creams or sponges, provide protection, the extent of which is not well documented.
- Early medical care with occurrence of genital lesions or abnormal discharge
- Intrauterine device (IUD) insertion is contraindicated in women with active (acute) cervical or pelvic infection.
- Annual chlamydia screening of all sexually active women aged <25 years and of older women with risk factors (e.g., those who have a new sex partner or multiple sex partners
- Routine STI screening in pregnancy
- Evaluation and treatment of sexual partners after diagnosis with STI

PATHOPHYSIOLOGY

- The precise mechanism by which microorganisms ascend from the lower genital tract is unknown. One possibility is that chlamydial or gonococcal endocervicitis disturbs the vaginal ecosystem, allowing ascent of the vaginal flora with or without the original pathogen. Thus, polymicrobial infection can occur without *Neisseria gonorrhoeae* or *C. trachomatis* infection.
- 75% of cases occur within 7 days of menses, when cervical mucus favors ascension of organisms.

ETIOLOGY

Multiple organisms act as etiologic agents in PID. Most cases are polymicrobial:

- *C. trachomatis*, *N. gonorrhoeae*, and a wide variety of aerobic and anaerobic bacteria are recognized as etiologic agents.
- The proportion of cases infected with chlamydia or gonorrhea varies widely depending on the population studied.
- The most common organisms include *H. influenzae, streptococcus pyogenes, Bacteroides, E. coli, Peptococcus, and Peptostreptococcus* sp.
- Bacterial vaginosis is more common among women with PID but does not confer an increased risk of PID.
- Mycoplasmas, cytomegalovirus (CMV), and *U. urealyticum* also have been implicated, but their role is less clear (1).

COMMONLY ASSOCIATED CONDITIONS

- If PID is suspected in a patient with an IUD and a pelvic abscess is present, an *Actinomyces* infection requiring penicillin treatment may be present.
- Rupture of an adnexal abscess is rare but life threatening. Early surgical exploration is mandatory.
- Chlamydial or gonococcal perihepatitis may occur with PID. This combination is called Fitz-Hugh-Curtis (FHC) syndrome and is characterized by severe pleuritic right upper quadrant pain:
  - FHC syndrome complicates 10% of PID cases.

DIAGNOSIS

- May present as new onset pelvic/lower abdominal pain, especially in women <25 years old. Have low threshold for empiric antibiotic treatment among at-risk women.
- The CDC recommends empiric treatment for PID based on clinical criteria of cervical motion tenderness and uterine or adnexal tenderness in the presence of lower abdominal or pelvic pain.

HISTORY

- Diagnosis may be challenging, and even asymptomatic patients are at risk for sequelae.
- Fever (50%)
- Nausea and vomiting
- Lower abdominal pain, worse with coitus and jarring movements
- New/abnormal vaginal discharge
- Irregular bleeding occurs in ≥1/3 patients
- Urinary discomfort
- Proctitis
- Recent hysterosalpingogram (HSG)
- IUD insertion within the last 21 days

PHYSICAL EXAM

- Criteria for diagnosis:
  - Lower abdominal/suprapubic pain (± rebound)
  - Adnexal tenderness (unilateral or bilateral)
  - Cervical motion tenderness (CMT)
- Supports diagnosis:
  - Temperature ≥38.3°C
  - Cervical or vaginal mucopurulent discharge
  - Cervical friability

DIAGNOSTIC TESTS & INTERPRETATION

Lab

Initial lab tests

- Pregnancy test: Must be performed to rule out ectopic pregnancy and complications of an intrauterine pregnancy
- CBC: WBC count ≥10,500/mm^3, ≤50% of PID cases present with leukocytosis.
- Chlamydia and gonorrhea cultures
- Urinalysis
- Saline microscopy of vaginal fluid with increased WBC

Follow-Up & Special Considerations

- ESR >15 mm/hr
- Elevated C-reactive protein
- Consider HIV testing in patients with PID.

Imaging

Not necessary for diagnosis, although supports diagnosis

Initial approach

Transvaginal ultrasound: May show thickened, fluid-filled tubes (hydrosalpinges) ± free fluid or tubo-ovarian abscess (TOA)

Follow-Up & Special Considerations

TOA will not resolve immediately after medical treatment. Follow-up ultrasound can be followed as outpatient for resolution of adnexal abscess.

Diagnostic Procedures/Surgery

- Culdocentesis with culture is rarely necessary.
- Laparoscopy is best used for confirming as opposed to making the diagnosis of PID and should be reserved for the following situations:
  - Ill patient with competing diagnosis (e.g., appendicitis)
  - Ill patient who has failed outpatient treatment
  - Any patient not improving after 72 hours of inpatient treatment
- Endometrial biopsy

Pathological Findings

Endometrial biopsy reveals endometritis/plasma cells.

DIFFERENTIAL DIAGNOSIS

- Appendicitis
- Ectopic pregnancy
- Ovarian torsion
- Hemorrhagic or ruptured ovarian cyst

- Endometriosis/dysmenorrhea
- Inflammatory bowel disease
- Diverticulitis
- Pyelonephritis

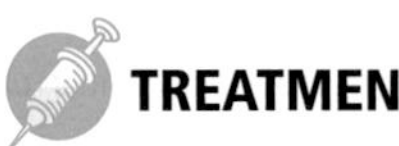

TREATMENT

- Outpatient treatment if appropriate
- Criteria for hospitalization and parenteral treatment are described below.

MEDICATION

First Line

- Several antibiotic regimens are highly effective, with no single regimen of choice. Broad coverage should include *Chlamydia*, gonorrhea, anaerobes, gram-negative rods, and streptococci. CDC regimens that follow are recommendations, and the specific antibiotics named are examples.
- Parenteral regimen A:
  - Cefotetan 2 g IV q12h or Cefoxitin 2 g IV q6h plus doxycycline 100 mg PO or IV q12h
  - Parenteral therapy × 24 hours after clinical improvement; continue doxycycline for a total of 14 days
- Parenteral regimen B:
  - Clindamycin 900 mg IV q8h plus gentamicin loading dose IV or IM (2 mg/kg of body weight) followed by a maintenance dose (1.5 mg/kg) q8h
  - Parenteral therapy for 24 hours after clinical improvement; continue doxycycline as above or clindamycin 450 mg PO q.i.d. for a total of 14 days
- Outpatient treatment regimen A:
  - Ceftriaxone 250 mg IM or Cefoxitin 2 g IM in a single dose
  - Plus doxycycline 100 mg PO b.i.d. × 14 days
  - ± metronidazole 500 mg PO b.i.d. × 14 days
- On the basis of the recent emergence of fluoroquinolone-resistant gonococci, the CDC no longer recommends the use of these agents for the treatment of gonococcal infections and associated conditions such as PID (2).
- Metronidazole should be considered in cases where risk of infection with anaerobic organisms is considered high (3).

Second Line

- Many other antibiotic regimens have been proposed and used with success. Examples:
  - Tobramycin in place of gentamicin
  - Tetracycline in place of doxycycline (4)
- In persons with documented severe allergic reactions to penicillins or cephalosporins, azithromycin or spectinomycin might be an option for therapy of uncomplicated gonococcal infections (3)[A].

ADDITIONAL TREATMENT

General Measures

Avoid intercourse until treatment is completed.

Issues for Referral

- Refer sex partners for appropriate evaluation and treatment:
  - Partners should be treated, irrespective of evaluation, with regimens effective against *Chlamydia* and gonorrhea.

SURGERY/OTHER PROCEDURES

- Reserved for failures of medical treatment and for suspected ruptured adnexal abscess with resulting acute surgical abdomen
- Conservative surgery preferred
- Failure of medical therapy is associated with adnexal abscess, which may be amenable to transabdominal or transvaginal drainage under guidance by ultrasonography, CT scan, or laparoscopy.

IN-PATIENT CONSIDERATIONS

Initial Stabilization

Manage fever, infection, and pelvic pain.

Admission Criteria

Hospitalization recommended in the following:

- Surgical emergencies (e.g., appendicitis)
- Suspected pelvic abscess
- Pregnancy
- Patient with uncertain compliance with therapy
- Severe illness
- Intolerance to outpatient regimen
- Failure to respond to outpatient therapy
- Inability to arrange clinical follow-up within 72 hours of starting antibiotics

IV Fluids

Maintenance

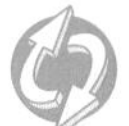

ONGOING CARE

FOLLOW-UP RECOMMENDATIONS

Patient Monitoring

- Close observation of clinical status, particularly for fever, symptoms, level of peritonitis, WBCs
- Retest for gonorrhea and chlamydia in 3–6 months. The likelihood of reinfection is high.
- Follow adnexal abscess size and position with serial US.

PATIENT EDUCATION

- Abstinence from any type of sexual contact until treatment of patient/partner (if necessary) is complete
- Consistent and correct condom use should be enforced.
- Hepatitis B and human papilloma virus (HPV) vaccines should be given to patients who meet criteria.
- Advise comprehensive STI screening.

PROGNOSIS

- Wide variation with good prognosis if early, effective therapy is instituted and further infection is avoided
- Poor prognosis related to late therapy and continued high-risk sexual behavior

COMPLICATIONS

- Tubo-ovarian abscess will develop in ~7–16% of patients with PID (5).
- Recurrent infection occurs in 20–25% of patients.
- Risk of ectopic pregnancy is increased 7–10-fold among women with a history of PID.
- Tubal infertility occurs in 15%, 35%, and 55% of women after 1, 2, and 3 episodes of PID, respectively (6).
- Chronic pelvic pain occurs in 20% of cases and is related to adhesion formation, chronic salpingitis, or recurrent infection.

REFERENCES

1. Weinstein SA, Stiles BG, et al. A review of the epidemiology, diagnosis and evidence-based management of *Mycoplasma genitalium*. *Sex Health*. 2011;8:143–58.
2. Centers for Disease Control and Prevention (CDC), et al. Update to CDC's sexually transmitted diseases treatment guidelines, 2006: Fluoroquinolones no longer recommended for treatment of gonococcal infections. *MMWR*. 2007;56:332–6.
3. Haggerty CL, Ness RB. Newest approaches to treatment of pelvic inflammatory disease: A review of recent randomized clinical trials. *Clin Infect Dis*. 2007;44:953–60.
4. Sexually transmitted disease treatment guidelines, 2006. *MMWR*. 2006;55(RR-11).
5. Lareau SM, Beigi RH. Pelvic inflammatory disease and tubo-ovarian abscess. *Infect Dis Clin North Am*. 2008;22:693–708.
6. Pellati D, Mylonakis I, Bertoloni G, et al. Genital tract infections and infertility. *Eur J Obstet Gynecol Reprod Biol*. 2008;140(1):3–11.

ADDITIONAL READING

- Haggerty CL, Ness RB. Diagnosis and treatment of pelvic inflammatory disease. *Womens Health (Lond Engl)*. 2008;4:383–97.
- Kruszka PS, Kruszka SJ, et al. Evaluation of acute pelvic pain in women. *Am Fam Physician*. 2010; 82:141–7.
- Risser JM, Risser WL. Purulent vaginal and cervical discharge in the diagnosis of pelvic inflammatory disease. *Int J STD AIDS*. 2009;20:73–6.
- Tarr ME, et al. Sexually transmitted infections in adolescent women. *Clin Obstet Gyn*. 2008;51(2): 306–18.
- Workowski KA, Berman S, Centers for Disease Control and Prevention (CDC), et al. Sexually transmitted diseases treatment guidelines, 2010. *MMWR Recomm Rep*. 2010;59:1–110.

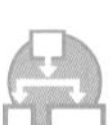

See Also (Topic, Algorithm, Electronic Media Element)

Algorithm: Pelvic Girdle Pain

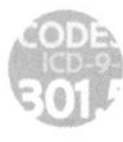

CODES

ICD9

- 614.0 Acute salpingitis and oophoritis
- 614.1 Chronic salpingitis and oophoritis
- 614.9 Unspecified inflammatory disease of female pelvic organs and tissues

CLINICAL PEARLS

- Most often PID starts with gonorrhea or *Chlamydia*, but it can be polymicrobial.
- History of lower abdominal pain, cervical motion tenderness, and adnexal tenderness is sufficient for a diagnosis of PID in an at-risk woman.
- Complications include hydrosalpinx, adhesions, pelvic pain, and 10-fold increased risk of ectopic pregnancy.
- PID is a common cause of infertility.

PEMPHIGOID, BULLOUS

Felix B. Chang, MD
Amanda Iantosca, DO

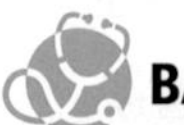

BASICS

DESCRIPTION
- Bullous pemphigoid (BP) is an antibody-mediated blistering skin disease.
- Intraepidermal blistering with widespread eruption of tense, symmetric, pruritic blisters on apparently normal skin or mucous membranes
- Common sites are the oral cavity (10–20% of cases) and the skin of the inner thighs, flexor surface of the forearm, groin, axilla, and lower abdomen.

EPIDEMIOLOGY
- ~61% of affected persons are females.
- Laryngeal mucous membrane pemphigoid disease has similar frequency in men and women.
- Most common in persons >60 years old.
- Childhood BP is very rare, and it most commonly involves acral regions. It is most often a benign, short course <1 year.

Incidence
In the UK, occurrence is 4.28 per 100,000 person-years.

Prevalence
There are 4.8 new cases per 100 elder-years.

RISK FACTORS
- Association with autoimmune disorders and inflammatory dermatoses, such as lichen planus and psoriasis
- Association with neurologic disorders, such as multiple sclerosis, stroke, Parkinson disease, and psychiatric disorders
- Drug-induced BP is rare: Furosemide, NSAIDs, captopril, aldosterone antagonists, penicillin, sulfasalazine, salicylazosulfapyridine, phenacetin, nalidixic acid, topical fluorouracil.
- Less frequent: Trauma, burns, surgical scars, ultraviolet (UV) radiation, and X-ray therapy

Genetics
Expression of the major histocompatibility complex (MHC) class II allele DQB1*0301 appears to be a marker for enhanced susceptibility.

PATHOPHYSIOLOGY
- Autoantibodies are formed against the protein components BP180 and BP230 of the hemidesmosomes in the dermoepidermal junction (1).
- IgG autoantibodies bind to these antigenic proteins, activating complement, which attracts inflammatory cells; inflammatory cells release proteases, which degrade the hemidesmosomes, leading to disruption of the dermoepidermal junction.
- BP180 appears to be the main pathogenic antigen causing subepidermal blister formation (2).
- A link between autoimmunity to BP230 and neurologic disease has been suggested (3).
- IgE autoantibodies against BP180 seem to be associated with the early urticarial phase of the disease and are detected in 86% of untreated patients with BP. The presence of IgE autoantibodies correlates with a more severe form of BP that requires longer and more intensive treatments for remission and higher doses of corticosteroids (4).

ETIOLOGY
Autoimmune

COMMONLY ASSOCIATED CONDITIONS
Multiple sclerosis, hypereosinophilic syndrome, ulcerative colitis

DIAGNOSIS

HISTORY
- Pruritus is a common and characteristic feature.
- Inquire about medication use, skin trauma, and history of autoimmune, neurologic, or skin disorders.
- Types:
  - Generalized bullous: Most common. Tense bullae arise on normal-appearing or erythematous skin. Oral lesions occur in ~10–20% of cases. The bullae usually heal without scarring (3).
  - Urticarial variant: Presents initially with mild to intractable pruritus and urticarial lesions. This form may persist for several weeks or months, then resolve or evolve into the generalized bullous form of BP.
  - Vesicular form: Less common, presenting as small tense blisters with an urticarial or erythematous base.
  - Vegetative form: Very uncommon, presenting as vegetating plaques in intertriginous areas.

PHYSICAL EXAM
- Large, tense bullae, often in conjunction with urticarial plaques, commonly involving the flexural aspects of the limbs, axillae, abdomen, and groin
- Bullae are typically symmetrically distributed.
- Oral lesions are present in 1/3 of patients. Ocular involvement and lesions of other mucosal surfaces are rare (3).
- The Nikolsky sign is absent. There is no exfoliation of the outermost layer of skin with the application of lateral pressure.
- The Asboe-Hansen sign is negative. No extension of bullae into the surrounding, unblistered skin when vertical pressure is applied to the top of the bulla.

DIAGNOSTIC TESTS & INTERPRETATION

Lab

Initial lab tests
- Skin biopsy
- ANA to rule out bullous lupus erythematosus
- Electrolyte panel in extensive BP

Follow-Up & Special Considerations
- Consider an age-related cancer screen on patients diagnosed below the age of 60, as there have been some studies demonstrating that these patients may be at higher risk for underlying malignancy.
- ELISA for the NC16A domain of BP180 is available at some centers, reported sensitivity 82–94%, and specificity 93–99.9%

Diagnostic Procedures/Surgery
- Obtain 4-mm punch biopsies: One for histologic examination and one for immunofluorescence
- For histopathology: Biopsy the edge of an intact bulla. Staining shows subepidermal blister formation with a discrete dermal inflammatory infiltrate rich in eosinophils.
- Direct immunofluorescence (DIF) is the gold standard for diagnosis. A perilesional biopsy of normal-appearing skin will show linear deposition of IgG and C3 (as well as other immunoglobulins, commonly) at the dermoepidermal junction. This linear pattern of deposition is common to most pemphigoid disorders.
- Salt-split technique using DIF may be performed to help distinguish BP from other pemphigoid disorders:
  - IgG autoantibodies will deposit on the epidermal side of the skin split, whereas dermal-side deposition is seen with other pemphigoid disorders and in epidermolysis bullosa acquisita.
  - Indirect immunofluorescence serum and skin from a normal human donor will show linear binding of IgG autoantibodies along the epidermal side of salt-split skin in 80–85% of cases (3).

DIFFERENTIAL DIAGNOSIS
- Drug-induced bullous
- Pemphigus vulgaris
- Cicatricial pemphigoid
- Pemphigoid gestationis
- Bullous lupus erythematosus
- Dermatitis herpetiformis
- Bullous erythema multiforme
- Epidermolysis bullosa acquisita
- Linear IgA dermatosis
- Contact or allergic dermatitis
- Prurigo
- Lichen planus pemphigoides
- Drug eruption
- Stevens-Johnson syndrome
- Impetigo
- Erythema multiforme
- Staphylococcal scaled-skin syndrome

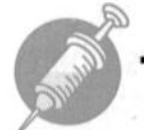

TREATMENT

MEDICATION
Treatment is directed at reducing inflammatory response and autoantibody production.

First Line
- The mainstay of therapy in most patients is oral glucocorticoids. However, these are poorly tolerated, particularly in the elderly (5).
- High-potency topical corticosteroids are considered first-line treatment:
  - Clobetasol ointment or emollient cream (applied b.i.d.) (5)[A]
  - Smaller amounts (30 g) of 0.05% Clobetasol propionate have been found to be just as effective as larger amounts (40 g) applied b.i.d. (5)[A].
- Extensive disease often requires systemic glucocorticoid therapy (6) because of patient difficulties with applying topical creams to large surface areas. However, topical corticosteroids have shown significantly more disease control than oral prednisolone in patients with extensive and moderate disease, with significantly reduced adverse events and mortality (5)[A].

- The goal is to achieve the lowest maintenance dosage that will prevent new lesion formation.
- Oral prednisolone (0.3–0.75 mg/kg/d starting dose); increase dose until new blisters stop developing. New evidence suggests that starting doses of prednisolone >0.75 mg/kg/d do not provide additional benefit and lower doses (0.5 mg/kg/d) may be adequate for disease control in more patients than previously thought (5)[A].
- Taper dose gradually within 1–2 years to avoid relapse. More rapid taper may be used in drug-induced BP.

- Steroid-sparing agents should be considered in patients taking systemic corticosteroids: Cyclophosphamide (5 mg/kg/d), mycophenolate mofetil (0.5–2 g/d), or azathioprine (0.5–2.5 mg/kg/d).
  - Azathioprine (Imuran) (2–3 mg/kg/d) and mycophenolate mofetil (1 g b.i.d.) appear to have similar efficacy when given with methylprednisolone (0.5 mg/kg/d). However, the time needed to achieve complete remission in 100% of patients was ~90 days in the azathioprine group vs. ~280 days in the mycophenolate mofetil group (7)[B]. Mycophenolate mofetil showed a significantly lower liver toxicity profile than azathioprine therapy.
- Methotrexate has been shown to have equivalent or even higher rates of remission than therapy with methotrexate plus prednisone, and it may be considered for the management of moderate to severe disease (8,9)[B].
- Tetracycline (500 mg t.i.d.) in combination with nicotinamide (500 mg t.i.d.) has been shown to have comparable response rates to prednisone therapy alone (2).
- Oral or topical treatment usually can be tapered gradually within 1–2 years.

Second Line

- Up to 24% of patients with BP do not respond to first-line therapies (2).
- IVIG may be an effective alternative for those patients not responsive to first-line therapy or at risk of potentially fatal side effects from conventional immunosuppressive therapy if started early. The recommended dose is 1–2 g/kg divided over a 3- or 5-day cycle every 3–4 weeks (10)[B].
- Plasmapheresis may be considered in patients resistant to conventional therapy (2)[B].

ADDITIONAL TREATMENT

Issues for Referral

- Ophthalmologic exam when ocular involvement is suspected or with prolonged courses of high-dose glucocorticoids
- Dental or otolaryngology evaluation for the care of oral disease

IN-PATIENT CONSIDERATIONS

Admission Criteria

- Septicemia
- Extensive denuding of skin
- Fluid balance derangement
- Inability to maintain temperature control

IV Fluids

In fluid balance derangement or electrolyte abnormalities, which are often associated with extensive denuding of skin

ONGOING CARE

FOLLOW-UP RECOMMENDATIONS

Patient Monitoring

- Perform periodic skin examination for new lesions.
- Maintain an up-to-date medication list if the patient has multiple prescribing physicians.
- Taper steroids slowly to avoid relapse.
- Adjust doses of corticosteroids as necessary for flares or relapse.
- Monitor for side effects of therapy (in a regular ophthalmologic exam, DEXA scan) to evaluate bone density.

DIET

- Consider a liquid or soft diet with active oral lesions. Once lesions are resolving, advance diet, avoiding hard or crunchy foods, such as nuts, chips, and raw vegetables, as these foods may cause flare-ups.
- Supplement with calcium and vitamin D for patients on systemic corticosteroids.

PATIENT EDUCATION

- Provide education on wound care, treatment side effects, and stress reduction.
- Avoid prolonged direct sun exposure and physical trauma to the skin.
- In drug-induced BP, educate on medications to avoid.

PROGNOSIS

- Spontaneous exacerbations and temporary remissions
- ~50% of patients achieve remission within 2.5–6 years.
- Mortality: 20–40% during the first year after diagnosis.
- Old age and poor general condition are the 2 major detrimental prognostic factors of BP. In one study, patients older than 83 years who were less autonomous had a more than 9-fold increase in their risk of dying during the first year of treatment relative to younger patients who were more autonomous. The 1-year survival rate was 90% for the younger, more autonomous patients and 38% for the older, less autonomous patients. Survival was not based on disease severity in this study.
- Patients who develop BP at <60 years of age are found to have a higher risk of underlying malignancy.
- Mortality associated with BP is often the result of prolonged immunosuppressive therapy.
- Risk factors for lethal outcome in the first year after diagnosis have been identified:
  - Age >80–82 years, daily prednisolone dose of more than 37 mg after hospitalization, serum albumin levels of <3.6 g/dL, ESR >300 mm/hr, Karnofsky score of functional impairment of ≤40.

COMPLICATIONS

- Superimposed infection from comorbid conditions in elderly persons, such as decubitus ulcers
- Malignancies and bone marrow suppression from immunosuppressants
- Osteoporosis, cataracts, and adrenal insufficiency from prolonged use of systemic glucocorticoids

REFERENCES

1. Ujiie H, Nishie W, Shimizu H. Pathogenesis of bullous pemphigoid. *Dermatol Clin*. 2011;29: 439–46.
2. Khandpur S, Verma P. Bullous pemphigoid. *Indian J Dermatol Venereol Leprol*. 2011;77:450–5.
3. Schmidt E, della Torre R, Borradori L. Clinical features and practical diagnosis of bullous pemphigoid. *Dermatol Clin*. 2011;29:427–38.
4. Iwata Y, Komura K, Kodera M, et al. Correlation of IgE autoantibody to BP180 with a severe form of bullous pemphigoid. *Arch Dermatol*. 2008;144: 41–8.
5. Kirtschig G, Middleton P, Bennett C, et al. Interventions for bullous pemphigoid. *Cochrane Database Syst Rev*. 2010;CD002292.
6. Mutasim DF. Autoimmune bullous dermatoses in the elderly: An update on pathophysiology, diagnosis and management. *Drugs Aging*. 2010;27:1–19.
7. Beissert S, Werfel T, Frieling U. A comparison of oral methylprednisolone plus azathioprine or mycophenolate mofetil for the treatment of bullous pemphigoid. *Arch Dermatol*. 2007;143: 1536–42.
8. Gurcan HM, Ahmed AR. Efficacy of dapsone in the treatment of pemphigus and pemphigoid: Analysis of current data. *Am J Clin Dermatol*. 2009;10:383–96.
9. Gürcan HM, Razzaque Ahmed A. Analysis of current data on the use of methotrexate in the treatment of pemphigus and pemphigoid. *Br J Dermatol*. 2009;161(4):723–31.
10. Dhar S. Intravenous immunoglobulin in dermatology. *Indian J Dermatol*. 2009;54:77–9.

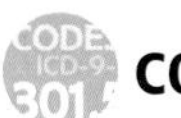

CODES

ICD9

694.5 Pemphigoid

CLINICAL PEARLS

- Bullous pemphigoid antibodies also can be detected in individuals without bullous pemphigoid.
- The detection of anti-BP 180 serum antibodies in patients with remission may be an indicator of subclinical active disease.
- Skin biopsy for routine and direct immunofluorescence is needed to differentiate pemphigus vulgaris from bullous pemphigoid.
- Close management of fluid loss and good topical care are mandatory in severe and extensive involvement.

PEMPHIGUS VULGARIS

Michelle A. Tinitigan, MD
Richard P. Usatine, MD

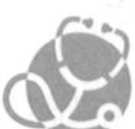

BASICS

Pemphigus is derived from the Greek word *pemphix* meaning "bubble" or "blister."

DESCRIPTION

- Rare, potentially fatal autoimmune vesiculobullous disease characterized by a loss of cell adhesion and blister formation within the epidermis in the skin and/or the mucosal surfaces.
- Flaccid bullae appear spontaneously that typically begin in the oropharynx and then may spread to the skin, having a predilection for the scalp, face, chest, axillae, groin, and pressure points. Bullae are tender and painful when they rupture.
- Patient often presents with erosions and no intact bullae.
- System(s) affected: Skin; Gastrointestinal; Genitourinary

EPIDEMIOLOGY

Incidence

- Increasing incidence with increasing age; median age of presentation 71 years (1)
- Predominant sex: Female > Male (66% vs. 34%) (1); female-to-male ratio 1.4/1

Prevalence

- Uncommon, affects <200,000 people in the US
- More prevalent in people of Mediterranean or Ashkenazi Jewish ancestry (2)

RISK FACTORS

Genetics

Strong association with certain human leukocyte antigens (HLA), especially HLA DR4, DR14, DQ1, and DQ3, though the susceptibility gene differs depending on ethnic origin.

PATHOPHYSIOLOGY

- Autoantibodies (IgG) are directed against desmoglein (Dsg) 1 and 3 adhesion molecules. Desmogleins interact with desmosomes, which hold epidermal cells together. The antibodies against Dsg molecules result in intraepidermal blister formation and acantholysis.
- Dsg3 is expressed in deeper epidermal layers than Dsg1. Dsg3 is found in mucous membranes.
- Patients with limited mucosal disease primarily have autoantibodies directed against Dsg3, whereas those with more extensive cutaneous disease have antibodies directed against both Dsg1 and Dsg3.

ETIOLOGY

- Autoimmune; stimulus is unknown.
- Inducing factors include physical trauma such as thermal burns, UV light and ionizing radiation, neoplasm, emotional stress, drugs, and infections. Nevertheless, most of the patients lack a recognized inducing factor.

COMMONLY ASSOCIATED CONDITIONS

- Thymoma
- Myasthenia gravis
- Paraneoplastic pemphigus is a type of pemphigus defined by the fact that the patient must have a malignancy at the time that the pemphigus is diagnosed.
- Gastric adenocarcinoma

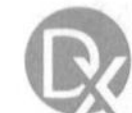

DIAGNOSIS

HISTORY

- Hoarseness, sore mouth
- Mucosal lesions (in 50–70% of patients) may be the sole sign for an average of 5 months before skin lesions or may be the sole manifestations of the disease.
- Cutaneous lesions: Primary lesion is a flaccid blister developed by most patients; affected skin is often painful but rarely pruritic.
- Drug-induced: Penicillamine, ACE inhibitors, thiol-containing compounds, rifampin

PHYSICAL EXAM

- Mucosal lesions: Intact bullae rare; commonly are ill defined, irregularly shaped gingival, buccal, or palatine erosions that are painful and slow healing; most often affected area is the oral cavity; may involve conjunctiva, oropharynx esophagus, labia, vagina, cervix, penis, urethra, and anus
- Cutaneous lesions: Painful, flaccid blisters with clear fluid found on normal skin or on erythematous base; fragile bullae rupture easily, leading to painful, open, denuded areas that can become secondarily infected
- Nails: Acute or chronic paronychia, onychomadesis, subungual hematomas, and nail dystrophies may be present.
- Nikolsky sign: Involves application of pressure to skin causing intraepidermal cleavage that allows the superficial skin to slip free from the deeper layers, producing an erosion; can be elicited on normal skin or at the margin of a blister
- Asboe-Hansen sign: Lateral pressure on the edge of a blister may spread the blister into clinically unaffected skin.

DIAGNOSTIC TESTS & INTERPRETATION

Diagnosis is achieved via 3 different parameters: Perilesional tissue biopsy, histological, and immunological examinations.

Lab

Initial lab tests

- Shave or 4-mm punch biopsy of edge of fresh bullous lesion
- A second 4-mm punch biopsy of the perilesional skin is sent for direct immunofluorescence (DIF).
- Serum for indirect immunofluorescence (IDIF) is positive for circulating autoantibodies against desmogleins in 80–90% if DIF is positive.

Follow-Up & Special Considerations

IDIF corresponds loosely to disease activity and may be useful to gauge disease activity.

Pathological Findings

- Light microscopy: Intradermal blister; loss of cohesion between epidermal cells (acantholysis) with an intact basement membrane; "row of tombstones appearance"
- DIF looking for deposits of IgG between epidermal cells

DIFFERENTIAL DIAGNOSIS

- Predominance of oral mucous lesions: Herpes simplex virus (HSV), aphthous ulcers, lichen planus, erythema multiforme
- Predominance of widespread cutaneous lesions: Bullous pemphigoid, cicatricial pemphigoid, bullous drug eruptions, pemphigus erythematosus, pemphigus foliaceus, paraneoplastic pemphigus, impetigo, contact dermatitis, dermatitis herpetiformis, erythema multiforme, Stevens-Johnson syndrome, toxic epidermal necrolysis, pemphigoid gestationis, and linear IgA dermatosis

TREATMENT

Reduce inflammatory response and autoantibody production by suppression of the immune system to decrease blister formation and promote healing of blisters and erosions.

MEDICATION

First Line

- High-dose systemic glucocorticoids (e.g., prednisone 1–2 mg/kg/d) are the mainstay of treatment.
- Other steroid-sparing immunosuppressive drugs (azathioprine [4 mg/kg/d], cyclophosphamide [2–3 mg/kg/d], dapsone, mycophenolate mofetil [MMF]) are used alone or in combination with systemic glucocorticoids.
- Combination therapy with steroid-sparing agents are particularly useful within the first 6 months and indicated if uncontrolled on relatively low doses of prednisone (5–10 mg/d to every other day) within a year of starting therapy.
- Dexamethasone-cyclophosphamide pulse therapy is a beneficial treatment, sparing the adverse effects of conventional regimens, and has claim to induce remission in many patients (3).
- For mild-to-moderate disease: Combination therapy of MMF and prednisone is an effective treatment regimen to achieve rapid and complete control of PV. For those patients who fail treatment with MMF and prednisone, rituximab is an efficacious alternative therapy (4).
- For oropharyngeal disease: Perilesional/intralesional triamcinolone acetonide injections combined with conventional immunosuppressive therapy shortened the time of complete clinical remission and reduced the total amount of corticosteroids used.
- Oral analgesics: Use before eating for painful oral lesions (viscous lidocaine, Benadryl).

Second Line
For refractory disease:
- Anti-CD20 monoclonal antibodies: Rituximab (5): Alone or in combination with IVIG appears to be an effective therapy for patients with refractory PV. This is the treatment of choice for patients with severe PV that is refractory to conventional therapy with systemic corticosteroids and immunosuppressives.
- Other options: Methotrexate, dapsone, hydroxychloroquine, gold, mycophenolate, and cyclosporine
- Tumor necrosis factor (TNF)-alpha antagonist, etanercept, may be an effective therapeutic agent and should be considered as an alternative treatment option for patients presenting with recalcitrant disease.
- Plasmapheresis in aggressive disease if combined with systemic steroids and immunosuppressant drugs
- IVIG is a promising therapeutic agent. It may be useful as monotherapy in patients who do not respond to steroids or who have contraindications. Experience with IVIG in patients with autoimmune skin blistering disease is limited (6).
- Pulsed therapy with IV methylprednisolone and cyclophosphamide can be an effective therapy for refractory PV.

ADDITIONAL TREATMENT
General Measures
- Minimize activities that may cause trauma to skin and precipitate blisters.
- Avoid use of dental plates, dental bridges, or contact lenses that may precipitate or exacerbate mucosal disease.
- Wound care: Daily gentle cleaning, topical agents to promote wound healing, and use of nonadhesive dressings

Issues for Referral
- Ophthalmologist referral in suspected ocular involvement and prolonged use of high-dose steroids
- Referral to a dentist and/or otolaryngologist for patients with extensive oral disease.

IN-PATIENT CONSIDERATIONS
Admission Criteria
- Secondary infections requiring IV antibiotics
- Severe oral lesions leading to dehydration requiring fluid resuscitation

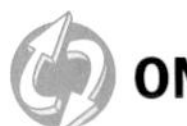

ONGOING CARE

A minority (10%) achieve complete remission after initial treatment and do not need continued drug therapy; most require maintenance therapy to stay in remission.

FOLLOW-UP RECOMMENDATIONS
Patients taking steroids long term should be screened for osteopenia/osteoporosis, avascular necrosis, HPA-axis suppression, cataract, cushingoid features, hyperlipoproteinemia, myopathy, mood changes, and immunosuppression (7). Patients on systemic steroids should maintain adequate vitamin D and calcium intake through diet and supplements.

Patient Monitoring
Seek medical care for any unexplained blisters and if you have been treated for PV and develop any of the following symptoms:
- Fever, chills
- General ill feeling
- Myalgias, joint pain
- New blisters or ulcers

DIET
- Patients with active oral lesions may benefit from liquid or soft diet and then advance as tolerated.
- Avoid spicy and acidic food when oral ulcers are present.
- Hard food that may cause mechanical trauma to epithelium such as nuts, chips, and hard vegetables and fruits may be best avoided with active oral disease.

PATIENT EDUCATION
- Minimize activities that may cause trauma to skin and precipitate blisters, such as contact sports. Nontraumatic exercises, such as swimming, may be helpful.
- Explain wound care of erosions: Daily gentle cleaning, covering open areas with clean petrolatum and nonadhesive dressings
- Educate patients about the chronicity of the disease and the need for long-term follow-up.
- For oral pemphigus:
  - Soft diets and soft toothbrushes help to minimize local trauma.
  - Explain the need for meticulous oral hygiene to prevent dental decay. Encourage gentle toothbrushing, dental flossing, and visits to the dentist/dental hygienist at least every 6 months.
  - Discuss how dental plates, dental bridges, or contact lenses may precipitate or exacerbate mucosal disease.
  - Topical analgesics or anesthetics (e.g., benzydamine hydrochloride 0.15% or viscous lidocaine) may be useful in alleviating oral pain, particularly prior to eating or toothbrushing.

PROGNOSIS
- Mortality rate with combination therapy is ~5%, with most deaths due to drug-induced complications, including sepsis.
- 10% of patients achieve complete remission after initial treatment; the majority require maintenance therapy to stay in remission.
- Morbidity and mortality are related to extent of disease, the maximum dose of oral steroids required to induce remission, and the presence of other diseases. Prognosis is worse in older persons and patients with extensive disease.
- Most deaths occur during the first few years of the disease, and if a patient survives 5 years, prognosis is good.

COMPLICATIONS
- Secondary infection, localized to skin or systemic, may occur because of impaired immune response due to use of immunosuppressive drugs. Most frequent cause of death is *Staphylococcus aureus* septicemia.
- Osteoporosis in patients requiring long-term systemic steroids
- Adrenal insufficiency has been reported following prolonged use of glucocorticoids.
- Bone marrow suppression and malignancies have been reported in patients receiving immunosuppressants, with an increased incidence of leukemia and lymphoma.
- Growth retardation has been reported in children taking systemic corticosteroids and immunosuppressants.

REFERENCES

1. Langan SM, Smeeth L, Hubbard R, et al. Bullous pemphigoid and pemphigus vulgaris–incidence and mortality in the UK: Population based cohort study. *BMJ*. 2008;337:a180.
2. Meyer N, Misery L, et al. Geoepidemiologic considerations of auto-immune pemphigus. *Autoimmun Rev*. 2010;9:A379–82.
3. Zivanovic D, Medenica L, Tanasilovic S, et al. Dexamethasone-cyclophosphamide pulse therapy in pemphigus: A review of 72 cases. *Am J Clin Dermatol*. 2010;11:123–9.
4. Strowd LC, Taylor SL, Jorizzo JL, et al. Therapeutic ladder for pemphigus vulgaris: Emphasis on achieving complete remission. *J Am Acad Dermatol*. 2011;64:490–4.
5. Schmidt E, Goebeler M, Zillikens D, et al. Rituximab in severe pemphigus. *Ann NY Acad Sci*. 2009; 1173:683–91.
6. Ishii N, Hashimoto T, Zillikens D, et al. High-dose intravenous immunoglobulin (IVIG) therapy in autoimmune skin blistering diseases. *Clin Rev Allergy Immunol*. 2010;38:186–95.
7. Chmurova N, Svecova D, et al. Pemphigus vulgaris: A 11-year review. *Bratisl Lek Listy*. 2009;110:500–3.

ADDITIONAL READING

Dermatology Section 16 on Bullous Disease. In Usatine R, Smith M, Mayeaux EJ, et al., eds. *The Color Atlas of Family Medicine*. McGraw-Hill, New York; 2009.

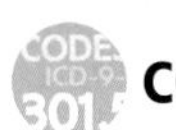

CODES

ICD9

694.4 Pemphigus

CLINICAL PEARLS

- Rare, chronic, potentially fatal autoimmune vesiculobullous disease of the mucous membranes and skin.
- Biopsy immediately with rush processing.
- When clinical suspicion is high, initiate therapy without delay using systemic corticosteroids.
- Minimize activities that may cause trauma to skin and precipitate blisters, such as contact sports.

PEPTIC ULCER DISEASE

Kelly O'Callahan, MD

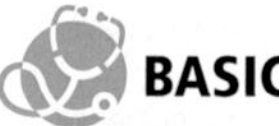

BASICS

DESCRIPTION

- Duodenal ulcer:
  - Most common form of peptic ulcer
  - Usually located in the proximal duodenum
  - Multiple ulcers or ulcers distal to the second portion of duodenum raise possibility of Zollinger-Ellison syndrome.
- Gastric ulcer:
  - Less common than duodenal ulcer in absence of NSAIDs
  - Commonly located along lesser curvature of the antrum
- Esophageal ulcers: Located in the distal esophagus; usually secondary to gastroesophageal reflux disease (GERD); also seen with Zollinger-Ellison syndrome
- Ectopic gastric mucosal ulceration: May develop in patients with a Meckel's diverticulum

EPIDEMIOLOGY

Incidence

- Predominant sex: Equal
- Predominant age:
  - 70% of ulcers occur in patients ages 25–64.
  - Ulcer incidence increases with age.
- Peptic ulcer: 500,000 new cases/yr
- Recurrence: 4 million/yr
- Global incidence rate: 0.1–0.19%

Prevalence

- Peptic ulcer: 1.8% in the US
- Lifetime prevalence is 5–10% for patients not infected with *Helicobacter pylori;* 10–20% if infected.

RISK FACTORS

- *H. pylori* infection
- NSAID use
- Smoking cigarettes
- Family history of ulcers
- Zollinger-Ellison syndrome
- Medications: Corticosteroids (high-dose and/or prolonged therapy), bisphosphonates, potassium chloride, chemotherapeutic agents (e.g., IV fluorouracil)

Genetics

Increased incidence of peptic ulcer disease (PUD) in families; familial clustering of *H. pylori* infection and inherited genetic factors reflecting response to the organism

GENERAL PREVENTION

- NSAID ulcers: Avoid salicylates and NSAIDs:
  - Alternatives include acetaminophen and tramadol. COX-2 inhibitor use (e.g., celecoxib) is controversial due to potential cardiac safety risks (also not clear that COX-2-selective agents reduce major GI bleeding).
  - If NSAIDs are needed, adjust the ibuprofen dose to <1,200 mg/d to decrease risk of ulcerogenesis, and add a proton pump inhibitor (PPI) or H_2 blockers.
  - To reduce ulcer risk, consider testing for and eradicating *H. pylori* before starting therapy with NSAIDs.
- Maintenance therapy with PPIs or H_2 blockers is indicated for patients with a history of ulcer complications or recurrences, refractory ulcers, or persistent *H. pylori* infection.

PATHOPHYSIOLOGY

Imbalance between aggressive factors (e.g., gastric acid, pepsin, bile salts, pancreatic enzymes) and defensive factors maintaining mucosal integrity (e.g., mucus, bicarbonate, blood flow, prostaglandins, growth factors, cell turnover)

ETIOLOGY

- May be multifactorial
- *H. pylori* infection: 90% of duodenal ulcers and 70–90% of gastric ulcers:
  - Lifetime risk for PUD in *H. pylori*–infected people: 10–20%
  - Annual risk of developing duodenal ulcer in *H. pylori*–infected people is ≤1%.
- Ulcerogenic drugs (e.g., NSAIDs)
- Hypersecretory syndromes (e.g., Zollinger-Ellison syndrome)
- Retained gastric antrum
- Less common: Crohn disease, vascular insufficiency, radiation therapy, cancer chemotherapy, smoking

COMMONLY ASSOCIATED CONDITIONS

- Zollinger-Ellison syndrome (gastrinoma)
- Multiple endocrine neoplasia type 1
- Carcinoid syndrome
- Chronic illness: Crohn disease, chronic obstructive pulmonary disease (COPD), chronic renal failure, hepatic cirrhosis, cystic fibrosis
- Hematopoietic disorders (rare): Systemic mastocytosis, myeloproliferative disease, hyperparathyroidism, polycythemia rubra vera

DIAGNOSIS

HISTORY

- Signs and symptoms:
  - Episodic gnawing or burning epigastric pain
  - Pain occurring after meals or on an empty stomach
  - Nocturnal pain
  - Pain relieved by food intake, antacids, or antisecretory agents
  - Nonspecific dyspeptic complaints: Indigestion, nausea, vomiting, loss of appetite, and heartburn
- Alarm symptoms:
  - Anemia, hematemesis, melena, or heme-positive stool suggests bleeding.
  - Vomiting and early satiety suggests obstruction.
  - Anorexia or weight loss
  - Persisting upper abdominal pain radiating to the back suggests penetration.
  - Severe, spreading upper abdominal pain suggests perforation.
- NSAID-induced ulcers are often silent; perforation or bleeding may be the initial presentation.

PHYSICAL EXAM

Physical exam for uncomplicated peptic ulcer may be unreliable and nonspecific: Epigastric tenderness (absent in at least 30% of older patients); guaiac-positive stool from occult blood loss

DIAGNOSTIC TESTS & INTERPRETATION

Lab

Initial lab tests

- Routine lab tests to consider when evaluating PUD:
  - CBC: Rule out anemia.
  - Fecal occult blood test
  - If multiple or refractory ulcers, consider serum gastrin to rule out Zollinger-Ellison syndrome.
- Indications for *H. pylori* testing: New-onset PUD, history of PUD, persistent symptoms after empirical antisecretory therapy, gastric mucosa–associated lymphoid tissue (MALT) lymphoma, uninvestigated dyspepsia in patients <50 years of age without alarm symptoms
- *H. pylori* diagnostic tests: False-negative results may occur if patient was recently treated with antibiotics, bismuth, or PPIs; or in patients with active bleeding. Diagnostic yield improved by checking 2 different tests in a patient with an ulcer to be sure *H. pylori* is not present:
  - Noninvasive tests:
    - Serology antibody: Most commonly used for testing in primary care but slow to normalize after treatment, so it cannot be used to document successful eradication (sensitivity 85%, specificity 79%) (1)[A]
    - Urea breath test: Identifies active *H. pylori* infection; also used for posttreatment testing (sensitivity >95%, specificity >90%) (1)[A]
    - Stool antigen: Can be used for screening and posttreatment testing (sensitivity 91%, specificity 94%) (1)[A]
  - Invasive tests:
    - Upper endoscopy with gastric biopsy, which can be evaluated with Steiner stain for direct visualization of organism (sensitivity >95%, specificity >95%) (1)[A]
    - Rapid urease test: Conducted on gastric biopsies (sensitivity 93–97%, specificity 95%) (1)[A]

Imaging

Initial approach

Barium or Gastrografin contrast radiography (double-contrast hypotonic duodenography): Indicated when endoscopy is unsuitable or not feasible

Diagnostic Procedures/Surgery

Indications for upper endoscopy: Patients with suspected peptic ulcers who are >55 years of age, those who have alarm symptoms, and those with ulcers that do not respond to treatment (2)[A]

DIFFERENTIAL DIAGNOSIS

Functional dyspepsia, gastritis, GERD, biliary colic, pancreatitis, cholecystitis, Crohn disease, intestinal ischemia, cardiac ischemia, GI malignancy

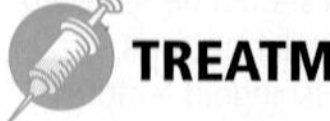

TREATMENT

MEDICATION

First Line

- Acid suppression: PPIs:
  - Omeprazole, 20 mg/d PO; lansoprazole, 30 mg/d PO; rabeprazole, 20 mg/d PO; esomeprazole, 40 mg/d PO; *or* pantoprazole, 40 mg/d PO
  - Administer PPIs before breakfast.

Pregnancy Considerations

PPIs are *not* associated with an increased risk for major congenital birth defects, spontaneous abortions, or preterm delivery (3)[A]:

- H_2 blockers: Ranitidine or nizatidine, 150 mg PO b.i.d. or 300 mg PO at bedtime; cimetidine, 400 mg PO b.i.d. or 800 mg PO at bedtime; famotidine, 150 mg PO b.i.d. or 300 mg PO at bedtime
- Treat ulcers for 6–8 weeks or until healing is confirmed in patients with complicated ulcers.
- PPIs heal peptic ulcers more rapidly and should not be taken with H_2 blockers.
- Optimal *H. pylori* eradication regimens (1)[A]: Triple therapy: 2 antibiotics plus a PPI × 14 days: Omeprazole, 20 mg PO b.i.d., or lansoprazole, 30 mg PO b.i.d., or pantoprazole, 40 mg PO b.i.d., or rabeprazole, 20 mg PO b.i.d., or esomeprazole plus clarithromycin, 500 mg PO b.i.d. plus amoxicillin, 1 g PO b.i.d. or metronidazole, 500 mg PO b.i.d. in patients with allergy to amoxicillin:
  - Triple and quadruple therapy have similar eradication rates for primary infection (4)[A].
- Bacterial resistance: Clarithromycin, 10%; amoxicillin, 1.4%; metronidazole, 37%: Culture-guided choice of triple therapy is more clinically and cost-effective.
- Treatment of *H. pylori*–negative ulcers (usually due to NSAIDs):
  - Discontinue NSAID use
  - Treat acutely with PPIs for 4–8 weeks; may use longer as maintenance for patients with recurrent or complicated ulcers or in patients who require long-term aspirin or NSAID use.
- Precautions:
  - Renal insufficiency: Decrease H_2 blocker dosage by 50%.
  - Cimetidine: Avoid with theophylline, warfarin, phenytoin, and lidocaine.
  - PPIs may decrease bone density. Obtain interval bone densitometry with long-term PPI use.
  - PPIs may cause hypomagnesemia. Consider baseline and interval levels in patients, especially for long-term use and in patients taking diuretics.
  - In spite of earlier concerns, PPIs do not appear to decrease the efficacy of clopidogrel (5).

Second Line

- For *H. pylori* eradication: Use second-line therapy if first line fails (1)[A]:
  - Bismuth quadruple therapy × 14 days:
    - Bismuth subsalicylate, 525 mg PO q.i.d. *plus*
    - Metronidazole, 500 mg PO q.i.d. *plus*
    - Tetracycline, 500 mg PO q.i.d. *plus*
    - PPI × 14 days
  - Alternative second-line therapy:
    - Levofloxacin, 250 mg PO b.i.d. *plus*
    - Amoxicillin, 1,000 mg PO b.i.d. *plus*
    - PPI PO b.i.d.
  - Another alternative salvage therapy:
    - Rifabutin, 300 mg PO daily *plus*
    - Amoxicillin, 1,000 mg PO b.i.d. *plus*
    - PPI PO b.i.d.
- Alternative ulcer-healing drugs: Sucralfate, 1 g PO q.i.d. or 2 g PO b.i.d. × 4–8 weeks
- Precautions: Renal insufficiency:
  - Reduce H_2 blocker dosage by 50%.
  - Avoid magnesium-containing antacids.
- Significant possible interactions:
  - Cimetidine inhibits cytochrome P450 isozymes (avoid with theophylline, warfarin, phenytoin, and lidocaine).
  - Omeprazole may prolong elimination of diazepam, warfarin, and phenytoin.
  - Sucralfate reduces absorption of tetracycline, norfloxacin, ciprofloxacin, and theophylline; it leads to subtherapeutic levels.

SURGERY/OTHER PROCEDURES

- Endoscopy indicated for patients over the age of 50 with new onset of dyspeptic symptoms, those who do not respond to treatment, and those of any age with alarm symptoms such as bleeding and weight loss (6)[A]
- At endoscopy:
  - Biopsy of stomach for *H. pylori* testing
  - Biopsy of margin of gastric ulcer to confirm benign etiology
  - Interventions to stop active bleeding, or prevent rebleeding in those with certain stigmata, include injection with epinephrine, heater probe treatment, or placement of endoscopic clips.
- Indications for surgery: Ulcers that are refractory to treatment and patients at high risk for complications (e.g., transplant recipients, patients dependent on steroids or NSAIDs); surgery also may be needed acutely for treatment of perforation and bleeding that is refractory to endoscopic therapy.
- Surgical options:
  - Duodenal ulcers: Truncal vagotomy and drainage (pyloroplasty or gastrojejunostomy), selective vagotomy (preserving the hepatic and/or celiac branches of the vagus) and drainage, or highly selective vagotomy
  - Gastric ulcers: Partial gastrectomy, Billroth I or II
  - Perforated ulcers: Laparoscopy or open patching (7)

IN-PATIENT CONSIDERATIONS

Initial Stabilization

- Discontinue ulcerogenic agents (e.g., NSAIDs).
- Bleeding peptic ulcers:
  - Stable: Give PPI to reduce transfusion requirements, need for surgery, and duration of hospitalization (2)[A].
  - Unstable: Fluid or packed RBC resuscitation followed by emergent EGD; use IV PPI
- Perforated peptic ulcers: Free peritoneal perforation with bacterial peritonitis is a surgical emergency.

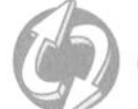

ONGOING CARE

FOLLOW-UP RECOMMENDATIONS

Patient Monitoring

- *H. pylori* eradication: Expected in >90% (with double antibiotic regimen): Confirm eradication by urea breath test.
- Acute duodenal ulcer: Monitor clinically.
- Acute gastric ulcer: Confirm healing via endoscopy after 12 weeks if biopsy is not done initially to confirm that the lesion is benign.

PROGNOSIS

After *H. pylori* eradication:

- Low ulcer relapse rate; if relapse, consider surreptitious use of NSAIDs
- Reinfection rates <1% per year
- Low risk of rebleeding
- Decreased NSAID ulcer recurrence

COMPLICATIONS

- Hemorrhage: Up to 25% of patients (initial presentation in 10%)
- Perforation: <5% of patients
- Gastric outlet obstruction: Up to 5% of duodenal or pyloric channel ulcers; male predilection found
- Risk of gastric adenocarcinoma increased in *H. pylori*–infected patients

REFERENCES

1. Saad R, Chey WD. A clinician's guide to managing Helicobacter pylori infection. *Cleve Clin J Med.* 2005;72:109–10, 112–3, 117–8 passim.
2. Ramakrishnan K, Salinas RC. Peptic ulcer disease. *Am Fam Physician.* 2007;76:1005–12.
3. Gill SK, O'Brien L, Einarson TR. The safety of proton pump inhibitors (PPIs) in pregnancy: A meta-analysis. *Am J Gastroenterol.* 2009;104: 1541–5.
4. Luther J, Higgins PD, Schoenfeld PS, et al. Empiric quadruple vs. triple therapy for primary treatment of Helicobacter pylori infection: Systematic review and meta-analysis of efficacy and tolerability. *Am J Gastroenterol.* 2010;105:65–73.
5. Rossini R, Capodanno D, Musumeci G, et al. Safety of clopidogrel and proton pump inhibitors in patients undergoing drug-eluting stent implantation. *Coron Artery Dis.* 2011;22:199–205.
6. ASGE Standards of Practice Committee, Banerjee S, Cash BD, et al. The role of endoscopy in the management of patients with peptic ulcer disease. *Gastrointest. Endosc.* 2010;71:663–8.
7. Bertleff MJ, Lange JF. Perforated peptic ulcer disease: A review of history and treatment. *Dig Surg.* 2010;27:161–9.
8. Lau JY, Sung J, Hill C, et al. Systematic review of the epidemiology of complicated peptic ulcer disease: Incidence, recurrence, risk factors and mortality. *Digestion.* 2011;84:102–13.

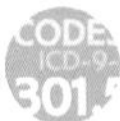

CODES

ICD9

- 530.20 Ulcer of esophagus without bleeding
- 531.90 Gastric ulcer, unspecified as acute or chronic, without mention of hemorrhage or perforation, without mention of obstruction
- 533.90 Peptic ulcer of unspecified site, unspecified as acute or chronic, without mention of hemorrhage or perforation, without mention of obstruction

CLINICAL PEARLS

- In patients with PUD, *H. pylori* should be eradicated to assist in healing and to reduce the risk of gastric and duodenal ulcer recurrence (2)[A].
- Upper endoscopy is indicated in patients with suspected peptic ulcers who are >55 years of age, those who have alarm symptoms, and those who do not respond to treatment (2)[A].

PERFORATED TYMPANIC MEMBRANE

Nedim Durakovic, MD
Daniel J. Lee, MD

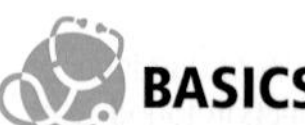

BASICS

DESCRIPTION

- The tympanic membrane, or eardrum, is a thin barrier that separates the external auditory canal from the middle ear and vibrates in response to sound waves, thus providing an important link in the hearing pathway.
- Rupture of the tympanic membrane disrupts hearing and creates an opening into the middle ear.
- Classification of perforations by location:
  - *Central* or those not involving the annulus are typical after a case of acute otitis media that leads to perforation.
  - *Marginal* involve the annulus and are frequently associated with cholesteatoma and are thus less likely to heal spontaneously.
  - *Subtotal*: A large defect surrounded with an intact annulus; often requires surgery to close
- Classification of perforations by etiology:
  - Acute/chronic suppurative otitis media
  - Traumatic (barotraumas, such as diving, and acoustic trauma, such as explosion)
  - Cholesteatoma
  - Iatrogenic (after extrusion of pressure equalization tubes)
- Spontaneous closure results in formation of a double skin layer (outer epidermal and inner mucosal), while inability to do so results in a chronic perforation.

EPIDEMIOLOGY

Incidence in the general population is unknown, since many perforations heal spontaneously.

RISK FACTORS

- Chronic eustachian tube dysfunction leading to OME
- Insertion of foreign objects into external ear canal (e.g., Q-tips, pressure equalization tubes)

GENERAL PREVENTION

- Avoid ear trauma and foreign object insertion into external ear canal.
- Treat otitis media in a timely fashion.

PATHOPHYSIOLOGY

- Chronic eustachian tube dysfunction or chronic negative middle-ear pressure
- Insertion of foreign objects into ear (Q-tips)
- Otitis media: A purulent, serous, or mucoid fluid builds up behind the tympanic membrane.
- A ruptured tympanic membrane that does not heal is often due to cholesteatoma.

ETIOLOGY

- Suppurative otitis media or middle ear infection leading to pressure buildup from pus and the resulting rupture of the tympanic membrane
- Direct trauma from foreign body (Q-tips, pencils, direct blows to the head, etc.), barotraumas, or temporal bone fracture
- Insertion of foreign objects into ear (Q-tips)
- Iatrogenic: For the treatment of chronic eustachian tube dysfunction, a myringotomy is performed and tympanostomy tubes are placed; after tubes are extruded, a chronic perforation may result.

COMMONLY ASSOCIATED CONDITIONS

- Chronic eustachian tube dysfunction
- OME
- Cholesteatoma
- Tympanosclerosis
- Ossicular chain damage

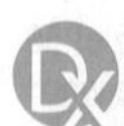

DIAGNOSIS

HISTORY

- Otorrhea or drainage from the ear (pus, blood, or clear fluid; malodorous pus is associated with cholesteatoma)
- Otalgia or earache consistent with AOM, followed by sudden relief of symptoms (perforation)
- Tinnitus or ear noise, buzzing
- Pressure/fluid/blocked feeling in the ears (OME)
- Audible whistling from the ear with Valsalva maneuver or nose-blowing
- Hearing loss
- Vertigo
- History of ear infections as a child or difficulty equalizing pressure with flights (chronic eustachian tube dysfunction)
- Ear surgery
- Recurrent ear infections

PHYSICAL EXAM

- External ear examination for tenderness consistent with OE
- Otoscopic exam
- Weber (tuning fork to center of forehead; sound should be equally loud on each side) and Rinne tests (tuning fork to mastoid, when no longer heard, just outside ear canal; air conduction should be greater than bone conduction)
- Conductive hearing loss (due to damage to tympanic membrane, ossicles, etc.)
- Sensorineural hearing loss (due to damage or defect in cranial nerve VIII, the inner ear, or brain defect)
- A perforated tympanic membrane is a conductive hearing loss (Weber will lateralize to bad ear, negative Rinne).
- Facial nerve palsy (ominous sign)
- Inspection of oropharynx noting tonsillar asymmetry and size
- Note foreign bodies (Q-tips, PE tubes).
- Presence of perforation
- Inflammation in the EAC consistent with OE
- Retraction pocket (chronic eustachian tube dysfunction)
- Thinned tympanic membrane (prior perforations)
- Keratin debris consistent with cholesteatoma
- Otorrhea (pus, blood, clear) can mask a perforation.
- Fluid or mass in the middle-ear space behind the tympanic membrane (cholesteatoma, fluid)

DIAGNOSTIC TESTS & INTERPRETATION

- Audiogram can reveal normal hearing or a mild conductive hearing loss:
  - A simple perforation will typically result in a low-frequency conductive hearing loss.
  - An audiogram that demonstrates a worse-than-expected conductive hearing loss or sensorineural hearing loss would be more suspicious for ossicular chain damage or middle-ear pathology.
- Tympanometry demonstrates an increased volume in the ear, decreased pressure (can demonstrate perforation even if not present on otoscopic exam); acoustic immittance demonstrates a volume >2 mL.
- MRI and CT imaging are only indicated if there is suspicion for cholesteatoma or a worsening clinical picture (CN VII palsy).
- Follow-up should be established with an otolaryngologist for proper debridement, identification of cholesteatoma, and possible surgery for chronic perforations.

DIFFERENTIAL DIAGNOSIS

- Tympanosclerosis
- Otitis externa (can mask perforation or cholesteatoma)
- AOM/OME
- Otosclerosis (conductive hearing loss without perforation)
- Cholesteatoma
- Sudden sensorineural hearing loss

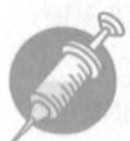

TREATMENT

- Most perforations are uncomplicated (hearing loss <40 dB and no vestibular symptoms), and will heal spontaneously within 4 weeks.
- All patients with perforations should avoid getting water into the external auditory canal and on the eardrum.
- Treatment of perforations with topical antibiotics will reduce otorrhea.
- Perforations with hearing loss >40 dB, those associated with vestibular symptoms, or those associated with cholesteatoma require referral to ENT; for traumatic perforation, obtain evaluation within 48 hours.

MEDICATION

- Some topical antibiotics (gentamicin, neomycin sulfate, or tobramycin) may rarely cause ototoxicity in the setting of a perforated tympanic membrane; nonototoxic drops are preferred, but cost and availability may be relevant considerations given the rarity of oto- and vestibulotoxicity (1).
- Oral antibiotics can be used if ear is severely infected or otorrhea prevents topical treatment.

First Line

- Ciprofloxacin ear drops
- Ofloxacin ear drops

ADDITIONAL TREATMENT

Maintain dry ear precautions (cotton ball with petroleum jelly while showering and use of hairdryer to dry out ear if water enters the EAC).

General Measures

- For some patients with chronic eustachian tube dysfunction, having a perforated tympanic membrane is a favorable situation since it allows for the equalization of pressure in the middle ear that would otherwise be more difficult because of the decreased eustachian tube function, thus obviating the need for tympanostomy tube placement later. For these patients, dry ear precautions are necessary.
- For patients who participate in water sports as a part of their daily life, such as swimmers and divers, repair would be indicated.
- Since there is a connection from the outer ear to the middle ear, dry ear precautions are needed to prevent a nidus of infection, such as using cotton swab in ear during showers and gentle hairdryer use over ear if water enters the ear canal.
- A case-by-case risk–benefit analysis must be performed in cases of conductive hearing loss, since surgery entails the risk of hearing loss.
- Prevent infection via eardrops or oral antibiotics.

SURGERY/OTHER PROCEDURES

- Nonhealing perforations are repaired through myringoplasty if the perforation is small, whereas a tympanoplasty is performed for larger perforations. Perichondrium or temporalis fascia are often used in reconstructing the tympanic membrane.
- A combined tympanoplasty/mastoidectomy surgery might be required for large perforations, chronic draining ears, presence of cholesteatoma, damage to the ossicular chain, or with evidence of mastoid disease.
- Ossiculoplasty might also be performed if pathology involves the ossicular chain; full repair of the ossicular chain might necessitate a second procedure:
  - Surgery is a same-day procedure, is usually done under general anesthesia, and generally does not require inpatient care.
  - Patients can expect to do no heavy lifting for 4 weeks after surgery.
  - Maintenance of dry ear precautions and the use of eardrops are important in the postoperative period.
  - Ear drainage, ear numbness, ear fullness/tinnitus, change in taste, and vertigo occur in the postoperative period.
  - Potential risks of surgery include inability to improve hearing, potentially worsened hearing, and facial nerve palsy.

IN-PATIENT CONSIDERATIONS

Inpatient care is generally not required for tympanic membrane perforation. The presence of comorbid disease like mastoiditis or meningitis would require inpatient stabilization with IV antibiotics and the appropriate care for those disorders.

ONGOING CARE

FOLLOW-UP RECOMMENDATIONS

Patient Monitoring

- Follow-up should be established with an ENT to confirm tympanic membrane healing and get a baseline audiogram.
- Since this condition is often associated with cholesteatoma, it is vital to re-examine the ear, especially after an episode of infection associated with a perforation, because an underlying cholesteatoma or chronic eustachian tube dysfunction might be contributing to the perforation.
- Follow-up after surgery is necessary to ensure that there is no cholesteatoma formation.

DIET

There are no dietary restrictions.

PATIENT EDUCATION

- Dry ear precautions
- Avoid Q-tips.
- Call physician for worsening hearing loss, vertigo, facial nerve palsy, fever, or persistent drainage.

PROGNOSIS

- Most perforations will heal spontaneously; however, large perforations and those associated with a chronic draining ear often require surgery.
- Mortality associated with this condition is low, but there is a potential for infection to spread to the mastoid, leading to meningitis, if proper aural care is not maintained.

COMPLICATIONS

- Nonhealing perforation
- Infection (otitis media, mastoiditis, meningitis)
- Hearing loss
- Facial paralysis
- Ossicular chain disruption

REFERENCE

1. Haynes DS, Rutka J, Hawke M, et al. Ototoxicity of ototopical drops—an update. *Otolaryngol Clin North Am*. 2007;40:669–83, xi.

ADDITIONAL READING

- Jensen RG, Koch A, Homøe P, et al. Long-term tympanic membrane pathology dynamics and spontaneous healing in chronic suppurative otitis media. *Pediatr Infect Dis J*. 2011;31(2):139–44.
- Morris PS, Leach AJ, et al. Acute and chronic otitis media. *Pediatr Clin North Am*. 2009;56:1383–99.

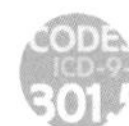

CODES

ICD9

- 381.01 Acute serous otitis media
- 382.01 Acute suppurative otitis media with spontaneous rupture of eardrum
- 384.20 Perforation of tympanic membrane, unspecified

CLINICAL PEARLS

- To evaluate a patient with a suspected tympanic membrane perforation, history and physical exam will usually suffice.
- Nonhealing perforations associated with malodorous or recurrent infections are often associated with cholesteatoma.
- Retraction pockets and history of AOM are suspicious for chronic eustachian tube dysfunction.
- It is vital to establish a follow-up with an otolaryngologist to ensure that more worrisome etiology like a cholesteatoma did not cause the perforation.
- Tympanoplasty surgery might be required for a perforation that does not spontaneously heal.
- If the presentation is a sudden sensorineural hearing loss, this should warrant referral and initiation of steroid therapy the same day or the following day.
- Normal physical exam with history of ear pain should also warrant otolaryngology referral for investigation of referred pain via fiber-optic exam.

PERICARDITIS

Kim-Lien Nguyen, MD

BASICS

DESCRIPTION

- Inflammatory process of the pericardium, with or without associated pericardial effusion; a broad spectrum of etiologies, with most common causes being idiopathic or viral
- System(s) affected: Cardiovascular
- Synonym(s): Acute suppurative pericarditis

EPIDEMIOLOGY

Incidence

- Epidemiologic studies lacking
- Exact incidence unknown, but occurs in up to 5% of patients evaluated in emergency room for chest pain without myocardial infarction (MI) (1)

RISK FACTORS

Genetics

No known genetic factors

PATHOPHYSIOLOGY

Acute inflammation that can produce serous or purulent fluid or dense fibrinous material (depending on etiology)

ETIOLOGY

- Idiopathic: 85–90% of cases. Likely related to viral infection (2)[B].
- Infectious:
  - Viral: Coxsackievirus, echovirus, adenovirus, Epstein-Barr virus, cytomegalovirus, hepatitis viruses, influenza virus, HIV, measles, mumps, varicella
  - Bacterial: Gram-positive and gram-negative organisms
  - Fungal (more common in immunocompromised populations): *Blastomyces dermatitidis, Candida* sp., *Histoplasma capsulatum*
  - Mycobacterial: *Mycobacterium tuberculosis*
  - Parasites: *Echinococcus*
- Noninfectious causes:
  - Acute MI (2–4 days after MI), Dressler syndrome (weeks–months after MI)
  - Aortic dissection
  - Renal failure, uremia
  - Malignancy (e.g., breast cancer, lung cancer, Hodgkin disease, leukemia, lymphoma)
  - Radiation therapy
  - Trauma
  - Postpericardiotomy
  - After cardiac procedures (e.g., catheterization, pacemaker placement, ablation) (3)[B]
  - Autoimmune disorders: Connective tissue disorders, systemic lupus erythematosus (SLE), rheumatoid arthritis, scleroderma, hypothyroidism, inflammatory bowel disease, spondyloarthropathies, Wegener granulomatosis
  - Sarcoidosis
- Medication-induced: Dantrolene, doxorubicin, hydralazine, isoniazid, mesalamine, methysergide, penicillin, phenytoin, procainamide, rifampin (1)[B]

COMMONLY ASSOCIATED CONDITIONS

Depends on etiology

DIAGNOSIS

HISTORY

- Prodrome of fever, malaise, myalgias
- Acute, sharp, stabbing chest pain
- Duration typically hours to days
- Pleuritic pain
- Pain improved by leaning forward, worsened by lying supine

PHYSICAL EXAM

- Heart rate is usually rapid and regular.
- Pericardial friction rub:
  - Coarse, high-pitched sound best heard during end expiration at left lower sternal border with patient leaning forward
  - Highly specific for diagnosis (but not sensitive)
  - May be transient and mono-, bi-, or triphasic (1)[B]
- New S_3 may suggest myopericarditis.
- Cardiac tamponade suggested by the presence of:
  - Systemic arterial hypotension
  - Elevated jugular venous pressure
  - Pulsus paradoxus (inspiratory fall in arterial pressure of at least 10 mm Hg)

DIAGNOSTIC TESTS & INTERPRETATION

Lab

Initial lab tests

- CBC: Typically shows leukocytosis
- Inflammatory markers: Elevated ESR, C-reactive protein (CRP)
- Cardiac biomarkers: Typically elevated creatine kinase, troponins:
  - Elevated troponins associated with younger age, male gender, pericardial effusion at presentation, and ST-segment elevation on ECG
  - Adverse outcomes not predicted by elevated troponin (4)[B]
- ECG: Findings include widespread upward concave ST-segment elevation and PR-segment depression that may evolve through 4 stages (but ECG may be normal or show nonspecific abnormalities) (1)[B]:
  - Stage 1: Diffuse ST-segment elevation and PR-segment depression
  - Stage 2: Normalization of the ST and PR segments
  - Stage 3: Widespread T-wave inversions
  - Stage 4: Normalization of T waves; may have persistent inversions if chronic pericarditis
  - ECG may demonstrate low voltage and electrical alternans with tamponade.
- Additional testing includes tuberculin skin test, sputum cultures, rheumatoid factor, antinuclear antibody, and HIV serology if clinically appropriate based on history or atypical presentation or course.
- Viral cultures and antibody titers rarely clinically useful

Imaging

Initial approach

- Chest x-ray (CXR) is performed to rule out pulmonary/mediastinal pathology. Enlarged cardiac silhouette suggests large pericardial effusion (at least 200 mL).
- Transthoracic echocardiogram recommended to evaluate for the presence of pericardial effusion, tamponade, or myocardial disease (presence of effusion helps to confirm diagnosis of pericarditis) (5)[B].
- CT and MRI permit visualization of pericardium to assess for complications or if initial workup is inconclusive.

Diagnostic Procedures/Surgery

- Pericardiocentesis indicated for cardiac tamponade and for suspected purulent, tuberculous, or neoplastic pericarditis
- Surgical drainage with pericardial biopsy recommended if recurrent tamponade or ineffective pericardiocentesis

Pathological Findings

- Microscopic examination may reveal hyperemia, leukocyte accumulation, or fibrin deposition.
- Purulent fluid with neutrophilic predominance if bacterial etiology
- Lymphocytic predominance in viral, tuberculous, and neoplastic pericarditis

DIFFERENTIAL DIAGNOSIS

- Acute MI
- Pneumonia with pleurisy
- Pulmonary embolism
- Aortic dissection
- Pneumothorax
- Mediastinal emphysema
- Cholecystitis
- Pancreatitis
- Esophageal inflammation, perforation, or rupture

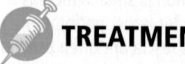

TREATMENT

- Goal of treatment is to relieve pain and reduce complications (e.g., recurrence, tamponade, chronic restrictive pericarditis).
- Outpatient therapy is reported to be successful in 85% patients with low-risk features (3)[B].

MEDICATION

First Line

- NSAIDs are considered the mainstay of therapy; dosage is tapered every 1–2 weeks to reduce recurrence rate:
  - Ibuprofen 600 mg t.i.d. Wean to 600 mg b.i.d. or 400 mg t.i.d., then 600 mg/d.
  - Aspirin 750–1,000 mg t.i.d. Wean to 750–1,000 mg b.i.d., then 750–1,000 mg/d. Preferable for patients with recent MI because other NSAIDs impair scar formation in animal studies.
  - Indomethacin 50 mg t.i.d. Wean by decreasing total daily dose by 25 mg every 1–2 weeks.
  - GI protection should be provided.
- Colchicine 0.6 mg b.i.d. (<70 kg patient) × 3 months (6–12 months for recurrences). Taper over 2–4 weeks. A higher initial loading dose is associated with adverse GI events (3)[B]. More effective as an adjunct to NSAID or steroids than monotherapy for initial attack and prevention of recurrences (6)[B].
- Tapering should only be done if the patient is asymptomatic and CRP/ESR are normal and is done every 1–2 weeks.
- Treatment duration using NSAIDs for initial attacks is 1–2 weeks, but for recurrences, consider 2–4 weeks of therapy

- Monitoring: NSAIDs: CBC and CRP at baseline and weekly until CRP normalizes; colchicine: Consider CBC, CRP, transaminases, creatine kinase, and creatinine at baseline and at least after 1 month (3)[B].
- Contraindications: Hypersensitivity to aspirin or NSAID, active peptic ulcer or GI bleeding
- Precautions: Use with caution in patients with asthma, third-trimester pregnancy, coagulopathy, and renal or hepatic dysfunction.
- Pregnant: <20 weeks' gestation: Aspirin is first choice, but NSAID and prednisone are also allowed; >20 weeks' gestation: Prednisone is allowed with avoidance of NSAIDs, aspirin, and colchicine (5)[B].

Second Line

- Corticosteroid treatment is indicated in connective tissue disease, uremic or tuberculous pericarditis, or severe recurrent symptoms unresponsive to NSAIDs or colchicine (4)[B]; should be avoided in uncomplicated acute pericarditis. *Corticosteroid use alone has been found to be an independent risk factor for recurrence.*
- If steroids are used, consider low dose (0.2–0.5 mg/kg/d × 2 weeks for first attack, 0.2–0.5 mg/kg/d × 2–4 weeks for recurrence) with slow taper (*>50 mg:* 10 mg/d every 1–2 weeks; *50–25 mg:* 5–10 mg/d every 1–2 weeks; *25–15 mg:* 2.5 mg/d every 2–4 weeks; *<15 mg/d:* 1–2.5 mg/d every 2–6 weeks) following remission with symptom resolution and normalization of CRP. Remember to use adequate prophylaxis treatment for osteoporosis prevention (3)[B].
- Intrapericardial administration of steroids may be effective and limits systemic side effects (4)[B].

ADDITIONAL TREATMENT

General Measures

Specific therapy directed toward underlying disorder for patients with identified cause other than viral or idiopathic disease

Issues for Referral

- Refractory cases include those on unacceptably high long-term steroid doses (>25 mg/d).
- Consider trial of aspirin and/or NSAID plus steroid and colchicine (3)[C].

SURGERY/OTHER PROCEDURES

- Pericardiocentesis is indicated in cases of cardiac tamponade, high likelihood of tuberculous/purulent/neoplastic pericarditis, and large symptomatic effusions refractory to medical therapy (3)[B].
- Pericardial biopsy may be considered for diagnosis in those with persistent worsening pericarditis without a definite diagnosis (3)[B].
- Pericardioscopy for targeted diagnostic imaging may be performed at experienced tertiary referral centers in refractory and difficult cases (3)[B].
- Pericardial window may be performed in cases of recurrent cardiac tamponade with large pericardial effusion despite medical therapy and severe symptoms (3)[B].
- Pericardiectomy can be considered for frequent and highly symptomatic recurrences with cardiac tamponade and constrictive pericarditis (3)[B]. The 2004 European Society of Cardiology guidelines recommend pericardiectomy (class IIa) for frequent and highly symptomatic recurrences of pericarditis refractory to medical therapy (4)[B]. However, this is rarely performed in the US.

IN-PATIENT CONSIDERATIONS

Admission Criteria

Inpatient therapy recommended for pericarditis associated with clinical predictors of poor prognosis (3)[B]:

- MAJOR predictors:
  - Fever >38°C
  - Subacute onset
  - Large pericardial effusion
  - Cardiac tamponade
  - Lack of response to NSAID/aspirin therapy after at least 1 week
- MINOR predictors:
  - Immunosuppressed state
  - Trauma
  - Oral anticoagulation therapy
  - Myopericarditis

IV Fluids

No specific therapy recommended; IV fluids considered for hypotension in the setting of pericardial tamponade

Nursing

No specific therapies

Discharge Criteria

- Response to therapy with symptom improvement
- Hemodynamic stability

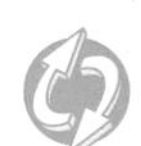

ONGOING CARE

FOLLOW-UP RECOMMENDATIONS

- 7–10 days to assess response to treatment
- 1 month to check CBC and CRP and thereafter if symptoms continue to be present
- Those with clinical predictors of poor prognosis may require closer follow up based on lab data and echocardiographic findings.

Patient Monitoring

Myopericarditis (3)[B]:

- Use lower doses of anti-inflammatory drugs to control symptoms for 1–2 weeks while minimizing deleterious effects on myocarditic process.
- Exercise restrictions for 4–6 weeks
- Echocardiographic monitoring at 1, 6, and 12 months (especially in those with left ventricular dysfunction)

DIET

No restrictions

PROGNOSIS

Overall good prognosis; disease usually benign and self-limiting

COMPLICATIONS

- Recurrent pericarditis (1):
  - Occurs in ~24% of patients, with most instances resulting from idiopathic, viral, or autoimmune pericarditis; inadequate treatment of the initial attack; and less commonly neoplastic etiologies
  - Recurrence usually within first weeks following initial episode, but may occur months to years later
  - Rarely associated with tamponade or constriction
- Cardiac tamponade: Rare complication with increased incidence in neoplastic, purulent, and tuberculous pericarditis
- Effusive-constrictive pericarditis (5):
  - Reported in 24% of patients undergoing surgery for constrictive pericarditis and in 8% of patients undergoing pericardiocentesis and cardiac catheterization for cardiac tamponade
  - Failure of right atrial pressure to fall by 50% or to a level below 10 mm Hg after pericardiocentesis is diagnostic
- Constrictive pericarditis:
  - Rare complication in which rigid pericardium produces abnormal diastolic filling with elevated filling pressures
  - Pericardiectomy remains definitive therapy.

REFERENCES

1. Tingle LE, Molina D, Calvert CW. Acute pericarditis. *Am Fam Physician*. 2007;76:1509–14.
2. Khandaker MH, Espinosa RE, Nishimura RA, et al. Pericardial disease: Diagnosis and management. *Mayo Clin. Proc*. 2010;85:572–93.
3. Imazio M, Spodick DH, Brucato A, et al. Controversial issues in the management of pericardial diseases. *Circulation*. 2010;121: 916–28.
4. Maisch B, Seferovi PM, Risti AD, et al. Guidelines on the diagnosis and management of pericardial diseases executive summary: The task force on the diagnosis and management of pericardial diseases of the European society of cardiology. *Eur Heart J*. 2004;25:587–610.
5. Imazio M, Brucato A, Trinchero R, et al. Diagnosis and management of pericardial diseases. *Nat Rev Cardiol*. 2009;6:743–51.
6. Imazio M, Bobbio M, Cecchi E, et al. Colchicine in addition to conventional therapy for acute pericarditis: Results of the COlchicine for acute PEricarditis (COPE) trial. *Circulation*. 2005;112: 2012–6.

CODES

ICD9

- 420.91 Acute idiopathic pericarditis
- 420.99 Other acute pericarditis
- 423.9 Unspecified disease of pericardium

CLINICAL PEARLS

- Common cause of chest pain with many possible etiologies, viral and idiopathic being most likely
- Typical presentation includes acute chest pain, pericardial friction rub, ECG changes with widespread PR-interval depression or ST-segment elevation, and evidence of pericardial effusion on echocardiogram.
- Therapy aimed at symptomatic relief, and NSAIDs are first-line treatment.
- Colchicine is recommended as adjunct to NSAIDs and has been found to reduce recurrences.
- Pericardiocentesis is recommended in the setting of cardiac tamponade or possible purulent pericarditis.

PERIODIC LIMB MOVEMENT DISORDER

Donald E. Watenpaugh, PhD
John R. Burk, MD

BASICS

DESCRIPTION

- Sleep-related movement disorder with these features (1)[A]:
  - Episodes of periodic limb movements (PLMs) during sleep
  - Movements consist of bilateral ankle dorsiflexion, sometimes with knee and hip flexion.
  - Arm or more generalized movements occur less commonly.
  - Movements may cause brief microarousals from sleep unbeknownst to the patient.
  - Complaints include insomnia, unrestorative sleep, daytime fatigue, and/or somnolence.
  - Bed partner may complain of movements.
  - Another sleep disorder (e.g., obstructive sleep apnea) does not cause the PLMs.
- System(s) affected: Musculoskeletal; Nervous
- Synonym(s): Nocturnal myoclonus; Sleep myoclonus; Periodic leg movements of sleep

EPIDEMIOLOGY

Incidence

- Increases with age: 1/3 of patients >age 60 exhibit PLMs, but not necessarily periodic limb movement *disorder* (PLMD) (1)[A].
- Predominant sex: Male = Female
- PLMs in 15% of insomnia patients

Prevalence

- PLMs in sleep: Common and often of no clinical consequence
- PLMs constituting PLMD (causing sleep complaints and/or daytime consequences) much less common: <5% of adults (but underdiagnosed)

RISK FACTORS

- Family history of restless legs syndrome (RLS) (2)[A]
- Iron deficiency and associated conditions (e.g., pregnancy, gastric surgery, renal disease)
- Attention-deficit hyperactivity disorder (ADHD) (3,4)[B]
- Aging
- Peripheral neuropathy
- Arthritis, orthopedic problems
- Chronic limb pain or discomfort

Genetics

Unstudied, but see RLS

GENERAL PREVENTION

- Regular physical activity
- Adequate nightly sleep
- Avoid causes of secondary PLMD.
- Avoid causes of RLS.

PATHOPHYSIOLOGY

Unstudied, but see RLS

ETIOLOGY

- Primary: Probable CNS dopaminergic impairment
- Secondary:
  - Iron deficiency
  - Peripheral neuropathy
  - Arthritis
  - Renal failure
  - Synucleinopathies (multiple-system atrophy)
  - Spinal cord injury
  - Pregnancy
  - Medications:
    - Most antidepressants (not bupropion or desipramine)
    - Some antipsychotic and antidementia medications
    - Antiemetics (metoclopramide)
    - Antihistamines

COMMONLY ASSOCIATED CONDITIONS

- RLS
- Rapid eye movement (REM) sleep behavior disorder
- Narcolepsy
- Iron deficiency
- Renal failure
- Cardiovascular disease; stroke
- Gastric surgery
- Pregnancy
- Arthritis
- Synucleinopathies (multiple-system atrophy)
- Lumbar spine disease; spinal cord injury
- Peripheral neuropathy
- Insomnia, insufficient sleep
- ADHD
- Depression

Pediatric Considerations

- PLMD may precede overt RLS by years.
- Association with RLS is more common than in adults.
- Symptoms may be more consequential than in adults
- Associated with ADHD (3,4)[B]

Pregnancy Considerations

- May be secondary to iron or folate deficiency
- Most severe in third trimester
- Usually subsides after delivery

Geriatric Considerations

- May become a significant source of sleep disturbance
- May cause or exacerbate circadian disruption and "sundowning"
- Many medications given to the elderly cause or exacerbate PLMs, which can lead to PLMD or RLS.

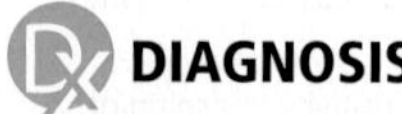

DIAGNOSIS

HISTORY

- Insomnia: Difficulty maintaining sleep
- Unrestorative sleep
- Daytime fatigue, tiredness, and/or somnolence
- Oppositional behaviors
- Memory impairment
- Depression
- ADHD, particularly in children (3,4)

DIAGNOSTIC TESTS & INTERPRETATION

Polysomnography with finding of repetitive, stereotyped limb movements:

- Tibialis anterior electromyographic (EMG) activity lasting 0.5–10 seconds
- EMG amplitude increases >8 μV from baseline.
- Movements occur in a sequence of 4 or more at intervals of 5–90 seconds
- Children: 5 or more movements/hr; adults: 15
- Associated with heart rate variability from autonomic-level arousals
- Most PLM episodes occur in the first hours of non-REM sleep.
- Significant night-to-night PLM variability

Lab

Serum ferritin to assess for iron deficiency

Diagnostic Procedures/Surgery

- Ankle actigraphy for in-home use
- EMG or nerve conduction studies for peripheral neuropathy/radiculopathy

Pathological Findings

Serum ferritin <75 ng/mL

DIFFERENTIAL DIAGNOSIS

- When PLMs occur along with RLS, REM sleep behavior disorder, or narcolepsy, those disorders are diagnosed as "with PLMs," and PLMD is not diagnosed separately.
- Obstructive sleep apnea: LMs occur during microarousals from apneas; treatment of sleep apnea eliminates these LMs (1).
- Sleep starts: Nonperiodic, generalized, occur only at wake–sleep transition, <0.2 seconds duration
- Sleep-related leg cramps: Isolated and painful
- Fragmentary myoclonus: 75–150 ms of EMG activity, minimal movement, no periodicity
- Nocturnal seizures: Epileptiform EEG, motor pattern incongruent with PLMs
- Fasciculations, tremor: No sleep association
- Sleep-related rhythmic movement disorder: Voluntary movement during wake–sleep transition; higher frequency than PLMs

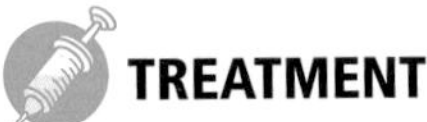

TREATMENT

- Daily exercise
- Adequate nightly sleep
- Treatment paradigm similar to that for RLS (5,6)[A], except that all medications are off-label for PLMD

MEDICATION

- Use minimum effective dose.
- Consider risks, side effects, and interactions individually (e.g., benzodiazepines in elderly).
- Daytime sleepiness is unusual with the doses and timing employed for PLMD.

First Line

- Dopamine agonists: Take 1 hour before bed; titrate weekly to optimal dose (5,6)[A]:
  - Pramipexole (Mirapex): 0.125–1.5 mg; titrate by 0.125 mg
  - Ropinirole (Requip): 0.25–4 mg; titrate by 0.25 mg
  - Cabergoline (Dostinex and Cabaser): 0.25–3 mg (*Warning:* Valvulopathy risk)
- Avoid dopamine agonists in psychotic patients, especially if taking dopamine antagonists.

Second Line

- Anticonvulsants: Useful for associated neuropathy:
  - Gabapentin enacarbil (Horizant): 600 mg/d
  - Pregabalin (Lyrica): 50–300 mg/d
- Opioids: Low risk for tolerance with bedtime dose:
  - Hydrocodone: 5–20 mg/d
  - Oxycodone: 2.5–20 mg/d
- Benzodiazepines and agonists:
  - Zaleplon, zolpidem, temazepam, triazolam, alprazolam, diazepam
  - Clonazepam (Klonopin): 0.5–3 mg/d

Pediatric Considerations

- First-line treatment is nonpharmacologic (4)[A].
- Low-dose clonidine or clonazepam may be considered.

Pregnancy Considerations

- Initial approach: Fe supplementation, nonpharmacologic therapies
- Most medications Class C or D and should be avoided
- In third trimester, low-dose opioids or clonazepam may be considered.

Geriatric Considerations

In weak or frail patients, avoid medications that may cause dizziness or unsteadiness.

ADDITIONAL TREATMENT

- If iron-deficient, iron supplementation:
  - 325 mg ferrous sulfate with 200 mg vitamin C between meals t.i.d.
  - Repletion may require months
  - Symptoms continue without other treatment
- Vitamin/mineral supplements, including calcium, magnesium, B_{12}, folate
- Clonidine: 0.1–0.7 mg/d

General Measures

- Daily exercise
- Adequate nightly sleep
- Warm the legs (long socks, leg warmers, electric blanket, etc.).
- Hot bath before bedtime
- Avoid nicotine and evening caffeine and alcohol.

SURGERY/OTHER PROCEDURES

Correction of orthopedic, neuropathic, or peripheral vascular problems

IN-PATIENT CONSIDERATIONS

- Control during recovery from orthopedic procedures
- Addition or withdrawal of medications that affect PLMD
- Changes in medical status may require medication changes, e.g.:
  - Renal failure: Mirapex contraindicated
  - Liver disease: Requip contraindicated

IV Fluids

- Consider iron infusion when oral supplementation is ineffective, not tolerated, or contraindicated.
- When NPO, consider IV opiates.

Nursing

- Evening walks, hot baths, leg warming
- Sleep interruption risks prolonged wakefulness.

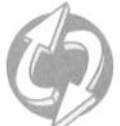

ONGOING CARE

FOLLOW-UP RECOMMENDATIONS

Patient Monitoring

- At monthly intervals until stable
- Annual and PRN follow-up thereafter
- If Fe-deficient, remeasure ferritin to assess repletion.

DIET

Avoid caffeine and alcohol late in the day.

PATIENT EDUCATION

- WE MOVE (Worldwide Education & Awareness for Movement Disorders): www.wemove.org; e-mail: wemove@wemove.org; 212-875-8312; fax: 212-875-8389
- National Sleep Foundation: www.sleepfoundation.org; e-mail: nsf@sleepfoundation.org; 202-347-3471; fax: 202-347-3472

PROGNOSIS

- Primary PLMD: Lifelong condition with no current cure
- Secondary PLMD: May subside with resolution of cause(s)
- Current therapies usually control symptoms.
- PLMD often precedes emergence of RLS.

COMPLICATIONS

- Tolerance to medications requiring increased dose or alternatives
- Augmentation (increased PLMs and sleep disturbance, emergence of RLS) from prolonged use of dopamine agonists:
  - Higher doses increase risk.
  - Iron deficiency increases risk.
  - Add alternative medication, then detitrate dopaminergic agent (6)[B].
- Iatrogenic PLMD (from antidepressants, etc.)

REFERENCES

1. Natarajan R, et al. Review of periodic limb movement and restless leg syndrome. *J Postgrad Med*. 2010;56:157–62.
2. Picchietti DL, Rajendran RR, Wilson MP, et al. Pediatric restless legs syndrome and periodic limb movement disorder: Parent-child pairs. *Sleep Med*. 2009;10(8):925–31.
3. Walters AS, Silvestri R, Zucconi M, et al. Review of the possible relationship and hypothetical links between attention deficit hyperactivity disorder (ADHD) and the simple sleep related movement disorders, parasomnias, hypersomnias, and circadian rhythm disorders. *J Clin Sleep Med*. 2008;4:591–600.
4. Picchietti MA, Picchietti DL. Restless legs syndrome and periodic limb movement disorder in children and adolescents. *Semin Pediatr Neurol*. 2008; 15:91–9.
5. Ferini-Strambi L. Treatment options for restless legs syndrome. *Expert Opin Pharmacother*. 2009;10: 545–54.
6. Trenkwalder C, Hening WA, Montagna P, et al. Treatment of restless legs syndrome: An evidence-based review and implications for clinical practice. *Mov Disord*. 2008;23:2267–302.

ADDITIONAL READING

- Imamura S, Kushida C. Gabapentin enacarbil (XP13512/GSK1838262) as an alternative treatment to dopaminergic agents for restless legs syndrome. *Expert Opin Pharmacother*. 2010;11(11):1925–32.
- Sateia MJ. Periodic limb movement disorder. In: *International Classification of Sleep Disorders Diagnostic & Coding Manual*, 2nd ed. Westchester, IL: American Academy of Sleep Medicine; 2005;182–6.

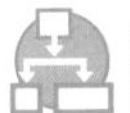

See Also (Topic, Algorithm, Electronic Media Element)

Restless Legs Syndrome

CODES

ICD9

327.51 Periodic limb movement disorder

CLINICAL PEARLS

- Many patients with PLMs may not require treatment. When sleep disturbance from PLMs causes insomnia and/or daytime consequences, PLMD exists and should be treated.
- Many antidepressants and some antihistamines cause or exacerbate PLMs.
- Accumulating data indicate that sleep disturbance, including that from PLMs, may cause or exacerbate ADHD (3,4)[B].

PERIORAL DERMATITIS

Heather Summe, MD
Nikki A. Levin, MD, PhD

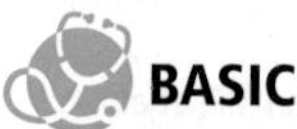

BASICS

DESCRIPTION

- A common facial eruption of women and children that presents as tiny, flesh-colored or erythematous monomorphic papules or pustules around the mouth with characteristic sparing of the area immediately adjacent to the vermillion border
- May also involve the periocular, perinasal, and glabellar regions of the face
- Without treatment, the course is usually fluctuating and chronic.
- Variants in children include granulomatous periorificial dermatitis (GPOD) and facial Afro-Caribbean childhood eruption (FACE)
- Etiology is unknown, but a relationship with topical steroid use has been suggested.
- Synonyms: Periorificial dermatitis; Chronic papulopustular facial dermatitis; Granulomatous perioral dermatitis; Light-sensitive seborrheid; Lupuslike perioral dermatitis; Papulopustular facial dermatitis; Rosacealike dermatitis; Stewardess disease

EPIDEMIOLOGY

- Occurs worldwide, especially in fair-skinned populations
- Predominantly affects children between 6 months and 16 years of age and women between 17 and 45 years of age
- ~90% of adult cases are in women (1).
- Childhood cases may be more common in boys.
- All races are affected, but the granulomatous form is more common in African American children.
- Some authors believe the number of cases peaked in the 1960s and 1970s and decreased in the 1980s and 1990s when the side effects of topical steroids were recognized. Others believe that cases are still increasing.

Incidence

- Peak incidence is in second and third decades of life.
- In children, peak incidence is in prepubertal period.

Prevalence

Represents about 2% of patients presenting to dermatology clinics (2)

RISK FACTORS

See "Etiology."

Genetics

55% of pediatric patients with POD have a family history of atopy (3).

GENERAL PREVENTION

- Avoid using potent topical corticosteroids on the face.
- Avoid using excessive foundation, moisturizer, and night cream.
- Avoidance of tartar control and whitening toothpastes may also be helpful.

PATHOPHYSIOLOGY

- Exposure to an irritant results in breakdown of the epidermal barrier and subsequent water loss and sensation of dryness, and encourages use of facial products and corticosteroids, which may worsen the condition.
- This inflammatory cycle eventually leads to clinical features of the disease.

ETIOLOGY

- The exact cause is unknown, and there may be more than 1 contributing factor.
- The most widely cited factor implicated in perioral dermatitis is use of potent topical corticosteroids on the face.
- Use of foundation, moisturizer, and night cream was associated with a 13-fold increased risk of POD in 1 study (3).
- Other factors that have been implicated but not proven include:
  - Drugs: Oral contraceptives
  - Toothpastes: Fluoridated, tartar control, whitening
  - Physical factors: Ultraviolet (UV) light, heat, wind, salivary leakage
  - Infectious factors: Fusiform bacteria, *Candida* species, *Demodex folliculorum*
  - Miscellaneous factors: Atopy, GI disturbances, stress, contact allergy, lip-licking, immunosuppression

COMMONLY ASSOCIATED CONDITIONS

Atopic dermatitis

DIAGNOSIS

HISTORY

- Patient reports a history of facial rash, which may improve with use of topical corticosteroids and flare with discontinuation
- Affected skin may be pruritic or have a burning sensation.
- Course may be chronic and fluctuating.
- Recent topical, inhaled, or systemic steroid use in 72% of patients (4)[C]
- May worsen with sun exposure

PHYSICAL EXAM

- Monomorphic, minute, flesh-colored-to-erythematous papules or pustules, sometimes surmounted with scale, in a perioral distribution, often asymmetrical, with sparing of the vermillion border 3–5 mm around the lips
- Common locations are alar creases, nasolabial folds, chin, periocular skin, eyelids, and glabella.
- Diameter of lesions usually 1–2 mm
- Distribution (2)[C]:
  - Perioral area (39%)
  - Perinasal (13%)
  - Periocular (1%)
  - Perioral and perinasal (14%)
  - Perioral and periocular (6%)
  - Perinasal and periocular (6%)
  - Perioral, perinasal, and periocular (10%)
- Lupuslike variant diagnosed by yellowish discoloration of lesions on diascopy

DIAGNOSTIC TESTS & INTERPRETATION

Diagnosis is usually clinical.

Lab

- No laboratory abnormalities expected
- Prick tests and IgE testing may show evidence of atopy, but are not routinely done.
- Patch testing may be used to rule out contact dermatitis.
- Scrapings for *Demodex* mites

Diagnostic Procedures/Surgery

Skin biopsy is not routinely performed, but can be helpful in atypical cases.

Pathological Findings

- Mild, nonspecific inflammation with variable perifollicular or perivascular lymphohistiocytic infiltrate
- Eczematous changes, acanthosis, parakeratosis, and spongiosis
- Occasionally, follicular abscesses are seen.
- Older lesions may contain diffuse hypertrophy of connective tissue and hyperplasia of sebaceous follicles with occasional noncaseating granulomas in the dermis (1).
- Caseating granulomas are seen with granulomatous variant.

DIFFERENTIAL DIAGNOSIS

- Acne vulgaris
- Contact dermatitis
- Rosacea
- Seborrheic dermatitis
- Lip licker's dermatitis
- Papular sarcoidosis
- *Demodex* infestation
- Acrodermatitis enteropathica
- Biotin deficiency
- Glucagonoma syndrome
- Xanthomas
- Eruptive syringomas
- Polymorphous light eruption
- Acne agminata
- Lupus miliaris disseminatus faciei
- Haber syndrome (familial rosacealike dermatosis)

TREATMENT

MEDICATION

Based on disease severity and patient's tolerance for adverse effects

First Line

- Severe disease:
  - Oral antibiotics:
    - Tetracycline has been proven an effective treatment (2)[A]:
      - 250–500 mg b.i.d. for 8–10 weeks
      - Dose may be halved after 3–4 weeks if improvement noted
      - NOTE: Contraindicated in children and pregnant women
      - Common side effects: Photosensitivity, GI upset, rash, candidiasis, headache, dizziness, tinnitus

- Doxycycline or minocycline (3)[C]:
  - 100 mg b.i.d. for 6–8 weeks
  - Dose may be halved after 3–4 weeks if improvement noted
  - NOTE: Contraindicated in children and pregnant women
  - Common side effects of doxycycline: GI upset, esophagitis, joint pain, upper respiratory infection (URI) symptoms, rash, dysmenorrhea, candidiasis, headache, dizziness, photosensitivity, elevated BUN
  - Common side effects of minocycline: GI upset, lightheadedness, vertigo, ataxia, headache, fatigue, tinnitus, rash, urticaria, candidiasis, hyperpigmentation
- Erythromycin (3)[C] may be used when tetracyclines are contraindicated or not tolerated:
  - 250 mg b.i.d.–t.i.d. for 6–8 weeks
  - Dose may be halved after 3–4 weeks if improvement noted
  - May be used in children or pregnant women
  - Common side effects: GI upset, diarrhea, rash, urticaria
  - Rarer serious side effects: Erythema multiforme, pancreatitis, convulsions, QT prolongation, and ventricular arrhythmias

- Moderate disease:
  - Topical antibiotics:
    - May be slower than systemic antibiotics in clearing lesions
    - Metronidazole cream 0.75% b.i.d. (2)[B]
    - Erythromycin 2% gel, solution, or ointment b.i.d. (2)[B]
    - Clindamycin 1% gel, lotion, or cream b.i.d.
- Mild disease:
  - "Zero therapy" (see "General Measures") (2)[B]

Second Line

- Severe disease:
  - Clarithromycin (250 mg daily) may be used when tetracyclines are contraindicated or not tolerated (2)[C]:
    - Common side effects: GI upset, headache, rash, abnormal taste sensation, urticaria
  - Oral isotretinoin may be useful in granulomatous cases that are not responsive to a full dose of tetracyclines (1)[C]:
    - 0.2 mg/kg initially followed by 0.1 mg/kg after notable improvement
    - NOTE: Isotretinoin is a pregnancy Category X drug and may cause severe birth defects. Use in caution with women of reproductive age. Physician and patient must register with iPLEDGE program.
    - Common side effects: Dry skin, cheilitis, arthralgias/myalgias, hypertriglyceridemia, elevated liver function tests (LFTs), hair loss, visual disturbances, depression, tinnitus
  - Pimecrolimus 1% cream may accelerate healing (2)[A] and tacrolimus 0.1% ointment use has been reported with success (2):
    - NOTE: Rare cases of lymphoma and skin malignancies have been reported. Avoid long-term use.
- Moderate disease:
  - Topical therapies:
    - Antiacne drugs such as azelaic acid and adapalene may be helpful (2).
    - Ichthyol (ammonium bituminosulfonate) (2)

ADDITIONAL TREATMENT

General Measures

"Zero therapy" can be an effective treatment in adherent patients (2)[B]:

- Reduce use of facial soaps, make-up, and moisturizers and wash with only water.
- Discontinue use of potent topical corticosteroids on the face:
  - This may result in a flare.
  - Flares may be decreased with use of less-potent topical steroids, calcineurin inhibitors, or IM steroid injection.
- Discontinue use of fluoridated, whitening, and tartar-control toothpaste.

Additional Therapies

A number of other therapies have been reported in the literature, including photodynamic therapy with 5-aminolevulenic acid (2)[B], radiotherapy, and liquid nitrogen.

COMPLEMENTARY AND ALTERNATIVE MEDICINE

Compress with chamomile tea or physiological solution may be used if the patient struggles with "zero therapy" (1)[C].

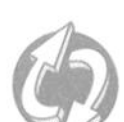

ONGOING CARE

DIET

No restrictions

PATIENT EDUCATION

- Lesions may take many weeks to resolve.
- Symptoms may temporarily worsen, especially with discontinuance of steroids.
- Recurrence is rare.
- Topical corticosteroid use on the face should be avoided in the future.

PROGNOSIS

- Most cases resolve without recurrence.
- Untreated disease may persist for months to years and be characterized by unpredictable flares.
- Oral or topical antibiotics usually lead to remission within 6–10 weeks.
- Disease is not associated with significant morbidity.

COMPLICATIONS

- Most cases resolve without complications.
- Emotional stress can result from bothersome appearance of lesions and chronic course of disease.
- Scarring may be problematic with lupuslike variant.

REFERENCES

1. Lipozencic J, Ljubojevic S, et al. Perioral dermatitis. *Clin Dermatol*. 2011;29:157–61.
2. Wollenberg A, Bieber T, Dirschka T, et al. Perioral dermatitis. *J Dtsch Dermatol Ges*. 2011;9:422–7.
3. Vanderweil SG, Levin NA, et al. Perioral dermatitis: It's not every rash that occurs around the mouth. *Dermatol Nurs*. 2009;21:317–20, 353; quiz 321.
4. Nguyen V, Eichenfield LF. Periorificial dermatitis in children and adolescents. *J Am Acad Dermatol* 2006;55(5):781–5.

ADDITIONAL READING

- Hafeez ZH, et al. Perioral dermatitis: An update. *Int J Dermatol*. 2003;42:514–7.
- Weber K, Thurmayr R. Critical appraisal of reports on the treatment of perioral dermatitis. *Dermatology*. 2005;210(4):300–7.

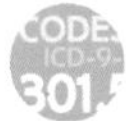

CODES

ICD9

695.3 Rosacea

CLINICAL PEARLS

- Suspect perioral dermatitis when an acneiform eruption involves the perioral, perinasal, and periocular areas with characteristic sparing of the skin immediately adjacent to the vermillion border.
- Ask patients about a history of recent corticosteroid use, facial product use, and use of whitening or tartar-control toothpastes.
- Substitution of low-potency steroids may allow patients to discontinue higher-potency steroids while avoiding a rebound flare.

PERIPHERAL ARTERIAL DISEASE

Zhen Lu, MD

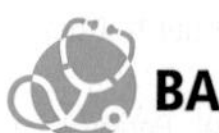

BASICS

DESCRIPTION

Peripheral arterial disease (PAD) is a manifestation of systemic atherosclerosis in which there is partial or total blockage in the arteries, exclusive of the coronary and cerebral vessels. Objectively, PAD is defined as a resting ankle-brachial index (ABI) of <0.90.

EPIDEMIOLOGY

- Predominant age: >40 years
- Predominant sex: Male > Female (2:1), based on the Framingham study
- Patients with symptomatic PAD have a 5-year mortality rate of 30%.
- Highly prevalent syndrome that affects 8–12 million individuals in the US

Incidence

Incidence per year overall: 1–2.7 in 1,000 per year

Prevalence

- US prevalence: 2.7–4.1%
- Age-adjusted prevalence of PAD is close to 12%.
- Up to 29% among patients in primary care practices

RISK FACTORS

- Age >40 years
- Cigarette smoking
- Diabetes mellitus
- Obesity
- Hypertension
- Hyperlipidemia
- Hyperhomocysteinemia

Genetics

Current National Institutes of Health–funded research focuses on single-nucleotide polymorphisms in candidate genes that are regulated in the vasculature in an attempt to explore genetic factors responsible for PAD.

GENERAL PREVENTION

Control risk factors.

PATHOPHYSIOLOGY

In patients with PAD, arterial stenoses cause inadequate blood flow in distal limbs, which fails to meet the metabolic demand during exertion:

- The degree of ischemia is proportional to the size and proximity of the occlusion to the end organ.
- The acidic products of anaerobic metabolism build up within the muscle and result in claudication clinically.
- Arterial occlusion also causes significantly diminished distal pressure in patients with PAD due to atherosclerotic lesions.

ETIOLOGY

The most common cause of arterial stenoses is atherosclerosis.

COMMONLY ASSOCIATED CONDITIONS

- See "Risk Factors."
- Associated with other common complications of atherosclerosis, including myocardial infarction, transient ischemic attack, stroke, and limb amputation
- Occurs in ~40% of patients with cardiovascular disease

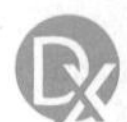

DIAGNOSIS

HISTORY

- Intermittent claudication, with symptoms typically resolving within 2–5 minutes of rest (although it is regarded as the classic symptom for PAD, intermittent claudication is present in only 10% of patients with PAD)
- Rest leg pain (especially in a supine position)
- Skin ulceration (in advanced PAD)
- Gangrene (in advanced PAD)
- Impotence

PHYSICAL EXAM

- Skin pallor when leg is elevated above the level of the heart (in mild PAD)
- Dependent rubor
- Dry and scaly skin
- Poor nail growth
- Hair loss
- Reduced or absent extremity pulses (in advanced PAD)

DIAGNOSTIC TESTS & INTERPRETATION

Lab

Serum glucose is recommended for screening for diabetes mellitus in suspected or confirmed PAD.

Initial lab tests

Fasting lipid profile is indicated for risk assessment of hyperlipidemia.

Imaging

- Magnetic resonance angiography, coupled with 3D reconstruction, is highly sensitive and specific for the localization of occluded lesions.
- CT scanning has a limited role in the evaluation of PAD.
- Angiography remains the gold standard in the diagnosis of PAD.

Initial approach

Duplex ultrasonography and Doppler color-flow imaging are useful in detecting stenosed segments and assessing lesion severity and are initial imaging test of choice.

Diagnostic Procedures/Surgery

- Doppler ABI measures the ratio the higher systolic BPs between the dorsalis pedis and the posterior tibial artery vs. the higher of the systolic BPs in the 2 brachial arteries: Values for the ankle-brachial index (ABI) should be reported as "incompressible" if over 1.40; "normal" if 1.00 to 1.40; "borderline" if 0.91 to 0.99; and "abnormal" if 0.90 or less (1). ABI <0.4: Severe ischemia
- Segmental limb pressures: Usually obtained if abnormal ABI measurement is identified; a 20-mm Hg or greater reduction in pressure is considered significant for PAD.
- Treadmill exercise test assesses the severity of claudication and the response to treatment.
- Segmental volume plethysmography: Often used in conjunction with segmental limb pressures to measure the volume change in an organ or limb; the study is indicated for calcified vessel when the ABI cannot be applied diagnostically.

DIFFERENTIAL DIAGNOSIS

- Arterial embolism
- Deep venous thrombosis
- Thromboangiitis obliterans (Buerger disease)
- Osteoarthritis
- Restless legs syndrome
- Peripheral neuropathy
- Spinal stenoses (pseudoclaudication)
- Intervertebral disc prolapse

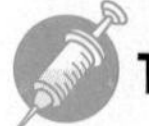

TREATMENT

MEDICATION

First Line

Antiplatelet therapy has been the mainstay treatment to prevent ischemic events in patients with PAD. However:

- The effect of aspirin on the risk reduction of overall ischemic events is inconclusive. Some suggest that aspirin delays disease progression and reduces the need for surgical intervention. AHA/ACCF Guidelines (1) note that the utility of antiplatelet therapy to reduce cardiovascular risks in asymptomatic patients with borderline ABIs is characterized as "not well established." Aspirin is recommended to reduce the risk of MI, stroke, and vascular death in symptomatic patients with PAD (1)[A]
- Low-dose aspirin (75–150 mg/d) is as effective as higher doses of aspirin (2).
- Ticlopidine (250 mg b.i.d.) reduces the risk of myocardial infarction (MI), stroke, and death by 1/3 in patients with PAD, but it has a complication of thrombocytopenia in 2–3% of patients (2)[A].

Second Line

- Clopidogrel (75 mg/d) is approved by the FDA for the secondary prevention of thrombotic events in patients with symptomatic lower-extremity PAD (3)[A], and is recommended as an alternative to aspirin (1)[A].
- Neither vasodilators nor anticoagulant therapy (e.g., heparin, low-molecular-weight heparin, or oral anticoagulant) has shown any clinically proven efficacy for the treatment of claudication (2)[B] and may be harmful.
- Other medications that may improve claudication include pentoxifylline (1.2 g/d), cilostazol (100 mg b.i.d.), naftidrofuryl (600 mg/d), and prostaglandins (120 μg/d).

ADDITIONAL TREATMENT

- Weight reduction, smoking cessation, and BP control are essential in treating claudication.
- A walking program should include at least 3 times per week for 30–60 minutes each time and has been shown to improve quality of life as much as or more so than medication (see below).
- A healthy diet high in complex carbohydrates (such as whole grains and pastas), fruits, and vegetables and low in salt and animal fats

General Measures

- Claudication exercise rehabilitation program: Patient to walk until symptoms develop, then rest and start again, for a total of 30 minutes initially; walking then is increased by 5 minutes until 50 minutes of intermittent walking is achieved.
- Modification of risk factors including smoking, diabetes mellitus, hypertension, and hyperlipidemia:
  - Weight loss is associated with a decrease in the risk of cardiovascular disease but has not been shown to improve PAD (2)[C].
  - Antiplatelet therapy (aspirin) is recommended for patients with PAD when there is no other contraindication; however, neither the addition of an anticoagulant nor anticoagulant therapy alone has demonstrated superior outcome in PAD patients (4)[A].
  - Simvastatin (20–40 mg/d) has been shown to reduce the incidence of new intermittent claudication from 3.6–2.3% in patients with CAD (3)[A].
  - No statistical significance for overall improvement of exercise performance or claudication symptoms for patients on Niacin ER/lovastatin combined therapy.
  - β-adrenergic antagonists should be used with caution in individuals with severe PAD (2)[B].
  - Smoking cessation is likely to reduce the severity of claudication (2)[C].

COMPLEMENTARY AND ALTERNATIVE MEDICINE

- Acupuncture, biofeedback, chelation therapy, and supplements such as *Ginkgo biloba,* omega-3 fatty acids, and vitamin E have been studied.
- *G. biloba* modestly improves the symptoms of intermittent claudication (120 mg/d for up to 6 months) and can be considered as an adjunct to exercise therapy. Inconclusive evidence exists for the use of vitamin E.

SURGERY/OTHER PROCEDURES

Surgical interventions, such as revascularization, are warranted for individuals who have debilitating intermittent claudication, ischemic rest pain, or tissue loss:

- Transluminal balloon angioplasty is a percutaneous method of dilating arterial stenoses or recanalizing occluded vessels with or without stents (reserved for short, isolated, and hemodynamically significant lesions of the iliac or proximal superficial femoral artery).
- Bypass surgery is the standard operative treatment for lower extremity peripheral occlusive disease.

ONGOING CARE

FOLLOW-UP RECOMMENDATIONS

- An exercise training program comprising walking or bicycle riding improves maximal treadmill walking distance and, therefore, enhances functional capacity (3)[A].
- However, there is little added benefit from *G. biloba* treatment when added to supervised exercise training in patients with peripheral arterial disease as compared with patients in exercise training program alone (5)[C].

DIET

A low-fat cardiac diet is recommended.

PROGNOSIS

- Among patients with intermittent claudication, 15–20% will experience worsening claudication, 5–10% will undergo lower extremity bypass surgery, and 2–5% will need primary amputation. (Rates for smokers and diabetics are much higher.)
- 30,000–50,000 people in the US undergo amputations annually because of PAD.

REFERENCES

1. Rooke TW, Hirsch AT, et al. 2011 ACC/ACCF Focused Update of the Guideline for the Management of Patients with Peripheral Arterial Disease (Updating the 2005 Guideline). *J Am Coll Cardiol*. 2011;58:2020–45.
2. Hankey GJ, Norman PE, Eikelboom JW. Medical treatment of peripheral arterial disease. *JAMA*. 2006;295:547–53.
3. Gey DC, Lesho EP, Manngold J. Management of peripheral arterial disease. *Am Fam Physician*. 2004;69:525–32.
4. Duprez DA. Pharmacological interventions for peripheral artery disease. *Expert Opin Pharmacother*. 2007;8:1465–77.
5. Wang J, Zhou S, Bronks R, et al. Supervised exercise training combined with ginkgo biloba treatment for patients with peripheral arterial disease. *Clin Rehabil*. 2007;21:579–86.

ADDITIONAL READING

Hiatt WR, Hirsch AT, Creager MA, et al. Effect of niacin ER/lovastatin on claudication symptoms in patients with peripheral artery disease. *Vasc Med*. 2010;15(3):171–9.

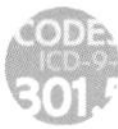

CODES

ICD9

- 440.20 Atherosclerosis of native arteries of the extremities, unspecified
- 443.9 Peripheral vascular disease, unspecified

CLINICAL PEARLS

- Screening of a general medical population for PAD is not recommended. Studies have indicated that screening for PAD among asymptomatic adults in the general population could lead to false-positive results and unnecessary workups. The prevalence among the general public who are asymptomatic is low.
- A patient already receiving medical treatment should be referred for further surgical evaluation for any of the following scenarios:
  - Unsatisfactory results despite medical therapy
  - No definitive diagnosis can be made
  - Critical limb ischemia is present, such as rest pain, gangrene, or ulceration
- In the clopidogrel (75 mg/d) vs. aspirin (325 mg/d) study in the Patients at Risk of Ischemic Events (CAPRIE) trial, there was a 23.8% relative risk ratio for MI, stroke, or cardiovascular death in PAD patients treated with clopidogrel compared with aspirin but no statistically significant difference in overall mortality reduction. Clopidogrel is much more expensive than aspirin.

PERITONITIS, ACUTE

Brenna Brucker, MSIV
Daithi S. Heffernan, MD

BASICS

DESCRIPTION

- Acute inflammation of the visceral and parietal peritoneum.
- Types:
  - Spontaneous (primary) bacterial peritonitis (SBP): Spontaneous infection of initially sterile ascitic fluid without detectable infectious source; associated with pre-existing ascites. The most common bacterial infection in cirrhosis, defined as a positive bacterial finding in ascites with increased PMN in ascites >250 cells/mm^3; typically monomicrobial.
  - Secondary bacterial peritonitis (2BP): Infection of peritoneal fluid from visceral inflammation, necrosis, or perforation, leading to a detectable abdominal infection. PMN in ascites >250 cells/mm^{3}or WBCs ≥500 cells/mm^3. Usually will have more than 2 of the following: Total ascites protein >1 g/dL, glucose concentration <50 mg/dL, elevated lactate dehydrogenase ≥225 units/L (1); typically polymicrobial.
  - Tertiary bacterial peritonitis (3BP): "Recurrent peritonitis"; infection or inflammation remains despite adequate treatment; can be due to failure of source control or patient immune response inadequacies.
  - These divisions derive from etiology. Treatment for and prognosis of each form of peritonitis are largely distinct from each other.

EPIDEMIOLOGY

Incidence

- SBP: 10–30% of patients with cirrhosis and ascites develop. 30% mortality due to multiorgan failure within days to weeks.
- 2BP: Directly related to the incidence of the underlying pathology, such as appendicitis, diverticulitis, colitis, or perforated peptic ulcer disease. <10% of inflamed visceral organs (e.g., appendicitis, diverticulitis).

Prevalence

- SBP and 2BP: Usually equates to incidence because incident cases typically necessitate rapid resolution or result in early death. 4.5% of all episodes of peritonitis in patients with cirrhosis and concomitant ascites will be from 2BP and not SBP (2).
- 3BP: 5–40% of 2BP, with rates increasing in direct proportion to the degree of illness upon presentation of the initial episode of 2BP. APACHE II scores upon initial presentation most directly correlate to 3BP risk.

RISK FACTORS

- SBP: Cirrhosis with large volume ascites (low volume rarely gives rise to SBP) (3), ascitic fluid total protein >1 g/dL, elevated bilirubin, prior SBP, malnutrition, high Model for End Stage Liver Disease (MELD) score, upper GI bleed
- 2BP: Relates to the underlying disease process, such as *H. pylori* infection and perforated peptic ulcer disease, diet/constipation and diverticulitis, underlying vascular disease, and intestinal ischemia
- 3BP: Malnutrition, APACHE II score >15 on presentation of 2BP, perioperative shock, and/or massive transfusion, organ system failure, and presence of antibiotic-resistant organisms

GENERAL PREVENTION

- SBP: Prophylactic antibiotics are indicated in cirrhotic patients with acute GI hemorrhage, given that 22% of cirrhotics with GI bleed have a risk of SBP. The role of long-term prophylactic antibiotics in cirrhotics remains very controversial; however, they may have a role in patients with ascitic fluid total protein levels <1 g/dL.
- 3BP: Open abdomen and scheduled abdominal washout within 48 hours following initial presentation of 2BP, especially in patients with an APACHE II score >15. For patients with foregut perforations, add antifungal therapy to the postoperative antimicrobial regime.

PATHOPHYSIOLOGY

- SBP: Key mechanism is bacterial translocation with ascitic fluid as a supportive growth medium. There is high incidence in cirrhotics due to their reduced humoral and local immunity (thus allowing bacteria and endotoxins to easily enter mesenteric lymph nodes). Portal hypertension also allows bacteria to bypass the liver's reticuloendothelial system.
- 2BP: Occurs due to inflamed, necrotic, or perforated intraperitoneal hollow viscus or because of traumatic injury of the intestinal tract, leading to spillage or translocation of the intestinal contents, thereby contaminating the peritoneal cavity with bacteria.
- 3BP: Most commonly, persistence of 2BP due to poor source control or multidrug-resistant organisms rather than a true recurrence of initial infection.

ETIOLOGY

- SBP: Related to ascites most commonly from cirrhosis, but also may be cardiac, nephritic, or malignant in origin. Organisms: *E. coli* (40)%, *Streptococcus* spp. (15%) Klebsiella (7%), *Pseudomonas* spp. (5%), *Proteus* spp. (5%). Gram-positive cocci most commonly are involved in nosocomial infection.
- 2BP: Related to bowel perforation, appendicitis, diverticulitis, acute cholecystitis, colitis (infectious or inflammatory), peptic ulcer perforation, ischemic bowel, pelvic inflammatory disease, iatrogenic causes (endoscopy, anastomotic dehiscence, mechanical or thermal bowel injury), or direct abdominal trauma. Organisms: *E. coli*, *Klebsiella*, *Proteus*, *Streptococcus*, *Enterococcus*, *Bacteroides*, *Clostridium* spp.
- 3BP: Often related to causative organism from 2BP: *Enterobacter*, *Pseudomonas*, *Enterococcus*, *Staphylococcus*, *Candida* spp.

DIAGNOSIS

HISTORY

- SBP: History of liver disease, recent GI bleed
- 2BP: Acute onset of abdominal pain, nausea, vomiting, anorexia, altered mental status

PHYSICAL EXAM

- Abdomen that does not move with respiration, abdominal distention, abdominal wall guarding and rigidity, rebound tenderness, hypoactive or absent bowel sound
- Tachycardia, fever >37.8°C (100°F), tachypnea; patients who are very young or very old may present with minimal physical examination findings
- 40% of 3BP can be diagnosed by history and physical alone and do not need imaging.

DIAGNOSTIC TESTS & INTERPRETATION

Lab

Initial lab tests

- CBC with differential: Leukocytosis >12 or leukopenia <4 (WBCs may migrate to peritoneum, causing peripheral leukopenia)
- SBP: Paracentesis to obtain ascitic fluid for analysis (4); cell count with differential, culture (only obtains organisms in 70% of cases), gram-stain, total protein, LDH, glucose, amylase, albumin. Ideally, complete ascitic fluid analysis before empiric antibiotics; a single dose of antibiotics prevents bacterial culture growth in 86% of cases (5)
- 2BP: Ascitic fluid analysis: PMN >250 cells/mm^3 or WBC count >500 cells/mm^3. Typically will have more than 2 of the following: Total ascites protein >1 g/dL, glucose concentration <50 mg/dL, elevated lactate dehydrogenase >225 units/L.

Follow-Up & Special Considerations

If no clinical improvement in 48–72 hours, repeat paracentesis to monitor treatment success (decrease in neutrophil count <50% original value and negative cultures).

Imaging

Initial approach

- Supine/upright abdominal films and chest x-ray: Free air in peritoneal cavity, large/small bowel dilatation, intestinal wall edema
- Sonograph or CT scan with enteral and IV contrast material: Intra-abdominal mass, ascites, abscess, extravasation of water-soluble gut contrast material
- For 3BP: Yield of CT is very low in the first 7 days following operative intervention for 2BP due to the inability to distinguish postoperative fluid from intra-abdominal abscess

DIFFERENTIAL DIAGNOSIS

- Alcoholic hepatitis: Fever, leukocytosis, and abdominal pain mimic SBP; fever from alcoholic has normal ascitic fluid PMN count, unlike the ascite fluid in SBP (3)
- Abscess formation (peritoneal, pelvic, subhepatic, subdiaphragmatic), ileus (volvulus, intussusception), mesenteric adenitis, pancreatitis, cholecystitis
- Ruptured ectopic pregnancy, tubo-ovarian abscess, pelvic inflammatory disease, severe UTI and/or pyelonephritis, pneumonia, myocardial infarction, porphyria

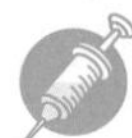

TREATMENT

MEDICATION

- SBP: No one antibiotic proven to be more efficacious than others:
  - Cefotaxime 2 g IV q8h × 5–14 days; excellent penetration into ascites
  - Ceftriaxone 1 g q24h × 5–14 days
  - Ampicillin-sulbactam 3 g IV q6h × 5–14 days
  - Quinolones (e.g., norfloxacin, ofloxacin, ciprofloxacin) for 7 days

- 2BP:
  - Source control is central to management, predominately with operative intervention, laparotomy with resection of the perforated viscus
  - If APACHE II score >15: Consider open abdomen with second look laparotomy at 24–48 hours. Need both aerobic and anaerobic coverage. Majority of cases can be managed with single-agent antimicrobial, most commonly piperacillin-tazobactam 3.375 g q8h for 7 days. Alternative agents include ampicillin-sulbactam, ticarcillin-clavulanate, or imipenem. Consider an antifungal agent such as fluconazole in cases of upper intestinal perforation.
- 3BP: Repeat source control; drug choice should be based on original culture data coupled with potential administration of an antimicrobial agent to which the patient has not previously been exposed.

ADDITIONAL TREATMENT

General Measures

- SBP: General measures to control the effects of the cirrhosis, such as lactulose for encephalopathy, aldosterone, and beta-blockers.
- 2BP: If peptic ulcer perforation, test for and treat possible underlying *H. pylori* and rule out malignancy. Diverticulitis requires diet modification education.
- 3BP: Consider potential underlying immunocompromised states.

SURGERY/OTHER PROCEDURES

- SBP: Rarely indicated, but remember that potentially 5% of cirrhotics have 2BP that would need operative intervention.
- 2BP: Emergent operative intervention remains the cornerstone of treatment: Peptic ulcer perforation—managed with omental patch; perforated small intestine—resection, often with primary anastomosis; perforated appendix—appendicectomy; perforated colon—colectomy with ostomy formation. A primary anastomosis in patients who present with peritonitis from perforated colon often leaks, leading to prolonged sepsis and severe 3BP. Patients with septic shock, acidosis, and/or severe illness as denoted by an APACHE II score >15 benefit from an open abdomen with planned return to the operating room for further washout within 48 hours.
- 3BP: Laparotomy, washout, and resection of any source such as missed or iatrogenic enterotomy

IN-PATIENT CONSIDERATIONS

Initial Stabilization

- Initial stabilization: Patients who present with peritonitis are severely hypovolemic. IV fluid resuscitation is critical to diminish the risk of secondary organ dysfunction. Large-bore IV access should be obtained rapidly upon presentation. Nasogastric tube placement will prevent aspiration in patients with nausea and/or vomiting.
- SBP: Fluid choice can be difficult because each has its complications. Normal saline can worsen ascites, lactated Ringer solution often is mal-metabolized, and the carrying agent for albumin has a large salt load.
- 2BP: Electrolyte deficits need to be accounted for and corrected using either lactated Ringer solution or normal saline. Large-volume resuscitation often is indicated, titrating to improving tachycardia, hypotension, and adequate urine output.
- Failure to respond to large-volume resuscitation necessitates consideration of vasoactive agents such as norepinephrine and vasopressin, or consideration of sepsis-induced adrenal insufficiency.
- In patients with septic shock and/or complex cardiopulmonary comorbidities, invasive monitoring may be required, with early goal-directed fluid therapy.

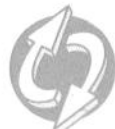

ONGOING CARE

FOLLOW-UP RECOMMENDATIONS

Patient Monitoring

Patients should be admitted to a close observation unit such as an ICU, as the patient will often require invasive BP monitoring such as an arterial line. Hourly monitoring of vital signs and urinary output will aid in judging patient response to treatment:

- Improvement is considered as a normalization of vital signs with resolution of leukocytosis.
- Development of leukopenia is a very concerning finding for immune exhaustion and is associated with a poor prognosis.
- SBP: If no clinical improvement in 48–72 hours, consider repeat paracentesis to follow treatment success (decrease in ascitic PMN count <50% of original value and negative cultures)
- 2BP: Need close patient follow-up for compliance with antiulcer medications and diet modification

DIET

- NPO; total parental nutrition may be necessary.
- After return of bowel function, may resume enteral feeding.

PROGNOSIS

General poor prognostic factors for SBP, 2BP, and 3BP include older age, high Child-Pugh-Turcotte score, high MELD score, malnutrition, malignancy, and peripheral leucopenia at presentation.

- SBP: Mortality rate is 10–30%, with highest rates in patients presenting with both SBP and GI bleed concomitantly. Recurrence in 6 months: 43%. Recurrence in 1 year- 69%, with mortality of ~50%. Renal insufficiency is the strongest prognostic factor for mortality because SBP leads to reduced effective circulating volume. Hospital-associated SBP has an overall 30-day mortality rate of nearly 58% (antibiotic-resistant bacterial strains) (6).
- 2BP: Mortality often is heavily related to the underlying 2BP etiology, with appendicitis linked with the lowest risk and perforated gastric or colon malignancy associated with the highest inhospital mortality. Overall uncomplicated 2BP <5% mortality. Complicated 2BP 30–50% mortality.
- 3BP: Prognosis varies widely depending on initial 2BP and the resultant patient immune dysfunction that led to the 3BP. Associated with prolonged hospitalization and NPO status requiring long-term TPN.

COMPLICATIONS

- Encephalopathy from worsening liver failure
- Respiratory failure, ARDS, secondary infection such as pneumonia
- Sepsis/septic shock, adrenal insufficiency, cardiovascular collapse
- Renal failure, liver failure, coagulopathy
- Abscess, abdominal compartment syndrome, failure to close the open abdomen, fistula formation

REFERENCES

1. Alaniz C, Regal RE, et al. Spontaneous bacterial peritonitis: A review of treatment options. *P T*. 2009;34:204–210.
2. Soriano G, Castellote J, Alvarez C, et al. Secondary bacterial peritonitis in cirrhosis: A retrospective study of clinical and analytical characteristics, diagnosis and management. *J Hepatol* 2010; 52:7–9.
3. Koulaouzidis A, Bhat S, et al. Spontaneous bacterial peritonitis. *Postgrad Med J*. 2007;83: 379–83.
4. Sheer TA, Runyon BA. Spontaneous bacterial peritonitis. *Dig Dis*. 2005;23:39–46.
5. Jain P, et al. Spontaneous bacterial peritonitis: Few additional points. *World J Gastroenterol*. 2009; 15(45):5754–5.
6. Cheong HS, Kang CI, Lee JA, et al. Clinical significance and outcome of nosocomial acquisition of spontaneous bacterial peritonitis in patients with liver cirrhosis. *Clin Infect Dis*. 2009;48:1230–6.

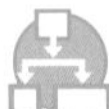

See Also (Topic, Algorithm, Electronic Media Element)

Appendicitis, Acute; Cirrhosis of the Liver; Diverticular Disease

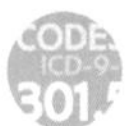

CODES

ICD9

- 567.9 Unspecified peritonitis
- 567.21 Peritonitis (acute) generalized
- 567.23 Spontaneous bacterial peritonitis

CLINICAL PEARLS

- SBP: Always maintain a high index of suspicion in a cirrhotic patient with ascites. SPB occurs in pre-existing ascites, it does not cause ascites. SBP carries a high mortality, especially if associated with a presenting GI bleed.
- SBP: Paracentesis is necessary to establish the diagnosis. One cannot make a clinical diagnosis of SBP.
- Distinguishing SBP from 2BP is vital. SBP generally requires only antibiotics and operating unnecessarily on SBP leads to very high mortality. 2BP often requires surgery, and giving the patient antibiotics alone often leads to high mortality.
- 2BP: Source control (usually operatively) and aggressive IV fluid resuscitation are critical.
- 2BP: For perforated viscus, always consider malignancy as an underlying cause of the perforation.
- 3BP: Consider poor source control, missed or iatrogenic enterotomy, and underlying immune dysfunction.

PERITONSILLAR ABSCESS

Matthew R. Leibowitz, MD

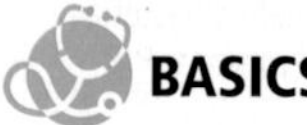

BASICS

DESCRIPTION

- Peritonsillar abscess results in infection with abscess formation and collection of pus in the space between the anterior and posterior tonsillar pillars and the superior pharyngeal constrictor muscle:
  - Usually follows an episode of acute pharyngitis or tonsillitis
- System(s) affected: Gastrointestinal; Pulmonary
- Synonym(s): Quinsy

EPIDEMIOLOGY

Incidence

- In the US, estimated 45,000 new cases yearly (30/100,000 person-years)
- Predominant age: All age groups, with greatest incidence in adolescents and young adults. 15–30 years of age
- Predominant sex: Male = Female

RISK FACTORS

- Prior episodes of tonsillitis
- Age (young more susceptible)

ETIOLOGY

- Polymicrobial infection is the rule in peritonsillar abscess, and multiple bacteria likely will be grown from cultures of drained pus. *Streptococcus* sp. are the most common pathogens.
- Aerobic bacteria:
  - *Streptococcus pyogenes* (group A *Streptococcus*)
  - *S. milleri* group
  - *Haemophilus influenzae*
  - *S. viridans*
  - *Neisseria* sp.
  - *Staphylococcus aureus*
- Anaerobic bacteria:
  - *Fusobacterium*
  - *Peptostreptococcus*
  - *Porphyromonas*
  - *Prevotella*
  - *Bacteroides*

COMMONLY ASSOCIATED CONDITIONS

- Pharyngitis
- Tonsillitis
- Peritonsillar cellulitis
- Retropharyngeal abscess
- Lateral space abscess
- Septic jugular vein thrombophlebitis (Lemierre syndrome)

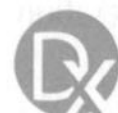

DIAGNOSIS

HISTORY

- Extreme sore throat or neck pain
- Odynophagia
- Dysphagia

PHYSICAL EXAM

- Fever >38°C
- Trismus
- "Hot potato voice" (thickened, muffled voice)
- Drooling and pooling of saliva in the mouth
- Tonsillar exudates seen uncommonly
- Erythematous, edematous tonsil
- Asymmetry of the oropharynx with inferior and medial displacement of the infected tonsil, often with contralateral deviation of the uvula
- Cervical adenopathy

DIAGNOSTIC TESTS & INTERPRETATION

Diagnosis is made based on history and limited exam; testing/imaging is needed only if the diagnosis is unclear and patient is stable.

Lab

- Leukocytosis
- Culture of pathogens from aspirated or drained pus to identify organism(s)

Imaging

- Intraoral ultrasonography often will show a discrete abscess cavity if present.
- CT scan, best performed with contrast material, also will show a discrete abscess cavity if present. Edema of the surrounding tissues also can be seen on CT scan.

Diagnostic Procedures/Surgery

Incision and drainage of pus via needle aspiration or an operative procedure under general anesthesia or conscious sedation

DIFFERENTIAL DIAGNOSIS

- Peritonsillar cellulitis
- Tonsillar abscess
- Retropharyngeal abscess
- Lateral space abscess
- Infectious mononucleosis (Epstein-Barr virus infection)
- Aspiration of foreign body
- Dental infection
- Salivary gland infection
- Cervical adenitis
- Mastoiditis
- Internal carotid artery aneurysm

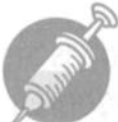

TREATMENT

Drainage of the abscess, antibiotics, and pain control are the most important aspects of treatment.

MEDICATION

First Line

- Penicillin remains the standard antimicrobial therapy, with initial therapy delivered parenterally, although some now consider clindamycin to be first line. Tailor therapy to cultured pathogens as much as possible. If organisms other than oral streptococci are suspected, expanded therapy may be indicated. With growing concern for β-lactamase-producing organisms, antibiotics with β-lactamase inhibitors or cephalosporins may be preferred. If *Fusobacterium* or *Bacteroides* are implicated, then additional anaerobic therapy with metronidazole may be indicated with increasing resistance to penicillin among these pathogens (1)[C]:
  - Penicillin G 1–4 million units IV q4h *or*
  - Benzathine penicillin G 1.2 million units IM 1 time *or*
  - Benzathine penicillin G 900,000 units and procaine penicillin G 300,000 units IM 1 time, followed by
  - Penicillin V 500 mg (25–50 mg/kg for children) PO t.i.d. to complete 10–14 days of total therapy
- For penicillin-allergic patients:
  - Erythromycin ethyl succinate 300–400 mg PO t.i.d. *or*
  - Cephalexin 250–500 mg PO t.i.d.
- If resistant organisms (including oral anaerobes) are suspected, add to the above oral therapy:
  - Metronidazole 500 mg PO t.i.d.–q.i.d. *or*
  - Clindamycin 150–450 mg PO t.i.d.–q.i.d. Some consider clindamycin alone to be first-line therapy.
- Alternatively:
  - Ampicillin-sulbactam (Unasyn) 3 g IV q6h *or*
  - Ticarcillin-clavulanate (Ticar) 3–4 g IV q4–6h *or*
  - Amoxicillin-clavulanate (Augmentin) 500 mg PO t.i.d. or 875 mg PO b.i.d. *or*
  - Cefuroxime 500 mg PO b.i.d. (or another second- or third-generation cephalosporin) and metronidazole 500 mg PO t.i.d.–q.i.d.

Second Line

The role of adjunctive corticosteroids in the treatment of peritonsillar abscess is controversial. A recent small randomized study suggests that a single high dose of methylprednisolone (2–3 mg/kg up to 250 mg) administered after needle drainage and before antimicrobial therapy may improve a patient's ability to open the mouth and drink water earlier, speed resolution of fever, and decrease length of hospital stay (2)[C].

ADDITIONAL TREATMENT

General Measures

- Same-day surgery is possible in some cases with outpatient management.
- IV rehydration
- Pain control

Issues for Referral

Follow up with ENT surgeon, especially if symptoms recur or do not improve.

SURGERY/OTHER PROCEDURES

- Small studies indicate that rates of success are equivalent between needle aspiration and operative incision and drainage:
  - Needle aspiration with intraoral ultrasound or CT guidance
  - Operative incision and drainage when needle aspiration is too difficult due to trismus or lack of patient cooperation
- Immediate tonsillectomy at the time of incision and drainage (known as *quinsy tonsillectomy*) has decreased in favor due to increased risk of hemorrhage and overall low rates of abscess recurrence without tonsillectomy.
- Delayed tonsillectomy (known as *interval tonsillectomy*) is also performed less commonly due to the low rates of recurrent abscess (1)[C].

IN-PATIENT CONSIDERATIONS

Admission Criteria

- Inability to swallow
- Trismus
- Need for parenteral analgesia
- Planned operative incision and drainage

IV Fluids

May be required if oral intake of fluids not possible

Discharge Criteria

- Ability to swallow
- Able to take oral antimicrobial therapy
- Oral analgesia effective

ONGOING CARE

FOLLOW-UP RECOMMENDATIONS

Patient Monitoring

- Follow up within 48 hours to ensure resolution of symptoms and tonsillar inflammation.
- Lack of improvement may indicate antibiotic-resistant pathogens or residual abscess necessitating repeat drainage.

DIET

No restrictions following decompressing abscess; liquid diet may be tolerated best until pain improves.

PATIENT EDUCATION

Important to complete course of antibiotics

PROGNOSIS

- Symptoms will improve rapidly after incision and drainage and appropriate antibiotics.
- Pain and inflammation may persist for up to a week after treatment.
- Recurrent peritonsillar abscess does occur but is rare.

COMPLICATIONS

- Airway obstruction
- Spread to parapharyngeal (lateral) or retropharyngeal spaces
- Septic jugular vein thrombosis
- Brain abscess
- Sepsis
- Possible complications of incision and drainage:
  - Pulmonary aspiration of blood and pus with bronchopneumonia
  - Tonsillar hemorrhage
  - Perforation of the carotid artery

REFERENCES

1. Schraff S, McGinn JD, Derkay CS. Peritonsillar abscess in children: A 10-year review of diagnosis and management. *Int J Pediatr Otorhinolaryngol*. 2001;57:213–8.
2. Ozbek C, Aygenc E, Tuna EU, et al. Use of steroids in the treatment of peritonsillar abscess. *J Laryngol Otol*. 2004;118:439–42.

ADDITIONAL READING

- National Guideline Clearinghouse. Sore throat and tonsillitis. Available at: www.guideline.gov/content.aspx?id=11045. Accessed February 14, 2012.
- Galioto NJ. Peritonsillar abscess. *Am Fam Physician*. 2008;77(2):199–202.
- Herzon FS, Martin AD, et al. Medical and surgical treatment of peritonsillar, retropharyngeal, and parapharyngeal abscesses. *Curr Infect Dis Rep*. 2006;8:196–202.

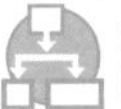

See Also (Topic, Algorithm, Electronic Media Element)

Epiglottitis; Pharyngitis

CODES

ICD9

475 Peritonsillar abscess

CLINICAL PEARLS

- Needle drainage is likely to be as effective as operative drainage.
- Penicillin remains the drug of choice for most cases.

PERSONALITY DISORDERS

Moshe S. Torem, MD, DLFAPA

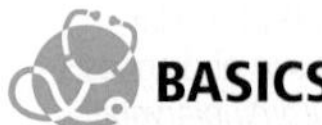

BASICS

DESCRIPTION

- Personality disorders (PDs) are a group of conditions, with onset at or before adolescence, characterized by enduring patterns of maladaptive and dysfunctional behavior that deviates markedly from one's culture and social environment, leading to functional impairment and distress to the individual, coworkers, and family:
  - These behaviors are perceived by patients to be "normal" and "right," and they have little insight as to their ownership, responsibility, and abnormal nature of these behaviors.
  - These conditions are classified based on the predominant symptoms and their severity.
- System(s) affected: Nervous/Psychiatric
- Synonym(s): Character disorder; Character pathology (1)

Geriatric Considerations

Coping with the stresses of aging is challenging.

Pediatric Considerations

A history of childhood neglect, abuse, and trauma is not uncommon.

Pregnancy Considerations

Pregnancy adds pressure in coping with the activities of daily living (ADLs).

EPIDEMIOLOGY

Prevalence

- General population: 1–5%
- Outpatient psychiatric clinic: 3–30%
- In the US: 12%
- In male prisoners, the prevalence of antisocial personality disorder is ~60%.
- Predominant age: Starts in adolescence and early 20s and persists throughout patient's life
- Predominant sex: Male = Female; some personality disorders are more common in females, and others are more common in males.

RISK FACTORS

- Positive family history
- Pregnancy risk factors:
  - Nutritional deprivation
  - Use of alcohol or drugs
  - Viral and bacterial infections
- Dysfunctional family with child abuse/neglect

Genetics

Major character traits are inherited; others result from a combination of genetics and environment.

PATHOPHYSIOLOGY

- Criteria for a PD includes an enduring pattern of:
  - Inner experience and behavior that deviate markedly from the expectations of one's culture in ≥2 of the following areas: Cognition, affectivity, interpersonal functioning, or impulse control
  - Inflexibility and pervasiveness across a broad range of personal and social situations
  - Significant distress or impairment in social or occupational functioning
- PDs are classified into 3 major clusters:
  - Cluster A: Eccentricism and oddness:
    - *Paranoid PD*: Unwarranted suspiciousness and distrust of others, defensive, guarded, and overly sensitive
    - *Schizoid PD*: Emotional, cold, or detached; apathetic to criticism or praise; socially isolated
    - *Schizotypal PD*: Eccentric behavior, odd belief system/perceptions, social isolation, and general suspiciousness
  - Cluster B: Dramatic, emotional, or erratic behavioral patterns:
    - *Antisocial PD*: Aggressive, impulsive, irritable, irresponsible, dishonest, deceitful
    - *Borderline PD:* Unstable interpersonal relationships, high impulsivity from early adulthood, intense fear of abandonment, mood swings, poor self-esteem, chronic boredom, and feelings of inner emptiness
    - *Histrionic PD:* Needs to be the center of attention, with self-dramatizing behaviors and attention seeking in a variety of contexts
    - *Narcissistic PD*: Grandiose sense of self-importance and preoccupation with fantasies of success, power, brilliance, beauty, or ideal love; lack of empathy for other people's pain or discomfort
  - Cluster C: Anxiety, excessive worry, fear, and unhealthy patterns of coping with emotions:
    - Avoidant PD: Social inhibition, feelings of inadequacy, hypersensitivity to negative evaluation, avoidance of occupational and interpersonal activities that involve the risk of criticism by others, views self as socially inept and personally unappealing or inferior to others
    - Dependent PD: Excessive need to be taken care of, leading to submissive and clinging behavior with fears of separation, avoids expressing disagreements with others due to fear of losing support and approval, usually seeks out strong and confident people as friends or spouses and feels more secure in such relationships
    - Obsessive–compulsive PD: Preoccupation with cleanliness, orderliness, perfectionism; preoccupation with excessive details, rules, lists, order, organization, and schedules to the extent that the major point of the activity is lost
    - PD not otherwise specified: A mixture of characteristics from other PDs without a predominant pattern compatible with preceding categories; it also can be used for specific PDs not mentioned in the American Psychological Association classification (*DSM-IV-TR)* such as depressive PD, passive-aggressive PD, masochistic PD, dangerous and severe PD (2), etc.

ETIOLOGY

Environmental and genetic factors (3)

COMMONLY ASSOCIATED CONDITIONS

Depression, other psychiatric disorders in patient and family members

DIAGNOSIS

HISTORY

- Comprehensive interview and mental status examination
- Screen to rule out alcohol and drug abuse.
- Interview of relatives and friends helpful in establishing an enduring pattern of behavior

DIAGNOSTIC TESTS & INTERPRETATION

Psychological testing (e.g., MMPI-II)

Lab

Initial lab tests

- CBC
- Comprehensive metabolic panel
- Thyroid-stimulating hormone
- HIV
- Toxicology screen for substance abuse
- ECG to rule out a chronic seizure disorder

Imaging

Initial approach

CT and MRI of the brain may be necessary in newly developed symptoms to rule out organic brain disease (e.g., frontal lobe tumor).

DIFFERENTIAL DIAGNOSIS

- Medical disorders with behavioral changes
- Other psychiatric disorders with similar symptoms:
  - In obsessive–compulsive disorder (OCD), symptoms are egodystonic (i.e., perceived as foreign and unwanted). In addition, OCD has a pattern of relapse and partial remission.
  - In obsessive–compulsive personality disorder (OCPD), symptoms are perceived as desirable behaviors (egosyntonic) that the patient feels proud of and wants others to emulate. In addition, OCPD has a lifelong pattern (i.e., without significant relapse or remission).

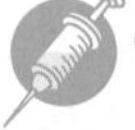

TREATMENT

Psychotherapy with family involvement is the foundation of treatment. No specific drugs are indicated to treat PDs; some medications can reduce the intensity, frequency, and dysfunctionality of certain behaviors (4).

MEDICATION

Medications are effective in the treatment of comorbid conditions such as anxiety and depression.

First Line

- Symptom management (5):
  - Minipsychosis (associated with paranoid, schizoid, borderline, and schizotypal PDs): Atypical antipsychotics: Risperidone (Risperdal), quetiapine (Seroquel), olanzapine (Zyprexa), ziprasidone (Geodon), aripiprazole (Abilify), asenapine (Saphris); start with a low dose, gradually adjusting to the patient's needs
  - Anxiety: Anxiolytics (benzodiazepines, buspirone [BuSpar], and serotonin reuptake inhibitors)
  - Depressed mood: Antidepressants
  - Many patients with borderline PD respond well to small doses of atypical neuroleptics and mood stabilizers (8)[A].

- Precautions: Some atypical neuroleptic drugs may be associated with hyperglycemia and insulin-resistant metabolic syndrome.

Second Line

Mood stabilizers: Lithium carbonate, lamotrigine (Lamictal), carbamazepine (Tegretol, Equetro), and valproate (Depacon, Depakene, Depakote) (6)

ADDITIONAL TREATMENT

General Measures

- Long-term psychotherapy and cognitive-behavioral therapy (7)
- Group therapy is helpful in the use of therapeutic confrontation and increasing one's awareness of and insight regarding the damaging effects of dysfunctional behavior patterns.

Issues for Referral

- When psychiatric comorbidity of Axis I disorders is present (e.g., mood disorders, anxiety disorders, substance abuse, etc.)
- Suicidal ideation or attempts

Additional Therapies

- Dialectical behavior therapy
- Psychoanalytic therapy
- Interactive psychotherapy
- Group therapy

IN-PATIENT CONSIDERATIONS

Admission Criteria

Disorders with complications of suicide attempts

ONGOING CARE

FOLLOW-UP RECOMMENDATIONS

Continue outpatient treatment, potentially long term.

Patient Monitoring

- Regular physical exercise, e.g., 30–45 minutes a day, helps with stress and the ADLs.
- If substance abuse is suspected, check drug screens.
- Infrequent sessions with relatives or friends are helpful in monitoring behavioral progress.

DIET

Emphasize variety of healthy foods; avoid obesity.

PATIENT EDUCATION

- Bibliotherapy and writing therapy, specific assignments, and watching certain movies to better understand the nature and origin of one's specific condition are helpful:
  - Kreger R. *The Essential Family Guide to Borderline Personality Disorder*. Center City, MN: Hazelden; 2008.
  - Mason PT, Kreger R. *Stop Walking on Eggshells*. Oakland, CA: New Harbinger Publishers; 2010.
- The movie *As Good As It Gets* illustrates someone with obsessive–compulsive behaviors and its impact on ADLs and relationships with family and friends.
- The movie series *The Godfather* includes several characters with antisocial PD and shows how this affects their interpersonal relationships and their own physical and mental health.
- The movie *What About Bob?* illustrates the challenges involved in treating certain patients with a borderline PD, especially in the management of boundaries in the doctor–patient relationship.
- The movie *A Streetcar Named Desire* illustrates an example of a woman with a histrionic PD.
- The movie *Wall Street* illustrates an example of a person with a narcissistic PD.
- The movie *The Caine Mutiny* illustrates an example of a person with a paranoid PD.
- The movie *Four Weddings and a Funeral* illustrates an example of a person with an avoidant PD.

PROGNOSIS

PDs are enduring patterns of behavior throughout one's lifetime and are not easily responsive to treatment.

COMPLICATIONS

- Disruptive family life with frequent divorces and separations, alcoholism, substance abuse, and drug addiction
- Disruptive behaviors in the workplace may cause absenteeism and loss of productivity.
- Violation of the law and disregard for the concerns and rights of others

REFERENCES

1. American Psychiatric Association. *Diagnostic and Statistical Manual of Mental Disorders: Text Revision*. 4th ed. Washington, DC: American Psychiatric Press; 2000.
2. Ullrich S, et al. Dangerous and severe personality disorder: An investigation of the construct. *Int J Law Psychiatry*. 2010;33:84–8.
3. Reichborn-Kjennerud T. Genetics of personality disorders. *Clin Lab Med*. 2010;30:893–910.
4. Hadjipavlou G, et al. Promising psychotherapies for personality disorders. *Can J Psychiatry*. 2010;55: 202–10.
5. Howland RH. Pharmacotherapy in personality disorders. *Psychosoc Nurs Ment Health Serv*. 2007;45:15–9.
6. Díaz-Marsá M, González Bardanca S, Tajima K, et al. Psychopharmacological treatment in borderline personality disorder. *Actas Esp Psiquiatr*. 2008;36:39–49.
7. Morana HC, Câmara FP. International guidelines for the management of personality disorders. *Curr Opin Psychiatry*. 2006;19:539–43.
8. Lieb K, et al. Pharmacotherapy for borderline personality disorder: Cochrane systematic review of randomised trials. *Br J Psychiatry*; 2010;196:4–12.

ADDITIONAL READING

- Abbass A, Sheldon A, Gyra J, et al. Intensive short-term dynamic psychotherapy for DSM-IV personality disorders: A randomized controlled trial. *J Nerv Ment Dis*. 2008;196:211–6.
- Eizirik M, Fonagy P. Mentalization-based treatment for patients with borderline personality disorder: An overview. *Rev Bras Psiquiatr*. 2009;31:72–5.
- Feurino L 3rd, Silk KR. State of the art in pharmacologic treatment of borderline personality disorder. *Curr Psychiatry Rep*. 2011;13:69–75.
- Ingenhoven T, et al. Effectiveness of pharmacotherapy for severe personality disorders: Meta-analysies of randomized controlled trials. *J Clin Psychiatry*. 2010;71:14–25.
- Kendall T, et al. Borderline and antisocial personality disorders: Summary of NICE guidelines. *BMJ*. 2009;338:b93.
- Leichsenring F, et al. Borderline personality disorder. *Lancet*. 2011;377:74–84.
- Lynch TR, Cheavens JS. Dialectical behavior therapy for comorbid personality disorders. *J Clin Psychol*. 2008;64:154–67.
- Matusiewicz AK, et al. The effectiveness of cognitive behavioral therapy for personality disorders. *Psychiatr Clin North Am*. 2010;33:657–85.
- Mauchnik J, et al. The latest neuroimaging findings in borderline personality disorder. *Curr Psychiatry Rep*. 2010;12:46–55.
- Mellos E, et al. Comorbidity of personality disorders with alcohol abuse. *In Vivo*. 2010;24:761–9.
- Molina JD, et al. Borderline personality disorder: A review and reformulation from evolutionary theory. *Med Hypotheses*. 2009;73:382–6.
- Ronningstam E. Narcissistic personality disorder: A current review. *Curr Psychiatry Rep*; 2010;12:68–75.
- Russ E, et al. Refining the construct of narcissistic personality disorder: Diagnostic criteria and subtypes. *Am J Psychiatry*. 2008;165:1473–81.
- Stanley B, Siever LJ. The interpersonal dimension of borderline personality disorder: Toward a neuropeptide model. *Am J Psychiatry*. 2010;167: 24–39.
- Stoffers J, et al. Pharmacological interventions for borderline personality disorder. *Cochrane Database Syst Rev*. 2010;16:CD005653.

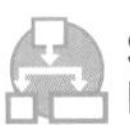

See Also (Topic, Algorithm, Electronic Media Element)

Obsessive–Compulsive Disorder

CODES

ICD9

- 301.0 Paranoid personality disorder
- 301.20 Schizoid personality disorder, unspecified
- 301.9 Unspecified personality disorder

CLINICAL PEARLS

- PDs are enduring patterns of behavior throughout one's lifetime and are not easily responsive to treatment.
- No specific drugs treat PDs; however, specific medications can reduce the intensity, frequency, and dysfunctionality of certain behaviors, thoughts, and feelings.
- Most patients with a PD require a well-trained and experienced mental health professional.
- A stable, trustful alliance with the patient is the foundation for any therapeutic progress.

PERTUSSIS

Mary Cataletto, MD

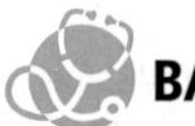

BASICS

Highly contagious bacterial infection

DESCRIPTION

- Exclusively human pathogen
- Seen worldwide
- Endemic in the US with epidemic cycles
- High secondary attack rate in households
- Transmission: Respiratory droplets
- Synonym(s): Whooping cough

EPIDEMIOLOGY

Incidence

- Estimated 48.5 million cases/year
- Case fatality rate up to 4% in low-income countries

Prevalence

- In 2004, more cases of pertussis occurred in adolescents and adults than in children.

RISK FACTORS

- Exposure to a confirmed case: Infects 80–90% of susceptible contacts
- Non- or underimmunized children
- Pregnancy
- Premature birth
- Age <4 months; these infants have the highest morbidity rate, complication rate, rate of hospitalization, and mortality rate.
- Smokers
- Patients with asthma
- Immunodeficiency (e.g., AIDS)

GENERAL PREVENTION

Immunization:

- Universal immunization with pertussis vaccine is recommended for children <7 years of age and those between 11 and 18 years of age and into adulthood (Tdap). See Red Book for immunization schedule and recommendations. average length of immunity ~10 years
- BOOSTRIX is licensed for use in persons aged 10–18 years; ADACEL, for persons 11–64 years.

Geriatric Considerations

Currently, there is no vaccine for those >64 years of age.

Pregnancy Considerations

- Recommendations for vaccination during pregnancy can be reviewed in a 2008 MMWR report: Tdap may be administered to a pregnant woman after an informed discussion. However, current practice is to administer Tdap to appropriate candidates in the immediate postpartum period.
- Early case reporting
- Early treatment with strong suspicion or confirmation: Quarantine (students and school staff members):
  - Keep out of school until they have completed 5 days of the recommended course of antibiotics.
  - Persons who do not receive antibiotic therapy should be excluded from school for 21 days after onset of symptoms.
- See Red Book for recommendations for childcare and hospital-based exposures and for older children and adults. Protection of contacts:
  - Chemoprophylaxis close contacts, including all household contacts and other close contacts such as young infants and pregnant women.
  - Observe all close contacts for symptoms for 21 days after exposure.
  - Evaluate symptomatic patients, and treat for pertussis when appropriate.
  - Initiate or continue scheduled immunization of all close unimmunized or underimmunized contacts <7 years of age.

PATHOPHYSIOLOGY

- Toxin-mediated
- Infectious process with predilection for ciliated respiratory epithelium

ETIOLOGY

- *Bordetella pertussis* (responsible for ~95% cases)
- *B. parapertussis*

COMMONLY ASSOCIATED CONDITIONS

- Sinusitis and otitis
- Urinary incontinence
- Apnea in young infants
- Seizures

DIAGNOSIS

HISTORY

- Incubation period: 5–21 days
- Classic symptoms, more common in adolescent and adult cases, include paroxysmal cough, posttussive whoop, and/or vomiting.
- Infants with pertussis may present with apnea or sudden death.

PHYSICAL EXAM

3 stages have been described:

- Catarrhal stage: Rhinorrhea, mild cough, low-grade fever
- Paroxysmal stage: Cough becomes paroxysmal, worsening in both frequency and severity. Posttussive whoop and vomiting may occur.
- Convalescent stage: Lasts 1–2 weeks with decreasing severity and frequency of coughing paroxysms
- In the absence of paroxysm or complications, a patient may have an essentially normal physical exam.

DIAGNOSTIC TESTS & INTERPRETATION

Lab

Initial lab tests

- If within 3 weeks of onset of cough, send nasopharyngeal aspirate for both polymerase chain reaction (PCR) and culture:
  - PCR results will come back sooner. Culture remains the gold standard.
  - Transport specimen to laboratory immediately:
    - Isolation of *B. pertussis* by PCR: Detection of paired genomic sequences by PCR is likely more sensitive. Sensitivity and specificity may vary from lab to lab. Lacks sensitivity in previously immunized individual. When sending nasopharyngeal specimen for detection by PCR, Dacron swabs are preferred, and calcium alginate swabs should *not* be used (because of inhibitory factors in the fibers).
    - Isolation of *B. pertussis* by culture (gold standard): Culture is highly specific but with variable sensitivity that may be related to techniques of swabbing and culture. When sending nasopharyngeal specimen for culture of *B. pertussis,* calcium alginate swabs are preferred. Dacron swabs are acceptable.
- If >2 weeks from onset of symptoms, consider serum pertussis toxin IgG.

Follow-Up & Special Considerations

Antipertussis toxin IgG: In adolescents and adults, high titer has good predictive value for current infection (sensitivity 76%, specificity 99% for acute pertussis).

Imaging

Initial approach

A chest x-ray (CXR) may be normal or show signs of hyperinflation with increased anteroposterior diameter and flattened diaphragm, focal atelectasis, and peribronchial cuffing. Pneumonia also may be present.

Follow-Up & Special Considerations

Follow-up CXRs as clinically indicated.

Pathological Findings

- Focal emphysema
- Mucopurulent exudate
- Patchy ulceration of respiratory epithelium

DIFFERENTIAL DIAGNOSIS

- Includes wide range of respiratory viruses, including *B. parapertussis* and respiratory syncytial virus
- Other infectious causes of prolonged cough include *M. pneumoniae. Chlamydia trachomatis, C. pneumoniae, B. bronchiseptica*, and adenovirus.
- Sinusitis
- Airway foreign body

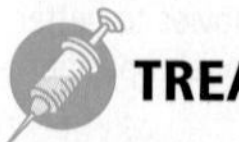

TREATMENT

MEDICATION

First Line

Short-term treatment with azithromycin (3–5 days) or clarithromycin or erythromycin (7 days) has been found to be as effective as 10–14 days of erythromycin in eradicating the virus from the nasopharynx. Fewer side effects were seen and there was no significant difference in clinical outcomes or relapse. Consultation with a pediatric infectious disease specialist should be considered for infants younger than 6 months of age (1)[A].

Second Line

For children older than 2 months of age for whom macrolides are not appropriate, trimethoprim-sulfamethoxazole can be considered as an alternative.

ADDITIONAL TREATMENT

General Measures

- Contact prophylaxis in individuals older than 6 months of age with antibiotics may not improve clinical symptoms or change the likelihood of developing a positive culture.
- Hospitalization for severely ill, very young, or high-risk infants; outpatient management for less ill patients
- Skilled nursing care with careful respiratory monitoring
- Avoid excessive stimulation of infants that may trigger paroxysms.
- Supplemental oxygen to prevent hypoxia
- Standard and respiratory droplet precautions
- Mechanical ventilation when necessary
- Supportive treatment:
  - Ensure adequate hydration and nutrition.
  - Clinical monitoring

Issues for Referral

- Infants <1 month: Pulmonology and/or ICU consult for patients hospitalized with respiratory distress or pneumonia
- Children <6 months: Consider pediatric infectious disease consultation.
- Apnea or seizures at the time of illness may be associated with subsequent impairment. Consultation with a pediatric neurologist or neurodevelopmental pediatrician may be indicated.

Additional Therapies

The Cochrane Database of Systematic Reviews (2010) found no significant evidence to support the use of corticosteroids, salbutamol, antihistamines, or pertussis-specific immunoglobulins to reduce symptoms (2)[A].

IN-PATIENT CONSIDERATIONS

Initial Stabilization

- Small, frequent meals may be necessary to ensure adequate nutrition.
- Correct fluid and electrolyte abnormalities
- Infants may require IV fluids.

Admission Criteria

- Consider for infants <6 months of age, especially preterms and unimmunized or underimmunized infants
- Patients with underlying diseases, especially neuromuscular disorders
- Infants with apnea, hypoxia, feeding difficulty
- Any patient with serious complications
- For supportive care or accelerating symptoms: Intensive care facilities may be required.

IV Fluids

Indicated for dehydration and when oral fluids are either contraindicated or poorly tolerated

Nursing

- Isolation of hospitalized patients with respiratory precautions for 5 days after the initiation of effective antibiotic treatment; for 3 weeks after onset of paroxysms in older patients if antibiotics are not used
- Gentle suctioning of nasal secretions
- Avoid stimuli that trigger paroxysms.
- Educate each family about the importance of vaccination.
- Discuss chemoprophylaxis with each family.

Discharge Criteria

- Clinically stable
- Able to tolerate oral feed

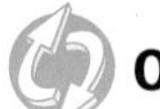

ONGOING CARE

FOLLOW-UP RECOMMENDATIONS

- Infants <1 month of age who receive treatment with a macrolide antibiotic should be monitored for 1 month for idiopathic hypertrophic pyloric stenosis.
- Neurologic and/or pulmonary follow-up as necessary

Patient Monitoring

- The ICU may be necessary for severely ill infants.
- Older children and adults with mild cases and no additional risk factors do not require hospital admission.

DIET

IV therapy is indicated with dehydration and/or when oral fluids are either not indicated or poorly tolerated.

PATIENT EDUCATION

- American Academy of Pediatrics: www.aap.org
- Centers for Disease Control: www.cdc.gov

PROGNOSIS

- Complete recovery in most cases
- Most severe morbidity and highest mortality in infants <4 months of age

COMPLICATIONS

- Highest and most severe in infants
- More frequent in adults than adolescents:
  - Sinusitis
  - Otitis media
  - Pneumonia
  - Weight loss
  - Fainting
  - Rib fracture
  - Urinary incontinence
  - Seizures
  - Encephalopathy
  - Death
  - ICD 9 Code 033.9

REFERENCES

1. Altunaiji SM, Kukuruzov RH, Curtis NC, et al. Antibiotics for whooping cough (pertussis). *Cochrane Database Syst Rev.* 2007;18(3): CD004404.
2. Bettiol S, Thompson MJ, Roberts NW, et al. Symptomatic treatment of the cough in whooping cough. *Cochrane Database Syst Rev.* 2010;(1): CD003257.

ADDITIONAL READING

- American Academy of Pediatrics. Pertussis. In Pickering L, et al., eds., *Red Book 2009 Report of the Committee in Infectious Diseases*, 28th ed. Elk Grove, IL: AAP; 2009:504–20.
- American Academy of Pediatrics Committee on Infectious Diseases. Prevention of pertussis among adolescents: Recommendations for use of tetanus toxoid, reduced diphtheria toxoid, and acellular pertussis (Tdap) vaccine. *Pediatrics*. 2006;117: 965–78.
- Centers for Disease Control and Prevention. Pertussis—United States, 2001–2003. *Morb Mortal Wkly Rep.* 2005;54:1283–6.
- Centers for Disease Control and Prevention. Recommended adult immunization schedule—United States 2009. *MMWR*. 2008;57(53).
- Crowcroft NS, Pebody RG. Recent developments in pertussis. *Lancet*. 2006;367:1926–36.
- Gerbie M, Tan T. Pertussis disease in new mothers: Effect on young infants and strategies for prevention. *Obstet Gynecol*. 2009;113:399–401.
- Mattoo S, Cherry JD. Molecular pathogenesis, epidemiology, and clinical manifestations of respiratory infections due to *Bordetella pertussis* and other *Bordetella* subspecies. *Clin Microbiol Rev.* 2005;18:326–82.
- Murphy TV, et al. Prevetntion of pertussis, tetanus and diphtheria among pregnant and postpartum women and their infants. *MMWR Recomm Rep.* 2008;57(04):1–47, 51.
- National Immunization Program, CDC. Recommended antimicrobial agents for the treatment and postexposure prophylaxis of pertussis 2005 CDC guidelines. *MMWR*. 2005;1–15.

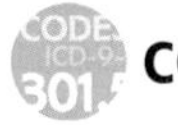

CODES

ICD9

033.9 Whooping cough, unspecified organism

CLINICAL PEARLS

- The physical exam in pertussis may be normal in the absence of paroxysms and clinical complications.
- When sending nasopharyngeal specimen for culture of *B. pertussis*, calcium alginate swabs are preferred. Dacron swabs are acceptable.
- When sending nasopharyngeal specimen for detection by PCR, Dacron swabs are preferred, and calcium alginate swabs should *not* be used (because of inhibitory factors in the fibers).
- Macrolides are first-line antibiotics.
- Prevention of transmission via immunization, isolation, and chemoprophylaxis is key.

PHARYNGITIS

David E. Burtner, MD

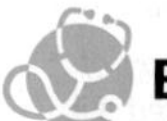

BASICS

DESCRIPTION

- Inflammation of the pharynx most commonly caused by acute viral infection
- Group A *Streptococcus* is a focus due to its potential for preventable rheumatic sequelae.
- Chronic low-grade symptoms usually are related to reflux disease or vocal abuse.
- System(s) affected: Respiratory
- Synonym(s): Sore throat; Tonsillitis; Streptococcal throat

EPIDEMIOLOGY

- Estimated 30 million cases diagnosed yearly
- 12–25% of all sore throats are thought to prompt visits to physicians.
- Predominant age: All age groups
- Predominant sex: Male = Female

Incidence

- Respiratory infections account for 38% of the 129 million visits per year to physicians in the US. This is ~200 visits to a physician per 1,000 population in the US annually (1).
- The etiology of the vast majority of these infections is viral.
- Group A *Streptococcus* is the most common bacterial cause of acute pharyngitis, accounting for ~15–30% of cases in children and 5–10% of cases in adults.
- Rheumatic fever is rare in the US. There were 112 cases reported to the CDC in 1994, the last year this was a reportable disease.

Pediatric Considerations

Rheumatic fever has its greatest incidence in children aged 5–18 years, but is currently a rare sequelae of streptococcal pharyngitis in the US.

Prevalence

Prevalence is quite variable in this acute, self-limited disease of short duration.

RISK FACTORS

- Epidemics of group A β-hemolytic streptococcal disease occur.
- Age (i.e., young people are more susceptible)
- Family history
- Close quarters, such as in new military recruits
- Immunosuppression
- Fatigue
- Smoking
- Excess alcohol consumption
- Receptive oral sex
- Diabetes mellitus
- Recent illness

Genetics

Patients with a positive family history of rheumatic fever have a higher risk of rheumatic sequelae following an untreated group A β-hemolytic streptococcal infection.

GENERAL PREVENTION

Avoid contact with infected people.

ETIOLOGY

- Acute, viral:
  - Rhinovirus
  - Adenovirus
  - Parainfluenza virus
  - Coxsackievirus
  - Coronavirus
  - Echovirus
  - Herpes simplex virus
  - Epstein-Barr virus (EBV) (mononucleosis)
  - Cytomegalovirus
- Acute, bacterial:
  - Group A β-hemolytic streptococci <10% of adult pharyngitis
  - *Neisseria gonorrhoeae*
  - *Corynebacterium diphtheriae* (diphtheria)
  - *Haemophilus influenzae*
  - *Moraxella (Branhamella) catarrhalis*
  - Groups C and G *Streptococcus*, rarely
- Chronic:
  - More likely noninfectious
  - Irritation from postnasal discharge of chronic allergic rhinitis or reflux
  - Chemical irritation or smoking
  - Neoplasms and vasculitides

DIAGNOSIS

Modified Centor clinical prediction rule for group A streptococcal infection (2)[A]:

- +1 point: Tonsillar exudates
- +1 point: Tender anterior chain cervical adenopathy
- +1 point: Fever by history
- +1 point: Age <15 years
- 0 points: Age 15–45 years
- –1 point: Age >45 years
- –1 point: Cough (presence of cough almost always *excludes* the diagnosis of group A strep.)
- Scoring:
  - If 3–4 points, positive predictive value of ~80%; treat empirically.
  - If 2 points, positive predictive value of ~50%, rapid strep antigen + culture; treat if either positive.
  - If 1 point, positive predictive value <50%, positive rapid strep. antigen or culture likely falsepositive
  - If 0 or –1 points, positive predictive value <20%; do not test; close follow-up PRN.
- Coryza (nasal congestion), hoarseness, cough, diarrhea, conjunctivitis, or viral rash highly suggests viral cause.

HISTORY

- Sore throat
- Cough, hoarseness, lower respiratory symptoms
- Fever
- Anorexia
- Chills
- Malaise
- Headache
- Contacts with similar symptoms or diagnosed infection

PHYSICAL EXAM

- Enlarged tonsils
- Pharyngeal erythema
- Tonsillar exudates
- Soft palate petechiae
- Cervical adenopathy
- Fever >102.5°F (>39.1°C)
- Scarlet fever rash: Punctate erythematous macules with reddened flexor creases and circumoral pallor (streptococcal pharyngitis)
- Gray pseudomembrane found in diphtheria and, occasionally, mononucleosis
- Characteristic erythematous-based clear vesicles are found in herpes stomatitis.
- Conjunctivitis is found more commonly with adenovirus infections.

DIAGNOSTIC TESTS & INTERPRETATION

Lab

- Testing, if performed, is usually for the presence of group A β-hemolytic streptococci (GAS). Options include:
  - Blood agar throat culture from swab. Bacitracin disk sensitivity of hemolytic colonies suggests group A streptococci. Specific antibody identification is available.
  - Rapid screening for streptococci can be done from throat swab with antigen agglutination kits; 5–10% false-negative results lead some clinicians to suggest routine backup of all negative results with blood agar culture (but which also has 5–10% false-negative rate). Newer optic immunoassay tests are more sensitive.
  - RNA screening assay has high sensitivity and specificity and rapid turnaround compared with culture.
- Special tests usually are done only if history is suggestive of a different diagnosis.
- Screening for gonococcal infection requires warm Thayer-Martin plate or antigen testing.
- Viruses can be cultured in special media (e.g., herpes simplex).
- Mono spot test for EBV
- Recent AHA scientific statement is "some form of microbiological confirmation, with either a throat culture or a rapid antigen detection test, is required for the diagnosis of GAS pharyngitis" (3).

Pathological Findings

Culture of pathogens may help to identify which is causative, but may not be cost-effective or influence outcome.

DIFFERENTIAL DIAGNOSIS

- Viral syndrome, including EBV infection (mononucleosis)
- Strep "carrier state": Absence of acute infection but persistence of bacteria; will result in positive rapid antigen testing but is not acute GAS. If suspected, have patient return when well, and repeat test.
- Secondary to allergic rhinitis, gastroesophageal reflux disease (GERD), cough from upper respiratory infection (URI), or asthma
- Nervous tic
- Peritonsillar abscess (rare)
- Nonstrep. bacterial causes: Gonococcal, etc.
- Fungal in immunocompromised patient

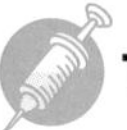

TREATMENT

- Acute pharyngitis is caused considerably more often by viruses than by bacteria.
- Empirical therapy leads to overuse of antibiotics in adults (4).

MEDICATION

First Line

For streptococcal pharyngitis, penicillin is the standard therapy. Only penicillin has been proven to prevent rheumatic fever. Penicillin courses <10 days are not as effective (7)[A]. Other antibiotics use streptococcal eradication as a proxy of effectiveness due to the low incidence of rheumatic fever and the ethics of further controlled studies:

- Penicillin V 250 mg PO t.i.d. or 500 mg b.i.d. (25–50 mg/kg/d) (7)[A] *or*
- Amoxicillin 20 mg/kg up to 750 mg divided t.i.d. Use with caution if diagnosis is unclear because amoxicillin and EBV infection may induce rash.
- For patients allergic to penicillin, erythromycin ethylsuccinate 300–400 mg PO t.i.d. (30 mg/kg/d) (7)[B] *or*
- Cephalexin 250 mg PO t.i.d. (30 mg/kg/d) (7)[C]

Second Line

- Treatment of carrier state is difficult, usually requiring the addition of rifampin or clindamycin to penicillin regimen.
- Penicillin is the most documented treatment to prevent rheumatic sequelae, but cephalosporins have a lower rate of bacteriologic failure.
- Bacterial eradication rates of 10 or more days' therapy with penicillin have been achieved with 6 days of amoxicillin and 5 days with various cephalosporins (6).
- The newer macrolides, azithromycin and clarithromycin, are also effective against streptococcal pharyngitis but are more expensive. The chief advantage of azithromycin is its 5-day course with 10-day effective duration.
- Macrolide-resistant strains of GAS are currently <10% in the US but more prevalent worldwide.
- Other cephalosporins generally are effective for streptococcal pharyngitis but more expensive than cephalexin.

ADDITIONAL TREATMENT

General Measures

- Salt water gargles
- Acetaminophen 15–20 mg/kg (pediatric) q4h gives more rapid relief than antibiotic therapy for strep. infection.
- Anesthetic lozenges
- Cool-mist humidifier

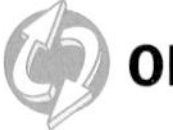

ONGOING CARE

FOLLOW-UP RECOMMENDATIONS

- Patient must complete antibiotic course for strep. regardless of symptom response.
- Patients may consider themselves noninfectious after 24 hours of antibiotic therapy.
- Usually, follow-up culture is not recommended.

DIET

As tolerated; encourage the consumption of fluids.

PROGNOSIS

- Streptococcal pharyngeal infection runs a 5–7-day course with peak fever at 2–3 days.
- Symptoms will resolve spontaneously without treatment, but rheumatic complications are still possible.
- Suppurative complications (e.g., peritonsillar abscess) often require surgical intervention.
- Immunologic complications (e.g., glomerulonephritis) may not be prevented by antibiotic treatment of group A β-hemolytic streptococci infection.

COMPLICATIONS

- Rheumatic fever (carditis, valve disease, arthritis, etc.)
- Poststreptococcal glomerulonephritis
- Peritonsillar abscess
- Systemic infection
- Otitis media
- Mastoiditis
- Septicemia
- Rhinitis
- Sinusitis
- Pneumonia

REFERENCES

1. Armstrong GL, Pinner RW. Outpatient visits for infectious diseases in the United States, 1980 through 1996. *Arch Intern Med*. 1999;159:2531–6.
2. McIsaac WJ, Kellner JD, Aufricht P, et al. Empirical validation of guidelines for the management of pharyngitis in children and adults. *JAMA*. 2004;291:1587–95.
3. Gerber MA, Baltimore RS, Eaton CB, et al. Prevention of rheumatic fever and diagnosis and treatment of acute streptococcal pharyngitis. A scientific statement from the American Heart Association Rheumatic Fever, Endocarditis, and Kawasaki Disease Committee of the Council on Cardiovascular Disease in the Young, the Interdisciplinary Council on Functional Genomics and Translational Biology, and the Interdisciplinary Council on Quality of Care and Outcomes Research. *Circulation*. 2009;119(11):1541–51.
4. Humair JP, Revaz SA, Bovier P, et al. Management of acute pharyngitis in adults: Reliability of rapid streptococcal tests and clinical findings. *Arch Intern Med*. 2006;166:640–4.
5. Denny FW, et al. Prevention of rheumatic fever. Treatment of the preceding streptococcic infection. *JAMA*. 1950;143:151–3.
6. Pichichero ME, Cohen R. Shortened course of antibiotic therapy for acute otitis media, sinusitis and tonsillopharyngitis. *Pediatr Infect Dis*. 1997;16:680–95.
7. Del Mar CB, Glasziou PP, Spinks AB. Antibiotics for sore throat. *Cochrane Database of Systematic Reviews*. 2006;4:CD000023.

ADDITIONAL READING

- Bisno AL. Acute pharyngitis. *N Engl J Med*. 2001;344:205–11.
- Bisno AL, Gerber MA, Gwaltney JM, et al. Diagnosis and management of group A streptococcal pharyngitis: A practice guideline. Infectious Diseases Society of America. *Clin Infect Dis*. 1997;25:574–83.
- Choby BA. Diagnosis and treatment of streptococcal pharyngitis. *Am Fam Physician*. 2009;79:383–90.
- Cooper RJ, Hoffman JR, Bartlett JG, et al. Principles of appropriate antibiotic use for acute pharyngitis in adults: Background. *Ann Intern Med*. 2001;134:509–17.
- Ebell MH. Making decisions at the point of care: Sore throat. *Fam Pract Manag*. 2003;10:68–9.
- Vincent MT, Celestin N, Hussain AN. Pharyngitis. *Am Fam Physician*. 2004;69:1465–70.

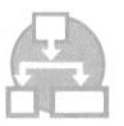

See Also (Topic, Algorithm, Electronic Media Element)

- Herpes Simplex; Mononucleosis; Rheumatic Fever
- Algorithm: Pharyngitis

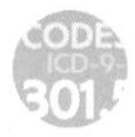

CODES

ICD9

- 034.0 Streptococcal sore throat
- 462 Acute pharyngitis
- 472.1 Chronic pharyngitis

CLINICAL PEARLS

- Most cases of pharyngitis are viral.
- Risk of missed case of group A beta hemolytic strep is rheumatic fever, a very rare complication (112 cases reported to CDC in 1994; last year it was reported)
- Use Modified Centor Score to guide testing and treatment.
- Presence of: Coryza (nasal congestion), hoarseness, cough, diarrhea, conjunctivitis, or viral rash highly suggests viral cause.

PHEOCHROMOCYTOMA

Maya Campara, PharmD, BCPS
Anna Porter, MD

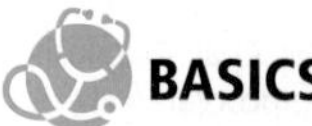

BASICS

DESCRIPTION

- A pheochromocytoma is a rare neuroendocrine tumor arising from the adrenal or extra-adrenal chromaffin tissue, and less commonly the sympathetic ganglia:
  - Catecholamine-producing tumor: Norepinephrine (NE) > epinephrine (EPI) >>> dopamine (DA)
- System(s) affected: Endocrine; Nervous; Cardiovascular
- Synonym(s): Chromaffin tumors and paraganglionomas

EPIDEMIOLOGY

Incidence

- 500–1,000 cases diagnosed in the US per year
- <0.2% of people with severe hypertension (HTN)

Prevalence

- 1:6,500–1:2,500 in Western countries
- Affects all genders and ages; usually diagnosed in fourth to fifth decade of life, familial cases diagnosed 1 decade earlier

RISK FACTORS

- Familial pheochromocytoma
- Familial paraganglioma
- Multiple endocrine neoplasia type 2 (MEN 2)
- von Hippel-Lindau disease (VHL)
- von Recklinghausen neurofibromatosis type 1 (NF 1)

Genetics

- Genetic testing is recommended for all patients.
- Genes identified in the pathogenesis:
  - REarranged during Transfection (RET) proto-oncogene
  - von Hippel-Lindau disease tumor suppressor gene (VHL)
  - Neurofibromatosis type 1 tumor suppressor gene (NH 1)
  - Genes encoding 4 succinate dehydrogenase complex (SDH) subunits
  - Gene encoding the enzyme responsible for flavination of the SDHA subunit
  - Tumor suppressor TMEM127 gene

PATHOPHYSIOLOGY

Pheochromocytoma is a tumor that releases catecholamines into circulation. Catecholamines interact with adrenergic receptors to produce various effects that could induce severe lethal cardiovascular and cerebrovascular complications:

- Stimulation of alpha-1 receptors (NE > EPI) causes smooth muscle constriction resulting in high BP (arteriolar vasoconstriction).
- Stimulation of alpha-2 receptors (EPI > NE) causes smooth muscle contraction, cardiac muscle relaxation, and inhibition of hormones like insulin resulting in elevated blood glucose levels.
- Stimulation of beta-1 receptors (EPI = NE) causes heart muscle contraction resulting in increased heart rate.
- Stimulation of beta-2 receptors (EPI >> NE) causes smooth muscle relaxation.

ETIOLOGY

- In 80% of cases, it is a sporadic disease of an unknown etiology.
- In 20% of cases, it has familial origin and is a component of 1 of the following 4 autosomal-dominant diseases:
  - Multiple endocrine neoplasia type 2 (MEN2)
  - von-Hippel-Lindau disease (VHL)
  - Hereditary paraganglioma syndrome (PGL)
  - Neurofibromatosis type 1 (NF1)
- Tumor location:
  - 80% of tumors are solitary and unilateral.
  - 20% are divided between bilateral lesions and extra-adrenal masses (organ of Zuckerkandl, neck, mediastinum, abdomen, pelvis)

COMMONLY ASSOCIATED CONDITIONS

- Multiple endocrine neoplasia type IIA (medullary thyroid carcinoma and primary hyperparathyroidism)
- Multiple endocrine neoplasia type IIB (medullary thyroid carcinoma and mucosal neuromas)
- von-Hippel-Lindau disease (retinal angiomas, cerebellar hemangioblastomas, renal cysts, carcinomas, pancreatic cysts, epididymal cystadenomas)
- Neurofibromatosis type 1
- Sturge-Weber syndrome
- Tuberous sclerosis
- Carney syndrome (gastric epithelioid leiomyosarcoma, pulmonary chondroma, extra-adrenal paraganglioma)
- Familial paraganglioma
- Ataxia-telangiectasia
- Renal artery stenosis

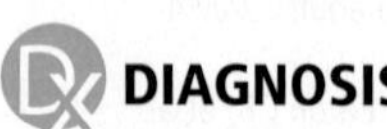

DIAGNOSIS

HISTORY

- Classic "triad" of symptoms includes headache, palpitations, and diaphoresis.
- 5 P's mnemonic:
  - Paroxysmal spells
  - Pressure: Sudden increase in BP
  - Pain: Headache, chest, abdominal pain
  - Perspiration (profuse sweating common in children)
  - Palpitations and Pallor
- Additional symptoms: Constipation, tremor, weight loss, anxiety, paresthesias, flushing, shortness of breath, nausea/vomiting
- Sudden death may occur in patients with an undiagnosed tumor who undergo surgery or biopsy due to lethal hypertensive crises and multiorgan failure.
- Dopamine-secreting pheochromocytomas lack the classic presentation of catecholamine excess.

PHYSICAL EXAM

- Hypertension (HTN): Paroxysmal in 1/2 of affected patients; most common clinical sign
- Tachyarrhythmias
- Orthostatic hypotension
- Café au lait spots
- Lisch nodules of the eye
- Grade II–IV retinopathy
- Transient ischemic attacks/stroke
- Cardiomyopathy
- GI crisis
- Diabetes mellitus or insipidus
- Fever
- Hypercalcemia
- Erythrocytosis

DIAGNOSTIC TESTS & INTERPRETATION

Lab

Initial lab tests

Diagnosis is typically confirmed by measurements of urinary catecholamines and their metabolites (NE/EPI → [nor]metanephrine, NE/EPI → vanillylmandelic acid (VMA), dopamine → homovanillic acid). Their amount in the urine correlates with the size of the pheochromocytoma tumor:

- Elevated metanephrine and catecholamines in 24-hour urine collection (sensitivity = 90%, specificity = 98%):
  - A positive test is considered to be a 2-fold elevation above the upper limit of normal in urine.
- Elevated plasma fractionated metanephrine (sensitivity = 97%, specificity = 85%):
  - Must be measured while patient is at rest (1)[A]
  - BP must be recorded during plasma sampling for catecholamines (1)[A].
  - Pheochromocytoma cannot be excluded if normal catecholamine values are obtained when the patient is normotensive and asymptomatic (1)[A].
- Elevated VMA in 24-hour urine collection (sensitivity = 64%, specificity = 95%)
- Dopamine-secreting pheochromocytomas are often missed if urinary or plasma dopamine is not included as part of the catecholamine screening. Urinary and plasma dopamine are the most widely used methods in the diagnosis of dopamine-secreting tumors.

Follow-Up & Special Considerations

- Drugs that may increase measured levels of catecholamines and metabolites and should be discontinued at least 2 weeks before assessment:
  - Tricyclic antidepressants
  - Monoamine oxidase inhibitors (MAOIs)
  - Levodopa, methyldopa
  - Drugs containing adrenergic receptor agonists (e.g., decongestants)
  - Amphetamines
  - Cocaine
  - Buspirone and most psychoactive agents (but not SSRIs)
  - Prochlorperazine
  - Reserpine
  - Withdrawal from clonidine and other drugs
  - Ethanol
  - Acetaminophen (may increase measured levels of fractionated plasma metanephrines in some assays)
- Drugs that may decrease measured levels of catecholamines and metabolites:
  - Reserpine
  - Centrally acting alpha-2 receptor agonists (dexmedetomidine, clonidine, tizanidine, guanfacine)
- Conditions that may alter lab results include major physical stress due to surgery, stroke, myocardial infarction, congestive heart failure, etc.

Imaging

Initial approach

Proceed with imaging after positive laboratory evaluation:

- Abdominal imaging with MRI or CT has similar specificity and sensitivity; MRI is more expensive but does not involve radiation or contrast dye exposure.
- If CT or MRI is negative but clinical suspicion is high, imaging can be done with 123-I-metaiodobenzylguanidine (MIBG) scan or pentetreotide scan.

Diagnostic Procedures/Surgery

Clonidine-suppression test distinguishes between pheochromocytoma and essential HTN when urine and plasma tests are equivocal. In essential hypertension, plasma and urine catecholamines decrease 3 hours after oral clonidine; in pheochromocytoma, they do not.

Pathological Findings

Pathology shows a tumor that demonstrates staining for chromogranin-A (catecholamine secretory granules).

DIFFERENTIAL DIAGNOSIS

- Labile essential hypertension
- Anxiety and panic attacks
- Paroxysmal cardiac arrhythmia
- Thyrotoxicosis
- Menopausal syndrome
- Hypoglycemia
- Withdrawal of adrenergic-inhibiting medications
- Angina
- Hyperventilation
- Migraine headache
- Amphetamine or cocaine use
- Sympathomimetic ingestion/overdose

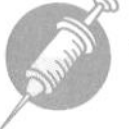

TREATMENT

MEDICATION

First Line

Surgical resection of the tumor is the treatment of choice. Medical management of BP is essential prior to surgery. Target preoperative BP <120/80 mm Hg:

- Preoperative control of BP is achieved first with alpha-adrenergic blockade followed by beta-adrenergic blockade starting 1 week before surgical removal of pheochromocytoma (longer for patients with recent history of CV complication). Never initiate beta-adrenergic blockade before alpha-adrenergic blockade, as unopposed alpha stimulation will result in worsened hypertension:
  - Alpha-adrenergic blockade is achieved by administering nonselective alpha-blocker phenoxybenzamine starting at a dose of 10 mg PO b.i.d. and increasing by 10–20 mg every 2 days as needed and tolerated for BP control (normal dose 100 mg/d but up to 240 mg/d have been reported). Warn patient of postural hypotension.
  - After adequate alpha-adrenergic blockade, beta blockade is initiated at low doses using short-acting agent propranolol 10 mg PO q 6 hours that can be titrated up until resting heart rate of 60–80 beats/min is achieved (maximum dose is 120 mg/d). Avoid beta-blockers in acute decompensated heart failure, bradycardia, and patients with uncontrolled asthma.

Second Line

- Treat hypertensive crisis with nitroprusside, nicardipine, or phentolamine.
- For inoperable tumors requiring long-term medical management, specific alpha-1 blocking agents can be used due to a more favorable side effect profile: Prazosin, terazosin, doxazosin
- Selective beta-1 blockers (no beta-2 activity): Atenolol, metoprolol, nadolol
- Combined beta- and alpha-blockers: Labetalol and carvedilol
- Catecholamine synthesis inhibitor: Metyrosine only if intolerant to first-line treatment (Mayo Clinic protocol). Avoid long-term use due to adverse reactions (sedation, depression, diarrhea, crystalluria or urolithiasis, and extrapyramidal signs).

SURGERY/OTHER PROCEDURES

- Removal of pheochromocytoma is treatment of choice.
- It is a high-risk surgical procedure requiring experienced surgical and anesthesia teams.
- Laparoscopic approach for tumors in the adrenal gland may result in shorter hospitalization.
- Cortical-sparing subtotal adrenalectomy may preserve adrenocortical function in those with bilateral disease.

IN-PATIENT CONSIDERATIONS

Initial Stabilization

Control of HTN and replacement of volume with IV normal saline

Admission Criteria

Severe or refractory HTN

Nursing

Monitor BP closely.

Discharge Criteria

When hemodynamically stable and blood glucose normalized

ONGOING CARE

FOLLOW-UP RECOMMENDATIONS

Patient Monitoring

- Monitor BP daily before surgery.
- Invasive hemodynamic monitoring intraoperatively
- Monitor urine metanephrines and catecholamine 2 weeks postoperatively and, if normal, recheck annually.
- Assure resolution of HTN and normalization of blood glucose.

DIET

- Preoperatively, after initiation of alpha-blocker, encourage high-sodium diet (>5,000 mg/d) to increase blood volume and prevent orthostasis. May be contraindicated in setting of renal or heart failure.
- Postoperatively, resume general diet.

PATIENT EDUCATION

Patient educational materials from National Adrenal Disease Foundation (NADF), 505 Northern Blvd., Great Neck, NY 11021; 516-487-4992; e-mail: nadfmail@aol.com

PROGNOSIS

- Survival after surgical removal of a benign tumor is similar to age-matched controls.
- Recurrence rate is 8–15%.
- 5-year survival for malignant disease is <50%.

COMPLICATIONS

- The most common lethal complications are myocardial infarction (MI) and cerebrovascular accident (CVA).
- Postural hypotension due to alpha-blockade can be ameliorated with volume expansion/high-sodium diet.
- Intraoperative hypertensive crisis can be managed with IV nitroprusside, nicardipine, and phentolamine.

REFERENCE

1. Karagiannis A, Mikhailidis DP, Athyros VG, et al. Pheochromocytoma: An update on genetics and management. *Endocr Relat Cancer*. 2007;14:935–56.

ADDITIONAL READING

- Bruynzeel H, Feelders RA, Groenland TH, et al. Risk factors for hemodynamic instability during surgery for pheochromocytoma. *J Clin Endocrinol Metab*. 2010;95:678–85.
- Scholz T, Eisenhofer G, Pacak K, et al. Clinical review: Current treatment of malignant pheochromocytoma. *J Clin Endocrinol Metab*. 2007;92:1217–25.

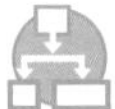

See Also (Topic, Algorithm, Electronic Media Element)

Hypertension, Essential; Multiple Endocrine Neoplasia (MEN)

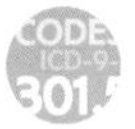

CODES

ICD9

- 194.0 Malignant neoplasm of adrenal gland
- 227.0 Benign neoplasm of adrenal gland

CLINICAL PEARLS

- Rare catecholamine-secreting tumor with serious and potentially lethal cardiovascular complications
- Clinical presentation is variable, but classic triad consists of episodic headaches, diaphoresis, and tachycardia/palpitations in association with hypertension.
- Diagnosis by urine screen for catecholamines and their metabolites followed by imaging studies (CT, MRI)
- Surgical removal of tumor is standard therapy that must be preceded by a period of BP stabilization with nonselective alpha-adrenergic blockade followed by beta-adrenergic blockade several days later.
- High-salt diet is initiated after alpha-blockade to minimize orthostasis and ensure fluid expansion.
- Never initiate beta-blocker before adequate alpha-blockade is achieved.

PHIMOSIS AND PARAPHIMOSIS

James P. Miller, MD

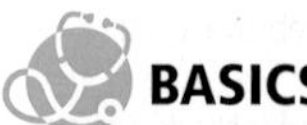

BASICS

DESCRIPTION

- Phimosis: Tightness of the distal penile foreskin that prevents it from being drawn back from over the glans
- Paraphimosis: Constriction of foreskin of an uncircumcised penis, preventing the foreskin from returning to its position over the glans; occurs after the retracted foreskin becomes swollen and engorged
- System(s) affected: Renal/Urologic; Reproductive; Skin/Exocrine

Geriatric Considerations

Recurrent infection and irritations (condom catheters) can lead to phimosis.

Pediatric Considerations

- Recurrent balanitis, either chemical or infectious, can lead to an acquired phimosis.
- Forced reduction of a physiologic foreskin can lead to chronic scarring and acquired phimosis.

EPIDEMIOLOGY

- Predominant age: Infancy and adolescence; unusual in adults; risk returns in geriatrics
- Predominant sex: Men only

Prevalence

In the US: 1% of men >16 years of age

RISK FACTORS

- Phimosis:
  - Poor hygiene
  - Diabetes
  - Frequent diaper rash in infants
- Paraphimosis:
  - Presence of foreskin
  - Inexperienced health care provider (leaving foreskin retracted after catheter placement)

GENERAL PREVENTION

- Good patient and parental education
- If the patient is uncircumcised, appropriate hygiene and care of the foreskin are necessary to prevent phimosis and paraphimosis.

ETIOLOGY

- Phimosis:
  - Physiologic: Present at birth and resolves spontaneously during the first 2–3 years of life through nocturnal erections, which slowly dilate the phimotic ring
  - Congenital: Unresolved physiologic phimosis
  - Acquired: Recurrent infection, irritation, or trauma from forced reduction of infants "physiologic" phimosis
- Paraphimosis:
  - Foreskin not pulled back over the glans after cleaning, cystoscopy, or catheter insertion

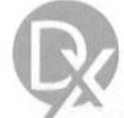

DIAGNOSIS

HISTORY

- Phimosis:
  - Painful erections
  - Recurrent balanitis
  - Foreskin balloons when voiding
- Paraphimosis:
  - Uncircumcised
  - Pain
  - Drainage

PHYSICAL EXAM

- Phimosis:
  - Foreskin cannot retract.
  - Secondary balanitis
- Paraphimosis:
  - Edema
  - Drainage
  - Ulceration

DIFFERENTIAL DIAGNOSIS

- Penile lymphedema, which can be related to insect bites, trauma, or allergic reactions
- Penile tourniquet syndrome: Foreign body around penis, most commonly a hair

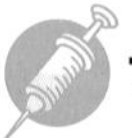

TREATMENT

MEDICATION

Topical 0.05% betamethasone b.i.d. for 1 month to soften phimosis

ADDITIONAL TREATMENT

General Measures

- Phimosis:
  - 0.05% betamethasone b.i.d. with gradual traction placed on foreskin. Over 4–6 weeks, the phimotic ring should open (1)[C].
- Paraphimosis:
  - Manual reduction if possible (should be done with the patient sedated). Place the middle and index fingers of both hands on the engorged skin proximal to the glans. Place both thumbs on glans and, with gentle pressure, push on the glans, and pull on the foreskin to attempt reduction. If unsuccessful, a dorsal slit will be necessary with eventual circumcision after the edema resolves.
  - Osmotic agents: Granulated sugar placed on edematous tissue for several hours to reduce edema (2)[C]
  - Puncture technique: Multiple punctures of foreskin with a 21-gauge needle will allow edematous fluid to escape and thus allow reduction (3)[C].
- Appropriate health care: Outpatient except when there are complications
- Pain control

Issues for Referral

Consider circumcision for recurrent balanitis and paraphimosis.

SURGERY/OTHER PROCEDURES

- Phimosis: Circumcision
- Paraphimosis:
  - Represents a true surgical emergency to avoid necrosis of glans
  - Dorsal slit with delayed circumcision if reduction is not possible
  - Operative exploration if the possibility of penile tourniquet syndrome cannot be eliminated. Hair removal cream can be applied if a hair is thought to be the cause of the tourniquet.

IN-PATIENT CONSIDERATIONS

Admission Criteria

Tissue loss with paraphimosis

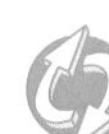

ONGOING CARE

FOLLOW-UP RECOMMENDATIONS

No sexual activity following circumcision until healing is complete

Patient Monitoring

Monitor for 1 week after the reduction of paraphimosis and for 1–2 weeks after a circumcision.

DIET

No limitations

PATIENT EDUCATION

Appropriate foreskin care should be discussed with parents of a child and with the patient once he is old enough to understand how to avoid the occurrence of paraphimosis.

PROGNOSIS

Complete resolution if treatment is carried out effectively

COMPLICATIONS

- Unreduced paraphimosis can lead to gangrene of the glans.
- Posthitis (inflammation of the prepuce)

REFERENCES

1. Palmer LS, Palmer JS. The efficacy of topical betamethasone for treating phimosis: A comparison of two treatment regimens. *Urology*. 2008;72(1): 68–71.
2. Cahill D, Rome A. Reduction of paraphimosis with granulated sugar. *BJU Int*. 1999;83:362.
3. Reynard JM, Barua JM. Reduction of paraphimosis the simple way—the Dundee technique. *BJU Int*. 1999;83:859–60.

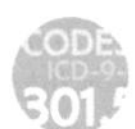

CODES

ICD9

605 Redundant prepuce and phimosis

CLINICAL PEARLS

- Physiologic phimosis usually will resolve during the first few years of life. As the child experiences nocturnal erections, the phimotic ring will dilate, and only then should it be retracted to clean. There is *no* reason to reduce a newborn's foreskin to clean underneath. The forced reduction will only predispose the infant to acquired phimosis.
- No controlled studies compare the various methods of reduction.

PHOBIAS

Thomas G. Zimmerman, DO, FACOFP

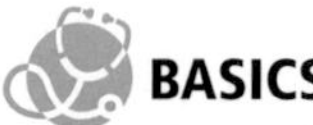

BASICS

DESCRIPTION

- A marked, persistent, excessive, and unreasonable fear of an object, activity, place, or situation. Symptoms develop in the presence or anticipation of the triggering factor(s). These factors are actively avoided or endured with extreme anxiety and dread. Adolescents and adults with phobias are usually aware that their reactions are abnormal.
- To qualify as a true disorder, symptoms must cause significant distress, interfere with normal social and vocational functioning, and result in a perceived loss of freedom.
- The American Psychiatric Association (*DSM-IV-TR*) classifies phobias as anxiety disorders and divides them into 3 categories:
  - Agoraphobia: Fear and avoidance of situations that may be difficult or embarrassing to escape in the event of paniclike symptoms. May involve fear of crowds, enclosed spaces (e.g., elevators, automobiles, or airplanes), or simply being alone (at home or away from home). Usually secondary to a coexisting panic disorder but may be a primary condition. See the topic "Panic Disorder."
  - Specific phobia (formerly *simple phobia*):
    - Fear and avoidance of clearly discernible, circumscribed objects or situations. Often divided into animal-type (e.g., snakes, spiders), environmental-type (e.g., storms, height), blood-injection/injury type, or situational type (e.g., enclosed spaces, flying, crowds).
    - Common specific phobias: Zoophobia (animals), brontophobia (thunderstorms), acrophobia (heights), nosophobia (disease), thanatophobia (death)
    - Blood-injection/injury phobia associated with a strong vasovagal reaction
  - Social phobia (social anxiety disorder): Fear and avoidance of certain social or performance situations where embarrassment or humiliation may occur under scrutiny of others. Individuals may experience marked anticipatory anxiety in advance of upcoming feared events. One of the most common (and underdiagnosed) phobias.

Pediatric Considerations

- Anxiety may be expressed by crying, tantrums, freezing, or clinging. Fears of animals and other objects in the natural environment are common and usually transitory in childhood.
- Preadolescent children are often not aware that their fears are excessive or unreasonable.

EPIDEMIOLOGY

Incidence

- Predominant age: Median age of onset 20 years for agoraphobia, 7 years for specific phobias, and 13 years for social phobia
- Predominant sex: Female > Male

Prevalence

In the general US population, the 12-month and lifetime prevalence (respectively):

- Agoraphobia without panic: 0.8% and 1.4%
- Specific phobia: 8.7% and 12.5%
- Social phobia: 6.8% and 12.1%

RISK FACTORS

- Female sex (phobias are the most common psychiatric disorders among women)
- First-degree relatives with the disorder
- Traumatic experience
- In children, observation of others with phobic reactions
- Social phobia is strongly associated with a perceived lack of control over one's own life. Other risk factors include low self-esteem, low education level, emotional neglect, major depression, and significant recent life stressors.

Genetics

Social phobia and agoraphobia are correlated with genetically influenced introversion and neuroticism.

PATHOPHYSIOLOGY

- Not well-understood but exaggerated amygdala, anterior cingulate, and insular activity increase fear and create mental-stress-induced heart rate and BP increases that can be decreased by evidence-based exposure treatment
- Fear of blood draws and severe public-speaking anxiety can create vasovagal syncope.

ETIOLOGY

Evidence suggests a complex interplay among genetic vulnerability, development neurobiology, and environment. Vulnerability may lead to persistence or exaggeration of a learned response, perhaps learned initially as a protective mechanism (such as avoidance of large dogs by small children).

COMMONLY ASSOCIATED CONDITIONS

- Other anxiety and mood disorders, as well as abuse of alcohol and other substances
- Most patients with agoraphobia experience panic disorder as well.

DIAGNOSIS

HISTORY

A major finding is the presence of irrational or ego-dystonic fear of a specific situation, activity, or object with associated avoidant behavior.

PHYSICAL EXAM

- Symptoms associated with exposure to phobic stimuli may include signs of sympathetic activation, pallor, dizziness, or paresthesias.
- A mental status exam should be performed.

DIAGNOSTIC TESTS & INTERPRETATION

Lab

Initial lab tests

No diagnostic laboratory tests for phobias

DIFFERENTIAL DIAGNOSIS

- Psychiatric differential diagnosis includes the following:
  - Other anxiety disorders (panic disorder, obsessive–compulsive disorder [OCD], generalized anxiety disorder [GAD], posttraumatic stress disorder [PTSD])
  - Mood disorders (unipolar or bipolar): Treat mood state first
  - Schizophrenia and psychoses
  - Schizoid personality disorder: Ego syntonic state (patient is happier by himself)
  - Avoidant personality disorder: History since childhood of fear of scrutiny by others
  - Alzheimer disease and autism: Fears are of new places and new things because of difficulty learning
- Consider underlying medical causes such as thyroid dysfunction, alcohol/benzodiazepine withdrawal, alcoholism and substance use (particularly hallucinogens, sympathomimetics, dextromethorphan), hypoglycemia, steroids, interferon, myocardial infarction, hypoxia, preictal and postictal states, pheochromocytoma, hyperparathyroidism, cerebrovascular disease, and CNS tumors.
- Agoraphobia is almost always preceded by panic or a paniclike state. The key feature of social phobia is fear of scrutiny by others. A specific phobia is a narrowly focused fear (e.g., a fear of needles).

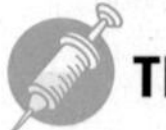

TREATMENT

Treat major psychiatric disorders first (bipolar, schizophrenia, alcoholism) as phobic symptoms may resolve. Benzodiazepines may make first-line treatments like cognitive-behavioral therapy and exposure therapy less effective.

MEDICATION

First Line

- Studies show effectiveness of SSRIs for agoraphobia (1)[A] and social phobia (2)[A]. If the patient has bipolar disorder, treat this first because antidepressants (like SSRIs) can make bipolar disorder worse:
  - Citalopram (10–60 mg/d), escitalopram (5–20 mg/d), fluoxetine (10–80 mg/d), fluvoxamine (50–300 mg/d), paroxetine (10–60 mg/d), and sertraline (25–200 mg/d). In patients with panic disorder, start lower than the FDA recommendations to enable patients to tolerate medications.
- Venlafaxine XR (75–300 mg/d), a serotonin-norepinephrine reuptake inhibitor (SNRI), has been shown to be as effective and well tolerated as SSRIs for social phobia (3,4)[A].
- Buspirone (15–60 mg/d), a serotonin-receptor agonist, also may be used in the treatment of social phobia; can be used to augment SSRIs.
- Taper treatment after 6–12 months if possible; can be restarted if symptoms recur (1,5)
- Medications are not known to help chronically with specific phobias. A short-acting benzodiazepine (alprazolam, 0.5–2 mg) may be helpful in treating acute fears (e.g., of flying)

Second Line

- Benzodiazepines quickly reduce fears associated with panic (1,6)[A], but they are second line due to long-term tolerance and abuse potential. May be first line in patients with bipolar disorder. Contraindicated in most patients with alcoholism:
  - Also useful in treatment of social phobia (7)[A]
  - Alprazolam (0.5–4 mg/d), lorazepam (2–6 mg/d), clonazepam (0.5–6 mg/d)
  - Discontinue gradually because of the risk for withdrawal seizures and rebound panic/anxiety.
- β-Blockers decrease sympathetic stimulation and can be used for performance anxiety:
  - Choices include propranolol (10–80 mg) and atenolol (25–100 mg) 30–60 minutes before activity (fewer CNS side effects).
  - Monitor for hypotension and bradycardia.
- Tricyclic antidepressants (TCAs) are as effective as SSRIs for panic symptoms associated with agoraphobia (though not as well tolerated) (8)[A]:
  - Start with 25 mg of a tricyclic (or less). May increase 25 mg every 3 days to target dose:
    - Imipramine (50–300 mg/d), desipramine (50–300 mg/d), nortriptyline (25–150 mg/d), and clomipramine (25–150 mg/d)
    - Anticholinergic, antihistaminic, orthostatic side effects common. Increased risk of death after MI if on TCAs.
- The monoamine oxidase inhibitor (MAOI) phenelzine (45–90 mg/d) is effective in the treatment of social phobia but less well tolerated (7)[A]. Do not use with other antidepressants, decongestants, diet pills, meperidine (Demerol), dextromethorphan, levodopa, and sympathomimetics. A special tyramine-elimination diet is needed.

ADDITIONAL TREATMENT

General Measures

- Cognitive-behavioral therapy (CBT), including exposure, cognitive restructuring, and relaxation techniques, has been shown to be effective for social phobia and agoraphobia (9)[A].
- Exposure-based treatment is superior to pharmacology and alternative psychotherapeutic approaches and placebo in the treatment of specific phobias (10)[A].

Issues for Referral

Consider a neurology consult if seizures are suspected.

COMPLEMENTARY AND ALTERNATIVE MEDICINE

- Inositol (12–18 g/d) may benefit those with panic disorder and possibly agoraphobia.
- There is no good evidence to support the use of St. John's wort, valerian, Sympathyl, passionflower, or cannabis in the treatment of anxiety disorders (11).

IN-PATIENT CONSIDERATIONS

Monitoring or treatment may be indicated in the setting of acute suicidality or comorbid alcohol and substance abuse.

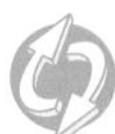

ONGOING CARE

FOLLOW-UP RECOMMENDATIONS

Patient Monitoring

Outpatient as needed

DIET

- Consider the restriction of stimulants, such as caffeine, that can exacerbate anxiety.
- If taking phenelzine or other MAOIs, a tyramine-free diet must be followed to decrease the risk of a hypertensive crisis.

PATIENT EDUCATION

- Many resources are available. Understanding the diagnosis and treatment is important not only for the patient but also for friends and family, who can provide a caring support system.
- Anxiety Disorders Association of America: http://adaa.org
- The Social Phobia/Social Anxiety Association: http://socialphobia.org
- Patient education on understanding social phobia: www.aafp.org/afp/991115ap/991115b.html

PROGNOSIS

- Most patients will experience resolution of symptoms with appropriate treatment.
- Even after successful treatment of agoraphobia and social phobia, residual symptoms or relapses may occur.

COMPLICATIONS

- Avoidance behavior may lead to significant impairment in social and vocational life.
- Morbidity is often more severe in agoraphobia and social phobia than in specific phobia.
- Alcohol and substance abuse is common.

REFERENCES

1. Ham P, Waters DB, Oliver MN. Treatment of panic disorder. *Am Fam Physician*. 2005;71:733–9.
2. Schneier F. Pharmacotherapy of social anxiety disorder. *Expert Opin Pharmacother*. 2011;12(4): 615–25.
3. Liebowitz MR. A randomized controlled trial of venlafaxine extended release in generalized social anxiety disorder. *J Clin Psychiatr*. 2005;66(2): 238–47.
4. Liebowitz MR, Gelenberg AJ, Munjack D. Venlafaxine extended release vs placebo and paroxetine in social anxiety disorder. *Arch Gen Psychiatry*. 2005;62:190–8.
5. Van Ameringen M, Allgulander C, Bandelow B. WCA recommendations for the long-term treatment of social phobia. *CNS Spectr*. 2003; 8:40–52.
6. Pollack MH, Allgulander C, Bandelow B. WCA recommendations for the long-term treatment of panic disorder. *CNS Spectr*. 2003;8:17–30.
7. Blanco C. Pharmacological treatment of social anxiety disorder: A meta-analysis. *Depress Anxiety*. 2003;18(1):29–40.
8. Bakker A, van Balkom AJ, Spinhoven P. SSRIs vs. TCAs in the treatment of panic disorder: A meta-analysis. *Acta Psychiatr Scand*. 2002;106: 163–7.
9. Rodebaugh TL, Holaway RM, Heimberg RG. The treatment of social anxiety disorder. *Clin Psychol Rev*. 2004;24:883–908.
10. Wolitzky-Taylor KB, Horowitz JD, Powers MB. Psychological approaches in the treatment of specific phobias: A meta-analysis. *Clin Psychol Rev*. 2008;28(6):1021–37.
11. Saeed SA, Bloch RM, Antonacci DJ. Herbal and dietary supplements for treatment of anxiety disorders. *Am Fam Physician*. 2007;76:549–56.

ADDITIONAL READING

- American Psychiatric Association. *Diagnostic and Statistical Manual of Mental Disorders (DSM-IV-TR)*, 4th ed. Washington, DC: American Psychiatric Association, 2000.
- Hudson C, Hudson S, MacKenzie J. Protein-source tryptophan as an efficacious treatment for social anxiety disorder: A pilot study. *Can J Physiol Pharmacol*. 2007;85:928–32.

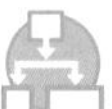

See Also (Topic, Algorithm, Electronic Media Element)

Anxiety; Depression; Dissociative Disorders; Obsessive–Compulsive Disorder; Posttraumatic Stress Disorder (PTSD); Schizophrenia

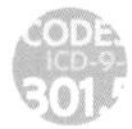

CODES

ICD9

- 300.20 Phobia, unspecified
- 300.21 Agoraphobia with panic disorder
- 300.22 Agoraphobia without mention of panic attacks

CLINICAL PEARLS

- CBT is a first-line, long-term effective treatment of panic with agoraphobia and social phobia. Behavioral exposure therapies are first-line, long-term effective treatments for specific phobias.
- You must rule out more serious psychiatric diagnoses and underlying medical conditions.
- For acute agoraphobic/panic reactions, rapid initiation of aerobic exercise (e.g., jogging in place) can be useful in patients without comorbid medical contraindications.

PHOTODERMATITIS

Aamir Siddiqi, MD

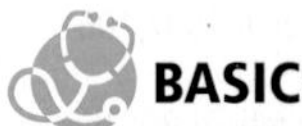

BASICS

DESCRIPTION
- Light-induced eruptions seen in a pattern of photodistribution:
  - Phototoxic reactions: Result of the acute toxic effect on skin of ultraviolet (UV) light alone (sunburn) or together with a photosensitizing substance (nonallergic)
  - Photoallergic eruptions: A form of allergic dermatitis resulting from combined effects of a photosensitizing substance (drugs or chemical) plus UV light (immunologic/delayed hypersensitivity)
  - Polymorphous light eruption (PLE): Chronic, intermittent, light-induced eruption with erythematous papules, urticaria, or vesicles on areas exposed to sunlight
- System(s) affected: Skin/Exocrine
- Synonym(s): Sun poisoning; Sun allergy

EPIDEMIOLOGY
Incidence
- Usually occurs after the first intense exposure in the spring or summer.
- Predominant age: All ages
- Predominant sex: Male = Female

Prevalence
May be as high as 20% in some areas

RISK FACTORS
- Job-related exposure to sunlight
- Light- and fair-colored skin

Genetics
Predisposition occurs in inbred populations (e.g., Pima Indians)

GENERAL PREVENTION
- Sunlight avoidance/protective clothing
- Identification and avoidance of causative drugs (see "Etiology")
- Sunscreens: Apply before exposure:
  - Zinc oxide: Opaque, cosmetically less acceptable
  - Chemical: Use sun-protective factor (SPF) >30 for maximum protection; substantively resistant to sweat and swimming; cosmetically more acceptable (1)[C]
- Avoid direct sun exposure.
- Wear appropriate gear to avoid sunlight exposure.

ETIOLOGY
- Sunlight
- Phenothiazines
- Diuretics
- Tetracyclines, sulfonamides
- Oral contraceptives
- Topicals: Psoralens, coal tars, photoactive dyes (eosin, acridine orange)
- 5-fluorouracil
- Quinine
- Sunscreens containing *para*-aminobenzoic acid (PABA)
- In the US, ~115 chemical agents used topically are known to cause photodermatitis.

COMMONLY ASSOCIATED CONDITIONS
- Sunlight aggravation of systemic lupus
- Persistent light reactivity
- Actinic reticuloid

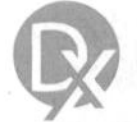

DIAGNOSIS

HISTORY
Pruritic and often painful rash developing in sun-exposed areas

PHYSICAL EXAM
- Phototoxic:
  - Erythema
  - With increasing severity: Vesicles and bullae
  - Classic example: Sunburn
  - Nails may exhibit onycholysis.
  - Chronic: Epidermal thickening, elastosis, telangiectasia, and pigmentary changes
  - Sharp lines of demarcation between involved and uninvolved skin (sunlight exposure)
  - Phototoxic eruption due to topicals: Area of application
  - Usually develops shortly after sun exposure
  - Hyperpigmentation may follow resolution.
  - Pain
- Photoallergic (1)[C]:
  - Papules with erythema and occasionally vesicles
  - Area exposed to light with less distinct borders
  - Usually delayed 24 hours or more after exposure
  - May spread to unexposed areas
  - Pruritus
- PLE:
  - Erythematous papules
  - Occasionally urticaria or vesicles
  - Scattered over sun-exposed areas with normal skin in between
  - Can spread to nonexposed areas
  - Often flares in spring or early summer
  - Desensitization effect (less over the course of the summer)
  - Burning or pruritus may precede lesions.

DIAGNOSTIC TESTS & INTERPRETATION

Lab

Follow-Up & Special Considerations

Antinuclear antibody to rule out systemic lupus erythematosus if suspected

Diagnostic Procedures/Surgery

- Phototesting: Exposing patient to UV light
- Photopatch testing: Applying suspected agents and chemicals to patient's skin
- Skin biopsy: To rule out other disorders if necessary

DIFFERENTIAL DIAGNOSIS

Systemic lupus erythematosus

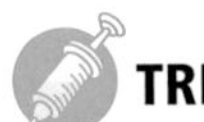

TREATMENT

MEDICATION

Topical corticosteroids (triamcinolone 0.25%, 0.1%, 0.5%; betamethasone valerate 0.1% cream, others)

ALERT

Limit use of fluorinated steroids on face; use hydrocortisone ointments.

- NSAIDs (ibuprofen 600 mg q.i.d., indomethacin 25 mg PO t.i.d., aspirin, others)
- Prednisone for severe reactions (0.5–1 mg/kg PO daily) × 3–10 days
- Antihistamines for pruritus (hydroxyzine 25–50 mg PO q.i.d.)
- Sunscreens (>30 SPF) for prevention: Use broad-spectrum sunscreen to block both UVA and UVB. PABA may aggravate photodermatitis in sensitized patients (due to the sulfa moiety) (1)[C].
- Contraindications: Refer to the manufacturer's profile for each drug.
- Precautions: Refer to the manufacturer's profile for each drug.
- Significant possible interactions: Refer to the manufacturer's profile for each drug.

Geriatric Considerations

More likely to experience adverse reactions to causative drugs

ADDITIONAL TREATMENT

General Measures

- Appropriate health care: Outpatient
- Avoid sunlight/limit exposure.
- Protective clothing/sunscreens
- Ice packs/cold water compresses

COMPLEMENTARY AND ALTERNATIVE MEDICINE

- Taking β-carotene orally seems to modestly reduce the risk of sunburn in individuals who are sensitive to sun exposure (2).
- Omega-3 fatty acid intake may decrease the sensitivity of skin to UV exposure (3).

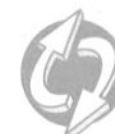

ONGOING CARE

FOLLOW-UP RECOMMENDATIONS

Avoid direct sunlight.

PATIENT EDUCATION

- Avoidance of direct sunlight exposure
- Avoidance of photosensitizing drugs
- Protective clothing (e.g., hats, long sleeves)
- Sunscreens >30 SPF

PROGNOSIS

Good with avoidance/protection measures

COMPLICATIONS

Rare (secondary bacterial infection)

REFERENCES

1. Deleo V. Sunscreen use in photodermatoses. *Dermatol Clin*. 2006;24:27–33.
2. Morison WL. Clinical practice. Photosensitivity. *N Engl J Med*. 2004;350:1111–7.
3. Rhodes LE, Durham BH, Fraser WD, et al. Dietary fish oil reduces basal and ultraviolet B-generated PGE2 levels in skin and increases the threshold to provocation of polymorphic light eruption. *J Invest Dermatol*. 1995;105:532–5.

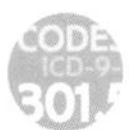

CODES

ICD9

- 692.70 Unspecified dermatitis due to sun
- 692.72 Acute dermatitis due to solar radiation
- 692.74 Other chronic dermatitis due to solar radiation

CLINICAL PEARLS

- Choose a sunscreen with an SPF of at least 30 with full-spectrum protection (UVA and UVB) for the best efficacy.
- The most common medications that predispose to photosensitivity include tetracyclines and sulfonamide. However, there are many other medications that may cause photosensitivity.

PILONIDAL DISEASE

Michael Rousse, MD, MPH

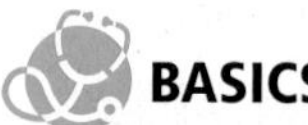

BASICS

DESCRIPTION
- Pilonidal disease results from an abscess, or sinus tract, in the upper part of the natal cleft.
- Synonym(s): Jeep disease

EPIDEMIOLOGY
Incidence
- 0.7%: 1.1% males, 0.1% females
- Predominant sex: Male > Female (3–4:1)
- Predominant age: Second to third decade, rare >45 years old
- Ethnic consideration: Whites > Blacks > Asians

Prevalence
Surgical procedures show male:female ratio of 4:1, yet incidence data are 10:1.

RISK FACTORS
- Sedentary/prolonged sitting
- Excessive body hair
- Obesity/increased sacrococcygeal fold thickness
- Congenital natal dimple
- Trauma to coccyx

Genetics
- Congenital dimple in the natal cleft/spina bifida occulta
- Follicular-occluding tetrad: Acne conglobata, dissecting cellulitis, hidradenitis suppurativa, pilonidal

GENERAL PREVENTION
- Weight loss
- Trim hair in/around gluteal cleft weekly
- Hygiene
- Ingrown hair prevention/follicle unblocking

PATHOPHYSIOLOGY
Pilonidal = "nest of hair"; excoriation by hair in the natal cleft allows hair to be drawn into the deeper tissues via negative pressure caused by movement of the buttocks (50%); follicular occlusion from stretching and blocking of pores with debris (50%)

ETIOLOGY
- Inflammation of SC gluteal tissues with secondary infection and sinus tract formation
- Polymicrobial, likely from enteric pathogens given proximity to anorectal contamination

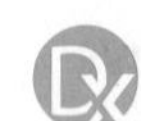

DIAGNOSIS

HISTORY
3 distinct clinical presentations:
- Asymptomatic: Painless cyst or sinus at the top of the gluteal cleft
- Acute abscess: Severe pain, swelling, discharge from the top of the gluteal cleft that may or may not have drained spontaneously
- Chronic abscess: Persistent drainage from a sinus tract at the top of the gluteal cleft

PHYSICAL EXAM
- Common: Inflamed cystic mass at the top of the gluteal cleft with limited surrounding erythema ± drainage or a sinus tract
- Less common: Significant cellulitis of the surrounding tissues near the gluteal cleft

DIAGNOSTIC TESTS & INTERPRETATION
Lab
Initial lab tests

CBC and wound culture

Imaging
Initial approach

MRI might be considered to differentiate between perirectal abscess and pilonidal disease.

DIFFERENTIAL DIAGNOSIS
- Furunculosis
- Hydradenitis suppurativa
- Anal fistula
- Perirectal abscess
- Crohn disease

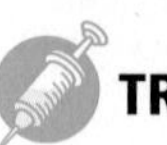

TREATMENT

MEDICATION
- Antibiotics not indicated unless there is significant cellulitis
- If antibiotics are needed, a culture to direct therapy might be useful.
- Cefazolin and metronidazole used empirically

ADDITIONAL TREATMENT
General Measures
Shave area; remove hair from crypts weekly.

Issues for Referral
- Patients who cannot comply with frequent dressing changes required after incision and drainage (I&D)
- Patients who have recurrence after I&D
- Patients who have complex disease with multiple sinus tracts

Additional Therapies
- I&D with only enough packing to allow the cyst to drain; overpacking not indicated
- Antibiotics only if significant cellulitis, temporizing, not curative

SURGERY/OTHER PROCEDURES

6 levels of care based on severity or recurrence of disease; recent innovations in technique are aimed at expediting healing and minimizing recurrence (1,2)[C]:

- I&D, remove hair, curette granulation tissue
- Excision of midline "pits" allows drainage of lateral sinus tracts (pit picking) (3)[C].
- Pilonidal cystotomy: Insert probe into sinus tract, excise overlying skin, and close wound (4)[B].
- Marsupialization: Excise overlying skin and roof of cyst, and suture skin edges to cyst floor.
- Excision: Use of flap closure (5)[B]
- Off-midline surgical excision (cleft lift or modified Karydakis procedure) (2,6)[B]

IN-PATIENT CONSIDERATIONS

Admission Criteria

- Severe cellulitis
- Large area excision

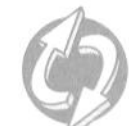

ONGOING CARE

FOLLOW-UP RECOMMENDATIONS

- Frequent dressing changes required after I&D
- Follow-up wound checks to assess for recurrence.

Patient Monitoring

Monitor for fever, more extensive cellulitis.

PATIENT EDUCATION

- Wash area briskly with washcloth daily.
- Shave the area weekly.
- Remove any embedded hair from the crypt.
- Avoid prolonged sitting.

PROGNOSIS

- Simple I&D has a 55% failure rate; median time to healing is 5 weeks.
- More extensive surgical excisions involve hospital stays and longer time to heal.

COMPLICATIONS

Malignant degeneration is a rare complication of untreated chronic pilonidal disease.

REFERENCES

1. Kement M, Oncel M, Kurt N, et al. Sinus excision for the treatment of limited chronic pilonidal disease: Results after a medium-term follow-up. *Dis Colon Rectum*. 2006;49:1758–62.
2. Theodropoulos GE, et al. Modified Bascom's asymmetric midgluteal cleft closure technique for recurrent pilonidal disease: Early experience in a military hospital. *Dis Colon Rectum*. 2003;49(11): 1755–7.
3. Iesalnieks I, Deimel S, Kienle K, et al. [Pit-picking surgery for pilonidal disease.] *Der Chirurg; Zeitschrift fur alle Gebiete der operativen Medizen*. 2011;82(10):927–31.
4. Rao MM, Zawislak W, Kennedy R, et al. A prospective randomised study comparing two treatment modalities for chronic pilonidal sinus with a 5-year follow-up. *Int J Colorectal Dis*. 2010;25:395–400.
5. Washer JD, Smith DE, Carman ME, et al. Gluteal fascial advancement: An innovative, effective method for treating pilonidal disease. *Am Surg*. 2010;76:154–6.
6. Rushfeldt C, Bernstein A, Norderval S, et al. Introducing an asymmetric cleft lift technique as a uniform procedure for pilonidal sinus surgery. *Scand J Surg*. 2008;97:77–81.

ADDITIONAL READING

- Ates M, Dirican A, Sarac M, et al. Short and long-term results of the Karydakis flap versus the Limberg flap for treating pilonidal sinus disease: A prospective randomized study. *Am J Surg*. 2011; 202(5):568–73.
- Aygen E, Arslan K, Dogru O, et al. Crystallized phenol in nonoperative treatment of previously operated, recurrent pilonidal disease. *Dis Colon Rectum*. 2010;53:932–5.
- Balik O, Balik AA, Polat KY, et al. The importance of local subcutaneous fat thickness in pilonidal disease. *Dis Colon Rectum*. 2006;49:1755–7.
- Harlak A, Mentes O, Kilic S, et al. Sacrococcygeal pilonidal disease: Analysis of previously proposed risk factors. *Clinics (Sao Paulo)*. 2010;65:125–31.
- Humphries AE, Duncan JE, et al. Evaluation and management of pilonidal disease. *Surg Clin North Am*. 2010;90:113–24, Table of Contents.
- Mohamed HA, Kadry I, Adly S. Comparison between three therapeutic modalities for non-complicated pilonidal sinus disease. *Surgeon*. 2005;3:73–7.
- Oram Y, Kahraman F, Karincaolu Y, et al. Evaluation of 60 patients with pilonidal sinus treated with laser epilation after surgery. *Dermatol Surg*. 2010; 36:88–91.

CODES

ICD9

- 685.0 Pilonidal cyst with abscess
- 685.1 Pilonidal cyst without mention of abscess

CLINICAL PEARLS

- Avoid prolonged sitting.
- Weight loss
- Trim hair in gluteal cleft weekly.

PINWORMS

Jonathan MacClements, MD

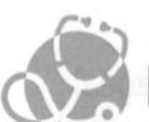

BASICS

DESCRIPTION
- Intestinal infection with *Enterobius vermicularis*, characterized by perineal and perianal itching, usually worse at night
- System(s) affected: Gastrointestinal; Skin/Exocrine
- Synonym: Enterobiasis

EPIDEMIOLOGY
Predominant age: 5–14 years

Prevalence
- Most common helminthic infection in the US, with 20–42 million people harboring the parasite
- ~30% of children are infected throughout the world.

Pediatric Considerations
More common in children, who are more likely to become reinfected

RISK FACTORS
- Institutionalization
- Crowded living conditions
- Poor hygiene
- Warm climate
- Handling of infected children's clothing or bedding

GENERAL PREVENTION
- Careful hand washing, especially after bowel movements; clip and maintain short fingernails.
- Wash anus and genitals at least once a day, preferably during a shower.
- Do not scratch anus or put fingers near nose or mouth.

PATHOPHYSIOLOGY
- Small white worms (2–13 mm) inhabit the cecum, appendix, and adjacent portions of the ascending colon following ingestion.
- Female worms migrate to the perianal and perineal areas at night, depositing ~11,000 eggs, resulting in irritation and itching of the perianal area.
- Scratching of the perianal and perineal areas followed by touching of the mouth can lead to ingestion of the eggs and continuation of pinworm's life cycle in the host.

ETIOLOGY
Infestation by the intestinal nematode *E.* (*Oxyuris*) *vermicularis*

COMMONLY ASSOCIATED CONDITIONS
Pruritus ani (1)

DIAGNOSIS

HISTORY
- Many patients are asymptomatic.
- Perianal itching
- Perineal itching
- Vulvovaginitis
- Dysuria
- Abdominal pain (rare)
- Insomnia
- Restless sleep

PHYSICAL EXAM
Perineal and perianal exam

DIAGNOSTIC TESTS & INTERPRETATION

Diagnostic Procedures/Surgery
- Adhesive tape test: A piece of transparent cellophane tape is stuck to the perianal skin in the early morning before bathing and then affixed to a microscope slide after removal. This procedure must be performed at least 3 times to achieve 90% sensitivity. Alternatively, anal swabs or a pinworm paddle coated with adhesive material also can be useful (2,3,4)[C].
- Digital rectal exam with saline slide preparation of stool on gloved finger (2)[C]
- *Routine stool examination for ova and parasites is positive in only 10–15% of infected patients.*

Pathological Findings
Identification of ova on low-power microscopy or direct visualization of the female worm (10 mm long); ova are asymmetric, flattened on 1 side, and measure 56 × 27 μm.

DIFFERENTIAL DIAGNOSIS
- Idiopathic pruritus ani
- Atopic dermatitis
- Contact dermatitis
- Psoriasis
- Lichen planus
- Infection with human papillomavirus
- Herpes simplex
- Fungal infections
- Erythrasma
- Scabies
- Vaginitis
- Hemorrhoids

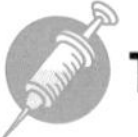

TREATMENT

MEDICATION

- Treatment options include any of the following (2,5)[A]:
  - Mebendazole (Vermox): Chewable 100-mg tablet as a single dose in adults and children >2 years of age; use with caution in children <2 years of age
  - Albendazole (Albenza): 400 mg PO as a single dose in adults and children >2 years of age; 100 mg PO as a single dose repeated in 7 days in children ≤2 years of age
  - Pyrantel pamoate (Pin-X, Reese's Pinworm Medicine): Oral liquid or tablet 11 mg/kg as a single dose in adults and children >2 years of age; maximum dose 1 g. Use with caution in children <2 years of age.
- Many clinicians recommend repeat treatment after 2 weeks due to the high frequency of reinfection and autoinfection. Occasionally, refractory cases may require re-treatment every 2 weeks for 4–6 cycles.
- All symptomatic family members should be treated.

Pregnancy Considerations

Drug therapy should be avoided in pregnancy. Treatment should be delayed until after delivery (6)[C].

ONGOING CARE

FOLLOW-UP RECOMMENDATIONS

Unnecessary unless symptoms do not abate following drug therapy

PATIENT EDUCATION

- Take medicine with food.
- Practice good hygiene.
- Encourage frequent and careful hand washing.
- Clip fingernails short.
- All clothing and bedding should be washed to prevent reinfection.
- Do not shake linen and clothing before laundering because this may spread the eggs.

PROGNOSIS

- Asymptomatic carriers are common.
- Symptomatic infections are cured >90% of the time by pharmacotherapy.
- Reinfection is common, especially among children.

COMPLICATIONS

- Perianal scratching may lead to bacterial superinfection.
- Females: Vulvovaginitis, urethritis, endometritis, salpingitis
- UTIs
- Rarely, ectopic disease involving granulomas of the pelvis, urinary tract, female genitourinary tract, and appendix

REFERENCES

1. Stermer E, Sukhotnic I, Shaoul R. Pruritus ani: An approach to an itching condition. *J Pediatr Gastroenterol Nutr*. 2009;48:513–6.
2. Jones JE. Pinworms. *Am Fam Phys*. 1988;38: 159–64.
3. Cram EB. Studies on oxyuriasis, 28. Summary and conclusions. *Am J Dis Child*. 1943;65:46–59.
4. Kucik CJ, et al. Common intestinal parasites. *Am Fam Phys*. 2004;69:1161–8.
5. *Enterobius vermicularis*. In: Drugs for Parasitic Infections. Treatment Guidelines from The Medical Letter Vol. 8 (Suppl), 2010.
6. Hamblin J, et al. Pinworms in pregnancy. *J Am Board Fam Practice*. 1995;8:321–4.

ADDITIONAL READING

- CDC Patient Education materials: www.cdc.gov/parasites/pinworm/.
- Jardine M, Kokai GK, Dalzell AM, et al. *Enterobius vermicularis* and colitis in children. *J Pediatr Gastroenterol Nutr*. 2006;43:610–2.
- Lamps LW, et al. Infectious causes of appendicitis. *Infect. Dis. Clin. North Am*. 2010;24:995–1018.

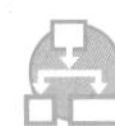

See Also (Topic, Algorithm, Electronic Media Element)

Pruritus Ani

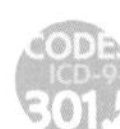

CODES

ICD9

127.4 Enterobiasis

CLINICAL PEARLS

- Treatment for pinworms includes use of mebendazole, albendazole, or pyrantelpamoate (2,5)[A].
- Close contacts should be treated as well.
- Retreatment after 2 weeks is recommended by many experts due to the difficulty in eradicating this parasite (2)[C].

PITUITARY ADENOMA

Anup K. Sabharwal, MD, FACE
Lewis S. Blevins, Jr., MD

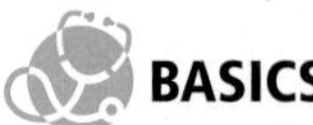

BASICS

DESCRIPTION

Typically benign, slow-growing tumors that arise from cells in the pituitary gland:

- Pituitary adenomas have been identified as the third most frequent intracranial tumor, and account for 10–25%.
- Autopsy and radiological data suggest that 1 in 6 have pituitary incidentalomas.
- Subtypes (hormonal): Prolactinoma (PRL) 50%, nonfunctioning pituitary adenomas 30%, somatotroph adenoma (growth hormone [GH]) 15–20%, corticotroph adenoma (adrenocorticotrophic hormone [ACTH]) 5–10%, thyrotroph adenoma (thyroid-stimulating hormone [TSH]) <1%, gonadotropinoma (luteinizing hormone/follicle-stimulating hormone [LH/FSH]), mixed
- Defined as microadenoma <10 mm and macroadenoma ≥10 mm
- May secrete hormones and/or cause mass effects

EPIDEMIOLOGY

- Predominant age: Age increases incidence
- Predominant sex: Female > Male (3:2) for microadenomas (often delayed diagnosis in men)

Incidence

- Autopsy studies: Pituitary microadenomas have been found in 3–27% of those without any pituitary disorders.
- Macroadenomas have been found in fewer than 0.5% of people.
- Clinically apparent pituitary tumors are seen in 18 per 100,000 persons.

RISK FACTORS

- Multiple endocrine neoplasia I
- Carney complex
- Familial isolated pituitary adenomas: ~15% have mutations in the aryl hydrocarbon receptor-interacting protein gene (AIP). Present at a younger age and are larger in size.
- McCune-Albright syndrome
- Multiple endocrine neoplasia (MEN) 1-like phenotype (MEN 4): Germline mutation in the cyclin-dependent kinase inhibitor 1B (CDKN1B)

Genetics

See "Diagnosis" and "Risk Factors" for syndromes.

PATHOPHYSIOLOGY

- Monoclonal adenohypophysial cell growth
- Hormonal effects of functional microadenomas often prompt diagnosis before mass effect
- Prolactin increased by functional prolactinomas or inhibited dopaminergic suppression by stalk effect

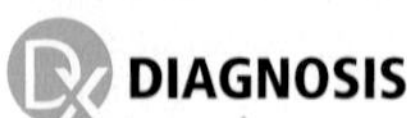

DIAGNOSIS

HISTORY

- Common:
  - Hyperprolactinemia: Infertility, amenorrhea, galactorrhea, gynecomastia, impotence
  - Headache (sellar expansion)
  - Visual disturbances: Bitemporal hemianopsia
- Less common:
  - Hypersomatotropinemia: Acromegaly (coarse facial features, hand/foot swelling, carpal tunnel syndrome, hyperhidrosis, left ventricular hypertrophy)
  - Hyposomatotropinemia: Failure to thrive (FTT) (children), asymptomatic (adults)
  - Intracranial pressure (ICP) elevation: Headache, nausea, seizures
  - Hypercorticotropinemia: Cushing disease (supraclavicular/dorsocervical fat pad thickening, moon face, hirsutism, acne, plethora, abdominal striae, centripetal obesity with thin limbs, easy bruising and bleeding, hyperglycemia)
- Rare:
  - Apoplexy: Headache, sudden collapse
  - Secondary hyperthyroidism: Palpitations, diaphoresis, heat intolerance, diarrhea
  - Secondary adrenal insufficiency: Weakness, irritability, anorexia, nausea/vomiting
- Hypothalamic compression: Temperature, thirst/appetite disorders

PHYSICAL EXAM

- Common:
  - Visual disturbances: Bitemporal hemianopsia
  - Hyperprolactinemia: Hypogonadism, galactorrhea, gynecomastia
  - Hypersomatotropinemia: Acromegaly (coarse features, hand/foot swelling, diaphoresis)
  - Hyposomatotropinemia: FTT (children)
- Less common:
  - ICP elevation: Papilledema, dementia
  - Cushing disease: Centripetal obesity, supraclavicular fat pad thickening, moon face, hirsutism, acne
- Rare:
  - Apoplexy: Hypotension, hypoglycemia, tachycardia, oliguria
  - Secondary hyperthyroidism: Tachycardia, tachypnea, diaphoresis, warm/moist skin, tremor
  - Adrenal crisis: Orthostatic hypotension
- Hypothalamic compression: Temperature dysregulation, obesity, increased urination

DIAGNOSTIC TESTS & INTERPRETATION

Lab

Select based on dysfunction(s) suspected.

- Somatotrophic (GH secreting: 40–130/million):
  - Acromegaly/hypersomatotropinemia: Serum IGF-1 elevated; oral glucose tolerance test with GH given at 0, 30, and 60 minutes (normally suppresses GH to <1 g/L)
  - Hyposomatotropinemia: Low growth hormone–releasing hormone response
- Corticotrophic:
  - Cushing disease/hypercorticotropinemia
  - 24-hour urinary-free cortisol >50 mcg
  - Overnight low-dose dexamethasone suppression test (DMST): Normal plasma cortisol (FPC) >1.8 μg/dL at 8 a.m. (after 1 mg given at 11 p.m. on night prior)
  - ACTH level assay (if DMST results abnormal): <20 pg/mL = adrenal tumor; ≥20 pg/mL = ectopic/pituitary source
  - Hypocorticotropinemia/secondary glucocorticoid deficiency: High-dose corticotropin stimulation test: FPC <10 g/dL at baseline with an increase of <25% 1 hour after 250 mcg; metyrapone test: 11-deoxycortisol <150 ng/L after 2 g given (prepare to give steroids because test may worsen insufficiency)
- Gonadotrophic: Hypogonadotropinism: Gonadotropin-releasing hormone stimulation of LH/FSH blunted in pituitary hypergonadism but increased in primary hypogonadism
- Lactotrophic (Prolactin secreting): Hyperprolactinemia: Serum PRL >20 ng/mL
- Thyrotrophic (TSH secreting): Hyper-/hypothyroidism: TSH and free T_4 both increased for pituitary hyperthyroidism and both decreased for pituitary hypothyroidism

Initial lab tests

- A typical panel for asymptomatic tumors: PRL, GH, IGF-1, ACTH, 24-hour urinary-free cortisol or overnight DMST, β-subunit FSH, LH, TSH, free T_4
- Screening for *AIP* mutations (see "Genetics") may be offered to families of patients with pituitary adenoma, where available (1)[B].

Imaging

- MRI preferred (>90% sensitivity/specificity) after biochemically confirmed
- Octreotide scintigraphy is useful in identifying tumors with somatostatin receptors.

Diagnostic Procedures/Surgery

Inferior petrosal sinus sampling: ACTH sampled from inferior petrosal sinuses to distinguish Cushing disease (pituitary source) from ectopic ACTH

Pathological Findings

- Cell types identified by immunohistochemistry
- Light microscope: Eosinophilic (GH, PRL), basophilic (FSH/LH, TSH, ACTH), chromophobic

DIFFERENTIAL DIAGNOSIS

Pituitary hyperplasia (e.g., pregnancy), Rathke cleft cyst, granulomatous disease (e.g., tuberculosis), lymphocytic hypophysitis, metastatic tumor, germinoma, craniopharyngioma

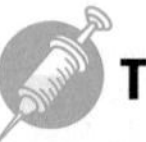

TREATMENT

Medical therapy is primary therapy for prolactinomas and adjunct for other tumors (2,3)[A].

MEDICATION

First Line

- Hyperprolactinemia: Dopamine agonists increase dopaminergic suppression of PRL:
  - Cabergoline (Dostinex): D_2 receptor-specific:
    - Initial dose: 0.25 mg PO once or twice weekly
    - Maintenance dose: Increase q4wk by 0.25 mg 2 ×/wk per PRL (maximum 2 mg/wk)
    - Contraindications: Hypersensitivity (ergots), hypertension (HTN), pregnancy
    - Precautions: Caution with liver impairment
    - Interactions: May be inhibited by tricyclic antidepressants, phenothiazines, opiates
    - Adverse reactions: Orthostatic hypotension, vertigo, dyspepsia, hot flashes
  - Bromocriptine (Parlodel): D_2 receptor-specific:
    - Initial dose: 1.25–2.5 mg PO daily (give with food)
    - Maintenance dose: Increase by 2.5 mg/d q2–7d (maximum 100 mg/d)

- Contraindications: Hypersensitivity (ergots), HTN, pregnancy; preferred over cabergoline if required
- Precautions: Caution with liver impairment
- Interactions: May be inhibited by tricyclic antidepressants, phenothiazines, opiates
- Adverse reactions: Orthostatic hypotension, seizures, hallucinations, stroke, myocardial infarction

- Somatotropinoma:
  - Long-acting analogues of somatostatin (Sandostatin LAR and Lanreotide Autogel):
    - Sandostatin LAR: 20 mg every 28 days; Lanreotide Autogel 90 mg every 28 days; titrate per package insert.
    - Contraindication: Hypersensitivity
    - Precautions: Caution with biliary, thyroid, cardiac, liver, or kidney disease
    - Interactions: Pimozide increases risk of QT prolongation; variable effects with β-blockers, diuretics, oral glycemic agents
    - Adverse reactions: Ascending cholangitis, arrhythmias, congestive heart failure, glycemic instability
    - More effective as adjuvant than as primary treatment for somatotropinomas (2)[A]
  - Pegvisomant (Somavert): Growth hormone receptor antagonist:
    - Initial dose: 40 mg SC × 1, then 20 mg daily and titrate by 5 mg every 4–6 weeks based on IGF-1 levels (maximum 30 mg/d maintenance dose)
    - Contraindication: Hypersensitivity
    - Precautions: Caution if GH-secreting tumors, diabetes mellitus, impaired liver function
    - Interactions: NSAIDs, opiates, insulins, oral glycemic agents
    - Adverse reactions: Hepatitis, tumor growth, GH-secreting
- Corticotropinemia: Peripheral inhibitors:
  - Mitotane (Lysodren):
    - Initial dose: 2–6 g PO t.i.d. (maximum 19 g/d)
    - Maintenance dose: 2–16 g t.i.d.
    - Contraindication: Hypersensitivity
    - Precautions: Caution with liver dysfunction and brain damage
    - Interactions: Contraindicated with rotavirus vaccine; caution with other vaccines
    - Adverse reactions: HTN, orthostatic hypotension, hemorrhagic cystitis, rash
  - Ketoconazole:
    - Dosing: 200 mg PO t.i.d. (maximum 1,200 mg/d)
    - Contraindications: Hypersensitivity, achlorhydria, fungal meningitis, impaired liver function
    - Precautions: Caution with liver dysfunction
    - Interactions: Contraindicated with cisapride, niacin, statins, pimozide, sirolimus; caution with other antifungals
    - Adverse reactions: Adrenal insufficiency, thrombocytopenia, hepatic failure, hepatotoxicity, anaphylaxis, leukopenia, hemolytic anemia
- Gonadotropinemia:
  - Bromocriptine: See above:
    - Initial dose: 1.25–2.5 mg PO daily (give with food), increase by 2.5 mg/d q2–7d (maximum 100 mg/d)
- Thyrotropinemia:
  - Somatostatin analogues: See above.

Second Line

- Corticotropinemia: Peripheral inhibitors:
  - Metyrapone:
    - Dose: 250–600 mg/d PO
    - Contraindication: Porphyria
    - Precautions: Caution in liver/thyroid disease
    - Interactions: Dilantin increases metabolism.
    - Adverse reactions: Nausea, hypotension
- Gonadotropinemia:
  - Octreotide: See above.

ADDITIONAL TREATMENT

Issues for Referral

- Neurosurgery consultation as soon as tumor with symptoms identified (except for prolactinoma)
- Ophthalmologist evaluation prior to surgery

Additional Therapies

- Fractionated radiotherapy: Often effective as adjunctive when surgery is inadequate (4)[A]
- Stereotactic radiosurgery: Alternative to surgery in high-risk patients or as adjunct (4)[B]

SURGERY/OTHER PROCEDURES

- Most are now done endoscopically via translabial/transsphenoidal approach
- Indications: Symptoms or treatment-resistant
- Follow-up: Serial neuro/hormonal evaluations to evaluate complications (e.g., diabetes insipidus, CNS damage) and need for more treatment (5)
- Remission rates: 72–87% for microadenoma but only 50–56% for macroadenomas (5)

IN-PATIENT CONSIDERATIONS

Initial Stabilization

- Pituitary apoplexy (see "Complications"): Must treat immediately to prevent death.
- Consider stress-dose steroids in frail or hemodynamically unstable patients.
- Maintain BP with fluids and/or pressor agents.
- Check serum sodium, serum osmolality, and urine specific gravity if polyuric or electrolytes are imbalanced.
- Contact neurosurgery.

Admission Criteria

Outpatient management unless apoplexy (see "Complications") or adrenal crisis

IV Fluids

- Diabetes insipidus: Hyposmolar IV fluids
- Adrenal crisis: Normal saline

Nursing

- Pituitary apoplexy: Monitor inputs/outputs (I/Os), central venous pressure, and ICP monitoring, and do frequent neurologic checks.
- Adrenal crisis: Monitor BP and I/Os.

Discharge Criteria

Keep as inpatients postoperatively until diabetes insipidus and/or adrenal insufficiency is managed.

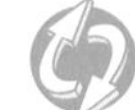

ONGOING CARE

FOLLOW-UP RECOMMENDATIONS

Patient Monitoring

- Follow-up MRIs at 6 and 12 months after discharge
- Involved hormone(s) are followed postoperatively, especially after radiation, because hypopituitarism may develop as late as 10–15 years later (2).

PROGNOSIS

- Depends on type, size, symptoms, therapy
- Acromegaly's 10-year life-expectancy reduction is prevented when GH <2.5 g/L (3).

COMPLICATIONS

- Postoperative diabetes insipidus and/or hypogonadism (usually transient/common)
- Pituitary apoplexy (acute/uncommon): Acute hemorrhagic pituitary infarction; adrenal crisis with severe headache; surgical decompression required to prevent shock, coma, and death
- Nelson syndrome (subacute/uncommon): Rapid adenoma growth postadrenalectomy
- Pituitary hormone insufficiency (chronic/uncommon): Often years after treatment
- Optic nerve neuropathy and brain necrosis after >60 Gy radiotherapy (chronic/rare)

REFERENCES

1. Georgitsi M, Raitila A, Karhu A. Molecular diagnosis of pituitary adenoma predisposition caused by aryl hydrocarbon receptor-interacting protein gene mutations. *Proc Natl Acad Sci U S A*. 2007;104:4101–5.
2. Tichomirowa MA, Daly AF, Beckers A. Treatment of pituitary tumors: Somatostatin. *Endocrine*. 2005; 28:93–100.
3. Drangé MR. Pituitary tumor registry: A novel clinical resource. *J Clin Endo Met*. 2000;85:168–74.
4. Mondok A, Szeifert GT, Mayer A. Treatment of pituitary tumors: Radiation. *Endocrine*. 2005;28: 77–85.
5. Buchfelder M. Treatment of pituitary tumors: Surgery. *Endocrine*. 2005;28:67–75.

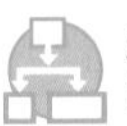

See Also (Topic, Algorithm, Electronic Media Element)

Cushing Disease and Cushing Syndrome; Galactorrhea

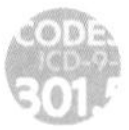

CODES

ICD9

227.3 Benign neoplasm of pituitary gland and craniopharyngeal duct

CLINICAL PEARLS

- An incidentaloma is an asymptomatic microadenoma found on imaging. General labs include PRL, GH, IGF-1, ACTH, 24-hour urinary-free cortisol or overnight DMST, β-subunit FSH, LH, TSH, and free T_4. Obtain follow-up MRIs at 6 and 12 months if normal, but consult endocrinology if not.
- The initial treatment selected for symptomatic pituitary adenoma includes a dopamine agonist for prolactinomas and surgical resection for all others.
- Pituitary apoplexy is a rapid hemorrhagic pituitary infarction due to compression of the blood supply. It is fatal within hours unless surgically decompressed.

PITYRIASIS ALBA

Brian B. Freniere, MD
Robert A. Baldor, MD

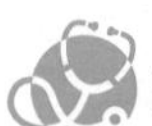

BASICS

DESCRIPTION

- A chronic skin disorder characterized by 1 or more groups of poorly marginated, pale pink or tan/white patches and plaques that appear on the cheeks, neck, and lateral arms of children and young adults
- System(s) affected: Skin/Exocrine
- Synonym(s): Pityriasis streptogenes; Pityriasis simplex; Pityriasis sicca faciei; Erythema streptogenes

Geriatric Considerations

Rare in this age group

Pediatric Considerations

More common in children aged 3–16 years

EPIDEMIOLOGY

Incidence

- Common; exact incidence unknown, but seen frequently in people with dark skin in sunnier climates
- Predominant age: 90% of affected patients are ages 6–12 years; rare >25 years
- Predominant sex: Male = Female

RISK FACTORS

Children with a genetic predisposition to atopic disease

Genetics

Unknown, but condition is seen primarily in children with a genetic predisposition to atopic disease

GENERAL PREVENTION

No known preventive measures (sun protection may minimize visibility of lesions)

ETIOLOGY

- Unknown; may be part of an atopic diathesis
- Possibly defects in melanin production or transfer

COMMONLY ASSOCIATED CONDITIONS

Atopic dermatitis

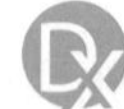

DIAGNOSIS

HISTORY

- Usually asymptomatic
- Pruritus (rare)
- More apparent in summertime in light-skinned people
- Lesions do not tan in summer.
- Even a small amount of sunlight exposure causes lesions to redden.

PHYSICAL EXAM

- Description: Small, ill-defined, pale pink or tan/white patches 0.5–5 cm
- Rash evolves from pink patch to white macule with fine scale to smooth hypopigmented macule
- Location: Cheeks, forehead, and lateral arms
- Number: 1–12 or more patches
- Palpation: Smooth or slightly rough, but dry
- Appearance: Pinpoint white papules (representing accentuation and keratinization of follicular orifices)
- Scale is either invisible or fine and light.

DIAGNOSTIC TESTS & INTERPRETATION

- Negative finding on potassium hydroxide (KOH) skin scraping
- Wood lamp exam can help demonstrate lesion borders and differentiate from fungal infection.

Pathological Findings

- Irregular melanin pigmentation of basal layer, follicular plugging, follicular spongiosis, and atrophic sebaceous glands
- Uncertain whether number of melanocytes is reduced in affected skin

DIFFERENTIAL DIAGNOSIS

- Tinea versicolor
- Vitiligo
- Postinflammatory hypomelanosis
- Chemical leukoderma
- Indeterminate or uncharacteristic leprosy
- T-cell lymphoma
- Sarcoidosis

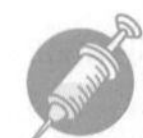

TREATMENT

MEDICATION

First Line

- Treatment is primarily symptomatic, as lesions tend to resolve spontaneously.
- Topical emollients and lubricants can be used to relieve dryness and/or roughness.
- Topical steroids (e.g., hydrocortisone acetate 1%) if needed to reduce redness and/or pruritus due to sunburn or spontaneous inflammation

Second Line

- Limited evidence to support the use of topical corticosteroids for resolution or treatment of extensive disease. Corticosteroids are not FDA approved for use in this condition (1)[C]. Long-term use has the potential to cause further depigmentation.
- Calcineurin inhibitors, pimecrolimus cream 1% applied topically b.i.d. (2)[C] and tacrolimus ointment 0.1% applied topically b.i.d. (3)[C] have been used with good effect for pityriasis alba associated with atopic dermatitis or more extensive involvement. Neither are currently FDA approved.
- Coal tar preparations (e.g., Alphosyl, Estar, Balnetar) applied topically once daily or b.i.d. for symptomatic relief

ALERT

- Extended duration or potent topical corticosteroid use on the face should be avoided.
- Use precaution in pediatric populations.
- Precautions: Refer to the manufacturer's literature for each drug.

ADDITIONAL TREATMENT

General Measures

Sun protection, including protective apparel and sunscreen, is essential.

Additional Therapies

Psoralen plus UVA (PUVA) considered for extensive involvement only (4)[C]

IN-PATIENT CONSIDERATIONS

Initial Stabilization

Outpatient

ONGOING CARE

FOLLOW-UP RECOMMENDATIONS

Patient Monitoring

As needed, only if lesions become symptomatic

DIET

No special diet

PATIENT EDUCATION

- Stress long-term chronicity and likely permanent resolution of condition in second or third decade of life.
- Sun protection

PROGNOSIS

- Permanent resolution during second or third decade of life in almost all cases
- Worse prognosis in patients with higher Fitzpatrick skin types

COMPLICATIONS

None expected

REFERENCES

1. Lin RL, Janniger CK, et al. Pityriasis alba. *Cutis*. 2005;76:21–4.
2. Fujita WH, McCormick CL, Parneix-Spake A, et al. An exploratory study to evaluate the efficacy of pimecrolimus cream 1% for the treatment of pityriasis alba. *Int J Dermatol*. 2007;46:700–5.
3. Rigopoulos D, Gregoriou S, Charissi C, et al. Tacrolimus ointment 0.1% in pityriasis alba: An open-label, randomized, placebo-controlled study. *Br J Dermatol*. 2006;155:152–5.
4. Di Lernia V, Ricci C, et al. Progressive and extensive hypomelanosis and extensive pityriasis alba: Same disease, different names? *J Eur Acad Dermatol Venereol*. 2005;19:370–2.

ADDITIONAL READING

- Halder RM, Nandedkar MA, Neal KW. Pigmentary disorders in ethnic skin. *Dermatol Clin*. 2003;21: 617–28, vii.
- Hall BJ, Hall JC. *Sauer's Manual of Skin Diseases*, 10th ed. Philadelphia: Lippincott Williams & Wilkins; 2010.
- In SI, Yi SW, Kang HY, et al. Clinical and histopathological characteristics of pityriasis alba. *Clin Exp Dermatol*. 2009;34:591–7.
- Jadotte YT, Janniger CK, et al. Pityriasis alba revisited: Perspectives on an enigmatic disorder of childhood. *Cutis*. 2011;87:66–72.
- Miller DC. Pigmentation disorders in adults. *Clin Fam Pract*. 2003;5(3):691.
- Plensdorf S, Martinez J, et al. Common pigmentation disorders. *Am Fam Physician*. 2009;79:109–16.

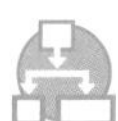

See Also (Topic, Algorithm, Electronic Media Element)

Keratosis, Actinic; Tinea Versicolor; Vitiligo

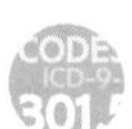

CODES

ICD9

696.5 Other and unspecified pityriasis

CLINICAL PEARLS

- More common in patients with atopic dermatitis
- Use of KOH preparation and Wood lamp is a quick way to differentiate this from a fungal infection (see "Tinea Versicolor").
- Treatment is largely symptomatic, and sun protection is essential.
- Topical calcineurin inhibitor therapy may become primary treatment for extensive pityriasis alba or when associated with atopic dermatitis.

PLACENTA PREVIA

Janelle M. Evans, MD

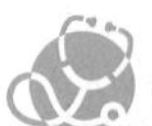

BASICS

DESCRIPTION
- Placental implantation in the lower uterine segment in advance of presenting fetal part and in proximity to or covering the internal os
- Complete previa: Placenta covers entire internal cervical os.
- Partial previa: Placenta covers part of internal cervical os.
- Marginal previa: No exact definition; commonly means placental edge is adjacent to cervical os by ultrasound but not overlapping
- Low-lying placenta: Placental edge located in the lower uterine segment but does not encroach on or cover the os; has been defined as within 2–3 cm of cervical os by ultrasound
- System(s) affected: Cardiovascular; Reproductive

EPIDEMIOLOGY
- Average gestational age of first bleed, 27–36 weeks
- Most common cause of minimally painful bleeding after 20 weeks' gestational age
- ~10% of low-lying placentas at 10–20 weeks persist to term.
- Some evidence that shortened cervical length in the third trimester is associated with increased risk of bleeding

Incidence
- ~0.4% of primiparous pregnancies, with increasing incidence with cesarean deliveries or other uterine scarring in future pregnancies
- Up to 5% incidence in grand multiparous women

RISK FACTORS
- History of placenta previa (relative risk [RR] = 8)
- Advanced maternal age (RR = 9 if >40 years of age)
- Multiparity (5% if >5 deliveries) (RR = 1.1–1.7)
- Assisted reproductive technology (RR = 2)
- Multiple gestation
- Smoking (RR = 1.4–3)
- Cocaine use
- Male fetus (RR = 1.4)
- Asian (RR = 1.9)
- Previous cesarean deliveries:
  - 1 previous C-section: RR = 1.5 (95% confidence interval [CI] 1.3–1.8)
  - 2 previous C-sections: RR = 2 (95% CI 1.3–3)
  - 4 previous C-sections: RR = 44.9 (95% CI 13.5–15)
- Induced or spontaneous abortion/curettage (Ashermans) (RR = 1.6)
- Leiomyoma or history of lower uterine segment surgery

Genetics
No genetic links have been identified.

GENERAL PREVENTION
Once pregnancy is diagnosed, risk factors are not modifiable. If patient has any risk factors for previa and anatomic survey is suggestive of previa, serial ultrasounds should be performed for monitoring purposes. Patient should be counseled regarding potential bleeding and should be triaged with all bleeding episodes.

PATHOPHYSIOLOGY
- Invasion of trophoblastic giant cells into the decidua, myometrium, and myometrial spiral arteries
- Increased inflammatory cell infiltration compared with women with normal implantation sites
- As lower uterine segment expands and the trophoblastic tissue expands toward the fundus, many marginal or low-lying placentas will resolve to a safe distance from the cervix to allow vaginal delivery (1).

ETIOLOGY
Prior endometrial insult/injury/scar or other unknown uterine factors, as listed previously

COMMONLY ASSOCIATED CONDITIONS
- Abnormal presentations (e.g., oblique and/or transverse fetal lie)
- Antepartum/intrapartum/postpartum hemorrhage
- Small for gestational age or intrauterine growth restriction (up to 16% in some reports after controlling for confounders)
- Vasa previa or velamentous insertion of the cord
- Premature rupture of membranes due to antepartum bleeding
- 5–10% of previas are associated with placenta accreta:
  - Placenta accreta encompasses various types of abnormal placentations in which chorionic villi attach directly to or invade the myometrium but do not cross the uterine serosa.
  - Placenta accreta affects ~1/2,500 pregnancies with increasing prevalence due to increased rates of cesarean section.
  - Risk greater with increasing number of cesarean deliveries
  - Associated with an increased risk of hemorrhage necessitating cesarean hysterectomy

DIAGNOSIS

HISTORY
- Painless, bright-red vaginal bleeding in second or third trimester (classic presentation)
- Contractions also may be present.
- Decreased fetal movement or nonreassuring fetal heart tracing

PHYSICAL EXAM

ALERT
- Do not perform digital cervical exam until placental position has been verified in any woman with a complaint of bleeding.
- Careful sterile speculum exam not contraindicated
- Check for vaginal or cervical source of bleeding.
- Check for rupture of membranes with standard tests.
- Perform cultures: *Gonorrhea*, *Chlamydia*, group B *Streptococcus*

DIAGNOSTIC TESTS & INTERPRETATION
- If patient is Rh-negative, Kleihauer-Betke test for maternal–fetal hemorrhage to determine if Rho(D) immunoglobulin (RhoGAM) is needed
- Ultrasound to confirm presence of previa
- Rule out accreta, percreta if suspicious findings on ultrasound
- Fetal testing and monitoring during all active bleeding

Lab
Initial lab tests
- Maternal blood type and antibody screen
- CBC: Normocytic, normochromic anemia with acute bleeding
- Prothrombin time (PT)/international normalization ratio (INR), and partial thromboplastin time (PTT): Coagulopathy is rare but may occur.
- Fibrinogen is optional, and DIC panel is often inconclusive.
- Kleihauer-Betke test: Positive test indicates fetal–maternal transfusion may be present.
- Cross-match at least 4 units of packed RBCs if bleeding ≥1 soaked pad/hr

Follow-Up & Special Considerations
Repeat hemoglobin/hematocrit determinations as needed to assess blood loss.

Imaging
Development of ultrasound, especially the transvaginal scan, has helped in the definitive diagnosis and management of placenta previa (2).

Initial approach
- External abdominal sonography with full, then empty bladder. Full bladder can cause compression of lower uterine segment causing a false appearance of previa.
- Careful assessment may still miss some posterior previas if fetal vertex is low.
- Vaginal probe sonography using 8.4 MHz transducer to further define placental position. Translabial ultrasound may also be utilized, but may not be able to specifically discern characteristics of previas.
- Given increased risk of accreta, the placental-uterine interface should be closely examined for evidence of lakes or other abnormal vasculature.
- MRI if concerned for placenta accreta without definitive ultrasound diagnosis; important also for surgical planning

Follow-Up & Special Considerations
- Previas found on ultrasound before 35 weeks should have a repeat ultrasound prior to delivery:
  - 12% of previas at 10–20 weeks persist until term.
  - 62% of previas at 28–31 weeks persist until term.
  - 75% of previas at 32–35 weeks persist until term.
- Anterior previas are more likely to resolve than posterior previas, since the anterior lower uterine segment expands more quickly.

Pathological Findings
Placental pathology often shows giant trophoblasts at placental interface, evidence of abruption.

DIFFERENTIAL DIAGNOSIS
- Abruptio placentae
- Vasa previa
- Varicosities
- Vaginal and cervical pathology, including erosion, cancer, trauma, or infections

TREATMENT

MEDICATION

First Line

- Oxygen supplementation if needed
- Aggressive IV fluids/blood products as needed: Fresh-frozen plasma, platelets, and packed RBCs
- Tocolytics for uterine contractions may be used with caution, especially to allow for steroids for fetal lung maturity if possible (3)[A]. Calcium channel blockers such as nifedipine, loading dose of 10 mg PO q20min × 3, then q4–6h:
  - Watch for placental hypoperfusion (nonreassuring fetal heart tracing).
  - Contraindications: Term fetus or unstable maternal or fetal cardiovascular status

Second Line

Alternative tocolytics:

- β-agonists such as terbutaline 0.25 mg SC q3–4h; watch for maternal–fetal tachycardia and maternal hypertension and pulmonary edema.
- Magnesium sulfate 4–6 g IV load over 20 minutes, then 2–3 g/hr continuous infusion (4)[A]; watch for toxicity: loss of reflexes, pulmonary edema, cardiac arrest

ADDITIONAL TREATMENT

General Measures

- Decrease physical activity to avoid bleeding.
- Avoid vaginal exams, sexual intercourse, douching, or other vaginal manipulation.
- If stable maternal–fetal status, delay delivery until 38 weeks (5)[C].
- Amniocentesis to determine fetal lung maturity for elective delivery <38 weeks
- A trial of labor may be considered with anterior previa >2 cm away from the cervix (6)[B].
- Transfuse platelets at <20,000 (or <50,000–100,000 depending on institutional guidelines prior to surgery).
- Blood volume is increased in pregnancy; patient can lose >30% maternal blood volume before shock develops.
- Central line placement as needed after checking coagulation studies
- With significant hemorrhage, Rh-negative women should receive 300 μg Rho(D) immunoglobulin (RhoGAM).

Issues for Referral

- Maternal–fetal medicine consult for delivery decisions regarding stable patients
- Neonatal ICU team should be alerted for high-risk delivery and consulted for preterm delivery.
- Appropriate interdisciplinary planning with blood bank, anesthesia, staff regarding plans if massive hemorrhage ensues intraoperatively or if unanticipated accreta encountered

Additional Therapies

Recombinant factor VII is an alternative blood product for disseminated intravascular coagulopathy when fresh-frozen plasma and cryoprecipitate fail (7)[C].

SURGERY/OTHER PROCEDURES

Cesarean delivery is indicated for partial or complete previa when fetal lung maturity is demonstrated or when patient becomes unstable secondary to blood loss prior to fetal maturity.

IN-PATIENT CONSIDERATIONS

Initial Stabilization

- Bed rest and NPO until delivery decision made
- 2 large-bore IV sites and IV fluids as needed for resuscitation
- Continuous fetal heart and contraction monitoring

Admission Criteria

- Heavy vaginal bleeding warrants inpatient observation at least until hemodynamically stable
- First bleed usually is self-limited. Patients should be observed and steroids for fetal lung maturity administered. Once stable, preterm patients may be observed on an outpatient basis without difference in outcome (5)[B].
- Multiple large bleeds may necessitate admission until scheduled delivery between 34 and 36 weeks depending on institutional guidelines.
- May consider transfer to high-risk perinatology service based on patient condition, local services, and concern for accreta
- Evidence that shortened cervical length in the third trimester is an independent risk factor for bleeding episodes (8)

IV Fluids

Lactated Ringer's or normal saline solution

Nursing

- Continuous fetal heart and contraction monitoring
- Frequent vital signs, including fluid intake and output

Discharge Criteria

- Demonstration of fetal well-being by fetal heart tracing or biophysical profile
- Demonstration of maternal hemodynamic stability: No active bleeding for >48 hours
- Proximity of patient to health care facility and patient reliability

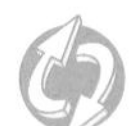

ONGOING CARE

FOLLOW-UP RECOMMENDATIONS

- Repeat ultrasound of placenta location if last ultrasound was done at <37 weeks gestational age.
- Placentas should be sent for pathologic evaluation.

DIET

No restrictions once stable; NPO if delivery possible

PATIENT EDUCATION

www.nlm.nih.gov/medlineplus/ency/article/000900.htm

PROGNOSIS

- Maternal death is rare with cesarean section (<1%).
- Greatest fetal risk is preterm delivery and consequences of hypoxemia if delay in delivery with fetal tracing abnormalities.
- Perinatal mortality is <10%.

COMPLICATIONS

- History of prior cesarean section and/or general anesthesia increases risk of needing a blood transfusion.
- Placenta accreta is associated with increased risk of hemorrhage and need for cesarean hysterectomy.
- Disseminated intravascular coagulation risk is low unless massive bleeding is present. Follow coagulation studies, and replenish FFP and clotting factors as needed.
- Fetal anemia and Rh isoimmunization

REFERENCES

1. Predanci M, et al. A sonographic assessment of different patterns of placenta previa "migration" in the third trimester of pregnancy. *J Ultrasound Med*. 2005;24:773.
2. Sinha P, Kuruba N. Ante-partum haemorrhage: An update. *J Obstet Gynaecol*. 2008;28:377–81.
3. Sharma A, Suri V, Gupta I. Tocolytic therapy in conservative management of symptomatic placenta previa. *Int J Gynaecol Obstet*. 2004;84:109–13.
4. Briggs GG, Wan SR. Drug therapy during labor and delivery, part 2 [Review]. *Am J of Health-System Pharm*. 2006;63(12):1131–9.
5. Oyelese Y, Smulian JC. Placenta previa, placenta accreta, and vasa previa. *Obstet Gynecol*. 2006; 107:927–41.
6. Bhide A, Prefumo F, Moore J, et al. Placental edge to internal os distance in the late third trimester and mode of delivery in placenta praevia. *BJOG*. 2003;110:860–4.
7. Alfirevic Z, Elbourne D, Pavord S, et al. Use of recombinant activated factor VII in primary postpartum hemorrhage: The Northern European registry 2000–2004. *Obstet Gynecol*. 2007;110: 1270–8.
8. Stafford IA, Dashe JS, Shivvers SA, et al. Ultrasonographic cervical length and risk of hemorrhage in pregnancies with placenta previa. *Obstet Gynecol*. 2010;116:595–600.

ADDITIONAL READING

Creasy RK, Resnik R, Iams J, et al. Placenta previa and abruptio placentae. In: *Creasy and Resnik's Maternal-Fetal Medicine: Principles and Practice: Expert Consult*, 6th ed. Philadelphia: WB Saunders; 2008:725–29.

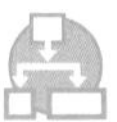

See Also (Topic, Algorithm, Electronic Media Element)

Abruptio Placentae

CODES

ICD9

- 641.00 Placenta previa without hemorrhage, unspecified as to episode of care or not applicable
- 641.01 Placenta previa without hemorrhage, delivered, with or without mention of antepartum condition
- 641.03 Placenta previa without hemorrhage, antepartum condition or complication

CLINICAL PEARLS

- Placenta previa is a major cause of antepartum bleeding in the second and third trimesters.
- Do *not* perform digital cervical exam, only careful speculum exam.
- Ultrasound, both transvaginal and transabdominal, is used to verify placenta location and diagnosis.
- Delivery is by cesarean section with rare exceptions.

PLANTAR FASCIITIS

Katie Crowder, MD
Alan Williamson, MD

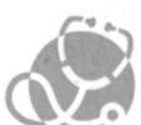

BASICS

DESCRIPTION
- Degenerative change of plantar fascia at origin from medial tuberosity of calcaneus
- Pain on plantar surface, usually at calcaneal insertion of plantar fascia upon weight-bearing, especially in morning or initiation of walking after prolonged rest

EPIDEMIOLOGY
Prevalence
- Lifetime: 10–15% of population
- Data suggest persistence with BMI >30.
- Condition is self-limiting; typically resolves within 10 months.

RISK FACTORS
- Dancers, runners, aerobic exercisers
- Obesity
- Pes planus (flat feet)
- Systemic connective tissue disorders
- Occupations with prolonged standing, especially on hard surfaces (RNs, letter carriers, warehouse/factory workers)
- Female, pregnancy
- >40–60 years

GENERAL PREVENTION
- Maintain normal body weight. Higher prevalence with BMI >30.
- Avoid prolonged standing on bare feet, sandals, or slippers.

PATHOPHYSIOLOGY
- Repetitive partial tearing of plantar fascia
- Chronic degenerative change (-osis/opathy rather than -itis) of plantar fascia generally at insertion on medial tuberosity of calcaneus

ETIOLOGY
- Excessive pronation
- Decreased ankle range of motion in dorsiflexion (tight heel chord; <10° dorsiflexion)

COMMONLY ASSOCIATED CONDITIONS
- Usually isolated
- Heel spurs common, but not marker of severity
- Posterior tibial neuropathy

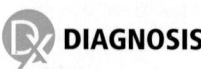

DIAGNOSIS

HISTORY
- Pain on plantar surface of foot, usually at fascial insertion at calcaneus, but can have pain anywhere along length of plantar fascia. Pain is typically worse on arising from sleep; first few steps in the morning or after prolonged rest ("poststatic dyskinesia").
- Pain with prolonged ambulation or standing
- Limp with excessive toe walking
- Numbness and burning of medial hindfoot when associated with posterior tibial nerve compression
- Pain can be dull and constant in chronic plantar fasciitis.

PHYSICAL EXAM
- Point tenderness on medial tuberosity of calcaneus at insertion of plantar fascia
- Pain along plantar fascia with foot dorsiflexion
- Decreased passive range of motion in dorsiflexion of ankle
- Spasm in foot muscles that compensate for injury

DIAGNOSTIC TESTS & INTERPRETATION
Imaging
- None necessary for the diagnosis
- 2 radiographic views of foot to rule out fracture, tumor, cyst, periostitis, bony erosions; prefer weightbearing
- Ultrasound (US): Demonstrates signs of inflammation at insertion (hypoechoic), including thickened plantar fascia (≥4 mm)
- Consider MRI for complex conditions or if concerned about other soft tissue etiologies.
- CT or technetium 99 bone scan to rule out calcaneal stress fracture

DIFFERENTIAL DIAGNOSIS
- Posterior tibial nerve compression (also known as tarsal tunnel syndrome) diagnosed if compression of region between medial malleolus and calcaneous results in numbness in first 3 toes
- Painful or atrophic heel pad
- Tendonitis of posterior tibialis
- Calcaneal stress fracture
- Plantar calcaneal bursitis
- Calcaneal contusion
- Plantar fascia tear
- Pain from neoplasm or infection
- Spondyloarthropathy (Reiter syndrome)
- In association with connective tissue disorder:
  - RA
  - Polymyositis

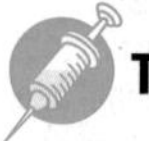

TREATMENT

Nonoperative management is mainstay of treatment.

MEDICATION
First Line
NSAIDS (1): Naprosyn 500 mg PO b.i.d. or ibuprofen 600–800 mg PO t.i.d. PRN for pain (6)[A]

Second Line
Limited evidence for topical NSAIDS

ADDITIONAL TREATMENT
General Measures
- Supportive footwear with stable midfoot; avoid wearing sandals or walking barefoot.
- Relative rest/activity modification
- Ice (frozen water bottle roll)
- Massage (golf ball roll)
- Weight reduction
- Stretching: Plantar fascial stretches more effective than Achilles tendon stretches (2)[B]
- Interosseous muscle strengthening utilizing the towel drag/pick-up exercise

Issues for Referral
- Consider referral for more invasive treatments if conservative measures (stretching, icing, massage, NSAIDs, OTC orthotics, night splints) fail after 3–6 months.
- Podiatry
- Custom orthotics
- Physical therapy
- Surgical intervention

Additional Therapies
- Taping (3)[B]:
  - Low-dye taping
  - Calcaneal taping more effective than stretching
  - Less effective in severe cases
- Night splints: Can be uncomfortable for the first few nights, but generally become less bothersome with time
- Corticosteroid injections (4)[B]:
  - Short-term pain relief
  - Recommend US guidance.
  - Risk for plantar fascial rupture and calcaneal fat pad atrophy with resultant permanent heel pain
  - Can cause injection pain and postinjection pain for up to 5–7 days
- Orthotics (5)[B]:
  - Custom orthotics show no benefit over prefabricated orthotics.
  - Improved effectiveness of night splints when used in association with orthotics
- Extracorporeal shock wave therapy (ESWT) of unclear benefit in large trials:
  - Newer ESWT devices show more promise.
  - Randomized trial demonstrated reduction in pain after 3 months compared with placebo.
  - Randomized trial in 2006 showed improvement in walking 3 months following a single treatment.
  - Randomized trial in 2009 showed improvement in pain at 12 weeks and 12 months compared with placebo.
  - Majority of studies focused on chronic plantar fasciitis.
  - Uncomfortable to patients
- Some orthopedic surgeons prefer casting in severe cases.
- Promising therapies:
  - Platelet-rich plasma injections
  - Intralesional autologous blood injection
  - Intracorporeal pneumatic shock application
  - Low-level laser therapy (LLLT)

COMPLEMENTARY AND ALTERNATIVE MEDICINE
- Botulinum toxin injection: RCT demonstrated improvement in pain and gait at 3 weeks and 3 months compared with placebo.
- Heel cup with magnet has proven ineffective.

SURGERY/OTHER PROCEDURES

- Only necessary in a small percentage of patients (10%)
- Recommended after resistance to conservative treatment of 6–12 months
- Open/endoscopic plantar fasciotomy (less complications with endoscopic technique)
- Calcaneal spur resection
- Other: Cryosurgery (leads to long-term heel numbness), radiofrequency nerve ablation (uses heat), Coblation therapy (uses Topaz wand)
- More likely beneficial in severely obese

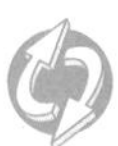

ONGOING CARE

FOLLOW-UP RECOMMENDATIONS

- Ensure patient is adhering to proper stretching exercises.
- Following 6 weeks of conservative treatment, consider formal physical therapy program if conservative measures do not show improvement.

PATIENT EDUCATION

- Weight reduction
- Stretch plantar fascia by pulling toes into dorsiflexion upon rising from prolonged sitting to standing prior to walking
- Ice the foot using a frozen water bottle, rolling foot over bottle for 10 minutes in morning and after work.
- Massage plantar fascia by rolling foot over a golf ball.
- Grab cloth or carpet by plantar flexing of toes.
- For athletes, back off on repetitive stress.
- Taping may help athletes.
- Video overview for patients: www.youtube.com/watch?v=Pnithn4EYQk

PROGNOSIS

- Excellent
- Self-limited condition in up to 85–90% of patients

COMPLICATIONS

- Rupture of plantar fascia (more common with repeated corticosteroid injections)
- Chronic pain
- Gait abnormality

REFERENCES

1. Donley BG, Moore T, Sferra J, et al. The efficacy of oral nonsteroidal anti-inflammatory medication (NSAID) in the treatment of plantar fasciitis: A randomized, prospective, placebo-controlled study. *Foot Ankle Int*. 2007;28:20–3.
2. Digiovanni BF, Nawoczenski DA, Malay DP, et al. Plantar fascia-specific stretching exercise improves outcomes in patients with chronic plantar fasciitis. A prospective clinical trial with two-year follow-up. *J Bone Joint Surg Am*. 2006;88:1775–81.
3. Speksnijder C, van de Water A. Efficacy of taping for the treatment of plantar fasciosis. A systematic review of controlled trials. *J Am Podiatr Med Assoc*. 2010;100(1):41–51.
4. Thomas J, Christensen J, Kravitz S, et al. The diagnosis and treatment of heel pain: A clinical practice guideline—Revision 2010. *J Foot Ankl Surg*. 2010;49:S1–S19.
5. Burns J, du Toit V, Hawke F, et al. Custom-made foot orthoses for the treatment of foot pain. *Cochrane Database Sys Rev*. 2008;(3):CD006801.
6. Crawford F, et al. Interventions for treating plantar heel pain. *Cochrane Database Sys Rev*. 2006;1:CD000416.

ADDITIONAL READING

- Dogramaci Y, Emir A, Gokce A. Intracorporeal pneumatic shock application for the treatment of chronic plantar fasciitis: A randomized, double blind prospective clinical trial. *Arch Orthop Trauma Surg*. 2009;130(4):541–6.
- Furia J. Maffulini N, Rompe J, et al. Shock wave therapy for chronic plantar fasciopathy. *Br Med Bull*. 2007;81/82:183–208.
- Hayley U, Boesch E, Kumar S. Plantar fasciitis-to jab or to support? A systematic review of the current best evidence. *J Multidiscip Healthc*. 2011;4:155–64.
- Healy K, Chen K. Plantar fasciitis: Current diagnostic modalities and treatments. *Clin Podiatr Med Surg*. 2010;27:369–80.
- Huang YC, Wei SH, Wang HK, et al. Ultrasonographic guided botulinum toxin type A treatment for plantar fasciitis: An outcome-based investigation for treating pain and gait changes. *J Rehab Med*. 2010;42(2):136–40.
- Ibrahim M, Donatelli R, Schmitz C, et al. Chronic plantar fasciitis treated with two sessions of radial extracorporeal shock wave therapy. *Foot Ankle Int*. 2010;31(5):391–7.
- Kiritsi O, Tsitas K, Malliaropoulos N, et al. Ultrasonographic evaluation of plantar fasciitis after low-level laser therapy: Results of a double-blind, randomized, placebo-controlled trial. *Lasers Med Sci*. 2010;25:275–81.
- Lee T, Ahmad T. Intralesional autologous blood injection compared to corticosteroid injection for treatment of chronic plantar fasciitis. A prospective, randomized, controlled trial. *Foot Ankle Int*. 2007;28(9):984–90.

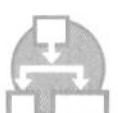

See Also (Topic, Algorithm, Electronic Media Element)

Algorithm: Heel Pain

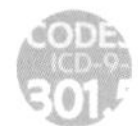

CODES

ICD9

728.71 Plantar fascial fibromatosis

CLINICAL PEARLS

- Degeneration of plantar fascia at origin from plantar tuberosity of calcaneum
- Pain on plantar surface on weightbearing, especially first few steps in the morning or after prolonged rest
- Conservative treatment is the mainstay of therapy:
  - Wear supportive footwear, particularly rigid shoes, to help avoid excess pronation.
  - Arch supports and/or athletic taping may be of benefit.
  - Activity modification, weight reduction
  - Stretching, NSAIDs
  - Ice (frozen water bottle roll), massage (golf ball roll)

PLEURAL EFFUSION

Felix B. Chang, MD

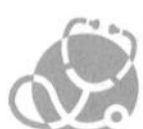

BASICS

A pleural effusion is an abnormal accumulation of fluid in the pleural space.

DESCRIPTION

- Pneumonia (25%), malignancy (15%), and pulmonary embolism (10%) account for exudative effusions.
- Malignant: Lung cancer and metastases of breast, ovary, and lymphoma constitute ~75–80%

EPIDEMIOLOGY

Incidence

Estimated 1.3 million cases/yr in the US; congestive heart failure (CHF), 500,000; pneumonia, 300,000; malignancy, 200,000; pulmonary embolus, 150,000; cirrhosis with ascites, 150,000; tuberculosis, 2,500; pancreatitis, 20,000; and collagen-vascular disease, 6,000 (1)

Prevalence

- Estimated 320 cases/1 million people in industrialized countries
- No gender predilection: About 2/3 of malignant pleural effusions occur in women.
- The prevalence of pleural effusion in hospitalized patients with AIDS is 7–27%.

RISK FACTORS

- Occupational exposures and drugs
- Risk factors for pulmonary embolism (PE) and tuberculosis (TB)
- Opportunistic infections (in HIV patients when the CD4 count is <150 cells/μL)
- Bacterial pneumonias (40%)

PATHOPHYSIOLOGY

Pleural fluid formation exceeds pleural fluid absorption. Transudates result from imbalances in hydrostatic and oncotic forces.

- Increase in hydrostatic and/or low oncotic pressures
- Increase in pleural capillary permeability
- Lymphatic obstruction or impaired drainage
- Movement of fluid from the peritoneal or retroperitoneal space

ETIOLOGY

- Transudates:
  - CHF: 40% of transudative effusions; 80% bilateral. Constrictive pericarditis, atelectasis
  - Cirrhosis (hepatic hydrothorax): 2/3 right side; nephrotic syndrome, hypoalbuminemia
  - Trapped lung, peritoneal dialysis; myxedema, superior vena cava obstruction
  - Urinothorax, central line misplacement; peritoneal dialysis
- Exudates:
  - Lung parenchyma infection, bacterial: Parapneumonic, tuberculous pleurisy, fungal, viral
  - Parasitic (amebiasis, *Echinococcus*)
  - Malignancy: Lung cancer, metastases (breast, lymphoma, ovaries), mesothelioma
  - Pulmonary embolism (although 25% of PEs are transudate)
  - Collagen-vascular disease: Rheumatoid arthritis, systemic lupus erythematosus (SLE), Wegener granulomatosis, sarcoidosis
  - GI: Pancreatitis, esophageal rupture, abdominal abscess, after liver transplant
  - Chylothorax: Thoracic duct tear, malignancy
  - Hemothorax: Trauma, PE, malignancy, coagulopathy, aortic aneurysm
  - Others: After coronary artery bypass grafting (CABG); Dressler syndrome: pericarditis and pleuritis after myocardial infarction (MI); uremia, asbestos exposure, radiation; drug-induced: nitrofurantoin, bromocriptine, amiodarone, procarbazine, methysergide, hydralazine, procainamide, quinidine, methotrexate, and methysergide; Meigs syndrome: benign ovarian tumor, ascites, and pleural effusion; yellow-nail syndrome: yellow nails, lymphedema, pleural effusion, and bronchiectasis; atelectasis, cholesterol effusion; ovarian stimulation syndrome; lymphangiomatosis; acute respiratory distress syndrome (ARDS)

COMMONLY ASSOCIATED CONDITIONS

- Hypoproteinemia
- Heart failure

DIAGNOSIS

- Presumptive diagnosis based on clinical impression in 50%.
- Small pleural effusions are asymptomatic.

HISTORY

- The degree of dyspnea is related to the associated lung disease, respiratory function, and the size of the pleural effusion.
- Fever, malaise, and weight loss with empyema; chest pain, either constant or pleuritic; nonproductive or purulent cough, hemoptysis

PHYSICAL EXAM

- Pleural effusion >300 mL: No voice transmission; tachypnea; asymmetric expansion of the thoracic cage; mediastinal shift (>1,000 mL)
- Pulmonary: Decreased or inaudible breath sounds; dullness to percussion; decreased or absent tactile fremitus; egophony; pleural friction rub

DIAGNOSTIC TESTS & INTERPRETATION

Lab

Initial lab tests

- Pleural fluid: Appearance, pH, WBC differential, total protein, lactate dehydrogenase (LDH), glucose, Gram stain and culture, acid-fast bacilli staining
- By clinical scenario: Amylase, triglycerides, cholesterol, LE cells, cytology, antinuclear antibodies (ANAs), adenosine deaminase, tumor markers, rheumatoid factor, cytology
- Transudate vs. exudate:
  - Light criteria for exudate: 98% sensitivity, 80% specificity (2)[B]:
    - Ratio of pleural fluid/serum protein levels >0.5
    - Ratio of pleural fluid/serum LDH levels >0.6
    - Pleural fluid LDH level >2/3 the upper limit for serum LDH level
  - Exudate criteria:
    - Serum-effusion albumin gradient ≤1.2; sensitivity 87%, specificity 92% (3)[B]
    - Cholesterol effusion >45 mg/dL and LDH effusion >200 mg/dL; sensitivity 90%, specificity 98%

Follow-Up & Special Considerations

- 75% of patients with exudative effusions have a non-CHF cause.
- 30% of cases of PE in AIDS patients are due to bacterial pneumonia.

Imaging

Initial approach

- Chest x-ray (CXR): Posteroanterior–anteroposterior (PA-AP) views:
  - Upright x-rays show a concave meniscus in the costophrenic angle that suggests >250 mL of pleural fluid; homogeneous opacity and diffuse haziness, visibility of pulmonary vessels through the haziness, and an absence of air bronchogram; 75 mL of fluid will obliterate the posterior costophrenic sulcus.
  - Lateral x-rays show blunting of the posterior costophrenic angle and the posterior gutter.
  - Decubitus x-rays to exclude a loculated effusion and underlying pulmonary lesion or pulmonary thickening.
  - Supine x-rays show costophrenic blunting, haziness, obliteration of the diaphragmatic silhouette, decreased visibility of the lower lobe vasculature, widened minor fissure.
- Ultrasonography (US): Detects as little as 5–50 mL of pleural fluid; identifies loculated effusions; useful to determine site for thoracocentesis, pleural biopsy, or pleural drainage
- Chest CT scan with contrast for patients with undiagnosed pleural effusion
- CT pulmonary angiography if pulmonary embolism is suspected
- Positron-emission tomographic (PET)/CT scan: Focal increased uptake of 18-fluorodeoxyglugose (FDG) in the pleura and the presence of solid pleural abnormalities on CT scan are suggestive of malignant pleural disease. A negative PET/CT scan favors a benign cause.

Follow-Up & Special Considerations

Observation in uncomplicated asymptomatic patients (i.e., CHF, cirrhosis), viral pleurisy, thoracic or abdominal surgery

Diagnostic Procedures/Surgery

Diagnostic thoracentesis indicated for:

- Clinically significant pleural effusion (>10 mm thick on US or lateral decubitus x-ray with no known cause);
- CHF: Asymmetric effusion, fever, chest pain, or failure to resolve after diuretics
- Parapneumonic effusions

DIFFERENTIAL DIAGNOSIS

- Empyema: Pus, putrid odor; culture; a putrid odor suggests an anaerobic empyema: LDH levels >1,000 IU/L (normal serum = 200 IU/L); glucose, <60 mg/dL; low pH
- Malignancy: Cytology, red, bloody; glucose normal to low depending of the tumor burden; RBCs, >100,000/mm^3
- Lupus pleuritis: LE cells present; pleural fluid serum ANAs >1; glucose, <60 mg/dL; pleural fluid/serum glucose ratio <0.5
- Fungal: Positive KOH, culture; peritoneal dialysis: protein, <1 g/dL; glucose, 300–400 mg/dL
- Urinothorax: Creatinine pleural/blood >0.5; high LDH pleural fluid with low protein levels

- Hemothorax: Hematocrit pleural/blood >0.5; benign asbestos effusion: unilateral, exudative; 1/3 have an elevated eosinophil count.
- TB pleuritis: Lymphocytes >80% predominance effusion; elevated levels of adenosine deaminase >50 units/L and interferon-γ >140 pg/mL; positive AFB stain, culture; total protein >4 g/dL
- Chylothorax: Milky; triglycerides >110 mg/dL; lipoprotein electrophoresis (chylomicrons)
- Amebic liver abscess: Anchovy paste effusion; Waldenström macroglobulinemia and multiple myeloma: Protein >7 g/dL
- Esophageal rupture: High salivary amylase; pleural fluid acidosis, pH <6; amylase-rich: Acute pancreatitis, chronic pancreatic pleural effusion, malignancy, esophageal rupture; rheumatoid pleurisy: Glucose <60 mg/dL; pleural fluid/serum glucose <0.5
- Pleural fluid lymphocytosis: Tuberculous pleurisy, lymphoma, sarcoidosis, chronic rheumatoid pleurisy, yellow-nail syndrome, or chylothorax (80–95% of the nucleated cells):
  - Carcinomatosis in 1/2 of cases (50–70% lymphocyte)
  - Pleural fluid eosinophilia (>10% of total nucleated cells): Pneumothorax, hemothorax, malignancy (carcinoma, lymphoma), drugs, fungal (coccidiomycosis, cryptococcosis, histoplasmosis), benign asbestos pleural effusion, pulmonary infarction
  - Low glucose (<60 mg/dL): TB, malignancy, rheumatoid pleurisy, complicated parapneumonic effusion, empyema, hemothorax, paragonimiasis, Churg-Strauss syndrome
  - RBC count >100,000/mm^3: Trauma, malignancy, PE, injury after cardiac surgery, asbestos pleurisy, pancreatitis, TB
  - Pleural fluid LDH >1,000 IU/L: Suggests empyema, malignant effusion, rheumatoid effusion, or pleural paragonimiasis
  - pH >7.3: Rheumatoid pleurisy, empyema, malignant effusion, TB, esophageal rupture, or lupus nephritis
  - Mesothelial cells in exudates: TB is unlikely if there are more than 5% of mesothelial cells.
- *Streptococcus pneumoniae* accounts for 50% of cases of parapneumonic effusions in AIDS patients, followed by *Staphylococcus aureus*, *Haemophilus influenzae*, *Mycoplasma pneumoniae*, *Legionella*, *Nocardia asteroides*, and *Bordetella bronchiseptica*. Exudate with a low count of nucleated cells.
- *Pneumocystis jiroveci* is an uncommon cause in HIV. Usually it is a small effusion, unilateral or bilateral, that is serous to bloody in appearance. Demonstration of the trophozoite or cyst is mandatory.
- Less common pathogens involved in HIV pleural effusion patients are *Mycobacterium*, *Toxoplasma*, *Histoplasma capsulatum*, *Cryptococcus*, and *Leishmania*.
- Cancer-related HIV pleural effusion: Kaposi sarcoma, multicentric Castleman disease, and primary effusion lymphoma
- Kaposi sarcoma: Mononuclear predominance, exudate, pH >7.4; LDH, 111–330 IU/L; glucose >60 mg/dL.

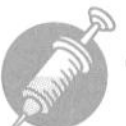

TREATMENT

Oxygen support as needed

MEDICATION

Therapy for breast, lymphoma, ovarian, prostate, and small cell lung cancer may control the effusion.

First Line

- CHF: Diuretics (75% clearing in 48 hours)
- Parapneumonic effusion: Antibiotics
- Rheumatologic conditions/inflammation: Steroids and NSAIDs

Second Line

Symptomatic nonmalignant effusions that are refractory to treatment may be managed with repeated therapeutic thoracentesis or pleurodesis.

ADDITIONAL TREATMENT

General Measures

- Therapeutic thoracentesis if symptomatic
- Chest tube thoracostomy drainage:
  - Indications: >1/2 hemithorax; complicated parapneumonic effusion (positive Gram stain or culture, pH <7.2, or glucose <60 mg/dL); empyema; hemothorax
  - The recommended limit is 1,000–1,500 mL in a single thoracentesis procedure.

Issues for Referral

- Uncertain etiology; thoracentesis technically difficult; high-risk diagnostic thoracentesis; malignant effusion; decortication
- Video-assisted thoracoscopy for sclerosis
- Peritoneal shunts for symptomatic recurrence

Additional Therapies

- Pleurodesis for symptomatic patients whose pleural effusion reaccumulates too quickly for repeat therapeutic thoracentesis (4)
- Sclerosing agents for malignant effusions: Doxycycline, bleomycin, talc, and minocycline; talc is more efficacious. The relative risk (RR) of nonrecurrent effusion was 1.34 (95% confidence interval 1.16–1.55) in favor of talc compared with bleomycin, tetracycline, or mustine (4)[A].

SURGERY/OTHER PROCEDURES

- Percutaneous pleural biopsy if a cause is not clear after thoracentesis:
  - Close pleural biopsy: When the pleura is diffusely involved (TB pleuritis, noncaseating granulomata in rheumatoid pleuritis)
  - CT-guided needle biopsy: Pleural mass; video-assisted thoracoscopic pleural biopsy: Negative percutaneous biopsy, patchy disease, or CT scan does not show obvious mass
- Parapneumonic effusion should be sampled if free-flowing but layer is >10 mm on a lateral decubitus film. Loculated, thickened pleura on a contrast-enhanced CT scan, clearly delineated by ultrasound. Open pleural biopsy by thoracotomy.
- Contraindications for thoracocentesis: Anticoagulation, bleeding diathesis, thrombocytopenia <20,000/mm^3, mechanical ventilation
- Bronchoscopy: When malignancy is likely; suggested by a pulmonary infiltrate or a mass on the chest x-ray or CT scan, hemoptysis, massive pleural effusion, or shift of the mediastinum toward the side of the effusion

IN-PATIENT CONSIDERATIONS

Initial Stabilization

Treat any underlying medical disorder.

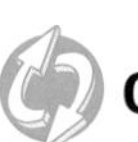

ONGOING CARE

FOLLOW-UP RECOMMENDATIONS

Patient Monitoring

- Check for the amount and quality of fluid drained, air leak (bubbling), oscillation.
- Repeat a chest x-ray when drainage decreases to <100 mL/d to evaluate complete clearing.
- For a large effusion, re-evaluate catheter position; if positioned appropriately, consider fibrinolytics (e.g., urokinase, streptokinase, alteplase).

DIET

- Cardiac diet in patients with heart failure
- Correct hypoproteinemia

PROGNOSIS

- Malignant effusion: Poor prognosis
- Patients with low-pH malignant effusions have a shorter survival and poorer response to chemical pleurodesis than those with a pH >7.3.
- Low pleural fluid pH (≤7.15): High likelihood of necessity for pleural space drainage

COMPLICATIONS

- Pleural effusion: Constrictive fibrosis, pleurocutaneous fistula
- Thoracentesis: Pneumothorax (5–10%); hemothorax (~1%); empyema; spleen/liver laceration; re-expansion pulmonary edema (if >1.5 L is removed)

REFERENCES

1. Light RW. Clinical practice. Pleural effusion. *N Engl J Med*. 2002;346:1971–7.
2. Light RW, Macgregor MI, Luchsinger PC. Pleural effusions: The diagnostic separation of transudates and exudates. *Ann Intern Med*. 1972;77:507–13.
3. Roth BJ, O'Meara TF, Cragun WH. The serum-effusion albumin gradient in the evaluation of pleural effusions. *Chest*. 1990;98:546–9.
4. Shaw P, Agarwal R. Pleurodesis for malignant pleural effusions. *Cochrane Database Syst Rev*. 2004;(1):CD002916.

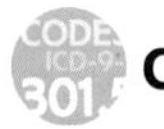

CODES

ICD9

- 511.1 Pleurisy with effusion, with mention of a bacterial cause other than tuberculosis
- 511.81 Malignant pleural effusion
- 511.9 Unspecified pleural effusion

CLINICAL PEARLS

- Primary effusion lymphoma is not associated with lymphadenopathy. It occurs in <1–4% of AIDS-related lymphomas. It may occur in the absence of HIV infection and is rarely seen after solid-organ transplantation.
- A chest CT scan with pleural phase contrast should be performed in all patients with undiagnosed pleural effusion.

PNEUMONIA, ASPIRATION

Jacob Kleinman, MD
Drew Grimes, MD

BASICS

DESCRIPTION

- Pneumonia due to macro-inhalation of microorganisms from the oral cavity or nasopharynx
- In contrast to typical pneumonia, which occurs by direct microinhalation of infectious particles from air
- Typically occurs in patients with dysphagia
- Can occur with any impairment of a mechanism that protects the lower airways. This may be a mechanical impairment or a defect in humoral and cellular immunity.
- System(s) affected: Pulmonary

EPIDEMIOLOGY

Geriatric Considerations

- Elderly with community-acquired pneumonia (CAP) have significantly higher incidence of aspiration than controls.
- Risk of aspiration pneumonia is highest among nursing home patients
- Risk of aspiration pneumonia is 6× higher if ≥75 years of age (1)

Prevalence

- Aspiration pneumonia is the cause of 5–15% of cases of CAP and healthcare-associated pneumonia (HCAP) is primarily due to aspiration pneumonia (1,2).
- Silent aspiration is extremely common in elderly patients but can occur even in normal individuals:
  - Up to 50% of normal adults aspirate during sleep.
  - Occurs in 40–70% of acute stroke patients
- In the US, ~300,000–600,000 people each year are affected by dysphagia resulting from neurological disorders. Aspiration pneumonia is the major cause of death in these patients (1).
- Pneumonia is the second most common infection in hospitalized patients.

RISK FACTORS

- Reduced consciousness, alcoholism, dementia, uremia, poor nutritional status (3)
- Mechanical ventilation, bronchoscopy, upper endoscopy
- Pulmonary diseases: Chronic obstructive pulmonary disease (COPD)
- Dysphagia: Due to stroke, neuromuscular diseases, radiation to the neck or oropharynx
- GI diseases: Gastroesophageal reflux disease, esophageal disease
- Diabetes mellitus
- Parkinson disease
- Use of proton pump inhibitors, antipsychotic drugs, and ACE inhibitors (4)
- Enteral feeding tubes, nasogastric tube feeding
- Immunosuppressed patients: Solid organ transplantation, steroid use >20 mg/d for >2 weeks, HIV

GENERAL PREVENTION

- Treatment of dysphagia, including new therapeutic sensory stimulation, can prevent aspiration (5).
- New evidence shows increased importance of aggressive oral hygiene in prevention of aspiration pneumonia (6).
- Aspiration prevention protocols, including bedside speech and swallow evaluations, progressive oral intake, sedation vacations, and ventilator-weaning protocols significantly reduce risk of aspiration pneumonia (7).
- Mechanical measures, such as semirecumbent or lateral-horizontal positioning, and a chin-down posture while eating are commonly used.
- A soft diet and nectar-thickened liquids are better than a pureed diet for preventing pneumonia.
- There is a lack of evidence to show that tube feeding will prevent aspiration.

PATHOPHYSIOLOGY

- Aspiration pneumonia occurs due to macroinhalation of microorganisms from the oral cavity or nasopharynx.
- Macroinhalation is increased with any pathologic process causing increased aspiration, particularly dysphagia.
- Mechanical factors:
  - Mechanical ventilation: Endotracheal tube is a direct path to lower respiratory tract, which also prevents clearance of bacteria and secretions from exiting lower airways
  - Reduced gag reflex due to sedation or stroke reduces spontaneous coughing and clearance of bacteria
- Increased colonization of bacteria in malnutrition, alcoholism, diabetes, COPD, etc., increase likelihood of infection with each aspiration event (1).
- If aspiration occurs while the patient is recumbent, infection is likely in the posterior segments of the upper lobes and the apical segments of the lower lobes. If aspiration occurs while upright or semirecumbent, the basal segments of the lower lobes are most likely to become infected.
- If untreated, patients appear to have a higher incidence of cavitation and lung abscess formation than in those with nonaspiration pneumonia.
- Must contrast to chemical pneumonitis, which is due to aspiration of contents toxic to lung, independent of bacterial involvement (e.g., gastric acid), which presents with an abrupt onset of symptoms and prominent dyspnea. Chest x-ray (CXR) changes are seen within 2 hours (8).

ETIOLOGY

- Pathogens vary according to setting:
  - CAP: Gram-positives and some gram-negatives (e.g., *Streptococcus pneumonia*, *Staphylococcus aureus*, *Haemophilus influenza*, and enterobacteria) (9)
  - Health care–associated (HCAP): Mostly polymicrobial, including gram-negative bacilli, such as *Pseudomonas aeruginosa*, and anaerobes, such as *Bacteroides fragilis*, and less commonly, gram-positives, including *S. aureus* (10)
  - Ventilator-associated (VAP): Common nosocomial bacteria, especially *P. aeruginosa*, *Acinetobacter baumannii*, methicillin-resistant *S. aureus* (MRSA) (10)
- Specific bacteria identified in minority of cases
- Most cases associated with predisposing factors (see "Risk Factors")

COMMONLY ASSOCIATED CONDITIONS

See "Risk Factors."

DIAGNOSIS

- There is no "gold standard" test for aspiration pneumonia. Most instances of aspiration are not observed. Diagnosis is inferred when a patient with risk factors for aspiration develops a pneumonia in a characteristic bronchopulmonary segment (1).
- After assessing for aspiration risk, other elements of history, physical, and diagnostic testing are similar to those used to diagnosis pneumonia of any cause.

HISTORY

- Common:
  - Fever and dyspnea
  - Delirium, change in mental status
  - Productive cough classically with putrid sputum
  - Pleuritic chest pain
  - Indolent course
- Less common: Rigors and weight loss

PHYSICAL EXAM

- Common:
  - Altered mental status
  - Periodontal disease, poor oral hygiene
  - Rhonchi
  - Decreased resonance on percussion, bronchovesicular breath sounds showing consolidation
- Less common: Wheezes, crackles, severe dyspnea, or acute respiratory failure

DIAGNOSTIC TESTS & INTERPRETATION

Lab

- Much new research has shown serum biomarkers, i.e., procalcitonin, to be significant indicators of aspiration. While increased serum levels are correlated with increased risk of aspiration pneumonia, they cannot be used to distinguish pneumonia from other types of aspiration injury (4,8)[B].
- CBC:
  - Leukocytosis: WBC >12,000
  - Anemia of chronic disease occasionally present
- Cultures:
  - Sputum cultures: Anaerobic oral flora notoriously difficult to culture, not uncommon to lack results
  - Blood cultures are low yield.
- Urine antigen test for pneumococcus and legionella (9)[B]
- Arterial blood gas if suspect acidosis

Imaging

Initial approach

CXR (posteroanterior and lateral):

- CXR may be entirely normal in early infection.
- Involvement of lower lobes favors aspiration as the cause.
- CXR may also show a bronchopneumonia pattern with segmental and subsegmental consolidation, usually in lower lobes.

Follow-Up & Special Considerations

Chest CT: More sensitive detection of infiltrates than CXR but should be used only if clinically indicated

Diagnostic Procedures/Surgery

- Bronchoscopy:
  - Bronchoscopic brush cultures show improved sensitivity of etiologic diagnosis but are affected by preprocedural administration of antibiotics.
  - Commonly used for VAP but controversial in clinical practice
- Swallowing evaluation, including possible videofluoroscopic evaluation with modified barium swallow, used in patients with suspected dysphagia

DIFFERENTIAL DIAGNOSIS

- Aspiration pneumonitis
- CAP
- Viral or fungal pneumonia
- Lung abscess
- Foreign-body aspiration
- Lung cancer

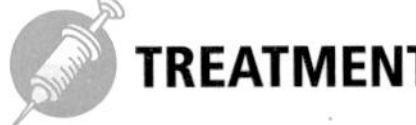

TREATMENT

MEDICATION

- Antibiotics are indicated for aspiration pneumonia, and should be tailored to the risk profile (CAP vs. HCAP) of the patient.
- It is important to initiate antibiotics early. Providers should empirically initiate broad-spectrum antibiotics with gram-negative coverage, until the results of cultures are known.
- Although commonly prescribed, new research has shown that antimicrobials with anaerobic coverage are not routinely warranted, unless there is evidence of severe periodontal disease, necrotizing pneumonia, or lung abscess (1,4)[B].
- New data have shown that a long duration of therapy may not be necessary. Treatment should last for 3–13 days, with more sources recommending 7–8 days, and be based on clinical response (4)[B].
- If no improvement after 3 days of antibiotic treatment, other diagnoses or resistant bacteria should be considered.
- *Outpatients or hospitalized patients without risk factors for resistant bacteria (9)[B]:*
  - First line: Ceftriaxone 1 g IV once daily plus azithromycin 500 mg IV/PO once daily
  - Second line: Levofloxacin 750 mg IV once daily or moxifloxacin 400 mg IV once daily
- *VAP or patients at risk for resistant bacteria:*
  - All patients should be treated with a β-lactam that is active against pseudomonas (10)[B].
  - First line: Cefepime 1–2 g IV q8–12h
  - Second line: Imipenem 500 mg IV q6h, meropenem 1 gm IV q8h, piperacillin-tazobactam 4.5 g IV q6h
- In addition, one should consider including a second agent active against *Pseudomonas*, especially in hemodynamically unstable patients (1,3)[B]:
  - First line: Ciprofloxacin 400 mg IV q12h
  - Second line: Gentamicin 4–7 mg/kg/d IV once q24h
- Either vancomycin or linezolid should be added for coverage against MRSA (10)[B]:
  - First line: Vancomycin 1g IV q12h
  - Second line: Linezolid 600 mg IV q12h
- If there is increased risk of anaerobic infection because of severe periodontal disease, necrotizing pneumonia, or lung abscess, then anaerobic coverage can be added. Not typically necessary in most cases of aspiration pneumonia (9)[B]:
  - First line: Clindamycin, 600 mg IV b.i.d. or 300 mg PO q.i.d.
  - Second line: Ampicillin/sulbactam, 3 g IV b.i.d.

ADDITIONAL TREATMENT

- If possible, avoid the use of medications that may increase the risk of aspiration pneumonia (see "Risk Factors").
- Optimize treatment of all comorbidities that may increase the risk of aspiration.
- If patient without dysphagia fails appropriate therapy or aspiration recurs, consider bronchoscopy to rule out neoplasm and other treatment-resistant microorganisms.
- Rarely, surgery may be necessary in the case of significant abscess, bronchopleural fistula, or empyema.

Issues for Referral

- Consider speech therapy evaluation.
- If patient without dysphagia fails appropriate therapy or aspiration recurs, consider pulmonology evaluation.

IN-PATIENT CONSIDERATIONS

Initial Stabilization

- Support ABCs.
- Assess for hypoxia with O_2 monitoring: O_2 saturation to determine need for supplemental O_2.
- Assess for signs of hemodynamic instability.

Admission Criteria

Admission recommended for anyone with signs of sepsis, immunosuppression, significant comorbid illness; poor functional or nutritional status

Nursing

- Aggressive oral hygiene and pulmonary toileting
- Elevate head of bed, semirecumbent position: 30–45°

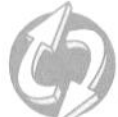

ONGOING CARE

DIET

- NPO if reduced consciousness
- Aggressive oral hygiene
- Soft diet with thickened liquids
- Encourage smaller bites
- Chin-down swallowing
- Mechanical strategies:
  - Elevated head 30–45° when eating; especially important if enteral feeding
- Tube feeding:
  - Usually reserved for continued aspiration despite other preventive measures, although this remains controversial
  - There is a lack of evidence that tube feeding prevents aspiration, but tube feeding does improve pulmonary toileting.

PROGNOSIS

- HCAP and VAP have greater morbidity and mortality than CAP. It is likely that the worse outcomes are associated with the increase in age and comorbidities of those at risk for HCAP and VAP (11).
- VAP has high morbidity and high mortality at 15–50%.
- Age, poor functional and nutritional status, and significant comorbid illness are independent predictors of increased mortality.

COMPLICATIONS

- Early: Sepsis, acute respiratory distress syndrome
- Late: Lung abscess, necrotizing pneumonia, bronchopleural fistula, empyema

REFERENCES

1. Marik PE, et al. Pulmonary aspiration syndromes. *Curr Opin Pulm Med*. 2011;17:148–54.
2. Teramoto S, Kawashima M, Komiya K, et al. Health-care-associated pneumonia is primarily due to aspiration pneumonia. *Chest*. 2009;136: 1702–3; author reply 1703.
3. van der Maarel-Wierink CD, Vanobbergen JN, Bronkhorst EM, et al. Risk factors for aspiration pneumonia in frail older people: A systematic literature review. *J Am Med Dir Assoc*. 2011;12: 344–54.
4. Raghavendran K, Nemzek J, Napolitano LM, et al. Aspiration-induced lung injury. *Crit Care Med*. 2011;39:818–26.
5. Paydarfar D, et al. Protecting the airway during swallowing: What is the role for afferent surveillance? *Head Neck*. 2011;33(Suppl 1): S26–9.
6. Tada A, Miura H, et al. Prevention of aspiration pneumonia (AP) with oral care. *Arch Gerontol Geriatr*. 2011. [Epub ahead of print].
7. Starks B, Harbert C, et al. Aspiration prevention protocol: Decreasing postoperative pneumonia in heart surgery patients. *Crit Care Nurse*. 2011; 31:38–45.
8. Niederman MS, et al. Distinguishing chemical pneumonitis from bacterial aspiration: Still a clinical determination. *Crit Care Med*. 2011; 39:1543–4.
9. Watkins RR, Lemonovich TL, et al. Diagnosis and management of community-acquired pneumonia in adults. *Am Fam Physician*. 2011;83:1299–306.
10. Labelle A, Kollef MH, et al. Healthcare-associated pneumonia: Approach to management. *Clin Chest Med*. 2011;32:507–15.
11. Chalmers JD, Taylor JK, Singanayagam A, et al. Epidemiology, antibiotic therapy, and clinical outcomes in health care-associated pneumonia: A UK cohort study. *Clin Infect Dis*. 2011;53:107–13.

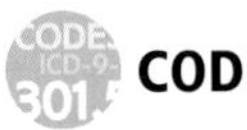

CODES

ICD9

- 507.0 Pneumonitis due to inhalation of food or vomitus
- 507.1 Pneumonitis due to inhalation of oils and essences
- 507.8 Pneumonitis due to other solids and liquids

CLINICAL PEARLS

- Aspiration pneumonia is usually a clinical diagnosis.
- Initial antibiotic treatment is empiric.
- Uncomplicated aspiration pneumonia no longer requires anaerobic coverage.
- Mechanical measures are the key to prevention.

PNEUMONIA, BACTERIAL

David Sapienza, MD
Frank J. Domino, MD

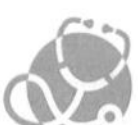

BASICS

Bacterial pneumonia is an infection of the pulmonary parenchyma by a bacterial organism.

DESCRIPTION

Bacterial pneumonia is further classified in these ways:

- Community-acquired pneumonia (CAP): Lower-respiratory tract infection not acquired in a hospital, long-term care facility, or during other recent contact with the health care system (1).
- Hospital-acquired pneumonia (HAP): Pneumonia that occurs 48 hours or more after admission and did not appear to be incubating at the time of admission (2).
- Ventilator-associated pneumonia (VAP): Pneumonia that develops more than 48–72 hours after endotracheal intubation (2).
- Health care–associated pneumonia (HCAP): Pneumonia that occurs in a nonhospitalized patient with extensive health care contact, such as:
  - IV therapy or wound care within the past 30 days
  - Residing in a nursing home or long-term care facility
  - Hospitalization in an acute care hospital for 2 or more days within the past 90 days
  - Visited a hospital or hemodialysis clinic within the past 30 days (2)

EPIDEMIOLOGY

- A combination of influenza and pneumonia is the eighth leading cause of death in the US, with about 52,700 deaths in 2007 (1).
- HAP is the leading cause of death among hospital-acquired infections, with mortality rates ranging from 20–50% (2).

Incidence

- CAP: 5–11 cases per 1,000 persons (1).
- HAP: 5–10 cases per 1,000 hospital admissions (2).

RISK FACTORS

- CAP (1):
  - Age older than 65
  - HIV or immunocompromised
  - Recent antibiotic therapy or resistance to antibiotics
  - Comorbidities such as asthma, CVD, COPD, chronic renal failure, CHF, diabetes, liver disease, neoplastic disease
- VAP, HAP, HCAP (2):
  - Hospitalization for 2 days or more during past 90 days
  - Severe illness
  - Antibiotic therapy in the last 6 months
  - Poor functional status as defined by activities of daily living score
  - Immunosuppression

GENERAL PREVENTION

- 23-valent pneumococcal polysaccharide vaccine is recommended for the following (3):
  - Age 65 and older. Second dose recommended if patient received vaccine 5 years prior and was younger than 65 at the time of the first vaccination.
  - Age 19–64 with chronic cardiovascular disease, chronic pulmonary disease (including asthma), diabetes mellitus, chronic liver disease, CSF leaks, cochlear implants, alcoholism, or who smoke cigarettes or live in chronic care facilities. Revaccination not recommended under age 65.
  - Age 19–64 who are immunocompromised. Second dose recommended if 5 years or more have elapsed since receipt of first dose.
- Annual influenza vaccine is recommended according to current guidelines (1).

ETIOLOGY

- Adults, CAP (1):
  - Typical: *Streptococcal pneumoniae, Haemophilus influenzae, Staphylococcus aureus,* group A *Streptococcus, Moraxella catarrhalis*
  - Atypical: *Legionella* sp., *Mycoplasma pneumoniae, Chlamydophila pneumoniae*
- Adults, HCAP/HAP/VAP (2):
  - Aerobic gram-negative bacilli: *Pseudomonas aeruginosa, Escherichia coli, Klebsiella pneumoniae,* and *Acinetobacter* sp.
  - Gram-positive cocci: *Streptococcus* sp. and *S. aureus* (including MRSA)
- Children (4):
  - Birth to 20 days: *E. coli,* group B streptococci, *Listeria monocytogenes*
  - 3 weeks to 3 months: *Chlamydia trachomatis, S. pneumoniae*
  - 4 months to 18 years:
    - Typical: *S. pneumoniae*
    - Atypical: *C. pneumoniae, M. pneumoniae*

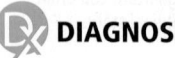

DIAGNOSIS

HISTORY

- Fever, chills, rigors, malaise, fatigue
- Dyspnea
- Cough, with or without sputum
- Pleuritic chest pain
- Myalgias
- GI symptoms

Pediatric Considerations

Atypical pneumonia in children is characteristically slowly progressing with malaise, low-grade fever, sore throat, and cough developing over 3–5 days (5).

Geriatric Considerations

Older adults with pneumonia often present with weakness and mental status change (1).

PHYSICAL EXAM

- Fever >100.4°F (38°C), tachypnea, tachycardia
- Lungs: Rales, rhonchi, egophony, increased fremitus, bronchial breath sounds, dullness to percussion, asymmetric breath sounds
- Abdominal tenderness

DIAGNOSTIC TESTS & INTERPRETATION

Lab

Initial lab tests

- Historically, for hospitalized patients with CAP, CBC, sputum Gram stain, and 2 sets of blood cultures are obtained.
  - These tests are optional for outpatients and uncomplicated hospitalized patients (6)[C].
- More extensive diagnostic testing in patients with CAP is recommended in the following clinical settings (6)[C]:
  - Blood cultures: ICU admission, cavitary infiltrates, leukopenia, alcohol abuse, chronic severe liver disease, asplenia, positive pneumococcal urine antigen test (UAT), pleural effusion
  - Sputum Gram stain and cultures: ICU admission, failure of outpatient treatment, cavitary infiltrates, alcohol abuse, severe chronic obstructive pulmonary disease (COPD) or structural lung disease, positive legionella UAT, positive pneumococcal UAT, pleural effusion
  - Legionella UAT: ICU admission, failure of outpatient treatment, alcohol abuse, travel in past 2 weeks, pleural effusion
  - Pneumococcal UAT: ICU admission, failure of outpatient treatment, leukopenia, alcohol abuse, chronic severe liver disease, asplenia, pleural effusion

Imaging

Initial approach

- A chest x-ray (CXR) is indicated when pneumonia is suspected, or in patients who present with an acute respiratory infection and meet certain criteria (1)[C]:
  - Any patient with at least one of the following abnormal vital signs: T >100°F (37.8°C); HR >100 beats/min; RR rate >20 breaths/min.
  - Any patient with at least 2 of the following clinical findings: Decreased breath sounds, rales, absence of asthma
- Early in the course of the disease, a CXR may be negative (6).

Follow-Up & Special Considerations

Chest CT scan if failing to improve

DIFFERENTIAL DIAGNOSIS

Bronchitis, asthma exacerbation, pulmonary edema, lung cancer, influenza, pulmonary tuberculosis

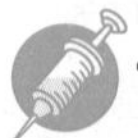

TREATMENT

MEDICATION

First Line

- Adults:
  - CAP, outpatient:
    - There are no significant differences in efficacy between different antibiotics in outpatient treatment of CAP in adults (7)[A]:
      - Previously healthy, no antibiotics in past 3 months:
        - Macrolide: Azithromycin 500 mg PO one time, then 250 mg PO daily for 4 days; clarithromycin 500 mg PO b.i.d. for 10 days; erythromycin 500 mg PO b.i.d. for 10 days (6)[A], or
        - Tetracycline: Doxycycline 100 mg PO b.i.d. for 10 days (6)[C]
      - Comorbidities, immunosuppressed, antibiotic use in past 3 months:
        - Fluoroquinolone: Levofloxacin 750 mg PO daily for 5 days; moxifloxacin 400 mg PO daily for 10 days; gatifloxacin 400 mg PO daily for 10 days (6)[A], or
        - β-Lactam (Amoxicillin 1 g PO t.i.d.; Amoxicillin-clavulanate 2 g PO b.i.d.) + macrolide (6)[A]

- CAP, inpatient (non-ICU):
  - IV antibiotics initially, then switch to oral antibiotics after clinical improvement and ability to tolerate oral medications.
  - β-Lactam (Cefotaxime; ceftriaxone; ampicillin-sulbactam) + macrolide (clarithromycin; erythromycin) for 14 days (6)[A], or
  - Fluoroquinolone (gatifloxacin; levofloxacin) for 14 days (6)[A]
  - If *pseudomonas* is a consideration:
    - β-Lactam (piperacillin-tazobactam; cefepime; imipenem; meropenem) + fluoroquinolone (levofloxacin) (6)[C], or
    - β-Lactam (piperacillin-tazobactam; cefepime; imipenem; meropenem) + aminoglycoside + azithromycin (6)[C], or
    - β-Lactam (piperacillin-tazobactam; cefepime; imipenem; meropenem) + aminoglycoside + fluoroquinolone (levofloxacin) (6)[C]
  - If MRSA is a consideration:
    - Add vancomycin or linezolid
- HCAP/HAP/VAP:
  - Use IV antibiotics.
  - Early onset (<5 days), and no risk factors for multidrug-resistant pathogens:
    - β-Lactam (ceftriaxone; ampicillin-sulbactam; ertapenem) (2)[C], or
    - Fluoroquinolone (levofloxacin; moxifloxacin) (2)[C]
  - Late onset (≥ 5 days) or risk factors for multidrug-resistant pathogens (antibiotic therapy in preceding 90 days; high frequency of antibiotic resistance in community or hospital; immunosuppressive disease or therapy; risk factors for HCAP):
    - MRSA coverage (linezolid or vancomycin) + β-Lactam (cefepime; ceftazidime; imipenem; meropenem; piperacillin-tazobactam) + either fluoroquinolone (levofloxacin) or aminoglycoside (amikacin; gentamicin; tobramycin) (2)[C]
- Adult IV antibiotic doses:
  - β-Lactams (ampicillin-sulbactam 3 g q6h; aztreonam 2 g q6h; cefepime 1–2 g q8–12h; cefotaxime 1 g q6–8h; ceftazidime 2 g q8h; ceftriaxone 1 g daily; imipenem 500 mg q6h; meropenem 1 g IV q8h)
  - Aminoglycosides (amikacin 20 mg/kg daily; gentamicin 7 mg/kg daily; tobramycin 7 mg/kg daily)
  - Fluoroquinolones (levofloxacin 750 mg daily; gatifloxacin 500 mg daily)
  - Macrolides (azithromycin 500 mg daily; clarithromycin 500 mg daily; erythromycin 500–1,000 mg q6h)
  - Vancomycin 15 mg/kg q12h
  - Linezolid 600 mg q12h

- Pediatric, outpatient (≥ 3 months):
  - Antibiotic treatment in preschool-aged children is not routinely required because viral pathogens are more common (5)[A].
  - Typical bacterial pneumonia:
    - Amoxicillin 90 mg/kg/d PO b.i.d. (max 4 g/d) (5,8)[A]
    - Amoxicillin-clavulanate 90 mg/kg/d PO b.i.d. (max 4 g/d) (5,8)[A]
    - Alternative: Levofloxacin 16–20 mg/kg/d PO b.i.d. for children 6 months to 5 years, 8–10 mg/kg/d daily for children ≥ 5 years (max 750 mg/d) (5)[C]
  - Atypical bacterial pneumonia:
    - Azithromycin 10 mg/kg PO on day 1, then 5 mg/kg/d on days 2–5 (max 500 mg day 1, 250 mg days 2–5) (5)[C]
    - Clarithromycin 15 mg/kg/d PO b.i.d. (max 1 g/d) (5)[C]
    - Erythromycin 40 mg/kg/d PO daily (5)[C]

IN-PATIENT CONSIDERATIONS

Admission Criteria

Clinical judgment and the use of a validated severity-of-illness score are recommended to determine when adult inpatient management is indicated (6)[C]:

- The Pneumonia Severity Index is a clinical prediction rule used to calculate the probability of morbidity and mortality among patients with CAP (online calculator available at www.mdcalc.com/psi-port-score-pneumonia-severity-index-adult-cap) (9)[B].
- The CURB-65 Score is another easy-to-use severity-of-illness score for stratifying adults with CAP into different management groups (10)[B].

Pediatric Considerations

In-patient treatment of children is recommended in the following settings: Infants $\leq$3–6 months (5)[C]; presence of respiratory distress (tachypnea, dyspnea, retractions, grunting, nasal flaring, apnea, altered mental status, O_2 sat $<90\%$) (5)[A]

Discharge Criteria

Clinical stability: T $\leq 37.8°C$; HR ≤ 100 beats/min; RR ≤ 24 beats/min; SBP ≥ 90 mm Hg; O_2 sat $\geq 90\%$ or pO_2 ≥ 60 mm Hg on room air; ability to maintain oral intake; normal mental status (6)[C].

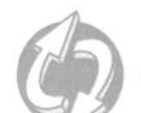

ONGOING CARE

PATIENT EDUCATION

Smoking cessation, vaccination

COMPLICATIONS

Necrotizing pneumonia, respiratory failure, empyema, abscesses, cavitation, bronchopleural fistula, sepsis

REFERENCES

1. Watkins RR, Lemonovich TL, et al. Diagnosis and management of community-acquired pneumonia in adults. *Am Fam Physician*. 2011;83:1299–306.
2. Guidelines for the management of adults with hospital-acquired, ventilator-associated, and healthcare-associated pneumonia. *Am J Respir Crit Care Med*. 2005;171:388–416.
3. Fisman DN, Abrutyn E, Spaude KA, et al. Prior pneumococcal vaccination is associated with reduced death, complications, and length of stay among hospitalized adults with community-acquired pneumonia. *Clin Infect Dis*. 2006;42:1093–101.
4. Ostapchuk M, Roberts DM, Haddy R. Community-acquired pneumonia in infants and children. *Am Fam Physician*. 2004;70(5):899–908.
5. Bradley JS, Byington CL, Shah SS, et al. The management of community-acquired pneumonia in infants and children older than 3 months of age: clinical practice guidelines by the Pediatric Infectious Diseases Society and the Infectious Diseases Society of America. *Clin Infect Dis*. 2011;53:e25–76.
6. Mandell LA, Wunderink RG, Anzueto A, et al. Infectious Diseases Society of America/American Thoracic Society consensus guidelines on the management of community-acquired pneumonia in adults. *Clin Infect Dis*. 2007;44 (Suppl 2):S27–72.
7. Bjerre LM, Verheij TJ, Kochen MM, et al. Antibiotics for community acquired pneumonia in adult outpatients. *Cochrane Database Syst Rev*. 2009;7(4):CD002109.
8. Kabra SK, Lodha R, Pandey RM, et al. Antibiotics for community-acquired pneumonia in children. *Cochrane Database Syst Rev*. 2010;(3):CD004874.
9. Fine MJ, Auble TE, Yealy DM. A prediction rule to identify low-risk patients with community-acquired pneumonia. *N Engl J Med*. 1997;336:243–50.
10. Lim WS, van der Eerden MM, Laing R, et al. Defining community acquired pneumonia severity on presentation to hospital: an international derivation and validation study. *Thorax*. 2003;58:377–82.

CODES

ICD9

- 482.1 Pneumonia due to *Pseudomonas*
- 482.2 Pneumonia due to *Streptococcus*, Pneumonia due *Haemophilus influenzae [H. influenzae]*
- 482.9 Pneumonia due to Bacterial pneumonia, unspecified

CLINICAL PEARLS

- Bacterial pneumonia can usually be treated empirically based on its classification as CAP or HCAP/HAP/VAP.
- A severity-of-illness score is helpful in determining the need for hospitalization of adult patients.

PNEUMONIA, MYCOPLASMA

Alyssa H. Tran, DO

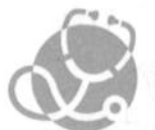

BASICS

DESCRIPTION

- Bronchopulmonary infection caused by infection of the lungs and bronchi with *Mycoplasma pneumoniae*, a fastidious and slow-growing organism
- Infection may be asymptomatic, confined to the upper respiratory tract, or it can progress to pneumonia. Usual course is acute. Incubation period is 1–4 weeks and includes prodromal symptoms.
- Peaks late summer/fall; most frequent in children/young adults but also elderly; may cause epidemics (schools, barracks)
- Synonym(s): Primary atypical pneumonia (PAP); Eaton agent pneumonia; Cold agglutinin-positive pneumonia; Walking pneumonia

Geriatric Considerations

Somewhat unusual as an isolated agent in elderly patients

Pediatric Considerations

- Unusual in infants and children <5 years as most pneumonia in this age group is viral in etiology
- All pediatric patients >6 months should be immunized annually against influenza to prevent community-aquired pneumonia (CAP) (1).
- *M. pneumoniae* is associated with increased incidence of asthma exacerbation in older children.
- All infants 3–6 months with suspected bacterial pneumonia should be hospitalized even if the pneumonia is not confirmed by blood tests (1).
- First-line treatment is macrolides. Tetracyclines may be used in patients older than 8 years. Fluoroquinolones are not approved by the FDA for use in patients younger than 18 years.

Pregnancy Considerations

- Azithromycin: Pregnancy class B (preferred treatment)
- Clarithromycin and levofloxacin: Pregnancy class C
- Doxycycline: Pregnancy class D (contraindicated)

EPIDEMIOLOGY

Incidence

- Estimated 2 million cases/yr in the US. Responsible for 20% of CAP requiring hospitalizations annually in the US
- Incidence does not vary greatly by season but accounts for higher proportion of pneumonia in the summer (up to 50%)

Prevalence

- Predominant sex: Male = Female
- Predominant age: 5–20 years:
  - May occur at any age
  - Rare in children <5 years of age
- Responsible for 15–20% of all cases of CAP:
  - The most common cause of pneumonia in schoolchildren and young adults who do not have a chronic underlying condition

RISK FACTORS

- Close community living (e.g., hospitals, prisons, military bases, fraternity houses, household contacts)
- Immunocompromised state
- Smoking

GENERAL PREVENTION

- Highly contagious, *M. pneumoniae* is transmitted by contact and aerosol.
- Consider the isolation of active cases in closed communities (e.g., schools, camps, military bases) and hospitals.
- Azithromycin prophylaxis (standard 5-day course) may lower the attack rate but is not routinely recommended.

PATHOPHYSIOLOGY

- *M. pneumoniae* is a mucosal pathogen, an exclusively human parasite.
- Prolonged paroxysmal, hacking cough seen in this disease is thought to be due to the inhibition of ciliary movement. The organism has a remarkable gliding motility and specialized filamentous tip ends (adhesin proteins) that allow it to burrow between cilia within the respiratory epithelium, eventually causing sloughing of the respiratory epithelial cells.
- H_2O_2 is an important virulence factor, causing oxidative damage to host cells and the loss of cilia.
- Pathogenicity of *M. pneumoniae* is linked to the activation of inflammatory mediators, including cytokines.

ALERT

Macrolide-resistant *M. pneumoniae* has emerged in adult CAP and pediatric pneumonia.

ETIOLOGY

Infection by *M. pneumoniae* has come to be recognized as a worldwide cause of CAP (2).

COMMONLY ASSOCIATED CONDITIONS

- Asthma: May be exacerbated by associated release of proinflammatory cytokines
- Chronic obstructive pulmonary disease

DIAGNOSIS

HISTORY

- Gradual onset with upper respiratory infection symptoms that progress
- Most patients will develop fever, nasal congestion, cough, headache, and sore throat. Some will develop dyspnea. Pleuritic chest pain is rare.
- Many patients will develop extrapulmonary findings, including myalgias, chest pain, cervical adenopathy, skin rash, and bullous myringitis.
- Neurologic symptoms may include cranial nerve palsies, diplopia, confusion, psychosis, ataxia, ascending paralysis, and coma.
- Persistent cough is common during convalescence; other sequelae are rare.

PHYSICAL EXAM

- Patients generally appear nontoxic.
- Hacking or pertussislike cough may be present along with fever and lassitude.
- Erythematous tympanic membranes or bullous myringitis in patients >2 years of age is an uncommon but unique sign.
- Mild pharyngeal injection without exudate
- Minimal or no cervical adenopathy
- Normal lung findings with early infection but rhonchi, rales, and/or wheezes several days later
- Some patients develop a pleural friction rub.
- Various exanthems, including erythema multiforme and Stevens-Johnson syndrome

DIAGNOSTIC TESTS & INTERPRETATION

Lab

- Labs are typically not necessary to make a diagnosis, but they may be indicated depending on clinical presentation.
- EIA serology of acute and convalescent sera is the mainstay of laboratory diagnosis.

Initial lab tests

- WBC count is generally not helpful in mycoplasmal pneumonia because results may be normal or elevated. Hemolytic anemia has been described but is rare.
- Elevated ESRs may be present but are nonspecific.
- Polymerase chain reaction testing for *M. pneumoniae* DNA in respiratory secretions, CSF, and tissue samples; when available, this may be the most sensitive and specific.

Follow-Up & Special Considerations

- Sputum Gram stains and cultures are usually not helpful because *M. pneumoniae* lacks a cell wall and cannot be stained.
- *M. pneumoniae* is difficult to culture and requires 7–21 days to grow; culturing is successful in only 40–90% of cases and does not provide information to guide patient management. Therefore, culturing is infrequently performed.
- A complement fixation serologic assay shows 4-fold rise in IgM antibody titer at 2–4 weeks after symptom onset; this is an older technique. Positive cold agglutinins (titer of 1:128 or greater or rising 4-fold) in 50% of infections but can take 1–2 weeks to develop; not sensitive or specific; not routinely recommended.

Imaging

Initial approach

CXR: Peribronchial pneumonia pattern with bronchial shadow, interstitial infiltrates, areas of atelectasis; pleural effusion present in up to 20% of patients

Follow-Up & Special Considerations

Chest CT scan findings: Combination of bronchial wall thickening and centrilobular nodules; however, these CT scan findings are not observed in progressed severe *M. pneumoniae* pneumonia patients.

DIFFERENTIAL DIAGNOSIS

- Viral/bacterial/fungal pneumonia
- Tuberculosis
- Other atypical pneumonias, including *Chlamydia pneumoniae*, *C. psittaci*, *Coxiella burnetii* (Q fever), *Francisella tularensis* (tularemia), *Pneumocystis jiroveci*, *Legionella pneumophila*

TREATMENT

- The treatment generally is empirical and must be comprehensive to cover all likely pathogens in the context of the clinical setting.
- Pediatric patients should receive a macrolide and amoxil to cover *M. pneumoniae* and other likely agents causing CAP.

MEDICATION

First Line

- Azithromycin:
  - Children: <6 months of age: Not established. Patients >6 months of age, day 1: 10 mg/kg PO once, not to exceed 500 mg/d; days 2–5: 5 mg/kg/d PO, not to exceed 250 mg/d

- Adults: Day 1: 500 mg PO; days 2–5: 250 mg PO (3)[A]
- Erythromycin:
  - Children: 20–50 mg/kg/d PO divided q6–8h × 10–14 days
  - Adults: 250 mg PO q6h × 10–14 days (3)[A]
- Clarithromycin:
  - Children <6 months of age: Not established. Patients >6 months of age: 15 mg/kg/d PO divided q12h × 10–14 days
  - Adults: 250–500 mg PO b.i.d. × 10–14 days (3)[A]
- Doxycycline:
  - Children <8 years of age: Not recommended. Patients >8 years of age: 2–4 mg/kg/d up to 200 mg/d PO divided b.i.d.
  - Adults: 100 mg PO b.i.d. × 1–4 weeks (3)[C]

Second Line

- Levofloxacin:
  - Children <18 years of age: Not recommended
  - Adults: 500 mg/d PO × 7–10 days
- Telithromycin:
  - Children <18 years of age: Not recommended
  - Adults: 800 mg/d PO × 7–10 days
- Levofloxacin and moxifloxacin show good activity against *M. pneumoniae*. Consider use with comorbidities and other pneumonia pathogens (3)[A].

ALERT

Penicillin antibiotics are ineffective against *M. pneumoniae*.

ADDITIONAL TREATMENT

Additional Therapies

- Albuterol inhaler: 2 puffs q.i.d. (with spacer for pediatric patients) for wheezing
- Up to 10.9% of hospitalized patients may require mechanical ventilation.
- Acetaminophen or ibuprofen as needed for fever

IN-PATIENT CONSIDERATIONS

Initial Stabilization

Respiratory support; calculation of pneumonia severity score (CAP score) may be helpful in determining inpatient vs. outpatient treatment (4).

Admission Criteria

- Advanced age with comorbidities
- Complicating neoplastic disease
- Significant cerebrovascular, cardiac, renal, liver, or GI symptoms or coexisting conditions
- Altered mental status
- Inability to maintain oxygen saturation
- Tachycardia or tachypnea
- Hypotension
- Neurologic symptoms
- Signs of Stevens-Johnson syndrome
- Significant hemolysis (autoimmune hemolytic anemia, cold agglutinin disease)

Discharge Criteria

- Change from IV to PO antibiotic may be made when:
  - Respiratory distress and hypoxia have resolved.
  - Patients are tolerating oral hydration.
  - There are no significant complications.
- There is generally no need for 24 hours of observation on oral antibiotics prior to discharge.

ONGOING CARE

FOLLOW-UP RECOMMENDATIONS

- Worsening symptoms or development of rash or meningeal or neurologic signs should prompt immediate presentation to medical attention.
- Antibiotic prophylaxis for exposed contacts is not routinely recommended.
- However, macrolide or doxycycline prophylaxis should be used for household contacts who may be predisposed to severe mycoplasmal infection, such as those with sickle cell disease or antibody deficiencies.

Patient Monitoring

- Follow up either in person or by telephone.
- Clearing of condition on CXR should be documented in patients >50 years of age.
- In smokers, document a clear CXR in 6–8 weeks.

DIET

Keep well hydrated; otherwise, no special diet

PATIENT EDUCATION

- Smoking cessation
- Contact and droplet precautions
- Proper hand-washing techniques

PROGNOSIS

- *Mycoplasma* infection symptoms usually resolve in 2 weeks.
- Some constitutional symptoms may persist for several weeks.
- With correct therapy, even most severe cases can expect complete recovery.

COMPLICATIONS

- All complications are rare, except reactive airways disease, hemolytic anemia, and erythema multiforme (2).
- Reactive airways disease may persist indefinitely and may cause acute chest syndrome in sickle cell anemia patients.
- Hemolytic anemia
- Erythema multiforme
- Meningoencephalitis
- Aseptic meningitis
- Peripheral neuropathy
- Transverse myelitis/acute transverse myelitis
- Cerebellar ataxia
- Acute disseminated encephalomyelitis
- Guillain-Barré syndrome
- Encephalitis (especially in children)
- Polyneuritis/polyarthritis
- Stevens-Johnson syndrome
- Pericarditis/myocarditis
- Respiratory distress syndrome
- Cerebral ataxia
- Thromboembolic phenomena
- Pleural effusion
- Nephritis
- Occasional deaths occur primarily among the elderly and persons with sickle cell disease.

REFERENCES

1. Bradley JS, Byington CL, Shah SS, et al. The management of community-acquired pneumonia in infants and children older than 3 months of age: Clinical practice guidelines by the Pediatric Infectious Diseases Society and the Infectious Diseases Society of America. *Clin Infect Dis*. 2011;53:e25–76.
2. Atkinson TP, Balish MF, Waites KB. Epidemiology, clinical manifestations, pathogenesis and laboratory detection of *Mycoplasma pneumoniae* infections. *FEMS Microbiol Rev*. 2008;32(6):956–73.
3. Mandell LA, Wunderink RG, Anzueto A. Infectious Diseases Society of America/American Thoracic Society consensus guidelines on the management of community-acquired pneumonia in adults. *Clin Infect Dis*. 2007;44(Suppl 2):S27–72.
4. Metlay JP. Testing strategies in the initial management of patients with community-acquired pneumonia. *Ann Intern Med*. 2003;138:115.

ADDITIONAL READING

- Blasi F. Atypical pathogens and respiratory tract infections. *Eur Respir J*. 2004;24:171–81.
- Carbonara S, Monno L, Longo B. Community-acquired pneumonia. *Curr Opin Pulm Med*. 2009;15:261–73.
- Fine MJ, Auble TE, Yealy DM. A prediction rule to identify low-risk patients with community-acquired pneumonia. *N Engl J Med*. 1997;336:243–50.
- Forgie S, Marrie TJ. Healthcare-associated atypical pneumonia. *Semin Respir Crit Care Med*. 2009;30:67–85.
- Isozumi R, Yoshimine H, Morozumi M, et al. Adult community-acquired pneumonia caused by macrolide resistant *Mycoplasma pneumoniae*. *Respirology*. 2009;14(8):1206–8.
- Neher JO, Morton JR, Mouw D. Clinical inquiries. What is the best macrolide for atypical pneumonia? *J Fam Pract*. 2004;53:229–30.
- Talkington DF, Waites KB, Schwartz SB, et al. Emerging from obscurity: Understanding pulmonary and extrapulmonary syndromes, pathogenesis, and epidemiology of human *Mycoplasma pneumoniae* infections. In: Scheld WM, Craig WA, Hughes JM (Eds). *Emerging Infections 5*. Washington, DC: ASM Press, 2001:57–84.
- Waites KB, Talkington DF. *Mycoplasma pneumoniae* and its role as a human pathogen. *Clin Microbiol Rev*. 2004;17:697–728, table of contents.

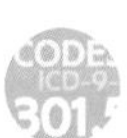

CODES

ICD9

483.0 Pneumonia due to *Mycoplasma pneumoniae*

CLINICAL PEARLS

- So-called atypical respiratory pathogens include *M. pneumoniae*, *C. pneumoniae*, and *L. pneumophila*.
- Atypical pneumonia is typically a clinical diagnosis; if labs are indicated, then the EIA serology of acute and convalescent sera is the mainstay of laboratory diagnosis.
- Watch closely for complicating symptoms that could indicate worsening disease.

PNEUMONIA, PNEUMOCYSTIS JIROVECI

Thomas J. Hansen, MD
Tejesh S. Reddy, MBBS

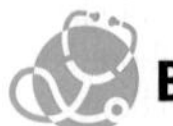

BASICS

DESCRIPTION

- The fungus that causes this pneumonia in humans was previously called *Pneumocystis carinii*.
- The name was formally changed to *Pneumocystis jiroveci* in 2001 following the discovery that the fungus that infects humans is unique and distinctive from the fungus that infects animals (1).
- *P. jiroveci* causes pneumonia primarily in immunocompromised patients.
- To prevent confusion, the term PCP, which used to represent *P. carinii* pneumonia, now represents *Pneumocystis* pneumonia (2).

ALERT

There is no combination of symptoms, signs, blood chemistries, or radiographic findings that is diagnostic of *P. jiroveci* pneumonia (3).

EPIDEMIOLOGY

- *P. jiroveci* has a worldwide distribution, and most children have been exposed to the fungus by age 2-4 years (4).
- The reservoir and mode of transmission for *P. jiroveci* is still unclear:
  - Human studies favor an airborne transmission model with person-to-person spread being the most likely mode of infection acquisition (3).

Incidence

- Infants with HIV infection have a peak incidence of PCP between the ages of 2 and 6 months (4).
- HIV-infected infants have a high mortality rate with a median survival of only 1 month.

Prevalence

- The prevalence of *P. jiroveci* colonization among healthy adults is between 0% and 20% (1).
- Recent studies have demonstrated the transient nature of *P. jiroveci* colonization in asymptomatic, immunocompetent patients (3).
- 50% of patients with PCP are coinfected with 2 or more strains of *P. jiroveci* (4).
- There is evidence that distinct strains are responsible for each episode in patients who develop multiple episodes of PCP (4).

RISK FACTORS

Individuals at risk (3):

- Patients with HIV/AIDS infection, especially if not receiving prophylactic treatment for PCP
- Patients who are receiving high doses of glucocorticoids
- Patients who have an altered immune system not due to HIV
- Patients who are receiving chronic immunosuppressive medications
- Patients who have hematologic or solid malignancies resulting in malignancy-related immune depression

GENERAL PREVENTION

- Medication:
  - Trimethoprim-sulfamethoxazole (TMP-SMX):
    - Adults: 1 double-strength tablet daily or 1 double-strength tablet 3 times per week
    - Children >2 months: 150 mg TMP/m^2/d in divided doses q12h for 3 times per week
  - Atovaquone suspension:
    - Adults: 1,500 mg PO once daily
    - Children: Not to exceed 1,500 mg daily:
      - 1–3 months: 30 mg/kg/d PO once daily
      - 4–24 months: 45 mg/kg/d PO once daily
      - >24 months: 30 mg/kg/d PO once daily
  - Dapsone:
    - Adults only: 50 mg b.i.d. or 100 mg once daily
  - Pentamidine:
    - Adults only: 300 mg aerosolized every 4 weeks
- Indications for prophylaxis:
  - HIV-infected adults (4):
    - Should start when CD4 count is <200 cells/μL or if the patient develops oropharyngeal candidiasis
  - HIV-infected children (4):
    - Prophylaxis should be provided for children 6 years or older based on adult guidelines.
    - For children aged 1–5 years, start when their CD4 count is <500 cells/μL.
    - For infants younger than 12 months, start when the CD4 percentage is <15%.
  - Non-HIV-infected adults receiving immunosuppressive medications or with underlying immune system deficits should receive PCP prophylaxis, but currently there are no specific guidelines as to when to start this.

ETIOLOGY

Mode of transmission is unknown; respiratory likely important

COMMONLY ASSOCIATED CONDITIONS

- HIV/AIDS
- Chronic obstructive lung disease (COPD)
- Interstitial lung disease
- Connective tissue diseases treated with corticosteroids
- Cancer and organ-transplant patients on immunosuppressive medication

DIAGNOSIS

HISTORY

- HIV-infected patients:
  - Subacute onset over several weeks:
    - Progressively worsening dyspnea
    - Tachypnea
    - Cough: Nonproductive or productive of clear sputum
    - Low-grade fever, chills
    - Weakness, fatigue, malaise
- Non–HIV-infected immunocompromised patients:
  - More acute onset with fulminant respiratory failure:
    - Abrupt tachypnea, dyspnea
    - Fever
    - Dry cough

PHYSICAL EXAM

- Fever
- Tachypnea
- Tachycardia
- Lung exam is normal or near normal.

DIAGNOSTIC TESTS & INTERPRETATION

P. jiroveci cannot be cultured. Therefore, a diagnosis relies on detection of the organism by colorimetric or immunofluorescent stains or by polymerase chain reaction (4)[C].

Lab

- Arterial blood gas reveals hypoxemia and increased alveolar–arterial (A-a) gradient that varies with severity of disease.
- Levels of serum lactate dehydrogenase are frequently increased (nonspecific, likely due to underlying lung inflammation and injury)
- CD4 cell count is generally <200 in HIV-infected patients with PCP.

Imaging

- Chest x-ray (CXR) (3)[C]:
  - Bilateral, symmetric, fine, reticular interstitial infiltrates involving perihilar areas. Becomes more homogeneous and diffuse as severity of infection progresses.
  - Less common patterns include upper lobe involvement in patients receiving aerosolized pentamidine, solitary or multiple nodular opacities, lobar infiltrates, pneumatoceles, and pneumothoraces.
  - Chest radiographs may be normal in up to 30% of patients with PCP (2)[C].
- High-resolution CT is more sensitive than CXRs.

Diagnostic Procedures/Surgery

- Fiber-optic bronchoscopy with bronchoalveolar lavage (BAL) is the preferred diagnostic procedure to obtain samples for direct fluorescent antibody staining:
  - Sensitivities range from 89% to >98%.
- *Pneumocystis* trophic forms or cysts obtained from induced sputum, BAL fluid, or lung tissue, which can be visualized using conventional stains
- Polymerase chain reaction (PCR) can detect *Pneumocystis* from respiratory sources, but the potential remains for false positives (3)[C].

DIFFERENTIAL DIAGNOSIS

- Tuberculosis
- Bacterial pneumonia
- Fungal pneumonia
- Viral pneumonia

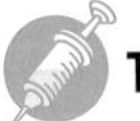

TREATMENT

The recommended duration of therapy differs in patients who have or do not have AIDS:

- In patients who have PCP who do not have AIDS, the typical duration of therapy is 14 days.
- Treatment of PCP in patients who have AIDS was increased to 21 days due to the risk for relapse after only 14 days of treatment (3)[C].

MEDICATION

Pediatric Considerations

Only medications that are FDA approved are listed for pediatric dosing.

First Line

- Trimethoprim-sulfamethoxazole (TMP-SMX) (3)[C]
- Adult dosing:
  - TMP: 15–20 mg/kg/d, PO or IV, divided into 3–4 doses
  - SMX: 75–100 mg/kg/d, PO or IV, divided into 3–4 doses
- Pediatric dosing (>2 months):
  - TMP: 15–20 mg/kg/d in divided doses q6–8h
- Reduce doses of TMP-SMX in patients with renal failure.
- Pregnancy risk factor: C
- Precautions:
  - History of sulfa allergy
  - There is an emergence of drug-resistant PCP, especially against TMP-SMX.

Second Line

- Pentamidine (for moderate to severe cases):
  - Adults and children: 4 mg/kg IV or IM once daily
- Dapsone + trimethoprim (adults only):
  - Dapsone, 100 mg PO once daily, plus
  - Trimethoprim, 5 mg/kg PO t.i.d.:
    - Check the glucose-6-phosphate dehydrogenase level before beginning dapsone, as hemolysis may result.
- Clindamycin + primaquine (adults only):
  - Clindamycin, 600 mg IV q8h or 300–450 mg PO q.i.d., plus
  - Primaquine, 30 mg PO once daily
- Atovaquone:
  - Adults: 750 mg PO b.i.d. (>13 years of age)
  - Children: 40 mg/kg/d PO divided b.i.d. (max 1,500 mg)
- Note: Pentamidine has greater toxicity than TMP-SMX: Hypotension, hypoglycemia, pancreatitis (3)[C]

ADDITIONAL TREATMENT

Adjunctive corticosteroid (prednisone or methylprednisolone) (3)[C]:

- Adjunctive corticosteroids are shown to provide benefits in patients who have AIDS and symptoms of moderate to severe PCP.
- Corticosteroids provide the greatest benefit to HIV patients who have hypoxemia manifested as a partial pressure of arterial oxygen under 70 mm Hg or an alveolar-arteriolar gradient >35 on room air.
- Adults and children >13 years of age: Prednisone, 40 mg PO b.i.d. on days 1–5; 40 mg daily on days 6–11; 20 mg daily on days 12–21

IN-PATIENT CONSIDERATIONS

- No set criteria for hospital admission
- 5 predictors of mortality in HIV-associated *Pneumocystis* pneumonia include the following (5):
  - Increased age of the patient
  - Recent IV drug use
  - Total bilirubin >0.6 mg/dL
  - Serum albumin <3 g/dL
  - Alveolar-arterial oxygen gradient ≥50 mm Hg (5)[C]

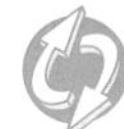

ONGOING CARE

FOLLOW-UP RECOMMENDATIONS

In patients with HIV/AIDS:

- Patients with previous episodes of PCP should receive lifelong secondary prophylaxis unless they respond well to highly active antiretroviral therapy (HAART) and have a CD4 count >200 cells/μL for at least 3 months.

Patient Monitoring

Serum lactate dehydrogenase levels, pulmonary function test results, and arterial blood gas measurements generally normalize with treatment.

DIET

No special diet needed

PATIENT EDUCATION

- Centers for Disease Control and Prevention at www.cdc.gov/ncidod/dpd/parasites/pneumocystis/default.htm
- Family Doctor.org at http://familydoctor.org/online/famdocen/home/common/sexinfections/hiv/475.html

REFERENCES

1. Catherinot E, Lanterneier F, Bougnoux ME. *Pneumocystis jirovecci* pneumonia. *Infect Dis Clin N Am*. 2010;24:107–38.
2. D'Avignon LC, Schofield CM, Hospenthal DR. *Pneumocystis* pneumonia. *Semin Repir Crit Care Med*. 2008;29:132–40.
3. Krajicek BJ, Thomas CF, Limper AH. Pneumocystis pneumonia: Current concepts in pathogenesis, diagnosis, and treatment. *Clin Chest Med*. 2009; 30:265–78, vi.
4. Kovacs JA, Masur H. Evolving health effects of Pneumocystis: One hundred years of progress in diagnosis and treatment. *JAMA*. 2009;301(24): 2578–85.
5. Fei WM, Kim EJ, Sant CA, et al. Predicting mortality from HIV-associated *Pneumocystis* pneumonia at illness presentation: An observational cohort study. *Thorax* 2009;64:1007–76.

ADDITIONAL READING

- Briel M, Bucher H, Boscacci R, et al. Adjunctive corticosteroids for *Pneumocystis jiroveci* pneumonia in patients with HIV-infection. *Cochrane Database Syst Rev*. 2006;3:CD006150.
- Centers for Disease Control. Guidelines for preventing opportunistic infections among HIV-infected persons—2002 recommendations of the US Public Health Service and the Infectious Disease Society of America. *MMWR*. 2002;51(No. RR-8).
- Centers for Disease Control. Treating opportunistic infections among HIV-infected adults and adolescents: Recommendations from CDC, the National Institutes of Health, and the HIV Medicine Association/Infectious Disease Society of America. *MMWR*. 2004;53(No. RR-15).
- Dohn MN, White ML, Vigdorth EM. Geographic clustering of *Pneumocystis carinii* pneumonia in patients with HIV infection. *Am J Respir Crit Care Med*. 2000;162:1617–21.
- Green H, Paul M, Vidal L, et al. Prophylaxis for *Pneumocystis pneumonia* (PCP) in non-HIV immunocompromised patients. *Cochrane Database Syst Rev*. 2007;(3):CD005590.
- Shankar SM, Nania JJ. Management of *Pneumocystis jiroveci* pneumonia in children receiving chemotherapy. *Paediatr Drugs*. 2007;9:301–9.
- Stringer JR, Beard CB, Miller RF. A new name (*Pneumocystis jiroveci*) for *Pneumocystis* from humans. *Emerg Infect Dis*. 2002;8:891–6.

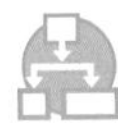

See Also (Topic, Algorithm, Electronic Media Element)

HIV Infection and AIDS

CODES

ICD9

136.3 Pneumocystosis

CLINICAL PEARLS

- Colonization with *P. jiroveci* is common in the pediatric population.
- PCP only occurs in immunocompromised patients.
- Patients with HIV are at risk once their CD4 count is <200. At that time, trimethoprim-sulfamethoxazole should be initiated as prophylaxis. Prophylaxis may end after HAART has been initiated and the CD4 count is above 200 for 3 months.
- Patients who are immunocompromised are also at risk. Currently there are no clear clinical guidelines as to when to initiate or end prophylaxis.
- The first-line treatment is trimethoprim-sulfamethoxazole. The typical duration of therapy is 14 days in non-AIDS-infected patients and 21 days in AIDS-infected patients.

PNEUMONIA, VIRAL

Bonnie Vallie, MD
Frank J. Domino, MD

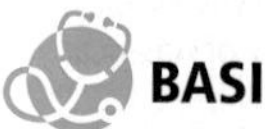

BASICS

DESCRIPTION

- Inflammatory disease of the lungs due to a viral infection
- Most viral pneumonia results from exposure of a susceptible nonimmune person to infection in the form of aerosolized secretions.

Geriatric Considerations

High rates of morbidity and mortality in the elderly

Pediatric Considerations

- The 2009 H1N1 influenza pandemic had higher rates of morbidity and mortality than seasonal influenza outbreaks in the pediatric population.
- Adenoviral infections in children are serious.
- More serious respiratory virus infections are almost always seen in infants and in immunocompromised patients.

Pregnancy Considerations

- Pregnant patients should avoid contact with anyone who has a viral infection.
- The 2009 H1N1 influenza pandemic had higher rates of morbidity and mortality than seasonal influenza outbreaks in the pregnant population.
- Vaccination is recommended for all pregnant women during the influenza season.

EPIDEMIOLOGY

Incidence

- Predominant age: Children
- Predominant sex: Male = Female

Prevalence

- Prevalence is unknown and varies with seasonal outbreaks, but the disease is more common during winter months.
- Around 90% of all cases of childhood pneumonias have a viral cause.
- In different published series, between 4% and 39% of pneumonia diagnosed in adults has been attributed to viral causes.

RISK FACTORS

- Immunocompromised state
- Living in close quarters
- Seasonal: Epidemic upper respiratory illness
- Elderly patients
- Pediatric patients, particularly those under 5 years of age or those born prematurely
- Cardiac disease
- Chronic pulmonary disease
- Recent upper respiratory infection
- Travel to endemic area (e.g., Southwest US, which has hantavirus)
- Nonvaccinated person
- Avian flu [influenza A (H1N1)] is currently not a risk for persons in the US, but it is a risk for those with poultry (chicken, duck, and turkey) contact in Asia, Europe, and the UK.

Genetics

No known genetic pattern has been recognized.

GENERAL PREVENTION

- General hand hygiene techniques are the first-line prevention in transmission of infectious particles.
- Influenza vaccination: Routine vaccination is now recommended for ALL persons aged 6 months and older. This represents an expansion of prior recommended populations (1):
  - Children who are 6 months to 8 years of age and receiving seasonal vaccination for the first time should receive 2 doses rather than 1.
  - Children who are 6 months to 8 years of age who received 1 or more doses of the 2010–2011 seasonal influenza vaccine should receive 1 dose of the 2011–2012 seasonal influenza vaccine (2).
  - The 2011–2012 influenza vaccine includes coverage for H1N1 (2).
  - See the CDC guidelines regarding the use of live, attenuated vaccine vs. inactivated vaccine.
- For those patients who are unable to receive influenza vaccine (e.g., with an egg allergy or other) and are at very high risk because of age, comorbid illness, or another risk factor, oseltamivir or zanamivir may be used for the duration of the season with special recognition for potential viral resistance (1).
- For those who did not receive the vaccine and have been exposed to influenza, use of oseltamivir or zanamivir is recommended for 7 days following exposure (1).

ETIOLOGY

Overall: Influenza A and respiratory syncytial virus (RSV) are leading causes followed by adenovirus and the parainfluenza viruses (3):

- Adults:
  - Influenza A, B, and C
  - Influenza H1N1
  - Adenovirus
  - Parainfluenza
  - Coronavirus
- Children:
  - Influenza A, B, and C
  - Influenza H1N1
  - Rhinovirus
  - Adenovirus
  - Parainfluenza
  - Rubeola (measles)
  - RSV (particularly for those born prematurely)
- Miscellaneous:
  - Cytomegalovirus (particularly in immunocompromised patients)
  - Varicella
  - Herpes simplex
  - Enterovirus
  - Rubeola
  - Epstein-Barr virus
  - Hantavirus
  - Human metapneumovirus
  - Avian influenza A (H1N1) is currently not a risk for persons in the US, but it is a risk for those with poultry (chicken, duck, and turkey) contact in Asia, Europe, and the UK.
  - Coinfection with bacterial pathogens is common.

COMMONLY ASSOCIATED CONDITIONS

- Bacterial forms of pneumonia
- Fungal infection and *Pneumocystis jiroveci* pneumonia in immunocompromised patients

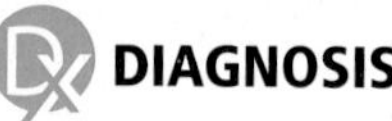

DIAGNOSIS

HISTORY

- Fever
- Chills
- Headache
- Myalgias
- Malaise
- Anorexia
- Cough (with or without purulent sputum production)
- Dyspnea
- Rhinorrhea
- Pharyngitis
- Pleurisy

PHYSICAL EXAM

- Fever
- Tachypnea
- Tachycardia
- Hypoxemia with severe disease
- Altered breath sounds
- Pulmonary rales and rhonchi
- Friction rub

DIAGNOSTIC TESTS & INTERPRETATION

Lab

- There are no standard labs to diagnose viral pneumonia.
- Specific laboratory investigations should be based upon the clinical scenario. For instance, in a patient with underlying pulmonary disease, a clinician may order an arterial blood gas to assess oxygenation.

Initial lab tests

CBC:

- Normal or near normal granulocyte count, occasionally leukopenic with increased lymphocyte percentage
- Hemoconcentration (hantavirus)

Follow-Up & Special Considerations

Clinicians can also consider additional testing, as clinically indicated:

- Appropriate direct fluorescent antibody or enzyme immunoassay from throat nasopharyngeal washings (children) or swab (adults), tracheal aspirate, or bronchoalveolar lavage specimens (HSV, varicella-zoster virus, influenza viruses A and B, RSV, adenovirus)
- Viral culture (3,4):
  - Limitations: Results take 3–14 days. False-negative results occur with lower viral titers.
  - Rapid antigen detection: Nasopharyngeal swab for rapid influenza testing
  - Cytopathology (cytoplasmic inclusion bodies [CMV], HSV, measles virus)

- Serology (4-fold rise in acute compared with convalescent titers): Confirm diagnosis retrospectively but not clinically useful
- Serologic testing for hantavirus: Enzyme immunoassay if available from health departments
- PCR detection if modality available (3):
  - Highly sensitive and specific but a positive result does not imply causality
- Sputum Gram stain and culture to identify bacterial copathogens if present

Imaging

Chest x-ray: Interstitial or alveolar infiltrates, peribronchial thickening, pleural effusion

Diagnostic Procedures/Surgery

Bronchoscopy with bronchoalveolar lavage

Pathological Findings

- Heavy lungs
- Enlarged regional lymph nodes
- CMV
- Intranuclear inclusion bodies (adenovirus, CMV, herpes virus, varicella virus)
- Intense inflammatory reaction with mononuclear cells
- Multinucleated giant cells (parainfluenza virus, measles virus, HSV, varicella virus)

DIFFERENTIAL DIAGNOSIS

- Bacterial pneumonia (especially atypical etiologies: *Chlamydophila pneumoniae* and *C. psittaci*, *Mycoplasma pneumoniae*, *Legionella pneumophila*)
- Pulmonary edema
- *Pneumocystis pneumonia/Pneumocystis jiroveci* pneumonia
- Aspiration pneumonia
- Hypersensitivity pneumonitis
- Bronchiolitis obliterans with organizing pneumonia
- Pulmonary embolus/infarction
- Cystic fibrosis (in infants)
- Severe acute respiratory syndrome or severe acute respiratory syndrome–associated coronavirus

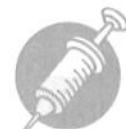

TREATMENT

- Outpatient treatment for most patients
- Inpatient treatment for infants <4 months of age or older people or for any patient with diffuse, severe infection (e.g., hypoxemia, hypercarbia, hypotension or shock, ARDS) or significant comorbidity (e.g., CHF, coronary artery disease, chronic obstructive pulmonary disease)
- The Pneumonia Severity Index Calculator (http://pda.ahrq.gov/clinic/psi/psicalc.asp) from the Agency for Healthcare Research and Quality may be used to assess the need for hospitalization as well as mortality risk (5)[A].

MEDICATION

First Line

- Influenza viruses A and B:
  - Oseltamivir (Tamiflu): Patients >18, 75 mg PO q12h for 5 days; dosage adjusted to 75 mg PO q24h in cases where creatinine clearance rate is <30 mL/min. Effectiveness is maximal when started within 48 hours of symptom onset (1)[A].
- Varicella-zoster virus:
  - Acyclovir:
    - Adults: For immunocompetent patients, 800 mg PO q6h for 5–7 days; use IBW for dosing (3)[B]
    - Children >2 years: For immunocompetent patients, 80 mg/kg/d PO divided q6h for 5 days. Start within 24 hours of symptom onset; immunocompromised patients, 30 mg/kg/d PO divided q6h for 5 days. Start within 24 hours of symptom onset; immunocompromised patients, 30 mg/kg/d IV div q8h for 7–10 days (3)[B]
- CMV or HSV:
  - Acyclovir:
    - Immunocompromised adults: 5 mg/kg IV q8h for 7 days (3)[B]
    - Children: Contact an infectious disease specialist or an experienced pharmacist regarding dosing.
  - Ganciclovir: Use should be in conjunction with infectious disease consultation (4)[B].
- RSV:
  - Ribavirin: Indicated in few, select cases (20 mg/mL via continuous aerosol administration for 12–18 hr/d for 3–7 days). Ribavirin is teratogenic and should not be administered by pregnant healthcare personnel: Its cost is high and benefits are marginal (3)[C].

Second Line

- Influenza: Amantadine and rimantadine are no longer recommended due to high levels of resistance among circulating influenza A viruses (1)[A].
- CMV, HSV, varicella virus infections:
  - Foscarnet (Foscavir): 60 mg/kg IV q8h in conjunction with infectious disease consultation (3,4)[C]

ADDITIONAL TREATMENT

General Measures

- Most healthy individuals will only require symptomatic treatment.
- Encourage coughing and deep breathing exercises to clear secretions.
- Careful disposal of secretions/universal precautions
- Hydration
- Respiratory isolation for varicella virus, which is highly contagious (i.e., negative pressure)

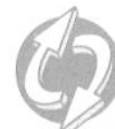

ONGOING CARE

FOLLOW-UP RECOMMENDATIONS

Patient Monitoring

- Physical exams
- Repeat a chest x-ray only if warranted by clinical presentation. A chest x-ray may take weeks to resolve after clinical illness has resolved.
- Oxygenation if illness severe enough for hospitalization

PATIENT EDUCATION

- For patient education materials on this topic, contact American Lung Association, 1301 Pennsylvania Avenue, NW, Suite 800, Washington, DC 20004; (800) LUNG-USA
- Centers for Disease Control and Prevention. Seasonal influenza (flu). Available at: www.cdc.gov/flu.

PROGNOSIS

- Usually favorable prognosis, with illness lasting several days to a week
- Postviral fatigue is common.
- Death can occur, especially in pediatric or bone marrow transplant patients with adenovirus infections or in older people with influenza.
- The 2009 H1N1 influenza pandemic resulted in higher-than-usual mortality rates among the pediatric, young adult, and pregnant populations.

COMPLICATIONS

- Superimposed bacterial infections such as *Streptococcus pneumoniae*, *Staphylococcus aureus*, *Haemophilus influenzae*, and others
- Respiratory failure requiring mechanical ventilation
- ARDS
- Reye syndrome after influenza in children

REFERENCES

1. Prevention & Control of Influenza with Vaccines—Recommendations of the Advisory Committee on Immunization Practices (ACIP) 2010. *MMWR*. 2010;59(RR08):1–62.
2. Prevention & Control of Influenza with Vaccines—Recommendations of the Advisory Committee on Immunization Practices (ACIP) 2011. *MMWR*. 2011;60(33):1128–32.
3. Marcos MA, et al. Viral pneumonia. *Curr Opin Infect Dis*. 2009;22:143–7.
4. Ruuskanen O, et al. Viral pneumonia. *Lancet*. 2011;377:1264–75.
5. *Pneumonia Severity Index Calculator: About*. December 2003. Agency for Healthcare Research and Quality. Rockville, MD. http://pda.ahrq.gov/psiabout.htm.

ADDITIONAL READING

Centers for Disease Control and Prevention. Seasonal influenza (flu). Available at: www.cdc.gov/flu.

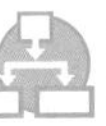

See Also (Topic, Algorithm, Electronic Media Element)

Bronchiolitis Obliterans and Organizing Pneumonia; Respiratory Distress Syndrome, Acute

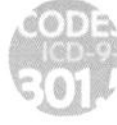

CODES

ICD9

- 480.1 Pneumonia due to respiratory syncytial virus
- 480.2 Pneumonia due to parainfluenza virus
- 480.9 Viral pneumonia, unspecified

CLINICAL PEARLS

- Laboratory testing may confirm the diagnosis of viral pneumonia but this must not replace clinical judgment.
- Influenza vaccination is now recommended for all persons age 6 months and older.
- Amantadine and rimantadine are no longer recommended for use against influenza.

PNEUMOTHORAX

Rocio Nordfeldt, MD
Felix B. Chang, MD

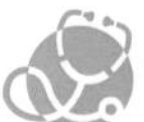

BASICS

DESCRIPTION

- Gas within the pleural space
- Primary spontaneous pneumothorax (PSP): This does not have a precipitating event in a person who does not have known lung disease.
- Secondary spontaneous pneumothorax (SSP): Associated with underlying lung disease. The most common: COPD, cystic fibrosis, pneumocystic jiroveci infection, and TB.

EPIDEMIOLOGY

Incidence

- PSP: 7.4 and 1.2 per 100,000/yr in men and women in the US, respectively.
- SSP: 6.3 and 2 per 100,000/yr in men and women in the US, respectively.

Prevalence

- 70% of cases of SSP occur with COPD.
- Rupture of apical blebs
- 30% of patients with pneumocystic pneumonia develop SSP.
- 6% of all patients with cystic fibrosis will have an episode of SSP.
- 1–3% of patients hospitalized with TB

RISK FACTORS

- PSP: Smoking, family history, Marfan syndrome, homocystinuria, and thoracic endometriosis
- SSP:
  - Airway disease: COPD, asthma, cystic fibrosis, alpha 1-antitrypsin deficiency
  - Infection: *Pneumocystis* pneumonia, TB, necrotizing pneumonia
  - Malignancy: Lung cancer, synovial sarcoma
  - Connective tissue disorder: Marfan or Ehlers-Danlos syndromes, scleroderma, rheumatoid arthritis, ankylosing spondylitis, polymyositis/dermatomyositis
  - Interstitial lung disease: Sarcoidosis, idiopathic pulmonary fibrosis, histiocytosis X, lymphangioleiomyomatosis, esophageal rupture, bronchial obstruction or foreign body (also complications from scuba diving or a loss of airplane cabin pressure)
  - Traumatic pneumothorax:
    - Trauma (penetrating injury, broken rib, ruptured bronchus, perforated esophagus)
    - Iatrogenic/postprocedure: Intubation, central line placement, liver biopsy, mechanical ventilation, thoracentesis, cardiopulmonary resuscitation
    - IV drug abusers (who attempt to access the internal jugular vein)

Genetics

- PSP: A family history of autosomal-dominant, autosomal-recessive, polygenic, and X-linked recessive inheritance has been proposed.
- Birt-Hogg-Dubé syndrome: Autosomal-dominant, associated with lung cysts, benign skin tumor, renal cancer; the *FLCN* mutation has been mapped to chromosome 17p11.2
- Marfan syndrome: Some patients develop lung bullae, which predispose them to PSP. Genes implicated: Mutations in fibrillin-1 (FBN1), transforming growth factor-beta receptor (TGFBR)

GENERAL PREVENTION

Patients should cease smoking and wear seatbelts while driving.

PATHOPHYSIOLOGY

- Loss of negative intrapleural pressure, lung collapse
- Simple pneumothorax: The pleural pressure in the affected hemithorax remains subatmospheric and is only more positive than the pleural pressure in the contralateral hemithorax.
- Tension pneumothorax: The pleural pressure in the affected hemithorax exceeds atmospheric pressure, particularly during expiration.
- Open pneumothorax: The traumatic chest wall defect persists, and ambient air enters the pleural space during inspiration. The mediastinum shifts to the normal hemithorax, and the lung within the injured hemithorax remains collapsed. During expiration, the air exits the pleural space through the chest wall defect, and the mediastinum swings back toward the injured hemithorax.
- Pneumothorax ex vacuo: This is the result of rapid atelectasis, producing an abrupt decrease in the intrapleural pressure with the subsequent release of nitrogen from pleural capillaries.

ETIOLOGY

- Perforation of the visceral pleura and entry of gas from the lung; penetration of the chest wall, diaphragm, mediastinum, or esophagus
- Blunt thoracic trauma: Gas generated by microorganisms in an empyema
- Spontaneous rupture of pulmonary or subpleural bleb into pleural space
- The rupture of large subpleural cysts caused by subpleural necrosis is the cause of most SSP in pneumocystic jiroveci patients.
- Cystic fibrosis: Rupture of apical subpleural cysts, coinfection with *Pseudomonas aeruginosa*, *Burkholderia cepacia* complex, or *Aspergillus* species, or a prior episode of massive hemoptysis.
- TB: Rupture of a tuberculous cavity into the pleural space
- Pulmonary barotrauma: 10% on mechanical ventilation

COMMONLY ASSOCIATED CONDITIONS

See "Risk Factors."

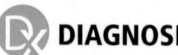

DIAGNOSIS

HISTORY

- Chest pain (sudden onset, maximum intensity, sharp, usually lateral and pleuritic), dyspnea; cough, palpitations, and Horner syndrome are less common.
- Moderate to severe: Profound respiratory distress, shock, circulatory collapse; referred pain to shoulder or back; history of chest trauma, lung disease, family history, previous hemothorax

PHYSICAL EXAM

- Asymmetry of respirations: Diminished or absent breath sounds on the affected side
- Decreased fremitus: Absent egophony and bronchophony on the affected side
- Hyperresonance to percussion: Crepitus over the chest wall and neck (SC emphysema), tachycardia, respiratory distress, cyanosis
- Tension pneumothorax: Hypotension, cyanosis, tachycardia. The tracheal deviation is away from the affected side. The patient usually has a weak, rapid pulse; pallor; neck vein distention; anxiety; and an altered mental status.
- Consider TP with the sudden onset of tachycardia and hypotension in patients on a ventilator.

DIAGNOSTIC TESTS & INTERPRETATION

Lab

Initial lab tests

- Arterial blood gases (ABGs): Elevated A–a gradient and acute respiratory alkalosis, hypoxemia
- ECG: May show axis deviation, nonspecific ST-segment changes, T-wave inversion

Imaging

Initial approach

- CXRs:
  - White visceral pleural line outlines the edge of lung, separated by a space with no lung/vascular markings adjacent to chest wall
  - Upright: ~50 mL of pleural gas; mostly apicolateral location
  - Supine: ~500 mL of pleural gas; most pleural gas accumulates in subpulmonic location; anterior pleural reflexion
  - Deep sulcus sign: Low lateral costophrenic angle on the affected side
  - Lateral decubitus: ~5 mL of pleural gas; gas in nondependent lateral location
- CT scan: This is the most sensitive technique and is valuable for locating small collections of gas, loculated pneumothoraces, atypical collections, and pleural pathology.
  - Occult pneumothorax (OP) is not suspected on the basis of a clinical exam or plain radiography but is detected with thoracoabdominal CT scanning.
- Ultrasound: Sliding lung sign: Visceral and parietal pleura move relative to one another during the respiratory cycle. Comet-tail artifacts are echogenic lines that originate at the visceral-parietal-pleural interface and extend to the bottom of the sonographic image (1).
- Simple pneumothorax: No mediastinal shift
- Tension pneumothorax: Radiograph shows the shift of the mediastinum to the contralateral side and flattening or inversion of the ipsilateral hemidiaphragm
- Open pneumothorax: Radiograph shows a visible chest wall defect and massive expiratory mediastinal shift toward the injured side
- Pneumothorax ex vacuo: Forms adjacent to an atelectasis lobe

DIFFERENTIAL DIAGNOSIS

- Acute coronary syndrome
- Pericarditis
- Congestive heart failure
- Pulmonary edema
- Aortic dissection
- Pneumonia
- Pulmonary embolism
- Pleural effusion
- Flail chest
- Hemothorax
- Asthma/COPD

- Airway obstruction/foreign body
- Esophageal perforation
- Diaphragmatic hernia
- Should be differentiated from bullae, skin folds, stomach herniation into chest following rupture of the left hemidiaphragm

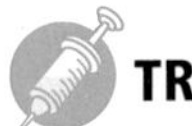

TREATMENT

MEDICATION

First Line

- Providing 100% O_2 accelerates the rate of pleural air absorption.
- TP: Within the second or third intercostal space of the midclavicular line, use needle decompression with a 14-gauge needle.

SURGERY/OTHER PROCEDURES

- For first-time PSP:
  - If small (<2–3 cm, <20%) and few symptoms: Patient may be observed in the emergency department for 3–6 hours and discharged if repeat x-ray shows no progression (2).
  - If larger and/or patient is symptomatic:
    - Aspiration technique: (i) Position patient semisupine at 45°, (ii) prep and anesthetize the skin, (iii) insert a 16-gauge over-the-needle catheter into the second anterior intercostal space and aspirate air, (iv) extract the needle and connect a 3-way stopcock and 60-mL syringe, and (v) aspirate until no more air can be removed. There is disagreement as to whether a failed aspiration should be reattempted (3)[A].
    - Radiologists can place small-bore catheters or small-caliber chest tubes over a guide wire and connect to a Heimlich valve or water seal. However, no RTCs have compared their effectiveness.
    - One RTC has shown no difference between aspiration and a chest tube in outcomes, and fewer hospitalizations with aspiration, but this should be accepted with caution owing to the small sample size in the study.
- TP (a medical emergency):
  - Needle decompression: Insert a 19F or larger needle (14–16-gauge, 5-cm needle) into the second intercostal space at the midclavicular line over the superior aspect of the rib to avoid vessels, and attach a 3-way stopcock. (Failure rate is 10–35%; longer needles are needed for patients with increased chest wall thickness.) Use a large syringe to withdraw air. Follow with a chest tube.
  - Insert a thoracostomy tube (16–22F) into the fourth, fifth, or sixth intercostal space at the midaxillary line and connect to a water seal device. Clamp the tube after 12 hours of no further air leakage.
- If the pneumothorax is large, the patient is unstable, or prior treatment has failed:
  - Insert a thoracostomy tube (16–22F) into the fourth, fifth, or sixth intercostal space at the midaxillary line and connect to a water seal device. Clamp the tube after 12 hours of no further air leakage.
- VATS can be used for persistent air leakage and when the lung is <90% expanded.
- For recurrent PSP:
  - Options: Pleurodesis via VATS, chemical pleurodesis via tube thoracostomy, and thoracotomy
  - VATS pleurodesis: The rate of recurrent pneumothorax is <5% after VATS with bleb/bullae resection and pleurodesis.
  - Pleurodesis with sclerosing agent via chest tube or thoracostomy: Superior to simple drainage in reducing recurrence rate; by symphysis between parietal and visceral pleura:
    - Intrapleural talc: 5 g in 250 mL of isotonic saline; more effective than tetracycline derivatives, but safety concerns still exist (4).
    - Intrapleural doxycycline: 5 mg/kg or 500 mg in total of 50 mL
    - Sclerosing agents are contraindicated if the patient is a possible candidate for a future lung transplant because the agents increase the risk of bleeding during surgery. Side effects are fever, pain, and acute lung injury.
    - VATS with pleurodesis is recommended for:
      - Recurrent PSP, initial SSP, with persistent air leakage after 3 days
      - Persistent bronchopleural fistula
      - Patient preference or patient with a high-risk occupation (e.g., pilot, diver)
      - Open thoracotomy if failed or unavailable VAT
- For traumatic/OP:
  - Usually both overt and occult pneumothorax patients get chest tubes.
  - Small to moderate OP can be treated conservatively.
- Aspiration is done with an 18-gauge needle with an 8–9F catheter inserted into the pleural space, the catheter is threaded deeper into the pleural space, and then the needle is withdrawn.
- A 16–24F chest tube is generally used for spontaneous or iatrogenic pneumothorax.
- For traumatic pneumothoraces, 28–40F tubes are used to drain blood as well as add air if necessary.

IN-PATIENT CONSIDERATIONS

Admission Criteria

Admit all patients with large PSPs that do not resolve completely with simple aspiration; recurrent pneumothorax; SSP; or traumatic pneumothorax.

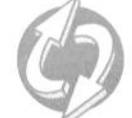

ONGOING CARE

FOLLOW-UP RECOMMENDATIONS

- A follow-up CXR showing a stable or smaller pneumothorax in 24 hours suggests adequate treatment.
- No air travel should be taken until radiographs are normal.
- Athletes with pneumothorax may return to sports after 2–3 weeks of rest as symptoms permit; athletes who require inpatient care should have a normal CXR before resuming sports activity.
- Deep-sea diving is contraindicated in patients with PSP until bilateral surgical pleurodectomy is performed.

Patient Monitoring

- Aspiration: A closed stopcock can be attached and the in-dwelling catheter is secured to the chest wall. Obtain a CXR 4 hours later. If adequate lung expansion had occurred, the catheter can be removed. Following 2 hours of observation, another chest radiograph should be performed. The patient can be discharged if the lung remains expanded on this chest radiograph. If not, the catheter can be left in place and attached to a Heimlich valve. The patient can then be discharged with follow-up within 2 days.
- Bed rest while chest tube is in place
- The chest tube might be clamped 12 hours after the last evidence of an air leak and a chest radiograph should be performed 24 hours after the last evidence of an air leak. The tube can be removed if the pneumothorax has not reaccumulated.
- If the lung has not fully re-expanded after 7 days, consider persistent bronchopleural fistula.
- Outpatient management should include a follow-up CXR to document the resolution of the pneumothorax, typically within several days after discharge.

PROGNOSIS

- Air is reabsorbed in days to weeks. Chest pain typically resolves in 24 hours in PSP.
- The prognosis is worse depending on comorbidities. It is more severe with SSP.
- The occurrence of SSP due to PCP has a poor prognosis.

COMPLICATIONS

- Recurrent PSP: 25–50%, with most recurrences occurring within the first year
- Failure of lung re-expansion; persistent air leak

REFERENCES

1. Havelock T, Teoh R, et al. Pleural procedures and thoracic ultrasound: British Thoracic Society Pleural Disease Guideline 2010. *Thorax*. 2010; 65(Suppl 2):ii61–76.
2. Management of spontaneous pneumothorax: an American College of Chest Physicians Delphi consensus statement. *Chest*. 2001;119(2):590.
3. Wakai A, O'Sullivan RG, McCabe G. Simple aspiration versus intercostal tube drainage for primary spontaneous pneumothorax in adults. *Cochrane Database Syst Rev*. 2007;CD004479.
4. Management of spontaneous pneumothorax. British Thoracic Society Pleural Disease Guideline 2010. *Thorax*. 2010;65(Suppl 2):ii18.

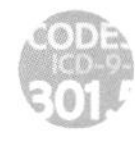

CODES

ICD9

- 512.0 Spontaneous tension pneumothorax
- 512.8 Other spontaneous pneumothorax
- 860.0 Traumatic pneumothorax without mention of open wound into thorax

CLINICAL PEARLS

- PSP is rare in patients over age 40; consider more aggressive workup if this occurs.
- Do not wait for a chest x-ray if there is a respiratory or hemodynamic compromise.
- If there is tension pneumothorax, use needle decompression. Insert a 19F or larger needle (14–16-gauge, 5-cm needle) into the second intercostal space at the midclavicular line over the superior aspect of the rib to avoid vessels, and attach a 3-way stopcock. Use a large syringe to withdraw air. Follow with a chest tube.

POLIOMYELITIS

Omar A. Khan, MD, MHS, FAAFP

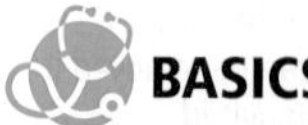

BASICS

DESCRIPTION

- Poliomyelitis describes the acute illness:
  - Most patients contracting the poliovirus are asymptomatic.
  - Around 5% develop symptoms, and 0.1% develop the paralytic form.
- Patients may present with GI symptoms.
- A subset will develop neurologic disease.
- Illness is biphasic; paralysis occurs in the second phase:
  - Paralytic disease occurs with rapid onset.
- Spread by direct fecal–oral contact; more common in warm months
- Virus secreted for weeks in stool:
  - Poliomyelitis syndromes: Encephalitic; bulbar (which produces cranial nerve paralysis); spinal (causing weakness in the extremities, particularly the legs)
  - Postpolio syndrome (PPS): A distinct entity affecting those previously diagnosed with poliomyelitis; involves atrophy of muscle groups unaffected by original illness (1)
- System(s) affected: Nervous; Musculoskeletal
- Synonym(s): Infantile paralysis; Acute anterior poliomyelitis; acute lateral poliomyelitis

Geriatric Considerations

Extremely rare; primary vaccination not recommended (except if a patient is traveling to endemic areas)

Pediatric Considerations

Most common in this age group. Infection is extremely rare in the US since the introduction of effective vaccines (see "Immunizations").

Pregnancy Considerations

A risk factor for developing polio (incidence and severity of polio are increased in pregnant women)

EPIDEMIOLOGY

Incidence

- Predominant age: 3 months–16 years; rare in adults
- Now rare but not yet eradicated; present in endemic settings; small outbreaks in areas where polio eradication has occurred, and rarely as vaccine-associated paralytic polio (VAPP) cases
- PPS can manifest years to decades after initial infection.

Prevalence

- In 2010, there were only 4 remaining polio-endemic countries: Afghanistan, India, Nigeria, and Pakistan. Importation cases are present in some others as well (sub-Saharan Africa, Nepal, and Tajikistan) (2).
- Worldwide: 1,595 cases in 2009 (1,247 from 4 endemic countries; 348 from 19 countries where the disease was imported or possibly re-established)
- Previous worldwide numbers were 1,660 cases in 2008; 1,315 cases in 2007
- Highest numbers in 2009 were in India (741) and Nigeria (388)
- No wild-virus cases of polio in the US

RISK FACTORS

- Poor sanitation and hygiene
- Poverty
- Unimmunized status, especially if <5 years of age

GENERAL PREVENTION

- Vaccination via the inactivated poliovirus vaccine (IPV) in developed settings (3)
- Oral vaccine (OPV) in endemic or at-risk countries
- No causal link between the polio vaccine and Guillain-Barré
- In developing countries, safe water treatment to avoid contaminated water and food sources

PATHOPHYSIOLOGY

- Poliovirus initially infects the GI tract. It may spread to lymph nodes and rarely to CNS.
- Pharyngeal spread is less common, but it is the prevalent mode of transmission in areas of good hygiene.
- Person-to-person spread is the most common means of transmission, followed by contaminated water and sewage.

ETIOLOGY

3 serotypes of poliovirus (genus *Enterovirus*):

- Type 1 most frequently associated with epidemics
- Types 2 and 3 usually associated with VAPP

COMMONLY ASSOCIATED CONDITIONS

- IM injections or trauma during the prodrome of paralytic polio can precipitate paralysis.
- Tonsillectomy is considered a risk factor for bulbar paralysis.

DIAGNOSIS

- Virus culture from stool, pharynx, or CSF
- An antibody response is useful for ruling out rather than ruling in polio, because immunization also may provoke such a response.

HISTORY

If the affected person is from a nonendemic country, then *travel history* is important.

- Most patients are asymptomatic:
- ~10% will show symptoms of a minor GI illness:
  - Fever
  - Headache
  - Malaise
  - Nausea and vomiting
- A minority of these patients will progress to the major illness, which includes asymmetric paralysis of extremities (usually lower).
- Aseptic meningitis occurs in a minority of patients with the major illness.

PHYSICAL EXAM

- Fever
- Significant motor loss on affected side or limb
- Meningeal signs may be present in the minor illness or early phases of paralytic polio.
- Decreased deep tendon reflexes
- Muscle atrophy in affected areas

DIAGNOSTIC TESTS & INTERPRETATION

CSF and pharynx virus isolation (early in disease) and/or feces (early and late in disease)

Lab

- Increased CSF protein
- Lymphocytosis, especially of CSF
- Normal CSF glucose
- Serology
- Virus culture from stool or pharynx

Imaging

An MRI may be helpful to evaluate the involvement of the anterior horn of the spinal cord or other findings.

Diagnostic Procedures/Surgery

An EMG may be useful to assess the progress of paralysis and of PPS.

Pathological Findings

Spinal cord: Perivascular cuffing, abnormal motor nuclei, chromatolysis of motor neurons, intermediate and posterior column inflammation

DIFFERENTIAL DIAGNOSIS

- For acute flaccid paralysis and paralytic polio:
  - Guillain-Barré syndrome
  - Transverse myelitis
  - Acute motor axonal neuropathy (China paralytic syndrome)
  - Traumatic neuritis
  - Myasthenia gravis
  - Polymyositis
  - Periodic paralysis
  - Trichinosis
  - Aseptic, bacterial, and tuberculous meningitis/encephalitis
  - Toxic encephalopathies
  - Tick paralysis
- For nonparalytic acute polio infection:
  - Enteroviruses, echoviruses, and coxsackieviruses

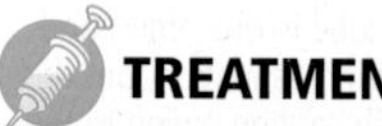

TREATMENT

The European Federation of Neurological Societies has guidelines on PPS describing muscular training, targeted physical therapy, and assistive devices as needed.

MEDICATION

- Nonnarcotic analgesics (aspirin should not be used for children due to the suggested, small risk of Reye syndrome)
- Antibiotics, only if concurrent infection develops
- Parasympathomimetic pharmacotherapy for urinary retention may be required.
- Preliminary investigations suggest that IVIG may improve the quality of life for PPS patients (4).
- Small studies on lamotrigine, modafinil, amantadine, and pyridostigmine suggest benefits, but no conclusive evidence is available to recommend these as therapy.
- Contraindications and precautions: Refer to the manufacturers' literature.
- Significant possible interactions: Refer to the manufacturers' literature.

First Line

None available for curative treatment

ADDITIONAL TREATMENT

General Measures

- Mechanical ventilation, if required
- Public health: With all suspected cases, report immediately to the local health authority, such as a public health department in the US or a WHO affiliate in developing countries.
- Any case of polio is considered an emergency.

Issues for Referral

- Referral to a neurologist is indicated in the case of the major illness.
- Infectious disease referral is warranted at the time of diagnosis.
- After discharge, referral to physical therapy (PT), neurology, or physical medicine and rehabilitation is indicated, especially for PPS.
- Psychiatry or clinical psychology referral can be helpful for the patient and caregivers.

Additional Therapies

- Early PT in acute paralytic polio may help a child to regain function and develop adaptations.
- With paralysis (acute or postpolio), extended PT may be required.
- Long-term rehabilitation plan: PT, braces, special shoes, possibly orthopedic surgery; team effort with doctors, physical and occupational therapists, and social worker or psychiatrist, if necessary

SURGERY/OTHER PROCEDURES

- Tracheostomy for respiratory paralysis
- Surgery may be required in patients with muscle contractures or to relieve severe deformity resulting from muscle atrophy and paralysis.

IN-PATIENT CONSIDERATIONS

Initial Stabilization

Inpatient admission for acute phase or if concern for respiratory/bulbar paralysis exists; outpatient or rehabilitation facility for therapy

Admission Criteria

- New-onset neurologic symptoms such as stiff neck, seizures, and paralysis
- Once diagnosed, cases of paralytic polio may need admission to observe for bulbar paralysis.
- Dehydration resulting from the minor illness

Nursing

The main concerns relate to mobilization to regain function, assurance of hygiene if bowel/bladder incontinence exists, skin care if mobility is severely restricted, and pain control in case of contractures:

- Provide a bed that has a firm mattress, footboard, foam-rubber pads, or sandbags. Change the patient's positions frequently. Ensure good skin care.
- Manage fecal impaction and urinary retention; catheterization may be necessary.

Discharge Criteria

- In case of the minor form of the illness, self-limited resolution
- In case of the major form of the illness, criteria include a plan for outpatient follow-up by the family physician, a specialist in orthopedics or neurology, and a physical therapist.

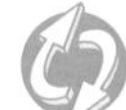

ONGOING CARE

FOLLOW-UP RECOMMENDATIONS

- PT is essential for patients with paralytic polio.
- Counseling for the patient, caregivers, and family is useful in managing lifetime sequelae.
- Bed rest is necessary during the active phase of the disease as per patient tolerance; as noted, PT and nonfatiguing exercises may help.

DIET

- May require tube feedings if patient is paralyzed
- Unrestricted except for conditions determined by patient's ability to swallow

PATIENT EDUCATION

For patient education materials, contact:

- International Polio Network, 4502 Maryland Avenue, St. Louis, MO 63108, (314) 361-0475
- Educational presentation on polio from the CDC: www.cdc.gov/vaccines/pubs/pinkbook/downloads/Slides/Polio10.ppt
- PPS patient materials via Post-Polio Health International: www.post-polio.org/
- The Global Polio Eradication Initiative, coordinated by the WHO: www.polioeradication.org
- Brain Resources and Information Network (BRAIN), National Institute of Neurological Disorders and Stroke (NINDS), National Institutes of Health, Bethesda, MD: www.ninds.nih.gov

PROGNOSIS

- Often irreversible paralysis; <5% mortality during acute phase of disease
- Increased mortality in patients >40 years of age
- Poor recovery for totally paralyzed muscle groups; good recovery for partially paralyzed muscle groups
- Variable recovery for PPS; can be facilitated by appropriate PT

COMPLICATIONS

- UTI
- Skin ulcers
- Traumatic injuries to affected limb(s)
- Atelectasis
- Pneumonia
- Myocarditis
- Postpoliomyelitis progressive muscular atrophy: Progressive weakness 30 years or more after an attack of poliomyelitis. Adult survivors of childhood polio now suffer late complications.
- Postpoliomyelitis motor neuron disease: Occurs years after acute poliomyelitis; less common than postpoliomyelitis progressive muscular atrophy
- VAPP is a rare complication of the oral poliovirus vaccine.

REFERENCES

1. Gonzalez H, Olsson T, Borg K, et al. Management of postpolio syndrome. *Lancet Neurol*. 2010;9:634–42.
2. Adams T. Global eradication of poliomyelitis: Is the end of the campaign in sight? *J Paediatric Child Health*. 2010;46(11):619–22.
3. Mayer CA, Neilson AA. Poliomyelitis—prevention in travellers. *Aust Fam Physician*. 2010;39:122–5.
4. Koopman FS, Uegaki K, Gilhus NE, et al. Treatment for postpolio syndrome. *Cochrane Database Syst Rev*. 201116;(2):CD007818.

ADDITIONAL READING

- Centers for Disease Control and Prevention. Polio. Available at: www.cdc.gov/polio/
- Global Polio Eradication Initiative www.polioeradication.org/
- Nathanson N, Kew OM, et al. From emergence to eradication: The epidemiology of poliomyelitis deconstructed. *Am J Epidemiol*. 2010;172:1213–29.
- Thompson KM, Tebbens RJ, Pallansch MA, et al. The risks, costs, and benefits of possible future global policies for managing polioviruses. *Am J Public Health*. 2008;98:1322–30.

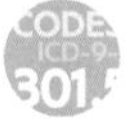

CODES

ICD9

- 045.90 Unspecified acute poliomyelitis, unspecified type poliovirus
- 045.91 Unspecified acute poliomyelitis, poliovirus type i
- 045.92 Unspecified acute poliomyelitis, poliovirus type ii

CLINICAL PEARLS

- VAPP has been eliminated from the US since the implementation of the IPV-only vaccine in 2000 (ending the use of the live oral poliovirus vaccine).
- VAPP occurred in roughly 1 of 2.9 million doses of the vaccine in the 1990s.
- About 95% of wild-virus polio cases are asymptomatic, and <1% will develop paralysis. Wild-type polio no longer exists in the United States. Polio remains in wild-type strains in 4 countries in Asia and Africa. The WHO goal to eradicate the disease likely will be pushed back beyond 2012.

POLYARTERITIS NODOSA

Prachaya Nitichaikulvatana, MD
Katherine Upchurch, MD

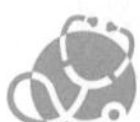

BASICS

DESCRIPTION

- Polyarteritis nodosa (PAN) is a necrotizing vasculitis that typically affects medium-sized arteries, with occasional involvement of small-sized arteries.
- Systemic symptoms are prominent at presentation.
- Most common organ involvement: GI tract, peripheral nervous system (sensory and motor), kidney, skin, testes and epididymis, cardiac, CNS
- PAN formerly encompassed several distinct clinical entities (classic PAN, microscopic PAN, and cutaneous PAN). With the advent of antineutrophilic antibody (ANCA) testing has come the understanding that microscopic PAN may not be related to the other 2 pathophysiologically. In particular, patients with microscopic PAN have ANCAs directed against myeloperoxidase (MPO) and generally involvement of small arterioles. This disease is also known as *microscopic polyangiitis* and is now classified as one of the ANCA-associated vasculitides.
- Classic PAN (now commonly referred to as PAN), in contrast, is *not typically associated with ANCA positivity*.
- Cutaneous (or limited) PAN is a disease in which patients have largely cutaneous and neurologic manifestations with characteristic histopathologic features but few systemic features. ANCA positivity is variable.
- Synonym(s) for PAN: Periarteritis; Panarteritis; Necrotizing arteritis

Pregnancy Considerations

One case report suggests that if a woman of childbearing age with PAN attains remission before becoming pregnant, there is a reasonable chance of a successful pregnancy.

EPIDEMIOLOGY

Incidence

- Predominant age: All ages; peak onset is in the fifth to sixth decade
- Predominant sex: Male > Female (2.5:1)

Prevalence

Rare; 31 cases/1 million adults in European study

RISK FACTORS

Hepatitis B infection

Genetics

Unknown

ETIOLOGY

- Unknown
- Immune-complex mediation has been postulated.
- In patients with PAN and hepatitis B, studies have shown immune complexes containing the hepatitis B antigen in involved vessel walls.

COMMONLY ASSOCIATED CONDITIONS

- Hepatitis B (most strongly in classic PAN)
- Hepatitis C (linked to cutaneous PAN)
- Hairy cell leukemia
- 27 case reports of systemic PAN following hepatitis B vaccination (1)
- Case reports of various drugs such as amphetamines, minocycline, and interferon

DIAGNOSIS

- Acute multisystem disease with a relatively short prodrome (i.e., weeks to months); delays in diagnosis are common.
- The spectrum of disease ranges from single-organ involvement to fulminant polyvisceral failure.

HISTORY

General: Systemic symptoms with multiorgan involvement (2,3):

- Constitutional symptoms (e.g., fever, weight loss, malaise)
- Symptoms highly dependent on specific organ system involved:
  - Focal muscular weakness or extremity numbness
  - Myalgia and arthralgia
  - Rash
  - Recurrent postprandial pain, intestinal angina, nausea, vomiting, and bleeding
  - Altered mental status, headaches

PHYSICAL EXAM

Related to organ system involved by vasculitic process (may dominate clinical picture and course):

- Peripheral nervous system: Mononeuritis multiplex, peripheral neuropathy
- Renal: Hypertension, proteinuria, progressive renal failure, hematuria (usually microscopic) but no RBC casts
- Skin: Purpura, urticaria, SC hemorrhages, polymorphic rashes, SC nodules (uncommon but characteristic), persistent livedo reticularis, deep skin ulcers, especially in lower extremities, Raynaud phenomenon (rare)
- GI: Acute abdomen due to bowel infarction and perforation, cholecystitis, and gallbladder infarctions; asymptomatic microaneurysm in the liver (4)
- CNS: Seizures, altered mental status, thrombotic stroke (with cerebral artery involvement), papillitis
- Lung: Pleural effusion, rarely bronchial arteritis:
  - Capillaritis or other lung parenchymal involvement by vasculitis strongly suggests another process (microscopic PAN, Wegener granulomatosis, Churg-Strauss syndrome) or antiglomerular basement membrane disease.
- Cardiac: Congestive heart failure (CHF) associated with hypertension (HTN) and/or myocardial infarction; pericarditis (rare)
- Genitourinary: Testicular, epididymal; ovarian involvement; neurogenic bladder (rare)
- Musculoskeletal: Arthritis (usually large joint in lower extremities)

DIAGNOSTIC TESTS & INTERPRETATION

- Diagnosis should be confirmed by biopsy whenever possible.
- Angiography may be helpful to reveal microaneurysms of blood vessels.
- CT angiography and MR angiography may be substituted for conventional angiography.

Lab

- Specific: Mainly based on pathologic findings of biopsy material from involved organs
- Nonspecific (2):
  - ESR and C-reactive protein (CRP)
  - Hepatitis B surface antigen positive in 10–50% of patients (strong circumstantial evidence)
  - Hepatitis C antibody or hepatitis C virus RNA
  - Antineutrophilic cytoplasmic antibody (ANCA) is usually negative.
  - Negative proteinase-3 (PR3) or MPO antibodies
  - Rheumatoid factor may be positive.
  - Anemia of chronic disease
  - Hypergammaglobulinemia
  - Mild proteinuria
  - Elevated creatinine

Initial lab tests

Laboratory studies with abnormalities:

- CBC (anemia of chronic disease)
- Chemistries: Elevated creatinine/BUN
- Hepatitis B serology: Often positive
- Liver function tests: Abnormal in unusual cases such as PAN involving the liver or gallbladder
- Urinalysis may show proteinuria but generally no cellular casts or active urinary sediment.
- ANCA antibody testing as well as specific tests for anti-MPO and anti-PR3

Imaging

Angiographic demonstration of aneurysmal changes in small and medium-sized arteries: Mesenteric, renal, hepatic artery aneurysm

Diagnostic Procedures/Surgery

- Electromyography (EMG) and nerve conduction studies (NCSs) can be useful in patients with suspected mononeuritis multiplex. EMG/NCSs can be used to guide a sural nerve biopsy, if necessary.
- Arterial or tissue biopsy wherever involvement suspected; biopsy feasible
- Skin biopsy: The biopsy should be collected at the edges of ulcer and include deep dermis and SC fat for high yield of diagnosis.

Pathological Findings

- Necrotizing inflammation with fibrinoid necrosis, in various stages, of small and medium-sized muscular arteries; segmental in distribution, it is often seen at bifurcations and branchings. Involvement of venules is not seen in classic PAN.
- Acute lesions show infiltration of polymorphonuclear cells through vessel walls and perivascular area.
- Subsequent proliferation, degeneration, appearance of monocytes, necrosis with thrombosis, and infarction of the involved tissue; aneurysmal dilatations are characteristic.
- Aortic dissection is reported to be attributed to necrotizing vasculitis of the vasa vasorum.
- Peripheral nerves: 50–70% (vasa nervorum with necrotizing vasculitis)
- GI vessels: 50% (at autopsy); gallbladder and appendix: 10%
- Muscle vessels: 50%
- Testicular vasculature is often positive when males are symptomatic.

- The key differences from other necrotizing vasculitides are lack of granuloma formation and sparing of veins and pulmonary arteries.

DIFFERENTIAL DIAGNOSIS

- Other forms of vasculitis; ANCA-associated vasculitis such as Wegener granulomatosis, Churg-Strauss syndrome, and microscopic polyangiitis; Henoch-Schönlein purpura
- Cryoglobulinemia
- Buerger disease
- Systemic lupus erythematosus (SLE)
- Amyloidosis
- Multiple sclerosis
- Embolic disease such as atrial myxoma, cholesterol emboli
- Dissecting aneurysm
- Subacute endocarditis
- Trichinosis
- Some rickettsial diseases

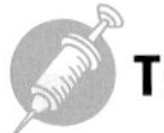

TREATMENT

MEDICATION

First Line

- **Corticosteroids** (high-dose prednisone or parenteral solumedrol ± pulse for stabilization)
  - Only 50% of patients achieved and maintained remission with corticosteroid alone, and 40% of patients required additional immunosuppressive therapy (5).
- Cyclophosphamide in combination with corticosteroids (improved survival and steroid-sparing) in moderate or severe PAN (5)
  - Cyclophosphamide can have long-term sequelae of infertility and malignancy (6)[A].
- Other immunosuppressive agents: Azathioprine (Imuran) (5), methotrexate
- Plasma exchange (efficacy not established)
- Small study of short-term steroids followed by lamivudine and plasma exchanges suggests effectiveness of this regimen in hepatitis B–related PAN (unconfirmed) (7).

Second Line

Tumor necrosis factor inhibitors (anecdotal evidence)

ADDITIONAL TREATMENT

- For patients receiving IV cyclophosphamide, suggest concurrent administration of mercaptoethane sulfonate (MESNA).
- For patients on cyclophosphamide, we recommend prophylactic treatment against *Pneumocystis jiroveci* (*carinii*) pneumonia with trimethoprim sulfamethoxazole or atovaquone in patients who are intolerant or allergic to trimethoprim sulfamethoxazole.

IN-PATIENT CONSIDERATIONS

Initial Stabilization

Depends on extent and involvement of specific organs

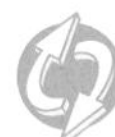

ONGOING CARE

FOLLOW-UP RECOMMENDATIONS

Patient Monitoring

- CBC, urinalysis, and renal and hepatic profiles
- Careful monitoring for infection
- Delayed appearance of neoplasms (especially in patients who were treated with cyclophosphamide)
- Acute-phase reactants such as CRP may be helpful in monitoring activity level during treatment and follow-up.

DIET

Low salt if patient has attendant HTN

PATIENT EDUCATION

Advise patient that materials are available from Arthritis Foundation, 1314 Spring St, N.W., Atlanta, GA 30309; (800) 283-7800.

PROGNOSIS

- Expected course of untreated PAN is poor, with an estimated 5-year survival of 13%.
- Steroid and cytotoxic therapy treatment may increase survival rate significantly (8), with a 5-year survival rate of 75–80% (9).
- Survival is greater for hepatitis B–related PAN as a result of the introduction of antiviral treatments (10)[A].
- Patients presenting with proteinuria, renal insufficiency, GI tract involvement, cardiomyopathy, or CNS involvement have a poorer prognosis than those without.
- Rate of mortality from PAN remains high for the elderly patients (3).

COMPLICATIONS

- Renal failure
- Thrombosis of involved vessels
- Tissue/organ necrosis
- Stroke
- Myocardial infarction
- Mononeuritis multiplex
- Peripheral neuropathy
- Perforated viscous (bowel)

REFERENCES

1. Carvalho JF, Pereira RM, Shoenfeld Y. Systemic polyarteritis nodosa following hepatitis B vaccination. *Eur J Intern Med*. 2008;19:575–8.
2. Gayraud M, Guillevin L, le Toumelin P, et al. Long-term followup of polyarteritis nodosa, microscopic polyangiitis, and Churg-Strauss syndrome: Analysis of four prospective trials including 278 patients. *Arthritis Rheum*. 2001;44:666–75.
3. Pagnoux C, Seror R, Henegar C, et al. Clinical features and outcomes in 348 patients with polyarteritis nodosa: A systematic retrospective study of patients diagnosed between 1963 and 2005 and entered into the French Vasculitis Study Group Database. *Arthritis Rheum*. 2010;62: 616–26.
4. Ebert EC, Hagspiel KD, Nagar M, et al. Gastrointestinal Involvement in polyarteritis nodosa. *Clin Gastroenterol Hepatol*. 2008;6(9): 960–6.
5. Ribi C, Cohen P, Pagnoux C, et al. Treatment of polyarteritis nodosa and microscopic polyangiitis without poor-prognosis factors: A prospective randomized study of one hundred twenty-four patients. *Arthritis Rheum*. 2010;62:1186–97.
6. Chan M, Luqmani R. Pharmacotherapy of vasculitis. *Expert Opin Pharmacother*. 2009;10(8):1273–89.
7. Guillevin L, Mahr A, Cohen P, et al. Short-term corticosteroids then lamivudine and plasma exchanges to treat hepatitis B virus-related polyarteritis nodosa. *Arthritis Rheum*. 2004; 51:482–7.
8. Bourgarit A, Le Toumelin P, Pagnoux C, et al. Deaths occurring during the first year after treatment onset for polyarteritis nodosa, microscopic polyangiitis, and Churg-Strauss syndrome: A retrospective analysis of causes and factors predictive of mortality based on 595 patients. *Medicine (Baltimore)*. 2005;84:323–30.
9. Phillip R, Luqmani R. Mortality in systemic vasculitis: A systematic review. *Clin Exp Rheumatol*. 2008;26:94–104.
10. de Menthon M, Mahr A, et al. Treating polyarteritis nodosa: Current state of the art. *Clin Exp Rheumatol*. 2011;29:S110–6.

ADDITIONAL READING

- Kallenberg CG, et al. The last classification of vasculitis. *Clin Rev Allergy Immunol*. 2008;35:5–10.
- Villa-Forte A, European League Against Rheumatism, European Vasculitis Study Group, et al. European League Against Rheumatism/European Vasculitis Study Group recommendations for the management of vasculitis. *Curr Opin Rheumatol*. 2010;22:49–53.

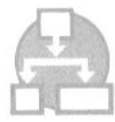

See Also (Topic, Algorithm, Electronic Media Element)

Hepatitis B; Hepatitis C

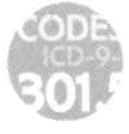

CODES

ICD9

446.0 Polyarteritis nodosa

CLINICAL PEARLS

- PAN is a necrotizing vasculitis of primarily medium-sized arteries with lack of granuloma formation and sparing of veins and pulmonary arteries.
- Skin biopsy should be collected at the edges of ulcer and include deep dermis and SC fat for high yield of diagnosis.
- Check hepatitis B and C serologies.

POLYCYSTIC KIDNEY DISEASE

Maricarmen Malagon-Rogers, MD

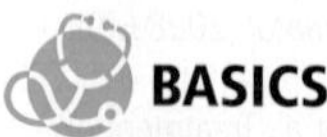

BASICS

DESCRIPTION

- A group of monogenic disorders that result in renal cyst development
- The most frequent ones are 2 genetically distinct conditions: Autosomal-dominant polycystic kidney disease (ADPKD) and autosomal-recessive polycystic kidney disease (ARPKD).
- ADPKD is one of the most common human genetic disorders.

EPIDEMIOLOGY

- ADPKD is generally late onset:
  - Mean age of end-stage kidney disease (ESKD) 57–69 years
  - More progressive disease in men than in women
  - Up to 90% of adults have cysts in the liver.
- ARPKD usually presents in infants:
  - A minority in older children and young adults may manifest as liver disease.
  - Nonobstructive intrahepatic bile dilatation is sometimes seen.
  - Found on all continents and in all races

Incidence

As ESKD:

- ADPKD: 8.7/1 million in the US; 7/1 million in Europe
- Mean age of ESRD: PKD1, 54.3 years vs. PKD2, 74 years

Prevalence

- ADPKD affects 1/400–1,000 live births.
- ARPKD affects 1/20,000 live births; carrier level 1/70.

RISK FACTORS

- Large inter- and intrafamilial variability
- A more rapid clinical course increased by onset of hypertension (HTN) <35 years, male gender, in PKD2, diagnosis <30 years, hyperlipidemia

Genetics

- ADPKD:
  - Autosomal-dominant inheritance
  - 50% of children of an affected adult are affected.
  - 100% penetrance; genetic imprinting and genetic anticipation are seen as well.
  - 2 genes isolated:
    - *PKD1* on chromosome 16p13.3 (85% of patients)
    - *PKD2* on chromosome 4q21 (15% of patients)
    - Presumed *PKD3* not yet identified
- ARPKD:
  - Autosomal-recessive inheritance
  - Siblings have a 1:4 chance of being affected; gene *PKHD1* on chromosome 6p21.1–p12

GENERAL PREVENTION

Genetic counseling

PATHOPHYSIOLOGY

- ADPKD:
  - Protein product of *PKD1:* Polycystin-1 mechanosensor in cilia; detects changes in flow, interacts with surrounding matrix and cell membrane proteins, and influences Ca^{2+} influx through *PKD2* product, polycystin-2 channel
  - Intracellular Ca^{2+} is reduced in cyst-derived cells, decreasing the Ca^{2+} inhibition of adenyl cyclase and increasing the concentration of cAMP.
  - cAMP stimulates cell proliferation and fluid secretion with cyst expansion.
  - Abnormal extracellular matrix and cell–cell interactions cause cells to detach and form cysts.
- ARPKD:
  - *PKHD1* product fibrocystin is also located in cilia; might be a cell surface receptor implicated in protein–protein interactions and is capable of enhancing the channel function of polycystin-2.
  - An alteration also occurs in intracellular calcium homeostasis.

ETIOLOGY

- ADPKD: Cysts arise from only 5% of nephrons:
  - Autosomal-dominant pattern of inheritance, but a molecularly recessive disease with the 2-hit hypothesis
  - Requires genetic and environmental factors
- ARPKD: Mutations are scattered throughout the gene with genotype–phenotype correlation.

COMMONLY ASSOCIATED CONDITIONS

- ADPKD:
  - Cysts in other organs:
    - Polycystic liver disease in 58% of young age group to 94% of 45-year-olds
    - Pancreatic cysts: 5%
    - Seminal cysts: 40%
    - Arachnoid cysts: 8%
  - Vascular manifestations:
    - Intracerebral aneurysms in 6% of patients without family history, and in 16% with family history
    - Aortic dissections
  - Cardiac manifestations: Mitral valve prolapse: 25%
  - Diverticular disease
- ARPKD: Liver involvement: Affected in inverse proportion to renal disease; congenital hepatic fibrosis with portal HTN

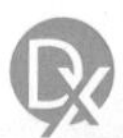

DIAGNOSIS

HISTORY

- ADPKD:
  - Positive family history
  - Flank pain: 60%
  - Hematuria
  - UTI
  - HTN: 50% aged 20–34 years; 100% with ESRD
  - Renal failure
- ARPKD:
  - 30% of affected neonates die:
    - Enlarged echogenic kidneys and oligohydramnios are diagnosed in utero.
    - Later in childhood: HTN
  - Adolescents and adults present with complications of portal HTN: Esophageal varices
  - Hypersplenism

PHYSICAL EXAM

- HTN
- Flank masses

DIAGNOSTIC TESTS & INTERPRETATION

Lab

Electrolytes, BUN/creatinine, urine analysis plus urinary citrate

Initial lab tests

- ADPKD:
  - Renal dysfunction:
    - Impaired renal concentration, hypocitraturia aciduria
    - Elevated creatinine
  - Urinalysis: Hematuria and mild proteinuria
- ARPKD:
  - Electrolyte abnormalities and renal insufficiency
  - Anemia, thrombocytopenia, leukopenia

Follow-Up & Special Considerations

- Diagnosis and prevention of secondary problems because of renal and liver abnormalities
- Follow-up of combined renal volume to assess disease severity (1)

Imaging

Initial approach

- ADPKD:
  - US: Diagnostic method of choice:
    - Renal enlargement is universal.
    - In at-risk patients: By age 30, 2 renal cysts (bilateral or unilateral) are 100% diagnostic. In children, it sometimes appears similar to ARPKD; may be diagnosed in utero.
    - Presence of hepatic cysts in young adults is pathognomonic for ADPKD.
    - In the absence of family history, bilateral renal enlargement and cysts make the diagnosis.
  - CT scan/MRI:
    - Kidney volume assessed by CT or MRI is a main predictor of progression (2).
    - Helpful in identifying cysts in other organs
- ARPKD:
  - US: Kidneys are enlarged, homogeneously hyperechogenic (cortex and medulla)
  - CT scan is more sensitive if diagnosis is in doubt.
  - Presence of hepatic fibrosis helps the diagnosis.

Follow-Up & Special Considerations

- Beyond age 2, renal size decreases in ARPKD but continues to grow in ADPKD at an average rate of 5.27%/year.
- Diagnosis of ADPKD in at-risk asymptomatic children may not need to be done because of psychological and insurance issues.
- Counseling should be done before testing.

Diagnostic Procedures/Surgery

- Genetic testing is available for the *PKD1* and *PKD2* in ADPKD when imaging results are equivocal and for potential living related donors (3).
- For the *PKHD1* gene in ARPKD, a prenatal diagnosis is feasible in about 72% of patients.

Pathological Findings

- ADPKD:
  - Kidneys are diffusely cystic and, although enlarged, retain their general shape.
  - Cysts range from a few millimeters to several centimeters and are distributed evenly throughout the cortex and medulla.
  - They arise in all segments of the nephron, although they are initially from the collecting ducts.
  - 1 kidney may be larger than the other.

- ARPKD:
  - Disease is a spectrum, ranging from severe renal disease with mild liver damage to mild renal disease with severe liver damage.
  - Renal enlargement is due to fusiform dilatation of the collecting ducts in the cortex and medulla in the newborn period.
  - Liver lesion is diffuse but limited to fibrotic portal areas.

DIFFERENTIAL DIAGNOSIS

- ADPKD and ARPKD
- Tuberous sclerosis: Prevalence 1/6,000
- Von Hippel–Lindau syndrome: Prevalence 1/36,000
- Nephronophthisis: Accounts for 10–20% cases of renal failure in children; medullary cystic kidney disease
- Renal cystic dysplasias: Multicystic dysplastic kidneys: Grossly deformed kidneys; most common type of bilateral cystic diseases in newborns: Prevalence: 1/4,000
- Simple cysts: Most common cystic abnormality:
  - Localized or unilateral renal cystic disease
  - Medullary sponge kidney
  - Acquired renal cystic disease
- Renal cystic neoplasms: Benign multilocular cyst (cystic nephroma)

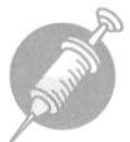

TREATMENT

MEDICATION

- No specific drug therapy is yet available for polycystic kidney disease.
- HTN: Should be very well controlled to prevent complications. ACE inhibitors may have an advantage (4).
- The use of antihypertensive medications has been found to decrease mortality (5).

ADDITIONAL TREATMENT

General Measures

- HTN: Moderate sodium restriction, weight control, and regular exercise
- Medications: ACE inhibitors; angiotensin receptor blockers (ARBs)
- Pain: Narcotics and other analgesics; bed rest; limit NSAIDs (they worsen renal function)
- Urolithiasis: Treated with alkalinization of urine and hydration therapy; surgery as needed
- UTIs/infections of cysts: Lipid-soluble antibiotics more effective (e.g., trimethoprim-sulfamethoxazole and chloramphenicol); fluoroquinolones also useful
- Dialysis for ESRD patients
- Hematuria: Reduce physical activity.

Issues for Referral

- Nephrologist primary management
- Urologic consultation for management of symptomatic/infected cysts
- Genetic counseling is critical.

SURGERY/OTHER PROCEDURES

- Indications for surgical intervention:
  - Uncontrollable HTN
  - Severe back and loin pain, abdominal fullness
  - Renal deterioration due to enlarging cysts
  - Hematuria/hemorrhage or recurrent UTI
- Open and laparoscopic cyst unroofing: May decrease pain and narcotics requirements; has not been proven to prevent renal failure or to prolong current renal function
- Percutaneous cyst aspiration ± injection of sclerosing agent; not usually performed secondary to recurrent fluid accumulation
- Renal transplant for ESRD
- Several trials are currently underway that may provide future treatments:
  - HALT-PKD: Combination therapy of ACE inhibitors and ARBs
  - Vasopressin V2 receptor inhibitors: Decrease cAMP
  - Somatostatins: Decrease cAMP
  - mTOR inhibitors (i.e., sirolimus): May reduce cyst growth

IN-PATIENT CONSIDERATIONS

Admission Criteria

Severe pain, gross hematuria with clots

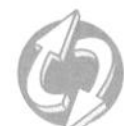

ONGOING CARE

FOLLOW-UP RECOMMENDATIONS

None in early stages of the disease; avoid vigorous activity if disease advances. Recurrent gross hematuria is secondary to trauma, associated with faster decline of renal function.

Patient Monitoring

- Monitor BP and renal function. Encourage hydration. Treat UTI and stone disease aggressively.
- Avoid nephrotoxic drugs
- Creatinine and BP monitoring at least twice a year; more often as needed

DIET

- Low-protein diet may retard renal insufficiency.
- Limit caffeine, since this might increase cyst's growth.

PROGNOSIS

- Renal failure in 2% by age 40 years; 23% by age 50; 48% by age 73
- ADPKD accounts for 10–15% of dialysis patients.
- No increased incidence of renal cell cancer

COMPLICATIONS

- Cyst rupture, infection, or hemorrhage
- Progression to renal failure
- Renal calculi

REFERENCES

1. Bae KT, Grantham JJ, et al. Imaging for the prognosis of autosomal dominant polycystic kidney disease. *Nat Rev Nephrol*. 2010;6:96–106.
2. Myrvang H, et al. Polycystic kidney disease: Imaging without contrast to improve safety in patients with impaired renal function. *Nat Rev Nephrol*. 2011;7:185.
3. Harris PC, Rossetti S, et al. Molecular diagnostics for autosomal dominant polycystic kidney disease. *Nat Rev Nephrol*. 2010;6:197–206.
4. Jia G, Kwon M, Liang HL, et al. Chronic treatment with lisinopril decreases proliferative and apoptotic pathways in autosomal recessive polycystic kidney disease. *Pediatr Nephrol*. 2010;25:1139–46.
5. Patch C, Charlton J, Roderick PJ, et al. Use of antihypertensive medications and mortality of patients with autosomal dominant polycystic kidney disease: A population-based study. *Am J Kidney Dis*. 2011;57(6):856–62.

ADDITIONAL READING

- Avner ED, et al. Renal cystic disease: New insights for the clinician. *Pediatr Clin N Am*. 2006;53: 889–909.
- Badani KK, Hemal AK, Menon M. Autosomal dominant polycystic kidney disease and pain—a review of the disease from aetiology, evaluation, past surgical treatment options to current practice. *J Postgrad Med*. 2004;50:222–6.
- Harris PC, Torres VE. Polycystic kidney disease. *Annu Rev Med*. 2009;60:321–37.
- Torres VE, Harris PC, Pirson Y. Autosomal dominant polycystic kidney disease. *Lancet*. 2007;369: 1287–301.
- Wilson PD. Polycystic kidney disease. *N Engl J Med*. 2004;350:151–64.

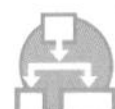

See Also (Topic, Algorithm, Electronic Media Element)

Kidney Failure, Chronic; Nephrolithiasis

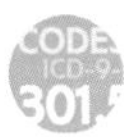

CODES

ICD9

- 753.12 Polycystic kidney, unspecified type
- 753.13 Polycystic kidney, autosomal dominant
- 753.14 Polycystic kidney, autosomal recessive

CLINICAL PEARLS

- Although many PKD patients eventually develop ESRD, many do not. See "Prognosis" to determine whether patient needs dialysis.
- No specific treatment has been proven to prevent ESRD, but hydration and control of BP are reasonable goals.
- Patients may benefit from a nephrology consultation after the initial diagnosis to counsel regarding disease progression prevention. They then can be followed by primary care if the disease was an incidental finding or no significant kidney dysfunction is present.

POLYCYSTIC OVARIAN SYNDROME (PCOS)

Maria de La Luz Nieto, MD
Shaila V. Chauhan, MD

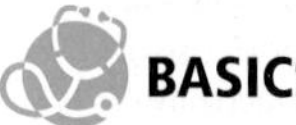

BASICS

DESCRIPTION

- Polycystic ovarian syndrome (PCOS) is a common heterogeneous endocrine disorder that affects up to 7% of US population.
- It is an endocrine stage of hyperandrogenism leading to anovulation, typically presenting as amenorrhea or oligomenorrhea.
- The diagnosis is based on clinical assessment and ultrasound finding.
- The diagnostic clinical characteristics include menstrual dysfunction, infertility, hirsutism, acne, obesity, and metabolic syndrome. In imaging, the ovaries are polycystic.
- The etiology of PCOS is unknown, but studies suggest a large genetic component modified by lifestyle factors.
- System(s) affected: Reproductive; Endocrine/Metabolic; Skin/Exocrine
- Synonym(s): Stein-Leventhal syndrome; Polycystic ovary disease

ALERT

- Condition may begin at puberty.
- Pregnancy does not resolve the syndrome.
- Predisposes to and associated with obesity, hypertension, diabetes, metabolic syndrome, hyperlipidemia, infertility, insulin-resistance syndrome

EPIDEMIOLOGY

Prevalence

- Incidence and prevalence are still highly debated due to a wide spectrum of diagnostic features:
  - The National Institutes of Health (NIH) criteria requires chronic anovulation in addition to clinical or biochemical signs of hyperandrogenism. The prevalence based on NIH criteria is 6.5–8%.
- Predominant age: Reproductive age
- Predominant sex: Females only

RISK FACTORS

See "Commonly Associated Conditions"; cause and effect are difficult to disentangle in this disorder.

Genetics

Ultimate expression is likely a combination of polygenic and environmental factors.

GENERAL PREVENTION

None known; focus on early diagnosis and treatment to prevent long-term complications.

PATHOPHYSIOLOGY

- PCOS is a multifactorial functional disorder of unclear etiology.
- Recent evidence points to a primary role for insulin resistance with hyperinsulinemia (1).

ETIOLOGY

- Androgenism: Ovaries are the main source of excess androgens. Polycystic ovaries have thickened thecal layers, which secrete excess androgens in response to LH. LH receptors are overexpressed in thecal and granulosa cells of polycystic ovaries.
- Ovarian follicles: Abnormal androgen signaling may account for abnormal folliculogenesis causing polycystic ovaries. The mechanism that determines abnormal number of follicles is unknown, but may be due to abnormal androgen signaling on the ovarian stroma.
- Insulin resistance: Women with PCOS have insulin resistance similar to type 2 diabetes. Elevated levels of insulin decreased sex hormone binding protein (SHBG) increasing bioavailability of testosterone. Insulin may also act directly on adrenal, ovary, and hypothalamus to regulate androgen and gonadotropin release. Insulin resistance causes elevated insulin levels.
- Insulin resistance may cause the frequently associated metabolic syndrome and frank diabetes mellitus (DM).

COMMONLY ASSOCIATED CONDITIONS

- Infertility
- Obesity
- Obstructive sleep apnea
- Hypertension
- Diabetes mellitus
- Endometrial hyperplasia/carcinoma
- Fatty liver disease
- Mood disturbances and depression

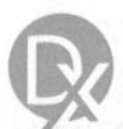

DIAGNOSIS

HISTORY

- A comprehensive history, including a family history of diabetes and premature onset of cardiovascular disease, is important in the differential diagnosis.
- Focus on the onset and duration of the various signs of androgen excess, menstrual history, and concomitant medications, including the use of exogenous androgens.

PHYSICAL EXAM

- Vital signs: Body mass index (BMI), high BP
- General appearance: Central obesity, deepened voice, hirsutism, acne
- Skin: Hair pattern and growth, acne, seborrhea, acanthosis nigricans
- Genitalia: Clitoromegaly and ovarian enlargement

ALERT

Look specifically for signs of virilization such as hair pattern, deepened voice, and clitoromegaly.

DIAGNOSTIC TESTS & INTERPRETATION

- The measurement of circulating androgens to document PCOS is uncertain but should include measuring free testosterone concentration directly by equilibrium dialysis.
- Most commonly diagnostic criteria used is Rotterdam criteria (need 2 of 3):
  - Oligo- or anovulation
  - Clinical and/or biochemical signs of hyperandrogenism
  - Transvaginal ultrasonographic polycystic ovaries and exclusion of other etiologies; therefore, consider exclusion of Cushing disease, congenital adrenal hyperplasia, and androgen-secreting tumors.
- More recent criteria also focus on similar criteria while acknowledging that there may be forms of PCOS without overt evidence of hyperandrogenism (2).

Lab

Initial lab tests

- Screening workup should include human chorionic gonadotropin (hCG), TSH, prolactin, and FSH (exclude premature ovarian failure).
- LH determination may be ordered but is not usually necessary:
  - Hirsute women should have a testosterone or free testosterone determination and a DHEAS determination.
  - Consider 17-OH progesterone if congenital adrenal hyperplasia is a possibility.
- LH/FSH level $\geq$2.5–3/L in $\sim$50% of women with PCOS, but LH testing is not generally necessary.
- Testosterone increased but <200 ng/dL (6.94 nmol/L)
- Typical findings in PCOS include mild elevation in DHEAS but <800 μg/dL (20.8 μmol/L), mild increase in 17-OH progesterone level, increased estrogen level, and decreased SHBG.
- Drugs that may alter lab results:
  - Oral contraceptives (OCs)
  - Steroids
  - Antidepressants

Follow-Up & Special Considerations

- Consider fasting serum glucose, insulin level, and plasminogen activator inhibitor-1 determinations to establish presence of insulin resistance and glucose intolerance, especially if diagnosis is in doubt.
- Overnight dexamethasone suppression test (Decadron 1 mg PO at 11:00 p.m. and fasting serum cortisol at 8:00 a.m. the next morning) to rule out Cushing syndrome in the appropriate setting.
- Endometrial biopsy to rule out hyperplasia and/or carcinoma if indicated
- If the syndrome is diagnosed, determination of fasting glucose and fasting lipid levels should be performed, and formal glucose tolerance test considered.

Imaging

Transvaginal ultrasound: Findings 1 or both ovaries with 12 or more follicles measuring 2–9 mm or increased ovarian volume to 10 cm^3

Pathological Findings

- Ovary usually enlarged with a smooth white glistening capsule
- Ovarian cortex lined with follicles in all stages of development but most atretic
- Thecal cell proliferation with an increase in the stromal compartment

DIFFERENTIAL DIAGNOSIS

- Cushing syndrome
- HAIRAN syndrome
- Testosterone-producing ovarian or adrenal tumor
- Prolactin-producing pituitary adenoma
- Hyperthecosis
- Adult-onset adrenal hyperplasia
- Partial congenital adrenal hyperplasia (21-hydroxylase deficiency)
- 11β-hydroxylase deficiency
- 17β-hydroxysteroid dehydrogenase deficiency

- Acromegaly
- Drug-induced hirsutism, oligo-ovulation (e.g., danazol, steroids, valproic acid)
- Thyroid disease

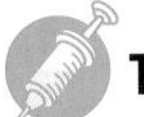

TREATMENT

MEDICATION

Drug costs related to this condition are high.

First Line

- The goal of treatment in PCOS depends on symptoms and patient's goals for fertility.
- Treatment can be divided into 5 main categories: Lifestyle changes; appropriate nutrition and exercise to decrease body weight can restore ovulation and increase insulin sensitivity.
- Menstrual irregularity when pregnancy not desired:
  - Low-dose OCs (30–35 μg); newer formulations containing progestins with lower androgenicity (e.g., norethindrone, desogestrel, norgestimate, drospirenone) may be particularly beneficial, but all OCs increase SHBG and decrease excess androgen and estrogen. If unable to tolerate OCPs, then intermittent medroxyprogesterone (Provera) 10 mg PO × 10 days given every 1–2 months.
  - Metformin may help to correct metabolic abnormalities in women who are shown to be insulin-resistant. Initial dose is 500 mg at dinner time × 1 week, increasing by 500 mg/wk to a total of 1,500–2,000 mg/d divided b.i.d.; take with food:
    - Overall, data support the usefulness of metformin on both cardiometabolic risk and reproduction assistance in PCOS women (3)[B].
    - Thiazolidinediones may increase likelihood of ovulation and treat insulin resistance.
- If pregnancy desired:
  - Ovulation induction with clomiphene (Clomid, Serophene) and/or exogenous gonadotropins: see "Infertility." Birth rate with Clomid is 22.5%, 7.2% with metformin, and 26.8% in women who use both medications (4)[B].
  - Metformin (Glucophage): 500–2,000 mg PO divided b.i.d. has been shown to improve hyperandrogenism and restore ovulation. Many times the drug is continued throughout the first trimester or the entire pregnancy if there is a history of spontaneous abortion or glucose intolerance. It does improve clinical pregnancy rates, but does not improve live birth rates alone or in combination with clomiphene when used for ovulation induction (5)[B].
  - Has been demonstrated that metformin reduces the incidence of gestational diabetes

Second Line

- Spironolactone for androgen-excess hirsutism not addressed by OC therapy
- Cosmetic issues due to hyperandrogenism: Acne may respond best with OCPs with low doses of cyproterone or drospirenone.
- Eflornithine hydrochloride cream 13% to inhibit hair growth

ADDITIONAL TREATMENT

General Measures

- No ideal treatment exists.
- Therapy must be individualized according to the needs and desires of each patient.
- Weight loss in overweight women results in biochemical and symptomatic improvement in most.

Issues for Referral

- To reproductive endocrinologist for all women who cannot achieve pregnancy with Clomid
- High-risk pregnancies
- To endocrinologist if Cushing syndrome, congenital adrenal hyperplasia, or adrenal or ovarian tumors are found during the workup

COMPLEMENTARY AND ALTERNATIVE MEDICINE

Acupuncture assists with cycle normalization and weight loss (6)[B].

SURGERY/OTHER PROCEDURES

- Ovarian wedge resection and laparoscopic laser drilling are controversial and rarely used today.
- Mechanical means of hair removal, including electrolysis, waxing, and depilatory, may improve cosmesis.

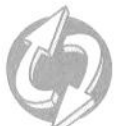

ONGOING CARE

FOLLOW-UP RECOMMENDATIONS

Follow up at 6-month intervals to evaluate response to therapy and to monitor weight as well as medication side effects.

Patient Monitoring

- Counsel patient about the risk of endometrial and breast carcinoma, insulin resistance, and diabetes, as well as obesity and its role in infertility.
- See patient frequently throughout the menstrual cycle, depending on which drug combination is used to induce ovulation.

DIET

In overweight patients, weight loss is the most successful therapy because it improves cardiovascular risk, insulin sensitivity, and menstrual patterns:

- Counsel on lifestyle dietary changes; consider referral to nutritionist and weight center.

PATIENT EDUCATION

- Provide patient with information about PCOS, such as from www.acog.org.
- Discuss the chronic nature of this condition and the risks and benefits and side effects of potential treatments.
- Review the importance of weight loss if applicable. Modest weight loss of 5–10% of initial body weight has been demonstrated to improve many of the features of PCOS.

PROGNOSIS

- Fertility prognosis is good, but may need assisted reproductive technologies.
- Proper follow-up and screening can prevent endometrial carcinoma.
- Early detection of diabetes may decrease morbidity and mortality associated with cardiovascular risk factor.

COMPLICATIONS

- Reproductive: Infertility
- Metabolic: Insulin resistance, diabetes mellitus, cardiovascular disease
- Psychosocial: Increased anxiety, mood disorder, eating disorder, depression

REFERENCES

1. Moran LJ, Misso ML, Wild RA, et al. Impaired glucose tolerance, type 2 diabetes and metabolic syndrome in polycystic ovary syndrome: A systematic review and meta-analysis. *Hum Reprod Update*. 2010;16:347–63.
2. Azziz R, Carmina E, Dewailly D, et al. The Androgen Excess and PCOS Society criteria for the polycystic ovary syndrome: The complete task force report. *Fertil Steril*. 2009;91(2):456–88.
3. Diamanti-Kandarakis E, Economou F, Palimeri S, et al. Metformin in polycystic ovary syndrome. *Ann N Y Acad Sci*. 2010;1205:192–8.
4. Legro RS, Barnhart HX, Schlaff WD, et al. Clomiphene, metformin, or both for infertility in the polycystic ovary syndrome. *N Engl J Med*. 2007;356:551–66.
5. Tang, et al. Insulin-sensitising drugs (metformin, rosiglitazone, pioglitazone, D-chiro-inositol) for women with polycystic ovary syndrome, oligo amenorrhoea and subfertility. *Cochrane Database Syst Rev*. 2010;5.
6. Lim CE, Wong WS, et al. Current evidence of acupuncture on polycystic ovarian syndrome. *Gynecol. Endocrinol*. 2010;26:473–8.

ADDITIONAL READING

- Carmina E, Oberfield SE, Lobo RA, et al. The diagnosis of polycystic ovary syndrome in adolescents. *Am J Obstet Gynecol*. 2010;203:201.e1–5.
- Chang RJ. A practical approach to the diagnosis of polycystic ovary syndrome. *Am J Obstet Gynecol*. 2004;191:713–7.
- Cibula D, et al. The effect of combination therapy with metformin and combined oral contraceptives (COC) versus COC alone on insulin sensitivity, hyperandrogenaemia, SHBG and lipids in PCOS patients. *Human Reprod*. 2005;20(1):180–4.
- Hirschberg AL, et al. Polycystic ovary syndrome, obesity and reproductive implications. *Womens Health (Lond Engl)*. 2009;5:529–40; quiz 541–2.
- Rotterdam ESHRE/ASRM Sponsored PCOS Consensus Workshop Group. Revised 2003 Consensus on diagnostic criteria and long-term health risks related to polycystic ovary syndrome. *Fertil Steril*. 2004;81:19–25.

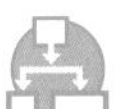

See Also (Topic, Algorithm, Electronic Media Element)

Algorithm: Amenorrhea

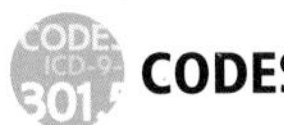

CODES

ICD9

256.4 Polycystic ovaries

CLINICAL PEARLS

- In the US, 40% of women with PCOS are not obese.
- Chronic anovulation should be treated because chronic estrogen stimulation in absence of progesterone may lead to endometrial hyperplasia.
- Specific therapies must be individualized according to the needs and desires of each patient.

POLYCYTHEMIA VERA

Michael S. Furman, MD
Nathan T. Connell, MD

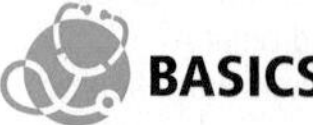

BASICS

DESCRIPTION

- Clonal cell hematologic malignant disorder whose hallmark is increased red cell mass (RCM) with excessive erythroid, myeloid, and megakaryocytic elements in the bone marrow
- One of a group of myeloproliferative disorders
- Synonym(s): Primary polycythemia; Vaquez disease; Polycythemia, splenomegalic; Vaquez-Osler disease

EPIDEMIOLOGY

Incidence

- Predominant age: Middle to late years; mean is 60 years (range 15–90 years)
- Predominant sex: Male > Female (slightly)

Prevalence

Incidence in the US: 1.9/100,000 person-years

RISK FACTORS

- Ashkenazi Jewish ancestry (may have increased frequency)
- Familial history (rare)

Genetics

JAK2 V617F (tyrosine kinase) mutation: Prevalence of 95–99%; is helpful for differentiating from secondary polycythemia. Homozygote carriers will have higher incidence of symptoms such as pruritus, but will not have higher incidence of disease than heterozygotes (1)[A].

ETIOLOGY

Unknown; all 3 hematopoietic cell lines originate in a single clone.

COMMONLY ASSOCIATED CONDITIONS

- May present as thrombosis in any organ, such as Budd-Chiari syndrome
- Mesenteric artery thrombosis
- Myocardial infarction
- Cerebrovascular accident
- Deep vein thrombosis/pulmonary embolism

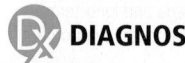

DIAGNOSIS

HISTORY

- Early stages may produce no symptoms.
- Burning pain of feet or hands, occasionally with erythema, pallor, cyanosis, or acral paresthesias
- Headaches
- Tinnitus
- Vertigo
- Blurred vision
- Epistaxis
- Increased blood viscosity
- Spontaneous bruising
- Upper GI bleeding
- Peptic ulcer disease
- Arterial and venous occlusive events
- Pruritus
- Sweating
- Weight loss
- Plethora (face, hands, feet)
- Hyperhistaminemia
- Bone pain (ribs and sternum)

PHYSICAL EXAM

- Bone tenderness (ribs and sternum)
- Splenomegaly
- Hepatomegaly

DIAGNOSTIC TESTS & INTERPRETATION

Lab

CBC; if suspicion is high, obtain erythropoietin and gene testing for JAK2 V617F

Initial lab tests

- PV Study Group (PVSG) (1960s) major (A) and minor criteria (B):
  - A_1: Increased RCM: Female ≥32 mL/kg; male ≥36 mL/kg
  - A_2: Normal arterial oxygen saturation (≥92%)
  - A_3: Splenomegaly
  - B_1: Thrombocytosis (platelet count >400,000/L)
  - B_2: Leukocytosis >12,000/L
  - B_3: Leukocyte alkaline phosphatase increased
  - B_4: Increased serum vitamin B_{12} or increased unsaturated vitamin B_{12} binding capacity
- PVSG diagnosis acceptable with following combinations:
  - $A_1 + A_2 + A_3$
  - $A_1 + A_2$ + any 2 from B category (splenomegaly absent in ~25% of patients)
- Recent advances have prompted development of other diagnostic models, namely, the discovery of *JAK2* V617F and improved assays for erythropoietin (EPO) measurement. Although the RCM was traditionally included in diagnostic criteria, it is difficult to perform and has been shown to no longer be a necessary component of diagnosis, given that additional laboratory tests and clinical evaluation are easily attainable.
- 2008 World Health Organization diagnostic criteria: Requires both major criteria or 1 major criterion and 2 minor criteria (1):
  - Major criteria:
    - Hemoglobin (Hgb) >18.5 g/dL (men); Hgb >16.5 g/dL (women); Hgb >17 g/dL (men) or Hgb >15 g/dL (women) if there is a sustained increase of 2 g/dL or more above baseline that cannot be attributed to iron-deficiency correction
    - Presence of *JAK2* V617F or similar mutation
  - Minor criteria:
    - BM trilineage myeloproliferation
    - Subnormal serum EPO level
    - Endogenous erythroid colony growth
- Some authors feel that diagnosis can be made reliably based on clinical symptoms, presence of *JAK2* V617 mutation, and low EPO (2).
- Other lab findings:
  - Hyperuricemia
  - Hypercholesterolemia
  - Elevated blood histamine level
- Conditions that can be confused with polycythemia vera (actual false-positive rate is <1%):
  - Cirrhosis
  - Tobacco use
  - Diuretic use
  - Other myeloproliferative disorders
- Conditions in which patients with polycythemia vera may not be recognized:
  - GI bleeding (dilution of hemoglobin)
  - Early in disease course
  - Obesity (leads to low RCM)

Imaging

Initial approach

CT to assess for splenomegaly (if not palpable), although imaging is not necessarily needed

Diagnostic Procedures/Surgery

- Bone marrow aspiration and biopsy
- Bone marrow aspiration (RBC hyperplasia, panmyelosis, clustering/clumping of pleomorphic megakaryocytes, absent iron stores, no pronounced inflammatory reaction): Cytogenetic testing (*JAK2* V617F)
- Biopsy: Fibrosis during spent phase of the disease (characterized by increased presence of reticulin)

Pathological Findings

- Plethoric congestion in all organs and tissues
- Major vessels contain thick, viscous blood.
- Sinuses of spleen packed with RBCs

DIFFERENTIAL DIAGNOSIS

- Secondary polycythemias
- Hemoglobinopathy
- Spurious polycythemia

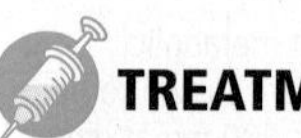

TREATMENT

MEDICATION

First Line

- Myelosuppression:
  - Low-dose aspirin (81 mg PO) has been demonstrated in 1 study to reduce the risk of thrombotic events without increasing bleeding complications when used in conjunction with phlebotomy. A follow-up meta-analysis, however, did not show a statistically significant benefit to aspirin therapy but did not show an increase in major bleeding either (3)[A].
  - Hydroxyurea if unable to maintain on phlebotomy alone or if at high risk for thrombosis (start 15–20 mg/kg/d). Be aware that hydroxyurea can lead to leukemic transformation (4).
  - Radioactive phosphorous in selected patients when life expectancy is <10 years given mutagenic potential
  - Refer to hematologist/oncologist for further dosing and instructions. Use of the novel tyrosine kinase inhibitor imatinib has been explored. This has been reported to reduce the amount of phlebotomy needed but ultimately has little effect on the course of the disease.
- Symptomatic/adjunctive:
  - Allopurinol 300 mg/d PO for uric acid reduction
  - Cyproheptadine 4–16 mg PO as needed for pruritus
  - H_2-receptor blockers or antacids for GI hyperacidity; cimetidine is also used for pruritus.
  - Other pruritus therapy: SSRIs have shown some efficacy in controlling pruritus in setting of PV.

Second Line

- Myelosuppression: Chlorambucil; some authors believe this is contraindicated.
- Pegylated interferon-α-2a has shown promise in inducing complete hematologic and molecular responses (5). This pharmacologic treatment should be considered only in consultation with a hematologist.

ADDITIONAL TREATMENT

General Measures

- Individualized management necessary by considering the patient's risk factors and comorbidities (4)
- Depend on many factors: Age, disease duration, disease phenotype, complications, disease activity
- Currently, phlebotomy is the mainstay of therapy. Beyond this, differences exist among authorities about use and effectiveness of myelosuppressives.
- Phlebotomy:
  - To reduce hematocrit to ~45%
  - Performed as often as every 2–3 days until normal hematocrit reached; phlebotomies of 250–500 mL. Reduce to 250–350 mL in elderly patients or patients with cerebrovascular disease.
  - Concomitant therapy possibilities; for example, some form of myelosuppression, radioactive phosphorus (in elderly patients), hydroxyurea
  - Phlebotomy repeated as necessary for maintenance
  - If patient cannot tolerate phlebotomy, then chemotherapy (hydroxyurea is the least mutagenic agent) or radiation therapy
- Other therapy:
  - Maintain hydration
  - Pruritus therapy
  - Manage thrombotic or hemorrhagic complications the same as with nonpolycythemic patient
- Uric acid reduction therapy

Issues for Referral

It is recommended that patients be referred to an experienced hematologist to assist in management.

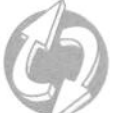

ONGOING CARE

FOLLOW-UP RECOMMENDATIONS

Patient Monitoring

- Frequent monitoring during early treatment until target hematocrit is reached
- Monitor hematocrit often and phlebotomize as needed to maintain target goal.

DIET

Avoid iron supplements.

PATIENT EDUCATION

- Stress the importance of lifelong maintenance.
- Continuous education regarding possible complications and importance of seeking treatment early should complications appear

PROGNOSIS

- Currently, survival is >15 years with treatment (1).
- Patients are at risk for developing postpolycythemic myelofibrosis (PPMF). One study showed that the risk of developing PPMF was 16% at 10 years and 34% at 15 years (6).

COMPLICATIONS

- Uric acid stones
- Secondary gout
- Vascular thromboses (major cause of death)
- Transformation to leukemia
- Transformation to myelofibrosis
- Hemorrhage
- Peptic ulcer
- Increased risk for complications and mortality from surgery procedures. Assess risk/benefits and ensure optimal control of disorder before any elective surgery.

REFERENCES

1. Tefferi A. Essential thrombocythemia, polycythemia vera, and myelofibrosis: Current management and the prospect of targeted therapy. *Am J Hematol*. 2008;83:491–7.
2. Tefferi A. The diagnosis of polycythemia vera: New tests and old dictums. *Best Prac Res Clin Haematol*. 2006;19:455.
3. Squizzato A, Romualdi E, Middeldorp S, et al. Antiplatelet drugs for polycythaemia vera and essential thrombocythaemia. *Cochrane Database Syst Rev*. 2008;CD006503.
4. Finazzi G, Barbui T, et al. Evidence and expertise in the management of polycythemia vera and essential thrombocythemia. *Leukemia*. 2008;22:1494–502.
5. Kiladjian JJ, Cassinat B, Chevret S, et al. Pegylated Interferon-alfa-2a induces complete hematological and molecular responses with low toxicity in polycythemia vera. *Blood*. 2008;112(8):3065–72.
6. Alvarez-Larrán A, Bellosillo B, Martínez-Avilés L, et al. Postpolycythaemic myelofibrosis: Frequency and risk factors for this complication in 116 patients. *Br J Haematol*. 2009;146:504–9.

ADDITIONAL READING

- James C, Ugo V, Le Couédic JP, et al. A unique clonal JAK2 mutation leading to constitutive signalling causes polycythaemia vera. *Nature*. 2005;434: 1144–8.
- Landolfi R, Marchioli R, Kutti J, et al. Efficacy and safety of low-dose aspirin in polycythemia vera. *N Engl J Med*. 2004;350:114–24.
- Levine RL, Gilliland DG, et al. Myeloproliferative disorders. *Blood*. 2008;112:2190–8.
- Nussenzveig RH, Cortes J, Sever M, et al. Imatinib mesylate therapy for polycythemia vera: Final result of a phase II study initiated in 2001. *Int J Hematol*. 2009;90:58–63.
- Tefferi A, Fonseca R. Selective serotonin reuptake inhibitors are effective in the treatment of polycythemia vera-associated pruritus. *Blood*. 2002;99:2627.

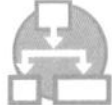

See Also (Topic, Algorithm, Electronic Media Element)

Myeloproliferative Neoplasms

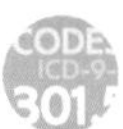

CODES

ICD9

238.4 Polycythemia vera

CLINICAL PEARLS

- *JAK2* mutations are an important component of myeloproliferative disorders.
- Multiple therapies exist, and consultation with an experienced hematologist is recommended.

POLYMYALGIA RHEUMATICA

Elise H. Pyun, MD

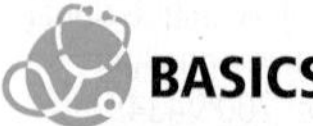

BASICS

DESCRIPTION

- Polymyalgia rheumatica (PMR) is a clinical syndrome characterized by pain and stiffness of the shoulder and hip girdles and neck:
  - Disease of the elderly, associated with morning stiffness and elevated markers of inflammation
- System(s) affected: Musculoskeletal; Hematologic/Lymphatic/Immunologic
- Synonym(s): Senile rheumatic disease; Polymyalgia rheumatica syndrome; Pseudo-polyarthrite rhizomélique

Geriatric Considerations

- Incidence increases with age
- Average age of onset ~70 years

Pediatric Considerations

Does not occur in patients <50 years of age

EPIDEMIOLOGY

Incidence

- Predominant age: Peak incidence between 70 and 80 years of age
- Incidence increases after age 50. Incidence in the US population >50 years old: 60 per 100,000 people
- Predominant sex: Female > Male (2:1)
- Most common in Caucasians, especially those of northern European ancestry

Prevalence

Prevalence in population >50 years old: 700 per 100,000 people

RISK FACTORS

- Age >50 years
- Presence of giant cell arteritis

Genetics

Associated with human leukocyte antigen determinants (HLA-DRB1*04 and DRB1*01 alleles)

ETIOLOGY

Unknown

COMMONLY ASSOCIATED CONDITIONS

Giant cell arteritis (temporal arteritis) may occur in 15–30% of patients with PMR.

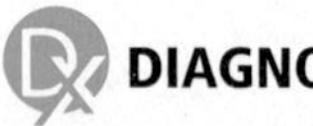

DIAGNOSIS

- No universally accepted diagnostic criteria
- Suspect PMR in an elderly patient with new onset of proximal limb pain and stiffness.

HISTORY

- Insidious, subacute, or acute onset of pain and stiffness
- Proximal symptoms: Shoulders, hip girdle, neck
- Symptoms usually symmetric
- Prominent morning stiffness (lasting at least 1 hour), sometimes impairing patient's ability to get out of bed
- Nighttime pain
- Prominent gelling (stiffening); difficulty arising from a chair or raising the arms
- Systemic symptoms in ~25% (fatigue, weight loss, low-grade fever)

PHYSICAL EXAM

- Decreased range of motion (ROM) of shoulders, neck, and hips may be seen.
- Muscle strength is usually normal, although it may be limited by pain.
- Disuse atrophy of muscles may be seen.
- Synovitis of the small joints may be seen.
- Coexisting carpal tunnel syndrome

DIAGNOSTIC TESTS & INTERPRETATION

Temporal artery biopsy if symptoms of giant cell arteritis are present

Lab

- ESR (Westergren) elevation >40 mm/hr:
  - ESR is elevated in most patients, sometimes >100 mm/h.
  - ESR may be normal (<40 mm/hr) in 7–22% of patients.
- Elevated C-reactive protein
- Normochromic/normocytic anemia common
- Anti-CCP antibodies usually negative (in contrast to elderly-onset rheumatoid arthritis [RA])
- Rheumatoid factor: Negative (5–10% of patients >60 years of age will have positive rheumatoid factor without RA)
- Mild elevations in liver function tests, especially alkaline phosphatase
- Drugs that may alter lab results: Prednisone
- Disorders that may alter lab results: Other disorders causing elevation of the sedimentation rate (e.g., infection, neoplasm, renal failure)

Initial lab tests

- ESR
- C-reactive protein
- CBC

Imaging

- MRI of the joints may show periarticular inflammation, tenosynovitis, and bursitis. However, MRI typically is not necessary for diagnosis.
- Ultrasound of the shoulder or hip may show bursitis, tendinitis, and synovitis.

Initial approach

Consider PMR in a patient >50 years old with proximal pain and stiffness. Obtain laboratory work recommended above. Consider a diagnostic and therapeutic trial of low-dose steroids.

Diagnostic Procedures/Surgery

If patients have symptoms suggestive of giant cell arteritis, a temporal artery biopsy is indicated.

Pathological Findings

Mild nonspecific synovitis

DIFFERENTIAL DIAGNOSIS

- RA
- Palindromic rheumatism
- Late-onset seronegative spondyloarthropathies (e.g., psoriatic arthritis, ankylosing spondylitis)
- Systemic lupus erythematosus
- Sjögren syndrome
- Fibromyalgia
- Depression
- Polymyositis-dermatomyositis (check creatine phosphokinase, aldolase)
- Thyroid disease
- Hyperparathyroidism, hypoparathyroidism
- Hypovitaminosis D
- Viral myalgia
- Osteoarthritis
- Rotator cuff syndrome
- Adhesive capsulitis
- RS3PE syndrome (remitting seronegative symmetrical synovitis with pitting edema)
- Occult infection
- Occult malignancy (e.g., lymphoma, leukemia, myeloma, solid tumor)
- Myopathy (e.g., steroid, alcohol, electrolyte depletion)

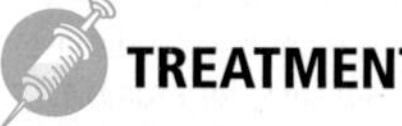

TREATMENT

MEDICATION

First Line

- Prednisone, 10–20 mg/d PO initially; typically, expect a dramatic (diagnostic) response within days. 15 mg/d is effective in almost all patients (1)[A]:
  - May increase to 20 mg/d if no immediate response
  - If no response to 10–20 mg/d, reconsider diagnosis.
- Divided-dose steroids (b.i.d. or t.i.d.) may be useful initially (especially if symptoms recur in the afternoon).
- Begin slow taper by 2.5-mg decrements every 2–4 weeks to a dose of 7.5–10 mg/d. Below this dose, taper by 1 mg/mo.
- Increase prednisone for recurrence of symptoms (relapse common).
- Corticosteroid treatment often lasts at least 2 years (2).
- Contraindications:
  - Use steroids with caution in patients with chronic heart failure, diabetes mellitus, and systemic fungal or bacterial infection.
  - Must treat infections concurrently if steroids are absolutely necessary.
- Precautions:
  - Long-term steroid use associated with several significant adverse effects, including sodium and water retention, exacerbation of chronic heart failure, hypokalemia, increased susceptibility to infection, osteoporosis, cataracts, glaucoma, avascular necrosis, depression, and weight gain
  - Patients may develop temporal arteritis while on low-dose corticosteroid treatment for polymyalgia. This requires an immediate increase in dose to 40–60 mg.
  - Alternate-day steroids are not effective.

Second Line

- NSAIDs usually are not adequate for pain relief (3)[B].
- Methotrexate may be used as a steroid-sparing drug, but studies supporting its use are not robust (4,5)[B].
- Antitumor necrosis factor agents (infliximab) have not been shown to add any steroid-sparing effects (6)[B].

ADDITIONAL TREATMENT

General Measures

- Address risk of steroid-induced osteoporosis: Obtain dual energy x-ray absorptiometry, check 25-OH vitamin D levels, and consider antiresorptive therapies (bisphosphonates) based on recommendations for treatment of corticosteroid-induced osteoporosis.
- Advise patient on adequate calcium (1,500 mg/d) and vitamin D (800–1,000 U/d) supplementation.
- Physical therapy for ROM exercises, if needed

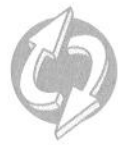

ONGOING CARE

FOLLOW-UP RECOMMENDATIONS

Patient Monitoring

- Follow monthly initially and during taper of medication, every 3 months otherwise.
- Follow ESR as steroids are tapered; both ESR and CRP should decline as symptoms improve.
- Follow up with patient for symptoms of giant cell arteritis. Educate patient to report such symptoms immediately (e.g., headache, visual loss, and diplopia).
- If the patient is asymptomatic, do not treat the ESR (i.e., do not increase the steroid dose in an attempt to normalize the ESR).

DIET

- Regular diet
- Aim for adequate calcium and vitamin D.

PATIENT EDUCATION

- Review adverse effects of corticosteroids.
- Discuss the symptoms of giant cell arteritis; instruct the patient to contact the physician immediately if any occur.
- Instruct patient to contact physician if symptoms recur during the steroid taper.
- Instruct the patient to never abruptly stop taking steroids without a taper.
- Counsel patients on calcium and vitamin D requirements.
- Resources for patients: Arthritis Foundation: www.arthritis.org/
- Resources for patients: American College of Rheumatology: www.rheumatology.org/public/factsheets/diseases_and_conditions/polymyalgiarheumatica.asp?aud=pat

PROGNOSIS

- Most patients require at least 2 years of corticosteroid treatment.
- Exacerbation if steroids are tapered too fast (7)
- Prognosis is very good if treated.
- Relapse is common (in 25–50% of patients).

COMPLICATIONS

- Medication: Complications related to steroid use
- Disease: Exacerbation of disease with taper of steroids; development of giant cell arteritis (may occur when polymyalgia rheumatica is being treated adequately)

REFERENCES

1. Hernández-Rodríguez J, Cid MC, López-Soto A, et al. Treatment of polymyalgia rheumatica: A systematic review. *Arch Intern Med*. 2009;169: 1839–50.
2. Narváez J, Nolla-Solé JM, Clavaguera MT, et al. Longterm therapy in polymyalgia rheumatica: Effect of coexistent temporal arteritis. *J Rheumatol*. 1999;26:1945–52.
3. Michet CJ, Matteson EL. Polymyalgia rheumatica. *BMJ*. 2008;336:765–9.
4. Caporali R, Cimmino MA, Ferraccioli G, et al. Prednisone plus methotrexate for polymyalgia rheumatica: A randomized, double-blind, placebo-controlled trial. *Ann Intern Med*. 2004;141: 493–500.
5. van der Veen MJ, Dinant HJ, van Booma-Frankfort C, et al. Can methotrexate be used as a steroid sparing agent in the treatment of polymyalgia rheumatica and giant cell arteritis? *Ann Rheum Dis*. 1996;55:218–23.
6. Salvarani C, Macchioni P, Manzini C, et al. Infliximab plus prednisone or placebo plus prednisone for the initial treatment of polymyalgia rheumatica: A randomized trial. *Ann Intern Med*. 2007;146:631–9.
7. Kremers HM, Reinalda MS, Crowson CS, et al. Relapse in a population based cohort of patients with polymyalgia rheumatica. *J Rheumatol*. 2005; 32:65–73.

ADDITIONAL READING

- Dasgupta B, Borg FA, Hassan N, et al. BSR and BHPR guidelines for the management of polymyalgia rheumatica. *Rheumatology (Oxford)*. 2010;49: 186–90.
- Hernández-Rodríguez J, Cid MC, López-Soto A, et al. Treatment of polymyalgia rheumatica: A systematic review. *Arch Intern Med*. 2009;169(20):1839–50.
- Salvarani C, Cantini F, Hunder GG. Polymyalgia rheumatica and giant-cell arteritis. *Lancet*. 2008; 372:234–45.

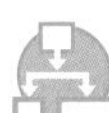

See Also (Topic, Algorithm, Electronic Media Element)

Arteritis, Temporal; Arthritis, Osteo; Arthritis, Rheumatoid; Depression; Fibromyalgia; Polymyositis/Dermatomyositis

CODES

ICD9

725 Polymyalgia rheumatica

CLINICAL PEARLS

- Consider PMR in an elderly patient with proximal limb girdle pain and stiffness.
- Markers of inflammation are usually elevated, but a normal ESR does not exclude the diagnosis.
- If the patient does not report a dramatic and rapid response to low-dose steroids, reconsider the diagnosis.
- Adjust steroids according to patient's symptoms, not based on their ESR.

POLYMYOSITIS/DERMATOMYOSITIS

Christopher M. Wise, MD

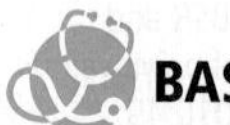

BASICS

DESCRIPTION

- Systemic connective tissue disease characterized by inflammatory and degenerative changes in proximal muscles, sometimes accompanied by characteristic skin rash:
  - If skin manifestations (Gottron sign: Symmetric, scaly, violaceous, erythematous eruption over the extensor surfaces of the metacarpophalangeal and interphalangeal joints of the fingers; heliotrope: Reddish violaceous eruption on the upper eyelids) are present, it is designated as dermatomyositis (1).
  - Different types of myositis include:
    - Idiopathic polymyositis
    - Idiopathic dermatomyositis
    - Polymyositis/dermatomyositis as an overlap (usually with lupus or systemic sclerosis or as part of mixed connective-tissue disease)
    - Myositis associated with malignancy
    - HIV-associated myopathy
- Inclusion-body myositis (IBM), a variant with atypical patterns of weakness and biopsy findings (2)
- System(s) affected: Cardiovascular; Musculoskeletal; Pulmonary; Skin/Exocrine
- Synonym(s): Myositis; Inflammatory myopathy; Antisynthetase syndrome (subset with certain antibodies)

EPIDEMIOLOGY

Incidence

- Estimated at 0.5–0.8/100,000 population
- Predominant age: 5–15 years, 40–60 years, peak incidence in mid-40s
- Predominant sex: Female > Male (2:1)

Prevalence

1–2 patients/100,000 population

Geriatric Considerations

Elderly patients with myositis or dermatomyositis are at increased risk of neoplasm.

Pediatric Considerations

Childhood dermatomyositis is likely a separate entity associated with cutaneous vasculitis and muscle calcifications.

RISK FACTORS

Family history of autoimmune disease (e.g., systemic lupus, myositis) or vasculitis

Genetics

Mild association with human leukocyte antigen (HLA)–DR3, HLA-DRw52

PATHOPHYSIOLOGY

- Inflammatory process, mediated by T cells and cytokine release, leading to damage to muscle cells (predominantly skeletal muscles)
- In patients with IBM, degenerative mechanisms may be important.

ETIOLOGY

Unknown; potential viral, genetic factors

COMMONLY ASSOCIATED CONDITIONS

- Malignancy (in 15–25%)
- Progressive systemic sclerosis
- Vasculitis
- Systemic lupus erythematosus
- Mixed connective-tissue disease

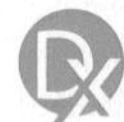

DIAGNOSIS

HISTORY

- Symmetric proximal muscle weakness causing difficulty when:
  - Arising from sitting or lying positions
  - Climbing stairs
  - Raising arms
- Joint pain/swelling
- Dysphagia
- Dyspnea
- Rash on face, eyelids, hands, arms

PHYSICAL EXAM

Proximal muscle weakness:

- Shoulder muscles
- Hip girdle muscles (trouble standing from seated or squatting position, weak hip flexors in supine position)
- Muscle swelling, stiffness, induration
- Distal muscle weakness is seen only in patients with IBM.
- Rash over face (eyelids, nasolabial folds), upper chest, dorsal hands (especially knuckle pads), fingers ("mechanic's hands")
- Periorbital edema
- Calcinosis cutis (childhood cases)
- Mesenteric arterial insufficiency/infarction (childhood cases)
- Cardiac impairment; arrhythmia, failure

DIAGNOSTIC TESTS & INTERPRETATION

- Diagnosis of muscle component (myositis) usually relies on 4 findings:
  - Weakness
  - Creatine kinase and/or aldolase elevation
  - Abnormal electromyogram
  - Findings on muscle biopsy
- Presence of compatible skin rash of dermatomyositis

Lab

Initial lab tests

- Increased creatine kinase (CK), aldolase
- Increased serum glutamic-oxaloacetic transaminase/aspartate aminotransferase
- Increased lactate dehydrogenase
- Myoglobinuria
- Increased ESR
- Positive rheumatoid factor (<50% of patients)
- Positive antinuclear antibody (>50% of patients)
- Leukocytosis (<50% of patients)
- Anemia (<50% of patients)
- Hyperglobulinemia (<50% of patients)
- Myositis-specific antibodies (antisynthetase antibodies) described in a minority of patients:
  - Anti-Jo-1 is the most common, but has been found in <20% of patients.
  - Associated with an increased incidence of interstitial lung disease

Follow-Up & Special Considerations

Changes in muscle enzymes (CK or aldolase) correlate with improvement and worsening.

Imaging

Initial approach

Chest radiograph part of initial evaluation to assess for associated pulmonary involvement or malignancy

Follow-Up & Special Considerations

MRI to assess muscle edema and inflammation may be used in some patients to determine best biopsy site or response to therapy.

Diagnostic Procedures/Surgery

- EMG: Muscle irritability, low-amplitude potentials, polyphasic action potentials, fibrillations
- Muscle biopsy (deltoid or quadriceps femoris)

Pathological Findings

- Microscopic findings:
  - Muscle fiber degeneration
  - Phagocytosis of muscle debris
  - Perifascicular muscle fiber atrophy
  - Inflammatory cell infiltrates in adult form
  - Via electron microscopy: Inclusion bodies (IBM only)
  - Sarcoplasmic basophilia
- Muscle fiber increased in size
- Vasculopathy (childhood polymyositis/dermatomyositis)

DIFFERENTIAL DIAGNOSIS

- Vasculitis
- Progressive systemic sclerosis
- Systemic lupus erythematosus
- Rheumatoid arthritis
- Muscular dystrophy
- Eaton-Lambert syndrome
- Sarcoidosis
- Amyotrophic lateral sclerosis
- Endocrine disorders:
  - Thyroid disease
  - Cushing syndrome
- Infectious myositis (viral, bacterial, parasitic)
- Drug-induced myopathies:
  - Cholesterol-lowering agents
  - Colchicine
  - Corticosteroids
  - Ethanol
  - Chloroquine
  - Zidovudine
- Electrolyte disorders (magnesium, calcium, potassium)
- Heritable metabolic myopathies
- Sleep-apnea syndrome

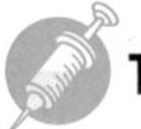

TREATMENT

MEDICATION

First Line

- Prednisone (3)[B],(4):
  - 40–80 mg/d PO in divided doses
  - Consolidate doses and reduce prednisone slowly when enzyme levels are normal.
  - Probably need to continue 5–10 mg/d for maintenance in most patients
- For steroid refractory or dependent patients (3)[B]:
  - Azathioprine: 1 mg/kg PO (arthritis dose) once daily or b.i.d.
  - Methotrexate: 10–25 mg PO weekly, useful in most steroid-resistant patients
- Rash of dermatomyositis may require topical steroids or oral hydroxychloroquine.
- Patients with IBM have very poor response to steroids and other first- and second-line drugs in general.

Second Line

- Other immunosuppressant drugs (e.g., cyclophosphamide, chlorambucil, cyclosporine, mycophenolate, tacrolimus) can be added to steroids.
- Combination methotrexate and azathioprine also may be useful in refractory cases (3)[B].
- IVIG, tumor necrosis factor (TNF) inhibitors (e.g., etanercept), and rituximab have been reported to be helpful in small series of patients with refractory disease.
- Contraindications: Methotrexate is contraindicated with previous liver disease, alcohol use, pregnancy, and underlying renal disease (use with extreme caution in patients with serum creatinine >1.5 mg/dL in general).
- Precautions:
  - Prednisone: Adverse effects associated with long-term steroid use include adrenal suppression, sodium and water retention, hypokalemia, osteoporosis, cataracts, and increased susceptibility to infection.
  - Azathioprine: Adverse effects include bone marrow suppression, increased liver function tests, and increased risk of infection.
  - Methotrexate: Adverse effects include stomatitis, bone marrow suppression, pneumonitis, and risk of liver fibrosis and cirrhosis with prolonged use.

ADDITIONAL TREATMENT

General Measures

General evaluation for malignancy in all adults, particularly with dermatomyositis, at initial evaluation, and during follow-up

Issues for Referral

- Diagnostic uncertainty, usually related to elevated muscle enzymes without typical symptoms of findings of muscle weakness
- Poor response to initial steroid therapy
- Excessive steroid requirement (unable to taper prednisone to <20 mg daily after 4–6 months)

SURGERY/OTHER PROCEDURES

None indicated, other than initial biopsy

IN-PATIENT CONSIDERATIONS

Initial Stabilization

Inpatient evaluation seldom needed

Admission Criteria

- Inability to stand, ambulate
- Respiratory difficulty
- Fever or other signs of infection

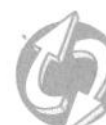

ONGOING CARE

FOLLOW-UP RECOMMENDATIONS

Patient Monitoring

- Follow muscle enzymes along with muscle strength and functional capacity.
- Monitor for steroid-induced complications (e.g., hypokalemia, hypertension, and hyperglycemia).
- Bone densitometry and consideration of calcium, vitamin D, and bisphosphonate therapy
- If azathioprine, methotrexate, or other immunosuppressant is used, appropriate laboratory monitoring should be done periodically (e.g., hematology, liver enzymes, and creatinine).
- Attempt to decrease and/or discontinue steroid dose as patient responds to therapy.
- Maintain immunosuppression until patient's muscle strength stabilizes for prolonged period depending on individual patient parameters, risks of medication, risk of relapse; time period undefined (months, years).

DIET

Moderation of caloric and sodium intake to avoid weight gain from corticosteroid therapy

PATIENT EDUCATION

- Curtail excess physical activity in early phases when muscles enzymes are markedly elevated.
- Emphasis on range-of-motion exercises
- Gradually muscle strengthening when muscle enzymes are normal or improved and stable

PROGNOSIS

- Residual weakness 30%
- Persistent active disease 20%
- 5-year survival 65–75%
- Survival is worse for women and African Americans and those with dermatomyositis, IBM, or cancer.
- Most patients improve with therapy.
- Patients with IBM respond poorly to most therapies.
- 50% have full recovery (5,6).

COMPLICATIONS

- Pneumonia
- Infection
- Myocardial infarction
- Carcinoma (especially breast, lung)
- Severe dysphagia
- Respiratory impairment due to muscle weakness, interstitial lung disease
- Aspiration pneumonitis
- Steroid myopathy
- Steroid-induced diabetes, hypertension, hypokalemia, osteoporosis

REFERENCES

1. Khan S, Christopher-Stine L, et al. Polymyositis, dermatomyositis, and autoimmune necrotizing myopathy: clinical features. *Rheum Dis Clin North Am*. 2011;37:143–58, v.
2. Solorzano GE, Phillips LH, et al. Inclusion body myositis: Diagnosis, pathogenesis, and treatment options. *Rheum Dis Clin North Am*. 2011;37:173–83, v.
3. Choy EH, Hoogendijk JE, Lecky B, et al. Immunosuppressant and immunomodulatory treatment for dermatomyositis and polymyositis. *Cochrane Database Syst Rev*. 2005;CD003643.
4. Aggarwal R, Oddis CV, et al. Therapeutic approaches in myositis. *Curr Rheumatol Rep*. 2011;13:182–91.
5. Ponyi A, Borgulya G, Constantin T, et al. Functional outcome and quality of life in adult patients with idiopathic inflammatory myositis. *Rheumatology (Oxford)*. 2005;44:83–8.
6. Airio A, Kautiainen H, Hakala M. Prognosis and mortality of polymyositis and dermatomyositis patients. *Clin Rheumatol*. 2006;25:234–9.

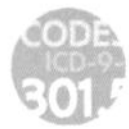

CODES

ICD9

- 710.3 Dermatomyositis
- 710.4 Polymyositis

CLINICAL PEARLS

- Corticosteroids alone may be sufficient in patients who have rapid improvement in weakness and muscle enzymes. However, most patients require azathioprine, methotrexate, or other immunosuppressive medications.
- The risk of associated malignancy is higher in patients over age 50 and those with cutaneous manifestations.
- Elevated muscle enzymes (e.g., CK and aldolase) are seen frequently as transient phenomena in patients with febrile illness and injuries; may return to normal on repeat.
- In patients with persistently elevated muscle enzymes and symptoms and findings of muscle weakness, EMG followed by muscle biopsy should be the initial studies considered.
- Suspect IBM in older patients with very slow onset and progression of symptoms, poor response to steroids and immunosuppressive therapy, and atypical patterns (asymmetric, sometimes distal) of muscle weakness.

PORPHYRIA

Jennifer Gao, MD
Nathan T. Connell, MD

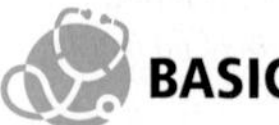

BASICS

Porphyria describes a variety of disorders of heme biosynthesis.

DESCRIPTION

- Heme: Primarily synthesized in erythropoietic cells for hemoglobin synthesis and liver parenchymal cells for cytochrome and hemoprotein synthesis (1):
  - Liver rate limiting step: 5-aminolevulinic acid synthase (ALAS)
  - Erythroid cell rate limiting step: Iron availability
- Porphyria: Inherited and acquired metabolic disorders due to defect in heme biosynthesis leading to accumulation and excessive excretion of porphyrins (2):
  - 8 enzymes involved in synthesis of heme: Defect at any step leads to porphyria
  - Complete enzyme deficiencies incompatible with life
- Classification:
  - Acute vs. chronic porphyrias (2,3)
  - Acute: AIP, HCP, VP, ALAD-P
  - Chronic: PCT, HEP, EPP, CEP
- System(s) affected: Gastrointestinal; Skin/Exocrine; Hematologic/Lymphatic/Immunologic; Nervous
- Abbreviations:
  - AIP = acute intermittent porphyria
  - HCP = hereditary coproporphyria
  - VP = variegate porphyria
  - ALAD-P = d-Aminolevulinate dehydratase deficiency porphyria
  - PCT = porphyria cutanea tarda
  - HEP = hepatoerythropoietic porphyria
  - EPP = erythropoietic protoporphyria
  - CEP = congenital erythropoietic porphyria
- Acute porphyrias:
  - Acute intermittent porphyria (AIP) (2):
    - Inheritance: Autosomal dominant
    - Classification: Acute
    - Deficiency of porphobilinogen deaminase
    - Symptoms: Purely neurologic (question whether ALA or PBG is neurotoxic)
  - Hereditary coproporphyria (HCP) (2):
    - Inheritance: Autosomal dominant
    - Classification: Acute
    - Deficiency of coproporphyrinogen oxidase
    - Symptoms: Neurovisceral, dermatologic (5%)
  - Variegate porphyria (VP) (2):
    - Inheritance: Autosomal dominant
    - Classification: Acute
    - Deficiency of protoporphyrinogen oxidase
    - Symptoms: Neurologic and dermatologic (60%) (1):
      - Dermatologic symptoms do not respond to phlebotomy or chloroquine.
      - Acute attacks peak in 20s and more common in women
    - Specific labs: Plasma fluorescence emission spectroscopy peak at 624–628 nm distinguishes VP from AIP and HCP (both have peaks at 620 nm).
  - d-Aminolevulinate dehydratase deficiency porphyria (ALAD-P) (2):
    - Rarest form of porphyria
    - Inheritance: Autosomal recessive
    - Classification: Acute
    - Deficiency of delta-aminolevulinic acid dehydratase (ALAD) causing unopposed ALAS expression in liver:
      - Acute attack due to overexpression of ALA synthetase (ALAS) in liver due to lack of negative feedback from deficient ALAD
      - Partial deficiency does not produce clinical symptoms.
    - Specific labs: Urinary coproporphyrin III and erythrocyte zinc-protoporphyrin
- Chronic porphyrias:
  - Porphyria cutanea tarda (PCT) (1,2):
    - Most common and readily treated porphyria
    - Inheritance: Autosomal dominant in 20%, may be acquired mutation
    - Classification: Chronic
    - Deficiency of uroporphyrinogen decarboxylase
    - Symptoms: Dermatologic: Blood vessels of papillary dermis site of injury:
      - Skin fragility: Negligible trauma causes superficial erosion that eventually forms crust; secondary infection common
      - Hypertrichosis
      - Increased pigmentation
    - Specific labs: Plasma fluorescent spectrum to differentiate VP and PCT
    - Specific treatment:
      - Phlebotomy in patients with hemochromatosis
      - Chloroquine (low dose) only if no hemochromatosis
- Erythropoietic protoporphyria (EPP) (1,2):
  - Inheritance: Autosomal dominant vs. coinheritance
  - Deficiency of mitochondrial ferrochelatase
  - Classification: Chronic
  - Symptoms: Dermatologic, GI
    - Dermatologic: Transient skin redness, swelling, pruritus, burning after sunlight exposure
    - GI: Liver dysfunction, gallstones, cholestatic liver failure due to accumulation of protoporphyrin
  - Specific labs: High protoporphyrin in RBCs, bone marrow, and plasma
  - Specific treatment:
    - Skin burning: Apply cold water
    - Afamelanotide: Alpha melanocyte-stimulating hormone analogue to induce photo-protective epidermal melanin formation
    - Oral beta carotene if nonsmoker
    - Cholestyramine or activated charcoal for liver dysfunction
    - Transplantation for liver failure
- Congenital erythropoietic porphyria (CEP) (1,2):
  - Rare and panethnic
  - Inheritance: Autosomal recessive
  - Classification: Chronic
  - Deficiency of uroporphyrinogen III cosynthase
  - Symptoms:
    - Dermatologic: Photosensitivity
    - Ocular: Chronic ulcerative keratitis, corneal scarring
- Hepatoerythropoietic porphyria (HEP) (1,2,3):
  - Inheritance: Autosomal recessive
  - Classification: Chronic
  - Deficiency of uroporphyrinogen decarboxylase
  - Symptoms: Presents in infancy or childhood with red urine, blistering, skin lesions, hypertrichosis, and scarring
  - Specific treatment: Phlebotomy and chloroquine not effective

EPIDEMIOLOGY

- More common in females than males (3)
- AIP (4):
  - Incidence: 1 per 100,000
  - Onset: 20–40 years old, rarely before puberty
- VP (4):
  - Incidence: 1 per 300 in South Africa, rare elsewhere
  - Onset: 20–30 years old, rare before puberty
- HCP (4):
  - Incidence: <50 total cases
  - Onset: Rare before puberty
- ALAD-P (4):
  - Incidence: <10 total cases
  - Onset: Bimodal in early and late years
- PCT (4):
  - Incidence: Most common porphyria worldwide
  - Onset: 30–40 years old, rare before puberty
- EPP (4):
  - Incidence: Second most common of cutaneous porphyrias
  - Onset: 1–4 years old
- CEP (4):
  - Incidence: ~150 total cases
  - Onset: Infancy to first decade of life
- HEP (4):
  - Incidence: ~25 total cases
  - Onset: Early infancy

Prevalence

- More common in whites than in Asians or individuals of African descent
- PCT: 1/10,000; most common of the porphyrias in the US and Europe
- AIP, HCP, VP: 1/10,000–1/100,000. The prevalence in Europe is ~1/75,000. In northern Sweden, because of a founder effect, the estimated prevalence is 1/1,000 (1).

RISK FACTORS

- Acute porphyria triggers (AIP, HCP, VP, ALAD-P) (3):
  - Viral infections
  - Hypocaloric diet
  - Alcohol
  - Drugs (e.g., barbiturates, sulfa)
  - Stress
  - Steroid hormones
  - Pregnancy
- Hexachlorobenzene exposure

Genetics

See within descriptions of each porphyria above.

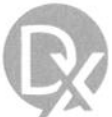

DIAGNOSIS

PHYSICAL EXAM

Symptoms of acute attacks (1):

- Duration: 1–2 weeks
- Mortality up to 10%
- Prodromic phase with behavioral changes (anxiety, restlessness, insomnia)
- GI: Abdominal pain, nausea, vomiting, constipation
- Psychiatric: Anxiety, depression, disorientation, hallucination, paranoia, confusion seen in 20–30%
- Cardiac: Tachycardia, hyperhydrosis, hypertension
- Imaging: Abdominal x-ray normal or with mild bowel ileus
- Labs: Dehydration, hyponatremia due to inappropriate antidiuretic hormone secretion in 40%, electrolyte imbalance
- Neurologic: Seizures due to hyponatremia or hypomagnesemia, neuropathy (mostly motor), normal CSF
- Urine: Excretion red or dark-colored urine

DIAGNOSTIC TESTS & INTERPRETATION

- Urinary porphobilinogen, porphyrins, 5-aminolevulinic acid
- Genetic studies when applicable

Lab

- Gold standard: DNA analysis to identify causative mutation (3):
  - ALAD-P: ALAD, chromosome 9q34
  - AIP: HMBS, chromosome 11q24
  - VP: PPOX, chromosome 3q19
  - HCP: CPOX, chromosome 1q22-23
  - CEP: UROS, chromosome 10q25.2
  - PCT: UROD, chromosome 1p34
  - EPP: FECH, chromosome 18q21.3
  - HEP: UROD, chromosome 1p34
- Urine: Assess for excess alanine (ALA) and porphobilinogen (1,3):
  - Acute attack confirmed by excretion > 10 times upper limit
- Serum: ALA levels to differentiate from other causes of abdominal pain (1,3)
- Plasma fluorescence emission spectroscopy (3)

DIFFERENTIAL DIAGNOSIS

- The differential diagnosis includes a spectrum of neurologic, psychiatric, and dermatologic disorders.
- Pseudoporphyria is a rare syndrome—indistinguishable from porphyria cutanea tarda—caused by some NSAIDs (e.g., nabumetone and naproxen) and flutamide

TREATMENT

MEDICATION

First Line

- Preventive: Avoid sun exposure, precipitating drugs, alcohol, smoking, cannabis, dieting, fasting (1)
- List of safe and unsafe drugs at www.drugs-porphyria.org (3)
- First-line treatment (1):
  - IV heme:
    - Monitor urinary porphobilinogen excretion to document response.
    - Administer with 1:1 dilution in 4–20% human serum albumin to increase solubility, stability, and lower risk of vein injury.
    - Can be used during pregnancy
    - Monitor for iron overload using iron studies.
  - Monitor fluids and electrolytes:
    - Avoid hyponatremia.
    - Maintain caloric intake with PO carbohydrate-rich food supplements or IV normal saline with 5% dextrose.
- Supportive treatment (1):
  - Abdominal pain: Opiates, aspirin
  - Vomiting: Antiemetics
  - Constipation: Laxatives
  - Hypertension and tachycardia: Beta-blockers
  - Neuropathy: Opiates, physiotherapy
  - Adrenergic symptoms: IV magnesium sulfate

ADDITIONAL TREATMENT

General Measures

- Neuropsychiatric–abdominal: Avoid precipitating drugs, alcohol, known toxins
- Dermatologic: Shade, protective clothing, avoid skin trauma; for porphyria cutanea tarda, weekly or monthly phlebotomy may help to prevent attacks
- Congenital erythropoietic porphyria: Consider bone marrow transplant.

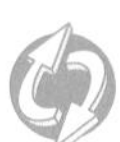

ONGOING CARE

DIET

Neuropsychiatric: Anecdotal evidence carbohydrates help to reduce symptoms or frequency of attacks

PATIENT EDUCATION

- The American Porphyria Foundation, P.O. Box 22712, Houston, TX 77227; (713) 266-9617 or 1-866-APF-3635 (toll-free); fax: (713) 840-9552; www.porphyriafoundation.com/
- The Drug Database for Acute Porphyria: www.drugs-porphyria.org/
- European Porphyria Network: www.porphyria-europe.com/

PROGNOSIS

- In all porphyrias:
  - Asymptomatic or minimally symptomatic: Unaffected longevity
  - Neurologic complications (e.g., peripheral neuropathy, neurosis, or hemiplegia) may be permanent.
- In AIP:
  - Acute attacks have 25% mortality.
  - Increased risk of hepatocellular carcinoma
- <10% of patients develop recurrent acute attacks (1).

REFERENCES

1. Puy H, Gouya L, Deybach JC, et al. Porphyrias. *Lancet*. 2010;375:924–37.
2. Antonello Pietrangelo. The porphyrias: pathophysiology. *Int Emerg Med*. 2010;5(S1): S65–71.
3. Cappellini M, Brancaleoni V, Graziadei G, et al. Porphyrias at a glance: Diagnosis and treatment. *Int Emerg Med*. 2010;5(S1):S73–80.
4. Siegesmund M, et al. The acute hepatic porphyrias: Current status and future challenges. *Best Pract Res Clin Gastroenterol*. 2010;24:593–605.

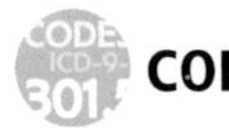

CODES

ICD9

277.1 Disorders of porphyrin metabolism

PORTAL HYPERTENSION

Walter M. Kim, MD, PhD
Jyoti Ramakrishna, MD

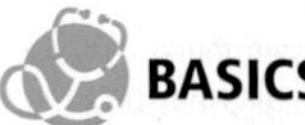

BASICS

DESCRIPTION

- Increased portal venous pressure >5–10 mm Hg that occurs in association with splanchnic vasodilatation, portosystemic collateral formation, and a hyperdynamic circulation
- Most commonly secondary to elevated hepatic venous pressure gradient (the gradient between the portal and central venous pressures)
- Course is generally progressive, with risk of complications including acute variceal bleeding, ascites, encephalopathy, and hepatorenal syndrome.

EPIDEMIOLOGY

Incidence

- Prevalence <200,000 persons in the US
- Predominant age: Adult
- Predominant sex: Male > Female

RISK FACTORS

See "Etiology."

Genetics

No known genetic patterns except those associated with specific hepatic diseases that cause portal hypertension (HTN)

ETIOLOGY

- Causes generally classified as:
  - Prehepatic (portal vein thrombosis or obstruction)
  - Intrahepatic (most commonly cirrhosis)
  - Posthepatic (hepatic vein thrombosis, Budd-Chiari syndrome, right-sided heart failure)
- Adult: May be intrahepatic or extrahepatic; cirrhosis accounts for 90% of cases; may be due to:
  - Virus (hepatitis B, hepatitis C, hepatitis D)
  - Alcoholism
  - Schistosomiasis
  - Wilson disease
  - Hemochromatosis
  - Primary biliary cirrhosis

Pediatric Considerations

In children, portal vein thrombosis is the most common extrahepatic cause; intrahepatic causes are more likely to be biliary atresia, viral hepatitis, and metabolic liver disease.

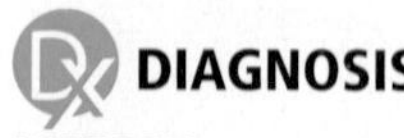

DIAGNOSIS

HISTORY

- Weakness/fatigue
- Jaundice
- Symptoms of heart failure including chest pain, shortness of breath, and/or edema
- Hematemesis
- Melena
- Oliguria
- History of chronic liver disease
- Alcoholic hepatitis
- Alcohol abuse

PHYSICAL EXAM

- Exam findings may be general or related to specific complications.
- General:
  - Pallor
  - Icterus
  - Digital clubbing
  - Palmar erythema
  - Splenomegaly
  - Caput medusa
  - Spider angiomata
  - Umbilical bruit
  - Hemorrhoids
  - Gynecomastia
  - Testicular atrophy
- Gastroesophageal varices:
  - Hypotension
  - Tachycardia
- Ascites:
  - Distended abdomen
  - Fluid wave
  - Shifting dullness with percussion
- Hepatic encephalopathy:
  - Confusion/coma
  - Asterixis
  - Hyperreflexia

DIAGNOSTIC TESTS & INTERPRETATION

Lab

Initial lab tests

Nonspecific changes associated with underlying disease:

- Hypersplenism: Anemia (also may be due to malnutrition or bleeding), leukopenia, thrombocytopenia
- Hepatic dysfunction:
  - Hypoalbuminemia
  - Hyperbilirubinemia
  - Elevated alkaline phosphatase
  - Elevated liver enzymes (AST, ALT)
  - Abnormal clotting (prothrombin time, partial thromboplastin time)
- GI bleeding:
  - Iron-deficiency anemia
  - Elevated serum ammonia
  - Fecal occult blood
- Hepatorenal syndrome:
  - Elevated serum creatinine (Cr), BUN
  - Urine Na <5 mEq/L (<20 mmol/L)

Imaging

Initial approach

- US and CT scan/MRI may detect cirrhosis, splenomegaly, ascites, and varices.
- US/duplex Doppler:
  - Can determine presence and direction of flow in portal and hepatic veins
  - Useful in diagnosing portal vein thrombosis, shunt thrombosis, or the presence of ascites
- CT scan/MRI: Angiographic measurement of hepatic venous wedge pressure via jugular or femoral vein:
  - Correlates with portal pressure
  - Risk of variceal bleeding is increased if hepatic venous pressure gradient >12 mm Hg
- Upper GI series may outline varices in esophagus and stomach.

Diagnostic Procedures/Surgery

Endoscopy can diagnose esophageal and gastric varices and portal hypertensive gastropathy.

Pathological Findings

Specific for underlying disease

DIFFERENTIAL DIAGNOSIS

Usually related to specific presentations:

- Gastroesophageal varices with hemorrhage:
  - Portal hypertensive gastropathy
  - Hemorrhagic gastritis
  - Peptic ulcer disease
  - Mallory-Weiss tear
- Ascites:
  - Spontaneous bacterial peritonitis
  - Pancreatic ascites
  - Peritoneal carcinomatosis
  - Tuberculous peritonitis
  - Nephrotic syndrome
  - Fluid overload from heart failure
- Hepatic encephalopathy:
  - Delirium tremens
  - Intracranial hemorrhage
  - Sedative abuse
  - Uremia
- Hepatorenal syndrome:
  - Drug nephrotoxicity
  - Renal tubular necrosis

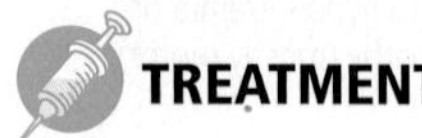

TREATMENT

MEDICATION

Therapy for encephalopathy: See "Hepatic Encephalopathy."

First Line

- Prophylaxis against variceal bleeding:
  - Nonselective β-blockade (1)[B]: Examples include:
    - Propranolol: Start with 10–20 mg/d PO 2–3 times daily; pediatric dose: 0.5–1 mg/kg/d divided q6–8h
    - Nadolol: 40–80 mg/d PO once-daily dosing
  - Doses may be titrated up as tolerated to maximum recommended doses.
- Therapy for acute variceal hemorrhage:
  - Vasopressin: Start with 0.2–0.4 U/min IV; increase to maximum dose 0.9 U/min as needed; pediatric dose: 0.002–0.005 U/kg/min; do not exceed 0.01 U/kg/min. After bleeding stops, continue at same dose for 12 hours and then taper off over 24–48 hours.
  - Somatostatin: 250-μg bolus, followed by 250 μg/hr continuous infusion; continue for 2–5 days if successful
  - Octreotide: 25–50 μg/hr continuous infusion; pediatric dose: 1 μg/kg bolus followed by 1 μg/kg/hr is used traditionally; treat for up to 5 days

- For prevention of recurrence and for overall reduction in mortality:
  - Propranolol: 10–60 mg/d PO 2–4×/day; pediatric dose: 0.5–1 mg/kg/d divided q6–8h
  - Nadolol: 40–80 mg/d orally reduces portal venous blood inflow by blocking the adrenergic dilatation of the mesenteric arterioles.
  - Tetrandrine, a calcium-channel blocker, also has been found to reduce the rate of rebleeding with fewer side effects.
- Treatment for ascites (along with salt and fluid restriction):
  - Furosemide: 20–40 mg/d; pediatric dose: 1–2 mg/kg/dose ± IV albumin infusion
  - Spironolactone: 50–100 mg/d; pediatric dose: 1–3 mg/kg/d

Second Line

- Terlipressin (1–2 mg IV q4–6h for up to 48 hours) is a more selective splanchnic vasoconstrictor and may be associated with fewer complications (1)[B]. It is currently used when standard therapy with somatostatin or octreotide fails.
- Addition of nitrates, such as nitroglycerin or isosorbide mononitrate, reduces portal pressures and bleeding rates, and has been shown to reduce mortality. Since the risk–benefit ratio is not clear, nitrates are not considered first-line treatment.

ADDITIONAL TREATMENT

General Measures

- Avoid sedatives that may precipitate encephalopathy.
- Limit sodium intake because cirrhotic patients avidly retain sodium.
- Restrict protein only if encephalopathic.

Issues for Referral

Patients with portal HTN should be managed longitudinally by both a primary care physician and a gastroenterologist.

SURGERY/OTHER PROCEDURES

- Treatments available for specific complications of portal HTN (in addition to or if refractory to medications):
  - Gastroesophageal varices with hemorrhage:
    - Endoscopic variceal sclerosis or banding (the first-line treatment in many cases for acute hemorrhage)
    - Balloon tamponade (not used commonly when endoscopic treatment is available)
    - Transjugular intrahepatic portosystemic shunt (TIPS)
    - Portocaval shunting
  - Ascites refractory to medical management:
    - Large-volume paracentesis
    - Peritoneovenous shunt
    - TIPS
- Liver transplantation should be considered for patients with advanced disease (1)[B].

IN-PATIENT CONSIDERATIONS

- Acute GI bleeding should be managed in the inpatient setting, either on the regular medical floor if the patient is hemodynamically stable or occasionally in the intensive care unit if the patient is unstable.
- Patients with mental status changes from encephalopathy need to be evaluated in the inpatient setting.

Initial Stabilization

- If acute variceal bleeding:
  - Type and cross
  - Initial resuscitation with isotonic fluid until packed RBCs are available
  - Correct coagulopathy with vitamin K and fresh-frozen plasma (FFP).
  - Endoscopy as soon as the patient is stabilized (for diagnosis and treatment)
- Avoid sedatives that may precipitate encephalopathy.
- Limit sodium administration because cirrhotic patients avidly retain sodium.
- Restrict protein only if encephalopathic.

ALERT

If the patient is an active alcohol drinker, watch for signs and symptoms of withdrawal. Follow inpatient protocols.

Admission Criteria

- Acute bleeding from the intestinal tract, either vomiting or per rectum
- Acute confusional state/mental status changes

IV Fluids

Use isotonic fluid.

Discharge Criteria

- For GI bleeding:
  - No active bleeding × 24 hours
  - Hemodynamically stable, especially pulse
  - Stable hemoglobin
- For encephalopathy: Improvement in or resolution of mental status changes

ONGOING CARE

DIET

- In patients with cirrhosis, sodium restriction is important because cirrhotic patients avidly retain sodium.
- Restrict protein only in patients who are encephalopathic.

PATIENT EDUCATION

Refrain from drinking alcohol. Resources for patients who have difficulty with not drinking alcohol can be obtained from Alcoholics Anonymous at www.aa.org.

PROGNOSIS

- Hepatic reserve defined by Child-Pugh classification: Rating based on encephalopathy, ascites, bilirubin, albumin, prothrombin
- Variceal bleeding:
  - 1/3 of patients with known varices will bleed eventually.
  - 50% rebleed, usually within 2 years, unless portal pressure is reduced by surgical or transjugular intrahepatic portosystemic shunt procedure.
  - 15–20% mortality rate
- Ascites and encephalopathy often recur.
- Prognosis of patients with ascites is poor: 50% 1-year survival without liver transplant (compared with 90% for patients with cirrhosis and no ascites).

REFERENCE

1. Abraldes JG, Angermayr B, Bosch J. The management of portal hypertension. *Clin Liver Dis*. 2005;9:685–713, vii.

ADDITIONAL READING

- Bosch J, et al. The management of portal hypertension: Rational basis, available treatments and future options. *J Hepatology*. 2008;48: S68–S92.
- Dib N, Oberti F, Calès P. Current management of the complications of portal hypertension: Variceal bleeding and ascites. *CMAJ*. 2006;174:1433–43.
- Samonakis DN, et al. Management of portal hypertension. *Postgrad Med*. 2004;80:634–41.
- Sanyal AJ, Bosch J, Blei A, et al. Portal hypertension and its complications. *Gastroenterology*. 2008; 134:1715–28.
- Sass DA, Chopra KB, et al. Portal hypertension and variceal hemorrhage. *Med Clin North Am*. 2009;93.
- Wright AS, Rikkers LF. Current management of portal hypertension. *J Gastrointest Surg*. 2005;9: 992–1005.

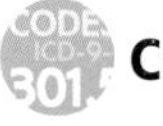

CODES

ICD9

572.3 Portal hypertension

CLINICAL PEARLS

- Endoscopic treatment is successful for acute variceal hemorrhage 85% of the time.
- Prognosis of patients with ascites is poor: 50% 1-year survival without liver transplant (compared with 90% for patients with cirrhosis and no ascites).
- Advantages and disadvantages of balloon tamponade for acute variceal bleed:
  - Advantages include rapid and often effective control of bleeding and common availability of device.
  - Disadvantages include recurrence of bleeding when balloon is deflated, patient discomfort, and risk of esophageal perforation.

POSTCONCUSSIVE SYNDROME

Ryung Suh, MD, MPP, MBA, MPH

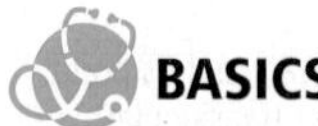

BASICS

DESCRIPTION
- Postconcussive syndrome (PCS) refers to the neurologic, cognitive, or behavioral symptoms that develop shortly after a concussion and persist for weeks or months, including:
  - Headache
  - Vertigo or dizziness
  - Fatigue
  - Memory impairment
  - Difficulty concentrating
  - Apathy
  - Anxiety
  - Depression
  - Irritability
  - Disordered sleep
  - New-onset seizures
  - Personality changes, inappropriateness
  - Sudden academic decline
  - Worsening of pre-existing symptoms
- Persistent PCS (PPCS) is defined as the same symptoms that last more than 6 months.
- Some people with mild traumatic brain injury (MTBI) develop PCS while others do not, and it is unclear what causes PCS symptoms to occur and persist.

EPIDEMIOLOGY
Incidence
- At 3 months after injury, 24–84% of MTBI patients exhibit PCS symptoms.
- At 1 year after injury, 10–15% exhibit PCS symptoms.

Prevalence
Predominant sex: Female > Male

RISK FACTORS
- Older than 40 years of age
- Low socioeconomic status
- Substance abuse
- Previous affective or anxiety disorder (1)[B]
- Repetitive head injury
- Premorbid physical conditions
- Noise sensitivity, anxiety, and trouble thinking during the 3–10 days following concussion have been identified as important predictors of PCS (2).

GENERAL PREVENTION
Avoid opiates, if possible, for analgesia in patients with TBI (3)[B].

PATHOPHYSIOLOGY
- Controversial; exact mechanism unknown
- There is debate about the actual diagnosis of PCS.
- MTBI can cause cortical contusions and axonal injury.
- It is postulated that microscopic axonal injury from shearing forces leads to inflammation that then causes the secondary injury responsible for persistent damage.
- One study showed an equal rate of PCS symptoms among both concussion and nonconcussion patients, implying that PCS is not driven by head injury alone (1)[B].
- A recent review of PPCS suggests that concomitant damage to eyes and ears during TBI plays a role in symptoms such as vertigo (4)[B].

ETIOLOGY
- Concussion is caused by direct blow to the head, face, or neck.
- Most commonly related to:
  - Motor vehicle accidents
  - Falls
  - Occupational accidents
  - Recreational accidents
  - Assaults

COMMONLY ASSOCIATED CONDITIONS
Posttraumatic stress disorder

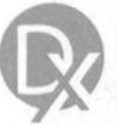

DIAGNOSIS

HISTORY
- Detailed history of recent impact or closed head injury, including:
  - Mechanism
  - Amount and type of force
  - Timing of injury related to symptoms
- Report of neurologic, cognitive, or behavioral symptoms by patient or family

PHYSICAL EXAM
Complete neurologic exam, including:
- Glasgow Coma Scale (GCS)
- Mini-Mental State Examination
- Memory testing

DIAGNOSTIC TESTS & INTERPRETATION
Lab
Initial lab tests

Rule out other causes of neurologic, cognitive, or behavioral symptoms if history and presentation suggest other possible etiologies. Consider ordering (but not necessary for most diagnoses and not helpful in the young):
- CBC with differential
- Electrolytes
- Urinalysis
- Toxicology screen

Imaging
Initial approach
- CT scan is the imaging modality of choice for the assessment of acute head trauma.
- The Canadian CT head rule requires a head CT scan for patients with MTBI and one of the following (to rule out more serious injury) (5)[B]:
  - GCS score <15 2 hours after injury
  - Open or depressed skull fracture
  - Signs of basilar skull fracture
  - 2 or more episodes of vomiting
  - ≥65 years of age
  - Prolonged anterograde amnesia >30 minutes
  - Dangerous mechanism
- Patients with concussion often have a negative head CT scan.
- Consider the use of cervical imaging when concomitant cervical spine injury is suspected.

Follow-Up & Special Considerations

Schedule regular follow-up to evaluate for persistent symptoms and the need for pharmacologic treatment.

Diagnostic Procedures/Surgery
Lumbar puncture if concerned about CNS infection

DIFFERENTIAL DIAGNOSIS
- Posttraumatic stress disorder
- Evolving intracranial hemorrhage
- Migraine headaches
- Affective disorders, anxiety, or depression
- Chronic fatigue syndrome, fibromyalgia
- Exposure to toxins

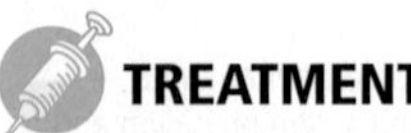

TREATMENT

MEDICATION
First Line
- Headache/neck pain:
  - Nonnarcotic pain control if possible, such as NSAIDs:
    - Sedation may obscure cognitive evaluation.
    - One study suggests a correlation between opiates and increased risk of depression and anxiety in PCS patients (3)[B].
- Depression/sleep disorders:
  - Tricyclic antidepressants
  - Selective serotonin reuptake inhibitors are not well supported.

Second Line
Cognition/psychiatric symptoms: Methylphenidate has been shown to improve cognition and alertness with fewer side effects compared with sertraline (6)[B].

ADDITIONAL TREATMENT

General Measures

Athletes with concussion should be restricted from sport activity until the clinical and cognitive symptoms of concussion resolve (7)[C].

Issues for Referral

- Psychiatric treatment, including behavioral therapy for anxiety and depression symptoms
- Occupational therapy for vocational rehabilitation, if needed
- Neurology referral if primary care interventions for seizures, headache, vertigo, or cognition are unsuccessful
- Comprehensive cognitive evaluation for potential TBI rehabilitation
- Cognitive-behavioral therapy
- Substance abuse counseling, if needed

COMPLEMENTARY AND ALTERNATIVE MEDICINE

Massage therapy or osteopathic manipulative treatment for headache and neck pain

IN-PATIENT CONSIDERATIONS

Initial Stabilization

- Follow Advanced Trauma Life Support algorithms immediately after injury to evaluate for additional injuries.
- If GCS score <8, support respirations until improved or consider definitive airway

Admission Criteria

If neurologic status prevents safe functioning at home:

- Decreased alertness
- Intractable nausea and vomiting
- Concern for respiratory status

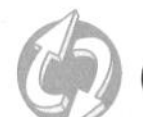

ONGOING CARE

FOLLOW-UP RECOMMENDATIONS

Return for further evaluation if symptoms worsen or persist longer than 3 months.

PATIENT EDUCATION

- Brain Injury Association of America: www.biausa.org; 800-444-6443
- Head and brain injuries: www.nlm.nih.gov/medlineplus/headandbraininjuries.html
- Explain the possibility of PCS symptoms and usual time course.
- Review "Return-to-Play" guidelines and the risks involved with second impact.

PROGNOSIS

- Prognosis generally is good.
- Young children may recover more slowly than young adults.

COMPLICATIONS

- Repeat head injury before resolution of PCS symptoms can worsen or prolong symptoms.
- Case studies of second-impact syndrome—a rare but fatal condition owing to a second head injury soon after the first, involving dysregulation of the brain's blood supply, causing vascular engorgement and herniation—have been reported.

REFERENCES

1. Meares S, Shores EA, Taylor AJ, et al. Mild traumatic brain injury does not predict acute postconcussion syndrome. *J Neurol Neurosurg Psychiatry*. 2008;79:300–6.
2. Dischinger PC, Ryb GE, Kufera JA, et al. Early predictors of postconcussive syndrome in a population of trauma patients with mild traumatic brain injury. *J Trauma*. 2009;66:289–96; discussion 296–7.
3. Meares S, Shores EA, Batchelor J, et al. The relationship of psychological and cognitive factors and opioids in the development of the postconcussion syndrome in general trauma patients with mild traumatic brain injury. *J Int Neuropsychol Soc*. 2006;12:792–801.
4. Bigler ED. Neuropsychology and clinical neuroscience of persistent post-concussive syndrome. *J Int Neuropsychol Soc*. 2008;14:1–22.
5. Stiell IG, Wells GA, Vandemheen K, et al. The Canadian CT head rule for patients with minor head injury. *Lancet*. 2001;357:1394.
6. Lee H, Kim S, Kim J, et al. Comparing effects of methylphenidate, sertraline and placebo on neuropsychiatric sequelae in patients with traumatic brain injury. *Hum Psychopharmacol Clin Exp*. 2005;20:97–104.
7. McCrory P, Meeuwisse W, Johnston K, et al. Consensus statement on Concussion in Sport 3rd International Conference on Concussion in Sport held in Zurich, November 2008. *Clin J Sport Med*. 2009;19:185–200.
8. Nampiaparampil DE. Prevalence of chronic pain after traumatic brain injury: A systematic review. *JAMA*. 2008;300(6):711–9.

ADDITIONAL READING

- McHugh T, Laforce R, Gallagher P, et al. Natural history of the long-term cognitive, affective, and physical sequelae of mild traumatic brain injury. *Brain Cogn*. 2006;60:209–11.
- Stulemeijer M, van der Werf S, Borm GF, et al. Early prediction of favourable recovery 6 months after mild traumatic brain injury. *J Neurol Neurosurg*. 2008;79:936–42.

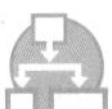

See Also (Topic, Algorithm, Electronic Media Element)

Concussion

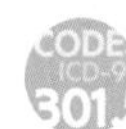

CODES

ICD9

310.2 Postconcussion syndrome

CLINICAL PEARLS

- Head CT scan is the test of choice for acute injury in which it is necessary to exclude intracranial bleeding.
- Coordinate multidisciplinary treatment plans for patients with persistent symptoms.
- Athletes may not return to practice until symptoms are completely cleared, nor can they play until they are able to practice fully without recurring symptoms.

POSTTRAUMATIC STRESS DISORDER (PTSD)

George Malcolmson, MD
Jeffrey G. Stovall, MD

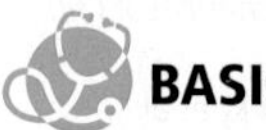

BASICS

DESCRIPTION

- Posttraumatic stress disorder (PTSD) is an anxiety disorder defined as a reaction that can occur after exposure to an extreme traumatic event involving death, threat of death, serious physical injury, or a threat to physical integrity.
- This reaction has 3 cardinal characteristics:
  - Re-experiencing the trauma
  - Avoidance of anything related to the traumatic event
  - Increased arousal
- Symptoms present for at least 1 month
- Traumatic events that may trigger PTSD include natural or human disasters, serious accidents, war, sexual abuse, rape, torture, terrorism, hostage-taking, or being diagnosed with life-threatening disease
- PTSD can be:
  - Acute: Symptoms lasting <3 months
  - Chronic: Symptoms lasting ≥3 months
  - Delayed onset: 6 months (from event to symptom onset) in 25% of diagnosed cases

EPIDEMIOLOGY

- ~30% of men and women who have spent time in a war zone experience PTSD.
- Current estimates of PTSD in military personnel who served in Iraq range from 12–20%.

Incidence

~7.7 million American adults aged ≥18 years (3.5% of this age group) are diagnosed with PTSD each year.

Prevalence

Lifetime prevalence for PTSD is 8–9%.

RISK FACTORS

- Pretrauma environment:
  - Female sex
  - Younger age
  - Psychiatric history
- Peritrauma environment:
  - Severity of the trauma
  - Peritrauma emotionality
- Posttrauma environment:
  - Perceived injury severity
  - Medical complications
  - Perceived social support

Genetics

- Monozygotic twins exposed to combat in Vietnam were at increased risk of the co-twin having PTSD compared to twins that were dizygotic.
- Some data suggest an association between dopamine transporter gene (DAT) SLC6A3 3′ (VNTR) polymorphism and PTSD (1).

GENERAL PREVENTION

- While there is some evidence suggestive of the benefit of pharmacologic interventions including morphine and propranolol, there is no standard pharmacologic intervention to prevent the onset of PTSD (2,3).
- Compulsory psychological debriefing immediately after a trauma (critical incident stress management) does not prevent PTSD and may be harmful (4).

PATHOPHYSIOLOGY

- During trauma, locus coeruleus mediates sympathetic outflows to amygdala (rapid effect) and adrenal medulla (sustained effect). Adrenal medulla then release catecholamines, which stimulate peripheral afferent vagal beta-receptors. Vagal afferents innervate the nucleus tractus solitarius (NTS) in brain-stem medulla. NTS fibers innervate the amygdala with norepinephrine (NE).
- With increase in NE, the amygdala mediates coupling of emotional valence to declarative memories via long-term potentiation, forming deeply engraved trauma memories and leading to intrusive memories and emotions, potentially leading to PTSD.
- Orbitoprefrontal cortex (which usually exerts an inhibiting effect on this activation) appears less capable of inhibiting this activation, due to stress-induced atrophy of specific nuclei in this region.

COMMONLY ASSOCIATED CONDITIONS

- Major depressive disorder
- Alcohol/substance abuse
- Panic disorder
- Obsessive compulsive disorder
- Agoraphobia and/or social phobia
- Traumatic brain injury
- Smoking (esp. with assaultive trauma)

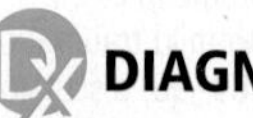

DIAGNOSIS

HISTORY

Diagnosis is based on *DSM-IV* criteria:

- Criterion A: Has 2 components, as follows:
  - Experiencing, witnessing, or being confronted with an event involving serious injury, death, or a threat to a person's physical integrity
  - A response involving helplessness, intense fear, or horror
- Criterion B: Persistent re-experiencing of the event: "flashbacks, nightmares, illusions, hallucinations"
- Criterion C: Avoidance of stimuli associated with the trauma (3 or more of the following):
  - Avoidance of thoughts, feelings, or conversations associated with the event
  - Avoidance of people, places, or activities that may trigger recollections of the event
  - Inability to recall important aspects of the event
  - Significantly diminished interest or participation in important activities
  - Feeling of detachment
  - Narrowed range of affect
  - Sense of having a foreshortened future
- Criterion D: Hyperarousal (2 or more of the following):
  - Difficulty sleeping or falling asleep
  - Decreased concentration
  - Hypervigilance
  - Outbursts of anger or irritable mood
  - Exaggerated startle response
  - Intense anxiety or hyperalertness to events that resemble the traumatic event (e.g., anniversaries of the trauma)
- Criterion E: The duration of the relevant criteria symptoms should be >1 month.
- Criterion F: Clinically significant distress or impairment in functioning

Pediatric Considerations

- Reactions can include a fear of being separated from a parent, crying, whimpering, screaming, immobility and/or aimless motion, trembling, frightened facial expressions, excessive clinging, and regressive behavior.
- Older children may show extreme withdrawal, disruptive behavior, and/or an inability to pay attention. Regressive behaviors, nightmares, sleep problems, irrational fears, irritability, refusal to attend school, outbursts of anger, and fighting are also common. Somatic complaints with no medical basis, in addition to schoolwork often suffering. Furthermore, depression, anxiety, feelings of guilt, and emotional numbing are often present.

PHYSICAL EXAM

- Patients may present with physical injuries from the traumatic event.
- Mental status examination:
  - Thoughts and perceptions may be affected (e.g., hallucinations, delusions, suicidal ideation, phobias)
  - General appearance may be affected: Disheveled, poor personal hygiene
  - Behavior: Agitation; startle reaction may be extreme.
  - Psychological numbness
  - Orientation may be affected.
  - Memory is usually affected: Forgetfulness, especially concerning the details of the traumatic event
  - Poor concentration
  - Poor impulse control
  - Altered speech rate and flow.
  - Mood and affect may be changed: Depression, anxiety, guilt, and/or fear

DIAGNOSTIC TESTS & INTERPRETATION

Lab

None are used in daily clinical practice

- Decreased urine cortisol (5)
- Increased catecholamine secretion (5)
- Increased norepinephrine/cortisol ratio (5)

Diagnostic Procedures/Surgery

Strong response to dexamethasone suppression test; however, there is not a standard diagnostic test employed (6).

DIFFERENTIAL DIAGNOSIS

- Acute stress disorder (symptoms <4 weeks)
- Generalized anxiety disorder
- Adjustment disorder
- Obsessive-compulsive disorder
- Schizophrenia
- Malingering
- Mood disorders: Depression
- Mood disorder with psychotic features
- Psychotic disorders caused by a general medical condition
- Substance abuse

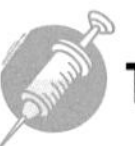

TREATMENT

- Treatment is often best accomplished with a combination of pharmacologic and nonpharmacologic therapies.
- The sooner therapy is initiated after the trauma, the better the prognosis.

MEDICATION

First Line

Sleep disruption: Sleep disruption due to hyperarousal is ubiquitous in PTSD. Standard sedatives such as trazodone (25–200 mg at bedtime), mirtazapine (7.5–30 mg at bedtime), or another sedating antidepressant can be used. Given the risk of substance abuse, it is recommended that benzodiazepines be used with caution.

- Nightmares or nighttime hyperarousal: Prazosin (Minipress) 2–15 mg at bedtime (7,8,9)

SSRIs: Depression, panic attacks, startle response, sleep disruption (11,12,13). All commonly used SSRIs have been shown to be effective in the treatment of PTSD and are the first-line treatment.

- Sertraline: 50–200 mg PO every day (FDA approved)
- Paroxetine: Starting dose: 20 mg PO every day; may be increased in 10–mg increments at intervals ≥1 week (FDA approved)
- Fluoxetine: 20 mg PO every day/b.i.d. not to exceed 80 mg/d (demonstrates some efficacy for all 3 symptom clusters) (11)

Second Line

Mirtazapine (Remeron): 15–45 mg/d (7)
Refractory or residual: Consider other monotherapy or augmentation (7)

- Hyperarousal: Clonidine, up to 0.45 mg/d divided doses; quetiapine, up to 65 mg/d; risperidone, 1.25–3.75 mg/d
- Antipsychotic medications (aripiprazole 5–30 mg daily, risperidone 0.5–4 mg daily, olanzapine 2.5–30 mg daily, quetiapine (25–800 mg daily) have been widely used but the evidence to support their use is equivocal.
- Psychotic symptoms after PTSD treated: Add an antipsychotic. Impulsivity-the use of anticonvulsants (valproic acid 500–2,000 mg daily, carbamazepine 200–1,200 mg daily, topiramate up to 200 mg daily, and lamotrigine up to 400 mg daily) has been effective in cases where impulsivity and irritability are prominent.
- Anxiety: Benzodiazepines including clonazepam, 1–4 mg/d for a limited duration. However, the risk of abuse and high rates of comorbidity limit the usefulness of benzodiazepines.

ADDITIONAL TREATMENT

- Psychotherapeutic interventions:
  - Behavioral and cognitive-behavioral therapy (CBT):
    - Early CBT has been shown to speed recovery (14).
    - CBT is currently considered the standard of care for PTSD by the US Department of Defense.
  - Prolonged exposure therapy: Re-experience distressing trauma-related memories and reminders in order to facilitate habituation and successful emotional processing of the trauma memory.
  - Eye movement desensitization and reprocessing has been shown to benefit some patients with PTSD (15)
  - Stress-reduction techniques:
    - Immediate symptom reduction (e.g., rebreathing in a bag for hyperventilation)
    - Early recognition and removal from a stress source
    - Relaxation, meditation, and exercise techniques are also helpful in reducing the reaction to stressful events.
- Interpersonal psychotherapy:
  - Supportive psychotherapy with an emphasis on the here and now
- Social:
  - Establish the framework of the problem. Clarifying the problem allows the patient to begin viewing it within the proper context (e.g., change of job or relocation of adult-dependent offspring)

COMPLEMENTARY AND ALTERNATIVE MEDICINE

In a recent study of service members with PTSD caused by the traumatic events of September 11, 2001, or Operation Iraqi Freedom, self-managed, Internet-based CBT led to a greater reduction in PTSD symptoms than Internet-based supportive counseling.

SURGERY/OTHER PROCEDURES

None

IN-PATIENT CONSIDERATIONS

Inpatient care is necessary only if the patient becomes suicidal or homicidal or for treatment of comorbid conditions (e.g., depression, substance abuse).

ONGOING CARE

PATIENT EDUCATION

National Center for PTSD: www.ptsd.va.gov

PROGNOSIS

- Varies significantly from patient to patient
- In ~50% of cases, the symptoms spontaneously remit after 3 months; however, in other cases symptoms may persist, often for many years, and cause long-term impairment in life functioning.
- Factors associated with a good prognosis include the following:
  - Rapid engagement of treatment
  - Early and ongoing social support
  - Avoidance of retraumatization
  - Positive premorbid function
  - Absence of other psychiatric disorders or substance abuse

COMPLICATIONS

- Individuals with PTSD may be at increased risk for panic disorder, agoraphobia, obsessive–compulsive disorder, social phobia, specific phobia, major depressive disorder, somatization disorder; and increased risk of impulsive behavior, suicide, and homicide. Victims of sexual assault are at especially high risk for developing mental health problems and committing suicide.
- Use of benzodiazepines can lead to abuse and dependence
- Avoidance of stimuli associated with the trauma can generalize to wide-ranging avoidance. This leads to a far greater negative impact on the patient's life.

REFERENCES

1. Segman RH, Cooper-Kazaz R, Macciardi F, et al. Association between the dopamine transporter gene and posttraumatic stress disorder. *Mol Psychiatry.* 2002;7:903–7.
2. Holbrook TL, Galarneau MR, Dye JL, et al. Morphine use after combat injury in Iraq and post-traumatic stress disorder. *N Engl J Med.* 2010;362:110–7.
3. Pitman RK, Sanders KM, Zusman RM, et al. Pilot study of secondary prevention of posttraumatic stress disorder with propranolol. *Biol Psychiatry.* 2002;51:189–92.
4. Rose S, Bisson J, Churchill R, et al. Psychological debriefing for preventing post traumatic stress disorder (PTSD). *Cochrane Database Syst Rev.* 2002;CD000560.
5. Mason JW, Giller EL, Kosten TR, et al. Elevation of urinary norepinephrine/cortisol ratio in posttraumatic stress disorder. *J Nerv Ment Dis.* 1988;176:498–502.
6. Yehuda R, Halligan SL, Golier JA, et al. Effects of trauma exposure on the cortisol response to dexamethasone administration in PTSD and major depressive disorder. *Psychoneuroendocrinology.* 2004;29:389–404.
7. Bajor LA, Ticlea AN, Osser DN, et al. The psychopharmacology algorithm project at the Harvard South shore program: An update on posttraumatic stress disorder. *Harv Rev Psychiatry.* 2011;19:240–58.
8. Shad MU, Suris AM, North CS, et al. Novel combination strategy to optimize treatment for PTSD. *Hum Psychopharmacol.* 2011 Feb 9. doi: 10.1002/hup.1171.
9. Raskind MA, Peskind ER, Hoff DJ, et al. A parallel group placebo controlled study of prazosin for trauma nightmares and sleep disturbance in combat veterans with post-traumatic stress disorder. *Biol Psychiatry.* 2007;61:928–34.
10. Pollack MH, Hoge EA, Worthington JJ, et al. Eszopiclone for the treatment of posttraumatic stress disorder and associated insomnia: A randomized, double-blind, placebo-controlled trial. *J Clin Psychiatry.* 2011;72:892–7.
11. Connor KM, Sutherland SM, Tupler LA, et al. Fluoxetine in post-traumatic stress disorder. Randomised, double-blind study. *Br J Psychiatry.* 1999;175:17–22.
12. Marshall RD, Pierce D, et al. Implications of recent findings in posttraumatic stress disorder and the role of pharmacotherapy. *Harv Rev Psychiatry.* 2000;7:247–56.
13. Stein DJ, Ipser JC, Seedat S, et al. Pharmacotherapy for post traumatic stress disorder (PTSD). *Cochrane Database Syst Rev.* 2006;CD002795.
14. Kornør H, Winje D, Ekeberg Ø, et al. Early trauma-focused cognitive-behavioural therapy to prevent chronic post-traumatic stress disorder and related symptoms: A systematic review and meta-analysis. *BMC Psychiatry.* 2008;8:81.
15. van der Kolk BA, Spinazzola J, Blaustein ME, et al. A randomized clinical trial of eye movement desensitization and reprocessing (EMDR), fluoxetine, and pill placebo in the treatment of posttraumatic stress disorder: Treatment effects and long-term maintenance. *J Clin Psychiatry.* 2007;68:37–46.

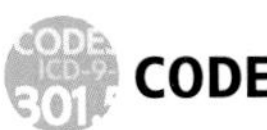

CODES

ICD9

309.81 Posttraumatic stress disorder

PREECLAMPSIA AND ECLAMPSIA (TOXEMIA OF PREGNANCY)

Konstantinos E. Deligiannidis, MD, MPH
Stacy E. Potts, MD

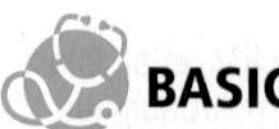

BASICS

DESCRIPTION

- Preeclampsia is a disorder of pregnancy developing at the 20th week (or beyond), with hypertension, proteinuria, and/or edema and poor perfusion of vital organs.
  - May progress from mild to life threatening in hours to days
  - The disease may include rapid weight gain and edema on the face and hands. The disorder is reversible by delivery if at term or, if maternal or fetal health are in danger, by preterm delivery.
  - Eclampsia is defined as seizure activity or coma in a patient with preeclampsia without underlying neurologic disease.
  - Most postpartum cases occur within 48 hours of delivery but can occur up to 4 weeks postpartum.
- System(s) affected: Cardiovascular; Renal; Reproductive; Feto-placental; Central Nervous System (CNS); hepatic
- Synonym(s): Toxemia of pregnancy

EPIDEMIOLOGY

Incidence

- Predominant age:
  - Most cases occur in younger women because of the higher incidence of preeclampsia in younger (nulliparous) women.
  - However, older (>40 years) preeclamptic patients have 4 times the incidence of seizures compared with patients in their 20s.
- Pregnancy-induced hypertension: 6% of pregnancies
- Preeclampsia: 5–7%
- Eclampsia develops in 1 in 2,000 deliveries in developed countries. In developing countries, estimates range from 1 in 100 to 1 in 1,700.
- 40% of eclamptic seizures occur before delivery; 16% occur more than 48 hours after delivery.

RISK FACTORS

- Nulliparity: 3:1 (relative risk [RR])
- Age >40 years: 2:1 (RR)
- High body mass index: 2:1 (RR)
- Antiphospholipid syndrome: 10:1 (RR)
- Diabetes: 3.5:1 (RR)
- Twin pregnancy: 3:1 (RR)
- Preeclampsia during a previous pregnancy
- Family history of preeclampsia: 3:1 (RR)
- Father of fetus previously experienced a preeclamptic pregnancy with another woman

Genetics

Increased incidence in pregnant women whose mothers or sisters had the disease

GENERAL PREVENTION

- Adequate prenatal care: Women who do not receive prenatal care are 7 times more likely to die from complications.
- Good control of pre-existing hypertension
- Recent systematic reviews and meta-analyses show that low-dose aspirin lowers the risk of developing preeclampsia in moderate- to high-risk patients, lowers the rate of preterm delivery and neonatal death, and has no significant effect on the rate of placental abruption or neonatal bleeding complications (1)[A].
- Calcium supplementation has been shown to reduce the risk of preeclampsia by 30%. The risk reduction seems to be greatest in women with a high risk of preeclampsia (RR = 0.22) (2)[A].
- Some evidence suggests vitamin C (1,000 mg/d) and vitamin E (400 units/d) reduce the risk for preeclampsia (3)[B], although some guidelines recommend against their use (4).

PATHOPHYSIOLOGY

Systemic derangements in eclampsia include:

- Cardiovascular: Generalized vasospasm
- Hematologic: Decreased plasma volume, increased blood viscosity, hemoconcentration, coagulopathy
- Renal: Decreased glomerular filtration rate
- Hepatic: Periportal necrosis, hepatocellular damage, subcapsular hematoma
- CNS: Cerebral vasospasm and ischemia, cerebral edema, cerebral hemorrhage

COMMONLY ASSOCIATED CONDITIONS

- Abruptio placenta
- Placental insufficiency
- Fetal growth restriction
- Preterm delivery
- Fetal demise
- Maternal seizures (eclampsia)
- Maternal pulmonary edema
- Maternal liver or kidney failure
- Maternal death

DIAGNOSIS

Diagnosis is dependent on new onset of elevated BP and proteinuria after 20 weeks of gestation.

HISTORY

May be asymptomatic. In some cases, rapid excessive weight gain (>5 lb/wk; >2.3 kg/wk); in more severe cases are associated with epigastric pain, headache, altered mental status, and visual disturbance.

PHYSICAL EXAM

- Preeclampsia:
  - Mild: Elevated BP ≥140 mm Hg systolic or 90 mm Hg diastolic on 2 BP readings 6 hours apart; proteinuria (>300 mg/24 hr or >1 g/L)
  - Severe: Elevated BP ≥160 systolic mm Hg or 110 mm Hg diastolic on 2 BP readings 6 hours apart
    - Proteinuria (>5 g/24 hr)
    - Facial or hand edema
    - Hyperreflexia
    - Retinal arteriolar spasm, papilledema
    - Epigastric/right upper quadrant (RUQ) pain
    - Oliguria or anuria
- Eclampsia:
  - Headache, visual disturbance, and epigastric or RUQ pain often precede seizure.
  - Tonic–clonic seizure activity (focal or generalized)
  - Seizures may occur once or repeatedly.
  - Postictal coma, cyanosis (variable)
  - Temperatures >39°C, consistent with CNS hemorrhage
  - Normal BP, even in response to treatment, does not rule out potential for seizures. Up to 30% may not have edema; 20% may not have proteinuria.

DIAGNOSTIC TESTS & INTERPRETATION

Lab

Initial lab tests

- Routine spot urine testing for protein should be done at each prenatal visit.
- CBC, including platelets
- Creatinine
- Serum transaminase levels
- Uric acid
- Coagulation profiles: Abnormalities suggest severe disease.
- 24-hour urine for protein/creatinine clearance: <90 mL/min/1.73 m^2 is abnormal.

Follow-Up & Special Considerations

Disseminated intravascular coagulation, thrombocytopenia, liver dysfunction, and renal failure can complicate preeclampsia associated with HELLP syndrome.

Imaging

- Daily fetal movement monitoring by mother ("kick counts")
- Nonstress test (NST) at diagnosis and then weekly until delivery
- Ultrasound is used to monitor growth and cord blood flow; perform as indicated based on clinical stability and laboratory findings.
- Ultrasound imaging for biophysical profile, estimation of fetal age, growth progress, amniotic fluid volume
  - Weekly for mild preeclampsia
  - Twice weekly in severe preeclampsia
- With seizures, CT scan and MRI should be considered if focal findings persist or uncharacteristic signs/symptoms are present.

Pathological Findings

CNS: Cerebral edema, hyperemia, focal anemia, thrombosis, and hemorrhage:

- Cerebral lesions account for 40% of eclamptic deaths.

DIFFERENTIAL DIAGNOSIS

- Chronic hypertension (HTN): HTN before pregnancy; high BP (HTN) before the 20th week; diagnosis during pregnancy but persisting beyond postpartum day 84
- Gestational HTN: Increased BP first discovered during pregnancy, with no proteinuria; normal BP by 12 weeks postpartum
- Seizures in pregnancy: Epilepsy, cerebral tumors, meningitis/encephalitis, ruptured cerebral aneurysm. Until other causes are proven, however, all pregnant women with convulsions should be considered to have eclampsia.

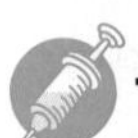

TREATMENT

- Mild:
  - Outpatient care
  - Maternal: Daily home BP monitoring; daily weights; weekly labs (24-hour protein, platelet count, creatinine, liver function tests [LFTs])
  - Fetal:
    - Patient-measured: Daily "kick counts"
    - Medical provider-measured: NST (see "Imaging" section)

- Severe:
  - Inpatient care if patient condition deteriorates (BP ≥160/110 mm Hg; severe headache; visual changes [scotoma or "flashing lights"]; impaired mentation; pulmonary edema; epigastric/RUQ pain; increasing LFTs; oliguria; thrombocytopenia) or if fetal status is deemed "nonreassuring"
  - Maternal: Daily labs, adding coagulation tests; IV magnesium sulfate as anticonvulsive prophylaxis; IV labetalol and oral nifedipine antihypertensive therapy titrated to keep systolic BP <155 mm Hg and diastolic BP <105 mm Hg. Keep diastolic BP >90 mm Hg to avoid hypoperfusing the uterus.
  - Fetal: Continuous heart monitoring; daily ultrasound with BP, amniotic fluid levels, fetal growth assessment as deemed necessary

ADDITIONAL TREATMENT

General Measures

- Management by gestational age of severe preeclampsia:
  - <23 weeks: Offer to terminate pregnancy.
  - At 23–32 weeks: Antihypertensives; evaluate maternal–fetal condition; steroids to enhance fetal lung maturity; plan delivery at 34 weeks with magnesium sulfate prophylaxis or for worsening maternal or fetal jeopardy.
  - At 33–34 weeks: Steroids, magnesium sulfate, and delivery
  - At >34 weeks: Magnesium sulfate and delivery

ALERT

- Regardless of gestational age, emergent delivery is recommended if there are signs of maternal hypertensive crisis, abruptio placentae, uterine rupture, or fetal distress (5)[B].
- Seizures:
  - Control of convulsions, correction of hypoxia and acidosis, lowering of BP, steps to effect delivery as soon as convulsions are controlled
  - See "Medication" section

MEDICATION

First Line

- For seizure prophylaxis: Magnesium sulfate (MgSO4): Loading dose 4 g IV in 200 mL normal saline over 20–30 minutes; maintenance dose 1–2 g/hr IV
- For HTN:
  - Nifedipine (PO): 40–120 mg/d *plus*
  - Labetalol (IV): 600–2,400 mg/d, both titrated to keep BP <155/105 mm Hg; antihypertensives are inadvisable for mild hypertension/preeclampsia.
- For eclampsia/seizures:
  - In recent randomized trials, $MgSO_4$ was found to be superior to phenytoin in the treatment and prevention of eclampsia and probably more effective and safer than diazepam.
  - Magnesium sulfate for seizures:
    - 2–4 g IV repeated q15min to a maximum of 6 g to achieve resolution of an ongoing convulsion
    - Magnesium then is continued at 1–3 g/hr, with the amount given based on the neurologic examination and patellar reflexes.
  - Levels of 6–8 mEq/mL are considered therapeutic, but clinical status is most important and must ensure that:
    - Patellar reflexes are present.
    - Respirations are not depressed.
    - Urine output is ≥25 mL/hr.
  - May be given safely, even in the presence of renal insufficiency
- Fluid therapy:
  - Ringer lactated solution with 5% dextrose at 60–120 mL/hr, with careful attention to fluid–volume status
- Hypertension, if present and severe (e.g., >160/110 mm Hg), also should be treated.
  - Hydralazine: 5 mg IV then 5–10-mg boluses as needed q20min *or*
  - Labetalol: 10–20 mg IV then double dose at 10-minute intervals up to 80 mg; maximum total cumulative dose of 220–230 mg (e.g., 20-40-80-80 or 10-20-40-80-80)
- Precautions: Do not use diuretics. Carefully monitor neurologic status, urine output, respirations, and fetal status.
- Calcium carbonate (1 g, administered slowly IV) may reverse magnesium-induced respiratory depression.

Second Line

- Diazepam 2 mg/min until resolution or 20 mg given *or*
- Lorazepam 1–2 mg/min up to total of 10 mg *or*
- Phenytoin 18–20 mg/kg at a rate of 20–40 mg/min *or*
- Phenobarbital 100 mg/min to a total of 20 mg/kg given

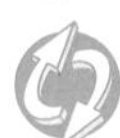

ONGOING CARE

FOLLOW-UP RECOMMENDATIONS

- Mild: Restricted activity
- Severe: Restricted activity, in hospital

DIET

- Salt restriction is inadvisable because the patient often is experiencing intravascular hypovolemia.
- Calcium supplementation is recommended for women who have low calcium intake (<600 mg/d) (4).

PATIENT EDUCATION

American College of Obstetricians and Gynecologists, 409 12th St. SW, Washington, DC 20024-2188; (800) 762-ACOG; www.acog.org

PROGNOSIS

- For nulliparous women with preeclampsia before 30 weeks of gestation, the recurrence rate for the disorder may be as high as 40% in future pregnancies (6).
- Multiparous women have higher rates of recurrence.
- 25% of eclamptic women will have hypertension during subsequent pregnancies, but only 5% of these will be severe and only 2% will be eclamptic again.
- Eclamptic, multiparous women may be at higher risk for subsequent essential hypertension; they also have higher mortality during subsequent pregnancies than do primiparous women.

COMPLICATIONS

- Most women do not have long-term sequelae from eclampsia, although many may have transient neurologic deficits.
- A history of preeclampsia is equivalent to traditional risk factors for cardiovascular disease. Women with a history of preeclampsia should be strongly advised to avoid obesity and smoking. Other signs of metabolic syndrome should be closely monitored, as well (7).
- Maternal and/or fetal death

REFERENCES

1. Gauer R, Atlas M, Hill J. Clinical inquiries. Does low-dose aspirin reduce preeclampsia and other maternal-fetal complications? *J Fam Pract*. 2008;57:54–6.
2. Hofmeyr GJ, Duley L, Atallah A, et al. Dietary calcium supplementation for prevention of pre-eclampsia and related problems: A systematic review and commentary. *BJOG*. 2007;114:933–43.
3. Rumbold A, Duley L, Crowther CA, et al. Antioxidants for preventing pre-eclampsia. *Cochrane Database Syst Rev*. 2008;CD004227.
4. Magee LA, Helewa M, Moutquin J-M, et al. Diagnosis, evaluation, and management of the hypertensive disorders of pregnancy. *JOGC*. 2008;30:3(S1–S48).
5. Sibai BM. Diagnosis and management of gestational hypertension and preeclampsia. *Obstet Gynecol*. 2003;102:181–92.
6. Report of the National High Blood Pressure Education Program Working Group on High Blood Pressure in Pregnancy. *Am J Obste Gynecol* 2000;183:S1–22.
7. Carty DM, Delles C, Dominiczak AF, et al. Preeclampsia and future maternal health. *J Hypertens*. 2010;28:1349–55.

ADDITIONAL READING

Churchill D, Duley L, et al. Interventionist versus expectant care for severe pre-eclampsia before term. *Cochrane Database Syst Rev*. 2002;CD003106.

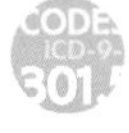

CODES

ICD9

- 642.40 Mild or unspecified preeclampsia, unspecified as to episode of care or not applicable
- 642.43 Mild or unspecified preeclampsia, antepartum condition or complication
- 642.53 Severe preeclampsia, antepartum condition or complication

CLINICAL PEARLS

- Prescribe 81 mg aspirin each day to 2 groups of pregnant women: Those who had severe preeclampsia in a prior pregnancy and those who develop signs of preeclampsia or strong risk factors for it before the third trimester in their current pregnancy.
- Management of preeclampsia depends on both the severity of the condition and the gestational age of the fetus.
- The disorder is reversible by delivery if at term or, if maternal or fetal health are in danger, by preterm delivery.

PREMENSTRUAL SYNDROME (PMS) AND PREMENSTRUAL DYSPHORIC DISORDER (PMDD)

Courtney I. Jarvis, PharmD
Jeremy Golding, MD

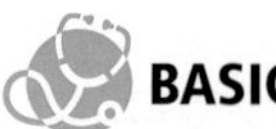

BASICS

DESCRIPTION

- Premenstrual syndrome (PMS) is defined as a symptom complex of physical and emotional symptoms severe enough to interfere with everyday life and occurring cyclically during the luteal phase of menses.
- Premenstrual dysphoric disorder (PMDD) is a severe form of PMS characterized by severe recurrent depressive and anxiety symptoms with premenstrual (luteal phase) onset that remit a few days after the start of menses.
- The American Psychiatric Association's *DSM-IV* revised diagnosis is PMDD when the dominant symptoms are emotional and severe enough to disrupt social and occupational functioning.
- System(s) affected: Endocrine/Metabolic; Nervous; Reproductive

EPIDEMIOLOGY

Prevalence

- Almost all women have some physical and psychic symptoms before menses (this is not premenstrual syndrome).
- ~30% of menstruating women suffer from PMS.
- ~5% of menstruating women have PMDD.

RISK FACTORS

- Age: Usually present in late 20s–mid-30s
- History of mood disorder (major depression, bipolar disorder), anxiety disorder, personality disorder, or substance abuse
- Family history
- Low parity
- Tobacco use
- Psychosocial stressors
- High body mass index (BMI)

Genetics

- Role of genetic predisposition is controversial; however, twin studies do suggest a genetic component.
- Involvement of gene coding for the serotonergic 5HT1A receptor and allelic variants of the estrogen receptor alpha gene (ESR1) is suggested.

PATHOPHYSIOLOGY

- Results from interaction of cyclic changes in ovarian steroids (estrogen, progesterone, allopregnanolone) with central neurotransmitters (serotonin, γ-endorphin, γ-aminobutyric acid [GABA]) and the autonomic nervous system
- Circadian rhythm alterations affecting secretion of melatonin, cortisol, thyroid-stimulating hormone (TSH), and prolactin reported
- Inconclusive evidence regarding low levels of vitamin D, magnesium, and calcium in women with PMDD

DIAGNOSIS

HISTORY

- Determine regularity of the menstrual cycle using prospective patient record of symptoms for 2 months, the Daily Record of Severity of Problems (available online at www.pmdd.factsforhealth.org/drsp/drsp_month.pdf), or similar inventory.
- *DSM-IV* criteria:
  - Symptoms occur 1 week before menses and resolve in the first few days after menses begin (over most menstrual cycles during the past year).
  - $\geq$5 of the following (1 must be among the first 4):
    - Markedly depressed mood with feelings of hopelessness
    - Marked anxiety or tension
    - Marked affective lability
    - Irritability and anger
    - Decreased interest in usual activities and social withdrawal
    - Lack of energy
    - Appetite change
    - Change in sleeping pattern
    - Feeling out of control or overwhelmed
    - Difficulty concentrating
    - Somatic symptoms such as abdominal bloating, breast tenderness, headaches, and joint pain
  - For PMDD, emotional symptoms must be severe enough to interfere with work, school, or usual activities.
  - Symptoms may be superimposed on an underlying psychiatric disorder but may not be an exacerbation of another condition.
  - Criteria must be confirmed by prospective daily charting for a minimum of 2 consecutive symptomatic menstrual cycles.

PHYSICAL EXAM

- Physiologic symptoms:
  - Food cravings
  - Weight gain
  - Fatigue
  - Headache
  - Sleep disturbance
  - Tension/muscle aches
  - Mastalgia/breast swelling
  - Abdominal bloating/pain
  - Edema
- Emotional symptoms:
  - Anger
  - Irritability/mood lability
  - Internal tension
  - Depressed mood
  - Anxiety
  - Insomnia

DIAGNOSTIC TESTS & INTERPRETATION

Lab

- The repetitive nature of symptoms precludes need for labs if a classic history is present.
- Hemoglobin may be helpful to rule out anemia.
- 25-OH vitamin D level to exclude deficiency, although precise relationship of deficiency with the disorder is unclear.
- Serum thyroid stimulating hormone (TSH) to rule out hypothyroidism

Imaging

Imaging to diagnose causes of pelvic pain and dysmenorrhea may be needed.

DIFFERENTIAL DIAGNOSIS

- Premenstrual exacerbation of underlying psychiatric disorder
- Psychiatric disorders (especially bipolar disorder, major depression, anxiety)
- Thyroid disorders
- Perimenopause
- Premenstrual migraine
- Chronic fatigue syndrome
- Irritable bowel syndrome (painful symptoms)
- Seizures
- Anemia
- Endometriosis (painful symptoms)
- Drug or alcohol abuse

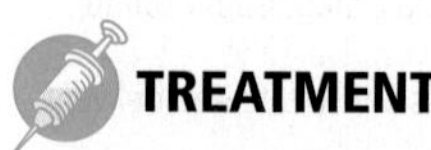

TREATMENT

- SSRIs (fluoxetine and sertraline most studied) are highly effective in the treatment of physical and behavioral symptoms of PMDD (odds ratio [OR] 0.40, 95% confidence interval [CI] 0.31–0.51) (1,2,3,4)[A]:
  - Intermittent luteal phase dosing (OR 0.55, 95% CI 0.45–0.68) is less effective than full-cycle dosing (OR 0.28, 95% CI 0.18–0.42) but has fewer adverse effects (4)[A].
  - Higher doses are not correlated with increased response (1,4)[A].
  - Other nonselective serotonergic agents (e.g., venlafaxine, clomipramine) also may be effective (3)[C].
- Alternative therapies should be considered if no response to SSRIs: Alprazolam, buspirone, gonadotropin-releasing hormone (GnRH) agonists, danazol, bromocriptine, spironolactone, oral contraceptives, meclofenamate, progesterone (2,3)[C]
- Oral contraceptive pills (OCPs) may improve physical symptoms but not mood (2,3)[C]:
  - OCPs can cause adverse effects similar to PMDD symptoms; monophasic preparations should be used continuously (daily without interruption) for PMDD (3)[C].
  - OCPs containing the progestin drospirenone (structurally similar to spironolactone) may improve physical symptoms and mood changes associated with PMDD (2,5)[A].
- Vitamin D supplementation, 2,000 IU/d, with no risk of toxicity (3)[C]
- Calcium carbonate 600 mg b.i.d. effectively reduces physical and emotional premenstrual symptoms (6)[B].
- Vitamin B_6 may reduce the severity of premenstrual symptoms (6)[B].

- Chasteberry (*Vitex agnus-castus*) may reduce physical premenstrual symptoms (6)[C].
- Cognitive-behavioral therapy (CBT) is as effective as drug therapy, but there is no additional benefit of combining CBT and drug therapy (2)[B].

MEDICATION

First Line

- Fluoxetine (Prozac, Sarafem) 20 mg/d every day, or 20 mg/d only during luteal phase, or 90 mg once a week × 2 weeks in luteal phase
- Sertraline (Zoloft) 50–150 mg/d every day or 50–150 mg/d only during luteal phase
- Citalopram (Celexa) 10–30 mg/d every day or 10–30 mg/d only during luteal phase
- Adverse effects:
  - GI upset
  - Jitteriness
  - Headache
  - Sexual dysfunction
  - Insomnia
  - Fatigue
- Contraindications: Patients taking monoamine oxidase inhibitors (MAOIs)
- Precautions:
  - Increased risk of suicidal thinking and behavior in children and adolescents with depressive disorders; uncertain if this risk applies to those taking SSRIs for PMDD
  - Bipolar disorder
  - Seizure disorder
  - Hepatic dysfunction
  - Renal dysfunction
- Possible interactions:
  - MAOIs (e.g., phenelzine, isocarbazine, tranylcypromine, linezolid)
  - Selegiline
  - Pimozide
  - Thioridazine

Second Line

- Spironolactone (Aldactone) 50–100 mg/d × 7–10 days during luteal phase; helpful for fluid retention. Adverse reactions: Lethargy, headache, irregular menses, hyperkalemia
- Oral contraceptives: Ethinyl estradiol/drospirenone (Yasmin/Yaz/Beyaz/Satyral): 1 tablet/d (Caution: Risk of venous thromboembolism may be higher than with other OCPs); although unstudied, other OCPs also may be effective.
- Alprazolam (Xanax) 0.25 mg t.i.d.–q.i.d. only during luteal phase; taper at onset of menses (other benzodiazepines not studied for PMDD). Caution: Addictive potential
- GnRH agonists:
  - Leuprolide (Lupron) depot 3.75 mg/mo IM
  - Precautions: Menopauselike side effects (e.g., osteoporosis, hot flashes, headaches, muscle aches, vaginal dryness, irritability) limit treatment to 6 months; if extended treatment is needed, supplement with estrogen and progesterone add-back therapy, minimizing frequency and dose of progestational agent.
- Danazol (Danocrine), 300–400 mg b.i.d.; adverse reactions: Androgenic and antiestrogenic effects (e.g., amenorrhea, weight gain, acne, fluid retention, hirsutism, hot flashes, vaginal dryness, emotional lability)

ADDITIONAL TREATMENT

Issues for Referral

Referral to psychiatrist may be indicated for mood or anxiety disorder if patient has no symptom-free period.

COMPLEMENTARY AND ALTERNATIVE MEDICINE

- Some data support the use of the following:
  - Calcium: 600 mg b.i.d.
  - Vitamin D: 2,000 IU/d
  - Vitamin B_6: 100 mg/d (usually 50 mg b.i.d.)
  - Magnesium: 200–400 mg/d
  - Vitamin E: 400 IU/d
  - Manganese: 1.8 mg/d
  - Chasteberry (*Vitex agnus-castus*): 4 mg/d of extract
  - St. John's wort: 900 mg/d (0.18% hypericin, 23.38% hyperforin)
- Evidence supporting efficacy and/or safety of herbal products is lacking; the following products/interventions have *not* been found useful for PMS/PMDD, although not all studies are of high quality and able to completely eliminate possibility of benefit:
  - Evening primrose oil
  - Black current oil
  - Black cohosh
  - Wild yam root
  - Dong quai
  - Kava kava
  - Light-based therapy
  - Acupuncture

SURGERY/OTHER PROCEDURES

Bilateral oophorectomy, usually with concomitant hysterectomy, is option for rare, refractory cases with severe, disabling symptoms.

ONGOING CARE

FOLLOW-UP RECOMMENDATIONS

Aerobic exercise is helpful in decreasing premenstrual symptoms (7)[C].

Patient Monitoring

Increased risk of suicidal thinking and behavior in children and adolescents with depressive disorders; uncertain if this risk applies to those taking SSRIs for PMDD

DIET

- Reduce consumption of salt, sugar, caffeine, dairy products, and alcohol (anecdotal reports).
- Eat small, frequent portions of food high in complex carbohydrates (limited data).

PATIENT EDUCATION

- Counsel patients to eat a balanced diet rich in calcium and omega-3 fatty acids and low in saturated fat and caffeine.
- Advise aerobic exercise.
- Counsel women that they are not "crazy." PMDD is a real disorder with a physiologic basis.
- Although incompletely understood, successful treatment is usually possible.

PROGNOSIS

- Many patients can have their symptoms adequately controlled. PMS disappears at menopause.
- PMS sometimes continues after hysterectomy.

REFERENCES

1. Brown J, O'Brien PM, Marjoribanks J, et al. Selective serotonin reuptake inhibitors for premenstrual syndrome. *Cochrane Database Syst Rev.* 2009: CD001396.
2. Cunningham J, Yonkers KA, O'Brien S, et al. Update on research and treatment of premenstrual dysphoric disorder. *Harv Rev Psychiatry.* 2009;17: 120–37.
3. Pearlstein T, Steiner M. Premenstrual dysphoric disorder: Burden of illness and treatment update. *J Psychiatry Neurosci.* 2008;33:291–301.
4. Shah NR, Jones JB, Aperi J, et al. Selective serotonin reuptake inhibitors for premenstrual syndrome and premenstrual dysphoric disorder: A meta-analysis. *Obstet Gynecol.* 2008;111:1175–82.
5. Lopez LM, Kaptein A, Helmerhorst FM. Oral contraceptives containing drospirenone for premenstrual syndrome. *Cochrane Database Syst Rev.* 2009:CD006586.
6. Whelan AM, Jurgens TM, Naylor H, et al. Herbs, vitamins and minerals in the treatment of premenstrual syndrome: A systematic review. *Can J Clin Pharmacol.* 2009;16:e407–29.
7. The American College of Obstetricians and Gynecologists. Practice Bulletin. Management of premenstrual syndrome. *Clinical Management Guidelines.* No. 15. April 2000.

ADDITIONAL READING

- Freeman EW. Therapeutic management of premenstrual syndrome. *Expert Opin Pharmacother.* 2010;11(17):2879–89.
- Thys-Jacobs S, McMahon D, Bilezikian JP. Cyclical changes in calcium metabolism across the menstrual cycle in women with premenstrual dysphoric disorder. *J Clin Endocrinol Metab.* 2007;92:2952–9.

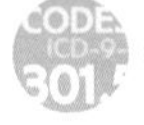

CODES

ICD9

625.4 Premenstrual tension syndromes

CLINICAL PEARLS

- Have the patient keep a daily log of her symptoms and menses. Symptoms beginning in the week before menses and abating before the end of menses, occurring over at least 2 months, and severe enough to interfere with daily functioning are diagnostic of PMS.
- The difference between PMS and PMDD is that PMDD is a severe form of PMS characterized by recurrent depressive and anxiety symptoms with premenstrual (luteal phase) onset, severe enough to disrupt social and occupational functioning. These symptoms remit a few days after the onset of menses.
- PMDD is not the same as more generalized depressive or anxiety disorders. PMDD-associated symptoms of depression and anxiety resolve within the first few days of menses.
- Treatment during the luteal phase only is somewhat less effective than continuous-cycle treatment with SSRIs but has fewer adverse effects.

PREOPERATIVE EVALUATION OF THE NONCARDIAC SURGICAL PATIENT

Drew Grimes, MD
Stacy Jones, MD

 BASICS

DESCRIPTION

- Preoperative medical evaluation should determine the presence of established or unrecognized disease or other factors that may increase the risk of perioperative morbidity and mortality in patients undergoing surgery.
- Specific assessment goals include:
  - Conducting a thorough medical history and physical examination to assess the need for further testing and/or consultation
  - Recommending strategies to reduce risk and optimize patient condition prior to surgery
  - Encouraging patients to optimize their health for possible improvement of both perioperative and long-term outcomes
- Synonym(s): Preoperative diagnostic workup; Preoperative preparation; Preoperative general health assessment

EPIDEMIOLOGY

Overall patient morbidity and mortality related to surgery is low. Multiple studies have shown an average mortality rate of ~1% for patients undergoing a full spectrum of surgical procedures. Preoperative patient evaluation and subsequent optimization of perioperative care can reduce both postoperative morbidity and mortality.

RISK FACTORS

- Functional capacity (1)[B]: Exercise tolerance is one of the most important determinants of cardiac risk:
  - Self-reported exercise tolerance may be an extremely useful predictive tool when assessing risk. Patients unable to meet a 4 metabolic equivalent (MET) demand (defined in the Diagnosis section) during daily activities have increased perioperative cardiac and long-term risks.
  - Patients who report good exercise tolerance require minimal, if any, additional testing.
- Levels of surgical risk:
  - High: Aortic, major vascular, and peripheral vascular surgery
  - Intermediate: Intraperitoneal, intrathoracic, carotid endarterectomy, head/neck, orthopedic, and prostate surgery
  - Low: Endoscopic, superficial, cataract, breast, and ambulatory surgery
- Clinical risk factors (2)[B]: History of ischemic heart disease, the presence of compensated heart failure or a history of prior congestive heart failure (CHF), cerebrovascular disease, diabetes mellitus (DM), and renal insufficiency; these risk factors plus surgical risk can dictate the need for further cardiac testing.
- Age: Patients >70 years of age are at higher risk for perioperative complications and mortality and have a longer length of stay in the hospital postoperatively. (Likely attributed to increasing medical comorbidities with increasing age.) Age alone should not be a deciding factor in the decision to proceed with surgery (3).

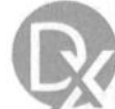 DIAGNOSIS

HISTORY

- Evaluate pertinent medical records and interview the patient. Many institutions provide standard patient questionnaires that screen for preoperative risk factors:
  - History of present illness and treatments
  - Past medical and surgical history
  - Patient and family anesthetic history and associated complications
  - Current medications (including over-the-counter [OTC] medications, vitamins, supplements, and herbals) as well as reasons for use
  - Allergies (including specific reactions)
  - Social history: Tobacco, alcohol, drug use, and cessation
  - Family history: Prior illnesses and surgeries
- Systems (both history and current status):
  - Cardiovascular: Inquire about exercise capacity:
    - 1 MET: Can take care of self, eat, dress, and use toilet; walk around house indoors; walk a block or 2 on level ground at 2–3 mi/hr
    - 4 METs: Can climb flight of stairs or walk up hill, walk on level ground at 4 mi/hr, run a short distance, do heavy work around house, participate in moderate recreational activities
    - 10 METs: Can participate in strenuous sports such as swimming, singles tennis, football, basketball, or skiing
  - Note presence of CHF, cardiomyopathy, ischemic heart disease (stable vs unstable), valvular disease, hypertension (HTN), arrhythmias, murmurs, pericarditis, history of pacemaker or implantable cardioverter defibrillator (ICD):
    - Rhythm management devices (pacemakers and automatic ICDs [AICD]) affect the perioperative course. Most importantly, patients need to know their type of device and bring that information with them for the procedure. Typically, the AICD tachyarrhythmia function is disabled during surgery and then restored postoperatively. Ideally, the device is interrogated postoperatively to confirm proper function (4).
    - Stents: Patients with coronary stents are maintained on antiplatelet therapy with a thienopyridine such as clopidogrel, frequently in combination with aspirin. Premature discontinuation of antiplatelet therapy markedly increases the risk of acute stent thrombosis, the results of which can be catastrophic. Elective surgery should be delayed and antiplatelet therapy continued for 4–6 weeks after bare metal stent placement, and for at least 12 months after placement of drug-eluting stents. Even after this time period, any perioperative disruption in the patient's antiplatelet regimen should be discussed with the patient's cardiologist and surgeon. The risk of perioperative bleeding must be weighed against the risks associated with discontinuation of antiplatelet drugs prior to surgery (5)[B].
  - Pulmonary: Chronic and active disease processes should be addressed: Chronic infections, bronchitis, emphysema, asthma, wheezing, shortness of breath, cough (productive or otherwise):
    - Sleep apnea: Patients with obstructive sleep apnea (OSA) are at increased risk for perioperative adverse events. It follows that preoperative diagnosis of OSA and institution of continuous positive airway pressure (CPAP) therapy should reduce that risk. Unfortunately, at present, the evidence is not clear on this point.
    - Patients with OSA frequently are at increased risk for obesity, coronary disease, HTN, atrial fibrillation, CHF, and pulmonary hypertension. Optimizing the management of these comorbidities may be the first important step in the preoperative management of patients with OSA. Often, patients with an existing diagnosis of OSA who use CPAP at night are asked to bring their CPAP machine to the hospital or surgery center when they are admitted for surgery (6)[C].
  - GI: Hepatic disease, gastric ulcer, inflammatory bowel disease, hernias (especially hiatal), significant weight loss, nausea, vomiting, history of postoperative nausea and vomiting:
    - Any symptoms consistent with gastroesophageal reflux disease (GERD) should be optimally treated.
  - Hematologic: Anemia, serious bleeding, clotting problems, blood transfusions, hereditary disorders
  - Renal: Kidney failure, dialysis, infections, stones, changes in bladder function
  - Endocrine: Nocturia, parathyroid, pituitary, adrenal disease, thyroid disease:
    - Diabetes: There is evidence that hyperglycemia in the perioperative period is associated with increased perioperative complications. Although recommendations vary, most experts recommend keeping perioperative blood glucose levels below 180 (7)[B].
  - Neurologic/psychiatric: Seizures, stroke, paralysis, tremor, migraine headaches, nerve injury, multiple sclerosis, extremity numbness, psychiatric disorders (anxiety, depression, etc.)
  - Musculoskeletal: Arthritis, lower back pain
  - Reproductive: Possibility of pregnancy in women of child-bearing potential
- Mouth/upper airway: Dentures, crowns, partials, bridges, teeth (loose, chipped, cracked, capped)

PHYSICAL EXAM

- Assess vital signs, including arterial BP bilaterally.
- Check carotid pulses; auscultate for bruits.
- Examine lungs by auscultating all lung fields, listening for rales, rhonchi, wheezes, or other sounds indicating disease.
- Examine cardiovascular system by auscultating heart and noting any irregular rhythms or murmurs. Precordial palpation.
- Palpate abdomen.
- Examine airway and mouth for ease of intubation, neck mobility, and size of tongue, and note any lesions or dental deformities.

- If a regional anesthesia technique is being contemplated, perform a relevant, focused neurologic exam.

DIAGNOSTIC TESTS & INTERPRETATION

Lab

Initial lab tests

- Laboratory testing should not be obtained routinely prior to surgery unless indicated (2)[C]. Specific tests should be requested if the evaluator suspects findings from the clinical evaluation that may influence perioperative patient management.
- Labs performed within the past 4 months prior to evaluation are reliable unless the patient has had an interim change in clinical presentation or is taking medications that require monitoring of plasma level or effect.
- CBC (2)[C]:
  - Hemoglobin: If patient has symptoms of anemia or is undergoing a procedure with major blood loss; extremes of age; liver or kidney disease
  - WBC count: If symptoms suggest infection or myeloproliferative disorder or the patient is at risk for chemotherapy-induced leukopenia
  - Platelet count: If history of bleeding, myeloproliferative disorder, liver or renal disease, or the patient is at risk for chemotherapy-induced thrombocytopenia
- Serum chemistries (electrolytes, glucose, renal and liver function tests) (2)[C]: Should be obtained for extremes of age; in known renal insufficiency, CHF, liver dysfunction, or endocrine abnormalities, or the patient is on medications that alter electrolyte levels, such as diuretics
- Prothrombin time (PT)/partial thromboplastin time (PTT) (2)[C]: If history of a bleeding disorder, chronic liver disease, or malnutrition, or those with recent or chronic antibiotic or anticoagulant use
- Urinalysis (2)[C]: Routine urinalysis is not recommended preoperatively.
- Pregnancy test: Controversial; should be *considered* for all female patients of child-bearing age

Imaging

Initial approach

Chest x-ray (CXR) is not generally indicated (2)[C]. It can be considered in patients with recent upper respiratory tract infection and in those with suspected cardiac or pulmonary disease (because there is a likelihood for unanticipated findings), but these indications are not considered unequivocal.

Diagnostic Procedures/Surgery

- ECG (2)[C]: There are various recommendations reported in the literature:
  - American Heart Association (AHA)/American College of Cardiology (ACC) recommends that a preoperative ECG be obtained for patients who are to undergo vascular surgery and have at least 1 clinical risk factor, and for patients undergoing intermediate-risk procedures who have a history of CHF, peripheral vascular disease (PVD), or cerebrovascular disease.
  - ECGs are reasonable in vascular surgery patients with no risk factors and patients having intermediate-risk procedures who have 1 clinical risk factor.
  - ECGs are not indicated for asymptomatic patients undergoing low-risk procedures (1).
- Further cardiac testing should be considered in patients with poor or unknown functional capacity and 3+ clinical risk factors if the surgery is high risk and testing will change management (e.g., dipyridamole-thallium scan).
- Pulmonary function tests: Definitive data regarding the efficacy of preoperative testing is lacking. The most important factor is preoperative optimization of patients with chronic obstructive pulmonary disease (COPD) or reactive airways disease with indicated use of antibiotics, bronchodilators, and inhaled corticosteroids. Spirometry can help guide therapy. Upper abdominal and thoracic surgery have a higher risk of postoperative pulmonary complications.

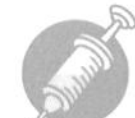

TREATMENT

MEDICATION

- Reducing cardiac risk:
  - Elective surgery should be delayed or canceled if the patient has any of the following: Unstable coronary syndromes (unstable or severe angina), recent myocardial infarction (MI) (<30 days), decompensated heart failure, significant arrhythmias, or severe valvular disease.
  - Active CHF should be treated with diuretics, afterload reduction, and β-adrenergic blockers.
  - Perioperative β-blockade has been shown to reduce mortality and the incidence of perioperative MIs in high-risk patients. Studies conflict, however, in what patients need to be treated, the dosage and timing of treatment, and for what surgeries. *Patients chronically on B-blockers need to have them continued in the perioperative period.* When B-blockers are discontinued in the perioperative period, 30-day mortality increases. B-blockers are reasonable for vascular surgery patients with at least 1 clinical risk factor (1)[C].
  - Perioperative statin use may have a protective effect on reducing cardiac complications. Currently the AHA has a class 1 indication for perioperative statin therapy for patients already on statins prior to their surgery. There is also evidence that vascular surgery patients benefit from perioperative statins (8).
- Reducing pulmonary risk:
  - Recommend *cigarette cessation* for at least *8 weeks prior to elective surgery*
  - Patients with asthma should not be wheezing and should have a peak flow of at least 80% of their predicted or personal-best value.
  - Treatment of COPD and asthma should focus on maximally reducing airflow obstruction and is identical to treatment of nonsurgical patients.
  - Lower respiratory tract infections (bacterial) should be treated with appropriate antibiotic therapy.

REFERENCES

1. American College of Cardiology Foundation/American Heart Association Task Force on Practice Guidelines, American Society of Echocardiography, American Society of Nuclear Cardiology, Heart Rhythm Society, et al. 2009 ACCF/AHA focused update on perioperative beta blockade. *J Am Coll Cardiol*. 2009;54:2102–28.
2. American Society of Anesthesiologists Task Force on Preanesthesia Evaluation. Practice advisory for preanesthesia evaluation: A report by the American Society of Anesthesiologists Task Force on Preanesthesia Evaluation. *Anesthesiology*. 2002; 96:485–96.
3. Carrillo PM, et al. Perioperative risk evaluation. *Internet J Anesthesiol*. 2004;8(2).
4. American Society of Anesthesiologists, et al. Practice advisory for the perioperative management of patients with cardiac implantable electronic devices: Pacemakers and implantable cardioverter-defibrillators: An updated report by the American Society of Anesthesiologists Task Force on Perioperative Management of Patients with Cardiac Implantable Electronic Devices. *Anesthesiology*. 2011;114:247–61.
5. Mauermann WJ, et al. Percutaneous coronary interventions and antiplatelet therapy in the perioperative period. *J Cardiothorac Vasc Anesth*. 2007;21(3):436–42.
6. Chung SA, Yuan H, Chung F. A Systematic review of obstructive sleep apnea and its implications for anesthesiologists. *Anesth Analg* 2008; 107(5):1543.
7. Akhtar S, Barash PG, Inzucchi SE et al. Scientific principles and clinical implications of perioperative glucose regulation and control. *Anesth Analg*. 2010;110:478–97.
8. Lander JS, Coplan NL, et al. Statin therapy in the perioperative period. *Rev Cardiovasc Med*. 2011; 12:30–7.

ADDITIONAL READING

- Menke H, Klein A, John KD, et al. Predictive value of ASA classification for the assessment of the perioperative risk. *Int Surg*. 1993;78:266–70.
- Polanczyk CA, Marcantonio E, Goldman L, et al. Impact of age on perioperative complications and length of stay in patients undergoing noncardiac surgery. *Ann Intern Med*. 2001;134:637–43.
- Reilly DF, McNeely MJ, Doerner D, et al. Self-reported exercise tolerance and the risk of serious perioperative complications. *Arch Intern Med*. 1999;159:2185–92.

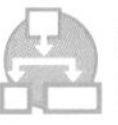

See Also (Topic, Algorithm, Electronic Media Element)

Algorithm: Preoperative Evaluation of the Noncardiac Surgical Patient

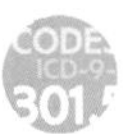

CODES

ICD9

- V72.83 Other specified pre-operative examination
- V72.84 Pre-operative examination, unspecified

CLINICAL PEARLS

- The preoperative evaluation should include medical record evaluation, patient interview, and physical exam.
- The minimum for the physical exam includes airway, pulmonary, and cardiovascular exams.
- Functional capacity, the level of surgical risk, and clinical risk factors determine if further cardiac testing is needed.
- No preoperative tests are routine.
- Active cardiac conditions should lead to delay or cancellation of nonemergent surgery.

PRESBYCUSIS

CPT Alain Michael P. Abellada, MD

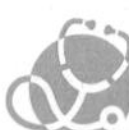

BASICS

DESCRIPTION

- Age-related, bilateral sensorineural hearing loss (HL)
- Represents the contributions of a lifetime of insults to the auditory system
- Initially presents as high-frequency hearing loss
- Later impacts ability to detect, identify, and localize sounds
- Due to mild and progressive nature, presbycusis is often untreated.
- Can lead to adverse effects of physical, cognitive, emotional, behavioral, and social function of the elderly
- 5 classifications:
  - Sensory
  - Neural
  - Strial (metabolic)
  - Cochlear conductive (mechanical)
  - Mixed
  - Indeterminate
- System(s) affected: Auditory, vestibular
- Synonym(s): Age-related hearing loss (ARHL)

EPIDEMIOLOGY

Incidence

According to recent community-based epidemiological study, the 5-year incidence of HL (1):

- Age 48–59: Male (19.1%), female (7%); all (11.6%)
- Age 60–69: Male (35%), female (18.1%); all (23.1%)
- Age 70–79: Male (59.1%), female (45.2%); all (4%)
- Age 80–92: Male (100%), female (94.7%); all (95.5%)
- All*: Male (27.4%), female (18.5%); all (21.4%)
  - Age adjusted*

Prevalence

- 10% of the population has a hearing loss great enough to impair communication
- Increases to 40% in the population older than 65 years
- 80% of HL cases occur in elderly people.
- Only 10–20% of older adults with HL have ever used hearing aids
- Predominant sex: Male > Female
- Hearing levels are poorer in industrialized societies than in isolated or agrarian societies.

RISK FACTORS

- Noise exposure
- Ototoxic substances:
  - Organic solvents
  - Heavy metals
  - Carbon monoxide
- Drugs:
  - Aminoglycosides
  - Cisplatin
  - Salicylates
- Tobacco smoking
- Alcohol
- Hunting and shooting
- Lower socioeconomic status
- Family history of presbycusis
- Head trauma
- Cardiovascular disease (hypertension, atherosclerosis, hyperlipidemia)
- Plasma hyperviscosity
- Diabetes mellitus
- Immune function impairment
- Metabolic bone disease
- Renal failure
- Endocrine medical conditions: Levels of aldosterone
- Alzheimer disease
- Bone mineral density
- Otological conditions such as Ménière disease or otosclerosis

Genetics

Presbycusis has a clear familiar aggregation (2):

- Heritability estimates show 35–55% of the variance of sensory presbycusis is from genetic factors; even greater percentage in strial presbycusis
- Heritability aggregation stronger among women than men.

GENERAL PREVENTION

- Avoidance of hazardous noise exposure
- Use of hearing protection
- Maintain healthy diet and exercise

PATHOPHYSIOLOGY

External ear resonates and enhances sound transmission to the tympanic membrane. The middle ear ossicles conduct the sound waves to the fluid-filled cochlea (inner ear). The Organ of Corti, located in the cochlea, contains hair cells that detect the vibrations and produce electrical signals. The stria vascularis is the cochlear tissue that generates endocochlear potential:

- Sensory presbycusis: Primary loss of the hair cells in the basal end of the cochlea
- Neural presbycusis: Loss of spiral ganglion cells
- Strial (metabolic) presbycusis: Atrophy of the stria vascularis
- Cochlear conductive (mechanical) presbycusis: No morphologic findings (presumed stiffening of the basilar membrane)
- Mixed presbycusis: Combinations of hair cell, ganglion cell, and stria vascularis loss
- Indeterminate presbycusis: No morphologic findings (presumed impaired cellular function)

ETIOLOGY

Presbycusis is caused by the accumulated effects of noise exposure, systemic disease, ototoxic drugs, and genetic susceptibility.

COMMONLY ASSOCIATED CONDITIONS

- Tinnitus
- Vertigo
- Dysequilibrium (3)
- Dementia (4)

DIAGNOSIS

HISTORY

- Reduced hearing sensitivity and speech understanding in noisy environments
- Impaired localization of sound sources
- Increased difficulty understanding conversations, especially with women, due to higher tone of spoken voice
- Presents bilaterally

PHYSICAL EXAM

- Whispered voice test:
  - Median positive LR of 5.1 and median negative LR of 0.03 for detection of >25- or >30-dB hearing loss when performed at 2 feet (5).
- Rinne and Weber test
- Otoscopy:
  - Rule out conductive hearing loss

DIAGNOSTIC TESTS & INTERPRETATION

- Single Question Screening ("Do you have difficulty with your hearing?"):
  - Median positive LR of 3 and median negative LR of 0.4 for detection of hearing loss >25 dB (5)
  - Median positive LR of 2.5 and median negative LR of 0.26 for detection of hearing loss >40 dB (5)
- Hearing Handicap Inventory for the Elderly—short form (HHIE-S):
  - Median positive LR of 3.5 and negative LR of 0.5 for detection of hearing loss >25 dB (5)
  - Median positive LR of 3.1 and median negative LR of 0.43 for detection of hearing loss >40 dB (5)
- Handheld audiometry
- Screening audiometry:
  - Audiometric patterns (6):
    - Abrupt high tone loss (sensory presbycusis)
    - Diminished word discrimination (neural presbycusis)
    - Gradual descending pattern (cochlear conductive presbycusis)
    - Combinations of flat, sloping, and abrupt high tone loss (mixed presbycusis)
    - Flat and/or abrupt high tone loss (indeterminate presbycusis)

DIFFERENTIAL DIAGNOSIS

- Noise-induced traumatic loss
- Autoimmune hearing loss
- Perilymph fistula
- Ménière disease
- Acoustic neuroma
- Complete canal occlusion
- Otitis externa
- Chronic otitis media
- Middle ear effusion
- Otosclerosis
- Glomus tumor
- Vascular anomaly
- Cholesteatoma

TREATMENT

ADDITIONAL TREATMENT

- Hearing aids (HA):
  - Types:
    - Analog HA: Pick up sound waves through a microphone; convert them into electrical signals, amplify, and send them through the ear canal to the tympanic membrane
    - Digital HA: Programmable; may reduce acoustic feedback, reduce background noise, detect and automatically accommodate different listening environments, control multiple microphones
  - HAs have an average decibel gain of 16.3 dB
  - Associated with hypersensitivity to loud sounds ("loudness recruitment")
- Hearing-assistive technologies (HATs) (7):
  - Can be used along or in combination with HAs (for difficult listening conditions)
  - Addresses face-to-face communication, broadcast or other electronic media (radio, TV), telephone conversation, sensitivity to alerting signals and environment stimuli (doorbell, baby's cry, alarm clock, etc.)
  - Includes personal FM systems, infrared systems, induction loop systems, hardwired systems, telephone amplifier, telecoil, TDD (telecommunication device for the deaf), situation-specific devices (e.g. television), alerting devices

Issues for Referral

Refer to audiologist for formal evaluation and optimal fitting of HAs and/or HATs:

- Individual receiving post-fitting orientation/education has significantly fewer HA returns
- Individuals receiving more than 2 hours of education and counseling report higher levels of satisfaction

SURGERY/OTHER PROCEDURES

- Cochlear implants (CI) (8):
  - Indications include hearing no better than identifying 50% or fewer key words in test sentences in the best aided condition in the worst ear and 60% in the better ear.
  - Works by bypassing the ear canal, middle ear, and hair cells in the cochlea to provide electric stimulation directly to the auditory nerve.
  - Incoming sounds are received through the microphone in the audio processor component (resembles a small HA that rests on the superior pinna), which converts them into electrical impulses and sends them to the magnetic coil (located on the skin). The impulses transmit these across intact skin via radio waves to the implanted component (direct subjacent to the coil). The pulses travel to the electrodes in the cochlea and stimulate the cochlea at high rates.
  - Receiving a unilateral CI is most common; some may receive bilateral CIs (either sequentially or in the same surgery). Others may wear a CI in 1 ear and an HA in the contralateral ear (bimodal fit).
- Active middle ear implants (AMEIs) (8):
  - Suitable for elderly adults who cannot wear conventional HAs for medical or personal (cosmetic reasons) and whose HL is not severe enough for a CI.
  - Comes in different models, and may include components that are implantable under the skin.
- Electric acoustic stimulation: Use of CI and HA together in 1 ear:
  - Addresses the specific needs of patients presenting with good low frequency hearing (a mild to moderate sensorineural HL in frequencies up to 1,000 Hz) but poorer hearing in the high frequencies (sloping to 60 dB or worse HL above 1,000 Hz) (8):
    - Contraindications: Progressive HL, autoimmune disease; HL related to meningitis, otosclerosis, or ossification; malformation of the cochlea; a gap in air conduction and bone conduction thresholds of >15 dB; external ear contraindications or unwillingness to use amplification devices (8).

ONGOING CARE

FOLLOW-UP RECOMMENDATIONS

Patient Monitoring

- During follow-up visits, check for compliance of HA use:
  - 25–40% of adults will either stop wearing them or use them only occasionally.
- Assess perceived benefit of HA, and, if ineffective, for indications for possible surgical treatments.

PATIENT EDUCATION

- Educate the patient that conversations should be face-to-face, spoken clearly and unhurriedly, without competing background noise (e.g., radio, TV), and include a confirmation that the message is received.
- Formal speech reading classes may be beneficial; however, availability may be limited.

REFERENCES

1. Nash SD, Cruickshanks KJ, Klein R, et al. The prevalence of hearing impairment and associated risk factors: The Beaver Dam Offspring Study. *Arch Otolaryngol Head Neck Surg*. 2011;137(5):432–9.
2. Huang Q, Tang J. Age-related hearing loss or presbycusis. *Eur Arch Otorhinolaryngol*. 2010;267(8):1179–91.
3. Belal A Jr., Glorig A. Dysequilibrium of ageing (presbyastasis). *J Laryngol Otol*. 1986;100(9):1037–41.
4. Lin FR, Metter RJ, O'Brien RJ, et al. Hearing loss and incident dementia. *Arch Neurol*. 2011;68(2):214–20.
5. Chou R, Dana T, Bougatsos C, et al. Screening adults aged 50 years or older for hearing loss: a review of the evidence for the U.S. preventive services task force. *Ann Intern Med*. 2011;154(5):347–55.
6. Nelson EG, Hinojosa R. Presbycusis: A human temporal bone study of individuals with downward sloping audiometric patterns of hearing loss and review of the literature. *Laryngoscope*. 2006;116(9 Pt 3 Suppl 112):1–12.
7. Valente M. Summary guidelines: Audiological management of adult hearing impairment. *Audio Today*. 2006;18:32–7.
8. Sprinzl GM, Riechelmann H. Current trends in treating hearing loss in elderly people: A review of the technology and treatment options—a mini-review. *Gerontology*. 2010;56:351–8.

ADDITIONAL READING

- Gates GA, Mills JH. Presbycusis. *Lancet*. 2005;366(9491):1111–20.
- Isaacson JE, Vora NM. Differential diagnosis and treatment of hearing loss. *Am Fam Physician*. 2003;68(6):1125–32.

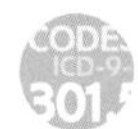

CODES

ICD9

388.01 Presbyacusis

CLINICAL PEARLS

- Presbycusis is age-related hearing loss, showing increased incidence with age. It is often bilateral and initially begins as high-frequency HL. It presents as difficulty communicating in noisy conditions.
- There are more affected males than females.
- Compliance is only from 25–40% for those who own HAs. A referral to an audiologist is key for optimal evaluation, fitting for HAs, and consideration for HATs or surgical treatment.
- Indication for CIs include hearing no better than identifying 50% or fewer key words in test sentences in the best aided condition in the worst ear and 60% in the better ear.

The views expressed in this chapter are those of the author and do not reflect the official policy or position of the Department of the Army, Department of Defense, or the U.S. Government. Opinions, interpretations, conclusions, and recommendations herein are those of the author and are not necessarily endorsed by the U.S. Army.

PRESSURE ULCER

Kim House, MD

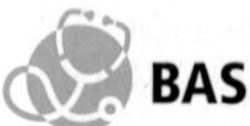

BASICS

DESCRIPTION

- A localized area of soft tissue breakdown resulting from pressure between an external surface and a bony prominence that causes local tissue ischemia and necrosis
- Synonym(s): Decubitus ulcer; Bed sores

EPIDEMIOLOGY

Incidence

- 2 million new patients each year
- Incidence is 43/100,000 population every year

Prevalence

- Hospitalized adults: 3–11%; long-term care facilities: 2.5–24%
- 65% of elderly with femoral fractures, 33% of critical-care patients, and over 60% prevalence among quadriplegic and orthopedic patients

RISK FACTORS

- Extended stay in hospital or nursing home, inadequate staffing (1)[B]
- Immobility (e.g., spinal cord injury, fracture, cerebrovascular accident)
- Malnutrition, recent weight loss, eating problems, vitamin C deficiency (1)[B]
- History of previous pressure ulcer
- Age-related skin changes
- Impairments of perfusion and oxygenation (anemia, peripheral vascular disease)
- Immunocompromise (e.g., diabetes)
- Decreased sensation (e.g., neuropathy, spinal cord injury)
- Impaired awareness (e.g., dementia, delirium, oversedation)
- Urinary or fecal incontinence
- For trauma and emergency patients, hard backboard should be removed as soon as possible after the secondary survey.
- Assessment scales for evaluating risk factors include Norton, Braden (Braden Q version for children), Waterlow, and Walsall.

GENERAL PREVENTION

- Up to 95% are preventable; identification of at-risk patients is essential, with early multidisciplinary care.
- Reposition frequently if immobile, hourly if wheelchair-bound and every 2 hours if bedridden.
- Initiate early mobilization when possible.
- Keep skin clean and dry by using mild soap, warm water, and moisturizer. Zinc oxide and petroleum products are advisable. Manage incontinence by scheduled toileting plans, or check and change diapers every 2 hours when turning patient.
- Use mattress overlays, thick air seat cushions, and beds that reduce pressure on pressure points, especially for hospitalized patients.
- Aggressive glycemic control (2)[B]
- Assess nutrient status and provide required macronutrients and micronutrients by oral, enteral, or parenteral route, if necessary.

PATHOPHYSIOLOGY

See "Etiology."

ETIOLOGY

- Sustained pressure causes occlusion of blood and lymphatic vessels; this occlusion of the microcirculation can cause ischemia and necrosis (3)[A]. This occurs when the tissue pressure exceeds capillary filling pressure (25 mm Hg).
- Skin is more resistant to pressure than is SC tissue.
- Moisture from incontinence or perspiration can increase the friction between 2 surfaces.

COMMONLY ASSOCIATED CONDITIONS

See "Risk Factors."

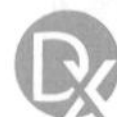

DIAGNOSIS

HISTORY

- Presence of risk factors
- Pain
- When was the ulcer first noticed?
- Prior treatment

PHYSICAL EXAM

- Do full skin examination on admission to hospital or extended-care facility.
- 83% of hospitalized patients with decubitus ulcers develop them in first 5 days of hospitalization (4)[B].
- National Pressure Ulcer Advisory Panel Classification: Deep tissue injury; may appear as a deep bruise over a bony prominence. Difficult to measure:
  - Stage I: Nonblanching erythema, warmth, induration
  - Stage II: May include dermis; appears as abrasion, blister, or superficial ulcer
  - Stage III: Extends through SC tissues but not fascia; may appear necrotic with changes in pigmentation
  - Stage IV: Ulcers extend beyond deep fascia into muscle or bone, decayed area may be larger than visibly apparent wound, osteomyelitis or sepsis may be present, and granulation tissue and epithelialization may be present at wound margins.

DIAGNOSTIC TESTS & INTERPRETATION

Lab

Initial lab tests

- Wound culture: Do not culture surface drainage. Do deep tissue culture/bone biopsy.
- WBC count and differential; blood cultures if fever is present (>37°C)
- ESR and C-reactive protein (CRP) if osteomyelitis is suspected
- Nutritional assessment: Albumin, prealbumin, transferrin

Follow-Up & Special Considerations

If poor nutritional status is known, consider vitamin C and zinc levels. If low, supplements are likely to be helpful (2)[B].

Imaging

Initial approach

Radiograph of bone for suspected osteomyelitis

Follow-Up & Special Considerations

CT/MRI: If plain films show inflammation, reaction; can document progress/effectiveness of treatment

DIFFERENTIAL DIAGNOSIS

- Stasis or ischemic ulcers
- Vasculitides
- Diabetic ulcers
- Cancers
- Radiation injury
- Pyoderma gangrenosum and other dermatologic conditions

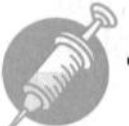

TREATMENT

MEDICATION

First Line

- See "General Measures" for first-line treatment.
- Silver dressings, triple antibiotic ointment can be tried for 2 weeks to treat bacterial overgrowth. Consider the following medications for specific indications:
  - Cellulitis: Requires oral vs. parenteral antibiotics. Treat for 7–10 days. Expect clinical response in 2–3 days.
  - Deep tissue culture should guide antibiotic selection, not surface swab.
  - Osteomyelitis: Radiology-proven or visualized bone; treat for 6 weeks, usually with parenteral antibiotics.

Second Line

Zinc and vitamin C: Use if dietary deficiency is noted (lab test).

ADDITIONAL TREATMENT

- Reduce pressure and prevent additional ulcers: Padding, frequent repositioning, mobilization if possible (4)[B]:
  - Static surfaces for stage I and II ulcers: Air, foam, and water mattress overlays
  - Dynamic surfaces for stage III and IV ulcers: Alternating air overlays, low-air-loss beds
  - Improve overall nutritional status (adequate protein intake, micronutrients).

- Wound management (4)[B]:
  - Remove dead tissue chemically (collagenase), via sharp debridement with a scalpel, or autolytically (hydrocolloid).
  - Dressing to manage drainage (e.g., calcium alginate, foam dressing, gauze dressing)
  - Dressing to protect from contamination, mechanical forces
  - Silver dressing used to reduce bacterial overgrowth; consider in wounds not responding to other therapy
  - Stimulate new tissue growth when slough removed: Collagen-containing products
  - Hydrogel can keep wound moist.
  - Advanced wound care therapies: In nonhealing wounds that have appropriate nutrition, vascular supply, and pressure relief, can consider skin substitutes developed in laboratory from human fibroblasts, extracellular matrix material derived from submucosal layer of porcine small intestines, or genetically engineered platelet-derived growth factors produced in yeast and then formulated into a gel.
- Vacuum-assisted closure is used increasingly for difficult wounds:
  - Negative pressure reduces wound edema and improves local tissue perfusion.
  - Removes necrotic debris and reduces bacterial load
  - Literature review shows that 2 of 5 randomized, controlled trials and 2 of 4 nonrandomized, controlled trials favor negative-pressure wound therapy (5)[A].
  - Consider cost vs. clinical efficacy.

Issues for Referral

- Vascular surgery is a consideration for improvement of blood flow to wound via vascular bypass.
- Plastic surgery is a consideration for skin graft or flap.

Additional Therapies

Whirlpool/PulseVac aids in wound debridement (4)[C].

COMPLEMENTARY AND ALTERNATIVE MEDICINE

- Zinc and vitamin C: Use if dietary deficiency is noted (lab test).
- Electrical stimulation creates new vasculature in affected region (5)[C].

IN-PATIENT CONSIDERATIONS

Admission Criteria

- Cellulitis/osteomyelitis that has not responded to oral antibiotics as outpatient
- Abnormal vital signs due to infectious process

Nursing

- Dressing changes 1–3× daily
- Wet-to-dry dressings not standard of care unless 100% of wound is necrotic tissue.

Discharge Criteria

Clinical improvement in WBC count, appearance of wound and/or surrounding tissue, resolution of vital sign abnormalities

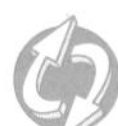

ONGOING CARE

FOLLOW-UP RECOMMENDATIONS

Weekly assessment by nurse with wound experience; biweekly assessment by physician

Patient Monitoring

- Home health nursing
- Change in plan of care if no improvement in 2–3 weeks

DIET

- 1–1.5 kg/d of protein
- Good glycemic control
- Include supply of micronutrients in diet or as supplements

PATIENT EDUCATION

- Signs and symptoms of infection
- Report new or increase in pain.
- Prevention of new wound where old wound healed

PROGNOSIS

Variable, depending on:

- Removal of pressure
- Nutrition
- Wound care

COMPLICATIONS

- Infection
- Amputation

REFERENCES

1. Horn SB, et al. The National Pressure Ulcer Long-Term Study. *J Am Geriatric Soc*. 2004;52: 359–67.
2. Mechanick JI. Practical aspects of nutritional support for wound-healing patients. *Am J Surgery*. 2004;188:525–65.
3. Grey JE, Harding KG, Enoch S. Pressure ulcers. *BMJ*. 2006;332:472–5.
4. Bansal C, Scott R, Stewart D, et al. Decubitus ulcers: A review of the literature. *Int J Dermatol*. 2005;44: 805–10.
5. Gregor S, Maegele M, Sauerland S, et al. Negative pressure wound therapy: A vacuum of evidence? *Arch Surg*. 2008;143:189–96.

ADDITIONAL READING

Ramundo J, Gray M. Enzymatic wound debridement. *J Wound Ostomy Continence Nurs*. 2008;35:273–80.

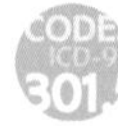

CODES

ICD9

- 707.00 Pressure ulcer, unspecified site
- 707.09 Pressure ulcer, other site
- 707.20 Pressure ulcer, unspecified stage

CLINICAL PEARLS

- Maximize nutrition of all hospitalized patients.
- Focus on reducing pressure to an area rather than on an expensive dressing.
- Assess wounds weekly or biweekly, and document clinical improvement or deterioration.

PRETERM LABOR

Kara M. Coassolo, MD
John C. Smulian, MD, MPH

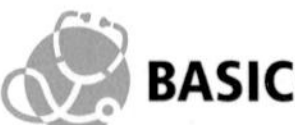

BASICS

DESCRIPTION
Contractions occurring between 20 and 36 weeks' gestation at a rate of 4 in 20 minutes or 8 in 1 hour with at least 1 of the following: Cervical change over time or dilation ≥2 cm (1)

EPIDEMIOLOGY
Preterm birth is the leading cause of perinatal morbidity and mortality in the US.

Incidence
10–15% of pregnancies experience at least 1 episode of preterm labor.

Prevalence
~12% of all births in the US are preterm (9% spontaneous preterm births and 3% indicated preterm births).

RISK FACTORS
- Demographic factors, including single parent, poverty, and black race
- Short interpregnancy interval
- No prenatal care
- Prepregnancy weight <45 kg (100 lb), body mass index <20
- Substance abuse (e.g., cocaine, tobacco)
- Prior preterm delivery (common)
- Previous second-trimester dilation and evacuation (D&E)
- Cervical insufficiency or prior cervical surgery (cone biopsy or LEEP)
- Abdominal surgery/trauma during pregnancy
- Uterine anomalies such as large fibroids or müllerian abnormalities
- Serious maternal infections/diseases
- Bacterial vaginosis
- Bacteriuria
- Vaginal bleeding during pregnancy
- Multiple gestation
- Fetal abnormalities
- Intrauterine growth restriction
- Placenta previa
- Premature placental separation (abruption)
- Polyhydramnios
- Ehler-Danlos syndrome

Genetics
Familial predisposition

GENERAL PREVENTION
- Patient education at each visit in second and third trimesters for those at risk and periodically in the last 2 trimesters for the general population
- If previous preterm birth, evaluate if etiology is likely to recur, and target intervention to specific condition:
  - Weekly injections of 17α-hydroxyprogesterone (250 mg IM every week) from 16–36 weeks if previous spontaneous preterm birth (2,3)[A]
  - Consider cerclage placement before 24 weeks' gestation for those at high risk because of cervical insufficiency or significant or progressive cervical shortening (4)[A].
- For women with a short cervix in the second trimester (<20 mm on transvaginal ultrasound), progesterone 200 mg/d per vagina × 24–34 weeks may decrease the risk of preterm delivery (5,6)[A].

PATHOPHYSIOLOGY
- Premature formation and activation of myometrial gap junctions
- Inflammatory mediator–stimulated contractions
- Weakened cervix (structural defect or extracellular matrix defect)
- Abnormal placental implantation

ETIOLOGY
- Systemic inflammation/infections (e.g., UTI, pyelonephritis, pneumonia)
- Local inflammation/infections (intra-amniotic infections from aerobes, anaerobes, *Mycoplasma, Ureaplasma*)
- Uterine abnormalities (e.g., cervical insufficiency, leiomyomata, septa, diethylstilbestrol exposure)
- Overdistension (by multiple gestation or polyhydramnios)
- Preterm premature rupture of membranes
- Trauma
- Placental abruption
- Immunopathology (e.g., antiphospholipid antibodies)
- Placental ischemic disease (preeclampsia and fetal growth restriction)

DIAGNOSIS

Diagnosis is generally based on a combination of significant cervical changes (such as dilation, effacement) with regular contractions. However, there is no single test that will reliably diagnose or predict true preterm labor. The diagnosis is based on a combination of physical findings and diagnostic tests that are interpreted in the context of the degree of risk to the patient.

HISTORY
- Address risk factors, especially etiologies of previous preterm birth.
- Regular uterine contractions or cramping
- Dull, low backache or pain
- Intermittent lower abdominal pain
- Increased low pelvic pressure
- Change in vaginal discharge
- Vaginal bleeding
- Fluid leakage

PHYSICAL EXAM
- Sterile speculum exam for membrane rupture evaluation, cultures, cervical inspection
- Bimanual cervical exam if intact membranes: Dilation of the cervix >1 cm and/or effacement of the cervix >50%

ALERT
Avoid bimanual examination when possible if rupture of the membranes is suspected.

DIAGNOSTIC TESTS & INTERPRETATION

Lab

Initial lab tests
- In symptomatic women from 22–34 weeks' gestation with intact membranes and no intercourse or bleeding in past 24 hours, obtain a fetal fibronectin swab (FFN) from the posterior vaginal fornix. FFN must be obtained prior to digital cervical exam:
  - If results are positive (≥50 ng/mL), patient is at a modest increased risk of preterm birth (positive predictive value [PPV] 13–30% for delivery within 2 weeks).
  - If results are negative, more than 97% of patients will not deliver in 14 days, so can consider avoiding complicated or high-risk interventions (7)[A].
- Urinalysis and urine culture
- Cultures for gonorrhea and chlamydia
- Wet prep for bacterial vaginosis evaluation (although evidence for improved outcomes with treatment is weak)
- Vaginal introitus and rectal culture for group B *Streptococcus*
- pH and Ferning test of vaginal fluid to evaluate for rupture of membranes
- CBC with differential
- Drug screen when appropriate

Follow-Up & Special Considerations
Repeat FFN as indicated by symptoms.

Imaging

Initial approach
- Ultrasound to identify number of fetuses and fetal position, confirm gestational age, estimate fetal weight, quantify amniotic fluid, and look for conditions making tocolysis contraindicated
- Transvaginal ultrasound to evaluate cervical length, funneling, and dynamic changes after obtaining FFN and if clinical assessment of the cervix is uncertain or if the cervix is closed on digital exam (4)[B]

Follow-Up & Special Considerations
After successful treatment, progressive changes of the cervix on repeat examination or ultrasound (in 1–2 weeks) may indicate need for hospitalization.

Diagnostic Procedures/Surgery
- Monitor contractions with external tocodynamometer.
- Consider amniocentesis at any preterm gestational age to evaluate for intra-amniotic infection (cell count with differential, glucose, Gram stain, aerobic, anaerobic, *Mycoplasma, Ureaplasma* cultures).
- Consider amniocentesis if ≥32 weeks' gestation for evaluation of fetal lung maturity (e.g., lecithin/sphingomyelin [L:S] ratio and phosphatidylglycerol [PG]). If L:S ratio >2:1 (nondiabetic) and PG is present, hyaline membrane disease is unlikely, so tocolysis is contraindicated.

Pathological Findings
- Placental inflammation:
  - Acute inflammation usually caused by infection
  - Chronic inflammation caused by immunopathology
- Abruption

DIFFERENTIAL DIAGNOSIS
- Braxton-Hicks contractions/false labor
- Round ligament pain
- Lumbosacral muscular back pain
- Urinary tract or vaginal infections
- Adnexal torsion
- Degenerating fibroid
- Appendicitis
- Dehydration
- Viral gastroenteritis

TREATMENT

MEDICATION

Tocolysis may allow time for interventions such as transfer to tertiary care facility and administration of corticosteroids, but may not prolong pregnancy significantly (2)[A].

First Line

- Tocolysis:
  - Nifedipine: 10 mg PO q10min up to 30 mg total; then 10–20 mg q6h × 24 hours; then 10–20 mg PO q8h (do not use sublingual route); check BP often, and avoid hypotension. Concurrent use with magnesium sulfate should be avoided to avoid theoretic risk of neuromuscular blockade.
  - Indomethacin: 50–100 mg PO initial dose; then 50 mg q6–8h × 24 hours (or, if available, 100-mg suppository per rectum q12h for 2 doses); then 25 mg q6–8h; use for no longer than 72 hours due to risk of premature closure of ductus arteriosus, oligohydramnios, and possibly neonatal necrotizing enterocolitis.
  - Contraindications to tocolysis: Severe preeclampsia, hemorrhage, chorioamnionitis, advanced labor, intrauterine growth retardation, fetal distress, or lethal fetal abnormalities
- Antibiotics: Antibiotics for group B *Streptococcus* prophylaxis if culture positive or unknown
- Steroids: If mother is at 23–34 weeks' gestation with no evidence of systemic infection, give glucocorticoids to decrease neonatal respiratory distress, intraventricular hemorrhage, necrotizing enterocolitis, and overall perinatal mortality (8)[A]. Betamethasone 12 mg IM × 2 doses 24 hours apart (preferred choice) *or* dexamethasone 6 mg IM q12h for 4 doses.

Second Line

- In the past, magnesium sulfate by IV infusion has been used as a first-line tocolytic agent. Recent data are conflicting as to whether it has a benefit for prolongation of pregnancy beyond 48 hours and whether it increases the risk for complications. Therefore, this agent should be used cautiously. (Standard dosages for tocolysis start with a 4–6-g IV bolus over 20 minutes and then 2–3 g/hr until contractions stop.):
  - Magnesium may decrease the risk of cerebral palsy when given prior to an anticipated preterm birth (9)[B].
  - Relative contraindications to magnesium sulfate include myasthenia gravis, hypocalcemia, renal failure, or concurrent use of calcium channel blockers.
- Terbutaline 0.25 mg SC q30min for up to 3 doses until contractions stop, then 0.25 mg SC q6h for 4 doses (optional); if contractions persist or pulse >120 beats/min, change to another tocolytic agent (may be poorly tolerated by mothers)
- Terbutaline by oral therapy or infusion pump has been used in the past for treatment or prevention of preterm labor. Due to reports of serious cardiovascular events and maternal deaths, PO or long-term SC administration of terbutaline should not be given (10).
- Significant possible interactions include pulmonary edema from crystalloid fluids and tocolytic agents, especially magnesium sulfate.
- Oral maintenance therapy with any agent is controversial, and its use is limited.

ADDITIONAL TREATMENT

General Measures

- Treat underlying risk factors (e.g., antibiotics for infections, hydration for dehydration).
- Liquids only or nothing by mouth if delivery imminent
- Hospitalization is necessary if the patient is on IV tocolysis or if bed rest is impossible at home.

Issues for Referral

- If delivery is inevitable but not immediate, consider transport to a tertiary care center or hospital equipped with a neonatal ICU.
- Consider consultation with maternal–fetal medicine specialist.

Additional Therapies

- Treating symptomatic bacterial vaginosis in second trimester with clindamycin 300 mg PO b.i.d. × 7 days or metronidazole 250 mg PO t.i.d. × 7 days might reduce risk of preterm delivery in high-risk symptomatic women.
- Pelvic rest (e.g., no douching or intercourse)
- Discontinue work and strenuous physical activity.
- Strict bed rest is not demonstrated to be effective in most situations.

SURGERY/OTHER PROCEDURES

- For malpresentation or fetal compromise, consider cesarean delivery if labor is progressing.
- Cerclage for incompetent cervix (until 24 weeks)

IN-PATIENT CONSIDERATIONS

Initial Stabilization

- IV access
- Continuous fetal and contraction monitoring
- Assess cervix for dilatation and effacement

Admission Criteria

Suspected/threatened preterm labor

IV Fluids

Hydrate with 500 mL 5% dextrose normal saline solution or 5% dextrose lactated Ringer solution for first half-hour; then at 125 mL/hr.

Nursing

Monitor for fluid overload (input/output monitoring, symptoms, lung auscultation, pulse oximetry), especially with tocolysis and multiple gestations.

Discharge Criteria

- Regular contractions and cervical change resolve
- If cervix is dilated ≥3 cm or FFN is positive, individualize decision to discharge by gestational age and patient circumstances

ONGOING CARE

FOLLOW-UP RECOMMENDATIONS

Patient Monitoring

- Weekly office visits with contraction monitoring, cervical checks, or cervical ultrasound if at high risk for recurrence
- Routine use of maintenance tocolysis has not been proven beneficial.

DIET

Regular

PATIENT EDUCATION

Call physician or proceed to hospital whenever contractions last >1 hour, bleeding, increased vaginal discharge or fluid

PROGNOSIS

- If membranes are ruptured and no infection is confirmed, delivery often occurs within 3–7 days.
- If membranes are intact, 20–50% deliver preterm.

COMPLICATIONS

Labor resistant to tocolysis, pulmonary edema, infection with preterm rupture of membranes

REFERENCES

1. Management of Preterm Labor. Summary, Evidence Report/Technology Assessment: Number 18. AHRQ Publication No. 01-E020, October 2000. Agency for Healthcare Research and Quality, Rockville, MD. http://archive.ahrq.gov/clinic/tp/pretermtp.htm.
2. Simhan HN, Caritis SN. Prevention of preterm delivery. *N Engl J Med*. 2007;357:477–87.
3. Tita AT, Rouse DJ. Progesterone for preterm birth prevention: An evolving intervention. *Am J Obstet Gynecol*. 2009;200:219–24.
4. Berghella V, Rafael TJ, Szychowski JM, et al. Cerclage for short cervix on ultrasonography in women with singleton gestations and previous preterm birth. *Obstet Gynecol*. 2011;117(3): 663–71.
5. Fonseca FB, Celik E, Parra M, et al. Progesterone and the risk of preterm birth among women with a short cervix. *NEJM*. 2007;357(5):462–9.
6. Hassan SS, Romero R, Vidyadhari D, et al. PREGNANT Trial. Vaginal progesterone reduces the rate of preterm birth in women with a sonographic short cervix: A multicenter, randomized, double-blind, placebo-controlled trial. *Ultrasound Obstet Gynecol*. 2011;38(1): 18–31.
7. Goldenberg RL, Goepfert AR, Ramsey PS. Biochemical markers for the prediction of preterm birth. *Am J Obstet Gynecol*. 2005;192(5 Suppl): S36–46.
8. Roberts D, Dalziel S. Antenatal corticosteroids for accelerating fetal lung maturation for women at risk of preterm birth. *Cochrane Database Syst Rev*. 2006;3:CD004454.
9. Magnesium sulfate before anticipated preterm birth for neuroprotection. Comm Opin No 455. *ACOG. Obstet Gynecol*. 2010;115:669–71.
10. FDA Drug Safety Communication: New warning against use of terbutaline to treat preterm labor. www.fda.gov/Drugs/DrugSafety/ucm243539.htm Accessed 28 June 2011.

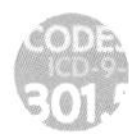

CODES

ICD9

- 644.03 Threatened premature labor, antepartum condition or complication
- 644.13 Other threatened labor, antepartum condition or complication

CLINICAL PEARLS

- Steroids improve neonatal outcomes.
- Progesterone therapy can prevent recurrence of preterm birth in next pregnancy.

PRIAPISM

Andrew Leone, MD
Kyle D. Wood, MD

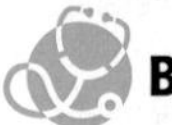

BASICS

DESCRIPTION

- Penile erection that lasts for >4 hours and is unrelated to sexual stimulation or excitement
- Classified into ischemic and nonischemic variants
- Ischemic (low-flow) priapism is painful and requires urgent clinical intervention.
- Stuttering priapism is recurrent ischemic priapism over an extended period.
- Nonischemic (high-flow) priapism could be related to prior trauma and does not require urgent treatment.
- System(s) affected: Reproductive

Pediatric Considerations

In children, nearly all priapism is caused either by sickle cell anemia or trauma (1).

EPIDEMIOLOGY

Incidence

In the Netherlands, the incidence is 1.5 cases of ischemic priapism per 100,000 person-years in the general male population (data not available for the US) (1). After exclusion of cases associated with intracavernous vasoactive drug use, incidence is 0.9 cases per 100,000 person-years (2).

RISK FACTORS

- Sickle cell anemia, lifetime risk of ischemic priapism 29–42% (1)
- Dehydration

GENERAL PREVENTION

- Avoid dehydration.
- Avoid excessive sexual stimulation.
- Avoid causative drugs (see "Causes") when possible.
- Avoid genital and pelvic trauma.

PATHOPHYSIOLOGY

- In ischemic priapism, decreased venous outflow results in increased intracavernosal pressure. This leads to erection, decreased arterial inflow, stasis of blood, local hypoxia, and acidosis (a compartment syndrome). Eventually penile tissue necrosis and fibrosis may occur. The exact mechanism is unknown and may involve trapping of erythrocytes in the veins draining the erectile bodies.
- In nonischemic priapism, there is increased arterial flow without decreased venous outflow. There is increased inflow and outflow, which result in a sustained, nonpainful, partially rigid erection.
- Aberrations in the phosphodiesterase (PDE-5A) pathway has been proven in mice to be one mechanism of priapism (3).

ETIOLOGY

- Ischemic priapism:
  - Idiopathic, estimated to about 50% (1)
  - Intracavernosal injections of vasoactive drugs for erectile dysfunction
  - Oral agents for erectile dysfunction
  - Pelvic vascular thrombosis
  - Prolonged sexual activity
  - Sickle cell disease and trait
  - Leukemia from infiltration of the corpora
  - Other blood dyscrasias (G6PD deficiency, thrombophilia)
  - Pelvic hematoma or neoplasia (penis, urethra, bladder, prostate, kidney, rectal)
  - Cerebrospinal tumors
  - Asplenism
  - Fabry disease
  - Tertiary syphilis
  - Total parenteral nutrition, especially 20% lipid infusion (results in hyperviscosity)
  - Bladder calculus
  - Trauma to penis
  - UTIs, especially prostatitis, urethritis, cystitis
  - Several drugs suspected as causing priapism (e.g., chlorpromazine, prazosin, cocaine, trazodone, and some corticosteroids); anticoagulants (heparin and Coumadin); phosphodiesterase inhibitors (Viagra, others); testosterone; immunosuppressants (tacrolimus); and antihypertensives (hydralazine, propranolol, guanethidine)
  - Intracavernous fat emulsion
  - Hyperosmolar IV contrast
  - Spinal cord injury
  - General or spinal anesthesia
  - Heavy alcohol intake or cocaine use
- Nonischemic priapism:
  - The most common cause is penile or perineal trauma resulting in a fistula between the cavernous artery and the corpora.
  - Rarely, iatrogenic causes for the management of ischemic priapism can result in nonischemic priapism.
  - Certain urological surgeries have also resulted in nonischemic priapism.

COMMONLY ASSOCIATED CONDITIONS

- Sickle cell anemia
- G6PD deficiency
- Leukemia
- Neoplasm

DIAGNOSIS

HISTORY

- Penile erection that is persistent, prolonged, painful, and tender (ischemic)
- Duration of erection, degree of pain
- Perineal or penile trauma
- Prior episodes of priapism
- Urination difficult during erection
- History of any hematological abnormalities
- Cardiovascular disease
- Medications
- Recreational drugs
- Loss of erectile function if treatment is not prompt and effective

PHYSICAL EXAM

- Ischemic priapism:
  - Penis is fully erect, corpora cavernosa are rigid and tender, and corpora spongiosum and glans are flaccid. Usually associated with tenderness and pain.
- Nonischemic priapism:
  - Penis is partially erect, and the corpora cavernosa are semirigid and nontender, with the glans and corpora spongiosum flaccid. Usually not tender or painful.
- Perineum, abdomen, and lymph node exam also valuable to rule out underlying condition
- A complete penile and scrotal exam is necessary. Determine if a penile prosthesis is present.

DIAGNOSTIC TESTS & INTERPRETATION

Lab

- CBC with reticulocyte count to detect leukemia or platelet abnormalities
- Sickling hemoglobin (Hgb) solubility test and Hgb electrophoresis
- Coagulation profile
- Platelet count
- Urinalysis
- Urine toxicology if illicit drugs suspected
- Corporal blood gas can be used to distinguish ischemic from nonischemic priapism.

Imaging

- A color duplex ultrasound of the penis and perineum may be necessary to differentiate ischemic from nonischemic priapism. In ischemic priapism, there is no blood flow in the cavernosal arteries, whereas in nonischemic patients there is high blood flow (1); may also see fistulas or pseudoaneurysms suggestive of nonischemic priapism.
- Penile arteriography can be used to identify the presence and site of fistulas in patients with nonischemic priapism.

Diagnostic Procedures/Surgery

A physical exam is usually able to distinguish ischemic from nonischemic priapism.

Pathological Findings

- Pelvic vascular thrombosis
- Partial thrombosis of corpora cavernosa of the penis
- Corpus spongiosum, glans penis: No involvement
- Arterial priapism will show arteriocavernous fistula.

TREATMENT

- Ischemic priapism requires immediate treatment in order to preserve future erectile function (a longer delay in treatment means a higher chance of future impotence):
  - Cavernosal aspiration with irrigation (success rate ~30%) (1,4)
  - Cavernosal injection of phenylephrine (α adrenergic sympathomimetic) with monitoring of patient's BP and pulse (success rate ~65 %) (4). Inject q5–10min until detumescence.
  - Continue aspiration, irrigation, and phenylephrine for several hours. If this fails, shunt procedures are considered (first a distal shunt).
- Nonischemic priapism:
  - Initial observation
  - If this fails, arteriography and embolization with absorbable materials (5% rate of impotence vs. 39% with permanent materials) or surgical ligation as a last resort (4)
- Treat the underlying condition (i.e., sickle cell disease). Do not delay intracavernous treatment.

MEDICATION

- Narcotics for pain if needed
- Pseudoephedrine is not recommended by the American Urological Association (4):
  - Efficacy is reported in nonrandomized studies as 28–36% (1).
  - No randomized studies have been conducted to date.
- Terbutaline has been studied and may be effective (uncontrolled trials showed a 65% resolution rate) for priapism caused by self-injection of agents to treat erectile dysfunction (4).
- For stuttering priapism, a trial of GnRH agonists or antiandrogens is effective; self-injection of phenylephrine is also effective.
- PDE-5 inhibitors also have a role in the prevention of priapism in patients suffering from stuttering priapism (5).

ADDITIONAL TREATMENT

General Measures

- Reassure the patient about the outcome if warranted.
- Provide continuous caudal or spinal anesthesia if the etiology is neurogenic.
- Treat any underlying cause.
- In sickle cell anemia: IV hydration; partial exchange or repeated transfusions to reduce percentage of sickle to <50%
- Relieve the patient's pain.

Issues for Referral

A urologist should be consulted in all cases of suspected priapism to ensure the highest likelihood of preserved erectile function.

SURGERY/OTHER PROCEDURES

- Introduction of 18- or 19-gauge needle into corpora cavernosa (best done by urologist if available) at 9 o'clock and 3 o'clock positions with aspiration of 20–30 mL of blood from corpus cavernosum. May follow with intracavernous injection of 100–500 mcg phenylephrine. (Mix 0.2 mL [200 mcg]) of 1% phenylephrine in 9.8 cc of normal saline.) If this fails, consider shunts.
- Distal shunt:
  - Winter shunt: Biopsy needle inserted in glans penis to create shunt between glans and corpora
  - Al-Ghorab shunt: Excision of tunica albuginea
- Proximal shunts

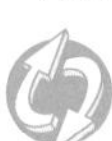

ONGOING CARE

FOLLOW-UP RECOMMENDATIONS

Bed rest until priapism resolves

Patient Monitoring

Close follow-up with a urologist is required after surgical treatments for priapism.

PATIENT EDUCATION

- Information about long-term outlook, referral for counseling
- Reduction of vasoactive drug therapy if responsible for priapism and elimination of offending drugs if causal

PROGNOSIS

- Even with excellent treatment for a prolonged priapism, detumescence may require several weeks secondary to edema (1).
- Impotence is likely in ischemic priapism and is up to 90% if the priapism lasts longer than 24 hours.
- Despite early intervention, ischemic priapism is likely to result in impotence in up to 50% of men.

COMPLICATIONS

Erectile dysfunction (i.e., impotence)

REFERENCES

1. Huang YC, Harraz AM, Shindel AW. Evaluation and management of priapism: 2009 update. *Nat Rev Urol*. 2009;6:262–71.
2. Eland IA, van der Lei J, Stricker BH, et al. Incidence of priapism in the general population. *Urology*. 2001;57:970–2.
3. Champion HC, Bivalacqua TJ, Takimoto E. Phosphodiesterase-5A dysregulation in penile erectile tissue is a mechanism of priapism. *Proc Natl Acad Sci USA*. 2005;102:1661–6.
4. Montague DK, Jarow J, Broderick GA. American Urological Association guideline on the management of priapism. *J Urol*. 2003;170: 1318–24.
5. Muneer A, Minhas S, Arya M, Ralph DJ, et al. Stuttering priapism--a review of the therapeutic options. *Int J Clin Pract*. 2008;62:1265–70.

ADDITIONAL READING

- Burnett AL. Pathophysiology of priapism: Dysregulatory erection physiology thesis. *J Urol*. 2003;170:26–34.
- Pryor J, Akkus E, Alter G. Priapism. *J Sex Med*. 2004;1:116–20.

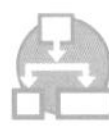

See Also (Topic, Algorithm, Electronic Media Element)

Anemia, Sickle Cell; Erectile Dysfunction

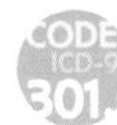

CODES

ICD9

607.3 Priapism

CLINICAL PEARLS

- Priapism is a prolonged penile erection that lasts longer than 4 hours and is unrelated to sexual stimulation.
- In evaluating priapism, the clinician must distinguish ischemic from nonischemic priapism by history and physical, as well as blood gas and possibly ultrasound, if needed.
- Ischemic priapism is an emergent condition that requires immediate urological evaluation and treatment.
- The most common causes of ischemic priapism are idiopathic, related to treatments for erectile dysfunction, or related to use of substances (medicinal or recreational).
- If an underlying medical condition is identified (sickle cell anemia), proper concomitant treatment is necessary to increase the efficacy of treatment.

PROCTITIS

Walter M. Kim, MD, PhD
Jyoti Ramakrishna, MD

BASICS

DESCRIPTION

- Acute or chronic inflammation of the rectal mucosa
- System(s) affected: Gastrointestinal

EPIDEMIOLOGY

Incidence

- Predominant age: Adult
- Predominant sex: Male > Female
- Radiation proctitis usually is encountered following pelvic radiation for cancers of the rectum, cervix, uterus, prostate, bladder, and testes; 2–20% incidence
- Ulcerative proctitis: 0.5–3 of 100,000 persons
- Gonococcal proctitis most common in individuals <25 years old

RISK FACTORS

- Pelvic radiation
- Receptive anal intercourse
- Rectal injury
- Rectal medications
- Inflammatory bowel disease (IBD)
- Jewish ancestry

Genetics

Higher incidence among the Jewish population

GENERAL PREVENTION

Safe sex practices including condom use during anal intercourse (if an STI is causative)

ETIOLOGY

- Infectious (sexually transmitted):
  - Gonorrhea
  - Chlamydia
  - Syphilis
  - Herpes simplex virus (HSV; 90% of cases due to HSV2)
  - Lymphogranuloma venereum (LGV)
  - Chancroid
  - Cytomegalovirus
  - Human papillomavirus
- Other infections:
  - *Clostridium difficile* (after antibiotics)
  - Enteric infections, including *Campylobacter, Shigella, Escherichia coli, Salmonella,* and amebiasis
- Inflammatory:
  - IBD (mostly ulcerative colitis)
  - Radiation therapy
- Other:
  - Ischemia
  - Vasculitis
  - Idiopathic
  - Toxins (e.g., hydrogen peroxide enemas)

COMMONLY ASSOCIATED CONDITIONS

- If an STI is causative, test accordingly, including HIV serology
- Treatment with pelvic radiation (e.g., for prostate, bladder, testicular, or gynecologic cancers)

DIAGNOSIS

HISTORY

- Anorectal pain or discomfort
- Rectal bleeding
- Purulent rectal discharge
- Passing of blood or mucous through rectum
- Urgency
- Tenesmus
- Diarrhea or constipation
- Abdominal cramps
- Fever
- Weight loss
- Radiation proctitis:
  - Acute radiation injury: Occurs within 6 weeks of therapy
  - Chronic radiation proctitis: Delayed onset; first sign most commonly occurs 9–14 months following radiation

PHYSICAL EXAM

- STI-associated proctitis:
  - Perianal or rectal vesicles and/or ulcers
  - Mucopurulent discharge
  - Rectal bleeding
  - Chancre
  - Condylomata lata or acuminata
  - May have tender inguinal lymphadenopathy with LGV infection
- IBD-associated proctitis
  - Perianal abscess
  - Fistula or fissures
  - Rectal bleeding

DIAGNOSTIC TESTS & INTERPRETATION

Lab

- STI proctitis
  - Rectal swab for gonococcal and chlamydial culture
  - Serology for syphilis
  - LVG culture
  - Viral culture for HSV
- IBD:
  - CBC
  - ESR
  - C-reactive protein
  - albumin
  - liver function tests (AST, ALT, AP)
- Enteric infections: Stool culture for *E. coli* O157:H7, *Salmonella, Shigella,* amebiasis
- Stool study for *C. difficile* toxin

Diagnostic Procedures/Surgery

- Proctosigmoidoscopy
- Colonoscopy to exclude more proximal involvement and rectal biopsy if IBD is suspected

Pathological Findings

- Radiation proctitis:
  - Proctosigmoidoscopy reveals friable, edematous mucosa, spontaneous or contact bleeding, telangiectasias, strictures, or fistulas.
- STI proctitis:
  - Ulceration, inflammation, mucopurulent discharge, or bleeding seen on proctoscopy may be present.
- Ulcerative proctitis:
  - Endoscopy reveals friable mucosa and pseudopolyps.
  - Biopsy reveals cryptitis and crypt abscesses.

DIFFERENTIAL DIAGNOSIS

- Traumatic proctitis
- Radiation proctitis
- IBD (ulcerative colitis, Crohn disease)
- Recurrent malignancies
- Enteric infections such as *Salmonella, Shigella, Campylobacter, E. coli, C. difficile,* or amebiasis

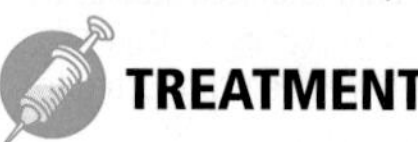

TREATMENT

- Gonorrhea:
  - Ceftriaxone 250 mg IM in a single dose (1)[A] *or*
  - Cefixime 400 mg PO in a single dose or
  - Single-dose cephalosporin regimen *plus* azithromycin 1 g in a single dose or doxycycline 100 mg PO b.i.d. for 7 days (to cover coinfection with chlamydia)
- Chlamydia:
  - Doxycycline 100 mg PO b.i.d. for 7 days *or* azithromycin 1 g PO single dose
- Herpes:
  - Acyclovir 400 mg PO t.i.d. for 7–10 days
- *C. difficile*:
  - Metronidazole 250–500 mg PO t.i.d. or vancomycin 125 mg PO q.i.d. for 7–10 days
- Ulcerative proctitis:
  - Mild to moderate (up to 8 bloody stools per day): Topical 5-aminosalicylic acid (5-ASA, Mesalamine) suppository or enema (Rowasa), topical steroids (hydrocortisone-containing foam, suppository, or enema), or a combination of oral 5-ASA (Pentasa or Asacol) and topical 5-ASA (2)[B],(3)[A]
  - Severe: Systemic corticosteroids may be needed for patients who do not tolerate or do not respond to the aforementioned therapies.
  - Chronic (moderate to severe steroid-refractory or dependent disease): 6-Mercaptopurine, azathioprine

- Radiation proctitis:
  - Topical hydrocortisone foam or enemas; mesalamine (5-ASA) enema alone or in combination with oral mesalamine; sucralfate enemas (20 mL of a 10% sucralfate suspension in water b.i.d.)
  - Systemic corticosteroids may be used if the aforementioned therapies are ineffective
  - Experimental treatments: Hyperbaric oxygen (4)[B], metronidazole, vitamin A, WF10 macrophage-regulating agent, argon plasma coagulation for bleeding telangiectasias

Single-dose injectable cephalosporin regimens
plus
Azithromycin 1 g PO in a single dose
or
Doxycycline 100 mg PO b.i.d. for 7 days

ADDITIONAL TREATMENT

General Measures

- Treatment depends on the cause.
- Rectal Gram stains have a significant false-negative rate, and if the clinician has a strong suspicion of gonorrheal proctitis, empirical treatment is warranted while culture results are still pending.
- Encourage sexual partners of patients diagnosed with STI-associated proctitis to be tested and treated.
- Sitz baths may provide some relief.

IN-PATIENT CONSIDERATIONS

Initial Stabilization

- Outpatient, unless severe and refractory to usual measures
- Hospitalization may be necessary in cases of severe ulcerative proctitis, especially with more proximal colon involvement.

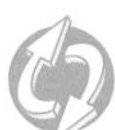

ONGOING CARE

FOLLOW-UP RECOMMENDATIONS

Patient Monitoring

Follow until completely healed.

DIET

No special diet

PATIENT EDUCATION

Counsel about safe sex practices, including condom use during every sexual encounter and additional barrier methods such as dental dams and gloves for alternative intimacy practices.

PROGNOSIS

- Satisfactory cure or control with appropriate treatment
- In patients with ulcerative proctitis, 10% will not experience a recurrent attack.
- Radiation proctitis may be associated with a significant decrease in health-related quality of life in up to 30% of patients.

COMPLICATIONS

- Chronic ulcerative colitis
- Fistula/abscess formation
- Treatment failure (may be as high as 35% in gonorrheal proctitis; check cultures and sensitivities)
- Perforation
- Radiation injury: Fistulas, strictures, obstruction, continued rectal mucosal bleeding, cystitis
- LGV infection: Hemorrhagic proctitis, rectal stricture
- Fecal incontinence

REFERENCES

1. CDC Sexually Transmitted Diseases Treatment Guidelines 2010; www.cdc.gov/std/treatment/2010/gonococcal-infections.htm.
2. Denton A, et al. Nonsurgical interventions for late radiation proctitis in patient who have received radical radiotherapy to the pelvis. *Cochrane Database Sys Rev*. 2002;1:CD003455.
3. Lawrance IC, et al. Topical agents for idiopathic distal colitis and proctitis. *J Gastroenterol Hepatol*. 2011;26:36–43.
4. Bennett MH, Feldmeier J, Hampson N, et al. Hyperbaric oxygen therapy for late radiation tissue injury. *Cochrane Database Syst Rev*. 2005; CD005005.

ADDITIONAL READING

- Cohen RD, Woseth DM, Thisted RA, et al. A meta-analysis and overview of the literature on treatment options for left-sided ulcerative colitis and ulcerative proctitis. *Am J Gastroenterol*. 2000;95: 1263–76.
- Hamlyn E, Taylor C. Sexually transmitted proctitis. *Postgrad Med J*. 2006;82:733–6.
- McMillan A, van Voorst Vader PC, de Vries HJ. The 2007 European Guideline (International Union against Sexually Transmitted Infections/World Health Organization) on the management of proctitis, proctocolitis and enteritis caused by sexually transmissible pathogens. *Int J STD AIDS*. 2007;18: 514–20.
- Regueiro MD, et al. Diagnosis and treatment of ulcerative proctitis. *J Clin Gastroenterol*. 2004;38: 733–40.
- Sutherland L, MacDonald JK, et al. Oral 5-aminosalicylic acid for maintenance of remission in ulcerative colitis. *Cochrane Database Syst Rev*. 2006;2:CD000544.

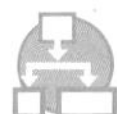

See Also (Topic, Algorithm, Electronic Media Element)

Crohn Disease; Gonococcal Infections; Herpes Simplex; Lymphogranuloma Venereum; Syphilis; Ulcerative Colitis

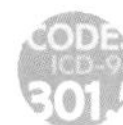

CODES

ICD9

- 556.2 Ulcerative (chronic) proctitis
- 569.49 Other specified disorders of rectum and anus

CLINICAL PEARLS

- Gonorrhea increasingly is resistant to antibiotics, and, as of April 2007, the CDC no longer recommends treatment with fluoroquinolones.
- If a patient has a true allergy to ceftriaxone, consider azithromycin 2 g PO in a single dose, but limit use. Do *not* use for simply a penicillin allergy (owing to concerns of the theoretical 5–10% cross-reactivity).
- For STI-related proctitis, consider expedited partner therapy (as permitted in your location).

PROSTATE CANCER

Kyle D. Wood, MD
Ilya Gorbachinsky, MD

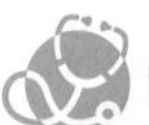

BASICS

DESCRIPTION

- The prostate is composed of acinar glands with their ducts arranged in a radial fashion and the stroma containing blood vessels, lymphatics, and nerves. Of prostate cancers (CaP), 95% are acinar adenocarcinomas.
- Only 3% of men with CaP die from the disease. Common metastatic locations (most to least common) are the pelvic lymph nodes, bone, lung, and liver.
- Staging: TNM classification (1)[C]:
  - Tx: Primary tumor cannot be assessed. T0: No evidence of primary tumor.
  - T1: Clinically inapparent tumor not palpable or visible by imaging. T1a: Tumor incidental histologic finding in ≤5% of tissue resected (by transurethral resection of prostate [TURP]). T1b: Tumor incidental histologic finding in >5% of tissue resected (by TURP). T1c: Tumor identified by needle biopsy (e.g., because of elevated prostate-specific antigen [PSA])
  - T2: Tumor confined within the prostate (*note:* Tumor found in one or both lobes by needle biopsy but not palpable or visible by imaging is classified as T1c). T2a: Tumor involves ≤1/2 of one lobe. T2b: Tumor involves >1/2 of one lobe, not both. T2c: Tumor involves both lobes.
  - T3: Tumor extends through the prostatic capsule (*Note:* Invasion into the prostatic apex or into [but not beyond] the prostatic capsule is still T2). T3a: Extracapsular extension (unilateral or bilateral). T3b: Tumor invades seminal vesicle(s).
  - T4: Tumor is fixed or invades adjacent structures other than seminal vesicles (e.g., bladder neck, external sphincter, rectum, levator muscles, and/or pelvic wall).
- Gleason grade: Tumors are graded from 1–5 based on the degree of glandular differentiation and structural architecture. Grade 1 represents the most well-differentiated appearance, and grade 5 represents the most poorly differentiated. Primary and secondary scores are reported and combined to form the combined Gleason score.
- System(s) affected: Reproductive; Urologic.
- Synonym(s): Carcinoma of the prostate (CaP)

EPIDEMIOLOGY

Mortality from CaP is decreasing.

Incidence

In the US, 200/100,000 men/yr

Prevalence

- The mean age at diagnosis is 71 years.
- Most common cancer in men (~17% lifetime risk) and second leading cause of cancer death in men (~3% of all CaP results in CaP-related death); however, autopsy studies find foci of latent CaP in 50% of men in their eighth decade.

RISK FACTORS

- Age >50 years, African American race, family history, baseline PSA above median for age group
- No increased risk of CaP postvasectomy per American Urological Association (AUA) policy statement
- Mixed data for CaP risk and presence of metabolic syndrome or coffee and alcohol consumption

ALERT

Obesity may be an indirect risk factor as obese men tend to have ↓ PSA levels and may subsequently undergo less PSA-driven biopsies

Genetics

~2 times ↑ risk with first-degree relative affected at age <50 years

GENERAL PREVENTION

- No level I evidence for diet or supplementation in CaP prevention:
  - Best available evidence:
    - May ↑ risk: Vitamin E supplementation, high calcium consumption
  - No dietary supplements reduce risk
- Reduction of risk of CaP with finasteride treatment
- Reduction by dutasteride of prostate cancer events (REDUCE) trial showed decreased risk of Gleason 5/6 CaP in treatment group.
- 5-α-reductase inhibitors are currently not FDA approved for CaP prevention; lower risk of low-grade disease but increases risk of high-grade CaP (2).

ALERT

- USPSTF: Screening for prostate cancer "D" recommendation; against screening for prostate cancer using PSA and DRE (digital rectal exam) as risks of morbidity and mortality outweigh survival benefit.
- Risk of dying from screening is greater than prior to screening. In the US in 1985 (before PSA), lifetime risk of prostate cancer diagnosis was 8.7% and a lifetime risk of 2.5% of dying from prostate cancer. In 2005, the risk of diagnosis is 17% and an increased (3% risk) of dying from prostate cancer (3)[B]

PATHOPHYSIOLOGY

- Adenocarcinoma: >95%
- Nonadenocarcinoma: <5% (most common transitional cell carcinoma)
- Cells often stain positive for PSA and PAP (prostatic acid phosphatase)
- Location of CaP: 70% peripheral zone, 20% transitional zone, 5–10% central zone, rarely in anterior fibromuscular zone
- Capsular penetration is most common near the neurovascular bundle.

DIAGNOSIS

HISTORY

- Inquire about family history of CaP, symptoms of bladder outlet obstruction (e.g., urinary retention), other voiding symptoms (e.g., frequency, hesitancy, etc.)
- Anorexia and weight loss, bone pain (with metastasis)
- Hematuria, hematospermia (rare)

PHYSICAL EXAM

If symptomatic, a DRE to assess for prostatic masses/firmness

DIAGNOSTIC TESTS & INTERPRETATION

Lab

- PSA is produced by prostatic epithelial cells.
- CaP and other conditions can distort the prostatic architecture, allowing more PSA to enter the bloodstream.

Initial lab tests

- Total PSA ≥4 ng/mL (sensitivity ~80%, specificity ~65% for CaP):
  - Rectal manipulation will not significantly increase PSA.
  - Ejaculation can alter total and free PSA levels. Men should abstain from sex for 24 hours prior to blood draw.
  - 5-α-reductase inhibitors (e.g., finasteride) decrease PSA ~50%; double result to compare with premedication results
  - Prostatitis/benign prostatic hyperplasia (BPH) can cause a PSA increase
- Patient-specific models to predict pathologic stage based on PSA, transrectal ultrasound (TRUS) biopsy results, and estimated clinical stage have been validated (4)[B].
- Age/race-adjusted "normal" PSA values:

Age	Asians	Blacks	Whites
40–49	0–2.0	0–2.0	0–2.5
50–59	0–3.0	0–4.0	0–3.5
60–69	0–4.0	0–4.5	0–4.5
70–79	0–5.0	0–5.5	0–6.5

Follow-Up & Special Considerations

- Total PSA velocity: ≥0.75 ng/mL/yr ↑ CaP suspicion
- Free PSA and age/race-adjusted PSA may be helpful in evaluating risk of CaP when total PSA is 4–10 ng/mL.
- Alkaline phosphatase associated with bony metastasis
- Consider prostate cancer if PSAD (PSA density) ≥0.15 or if PSA rises even while on 5-α-reductase inhibitors
- PSA/free PSA and probability of cancer:

PSA (ng/dL)	Cancer rate	% Free PSA	Cancer rate
0–2	1%	0–10%	56%
2–4	15%	10–15%	28%
4–10	25%	15–20%	20%
>10	>50%	20–25%	16%
		>25%	8%

Imaging

Initial approach

- Ultrasound-guided prostate biopsy: Indication: Abnormal DRE and/or ↑ PSA
- Bone scan: Positive with metastasis; indication: PSA ≥20 ng/mL, Gleason ≥8, or bone pain (5)[B].
- If PSA >20, locally advanced, or high-grade (Gleason ≥8) disease: CT scan to assess pelvic lymph nodes or MRI (with or without endorectal coil) to assess extracapsular extension may assist treatment planning.

Pathological Findings

Small, closely packed glandular tissue, loss of basement membrane, perineural invasion, and smaller prostate size are associated with higher grade disease.

DIFFERENTIAL DIAGNOSIS

- BPH, benign nodule prostate growth, subacute prostatitis, prostatic intraepithelial neoplasia
- Prostate stones

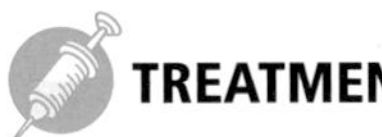

TREATMENT

A treatment decision should be reached after a long discussion about options, risks, and benefits:

- Treatment options:
  - T1a: Active surveillance may be appropriate
  - T1b, T1c: Candidate for prostatectomy, external-beam radiation, brachytherapy
  - T2a, T2b: Prostatectomy, external-beam radiation, brachytherapy
  - T3: Possible prostatectomy, possible radiation (generally with androgen ablation)
  - T4: Hormonal (androgen ablation) and/or radiation; chemotherapy at this time is reserved for hormone-refractory disease.
- Localized CaP:
  - Surveillance
  - Radical prostatectomy: Best overall survival, greatest survival benefit seen in patients <65 years old
  - External beam radiation
  - Brachytherapy: Not used to treat high-risk prostate cancer alone
  - Cryotherapy: Not used to treat high-risk prostate cancer alone
- Advanced or metastatic CaP:
  - Androgen deprivation by medical or surgical castration
  - Numerous ongoing trials evaluating surveillance vs. treatment: PIVOT, ProTeCT, StART

MEDICATION

First Line

- In androgen-dependent tumors, a reduction in serum testosterone reduces tumor size and bone pain and improves survival. Medical castration with gonadotropin-releasing hormone (GnRH) agonists (e.g., leuprolide or goserelin) is most commonly used. Bilateral orchiectomy is another option but is rarely done. Indication: ≥T3 at diagnosis, poor physical status, metastatic disease, patient preference (5)
- Side effects: Osteoporosis, gynecomastia, erectile dysfunction/decreased libido; flare phenomenon (disease flare) can occur owing to transient increase in testosterone levels on initiation of GnRH agonist therapy. It can be avoided by giving concurrent antiandrogen therapy for 21 days. Hot flashes, fatigue. May increase risk for metabolic syndrome, diabetes, and cardiovascular disease

Second Line

- Combined androgen blockade with GnRH agonist and antiandrogen (e.g., bicalutamide, nilutamide, or flutamide)
- Systematic androgen suppression: Ketoconazole has a 30% response rate in those failing other antiandrogens (via suppression of adrenal androgens).
- Castration-resistant disease: Most patients develop continued disease after androgen deprivation (either castration or GnRH therapy); continued hormonal treatment may be beneficial
- Chemotherapy with a docetaxel-based regimen has shown survival benefit and is the preferred first-line chemotherapy in castration-resistant metastatic prostate cancer. Mitoxantrone-based regimen is another option.
- Abiraterone (Zytiga): 1,000 mg/d PO given with prednisone 5 mg b.i.d. (NNT 25 for additional 4 months of overall survival)
- Bisphosphonate (zoledronic acid) every 4 weeks is recommended together with androgen-deprivation therapy or systemic chemotherapy for castration-recurrent metastatic prostate cancer. This may prevent disease-related skeletal complications such as pathologic fractures and spinal cord compression.

ADDITIONAL TREATMENT

Additional Therapies

- External-beam radiation therapy (XRT) for symptomatic bone metastasis
- Radioisotopes (e.g., samarium-153 and strontium-89) are approved for patients with multifocal symptomatic osteoblastic bone metastases that are not controllable with systemic therapy or local field XRT.

SURGERY/OTHER PROCEDURES

- Treatment options for localized CaP:
  - Active surveillance (6)[C]
  - Prostatectomy: Retropubic, robotic-assisted laparoscopic ± lymph node dissection; nerve-sparing surgery is possible if there is no extracapsular extension
  - Radiation therapy: External beam and/or brachytherapy—seed implantation
  - Cryoablation: Argon gas–based freezing of tissue; first for progression after failed XRT
- For clinically localized CaP (T1/T2), no data definitively proving the superiority among surgery, XRT, or brachytherapy. Consider age, physical status, side-effect profile, and patient preference (7)[B].

ONGOING CARE

FOLLOW-UP RECOMMENDATIONS

- CT/bone scan if suspected recurrence
- Prostatectomy: PSA/DRE every 6 months for 5 years; yearly thereafter; PSA >0.2 ng/mL after surgery is suggestive of recurrence
- XRT: PSA/DRE every 3 months for 1 year; every 3–6 months for 4 years; yearly thereafter; PSA ≥2 ng/mL from post-XRT nadir is suggestive of recurrence.

DIET

A low-fat diet, if strictly adhered to, may slow progression of prostate cancer.

PROGNOSIS

- Localized disease should be curable.
- Advanced disease has a favorable prognosis if lesions are hormone-sensitive.
- Advanced unresponsive disease progresses in 18 months, on average.
- Prostate cancer survival by stage:

Stage	TNM	10-year survival
A	T1	NC
B	T2	75%
C	T3	55%
D	N1–2	(70% at 7 years)
D	M1	15%

- Postoperative nomograms to predict patient-specific CaP recurrence rates after prostatectomy and XRT have been validated.

COMPLICATIONS

- Urinary incontinence, mild colitis, and erectile dysfunction are the most common.
- Treatment options for postoperative erectile dysfunction include phosphodiesterase inhibitors, intracavernosal/urethral injections, and an implantable penile prosthesis.

REFERENCES

1. Makarov DV, Trock BJ, Humphreys EB, et al. Updated nomogram to predict pathologic stage of prostate cancer given prostate-specific antigen level, clinical stage, and biopsy Gleason score (Partin tables) based on cases from 2000 to 2005. *Urology*. 2007;69:1095–101.
2. Kramer BS, Hagerty KL, Justman S, et al. Use of 5alpha-reductase inhibitors for prostate cancer chemoprevention: American Society of Clinical Oncology/American Urological Association 2008 Clinical Practice Guideline. *J Urol*. 2009;181: 1642–57.
3. Boyle P, Brawley OW, et al. Prostate cancer: Current evidence weighs against population screening. *CA Cancer J Clin*. 2009;59:220–4.
4. Partin AW. Combination of prostate specific antigen, clinical stage and Gleason score to predict pathological stage of localized prostate cancer: A multi-institutional update. *JAMA*. 1999;277: 1445–51.
5. National Comprehensive Cancer Network. Clinical practice guidelines: Prostate cancer. 2009. www.nccn.org.
6. Klotz L. Active surveillance versus radical treatment for favorable-risk localized prostate cancer. *Curr Treat Options Onc*. 2006;7(5):355–62.
7. Thompson I, et al. Guideline for the management of clinically localized prostate cancer: 2007 update. 2007. www.auanet.org.

ADDITIONAL READING

Agency for Healthcare Research and Quality. Available at: www.ahrq.gov.

CODES

ICD9

185 Malignant neoplasm of prostate

CLINICAL PEARLS

- Most men with CaP are asymptomatic.
- In patients taking 5-α-reductase inhibitors, multiply the measured PSA level by 2 to estimate the actual PSA.
- After nerve-sparing prostatectomy, urinary continence returns in <6 months (>50%), <9 months (~75%), and >12 months (~95%).
- The rate of erectile dysfunction:
  - After XRT: (~10–80%), brachytherapy (~15–60%).
  - After prostatectomy: Depends on age and if nerve-sparing surgery was performed. PDE5 drugs improve recovery.

PROSTATIC HYPERPLASIA, BENIGN (BPH)

David Longstroth, MD

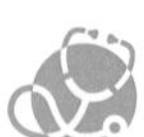

BASICS

- Increase in number of cells (both stroma and epithelial cell lines) within prostate, ultimately increasing its size.
- As it grows in volume, the central urethra may become compressed and narrowed, causing symptoms of obstruction and results in clinical symptoms (difficulty initiating urination, frequency, dysuria).
- May result in increased risk for upper and lower tract infections, and may progress to acute renal failure causing partial, or sometimes virtually complete, obstruction of the urethra, which interferes with the normal flow of urine

DESCRIPTION

- Benign prostatic hyperplasia (BPH) is one of the most common diseases of older men.
- Diagnosed histologically, characterized by an increase in the total number of stromal and epithelial cells within the prostate gland
- Associated with bothersome lower urinary tract symptoms (LUTS) that affect quality of life
- Disease affects the renal, urologic, and reproductive systems

EPIDEMIOLOGY

- In the US, near universal development in men, age-dependent
- Average prostate weighs 20 g in a normal 20–30-year-old male

Incidence

- No clear identifying characteristics
- Commonly involves prostate volume >30 mL and high prostate symptom score

Prevalence

From 8% in men aged 31–40; to 40–50% in men 51–60; and over 80% in men <80 years old

RISK FACTORS

- Increased risk of BPH with higher free prostate-specific antigen (PSA) levels, heart disease, and use of β-blockers
- Decreased risk with cigarette smoking, higher physical activity
- Intact testes (BPH rare in eunuchs)
- No evidence of increased or decreased risk with smoking, alcohol, or any dietary factors
- Low androgen levels from cirrhosis/chronic alcoholism can reduce the risk of BPH

Genetics

- Males who had a first-degree relative with BPH are at increased risk.
- Race has some influence on the risk for BPH severe enough to require surgery.
- Black men who are younger than 65 may need treatment more often than white men.
- Asians have a lower risk for nocturia, while risks for blacks and whites are similar.

GENERAL PREVENTION

The disease appears to be part of the aging process.

PATHOPHYSIOLOGY

- Older age and functional Leydig cells in testes are determinant.
- BPH is rare in men with hypogonadism onset before 40 years not treated with androgens.

ETIOLOGY

- BPH develops in the periurethral or transition zone of the prostate.
- Hyperplastic nodules of stromal and epithelial components increase glandular components.

COMMONLY ASSOCIATED CONDITIONS

- Lower urinary tract symptoms (LUTS):
  - LUTS can be divided into 3 groups: Filling/storage symptoms, voiding symptoms, and postmicturition symptoms
  - Filling/storage symptoms include frequency, nocturia, urgency, and urge incontinence.
  - Voiding: Irritative: Frequency, urgency, dysuria, nocturia; Obstructive symptoms: Poor stream, hesitancy, terminal dribbling, incomplete voiding, overflow incontinence
  - Post micturition: Leakage
- BPH symptoms are strong and independent risk factors for sexual dysfunction, including erectile dysfunction and ejaculatory disorders (1)[C].

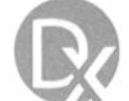

DIAGNOSIS

HISTORY

- Symptom scores such as American Urological Association (AUA). It consists of 7 questions, each of which is scored on a scale of 0 (not present) to 5 (almost always present). Symptoms are classified as mild (total score 0–7), moderate (total score 8–19), and severe (total score 20–35):
  - Frequency
  - Nocturia
  - Weak urinary stream
  - Hesitancy
  - Intermittence
  - Incomplete emptying
  - Urgency
- Gross hematuria
- History of type 2 diabetes, which can cause nocturia and is a risk factor for BPH
- Symptoms of neurologic disease that would suggest a neurogenic bladder
- Sexual dysfunction, which is correlated with LUTS
- History of urethral trauma, urethritis, or urethral instrumentation that could lead to urethral stricture
- Family history of BPH and prostate cancer
- Treatment with drugs that can impair bladder function (anticholinergic drugs) or increase outflow resistance (sympathomimetic drugs)

PHYSICAL EXAM

- Digital rectal exam finding of enlarged prostate, but *size does not always correlate with symptoms*
- Percussion to detect distended bladder, particularly if post-void
- Signs of renal failure due to obstructive uropathy (edema, pallor, pruritus, ecchymoses, nutritional deficiencies)

DIAGNOSTIC TESTS & INTERPRETATION

Lab

Initial lab tests

- PSA may be elevated, but usually <10 ng/mL (10 μg/L). Acute urinary retention, prostatitis, urinary tract instrumentation, or prostatic infarction may elevate PSA.
- Urinalysis: Pyuria if stones or infection present, pH changes due to chronic residual urine
- Urine culture positive (sometimes due to chronic residual urine)
- BUN and creatinine (if concerns for uremia)

Follow-Up & Special Considerations

- Uroflow: Volume voided per unit time (peak flow <10 mL/sec is abnormal)
- Post-void residual: Either with catheterization or bladder ultrasound (>100 mL demonstrates incomplete emptying)

Imaging

Initial approach

Postvoid residual in order to detect obstruction/distended bladder

Follow-Up & Special Considerations

- Transrectal ultrasound: Assessment of gland size; not necessary in the routine evaluation
- Abdominal ultrasound: Can demonstrate increased postvoid residual or hydronephrosis; not necessary in the routine evaluation

Geriatric Considerations

Drugs to be avoided include anticholinergics, antihistamines, sympathomimetics, tricyclic antidepressants, narcotics, and skeletal muscle relaxants when possible.

Diagnostic Procedures/Surgery

- Pressure-flow studies (urine flow vs. voiding pressures):
  - Best test to determine etiology of voiding symptoms
  - Obstructive pattern shows high voiding pressures with low flow rate
- Cystoscopy:
  - Demonstrates presence, configuration, cause (stricture, stone), and site of obstructive tissue
  - May help determine best minimally invasive therapeutic option
  - Not recommended in initial evaluation unless other factors such as hematuria are present

Pathological Findings

Confirmation obtained by biopsy, resection, or surgical removal

DIFFERENTIAL DIAGNOSIS

- Obstructive:
  - Prostate cancer
  - Urethral stricture or valves
  - Bladder neck contracture (usually secondary to prostate surgery)
  - Prostatitis
  - Inability of bladder neck or external sphincter to relax appropriately during voiding
- Neurologic:
  - Spinal cord injury
  - Stroke
  - Parkinsonism
  - Multiple sclerosis
- Medical:
  - Poorly controlled diabetes mellitus
  - Congestive heart failure (CHF)
- Pharmacologic:
  - Diuretics
  - Sympathomimetics (e.g., cold medications)
  - Anticholinergics
- Other:
  - Bladder carcinoma
  - Overactive bladder
  - Bladder calculi
  - UTI

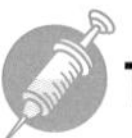

TREATMENT

MEDICATION

The AUA recommends watchful waiting for patients with mild symptoms or without bothersome LUTS who have not developed a serious complication.

First Line

- α-adrenergic antagonists more effective than other methods alone (2)[A]:
  - Nonselective, reduce prostatic smooth muscle tone, improving urinary flow (3):
    - Terazosin (Hytrin): 1–10 mg/d PO (4)[A]
    - Doxazosin (Cardura): 1–8 mg/d PO
  - Selective, may produce fewer side effects. Generally more expensive:
    - Tamsulosin (Flomax): 0.4 mg/d PO (5)[A]
    - Alfuzosin (Uroxatral): 10 mg/d PO
- 5-α-reductase inhibitors reduce prostatic volume (useful if prostatic enlargement) (6)[A]:
  - Finasteride (Proscar): 5 mg/d PO
  - Dutasteride (Avodart): 0.5 mg/d PO
  - Also useful in controlling prostatic bleeding
- Combination therapy of α-blocker plus 5-α-reductase inhibitor is superior to monotherapy when used for very large prostates and evaluated over at least 4.5 years (7):
  - Dutasteride and tamsulosin combination known as Jalyn
- Contraindications:
  - α-blockers can cause orthostatic hypotension; less risk with tamsulosin and alfuzosin
  - See specific recommendations for α-blocker use with phosphodiesterase type-5 inhibitors (for erectile dysfunction).

ALERT

5-α-reductase inhibitors reduce PSA by 1/2, so the PSA result should be doubled for purposes of screening for prostate cancer.

ADDITIONAL TREATMENT

General Measures

- Patients in urinary retention require bladder drainage.
- If catheterization is difficult, consider coude catheter or flexible cystoscopy.
- Consider possible postobstructive diuresis; if present, monitor electrolytes.
- Avoid prolonged periods of not voiding.
- Avoid sympathomimetic and anticholinergic medications.

Issues for Referral

- Recurrent UTIs
- Hematuria
- Failure to respond to medical therapy
- Bladder stones

COMPLEMENTARY AND ALTERNATIVE MEDICINE

- Phytotherapy
- Saw palmetto (Serenoa repens) may provide mild improvement of peak flow rates and appears to work by blocking 5-α-reductase.

SURGERY/OTHER PROCEDURES

- Indications for surgery:
  - Urinary retention due to prostatic obstruction, recurrent
  - Intractable symptoms due to prostatic obstruction AUA score >8 and symptoms
  - Obstructive uropathy (renal insufficiency)
  - Recurrent or persistent UTIs due to prostatic obstruction
  - Recurrent gross hematuria due to enlarged prostate
  - Bladder calculi
- Surgical procedures:
  - Transurethral resection of the prostate (TURP): Gold standard
  - Open prostatectomy: Treatment of choice for patients with extremely large prostates (>100 g)
  - Transurethral incision of the prostate: Treatment of choice for men with obstruction and small prostates
  - Transurethral laser ablation: Holmium laser ablation of the tissue; useful in patients on anticoagulant therapy
  - Transurethral needle ablation: Office-based minimally invasive approach usually used with small prostates
  - Transurethral microwave thermotherapy: Office-based minimally invasive approach usually used with small prostates
  - Transurethral laser resection/enucleation
  - UroLume stent placement: Not a primary treatment alternative for the standard patient, but considered in those too ill for other surgical procedures
- Complications of TURP:
  - Bleeding can be significant.
  - TUR syndrome: Hyponatremia secondary to absorption of hypotonic irrigant
  - Retrograde ejaculation
  - Urinary incontinence

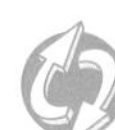

ONGOING CARE

FOLLOW-UP RECOMMENDATIONS

The patient is more likely to void after surgery or illness when ambulatory/able to stand over toilet.

Patient Monitoring

- Symptom index (IPSS) monitored every 3–12 months
- Digital rectal exam yearly
- PSA yearly: Should not be checked while patient is in retention, recently catheterized, or within a week of any surgical procedure to the prostate
- Consider monitoring postvoid residual if elevated.

DIET

Avoid large boluses of oral or IV fluids or alcohol intake.

PATIENT EDUCATION

National Kidney and Urologic Diseases Information Clearinghouse, Box NKUDIC, Bethesda, MD 20893; (301) 468-6345

PROGNOSIS

- Symptoms improve or stabilize in 70–80% of patients; 20–30% require treatment because of worsening symptoms.
- 25% of men with LUTS will have persistent storage symptoms after prostatectomy.
- Of men with BPH, 11–33% have occult prostate cancer.

COMPLICATIONS

- Urinary retention (acute or chronic)
- Bladder stones
- Prostatitis
- Renal failure
- Hematuria

REFERENCES

1. Rosen R, Altwein J, Boyle P. Lower urinary tract symptoms and male sexual dysfunction: The multinational survey of the aging male (MSAM-7). *Eur Urol*. 2003;44:637–49.
2. Rich KT. FPIN's clinical inquiries. Medical treatment of benign prostatic hyperplasia. *Am Fam Physician*. 2008;77:665–6.
3. Neal RH, Keister D. What's best for your patient with BPH? *J Fam Pract*. 2009;58:241–7.
4. Wilt TJ. Terazosin for benign prostatic hyperplasia. *Cochrane Database Syst Rev*. 2002;4:CD003851.
5. Wilt TJ. Tamsulosin for benign prostatic hyperplasia. *Cochrane Database Syst Rev*. 2003;1:CD002081.
6. AUA Guidelines: Guideline on the Management of Benign Prostatic Hyperplasia (BPH): Updated 2006. www.AUAnet.org.
7. Hollingsworth JM, Wei JT. Does the combination of an alpha1-adrenergic antagonist with a 5alpha-reductase inhibitor improve urinary symptoms more than either monotherapy? *Curr Opin Urol*. 2010;20:1–6.

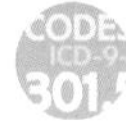

CODES

ICD9

- 600.20 Benign localized hyperplasia of prostate without urinary obstruction and other LUTS
- 600.21 Benign localized hyperplasia of prostate with urinary obstruction and other LUTS

CLINICAL PEARLS

- Although medical therapy has changed the management of BPH, it has only delayed the need for TURP by 10–15 years, not eliminated it.
- Urinary retention, obstructive uropathy, recurrent UTIs, bladder calculi, and recurrent hematuria are indications for surgical management of BPH.
- Indications for referral include recurrent UTIs, elevated PSA, failure of medical therapy, hematuria, retention, and patient desire.

PROSTATITIS

Alfred Chege Gitu, MD

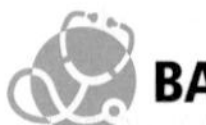

BASICS

DESCRIPTION

- Inflammatory or painful condition affecting the prostate gland; variety of etiologies
- National Institutes of Health's (NIH) prostatitis classification:
  - Acute infection (NIH class I): Febrile illness with perineal pain, dysuria, and obstructive symptoms
  - Chronic bacterial prostatitis (NIH class II): Recurrent infection with pain and voiding disturbances
  - Chronic abacterial prostatitis/chronic pelvic pain syndrome (NIH class III):
    - Inflammatory (NIH class IIIa): Significant inflammatory cells in prostatic secretions, postprostatic massage urine or semen
    - Noninflammatory (NIH class IIIb): Insignificant number of inflammatory cells (prostatosis)
  - Asymptomatic inflammatory prostatitis (NIH class IV): Incidental finding during prostate biopsy for infertility, cancer workup
- System(s) affected: Renal/Urologic; Reproductive

EPIDEMIOLOGY

Incidence

- 2 million cases annually in the US
- Predominant age: 30–50 years, sexually active; chronic more common in ages >50 years of age
- Bacterial prostatitis occurs more frequently in patients with HIV.

Prevalence

2.2–9.7% of male population

RISK FACTORS

- Age >50 years
- Prostate biopsy (especially in patients with prior exposure to quinolones) (1)
- Prostatic calculi
- UTI
- Trauma (e.g., bicycle, horseback riding)
- Dehydration
- Sexual abstinence
- Chronic indwelling catheter
- Intermittent catheterization
- HIV infection
- Urethral stricture
- Cystoscopy
- Urethral dilatation
- Transurethral resection of prostate

GENERAL PREVENTION

- Suppression therapy may benefit patients with chronic bacterial prostatitis.
- Antibiotic prophylaxis and enema prior to prostatic biopsy

PATHOPHYSIOLOGY

- Extension of UTI
- May occur following manipulation/biopsy of prostate or urethra
- Ascending infection through urethra

ETIOLOGY

- Infectious: NIH classes I and II:
  - Aerobic gram-negative bacteria (e.g., *E. coli, Klebsiella, Proteus, Pseudomonas, N. gonorrhoeae, B. pseudomallei*)
  - Miscellaneous: *C. trachomatis, Ureaplasma*, trichomoniasis
  - Gram-positive bacteria (*S. faecalis, S. aureus*)
  - Organisms suspected but unproven (*S. epidermidis, S. micrococci*, non–group D *Streptococcus*, diphtheroids)
  - Uncommon: *M. tuberculosis*, parasitic, mycoses (blastomycosis, coccidioidomycosis, cryptococcus, histoplasmosis, paracoccidiomycosis, candidiasis)
- Nonbacterial: Cause unknown: Leading theory suggests nonrelaxation (spasm) of the internal urinary sphincter and pelvic floor striated muscles leading to increased prostatic urethral pressure and intraprostatic urinary reflux.

COMMONLY ASSOCIATED CONDITIONS

- Prostatic hypertrophy
- Cystitis
- Urethritis
- Pyelonephritis
- Sexual dysfunction

DIAGNOSIS

HISTORY

- Acute prostatitis (NIH class I):
  - Fever, chills, malaise
  - Low back pain, myalgias
  - Prostatodynia, perineal pain
  - Obstructive voiding symptoms
  - Frequency, urgency, dysuria, nocturia
- Chronic prostatitis (NIH classes II and III):
  - Prostatodynia, perineal pain
  - Dysuria, irritative voiding
  - Lower abdominal pain
  - Low back, scrotal, and/or penile pain
  - Pain on ejaculation
  - Hematospermia

PHYSICAL EXAM

- Very tender boggy prostate on rectal exam
- Prostate may be warm, swollen, firm, or irregular.

ALERT

Avoid massage of the prostate in acute bacterial prostatitis; may induce iatrogenic bacteremia.

DIAGNOSTIC TESTS & INTERPRETATION

Lab

Initial lab tests

- Suspected acute prostatitis (NIH class I):
  - Urinalysis (UA), urine and blood cultures, urine Gram stain
  - CBC with differential
- Suspected chronic bacterial prostatitis or abacterial prostatitis (NIH class II or III):
  - Fractional urine exam (4-glass test) (2)[B],(3)[A]:
    - VB1 (voided bladder 1): Initial 10 mL urine from urethra
    - VB2: Next 200 mL discarded; then midstream urine from bladder
    - EPS: Expressed prostate secretion after prostate massage
    - VB3: Urine *after* prostate massage
  - Post-VB3 semen culture increases sensitivity and specificity (3)[A].
  - Many clinicians employ 2-glass test (VB2 and VB3) only (2)[B].
  - Specimen handling:
    - UA, culture, sensitivities, Gram stain on all samples
    - pH of EPS
    - Bacterial antigen-specific IgA and IgG levels in EPS
    - Wet mount of EPS
  - Interpretation:
    - 10–15 WBCs per high-powered field in VB3 suggest bacterial prostatitis.
    - Macrophages containing fat (oval bodies) suggest bacterial prostatitis.
    - A positive culture in EPS, VB3, or post a VB3 semen sample but not VB1 or VB2 is diagnostic of bacterial prostatitis.
    - In acute bacterial prostatitis, serum and EPS fluid bacterial antigen-specific IgA and IgG can be detected immediately after the onset of the infection. Level declines over 6–12 months after successful antibiotic therapy.
    - Bacteria count is less in chronic prostatitis.
    - In chronic bacterial prostatitis, no serum IgG elevation is seen, whereas EPS fluid IgA and IgG levels are increased. With antibiotic therapy, IgG levels return to normal in several months, but IgA levels remain elevated for 2 years.
    - Prostatic fluid is alkaline in chronic bacterial prostatitis.
    - Inflammatory cells (WBCs) with a negative culture (although false-negative cultures are not uncommon) suggest abacterial prostatitis.
    - No abnormal findings with chronic prostatitis without inflammation (this misnomer refers to patients with symptoms such as perineal pain, ejaculatory pain, and lower abdominal pain but no inflammatory changes on lab studies).
    - Prostate-specific antigen (PSA) level is increased with acute prostatitis (do not order until at least 1 month after prostatitis is treated).
- Drugs that may alter lab results: Antibiotics

Follow-Up & Special Considerations

- Acute bacterial: Urinalysis and culture 30 days after initiating treatment
- Chronic bacterial: Urinalysis and culture every 30 days (may take several months of treatment to clear)

Imaging

Initial approach

- Imaging not required in most cases
- CT or MRI if malignancy or abscess suspected
- Transrectal ultrasound if prostatic calculi or abscess suspected

Diagnostic Procedures/Surgery

- Needle biopsy or aspiration for culture
- Urodynamic testing (prostatodynia)
- Cystoscopy (in persistent nonbacterial prostatitis to rule out bladder cancer, interstitial cystitis)

DIFFERENTIAL DIAGNOSIS

- Cystitis (bacterial, interstitial)
- Urethritis
- Pyelonephritis
- Malignancy
- Obstructive calculus
- Foreign body
- Acute urinary retention

TREATMENT

MEDICATION

First Line

- Acute bacterial (outpatient) (4)[A]:
  - Fluoroquinolone (ciprofloxacin 500 mg PO q12h or levofloxacin 500 mg PO once daily) × 4–6 weeks or
  - Trimethoprim-sulfamethoxazole, 1 DS tab b.i.d. PO × 4–6 weeks or
  - If gram-positive cocci are seen in initial urine Gram stain, start with amoxicillin 500 mg PO q8h. Adjust antibiotics once culture and sensitivities report is available.
  - Local sensitivity pattern should guide therapy.
- Acute bacterial (inpatient):
  - Ampicillin 1–3 g IV divided q6h or fluoroquinolone (ciprofloxacin 400 mg IV q12h or levofloxacin 750 mg q24h) PLUS aminoglycoside, gentamicin 2 mg/kg IV loading dose, 1.7 mg/kg IV q8h maintenance; begin oral therapy after afebrile for 24–48 hours.
- Chronic bacterial (NIH class II) (5)[B]:
  - Fluoroquinolone (e.g., levofloxacin 500 mg PO once daily for 4 weeks (6,7)[A], or ciprofloxacin 500 mg b.i.d. PO for 4–12 weeks
  - Combination therapy with azithromycin may help to eradicate unusual pathogens.
  - Anti-inflammatory agents for pain symptoms and alpha-adrenergic receptor antagonists for urinary symptoms
- Chronic abacterial prostatitis (NIH class III):
  - No universally effective treatment
  - Treatment choice is usually by trial and error (8):
    - α-blockers, antibiotics, and combinations of these therapies achieve greatest improvement in clinical symptom scores (9)[A].
    - α-blockers better than placebo in some trials (10)[A]
    - Tamsulosin 0.2 mg PO once daily at bedtime for at least 6 months. Continue if there is a response (11)[A].
- Contraindications: Drug allergies
- Precautions:
  - Renal disease
  - Hepatic disease
  - Glucose-6-phosphate dehydrogenase deficiency may manifest with sulfonamides or NSAIDs.
  - Significant possible interactions: Fluoroquinolones, magnesium/aluminum antacids, theophylline, probenecid, NSAIDs, warfarin

Second Line

- Piperacillin or ticarcillin with aminoglycoside, erythromycin, tetracycline, cephalexin, fluoroquinolones, dicloxacillin, nafcillin IV, vancomycin IV
- Finasteride (in patients >45 years of age, category IIIa inflammatory chronic prostatitis/chronic pelvic pain syndrome, and enlarged prostate glands)
- Nonbacterial: May benefit from erythromycin, doxycycline, trimethoprim-sulfamethoxazole

ADDITIONAL TREATMENT

General Measures

- Analgesics/antipyretics/stool softeners
- Some anecdotal data suggest that elimination of caffeine may reduce symptoms of chronic prostatitis in younger men.
- Hydration
- Sitz baths to relieve pain and spasm
- Suprapubic catheter for urinary retention
- Anxiolytics, antidepressants

Issues for Referral

Urology referral for surgical drainage if an abscess is persistent after ≥1 week of therapy

Additional Therapies

Psychotherapy if sexual dysfunction

COMPLEMENTARY AND ALTERNATIVE MEDICINE

Neuromodulation, acupuncture, heat therapy; limited data to support

SURGERY/OTHER PROCEDURES

Surgical resection for intractable chronic disease or to drain an abscess

IN-PATIENT CONSIDERATIONS

Admission Criteria

- Proven or suspected abscess
- Unstable vital signs (sepsis)
- Immunocompromised

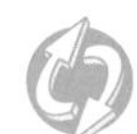

ONGOING CARE

FOLLOW-UP RECOMMENDATIONS

- Most improve in 3–4 weeks.
- Consider prostatic abscess in patients who do not respond well to therapy.

Patient Monitoring

- NIH Chronic Prostatitis Symptom Index: 13 items tabulated into 3 domain scores:
  - Pain
  - Urinary symptoms
  - Quality of life
- See www2.niddk.nih.gov

PROGNOSIS

- Often prolonged and difficult to cure; 55–97% cure rate depending on population and drug used
- 20% have reinfection or persistent infection.

COMPLICATIONS

- Prostatic abscess (common in HIV-infected)
- Gram-negative sepsis, bacteremia
- Urinary retention
- Epididymitis
- Chronic bacterial prostatitis (with acute prostatitis)
- Metastatic infection (spinal, sacroiliac)

REFERENCES

1. Mosharafa AA, Torky MH, Said WM, et al. Rising incidence of acute prostatitis following prostate biopsy: Fluoroquinolone resistance and exposure is a significant risk factor. *Urology*. 2011;78(3):511–4.
2. Benway BM, Moon TD, et al. Bacterial prostatitis. *Urol Clin North Am*. 2008;35:23–32; v.
3. Magri V, Wagenlehner FM, Montanari E, et al. Semen analysis in chronic bacterial prostatitis: Diagnostic and therapeutic implications. *Asian J Androl*. 2009;11:461–77.
4. Lipsky BA, Byren I, Hoey CT, et al. Treatment of bacterial prostatitis. *Clin Infect Dis*. 2010;50:1641–52.
5. Murphy AB, Macejko A, Taylor A, et al. Chronic prostatitis: Management strategies. *Drugs*. 2009;69:71–84.
6. Paglia M, Peterson J, Fisher AC, et al. Safety and efficacy of levofloxacin 750 mg for 2 weeks or 3 weeks compared with levofloxacin 500 mg for 4 weeks in treating chronic bacterial prostatitis. *Current Med Res Opin*. 2010;26(6):1433–41.
7. Naber KG, Roscher K, Botto H, et al. Oral levofloxacin 500 mg once daily in the treatment of chronic bacterial prostatitis. *Int J Antimicrob Agents*. 2008;32:145–53.
8. McNaughton CM, et al. Interventions for abacterial prostatitis. *Cochrane Database Sys Rev*. 2006:4.
9. Anothaisintawee T, Attia J, Nickel JC, et al. Management of chronic prostatitis/chronic pelvic pain syndrome: A systematic review and network meta-analysis. *JAMA*. 2011;305(1):78–86. Review.
10. Dimitrakov, et al. Management of chronic prostatitis/chronic pelvic pain syndrome: An evidence based approach. *Urology*. 2006;67(5).
11. Chen Y, Wu X, Liu J, et al. Effects of a 6-month course of tamsulosin for chronic prostatitis/chronic pelvic pain syndrome: A multicenter, randomized trial. *World J Urol*. 2011;29(3):381–5.

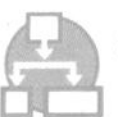

See Also (Topic, Algorithm, Electronic Media Element)

- Prostate Cancer; Prostatic Hyperplasia Benign (BPH); Urinary Tract Infection (UTI) in Males
- Algorithm: Hematuria

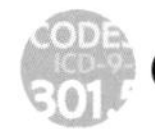

CODES

ICD9

- 601.0 Acute prostatitis
- 601.1 Chronic prostatitis
- 601.9 Prostatitis, unspecified

CLINICAL PEARLS

- Prostatic massage is contraindicated in acute prostatitis.
- Antibiotic therapy is not proven to be effective in chronic abacterial prostatitis (NIH class III).
- At least 30 days of antibiotic therapy is required for acute prostatitis.

PROTEIN C DEFICIENCY

Marc Jeffrey Kahn, MD, MBA
Rebecca Kruse-Jarres, MD, MPH

BASICS

DESCRIPTION

- Protein C is a vitamin K–dependent factor made by the liver that becomes activated when thrombin binds to the endothelial receptor thrombomodulin.
- Activated protein C, with protein S as a cofactor, inactivates factors Va and VIIIa.
- Patients with protein C deficiency have a thrombotic disorder that primarily affects the venous system, but can also affect the arterial system.
- System(s) affected: Cardiovascular; Hemic/Lymphatic/Immunologic; Pulmonary

EPIDEMIOLOGY

Prevalence

- 0.3% of normal individuals
- 4–5% of persons with VT
- Predominant age: Mean age of first thrombosis is 45 years.
- Predominant sex: Male = Female

RISK FACTORS

Genetics

Patients heterozygous for protein C deficiency who start warfarin without concomitant heparin can develop warfarin-induced skin necrosis because the half-life of other vitamin K–dependent clotting factors, prothrombin, factor IX, and factor X is much longer than that of protein C (4–8 hours). These patients develop extremely low levels of protein C and develop necrosis of the skin over central areas of the body such as the breast, abdomen, buttocks, and genitalia (1)[A].

GENERAL PREVENTION

Since protein C deficiency is a congenital disease, there are no preventive measures.

ETIOLOGY

- Polymorphisms in the promoter region of the protein C gene can affect antigen levels. At least 150 mutations have been described in the protein C gene that can lead to functional deficiency.
- Acquired protein C deficiency can occur with liver disease, and rare patients can develop inhibitors to activated protein C. Neonates have lower levels of protein C than adults.

COMMONLY ASSOCIATED CONDITIONS

- Deep and superficial venous thrombosis, often spontaneous
- Up to 50% of homozygotes will have thrombosis.
- Homozygosity is associated with catastrophic thrombotic complications at birth: *Purpura fulminans*
- Sites of thrombosis can be unusual, including the mesentery and cerebral veins.
- Arterial thrombosis is rare.
- Skin necrosis can be seen in patients on warfarin.

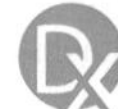

DIAGNOSIS

HISTORY

- Venous thrombosis at age <40 year without another etiology
- Thrombosis in unusual locations (e.g., mesentery, sagittal sinus, portal vein)
- Family history of thrombosis or spontaneous abortion

PHYSICAL EXAM

Normal

DIAGNOSTIC TESTS & INTERPRETATION

Lab

Initial lab tests

- For evaluation of new clot in patient at risk (see "History"): CBC with peripheral smear, PT/INR, aPTT, thrombin time, lupus anticoagulant, antiphospholipid antibodies, factor VIII, anticardiolipin antibody, anti-B2 glycoprotein I antibody, activated protein C resistance, protein S antigen and resistance, antithrombin III assay, fibrinogen, factor V Leiden, prothrombin G20210A, homocysteine
- Protein C activity assay using a snake venom protease to activate protein C
- Immunoassay for quantitative assessment of protein C level
- Drugs that may alter lab results:
  - Oral contraceptives can raise protein C levels.
  - Warfarin reduces protein C levels.
  - Patients should be off warfarin for 2–3 weeks before reliable testing (2)[C].
- Disorders that may alter lab results:
  - Liver disease reduces protein C levels.
  - Acute thrombosis can lower protein C levels. Repeat confirmatory test of low protein C level at a separate time is advisable.

DIFFERENTIAL DIAGNOSIS

- Factor V Leiden (causes resistance to activated protein C, not a deficiency of protein C)
- Protein S deficiency
- Antithrombin deficiency
- Dysfibrinogenemia
- Dysplasminogenemia
- Homocystinemia
- Prothrombin 20210 mutation
- Elevated factor VIII levels

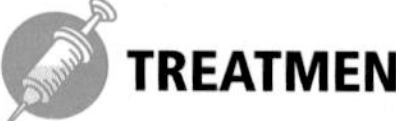

TREATMENT

Of active thrombosis and follow-up period

MEDICATION

First Line

- Low-molecular-weight heparin (LMWH) (1)[A]: Continue until therapeutic on warfarin and for at least 5 days:
  - Enoxaparin (Lovenox) 1 mg/kg SC b.i.d.
- Alternatively, enoxaparin 1.5 mg/kg/d SC, which is slightly less effective. Continue until therapeutic on warfarin and for at least 5 days:
  - Fondaparinux (Arixtra): 7.5 mg SC every day
  - Tinzaparin (Innohep): 175 anti-Xa IU/kg/d SC
  - Dalteparin (Fragmin): 200 units/kg/d
- Oral anticoagulant: Warfarin (Coumadin) 5 mg/d PO initially and maintained on warfarin with an INR of 2–3 for at least 3–6 months (1)[A]
- Contraindications:
  - Active bleeding precludes anticoagulation; risk of bleeding is a relative contraindication to long-term anticoagulation.
  - Warfarin is contraindicated in patients with a prior history of warfarin-induced skin necrosis.
- Precautions:
  - Observe patient for signs of embolization, further thrombosis, or bleeding.
  - Avoid IM injections.
  - Periodically check stool and urine for occult blood, monitor CBC, including platelets.
  - Heparin: Thrombocytopenia and/or paradoxical thrombosis with thrombocytopenia
  - Warfarin: Necrotic skin lesions (typically breasts, thighs, and buttocks)
  - LMWH: Adjust dose in renal insufficiency.
- Significant possible interactions:
  - Agents that intensify the response to oral anticoagulants: Alcohol, allopurinol, amiodarone, anabolic steroids, androgens, many antimicrobials, cimetidine, chloral hydrate, disulfiram, all NSAIDs, sulfinpyrazone, tamoxifen, thyroid hormone, vitamin E, ranitidine, salicylates, acetaminophen
  - Agents that diminish the response to oral anticoagulants: Aminoglutethimide, antacids, barbiturates, carbamazepine, cholestyramine, diuretics, griseofulvin, rifampin, oral contraceptives

Second Line

- Heparin 80 mg/kg IV bolus followed by 18 mg/kg/hr; adjust dose depending on PPT.
- In patients requiring large daily doses of heparin, measure an anti-Xa level for dose guidance.
- Alternatively, unfractionated heparin can be given at 35,000 U/24 hr SC, with subsequent dosing to maintain a therapeutic aPTT (3)[C].

ADDITIONAL TREATMENT

General Measures

- Routine anticoagulation for asymptomatic patients with protein C deficiency is not recommended (1)[A].
- Anticoagulation for 6–12 months is recommended for patients with protein C deficiency and a first thrombosis.
- Some argue for lifetime anticoagulation; data are limited.
- Anticoagulation for life is indicated for patients with protein C deficiency and recurrent thromboses.
- The role of family screening for protein C deficiency is unclear because most patients with this mutation do not have thrombosis. Screening should be considered for women considering using oral contraceptives or pregnancy with a family history of protein C deficiency (4)[B].
- Treatment with LMWH is recommended over unfractionated heparin, unless the patient has severe renal failure (3)[B].
- Treat as outpatient, if possible (3)[B].
- Initiate warfarin together with heparin on the first treatment day and discontinue heparin after 5 days and when INR >2 (3)[A].

Issues for Referral

Patients with suspected protein C deficiency should be seen by a hematologist.

SURGERY/OTHER PROCEDURES

- Anticoagulation must be held for surgical interventions.
- For most patients with DVT, recommendations are against routine use of vena cava filter in addition to anticoagulation (3)[A].

IN-PATIENT CONSIDERATIONS

Admission Criteria

- Life-threatening VT
- Significant bleeding while on anticoagulant therapy

Nursing

Look for signs of bleeding while on anticoagulation therapy.

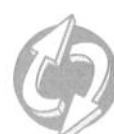

ONGOING CARE

FOLLOW-UP RECOMMENDATIONS

Patient Monitoring

- Warfarin requires periodic (monthly after initial stabilization) monitoring of the INR to maintain a range of 2–3.
- LMWH is the treatment of choice in pregnancy. Periodic monitoring with anti-Xa levels is recommended in these patients.

DIET

Unrestricted

PATIENT EDUCATION

- Patients should be educated about use of oral anticoagulant therapy if taking such.
- Avoid NSAIDs while on warfarin.

PROGNOSIS

- When compared with normal individuals, persons with protein C deficiency have normal life spans.
- By age 45, 50% of the people heterozygous for protein C deficiency will have VT that is spontaneous half the time.

COMPLICATIONS

Recurrent thrombosis (requires indefinite anticoagulation)

REFERENCES

1. Bick RL. Prothrombin G20210A mutation, antithrombin, heparin cofactor II, protein C, and protein S defects. *Hematol Oncol Clin North Am*. 2003;17:9–36.
2. Moll S. Thrombophilias–practical implications and testing caveats. *J Thromb Thrombolysis*. 2006; 21:7–15.
3. Büller HR, Agnelli G, Hull RD, et al. Antithrombotic therapy for venous thromboembolic disease: The Seventh ACCP Conference on Antithrombotic and Thrombolytic Therapy. *Chest*. 2004;126: 401S–428S.
4. Langlois NJ, Wells PS. Risk of venous thromboembolism in relatives of symptomatic probands with thrombophilia: A systematic review. *Thromb Haemost*. 2003;90:17–26.

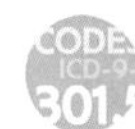

CODES

ICD9

289.81 Primary hypercoagulable state

CLINICAL PEARLS

- Asymptomatic patients with protein C deficiency do not need prophylactic anticoagulation because the risk of thrombosis is low.
- Patients with protein C deficiency who have DVT should be anticoagulated for at least 6 months.

PROTEIN ENERGY MALNUTRITION

Melissa Phillips Black, MD
Thomas Price, MD

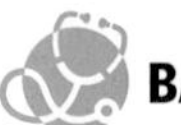

BASICS

DESCRIPTION

- Protein–energy malnutrition (PEM) is present when sufficient energy and/or protein is not available to meet metabolic demands, leading to impairment in normal physiologic processes. It highly associated with systemic inflammation (1).
- PEM affects all age groups and is often due to impaired access to proper nutrition.
- Malnutrition in children is a major underlying factor in ~5 million preventable deaths annually, with 2 distinct phenotypes:
  - *Marasmus* is a wasting condition resulting from deficiency of calories and protein. Weight is decreased relative to that expected for the patient's height/length.
  - *Kwashiorkor* is distinguished by generalized edema and is associated with low protein relative to caloric intake. Resulting fat deposition in liver results in ascites. Weight is normal or elevated due to increased body fluid.
- System(s) affected: Immunologic; Gastrointestinal; Endocrine/Metabolic; Hematologic; Musculoskeletal; Integumentary; Neurologic

EPIDEMIOLOGY

- Children:
  - Most commonly <5 years of age; both sexes are affected equally.
  - Globally, malnutrition increases morbidity and mortality from other common childhood diseases.
- Older patients:
  - Highest risk in population >75 years of age
  - Increased mortality and morbidity, including pressure ulcers, infection, and cognitive status changes (see "Delirium" topic).
- Malnutrition may be common, but it is difficult to recognize in hospital populations

Prevalence

- Worldwide, >70 million children suffer from moderate and severe acute malnutrition.
- Prevalence in older patients is between 29% and 61% of population.

RISK FACTORS

- Nutritional:
  - Prolonged and severe reduction of intake
  - Anorexia nervosa
- Underlying illnesses:
  - Fever, infection, trauma, burns, and other hypercatabolic states
  - Malabsorptive and maldigestive states
  - Protein-losing enteropathy, nephrotic syndrome, enteric fistulas
  - Metabolic disorders (diabetes, hyperthyroidism)
  - Chronic cardiac or lung disease, chronic inflammatory states
  - Psychiatric disorders (dementia, depression)
  - Any prolonged hospitalization (2)
- Other states in which requirements are increased:
  - Pregnancy and lactation
  - Growth and development during infancy, childhood, and adolescence

ALERT

Functional, financial, and social limitations may obstruct access to a nutritionally sound diet, particularly in geriatric and pediatric populations.

GENERAL PREVENTION

- Observation and recording of patients' nutritional intake and body mass index (BMI)
- In children, routine record of anthropomorphic measurements and developmental milestones
- Early recognition of increased nutritional requirements during stress, infection, and other medical illness
- Frequent interactions among physician, nurse, and dietitian to assess nutritional needs
- Emphasis on food security and nutritional education

ETIOLOGY

- Inadequate dietary intake
- Increased metabolic demands
- Increased nutrient losses

COMMONLY ASSOCIATED CONDITIONS

- Infection: Weakened immune system, predisposing to bacterial, viral, and parasitic infections
- Electrolyte disturbances: Loss of cellular integrity and diminished transmembrane pump activity; renal dysfunction
- Hypoglycemia: Decreased glycogen stores and increased glucose utilization (as in infection or trauma)
- Micronutrient deficiencies: Vitamins, including B complex, folic acid, iron, magnesium
- Wounds: Pressure ulcers in older patients (increased incidence if reduced mobility)

DIAGNOSIS

HISTORY

- Quantity and quality of nutritional intake
- Presence of GI tract disorders:
  - Early satiety, constipation, vomiting, diarrhea, dysphagia, dental and oral health problems
- Urine output (assess for dehydration)
- Chronic medical illness
- Weight loss, stunted growth, SC fat and muscle wasting
- Impaired work capacity, endurance, and muscle strength
- Falls and/or reduced physical activity
- Impaired concentration/cognitive function, delirium, or lethargy
- Delayed wound healing and recovery
- Subnormal heart rate, BP, and core body temperature
- In children:
  - Delayed puberty
  - Diminished cognitive and psychosocial development
- Medications that cause nausea, dry mouth, loss of appetite or taste distortion

PHYSICAL EXAM

- Clinical signs: Muscle wasting, peripheral edema, glossitis, cheilosis, loss of vibratory or position sense, sparse hair, nail spooning, night blindness, Bitot spots, loss of taste (2)
- Anthropomorphic measurements:
  - Weight (W) and height (H): In children, measure W:H; in adults, BMI <18.5 kg/m^2 in PEM.
  - Mid–upper arm circumference (MUAC):
    - In children 1–5 years of age, MUAC >125 mm is normal.
    - 110–125 mm corresponds to a state of mild or moderate malnutrition.
    - <110 mm corresponds to severe malnutrition.
    - In adults, MUAC <200 mm is suggestive of PEM.
  - Triceps skin-fold thickness
- Decreased hand grip strength
- Bioelectrical impedance analysis to estimate total body water and fat-free body mass
- Marasmic children: Thin, little SC fat. Wasting is evident at the shoulders, buttocks, arms, and thighs.
- Children with Kwashiorkor are irritable, with anasarca, sparse and brittle hair:
  - They can develop a "flaky paint" dermatosis characterized by blackish discoloration and excoriation.
  - Hepatomegaly from fatty infiltration may be present.
- Decreased SC tissue; with serum albumin <1 g/dL, anasarca

ALERT

- Commonly used markers of dehydration (i.e., dry mucous membranes, lack of tears, skin tenting) are not reliable in PEM.
- Poor immune function may make identification of superimposed infection difficult. Fevers, swelling, and redness are often absent.

DIAGNOSTIC TESTS & INTERPRETATION

Lab

Initial lab tests

- Diagnosis is often clinical in PEM-endemic countries (lack of laboratory resources).
- Pediatric patients:
  - Serum chemistries: Hypernatremia, hypokalemia, hypocalcemia, hypophosphatemia, hypomagnesemia
  - Hypoglycemia
  - Anemia, decreased lymphocyte count
  - Plasma albumin: Decreased
  - BUN: Decreased
  - Plasma transferrin: Decreased
  - Plasma cortisol, growth hormone: Increased, but insulin is low.
- Adult and elderly patients:
  - Serum albumin is affected by acute illness, and while not a specific marker of PEM, lower levels correlate with increased mortality.
  - Serum prealbumin measures PEM risk level:
    - >15 mg/dL: Normal
    - <15 to >11 mg/dL: Increased risk
    - <11 to >5 mg/dL: Significant risk
    - <5 mg/dL: Poor prognosis, high mortality

- Mild elevation of serum alkaline phosphatase
- Elevated CRP as a marker of inflammation (1)

Follow-Up & Special Considerations

- Prealbumin trends can be used to determine response to therapy. Biweekly measurements, in conjunction with monitoring body weight, are often recommended.
- In critically ill patients, blood glucose levels exceeding 180 mg/dL are associated with increased morbidity and mortality (3)[C].

Imaging

Initial approach

CXR: Evaluate for coexisting pneumonia, neoplasm, or tuberculosis. Cardiomegaly may be present (suggestive of cardiac failure; may result from marked anemia).

DIFFERENTIAL DIAGNOSIS

- In children, secondary growth failure due to malabsorption, congenital defects, or deprivation
- Pellagra (niacin deficiency = "4 Ds"): Diarrhea, dermatitis, dementia, death
- Nephritis or nephrosis
- Hypo- or hyperthyroidism
- Hyperparathyroidism
- Cardiac failure
- Neoplasm
- Viral or parasitic infection

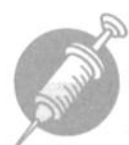

TREATMENT

MEDICATION

- Diet prescription in conjunction with a dietician or nutritionist
- Appetite stimulants (e.g., megestrol acetate, mirtazapine, oxandrolone, others) may be appropriate for short-term treatment of anorexia in adults but increase thromboembolic risk.
- Medications that have weight gain as a side effect (atypical antipsychotics, carbamazepine, gabapentin, corticosteroids, valproic acid, SSRIs, sulfonylureas, injectable medroxyprogesterone) may be used if otherwise indicated in patients with comorbid conditions.

ADDITIONAL TREATMENT

General Measures

- Slowly restore and maintain fluid and electrolyte balance.
- Initiate oral iron and folate supplements (begin iron therapy ~2 weeks after initiation of dietary treatment to avoid promotion of bacterial infection).
- Administer blood transfusion in the presence of severe anemia (hemoglobin <4–6 g/dL) or symptomatic moderate anemia.
- Ensure that immunizations are up to date (PEM is not a contraindication to vaccination).

Issues for Referral

Consider dentistry referral for oral disorders and speech therapy referral for dysphagia.

IN-PATIENT CONSIDERATIONS

Initial Stabilization

- Reversal of fluid and electrolyte imbalance should occur before IV nutrition, if any, is started.
- Continuous cardiac rhythm monitoring (telemetry) is recommended when electrolyte imbalance or acidosis is found on initial assessment.

Admission Criteria

- Hemodynamic instability
- Alteration of consciousness (delirium)
- Unsafe living environment (evidence of child/elder mistreatment)
- Profound hypokalemia or hypocalcemia
- Cardiac abnormalities/arrhythmia
- Anemia (hemoglobin <10 g/dL in older patients)

IV Fluids

Parenteral (IV) nutrition, which carries a high risk of associated infection, should be reserved for use in patients with severe GI tract dysfunction or anatomic disturbance (2).

Nursing

- Patients should be assessed for risk of pressure ulcer (using a Braden scale or other tool) and a skin care protocol initiated.
- Any patient admitted to hospital with malnutrition should have a nutritionist consult, if available.
- Physical therapy should be initiated once the patient is stable for assessment.

Geriatric Considerations

Older patients may require assistance with basic activities of daily living (ADLs) and are at high risk of injury due to falls.

Discharge Criteria

- Basic electrolyte abnormalities corrected to tolerance
- Patient demonstrates ability to maintain adequate oral intake of a nutritionally sound diet.
- Social and financial considerations have been identified and addressed.

Geriatric Considerations

Patient may need transfer to alternative level of care (e.g., skilled nursing home, rehabilitation center, etc.) temporarily for continued care depending on level of disability before returning safely home.

ONGOING CARE

FOLLOW-UP RECOMMENDATIONS

Children are discharged from a nutritional rehabilitation program when W:H ratio is >85%, at least 1 week of consistent weight gain has been achieved, and all disease conditions associated with PEM have been addressed.

Patient Monitoring

Frequent assessment until weight has stabilized (BMI >18.5 kg/m^2)

DIET

- Amino acid constituent and calorie-to-BMI-adjusted diet per dietician
- Refeeding of adults should occur slowly and, if possible, in consultation with a nutritionist.
- For children, initially provide 100 kcal/kg/d with 3 g/kg/d protein. When tolerated, advance to at least 200 kcal/kg/d with 5 g/kg/d protein:
  - Small, frequent feedings are preferred.
  - Consider low-lactose formulas to decrease diarrhea from disaccharidase deficiency.
  - Target growth: 10–15 g/kg/d
  - Supplement with vitamins and micronutrients, especially vitamin A and zinc.

PATIENT EDUCATION

- Emphasis on diet education
- In older patients, caregiver education and supervision may be relevant.

PROGNOSIS

- Excellent when PEM is identified early and managed aggressively
- Mortality varies between 15% and 40%.
- Compromised immune function returns to normal with recovery.
- Behavioral and mental issues may persist following treatment of severe cases.
- There is insufficient evidence that enteral tube feeding in patients with advanced dementia improves survival or lowers the prevalence of pressure ulcers (3)[A].

COMPLICATIONS

- Fatalities in the early days of treatment usually result from electrolyte imbalance, infection, hypothermia, or circulatory failure. Lethargy, anorexia, stupor, and petechiae are ominous signs.
- Patients who develop PEM have greater risk of hospital-acquired infection (2).

Pregnancy Considerations

Pregnant women with PEM are at risk of delivering a growth-restricted infant.

REFERENCES

1. Soeters PB, Schols AM, et al. Advances in understanding and assessing malnutrition. *Curr Opin Clin Nutr Metab Care*. 2009;12:487–94.
2. Ziegler TR, et al. Parenteral nutrition in the critically ill patient. *N Engl J Med*. 2009;361:1088–97.
3. Sampson EL, Candy B, Jones L, et al. Enteral tube feeding for older people with advanced dementia. *Cochrane Database Syst Rev*. 2009;CD007209.

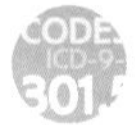

CODES

ICD9

- 260 Kwashiorkor
- 261 Nutritional marasmus
- 263.9 Unspecified protein-calorie malnutrition

CLINICAL PEARLS

- Malnutrition in children is a major underlying factor in ~5 million preventable deaths annually, with 2 distinct phenotypes:
  - Marasmus is a wasting condition resulting from deficiency of calories and protein. Weight is decreased relative to that expected for the patient's height/length.
  - Kwashiorkor is distinguished by generalized edema and is associated with low protein relative to caloric intake. Resulting fat deposition in liver causes ascites. Weight is normal or elevated due to increased body fluid.
- Older patients may experience elevated BUN levels if excessive protein supplementation is added to their diet; routine monitoring is suggested.

PROTEIN S DEFICIENCY

Marc Jeffrey Kahn, MD, MBA
Rebecca Kruse-Jarres, MD, MPH

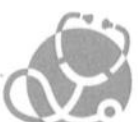

BASICS

DESCRIPTION

- Protein S is a vitamin K–dependent factor made principally by the liver that acts as a cofactor for protein C.
- Protein C becomes activated when thrombin binds to the endothelial receptor, thrombomodulin.
- Activated protein C, with protein S as a cofactor, inactivates clotting factors Va and VIIIa.
- Protein S is also able to directly inhibit factors Va, VIIa, and Xa independently of activated protein C.
- Patients with protein S deficiency have a thrombotic disorder that primarily affects the venous system.
- System(s) affected: Cardiovascular; Hematologic/Lymphatic/Immunologic; Pulmonary

EPIDEMIOLOGY

Incidence

- Predominant age: Mean age of first thrombosis is the second decade.
- Predominant sex: Male = Female

Prevalence

- 0.3% of normal individuals
- Found in 3% of persons with VT

RISK FACTORS

- Oral contraceptives, pregnancy, and the use of HRT increase the risk of VT in patients with protein S deficiency (1)[A].
- Patients with protein S deficiency and another prothrombotic state, such as factor V Leiden, have further increased rates of thrombosis (1)[A].
- Patients heterozygous for protein S deficiency who are begun on warfarin without concomitant heparin can develop warfarin-induced skin necrosis because the half-life of other vitamin K–dependent clotting factors (e.g., prothrombin, factor IX, and factor X) is much longer than the anticoagulant protein S (4–8 hours), leading to a transient hypercoagulable state when protein S becomes depleted. These patients develop extremely low levels of protein S and develop necrosis of the skin over central areas of the body such as the breast, abdomen, buttocks, and genitalia (1)[A].

Genetics

Autosomal dominant. Heterozygotes have an OR of VT of 1.6–11.5. Arterial thrombosis is more frequent in patients with protein S deficiency who smoke. Homozygotes can have a fulminant thrombotic event in infancy, termed *neonatal purpura fulminans*. Homozygosity or compound heterozygosity, if untreated, is usually incompatible with adult life.

Pregnancy Considerations

Increased thrombotic risk in patients with protein C deficiency

GENERAL PREVENTION

Since protein S deficiency is a congenital disease, there are no preventive measures.

ETIOLOGY

- >131 mutations in the protein S gene leading to an inherited protein S deficiency have been described. Protein S reversibly binds to the C4b-binding protein. Only the free form acts as a cofactor for activated protein C. This leads to conditions where free protein S is low, but total protein S is normal. These individuals are prone to thrombosis.
- Acquired protein S deficiency from decreased free protein S can occur during pregnancy; in patients taking oral contraceptives or warfarin; and in DIC, liver disease, nephrotic syndrome, inflammation, and acute thrombosis.
- Autoantibodies can develop to protein S in patients with acute varicella (2)[C].

COMMONLY ASSOCIATED CONDITIONS

- Deep and superficial VT, often spontaneous
- Up to 50% of homozygotes will have thrombosis.
- Homozygosity is associated with catastrophic thrombotic complications at birth: *Purpura fulminans*
- Sites of thrombosis can be unusual, including the mesentery and cerebral veins.
- Arterial thrombosis is rare.
- Skin necrosis can be seen in patients on warfarin.

DIAGNOSIS

HISTORY

Order testing for patients with VT at age <40 without another etiology; thrombosis in unusual locations (e.g., mesentery, sagittal sinus, portal vein) with a family history of thrombosis or spontaneous abortion.

PHYSICAL EXAM

Normal

DIAGNOSTIC TESTS & INTERPRETATION

Lab

Initial lab tests

- For evaluation of new clot in patient at risk: CBC with peripheral smear, PT/INR, aPTT, thrombin time, lupus anticoagulant, antiphospholipid antibodies, factor VIII, anticardiolipin antibody, anti-B2 glycoprotein I antibody, activated protein C resistance, protein S antigen and resistance, antithrombin III assay, fibrinogen, factor V Leiden, prothrombin G20210A, homocysteine
- Protein S activity assay
- Immunoassay for quantitative assessment of protein S level
- Disorders that may alter lab results: Liver disease and pregnancy reduce protein S levels.

DIFFERENTIAL DIAGNOSIS

- Factor V Leiden
- Protein C deficiency
- Antithrombin deficiency
- Dysfibrinogenemia
- Dysplasminogenemia
- Homocystinemia
- Prothrombin 20210 mutation
- Elevated factor VIII levels

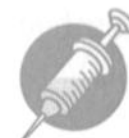

TREATMENT

MEDICATION

First Line

- Low-molecular-weight heparin (LMWH) (1)[A] initially for at least 5 days and until INR is 2–3, at which time it can be stopped:
  - Enoxaparin (Lovenox): 1 mg/kg SC b.i.d.:
    - Alternatively, 1.5 mg/kg/d SC. Initially for at least 5 days and until INR is 2–3, at which time it can be stopped.
  - Fondaparinux (Arixtra): 7.5 mg SC every day
  - Tinzaparin (Innohep): 175 anti-Xa IU/kg/d SC
  - Dalteparin (Fragmin): 200 IU/kg/d
- Oral anticoagulant: Warfarin (Coumadin): 5 mg/d PO initially and maintained on warfarin with an INR of 2–3 for at least 6 months (1)[A]
- Contraindications:
  - Active bleeding precludes anticoagulation; risk of bleeding is a relative contraindication to long-term anticoagulation.
  - Warfarin is contraindicated in patients with a prior history of warfarin-induced skin necrosis.
- Precautions:
  - Observe patient for signs of embolization, further thrombosis, or bleeding.
  - Avoid IM injections.
  - Periodically check stool and urine for occult blood, monitor CBC, including platelets.
  - Heparin: Thrombocytopenia and/or paradoxical thrombosis with thrombocytopenia
  - Warfarin: Necrotic skin lesions (typically breasts, thighs, and buttocks)
  - LMWH: Adjust dose in renal insufficiency.
- Significant possible interactions:
  - Agents that intensify the response to oral anticoagulants: Alcohol, allopurinol, amiodarone, anabolic steroids, androgens, many antimicrobials, cimetidine, chloral hydrate, disulfiram, all NSAIDs, sulfinpyrazone, tamoxifen, thyroid hormone, vitamin E, ranitidine, salicylates, acetaminophen
  - Agents that diminish the response to oral anticoagulants: Aminoglutethimide, antacids, barbiturates, carbamazepine, cholestyramine, diuretics, griseofulvin, rifampin, oral contraceptives

Second Line

Heparin 80 mg/kg IV bolus, followed by 18 mg/kg/hr; adjust dose depending on aPTT:

- In patients requiring large daily doses of heparin, measure an anti-Xa level for dose guidance.
- Alternatively, unfractionated heparin can be given at 35,000 U/24 hours SC, with subsequent dosing to maintain a therapeutic aPTT (3)[C].

ADDITIONAL TREATMENT

General Measures

- Routine anticoagulation for asymptomatic patients with protein S deficiency is not recommended (1)[A].
- Anticoagulation for 6–12 months is recommended for patients with protein S deficiency and a first thrombosis.
- Some argue for lifetime anticoagulation; data are limited.
- Anticoagulation for life is indicated for patients with protein S deficiency and recurrent thromboses.
- The role of family screening for protein S deficiency is unclear because most patients with this mutation do not have thrombosis. Screening should be considered for women considering using oral contraceptives or pregnancy with a family history of protein S deficiency (4)[B].
- Treatment with LMWH is recommended over unfractionated heparin, unless the patient has severe renal failure (3)[B].
- Treat as outpatient, if possible (3)[B].
- Initiate warfarin together with heparin on the first treatment day, and discontinue heparin after a minimum of 5 days and when INR >2 (3)[A].

Issues for Referral

Patients with suspected protein S deficiency should be seen by a hematologist.

SURGERY/OTHER PROCEDURES

- Anticoagulation must be held for surgical interventions.
- For most patients with DVT, recommendations are against routine use of vena cava filter in addition to anticoagulation (3)[A].

IN-PATIENT CONSIDERATIONS

Admission Criteria

- Life-threatening VT
- Significant bleeding while on anticoagulant therapy

Nursing

Look for signs of bleeding while on anticoagulation therapy.

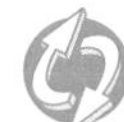

ONGOING CARE

FOLLOW-UP RECOMMENDATIONS

Patient Monitoring

- Warfarin requires periodic (monthly after initial stabilization) monitoring of the INR.
- Periodic measurement of INR to maintain a range of 2–3
- LMWH is the treatment of choice in pregnancy. Periodic monitoring with anti-Xa levels is recommended.

DIET

Unrestricted

PATIENT EDUCATION

- Patients should be educated about use of oral anticoagulant therapy if taking such.
- Avoid NSAIDs while on warfarin.

PROGNOSIS

- Persons with protein S deficiency have normal life spans.
- By age 45, 50% of the people heterozygous for protein S deficiency will have VT that is spontaneous half the time.

COMPLICATIONS

Recurrent thrombosis (requires indefinite anticoagulation)

REFERENCES

1. Bick RL. Prothrombin G20210A mutation, antithrombin, heparin cofactor II, protein C, and protein S defects. *Hematol Oncol Clin North Am*. 2003;17:9–36.
2. Moll S. Thrombophilias–practical implications and testing caveats. *J Thromb Thrombolysis*. 2006;21: 7–15.
3. Büller HR, Agnelli G, Hull RD, et al. Antithrombotic therapy for venous thromboembolic disease: The Seventh ACCP Conference on Antithrombotic and Thrombolytic Therapy. *Chest*. 2004;126: 401S–28S.
4. Langlois NJ, Wells PS. Risk of venous thromboembolism in relatives of symptomatic probands with thrombophilia: A systematic review. *Thromb Haemost*. 2003;90:17–26.

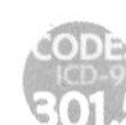

CODES

ICD9

289.81 Primary hypercoagulable state

CLINICAL PEARLS

- Asymptomatic patients with protein S deficiency do not need to have prophylactic anticoagulation because the risk of thrombosis is low; asymptomatic patients do not require anticoagulation.
- Patients with protein S deficiency and DVT should be anticoagulated for at least 6 months.

PROTEINURIA

Andrew Allegretti, MD
Douglas Shemin, MD

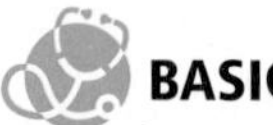

BASICS

DESCRIPTION

Proteinuria: Urinary protein excretion of more than 150 mg/d:

- Nephrotic-range proteinuria: Urinary protein excretion of more than 3.5 g/d; also called *heavy proteinuria*

Pediatric Considerations

- Proteinuria: Normal is daily excretion of up to 100 mg/m^2 (body surface area)
- Nephrotic-range proteinuria: Daily excretion of >1,000 mg/m^2 (body surface area)
- 3 pathologic types:
  - Glomerular proteinuria: Increased permeability of proteins across glomerular capillary membrane
  - Tubular proteinuria: Decreased proximal tubular reabsorption of proteins
  - Overflow proteinuria: Increased production of low-molecular-weight proteins

Pregnancy Considerations

- Proteinuria in pregnancy beyond 20 weeks' gestation is a hallmark of pre-eclampsia/eclampsia and demands further workup.
- Proteinuria in pregnancy before 20 weeks' gestation is suggestive of underlying renal disease.

RISK FACTORS

- Hypertension
- Diabetes
- Obesity
- Excessive exercise
- Congestive heart failure (CHF)
- UTI
- Fever

Genetics

No known genetic pattern

GENERAL PREVENTION

Control of weight, BP, and blood glucose reduces the risk of proteinuria.

PATHOPHYSIOLOGY

- Glomerular proteinuria: Increased filtration or larger proteins (albumin) due to:
  - Increased size of glomerular basement membrane pores and
  - Loss of proteoglycan negative charge barrier
- Tubular proteinuria: Tubulointerstitial disease prevents proximal tubular reabsorption of smaller proteins (β_2-microglobulin, immunoglobulin (Ig) light chains, retinol-binding protein, amino acids).
- Overflow proteinuria: Proximal tubular reabsorption overwhelmed by increased production of smaller proteins

ETIOLOGY

- Glomerular proteinuria:
  - Primary glomerulonephropathy:
    - Minimal-change disease
    - Idiopathic membranous glomerulonephritis
    - Focal segmental glomerulonephritis
    - Membranoproliferative glomerulonephritis
    - IgA nephropathy
  - Secondary glomerulonephropathy:
    - Diabetic nephropathy
    - Autoimmune/collagen-vascular disorders (e.g., lupus nephritis, Goodpasture syndrome)
    - Amyloidosis
    - Preeclampsia
    - Infection (HIV, hepatitis B and C, poststreptococcal, endocarditis, syphilis, malaria)
    - Malignancy (GI, lung, lymphoma)
    - Renal transplant rejection
    - Structural (reflux nephropathy, polycystic kidney disease)
    - Drug-induced (NSAIDs, penicillamine, lithium, heavy metals, gold, heroin)
- Tubular proteinuria:
  - Hypertensive nephrosclerosis
  - Tubulointerstitial disease (uric acid nephropathy, hypersensitivity, interstitial nephritis, Fanconi syndrome, heavy metals, sickle-cell disease, NSAIDs, antibiotics)
  - Acute tubular necrosis
- Overflow proteinuria:
  - Multiple myeloma (light chains also tubulotoxic)
  - Hemoglobinuria
  - Myoglobinuria (in rhabdomyolysis)
  - Lysozyme (in acute monocytic leukemia)
- Benign proteinuria:
  - Functional (fever, exercise, cold exposure, stress, CHF)
  - Idiopathic transient
  - Orthostasis (postural)

COMMONLY ASSOCIATED CONDITIONS

- Hypertension (common)
- Diabetes mellitus (common)
- Preeclampsia (common)
- Multiple myeloma (rare)

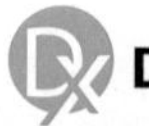

DIAGNOSIS

HISTORY

- Frothy or foamy urine
- Change in urine output
- Blood- or cola-colored urine
- Recent weight change
- Swelling
- Rule out systemic illness: Diabetes, heart failure, autoimmune, poststreptococcal infection

PHYSICAL EXAM

- BP
- Weight
- Peripheral edema
- Periorbital/facial edema
- Ascites
- Palpation of kidneys
- Check lungs, heart for signs of CHF

DIAGNOSTIC TESTS & INTERPRETATION

Lab

Screening for proteinuria is not cost effective unless directed at groups with hypertension or diabetes, older persons, etc. (1)[B].

Initial lab tests

- Urinalysis (UA) quantitatively estimates proteinuria:
  - Only sensitive to albumin; will not detect smaller proteins of overflow/tubular etiologies
  - False-positive if urine pH >7, highly concentrated (specific gravity [SG] >1.015), gross hematuria, mucus, semen, leukocytes, iodinated contrast agents, penicillin analogues, sulfonamide metabolites
  - False-negative if urine is dilute (SG >1.005), albumin excretion <20–30 mg/dL, protein is nonalbumin
  - Sensitivity 32–46%; specificity 97–100%
  - Also can perform sulfosalicylic acid test to detect nonalbumin protein
- If UA positive, perform urine microscopy. Refer to nephrologist if positive for signs of glomerular disease.
- If UA shows trace to 2+ protein, rule out transient proteinuria with repeat UA at another visit:
  - More common than persistent proteinuria
  - Causes include exercise, fever, CHF, UTI, and cold exposure.
  - Should reassure patient that transient proteinuria is benign and requires no further workup
- If initial UA shows 3+ to 4+ protein or repeat UA is positive, measure creatinine clearance and quantify proteinuria with 24-hour urine collection (gold standard) or spot urine protein/creatinine (P/C) ratio (acceptable practice) (2)[A]:
  - Numerical P/C ratios correlate with total protein excreted in grams per day (i.e., ratio of 0.2 correlates with 0.2 g during a 24-hour collection).
  - Patients younger than age 30 with 24-hour urine excretion of <2 g/d and normal creatinine clearance should be tested for orthostatic proteinuria:
    - Benign condition is present in 2–5% of adolescents
    - Diagnosed with a normal urine P/C ratio in first morning void and an elevated urine P/C ratio in a second specimen taken after standing for several hours
- If protein excretion >2 g/d, consider nephrology referral and begin workup for systemic or renal disease.

Follow-Up & Special Considerations

Renal or systemic disease workup can include:

- CBC, ferritin, ESR, serum iron
- Electrolytes, liver function tests
- Lipid profile (ideally, fasting)
- Prothrombin time/international normalized ratio
- Antinuclear antibodies: Elevated in lupus
- Antistreptolysin O titer: Elevated after streptococcal glomerulonephritis
- Complement C3 and C4: Low in glomerulonephritis
- HIV, Venereal Disease Research Laboratory, and hepatitis serologies: All associated with glomerular proteinuria
- Serum and urine protein electrophoresis: Abnormal in multiple myeloma

- Blood glucose: Elevated in diabetes
- All patients with diabetes should be screened for microalbuminuria.
- Patients with nephrotic-range proteinuria are at increased risk for hypercholesterolemia and thromboembolic events. Optimal duration of prophylactic anticoagulation is unknown (Cochrane Review is ongoing) but may extend for the duration of the nephrotic state (3)[C].
- Proteinuric pregnant patients beyond 20 weeks' gestation should be examined for other signs/symptoms of preeclampsia (e.g., hypertension, thrombocytopenia, elevated liver transaminases).

Imaging

Patients with persistent proteinuria not explained by orthostatic changes should undergo renal ultrasound to rule out structural abnormalities (e.g., reflux nephropathy, polycystic kidney).

DIFFERENTIAL DIAGNOSIS

Includes all causes listed under "Etiology."

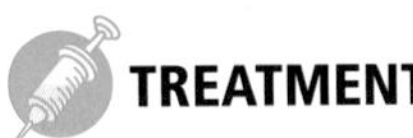

TREATMENT

- Systolic BP goal is in the 120s or lower, if tolerated (4)[A].
- Proteinuria goal is <0.5 g/d (4)[A].

MEDICATION

First Line

- ACE inhibitors: First choice; use maximally tolerated doses; use even if normotensive (4)[A]
- Angiotensin receptor blockers (ARBs): Proven antiproteinuric and renoprotective; studies ongoing to assess cardioprotection vs. ACE inhibitors; ARBs are first choice if ACE inhibitors are not tolerated (4)[A]
- Combination ACE inhibitor and ARB: Shown to reduce proteinuria; may not further reduce BP (4)[A]
- Statins: In addition to cardioprotection (4)[A], may be antiproteinuric and renoprotective (4)[B]

Second Line

- β-Blockers: Antiproteinuric and cardioprotective (4)[A]
- Dihydropyridine calcium channel blockers (DHCCB): Should be avoided unless needed for BP control; not antiproteinuric (4)[A]
- Non-DHCCB: Antiproteinuric, may be renoprotective (4)[B]
- Aldosterone antagonists: Antiproteinuric independent of BP control (4)[B]
- NSAIDs: Antiproteinuric but also nephrotoxic; generally should be avoided and reserved for refractory nephrotic syndrome (4)[C]

ADDITIONAL TREATMENT

General Measures

- Limit protein intake to 0.7 mg/kg/d. Soy protein may be renoprotective. Monitor protein intake with 24-hour urine urea excretion (4)[A].
- Limit sodium chloride intake to 2–3 g/d to optimize antiproteinuric medications (4)[B]. Effect on BP is further protective (4)[A].
- Limit fluid intake for urine output goal of <2 L/d. Larger urine volumes are associated with increased proteinuria and later glomerular filtration rate (GFR) decline (4)[B].
- Smoking cessation: Smoking is associated with increased proteinuria and faster kidney disease progression (4)[B].
- Encourage supine posture (up to 50% reduction vs. upright) (4)[B].
- Discourage severe exertion (4)[B].
- Encourage weight loss (4)[B].

Issues for Referral

Consider nephrology referral for possible renal biopsy if:

- Impaired creatinine clearance
- Nephrotic-range proteinuria
- Unclear etiology of nonnephrotic-range proteinuria
- Diabetics with microalbuminuria

COMPLEMENTARY AND ALTERNATIVE MEDICINE

- Corticosteroids: No proven benefit in mortality or need for renal replacement in adults with nephrotic syndrome, though steroids are recommended in some patients who do not respond to conservative treatment. Classically, children with nephrotic syndrome respond better than adults, especially those with minimal-change disease (5)[A].
- Estrogen/progesterone replacement: May be renoprotective in premenopausal women but should be avoided in postmenopausal women (4)[B]
- Decrease elevated homocysteine: Associated with microalbuminuria and cardiovascular risk; folic acid, vitamin B_6, and vitamin B_{12} may be effective (4)[C]
- Antioxidant therapy: May be antiproteinuric in diabetic nephropathy (4)[C]
- Sodium bicarbonate: Not antiproteinuric but may block tubular injury caused by proteinuria; correcting metabolic acidosis may decrease protein catabolism (4)[C]
- Avoid excessive caffeine consumption: Antiproteinuric in diabetic rat models (4)[C]
- Avoid iron overload (4)[C].
- Pentoxifylline: Prevents progression of renal disease by unclear mechanisms (4)[C]
- Mycophenolate mofetil: Antiproteinuric and renoprotective in animal models (4)[C]

ONGOING CARE

FOLLOW-UP RECOMMENDATIONS

Patient Monitoring

All patients with persistent proteinuria should be followed with serial BP checks, urinalysis, and renal function tests in the outpatient setting. Intervals depend on underlying etiology.

DIET

See "Additional Treatment."

PATIENT EDUCATION

See "Additional Treatment."

PROGNOSIS

- Transient and orthostatic proteinuria are benign conditions that do not convey a poor prognosis.
- Clinical significance of persistent proteinuria varies greatly and depends on underlying etiology.
- Degree of proteinuria is associated with disease progression in chronic kidney disease.
- Independent of GFR, higher levels of proteinuria likely convey an increased risk of mortality, myocardial infarction, and progression to kidney failure (6).

COMPLICATIONS

- Progression to chronic renal failure and the need for dialysis or renal transplant
- Hypercholesterolemia
- Hypercoagulable state

REFERENCES

1. Boulware LE, Jaar BG, Tarver-Carr ME, et al. Screening for proteinuria in US adults: A cost-effectiveness analysis. *JAMA*. 2003;290: 3101–14.
2. DOQI: Clinical practice guidelines for chronic kidney disease: Evaluation classification, and stratification: Guideline 5. Assessment of proteinuria. www.kidney.org/Professionals/Kdoqi/guidelines_ckd/p5_lab_g5.htm.
3. Glassock RJ, et al. Prophylactic anticoagulation in nephrotic syndrome: A clinical conundrum. *J Am Soc Nephrol*. 2007;18:2221–5.
4. Wilmer WA, Rovin BH, Hebert CJ, et al. Management of glomerular proteinuria: A commentary. *J Am Soc Nephrol*. 2003;14:3217–32.
5. Kodner C, et al. Nephrotic syndrome in adults: Diagnosis and management. *Am Fam Physician*. 2009;80:1129–34.
6. Tonelli M, Muntner P, Lloyd A, et al. Using proteinuria and estimated glomerular filtration rate to classify risk in patients with chronic kidney disease: A cohort study. *Ann Intern Med*. 2011; 154:12–21.

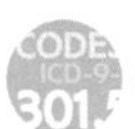

CODES

ICD9

791.0 Proteinuria

CLINICAL PEARLS

- Transient and orthostatic proteinuria are benign conditions that do not convey a poor prognosis.
- Proteinuria >2 g/d likely represents glomerular malfunction and warrants a nephrology consultation.
- Clinical course varies greatly but, in general, the amount of proteinuria correlates with kidney disease progression.
- First-line therapy for persistent proteinuric patients is high-dose ACE inhibitors/ARBs.

PROTHROMBIN 20210 (MUTATION)

Marc Jeffrey Kahn, MD, MBA
Rebecca Kruse-Jarres, MD, MPH

BASICS

DESCRIPTION

- Prothrombin 20210 mutation is the second most common inherited risk factor for venous thromboembolism after factor V Leiden mutation.
- Polymorphism (replacement of G by A) in the 3′ untranslated end of the prothrombin gene causes increased translation, resulting in elevated synthesis and secretion of prothrombin. This leads to a 2.8-fold increased risk for venous thrombosis.
- System(s) affected: Cardiovascular; Hemic/Lymphatic/Immunologic; Nervous; Pulmonary; Reproductive
- Synonym(s): Prothrombin G20210A mutation; Prothrombin G20210 gene polymorphism; Prothrombin gene mutation; FII A^{20210} mutation

EPIDEMIOLOGY

- Found largely in Caucasian populations. Found in 2–5% of European and Middle Eastern populations, but rarely in nonwhites. Found in 4–8% of persons with venous thromboembolism and in up to 18% of patients with recurrent thrombosis.
- Predominant age: Mean age of first thrombosis is in the second decade
- Predominant gender: Male = Female

Prevalence

3–5% of the population

RISK FACTORS

- Oral contraceptives, pregnancy, and the use of hormone replacement therapy increase the risk of venous thrombosis in patients with prothrombin 20210 (1).
- Patients with prothrombin 20210 and another prothrombotic state such as factor V Leiden have increased rates of thrombosis (1).

Pregnancy Considerations

Increased thrombotic risk in patients with prothrombin 20210

Genetics

Autosomal dominant

GENERAL PREVENTION

Patients with prothrombin 20210 without thrombosis do not require prophylactic treatment with full anticoagulation (2)[A].

PATHOPHYSIOLOGY

Replacement of G for A in the 3′ untranslated region of the prothrombin gene resulting in relatively higher plasma prothrombin activity, leading to increased risk for venous thrombosis

ETIOLOGY

Gene mutation

COMMONLY ASSOCIATED CONDITIONS

Venous thromboembolism

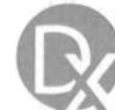

DIAGNOSIS

HISTORY

- Previous thrombosis
- Family history of thrombosis
- Family history of factor prothrombin 20210 mutation

PHYSICAL EXAM

Arterial thrombosis is rare in adults with prothrombin 20210 gene mutation.

DIAGNOSTIC TESTS & INTERPRETATION

Test patients with thrombosis at age <50, history of recurrent idiopathic thrombosis, those with thrombosis in unusual locations, or those with strong family history.

Lab

Initial lab tests

- For evaluation of new clot in patient at risk: CBC with peripheral smear, PT/INR, aPTT, thrombin time, lupus anticoagulant, antiphospholipid antibodies, factor VIII, anticardiolipin antibody, anti-B2 glycoprotein I antibody, activated protein C resistance, protein S antigen and resistance, antithrombin III assay, fibrinogen, factor V Leiden, prothrombin G20210A, homocysteine
- DNA analysis for mutation
- Testing is reliable during acute thrombosis and on any kind of anticoagulation (3).

Follow-Up & Special Considerations

Although prothrombin levels are elevated, this is not a sensitive test to make the diagnosis.

Imaging

Initial approach

As appropriate for suspected site of thrombosis: Ultrasound, CT scan, and V/Q scan

Diagnostic Procedures/Surgery

Magnetic resonance angiography (MRA), venography, or arteriography to detect thrombosis

Pathological Findings

Venous thrombus

DIFFERENTIAL DIAGNOSIS

- Factor V Leiden mutation
- Protein C deficiency
- Protein S deficiency
- Antithrombin deficiency
- Other causes of activated protein C resistance (e.g., antiphospholipid antibodies)
- Dysfibrinogenemia
- Dysplasminogenemia
- Homocystinemia
- Elevated factor VIII levels

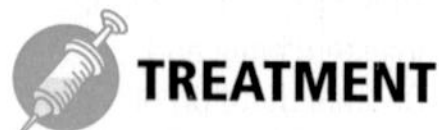

TREATMENT

For acute thrombosis

MEDICATION

First Line

- Low-molecular-weight heparin (2)[A]:
  - Enoxaparin (Lovenox): 1 mg/kg SC b.i.d., start warfarin simultaneously, continue Lovenox for at least 5 days and until international normalized ratio (INR) is >2, at which time it can be stopped
  - Fondaparinux (Arixtra): 7.5 mg SC every day
  - Tinzaparin (Innohep): 175 anti-Xa IU/kg SC daily for 6 days and patient is adequately anticoagulated with warfarin (INR of at least 2 for 2 consecutive days)
  - Dalteparin (Fragmin): 200 IU/kg SC daily
- Oral anticoagulant:
  - Warfarin (Coumadin) 5 mg PO daily initially and adjusted to an INR of 2–3
- Contraindications:
  - Active bleeding precludes anticoagulation (2)[A].
  - Risk of bleeding is a relative contraindication to long-term anticoagulation (2)[A].
  - Warfarin is contraindicated in patients with history of warfarin skin necrosis (2)[A].
- Precautions:
  - Observe patient for signs of embolization, further thrombosis, or bleeding.
  - Avoid IM injections. Periodically check stool and urine for occult blood; monitor CBCs, including platelets.
  - Heparins: Thrombocytopenia and/or paradoxic thrombosis with thrombocytopenia
  - Warfarin: Necrotic skin lesions (typically breasts, thighs, or buttocks)
  - Low-molecular-weight heparin (LMWH): Adjust dosage in renal insufficiency.
- Significant possible interactions:
  - Agents that intensify the response to oral anticoagulants: Alcohol, allopurinol, amiodarone, anabolic steroids, androgens, many antimicrobials, cimetidine, chloral hydrate, disulfiram, all NSAIDs, sulfinpyrazone, tamoxifen, thyroid hormone, vitamin E, ranitidine, salicylates, acetaminophen
  - Agents that diminish the response to anticoagulants: Aminoglutethimide, antacids, barbiturates, carbamazepine, cholestyramine, diuretics, griseofulvin, rifampin, oral contraceptives

Second Line

- Heparin 80 mg/kg IV bolus followed by 18 g/kg/hr continuous infusion
- Adjust dose depending on activated partial thromboplastin time (aPTT).
- In patients requiring large daily doses of heparin, measure an anti-Xa level for dose guidance.
- Alternatively, unfractionated heparin can be given at 35,000 U/24 hours SC, with subsequent dosing to maintain a therapeutic aPTT (3)[C].

ADDITIONAL TREATMENT

General Measures

- Patients with prothrombin 20210 mutation, and a first thrombosis should be anticoagulated initially with heparin or LMWH (1)[A].
- Treatment with LMWH is recommended over unfractionated heparin, unless the patient has severe renal failure (3)[B].
- Treat as outpatient, if possible (3)[B].
- Initiate warfarin together with heparin on the first treatment day, and discontinue heparin after 5 days if INR >2 (3)[A].
- Patients should be maintained on warfarin with an INR of 2–3 for at least 6 months (1)[A].
- Recurrent thrombosis requires indefinite anticoagulation (1)[B].

Issues for Referral

- Recurrent thrombosis on anticoagulation
- Difficulty anticoagulating
- Genetic counseling

COMPLEMENTARY AND ALTERNATIVE MEDICINE

Compression stockings for prevention

SURGERY/OTHER PROCEDURES

- Anticoagulation must be held for surgical interventions.
- For most patients with DVT, recommendations are against routine use of vena cava filter in addition to anticoagulation (3)[A].
- Thrombectomy may be necessary in some cases.

IN-PATIENT CONSIDERATIONS

Initial Stabilization

Heparin

Admission Criteria

Complicated thrombosis, such as pulmonary embolus

Nursing

- Teach LMWH and warfarin use.
- See above for drug interactions.

Discharge Criteria

Stable on anticoagulation

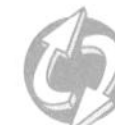

ONGOING CARE

FOLLOW-UP RECOMMENDATIONS

Patient Monitoring

- Warfarin use requires periodic (monthly after initial stabilization) INR measurements, with a goal of 2–3 (2)[A].
- Heterozygous prothrombin 20210 mutations increase the risk for recurrent venous thromboembolism (VTE) only slightly once anticoagulation is stopped, and should have the same length of anticoagulation as someone without the mutation.

DIET

- No restrictions
- Foods rich in vitamin K may interfere with warfarin anticoagulation.

PATIENT EDUCATION

- Patients should be educated about:
  - Use of oral anticoagulant therapy
  - Avoidance of NSAIDs while on warfarin
- The role of family screening is unclear, as most patients with this mutation do not have thrombosis. In a patient with a family history of prothrombin 20210, consider screening during pregnancy or if considering oral contraceptive use.

PROGNOSIS

When compared to normal individuals, persons with prothrombin 20210 have normal life spans.

COMPLICATIONS

- Recurrent thrombosis
- Bleeding on anticoagulation

REFERENCES

1. Girolami A, Simioni P, Scarano L, et al. Prothrombin and the prothrombin 20210 G to A polymorphism: Their relationship with hypercoagulability and thrombosis. *Blood Rev*. 1999;13:205–10.
2. Girolami A, Scarano L, Tormene D, et al. Homozygous patients with the 20210 G to A prothrombin polymorphism remain often asymptomatic in spite of the presence of associated risk factors. *Clin Appl Thromb Hemost*. 2001;7: 122–5.
3. Moll S. Thrombophilias–practical implications and testing caveats. *J Thromb Thrombolysis*. 2006;21: 7–15.

ADDITIONAL READING

- American College of Chest Physicians Evidence-Based Clinical Practice Guidelines (8th Edition). *Chest*. 2008;133(6 Suppl).
- Büller HR, Agnelli G, Hull RD, et al. Antithrombotic therapy for venous thromboembolic disease: The Seventh ACCP Conference on Antithrombotic and Thrombolytic Therapy. *Chest*. 2004;126:401S–28S.
- Seligsohn U, Lubetsky A. Genetic susceptibility to venous thrombosis. *N Engl J Med*. 2001;344: 1222–31.

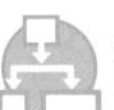

See Also (Topic, Algorithm, Electronic Media Element)

Antithrombin Deficiency; Deep Vein Thrombophlebitis (DVT); Factor V Leiden; Protein C Deficiency; Protein S Deficiency

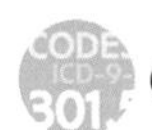

CODES

ICD9

289.81 Primary hypercoagulable state

CLINICAL PEARLS

- Prothrombin 20210 mutation is the second most common inherited risk factor for venous thromboembolism after factor V Leiden mutation.
- Asymptomatic patients with prothrombin 20210 mutation do not need anticoagulation.
- Testing for the prothrombin G20210 mutation may be done while the patient is anticoagulated, as it is a genetic assay.

PRURITUS ANI

Katharine Barnard, MD

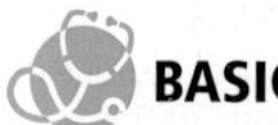

BASICS

DESCRIPTION
- Intense anal and perianal itching
- Usually acute
- Must be differentiated from other primary dermatologic disorders

EPIDEMIOLOGY
Incidence
- Common
- Predominant age: 40–70
- Predominant sex: Male > Female (4:1)

Prevalence
Difficult to estimate because condition is thought to be underreported and because almost any anorectal discomfort is often attributed to symptomatic hemorrhoids

RISK FACTORS
- Overweight
- Hairy, excessive perspiration
- Underlying anorectal pathology
- Underlying anxiety disorder

GENERAL PREVENTION
- Practice good perianal hygiene. Absorb excess sweating with talcum powder or cornstarch.
- Avoid mechanical irritation of skin (excessive cleaning or rubbing, harsh soaps or perfumed products, or tight or synthetic undergarments).
- Avoid laxative use (loose stool is an irritant).
- Eat yogurt or take *Acidophilus* supplements when taking broad-spectrum antibiotics; malt extract also may help.

PATHOPHYSIOLOGY
- Perianal itching usually due to fecal irritants.
- Itch–scratch cycle may be initiated via other mechanical or inflammatory factors and perpetuated by the resulting lichenification caused by scratching.

ETIOLOGY
- 25% idiopathic vs. 75% associated with colonic or anorectal pathology (e.g., hemorrhoids, anal fissures, skin tags, rectal prolapse, polyps, or—rarely—cancers of the colon, rectum, or anus)
- In 50–75% of cases, skin irritation is from feces (due to poor hygiene, loose or leaking stool, pathology that makes cleansing difficult, or laxity of the internal sphincter mechanism).
- In the remaining 25–50% of cases, the inciting irritation may be caused by:
  - Dermatologic disorders:
    - Allergic contact dermatitis (e.g., to soaps, perfumes or dyes in toilet paper, topical anesthetics [especially -caines], oral antibiotics [especially tetracyclines])
    - Excess skin moisture due to hyperhydrosis
    - Psoriasis
    - Erythrasma (*Corynebacterium* infection)
    - Atopic dermatitis ± lichen simplex chronicus
    - Eczema due to dietary components: Citrus, vitamin C supplements, milk products, coffee, tea, cola, chocolate, beer, wine
  - Infection with dermatophytes (*Tinea*), *Candida*, or seborrheic dermatitis
  - Bacterial and viral infections (either primary infections such as STIs, or secondary *Staphylococcus* or *Streptococcus* infections); especially a concern for immune-suppressed patients
  - Parasitic infections, most commonly pinworms, and rarely scabies or pediculosis
  - Mechanical factors: Vigorous cleaning and rubbing, tight-fitting clothes, or synthetic undergarments
  - Systemic disease: Diabetes mellitus, chronic liver disease, renal failure, leukemia or lymphoma, hyperthyroidism, or anemia
  - Psychogenic: Anxiety–itch–anxiety cycle
  - Chemical irritation from chemotherapy or alkaline diarrhea

COMMONLY ASSOCIATED CONDITIONS
See above listing of conditions causing perianal irritation.

DIAGNOSIS

HISTORY
- Patient presents with complaint of anal and/or perianal itching.
- Inquire about melena or hematochezia, change in bowel habits, or a family history of colorectal cancer; anal receptive intercourse; antecedent change in toiletry products; household members with itching (think pinworms); and clothing preference (tight, synthetic).

PHYSICAL EXAM
- Perianal inspection for erythema, hemorrhoids, anal fissures, maceration, lichenification, rashes, warts, or excoriations
- Digital rectal exam to check for masses and to evaluate internal sphincter tone
- Anoscopy to evaluate for hemorrhoids, fissures, other internal lesions

DIAGNOSTIC TESTS & INTERPRETATION
Lab

Initial lab tests

Depending on patient's history and exam, consider the following:
- Blood glucose and urine dip for glycosuria (association with diabetes)
- Test for pinworms via cellophane tape to area; check stool for ova and parasites

Pediatric Considerations
Pinworms are more common in children than in adults; therefore, testing is always indicated:
- Skin scraping with KOH prep for dermatophytes or candidiasis (as etiology or as superinfection) and mineral oil prep for scabies
- Perianal skin culture (bacterial superinfection)
- Hemoccult testing of stool (though may be positive due to excoriations)

Follow-Up & Special Considerations
- Anal DNA polymerase chain reaction (PCR) probe for gonorrhea and chlamydia and anal Pap smear (*if receptive anal intercourse*)
- Consider lab evaluation of liver and renal function, glucose, hematocrit (Hct), thyroid-stimulating hormone (TSH), and CBC.

Diagnostic Procedures/Surgery
- Suspicious lesions (e.g., lichenification, ulcerated epithelium, refractory cases) should be biopsied to exclude neoplasia.
- Consider colonoscopy if history suggests colorectal pathology (preceding historical elements, especially if age >40).

DIFFERENTIAL DIAGNOSIS
- Dermatologic conditions
- Infections, including condylomata acuminata
- Allergies (topical agents)
- Colorectal pathology: Fistulas (e.g., associated with inflammatory bowel disease [IBD]), fissures, rectal prolapse, sphincter weakness, hemorrhoids, tumor/malignancy
- Skin cancer: Squamous cell cancer, extramammary Paget disease, Bowen disease, melanoma
- Systemic illness such as diabetes

Geriatric Considerations
- Stool incontinence may be a predisposing factor.
- Consider possible systemic disease.
- Higher likelihood of colorectal pathology

TREATMENT

MEDICATION
First Line
- Treat underlying and associated conditions: Fungal or dermatophyte infection with topical imidazoles, bacterial infection with topical antibacterials (or oral erythromycin if itch >1 year)
- Break itch–scratch cycle with low-potency steroid cream (not ointment) applied sparingly up to q.i.d. Discontinue when itching subsides. Recommended not to use >12 weeks due to risk of skin atrophy.
- If lichenification or no response with low-potency steroid, use high-potency steroid cream sparingly to area b.i.d., totaling <8 weeks of steroid treatment (1).
- Antihistamines may be useful until local measures take effect, particularly sedating antihistamines, which will reduce nighttime itching. Psychotropic medications may be added for additional sedation (2,3).
- Zinc oxide can be used after completing steroid course; petroleum jelly as barrier during treatment period (4)
- Topical capsaicin cream also may be used in combination with steroid cream or if refractory itch or hypersensitized skin (5,6).
- Use a hair dryer on the cool setting to dry the area after cleansing (7)[C].
- Treat comorbid anxiety or depression.

Second Line

Radiation or methylene blue injections may be used to destroy nerve endings (create permanent anesthesia) in intractable cases. This is almost never indicated, but is close to 100% effective for those who require it (1,8).

ADDITIONAL TREATMENT

Issues for Referral

- Intractable pruritus: Consider referral to gastroenterology (for colonoscopy) or dermatology (for additional treatment, possibly injections). Refractory or persistent symptoms should signal the possibility of underlying neoplasia because pruritus ani of long duration is associated with a greater likelihood of colorectal pathology (9,10).
- If risks or red flags for colonic malignancy, refer for colonoscopy.
- If neoplasia on biopsy, refer to colorectal surgery.

COMPLEMENTARY AND ALTERNATIVE MEDICINE

Self-hypnosis using relaxation and imagery has been shown to be effective in at least 1 case of refractory idiopathic pruritus ani (11).

SURGERY/OTHER PROCEDURES

None unless neoplasia

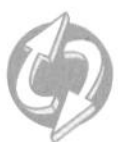

ONGOING CARE

FOLLOW-UP RECOMMENDATIONS

See patient in 2 weeks if not improving. Check for persistent lichenification. Biopsy persistent or refractory pruritus or lichenification that does not resolve (9,12).

DIET

- Trial elimination of foods and beverages known or suspected to exacerbate symptoms: Coffee, tea, chocolate, beer, cola, vitamin C tablets in excessive doses, citrus fruits, tomatoes, or spices (4)
- Eliminate foods or drugs contributing to loose bowel movements. Add fiber supplementation to bulk stools and prevent fecal leakage in patients who have fecal incontinence or partially formed stools.

PATIENT EDUCATION

- Resist overuse of soap and rubbing.
- Avoid toiletry products with irritating perfumes and dyes.
- Avoid use of ointments to the area.
- Wear loose, light clothing.
- If moisture is a problem, unmedicated talcum powder or cornstarch may be used to keep the area dry.
- Cleanse perianal area after bowel movements with cotton moistened with water or witch hazel.
- Following bathing, the area should be dried by patting with a soft towel or with a hair drier.
- Avoid medications that cause diarrhea or constipation.
- If taking antibiotics, eat yogurt with active cultures or take *Acidophilus* supplements.
- Use barrier protection if engaging in anal intercourse.
- If unable to completely empty rectum with defecation, use small plain-water enema (infant bulb syringe) after each bowel movement to prevent soiling and irritation.

PROGNOSIS

- Conservative treatment and reassurance are successful in ~90% of patients.
- Idiopathic form often is chronic, waxing and waning, but regardless of etiology, the condition may be persistent and recurrent.

COMPLICATIONS

- Bacterial superinfection at site of excoriations, and potentially abscess formation or penetrating infection via self-inoculation with colonic pathogens
- Lichenification, which makes cure more difficult

REFERENCES

1. Weichert GE. An approach to the treatment of anogenital pruritus. *Dermatol Ther*. 2004;17:129–33.
2. Crownover BK, Jamieson B, Mott TF. Clinical inquiries. First- or second-generation antihistamines: Which are more effective at controlling pruritus? *J Fam Pract*. 2004;53:742–4.
3. Southerland AD, et al. Intradermal injection of methylene blue for the treatment of refractory pruritus ani. *Colorectal Dis*. 2009;11(3):282–7.
4. Siddiqi S, Vijay V, Ward M, et al. Pruritus ani. *Ann R Coll Surg Engl*. 2008;90:457–63.
5. Heard S. Pruritus ani. *Aus Fam Physician*. 2004;33(7):511–3.
6. Lysy J, Sistiery-Ittah M, Israelit Y, et al. Topical capsaicin–a novel and effective treatment for idiopathic intractable pruritus ani: A randomised, placebo controlled, crossover study. *Gut*. 2003;52:1323–6.
7. Markell KW, Billingham RP, et al. Pruritus ani: Etiology and management. *Surg Clin North Am*. 2010;90:125–35, Table of Contents.
8. Mentes BB, Akin M, Leventoglu S, et al. Intradermal methylene blue injection for the treatment of intractable idiopathic pruritus ani: Results of 30 cases. *Tech Coloproctol*. 2004;8:11–4.
9. Daniel GL, Longo WE, Vernava AM. Pruritus ani. Causes and concerns. *Dis Colon Rectum*. 1994;37:670–4.
10. Longo WE, Dean PA, Virgo KS, et al. Colonoscopy in patients with benign anorectal disease. *Dis Colon Rectum*. 1993;36:368–71.
11. Rucklidge JJ, Saunders D. Hypnosis in a case of long-standing idiopathic itch. *Psychosom Med*. 1999;61:355–8.
12. Handa Y, Watanabe O, Adachi A, et al. Squamous cell carcinoma of the anal margin with pruritus ani of long duration. *Dermatol Surg*. 2003;29:108–10.

ADDITIONAL READING

- *Evidence-Based Medicine*. 2004;9(3):86.
- Pfenninger JL, Zainea GG. Common anorectal conditions: Part I. Symptoms and complaints. *Am Fam Physician*. 2001;63:2391–8.
- Zuccati G, Lotti T, Mastrolorenzo A, et al. Pruritus ani. *Dermatol Ther*. 2005;18:355–62.

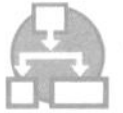

See Also (Topic, Algorithm, Electronic Media Element)

Pinworms; Pruritus Vulvae

CODES

ICD9

698.0 Pruritus ani

CLINICAL PEARLS

- In over 50% the cases of pruritus ani, the irritant is feces.
- Vigorous cleansing can potentiate the problem.
- Consider infection in immunosuppressed patients.
- Chronic tetracycline use (such as for acne) can cause pruritus ani.
- Consider trial of dietary elimination of citrus, vitamin C supplements, milk products, coffee, tea, cola, chocolate, beer, and wine.

PRURITUS VULVAE

Michael P. Hopkins, MD, MEd
Jennifer L. Rogers, MD

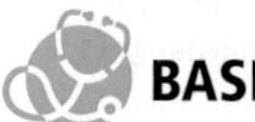

BASICS

DESCRIPTION

- Pruritus vulvae is a symptom as well as a primary diagnosis:
  - The symptom may indicate an underlying pathological process.
  - Only when no underlying disease is identified may this be used as a primary diagnosis.
- Pruritus vulvae as a primary diagnosis may also be more appropriately documented as vulvodynia (see "Vulvodynia" topic) and burning vulva syndrome.

EPIDEMIOLOGY

Symptoms may occur at any given age during a woman's lifetime:

- Young girls most commonly have infectious etiology.
- The primary diagnosis is more commonly seen in postmenopausal women.

Incidence

The exact incidence is unknown. However, the majority of women complain of vulvar pruritus at some point in their lifetime.

RISK FACTORS

- High-risk sexual behavior
- Immunosuppression
- Obesity

GENERAL PREVENTION

- Attention should be paid to personal hygiene and avoidance of possible environmental factors.
- Tight-fitting clothing should be avoided.
- Only cotton underwear should be worn.

ETIOLOGY

Local irritants:

- Perfumes
- Soaps
- Laundry detergent
- Douches
- Toilet paper
- Sanitary napkins

COMMONLY ASSOCIATED CONDITIONS

- Infectious etiology:
  - Vaginal or vulvar candida
  - *Gardnerella vaginalis*
  - *Trichomonas*
  - Human papillomavirus
  - Herpes simplex virus
- Vulvar vestibulitis
- Lichen sclerosis
- Hyperkeratosis
- Malignant or premalignant conditions
- Psoriasis
- Fecal or urinary incontinence
- Excessive heat with sweat
- Dietary: Methylxanthines (e.g., coffee, cola), tomatoes, peanuts

DIAGNOSIS

Pruritus vulvae is a diagnosis of exclusion.

HISTORY

- Persistent itching
- Persistent burning sensation over the vulva or perineum
- Change in vaginal discharge
- Postcoital bleeding
- Dyspareunia

PHYSICAL EXAM

- Visual inspection of the vulva, vagina, perineum, and anus
- Light touch identification of affected areas
- Q-tip-applied pressure to vestibular glands

DIAGNOSTIC TESTS & INTERPRETATION

- Sodium chloride: *Gardnerella* or *Trichomonas*
- 10% potassium hydroxide: *Candida*
- Tzanck smear: Herpes simplex virus
- Directed biopsy: Human papillomavirus, lichen, malignancy

Lab

Follow-Up & Special Considerations

A patch test may be performed by a dermatologist to assist in identifying a causative agent if contact dermatitis is suspected.

Imaging

Initial approach

Colposcopy with acetic acid of Lugol's solution of vagina and vulva

Follow-Up & Special Considerations

Exam-directed biopsies are essential in the postmenopausal population to rule out malignancy (1).

Diagnostic Procedures/Surgery

Biopsies should be collected from any ulceration, discoloration, raised areas, macerated areas, and the area of most intense pruritus.

Pathological Findings

Only in the absence of pathological findings can the primary diagnosis of pruritus vulvae be made.

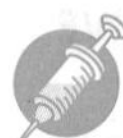

TREATMENT

Initial treatment is conservative (2)[C]:

- Treatment of etiology beyond the primary diagnosis of vulvae pruritus
- Avoidance of environment and dietary irritants
- Sitz baths
- Cool compresses or ice packs (gel packs or frozen vegetables)

MEDICATION

First Line

- Antihistamines:
  - Hydroxyzine 10–50 mg 2 hours before bedtime
  - Diphenhydramine 25–50 mg at bedtime
- Topical steroids (3)[C]:
  - Triamcinolone 0.1% applied daily for 2–4 weeks then twice weekly
  - Hydrocortisone 1–2.5% cream applied 2–4 times daily (4)
  - Avoid long-term use due to risk of atrophy.
  - One randomized controlled trial (RCT) showed no difference between topical triamcinolone and placebo cream (5)
- SSRIs (citalopram, fluoxetine, or sertraline):
  - Citalopram 20–40 mg daily

Second Line

Topical pimecrolimus 1% cream applied b.i.d. for 3 weeks (6)[B]

ADDITIONAL TREATMENT

- SC triamcinolone injections (7)[B]
- Alcohol nerve block (8)[B]
- Laser therapy (9)[B]

Issues for Referral

- Persistent symptoms should prompt additional investigation and referral to a gynecologist or gynecologist oncologist.
- Gynecology oncology referral for proven or suspected malignancy
- Dermatology referral for patch testing to evaluate for contact dermatitis

ONGOING CARE

- Frequent evaluation, repeat cultures, and biopsies are necessary for cases resistant to treatment.
- Refractory cases may require referral to gynecologist or gynecology oncology for further management.

DIET

Dietary alterations include avoidance of the following:

- Coffee and other caffeine-containing beverages
- Tomatoes
- Peanuts

PATIENT EDUCATION

- American Congress of Obstetricians and Gynecologists: www.acog.org
- National Vulvodynia Foundation: www.nva.org

PROGNOSIS

Conservative measures and short-term topical steroids control most patients' symptoms.

COMPLICATIONS

Malignancy

REFERENCES

1. Sener AB, Kuscu E, Seckin NC. Postmenopausal vulvar pruritus—colposcopic diagnosis and treatment. *J Pak Med Assoc.* 1995;45:315–7.
2. Boardman LA, Botte J, Kennedy CM. Recurrent vulvar itching. *Obstet Gynecol.* 2005;100(6): 1451–5.
3. Weichert GE. An approach to the treatment of anogenital pruritus. *Dermatol Ther.* 2004;17: 129–33.
4. Pincus SH. Vulvar dermatoses and pruritus vulvae. *Dermatol Clin.* 1992;10(2):297–308.
5. Lagro-Janssen AL, Sluis S, et al. Effectiveness of treating non-specific pruritus vulvae with topical steroids: A randomized controlled trial. *Eur J Gen Pract.* 2009;15:29–33.
6. Sarifakioglu E, Gumus II. Efficacy of topical pimecrolimus in the treatment of chronic vulvar pruritus: A prospective case series—a non-controlled, open-label study. *J Dermatolog Treat.* 2006;17(5):276–8.
7. Kelly RA, Foster DC, Woodruff JD. Subcutaneous injection of triamcinolone acetonide in the treatment of chronic vulvar pruritus. *Am J Obstet Gynecol.* 1993;169(3):568–70.
8. Woodruff JD, Babaknia A. Local alcohol injection of the vulva: Discussion of 35 cases. *Obstet Gynecol.* 1979;54:512–4.
9. Ovadia J, Levavi H, Edelstein T. Treatment of pruritus vulvae by means of CO_2 laser. *Acta Obstet Gynecol Scand.* 1984;63:265–7.

ADDITIONAL READING

- Bohl TG. Overview of vulvar pruritus through the life cycle. *Clin Obstet Gynecol.* 2005;48:786–807.
- Farage MA, Miller KW, Ledger WJ. Determining the cause of vulvovaginal symptoms. *Obstet Gynecol Surv.* 2008;63:445–64.
- Foster DC. Vulvar disease. *Obstet Gynecol.* 2002; 100:145–63.
- Petersen CD, Lundvall L, Kristensen E. Vulvodynia. Definition, diagnosis and treatment. *Acta Obstet Gynecol Scand.* 2008;87:893–901.

CODES

ICD9

698.1 Pruritus of genital organs

CLINICAL PEARLS

- The majority of women complain of pruritus vulvae at some point in their lifetime.
- Pruritus vulvae is a diagnosis of exclusion once other causes of itching have been ruled out.
- Exam-directed biopsies from any ulceration, discoloration, raised areas, macerated areas, and the area of most intense pruritus are essential to rule out malignancy.
- Initial treatment is conservative.

PSEUDOFOLLICULITIS BARBAE

Michelle St. Fleur, MD
Anna Doubeni, MD

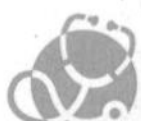

BASICS

DESCRIPTION

- Foreign-body inflammatory reaction surrounding an ingrown hair (usually in beard area, especially in submandibular region, but may occur on scalp, axilla, or pubic area if these sites are shaved or plucked)
- Characterized by red papule/pustule at point of entry
- A mechanical problem
- System(s) affected: Skin/Exocrine
- Synonym(s): Chronic sycosis barbae; Pili incarnate; Folliculitis barbae traumatica; Razor bumps; Shaving bumps; Tinea barbae

EPIDEMIOLOGY

- Predominant age: Postpubertal, middle age (40–75 years of age)
- Predominant sex: Male > Female (can be seen in females of all races who wax/shave axillary and pubic areas) (1).

Incidence

- Adult male African Americans: 50,000/100,000
- Adult male whites: 3,000–5,000/100,000

Prevalence

- Widespread
- 45–83% of African American soldiers who shave

RISK FACTORS

- Curly hair
- Shaving too close with multiple razor strokes
- Plucking hairs
- Black and Hispanic races

Genetics

- People with curly hair, especially African Americans and Hispanics (2)
- Single-nucleotide polymorphism (disruption Ala12Thr substitution) affects keratin of hair follicle (3).

GENERAL PREVENTION

- Use tiny plastic hook to remove ingrown hairs before shaving.
- Prior to shaving, rinse and compress face with warm water.
- Shave with either a manual adjustable razor at coarsest setting (avoids close shaves), a single-edge blade razor (e.g., Bump Fighter), a foil-guarded razor (e.g., PFB razor), electric triple "O-head" razor, or electric hair clipper with polyester skin-cleansing pad (e.g., Buf-Puf by Riker Laboratories).
- Shave in the direction of hair growth. Do not stretch skin when shaving.
- Use a generous amount of the correct shaving cream/gel (e.g., Ef-Kay Shaving Gel, Edge Shaving Gel, Aveeno Therapeutic Shave Gel, Easy Shave Medicated Shaving Cream).
- Use "collar extender" (JCPenney).

PATHOPHYSIOLOGY

- Because of its curvature, the advancing hair's sharp-tipped free end after shaving causes an epidermal invagination as it approaches the skin. This is accompanied by inflammation and often an intraepidermal abscess (4).
- As the hair enters the dermis, more severe inflammation occurs, with downgrowth of the epidermis in an attempt to sheath the hair.
- An abscess forms within the pseudofollicle, and a foreign-body reaction forms at the tip of the invading hair.

ETIOLOGY

- Re-entry penetration of skin by external pointed tip of growing curved whisker or sharp-tipped whisker may grow into follicular wall if shaved too close
- Plucking of hair may cause abnormal hair growth in injured follicles.

COMMONLY ASSOCIATED CONDITIONS

Keloidal folliculitis

DIAGNOSIS

HISTORY

Pain on shaving; irritated "razor bumps"

PHYSICAL EXAM

- Tender exudative, erythematous follicular papules or pustules in beard area (less commonly in scalp, axilla, and pubic areas); range from 2–4 mm (2)
- Hyperpigmented "razor or shave bumps"
- Alopecia
- Lusterless, brittle hair

DIAGNOSTIC TESTS & INTERPRETATION

Lab

Initial lab tests

- Clinical diagnosis
- Culture of pustules: Usually sterile; may show coagulase-negative staphylococcal epidermidis (normal skin flora)
- Additional hormonal testing may be indicated in females with hirsutism: PCOS, DHEA, luteinizing hormone (LH)/follicle-stimulating hormone (FSH), and free and total testosterone (3).

Pathological Findings

Follicular papules and pustules (4)

DIFFERENTIAL DIAGNOSIS

- Bacterial folliculitis
- Impetigo
- Acne vulgaris
- Tinea barbae
- Sarcoidal papules

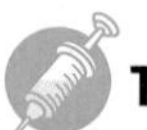

TREATMENT

- Mild cases:
  - Consider 5% benzoyl peroxide after shaving and application of 1% hydrocortisone cream at bedtime (or LactiCare HC lotion after shaving).
  - Tretinoin cream 0.025%; apply daily
- Moderate cases:
  - Chemical depilatories (barium sulfide; Magic Shave powder); first test on forearm for 48 hours (for irritation).
  - Consider eflornithine HCl cream (Vaniqa), but it can cause pseudofolliculitis barbae (PFB) (5).
- Severe cases:
  - Laser therapy (6,7)[A]: Longer-wavelength laser (e.g., Nd:YAG) is safer for dark skin (1).
  - Avoid shaving; completely grow beard.

MEDICATION

First Line

- Topical or systemic antibiotic for secondary infection:
  - Application of clindamycin (Cleocin T) solution b.i.d. or topical erythromycin if mild
  - Low-dose erythromycin or tetracycline, 250–500 mg PO b.i.d., if more severe inflammation (8)
  - Benzoyl peroxide 5%–clindamycin 1% gel b.i.d. (9)[C]: Administer until papule/pustule resolves.
- Mild cases: Tretinoin cream 0.025% at bedtime (8)
- Moderate disease/chemical depilatories:
  - Disrupt cross-linking of disulfide bonds of hair, causing blunt hair tip.
  - Apply no more frequently than every third day: 2% barium sulfide (Magic Shave) or calcium thioglycolate (Surgex)
- Contraindications:
  - Clindamycin: History of regional enteritis or ulcerative colitis; history of antibiotic-associated colitis
  - Erythromycin, tetracycline, tretinoin hypersensitivity only

- Precautions:
  - Clindamycin: Colitis, eye burning and irritation, skin dryness; pregnancy category B
  - Erythromycin: Use cautiously in patients with impaired hepatic function; GI side effects, especially abdominal cramping; pregnancy category B.
  - Chemical depilatories: Use cautiously; frequent use and prolonged application may lead to irritant contact dermatitis and chemical burns.
  - Tetracycline: Permanent discoloration of teeth if given during last half of pregnancy
  - Tretinoin: Severe skin irritation; pregnancy category C
  - Benzoyl peroxide: Skin irritation and dryness, allergic contact dermatitis
  - Hydrocortisone cream: Local skin irritation, skin atrophy with prolonged use
- Significant possible interactions:
  - Erythromycin: Increases theophylline and carbamazepine levels; decreases clearance of warfarin; cardiac toxicity with terfenadine and astemizole
  - Tetracycline: Depresses plasma prothrombin activity (therefore, warfarin dosage must be decreased)

Second Line

Topical application of glycolic acid lotion (8% buffered glycolic acid in a suitable carrier, either oil-in-water lotion or a nonlipid soap) b.i.d.; this treatment may allow comfortable shaving every day (10)[C].

ADDITIONAL TREATMENT

General Measures

Acute treatment:

- Dislodge embedded hair with sterile needle/tweezers.
- Discontinue shaving until red papules have resolved (minimum 3–4 weeks; longer if moderate or severe); can trim to length >0.5 cm during this time (8).
- Massage beard area with washcloth, coarse sponge, or brush several times daily.
- Hydrocortisone 1% cream to relieve inflammation
- Systemic antibiotics if secondary infection is present

Pregnancy Considerations

Do not use tretinoin (Retin-A), tetracycline, or benzoyl peroxide.

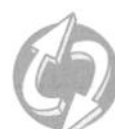

ONGOING CARE

FOLLOW-UP RECOMMENDATIONS

Patient Monitoring

- As needed
- Educate patient on curative and preventive treatment.

DIET

No restrictions

PATIENT EDUCATION

- Dunn JF Jr. Pseudofolliculitis barbae. *Am Fam Physician*. 1988;38:170–2.
- See section "General Prevention."

PROGNOSIS

- Course is recurrent if preventive measures are not followed.
- Prognosis is poor in the presence of progressive scarring and foreign-body granuloma formation.

COMPLICATIONS

- Scarring (occasionally keloidal)
- Foreign-body granuloma formation
- Disfiguring postinflammatory hyperpigmentation (use sunscreens; can treat with hydroquinone 4% cream, Retin A, clinical peels) (3)
- Impetiginization of inflamed skin
- Epidermal (erythema, crusting, burns with scarring) and pigmentary changes with laser (1,2,8)

REFERENCES

1. Bridgeman-Shah S. The medical and surgical treatment of pseudofolliculitis barbae. *Dermatol Ther*. 2004;17:158–63.
2. Perry PK, et al. Defining pseudofolliculitis barbae in 2001: A review of the literature and current trends. *J Am Acad Dermatol*. 2002;46(suppl 2): S113–9.
3. Quarles FN, Brody H, Johnson BA, et al. Pseudofolliculitis barbae. *Dermatol Ther*. 2007;20:133–6.
4. Lever WF, Schaumburg-Lever G. *Histopathology of the Skin*. Philadelphia, PA: JB Lippincott; 1990.
5. Shenenberger DW, et al. Removal of unwanted facial hair. *Am Fam Phys*. 2002;66(10):1907–11.
6. Rogers CJ, Glaser DA. Treatment of pseudofolliculitis barbae using the Q-switched Nd:YAG laser with topical carbon suspension. *Dermatol Surg*. 2000;26:737–42.
7. Weaver SM, Sagaral EC. Treatment of pseudofolliculitis barbae using the long-pulse Nd:YAG laser on skin types V and VI. *Dermatol Surg*. 2003;29:1187–91.
8. Pseudofolliculitis barbae. *Up To Date*. 2007;
9. Cook-Bolden FE, et al. Twice daily application of benzoyl peroxide 5% clindamycin 1% gel versus vehicle in treatment of pseudofolliculitis barbae. *Cutis*. 2004;73(6 suppl):13–24.
10. Perricone NV. Treatment of pseudofolliculitis barbae with topical glycolic acid: A report of two studies. *Cutis*. 1993;52:232–5.

ADDITIONAL READING

Dunn JF Jr. Pseudofolliculitis barbae. *Am Fam Physician*. 1988;38:169–74.

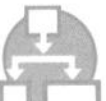

See Also (Topic, Algorithm, Electronic Media Element)

Folliculitis; Impetigo

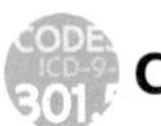

CODES

ICD9

704.8 Other specified diseases of hair and hair follicles

CLINICAL PEARLS

- Electrolysis is not recommended as a treatment. It is expensive, painful, and often unsuccessful (8).
- Curable by not shaving or complete hair removal (via laser)
- ~3–5% of white men who shave are affected.
- Bump Fighter razor from American Safety Razor Company (www.asrco.com)

PSEUDOGOUT (CPPD)

Dylan C. Kwait, MD
Paul T. Cullen, MD

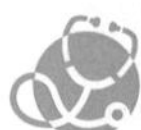

BASICS

DESCRIPTION

- Acute inflammatory arthritis caused by calcium pyrophosphate dihydrate (CPPD) crystal deposition in joints:
  - Primarily affects the elderly
  - Usually involves large joints
  - Associated with chondrocalcinosis
- Symptom onset is insidious, resulting in symmetric polyarthritis similar to rheumatoid arthritis (RA).
- CPPD crystal deposition may cause a progressive degenerative arthritis in numerous joints.
- Definitive CPPD diagnosis requires the presence of CPPD crystals in synovial fluid (1)[A].
- System(s) affected: Endocrine/Metabolic; Musculoskeletal
- Synonym(s): Calcium pyrophosphate deposition disease

EPIDEMIOLOGY

Prevalence

- Predominant age: 80% of patients >60 years of age
- Predominant sex: Male = Female
- Chondrocalcinosis is present in 1 in 10 adults age 60–75 years and 1 in 3 by >80 years; only a small percentage develop pseudogout (2).

RISK FACTORS

- Advanced age
- Traumatic injury
- Pseudogout often occurs as a complication in patients hospitalized for other medical and surgical illnesses.

Genetics

Uncommonly seen in familial pattern with autosomal-dominant inheritance (<1% of patients); most cases are sporadic.

GENERAL PREVENTION

Colchicine 0.6 mg b.i.d. may reduce frequency of episodes in recurrent monoarthritic CPPD.

ETIOLOGY

- Arthropathy results from an acute inflammatory reaction to CPPD crystals shed into synovial cavity.
- Physical and chemical changes in aging cartilage favor crystal growth.

COMMONLY ASSOCIATED CONDITIONS

- Hyperparathyroidism
- Hemochromatosis
- Gout
- Hypophosphatasia
- Hypothyroidism
- Ochronosis
- Wilson disease
- Amyloidosis
- Hypomagnesemia

DIAGNOSIS

HISTORY

- Acute pain and swelling of ≥1 or more joints; knee involved in 1/2 of all attacks; ankle, wrist, and shoulder are also commonly involved.
- May present as a chronic progressive arthritis with superimposed acute inflammatory attacks
- Progressive degenerative arthritis in numerous joints, including wrists, metacarpophalangeal, hips, shoulders, elbows, and ankles
- Low-grade inflammatory arthritis with multiple symmetric joint involvement (mimics RA) <5% of cases
- Can present in proximal joints mimicking polymyalgia rheumatica, often accompanied by tibiofemoral and ankle arthritis and tendinous calcifications (3)[C]
- May develop after intra-articular injection of hyaluronic acid (Hyalgan, Synvisc) (4)[C]

PHYSICAL EXAM

- Inflammation, joint effusion, decreased range of motion
- 50% associated with fever
- Any other synovial joint may be involved, including first metatarsophalangeal joint.

DIAGNOSTIC TESTS & INTERPRETATION

Lab

Initial lab tests

Synovial fluid analysis consistent with an inflammatory effusion:

- Cell count from 2,000–100,000 WBCs/mL
- Differential predominantly neutrophils (80–90%)
- >50,000 WBC count increases likelihood of septic arthritis, 11% prevalence; number needed to treat (NNT) = 9; >100,000 WBCs/mL, 22% prevalence (5)[C]
- Wet prep with polarized microscopy may demonstrate small numbers of weakly *positively birefringent* crystals in the fluid and within neutrophils; false-negative rate is high.
- Metabolic studies to exclude an underlying cause always should be obtained in patients <50 years of age and should be considered in the elderly:
  - Serum calcium
  - Serum phosphorus
  - Serum alkaline phosphatase
  - Serum parathormone (i-PTH)
  - Serum iron, total iron-binding capacity, and serum ferritin
  - Serum magnesium
  - Serum thyroid-stimulating hormone (TSH) level

Imaging

Initial approach

- Joint radiographs:
  - Radiographic findings in pseudogout are not sensitive or specific (1)[A].
  - Punctate and linear calcifications may be visualized in articular hyaline or fibrocartilage.
  - Knees, hips, symphysis pubis, and wrists are most commonly affected.
  - Patients with chronic CPPD may demonstrate subchondral cysts and loose bodies (i.e., osseous fragmentation with formation of intra-articular radiodense bodies) in joints not typically affected by degenerative joint disease (e.g., osteoarthritis).
- Ultrasound:
  - Ultrasound may be more useful than plain radiography for the diagnosis of pseudogout in peripheral joints (1)[A], with a positive predictive value of 92% and negative predictive value of 93% (6)[C].
  - The ultrasonographic imaging characteristics of pseudogout include: Joint effusion, synovial thickening, and hyperechoic deposits (6)[C].

Diagnostic Procedures/Surgery

Aspiration of joint fluid with synovial fluid analysis and demonstration of CPPD crystals is required for diagnosis (1)[A]; aspiration may relieve symptoms and speed resolution of inflammatory process.

Pathological Findings

CPPD crystal deposition in articular cartilage, synovium, ligaments, and tendons

DIFFERENTIAL DIAGNOSIS

- Illnesses that may cause acute inflammatory arthritis in a single or multiple joint(s):
  - Gout
  - Septic arthritis
  - Trauma
- Other illnesses that may present with an acute inflammatory arthritis:
  - Reiter syndrome
  - Lyme disease
  - Acute RA

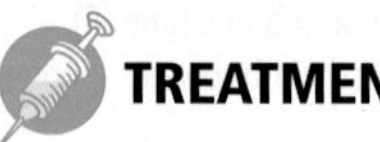

TREATMENT

MEDICATION

First Line

- A combination of pharmacologic and nonpharmacologic measures is recommended for optimal treatment (7)[A].
- Acute attacks should be treated with cool packs, rest, and joint aspiration/steroid injection (7)[A].
- Chronic inflammatory CPPD arthropathy should be managed prophylactically with oral NSAIDs and/or colchicine (7)[A].
- Oral NSAIDs:
  - Ibuprofen (Motrin): 600–800 mg PO t.i.d.–q.i.d. with food; maximum 3.2 g/d
  - Naproxen (Naprosyn): 500 mg PO b.i.d. with food
  - Other NSAIDs at anti-inflammatory doses are effective, although indomethacin has higher complication rates (relative risk [RR] = 2.2) compared with ibuprofen (RR = 1.2) (8)[B].
- Intra-articular steroid injection:
  - Prednisolone–sodium phosphate 4–20 mg or triamcinolone diacetate 2–40 mg administered with local anesthetic.

- Oral colchicine (9)[C]:
  - 0.6 mg q.i.d. or 0.6 mg hourly until symptoms relieved or vomiting/diarrhea develops; maximum dose per attack 4–6 mg; 0.5–1 mg/d may be used (7)[A]; avoid with significant renal insufficiency.
- Contraindications:
  - History of hypersensitivity to NSAIDs or aspirin
  - Active peptic ulcer disease or history of recurrent upper GI lesions
  - Avoid in renal insufficiency if serum creatinine >1.6 mg/dL.
  - Serious GI bleeding can occur without warning; follow the patient carefully for internal bleeding. Administer proton pump inhibitor (PPI) or misoprostol 200 μg PO q.i.d. in patients with peptic ulcer disease history.

ALERT

Significant possible interactions:

- May elevate BP in treated hypertensives
- May blunt antihypertensive effects of ACE inhibitors
- May prolong prothrombin time (PT) in patients taking oral anticoagulants
- Avoid concomitant aspirin use.
- May blunt diuretic effect of furosemide and hydrochlorothiazide
- May increase plasma lithium level in patients taking lithium carbonate

Second Line

- Oral prednisone: Begin at 40–60 mg/d and taper over 10 days.
- IM triamcinolone acetonide 60 mg; may repeat in 1–4 days (5)[B]
- Methotrexate may have a role in severe disease resistant to traditional therapy (9,10)[C].

ADDITIONAL TREATMENT

General Measures

- Rest and elevate affected joint(s).
- Apply ice/cool compresses to affected joints.
- Non–weight-bearing on affected joint while painful; use crutches or walker.

Issues for Referral

Consider consultation with orthopedist or rheumatologist if septic joint is a serious consideration or patient is not responding.

Additional Therapies

Physical therapy:

- Isometric exercises to maintain muscle strength during the acute stage (e.g., quadriceps isometric contractions, and leg lifts if knee affected)
- Begin joint range-of-motion (ROM) exercises as inflammation and pain subside.
- Resume weight-bearing when pain subsides.

SURGERY/OTHER PROCEDURES

Perform arthrocentesis and joint fluid analysis.

IN-PATIENT CONSIDERATIONS

Admission Criteria

Consider admission for septic arthritis if synovial fluid WBC count >50,000/mL; strongly consider if >100,000/mL; treat with appropriate antibiotics pending culture results.

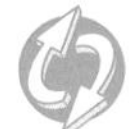

ONGOING CARE

FOLLOW-UP RECOMMENDATIONS

Patient Monitoring

Re-evaluate patient for response to therapy 48–72 hours after treatment instituted; re-examine 1 week later and then as needed.

DIET

No known relationship to diet

PATIENT EDUCATION

- Rest affected joint.
- Symptoms usually resolve in 7–10 days.

PROGNOSIS

- Acute attack usually resolves in 10 days; prognosis for resolution of acute attack is excellent.
- Some patients experience progressive joint damage with functional limitation.

COMPLICATIONS

- Erosive destructive arthritis in a pattern of joints not usually affected by degenerative joint disease (e.g., metacarpophalangeal joints, wrists)
- Recurrent acute attacks

Geriatric Considerations

Elderly patients treated with NSAIDs require careful monitoring and are at higher risk for GI bleeding and acute renal insufficiency.

REFERENCES

1. Zhang W, Doherty M, Bardin T, et al. European League Against Rheumatism recommendations for calcium pyrophosphate deposition. Part I: Terminology and diagnosis. *Ann Rheum Dis*. 2011;70:563–70.
2. Richette P, Bardin T, Doherty M. An update on the epidemiology of calcium pyrophosphate dihydrate crystal deposition disease. *Rheumatology (Oxford)*. 2009;48(7):711–5.
3. Pego-Reigosa JM, Rodriguez-Rodriguez M, Hurtado-Hernandez Z, et al. Calcium pyrophosphate deposition disease mimicking polymyalgia rheumatica: A prospective followup study of predictive factors for this condition in patients presenting with polymyalgia symptoms. *Arthritis Rheum*. 2005;53:931–8.
4. Hamburger MI, Lakhanpal S, Mooar PA, et al. Intra-articular hyaluronans: A review of product-specific safety profiles. *Semin Arthritis Rheum*. 2003;32:296–309.
5. Shah K, Spear J, Nathanson LA, et al. Does the presence of crystal arthritis rule out septic arthritis? *J Emerg Med*. 2007;32:23–6.
6. Filippou G, Frediani B, Gallo A, et al. A "new" technique for the diagnosis of chondrocalcinosis of the knee: Sensitivity and specificity of high-frequency ultrasonography. *Ann Rheum Dis*. 2007;66(8):1126–8.
7. Zhang W, Doherty M, Pascual E, et al. EULAR recommendations for calcium pyrophosphate deposition. Part II: Management. *Ann Rheum Dis*. 2011;70:571–5.
8. Richy F, Bruyere O, Ethgen O, et al. Time dependent risk of gastrointestinal complications induced by non-steroidal anti-inflammatory drug use: A consensus statement using a meta-analytic approach. *Ann Rheum Dis*. 2004;63:759–66.
9. Lioté F, Ea HK, et al. Recent developments in crystal-induced inflammation pathogenesis and management. *Curr Rheumatol Rep*. 2007;9: 243–50.
10. Chollet-Janin A, Finckh A, Dudler J, et al. Methotrexate as an alternative therapy for chronic calcium pyrophosphate deposition disease: An exploratory analysis. *Arthritis Rheum*. 2007;56:688–92.

ADDITIONAL READING

- Announ N, Guerne PA, et al. Treating difficult crystal pyrophosphate dihydrate deposition disease. *Curr Rheumatol Rep*. 2008;10:228–34.
- Wise CM. Crystal-associated arthritis in the elderly. *Clin Geriatr Med*. 2005;21:491–511, v-vi.

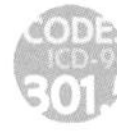

CODES

ICD9

- 275.49 Other disorders of calcium metabolism
- 712.20 Chondrocalcinosis, due to pyrophosphate crystals, site unspecified
- 712.26 Chondrocalcinosis, due to pyrophosphate crystals, lower leg

CLINICAL PEARLS

- Perform joint fluid aspiration and analysis to evaluate acute arthritis.
- If septic arthritis is considered, treat presumptively with antibiotics until culture results are available.
- NSAID therapy is preferred treatment.
- Oral steroids are useful if NSAIDs are contraindicated.
- Intra-articular steroids can be used *if* septic arthritis has been excluded.

PSORIASIS

Debora B. Sternaman, PharmD
Edward C. Sternaman II, MD

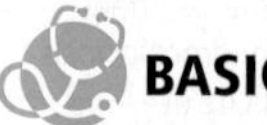

BASICS

DESCRIPTION

- A proliferative rash characterized by well-defined brick-red papulosquamous plaques with a silvery scale
- A T-cell–mediated immunologic genetic disorder of the skin characterized by flares (related to systemic, emotional, and environmental factors) and remissions
- Usual course: Acute; chronic; unpredictable
- Clinical forms:
  - Plaque: Most common; patches on scalp, trunk, limbs (extensor surfaces); nails may be pitted and/or thickened
  - Guttate: Usually presents <20 years of age; numerous small papules over wide area of skin, greatest on trunk
  - Inverse or flexural: Affects intertriginous areas; lesions moist ± scales
  - Pustular (von Zumbusch): True emergency: Severe form characterized by widespread erythema, scaling, pustule formation
  - Erythrodermic: Severe form, skin turns red; often presents with chronic disease and/or precipitated by high use of topical steroids
  - Nail disease: Can occur in all subtypes; fingernails involved in ~50% of cases and toenails in 35%
  - Psoriatic arthritis: Inflammatory arthropathy; see "Arthritis, Psoriatic" topic

EPIDEMIOLOGY

Incidence

- Predominant sex: Male = Female
- Greater incidence in whites

Prevalence

- 2–4%
- Predominant age: Mean age of onset 33 years of age; earlier in women; most occur <46 years of age
- ~80% of patients have mild to moderate disease with 20% having severe disease (1).

RISK FACTORS

- Family history
- Local trauma; local irritation
- Infection (β-hemolytic streptococcal or viral infection can stimulate acute guttate psoriasis)
- HIV
- Stress (physical and emotional)
- Withdrawal of steroid therapy
- Folate and vitamin B_{12} deficiency
- Medications (see "General Prevention")
- Alcohol use, smoking
- Diabetes, obesity, metabolic syndrome

Genetics

- Genetic predisposition (probably polygenic)
- 20–30% have psoriasis in a first-degree relative.
- Type I psoriasis (onset <40 years) theorized to have a strong familial pattern and more severe course than type 2 (onset >40 years)
- Increased incidence of specific human leukocyte antigens

GENERAL PREVENTION

Avoid trauma/sunburns, irritating drugs, stimulating drugs, antimalarial medications (aminoquinolines), and alcoholic beverages.

PATHOPHYSIOLOGY

- Multisystem inflammatory autoimmune condition affecting primarily the skin and joints
- Characterized by disfiguring, scaly, erythematous patches, papules, and plaques, which may be painful, leading to quality-of-life (QOL) issues

ETIOLOGY

- T-cell–mediated: Triggered by some environmental antigen (e.g., trauma) or internal antigen (HIV) that promotes a cycle of cytokine production and cell proliferation

COMMONLY ASSOCIATED CONDITIONS

- Autoimmune: Crohn disease, ulcerative colitis, multiple sclerosis (MS)
- Cardiovascular: Inflammatory process
- Metabolic syndrome
- Psychiatric/psychologic: Depression, suicide, psychologic, and emotional burden/anxiety
- Psoriatic arthritis
- Atopic dermatitis
- May be among first signs of AIDS
- Nonmelanoma skin cancer (unclear whether related to disease process or treatment)
- Hepatic abnormalities (pustular psoriasis)

DIAGNOSIS

HISTORY

- History of trauma, previous treatment, pruritus
- Family history

PHYSICAL EXAM

- Rash: Color, size, morphology, distribution, scale; Auspitz sign: Underlying pinpoints of bleeding following scraping (2)[C]
- Special attention to scalp, umbilicus, intergluteal cleft, and nails
- Well-defined red papules coalescing to plaques; sharply demarcated silvery scales on red plaques (3)[C]
- Knee-elbow-scalp-sacral-groin distribution
- Koebner phenomenon: Psoriatic response in traumatic area (2)[C]
- Stippled nails and pitting
- Sebopsoriasis: Greasy scales in the eyebrows, nasolabial folds, and postauricular and presternal areas (3)

DIAGNOSTIC TESTS & INTERPRETATION

Lab

Initial lab tests

- Diagnosis by history and physical (4)[C]
- Negative rheumatoid factor (5)[C]
- Increased ESR and C-reactive protein (CRP) (5)[C]
- Fungal studies may show a superimposed infection.

Diagnostic Procedures/Surgery

- Psoriasis Area and Severity Index evaluates overall severity and body surface area (BSA) involvement.
- Physicians Global Assessment: Target plaque score and the percent BSA together
- Biopsy is rarely required (2).

Pathological Findings

- Epidermal hyperplasia
- Parakeratotic scale
- Loss of granular cell layer
- Mitotic figures in basal cell layer
- Elongation and thickening of rete ridges
- Dilated tortuous surface capillary loops
- Inflammatory infiltrate with T cells, neutrophils, mast cells, and macrophages

DIFFERENTIAL DIAGNOSIS

- Scalp: Seborrheic dermatitis
- Chronic/nummular eczema
- Lichen simplex chronicus
- Trunk: Pityriasis rosea, pityriasis rubra pilaris, tinea corporis

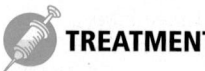

TREATMENT

MEDICATION

First Line

- Mild-to-moderate disease:
  - Emollients b.i.d.: Petrolatum or thick creams
  - Topical corticosteroids (1,2,3,5)[A]:
    - Tachyphylaxis develops over time; may alternate to prevent
    - Side effects include skin thinning, hypopigmentation, and increased chance of local infection.
    - Occlusive dressing increases effectiveness but also increases chance of side effects.
    - For scalp: Strong potency in alcohol base
    - Face, intertriginous areas: Low-potency corticosteroids; infants, 1% hydrocortisone
    - Medium-potency corticosteroids daily (e.g., 0.1% mometasone or triamcinolone)
    - Strong-potency corticosteroids: 0.05% betamethasone or fluocinonide daily; good initial plaque treatment (4)[A]
    - Superpotency corticosteroids: Clobetasol, halobetasol; limit use to 2 weeks; avoid occlusive dressings; reserved for recalcitrant plaques (2,4)[A]
  - Vitamin D analogues: Calcipotriene ointment 0.005% b.i.d. limits keratinocyte hyperproliferation; monitor calcium (2,4)[A].
  - Topical retinoids: Tazarotene (Tazorac) 0.05% or 0.1% daily; local irritation; solar sensitivity; avoid in pregnancy (4,5)[A].
  - Adjunctive therapy with low-dose prednisone (<10 mg/d) in patients with psoriasis and concurrent psoriatic arthritis (1)
- Moderate-to-severe disease: Combination therapy may be required to control appropriately.
  - Light therapy: Natural sunlight improves symptoms, office-administered light available as ultraviolet B (broad or narrow band) or PUVA (PO or bath psoralen + ultraviolet A [UVA]). Narrowband ultraviolet B (UVB) may be more effective (2,4)[C]:
    - Broadband UVB up to 20–25 treatments 2–3 times weekly with or without topical tar or anthralin (may increase effectiveness); after initial treatment, treat weekly to maintain.
    - UVA administered within 2 hours of receiving psoralen; initially 3 times weekly, then 1 or 2 times weekly

- Systemic therapies:
  - Methotrexate: Blocks DNA synthesis in rapidly dividing epithelial cells and suppresses T cells. Start 7.5–15 mg/wk IV, PO, IM, or SC. Increase 2.5 mg every 2–3 weeks, up to 25 mg with folic acid 1–5 mg/d (2,4)[C]:
    - Side effects: Teratogenic, hepatotoxic
    - Monitor liver function tests (LFTs), renal function, and CBC; liver biopsy when cumulative dose reaches 1.5 g; no alcohol; avoid Bactrim, retinoids, sulfamethoxazole (2)[C]
  - Cyclosporine: Inhibits T cells; start high dose, 5 mg/kg/d, and taper; 0.5–1 mg/kg/d for maintenance; pregnancy class C. Side effects: Monitor renal function, CBC with Mg^{2+} and K^{+}, and BP (3)[C]
  - Acitretin (Soriatane): Oral retinoid; for plaque psoriasis, only moderately effective as monotherapy; sometimes combined with PUVA; start 25–50 mg/d:
    - Teratogenic: Pregnancy test before starting; 2 forms of contraception needed 1 month before, during, and for at least 3 years after treatment; avoid alcohol (may convert acitretin to etretinate) (1,2,3)[C]; check FDA monitoring guidelines.
    - Side effects: Hepatotoxicity, hyperlipidemia, myalgias; monitor LFTs, renal functions, CBC, creatine phosphokinase (2,3)[C].
  - Oral corticosteroids only for severe or life-threatening disease (risk of rebound)
- Biologics:
  - Etanercept (Enbrel): Blocks tumor necrosis factor α (TNF-α); begin at 50 mg SC twice a week × 3 months; then maintenance of 50 mg/wk (2,4)[B],(6). Side effects: Reactivation of tuberculoses, drug-induced lupus, some concern of lymphoma, CNS demyelinating disorder (resolves on stopping), rarely, heart failure; pregnancy Category B (2,4,7)[C]
  - Adalimumab (Humira): First fully human anti-TNF-α monoclonal antibody; specifically binds to soluble membrane-bound TNF-α. Dosing starts at 80 mg SC × 1 week; then 40 mg SC every other week (2,4,6)[B]. Side effects: Rare reports of serious infections and malignancies, rare drug-induced reversible conditions (i.e., lupus, cytopenia, MS, and congestive heart failure) (2,4)[C]
  - Alefacept (Amevive): Interferes with CD2 on memory T cells and inhibits activation; 15 mg IM weekly × 12 weeks; can do an additional round after 12 weeks of rest (2,4)[B]. Side effects: Lymphopenia; monitor CD4 cell counts weekly; discontinue when $<250/\mu L$.
  - Efalizumab (Raptiva): Inhibits T cells and their adhesion to endothelial cells; initial dose 0.7 mg/kg; then 1 mg/kg weekly; maximum single dose of 200 mg; patient can administer (2,4,5)[B]. Side effects: Monitor platelets monthly for 3 months, then every 3 months. Up to 14% of patients develop rebound or flare.
  - Infliximab (Remicade): Like etanercept, blocks TNF-α; 3–10 mg/kg IV at weeks 0, 2, and 6; maintenance doses of 5 mg/kg every 6–8 weeks; adjust interval as needed (2,4,7)[B]. Side effects (see etanercept): To increase efficacy and limit toxicity, combine, rotate, or use sequentially.
  - Golimumab (Simponi): Like etanercept, blocks TNF-α; 50 mg SQ monthly. Side effects (see etanercept): pregnancy Category B; can be self-administered.
  - Ustekinumab (Stelara): Selectively targets cytokines interleukin 12 and 23 (IL12, IL23), which mediate inflammation; dosing based on weight <100 kg 45 mg SC at weeks 0 and 4, then 45 mg every 12 weeks, >100 kg 90 mg SQ at weeks 0, and 4, then 90 mg every 12 weeks. Side effects: May increase risk of malignancy; monitor for reversible posterior leukoencephalopathy syndrome, which was suspected in 1 case.

Second Line

- Topical immunosuppressants: Tacrolimus (Prograf) or pimecrolimus (Elidel); dermatology consult recommended (4)[C]
- Topicals: Salicylic acid; coal tar; anthralin (2,4)[C]

ADDITIONAL TREATMENT

General Measures

- Adequate topical hydration (emollients)
- Solar radiation (but avoid excessive exposure)
- Tar shampoos

Issues for Referral

- Psoriasis >20% of BSA (2,4)
- Severe extremity involvement, particularly hands and feet

SURGERY/OTHER PROCEDURES

- Psoriasis and psoriatic medications can affect wound healing postoperatively.
- Perioperative considerations include:
  - Aspirin, NSAIDs, COX-2 inhibitors, and glucocorticoids; use sparingly.
  - Methotrexate: Monitor for postoperative infections.
  - Hold cyclosporine for 1 week before and after.

IN-PATIENT CONSIDERATIONS

Initial Stabilization

- Intensive topical therapy
- Phototherapy
- Systemic therapy

Admission Criteria

- Generalized pustular psoriasis; von Zumbusch
- Erythrodermic psoriasis
- Debilitation; patient-specific

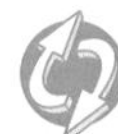

ONGOING CARE

FOLLOW-UP RECOMMENDATIONS

Measure BSA involvement to determine if therapy is working; change therapy if no improvement is seen, or add an agent (2,3).

DIET

- No evidence-based information; suggestions of gluten-free diet to minimize food allergies (3)
- Good fats, whole grains, legumes, vegetables, fruits, omega-6 fatty acid
- Herbs and seasonings such as turmeric, red pepper, cloves, ginger, basil, and garlic can block activation of inflammatory cytokines.
- Essential fatty acid supplements

PATIENT EDUCATION

- American Academy of Family Physicians: www.aafp.org; (800) 274-2237
- National Psoriasis Foundation: www.psoriasis.org; (800) 723-9166

PROGNOSIS

- Benign, but life-threatening forms do occur.
- May be refractory to treatment

COMPLICATIONS

- Psoriatic arthritis
- Pustular psoriasis
- Erythrodermic psoriasis

REFERENCES

1. Menter A, Korman NJ, Elmets CA, et al. Guidelines of care for the management of psoriasis and psoriatic arthritis: Section 6. Guidelines of care for the treatment of psoriasis and psoriatic arthritis: Case-based presentations and evidence-based conclusions. *J Am Acad Dermatol*. 2011;65: 137–74.
2. Menter A, Gottlieb A, Feldman SR, et al. Guidelines of care for the management of psoriasis and psoriatic arthritis: Section 1. Overview of psoriasis and guidelines of care for the treatment of psoriasis with biologics. *J Am Acad Dermatol*. 2008;58: 826–50.
3. Traub M, Marshall K. Psoriasis–pathophysiology conventional, and alternative approaches to treatment. *Altern Med Rev*. 2007;12:319–30.
4. Luba KM, et al. Chronic plaque psoriasis. *Am Fam Phys*. 2006;73(4):636–44.
5. Heymann WR. Psoriasis: The heart of the matter. *J Am Acad Dermatol*. 2008;58:477–8.
6. Sobell JM, Kalb RE, Weinberg JM. Management of moderate to severe plaque psoriasis (part 2): Clinical update on T-cell modulators and investigational agents. *J Drugs Dermatol*. 2009; 8:230–8.
7. Sobell JM, Kalb RE, Weinberg JM. Management of moderate to severe plaque psoriasis (part I): Clinical update on antitumor necrosis factor agents. *J Drugs Dermatol*. 2009;8:147–54.

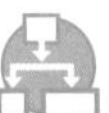

See Also (Topic, Algorithm, Electronic Media Element)

Arthritis, Psoriatic

CODES

ICD9

- 696.1 Other psoriasis
- 696.8 Other psoriasis and similar disorders

CLINICAL PEARLS

- Chronic life-long condition
- Disease-state severity cycles in many patients.
- May need multiple medications to treat; if one does not work, use or add another.

PSYCHOSIS

Michael Golding, MD

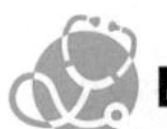

BASICS

DESCRIPTION
Syndrome seen with schizophrenia, schizoaffective disorder, mood disorder, substance use, medical problems, delirium, and dementia; symptoms include:
- Positive symptoms: Hallucinations and delusions (fixed false beliefs that the person does not recognize as untrue), often paranoid delusions
- Negative symptoms: Apathy, avolition, withdrawal, paucity of speech
- Disorganized speech or behavior

EPIDEMIOLOGY
Prevalence
- Schizophrenia: Men peak onset 18–25 years; women peak onset 25–35 years
- Schizophrenia: 1% of the US population; thought to be similar worldwide
- Delusional disorder: 0.03% of population
- Bipolar type I: 1% of population
- Prevalence of psychosis in major depression not known, likely underrecognized

RISK FACTORS
Substance abuse (particularly marijuana), family history of psychosis, lower socioeconomic status

Genetics
Schizophrenia: 50% concordance for monozygotic twins, little or no shared environmental effect. Multiple candidate genes involving disruption of neurodevelopment.

GENERAL PREVENTION
Community interventions for early detection and treatment of prodromal symptoms show promise.

PATHOPHYSIOLOGY
Neurodevelopmental predisposition plus first or third trimester in-utero insult (e.g., first trimester infection or third trimester birth hypoxia) leads to exaggerated neuronal apoptosis in late adolescence with subsequent thalamic sensory overload. Increased dopaminergic mesolimbic transmission may contribute to delusions and hallucinations in schizophrenia. Dopamine deficiency in mesocortical pathways may contribute to frontal lobe hypoactivity often associated with apathy and withdrawal in schizophrenia. Glutamate, neurosteroids, and neurodevelopmental abnormalities are active areas of research.

ETIOLOGY
Postulated stress-diathesis model: Individuals biologically at risk develop psychosis when under stress.

COMMONLY ASSOCIATED CONDITIONS
- Cardiovascular diseases: Serious mental illness is associated with metabolic syndrome, autonomic dysfunction, sudden cardiac death
- Cancer mortality: Particularly breast and lung cancer
- Substance abuse disorders, including nicotine dependence

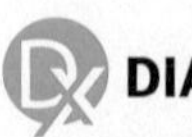

DIAGNOSIS

First rule out delirium: Psychosis should not have fluctuating consciousness or reduced clarity of awareness.

HISTORY
- Delusions (fixed false beliefs): Persecutory (being monitored), bizarre (involving impossible states), somatic (fixed belief in nonexistent serious illness), referential (getting messages from TV, radio, or thoughts inserted or deleted by others), grandiose (belief that one has special powers)
- Hallucinations: Auditory, visual, tactile
- Bipolar illness, depression, and dementia are all associated with psychosis, so screen for symptoms of depression, mania, and memory loss.
- Screen for toxidromes of drugs of abuse.
- Screen for history of epileptiform activity.
- Suicidality: Higher risk with comorbid depression or mania, previous suicide attempts, drug abuse, agitation/akathisia, poor compliance

PHYSICAL EXAM
- Schizophrenia and schizoaffective disorder are associated with negative symptoms (e.g., social withdrawal, lack of initiative, poverty of thought) and disorganized speech or behavior.
- Attention to neurologic focalities, antipsychotic-induced parkinsonism, tardive dyskinesia, and akathisia
- May rarely present with catatonia: Extreme excitement or lack of movement, posturing, mutism, grimacing, waxy flexibility
- Mental status exam

DIAGNOSTIC TESTS & INTERPRETATION
Test for causes of delirium mimicking psychosis, if uncertain.

Lab
- Broad screen for medical causes: CBC, metabolic panel, liver function tests, thyroid-stimulating hormone, RPR, HIV, B_{12}, U/A, and screens for subclinical infection in elderly
- Screen for drugs of abuse.

Follow-Up & Special Considerations
Because of elevated risk related to schizophrenia and psychotropic medications, screen for metabolic syndrome.

Imaging
No imaging necessary for diagnosis. Consider MRI or CT to evaluate for medical cause of symptoms, especially if new onset or in elderly. In research studies, schizophrenia is associated with enlarged lateral ventricles and less frontal activity.

Follow-Up & Special Considerations
- Consider: Wilson disease, porphyria, metachromatic leukodystrophy, inflammatory conditions
- Consider ECG: Antipsychotics can prolong corrected QT (QTc) interval, particularly ziprasidone, thioridazine, droperidol, IV haloperidol
- Consider LP if unable to distinguish from delirium and/or unexplained rapid-onset psychosis.
- Consider EEG for partial complex seizures and psychosis associated with preictal and postictal events.

DIFFERENTIAL DIAGNOSIS
- Schizophrenia: Positive symptoms (psychosis) and negative symptoms (flat affect), prodrome of social withdrawal, cognitive impairment; schizophreniform disorder: Psychotic/prodromal symptoms in fewer than 6 months; schizoaffective disorder: Manic or depressive mood disorder with hallucinations or delusions that persist when mood improves; schizotypal personality disorder: No true psychosis, but distance in relationships and odd beliefs; delusional disorder: Nonbizarre delusion (e.g., erotomanic, grandiose, jealous, persecutory, somatic), no negative or mood symptoms
- Mood disorder with psychotic features: Can occur in mania or depression. Delusions often mood-congruent; psychosis remits when mood improves.
- Substance-induced psychosis: Establish timeline of substance use vs. timeline of psychosis; most common: Alcohol and benzodiazepine withdrawal, intoxication with cocaine, PCP, cannabis, amphetamines, hallucinogens, and alcohol. May persist beyond acute intoxication.
- Borderline personality disorder: During extreme stress, patients often experience auditory/visual hallucinations (psychosis NOS)
- Posttraumatic stress disorder: Psychosis associated with traumatic recollections. Often visual hallucinations (vs. more auditory in schizophrenia).
- Psychosis due to general medical condition: Delirium, stroke, infection, collagen vascular disease, head injury, tumor, interictal, porphyria, syphilis, Wilson disease, hypo- or hyperthyroidism, metachromatic leukodystrophy, dementia, HIV
- Medication-induced psychosis: Common causes: Steroids, L-dopa, anticholinergic medication, antidepressants in bipolar patients, interferon, digoxin, stimulants

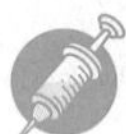

TREATMENT

Before antipsychotic treatment, lipid profile, fasting blood sugar, LFTs, metabolic panel, weight

MEDICATION
- Antipsychotics are the mainstay of treatment. Classified as typical vs. atypical. Dopamine-2 (D_2) antagonists with varied affinity for the receptor. Atypicals also block serotonin 5-HT2A receptors. Help positive symptoms more than negative. Nonspecific effect on agitation begins early; antipsychotic effect takes 1–6 weeks.
- For mania with psychotic features, a mood stabilizer may be used with antipsychotic
- For major depression with psychotic features, antidepressant and antipsychotic medications yield better response rate than either medication alone.
- In delirium, must treat underlying cause.
- Risks of antipsychotic medications include:
  - Acute dystonia: Utilize 1–3 mg IM/IV benztropine initially, then 0.5–2 mg b.i.d.–t.i.d. and/or diphenhydramine 50–100 mg IM/IV b.i.d.–t.i.d. max 400 mg/d.
  - Parkinsonism: Lower medication dose; switch to atypical (particularly quetiapine, olanzapine or clozapine) or add benztropine 0.5–2 mg PO b.i.d.–t.i.d., diphenhydramine 25–50 mg b.i.d.–t.i.d.
  - Akathisia: Intense restlessness, especially legs. Lower dose; switch or beta-blocker, anticholinergic, antihistaminic or benzodiazepine, or utilize quetiapine, olanzapine, or clozapine.
  - Tardive dyskinesia: 20% of those treated long-term with typicals. Switch to clozapine or quetiapine. If can't, minimize dose.

- Neuroleptic malignant syndrome: Potentially fatal; rigidity, tremor, fever, autonomic instability, mental status changes; discontinue neuroleptic; ICU; volume resuscitation; cooling blankets; no anticholinergics/antihistaminics; Consider dantrolene, amantadine, bromocriptine, ECT
- Metabolic syndrome, sudden cardiac death (risk higher IM/IV droperidol, IV haloperidol), stroke (elderly), QTc prolonged, pulmonary embolus

First Line

- Benefits of some of the atypical antipsychotics include low risk of extrapyramidal symptoms (quetiapine, olanzapine, iloperidone, or clozapine) and tardive dyskinesia (quetiapine, clozapine); and possibly more effective for negative symptoms
- Compared with typicals and some of the atypicals (ziprasidone, aripiprazole), there is more risk of weight gain, new-onset diabetes, and hyperlipidemia with olanzapine and clozapine.
- Acute psychotic agitation: Olanzapine 5–10 mg IM with up to three 10-mg injections over a 24-hour period, care with subsequent benzodiazepines; ziprasidone 5–20 mg IM q4–6h maximum 40 mg over a 24-hour period; haloperidol/lorazepam 5 mg/2 mg IM often with 1 mg IM benztropine, maximum 20 mg haloperidol, and 8 mg lorazepam over a 24-hour period
- Psychosis in schizophrenia:
  - Olanzapine start 5–10 mg at bedtime, target dose 5–20 mg/d within 2 days and up to 40 mg/d in treatment-refractory schizophrenia. More likely weight gain, hyperlipidemia, and hyperglycemia than other oral atypicals except clozapine (1)[B], but may have lower rates of discontinuation and rehospitalization than several other atypicals (1)[B], but likely not more efficacy than clozapine (2)[B]. Sedation initially.
  - Quetiapine start 25 mg b.i.d. 25–50 mg b.i.d.–t.i.d. on days 2 and 3, up to 300–400 mg in divided doses by day 4. Within 2 weeks up to 400–800 mg/d divided b.i.d.–t.i.d.; less parkinsonism, useful in Parkinson disease psychosis; more weight gain than aripiprazole and ziprasidone. Sedation can be a problem initially; more gradual titration tolerated better.
  - Quetiapine XR can start 300 mg/d. Dose increases can be within 1 day and up to 300 mg/d, but slower start and titration may be better; target dose 300–800 mg at bedtime; lower parkinsonism but more weight gain than aripiprazole and ziprasidone. Sedation initially.
  - Risperidone start 1–2 mg/d; target dose of 1–4 mg/d to be reached over 1–2 weeks; 5–8 mg rarely more effective and higher risk of parkinsonism. Higher risk of prolactinemia/parkinsonism than quetiapine, olanzapine, clozapine.
  - Paliperidone start 3 mg/d target dose 3–12 mg/day; titrate over 1–2 weeks. Higher risk of prolactinemia/parkinsonism than quetiapine, olanzapine, clozapine.
  - Ziprasidone start 40 mg PO b.i.d., with target dose of 100–200 mg/d in divided doses over 2 weeks; prolongs QTc; less likely to cause weight gain than other atypicals; higher risk of akathisia/parkinsonism than quetiapine, olanzapine, clozapine. Requires meal. Often sedation.
  - Aripiprazole start 5–15 mg every day, increase to 10–30 mg/d over a week or 2; less weight gain but higher rates of akathisia/parkinsonism than quetiapine, olanzapine, clozapine
  - Asenapine start 5 mg at bedtme or b.i.d. sublingually, increase to 10 b.i.d. if needed over a week or 2; less weight gain than some, higher rates of akathisia/parkinsonism than quetiapine, olanzapine, clozapine. Sedation, numb tongue, nausea, bad taste. Black cherry flavor preferred to plain.
  - Lurasidone start 40 mg at bedtime with 350 calories, increase to 80 or 120 mg at bedtime if needed over a week or 2. Less weight gain than some, but higher rates of akathisia/parkinsonism that quetiapine, olanzapine, clozapine. Not antihistaminic, but serotonergic sedation, nausea.
  - Iloperidone start 1 mg b.i.d. may increase by 2 mg b.i.d. each day, but slower can be better due to significant orthostasis. Increase to max 12 mg b.i.d. Little akathisia/parkinsonism, less weight gain than olanzapine or clozapine, but slower efficacy due to long titration, dizziness, sedation.

Geriatric Considerations

Increased risk of cerebrovascular accident when antipsychotics are used in the elderly with dementia. Caution is advised in this population (3)[B].

Second Line

- Clozapine: More effective for reducing symptoms, preventing relapse, decreasing tardive dyskinesia, and decreasing suicidality than other antipsychotics (2), but second line given risk of fatal agranulocytosis. National registry for all patients on clozapine, weekly CBC and absolute neutrophil count (ANC) for 6 months then every 2 weeks for 6 months then every 4 weeks. More weight gain, hyperlipidemia, hyperglycemia, seizures, myocarditis, pulmonary embolus, and sedation, but low rate of parkinsonism, tardive dyskinesia. Useful in treatment-refractory psychosis and in Parkinson disease psychosis.
- Despite precipitating more weight gain than other antipsychotics, clozapine and olanzapine do not appear to increase risk of cardiac and all-cause mortality (4,5).
- Long-acting preparations: Available for 2 typicals (haloperidol and fluphenazine) and 3 atypicals (risperidone, paliperidone, olanzapine; olanzapine requires registry due to rare delirium syndrome). Test tolerability with oral medication first. Long-acting neuroleptics promote compliance.
- Long-acting haloperidol, paliperidone, olanzapine administered every 4 weeks; long-acting risperidone and fluphenazine administered every 2 weeks

ADDITIONAL TREATMENT

Issues for Referral

Encourage contact with advocacy groups for families and patients (National Alliance for the Mentally Ill).

Additional Therapies

Cognitive-behavioral therapy is an effective adjuvant to antipsychotics.

IN-PATIENT CONSIDERATIONS

Admission Criteria

At risk for harm to self or others; extreme functional impairment; unable to care for self; new-onset psychosis

Discharge Criteria

No longer a danger to self or others and adequate outpatient treatment in place

ONGOING CARE

FOLLOW-UP RECOMMENDATIONS

Close follow-up for inpatient discharge (high risk for suicide), utilize cognitive-behavioral therapy, exercise, teach smoking cessation

PATIENT EDUCATION

National Alliance on Mental Illness: www.nami.org/

PROGNOSIS

Schizophrenia: Fluctuating course, 70% first-episode psychosis patients improve in 3–4 months; 7% will die of suicide; 20–40% attempt

REFERENCES

1. Komossa K, Rummel-Kluge C, Hunger H, et al. Olanzapine versus other atypical antipsychotics for schizophrenia. *Cochrane Database Syst Rev.* 2010;3:CD006654.
2. McEvoy JP, Lieberman JA, Stroup TS, et al. Effectiveness of clozapine versus olanzapine, quetiapine, and risperidone in patients with chronic schizophrenia who did not respond to prior atypical antipsychotic treatment. *Am J Psychiatry.* 2006; 163:600–10.
3. van Iersel MB, Zuidema SU, Koopmans RT, et al. Antipsychotics for behavioural and psychological problems in elderly people with dementia: A systematic review of adverse events. *Drugs Aging.* 2005;22:845–58.
4. Tilhonen J, Lonnqvist J, Wahlbeck K, et al. 11-year follow-up mortality in patients with schizophrenia: A population-based cohort study. *Lancet.* 2009; 22(9690):620–7.
5. Strom BL, Faich G, Eng SM, et al. Comparative mortality associated with ziprasidone vs. olanzapine in real-world use: The ziprasidone observational study of cardiac outcomes (zodiac). *European Psychiatry.* 2008;23:158.
6. Fayek M, Flowers C, Signorelli D, et al. Psychopharmacology: Underuse of evidence-based treatments in psychiatry. *Psychiatr Serv.* 2003;54: 1453–6.

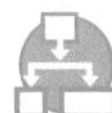

See Also (Topic, Algorithm, Electronic Media Element)

Delirium; Schizophrenia

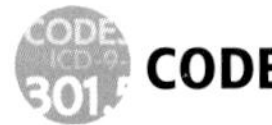

CODES

ICD9

- 295.70 Schizoaffective disorder, unspecified
- 295.90 Unspecified schizophrenia, unspecified
- 298.9 Unspecified psychosis

CLINICAL PEARLS

- Antipsychotics are the mainstay of treatment; evidence corroborates decreased all-cause mortality in patients who are adherent to antipsychotic medications (4).
- Clozapine and long-acting preparations are likely underutilized in schizophrenia in the US and may increase adherence (6), while newer atypicals (quetiapine XR, olanzapine-fluoxetine combination, Abilify, lurasidone) may help with depressive symptoms in psychosis.

PULMONARY ARTERIAL HYPERTENSION

Lisa Laskiewicz, MD
Joseph F. Yammine, MD

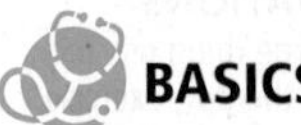

BASICS

DESCRIPTION

- Pulmonary arterial hypertension (PAH) is a category of pulmonary hypertension (PH) characterized by abnormalities in the small pulmonary arteries that produce increased pulmonary arterial pressure (PAP) and vascular resistance, eventually resulting in right heart failure. PAH is a progressive disorder associated with increased mortality:
  - PAH is defined by all 3 of the following measurements (1):
    - Mean PAP ≥25 mm Hg
    - Pulmonary capillary wedge pressure ≤15 mm Hg
    - Pulmonary vascular resistance >3 Wood units
  - Classified as primary (without cause) or secondary (with cause or associated condition)
  - Also classified into 5 main categories:
    - Idiopathic: Sporadic, with no family history or risk factors
    - Heritable: Idiopathic PAH (IPAH) with mutations or familial cases with or without mutations
    - Drug or toxin induced: Mostly associated with anorectics
    - Associated: Connective tissue diseases (e.g., systemic lupus erythematosus, rheumatoid arthritis, scleroderma); HIV infection; portal hypertension; congenital heart disease; schistosomiasis; chronic hemolytic anemia (e.g., sickle cell disease)
    - Persistent PH of the newborn
- System(s) affected: Pulmonary; Cardiovascular

EPIDEMIOLOGY

- Age: Can occur at any age; mean age, 37 years.
- Sex (IPAH): Female > Male (~2:1)

Incidence

- IPAH: Low, ~1–2 per million
- Drug-induced PAH: 1 per 25,000 with >3 months of anorectic use
- HIV associated: 0.5 per 100
- Portal hypertension associated: 1–6 per 100
- Scleroderma associated: 10–50%

Prevalence

- PAH: ~15–50 cases per million
- IPAH: ~6 cases per million

RISK FACTORS

- Female sex
- Previous anorectic drug use
- Recent acute pulmonary embolism
- Commonly associated conditions
- First-degree relatives of patient with familial PAH

Genetics

- 75% of HPAH cases and 25% of IPAH cases have mutations in BMPR2 (autosomal dominant)
- Mutations in ALK1 and endoglin (autosomal dominant) also are associated with PAH.

PATHOPHYSIOLOGY

- Pulmonary: Inflammation, vasoconstriction, endothelial dysfunction, and remodeling of pulmonary arteries produced by increased cell proliferation and reduced rates of apoptosis lead to obstruction.
- Cardiovascular: Right ventricular hypertrophy (RVH), eventually leading to right heart failure

ETIOLOGY

- IPAH: By definition, unknown. True IPAH is mostly sporadic or sometimes familial in nature.
- Pulmonary arteriolar hyperactivity and vasoconstriction, occult thromboembolism, or autoimmune (high frequency of antinuclear antibodies)

COMMONLY ASSOCIATED CONDITIONS

See Associated PAH, above.

DIAGNOSIS

Symptoms of PAH are nonspecific, which can lead to missed or delayed diagnosis of this serious disease.

HISTORY

Fatigue, syncope, dizziness, dyspnea, chest pain, palpitations, lower extremity edema

PHYSICAL EXAM

- Pulmonary component of S2 (at apex in more than 90% of patients)
- Right ventricular lift
- Early systolic click of pulmonary valve
- Pansystolic murmur of tricuspid regurgitation
- Diastolic murmur of pulmonic insufficiency
- Right ventricular S3 or S4
- Edema as jugular vein distention, ascites, hepatomegaly, or peripheral edema

DIAGNOSTIC TESTS & INTERPRETATION

- EKG: RVH and right axis deviation
- Pulmonary function testing and/or arterial blood gas: Arterial hypoxemia, reduced diffusion capacity, hypocapnia
- Ventilation-perfusion ratio (V/Q) scan: Must rule out proximal pulmonary artery emboli
- Exercise test: Reduced maximal O_2 consumption, high minute ventilation, low anaerobic threshold, increased PO_2 alveolar-arterial gradient; correlation to severity of disease with 6-minute walk test.

Lab

- Antinuclear antibody positive (up to 40% of patients):
- Liver function tests to evaluate for portopulmonary hypertension, a complication of chronic liver disease
- HIV test, thyroid function tests, sickle cell disease screening
- Elevated brain natriuretic peptide (BNP) and N-terminal-proBNP may be useful for early detection of PAH in young, otherwise healthy patients with mild symptoms

Imaging

- Chest radiograph:
  - Prominent central pulmonary arteries with peripheral hypovascularity of pulmonary arterial branches
  - Right ventricular enlargement is a late finding.
- Echo Doppler:
  - Should be performed if suspicion of PAH is present; recent studies show some inaccuracy compared with right-heart catheterization.
  - Most commonly used screening tool:
    - Estimates mean PAP and assesses cardiac structure and function
    - Echo suggests, but does not diagnose, PAH. Invasive hemodynamic evaluation confirms PAH diagnosis.
  - Right atrial and ventricular enlargement; tricuspid regurgitation
  - Important to rule out underlying cardiac disease, such as atrial septal defect with secondary PH or mitral stenosis
- Cardiac magnetic resonance is not commonly used.

Diagnostic Procedures/Surgery

- V/Q scan to rule out chronic thromboembolic PH (CTEPH)
- Pulmonary angiography:
  - Should be done if V/Q scan suggests CTEPH
  - Use caution; can lead to hemodynamic collapse; use low osmolar agents, subselective angiograms
- Right-sided cardiac catheterization (gold standard for diagnosis of PAH):
  - Essential first step to confirm diagnosis and determine severity and prognosis by measuring pulmonary arterial pressures and hemodynamics
  - Rule out underlying cardiac disease (e.g., left heart disease) and response to vasodilator therapy.
- Lung biopsy: Not recommended unless primary pulmonary parenchymal disease exists
- 6-minute walk test: Classifies severity of PAH and estimates prognosis

Pathological Findings

- Distal arterioles show medial hypertrophy, proliferative/fibrotic intima, complex lesions, and thrombosis.
- Pulmonary veins usually are not affected.

DIFFERENTIAL DIAGNOSIS

Other causes of dyspnea:

- Pulmonary parenchymal disease such as chronic obstructive pulmonary disease
- Pulmonary vascular disease such as pulmonary thromboembolism
- Cardiac disease such as cardiomyopathy
- Other disorders of respiratory function such as sleep apnea

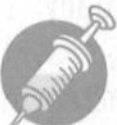

TREATMENT

- PAH remains incurable. Treat underlying diseases/conditions that may cause PAH to relieve symptoms and improve quality of life and survival.
- PAH-specific treatment has been studied mostly in IPAH.

MEDICATION

- Acute vasodilator test (performed during cardiac catheterization) for all IPAH patients who are potential candidates for long-term oral calcium channel blocker (CCB) therapy.
  - Screens for pulmonary vasoreactivity/responsiveness using inhaled nitrous oxide; IV epoprostenol, or IV adenosine. Positive response may be a prognostic indicator.
  - Contraindicated in right heart failure or hemodynamic instability
- Chronic vasodilator therapy:
  - If IPAH with positive response to acute vasodilator test (a fall in mean PAP with unchanged/increased cardiac output), use CCBs:
    - ~13% will initially respond. Unfortunately, long-term clinical response to CCB therapy is small (~7%) (2)[C].

- CCBs include Nifedipine (long-acting); diltiazem; amlodipine.
- Avoid verapamil due to its significant negative inotropic effect.

– PAH with negative response to acute vasodilator test or worsening on therapy; specific vasodilator choice based on risk stratification (2)[C]:
- Higher risk:
  - Prostanoids: Improve exercise capacity, cardiopulmonary hemodynamics: Epoprostenol (IV) (only drug with demonstrated survival benefit and preferred for most ill class IV patients); treprostinil (IV, SC, or inhaled); iloprost (inhaled)
- Lower risk:
  - Endothelin receptor antagonists: Improve exercise capacity; trend toward reducing mortality has been noted (3)[A]: Bosentan (PO); ambrisentan (PO). Monitor liver function tests monthly.
  - Phosphodiesterase-5 inhibitors: Suggested improvement in exercise capacity, cardiopulmonary hemodynamics, and symptoms (1)[C]: Sildenafil (PO); tadalafil (PO)
- It is unclear whether any of the above 3 separate classes of drugs significantly reduce mortality; however, pooling all the vasodilators in a recent systematic review shows 39% reduction in mortality (4)[A]; another recent meta-analysis shows that only prostanoid class has survival benefit, particularly IV prostacyclins (5)[A].
- If one agent fails, vasodilator combination therapy (CT) using a combination of 2 vasodilators (e.g., epoprostenol + sildenafil) is currently being studied (1)[C]. A recent meta-analysis found that CT did not improve outcomes compared to monotherapy (MT). Only 6-minute walk distance was significantly improved when using CT vs. MT (6)[A].

- Anticoagulation:
  - Improved survival originally suggested in patients with IPAH only. Newer studies show some evidence for favorable effects of anticoagulation on survival in IPAH, HPAH, or PAH associated with anorexigens (7)[C].
  - Warfarin with international normalized ratio of 1.5–2.5:
    - Contraindications: Avoid in patients with syncope or significant hemoptysis; consider drug interactions
- Diuretics indicated in patients with right ventricular volume overload (e.g., peripheral edema or ascites)
- Digoxin has little long-term data in PAH:
  - Utilized in right ventricular failure and/or atrial dysrhythmias, increases cardiac output and preserves right ventricle contractility

ADDITIONAL TREATMENT

General Measures

Oxygen supplementation to O_2 >90% is indicated for rest, exercise, or nocturnal hypoxemia.

Issues for Referral

Refer to a pulmonologist and/or a cardiologist for further evaluation/treatment if PAH is suspected or known.

SURGERY/OTHER PROCEDURES

- Patients with documented large-vessel thromboembolic disease should be considered for pulmonary thrombectomy.
- Balloon atrial septostomy for severe PAH with right heart failure despite optimized medical therapy to relieve symptoms prior to lung transplant or as a treatment on its own
- Heart-lung or lung transplantation

IN-PATIENT CONSIDERATIONS

Initial Stabilization

- Medical therapy is first line and primarily palliative.
- Hospitalization with invasive monitoring is needed to screen vasodilator responsiveness and initiate vasodilator therapy.
- National registry has been established by the National Heart, Lung, and Blood Institute

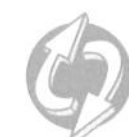

ONGOING CARE

FOLLOW-UP RECOMMENDATIONS

- Pneumococcal and influenza vaccines
- Exercise: Walking or low-level aerobic activity as tolerated once stable; respiratory training

Patient Monitoring

Frequently evaluate disease progression and therapeutic efficacy. Objective tests to measure treatment response include 6-minute walk test and cardiopulmonary exercise test.

DIET

Fluid and salt restrictions, especially with right ventricle failure

PATIENT EDUCATION

Discuss disease, prognosis, lifestyle changes, and all therapeutic options (including transplant).

PROGNOSIS

- Median survival is 2–3 years from diagnosis; 5-year survival rate is 34% for National Institute of Health registry; newer studies show 5-year survival near 70% with new treatment.
- Mode of death: Right heart failure (most common), pneumonia, sudden death, cardiac death
- Poor prognostic factors:
  - Rapid symptom progression
  - Clinical evidence of right ventricular failure
  - World Health Organization functional PAH class 4 (or NYHA functional class 3 or 4)
  - 6-minute walk distance <300 m
  - Peak VO_2 during cardiopulmonary exercise testing <10.4 mL/kg/min
  - Echocardiography with pericardial effusion, significant right ventricle enlargement/dysfunction, right atrial enlargement
  - Mean right atrial pressure >20 mm Hg
  - Cardiac index <2 L/min/m^2
  - Elevated mean PAP
  - Significantly elevated BNP and NT-proBNP; other markers also show promise in predicting survival: RDW, GDF-15, interleukin-6, creatinine (8)[B]
  - Scleroderma spectrum of diseases

COMPLICATIONS

- Thromboembolism, heart failure, and sudden death
- Pregnancy should be avoided due to high maternal mortality (30–50%) and fetal wastage.

REFERENCES

1. McLaughlin VV, Archer SL, Badesch DB, et al. ACCF/AHA 2009 expert consensus document on pulmonary hypertension a report of the American College of Cardiology Foundation Task Force on Expert Consensus Documents and the American Heart Association developed in collaboration with the American College of Chest Physicians; American Thoracic Society, Inc.; and the Pulmonary Hypertension Association. *J Am Coll Cardiol*. 2009;53:1573–619.
2. Badesch DB, Abman SH, Simonneau G, et al. Medical therapy for pulmonary arterial hypertension: Updated ACCP evidence-based clinical practice guidelines. *Chest*. 2007;131: 1917–28.
3. Liu C, Chen J, Gao Y, et al. Endothelin receptor antagonists for pulmonary arterial hypertension. *Cochrane Database Syst Rev*. 2009;CD004434.
4. Macchia A, Marchioli R, Tognoni G, et al. Systematic review of trials using vasodilators in pulmonary arterial hypertension: Why a new approach is needed. *Am Heart J*. 2010;159: 245–57.
5. Ryerson CJ, Nayar S, Swiston JR, et al. Pharmacotherapy in pulmonary arterial hypertension: A systematic review and meta-analysis. *Respir Res*. 2010;11:12.
6. Fox BD, Shimony A, Langleben D, et al. Meta-analysis of monotherapy versus combination therapy for pulmonary arterial hypertension. *Am J Cardiol*. 2011;108:1177–82.
7. Barst RJ, Gibbs JS, Ghofrani HA, et al. Updated evidence-based treatment algorithm in pulmonary arterial hypertension. *J Am Coll Cardiol*. 2009;54: S78–84.
8. Rhodes CJ, Wharton J, Howard LS, et al. Red cell distribution width outperforms other potential circulating biomarkers in predicting survival in idiopathic pulmonary arterial hypertension. *Heart*. 2011;97:1054–60.

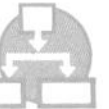

See Also (Topic, Algorithm, Electronic Media Element)

Cor Pulmonale; Pulmonary Embolism

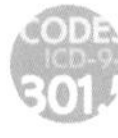

CODES

ICD9

416.0 Primary pulmonary hypertension

CLINICAL PEARLS

- In patients with PAH, a V/Q scan should be performed to rule out CTEPH; a normal scan effectively excludes a diagnosis of CTEPH.
- CCBs are first-line agents to manage IPAH.

PULMONARY EDEMA

Brandon Maughan, MD, MHS
Francesca L. Beaudoin, MS, MD

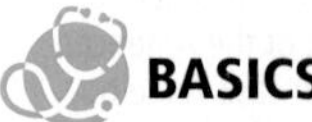

BASICS

DESCRIPTION

- Fluid from pulmonary capillaries leaks into the lung interstitium and alveoli, leading to hypoxia and respiratory distress.
- Fluid accumulation results from cardiogenic causes (e.g., heart failure) that lead to imbalanced hydrostatic and oncotic pressures within the pulmonary capillaries or from noncardiogenic causes (e.g., acute lung injury) that increase alveolar-capillary membrane permeability.

EPIDEMIOLOGY

Incidence

- Heart failure: Annual incidence increases with age:
  - Patients age 35–64: 2 cases per 1,000
  - Patients over age 70: 13.6 cases per 1,000:
    - Higher rates among blacks (16.3 per 1,000) than whites (11.9 per 1,000)
    - Higher rates among men (15.8 per 1,000) than women (11.7 per 1,000)
- Acute lung injury (ALI): 86 cases per 100,000 per year (about 190,000 cases annually in the US)
- Acute respiratory distress syndrome (ARDS): 64 cases per 100,000 per year

Prevalence

Heart failure syndromes: 5.8 million US adults

RISK FACTORS

- Cardiogenic: Hypertension, ischemic heart disease, valvular disease, left ventricular hypertrophy (LVH)
- Noncardiogenic: Sepsis, severe systemic inflammatory states, aspiration, pneumonia, trauma

Genetics

Multifactorial

GENERAL PREVENTION

Early detection and treatment of predisposing condition

PATHOPHYSIOLOGY

- Cardiogenic causes will increase hydrostatic pressure in the pulmonary capillaries, leading to increased transvascular filtration of a protein-poor fluid into lung interstitium.
- Systolic dysfunction is due to decreased contractility of the left ventricle, leading to decreased cardiac output, which in turn stimulates the renin–angiotensin system and increases fluid retention. Diastolic dysfunction is often due to decreased LV compliance secondary to hypertrophy.
- Noncardiogenic causes will increase permeability of the lung vasculature, leading to accumulation of protein-rich fluid in the lung interstitium and air spaces. Many causes of this vascular permeability are associated with ALI/ARDS.

ETIOLOGY

- Cardiogenic (left-sided heart failure):
  - Impaired contractility:
    - Ischemic heart disease
    - Dilated cardiomyopathy
    - Myocarditis
    - Volume overload
    - Alcoholic cardiomyopathy
  - Increased LV afterload:
    - Systemic hypertension
    - Aortic stenosis
    - Cocaine abuse
  - Poor diastolic filling:
    - Left ventricular hypertrophy
    - Hypertrophic cardiomyopathy
    - Mitral stenosis
    - Atrial fibrillation
  - High cardiac output states:
    - Thyrotoxicosis
    - Systemic arteriovenous fistulas
    - Anemia
  - Noncompliance with medications or diet
- Noncardiogenic:
  - Severe systemic inflammatory states:
    - Sepsis
    - Severe trauma
    - Severe burns
    - Pancreatitis
    - DIC
  - Pneumonia
  - Aspiration or near-drowning
  - Inhalation of smoke or toxic gases
  - Blood product transfusion
  - Preeclampsia
  - Rapid ascent to high altitude (>2,500 m)
  - Drug toxicity (salicylates, opiates)
  - Embolism (thrombus, fat, air, amniotic fluid)
  - Rapid ascent to high altitude
  - Neurogenic (after head trauma/surgery)
  - Re-expansion (after pneumothorax/paracentesis)

COMMONLY ASSOCIATED CONDITIONS

See "Etiology."

DIAGNOSIS

HISTORY

- Past medical history:
  - Underlying comorbidities, including prior heart failure or prior MI
  - Fever or other symptoms of infection
  - Recent trauma
  - Drug or alcohol abuse
  - Dietary or medication noncompliance
  - Recent weight gain or increasing edema
  - Recent use of negative inotropic agents (calcium channel blockers)
  - Recent use of NSAIDs
- Symptoms:
  - Progressive dyspnea
  - Orthopnea and paroxysmal nocturnal dyspnea
  - Cough
  - Fatigue and generalized weakness
  - Pink frothy sputum
  - Chest pain

PHYSICAL EXAM

- Vital signs: Tachypneic, tachycardic, and hypoxemic. Patients may be hypotensive or hypertensive.
- General: Respiratory distress, diaphoresis
- HEENT: Cyanosis, frothy oral secretions
- Cardiac: S3, murmurs corresponding to valvular lesions, JVD
- Pulmonary: Crackles or wheezing
- Extremities: Edema, cyanosis, mottled skin

DIAGNOSTIC TESTS & INTERPRETATION

Lab

Initial lab tests

- CBC with differential to screen for infection or anemia
- Chemistry panel to screen for acute kidney injury, hyponatremia (associated with severe heart failure), or electrolyte disturbances associated with dysrhythmias
- Troponin may be elevated from recent infarction causing acute heart failure, or may be from myocyte ischemia secondary to elevated ventricular strain. Elevated cardiac enzymes carry a strongly negative prognosis in heart failure.
- Brain natriuretic peptide (BNP) can add to clinical judgment in patients with intermediate risk of heart failure. BNP >500 pg/mL suggests heart failure, and BNP <100 pg/mL suggests alternative causes (1,2,3)[A]. Less useful in setting of atrial fibrillation or renal failure.
- Liver function tests (LFTs) to check for elevated transaminases, which can suggest hepatic congestion from heart failure or may indicate heavy alcohol use contributing to cardiomyopathy
- Drug screens (aspirin, opiates, cocaine, alcohol)
- Consider arterial blood gas to determine pH and A-a gradient for moderate-severe respiratory distress or persistent hypoxemia
- Serum lipase if suspicious for pancreatitis
- TSH if suspicious for thyrotoxicosis
- Blood cultures, urine cultures, and lactic acid if concerned for sepsis
- Urinalysis to check for nephrotic syndrome or UTI

Imaging

Initial approach

- Chest x-ray (CXR):
  - Rule out pneumothorax.
  - Evaluate for focal infiltrate suggestive of pneumonia.
  - Look for signs of edema such as increased interstitial markings, cardiomegaly, perihilar alveolar edema, or pleural effusions.
- ECG to evaluate for cardiac ischemia or signs of pericardial effusion
- Echocardiography with Doppler to evaluate for systolic dysfunction and wall motion abnormalities

Follow-Up & Special Considerations

Emergent echocardiography if suspicious for cardiogenic shock or tamponade physiology

Pathological Findings

- Expansion of perivascular, peribronchiolar, and interstitial space by fluid
- Alveolar wall thickening with capillary congestion and alveolar filling
- Hyaline membrane formation

DIFFERENTIAL DIAGNOSIS

- COPD
- Pneumonia
- Pulmonary embolism
- Asthma/reactive airway disease
- Pneumothorax
- Cardiac tamponade

TREATMENT

MEDICATION

First Line

- All treatment should be tailored to the suspected cause.
- Preload reduction for acute cardiogenic edema:
  - Loop diuretics: Furosemide 40–80 mg IV, torsemide 10 mg IV, or bumetanide 1 mg IV. If on chronic diuretics, start IV dose at home dose and titrate. Onset 15–30 minutes (1,2,3)[B]
  - IV nitrate vasodilators: Rapid onset. Start IV nitroglycerin 20 mcg/min, titrate 20 mcg/min q3–5min to max 200 mcg/min until distress resolved or onset of hypotension.
  - For severe hypertension, consider IV nitroprusside 5–10 mcg/min, titrate. Max 400 mcg/min. Use <48 hours due to risk of cyanide toxicity (3)[C].
- Afterload reduction for systolic heart failure:
  - Angiotensin-converting enzyme inhibitors (ACEI): lisinopril 2.5–5 mg PO daily, enalapril 2.5 mg PO b.i.d., or captopril 6.25 mg PO t.i.d. Avoid in acutely ill patients with hypotension, acute renal failure, hyperkalemia, or poor diuresis (1)[A].
  - Angiotensin receptor blockers (ARB) for ACEI-intolerant patients: candesartan 4 mg PO daily, losartan 25 mg PO daily, or valsartan 20 mg PO b.i.d. Use the same precautions as with ACEI.
  - Beta blockers: carvedilol 3.125 mg PO b.i.d., bisoprolol 1.25 mg PO daily, or metoprolol CR/XL 12.5 mg PO daily. Avoid if patients are hypotensive or recently required inotropes.
- Improve contractility in hypotensive patients with severe systolic heart failure (1,2,3)[C]:
  - Dobutamine: 5–10 mcg/kg/min IV, titrate.
  - Milrinone: Load 50 mcg/kg IV over 10 minutes, then infuse 0.375–0.75 mcg/kg/min, titrate.
  - Dopamine: 5–10 mcg/kg/min IV, titrate.
  - Norepinephrine: 2–4 mcg/min IV for acute cardiogenic shock following acute MI. Not for use in acute decompensated heart failure.
- High altitude pulmonary edema:
  - Adjunctive therapy: Consider nifedipine ER 30 mg PO q12h or sildenafil 50 mg PO q8h in conjunction with oxygen, descent, and hyperbarics.
- Chronic heart failure: Gradually titrate daily oral therapy, maximum daily doses listed (1,2):
  - Loop diuretics: Furosemide 20–80 mg t.i.d.–q.i.d., torsemide 20 mg daily, bumetanide 1 mg b.i.d. (1,2)[C]
  - ACEIs: Lisinopril 20–40 mg PO daily, enalapril 10–20 mg b.i.d., captopril 50 mg t.i.d. (1,2)[A]
  - ARBs: Candesartan 32 mg daily, valsartan 160 mg b.i.d., losartan 100 mg (1,2)[A]
  - Beta-blockers: Carvedilol 25 mg b.i.d., metoprolol CR/XL 200 mg daily, bisoprolol 10 mg daily (1,2)[A]
  - Nitrates: Isosorbide dinitrate 10–60 mg t.i.d. (1,2)[B]
- Precautions:
  - Diuretics: Monitor for electrolyte derangement and renal dysfunction. Use very carefully in patients with aortic stenosis.
  - Inotropes increase myocardial oxygen demand and may damage the ischemic myocardium.
  - Monitor the additive hypotensive effects of diuretics, nitrates, and afterload reducers.

Second Line

- Thiazide diuretics: HCTZ 25–50 mg PO daily, metolazone 2.5–10 mg PO daily
- Spironolactone: 25–50 mg PO daily; patients need follow-up renal testing
- Digoxin: 125 mcg PO daily, titrate to serum concentration of 0.5–0.8 ng/mL

ADDITIONAL TREATMENT

Issues for Referral

Cardiology referral for underlying cardiac disease

Additional Therapies

Nesiritide is no longer recommended; new data show no effect on hospitalization or mortality (4)[B]

SURGERY/OTHER PROCEDURES

- Cardiac catheterization for cardiac ischemia/ACS
- ECMO for severe refractory hypoxia/ARDS
- Intra-arterial balloon pump for cardiogenic shock
- ICD for sudden cardiac death prevention in patients with prior cardiac arrest or ischemic/dilated cardiomyopathy and LVEF <30% (2)[A]
- Cardiac resynchronization therapy (CRT) for severe systolic heart failure and QRS >0.12 ms
- Left ventricular assist device (LVAD) for severe systolic dysfunction as bridge to a heart transplant

IN-PATIENT CONSIDERATIONS

Initial Stabilization

- Mild distress: Oxygen by nonrebreather mask
- Significant hypoxia: Noninvasive positive pressure ventilation (BiPAP/CPAP) to improve oxygenation and decrease LV afterload (5)[A]
- Intubation for patients with apnea, altered mental status, or hypoxia despite NPPV.
- High altitude pulmonary edema: Supplemental oxygen, descent, hyperbaric therapy

Admission Criteria

- Hypotension
- Acute kidney injury
- Altered mental status
- Dyspnea at rest
- O_2 saturation <90%
- Acute coronary syndromes
- Arrhythmias (i.e., new-onset atrial fibrillation)

IV Fluids

Use crystalloid infusions cautiously.

Nursing

- Daily weights, strict input/output
- Assess for functional improvement

Discharge Criteria

- Underlying condition treated, fluid status optimized
- Started beta-blocker and ACEI in heart failure patients
- Family and patient education completed

ONGOING CARE

FOLLOW-UP RECOMMENDATIONS

Patient Monitoring

- Strict input/output measurement, daily weights
- Posthospitalization appointment in 7–10 days

DIET

- Low-sodium diet (<2 g/d), fluid restriction <2 L/d

PATIENT EDUCATION

- Early signs and symptoms of fluid overload
- Adjust diuretic dose based on recent weight gain

PROGNOSIS

- Mortality: 30–60% for noncardiogenic edema/ARDS and up to 80% for cardiogenic causes

COMPLICATIONS

- Pulmonary fibrosis/hypertension (ARDS)
- Dysrhythmias and sudden cardiac death

REFERENCES

1. Hunt SA, Abraham WT, Chin MH, et al. 2005 Guideline Update for the Diagnosis and Management of Chronic Heart Failure in the Adult: A report of the American College of Cardiology/American Heart Association Task Force on Practice Guidelines (Writing Committee to Update the 2001 Guidelines for the Evaluation and Management of Heart Failure): Developed in collaboration with the American College of Chest Physicians and the International Society for Heart and Lung Transplantation: Endorsed by the Heart Rhythm Society. *Circulation*. 2005;112:e154–235.
2. Jessup M, et al. 2009 focused update: ACCF/AHA Guidelines for the Diagnosis and Management of Heart Failure in Adults: A Report of the American College of Cardiology Foundation/American Heart Association Task Force on Practice Guidelines: Developed in Collaboration With the International Society for Heart and Lung Transplantation. *Circulation*. 2009;119:1977–2016.
3. Heart Failure Society of America, Lindenfeld J, Albert NM, et al. HFSA 2010 Comprehensive Heart Failure Practice Guideline. *J Card Fail*. 2010;16:e1–194.
4. O'Connor CM, Starling RC, Hernandez AF, et al. Effect of nesiritide in patients with acute decompensated heart failure. *N Engl J Med*. 2011;365:32–43.
5. Vital FM, Saconato H, Ladeira MT, et al. Non-invasive positive pressure ventilation (CPAP or bilevel NPPV) for cardiogenic pulmonary edema. *Cochrane Database Syst Rev*. 2008;CD005351.

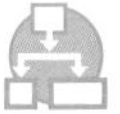

See Also (Topic, Algorithm, Electronic Media Element)

Altitude Illness; Congestive Heart Failure; Respiratory Distress Syndrome, Acute (ARDS)

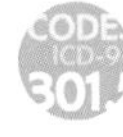

CODES

ICD9

- 514 Pulmonary congestion and hypostasis
- 518.4 Acute edema of lung, unspecified

CLINICAL PEARLS

- The identification of the underlying etiology is essential.
- Provide NPPV for alert patients with respiratory distress.
- The initial treatment is with IV diuretics and nitrates in acute cardiogenic edema.
- Home dietary and medication management is critical.

PULMONARY EMBOLISM

Alfonso J. Tafur, MD, RPVI
Ana Isabel Casanegra, MD

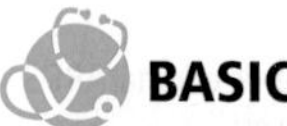

BASICS

DESCRIPTION

- Pulmonary embolism (PE) is the obstruction of the pulmonary arteries typically due to a thrombus that formed at another site and traveled in the bloodstream until it lodges.
- Venous thromboembolism (VTE) refers to both pulmonary embolism and deep vein thrombosis.

EPIDEMIOLOGY

The case fatality rate ranges from 1–60% depending on the severity of the clinical presentation.

Incidence

- Incidence increases with age.
- ~23–69 new PE cases per 100,000 per year
- 25,000 hospitalizations per year in the US, 10–60% in hospitalized patients:
  - Highest risk for orthopedic patients
  - 1 in 1,000 pregnancies (including postpartum)

RISK FACTORS

- Acquired: Age, immobilization, surgery, cancer, oral contraceptives, hormonal replacement therapy, pregnancy/puerperium, previous thrombosis, paroxysmal nocturnal hemoglobinuria, antiphospholipid syndrome, prolonged travel
- Inherited: Antithrombin deficiency, protein C deficiency, protein S deficiency, factor V Leiden, prothrombin gene mutation G20210A, dysfibrinogenemia

Genetics

- Factor V Leiden: The most common thrombophilia. In population studies: 5.5% in Caucasian, 2.2% in Hispanics, 1.2% in African American, 0.5% in Asian. 20% of all the patients with VTE (1,2).
- Prothrombin G20210A: 3% of Caucasians, rare in African American, Asian, and Native American. 6% in patients with VTE (1).

GENERAL PREVENTION

- Prevention strategies should be tailored to the patient VTE risk and the patient bleeding risk (3).
- Mechanical thromboprophylaxis includes: Early ambulation after surgery, graduated compression stockings, and intermittent pneumatic compression
- Intermediate risk: Medical patients, general surgery, gynecologic or urologic surgery. Pharmacologic prophylaxis is recomended with low-molecular-weight heparin (LMWH), unfractionated heparin (UFH) or fondaparinux.
- High risk: Hip or knee arthroplasty, hip fracture surgery, major trauma, spinal cord injury. Pharmacologic prophylaxis is recommended with LMWH, fondaparinux, or vitamin K antagonists (VKA).
- Long-distance travel (>8 hours): Adequate hydration, avoidance of constrictive clothing and frequent calf exercises. If additional risk factors are present, graduate compression stockings below knee or single dose of LMWH if risk is very high.

PATHOPHYSIOLOGY

- Venous stasis, endothelial damage, and changes in the coagulation properties of the blood trigger the formation of thrombus.
- PE causes increased pulmonary vascular resistance, impaired gas exchange, and decreased pulmonary compliance.

ETIOLOGY

- DVT in the proximal veins is the most common source of PE.
- Upper extremity DVT and pelvic vein thrombi can also cause PE.

DIAGNOSIS

Establish a pretest probability based on clinical criteria such as Wells score or Geneva score (4):

- Wells score:
  - Clinical signs and symptoms of DVT +3
  - Alternative diagnosis is less likely than PE +3
  - Heart rate >100 +1.5
  - Immobilization/surgery in previous 4 weeks +1.5
  - Previous DVT/PE +1.5
  - Hemoptysis +1
  - Malignancy +1:
    - Fewer than 2 points: Low clinical probability; 2–6 points: Moderate; more than 6 points: High

HISTORY

- Provoked or idiopathic
- Presence of risk factors and family history
- Bleeding risk (previous anticoagulation, history of bleeding, recent interventions/surgeries, liver disease)
- Dyspnea (82%), chest pain (49%), cough (20%), syncope (14%), hemoptysis (7%) (5)

PHYSICAL EXAM

- Tachycardia, tachypnea, accentuated pulmonary component in S2
- Pleuritic chest pain, pleural friction rub, râles
- Leg swelling, tenderness along a vein, visible collateral veins
- Signs of right ventricular failure may be present (rare): Jugular vein distention, third or fourth sound, audible systolic murmur at left sternal edge, hepatomegaly

ALERT

- Massive PE: Acute PE with sustained hypotension, pulselessness, or persistent profound bradycardia (6)
- Submassive PE: Acute PE without systemic hypotension but with either RV dysfunction or myocardial necrosis (6):
  - RV dysfunction is defined as: RV dilation or RV systolic dysfunction on echocardiography, RV dilation (4-chamber RV diameter divided by LV diameter 0.9) on CT, elevation of BNP, elevation of N-terminal pro-BNP (500 pg/mL), or consistent ECG changes
  - Myocardial necrosis is evidenced by troponin elevation.
- Low-risk PE: Acute PE and the absence of the clinical markers of adverse prognosis that define massive or submassive PE

DIAGNOSTIC TESTS & INTERPRETATION

Lab

- D-dimer: In patients with low pretest probability, it can rule out PE if it is negative (high NPV). It is not diagnostic if it is positive (low PPV), and it is not helpful if pretest probability is intermediate or high (4).
- CBC, including platelets, creatinine, aPTT and PT, ABG.
- In young patients with idiopathic VTE, recurrent VTE, or significant family history of VTE, consider testing for hypercoagulable tests:
  - Do not test for protein C, S, factor VIII, and antithrombin in the acute setting or while on treatment, as results may be falsely abnormal.

Follow-Up & Special Considerations

Elevated troponin I or T and elevated BNP are markers for higher-risk patients.

Imaging

All patients with intermediate or high pretest probability and low probability with abnormal D-dimer, need further diagnostic testing:

- Chest x-ray (CXR): Suggestive findings include: Westermark (lack of vessels in an area distal to the embolus), Hampton hump (wedge-shaped opacity with base in pleura), Fleischner sign (enlarged pulmonary arteries), atelectasis, pleural effusion, pulmonary infarct, elevation of hemidiaphragm
- EKG: Right heart strain, nonspecific rhythm abnormalities, S1Q3T3
- CT pulmonary angiography: Sensitivity 96–100%, specificity 86–89%. NPV 99.8%. Requires IV iodine contrast (7).
- Ventilation/perfusion scintigraphy (V/Q scan): Use if CTA is not available or contraindicated. A high-probability V/Q scan makes the diagnosis of PE; a normal V/Q scan excludes PE.
- Pulmonary angiogram: Gold standard but invasive and technically difficult. 2% morbidity and <0.01 mortality risk.
- Echocardiogram: Helpful to asses right ventricle function
- Magnetic resonance angiography: Lower sensitivity and specificity than CTA
- Compression ultrasound (CUS): Noninvasive. 1/3 of the patients with PE will have a DVT.
- CT venography: Can be done at the same time of the CTA, increases diagnostic yield. Requires IV iodinated contrast.

ALERT

If your preclinical probability is intermediate or high and the patient has a low bleeding risk, start the treatment while you wait for the diagnostic results.

DIFFERENTIAL DIAGNOSIS

- Pulmonary: Pneumonia, bronchitis, pneumonitis, COPD exacerbation, pulmonary edema, pneumothorax
- Cardiac: Myocardial infarction (angina pectoris), pericarditis, CHF
- Vascular: Dissection of the aorta
- Musculoskeletal: Rib fracture(s), musculoskeletal chest wall pain

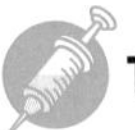

TREATMENT

MEDICATION

- If the clinical suspicion is high and there are no contraindications, start treatment as soon as possible (8).
- LMWH, UFH, fondaparinux, as initial therapy. VKA can be started the first day, and need to overlap with parenteral treatment a minimum of 5 days, and until the INR is 2–3 for 24 hours (8).
- Patients with massive PE with low bleeding risk consider thrombolytics if they have no contraindications (6,8)

First Line

- Unfractionated heparin (UFH) (8):
  - IV bolus of 80 U/kg or 5,000 U followed by continuous infusion (initially at 18 U/kg/hr or 1,300 U/hr) with dose adjustments to maintain an aPTT that corresponds to antiactivated factor X (anti-Xa) levels of 0.3–0.7
  - SC injection: 2 options:
    - Monitored: 17,500 U or 250 U/kg b.i.d. with dose adjustments to maintain an aPTT that corresponds to anti-Xa levels of 0.3–0.7 measured 6 hours after a dose
    - Fixed dose: 333 U/kg initial dose, followed by 250 U/kg b.i.d.
- Low-molecular-weight heparin (LMWH) (8):
  - Enoxaparin (Lovenox): 1 mg/kg/dose SC q12h or 1.5 mg/kg q24h
  - Dalteparin (Fragmin): 200 U/kg SC q24h
- Fondaparinux (Arixtra):
  - 5 mg (body weight <50 kg), 7.5 mg (body weight 50–100 kg) or 10 mg (body weight >100) SC q24h
- Maintenance therapy: VKA:
  - Warfarin: Start on day 1, if possible. 5 mg daily for 3 days, and adjust dose to maintain an INR of 2–3.

ALERT

Contraindications:

- Active bleeding is a contraindication for anticoagulation. Heparin: Heparin-induced thrombocytopenia (HIT)
- LMWH: HIT, renal failure
- Fondaparinux: Renal failure
- Warfarin: Pregnancy

Pregnancy Considerations

- Warfarin is teratogenic and should not be used in pregnant patients (especially in first trimester); safe while breast-feeding
- Dalteparin, enoxaparin, and fondaparinux are Category B for pregnancy; heparin is Category C.

Second Line

- Massive PE: Evaluate carefully the risks and benefits. Thrombolytics are considered if the patient has hemodynamic compromise and a low bleeding risk (6,8,9):
  - Tissue plasminogen activator (tPA) 100 mg infused through a peripheral vein over 2 hours
  - Absolute contraindications: Intracranial hemorrhage, known intracranial cerebrovascular or malignant disease, ischemic stroke within 3 months, suspected aortic dissection, bleeding diathesis, active bleeding, recent neuro surgery, recent major trauma

SURGERY/OTHER PROCEDURES

- IVC filter placement in patients with contraindication for anticoagulation (6,8)
- Emergency surgical embolectomy can be considered if the patient has massive PE with contraindications for thrombolysis (6).
- Consider catheter-based interventions if the patient has massive PE and either contraindications to thrombolytics or if they remain unstable despite the use of thrombolytics (6)[C].

IN-PATIENT CONSIDERATIONS

Initial Stabilization

May require ICU-level care if hemodynamically unstable

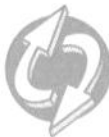

ONGOING CARE

Duration of anticoagulation:

- Provoked PE (and the trigger is no longer present): 3 months
- Unprovoked (idiopathic) PE: A minimum of 3 months, but consider long-term or prolonged secondary prophylaxis if the bleeding risk is low
- Cancer-related PE: LMWH for the first 3–6 months, followed by long-term anticoagulation with LMWH or VKA
- Recurrent PE: Long-term anticoagulation

FOLLOW-UP RECOMMENDATIONS

- If concomitant DVT, knee height compression stockings 30–40 mm Hg knee height
- Consider retrieval of retrievable IVC filters in anticoagulated patients.

Patient Monitoring

- INR should be checked at regular intervals. Target INR: 2–3 for therapy.
- aPTT needs to be monitored if the patient is on adjustable SC UFH.
- Anti-Xa can be checked in special circumstances in patients treated with LMWH.

DIET

Patients taking VKA need to receive education on food content of vitamin K to keep a consistent diet and avoid INR fluctuations.

PATIENT EDUCATION

Risks, monitoring, and compliance

PROGNOSIS

Severity at presentation affects mortality: Massive PE 50% vs. nonmassive PE 8–14%

COMPLICATIONS

- 1 in 25 PE patients will develop chronic thromboembolic pulmonary hypertension.
- Recurrent DVT or PE
- Postphlebitic syndrome
- Complications of the treatment, such as anticoagulation-associated bleeding. Incidence of major hemorrhage associated with thrombolytics is 8%; intracerebral bleed is 2% (fatal in half of the cases).

REFERENCES

1. Lindhoff-Last E, Luxembourg B, et al. Evidence-based indications for thrombophilia screening. *VASA*. 2008;37:19–30.
2. Walker P, Gregg AR, et al. Screening, testing, or personalized medicine: Where do inherited thrombophilias fit best? *Obstet Gynecol Clin North Am*. 2010;37:87–107, Table of Contents.
3. Geerts WH, Bergqvist D, Pineo GF, et al. Prevention of venous thromboembolism: American College of Chest Physicians Evidence-Based Clinical Practice Guidelines (8th Edition). *Chest*. 2008;133:381S–453S.
4. Douma RA, Mos IC, Erkens PM, et al. Performance of 4 clinical decision rules in the diagnostic management of acute pulmonary embolism: A prospective cohort study. *Ann Intern Med*. 2011;154:709–18.
5. Goldhaber SZ, Visani L, De Rosa M. Acute pulmonary embolism: Clinical outcomes in the International Cooperative Pulmonary Embolism Registry (ICOPER). *Lancet*. 1999;353(9162): 1386–9.
6. Jaff MR, McMurtry MS, Archer SL, et al. Management of massive and submassive pulmonary embolism, iliofemoral deep vein thrombosis, and chronic thromboembolic pulmonary hypertension: A scientific statement from the American Heart Association. *Circulation*. 2011;123:1788–830.
7. Sadigh G, Kelly AM, Cronin P, et al. Challenges, controversies, and hot topics in pulmonary embolism imaging. *AJR Am J Roentgenol*. 2011;196:497–515.
8. Kearon C, Kahn SR, Agnelli G, et al. Antithrombotic therapy for venous thromboembolic disease: American College of Chest Physicians Evidence-Based Clinical Practice Guidelines (8th Edition). *Chest*. 2008;133: 454S–545S.
9. Dong BR, Hao Q, Yue J, et al. Thrombolytic therapy for pulmonary embolism. *Cochrane Database Syst Rev*. 2009;CD004437.
10. Konstantinides S. Clinical practice. Acute pulmonary embolism. *N Engl J Med*. 2008;359: 2804–13.

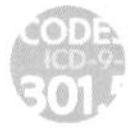

CODES

ICD9

415.19 Other pulmonary embolism and infarction

CLINICAL PEARLS

- PE can be excluded in patients who have a low pretest probability and negative D-dimer testing.
- Unless contraindicated, CT angiogram can reliably be used to diagnose or rule out PE in the majority of cases (10).
- Cancer-oriented review of systems and age- and gender-appropriate cancer screening in patients >40, recurrent VTE, upper extremity DVT (not related to catheter or lines), bilateral lower extremity DVT, intra-abdominal DVT, resistance to treatment
- In patients with a prolonged baseline aPTT, adjust the heparin dose with anti-Xa levels (therapeutic range 0.3–0.7).

PULMONARY VALVE STENOSIS

Kevin Engelhardt, MD
Brent J. Barber, MD

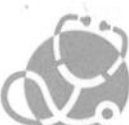

BASICS

DESCRIPTION

Congenital deformity consisting of obstruction to right ventricular (RV) outflow at the level of the pulmonic valve

EPIDEMIOLOGY

Incidence

- Predominant age: Present in newborns but often asymptomatic for years
- Predominant sex: Male < Female (slight)
- Small increase in black male/female relative to white male/female (1)

Prevalence

- 10% of all cases of congenital heart disease
- In association with other lesions, may be as high as 25–30% of congenital heart disease

Pediatric Considerations

This is a congenital disorder.

Pregnancy Considerations

In asymptomatic young women with mild to moderate pulmonic stenosis, pregnancy is generally well tolerated.

RISK FACTORS

Family history

Genetics

- Genetic cause is likely, with numerous familial and syndromic cases
- Associated with Noonan, LEOPARD, and Williams syndromes and neurofibromatosis

PATHOPHYSIOLOGY

- Valvular
- Subvalvular
- Supravalvular

ETIOLOGY

- Abnormal development of distal bulbus cordis secondary to:
  - Congenital/genetic
  - Rubella embryopathy
- Acquired:
  - Stenosis of bioprosthetic valve
  - Rarely, rheumatic fever
  - Very rarely, carcinoid syndrome

COMMONLY ASSOCIATED CONDITIONS

- Tetralogy of Fallot
- Noonan syndrome
- LEOPARD syndrome
- Ventricular septal defect and atrial septal defect
- Neurofibromatosis
- Williams syndrome
- Alagille syndrome

DIAGNOSIS

HISTORY

- History of heart murmur since birth
- Usually asymptomatic; exercise tolerance is normal unless stenosis is severe.
- Most frequent symptoms are dyspnea and fatigue.
- Other symptoms include chest pain and occasionally dizziness or syncope, particularly exertional, owing to low fixed cardiac output.
- Myocardial infarction (MI) of the hypertrophied right ventricle has been noted.

PHYSICAL EXAM

- Acyanotic, unless septal defect allows right-to-left shunting
- Prominent A wave of the jugular venous pulse
- RV heave
- Thrill; does not correlate with stenosis severity; often present in mild to moderate stenosis
- Pulmonic ejection sound/click: Louder during expiration; may be absent in patients with severe stenosis or dysplastic valve
- Midsystolic murmur (increased duration and later peaking with increased severity); heard best at left upper sternal border; may radiate throughout precordium and to left upper back
- Delay in P2; P2 becomes softer in severe stenosis.

DIAGNOSTIC TESTS & INTERPRETATION

Lab

Initial lab tests

Echocardiography:

- Generally sinus rhythm, occasionally supraventricular arrhythmias
- Rightward axis
  - Right ventricular hypertrophy (RVH)
  - RVH severity correlates with R:S ratio in leads V1 and V6 (R in V1 >30 mV correlates with severe stenosis)
- Tall peaked P waves (right atrial enlargement)
- Abnormal T waves in V1 also a sign of RVH (upright in children, inverted in adults)

Imaging

Initial approach

- Radiograph: Poststenotic dilatation of the pulmonary trunk, prominence of right atrium and ventricle
- Echocardiography: Mobile, doming, thickened pulmonic valve; poststenotic dilatation of the pulmonary trunk (does not correlate with degree of stenosis)
- Continuous-wave Doppler: Provides an estimate of the transvalvular gradient (<35–40 mm Hg = mild; 40–60 mm Hg = moderate; >60–70 mm Hg = severe)
- Color-flow Doppler: Delineation of areas of obstruction; assesses for pulmonary regurgitation

Diagnostic Procedures/Surgery

Cardiac catheterization:

- Not indicated in mild pulmonic stenosis
- Perform prior to planned valvuloplasty for moderate to severe stenosis
- Assesses morphology of the right ventricle, pulmonary outflow tract, and pulmonary arteries
- Rules out associated lesions (e.g., atrial septal defect), although echocardiogram usually will suffice

Pathological Findings

- Trileaflet valve with fibrous thickening and fusion of commissures
- Markedly dysplasia of valve with hypoplastic annulus and increased leaflet thickening (especially seen in patients with Noonan syndrome)

DIFFERENTIAL DIAGNOSIS

- Dysplastic pulmonic valve stenosis
- Discrete infundibular stenosis
- Subinfundibular obstruction
- Isolated pulmonary artery stenosis
- Supravalvar pulmonary stenosis
- Tetralogy of Fallot (Pink)

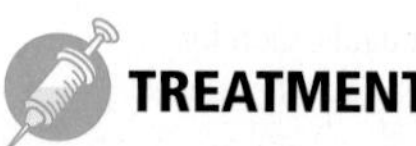

TREATMENT

Pulmonary balloon valvuloplasty is the treatment of choice (2)[A], recommended for the following patients:

- Symptomatic patients with peak-to-peak catheter gradient >30 mm Hg
- Asymptomatic patients with peak-to-peak catheter gradient >40 mm Hg

MEDICATION

No specific regimen in the absence of congestive heart failure

ADDITIONAL TREATMENT

General Measures

Prophylaxis for subacute bacterial endocarditis is no longer recommended for pulmonary valve stenosis unless the patient has associated congenital heart disease with cyanosis or a prosthetic cardiac valve/conduit (3)[A].

Issues for Referral

Patients should be followed longitudinally by a cardiologist.

Additional Therapies

Penicillin prophylaxis if rheumatic fever is the cause

SURGERY/OTHER PROCEDURES

- Surgical pulmonic valvuloplasty in patients with obstruction that is not amenable to balloon valvuloplasty; most frequently supravalvular pulmonary stenosis or dysplastic pulmonary valve (4)[B]
- Patients may manifest dynamic subvalvular gradient after balloon valvuloplasty or surgical repair, which typically regresses with time.
- Future directions include percutaneous pulmonary valve placement currently in clinical trials for indications of RV-pulmonary artery conduit dysfunction with moderate to severe PR , age >5 and size limitations. Early results and expanded multicenter trials both indicate promising safety and short-term effectiveness (5,6).

ONGOING CARE

FOLLOW-UP RECOMMENDATIONS

Regular follow-up assessment for patients not undergoing surgical correction

Patient Monitoring

- Postoperative (or after balloon valvuloplasty) Doppler ultrasound to follow gradient and pulmonic insufficiency
- Cardiac MRI allows for accurate quantification of RV volumes and ejection fraction postoperatively (7)[C].

DIET

No specific regimen mandated

PATIENT EDUCATION

Information is available from the American Heart Association, 7320 Greenville Avenue, Dallas, TX 75231; (214) 373-6300 or www.americanheart.org.

PROGNOSIS

Outcome after either balloon or surgical valvotomy is generally excellent.

COMPLICATIONS

- Up to 10% late mortality following valvotomy in critical pulmonary stenosis in neonates
- Slower recovery in those with chronic severe RVH
- Postvalvotomy pulmonic regurgitation reported in up to 50% (variable severity)
- Residual atrial septal defect or patent foramen ovale
- Persistent repolarization abnormalities on ECG associated with severe postoperative pulmonic regurgitation
- Late atrial arrhythmias
- Rare risk of aneurysms after balloon valvuloplasty
- Long-term associated reduction in exercise capacity and peak VO_2 after valvuloplasty related to degree of PR (8)

REFERENCES

1. Nembhard WN, Wang T, Loscalzo ML. Variation in the prevalence of congenital heart defects by maternal race/ethnicity and infant sex. *J Pediatr.* 2010;156:259–64.
2. Perterson C. Comparative long-term results of surgery versus balloon valvuloplasty for pulmonary valve stenosis in infants and children. *Ann Thoracic Surg.* 2003;76:1078–82.
3. Nishimura RA, Carabello BA, Faxon DP. ACC/AHA 2008 guideline update on valvular heart disease: Focused update on infective endocarditis: A report of the American College of Cardiology/American Heart Association Task Force on Practice Guidelines endorsed by the Society of Cardiovascular Anesthesiologists, Society for Cardiovascular Angiography and Interventions, and Society of Thoracic Surgeons. *Catheter Cardiovasc Interv.* 2008;72:E1–12.
4. Sharieff S, Shah-e-Zaman K, Faruqui AM. Short- and intermediate-term follow-up results of percutaneous transluminal balloon valvuloplasty in adolescents and young adults with congenital pulmonary valve stenosis. *J Invasive Cardiol.* 2003;15:484–7.
5. Zahn EM, Hellenbrand WE, Lock JE, et al. Implantation of the melody transcatheter pulmonary valve in patients with a dysfunctional right ventricular outflow tract conduit early results from the U.S. Clinical trial. *J Am Coll Cardiol.* 2009; 54:1722–9.
6. McElhinney DB, Hellenbrand WE, Zahn EM, et al. Short- and medium-term outcomes after transcatheter pulmonary valve placement in the expanded multicenter US melody valve trial. *Circulation.* 2010;122:507–16.
7. Vliegen HW, van Straten A, de Roos A. Magnetic resonance imaging to assess the hemodynamic effects of pulmonary valve replacement in adults late after repair of tetralogy of fallot. *Circulation.* 2002;106:1703–7.
8. Harrild DM, Powell AJ, Tran TX, et al. Long-term pulmonary regurgitation following balloon valvuloplasty for pulmonary stenosis. *J Am Coll Cardiol.* 2010;55:1041–7.

ADDITIONAL READING

American College of Cardiology, American Heart Association Task Force on Practice Guidelines (Writing Committee to revise the 1998 guidelines for the management of patients with valvular heart disease), Society of Cardiovascular Anesthesiologists, et al. ACC/AHA 2006 guidelines for the management of patients with valvular heart disease: A report of the American College of Cardiology/American Heart Association Task Force on Practice Guidelines (writing Committee to revise the 1998 guidelines for the management of patients with valvular heart disease) developed in collaboration with the Society of Cardiovascular Anesthesiologists endorsed by the Society for Cardiovascular Angiography and Interventions and the Society of Thoracic Surgeons. *J Am Coll Cardiol.* 2006;48:e1–148.

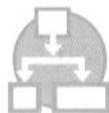

See Also (Topic, Algorithm, Electronic Media Element)

Noonan Syndrome; Tetralogy of Fallot

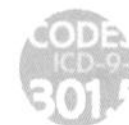

CODES

ICD9

- 424.3 Pulmonary valve disorders
- 746.02 Stenosis of pulmonary valve, congenital

CLINICAL PEARLS

- A pulmonary ejection click denotes mild to moderate stenosis.
- Echocardiography is the preferred test to evaluate the severity of pulmonic stenosis.
- Mild pulmonary valve stenosis is unlikely to progress in severity or cause symptoms.

PYELONEPHRITIS

Stephen A. Martin, MD, EdM

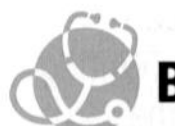

BASICS

DESCRIPTION

- Acute pyelonephritis is a syndrome caused by an infection of the renal parenchyma and renal pelvis, often producing localized flank or back pain combined with systemic symptoms such as fever, chills, and nausea. It has a wide spectrum of presentation, from mild illness to septic shock.
- Chronic pyelonephritis is the result of progressive inflammation of the renal interstitium and tubules, presumed to be caused by recurrent infection, vesicoureteral reflux, or both.
- Uncomplicated vs. complicated: The presentation is considered uncomplicated if the infection is caused by a typical pathogen in an immunocompetent patient who has normal urinary tract anatomy and renal function.
- System(s) affected: Renal; Urologic
- Synonym(s): Acute upper urinary tract infection (UTI)

Geriatric Considerations

- May present only as confusion; absence of fever is common in this age group.
- Elderly patients with diabetes and pyelonephritis are at higher risk of bacteremia, long hospitalization, and mortality.

Pregnancy Considerations

- The most common medical complication requiring hospitalization
- Affects 1–2% of all pregnancies. Morbidity does not differ between trimesters.
- Urine culture follow-up 1–2 weeks after therapy

Pediatric Considerations

- UTI is present in ~5% of patients 2 months to 2 years old with fever and no source evident from history and physical exam.
- The route for antibiotics and location of care should be based on the clinical situation.

EPIDEMIOLOGY

Incidence

Community-acquired acute pyelonephritis: 28/10,000/yr

Prevalence

Adult cases/yr: 250,000, with 100,000 hospitalizations

RISK FACTORS

- Underlying urinary tract abnormalities
- Indwelling catheter
- Recent urinary tract instrumentation
- Nephrolithiasis
- Immunocompromise, including diabetes
- Elderly, institutionalized women
- Prostatic enlargement
- Childhood UTI
- Acute pyelonephritis within the prior year
- Frequency of recent sexual intercourse
- Spermicide use
- Stress incontinence
- Pregnancy
- Hospital-acquired infection
- Symptoms >7 days at presentation

ETIOLOGY

- Infection with *E. coli* (>80%)
- Other gram-negative pathogens: *Proteus, Klebsiella, Serratia, Clostridium, Pseudomonas*, and *Enterobacter*
- *Enterococcus*
- *Staphylococcus*: *S. epidermis*, *S. saprophyticus* (number 2 cause in young women), and *S. aureus*
- *Candida*

COMMONLY ASSOCIATED CONDITIONS

- Indwelling catheters
- Renal calculi
- Benign prostatic hyperplasia

DIAGNOSIS

HISTORY

- In adults (1)[C]:
  - Flank pain
  - Nausea ± vomiting
  - Malaise
  - Myalgia
  - Anorexia
  - Dysuria, urinary frequency, urgency
  - Suprapubic discomfort
- In infants and children:
  - Irritability
  - GI symptoms

PHYSICAL EXAM

- In adults (1)[C]:
  - Fever: ≥37.8°C (100°F)
  - Costovertebral angle tenderness
  - From no physical findings to septic shock
  - A pelvic exam may be needed in female patients to assess for pelvic inflammatory disease (PID)
- In infants and children:
  - Sepsis
  - Fever
  - Poor skin perfusion
  - Inadequate weight gain or weight loss
  - Jaundice to gray skin color

DIAGNOSTIC TESTS & INTERPRETATION

Lab

Initial lab tests

- Urinalysis: Pyuria ± leukocyte casts, hematuria, nitrites, and mild proteinuria
- Urine leukocyte esterase test positive
- Urine Gram stain
- Urine culture (>10,000 colony-forming units/mL) and sensitivities
- CBC, BUN, and creatinine (2)[C]
- In 1 study of hospitalized patients, C-reactive protein levels were found to correlate with prolonged hospitalization and infection recurrence.

Follow-Up & Special Considerations

- Blood culture(s): Indicated in diagnostic uncertainty, immunosuppression, or a suspected hematogenous source (1)[B]
- Drugs that may alter lab results: Antibiotics

Imaging

Initial approach

- Imaging generally not indicated in straightforward cases
- Pediatrics: Practice is evolving based on recent studies; imaging generally has involved an ultrasound and voiding cystourethrogram or radionucleotide cystogram after initial treatment.

Follow-Up & Special Considerations

If patient's condition does not respond in >72 hours or if obstruction/anatomic abnormality suspected:

- CT scan of abdomen and pelvis ± contrast material
- Ultrasound, renal with kidneys, ureter, bladder
- Cystoscopy with ureteral catheterization

Pathological Findings

- Acute: Abscess formation with neutrophils
- Chronic: Fibrosis with reduction in renal tissue

DIFFERENTIAL DIAGNOSIS

- Obstructive uropathy
- Acute bacterial pneumonia (lower lobe)
- Cholecystitis
- Acute pancreatitis
- Appendicitis
- Perforated viscus
- Aortic dissection
- PID
- Kidney stone
- Ectopic pregnancy
- Diverticulitis

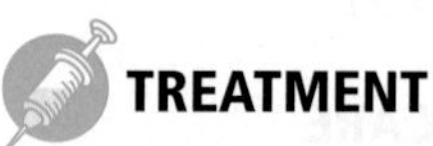

TREATMENT

- Total duration of antibiotic use is guided by the clinical situation. Shorter treatment times have been validated for uncomplicated oral outpatient management (3)[A].
- IV antibiotics are indicated for inpatients.

MEDICATION

- For empirical oral therapy, a fluoroquinolone is recommended. These recommendations are evolving due to increasing fluoroquinolone resistance and they should be used when the resistance of community uropathogens to fluoroquinolones is not known to exceed 10%. Should it exceed 10%, a single initial IV dose of a long-acting antibiotic such as ceftriaxone 1 g is recommended (3)[C].
- For parenteral therapy, a fluoroquinolone, aminoglycoside ± ampicillin, or an extended-spectrum cephalosporin ± an aminoglycoside can be used (3)[B].
- Contraindications:
  - Allergies to agents listed
  - Fluoroquinolones are contraindicated in children, adolescents, and pregnant women.
  - Nitrofurantoin does not achieve reliable tissue levels for pyelonephritis treatment.
- Precautions:
  - Most antibiotics require adjustments in dosage in patients with renal insufficiency.
  - Test for aminoglycoside levels and renal function.
  - If *Enterococcus* is suspected based on Gram stain, ampicillin plus gentamicin is a reasonable empirical choice, unless patient is penicillin-allergic; then use vancomycin. If outpatient, add amoxicillin to fluoroquinolone pending culture results and sensitivity. Do not use a third-generation cephalosporin for suspected or proven enterococcal infection.

First Line

- Adults:
  - Severe illness: IV therapy until afebrile 24–48 hours and tolerating oral hydration and medications, then oral agents to complete 2 weeks. Adult doses (3)[B].
  - IV agents (assuming normal CrCl):
    - Ciprofloxacin: 400 mg q12h
    - Levofloxacin: 500 mg/d
    - Gatifloxacin: 400 mg/d
    - Cefotaxime: 1 g q8–12h up to 2 g q4h
    - Ceftriaxone: 1–2 g/d
    - Cefoxitin: 2 g q4–8h
    - Gentamicin: 5–7 mg/kg of body weight daily (± ampicillin 2 g q6h for enterococcus)
  - Oral agents (initial outpatient treatment):
    - Ciprofloxacin: 500 mg q12h for 7 days
    - Ciprofloxacin XR: 1,000 mg/d for 7 days
    - Levofloxacin: 750 mg/d for 5 days
    - Trimethoprim/Sulfamethoxazole (160/800 mg): 1 tab PO b.i.d. for 14 days provided uropathogen known to be susceptible and ceftriaxone 1 g initial IV dose given
- Pediatric:
  - IV agents (general indication is for age <2 months or clinical concern in other ages):
    - Ceftriaxone: 50–100 mg/kg/d (also can be used IM in outpatient setting)
    - Ampicillin: 100 mg/kg/d IV divided in 4 doses + gentamicin 7.5 mg/kg/d divided in 3 doses
  - Oral agents: Cefixime: 16 mg/kg/d PO in 2 divided doses on the first day, followed by 8 mg/kg once per day to complete therapy
  - IV agents (general indication is for age <2 months or clinical concern in other ages):
    - Ceftriaxone: 50–100 mg/kg/d (also can be used IM in outpatient setting)
    - Ampicillin: 100 mg/kg/d IV divided in 4 doses + gentamicin 7.5 mg/kg/d divided in 3 doses
  - Oral agents: Cefixime: 16 mg/kg/d PO in 2 divided doses on the first day, followed by 8 mg/kg once per day to complete therapy

Second Line

Adults:

- IV agents:
  - Piperacillin–tazobactam: 3.375 g q6–8h
  - Ticarcillin–clavulanate: 3.1 g q4–6h
- Oral agents:
  - Cefixime: 400 mg PO q12h
  - Cefpodoxime (Proxetil): 200 mg q12h
  - Amoxicillin–clavulanate: 875/125 mg q12h or 500/125 mg t.i.d.
  - Trimethoprim–sulfamethoxazole (TMP-SMX): 60–800 mg q12h (up to 30% *E. coli* strains are resistant to ampicillin and TMP-SMX in community-acquired infections)

Pediatric Considerations

- Children <2 years of age and children with febrile or recurrent UTI are usually treated for 10 days.
- Empirical coverage should include *E. coli*. Ampicillin should be added if *Enterococcus* is suspected:
  - Oral antibiotics (cefixime, ceftibuten, and amoxicillin/clavulanic acid) may be used alone, or
  - IV antibiotics (single daily dosing with aminoglycoside) for 2–4 days, followed by oral antibiotics (4)[A]
- If patient is treated as an outpatient, antibiotic course must be completed successfully.

ADDITIONAL TREATMENT

General Measures

- Broad-spectrum antibiotics initially, tailoring therapy to culture and sensitivity results
- Analgesics and antipyretics
- Consider urinary analgesics (e.g., phenazopyridine 200 mg t.i.d.) for severe dysuria.

Issues for Referral

- Acute pyelonephritis unresponsive to therapy
- Chronic pyelonephritis

SURGERY/OTHER PROCEDURES

Perinephric abscess drainage as indicated

IN-PATIENT CONSIDERATIONS

Initial Stabilization

Outpatient therapy if mild–moderate illness (not pregnant, no nausea or vomiting; fever and pain not severe), uncomplicated, and tolerating oral hydration and medications; up to 70% of patients can be selected for outpatient management (1)[B]

Admission Criteria

In-patient therapy for severe illness (e.g., high fevers, severe pain, marked debility, intractable vomiting, possible urosepsis), risk factors for complicated pyelonephritis, or extremes of age

IV Fluids

As indicated for dehydration or renal calculi

Discharge Criteria

Discharge on oral agent (see above) after patient is afebrile 24–48 hours to complete 2 weeks

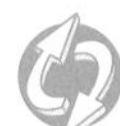

ONGOING CARE

FOLLOW-UP RECOMMENDATIONS

- Women: Routine follow-up cultures not recommended unless symptoms resolve but recur within 2 weeks; obtain urine culture, sensitivity, Gram stain, and CT scan, or renal ultrasound. If symptoms resolve but recur after 2 weeks, treat as sporadic episode of pyelonephritis unless ≥2 recurrences; then urologic evaluation is necessary.
- Men, children, adolescents, patients with recurrent infections, patients with risk factors: Repeat cultures 1–2 weeks after completing therapy; do a urologic evaluation after first episode of pyelonephritis and with recurrences.

Patient Monitoring

- No response within 48 hours (5% of patients): Re-evaluate and review cultures, CT scan, or ultrasound, and adjust therapy as needed; may need urologic consult. The 2 most common causes are a resistant organism and nephrolithiasis.
- Mild–moderate illness: Oral therapy for 2 weeks as outpatient
- Close contact should be maintained with children's families to monitor their response.

DIET

Encourage fluid intake.

PROGNOSIS

95% of treated patients respond within 48 hours.

COMPLICATIONS

- Kidney abscess
- Metastatic infection: Skeletal system, endocardium, eye, meningitis with subsequent seizures
- Septic shock and death
- Acute or chronic renal failure
- Complications of antibiotics

REFERENCES

1. Ramakrishnan K, Scheid DC. Diagnosis and management of acute pyelonephritis in adults. *Am Fam Physician*. 2005;71:933–42.
2. Nicolle LE. Uncomplicated urinary tract infection in adults including uncomplicated pyelonephritis. *Urol Clin North Am*. 2008;35:1–12, v.
3. Gupta K, Hooton TM, Naber KG, et al. International clinical practice guidelines for the treatment of acute uncomplicated cystitis and pyelonephritis in women: A 2010 update by the Infectious Diseases Society of America and the European Society for Microbiology and Infectious Diseases. *Clin Infect Dis*. 2011;52:e103–20.
4. Hodson EM, Willis NS, Craig JC, et al. Antibiotics for acute pyelonephritis in children. *Cochrane Database Syst Rev*. 2007;CD003772.

ADDITIONAL READING

- 2010 IDSA Guidelines for Catheter-Associated UTIs.
- American College of Obstetricians and Gynecologists. ACOG Practice Bulletin No. 91: Treatment of urinary tract infections in nonpregnant women. *Obstet Gynecol*. 2008;111:785–94.
- Bader MS, Hawboldt J, Brooks A, et al. Management of complicated urinary tract infections in the era of antimicrobial resistance. *Postgrad Med*. 2010;122:7–15.
- Jolley JA, Wing DA, et al. Pyelonephritis in pregnancy: An update on treatment options for optimal outcomes. *Drugs*. 2010;70:1643–55.

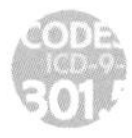

CODES

ICD9

- 590.01 Chronic pyelonephritis with lesion of renal medullary necrosis
- 590.10 Acute pyelonephritis without lesion of renal medullary necrosis
- 590.80 Pyelonephritis, unspecified

CLINICAL PEARLS

- Pyelonephritis can be classic or subtle in its presentation. Early diagnosis can help to prevent clinical deterioration.
- Keep pyelonephritis in mind with less common populations (e.g., children and men).
- The most common causes of poor response to antibiotics are antibiotic resistance and kidney stones.

PYLORIC STENOSIS

Ruben Peralta, MD, FACS

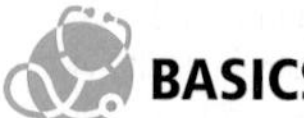

BASICS

DESCRIPTION
- Progressive narrowing of the pyloric canal occurring in infancy
- Synonym(s): Infantile hypertrophic pyloric stenosis (IHPS)

EPIDEMIOLOGY
- Predominant age: Infancy:
  - Onset usually at 3–6 weeks of age, rarely in the newborn period or as late as 5 months of age
- Considered the most common condition requiring surgical intervention in the first year of life
- A recent decline in its incidence has been reported in a number of countries (1).
- Predominant sex: Male > Female (4:1)

Incidence
In Caucasian population, 2–5:1,000 babies; less common in African American and Asian populations

Prevalence
National prevalence level is 1–2 per 1,000 infants, ranging from 0.5–4.21 per 1,000 live births.

RISK FACTORS
- Incidence higher in first-born boys
- 5 times increased risk with affected first-degree relative
- Strong familial aggregation and heritability (2)

Genetics
Recent studies have identified linkage to chromosome 11 and multiple loci and chomosone 16 (3).

PATHOPHYSIOLOGY
- Abnormal relaxation of the pyloric muscles leads to hypertrophy.
- Redundant mucosa fills the pyloric canal.
- Gastric outflow is obstructed, leading to gastric distension and vomiting.

ETIOLOGY
- The exact cause remains unknown, but multiple genetic and environmental factors have been implicated (3,4).
- A recent surveillance study of a population-based birth defects registry identified an association between pyloric stenosis and the use of fluoxetine in the first trimester of pregnancy, even after adjustment for maternal age and smoking. The adjusted odds ratio was 9.8 (95% confidence interval: 1.5–62) (5).

COMMONLY ASSOCIATED CONDITIONS
Associated anomalies present in ~4–7% of infants with pyloric stenosis:
- Hiatal and inguinal hernias (most commonly)
- Other anomalies include:
  - Congenital heart disease
  - Esophageal atresia
  - Tracheoesophageal fistula
  - Renal abnormalities
  - Turner syndrome and trisomy 18
  - Cornelia de Lange syndrome
  - Smith-Lemli-Opitz syndrome
- A common proposed genetic link between breast cancer, endometriosis, and pyloric stenosis has been observed in families.

DIAGNOSIS

HISTORY
- Nonbilious projectile vomiting after feeding, increasing in frequency and severity
- Emesis may become blood-tinged from vomiting-induced gastric irritation.
- Hunger due to inadequate nutrition
- Decrease in bowel movements
- Weight loss

PHYSICAL EXAM
- Firm, mobile ("olivelike") mass palpable in the right upper quadrant (70–90% of the time)
- Epigastric distention
- Visible gastric peristalsis after feeding
- Late signs: Dehydration, weight loss
- Rarely, jaundice when starvation leads to decreased glucuronyl transferase activity resulting in indirect hyperbilirubinemia

DIAGNOSTIC TESTS & INTERPRETATION
Metabolic disturbances are late findings and are uncommon in present time of early diagnosis and intervention.

Lab
- If prolonged vomiting, then check electrolytes for:
  - Hypokalemia
  - Hypochloremia
  - Metabolic alkalosis
- Elevated unconjugated bilirubin level (rare)
- Paradoxical aciduria: The kidney tubules excrete hydrogen to preserve potassium in face of hypokalemic alkalosis.

Imaging
- Abdominal ultrasound is the study of choice:
  - Ultrasound shows thickened and elongated pyloric muscle and redundant mucosa.
- Upper GI series reveals strong gastric contractions; elongated, narrow pyloric canal (string sign); and parallel lines of barium in the narrow channel (double tract sign or railroad track sign).

Pathological Findings
Concentric hypertrophy of pyloric muscle

DIFFERENTIAL DIAGNOSIS
- Inexperienced or inappropriate feeding
- GERD
- Gastritis
- Congenital adrenal hyperplasia, salt-losing
- Pylorospasm
- Gastric volvulus
- Antral or gastric web

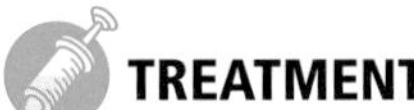

TREATMENT

SURGERY/OTHER PROCEDURES

- Ramstedt pyloromyotomy is curative. The entire length of hypertrophied muscle is divided with preservation of the underlying mucosa.
- Frequent surgical approaches include open (traditional right upper quadrant transverse incision), more contemporary circumumbilical incision, and laparoscopic techniques.
- A recent review concluded that the laparoscopic approach results in less postoperative pain and can be performed with no increase in operative time or complications (6).

IN-PATIENT CONSIDERATIONS

Initial Stabilization

- Prompt treatment to avoid dehydration and malnutrition
- Correct acid–base and electrolyte disturbances. Surgery should be delayed until the alkalosis is corrected.
- Patients need pre- and postop apnea monitoring. They have a tendency toward apnea to compensate with respiratory acidosis for their metabolic alkalosis.

IV Fluids

To correct dehydration and metabolic abnormalities

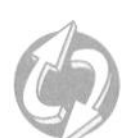

ONGOING CARE

FOLLOW-UP RECOMMENDATIONS

Patient Monitoring

- Routine pediatric health maintenance
- Postoperative monitoring, including monitoring for pain, emesis, apnea

DIET

- No preoperative feeding
- Initiate feeding 12–24 hours after surgery, with goal of advancing to full oral feedings within 36–48 hours of surgery.

PROGNOSIS

Surgery is curative.

COMPLICATIONS

No long-term morbidity. Duodenal perforation is a known, but uncommon, complication of surgery.

REFERENCES

1. Sommerfield T, Chalmers J, Youngson G, et al. The changing epidemiology of infantile hypertrophic pyloric stenosis in Scotland. *Arch Dis Child*. 2008; 93(12):1007–11.
2. Krogh C, Fischer TK, Skotte L, et al. Familial aggregation and heritability of pyloric stenosis. *JAMA*. 2010;303:2393–9.
3. Everett KV, Capon F, Georgoula C, et al. Linkage of monogenic infantile hypertrophic pyloric stenosis to chromosome 16q24. *Eur J Hum Genet*. 2008;16: 1151–4.
4. Ranells JD, Carver JD, Kirby RS, et al. Infantile hypertrophic pyloric stenosis: Epidemiology, genetics, and clinical update. *Adv Pediatr*. 2011;58: 195–206.
5. Bakker MK, De Walle HE, Wilffert B, et al. Fluoxetine and infantile hypertrophic pylorus stenosis: A signal from a birth defects-drug exposure surveillance study. *Pharmacoepidemiol Drug Saf*. 2010;19(8):808–13.
6. Sola JE, Neville HL, et al. Laparoscopic vs open pyloromyotomy: A systematic review and meta-analysis. *J Pediatr Surg*. 2009;44:1631–7.

ADDITIONAL READING

- Colletti JE. Pyloric stenosis. *CJEM*. 2004;6:444–5.
- Everett KV, Chioza BA, Georgoula C, et al. Genome-wide high-density SNP-based linkage analysis of infantile hypertrophic pyloric stenosis identifies loci on chromosomes 11q14-q22 and Xq23. *Am J Hum Genet*. 2008;82:756–62.
- National Birth Defects Prevention Network. Selected birth defects data from population-based birth defects surveillance programs in the United States, 2003–2007. *Birth Defects Res A Clin Mol Teratol*. 2010;88(12):1062–174.
- St Peter SD, Holcomb GW, Calkins CM, et al. Open versus laparoscopic pyloromyotomy for pyloric stenosis: A prospective, randomized trial. *Ann Surg*. 2006;244:363–70.

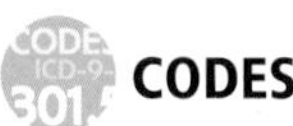

CODES

ICD9

750.5 Congenital hypertrophic pyloric stenosis

CLINICAL PEARLS

- Pyloric stenosis is the most common condition requiring surgical intervention in the first year of life.
- The condition classically presents between 1 and 5 months of life, with projectile vomiting after feeds and a firm, mobile mass in the right upper quadrant.
- Abdominal ultrasound is the study of choice.
- Surgery (Ramstedt pyloromyotomy, laparoscopically is the preferred method) is curative.

RABIES

Alan M. Ehrlich, MD

BASICS

DESCRIPTION
- A rapidly progressive CNS infection caused by a ribonucleic acid (RNA) rhabdovirus affecting mammals, including humans
- The disease is generally considered to be 100% fatal once symptoms develop.
- System(s) affected: Nervous
- Synonym(s): Hydrophobia (due to inability to swallow water)

EPIDEMIOLOGY
Incidence
- Most cases are in developing countries.
- Estimated 55,000 deaths worldwide per year
- Only 1 death in the US in 2007.
- Only 3 cases in the US in 2006.
- Predominant age: Any
- Predominant sex: Male = Female

RISK FACTORS
- Professions or activities that may expose a person to wild or domestic animals (e.g., animal handlers, lab workers, veterinarians, spelunkers [cave explorers])
- In the US, most cases due to exposure to bats
- Internationally, many countries still have rabies widespread in both domestic and feral dogs.
- Human-to-human transmission has occurred through cornea and other tissue transplants.
- International travel to countries where canine rabies is endemic

GENERAL PREVENTION
- Pre-exposure vaccination if at risk of unapparent or unrecognized exposure to rabies, such as traveling to endemic areas
- Pre-exposure vaccination for high-risk groups such as veterinarians, animal handlers, and certain laboratory workers
- Consider pre-exposure vaccination for travelers visiting relatives in areas such as North Africa that have increased risk of rabies from domestic animals.
- Immunization of dogs and cats
- People who observe abnormal behavior in any wildlife species should contact animal control and should avoid approaching or handling those animals.
- Avoid wild and unknown domestic animals.
- Seek treatment promptly if bitten, scratched, or in contact with saliva.
- Infection can be prevented by prompt postexposure treatment of persons bitten by or otherwise exposed to animals known or suspected to be carrying the disease.
- Postexposure prophylaxis should be considered for any person who reports direct contact with bats, unless it is known that an exposure did not occur.

PATHOPHYSIOLOGY
Lyssavirus, which is an RNA virus in the family *Rhabdoviridae*

ETIOLOGY
- Rabies virus, a neurotropic virus present in saliva of infected animals
- Transmission occurs via bites from infected animals or rarely via saliva coming in contact with open wound or mucous membranes.
- In the US, bats are the most common source of rabies.

DIAGNOSIS

HISTORY
- It is important to elicit history of animal exposure, because early diagnosis and treatment are necessary for survival.
- Diagnosis should be considered if there is a bite by an animal capable of transmitting the disease or travel to a rabies-endemic country; however, most patients in the US do not recall exposure.
- 5 stages (may overlap):
  - Incubation period: Time between bite and first symptoms of disease: Usually 10 days–1 year, with average of 20–60 days. It is shortest in patients with extensive bites about the head and trunk.
  - Prodrome: Lasts 1–14 days; symptoms include pain or paresthesia at bite site and nonspecific flulike symptoms, including fever and headache.
  - Acute neurologic period: Lasts 2–10 days. CNS symptoms dominate clinical picture; generally takes 1 of 2 forms: Furious rabies: Episodes of hyperactivity last about 5 minutes and include hydrophobia, aerophobia, hyperventilation, hypersalivation, and autonomic instability interspersed with periods of normalcy. Paralytic rabies: Paralysis dominates clinical picture; may be ascending (as in Guillain-Barré syndrome) or may affect 1 or more limbs differentially.
  - Coma: Lasts hours to days; with intensive care, rarely may last months. May evolve over a few days following acute neurologic period. May be sudden, with respiratory arrest.
  - Death: Usually occurs within 3 weeks of onset as result of complications. Only 6 survivors have been reported in the literature (1)[C].

PHYSICAL EXAM
Findings can range from normal exam up to severe neurologic findings, including paralysis and coma, depending on the stage of rabies at the time of presentation.

DIAGNOSTIC TESTS & INTERPRETATION
Lab
Initial lab tests
- Spinal tap
- WBC count in CSF examination may be normal or show moderate pleocytosis.
- CSF protein may be normal or moderately elevated.
- Skin biopsy to detect rabies antigen in hair follicles
- Available at state and federal reference labs
- Rabies antibody titer on serum and CSF
- Skin biopsy from nape of neck for direct fluorescent antibody examination
- Viral isolation from saliva or CSF
- Corneal smear stains are positive by immunofluorescence in 50% of patients.

Follow-Up & Special Considerations
For wild animals, the brain of the biting animal, if available, should be submitted for laboratory testing.

Imaging
Initial approach
- Head CT scan: Normal or nonspecific findings consistent with encephalitis
- MRI may allow early diagnosis and can be used to rule out other forms of encephalitis.

Diagnostic Procedures/Surgery
Spinal tap

Pathological Findings
Encephalitis may be found on brain biopsy, but abnormal findings may be confined to parts (e.g., brain stem, midbrain, cerebellum) examined only postmortem.

DIFFERENTIAL DIAGNOSIS
- Any rapidly progressive encephalitis; important to exclude treatable causes of encephalitis, especially herpes
- Only 2007 case in the US was diagnosed initially as transverse myelitis

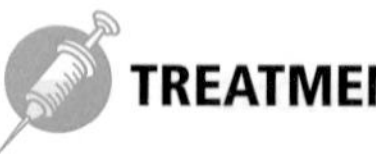

TREATMENT

Thorough wound cleansing with soap and water is the first line of treatment. Irrigate wound with virucidal agent, such as povidone-iodine, if available (2).

MEDICATION
ALERT
- Immunosuppression, either by medications or disease, can interfere with the development of immunity after vaccination. Immunosuppressive drugs should be avoided during postexposure prophylaxis unless absolutely necessary for the treatment of other conditions. If postexposure prophylaxis is given to an immunosuppressed person, serum samples should be checked for the presence of rabies virus–neutralizing antibody in response to vaccination (3)[B].
- All wounds should be thoroughly cleansed, regardless of whether postexposure prophylaxis was given.
- Assessment of need for postexposure prophylaxis based on circumstances of possible exposure
- Increased risk associated with:
  - Bites involving any puncture of the skin constitute a significant risk, while saliva is only a risk if in contact with an open wound.
  - Wild animals or domestic animals that cannot be quarantined
  - Any potential exposure to bats
  - Hybrid animals of wild and domestic species (e.g., wolf-dog)
  - Unprovoked attack (feeding a wild animal is considered a provoked attack)
- Management based on type of animal:
  - Bites from cats, dogs, and ferrets that can be watched for 10 days do not require prophylaxis unless animal shows signs of illness.
  - Skunks, foxes, bats, raccoons, and most carnivores are high risk, and prophylaxis should begin promptly unless animal can be captured and euthanized for pathological evaluation.
  - For rodents or livestock, consult local public health authorities before initiating prophylaxis.
- Postexposure prophylaxis regimen consists of (2):
  - Passive vaccination: Rabies immunoglobulin (RIG, Hyperab) administered once: 20 IU/kg of body weight. If anatomically feasible, all the RIG should be thoroughly infiltrated in the area around the wound. Any remaining RIG should be administered IM. RIG never should be administered in the same syringe or into the same anatomic site as vaccine.

R

- – Active vaccination: Rabies vaccine, human diploid cell (HDCV) or rabies vaccine adsorbed (RVA) or purified chick embryo cell vaccine IM in the deltoid. For children, the anterolateral aspect of the thigh is acceptable. The gluteal area never should be used for vaccine injections. Give the first dose, 1 mL, as soon as possible after exposure. The day of the first dose is designated Day 0. Give an additional 1-mL dose on days 3, 7, and 14. If immunocompromised, give fifth dose on day 28.
- For previously vaccinated patients, a 1-mL IM dose of vaccine should be administered immediately and an additional 1-mL dose 3 days later. RIG is not necessary in these patients (2).
- Pre-exposure vaccination: For people in high-risk groups, such as veterinarians, animal handlers, certain laboratory workers, and those spending time in foreign countries where rabies is enzootic (2):
  - – Primary pre-exposure: IM vaccination regimen consists of 3 1-mL injections of HDCV or RVA given in deltoid area, 1 each on days 1, 7, and 28. HDCV also may be given in intradermal doses, administered with a special syringe developed for that purpose (Imovax Rabies ID Vaccine); the 0.1-mL IM dose is administered in the deltoid area; follow the same schedule as for IM doses. Recently, the manufacturer discontinued production of Imovax Rabies ID Vaccine.
  - – Pre-exposure boosters: For people at frequent risk of exposure to rabies, serum should be tested every 2 years. A pre-exposure booster (1.0 mL IM) should be administered if this is less than acceptable level. If titer cannot be obtained, a booster can be administered instead.
- Contraindications: None for postexposure treatment

Pregnancy Considerations

- Pregnancy is not a contraindication to postexposure prophylaxis.
- Rabies vaccination is not associated with a higher incidence of abortion, premature births, or fetal abnormalities.

ADDITIONAL TREATMENT

General Measures

- Physicians should evaluate each possible exposure to rabies and consult local or state public health officials about the need for rabies prophylaxis. In the US, raccoons, skunks, bats, foxes, and coyotes are the animals most likely to be infected, but any carnivore can carry the disease.
- Before specific antirabies treatment is initiated, consider:
  - – Type of exposure (bite or nonbite)
  - – Epidemiology of rabies in species involved
  - – Circumstances of biting incident (provoked vs. unprovoked)
  - – Vaccination status of exposing animal

IN-PATIENT CONSIDERATIONS

Initial Stabilization

- For diagnosed rabies, comfort care and sedation are indicated for all patients.
- Milwaukee Protocol: Experimental treatment using ketamine, midazolam, amantadine, and ribavirin (4)[C] (see "Prognosis")

Admission Criteria

Clinical rabies

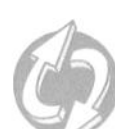

ONGOING CARE

FOLLOW-UP RECOMMENDATIONS

After primary vaccination, serologic testing is necessary only if the patient has a disease or takes a medication that may suppress the immune system.

PATIENT EDUCATION

Homes should be secured from bats by using screens over ventilation areas in the roof.

PROGNOSIS

- No postexposure failures reported in the US since the 1970s
- Rabies has the highest case-fatality rate of any infectious disease.
- The disease is generally considered to be 100% fatal once symptoms develop.
- Survival has been well documented for only 6 patients. In 5 of these, the persons had received rabies vaccination before the onset of disease.
- There was 1 documented recovery from clinical rabies in 2004 in a patient who did not receive pre- or postexposure prophylaxis, and this patient was treated with the Milwaukee Protocol (4)[C]. 2 years after treatment, there were some persistent neurologic deficits, but overall functioning was normal enough for the patient to finish high school and enroll in college (5)[C]. However, other patients treated similarly since have not survived (6,7)[C].

COMPLICATIONS

0.6% of people develop mild serum sickness reaction following HDCV boosters. Mild local and systemic reactions are common following vaccination. Mild reactions should not be a cause for interruption of immunization.

REFERENCES

1. Hankins DG, Rosekrans JA. Overview prevention, and treatment of rabies. *Mayo Clin Proc.* 2004;79: 671–6.
2. Rupprecht CE, Briggs D, Brown CM, et al. Use of a reduced (4-dose) vaccine schedule for postexposure prophylaxis to prevent human rabies: Recommendations of the advisory committee on immunization practices. *MMWR Recomm Rep.* 2010;59:1–9.
3. Manning SE, et al. Human rabies prevention–United States, 2008: Recommendations of the advisory committee on immunization practices. *MMWR Recomm Rep.* 2008;57(RR-3):1–28.
4. Willoughby R, et al. Survival after treatment of rabies with induction of coma. *NEJM.* 2005; 352(24):2508–14.
5. Hu WT, et al. *NEJM.* 2007;357(9):945–6.
6. McDermid RC, et al. Human rabies encephalitis following bat exposure: Failure of therapeutic coma. *CMAJ.* 2008;178(5):557–61.
7. Maier T, Schwarting A, Mauer D, et al. Management and outcomes after multiple corneal and solid organ transplantations from a donor infected with rabies virus. *Clin Infect Dis.* 2010;50:1112–9.
8. De Serres G, Skowronski DM, Mimault P, et al. Bats in the bedroom, bats in the belfry: Reanalysis of the rationale for rabies postexposure prophylaxis. *Clin Infect Dis.* 2009;48(11):1493–9.

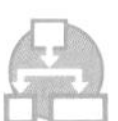

See Also (Topic, Algorithm, Electronic Media Element)

Bites

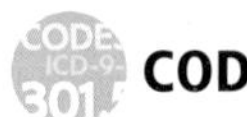

CODES

ICD9

071 Rabies

CLINICAL PEARLS

- Rare in the US, but quite common in other areas of the world
- Seek treatment if exposed to scratch, bite, or saliva of potentially infected animal (e.g., feral dog, bat, fox, raccoon, or other wild animals).
- Postexposure prophylaxis consists of 3 steps: Local wound cleansing, passive immunization with rabies immunoglobulin, and active immunization with human diploid cell vaccine.
- Postexposure prophylaxis should be considered for any person who reports direct contact with bats, unless it is known that an exposure did not occur.
- Exposure to bats in bedrooms while sleeping is not uncommon, but contraction of rabies in this circumstance is rare (8)[B].

RADIATION ENTERITIS

Eric J. Mao, MD
Edward Feller, MD

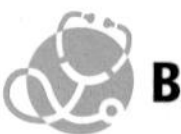

BASICS

- Radiation therapy (RT) to treat abdominal, pelvic, and retroperitoneal cancers is used in as many as 200,000 patients yearly in the US.
- Toxicity to normal tissues is a common, potentially devastating complication of this treatment.
- Radiation enteritis (RE) is a barrier to curability of abdomino-pelvic malignancy and is the leading cause of postirradiation toxicity.

DESCRIPTION

- Radiation enteritis is injury to the colon and small intestine secondary to radiation therapy.
- Acute RE can occur in the first hours of treatment, but usually presents 1–2 weeks after initiation of RT:
  - Most cases will present within 3 months of RT (1).
- Chronic RE occurs more than 3 months after RT (usually between 1.5 and 6 years) (1,2).
- Chronic RE is commonly progressive with potential for significant long-term morbidity and mortality; therapeutic options other than symptomatic treatment are limited.
- Recent introduction of radioembolization of liver tumors using yttrium-90 microspheres has produced gastroduodenal and other toxicities caused by ectopic distribution of radioactive microspheres.

EPIDEMIOLOGY

Incidence

- Incidence of acute RE: 60–80% of patients receiving intra-abdominal or pelvic RT (1)
- Incidence of chronic RE: 20% receiving pelvic RT for gynecologic or urologic tumors (2)

Prevalence

Prevalence of RE in the US: 1.5–2 million people (1)

RISK FACTORS

- Patient factors:
  - Older age
  - Low body mass index
  - Comorbidities (diabetes, hypertension, atherosclerosis, collagen vascular disease, inflammatory bowel disease, occlusive vascular disease)
  - Smoking history
  - Prior abdominal or pelvic surgery
  - Prior intra-abdominal infection
- Treatment factors:
  - Volume of bowel exposure
  - Radiation dose and duration
  - Fractionation and technique
  - Concurrent chemotherapy
  - Errors in dose calibration, equipment, or radiation field

GENERAL PREVENTION

- Physical measures:
  - Belly board device
  - Surgical placement of intestinal sling
  - Bladder distension during RT
  - Trendelenburg position in pelvic RT
- Treatment measures:
  - Reduce field size
  - Multiple field arrangements
  - Conformal RT techniques
  - Intensity-modulated RT (3)
- Other: Acts of terror can also lead to radiation injury; coordination of public health resources such as hospitals, health departments, and regional services is essential to prepare for potential disasters (4).

PATHOPHYSIOLOGY

- Radiation injury can lead to impaired cell division or immediate cell death from absorption of energy from incident radiation; indirectly, injury may be mediated by release of free radicals, which may damage DNA (2).
- Acute RE: Mucosal atrophy and inflammation leading to nutrient and fluid loss with possible blood loss
- Chronic RE: Obliterative endarteritis causing tissue ischemia and necrosis leading to transmural fibrosis
- Result: Vascular degeneration, telangiectatic vessel formation, mucosal ulceration, intestinal wall necrosis, serosal adhesion formation

COMMONLY ASSOCIATED CONDITIONS

Radiation injury to other organs

DIAGNOSIS

- All patients with history of RT should be questioned; many patients do not seek medical care for chronic morbidity.
- Diagnosis may be difficult and unsuspected because of the complicated, multifactorial causality of these nonspecific symptoms in cancer patients.

HISTORY

Clinical presentation:

- Onset: Acute RE within 1–2 weeks of RT; chronic RE within 1–2 years of RT
- Small bowel symptoms: Nausea, vomiting, abdominal bloating, dyspepsia
- Large bowel symptoms: Constipation, diarrhea, abdominal pain, intestinal bleeding manifested as hematochezia, melena, occult blood positivity in stools, or iron deficiency anemia
- Rectal symptoms: Defecation urgency, tenesmus, mucus, incontinence, bleeding
- Malabsorption symptoms: Diarrhea, steatorrhea, weight loss, wasting illness
- Nonspecific symptoms: Weight loss, lethargy, fever, abdominal pain
- Associated conditions may present as osteoporosis, anemia, bone marrow suppression, dermatitis, cardiac injury depending on the nature of RT utilized

PHYSICAL EXAM

- Nonspecific; may mimic diverse, common abdominal disorders
- Clues suggestive of RE: Abdominal tenderness, blood in stool, evidence of malnutrition in a patient with prior RT

DIAGNOSTIC TESTS & INTERPRETATION

- Acute RE: Diagnostic tests not indicated except to exclude other pathology or if clinical presentation suggests serious disease
- Chronic RE: Diagnostic tests indicated

Lab

- Initial labs:
  - CBC
  - Comprehensive metabolic panel
  - Serum albumin and globulin
  - Fecal occult blood test
- First-line investigations:
  - If small bowel symptoms:
    - Esophagogastroduodenoscopy for upper GI involvement
    - Upper GI series with small bowel follow-through to visualize distal segments
    - Video capsule endoscopy, small bowel enteroscopy, and MR enterography are increasingly used because of the relative inaccessibility of small bowel.
  - If large bowel symptoms:
    - Colonoscopy with terminal ileal intubation and potential for endoscopic control of bleeding with thermal or laser methodology
  - If nonspecific symptoms (i.e., weight loss or abdominal pain):
    - Abdominopelvic CT or MRI imaging to assess bowel wall thickening, stricture, or alternative diagnosis

Initial lab tests

If first-line investigation is negative:

- Reassess symptoms .
- Stool studies (in selected cases) for pathogens, fecal leukocytes, spot stool for fat and muscle fibers
- Reconsider other first-line investigations.

R

Follow-Up & Special Considerations

Second-line investigations:

- Diarrhea may be due to: Accelerated bowel transit time; medication effect; malabsorption of bile salts, fat, or carbohydrates; bacterial overgrowth; pancreatic insufficiency; ischemic colitis; mucosal inflammation:
  - Vitamin deficiency: Serum vitamin $B_{12}$and folate, serum carotene, D-xylose test, prothrombin time, 25-hydroxy vitamin D; serum iron/iron-binding capacity ratio
  - Carbohydrate: Hydrogen breath test after carbohydrate challenge
  - Pancreatic exocrine or endocrine insufficiency: Spot stool sample for fat and muscle fibers; glucose tolerance test, fasting plasma glucose or hemoglobin A1c
- If evidence of GI bleeding or iron deficiency with negative first-line tests, investigate small bowel:
  - Small bowel enteroscopy or capsule endoscopy (if strictures excluded)

DIFFERENTIAL DIAGNOSIS

- Postsurgical adhesions
- Inflammatory bowel disease
- Irritable bowel syndrome
- New or recurrent neoplasia or metastatic lesions
- Ischemic colitis
- Infectious colitis
- Malabsorption syndromes
- Lymphoma
- Gynecologic disorders
- Medication toxicity

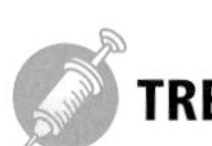

TREATMENT

- Evidence-based treatment of RE is limited.
- Acute RE: Treat symptomatically; spontaneous resolution is common.
- 1/3 of patients with chronic RE will require surgery for RE complications and must be counseled on likely impaired quality of life.

MEDICATION

First Line

- Acute RE:
  - First-line (antidiarrheal):
    - Loperamide 2–4 mg/d PO (5)[B]
    - Diphenoxylate 5 mg PO t.i.d. (5)[B]
  - First-line (antiemetic):
    - Prochlorperazine 5–10 mg PO or by rectal suppository t.i.d.
    - Ondansetron 8 mg PO b.i.d. (1)[B]
  - Second-line (antidiarrheal):
    - Octreotide 150 mcg SC t.i.d. for diarrhea (1)[B]
- Chronic RE:
  - Treatment options with good evidence:
    - Loperamide 2–4 mg PO b.i.d. for symptomatic treatment of diarrhea (obstruction must be excluded prior to use) (2,5)[B]
    - Diphenoxylate 5 mg PO q.i.d. for symptomatic treatment of diarrhea (obstruction must be excluded prior to use) (2,5)[B]
    - Cholestyramine 4 g PO 1–2 times per day for bile acid malabsorption (2)[C]
    - Doxycycline 100 mg/d PO and metronidazole 400 mg PO t.i.d. for 7–10 days for bacterial overgrowth (2)[C]
  - Treatment options with weak evidence:
    - Hyperbaric oxygen (2,5)[C] posttreatment failure

SURGERY/OTHER PROCEDURES

- Endoscopy:
  - Thermal or laser modalities useful for radiation-induced colonic telangiectasia or hemorrhagic duodenitis or ileitis (2)[C]
- Surgery:
  - May be more difficult and complicated because of poor nutrition, comorbidities, prior surgery, and dense intra-abdominal adhesions from prior radiotherapy
  - Indications:
    - Obstruction secondary to strictures or adhesions
    - Fistula (colovesical in men, rectovaginal in women)
    - Perforation
  - Wide excision preferable to bypass operations due to higher risk of anastomotic leak, bacterial overgrowth, perforation, fistula formation (6)
  - Stricturoplasty for patients with limited intestinal reserve and strictures within long segments of diseased intestine (6)
  - Risk factors for complications: Poor nutritional status, >1 abdominal or pelvic surgery prior to RT, <12 months between RT and surgery; advanced malignancy
  - Postoperative complications (30%); 40–60% will require >1 laparotomy (2,5)

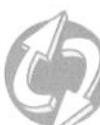

ONGOING CARE

DIET

- Total parenteral nutrition (TPN) is commonly used for malnourishment.
- TPN can be therapeutic in chronic RE as "intestinal rest" (2,6)[C].
- Exclusion diets useful only in selected cases (lactose-free or low fat)

REFERENCES

1. Hauer-Jensen M, Wang J, Boerma M, et al. Radiation damage to the gastrointestinal tract: Mechanisms, diagnosis, and management. *Current opinion in supportive and palliative care*. 2007;1: 23–9.
2. Theis VS, Sripadam R, Ramani V, et al. Chronic radiation enteritis. *Clin Oncol (R Coll Radiol)*. 2010; 22:70–83.
3. Samuelian JM, Callister MD, Ashman JB, et al. Reduced acute bowel toxicity in patients treated with intensity-modulated radiotherapy for rectal cancer. *Int J Radiat Oncol Biol Phys*. 2011 Apr 6. Epub ahead of print.
4. Chambers JA, Purdue GF, et al. Radiation injury and the surgeon. *J Am Coll Surg*. 2007;204:128–39.
5. Zimmerer T, Böcker U, Wenz F, et al. Medical prevention and treatment of acute and chronic radiation induced enteritis—is there any proven therapy? A short review. *Z Gastroenterol*. 2008;46: 441–8.
6. Bismar MM, Sinicrope FA, et al. Radiation enteritis. *Curr Gastroenterol Rep*. 2002;4:361–5.

ADDITIONAL READING

Kim HM, Kim YJ, Kim HJ, et al. A pilot study of capsule endoscopy for the diagnosis of radiation enteritis. *Hepatogastroenterology*. 2011;58:459–64.

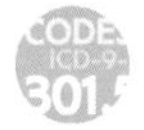

CODES

ICD9

558.1 Gastroenteritis and colitis due to radiation

CLINICAL PEARLS

- Radiation injury is common, nonspecific, and can occur at any time, even decades after irradiation.
- Index of suspicion is vital, since radiation injury may be mimicked by medications, advanced or ongoing malignancy, or more common GI disorders.
- Acute RE is transient and usually resolves spontaneously.
- Chronic RE is very common, has late onset, and is progressive.
- RE has multifactorial causes; always consider recurrent malignancy.

RAPE CRISIS SYNDROME

Jocelyn F. Blackwell, MD, MAJ, MC

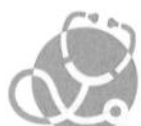

BASICS

DESCRIPTION
- Definitions (legal definitions may vary from state to state):
  - Sexual contact: Intentional touching of a person's intimate parts (including thighs) or the clothing covering such areas, if it is construed as being for the purpose of sexual gratification
  - Sexual conduct: Vaginal intercourse between a male and female, or anal intercourse, fellatio, or cunnilingus between persons, regardless of sex
  - Rape: Any sexual penetration, however slight, using force or coercion against the person's will
  - Sexual imposition: Similar to rape but without penetration or the use of force (i.e., nonconsensual sexual contact)
  - Gross sexual imposition: Nonconsensual sexual contact with the use of force
  - Corruption of a minor: Sexual conduct by an individual ≥18 years old with an individual <16 years of age
- Most states have expanded rape statutes to include marital rape, date rape, and shield laws.
- System(s) affected: Nervous; Reproductive
- Synonym(s): Sexual assault; Rape trauma

EPIDEMIOLOGY
- Anyone can be sexually assaulted, but some populations are especially vulnerable (1):
  - Adolescents and young women
  - People with disabilities
  - Poor and homeless people
  - Sex workers
  - Those living in institutions or areas of conflict
- Predominant age:
  - The incidence of sexual assault peaks in the 16–19-year-old age group, with the mean occurring at 20 years of age:
    - Adolescent sexual assault has a greater frequency of anogenital injuries.
- Predominant sex: Female > Male:
  - For males:
    - 69% of male victims were first raped before age 18.
    - 41% of male victims were raped before age 12.

Incidence
- There were 208,830 rapes and sexual assaults reported in 2008 in the US.
- Estimated that only 1:3–1:5 of adult cases are reported:
  - In 2005, only 38% of rape or sexual assaults were reported to the police.
- 1/5 American women report being raped during their lifetime (2):
  - Between 20% and 25% of females will experience rape or attempted rape during their college years.
- 1/7 males will be sexually assaulted during a lifetime.
- ~2/1,000 children in the US were confirmed by child protective agencies as having experienced sexual assault in 2003.
- The majority of rape victims either know or have some acquaintance with their attacker.

RISK FACTORS
- Numerous, and include multiple individual, relationship, community, and societal factors
- In general, adults are assaulted in their own homes, while adolescents are assaulted in their assailant's residence.
- Most perpetrators of sexual violence are males, with all acts against females >90%.
- Most acts against males are >65% male perpetrators.

GENERAL PREVENTION
- Scope of rape prevention is very complex and broad.
- The public health approach should include both prevention/avoidance of vulnerability factors and implementation of protective factors.
- Females may benefit from assertiveness training and self-defense training.
- Universal screening by health care providers for interpersonal violence does assist in identifying victims (2).

DIAGNOSIS

- In adults:
  - History of sexual penetration
  - Sexual contact or sexual conduct without consent and/or with the use of force
- In children:
  - Actual observation or suspicion of sexual penetration, sexual contact, or sexual conduct
  - Signs include evidence of the use of force and/or evidence of sexual contact (e.g., presence of semen and/or sperm).

HISTORY
- Avoid questioning that implies the patient is at fault.
- Record answers in patient's own words insofar as possible. Include date, approximate time, and general location as best as possible. Document physical abuse other than sexual. Describe all types of sexual contact, whether actual or attempted. Take history of alcohol and/or drugs before or after alleged incident.
- Document time of last activity that could possibly alter specimens (e.g., bath, shower, or douche). Thorough gynecologic history is mandatory, including last menstrual period, last consenting sexual contact, contraceptive practice, and prior gynecologic surgery.

PHYSICAL EXAM
- Use of drawings and/or photographs is encouraged.
- Document all signs of trauma or unusual marks.
- Document mental status/emotional state.
- Use UV light (Wood lamp) to detect seminal stains on clothing or skin.

ALERT
- A forensic kit or "rape kit" contains swabs that are collected from the vagina and rectum, and instructions are given with the kit as to proper collection.
- Many states and emergency departments across the country are utilizing Sexual Assault Nurse Examiner (SANE) when available. This has led to more consistent and more accurate collection of evidence in alleged rape cases.

- Complete genital-rectal examination, including evidence of trauma, secretions, or discharge:
  - Use of a nonlubricated, water-moistened speculum is mandatory because commonly used lubricants may destroy evidence.
  - Testing and/or specimen collection as indicated and in compliance with state requirements

DIAGNOSTIC TESTS & INTERPRETATION
Lab
- In females, obtain a serum or urine pregnancy test.
- Record results of wet mount, screening for vaginitis, but also note the presence or absence of sperm and, if present, whether it is motile or immotile.
- Drug/alcohol testing as indicated by history and/or physical findings

DIFFERENTIAL DIAGNOSIS
Consenting sex among adults

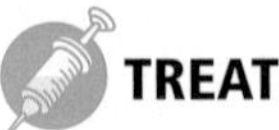

TREATMENT

MEDICATION
First Line
- Gonorrhea: Ceftriaxone 250 mg IM once or cefixime 400 mg PO once.
- Chlamydia: Azithromycin 1 g PO single dose, or doxycycline 100 mg PO b.i.d. × 7 days, or erythromycin base 500 mg PO q.i.d. × 7 days, or erythromycin ethylsuccinate 800 mg PO q.i.d. × 7 days, or ofloxacin 300 mg PO b.i.d. × 7 days or levofloxacin 300 mg PO b.i.d. × 7 days.
- Syphilis: Benzathine penicillin G 2–4 million units IM once, or doxycycline 100 mg PO b.i.d. × 14 days. Some suggest ceftriaxone 1 g daily either IM/IV × 8–10 days, or azithromycin 2 g PO single dose, but treatment failures have been reported in several geographic areas.
- Trichomoniasis and bacterial vaginosis, if present: Metronidazole 2 g PO once, or metronidazole 500 mg PO b.i.d. × 7 days (consider single dose to maximize compliance), or metronidazole gel 0.75% 1 full applicator (5 g) intravaginally every day × 5 days; or clindamycin cream 2% 1 full applicator (5 g) intravaginally at bedtime × 7 days (considered less efficacious than PO metronidazole)
- If pregnancy prophylaxis is indicated, use levonorgestrel 1.5 mg once (Plan B, progestin-only), efficacious for up to 5 days after the incident:
  - Levonorgestrel has proved more effective than the Yuzpe regimen, a method of emergency contraception using a combination of estrogen and progesterone (3)[A].
  - Alternatively, an intrauterine device can be inserted up to 5 days after the earliest predicted date of ovulation in that cycle.
- HIV: Currently, there is a low likelihood of HIV transmittance, but the CDC still recommends postexposure prophylaxis for victims of sexual assault. Regimen is lamivudine–zidovudine (Combivir) 1 tablet PO b.i.d. × 28 days or zidovudine 300 mg plus lamivudine 150 mg PO b.i.d. × 28 days:
  - Medications most effective if started within 24 hours, and could reduce transmission of HIV by as much as 80%
  - Unlikely to be beneficial if started after 72 hours

R

- Hepatitis B: If prevalent in area or assailant known to be high risk—hepatitis B immunoglobulin 0.06 mL/kg IM, single dose, and initiate 3-dose hepatitis B virus immunization series. No treatment is indicated if the victim has had a complete hepatitis B vaccine series, with documented levels of immunity.
- Note: Gonorrhea and chlamydia medications may be given concomitantly.

Second Line

Gonorrhea: Cefotaxime 500 mg IM once *plus* probenecid 1 g PO once. Note: Be aware that drug resistance is on the rise in several major cities. Quinolones are no longer recommended for treatment of gonorrhea.

ADDITIONAL TREATMENT

General Measures

- Providing health care to victims of sexual assault/abuse requires special sensitivity and privacy.
- All such cases *must* be reported immediately to the appropriate law enforcement agency.
- With the victim's permission, enlist the help of personnel from local support agencies (e.g., rape crisis center). When available, use of in-house social services is extremely helpful to victim and family.
- Sexual Assault Nurse Examiner (SANE) programs have been shown to be beneficial, especially in large cities and metropolitan areas with multiple emergency departments of varying capability and staff training/experience.
- Give sedation and tetanus prophylaxis when indicated.
- Discuss possible pregnancy and pregnancy termination with the victim. If hospital policy precludes such a discussion, then information about this option should be offered to the victim via follow-up mechanisms.
- Discuss suspected HIV and hepatitis B exposure and testing with the victim in accordance with hospital, regional, and state policies/protocols. The initial HIV test should be completed within 7 days of the suspected exposure.

Pregnancy Considerations

Conduct baseline pregnancy test; discuss pregnancy prevention and termination with patient.

Pediatric Considerations

Assure the child that s/he is a good person and was not the cause of the incident.

IN-PATIENT CONSIDERATIONS

Initial Stabilization

- Contact appropriate social services agency.
- Majority of adult victims can be treated as outpatients, unless associated trauma (physical or mental) requires admission.
- Majority of pediatric sexual assault/abuse victims will require admission or outside placement until appropriate social agency can evaluate home environment.

ONGOING CARE

FOLLOW-UP RECOMMENDATIONS

Patient Monitoring

- The patient should be seen in 7–10 days for follow-up care, including pregnancy testing and counseling.
- Close examination for vaginitis, and treatment if necessary
- Follow-up test for gonorrhea should occur in 1–2 weeks.
- Follow-up testing for syphilis, HIV, and hepatitis B should occur at 6 weeks, 3 months, and 6 months.
- Provide telephone numbers of counseling agency(ies) that can provide counseling/legal services to the patient.
- Strongly consider Sexual Assault Nurse Examiner (SANE), if available in area.

PATIENT EDUCATION

- Information and help are available from local rape crisis support organizations.
- National Institute of Mental Health, Public Inquiries Branch, Office of Scientific Information, Department of Health and Human Services, Parklawn Bldg., Room 15C-05, 5600 Fishers Lane, Rockville, MD 20857; (301) 443-4513
- National Sexual Violence Resource Center, 123 Enola Drive, Enola, PA 17025; 1-877-739-3895; www.nsvrc.org
- National Domestic Violence Hotline at 1-800-799-SAFE(7233) or TTY 1-800-787-3224 or www.ndvh.org

PROGNOSIS

- Acute phase (usually 1–3 weeks following rape): Shaking, pain, wound healing, mood swings, appetite loss, crying. Also feelings of grief, shame, anger, fear, revenge, or guilt.
- Late or chronic phase (also called "reorganization"): Female victim may develop fear of intercourse, fear of men, nightmares, sleep disorders, daytime flashbacks, fear of being alone, loss of self-esteem, anxiety, depression, posttraumatic stress syndrome, and somatic complaints (e.g., nonspecific abdominal pain).
- Recovery may be prolonged. Patients who are able to talk about their feelings seem to have a faster recovery. It is unclear if pharmaco- or psychotherapy result in better outcomes.

COMPLICATIONS

Sequelae include (1):

- Trauma (physical and mental)
- STIs, including HIV
- Unwanted pregnancy (with the possibility of abortion):
  - The rape-related pregnancy rate in the US is 5% per rape among victims of reproductive age, resulting in more than 32,000 unwanted pregnancies each year (2).
  - Adolescents are at highest risk of pregnancy.
- Depression
- Posttraumatic stress disorder
- Substance abuse

REFERENCES

1. Welch J, Mason F. Rape and sexual assault. *BMJ*. 2007;334:1154–8.
2. Toohey JS. Domestic violence and rape. *Med Clin North Am*. 2008;92:1239–52, xii.
3. Cheng L, Gülmezoglu AM, Piaggio G, et al. Interventions for emergency contraception. *Cochrane Database Syst Rev*. 2008:CD001324.

ADDITIONAL READING

- A National Protocol for Sexual Assault Medical Forensic Examinations (Adults/Adolescents). *U.S. Department of Justice, Office on Violence Against Women; September* 2004.
- Bullock CM, Beckson M. Male victims of sexual assault: Phenomenology, psychology, physiology. *J Am Acad Psychiatry Law*. 2011;39(2):206–8.
- Bureau of Justice Statistics. National Center for Injury Prevention and Control. *Criminal Vicitimization in the United States, Statistical Tables*. 2008.
- Centers for Disease Control and Prevention. *Sexual Violence: Facts at a Glance*. 2008.
- Devorett K, Sachs CJ. Sexual assault. *Emerg Med Clin North Am*. 2011;9(3):605–20.
- Hogan TM, Uyanishi AA. Sexual Assault: Medical and legal implications of the emergency care of adult victims. *Emerg Med Pract*. 2003;10:872–7.

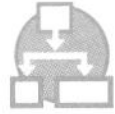

See Also (Topic, Algorithm, Electronic Media Element)

Chlamydial Sexually Transmitted Diseases; Gonococcal Infections; Hepatitis B; Hepatitis C; HIV Infection and AIDS; Posttraumatic Stress Disorder (PTSD); Syphilis

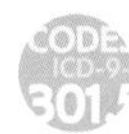

CODES

ICD9

- 995.83 Adult sexual abuse
- V71.5 Observation following alleged rape or seduction

CLINICAL PEARLS

- *Rape* is a legal term, and the examining physician is encouraged to use terminology such as *alleged rape* or *alleged sexual conduct*.
- Marital rape is a federal offense in all 50 states and the District of Columbia, and in some states also applies to unmarried cohabitating couples.
- Because "consent defense" is common, documentation of evidence supporting the use of force or the administration of drugs/alcohol is imperative.
- The use of a protocol is encouraged to assure every victim a uniform, comprehensive evaluation, regardless of the expertise of the examining physician. The protocol must ensure that all evidence is properly collected and labeled, chain of custody is maintained, and the evidence is sent to the most appropriate forensic laboratory.
- All medical records must be well documented and legible.
- All medical personnel must be willing and able to testify on behalf of the patient.

The views expressed in this chapter are those of the author and do not reflect the official policy or position of the Department of the Army, Department of Defense, or the US Government. Opinions, interpretations, conclusions, and recommendations herein are those of the author and are not necessarily endorsed by the US Army.

RAYNAUD PHENOMENON

Herbert L. Muncie, Jr., MD

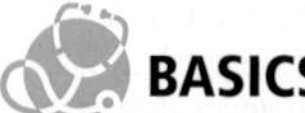

BASICS

DESCRIPTION

- Idiopathic intermittent episodes of vasoconstriction of digital arteries, precapillary arterioles, and cutaneous arteriovenous shunts in response to cold temperatures or emotional stress:
  - A triphasic color change of the fingers (occasionally, of the toes) is the physical manifestation of the episodes:
    - Thumbs are rarely involved.
    - The initial color is white from extreme pallor, then blue from cyanosis, and finally with warming and vasodilatation intense redness develops.
  - Swelling, throbbing, and paresthesias are the final symptoms.
  - Primary (idiopathic Raynaud disease):
    - 80% of patients with Raynaud phenomenon have primary disease.
    - Episodes are bilateral and nonprogressive.
    - Diagnosis confirmed only if after >2 years of symptoms, no underlying associated disease develops
  - Secondary (Raynaud syndrome):
    - Progressive and asymmetric
    - Spasm is more frequent and more severe with time. No gangrene; rarely, ulceration; 13% may progress to atrophy of digital fat pads and ischemic ulcers of fingertips.
- System(s) affected: Hematologic; Lymphatic; Immunologic; Musculoskeletal; Dermatologic; Exocrine

Pregnancy Considerations

- Raynaud phenomenon can appear as breast pain in lactating women.
- Bacterial culture of breast milk can distinguish mastitis from Raynaud phenomenon.

Geriatric Considerations

Initial appearance of Raynaud phenomenon at >40 years of age frequently indicates an underlying connective tissue disease.

Pediatric Considerations

Associated with SLE and scleroderma

EPIDEMIOLOGY

Incidence

- Primary:
  - Predominant age: 14 years; ~1/4 begin >40 years of age
  - Predominant sex: Female > Male (4:1)
- Secondary:
  - Predominant age: >40 years of age
  - Predominant sex: No gender predilection

Prevalence

- Primary: ~3–16% of population (based on reporting of characteristic skin color changes, intolerance to cold)
- Secondary: Less common, only about 1% of population

RISK FACTORS

- Smoking may reduce digital blood flow but is not associated with increased risk of Raynaud phenomenon.
- Existing autoimmune or connective tissue disorder
- End-stage renal disease with hemodialysis may increase the risk due to a steal phenomenon complicating the arterial-venous shunt.
- An elevated homocysteine level has been associated with primary and secondary disease.

Genetics

Little information is available, but some studies suggest a dominant inheritance pattern. ~1/4 of primary patients have a first-degree relative with Raynaud phenomenon.

GENERAL PREVENTION

- Avoid exposure to cold.
- Stop smoking.
- Avoid trauma and vibration to hands and fingertips; however, no relationship has been established between etiology of Raynaud phenomenon and occupational vibratory tool use.

ETIOLOGY

Unknown. May involve increased sensitivity of β_2-adrenergic receptors in digital vessels in primary type. Serotonin receptors (5-HT_2 type) may be involved in secondary Raynaud phenomenon. Dysregulation of control mechanisms of vascular motility leading to imbalance between vasodilation and vasoconstriction. Platelet and blood viscosity abnormalities are also implicated.

COMMONLY ASSOCIATED CONDITIONS

Secondary Raynaud:

- Scleroderma
- Systemic lupus erythematosus (SLE)
- Polymyositis
- Sjögren syndrome
- Occlusive vascular disease
- Cryoglobulinemia
- Use of vibrating tools

DIAGNOSIS

HISTORY

- Primary:
  - Symmetric attacks
  - Absence of tissue necrosis, ulceration, or gangrene
  - Absence of secondary cause after history and general physical examination
  - If after >2 years of symptoms no abnormal clinical or laboratory signs have developed, secondary disease is highly unlikely.
- Secondary:
  - Onset typically >40 years of age
  - Asymmetric episodes more intense and painful
  - Inquire regarding arthritis, myalgias, fever, dry eyes and/or mouth, rash, or cardiopulmonary symptoms.
  - Inquire about past or current drug use.
  - Any exposure to toxic agents
  - Any repetitive trauma

PHYSICAL EXAM

Pallor/whiteness of fingertips with cold exposure, followed by cyanosis, then redness and pain with warming:

- Ischemic attacks evidenced by demarcated or cyanotic skin limited to digits usually starts on 1 digit and spreads symmetrically to all fingers of both hands; however, the thumb is often spared.
- Beau lines: Transverse linear depressions in nail plate of most or all fingernails, which can occur after exposure to cold temperature or any disease serious enough to disrupt normal nail growth
- Livedo reticularis: Mottling of the skin of the arms and legs may occur but is completely benign and reversible with warming.
- Primary:
  - Normal general physical exam
  - Nail bed capillaries: Place 1 drop of grade B immersion oil on skin at base of fingernail, and view capillaries with handheld ophthalmoscope at 10–40 diopters. Normal appearance.
- Secondary:
  - Clinical features suggestive of connective tissue disease (e.g., arthritis, abnormal lung function)
  - Ischemic skin lesions: Ulceration of finger pads, progressing to autoamputation in severe, prolonged cases
  - Nail bed capillaries distorted and anatomically abnormal (1)[C]

DIAGNOSTIC TESTS & INTERPRETATION

Unnecessary to perform provocative test (e.g., immersion of patient's hand in ice water)

Lab

- Primary:
  - Antinuclear antibody: Negative
  - ESR: Normal
- Secondary:
  - Tests for underlying secondary causes (e.g., CBC, ESR)
  - Positive autoantibody has low positive predictive value for an associated connective tissue disease (30%).
  - Antibodies to specific autoantigens more suggestive of secondary disease (e.g., scleroderma with anticentromere or antitopoisomerase antibodies)

Imaging

Rarely necessary; patients may demonstrate osteolysis of distal metaphysial portions of phalanges with tapering and calcification of soft tissue

Follow-Up & Special Considerations

Periodic assessments could be helpful during the initial years after the diagnosis is made to determine if a connective tissue disease has become manifest.

Diagnostic Procedures/Surgery

Diagnosis is determined by history and physical exam.

DIFFERENTIAL DIAGNOSIS

- Thromboangiitis obliterans (Buerger disease): Primarily affects men; involves legs and feet; <5% have hand involvement; smoking-related
- Rheumatoid arthritis (RA)
- Progressive systemic sclerosis (scleroderma): Raynaud phenomenon may precede other symptoms by years.
- SLE
- Carpal tunnel syndrome
- Thoracic outlet syndrome
- Hypothyroidism
- CREST syndrome (calcinosis cutis, Raynaud phenomenon, esophageal dysmotility, sclerodactyly, and telangiectasias)

- Cryoglobulinemias
- Waldenström macroglobulinemia
- Acrocyanosis
- Polycythemia
- Occupational (e.g., especially from vibrating tools, masonry work, exposure to polyvinyl chloride)
- Drugs (e.g., clonidine, ergotamine, methysergide, amphetamines, bromocriptine, bleomycin, vinblastine, cisplatin, cyclosporine)

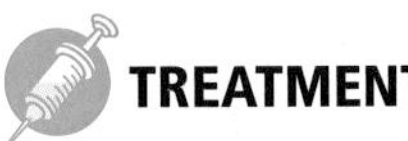

TREATMENT

The effects of treatment can be assessed using a Raynaud Condition Score (2).

MEDICATION

Calcium-channel blockers (CCBs) have been the primary treatment for many years. Nifedipine has been best studied and is the most frequently used drug in this group.

First Line

- Nifedipine: 30–180 mg/d (sustained-release form); may be needed only during winter; up to 75% experience improvement (8)[A]
- Symptomatic responses do not correlate with objective evidence of improvement.
- Contraindications: Allergy to drug, pregnancy, CHF
- Precautions: May cause headache, dizziness, lightheadedness, edema, or hypotension
- Significant possible interactions:
  - Increases serum level of digoxin; monitor digoxin levels closely after nifedipine is added
  - May increase PT in patients taking warfarin

Second Line

- Amlodipine (5–20 mg/d) and nicardipine appear to be effective and may have fewer adverse effects.
- No data exist to support use of another CCB if initial one is ineffective.
- Prazosin (1–2 mg t.i.d.) is the only well-studied α_1-adrenergic receptor blocker with modest effect.
- Small studies support benefit from losartan, fluoxetine, and phosphodiesterase type 5 inhibitors (3).
- Parenteral iloprost, a prostacyclin, even in low doses (0.5 ng/kg/min over 6 hours) has improved ulcerations with severe Raynaud phenomenon (4)[B]. Oral prostacyclin has not proved useful.
- Nitroglycerin patches may be helpful, but use is limited by the occurrence of severe headache. Nitroglycerin gel has shown promise as a topical therapy (5)[B].

ADDITIONAL TREATMENT

General Measures

- Dress warmly, wear gloves, and avoid cold.
- Stop smoking.
- Avoid beta-blockers, amphetamines, ergot alkaloids, and sumatriptan.
- Temperature-related biofeedback may help patients to increase hand temperature, but at the 1-year follow-up no better than control
- Use finger guards over ulcerated fingertips.

Issues for Referral

If an underlying disease is strongly suspected, consider rheumatology consultation for evaluation and treatment.

Additional Therapies

- Short-acting CCBs such as nifedipine
- Aspirin
- Digital or wrist block with lidocaine or bupivacaine (without epinephrine)
- Short-term anticoagulation with heparin if persistent critical ischemia, evidence of large-artery occlusive disease, or both

COMPLEMENTARY AND ALTERNATIVE MEDICINE

- Although well-designed studies have not been done yet for complementary medicine, some treatments have shown an effect (6).
- *Ginkgo biloba* has been found to reduce the frequency of attacks (7)[B].
- Fish oil supplements may increase digital systolic pressure and time to onset of symptoms after exposure to cold but was not proven in controlled trials.
- Oral arginine is no better than placebo.
- Biofeedback is not helpful (6)[A].

SURGERY/OTHER PROCEDURES

Effect of cervical sympathectomy is transient; symptoms return in 1–2 years.

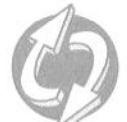

ONGOING CARE

FOLLOW-UP RECOMMENDATIONS

Avoid exposure to cold situations; avoid use of vibrating tools.

Patient Monitoring

Management of fingertip ulcers, including rapid treatment of infection

DIET

No special diet

PATIENT EDUCATION

- Emphasize cessation of smoking.
- Discuss avoiding aggravating factors (e.g., trauma, vibration, cold).
- Dress warmly; wear gloves.
- Warm hands when experiencing vasospasm.

PROGNOSIS

- Attacks may last from several minutes to a few hours.
- 2/3 are likely to have spontaneous resolution.
- In cases of secondary Raynaud phenomenon, affected patients develop the hallmarks of underlying disease.
- ~13% of Raynaud phenomenon patients develop a secondary disorder, many of which are connective tissue diseases.

COMPLICATIONS

- Primary: Very rare
- Secondary: Gangrene, autoamputation of fingertips

REFERENCES

1. Herrick AL, Cutolo M, et al. Clinical implications from capillaroscopic analysis in patients with Raynaud's phenomenon and systemic sclerosis. *Arthritis Rheum*. 2010;62:2595–604.
2. Khanna PP, Maranian P, Gregory J, et al. The minimally important difference and patient acceptable symptom state for the Raynaud's condition score in patients with Raynaud's phenomenon in a large randomised controlled clinical trial. *Ann Rheum Dis*. 2010;69:588–91.
3. De LaVega AJ, Derk CT, et al. Phosphodiesterase-5 inhibitors for the treatment of Raynaud's: A novel indication. *Expert Opin Investig Drugs*. 2009;18: 23–9.
4. Kawald A, Burmester GR, Huscher D, et al. Low versus high-dose iloprost therapy over 21 days in patients with secondary Raynaud's phenomenon and systemic sclerosis: A randomized, open, single-center study. *J Rheumatol*. 2008;35:1830–7.
5. Chung L, Shapiro L, Fiorentino D, et al. MQX-503, a novel formulation of nitroglycerin, improves the severity of Raynaud's phenomenon: A randomized, controlled trial. *Arthritis Rheum*. 2009;60:870–7.
6. Malenfant D, Catton M, Pope JE, et al. The efficacy of complementary and alternative medicine in the treatment of Raynaud's phenomenon: A literature review and meta-analysis. *Rheumatology (Oxford)*. 2009;48:791–5.
7. Choi WS, Choi CJ, Kim KS, et al. To compare the efficacy and safety of nifedipine sustained release with Ginkgo biloba extract to treat patients with primary Raynaud's phenomenon in South Korea; Korean Raynaud study (KOARA study). *Clin Rheumatol*. 2009;28:553–9.
8. Huisstede BM, Hoogvliet P, Paulis WD, et al. Effectiveness of interventions for secondary Raynaud's phenomenon: A systematic review. *Arch Phys Med Rehabil*. 2011;92:1166–80.

ADDITIONAL READING

Pope JE. The diagnosis and treatment of Raynaud's phenomenon: A practical approach. *Drugs*. 2007;67: 517–25.

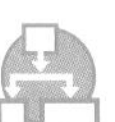

See Also (Topic, Algorithm, Electronic Media Element)

Algorithm: Raynaud Phenomenon

CODES

ICD9

443.0 Raynaud's syndrome

CLINICAL PEARLS

- Initial presentation of Raynaud phenomenon after age 40 suggests underlying disease.
- Remember Raynaud in differential diagnosis of a lactating woman with breast pain (vs. mastitis).
- Primary Raynaud phenomenon is symmetric, whereas secondary is asymmetric.

RECTAL PROLAPSE

Timothy L. Black, MD
James P. Miller, MD

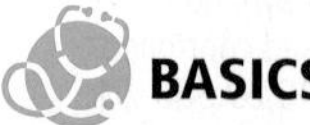

BASICS

Protrusion of the rectum through the anus

DESCRIPTION

- Partial prolapse:
  - Involves only mucosa
  - frequently follows anal operative procedures (radial rectal folds prolapsed through anus)
- Complete prolapse:
  - Involves the entire rectal wall (procidentia)
  - Occurs most commonly as a spontaneous event in children and as a complication of other disorders in the elderly (concentric rectal folds prolapsed through anus)
- System(s) affected: Gastrointestinal

EPIDEMIOLOGY

Incidence

- Predominant age: <3 years in children, fifth decade in adults
- Predominant sex: Female > Male in adults; females represent 80–90% of adult patients; Male = Female in children (1)[B]
- 4.2/1,000 overall; 10/1,000 >65 years of age

Geriatric Considerations

Common problem in the elderly

Pediatric Considerations

Idiopathic type most common in children

RISK FACTORS

- Myelomeningocele
- Exstrophy of the bladder
- Cystic fibrosis (CF)
- Chronic constipation or diarrhea
- Imperforate anus (2)[C]
- Multiple sclerosis
- Stroke/paralysis
- Mental retardation

Genetics

Unknown

GENERAL PREVENTION

Avoid constipation and diarrhea.

PATHOPHYSIOLOGY

The anatomic basis for rectal prolapse is a deficient pelvic floor through which the rectum herniates.

ETIOLOGY

- Children:
  - Idiopathic (most common)
  - Abnormal innervation of levator ani muscle complex or puborectalis or anal sphincter, or abnormal anatomic relationships of these muscle groups
- Adults:
  - Diastasis of levator ani
  - Loose endopelvic fascia
  - Loss of normal horizontal position of rectum
  - Weak anal sphincter
  - Pudendal neuropathy
  - Redundant sigmoid colon
  - Loss of rectal-sacral attachments

COMMONLY ASSOCIATED CONDITIONS

- CF
- Myelomeningocele
- Exstrophy of the bladder
- Chronic constipation or diarrhea
- Imperforate anus
- Paraplegia
- Stroke
- Fecal incontinence
- Vaginal vault or uterine prolapse
- Mental retardation
- Marfan syndrome
- Ehlers-Danlos disease
- Urinary incontinence (may be found in 58% of patients operated on for rectal prolapse) (3)[B]
- Bladder stones
- Nutritional disorders
- Progressive systemic sclerosis

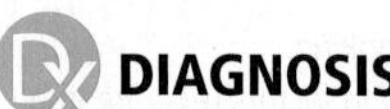

DIAGNOSIS

HISTORY

- History of:
  - Visible mass
  - Rectal bleeding or soiling
  - Rectal pain
  - Prior anorectal surgery
  - Spinal cord injury or defect
  - Constipation and straining

Pediatric Considerations

- Sensation of anal mass in children
- Adults:
  - Feeling of incomplete evacuation
  - Rectal and urinary incontinence (50–75% of adult patients)
  - Rectal bleeding or discharge

PHYSICAL EXAM

- Children:
  - Protruding mass
- Adults:
  - Visible mass of rectal mucosa or full thickness of rectal wall
  - Poor anal sphincter tone on rectal exam
  - Reproduce prolapse with straining

DIAGNOSTIC TESTS & INTERPRETATION

- Anorectal manometry (3)[B]
- Cinedefecography
- Electromyography
- Colon transit study

Lab

Evaluate for CF with genetic screening and sweat chloride evaluation.

Imaging

Barium enema is useful in selected cases of recurrent rectal prolapse.

Diagnostic Procedures/Surgery

- Sigmoidoscopy is useful in recurrent prolapse to rule out rectal lesions.
- MRI of lumbosacral spine to evaluate for spinal canal defects if not already diagnosed
- Anal manometry
- Pudendal nerve terminal latencies

DIFFERENTIAL DIAGNOSIS

- Intussusception
- Rectal polyps
- Hemorrhoids

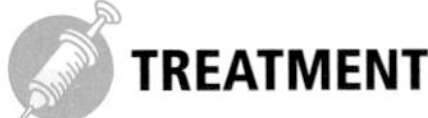

TREATMENT

MEDICATION

Medications to soften stools; avoid constipation and straining:

- Mineral oil
- Stool softeners
- Lactulose
- Polyethylene glycol (MiraLAX, GlycoLax)

ADDITIONAL TREATMENT

General Measures

- For acute cases: Prompt manual reduction of prolapse
- Treatment of diarrhea or constipation
- Conservative management in children is successful in most cases (4)[C], with resolution reported in 92% of children followed 2 years

SURGERY/OTHER PROCEDURES

- Abdominal procedures:
  - Suture rectopexy
  - Transabdominal proctopexy; also may be done laparoscopically (suture material, absorbable mesh, and nonabsorbable mesh may be used) (1,5)[B],(4)[C]:
    - Laparoscopic rectopexy may give equivalent results with shorter hospital stay and decreased cost (6)[B],(7)[A].
    - Advantages of laparoscopic rectopexy are all short term, with long-term outcomes equal to those of the abdominal approach (8)[A].
  - Transabdominal Ripstein procedure (suspension of rectum from sacrum by means of artificial material) (1)[B]
  - Anterior resection of rectum (rarely used)
  - Diverting colostomy occasionally may be required in the most severe cases.
- Perineal procedures:
  - Submucosal injection (sclerotherapy) of 5% phenol, 30% saline, or 25% glucose (or other sclerosants) in 4 quadrants under general anesthesia (outpatient)
  - Linear electrocauterization (inpatient or outpatient)
  - Posterior sagittal rectal suspension and levator repair
  - Delorme procedure (mucosal stripping of prolapsed rectum with plication of underlying muscle)
  - Perineal rectosigmoidectomy (1)[B]
  - Thiersch wire (outpatient procedure; may be modified by using Marlex or Silastic strip or other strong suture material instead of wire); used more commonly in children, older patients, and poor-risk adults
  - Gracilis sling procedure
  - Stapled transanal resection

IN-PATIENT CONSIDERATIONS

Initial Stabilization

Outpatient care unless complications occur or surgical intervention is required

Admission Criteria

- Inpatient care required for patients treated with laparotomy
- Inpatient care may be required after extensive perineal dissection or for pain control.

ONGOING CARE

Biofeedback has been used to improve postoperative function (3)[B].

FOLLOW-UP RECOMMENDATIONS

Patient Monitoring

Monthly visits until possible need for surgery has been determined or until prolapse has resolved

DIET

- High fiber (25 g/d)
- 100% bran granules
- Keep well hydrated.

PATIENT EDUCATION

- Particular reassurance to parents of infants with prolapse regarding benign nature of problem and high rate of spontaneous resolution
- Diet instructions
- Teach measures to avoid constipation.
- Teach family/patient to reduce prolapse.

PROGNOSIS

- Spontaneous resolution is expected in most children with idiopathic prolapse.
- Recurrence rate is 5–10% for most procedures.
- Sclerotherapy frequently needs to be repeated.
- Good prognosis with treatment

COMPLICATIONS

- Mucosal ulcerations
- Necrosis of rectal wall
- Persistent or recurrent prolapse
- Constipation and pain if Thiersch wire is too tight
- Recurrence of rectal prolapse
- Fecal incontinence

REFERENCES

1. Madiba TE, Baig MK, Wexner SD. Surgical management of rectal prolapse. *Arch Surg*. 2005; 140:63–73.
2. Belizon A, et al. Rectal prolapse following posterior sagittal anorectoplasty for anorectal malformations. *J Ped Surg*. 2005;40:192–6.
3. Gourgiotis S, Baratsis S, et al. Rectal prolapse. *Int J Colorectal Dis*. 2007;22:231–43.
4. Shalaby R, Ismail M, et al. Laparoscopic mesh rectopexy for complete rectal prolapse in children: A new simplified technique. *Pediatr Surg Int*. 2010; 26:807–813.
5. Brazzelli M, Bachoo P, Grant A. Surgery for complete rectal prolapse in adults (review). *Cochrane Database Syst Rev*. 2006;1.
6. Boccasanta P, Rosati R, Venturi M, et al. Comparison of laparoscopic rectopexy with open technique in the treatment of complete rectal prolapse: Clinical and functional results. *Surg Lap Endoscopy*. 1998;8:460–5.
7. Sajid M, Siddiqui M, Baig M. Open versus laparoscopic repair of full thickness rectal prolapse: A re-meta-analysis. *Colorectal Dis*. 2009 Apr 13. Epub ahead of print.
8. Solomon MJ, Young CJ, Eyers AA, et al. Randomized clinical trial of laparoscopic versus open abdominal rectopexy for rectal prolapse. *Br J Surg*. 2002;89:35–9.

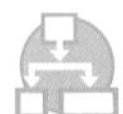

See Also (Topic, Algorithm, Electronic Media Element)

Hemorrhoids; Intussusception

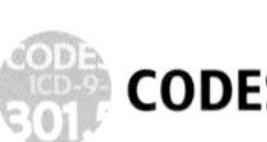

CODES

ICD9

569.1 Rectal prolapse

CLINICAL PEARLS

- Most common in females in their fifth decade
- In children, rectal prolapse occurs most often under the age of 3 and often resolves spontaneously.
- High-fiber diet and good hydration may prevent recurrences.

REFRACTIVE ERRORS

Robert M. Kershner, MD, MS, FACS

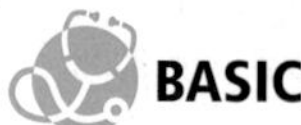

BASICS

DESCRIPTION

- Inability of the eye to produce a focused image on the fovea or central part of the retina
- Emmetropia: When light rays are in perfect focus, the image being viewed is seen clearly.
- Ametropia: Any refractive error of the eye that prevents normal focusing of the image
- Hyperopia: When the cornea of the eye is too flat or the eye is too short, light rays fall in focus behind the retina, and the individual is "farsighted."
- Myopia: When the cornea is too steep or the length of the eyeball is too long, the focal point for light rays lies short of the retina, and the individual is "nearsighted."
- Presbyopia: The natural tendency of the crystalline lens to harden or become sclerotic, limiting the focusing of the eye on near objects (accommodation):
  - The human crystalline lens thickens with age. By the age of 40 years, most people do not have enough room within the eye to allow normal excursion of the lens and accommodation; viewing of near objects is blurred, and reading glasses are required.
- Astigmatism: When the cornea is steeper in 1 meridian more than the other or the globe is not round (i.e., is oval or almond-shaped), visual blurriness occurs.
- System(s) affected: Nervous

Geriatric Considerations

Presbyopia occurs in later life.

Pediatric Considerations

Refractive errors can be detected early in life.

EPIDEMIOLOGY

- Predominant age: Refractive errors are present at birth, but usually are not detected until puberty.
- Predominant gender: Male = Female
- Individuals >40 years of age are more likely to experience presbyopia or normal loss of accommodation that occurs with age, necessitating the use of reading glasses for close work.

Prevalence

Of the general US population, 70% have some form of ametropia.

RISK FACTORS

Genetics

Inherited

ETIOLOGY

- Developmental (most common)
- Ocular trauma
- Iatrogenic (e.g., postcataract removal)

COMMONLY ASSOCIATED CONDITIONS

Patients with diabetes mellitus have fluctuating myopia as a result of poorly controlled blood glucose and concomitant swelling of the crystalline lens.

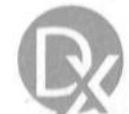

DIAGNOSIS

HISTORY

- Difficulty seeing objects at a distance
- Difficulty focusing on near objects
- Difficulty reading
- Squinting
- Headaches (from squinting)
- In children:
  - Rubbing of the eyes
  - Sitting close to TV or computer screen
  - Problems in sports, particularly declining performance
  - Declining grades
  - Preference for front-row seating
  - Covering of an eye while reading

PHYSICAL EXAM

Snellen Eye Chart (developed by Dr. Hermann Snellen in 1862):

- Test each eye separately.
- The smallest row of letters that the patient can read determines visual acuity in the uncovered eye.

DIAGNOSTIC TESTS & INTERPRETATION

- Pinhole vision test: To distinguish a refractive error from an organic cause of visual blurring, have the patient look through a pinhole in a card without a corrective lens.
- Patients with a pure refractive error have improved vision because the pinhole blocks nonparallel and unfocusable rays of light.

Diagnostic Procedures/Surgery

- Methods:
  - Objective streak retinoscopy may be used to measure the degree of refractive error in spherocylinder correction for the proper spectacle or contact lens.
  - Antimuscarinic agents such as cyclopentolate (Cyclogyl) or tropicamide (Mydriacyl) applied topically paralyze the ciliary body, preventing accommodation. Cycloplegic refraction can then be performed.
- Age-related testing:
  - Newborns should be examined for general eye health; ophthalmologic evaluation is indicated for any problems discovered.
  - Vision screening should occur at each well-child visit.
  - Visual acuity testing should be performed at ~3.5 years of age.
  - Visual acuity and motility testing should be performed at age 5 years:
    - Visual acuity should be retested prior to obtaining a driver's license, at age 40 years, and every 2–4 years until age 65, after which age evaluations are recommended every 1–2 years.

DIFFERENTIAL DIAGNOSIS

- Corneal disease
- Cataract
- Retinal abnormalities
- Diseases of the optic nerve

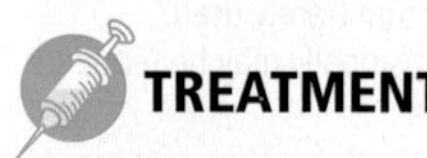

TREATMENT

MEDICATION

Precaution: Antimuscarinic agents may induce acute glaucoma via acute-angle closure.

ADDITIONAL TREATMENT

General Measures

- Spectacle lenses (glasses)
- Soft or hard contact lenses

SURGERY/OTHER PROCEDURES

- Laser-assisted in-situ keratomileusis (LASIK), approved by the FDA in 1997. A superficial corneal flap is created with the keratome, and the excimer laser removes a small amount of tissue, thus reshaping the cornea. Corrects all refractive errors. Healing is rapid because re-epithelialization is not needed. Considered an adjunctive procedure for use with the excimer laser.
- Other modifications:
  - LASIK and EPI LASIK involve removing just the superficial epithelium before laser application.
  - IntraLASIK is a laser used to create the flap.
  - Custom ablation: Wavefront maps of the cornea and eye for ablation
- Older methods now superseded by LASIK:
  - Radial keratotomy: With topical anesthesia, using a surgical keratome, multiple (4–8) radial incisions are placed onto the surface of the peripheral cornea to flatten the central, optical zone. The length, depth, and proximity of the incision to the central optical zone determine its effect and degree of correction obtained. Radial keratotomy is safe and effective, and corrects nearsightedness, astigmatism, or a combination of both, after the age of 18 years when the prescription has stabilized.
  - Photorefractive keratectomy: Surface corneal tissue is removed with the excimer laser to reshape the cornea, thus correcting nearsightedness, farsightedness, or astigmatism. Risks and disadvantages include pain, keratitis, and potential scarring. Healing requires 3 months with topical antibiotics and steroids, with associated risks of glaucoma, cataract, and chronic inflammation.
  - Automated lamellar keratoplasty: A microsurgical dermatome removes a layer of the superficial cornea to induce flattening; investigational.
- Excimer laser: The laser photo ablates corneal tissue from the central visual axis, thus flattening it. Following the procedure, the cornea must re-epithelialize. Healing takes several months, during which there is a mild haze and blurring of vision. FDA approved October 1995.
- Implantable contact lens: A thin plastic lens is permanently implanted either in the anterior chamber and anchored to the iris (FDA approved in 2005, VERISYES) or in the posterior chamber (Vision Lens, FDA approved 2006) between the iris and the human crystalline lens. All refractive errors can be corrected. Risks include damage to the natural lens during surgery, cataract formation, and intraocular inflammation or infection; investigational anterior–chamber intraocular lens.
- Several scleral expansion procedures presently under investigation increase the space within the ciliary body by surgical means to restore lens movement and accommodation. The results have been unsatisfactory.
- Bifocal intraocular lenses (several types have been approved by the FDA: ReSTOR_Alcon, ReZOOM-AMO, Tecnis_AMO) implanted in the posterior chamber. They increase the depth of field to allow viewing objects both at near and at distance. Side effects include decreased contrast, glare, ghosting of images, and problems with night vision.
- Accommodative intraocular lenses (Crystalens). First FDA-approved intraocular lens; several others under clinical investigation. The accommodative intraocular lens moves in response to ciliary body movement to allow focusing at different focal lengths. Side effects are minimal. Present lenses have limited range of focus.

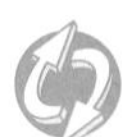

ONGOING CARE

FOLLOW-UP RECOMMENDATIONS

Patient Monitoring

- Examinations recommended when starting school, entering college, any change in vision quality, and at the age of onset of presbyopia (the need for reading glasses)
- Individuals with any of the known risks of eye disease or conditions that could affect the eyes (such as diabetes) need annual ocular examinations.

PATIENT EDUCATION

- All patients should have their eyes examined when starting school and periodically thereafter.
- The options of eyeglasses, contact lenses, and permanent surgical correction of refractive errors can be considered.
- Encourage aggressive control of diabetes mellitus. These individuals are most likely contraindicated to undergo refraction corrective surgery.

PROGNOSIS

- Good, if discovered early and corrected appropriately
- It is not unusual for refractive errors to be temporarily worsened during pregnancy because of hormonal changes in tear function and corneal swelling.
- It is common that refractive errors worsen as a child ages until complete adult growth has been achieved. This is a common source of concern for parents. Reassurance that refractive change is often seen with growth spurts, especially at puberty, is advised.

COMPLICATIONS

- Amblyopia
- Poor school performance

ADDITIONAL READING

- Fax-on-Demand service of American Academy of Ophthalmology for policy statement and patient education materials: (908) 935-2761.
- Frequency of Ocular Exams. *Policy Statement*. San Francisco: American Academy of Ophthalmology; 2009.
- Kershner RM. Lessons from the Practice: The Gift of Sight. *A Guide to Understanding Your Eyes*. Thorofare, NJ: Slack; 1994.
- Vision Screening for Infants and Children. *Policy Statement*. San Francisco: American Academy of Ophthalmology; 2007.

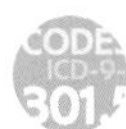

CODES

ICD9

- 367.1 Myopia
- 367.9 Unspecified disorder of refraction and accommodation
- 367.20 Astigmatism, unspecified

CLINICAL PEARLS

- Vision screening should occur at each well-child visit.
- Visual acuity testing should be performed at ~3.5 years of age.

REITER SYNDROME

Douglas W. MacPherson, MD, MSc(CTM), FRCPC

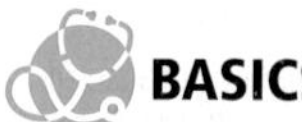

BASICS

Reiter syndrome is a seronegative, multisystem, inflammatory disorder classically involving joints, the eye, and the lower genitourinary (GU) tract. Axial joint involvement (e.g., spine, sacroiliac joints) is also common. Dermatologic manifestations are also seen frequently.

DESCRIPTION

A classic triad of features including arthritis, conjunctivitis/iritis, and either urethritis or cervicitis:

- The epidemiology is similar to other reactive arthritis syndromes, characterized by sterile inflammation of joints associated with infections originating at nonarticular sites. A fourth feature of dermatologic manifestations may include buccal ulceration or balanitis or a psoriaform skin eruption. (Having only 2 features present does not rule out the diagnosis.)
- It has 2 forms: Sexually transmitted, in which symptoms generally emerge between 7 and 14 days after exposure to *Chlamydia trachomatis* and other urethral/cervical pathogens acquired during sexual contact and postdysenteric or other bacterial enteric infections.
- System(s) affected: Musculoskeletal; Renal/Urologic; Dermatologic/Exocrine
- Synonym(s): Idiopathic blennorrheal arthritis; Arthritis urethritica; Urethro-oculosynovial syndrome; Fiessinger-Leroy-Reiter disease

Geriatric Considerations

In a demographic group associated with new or frequent sexual partners, the antecedent triggering infection is more likely to be sexually transmitted than enteric.

Pediatric Considerations

With a preceding history of enteric illness, the antecedent triggering event is more likely to be a bacterial enteric infection than sexually transmitted.

Pregnancy Considerations

There are no special considerations except as related to the usual precautions concerning pharmaceutical therapies.

EPIDEMIOLOGY

Incidence

- Predominant age: 20–40 years
- Predominant sex: Male > Female
- 0.24–1.5% incidence after epidemics of bacterial dysentery
- Complicates 1–2% of all cases of nongonococcal urethritis (1,2)

RISK FACTORS

- New or high-risk sexual contacts occurring 7–14 days before the onset of clinical presentation; for sexually acquired precipitants of Reiter syndrome, the primary infection may be subclinical and undiagnosed.
- Food poisoning or bacterial dysentery

Genetics

HLA-B27 tissue antigen present in 60–80% of patients

GENERAL PREVENTION

- The immune-response characteristics of this syndrome make specific avoidance of infectious precipitants the most important general precaution and potentially the most difficult to achieve.
- Safer sexual exposures and good food and water handling for personal consumption are essential for all persons at all times to maintain health and to avoid infections and the chronic inflammatory consequences of a previous infection.
- A family history of seronegative or reactive arthritis syndromes may suggest a genetic predisposition.

PATHOPHYSIOLOGY

- The pathophysiology of all the seronegative reactive arthritis syndromes and the immunologic role of infectious diseases as precipitants for clinical illness remain incompletely understood.
- Avoidance of precipitant infections and early management of the multiorgan system inflammatory consequences are important. Scientific evidence does not suggest that antibiotic treatment following onset of syndrome will benefit inflammatory joint, eye, or urinary tract symptoms.

ETIOLOGY

- *C. trachomatis* is the usual causative organism of the postvenereal variety.
- Dysentery-associated form follows enteric bacterial infection owing to *Shigella, Salmonella, Yersinia,* and *Campylobacter* spp. This form is more likely to be seen in women, children, and the elderly than the postvenereal form.

COMMONLY ASSOCIATED CONDITIONS

Recent case of:

- Enteric disease from:
  - Shigellosis or,
  - Salmonellosis or,
  - Campylobacteriosis or,
  - Enteric infection with *Yersinia* spp.
- Urogenital infection from:
  - *Mycoplasma* or *Ureaplasma* spp. or,
  - *Chlamydia* urethritis
- Infection with HIV

DIAGNOSIS

- The diagnosis of Reiter syndrome is based on the clinical presentation of the classic triad of joint, eye, and GU inflammation and negative serologic testing for rheumatoid factor.
- These 3 symptoms and signs may not all be evident at the same time.
- HLA-B27 testing is not required for diagnosis.
- Treatable STIs should be sought when clinically indicated.
- Screening for enteric infections is rarely useful and generally is not indicated diagnostically.

HISTORY

The presence of the clinical syndrome plus:

- Diarrhea, dysentery, urethritis, or genital discharge and risk events for enteric or sexually acquired infections
- Include a risk history, including travel or migration history and potential exposure to a precipitating infectious agent.

PHYSICAL EXAM

- Musculoskeletal:
  - Asymmetric arthritis (especially knees, ankles, and metatarsophalangeal joints)
  - Enthesopathy (inflammation at tendinous insertion into bone, such as plantar fasciitis, digital periostitis, and Achilles tendinitis)
  - Spondyloarthropathy (spine and sacroiliac joint involvement)
- Urogenital tract:
  - Urethritis
  - Prostatitis
  - Occasionally cystitis
  - Balanitis
  - Cervicitis: Usually asymptomatic
- Eye:
  - Conjunctivitis of one or both eyes
  - Occasionally scleritis, keratitis, and corneal ulceration
  - Rarely uveitis and iritis
- Skin:
  - Mucocutaneous lesions (small, painless, superficial ulcers on oral mucosa, tongue, or glans penis)
  - Keratoderma blennorrhagica (hyperkeratotic skin lesions of palms and soles and around nails—can be mistaken for psoriasis)
- Cardiovascular: Occasionally pericarditis, murmur, conduction defects, and aortic incompetence
- Nervous system: Rarely peripheral neuropathy, cranial neuropathy, meningoencephalitis, and neuropsychiatric changes
- Constitutional:
  - Fever, malaise, anorexia, and weight loss
  - Patient can appear seriously ill (e.g., fever, rigors, tachycardia, and exquisitely tender joints).

DIAGNOSTIC TESTS & INTERPRETATION

Lab

- Blood:
  - Negative rheumatoid factor
  - Leukocyte count: 10,000–20,000 cells/mm^3
  - Neutrophilic leukocytosis
  - Elevated ESR
  - Moderate normochromic anemia
  - Hypergammaglobulinemia
- Synovial fluid:
  - Leukocyte count: 1,000–8,000 cells/mm^3
  - Bacterial culture negative
- Supportive test results (3):
  - Cultures, antigens, or serology positive for *C. trachomatis* or stool test positive for *Salmonella, Shigella, Yersinia,* or *Campylobacter* spp. supports the diagnosis.
  - HLA-B27-positive status (*not required or recommended for diagnosis)*
- Drugs that may alter lab results: Antibiotics may affect isolation of the bacterial pathogens.

Imaging

X-ray:

- Periosteal proliferation, thickening
- Spurs
- Erosions at articular margins
- Residual joint destruction
- Syndesmophytes (spine)
- Sacroiliitis

Diagnostic Procedures/Surgery

HLA-B27 histocompatibility antigen: Positive result in 60–80% of cases in non–HIV-related Reiter syndrome; HLA testing is not required or recommended for diagnosis. Rheumatoid factor is negative.

Pathological Findings

- A seronegative spondyloarthropathy (similar to ankylosing spondylitis, enteric arthritis, and psoriatic arthritis)
- Villous formation in joints
- Joint hyperemia
- Joint inflammation
- Prostatitis
- Seminal vesiculitis
- Skin biopsy similar to psoriasis
- Nonspecific conjunctivitis

DIFFERENTIAL DIAGNOSIS

- For specific diagnosis, arthritis associated with urethritis for >1 month
- Rheumatoid arthritis (RA)
- Ankylosing spondylitis
- Arthritis associated with inflammatory bowel disease
- Psoriatic arthritis
- Juvenile RA
- Bacterial arthritis, including gonococcal

TREATMENT

MEDICATION

First Line

- Symptomatic management: NSAIDs including indomethacin, naproxen, and others; intraarticular or systemic corticosteroids for refractory arthritis and enthesitis (4):
  - Contraindications:
    - GI bleeding
    - Patients with peptic ulcer, gastritis, or ulcerative colitis
    - Renal insufficiency
- Specific treatment of pathogenic microorganism may be attempted if isolated:
  - *C. trachomatis*: Doxycycline 100 mg PO b.i.d. × 7–14 days (*Note:* All STDs should be treated whether associated with Reiter syndrome or not.)
  - *Salmonella*, *Shigella*, *Yersinia*, and *Campylobacter* infections: Ciprofloxacin 500 mg PO b.i.d. × 5–10 days (*Note:* Emerging antimicrobial resistance may limit this agent's effectiveness in treatment and bacterial clearance. Antibiotic treatment does not improve GI symptoms or duration of infection or prevent carrier state.)
- GI upset: Antacids
- Iritis: Intraocular steroids
- Keratitis: Topical steroids

Second Line

- Aspirin or other NSAIDs
- Sulfasalazine is promising but not approved for this indication by the FDA.
- Methotrexate or azathioprine in severe cases (such usage is still experimental and not approved or agreed to be effective); immunosuppressive therapy is relatively contraindicated if patient suffers from HIV-related Reiter syndrome.
- Consultation with specialist is recommended, particularly when considering immunomodulatory agents such as sulfasalazine, methotrexate, or azathioprine.
- Role of antibiotics have been under investigation. They are currently unproven in effectiveness in seronegative arthritis syndromes.
- No published evidence supports the beneficial effect of antibiotics on development of this syndrome or the long-term outcome in patients with Reiter syndrome.

ADDITIONAL TREATMENT

General Measures

Treatment is determined by symptoms.

- Conjunctivitis does not require treatment.
- Iritis requires treatment.
- Mucocutaneous lesions do not require treatment.
- Physical therapy (PT) is needed during recovery.
- Arthritis may become prominent and disabling during the acute phase.

Issues for Referral

Joint and eye complications; complex management

IN-PATIENT CONSIDERATIONS

Initial Stabilization

Inpatient care may be needed during acute phase.

Admission Criteria

Severity, complications, and degree of disability

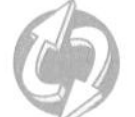

ONGOING CARE

FOLLOW-UP RECOMMENDATIONS

Bed rest until joint inflammation subsides

Patient Monitoring

Monitor clinical response to anti-inflammation medications. Observe for complications of therapy, particularly sulfasalazine and immunosuppressive drugs.

PATIENT EDUCATION

- Educate on risk factors for exposure, occurrence, and recurrence.
- Teach home PT techniques.
- For a listing of sources for patient education materials favorably reviewed on this topic, physicians may contact American Academy of Family Physicians Foundation, P.O. Box 8418, Kansas City, MO 64114, (800) 274-2237, ext. 4400.
- Arthritis Foundation, 1314 Spring Street NW, Atlanta, GA 30309, (404) 872-7100

PROGNOSIS

- Urethritis occurs 1–15 days after sexual exposure to causative agent.
- Reiter syndrome onset within 10–30 days of either enteric infection or STD
- Mean duration of symptoms is 19 weeks.
- Prognosis is poor in cases involving the heel, eye, or heart.

COMPLICATIONS

- Chronic or recurrent disease in 5–50% of patients (5)[A]
- Ankylosing spondylitis develops in 30–50% of patients who test positive for HLA-B27 antigen.
- Urethral strictures
- Cataracts and blindness
- Aortic root necrosis

REFERENCES

1. Siegel DM. Chronic arthritis in adolescence. *Adolesc Med State Art Rev*. 2007;18:47–61, viii.
2. Kim PS, Klausmeier TL, Orr DP, et al. Reactive arthritis: A review. *J Adolesc Health*. 2009;44: 309–15.
3. Contini C, Grilli A, Badia L, et al. Detection of Chlamydophila pneumoniae in patients with arthritis: Significance and diagnostic value. *Rheumatol Int*. 2011;31(10):1307–13.
4. National Guideline Clearinghouse 2009 July 13:13596; British Association of Sexual Health and HIV (BASHH) United Kingdom national guideline on management of sexually acquired reactive arthritis. Available at: www.bashh.org/guidelines.
5. Pope JE, et al. *Campylobacter* reactive arthritis: A systematic review. *Semin Arthritis Rheum*. 2007 Mar 20. [Epub ahead of print].

ADDITIONAL READING

Curry JA, Riddle MS, Gormley RP, et al. The epidemiology of infectious gastroenterology related reactive arthritis in U.S. military personnel: A case control study. *BMC Infect Dis*. 2010;10:266.

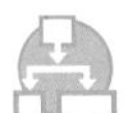

See Also (Topic, Algorithm, Electronic Media Element)

Ankylosing Spondylitis; Arthritis, Psoriatic; Behçet Syndrome

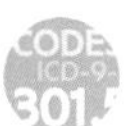

CODES

ICD9

099.3 Reiter's disease

CLINICAL PEARLS

- To differentiate Reiter syndrome from other seronegative arthritis syndromes, keep in mind that many of these syndromes may have similar clinical components and overlap in the presenting symptoms. Seek the opinion of a specialist if unsure.
- When the history points toward a sexually acquired infection as a cause, including HIV, associated treatable infectious precipitants of Reiter syndrome must be tested for both personal and public health reasons. Enteric investigations are rarely indicated clinically nor justify a therapeutic response.
- Some patients have a chronic course, experience recurrences, or have clinical complications. If the inflammatory symptoms do not settle down quickly on NSAID agents, consider referral to a specialist.

RENAL CELL CARCINOMA

Jonathon M. Firnhaber, MD

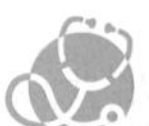

BASICS

DESCRIPTION

- Renal cell carcinoma (RCC), (aka *hypernephroma* or *Grawitz tumor),* accounts for 3–4% of all cancers and 2.3% of all cancer deaths; seventh most common malignant tumor in men and ninth in women
- Characterized by obscure and varied presentations, including paraneoplastic syndromes, vascular findings, and uncommon metastatic sites
- Early, aggressive surgical management provides the best opportunity for cure.
- System(s) affected: Renal/Urologic

EPIDEMIOLOGY

Incidence

- Predominant age: Patients in fifth to seventh decades; median age at diagnosis is 66 years.
- Predominant sex: Male > Female (1.6:1)
- Age-adjusted incidence increasing 3% per year, likely due in part to increased detection as an incidental finding on imaging studies
- In males, 10.7 new cases of RCC per 100,000 population per year vs. 6.5 in females
- Between 1975 and 1998, incidence among blacks increased by 4.5% compared with 2.9% among whites; reasons are unclear.

RISK FACTORS

- Smoking, active and passive (increases relative risk by 2–3)
- Obesity (linear relationship in women)
- Hypertension (antihypertensive medications are not independently associated with RCC)
- End-stage renal failure
- Acquired renal cystic disease
- Tuberous sclerosis
- HIV infection
- Urban environment
- Heavy metal exposure (cadmium, lead)
- Environmental toxin exposure (asbestos, petroleum by-products, chlorinated solvents)

Genetics

- 2–3% of cases are familial, with several autosomal-dominant syndromes described.
- Oncogenes localized to the short arm of chromosome 3 may have etiologic implications. Chromosome 3p12–p26 is specific for clear cell RCC.
- People with human leukocyte antigen (HLA) types Bw44 and DR8 are prone to develop RCC. These are rare familial RCCs.
- Hereditary papillary RCC is an autosomal dominant form of disease associated with multifocal papillary renal tumors and a 5:1 male predominance.

GENERAL PREVENTION

Smoking may contribute to 1/3 of all cases.

ETIOLOGY

Unknown

COMMONLY ASSOCIATED CONDITIONS

- Von Hippel–Lindau disease: 30–45% of these patients develop clear cell tumors.
- Tuberous sclerosis: Associated primarily with angiomyolipoma and clear cell tumors
- Sickle-cell trait: With few exceptions, renal medullary tumor is seen in young African American males with sickle-cell trait.
- Adult polycystic kidney disease
- Horseshoe kidney
- Acquired renal cystic disease from chronic renal failure

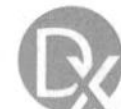

DIAGNOSIS

HISTORY

- Diverse and obscure presentations
- > 70% of RCC are incidentally discovered in asymptomatic patients due to increased use of ultrasound, CT scanning, and MRI

PHYSICAL EXAM

- Classic triad of hematuria, abdominal mass, and flank pain in fewer than 10% of patients
- Hematuria: 50–60%
- Flank pain: 35–40%
- Palpable mass: 25%
- Hypertension: 22–38%
- Weight loss: 28–36%
- Pyrexia: 7–17%
- Nonmetastatic hepatic dysfunction (Stauffer syndrome): 10–15%
- Neuromyopathy: 3%
- Scrotal varicoceles: 2–11% (most are left-sided)
- Patients with vena cava thrombus present with lower extremity edema, new varicocele, dilated superficial abdominal veins, albuminuria, pulmonary emboli, right atrial mass, or nonfunction of the involved kidney.

DIAGNOSTIC TESTS & INTERPRETATION

Lab

Initial lab tests

- Increased ESR: 50–60%
- Anemia: 21–41%
- Hypercalcemia: 3–6%
- Erythrocytosis: 3–4%
- Hematuria
- Urinary neoplastic cells
- Alkaline phosphate may be elevated.
- Increased renin
- Increased plasma fibrinogen

Imaging

Initial approach

- Ultrasonography: Can determine whether mass is solid or cystic; simple cystic lesions may be observed or subjected to percutaneous aspiration; solid lesions require further imaging.
- Abdominal/pelvic CT, using 3-phase imaging, with and without IV contrast, is the optimal imaging modality to evaluate the kidneys, and is nearly 100% sensitive for detecting a renal mass greater than 15 mm in diameter. A solid renal mass with >15–20 Hounsfield units change on multiphase CT has an 80% likelihood of being RCC. A predominantly cystic mass with an irregular, nodular or enhancing wall, calcifications, and/or septa >2 mm thick has a >70% likelihood of being cystic RCC.

Follow-Up & Special Considerations

- MRI with pre- and postgadolinium phases, is superior to ultrasound in evaluating adenopathy, diagnosing intracaval and renal venous thrombus, and demonstrating bony metastases.
- Chest CT scan if initial chest x-ray suggests metastatic disease; brain CT scan is indicated if the patient has neurologic symptoms.
- Bone scan is indicated if the alkaline phosphatase level is elevated or the patient has bone pain.
- CT or MR angiography for staging evaluation; vascular information helpful in planning resection
- Positron-emission tomography does not yet have an established role in staging RCC.

Diagnostic Procedures/Surgery

- No need to aspirate simple cyst unless symptomatic
- Calcified cysts may contain RCC and, therefore, require open renal biopsy of the wall of the cyst or partial nephrectomy.
- Hemorrhagic cyst: Aspiration cytology may be helpful, but needle biopsy of solid masses is to be discouraged, particularly if the patient has a normal contralateral kidney.
- Doppler-flow ultrasound of the renal veins or CT scan that shows the renal vein entering the vena cava can be used to rule out tumor thrombus.

Pathological Findings

- RCC tends to bulge out from the cortex, producing a mass effect.
- 48% of RCCs measure <5 cm and are grossly yellow to yellow–orange due to high lipid content in the clear cell variety. Average size has been decreasing due to incidental discovery, and is now ~3.6 cm.
- Small tumors are typically homogeneous.
- Large tumors may have areas of necrosis and hemorrhage.
- About 5–10% of RCCs extend into the venous system as tumor thrombi.
- 5 distinct subtypes:
  - Clear cell: 70–80%; proximal tubule, typically solitary
  - Papillary renal cell (previously termed *chromophilic*): 10–15%; proximal tubule; tumors tend to be bilateral and multifocal; type 1 and more aggressive type 2 variant
  - Chromophobic: 3–5%; intercalated cells; tend to have a less aggressive course
  - Medullary: <1%; typically affect younger patients; most are at an advanced stage with metastases at time of diagnosis; occur almost exclusively in patients with sickle-cell trait
  - Collecting duct: <1%

DIFFERENTIAL DIAGNOSIS

- Benign renal masses (e.g., renal hamartomas)
- Hydronephrosis
- Pyelonephritis
- Renal abscess
- Polycystic kidneys
- Renal tuberculosis
- Renal calculi
- Renal infarction
- Benign renal cyst
- Transitional cell carcinoma of the renal pelvis
- Wilms tumor
- Metastatic disease, especially melanoma

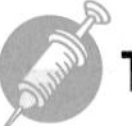

TREATMENT

Among small (<4 cm) renal masses, about 20% are benign, 60% represent indolent variants of RCC, and only 20% are potentially aggressive tumors.

MEDICATION

First Line

- Sunitinib represents front-line standard treatment for the good and intermediate prognosis groups of patients with clear cell RCC (1)[C].
- In fit patients with metastatic disease and minimal symptoms, nephrectomy followed by interferon-alfa gives the best survival strategy for fully validated therapies (2)[A]. Interferon is the standard comparator for the assessment of new treatments in metastatic RCC.
- Sunitinib and sorafenib are both oral inhibitors of the tyrosine kinase portion of the VEGF family of receptors. Sunitinib is considered first-line treatment in advanced RCC and in patients refractory or intolerant to cytokine therapy. Sunitinib demonstrated improved response (31% vs. 6%; number needed to treat [NNT] = 4) and longer median progression-free survival (11 vs. 5 months) over interferon-alfa in a randomized study of 750 patients (3)[B]. Sorafenib is considered a second-line option.
- Bevacizumab is a monoclonal antibody that binds and neutralizes circulating VEGF protein. Combined with interferon-alfa, bevacizumab offers patients with metastatic RCC a hazard ratio for progression-free survival of 0.63 (95% confidence interval 0.52–0.75; $p = .0001$) compared with interferon alone (4)[B].
- Temsirolimus, an IV mTOR inhibitor, is also approved for advanced RCC and is the frontline choice for patients with non-clear cell histology. It has shown improved response (32% vs. 16%; NNT = 6) and longer median survival (10.9 vs. 7.3 months) over interferon-alfa in a comparative clinical trial of 626 patients.
- A 2008 phase 3 trial of 410 patients comparing everolimus, another mTOR inhibitor, with placebo was stopped early after disease progression was seen in 37% of patients receiving everolimus vs. 65% receiving placebo (hazard ratio = 0.30, 95% confidence interval 0.22–0.40; $p < .0001$) (5)[B].

Second Line

- Response rates with traditional chemotherapeutic agents are typically <15%.
- Despite occasional reports of responses, a review of medroxyprogesterone, the most widely studied progestational agent, concluded that RCCs are neither hormone-dependent nor hormone-responsive.

ADDITIONAL TREATMENT

Additional Therapies

While RCC is typically characterized as radioresistant, radiation therapy may be useful to treat a single or limited number of metastases, particularly brain or painful bone metastases or painful recurrences in the renal bed.

SURGERY/OTHER PROCEDURES

- Surgery is curative in most patients with nonmetastatic RCC and is the preferred treatment for all but the most extensive disease.
- Assuming a normal contralateral kidney, radical nephrectomy, which can be done laparoscopically and involves node dissection and complete removal of the kidney and Gerota fascia, is the typical preferred approach.
- Partial nephrectomy has shown equal long-term cancer-specific survival for small-to-medium (<7 cm) tumors when compared to radical nephrectomy. Partial nephrectomy, however, is a more technically challenging procedure and is not available at all centers.
- Surgical intervention in metastatic disease: Metastasectomy in those with limited metastatic disease vs. cytoreductive nephrectomy (debulking) prior to systemic therapy
- Transitional cell carcinoma of the renal pelvis or calyces: Nephroureterectomy
- Wilms tumor in adults: Radical nephrectomy for unilateral disease
- Cortical adenoma <3 cm (7–22% at autopsy): Wedge resection
- Image-guided radiofrequency or cryoablation has been successful in limited studies for the treatment of small (average 2 cm) peripheral renal tumors; long-term efficacy data are limited (6)[C].

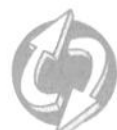

ONGOING CARE

FOLLOW-UP RECOMMENDATIONS

Patient Monitoring

- CT scan of the abdomen and renal fossa 3–6 months after surgery, particularly if capsule or lymph nodes are positive, to monitor recurrences and repeat resection if needed for flank pain or mass
- For partial nephrectomy: Renal ultrasound every 6 months for 3 years, then annually
- Since most pulmonary metastases are asymptomatic, routine imaging of the chest with x-ray or CT scan is performed quarterly for 2 years and periodically thereafter.
- Skeletal x-rays and bone scan can be useful in detecting skeletal metastasis but should be obtained only if patient complains of bone pain or if alkaline phosphatase is elevated.
- Postoperative follow-up may be possible with plasma transcobalamin II or serum haptoglobin level to detect or monitor recurrences.
- Small (<3 cm), incidentally detected tumors may have an indolent behavior; immediate treatment in poor-risk patients may not be of benefit, and active surveillance may be a viable management strategy.

DIET

Patients with proteinuria should follow a low-protein diet.

PROGNOSIS

- The 5-year survival following treatment correlates well with the anatomic extent of disease.
- 5-year survival in the absence of metastases exceeds 50%; in the presence of distant metastases, 5-year survival decreases to 10%.
- Median survival for metastatic RCC is in the range of 10–12 months.
- Performance status at diagnosis and histologic grade of tumor also influence prognosis.

COMPLICATIONS

- Paraplegia can result with little warning from spinal vertebral metastasis.
- CNS metastases are not uncommon.
- ~30% of patients with RCC have metastatic disease when the diagnosis is established. The most common sites of metastasis are the lung (50–60%), bone (30–40%), regional nodes (15–30%), brain (10%), and adjacent organs (10%).

REFERENCES

1. Di Lorenzo G, Buonerba C, Biglietto M, et al. The therapy of kidney cancer with biomolecular drugs. *Cancer Treat Rev*. 2010;36(Suppl 3):S16–20.
2. Coppin C, et al. Immunotherapy for advanced renal cell cancer (Cochrane Review). *Cochrane Database Syst Rev*. 2006;(2).
3. Motzer RJ, Hutson TE, Tomczak P, et al. Sunitinib versus interferon alfa in metastatic renal-cell carcinoma. *N Engl J Med*. 2007;356:115–24.
4. Escudier B, Bellmunt J, Négrier S, et al. Phase III trial of bevacizumab plus interferon alfa-2a in patients with metastatic renal cell carcinoma (AVOREN): Final analysis of overall survival. *J Clin Oncol*. 2010;28:2144–50.
5. Motzer RJ, Escudier B, Oudard S, et al. Efficacy of everolimus in advanced renal cell carcinoma: A double-blind, randomised, placebo-controlled phase III trial. *Lancet*. 2008;372:449–56.
6. Sabharwal R, Vladica P. Renal tumors: Technical success and early clinical experience with radiofrequency ablation of 18 tumors. *Cardiovasc Intervent Radiol*. 2006;29:202–9.

ADDITIONAL READING

- Chen DY, Uzzo RG, et al. Evaluation and management of the renal mass. *Med Clin North Am*. 2011;95:179–89.
- Rini BI, Campbell SC, Escudier B, et al. Renal cell carcinoma. *Lancet*. 2009;373:1119–32.

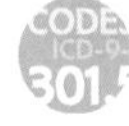

CODES

ICD9

189.0 Malignant neoplasm of kidney, except pelvis

CLINICAL PEARLS

- RCC represents 3–4% of all cancers and 2% of all cancer deaths; most patients have clear cell histology and do not respond to standard chemotherapy.
- Diverse and obscure presentations are typical; most RCCs are found incidentally during radiologic studies.
- At presentation, up to 30% of patients with RCC have metastatic disease; recurrence develops in ~40% treated for localized disease.
- Only 20% of renal masses <4 cm represent potentially aggressive tumors.
- Surgery is curative in most patients with nonmetastatic RCC and is the preferred treatment for all but the most extensive disease.
- Multiple pharmacologic options are considered first-line for metastatic RCC; sequential treatments are likely to be pursued for most patients.

RENAL FAILURE, ACUTE

Rasai L. Ernst, MD
Mazen Albeldawi, MD

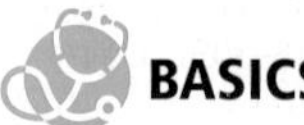

BASICS

DESCRIPTION

Sudden loss of kidney function resulting in retention of nitrogenous waste as well as electrolyte and volume homeostasis abnormalities, with or without oliguria (urine output <500 mL/d).

EPIDEMIOLOGY

Incidence

5% of hospital and 30% of ICU admissions have a diagnosis of acute renal failure (ARF). 25% of patients develop ARF while in the hospital, and 50% of those cases are iatrogenic.

RISK FACTORS

- Comorbidities (e.g., liver failure, heart failure, diabetes)
- Advanced age
- Radiographic contrast material exposure
- Nephrotoxic medications (e.g., NSAIDs, ACE inhibitors)
- Volume depletion (e.g., sepsis, hemorrhage)
- Surgery
- Rhabdomyolysis
- Solitary kidney (risk in nephrolithiasis)
- Benign prostatic hypertrophy (BPH)
- Malignancy

Genetics

No known genetic pattern.

GENERAL PREVENTION

See "Treatment."

PATHOPHYSIOLOGY

Can be divided into 3 categories: Prerenal, intrarenal, and postrenal:

- Prerenal: Pathology secondary to decreased renal perfusion (often due to hypovolemia) leading to a decrease in glomerular filtration rate (GFR); reversible if factors decreasing perfusion are corrected; otherwise, it can progress to an intrarenal pathology known as *ischemic acute tubular necrosis (ATN)*.
- Intrarenal: Pathology secondary to pathology within the kidney; ATN is the most common cause via ischemic or nephrotoxic injury to the kidney; 75% of ATN is a complication of prerenal etiology (1).
- Postrenal: Pathology secondary to extrinsic or intrinsic obstruction (e.g., BPH) of the urinary collection system.

ETIOLOGY

- Prerenal (~55%): Hypotension, volume contraction, severe heart failure, or liver failure
- Intrarenal (~40%): ATN (from prolonged prerenal failure, radiographic contrast material, aminoglycosides, or nephrotoxic substances), glomerulonephritis, acute interstitial nephritis (drug-induced), arteriolar insults, vasculitis, accelerated hypertension, cholesterol embolization (common after arterial procedures), intrarenal deposition or sludging (seen in increased uric acid and multiple myeloma—Bence-Jones proteins)
- Postrenal (~5%): Extrinsic compression (prostatic hypertrophy, carcinoma), intrinsic obstruction (calculus, tumor, clot, stricture, sloughed papillae), decreased function (neurogenic bladder)

COMMONLY ASSOCIATED CONDITIONS

Hyperphosphatemia, hypercalcemia, hyperuricemia, hydronephrosis, BPH, nephrolithiasis, congestive heart failure (CHF), pericarditis, cirrhosis, chronic renal insufficiency, malignant hypertension, vasculitis, drug reactions, sepsis, severe trauma, burns, transfusion reactions, recent chemotherapy, muscle injury, internal bleeding

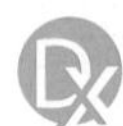

DIAGNOSIS

HISTORY

- General: PO intake, urine output, body weight, and baseline creatinine measurement (to assess how far from baseline the current creatinine is), medication use
- Prerenal: Thirst, orthostatic dizziness
- Intrarenal: Nephrotoxic medications, radiocontrast material, other toxins; fever, arthralgias, and pruritic rash suggest allergic interstitial nephritis, although systemic effects are not always seen in this pathology. Edema, hypertension, and oliguria with nephritic urine sediment point to glomerulonephritis or vasculitis. Livedo reticularis, SC nodules, and ischemic toes and fingers despite good pulses suggest atheroembolization. Flank pain suggests occlusion of the renal artery or vein.
- Postrenal: Colicky flank pain that radiates to the groin suggests a ureteric obstruction such as a stone. Nocturia, frequency, and hesitancy suggest prostatic disease. Suprapubic and flank pain are usually secondary to distension of the bladder and collecting system. Ask about anticholinergic drugs that could lead to neurogenic bladder.

PHYSICAL EXAM

- General uremic signs: Lethargy, seizures, asterixis, myoclonus, pericardial friction rub, peripheral neuropathies
- Prerenal signs: Tachycardia, decreased jugular venous pressure (JVP), orthostatic hypotension, dry mucous membranes, decreased skin turgor; look for stigmata of associated comorbidities such as liver and heart failure, as well as sepsis.
- Intrinsic renal signs: Pruritic rash, livedo reticularis, SC nodules, ischemic digits despite good pulses
- Postrenal signs: Suprapubic distension, flank pain, and enlarged prostate

DIAGNOSTIC TESTS & INTERPRETATION

Lab

Initial lab tests

- Urinalysis: Dipstick for blood and protein; microscopy for cells, casts, and crystals
- Casts: Transparent hyaline casts—prerenal etiology; pigmented granular/muddy brown casts—ATN; WBC casts—acute interstitial nephritis; RBC casts—glomerulonephritis
- Urine eosinophils: Interstitial nephritis
- Urine electrolytes in an oliguric state:
  - $FE_{Na} = [(U_{Na} \times P_{Cr})/(P_{Na} \times U_{Cr})] \times 100$, where U = urine, P = plasma, Na = sodium, Cr = creatinine. If $Fe_{Na} < 1$, then likely prerenal; >2, then likely intrarenal; >4, then likely postrenal
  - If patient is on diuretics, use FE_{urea} instead of FE_{Na}. $FE_{urea} = [(U_{urea} \times P_{Cr})/(P_{BUN} \times U_{Cr}) \times 100$ FE_{urea} <35% suggests prerenal (2).
  - In 1 study, low FE_{urea} (<35%) was found to be more sensitive and specific than FE_{Na} in differentiating between prerenal and intrarenal etiologies of renal failure, especially if diuretics were administered (3)[A].
- CBC, BUN, creatinine, arterial blood gases (ABGs)
- Common lab abnormalities in ARF:
  - Increased: K^+, phosphate, Mg, uric acid
  - Decreased: Hematocrit (Hct), Na, Ca
- Calculate creatinine clearance to ensure that medications are dosed appropriately:
  - Cockcroft-Gault equation creatinine clearance (mL/min) = (140-age)* (weight in kilograms)* (0.85 if female) / (72* serum creatinine)

Follow-Up & Special Considerations

Consider creatine kinase (CK) and immunology antibodies.

Imaging

Initial approach

- Renal ultrasound (US): Excludes postrenal causes if negative; identifies presence of kidneys, hydronephrosis, and nephrolithiasis
- Doppler-flow kidney US: Rules out renal artery stenosis/thrombosis
- Abdominal x-ray (KUB): Rules out renal calculi

Follow-Up & Special Considerations

More advanced imaging techniques should be considered if initial tests do not reveal etiology:

- Radionucleotide renal scan: Evaluates renal flow, function, and presence of obstructive uropathy and extravasation
- CT scan: Limited use due to need for radiographic contrast material, which can worsen ARF
- MRI: Acute tubulointerstitial nephritis can show an increased T_2-weighted signal.

Diagnostic Procedures/Surgery

Cystoscopy with retrograde pyelogram evaluates for bladder tumor, hydronephrosis, obstruction, and upper tract abnormalities, and poses no threat of contrast material toxicity.

Pathological Findings

Kidney biopsy: Used only as a last resort when all other tests do not reveal a diagnosis; most useful for suspicion of rapidly progressive glomerulonephritis or kidney transplant patients

DIFFERENTIAL DIAGNOSIS

See "Etiology."

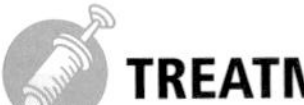

TREATMENT

MEDICATION

First Line

- Current treatment is focused on treating the underlying cause and associated complications.
- If patient is found to be oliguric and not volume overloaded, a fluid challenge may be appropriate with diligent monitoring for volume overload (4)[C].
- Studies show Furosemide is ineffective in preventing and treating ARF (4)[A]. Dopamine, natriuretic peptides, insulinlike growth factor, and thyroxine also have no benefit in the treatment of ARF (2,4)[A].
- If a patient is found to be hyperkalemic with ECG changes, IV calcium, sodium bicarbonate, and glucose with insulin should be given. These measures drive K^+ into cells and can be supplemented with Kayexalate, which removes K^+ from the body. Hemodialysis is also an emergency method of removal (5)[A].
- Oliguric patients should have a fluid restriction of 400 mL + yesterday's urine output (unless there are signs of volume depletion or overload) (5)[A].
- Acidosis: Serum bicarbonate <15–18 mmol/L; small amounts of sodium bicarbonate can be given. Be aware of volume overload (5)[A].
- Certain strategies have been investigated in the prevention of ARF: Those likely to be effective are IV isotonic hydration, once-daily dosing of aminoglycosides, use of lipid formulations of amphotericin B, use of isoosmolar nonionic contrast media (6)[A].
- Contrast-induced ARF (CIARF) can be prevented by *N*-acetylcysteine 600 mg PO b.i.d. on day prior to and day of contrast (7)[A] and isotonic $NaHCO_3$ 3 mL/kg/hr × 1 hour before administration of contrast material and 1 mL/kg/hr × 6 hours after contrast material (8)[B].

Second Line

- Flomax or other selective α-blockers for bladder outlet obstruction secondary to BPH
- Calcium channel blockers may have a protective effect in posttransplant ATN.

ADDITIONAL TREATMENT

General Measures

Identify and correct all prerenal and postrenal causes:

- Review drug list: Stop nephrotoxic drugs and renally adjust others.
- Always record ins and outs and daily weights.
- Watch for complications, including hyperkalemia, pulmonary edema, and acidosis—all potential reasons to start dialysis.
- Ensure good cardiac output and subsequent renal blood flow.
- Follow nutrition suggestions and be aware of infections; treat aggressively if they occur.
- Start patients on H_2 inhibitors or proton pump inhibitors; avoid aspirin to reduce bleeding tendency (4)[A].

Issues for Referral

- Nephrology should be consulted for all cases as soon as patient is found to be in ARF.
- Urology consult for obstructive nephropathies

COMPLEMENTARY AND ALTERNATIVE MEDICINE

Many supplements not approved by the FDA can be nephrotoxic.

SURGERY/OTHER PROCEDURES

- Relief of obstruction with retrograde ureteral catheters or percutaneous nephrostomy
- Hemodialysis catheter placement

IN-PATIENT CONSIDERATIONS

Initial Stabilization

- ABCs of resuscitation
- Treat hyperkalemia emergently, especially with ECG changes.
- If volume depleted, give IV fluids.
- Place a Foley catheter.

Admission Criteria

All patients with ARF should be admitted.

IV Fluids

Should be used in patients with volume depletion

Nursing

Place a Foley catheter; strict recording of ins and outs

Discharge Criteria

Stabilization of renal function and a concrete plan for continued treatment if necessary

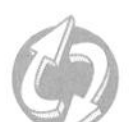

ONGOING CARE

FOLLOW-UP RECOMMENDATIONS

Patient Monitoring

As needed

DIET

- Total caloric intake should be 35–50 kcal/kg/d to avoid catabolism.
- Sodium should be restricted to 2 g/d (5)[A].
- Potassium intake should be restricted to 40 mEq/d.
- Phosphorus should be restricted to 800 mg/d. If it becomes high, treat with calcium carbonate or other phosphate binder (5)[A].
- Magnesium compounds should be avoided.

PATIENT EDUCATION

Keep well hydrated. Avoid nephrotoxic drugs such as NSAIDs, ACE inhibitors, and aminoglycosides.

PROGNOSIS

- Depending on the cause, comorbid conditions, and age of patient, mortality ranges from 5–80%.
- In cases of prerenal and postrenal failure, there are very good rates of recovery positively correlated with shorter duration of renal failure. Intrarenal etiologies usually take more time to recover from. Overall, average recovery takes from days to a few months.

COMPLICATIONS

Death, sepsis, infection, seizures, paralysis, peripheral edema, CHF, pulmonary edema, arrhythmias, uremic pericarditis, bleeding, GI bleed, hypotension, anemia, hyperkalemia, uremia

REFERENCES

1. Lameire N. The pathophysiology of acute renal failure. *Crit Care Clin*. 2005;21:197–210.
2. Schrier R. Acute renal failure: Definitions, diagnosis, pathogenesis, and therapy. *J Clin Invest*. 2004;114:5–14.
3. Carvounis CP, Nisar S, Guro-Razuman S. Significance of the fractional excretion of urea in the differential diagnosis of acute renal failure. *Kidney Int*. 2002;62:2223–9.
4. Hilton R. Acute renal failure. *BMJ*. 2006;333:786–90.
5. Lameire N, Van Biesen W, Vanholder R. Acute renal failure. *Lancet*. 2005;365:417–30.
6. Venkataraman R. Prevention of acute renal failure. *Chest*. 2007;131:300–8.
7. Birck R, Krzossok S, Markowetz F. Acetylcysteine for prevention of contrast nephropathy: Meta-analysis. *Lancet*. 2003;362:598–603.
8. Merten GJ, Burgess WP, Gray LV. Prevention of contrast-induced nephropathy with sodium bicarbonate: A randomized controlled trial. *JAMA*. 2004;291:2328–34.

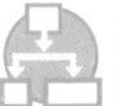

See Also (Topic, Algorithm, Electronic Media Element)

- Glomerulonephritis, Acute; Hepatorenal Syndrome; Hyperkalemia; Prostatic Hyperplasia, Benign (BPH); Renal Failure, Chronic; Reye Syndrome; Rhabdomyolysis; Sepsis
- Algorithm: Anuria or Oliguria

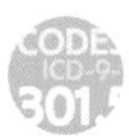

CODES

ICD9

584.9 Acute kidney failure, unspecified

CLINICAL PEARLS

- Can be divided into 3 categories: Prerenal, intrarenal, and postrenal:
  - Prerenal: Pathology secondary to decreased renal perfusion (often from hypovolemia) leading to a decrease in GFR; reversible if factors decreasing perfusion are corrected; otherwise, it can progress to an intrarenal pathology known as ischemic ATN.
  - Intrarenal: Pathology secondary to pathology within the kidney; ATN is the most common cause via ischemic or nephrotoxic injury to the kidney. 75% of ATN is a complication of prerenal etiology (1).
  - Postrenal: Pathology secondary to extrinsic or intrinsic obstruction of the urinary collection system (e.g., BPH, etc.).
- Recognize the need for emergent hemodialysis: Severe hyperkalemia, acidosis, or volume overload refractory to conservative therapy, uremic pericarditis, encephalopathy, neuropathy, and alcohol and drug intoxications.

RENAL TUBULAR ACIDOSIS

Jason M. Kurland, MD

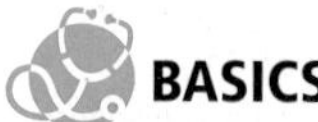

BASICS

DESCRIPTION

- Renal tubular acidosis (RTA): A group of disorders characterized by an inability of the kidney to resorb bicarbonate or secrete hydrogen ions, resulting in hyperchloremic, normal anion gap acidosis. Renal function (glomerular filtration rate [GFR]) must be normal or near normal.
- Several types have been identified:
  - Type I (distal) RTA: Inability of the distal tubule to acidify the urine. Due to impaired hydrogen ion secretion, increased backleak of secreted hydrogen ions, or impaired sodium reabsorption (interfering with the generation of negative luminal charge required for hydrogen/potassium secretion). Urine pH >5.5.
  - Type II (proximal) RTA: Defect of the proximal tubule in bicarbonate (HCO_3) reabsorption. HCO_3 fully reabsorbed only when plasma HCO_3 concentration <15–16 mEq/L (compared with normal threshold of 24 mEq/L). Urine pH <5.5 unless plasma HCO_3 above reabsorptive threshold.
  - Type III RTA: Extremely rare autosomal-recessive syndrome with features of both type I and type II (may be due to carbonic anhydrase II deficiency)
  - Type IV RTA (hyporeninemic hypoaldosteronism): Due to aldosterone resistance or deficiency that results in hyperkalemia. Urine pH usually <5.5.

EPIDEMIOLOGY

Incidence

- Predominant age: All ages
- Predominant sex: Male > Female (with regard to type II RTA with isolated defect in bicarbonate reabsorption)

RISK FACTORS

Genetics

- Type I RTA: Autosomal dominant or recessive. May occur in association with other genetic diseases (e.g., Ehlers-Danlos syndrome, hereditary elliptocytosis, or sickle cell nephropathy). The autosomal-recessive form is associated with sensorineural deafness.
- Type II RTA: Autosomal-dominant form is rare. Autosomal-recessive form is associated with ophthalmologic abnormalities and mental retardation. Occurs in Fanconi syndrome, which is associated with several genetic diseases (e.g., cystinosis, Wilson disease, tyrosinemia, hereditary fructose intolerance, Lowe syndrome, galactosemia, glycogen storage disease, and metachromatic leukodystrophy).
- Type IV RTA: Some cases are familial, such as pseudohypoaldosteronism type I (autosomal dominant).

GENERAL PREVENTION

Careful use or avoidance of agents listed here as causative

ETIOLOGY

- Type I RTA:
  - Genetic: Autosomal dominant, autosomal recessive associated with sensorineural deafness
  - Sporadic
  - Other familial disorders: Ehlers-Danlos syndrome, glycogenosis type III, Fabry disease, Wilson disease
  - Autoimmune diseases: Sjögren syndrome, rheumatoid arthritis (RA), systemic lupus erythematosus
  - Hematologic diseases: Sickle cell disease, hereditary elliptocytosis
  - Medications: Amphotericin B, lithium, ifosfamide, foscarnet, analgesics, K^+-sparing diuretics (amiloride, triamterene), trimethoprim
  - Toxins: Toluene, glue
  - Hypercalciuria, diseases causing nephrocalcinosis
  - Vitamin D intoxication
  - Medullary cystic disease
  - Hypergammaglobulinemic syndrome
  - Obstructive uropathy
  - Chronic pyelonephritis
  - Chronic renal transplant rejection
  - Leprosy
  - Hepatic cirrhosis
  - Malnutrition
- Type II RTA:
  - Familial disorders (cystinosis, tyrosinemia, hereditary fructose intolerance, galactosemia, glycogen storage disease type I, Wilson disease, Lowe syndrome, inherited carbonic anhydrase deficiency)
  - Sporadic
  - Multiple myeloma and other dysproteinemic states
  - Amyloidosis
  - Heavy-metal poisoning (e.g., cadmium, lead, mercury, copper)
  - Medications: Acetazolamide, ifosfamide, tenofovir, sulfanilamide, outdated tetracycline, topiramate, aminoglycosides
  - Interstitial renal disease
  - Paroxysmal nocturnal hemoglobinuria
  - Defects in calcium metabolism (hyperparathyroidism)
- Type IV RTA:
  - Medications: NSAIDs, ACE inhibitors, angiotensin receptor blockers, heparin/LMW heparin, calcineurin inhibitors (tacrolimus, cyclosporine) (1)
  - Diabetic nephropathy
  - Obstructive nephropathy
  - Nephrosclerosis due to hypertension
  - Tubulointerstitial nephropathies
  - Primary adrenal insufficiency
  - Pseudohypoaldosteronism (end-organ resistance to aldosterone)
  - Gordon syndrome (2)[C]
  - Sickle cell nephropathy

COMMONLY ASSOCIATED CONDITIONS

- Type I RTA in children: Hypercalciuria leading to rickets, nephrocalcinosis
- Type I RTA in adults: Autoimmune diseases (Sjögren syndrome, RA), hypercalciuria
- Type II RTA: Fanconi syndrome (generalized proximal tubular dysfunction resulting in glycosuria, aminoaciduria, hyperuricosuria, phosphaturia, bicarbonaturia)
- Type II RTA in adults: Multiple myeloma, carbonic anhydrase inhibitors (acetazolamide)
- Type IV RTA: Obstructive uropathy, renal insufficiency, diabetic nephropathy

DIAGNOSIS

HISTORY

- Often asymptomatic (particularly type IV)
- Failure to thrive in children
- Anorexia, nausea/vomiting, constipation
- Weakness or polyuria (due to hypokalemia)
- Rickets in children
- Osteomalacia in adults
- Polydipsia

DIAGNOSTIC TESTS & INTERPRETATION

Lab

- Electrolytes reveal hyperchloremic metabolic acidosis.
- Plasma anion gap normal (anion gap = Na – [Cl + HCO_3]). Normal values (in mEq/L): Neonates ≤16; infants/children ≤14–16; adolescents/adults 8 ± 4). Must correct calculated anion gap for hypoalbuminemia. Increase calculated anion gap by 2.5 mEq/L for each 1 g/dL decrease in albumin below 4 g/dL.
- Hypokalemia or normokalemia: Type I (if due to impaired distal H^+ secretion or increased H^+ backleak), type II
- Hyperkalemia: Type IV, type I (if due to impaired distal Na^+ reabsorption)
- Plasma HCO_3 (in untreated RTA): Type I: <15 mEq/L; type II: 12–20 mEq/L; type IV: >17 mEq/L
- BUN and creatinine usually normal (rules out renal failure as cause of acidosis)
- Urinalysis: Urine microscopy can help to discern between prerenal and renal tubular acidosis:
  - In prerenal ATN, microscopy will show renal tubular epithelial cells, epithelial cell casts, and muddy brown granular casts (3)[A].
- Urine pH: Inappropriately alkaline (pH >5.5) despite metabolic acidosis in type I or in type II when HCO_3 above reabsorptive threshold (15–16 mEq/L)
- Urine culture: Rule out UTI with urea-splitting organism (may elevate pH) and chronic infection
- Urine anion gap (urine Na^+, K^+, and Cl^- on random urine): Reflects unmeasured urine anions, so inversely related to urine NH_4^+ (or acid) excretion. Positive urine anion gap in an acidemic patient indicates impaired renal acid excretion. Urine Na^+ > 25 mEq/L required for accurate interpretation of urine anion gap (reabsorption of Na^+ in collecting tubule generates net negative luminal charge, facilitating H^+ secretion). Results tend to be:
  - Negative in HCO_3 losses due to diarrhea, or UTI caused by urea-splitting organisms
  - Negative in other extrarenal causes of normal anion gap metabolic acidosis
  - Variable in type II RTA
  - Positive in type I RTA, type IV RTA (4)[C]
  - Positive in impaired acid excretion due to renal failure
- Urine calcium:
  - High in type I
  - Typically normal in type II

- Drugs that may alter lab results:
  - Diuretics
  - Sodium bicarbonate (and other alkali)
  - Cholestyramine

Initial lab tests

Serum electrolytes, urinalysis, urine culture

Imaging

Not needed except to rule out associated conditions (e.g., nephrocalcinosis)

Diagnostic Procedures/Surgery

- Helpful to measure urine pH on fresh sample with pH meter for increased accuracy instead of dipstick. Pour film of oil over urine to avoid loss of CO_2 if pH cannot be measured quickly.
- Urine NH_4^+ excretion (anion gap is indirect measurement of this but not as accurate)
- Ammonium chloride (NH_4^+) loading to evaluate acid excretion
- Fractional excretion of HCO_3 $>15\%$ during HCO_3 infusion (type II RTA)

Pathological Findings

- Nephrocalcinosis
- Nephrolithiasis
- Rickets
- Osteomalacia
- Findings of an underlying disease causing renal tubular acidosis

DIFFERENTIAL DIAGNOSIS

- Plasma anion gap should be normal. If not, evaluate for causes of anion-gap metabolic acidosis. (MUDPILES: *M*etabolic disease or methanol ingestion, *u*remia, *d*iabetic ketoacidosis, *p*araldehyde ingestion, *i*ron or isoniazid ingestion, *l*actic acidosis, *e*thylene glycol ingestion, *s*alicylate ingestion)
- Extrarenal HCO_3 losses:
  - Diarrhea
  - Small bowel, pancreatic, or biliary fistulas (4)[C]
  - Urinary diversion (e.g., ureterosigmoidostomy, ileal conduit)
- Acidosis of chronic renal failure (develops when GFR $\leq$20–30% of normal) (5)[C]
- Excessive administration of acid load via chloride salts (NaCl, HCl, NH_4Cl, lysine hydrogen chloride, $CaCl_2$, $MgCl_2$)

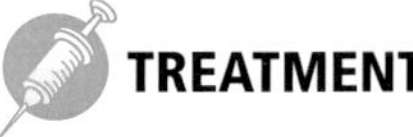

TREATMENT

MEDICATION

First Line

- Provide oral alkali to raise serum HCO_3 to normal. Start at a low dose and increase until HCO_3 is normal. Give as sodium bicarbonate or citrate mixtures (1 mEq citrate = 1 mEq HCO_3) such as Bicitra (1 mEq Na, 1 mEq citrate/mL, no K) or Polycitra (1 mEq Na, 1 mEq K, 2 mEq citrate/mL) depending on need for potassium. Sodium bicarbonate tablets are available (7.7 mEq $NaHCO_3$/650 mg tab) (6)[C].
- Type I RTA: Typical doses 1–4 mEq/kg/d PO alkali divided 3–4×/d (require much higher doses if HCO_3 wasting is present). May require K^+ supplementation for hypokalemia (7)[C].
- Type II RTA: Typical doses 10–15 mEq/kg/d alkali, divided 4–6×/d. Very difficult to restore plasma HCO_3 to normal because renal HCO_3 losses increase once plasma HCO_3 is corrected above the resorptive threshold. Exogenous HCO_3 increases K^+ losses, requiring K^+ supplementation. Often need PO_4 and vitamin D supplementation due to proximal PO_4 losses. May add thiazide diuretic to induce mild hypovolemia, which increases proximal Na^+/HCO_3^- reabsorption.
- Type IV RTA: Avoid inciting medications; restrict dietary K^+. May augment K^+ excretion with loop diuretic, thiazide diuretic, or Kayexalate. Correcting hyperkalemia will actually increase activity of the urea cycle, augmenting renal ammoniagenesis and providing more substrate for renal acid excretion. If necessary, 1–5 mEq/kg/d alkali divided 2–3×/d. If mineralocorticoid deficiency, fludrocortisone: 0.1–0.3 mg/d.
- Contraindications: Refer to the manufacturers' literature.
- Precautions: Sodium bicarbonate may cause flatulence because CO_2 is formed, whereas citrate mixtures are metabolized to HCO_3 in the liver, thereby avoiding gas production. The use of sodium-containing compounds or mineralocorticoids may lead to hypertension and/or edema.

Second Line

Thiazide diuretics may be used as adjunctive therapy in type II RTA (after maximal alkali replacement), but are likely to further increase urinary K^+ losses.

ADDITIONAL TREATMENT

General Measures

Treatment with appropriate medications to correct acidosis

SURGERY/OTHER PROCEDURES

If distal RTA is due to obstructive uropathy, surgical intervention may be required.

IN-PATIENT CONSIDERATIONS

Initial Stabilization

- Generally managed as outpatient
- Inpatient if acidosis severe, patient unreliable, emesis persistent, or infant with severe failure to thrive

ONGOING CARE

FOLLOW-UP RECOMMENDATIONS

Patient Monitoring

- Varies with patient response. Suggested: Electrolytes every 2–4 weeks at onset of therapy, every 2 weeks for 1–2 months after bicarbonate concentration normal, then monthly for several months.
- Monitor underlying disease as indicated.
- Poor compliance common due to 3–6×/d alkali dosing schedule

DIET

Varies based on serum K^+ level and volume status

PATIENT EDUCATION

- National Kidney & Urologic Diseases Information Clearinghouse, Box NKUDIC, Bethesda, MD 20893, (301) 468-6345; www.niddk.nih.gov/health/kidney
- National Kidney Foundation: www.kidney.org

PROGNOSIS

- Depends on associated disease; otherwise, good with therapy
- Transient forms of all types of RTA may occur.

COMPLICATIONS

- Nephrocalcinosis, nephrolithiasis (type I)
- Hypercalciuria (type I)
- Hypokalemia (type I, type II if given bicarbonate)
- Hyperkalemia (type IV, some causes of type I)
- Osteomalacia (type II due to phosphate wasting)

REFERENCES

1. Heering P, Ivens K, Aker S, et al. Distal tubular acidosis induced by FK506. *Clin Transplant*. 1998; 12:465–71.
2. Rodríguez-Soriano J. New insights into the pathogenesis of renal tubular acidosis–from functional to molecular studies. *Pediatr Nephrol*. 2000;14:1121–36.
3. Kanbay M, Kasapoglu B, Perazella MA, et al. Acute tubular necrosis and pre-renal acute kidney injury: Utility of urine microscopy in their evaluation—a systematic review. *Int Urol Nephrol*. 2010;42: 425–33.
4. Casaletto J. Differential diagnosis of metabolic acidosis. *Emer Med Clin N Am*. 2005;23(3): 771–87.
5. Kurtzman NA. Renal tubular acidosis syndromes. *South Med J*. 2000;93:1042–52.
6. Chan JC, Scheinman JI, Roth KS. Consultation with the specialist: Renal tubular acidosis. *Pediatr Rev*. 2001;22:277–87.
7. Domrongkitchaiporn S, Khositseth S, Stitchantrakul W, et al. Dosage of potassium citrate in the correction of urinary abnormalities in pediatric distal renal tubular acidosis patients. *Am J Kidney Dis*. 2002;39:383–91.

ADDITIONAL READING

Izzedine H, Launay-Vacher V, Deray G. Topiramate-induced renal tubular acidosis. *Am J Med*. 2004; 116:281–2.

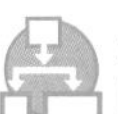

See Also (Topic, Algorithm, Electronic Media Element)

- Hyperkalemia
- Algorithm: Anuria or Oliguria

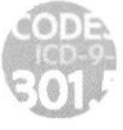

CODES

ICD9

588.89 Other specified disorders resulting from impaired renal function

CLINICAL PEARLS

- Consider RTA in cases of nonanion gap metabolic acidosis with normal or near-normal renal function.
- Type I RTA: Urine pH >5.5 in setting of acidemia; positive urine anion gap; HCO_3 <15 mEq/L
- Type II RTA: Urine pH <5.5 unless HCO_3 raised above reabsorptive threshold (15–16 mEq/L)
- Type IV RTA: Most common subtype; hyperkalemia; urine pH <5.5; acidemia usually mild
- Treatment includes avoidance of inciting causes, provision of oral alkali (HCO_3 or citrate), and measures to supplement (type II, many type I) or restrict (type IV) potassium.

RESPIRATORY DISTRESS SYNDROME, ACUTE (ARDS)

Patrick J. Worth, MD
Sean Monaghan, MD
Daithi S. Heffernan, MD

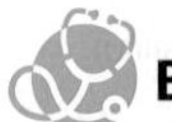

BASICS

DESCRIPTION

- Syndrome characterized by abrupt onset of diffuse lung injury with severe hypoxemia and bilateral pulmonary infiltrates:
  - Absence of left atrial hypertension (HTN)
  - By consensus, $PaO_2/FiO_2 < 200$
  - Most severe form of acute lung injury
- System(s) affected: Pulmonary; Cardiovascular
- Synonym(s): Shock lung; Wet lung; Noncardiac pulmonary edema

EPIDEMIOLOGY

Incidence

Acute lung injury: 40–75 cases/100,000 annually

RISK FACTORS

- Severe infection (localized or systemic) most common
- Aspiration of gastric contents
- Shock
- Infection
- Lung contusion
- Nonthoracic trauma
- Toxic inhalation
- Near-drowning
- Multiple blood transfusions

GENERAL PREVENTION

No effective measures have been identified.

PATHOPHYSIOLOGY

3 phases:

- Acute exudative phase: Characterized by profound hypoxia and associated with inflammation with infiltration of inflammatory and proinflammatory mediators and diffuse alveolar damage
- Fibrosing alveolitis phase: Coincides with recovery or after ~1–2 weeks; patients continue to be hypoxic and have increased dead space and decreased compliance.
- Resolution may require 6–12 months.

ETIOLOGY

- Several mediators are involved in the initiation and perpetuation of acute respiratory distress syndrome (ARDS):
  - Cytokines
  - Complement activation
  - Coagulation activation
  - Platelet-activating factor
  - Oxygen free radicals
  - Lipoxygenase pathways
  - Neutrophil proteases
  - Nitric oxide
  - Endotoxin
  - Cyclo-oxygenase pathway products
- Systemic inflammatory response with activation of the previous mediators can occur with direct or indirect injury to the lung:
  - Direct:
    - Aspiration
    - Pulmonary infections
    - Air, fat, or amniotic fluid emboli
    - Near-drowning
    - Pulmonary contusion
    - Inhalation of toxic gases and dusts
  - Indirect:
    - Sepsis
    - Shock
    - Transfusion
    - Trauma
    - Overdose
    - Pancreatitis, severe
    - Eclampsia

COMMONLY ASSOCIATED CONDITIONS

- Severe sepsis
- Trauma
- Shock

DIAGNOSIS

HISTORY

- No history of heart disease
- Precipitating event (see "Commonly Associated Conditions"): Abrupt onset of respiratory distress

PHYSICAL EXAM

- Tachypnea and tachycardia during the first 12–24 hours; respiratory distress
- Lethargy, obtundation
- Flat neck veins
- Hyperdynamic pulses
- Physiologic gallop
- Absence of edema
- Moist, cyanotic skin
- Manifestations of underlying disease

DIAGNOSTIC TESTS & INTERPRETATION

Lab

Initial lab tests

- Arterial blood gases (ABGs) show evidence of severe hypoxemia.
- $PaO_2/FiO_2 < 200$
- ECG: Sinus tachycardia; nonspecific ST-T-wave changes
- Pulmonary artery wedge pressure (PAWP) <15 mm Hg
- Cardiac index >3.5 L/min/m^2

Follow-Up & Special Considerations

- Serial blood gases
- Monitor for and treat multisystem organ failure when it occurs.

Imaging

Initial approach

- Chest x-ray (CXR): Normal heart size; fluffy, bilateral infiltrates; air bronchograms common
- Chest CT scan: Diffuse interstitial opacities and bullae

Follow-Up & Special Considerations

Serial CXRs

Diagnostic Procedures/Surgery

Invasive monitoring of vital signs, cardiac output, and PAWP has been questioned by large clinical trials.

Pathological Findings

- Lungs show exudative, early proliferative, or late proliferative phases.
- Interstitial and alveolar edema is present.
- Inflammatory cells and erythrocytes spill into the interstitium and the alveolus.
- Type 1 cells are destroyed, leaving a denuded basement membrane.
- Protein-rich fluid fills the alveoli.
- Type 2 alveolar cells initially appear unaltered.
- Type 2 cells begin to proliferate within 72 hours of initial insult.
- Type 2 cells cover the denuded basement membrane.
- Aggregates of plasma proteins, cellular debris, fibrin, and surfactant remnants form hyaline membranes.
- Over the next 3–10 days, alveolar septum thickens by proliferating fibroblasts, leukocytes, and plasma cells.
- Capillary injury begins to occur.
- Hyaline membranes begin to reorganize.
- Fibrosis becomes apparent in respiratory ducts and bronchioles.

DIFFERENTIAL DIAGNOSIS

- Left ventricular failure
- Interstitial and airway diseases
- Venoocclusive disease
- Mitral stenosis: Intravascular volume overload

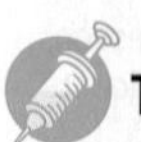

TREATMENT

MEDICATION

- No single drug or combination of drugs prevents or treats full-blown ARDS. Treatment is supportive while addressing the underlying cause.
- Supplemental oxygen
- Ventilatory support:
  - Most often requires endotracheal intubation with emphasis on lower tidal volumes per weight and optimization of positive end-expiratory pressure (PEEP).
  - High-frequency oscillation might improve survival and is unlikely to cause harm (1)[A].

ADDITIONAL TREATMENT

- Inotropic agents: Dobutamine to maintain adequate cardiac output after appropriate fluid resuscitation fails to restore perfusion
- Corticosteroids: Short-term use during the acute phase has not been shown to be effective. However, recent data suggest that sustained therapy in patients with full-blown, established ARDS may be beneficial (2)[A].
- Vasodilators: Inhaled nitric oxide (INO) is not recommended for patients with ARDS. INO results in a transient improvement in oxygenation but does not reduce mortality and may be harmful (3)[A].
- Pulmonary surfactant: Successful in neonatal respiratory distress syndrome; investigational outside this age group

- Inhaled β_2 agonists may be helpful during the resolution phase.
- There is no current evidence to support or refute the routine use of aerosolized prostacyclin for patients with ARDS (4)[A].
- Antioxidants (e.g., procysteine) have produced conflicting results.
- Activated protein C may be helpful in patients with sepsis.
- Deep vein thrombosis (DVT) prophylaxis
- Ulcer prophylaxis

Pregnancy Considerations

Supportive care while identifying the underlying cause of ARDS continues to be important in the management of pregnant women with ARDS. However, fetal well-being, possible need for delivery, and physiologic changes associated with pregnancy must be considered (5).

General Measures

- Ensure adequate oxygenation.
- Ventilatory support generally requires endotracheal intubation and use of PEEP (6).
- Provide appropriate cardiorespiratory monitoring.
- Fluid management

Issues for Referral

- All patients with ARDS should be cared for in an ICU with appropriately trained staff.
- Pregnant patients with ARDS also should be followed by a high-risk perinatologist or obstetrician.

IN-PATIENT CONSIDERATIONS

Initial Stabilization

- Consider prone positioning.
- Identify and treat underlying condition.
- Circulatory support, adequate fluid volume, and nutritional support
- Supplemental oxygen
- Monitoring blood gases, pulse oximetry, bedside pulmonary function test
- Support ventilation using lung-protective strategies and PEEP.
- Monitor for systemic hypotension and hypovolemia without fluid overload.
- BP support, if necessary
- Vasopressor agents
- Fluid management with IV crystalloid solutions while monitoring pulmonary status
- Pulmonary catheter pressure monitoring
- Treat underlying disease process.
- Prevent complications.

Admission Criteria

All patients with ARDS should be managed in an ICU setting.

IV Fluids

- Maintain the intravascular volume at the lowest level consistent with adequate perfusion (assessed by metabolic acid–base balance and renal function).
- If perfusion is inadequate after restoration of intravascular volume (e.g., septic shock), vasopressor therapy is indicated.
- Increase oxygen content with packed erythrocyte transfusions as necessary.
- Provide appropriate nutritional support with enteral or parenteral nutrition.
- Steroid therapy

Nursing

May include any or all of the following:

- Skin care, eye and mouth care
- DVT prophylaxis
- GI prophylaxis
- Suctioning
- Ensure adequate level of sedation and/or paralysis while on mechanical ventilation.
- Oxygen supplementation
- Nebulizer therapy
- Chest physiotherapy
- Tracheostomy care
- Explain all procedures to patient and family; reduce anxiety.

Discharge Criteria

- Supplemental oxygen
- Nutrition counseling
- Family monitoring of signs and symptoms of respiratory distress

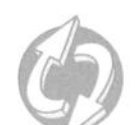

ONGOING CARE

FOLLOW-UP RECOMMENDATIONS

Patient Monitoring

- Vital capacity and static lung compliance are important measures of lung mechanics.
- Daily labs are needed until the patient is no longer critical.
- CXRs to assess endotracheal tube placement, the presence of progressing infiltrates, catheter placement, and complications of mechanical ventilation (e.g., air leaks)
- A Swan-Ganz catheter to help assess oxygen delivery, oxygen consumption, and cardiac output may be helpful but has not been shown to improve survival.

DIET

- Nutritional support
- Conservative fluid management shortens ventilator and ICU time but does not affect survival.

PATIENT EDUCATION

www.ards.org has ARDS support center and brochure entitled "Learn About ARDS."

PROGNOSIS

- Mortality rate is 43% (7).
- Survivors may have pulmonary sequelae with mild abnormalities in oxygenation, diffusion, and lung mechanics, as well as some pulmonary symptoms of cough and dyspnea.

COMPLICATIONS

- Permanent lung disease
- Oxygen toxicity
- Barotrauma
- Superinfection
- Multiple organ dysfunction syndrome
- Death

REFERENCES

1. Sud S, Sud M, Friedrich JO, et al. High frequency oscillation in patients with acute lung injury and acute respiratory distress syndrome (ARDS): Systematic review and meta-analysis. *BMJ*. 2010; 340:c2327.
2. Peter JV, John P, Graham PL, et al. Corticosteroids in the prevention and treatment of acute respiratory distress syndrome (ARDS) in adults: Meta-analysis. *BMJ*. 2008;336:1006–9.
3. Afshari A, Brok J, Møller AM, et al. Inhaled nitric oxide for acute respiratory distress syndrome (ARDS) and acute lung injury in children and adults. *Cochrane Database Syst Rev*. 2010;7:CD002787.
4. Afshari A, Brok J, Møller AM, et al. Aerosolized prostacyclin for acute lung injury (ALI) and acute respiratory distress syndrome (ARDS). *Cochrane Database Syst Rev*. 2010;8:CD007733.
5. www.ardsnet.org for ARDS Net ventilatory management protocol.
6. Petrucci N. Ventilation with lower tidal volumes vs. traditional tidal volumes in adults for acute lung injury and acute respiratory distress syndrome. *Cochrane Database Syst Rev*. 2007;2:CD003844.
7. Zambon M, Vincent JL. Mortality rates for patients with acute lung injury/ARDS have decreased over time. *Chest*. 2008;133:1120–7.

ADDITIONAL READING

- Cole DE, Taylor TL, McCullough DM. Acute respiratory distress syndrome in pregnancy. *Crit Care Med*. 2005;33:S269–78.
- Piantadosi CA, Schwartz DA. The acute respiratory distress syndrome. *Ann Intern Med*. 2004;141: 460–70.
- Ware LB, Matthay MA. The acute respiratory distress syndrome. *N Engl J Med*. 2000;342:1334–49.
- Wheeler AP, Bernard GR. Acute lung injury and the acute respiratory distress syndrome: A clinical review. *Lancet*. 2007;369:1553–64.

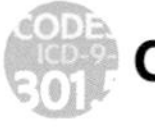

CODES

ICD9

518.5 Pulmonary insufficiency following trauma and surgery

CLINICAL PEARLS

- ARDS is a syndrome characterized by an abrupt onset of diffuse lung injury with severe hypoxemia and bilateral pulmonary infiltrates.
- Treatment of ARDS requires aggressive supportive care in an ICU setting while also addressing the underlying cause.
- The benefit of invasive monitoring of vital signs, cardiac output, and PAWP has been questioned by large clinical trials.

RESPIRATORY DISTRESS SYNDROME, NEONATAL

Mary Cataletto, MD

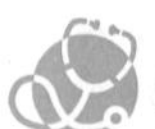

BASICS

DESCRIPTION

- Neonatal respiratory distress syndrome (RDS) is a serious disorder of prematurity with a clinical manifestation of respiratory distress.
- Pulmonary surfactants that are deficient at birth and an overly compliant chest wall cause diffuse lung atelectasis.
- Must differentiate from pneumonia, transient tachypnea of the newborn (TTN), sepsis, meconium aspiration
- System(s) affected: Pulmonary
- Synonym: Hyaline membrane disease

ALERT

A disorder of the neonatal period

EPIDEMIOLOGY

Incidence

- Affects 40,000 neonates each year in the US and accounts for ~6% of neonatal deaths
- Predominant age: Neonatal
- Predominant sex: Slight male predominance
- About 50% of neonates with birth weights of 501–1,500 g
- Inversely proportional to gestational age and birth weight
- In 1 study, rates of RDS, regardless of mode of delivery, increased between 1997 and 2005 from 2.1–2.4% (1).

Prevalence

Common

RISK FACTORS

- Neonatal complication rates vary by mode of delivery and decrease with gestational age (1):
  - Premature neonates born <37 weeks' gestation
  - Cesarean section without labor
- Neonates born of diabetic mothers
- Perinatal asphyxia
- History of RDS in a sibling

Genetics

No known genetic pattern

GENERAL PREVENTION

- Prevention of premature birth with education, regular prenatal care, and tocolytics
- Antenatal corticosteroids given to mother when fetal lung profile is immature, at least 24 hours before delivery; 2 doses of betamethasone 12 mg IM separated by a 24-hour interval (contraindications: Chorioamnionitis or other indications for immediate delivery)
- Prenatal amniotic fluid testing looking for indications of immature lungs/deficient surfactant production:
  - Lecithin:sphingomyelin (L:S) ratio <2:1
  - Absence of phosphatidyl glycerol
  - TDx fetal lung maturity (FLM) <70 (measures surfactant:albumin ratio)

PATHOPHYSIOLOGY

- Structurally immature lungs and surfactant deficiency lead to diffuse atelectasis.
- Exposure to high FiO_2 and barotrauma associated with mechanical ventilation trigger proinflammatory cytokines that further damage alveolar epithelium.
- Decreased lung compliance leads to alveolar hypoventilation and ventilation–perfusion mismatch.
- Shunting of blood (R → L) at patent ductus arteriosus (PDA), PFO causes further hypoxemia

DIAGNOSIS

HISTORY

Preterm neonates with worsening respiratory distress beginning shortly after birth and progressing over first few hours of life

PHYSICAL EXAM

- Tachypnea
- Expiratory grunting
- Nasal flaring
- Sub- and intercostal retractions
- Decreased breath sounds
- Cyanosis

DIAGNOSTIC TESTS & INTERPRETATION

Lab

- CBC and blood culture to rule out sepsis, pneumonia
- Electrolytes: Monitor for hypoglycemia, hypocalcemia
- Arterial blood gases (ABGs):
  - Hypoxemia (which responds to supplemental oxygen)
  - Features of respiratory and metabolic acidosis

Imaging

Chest x-ray (CXR):

- Diffuse reticulogranular pattern (ground-glass appearance)
- Air bronchograms
- Low lung volumes

Diagnostic Procedures/Surgery

Echocardiogram: Consider if murmur present to evaluate for PDA and contribution to lung disease due to L → R shunting (2)

Pathological Findings

- Macroscopically: Uniformly ruddy, airless appearance of lungs
- Microscopically: Diffuse atelectasis and hyaline membranes (eosinophilic and fibrinous membrane lining airspaces)
- Dilatation of right ventricle
- Possible PDA

DIFFERENTIAL DIAGNOSIS

- Early-onset group B streptococcal pneumonia and/or sepsis
- Transient tachypnea of newborn
- Meconium aspiration pneumonia

TREATMENT

Along with antenatal steroids, surfactants improve survival for preterm babies, and they are now recommended routinely as early in the course of RDS as possible (3)[A].

MEDICATION

- Surfactant via endotracheal tube (ETT):
  - Prophylactic surfactant administration: Given at birth to neonates <30 weeks' gestation (if it can be done safely at the same time as resuscitation)
  - Rescue surfactant administration: Given to neonates after RDS diagnosis
- Initial dosage of animal-derived surfactant preparations:
  - Poractant alfa (Curosurf): 2.5 mL/kg
  - Calfactant (Infasurf): 3 mL/kg
  - Beractant (Survanta): 4 mL/kg
- Continued therapy: After initial dose of chosen surfactant, if clinical evidence of persistent disease after initial improvement (recurrent O_2 requirement of >30–40%)
- Repeated dosages:
  - Poractant alfa: 1.25 mL/kg q12h for up to a total of 3 doses
  - Calfactant: 3 mL/kg q12h for up to a total of 3 doses
  - Beractant: 4 mL/kg repeated q6h for up to a total of 4 doses
- Side effects: Bradycardia, hypotension, airway obstruction/endotracheal tube blockage with administration; rapid changes in tidal volume due to increased compliance can cause a pneumothorax and small risk of pulmonary hemorrhage
- Precautions: Transient adverse effects seen with the administration of surfactant may require stopping administration and alleviating situation; may proceed with dosing when stable.

- Contraindications: Presence of congenital anomalies incompatible with life beyond neonatal period; infant with laboratory evidence of lung maturity
- Perform frequent clinical and laboratory checks so that oxygen and ventilatory support can be modified to respond to respiratory changes.

ADDITIONAL TREATMENT

General Measures

- Warm, humidified, oxygen-enriched gases by hood if the neonate is ventilating effectively
- Continuous positive airway pressure (CPAP) if infant is active and breathing spontaneously
- Positive-pressure ventilation per ETT via conventional mechanical ventilator (CMV) or high-frequency oscillation ventilator (HFOV) if respiratory failure occurs (i.e., respiratory acidosis, apnea, or hypoxia despite nasal CPAP)
- Transcutaneous monitors to measure O_2 and CO_2 tension
- Pulse oximetry
- Umbilical artery catheter placement for continuous BP monitoring and sampling ABGs
- Umbilical vein catheter placement for fluid and total parenteral nutrition (TPN) administration
- Tube feedings or hyperalimentation
- Optimize thermoneutral environment with radiant warmer or isolette.
- Sedation and analgesia with phenobarbital, fentanyl, or morphine may be required while the patient is intubated.
- Muscle paralysis is controversial.
- Inhaled nitric oxide and administration of postnatal glucocorticoids not recommended at this time

Additional Therapies

- Empirical therapy for sepsis (i.e., ampicillin and gentamicin) can be discontinued if CBC has normalized and blood culture has no growth after 48 hours.
- Consider medical or surgical closure of PDA if it is contributing to lung disease.

IN-PATIENT CONSIDERATIONS

Admission Criteria

All neonates with respiratory distress require inpatient treatment.

Discharge Criteria

Should have stable vital signs and pulse oximetry before discharge in addition to other premature considerations

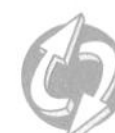

ONGOING CARE

DIET

Special premature formula and parenteral alimentation

PATIENT EDUCATION

For patient education materials favorably reviewed on this topic, go to Boston Children's Hospital Web site (www.childrenshospital.org) and search for respiratory distress syndrome in the "My Child Has" window.

PROGNOSIS

- Prognosis and outcome highly dependent on gestational age and birth weight
- Survival for neonates with birth weight of $\leq$500 g is 10%; >500 g, upwards of 75%.
- Complications of RDS decrease as birth weight increases.

COMPLICATIONS

- Some due to therapeutic interventions; others due to complications related to prematurity
- Pneumothorax
- Chronic lung disease, bronchopulmonary dysplasia (BPD)
- Intraventricular hemorrhage
- Retinopathy of prematurity
- Necrotizing enterocolitis
- Pulmonary interstitial edema (PIE)

REFERENCES

1. Jain NJ, Kruse LK, Demissie K. Impact of mode of delivery on neonatal complications: Trends between 1997 and 2005. *J Matern Fetal Neonatal Med.* 2009:1–10.
2. Hamrick SE, Hansmann G. Patent ductus arteriosus of the preterm infant. *Pediatrics.* 2010;125: 1020–30.
3. Sweet DG, Halliday HL. The use of surfactants in 2009. *Arch Dis Child Educ Pract Ed.* 2009;94: 78–83.

ADDITIONAL READING

- Engle WA, American Academy of Pediatrics Committee on Fetus and Newborn. Surfactant-replacement therapy for respiratory distress in the preterm and term neonate. *Pediatrics.* 2008;121: 419–32.
- Moya F. Synthetic surfactants: Where are we? Evidence from randomized, controlled clinical trials. *J Perinatol.* 2009;29(Suppl 2):S23–8.
- Ramachandrappa A, Jain L. Health issues of the late preterm infant. *Pediatr Clin North Am.* 2009;56: 565–77, Table of Contents.
- Sekar KC, Corff KE. To tube or not to tube babies with respiratory distress syndrome. *J Perinatol.* 2009; 29(Suppl 2):S68–72.
- Soll RF. Multiple versus single dose natural surfactant extract for severe neonatal respiratory distress syndrome. *Cochrane Database Sys Rev.* 1999;2:CD000141.

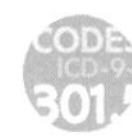

CODES

ICD9

769 Respiratory distress syndrome in newborn

CLINICAL PEARLS

- Surfactants are used routinely as early in the course of RDS as possible.
- If an infant has a murmur, consider an echocardiogram to rule out PDA and shunting.
- Prognosis and outcome are highly dependent on gestational age and birth weight.

RESPIRATORY SYNCYTIAL VIRUS INFECTION

Elizabeth Colman McKeen, MD

BASICS

Respiratory syncytial virus (RSV) is a medium-sized, membrane-bound ribonucleic acid (RNA) virus that causes acute respiratory tract illness in all ages, with most clinically significant disease in infants and young children.

DESCRIPTION

A major cause of respiratory illness, either of the upper respiratory tract (URT) or of the lower respiratory tract (LRT/bronchiolitis):

- In adults, RSV causes URT infections (URTIs).
- In infants and children, RSV causes URTIs and LRT infections (bronchiolitis).

Pediatric Considerations

- 90–95% of children are infected at least once by the age of 24 months; reinfection is common.
- Leading cause of pediatric bronchiolitis (50–90%)
- Premature infants are at increased risk for severe acute RSV infection.

EPIDEMIOLOGY

- Seasonality: Highest incidence of RSV infection in the US is between December and March.
- Morbidity: RSV infection leads to 75–125,000 hospitalizations annually nationwide.

RISK FACTORS

- Risk factors for severe disease:
  - History of prematurity
  - Age <12 weeks
  - Underlying cardiopulmonary disease
  - Immunodeficiency
- Other risk factors:
  - Low socioeconomic status
  - Exposure to environmental air pollutants
  - Childcare attendance
  - Severe neuromuscular disease
  - In adults, occupational exposure: Pediatric hospital staff, teachers, and daycare workers

Genetics

- A genetic predisposition to severe RSV infections may be associated with polymorphisms in cytokine- and chemokine-related genes, including *CCR5*, *IL4* and its receptor, *IL8*, *IL10*, and *IL13*.
- Infants with transplacentally acquired antibody against RSV are not protected against infection, but may have milder symptoms.

GENERAL PREVENTION

- Hand decontamination is the most important step in preventing nosocomial spread of RSV:
  - Alcohol-based rubs are preferred; an alternative is hand washing with antimicrobial soap (1)[B].
  - In patients with proven or suspected RSV, infection should be isolated or cohorted.
- Exposure to passive tobacco smoke should be avoided, especially in infants and children.
- Palivizumab (Synagis), a monoclonal antibody directed against the F (fusion) protein of RSV, is indicated as prophylaxis for the following groups:
  - Infants and children <24 months of age with:
    - Chronic lung disease of prematurity requiring medical therapy within 6 months of the start of RSV season
    - Hemodynamically significant cyanotic or acyanotic congenital heart disease
    - Prematurity <32 weeks' gestation, even in the absence of chronic lung disease. Those born at ≤28 weeks should receive prophylaxis during their first RSV season whenever that occurs during the first 12 months of life. Those born at 29–32 weeks benefit most from prophylaxis up to 6 months of age.
    - Prematurity 32 0/7–34 6/7 weeks' gestation *and* at least 1 of 2 risk factors born within 3 months before the start of RSV season or at any time throughout the RSV season:
      - Infant attends childcare, or
      - 1 or more siblings or other children younger than 5 years live permanently in the child's household
  - Dosage: 5 monthly doses beginning in November or December at 15 mg/kg per dose administered IM

PATHOPHYSIOLOGY

RSV-induced bronchiolitis causes acute inflammation, edema, and necrosis of the epithelial cells lining the small airways, air trapping, bronchospasm, and increased mucus production.

ETIOLOGY

- RSV is a medium-sized, membrane-bound RNA virus. It develops in the cytoplasm of infected cells and matures by budding from the plasma membrane.
- Infection spreads via infected droplets, either airborne or conveyed on hands, that are inoculated in the nose or conjunctivae of a susceptible subject.

COMMONLY ASSOCIATED CONDITIONS

- Asthma
- Serious bacterial infection (SBI) in infants and children with concurrent RSV infection is rare. When it occurs, the most likely etiology is URTI, followed by acute otitis media.

DIAGNOSIS

ALERT

In most cases, diagnosis should be made by history and physical exam alone. Laboratory and radiologic studies should not be ordered routinely (1)[B].

HISTORY

Patients may present with a variety of symptoms, including but not limited to, upper respiratory congestion, respiratory distress, cough, and fever.

PHYSICAL EXAM

- Fever
- Rhinorrhea
- Cough
- Wheezing
- Crackles
- Increased work of breathing, manifested as tachypnea, retractions, nasal flaring, and/or grunting
- In infants and children, evidence of poor hydration status, such as feeding difficulty, dry mucous membranes, poor skin turgor
- Repeat examinations over time are most helpful in providing the best overall assessment.

Pediatric Considerations

Young infants with bronchiolitis may develop apnea, which is associated with increased risk of prolonged hospitalization, ICU admission, and mechanical ventilation.

DIAGNOSTIC TESTS & INTERPRETATION

Lab

Initial lab tests

- *Routine laboratory testing is not necessary:*
  - If obtained, WBC count may be normal or elevated.
  - Virologic tests for RSV, despite high predictive value, rarely change management decisions or outcomes for patients with clinically diagnosed bronchiolitis.
- Given the low risk of SBI, full septic workups in these patients should not be undertaken routinely.

Imaging

- Chest x-ray (CXR) has not been proven to affect patient outcomes or predict disease severity.
- A CXR may be most helpful when a patient does not improve as expected, if the severity of the disease requires further investigation, or if another diagnosis is suspected.
- If obtained, typical findings on CXR can include:
  - Hyperinflation and peribronchiolar thickening
  - Atelectasis
  - Interstitial infiltrates
  - Segmental or lobar consolidation
  - Pleural fluid (rare)

DIFFERENTIAL DIAGNOSIS

- Mild illness/URTI:
  - Other (non-RSV) respiratory viral infections such as rhinovirus, human metapneumovirus, influenza virus, human bocavirus
  - Allergic rhinitis
  - Sinusitis
- Severe illness/LRTI:
  - Bronchiolitis
  - Asthma
  - Pneumonia
  - Foreign-body aspiration

TREATMENT

MEDICATION

- No first-line medication for RSV infections; treatment is usually supportive.
- Bronchodilators show small short-term improvements in clinical scores, but this small benefit should be weighed against the costs and adverse effects of these agents:
  - Bronchodilators do not improve oxygen saturation, do not reduce hospital admission after outpatient treatment, do not shorten the duration of hospitalization, and do not reduce the time to resolution of illness at home.
  - Routine use not recommended
- Epinephrine is superior compared to placebo for short-term outcomes for outpatients, particularly in the first 24 hours of care:
  - Evidence shows the effectiveness and superiority of adrenaline for outcomes of most clinical relevance among outpatients with acute bronchiolitis, and evidence from a single precise trial for combined adrenaline and dexamethasone (2)[A].
- Current evidence does not support a clinically relevant effect of systemic or inhaled glucocorticoids on admissions or length of hospitalization (3)[A]:
  - However, combined dexamethasone and epinephrine may reduce outpatient admissions, but results are exploratory and safety data limited (3)[A].
- A recent study found that montelukast (Singulair) has no effect on the clinical course of acute bronchiolitis (4)[C].
- Ribavirin, a nucleoside analogue and antiviral agent, has not been shown to be efficacious in the treatment of RSV (5)[C].
- Use of antibacterial agents should be reserved for patients who have specific signs of a coexisting SBI. When such an infection is present, it should be treated in the same manner as in the absence of RSV infection (6)[B].
- Current evidence suggests nebulized 3% saline may significantly reduce the length of hospital stay and improve the clinical severity score in infants with acute viral bronchiolitis (7)[A].

ADDITIONAL TREATMENT

General Measures

- Clinicians must promptly assess hydration status and ability to take fluids orally. Dehydration must be treated adequately with an oral or IV fluid, with special attention to infants.
- Supplemental O_2 is indicated if the saturation of peripheral oxygen (SpO_2) falls persistently below 90% in previously healthy patients:
  - An SpO_2 of 90% is an approximate cutoff and should be adjusted in the context of the patient.
  - Continuous O_2 monitoring can be discontinued in a patient whose clinical status is improving.

Additional Therapies

Bulb suctioning of the nares may provide some comfort to infants and allow for easier feeding.

Pediatric Considerations

Parents must be reminded that the American Academy of Pediatrics strongly recommends against the use of over-the-counter (OTC) cough and cold medications in children <6 years of age due to lack of efficacy and the risk of life-threatening side effects.

COMPLEMENTARY AND ALTERNATIVE MEDICINE

Clinicians should inquire about patients' use of complementary and alternative therapies, such as echinacea and zinc.

IN-PATIENT CONSIDERATIONS

Initial Stabilization

- A full history and physical exam should be completed, including the ABCs. Special attention should be paid to respiratory and hydration status.
- Mechanical ventilation is required in about 5% of infants hospitalized with RSV and 20% of children with underlying congenital heart disease, chronic lung disease, or immunosuppression, and should be instituted in the case of respiratory failure.

Admission Criteria

- Clinical judgment of the patient's degree of respiratory distress is the most important consideration.
- Significant respiratory distress and/or O_2 requirement to keep SpO_2 >90%
- Inability to hydrate orally

IV Fluids

See "Treatment."

Discharge Criteria

No set criteria for discharge exists, but the following guidelines may be helpful:

- Respiratory distress resolving or resolved
- Patient oxygenating well without O_2 therapy
- Adequate oral intake for sustained hydration
- Caretaker able to clear the infant's airway with bulb suctioning
- Home resources adequate to support use of any necessary home therapies
- Education of family complete

ONGOING CARE

FOLLOW-UP RECOMMENDATIONS

Close follow-up with the patient's primary health care provider is essential.

PATIENT EDUCATION

- See "General Prevention."
- *Bronchiolitis and Your Child,* available at http://familydoctor.org/online/famdocen/home/children/parents/common/common/020.html.

PROGNOSIS

Most patients with RSV infection recover fully within 7–10 days, although reinfection is common.

COMPLICATIONS

- Infants hospitalized for RSV may be at increased risk for recurrent wheezing and reduced pulmonary function, particularly during the first decade of life.
- Overall mortality for infants and children <24 months of age is <1%.

REFERENCES

1. American Academy of Pediatrics Subcommittee on Diagnosis and Management of Bronchiolitis. *Pediatrics*. 2006;118:1774–93.
2. Hartling L, Fernandes RM, Bialy L, et al. Steroids and bronchodilators for acute bronchiolitis in the first two years of life: Systematic review and meta-analysis. *BMJ*. 2011;342:d1714.
3. Fernandes RM, Bialy LM, Vandermeer B, et al. Glucocorticoids for acute viral bronchiolitis in infants and young children. *Cochrane Database Syst Rev*. 2010;(10):CD004878.
4. Amirav I, Luder AS, Kruger N, et al. A double-blind, placebo-controlled, randomized trial of montelukast for acute bronchiolitis. *Pediatrics*. 2008;122:e1249–55.
5. Ventre K, et al. Ribavirin for respiratory syncytial virus infection of the lower respiratory tract in infants and young children. Cochrane Acute Respiratory Infections Group. *Cochrane Database Sys Rev*. 2009;1:CD000181.
6. Spurling GKP, et al. Antibiotics for bronchiolitis in children. Cochrane Acute Respiratory Infections Group. *Cochrane Database Sys Rev*. 2007;1: CD005189.
7. Zang L. Nebulized hypertonic saline solution for acute bronchiolitis in infants. *Cochrane Database Syst Rev*. 2008;(4):CD006458.

ADDITIONAL READING

- AAP Policy Statements: Modified recommendations for use of palivizumab for prevention of respiratory syncytial virus infections. Committee on Infectious Diseases. *Pediatrics*. 2009;124(6):1694–701.
- Bourke T, Shields M. Bronchiolitis. *Clin Evid (Online)*. 2011;2011. pii:0308.
- Gadomski AM, Brower M, et al. Bronchodilators for bronchiolitis. *Cochrane Database Syst Rev*. 2010; CD001266.

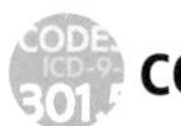

CODES

ICD9

- 079.6 Respiratory syncytial virus (RSV)
- 465.9 Acute upper respiratory infections of unspecified site
- 466.11 Acute bronchiolitis due to respiratory syncytial virus (RSV)

CLINICAL PEARLS

- RSV causes 50–90% of pediatric bronchiolitis.
- Hand sanitation is key for prevention in the general population.
- Palivizumab is key for prevention in the high-risk population.
- Diagnosis is clinical in most cases.
- Treatment is usually supportive.

RESTLESS LEGS SYNDROME

Donald E. Watenpaugh, PhD
John R. Burk, MD

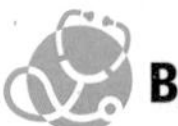

BASICS

DESCRIPTION

- Sensorimotor disorder defined by 4 criteria (1):
  - A strong urge to move the legs, usually with paresthesia
  - Symptoms emerge during inactivity.
  - Movement relieves symptoms, but they soon recur with inactivity.
  - Symptoms occur in the evening/night.
- Symptoms may involve the arms or be more generalized.
- Patient may also report involuntary leg jerks.
- System(s) affected: Musculoskeletal; Nervous
- Synonym(s): Willis-Ekbom disease; Ekbom syndrome

EPIDEMIOLOGY

Incidence

- Onset at any age; increases with age (2)
- Predominant sex: Male = Female (nulliparous); Female (parous) 2 × > Male

Prevalence

- 4–15% of Caucasian adults; underdiagnosed
- 1–3% in children and adolescents
- Increases with age
- Lower in non-Caucasians

Pregnancy Considerations

10–30% prevalence; exacerbates existing restless legs syndrome (RLS)

RISK FACTORS

- Family history (1,2)[A]
- Aging
- Chronic inactivity
- Inadequate sleep
- Associated conditions (see below)
- Certain medications (see "Etiology")

Genetics

- Primary RLS heritability: ~50%
- Genetically heterogenous (1):
  - Susceptibility loci: 2p14, 2q, 6p21.2, 9p, 12q, 14q, 15q23, and 20p
  - Genes: MEIS1, MAP2K5/LBXCOR1, and BTBD9

GENERAL PREVENTION

- Regular physical activity/exercise
- Adequate sleep
- Avoid evening caffeine, alcohol, tobacco

PATHOPHYSIOLOGY

- CNS iron or dopamine deficiency/dysmetabolism
- Chronic extremity tissue pathology/inflammation

ETIOLOGY

- Primary RLS: Subcortical dopamine deficiency (1)
- Secondary RLS:
  - Iron deficiency and associated conditions
  - Chronic extremity tissue irritation
  - Medications:
    - Most antidepressants (exceptions: Bupropion and desipramine)
    - Dopamine-blocking antiemetics (e.g., metoclopramide)
    - Some antiepileptic agents (e.g., phenytoin)
    - Phenothiazine antipsychotics; donepezil
    - Theophylline
    - Antihistamines/over-the-counter (OTC) cold preparations (e.g., pseudoephedrine)
    - Stimulants

COMMONLY ASSOCIATED CONDITIONS

- Periodic limb movements of sleep; insomnia; sleep walking and other parasomnias; delayed sleep phase
- Iron deficiency; renal disease/uremia/dialysis; gastric surgery; liver disease
- Parkinson disease; multiple sclerosis; peripheral neuropathy; migraine
- Orthopedic problems; arthritis; fibromyalgia
- Venous insufficiency/peripheral vascular disease; erectile dysfunction
- Pulmonary hypertension; lung transplantation; chronic obstructive pulmonary disease (COPD)
- ADHD; anxiety/depression; "sundowning"
- Pregnancy (especially if Fe- or folate-deficient)

DIAGNOSIS

- Dependent on history, yet often "difficult to describe"
- May go undiagnosed for years and by multiple doctors

HISTORY

- Signs/symptoms (see also "Description") (1):
  - Example descriptions: Burning, achy, itching, antsy, "can't get comfortable"
  - Painful in ~35% of patients
  - Discomfort associated with overwhelming urge to move and relieved by movement
  - Urge to move may be the only "discomfort."
  - Movement frequency every 10–90 seconds (mean ~25 seconds)
  - Some patients must get up and walk.
  - May involve arms or, rarely, whole body
  - Periodic movements in sleep in ~80% of patients
  - Insomnia, fatigue, anxiety
- Severity range: From rare, minor problem to daily severe impact on quality of life
- Primary RLS presents early and progresses slowly.
- Secondary RLS:
  - Precipitated by other conditions/medications
  - Tends to progress rapidly
  - Resolves to extent that cause(es) resolve

Pediatric Considerations

If all 4 diagnostic criteria not met, apply first 3 along with 2 of the following (2)[A]:

- Insomnia or sleep disturbance
- RLS in immediate biological relative
- Periodic limb movements during sleep

Geriatric Considerations

For diagnosis in the cognitively impaired (1,3)[A]:

- Rubbing or kneading the legs in evening
- Evening hyperactivity (foot tapping, pacing, fidgeting, tossing/turning in bed)

PHYSICAL EXAM

Patient may be fidgety, unable to sit still.

DIAGNOSTIC TESTS & INTERPRETATION

Lab

Serum ferritin to assess for iron deficiency

Diagnostic Procedures/Surgery

- Sleep study helpful but not required:
  - Frequent, periodic movements during wake
- Suggested immobilization test:
  - Conducted before nocturnal polysomnography
  - Patient attempts to sit still in bed for 1 hour.
  - >40 movements per hour suggests RLS.
- Ankle actigraphy for in-home use
- Electromyography, nerve conduction studies for peripheral neuropathy, radiculopathy

Pathological Findings

- Serum ferritin: <75 ng/mL
- Transferrin saturation: <16%

DIFFERENTIAL DIAGNOSIS

- Claudication: Movement does not relieve pain and may worsen it.
- Motor neuron disease fasciculation/tremor: No discomfort or circadian pattern
- Dermatitis/pruritus: Movement only to scratch; no circadian pattern
- Sleep-related leg cramps: Isolated and very painful muscle contracture
- Periodic limb movement disorder: No wakeful movement
- Sleep starts: Isolated involuntary events
- Rhythmic movement sleep disorder: Movement periodicity faster than RLS
- Growing pains: No urge to move or relief by movement; circadian pattern opposite RLS
- ADHD: No sleep disorders or complaints in diagnostic criteria.

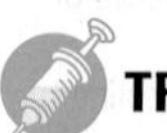

TREATMENT

First-line treatments (1,2,4,5,6)[A]:

- Prescribed daily exercise; adequate sleep
- Dopaminergic medications
- Correct iron deficiency
- For secondary RLS, treat cause(s); multiple possible causes are *not* mutually exclusive.

MEDICATION

- Use minimum effective dose (1,5,6)[A].
- Daytime sleepiness unusual with doses and timing for RLS.
- Severe/refractory RLS may require combination therapy.

First Line

- Dopamine agonists (6)[A]; titrate every 3 days to minimum necessary dose (1)[A]:
  - Pramipexole (Mirapex): 0.125–1.5 mg 1 hour before symptoms; titrate by 0.125 mg

R

– Ropinirole (Requip): 0.25–4 mg 1 hour before symptoms; titrate by 0.25 mg
– Divide dose for evening and bedtime symptoms.
– Liver disease: Pramipexole (renal clearance)
– Renal insufficiency: Ropinirole (hepatic catabolism)

- Gabapentin enacarbil (Horizant) (7)[A]: 600 mg every day ~5:00 PM
- Avoid dopamine agonists in psychotic patients, particularly if taking dopamine antagonists.
- All other medications off-label

Second Line

- Dopamine agonists:
  – Carbidopa-levodopa (Sinemet or Sinemet CR): 25/100–100/400; PRN for sporadic symptoms
  – Cabergoline: 0.25–3 mg (warning: Valvulopathy)
- Anticonvulsants (for neuropathic RLS):
  – Pregabalin (Lyrica): 50–300 mg/d
  – Carbamazepine: 200–800 mg/d
- Opioids (low risk of tolerance/addiction at bedtime):
  – Hydrocodone: 5–20 mg/d
  – Tramadol: 50 mg/d
  – Oxycodone: 2.5–20 mg/d
- Benzodiazepines and agonists (for associated insomnia or anxiety):
  – Temazepam, triazolam, alprazolam, zaleplon, zolpidem, and diazepam
  – Clonazepam (Klonopin): 0.5–3 mg/d

Pregnancy Considerations

- Initial approach: Nonpharmacologic therapies, iron supplements
- Avoid medications Class C or D.
- In third trimester, low-dose opioids or clonazepam may be considered.

Pediatric Considerations

- First-line treatment: Nonpharmacologic (2)[C]
- Low-dose clonidine or clonazepam may be considered.

Geriatric Considerations

- Avoid medications that cause dizziness or unsteadiness.
- Many medications given to elderly cause/ exacerbate RLS (3)[B].

ADDITIONAL TREATMENT

General Measures

- If iron deficient, supplement:
  – 325 mg $FeSO_4$ with vitamin C between meals t.i.d.
  – Repletion requires months.
- Daily exercise (2,4)[B]
- Unusual activity may exacerbate symptoms.
- Regular and replete sleep
- Hot bath and leg massage
- Warm the legs (long heavy socks, electric blanket)
- Intense mental activity (games, puzzles, etc.)

Issues for Referral

- Severe symptoms/augmentation; peripheral neuropathy; orthopedic problems
- Peripheral vascular disease; intransigent iron deficiency

Additional Therapies

- Vitamin, mineral supplements: Ca, Mg, B_{12}, folate
- Clonidine: 0.1–0.7 mg/d
- Baclofen: 20–80 mg/d
- Quinine
- Methadone
- Prescription or OTC hypnotics

COMPLEMENTARY AND ALTERNATIVE MEDICINE

- Sequential pneumatic leg compression
- Enhanced external counterpulsation
- Acupuncture
- MicroVas therapy

SURGERY/OTHER PROCEDURES

For orthopedic, neuropathic, or leg vascular disease (laser ablation, sclerotherapy, etc.)

IN-PATIENT CONSIDERATIONS

- Control RLS after orthopedic procedures.
- Addition/withdrawal of medications affecting RLS (e.g., narcotics)
- Changes in medical status may require medication changes.

IV Fluids

- Iron infusion when oral Fe fails
- When NPO, consider IV opiates.

Nursing

- Evening walks, hot baths, leg massage and warming
- Sleep interruption risks prolonged wakefulness.

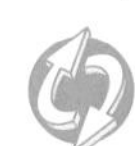

ONGOING CARE

FOLLOW-UP RECOMMENDATIONS

Patient Monitoring

- At 2-week intervals until stable, then annually
- If taking iron, remeasure ferritin.
- If status changes, assess for associated conditions and medications.

DIET

Avoid evening caffeine and alcohol.

PATIENT EDUCATION

- Restless Legs Syndrome Foundation: www.rls.org; e-mail: rlsfoundation@rls.org; Tel: 507-287-6465; Fax: 507-287-6312
- Worldwide Education & Awareness for Movement Disorders (WE MOVE): www.wemove.org; e-mail: wemove@wemove.org; Tel: 212-875-8312; Fax: 212-875-8389
- National Sleep Foundation: www.sleepfoundation.org; e-mail: nsf@sleepfoundation.org; Tel: 202-347-3471

PROGNOSIS

- Primary RLS: Lifelong condition with no current cure
- Secondary RLS: May subside with resolution of precipitating factors
- Current therapies usually control symptoms.

COMPLICATIONS

- Augmentation of symptoms from prolonged dopaminergic therapy:
  – Symptoms increase in severity, occur earlier, and/or spread.
  – Higher doses increase risk.
  – Highest risk from daily levodopa or Sinemet
  – Iron deficiency increases risk.
  – Add alternative medication, then slowly detitrate dopamine agonist (1,5)[B].
- Obsessive–compulsive or impulse-control disorders from dopamine agonists
- Vicious cycle between sleep loss from RLS and exacerbation of RLS by sleep loss
- Iatrogenic RLS (from antidepressants, etc.)

REFERENCES

1. Satija P, Ondo WG. Restless legs syndrome: Pathophysiology, diagnosis and treatment. *CNS Drugs*. 2008;22:497–518.
2. Picchietti MA, Picchietti DL, et al. Advances in pediatric restless legs syndrome: Iron, genetics, diagnosis and treatment. *Sleep Med*. 2010;11: 643–51.
3. Spiegelhalder K, Hornyak M. Restless legs syndrome in older adults. *Clin Geriatr Med*. 2008;24:167–80.
4. Aukerman MM, Aukerman D, Bayard M, et al. Exercise and restless legs syndrome: A randomized controlled trial. *J Am Board Fam Med*. 2006;19: 487–93.
5. Ferini-Strambi L. Treatment options for restless legs syndrome. *Expert Opin Pharmacother*. 2009;10: 545–54.
6. Scholz H, Trenkwalder C, Kohnen R, et al. Dopamine agonists for restless legs syndrome. *Cochrane Database Syst Rev*. 2011;16(3):CD006009.
7. Imamura S, Kushida C. Gabapentin enacarbil (XP13512/GSK1838262) as an alternative treatment to dopaminergic agents for restless legs syndrome. *Expert Opin Pharmacother*. 2010;11(11): 1925–32.

ADDITIONAL READING

- Thomas K, Watson CB. Restless legs syndrome in women: A review. *J Womens Health (Larchmt)*. 2008;17:859–68.
- Trotti LM, Bhadriraju S, Rye DB. An update on the pathophysiology and genetics of restless legs syndrome. *Curr Neurol Neurosci Rep*. 2008;8: 281–7.

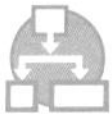

See Also (Topic, Algorithm, Electronic Media Element)

- Periodic Limb Movement Disorder
- Algorithm: Restless Leg Syndrome (RLS)

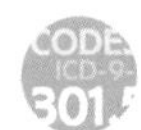

CODES

ICD9

333.94 Restless legs syndrome (RLS)

CLINICAL PEARLS

- Insomnia with frequent tossing/turning and difficulty "getting comfortable" is often RLS.
- Many antidepressants, antipsychotics, antiemetics, and antihistamines cause or exacerbate RLS.
- RLS may interfere with use of positive airway pressure to treat obstructive sleep apnea.
- RLS and other sleep disorders may cause ADHD.

RETINAL DETACHMENT

Richard W. Allinson, MD

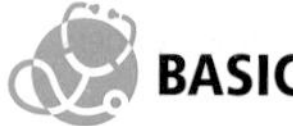

BASICS

DESCRIPTION

- Separation of the sensory retina from the underlying retinal pigment epithelium
- Rhegmatogenous retinal detachment (RRD): Most common type; occurs when the fluid vitreous gains access to the subretinal space through a break in the retina (Greek *rhegma*, "rent")
- Exudative or serous detachment: Occurs in the absence of a retinal break, usually in association with inflammation or a tumor
- Traction detachment: Vitreoretinal adhesions mechanically pull the retina from the retinal pigment epithelium. The most common cause is proliferative diabetic retinopathy.
- System(s) affected: Nervous

EPIDEMIOLOGY

Incidence

- Predominant age: Incidence increases with age.
- Predominant sex: Male > Female (3:2)
- Per year: 1/10,000 in patients who have not had cataract surgery

Prevalence

After cataract surgery, 1–3% of patients will develop a retinal detachment.

RISK FACTORS

- Myopia (>5 diopters)
- Aphakia or pseudophakia: In patients undergoing small-incision coaxial phacoemulsification with high myopia (axial length ≥26 mm), the incidence of retinal detachment is 2.7%.
- Posterior vitreous detachment (PVD) and associated conditions (e.g., aphakia, inflammatory disease, and trauma)
- Trauma
- Retinal detachment in fellow eye
- Lattice degeneration: A vitreoretinal abnormality found in 6–10% of the general population
- Glaucoma: 4–7% of patients with retinal detachment have chronic open-angle glaucoma.
- Vitreoretinal tufts: Peripheral retinal tufts are caused by focal areas of vitreous traction.
- Meridional folds: Redundant retina usually is found in the supranasal quadrant.

Genetics

- Most cases are sporadic.
- There is an increased risk of RRD if a sibling has been affected by this condition. The risk increases with higher levels of myopia in the family history (1)[B].

GENERAL PREVENTION

Patients at risk for retinal detachment should have regular ophthalmologic examinations.

ETIOLOGY

- Traction from a PVD causes most retinal tears. With aging, vitreous gel liquefies, leading to separation of the vitreous from the retina. The vitreous gel remains attached at the vitreous base, in the retinal periphery, resulting in vitreous traction that produces tears in the retinal periphery. There is an ~15% chance of developing a retinal tear from a PVD.
- PVD associated with vitreous hemorrhage has a high incidence of retinal tears.
- Exudative detachment:
  - Tumors
  - Inflammatory diseases (Harada, posterior scleritis)
  - Miscellaneous (central serous retinopathy, uveal effusion syndrome, malignant hypertension)
- Traction detachment:
  - Proliferative diabetic retinopathy
  - Cicatricial retinopathy of prematurity
  - Proliferative sickle-cell retinopathy
- Penetrating trauma

Geriatric Considerations

- Posterior vitreous detachment
- Cataract surgery

Pediatric Considerations

Usually associated with underlying vitreoretinal disorders and/or retinopathy of prematurity

COMMONLY ASSOCIATED CONDITIONS

- Lattice degeneration
- High myopia
- Cataract surgery
- Glaucoma
- History of retinal detachment in the fellow eye
- Trauma

Pregnancy Considerations

Preeclampsia/eclampsia may be associated with exudative retinal detachment. No intervention is indicated, provided hypertension is controlled. Prognosis is usually good.

DIAGNOSIS

HISTORY

- Sudden flashes (photopsia)
- Shower of floaters
- Visual field loss: "Curtain coming across vision"
- Central vision will be preserved if the macula is not detached.
- Poor visual acuity (20/200 or worse), with loss of central vision when macula is detached

PHYSICAL EXAM

- Slit-lamp exam
- Dilated fundus exam with binocular indirect ophthalmoscopy

DIAGNOSTIC TESTS & INTERPRETATION

Visual field testing: Differentiates RRD from retinoschisis. An absolute scotoma is seen in retinoschisis, whereas RRD causes a relative scotoma.

Imaging

- Ultrasound can demonstrate a detached retina and may be helpful when the retina cannot be visualized directly (e.g., with cataracts).
- Fluorescein dye leakage can be seen in exudative retinal detachment; caused by central serous retinopathy and other inflammatory conditions.

Pathological Findings

- Elevation of the neurosensory retina from the underlying retinal pigment epithelium
- Elevation of retina associated with ≥1 retinal tears in RRD or elevation of the retina without tears in exudative detachment
- In 3–10% of patients with presumed RRD, no definite retinal break is found.
- Tenting of the retina without retinal tears in traction detachment
- Pigmented cells within the vitreous ("tobacco dust")

DIFFERENTIAL DIAGNOSIS

Retinoschisis (splitting of the retina):

- Vitreous cells and vitreous hemorrhage are found rarely in the vitreous with retinoschisis, whereas they are seen commonly in RRD.
- Retinoschisis usually has a smooth surface and is dome shaped, whereas RRD often has a corrugated, irregular surface.

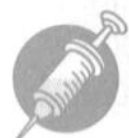

TREATMENT

MEDICATION

First Line

- Intraocular gases:
  - Air
  - Perfluoropropane (C_3F_8)
  - Sulfur hexafluoride (SF_6)
- Perfluorocarbon liquids
- Silicone oil
- Contraindications to intraocular gas: Patients with poorly controlled glaucoma
- Precautions with intraocular gas: Expanding intraocular gas bubble increases intraocular pressure; therefore, avoid higher altitudes.
- Significant possible interactions with intraocular gas: Nitrous oxide used in general anesthesia can expand an intraocular gas bubble.

Second Line

Steroids may cause worsening of central serous retinopathy.

ADDITIONAL TREATMENT

General Measures

- Not all retinal tears or breaks need to be treated:
  - Flap or horseshoe tears in symptomatic patients (e.g., patients with flashes or floaters) are treated frequently.
  - Operculated holes in symptomatic patients are treated sometimes.
  - Atrophic holes in symptomatic patients are treated rarely.
- Lattice degeneration with or without holes within the lattice in an asymptomatic patient with prior retinal detachment in the fellow eye may be treated prophylactically.
- Flap retinal tears in asymptomatic patients frequently are treated prophylactically.
- Exudative detachments usually are managed by treating underlying disorder.
- Traction detachments usually are managed by observation. If the fovea is involved, a vitrectomy is needed.

SURGERY/OTHER PROCEDURES

- Timing of repairs:
  - Macula attached: Within 24 hours. If the detachment is peripheral and does not have features suggestive of rapid progression (e.g., large and/or superior tears), repair can be performed within a few days.
  - Macula recently detached: Within 10 days of development of a macula-off retinal detachment (2)[B]
  - Old macular detachment: Elective repair within 2 weeks

- If a retinal break has led to the development of a retinal detachment, surgery is needed. Surgical options (and combinations) include:
  - Demarcation laser treatment (3)[C]
  - Pneumatic retinopexy: Head positioning is required postoperatively.
  - Scleral buckle
  - Vitrectomy
  - Perfluorocarbon liquids for giant tears (circumferential tears ≥90°)
  - Silicone oil for complex repairs
- Anesthesia: Local or general
- RRD may have >1 break. If any retinal break is not closed at the time of surgery, the surgery will fail.
- Additional surgery may be required if the retina redetaches secondary to a new retinal break or because of proliferative vitreoretinopathy (PVR).
- Adjuvant combination therapy using 5-fluorouracil (5-FU) and low-molecular-weight heparin (LMWH) can reduce the incidence of PVR in patients undergoing vitrectomy for RRD who are at a greater risk of developing PVR, such as patients with uveitis.
- If a vitreous hemorrhage is present, presumably from a retinal tear, and the fundus cannot be well visualized, consideration can be given for early vitrectomy (4)[C].
- There is a trend toward primary vitrectomy in the management of RRD. Eyes undergoing PPV for primary RRD repair may not need the addition of a scleral buckle (5)[B].

IN-PATIENT CONSIDERATIONS

Initial Stabilization

- Recognition of condition is key (see "Diagnosis").
- Referral to an ophthalmologist for examination and treatment, if indicated

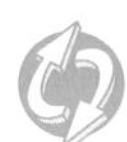

ONGOING CARE

FOLLOW-UP RECOMMENDATIONS

- Bed rest prior to surgery
- Postoperatively, if intraocular gas has been used, the patient may need specific head positioning and should not travel to high altitudes.

Patient Monitoring

- Alert ophthalmologist if there is new onset of floaters or flashes, increase in floaters or flashes, sudden shower of floaters, curtain or shadow in the peripheral visual field, or reduced vision.
- Patients with acute symptomatic PVD should be re-examined by the ophthalmologist in 3–4 weeks. The development of a retinal detachment is unlikely if no retinal tears are present on re-examination in 3–4 weeks.
- If acute symptomatic PVD is associated with gross vitreous hemorrhage that interferes with complete visualization of the retinal periphery by indirect ophthalmoscopy, the patient should be re-examined at short intervals with indirect ophthalmoscopy until the entire retinal periphery can be observed.
- If the examiner is not certain whether the retina is detached in the presence of opaque medium, US should be performed.

DIET

NPO if surgery is imminent

PATIENT EDUCATION

American Academy of Ophthalmology, 655 E. Beach Street, San Francisco, CA 94109-1336

PROGNOSIS

- RRD:
  - 90% of retinal detachments can be reattached successfully after ≥1 surgical procedures. Postoperative visual acuity depends primarily on the status of the macula preoperatively. Also important is the length of time between the detachment and the repair (75% of eyes with macular detachments of <1 week will obtain a final visual acuity of 20/70 or better).
  - 87% of eyes with a retinal detachment not involving the macula attain a visual acuity of 20/50 or better postoperatively. 37% of eyes with a detached macula preoperatively attain 20/50 or better vision postoperatively.
  - In 10–15% of successfully repaired retinal detachments not involving the macula preoperatively, visual acuity does not return to the preoperative level. This decrease is secondary to complications such as macular edema and macular pucker.
- Tractional retinal detachment: When not involving the fovea, the patient usually can be observed because it is uncommon for these to extend into the fovea.
- Exudative retinal detachment:
  - Management is usually nonsurgical.
  - The presence of shifting fluid is highly suggestive of an exudative retinal detachment. Fixed retinal folds, which are indicative of PVR, are seen rarely in exudative retinal detachment. If the underlying condition is treated, the prognosis generally is good.

COMPLICATIONS

- PVR is the most common cause of failed retinal detachment repair; 10–15% of retinas that reattach initially after retinal surgery will redetach subsequently, usually within 6 weeks, as a result of cellular proliferation and contraction on the retinal surface.
- Partial or total loss of vision due to macular detachment and/or PVR
- Moderate-to-severe forms of PVR usually are treated with pars plana vitrectomy and fluid–gas exchange (6)[A]. If a segmental scleral buckle was placed at the initial procedure, it may need to be revised.
- Primary retinectomy can be used in cases of PVR without a scleral buckle (7)[C].
- Scleral buckles may erode the overlying conjunctiva and lead to an infection.

REFERENCES

1. Mitry D, Williams L, Charteris DG, et al. Population-based estimate of the sibling recurrence risk ratio for rhegmatogenous retinal detachment. *Invest Ophthalmol Vis Sci*. 2011;52:2551–5.
2. Hassan TS, Sarrafizadeh R, Ruby AJ, et al. The effect of duration of macular detachment on results after the scleral buckle repair of primary, macula-off retinal detachments. *Ophthalmology*. 2002;109:146–52.
3. Vrabec TR, Baumal CR. Demarcation laser photocoagulation of selected macula-sparing rhegmatogenous retinal detachments. *Ophthalmology*. 2000;107:1063–7.
4. Tan HS, Mura M, Bijl HM. Early vitrectomy for vitreous hemorrhage associated with retinal tears. *Am J Ophthalmol*. 2010;150:529–33.
5. Kinori M, Moisseiev E, Shoshany N, et al. Comparison of pars plana vitrectomy with and without scleral buckle for the repair of primary rhegmatogenous retinal detachment. *Am J Ophthalmol*. 2011;152(2):291–7.
6. Vitrectomy with silicone oil or perfluoropropane gas in eyes with severe proliferative vitreoretinopathy: Results of a randomized clinical trial. Silicone Study Report 2. *Arch Ophthalmol*. 1992;110:780–92.
7. Tan HS, Mura M, Oberstein SY. Primary retinectomy in proliferative vitreoretinopathy. *Am J Ophthalmol*. 2010;149:447–52.

ADDITIONAL READING

Alio JL, Ruiz-Moreno JM, Shabayek MH, et al. The risk of retinal detachment in high myopia after small incision coaxial phacoemulsification. *Am J Ophthalmol*. 2007;144:93–98.

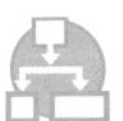

See Also (Topic, Algorithm, Electronic Media Element)

Retinopathy, Diabetic

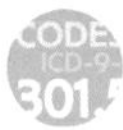

CODES

ICD9

- 361.2 Serous retinal detachment
- 361.9 Unspecified retinal detachment
- 361.81 Traction detachment of retina

CLINICAL PEARLS

- If a patient complains of the new onset of floaters or flashes of light, the patient should undergo a dilated eye examination to rule out a retinal tear or retinal detachment.
- There is an increased risk of retinal detachment after cataract surgery.
- Proliferative vitreoretinopathy can result in redetachment of the retina after an initially successful repair.

RETINITIS PIGMENTOSA

Richard W. Allinson, MD

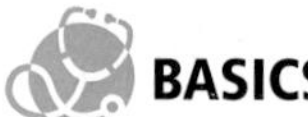

BASICS

DESCRIPTION

- An eye disease in which there is progressive damage to the retina with gradual loss of peripheral vision that eventually leads to significant visual impairment; signs often seen in childhood, but severe vision problems do not develop until adulthood.
- Characterized by poor night vision, constricted visual fields, bone spiculelike pigmentation of the fundus, and electroretinographic evidence of photoreceptor cell dysfunction
- System(s) affected: Nervous
- Synonym(s): Rod-cone dystrophy; Retinal dystrophy

EPIDEMIOLOGY

Incidence

- Predominant age:
  - X-linked retinitis pigmentosa (RP) has the earliest onset of the major hereditary types; many X-linked patients are legally blind by age 30.
  - Autosomal-dominant RP has a later onset than autosomal-recessive or X-linked-recessive RP.
  - Leber's congenital amaurosis, which is a variant of RP, presents at birth.
  - Late-onset RP typically is asymptomatic and unrecognized until age 40–50 years.
- Predominant sex: Male > Female

Prevalence

Affects ~1/4,000 people in the US

Pediatric Considerations

Leber's congenital amaurosis is characterized by severely reduced vision from birth and impaired electroretinogram responses from both cones and rods. Most cases are autosomal recessive.

Geriatric Considerations

Late-onset RP is asymptomatic and generally unrecognized until age >40 years.

RISK FACTORS

Family history

Genetics

- Autosomal dominant: 20%
- Autosomal recessive: 37%
- X-linked recessive: 4.5%
- Sporadic: 38.5%

GENERAL PREVENTION

- Genetic counseling
- No conclusive evidence demonstrates that the amount of light modifies the course of RP. A study in which 1 eye was covered with an opaque lens did not show any difference in disease progression compared with the fellow eye.
- Ultraviolet (UV)–absorbing sunglasses and brimmed hats are recommended when patients are at the beach or in the snow.

ETIOLOGY

- The genetic mutations responsible for RP have been identified in some families with RP, primarily those with the autosomal-dominant form.
- Mutations in the rhodopsin gene account for ~30% of cases of autosomal-dominant RP.
- Another 4–6% of autosomal-dominant RP is caused by a mutation in the gene for a photoreceptor protein peripherin/rds.

COMMONLY ASSOCIATED CONDITIONS

With systemic disorders:

- Usher syndrome: RP and congenital sensorineural hearing impairment
- Laurence-Moon-Biedl syndrome (also called *Bardet-Biedl syndrome*): Autosomal-recessive disorder associated with retinal dystrophy, mental retardation, obesity, hypogonadism, and postaxial polydactyly
- Cockayne syndrome: Autosomal-recessive disorder in which children at the age of 1–2 years present with retinal dystrophy, sensorineural deafness, cerebellar dysfunction, dementia, and UV light photosensitivity

DIAGNOSIS

HISTORY

- Headache and light flashes are the most common initial complaints.
- Night blindness (nyctalopia)
- Progressive visual field loss
- Central visual acuity is usually preserved until the end stages.

PHYSICAL EXAM

- Bone spicule pigmentation in the retina
- Retinal arteriolar narrowing
- Optic nerve head pallor, "waxy pallor"
- Most patients are myopic.
- Posterior subcapsular cataracts are common in all forms.
- Cystoid macular edema
- Optic nerve head drusen
- Electroretinogram changes
- Retinal neovascularization
- RP is associated with an exudative retinal vasculopathy. Fundus findings include serous retinal detachment, lipid deposition in the retina, and telangiectatic vascular anomalies.
- Variants of RP exist with unusual or regional distribution, including:
  - Sectorial RP
  - Pigmented paravenous atrophy
  - Unilateral RP

DIAGNOSTIC TESTS & INTERPRETATION

- Electroretinography: Photoreceptors generate reduced-amplitude A and B waves in RP. Rod and cone responses may be undetectable in advanced RP.
- Visual field testing: A ring scotoma in the midperiphery may be identified. The ring scotoma generally starts as a group of isolated scotomas in the area 20–25° from fixation. Long after the entire peripheral field is gone, a small island of intact central visual field remains.
- Fluorescein angiography can demonstrate cystoid macular edema.
- Fundus photography to document the status of the retina
- Hearing tests in patients complaining of hearing loss, such as those with Usher syndrome (RP with hearing loss)
- Optical coherence tomography can be used to detect and monitor cystoid macular edema.

Lab

Follow-Up & Special Considerations

- Elevated plasma levels of phytanic acid in Refsum disease
- Acanthocytosis of red blood cells in peripheral blood smear in abetalipoproteinemia, an autosomal-recessive disorder in which apolipoprotein B is not synthesized, leading to fat malabsorption and deficiencies of fat-soluble vitamins; therapy with vitamins A and E may improve retinal function.
- Syphilitic neuroretinitis can be diagnosed by performing a fluorescent treponemal antibody absorption or microhemagglutination *Treponema pallidum* test.
- Elevated plasma ornithine levels in gyrate atrophy of the choroid and retina; usually a 10–20-fold elevation of plasma ornithine levels

Pathological Findings

- Disappearance of the rods, cones, and outer nuclear layers of the retina
- Bone spicule formation in the retina is secondary to the migration of retinal pigment epithelial cells into the overlying retina.

DIFFERENTIAL DIAGNOSIS

- Bone spiculelike retinal pigmentation and retinal atrophy are nonspecific findings and may result from conditions other than RP.
- Infections
- Syphilis
- Rubella
- Inflammation (severe uveitis)
- Choroidal vascular occlusion
- Toxicity (chloroquine or thioridazine)
- Choroideremia
- Gyrate atrophy of choroid and retina (10–20-fold elevation of plasma ornithine levels)
- Systemic metabolic disorders such as Refsum disease and abetalipoproteinemia
- Kearns-Sayre syndrome: Usually presents in adolescents; characterized by progressive external ophthalmoplegia—the first sign usually being ptosis—pigmentary degeneration of the retina, and a cardiac conduction defect, which may cause complete heart block

R

- Cone-rod dystrophy: Characterized by bilateral and symmetric loss of cone function in the presence of reduced rod function
- Cone dystrophy: Characterized by marked abnormality in cone function with some or no rod involvement
- Congenital stationary night blindness
- Oguchi disease
- Fundus albipunctatus
- Trauma

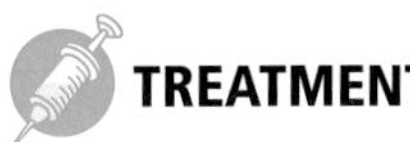

TREATMENT

MEDICATION

- Vitamin A 15,000 IU/d (retinal degeneration slowed, as measured by electroretinogram/visual fields); β-carotene is not a suitable substitute; has not been studied in patients <18 years of age (1)[A]
- Vitamin E 400 IU/d results in faster retinal degeneration and is not recommended (1)[A].
- Lutein supplementation at a dose of 12 mg/d slowed visual field loss among nonsmoking adults with RP taking vitamin A (2)[B].
- Acetazolamide may be of benefit in the treatment of cystoid macular edema, which may occur in RP; 500 mg/d in a sustained-release capsule was found to be more effective than 250 mg/d.
- Topical dorzolamide may be of benefit in the treatment of cystoid macular edema associated with RP (3)[C].
- Intravitreal bevacizumab and ranibizumab injection may be of benefit in the treatment of cystoid macular edema associated with RP (4)[C].
- Contraindications: Women who are pregnant or considering pregnancy should not take >8,000 IU/d of vitamin A. There is an increased incidence of birth defects in babies born to women who ingest higher dosages of vitamin A during pregnancy. Women should consult their obstetrician (5)[A].
- Precautions: Avoid vitamin A supplement dosages >15,000 IU/d because higher dosages may cause liver damage.

Pregnancy Considerations

Risk of teratogenicity with a high intake of vitamin A during pregnancy

ADDITIONAL TREATMENT

General Measures

- Supportive care
- Genetic counseling
- Low-vision aids
- Patient education

SURGERY/OTHER PROCEDURES

- The efficacy of the "Cuban therapy"—electric stimulation, autotransfused ozonized blood, and ocular surgery—has not been proven.
- Macular grid laser photocoagulation may be of benefit in patients with cystoid macular edema secondary to RP.
- Research is being done on photoreceptor and retinal pigment epithelium transplantation, gene therapy, and implantation of a visual prosthesis. The inner retinal neurons may be preserved after death of photoreceptors in RP, which could make some of these experimental procedures feasible (6)[C].
- Gene therapy has been successful in treating patients with Leber's congenital amaurosis due to defects in the RPE65 gene (7,8)[C].

IN-PATIENT CONSIDERATIONS

Initial Stabilization

Outpatient care

ONGOING CARE

FOLLOW-UP RECOMMENDATIONS

Caution should be exercised because of reduced peripheral vision and poor night vision.

Patient Monitoring

- Ophthalmic examinations every 1–2 years
- Check for complications (e.g., cataracts).

PATIENT EDUCATION

- Counsel patients to help them understand RP and its genetics.
- RP is a slowly progressive, chronic disease; patients do not go blind rapidly, and total blindness is not a frequent endpoint of this disease.
- RP Foundation Fighting Blindness, Executive Plaza One, Suite 800, 11350 McCormick Road, Hunt Valley, MD 21031-1014, (800) 683-5555
- The American Academy of Ophthalmology, 655 E. Beach Street, San Francisco, CA 94109-1336, (415) 561-8540

PROGNOSIS

- Reassurance about the slow course of RP
- Most of the deafness in Usher syndrome is congenital. It is unlikely that an RP patient who is not born deaf will become deaf later in life.
- RP severity varies with inheritance pattern.
- Autosomal-recessive form has an early age of onset and may have severely constricted visual fields by age 20 years. Tends toward more rapid progression compared with autosomal-dominant RP; also increased incidence of cataracts.
- X-linked RP is similar in clinical presentation to autosomal-recessive RP.
- Autosomal-dominant RP generally has less severe findings initially than does autosomal-recessive RP; symptoms may not occur until 30 years of age.
- Good central vision is usually preserved. If the central visual field radius is >30°, >90% of patients will have visual acuities of 20/40 or better. If the central visual field radius is <10°, 30% of patients will have a visual acuity of 20/40 or better.

COMPLICATIONS

- Cataract
- Cystoid macular edema
- Loss of visual field
- Poor night vision
- Blindness

REFERENCES

1. Berson EL, Rosner B, Sandberg MA, et al. A randomized trial of vitamin A and vitamin E supplementation for retinitis pigmentosa. *Arch Ophthalmol*. 1993;111:761–72.
2. Berson EL, Rosner B, Sandberg MA, et al. Clinical trial of lutein in patients with retinitis pigmentosa receiving vitamin A. *Arch Ophthalmol*. 2010;128:403–11.
3. Grover S, Apushkin MA, Fishman GA. Topical dorzolamide for the treatment of cystoid macular edema in patients with retinitis pigmentosa. *Am J Ophthalmol*. 2006;141:850–8.
4. Artunay O, Yuzbasioglu E, Rasier R, et al. Intravitreal ranibizumab in the treatment of cystoid macular edema associated with retinitis pigmentosa. *J Ocul Pharmacol Ther*. 2009;25:545–50.
5. Rothman KJ, Moore LL, Singer MR, et al. Teratogenicity of high vitamin A intake. *N Engl J Med*. 1995;333:1369–73.
6. Yanai D, Weiland JD, Mahadevappa M, et al. Visual performance using a retinal prosthesis in three subjects with retinitis pigmentosa. *Am J Ophthalmol*. 2007;143:820–7.
7. Bainbridge JW, Smith AJ, Barker SS, et al. Effect of gene therapy on visual function in Leber's congenital amaurosis. *N Engl J Med*. 2008;358:2231–9.
8. Maguire AM, Simonelli F, Pierce EA, et al. Safety and efficacy of gene transfer for Leber's congenital amaurosis. *N Engl J Med*. 2008;358:2240–8.

CODES

ICD9

362.74 Pigmentary retinal dystrophy

CLINICAL PEARLS

- Characterized by poor night vision, constricted visual fields, bone spiculelike pigmentation of the fundus, and electroretinographic evidence of photoreceptor cell dysfunction
- Vitamin E 400 IU/d results in faster retinal degeneration and is not recommended.
- RP severity varies with inheritance pattern.

RETINOPATHY OF PREMATURITY

Richard W. Allinson, MD

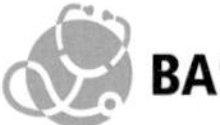

BASICS

DESCRIPTION

- Proliferative disorder of the retinal blood vessels in premature infants: The normal retinal vascularization occurs nasally at ~36 weeks' gestational age and temporally at ~40 weeks' gestational age.
- System(s) affected: Nervous
- Synonym(s): Retinopathy of prematurity (ROP); Retrolental fibroplasia

EPIDEMIOLOGY

Incidence

- 65.8% of infants weighing <1,251 g at birth and 81.6% of those weighing <1,000 g
- Predominant age: Premature infants
- Predominant sex: Male = Female

RISK FACTORS

- Low birth weight
- Prematurity
- Supplemental oxygen; once the retina becomes fully vascularized, oxygen does not affect the retina.
- Supplemental oxygen given to premature infants with moderate ROP will not make the retinopathy worse.

Genetics

African American infants appear less susceptible.

ETIOLOGY

Oxidative processes (influenced by high levels of arterial oxygen) in immature retina may be an important causative factor.

COMMONLY ASSOCIATED CONDITIONS

Neonatal respiratory distress syndrome

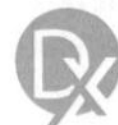

DIAGNOSIS

PHYSICAL EXAM

- Acute ROP classification:
  - Location:
    - Zone I: Posterior retina within a 60° circle centered on the optic nerve
    - Zone II: Extends from the edge of zone I to the nasal ora anteriorly
    - Zone III: The residual temporal crescent of retina anterior to zone II
  - Extent: Number of clock hours involved
  - Degree of abnormal vascular response observed:
    - Stage 1: The development of a demarcation line between the vascularized and nonvascularized retina
    - Stage 2: The presence of a demarcation line that extends out of the plane of the retina (ridge)
    - Stage 3: A ridge with extraretinal fibrovascular proliferation
    - Stage 4: Subtotal retinal detachment
    - Stage 5: Total retinal detachment
  - *Plus disease* is characterized by the tortuosity of the retinal vasculature in the posterior fundus. *Preplus disease* denotes retinal vascular abnormalities not of sufficient degree for plus disease but demonstrating more arterial tortuosity and more venous dilatation than normal (1).
- Aggressive posterior ROP (AP-ROP) represents an uncommon, aggressive posterior ROP that is rapidly progressive (1).

DIAGNOSTIC TESTS & INTERPRETATION

Lab

Possible serum markers to monitor ROP include insulinlike growth factor 1 and insulinlike growth factor–binding protein 3.

Diagnostic Procedures/Surgery

- Infants with a birth weight <1,500 g or gestational age ≤30 weeks and selected infants with birth weight 1,500–2,000 g or gestational age >30 weeks with an unstable clinical course, including those requiring cardiorespiratory support, should have screening examinations performed after pupillary dilation using binocular indirect ophthalmoscopy (2)[A].
- Joint recommendations are for an initial eye examination between 4 and 6 weeks of chronologic age or between 31 and 33 weeks of postconceptional age (gestational age at birth plus chronologic age) (3)[B].
- The preceding joint statement had its limitations, and some patients would have been diagnosed with threshold disease at their initial examination if postconceptional age criteria from the joint statement had been followed. Analysis of the natural history data from the Multicenter Trial of Cryotherapy for Retinopathy of Prematurity (CRYO-ROP) and the Light Reduction in Retinopathy Study provided evidenced-based screening criteria and the following updated recommendations:
  - Eye examinations for infants at risk for ROP should commence at 31 weeks' postmenstrual age (gestational age at birth plus chronological age) for infants with a gestational age of less than 27 weeks and at 4 weeks' chronologic (postnatal) age for infants with a gestational age of 27 weeks or greater (4)[B].
  - Findings that suggest that acute-phase ROP screening may be curtailed include the following:
    - Infant's attainment of 45 weeks' postmenstrual age without the development of prethreshold ROP or worse
    - Progression of retinal vascularization into zone III without previous zone I or zone II ROP
    - Full retinal vascularization
    - Regression of ROP (2)[A]
- Longitudinal assessment of postnatal weight gain may help predict severity of ROP. Infants entered into a computer-based surveillance system, WINROP (weight, insulinlike growth factor, neonatal ROP). A persistent reduction in insulinlike growth factor (IGF-1) is associated with reduced postnatal weight gain and the subsequent development of ROP (5)[A].
- Follow-up examinations are performed until the retina is fully vascularized.
- Telemedicine using the RetCam may be more cost-effective than standard ophthalmoscopy for ROP management.

Pathological Findings

- Peripheral retinal nonperfusion
- Retinal neovascularization
- Retinal hemorrhages
- Retinal detachment

DIFFERENTIAL DIAGNOSIS

- Retinoblastoma
- Congenital cataracts
- Norrie disease
- Incontinentia pigmenti
- Familial exudative vitreoretinopathy
- Ocular toxocariasis
- Coats disease
- Persistent hyperplastic primary vitreous
- X-linked retinoschisis

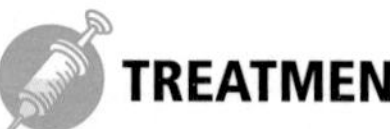

TREATMENT

MEDICATION

Vascular endothelial growth factor (VEGF) has been demonstrated in the subretinal fluid of patients with advanced ROP:

- Bevacizumab (Avastin) is a full-length antibody to VEGF that inhibits VEGF.
- There are case reports of the off-label intravitreal administration of Avastin in the treatment of ROP.
- The off-label administration of intravitreal bevacizumab demonstrated a significant benefit over conventional laser therapy for the treatment of stage 3+ ROP with zone I involvement (6)[C]:
  - ROP recurred in 4% of the bevacizumab-treated eyes and in 22% of eyes receiving standard laser treatment. The difference was statistically significant for zone I ROP, but not for zone II disease.
  - In addition peripheral retinal vessel development continued after bevacizumab administration; in contrast, there was permanent destruction of the peripheral retina with conventional laser therapy.

ADDITIONAL TREATMENT

General Measures

- The CRYO-ROP study demonstrated a favorable outcome for eyes treated at threshold vs. control eyes. Threshold ROP is defined as zone I or II, stage 3 (≥5 contiguous or 8 total clock hours with plus disease).
- Stage 3 retinopathy is defined as a ridge of extraretinal fibrovascular proliferation.
- A plus sign is added to the ROP stage number when retinal vascular tortuosity is noted in the posterior fundus.
- *Threshold disease* was defined as at least 5 contiguous or 8 cumulative clock hours of stage 3 associated with retinal vascular tortuosity in the posterior segment of the eye (plus disease) in zone I or II.
- When threshold disease is detected in infants, ablative therapy should be considered in at least 1 eye within 72 hours of diagnosis.
- The Early Treatment for Retinopathy of Prematurity (ETROP) study demonstrated that premature infants at high risk of vision loss from ROP retain better vision when therapy is administered early than when treatment is held until the traditional threshold (7)[A]:
  - In the ETROP study, patients received treatment with laser therapy, but cryotherapy also was allowed.
  - Eyes with high-risk prethreshold ROP or type 1 ROP were treated. Type 1 ROP was defined as zone I with any stage of ROP with plus disease (dilatation and tortuosity of posterior pole retinal vessels in at least 2 quadrants, usually ≥6 clock hours); zone I, stage 3 ROP without plus disease; or zone II, stage 2 or 3 ROP with plus disease.

- Serial examinations should be performed on eyes with prethreshold type 2 ROP, defined as zone I, stage 1 or 2 ROP without plus disease or zone II, stage 3 ROP without plus disease. Treatment should be considered for an eye with prethreshold type 2 ROP when progression to high-risk prethreshold type 1 ROP or threshold ROP occurs. Eyes with low-risk prethreshold type 2 ROP receive follow-up every 2–4 days for at least 2 weeks until the ROP regresses or progresses to high-risk prethreshold disease:
  - The risk of progression from type 2 ROP to type 1 ROP in <7 days is greatest between 33 and 36 weeks postmenstrual age, regardless of zone of retinopathy (8)[A].

SURGERY/OTHER PROCEDURES

- Transscleral cryotherapy to the avascular retina when applied to high-risk eyes may reduce the incidence of sight-threatening complications. The CRYO-ROP study has shown that treatment of high-risk eyes reduces the incidence of unfavorable outcomes by 46%.
- The results at 1 year from CRYO-ROP demonstrated an unfavorable outcome in 25.7% of eyes that received cryotherapy compared with 47.4% of control eyes.
- The results at 15 years from CRYO-ROP for retinopathy of prematurity demonstrated the following: Vision rated 20/200 or worse occurred in 44.7% of treated eyes vs. 64.3% of control eyes, and an unfavorable outcome for fundus status was found in 30% of treated eyes vs. 51.9% of control eyes.
- Laser treatment applied to the avascular retina in high-risk eyes may reduce the incidence of sight-threatening complications; cataract formation and serous retinal detachment are possible complications of laser treatment.
- Diode laser treatment is becoming the primary treatment modality because it may be better tolerated and probably results in better vision, less myopia, and less retinal dragging compared with eyes treated with cryotherapy.
- Threshold ROP had a reduced rate of progression in eyes with zone 2 disease when a dense, near-confluent pattern of diode laser treatment was applied vs. a less-dense pattern of diode laser treatment.
- After 10 years of follow-up, eyes treated with laser were 5.2 times more likely to have 20/50 or better vision than eyes treated with cryotherapy.
- Scleral buckling may reduce progression from stage 4 to stage 5 ROP. The encircling 240 band can be divided at 3 months after surgery if it is felt that the retina will remain attached.
- Vitrectomy and/or scleral buckling may be used to treat retinal detachment associated with ROP. Lens-sparing vitrectomy may be used to treat stage 4 ROP. Emphasis should be placed on prevention of retinal detachment in premature infants because of the poor visual outcome after a lensectomy/vitrectomy procedure for retinal detachment due to ROP.

IN-PATIENT CONSIDERATIONS

Initial Stabilization

Treatment usually is performed in the neonatal ICU or as an outpatient or inpatient as the child grows older.

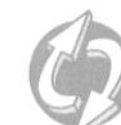

ONGOING CARE

FOLLOW-UP RECOMMENDATIONS

Patient Monitoring

- Close follow-up of patients with ROP is required.
- Eyes with low-risk prethreshold type 2 ROP receive follow-up every 2–4 days for at least 2 weeks until the ROP regresses or progresses to high-risk prethreshold type 1 ROP (7)[A].
- Schedule for follow-up examinations:
  - 1-week or less follow-up:
    - Stage 1 or 2 ROP: Zone I
    - Stage 3 ROP: Zone II
  - 1–2-week follow-up:
    - Immature vascularization: Zone I, no ROP
    - Stage 2 ROP: Zone II
    - Regressing ROP: Zone I
  - 2-week follow-up:
    - Stage 1 ROP: Zone II
    - Regressing ROP: Zone II
  - 2–3-week follow-up:
    - Immature vascularization: Zone II, no ROP
    - Stage 1 or 2 ROP: Zone III
    - Regressing ROP: Zone III (2)[A]
- In some cases of regressed ROP, cicatrization may develop and is associated with variable degrees of fibrosis. This may lead to vitreoretinal traction and subsequent retinal detachment from formation of a retinal hole.
- Retinal detachment secondary to cicatricial ROP may occur during the midteens; long-term follow-up of ROP cicatricial patients is indicated.

PROGNOSIS

- Spontaneous regression occurs over a period of weeks or months in most cases.
- Some cases of ROP do not regress spontaneously without sequelae, but rather progress. A gradual transition then occurs from active ROP to cicatricial ROP, which is associated with varying degrees of fibrosis and vitreoretinal traction that may lead to retinal detachment.
- ETROP study subjects at 6 years of age demonstrated that early treatment preserves peripheral vision and that there is only a small reduction in the extent of the visual field compared to eyes that underwent conventional management (9)[A].
- When compared to conventional management, early treatment for type 1 high-risk prethreshold eyes in subjects at 6 years of age had improved visual acuity outcomes (10)[A].

COMPLICATIONS

- Retinal detachment
- Retinal fold involving the macula
- Vitreous hemorrhage
- Angle-closure glaucoma
- Amblyopia
- Strabismus
- Myopia

REFERENCES

1. International Committee for the Classification of Retinopathy of Prematurity. The International Classification of Retinopathy of Prematurity revisited. *Arch Ophthalmol*. 2005;123:991–9.
2. Section on Ophthalmology American Academy of Pediatrics, American Academy of Ophthalmology, American Association for Pediatric Ophthalmology and Strabismus. Screening examination of premature infants for retinopathy of prematurity. *Pediatrics*. 2006;117:572–6. Erratum in: *Pediatrics* 2006;118:1324.
3. Screening examination of premature infants for retinopathy of prematurity: A joint statement of the American Academy of Pediatrics, the American Association for Pediatric Ophthalmology and Strabismus, and the American Academy of Ophthalmology. *Ophthalmol*. 1997;104:888–9.
4. Reynolds JD, Dobson V, Quinn GE, et al. Evidence-based screening criteria for retinopathy of prematurity: Natural history data from the CRYO-ROP and LIGHT-ROP studies. *Arch Ophthalmol*. 2002;120:1470–6.
5. Wu C, Vanderveen DK, Hellström A, et al. Longitudinal postnatal weight measurements for the prediction of retinopathy of prematurity. *Arch Ophthalmol*. 2010;128:443–7.
6. Mintz-Hittner HA, Kennedy KA, Chuang AZ, for the BEAT-ROP Cooperative Group. Efficacy of intraviteal bevacizumab for stage 3+ retinopathy of prematurity. *N Engl J Med*. 2011;364:603–15.
7. Early Treatment for Retinopathy of Prematurity Cooperative Group. Revised indications for the treatment of retinopathy of prematurity: Results of the early treatment for retinopathy of prematurity randomized trial. *Arch Ophthalmol*. 2003;121:1684–94.
8. Christiansen SP, Dobson V, et al. Progression of type 2 to type 1 retinopathy of prematurity in the Early Treatment for Retinopathy of Prematurity Study. *Arch Ophthalmol*. 2010;128:461–5.
9. Early Treatment for Retinopathy of Prematurity Cooperative Group. Visual field extent at 6 years of age in children who had high-risk prethreshold retinopathy of prematurity. *Arch Ophthalmol*. 2011;129:127–32.
10. The Early Treatment for Retinopathy of Prematurity Cooperative Group. Final visual acuity results in the early treatment for retinopathy of prematurity study. *Arch Ophthalmol*. 2010;128:663–71.

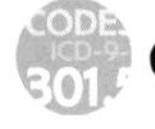

CODES

ICD9

- 362.20 Retinopathy of prematurity, unspecified
- 362.21 Retrolental fibroplasia
- 362.22 Retinopathy of prematurity, stage 0

CLINICAL PEARLS

- Infants with birth weight <1,500 g or gestational age ≤ 30 weeks and selected infants with birth weight 1,500–2,000 g or gestational age >30 weeks with an unstable clinical course should have retinal screening examinations performed after pupillary dilation using binocular indirect ophthalmoscopy.
- Diode laser treatment is becoming the primary treatment modality.
- The ETROP study demonstrated that premature infants at high risk of vision loss from ROP retain better vision when therapy is administered early than when treatment is held until the traditional threshold.

RETINOPATHY, DIABETIC

Richard W. Allinson, MD

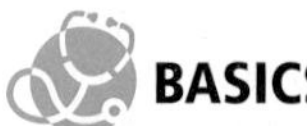

BASICS

DESCRIPTION

- Noninflammatory retinal disorder characterized by retinal capillary closure and microaneurysms. Retinal ischemia leads to release of a vasoproliferative factor stimulating neovascularization on retina, optic nerve, or iris.
- Most patients with diabetes mellitus (DM) will develop diabetic retinopathy (DR). It is the leading cause of new cases of legal blindness among residents in the US between the ages of 20 and 64 years.
- Diabetic retinopathy can be divided into 3 stages:
  - Nonproliferative (background) diabetic retinopathy
  - Severe nonproliferative (preproliferative) diabetic retinopathy
  - Proliferative diabetic retinopathy
- System(s) affected: Nervous

Geriatric Considerations

Prevalence will increase as population generally ages and patients with diabetes live longer.

Pregnancy Considerations

- Pregnancy can exacerbate condition.
- Pregnant diabetic women should be examined in first trimester, then every 3 months until delivery.

EPIDEMIOLOGY

Incidence

- Peak incidence of type I, juvenile-onset DM is between the ages of 12 and 15 years.
- Peak incidence of type II, adult-onset DM is between the ages of 50 and 70 years.
- Incidence of diabetic retinopathy is directly related to the duration of diabetes.
- <10 years of age, it is unusual to see diabetic retinopathy, regardless of DM duration.

Prevalence

- 6.6% of the US population between ages of 20 and 74 has DM.
- ~25% of the diabetic population has some form of diabetic retinopathy.
- Predominant age:
  - The risk increases after puberty.
  - 2/3 of juvenile-onset diabetics who have had DM for at least 35 years will develop proliferative diabetic retinopathy, and 1/3 will develop macular edema. Proportions are reversed for adult-onset diabetes.
- Predominant sex: Male = Female (juvenile-onset DM); Female > Male (type II)

RISK FACTORS

- Duration of DM (usually >10 years)
- Poor glycemic control
- Pregnancy
- Renal disease
- Systemic hypertension (HTN)
- Smoking
- Elevated lipid levels associated with increased risk of retinal lipid deposits (hard exudates)
- Myopic eyes have a lower risk of DR (1)[B].

GENERAL PREVENTION

- Monitor and control of blood glucose
- Schedule yearly ophthalmologic eye examinations.

ETIOLOGY

- Related to development of diabetic microaneurysms and microvascular abnormalities
- Reduction in perifoveal capillary blood flow velocity, perifoveal capillary occlusion, and increased retinal thickness at the central fovea in diabetic patients are associated with visual impairment in patients with diabetic macular edema.

COMMONLY ASSOCIATED CONDITIONS

- Glaucoma
- Cataracts
- Retinal detachment
- Vitreous hemorrhage
- Disc edema (diabetic papillopathy); may occur in type I or type II DM

DIAGNOSIS

HISTORY

Diabetic patients should be encouraged to undergo an annual ophthalmologic examination yearly, as early changes are asymptomatic.

PHYSICAL EXAM

- Eye examination: Measurement of visual acuity and documentation of the status of the iris, lens, vitreous, and fundus
- Nonproliferative (background) diabetic retinopathy:
  - Microaneurysms
  - Intraretinal hemorrhage
  - Macular edema causing decrease in central vision
  - Lipid deposits
- Severe nonproliferative (preproliferative) diabetic retinopathy:
  - Nerve fiber layer infarctions ("cotton wool spots")
  - Venous beading
  - Venous dilatation
  - Intraretinal microvascular abnormalities
  - Extensive retinal hemorrhage
- Proliferative diabetic retinopathy:
  - New blood vessel proliferation (neovascularization) on the retinal surface, optic nerve, and iris
  - Visual loss caused by vitreous hemorrhage, traction retinal detachment

DIAGNOSTIC TESTS & INTERPRETATION

Diagnostic Procedures/Surgery

- Fluorescein angiography demonstrates retinal nonperfusion, retinal leakage, and proliferative diabetic retinopathy.
- Optical coherence tomography (OCT) can be used to help detect diabetic macular edema by measuring retinal thickness.

Pathological Findings

- Increased capillary permeability
- Microaneurysms
- Hemorrhages in retina
- Exudates in retina
- Capillary nonperfusion

DIFFERENTIAL DIAGNOSIS

Other causes of retinopathy (e.g., radiation, retinal venous obstruction, HTN)

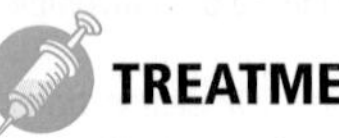

TREATMENT

MEDICATION

- Treatment with the angiotensin-receptor blocker candesartan has been shown to result in regression of diabetic retinopathy in some patients (2)[B].
- Under evaluation: Protein kinase C-β is activated by hyperglycemia and is associated with the development of vascular dysfunction. Inhibition of this enzyme could help to reduce the retinal vascular complications from DM.
- Nutritional antioxidant intake of vitamins C and E and of β-carotene has no protective effect on diabetic retinopathy.
- Atorvastatin may reduce the severity of lipid deposits with clinically significant diabetic macular edema in type II DM and dyslipidemia.

ADDITIONAL TREATMENT

General Measures

- The Diabetes Control and Complications Trial (DCCT) recommended that for most patients with insulin-dependent DM, blood glucose levels should be as close to the nondiabetic range as is safe to reduce the risk and rate of progression of diabetic retinopathy:
  - In the DCCT, insulin-dependent DM patients were randomly assigned into either conventional or intensive insulin treatment. Conventional treatment consisted of 1–2 daily insulin injections, with daily self-monitoring of urine or blood glucose. Intensive treatment consisted of insulin administered 3 or more times daily by injection or an external pump, with self-monitored blood glucose levels measured at least 4×/d.
  - The DCCT demonstrated that intensive insulin therapy reduced the risk of macular edema and retinal neovascularization. The benefit of intensive insulin therapy and the reduced risk of diabetic retinopathy–associated microvascular complications persist for at least 10 years (3)[A].

– In the DCCT, intensive insulin therapy was more effective in reducing the risk of progression of diabetic retinopathy in the less advanced stages. However, advanced diabetic retinopathy also benefited from the intensive insulin therapy.

- The Early Treatment Diabetic Retinopathy Study demonstrated that aspirin therapy did not prevent the development of proliferative diabetic retinopathy or reduce the risk of visual loss associated with diabetic retinopathy.
- Microvascular complications, including proliferative diabetic retinopathy, are increased when blood sugar levels ≥200 mg/dL.
- Poor glycemic control is associated with an increased risk both for developing diabetic retinopathy and its progression, regardless of the type of DM; that hyperglycemia itself is causative is not established, especially for type II DM.
- Cataracts are more common among those with DM. Try to delay cataract surgery in DM patients with retinopathy until the symptoms are severe; cataract surgery can cause retinopathy to worsen.
- HTN has a detrimental effect on diabetic retinopathy and must be controlled.

SURGERY/OTHER PROCEDURES

- Laser photocoagulation treatment: Recommended for patients with proliferative diabetic retinopathy and for those with clinically significant macular edema; destroys leaking blood vessels and areas of neovascularization.
- The Diabetic Retinopathy Study demonstrated that panretinal photocoagulation reduced overall rate of severe visual loss from 15.9% in untreated eyes to 6.4% in treated eyes. In certain subgroups, the incidence of severe visual loss in untreated eyes was as high as 36.9% within 2 years.
- The Early Treatment Diabetic Retinopathy Study demonstrated that eyes with significant diabetic macular edema benefited from focal laser treatment. Clinically significant diabetic macular edema (CSDME) is defined as:
  - Thickening of the retina within 500 μm of the center of the macula
  - Hard exudates within 500 μm of the center of the macula associated with thickening of the adjacent retina
  - Zone of retinal thickening 1 disc area or larger within 1 disc diameter of the center of the macula
- Patients with clinically significant diabetic macular edema and high-risk proliferative disease can have simultaneous focal and panretinal photocoagulation without adversely affecting the visual outcome.
- Vitrectomy may benefit some with diffuse macular edema. This may apply especially to eyes with vitreomacular traction found on OCT and with persistent clinically significant diabetic macular edema.
- Intravitreal triamcinolone may be used for DM-related macular edema that fails laser treatment. There is no long-term benefit of intravitreal triamcinolone relative to focal/grid photocoagulation in patients with CSDME. This is an off-label usage (4)[C].
- Ranibizumab, an antibody fragment that binds vascular endothelial growth factor (VEGF), can be used to treat CSDME when injected intravitreally. This is an off-label use (5)[B].
- Bevacizumab, a full-length antibody that binds VEGF, can be used to treat CSDME. This is an off-label use (6)[C].
- Preoperative bevacizumab can be used as an adjuvant to vitrectomy for complications of proliferative diabetic retinopathy. This is an off-label use:
  - At ~10 days postintravitreal injection of bevacizumab, the vascular component of proliferation is markedly reduced, and the contractile components are not yet very significant. Patients with dense fibrovascular proliferation need to be monitored closely for evidence of traction retinal detachment (7)[C].
- Cryoretinopexy can be used instead of laser treatment in certain patients to decrease the neovascular stimulus and treat proliferative diabetic retinopathy.
- Vitrectomy: Recommended for patients with severe proliferative diabetic retinopathy, traction retinal detachment involving the macula, and nonclearing vitreous hemorrhage.

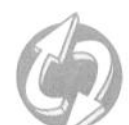

ONGOING CARE

FOLLOW-UP RECOMMENDATIONS

Patient Monitoring

Scheduled ophthalmologic eye examinations:

- Yearly follow-up if no retinopathy
- Every 6 months with background diabetic retinopathy
- At least every 3–4 months with preproliferative diabetic retinopathy
- Every 2–3 months with active proliferative diabetic retinopathy

DIET

Follow prescribed diet for patients with diabetes.

PATIENT EDUCATION

- Patient education should include regular ophthalmic examinations.
- Stress importance of strict blood glucose control through diet, exercise, drugs/insulin, and monitoring of blood glucose.

PROGNOSIS

If the condition is diagnosed and treated early in development, outlook is good. If treatment is delayed, blindness may result.

COMPLICATIONS

Blindness

REFERENCES

1. Lim LS, Lamoureux E, Saw SM, et al. Are myopic eyes less likely to have diabetic retinopathy? *Ophthalmology*. 2010;117:524–30.
2. Sjølie AK, Klein R, Porta M, et al. Effect of candesartan on progression and regression of retinopathy in type 2 diabetes (DIRECT-Protect 2): A randomised placebo-controlled trial. *Lancet*. 2008;372:1385–93.
3. White NH, Sun W, Cleary PA, et al. Prolonged effect of intensive therapy on the risk of retinopathy complications in patients with type 1 diabetes mellitus: 10 years after the Diabetes Control and Complications Trial. *Arch Ophthalmol*. 2008;126: 1707–15.
4. Diabetic Retinopathy Clinical Research Network (DRCR.net), Beck RW, Edwards AR, et al. Three-year follow-up of a randomized trial comparing focal/grid photocoagulation and intravitreal triamcinolone for diabetic macular edema. *Arch Ophthalmol*. 2009;127:245–51.
5. Nguyen QD, Shah SM, Khwaja AA, et al. Two-year outcomes of the ranibizumab for edema of the macula in diabetes (READ-2) study. *Ophthalmology*. 2010;117:2146–51.
6. Michaelides M, Kaines A, Hamilton RD, et al. A prospective randomized trial of intravitreal bevacizumab or laser therapy in the management of diabetic macular edema (BOLT Study): 12-month data: Report 2. *Ophthalmology*. 2010;117: 1078–86.
7. El-Sabagh HA, Abdelghaffar W, Labib AM, et al. Preoperative intravitreal bevacizumab use as an adjuvant to diabetic vitrectomy: Histopathologic findings and clinical implications. *Ophthalmology*. 2011;118:636–641.

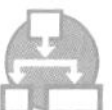

See Also (Topic, Algorithm, Electronic Media Element)

Diabetes Mellitus, Type 1; Diabetes Mellitus, Type 2.

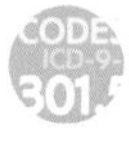

CODES

ICD9

- 250.50 Diabetes mellitus with ophthalmic manifestations, type II or unspecified type, not stated as uncontrolled
- 250.51 Diabetes mellitus with ophthalmic manifestations, type I (juvenile type) not stated as uncontrolled
- 362.01 Background diabetic retinopathy

CLINICAL PEARLS

- Options for the treatment of diffuse macular edema include focal laser treatment, intravitreal triamcinolone, intravitreal ranibizumab, intravitreal bevacizumab, and vitrectomy.
- High BP should be controlled to reduce the risk of diabetic eye complications.
- Blood glucose levels should be well controlled to help reduce the risk and rate of progression of diabetic retinopathy.
- Schedule yearly ophthalmologic eye examinations.

REYE SYNDROME

William A. Primack, MD

BASICS

DESCRIPTION

- An acute encephalopathy with cerebral edema and fatty infiltration of the liver
- Occurs in previously healthy children and is often associated with an antecedent viral infection such as varicella or influenza (1)[C]
- Markedly decreased in incidence since the late 1970s, when association with aspirin use was determined (2,3)[B]
- Most current cases are actually Reye-like syndrome caused by an inborn error of metabolism or toxin (see "Differential Diagnosis").
- System(s) affected: Gastrointestinal; Nervous
- Synonym(s): White liver disease

EPIDEMIOLOGY

Incidence

- Predominant age:
  - Infants, children, adolescents
  - Peak incidence at 6 years of age
  - Most cases between 4 and 12 years of age
- Predominant sex: Male = Female
- Currently very rare

RISK FACTORS

- Pediatric age group
- Rural and suburban areas
- Viral illnesses such as varicella and influenza A
- Use of preparations containing aspirin, salicylates, and/or salicylamides (4)[C]

Genetics

No known genetic pattern

GENERAL PREVENTION

- Avoid salicylates in children with viral illnesses because the drug appears to act as a cofactor in susceptible individuals.
- A physician should be consulted before giving any child aspirin or antinausea medicines during a viral illness, especially influenza A.
- Recognize early symptoms of the disease.

ETIOLOGY

Unknown; mitochondrion is major site of injury

DIAGNOSIS

Symptoms reflected in clinical staging system:

- I: Vomiting, sleepiness, lethargy
- II: Confusion, delirium, hyperpnea, irritability, combativeness, hyperreflexia, altered muscle tone
- III: Obtundation, light coma and seizures, decorticate rigidity, loss of oculocephalic reflexes, intact pupillary reflex
- IV: Coma, decerebrate posturing spontaneously or in response to painful stimuli, seizures, fixed pupils
- V: Coma, flaccid paralysis, loss of deep tendon reflexes, seizures, respiratory arrest, isoelectric EEG (2)[C]

HISTORY

- Recent aspirin use
- Sleepiness, lethargy, or confusion
- Vomiting

PHYSICAL EXAM

- Vital signs
- Complete physical exam, especially a thorough neurologic exam, to evaluate different criteria in the clinical staging system

DIAGNOSTIC TESTS & INTERPRETATION

Lab

- Hypoglycemia
- Severe elevations of aspartate aminotransferase/alanine aminotransferase
- Normal or slightly elevated bilirubin or alkaline phosphatase
- Elevated ammonia
- Prolonged prothrombin time: Often not responsive to vitamin K
- Mixed respiratory alkalosis and metabolic acidosis
- Hyperaminoacidemia (glutamine, alanine, lysine)

Diagnostic Procedures/Surgery

- Lumbar puncture with CSF pressure measurement: Increased CSF pressure without pleocytosis (<8 leukocytes/mm^3)
- Liver biopsy

Pathological Findings

- Slightly enlarged, firm, yellow liver with fat droplets throughout
- Characteristic liver biopsy (may need special preparation) shows foamy cytoplasm with microvesicular fat
- Uniformly severe mitochondrial injury

DIFFERENTIAL DIAGNOSIS

- Acute encephalopathy without hepatic abnormalities:
  - Encephalitis
  - Meningitis
  - Drug overdose
  - Poisoning
  - Psychiatric illness
  - Diabetes mellitus
- Reye-like syndrome: Acute toxic encephalopathy with hepatic abnormalities (4)[C] due to either metabolic disorders or drug or toxin ingestions, including:
  - Inherited metabolic disorders: Organic acidurias with defects in hepatic fatty acid oxidation; fatty acid metabolism defects
  - Acyl-CoA dehydrogenase, carnitine deficiency:
    - Urea cycle defects
    - Carbamyl phosphate synthetase, ornithine transcarbamylase
    - Fructosemia
  - The most commonly diagnosed metabolic disorder in association with Reye syndrome (RS) is medium-chain acyl coenzyme A dehydrogenase deficiency.
  - Drug ingestions: Valproate, aspirin
  - Toxin ingestions: Margosa oil, hopantenate, aflatoxin, hypoglycin (akee fruit; Jamaican vomiting sickness)

Pediatric Considerations

- It is essential to make the correct diagnosis, especially in infants <2 years of age.
- Rule out other causes of Reye-like syndrome (3,4)[C].

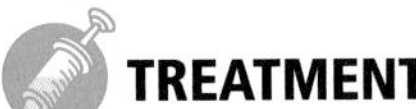

TREATMENT

MEDICATION

- All treatment is supportive and may include:
  - Glucose 10–15% IV
  - Vitamin K
  - For increased intracranial pressure:
    - Mannitol 0.5–1 g/kg IV as long as there is adequate urine output
    - Dexamethasone 0.5 mg/kg/d
    - Barbiturates
- Contraindications: Do not use mannitol if patient has no renal output.
- Precautions: Mannitol and poor renal output may result in vascular overload and pulmonary edema.
- Significant possible interactions: Refer to the manufacturers' literature.

ADDITIONAL TREATMENT

General Measures

- Supportive care dictated by the severity of illness
- IV glucose and frequent monitoring of serum glucose (to prevent severe hypoglycemia)
- Hyperventilation, mannitol, and barbiturates to reduce intracranial pressure (ICP)
- Minimization of noise and other CNS stimulation to prevent increases in ICP
- Vitamin K, fresh-frozen plasma, and platelets as needed
- Mechanical ventilation as needed
- Dialysis to reduce high ammonia levels and/or residual salicylate

SURGERY/OTHER PROCEDURES

Decompression craniotomy may be necessary.

IN-PATIENT CONSIDERATIONS

Initial Stabilization

Medical emergency requiring immediate hospitalization and frequent monitoring, often in an intensive care setting

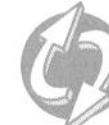

ONGOING CARE

FOLLOW-UP RECOMMENDATIONS

Complete bed rest

Patient Monitoring

Depends on specific residual effects; may require care of physicians, nurses, psychologists, and/or physical, occupational, and/or speech therapists

DIET

NPO during the acute phase

PATIENT EDUCATION

- National Reye Syndrome Foundation, P.O. Box 829, Byron, OH 43506-0829, (800) 233-7393; www.reyessyndome.org
- National Institutes of Health: www.ninds.nih.gov/disorders/reyes_syndrome/reyes_syndrome.htm

PROGNOSIS

- Overall prognosis is related to degree of cerebral edema and ammonia level on admission.
- Outcomes range from a mild illness without progression and complete resolution to a critical illness with significant lasting sequelae.
- Possible neurologic sequelae include brain damage and disability, including problems with attention, concentration, speech, language, and fine and gross motor skills.
- Sequelae are more common with higher stages.

COMPLICATIONS

- Aspiration pneumonia
- Respiratory failure
- Cardiac dysrhythmia/arrest
- Inappropriate vasopressin excretion
- Diabetes insipidus
- Cerebral edema
- Seizures
- Death

REFERENCES

1. Schror K. Aspirin and Reye syndrome: A review of the evidence. *Pediatr Drugs*. 2007;9:195–204.
2. Monto AS. The disappearance of Reye's syndrome–a public health triumph. *N Engl J Med*. 1999;340:1423–4.
3. Belay ED, Bresee JS, Holman RC, et al. Reye's syndrome in the United States from 1981 through 1997. *N Engl J Med*. 1999;340:1377–82.
4. Glasgow JF, Middleton B. Reye syndrome–insights on causation and prognosis. *Arch Dis Child*. 2001; 85:351–3.

ADDITIONAL READING

- Gosalakkal JA, Kamoji V. Reye syndrome and Reye-like syndrome. *Pediatr Neurol*. 2008;39: 198–200.
- Green A, Hall SM. Investigation of metabolic disorders resembling Reye's syndrome. *Arch Dis Child*. 1992;67:1313–7.
- Pugliese A, Beltramo T, Torre D, et al. Reye's and Reye's-like syndromes. *Cell Biochem Funct*. 2008;26: 741–6.

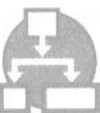

See Also (Topic, Algorithm, Electronic Media Element)

Encephalitis, Viral; Hepatic Encephalopathy

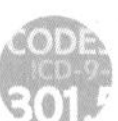

CODES

ICD9

331.81 Reye's syndrome

CLINICAL PEARLS

- RS is a rare acute metabolic encephalopathy largely affecting children and adolescents.
- Associations include antecedent viral infection and aspirin use.
- Most current cases of RS are actually Reye-like syndrome, caused by an inborn error of metabolism or a toxin.
- All treatment is supportive.
- Prognosis is related to the degree of cerebral edema and ammonia level on admission, and ranges from complete resolution to persistent neurologic sequelae.

RH INCOMPATIBILITY

Donald A.F. Nelson, MD

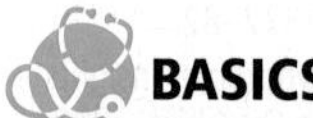

BASICS

DESCRIPTION

- Antibody-mediated destruction of RBCs that bear Rh surface antigens in individuals who lack the antigens and have become isoimmunized (sensitized) to them
- System(s) affected: Hematologic/Lymphatic/Immunologic
- Synonym(s): Rh isoimmunization; Rh alloimmunization; Rh sensitization

EPIDEMIOLOGY

Incidence

Predominant age and sex: Affects fetuses/neonates of isoimmunized child-bearing females

RISK FACTORS

- Of white population, 15% and smaller fractions of other races are Rh-negative and susceptible to sensitization (1).
- Any Rh-positive pregnancy in an Rh-negative woman can result in sensitization.
- Native risk of isoimmunization after Rh-positive pregnancy had been estimated to be ≤15%, but it seems to be decreasing.
- The risk of isoimmunization antepartum is only 1–2%.
- The risk of isoimmunization is 1–2% after spontaneous abortion and 4–5% after induced abortion (2).
- Use of Rho(D) immunoglobulin prophylaxis has reduced incidence of isoimmunization to <1% of susceptible pregnancies.

Genetics

- Complex autosomal inheritance of polypeptide Rh antigens; 3 genetic loci with closely related genes carry an assortment of alleles: Dd, Cc, and Ee (3).
- Individuals who express the D antigen (also called *Rho* or *Rho[D]*) or its weak D (D^u) variant are considered Rh-positive. Individuals lacking the D antigen are Rh-negative. (There is no antigen identified with the d allele.)
- Another variant D antigen, DEL, has been identified in some individuals (predominantly Asians) who are classified as Rh-negative by the usual assays. While testing Rh-negative, these individuals are not likely to be sensitized by exposure to Rh-D antigens by pregnancy or transfusion (4).
- Antibodies may be produced to C, c, D, E, or e in individuals lacking the specific antigen; only D is strongly immunogenic (5).
- Isoimmunization to Rh antigens in susceptible individuals is acquired, not inherited.

GENERAL PREVENTION

- Blood typing (ABO and Rh) on all pregnant women and prior to blood transfusions
- Antibody screening early in pregnancy
- Rh immunoglobulin prevents only sensitization to the D antigen.
- For prophylaxis, Rho(D) immunoglobulin (RhIG, RhoGAM, HyperRHO, RHOphylac) given to unsensitized, Rh-negative women after the following:
  - Spontaneous abortion
  - Induced abortion
  - Ectopic pregnancy
  - Antepartum hemorrhage
  - Trauma to abdomen
  - Amniocentesis
  - Chorionic villus sampling
  - Routinely at 28 weeks' gestation
  - Within 72 h of delivery of an Rh-positive infant
- Dose for prophylaxis:
  - 50-μg dose for events up to 12 weeks' gestation
  - 300-μg dose for events after 12 weeks' gestation
  - Higher doses may be required in the event of a large fetal–maternal hemorrhage (>30 mL of whole blood).

PATHOPHYSIOLOGY

- Circulating antibodies to Rh antigens (transplacentally transferred antibodies in the case of a fetus/newborn) attach to Rh antigens on RBCs.
- Immune-mediated destruction of RBCs leads to hemolysis, anemia, and increased bilirubin production.

ETIOLOGY

- Transfusion of Rh-positive blood to Rh-negative recipient
- Maternal exposure to fetal Rh antigens, either antepartum or intrapartum
- Most commonly seen in the Rh-positive fetus or infant of an Rh-negative mother

COMMONLY ASSOCIATED CONDITIONS

- Hemolytic disease of newborn
- Hydrops fetalis
- Neonatal jaundice
- Kernicterus
- See "Erythroblastosis Fetalis" topic.

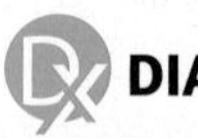

DIAGNOSIS

PHYSICAL EXAM

- Jaundice of newborn
- Kernicterus
- Fetal hydrops or fetal death in utero if severe (see "Erythroblastosis Fetalis" topic)

DIAGNOSTIC TESTS & INTERPRETATION

Lab

Initial lab tests

- Positive indirect Coombs test (antibody screen) during pregnancy
- Paternal blood type
- Kleihauer-Betke (fetal hemoglobin acid elution, Hb F slide elution) test to quantify an acute fetal–maternal bleed
- Congenital or fetal anemia
- Blood type, direct Coombs test in newborn

Follow-Up & Special Considerations

Prior administration of IgD may lead to weakly (false-) positive indirect Coombs test in mother and direct Coombs test in infant.

DIFFERENTIAL DIAGNOSIS

- ABO incompatibility
- Other blood group (non-Rh) isoimmunization
- Nonimmune fetal hydrops
- Hereditary spherocytosis
- RBC enzyme defects

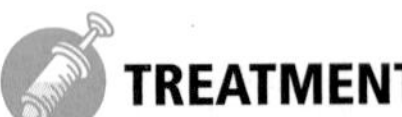

TREATMENT

ADDITIONAL TREATMENT

General Measures

- Depending on severity of involvement, treatment of fetus may include:
  - Intrauterine transfusion
  - Early delivery
- Treatment of newborn may include:
  - Exchange transfusion
  - Transfusion after delivery
  - Phototherapy
  - Diuretics and digoxin for hydrops
  - Immunoglobulin infusion has reduced the need for exchange transfusion in a few studies (6)[A].

Issues for Referral

Because of the specialized, somewhat hazardous treatment measures involved, pregnancies in Rh-sensitized women are usually managed at tertiary-care level.

IN-PATIENT CONSIDERATIONS

Initial Stabilization

Initial monitoring of the newborn is inpatient or in special care nursery if treatment interventions are needed.

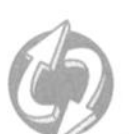

ONGOING CARE

FOLLOW-UP RECOMMENDATIONS

Patient Monitoring

- In most cases, outpatient ambulatory management is appropriate during the antepartum period.
- Antibody titer measured at 20 weeks and every 4 weeks thereafter during pregnancy; a titer of ≥1:16 indicates the need for further testing (3).
- If the patient had a previously affected infant, an Rh-positive fetus in the current pregnancy should be considered at risk regardless of antibody titers (7):
  - Fetal heart rate testing/ultrasonography to assess fetal status
  - Doppler ultrasonography measurement of cerebral blood flow is now a suitable alternative to invasive tests (amniocentesis, cordocentesis) for diagnosing fetal anemia (7).
  - Umbilical blood sampling (cordocentesis) for fetal blood type, hematocrit, reticulocyte count, and presence of erythroblasts (3).
  - Amniocentesis for amniotic fluid bilirubin levels (3).
  - Amniocentesis for fetal lung maturity if early delivery is a treatment option (3).

PROGNOSIS

- With appropriate monitoring and treatment, infants born of severely affected pregnancies have a survival rate of >80% (3).
- Fetuses with hydrops have a higher mortality rate.
- Even with severe disease, the neurologic outcome of survivors is generally good.
- Disease is likely to be more severe in affected subsequent pregnancies.

COMPLICATIONS

- Pregnancy loss from umbilical blood sampling
- Pregnancy loss from intrauterine transfusion
- Fetal distress requiring emergent delivery (3)

REFERENCES

1. Bianchi DW, Avent ND, Costa JM, et al. Noninvasive prenatal diagnosis of fetal Rhesus D: Ready for Prime(r) Time. *Obstet Gynecol*. 2005;106:841–4.
2. Bowman J. Thirty-five years of Rh prophylaxis. *Transfusion*. 2003;43:1661–6.
3. Management of alloimmunization during pregnancy. ACOG Practice Bulletin. 75. Aug 2006, reaffirmed 2008.
4. Shao C, Xu H, Xu Q, et al. Antenatal Rh prophylaxis is unnecessary for "Asia type" DEL women. *Transfus Clin Biol*. 2010;17:260–4.
5. Agre P, Cartron JP. Molecular biology of the Rh antigens. *Blood*. 1991;78:551–63.
6. Alcock GS, Liley H. Immunoglobulin infusion for isoimmune haemolytic jaundice in neonates. *Cochrane Database Syst Rev*. 2006;1.
7. Moise KJ. Management of rhesus alloimmunization in pregnancy. *Obstet Gynecol*. 2008;112:164–76.

ADDITIONAL READING

Prevention of Rh D alloimmunization. ACOG Practice Bulletin 4. May 1999, reaffirmed 2009.

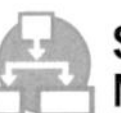

See Also (Topic, Algorithm, Electronic Media Element)

Anemia, Autoimmune Hemolytic; Erythroblastosis Fetalis; Jaundice

CODES

ICD9

- 656.11 Rhesus isoimmunization, delivered, with or without mention of antepartum condition
- 656.13 Rhesus isoimmunization, antepartum condition or complication
- 773.0 Hemolytic disease of fetus or newborn due to Rh isoimmunization

CLINICAL PEARLS

- If paternity is certain, determining that the father does not carry the Rh(D) blood group antigen eliminates the need to give RhIG prophylaxis during pregnancy or the need for special fetal surveillance if the mother is already sensitized.
- Attempts have been made to determine the fetal blood type noninvasively by detecting fetal DNA in the maternal blood. Because Rh antigens are polymorphic among racial groups, this technique has both false-positive and false-negative results and should be considered experimental.
- The weak D antigen, formerly called D^u, is a weakly reacting variant of the D antigen. A "weak D–positive" mother or infant should be managed as any other D-positive mother or infant, respectively.
- The dose of RhIG for prophylaxis is affected by gestational age. The fetal blood volume is only a few milliliters at 12 weeks' gestation. Therefore, a 50-μg dose of RhIG may be used for threatened, spontaneous, or induced abortions up to 12 weeks' gestation instead of the standard 300-μg dose.

RHABDOMYOLYSIS

Caroline Tschibelu, MD
Joao Tavares, MD

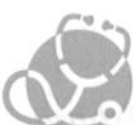

BASICS

DESCRIPTION

- Breakdown of skeletal muscle cells and release of intracellular contents into the circulation
- Rhabdomyolysis typically manifests with muscle aches, pains and weakness, and reddish brown (tea-colored) urine, but up to 50% of patients are asymptomatic.

EPIDEMIOLOGY

Incidence

Annually in the US: 26,000 hospitalized cases

RISK FACTORS

See "Etiology."

Genetics

- Hereditary causes of rhabdomyolysis are rare but should be suspected for children, patients with recurrent attacks, or patients who have attacks after minimal exertion, mild illness, or starvation.
- The main inherited disorders are described below in "Etiology."

GENERAL PREVENTION

- Avoid excessive exertional muscle injury. Preventing hypovolemia is important to prevent renal hypoperfusion, acidemia, and subsequent renal failure.
- Avoid precipitating drugs, metabolic and electrolyte abnormalities.

ETIOLOGY

- Direct muscle trauma (most common cause):
  - Crush injuries
  - Extended periods of muscle pressure (during surgery, unconscious from alcohol ingestion)
  - Burns, electrocution, lightning strike
- Muscle exertion:
  - Intense and/or prolonged physical exercise (marathon runners, athletes, contact sports)
  - Seizures
  - Delirium tremens
- Drugs and toxins:
  - Alcohol
  - Cocaine (most common recreational drug), methamphetamine, phencyclidine
  - Antipsychotics (due to neuroleptic malignant syndrome, malignant hyperthermia, and severe dystonia)
  - Zidovudine
  - Antimalarials
  - Heroin
  - HMG-CoA reductase inhibitors (statins) (risk <0.01%), higher with high dose and in combination with fibrates
  - Fibrates
  - Colchicine
  - Corticosteroids
  - Carbon monoxide
  - Snake envenomation
- Muscle ischemia:
  - Thrombosis, embolism, sickle cell disease
  - Compartment syndrome
  - Tourniquets
- Infections:
  - Viral: Influenza A and B, coxsackievirus, HIV, varicella
  - Bacterial: *Streptococcus* or *Staphylococcus* sepsis, gas gangrene, necrotizing fasciitis, *Salmonella, Legionella*
  - Malaria
- Hypothermia
- Hyperthermia:
  - Heat stroke
  - Neuroleptic malignant syndrome
  - Malignant hyperthermia
- Autoimmune and genetic disorders:
  - Polymyositis, dermatomyositis
  - Muscular dystrophies
  - Disorders of lipid metabolism (e.g., carnitine palmitoyltransferase deficiency and carnitine deficiency)
  - Disorders of carbohydrate metabolism (i.e., phosphofructokinase deficiency, phosphoglycerate mutase, myophosphorylase deficiency, aka McArdle disease/deficiency)
  - Glycogen storage diseases (e.g., phosphorylase B kinase deficiency) and others (e.g., lactate dehydrogenase A deficiency)
- Metabolic and endocrinologic:
  - Hypothyroidism or thyrotoxicosis
  - Electrolyte imbalances (e.g., hyponatremia, hypernatremia, hypokalemia, hypocalcemia, hypophosphatemia)
  - Diabetic ketoacidosis
  - Hyperosmolar state

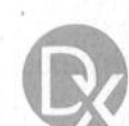

DIAGNOSIS

HISTORY

- Crush injury: Direct trauma, prolonged compression or immobility. Causes include MVA, entrapment in collapsed buildings. The elderly are more susceptible to crush injury due to immobility and falls. Rhabdomyolysis usually occurs after 1 hour of immobilization, but cases reported with compression lasting <20 minutes.
- Possible history of overexertion or use of drug or toxin (e.g., cocaine, amphetamine, statins)
- Patient may complain of muscle aches, cramps, or fatigue.

PHYSICAL EXAM

- May have obvious muscle tenderness or injury and swelling on exam (e.g., crush injury, compartment syndrome), or muscle exam may be completely normal
- Tea-colored urine is indicative of myoglobinuria.
- Decreased urine output may indicate renal failure.

DIAGNOSTIC TESTS & INTERPRETATION

Lab

Initial lab tests

- CK is the most important diagnostic enzyme: elevated >5 times the upper limit of normal or >1,000 units/L. CK levels >5,000 units/L are causally related to acute renal failure (ARF) (1) and should prompt aggressive fluid resuscitation. Other elevated muscle enzymes are aldolase and lactic dehydrogenase [LDH]).
- CK levels peak at ~24 hours and return to normal after 3–5 days, making it a more sensitive marker than myoglobin. CK is also a cheaper and easier surrogate than myoglobin. Myoglobin, however, is the enzyme responsible for kidney failure (1).
- Serum myoglobin levels peak within a few hours and return to normal after ~24 hours as it is cleared quickly from the circulation. Urine or serum myoglobin levels may be useful markers early on, but normal levels do not rule out rhabdomyolysis because of its rapid clearance.
- Urinalysis: Dipstick test positive for blood without erythrocytes in sediment is suggestive of injury from either hemoglobin or myoglobin. However, rhabdomyolysis often presents with hematuria, which is a limitation to using dipstick due to false-positive results.
- Marked elevations of potassium from the muscle injury sometimes are compounded by ARF.
- Initial hypocalcemia: Calcium enters the injured muscle cells and precipitates as calcium phosphate leading to calcification of ischemic muscle cells. Only correct initial hypocalcemia if patient is symptomatic/has EKG changes; it will self-resolve during the renal recovery phase.
- Hypercalcemia during renal recovery phase: Unique to rhabdomyolysis-induced ARF for 20–30% of patients (2). As renal function improves, there is mobilization of the precipitated calcium, increase in calcitriol, and hyperphosphatemia resolves.
- Extreme hyperuricemia may be present and can cause acute uric acid nephropathy in the setting of rhabdomyolysis.
- Elevations in BUN and creatinine are indicative of acute renal failure.
- Reversible hepatic dysfunction can occur. However, elevations in ALT, AST, and LDH may be due to muscle injury and may not indicate any hepatic injury.
- Disseminated intravascular coagulation (DIC) can occur, with increase in coagulation times, fibrin degradation products, and D-dimer; decreases in platelets and fibrinogen.

Follow-Up & Special Considerations

- Delayed renal failure or electrolyte abnormalities despite normal initial levels
- Ongoing muscle injury is manifested by rising creatine phosphokinase (CPK).

Imaging

Initial approach

No routine approach

Follow-Up & Special Considerations

Any renal imaging is similar to other evaluations of acute renal failure.

Diagnostic Procedures/Surgery

Muscle compartment pressures if compartment syndrome suspected

Pathological Findings

- Muscle necrosis
- Myoglobin-related renal injury may resemble acute tubular necrosis from other causes.

DIFFERENTIAL DIAGNOSIS

- For acute renal failure with rhabdomyolysis: Any disease that causes acute tubular necrosis may be confused with rhabdomyolysis.
- Renal pigment injury from hemoglobin resembles pigment injury from myoglobin.

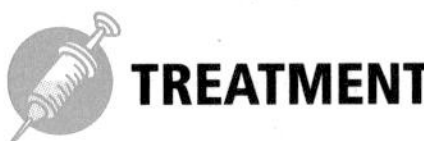

TREATMENT

MEDICATION

First Line

- When rhabdomyolysis is identified, appropriate intervention may prevent renal failure.
- Aggressive fluid resuscitation is the most important intervention: Normal saline (NS) and 5% glucose solution with a target urine output of 200 mL/hr. Alternating NS and 5% glucose is recommended to prevent volume overload. Infusion rate should be 500 mL/hr (3).
- Alkalinization of the urine is thought to decrease myoglobin-induced nephrotoxicity in the tubules (sodium bicarbonate to increase urine pH >6.5):
  - Use is controversial without strong evidence of efficacy
  - Side effects include worsening hypocalcemia.
  - Sodium bicarbonate may be of use in patients with very high CK levels, an acidotic state, or coexisting hyperkalemia.
- IV mannitol as a bolus, 1–2 g/kg, not to exceed 200 g in 24 hours and cumulative dose up to 800 g. It is used by some to prevent ARF. Plasma osmolality should be closely monitored and stopped if diuresis is not adequate (>20 mL/hr):
  - Causes renal vasodilation and diuresis, making the kidneys less susceptible to myoglobin injury. As an osmotic agent, may also remove fluids trapped in damaged muscle cells preventing rise in compartment pressure and potential compartment syndrome.
  - Use of mannitol is controversial in this setting because there is no good evidence that it improves outcomes more than aggressive IV hydration. Doses >800 g associated with osmotic nephrosis (acute kidney injury due to renal vasoconstriction and tubular injury).
  - Consider adding furosemide to force diuresis if necessary (40–120 mg/d) .
  - Diuresis should not be used in anuric renal failure. Customize the regimen for elderly and patients with heart disease.

Second Line

- Hyperkalemia can result from massive release of intracellular potassium stores or acute renal failure. Severe hyperkalemia may be life threatening. Treatment is warranted when ECG changes are present (tall, thin T waves; P-R prolongation; QRS widening; P-wave flattening).
- Treatments aiming at resolving hyperkalemia:
  - Calcium gluconate: To stabilize the cardiac membrane. IV 1–2 ampules (0.5 mL 10% calcium gluconate = 4 mg elemental calcium; give 4 mg/kg/hr × 4 hours)
  - If acidosis is present: 1–2 ampules (2–3 mL/kg) sodium bicarbonate IV. Remember that bicarbonate administration may lead to alkalosis and worsening hypocalcemia.
  - If tolerated: Oral sodium polystyrene sulfonate (Kayexalate) as much as 20 g (1 g/kg); also can be given via enema if oral intake is not tolerated or not indicated.
  - Insulin and albuterol will transiently drive potassium into the cells. Administration of glucose can prevent the hypoglycemic effects of insulin.
  - Precautions: See "Etiology," especially drug combinations. Continuous monitoring of potassium levels to prevent overcorrecting with potential hypokalemia and arrhythmias.
  - Indications for dialysis include resistant and symptomatic hyperkalemia (EKG), oliguria (<0.5 mL/kg over 12-hour period), anuria, volume overload, or persistent acidosis (PH <7.1).

ADDITIONAL TREATMENT

General Measures

- Aggressive hydration is often necessary. With severe muscle trauma (crush injuries), up to 12 L of fluid may be sequestered in the muscles, leading to intravascular volume depletion and explaining the low urine output despite fluid resuscitation. Those increase the risk for renal failure.
- Monitor CK levels to ensure that rhabdomyolysis has ended.
- Monitor renal function and electrolytes.
- Continuous monitoring of potassium levels to prevent hyperkalemic arrhythmias and potential hypokalemia and arrhythmias.
- If DIC or hepatic dysfunction occurs, patients will need treatment and monitoring appropriate to these conditions.

Issues for Referral

- Usually managed as an inpatient
- Diagnosis of muscle entrapment or compartment syndromes may require surgical intervention (fasciotomy) to stop rhabdomyolysis
- Early escharotomy for compartment syndrome related to burn
- Renal dialysis may be indicated in ARF.

Additional Therapies

Severe hypocalcemia with symptoms (perioral paresthesia, Chvostek and Trousseau signs present) during the oliguric phase may benefit from IV calcium gluconate. Symptomatic hypocalcemia is rare.

SURGERY/OTHER PROCEDURES

For muscle entrapment or compartment syndrome

IN-PATIENT CONSIDERATIONS

Admission Criteria

- Patients with significant elevations of CK should be admitted for IV hydration and serial laboratory monitoring.
- Usually required for symptomatic patients or other complications

IV Fluids

Volume expansion with normal saline to increase urine output to at least 150 mL/hr

Nursing

Monitoring of vital signs and urine output

Discharge Criteria

CK usually peaks 24–36 hours after muscle injury, so monitoring should confirm that the CK is trending down. Renal function should be stable or improving. Electrolytes should be normal. Patients with mild CK elevation, trending down, and normal renal function may be discharged after observation phase.

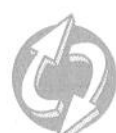

ONGOING CARE

FOLLOW-UP RECOMMENDATIONS

Outpatient assessment within a few days to recheck CPK, electrolytes, and renal function

Patient Monitoring

- Contingent on disease: Essential for metabolic myopathies
- Myotoxic drugs should be discontinued or monitored closely.

DIET

- When rhabdomyolysis causes renal failure, restrict protein intake to lower BUN level.
- Potassium intake must be limited.
- With anuria, essential to restrict volume intake; once resolved, no restrictions

PROGNOSIS

Contingent on primary cause of rhabdomyolysis and on recovery from ARF without complications

COMPLICATIONS

- Death, especially from hyperkalemia or renal failure
- With dialysis and supportive care, the prognosis is very good.

REFERENCES

1. Huerta-Alardín AL, Varon J, Marik PE, et al. Bench-to-bedside review: Rhabdomyolysis—an overview for clinicians. *Crit Care*. 2005;9:158–69.
2. Bosch X, Poch E, Grau JM. Rhabdomyolysis and acute kidney injury. *N Engl J Med*. 2009;361: 62–72.
3. Cervellin G, Comelli I, Lippi G. Rhabdomyolysis: Historical background, clinical, diagnostic and therapeutic features. *Clin Chem Lab Med*. 2010;48: 749–56.

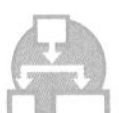

See Also (Topic, Algorithm, Electronic Media Element)

Renal Failure, Acute

CODES

ICD9

728.88 Rhabdomyolysis

CLINICAL PEARLS

- Acute CPK elevation into the thousands (often tens of thousands) is necessary before one sees myoglobinuric renal failure.
- The cornerstone of treatment of rhabdomyolysis is aggressive fluid administration.
- Frequent monitoring of potassium, calcium, and creatinine is necessary in the acute period.

RHABDOMYOSARCOMA

Richard Hinds, MD
Richard Terek, MD

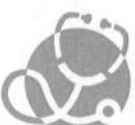

BASICS

DESCRIPTION

- Rhabdomyosarcoma (RMS) is the most common soft tissue sarcoma in patients younger than 20 years of age. Overall, it is a relatively uncommon malignancy that arises from embryonal skeletal muscle (mesenchymal) cells.
- Common anatomic sites:
  - Head and neck
  - Genitourinary
  - Musculoskeletal
- Subtypes:
  - Alveolar (ARMS): Comprises 21% of all cases of RMS
  - Embryonal (ERMS): Early onset. Comprises 59% of all cases of RMS:
    - Classic: Comprises 50% of all cases of RMS
    - Botryoid: Sarcoma botryoids is typically seen in girls <4 years of age. Comprises 6% of all RMS
    - Spindle cell: Comprises 3% of all cases of RMS
  - Pleomorphic: Usually occurs in adults. Comprises 1% of all cases of RMS
  - Sarcoma (not otherwise specified): Comprises 11% of all cases of RMS
  - Undifferentiated: Comprises 8% of all cases of RMS
- Associated term(s): Soft tissue sarcoma

EPIDEMIOLOGY

Incidence

4.5 cases of RMS per 1,000,000 patients younger than 20 years of age per year (1)[A]

Prevalence

- RMS comprises 3% of all childhood cancers.
- 59% of RMS occurs in males.

RISK FACTORS

Most cases are sporadic.

Genetics

- Alveolar: *PAX3-FOXO1* or *PAX7-FOXO1* fusion genes as a result of t(2;13) and t(1;13), respectively; found in 80% of ARMS (2)[B]
- Embryonal: Loss of alleles on chromosome 11 may be seen.

COMMONLY ASSOCIATED CONDITIONS

- Neurofibromatosis (NF) 1: 20-fold increased risk of RMS in patients with NF1
- Li-Fraumeni syndrome: p53 mutations predispose to multiple tumors, including RMS
- Some congenital defects

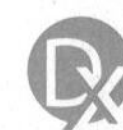

DIAGNOSIS

HISTORY

- May present as a nontender mass of the head and neck, genitourinary tissue, trunk, or extremities; often a nonspecific presentation.
- RMS of genitourinary tissue may present as vaginal bleeding in females.
- Other symptoms may be noted due to mass effect of the primary or metastatic lesions.

PHYSICAL EXAM

- Painless, enlarging mass
- Exophthalmos
- Abdominal pain

DIAGNOSTIC TESTS & INTERPRETATION

- Staging: Based on site, size, regional nodal involvement and distance spread (3)[A]
- Treatment is determined by clinical grouping:
  - Group I: Localized disease, completely resected
  - Group II: Total gross resection with evidence of regional spread:
    - A: Grossly resected tumor with microscopic residual disease
    - B: Regional disease with involved nodes, completely resected with no microscopic residual disease
    - C: Regional disease with involved nodes, grossly resected but with evidence of microscopic residual disease and/or histologic involvement of the most distal regional node in the dissection
  - Group III: Incomplete resection with gross residual disease
  - Group IV: Distant metastatic disease present at onset

Imaging

Initial approach

- Ultrasound: Used for differentiation of cystic vs. solid mass.
- MRI: Used to evaluate extent of primary tumor.
- Staging test: Total body bone scan, chest CT scan, FDG positron emission tomography (4)[B]

Diagnostic Procedures/Surgery

- Open biopsy of primary and regional lymph nodes, bone marrow biopsy:
  - The presence of rhabdomyoblast indicates the diagnosis.
- Immunohistochemical markers (5)[B]:
  - Myogenin: Commonly expressed in ARMS
  - Desmin: Associated with multiple subtypes of RMS

Pathological Findings

- Alveolar: Rhabdomyoblasts arranged in what grossly appears to mimic pulmonary alveoli
- Embryonal:
  - Classic: Rhabdomyoblasts configured in sheets without alveolar pattern
  - Botryoid: "Grape like" appearance of rhabdomyoblasts with notable clustering in the subepithelium forming the cambium layer
  - Spindle cell: Rhabdomyoblasts with a spindlelike appearance
- Undifferentiated: Rhabdomyoblast arrangement that cannot be classified as any other subtype

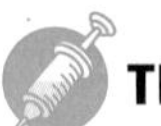

TREATMENT

The 3 tenets of treatment consist of surgical resection, radiation therapy, and chemotherapy. Patients should be referred to a multidisciplinary treatment team with expertise in pediatric oncology for definitive treatment.

MEDICATION

- Multiagent chemotherapy typically consists of the standard agents vincristine, dactinomycin, and cyclophosphamide (6)[B]:
  - Vincristine:
    - Adverse reactions: Alopecia, constipation, peripheral neuropathy
  - Actinomycin-D:
    - Adverse reactions: Pancytopenia, hepatotoxicity
  - Cyclophosphamide:
    - Adverse reactions: Hemorrhagic cystitis, sterility, transitional cell carcinoma
- In addition, ifosfamide, doxorubicin, etoposide, and irinotecan may also be used.
- Duration of chemotherapy is ~1 year.

ADDITIONAL TREATMENT

Radiation therapy:

- May be given for primary tumor and/or metastatic sites

SURGERY/OTHER PROCEDURES

Surgery:

- Wide resection of primary tumor and metastatic sites is ideal. However, wide resection may not be feasible in cases where grossly impaired functionality results.

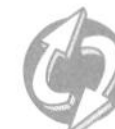

ONGOING CARE

FOLLOW-UP RECOMMENDATIONS

Patients should follow up with their multidisciplinary treatment team. Long-term follow up is necessary for detection of recurrence, metastatic disease, and development of secondary malignancies. Follow-up consists of physical exam, chest x-ray, and imaging of the primary tumor site.

PROGNOSIS

- RMS (all cases): 62% 5-year survival (1)[A]
- ARMS: 48% 5-year survival
- ERMS: 73% 5-year survival

COMPLICATIONS

- Recurrence
- Secondary neoplasm
- Growth abnormalities
- Treatment side effects

REFERENCES

1. Ognjanovic S, Linabery AM, Charbonneau B, et al. Trends in childhood rhabdomyosarcoma incidence and survival in the United States, 1975–2005. *Cancer*. 2009;115(18):4218–26.
2. Wexler LH, Ladanyi M, et al. Diagnosing alveolar rhabdomyosarcoma: Morphology must be coupled with fusion confirmation. *J Clin Oncol*. 2010;28: 2126–8.
3. Meza JL, Anderson J, Pappo AS, et al. Analysis of prognostic factors in patients with nonmetastatic rhabdomyosarcoma treated on intergroup rhabdomyosarcoma studies III and IV: The Children's Oncology Group. *J Clin Oncol*. 2006;24: 3844.
4. Klem ML, Grewal RK, Wexler LH, et al. PET for staging in rhabdomyosarcoma: An evaluation of PET as an adjunct to current staging tools. *J Pediatr Hematol Oncol*. 2007;29:9–14.
5. Dias P, Chen B, Dilday B, et al. Strong immunostaining for myogenin in rhabdomyosarcoma is significantly associated with tumors of the alveolar subclass. *Am J Pathol*. 2000;156:399–408.
6. Arndt CA, Stoner JA, Hawkins DS, et al. Vincristine, actinomycin, and cyclophosphamide compared with vincristine, actinomycin, and cyclophosphamide alternating with vincristine, topotecan, and cyclophosphamide for intermediate-risk rhabdomyosarcoma: Children's oncology group study D9803. *J Clin Oncol*. 2009; 27(31):5182–8.

ADDITIONAL READING

Grufferman S, Ruymann F, Ognjanovic S, et al. Prenatal X-ray exposure and rhabdomyosarcoma in children: A report from the children's oncology group. *Cancer Epidemiol Biomarkers Prev*. 2009;18:1271–6.

CODES

ICD9

171.9 Malignant neoplasm of connective and other soft tissue, site unspecified

CLINICAL PEARLS

- All soft tissue masses should be evaluated with imaging and possibly a biopsy.
- RMS is the most common soft tissue sarcoma in children.

RHEUMATIC FEVER

Payal Modi, MD, MScPH
Francesca L. Beaudoin, MS, MD

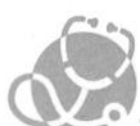

BASICS

DESCRIPTION

- Acute rheumatic fever (ARF) is a recurrent inflammatory disease, possibly autoimmune in nature, that affects multiple organ systems.
- Delayed nonsuppurative sequelae of pharyngeal infection with group A streptococci
- Can cause permanent cardiac valvular disease as well as acute cardiac decompensation
- Recurrences in both adults and children are common if not prevented with prophylactic antibiotic treatment.
- System(s) affected: Cardiovascular; Hematologic/Lymphatic/Immunologic; Musculoskeletal; Nervous; Skin/Exocrine

Pediatric Considerations

- More common in children
- In early studies, ARF developed in 3% of children with untreated group A β-hemolytic streptococcal pharyngitis (1).

EPIDEMIOLOGY

Incidence

- ARF and rheumatic heart disease (RHD) are now largely restricted to developing countries and some poor, mainly indigenous populations of wealthy countries.
- Predominant age: Most common in children ages 5–15 years
- Predominant sex: Male = Female. Females are more prone to develop chorea.
- Worldwide, the incidence of rheumatic fever has been declining for decades due to improved living conditions, better access to health care, and the increasing use of antibiotics.
- In the US, ARF had an incidence rate of 10.2/100,000 in the 1970s and currently is less than 1/100,000. However, since the mid-1980s, a resurgence of cases has occurred, with multiple outbreaks likely due to immigration from high-incidence countries (1)[A].
- Currently, the incidence of ARF is highest in developing countries, exceeding 50 per 100,000 children in some and accounting for 95% of ARF cases worldwide (1,2)[A].

Prevalence

- Prevalence of RHD in the US is now <0.05/1,000 population, with rare regional outbreaks.
- Worldwide, 15.6 million people have RHD. There are 470,000 new cases of rheumatic fever and 233,000 deaths attributable to rheumatic fever or RHD each year (1).
- The overall prevalence worldwide is rising due to advancements in medical care and longer life expectancies.

RISK FACTORS

Possible increased incidence with iron deficiency and low albumin concentrations (3)[C]

Genetics

- Certain human leukocyte antigen (HLA) class II DR and DQ genotypes and haplotypes, particularly DR7 and DR4. Additionally, polymorphisms in the promoter region of the TNFα, IL-10, and IL-6 genes (1).
- Increased susceptibility in certain populations including Australian Aborigines and Pacific Islanders, likely due to genetic predisposition.

GENERAL PREVENTION

- Primary prevention: Antibiotics are effective at reducing the incidence of ARF after known or suspected group A streptococcal pharyngitis. To achieve clinical and bacteriologic cures, treat streptococcal pharyngitis with 10 days of penicillin, an oral cephalosporin, or an oral macrolide in patients who are allergic to penicillin. Number needed to treat: 100 for 1.2 (4)[A]
- Secondary prevention: Long-term prophylaxis (with penicillin G or a macrolide) in selected populations

PATHOPHYSIOLOGY

- Presents 1–4 weeks following an untreated group A β-hemolytic streptococcal pharyngitis or tonsillitis
- Molecular mimicry: Antibodies created against the M protein on cells of group A streptococcus also crossreact with various proteins in the heart and vessel walls. They subsequently attack self-cells initiating an inflammatory cascade causing the symptoms of rheumatic fever.

ETIOLOGY

- Preceding infection of the upper respiratory tract with group A streptococcus
- Autoimmune mechanisms

DIAGNOSIS

- Evidence of preceding group A streptococcal (GAS) infection (positive throat culture for GAS, positive streptococcal antigen test, or elevated/rising streptococcal antibody titer)
- Modified Jones Criteria for diagnosis of ARF: 2 major manifestations or 1 major and 2 minor manifestations
- Major criteria: Carditis, migratory polyarthritis, Sydenham chorea, erythema marginatum, and SC nodules
- Minor criteria: Fever, arthralgia, leukocytosis, ECG findings (prolonged PR interval, heart block), increased inflammatory marker (elevated ESR or C-reactive protein), and history of rheumatic fever or heart disease

HISTORY

- Pharyngitis usually 1–4 weeks prior
- Acute febrile illness with malaise and muscle weakness
- Migratory large joint polyarthritis and arthralgia (75%) with dramatic response to small doses of salicylates or NSAIDs.
- Lower extremity joints typically involved first; symptoms are usually transient
- In patients treated with anti-inflammatory drugs, arthritis may be monoarticular, nonmigratory, or of short duration
- Chest discomfort, pleuritic chest pain
- Rash
- Choreiform movements: Late manifestation 2–6 months after infection
- Emotional disturbances, outbursts of inappropriate behavior, crying, restlessness

PHYSICAL EXAM

- Pericardial frictional rub
- Pancarditis (50%): Blowing pansystolic murmur, rarely diastolic or new or changing murmurs
- Evidence of heart failure
- SC nodules (<1%): Firm, painless, up to 2 cm; over bony surface, prominences, or near tendons present for a few weeks
- Erythema marginatum (5–13%): Nonpruritic erythematous rings on trunk that transiently appear and disappear over months, can be accentuated by warming the skin
- Sydenham chorea (10–15%): Nonrhythmic involuntary movements, more marked on one side, cease during sleep, may last up to 8 months
- "Milking sign": Diffuse hypotonia with no sensory losses

DIAGNOSTIC TESTS & INTERPRETATION

Lab

Initial lab tests

- Prior treatment with aspirin or steroids may alter lab results.
- CBC with differential: Can show elevated WBC count and normochromic normocytic anemia
- Increased acute-phase reactants: ESR and CRP
- Throat culture for group A hemolytic streptococci (75% are negative)
- Bacteriologic or serologic evidence of GAS infection
  – Antistreptolysin O titers (ASO, 80%): peak at 4–5 weeks
  – if negative, check ASO antideoxyribonuclease (DNase B:detectable for 6–9 months), streptokinase, and antihyaluronidase.
- No changes in complement levels
- ECG: All degrees of heart block, including prolonged PR interval, A-V dissociation, evidence of pericarditis
- Joint aspiration of affected joints reveals sterile inflammatory fluid with 10–100,000 WBC/mm^3

Follow-Up & Special Considerations

- Repeat ASO titers every 1–2 weeks until normalized (cannot be used as a measure of rheumatogenic activity).
- CRP and ESR are useful in monitoring rebounds of inflammation.

Imaging

Initial approach

- Chest x-ray (CXR): The most common radiologic manifestation of carditis is cardiomegaly.
- Echocardiogram: Assess for chamber size and function, valvular disease including silent mitral regurgitation, and pericardial effusion; comprehensive echocardiographic screening identified ~10 times as many children with RHD as were identified by the traditional strategy of clinical screening with echocardiographic confirmation (2)
- Antimyosin scintigraphy for detection of carditis (80% sensitive, limited specificity) (5)
- Radiographs of affected joints rarely may show slight effusion.

Follow-Up & Special Considerations

- Serial CXRs to monitor carditis
- Serial echocardiograms to document the course of valvular lesions

Pathological Findings
- Fibrinous pericardium and Anitschkow cells: Cardiac histiocytes
- Aschoff bodies: Focal inflammation surrounding fibrinoid necrosis
- Aschoff cells: Multinucleated giant cells in mass of fragmented swollen collagen fibers
- SC nodules have a characteristic histologic appearance.

DIFFERENTIAL DIAGNOSIS
- Systemic lupus erythematosus (SLE)
- Poststreptococcal reactive arthritis
- Juvenile rheumatoid arthritis (JRA)
- Infectious arthritis
- Viral myocarditis
- Innocent cardiac murmurs
- Tourette syndrome
- Kawasaki syndrome
- Pediatric autoimmune neuropsychiatric disorders associated with streptococcal infections (PANDAS)

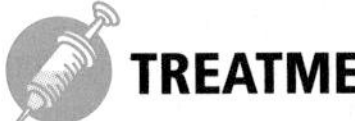

TREATMENT

MEDICATION
First Line
- Symptomatic relief
- Eradication: Treat initially with penicillin as if active streptococcal infection is present; then begin prophylaxis (see "Follow-Up"):
  - Penicillin × 10 days IM or IV
  - If the patient is allergic to penicillin, use a narrow-spectrum cephalosporin or a macrolide such as erythromycin.
- If patient has moderate-severe carditis with cardiomegaly/CHF, treat with prednisone 2 mg/kg/d (60 mg/d max) × 2 weeks; then taper over 2 weeks. Data on use of steroids are inconclusive (6)[C].
- If no cardiomegaly, start aspirin 80–100 mg/kg/d in children and 4–8 g/d in adults × 4–6 weeks. Start aspirin at beginning of steroid taper, and continue until symptoms are absent and ESR and CRP are normal (may be ~6 weeks).
- For severe cases of chorea, sedation may be required with valproic acid as first-line, then haloperidol or carbamazepine. IVIG may be beneficial as well (7).
- Household contacts should be screened with a throat culture and treated with appropriate antibiotics even if asymptomatic.
- Contraindications: Specific drug allergies
- Significant possible interactions: Refer to the manufacturer's profile of each drug.

Second Line
For children, naproxen at a dose of 15–20 mg/kg/d divided b.i.d. has been found to be safe and effective in ARF and has fewer adverse reactions than aspirin (8).

ADDITIONAL TREATMENT
General Measures
- The mainstay of therapy is anti-inflammatory, especially for patients with carditis.
- Treat arrhythmias with appropriate agents
- Pain relief for patients with arthritis
- Heart failure therapy as needed

Issues for Referral
Patients should be managed or comanaged by a cardiologist.

SURGERY/OTHER PROCEDURES
Mitral stenosis is a manifestation of late scarring and calcification of damaged valves that often requires surgical correction (valve repair preferred over replacement), especially in the presence of left atrial enlargement.

IN-PATIENT CONSIDERATIONS
Initial Stabilization
- Initial hospitalization may be helpful for diagnosis and to establish stability of the patient.
- Congestive heart failure (CHF) requires prompt hospitalization.

IV Fluids
Only if signs of dehydration present. Use cautiously in patients with carditis/CHF.

Nursing
- Gradual activity as tolerated.
- Bed rest initially for arthralgia and heart failure. Once symptoms are improved, advance activity cautiously.

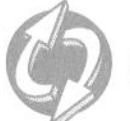

ONGOING CARE

FOLLOW-UP RECOMMENDATIONS
- ARF patients should be on prophylactic antibiotics throughout childhood and possibly indefinitely during adulthood:
  - The preferred treatment regimen is monthly IM injections of 1.2 million units of benzathine penicillin.
  - Oral penicillin V-K 250 mg b.i.d. is an alternative to monthly injections for patients at lower risk for recurrence.
  - Patients should be treated for a minimum of 5 years after an attack or until age 18.
  - In adults with valvular disease, consider treating indefinitely.
  - If the patient is allergic to penicillin, treat with sulfadiazine 500 mg/d for children weighing <27 kg up to a maximum dose of 1 g/d for adults. Fluid intake should be maintained ≥1,500 mL/d to guard against sulfadiazine crystalluria.
- If patients have valvular damage from ARF, they also require bacterial endocarditis prophylaxis for dental and other high-risk procedures.
- Low threshold to test and treat acute episodes of GAS pharyngitis

Patient Monitoring
Initially each week, then every 6 months

Pediatric Considerations
Use aspirin with great caution in children, given the potential risk of Reye syndrome.

Pregnancy Considerations
Residual valvular disease may be exacerbated by pregnancy. Refer preconception and pregnant patients to a cardiologist for assistance in management.

DIET
- Regular diet
- Low-sodium diet if the patient has carditis

PATIENT EDUCATION
American Heart Association at www.heart.org

PROGNOSIS
Sequelae are limited to the heart and depend on the severity of carditis during an acute attack.

COMPLICATIONS
- Subsequent attacks of ARF secondary to streptococcal reinfection
- Cardiac sequelae including carditis, RHD (specifically mitral stenosis, more likely in patients with carditis), and CHF

REFERENCES

1. Chang C, et al. Cutting edge issues in rheumatic fever. *Clin Rev Allergy Immunol*. 2011. [Epub ahead of print].
2. Seckeler MD, Hoke TR, et al. The worldwide epidemiology of acute rheumatic fever and rheumatic heart disease. *Clin Epidemiol*. 2011;3: 67–84.
3. Zaman MM, Yoshiike N, Rouf MA, et al. Association of rheumatic fever with serum albumin concentration and body iron stores in Bangladeshi children: Case-control study. *BMJ*. 1998;317: 1287–8.
4. Del Mar CB, Glasziou PP, Spinks AB, et al. Antibiotics for sore throat. *Cochrane Database Syst Rev*. 2006;CD000023.
5. Narula J, Malhotra A, Yasuda T. Usefulness of antimyosin antibody imaging for the detection of active rheumatic myocarditis. *Am J Cardiol*. 1999; 84:946–50, A7.
6. Cilliers AM, Manyemba J, Saloojee H. Anti-inflammatory treatment for carditis in acute rheumatic fever. *Cochrane Database Syst Rev*. 2003:CD003176.
7. Weiner SG, Normandin PA, et al. Sydenham chorea: A case report and review of the literature. *Pediatr Emerg Care*. 2007;23:20–4.
8. Hashkes PJ, Tauber T, Somekh E, et al. Naproxen as an alternative to aspirin for the treatment of arthritis of rheumatic fever: A randomized trial. *J Pediatr*. 2003;143:399–401.

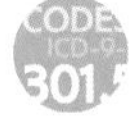

CODES

ICD9
- 390 Rheumatic fever without mention of heart involvement
- 391.0 Acute rheumatic pericarditis
- 391.1 Acute rheumatic endocarditis

CLINICAL PEARLS
- ARF is a recurrent inflammatory disease, possibly autoimmune in nature, that affects multiple organ systems including the heart.
- The modified Jones criteria for the diagnosis of ARF include 2 major manifestations or 1 major and 2 minor manifestations in the context of a preceding documented GAS infection.
- ARF patients should be on prophylactic antibiotics throughout childhood.

RHINITIS, ALLERGIC

Naureen B. Rafiq, MBBS, MD

BASICS

Allergic rhinitis is the collection of symptoms, involving mucous membranes of nose, eyes, ears, and throat after an exposure to allergens like pollen, dust, or dander.

DESCRIPTION

- IgE-mediated inflammation of the nasal mucosa following exposure to an extrinsic protein. An immediate symptomatic response is characterized by sneezing, congestion, and rhinorrhea followed by persistent late phase dominated by congestion and mucosal hyperreactivity.
- Allergic rhinitis can be classified into seasonal or perennial and can be intermittent or persistent.
- Seasonal responses are usually due to outdoor allergens like tree pollen, flowering shrubs in spring, grasses and flowering plants in summer, and ragweed and mold in fall.
- Perennial responses, or the year-round symptoms, are usually associated with indoor allergens like dust mites, mold, and animal dander.
- Occupational allergic rhinitis is caused by allergens at the workplace and can be sporadic or year round.
- Nonallergic rhinitis (e.g., vasomotor, rhinitis of pregnancy, and rhinitis medicamentosa) can occur.

Pediatric Considerations

Chronic nasal obstruction can result in facial deformities, dental malocclusions, and sleep disorders.

Pregnancy Considerations

Physiologic changes during pregnancy may aggravate all types of rhinitis, frequently in the second trimester.

EPIDEMIOLOGY

- Onset usually in first 2 decades, rarely before 6 months of age, with tendency declining with advancing age.
- The mean age of onset is 8–11 years, and about 80% of cases have established allergic rhinitis by age 20.

Prevalence

- ~10–25% of the US adult population and 9–42% of the US pediatric population are affected.
- 44–87% of patients with allergic rhinitis have mixed allergic and nonallergic rhinitis, which is more common than either pure form (1).
- Scandinavian studies have demonstrated cumulative prevalence rate of 14% in men and 15% in women.

RISK FACTORS

- Family history of atopy, with a greater risk if both parents have atopy than one
- Higher socioeconomic status
- Tobacco smoke can exacerbate symptoms and increase risk of developing asthma in patients with allergic rhinitis
- Having other allergies like asthma
- Unclear evidence regarding risk due to early, repeated exposure to offending allergen and early introduction of solid food
- Pets in house and houses infested with cockroaches can cause perennial allergic rhinitis.

Genetics

Complex but strong genetic predilection present (80% have family history of allergic disorders)

GENERAL PREVENTION

- Primary prevention of atopic disease has not been proven effective by maternal diet or maternal allergen avoidance (2).
- Symptomatic control or secondary prevention by environmental avoidance by patient is the "first-line treatment."
- Use of acaricides along with mite-proof mattress and pillow covers, carpet and drape removal, removal of plants in the home, pet control (2,3)[B]
- Air conditioning and limited outside exposure during allergy season (1)[B]
- HEPA air cleaners and vacuum bags are of unclear efficacy.
- Close doors and windows during allergy season.
- Use a dehumidifier to reduce indoor humidity.

PATHOPHYSIOLOGY

Aeroallergen-driven mucosal inflammation due to resident and infiltrating inflammatory cells, as well as vasoactive and proinflammatory mediators (e.g., cytokines)

ETIOLOGY

Inhalant allergens:

- Perennial: House dust mites, indoor molds, animal dander, cockroach/insect detritus
- Seasonal: Tree, grass, and weed pollens; outdoor molds
- Occupational: Latex, plant products (e.g., baking flour), sensitizing chemicals, and certain animals for people working in farms and vet clinics

COMMONLY ASSOCIATED CONDITIONS

Other IgE-mediated conditions: Asthma, atopic dermatitis, allergic conjunctivitis, food allergy

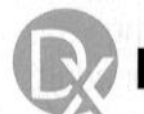

DIAGNOSIS

Diagnosis is made primarily by history and physical examination.

HISTORY

- Evaluation of nature, duration, and time course of symptoms
- History of atopic dermatitis and/or food allergies
- History of nasal congestion; rhinorrhea; pruritus of nose, eyes, ears, and/or palate; sneezing; itching; and watering of eye
- Family history of allergic diseases
- History of environmental and occupational exposure and various nasal stimuli can help differentiate between allergic and vasomotor rhinitis.

PHYSICAL EXAM

Many findings are suggestive of but not specific for allergic rhinitis:

- Dark circles under eyes, "allergic shiners" (infraorbital venous congestion)
- Transverse nasal crease from rubbing nose upward; typically seen in children
- Rhinorrhea, usually with clear discharge
- Pale, boggy, blue–gray nasal mucosa
- Postnasal mucus discharge
- Oropharyngeal lymphoid tissue hypertrophy

DIAGNOSTIC TESTS & INTERPRETATION

- Lab tests rarely needed
- Skin testing is done to identify the allergen for immunotherapy.

Lab

Initial lab tests

- CBC with differential may show elevated eosinophils.
- Increased total serum IgE level
- Nasal probe smear may show elevated eosinophils.
- Medications that may alter lab results:
  - Corticosteroids may decrease eosinophilia.
  - Antihistamines suppress reactivity to skin tests; stop antihistamines 7 days before testing.

Imaging

CT scan of sinuses is not routinely done, but can be used to check for complete opacity, fluid level, and mucosal thickening.

Diagnostic Procedures/Surgery

- Specific allergen sensitivity with allergen skin testing or radioallergosorbent testing (RAST); clinical correlation based on history is essential in interpreting results.
- Diagnostic allergen prick tests are used to select agent to determine appropriate environmental control measures, as well as to direct immunotherapy:
  - Prick or puncture: Superficial injury to epidermis with application of test antigen
  - Intradermal
- RAST: More expensive and less sensitive than skin testing; typically used in patients in whom skin testing is not practical or a severe reaction is possible
- Rhinoscopy: Useful to visualize intranasal anatomy and posterior pharyngeal structures, including adenoids, polyps, and larynx

Pathological Findings

- Nasal washing/scraping: Eosinophils predominate but may see basophils, mast cells
- Nasal mucosa: Submucosal edema but without destruction; eosinophilic infiltration; congested mucous glands and goblet cells

DIFFERENTIAL DIAGNOSIS

- Infectious rhinitis: Usually viral, commonly with secondary bacterial infection:
  - Usually associated with sinusitis and is known as rhinosinusitis
  - Viral rhinitis averages 6 episodes/yr from ages 2–6 years.
  - IgA deficiency with recurrent sinusitis
  - Rhinitis medicamentosa:
    - Rebound effect associated with continued use of topical decongestant drops and sprays
    - ACE inhibitors, reserpine, β-blockers, oral contraceptive pills (OCPs), guanethidine, methyldopa
    - Aspirin, NSAIDs
  - Vasomotor (idiopathic) rhinitis caused by numerous nasal stimuli like warm or cold air, scents and odors, light or particulate matter
  - Hormonal: Pregnancy, thyroid, OCPs
  - Nonallergic rhinitis with eosinophilia syndrome (NARES)

R

– Gustatory: Watery rhinorrhea in response to alcohol or food
– "Skier's nose": Watery rhinorrhea in response to cold air
- Conditions associated with rhinitis:
  – Nasal polyps, tumor
  – Septal/anatomic obstruction:
    ○ Adenoidal hypertrophy, particularly in children
    ○ Septal abnormality or deflected nasal septum (DNS) in adults

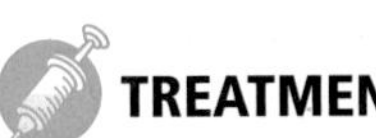

TREATMENT

There are 3 mainstays of treatment of allergic rhinitis:
- Allergen avoidance
- Medication
- Allergy immunotherapy

MEDICATION

Oral medication and intranasal sprays are commonly used.

First Line

- Second-generation nonsedating antihistamines are first-line therapy for mild-to-moderate allergic rhinitis (1,4).
- Adverse effects: Mild sedation, mild anticholinergic effects
- Generic: Cetirizine, fexofenadine, loratadine
- Intranasal corticosteroids are first-line therapy for moderate-to-severe allergic rhinitis (1,4)[A]:
  – Most effective drug class for symptoms of allergic rhinitis.
  – Use nasal sprays after showering, and direct spray away from septum to improve deposition on mucosal surface.
  – May be used as needed; however, less effective than regular use (1)
  – Adverse effects: Nosebleed, nasal septal perforation, and systemic corticosteroid effects
- Systemic steroids should be considered only in urgent cases and only for short-term use.
- Generic: Fluticasone

Second Line

- First-generation antihistamines, such as:
  – Brompheniramine 12–24 mg PO b.i.d.
  – Chlorpheniramine 4 mg PO q4–6h PRN
  – Clemastine 1–2 mg PO b.i.d. PRN
  – Diphenhydramine 25–50 mg PO q4–6h PRN:
    ○ May precipitate urinary retention in men with prostatism and/or hypertrophy
    ○ Adverse effects: Sedation, prolonged QT interval, performance impairment, and anticholinergic effect:
      ▪ Nasal antihistamines may be systemically absorbed and thus may cause sedation: Azelastine, olopatadine
      ▪ Decongestants:
        ▫ Phenylephrine 10 mg PO q4h PRN
        ▫ Pseudoephedrine 60 mg PO q4–6h PRN
        ▫ Oxymetazoline nasal spray (Afrin) 2–3 sprays per nostril q10–12h PRN (max 3 days). Intranasal agents should not be used for >3 days due to rebound rhinitis. Discourage use in patients with hypertension (HTN) or cardiac arrhythmia.
      ▪ Intranasal anticholinergics such as ipratropium nasal spray 2 sprays per nostril b.i.d.–t.i.d.:
        ▫ Intranasal anticholinergics can increase efficacy in combination with steroid use (1).
      ▪ Leukotriene antagonists such as montelukast 10 mg PO every day:
        ▫ Should generally be used as an adjunct, not monotherapy
      ▪ Mast cell stabilizers such as Cromolyn nasal spray 1 spray per nostril t.i.d.–q.i.d.:
        ▫ May take 2–4 weeks of therapy for optimal efficacy
        ▫ May be ineffective in patients with nonallergic rhinitis and nasal polyps

ADDITIONAL TREATMENT

Immunotherapy, either by injection (5)[A] or sublingually, which may be better tolerated by children (6)[A]

General Measures

- Establish specific cause(s) by history and appropriate testing.
- Limit exposure to offending allergen.
- Allergen immunotherapy (desensitization):
  – Reserved when symptoms are uncontrollable with medical therapy or have a comorbidity (e.g., asthma)
  – Specific allergen extract is injected SC in increasing doses to induce patient tolerance.

Issues for Referral

Refer to allergist for consideration of immunotherapy.

Additional Therapies

Nasal saline use has evidence of efficacy as sole agent or as adjunctive treatment (1,7)[A].

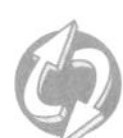

ONGOING CARE

FOLLOW-UP RECOMMENDATIONS

No specific restrictions on activity; emphasize avoiding activity where exposure to the allergen is likely.

Patient Monitoring

Initiation of patient education is critical.

DIET

- No special diet unless concomitant food reactions are suspected and evaluated
- Some patients with severe sensitivity to seasonal pollens may have oral allergy syndrome, which is associated with itching in the mouth with the ingestion of fresh fruits that may cross-react with the allergens.

PATIENT EDUCATION

- Asthma & Allergy Foundation of America, 1717 Massachusetts Ave., Suite 305, Washington, DC 20036; (800) 7-ASTHMA; www.aafa.org.
- Other helpful information available at www.acaai.org and www.aaaai.org.

PROGNOSIS

- Acceptable control of symptoms is the goal.
- Treatment is helpful to reduce the risk of comorbidities, such as sinusitis and asthma.

COMPLICATIONS

- Secondary infection such as otitis media or sinusitis
- Epistaxis
- Nasopharyngeal lymphoid hyperplasia
- Airway hyperreactivity with allergen exposure
- Asthma
- Facial changes, especially in children who are mouth breathers
- Sleep disturbance

REFERENCES

1. Wallace DV. The diagnosis and management of rhinitis: An updated practice parameter. *J Allergy Clin Immunol*. 2008;122:S1–84.
2. Kramer MS, Kakuma R. Maternal dietary antigen avoidance during pregnancy or lactation, or both, for preventing or treating atopic disease in the child. *Cochrane Database Syst Rev*. 2009;1.
3. Sheikh A, Hurwitz B, Shehata YA. House dust mite avoidance measures for perennial allergic rhinitis. *Cochrane Database Syst Rev*. 2009;1.
4. Plaut M, Valentine MD. Clinical practice. Allergic rhinitis. *N Engl J Med*. 2005;353:1934–44.
5. Calderon MA, Alves B, Jacobson M, et al. Allergen injection immunotherapy for seasonal allergic rhinitis. [Systematic Review]. Cochrane Ear, Nose and Throat Disorders Group. *Cochrane Database Syst Rev*. 2009;1.
6. Wilson D, Torres-Lima M, Durham S. Sublingual immunotherapy for allergic rhinitis. *Cochrane Database Syst Rev*. 2009;1.
7. Harvey R, Hannan SA, Badia L, et al. Scadding Glenis. Nasal saline irrigations for the symptoms of chronic rhinosinusitis. *Cochrane Database Syst Rev*. 2009;1.

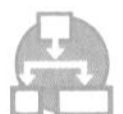

See Also (Topic, Algorithm, Electronic Media Element)

Conjunctivitis, Acute

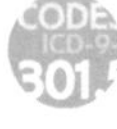

CODES

ICD9

- 477.0 Allergic rhinitis due to pollen
- 477.8 Allergic rhinitis due to other allergen
- 477.9 Allergic rhinitis, cause unspecified

CLINICAL PEARLS

- Nasal saline irrigation (flushing 6–8 oz) may be very helpful in clearing upper airway of secretions and may precede the use of nasal corticosteroids.
- Second-generation antihistamines and intranasal corticosteroids are first-line therapies for allergic rhinitis.
- Referral to allergist is appropriate for identification of offending allergens and consideration of immunotherapy for inadequate symptom control.

ROCKY MOUNTAIN SPOTTED FEVER

Lawren Wellisch, MD
Michael Koster, MD

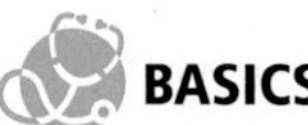

BASICS

DESCRIPTION

- Rocky Mountain spotted fever (RMSF) is a potentially fatal vectorborne illness caused by *Rickettsia rickettsii*, transmitted by the *Dermacentor* spp. tick, and characterized by fever, headache, and centripetal rash.
- Systems affected: Cardiovascular; Musculoskeletal; Central Nervous System (CNS); Skin; Exocrine

EPIDEMIOLOGY

Incidence

- In the US, the incidence of RMSF has increased over the last decade from <2 cases per million persons in 2000 to over 8 per million in 2008.
- RMSF has been reported in almost all states, but North Carolina, Oklahoma, Arkansas, Tennessee, and Missouri account for ~60% of cases. It is also endemic to some areas of Canada and South America.
- Predominant age: All ages are susceptible, but highest prevalence is in persons aged 50–69. Children aged 0–9 are at higher risk of fatal outcomes.
- Predominant sex: Male > Female
- Peak incidence is in late spring and summer, highest in June and July.

Prevalence

In the US, ~2,000–2,500 cases are reported per year.

RISK FACTORS

- Known tick bite, especially if engorged or present >20 hours
- Outdoor activity, particularly, although not exclusively, during spring and summer months in an endemic area
- Contact with outdoor pets or wild animals

GENERAL PREVENTION

People who frequent tick-infested areas can take measures to prevent infection (1)[B]:

- When in or near a wooded area, cover exposed skin with long pants and sleeves; pants should be tucked into socks.
- Insect repellents containing DEET should be used on exposed skin, avoiding eyes and mouth. Permethrin is an insecticide that can be used on clothing.
- After possible exposure, all body areas should be carefully inspected for ticks, especially legs, groin, external genitalia, and belt lines.
- *Likelihood of infection increases with the duration of tick attachment*
- Attached ticks should be removed immediately using tweezers and wearing gloves if possible:
  - *It is vital that hands be washed thoroughly after tick removal.*

PATHOPHYSIOLOGY

- Rickettsiae are injected into the body from tick salivary glands during a prolonged feeding (at least 6–10 hours) and spread hematogenously.
- They invade contiguous endothelial cells, causing a small-vessel vasculitis.
- Subsequent increased vascular permeability can lead to life-threatening damage to the brain, lungs, and other viscera.
- Incubation time is ~7–12 days.

ETIOLOGY

- RMSF is caused by *R. rickettsii* and is transmitted by attachment and prolonged feeding of an infected tick, primarily the wood tick, *Dermacentor andersoni*, in the western US and dog tick, *Dermacentor variabilis*, in the eastern US.
- Rarely, RMSF is caused by direct inoculation of tick blood into open wounds or conjunctivae, but it can be caused by removing ticks without gloves or good hand washing.

DIAGNOSIS

Delay in presentation and initiation of therapy can increase long-term sequelae and mortality.

HISTORY

Should be suspected in cases of acute febrile illness, especially with history of potential tick exposure within previous 14 days, travel to endemic area, and presentation in the spring or fall. *Many patients will not recall tick bite.*

PHYSICAL EXAM

- Early disease (days 1–3) presents like many viral illnesses with features including headache, fever, malaise, nausea, and vomiting.
- Many patients will go on to exhibit a centripetal rash (involves the palms and soles and spreads centrally to arms, legs, and trunk), which is often petechial, and usually presents on days 3–5 of illness:
  - Roughly 1/3 of patients will never develop this "classic" rash and may suffer from subsequent delay in diagnosis.
  - Pruritus and urticaria are not features of RMSF, and their presence make the diagnosis less likely.
- Signs and symptoms associated with RMSF and their frequency of occurrence:
  - Fever (99–100%)
  - Rash (macular, maculopapular, petechial; 88–90%)
  - Headache (79–91%)
  - "Classic triad": Headache, fever, and rash (50–60%)
  - Myalgias (72–83%)
  - Nausea, vomiting (56–60%)
  - Abdominal pain (35–52%)
  - Hepatosplenomegaly (12–16%)
  - Lymphadenopathy (27%)
  - Cough (33%)
  - CNS dysfunction (e.g., stupor, confusion, coma, focal abnormalities; 10–30%)

DIAGNOSTIC TESTS & INTERPRETATION

Lab

- Diagnosis is usually presumptive and based on a compatible syndrome in a patient with exposure history in an endemic area. Confirmation is obtained by subsequent serology. *Treatment should not be delayed awaiting confirmatory serology.*
- Specific laboratory diagnosis:
  - Serum indirect fluorescent antibody (IFA): 4-fold increase of acute vs. convalescent titers confirms an active case of RMSF, but any positive titer (>1:64, minimum detectable concentration) is considered diagnostic.
  - IFA may not be positive for at least 7–10 days after onset of symptoms; optimal time for testing is 14–21 days. Do not delay treatment waiting for titer confirmation.
  - Early treatment may blunt antibody response.
- Nonspecific laboratory changes (incidence):
  - WBC count: Variable; may be increased or decreased
  - Thrombocytopenia (32–52%)
  - Anemia, mild (5–24%)
  - Hyponatremia, mild (19–56%)
  - Azotemia (12–14%)
  - Elevated aspartate aminotransferase (AST) (36–62%)
  - Prolonged prothrombin time and partial thromboplastin time; decreased fibrinogen; elevated fibrin degradation products uncommon
  - CSF protein and WBC count modestly elevated with lymphocytic or polymorphonuclear predominance; glucose usually normal

Imaging

Other than nonspecific pneumonic infiltrates, which may be seen on routine chest radiograph, imaging procedures are rarely helpful.

Diagnostic Procedures/Surgery

Tissue biopsy, usually skin, can offer definitive diagnosis. A 3-mm punch biopsy of a skin lesion is sufficient to perform a rapid direct fluorescent antibody (DFA) test (sensitivity 70%, specificity 100%). Polymerase chain reaction (PCR) and electron microscopy (EM) can also identify rickettsiae within endothelial cells.

Pathological Findings

- Rickettsiae may be demonstrated within endothelial cells by DFA, PCR, or electron microscopy.
- Petechiae due to the vasculitis may be seen on various organ surfaces (e.g., liver, brain, or epicardium).
- Secondary thromboses and tissue necrosis may be seen.

R

DIFFERENTIAL DIAGNOSIS

- Viral exanthems (e.g., measles, rubella, roseola)
- Meningoencephalitis (viral meningitis or encephalitis, bacterial meningitis)
- Meningococcemia
- Typhus
- Ehrlichiosis
- Lyme disease
- Leptospirosis
- Toxic shock syndrome

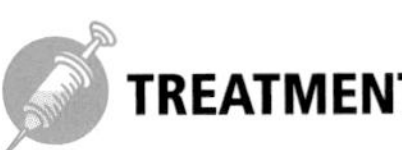

TREATMENT

MEDICATION

First Line

- Doxycycline is the treatment of choice in children and adults (2,3,4)[A]:
  - For adults, doxycycline 100 mg PO or IV q12h until including 3 days after fever resolution; 100 mg q24h in renal failure
  - For children weighing <45kg: 2.2 mg/kg/dose q12h
- Side effects:
  - Patients taking doxycycline should be counseled about possible dyspepsia. Encourage patients to take medication with full glass of water and food and remain upright for 30 minutes after ingestion.
  - Absorption of doxycycline may be inhibited by dairy products, iron preparations, or antacids.
  - Doxycycline increases photosensitivity. Patients should minimize sun exposure.
  - Doxycycline may cause staining of permanent teeth when given to children <9 years of age. This risk appears to be minimal if no more than 5 courses of therapy are administered before age 9.

Second Line

- Use second-line treatment *only* in pregnant or tetracycline-allergic patients.
- Chloramphenicol 20 mg/kg IV q6h (4 g/d maximum); same dose in renal failure (oral chloramphenicol is not available in the US); chloramphenicol may be less effective than doxycycline.
- Modern fluoroquinolones have in vitro activity against *R. rickettsii* and have been evaluated in other spotted-fever-group rickettsioses but have not been evaluated clinically in RMSF.

Pregnancy Considerations

- Brief course of doxycycline is appropriate for this life-threatening infection if suspicion is high, despite the potential risk to fetal bones and teeth.
- Chloramphenicol may be preferred during the first 2 trimesters but should be avoided in the third trimester because of potential gray baby syndrome.
- Transplacental transmission of infection has not been demonstrated.

ADDITIONAL TREATMENT

Issues for Referral

Consider consultation with infectious disease specialist.

Additional Therapies

Patients with neurologic injury may require prolonged physical and cognitive therapy.

IN-PATIENT CONSIDERATIONS

Admission Criteria

- Severe illness
- Obtundation
- Nausea/vomiting preventing oral antibiotic therapy
- Acutely ill patients with signs and symptoms of shock should be treated in an ICU.

IV Fluids

Aggressive fluid resuscitation may be required in critically ill patients.

Discharge Criteria

- Resolution of fever
- Able to take oral therapy and nutrition

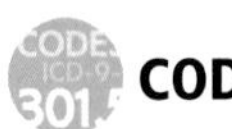

ONGOING CARE

FOLLOW-UP RECOMMENDATIONS

- Patients moderately ill usually should be hospitalized.
- Patients with mild disease are treated presumptively as outpatients. Close follow-up is important in identifying complications.
- Bed rest until symptoms subside.
- Infection does not confer lifelong immunity, and patients should be counseled on general prevention measures.

Patient Monitoring

- If patients are not hospitalized, then they should be seen every 2–3 days until symptoms have fully resolved.
- CBC and electrolytes (including BUN/creatinine) should be monitored.

DIET

Consider nutritional supplementation if appetite is poor.

PROGNOSIS

- When treated promptly, the usual prognosis is excellent with the resolution of symptoms over several days and no sequelae.
- Death is rare with prompt institution of appropriate therapy.
- If complications develop (see "Complications"), the course may be more severe, and long-term sequelae may be present, particularly neurologic sequelae.
- Mortality risk is significantly higher in the elderly and in young children.

COMPLICATIONS

- Encephalopathy, usually transient (30–40%)
- Seizures, focal neurologic signs (10%)
- Renal insufficiency (10%)
- Hepatitis (10%)
- Congestive heart failure (CHF) (5%)
- Respiratory failure (5%)

REFERENCES

1. Minniear TD, Buckingham SC, et al. Managing Rocky Mountain spotted fever. *Expert Rev Anti Infect Ther*. 2009;7:1131–7.
2. Centers for Disease Control and Prevention. Nonfatal, unintentional medication exposures among young children—United States, 2001–2003. *MMWR Morb Mortal Wkly Rep*. 2006;55:1–5.
3. Elston DM, et al. Tick bites and skin rashes. *Curr Opin Infect Dis*. 2010;23:132–8.
4. Botelho-Nevers E, Raoult D, et al. Host, pathogen and treatment-related prognostic factors in rickettsioses. *Eur J Clin Microbiol Infect Dis*. 2011;30(10):1139–50.

ADDITIONAL READING

- Chapman AS, Bakken JS, Folk SM, et al. Diagnosis and management of tickborne rickettsial diseases: Rocky Mountain spotted fever, ehrlichioses, and anaplasmosis–United States: A practical guide for physicians and other health-care and public health professionals. *MMWR Recomm Rep*. 2006;55:1–27.
- Chen LF, Sexton DJ. What's new in Rocky Mountain spotted fever? *Infect Dis Clin North Am*. 2008;22(3): 415–32, vii–viii.
- Salinas LJ, Greenfield RA, Little SE, et al. Tickborne infections in the southern United States. *Am J Med Sci*. 2010;340:194–201.
- Stallings SP. Rocky Mountain spotted fever and pregnancy: A case report and review of the literature. *Obstet Gynecol Surv*. 2001;56:37–42.

CODES

ICD9

082.0 Spotted fevers

CLINICAL PEARLS

- Initiate treatment based on clinical suspicion; do not delay for serologic confirmation or development of characteristic rash.
- While prevalence is highest in central and southeastern US, cases have been reported in almost all states.
- 70% of patients recall a tick bite in the preceding 14 days.

ROSEOLA

Jeffery T. Kirchner, DO, FAAFP, AAHIVS

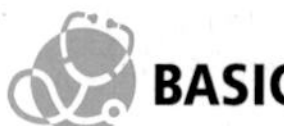

BASICS

DESCRIPTION

- Acute infection of infants or very young children
- Characteristically, it causes a high fever followed by an eruption similar in appearance to that of measles as the fever resolves.
- Transmission now believed to be via contact of salivary secretions from adults shedding HHV-6.
- Perinatal transmission has been suggested with newborn infections but not definitively proven.
- Virus establishes lifelong infection, including in the CNS.
- Incubation period of ~5–15 days
- System(s) affected: Endocrine/Metabolic; Skin/Exocrine; Brain/Neurologic
- Synonym(s): Exanthem subitum; Pseudorubella; Sixth disease; 3-day fever

Pediatric Considerations

A disease of infants and very young children

EPIDEMIOLOGY

- Predominant age:
  - Infants and very young children (6 months–3 years)
  - 90% before age 2 years (1,2)
- Predominant sex: Male = Female

Incidence

- Unknown
- More likely to occur in spring and fall

Prevalence

Peak prevalence is between 7 and 13 months of age

RISK FACTORS

- Daycare center
- Exposure to infected infant

Genetics

No known genetic pattern

ETIOLOGY

A communicable DNA virus: HHV-6B (1,3)

DIAGNOSIS

HISTORY

- Anorexia
- Irritability
- Abrupt fever without apparent cause (39.4–40.5°C [103–105°F]) for 3–5 days

PHYSICAL EXAM

- Child usually does not appear seriously ill, but may be listless
- Febrile convulsions during height of fever (10–15%)
- Sudden drop of fever:
  - As fever disappears, skin rash begins (lasts hours–days).
- Rash (exanthem subitum):
  - Nonpruritic, maculopapular, blanching rash appears as very slightly elevated, rose-pink papules.
  - First appears on the neck and trunk
  - Appears profusely on trunk, arms, and neck, but mildly on face and legs
  - Fades within a few hours to 2 days
- Inflammation of the tympanic membranes
- Lymphadenopathy in cervical and posterior auricular regions (often a later finding)
- Spleen enlarged (uncommon)

DIAGNOSTIC TESTS & INTERPRETATION

Lab

- Typically a clinical diagnosis
- Consider labs only if concerned about the patient's overall condition.

Initial lab tests

- CBC:
  - Leukopenia with relative (atypical) lymphocytosis
  - Thrombocytopenia
- Urinalysis (rule out UTI as source of fever)
- IgM; poor sensitivity/specificity
- Paired sera for IgG (4-fold increase IgG for diagnosis) for HHV-6 (but can cross-react with HHV-7)
- Serum polymerase chain reaction (PCR) for HHV-6, qualitative and quantitative, can be performed:
  - Serological confirmation should only be considered if there is evidence of neurological sequelae (4).
  - Quantitative is more accurate than qualitative.
  - Typically, results take 2–7 days, depending on the lab.
- Blood culture (peripheral blood mononuclear cells [PMBC]) for HHV-6

Imaging

Initial approach

- Consider chest x-ray (CXR) if a child is exhibiting respiratory symptoms such as tachypnea or wheezing.
- When ordered, a CXR is typically negative.

Diagnostic Procedures/Surgery

- HHV-6-IgM: Diagnostic for acute infection (but limited sensitivity and specificity)
- HHV-6 by qualitative or quantitative PCR found in serum, CSF, and saliva

DIFFERENTIAL DIAGNOSIS

- Enterovirus infection
- Fifth disease
- Rubella
- Measles (rubeola)
- Scarlet fever
- Sepsis
- Drug eruption (including medication hypersensitivity syndrome)

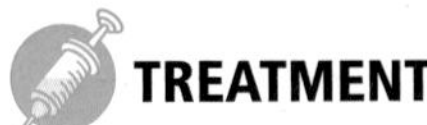

TREATMENT

Is usually supportive

MEDICATION

First Line

- Acetaminophen for excessively high fever, 10–15 mg/kg q4h to a maximum of 2.6 g/24-hour period
- Avoid aspirin as it may enhance the risk of Reye syndrome (1)[C].
- Phenobarbital may be considered for seizure (1)[C].

Second Line

- Medications for use in immunocompromised children:
  - Foscarnet active against HHV-6A and -6B
  - Acyclovir has very little activity.
  - Ganciclovir active against HHV-6B, but -6A is relatively resistant.
- No clinical trials evaluating these antiviral agents. Most evidence is from in vitro studies.

ADDITIONAL TREATMENT

General Measures

- Symptomatic
- Tap water baths to cool excess temperature elevation
- Lightweight clothing
- Maintain normal room temperature.

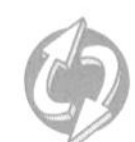

ONGOING CARE

FOLLOW-UP RECOMMENDATIONS

Patient Monitoring

- None after typical rash appears and fever resolves
- If seizures occur, they will cease after fever subsides and will not cause brain damage.

DIET

Encourage fluids.

PATIENT EDUCATION

Parental reassurance

PROGNOSIS

- Course: Acute, benign, complete recovery without sequelae
- One attack usually confers permanent immunity.
- Reactivation in immunocompromised patients is possible.

COMPLICATIONS

- Febrile seizures
- Encephalitis (rare)
- Meningitis
- Hepatitis
- Medication hypersensitivity syndromes
- Possible association with temporal lobe epilepsy and multiple sclerosis (5)

REFERENCES

1. Leach CT. Human herpesvirus-6 and -7 infections in children: Agents of roseola and other syndromes. *Curr Opin Pediatr*. 2000;12:269–74.
2. Zerr DM, Meier AS, Selke SS, et al. A population-based study of primary human herpesvirus 6 infection. *N Engl J Med*. 2005;352: 768–76.
3. Zerr DM. Human herpesvirus 6: A clinical update. *Herpes*. 2006;13:20–4.
4. Ward KN. The natural history and laboratory diagnosis of human herpesviruses-6 and -7 infections in the immunocompetent. *J Clin Virol*. 2005;32:183–93.
5. Gewurz BE, Marty FM, Baden LR, et al. Human herpesvirus 6 encephalitis. *Curr Infect Dis Rep*. 2008;10:292–9.

ADDITIONAL READING

- Ablashi DV, Devin CL, Yoshikawa T, et al. Review part 3: Human herpesvirus-6 in multiple non-neurological diseases. *J Med Virol*. 2010;82: 1903–10.
- Asano Y, Yoshikawa T, Suga S, et al. Clinical features of infants with primary human herpesvirus 6 infection (exanthem subitum, roseola infantum). *Pediatrics*. 1994;93:104–8.
- Caselli E, Di Luca D. Molecular biology and clinical associations of Roseoloviruses human herpesvirus 6 and human herpesvirus 7. *New Microbiol*. 2007;30: 173–87.
- Dockrell DH, Smith TF, Paya CV. Human herpesvirus 6. *Mayo Clin Proc*. 1999;74:163–70.
- Theodore WH, Epstein L, Gaillard WD, et al. Human herpes virus 6B: A possible role in epilepsy? *Epilepsia*. 2008;49(11):1828–37.
- Vianna RA, de Oliveira SA, Camacho LA, et al. Role of human herpesvirus 6 infection in young Brazilian children with rash illnesses. *Pediatr Infect Dis J*. 2008;27:533–7.

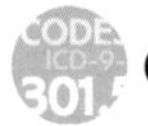

CODES

ICD9

- 057.8 Other specified viral exanthemata
- 058.10 Roseola infantum, unspecified

CLINICAL PEARLS

- Roseola infection should be suspected if it is known to be in the community and a young child presents with a high temperature.
- As the fever abates, a blanching macular rash will be seen on the neck and trunk, with eventual spread to the face and extremities.
- Laboratory testing is not necessary for most children with classic roseola.
- For atypical presentations, complications, and immunocompromised hosts, several laboratory tools are available, including serologic testing for antibody and viral PCR testing.
- Infection is typically self-limiting and without sequelae.

R

ROTATOR CUFF IMPINGEMENT SYNDROME

Derek M. Richardson, Capt USAF AMC 60 MDOS/SGOF

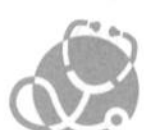

BASICS

DESCRIPTION

- Compression of the rotator cuff tendons and subacromial bursa between the humeral head and the structures that make up the coracoacromial arch and humeral tuberosities
- Most common cause of atraumatic shoulder pain in patients >25 years old
- Typical symptom is pain that is most severe with arm abducted between 40° and 120°.
- Classically divided into 3 stages:
  - Stage I: Acute inflammation, edema, or hemorrhage of the underlying tendons due to overuse (typically <25 years old)
  - Stage II: Progressive tendinosis that leads to partial rotator cuff tear along with underlying thickening or fibrosis of surrounding structures (commonly, ages 25–40 years)
  - Stage III: Full-thickness tear (typically in patients aged >40 years)

EPIDEMIOLOGY

Incidence

- Shoulder pain in primary care practices averages around 11.2/1,000 patients per year.
- Peak incidence of 25/1,000 patients per year in those aged 42–46
- Shoulder pain accounts for 1.2% of all primary care visits.
- Impingement cited as cause in 18–74% of shoulder pain patients.

Prevalence

Prevalence of shoulder pain in general population thought to range from ~7–36%.

RISK FACTORS

- Repetitive overhead motions, including throwing
- Glenohumeral joint instability or muscle imbalance
- Hooked acromion
- Acromioclavicular (AC) spurs, osteophytes
- Thickened coracoacromial ligament
- Shoulder trauma
- Os acromiale
- Increasing age
- Smoking

GENERAL PREVENTION

- Proper throwing and lifting techniques
- Proper development of rotator cuff and scapula stabilizer muscles

PATHOPHYSIOLOGY

- The exact pathophysiology is still not entirely clear.
- Originally described by Neer as pinching of the soft-tissue structures (such as rotator cuff tendons or subacromial bursa) between humerus and the anteroinferior portion of the acromion, which is exacerbated by repetitive shoulder forward flexion and internal rotation.
- Commonly believed that intrinsic degeneration of the rotator cuff tendons with age combines with repetitive microtrauma.
- Also possible that any abnormal reduction in the subacromial outlet volume may predispose or cause this syndrome.

ETIOLOGY

- Compression and irritation of a rotator cuff tendon (typically supraspinatus) and subacromial bursa due to:
  - Repetitive overhead activities (e.g., throwing, swimming) and shoulder instability
  - Direct trauma that compresses the humerus and the coracoacromial arch
  - Narrowing of the subacromial space secondary to AC joint spurring, thickened coracoacromial ligament, and sloped acromion
- Sudden rotator cuff tears can create impingement syndrome because the humeral head depressors (rotator cuff muscles) fail to keep the humeral head from riding upward into the coracoacromial arch.

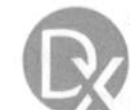

DIAGNOSIS

HISTORY

- Gradual increase in shoulder pain with overhead activities (sudden onset of sharp pain is more suggestive of a tear)
- Waking up with nighttime pain is a typical complaint.
- Common complaint of anterolateral shoulder pain with overhead activities
- May progress to weakness and decreased range of motion

PHYSICAL EXAM

- Positive impingement tests suggest impingement syndrome:
  - Neer impingement sign: Stabilize the patient's scapula and passively flex the arm until the patient reports pain or has full elevation.
  - Hawkins-Kennedy impingement sign: The patient's arm is placed in 90° of forward flexion, and the examiner stabilizes the scapula and internally rotates the shoulder. Pain signifies a positive test.
- Sensitivity and specificity of Neer test for impingement are 79% and 53%, respectively (1)[A].
- Sensitivity and specificity of Hawkin's test for impingement are 79% and 59%, respectively (1)[A].
- Empty-can test: Evaluates for weakness of supraspinatus muscle by placing arm in 90° of forward flexion and internal rotation; examiner provides downward pressure, testing for weakness of supraspinatus strength between sides.
- Lift-off test: Have patient place hand of affected limb on back with palm facing out. Resist patient's attempts to push hand off the back. Weakness or pain is suggestive of subscapularis tendon involvement.
- Resisted external rotation: Suggestive of infraspinatus and/or teres minor tendon involvement
- Evaluate C-spine to rule out cervical pathology.

DIAGNOSTIC TESTS & INTERPRETATION

Imaging

Initial approach

- Plain-film radiographs of the shoulder (4 views): anteroposterior, axillary, lateral, and supraspinatus outlet views
- Plain film may reveal:
  - Osteophytes or hooked acromion (leading to irritation)
  - Cephalad migration of the humerus (from torn rotator cuff muscles that usually depress the humerus)
  - Decreased subacromial space (if worn bursa)
- MRI used to evaluate rotator cuff integrity and possible sources of impingement in those patients willing to undergo surgery
- MR arthrogram increases sensitivity for detecting partial-thickness tears of the rotator cuff and labral pathology.
- Ultrasound is shown to have high accuracy for diagnosis in full-thickness tears but is limited with respect to impingement.

Diagnostic Procedures/Surgery

- Lidocaine injection test:
  - Inject lidocaine into the subacromial space:
    - Repeat impingement tests; if pain is completely relieved and range of motion is improved, likely impingement syndrome.
  - Allows for more accurate strength testing on physical examination:
    - If strength is intact, rules out rotator cuff tear
    - If range of motion does not improve at all, more likely adhesive capsulitis
  - Some pain relief and improved range of motion occurs after lidocaine injection with:
    - Glenoid labral tear
    - Capsular strain
    - Glenohumeral osteoarthritis
    - Glenohumeral instability
- A lack of any pain relief suggests other sources or inappropriate placement of injection.

Pathological Findings

May have tendinosis, tendonitis, or tear of the muscle or its tendon

DIFFERENTIAL DIAGNOSIS

- Labral injury (labrum of glenoid is a cartilage cuff that assists in supporting the head of the humerus; tears usually due to trauma)
- Acromioclavicular arthritis (more common as age increases; likely to have pain with cross-arm testing)
- Adhesive capsulitis (rotator cuff tendonitis leads to decreased use and atrophy of rotator cuff muscles, followed by contracture of joint; has been linked to diabetes)
- Anterior shoulder instability (owing to trauma; more common <25 years of age)
- Multidirectional instability
- Biceps tendonitis or rupture (perform Speed's and Yergeson's tests and look for visible or palpable defect of biceps)
- Calcific tendonitis
- Cervical radiculopathy (spinal or foraminal stenosis, can test with Spurling's maneuver)
- Glenohumeral arthritis (evaluate with plain films)
- Suprascapular nerve entrapment
- Thoracic outlet syndrome
- Traumatic rotator cuff tear

TREATMENT

Anti-inflammatory agents plus aggressive rehabilitation can improve and fully resolve rotator cuff tendonitis in most patients.

MEDICATION

NSAIDs or other analgesic, often for 6–12 weeks

ADDITIONAL TREATMENT

General Measures

- Rest
- Ice or heat for symptom relief
- Activity modification with avoidance of aggravating activities which are typically overhead motions
- Range-of-motion exercises
- Rotator-cuff strengthening to prevent further injuries

Issues for Referral

Failure of conservative treatment, persistent pain, weakness, or complete tear of rotator cuff

Additional Therapies

- Supervised- or home-exercise regimens have been shown to provide clinically significant pain reduction and improved function. However, these measures have no effect on range of motion or strength (2)[A].
- Physical therapy has shown evidence of effectiveness for both short-term and long-term recovery with respect to function (3)[A]:
  - Initial goal is to restore range of motion.
  - After pain resolves, gradually strengthen rotator cuff muscles in internal rotation, external rotation, and abduction.

COMPLEMENTARY AND ALTERNATIVE MEDICINE

- Little evidence to support or refute acupuncture as treatment; it possibly provides some short-term benefit with regard to pain and function (4)[A].
- Some evidence that 5 mg of topical glyceryl trinitrate is more effective than placebo for acute rotator cuff symptoms (5)[A].

SURGERY/OTHER PROCEDURES

- Little overall evidence regarding steroid injections; studies suggest they may be beneficial, although effects may be small and short-lived (6)[A].
  - No apparent significantly increased risk for rotator cuff tears in those receiving subacromial steroid injections (7)[C]
- No significant differences between open versus arthroscopic subacromial decompression and active nonoperative treatment for impingement (8)[A].

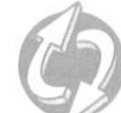

ONGOING CARE

PATIENT EDUCATION

- Patient must understand that physical rehabilitation will be necessary both in conservative course of treatment (i.e., NSAIDs, physical therapy) and with surgical decompression. An aggressive trial of rehabilitation should be encouraged prior to extensive testing or surgical intervention.
- Symptoms often recur if not fully addressed.

PROGNOSIS

- Variable
- Most patients improve with conservative management.

COMPLICATIONS

- Progression of injury
- Tendon retraction in complete rotator cuff tear

REFERENCES

1. Hegedus EJ, Goode A, Campbell S, et al. Physical examination tests of the shoulder: A systematic review with meta-analysis of individual tests. *Br J Sports Med*. 2008;42:80–92.
2. Kuhn JE. Exercise in the treatment of rotator cuff impingement: A systematic review and a synthesized evidence-based rehabilitation protocol. *J Shoulder Elbow Surg*. 2009;18(1):138–60.
3. Green S, Buchbinder R, Hetrick S. Physiotherapy interventions for shoulder pain. *Cochrane Database Syst Rev*. 2008;3.
4. Green S, Buchbinder R, et al. Accupuncture for shoulder pain. *Cochrane Database Syst Rev*. 2008;4.
5. Cumpston M, Johnston R, Wengier L, et al. Topical glyceryl trinitrate for rotator cuff disease. *Cochrane Database Syst Rev*. 2009;3.
6. Buchbinder R, Green S, Youd J. Corticosteroid injections for shoulder pain. *Cochrane Database Syst Rev*. 2009;1.
7. Bhatia M, Singh B, et al. Correlation between rotator cuff tears and repeated subacromial steroid injections: A case-controlled study. *Ann R Coll Surg Engl*. 2009;91(5):414–6.
8. Coghlan J, Buchbinder R, et al. Surgery for rotator cuff disease. *Cochrane Database Syst Rev*. 2009;1.

ADDITIONAL READING

- Baumgarten KM, Gerlach D, et al. Cigarette smoking increases the risk for rotator cuff tears. *Clin Orthop Relat Res*. 2010;468(6):1534–41.
- Bytomski JR, Black D. Conservative treatment of rotator cuff injuries. *J Surg Orthop Adv*. 2006;15(3): 126–31.
- Hanchard N, Handoll H. Phsyical tests for shoulder impingements and local lesions of bursa, tendon or labrum that may accompany impingement. *Cochrane Database Syst Rev*. 2008;4.
- Kennedy DJ, Visco CJ, Press J. Current concepts for shoulder training in the overhead athlete. *Curr Sports Med Rep*. 2009;8(3):154–60.
- Meislin RJ, Sperling JW, Stitik TP. Persistent shoulder pain: Epidemiology, pathophysiology, and diagnosis. *Am J Orthop*. 2005;35(12):5–9.
- Ostor AJ, Richards CA, et al. Diagnosis and relation to general health of shoulder disorders presenting to primary care. *Rheumatology*. 2005;44(6):800–5.

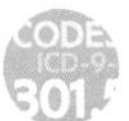

CODES

ICD9

726.10 Disorders of bursae and tendons in shoulder region, unspecified

CLINICAL PEARLS

- Consider impingement syndrome in patients with repetitive overhead arm motion (e.g., swimming, throwing).
- Shoulder pain after age 25 without trauma is most likely secondary to rotator cuff tendonitis.
- Supraspinatus tendon most commonly affected
- Use Neer and Hawkins tests as confirmatory impingement tests.
- Use empty-can test to test for weakness of supraspinatus muscle.
- Lidocaine injection test can aid in identification of type of shoulder pathology.
- Physical therapy over 6–12 weeks promotes return to function.

RUPTURED BOWEL

William J. Brucker, MD
Daithi S. Heffernan, MD

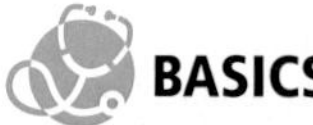

BASICS

DESCRIPTION
- A perforation of the alimentary canal resulting in spillage of intestinal contents; perforations are divided into iatrogenic, pathologic, and traumatic (1)
- Perforations may also be divided by anatomy:
  - Oesophageal
  - Gastric/duodenal
  - Small bowel
  - Appendix
  - Colon

EPIDEMIOLOGY
- Traumatic perforations
  - Small bowel:
    - Injured in 80% of abdominal gunshot wounds
    - Injured in 30% of abdominal stab wounds
    - Injured in 5% of blunt abdominal trauma
  - Colon:
    - Injured in 20% of penetrating abdominal trauma
    - Injured in 7% of transpelvic gunshot wounds
- Perforated duodenal ulcer:
  - Incidence has decreased in recent long-term studies from 14 in 1,000 to 8 in 1,000 person years; perforated duodenal ulcer comprises 5% of all abdominal emergencies.
- Perforated appendicitis:
  - Occurs in 4% of patients with appendicitis
- Perforated colonic diverticulitis:
  - 3.5 cases per 100,000 per year
- Iatrogenic: Varies by underlying disease and reason for intervention
- Infection induced perforation: Typhoid is the most common etiological organism. Consider HIV- or tuberculosis-related bowel perforation.
- Radiation/medication induced:
  - NSAIDs, steroids
  - Cancer chemotherapy, especially bevacizumab used in colorectal, ovarian, or breast cancer: Risk of duodenal ulcer perforation as well as small bowel and colonic perforation

Incidence
- Rapid decrease in incidence of perforated peptic ulcer disease due to use of proton pump inhibitors and *Helicobacter pylori* eradication strategies.
- Annual incidence estimated to be 10 per 100,000 individuals.
- Diverticular perforation incidence of 4 per 100,000 population; incidence is rising among young patients

RISK FACTORS
- Trauma: Both penetrating and blunt
- Iatrogenic: Open, laparoscopic, or endoscopic procedures
- Peptic ulcer disease
- Diverticular disease
- Appendicitis
- Malignancies, especially colon cancer
- Inflammatory bowel disease
- Parasitic infestation

Genetics
Collagen vascular diseases such as Ehlers-Danlos syndrome and osteogenesis imperfecta

GENERAL PREVENTION
- Peptic ulcer disease:
  - Eradication of *H. pylori* and/or the use of proton pump inhibitors in patients with peptic ulcer disease
- Diverticulitis:
  - Diet modification and high-fiber diet
- Iatrogenic:
  - Meticulous attention to detail with gentle tissue handling

PATHOPHYSIOLOGY
- Peptic ulcer disease: *H. pylori*, NSAID use
- Zollinger-Ellison syndrome: Hyperacidity and gastric/duodenal mucosal erosion
- Appendicitis: Appendiceal occlusion with fecalith
- Diverticulitis: Constipation, low-fiber diet
- Malignancy: Cancerous erosion of the bowel wall
- Crohn disease: Excessive and prolonged transmural inflammation of the bowel wall
- Any mechanism that results in the increase in intraluminal pressure can, by definition, perforate the lumen of the intestines according to the Law of La Place.
- Iatrogenic:
  - Greater risk of colonic perforation during colonoscopy in patients with diverticulitis
  - Greater risk of bowel injury or perforation during reoperative surgery or in patients with adhesions

COMMONLY ASSOCIATED CONDITIONS
- One must remain vigilant for the possibility of an underlying malignancy that has eroded through the bowel wall, leading to perforation.
- Zollinger-Ellison syndrome in patients with treatment-resistant peptic ulcer disease
- Appendiceal carcinoid tumors
- Peritonitis: An inflammatory process of the abdominal peritoneum caused by any irritant:
  - Any interruption in the intestinal wall that results in leakage of intestinal contents into the peritoneum can result in peritonitis.
  - If the diagnosis is suspected clinically but cannot be confirmed, peritonitis is the indication to operate.

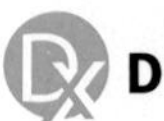

DIAGNOSIS

> **ALERT**
> A diagnosis of ruptured bowel with peritonitis is a surgical emergency, requiring immediate fluid resuscitation and stabilization coupled with surgical consultation. Definitive treatment should not be delayed by extensive workup in the setting of generalized peritonitis.

HISTORY
- Abdominal pain: Often sudden onset
- Abdominal distention, nausea, and/or vomiting
- Preference for supine position; pain worse with movement
- In patients with suspected appendicitis, a right lower quadrant pain that suddenly lessens is highly suspicious for ruptured appendicitis.
- Pain may become more insidious and more generalized as the hours progress.
- Symptoms may be more subtle in the elderly and very young; physicians need to maintain a higher index of suspicion.

PHYSICAL EXAM
- Fever
- Tachycardia, hypotension
- Abdominal guarding
- Rigid abdomen
- Absent bowel sounds

DIAGNOSTIC TESTS & INTERPRETATION

Lab
- CBC with differential, looking for a leukocytosis with left shift
- Chemistries may show a metabolic acidosis.
- Liver function tests
- Amylase and lipase
- Urinalysis may be normal.
- Pregnancy test
- Type and screen and type and cross in case transfusion may be necessary

Imaging
- Plain films:
  - Upright chest x-ray and/or upright abdominal x-ray: Free air under the diaphragm
  - Seen in 80% of duodenal perforations
- CT:
  - Not needed if diagnosis can be made clinically in patient with peritonitis, and it may delay appropriate operative intervention.
  - May help localize an intra-abdominal abscess around a perforation, which may be amenable to radiographically placed drainage catheters.

Diagnostic Procedures/Surgery
Diagnostic peritoneal lavage: When clinical diagnosis cannot be made; suggests peritonitis if >500 WBCs or >100,000 RBCs; difficult to interpret if patient is immunocompromised

DIFFERENTIAL DIAGNOSIS
- Varies based on the location of the abdominal pain
- Pancreatitis: Can mimic an acute abdomen, especially peptic ulcer disease
- Ruptured ovarian cyst
- Strangulated hernias
- Bowel obstruction
- Sickle cell crisis
- Men: Testicular torsion
- Women:
  - Ectopic pregnancy
  - Pelvic inflammatory disease (may mimic ruptured appendicitis)

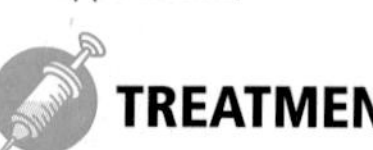

TREATMENT

General resuscitation:
- Patients with suspected bowel perforation should be admitted to the hospital.
- Commence crystalloid fluid resuscitation.

- Fluids should be administered to achieve early goal-directed therapy if the patient is in septic shock due to peritonitis:
  - Mean arterial pressure: >65 mm Hg
  - Urine output >0.5 mL/kg/hr
  - Mixed venous O_2 saturation of 65–75%
- Early operative intervention for source control is essential

MEDICATION

First Line

Antibiotics (2)

- Antibiotics cannot supplant proper source control of a perforated viscus.
- Start with empiric and broad-spectrum coverage (e.g., piperacillin/tazobactam or a carbapenem)
- Tailor to operative culture results
- In cases of typhoid, ciprofloxacin has largely replaced chloramphenicol.
- Typically will need polymicrobial coverage:
  - *Escherichia coli* is the most common bacteria implicated in a perforated abdominal viscus.
  - *Streptococcus* is the most common gram-positive organism.
  - Bacteroides is the most common anaerobe.
  - Other common organisms: *Klebsiella*, *Proteus*, *Enterobacter*, *Clostridium*, *Enterococcus*, *Pseudomonas*
  - Further consideration should be given to adding an antifungal agent in perforated peptic ulcer disease.

SURGERY/OTHER PROCEDURES

- For perforated gastric ulcer:
  - Antrectomy and pyloroplasty
  - Billroth I versus II gastrectomy, depending on the amount of scar tissue in the duodenal region
- For perforated duodenal ulcer:
  - Omental patch repair in the fashion of a Graham patch
  - May require proximal, selective, or highly selective gastric vagotomy for stable patients who have failed or are noncompliant with medical therapy
  - If the patient has not used proton pump inhibitor previously, then one may forgo vagotomy and attempt long-term proton pump inhibitors postoperatively.
- Perforated appendicitis:
  - Operation of choice: Appendicectomy
  - Open versus laparoscopic, depending on anatomy, body habitus, and surgeon preference
  - In older patients, clinicians must consider possibility of a perforated malignancy masking as appendicitis.
- Perforated diverticulitis (open surgery) (2):
  - Resection of perforated portion with end-colostomy (Hartmann procedure)
  - If hemodynamically stable with minimal abdominal contamination, the resection, primary anastomosis, protecting diverting ileostomy may be safe
  - Laparoscopic explorations: Only few surgeons have expertise with this in the emergent setting.
- Trauma:
  - If hemodynamically unstable: Immediate laparotomy
  - If hemodynamically unstable, gross contamination, >6 hours from the time of the trauma, or patient requiring more than 4 units of blood: Resection with end-colostomy
  - If patient presents early and is hemodynamically stable: May be amenable to resection with primary anastomosis

IN-PATIENT CONSIDERATIONS

Initial Stabilization

- Patients with perforated viscus may present in septic shock; therefore, early aggressive fluid management is critical with resuscitative normal saline or lactated Ringer solution (3).
- Placement of a sepsis catheter with measurement of central venous pressure and mixed venous saturations will aid in fluid resuscitation.

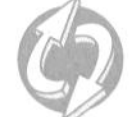

ONGOING CARE

FOLLOW-UP RECOMMENDATIONS

- Peptic ulcer disease:
  - Patient needs to stay compliant with acid-reducing medications if they were prescribed.
  - If ulcers do not heal, need to consider Zollinger-Ellison syndrome or malignancy; patient should undergo repeat endoscopy.
- Diverticulitis:
  - High-fiber diet and avoid straining during bowel movements
  - If the patient did not have a colonoscopy before the perforation, then one is recommended within 6 months to assess for a potential colonic mass, and probably it should be undertaken prior to reversal of stoma.

PROGNOSIS

- Perforated peptic ulcer (4):
  - Nonsurgical management:
    - Check contrast studies to document closure.
    - Interval endoscopy to rule out gastric cancer
- Surgical management:
  - 6–10% postoperative mortality
  - Factors that increase the risk of death:
    - Age >60 years
    - Delay in treatment >24 hours
    - Shock on presentation
    - Comorbid conditions
    - Can use Boey score to predict morbidity and mortality outcome
- Perforated appendicitis:
  - 1.7% mortality rate
- Perforated diverticulitis:
  - 7–15% mortality depending on delay of presentation and underlying comorbidities
- Trauma:
  - Prognosis and follow-up depends on the mechanism of trauma, extent of injury, and success of the operation.

COMPLICATIONS

- Following operative repair, one must remain vigilant for the possible development of a complicating intra-abdominal abscess.
- Signs and symptoms that would alert the physician to a possible intra-abdominal abscess include:
  - Prolonged postoperative ileus
  - New onset of intolerance of diet after initially tolerating diet
  - Persistent fevers
  - Persistent leukocytosis
  - Pain out of proportion to expected postoperative pain
  - Wound infection may be a sign of an intra-abdominal infectious process.
- Ileus
- Wound infection
- Enterocutaneous fistula
- Long-term complications of operative management of perforated peptic ulcer disease:
  - Diarrhea: 30% after vagotomy
  - Dumping syndromes: 10% after vagotomy and drainage procedures
  - Gastric outlet obstruction
  - Recurrent peptic ulcer

REFERENCES

1. Mazuski JE, Solomkin JS, et al. Intra-abdominal infections. *Surg Clin North Am*. 2009;89:421–37, ix.
2. Trenti L, Biondo S, Golda T, et al. Generalized peritonitis due to perforated diverticulitis: Hartmann's procedure or primary anastomosis? *Int J Colorectal Dis*. 2011;26:377–84.
3. Ordonez CA, Puyana JC. Management of peritonitis in the critically ill patient. *Surg Clin North Am*. 2006;86:1323–49.
4. Bertleff MJ, Lange JF, et al. Perforated peptic ulcer disease: A review of history and treatment. *Dig Surg*. 2010;27:161–9.

ADDITIONAL READING

Solomkin JS, Mazuski JE, Bradley JS, et al. Diagnosis and management of complicated intra-abdominal infection in adults and children: Guidelines by the Surgical Infection Society and the Infectious Diseases Society of America. *Surg Infect*. 2010;11(1):79–109.

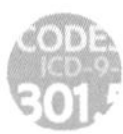

CODES

ICD9

- 532.50 Chronic or unspecified duodenal ulcer with perforation, without mention of obstruction
- 540.0 Acute appendicitis with generalized peritonitis
- 569.83 Perforation of intestine

CLINICAL PEARLS

- Perforation is most often a clinical diagnosis.
- Maintain a high index of suspicion in patients of extremes of age and with high comorbidities to avoid delays in diagnosis and intervention.
- Stabilizing the patient with aggressive, large-volume fluid resuscitation should be the first priority.
- Source control is paramount.
- Use broad-spectrum antibiotics such as piperacillin/tazobactam or a carbapenem.

SALICYLATE POISONING

Lars C. Larsen, MD

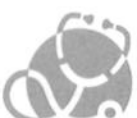

BASICS

DESCRIPTION

Systemic disorder caused by acute and/or chronic intoxication from salicylate-containing medications:

- Following accidental or intentional exposure, toxic actions of salicylates include:
  - Stimulation of CNS respiratory center
  - Uncoupling of oxidative phosphorylation
  - Inhibition of Krebs cycle dehydrogenases
  - Stimulation of gluconeogenesis
  - Increased lipolysis and lipid metabolism
  - Inhibition of aminotransferases
  - Cyclo-oxygenase inhibition and decreased production of clotting factors
  - Irritation of the gastric mucosa and stimulation of the CNS chemoreceptor trigger zone
- These actions cause sequential and progressively severe physiologic abnormalities with increasing doses of salicylates, time following exposure, duration of chronic exposure, extremes of age, and presence of concurrent medical conditions; abnormalities include:
  - Respiratory alkalosis accompanied by progressive metabolic acidosis
  - Hyperpyrexia
  - GI, renal, pulmonary, and skin losses of body fluids and electrolytes
  - Initial hyperglycemia followed by hypoglycemia, particularly CNS hypoglycemia
  - Abnormal hemostasis and coagulation
- Clinical presentation of patients with salicylate toxicity can range from minor symptoms to a syndrome initially indistinguishable from septic shock with multiple organ failure, including encephalopathy and acute respiratory distress syndrome (ARDS).
- The very young and elderly are particularly prone to develop severe toxicity, as are those with chronic intoxication.
- Conditions causing concurrent acidosis may increase tissue concentrations of salicylate and result in greater morbidity and mortality.
- System(s) affected: Cardiovascular; Endocrine/Metabolic; Gastrointestinal; Hematologic/Lymphatic/Immunologic; Musculoskeletal; Nervous; Pulmonary; Renal/Urologic; Skin/Exocrine

Geriatric Considerations

- Increased risk for chronic toxicity because of decreased renal function
- Increased risk for bleeding or perforated gastric ulcers in patients >70 years of age

Pediatric Considerations

Acidosis is often more severe in the very young, particularly in chronic or repeated therapeutic-dose poisonings.

Pregnancy Considerations

- Salicylates may cause premature closure of ductus arteriosus in the fetus.
- Increased risk of ante- and intrapartum hemorrhage

EPIDEMIOLOGY

Incidence/prevalence in the US:

- More than 11,280 single-substance ingestions of acetylsalicylic acid (ASA) or ASA combination products reported by poison control centers in 2009.
- 22 deaths in 2009, none in children <6 years of age
- Occurs in children and adults at any age

RISK FACTORS

- Dehydration
- Conditions causing metabolic or respiratory acidosis
- Extremes of age—very young and elderly
- Psychiatric illness
- History of previous toxic ingestions or suicide attempts
- Concurrent oral poisoning with other substances
- Concurrent use of acetazolamide (Diamox)

GENERAL PREVENTION

- Patient and parent/caregiver education essential; see "Patient Education"
- Emergency telephone numbers (poison control centers): (800) 222-1222

ETIOLOGY

- Accidental or intentional ingestion of salicylates or salicylate-containing medications
- Percutaneous absorption of dermatologic medications containing salicylate
- Breast-feeding by mothers ingesting salicylate-containing medications
- Teething gels containing salicylates

COMMONLY ASSOCIATED CONDITIONS

Reye syndrome with salicylate use and varicella or influenza viral infection

DIAGNOSIS

PHYSICAL EXAM

- Signs and symptoms may differ when the intoxication is acute or chronic.
- Acute intoxication:
  - Symptoms vary with amount ingested, usually begin within 3–8 hours of ingestion, and progress more rapidly in children:
    - <150 mg/kg, minimal symptoms
    - 150–300 mg/kg, moderate symptoms
    - 300–500 mg/kg, severe symptoms
    - >500 mg/kg, potentially fatal
  - Nausea and vomiting
  - Hyperpnea, tachypnea
  - Hyperpyrexia
  - Tinnitus
  - Disorientation, coma, convulsions
  - Cardiac arrhythmias
  - Hypotension
  - Pulmonary edema
- Chronic intoxication:
  - Onset of symptoms is usually gradual.
  - Signs and symptoms similar to acute intoxication may occur and may be advanced at diagnosis and include severe hypotension and ARDS.
  - Neurologic symptoms often predominate, particularly in the elderly, and include agitation, confusion, stupor, hyperactivity, paranoia, bizarre behavior, dysarthria, and restlessness.

DIAGNOSTIC TESTS & INTERPRETATION

Lab

- Serum salicylate levels initially on all patients to confirm diagnosis; following acute ingestions, check levels ≥6 h after ingestion and repeat q2h until the levels are declining and patient's condition has stabilized.
- Acid–base abnormalities common:
  - Usually respiratory alkalosis or mixed respiratory alkalosis and metabolic acidosis
  - Metabolic acidosis often predominates in chronic or severe acute poisonings and in poisonings in young children.
- Increased anion gap, especially in acute poisonings and salicylate-only poisonings
- Initial hyperglycemia may be followed by hypoglycemia.
- Electrolyte abnormalities, such as hypernatremia or hyponatremia and hypokalemia, are common.
- Dehydration findings are common, including an increased BUN:creatinine ratio.
- Prothrombin time (PT)/international normalization ratio (INR) may be increased.
- Liver function abnormalities may be present.
- Proteinuria and renal function abnormalities may be present.
- Stool guaiac testing may be positive.
- Occasional hypouricemia
- Drugs that may alter lab results:
  - Diflunisal (Dolobid) may cross-react with assay of salicylate concentration.
  - Medications affecting similar organ systems, including oral anticoagulants and hypoglycemic agents
- Disorders that may alter lab results: Concurrent medical conditions involving similar organ systems

Initial lab tests

- Serum salicylate levels initially and ≥6 hours after ingestion, then repeat q2h until the levels are declining and patient's condition has stabilized
- Electrolytes, BUN, creatinine, glucose, liver function tests, uric acid
- Arterial blood gases
- PT/INR
- Urinalysis
- Stool guaiac testing may be positive.

Imaging

- Chest radiograph:
  - Noncardiogenic pulmonary edema
  - Variable severity, from mild to ARDS
- Abdominal plain film: Nonspecific bowel gas pattern with retained contrast material in chronic bismuth subsalicylate ingestion

Diagnostic Procedures/Surgery

- None, other than correlating serum salicylate concentration with clinical presentation
- Use of the Done nomogram in managing patients following acute ingestion is not recommended because it may underestimate the severity of poisonings in patients with:
  - Illnesses accompanied by dehydration and/or acidosis
  - Chronic exposure to salicylates
  - Ingestion of enteric-coated or sustained-release medications
  - Unknown time of ingestion

Pathological Findings
None specific for salicylate intoxication; associated findings include:
- GI:
  - Antral and prepyloric ulcers
  - Small bowel ulcerations with enteric-coated salicylates
- Renal:
  - Interstitial nephritis
  - Acute tubular necrosis
  - Minimal-change nephrotic syndrome
- Pulmonary:
  - Noncardiogenic pulmonary edema

DIFFERENTIAL DIAGNOSIS
- All ages:
  - Infection
  - Sepsis
  - Diabetic ketoacidosis
  - Other causes of metabolic acidosis
- In the elderly:
  - Delirium
  - Cerebral vascular accident
  - Myocardial infarction
  - Ethyl alcohol intoxication
  - Congestive heart failure

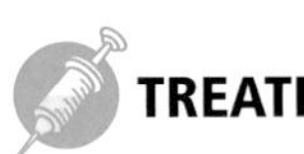

TREATMENT

MEDICATION
- Prevent further absorption if the ingestion is felt to be life threatening:
  - Gastric lavage is rarely indicated.
  - Activated charcoal may be given within 1 hour of toxic ingestion (immediately after gastric lavage if performed (1,2)[C].
  - Ipecac is no longer recommended for use at home or in health care facilities (3)[C].
- Emergency facility/hospital:
  - Activated charcoal 1 g/kg, single dose
  - Fluid/electrolyte balance: IV fluids to restore intravascular volume and prevent hypoglycemia
  - With hypotension, give isotonic fluid until orthostatic changes are no longer present.
  - Fluids should contain ≥5% dextrose unless hyperglycemia is a problem.
  - Normal saline or a mixture of 0.45% NaCl with 1 ampule of sodium bicarbonate (43 mEq $NaHCO_3$) may be administered at 10–15 mL/kg/hr × 1–2 hours depending on the degree of acidosis.
  - When BP is stable, fluid management is directed toward alkalinizing the urine to enhance salicylate excretion, prevent CNS hypoglycemia, and treat fluid and electrolyte abnormalities.
  - Enhance elimination by alkaline diuresis (4)[C]:
    - Alkaline diuresis (urine pH >7.5) and prevention of hypoglycemia usually can be accomplished by initial bolus of $NaHCO_3$ 1–2 mEq/kg IV given over 1 hour, followed by infusion of 1,000 mL D_5W plus 2–3 ampules of $NaHCO_3$ (43 mEq $NaHCO_3$/ampule) at 1.5–2 times maintenance rate (or, at 2–3 mL/kg/hr). Consider adding 40 mEq of potassium chloride to each liter; monitor potassium levels closely.
    - Goal: Bicarbonate to alkalinize the urine (pH >7.5) and, when appropriate, to correct severe systemic acidosis (for pH <7.1)
    - Potassium should be added for potassium levels <4 mEq/L.
    - Patients with cardiovascular compromise should be monitored closely for fluid overload.
    - Alkalinization can be discontinued when the salicylate level decreases into the therapeutic range.
  - Serum electrolytes and glucose should be monitored frequently and urine pH checked hourly until stable at >7.5. Arterial blood gases should be monitored >2–4 hours to ensure blood pH ≤7.5.
  - Hemodialysis should be considered in poisonings with markedly elevated salicylate levels (>100 mg/dL in acute poisonings, >40 mg/dL in chronic poisonings), acidosis unresponsive to alkalinization and diuresis, renal and/or hepatic dysfunction with impaired salicylate clearance, endotracheal intubation (excluding for coingestants), noncardiac pulmonary edema, and persistent, severe CNS symptoms.
  - Dextrose-containing IV solution to prevent hypoglycemia; CNS hypoglycemia may be present despite a normal serum glucose level.
- Contraindications: Medication allergies
- Precautions:
  - Intravascular overload may result from injudicious use of sodium bicarbonate.
  - Dextrose should not be given to patients with severe hyperglycemia.

ADDITIONAL TREATMENT
Issues for Referral
Psychiatric and psychological evaluation in emergency department and in close follow-up for intentional overdose

IN-PATIENT CONSIDERATIONS
Initial Stabilization
- Evaluate all patients at a health care facility.
- Outpatient for nontoxic accidental ingestions
- Inpatient for toxic and intentional ingestions (3)[C]

ONGOING CARE

FOLLOW-UP RECOMMENDATIONS
Patient Monitoring
- Fluid, acid–base, blood glucose, and electrolyte status until stable; urine pH (to enhance elimination of salicylate)
- Psychiatric follow-up after intentional ingestions

DIET
No special diet

PATIENT EDUCATION
- Education of parents/caregivers during well-child visits
- Education of patients about chronic salicylate therapy
- Anticipatory guidance for caregivers, family, and cohabitants of potentially suicidal patients
- Patient brochure (item 1515): *Child Safety: Keeping Your Home Safe for Your Baby;* available from American Academy of Family Physicians or: http://familydoctor.org/online/famdocen/home/healthy/safety/kids-family/027.html
- Poison control: (800) 222-1222

PROGNOSIS
- Complete recovery with early therapy
- Clinical course and prognosis are worse in the very young and elderly, chronic intoxications, and in patients with concurrent conditions that cause dehydration and/or acidosis.

COMPLICATIONS
- Rare following recovery from poisoning
- Noncardiogenic pulmonary edema
- ARDS

REFERENCES

1. Gaudreault P. Activated charcoal revisited. *Clin Pediatr Emerg Med*. 2005;6:76–80.
2. Heard K. Gastrointestinal decontamination. *Med Clin North Am*. 2005;89:1067–78.
3. Chyka PA, et al. *Salicylate Poisoning: An Evidence-based Consensus Guideline for Out-of-Hospital Management*. Washington, DC: American Association of Poison Control Centers; 2006.
4. Proudfoot AT, Krenzelok EP, Vale JA. Position Paper on urine alkalinization. *J Toxicol Clin Toxicol*. 2004; 42:1–26.

ADDITIONAL READING

Bronstein AC, Spyker DA, Cantilena LR, et al. 2009 Annual Report of the American Association of Poison Control Centers' National Poison Data System (NPDS): 27th Annual Report. *Clin Toxicol*. 2010;48:979–1178.

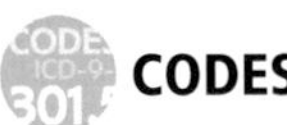

CODES

ICD9
965.1 Poisoning by salicylates

CLINICAL PEARLS
- Gastric decontamination should not be done in all poisonings, only in potentially life-threatening ingestions.
- Think of salicylate toxicity with mixed metabolic acidosis and respiratory alkalosis, especially if anion gap.
- Activated charcoal within 1 hour of toxic ingestion (immediately after gastric lavage, if performed) (1,2)[C]
- Ipecac is no longer recommended for use at home or in health care facilities.
- There is a bedside test to evaluate for the presence of salicylates. A few drops of 10% ferric chloride solution added to 1 mL of urine usually will produce a purple color if salicylates are present.

SALIVARY GLAND CALCULI/SIALADENITIS

Richard Gacek, MD

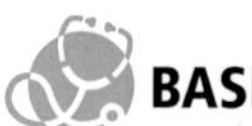

BASICS

DESCRIPTION

- Inflammation or stones involving 1 or more than 1 salivary gland
- The submandibular gland is more commonly affected by sialolithiasis and infection than the parotid gland.
- Chronicity:
  - Acute
  - Chronic
- Types:
  - Infectious
  - Obstructive (sialolithiasis)
  - Autoimmune
- System(s) affected: Gastrointestinal

EPIDEMIOLOGY

Incidence

- A review of British patients showed an incidence of symptomatic sialolithiasis of 27–59/1,000,000 population per year (1).
- Most common in debilitated patients
- Rare in children
- Predominant sex: Male = Female

RISK FACTORS

- Dehydration
- Anticholinergic use
- Antihistamine use
- Diuretic use
- Poor oral hygiene
- Malnutrition
- Head/neck radiation
- Tuberculosis (TB)
- HIV
- Failure to immunize (mumps)

Genetics

- Sjögren syndrome
- Polygenic cause, with several loci under investigation (2)

GENERAL PREVENTION

- Adequate postop hydration
- Maintain oral care.
- Avoid antihistamines, anticholinergics, and other causes of xerostomia.

PATHOPHYSIOLOGY

Decreased salivary outflow from anticholinergics, dehydration, or radiation is thought to allow bacterial infection of salivary glands.

ETIOLOGY

- Bacterial:
  - *Staphylococcus aureus*
  - *Streptococcus viridans*
  - *Streptococcus pyogenes*
  - *Haemophilus influenza*
  - *Escherichia coli*
- Viral:
  - Mumps
  - Cytomegalovirus (CMV), Epstein-Barr virus (EBV)
  - HIV
  - Enteroviruses

COMMONLY ASSOCIATED CONDITIONS

- Postop dehydration
- Radiation-induced xerostomia
- Drug-induced xerostomia
- Sjögren syndrome
- Hypercalcemia

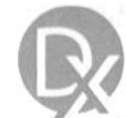

DIAGNOSIS

HISTORY

- Onset, duration of symptoms, previous episodes
- Dental pain, discharge, foul breath, pain with chewing
- Fever, unintentional weight loss
- Recent dental work, surgery
- Immunization history
- Radiation, TB, and HIV exposure
- History of alcoholism, bulimia, malnutrition (suggest sialadenosis)

PHYSICAL EXAM

- Palpate all salivary glands, floor of mouth, tongue, and neck to assess symmetry, tenderness, presence of stones, and lymphadenopathy.
- Examine duct openings for purulent discharge. Palpate gland gently to express purulent material.
- Examine eyes for keratitis.

DIAGNOSTIC TESTS & INTERPRETATION

Lab

Initial lab tests

- CBC, electrolytes (3)[B]
- Culture and sensitivity of any expressed pus (3)[B]

Follow-Up & Special Considerations

If autoimmune process is suspected, consider ordering appropriate labs.

Imaging

Initial approach

- CT scan with IV contrast is the preferred imaging modality (4)[B].
- Ultrasound can localize abscesses, differentiate between solid and cystic disease, and extraglandular disease (5)[B].

Follow-Up & Special Considerations

Consider serial CT scans with contrast to evaluate disease resolution.

Diagnostic Procedures/Surgery

- Sialography to evaluate sialolithiasis and other obstructive lesions
- Sialoscopy to find and remove sialoliths (6)[B]

Pathological Findings

In chronic sialadenitis, loss of acini, fibrosis, and periductal lymphocytosis are evident. Degree indicates chronicity.

DIFFERENTIAL DIAGNOSIS

- Acute bacterial parotitis
- Chronic bacterial parotitis
- Dental abscess
- Mumps
- TB
- HIV (in pediatric populations)
- EBV, CMV, enteroviruses
- Tularemia
- Sialolithiasis
- Cystic fibrosis
- Lupus
- Sjögren syndrome
- Alcoholism
- Bulimia
- Hypothyroidism
- Pleomorphic adenoma
- Lymphoma
- Sarcoidosis
- Collagen-vascular disease
- Metal poisoning

TREATMENT

MEDICATION

First Line

- As *S. aureus* is the most common agent, antistaphylococcal penicillins (nafcillin, oxacillin, Unasyn, Augmentin) are indicated in areas where methicillin-resistant *Staphylococcus aureus* (MRSA) is not predominant.
- For PCN-allergic: Use clindamycin 300 mg PO q8h.
- Antibiotic coverage should be narrowed once culture and sensitivity are available.
- Continue antibiotic therapy for 10–14 days (3)[B].

Second Line

First-generation cephalosporin (cephazolin) or clindamycin is also indicated for empiric coverage (3)[B].

ADDITIONAL TREATMENT

General Measures

- Maintain hydration.
- Apply warm compresses.
- Maintain good oral hygiene.

Issues for Referral

In the case of poor dentition, dental abscess, refer patients to a dentist.

Additional Therapies

In the case of chronic sialadenitis with strictures, consider sialostent placement (6)[B].

COMPLEMENTARY AND ALTERNATIVE MEDICINE

Consider lemon drops or other sialogogues to promote salivation. In one study, postop use of sialogogues nearly halved rates of sialadenitis (7)[B].

SURGERY/OTHER PROCEDURES

- Incision and drainage of parotid abscess is indicated after failing 3–5 days of medical management (3)[B].
- In the case of sialolithiasis, sialoscopy may be indicated for stone removal (3)[B].
- Patients with chronic sialadenitis refractory to medical management may be eligible for salivary gland removal (8)[B].

IN-PATIENT CONSIDERATIONS

Initial Stabilization

- Check vital signs, with particular attention to BP, as patient may be septic secondary to abscess formation.
- Evaluate airway patency.

Admission Criteria

- Parotid abscess
- Sepsis
- Inability to tolerate PO intake

Nursing

Responsibilities may include ensuring excellent oral hygiene, avoiding administration of sialogogues.

Discharge Criteria

- Exclude abscess, sepsis.
- Ensure ability to tolerate PO intake.

ONGOING CARE

FOLLOW-UP RECOMMENDATIONS

- Provide regular follow-up visits for patients with chronic sialadenitis.
- Avoid prescribing medications that cause xerostomia.

Patient Monitoring

Monitor patients with chronic sialadenitis, as decreased salivary gland function due to fibrosis and loss of acini can lead to acute exacerbations.

DIET

- Avoid sialogogues during acute attacks.
- Maintain adequate hydration on an outpatient basis.

PATIENT EDUCATION

- Educate patients on maintaining excellent oral hygiene.
- Educate patients on maintaining good hydration.

PROGNOSIS

Generally excellent, with acute symptoms resolving in about a week with appropriate treatment.

COMPLICATIONS

- Abscess
- Dental caries
- Recurrent sialadenitis
- Facial nerve impingement (rare)
- Ludwig angina

REFERENCES

1. Escudier MP, McGurk M. Symptomatic sialoadenitis and sialolithiasis in the English population, an estimate of the cost of hospital treatment. *Br Dent J*. 1999;186:463–6.
2. Williams PH, Cobb BL, Namjou B, et al. Horizons in Sjögren's syndrome genetics. *Clin Rev Allerg Immunol*. 2007;32:201–9.
3. Fattahi TT, Lyu PE, Van Sickels JE. Management of acute suppurative parotitis. *J Oral Maxillofac Surg*. 2002;60:446–8.
4. Yousem DM, Kraut MA, Chalian AA. Major salivary gland imaging. *Radiology*. 2000;216:19–29.
5. Alyas F, Lewis K, Williams M, et al. Diseases of the submandibular gland as demonstrated using high resolution ultrasound. *Br J Radiol*. 2005;78:362–9.
6. Nahlieli O, Bar T, Shacham R, et al. Management of chronic recurrent parotitis: Current therapy. *J Oral Maxillofac Surg*. 2004;62:1150–5.
7. Nakada K, Ishibashi T, Takei T, et al. Does lemon candy decrease salivary gland damage after radioiodine therapy for thyroid cancer? *J Nucl Med*. 2005;46:261–6.
8. Patel RS, Low TH, Gao K, et al. Clinical outcome after surgery for 75 patients with parotid sialadenitis. *Laryngoscope*. 2007;117:644–7.

ADDITIONAL READING

Ship JA. Diagnosing, managing, and preventing salivary gland disorders. *Oral Dis*. 2002;8:77–89.

CODES

ICD9

- 527.2 Sialoadenitis
- 527.5 Sialolithiasis

CLINICAL PEARLS

- Sialadenitis occurs mainly in debilitated patients.
- Mainstay of treatment is hydration, good oral hygiene.
- Salivary gland abscess must be drained surgically.

SALIVARY GLAND TUMORS

Sagar C. Patel, MD
Edward Feller, MD

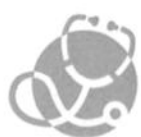

BASICS

Salivary gland tumors consist of benign or malignant neoplasms of the major and minor salivary glands. Tumors may be mimicked clinically by a variety of inflammatory or infectious disorders:

- Major: Parotid, submaxillary, sublingual glands
- Minor: Intraoral, pharyngeal, and nasal glands (600–1,000 glands distributed throughout the upper aerodigestive tract)

DESCRIPTION

- Adult neoplasms:
  - Benign: Pleomorphic adenoma, Warthin tumor, oncocytoma, and monomorphic adenoma
  - Malignant: Mucoepidermoid carcinoma, adenoid cystic carcinoma, acinic cell carcinoma, carcinoma ex-pleomorphic adenoma, squamous cell carcinoma (SCC), adenocarcinoma
- Total distribution of salivary gland neoplasms by type:
  - Pleomorphic adenoma (most common): 45% overall
  - Monomorphic adenoma: 12% overall
  - Mucoepidermoid carcinoma: 12% overall
  - Adenoid cystic carcinoma: 6% overall
  - Remaining neoplasms: 15% overall
- Distribution: Parotid (80%); submandibular (10–15%); sublingual and minor (5–10%):
  - Parotid (80% benign; 20% malignant):
    - Pleomorphic adenoma: 60%
    - Monomorphic adenoma: 8%
    - Warthin tumor: 8%
    - Mucoepidermoid carcinoma: 12%
    - Adenoid cystic carcinoma: 5%
    - Adenocarcinoma and SCC: 5%
  - Submandibular (60% benign; 40% malignant):
    - Pleomorphic adenoma: 40%
    - Mucoepidermoid carcinoma: 10%
    - Adenoid cystic carcinoma: 20%
  - Lingual a minor salivary glands (40% benign; 60% malignant):
    - Pleomorphic adenoma: 40%
    - Mucoepidermoid carcinoma: 25%
    - Adenoid cystic carcinoma: 25%; generally, as the size of the neoplasm decreases, the incidence of malignancy increases.
- Pediatric neoplasms:
  - Incidence is rare in children but much more likely to be malignant.
  - Benign: 65% of overall cases; the most common types are hemangiomas and pleomorphic adenomas.
  - Malignant: 35% of overall cases; most common type is mucoepidermoid carcinoma

EPIDEMIOLOGY

Incidence

- 1.5 cases per 100,000 individuals in the US
- ~700 deaths annually
- Median age:
  - Benign: Age 45
  - Malignant: Age 60
- Gender predilection:
  - Benign: Female > Male
  - Malignant: Male = Female

Prevalence

Make up 6% of all head and neck neoplasms

RISK FACTORS

- Tobacco and alcohol abuse associated with Warthin tumor, but not with SCC
- Alcohol increases likelihood ratio by 2:1 (1,2).
- Radiation has shown a 4-fold increased dose-related response in salivary gland cancer 15–20 years after treatment. Increased risk has also been reported in atomic bomb survivors (1,2).
- Epstein-Barr virus has been associated with lymphoepithelial carcinoma in Asians, but there is no evidence of causal association in other tumors (1,2).
- Silica dust has been associated with a 2.5-fold increase in salivary gland neoplasia (1,2).
- Kerosene cooking fuel exposure (1,2)
- Nitrosamine exposure in rubber workers (1,2)
- Early menarche and nulliparity (1,2)

Genetics

Increased incidence of adenocarcinoma of parotid in Eskimos; otherwise, no known genetic pattern

GENERAL PREVENTION

- Tobacco cessation
- Alcohol cessation

PATHOPHYSIOLOGY

Pathophysiology is not fully understood. Certain pathways and oncogenes have been implicated, such as *p53*, *Bcl-2*, *PI3K/Akt*, *MDM2*,*VEGF*, *HGF*, and *ras*.

ETIOLOGY

- Etiology is not fully understood.
- Predominant theory: Tumors arise from either the excretory duct reserve cell or the intercalated duct reserve cell.

DIAGNOSIS

HISTORY

- Focused inquiry:
  - Specific presentation of mass: Initial recognition; rate of growth; change in size with actions, especially with food consumption; xerostomia (Sjögren syndrome, prior irradiation, medication)
  - Intermittent, recurrent gland enlargement suggests sialolithiasis (calculi in salivary duct); rarely, can be due to malignancy.
  - Pain: Type, degree, accentuating and/or alleviating factors, temporality
  - Location and spread
  - Effect on associated structures with relevant review of systems: Larynx (airway obstruction, hoarseness, dysphagia); nasal cavity/paranasal sinuses (nasal obstruction, sinusitis); pharyngeal wall invasion (dysphagia, muffled voice)
- Common presentations:
  - Overall: Typically, a slow-growing, painless, discrete mass
  - Parotid neoplasm: Discrete mass typically at the tail of the gland
  - Submandibular neoplasm: Associated with diffuse enlargement of the gland itself
  - Sublingual neoplasm: Tends to produce palpable fullness in the floor of the mouth
  - Minor gland neoplasm: Depends on initial site of origin
- Indicator of malignancy:
  - Facial paralysis, paresthesias, or other neurologic deficit associated with mass
  - Pain is not a clear indicator of malignancy; may be associated with both benign and malignant neoplasms; exquisite pain is more likely due to infectious cause.

PHYSICAL EXAM

- Complete HEENT examination with emphasized focus:
  - Evaluate the size, mobility, tenderness and extent of the mass, and fixation to surrounding structures.
  - If tenderness present, massage gland to express purulent material due to infection.
  - Lymphadenopathy, especially, in neck levels I–V
  - Referred pain (otalgia)
- Complete neurologic exam with focus on cranial nerves:
  - Facial nerve palsy or paralysis may indicate a malignant lesion with perineural invasion.

DIAGNOSTIC TESTS & INTERPRETATION

- Technetium-99m (Warthin tumor): Follow patient closely; Warthin tumor has low chance of metastasis.
- Sialography (for calculi or chronic parotitis)

Lab

- Autoimmune studies (ESR, CRP, ANA)
- Fractionated amylase (inflammation)
- Drugs that may alter lab results: None known
- Disorders that may alter lab results: None known

Imaging

- CXR:
  - Sjögren syndrome
  - Metastases
- Ultrasound: Inflammatory or malignant
- CT scan: Provides detail of tumor invasion and temporal bone or mandibular destruction
- MRI:
  - Provides definition of soft tissue and any evidence of perineural invasion or intracranial extension
  - Discriminates tumor from mucus and bone marrow invasion
- PET scan: Useful for detecting malignancy in early stages and for detecting recurrences and differentiating soft tissue damage secondary to radiation from inflammatory changes
- Staging (2002 AJCC):
  - TNM (tumor size, nodal status, and metastasis)
  - Stage I–IVc

Diagnostic Procedures/Surgery

- Fine-needle aspiration:
  - Concern for possible tumor seeding via needle track; however, tumor spread from tumor seeding is rare.
  - Sensitivity 92%, specificity 100%, but false-negative rate up to 53% (3)
- Superficial parotidectomy with identification and preservation of facial nerve

DIFFERENTIAL DIAGNOSIS

- Metabolic causes (diabetes, vitamin deficiencies, alcohol, gout)
- Drugs (thiourea, iodine)
- Inflammatory masses
- Parotid and submandibular lymph nodes
- Mikulicz syndrome
- Salivary gland stones
- Torus palatinus (minor)
- Necrotizing sialometaplasia (minor)
- Cervical lymph nodes
- Sjögren syndrome
- Sarcoidosis
- HIV-associated enlargement (lymphoepithelial cyst)
- Actinomycosis
- Cat-scratch disease
- Tuberculosis

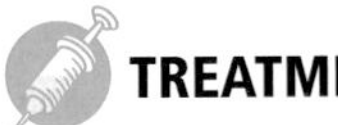

TREATMENT

- Surgical excision is the primary treatment for all salivary gland tumors.
- Facial nerve is spared unless it is directly involved or highly suspicious.
- Poor general response to chemotherapy
- Adjuvant chemotherapy is currently indicated for palliation.
- Radiotherapy is currently used for nonresectable, extensive, large tumors.
- No level 1 trials have shown efficacy for postoperative radiotherapy.

MEDICATION

Cisplatin-, fluorouracil-, or paclitaxel-based regimens for recurrent or nonoperable disease (4)

ADDITIONAL TREATMENT

General Measures

Postoperative care:

- Elevate head of bed postoperatively.
- Suction drainage for 1–2 days
- Suture-line care with antibiotic ointment
- Examination for facial nerve function
- Monitor for signs of hematoma and drain if present.
- Usually 1–2-day hospitalization

Additional Therapies

- Postoperative irradiation (via fast neutron beam) for larger and high-grade carcinomas
- Chemotherapy reserved for metastases or locally advanced and unresectable tumors

SURGERY/OTHER PROCEDURES

- Benign tumors: Superficial or total conservative (nerve-sparing) parotidectomy
- Malignant tumors:
  - Total parotidectomy or sialadenectomy with adjuvant radiotherapy to parotid base of skull ± neck dissection
  - Preservation of facial nerve unless involved by tumor
- Cervical lymphadenectomy if palpable nodes or elective neck dissection in SCC, high-grade mucoepidermoid carcinoma, or high-grade adenocarcinoma

IN-PATIENT CONSIDERATIONS

Admission Criteria

Airway impingement

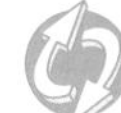

ONGOING CARE

FOLLOW-UP RECOMMENDATIONS

Patient Monitoring

- For malignancy: Once every 6–8 weeks the first year, every 8–12 weeks the second year, every 4 months the third year, every 6 months the fourth year, and then yearly visits
- For benign tumors: Once a year for 5 years

DIET

Nonstimulating liquid diet

PATIENT EDUCATION

- Xerostomia treatment and mouth care
- Tobacco cessation
- Alcohol abstinence
- Sensorineural hearing loss

PROGNOSIS

- By tumor type:
  - Parotid pleomorphic adenoma: Untreated will demonstrate malignant degeneration in 2–10% over 20 years. Treated adequately, parotid pleomorphic adenoma has 1.5% recurrence rate. Extension of pseudopods of tumor beyond the tumor mass increases the risk of recurrent disease.
  - Adenoid cystic:
    - Parotid: 5-year survival, 73%; 15-year survival, 21%
    - Submandibular: 5-year survival, 50%; 15-year survival, 0%;
    - Palate: 5-year survival, 80%; 15-year survival, 38%
  - Adenocarcinoma:
    - Aggressive tumors with a tendency for local recurrence (38%); regional lymph node metastasis (33%); and dissemination to lungs, bone, and liver
    - 5-year survival, 78%; 20-year survival, 41%
  - Mucoepidermoid:
    - Low-grade: 5-year survival, 81%; 15-year survival, 48%
    - High-grade: 5-year survival, 46%; 15-year survival, 25%
  - SCC:
    - Rare tumor with 50% incidence of cervical lymph node metastasis and local recurrence
    - 5-year survival, 18%; 15-year survival, 0%
  - Lymphoma:
    - Rare, accounting for 1.7% of salivary neoplasms
    - 5-year survival: Hodgkin-type, 90%; non-Hodgkin-type, 43%
- 5-year survival rate for stages I–IV and cause-specific survival (CSS):
  - Stage I: 75% (CSS 86%)
  - Stage II: 59% (CSS 66%)
  - Stage III: 57% (CSS 53%)
  - Stage IV: 28% (CSS 32%)

COMPLICATIONS

- Frey syndrome (gustatory sweating) occurs symptomatically in ~20% of patients undergoing parotidectomy.
- Hematoma with possible posterior displacement of tongue and airway obstruction
- Facial neurapraxia from surgery should resolve within 6 months, even with radiotherapy.
- Cosmetic deformity of moderate facial flattening on side of parotidectomy
- Injury to hypoglossal or lingual nerve
- If inadequately excised, pleomorphic adenoma may recur due to pseudopods in the lobe.
- Wound infection of surgical site

REFERENCES

1. Spitz MR. Epidemiology and risk factors for head and neck cancer. *Semin Oncol*. 1994;21:281–8.
2. Zheng W, et al. Diet and other risk factors for cancer of the salivary glands: A population-based case-control study. *Intern J Cancer*. 1996;67(2): 194–8.
3. Cohen EG, Patel SG, Lin O, et al. Fine-needle aspiration biopsy of salivary gland lesions in a selected patient population. *Arch Otolaryngol Head Neck Surg*. 2004;130:773–8.
4. Surakanti SG, Agulnik M. Salivary gland malignancies: The role for chemotherapy and molecular targeted agents. *Semin Oncol*. 2008;35: 309–19.

ADDITIONAL READING

- de Bree R, van der Waal I, Leemans CR. Management of frey syndrome. *Head Neck*. 2007; 29(8):773–8.
- Guzzo M, Ferrari A, Marcon I, et al. Salivary gland neoplasms in children: The experience of the Istituto Nazionale Tumori of Milan. *Pediatr Blood Cancer*. 2006;47:806–10.
- Tiselius HG. Epidemiology and medical management of stone disease. *BJU Int*. 2003;91:758–67.
- Worster A, Preyra I, Weaver B, et al. The accuracy of noncontrast helical computed tomography versus intravenous pyelography in the diagnosis of suspected acute urolithiasis: A meta-analysis. *Ann Emerg Med*. 2002;40:280–6.

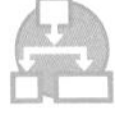

See Also (Topic, Algorithm, Electronic Media Element)

Sjögren Syndrome

CODES

ICD9

- 142.0 Malignant neoplasm of parotid gland
- 142.1 Malignant neoplasm of submandibular gland
- 142.2 Malignant neoplasm of sublingual gland

CLINICAL PEARLS

- Delay in diagnosis is common in rare disease, especially with diverse, nonspecific presentation of minor salivary gland tumors.
- To evaluate a patient with a suspected salivary gland malignancy, complete history, physical, and consider either CT scan or MRI; fine-needle aspiration likely will yield a working diagnosis
- A neck lymphadenectomy is required with tumors ≥4 cm in size, SCC, adenocarcinoma, undifferentiated carcinoma, and high-grade mucoepidermoid carcinoma.

SALMONELLA INFECTION

April Wilhelm, MD
David Anthony, MD

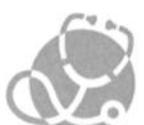

BASICS

DESCRIPTION

- Disease caused by any serotype of the bacterial genus *Salmonella*
- *S. enterica*, which has 2,500 different serotypes, is the most pathogenic species in humans.
- Nontyphoidal *Salmonella* has a number of agricultural animal hosts and is an important cause of foodborne infection.
- Clinical syndromes include:
  - Enterocolitis (75%)
  - Bacteremia (10%)
  - Enteric fever (10%) (see "Typhoid Fever")
  - Localized infection outside GI tract (5%)
  - Asymptomatic carrier state (<1%)
- Pathogenesis: Organisms are ingested, invade gut mucosa, and produce an inflammatory, cytotoxic response. They can then disseminate into systemic circulation via lymphatics.
- Infective dose and host defenses (e.g., gastric acidity) dictate extent of disease.
- System(s) affected: Primarily GI
- Synonym: Nontyphoidal salmonellosis (NTS)

Geriatric Considerations

- Patients over 65 years of age have increased risk of developing invasive disease (1). This population often has comorbidities (atherosclerotic endovascular lesions, prostheses, etc.) that increase risk of seeding and bacteremia.
- Antibiotics should be considered for uncomplicated gastroenteritis due to *Salmonella* infection in patients >50 years of age.

Pediatric Considerations

Neonates (<3 months of age) are more susceptible to invasive disease and subsequent complications, including CNS infection; treat with antibiotics for uncomplicated infection.

Pregnancy Considerations

- Pregnancy has not been demonstrated to increase the risk or severity of infection.
- Routine antibiotic treatment is unnecessary in mild, uncomplicated gastroenteritis early in pregnancy. Antibiotic treatment is indicated in the following clinical settings:
  - Febrile patients with severe disease or bacteremia
  - Infection near term (to limit risk of transmission during childbirth)

EPIDEMIOLOGY

Incidence

- Incidence of laboratory-confirmed *Salmonella* infection in 2009 in the US (2):
  - 15.19 cases/100,000 population
  - Highest incidence in children <4 years of age: 72.93 cases/100,000 population
  - Hospitalization rates for infection are high among patients ≥50 years old (45.2%).
- Peak frequency: July–November
- *Salmonella* isolations represent only 1–10% of the actual yearly incidence.
- A less common cause of traveler's diarrhea (3), but second only to *Campylobacter* as the cause of bacterial diarrhea illness in the US.
- Foodborne outbreak updates: www.cdc.gov

RISK FACTORS

- Recent travel outside the US
- Alteration of endogenous bowel flora (e.g., after antimicrobial therapy or surgery)
- Impaired gastric acidity: H2 receptor blockers, antacids, PPIs, gastrectomy, achlorhydria
- Reticuloendothelial blockade: Sickle cell, malaria, bartonellosis
- Malignancy
- Rheumatologic conditions
- Immunosuppression: AIDS, DM, steroids, other immunosuppressants, chemotherapy, radiation

GENERAL PREVENTION

- Proper hygiene in production, transport, and storage of food (e.g., refrigerating eggs to minimize multiplication of the bacteria if present, then cooking them thoroughly prior to consumption)
- Control of animal reservoir, especially by avoiding contact with animal feces.
- Hand hygiene

ETIOLOGY

- Ingestion of contaminated food (e.g., poultry, beef, eggs, tomatoes, dairy products, commercially prepared nuts and nut products) or water accounts for 95% of cases (4).
- Person-to-person and/or fecal–oral spread
- Contact with asymptomatic chronic carrier (e.g., daycare center)
- Contact with exotic pets with high fecal carriage rates for *Salmonella*, especially reptiles
- Iatrogenic contamination (e.g., blood transfusion, endoscopy)

COMMONLY ASSOCIATED CONDITIONS

- Gastroenteritis: Typically associated with normal immune function
- Bacteremia with: Immunocompromised, anatomic disruptions (e.g. cholelithiasis, prostheses)

DIAGNOSIS

HISTORY

- *Salmonella* infections typically result in mild, self-limited gastroenteritis or asymptomatic carriage.
- Symptoms usually occur 12–72 hours after contaminated ingestion and resolve within 4–10 days.
- Clinical presentation cannot be reliably distinguished from other bacterial enteric infections.
- Acute uncomplicated illness (4)[C]:
  - Sudden onset of nausea, vomiting, diarrhea (rarely bloody), and abdominal cramping
  - Headache, myalgias
  - Fever to 102°F (39°C)
- The median duration of fecal shedding of nontyphoidal *Salmonellae* after gastroenteritis is ~1 month in adults and 7 weeks in children <5 years of age.

PHYSICAL EXAM

- Fever, tachycardia, tachypnea
- Evidence of hypovolemia
- Severe abdominal pain (may mimic acute appendicitis)
- Heme-positive stool
- Rash (subtle rash possible if bacteremic)
- Evidence of localized infection: Arthritis, soft tissue abscesses, UTIs

DIAGNOSTIC TESTS & INTERPRETATION

Lab

Initial lab tests

- Enterocolitis:
  - Stool cultures are not routinely recommended for watery or traveler's diarrhea because of the low yield of bacterial pathogens (4)[C].
  - If ordered, conventional stool culture should evaluate for *Salmonella*, *E. coli*, *Shigella*, and *Campylobacter* species.
  - Indications for stool culture include (4)[C]:
    - Severe diarrhea (6+ unformed stools/d)
    - Diarrhea >1 week in duration
    - Fever
    - Dysentery (diarrhea containing blood or mucous)
    - Multiple cases of illness suggesting an outbreak
  - Fecal leukocytes: Positive
  - CBC: WBC normal or decreased
- Bacteremia:
  - Blood cultures: Positive for *Salmonella*
  - Stool cultures: Negative
- Local infections:
  - CBC: Polymorphonuclear leukocytosis
  - Wound culture: Positive for *Salmonella*
- Asymptomatic carrier state:
  - Stool culture positive for >1 year
  - Urine culture may be positive.

Follow-Up & Special Considerations

- Serotyping of isolates can be performed at public health laboratories.
- PCR-based tests can be used in outbreaks to determine the relationship between strains.
- A positive stool culture for *Salmonella* may be due to asymptomatic carriage of the bacteria and thus may not accurately identify the diarrhea etiology.
- Early, empiric antibiotics may lead to false-negative culture and blunted immunologic response.

Imaging

Consider angiography in patients >50 years of age with bacteremia to rule out presence of infected aneurysm, particularly of aortoiliac vessels.

Pathological Findings

- Mucosal ulceration, hemorrhage, and necrosis
- Reticuloendothelial hyperplasia and hypertrophy
- Focal organ and soft-tissue abscesses

DIFFERENTIAL DIAGNOSIS

- Viral gastroenteritis
- Other bacterial enteritis (e.g., shigellosis, cholera)
- Other bacterial sources of systemic and localized sepsis (e.g., meningococci, staphylococci)
- Pseudomembranous colitis
- Inflammatory or granulomatous bowel disease
- Appendicitis
- Cholecystitis
- Perforated viscus

TREATMENT

- Nonsevere enterocolitis and asymptomatic carriage of *Salmonella* is typically self-limited and does not require antibiotic therapy in the immunocompetent patient (5)[A].
- Antibiotic courses of 1–14 days do not decrease the positive rates of *Salmonella* after 2–3 weeks, but prolong bacterial excretion and increase the risk of relapse (5)[A].
- Bacteremia complicates *Salmonella* infection in ~8% of healthy people (4)[C].
- Certain populations at increased risk of developing bacteremia benefit from antibiotics for acute enterocolitis and *Salmonella* carrier state:
  - Infants <3 months of age
  - Persons >50 years of age
  - Patients with immunosuppression, hemoglobinopathies, underlying atherosclerotic lesions, and prosthetic valves, grafts, or joints

MEDICATION

First Line

- Enterocolitis, uncomplicated: None advised (5)[A]
- Enterocolitis, complicated (risk factors above) (4)[C]:
  - Adults (treat for 14 days if immunocompromised):
    - Levofloxacin (or other fluoroquinolone): 500 mg PO every day × 7–10 days; *or*
    - Azithromycin: 500 mg PO every day for 7 days
  - Children:
    - Ceftriaxone: 100 mg/kg/d IV or IM in 2 equally divided doses × 7–10 days; *or*
    - Azithromycin: 20 mg/kg/d PO daily × 7 days
- Bacteremia: Due to resistance trends, life-threatening infections in adults should be treated with a fluoroquinolone *and* a third-generation cephalosporin until susceptibilities are determined.
  - Adults:
    - Ciprofloxacin (or other fluoroquinolone): 400 mg IV b.i.d. or 500 mg PO b.i.d. × 7–10 days; *or*
    - Ceftriaxone: 2 g IV or IM every day × 7–14 days
  - Children:
    - Ampicillin: 200 mg/kg/d in 4 divided doses × 10–14 days; *or*
    - Trimethoprim-sulfamethoxazole: 10–50 mg/kg/d in 2 divided doses × 10–14 days; *or*
    - Ceftriaxone: 50–75 mg/kg/d once per day × 10–14 days
- Localized infection (e.g., septic arthritis, osteomyelitis, cholangitis, and pneumonia):
  - Same as for bacteremia
  - In sustained bacteremia, prolonged local infection, or immunocompromised patients, antibiotics can be given PO for 4–6 weeks.
- Chronic carrier state (shedding >1 year duration):
  - Amoxicillin: 1 g/d PO t.i.d. × 12 weeks; *or*
  - Trimethoprim: 160 mg *and* sulfamethoxazole 800 mg PO b.i.d. × 12 weeks; *or*
  - Ciprofloxacin: 750 mg PO b.i.d. × 4 weeks, or norfloxacin 400 mg PO b.i.d. × 4 weeks if gallstones are present.
- Antimicrobial resistance rates:
  - Strains resistant to ampicillin, chloramphenicol, and trimethoprim-sulfamethoxazole have been increasing over the last 15 years. Some strains are rapidly becoming multidrug-resistant (1)[B].
  - Fluoroquinolone resistance has been observed in serotypes common to swine and humans
  - Extended-spectrum cephalosporin resistance has been reported in the US with increasing frequency. 2.5% of invasive serotypes isolated from 1996–2007 in the US demonstrated resistance to ceftriaxone (1)[B].

Second Line

- Aztreonam is an alternative agent that may be useful in patients with multiple allergies or organisms with unusual resistance patterns
- Fluoroquinolones are now routinely given to children for 5–7 days in areas of the world where multidrug-resistant *Salmonella typhi* is common

ADDITIONAL TREATMENT

General Measures

- Precautions: Do NOT use bowel motility inhibitors (Lomotil, Imodium). Antimotility drugs may lead to increased contact time of the enteropathogen with the gut mucosa (4)[C].

SURGERY/OTHER PROCEDURES

- Surgical excision and drainage for infected tissue sites, followed by a minimum of 2 weeks antimicrobial therapy
- If biliary tract disease is present, a preoperative 10–14-day course of parenteral antibiotics followed by cholecystectomy is the standard.

ONGOING CARE

FOLLOW-UP RECOMMENDATIONS

Patient Monitoring

- Follow-up fecal cultures are generally not indicated for the typical patient with uncomplicated enterocolitis. Requirements may differ during a *Salmonella* outbreak.
- Cessation of diarrhea and good hand hygiene are appropriate criteria for return of health care workers to their duties.
- Criteria may vary by state and local regulations. For example, some public health departments require negative stool cultures for health workers and food handlers prior to returning to work. Shedding may last 4–8 weeks.

DIET

Give oral rehydration solution during diarrhea phase; advance to normal, easily digestible diet as tolerated.

PATIENT EDUCATION

- Meticulous hand hygiene to prevent primary and secondary infections; caution when handling raw meat, poultry, and eggs
- Fruits and vegetables should be thoroughly washed prior to consumption.
- For more details, visit: www.cdc.gov/salmonella/general/prevention.html

PROGNOSIS

- Most cases of *Salmonella* enterocolitis are self-limited with an excellent prognosis.
- Increased mortality is seen in the very young (<3 months of age), the very old (>65 years of age), and the immunocompromised.
- Complications of meningitis and endocarditis have a poor prognosis, with fatality approaching 50% of cases.
- Mortality is increased with multidrug-resistant strains.

COMPLICATIONS

Toxic megacolon, hypovolemic shock, metastatic abscess formation, endocarditis, infectious endarteritis, meningitis, septic arthritis, osteomyelitis, pneumonia

REFERENCES

1. Crump JA, Medalla FM, Joyce KW, et al. Antimicrobial resistance among invasive nontyphoidal Salmonella enterica isolates in the United States: National Antimicrobial Resistance Monitoring System, 1996 to 2007. *Antimicrob. Agents Chemother*. 2011;55:1148–54.
2. Centers for Disease Control and Prevention (CDC), et al. Preliminary FoodNet data on the incidence of infection with pathogens transmitted commonly through food - 10 states, 2009. *MMWR*. 2010;59: 418–22.
3. Shah N, DuPont HL, Ramsey DJ. Global etiology of travelers' diarrhea: systematic review from 1973 to the present. *Am J Trop Med Hyg*. 2009;80:609–14.
4. DuPont HL, et al. Clinical practice. Bacterial diarrhea. *N Engl J Med*. 2009;361:1560–9.
5. Sirinavin S, Garner P. Antibiotics for treating salmonella gut infections. *Cochrane Database Syst Rev*. 2000;93:CD991167.

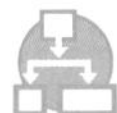

See Also (Topic, Algorithm, Electronic Media Element)

Gastroenteritis; Typhoid Fever

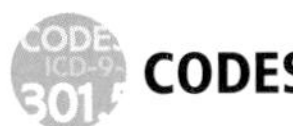

CODES

ICD9

- 003.0 *Salmonella* gastroenteritis
- 003.1 *Salmonella* septicemia
- 003.9 *Salmonella* infection, unspecified

CLINICAL PEARLS

- Nontyphoidal *Salmonella* is a foodborne infection strongly associated with poultry, eggs, and fresh produce.
- If 1 member of a household becomes infected with *Salmonella*, the chance of at least 1 other member becoming infected is 60%.
- In outbreaks, >50% of individuals infected may remain asymptomatic.
- Symptoms usually occur 6–72 hours after a contaminated ingestion.
- Acute uncomplicated enterocolitis is manifested by: Nausea, vomiting, abdominal cramping, headache, myalgias, fever, and possibly bloody diarrhea.
- Those at greatest risk of death from *Salmonella* infection include the very young and the very old.
- Treatment of uncomplicated gastroenteritis in healthy populations generally is unnecessary due to its self-limited nature. Antibiotic treatment has been shown to prolong the carrier state.

SARCOIDOSIS

Donnah Mathews, MD

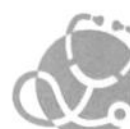

BASICS

DESCRIPTION

- Sarcoidosis is a noninfectious, multisystem granulomatous disease of unknown cause, commonly affecting young and middle-aged adults:
  - Frequently presents with hilar adenopathy, pulmonary infiltrates, ocular and skin lesions
  - In ~50% of cases, it is diagnosed in asymptomatic patients with abnormal chest x-rays (CXRs).
  - Almost any organ may be involved.
- System(s) affected: Primarily Pulmonary, but also Cardiovascular; Gastrointestinal; Hematologic/Lymphatic; Endocrine; Renal; Neurologic; Dermatologic; Ophthalmologic; Musculoskeletal
- Synonyms: Löfgren syndrome (erythema nodosum, hilar adenopathy plus uveitis); Heerfordt syndrome (uveitis, parotid enlargement, facial palsy, fever); Besnier-Boeck disease; Boeck sarcoid; Schaumann disease) (1,2)[C]

EPIDEMIOLOGY

Incidence

Estimated 6/100 person-years (3)

Prevalence

- Estimated 10–20/100,000 persons
- <15% of patients with active disease >60 years of age
- Rare in children (3,4)

RISK FACTORS

Exact etiology and pathogenesis remain unknown.

Genetics

- Reports of familial clustering
- 3–4× more common in African Americans
- Although worldwide in distribution, there is increased prevalence in Scandinavians, Japanese, and Black women (3,4).

GENERAL PREVENTION

None

PATHOPHYSIOLOGY

- Thought to be due to exaggerated cell-mediated immune response to unknown antigen(s)
- In the lungs, the initial lesion is CD4+ T-cell alveolitis, causing noncaseating granulomata, which may resolve or undergo fibrosis.
- "Immune paradox" with affected organs showing an intense immune response and yet anergy exists elsewhere (5).

ETIOLOGY

Unknown

COMMONLY ASSOCIATED CONDITIONS

None

DIAGNOSIS

HISTORY

- Patients may be asymptomatic.
- Patients may have nonspecific complaints, such as:
  - Nonproductive cough
  - Shortness of breath
  - Fever
  - Night sweats
  - Weight loss
  - General fatigue
  - Eye pain
  - Chest pain or palpitations
  - Skin lesions
  - Polyarthritis
  - Renal calculi (5)
  - Facial droop due to Bell palsy (6)
  - Encephalopathy, seizures, hydrocephalus (rare)

PHYSICAL EXAM

- Many patients have a normal physical exam.
- Lungs may reveal wheezing or fine interstitial crackles in advanced disease.
- Extrapulmonary manifestations may include:
  - Uveitis
  - Other eye findings: Conjunctival nodules, lacrimal gland enlargement, cataracts, glaucoma, papilledema
  - Cranial nerve palsies
  - Salivary gland swelling
  - Lymphadenopathy
  - Arrhythmias
  - Hepatosplenomegaly
  - Polyarthritis
  - Rashes: Maculopapular, nodular, plaques, or erythema nodosum

DIAGNOSTIC TESTS & INTERPRETATION

Lab

No definitive test for diagnosis, but diagnosis is suggested by the following:

- Clinical and radiographic manifestations
- Exclusion of other diagnoses
- Histopathologic detection of noncaseating granulomas

Initial lab tests

- CBC: Anemia or leukopenia ± eosinophilia can be seen.
- Hypergammaglobulinemia can exist.
- Liver function tests (LFTs): Abnormal liver function and increased alkaline phosphatase are encountered frequently.
- Calcium: Hypercalciuria occurs in up to 10% of patients, with hypercalcemia less frequent.
- Serum ACE is elevated in >75% of patients but is not diagnostic or exclusionary:
  - Drugs that may alter lab results: Prednisone will lower serum ACE and normalize gallium scan. ACE inhibitors will lower serum ACE level.
  - Disorders that may alter lab results: Hyperthyroidism and diabetes will increase serum ACE level (6)[C].

Imaging

Initial approach

- CXR or CT scan may reveal granulomas or hilar adenopathy. Routine CXRs are staged using Scadding classification (7):
  - Stage 0 = normal
  - Stage 1 = bilateral hilar adenopathy alone
  - Stage 2 = bilateral hilar adenopathy plus parenchymal infiltrates
  - Stage 3 = parenchymal infiltrates alone (primarily upper lobes)
  - Stage 4 = pulmonary fibrosis
- Chest CT scan may enhance appreciation of lymph nodes.
- High-resolution chest CT scan shows peribronchial disease.
- Gallium scan will be positive in areas of acute disease or inflammation, but is not specific.
- Positron emission tomography (PET) scan can indicate areas of disease activity in lungs, lymph nodes, and other areas of the body.
- Cardiac PET scan may detect cardiac sarcoidosis (6)[B].

Diagnostic Procedures/Surgery

- Pulmonary function testing may reveal restrictive pattern with decreased carbon monoxide diffusing capacity (DLCO).
- Characteristically in active disease, bronchioalveolar lavage fluid has an increased CD4/CD8 ratio.
- Ophthalmologic examination may reveal uveitis, retinal vasculitis, or conjunctivitis.
- ECG
- Tuberculin skin test
- Biopsy of lesions should reveal noncaseating granulomas.
- If lungs are affected, bronchoscopy with biopsy of central and peripheral airways is helpful. Endobronchial ultrasound (EBUS)-guided transbronchial needle aspiration may potentially have a better diagnostic yield (8)[B].

ALERT

If signs indicate Löfgren syndrome, it is not necessary to perform a biopsy because prognosis is good with observation alone, and biopsy would not change management.

Pathological Findings

Noncaseating epithelioid granulomas without evidence of fungal or mycobacterial infection

DIFFERENTIAL DIAGNOSIS

- Infectious granulomatous disease, such as tuberculosis and fungal infections
- Hypersensitivity pneumonitis
- Lymphoma
- Other malignancies associated with lymphadenopathy
- Berylliosis

TREATMENT

- A large portion of patients undergo spontaneous remission. It is difficult to assess disease activity and severity, however, making it challenging to develop guidelines.
- No treatment may be necessary in asymptomatic individuals, but treatment may be needed for specific indications, such as cardiac, CNS, or ocular involvement.
- Treatment of pulmonary and skin manifestations is done on the basis of impairment. The symptoms that necessitate systemic therapy remain controversial:
  - Worsening pulmonary symptoms
  - Deteriorating lung function
  - Worsening radiographic findings

MEDICATION

Systemic therapy is clearly indicated for hypercalcemia, cardiac disease, neurologic disease, and eye disease not responding to topical therapy.

First Line

- Systemic corticosteroids in the symptomatic individual:
  - Usually prednisone initially, 40–60 mg/d × first 6 weeks
  - If stable, taper by 5 mg/wk to 15–20 mg/d over the next 6 weeks
  - If no relapse, 15–20 mg/d × 8–12 months
  - Relapse is common.
  - Higher doses may be warranted in patients with cardiac, neurologic, or ocular disease.
- In patients with skin disease, topical steroids may be effective.
- Inhaled steroids (budesonide 800–1,600 mcg b.i.d.) may be of some clinical benefit in early disease with mild pulmonary symptoms:
  - Contraindications: Patients with known problems with corticosteroids
  - Precautions: Careful monitoring in patients with diabetes mellitus and/or hypertension
  - Significant possible interactions: Refer to the manufacturer's profile of each drug (3,9).

Second Line

- Methotrexate: 10–15 mg/wk
- Cyclophosphamide: 25–50 mg/d, increasing to goal WBC count of 4,000–7,000/mm^3
- Hydroxychloroquine (Plaquenil): 100–400 mg/d
- Azathioprine: 50–100 mg/d
- Use of immunosuppressants such as methotrexate or azathioprine will require regular monitoring of CBC and LFTs.
- Infliximab, a chimeric monoclonal antibody, has been useful in refractory cases. Dose is 3–5 mg/kg IV initially, 2 weeks later, then q4–6wk.
- Thalidomide has been used for chronic skin lesions. The anti-tumor necrosis factor (TNF) agent infliximab also has been used in some refractory cases (3)[C].

ADDITIONAL TREATMENT

Issues for Referral

- Patients with sarcoidosis are typically followed longitudinally by a pulmonologist.
- Referrals to other specialists as dictated by involvement of other organ systems

COMPLEMENTARY AND ALTERNATIVE MEDICINE

None known to be effective

SURGERY/OTHER PROCEDURES

Lung transplantation in severe, refractory cases; long-term outcomes unknown (3)[C]

ONGOING CARE

FOLLOW-UP RECOMMENDATIONS

There is limited data on indications for the specific tests and optimal frequency of monitoring of disease activity. Suggestions are below.

Patient Monitoring

- Patients on prednisone for symptoms should be seen every 1–2 months while on therapy.
- Patients not requiring therapy should be seen regularly (every 3 months) for at least the first 2 years after diagnosis.
- If active disease, follow annually: Eye exam, CBC, creatinine, calcium, LFTs, ECG, CXR
- Other testing per individual patient's symptoms
- The serum ACE level is used by some physicians to follow the disease activity. In patients with an initially elevated ACE level, it should fall toward normal while on the therapy or when the disease resolves (9)[C].

DIET

No special diet

PATIENT EDUCATION

- The American Lung Association at www.lungusa.org/lung-disease/sarcoidosis/?gclid=CPX6zuipm6MCFQxW2godISFepQ
- Sarcoidosis by Medline Plus at www.nlm.nih.gov/medlineplus/sarcoidosis.html

PROGNOSIS

- 50% of patients will have spontaneous resolution within 2 years.
- 25% of patients will have significant fibrosis but no further worsening of the disease after 2 years.
- 25% of patients (higher in some populations, including blacks) will have chronic disease.
- Patients on corticosteroids for >6 months have a greater chance of having chronic disease.
- Overall death rate <5%

COMPLICATIONS

- Patients may develop significant respiratory involvement, including cor pulmonale.
- Pulmonary hemorrhage from infection with aspergillosis in the damaged lung is possible.
- Other organs, especially the heart (congestive heart failure, arrhythmias), eyes (rarely blindness), and CNS can be involved with serious consequences. Cardiac, ocular, and CNS involvement usually manifests early on in patients with these complications of the disease.

REFERENCES

1. Holmes J, Lazarus A, et al. Sarcoidosis: Extrathoracic manifestations. *Dis Mon*. 2009;55:675–92.
2. King CS, Kelly W, et al. Treatment of sarcoidosis. *Dis Mon*. 2009;55:704–18.
3. Iannuzzi MC, Rybicki BA, Teirstein AS. Sarcoidosis. *N Engl J Med*. 2007;357:2153–65.
4. Rybicki BA, Iannuzzi MC, Frederick MM, et al. Familial aggregation of sarcoidosis. A case-control etiologic study of sarcoidosis (ACCESS). *Am J Respir Crit Care Med*. 2001;164:2085–91.
5. Dempsey OJ, Paterson EW, Kerr KM, et al. Sarcoidosis. *BMJ*. 2009;339:b3206.
6. Baughman RP. Pulmonary sarcoidosis. *Clin Chest Med*. 2004;25:521–30, vi.
7. Statement on sarcoidosis. Joint Statement of the American Thoracic Society (ATS), the European Respiratory Society (ERS) and the World Association of Sarcoidosis and Other Granulomatous Disorders (WASOG) adopted by the ATS Board of Directors and by the ERS Executive Committee, February 1999. *Am J Respir Crit Care Med*. 1999;160: 736–55.
8. Tremblay A, Stather DR, Maceachern P, et al. A randomized controlled trial of standard vs endobronchial ultrasonography-guided transbronchial needle aspiration in patients with suspected sarcoidosis. *Chest*. 2009;136:340–6.
9. Weinberger SE. A 47-year-old woman with sarcoidosis. *JAMA*. 2006;296:2133–40.

ADDITIONAL READING

- Hoang DQ, Nguyen ET, et al. Sarcoidosis. *Semin Roentgenol*. 2010;45:36–42.
- Mock B, Richter S, Hein G, Wollina U, et al. [Recurrent panuveitis. First manifestation of Behçet disease in childhood]. *Ophthalmologe*. 1998;95: 784–7.
- Polychronopoulos VS, Prakash UB, et al. Airway involvement in sarcoidosis. *Chest*. 2009;136: 1371–80.

CODES

ICD9

135 Sarcoidosis

CLINICAL PEARLS

- Sarcoidosis is a noninfectious, multisystem granulomatous disease of unknown cause, typically affecting young and middle-aged adults.
- Any organ can be affected.
- Diagnosis is based on clinical findings, exclusion of other disorders, and pathologic detection of noncaseating granulomas.
- Most patients do not need systemic treatment and the disease resolves spontaneously; a minority will have life-threatening progressive organ dysfunction.

SCABIES

Kaelen C. Dunican, PharmD
Robert A. Baldor, MD

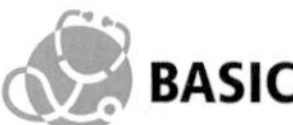

BASICS

DESCRIPTION

- A contagious parasitic infection of the skin caused by the mite *Sarcoptes scabiei*, var. *hominis*
- System(s) affected: Skin/Exocrine
- Synonym(s): Sarcoptic mange

EPIDEMIOLOGY

Incidence

Predominant age: Children and young adults

Prevalence

- Global prevalence is estimated at 300 million cases.
- May be more prevalent in urban areas and areas of overcrowding

RISK FACTORS

- Personal skin-to-skin contact (e.g., sexual promiscuity, crowding, nosocomial infection)
- Poor nutritional status, poverty, homelessness, and poor hygiene
- Seasonal variation: Incidence may be higher in the winter than in the summer (may be due to overcrowding).
- Immunocompromised patients, including those with HIV/AIDS, are at increased risk of developing severe (crusted/Norwegian) scabies.

GENERAL PREVENTION

Prevent outbreaks by prompt treatment and cleansing of fomites (see "Additional Treatment").

PATHOPHYSIOLOGY

Itching is a delayed hypersensitivity reaction to the mite saliva, eggs, or excrement.

ETIOLOGY

S. scabiei, var. *hominis*:

- An obligate human parasite
- Female mite lays eggs in burrows in the stratum corneum and epidermis.
- Primarily transmitted by human-to-human direct skin contact
- Infrequently transmitted via fomites (e.g., bedding, clothing, or furnishings)

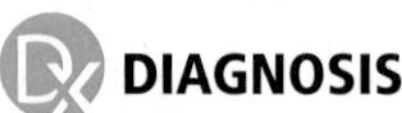

DIAGNOSIS

HISTORY

- Generalized itching is often severe and worse at night.
- Determine any contact with infected individuals.
- Initial infection may be asymptomatic.
- Symptoms may develop after 3–6 weeks.

PHYSICAL EXAM

- Lesions (inflammatory, erythematous, pruritic papules) most commonly located in the finger webs, flexor surfaces of the wrists, elbows, axillae, buttocks, genitalia, feet, and ankles
- Burrows (thin, curvy, elevated lines in the upper epidermis that measure 1–10 mm) may be seen in involved areas—a pathognomic sign of scabies.
- Secondary erosions or excoriations from scratching
- Pustules (if secondarily infected)
- Pruritic nodules in covered areas (buttocks, groin, axillae) resulting from an exaggerated hypersensitivity reaction.
- Crusted scabies (Norwegian scabies) is a psoriasiform dermatosis occurring with hyperinfestation with thousands of mites (more common in immunosuppressed patients).

Geriatric Considerations

The elderly often itch more severely despite fewer cutaneous lesions and are at risk for extensive infestations, perhaps related to a decline in cell-mediated immunity. There may be back involvement in those who are bedridden.

Pediatric Considerations

Infants and very young children often present with vesicles, papules, and pustules and have more widespread involvement, including the hands, palms, feet, soles, body folds, and head (rare for adults).

DIAGNOSTIC TESTS & INTERPRETATION

- Definitive diagnosis requires microscopic identification of mites, eggs, or feces.
- A failure to find mites does not rule out scabies (1)[C].

Lab

Initial lab tests

CBC is rarely needed but may show eosinophilia.

Diagnostic Procedures/Surgery

- Examination of skin with magnifying lens:
  - Look for typical burrows in finger webs and on flexor aspects of the wrists and penis.
  - Look for a dark point at the end of the burrow (the mite).
  - Presumptive diagnosis is based on clinical presentation, skin lesions, and identification of burrow (1,2)[C].
  - The mite can be extracted with a 25-gauge needle and examined microscopically.
- Mineral oil mounts (3)[C]:
  - Place a drop of mineral oil over a suspected lesion. Nonexcoriated papules or vesicles also may be sampled.
  - Scrape the lesion with a no. 15 surgical blade.
  - Examine under a microscope for mites, eggs, egg casings, or feces.
  - Scraping from under fingernails often may be positive.
- Potassium hydroxide (KOH) wet mount not recommended because it can dissolve mite pellets (1)[C].
- Burrow ink test (3)[C]:
  - If burrows are not obvious, apply blue–black ink to an area of rash. Wash off the ink with alcohol. A burrow should remain stained and become more evident.
  - Then apply mineral oil, scrape, and observe microscopically, as noted previously.
- Epiluminescence microscopy and high-resolution video dermatoscopy are expensive and have not been proven to be more sensitive than skin scraping (2)[C]

Pathological Findings

Skin biopsy of a nodule (although performed rarely) will reveal portions of the mite in the corneal layer.

DIFFERENTIAL DIAGNOSIS

- Atopic dermatitis
- Contact dermatitis
- Folliculitis/impetigo
- Tinea corporis
- Dermatitis herpetiformis
- Eczema
- Insect bites
- Papular urticaria
- Pediculosis corporis
- Pityriasis rosea
- Prurigo
- Psoriasis (crusted scabies)
- Pyoderma
- Seborrheic dermatitis
- Syphilis

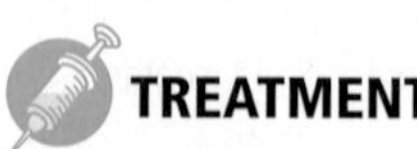

TREATMENT

MEDICATION

First Line

Permethrin is the most effective topical agent for scabies (4,5,6)[A]. 5% cream (Elimite):

- After bathing or showering, apply cream from the neck to the soles of the feet paying particular attention to areas that are most involved; then wash off after 8–14 hours. A second application 1 week later is recommended if new lesions develop.
- The adult dose is usually 30 g.
- Side effects include itching and stinging (minimal absorption).
- Crusted scabies may require more frequent application (every 2–3 days for 1–2 weeks) in combination with oral ivermectin (7)[C]

Pediatric Considerations

Permethrin may be used on infants >2 months of age. In children <5 years of age, the cream should be applied to the head and neck as well as to the entire body.

Second Line

- Crotamiton (Eurax) 10% cream:
  - Apply from the neck down for 24 hours, rinse off, then reapply for an additional 24 hours, and then thoroughly wash off.
  - Nodular scabies: Apply to nodules for 24 hours, rinse off, then reapply for an additional 24 hours, and then thoroughly wash off.
- Ivermectin (Stromectol):
  - Not FDA approved for scabies; 200–250 μg/kg as single dose; repeated in 1 week
  - Take with food to improve bioavailability and enhance penetration into the epidermis.
  - May need higher doses or may need to use in combination with topical scabicide for HIV-positive patients

- Precipitated sulfur 5–10% in petrolatum:
  - Not FDA approved for scabies.
  - Apply to the entire body from the neck down for 24 hours, rinse by bathing, then repeat for 2 more days (3 days total). It is malodorous and messy but is thought to be safer than lindane, especially in infants <6 months of age, and safer than permethrin in infants <2 months of age.
- Lindane (Kwell) 1% lotion:
  - Apply to all skin surfaces from the neck down and wash off 6–8 hours later.
  - 2 applications 1 week apart are recommended but may increase the risk of toxicity.
  - 2 oz is usually adequate for an adult:
    - Side effects: Neurotoxicity (seizures, muscle spasms), aplastic anemia
    - Contraindications: Uncontrolled seizure disorder, premature infants
    - Precautions: Use on excoriated skin, immunocompromised patients, conditions that may increase risk of seizures, or medications that decrease seizure threshold
    - Possible interactions: Concomitant use with medications that lower the seizure threshold

ALERT

Lindane: FDA black box warning of severe neurologic toxicity; use only when first-line agents have failed.

Pediatric Considerations

- The FDA recommends caution when using lindane in patients who weigh <50 kg. It is not recommended for infants and is contraindicated in premature infants.
- Ivermectin should be avoided in children <5 years of age and in those weighing <15 kg.

Pregnancy Considerations

- Permethrin is pregnancy category B, and lindane, ivermectin, and crotamiton are category C.
- Permethrin is considered compatible with lactation, but if permethrin is used while breast-feeding, the infant should be bottle-fed until the cream has been thoroughly washed off.

ADDITIONAL TREATMENT

General Measures

- Treat all intimate contacts and close household and family members.
- Wash all clothing, bed linens, and towels in hot (60°C) water or dry-clean.
- Personal items that cannot be washed or dry cleaned should be sealed in a plastic bag for 3–5 days.
- Some itching and dermatitis commonly persists for 10–14 days and can be treated with antihistamines and/or topical or oral corticosteroids.

Additional Therapies

Crusted scabies may require use of keratolytics to improve penetration of permethrin.

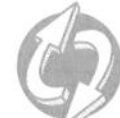

ONGOING CARE

FOLLOW-UP RECOMMENDATIONS

Patient Monitoring

Recheck patient at weekly intervals only if rash or itching persists. Scrape new lesions and retreat if mites or products are found.

PATIENT EDUCATION

- Patients should be instructed on proper application and cautioned not to overuse the medication when applying it to the skin.
- A patient fact sheet is available from the CDC: www.cdc.gov/parasites/scabies/

PROGNOSIS

- Lesions begin to regress in 1–2 days, along with the worst itching, but eczema and itching may persist for up to 6 weeks after treatment.
- Nodular lesions may persist for several weeks, perhaps necessitating intralesional or systemic steroids.
- Some instances of lindane-resistant scabies have now been reported. These do respond to permethrin.

COMPLICATIONS

- Poor sleep due to pruritus
- Social stigma
- Secondary bacterial infection
- Sepsis
- Glomerulonephritis
- Eczema
- Pyoderma
- Postscabetic pruritus
- Nodules (nodular scabies) may persist for weeks to months after treatment.

REFERENCES

1. Chosidow O. Scabies. *N Engl J Med*. 2006;354: 1718–27.
2. Leone PA. Scabies and pediculosis pubis: An update of treatment regimens and general review. *Clin Infect Dis*. 2007;44(Suppl 3):S153–59.
3. Hengge UR, Currie BJ, Jäger G. Scabies: A ubiquitous neglected skin disease. *Lancet Infect Dis*. 2006;6:769–79.
4. Hu S, Bigby M. Treating scabies: Results from an updated Cochrane review. *Arch Dermatol*. 2008; 144:1638–40.
5. Stong M, Johnstone PW. Interventions for treating scabies. *Cochrane Database Sys Rev*. 2007:3.
6. Hicks MI, Elston DM. Scabies. *Dermatol Ther*. 2009;22:279–92.
7. Currie BJ, McCarthy JS. Permethrin and ivermectin for scabies. *N Engl J Med*. 2010;362:717–24.

ADDITIONAL READING

- Flinders DC, De Schweinitz P. Pediculosis and scabies. *Am Fam Physician*. 2004;69:341–8.
- Heukelbach J, Feldmeier H. Scabies. *Lancet*. 2006;367:1767–74.
- Orien E, Marcos B, Davidovici B, et al. Itch and scratch: Scabies and pediculosis. *Clin Dermatol*. 2006;24:168–75.

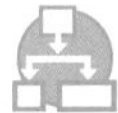

See Also (Topic, Algorithm, Electronic Media Element)

Arthropod Bites and Stings; Pediculosis (Lice)

CODES

ICD9

133.0 Scabies

CLINICAL PEARLS

- Prior to diagnosis, use of a topical steroid to treat pruritic symptoms may mask symptoms and is termed *scabies incognito*.
- Environmental control is essential. All linens, towels, and clothing used in the previous 4 days should be washed in hot water or dry cleaned. Personal items that cannot be washed or dry cleaned should be sealed in a plastic bag for 3–5 days.
- All members of the affected household may require treatment, especially close contacts (those sharing the same bed or who have intimate contact). It may be advisable to provide prescriptions for all household members.
- Eczema and itching may persist for up to 6 weeks after treatment, causing many patients to falsely believe that they have failed treatment or are being reinfected.
- In patients with actual reinfection, either the patient has not applied the medication properly or, more likely, the index patient has not been identified and treated.
- Some experts recommend routine reapplication of permethrin between days 8 and 15.

SCHIZOPHRENIA

Jeffrey Scott Anderson, MD
Jeffrey G. Stovall, MD

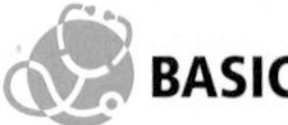

BASICS

Schizophrenia is a chronic, severe, and disabling psychiatric disorder.

DESCRIPTION

- Major psychiatric disorder with prodrome, active, and residual symptoms involving disturbances (lasting) in appearance (deteriorated), speech (loosened association), behavior (grossly disorganized), perception (hallucinations), or thinking (delusions) that last for ≥6 months
- There are 5 types of schizophrenia: Paranoid, disorganized, catatonic, undifferentiated, and residual (1).
- System(s) affected: Nervous

EPIDEMIOLOGY

Incidence

- 0.15–0.42/1,000
- Predominant age: Onset typically <45 years
- Predominant sex: Male = Female; onset earlier in males (early to mid-20s) than females (late 20s)

Prevalence

- Lifetime (1%): Highest prevalence in lower socioeconomic classes
- 1.1% of the population >18 years; similar rates in all countries

RISK FACTORS

Genetics

Biologic relative with schizophrenia: If first-degree relative, risk is 8–10%, a 10-fold increase (2)[B]

GENERAL PREVENTION

- Currently, no known preventive measures decrease the incidence of schizophrenia.
- Interventions to prevent some of the associated comorbidities and to improve the long-term course and outcome are employed as approaches to prevention.

ETIOLOGY

- Unknown: Not initiated or maintained by an organic factor
- Probably a complex interaction between inherited and environmental factors

COMMONLY ASSOCIATED CONDITIONS

- Substance use disorders and nicotine dependence are common and lead to significant long-term medical and social complications (3).
- Metabolic syndrome, diabetes mellitus, obesity, and certain infectious diseases, including HIV, hepatitis B, and hepatitis C all occur in higher-than-expected rates in individuals with schizophrenia.

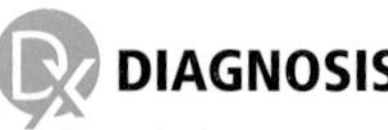

DIAGNOSIS

HISTORY

Focused on identifying an insidious social decline associated with the onset of characteristic signs and symptoms:

- Withdrawal from usual activities
- Presence of delusions
- Referential thoughts
- The belief that others can read one's mind or put thoughts into one's mind
- Hallucinations, most commonly auditory
- Affective flattening
- Altered thought processing seen as loose associations or illogical thought
- Abnormalities in motor functioning seen as periods of increased energy or catatonia (4)[B]

PHYSICAL EXAM

No characteristic physical findings

DIAGNOSTIC TESTS & INTERPRETATION

Lab

- No tests are available to indicate schizophrenia.
- Laboratory tests are needed to rule out other causes; these may include:
  - CBC, blood chemistries
  - Thyroid-stimulating hormone (TSH)
  - RPR
  - Urinalysis
  - Vitamin levels (B_{12}, folate, thiamine, vitamin D)
  - Drug/alcohol screen of blood and urine
  - Heavy-metal exposure: Ceruloplasmin, urine porphobilinogen as indicated

Initial lab tests

Laboratory tests are needed when starting antipsychotic medications; these may include:

- CBC, blood chemistries
- Blood glucose level, preferably fasting
- Hemoglobin A1C
- Lipid panel
- TSH
- ECG

Follow-Up & Special Considerations

Laboratory tests are needed, at least yearly, for routine monitoring, if using antipsychotic medications; these may include:

- CBC, blood chemistries
- Blood glucose level, preferably fasting
- Hemoglobin A1C
- Lipid panel
- TSH
- Prolactin level, if indicated
- ECG

Imaging

CT scan and MRI to rule out other causes

Diagnostic Procedures/Surgery

- Psychological: Not a routine part of assessment
- EEG to rule out seizure disorder
- Lumbar puncture if indicated by clinical presentation

Pathological Findings

No consistent or clinically useful pathologic findings

DIFFERENTIAL DIAGNOSIS

- Mental disorder due to medical illnesses:
  - Characterized by impaired judgment, orientation, memory, affect, and concentration in association with a known medical illness
  - Disorientation, in particular, indicates delirium.
  - Possible medical illnesses include trauma, infection, tumor, metabolic, endocrine, intoxication (psychoactive substance use), epilepsy, and withdrawal states.
- Organic delusional syndrome: Secondary to substance use/abuse, including cocaine, amphetamines, LSD, phencyclidine, and alcohol, which may have identical symptoms
- Mood disorders: Especially bipolar disorder (manic–depressive disorder), schizoaffective disorder, mood disorders with psychotic features
- Cultural belief system
- Medication-induced, including steroids, anticholinergics, and narcotics

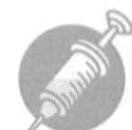

TREATMENT

MEDICATION

First Line

- 2 main groups of antipsychotics:
  - Conventional: Chlorpromazine, fluphenazine, trifluoperazine, perphenazine, thioridazine, haloperidol, thiothixene
  - Atypical: Risperidone, clozapine, olanzapine, quetiapine, ziprasidone, aripiprazole, paliperidone, iloperidone, asenapine, lurasidone
- Medication choice is based on clinical and subjective response and side effect profile:
  - For sensitivity to extrapyramidal adverse effects: Atypical
  - For tardive dyskinesia: Clozapine
  - For poor compliance/high risk of relapse: Injectable form of long-acting antipsychotic such as haloperidol, fluphenazine, risperidone, olanzapine, or paliperidone
- Usual oral daily dose (initial dose may be lower):
  - Chlorpromazine: 200 mg b.i.d.
  - Fluphenazine: 5 mg b.i.d.
  - Trifluoperazine: 10 mg b.i.d.
  - Perphenazine: 24 mg/d divided b.i.d. or t.i.d.
  - Haloperidol: 5 mg b.i.d.
  - Thiothixene: 10 mg b.i.d.
  - Risperidone: 3 mg/d
  - Clozapine: 200 mg b.i.d.
  - Olanzapine: 15–30 mg/d
  - Quetiapine: 200–300 mg b.i.d.
  - Ziprasidone: 60–80 mg b.i.d.
  - Aripiprazole: 10–30 mg/d
  - Paliperidone: 6–12 mg/d
  - Iloperidone: 6–12 mg b.i.d.
  - Asenapine: 5 mg b.i.d.
  - Lurasidone: 40-80 mg/d
- Precautions:
  - For acute side effects of antipsychotics: Dystonic reaction (especially of head and neck): Give diphenhydramine (Benadryl) 25–50 mg IM or benztropine (Cogentin) 1–2 mg IM.
  - For pseudoparkinsonism reaction: Trihexyphenidyl (Artane) 2 mg b.i.d. (may be increased to 15 mg/d if needed) or benztropine (Cogentin) 0.5 b.i.d. (range 1–4 mg/d)

- For neuroleptic malignant syndrome: Hyperthermia, severe extrapyramidal effect, and autonomic dysfunction (e.g., hypertension, tachycardia, diaphoresis, and incontinence): Stop antipsychotic. Acute hyperthermia is treated with dantrolene 1 mg/kg IV push and continued as needed until cumulative total dose is up to 10 mg/kg. Postcrisis management is with dantrolene 4–8 mg/kg/d PO in 4 divided doses × 1–3 days to prevent recurrence. Extrapyramidal effects are treated with bromocriptine 2.5 mg t.i.d. to q.i.d. PO/NG.

- Risperidone, olanzapine, quetiapine, and clozapine are associated with weight gain and development of metabolic syndrome.

Second Line

- In a recent Cochrane Review, clozapine was shown to be more effective in reducing symptoms of schizophrenia, producing clinically meaningful improvements and postponing relapse, than typical antipsychotic drugs, but data were weak and prone to bias (5)[B].
- Clozapine (Clozaril) 25 mg/d:
  - Increase slowly to a dose of 300–400 mg/d given b.i.d.; do not exceed 900 mg/d.
  - Serious toxicity of agranulocytosis mandates weekly CBC; reserve for therapy-resistant patients. Significant risk of seizure at higher doses.
  - Effective in treatment of refractory or suicidal patients
- Benzodiazepines:
  - May be effective adjuncts to antipsychotics during acute phase of illness
  - Withdrawal reactions can include psychosis or seizures.
  - Individuals with schizophrenia are vulnerable to abuse/addiction.
- Anticonvulsants: May be effective adjuncts for patients with EEG abnormalities suggestive of seizure activity and those with agitated/violent behavior (5,6)[A]

ADDITIONAL TREATMENT

General measures include family and patient education and engagement in the management of a chronic and severe illness. These include specific treatments to reduce the impact of psychotic symptoms and to enhance the social functioning and rehabilitation of the patient.

Issues for Referral

- Patients with schizophrenia should receive multidisciplinary ongoing care from both a primary care physician and a psychiatrist.
- Issues for referral include suicidality, the coexistence of an addiction, or difficulty in engagement.
- Additional therapies: Specific psychosocial rehabilitation programs are strongly encouraged.
- Supportive therapy and family and patient education are essential.
- Family members often benefit from referral to family advocacy organizations such as the National Alliance for the Mentally Ill (NAMI) (7)[A].

COMPLEMENTARY AND ALTERNATIVE MEDICINE

No other alternative therapies are validated.

SURGERY/OTHER PROCEDURES

Surgical interventions are not available.

IN-PATIENT CONSIDERATIONS

Initial stabilization focuses on maintaining a safe environment and reducing acute psychotic symptoms and agitation through the initiation of pharmacologic treatment.

Admission Criteria

The decision to admit is usually based on the patient's risk of harming himself or herself or someone else and the ability to care for himself or herself in the community.

Nursing

Monitor for safety concerns and establish a safe and supportive environment.

Discharge Criteria

The decision to discharge is based on the patient's ability to remain safe in the community and reflects a combination of suicide risk, level of psychotic symptoms, support systems, and the availability of appropriate outpatient services.

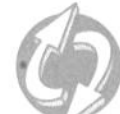

ONGOING CARE

FOLLOW-UP RECOMMENDATIONS

- Long-term symptom management and rehabilitation depend on engagement in ongoing pharmacologic and psychosocial treatment.
- Monitoring is based on evaluation of symptoms (including safety and psychotic symptoms), looking for the emergence of comorbidities and medication side effects, and prevention of complications.

DIET

- Newer atypical antipsychotics confer a higher risk of metabolic side effects such as diabetes, hypercholesterolemia, and weight gain.
- While there no specific dietary requirements, attention should be paid to the high risk of development of obesity, metabolic syndrome, and diabetes mellitus in individuals with schizophrenia.

PATIENT EDUCATION

- National Institute of Mental Health: *Schizophrenia,* at www.nimh.nih.gov/health/topics/schizophrenia/index.shtml
- *Helping a Family Member with Schizophrenia,* at www.aafp.org/afp/20070615/1830ph.html

PROGNOSIS

- Chronic course: Remission and exacerbations; complete remission not common
- Guarded prognosis
- The negative symptoms (consisting of decreased ambition, energy, and emotional responsiveness and social withdrawal) are often most difficult to treat.
- Excessive mortality occurs due to suicide, accidents, coronary artery disease, nicotine dependence, or substance abuse.

COMPLICATIONS

- Side effects from antipsychotic medications, including tardive dyskinesia and metabolic syndrome
- Self-inflicted trauma and suicide
- Combative behavior toward others
- Comorbid addictions, including nicotine (8)[A]

REFERENCES

1. Schultz SH, North SW, Shields CG. Schizophrenia: A review. *Am Fam Physician*. 2007;75:1821–9.
2. Norman RM, Manchanda R, Malla AK, et al. The significance of family history in first-episode schizophrenia spectrum disorder. *J Nerv Ment Dis*. 2007;195:846–52.
3. Fagerström K, Aubin HJ. Management of smoking cessation in patients with psychiatric disorders. *Curr Med Res Opin*. 2009;25:511–8.
4. American Psychiatric Association. *Diagnostic and Statistical Manual of Mental Disorders*, Text Revised, 4th ed. (DSM-IV-TR). Washington, DC: Author, 2000.
5. Essali A, Al-Haj Haasan N, Li C, et al. Clozapine versus typical neuroleptic medication for schizophrenia. *Cochrane Database Syst Rev*. 2009: CD000059.
6. Lieberman JA, Stroup TS, McEvoy JP, et al. Effectiveness of antipsychotic drugs in patients with chronic schizophrenia. *N Engl J Med*. 2005;353: 1209–23.
7. Mojtabai R, Nicholson RA, Carpenter BN. Role of psychosocial treatments in management of schizophrenia: A meta-analytic review of controlled outcome studies. *Schizophr Bull*. 1998;24:569–87.
8. Saha S, Chant D, McGrath J. A systematic review of mortality in schizophrenia: Is the differential mortality gap worsening over time? *Arch Gen Psychiatry*. 2007;64:1123–31.

ADDITIONAL READING

- Mala E. Schizophrenia in childhood and adolescence. *Neuro Endocrinol Lett*. 2008;29.
- Xia J, Grant TJ. Dance therapy for schizophrenia. *Cochrane Database Syst Rev*. 2009:CD006868.

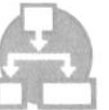

See Also (Topic, Algorithm, Electronic Media Element)

Algorithm: Delirium

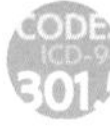

CODES

ICD9

295.90 Unspecified type schizophrenia, unspecified state

CLINICAL PEARLS

- A debilitating chronic mental illness that affects all cultures
- Schizophrenia is characterized by positive symptoms, including hallucinations, voices that converse with or about the patient, and delusions that are often paranoid, and negative symptoms, including flattened affect, loss of a sense of pleasure, loss of will or drive, and social withdrawal.
- Prominent mood symptoms are not common and can serve to differentiate schizophrenia from bipolar disorder.
- Multidisciplinary teams to prevent and treat comorbidities such as substance use, nicotine use, and obesity

SCIWORA SYNDROME (SPINAL CORD INJURY WITHOUT RADIOLOGIC ABNORMALITY)

Elizabeth Varadian, DO, MS
Tyler Cymet, DO

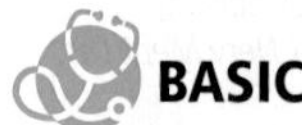

BASICS

DESCRIPTION

- SCIWORA occurs after trauma and is an acute spinal cord injury and nerve root trauma that results in sensory, motor, or combined sensorimotor deficits that can be either transient or permanent.
- These neural injuries occur without a fracture or misalignment visible on radiographic (x-ray, CT) imaging and without radiological explanations for the abnormal examination findings.
- MRI may be able to demonstrate neural and extra-neural injuries occurring primarily in the cervical region (C2–C6) due to fracture through cartilaginous end plates, edema, herniation, interspinous ligamentous injury, or other soft tissue damage.
- SCIWORA has a broad presentation from minor positive neurological symptoms to complete quadriplegia.
- It can occur in all populations but is primarily observed in the pediatric patients.

EPIDEMIOLOGY

Incidence

Variable: In trauma victims it has been reported to be 19–34%.

RISK FACTORS

- History of trauma
- Age <8 years old
- Location (upper cervical spine)

PATHOPHYSIOLOGY

Mechanism:

- The possible mechanisms of traumatic spinal cord injury causing SCIWORA are thought to include:
  - Hyperextension
  - Hyperflexion
  - Longitudinal distraction
  - Ischemic damage
- Neural injury: Edema
- Extraneural injury: Ligamentous injury

ETIOLOGY

Trauma:

- Motor vehicle accident (most common cause of SCIWORA); either unrestrained passengers, pedestrians, or bicyclists struck by motor vehicles
- Sports-related injury
- Significant fall
- Child abuse
- Age: Pediatric patients have a higher incidence of SCIWORA than adults due to several differences that permit increased mobility and flexibility:
  - Anatomy
    - Facet joints are oriented horizontally, which permits increased translational motion in the coronal (AP) plane.
    - Superior aspects of vertebral bodies demonstrate anterior wedging.
    - Ligaments and joint capsules have increased elasticity, permitting increased intersegmental movement and transient soft disc protrusion.
    - In patients <8 years old, head size to trunk ratio is disproportionately large.
    - Nuchal musculature is immature and lacking in strength.
    - Uncovertebral joints are absent.
  - Location: Mostly cervical region; thoracic spine is protected and splinted by the rib cage preventing forced flexion or extension.

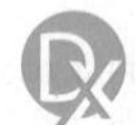

DIAGNOSIS

HISTORY

Trauma:

- Motor vehicle accident
- Sports-related injury
- Fall injury
- Child abuse injury

PHYSICAL EXAM

Assess for sensorimotor deficit:

- On neurological examination abnormal findings are not accounted for by known/visible injuries.
- Abnormalities on musculoskeletal exam leads one to suspect spinal cord injury causing motor function problems.

DIAGNOSTIC TESTS & INTERPRETATION

Lab

Follow-Up & Special Considerations

Adult considerations: Adults are less prone to SCIWORA due to decreased flexibility and mobility in comparison to pediatric patients, although SCIWORA is possible in the setting of acute trauma or cervical spondylosis

Imaging

Initial approach

- Depending on the affected area, radiographic images can rule out a fracture:
  - Lateral x-ray C-spine
  - CT scan C-spine
  - If negative and pathology still suspected, flexion/extension views of C-spine on plain films
- If there is no radiographic evidence of a fracture:
  - MRI imaging C-spine
  - Consider bone scan

Follow-Up & Special Considerations

- MRI imaging can also rule out reoccurrence of SCIWORA after the initial traumatic event.
- MRI abnormalities correlate closely with neurological injury.

Diagnostic Procedures/Surgery

Diagnosis is based on clinical findings of neurological changes, and radiographic or neuroimaging evidence of injury.

DIFFERENTIAL DIAGNOSIS

- Cervical fracture through end-plate (1)[A]
- Central cord syndrome (1)[A]
- Brown-Sequard syndrome (1)[A]
- Anterior spinal artery syndrome (1)[A]
- Partial spinal cord injury (1)[A]
- Complete spinal cord injury (1)[A]

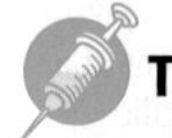

TREATMENT

MEDICATION

First Line

Supportive care and observation with serial neurological and musculoskeletal examinations. Corticosteroids to decrease inflammation

ADDITIONAL TREATMENT

Permanent rigid immobilization for 12 weeks (day and night)

General Measures

SCIWORA can present with a trauma history and no initial symptoms followed by subsequent neurological deterioration:

- SCIWORA should be suspected with a history of trauma even if there are no initial neurological exam findings.
- Unconscious patients should be immobilized until plain x-ray and CT radiographs are obtained or until consciousness improves and a neurological and pain assessment can be made.
- Transient findings, such as numbness, and a history of trauma should be treated following spinal cord injury protocol with immobilization.
- Immobilization should be implemented for 12 weeks even after the return of normal neurological function to minimize SCIWORA recurrence.
- If x-ray and CT scan are negative following a history of trauma, an MRI should be obtained as soon as possible to rule out neural injury and formulate a treatment plan.
- Treatment is nonoperative initially. Surgery may be required for spinal cord compression or spine instability secondary to extraneural injury.

IN-PATIENT CONSIDERATIONS

Initial Stabilization

- Trauma and spinal injury protocol
- Immobilization
- Consultation with a neurosurgeon once stable

Admission Criteria

- Unexplained neurological findings post trauma, MVC (motor vehicle collision)
- Neurologic injury demonstrated through MRI
- Suspected ligamentous lesion

Discharge Criteria

- Neurological examination without any deficits
- History of transient cervical neurological symptoms that have since resolved

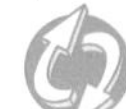

ONGOING CARE

FOLLOW-UP RECOMMENDATIONS

Patient Monitoring

- Reassessing neurological function within 24–48 hours if patients present with no initial symptoms after a traumatic event considering a possible latency period
- Follow up MRI before discharge.

PROGNOSIS

Initial clinical instability or severity, MRI findings, neurological features, location, age, and persistence of injury have a direct correlation with prognosis.

- Favorable:
  - Initial mild-to-moderate injury is associated with good recovery.
  - Resolution of changes as evidenced by follow-up MRI predicts favorable outcome.
- Unfavorable:
  - Initial severe neural injury is associated with a poor prognosis.
  - MRI findings of spinal cord transection and significant hemorrhage are associated with a poor prognosis.
  - MRI follow-up findings of persistent spinal cord injury result in a less favorable outcome.
  - Higher cervical injuries have greater neurological trauma and a worse prognosis.
  - Patients <8 years old have greater neurological trauma and a worse prognosis.

COMPLICATIONS

Recurrent SCIWORA has been reported and should be considered in trauma patients who present themselves to a health care provider.

REFERENCES

1. Buldini B, Amigoni A, et al. Spinal cord injury without radiographic abnormalities. *Eur J Pediatr*. 2006;165:108–11.

ADDITIONAL READING

- Launay F, Leet AI, Sponseller PD. Pediatric spinal cord injury without radiographic abnormality: A meta-analysis. *Clin Orthop Relat Res*. 2005;433:166–70.
- Kasimatis GB, Panagiotopoulos E, et al. The adult spinal cord injury without radiographic abnormalities syndrome: Magnetic resonance imaging and clinical findings in adults with spinal cord injuries having normal radiographs and computed tomography studies. *J Trauma*. 2008;65:86–93.
- Pillai A, Crane E, et al. Traumatic cervical hematomyelia: Report of a rare spinal cord injury without radiographic abnormality. *J Trauma*. 2008;65:938–41.
- Trigylidas T, Yuh SJ, et al. Spinal cord injuries without radiographic abnormality at two pediatric trauma centers in Ohio. *Pediatr Neurosurg*. 2010;46:283–89.

CODES

ICD9

- 952.9 Unspecified site of spinal cord injury without evidence of spinal bone injury
- 953.9 Injury to unspecified site of nerve roots and spinal plexus

CLINICAL PEARLS

If a child presents with a history of trauma and neurological symptoms, but has negative x-ray and CT findings, consider SCIWORA.

SCLERITIS

Birgit Khandalavala, MD

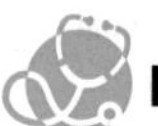

BASICS

DESCRIPTION

- Scleritis is a painful, inflammatory process of the sclera, part of the eye's outer coat
  - Commonly associated with systemic disorders and requires systemic anti-inflammatory therapy (1).
  - Potentially vision-threatening due to the deeper layer of the sclera being involved
- In contrast, episcleritis is self-limited inflammation of the eye with only mild discomfort.
- System(s) affected: Ocular

EPIDEMIOLOGY

- Predominant age: Most frequently occurs in fourth and sixth decades; mean age for all types of scleritis is 52 years
- Predominant sex: Female > Male (1.6:1)

Incidence

Occurs in 0.08–4% of patients (1):

- 94% of patients have anterior scleritis.
- The remaining 6% have posterior scleritis:
  - Anterior scleritis is further defined as diffuse anterior scleritis, nodular anterior scleritis, or necrotizing anterior scleritis, the latter having the worst prognosis.

Prevalence

Uncommon in the US

RISK FACTORS

Individuals with autoimmune disorders are most at risk.

ETIOLOGY

- ~50% of cases of scleritis are associated with autoimmune diseases such as rheumatoid arthritis.
- In 15% of cases, scleritis is the presenting manifestation of a systemic disorder, appearing 1 or more months before other symptoms of the condition.
- A recently described T-helper cell population, known as Th-17, has been implicated (2).
- Scleritis has been reported in patients taking bisphosphonate therapy.

COMMONLY ASSOCIATED CONDITIONS

- Rheumatoid arthritis
- Sjögren syndrome
- Ankylosing spondylitis
- Systemic lupus erythematosus
- Reactive arthritis
- Relapsing polychondritis
- Polyarteritis nodosa
- Wegener granulomatosis
- Sarcoidosis
- Inflammatory bowel disease
- Varicella zoster virus
- Syphilis
- Lyme disease
- Herpes zoster
- Tuberculosis

DIAGNOSIS

HISTORY

- Redness and inflammation of the sclera
- Can be bilateral in 1/3 of cases
- Pain ranging from mild discomfort to extreme localized tenderness.
  - May be described as constant, deep, boring, or pulsating.
  - Pain may be referred to the eyebrow, temple, or jaw.
- Photophobia and lacrimation may occur, but discharge is uncommon.
- Posterior scleritis tends to be less symptomatic, as is the variant scleromalacia perforans, due to associated pain fiber necrosis.

PHYSICAL EXAM

- Check visual acuity.
- Photophobia and tearing on exam
- Examine for pain with consensual constriction, which suggests uveal involvement.
- Engorged purplish red blood vessels
- Inspect for breadth and degree of injection
- A bluish hue may suggest thinning of the sclera.
- Scleral edema is often present.
- Deeper scleral blood vessels appear darker, follow a radial pattern, and do not move when manipulated with a cotton swab.
- A complete physical examination, particularly of the skin, joints, heart, and lungs, should be done to evaluate for associated conditions.

DIAGNOSTIC TESTS & INTERPRETATION

Lab

- Consider further testing if history, physical examination, CBC, serum chemistry, urinalysis, ESR, and/or C-reactive protein suggest a systemic cause.
- Rheumatoid factor, anticyclic citrullinated peptide antibodies, antineutrophil cytoplasmic antibody, and antinuclear antibody may aid in the diagnosis.
- FTA-ABS, rapid plasma reagin, and Lyme titers

Imaging

Initial approach

- Further imaging studies, such as a chest x-ray (CXR) and/or chest CT and sacroiliac joint films, may be useful if specific systemic illnesses are suspected.
- Ultrasound or CT scan of the orbit may be useful to determine the extent and location (especially posterior) of scleritis and the presence of local associated disease.

Diagnostic Procedures/Surgery

Biopsy is not routinely required unless diagnosis remains uncertain after above investigations.

Pathological Findings

- Adjacent inflammation may or may not be present.
- The scleritis may be diffuse, nodular, or necrotizing (with or without associated inflammation).
- If the posterior region of the globe is involved, adjacent swelling of orbital tissues may occur.

DIFFERENTIAL DIAGNOSIS

- Conjunctivitis
- Episcleritis
- Pink eye
- Iritis (anterior uveitis)
- Trauma
- Ocular rosacea
- Herpes zoster

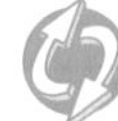

TREATMENT

MEDICATION

First Line

- Glucocorticoids are the mainstay of treatment, including topical, periocular, and systemic (2)[A]:
  - Recent data have confirmed excellent efficacy and tolerability to subconjunctival corticosteroids (2).
- Contraindications: Documented hypersensitivity; active peptic ulcer disease; untreated concomitant viral or bacterial infection
- Precautions: Scleritis can progress to ocular perforation, which may be hastened with periocular steroid injection.

Second Line

- The more clinically benign subtypes—diffuse and nodular anterior scleritis—may respond to NSAIDs alone.
- Necrotizing or posterior scleritis, on the other hand, may require immunosuppressive therapy in addition to systemic steroids:
  - Other immunosuppressive and immunomodulating agents may be indicated, depending on the systemic condition and include cyclophosphamide, cyclosporine, methotrexate, and mycophenolate mofetil:
    - Rarely, infliximab or rituximab has been effective in resistant cases (3,4)[C]

ADDITIONAL TREATMENT

Issues for Referral

- All patients with scleritis should be managed by an ophthalmologist familiar with this condition.
- Rheumatology referral for coexistent systemic diseases is helpful for long-term success.

Additional Therapies

Immunosuppressants used for autoimmune and collagen vascular disorders may be of help in active scleritis.

SURGERY/OTHER PROCEDURES

- In rare cases, scleral biopsy may be indicated.
- Ocular perforation requires scleral grafting.

ONGOING CARE

FOLLOW-UP RECOMMENDATIONS

- No restrictions
- Avoid contact lenses only if there is corneal involvement, which is rare.

Patient Monitoring

- The patient should be followed very closely by an ophthalmologist in the active stage of inflammation to assess the effectiveness of therapy.
- Medication use mandates close surveillance for adverse effects.

DIET

No special diet

PATIENT EDUCATION

Scleritis at PubMed Health: www.ncbi.nlm.nih.gov/pubmedhealth/PMH0001998/

PROGNOSIS

- Scleritis is indolent, chronic, and often progressive.
- Recurrent bouts of inflammation may occur.
- Scleromalacia perforans has the highest risk of perforation of the globe.

COMPLICATIONS

- Increased intraocular pressure
- Cataract and glaucoma can result from treatment.
- Visual loss due to posterior extension or adjacent structural involvement
- Ocular perforation can occur in severe stages.

REFERENCES

1. Kirkwood BJ, Kirkwood RA, et al. Episcleritis and scleritis. *Insight*. 2010;35:5–8.
2. Rachitskaya A, Mandelcorn ED, Albini TA, et al. An update on the cause and treatment of scleritis. *Curr Opin Ophthalmol*. 2010;21:463–7.
3. Jabbarvand M, Fard MA, et al. Infliximab in a patient with refractory necrotizing scleritis associated with relapsing polychondritis. *Ocul Immunol Inflamm*. 2010;18:216–7.
4. Iaccheri B, Androudi S, Bocci EB, et al. Rituximab treatment for persistent scleritis associated with rheumatoid arthritis. *Ocul Immunol Inflamm*. 2010;18:223–5.

ADDITIONAL READING

- DeCroos FC, Garg P, Reddy AK, et al. Optimizing diagnosis and management of nocardia keratitis, scleritis, and endophthalmitis: 11-year microbial and clinical overview. *Ophthalmology*. 2011;118:1193–200.
- Fong LP, Sainz de la Maza M, Rice BA. Immunopathology of scleritis. *Ophthalmology*. 1991;98:472–9.
- Fraunfelder FW, Fraunfelder FT. Bisphosphonates and ocular inflammation. *N Engl J Med*. 2003;348:1187–8.
- Galor A, Thorne JE, et al. Scleritis and peripheral ulcerative keratitis. *Rheum Dis Clin North Am*. 2007;33:835–54, vii.
- Smith JR, Mackensen F, Rosenbaum JT. Therapy insight: scleritis and its relationship to systemic autoimmune disease. *Nat Clin Pract Rheumatol*. 2007;3:219–26.

CODES

ICD9

- 379.00 Scleritis, unspecified
- 379.03 Anterior scleritis
- 379.07 Posterior scleritis

CLINICAL PEARLS

- Episcleritis is self-limited inflammation of the eye with mild discomfort. In contrast, scleritis is a painful, severe, and potentially vision-threatening condition due to the deeper layer of the sclera being involved for which active treatment is imperative.
- Uveitis, by definition, involves some combination of the iris, ciliary body, and choroid membrane and thus, generally, is associated with pain, with consensual constriction of the pupil. Scleritis can spread to involve these structures but may not always do so. Both conditions can be associated with underlying inflammatory diseases.
- ~50% of all cases of scleritis are associated with autoimmune diseases such as rheumatoid arthritis.

SCLERODERMA

Ann M. Lynch, PharmD, RPh, AE-C
Deborah DeMarco, MD

BASICS

DESCRIPTION

- Scleroderma (systemic sclerosis [SSc]) is a chronic disease of unknown cause characterized by diffuse fibrosis of skin and visceral organs and vascular abnormalities.
- Most manifestations have vascular features (e.g., Raynaud phenomenon), but frank vasculitis is rarely seen.
- Can range from a mild disease, affecting the skin, to a systemic disease that can cause death in a few months
- The disease is categorized into 2 major clinical variants:
  - Diffuse: Distal and proximal extremity and truncal skin thickening
  - Limited:
    - Restricted to the fingers, hands, and face
    - CREST syndrome (calcinosis, Raynaud phenomenon, esophageal dysmotility, sclerodactyly, telangiectasia)
- System(s) affected: Include but not limited to Skin; Renal; Cardiovascular; Pulmonary; Musculoskeletal; Gastrointestinal

Geriatric Considerations

Uncommon >75 years of age

Pediatric Considerations

Rare in this age group

Pregnancy Considerations

- Safe and healthy pregnancies are common and possible despite higher frequency of premature births.
- High-risk management must be standard care to avoid complications, specifically renal crisis.
- Diffuse scleroderma causes greater risk for developing serious cardiopulmonary and renal problems. Pregnancy should be delayed until disease stabilizes.

EPIDEMIOLOGY

Incidence

- In the US: 1–2/100,000/yr
- Predominant age:
  - Young adult (16–40 years); middle-aged (40–75 years), peak onset 30–50 years
  - Symptoms usually appear in the third to fifth decades.
- Predominant sex: Female > Male (4:1)

Prevalence

In the US: 1–25/100,000

RISK FACTORS

Unknown

Genetics

Familial clustering is rare but has been seen.

ETIOLOGY

- Unknown
- Possible alterations in immune response
- Possibly some association with exposure to quartz mining, quarrying, vinyl chloride, hydrocarbons, toxin exposure
- Treatment with bleomycin has caused a sclerodermalike syndrome, as has exposure to rapeseed oil.

DIAGNOSIS

HISTORY

- Raynaud phenomenon is generally the presenting complaint (differentiated from Raynaud disease, generally affecting younger individuals and without digital ulcers)
- Skin thickening, "puffy hands," and gastroesophageal reflux disease (GERD) are often noted early in the disease process.

PHYSICAL EXAM

- Skin:
  - Digital ulcerations
  - Tightness, swelling, thickening of digits
  - Hyperpigmentation/hypopigmentation
  - Narrowed oral aperture
  - Pruritus
  - Scaling of skin
  - SC calcinosis
- Peripheral vascular system:
  - Telangiectasia
- Joints, tendons, and bones:
  - Flexion contractures
  - Friction rub on tendon movement
  - Hand swelling
  - Joint stiffness
  - Polyarthralgia
  - Sclerodactyly
- Muscle:
  - Proximal muscle weakness
- GI tract:
  - Dysphagia
  - Esophageal reflux due to dysmotility (most common systemic sign in diffuse disease)
  - Malabsorptive diarrhea
  - Nausea and vomiting
  - Weight loss
  - Xerostomia
- Kidney:
  - Hypertension
  - May develop scleroderma renal crisis: Acute renal failure (ARF)
- Pulmonary:
  - Dry crackles at lung bases
  - Dyspnea
- Nervous system:
  - Peripheral neuropathy
  - Trigeminal neuropathy
- Cardiac (progressive disease):
  - Conduction abnormalities
  - Cardiomyopathy
  - Secondary cor pulmonale

DIAGNOSTIC TESTS & INTERPRETATION

Lab

Initial lab tests

- Nail fold capillary microscopy
- CBC
- Creatinine
- Urinalysis (albuminuria, microscopic hematuria)
- Antinuclear antibodies (ANA): Positive in >90% of patients
- Anti–Scl-70 (topoisomerase) antibody is highly specific for systemic disease.
- Anticentromere antibody usually associated with CREST variant

Follow-Up & Special Considerations

- Pulmonary function tests (PFTs):
  - Decreased maximum breathing capacity
  - Increased residual volume
  - Diffusion defect
- Hypergammaglobulinemia
- Positive rheumatoid factor test (33%)
- ECG (low voltage): Possible nonspecific abnormalities, arrhythmia, and conduction defects
- Echocardiography: Pulmonary hypertension or cardiomyopathy
- Nail fold capillary loop abnormalities

Imaging

Initial approach

- Chest radiograph:
  - Diffuse reticular pattern
  - Bilateral basilar pulmonary fibrosis
- Hand radiograph:
  - Soft tissue atrophy and acro-osteolysis
  - Can see overlap syndromes such as rheumatoid arthritis
  - SC calcinosis

Follow-Up & Special Considerations

- Upper GI:
  - Distal esophageal dilatation
  - Atonic esophagus
  - Esophageal dysmotility
  - Duodenal diverticula
- Barium enema:
  - Colonic diverticula
  - Megacolon
- High-resolution CT scan for detecting alveolitis, which has a ground-glass appearance or honeycomb pattern in fibrosis

Diagnostic Procedures/Surgery

- Skin biopsy:
  - Compact collagen fibers in the reticular dermis and hyalinization and fibrosis of arterioles
  - Thinning of epidermis with loss of rete pegs and atrophy of dermal appendages
  - Accumulation of mononuclear cells is also seen.
- Right-sided heart catheterization: Pulmonary hypertension is an ominous prognostic feature.

Pathological Findings

- Skin:
  - Edema, fibrosis, or atrophy (late stage)
  - Lymphocytic infiltrate around sweat glands
  - Loss of capillaries
  - Endothelial proliferation
  - Hair follicle atrophy

- Synovium:
  - Pannus formation
  - Fibrin deposits in tendons
- Kidney:
  - Small kidneys
  - Intimal proliferation in interlobular arteries
- Heart:
  - Endocardial thickening
  - Myocardial interstitial fibrosis
  - Ischemic band necrosis
  - Enlarged heart
  - Cardiac hypertrophy
- Lung:
  - Interstitial pneumonitis
  - Cyst formation
  - Interstitial fibrosis
  - Bronchiectasis
- Esophagus:
  - Esophageal atrophy
  - Fibrosis

DIFFERENTIAL DIAGNOSIS
- Sclerodermatomyositis
- Mixed connective tissue disease
- Toxic oil syndrome (Madrid, 1981, affecting 20,000 people)
- Eosinophilia–myalgia syndrome
- Diffuse fasciitis with eosinophilia
- Scleredema of Buschke

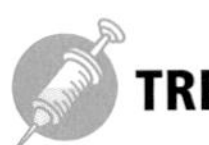

TREATMENT

MEDICATION
First Line
- ACE inhibitors for preservation of renal blood flow and for treatment of hypertensive renal crisis (1)[C]
- Corticosteroids: For disabling myositis, pulmonary alveolitis, or mixed connective tissue disease (not recommended in high doses due to increased incidence of renal failure) (1)[C]
- NSAIDs: For joint or tendon symptoms. Caution with long-term concurrent use with ACEIs (potential renal complications)
- Antibiotics: For secondary infections in bowel and active skin infections (1)
- Antacids, proton pump inhibitors: For gastric reflux (1)[B]
- Intestinal dysfunction: Metoclopramide (1)[C]
- Dipyridamole or aspirin: Antiplatelet therapy
- Hydrophilic skin ointments: Skin therapy
- Topical clindamycin, erythromycin, or silver sulfadiazine cream may prevent recurrent infectious cutaneous ulcers.
- Consider immunosuppressives for treatment of life-threatening or potentially crippling scleroderma or interstitial pneumonitis (1)[A].
- Avoidance of caffeine, nicotine, and sympathomimetics may ease Raynaud symptoms.
- Nitrates and dihydropyridine calcium channel blockers for Raynaud phenomenon (2)[A]
- Penicillamine: To reduce skin thickening and delay the rate of new visceral involvement (use is now controversial; newer therapies such as relaxin may be better)
- PDE-5 antagonists (e.g., sildenafil), prostanoids, and endothelin-1 antagonists are changing the management of pulmonary hypertension (1)[B].
- Alveolitis: Immunosuppressants and alkylating agents (e.g., cyclophosphamide) (1)[A]

ADDITIONAL TREATMENT
General Measures
- Treatment is symptomatic and supportive.
- Esophageal dilation may be used for strictures.
- Avoid cold; dress appropriately for the weather; be wary of air conditioning.
- Avoid smoking (crucial).
- For chronic digital ulcerations:
  - Débridement after soaking in 1/2-strength hydrogen peroxide solution
  - Digital plaster to immobilize
- Avoid finger sticks (e.g., blood tests).
- Elevate the head of the bed during sleep to help relieve GI symptoms.
- Use softening lotions, ointments, and bath oils to help prevent dryness and cracking of skin.
- Dialysis may be necessary in renal crisis.

Additional Therapies
- Physical therapy to maintain function and promote strength
- Heat therapy to relieve joint stiffness

SURGERY/OTHER PROCEDURES
- Some success with gastroplasty for correction of GERD
- Limited role for sympathectomy for Raynaud phenomenon

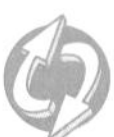

ONGOING CARE

FOLLOW-UP RECOMMENDATIONS
Patient Monitoring
- Monitor every 3–6 months for end-organ and skin involvement and medications. Provide encouragement.
- Cardiac echo and PFTs yearly

DIET
Drink plenty of fluids with meals.

PATIENT EDUCATION
- Stay as active as possible, but avoid fatigue.
- Printed patient information available from the Scleroderma Federation, 1725 York Avenue, No. 29F, New York, NY 10128; (212) 427-7040
- Advise the patient to report any abnormal bruising or nonhealing abrasions.
- Assist the patient about smoking cessation, if needed.

PROGNOSIS
- Possible improvement, but incurable
- Prognosis is poor if cardiac, pulmonary, or renal manifestations present early.

COMPLICATIONS
- Renal failure
- Respiratory failure
- Flexion contractures
- Disability
- Esophageal dysmotility
- Reflux esophagitis
- Arrhythmia
- Megacolon
- Pneumatosis intestinalis
- Obstructive bowel
- Cardiomyopathy
- Pulmonary hypertension
- Possible association with lung and other cancers
- Death

REFERENCES

1. Kowal-Bielecka O, Landewé R, Avouac J, et al. EULAR recommendations for the treatment of systemic sclerosis: A report from the EULAR Scleroderma Trials and Research group (EUSTAR). *Ann Rheum Dis*. 2009;68:620–8.
2. Harding SE, Tingey PC, Pope J, et al. Prazosin for Raynaud's phenomenon in progressive systemic sclerosis. *Cochrane Database Syst Rev*. 1998;2:CD000956.

ADDITIONAL READING

- Reveille JD, Solomon DH. American College of Rheumatology Ad Hoc Committee of Immunologic Testing Guidelines. Evidence-based guidelines for the use of immunologic tests: Anticentromere, Scl-70, and nucleolar antibodies. *Arthritis Rheum*. 2003;49:399–412.
- Steen VD. Pregnancy in scleroderma. *Rheum Dis Clin North Am*. 2007;33:345–58, vii.

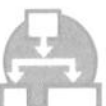

See Also (Topic, Algorithm, Electronic Media Element)

Morphea

CODES

ICD9
710.1 Systemic sclerosis

CLINICAL PEARLS

- Raynaud phenomenon is frequently the initial complaint.
- Skin thickening, "puffy hands," and GERD are often noted early in disease.
- Eosinophilic fasciitis can mimic scleroderma but differs with the absence of Raynaud symptoms and is responsive to corticosteroid treatment.

SEASONAL AFFECTIVE DISORDER

Christopher C. White, MD, JD, FCLM

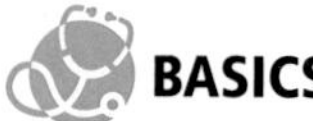

BASICS

DESCRIPTION

- Seasonal affective disorder (SAD) is a heterogeneous mood disorder with depressive episodes usually in winter months with full remissions in the spring and summer.
- Ranges from a milder form (winter blues) to a seriously disabling illness
- Must separate out patients with other mood disorders (such as major depressive disorder and bipolar affective disorder) whose symptoms persist during spring and summer months

EPIDEMIOLOGY

Incidence

- Affects up to 500,000 people every winter
- Up to 30% of patients visiting a primary care physician (PCP) during winter may report winter depressive symptoms.
- Predominant age: Occurs at any age; peaks in 20s and 30s
- Predominant sex: Female > Male (3:1)

Prevalence

- 1–9% of the general population
- 10–20% of patients identified as having mood symptoms will have a seasonal component.

RISK FACTORS

- Most common during months of January and February: Patients frequently visit PCP during winter months complaining of recurrent flu, chronic fatigue, and unexplained weight gain.
- Working in a building without windows or other environment without exposure to sunlight

Genetics

- Some twin studies have suggested a genetic component, but further study is needed.
- Increased incidence of depression, ADHD, and alcoholism in close relatives

GENERAL PREVENTION

- Consider use of light therapy at start of winter (if prior episodes begin in October), increase time outside during daylight, or move to a more southern location.
- Bupropion (Wellbutrin) is an FDA-approved antidepressant for the prevention of SAD.

PATHOPHYSIOLOGY

The major theories currently involve the interplay of phase-shifted circadian rhythms, genetic vulnerability, and serotonin dysregulation.

ETIOLOGY

- Melatonin produced by the pineal gland at increased levels in the dark has been linked to depressive symptoms; light therapy on the retina acts to inhibit melatonin secretion.
- Serotonin dysregulation, because it is secreted less during winter months, must be present for light therapy to work, and treatment with SSRIs appears to reverse SAD symptoms.
- Decreased levels of vitamin D, often occurring during low-light winter months, may be associated with depressive episodes in some individuals experiencing SAD symptoms.

COMMONLY ASSOCIATED CONDITIONS

Some individuals with SAD have a weakened immune system and may be more vulnerable to infections.

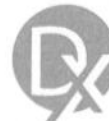

DIAGNOSIS

- Carefully document the presence or absence of prior manic episodes.
- Screen for the existence of any suicidal ideation and safety risk factors.
- Remission of symptoms during spring and summer
- Symptoms have occurred for the past 2 years.
- Seasonal episodes associated with winter months substantially outnumber any nonseasonal depressive episodes.

HISTORY

- Symptoms of depression meeting the criteria for major depressive disorder:
  - *S*leep disturbance—either too much or too little
  - *I*nterest (lack of)—in life and absence of pleasure from hobbies/activities
  - *G*uilt—feelings of guilt or worthlessness
  - *E*nergy—fatigue or constantly feeling tired
  - *C*oncentration—difficulty with concentration and memory
  - *A*ppetite—changes in appetite and weight
  - *P*sychomotor retardation—patients feeling slowed down with decreased activity
  - *S*uicidal thoughts—patients reporting thoughts of suicide
- In SAD, hypersomnia, hyperphagia (craving for carbohydrates and sweets), and weight gain usually predominate. Despite sleeping more, patients report daytime sleepiness and fatigue. Cravings may lead to binge eating and weight gains >20 lb.
- Obtain collateral history if patient is unable to provide insight into the seasonal component.

PHYSICAL EXAM

Use exam to exclude other organic causes for symptoms. Focal neurologic deficits, signs of endocrine dysfunction, or stigmata of substance abuse should prompt further testing.

DIAGNOSTIC TESTS & INTERPRETATION

Lab

- Thyroid-stimulating hormone to rule out hypothyroidism
- CBC to rule out anemia
- Rule out electrolyte and glucose dysregulation.
- 25-OH vitamin D level
- Pregnancy test for women of child-bearing potential
- Urine tox screen if substance abuse is a concern

Imaging

Generally not useful unless focal neurologic finding or looking to exclude an organic cause

DIFFERENTIAL DIAGNOSIS

- Similar to that of major depression, meaning that organic causes of low energy and fatigue, such as hypothyroidism, anemia, and mononucleosis (or other viral syndromes), need to be considered
- Other mood disorders without a seasonal component, such as major depression, bipolar disorder, adjustment disorder, or dysthymia
- Symptoms should not be better accounted for by seasonal psychosocial stressors, which often accompany the winter holiday seasons.
- Substance abuse

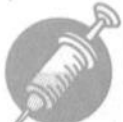

TREATMENT

MEDICATION

There is a lack of evidence to determine whether light therapy or medication should be the first-line agent. Both are supported by the literature and in some studies have equal efficacy. Medications typically have more side effects. Adherence to both treatments remains a critical issue. The ultimate choice depends on the acuity of the patient and the comfort level of the prescribing clinician with each treatment modality (1)[B]:

- SSRIs such as sertraline (Zoloft), paroxetine (Paxil), fluoxetine (Prozac), citalopram (Celexa), and escitalopram (Lexapro) in their traditional antidepressant doses (2)[B]
- Bupropion (Wellbutrin) is the only antidepressant currently approved by the FDA for the prevention of SAD (3)[A].

ADDITIONAL TREATMENT

Issues for Referral

- Patients with a history of ocular disease should be referred for an ophthalmologic exam before phototherapy and for serial monitoring.
- Patients who fail to respond or who develop manic symptoms or suicidal ideation once treatment is initiated should be considered for psychiatric referral.

Additional Therapies

Phototherapy using special light sources has been shown to be effective in 60–90% of patients, often providing relief with a few sessions (2,4)[A]:

- Variables that can regulate effect are:
  - Light intensity: Although the minimum light source intensity is under investigation, 2,500 lux is suggested (domestic lights emit, on average, 200–500 lux). There is good evidence for 10,000 lux as the recommended source (2)[B].
  - Treatment duration: Exposure time varies based on intensity of light source with daily sessions of 30 minutes to a few hours.
  - Time of treatment: Most patients respond better by using the light therapy early in the morning.
  - Color of light source: Emerging data suggest that lower-intensity light-emitting diodes in the blue spectrum may have equal efficacy to the traditional white light boxes with a decreased incidence of side effects, but these results are preliminary (5)[B].
- Light box is placed on table several feet away, and the light is allowed to shine onto the patient's eyes (sunglasses should be avoided). Ensure that the light box has an ultraviolet filter.
- Most common side effects are eye strain and headache. Insomnia can result if the light box is used too late in the day. Light boxes also can precipitate mania in some patients.
- Dawn simulation machines gradually increase illumination while the patient sleeps, simulating sunrise while using a significantly less intense light source.

COMPLEMENTARY AND ALTERNATIVE MEDICINE

- Work to reduce stress levels through meditation, progressive relaxation exercises, and/or lifestyle modification.
- The potential role of vitamin D supplementation is under investigation. A small study found it to be more effective than phototherapy, but a much larger and more rigorous study recently found no benefit in elderly women for SAD symptoms. Doses used are typically 400–800 IU/d (6)[B].

IN-PATIENT CONSIDERATIONS

Admission Criteria

If the patient develops suicidal ideation as part of his or her depression or mania after treatment is initiated

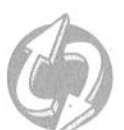

ONGOING CARE

FOLLOW-UP RECOMMENDATIONS

Regular monitoring by PCP or psychiatrist for response to treatment; patients may become manic when treated with SSRIs or light therapy.

Patient Monitoring

Patients should be seen in the outpatient clinic weekly to biweekly when initiating light or pharmacotherapy to monitor treatment results, side effects, and any increased suicidal thoughts if using SSRIs.

DIET

No specific diet modification needed

PATIENT EDUCATION

- Increase time outdoors during daylight.
- Rearrange home or work environment to get more direct sunlight through windows.

PROGNOSIS

Symptoms, if untreated, generally remit within 5 months with exposure to spring light, only to return in subsequent winters. If treated, patients usually respond within 3–6 weeks.

COMPLICATIONS

Development of suicidal ideation and mania are 2 outcomes the clinician needs to monitor.

REFERENCES

1. Lam RW, Levitt AJ, Levitan RD, et al. The Can-SAD study: A randomized controlled trial of the effectiveness of light therapy and fluoxetine in patients with winter seasonal affective disorder. *Am J Psychiatry*. 2006;163:805–12.
2. Lurie SJ, Gawinski B, Pierce D, et al. Seasonal affective disorder. *Am Fam Physician*. 2006;74:1521–4.
3. Modell JG, Rosenthal NE, Harriett AE, et al. Seasonal affective disorder and its prevention by anticipatory treatment with bupropion XL. *Biol Psychiatry*. 2005;58:658–67.
4. Terman M, Terman JS. Light therapy for seasonal and nonseasonal depression: Efficacy, protocol, safety, and side effects. *CNS Spectr*. 2005;10:647–63; quiz 672.
5. Anderson JL, Glod CA, Dai J, et al. Lux vs. wavelength in light treatment of seasonal affective disorder. *Acta Psychiatr Scand*. 2009.
6. Dumville JC, Miles JN, Porthouse J, et al. Can vitamin D supplementation prevent winter-time blues? A randomised trial among older women. *J Nutr Health Aging*. 2006;10:151–3.

ADDITIONAL READING

Howland RH. Somatic therapies for seasonal affective disorder. *J Psychosoc Nurs Ment Health Serv*. 2009; 47:17–20.

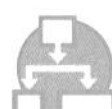

See Also (Topic, Algorithm, Electronic Media Element)

- Bipolar I Disorder; Bipolar II Disorder; Depression
- Algorithm: Depressive Episode, Major

CODES

ICD9

296.99 Other specified episodic mood disorder

CLINICAL PEARLS

- The difference between SAD and depression is that SAD is a subtype of major depressive disorder. Once someone has a diagnosed mood disorder such as depression or bipolar, one needs to ask whether the symptoms vary in a seasonal pattern to qualify for the diagnosis of SAD. Generally, these patients will report sleeping too much, eating too much (especially carbs and sweets), and gaining weight during winter months.
- As with all psychiatric diagnoses, ensure that the symptoms are not due to an organic process (e.g., anemia, hypothyroidism, mononucleosis) or better explained by substance abuse.
- There is a lack of good evidence to decide whether light therapy or SSRIs should be the first-line agent. Guidelines suggest that SSRIs should be used first if the patient is more acute or has contraindications to light therapy, or the clinician is not comfortable with light therapy.
- Light therapy boxes are available from numerous online suppliers, but they are not extensively regulated, and thus practitioners should take care to ensure that patients are using devices from reputable suppliers.
- If using SSRIs, there have been recent studies indicating that some patients may begin to experience increased suicidal thoughts on therapy, and thus these patients need to be monitored closely in your outpatient office every 1–2 weeks. Patients on light therapy also should be monitored closely initially in order to adjust treatment. Once stabilized, both groups of patients can be seen every 4–8 weeks during the winter months.
- All patients who demonstrate suicidal ideation or symptoms of mania should be referred for consideration of hospitalization.

SECRETION OF INAPPROPRIATE ANTIDIURETIC HORMONE (SIADH)

Ruben Peralta, MD, FACS

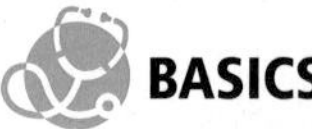

BASICS

DESCRIPTION

- A syndrome of abnormal production of antidiuretic hormone (ADH), despite low serum osmolality, leading to hyponatremia and inappropriately elevated urine osmolality:
  - The resulting abnormal urinary free water retention leads to dilutional hyponatremia (total body sodium levels may be normal or near normal, but the patient's total body water is increased).
  - Often secondary to medications, but may be associated with an underlying disorder such as neoplasm, pulmonary disorder, or CNS system disease
- Synonym(s): Syndrome of inappropriate secretion of ADH

EPIDEMIOLOGY

Incidence

- Usually found in the hospital setting, where incidence can be as high as 35%
- Predominant age: Elderly
- Predominate sex: Females > Males

RISK FACTORS

- Use of predisposing drugs
- Advanced age
- Postoperative status
- Institutionalization

Genetics

No known genetic pattern

GENERAL PREVENTION

- Search for cause, if unknown.
- Administration of 0.9% sodium chloride in adults during the perioperative period is recommended (if hypernatremia is not present) (1).
- Monitor electrolytes in postoperative patients to determine if fluid intake needs restriction.
- Reduce or change medications, if drug-induced.
- Lifelong restriction of fluid intake

ETIOLOGY

- Drugs:
  - Antidepressants (e.g., monoamine oxidase inhibitors [MAOIs], tricyclics, SSRIs)
  - Oral hypoglycemics (e.g., chlorpropamide, metformin)
  - Antineoplastic drugs (e.g., vincristine, vinblastine, cisplatin, cyclophosphamide)
  - Antipsychotic agents (e.g., phenothiazines, thioridazine, haloperidol)
  - Analgesics (e.g., NSAIDs)
  - Antiepileptics (e.g., carbamazepine, valproic acid)
  - Diuretics (thiazides and loop)
  - Others (e.g., vasopressin, DDAVP, ecstasy, oxytocin, α-interferon)
- Neoplasms (ectopic ADH production):
  - Small cell carcinoma of the lung
  - Oat cell carcinoma of the lung
  - Hodgkin disease
  - Pancreatic carcinoma
  - Thymoma
  - Mesothelioma
  - Bronchogenic carcinoma
- Infectious diseases:
  - Meningitis
  - Encephalitis
  - Pneumonia
  - Pulmonary tuberculosis (TB)
  - Rocky Mountain spotted fever
  - HIV infection
- Miscellaneous cardiopulmonary conditions:
  - Asthma
  - Atelectasis
  - Myocardial infarction
  - Vascular diseases
- Other:
  - CNS injury
  - Mechanical ventilation
  - Multiple sclerosis
  - Guillain-Barré syndrome
  - Lupus erythematosus
  - Porphyria
  - Hypothyroidism, myxedema
- Idiopathic

COMMONLY ASSOCIATED CONDITIONS

See "Etiology."

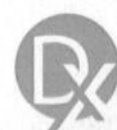

DIAGNOSIS

HISTORY

Early symptoms:

- Fatigue
- Anorexia
- Nausea
- Vomiting
- Diarrhea
- Headaches
- Myalgias
- Increased thirst

PHYSICAL EXAM

Late/severe hyponatremia (serum Na <100–115 mEq/L):

- Altered mental status
- Confusion
- Lethargy
- Seizures
- Psychosis
- Coma
- Death

DIAGNOSTIC TESTS & INTERPRETATION

Lab

- Serum Na level: Low
- Serum osmolality: Low
- Urine osmolality: High
- Urinary Na concentration: High (losing sodium, rather than retaining)
- Serum glucose; BUN; creatinine
- Thyroid function
- Morning cortisol
- Serum ADH level: High
- Uric acid

Imaging

Not usually required for diagnosis

DIFFERENTIAL DIAGNOSIS

- Postoperative complications:
  - Usually after major abdominal or thoracic surgery
  - Caused by nonosmotic release of ADH, probably mediated by pain afferents
  - ADH increased by pain and narcotics
- Postprostatectomy syndrome:
  - Irrigating solution must be nonconducting (i.e., electrolyte-free).
  - D_5W absorbed
- Psychogenic polydipsia:
  - Active therapy rarely is needed.
  - Diuresis occurs when intake is stopped.
  - Intake usually over 10 L/d
  - Interaction with other psychotropic drugs
- Acute (usually in children):
  - Swallowing water during swimming
  - Diluted formula
  - Tap-water enemas
- Endocrine:
  - Addison disease
  - Hypothyroidism
- Spurious hyponatremia: Caused by increased serum glucose, cholesterol, or proteins
- Appropriate ADH secretion and hyponatremia with decreased effective arterial blood volume (e.g., congestive heart failure [CHF], nephrotic syndrome, cirrhosis)
- Cerebral salt wasting syndrome (hyponatremia, extracellular fluid depletion, CNS insult)

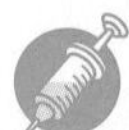

TREATMENT

MEDICATION

- Diuretics: Furosemide (Lasix) plus hourly NaCl and KCl replacement:
  - Requires frequent monitoring (see "Patient Monitoring")
  - Treatment of choice for acute management

- Hypertonic (3%) saline to cautiously increase serum Na (2):
  - By 10–12 mEq/L (10–12 mmol/L) q24h (in chronic hyponatremia)
  - 5% over first few hours
  - To only 120 mEq/L (120 mmol/L) acutely
  - By 0.5 mEq/h (0.5 mmol/hr)
- Contraindications: Avoid fluids in CHF, nephrotic syndrome, or cirrhosis.
- Precautions: Overly rapid correction (>12 mEq/L/d [>12 mmol/d]) can cause:
  - CHF
  - Subdural and intracerebral hemorrhage
  - Permanent CNS damage, especially with serum Na <120 mEq/L (<120 mmol/L)
  - Demyelination syndrome
- Demeclocycline:
  - Blocks ADH at renal tubule; produces nephrogenic diabetes insipidus
  - Dosage for long-term management: 600–1,200 mg/d
  - Onset of action within 1 week; therefore, not best for acute management
- Lithium:
  - Blocks ADH at renal tubule
  - Use with caution to avoid lithium toxicity.
- Vasopressin-2 receptor antagonist (the vaptans: Tolvaptan, conivaptan):
  - Good efficacy and safety profiles in the treatment of mild-to-moderate hyponatremia due to SIADH (1,2,3).

ADDITIONAL TREATMENT

General Measures

- Fluid restriction (800–1,000 mL/d) is the main form of treatment.
- Mildly symptomatic (serum Na >125 mEq/L [>125 mmol/L]): Restrict fluid to 800–1,000 mL/d.
- Acute (<48 hours duration) or symptomatic (altered mental status, seizure, coma):
  - Hypertonic saline (3% normal saline) bolus
  - Diuresis with loop diuretics
  - Decrease oral free water to 2/3 maintenance.
  - Increase oral salt.
  - Correct serum Na deficit (mEq Na deficit = [desired Na − actual Na] × 0.5 × body weight [kg]).
  - Increase serum Na slowly with hypertonic saline by 0.5 mEq/L/hr until it reaches 120 mEq/L.

ALERT

Increase Na levels slowly, no more than 0.5–1 mEq/L/hr, to prevent complications such as central pontine myelinosis (CPM).

ONGOING CARE

FOLLOW-UP RECOMMENDATIONS

Patient Monitoring

- Careful continuous clinical and laboratory monitoring of hyponatremic state during acute phase:
  - Hourly urine output
  - Urine Na
  - Serum Na and potassium (K)
- Chronic management: Monitor underlying cause as needed.

DIET

May need increased salt or decreased water intake, depending on cause

PATIENT EDUCATION

Diet and fluid restrictions

PROGNOSIS

- Depends on underlying cause, but in general, higher morbidity and mortality in hospitalized patients with hyponatremia
- If symptomatic (seizure, coma): High mortality due to cerebral edema if serum Na <120 mEq/L (<120 mmol/L)

COMPLICATIONS

- Osmotic demyelination: Central pontine and extrapontine irreversible myelinolysis (2,4)
- Chronic hyponatremia: Usually <120 mEq/L (<120 mmol/L)
- Complications of overly rapid correction (see "Treatment, Precautions")
- Chronic hyponatremia is associated with osteoporosis (5).

REFERENCES

1. Ellison DH, Berl T. Clinical practice. The syndrome of inappropriate antidiuresis. *N Engl J Med*. 2007;356: 2064–72.
2. Esposito P, Piotti G, Bianzina S, et al. The syndrome of inappropriate antidiuresis: Pathophysiology, clinical management and new therapeutic options. *Nephron Clinical Pract*. 2011;119:c62–c73.
3. Sherlock M, Thompson CJ, et al. The syndrome of inappropriate antidiuretic hormone: Current and future management options. *Eur J Endocrinol*. 2010;162(Suppl 1):S13–8.
4. Fleming JD, Babu S, et al. Images in clinical medicine. Central pontine myelinolysis. *N Engl J Med*. 2008;359:e29.
5. Verbalis JG, Barsony J, Sugimura Y, et al. Hyponatremia-induced osteoporosis. *J Bone Miner Res*. 2010;25:554–63.
6. Adrogué HJ, Madias NE. Hyponatremia. *N Engl J Med*. 2000;342:1581–9.

ADDITIONAL READING

- Holm EA, Bie P, Ottesen M, et al. Diagnosis of the syndrome of inappropriate secretion of antidiuretic hormone. *South Med J*. 2009;102:380–4.
- Moritz ML, Ayus JC, et al. 100 cc 3% sodium chloride bolus: a novel treatment for hyponatremic encephalopathy. *Metab Brain Dis*. 2010;25:91–6.
- Upadhyay UM, Gormley WB, et al. Etiology and management of hyponatremia in neurosurgical patients. *Intensive Care Med*. 2011 Feb 23. [Epub ahead of print]

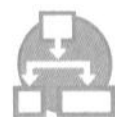

See Also (Topic, Algorithm, Electronic Media Element)

Hyponatremia

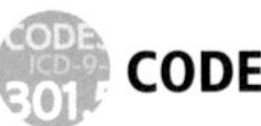

CODES

ICD9

253.6 Other disorders of neurohypophysis

CLINICAL PEARLS

- Fluid restriction to 600–800 mL/d × 2–3 days will result in weight loss and correction of hyponatremia and salt wasting in SIADH. Fluid restriction fails to correct hyponatremia and Na wasting in salt-losing renal disease (1,6).
- Cerebral salt wasting is a controversial disease entity and is similar to SIADH. However, patients with SIADH are euvolemic, whereas patients with cerebral salt wasting are hypovolemic. The only real way to establish the diagnosis is through fluid restriction. Serum urate and fractional excretion of urate will be corrected with fluid restriction in SIADH but will not correct in cerebral salt wasting.
- CPM is a cerebral demyelination syndrome that causes quadriplegia, pseudobulbar palsy, seizures, coma, and death. It is caused by an overly rapid rate of Na correction (2,4).
- Safe correction of hyponatremia is important; mathematical formulas such as the one of Androgue and Madias are helpful (6). Online calculators are available: www.medcal.com/sodium.html.

S

SEIZURE DISORDER, ABSENCE

Jane K. Louie, MD

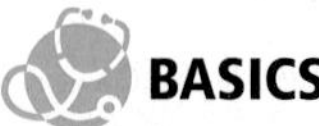

BASICS

DESCRIPTION

- Committee on Classification and Terminology of the International League Against Epilepsy divides epilepsy syndromes into 4 groups:
  - Localization-related: Focal or multifocal seizures
  - Generalized: Generalized seizures
  - Undetermined epilepsies: Both focal and generalized seizures where objective studies (e.g., EEG) do not indicate etiology or localization
  - Special syndromes: Now called "conditions with epileptic seizures that do not require a diagnosis of epilepsy" (e.g., febrile seizures)
- Epilepsy syndromes further classified by etiology:
  - Idiopathic: Presumed genetic etiology without structural brain lesion or other neurologic deficits
  - Symptomatic: Clearly identified cause (e.g., Mesial temporal lobe epilepsy with hippocampal sclerosis)
  - Cryptogenic: Etiology suspected but exact cause cannot be identified
- Absence seizures are a generalized epileptic seizure type, characterized by brief lapses of awareness.
- Typical absence:
  - Associated with pediatric idiopathic generalized epilepsy syndromes, namely, childhood absence epilepsy
  - Formerly called *petit mal seizures*
  - Abrupt-onset behavioral arrest, loss of awareness, and blank staring, sometimes with mild upward eye deviation, repetitive blinking
  - May include automatisms, tonic or atonic features, eyelid or facial clonus, autonomic features
  - Last 5–30 seconds
  - Immediate return to normal consciousness
- Atypical absence:
  - Associated with symptomatic generalized epilepsy syndromes such as Lennox-Gastaut
  - Onset and offset less abrupt than typical absence seizures
  - Last 10–45 seconds
  - Impairment of consciousness often incomplete with continued purposeful activity
  - Postictal confusion sometimes occurs.
  - Associated clinical features more pronounced and frequent than typical absence; atonia most common
- Myoclonic absence:
  - Additional proposed seizure type by the International League Against Epilepsy (1)
  - Seizure type in epilepsy with myoclonic absences, a cryptogenic generalized epilepsy syndrome
  - Rhythmic clonic jerking at 2–4 Hz
  - Last 5–10 seconds
  - Unlike myoclonic seizures with no impairment of consciousness, brief lapses of awareness are characteristic of myoclonic absence
- Rest of topic details idiopathic generalized epilepsy syndromes characterized by *typical absence seizures*, specifically childhood absence epilepsy (CAE)
- Juvenile absence epilepsy (JAE) is mentioned briefly here.
- CAE:
  - Also known as *pyknolepsy*
  - Typical absence seizures are the only seizure type in 90% of children.
  - 10% develop additional generalized tonic–clonic seizures.
  - Seizures last about 10 seconds and often occur hundreds of times per day.
  - Onset ages 4–10 years, with peak at ages 5–7 years (2)
  - Normal neurologic state and development
  - Spontaneous remission occurs in 65–70% of patients during adolescence.
- JAE:
  - Typical absence seizures are the main seizure type.
  - Seizures last longer than in CAE and occur usually less than once a day (3).
  - Onset ages 9–16 years, with peak at ages 10–13 years
  - Generalized tonic–clonic seizures occur in most patients, often in the first 1–2 hours after awakening.
  - Seizures often persist into adulthood.

EPIDEMIOLOGY

Incidence

6–8 per 100,000 per year

Prevalence

5–50 per 100,000

RISK FACTORS

Genetics

- 70–85% concordance occurs in monozygotic twins; 82% share EEG features.
- 33% concordance among first-degree relatives
- 15–45% have a family history of epilepsy.
- Girls are more often affected, with a 3:2–2:1 ratio.
- Complex multifactorial inheritance
- For childhood absence, genes/loci implicated include 6q, 8q24, and 5q14 (3).
- Mutations of $GABA_A$ receptor and voltage-gated Ca^{2+} channel are implicated.

PATHOPHYSIOLOGY

- Corticoreticular theory implicates abnormal activity in thalamocortical circuits.
- Thalamic reticular nucleus is responsible for both normal sleep spindles and pathologic slow-wave discharges; contains inhibitory GABAergic neurons.
- These neurons affect low-threshold calcium currents.
- These circuits can fire in oscillatory/rhythmic fashion:
  - Normally, activation of $GABA_A$ receptors causes 10-Hz oscillations in sleep spindle frequency.
  - If $GABA_B$ receptors strongly activated, oscillation frequency will be 3–4 Hz, similar to spike-and-wave typical absence seizure frequency.

COMMONLY ASSOCIATED CONDITIONS

- 3–8% of CAE cases evolve into juvenile myoclonic epilepsy.
- Associated with cognitive/learning problems

DIAGNOSIS

Seizures are often so brief that untrained observers are not aware of the occurrence.

HISTORY

- Frequently diagnosed in children being evaluated for poor school performance
- Teachers report that child seems to daydream or zone out frequently.
- Child will forget portions of conversations.
- Child with normal intelligence quotient (IQ) underperforms in school.

PHYSICAL EXAM

- Unless a child has another genetic or acquired abnormality, a neurologic exam usually is normal.
- Seizures may be frequent enough to be observed during physical exam:
  - Manifest by behavior arrest: Child will stop speaking in midsentence, stare blankly, etc.
  - Automatisms (repetitive stereotyped behaviors) may be present.
  - Child resumes previous activity.
- Seizures may be induced by hyperventilation:
  - Have child blow on pinwheel or similar exercise to provoke seizure.
  - Alternatively, ask the patient to perform hyperventilation with eyes closed and count. Patient will open eyes at onset of seizure and stop counting (3).
- Patient manifests unresponsiveness but retains postural tone in a typical absence seizure.

DIAGNOSTIC TESTS & INTERPRETATION

Lab

- No specific hematologic workup
- Follow blood chemistry, hepatic function, and blood counts specific to drug regimen.
- Drug levels are useful in evaluating symptoms of toxicity or for breakthrough seizures.

Initial lab tests

- EEG is standard for diagnosis:
  - Typical absence features: 3-Hz spike-and-wave activity on normal EEG background
  - Seizures feature bursts of 3–4-Hz spike-and-wave activity, which may slow to 2.5–3 Hz during seizure.
  - Seizure usually is evident clinically if bursts last >3 seconds; subtle changes of transient cognitive impairment may be evident with briefer seizures.
- Hyperventilation and occasionally photic stimulation may induce seizure, thus confirming diagnosis of typical absence epilepsy.

Imaging

- Not routinely indicated in children with typical absence and normal neurologic exam and IQ
- Brain MRI is indicated in atypical absence and in children with mixed seizure types when combined with abnormal neurologic exam or low IQ.

DIFFERENTIAL DIAGNOSIS

- Typical absence seizures frequently are misdiagnosed as complex partial seizures.
- Nonepileptic staring spells: Suggestive features include:
  – Events do not interrupt play.
  – Events are first noticed by professional such as schoolteacher, speech therapist, occupational therapist, or physician (rather than parent).
  – During a staring spell, child is responsive to touch or other external stimuli.

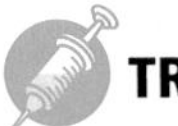

TREATMENT

MEDICATION

Certain common anticonvulsants may exacerbate absence: Carbamazepine, tiagabine, vigabatrin, and gabapentin.

First Line

- Ethosuximide blocks T-type calcium channels:
  – First-line, except in absence patients with tonic–clonic seizures (lacks efficacy)
  – Side effects: Headache, hiccups, behavior changes, tremor
  – Adverse effects: Rare blood dyscrasias (monitor CBC)
- Lamotrigine affects sodium channels:
  – Side effects: Headache, insomnia, dizziness
  – Adverse effects: Rare Stevens-Johnson rash, more often when coadministered with valproic acid
- Valproic acid has multiple mechanisms:
  – First choice in absence patients with tonic–clonic, myoclonic, mixed seizure types
  – Side effects: Weight gain, alopecia, sedation
  – Adverse effects: Thrombocytopenia, rare fulminant hepatic failure (especially in children <2 years of age)

Second Line

- Topiramate affects GABA and excitatory neurotransmission:
  – FDA approved for Lennox-Gastaut syndrome
  – Side effects: Psychomotor slowing
  – Adverse effects: Weight loss, renal stones, myopia, glaucoma (rare), anhidrosis
- Zonisamide and levetiracetam also are used off-label.

Pregnancy Considerations

Anticonvulsants, especially valproic acid, are associated with an increase in fetal malformations. Use of valproic acid in women who are or are likely to become pregnant generally is contraindicated. Obtain specialty consultation.

ADDITIONAL TREATMENT

- Most absence seizure patients respond to a single medication.
- Male sex and an early age at diagnosis are associated with the need for 2 medications to control the disease (4)[A].

IN-PATIENT CONSIDERATIONS

Admission Criteria

- Absence epilepsy rarely requires admission.
- Status epilepticus requires inpatient management.

Discharge Criteria

Resolution of status epilepticus

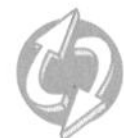

ONGOING CARE

FOLLOW-UP RECOMMENDATIONS

- Patients with associated tonic–clonic seizures should avoid high places and swimming alone.
- Absence rarely persists into adulthood, but affected adults may be restricted from driving, working over open flames, etc., as with other generalized and partial epilepsy subtypes.
- Patients should be monitored periodically by a neurologist for evolution of absence epilepsy into tonic–clonic or other seizure types.

PROGNOSIS

- Of those with childhood absence epilepsy without tonic–clonic seizures, 90% remit by adulthood (2).
- 35% of patients with tonic–clonic seizures experience complete remission of absence seizures.
- 15% of patients develop juvenile myoclonic epilepsy (5).

COMPLICATIONS

Reported frequencies of typical absence status epilepticus range from 5.8–9.4% of patients with CAE (6).

REFERENCES

1. Engel J. Report of the ILAE classification core group. *Epilepsia*. 2006;47:1558–68.
2. Valentin A, Hindocha N, Osei-Lah A, et al. Idiopathic generalized epilepsy with absences: Syndrome classification. *Epilepsia*. 2007;48: 2187–90.
3. Nordli DR. Idiopathic generalized epilepsies recognized by the International League Against Epilepsy. *Epilepsia*. 2005;46(Suppl 9):48–56.
4. Nadler B, Shevell MI. Childhood absence epilepsy requiring more than one medication for seizure control. *Can J Neurol Sci*. 2008;35:297–300.
5. Grosso S, Galimberti D, Vezzosi P, et al. Childhood absence epilepsy: Evolution and prognostic factors. *Epilepsia*. 2005;46:1796–801.
6. Shorvon S, Walker M. Status epilepticus in idiopathic generalized epilepsy. *Epilepsia*. 2005; 46(Suppl 9):73–9.
7. Kesselheim AS, Stedman MR, Bubrick EJ, et al. Seizure outcomes following the use of generic versus brand-name antiepileptic drugs: A systematic review and meta-analysis. *Drugs*. 2010;70:605–21.

ADDITIONAL READING

Commission on Classification and Terminology of the International League Against Epilepsy Proposal for revised classification of epilepsies and epileptic syndromes. *Epilepsia*. 1989;30(4):389–99.

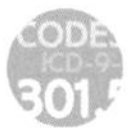

CODES

ICD9

345.00 Generalized nonconvulsive epilepsy, without mention of intractable epilepsy

CLINICAL PEARLS

- To help aid with diagnosis during an exam, try having child blow repetitively on pinwheel (causing hyperventilation) to attempt to trigger absence seizure.
- Alternatively, ask patient to perform hyperventilation with eyes closed and count. Patient will open eyes and stop counting at onset of the seizure (3).
- Concern regarding generic medications allowing more breakthrough seizures has not been supported in evidence-based studies (7)[A].

SEIZURE DISORDER, PARTIAL

Ruben Peralta, MD, FACS
Wynne Morgan, MD

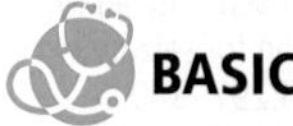

BASICS

DESCRIPTION

- Seizures occur when abnormal synchronous neuronal discharges in the brain cause transient cortical dysfunction.
- Generalized seizures involve bilateral cerebral cortex from the seizure's onset.
- Partial seizures originate from a discrete focus in the cerebral cortex.
- Partial seizures are further divided into simple and complex subtypes:
  - If consciousness is impaired during a partial seizure, it is classified as complex.
  - If consciousness is preserved, it is a simple partial seizure.

EPIDEMIOLOGY

Prevalence

Partial seizures occur in 20/100,000 persons in the US.

RISK FACTORS

- History of traumatic brain injury (1)
- Children exposed to a thiamine-deficient formula (2)

Genetics

Benign rolandic epilepsy, a form of partial seizure disorder, has an autosomal dominant inheritance pattern with penetrance depending on multiple factors.

ETIOLOGY

- Partial seizures begin when a localized seizure focus produces an abnormal, synchronized depolarization that spreads to a discrete portion of the surrounding cortex.
- The area of cortex involved in the seizure determines the symptoms; for example, an epileptogenic focus in motor cortex produces contralateral motor symptoms.
- In some cases, etiology is related to structural abnormalities that are prone to epileptogenesis. Most common etiologies vary by life stage:
  - Early childhood: Developmental/congenital malformation, trauma
  - Young adults: Developmental, infection, trauma
  - Adults 40–60 years of age: Cerebrovascular insult, infection, trauma
  - Adults >60 years of age: Cerebrovascular insult, trauma, neoplasm
- Complex partial seizures: A common cause is mesial temporal sclerosis.

COMMONLY ASSOCIATED CONDITIONS

Epilepsy patients have a higher incidence of depression than does the general population.

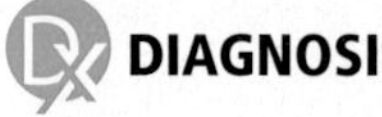

DIAGNOSIS

- Seizure activity usually stereotyped
- Duration: Seconds–minutes unless status epilepticus develops; status epilepticus may present as focal or generalized convulsions or altered mental status without convulsions.
- Simple partial seizures:
  - Simple partial seizures are characterized by localized symptoms. The patient is conscious. Symptoms may involve motor, sensory, or psychic systems.
  - Motor: Seizure activity in motor strip causes contraction (tonic) or rhythmic jerking (clonic) movements that may involve 1 entire side of body or may be more localized (i.e., hands, feet, or face):
    - Jacksonian march: As discharge spreads through motor cortex, tonic–clonic activity spreads in predictable fashion (i.e., beginning in hand and progressing up arm and to the face).
  - Sensory/psychic:
    - Todd paresis: After motor seizure, residual, temporary weakness in the affected area
    - Parietal lobe: Sensory loss or paresthesias, dizziness
    - Temporal lobe: Déjà vu, rising sensation in epigastrium, auditory hallucinations or forced memories, unpleasant smell or taste
  - Occipital: Visual hallucinations
- Complex partial seizures:
  - Impaired consciousness by definition
  - May have aura; this is start of seizure
- Amnesia for the event, postictal confusion:
  - Most often, focus in complex partial seizures is temporal or frontal.
  - Motor manifestations may include dystonic posturing or automatisms (i.e., simple, repetitive movements of face and hands such as lip smacking, picking, or more complex actions such as purposeless walking).
  - Frontal lobe seizure is characterized by brief, bilateral complex movements, vocalizations, often with onset during sleep.

HISTORY

- A detailed description of the seizure should be obtained from an observer.
- Review medication list for drugs that lower seizure threshold (e.g., tramadol, bupropion, theophylline).
- Drugs of abuse (e.g., cocaine) lower seizure threshold.
- History of traumatic brain injury (1)

PHYSICAL EXAM

Include neurologic exam, with attention to lateralizing signs suggestive of structural lesion.

DIAGNOSTIC TESTS & INTERPRETATION

EEG: Spikes/sharp waves over seizure focus:

- Yield of EEG is increased by obtained in first 24 hours following seizure and by sleep deprivation.
- Frontal lobe seizure focus may be difficult to detect by routine EEG.
- If difficulty with diagnosis, continuous video–EEG monitoring may be appropriate.

Lab

- Serum electrolytes, including calcium, magnesium, phosphorus; hepatic function panel; CBC; drugs of abuse
- If measured within 10–20 minutes of suspected seizure, an elevated prolactin level may help to differentiate generalized or complex partial seizure from psychogenic seizure.
- CSF exam if infection is suspected
- Urinalysis, chest x-ray, levels of antiepileptic drugs for breakthrough seizure

Imaging

- Technological advances in neuroimaging are usually directed at the diagnosis and prognosis for seizure control (3).
- Emergency evaluation of new seizure: CT scan to screen for hemorrhage, stroke
- After emergency evaluation, MRI with thin cuts through area of interest
- If planning epilepsy surgery, positron emission tomography scan and/or interictal single-photon emission computed tomography (SPECT) may be of value.
- Magnetoencephalography (MEG) is an evolving technology for localizing seizure focus.

DIFFERENTIAL DIAGNOSIS

- Nonepileptic seizure
- Syncope/postanoxic myoclonus
- Hypoglycemia
- For hemiparesis following event:
  - Transient ischemic attack
  - Hemiplegic migraine

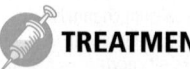

TREATMENT

MEDICATION

- Some physicians do not start medication after a single seizure if EEG and MRI are normal and/or a precipitant is clear and avoidable.
- Antiepileptic drugs (AEDs) act on voltage-gated ion channels, affect neuronal inhibition via enhancement of γ-aminobutyric acid (GABA, an inhibitory neurotransmitter), or decrease neuronal excitation. End result is to decrease the abnormal synchronized firing and to prevent seizure propagation.
- ~50% of those with newly diagnosed partial seizures respond to and tolerate first AED trial.
- Choose AED based on seizure type, side-effect profile, and patient characteristics. Increase dose until seizure control is obtained or side effects become unacceptable.
- Attempt monotherapy, but many patients will require adjunctive agents.
- *Refractory to medications* is defined as failure of at least 3 anticonvulsants to achieve adequate control.
- Several AEDs induce or inhibit cytochrome P450 enzymes (watch for drug interactions).

First Line

- Carbamazepine: Affects sodium channels; side effects include GI distress, hyponatremia, diplopia, dizziness, rare pancytopenia/marrow suppression, exfoliative rash
- Oxcarbazepine: Affects sodium channels; side effects include dizziness, diplopia, hyponatremia, headache
- Lamotrigine: Affects sodium channels:
  - Side effects include insomnia, dizziness, ataxia
  - Risk of Stevens-Johnson reaction (potentially fatal exfoliative rash) especially when given with valproate; requires slow titration
- Levetiracetam: Multiple mechanisms; side effects include sedation, ataxia, irritability

Second Line

- Phenytoin: Affects sodium channels; side effects include ataxia, dizziness, diplopia, tremor, GI upset, gingival hyperplasia, fever
- Phenobarbital: Multiple mechanisms; side effects include sedation, withdrawal seizures

- Valproate: Multiple mechanisms; side effects include GI upset, weight gain, alopecia, tremor; less common thrombocytopenia, hepatitis, pancreatitis
- Topiramate: Multiple mechanisms; side effects include anorexia, cognitive slowing, sedation, nephrolithiasis, anhidrosis
- Gabapentin: Multiple mechanisms; side effects include sedation, dizziness, ataxia
- Pregabalin: Affects calcium channels; side effects include sedation, dizziness, weight gain
- Zonisamide: Affects sodium channels:
  - Side effects include sedation, anorexia, nausea, dizziness, ataxia, anhidrosis, nephrolithiasis
  - Cross-reaction with sulfa allergy

Pregnancy Considerations

- Several AEDs induce hepatic metabolism of oral contraceptives, decreasing their efficacy. AED therapy during first trimester is associated with doubled risk for major fetal malformations (6% vs. 3%).
- Phenytoin in pregnancy may result in fetal hydantoin syndrome.
- Valproate is associated with neural tube defects.
- Fetal insult from seizures following withdrawal of therapy also may be severe. Risk–benefit balance should be evaluated with high-risk pregnancy and epileptology consultations. Most patients remain on anticonvulsants.
- Consider vagal nerve stimulator during pregnancy (4).

ADDITIONAL TREATMENT

General Measures

- Ask patient to maintain a seizure diary.
- Note potential triggers such as stress, sleep deprivation, drug use, discontinuation of alcohol or benzodiazepines, menses.

Issues for Referral

For refractory seizures, consider referral to an epilepsy specialist and/or epileptic center (5).

Additional Therapies

- Vagal nerve stimulator: Implanted in neck; provides periodic stimulation to vagus nerve; may induce hoarseness, cough, and dysphagia (6).
- New technologies under development include deep brain stimulation.

SURGERY/OTHER PROCEDURES

- For refractory partial complex seizures
- Should have identifiable focus
- Preoperative testing, such as Wada test, should be done to decrease likelihood of inducing aphasia and memory loss.
- Workup also may include MRI, video–EEG monitoring, electrocorticography, MEG, and ictal SPECT.
- 64% will be seizure-free after surgery (with continued medication treatment); 25% will have significant decrease in frequency; 1/3 continue to have disabling seizures.
- Goal of surgical intervention is to reduce reliance on medications; most patients remain on anticonvulsants postoperatively.

IN-PATIENT CONSIDERATIONS

Admission Criteria

Generally, outpatient treatment; admission for unremitting seizure (partial or secondary generalized status epilepticus)

ONGOING CARE

FOLLOW-UP RECOMMENDATIONS

- Most states have restrictions on driving for those with seizure disorders.
- Depending on seizure manifestation, may recommend against activities such as swimming, climbing to heights, working over open flames, or operating heavy machinery
- Outpatient follow-up with neurologist

Patient Monitoring

AED levels if concern over toxicity, noncompliance, or for breakthrough seizures

DIET

Ketogenic or low-glycemic-index diet may improve seizure control in some patients.

PATIENT EDUCATION

Avoid potential triggers such as alcohol or drug use, sleep deprivation.

PROGNOSIS

- Risk of seizure recurrence: ~30% after first seizure; 50% of these recurrences will occur in the first 6 months; 90% in the first 2 years.
- Depends on seizure type; rolandic epilepsy has a good prognosis; temporal lobe epilepsy is more likely to be persistent.
- ~25–30% of all seizures are refractory to current medications.
- AEDs initiated after an initial seizure have been shown to decrease the risk of seizure over the first 2 years but are not demonstrated to reduce long-term risk of recurrence.
- Long duration of uncontrolled seizure disorder associated with increased cognitive and functional impairments; early pharmacologic intervention is encouraged.
- The potential for AEDs to confer neuroprotection is under investigation.
- The risk of developing seizure after mild traumatic brain injury remains high for a long period (>10 years) (1).

COMPLICATIONS

Risk of accidental injury

REFERENCES

1. Christensen J, Pedersen MG, Pedersen CB, et al. Long-term risk of epilepsy after traumatic brain injury in children and young adults: A population-based cohort study. *Lancet*. 2009; 373(9669):1105–10.
2. Fattal-Valevski A, Bloch-Mimouni A, Kivity S, et al. Epilepsy in children with infantile thiamine deficiency. *Neurology*. 2009;73:828–33.
3. Gaillard WD, Cross JH, Duncan JS, et al. Epilepsy imaging study guideline criteria: Commentary on diagnostic testing study guidelines and practice parameters. *Epilepsia*. 2011;52(9):1750–6.
4. Houser MV, Hennessy MD, Howard BC, et al. Vagal nerve stimulator use during pregnancy for treatment of refractory seizure disorder. *Obstet Gynecol*. 2010;115:417–9.
5. Hemb M, Velasco TR, Parnes MS, et al. Improved outcomes in pediatric epilepsy surgery: The UCLA experience, 1986–2008. *Neurology*. 2010;74:1768–75.
6. Siddiqui F, Herial NA, Ali II, et al. Cumulative effect of vagus nerve stimulators on intractable seizures observed over a period of 3 years. *Epilepsy Behav*. 2010;18(3):299–302.

S

ADDITIONAL READING

- Adams SM, Knowles PD, et al. Evaluation of a first seizure. *Am Fam Physician*. 2007;75:1342–7.
- Auvin S, Vallée L. [Febrile seizures: Current understanding of pathophysiological mechanisms.] *Arch Pediatr*. 2009;16(5):450–6.
- Cross JH, Jayakar P, Nordli D, et al. Proposed criteria for referral and evaluation of children for epilepsy surgery: Recommendations of the Subcommission for Pediatric Epilepsy Surgery. *Epilepsia*. 2006;47: 952–9.
- Deprez L, Jansen A, De Jonghe P, et al. Genetics of epilepsy syndromes starting in the first year of life. *Neurology*. 2009;72:273–81.
- Sankar R, Ramsay E, McKay A, et al. A multicenter, outpatient, open-label study to evaluate the dosing, effectiveness, and safety of topiramate as monotherapy in the treatment of epilepsy in clinical practice. *Epilepsy Behav*. 2009;15(4):506–12.
- Ueda Y, Kitamoto A, Willmore LJ, et al. Hippocampal gene network analysis in an experimental model of posttraumatic epilepsy. *Neurochem Res*. 2011;36:1323–8.

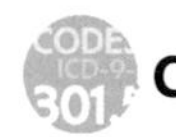

CODES

ICD9

- 345.40 Partial epilepsy, without mention of intractable epilepsy
- 345.50 Partial epilepsy, without mention of impairment of consciousness, without mention of intractable epilepsy

CLINICAL PEARLS

- It is controversial whether AED treatment is indicated after a first seizure. Treatment should be strongly considered when a clear structural cause is identified or risk of injury from seizure is high (e.g., osteoporosis, anticoagulation).
- Consider vagus nerve stimulation in pregnancy and in patients with medically refractory seizures.
- Postictal elevation in prolactin levels can help distinguish physiologic from psychogenic seizures.

SEIZURE DISORDERS

Ann M. Lynch, PharmD, RPh, AE-C
Stephanie Carinci, MD

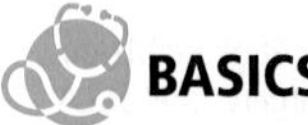

BASICS

DESCRIPTION

- Seizure: Sudden change in cortical electrical activity, manifested through motor, sensory, or behavioral changes, and/or an alteration in consciousness.
- System(s) affected: Nervous
- Synonym(s): Epilepsy; Convulsion; Attacks; Spells

Geriatric Considerations

Fractures from falls are more common in the osteopenic age range.

Pediatric Considerations

Breast-feeding is not contraindicated. Sedation of the infant should be monitored.

Pregnancy Considerations

- Monitor serum levels of antiepileptic drugs (AEDs).
- There is a 2-fold increase in congenital malformations in children born to mothers taking anticonvulsants, depending on the anticonvulsant. Some expectant mothers can stop taking anticonvulsants safely for the first trimester or initial 6-week period (organogenesis). Avoid Depakote. Epileptic patients should notify their neurologist before conception if possible.
- Recommend against use of category C or D AEDs during pregnancy/nursing.

EPIDEMIOLOGY

Incidence

- ~200,000 new cases of epilepsy are diagnosed in the US yearly, with 45,000 new cases in children <15 years of age.
- Pediatric (<2 years) and older adults (>65 years) more commonly present with new-onset seizures.
- Predominant sex: Male = Female

Prevalence

- 2.7 million with seizure disorder
- 4 million people have had 1 or more seizures.
- 326,000 children (≤14 years) and 600,000 adults (>65 years) have a seizure disorder.

RISK FACTORS

Children delivered breech have a prevalence rate of 3.8% compared with 2.2% in vertex deliveries.

Genetics

Family history increases risk 3-fold.

GENERAL PREVENTION

Take measures to prevent head injuries. Reduce exposure to lead-containing products. Avoid excessive alcohol use/abuse.

PATHOPHYSIOLOGY

Synchronous and excessive firing of neurons, resulting in impairment of normal control of CNS

ETIOLOGY

True seizures may be triggered by the following metabolic/medical conditions, but seizures occurring due to these conditions do not necessarily define the presence of a seizure disorder (see also "Differential Diagnosis"):

- CNS infection
- Hyperthyroidism
- Hypoglycemia or hyperglycemia
- Hyponatremia
- Uremia
- Porphyria
- Hypoxia
- Confusional migraine
- Transient ischemic attack
- Narcolepsy/sleep disorder
- Toxins (such as lead, picrotoxin, strychnine)
- Brain tumor
- Cerebral hypoxia
- Stroke/CVA
- Drug or alcohol overdose/withdrawal
- Eclampsia
- Head injury
- Heat stroke

COMMONLY ASSOCIATED CONDITIONS

Infections, tumors, drug abuse, alcohol and drug withdrawal, trauma, metabolic disorders

DIAGNOSIS

- Differentiate first between epileptiform seizures and nonepileptiform seizures (NESs).
- If NESs are psychogenic, they often are associated with history of sexual abuse. Psychogenic NESs usually are associated with a history of psychiatric conditions.
- Physiologic seizures are true cortical events and may require acute intervention.
- International classification of seizures:
  - Generalized seizures
  - Absence
  - Atonic
  - Juvenile myoclonic
    - Myoclonic: Repetitive muscle contractions
    - Tonic–clonic: Tonic phase: Sudden loss of consciousness; clonic phase: sustained contraction followed by rhythmic contractions of all 4 extremities; postictal phase: headache, confusion, fatigue; clinically hypertensive, tachycardic, and otherwise hypersympathetic
  - Febrile seizures:
    - Age between 3 months and 5 years
    - Fever without evidence of any other defined cause of seizures
    - Recurrent febrile seizures probably do not increase the risk of epilepsy
  - Symptomatic focal epilepsies
  - Complex partial seizures
  - Nonconvulsive status epilepticus: Most commonly seen in ICU patients; no tonic–clonic activity seen so must diagnose with bedside EEG
  - Status epilepticus: Repetitive generalized seizures without recovery between seizures; considered a neurologic emergency

HISTORY

- Eyewitness descriptions of event; patient impressions of what occurred before, during, and after the event
- Screen for etiologies, including provoking or ameliorating factors for the event such as sleep deprivation.
- Ask about bowel or bladder incontinence, tongue biting, other injury, or automatisms.

PHYSICAL EXAM

Thorough neurologic exam

DIAGNOSTIC TESTS & INTERPRETATION

A negative EEG does not rule out a seizure disorder. Interictal EEG sensitivity may be as low as 20%; multiple EEGs may increase sensitivity to 80%. Prognostically, EEG abnormality may predict likelihood of seizure recurrence:

- Sleep deprivation may be helpful prior to EEG, and hyperventilation and photic stimulation during recording may increase sensitivity for spike wave formations.
- Video EEG monitoring is used to differentiate psychomotor NES from true cortical events.

Lab

Initial lab tests

- Serum tests: Glucose, Na, K, calcium, phosphorus, magnesium, BUN, ammonia. Drug and toxic screens: Include alcohol.
- AED levels (if patient taking antiepileptic medication)
- CBC: Rule out infection.

Follow-Up & Special Considerations

- Consider an arterial blood gas determination.
- Drugs that may alter lab results: AED therapy may affect the EEG results dramatically.
- Inadequate AED levels: May be altered by many medications, such as erythromycin, sulfonamides, warfarin, cimetidine, and alcohol.
- Disorders that may alter lab results: Pregnancy decreases serum concentration.

Imaging

Imaging is recommended for new-onset seizures when localization-related epilepsy is known or suspected, when the epilepsy classification is in doubt, or when an epilepsy syndrome with remote symptomatic cause is suspected. MRI is preferred to CT because of its superior resolution, versatility, and lack of radiation.

Initial approach

- Brain MRI: Superior in evaluation of the temporal lobes (e.g., mesial temporal sclerosis)
- CT scan of brain: Indicated routinely as initial evaluation, especially in the ER
- Bone scan to determine BMD: Generally done if patients are taking older AEDs such as Dilantin and Tegretol

Diagnostic Procedures/Surgery

LP for spinal fluid analysis may be necessary, especially if fever or impairment of consciousness are present.

Pathological Findings

MRI may identify a nidus for seizure activity.

DIFFERENTIAL DIAGNOSIS

Below represents a differential diagnosis for the etiology of actual seizures, not for apparent seizures (see also "Etiology," above):

- Idiopathic
- Hippocampal sclerosis and other neurodevelopmental abnormalities of the brain
- Acute infection (meningitis, abscess, encephalitis)
- Metabolic and endocrine disorders
- Trauma
- Drug and alcohol withdrawal
- Tumor
- Conversion disorder: Pseudoseizure

- Vascular disease including vasculitis
- Familial/genetic, infantile and pediatric seizure syndromes (e.g., Lennox-Gastaut, benign familial, myoclonic epilepsy of infancy)
- Other etiologies (by age of onset):
  - Infancy (0–2 years):
    - Perinatal hypoxia or other injury to cerebral cortex
    - Metabolic: Hypoglycemia, hypocalcemia, hypomagnesemia, vitamin B_6 deficiency, phenylketonuria
  - Childhood (2–10 years): Febrile seizure
  - Adolescent (10–18 years): AVM
  - Late adulthood (>60 years):
    - Degenerative disease including dementia
    - Metabolic: Hypoglycemia, uremia, hepatic failure, electrolyte abnormality

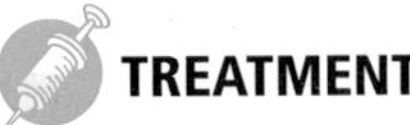

TREATMENT

- 50–60% presenting with an initial unprovoked seizure will not have a recurrence; 40–50% will have a recurrence within 2 years (1)[A].
- Starting antiepileptic medications reduces recurrences of seizures, but they do not alter long-term outcomes (2)[A].
- Evidence is conflicting whether or not to start AEDs routinely in patients with an initial seizure and no focal abnormalities on exam or imaging, though many recommend deferring treatment until a second seizure has occurred (3)[A].

MEDICATION

- AEDs of choice: Select from seizure groups below, with attention toward potential side effects.
- Choice of AED is based on type of seizure.
- Monotherapy is preferred whenever possible. Systemic reviews found insufficient evidence on which to base a first- or second-line choice among these drugs in terms of seizure control.
- Treatment options include:
  - Carbamazepine (Tegretol) 100–200 mg/d in 1–2 doses; therapeutic range, 4–12 mg/L
  - Phenytoin (Dilantin) 200–400 mg/d in 1–3 doses; therapeutic range, 10–20 mg/L
  - Valproic acid (Depakene) 750–3,000 mg/d in 1–3 doses to begin at 15 mg/kg/d; therapeutic range, 50–150 mg/L
  - Lamotrigine (Lamictal) 25–50 mg/d; adjust in 100-mg increments every 1–2 weeks to 300–500 mg/d in 2 divided doses.
  - Oxcarbazepine (Trileptal) 300 mg b.i.d., increase to 300 mg every 3 days; maintenance, 1,200 mg/d
  - Topiramate (Topamax) 50 mg/d; adjust weekly to effect; 400 mg/d in 2 doses, maximum 1,600 mg/d
  - Pregabalin (Lyrica)
  - Lacosamide (Vimpat), particularly if refractory seizures
- Alternative drugs (in addition to any of the preceding):
  - Phenobarbital: 50–100 mg b.i.d.–t.i.d.; therapeutic range, 15–40 mg/L
  - There is evidence to suggest long-term use of phenobarbital may impair cognitive ability.
  - Primidone (Mysoline) 100–125 mg at bedtime; adjust to maximum of 2,000 mg/d in 2 doses.
- Contraindications: Refer to manufacturer's profile of each drug.
- Precautions: Doses should be based on individual's response guided by drug levels.
- Consider cautioning about increased risk of suicide, but risk of untreated seizures is far greater than increased risk of suicide (4)[A].
- Patients are susceptible to sudden unexpected death in epilepsy, possibly due to cardiac arrhythmia.

ADDITIONAL TREATMENT

Issues for Referral

Patients should be referred to and followed by a specialist regularly. Frequency of visits is based on severity and patient's wishes; maximum of 1 year between visits.

COMPLEMENTARY AND ALTERNATIVE MEDICINE

- There is no evidence that any complementary medicines improve seizures, but they may induce serious drug interactions with prescribed AEDs.
- Psychological therapies may be used in conjunction with AED therapy. Cognitive-behavioral therapy, relaxation, biofeedback, and yoga all may be helpful as adjunctive therapy (5)[C].
- Patients with NES should be referred for psychotherapy.

SURGERY/OTHER PROCEDURES

- Resection for seizures that fail traditional therapy
- Vagus nerve stimulation

IN-PATIENT CONSIDERATIONS

Initial Stabilization

Protect the airway, and if possible, protect the patient from physical harm; do not restrain. Administer acute AEDs.

Admission Criteria

Outpatient therapy usually is sufficient except for status epilepticus.

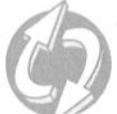

ONGOING CARE

FOLLOW-UP RECOMMENDATIONS

Maintain adequate drug therapy; ensure compliance and/or access to medication. Drug therapy withdrawal may be considered after a seizure-free 2-year period. Expect a 33% relapse rate in the following 3 years.

Patient Monitoring

- Monitoring of drug levels and seizure frequency
- CBC and lab values (e.g., calcium, vitamin D) as indicated; BMD
- Monitor for side effects and adverse reactions.
- All patients currently taking any AED should be monitored closely for notable changes in behavior that could indicate the emergence or worsening of suicidal thoughts or behavior or depression.

DIET

Ketogenic diet may be beneficial in children in conjunction with AED therapy.

PATIENT EDUCATION

- Stress the importance of medication compliance and the avoidance of alcohol and recreational drugs.
- Individuals with uncontrolled seizures should be encouraged to avoid heights and swimming.
- State driving laws: http://epilepsyfoundation.org; most states require a minimum of 6 months free of seizures
- http://epilepsy.org

PROGNOSIS

- Depends on type of seizure disorder: ~70% will become seizure-free with initial appropriate treatment, but 30% will continue to have seizures. The number of seizures within 6 months after first presentation is the most important factor for remission.
- ~90% who are seen for a first unprovoked seizure attain a 1–2-year remission within 4 or 5 years of the initial event (1)[A].
- Life expectancy is shortened in persons with epilepsy.
- The case-fatality rate for status epilepticus may be as high as 20%.

COMPLICATIONS

Drug toxicity

REFERENCES

1. Berg AT, et al. Risk of recurrence after a first unprovoked seizure. *Epilepsia*. 2008;49(1):13–8.
2. Arts WF, Geerts AT, et al. When to start drug treatment for childhood epilepsy: The clinical-epidemiological evidence. *Eur J Paediatr. Neurol*. 2009;13:93–101.
3. Haut SR, Shinnar S, et al. Considerations in the treatment of a first unprovoked seizure. *Semin Neurol*. 2008;28:289–96.
4. Hesdorffer DC, Kanner AM. The FDA alert on suicidality and antiepileptic drugs: Fire or false alarm? *Epilepsia*. 2009;50:978–86.
5. Marson A, Ramaratnam S. Epilepsy. *Clin Evid Concise*. 2005;13:362–4.
6. Wiebe S, Téllez-Zenteno JF, Shapiro M, et al. An evidence-based approach to the first seizure. *Epilepsia*. 2008;49(1):50–7.
7. Shih JJ, Ochoa JG. A systematic review of antiepileptic drug initiation and withdrawal. *Neurologist*. 2009;15:122–31.

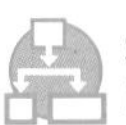

See Also (Topic, Algorithm, Electronic Media Element)

Seizures, Febrile; Status Epilepticus

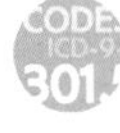

CODES

ICD9

- 345.90 Epilepsy, unspecified, without mention of intractable epilepsy
- 779.0 Convulsions in newborn
- 780.39 Other convulsions

CLINICAL PEARLS

- Encourage helmet usage to minimize head injuries.
- For the patient to be allowed to drive, he or she must be seizure-free from a minimum of 3 months and up to a year, depending on state requirements.
- Drug initiation after a single seizure will decrease risk of early seizure recurrence (6)[A] but does not affect long-term prognosis of developing epilepsy (7)[A].

SEIZURES, FEBRILE

Kinga K. Tomczak, MD, PhD
N. Paul Rosman, MD

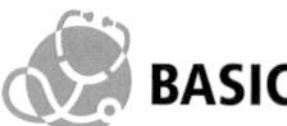

BASICS

DESCRIPTION

A seizure usually occurring between the ages of 6 months and 6 years of age associated with a febrile illness (fever of ≥100.4°F or 38°C) in the absence of CNS infection in a child that has no prior history of afebrile seizures; febrile seizures are classified as either simple or complex:

- Simple (70–75%; need all 3 criteria):
  - Duration <15 minutes *and*
  - Generalized seizure with no focal features *and*
  - No recurrence within 24 hours
- Complex (4–35%; need 1 or more criteria):
  - Duration >15 minutes *or*
  - Focal features *or*
  - >1 seizure in 24 hours

EPIDEMIOLOGY

Febrile seizures (FS) are the most common seizures seen in children under age 5 hours. They typically occur between the ages of 6 months and 36 months (peak at 18 months) (1).

Incidence

- ~500,000 febrile seizures occur yearly in the US (1).
- Incidence is between 2% and 5% of children/yr.

Prevalence

3–4% of all children in North America will experience an FS before age 5 years (most of these seizures are simple) (1).

RISK FACTORS

- For first FS (1):
  - Family history of febrile or afebrile seizures
  - Neurodevelopmental abnormality
  - Recent immunizations (increased risk following DTP and MMR).
  - Possibly increased risk with certain viral illnesses, including human herpesvirus type 6 (HHV-6) and influenza A infection
- For recurrent FS (1):
  - Onset at age <12 months
  - Family history of FS in first-degree relative
  - Temperature <40°C (104°F) at time of seizure
  - Complex FS at initial presentation
  - Brief duration between fever onset and seizure
- For subsequent epilepsy after FS (1–2.4%, slightly increased risk over that in general population) (2):
  - Complex FS
  - Neurodevelopmental abnormality
  - Family history of afebrile seizures or epilepsy in first-degree relative
  - Onset at age <12 months
  - Recurrent FS, especially if complex
  - Brief duration between fever onset and seizure

Genetics

- Genetic factors play a role, with susceptibility linked to several genetic loci.
- A history of FS in immediate family members is present in 7–40% of patients.
- Monozygotic twins have a much higher concordance rate than dizygotic twins.
- Sodium channels and gamma-aminobutyric acid A ($GABA_A$) receptor genes have been associated with a syndrome of generalized epilepsy and FS (GEFS+).

GENERAL PREVENTION

- Evidence exists that anticonvulsant therapy can reduce the risk of recurrence of FS, but in most instances neither continuous nor intermittent anticonvulsive therapy is recommended for children with 1 or more simple FS, as risks usually outweigh the benefits (2)[B].
- There is insufficient data to make a firm recommendation regarding AED prophylaxis in children with complex FS, and these cases need to be individualized based on underlying risk factors.
- Antipyretics help to improve comfort of the child, but neither dosing at regular intervals (e.g., acetaminophen every 4 hours) nor sporadic dosing based on temperature elevation has been shown to prevent FS recurrence (2)[B].

ETIOLOGY

- Any viral or bacterial infections can provoke FS.
- Increased risk found with HHV-6 and influenza A infection.
- MMR vaccine has been associated with up to a 3-fold increased risk of FS, with peak incidence 1–2 weeks after vaccination, but benefits of vaccination greatly outweigh risk of triggering an FS (1)[B].
- DTP vaccine also has been associated with a 4-fold increase risk of FS, with peak incidence 1–3 days after vaccination, but again, vaccine benefit greatly outweighs FS risk (1)[B].

DIAGNOSIS

HISTORY

- Description of convulsions, including any focal movements (simple FS are, by definition, generalized; focal seizures can be clonic and/or tonic; less frequently, they present with loss of muscle tone, beginning unilaterally, with or without secondary generalization, head and/or eye deviation to 1 side; occasionally, focal seizures are followed by transient unilateral paralysis) (3)[B].
- Duration of seizure
- Interventions to control seizures (most will resolve spontaneously)
- History of recent febrile illness (though seizure is often the presenting sign)
- Signs of CNS infection or inflammation (e.g., irritability, lethargy, decreased feeding, emesis)
- Signs of acutely increased intracranial pressure (altered mental state, emesis, strabismus with sixth or third cranial nerve palsy, "setting sun" eyes, and in the infant, a full fontanelle and/or separated cranial sutures) (3)[B].
- Recent immunization
- History of previous seizures (febrile and afebrile) in patient, family members
- Recent treatment with antibiotics (meningitis can be masked if partially treated)
- Look for other causes of seizures, such as trauma, toxin exposure, electrolyte imbalance, hypoglycemia, anticholinergic medications (e.g., diphenhydramine), discontinuance of previously prescribed anticonvulsants, or phakomatosis (e.g., tuberous sclerosis, neurofibromatosis) (3)[B].

PHYSICAL EXAM

- Vital signs:
  - Fever
  - Monitor for respiratory or circulatory compromise (with persistent seizure activity).
- Full neurologic exam:
  - Usually normal, though focal signs (e.g., eye deviation, upgoing toe) may be seen
  - May have transiently decreased alertness in postictal state; monitor for improvement
- Detailed exam to determine source of fever

DIAGNOSTIC TESTS & INTERPRETATION

Lab

- AAP recommendations with first simple FS (4)[A]:
  - Lumbar puncture (LP) should be *done* in any child with meningeal signs or symptoms (e.g., neck stiffness, Kernig and/or Brudzinski signs) or in any child whose history or exam suggests the presence of meningitis or other intracranial infection.
  - LP should be *considered* in any infant between 6 and 12 months of age who is deficient in *Haemophilus influenzae* type b (Hib) or *Streptococcus pneumoniae* immunizations or when immunization status cannot be determined.
  - LP should be *considered* in the child who is pretreated with antibiotics, because antibiotic treatment can mask the signs and symptoms of meningitis.
- Risk of bacterial meningitis is very low with first simple FS in whom this was not otherwise suspected clinically (5)[A].
- CSF more likely to show abnormalities when (6)[A]:
  - Abnormal physical/neurologic exam
  - Complex FS
  - Persistent seizures on arrival to emergency department
  - Prolonged postictal state
- In practice, the decision to perform LP should be tailored to each child's presentation.

Pediatric Considerations

In infants <18 months of age, clinical signs and symptoms of meningitis may be minimal or absent.

Initial lab tests

- If LP is indicated, blood culture and serum glucose testing should be performed concurrently.
- Measurement of serum electrolytes, calcium, phosphorus, magnesium; CBC; and serum glucose determination are low-yield and should not be performed routinely (4)[A].
- Serum glucose should be obtained if there is prolonged postictal obtundation (6)[A].

Imaging

Initial approach

- Routine neuroimaging is not indicated in the evaluation of simple FS (4)[A].
- Neuroimaging should be performed if the physical exam points to a possible structural lesion (e.g., signs of head trauma, micro-/macrocephaly, focal neurologic signs, evidence of increased intracranial pressure) (3)[B].

Diagnostic Procedures/Surgery

- EEG is not recommended as part of evaluation of a neurologically healthy child with a first simple FS. EEG does not predict the recurrence of FS or the development of later afebrile seizures/epilepsy (4)[A].
- EEG should be considered in children with complex FS and neurodevelopmental delay, abnormal neurologic signs and symptoms, or a family history of epilepsy.

DIFFERENTIAL DIAGNOSIS

- Rigors (shivering)
- Febrile delirium (confusional state associated with high fever)
- Syncope
- Breath-holding spell
- Reflex anoxic seizure

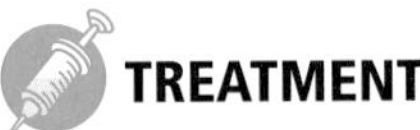

TREATMENT

MEDICATION

First Line

- Acute treatment:
  - Anticonvulsants: FS lasting >5 minutes should be treated with anticonvulsants (2)[B]:
    - Lorazepam: 0.05–0.1 mg/kg IV; if seizure persists can be repeated
    - Diazepam: 0.1–0.3 mg/kg IV; if seizure persists, can be repeated
    - Diastat (rectal gel): 0.5 mg/kg; if IV access is not established or when child is treated at home
    - Phenobarbital: 10–15 mg/kg IV
    - Valproic acid: 20 mg/kg IV
    - Fosphenytoin: 15–20 mg/kg IV
  - Antipyretics: Use acutely to reduce fever:
    - Acetaminophen: 15 mg/kg PO or PR
    - Ibuprofen: 10 mg/kg PO
- Long-term treatment to prevent FS recurrence (2)[B]:
  - Daily anticonvulsants (e.g., phenobarbital, primidone, valproate) may be effective in preventing FS, but the potential side effects usually outweigh the benefits; therefore, daily anticonvulsant therapy is rarely recommended for children with FS.
  - A better choice is intermittent oral diazepam (0.33 mg/kg q8h), given only at times of fever; accompanying drowsiness and ataxia are frequent but are transitory.
  - Antipyretics may be given for comfort, but have not been shown to reduce the risk of FS recurrence.

Second Line

Cooling blankets to reduce fever as needed

ADDITIONAL TREATMENT

General Measures

- Treat source of fever based on results of focused evaluation.
- Supportive care, as needed

Issues for Referral

Refer to pediatric neurologist with complex FS, or if suspicious for underlying seizure disorder, or with persisting focal neurologic signs and/or neurodevelopmental delay.

IN-PATIENT CONSIDERATIONS

Initial Stabilization

- Assessment of airway, breathing, and circulatory status (ABCs)
- FS of >5 minutes duration should be treated as outlined under "Acute Treatment"

Admission Criteria

Admission should be strongly considered if:

- Age <1 year
- Glasgow Coma Scale <13 (1 hour following seizure)
- Signs of increased intracranial pressure
- Any instability in vital signs
- With clinical suspicion for meningitis
- A first-time complex FS

IV Fluids

If child appears dehydrated, administer IV fluids as appropriate.

Nursing

- Nursing care should be provided, according to the patient's clinical needs.
- Precautionary measures to prevent secondary injuries from seizure activity
- Monitoring vital signs and watching for signs of FS recurrence

Discharge Criteria

Children with simple FS, with treated infection, and who appear well can be discharged home from the emergency department after a minimum of 2 hours of observation.

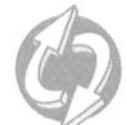

ONGOING CARE

FOLLOW-UP RECOMMENDATIONS

For any patient with simple FS, a follow-up appointment with the primary care physician should be scheduled within 1 week of discharge. Follow-up for complex FS should also be made, with the timing pending results of further evaluation.

Patient Monitoring

Families should call physician with FS recurrence or if child develops an afebrile seizure.

PATIENT EDUCATION

Parental education is important because of the significant caretaker anxiety surrounding the diagnosis (1)[B]:

- FS are common and occur in 3–5% of otherwise healthy children.
- FS recur in ~1/3 of children.
- No evidence indicates that simple FS cause neurologic sequelae or death.
- Complex FS are occasionally complicated by neurologic sequelae.
- Evaluation depends on the clinical presentation; there is no role for routine lab testing, imaging, or EEG.
- Simple FS usually do not have to be treated once the FS has stopped.
- Occasionally, intermittent prophylactic treatment is recommended for FS.
- Daily prophylactic treatment of FS is generally not recommended and has not been shown to prevent the development of later epilepsy.
- Referral to a pediatric neurologist is usually not required for a simple FS.

PROGNOSIS

- Overall, excellent prognosis
- No evidence of neurodevelopmental problems, learning disabilities, or increased mortality with simple FS
- Children with FS are at risk for developing recurrent FS:
  - Children <12 months of age have a recurrence rate of 50%.
  - Children >12 months of age have a recurrence rate of 30%.
  - Children with second FS have a 50% risk of having additional episodes.
- Risk of later epilepsy after a simple FS is slightly greater than in the general population, where the prevalence of epilepsy, in developed countries, ranges from 0.5–1%:
  - Factors that increase risk of later epilepsy in FS include neurodevelopmental abnormality, complex FS, and family history of epilepsy (2)[B].

COMPLICATIONS

- Secondary complications include injuries resulting from seizure activity, aspiration, and complications from prolonged complex FS (1)[B].
- There is some evidence that complex FS may contribute to later temporal lobe epilepsy.

REFERENCES

1. Jones T, Jacobsen SJ. Childhood febrile seizures: Overview and implications. *Int J Med Sci*. 2007;4:110–4.
2. Steering Committee on Quality Improvement and Management, Subcommittee on Febrile Seizures American Academy of Pediatrics. Febrile seizures: Clinical practice guideline for the long-term management of the child with simple febrile seizures. *Pediatrics*. 2008;121:1281–6.
3. Rosman NP. Evaluation of the child who convulses with fever. *Pediatr Drugs*. 2003;5:457–461.
4. Subcommittee on Febrile Seizures, Americal Academy of Pediatrics. Febrile seizures: Guideline for the neurodiagnostic evaluation of the child with a simple febrile seizure. *Pediatrics*. 2011;127:389.
5. Kimia AA, Capraro AJ, Hummel D, et al. Utility of lumbar puncture for first simple febrile seizure among children 6 to 18 months of age. *Pediatrics*. 2009;123:6–12.
6. Practice parameter: The neurodiagnostic evaluation of the child with a first simple febrile seizure. American Academy of Pediatrics. Provisional Committee on Quality Improvement, Subcommittee on Febrile Seizures. *Pediatrics*. 1996;97:769–72; discussion 773–5.

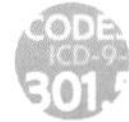

CODES

ICD9

780.31 Febrile convulsions (simple), unspecified

CLINICAL PEARLS

- FSs are common and account for 1% of all pediatric emergency department visits.
- Keystones of evaluation and treatment of FS are identifying and treating the underlying illness and, particularly, excluding CNS infection.
- Thorough neurodiagnostic workup (LP, EEG, and imaging) is usually not needed with simple FS.
- FS are associated with only a slightly increased risk of epilepsy compared with general population (risk greater with complex FS than simple FS).
- There is usually no need for long-term preventive treatment of FS.

SEPSIS

Tui A. Lauilefue, MD
Damon F. Lee, MD

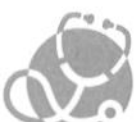

BASICS

DESCRIPTION

Sepsis: Infection, either documented or suspected, and some of the following characteristics (1):

- General variables:
  - Temperature >38.3°C or <36°C*
  - Heart rate >90 beats/min or >2 SD above the normal value for age*
  - Tachypnea (respiratory rate >20 breaths/min or PCO_2 <32 mm Hg)*
  - Altered mental status (AMS)
  - Significant edema or positive fluid balance (>20 mL/kg over 24 hours)
  - Hyperglycemia (plasma glucose >120 mg/dL or 7.7 mmol/L) in the absence of diabetes
- Inflammatory variables:
  - WBC count >12,000 cells/mm^3, or <4,000 cells/mm^3, or normal WBC count with >10% bands*
  - Plasma C-reactive protein >2 SD above normal
  - Plasma procalcitonin >2 SD above normal
- Hemodynamic variables:
  - Arterial hypotension (SBP <90 mm Hg; MAP <70; or SBP decrease >40 mm Hg in adults or <2 SD below age normal)
  - SVO_2 >70%
  - Cardiac index >3.5 L min^{-1} M^{-23}
- Organ dysfunction variables:
  - Arterial hypoxemia (PaO_2/FIO_2 <300)
  - Acute oliguria (urine output<0.5 mL kg^{-1}hr^{-1} or 45 mmol/L for at least 2 hours)
  - Creatinine increase >0.5 mg/dL
  - Coagulation abnormalities (INR >1.5 or aPTT >60 seconds)
  - Ileus (absent bowel sounds)
  - Thrombocytopenia (platelet <100,000)
  - Hyperbilirubinemia (plasma total bilirubin >4 mg/dL or 70 mmol/L)
- Hypoperfusion variables:
  - Hyperlactatemia (>1 mmol/L)
  - Decreased capillary refill or mottling

Systemic Inflammatory Response Syndrome (SIRS): An inflammatory reaction to a noninfectious insult (e.g., severe trauma or burn) manifested by 2 or more symptoms as denoted by * above (2).

Severe sepsis: Sepsis complicated by hypoperfusion or organ dysfunction variables (as above)

Septic shock/sepsis-induced hypotension: Persistent arterial hypotension unexplained by other causes of hypotension:

- Hypotension: Persistence of any of the following despite adequate fluid resuscitation:
  - Systolic arterial pressure <90 mm Hg
  - MAP <70 mm Hg
  - Reduction in SBP >40 mm Hg from baseline

Multiple organ dysfunction syndrome: Progressive organ dysfunction in an acutely ill patient necessitating intervention to maintain homeostasis; represents the end stage of both SIRS and sepsis:

- Synonym(s): Septicemia

Geriatric Considerations

Often more difficult to diagnose; change in mental status/behavior may be only early manifestation

Pediatric Considerations

Septic shock in children is defined as tachycardia with signs of decreased perfusion. Hypotension (<2 SD below normal for age) is a sign of late and decompensated shock in children (1).

EPIDEMIOLOGY

Incidence

- 3 per 1,000 population
- Increasing incidence, with 750,000 new cases annually in the US
- 2% of hospitalized patients; ~75% of ICU patients

RISK FACTORS

- Bacteremia
- Age extremes (very old or young)
- Immunosuppression (see "Associated Conditions")
- Community-acquired pneumonia
- Critically ill patients
- Indwelling catheters: Intravascular, urinary, biliary
- Complicated labor and delivery: Premature labor and/or PROM, untreated maternal group B strep colonization

Genetics

- Studies link polymorphisms in genes encoding tumor necrosis factor (TNF) to possibly greater susceptibility to and death from sepsis.
- Other candidate genes include the IL-1 receptor antagonist, heat-shock proteins, IL-6, IL-10, and toll-like receptors.

GENERAL PREVENTION

- Vaccination: Pneumococcal (geriatric patients, patients with certain chronic diseases), *Haemophilus influenzae* type B (infants, young children), influenza (H1N1 in pregnant women), meningococcal vaccine
- Gamma-globulin (for hypo- or agammaglobulinemia)
- Treat pregnant group B strep carriers during labor
- Cleanliness with regular hand washing, sterile technique for catheters, appropriate glove use
- Antibiotic prophylaxis for certain operations (bowel and GU; prosthetic device placement)

PATHOPHYSIOLOGY

- An imbalance between pro- and anti-inflammatory mediators yields widespread systemic inflammation that damages distant uninvolved tissues.
- Widespread endothelial damage leads to maldistribution of blood flow, causing impaired tissue oxygenation and resultant organ dysfunction.
- Dysregulated nitric oxide production and activation of the coagulation system cause maldistribution of organ blood flow.
- Initial, overexuberant inflammatory response can progress to significant immunosuppression.

ETIOLOGY

- Specific etiologic agents:
  - Gram-positive organisms (most common): *Staphylococcus* sp., *Streptococcus* sp., *Enterococcus* sp.
  - Gram-negative organisms: *Escherichia coli*, *Klebsiella* sp., *Proteus* sp., *Pseudomonas* sp.
  - Anaerobes
  - Fungi: *Candida* sp. (incidence increased 207% from 1976–2000)
- Common sources: Lungs (most common), urinary tract, abdomen (biliary tree, abscess, peritonitis), skin (cellulitis, decubitus ulcer, gangrene), heart valves, CNS (meningitis) and intravascular catheters
- Unknown source of infection in 20–30% of patients

COMMONLY ASSOCIATED CONDITIONS

- Immunologic: Neutropenia, HIV, hypo-/agammaglobulinemia, complement deficiency, splenectomy, immunomodulatory medication (corticosteroids, chemotherapy, TNF-alpha antagonists)
- Diabetes mellitus, alcoholism, malignancy, cirrhosis, burns, multiple trauma, IV drug abuse, malnutrition

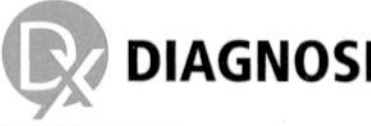

DIAGNOSIS

HISTORY

- General symptoms:
  - Fever, chills, rigors, myalgias
  - Mental status changes: Restlessness, agitation, confusion, delirium, lethargy, stupor, coma
- Specific symptoms (site of the primary infection):
  - Respiratory tract: Cough, sputum production, dyspnea, chest pain
  - Urinary tract: Dysuria, frequency, urgency, flank pain
  - Intra-abdominal source: Nausea, vomiting, diarrhea, constipation, abdominal pain
  - CNS: Stiff neck, headache, photophobia, focal neurologic signs
- End-organ failure symptoms: Shortness of breath, oliguria/anuria, mottled appearance of the skin

PHYSICAL EXAM

Hyper-/hypothermia, tachycardia, tachypnea, hypotension, poor capillary refill, cyanosis, jaundice, skin lesions (erythema, petechiae, embolic lesions, purpura)

DIAGNOSTIC TESTS & INTERPRETATION

Lab

Initial lab tests

- Blood cultures: Bacteremia (not required for diagnosis; 50% of blood cultures are negative in severe sepsis/septic shock)
- Cultures/Gram stains from other sources (sputum, urine, pleural fluid, ascites, CSF, wound)
- Prior antibiotic use may suppress the growth of organisms, causing a false-negative result.
- CBC with differential, C-reactive protein, coagulation profile, electrolytes, BUN, creatinine, glucose, liver function tests, lactic acid level, arterial blood gas (ABG), urinalysis
- Common findings: Leukocytosis, bandemia (above 10%), hyperglycemia, metabolic acidosis, mild hyperbilirubinemia, hypoxemia, respiratory alkalosis, proteinuria
- Less common findings (more severe): Leukopenia, anemia, thrombocytopenia, prolonged prothrombin time, azotemia, hypoglycemia, lactic acidosis

Imaging

Initial approach

Relevant radiographs, US, CT, and MRI should be performed promptly to confirm and sample any source of infection (3)[C].

Diagnostic Procedures/Surgery
- Aspiration of potentially infected body fluids (pleural, peritoneal, CSF)
- Biopsy, drainage of potentially infected tissues (abscess, biliary tree, others)
- EKG and cardiac enzymes

Pathological Findings
- Inflammation at primary site of infection
- Disseminated intravascular coagulation
- Noncardiogenic pulmonary edema

DIFFERENTIAL DIAGNOSIS
- Bacteremia without sepsis
- Viral, rickettsial, spirochetal, and protozoal diseases
- Collagen vascular diseases, vasculitides, pancreatitis, myocardial infarction, congestive heart failure, pulmonary embolism, TTP–HUS, thyrotoxicosis, adrenal insufficiency, poisoning, allergic reaction/drug eruption

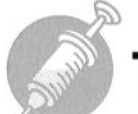

TREATMENT

MEDICATION
First Line
- Fluid resuscitation with natural or artificial colloids or crystalloids:
  - Initial therapy with fluid bolus (at least 20 mL/kg or 2 liters of crystalloid or 300–500 mL of colloid over 30 minutes) (3)[C].
- Vasopressors:
  - Norepinephrine or dopamine (3)[B] (dopamine has a greater incidence of adverse events; start with norepinephrine) (4)[B]
  - Low-dose dopamine for renal protection is not recommended (3)[A].
- Broad-spectrum antibiotic therapy as early as possible (<3 hours of ED or <1 hour of ICU admission) aimed at likely source (3)[A]:
  - Adult (*Pseudomonas* not suspected): Vancomycin plus gram-negative coverage (third-generation cephalosporin, β-lactamase/β-lactamase inhibitor, or carbapenem)
  - Adult (*Pseudomonas* suspected; e.g., neutropenic/burn): Vancomycin plus 2 agents aimed at resistant gram-negative bacteria (ceftazidime/cefepime/carbapenem); piperacillin-tazobactam plus either fluoroquinolone (ciprofloxacin) or aminoglycoside (gentamicin/amikacin), depending on local hospital sensitivities
  - Nonimmunocompromised child: Third-generation cephalosporin
  - Neonatal (<7 days old) sepsis: Ampicillin and gentamicin
  - After culture and sensitivity results: Treatment should be organism-specific for 7–10 days.
  - Antifungals if fungal infection suspected: Long-term antibiotic use, TPN, GI surgery

Pregnancy Considerations
β-lactam antibiotics and azithromycin/erythromycin generally are considered safe.

ALERT
- Adjust medication doses for impaired renal and/or hepatic function.
- Consider narrowing antibiotic regimen at 48–72 hours based on culture results and clinical course.
- Possible interactions:
  - Aminoglycosides: Increased nephrotoxicity with enflurane, cisplatin, and possibly vancomycin; increased ototoxicity with loop diuretics; increased paralysis with neuromuscular-blocking agents

Second Line
- Vasopressors, epinephrine, vasopressin, or phenylephrine, should be considered if unable to maintain goal MAP of >65 mm Hg on norepinephrine/dopamine (3)[C].
- Low-dose IV hydrocortisone should only be considered if the patients is poorly responsive to both IV fluid resuscitation and vasopressors (3)[C].
- Recombinant human-activated protein C (Xigris) was voluntarily withdrawn from the market in 2011 due to failure to improve survival in a critical trial.
- Inotropic therapy with dobutamine may benefit patients with myocardial dysfunction and evidence of oxygen deficit (low mixed venous oxygen saturation [below 70%]) (3)[C].

ADDITIONAL TREATMENT
General Measures
- O_2 monitoring/supplementation with intubation and invasive monitoring for respiratory failure or hemodynamic instability (3)
- Early goal-directed therapy with adequate volume resuscitation followed by vasopressors if required (within first 6 hours) targeted at (3)[C]:
  - Central venous pressure (CVP) 8–12 mm Hg, MAP ≥65 mm Hg, urine output ≥0.5 mL/kg/hr
  - Central/mixed venous O_2 saturation ≥70%:
    - If not achieved after fluid resuscitation (CVP 8–12 mm Hg) and vasopressors (MAP >65 mm Hg), transfuse pRBCs to achieve hematocrit >30%, and if still <70%, add dobutamine (3)[C]
- Early identification of etiology with appropriate removal/drainage of septic foci (3)[C]:
  - Early surgical consultation for acute abdomen, empyema, necrotizing fasciitis
- Transfusion of RBCs, platelets, and/or fresh frozen plasma for bleeding complications of coagulopathy or for planned procedures
- Stress ulcer and deep vein thrombosis prophylactic measures (3)[A].
- Glucose control (below 150 mg/dL) (3,5)[B]

Additional Therapies
Intermittent hemodialysis or CVVH

SURGERY/OTHER PROCEDURES
Debridement of necrotic tissues

IN-PATIENT CONSIDERATIONS
Initial Stabilization
ICU-level care

IV Fluids
- Colloid and crystalloid fluids are equally effective initially.
- Aggressive fluid resuscitation with normal saline can result in nongap metabolic acidosis; alleviated by lactated Ringer solution.

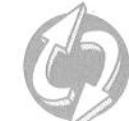

ONGOING CARE

FOLLOW-UP RECOMMENDATIONS
Patient Monitoring
- In unstable patients: Invasive hemodynamic monitoring, ABG, venous blood gas, central venous catheter placement, CVP monitoring
- Electrolytes, BUN, creatinine, and CBC daily; lactate, mixed venous oxygen saturation q2h in initial resuscitation, and daily INR/PTT if disseminated intravascular coagulation (DIC) is a consideration
- Antibiotic drug levels

DIET
NPO if intubation being considered; otherwise, enteral feeds are preferred to help preserve mucosal integrity of the GI tract.

PATIENT EDUCATION
www.nlm.nih.gov/medlineplus/sepsis.html

PROGNOSIS
Mortality is 10–50% overall. Poor prognostic factors: Inability to mount a fever, >40 years of age, nonurinary source of infection, nosocomial infection, inappropriate antibiotic coverage and certain comorbidities (e.g., AIDS, cancer, immunosuppression).

COMPLICATIONS
GI hemorrhage, DIC, hyperglycemia, new foci of infection, acute respiratory distress syndrome, multiorgan failure, death

REFERENCES

1. Levy MM, Fink MP, Marshall JC, et al. 2001 SCCM/ESICM/ACCP/ATS/SIS International Sepsis Definitions Conference. *Crit Care Med*. 2003;31:1250–6.
2. Annane D, Bellissant E, Cavaillon JM, et al. Septic shock. *Lancet*. 2005;365:63–78.
3. Dellinger RP, Levy MM, Carlet JM et al. Surviving Sepsis Campaign: International guidelines for management of severe sepsis and septic shock: 2008. *Crit Care Med*. 2008;36:296–327.
4. De Backer D, Biston P, Devriendt J, et al. Comparison of dopamine and norepinephrine in the treatment of shock. *N Engl J Med*. 2010;362:779–89.
5. Wiener RS, Wiener DC, Larson RJ. Benefits and risks of tight glucose control in critically ill adults: A meta-analysis. *JAMA*. 2008;300:933–44.

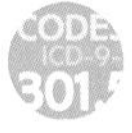

CODES

ICD9
- 038.9 Unspecified septicemia
- 995.91 Sepsis

CLINICAL PEARLS
- Appropriate treatment consists of rapid and appropriate antimicrobial therapy along with early goal-directed therapy aimed at maintaining adequate tissue perfusion.
- Despite aggressive treatment, overall mortality rates are still very high (10–50%) in patients with severe sepsis/septic shock.

SEROTONIN SYNDROME

Angela Camacho-Duran, MD
Mirjana Jojic, MD

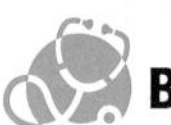

BASICS

DESCRIPTION

- A potentially life-threatening adverse drug reaction that results from excessive stimulation of central and peripheral nervous system serotonergic receptors
- It is a concentration-dependent toxicity that can develop in any individual who has ingested drug combinations that synergistically increase synaptic 5-HT.
- Serotonin toxicity occurs in 3 main settings: (i) Therapeutic drug use, which often results in mild-to-moderate symptoms; (ii) intentional overdose of a single serotonergic agent, which typically leads to moderate symptoms; and (iii) as the result of a drug interaction between numerous serotonergic agents (most commonly SSRIs and MAOIs), most often associated with severe serotonin toxicity.
- Classically characterized by a triad of mental status change, neuromuscular abnormalities, and autonomic hyperactivity
- Onset is usually within 24 hours, with 60% of cases occurring within 6 hours of exposure to or change in dosing of a serotonergic agent. Rarely, cases have been reported weeks after discontinuation of serotonergic agents.

Geriatric Considerations

The elderly can be at increased risk given their use of multiple medications.

Pediatric Considerations

- Serotonin syndrome has similar manifestations in children and adults.
- General management is unchanged in children, other than medication dosing.

Pregnancy Considerations

- 3rd-trimester exposure to serotonin reuptake inhibitors has been associated with transient neonatal complications that may reflect either acute drug withdrawal or serotonergic toxicity.
- Symptoms are generally mild, self-limited, and require only supportive care.
- Symptoms in neonates may include tremors, increased muscle tone, jitteriness, shivering, feeding or digestive disturbances, irritability, agitation, sleep disturbances, increased reflexes, excessive crying, and respiratory disturbances.

EPIDEMIOLOGY

- Due to the variability of presenting clinical features, many cases go unrecognized, and the true incidence is unknown. Seen in about 14–16% of SSRI overdose patients.
- Serotonin syndrome usually involves a combination of an SSRI, an MAOI, an antiparkinsonian agent, and/or lithium. Initially, patients can develop a peripheral tremor, confusion, and ataxia; systemic signs are next (e.g., agitation, diaphoresis, hyperreflexia, and shivering). If it worsens, the severe signs of fever, jerking, and diarrhea may develop. Serotonin syndrome can last from hours to days after the offending agents are stopped and support initiated.

Incidence

- In 2008 there were 106,336 adverse events reported with antidepressant use and 28 deaths. The majority of these were associated with SSRIs, either alone or in combination with other drugs. SSRIs alone were responsible for adverse events in 18.8% of cases, with 55.7% due to intentional causes, 39.5% unintentional, and remainder of causes unknown. 48.6% of patients reporting adverse effects with SSRIs had symptoms requiring hospitalization, and significant toxic effects occurred in 90 patients, with 2 resultant deaths (1).
- The incidence of serotonin syndrome is rising because serotonergic agents are increasingly used in clinical practice and in combination with other serotonergic agents.
- Predominant age: Affects all age groups
- Predominant sex: Male = Female

RISK FACTORS

- Serotonergic agents
- Reported following ingestion of a single agent. However, the greatest number of adverse events have shown to be associated with SSRIs in combination with other substances, and the combination of serotonin reuptake inhibitors and MAOIs carries the greatest risk for developing serotonin toxicity.

Genetics

Unknown

GENERAL PREVENTION

- Avoid multidrug regimens.
- Consider drug–drug interactions when a multidrug regimen is required.
- Caution patients about taking SSRIs with over-the-counter (OTC) medications or herbal supplements prior to consulting a physician.
- Clinician education
- Continual improvement in use of health information technology

PATHOPHYSIOLOGY

- The result of excessive stimulation in central and peripheral nervous system serotonergic receptors
- Risk is mediated in a dose-related manner to the action of 5-HT or 5-HT agonists on 5-HT2A receptors. The mechanism of development of the syndrome is unknown.
- It is hypothesized that the degree of serotonin elevation in blood plasma has to be 10–15% times above baseline levels to result in serotonin toxicity (2).
- 1 study found a relationship between paroxetine plasma levels and the risk of developing mild serotonin syndrome. However, these findings have not been validated by other researchers (3).

ETIOLOGY

- A number of drugs are associated with the serotonin syndrome. These include SSRIs; SNRIs; tricyclic antidepressants; MAOIs, other antidepressants (Trazodone, Wellbutrin); lithium; triptans; anticonvulsants (Depakote); opiate analgesics; antibiotics; OTC cough medications (dextromethorphan); some antipsychotics (Risperdal, Zyprexa); other meds, such as BuSpar, Zofran, Reglan, l-dopa; dietary supplements (tryptophan); herbal supplements (St. John's wort, nutmeg); methylene blue; and drugs of abuse (e.g., MDMA, cocaine, LSD, and amphetamine).
- Drug interactions are most often the cause of severe cases of serotonin syndrome. Many of the same classes of medications listed above are involved (e.g., phenelzine and meperidine, tranylcypromine and imipramine, linezolid and citalopram).

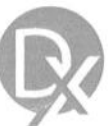

DIAGNOSIS

- Serotonin syndrome is a clinical diagnosis.
- Hunter Toxicity Criteria Decision Rules aid in the diagnosis of clinically significant serotonin toxicity (sensitivity 84%, specificity 97%).
- To fulfill Hunter Criteria, a patient must have taken a serotonergic agent and have 1 of the following:
  - Spontaneous clonus
  - Inducible clonus plus agitation or diaphoresis
  - Ocular clonus plus agitation or diaphoresis
  - Tremor and hyperreflexia
  - Hypertonia
  - Temperature above 38°C plus ocular clonus or inducible clonus (4)[B]

HISTORY

- Obtain a thorough drug history, including prescription medications, OTC remedies, dietary supplements, herbal supplements, and illicit drugs. Ask about dose, formulation, and recent changes.
- Address possibility of drug overdose, and obtain collateral information if intentional overdose is suspected.
- Elicit description of symptoms, including onset and progression of symptoms.

PHYSICAL EXAM

- Vital signs: Tachycardia, hypertension (HTN), hyperthermia, pulse and BP alterations (severe cases)
- Neuromuscular findings:
  - Hyperreflexia (greater in lower extremities)
  - Clonus (involuntary muscle contractions, most commonly tested by flexing foot upward rapidly; includes ocular)
  - Myoclonus (greater in lower extremities)
  - Tremor (greater in lower extremities)
  - Hypertonia
  - Bilateral Babinski sign
  - Akathisia
  - Tonic-clonic seizures (severe cases)
  - Autonomic signs:
    - Diaphoresis
    - Mydriasis
    - Flushing
    - Dry mucous membranes
    - Vomiting, diarrhea, increased bowel sounds
    - Mental status changes: Anxiety, disorientation, delirium (5)
    - Severe cases have led to disseminated intravascular coagulopathy, usually appear acutely ill with widespread hemorrhage, and may be in shock.

DIAGNOSTIC TESTS & INTERPRETATION

Lab

- Serum serotonin levels do not correlate with clinical findings.
- Nonspecific lab findings that may develop include:
  - Elevated WBC count
  - Elevated creatine phosphokinase (CK or CPK)

- Decreased serum bicarbonate
- Elevated hepatic transaminases
- In severe cases, the following complications may develop:
  - Disseminated intravascular coagulation (DIC)
  - Metabolic acidosis
  - Rhabdomyolysis
  - Renal failure
  - Myoglobinuria
  - Acute respiratory distress syndrome (ARDS) (5)

Imaging

None indicated

DIFFERENTIAL DIAGNOSIS

- Neuroleptic malignant syndrome (NMS)
- Anticholinergic delirium (e.g. Cogentin, Benadryl, Detrol, oxybutynin, nifedipine, Zantac; plant poisoning from belladonna/"deadly nightshade," datura, henbane, mandrake, brugmansia)
- Malignant hyperthermia
- Heat stroke
- CNS infection (meningitis, encephalitis)
- Sympathomimetic toxicity
- Nonconvulsive seizures
- Hyperthyroidism
- Tetanus
- Acute baclofen withdrawal (6)

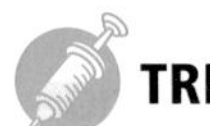

TREATMENT

- Discontinuation of all serotonergic agents
- Supportive care is the mainstay of therapy. This includes administration of oxygen and IV fluids, continuous cardiac monitoring, and correction of vital signs:
  - Benzodiazepines may be effective for the management of agitation in patients with serotonin syndrome.
  - Benzodiazepines should be used with caution in patients with delirium due to the risk of worsening delirium.
  - Administration of serotonin antagonists: Cyproheptadine may be useful if supportive measures and sedation are unable to control agitation and correct vital signs.
- Mild cases (afebrile, tachycardia, shivering, diaphoresis, mydriasis, hyperreflexia, intermittent tremor or myoclonus):
  - Discontinuation of precipitating agent(s)
  - Supportive care
  - Sedation
- Moderate cases (temperature >38°C, autonomic instability, mydriasis, hyperactive bowel sounds, diarrhea, diaphoresis, ocular clonus, hyperreflexia, tremor, mild agitation, or hypervigilance):
  - Discontinuation of precipitating agent(s)
  - Supportive care
  - Sedation
  - Aggressive treatment of autonomic instability
  - Treatment with cyproheptadine, a histamine and serotonin antagonist, should be initiated if agitation and vital sign abnormalities are unimproved with benzodiazepines and supportive care.
  - Hypotension from MAOI interactions should be treated with low doses of direct-acting sympathomimetics (e.g., norepinephrine, phenylephrine, epinephrine).
  - Avoid use of indirect serotonin agonists such as dopamine.
  - Severe HTN and tachycardia should be treated with short-acting agents such as nitroprusside or esmolol.
  - Avoid use of longer-acting agents such as proprandol.
- Severe cases (temperature >41.1°C, autonomic instability, delirium, muscular rigidity, and hypertonicity):
  - Immediate sedation
  - Paralysis (with nondepolarizing agents such as etomidate, succinylcholine, and vecuronium; avoid succinylcholine in patients with hyperkalemia)
  - Endotracheal intubation as clinically indicated
  - Treatment of hyperthermia is critical.
  - Antipyretic medications are not effective (5)[C]; the increased body temperature is due to muscle activity, not an alteration in the hypothalamic set point.

MEDICATION

- Activated charcoal: May be used in patients who intentionally overdose on serotonergic agents (4)[C]
- Benzodiazepines: May be used to manage agitation in serotonin syndrome and also may correct mild increases in BP and heart rate. Use with caution in patients with delirium given the known paradoxical effect of exacerbating delirium.
- Cyproheptadine (Periactin): Consider use if benzodiazepines and supportive measures are unable to control agitation and correct vital signs:
  - Adults: Initial dose of 12 mg PO (or crushed and given NG) followed by 2 mg q2h until clinical response observed. 12–32 mg of drug may be required in a 24-hour period.
  - Children:
    - <2 years: 0.06 mg/kg per dose q6h
    - 2–6 years: 2 mg q6h
    - 7–14 years: 4 mg q6h
- Propofol (Diprivan) may represent an effective therapy for controlling serotonergic signs in severely ill patients.
- Use of antipsychotics with 5-HT_{2A} antagonist activity, such as olanzapine and chlorpromazine, is not recommended (5)[C].

ADDITIONAL TREATMENT

Issues for Referral

- Psychiatry: For assistance with medication management and follow-up care (inpatient psychiatric care vs. outpatient psychiatric follow-up)
- Toxicology or clinical pharmacology service
- Poison control center

IN-PATIENT CONSIDERATIONS

Patients with known or suspected serotonin syndrome should be admitted to a medical inpatient unit for observation.

Discharge Criteria

- Mental status is returned to baseline.
- Stable vital signs
- No increase in clonus or DTR
- Close patient follow-up ensured

ONGOING CARE

FOLLOW-UP RECOMMENDATIONS

- In mild cases of serotonin toxicity, address risks and benefits of restarting offending agents. Serotonergic medications need to be titrated slowly, and patients must have close outpatient follow-up with physician.
- If patient developed severe serotonin syndrome, the offending agent should likely not be resumed unless precipitant for serotonin syndrome is found (i.e., combination with another serotonin agonist), the patient can be carefully monitored, or there is clear benefit vs. risk of restarting the medication.

PROGNOSIS

- Generally favorable with early recognition of the syndrome and prompt initiation of treatment
- Most cases resolve within 24 hours of discontinuation of serotonergic agents; this can be longer depending on the drug's half-life:
  - MAOIs can result in toxicity for several days.
  - SSRIs can result in toxicity for up to several weeks after discontinuation.
- ICU admission is often indicated in severe cases.

COMPLICATIONS

- Adverse outcomes, including death, are usually the consequence of poorly treated hyperthermia.
- Nonhyperthermic patients who survive typically do not have long-term sequelae.

REFERENCES

1. Bronstein AC, Spyker DA, Cantilena LR Jr, et al. 2008 Annual Report of the American Association of Poison Control Centers' National Poison Data System (NPDS): 26th Annual Report.
2. Ables AZ, Nagubilli R, et al. Prevention, recognition, and management of serotonin syndrome. *Am Fam Physician*. 2010;81:1139–42.
3. Hegerl U, Bottlender R, Gallinat J, et al. The serotonin syndrome scale: First results on validity. *Eur Arch Psychiatry Clin Neurosci*. 1998;248: 96–103.
4. Dunkley EJ, Isbister GK, Sibbritt D, et al. The Hunter Serotonin Toxicity Criteria: Simple and accurate diagnostic decision rules for serotonin toxicity. *QJM*. 2003;96:635–42.
5. Boyer EW, Shannon M. The serotonin syndrome. *N Engl J Med*. 2005;352:1112–20.
6. Isbister GK, Buckley NA, Whyte IM. Serotonin toxicity: A practical approach to diagnosis and treatment. *Med J Aust*. 2007;187:361–5.

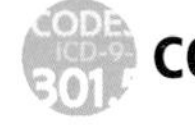

CODES

ICD9

333.99 Other extrapyramidal diseases and abnormal movement disorders

CLINICAL PEARLS

Consider serotonin syndrome in patients with recent use of a serotonergic agent (particularly if multiple proserotonergic agents are involved) presenting with unexplained tachycardia, hypertension, hyperthermia, clonus, hyperreflexia, and change in mental status.

SEXUAL DYSFUNCTION IN WOMEN

Teresa L. Knight, MD

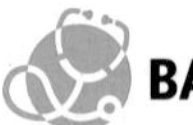

BASICS

- Sexual dysfunction may be a lifelong problem or may be acquired.
- Very common: ~40% of women surveyed in the US have sexual concerns.
- Female sexual dysfunction may present as a lack of sexual desire, impaired arousal, pain with sexual activity, or inability to achieve orgasm.

DESCRIPTION

The American Psychiatric Association guidelines for establishing a diagnosis of sexual dysfunction require that the problem be recurrent or persistent and that it cause personal distress or interpersonal difficulty:

- 5 major types:
  - Disorders of desire: Hypoactive sexual desire with deficient or absent sexual fantasies and desire for sexual activity
  - Disorder of arousal: Inability to attain or maintain adequate lubrication/engorgement in response to sexual excitement
  - Dyspareunia: Genital pain associated with intercourse
  - Vaginismus: Involuntary contractions of the perineal muscles in response to vaginal penetration
  - Disorders of orgasm: Delay or absence of orgasm following normal sexual excitement
- System(s) affected: Nervous; Reproductive; Genitourinary; Psychiatric
- Synonym(s): Hypoactive sexual desire disorder; Sexual aversion disorder; Female sexual arousal disorder; Inhibited female orgasm

EPIDEMIOLOGY

- In one international study, 40% of women aged 40–80 years reported sexual complaints (1).
- In the largest study of female sexual dysfunction in the US, 43% of over 30,000 women reported sexual dysfunction (2).
- Unfortunately, many studies do not assess whether the sexual issues are associated with distress, which is required to meet the criteria for the diagnosis of sexual dysfunction.

Incidence

Incidence is highest during the postpartum period and perimenopause:

- Postpartum: In a study of over 400 primiparous women, 83% reported sexual problems at 3 months postpartum and 64%, at 6 months (3). There was no difference between vaginal and cesarean delivery.
- Perimenopause: Sexual problems associated with distress are highest in women aged 45–64 years. Though sexual activity decreases with age, so does the distress, as well as the perception that it represents dysfunction.

Prevalence

- Overall prevalence of diagnosed sexual dysfunction is 15–30% among US women:
  - Orgasmic disorders are the most common: <10% are primary, and 65–80% are secondary.
  - Desire disorders are the complaint of 30–55% of individuals and 31% of couples presenting to clinics.
  - Arousal disorders are present in 14–48% of patients.
- There are many women who report some degree of dissatisfaction but do not meet clinical criteria for diagnosis for sexual dysfunction:
  - 1 out of 5 women report that they are sexually dissatisfied.
  - 2 out of 3 women report some degree of sexual dysfunction but do not meet criteria for diagnosis.
  - Of women who are anorgasmic, only 1 out of 3 perceive it as a problem causing significant personal distress.

RISK FACTORS

- Advancing age
- Previous sexual trauma
- Lack of knowledge about sexual stimulation and response
- Chronic medical problems (e.g., depression or other psychiatric disorders); cardiovascular disease; endocrine disorders (e.g., diabetes, hypertension); neurologic disorders
- Gynecologic issues such as childbirth, pelvic floor or bladder dysfunction, endometriosis, and uterine fibroids
- Medications such as hormonal contraception, SSRIs, β-blockers, and antipsychotic medications
- Relationship factors such as couple discrepancies in expectations and/or cultural backgrounds, attitudes toward sexuality in family of origin
- Substance abuse such as smoking, alcohol, and illicit drugs

PATHOPHYSIOLOGY

The pathophysiology of sexual dysfunction is complex and multifactorial since it can be the result of any etiology that interferes with the normal female sexual response cycle of desire, arousal, orgasm, and resolution.

ETIOLOGY

- Epilepsy: Higher rates of sexual dysfunction
- Diabetes (specifically anorgasmia)
- Anxiety or depression
- Spinal cord damage
- Thyroid disease
- Hormonal imbalance (including anovulation from the use of hormonal contraception)
- Drug use, including prescription medications (e.g., SSRIs, monoamine oxidase inhibitors [MAOIs], tricyclic antidepressants [TCAs], β-blockers)
- Interrelational difficulties and conflict regarding intimacy
- Control issues in the relationships
- Sexual frequency myths
- Survivor of sexual abuse, including incest
- Body image issues
- Alcohol
- Proximity of other people in household

COMMONLY ASSOCIATED CONDITIONS

- Marital discord
- Depression

DIAGNOSIS

- Female sexual dysfunction is diagnosed by identifying diagnostic criteria through both a medical and a sexual history.
- The diagnosis requires that the sexual problem be recurrent or persistent and cause personal distress or interpersonal difficulty.

HISTORY

- Complaint to health care provider:
  - If the clinician inquires, "Do you have any sexual concerns?" more than twice as many are revealed than if clinician waits for the patient to mention it.
- Pregnancy/childbirth history
- Infertility
- Menopausal status (natural, surgical, or postchemotherapy)
- STDs and vaginitis
- Pelvic surgery, injury, or cancer
- Chronic pelvic pain
- Abnormal genital tract bleeding
- Urinary/anal incontinence
- Marital conflict
- Family dysfunction

PHYSICAL EXAM

Most commonly, patients have a normal physical exam:

- Assess for scars or evidence of trauma.
- Assess for vaginal atrophy, adequate estrogenization.
- Assess for infection.
- Recognize signs of anxiety, apprehension, and pain during the speculum and pelvic exam.

DIAGNOSTIC TESTS & INTERPRETATION

Lab

- Neither estrogen nor androgen levels should be used to determine the cause of the sexual dysfunction, because there is no established serum hormone range that correlates with sexual dysfunction.
- Measurements of estrogen and androgen levels may be used to monitor hormone replacement therapy in perimenopausal women.

Initial lab tests

As needed to identify infections and other medical causes:

- Wet prep
- Thyroid-stimulating hormone
- Prolactin
- Follicle-stimulating hormone

Follow-Up & Special Considerations

Encourage counseling.

Imaging

Initial approach

Transvaginal ultrasound if indicated

DIFFERENTIAL DIAGNOSIS

- Medication side effects: SSRIs, TCAs, and other antidepressants; psychotropics; MAOIs; many antihypertensives
- Vaginitis
- Decreased vaginal lubrication secondary to hormonal imbalance
- Decreased sensation secondary to nerve injury
- Multiple sclerosis
- Anatomic abnormalities
- Abdominal surgery (which can interfere with pelvic innervation)
- Depression
- Marital dysfunction, including domestic violence
- Pregnancy
- Pseudodyspareunia (use of complaint of pain to distance self from partner)

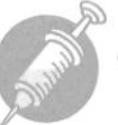

TREATMENT

- Assess patient goals.
- Treatment should address associated chronic conditions.
- Hormone therapy, alone or in conjunction with other therapies
- An increase in fitness and body image alone can improve libido.
- Consider couples therapy for women who complain of relationship conflicts.

MEDICATION

Sexual dysfunction is often a multifactorial psychosocial condition. Using medications does not usually address the cause of the problem and can, in some cases, make the condition worse.

First Line

- Bupropion: May be useful in treating sexual dysfunction or as an adjunct for SSRI-induced sexual dysfunction (4,5). Generally, Bupropion XL 300 mg/d is used.
- Premenopausal women:
  - Some data suggest that low circulating levels of testosterone may be associated with decreased libido.
  - No clear studies indicate testosterone replacement as beneficial in premenopausal women.
- Postmenopausal women:
  - Adding testosterone to hormone-replacement therapy may increase sexual desire (6)[B]. Unfortunately, the FDA has not approved the use of testosterone to treat sexual dysfunction in women. Current testosterone therapy for women must be compounded into an oral or topical form. Typical dosages range from 0.625–1.25 mg/d but have been safely used up to 3 mg/day. Testosterone therapy designed for men should not be used in women, as women require 1/10 the dose of men.
  - Estrogen replacement may help to improve sexual desire, vaginal atrophy, and clitoral sensitivity. Vaginal estrogen therapy is available in cream, vaginal tablet, or ring form (7)[B].

ADDITIONAL TREATMENT

Issues for Referral

Consider referral for marriage or sex therapy counseling.

Additional Therapies

- Vaginal lubricants
- Aerobic exercise
- Smoking cessation and reduction of alcohol intake
- For childhood trauma: Scripting, psychotherapy, cognitive restructuring
- For anorgasmia: Directed masturbation and "homework" with partners
- For prescription-drug causes: Reduced dosages or change to different medication
- Other: Family therapy, sensate conditioning; referral to specialized sex therapy

COMPLEMENTARY AND ALTERNATIVE MEDICINE

- Yohimbe: Not recommended, potentially dangerous
- Ginseng and St. John's wort have no evidence to support treatment of sexual dysfunction.
- DHEA: Androgenic effects; will decrease high-density lipoprotein cholesterol

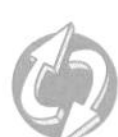

ONGOING CARE

DIET

Weight reduction if needed for either partner

PATIENT EDUCATION

- In the US, sex therapists and counselors can be found through the American Association of Sex Educators, Counselors and Therapists: www.assect.org.
- National Women's Health Resource Center: www.Healthwomen.org
- American Association of Sex Educators, Counselors, and Therapists: www.aasect.org
- Female Sexual Dysfunction Online: www.femlaesexualdysfunctiononline.org
- North American Menopause Society: www.menopause.org

PROGNOSIS

Lack of desire is most difficult type to treat, with <50% success.

REFERENCES

1. Laumann EO, Nicolosi A, Glasser DB, et al. Sexual problems among women and men aged 40–80 y: Prevalence and correlates identified in the Global Study of Sexual Attitudes and Behaviors. *Int J Impot Res*. 2005;17:39–57.
2. Shifren JL, Monz BU, Russo PA, et al. Sexual problems and distress in United States women: Prevalence and correlates. *Obstet Gynecol*. 2008; 112:970–8.
3. Barrett G, Pendry E, Peacock J, et al. Women's sexual health after childbirth. *BJOG*. 2000;107: 186–95.
4. Segraves RT, Clayton A, Croft H, et al. Bupropion sustained release for the treatment of hypoactive sexual desire disorder in premenopausal women. *J Clin Psychopharmacol*. 2004;24:339–42.
5. Ginzburg R, Wong Y, Fader JS. Effect of bupropion on sexual dysfunction. *Ann Pharmacother*. 2005; 39:2096–9.
6. Somboonporn W, Davis S, Seif MW, et al. Testosterone for peri- and postmenopausal women. *Cochrane Database Syst Rev*. 2005;CD004509.
7. Gast MJ, Freedman MA, Vieweg AJ, et al. A randomized study of low-dose conjugated estrogens on sexual function and quality of life in postmenopausal women. *Menopause*. 2009;16: 247.

ADDITIONAL READING

- Basaria S, Dobs AS. Safety and adverse effects of androgens: How to counsel patients. *Mayo Clin Proc*. 2004;79:S25–32.
- Blumel JE, Del Pino M, Aprikian D, et al. Effect of androgens combined with hormone therapy on quality of life in post-menopausal women with sexual dysfunction. *Gynecol Endocrinol*. 2008;24: 691.
- Braunstein GD. Safety of testosterone treatment in postmenopausal women. *Fertil Steril*. 2007;88:1.
- Davis SR, Moreau M, Kroll R, et al. Testosterone for low libido in postmenopausal women not taking estrogen. *N Engl J Med*. 2008;359:2005.
- El-Hage G, Eden JA, Manga RZ. A double-blind, randomized, placebo-controlled trial of the effect of testosterone cream on the sexual motiviation of menopausal hysterectomized women with hypoactive sexual desire disorder. *Climacteric*. 2007; 10:335.
- Goldstat R, Briganti E, Tran J, et al. Transdermal testosterone therapy improves well-being, mood, and sexual function in premenopausal women. *Menopause*. 2003;10:390.
- Leiblum SR, Rosen RC. *Principles and Practice of Sex Therapy: Update for the 1990s*. New York: Guilford Press; 1989.
- Modelska K. Female sexual dysfunction in postmenopausal women: Systematic review of placebo-controlled trials. *Am J Obstet Gynecol*. 2003;188:286.
- Osmanaaolu MA, Atasaral T, Baltac D, et al. Effect of different preparations of hormone therapy on sexual dysfunction in naturally postmenopausal women. *Climacteric*. 2006;9:464–72.
- Rudkin L, Taylor MJ, Hawton K. Strategies for managing sexual dysfunction induced by antidepressant medication. *Cochrane Database Syst Rev*. 2004:CD003382.
- The role of testosterone therapy in postmenopausal women: Position statement of The North American Menopause Society. *Menopause*. 2005;12:497.
- Wincze JP, Carey MP. *Sexual Dysfunction: A Guide for Assessment and Treatment*. New York: Guilford Press; 1991.

CODES

ICD9

- 302.70 Psychosexual dysfunction, unspecified
- 302.71 Hypoactive sexual desire disorder
- 302.79 Psychosexual dysfunction with other specified psychosexual dysfunctions

CLINICAL PEARLS

- Female sexual dysfunction is a common, complex, multifactorial problem.
- Most commonly, patients with sexual dysfunction have a completely normal physical exam.
- Symptoms of sexual dysfunction peak during perimenopause between the ages of 45 and 64, even though hormone levels of estrogen and testosterone may fall in the normal range; women often benefit from hormone supplementation with estrogen and/or testosterone.
- Encourage follow-up with counseling for marriage, individual, and/or sex therapy.
- Use of hormonal contraception in premenopausal women is commonly associated with complaints of decreased libido.

S

SHIN SPLINTS

Gary Yen, MD

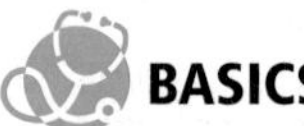

BASICS

DESCRIPTION

- American Medical Association defines shin splints as "pain or discomfort in the leg from repetitive running on hard surfaces or forcible excessive use of the foot flexors." Definition excludes stress fracture or pain from ischemic origin.
- Synonym(s): Medial tibial stress syndrome (preferred term); medial tibial periostalgia; Tibial periostitis; Shin soreness; Tibial stress syndrome; Medial tibial syndrome

EPIDEMIOLOGY

Prevalence

Can account for 6–16% of all running injuries (1)

RISK FACTORS

- Runners (particularly sprinters and hurdlers), dancers (particularly ballet), gymnasts, basketball players, military personnel
- Usually categorized into intrinsic (personal) and extrinsic (environmental) factors (2):
  - Intrinsic factors include overpronation, female sex, increased hip internal/external range of motion, higher body mass index, and leaner calf girth.
  - Extrinsic factors include training errors (increased mileage, increased intensity of workout), low calcium intake in female athletes, running on hard or inclined surfaces, and running while wearing worn-out footwear.

GENERAL PREVENTION

Suggested recommendations include (1)[C]:

- Screening for overpronation
- Designing appropriate training regimen/identifying training errors
- Regular stretching, strength, and flexibility exercises
- Rehabilitation of previous injuries
- Wearing proper footwear

PATHOPHYSIOLOGY

Somewhat controversial with many different theories, including bone stress reaction, periostitis, periostalgia, low bone mineral density, tendinopathy, periosteal remodeling with several structures possibly involved, including the soleus, deep crural fascia, flexor digitorum longus, and tibialis posterior

ETIOLOGY

Likely multifactorial, drawing from biomechanical, anatomic, and environmental causes

DIAGNOSIS

HISTORY

- Pain along the junction of the middle and distal thirds of the posteromedial tibia (most common) or anterior tibia, described as "dull ache" or "soreness"
- Pain with exercise (commonly bilateral) dissipates with rest
- Severe shin splints may cause persistent pain at rest or pain with only mild activity, and the character of the pain can become "sharp" or "penetrating."
- Pain subsides or is gone in shin splints compared with a stress fracture of the tibia, where the pain persists with rest.

PHYSICAL EXAM

- Generalized tenderness to palpation along the medial border of the tibia with possible mild swelling (see www.youtube.com/watch?v=7vZVq3ov914 for overview of muscular dysfunction)
- Pain with resisted plantar flexion or toe raises
- Clinical presentation may closely resemble that of stress fractures and exertional compartment syndrome, which can carry a far worse prognosis if undiagnosed:
  - Stress fracture tenderness usually is more localized.
  - Exertional compartment syndrome has characteristic physical findings of anterolateral leg pain (described as "cramplike, tight, squeezing ache"), most commonly over the anterior compartment; fascial hernias may be present. Depending on the compartment affected, characteristic weakness and/or paresthesias also can be present.

DIAGNOSTIC TESTS & INTERPRETATION

Imaging

- Serial plain radiographs are normal but are needed to rule out stress fractures, which usually are positive after 2 weeks of symptoms.
- A bone scan for shin splints reveals diffuse, linear uptake along the posteromedial border of the tibia on the delayed phase, whereas a bone scan for stress fracture reveals localized, more intense, fusiform, or transverse uptake in all phases.
- MRI also can be used to identify a stress fracture earlier.
- Compartment pressure measurement with exercise may be needed to diagnose exertional compartment syndrome if pain is anterolateral.

DIFFERENTIAL DIAGNOSIS

- Stress fractures
- Chronic exertional compartment syndrome
- Acute tendinitis/muscle strain/muscle tear/fascial defects
- Vascular disease
- Lumbar radiculopathy
- Hematoma
- Popliteal artery entrapment
- Peroneal nerve entrapment
- Deep vein thrombosis
- Tumor (sarcoma or osteosarcoma)

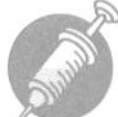

TREATMENT

- Acute phase treatment includes reducing training activity below symptom level or, if it is a serious case, the patient may need to stop activity altogether; ice the area of injury (3)[C].
- Recovery time is variable.
- Exercises to consider: www.youtube.com/watch?v=kv6ycmOWnq0
- Running in a pool or bicycling can aid in keeping up with conditioning while rehabilitation occurs.
- Options mostly based on expert opinion and clinical experience (3).
- Though exercising and modifying training schedules have been suggested as interventions to reduce injury, there is little to no evidence to support this (4)[A].

MEDICATION

- NSAIDs
- Analgesics

ADDITIONAL TREATMENT

Additional Therapies

- Physical therapy (3)[C]:
  - Therapist-determined modalities
  - Strengthening, stretching, and flexibility exercises after acute symptoms disappear
- Whirlpool, phonophoresis, electrical stimulation, ultrasound, augmented soft tissue mobilization, and acupuncture can be considered (3)[C].

COMPLEMENTARY AND ALTERNATIVE MEDICINE

- Orthotic or shoe modification if there is significant foot pronation
- Evidence for shock-absorbing orthotics reducing the incidence of shin splints is limited at best (4)[A].

SURGERY/OTHER PROCEDURES

- Only after a documented trial of maximal nonoperative treatment (for at least 6 months) has failed should posterior medial fascia release be considered. Consider if there is severe limitation of physical activity or frequent recurrence of pain despite proper rehabilitation (5)[C].
- Extracorporeal shock wave therapy is a possible alternative to surgical treatment, although more investigation is needed on this mode of therapy (6)[C].

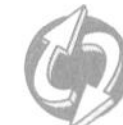

ONGOING CARE

PATIENT EDUCATION

- Identifying training errors and avoiding a rush back to preinjury pace will help to prevent recurrence.
- Emphasize the importance of modified activity followed by stretching and strengthening exercises.
- Resumption of activity should be done gradually, below the level of the symptoms.

PROGNOSIS

- Most patients respond well to nonoperative treatment.
- Gradual return to activity can be expected.

COMPLICATIONS

- If shin splints are not addressed, the degree of leg pain can interfere with activities of daily living, and stress fractures/true fractures may occur.
- Undiagnosed stress fracture can lead to complete fracture and displacement.
- Undiagnosed chronic compartment syndrome could develop into an acute syndrome with possible tissue necrosis.

REFERENCES

1. Thacker SB, Gilchrist J, Stroup DF, et al. The prevention of shin splints in sports: A systematic review of literature. *Med Sci Sports Exerc*. 2002;34:32–40.
2. Moen MH, Tol JL, Weir A, et al. Medial tibial stress syndrome: A critical review. *Sports Med*. 2009;39:523–46.
3. Galbraith RM, Lavallee ME, et al. Medial tibial stress syndrome: Conservative treatment options. *Curr Rev Musculoskelet Med*. 2009;2:127–33.
4. Yeung SS, Yeung EW, Gillespie LD, et al. Interventions for preventing lower limb soft-tissue running injuries. *Cochrane Database Syst Rev*. 2011;CD001256.
5. Yates B, Allen MJ, Barnes MR. Outcome of surgical treatment of medial tibial stress syndrome. *J Bone Joint Surg Am*. 2003;85-A:1974–80.
6. Rompe JD, Cacchio A, Furia JP, et al. Low-energy extracorporeal shock wave therapy as a treatment for medial tibial stress syndrome. *Am J Sports Med*. 2010;38:125–32.

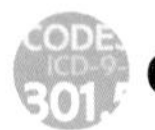

CODES

ICD9

844.9 Sprain of unspecified site of knee and leg

CLINICAL PEARLS

- *Medial tibial stress syndrome* is the much more anatomically accurate and preferred term.
- Diagnosis is usually made clinically by pain most commonly in the middle and distal thirds of the posteromedial border of the tibia that comes on with activity and reduces or resolves with rest; this is contrasted with a stress fracture, in which the pain persists with rest.
- Relative rest, ice, and NSAIDs are the generally agreed-upon mainstays of treatment.

SHOCK, CIRCULATORY

Felix B. Chang, MD

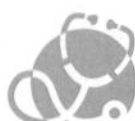

BASICS

DESCRIPTION

Inadequate tissue perfusion leading to hypoxia and organ dysfunction:

- Hypovolemic shock: Low preload
- Cardiogenic shock: Persistent systolic pressure <80–90 mm Hg or mean arterial pressure 30 mm Hg lower than baseline with severe reduction in the cardiac index and adequate or elevated filling pressures
- Septic shock: Severe sepsis plus systemic mean BP <60 mm Hg (or <80 mm Hg if the patient has baseline hypertension) despite fluid resuscitation. Maintaining the systemic mean BP >60 mm Hg (or >80 mm Hg if the patient has baseline hypertension) requires dopamine >5 mcg/kg/min, norepinephrine <0.25 mcg/kg/min, or epinephrine <0.25 mcg/kg/min despite adequate fluid resuscitation.
- Neurogenic shock: Vasodilation associated with loss of sympathetic tone; venous pooling in periphery

EPIDEMIOLOGY

Accidental injuries are the leading cause of death between 1 and 44 years. Cardiogenic shock: 5–10% in patients with acute myocardial infarction (MI). Over 750,000 cases/yr of sepsis in the US.

Incidence

Male > Female; sepsis is highest among African American males.

RISK FACTORS

- Hypovolemic shock: Hemorrhage, dehydration, burns
- Cardiogenic shock: Older age, anterior MI, hypertension, diabetes mellitus, multivessel coronary artery disease, prior MI or diagnosis of heart failure, STEMI, and left bundle branch block
- Septic shock: Bacteremia, age >65 years, immunosuppression, critical illness, malnutrition, cancer, pneumonia, genetic factors
- Neurogenic: Spinal anesthesia, spinal cord injury, anaphylactic shock, fainting (vasovagal reaction)

GENERAL PREVENTION

Prompt recognition and early treatment of underlying condition

ETIOLOGY

- Hypovolemic shock (hemorrhagic):
  - Blood loss: Trauma (e.g., injuries to liver, spleen, lung; fractures, wounds), GI bleeding (e.g., gastric and duodenal ulcer, colonic polyps, diverticulosis, or tumors), rupture of aortic or ventricular aneurysm, ectopic pregnancy, hemorrhagic ovarian cyst, DUB:
    - Class I: Blood loss up to 750 mL (15% blood volume), pulse <100, BP normal with normal or increased pulse pressure, normal capillary blanch test, respiratory rate 14–20, urine output >30 mL/hr, slightly anxious
    - Class II: Blood loss 750–1,500 mL (15–30% blood volume), pulse >100, BP normal with decreased pulse pressure, positive capillary blanch test, respiratory rate 20–30, urine output 20–30 mL/hr, mildly anxious
    - Class III: Blood loss 1,500–2,000 mL (30–40% blood volume), pulse >120, BP decreased with decreased pulse pressure, positive capillary blanch test, respiratory rate 30–40, urine output 5–15 mL/hr, anxious + confused
    - Class IV: Blood loss >2,000 mL (>40% blood volume), pulse >140, BP decreased with decreased pulse pressure, positive capillary blanch test, RR >35, urine output negligible, confused, lethargic
- Hypovolemic shock (nonhemorrhagic): Dehydration, vomiting, diarrhea, heat stroke, or burns; third-space loss of plasma volume
- Cardiogenic shock:
  - Acute MI (>40% of left ventricular myocardium), right ventricular infarction, β- and calcium channel blocker overdose
  - Dilated cardiomyopathies (e.g., viral, alcohol, Adriamycin toxicity)
  - Arrhythmias: Heart block, ventricular tachycardia/fibrillation, atrial fibrillation with rapid ventricular response, bradycardias, etc.
  - Mechanical difficulties: Valvular dysfunction, papillary muscle rupture, aortic or mitral valve dysfunction; ventricular septal rupture
  - Obstruction:
    - Pericardial tamponade, tension pneumothorax, constrictive pericarditis
    - Aortic dissection or pulmonary embolism
- Septic shock: UTI is the most common source in the elderly:
  - Bacteremia
  - Systemic inflammatory response syndrome: Requires 2 or more criteria. Temperature >38.5°C or <35°C, heart rate >90 beats/min, respiratory rate >20 breaths/min or $PaCO_2$, 32 mm Hg, WBC 12,000/mm^3, <4000 cells/mm^3, or >10% immature forms.
  - Sepsis: Requires 2 or more of the following criteria, and documented infection. Temperature >38.5°C or <35°C, heart rate >90 beats/min, respiratory rate > 20 breaths/min or $PaCO_2$ <32 mm Hg, WBC >12,000 cells/mm^3, <4000 cells/mm$_3$, or >10 % immature (band) forms. Documented infection requires positive culture or Gram stain of blood, sputum, urine, or normally sterile body fluid positive for pathogenic microorganism; or focus of infection identified by visual inspection.
  - Severe sepsis (sepsis plus at least 1 additional criterion): Mottled skin; capillary refill of ≥3 seconds, urinary output of <0.5 mL/Kg for at least 1 hour or requiring dialysis; lactate >2 mmol/L; abrupt change in mental status or abnormal EEG findings; platelet count of <100,000 cells/mL or disseminated intravascular coagulation; acute lung injury/ARDS; or cardiac dysfunction (echocardiography)
- Neurogenic shock: Acute spinal injury, general or spinal anesthesia, vasovagal reaction

COMMONLY ASSOCIATED CONDITIONS

Adrenal failure in septic shock

DIAGNOSIS

HISTORY

- Hypovolemic shock: Burns, trauma, bleeding, vomiting, melena, diarrhea
- Cardiogenic shock: Dizziness, chest pain, dyspnea, palpitations
- Septic shock: Fever, chills, rigors, malaise, myalgias, dysuria, shortness of breath
- Neurogenic shock: Spinal trauma

PHYSICAL EXAM

- Hypovolemic shock: Orthostatic hypotension, dry skin and mucosa, collapsed neck veins
- Cardiogenic shock: Cyanosis, cool, rapid and faint pulses, JVD, pulsus paradoxus, systolic murmur, crackles
- Neurogenic shock: Normal capillary refill, areflexia + weakness below level of lesion. Absent bulbocavernosus reflex.
- Septic shock:
  - Hyperdynamic state: Fever, tachycardia; warm, dry, flushed skin
  - Hypodynamic state: Hypotension, diminished sensorium, cold clammy skin
  - Temperature >38.3°C (100.9°F) or temperature <36°C (96.8°F), tachycardia with heart rate >90 beats/min or >2 standard deviations above normal value for age, tachypnea >30 breaths/min. Altered mental status (confusion, anxiety, agitation, coma). Edema. Skin: Erythema, petechiae, embolic lesions, purpura.
- Specific signs of underlying disease: Upper GI (UGI) tract bleeding (hematemesis, melena). MI (chest pain, diaphoresis, nausea, vomiting, S_4 or S_3 gallop, new heart murmur, rales). Pericardial tamponade (JVD and pulsus paradoxus). Urosepsis (suprapubic and/or costovertebral angle tenderness).

DIAGNOSTIC TESTS & INTERPRETATION

Lab

Initial lab tests

- Hypovolemic hemorrhagic: CBC with differential, PT/INR, PTT; LFTs, blood type and cross-match, DIC panel. Nonhemorrhagic: Creatinine and electrolytes; consider lipase and LFTs.
- Cardiogenic shock: ECG, cardiac enzymes, ABGs, tox screen, lactic acid, BNP
- Septic shock: CBC with differential, PT/INR/PTT, chem panel, lactic acid, ABGs, C-reactive protein, urinalysis, pan-cultures Gram stain, ACTH stimulation test
  (? adrenal insufficiency)
- Endocervical and high vaginal swabs in patients with low abdominal pain and vaginal discharge
- Procalcitonin levels safely reduce antibiotics use in elderly with community-acquired pneumonia (1)[A]. Procalcitonin <0.1 mcg/L antibiotics strongly discouraged. 0.1–0.25 mcg/L equivocal. Levels 0.25–0.5 mcg/L: Antibiotics recommended; procalcitonin >0.5 mc/L: antibiotics strongly recommended.

Imaging

Initial approach

Chest: CXR/CT scan as appropriate to evaluate for pneumonia, empyema, hemothorax, aortic aneurysm. Abdomen: KUB, CT scan, and/or ultrasound to evaluate intestinal obstruction, aortic aneurysm, liver abscess, peritoneal abscess, peritonitis, pancreatitis.

Diagnostic Procedures/Surgery

- Central venous pressure. Pulmonary artery pressure (Swan-Ganz catheter). Lumbar puncture.
- Upper/lower endoscopy for GI bleeding, cystoscopy for GU hemorrhage

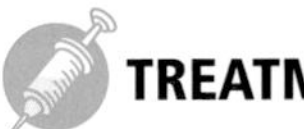

TREATMENT

MEDICATION

First Line

- Cardiogenic shock: Aspirin, β-blockers, nitroglycerin, morphine see STEMI and NSTEMI, and control arrhythmias with appropriate antiarrhythmic, if necessary
- Cultures, broad-spectrum antibiotic therapy as early as possible aimed at the likely source of infection

Second Line

- Vasopressors and inotropes are indicated for MAP <60 mm Hg or decrease SBP >30 mm Hg from baseline.
- Norepinephrine and dopamine have similar effects on mortality, but less arrhythmia is seen with norepinephrine (2)[A].
- Dopamine: Cardiogenic and hypodynamic septic shock that is refractory to fluids. Dopamine is also the first-line catecholamine for bradycardia refractory to atropine.
- Dobutamine for refractory heart failure and cardiogenic shock
- Epinephrine is the agent of choice in patients with anaphylaxis.
- Norepinephrine and phenylephrine are first-line agents for hyperdynamic septic shock. Norepinephrine acts on both alpha-1 and beta-1 adrenergic receptors, producing potent vasoconstriction and a less pronounced increase in cardiac output.
- Vasopressin is an alternative agent for patients refractory to inotropic agents.
- Norepinephrine is useful in cardiogenic shock unresponsive to dopamine or dobutamine and in refractory hypotension secondary to tricyclic acid overdose.
- Phenylephrine is indicated in refractory shock, spinal anesthesia, or drug-related hypotension. Phenylephrine has minimal cardiac inotropy or chronotropy. Potent vasoconstrictor (pure alpha-adrenergic agonist).
- Epinephrine, phenylephrine, or vasopressin should not be administered as the initial vasopressor in septic shock (3)[C].
- Naloxone might improve BP in patients with shock.
- Levosimendan may improve survival in patients with refractory cardiogenic shock.
- Isoproterenol has a potent chronotropic effect.
- IV hydrocortisone: Controversial
- There is no clear evidence suggesting the use of recombinant human-activated protein C (drotrecogin-alfa) in patients with sepsis or septic shock (4). Drotrecogin is not recommended for low-risk patients with severe sepsis; increases risk of serious bleeding in low-risk patients. Might be used in high-risk patients with APACHE II scores ≥25, multiple organ dysfunction syndrome (MODS), or sepsis-induced acute respiratory distress syndrome (ARDS) (5)[B].

ADDITIONAL TREATMENT

General Measures

First correct hypovolemia, maintain SaO_2 >92%. Control ongoing losses: Bleeding, diarrhea, third-space loss. Control glycemia (6)[A]. Identify and treat infections. Monitor urine output.

SURGERY/OTHER PROCEDURES

- Hemorrhage control. Revascularization: MI, thrombolysis. Pericardiocentesis for pericardial effusion.
- Surgical drainage or debridement as needed. Chest tube for empyema or pleural effusion.
- Mechanical ventilation of sepsis-induced acute lung injury (ALI)/ARDS

IN-PATIENT CONSIDERATIONS

Initial Stabilization

ABCs. IV access: 2 large IV catheters or central line. ICU-level care.

IV Fluids

- Initial 10–20 mL/kg IV bolus lactated Ringer's or normal saline if there is no sign of heart failure. Restore blood or fluid loss: 3 L of fluid per liter of blood loss.
- Colloids do not appear to reduce mortality compared with crystalloids in patients with trauma, burns, postoperatively (7)[A].
- Target in septic shock: Central venous pressure (CVP): 8–12 mm Hg; MAP ≥65 mm Hg; urine output ≥0.5 mL/kg/hr; superior vena cava or mixed venous oxygen saturation >70% or 65%, respectively (3)[C]

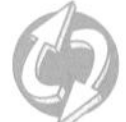

ONGOING CARE

FOLLOW-UP RECOMMENDATIONS

Patient Monitoring

ICU

PATIENT EDUCATION

Medline Plus: www.nlm.nih.gov/MEDLINEPLUS/ency/article/000039.htm

PROGNOSIS

- Cardiogenic shock: Worse prognosis with increasing age, prior MI, altered sensorium, cold, clammy skin, and oliguria. These are predictive factors of increased mortality (Gusto I trial). SHOCK trial: 38% overall mortality with early revascularization vs. 70% when rapid revascularization was not attempted.
- Septic shock: Sepsis 20–50% mortality rate. Higher mortality in patients at the age extremes and those with poor functional status; also in patients with immunosuppression due to neutropenia, diabetes, alcoholism, renal failure, respiratory failure, or hypogammaglobulinemia; positive blood cultures, certain etiologic agents (e.g., *P. aeruginosa*), or delay in appropriate antimicrobial therapy

COMPLICATIONS

Multiple organ dysfunction syndrome. Pulmonary edema, ARDS, ischemic hepatitis, ischemic bowel. Abdominal compartment syndrome. Acute tubular necrosis (ATN). Coagulopathy, DIC, thrombocytopenia. Acid–base disturbances (e.g., respiratory alkalosis, anion gap metabolic acidosis). Adrenal failure, osteomyelitis, death. Refractory septic shock.

REFERENCES

1. Schuetz P, Christ-Crain M, et al. Effect of procalcitonin-based guidelines vs standard guidelines on antibiotics use in lower respiratory tract infections: The ProHOSP randomized controlled trial. *JAMA*. 2009;302(10):1059–66.
2. De Backer D, Biston P, Devriendt J, et al. Comparison of dopamine and norepinephrine in the treatment of shock. *N Engl J Med*. 2010;362: 779–89.
3. Dellinger RP, Levy MM, Carlet JM, et al. Surviving Sepsis Campaign: International guidelines for management of severe sepsis and septic shock: 2008. *Crit Care Med*. 2008;36:296–327.
4. Marti-Carvajal AJ, Sola I, et al. Human recombinant activated protein C for severe sepsis. *Cochrane Database Syst Rev*. 2011;4:CD004388.
5. Laterre PF, Abraham E, Janes JM, et al. ADDRESS (ADministration of DRotrecogin alfa [activated] in Early stage Severe Sepsis) long-term follow-up: One-year safety and efficacy evaluation. *Crit Care Med*. 2007;35:1457–63.
6. Brunkhorst F, Enget C, et al. Intensive insulin therapy in patients with sepsis associated with higher risk of hypoglycemia and no reduction in mortality. *N Engl J Med*. 2008;358(2):125–39.
7. Perel P, Roberts I, et al. Colloids versus crystalloids for fluid resuscitation in critically ill patients. *Cochrane Database Syst Rev*. 2009;(3):CD000567.

ADDITIONAL READING

Lindenauer PK, Rothberg MB, et al. Activated protein C and hospital mortality in septic shock: A propensity-matched analysis. *Crit Care Med*. 2010; 38(4):1101.

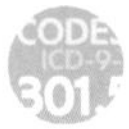

CODES

ICD9

- 785.50 Shock, unspecified
- 785.51 Cardiogenic shock
- 785.52 Septic shock

CLINICAL PEARLS

Hypovolemic shock, septic shock, neurogenic shock, and cardiogenic shock present somewhat differently, but are all characterized by inadequate tissue perfusion leading to hypoxia and organ dysfunction.

SHOULDER PAIN

Jennifer Schwartz, MD
J. Herbert Stevenson, MD

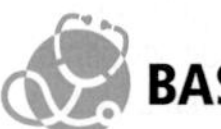

BASICS

DESCRIPTION

Shoulder pain is a common condition affecting patients of all ages. It can arise from acute trauma or overuse injuries from athletics or daily activities. Age plays an important role in determining the etiology of shoulder pain. Characteristics of pain or weakness, acuity of onset, mechanism of injury, and functional limitation also help in diagnosing and treating shoulder pain.

EPIDEMIOLOGY

- Shoulder pain accounts for 16% of all musculoskeletal complaints.
- The lifetime prevalence of shoulder pain is as high as 70% (1).
- Predominant age:
  - <30: Shoulder instability
  - >30: Rotator cuff (RTC) disorder:
    - 30–50: Tendinopathy
    - 40–60: Partial tear
    - >60 Full-thickness tear
  - >60: Osteoarthritis (OA) of the glenohumeral joint

Incidence

The incidence of shoulder pain is 6.6–25 cases/1,000 patients, with a peak incidence in the fourth to sixth decades.

RISK FACTORS

- Repetitive overhead activities
- Overhead and upper extremity weightbearing sports (baseball, softball, swimming)
- Weight lifting: Acromioclavicular (AC) disorders
- Rapid increases in training, improper technique
- Muscle weakness or imbalance
- Trauma or fall onto the shoulder
- Diabetes, thyroid disorders, female gender, age 40–60 years are risk factors for adhesive capsulitis.

GENERAL PREVENTION

- Maintenance of good shoulder strength and range of motion (ROM)
- Avoidance of repetitive overhead activities

PATHOPHYSIOLOGY

Depends on underlying etiology

ETIOLOGY

- Trauma (fracture, dislocation, ligament/tendon tear)
- Overuse (RTC pathology, biceps tenosynovitis, bursitis, muscle strain):
  - RTC disorders most commonly occur from repetitive overhead activity. This leads to impingement of the RTC that can progress through 3 stages:
    - Stage I: Tendinopathy
    - Stage II: Partial RTC tear
    - Stage III: Full-thickness RTC tear
  - Subacromial bursitis can occur with RTC disorders, but is rarely an isolated diagnosis.
- Age-related (AC and glenohumeral joint OA, adhesive capsulitis, RTC tear, instability)
- Rheumatologic (rheumatoid arthritis, polymyalgia rheumatica, fibromyalgia)
- Referred pain (neck, gallbladder)

DIAGNOSIS

Majority of shoulder pain is diagnosed in the outpatient setting.

HISTORY

- Characteristic of pain:
  - Superior shoulder pain: AC pathology, trapezius strain
  - Lateral/deltoid pain: RTC pathology (RTC pain typically does not extend past elbow)
  - Diffuse pain: RTC pathology, adhesive capsulitis, glenohumeral OA
  - Nighttime pain: RTC pathology (lying on affected side), adhesive capsulitis, glenohumeral OA
  - Stiff shoulder: Adhesive capsulitis
  - Pain with cross-body activities: AC pathology
  - Pain with abduction/external rotation (reaching behind): Shoulder instability
  - Pain with overhead activity: RTC pathology
  - Pain with tinging toward neck, pain past elbow: Cervical pathology
- Mechanism of injury:
  - Fall on outstretched hand: Traumatic shoulder instability/dislocation
  - Fall directly onto shoulder: AC joint sprain, clavicle fracture
  - Repetitive overhead activity: RTC pathology
- Age:
  - Shoulder instability (subluxation, dislocation, multidirectional instability) is most common cause of shoulder pain in the young athlete (<30 years old).
  - RTC disorders are the most common cause of shoulder pain in patients >30 years old. Severity of RTC disorder also increases with age:
    - Tendinopathy: 30–50 years old
    - Partial RTC tear: 40–60 years old
    - Full-thickness tear: >60 years old
  - Older patients (>60 years old) more likely to have OA
  - Trauma in a young person <40 more commonly associated with dislocation/subluxation; in a person >40 trauma more commonly associated with RTC tear.

PHYSICAL EXAM

- Observe as patient takes off jacket, moves arm.
- Inspect for malalignment, muscle atrophy, asymmetry, swelling. Scapular winging suggests long thoracic nerve or muscular (trapezius, serraticus anterior) dysfunction.
- Palpate for tenderness, warmth, bony step-offs.
- Evaluate for active and passive ROM and flexibility:
  - Decreased active AND passive ROM: Adhesive capsulitis:
    - Mildly decreased active and/or passive ROM can also indicate glenohumeral OA.
  - Decreased active, full passive ROM: RTC pathology
- Evaluate for muscle strength.
- Special tests:
  - Neer, Hawkins: RTC impingement
  - Pain with strength testing the supraspinatus (empty can test), infraspinatus/teres minor (resisted external rotation), subscapularis (lift-off test, resisted internal rotation): RTC pathology. Weakness could suggest tear.
  - Drop arm test: RTC tear
  - Cross-arm adduction test: AC joint arthritis
  - Speed, Yergason test: Biceps tendinopathy
  - Apprehension, relocation test: Anterior glenohumeral joint instability
  - Sulcus sign: Inferior glenohumeral joint instability
  - Obrien, clunk test: Labral pathology
  - Spurling test: Cervical pathology

DIAGNOSTIC TESTS & INTERPRETATION

- EMG study of the upper extremity may help differentiate cervical pain referred to the shoulder from a primary shoulder disorder.
- Obtain ECG if any suspicion for cardiac etiology of left shoulder pain.

Lab

Appropriate rheumatologic tests may be indicated if autoimmune etiology considered.

Imaging

Most shoulder pain can be diagnosed by history and physical exam:

- Adults with nontraumatic shoulder pain of <4 weeks may not require initial imaging.
- When diagnosis remains unclear, surgery is planned, history of significant trauma, prolonged symptoms, or red flags (older age, fever, rest pain), further imaging may be indicated:
  - Plain radiographs are first-line imaging:
    - Can assess for fracture, degenerative changes, signs of dislocation (Bankart, Hill-Sachs deformity), signs of large RTC tear (sclerosis, humeral head proximal migration), anatomic deformities contributing to impingement, occult tumor
    - Standard views: Anteroposterior, scapular Y, axillary
- CT scan may rule out occult fracture.
- MRI is gold standard for noninvasive imaging of soft tissue structures, including RTC, biceps tendon.
- MR arthrogram may be needed to assess for labral tears or small/partial RTC tears.
- Ultrasound is gaining recognition in screening for shoulder pathologies, including RTC tears, biceps tendinopathies, and AC joint disorders (1)[B].

Diagnostic Procedures/Surgery

Diagnostic arthroscopy may be used in the proper setting after noninterventional means have been exhausted and structural injury suspected.

Pathological Findings

Depends on underlying diagnosis:

- Tendinosis rather than tendonitis often found with stage I impingement.
- Scarring of the shoulder capsule hallmark of adhesive capsulitis.
- Calcifications can be found in rotator cuff tendons with calcific tendonitis.

DIFFERENTIAL DIAGNOSIS

- Fracture (clavicle, humerus, scapula), contusion
- RTC disorder: Impingement, tear, calcific tendonitis
- Subacromial bursitis
- AC joint pathology (sprain/OA)
- Biceps tenosynovitis or tear
- Glenohumeral joint OA
- Glenohumeral joint instability (acute dislocation or chronic multidirectional instability)
- Adhesive capsulitis
- Labral tear or associated bony pathology
- Muscle strain (trapezius, deltoid, bicep)
- Cervical radiculopathy
- Other: Autoimmune, rheumatologic, referred pain

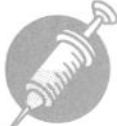

TREATMENT

Treatment is based on underlying pathology, but in general, conservative therapy includes relative rest, analgesics, and/or anti-inflammatory medicines:

- Little evidence to support or refute many common interventions for shoulder pain (2)[A].

MEDICATION

- Analgesics and anti-inflammatory medications may be required for symptomatic relief of shoulder pain:
  - Ibuprofen: 200–800 mg t.i.d.
  - Naprosyn: 250–500 mg b.i.d.
  - Acetaminophen: Up to 3–4 g/d
- Corticosteroid injections (subacromial, glenohumeral) may relieve pain acutely: RTC pathology, adhesive capsulitis, OA (3,4)[B]. Effect may be enhanced if ultrasound-guided (5)[B].

ADDITIONAL TREATMENT

Issues for Referral

Shoulder pain where etiology remains unclear, nonresponsive to conservative care, complicated or displaced fractures, large RTC tears

Additional Therapies

- Physical therapy may provide benefit if unimproved with conservative measures—consider for RTC disorders, adhesive capsulitis, shoulder instability (3,6)[B].
- Manual manipulative therapy by chiropractors, osteopathic physicians, or physical therapists can improve pain with adhesive capsulitis, RTC, and soft tissue disorders (7)[B].

COMPLEMENTARY AND ALTERNATIVE MEDICINE

There is no conclusive evidence to support or refute the use of acupuncture for shoulder pain, although there may be short-term improvement in pain (8)[A].

SURGERY/OTHER PROCEDURES

May be required for shoulder pain unresponsive to conservative care, acute displaced fractures, large rotator cuff tears, shoulder dislocation in patients <20 years of age

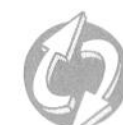

ONGOING CARE

FOLLOW-UP RECOMMENDATIONS

Limiting overhead activity may reduce the symptoms of impingement syndrome.

PATIENT EDUCATION

Refer to specific diagnosis for shoulder pain.

PROGNOSIS

Shoulder pain generally has a favorable outcome with conservative care, but recovery can be slow, with 40–50% with persistent pain or recurrence at 12 months (1).

REFERENCES

1. Cadagon A, Laslett M, et al. A prospective study of shoulder pain in primary care: Prevalance of imaged pathology and response to guided diagnostic blocks. *BMC Musculoskel Disord*. 2011;28(12):119.
2. Green S, Buchbinder R, Forbes A. Interventions for shoulder pain. *Cochrane Database Systematic Rev*. 2009:CD001156.
3. Favejee MM, Huisstede BM, Koes BW. Frozen shoulder: The effectiveness of conservative and surgical interventions: a systematic review. *Br J Sports Med*. 2011;45(1):49–56.
4. Buchbinder R, Green S, Youd JM. Corticosteroid injections for shoulder pain. *Cochrane Database Systematic Rev*. 2009:CD004016.
5. Soh E, Li W, et al. Image guided versus blind corticosteroid injections in adults with shoulder pain: A systematic review. *BMC Musculoskel Disord*. 2011;12(1):137.
6. Green S, Buchbinder R, Hetrick SE. Physiotherapy interventions for shoulder pain. *Cochrane Database of Systematic Reviews*. 2010:CD004258.
7. Brantingham JW, Cassa TK, et al. Manipulative therapy for shoulder pain and disorders: An expansion of a systematic review. *J Manipulative Ther*. 2011;34(5):314–16.
8. Green S, Buchbinder R, Hetrick SE. Acupuncture for shoulder pain. *Cochrane Database Systematic Rev*. 2009:CD005319.

ADDITIONAL READING

- Burbank KM, Stevenson JH, et al. Chronic Shoulder Pain: Part I and II. *Am Fam Physician*. 2008;77(4):453–60, 493–97.
- Bussieres AE, Peterson C, Taylor JA. Diagnostic imaging guidelines for musculoskeletal complaints in adults- an evidence based approach. Part 2-upper extremity disorders. *J Manipulative Physiol Ther*. 2008;31(1):2–32.
- Celik D, Sirmen B, Demirhan M. The relationship of muscle strength and pain in subacromial impingement. *Acta Orthop Traumatol Turk*. 2011; 45(2):79–84.
- Sipola P, Niemitukia L, et al. Detection and quantification of rotator cuff tears with ultrasonography and MRI-a prospective study in 77 consecutive patients with a surgical reference. *Ultrasound Med Biol*. 2010;36(12):1981–9.
- Urwin M, Symmons D, Allison T, et al. Estimating the burden of musculoskeletal disorders in the community: The comparative prevalence of symptoms at different anatomical sites, and the relation to social deprivation. *Ann Rheum Dis*. 1998;57:649–55.

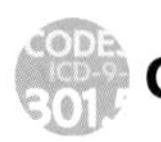

CODES

ICD9

- 719.41 Pain in joint involving shoulder region
- 726.0 Adhesive capsulitis of shoulder
- 840.4 Rotator cuff (capsule) sprain

CLINICAL PEARLS

- Rotator cuff disorders (tendinopathy, tears) are the most common source of shoulder pain in individuals >30 years of age.
- Shoulder instability (acute dislocation/subluxation or chronic instability) is the most common source of shoulder pain in individuals <30 years of age.

SINUSITIS

Adarsh K. Gupta, DO, MS

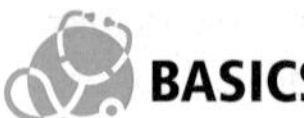

BASICS

DESCRIPTION

- Acute sinusitis is a symptomatic inflammation of 1 or more paranasal sinuses of <4 weeks' duration resulting from impaired drainage and retained secretions. Because rhinitis and sinusitis usually coexist, "rhinosinusitis" is the preferred term.
- Disease is subacute when symptomatic for 4–12 weeks and chronic when symptomatic for >12 weeks.
- System(s) affected: Head/Eyes/Ears/Nose/Throat (HEENT); Pulmonary

EPIDEMIOLOGY

- It affects 31 million individuals in the US each year with an estimated annual cost of $5.8 billion.
- Diagnosis of acute bacterial rhinosinusitis remains the fifth-leading reason for prescribing antibiotics.
- About 0.2–2% episodes of viral rhinosinusitis have bacterial superinfection.

Incidence

Incidence highest in early fall through early spring (related to incidence of viral upper respiratory infection [URI]). Adults have 2 or 3 viral URIs per year; 90% of these colds are accompanied by viral rhinosinusitis.

RISK FACTORS

- Viral URI
- Allergic rhinitis
- Asthma
- Cigarette smoking
- Dental infections and procedures
- Anatomic variations:
  - Tonsillar and adenoid hypertrophy
  - Turbinate hypertrophy, nasal polyps
  - Deviated septum
  - Cleft palate
- Immunodeficiency (e.g., HIV)
- Cystic fibrosis

Genetics

No known genetic pattern

GENERAL PREVENTION

Hand washing to prevent transmission of viral infection

PATHOPHYSIOLOGY

- Important features:
  - Inflammation and edema of the sinus mucosa
  - Obstruction of the sinus ostia
  - Impaired mucociliary clearance
- Secretions that are not cleared become hospitable to bacterial growth.
- Inflammatory response (neutrophil influx and release of cytokines) damages mucosal surfaces.

ETIOLOGY

- Viral: Vast majority of cases (rhinovirus, influenza A and B; parainfluenza virus; respiratory syncytial; adeno-, corona-, and enteroviruses)
- Bacterial (complicates 0.2–2% of viral cases):
  - More likely if symptoms worsen after 5–7 days or do not improve >10 days
  - *S. pneumoniae*, *H. influenzae*, and *M. catarrhalis* are the most common bacterial pathogens.
  - Often overdiagnosed, which leads to overuse of and increasing resistance to antibiotics
- Fungal: Seen in immunocompromised hosts (uncontrolled diabetes, neutropenia, use of corticosteroids) or as a nosocomial infection

DIAGNOSIS

History and physical exam suggest and establish the diagnosis, but are rarely helpful in distinguishing bacterial from viral causes.

ALERT

- Symptoms somewhat predictive of bacterial sinusitis:
  - Worsening of symptoms >5–7 days after initial improvement
  - Persistent symptoms for ≥10 days
  - Persistent purulent nasal discharge
  - Unilateral upper tooth or facial pain
  - Unilateral maxillary sinus tenderness
  - Fever
- Associated symptoms:
  - Headache
  - Nasal congestion
  - Retro-orbital pain
  - Otalgia
  - Hyposomia
  - Halitosis
  - Chronic cough
- Symptoms requiring urgent attention:
  - Visual disturbances, especially diplopia
  - Periorbital swelling or erythema
  - Altered mental status

HISTORY

Major challenge is to distinguish between viral and bacterial disease; use constellation of symptoms rather than a particular sign or symptom.

PHYSICAL EXAM

- Fever
- Edema and erythema of nasal mucosa
- Purulent discharge
- Tenderness to palpation over sinus(es)

Pediatric Considerations

- Sinuses are not fully developed until age 20. Maxillary and ethmoid sinuses, although small, are present from birth.
- Since children have an average of 6–8 colds per year, they are at risk for developing sinusitis.
- Diagnosis can be more difficult than in adults because symptoms are often more subtle.

DIAGNOSTIC TESTS & INTERPRETATION

Diagnostic tests are not routinely recommended; no diagnostic tests can adequately differentiate between viral and bacterial rhinosinusitis.

Lab

- None indicated in routine evaluation
- Transillumination of the sinuses may confirm fluid in sinuses (helpful if asymmetric; not helpful if symmetric exam).

Imaging

- Routine use of sinus radiography discouraged because:
  - ≥3 clinical findings have similar diagnostic accuracy as imaging.
  - Imaging does not distinguish viral from bacterial etiology.
- Limited coronal CT scan can be useful in recurrent infection or failure to respond to medical therapy.

Diagnostic Procedures/Surgery

- Value of imaging studies is limited because they do not distinguish between viral and bacterial etiology.
- Sinus CT scanning may be warranted if symptoms or signs suggest extrasinus involvement or for evaluation of chronic rhinosinusitis (1).

Pathological Findings

- Inflammation
- Edema
- Thickened mucosa
- Impaired ciliary function
- Metaplasia of ciliated columnar cells
- Relative acidosis and hypoxia within sinuses
- Polyps

DIFFERENTIAL DIAGNOSIS

- Dental disease
- Cystic fibrosis (CF)
- Wegener granulomatosis
- HIV infection
- Kartagener syndrome
- Immotile cilia syndrome
- Neoplasm
- Headache, tension, or migraine

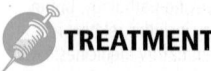

TREATMENT

Most cases of acute rhinosinusitis resolve with supportive care (treating pain, nasal symptoms). Antibiotics should be reserved for symptoms that persist more than 10 days or get worse in 5–7 days.

MEDICATION

First Line

- Decongestants:
  - Pseudoephedrine HCl
  - Phenylephrine nasal spray (limited use)
  - Oxymetazoline nasal spray (e.g., Afrin) (not to be used >3 days)
- Analgesics:
  - Acetaminophen
  - Aspirin
  - NSAIDs
  - Acetaminophen codeine (for severe cases)
- Antibiotics:
  - In large case series, antibiotics have a slight advantage over placebo, yet most patients improve without therapy (number needed to treat [NNT] ≈15 to prevent 1 persistent case at follow-up).
  - Reserve antibiotic use for patients with moderate-to-severe disease.
  - Treat for 10–14 days unless otherwise specified.
  - Choice should be based on understanding of antibiotic resistance in the community.
  - Initial therapy (narrow-spectrum antibiotics) (2,3)[A]:
    - Amoxicillin: 1 g t.i.d. (adults); 80–90 mg/kg/d divided q8h (children)
    - Trimethoprim-sulfamethoxazole (TMP/SMX): 160/800 mg q12h in adults and 8–12 mg/kg/d of trimethoprim component divided q12h for children
    - Doxycycline: 100 mg PO b.i.d. (adults only)

- Since allergies may be a predisposing factor, some patients may benefit from use of the following agents:
  - Oral antihistamines:
    - Loratadine (Claritin), fexofenadine (Allegra), cetirizine (Zyrtec), Clarinex (desloratadine), or Xyzal (levocetirizine)
    - Chlorpheniramine (Chlor-Trimeton)
    - Diphenhydramine (Benadryl)
  - Leukotriene inhibitors (Singulair, Accolate), especially in patients with asthma
  - Nasal steroids (i.e., fluticasone [Flonase])

Second Line

- Amoxicillin-clavulanate (Augmentin): 875/125 mg q12h (adults); 30 mg/kg/d of amoxicillin component divided b.i.d. in children
- High-dose amoxicillin-clavulanate (Augmentin XR) b.i.d. in adults and Augmentin ES-600 in children (for both β-lactam and penicillin-binding protein resistance)
- Cefpodoxime (Vantin): 200 mg q12h in adults and 10 mg/kg/d divided b.i.d. in children
- Cefuroxime axetil (Ceftin): 250 mg q12h in adults and 30 mg/kg/d divided q12h in children
- Azithromycin (Zithromax): 500 mg on day 1 and 250 mg on days 2–5 in adults; 10 mg/kg on day 1 and 5 mg/kg on days 2–5 in children
- Clarithromycin (Biaxin): 500 mg b.i.d. (regular) or 1,000 mg/d (extended release) in adults; 15 mg/kg/d divided b.i.d. in children
- Levofloxacin (Levaquin): 750 mg/d for 5 days (adults only)
- If no response to first-line therapy after 72 hours, or if patients have had antibiotics within the past 4–6 weeks, use or change to:
  - High-dose amoxicillin-clavulanate
  - Cephalosporins as above
  - Fluoroquinolones as above
- *Note:* Bacteriologic failure rates of up to 20–25% are possible with use of azithromycin and clarithromycin (2)[C].
- If lack of response to 3 weeks of antibiotics, consider:
  - CT scan of sinuses
  - Ear/nose/throat (ENT) referral

ADDITIONAL TREATMENT

ALERT

- When bacterial infection is present, patients recover somewhat more quickly with antibiotics, but the majority will recover with symptomatic treatment alone (3)[A].
- Multiple meta-analyses have demonstrated no benefit of newer antibiotics over amoxicillin, trimethoprim-sulfamethoxazole, or doxycycline (3)[A].
- Use of intranasal steroids produces modest improvement in symptoms when used alone or in combination with antibiotics (4)[B].
- Precautions:
  - Decongestants can exacerbate hypertension (HTN).
  - Intranasal decongestants might relieve nasal congestion but should be limited to 3 days to avoid rebound nasal congestion.
  - Sulfonamides may induce Stevens-Johnson syndrome (risk $\approx$ 1/2,000). Inform patients to report any mucous membrane ulcerations.
  - Significant possible interactions:
    - Warfarin (Coumadin): Increased effect of warfarin with macrolides or TMP/SMX, resulting in marked increase in international normalized ratio (INR) and prothrombin time (PT)
    - Statins should be stopped temporarily when macrolides are prescribed due to increased risk of myopathy and rhabdomyolysis.

Pregnancy Considerations

- Pregnancy Considerations
- Rhinitis of pregnancy predisposes to sinusitis.
- Nasal irrigation with saline, pseudoephedrine, most antihistamines, and some nasal steroids is safe during pregnancy and lactation.
- Antibiotics considered to be safe in pregnancy and lactation:
  - Amoxicillin and amoxicillin-clavulanate
  - Cephalosporins, azithromycin
  - Antibiotic contraindicated in pregnancy and lactation: Clarithromycin
  - Antibiotic safe in lactation but not during pregnancy: Levofloxacin

General Measures

- Hydration
- Steam inhalation 20–30 minutes t.i.d.
- Saline irrigation (Neti pot) or nose drops
- Sleep with head of bed elevated.
- Avoid exposure to cigarette smoke or fumes.
- Avoid caffeine and alcohol.
- Antibiotics indicated only when findings suggest bacterial infection
- Analgesics, NSAIDs (see below)
- Acute viral sinusitis is self-limiting, and antibiotics should not be used.

Issues for Referral

Complications or failure of treatment

SURGERY/OTHER PROCEDURES

- If medical therapy fails, consider sinus irrigation.
- Functional endoscopic sinus surgery is the preferred treatment for medically recalcitrant cases (2)[C].
- Absolute surgical indications:
  - Massive nasal polyposis
  - Acute complications: Subperiosteal or orbital abscess, frontal soft tissue spread of infection
  - Mucocele or mucopyocele
  - Invasive or allergic fungal sinusitis
  - Suspected obstructing tumor
  - CSF rhinorrhea

IN-PATIENT CONSIDERATIONS

- Most patients are treated in outpatient setting.
- Hospitalization for complications (e.g., meningitis, orbital cellulitis or abscess, brain abscess)

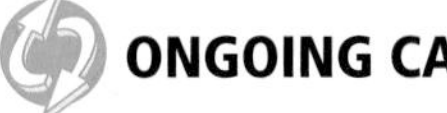

ONGOING CARE

FOLLOW-UP RECOMMENDATIONS

- Return if no improvement after 72 hours or no resolution of symptoms after 10 days of antibiotics.
- If symptoms resolve, no follow-up is needed.

PATIENT EDUCATION

- http://familydoctor.org
- http://medlineplus.gov

PROGNOSIS

Alleviation of symptoms within 72 hours with complete resolution within 10–14 days

COMPLICATIONS

- Serious complications are rare.
- Meningitis, orbital cellulitis, brain abscess
- Cavernous sinus thrombosis
- Osteomyelitis, subdural empyema

REFERENCES

1. Dykewicz MS, Hamilos DL, et al. Rhinitis and sinusitis. *J Allergy Clin Immunol*. 2010;125: S103–15.
2. Varonen H, Mäkelä M, Savolainen S, et al. Comparison of ultrasound, radiography, and clinical examination in the diagnosis of acute maxillary sinusitis: a systematic review. *J Clin Epidemiol*. 2000;53:940–8.
3. Williams JW Jr, et al. Antibiotics for acute maxillary sinusitis. *Cochrane Database Sys Rev*. 2003;2: CD000243.
4. Zalmanovici A, et al. Steroids for acute sinusitis. *Cochrane Database Sys Rev*. 2007;2:CD005149.

ADDITIONAL READING

- Anon JB, Jacobs MR, Poole MD, et al. Antimicrobial treatment guidelines for acute bacterial rhinosinusitis. *Otolaryngol Head Neck Surg*. 2004;130:1–45.
- Rosenfeld RM, Andes D, Bhattacharyya N, et al. Clinical practice guideline: Adult sinusitis. *Otolaryngol Head Neck Surg*. 2007;137:S1–31.
- Sande MA, Gwaltney JM. Acute community-acquired bacterial sinusitis: Continuing challenges and current management. *Clin Infect Dis*. 2004;39(Suppl 3):S151–8.

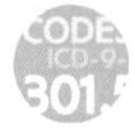

CODES

ICD9

- 461.3 Acute sphenoidal sinusitis
- 461.9 Acute sinusitis, unspecified
- 473.9 Unspecified sinusitis (chronic)

CLINICAL PEARLS

- When bacterial infection is present, patients recover somewhat more quickly with antibiotics, but the majority will recover with symptomatic treatment alone, and accurate diagnosis of bacterial sinusitis is very difficult (3)[A].
- Multiple meta-analyses have demonstrated *no* benefit of newer antibiotics over amoxicillin, trimethoprim-sulfamethoxazole, or doxycycline (3)[A].
- Overall NNT to prevent 1 persistent case at follow-up = 15; NNT-H (harm) due to antibiotic-associated diarrhea is similar.
- Significant patient symptom relief with nasal saline spray or drops or irrigation (Neti pot)

SJÖGREN SYNDROME

Katrina Darlene Zedan, MSPAS, PA-C
Alyssa H. Tran, DO

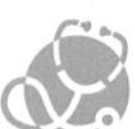

BASICS

- Chronic inflammatory disorder characterized by lymphocytic infiltrates in exocrine organs
- Typically presents with diminished salivary and lacrimal gland function, manifested as sicca symptoms such as:
  – Dry eyes, dry mouth, and enlargement of the parotid glands
  – Extraglandular symptoms may also be present, such as arthralgia, arthritis, Raynaud phenomenon, myalgia, pulmonary disease, GI disease, leukopenia, anemia, lymphadenopathy, neuropathy, vasculitis, renal tubular acidosis, and lymphoma.
- Primary Sjögren: Not associated with other diseases
- Secondary Sjögren: Complication of other rheumatologic conditions, most commonly rheumatoid arthritis
- The disease is named after Swedish ophthalmologist Henrik Sjögren (1899–1986), who first described it (1).

EPIDEMIOLOGY

Incidence

- Depending on the study, annual incidence is about 4/100,000–4.8% of population. Variability is likely due to the different criteria used in diagnosis.
- People of all races are affected.
- Predominant sex: Female > Male (9:1)
- Predominant age: Can affect patients of any age, but is most common in the elderly; onset typically occurs in the fourth to fifth decades of life

Prevalence

Sjögren syndrome (SS) affects 1–4 million people in the US.

RISK FACTORS

There are no known modifiable risk factors.

Genetics

Sjögren syndrome has a familial tendency and seems to be associated with family members with a wide variety of autoimmune diseases.

GENERAL PREVENTION

- No known prevention, but complications can be prevented by diagnosing and treating early.
- Dentists can play a key role in early detection of SS as well as management of oral symptoms that result from salivary dysfunction (2)[A].

PATHOPHYSIOLOGY

- Systemic autoimmune disease
- Characterized by infiltration of glandular tissue primarily by CD4 T-lymphocytes
- A theory is that glandular epithelial cells present antigen to the T cells. Cytokine production then occurs, and there is also evidence for B-cell activation, resulting in autoantibody production and increased incidence of B-cell malignancies.

ETIOLOGY

Etiology is unknown. Estrogen may play a role because SS is more common in women.

COMMONLY ASSOCIATED CONDITIONS

May be primary or secondary (associated with rheumatoid arthritis, scleroderma, systemic lupus erythematosus [SLE], polymyositis, HIV, hepatitis C)

DIAGNOSIS

- There is no single diagnostic test. Diagnosis is made by presence of compatible clinical signs and symptoms, as well as lab tests, and after exclusion of other causes.
- International consensus criteria for SS (3)[C]:
  – Ocular signs and symptoms (at least 1 present):
    ○ Persistent, troublesome dry eyes every day for longer than 3 months
    ○ Recurrent sensation of sand or gravel in the eyes *or*
    ○ Use of tear substitute >3 times/d
  – Oral signs and symptoms (at least 1 present):
    ○ Feeling of dry mouth every day for at least 3 months
    ○ Recurrent feeling of swollen salivary glands as an adult *or*
    ○ Need to drink liquids to aid in swallowing dry foods
  – Objective evidence of dry eyes (at least 1 present):
    ○ Schirmer test
    ○ Rose bengal
    ○ Lacrimal gland biopsy sample with focus score >1
  – Objective evidence of salivary gland involvement (at least 1 present):
    ○ Salivary gland scintigraphy
    ○ Parotid sialography
    ○ Unstimulated whole sialometry
  – Laboratory abnormality (at least 1 present):
    ○ Anti-SS-A or anti-SS-B
    ○ Antinuclear antibodies (ANAs)
    ○ IgM rheumatoid factor (anti-IgG Fc)
- Exclusion criteria: Prior head/neck irradiation, infection with hepatitis C, AIDS, lymphoma, sarcoidosis, graft-versus-host disease, recent use of anticholinergic medications (3)[C]
- Patients who fulfill 4 or more of the criteria likely have SS.

HISTORY

- Decreased tear production, burning, scratchy sensation in eyes
- Difficulty speaking/swallowing; dental caries; xerotrachea
- Enlarged parotid glands or intermittent swelling (bilateral)
- Dyspareunia

PHYSICAL EXAM

Common physical exam findings include:

- Eye exam: Dry eyes (keratoconjunctivitis sicca), decreased tear pool in the lower conjunctiva, dilated conjunctival vessels, mucinous threads, and filamentary keratosis can be detected during a slit-lamp examination.
- Mouth exam: Dry mouth (xerostomia), decreased sublingual salivary pool, tongue may stick to the tongue depressor, frequent caries—sometimes in unusual locations such as the incisor surface and the gum line, deep red tongue from prolonged xerostomia
- Ear, nose, and throat exam: Bilateral parotid gland enlargement, submandibular gland enlargement
- Skin exam: Nonpalpable or palpable vasculitic purpura with lesions that are typically 2–3 mm in diameter and located on the lower extremities
- Other manifestations: Chronic arthritis, interstitial nephritis (40%), type I rheumatoid arthritis (20%), vasculitis (25%), vaginal dryness, pleuritis, pancreatitis

DIAGNOSTIC TESTS & INTERPRETATION

In addition to history and physical exam, the following tests are recommended when SS is suspected:

- Schirmer test
- Rose bengal test
- Basic labs, special labs (see below)
- MRI with fat suppression, chest x-ray, minor salivary gland biopsy

Lab

- Most have autoantibodies: +ANAs (95%), +RF (75%)
- In primary SS: +anti-Ro (anti SS-A, 56%) and +anti-La (anti-SS-B, 30%)

Initial lab tests

Preliminary lab workup:

- Basic labs: CBC with differential, BUN/creatinine (Cr), AST/ALT, ESR, C-reactive protein (CRP), urinalysis (UA)
- Special labs: ANA, rheumatoid factor (RF), anti-Ro/SS-A, anti-La/SS-B, anti-Sm, anti-RNP, anti-dsDNA, serum C3 and C4, cryoglobulins, SPEP, UPEP, IgM, IgG, IgA
- Other: HIV, hepatitis C, CXR, minor salivary gland biopsy, MRI with fat suppression

Imaging

Initial imaging studies may include (4)[C]:

- Imaging for xerostomia: Salivary gland scintigraphy (insensitive but highly specific)
- Parotid gland sialography (should not be used in acute parotitis)
- MRI (correlates well with salivary gland biopsy)

Initial approach

MRI with fat suppression (4)[B]

Diagnostic Procedures/Surgery

- Salivary gland biopsy: Used to confirm suspected diagnosis of SS or exclusion of other causes of xerostomia and bilateral gland enlargement
- Schirmer test (3)[B]
- Rose bengal test (3)[B]
- Perform a biopsy on the parotid gland if malignancy is suggested.
- Perform a biopsy on an enlarged lymph node to help rule out pseudolymphoma or lymphoma.

Pathological Findings

Salivary gland biopsy: Histology shows focal collections of lymphocytes; immunocytology shows that most of the lymphocytes are CD4+ T cells.

DIFFERENTIAL DIAGNOSIS

- Causes of ocular dryness: Hypovitaminosis A, decreased tear production unrelated to autoimmune process, chronic blepharitis or conjunctivitis, impaired blinking (i.e., due to Parkinson disease or Bell palsy), working long hours at a computer, infiltration of lacrimal glands (i.e., amyloidosis, lymphoma, sarcoidosis), low estrogen levels
- Causes of oral dryness: Anticholinergic medications, sialadenitis due to chronic obstruction, chronic viral infections (i.e., hepatitis C or HIV), irradiation of head and neck
- Causes of salivary gland swelling: Unilateral: bacterial infection, neoplasm; bilateral: acute or chronic viral infection (i.e., mumps, Epstein–Barr virus [EBV], coxsackievirus, echovirus, HIV, hepatitis C), granulomatous diseases (i.e., tuberculosis, sarcoidosis), malnutrition, alcoholism, bulimia, acromegaly, diabetes

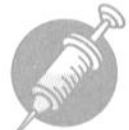

TREATMENT

- Treatment is primarily supportive care and treating symptoms that are problematic to patients.
- Treatment of dry eyes
- Topical therapy for dry mouth
- Treatment of systemic manifestations
- Addressing fatigue, vague complaints, and pain syndromes

MEDICATION

- Usually only requires local therapy for sicca symptoms: secretions and tears
- Immunosuppressive therapy such as hydroxychloroquine can be used for systemic symptoms; however, it has not shown any benefit in relieving refractory sicca symptoms.
- Topical therapy for dry mouth: Can be as simple as liberally drinking sips of water, trying sugar-free lemon drops or artificial saliva preparations such as Salivart, Saliment, Xero-Lube, Mouthkote (5)
- Depends on the severity of eye dryness, which is best determined by an ophthalmologist. Dry eyes are graded according to degree of symptoms, conjunctival injection and staining, corneal damage, tear quality, and lid involvement. Artificial tears may be used; however, artificial tears with hydroxymethylcellulose or dextran are more viscous and can last longer.
- Acetaminophen or NSAIDs can be taken for arthralgias.

First Line

- Xerostomia: Sugar-free lozenges, especially malic acid (4)[B], pilocarpine (4)[A], cevimeline (dose of 30 mg t.i.d. showed significant improvement (4)[A], artificial saliva
- Keratoconjunctivitis sicca: Artificial tears and ocular lubricants for symptomatic relief (4)[C], topical cyclosporine (4)[A]

Second Line

- Xerostomia: Interferon-alfa lozenges may enhance salivary gland flow (4)[B].
- Keratoconjunctivitis sicca: Emerging therapies include diquafosol (pending FDA approval) and topical NSAIDs (use with caution).
- Immunosuppressive therapy: Antimalarials (e.g., hydroxychloroquine) for arthralgias, lymphadenopathies, and skin manifestations (4)[B]; may then consider methotrexate or cyclosporine, which showed subjective improvement but no significant objective improvement
- Early studies show improvement in fatigue with rituximab (6)[B].
- For life-threatening extraglandular manifestations, cyclophosphamide (PO or IV), mycophenolate mofetil, and azathioprine are often used.

ADDITIONAL TREATMENT

- Patients should use vaginal lubricants, such as Replens, for vaginal dryness. Vaginal estrogen creams can be considered in postmenopausal women. Watch for and treat vaginal yeast infections (5).
- Xerostomia: Small sips of water, good dental care
- Keratoconjunctivitis sicca: Conservation of tears with side shields or ski/swim goggles, humidifiers, moist washcloths
- DHEA does not offer improvement in fatigue and well-being greater than placebo (7)[B].

Issues for Referral

- Systemic manifestations or resistant symptoms
- Rheumatology, as a rheumatologist is key in the management of patients with Sjögren syndrome
- Dentistry, for routine oral care is necessary
- Ophthalmology, for grading of severity of eye dryness

COMPLEMENTARY AND ALTERNATIVE MEDICINE

Studies show unclear and conflicting data on the efficacy of acupuncture.

SURGERY/OTHER PROCEDURES

Keratoconjunctivitis sicca: If refractory to artificial tears, punctal occlusion is the treatment of choice.

IN-PATIENT CONSIDERATIONS

May be required for extraglandular manifestations, such as cardiopulmonary disease, renal involvement, and CNS manifestations (e.g., optic neuritis, transverse myelitis, vasculitis, or ischemic stroke)

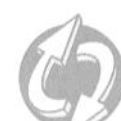

ONGOING CARE

FOLLOW-UP RECOMMENDATIONS

Frequency of follow-up depends on severity.

Patient Monitoring

- Monitor for complications, systemic manifestations, and relief of symptoms.
- Medicolegal pitfalls: Failure to monitor and evaluate for parotid tumor or lymphoma

PATIENT EDUCATION

Explanation of SS is essential. In most cases, simple measures are adequate, such as humidifiers, sips of water, chewing gum, or artificial tears.

PROGNOSIS

- Risk of lymphoma is increased.
- Hypocomplementemia is an independent risk factor for premature death.

COMPLICATIONS

Complications include dental caries, gum disease, dysphagia, salivary gland calculi, keratitis, conjunctivitis, and scarring of the ocular surface.

REFERENCES

1. Ramos-Casals M, Tzioufas AG, Stone JH, et al. Treatment of primary Sjögren syndrome: A systematic review. *JAMA*. 2010;304:452–60.
2. Stewart CM, Berg KM, Cha S, et al. Salivary dysfunction and quality of life in Sjogren syndrome: A critical oral-systemic connection. *J Am Dent Assoc*. 2008;139:291–9.
3. Fox RI. Sjogren's syndrome. *Lancet*. 2005;366:321.
4. von Bültzingslöwen I, Sollecito TP, Fox PC, et al. Salivary dysfunction associated with systemic diseases: Systematic review and clinical management recommendations. *Oral Surg Oral Med Oral Pathol Oral Radiol Endod*. 2007; 103(Suppl):S57.e1–15.
5. Miller AV, et al. Sjogren syndrome: Treatment & medications. Available at: http://emedicine.medscape.com/article/332125-treatment. Assessed: 8/21/2010.
6. Dass S, Bowman SJ, Vital EM, et al. Reduction of fatigue in Sjogren's syndrome with rituximab: Results of a randomised, double-blind, placebo controlled pilot study. *Ann Rheum Dis*. 2008; 67(11):1541–4.
7. Hartkamp A, Geenen R, Godaert GL, et al. Effect of dehydroepiandrosterone administration on fatigue, well-being, and functioning in women with primary Sjogren's syndrome. A randomized controlled trial. *Ann Rheum Dis*. 2008;67(1):91–7.
8. Fischer A, Swigris JJ, du Bois RM, et al. Minor salivary gland biopsy to detect primary Sjogren syndrome in patients with interstitial lung disease. *Chest*. 2009;136(4):1072–8.

ADDITIONAL READING

- Gálvez J, Sáiz E, López P, et al. Diagnostic evaluation and classification criteria in Sjögren's syndrome. *Joint Bone Spine*. 2009;76(1):44–9.
- Voulgarelis M, Tzioufas AG, Moutsopoulos HM. Mortality in Sjögren's syndrome. *Clin Exp Rheumatol*. 2008;26:S66–71.

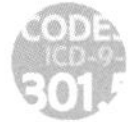

CODES

ICD9

710.2 Sicca syndrome

CLINICAL PEARLS

- Many symptoms can be treated with nonprescription interventions such as artificial tears and sugar-free lozenges.
- Consider lacrimal duct plugs for dry eyes (placed under local anesthetic by an ophthalmologist).
- Consider minor salivary gland biopsy to confirm diagnosis in the setting of interstitial lung disease (8)[B].

S

SLEEP APNEA, OBSTRUCTIVE

Anjali Koka, MD

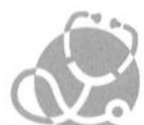

BASICS

DESCRIPTION

- Obstructive sleep apnea (OSA) is defined as repetitive episodes of cessation of airflow (apnea) at the nose and mouth during sleep due to obstruction at the level of the pharynx:
  - Apneas often terminate with a snort or gasp.
  - Repetitive apneas produce sleep disruption, leading to excessive daytime sleepiness.
  - Associated with oxygen desaturation and nocturnal hypoxemia
  - Usual course is chronic
- System(s) affected: Cardiovascular; Nervous; Pulmonary
- Synonym(s): Pickwickian syndrome; Sleep apnea syndrome; Nocturnal upper airway occlusion

EPIDEMIOLOGY

Incidence

- Predominant age: Middle-aged men and women
- Predominant sex: Male > Female (2–3:1)

Prevalence

- Up to 4% in men, 2% in women
- Prevalence is higher in obese or hypertensive patients.

RISK FACTORS

- Obesity
- Male sex
- Age >40 years
- Alcohol/sedative intake before bedtime
- Smoking
- Nasal obstruction (due to polyps, rhinitis, or deviated septum)
- Anatomic narrowing of nasopharynx (e.g., tonsillar hypertrophy, macroglossia, micrognathia, retrognathia, craniofacial abnormalities)
- Acromegaly
- Hypothyroidism
- Neurologic syndromes (e.g., muscular dystrophy, cerebral palsy)

GENERAL PREVENTION

Weight loss and avoidance of alcohol and sedatives at night can help to prevent airway collapse.

PATHOPHYSIOLOGY

OSA occurs when the naso- or oropharynx collapses passively during inspiration. Anatomic and neuromuscular factors contribute to pharyngeal collapse:

- Anatomic abnormalities, such as increased soft tissue in the palate, tonsillar hypertrophy, macroglossia, and craniofacial abnormalities, predispose the airway to collapse by decreasing the area of the upper airway or by increasing the pressure surrounding the airway.
- During sleep, decreased muscle tone in the naso- or oropharynx contributes to airway obstruction and collapse.

ETIOLOGY

Upper airway narrowing may be due to:

- Obesity, redundant tissue in the soft palate
- Enlarged tonsils or uvula
- Low soft palate
- Large or posteriorly located tongue
- Craniofacial abnormalities
- Neuromuscular disorders
- Alcohol or sedative use before bedtime

COMMONLY ASSOCIATED CONDITIONS

- Hypertension (common)
- Obesity (common)
- Daytime sleepiness (common)
- Metabolic syndrome (common)
- Cardiac arrhythmias (rare)
- Cardiovascular diseases such as myocardial infarction and stroke (rare)
- Congestive heart failure (rare)
- Pulmonary hypertension (rare)
- Nasal obstructive problems (rare)

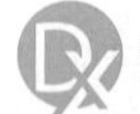

DIAGNOSIS

HISTORY

Be sure to elicit a complete history of daytime and nighttime symptoms. Symptoms can be insidious and present for years:

- Daytime symptoms:
  - Excessive daytime sleepiness (EDS) or fatigue (cardinal symptom):
    - Mild symptoms occur during quiet activities (e.g., reading, watching television).
    - Severe symptoms occur during dynamic activities (e.g., work, driving).
  - Tired on morning awakening
  - Sore or dry throat
  - Poor concentration, memory problems, irritability, mood changes
  - Morning headaches
  - Decreased libido
  - Depression
- Nighttime symptoms:
  - Loud snoring (present in 60% of people with OSA)
  - Snort or gasp that arouses patient from sleep
  - Disrupted sleep
  - Witnessed apneic episodes at night

PHYSICAL EXAM

- Most patients have a normal physical exam. However, OSA is commonly associated with hypertension, obesity, or sleepiness.
- Focused head and neck exam:
  - Short neck with large circumference
  - Oropharynx:
    - Narrowing of the lateral airway wall
    - Tonsillar hypertrophy
    - Macroglossia
    - Micrognathia or retrognathia
    - Soft palate edema
    - Long or thick uvula
    - High, arched hard palate
  - Nasopharynx:
    - Deviated nasal septum
    - Poor nasal airflow

DIAGNOSTIC TESTS & INTERPRETATION

Lab

Initial lab tests

When clinically indicated:

- Thyroid-stimulating hormone to evaluate hypothyroidism
- CBC to evaluate anemia and polycythemia, which can indicate nocturnal hypoxemia
- Fasting glucose in obesity to evaluate for diabetes
- Rare: Arterial blood gases to evaluate daytime hypercapnia

Imaging

Cephalometric measurements from lateral head and neck radiographs aid in surgical treatment.

Diagnostic Procedures/Surgery

- The gold standard for OSA is polysomnography (PSG), a nighttime sleep study:
  - Demonstrates severity of hypoxemia, sleep disruption, and cardiac arrhythmias associated with OSA and elevated end-tidal CO_2
  - Shows repetitive episodes of cessation or marked reduction in airflow despite continued respiratory efforts
  - Apneic episodes must last at least 10 seconds and occur 10–15×/hr to be considered clinically significant.
  - Complete PSG is expensive, and health insurance may not cover the cost.
- Multiple sleep latency testing is a diagnostic tool used to measure the time it takes from the start of a daytime nap period to the first signs of sleep (sleep latency). It provides an objective measurement of daytime sleepiness.
- The apnea/hypoapnea index (AHI) is defined as the total number of apneas and hypopneas divided by the total sleep time:
  - Mild OSA: AHI = 5–15
  - Moderate OSA: AHI = 15–30
  - Severe OSA: AHI >30
- Drugs that may alter the test results include benzodiazepines and other sedatives that can amplify the severity of apnea seen during the sleep study.

DIFFERENTIAL DIAGNOSIS

- Other causes of excessive daytime sleepiness, such as:
  - Narcolepsy
  - Idiopathic daytime hypersomnolence
  - Inadequate sleep time
  - Depressive episodes with excessive daytime sleepiness
  - Periodic limb movements disorder
- Respiratory disorders with nocturnal awakenings, such as:
  - Asthma
  - Chronic obstructive pulmonary disease
  - Congestive heart failure
- Central sleep apnea
- Sleep-related choking or laryngospasm
- Gastroesophageal reflux
- Sleep-associated seizures (temporal lobe epilepsy)

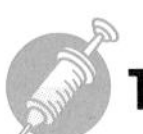

TREATMENT

- Weight loss
- Avoid alcohol, smoking, and sedatives, especially before bedtime.
- Significantly sleepy patients should not drive a motor vehicle or operate dangerous equipment.
- The most effective treatment for OSA is nasal continuous positive airway pressure (CPAP). The CPAP mask fits over the nose or nose and mouth and acts as a pneumatic stent to prevent soft tissue in the pharynx from collapsing, thus eliminating apneas and restoring oxygen saturation. CPAP restores regular nighttime breathing and not only reduces snoring and EDS, but also lowers BP over the short term (1)[A] and may also decrease the risk for stroke (2)[C] and atherosclerosis (2)[C].
- CPAP therapy initially can be difficult to tolerate and requires perseverance.
- If OSA is present only when supine, keep the patient off his or her back when sleeping (e.g., tennis ball worn on back of nightshirt).
- Dental appliances advance the mandible and tongue, helping the airway to stay open during sleep. When compared with nasal CPAP, dental appliances decreased AHI to a lesser extent (3)[C].
- CPAP has been shown to improve OSA symptoms better than dental appliances. However, patients who are unable to tolerate CPAP may benefit from dental appliances.
- Surgical treatments (described below) are directed at opening up the oropharynx to relieve airway obstruction.

MEDICATION

Medications are yet to be proven effective in treating OSA (4)[A]. Further studies in this area are needed.

First Line

Some short-term data found fluticasone nasal spray, mirtazapine, physostigmine, and nasal lubricant of some benefit; longer-term studies needed (4)[A].

ADDITIONAL TREATMENT

Issues for Referral

If sleep apnea is suspected, patient should be referred to a sleep specialist/neurologist for a sleep study evaluation.

SURGERY/OTHER PROCEDURES

Surgical corrections of the upper airway include uvulopalatopharyngoplasty (UPPP), tracheostomy, and craniofacial surgery. Studies to assess the efficacy of UPPP to improve symptoms of OSA are indeterminant (5)[C],6[A].

IN-PATIENT CONSIDERATIONS

On admission, patients should continue to use CPAP or dental devices if they do so at home. They should bring in their own appliance and know their CPAP settings.

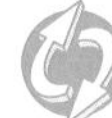

ONGOING CARE

Lifelong compliance with weight loss or CPAP is necessary for successful OSA treatment.

DIET

Overweight patients must lose weight, and all patients must avoid weight gain. Weight loss alone can relieve symptoms of OSA.

PATIENT EDUCATION

- Weight loss and avoidance of alcohol and sedatives can improve OSA symptoms.
- Avoid driving if excessive daytime sleepiness is significant.

PROGNOSIS

- EDS improves dramatically with appropriate apnea control.
- Lifelong compliance with weight loss or CPAP is necessary for effective treatment of OSA.
- If untreated, OSA is progressive.
- Significant morbidity and mortality due to OSA usually are due to motor vehicle accidents or secondary to cardiac complications, including arrhythmias, cardiac ischemia, and hypertension.

COMPLICATIONS

Untreated OSA may increase the risk for development of hypertension, stroke, myocardial infarction, diabetes, cardiovascular disease, and work-related and driving accidents.

Pediatric Considerations

- The prevalence of pediatric OSA is 1–2% in children 4–5 years of age, and the peak incidence is between 3 and 6 years of age. Predominant sex: Male = Female.
- Etiology: The most common cause is tonsillar hypertrophy. Additional causes are obesity and craniofacial abnormalities. OSA is also seen in children with neuromuscular diseases, such as cerebral palsy and spinal muscular atrophy, due to abnormal pharyngeal muscle control.
- Signs and symptoms:
  - Nighttime: Loud snoring, restlessness, and sweating
  - Daytime: Hyperactivity and decreased school performance
  - EDS is not a significant symptom.
- Diagnosis: Gold standard is PSG. Abnormal AHI is different in children: >1–2/h is abnormal.
- Treatment: Surgery is the first-line treatment in cases due to tonsillar enlargement (improves symptoms in 70%). Some data suggest improved academic performance if tonsillectomy is performed for OSA. For cases due to obesity or craniofacial abnormalities, patients can use CPAP treatment.

REFERENCES

1. Giles T, et al. Continuous positive airways pressure for obstructive sleep apnoea in adults. *Cochrane Database Syst Rev*. 2007;(1):CD001106.
2. Drager LF, Bortolotto LA, Figueiredo AC, et al. Effects of continuous positive airway pressure on early signs of atherosclerosis in obstructive sleep apnea. *Am J Respir Crit Care Med*. 2007;176: 706–12.
3. Petri N, Svanholt P, Solow B, et al. Mandibular advancement appliance for obstructive sleep apnoea: Results of a randomised placebo controlled trial using parallel group design. *J Sleep Res*. 2008;17:221–9.
4. Smith I, Lasserson TJ, Wright J. Drug therapy for obstructive sleep apnoea in adults. *Cochrane Database Syst Rev*. 2006:CD003002.
5. Shine NP, Lewis RH. Transpalatal advancement pharyngoplasty for obstructive sleep apnea syndrome: Results and analysis of failures. *Arch Otolaryngol Head Neck Surg*. 2009;135(5):434–8.
6. Sundaram S, Bridgman SA, Lim J, et al. Surgery for obstructive sleep apnoea. *Cochrane Database Syst Rev*. 2005:CD001004.

ADDITIONAL READING

- Kato M, Adachi T, Koshino Y, et al. Obstructive sleep apnea and cardiovascular disease. *Circ J*. 2009;73:1363–70.
- Lim J, Lasserson TJ, Fleetham J, et al. Oral appliances for obstructive sleep apnoea. *Cochrane Database Syst Rev*. 2004:CD004435.
- Redline S, Yenokyan G, Gottlieb DJ, et al. Obstructive sleep apnea-hypopnea and incident stroke: The sleep heart health study. *Am J Respir Crit Care Med*. 2010;182(2):269–77.

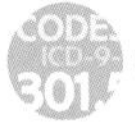

CODES

ICD9

327.23 Obstructive sleep apnea (adult) (pediatric)

CLINICAL PEARLS

- OSA is characterized by repetitive episodes of apnea at the pharynx often terminating in a snort or gasp.
- PSG is a key to diagnosis.
- CPAP is standard medical treatment.
- Central sleep apnea may mimic OSA.

SLEEP DISORDER, CIRCADIAN RHYTHM

Adam J. Sorscher, MD

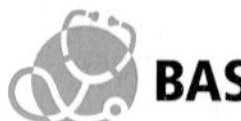

BASICS

DESCRIPTION

- Circadian rhythm sleep disorders (CRSDs) are a family of conditions that occur when an individual's preferred timing of sleep is not well synchronized with commitments to job, school, family, or social engagements. In CRSDs, intrinsic sleep is normal (i.e., there is no sleep fragmenting condition such as obstructive sleep apnea or periodic limb movement disorder). However, when forced by obligations to attempt sleep at nonpreferred times, individuals with CRSDs complain of both sleep-initiation insomnia and excessive daytime sleepiness. These symptoms resolve entirely *if the individual is allowed to sleep at his/her preferred time*. This topic addresses circadian rhythm disorder, delayed-phase type.
- Circadian rhythm sleep disorder, delayed-phase type (CRSD-DPT) is marked by a stable but persistent inability to initiate sleep at a desired time. Individuals are typically unable to initiate sleep until 3–6 hours later than societal norms (i.e., after 2 a.m.), and this frequently results in insufficient sleep/sleepiness in the day that follows.

EPIDEMIOLOGY

CRSD-DPT is the most common circadian rhythm disorder seen by referral in sleep medicine clinics (1).

Prevalence

CRSD-DPT has an estimated prevalence of 0.1–0.2% in the general population. It is most common in adolescents with a prevalence of 7–16%.

RISK FACTORS

CRSD-DPT primarily affects adolescents and young adults who have a biologic tendency to delay the onset of sleep yet often need to be up early for school or work responsibilities.

Genetics

There is emerging evidence of a genetic component to both CRSD-DPT and morning/evening preference. In 1 familial case report, CRSD-DPT was shown to occur in an autosomal dominant inheritance pattern. Polymorphisms in circadian rhythm genes such as *hPer3* and *clock* among individuals with CRSD-DPT constitute evidence of a genetic component to the disorder (2).

GENERAL PREVENTION

In CRSD-DPT (and all CRSDs), careful attention to sleep hygiene is necessary to establish and maintain a desired sleep schedule. A thorough list of sleep hygiene measures is downloadable from the Internet. The most important behavioral practices to prevent an undesirably late fall-asleep time are: Maintain a regular sleep/wake schedule 7 days per week, avoid napping, and minimize caffeine and stimulants. People with CRSD-DPT need to avoid stimulating activities in the evening, such as computer, TV, and social interactions, which may exacerbate the tendency to delay the onset of sleep. A 30-minute "wind-down" time prior to bedtime in which homework, socializing, and electronic devices are off-limits is helpful. Adolescents who sleep ad lib on the weekends (sometimes into the afternoon) often find that they have especially great difficulty initiating sleep on Sunday night and thus get the week off to a bad start; to prevent this, they should be advised to arise at a similar time on weekends as compared to the school/work mornings.

PATHOPHYSIOLOGY

In all mammals, an oscillating signal from the suprachiasmatic nucleus (SCN) in the anterior hypothalamus establishes circadian rhythms, including the propensity to be awake or asleep. The average period of this signal in humans is 24.2 hours. Certain factors, most significantly light, can shift the timing of the circadian rhythm and thereby synchronize it to the shorter environmental cycle day-by-day. CRSD-DPT and other circadian rhythm disorders occur when the circadian rhythm is not adequately synchronized to the shorter 24-hour environmental cycle creating a mismatch between the two. Some theories to account for inadequate synchronization are that it occurs in individuals who have an abnormally long circadian period (>25 hours) or whose circadian clock does not properly respond to synchronizing agents such as light.

ETIOLOGY

CRSD-DPT is the result of biologic, behavioral, and psychosocial factors. Release of melatonin from the pineal gland in the evening initiates a cascade of events that usually triggers sleep behavior several hours later. Studies suggest that the timing of melatonin release within the circadian cycle is delayed by 40–120 minutes in later adolescence compared to prepuberty. This suggests that the tendency for teenagers to delay sleep onset is largely a genetically programmed developmental phenomenon. In addition, behaviors such as ingestion of caffeine, physical activity and light exposure in the evening, and stimulating activities (computer, TV, texting, etc.) all exacerbate the innate tendency to delay sleep onset. The relative contributions of genetically ordained endogenous factors (the shifting of the circadian pattern) vs. voluntary behaviors that delay bedtime are not fully delineated. Finally, it can be argued that Western societies, in which high schools and jobs tend to start early in the morning are simply at odds with human circadian rhythms. CRSD-DPT would undoubtedly be less prevalent if school and work start times were later.

DIAGNOSIS

HISTORY

People with CRSD-DPT report both sleep initiation insomnia and excessive sleepiness in the daytime. They struggle to awaken for school/work in the morning. Careful questioning should explore for competing/comorbid causes of insomnia (poor sleep hygiene, significant mental health disorders, restless legs syndrome, and medical conditions/medication side effects) and for competing/comorbid causes of hypersomnolence (symptoms of narcolepsy and obstructive sleep apnea, voluntary insufficient sleep, and medication side effects). Individuals with psychophysiological insomnia (psychologically conditioned arousal when attempting to initiate sleep) do not usually experience genuine hypersomnolence in the daytime despite short sleep times overnight. Those who voluntarily stay up late and obtain insufficient sleep do not report insomnia when they do attempt to initiate sleep. In contrast to the other disorders in the differential, people with CRSD-DPT will usually assert that they would have no complaint about sleep or wakefulness if they were simply allowed to sleep at their preferred time (e.g., they do not have sleep/wakefulness issues when on summer vacation from school).

PHYSICAL EXAM

Explore for features of sleep apnea: Obesity/large neck circumference; hypertension, crowded oropharynx. Physical exam (PE) is otherwise unrevealing.

DIAGNOSTIC TESTS & INTERPRETATION

The diagnosis of CRSD-DPT is made primarily by thorough history-taking (see above). Sleep logs (downloadable from the Internet) completed over 3 weeks time graphically reveal fall-asleep times that are consistently 3–6 hours later than societal norms and much later wake-up times (not infrequently in the afternoon) on days off from school/work (3)[C]. Wrist actigraphy (using a wristwatch-like device with an accelerometer), worn for 3 weeks, also provides an accurate display of sleep and wake timing but is currently not reimbursable and is not needed if the individual can complete sleep logs (3)[B].

Lab

Testing in the sleep lab is not indicated unless there is suspicion of comorbid intrinsic disorders of sleep, such as sleep apnea, narcolepsy, or parasomnias (unusual behaviors arising out of sleep) (see also "Issues for Referral"). No other lab tests are necessary.

DIFFERENTIAL DIAGNOSIS

CRSDs are unique in that they are marked by the twin complaints of insomnia when attempting to sleep *and* hypersomnolence in the wake period. Usually, other sleep disorders cause either insomnia or hypersomnolence (see "History" section) but not both. In contrast to other sleep/wakefulness disorders, symptoms of CRSDs resolve entirely if the individual is allowed to sleep at their preferred time.

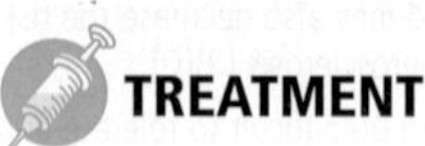

TREATMENT

- The goal of treatment in CRSD-DPT is to help the individual consistently initiate sleep at an earlier time. The principal therapies to achieve a shift in sleep/wake timing are light and melatonin (factors that shift the circadian rhythm are also called *zeitgebers)* (4)[A]. Comparatively, light is much more potent than melatonin in its phase-shifting ability. The phase-shifting effects of light and melatonin are depicted in the phase-response curve. Key points: Light will advance sleep onset to an earlier time if provided in the last 1/3 of the sleep period or for several hours immediately after arising. Proper timing is critical, since exposure to light in the evening or in the initial 2/3 of the sleep period will further delay sleep onset. For melatonin, the most potent phase-advancing occurs if it is provided in the evening, 5–6 hours before an individual's usual sleep onset time.
- Use the following rules to guide prescribing of light and melatonin in order to advance sleep phase (5)[A]:
  – There is no single rule for intensity, duration, or wavelength for light therapy. Most protocols employ a 2,500–10,000 lux full-spectrum light box, set 2–3 feet from the individual for 30–120 minutes. A common prescription is 10,000 lux box for 30 minutes upon awakening in the morning. Sunlight, when present in warm weather seasons, is also effective. Retailers for full-spectrum light boxes abound on the Internet.

– Prescribe exposure to full-spectrum light immediately upon awakening (Note: Though the phase-advancing effect of light is actually greatest if it is provided immediately after the body temperature nadir that occurs ~2/3 through the sleep period, the strategy of waiting until the habitual waking time is preferred for these reasons: (a) it acknowledges that it is onerous for the individual to wake up artificially early for light therapy and (b) it minimizes the risk of unintentionally providing light *before* the temperature nadir, which further delays the sleep phase).
– Light exposure in the evening has the effect of delaying sleep phase and worsening CRSD-DPT. Instruct individuals to limit light exposure in the evening (consider using sunglasses or curtailing outdoors activities in warm weather months).
– Contraindications to phototherapy include retinopathy, photosensitivity, and bipolar disorder.
– Prescribe melatonin to be taken 5–6 hours before the habitual (usual) fall-asleep time, not at bedtime. Melatonin in minute doses is as effective as higher doses in producing phase-shift; therefore, use the lowest dose available—usually 1 or 3 mg.
– Melatonin has a weak sedating effect, and individuals should be counseled not to drive or operate dangerous machines after taking the medication.
– Once earlier sleep onset and wake-up occurs, adjust the timing of therapies every 3–5 days—continue to use light directly upon awakening; provide melatonin earlier and earlier in the evening corresponding to 5–6 hours before the newly observed fall asleep time.

MEDICATION

See description for use of melatonin above.

ADDITIONAL TREATMENT

- Chronotherapy is an older strategy in which the individual is instructed to delay sleep and wake times by 2–3 hours every 2–3 days, shifting their sleep cycle across the 24-hour day, until they reach their desired bedtime. Carried out over several weeks, this protocol is extremely disruptive to daytime schedules and also has not been demonstrated to be effective. It is seldom used (3)[C].
- Some early reports suggested that vitamin B_{12} has circadian phase-shifting properties. This finding has not been confirmed in subsequent investigations, and there presently is no evidence of benefit to the use of this supplement in CRSDs (3).
- The use of sedative-hypnotic medications to treat the insomnia component and stimulant medications to treat daytime sleepiness has not been shown to be effective in the context of CRSD-DPT (5).

Issues for Referral

- Referral for evaluation and testing at a sleep clinic is not necessary in most cases of CRSD-DPT. The chief indications for referral are suspicion of the following comorbid disorders:
  – Obstructive sleep apnea: Indicated by loud snoring, obesity/large neck, witnessed apneas, and history of hypertension
  – Narcolepsy: Indicated by severe levels of daytime sleepiness despite adequate sleep quantity and sometimes accompanied by cataplexy (bouts of sudden muscular weakness triggered by strong emotions)
  – Parasomnias: Undesirable experiential or behavioral phenomena that arise out of sleep, such as dangerous sleepwalking or dream-enactment
- In addition, many individuals with the complaint of insomnia or sleepiness have comorbid mental health disorders, primarily depression and possibly substance abuse. Referral for mental health disorders or substance abuse treatment is indicated if these are present.

ONGOING CARE

CRSD-DPT is the product of both biologic and behavioral factors. Most individuals can successfully initiate sleep at an appropriate bedtime, but only if they are motivated to do so. Light and melatonin, provided at the proper time with respect to the circadian period, will cause an advance in the sleep phase. In addition to these measures, the primary care physician must remind the patient to practice healthy sleep behaviors (see "General Prevention") if they wish to maintain an earlier sleep/wake pattern.

REFERENCES

1. Weitzman ED, Czeisler CA, Coleman RM, et al. Delayed sleep phase syndrome. A chronobiological disorder with sleep-onset insomnia. *Arch Gen Psychiatry*. 1981;38:737–46.
2. Ebisawa T, Uchiyama M, Kajimura N, et al. Association of structural polymorphisms in the human period3 gene with delayed sleep phase syndrome. *EMBO Rep*. 2001;2:342–6.
3. Morgenthaler TI, Lee-Chiong T, Alessi C, et al. Practice parameters for the clinical evaluation and treatment of circadian rhythm sleep disorders. An American Academy of Sleep Medicine report. *Sleep*. 2007;30:1445–59.
4. Wilson SJ, Nutt DJ, Alford C, et al. British Association for Psychopharmacology consensus statement on evidence-based treatment of insomnia, parasomnias and circadian rhythm disorders. *J Psychopharmacol. (Oxford)*. 2010;24: 1577–601.
5. Sack RL, Auckley D, Auger RR, et al. Circadian rhythm sleep disorders: Part II, advanced sleep phase disorder, delayed sleep phase disorder, free-running disorder, and irregular sleep-wake rhythm. An American Academy of Sleep Medicine review. *Sleep*. 2007;30:1484–501.

ADDITIONAL READING

- Barion A, Zee PC, et al. A clinical approach to circadian rhythm sleep disorders. *Sleep Med*. 2007;8:566–77.
- Kanathur N, Harrington J, Lee-Chiong T, et al. Circadian rhythm sleep disorders. *Clin Chest Med*. 2010;31:319–25.

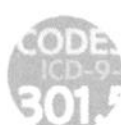

CODES

ICD9

- 327.30 Circadian rhythm sleep disorder, unspecified
- 327.31 Circadian rhythm sleep disorder, delayed sleep phase type
- 327.39 Other circadian rhythm sleep disorder

CLINICAL PEARLS

- The tendency to become night-owlish with adolescence is, to a large extent, a biologically programmed phenomenon, not strictly a behavioral choice. Enlightened public policy would recognize this and allow for later start times for high schools.
- CRSD-DPT can be diagnosed with careful history-taking and sleep logs; referral for formal sleep studies is usually not indicated.
- Use of light and melatonin can shift habitual sleep onset and offset time by their action on the human circadian rhythm.
- To maintain a desirable sleep phase, individuals with CRSD-DPT usually need to maintain meticulous attention to sleep hygiene, including a regular sleep/wake schedule 7 days per week, in order to avoid lapsing into a delayed phase pattern.

SLEEP DISORDER, SHIFT WORK

Lisa Shives, MD

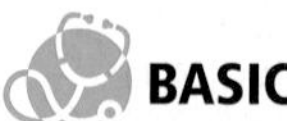

BASICS

DESCRIPTION

- The nomenclature of the *International Classifications of Sleep Disorders*, 2nd edition, calls this disorder circadian rhythm sleep disorder, shift work type, but in clinical practice, it is usually called shift work disorder (SWD). As the official name denotes, this is classified among the circadian rhythm sleep disorders.
- A universally accepted definition has not been consistently used in the research, but current best-practice standards require all the general criteria for circadian rhythm disorders be met (see below) and that the complaints are associated with night shifts, early morning shifts, or rotating shifts.
- General criteria for circadian rhythm disorders are the following:
  – There is a persistent or recurrent sleep disruption due to either an alteration in the circadian (24-hour) timekeeping system or due to a misalignment between endogenous circadian rhythm and exogenous factors that affect sleep.
  – There is a complaint of insomnia or excessive daytime sleepiness or both.
  – There is an impairment in occupational, educational, or social functioning.

EPIDEMIOLOGY

Incidence

Both incidence and prevalence depend on the number of shift workers in a given society, which can change over time. Therefore, the literature does not even estimate incidence.

Prevalence

- Epidemiologic data are rare but one study found that ~1/3 of night/rotating shift workers met the minimum criteria for SWD (1)[A].
- In the literature, it is often stated that ~20% of the population in industrialized countries performs shift work. Therefore, a rough estimate of the prevalence of SWD is 5%.

RISK FACTORS

Shift work, meaning night shifts, early morning shifts, or rotating shifts, is the obvious risk factor. There is great individual variability in tolerance for shift work that may indicate that certain individuals are at a greater risk for developing SWD is they perform shift work.

Genetics

No genetic predisposition has been described.

GENERAL PREVENTION

As shift work is surely here to stay in industrialized countries, it is best to focus on measures that make it more tolerable. They include the following:

- Limiting rotating shifts
- Using bright light during shifts
- Scheduling brief, 10–20-minute naps during the shifts if suitable

PATHOPHYSIOLOGY

- The common understanding is that every cell in the human body regulates its physiology according to a 24-hour (i.e., circadian) clock.
- The most powerful *zeitgeber*, or timekeeper, is light. It is not just a social convention that has us sleeping at night and up in the daytime; this is indeed the natural rhythm for most humans and it is difficult to work when both circadian and homeostatic forces are signaling sleep, and it is difficult to sleep when these forces are in alert mode.

ETIOLOGY

See above.

COMMONLY ASSOCIATED CONDITIONS

- Some evidence that SWD increases the risk of breast and prostate cancer such that the International Agency for Research on Cancer (IARC) has classified shift work that involves a circadian disruption as a probable carcinogen (2)[A].
- There are also association data that link SWD to increased risk of GI disease, specifically peptic ulcer disease, cardiovascular disease, infertility, and pregnancy complications.

DIAGNOSIS

This is primarily a clinical diagnosis. However, there are some useful diagnostic aids.

HISTORY

- A careful history is critical.
- Special attention should be paid to:
  – Sleep/wake habits
  – The sleep environment
  – Light exposure before, during, and after the shift
  – Medications as well as over-the-counter (OTC) stimulants such as caffeine and energy drinks
- It is also important to know patients' sleep/wake schedules when they have days off.
- It is essential to ask about other sleep disorders such as:
  – Snoring (obstructive sleep apnea [OSA])
  – Sudden sleep attacks and leg symptoms (restless legs syndrome [RLS])
  – Drop attacks and daytime fatigue (narcolepsy)

PHYSICAL EXAM

Evaluate for telltale signs of obstructive sleep apnea such as obesity, a large neck, and a tight oropharynx.

DIAGNOSTIC TESTS & INTERPRETATION

Although there is no real diagnostic test, there are some useful tools.

Lab

Because there is a possible increased risk for CVD and cancer among shift workers, consider appropriate screenings.

Initial lab tests

Fasting lipid panel, fasting glucose, age-appropriate cancer screenings

Imaging

None

Diagnostic Procedures/Surgery

- The 2 most widely used and recommended tools are sleep diaries and actigraphy (3)[A].
- Data should be collected for at least 1 week, but 2 weeks is preferable.
- There is no standard, validated sleep diary. Note that the terms "sleep diary" and "sleep log" are used interchangeably by sleep specialists.
- Some sleep specialists use actigraphy, which is a gross measure of time and amount of activity and rest.

Pathological Findings

Both the sleep diary and the actigraph data usually show the following:

- Increased sleep latency
- Decreased total sleep time
- Frequent awakenings
- They also usually show that most people revert to nocturnal sleeping on their days off, which means that every workweek, they start fresh in their attempts to shift their circadian rhythms in order to align with work schedules.

DIFFERENTIAL DIAGNOSIS

- Another primary sleep disorder such as OSA, RLS, narcolepsy, and psychophysiological insomnia. Keep in mind that shift workers often have another coexisting primary sleep disorder such as OSA in addition to and separate from their shift work disorder, which exacerbates symptoms.
- Another circadian rhythm sleep disorder such as delayed sleep phase disorder or jet lag syndrome. Distinguishing among these is challenging even for sleep specialists.

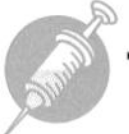

TREATMENT

- The American Academy of Sleep Medicine (AASM) published its most recent practice parameters for diagnosis and treatment of circadian rhythm sleep disorders, including SWD, in 2007.
- The only therapeutic modality deemed as "standard" treatment is planned (or prescribed) sleep schedules.
- Regular exercise on a schedule will help with sleep quality and daytime fatigue.
- The 2 most researched and commonly used treatments in clinical practice are bright light therapy and melatonin, although the research shows such mixed results that neither was ranked as a standard treatment (4)[A].

MEDICATION

- Much research has shown that melatonin may help shift circadian rhythms.
- Although melatonin has little soporific effect when given at night when endogenous levels are high anyway, some research has shown good results in its ability to shorten sleep latency when taken in the daytime, making it useful in treating SWD.
- Melatonin is not considered a medication by the FDA and its use in the treatment of SWD (or anything else) is not approved by the FDA.
- No reports of serious side effects have been reported with melatonin. There is a medication, ramelteon (Rozerem), which is a melatonin receptor agonist recently approved as a hypnotic.
- There is no good research on melatonin's use in circadian rhythm disorders.
- For excessive sleepiness, wakefulness-promoting medications (modafinil, armodafinil) may be very beneficial to the patient's quality of life.
- The use of hypnotics such as zolpidem received a "guideline" rating by the AASM.
- While stimulants are an "option" according to the AASM, modafinil, which is a wakefulness-promoting agent, received a guideline rating as a treatment modality.

First Line

Circadian shift/sleep promoting: Melatonin, 3 mg PO or sublingual, 30 minutes before daytime sleep period. It should be taken only when the patient is home and able to go to bed if the hypnotic effects begin.

Second Line

- Wakefulness-promoting:
  - Modafinil (Provigil) 100–200 mg PO 60 minutes before the shift begins.
  - Armodafinil (Nuvigil) 150–250 mg is long-acting (12–16 hours depending on food intake) and should be used judiciously in SWD so as to not impede a patient's ability to sleep after the shift.
- Hypnotic: Zolpidem (Ambien) 5–10 mg or eszopiclone (Lunesta) 2–3 mg 30 minutes before desired sleep period.

ADDITIONAL TREATMENT

General Measures

- Bright light therapy with conventional light or light boxes (10,000 lux preferable but >1,000 lux will help) should be given during the night or early morning shift.
- When night-shift workers are ending their shifts in the morning, bright light should be avoided. We recommend the use of dark sunglasses or special glasses that filter the blue wavelength, as well as a hat.

Issues for Referral

Reasons to refer to a sleep specialist: Suspicion of other primary sleep disorders; dependence on hypnotics, alcohol, or stimulants.

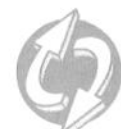

ONGOING CARE

PATIENT EDUCATION

- Health care providers should discuss good sleep hygiene and give advice on how to optimize the sleep environment.
- Shift workers who need to sleep in the daytime must take serious measures to ensure that their sleep environment is cool, dark, and quiet.
- Remove all telephones, including mobile phones, and disconnect the doorbell.
- Blackout shades are usually necessary in order to achieve the proper darkness. Patients need to understand that the single most powerful wake signal to the brain is light. They need to learn when to seek light and when to avoid it.

PROGNOSIS

Given how little the general public understands about good sleep habits and the importance of sleep, there is hope that with increased understanding, shift workers will learn the essential tactics needed to regulate their sleep/wake cycle. That said, there is certainly much individual variation in the ability to successfully manage shift work to the extent that some people simply cannot do it and maintain adequate function.

REFERENCES

1. Sack RL, Auckley D, Auger RR, et al. Circadian rhythm sleep disorders: Part I, basic principles, shift work and jet lag disorders. An American Academy of Sleep Medicine review. *Sleep.* 2007;30:1460–83.
2. Stevens RG, Hansen J, Costa G, et al. Considerations of circadian impact for defining "shift work" in cancer studies: IARC Working Group Report. *Occup Environ Med.* 2011;68: 154–62.
3. Morgenthaler TI, Lee-Chiong T, Alessi C, et al. Practice parameters for the clinical evaluation and treatment of circadian rhythm sleep disorders. An American Academy of Sleep Medicine report. *Sleep.* 2007;30:1445–59.
4. Bjorvatn B, Pallesen S, et al. A practical approach to circadian rhythm sleep disorders. *Sleep Med Rev.* 2009;13:47–60.

ADDITIONAL READING

Sleep Diary: http://www.helpguide.org/life/pdfs/sleep_diary.pdf.

CODES

ICD9

- 780.50 Sleep disturbance, unspecified
- 780.55 Disruption of 24 hour sleep wake cycle, unspecified

CLINICAL PEARLS

- Shift work is exceedingly and increasingly common in the industrialized world and is negatively impacting both the quality of life and the long-term health of many of those who perform shift work.
- Other primary sleep disorders commonly coexist (obstructive sleep apnea, restless leg syndrome) with and exacerbate shift work disorder, as do some OTC agents, like stimulants. There should be careful screening for OSA in particular among the shift-work population.
- It is essential to educate the shift worker about the effect that light has on his or her sleep/wake cycle.
- The most important first diagnostic step is to obtain a sleep diary.

S

SMELL AND TASTE DISORDERS

Beth Mazyck, MD
Daniel B. Kurtz, PhD

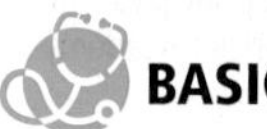

BASICS

DESCRIPTION

- The senses of smell and taste allow a full appreciation of the flavor and palatability of foods and also serve as a warning system against toxins, polluted air, smoke, and spoiled food.
- Physiologically, the chemical senses aid in normal digestion by triggering GI secretions. Smell or taste dysfunction may have a significant impact on quality of life.
- Loss of smell occurs more frequently than loss of taste, and patients frequently confuse the concepts of flavor loss (as a result of smell impairment) with taste loss (an impaired ability to sense sweet, sour, salty, or bitter).
- Smell depends on the functioning of CN I (olfactory nerve) and CN V (trigeminal nerve).
- Taste depends on the functioning of CNs VII, IX, and X. Because of these multiple pathways, total loss of taste (ageusia) is rare.
- System(s) affected: Nervous; Upper Respiratory

EPIDEMIOLOGY

Incidence

There are ~200,000 patient visits a year for smell and taste disturbances.

Prevalence

- Predominant sex: Male > Female. Men begin to lose their ability to smell earlier in life than women.
- Predominant age: Chemosensory loss is age-dependent:
  - Age >80 years: 80% have major olfactory impairment; nearly 50% are anosmic.
  - Ages 65–80 years: 60% have major olfactory impairment; nearly 25% are anosmic.
  - Age <65 years: 1–2% have smell impairment.
- Estimated >2 million affected in the US

RISK FACTORS

- Age >65 years
- Poor nutritional status
- Smoking tobacco products

Genetics

May be related to underlying genetically associated diseases (Kallmann syndrome, Alzheimer disease, migraine syndromes, rheumatologic conditions, endocrine disorders)

GENERAL PREVENTION

- Eat a well-balanced diet, with appropriate vitamins and minerals.
- Maintain good oral and nasal health, with routine visits to the dentist.
- Do not smoke tobacco products.
- Avoid noxious chemical exposures or unnecessary radiation.

Geriatric Considerations

- Elders are at particular risk of eating spoiled food or inadvertently being exposed to natural gas leaks owing to anosmia from aging.
- Anosmia also may be an early sign of degenerative disorders such as Alzheimer disease.

Pediatric Considerations

- Smell and taste disorders are uncommon in children in developed countries.
- In developing countries with poor nutrition (particularly zinc depletion), smell and taste disorders may occur.
- Delayed puberty in association with anosmia (± midline craniofacial abnormalities, deafness, or renal abnormalities) suggests the possibility of Kallmann syndrome (hypogonadotropic hypogonadism).

Pregnancy Considerations

- Pregnancy is an uncommon cause of smell and taste loss or disturbances.
- Many women report increased sensitivity to odors during pregnancy, as well as an increased dislike for bitterness and a preference for salty substances.

ETIOLOGY

- Smell and/or taste disturbances (1,2,3):
  - Nutritional factors (e.g., malnutrition, vitamin deficiencies, liver disease, anemia)
  - Endocrine disorders (e.g., thyroid disease, diabetes mellitus, renal disease)
  - Head trauma
  - Migraine headache (e.g., gustatory aura, olfactory aura)
  - Sjögren syndrome
  - Toxic chemical exposure
  - Industrial agent exposure
  - Aging
  - Medications (see below)
  - Neurodegenerative diseases (e.g., multiple sclerosis, Alzheimer disease, cerebrovascular accident, Parkinson disease)
  - Infections (e.g., upper respiratory infection [URI], oral and perioral infections, candidiasis, coxsackievirus, AIDS, viral hepatitis, herpes simplex virus)
- Possible causes of smell disturbance:
  - Nasal and sinus disease (e.g., allergies, rhinitis, rhinorrhea)
  - Cigarette smoking
  - Cocaine abuse (intranasal)
  - Hemodialysis
  - Radiation treatment of head and neck
  - Congenital conditions
  - Neoplasm (e.g., brain tumor, nasal polyps, intranasal tumor)
  - Systemic lupus erythematosus (SLE)
  - Bell palsy
  - Oral or perioral skin lesion
  - Damage to CN I or V
  - Possible association with psychosis and schizophrenia
- Possible causes of taste loss:
  - Oral appliances
  - Dental procedures
  - Intraoral abscess
  - Gingivitis
  - Damage to CN VI, IX, or X
  - Stroke (especially frontal lobe)
- Selected medications that reportedly alter smell and taste:
  - Antibiotics: Amikacin, ampicillin, azithromycin (Zithromax), ciprofloxacin (Cipro), clarithromycin (Biaxin), doxycycline, griseofulvin (Grisactin), metronidazole (Flagyl), ofloxacin (Floxin), tetracycline, terbinafine (Lamisil), beta-lactamase inhibitors
  - Anticonvulsants: Carbamazepine (Tegretol), phenytoin (Dilantin)
  - Antidepressants: Amitriptyline (Elavil), clomipramine (Anafranil), desipramine (Norpramin), doxepin (Sinequan), imipramine (Tofranil), nortriptyline (Pamelor)
  - Antihistamines and decongestants: Chlorpheniramine, loratadine (Claritin), pseudoephedrine, zinc-based cold remedies (Zicam)
  - Antihypertensives and cardiac medications: Acetazolamide (Diamox), amiloride (Midamor), betaxolol (Betoptic), captopril (Capoten), diltiazem (Cardizem), enalapril (Vasotec), hydrochlorothiazide (Esidrix) and combinations, nifedipine (Procardia), nitroglycerin, propranolol (Inderal), spironolactone (Aldactone)
  - Anti-inflammatory agents: Auranofin (Ridaura), colchicine, dexamethasone (Decadron), gold (Myochrysine), hydrocortisone, penicillamine (Cuprimine),
  - Antimanic drugs: Lithium
  - Antineoplastics: Cisplatin (Platinol), doxorubicin (Adriamycin), methotrexate (Rheumatrex), vincristine (Oncovin)
  - Antiparkinsonian agents: Levodopa (Larodopa, with carbidopa (Sinemet)
  - Antipsychotics: Clozapine (Clozaril), trifluoperazine (Stelazine)
  - Antithyroid agents: Methimazole (Tapazole), propylthiouracil
  - Lipid-lowering agents: Fluvastatin (Lescol), lovastatin (Mevacor), pravastatin (Pravachol)
  - Muscle relaxants: Baclofen (Lioresal), dantrolene (Dantrium)

COMMONLY ASSOCIATED CONDITIONS

URI, allergic rhinitis, dental abscesses

DIAGNOSIS

Smell and taste disturbances are symptoms; it is essential to look for possible underlying causes.

HISTORY

- Symptoms of URI, environmental allergies
- Oral pain, other dental problems
- Cognitive/memory difficulties
- Current medications
- Nutritional status, ovolactovegetarian
- Weight loss or gain
- Frequent infections (impaired immunity)
- Worsening of underlying medical illness
- Increased use of salt and/or sugar to increase taste of food

PHYSICAL EXAM

Thorough HEENT exam

DIAGNOSTIC TESTS & INTERPRETATION

Lab

Initial lab tests

Consider (not all patients require all tests):

- Hemoglobin
- WBC count
- BUN
- Blood glucose
- Creatinine
- Bilirubin
- Alkaline phosphatase
- Thyroid-stimulating hormone (TSH)
- serum IgE

Follow-Up & Special Considerations

Diagnosis of smell and taste disturbances is usually possible through history (1); however, the following tests can be used to confirm:

- Olfactory tests:
  - Smell identification test: Evaluates the ability to identify 40 microencapsulated scratch-and-sniff odorants
  - Brief smell identification test
- Taste tests (more difficult because no convenient standardized tests are presently available): Solutions containing sucrose (sweet), sodium chloride (salty), quinine (bitter), and citric acid (sour) are helpful.

Imaging

Initial approach

- Plain radiographs have substantial limitations (and are rarely useful).
- CT scanning is the most useful and cost-effective technique for assessing sinonasal disorders and is superior to an MRI in evaluating bony structures and airway patency. Coronal CT scans are particularly valuable in assessing paranasal anatomy.

Follow-Up & Special Considerations

An MRI is useful in defining soft tissue disease; therefore, a coronal MRI is the technique of choice to image the olfactory bulbs, tracts, and cortical parenchyma. Possible placement of an accessory coil (TMJ) over the nose to assist in imaging.

DIFFERENTIAL DIAGNOSIS

- Epilepsy (gustatory aura)
- Epilepsy (olfactory aura)
- Memory impairment
- Psychiatric conditions

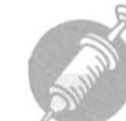

TREATMENT

MEDICATION

- Treat underlying causes as appropriate. 2/3 of idiopathic cases will resolve spontaneously.
- Corticosteroids topically (e.g., aqueous nasal spray) or systemically (e.g., oral prednisone) may be helpful. Prednisone 60 mg/d × 4 days, then taper by 10 mg/d thereafter.
- Artificial saliva (e.g., Xero-Lube) may be helpful in patients with xerostomia.
- Pilocarpine (Salagen), 5–10 mg PO t.i.d. may help with dry mouth/xerostomia; response may take 6–12 weeks.
- Chlorhexidine (Peridex) 0.12% oral rinse may help with gingivitis or dysgeusia.
- Zinc and vitamins (A, B complex) when deficiency is suspected

ADDITIONAL TREATMENT

General Measures

- Appropriate treatment for underlying cause
- Quit smoking.
- Some drug-related dysgeusias can be reversed with cessation of the agent, but it may take many months.
- Eliminate exposures (e.g., volatile gases, toxins, use of oxygen-liberating mouthwashes).
- Stop repeated oral trauma (e.g., appliances, tongue-biting behaviors).
- Proper nutritional and dietary assessment
- Formal dental evaluation

Issues for Referral

- Consider referral to an otolaryngologist or neurologist for persistent cases.
- Referral to a subspecialist at a smell and taste center if needed

SURGERY/OTHER PROCEDURES

If needed for treatment of underlying cause

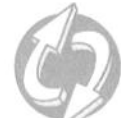

ONGOING CARE

DIET

- Weight gain or loss is possible because the patient may reject food or may switch to calorie-rich foods that are still palatable.
- Ensure a nutritionally balanced diet with appropriate levels of nutrients, vitamins, and essential minerals.

PATIENT EDUCATION

- Caution patients not to overindulge as compensation for the bland taste of food. For example, patients with diabetes may need help in avoiding excessive sugar intake as an inappropriate way of improving food taste.
- Patients with chemosensory impairments should use measuring devices when cooking and should not cook by taste.
- Optimizing food texture, aroma, temperature, and color may improve the overall food experience when taste is limited.
- Patients with permanent smell dysfunction must develop adaptive strategies for dealing with hygiene, appetite, safety, and health.
- Natural gas and smoke detectors are essential; check for proper function frequently.
- Check food expiration dates frequently; discard old food.

PROGNOSIS

- In general, the olfactory system regenerates poorly after a head injury. Most patients who recover smell function subsequent to head trauma do so within 12 weeks of injury.
- Patients who quit smoking typically recover improved olfactory function and flavor sensation.
- Many taste disorders (dysgeusias) resolve spontaneously within a few years of onset.
- Phantosmias that are flow-dependent may respond to surgical ablation of olfactory mucosa.
- Conditions such as radiation-induced xerostomia and Bell palsy generally improve over time.

COMPLICATIONS

- Permanent loss of ability to smell or taste
- Psychiatric issues with dysgeusias and phantosmia

REFERENCES

1. Bromley SM. Smell and taste disorders: A primary care approach. *Am Fam Physician*. 2000;61: 427–36, 438.
2. Nguyen-Khoa B, Goehring Jr EL, Vendiola RM. Epidemiologic study of smell disturbance in 2 medical insurance claims populations. *Arch Otolaryngol Head Neck Surg*. 2007;133(8)748–57.
3. Deems DA, Doty RL, Settle RG. Smell and taste disorders, a study of 750 patients from the University of Pennsylvania Smell and Taste Center. *Arch Otolaryngol Head Neck Surg*. 1991;117: 519–28.

ADDITIONAL READING

- Cullen MM, Leopold DA, et al. Disorders of smell and taste. *Med Clin North Am*. 1999;83:57–74.
- Lacroix JS, Landis BN et al. Future perspectives in smell and taste disorders. *B-ENT*. 2009;5 Suppl 13:133–6.

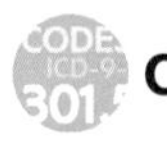

CODES

ICD9

781.1 Disturbances of sensation of smell and taste

CLINICAL PEARLS

- Smell disorders are often mistaken as decreased taste by patients.
- Actual taste disorders are often related to dental problems.
- Smell disorders are very common in the elderly; extensive workup in this population may not be indicated if no associated signs or symptoms are present.

S

SOMATIZATION DISORDER

Laurie A. Carrier, MD

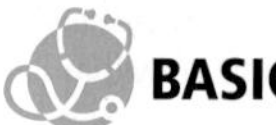

BASICS

DESCRIPTION

- A pattern of recurring, multiple, clinically significant somatic complaints beginning <30 years of age that occur over a period of several years and result in treatment being sought or significant impairment in social, occupational, or other important areas of functioning
- Each of the following criteria must be met, with individual symptoms occurring at any time during the course of the disturbance:
  - 4 pain symptoms: Different sites or functions
  - 2 GI symptoms: Other than pain
  - 1 sexual symptom
  - 1 pseudoneurologic symptom
- These symptoms are not intentionally produced or feigned.
- Chronic course, fluctuating in severity
- Affected individual rarely goes 1 year without seeking medical attention prompted by unexplained somatic complaints.
- System(s) affected: Multiple
- Synonym(s): Briquet syndrome

EPIDEMIOLOGY

Incidence

- Usually, first symptoms appear in adolescence; full criteria met by 30 years of age.
- Predominant sex: Female > Male (10:1)
- The type and frequency of somatic complaints may differ among cultures, so symptom reviews should be adjusted based on culture.

Prevalence

- Ranges from 0.2–2% among women and <0.2% among men
- 1/500 adults in the US
- Seen in up to 29% of patients presenting to primary care offices (1)

RISK FACTORS

- Child abuse, particularly sexual abuse, has been shown to be a risk factor.
- Symptoms begin or worsen after losses (e.g., job, close relative, or friend).
- Greater intensity of symptoms often occurs with stress.

Genetics

- Observed in 10–20% of female first-degree biologic relatives of women with somatization disorder (SD)
- Male relatives of women with this disorder show an increased risk of antisocial personality disorder and substance-related disorders.

ETIOLOGY

- Unknown
- Adoption studies indicate that both genetic and environmental factors contribute to the risk of SD.

COMMONLY ASSOCIATED CONDITIONS

Comorbid with other psychiatric conditions, including major depression (55% of patients), anxiety disorders (34%), personality disorders (61%), and panic disorders (26%)

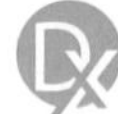

DIAGNOSIS

HISTORY

- Multiple somatic complaints, usually a grossly positive review of symptoms
- Pain symptoms (4 or more) related to different sites, such as head, abdomen, back, joints, extremities, chest, or rectum or related to body functions such as menstruation, sexual intercourse, or urination
- GI symptoms (2 or more, excluding pain) such as nausea, bloating, vomiting (not during pregnancy), diarrhea, intolerance of several foods
- Sexual symptoms (at least 1, excluding pain) such as indifference to sex, difficulties with erection or ejaculation, irregular menses, excessive menstrual bleeding, or vomiting throughout all 9 months of pregnancy
- Pseudoneurologic symptoms (at least 1) such as impaired balance or coordination, weak or paralyzed muscles, lump in throat or trouble swallowing, loss of voice, retention of urine, hallucinations, numbness (to touch or pain), double vision, blindness, deafness, seizures, amnesia or other dissociative symptoms, loss of consciousness (other than with fainting); none of these is limited to pain

PHYSICAL EXAM

Physical exam remarkable for absence of objective findings to fully explain the many subjective complaints

DIAGNOSTIC TESTS & INTERPRETATION

Several screening tools are available that help to identify symptoms as somatic:

- Patient Health Questionnaire (PHQ)-15 (screens and monitors symptoms) (2)[C]
- Minnesota Multiphasic Personality Inventory (MMPI) (identifies somatization) (3)[C]
- Perley-Guze Checklist (helps the physician to identify SD)

Lab

Initial lab tests

Laboratory test results do not support the subjective complaints.

Imaging

Initial approach

Imaging studies do not support the subjective complaints.

Pathological Findings

None are identified.

DIFFERENTIAL DIAGNOSIS

- Other psychiatric illnesses must be ruled out:
  - Depressive disorders
  - Anxiety disorders
  - Schizophrenia
  - Other somatoform disorders: Conversion disorder, factitious disorders, hypochondriasis, pain disorder
- General medical conditions, with vague, multiple, confusing symptoms, must be ruled out:
  - Systemic lupus erythematosus
  - Hyperparathyroidism
  - Hyper- or hypothyroidism
  - Lyme disease
  - Porphyria

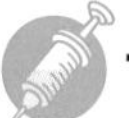

TREATMENT

MEDICATION

Antidepressants (e.g., SSRIs) help to treat comorbid depression and anxiety.

ADDITIONAL TREATMENT

General Measures

- The goal of treatment is to help the person learn to control the symptoms.
- A supportive relationship with a sympathetic health care provider is the most important aspect of treatment (4)[C]:
  - Regularly scheduled appointments should be maintained to review symptoms and the person's coping mechanisms (at least 15 minutes once a month) (4)[C].
  - Acknowledgment and explanation of test results should occur.
- The involvement of a single physician is important because a history of seeking medical attention and "doctor shopping" is common.
- Antidepressant or antianxiety medication and referral to a support group or psychiatrist can help patients who are willing to participate in their treatment.
- Patients usually receive the most benefit from primary care physicians who accept the limitations of treatment, listen to their patient's concerns, and provide reassurance.
- It is not helpful to tell patients that their symptoms are imaginary.

Issues for Referral

- Referrals to specialists for further investigation of somatic complaints should be discouraged.
- Referrals to support groups or to a psychiatrist may be helpful.

Additional Therapies

Treatment typically includes long-term therapy, which has been shown to decrease the severity of symptoms:

- Cognitive-behavioral therapy has been shown to be the most efficacious treatment in SD (5)[B],(6)[C].
- Psychotherapy
- Supportive therapy

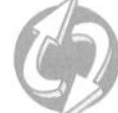

ONGOING CARE

FOLLOW-UP RECOMMENDATIONS

Patients should have regularly scheduled follow-up with a primary care doctor, psychiatrist, and/or therapist.

PATIENT EDUCATION

Interventions that decrease stressful elements of the patient's life should be encouraged:

- Psychoeducational advice
- Increase in exercise
- Pleasurable private time

PROGNOSIS

- Chronic course, fluctuating in severity
- Full remission is rare.
- Individuals with this disorder do not experience any significant difference in mortality rate or significant physical illness.
- Patients with this diagnosis do experience substantially greater functional disability and role impairment than nonsomatizing patients (7).

COMPLICATIONS

- May result from invasive testing and from multiple evaluations that are performed while looking for the cause of the symptoms
- A dependency on pain relievers or sedatives may develop.

REFERENCES

1. Roca M, Gili M, Garcia-Garcia M, et al. Prevalence and comorbidity of common mental disorders in primary care. *J Affect Disord*. 2009;119(1–3):52–8.
2. Kroenke K, Spitzer RL, Williams JB. The PHQ-15: Validity of a new measure for evaluating the severity of somatic symptoms. *Psychosom Med*. 2002;64:258–66.
3. Wetzel RD, Brim J, Guze SB, et al. MMPI screening scales for somatization disorder. *Psychol Rep*. 1999;85:341–8.
4. Servan-Schreiber D, Tabas G, Kolb R. Somatizing patients: Part II. Practical management. *Am Fam Physician*. 2000;61:1423–8, 1431–2.
5. Allen LA, Woolfolk RL, Escobar JI, et al. Cognitive-behavioral therapy for somatization disorder: A randomized controlled trial. *Arch Intern Med*. 2006;166:1512–8.
6. Kroenke K, Swindle R. Cognitive-behavioral therapy for somatization and symptom syndromes: A critical review of controlled clinical trials. *Psychother Psychosom*. 2000;69:205–15.
7. Harris AM, Orav EJ, Bates DW, et al. Somatization increases disability independent of comorbidity. *J Gen Intern Med*. 2008.

ADDITIONAL READING

- American Psychiatric Association. *Diagnostic and Statistical Manual of Mental Disorders*, 4th ed. Text revision. Washington, DC: American Psychiatric Association; 2000.
- Mai F. Somatization disorder: A practical review. *Can J Psychiatry*. 2004;49:652–62.

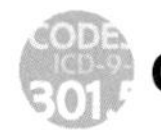

CODES

ICD9

300.81 Somatization disorder

CLINICAL PEARLS

- Acknowledge the patient's pain, suffering, and disability.
- Do not tell patients the symptoms are "all in their head."
- Emphasize that this is not a rare disorder.
- Discuss the limitations of treatment while providing reassurance that there are interventions that will lessen suffering and symptoms.

SPINAL STENOSIS

N. Wilson Holland, MD, FACP
Birju B. Patel, MD, FACP

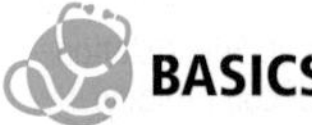

BASICS

DESCRIPTION

Spinal stenosis is a condition in which a narrowing of the spinal canal and foramen occurs. Spondylosis or degenerative arthritis is the most common etiology for spinal stenosis and results from compression of the spinal cord by disc degeneration, facet arthropathy, osteophyte formation, and ligamentum flavum hypertrophy. The L_4–L_5 level is involved most commonly, but other lumbar levels also can be affected.

EPIDEMIOLOGY

The prevalence of spinal stenosis increases with age because it is essentially an arthritic condition from "wear and tear" on the normal spine.

Incidence

The incidence of symptomatic spinal stenosis is as high as 8% of the general population.

Prevalence

- The prevalence increases with age and can be very high when assessed by imaging studies in elderly patients; however, not all patients with radiographic spinal stenosis are symptomatic.
- Predominant age: Symptoms develop in fifth and sixth decades (congenital stenosis becomes symptomatic much earlier).

RISK FACTORS

Increasing age and degenerative spondylolisthesis

Genetics

No definitive genetic links

GENERAL PREVENTION

There is no known way to prevent spinal stenosis. Symptoms can be alleviated with flexion at the waist:

- Leaning forward while walking
- Pushing a shopping cart
- Lying in flexed position
- Sitting
- Avoid provocative maneuvers that can cause pain (e.g., back extension, ambulating long distances without resting) (1)

PATHOPHYSIOLOGY

Disc dehydration leads to loss of height with bulging of the disc annulus and ligamentum flavum into the spinal canal, thus increasing joint loading of facets. This leads to reactive sclerosis and osteophytic bone growth, resulting in further compression of neural elements in the spinal canal and foramen.

ETIOLOGY

Spinal stenosis can result from congenital or acquired causes. Degenerative spondylosis is the most common cause. Acquired causes include:

- Disc degeneration and spondylosis
- Trauma
- Neoplasms
- Neural cysts and lipomas
- Postoperative changes
- Rheumatoid arthritis
- Diffuse idiopathic skeletal hyperostosis
- Ankylosing spondylitis
- Metabolic/endocrine:
  - Osteoporosis
  - Renal osteodystrophy
  - Paget disease

DIAGNOSIS

- Long-standing back pain that progresses to buttocks and lower extremity pain
- Neurogenic claudication (i.e., pain, tightness, numbness, and subjective weakness of lower extremities) may mimic arterial insufficiency–related claudication.

HISTORY

- The history is an extremely important aspect in distinguishing patients with spinal stenosis from those with other causes of back pain and peripheral vascular disease.
- Components of the history that should be considered include:
  - Insidious onset
  - Generally progresses slowly but may rarely have periods of remittance
  - Symptoms worsen with extension of the spine (prolonged standing, walking especially downhill or downstairs).
  - Symptoms improve with flexion (sitting, leaning forward while walking, walking uphill or upstairs, and lying in a flexed position).
  - Intermittent claudication
  - Urinary symptoms
  - Bilateral plantar numbness

PHYSICAL EXAM

Neurologic exam may be normal. There may be very few physical findings even in affected patients:

- Gait alteration (rule out cervical myelopathy or intracranial pathology)
- Loss of lumbar lordosis
- Decreased range of motion of lumbar spine
- Pain with extension of the lumbar spine
- Straight-leg-raise test may be positive if nerve root entrapment is present.
- Muscle weakness is usually mild or subtle and involves the L_4, L_5, and rarely, S_1 nerve roots.
- About 1/2 of patients with symptomatic stenosis have a reduced or absent Achilles reflex, and some have reduced or absent knee-jerk reaction.

DIAGNOSTIC TESTS & INTERPRETATION

Spinal stenosis generally is diagnosed with a combination of history, physical exam, and imaging studies (MRI is best).

Lab

Initial lab tests

Consider CBC, ESR, C-reactive protein (to look for infection or malignancy)

Imaging

- New back pain lasting longer than 2 weeks, or accompanied by neurologic findings in those over age 50 generally warrants neuroimaging.
- MRI is the modality of choice for the diagnosis of spinal stenosis. 3D MR myelography may be more sensitive but is more expensive at diagnosing lumbar spinal stenosis, as shown by a few studies.
- CT myelography is an alternative to MRI but is invasive with the potential risk of complications.
- Plain radiography may help to support the diagnosis but in general will not reveal the underlying pathology (but may be helpful to help exclude other causes of new back pain).
- Radiological abnormalities in general do not correlate with the clinical diagnosis (2)

Initial approach

Spinal stenosis generally does not lead to neurologic damage. Surgery may be required for pain relief, allowing patients to become more mobile and thus improving overall health.

Diagnostic Procedures/Surgery

Surgical decompression is the only definitive treatment in patients who continue to be symptomatic after nonoperative treatment.

Pathological Findings

- Decreased disc height
- Facet hypertrophy
- Spinal canal and/or foraminal narrowing

DIFFERENTIAL DIAGNOSIS

- Vascular claudication also can cause calf pain with ambulation. Symptoms of vascular claudication do not improve with leaning forward and should not persist with standing.
- Disc herniation
- Cervical myelopathy

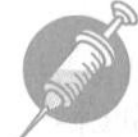

TREATMENT

- A few studies have shown improvement with decompressive surgery, but the duration of improvement is uncertain.
- In general, nonoperative interventions are tried prior to surgical interventions unless there are progressive or life-threatening neurologic symptoms.
- If decompressive surgery is performed, it is generally successful in alleviating symptoms of spinal stenosis.
- There is some controversy about whether a fusion should be performed with the decompression because of risk of future spondylolisthesis.
- A unilateral partial hemilaminectomy combined with transmedian decompression may adequately treat stenosis with less morbidity in the elderly population (3).

MEDICATION

First Line

- Acetaminophen
- NSAIDs: consider potential for GI side effects, fluid retention, and renal failure
- Tramadol

Second Line
- There is limited evidence for long-term efficacy of lumbar epidural steroid and/or anesthetic injections. Injections maybe less effective in those with more severe stenosis and those with stenosis involving more than 3 lumbar levels.
- Consider judicious use of opioids only when other treatments have failed to control severe pain.

Geriatric Considerations
- Anti-inflammatory medications should be used with caution in the elderly due to the risks of GI bleeding, fluid retention, renal failure, and cardiovascular risks.
- Side effects of opioids, including constipation, confusion, urinary retention, drowsiness, nausea, vomiting, and potential for dependence, should be considered.
- Over 10% of elderly lack Achilles reflexes.

ADDITIONAL TREATMENT

Issues for Referral
Refer to a spine surgeon when patients are in unremitting pain or have a neurologic deficit.

Additional Therapies
- General conditioning; these patients are able to ride an exercise bicycle without many problems because they can lean forward and relieve symptoms.
- Aquatic therapy (helpful for muscle and general conditioning)
- Back extensor muscle strengthening
- Abdominal muscle strengthening
- Gait training

SURGERY/OTHER PROCEDURES
- Surgery is indicated when symptoms persist despite conservative measures (4).
- Age alone should not be an exclusion factor for surgical intervention. However, cognitive impairment, multiple comorbidities, and osteoporosis may increase the risk of perioperative complications in the elderly (5).
- Decompression of neural elements is the mainstay of treatment. The traditional approach is laminectomy and partial facetectomy (6).
- Controversy exists about whether the decompression should be supplemented by a fusion procedure.
- A less invasive alternative, known as interspinous distraction (X STOP implant), is also available. Elderly patients with significant degenerative spondylolisthesis may have more postoperative neurologic sequelae with use of the X STOP implant at severely stenotic levels (7).

IN-PATIENT CONSIDERATIONS

Initial Stabilization
- A brace or corset may help for a short time but is not recommended long term because it leads to paraspinal muscle weakness.
- Patient should be encouraged to continue to be active despite pain to prevent deconditioning.
- Weight loss

Admission Criteria
Unremitting pain that prevents the ability to perform the activities of daily living (ADLs) or acute or progressive neurologic deficit

Discharge Criteria
Improved pain or after neurologic deficit has been addressed

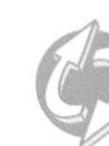

ONGOING CARE

FOLLOW-UP RECOMMENDATIONS
- Routine follow-up as needed
- No limitations to activity; patients may be as active as tolerated. Exercise should be encouraged.

Patient Monitoring
Patients are monitored for improvement of symptoms and development of any complications.

DIET
If undergoing surgery, optimize nutritional status.

PATIENT EDUCATION
- Activity as tolerated, as long as no other pathology is present (e.g., fractures)
- Patients should be alerted to possibility of progressive motor weakness and bladder/bowel dysfunction
- Patients should be educated about the natural history of the condition.

PROGNOSIS
- Spinal stenosis generally is benign, but the pain can lead to limitation in ADLs and progressive disability.
- Surgery is usually successful in improving pain and symptoms in patients who fail nonoperative treatment.
- Clinical outcomes in elderly patients after surgery are similar in terms of pain relief and functional improvement compared with younger patients (5).

COMPLICATIONS
- Severe spinal stenosis can lead to bowel and/or bladder dysfunction.
- Surgical complications include infection, neurologic injury, chronic pain, and disability.

REFERENCES

1. Suri P, Rainville J, Kalichman L, et al. Does this older adult with lower extremity pain have the clinical syndrome of lumbar spinal stenosis? *JAMA*. 2010;204(23):2628–36.
2. Li AL, Yen D. Effect of increased MRI and CT scan utilization on clinical decision-making in patients referred a surgical clinic for back pain. *Can J Surg*. 2011;54(2):128–32.
3. Morgalla MH, Noak N, Merkle M, et al. Lumbar spinal stenosis in elderly patients: Is a unilateral microsurgical approach sufficient for decompression? *J Neurosurg Spine*. 2011;14(3):305–12.
4. Weinstein JN, Tosteson TD, Lurie JD, et al. Surgical versus nonsurgical therapy for lumbar spinal stenosis. *N Engl J Med*. 2008;358:794–810.
5. Cloyd JM, Acosta FL, Ames CP, et al. Complications and outcomes of lumbar spine surgery in elderly people: A review of the literature. *J Am Geriatr Soc*. 2008;56:1318–27.
6. Katz JN, Harris MB. Clinical practice. Lumbar spinal stenosis. *N Engl J Med*. 2008;358:818–25.
7. Epstein NE et al. X-Stop: Foot drop. *Spine J*. 2009;9:e6–9.

S

ADDITIONAL READING

Devereaux M, et al. Low back pain. *Med Clin North Am*. 2009;93:477–501, x.

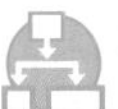

See Also (Topic, Algorithm, Electronic Media Element)

Algorithm: Low Back Pain, Acute

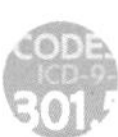

CODES

ICD9
- 724.00 Spinal stenosis, unspecified region
- 724.01 Spinal stenosis, thoracic region
- 724.02 Spinal stenosis, lumbar region, without neurogenic claudication

CLINICAL PEARLS
- Spinal stenosis may present as neurogenic claudication (pain, tightness, numbness, and subjective weakness of lower extremities) and may mimic arterial insufficiency–related claudication.
- Neurogenic claudication as opposed to vascular claudication is improved by uphill ambulation and lumbar flexion and is not alleviated by standing.
- Positions that cause flexion of the spine such as sitting, bending forward, walking uphill, or walking with a shopping cart generally relieve symptoms and can be helpful in making the diagnosis.
- Positions that cause spinal extension such as prolonged standing, walking downhill, and walking downstairs can worsen symptoms.
- Surgery should be considered urgently in patients who present with rapidly evolving cauda equina/conus medullaris syndrome or newly progressive bladder dysfunction.

SPOROTRICHOSIS

Raul Davaro, MD
Sumanth Gandra, MD, MPH

BASICS

DESCRIPTION

- Subacute or chronic *Sporothrix schenckii* fungal infection
- Most common and least severe of the deep mycoses
- Occurs in the following forms:
  - Cutaneous/lymphocutaneous (most common)
  - Disseminated:
    - Osteoarticular
    - Renal
    - Testicular
    - Mastitis
    - Meningeal
  - Pulmonary
- Most likely to occur in farmers, horticulturists, and gardeners
- System(s) affected: Hematologic/Lymphatic/Immunologic; Musculoskeletal; Skin/Exocrine; Renal; Respiratory
- Synonym(s): Schenck disease; Rose gardener disease

EPIDEMIOLOGY

Incidence

- <1/100,000 persons/yr
- Occurs worldwide, but is most common in tropics and subtropics; endemic in Central and South America and Africa

RISK FACTORS

- Gardening: Contact with mulch, sphagnum moss, hay, timber, or thorny bushes
- Occupations involving the handling of gardening materials: Nursery workers, landscapers, florists, carpenters
- Animal handlers (transmission from animals, especially cats and armadillos, to humans has been documented)
- Immunocompromised patients (e.g., HIV, hematologic malignancy, use of immunosuppressants), as well as patients with chronic obstructive pulmonary disease, alcoholism, and diabetes mellitus, are at risk for developing disseminated disease.

GENERAL PREVENTION

- Avoid areas where sporotrichosis is endemic.
- Wear gloves when working in soil.

PATHOPHYSIOLOGY

- Lymphocutaneous: Primary lesion forms within 3 weeks to 6 months of direct inoculation with mold and spreads along lymphatic channels.
- Disseminated: Via hematogenous spread
- Pulmonary: Via inhalation of spores

ETIOLOGY

- Traumatic inoculation of fungus through skin into SC fat or pulmonary inoculation via inhalation of conidia.
- *S. schenckii* is a dimorphic, aerobic fungus existing in hyphal form at temperatures below 37°C and yeast form above 37°C; a ubiquitous saprophyte found in soil, sphagnum peat moss, wood, marine animals, decaying vegetation, some insects, etc (1).

DIAGNOSIS

HISTORY

- Minor skin trauma involving contact with plants or plant products (rose thorns, hay, conifer needles, etc.) with subsequent delayed development of characteristic lesions
- Zoonotic transmission (animal to human) documented (dogs, cats, horses, rodents, pigs, armadillos, and insects)
- Pulmonary disease presents with high fever, night sweats, dyspnea, fatigue, hemoptysis, and cough productive of purulent sputum.

PHYSICAL EXAM

- Cutaneous/lymphocutaneous:
  - Characteristic skin lesions beginning as an inoculation chancre or erythematous plaque with satellite, small papules, and painless, movable, SC nodules in a linear distribution; lesions progress to larger nodules, which may ulcerate and drain; affects primarily upper extremities
  - Additional lesions spread proximally along lymphatics, giving linear appearance.
- Disseminated disease:
  - Widespread, multifocal, cutaneous lesions
  - Physical exam will depend on organ system involved.
- Osteoarticular:
  - Subacute or chronic inflammatory arthritis, often monoarticular; may persist for many years
  - Signs and symptoms of osteomyelitis
  - Generally afebrile
- Pulmonary: Physical exam nonspecific other than suggestive of cavitary lung disease

DIAGNOSTIC TESTS & INTERPRETATION

Lab

Initial lab tests

- Culture of *S. schenckii* is the gold standard for diagnosis of sporotrichosis.
- Fungal cultures from tissue biopsy or aspirated pus; cultures may be more difficult to grow from synovial fluid or sputum
- Incubate at 25°C on Sabouraud or potato dextrose agar, with creamy white colonies appearing in 3–5 days that then convert to characteristic brown-black leathery colonies within several days (2)

Follow-Up & Special Considerations

- Organisms may be difficult to find on light microscopy, and thus culture is vastly superior for diagnosis.
- Perform culture for atypical *Mycobacterium* spp. and/or acid-fast stain if considered in differential diagnosis.

Imaging

Chest x-ray if pulmonary symptoms present

Initial approach

- Careful history and physical exam
- Culture of draining lesions
- Culture of inflammatory joint effusions or sputum
- Tissue biopsy with culture if diagnosis not confirmed

Pathological Findings

- Nonspecific granulomata with central necrosis may be found on tissue biopsy.
- Periodic acid–Schiff staining rarely may reveal spores within the granuloma.
- Asteroid corpuscles may be seen on hematoxylin and eosin stain.

DIFFERENTIAL DIAGNOSIS

- Cutaneous or lymphocutaneous (1):
  - Sporotrichoid nocardiosis
  - Leishmaniasis
  - Paracoccidiomycosis
  - Chromoblastomycosis
  - Blastomycosis
  - Tuberculosis
  - Atypical mycobacterial infection (*Mycobacterium marinum, M. chelonae, M. kansasii*)
  - Cat-scratch disease
  - Tularemia
  - Plague
  - Primary syphilis
  - Pyoderma gangrenosum
- Pulmonary:
  - Tuberculosis
  - Sarcoidosis
  - Chronic fungal pneumonia
  - Neoplasm
  - Atypical mycobacterial infection (*M. avium* complex, *M. kansasii*)
  - *Rhodococcus equi* infection
  - *Nocardia* sp. infections
- Osteoarticular:
  - Rheumatoid arthritis
  - Bacterial arthritis/osteomyelitis

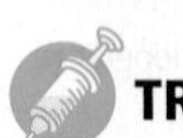

TREATMENT

MEDICATION

First Line

- Cutaneous/lymphocutaneous:
  - Itraconazole: 200 mg/d PO recommended for 2–4 weeks after all lesions have resolved, usually a total of 3–6 months (1)[A]
  - Patients who do not respond should be given a higher dosage of itraconazole, 200 mg b.i.d. (1)[A], terbinafine at a dosage of 500 mg PO b.i.d. (1)[A], or SSKI initiated at a dosage of 5 drops t.i.d., increasing as tolerated to 40–50 drops t.i.d. (1) although the role of SSKI is anecdotal as evidence is inconclusive (3).
  - Fluconazole at a dosage of 400–800 mg/d should be used only if the patient cannot tolerate the other agents (1)[A].
  - Local hyperthermia can be used for treating patients, such as pregnant and nursing women, who have fixed cutaneous sporotrichosis and who cannot safely take any of the above regimens (1)[C].

- Osteoarticular:
  - Itraconazole: 200 mg PO b.i.d. for at least 12 months is recommended (1)[A].
  - Amphotericin B lipid formulation: 3–5 mg/kg/d or amphotericin B deoxycholate 0.7–1 mg/kg/d can be used for initial therapy (1)[C].
  - After the patient has shown a favorable response, therapy can be changed to itraconazole 200 mg PO b.i.d. to complete a total of at least 12 months of therapy (1)[C].
  - Serum levels of itraconazole should be obtained after the patient has been on this agent for at least 2 weeks to ensure adequate drug exposure (1)[C].
- Pulmonary:
  - For severe or life-threatening pulmonary sporotrichosis, including patients with severe gas-exchange abnormality, severe toxicity, and rapid progression, amphotericin B is recommended (4)[B].
  - Amphotericin B deoxycholate: 0.7–1 mg/kg/d should be used until clinical improvement is observed or until a cumulative dose of 1–2 g of amphotericin B is reached (4)[B].
  - After the patient has shown a favorable response to amphotericin B, therapy can be switched to itraconazole 200 mg PO b.i.d. to complete a total of at least 3–6 months of therapy based on overall clinical response (4)[B].
  - For mild to moderately severe pulmonary sporotrichosis, based on the extent of radiographic involvement and oxygenation status, itraconazole 200 mg b.i.d., with a total duration of therapy generally of 3–6 months based on overall clinical response (4)[B].
  - Surgical resection combined with amphotericin B is recommended for localized pulmonary disease (1)[C].
- Disseminated disease or meningeal involvement:
  - Amphotericin B given as a lipid formulation at a dosage of 5 mg/kg/d × 4–6 weeks is recommended for initial treatment (1)[C].
  - Amphotericin B deoxycholate at 0.7–1 mg/kg/d also can be used but is not a preferred regimen (1)[C].
  - Itraconazole at 200 mg b.i.d. is recommended as step-down therapy after the patient responds to initial treatment with amphotericin B and should be given to complete a total of at least 12 months of therapy (1)[C].
  - Serum levels of itraconazole should be obtained after the patient has been on this agent for at least 2 weeks to ensure adequate drug exposure (1)[C].
  - For AIDS and other immunosuppressed patients, lifelong suppressive therapy with itraconazole 200 mg/d is recommended to prevent relapse (1)[C].

Pediatric Considerations

- Itraconazole at a dosage of 6–10 mg/kg/d to a maximum of 400 mg/d PO is recommended for children with cutaneous or lymphocutaneous sporotrichosis (1)[C].
- An alternative for children is SSKI initiated at a dosage of 1 drop (using a standard eye dropper) t.i.d., increasing as tolerated up to a maximum of 1 drop/kg or 40–50 drops t.i.d., whichever is lowest (1)[C].
- For children with disseminated sporotrichosis, amphotericin B 0.7 mg/kg/d should be the initial therapy, followed by itraconazole 6–10 mg/kg up to 400 mg/d maximum as step-down therapy (1)[C].

Pregnancy Considerations

- Amphotericin B given as a lipid formulation at a dosage of 3–5 mg/kg/d or amphotericin B deoxycholate given as 0.7–1 mg/kg/d is recommended for severe sporotrichosis that must be treated during pregnancy (1)[C].
- Azoles should be avoided.
- Local hyperthermia can be used for cutaneous sporotrichosis in pregnant women (1)[C].

Second Line

Terbinafine at 250 mg PO daily, although not approved for treatment of sporotrichosis, may be a reasonable alternative to itraconazole for cutaneous disease (5)[C].

ADDITIONAL TREATMENT

General Measures

- Local heat application is useful for cutaneous and lymphocutaneous disease.
- Keep cutaneous lesions clean.
- Repeated drainage of infected joints may be indicated.

Issues for Referral

Infectious diseases consultation is suggested for optimal management.

SURGERY/OTHER PROCEDURES

- Synovectomy of infected joints may be indicated.
- Surgical débridement of osteomyelitis is usually indicated.
- Surgical resection of pulmonary lesions may be indicated when feasible.

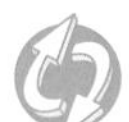

ONGOING CARE

FOLLOW-UP RECOMMENDATIONS

Patient Monitoring

- Check for compliance with long-term drug therapy (SSKI should be continued for 1–2 months after lesions heal).
- Hepatic enzyme tests should be monitored periodically in patients receiving itraconazole treatment for >1 month.

PROGNOSIS

- Excellent for complete recovery from cutaneous or lymphocutaneous infections
- Other disease forms demonstrate a chronic indolent course and are variably responsive to therapy.
- AIDS patients often have a poor outcome.

COMPLICATIONS

- Secondary bacterial infection
- Bone and joint deformities from osteoarticular disease

REFERENCES

1. Kauffman CA, Bustamante B, Chapman SW. Clinical practice guidelines for the management of sporotrichosis: 2007 update by the Infectious Diseases Society of America. *Clin Infect Dis.* 2007;45:1255–65.
2. Ramos-e-Silva M, Vasconcelos C, Carneiro S, et al. Sporotrichosis. *Clin Dermatol.* 2007;25(2):181–7.
3. Xue S, Gu R, Wu T, et al. Oral potassium iodide for the treatment of sporotrichosis. *Cochrane Database Syst Rev.* 2009;CD006136.
4. Limper AH, Knox KS, Sarosi GA, et al. An official American Thoracic Society statement: Treatment of fungal infections in adult pulmonary and critical care patients. *Am J Respir Crit Care Med.* 2011;183:96–128.
5. Francesconi G, Valle AC, Passos S, et al. Terbinafine (250 mg/day): An effective and safe treatment of cutaneous sporotrichosis. *J Eur Acad Dermatol Venereol.* 2009;23:1273–6.

ADDITIONAL READING

- Kauffman CA. Endemic mycoses: Blastomycosis, histoplasmosis, and sporotrichosis. *Infect Dis Clin North Am.* 2006;20:645–62, vii.
- Kauffman CA, Hajjeh R, Chapman SW. Practice guidelines for the management of patients with sporotrichosis. For the Mycoses Study Group. Infectious Diseases Society of America. *Clin Infect Dis.* 2000;30:684–7.
- Milby AH, Pappas ND, O'Donnell J, et al. Sporotrichosis of the upper extremity. *Orthopedics.* 2010;273–5.

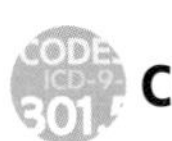

CODES

ICD9

117.1 Sporotrichosis

CLINICAL PEARLS

- Consider cutaneous/lymphocutaneous sporotrichosis in gardeners or those whose occupation puts them in contact with soil.
- Disseminated sporotrichosis may develop in immunocompromised individuals.
- Antifungal agents are frequently effective in the treatment of sporotrichosis.

SPRAIN, ANKLE

Salwa Khan, MD, MHS, FAAP

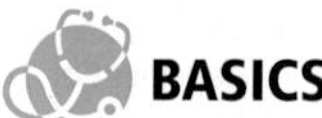

BASICS

DESCRIPTION

Ankle sprains are the most common cause of ankle injury and make up a significant proportion of sports injuries.

- There are several types of ankle sprains, including lateral, medial, and syndesmotic (or high ankle sprain):
  - The most common type of ankle sprain is a lateral ankle sprain, accounting for 85% of all ankle sprains. In lateral ankle sprains, the anterior talofibular ligament (ATFL) is the weakest ligament and, therefore, the most likely to be injured. The calcaneofibular ligament (CFL) is the second most likely ligament to be injured, and the posterior talofibular ligament (PTFL) is the least likely.
  - The medial deltoid ligament is the strongest ligament. Medial ankle sprains make up 5–10% of ankle sprains and result from an injury to the deltoid ligament.
  - Syndesmotic sprains are also rare; they account for 5–10% of ankle sprains.
- Ankle sprains can be classified based on degree of injury from grade I–III:
  - Grade I: Mild stretching of a ligament with possible microscopic tears
  - Grade II: Incomplete tear of a ligament
  - Grade III: Complete ligament tear

Geriatric Considerations

Increased risk of fracture occurring with a sprain secondary to weaker bones caused by osteoporosis or osteopenia

Pediatric Considerations

- Increased risk of physeal injuries instead of ligament sprain
- Ligaments are stronger than physes.
- Inversion ankle injuries in children may have a concomitant fibular physeal injury (Salter Harris type I fracture or higher fracture).

EPIDEMIOLOGY

Incidence

- Highest among basketball, soccer, and football players; cross-country runners; dancers
- Most common sports injury
- 2 million per year in the US

Prevalence

- 20% of sports injuries in the US (1)
- 75% of all ankle injuries are sprains.

RISK FACTORS

- Previous ankle sprain is the number 1 risk factor (2): Of people who have had a sprain, 3–34% will sustain another (3).
- Postural instability and talar tilting may be risk factors (2).
- Joint laxity was not found to be a risk factor (2).

GENERAL PREVENTION

- Conditioning before participating in sports and throughout the season (2)[B],(4)[A]:
  - Training in agility and flexibility
  - Single-leg balancing
- Taping or wearing ankle braces may help prevent reinjury to a sprained ankle (2)[B].

ETIOLOGY

- Lateral ankle sprains result from an inversion while plantarflexing the ankle.
- Medial ankle sprains are due to forced eversion while in dorsiflexion.
- Syndesmotic sprains result from eversion stress or extreme dorsiflexion along with internal rotation of tibia.

COMMONLY ASSOCIATED CONDITIONS

- Contusions
- Fractures:
  - Fibula head fracture or dislocation
  - Base of the fifth metatarsal fracture
  - Distal fibula fracture (including Salter Harris fractures in pediatric patients)

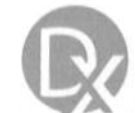

DIAGNOSIS

HISTORY

- Mechanism of injury (inversion versus eversion)
- Popping or snapping sensation during the injury
- Previous history of ankle injuries
- Ability to ambulate immediately after the injury
- Rapid onset of pain and swelling
- Ecchymosis
- Pain on lateral or medial ankle
- Weakness
- Difficulty bearing weight

PHYSICAL EXAM

- Compare to noninjured ankle for swelling and laxity.
- Palpate ATFL, CFL, PTFL, and deltoid ligament for tenderness.
- Palpate lateral and medial malleolus, base of fifth metatarsal, and entire fibula.
- Grade I sprain: Mild swelling and pain, no laxity
- Grade II sprain: Moderate swelling and pain, mild laxity with endpoint noted
- Grade III sprain: Severe swelling, pain, and bruising, laxity with no endpoint
- Special tests:
  - Anterior drawer test to check for laxity of ATFL
  - Talar tilt test to check laxity in CFL or deltoid ligament
  - Squeeze test of tibia and fibula midcalf to check for syndesmotic injury. Positive test is causing of pain isolated to the syndesmosis.
  - Dorsiflexion/external rotation test

DIAGNOSTIC TESTS & INTERPRETATION

Imaging

Initial approach

- Use the Ottawa ankle rules to determine whether radiographs are needed (patient must be aged 18–55 years):
  - Bony tenderness at tip or posterior edge of the lateral or medial malleolus *or*
  - Inability to bear weight (walk ≥4 steps) immediately and in the emergency department or office
  - Tenderness over the base of fifth metatarsal, navicular, or midfoot
- Obtain anteroposterior, lateral, and mortise views of the ankle.
- Small avulsion fractures are associated with grade III sprains.
- Consider CT if radiographs are negative, but have a high suspicion for occult fracture.
- MRI is gold standard for soft tissue, including ligaments, but is expensive and usually unnecessary.

Follow-Up & Special Considerations

If patient is not improving in 6 weeks, consider CT or MRI.

DIFFERENTIAL DIAGNOSIS

- Tendon injury:
  - Tendinopathy
  - Tendon tear
- Fracture of the ankle or foot
- Hindfoot or midfoot injuries
- Nerve injury
- Contusion
- Hematologic

TREATMENT

Short-term immobilization (10 days) for severe ankle sprains

MEDICATION

- NSAIDs
- Opioids if severe pain

ADDITIONAL TREATMENT

General Measures

- PRICE: *P*rotection, *r*est, *i*ce, *c*ompression, *e*levation
- Wrapping the ankle with an elastic bandage helps decrease swelling, but its use alone has a slower return to sports and work and provides less stability than an ankle brace (5)[A].
- Air-filled or gel-filled ankle brace or an ankle-stabilizing orthoses provides better support than elastic bandage or taping.

- Early mobilization and proper exercise are recommended rather than immobilization (6)[B].
- Short-term immobilization (10 days) has been shown to be beneficial for severe ankle sprains (7)[B].
- Do not use heat in an acute injury.
- Activity:
  - Weight-bearing as tolerated
  - Crutches may be needed if patient is unable to bear weight.
  - Exercises should be limited to pain-free range of motion.
  - Patient can start mobilization by tracing the alphabet with the foot in the air.
  - Elastic resistance exercises to improve balance

Issues for Referral

- Malleolar or talar dome fracture
- Syndesmotic sprain
- Tendon rupture

Additional Therapies

Physical therapy:

- After the acute phase of the injury, patients should start physical therapy.
- Physical therapy should include increasing range of motion, strength, flexibility, and proprioceptive balance (wobble board or ankle disk).
- Functional rehab is necessary to prevent chronic instability.
- Athletes should go through a sport-specific rehab before returning to play.

SURGERY/OTHER PROCEDURES

Syndesmotic sprains may require surgery. Patients with chronic ankle instability who fail functional rehabilitation or with poor tissue quality may need anatomic repair or reconstructive surgery (8).

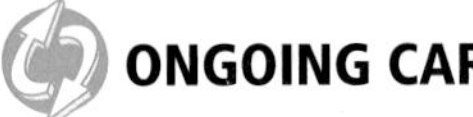

ONGOING CARE

FOLLOW-UP RECOMMENDATIONS

- Ankle-stabilizing orthoses should be worn for high-risk sports after a person has sustained an ankle sprain to prevent future ankle sprains (9)[A].
- Moderate and severe sprains require ankle orthoses for ≥6 months while participating in sports (2)[B].
- Return to play for athletes with a grade I lateral ankle sprain is generally 1–2 weeks; grade II sprain is 2–3 weeks; grade 3 sprain is 4 weeks.
- Return to play with medial or syndesmotic sprains is longer.

Patient Monitoring

If athletes continue to have symptoms when they return to play, consider further rehab.

PATIENT EDUCATION

- Training on how to use crutches
- Training on how to use elastic bandages, brace, and/or orthoses
- Demonstrate mobilization exercises for ankle.

PROGNOSIS

- Earlier mobilization with bracing allows for faster return to daily living and/or sports.
- Grade of ankle sprain does not relate to prognosis.
- Ligamentous strength does not return for months after the injury.

COMPLICATIONS

- Joint instability
- Intermittent swelling and pain if not treated properly
- Accumulation of cartilage damage leading to degenerative changes
- 5–33% will continue to have pain 1 year from the injury (3).

REFERENCES

1. Ivins D. Acute ankle sprain: An update. *Am Fam Physician*. 2006;74:1714–20; 1723–4; 1725–6.
2. Thacker SB, Stroup DF, Branche CM, et al. The prevention of ankle sprains in sports. A systematic review of the literature. *Am J Sports Med*. 1999;27: 753–60.
3. van Rijn RM. What is the Clinical Course of Acute Ankle Sprains? A Systematic literature review. *Am J Med*. 2008;121(4):324–31.e6.
4. Abernethy L. Strategies to prevent injury in adolescent sport: A systematic review. *Br J Sports Med*. 2007;41:627–38.
5. Kerkhoffs GMMJ, Struijs PAA, Marti RK, et al. Different functional treatment strategies for acute lateral ankle ligament injuries in adults. *Cochrane Database Syst Rev*. 2002;3:CD002938.
6. Jones MH. Acute treatment of inversion ankle sprains: Immobilization versus functional treatment. *Clin Orthop Relat Res*. 2007;455:169–72.
7. Lamb SE, Marsh JL, Hutton JL, et al. Mechanical supports for acute, severe ankle sprain: A pragmatic, multicentre, randomised controlled trial. *Lancet*. 2009;373:575–81.
8. Chan KW, Ding BC, Mroczek KJ. Acute and chronic lateral ankle instability in the athelete. *Bull NYU Hosp Jt Dis*. 2011;69(1):17–26.
9. Handoll HHG, Rowe BH, Quinn KM, et al. Interventions for preventing ankle ligament injuries. *Cochrane Database Syst Rev*. 2001;3:CD000018.

ADDITIONAL READING

- Ekman EF, Ruoff G, Kuehl K, et al. The COX-2 specific inhibitor Valdecoxib versus tramadol in acute ankle sprain: A multicenter randomized, controlled trial. *Am J Sports Med*. 2006;34:945–55.
- LaBella CR. Common acute sports-related lower extremity injuries in children and adolescents. *Clin Ped Emerg Med*. 2007;8:31–42.
- Mehallo CJ, Drezner JA, Bytomski JR. Practical management: Nonsteroidal antiinflammatory drug (NSAID) use in athletic injuries. *Clin J Sport Med*. 2006;16:170–4.
- Williams GN, Jones MH, Amendola A. Syndesmotic ankle sprains in athletes. *Am J Sports Med*. 2007;35: 1197–207.

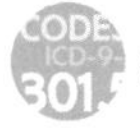

CODES

ICD9

- 845.00 Sprain of ankle, unspecified site
- 845.01 Deltoid (ligament), ankle sprain
- 845.02 Calcaneofibular (ligament) ankle sprain

CLINICAL PEARLS

- Increased risk of physeal injuries rather than ligament sprains in pediatric patients because ligaments are stronger than physes.
- Conditioning before participating in sports and throughout the season prevents ankle sprains.
- Taping or wearing ankle braces may help prevent reinjury to a sprained ankle, but does not help prevent initial ankle sprains.
- If patient is not improving in 6 weeks, consider CT or MRI.
- Short-term immobilization (10 days) using mechanical supports (e.g., Aircast) is superior to elastic bandages.
- Early mobilization is better than long-term immobilization.

SPRAINS AND STRAINS

Jennifer Schwartz, MD
J. Herbert Stevenson, MD

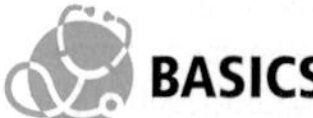

BASICS

DESCRIPTION

- Sprains are complete or partial ligamentous injuries either within the body of the ligament or at the site of attachment to bone:
  - May be classified as grade I, II, or III (AMA Ligament Injury Classification):
    - Grade I: Stretch injury without ligamentous laxity
    - Grade II: Partial tear with increased ligamentous laxity but firm endpoint on exam
    - Grade III: Complete tear with increased ligamentous laxity and no firm endpoint on exam
  - Physical exam is the key to diagnosis.
  - Usually secondary to trauma (e.g., falls, twisting injuries, motor vehicle accidents)
- Strains are partial or complete disruptions of the muscle, muscle-tendon junction, or tendon:
  - May be classified as:
    - First degree: Minimal damage to muscle, tendon, or musculotendinous unit
    - Second degree: Partial tear to the muscle, tendon, or musculotendinous unit
    - Third degree: Complete disruption of the muscle, tendon, or musculotendinous unit
  - Often associated with overuse injuries

Geriatric Considerations

More likely to see associated bony injuries due to decreased joint flexibility and prevalence of osteoporosis and osteopenia

Pediatric Considerations

- Sprains and strains have been found to account for 24% of injuries in pediatric patients.
- 3 million pediatric sports injuries occur annually.
- Must be concerned about physeal/apophyseal injuries in the skeletally immature

EPIDEMIOLOGY

Incidence

~80% of all US athletes at some time in their career will experience a sprain or strain that involves the upper or lower extremities or spine.

Prevalence

- Ankle sprains are among the most common injuries seen in the primary care setting and account for up to 30% of sports medicine clinic visits.
- Most ankle sprains are due to inversion injuries (lateral sprains).
- Predominant age:
  - Sprains: Any age when patient is physically active
  - Strains: Usually 15–40 years of age
- Predominant sex: Male > Female; Female > Male for sprain of acromioclavicular ligament

RISK FACTORS

- Prior history of sprain or strain is greatest risk factor for future sprain/strain.
- Change in or improper shoe gear, protective gear, or environment (e.g., surface)
- Inappropriate sudden increase in training schedule

GENERAL PREVENTION

- Use appropriate conditions, warm-up, and cool-down exercises.
- Use proper equipment for the activity.
- Balance training programs can improve joint position sense and reduce the risk of ankle sprains (1)[A].
- Semirigid orthoses or air casts may prevent ankle sprains during high-risk sports, especially in athletes with history of sprain (2,3)[A].

ETIOLOGY

- Trauma, falls, MVA
- Excessive exercise
- Improper footwear
- Inadequate warm-up and stretching before activity
- Poor conditioning
- Prior sprain or strain

COMMONLY ASSOCIATED CONDITIONS

- Effusions, hemarthrosis
- Stress, avulsion, or other fractures
- Syndesmotic injuries
- Contusions
- Wounds
- Dislocations/subluxations

DIAGNOSIS

HISTORY

- May describe feeling or hearing pop or snap
- May remember mechanism (key in diagnosis)

PHYSICAL EXAM

- Observe gait. Gait disturbances if severe.
- Inspect for swelling, asymmetry, ecchymosis.
- Palpate for tenderness.
- Evaluate for decreased range of motion (ROM) of joint and joint instability.
- Evaluate for strength.
- Sprains:
  - Grade I: Tenderness without laxity. Minimal pain, swelling. Little ecchymosis. Can bear weight.
  - Grade II: Tenderness with increased laxity on exam but firm endpoint. More pain, swelling. Often ecchymosis. Some difficulty bearing weight.
  - Grade III: Tenderness with increased laxity on exam and no firm endpoint. Severe pain, swelling. Obvious ecchymosis. Difficulty bearing weight.

DIAGNOSTIC TESTS & INTERPRETATION

- Examination under anesthesia and/or arthroscopy may be required in some cases.
- Ankle:
  - Anterior drawer test assesses integrity of anterior talofibular ligament.
  - Talar tilt test assesses integrity of calcaneofibular ligament.
- Knee:
  - Lachman test assesses integrity of anterior cruciate ligament. Posterior drawer assesses integrity of posterior cruciate ligament.
  - Valgus/varus stress tests assess integrity of collateral ligaments.
- Shoulder:
  - Positive apprehension test may indicate glenohumeral ligament sprain.

Imaging

- Radiographs may be needed to rule out bony injury; stress views may be helpful. Should obtain radiographs in children to rule out growth plate injuries.
- Use Ottawa ankles rules (age 18–55) to determine if radiograph necessary (3)[A].
- Ankle films: Required if pain in the malleolar zone *and*:
  - Bone tenderness in posterior aspect distal 6 cm of tibia *or* fibula *or*
  - Inability to bear weight immediately or in emergency department
- Foot films: Required if midfoot zone pain is present *and*:
  - Bone tenderness at base of fifth metatarsal *or*
  - Bone tenderness at navicular *or*
  - Inability to bear weight immediately or in emergency department
- CT scan of the affected area may be required if occult fracture is suspected.
- MRI is "gold standard" for imaging soft tissue structures, including muscle, ligaments, and intraarticular structures.

Diagnostic Procedures/Surgery

Surgery may be required for some partial and complete sprains. Need for surgery depends on the ability of ligaments or muscles to heal on their own or the ability to attain full ROM and stability of the affected joint.

DIFFERENTIAL DIAGNOSIS

- Tendonitis
- Bursitis
- Contusion
- Hematoma
- Fracture
- Rheumatologic process

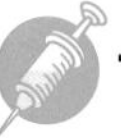

TREATMENT

MEDICATION

- Acetaminophen: Up to 3–4 g/d
- NSAIDs:
  - Ibuprofen: 200–800 mg t.i.d.
  - Naproxen: 250–500 mg b.i.d.
  - Diclofenac 75 mg b.i.d.
- Narcotics for severe pain, acute injury
- Acetaminophen and NSAIDs found to have similar efficacy in reducing pain after ankle sprains
- Topical diclofenac may reduce pain in acute ankle sprains (4)[B].
- Platelet-rich plasma injections may aid recovery in treatment of muscle strains, but more studies are needed (5)[C].
- Refer to manufacturer's profile of each drug for contraindications, precautions, and possible interactions.

ADDITIONAL TREATMENT

General Measures

- History and physical exam along with treatment of the worst possible suspected injury
- Acutely: PRICEMM therapy (*p*rotection, relative *r*est, *i*ce, *c*ompression, *e*levation, *m*edications, *m*odalities)
- Grade I, II ankle sprain: Functional treatment with brace, orthosis, taping, elastic bandage wrap (3)[A]:
  - Ankle braces (lace up, stirrup type, air cast) more effective functional treatment than elastic bandages or taping (3,6)[B]
- Grade III ankle sprain: Short period of immobilization with cast/crutches may be needed (3)[A].
- For high-level athletes with more extensive damage, consider surgery.

Issues for Referral

- ACL sprain in athletes/physically active
- Salter-Harris physeal fractures
- Lack of improvement with conservative measures
- Joint instability
- Tendon disruption (i.e., Achilles, biceps)

Additional Therapies

Physical therapy is a useful adjunct after a sprain, and early mobilization is crucial (7)[A]:

- Proprioception retraining
- Core strengthening
- Eccentric exercises

SURGERY/OTHER PROCEDURES

Casting and surgery are reserved for select grade III injuries.

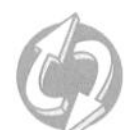

ONGOING CARE

FOLLOW-UP RECOMMENDATIONS

If affected joint has full strength and ROM, patient can advance activity as tolerated.

Patient Monitoring

After initial treatment, consider rehabilitation. Direct emphasis toward limiting swelling and providing a pain-free full ROM.

DIET

Weight loss if obesity is etiologic

PATIENT EDUCATION

- Instructions on how to wrap with elastic bandage
- Prevention of injury

PROGNOSIS

With appropriate treatment and rest, 1–8 weeks or longer for recovery, depending on the severity of injury

COMPLICATIONS

- Chronic joint instability
- Arthritis
- Muscle contracture

REFERENCES

1. Sefton JM, Yarar C, et al. Six weeks of balance training improved sensorimotor function in individuals with chronic ankle instability. *J Orthop Sports Phys Ther*. 2011;41(2):81–9.
2. Handoll MM, Rowe BH, et al. Interventions for preventing ankle ligament injuries. *Cochrane Database Systematic Rev*. 2011:CD000018.
3. Seah R, Mani-Babu S. Managing ankle sprains in primary care: what is the best practice? A systematic review of the last 10 years of evidence. *Br Med Bull*. 2011;97:105–35.
4. Lionberger DR, Joussellin E, Lanzarotti A. Diclofenac epolamine topical patch relieves pain associated with ankle sprain. *J Pain Res*. 2011;4:47–53.
5. Hamilton BH, Best TM. Platelet-rich plasma and muscle strain injuries-challenges imposed by the burden of proof. *Clin J Sports Med*. 2011;21(1): 31–6.
6. Kemler E, Van de port I, et al. A systematic review of acute ankle sprains: Brace versus other functional treatment types. *Sports Med*. 2011;41(3):185–97.
7. Bleakley CM, O'Connor SR, et al. Effect of accelerated rehabilitation on function after ankle sprain: A randomized control trial. *BMJ*. 2010;34: c1964.

ADDITIONAL READING

- Bachmann LH, Kolb E. Accuracy of the Ottawa Ankle Rules to excude fractures of the ankle and mid-foot: A systematic review. *BMJ*. 2003;326(7386):417.
- Dalton JD, Schweinle JE. Randomized controlled noninferiority trial to compare extended release acetaminophen and ibuprofen for the treatment of ankle sprains. *Ann Emerg Med*. 2006;48:615–23.
- Kerkoffs MMJ, Rowe BH, et al. Immobilisation and functional treatment for acute lateral ankle ligament injuries. *Cochrane Database Systematic Rev*. 2010: CD003762.
- Mahaffey D, Hilts M, Fields KB. Ankle and foot injuries in sports. *Clin Fam Pract*. 1999;1:233–50.
- McGuine TA, Keene JS. The effect of a balance training program on the risk of ankle sprains in high school athletes. *Am J Sports Med*. 2006;34: 1103–11.

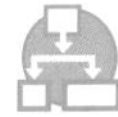

See Also (Topic, Algorithm, Electronic Media Element)

Tendinitis

CODES

ICD9

- 845.00 Unspecified site of ankle sprain
- 848.9 Unspecified site of sprain and strain

CLINICAL PEARLS

For acute injury, remember PRICEMM:

- Protection of the joint
- Rest as appropriate
- Apply ice
- Apply compression
- Elevate joint
- Medications for pain
- Other modalities as needed

S

STAPHYLOCOCCAL TOXIC SHOCK SYNDROME

Rebecca Feldman, MD
William J. Durbin, MD
Amanda Johnson, MD

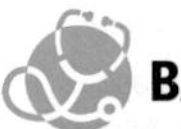

BASICS

DESCRIPTION

- An acute toxin-mediated illness associated with *Staphylococcus aureus* infection
- TSS (toxic shock syndrome) is characterized by sudden onset of high fever and rash with subsequent hypotension, desquamation, and involvement of ≥3 organ systems.
  - Menstrual (less common): Associated with menstruation and tampon use
  - Nonmenstrual (more common): Associated with postoperative wounds and barrier contraception
- Can occur in children and adults
- System(s) affected: All organ systems can be affected.

EPIDEMIOLOGY

- Predominant age: 15–35 years, but can occur at any age
- Predominant sex: Female > Male
- Nonmenstrual cases increasingly are associated with methicillin-resistant *S. aureus* (MRSA) infections and carry a higher mortality rate (1).
- Newborn population: Neonatal TSS-like exanthematous disease syndrome

Incidence

71–101 cases per year were reported to the CDC between 2005 and 2010 (2).

RISK FACTORS

- High:
  - Absence of antibody to TSS toxin-1 (TSST-1)
  - Infection with *S. aureus,* which produces TSST-1; only a small proportion of *S. aureus* isolates carry the gene encoding TSST-1
  - Focal: Abscess, sinusitis, bacterial tracheitis
  - Invasive: Pneumonia, osteomyelitis, bacteremia, endocarditis
  - Focus of infection may not be apparent:
    - Continuous use of super-absorbency tampons during menstruation
    - Nasal surgery with packing
- Moderate:
  - Use of regular-absorbency tampons during menstruation
  - Use of contraceptive sponge
- Low:
  - Alternating use of tampons and pads during menstruation
  - Surgical wound infections
  - Cellulitis
  - Early postpartum state, especially after cesarean section or episiotomy
- Pediatric considerations:
  - TSS may occur as a complication of:
    - Chickenpox
    - Burns: TSS is the most common cause of unexpected mortality after small burns among the pediatric population.

Genetics

- Patient's genetic composition may influence his or her inflammatory response to the toxins.
- Genetic polymorphisms leading to different human leukocyte antigen haplotypes may influence the susceptibility to the toxic effects of superantigens.

GENERAL PREVENTION

- Avoid continuous tampon use during menstruation.
- Avoid super-absorbency tampons.
- Change tampons frequently during the day.
- Use sanitary napkins at night.
- Early medical attention to infected wounds

PATHOPHYSIOLOGY

- In vivo production and release of staphylococcal superantigens in the absence of neutralizing antibodies. Superantigen simultaneously binds to APC MHC class II and V-beta region of T cell receptor. A large subset of T cells are then activated, resulting in massive release of cytokines (interleukin [IL]-1, IL-2, gamma interferon, tumor necrosis factor [TNF] alpha, TNF beta, IL-6). Capillary leak, hypotension, and shock ensue.
- Although both serum IgG and IgM antibodies bind to TSST-1 in vitro, only IgG1 and IgG4 isotype antibodies are protective (3).

ETIOLOGY

- *S. aureus* exotoxins, especially TSST-1 (etiology in >90% of menstrual cases)
- Staphylococcal enterotoxins A–E and G–I
- Enterotoxins B and C cause 50% of nonmenstrual TSS.

COMMONLY ASSOCIATED CONDITIONS

Staphylococcal infections

DIAGNOSIS

HISTORY

- Prodrome of 1–3 days that often includes malaise, myalgias, fever, chills, vomiting, and/or diarrhea
- Acute-onset fever and chills
- Lightheadedness or syncope
- Disorientation, confusion, or alteration in consciousness
- Myalgias
- Diffuse macular rash
- Other symptoms of multiorgan involvement

PHYSICAL EXAM

- Temperature >38.9°C (>102°F)
- Hypotension:
  - Systolic BP <90 mm Hg
  - Orthostatic drop in diastolic BP of ≥15 mm Hg
  - BP less than fifth percentile for age in children
- Tachycardia
- Tachypnea
- Diffuse erythroderma, initially appearing on trunk, spreading to arms and legs, including palms and soles:
  - Skin desquamation of palms and soles 1–2 weeks after rash onset
- Signs of multiorgan involvement, including:
  - Cardiac (arrhythmias, pericarditis, cardiomyopathy)
  - Pulmonary (acute respiratory distress syndrome [ARDS])
  - Renal (oliguria)
  - Disseminated intravascular coagulation (DIC)
  - CNS involvement (headache, confusion, agitation, photophobia, meningismus, seizure, loss of consciousness)
  - Mucosal inflammation (conjunctivitis, strawberry tongue, pharyngitis, vaginitis)

DIAGNOSTIC TESTS & INTERPRETATION

Lab

Initial lab tests

- Neutrophilic leukocytosis
- Thrombocytopenia may be present (platelet count ≤100,000/mm^3), increased prothrombin time and activated partial thromboplastin time.
- BUN and creatinine may be increased.
- Liver function tests, including total bilirubin, aspartate aminotransferase), and/or alanine aminotransferase, may be increased.
- Creatine phosphokinase may be increased.
- Urinary sediment may contain WBCs in absence of UTI.
- Culture and Gram stains of possible infection sites (vaginal and/or wound swabs)
- Blood culture is positive for *S. aureus* in <5% of cases; vaginal swab is positive in >90% of menstrual-related cases.
- Throat and CSF cultures usually are negative.
- If clinically plausible, serologies for Rocky Mountain spotted fever, leptospirosis, and measles should be negative.

Imaging

No unusual or characteristic findings

Diagnostic Procedures/Surgery

- No specific diagnostic test is currently available.
- Acute and convalescent anti–TSST-1 antibodies

Pathological Findings

- Subepidermal cleavage plane in skin
- Minimal inflammatory reaction in tissues
- Lymphocyte depletion in lymph nodes

DIFFERENTIAL DIAGNOSIS

- Requires high index of suspicion and active search for source of infection.
- Streptococcal scarlet fever

- Streptococcal TSS:
  - More often associated with severe pain and tenderness at a site of local trauma and infection, and more frequently accompanied by bacteremia
- Staphylococcal scalded-skin syndrome
- Necrotizing fasciitis
- Meningococcemia/sepsis (petechial/purpuric rash)
- Gram-negative sepsis (more likely in hospitalized patients)
- Rocky Mountain spotted fever (petechial rash beginning distally; often presents with severe headache)
- Leptospirosis
- Kawasaki disease
- Measles
- Drug reactions (i.e., Stevens Johnson syndrome)

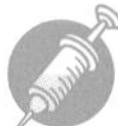

TREATMENT

Inpatient; typically requires admission to intensive care for close monitoring

MEDICATION

First Line

- Treatment of shock or hypotension (see "Shock, Circulatory" for details):
  - Aggressive fluid replacement with isotonic crystalloids or colloids
  - Oxygen support; if fail to achieve adequate oxygen delivery, packed RBCs if the hematocrit is <30%
  - Pressors, generally with norepinephrine or dopamine
  - Steroids have not proven to be of value, although low-dose steroids may be beneficial if sepsis is severe (4)[A].
- Antibiotics to eradicate *S. aureus* and inhibit toxin production; give within 1 hour of diagnosis (with blood cultures prior to start of antibiotics):
  - Oxacillin or nafcillin: 100 mg/kg/d IV divided q4h (bactericidal against susceptible *S. aureus*, but may induce more toxin production and release more toxins by bacterial lysis) (5)[B]
  - Clindamycin: 30–40 mg/kg/d IV divided q8h (more efficacious than beta-lactams in suppressing in vitro production of TSST-1 and other exotoxins) (5)[B]
  - Combination of clindamycin 25 mg/kg/d IV divided q8h plus oxacillin or nafcillin 100 mg/kg/d IV q4h (recommended for patients with deep-seated infections or bacteremia) (5)[B]
  - For patients infected with MRSA: Vancomycin 40 mg/kg/d IV divided q6h or linezolid 600 mg IV q12h
- Antimicrobial therapy should be continued for at least 10–14 days.

Second Line

- Toxin neutralization with IVIG 1 g/kg
- IVIG equivocal results; newer reviews suggest it may help.

ADDITIONAL TREATMENT

General Measures

- Ongoing fluid resuscitation
- Removal of tampon or other vaginal foreign bodies and irrigation of vaginal vault with saline or povidone-iodine
- Removal of nasal packing
- Local wound care; debridement of infected wound or drainage of focal collection
- Management of renal or cardiac insufficiency
- Mechanical ventilation if necessary

IN-PATIENT CONSIDERATIONS

IV Fluids

Crystalloids, up to 10–20 L/d, may be necessary.

Nursing

- Vital signs should be monitored closely.
- Foley catheter to monitor urine output

Discharge Criteria

- Hemodynamic stability
- Improvement in symptoms
- Tolerating oral alimentation

ONGOING CARE

FOLLOW-UP RECOMMENDATIONS

- Women can reduce the risk of recurrent TSS by avoiding continuous tampon use during menstruation.
- Wound care/hygiene

DIET

As tolerated

PATIENT EDUCATION

CDC: www.cdc.gov/ncidod/dbmd/diseaseinfo/toxicshock t.htm

PROGNOSIS

- Mortality: 4–22%; higher in older patients, nonmenstrual TSS, and delayed diagnosis
- Rare recurrence in both menstrual and nonmenstrual cases

COMPLICATIONS

- Common (>20%):
  - Acute renal failure
  - ARDS
  - Menorrhagia
  - Alopecia
  - Nail loss
- Rare (<20%):
  - DIC
  - Encephalopathy/memory impairment
  - Cardiomyopathy
  - Protracted malaise

REFERENCES

1. Descloux E, Perpoint T, Ferry T, et al. One in five mortality in non-menstrual toxic shock syndrome versus no mortality in menstrual cases in a balanced French series of 55 cases. *Eur J Clin Microbiol Infect Dis*. 2008;27:37–43.
2. Centers for Disease Control and Prevention (CDC): Notifiable diseases and mortality tables. *MMWR* 2010;59:398–411.
3. Kansal R, Davis C, Hansmann M, et al. Structural and functional properties of antibodies to the superantigen TSST-1 and their relationship to menstrual toxic shock syndrome. *J Clin Immunol*. 2007;27:327–38.
4. Minneci PC, Deans KJ, Eichacker PQ, et al. The effects of steroids during sepsis depend on dose and severity of illness: An updated meta-analysis. *Clin Microbiol Infect*. 2009;15:308–18.
5. Stevens DL, Ma Y, Salmi DB, et al. Impact of antibiotics on expression of virulence-associated exotoxin genes in methicillin-sensitive and methicillin-resistant *Staphylococcus aureus*. *J Infect Dis*. 2007;195:202–11.

ADDITIONAL READING

- Andrews JI, Shamshirsaz AA, Diekema DJ. Nonmenstrual toxic shock syndrome due to methicillin-resistant *Staphylococcus aureus*. *Obstet Gynecol*. 2008;112:933–8.
- Lin YC, Peterson ML. New insights into the prevention of staphylococcal infections and toxic shock syndrome. *Expert Rev Clin Pharmacol*. 2010; 3(6):753–67.
- Llewelyn M, Sriskandan S, Peakman M, et al. HLA class II polymorphisms determine responses to bacterial superantigens. *J Immunol*. 2004;172: 1719–26.
- Silversides, JA, Lappin E, Ferguson AJ. Staphylococcal toxic shock syndrome: Mechanisms and management. *Curr Infect Dis Rep*. 2010;12: 392–400.
- Walden A, Harriet H, Alyaqoobi M. Methicillin-resistant *Staphylococcus aureus* toxic shock syndrome. *J Infect*. 2008;56:161–2.

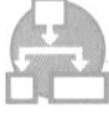

See Also (Topic, Algorithm, Electronic Media Element)

Measles (Rubeola); Pancreatitis; Rocky Mountain Spotted Fever; Scarlet Fever

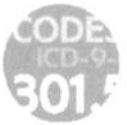

CODES

ICD9

- 040.82 Toxic shock syndrome
- 041.11 Methicillin susceptible Staphylococcus aureus

CLINICAL PEARLS

- TSS is a rare, acute, toxin-mediated illness caused by *S. aureus*.
- In women, TSS is associated with the continuous use of super-absorbency tampons during menstruation.
- Patients typically require ICU-level care and IV antibiotics.

STATUS EPILEPTICUS

Jeff Ray Gibson, Jr., MD

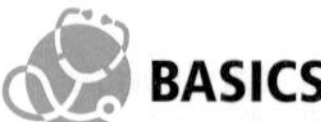

BASICS

ALERT
- Status epilepticus is a life-threatening emergency; rapid seizure control is critical, even before a definitive diagnosis is reached (like CPR).
- Begin drug treatment if seizure lasts >5 minutes or after 2 seizures without full recovery.

DESCRIPTION
- Established status epilepticus: Seizure lasting >30 minutes or absence of recovery of consciousness between seizures. Tonic–clonic (grand mal or generalized convulsive) status is the most common and most serious form.
- Refractory status epilepticus: Seizure that persists after treatment with first-line drugs.
- System affected: Nervous
- Synonym: Status convulsivus

EPIDEMIOLOGY
Incidence
- 18–50 cases per 100,000 per year:
  - 1/3 as unprovoked first seizure
  - 1/6 in patients with known epilepsy
  - 1/2 secondary to acute CNS insult
  - Incidence is 2 times higher in the elderly.
- Predominant age: >50% of new cases in the young
- Predominant sex: Male > Female

Prevalence
In the US, 100,000–150,000 patients per year present in generalized tonic–clonic status epilepticus, with 55,000 associated deaths.

RISK FACTORS
- Seizure disorder plus any precipitating insult
- Prior history of status epilepticus (recurrence rates: In children, 17%; in those with neurologic abnormality, 50%)
- Porphyria, autoimmune diseases, CNS lesion

Genetics
Links are suspected, but not defined.

GENERAL PREVENTION
Established maintenance therapy with anticonvulsant

PATHOPHYSIOLOGY
- Neuronal: Stress injury, autonomic activation
- Metabolic: Lactic acidosis, CO_2 narcosis, hyperkalemia, hyperglycemia followed by hypoglycemia
- Cardiac: Hypertension (followed by hypotension), ischemia, arrhythmias, high-output failure
- Respiratory: Increased secretions, lax tongue and possibly: Airway obstruction, pneumothorax, neurogenic pulmonary edema, or aspiration
- Renal: ATN from myoglobinuria after rhabdomyolysis
- Cerebrovascular: Loss of autoregulation, focal ischemia, cerebral edema

ETIOLOGY
- Adults: Usually from a known condition (epilepsy, alcohol withdrawal, anticonvulsant withdrawal/noncompliance) or acquired CNS pathology (especially frontal lobe)
- Children: Status epilepticus may present as the first seizure from febrile seizure, new-onset epilepsy, CNS infection, or metabolic derangement.
- Neonatal status: Meningitis or metabolic disorders (deficiencies of calcium, magnesium, or pyridoxine)
- CNS pathology (acute or chronic): Trauma, infection, stroke, hypoglycemia, mass or vascular lesion, metabolic disorder, encephalopathy (hypoxic, hypertensive, autoimmune or degenerative type)
- Intoxication: Reports include cocaine, tricyclic antidepressants, lead, isoniazid, chloroquine, cephalosporins, penicillins, ciprofloxacin, cyclosporine, theophylline, tacrolimus, tiagabine, or nerve-agent poisoning
- Idiopathic, cryptogenic

COMMONLY ASSOCIATED CONDITIONS
Premonitory status epilepticus: Increasing frequency of seizures, which may precede convulsive status epilepticus. Treat early to prevent status.

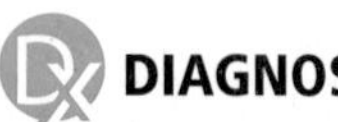

DIAGNOSIS

ALERT
- Rule out pseudo (psychogenic)-status epilepticus; usually atypical, e.g., pelvic thrusting, no self-injury
- Check the EEG; avoid dangerous therapy.
- Treat while searching for cause.

HISTORY
Previous seizures, drug history, toxic exposure?

PHYSICAL EXAM
- Signs and symptoms depend on the type of seizure; generalized (tonic–clonic) convulsion is most common:
  - May be preceded by aura
  - Tonic phase (stiffening) for 30–45 seconds
  - Clonic phase (rhythmic jerking) for 2–5 minutes
  - No intervening consciousness; seizure recurs
- Neurologic exam: Look for localizing signs of CNS lesion; rule out pseudo status.
- Postictal findings: Fever, tachycardia, mydriasis, conjugate deviation of eyes, decreased corneal reflex, positive Babinski sign, Todd paralysis, fecal/urinary incontinence, injury (to tongue, cheek, lips)

DIAGNOSTIC TESTS & INTERPRETATION
Lab
- Glucose (rapid determination); electrolytes, CBC, osmolarity, liver/renal function, troponin, CPK, calcium, magnesium, phosphate, coag profile
- Arterial blood gases, carboxyhemoglobin
- Anticonvulsant levels
- Toxicology screens (urine and blood)

Imaging
- Noncontrast CT scan in new-onset seizure
- MRI or PET for more anatomic detail
- CXR for ET tube position and check for aspiration

Diagnostic Procedures/Surgery
- Lumbar puncture: If meningitis is suspected. CAUTION: Intracranial pressure may be increased.
- EEG: To differentiate pseudoseizures; to reveal nonconvulsive status epilepticus in comatose or paralyzed patient; to confirm successful treatment

DIFFERENTIAL DIAGNOSIS
- Pseudo (psychogenic)–status epilepticus may occur with pseudo seizures; check EEG.
- Non-clonic–tonic status and nonconvulsive status (in comatose or paralyzed patients) require neurologic exam and EEG.
- Special Considerations
  - If patient is not awake 30 minutes after a seizure, check the EEG for nonconvulsive status.

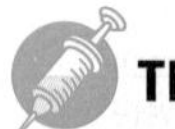

TREATMENT

Simultaneous goals are to stop the seizure, find the cause, and prevent complications (1,2,3,4)[B]:
- Support ABCs and watch vitals.
- Treat glucose if <60 mg/100 dL.
- Start IV or intraosseous (IO) line and draw labs.
- If seizure lasts >5 minutes, start first-line medication for established status epilepticus.
- IV or IO is preferred, but administer non-IV alternatives (below) rather than delay treatment.
- If seizure continues >30 minutes, treat as refractory status epilepticus with anesthesia/drug coma.
- Continue to pursue the underlying cause.

MEDICATION
First Line
- Start with lorazepam (Ativan): This is the preferred benzodiazepine (1,2,3,4,5,6)[A]:
  - Give 0.1 mg/kg IV or IO at 1–2 mg/min to a maximum of 10 mg.
  - May repeat q10min × 2:
    - For child: 0.05–0.1 mg/kg IV at <2 mg/min to a maximum of 4 mg
- Then add fosphenytoin (Cerebyx) after 5 minutes, if seizure persists: This is the preferred anticonvulsant and the prodrug of phenytoin (1,2,4)[B]:
  - Give 15–20 mg phenytoin equivalents (PE) per kg IV or IO at <150 mg PE/min (follow BP, ECG).
  - May add 5–10 mg PE/kg IV after 5 minutes.
  - Maintenance: 4–6 mg PE/kg/d IV or IM:
    - For child: Same dose as for an adult at <3 mg PE/kg/min

ALERT
If seizure lasts >30 minutes, move on to second-line (refractory) treatment.

- Non-IV alternatives:
  - Midazolam (Versed): 0.2 mg/kg IM or up to 0.5 mg/kg buccal or intranasal (onset 5–10 minutes) (3,5,7)[A]
  - Lorazepam (SL or intranasal) (5)[B]: Use IV dose.
  - Rectal diazepam (Valium) (6)[A]: 0.2–0.5 mg/kg (for child: 20 mg maximum). Use gel (Diastat) or IV solution.
- Alternative for IV lorazepam:
  - Diazepam (Valium) (4,6)[B]: 0.2–0.5 mg/kg IV or IO at 5 mg/min up to a dose of 40 mg:
    - For child: 0.3 mg/kg at <2 mg/min IV up to 10 mg total
    - May repeat q5min × 3
    - Antiseizure wears off quickly; sedation persists.
- Alternatives for IV fosphenytoin:
  - Phenytoin IV (4,6)[B] doses are the same (mg-for-mg phenytoin equivalents), but must be given more slowly (<1 mg/kg/min) to lessen cardiovascular depression and toxicity.
  - Fosphenytoin IM: Use IV dose (slowly).

S

Second Line

- To treat refractory status epilepticus:
  - When seizure persists >30 minutes, admit to ICU and induce anesthesia/drug coma (1,3,4)[B].
  - Consult neurologist, intensivist, or anesthesiologist.
  - Induce drug coma and adjust to keep EEG at burst suppression (drug choices listed below).
  - Often requires intubation, ventilation, and BP support (e.g., dopamine)
  - Maintain anesthetic for 12–48 hours; then withdraw gradually while adjusting maintenance anticonvulsant therapy.
  - Consider EEG and end-tidal CO_2 monitoring.
  - For muscle relaxation, use short-acting rocuronium bromide 0.6–1 mg/kg (to avoid hyperkalemia).
  - Cool and treat if febrile
- Drug choices (choose 1):
  - Propofol (Diprivan) (1,2,3,4)[C]:
    - 1–2 mg/kg IV (in elderly, halve initial dose)
    - Follow with 30–150 μg/kg/min IV; titrated to EEG
    - Less tissue accumulation
  - Midazolam (Versed) (1,2,3,4)[C]:
    - 0.2–0.5 mg/kg slow IV bolus injection
    - Follow with 0.75–10 μg/kg/min IV; titrate to EEG
    - Tachyphylaxis may develop.
  - Pentobarbital (1,3,4)[B]:
    - 5–15 mg/kg IV loading dose over 1 hour
    - Follow by continuous infusion of 0.5–10 mg/kg/hr; adjust based on EEG
  - Alternates: That may not require intubation (2,3)[C]:
    - Sodium valproate: 15–30 mg/kg bolus at <6 mg/kg/min, then maintenance at 500 mg t.i.d.
    - Phenobarbital: 20 mg/kg infused at a rate of 30–50 mg/min (slower with older populations; close monitoring of respiratory and cardiac status; causes prolonged sedation), then initial maintenance dosing of 60 mg t.i.d.
    - Levetiracetam: 20 mg/kg bolus over 15 minutes, then maintenance dosing of 1,500 mg b.i.d.
    - Topiramate: 300–1,600 mg/d PO (3)[C]
- Investigational or anecdotal drugs:
  - Isoflurane (by inhalation), desflurane (by inhalation), lidocaine, thiopental, lacosamide, ketamine, nimodipine, chlormethiazole, lamotrigine, propofol (by inhalation), immunologic therapy, ECT
- Contraindications:
  - Benzodiazepines in narrow-angle glaucoma
  - Propofol in allergy to soybean oil, egg, lecithin, or glycerol
  - Barbiturates in acute intermittent porphyria
  - Valproic acid in hepatic disease and pregnancy (risk of neural tube defects)
- Precautions:
  - Propofol: Prolonged use may cause propofol infusion syndrome (lactic acidosis, lipemia, heart failure, systemic collapse, and death) in both children and adults. Not for child <3 years old. Strict aseptic technique required.
  - Most drugs listed may exacerbate porphyria. Exceptions are lorazepam, midazolam, propofol.
  - Diazepam: May cause venous thrombosis/phlebitis
  - Fosphenytoin (Cerebyx) and phenytoin:
    - Safety not established for children. Abrupt withdrawal may precipitate status epilepticus. Overdose may cause paradoxical inefficacy.
    - Monitor for arrhythmias, prolonged QT interval, and hypotension. If these occur, decrease the rate of administration. Use caution in liver disease, hyperglycemia, the elderly, and pregnancy (increased risk of malformations and may lead to vitamin K–deficiency bleeding problems in both mother and newborn).
  - Phenytoin: Infiltration may cause local ischemia (purple glove syndrome).
  - Valproic acid: May decrease platelet function and cause hyperammonemic encephalopathy or pancreatitis
- Significant possible interactions:
  - Fosphenytoin/phenytoin: May increase serum levels and toxicity of warfarin, disulfiram, phenylbutazone, and isoniazid; decrease dose with renal insufficiency
  - Valproic acid: May increase toxicity of phenytoin/fosphenytoin

ADDITIONAL TREATMENT

General Measures

- Monitor: Pulse oximetry, end-tidal CO_2, BP, ECG, EEG, and temperature
- Give oxygen; intubate and hyperventilate if hypoventilation, hypoxia, or hypercarbia occur *or* if aspiration is a concern.
- Establish 2 IV lines (or an intraosseous line) and check labs.
- Protect from injury, clear/suction airway, prevent tongue laceration
- If comatose, place NG tube, urinary catheter

Additional Therapies

- In suspected alcoholism: Thiamine, 100 mg IV/IM
- If blood sugar is low or cannot be measured: 50% dextrose, 50 mL IV:
  - For child: Use $D_{25}W$; give 2 mL/kg slowly
- If pupils are myotic or drug overdose suspected: Naloxone (Narcan), 2 mg IV:
  - For child: 0.1 mg/kg IV, up to 2 mg slowly
- If isoniazid poisoning is suspected: Pyridoxine
- If meningitis is strongly suspected: Consider antibiotics
- For nerve-agent poisoning: Give atropine, benzodiazepine, and pralidoxime (2-PAM)

SURGERY/OTHER PROCEDURES

Experimental: Surgical excision of epileptic focus or propagation pathways, vagal nerve stimulator

IN-PATIENT CONSIDERATIONS

IV Fluids

Hemodynamic instability may require fluid boluses or vasopressors (e.g., dopamine).

Discharge Criteria

Seizures under control and therapeutic levels of maintenance anticonvulsants established

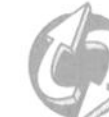

ONGOING CARE

PATIENT EDUCATION

Reinforce the importance of continuing anticonvulsant medications, regular medical care, avoiding alcohol, and seeking help if seizure frequency increases:

- Epilepsy Foundation: (800) EFA-1000, www.efa.org
- Epilepsy Therapy Development Project: www.epilepsy.com

PROGNOSIS

- Prolonged seizures (>30 min) may cause neurologic injury or death.
- Reported mortality is 16–25% in adults, 3–19% in children, extremely high in neonates, and up to 76% in the elderly.
- With seizure duration >4 hours, mortality is 50%; for >12 hours, mortality is 80%.

COMPLICATIONS

Morbidity/mortality is usually related to: Underlying CNS pathology; stress from repeated seizures (e.g., hyperthermia, acidosis, hypotension, cardiac arrest, rhabdomyolysis, renal failure or aspiration pneumonia); or from the treatment instituted

REFERENCES

1. Meierkord H, Boon P, Engelsen B, et al. EFNS guideline on the management of status epilepticus. *Eur J Neurol*. 2006;13:445–50.
2. Costello DJ, Cole AJ. Treatment of acute seizures and status epilepticus. *J Intensive Care Med*. 2007;22:319–47.
3. Cherian A, Thomas SV, et al. Status epilepticus. *Ann Indian Acad Neurol*. 2009;12:140–53.
4. Mirski MA, Varelas PN, et al. Seizures and status epilepticus in the critically ill. *Crit Care Clin*. 2008;24:115–47, ix.
5. Appleton R, Macleod S, Martland T. Drug management for acute tonic-clonic convulsions including convulsive status epilepticus in children. *Cochrane Database Syst Rev*. 2008;3:CD001905.
6. Prasad K, et al. Anticonvulsant therapy for status epilepticus. *Cochrane Database Syst Rev*. 2007: CD003723.
7. Sofou K, Kristjánsdóttir R, Papachatzakis NE, et al. Management of prolonged seizures and status epilepticus in childhood: A systematic review. *J Child Neurol*. 2009;24(8):918–26.

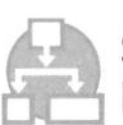

See Also (Topic, Algorithm, Electronic Media Element)

Seizure Disorders; Seizures, Febrile

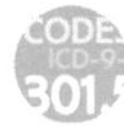

CODES

ICD9

- 345.2 Petit mal status, epileptic
- 345.3 Grand mal status, epileptic
- 345.80 Other forms of epilepsy, without mention of intractable epilepsy

CLINICAL PEARLS

- Status epilepticus is life-threatening; begin treatment if seizure lasts >5 minutes.
- Start with IV lorazepam or buccal midazolam.
- If not controlled in 30 minutes, admit to ICU and induce general anesthesia/drug coma.
- Morbidity/mortality increase with seizure duration.

STEVENS-JOHNSON SYNDROME

Matthew A. Silva, PharmD, RPh, BCPS
Pablo I. Hernandez Itriago, MD

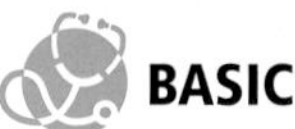

BASICS

DESCRIPTION

- A generalized hypersensitivity reaction, usually to a drug, in which skin and mucous membrane lesions are an early manifestation
- Once considered to be the same as erythema multiforme major, a severe form of erythema multiforme in which >1 mucosal surface was involved, many now consider it to be a different disease with a more difficult course and a more ominous prognosis.
- Stevens-Johnson syndrome (SJS) exists on a continuum with toxic epidermal necrolysis (TEN).
- SJS presents with characteristic targetoid cutaneous lesions when <10% of the body surface area (BSA) is involved.
- Targetoid cutaneous lesion involvement of 10–30% of BSA is considered an overlap between SJS and TEN. Involvement of >30% of BSA is TEN, which has a high morbidity and up to 70% mortality (1).
- System(s) affected: Cardiovascular; Hematologic/Lymphatic/Immunologic; Nervous; Renal/Urologic; Skin/Exocrine
- Synonym(s): Ectodermosis erosiva pluriorificialis; Febrile mucocutaneous syndrome; Herpes iris; Erythema polymorphe; Toxic epidermal necrolysis (TEN)

ALERT

- Dangerous progression
- Patients with discrete skin lesions and >10% epidermal detachment are at risk of rapid progression to TEN.

Geriatric Considerations

TEN has a greater mortality in older patients.

Pediatric Considerations

- Rare in children <3 years of age
- More common in children and young adults

Pregnancy Considerations

Pregnancy is a possible predisposing condition.

EPIDEMIOLOGY

Incidence

- Incidence/prevalence of SJS in the US is difficult to estimate because there is no universally accepted definition of SJS.
- 1.1–7.1 and 0.4–1.2 cases/1 million person-years for SJS and TEN, respectively (1)

Prevalence

- Predominant age: SJS is more common in children and young adults.
- Predominant sex: Male > Female (2:1)
- Sex (% range of females): 33–62% for SJS and 61.3–64.3% for TEN (1)
- Age (average range): 25–47 years for SJS and 46–63 years for TEN (1)

RISK FACTORS

- Previous history of SJS
- Immunocompromised status, including chronic viral infections with Epstein-Barr virus and HIV (2,3)
- Patients with HIV infection may be predisposed to developing SJS in response to their medications.
  - Human leukocyte antigen (HLA) subtypes A, B, and D
  - Diseases that cause immune compromise (e.g., deficiencies, malignancy)
  - Possibly radiation therapy or ultraviolet (UV) light

Genetics

Associations with HLA-A*3101 in Northern Europeans, HLA-B*1501, HLA-B*1502 , HLA-B*1511, HLA-B*5801 in patients of Asian ancestry, HLA-Bw44, HLA-B12, and HLA-DQB1*0601

GENERAL PREVENTION

Secondary prevention may be possible by avoiding exposure to offending medications or chemical agents.

PATHOPHYSIOLOGY

- Erythematous papular lesions and keratinocyte necrosis are a consequence of cell-mediated immunity.
- Occurs 1–2 weeks after initial exposure to offending drugs and within 48 hours on rechallenge.
- Accumulation and binding of reactive drug metabolites to mucocutaneous epithelial cells as haptens (4)
- Drug haptens signal drug-specific CD8+ T-lymphocyte and macrophages, which infiltrate and express interleukin 2 (IL-2), tumor necrosis factor α (TNF-α), and interferon-γ, leading to keratinocyte activation.
- Cytokines enhance keratinocyte expression of soluble Fas-ligand (sFasL) and Fas receptors, leading to apoptosis (5).

ETIOLOGY

- 50% of cases are idiopathic.
- Associated with metabolism of parent drugs and metabolites
- Slow intrinsic acetylation rates
- Sulfonamides are the drugs most strongly associated with SJS and TEN. Then:
  - Cephalosporins
  - Quinolones
  - Aminopenicillins
  - Tetracyclines
  - Macrolides
  - Imidazole antifungals
  - HIV antiretrovirals (e.g., protease inhibitors, efavirenz, abacavir, amprenavir, fosamprenavir, atazanavir, darunavir, etravirine) (2)
  - Anticonvulsants, especially carbamazepine
  - NSAIDs, especially oxicam
  - Allopurinol
  - Vaccines—dPT, BCG, oral polio
  - *Mycoplasma pneumoniae* infection

COMMONLY ASSOCIATED CONDITIONS

- SJS progressing to TEN is ominous prognostically.
- *Mycoplasma pneumoniae* may be an infectious precursor.

DIAGNOSIS

HISTORY

- Usually a preceding illness for which the medication was given 1–3 weeks before initial cutaneous manifestations
- Sudden onset with rapidly progressive pleomorphic rash that includes petechiae, vesicles, bullae
- Considered to be SJS if epidermal detachments affect <10% of the skin
- Classified as TEN if epidermal detachments affect >30% or >10% in the absence of discrete skin lesions
- Burning sensation of the skin and sometimes of the mucous membranes
- Usually no pruritus
- Fever 39–40°C (102–104°F)
- Headache, malaise, arthralgias
- Cough productive of thick, purulent sputum

PHYSICAL EXAM

- Recognized by the presence of several of the following features:
  - Vesicles and ulcers on the mucous membranes, especially of the mouth and throat
  - Erythematous macules with purpuric, necrotic centers and overlying blistering (5)
  - Epidermal detachment with light lateral pressure (Nikolsky's sign)
  - Fever 39–40°C (102–104°F)
  - Crusted nares
  - Conjunctivitis and/or corneal ulcerations
  - Erosive vulvovaginitis or balanitis
  - Cough productive of thick, purulent sputum
  - Tachypnea/respiratory distress
  - Arrhythmias
  - Pericarditis
  - Congestive heart failure (CHF)
  - Mental status changes
  - Seizures
  - Coma
- Sepsis:
  - Seen in SJS if epidermal detachment affects <10% of the skin
  - Seen in TEN if epidermal detachment exceeds 30% or if it exceeds 10% in the absence of discrete skin lesions
- Patients with discrete skin lesions and 10–30% epidermal detachment are an overlap between SJS and TEN.

DIAGNOSTIC TESTS & INTERPRETATION

Lab

Initial lab tests

- Culture or serologic tests for suspected sources of infection
- Electrolytes and creatinine
- Urine for albuminuria/hematuria

Follow-Up & Special Considerations

Skin biopsy

DIFFERENTIAL DIAGNOSIS

- Exfoliative dermatitis
- Linear IgA bullous dermatosis
- Staphylococcal scalded-skin syndrome
- Pemphigus (paraneoplastic)
- Generalized fixed drug eruption
- Erythema multiforme major
- Burns
- Pressure blisters (coma, barbiturates)

TREATMENT

MEDICATION

First Line

- Corticosteroids are controversial. Early high-dose IV steroids may attenuate disease progression, reduce skin detachment, decrease inflammatory cytokine activity, and improve patient comfort. Withdraw if no benefit is seen in the first few days.
- Experimental treatments that appear to have been useful include:
  - Recombinant granulocyte colony-stimulating factor
  - Cyclophosphamide
  - Cyclosporine (6)
  - IVIG in HIV-positive patients; IVIG is considered beneficial treatment (7) and prophylaxis, although not approved by the FDA (3). Interferes with Fas-ligand induced apoptosis.
- Contraindications: Avoid steroids in diabetic or immunosuppressed patients or those with chronic infections.

Second Line

- Acyclovir for herpetic infections
- Erythromycin or related antibiotic for *Mycoplasma* infections (empirical use of antibiotics is not recommended)

ADDITIONAL TREATMENT

General Measures

- Withdraw all suspected medications, and treat any underlying disease.
- Meticulous care of damaged skin
- Supportive care, including moisture-retentive ointment, petroleum jelly, and sterile saline compresses
- Catheter changing and culturing
- Reverse isolation and temperature control with extensive epidermal loss
- Maintenance of fluid, electrolyte, and protein balance
- Plasmapheresis
- Adequate calorie intake; parenteral nutrition, if necessary
- Mouthwashes of warm saline or a solution of diphenhydramine, lidocaine, and kaolin suspension
- Ophthalmologic consultation and monitoring for corneal damage
- Venous thromboembolism prophylaxis with unfractionated heparin or low-molecular-weight heparin

Additional Therapies

In severe ocular surface and eyelid inflammation due to acute SJS and TEN, amniotic membrane transplantation (AMT) is an effective treatment for severe ocular surface and eyelid inflammation, greatly decreasing the risk of significant ocular and visual sequelae.

SURGERY/OTHER PROCEDURES

- Sterile débridement of areas of extensive epidermal loss
- Application of biosynthetic dressings such as Biobrane to denuded areas
- Damage to the vulva, vagina, or cornea: Consider surgical repair.

IN-PATIENT CONSIDERATIONS

Admission Criteria

- This disease progresses rapidly; all patients should be admitted.
- Admission to a burn unit greatly improves the outcome for any patient who has sloughed skin over 10% or more of the body surface area.
- ICU for bronchiolitis, acute respiratory distress syndrome (ARDS), or multiorgan damage

IV Fluids

Fluid management with saline and macromolecules is necessary in the first 24 hours with decreasing IV fluid requirements as oral intake proceeds with nasogastric tube.

Nursing

- Bed rest until clinically stabilized
- Avoid administration of topical silver sulfadiazine owing to association with sulfonamide and SJS.
- Use a coordinated approach involving critical care, wound care, and burn specialists (8).

ONGOING CARE

FOLLOW-UP RECOMMENDATIONS

- Extensive documentation of all offending or suspected medications or chemical agents
- Education and strategies to limit exposure to offending or suspected medications or chemical agents

Patient Monitoring

- Observe carefully for secondary or concurrent infections
- Hydration, electrolytes, nutrition
- End-organ damage

DIET

- Oral fluid intake is recommended.
- Early oral nutrition by nasogastric tube as tolerated
- IV nutritional support with increased protein requirements; may need insulin for glycoregulation in this hypercatabolic state

PATIENT EDUCATION

- Discuss offending or suspected medications and chemical agents with patient and family as applicable.
- Plan to prevent repeated exposure.

PROGNOSIS

- Disease may have a rapid onset or may evolve slowly over 1–2 weeks with resolution over 4–6 weeks.
- Often scarring of the skin or mucous membranes occurs, especially of the vulva.
- Blindness or corneal opacities occur in 7–20% of patients.
- The risk of recurrence is as high as 37%.
- Death occurs in 5–15% of the patients with SJS and in up to 40% of patients with TEN.

COMPLICATIONS

- Secondary infections, sepsis, pneumonia, ARDS
- Bronchiolitis obliterans in children
- Dehydration/electrolyte disturbance, acute tubular necrosis
- Corneal ulceration or iritis, urethral erosions, and genitourinary strictures
- Arrhythmias
- Venous thromboembolism, disseminated intravascular coagulation (DIC)
- Death in 15% of untreated cases of SJS and up to 40% of TEN cases

REFERENCES

1. Letko E, Papaliodis DN, Papaliodis GN, et al. Stevens-Johnson syndrome and toxic epidermal necrolysis: A review of the literature. *Ann Allergy Asthma Immunol*. 2005;94:419–36; quiz 436–8, 456.
2. Borrás-Blasco J, Navarro-Ruiz A, Borrás C, et al. Adverse cutaneous reactions associated with the newest antiretroviral drugs in patients with human immunodeficiency virus infection. *J Antimicrob Chemother*. 2008;62(5):879–88.
3. Hazin R, Ibrahimi OA, Hazin MI, et al. Stevens-Johnson syndrome: Pathogenesis, diagnosis, and management. *Ann Med*. 2008;40: 129–38.
4. Pichler WJ, Naisbitt DJ, Park BK. Immune pathomechanism of drug hypersensitivity reactions. *J Allergy Clin Immunol*. 2011;127(3 Suppl):S60–6.
5. Murata J, Abe R, Shimizu H. Increased soluble Fas ligand levels in patients with Stevens-Johnson syndrome and toxic epidermal necrolysis preceding skin detachment. *J Allergy Clin Immunol*. 2008; 122(5):992–1000.
6. Reese D, Henning JS, Rockers K, et al. Cyclosporine for SJS/TEN: A case series and review of the literature. *Cutis*. 2011;87:24–9.
7. Chen J, Wang B, Zeng Y, et al. High-dose intravenous immunoglobulins in the treatment of Stevens-Johnson syndrome and toxic epidermal necrolysis in Chinese patients: A retrospective study of 82 cases. *Eur J Dermatol*. 2010;20:743–7.
8. Struck MF, Hilbert P, Mockenhaupt M, et al. Severe cutaneous adverse reactions: Emergency approach to non-burn epidermolytic syndromes. *Intensive Care Med*. 2010;36:22–32.

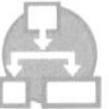

See Also (Topic, Algorithm, Electronic Media Element)

Burns; Cutaneous Drug Reactions; Dermatitis, Herpetiformis; Erythema Multiforme; Pemphigoid, Bullous; Pemphigus Vulgaris; Respiratory Distress Syndrome, Acute (ARDS)

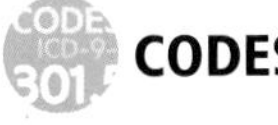

CODES

ICD9

695.13 Stevens-Johnson syndrome

CLINICAL PEARLS

- Corticosteroid treatment is controversial. If chosen and no response within first few days, discontinue.
- Recurrences are possible. Etiologic agents should be identified if possible and avoided indefinitely.

STOKES-ADAMS ATTACKS

Kelsey A. White, PharmD
Emmanouil Tampakakis, MD

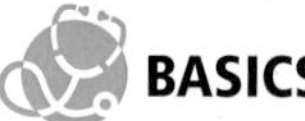

BASICS

DESCRIPTION

- Syncope due to cerebral hypoxia in patients with third-degree (complete) heart block. Syncope occurs following severe bradycardia or asystole.
- System(s) affected: Cardiovascular; Nervous
- Synonym(s): Drop attacks

EPIDEMIOLOGY

Incidence

Uncertain, although increasing age is a risk factor

Prevalence

- Unknown (0.04% prevalence of third-degree atrioventricular block) (1)
- Predominant age: Most common >40 years of age
- Predominant sex: Male = Female

Pediatric Considerations

Rare during pregnancy

RISK FACTORS

- Use of the medications listed under "Etiology"
- Coronary artery disease
- Endocarditis and myocarditis
- Mitral or aortic valve disease
- History of previous atrioventricular nodal dysfunction or cardiac surgery
- Bundle-branch and/or fascicular block
- Acute myocardial infarction (MI) (especially acute right coronary artery occlusion)
- Amyloidosis
- Chagas disease
- Lyme disease
- Connective tissue diseases involving the heart (e.g., systemic lupus erythematosus, rheumatoid arthritis, sarcoidosis)
- Hyperkalemia
- Acidosis

Genetics

- May be associated with complete congenital atrioventricular block (CCAVB)
- Forty percent of children with CCAVB experience syncopal episodes (2).

GENERAL PREVENTION

- Avoid negative chronotropic drugs (e.g., β-blockers, calcium channel blockers, digoxin) in at-risk patients.
- Prevention of cardiovascular disease through diet/exercise

PATHOPHYSIOLOGY

- The abrupt development of complete atrioventricular (AV) block, especially at His-bundle level, may result in a prolonged period of asystole because of a slow and delayed response of the quiescent subsidiary (escape) ventricular pacemaker.
- Marked bradycardia secondary to AV conduction abnormality may lead to prolonged QT interval and paroxysmal torsades de pointes.
- Abrupt termination of tachyarrhythmia leading to precipitous decrease in heart rate
- Degree of cerebral dysfunction related to duration of cardiac block and effect on cerebral circulation

ETIOLOGY

- Medications:
  - Digoxin (common)
  - Calcium channel blockers
  - β-Blockers (e.g., Sotalol)
  - Clonidine
  - Propafenone (Rythmol), a class IC antiarrhythmic
  - Isoproterenol
- Other causes:
  - Myocardial ischemia involving the AV node
  - Degenerative (fibrosing) and infiltrative diseases involving the heart and its conduction system (e.g., Lenègre, systemic sclerosis, valvular disease, infective endocarditis, sarcoidosis)
  - Degeneration of the AV node secondary to aging
  - Neuromuscular diseases (e.g., myotonic muscular dystrophy or Kearns-Sayre syndrome)
  - Postoperative cardiac damage

COMMONLY ASSOCIATED CONDITIONS

- Myocardial ischemia/acute MI
- High-degree AV conduction abnormality
- Atrial standstill
- Right bundle-branch block
- CCAVB
- Systemic manifestations of connective tissue disease
- Sick sinus syndrome
- Neuromuscular disease

DIAGNOSIS

HISTORY

- History of predisposing factor or related conditions
- Angina
- Acute bradycardia
- Hypotension
- Pallor
- Fatigue/exercise intolerance
- Dyspnea
- Altered sensorium or loss of consciousness unrelated to position or exertion
- Acute onset of syncopal or near-syncopal symptoms (± palpitations)

PHYSICAL EXAM

- Pallor
- Reactive hyperemia with recovery
- Convulsions or seizurelike activity without postictal state
- Pulse <50

DIAGNOSTIC TESTS & INTERPRETATION

Lab

Initial lab tests

- Cardiac enzymes
- EEG with cardiac monitoring (to differentiate between syncope and epilepsy) (3)
- ECG: Partial or complete heart block at onset of symptoms with slow or no ventricular escape:
  - Bradycardia
  - AV block 50–60%
  - Sinoatrial block 30–40%
  - Ventricular fibrillation/tachycardia <1%
- Serum digoxin level (other medication levels if appropriate)
- Thyroid-stimulating hormone level
- Hematocrit/hemoglobin
- Blood electrolyte levels (especially potassium)

Follow-Up & Special Considerations

- ECG, event monitor, or Holter monitor
- Renal failure may lead to falsely elevated creatinine kinase.

Imaging

Initial approach

Transthoracic echocardiogram if cardiomyopathy or valvular disease is suspected

Diagnostic Procedures/Surgery

- Coronary catheterization to rule out coronary ischemia if suspected
- Electrophysiologic testing to assess cardiac conduction system if ECG testing is ambiguous
- Tilt-table test to evaluate neurogenic etiology
- Myocardial biopsy if infiltrative disease suspected

Pathological Findings

- Myocardial ischemia
- Evidence of degenerative or infiltrative disease involving the AV node/His bundle

DIFFERENTIAL DIAGNOSIS

- Seizure
- Vertigo
- Transient ischemic attack
- Orthostatic hypotension
- Vasovagal syncope
- Hypoglycemia
- Neurocardiogenic syncope
- Cardiac arrhythmias:
  - Ventricular tachycardia
  - Supraventricular tachycardia
  - Re-entrant tachycardia
  - Wolff-Parkinson-White syndrome
  - Sinus arrest
  - Sinus exit block
  - Sick sinus syndrome
  - Transition from normal sinus rhythm to atrial fibrillation or vice versa

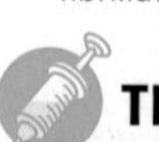

TREATMENT

MEDICATION

First Line

- No medication currently is recommended for long-term treatment of symptomatic arrhythmias (4)[A].
- For symptomatic bradyarrhythmias (5)[C]:
  - Atropine 0.5 mg IV push to be given during the complete heart block with hypotension; may be repeated q3–5min with a maximum total dose of 3 mg; less likely to be effective if atrial rate is already adequate and in patients who have undergone cardiac transplantation:
    - Precautions: Doses of atropine sulfate of <0.5 mg may paradoxically result in further slowing of the heart rate

- Contraindications: Narrow-angle glaucoma, reflux esophagitis, obstructive GI disease, unstable cardiovascular status in acute hemorrhage or thyrotoxicosis, myasthenia gravis
- Refer to package insert for additional precautions, contraindications, interactions, and adverse effects.

- Correction of precipitating conditions (e.g., hypokalemia, acidosis)

Second Line

- For symptomatic bradyarrhythmias (5)[C]:
  - Epinephrine 2–10 mcg/min IV infusion, titrate to patient response; use of epinephrine in normotensive patient with bradycardia may precipitate hypertensive crisis:
    - Precautions: Use with caution in the elderly, patients with cerebrovascular disease, cardiovascular disease, hypertension, diabetes, hyperthyroidism, psychoneurotic individuals, and pregnancy.
    - Contraindications: Labor, narrow-angle glaucoma, organic brain damage, shock (nonanaphylactic), sulfite hypersensitivity, heart failure, coronary insufficiency
  - Dopamine 2–10 mcg/kg/min IV infusion, titrate to patient response; add to epinephrine or administer alone:
    - Precautions: Avoid extravasation; infuse into a large vein if possible. Avoid infusion into leg veins. Watch IV site closely; use with caution in patients with cardiac disease, pre-existing vascular damage, or occlusive vascular disease. Avoid abrupt discontinuation.
    - Contraindications: Pheochromocytoma, tachyarrhythmias/ventricular fibrillation
  - Isoproterenol 2–10 mcg/min IV infusion, titrate to patient response:
    - Precautions: Some formulations contain sulfites: avoid use in patients with sulfite hypersensitivity; use with caution in the elderly, patients with coronary artery disease, cardiac disease, hypertension, diabetes, hyperthyroidism, pheochromocytoma, and pregnancy
    - Contraindications: Angina pectoris, digitalis-induced tachycardia or heart block, tachyarrhythmias
  - Possible interactions: Concurrent use of certain MAOIs and catecholamines may result in increased hypertensive effects or hypertensive crisis; concurrent use of dopamine and epinephrine with cyclopropane or halogenated hydrocarbon anesthetic may sensitize the heart to the arrhythmic action of sympathomimetic drugs
  - Refer to individual package inserts for additional precautions, contraindications, interactions, and adverse effects.

ADDITIONAL TREATMENT

General Measures

- Inpatient assessment in a monitored setting
- Continued treatment for prevention of future episodes in an ambulatory setting
- Cessation of precipitating medications

Issues for Referral

Syncope requires frequent and close follow-up

SURGERY/OTHER PROCEDURES

- Intracardiac pacing is the treatment of choice for patients with complete heart block and Stokes-Adams syncope (4)[A].
- Dual chamber may be more effective than single chamber pacing in AV block (6).
- Temporary external pacing or transvenous pacing as interim measure to stabilize
- See American College of Cardiology/American Heart Association/Heart Rhythm Society 2008 guidelines (4) for suggested intervention based on precipitating cause.
- Emergency insertion of a ventricular pacemaker is required when ventricular fibrillation or tachycardia is present.

IN-PATIENT CONSIDERATIONS

Initial Stabilization

See first-line treatments to be used when intracardiac pacing is not available. External pacing may be life-saving.

Admission Criteria

Syncope in the setting of known AV node conduction abnormality or of unknown cause

IV Fluids

Use caution in patients with congestive heart failure.

Nursing

- Telemetry
- Out of bed with assist if patient has history of falls due to syncope

Discharge Criteria

Institution of proper treatment with resolution of symptoms

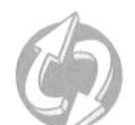

ONGOING CARE

FOLLOW-UP RECOMMENDATIONS

Routine follow-up with cardiologist

Patient Monitoring

- Routine pacemaker check if permanent pacemaker has been implanted
- Follow-up Holter and/or event monitoring for 2 weeks after causal medication has been discontinued
- Discontinuation of driving, heavy machinery operation; caution about fall risks

DIET

Regular

PATIENT EDUCATION

After the diagnosis has been made and a pacemaker has been implanted (if required), instruct patient as to pacemaker guidelines.

PROGNOSIS

Excellent with proper institution of exogenous pacing; further symptoms are not expected.

COMPLICATIONS

- Sudden death (uncommon)
- Cerebral hypoxic damage and other end-organ damage with protracted bradycardia with hypotension

REFERENCES

1. Kojic EM, Hardarson T, Sigfusson N, et al. The prevalence and prognosis of third-degree atrioventricular conduction block: The Reykjavik Study. *J Intern Med*. 1999;246(1):81–6.
2. Vukomanovic V, Stajevic M, Kosutic J. Age-related role of ambulatory electrocardiographic monitoring in risk stratification of patients with complete congenital atrioventricular block. *Europace*. 2007;9:88–93.
3. Diaz-Castro O. "Stokes-Adams epilepsy": Sometimes we need the electroencephalogram. *Circulation*. 2005;112:e101–2.
4. Epstein AE, Dimarco JP, Ellenbogen KA, et al. 2008 guidelines for device-based therapy of cardiac rhythm abnormalities: Executive summary. *Heart Rhythm*. 2008;5:934–55.
5. 2010 American Heart Association Guidelines for Cardiopulmonary Resuscitation and Emergency Cardiovascular Care Science. Part 8.3: Management of symptomatic bradycardia and tachycardia. *Circulation*. 2010;122:S729–67.
6. Dretzke J. Dual chamber versus single chamber ventricular pacemakers for sick sinus syndrome and atrioventricular block. *Cochrane Database Syst Rev*. 2004;(2):CD003710.

ADDITIONAL READING

- Elizari MV, Acunzo RS, Ferreiro M. Hemiblocks revisited. *Circulation*. 2007;115:1154–63.
- Hood R. Syncope in the elderly. *Clin Geriatric Med*. 2007;23(2):351–61, vi.
- Jensen G, Sigurd B, Sandoe E. Adams-Stokes seizures due to ventricular tachydysrhythmias in patients with heart block: Prevalence and problems of management. *Chest*. 1975;67:43–48.
- You C, Chong C, Wang T, et al. Unrecognized paroxysmal ventricular standstill masquerading as epilepsy: A Stokes Adams attack. *Epileptic Disord*. 2007;9(2):179–81.

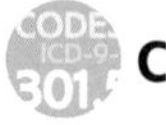

CODES

ICD9

426.9 Conduction disorder, unspecified

CLINICAL PEARLS

- Syncope due to Stokes-Adams attacks can be frequently confused for epilepsy.
- Stokes-Adams attacks usually require insertion of a pacemaker for definitive treatment unless due to a reversible condition such as medication toxicity.
- External pacing may serve as a bridge until more definitive management can be accomplished.

STOMATITIS

Hugh J. Silk, MD, MPH
Sheila O. Stille, DMD, MAGD

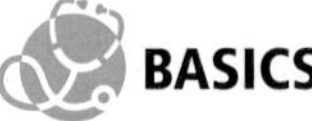

BASICS

Inflammation of mucous lining of any of the structures in the mouth, cheeks, lip, tongue, gingiva, and floor or roof of the mouth. It is usually painful and associated with redness, swelling, and sometimes bleeding. It affects people of all ages. Stomatitis can be result of localized injury/irritation, or the manifestation of systemic conditions.

DESCRIPTION

- Generalized inflammation of the oral mucosa of many possible etiologies
- System(s) affected: Skin/Exocrine; ENT; Oropharynx; Dental

EPIDEMIOLOGY

- Children:
  - Primary herpetic infections (6 months to 5 years old)
  - Hand-foot-mouth disease
  - Herpangina
  - Angular stomatitis
  - Aphthous stomatitis (peak onset 10–19 years old)
- Teenagers and adults:
  - Vincent stomatitis (also known as *Vincent disease* or *acute necrotizing ulcerative gingivitis*)
  - Behçet disease
  - Nicotinic stomatitis
  - Chronic ulcerative stomatitis (white women in late middle age) (1)

Prevalence

- Very common: Herpetic stomatitis, hand-foot-mouth disease, and recurrent aphthous stomatitis (RAS)
- Common: Herpangina, nicotinic stomatitis, and denture-related stomatitis
- The remaining causes are uncommon or rare.

RISK FACTORS

- Poor oral hygiene
- Dietary deficiencies and malnutrition
- Chronic systemic disease
- Immune deficiencies
- Poor denture
- Smoking
- Cancer therapies

Genetics

Polymorphisms causing high interleukin 1p (IL-1p) and tumor necrosis factor α (TNF-α) production increase risk for recurrent aphthous stomatitis (2).

GENERAL PREVENTION

- Avoid causative factors (see "Etiology").
- Good oral hygiene
- Good nutrition
- Avoid/discontinue smoking.
- Properly fitting dentures

ETIOLOGY

- Allergy: Foods, drugs, contact (some erythema multiforme)
- Nutritional deficiencies: Vitamin B_6 (angular stomatitis), vitamin B_{12}, folic acid, vitamin C, iron deficiencies
- Malnutrition (gangrenous stomatitis; internationally known as "noma")
- Viral: Herpes simplex I and II (herpetic stomatitis), coxsackie A (herpangina and hand-foot-mouth disease)
- Smoking (nicotinic stomatitis)
- Hormonal (possibly RAS)
- Uncertain (RAS, Vincent stomatitis, recurrent scarifying stomatitis, Behçet disease, erythema multiforme)
- RAS may be associated with vitamin B_{12}, folic acid, vitamin C, and iron deficiencies and toothpastes containing sodium lauryl sulfate.
- Bacterial (scarlatina)
- Traumatic (mechanical, chemical, or thermal)
- Uremic (uremic/nephritic)
- Ill-fitting dentures
- Chemotherapy or radiation

Pediatric Considerations

Common causes in the pediatric population (e.g., herpetic [primary], hand-foot-mouth disease, herpangina, traumatic ulcers)

Geriatric Considerations

Certain etiologies are more likely in the geriatric population (e.g., ill-fitting dentures, nutritional deficiencies).

COMMONLY ASSOCIATED CONDITIONS

- Pregnancy may bring on recurrent ulcerative stomatitis.
- AIDS: Associated with severe oral lesions
- Aphthous ulcers may be associated with Crohn disease or celiac disease.

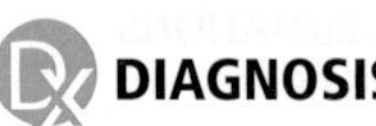

DIAGNOSIS

- General:
  - Depends on etiology
  - Varies from minimal to severe pain
  - Some with constitutional symptoms: Fever, malaise, headache
- Allergic stomatitis:
  - Intense shiny erythema
  - Slight swelling
  - Itching
  - Dryness
  - Burning
  - Usual allergens include: Nuts, shellfish, cinnamon, fruits, metals, dental materials, and ingredients in toothpaste, mouthwash, and chewing gum
- Vincent infection: Necrotic ulceration of interdental papillae and mucous membrane
- Thrush (candidiasis):
  - White patches, slightly raised (resembling milk curds)
  - Distribution: Tongue, buccal mucosa, palate, gums, tonsils, larynx, pharynx, GI tract, skin (skin folds); commonly seen in infants (oral cavity, diaper area, neck), immunocompromised patients, and patients on long-term antibiotics, corticosteroids, and antineoplastic treatment
- Pseudomembranous stomatitis: Membranelike exudate
- Mucous lesions accompanying systemic disease:
  - Mucous patches (syphilis)
  - Strawberry tongue (Kawasaki disease, scarlet fever, staphylococcal toxic shock syndrome)
  - Koplik spots (measles)
  - Ulcers (erythema multiforme)
  - Smooth, fire red, painful (pellagra)
  - Varicella zoster

HISTORY

The patient will complain of burning sensation, intolerance to temperature, and irritating foods.

PHYSICAL EXAM

The physical exam should include comprehensive oral examination. Examine and palpate the lips, tongue, cheeks, and hard and soft palate, as well as cervical, submandibular, and submental lymph nodes. Erythema and edema are the usual oral manifestations. When the gingiva is involved, the tissue of the affected area will appear uniformly red and erythematous.

DIAGNOSTIC TESTS & INTERPRETATION

The diagnosis relies on clinical symptoms and history. Testing is not routinely performed.

Lab

- Tzanck test of historic interest only; herpes simplex virus (HSV) culture
- Serologic test for syphilis
- CBC; cultures to determine secondary infection

Follow-Up & Special Considerations

If not resolving in 7–14 days or getting worse, consider CBC.

Diagnostic Procedures/Surgery

- Biopsy if persistent/recurrent/suspicious
- Immunofluorescence is useful in the differential diagnostic between RAS and bullous skin diseases (3).

Pathological Findings

Biopsy suspicious lesions or lesions that fail to heal or chronically recur to rule out oral or hematologic cancer or vasculitis.

DIFFERENTIAL DIAGNOSIS

- Herpetic stomatitis
- Hand-foot-mouth disease
- RAS
- Vincent stomatitis
- Nicotinic stomatitis
- Denture-related stomatitis
- Erythema multiforme/Stevens-Johnson syndrome
- Recurrent ulcerative stomatitis
- Recurrent scarifying stomatitis
- Behçet disease
- Angular stomatitis
- Noma (gangrenous stomatitis)
- Scarlatina (scarlet fever)
- Herpangina
- Uremic stomatitis
- Reactive arthritis
- Pemphigus/pemphigoid
- Squamous cell cancer
- Cyclic neutropenia
- Burning mouth syndrome

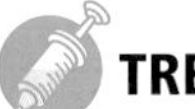

TREATMENT

Treatment of stomatitis depends on the causative factors. If cause is allergic, identification removal of the agent is critical. For infectious causes, antibiotic or antifungal regiments. Steroidal anti-inflammatory drugs for systemic conditions with stomatitis manifestation. If the cause of stomatitis is due to medical treatment or cancer therapy, treatment needs to be more aggressive.

MEDICATION

- Acetaminophen or ibuprofen for analgesia
- Steroids, colchicine, and cytotoxic drugs for Behçet disease
- 2% viscous lidocaine (Xylocaine) swish and spit for local discomfort
- Liquid diphenhydramine (Benadryl) by mouth or swish and spit, for allergic reactions
- Antibiotics for gangrenous stomatitis (penicillin and metronidazole are reasonable first-line agents; often start with IV)
- Antifungal ointment (e.g., nystatin [Mycostatin]) for candidiasis-complicating angular stomatitis
- For candidiasis: Nystatin oral suspension 400,000 units (4 mL) q.i.d. × 10 days; swish and swallow (1 mL q.i.d. for infants)
- Acyclovir 200–800 mg 5 times a day × 7–14 days for herpetic stomatitis
- Sucralfate (Carafate) suspension 1 tsp swish in mouth or place on ulcers q.i.d. (helpful)
- Topical 0.2% hyaluronic acid for recurrent aphthous ulcers
- "Miracle mouth rinses": Various combinations of the preceding in equal parts; use swish and spit out q.i.d.:
  – Maalox or Mylanta, diphenhydramine, lidocaine
  – Maalox or Mylanta, diphenhydramine, Carafate
  – Duke's: Nystatin, diphenhydramine, hydrocortisone
- Chemical cauterization with silver nitrate for aphthous stomatitis (treatment can cause burning sensation)
- Contraindications: Allergy to specific medication
- Precautions: Toxic dose of topical lidocaine is uncertain, but likely only 25–33% of dose may have significant absorption from open ulcers or mucous membrane.
- Topical minocycline for aphthous stomatitis (4)
- Steroid oral rinses (see "General") or topical preparations for aphthous ulcers (Kenalog in Orabase) or oral steroids injected into lesions for severe cases
- Thalidomide 20 mg 1–2× daily × 3–8 weeks in HIV-positive patients with nonhealing aphthous ulcers (extreme caution for birth defects)
- For prevention or reducing severity of mucositis with cancer treatments, these agents have some evidence of benefit: allopurinol, aloe vera, amifostine, cryotherapy, glutamine (IV), honey, keratinocyte growth factor, laser, and polymixin/tobramycin/amphotericin (PTA) antibiotic pastille/paste (5)

ADDITIONAL TREATMENT

General Measures

- In most cases, treatment of symptoms only
- Severe cases may require parenteral fluids, particularly children.
- Good oral hygiene
- Topical anesthesia
- Analgesics
- Oral rinses such as half-strength hydrogen peroxide
- Smoking cessation
- Refit dentures; daytime wear only
- Avoid specific allergens.
- Replace vitamin deficiencies.
- Treat malnutrition if present.

COMPLEMENTARY AND ALTERNATIVE MEDICINE

- Avoid toothpaste with sodium lauryl sulfate for prevention of aphthous ulcers.
- Replenish vitamin deficiencies.

IN-PATIENT CONSIDERATIONS

IV Fluids

In severe cases involving dehydration owing to oral ulcerations

Nursing

For infants with painful stomatitis, feeding can be particularly challenging. Topical analgesic agents should be used prior to bottle-feeding. Nasogastric feeds or parenteral as needed.

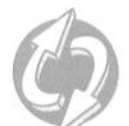

ONGOING CARE

FOLLOW-UP RECOMMENDATIONS

Patient Monitoring

Lesions need to be followed until resolved. If they fail to resolve, continuously recur, or appear suspicious, biopsy may be needed.

DIET

May need to avoid spicy, acidic, sharp, hard, and dry foods

PATIENT EDUCATION

Patient handouts:

- Aphthous ulcers (English and Spanish): www.aafp.prg/afp/20701/160ph.html
- Gingivostomatitis: www.nlm.nih.gov/medlineplus/ency/article/152.htm
- Mouth sores (English and Spanish): www.nlm.nih.gov/medlineplus/ency/article/003059.html
- Mouth problems in infants and children: http://familydoctor.org/online/famdocen/home/tools/symptom/510.html

PROGNOSIS

- Herpetic: Self-limited, with resolution in 7–14 days
- Hand-foot-mouth disease: Same as for herpetic
- RAS: 7–14-day course per episode
- Vincent: May progress to fascial space infection with airway compromise or sepsis
- Nicotinic: Resolves with cessation of smoking
- Denture: Resolves with proper fitting, careful oral hygiene, and daytime-only denture wear
- Erythema multiforme: Resolution in 2–3 weeks
- Stevens-Johnson: Resolution in about 6 weeks with adequate supportive care
- Recurrent ulcerative: As the name implies, recurs over time, but the overall prognosis is good
- Recurrent scarifying: Occasional patients suffer continuous ulcers; others have recurrence with eventual scarring. The prognosis is otherwise good.
- Behçet disease may recur for several years. Overall prognosis is related to other aspects of the disease.
- Angular: After correction of mechanical problems, allergic disorders, and nutritional deficiencies, the prognosis is good.
- Gangrenous: The most serious stomatitis, requiring aggressive treatment with IV antibiotics and débridement to avoid death
- Scarlatina: The prognosis is related to other manifestations of the disease.
- Herpangina: 7–14-day course with total resolution
- Uremic: Depends on the underlying renal disease

COMPLICATIONS

- Recurrent scarifying stomatitis may result in intraoral scarring with restriction of oral mobility.
- Behçet disease may result in visual loss, pneumonia, colitis, vasculitis, large-artery aneurysms, thrombophlebitis, or encephalitis.
- Gangrenous stomatitis may lead to facial disfigurement and even death.
- Scarlet fever may result in cardiac disease.
- Herpetic stomatitis may be complicated by ocular or CNS involvement.

REFERENCES

1. Solomon LW. Chronic ulcerative stomatitis. *Oral Dis*. 2008;14:383–9.
2. Guimaraes AL, Correia-Silva Jde F, Sá AR, et al. Investigation of functional gene polymorphisms IL-1 beta, IL-6, IL-10 and TNF-alpha in individuals with recurrent aphthous stomatitis. *Arch Oral Bio*. 2007;52(3):268–72.
3. Wilhelmsen NS, Weber R, Miziara ID. The role of immunofluorescence in the physiopathology and differential diagnosis of recurrent aphthous stomatitis. *Revista Brasileira de Otorrinolaringologia*. 2008;74(3):331–6.
4. Gorsky M, Epstein J, Raviv A, et al. Topical minocycline for managing symptoms of recurrent aphthous stomatitis. *Spec Care Dentist*. 2008;28: 27–31.
5. Worthington HV, Clarkson JE, Bryan G, et al. Interventions for preventing oral mucositis for patients with cancer receiving treatment. *Cochrane Database Syst Rev*. 2010:CD000978.

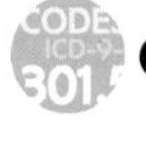

CODES

ICD9

- 074.3 Hand, foot, and mouth disease
- 528.00 Stomatitis and mucositis, unspecified
- 528.2 Oral aphthae

CLINICAL PEARLS

- Stomatitis is often self-limiting and requires only pain relief treatment.
- Consider broad differential diagnosis in order to consider etiology.
- Treat all underlying conditions.
- Depending on geographic location, age of patient, and comorbities, be prepared to aggressively treat worsening or severe causes.

STREPTOCOCCAL PHARYNGITIS AND SCARLET FEVER

John C. Huscher, MD
Mitchell S. King, MD

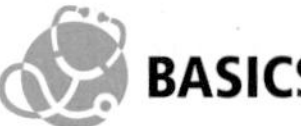

BASICS

DESCRIPTION
- Generally a childhood disease characterized by fever, pharyngitis, and rash caused by group A β-hemolytic *Streptococcus pyogenes* (GAS) that produces erythrogenic toxin
- Incubation period: 1–7 days
- Duration of illness: 4–10 days
- Rash usually appears on the second day of illness.
- Rash first appears in the upper chest and flexural creases and then spreads rapidly all over the body.
- Rash clears at the end of the first week and is followed by several weeks of desquamation.
- System(s) affected: Head, Eyes, Ears, Nose, Throat; Skin/Exocrine
- Synonym: Scarlatina

EPIDEMIOLOGY
Incidence
- Fairly common; rare in infancy because of maternal antitoxin antibodies
- Predominant age: 6–12 years
- Peak age: 4–8 years
- Predominant sex: Male = Female
- Rare in the US: Age >12 because of high rates (>80%) of lifelong protective antibodies to erythrogenic toxins

Prevalence
- 5–30% of pediatric sore throats are due to GAS.
- <10% of children with streptococcal pharyngitis develop scarlet fever.

RISK FACTORS
- Winter/spring seasons
- Age: School-aged children
- Contact with infected individual(s)
- Crowded living conditions (e.g., lower socioeconomic status, military, child care, schools)

GENERAL PREVENTION
- GAS is spread by contact with airborne respiratory particles.
- Asymptomatic contacts do not require cultures or prophylaxis.
- Symptomatic contacts may be treated ± cultures.
- Children should not return to school or daycare until they have received >24 hours of antibiotic therapy.

PATHOPHYSIOLOGY
- Erythrogenic toxin produced by phage is necessary for scarlet fever.
- 3 types: A, B, C
- These toxins damage capillaries (producing rash) and act as superantigens stimulating cytokine release.
- Antibodies to toxins prevent development of rash but do not protect against underlying infection.

ETIOLOGY
Site of streptococcal infection usually tonsils; may occur with infection of skin, surgical wounds, or uterus (puerperal scarlet fever)

COMMONLY ASSOCIATED CONDITIONS
- Pharyngitis
- Impetigo
- Puerperal sepsis
- Rheumatic fever
- Glomerulonephritis

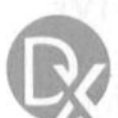

DIAGNOSIS

HISTORY
Prodrome 1–2 days:
- Sore throat
- Headache
- Myalgias
- Malaise
- Fever (>38°C [100.4°F])
- Vomiting
- Abdominal pain (may mimic acute abdomen)
- Rash
- Cough (coryza), more likely viral

PHYSICAL EXAM
- Oral exam:
  - Beefy red tonsils and pharynx with or without exudate
  - Petechiae on palate
  - White coating on tongue: White strawberry tongue appears on days 1–2. This sheds by days 4–5, leaving a red strawberry tongue, which is shiny and red with prominent papillae.
- Exanthem (appears within 1–5 days):
  - Scarlet macules over generalized erythema
  - Orange-red punctate skin eruption with sandpaperlike texture: Sunburn with goose pimples
  - Initially, chest and axillae; then spreads to abdomen and extremities; prominent in skin folds, flexural surfaces (e.g., axillae, groin, buttocks), with sparing of palms and soles
  - Flushed face with circumoral pallor, red lips
  - Pastia lines: Transverse red streaks in skin folds of abdomen, antecubital space, and axillae
  - Desquamation begins on face after 7–10 days and proceeds over trunk to hands and feet; may persist for 6 weeks
  - In severe cases, small vesicular lesions (miliary sudamina) may appear on abdomen, hands, and feet.
  - Rash: Blanches if pressed

DIAGNOSTIC TESTS & INTERPRETATION
Lab
Use Modified Centor prediction rule to determine risk of Streptococcal infection

Initial lab tests
- Modified Centor clinical prediction rule for group A Streptococcal infection:
  - +1 point: Tonsillar exudates
  - +1 point: Tender anterior chain cervical adenopathy
  - +1 point: Fever by history
  - +1 point: Age <15 years
  - 0 points: Age 15–45 years
  - −1 point: Age >45 years
  - −1 point: Cough (presence of cough almost always excludes the diagnosis of group A streptococcus)
  - Scoring:
    - If 3–4 points, positive predictive value of ~80%: Treat empirically
    - If 2 points, positive predictive value of ~50%, rapid streptococcus antigen + culture: Treat if either positive
    - If 1 point, positive predictive value <50%: Positive rapid streptococcus antigen or culture likely false positive
    - If 0 or −1 point, positive predictive value <20%: Do not test; close follow-up PRN
    - Coryza (nasal congestion), hoarseness, cough, diarrhea, conjunctivitis, or viral rash highly suggests viral cause.
- Rapid streptococcus antigen tests: Diagnostic if positive, 95% specific; sensitivity approaches that of culture
- Throat culture: Culture β-hemolytic colonies, catalase negative, sensitive to bacitracin; culture is gold standard for confirming streptococcal infection (99% specific, 90–97% sensitive, but 5–10% of healthy individuals are carriers).
- Serologic tests (includes antistreptolysin O titer and streptozyme tests, antihyaluronidase): Confirm recent GAS infection; not helpful for diagnosis of acute disease
- Gram stain: Positive cocci in chains
- Dick test: Injection of skin-test dose of erythrogenic toxin is positive in persons lacking antitoxin; not used clinically
- CBC may show elevated WBC count (12,000–16,000/mm^3); possible eosinophilia later (second week)

Follow-Up & Special Considerations
- Drugs that may alter lab results: Prior antibiotic therapy may result in negative throat culture.
- Within 5 days of symptoms, antibiotics can delay/abolish antistreptolysin O response.

Pathological Findings
Skin lesions reveal characteristic inflammatory reaction, specifically hyperemia, edema, and polymorphonuclear cell infiltration.

DIFFERENTIAL DIAGNOSIS
- Viral exanthem
- Measles
- Rubella
- Infectious mononucleosis
- Roseola
- *Mycoplasma* pneumonia
- Secondary syphilis
- *Arcanobacterium haemolyticum*
- Toxic shock syndrome
- Staphylococcal scalded-skin syndrome
- Kawasaki disease
- Drug hypersensitivity
- Severe sunburn

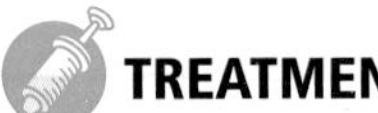

TREATMENT

MEDICATION

First Line

- Penicillin (oral; penicillin V and others) for 10 days (1,2)[A]:
  - 250 mg PO b.i.d. or t.i.d. for <27 kg (60 lb); 500 mg b.i.d. or t.i.d. for >27 kg (60 lb) adolescents and adults
  - If compliance is questionable, use penicillin G, benzathine: Single IM dose 600,000 U for <27 kg (60 lb); 1.2 mU for others
- Amoxicillin (oral) 50 mg/kg once daily (3) (use only for definitive GAS because it can induce rash with some viral infections) (1)[A]:
  - Contraindications: Penicillin allergy
- Acetaminophen for fever and pain
- Precautions: Refer to manufacturer's profile of each drug.
- Significant possible interactions: Refer to manufacturer's profile of each drug.

Second Line

- For patients allergic to penicillin:
- Azithromycin (Zithromax, Z pack): 12 mg/kg/d (maximum of 500 mg) for 5 days (1)[B]
- Clarithromycin (Biaxin): Children >6 months: 7.5 mg/kg b.i.d. for 10 days; adults: 250 mg b.i.d. for 10 days (1)[B]
- Oral cephalosporins: Many are effective, but first-generation cephalosporins are less expensive:
  - Cephalexin 40 mg/kg/d divided t.i.d.; maximum: 250 mg t.i.d. × 10 days (1)[B]
  - Cefadroxil 30 mg/kg/d divided b.i.d.; maximum: 500 mg b.i.d. × 10 days (1)[B]
- Clindamycin 20 mg/kg/d divided t.i.d. × 10 days (1)[B]
- Tetracyclines and sulfonamides should not be used.

ADDITIONAL TREATMENT

General Measures

Supportive care

Issues for Referral

Development of peritonsillar abscess or shock symptoms: Hypotension, disseminated intravascular coagulation (DIC), cardiac, liver, renal dysfunction

SURGERY/OTHER PROCEDURES

- Tonsillectomy may be recommended with recurrent bouts of pharyngitis (≥6 positive strep cultures in 1 year).
- Children still may get strep throat after a tonsillectomy, but for some children with recurring strep throat, tonsillectomy reduces the frequency and severity of strep throat infections.

ONGOING CARE

FOLLOW-UP RECOMMENDATIONS

Follow-up throat culture is not needed unless the patient is symptomatic.

Patient Monitoring

Because GAS is uniformly susceptible to penicillin, bacteriologic treatment failures are possible due to:

- Poor compliance
- β-Lactamase oral flora hydrolyzing penicillin
- GAS carrier state and concurrent viral rash (requires no treatment)
- Repeat exposure to carriers in family: Strep persists on unrinsed toothbrushes and orthodontic appliances for up to 15 days.

DIET

No special diet

PATIENT EDUCATION

- Brief delay in initiating treatment while awaiting throat culture results does not increase the risk of rheumatic fever.
- Must take antibiotics for full course
- Children should not return to school or daycare until they have received >24 hours of antibiotic therapy.
- Can spread person to person: Avoid contact, wash hands.
- "Recurring strep throat: When is tonsillectomy useful?" Available at www.mayoclinic.com/health/recurring-strep-throat/AN01626

PROGNOSIS

- Course may be shortened by 12–24 hours with penicillin.
- Recurrent attacks are possible (different erythrogenic toxins).
- Mild disease usually responds well to antibiotics.

COMPLICATIONS

- Suppurative:
  - Sinusitis
  - Otitis media/mastoiditis
  - Cervical adenitis
  - Peritonsillar abscess/retropharyngeal abscess
  - Pneumonia
  - Bacteremia with metastatic infectious foci: Meningitis, brain abscess, osteomyelitis, septic arthritis, endocarditis, intracranial venous sinus thrombosis, necrotizing fasciitis
- Nonsuppurative:
  - Rheumatic fever: Therapy prevents rheumatic fever when started as long as 10 days after onset of acute GAS infection.
  - Glomerulonephritis: Due to nephritogenic strain of *Streptococcus*; prevention even after adequate treatment of GAS is less certain.
  - Streptococcal toxic shock syndrome: Fever, hypotension, DIC, and cardiac, liver, and/or kidney dysfunction related to other toxin-mediated sequelae
  - Cellulitis
  - Weeks to months later may develop transverse grooves in nail plates and hair loss (telogen effluvium)

REFERENCES

1. Gerber MA, et al. Prevention of rheumatic fever and diagnosis and treatment of acute streptococcal pharyngitis: A statement from the American Heart Association Rheumatic Fever, Endocarditis, and Kawasaki Disease Committee of the Council on Cardiovascular Disease in the Young, the Interdisciplinary Council on Functional Genomics and Translational Biology, and the Interdisciplinary Council on Quality of Care and Outcomes Research: Endorsed by the American Academy of Pediatrics. *Circulation*. 2009;119:1541–51.
2. Spinks A. Antibiotics for sore throat (Review). *Cochrane Database of Systemic Reviews*. 2010;3.
3. Lennon DR, Farrell E, Martin DR. Once-daily amoxicillin versus twice-daily penicillin V in group A beta-haemolytic streptococcal pharyngitis. *Arch Dis Child*. 2008;93:474–8.

ADDITIONAL READING

Baltimore RS. Re-evaluation of antibiotic treatment of streptococcal pharyngitis. *Curr Opin Pediatr*. 2010;22:77–82.

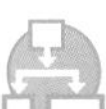

See Also (Topic, Algorithm, Electronic Media Element)

- Pharyngitis
- Algorithm: Tonsillar Exudates

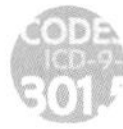

CODES

ICD9

- 034.0 Streptococcal sore throat
- 034.1 Scarlet fever

CLINICAL PEARLS

- Consider scarlet fever in the differential diagnosis of children with fever and a rash.
- Look for strawberry tongue, circumoral pallor (vs. hyperemic cracked lips as in Kawasaki disease), and a coarse sandpaper rash (especially helpful in dark-skinned individuals). Desquamation may last for several weeks following the illness.
- Perform throat swabs to document streptococcal illness vs. other etiologies.

S

STRESS FRACTURE

Jessica Devitt, MD
Morteza Khodaee, MD, MPH

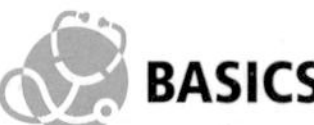

BASICS

DESCRIPTION

- Stress fractures are microscopic fractures that occur when repetitive stresses are applied to bone causing breakdown (via osteoclasts) faster than remodeling of new bone formation (via osteoblasts).
- Stress fractures can occur in different situations.
  - Fatigue fracture: Abnormal stress applied to normal bone (e.g., young college athletes or new military recruits with inadequate conditioning)
  - Insufficiency fracture: Normal stress applied to abnormal bone (e.g., femoral neck fracture in osteopenic elderly woman)
  - Combination: Abnormal stress applied to abnormal bone (e.g., female long-distance runners with premature osteoporosis from female athlete triad)
- Weight-bearing bones of the lower extremity are affected the most.
- Commonly affected sites:
  - Tibia
  - Metatarsus
  - Fibula
  - Navicular
  - Femoral neck
  - Pars interarticularis
- Less commonly affected sites:
  - Pelvis
  - Calcaneus
  - Ribs
  - Ulna
- High-risk stress fractures are defined as stress fractures that are more likely to result in fracture displacement and/or nonunion (1)[B]. High-risk sites include:
  - Femoral neck
  - Anterior tibial cortex
  - Sesamoids
  - Pars interarticularis
  - Fifth metatarsal metaphyseal
  - Proximal second metatarsal
  - Medial malleolus
  - Tarsal navicular
  - Body of the talus
- Synonym(s): March fracture; Fatigue fracture

EPIDEMIOLOGY

Incidence

- Predominant age: Can occur at any age
- Predominant sex: Female > Male
- High occurrence in running and jumping athletes
- Affects 8.7–21.1% of track and field athletes annually
- Accounts for as many as 7.8% of visits to sports medicine and orthopedic clinics

Prevalence

- Affects 5% of military recruits
- Affects 1–2.6% of college athletes

RISK FACTORS

- Sports involving running and jumping
- Rapid increase in physical training programs
- Female athlete triad (i.e., amenorrhea, eating disorder, premature osteoporosis)
- History of previous stress fracture
- Skeletal malalignment:
  - Pes cavus, pes planus
  - Excessive external rotation of the hip
- Inappropriate footwear
- Increased vertical loading rate (e.g., heel to toe running instead of forefoot striking in runners) (2)[C]
- Extremes of body size and composition
- Muscle fatigue and decreased lean muscle mass
- Low bone density
- Previous inactivity or low aerobic fitness

GENERAL PREVENTION

- Avoid abrupt increases in physical activity.
- Reduce intensity and duration of activity if new-onset pain.
- Use proper footwear.
- Decrease vertical loading rate either by switching to forefoot strike style running, or, if continuing with heel to toe strike, using a heel pad insert (2)[C].
- Shock-absorbing foot inserts may help.
- Increasing calcium, vitamin D, skim milk, and low-fat dairy product intake may reduce the rate of stress fractures in female runners/military recruits (3)[B].

PATHOPHYSIOLOGY

- Osteoblastic activities lag behind osteoclastic activities during the initial increase in exercise activity.
- Strong and repetitive stress transmits to bone when the surrounding muscles become fatigued.

COMMONLY ASSOCIATED CONDITIONS

- Osteoporosis/osteopenia
- Female athlete triad
- Metabolic bone disorders

DIAGNOSIS

HISTORY

- Insidious onset of vague, achy pain over period of weeks that occurs at the end or after physical activity
- Rest will relieve the pain initially.
- If untreated, pain will occur earlier during training sessions or even with daily walking and also become more localized.
- Eventual fracture of untreated stress fractures will cause pain at rest.
- More detailed history may reveal recent change in training intensity and/or footwear.

PHYSICAL EXAM

- Antalgic gait
- Point tenderness or percussion tenderness over injury site
- Placing a vibrating tuning fork over the fracture site may intensify pain.
- Swelling may be present.
- Specific tests may be helpful.
  - Hop test for tibia: Cannot hop on 1 leg 10 times; if able, consider shin splints (i.e., medial tibial stress syndrome)
  - Fulcrum test for femur: With patient seated, provoke pain by applying downward force on the distal femur while examiner uses other hand under the midthigh as fulcrum for femoral shaft
  - Single-leg hyperextension (Stork) test for pars interarticularis of lumbar spine: Stand on ipsilateral leg of symptomatic side, and extend lumbar spine.
- Anatomic malalignment may be present (e.g., leg-length discrepancy, pes planus/cavus).

DIAGNOSTIC TESTS & INTERPRETATION

Lab

None unless clinically indicated for suspected disease process (e.g., hyperparathyroidism and vitamin D deficiency)

Imaging

- Radiography:
  - First-line management in suspected stress fracture (4)[B]
  - Findings typically seen 2–8 weeks after onset of pain.
  - Sensitivity during early stages may be as low as 10%.
  - May see periosteal callus, "gray cortex" sign (cortical region of decreased intensity), osteopenia, endosteal reaction, or ill-defined cortical margin
  - Severe cases may show discrete partial or complete fracture.
- MRI:
  - "Gold standard" for imaging stress fractures (4)[B]
  - Very sensitive
  - Better evaluation of surrounding soft tissue
  - Allows for classification of the injury
  - T_2 weighting and short time inversion recovery (STIR) methods
- Bone scan:
  - Very sensitive, but lack of specificity may limit clinical utility.
  - Should not be used to assess healing process
- CT scan:
  - Less sensitive than MRI for early stress fractures, but has an important role in evaluating occult fractures in certain regions: Foot, tibia, carpal scaphoid, and pars interarticularis (4)[B]
  - Can distinguish diseases such as osteoid osteoma, malignancy, and osteomyelitis that mimic stress fracture on bone scan
  - Useful for evaluating lesions found to be equivocal on other imaging modalities (4)[B]
  - May also be used to determine whether a known stress fracture is complete or incomplete (4)[B]
- Ultrasound:
  - Not routinely used for the diagnosis of stress fractures
  - Able to detect cortical breaks and periosteal reactions
  - Of particular use in the evaluation of the foot; may distinguish between metatarsal stress fractures and other causes of metatarsalgia (e.g., Morton's neuroma) (4)[B]
- Classification by radiographic grading:
  - Grade I: Normal x-ray, positive STIR (MRI)
  - Grade II: Normal x-ray, positive STIR + positive T_2-weighted MRI
  - Grade III: Discrete line or discrete periosteal reaction on x-ray, positive T_1/T_2-weighted MRI but with no definite cortical break
  - Grade IV: Fracture or periosteal reaction on x-ray, positive T_1/T_2-weighted fracture line

DIFFERENTIAL DIAGNOSIS

- Fracture
- Shin splints (i.e., medial tibial stress syndrome) pain resolves with rest, whereas stress fracture pain does not.
- Infection (osteomyelitis)
- Soft tissue injury (e.g., sprain, tendonitis, and periostitis)
- Compartment syndrome
- Neoplasm (osteoid osteoma)
- Nerve or artery entrapment syndromes
- Intermittent claudication

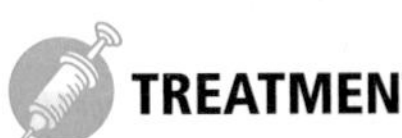

TREATMENT

- Protection, rest, ice, compression, and elevation (PRICE) for acute pain and edema
- Decrease activity below threshold of pain.
- Pain at rest or with range of motion (ROM) may require temporary immobilization.
- Painful ambulation is criterion for crutches with periodic walking trials.
- Gradually increase activity as long as patient remains pain-free.
- Early surgical management of high-risk fractures is indicated in the elite athlete secondary to the high risk of displacement and nonunion as well as the association with earlier return to sports (1)[C].

MEDICATION

- Acetaminophen
- NSAIDs are beneficial for pain and inflammation, but are controversial and discouraged by some authors because of negative impact on bone/tissue healing.
- Bisphosphonates theoretically could treat stress fractures, but their use should be limited because no randomized, controlled trials have been performed that show conclusive evidence (5)[B]. Currently, only case reports have shown benefit.

ADDITIONAL TREATMENT

- Electrical stimulator may be indicated in more severe injuries and/or elite athletes (6)[B].
- Low-intensity pulsed ultrasonography:
  - No evidence for improved healing in stress fracture
  - May improve healing with subsequent complete fracture

Issues for Referral

Referral and surgical intervention are reserved for high-risk stress fractures with potential for progression to complete fracture and possible delayed union or nonunion.

Additional Therapies

Physical therapy:

- Correct training errors predisposing to stress fracture.
- Correct inappropriate mechanics.
- Strengthen muscles around the site of stress fracture.
- Correct anatomic variations.

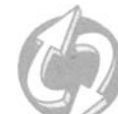

ONGOING CARE

FOLLOW-UP RECOMMENDATIONS

- After initial treatment, activity should be increased gradually.
- Once the patient is pain-free, low-impact training can be started and advanced as tolerated.
- Once running is resumed, mileage should be increased slowly.

Patient Monitoring

Radiographs every 4–6 weeks to document healing progress

PATIENT EDUCATION

- Gradually increase activity as tolerated as long as patient is pain-free.
- Rest if there is a recurrence of pain.
- Correct mechanical and training errors.
- Strengthen core muscles.

PROGNOSIS

- Stress fractures in young people have a good prognosis.
- Older patients or those with metabolic bone disease typically continue to develop insufficiency fractures in other bones.
- Time to return to full activity:
  - Grade I: 3+ weeks
  - Grade II: 5+ weeks
  - Grade III: 11+ weeks
  - Grade IV: 14+ weeks

COMPLICATIONS

Completion of fracture:

- Delayed union
- Nonunion
- May require surgery with internal fixation

REFERENCES

1. Anderson RB, Hunt KJ, McCormick JJ, et al. Management of common sports-related injuries about the foot and ankle. *J Am Acad Orthop Surg*. 2010;18:546–56.
2. Zadpoor AA, Nikooyan AA. The relationship between lower-extremity stress fractures and the groundreaction force: A systematic review. *Clin Biomech (Bristol, Avon)*. 2011;26(1):23–8.
3. Tenforde AS, Sayres LC, Sainani KL, et al. Evaluating the relationship of calcium and vitamin D in the prevention of stress fracture injuries in the young athlete: A review of the literature. *PM R*. 2010;2:945–9.
4. Dixon S, Newton J, Teh J, et al. Stress fractures in the young athlete: A pictorial review. *Curr Probl Diagn Radiol*. 2011;40:29–44.
5. Shima Y, et al. Use of bisphosphonates for the treatment of stress fractures in athletes. *Knee Surg Sports Traumatol Arthrosc*. 2009;5:542–50.
6. Beck B, et al. Do capacitively coupled electric fields accelerate tibial stress fracture healing?: A randomized controlled trial. *Am J Sports Med*. 2008;3:545–53.

ADDITIONAL READING

- Arendt EA, Griffiths HJ. The use of MR imaging in the assessment and clinical management of stress reactions of bone in high-performance athletes. *Clin Sports Med*. 1997;16:291–306.
- Armstrong DW, Rue JP, Wilckens JH, et al. Stress fracture injury in young military men and women. *Bone*. 2004;35:806–16.
- Boden BP, Osbahr DC. High-risk stress fractures: Evaluation and treatment. *J Am Acad Orthop Surg*. 2000;8:344–53.
- Busse JW, Kaur J, Mollon B, et al. Low intensity pulsed ultrasonography for fractures: Systematic review of randomised controlled trials. *BMJ*. 2009;338:b351.
- Fredericson M, Jennings F, Beaulieu C, et al. Stress Fractures in Athletes. *Top Magn Reson Imaging*. 2006;17:309–25.
- Manore MM, Kam LC, Loucks AB. The female athlete triad: Components, nutrition issues, and health consequences. *J Sports Sci*. 2007;25(Suppl 1): 61–71.
- Niva MH, Kiuru MJ, Haataja R, et al. Fatigue injuries of the femur. *J Bone Joint Surg Br*. 2005;87: 1385–90.
- Pepper M, Akuthota V, McCarty EC. The pathophysiology of stress fractures. *Clin Sports Med*. 2006;25:1–16, vii.
- Raasch WG, Hergan DJ. Treatment of stress fractures: The fundamentals. *Clin Sports Med*. 2006;25:29–36, vii.
- Snyder RA, Koester MC, Dunn WR. Epidemiology of stress fractures. *Clin Sports Med*. 2006;25:37–52, viii.

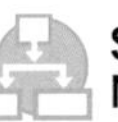

See Also (Topic, Algorithm, Electronic Media Element)

Algorithm: Foot Pain

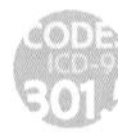

CODES

ICD9

- 733.93 Stress fracture of tibia or fibula
- 733.94 Stress fracture of the metatarsals
- 733.95 Stress fracture of other bone

CLINICAL PEARLS

- Diagnosis requires a high index of suspicion because x-rays are often negative initially.
- Emphasis must be placed on rest to allow for proper bone healing.
- Once the patient can walk pain-free, he/she can proceed to low-impact activity, and when low-impact activity can be performed pain-free, proceed to running.
- Gradually increase running mileage.
- Rest if there is a recurrence of pain.
- Recognize high-risk stress fracture for appropriate referral and possible surgery.

STROKE REHABILITATION

Jessica Lenore Wilson, MD

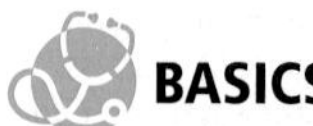

BASICS

DESCRIPTION

- Stroke is a compromise in blood supply to an area of the nervous system, secondary to hemorrhage or occlusion, with resultant infarction of nervous tissue.
- Rehabilitation refers to the process of restoration of a debilitated person toward baseline level of functionality.
- Stroke is the third leading cause of death and the leading cause of long-term disability in the US (1).
- $25.2 billion was the approximate direct medical cost of stroke in 2007 (2).

EPIDEMIOLOGY

Incidence

- Each year, about 795,000 people suffer a stroke, about 610,000 of which are first attacks and 185,000 are recurrent attacks (2).
- ~14% of survivors of stroke reach full recovery in physical function, but 25–50% require assistance post stroke (1).
- According to the World Health Organization, 15 million people suffer stroke worldwide each year. Of these, 5 million die and another 5 million are permanently disabled.

Prevalence

- About 7 million Americans ≥20 years old have had a stroke (~3%) (2).
- About 50 million stroke survivors worldwide (3)
- More than half of strokes under age 65 result in death within 8 years (1).

RISK FACTORS

Risk factors for stroke are discussed in the topics "Stroke, Acute" and "Atherosclerosis."

GENERAL PREVENTION

See "Stroke, Acute."

PATHOPHYSIOLOGY

Stroke involves a compromise in blood supply to an area, usually by either rupture or blockage of a vessel.

ETIOLOGY

Of all strokes, 87% are ischemic, 10% intracerebral hemorrhage, and 3% subarachnoid hemorrhage (2).

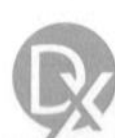

DIAGNOSIS

HISTORY

- In the setting of acute stroke, presentation can vary depending on the site of the stroke.
- History may include:
  - Acute onset, often unilateral, weakness of face, arm, or leg
  - Acute onset of sudden confusion, trouble speaking or difficulty understanding speech
  - Acute onset of monocular or binocular trouble seeing
  - Acute onset of trouble walking, dizziness, loss of balance or coordination
  - Acute onset of severe headache with no known cause (consider subarachnoid hemorrhage)

PHYSICAL EXAM

Neurologic manifestations based on location of stroke, but can include:

- Sensory or motor deficits, especially unilaterally (i.e., hemiparesis/hemiplegia)
- Dysarthria or aphasia
- Visual field deficits (i.e., hemianopsia)
- Dysphagia
- Apraxia
- Unilateral facial palsy

DIAGNOSTIC TESTS & INTERPRETATION

See "Stroke, Acute."

Lab

Follow-Up & Special Considerations

Monitor the coagulation profile of patients on anticoagulants.

Imaging

Initial approach

See topic "Stroke, Acute."

DIFFERENTIAL DIAGNOSIS

Seizure with postictal neurologic signs, infection, toxic/metabolic manifestations, intracranial mass (i.e., tumor), migraine with neurologic signs, trauma

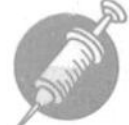

TREATMENT

The 3 major stroke rehabilitation goals are (1):

- Prevention/treatment of the various complications of prolonged inactivity
- Prevention of recurrent stroke and cardiovascular events
- Increase in aerobic fitness

MEDICATION

First Line

- Management of controllable risk factors, including BP reduction (A), diabetes (C), and cholesterol (initiate statin therapy, if history of TIA or stroke with evidence of atherosclerosis, LDL ≥100, and no CHD; A)
- Anticoagulation with warfarin for patients mechanical prosthetic heart valves and ischemic stroke or TIA (dosage of warfarin varies depending on optimum INR for pt in setting of comorbidities)
- Antiplatelet drugs (aspirin, aspirin/dipyridamole, clopidogrel, ticlopidine) decrease relative risk of stroke, MI, or death by ~22% (4). See topic "Stroke, Acute."

ADDITIONAL TREATMENT

General Measures

Prevention and/or treatment of the complications associated with stroke (3):

- Aspiration:
  - Immediately after stroke, up to 50% of patients have dysphagia; this resolves or improves in many
  - Patient should be kept NPO until initial bedside swallow to assess.
  - Prevention of aspiration involves postural changes, increased sensory input, swallowing maneuvers, active exercise programs, diet modifications, nonoral feeding (if indicated), psychological support, and supportive nursing interventions.
- Pulmonary embolism/deep venous thrombosis:
  - Risk highest during first 3–120 days post stroke
  - Pneumatic compression devices and compression stockings
  - Ambulation as soon as possible
  - DVT prophylaxis
- Skin breakdown:
  - Increased risk due to loss of sensation, impaired circulation, older age, decreased level of consciousness, inability to move oneself due to paralysis, and incontinence of urine or stool
  - Regularly assess patient's skin
  - In the inpatient setting, nurse assessment every shift and every time the patient is repositioned or sitting
  - Frequent repositioning (at least every 2 hours) with special care to avoid excessive friction
  - Keep skin clean and dry.
- Spasticity:
  - Occurs in ~35% of stroke survivors. Treated with a combination of physical and pharmacological modalities:
    - Range of motion exercises
    - Heat, cold, or electric stimulation
    - Splinting
    - Oral medications for spasticity of cerebral origin (e.g., dantrolene, tizanidine); phenol or botulinum toxin injections for targeting specific muscles or muscle groups
- Malnutrition:
  - At 2–3 weeks post stroke, 50% of severe stroke survivors are reported to be malnourished.
  - Nutritional assessment with a diet history and monitoring by a dietician
- Seizures:
  - More common after hemorrhagic stroke (11%) than after ischemic stroke (9%)
  - Treatment with antiepileptic drugs and elimination of disturbances (i.e., toxins, metabolic) that may lower seizure threshold
- Falls:
  - Lifestyle changes:
    - Avoid loose rugs; maintain a clear path without obstruction.
    - Avoid slippery surfaces (such as wet floors).
    - Maintain good lighting.
    - Shoes with nonskid soles
    - Slow down movements for transfers or walking.
- Severe sleep apnea:
  - Lifestyle changes:
    - Stop smoking.
    - Lose weight.
    - Sleep on side vs. back.
    - Mouthpieces
    - Breathing devices (i.e., CPAP)
    - Surgery
- Depression:
  - May be organic secondary to stroke or reactive to the stroke itself
  - Poststroke depression has been found to cause higher mortality, poorer functional recovery, and less activity socially (1).

- Treat with a combination of pharmacotherapy and psychotherapy:
  - Evidence suggests heterocyclic antidepressants are effective in the setting of poststroke depression but must be closely monitored in older adults due to side effects.
  - SSRIs are also effective in treating poststroke depression.
  - All stroke patients should be assessed for depression and treated with the appropriate antidepressant for 6 months.

Issues for Referral
For stroke survivors who require 24-hour care of medical comorbidities, close physician supervision, and specialized nursing care (RN with specialized training or rehabilitation experience), an inpatient rehabilitation facility (IRF) can offer hospital-level care.

Additional Therapies
- Physical therapy
- Occupational therapy
- Speech therapy
- Recreational therapy

IN-PATIENT CONSIDERATIONS
Initial Stabilization
See "Stroke, Acute"

Admission Criteria
- For stroke survivors who require 24-hour care of medical comorbidities, close physician supervision, and specialized nursing care (RN with specialized training or rehabilitation experience), an inpatient rehabilitation facility (IRF) can offer hospital-level care.
- Such patients must also require and receive a minimum of 3 hours daily for occupational or physical therapy for no less than 5 days each week; this can be combined with other skilled modalities, such as speech-language or prosthetic-orthotic services) to meet the 3-hours per day requirement.
- Either the aforementioned is required, or an IRF is the only reasonable setting in which a low-intensity rehab program may be executed.
- An alternative inpatient setting would be a skilled nursing facility, which is the primary function to provide nursing care or rehabilitation to residents needing daily rehab or nursing care on an inpatient basis.

IV Fluids
Avoid D5W in acute setting, to avoid hyperglycemia and its secondary effects.

Nursing
An alternative inpatient setting would be a skilled nursing facility, which is the primary function to provide nursing care or rehabilitation to residents needing daily rehab or nursing care on an inpatient basis.

Discharge Criteria
Chronic care settings support and help make external resources available to manage the patient's level of health; such services must be prescribed by a qualified health care professional, such as a physician.

ONGOING CARE

FOLLOW-UP RECOMMENDATIONS
Patient should follow up regularly with primary care physician for management of risk factors for stroke.

Patient Monitoring
Continue to monitor for risk factors. Lab studies monitored periodically may include: Hemoglobin A1c (and finger-stick glucose testing in diabetics), lipid panel, CBC including platelets, lipid profile, coagulation studies (PT/INR—of special importance in patients on anticoagulation)

DIET
Low salt, low calorie, low saturated and trans fat, low cholesterol

PATIENT EDUCATION
National Stroke Association: www.stroke.org

PROGNOSIS
- Strong evidence suggests an organized, interdisciplinary stroke care team of physicians, nurses, therapists, family, and patient can reduce mortality rates and the likelihood of institutional care and long-term disability. It can also enhance recovery and increase ADL (activities of daily living) independence.
- Aggressive rehabilitation beyond the time window of the first poststroke months, including treadmill with or without body weight support, can increase aerobic capacity and sensorimotor functionality.

COMPLICATIONS
- Aspiration
- Pulmonary embolism/deep venous thrombosis
- Greater exercise intolerance
- Muscle atrophy
- Osteoporosis
- Skin breakdown
- Spasticity
- Malnutrition
- Seizures
- Falls
- Severe sleep apnea

REFERENCES

1. Gordon NF, Gulanick M, Costa F, et al. Physical activity and exercise recommendations for stroke survivors: An American Heart Association scientific statement from the Council on Clinical Cardiology, Subcommittee on Exercise, Cardiac Rehabilitation, and Prevention; the Council on Cardiovascular Nursing; the Council on Nutrition, Physical Activity, and Metabolism; and the Stroke Council. *Circulation*. 2004;109:2031–41.
2. Roger VL, Go AS, Lloyd-Jones DM, et al. Heart disease and stroke statistics–2011 update: A report from the American Heart Association. *Circulation*. 2011;123:e18–e209.
3. Miller EL, Murray L, Richards L, et al. Comprehensive overview of nursing and interdisciplinary rehabilitation care of the stroke patient: A scientific statement from the American Heart Association. *Stroke*. 2010;41:2402–48.
4. Furie KL, Kasner SE, Adams RJ, et al. Guidelines for the prevention of stroke in patients with stroke or transient ischemic attack: A guideline for healthcare professionals from the american heart association/american stroke association. *Stroke*. 2011;42:227–76.

ADDITIONAL READING

Moskowitz MA, Lo EH, Iadecola C, et al. The science of stroke: Mechanisms in search of treatments. *Neuron*. 2010;67:181–98.

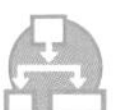

See Also (Topic, Algorithm, Electronic Media Element)

- Brain Injury—Post Acute Care Issues; Stroke, Acute; Dementia; Delirium
- Algorithm: Stroke

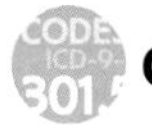

CODES

ICD9
434.91 Cerebral artery occlusion, unspecified with cerebral infarction

CLINICAL PEARLS

- Stroke is the third leading cause of death and the leading cause of long-term disability in the US.
- An essential part of poststroke management is the treatment of controllable risk factors, including BP reduction (A) and cholesterol control (initiate statin therapy, if history of TIA or stroke with evidence of atherosclerosis, LDL $\geq$100 (A)
- Strong evidence suggests an organized, interdisciplinary stroke care team of physicians, nurses, therapists, family, and patient can reduce mortality rates and the likelihood of institutional care and long-term disability. It can also enhance recovery and increase ADL independence.

STROKE, ACUTE

Nihal Patel, MD
Erik J. Garcia, MD

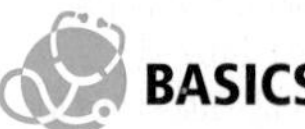

BASICS

A cerebrovascular accident (CVA) is an infraction in the brain.

DESCRIPTION

Stroke is the sudden onset of a focal neurologic deficit(s) resulting from either infarction or hemorrhage within the brain:

- 2 broad categories: Ischemic (thrombotic or embolic; 87%) and hemorrhagic (13%) (1)
- Hemorrhage can be intracerebral or subarachnoid.
- System(s) affected: Neurologic; Cardiovascular
- Synonym(s): Cerebrovascular accident; Cerebral infarct; brain attack
- Related terms: Transient ischemic attack (TIA), a transient episode of neurologic dysfunction due to focal ischemia without permanent infarction on imaging (see topic "Transient Ischemic Attack [TIA]")

Pediatric Considerations

- Cardiac abnormalities (congenital heart disease, paradoxical embolism, rheumatic fever, bacterial endocarditis)
- Metabolic: Homocystinuria, Fabry disease

EPIDEMIOLOGY

Incidence

Incidence in the US: 150 per 100,000 per year

Prevalence

- Prevalence in the US: 550 per 100,000
- Predominant age: Risk increases >45 years of age and is highest during the seventh and eighth decades
- Predominant sex: Male > Female (3:1), but equalizes after menopause

RISK FACTORS

- Uncontrollable: Age, sex, race, family history/genetics, prior stroke or TIA
- Controllable/modifiable/treatable:
  - Metabolic: Diabetes mellitus, obesity, metabolic syndrome, impaired glucose tolerance
  - Lifestyle: Smoking, heavy alcohol use, substance abuse, increased sodium intake, poor physical function
  - Cardiovascular: Hypertension, atrial fibrillation, valvular heart disease, severe carotid artery stenosis, hypercoagulable states (including use of OCP), pregnancy and postpartum states

Genetics

Stroke is a polygenic multifactorial disease, with some clustering within families.

GENERAL PREVENTION

Smoking cessation, regular exercise, weight control to maintain nonobese BMI and prevent type 2 diabetes, use of alcohol in moderation, control BP, and manage hyperlipidemia with appropriate statin therapy; use of antiplatelet agent such as aspirin in at-risk persons, treatment of nonvalvular atrial fibrillation with dose-adjusted warfarin or dabigatran

ETIOLOGY

- 87% of stroke is ischemic, secondary to cardioaortic embolism (including atrial fibrillation), large artery arthrosclerosis such as carotid artery stenosis, small vessel occlusion or dissection.
- 13% of stroke is hemorrhagic, most commonly due to hypertension. Other causes include intracranial vascular malformations (cavernous angiomas, AVMs), cerebral amyloid angiopathy (lobar hemorrhages in elderly), or secondary hemorrhage into previous infarcts.
- Other causes include fibromuscular dysplasia (rare), vasculitis, or drug use (cocaine, amphetamines).

COMMONLY ASSOCIATED CONDITIONS

Cardiac disease is the major cause of death during the first 5 years after a stroke.

DIAGNOSIS

HISTORY

Acute onset of focal arm/leg weakness, facial weakness, difficulty with speech or swallowing, vertigo, visual disturbances, diminished consciousness; presence of vomiting and severe headache favor diagnosis of hemorrhagic stroke

PHYSICAL EXAM

- Anterior (carotid) circulation: Hemiparesis/hemiplegia, neglect, aphasia, visual field defects
- Posterior (vertebrobasilar) circulation: Diplopia, vertigo, ataxia, facial paresis, Horner syndrome, dysphagia, dysarthria

DIAGNOSTIC TESTS & INTERPRETATION

Lab

Primarily used to narrow differential and identify etiology of stroke

Initial lab tests

- ECG
- Serum glucose level, including finger-stick testing (exclude hypo- and hyperglycemia)
- CBC including platelets
- Electrolytes including BUN and creatinine
- Coagulation studies: PT, PTT, INR
- Markers of cardiac ischemia

Follow-Up & Special Considerations

Consider LFT, tox screen, blood alcohol, ABG, lumbar puncture if suspected SAH, EEG if suspect seizures, blood type and cross

Imaging

Initial approach

- Emergent brain imaging with noncontrast CT or brain MRI with diffusion weighing (DW) MRI to exclude hemorrhage
- Subsequent multimodal CT (perfusion CT, CTA, unenhanced CT) or MRI to improve diagnosis of acute ischemic stroke (2)

Follow-Up & Special Considerations

- DW MRI is more sensitive than conventional CT for acute ischemic stroke (3); however, multimodal CT is equivalent to MRI. MRI also is better than CT for diagnosis of posterior fossa lesions.
- Emergent treatment (IV thrombolysis) should not be delayed to obtain imaging studies.
- Follow-up imaging of carotid vessels with Doppler ultrasound, CTA, or MRA should be completed.

Diagnostic Procedures/Surgery

Echocardiogram (transthoracic) in patients with increased suspicion for cardioembolic source

Pathological Findings

Early CT findings: Hyperdense MCA sign, loss of gray-white differentiation in cortical ribbon, sulcal effacement, loss of insular ribbon

DIFFERENTIAL DIAGNOSIS

- Migraine (complicated)
- Postictal state (Todd paralysis)
- Systemic infection, including meningitis or encephalitis (infection also may uncover or enhance previous deficits)
- Toxic or metabolic disturbance (hypoglycemia, acute renal failure, liver failure, drug intoxication)
- Brain tumor, primary or metastases
- Head trauma
- Intracranial hemorrhage (epidural, subdural, subarachnoid)
- Trauma, septic emboli

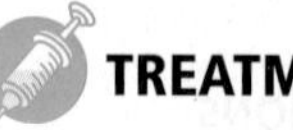

TREATMENT

- BP management: Hypertension should be cautiously managed due to spontaneous BP decline in the first 24 hours:
  - Antihypertensives should be withheld unless systolic BP >220 mm Hg or diastolic BP >120 mm Hg, with a goal to lower BP by ~15% during first 24 hours (2)[A].
  - If patient is eligible for thrombolysis, pressure may be reduced to <185/110 (2)[A].
  - In hemorrhagic stroke, goal for BP control is lower at 160/100 (see topic, "Subarachnoid Hemorrhage" for details on BP management)
  - Antihypertensive medications should be restarted 24 hours after stroke onset for patients with a history of hypertension who are neurologically stable (2)[A].
- Thrombolysis (2)[A]: IV thrombolysis should be started in patients with measurable neurologic deficits that do not clear spontaneously, presenting within 4.5 hours of stroke onset.
- Exclusion criteria for thrombolysis within 3 hours of onset include:
  - Symptoms suggestive of SAH
  - Head trauma or prior stroke within 3 months
  - MI within 3 months
  - GI or gastric ulcer hemorrhage within 21 days
  - Major surgery within 14 days
  - Arterial puncture at noncompressible site within 7 days
  - Any history of ICH persistently
  - Elevated BP (systolic >185 mm Hg and diastolic >110 mm Hg)
  - Active bleeding or acute trauma on examination
  - Taking anticoagulant and INR ≥1.7
  - Activated PTT not in normal range if heparin received during previous 48 hours; platelet count <100,000 mm^3
  - Blood glucose concentration <50 mg/dL
  - Seizure with postictal residual neurological impairment
  - Multilobar infarction on CT (hypodensity >1/3 cerebral hemisphere)
  - Patient or family members not able to weigh and understand potential risks and benefits of treatment

- Extended exclusion criteria for thrombolysis within 4.5 hours include:
  - Age >80 years
  - All patients taking oral anticoagulants
  - National Institute of Health (NIH) Stoke Scale >25
  - History of stroke and diabetes
- Antiplatelet agents: Oral aspirin (initial dose, 325 mg) should be started within 24–48 hours (2)[A]:
  - In the acute setting, clopidogrel alone or in combination with aspirin is not recommended.
  - Urgent anticoagulation with goal of preventing early recurrent stroke is not recommended.

MEDICATION

First Line

- BP management: Antihypertensive options include (2)[A]:
  - Labetalol 10–20 mg IV over 1–2 minutes, which may be repeated once
  - Nitropaste 1–2 inches
  - Nicardipine infusion 5 mg/hr, titrate up by 2.5 mg/hr at 5–15-minute intervals to maximum of 15 mg/hr; reduce to 3 mg/hr when target BP is reached
- Thrombolysis, IV administration of rtPA: Infuse 0.9 mg/kg, maximum dose 90 mg over 60 minutes with 10% of dose given as bolus over 1 minute (2)[A]:
  - Admit to ICU or stroke unit, with neurological exams every 15 minutes during infusion, every 60 minutes for next 6 hours, then hourly until 24 hours after treatment.
  - Discontinue infusion and obtain emergent CT scan if severe headache, angioedema, acute hypertension, or nausea and vomiting develop.
  - Measure BP every 15 minutes for first 2 hours, every 30 minutes for next 6 hours, then every hour until 24 hours after treatment. Maintain BP below 185/105. Follow-up CT at 24 hours before starting anticoagulants or antiplatelet agents.
- Antiplatelet: Aspirin 325 mg/d within 48 hours, or 24–48 hours after thrombolytic therapy

Second Line

Carotid endarterectomy (CEA) for carotid artery stenosis rarely is indicated emergently. CEA is indicated for stenosis >70% ipsilateral to TIA or incomplete stroke lesion, and may be indicated for 50–69% stenosis in carefully selected patients, depending on risk factors.

ADDITIONAL TREATMENT

- Prophylactic antibiotics are *not* recommended (2)[A].
- Deep vein thrombosis (DVT) prophylaxis should be instituted for immobilized patients.
- Corticosteroids are *not* recommended for cerebral brain edema (2)[A].
- Statin use should be continued without interruption following acute stroke.

Issues for Referral

Follow-up with neurologist 1 week after discharge, with subsequent follow-up based on individual circumstances.

Additional Therapies

Upon discharge, patient should be referred for physical therapy, occupational therapy, and speech therapy as necessary.

COMPLEMENTARY AND ALTERNATIVE MEDICINE

Acupuncture starting within 30 days from stroke onset may improve neurological functioning.

SURGERY/OTHER PROCEDURES

- Ventricular drain may be placed for patients with acute hydrocephalus secondary to stroke (most commonly due to cerebellar stroke).
- Decompressive surgery is recommended for major cerebellar infarction, and it may be considered for malignant edema in severely affected patients.
- Consider Mechanical Embolus Removal in Cerebral Infarction device.

IN-PATIENT CONSIDERATIONS

Initial Stabilization

- Observe closely within first 24 hours for neurological decline, particularly due to brain swelling.
- Keep head of bed at least 30° when elevated intracranial pressure is suspected. Patients with ischemic stroke may benefit from a horizontal bed position during the acute phase.
- Monitor cardiac rhythm for at least first 24 hours to identify any arrhythmias.
- Airway support and ventilatory assistance may be necessary due to diminished consciousness or bulbar involvement; supplemental oxygen should be reserved for hypoxic patients. Consider elective intubation for patients with malignant edema.
- Correct hypovolemia with normal saline.
- All patients should be kept NPO until a formal swallow evaluation has been performed; to reduce risk of aspiration pneumonia, maintain elevated head of bed to 30°.
- Hypoglycemia can cause neurological dysfunction; rapidly correct during initial evaluation.
- Hyperglycemia within first 24 hours after stroke is associated with poor functional outcomes and AHA/ASA guidelines: Insulin treatment for patients with glucose levels >140–185 mg/dL.
- In patients with ICH and anticoagulant use, correction of elevated INR is necessary with use of IV vitamin K and fresh frozen plasma. Consider neurosurgical intervention for hematoma evacuation if indicated.
- DVT prophylaxis

IV Fluids

IV hydration with normal saline until swallowing status is assessed; monitor fluid balance closely

Nursing

- Regular neurologic exams more frequent in first 24 hours (every 1–2 hours)
- Fall precautions; frequent repositioning to prevent skin breakdown

Discharge Criteria

Medically stable, adequate nutritional support, neurologic status stable or improving

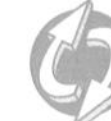

ONGOING CARE

FOLLOW-UP RECOMMENDATIONS

- Secondary prevention of stroke with aggressive management of risk factors
- Platelet inhibition using aspirin, clopidogrel, or aspirin plus extended-release dipyridamole (Aggrenox) based on physician and patient preference.

Patient Monitoring

Follow-up every 3 months for first year, then annually.

DIET

Patients with impaired swallowing should receive nasogastric or percutaneous endoscopic gastrostomy feedings to maintain nutrition and hydration.

PATIENT EDUCATION

National Stroke Association (800-STROKES or www.stroke.org)

PROGNOSIS

Variable depending on subtype and severity of stroke; NIH stroke scale may be used for prognosis.

COMPLICATIONS

- Acute: Brain herniation, hemorrhagic transformation, MI, congestive heart failure, dysphagia, aspiration pneumonia, UTI, DVT, pulmonary embolism, malnutrition, pressure sores
- Chronic: Falls, depression, dementia, orthopedic complications, contractures

REFERENCES

1. Yew KS, Cheng E, et al. Acute stroke diagnosis. *Am Fam Physician*. 2009;80:33–40.
2. Adams HP, del Zoppo G, Alberts MJ, et al. Guidelines for the early management of adults with ischemic stroke: A guideline from the American Heart Association/American Stroke Association Stroke Council, Clinical Cardiology Council, Cardiovascular Radiology and Intervention Council, and the Atherosclerotic Peripheral Vascular Disease and Quality of Care Outcomes in Research Interdisciplinary Working Groups: The American Academy of Neurology affirms the value of this guideline as an educational tool for neurologists. *Stroke*. 2007;38:1655–711.
3. Chalela JA, Kidwell CS, Nentwich LM, et al. Magnetic resonance imaging and computed tomography in emergency assessment of patients with suspected acute stroke: A prospective comparison. *Lancet*. 2007;369:293–8.

See Also (Topic, Algorithm, Electronic Media Element)

- Stroke Rehabilitation; Transient Ischemic Attack (TIA)
- Algorithm: Stroke

CODES

ICD9

- 430 Subarachnoid hemorrhage
- 431 Intracerebral hemorrhage
- 434.91 Cerebral artery occlusion, unspecified with cerebral infarction

CLINICAL PEARLS

- Unless stroke is hemorrhagic or patient is undergoing thrombolysis, BP should not be lowered acutely to maintain perfusion of penumbric region.
- DW MRI is more sensitive than conventional CT for acute ischemic stroke (3); however, multimodal CT is equivalent to MRI. MRI is also better than CT for diagnosis of posterior fossa lesions.

SUBARACHNOID HEMORRHAGE

Abir O. Kanaan, PharmD, RPh
Kristin A. Tuiskula, PharmD, RPh
George M. Abraham, MD, MPH, FACP

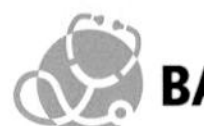

BASICS

1 in every 20 strokes is caused by subarachnoid hemorrhage from intracranial aneurysm. The disease often strikes at a young age and is often fatal.

DESCRIPTION

- Extravasation of blood into the subarachnoid space, particularly of the basal cisterns, and into CSF pathways, including the ventricles
- Accounts for 2–5% of new strokes
- Traumatic: Most common cause; related to head trauma
- Spontaneous: Less common; however, 85% of these are due to ruptured intracranial saccular aneurysms, and they have a worse prognosis than nonaneurysmal bleeds, which account for roughly 10% of spontaneous subarachnoid hemorrhages (SAHs).
- Also may occur from rupture of arteriovenous malformations (AVMs)
- System(s) affected: Nervous; Cardiovascular; Pulmonary

Pregnancy Considerations

Increased BP and blood volume may predispose pregnant women to hemorrhages.

EPIDEMIOLOGY

Incidence

- Spontaneous: Aggregate worldwide incidence is 10.5/100,000 person-years; 20/100,000 in Finland and Japan
- 1 in 100 ED patients presenting with headache has SAH.
- Although incidence increases with age, mean age of presentation is 55 years.
- Predominant age: Most occur in fourth to seventh decades.
- SAHs due to AVMs occur in second to fourth decades.
- Predominant sex: Female > Male (1.6:1)
- Blacks > Whites (2.1:1)

Prevalence

In the US: 21,000–33,000 new cases each year

RISK FACTORS

- Cigarette smoking
- Cocaine abuse
- Excessive alcohol intake
- Hypertension (HTN) is associated with rupture of aneurysms but not with saccular aneurysms.
- First-degree relatives with SAH
- AVMs

Genetics

Heritable connective tissue disorders:

- Polycystic kidney disease
- Fibromuscular dysplasia
- Pseudoxanthoma elasticum

GENERAL PREVENTION

- Incidentally identified aneurysms have risk of hemorrhage according to size and location; therefore, endovascular coiling or surgical clipping may be indicated, depending upon surgical risk.
- The 5-year cumulative rate of aneurysmal rupture in the internal carotid artery, anterior cerebral artery, middle cerebral artery, or anterior communicating artery is based on size:
  - <7 mm: 0%
  - 7–12 mm: 2.6%
  - 13–24 mm: 14.5%
  - >25 mm: 40%
- The 5-year cumulative rate of aneurysmal rupture in the posterior circulating and posterior communicating arteries is based on size:
  - <7 mm: 2.5%
  - 7–12 mm: 14.5%
  - 13–24 mm: 18.4%
  - >25 mm: 50% (1)
- In younger age groups, incidentally found AVMs have a 2% risk of rupture per year.

ETIOLOGY

- Trauma
- Intracranial saccular aneurysm
- Intracranial AVM
- HTN
- Rarely, tumors and blood dyscrasias

COMMONLY ASSOCIATED CONDITIONS

- Morbidity and mortality of SAH are determined by complications that develop after the initial bleed.
- Outcome predicted by the World Federation of Neurological Surgeons clinical grading: Based on sum score of Glasgow Coma Scale (GCS) and presence of focal neurologic signs
- Blood volume on initial CT scan is predictive of vasospasm.
- The following complications are common:
  - Cerebral vasospasm occurs within 4–12 days of initial bleed and is seen angiographically in 67%.
  - Cardiac arrhythmias occur in 35% of patients.
  - Seizures occur in up to 33% of patients.
  - Electrolyte disturbances (including syndrome of inappropriate antidiuretic hormone [SIADH] and cerebral salt wasting) occur in 28% of patients.
  - Pulmonary edema occurs in 23% of patients.
  - Hydrocephalus occurs in 20% of patients.
  - Rebleeding occurs in 7% of patients and has a 50% risk of permanent neurologic damage.

DIAGNOSIS

HISTORY

- Assess for recent head trauma, HTN, nicotine/EtOH/cocaine use, AVMs, family history of SAH, and current use of anticoagulants.
- Abrupt onset of headache ("worst headache of life") associated with stiff neck, nausea, vomiting, photophobia, and/or loss of consciousness
- Headache may be the only presenting symptom in up to 40% of patients and may disappear within hours (so-called thunderclap headaches, sentinel bleeds, or warning leaks).
- Seizures at onset of hemorrhage occur in 1/14 patients.

PHYSICAL EXAM

- Retinal hemorrhages
- Meningismus
- Diminished consciousness; calculate GCS on all patients.
- Focal neurologic signs, such as third-nerve palsy (posterior communicating artery aneurysm), sixth-nerve palsy (increased intracranial pressure [ICP]), bilateral leg weakness and/or abulia (anterior communicating artery aneurysm), hemiparesis and/or aphasia and/or visuospatial neglect (MCA aneurysm)
- Perform lumbar puncture if CT scan is negative and suspicion is high. Elevated opening pressure, xanthochromia (takes 12 hours to develop), or RBCs unchanged in tubes 1–4 are consistent with SAH.

DIAGNOSTIC TESTS & INTERPRETATION

Imaging

- Noncontrast-enhanced head CT scan with thin cuts through the base of the brain; sensitivity drops to 50% at 7 days but is 100% at 12 hours and 93% at 24 hours.
- CT scan may show hydrocephalus, cerebral edema, and intraparenchymal bleeds and can predict the site of rupture (particularly in the anterior circulation).
- CT scan is the most reliable predictor of vasospasm and poor outcome using the Fisher scale.
- CT scan can rule out mass effect to safely perform a necessary lumbar puncture (LP).
- If CT scan or LP is positive, check cerebral angiography (gold standard) or CT angiography; they have similar sensitivity and specificity.
- If second study is negative, high-definition MRI should be performed. MRI can be used but is not the standard for surgical planning.
- Important: If no source of SAH is found intracranially, obtain spinal MRI or myelography.
- Funduscopic exam to rule in intraocular hemorrhage

Initial approach

- If prehospital, stabilize ABCs, IV, O_2 monitor
- After stabilizing patient, consider transfer to neurovascular center.
- Strict bed rest, reduced noise level, and limited visitors until source of bleeding is secured
- Ideal BP management in the setting of acute SAH is uncertain because of incomplete and conflicting evidence and recommendations. Level of alertness is a rough indicator of adequate cerebral perfusion pressure. Generally, if the patient is alert, systolic BP (SBP) may be safely lowered below 140 mm Hg. If the patient's level of consciousness is severely affected, BP reduction should not be attempted. The American Heart Association 2010 guideline makes the following recommendations (2)[B]:
  - In patients presenting with a SBP of 150–220 mm Hg, acute lowering of SBP to 140 mm Hg is probably safe.
  - If SBP is >200 mm Hg or mean arterial pressure (MAP) is >150 mm Hg, then consider aggressive reduction of BP with continuous IV infusion, with frequent BP monitoring q5min.

- If SBP is >180 mm Hg or MAP is >130 mm Hg and there is the possibility of elevated ICP, then consider monitoring ICP and reducing BP using intermittent or continuous IV medications while maintaining a cerebral perfusion pressure (CPP) >60 mm Hg.
- If SBP is >180 mm Hg or MAP is >130 mm Hg and there is no evidence of elevated ICP, then consider a modest reduction of BP (e.g., MAP of 110 mm Hg or target BP of 160/90 mm Hg) using intermittent or continuous IV medications to control BP and clinically re-examine the patient q15min.

- Control pain.
- Provide venous thromboembolism prophylaxis.
- Correct fluid and electrolytes.

DIFFERENTIAL DIAGNOSIS

Traumatic SAH; aneurysmal rupture (including mycotic aneurysms associated with bacterial endocarditis); VM; arterial dissection with intracranial extension; pituitary apoplexy; drug abuse (e.g., cocaine) ± aneurysm as a result of vasculitis; coagulopathies; migraine (especially with aura)

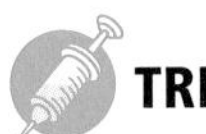

TREATMENT

MEDICATION

- Nimodipine: 60 mg PO (via nasogastric tube if necessary) q4h × 21 days for prevention of cerebral vasospasm; start immediately (3)[A].
- The use of antifibrinolytic therapy is controversial; cerebral ischemia may occur with these agents (3,4).
- Patients with a severe coagulation factor deficiency of severe thrombocytopenia should receive factor replacement therapy or platelets, respectively (2).
- Prophylactic anticonvulsant therapy is controversial; only clinical seizures or electrographic seizures in patients with a change in mental status should be treated with antiepileptic drugs (2):
  - Treat seizures with lorazepam 0.1 mg/kg IV at a 2 mg/min rate, followed by phenytoin 20 mg/kg IV bolus at <50 mg/min up to 30 mg/kg (5).
- SIADH vs. cerebral salt wasting *must* be distinguished with serum and urine electrolytes.
- Symptomatic vasospasm is currently treated with hypervolemia (central venous pressure [CVP] 8–12 mm Hg, pulmonary capillary wedge pressure 12–16 mm Hg) and/or induced hypertension (using phenylephrine, norepinephrine) (5)[A].

ADDITIONAL TREATMENT

General Measures

- Initial therapy in ICU. Treatment is directed toward preventing complications, including rebleeding, hydrocephalus, and cerebral vasospasm.
- If indicated, BP elevation is treated (see "Treatment") with small, frequent doses of IV labetalol or nicardipine, or with an IV drip.
- Continuous EEG monitoring is probably indicated in ICH patients with depressed mental status out of proportion to the degree of brain injury (2).
- Maintain euvolemia (CVP 5–8 mm Hg) *unless* cerebral vasospasm is present (see below).
- Evaluate and treat myocardial injury and/or arrhythmias.
- Distinguish cardiogenic vs. neurogenic pulmonary edema, and treat appropriately.
- Control pain with morphine sulfate 2–4 mg IV q2–4h.
- Maintain serum glucose at 80–120 mg/dL with insulin sliding scale or continuous infusion.
- Maintain core body temperature ≤37.2°C. APAP 325–650 mg PO q4–6h and cooling devices may be used.
- Deep vein thrombosis prophylaxis with thigh-high stockings and compressive devices; *after* aneurysm is secured, SC heparin 5,000 units SC q8h, or enoxaparin 40 mg SC q24h
- GI prophylaxis with ranitidine 150 mg PO b.i.d. (50 mg IV q8–12h) or lansoprazole 30 mg PO daily
- Stool softeners also may be used.

Additional Therapies

Aggressive physical, occupational, and speech therapies are recommended.

SURGERY/OTHER PROCEDURES

- Endovascular coiling and surgical clipping are options for securing aneurysms.
- Coiling appears to have better outcomes; clipping is a second choice for most patients.
- Rebleeding should be dealt with immediately by treatment of aneurysm.
- Of aneurysms, 25–30% will be multiple.
- Hydrocephalus should be treated with external ventricular drain, lumbar drain, or permanent CSF drainage.
- AVMs may be obliterated with embolization and surgery.

IN-PATIENT CONSIDERATIONS

Initial Stabilization

Stabilize ABCs, IV, O_2 monitor

IV Fluids

Give at least 3 L/d of 0.9% isotonic saline.

Nursing

Continuous observation (focal deficits, temperature, ECG, GCS)

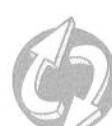

ONGOING CARE

FOLLOW-UP RECOMMENDATIONS

Perform neuropsychological testing before discharge and schedule cognitive rehabilitation.

Patient Monitoring

As needed

DIET

- If intact cough and swallowing reflexes, give PO diet; otherwise, diet should be advanced via a nasogastric tube.
- Parenteral nutrition should be used only when oral route is not feasible.

PROGNOSIS

- Average case-fatality rate is 50% overall: 10% before receiving care, 25% within the first 24 hours
- Highest morbidity secondary to cerebral vasospasm; 25–30% of patients die from spontaneous SAH caused by aneurysm.
- If aneurysm can be obliterated successfully and vasospasm treated effectively, satisfactory outcome occurs in 50–65% of patients.
- 46% of survivors report long-term cognitive impairment of varying degrees.
- Survivors who return to work after 1 year: 50–75%.
- Disabled after a rebleed: 80%.

COMPLICATIONS

- Temporary and permanent neurologic deficits and/or disorders (e.g., seizures [1/14 patients], headache, SIADH)
- Psychosocial dysfunction (60%)
- Death
- Systemic complications: Fever, anemia, cardiac failure and arrhythmias, pulmonary edema

S

REFERENCES

1. Jabbour PM, Tjoumakaris SI, Rosenwasser RH. Endovascular management of intracranial aneurysms. *Neurosurg Clin N Am.* 2009;20: 383–98.
2. Morgenstern LB, Hemphill JC, Anderson C, et al. Guidelines for the management of spontaneous intracerebral hemorrhage: A guideline for healthcare professionals from the American Heart Association/American Stroke Association. *Stroke.* 2010;41:2108–29.
3. Bederson JB, Connolly ES, Batjer HH, et al. Guidelines for the management of aneurysmal subarachnoid hemorrhage: A statement for healthcare professionals from a special writing group of the Stroke Council, American Heart Association. *Stroke.* 2009;40:994–1025.
4. Chwajol M, Starke RM, Kim GH, et al. Antifibrinolytic therapy to prevent early rebleeding after subarachnoid hemorrhage. *Neurocrit Care.* 2008;8:418–26.
5. Suarez JI, Tarr RW, Selman WR. Aneurysmal subarachnoid hemorrhage. *N Engl J Med.* 2006;354:387–96.

ADDITIONAL READING

- Rinkel GJE. Calcium antagonists for aneurysmal subarachnoid haemorrhage. *Cochrane Database Sys Rev.* 2007;3:CD000277.
- van Gijn J, Kerr RS, Rinkel GJ. Subarachnoid haemorrhage. *Lancet.* 2007;369:306–18.

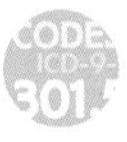

CODES

ICD9

- 430 Subarachnoid hemorrhage
- 852.00 Subarachnoid hemorrhage following injury, without mention of open intracranial wound, with state of consciousness unspecified

CLINICAL PEARLS

- Start nimodipine 60 mg PO q4h × 21 days.
- Headache may be the only symptom in 40% of patients with SAH and may disappear within hours.
- 1 in 100 ED patients presenting with headache has an SAH.
- Almost 1/3 of aneurysms are multiple.

SUBCLAVIAN STEAL SYNDROME

Alfonso J. Tafur, MD, RPVI
Angeline Opina, MD

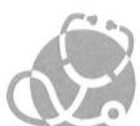

BASICS

DESCRIPTION

- A condition that results from stenosis or occlusion of the subclavian artery proximal to the origin of the vertebral artery; blood is drawn from the contralateral vertebral basilar or carotid artery regions into the low-pressure ipsilateral upper limb vessels, "stealing" the blood flow from the circle of Willis.
- The term was reported for the first time by Fisher in 1961. It is a normal pattern of collateral response to proximal subclavian artery occlusion.

EPIDEMIOLOGY

Incidence

- Predominant age:
  - Age >55 years—atherosclerotic etiology
  - Age <30 years—90% of patients with Takayasu arteritis
- Predominant sex: Male > Female

Prevalence

- Present in 6% of the patients with asymptomatic carotid bruit
- Hemodynamically significant left subclavian artery stenosis is present in ~2.5% of patients undergoing coronary revascularization (1).

RISK FACTORS

- Smoking
- Hypertension
- Diabetes
- Hyperlipidemia
- Radiotherapy

PATHOPHYSIOLOGY

- With a left subclavian occlusion, maintenance of blood flow to the left arm occurs with reversal of flow from the basilar artery via the left vertebral artery.
- Symptoms are associated with the degree and location of a second extracranial vessel occlusion.

ETIOLOGY

- Arteriosclerosis obliterans of the proximal subclavian artery in 95% of cases
- Lesions are 4:1 more common on the left side.
- Less common causes of obstruction:
  - Dissecting aneurysm of aortic arch
  - Trauma
  - Embolus
  - Radiotherapy induced
  - Takayasu arteritis
  - Giant cell arteritis
  - Fibromuscular dysplasia
  - May happen after Blalock-Taussig procedure for tetralogy of Fallot

COMMONLY ASSOCIATED CONDITIONS

- Carotid artery disease
- Coronary artery disease is present in 30–60% of patients.
- Arteriosclerosis

Geriatric Considerations

Older patients are more likely to have arteriosclerosis.

DIAGNOSIS

- Reduced BP of >20 mm Hg in involved arm
- Symptoms should be reproducible by exercising the arm.
- A variation of the syndrome is the coronary–subclavian steal syndrome, which can only occur after coronary artery bypass grafting (CABG); may present with symptoms of cardiac ischemia.

HISTORY

- Patients can present with:
  - Upper extremity claudication or muscle fatigue following minimal exercise, rest pain, ulcers, and digital necrosis.
  - Transient ischemic attacks (usually of the vertebrobasilar territory) often precipitated by exercise or work of the involved upper extremity.
  - Symptoms of vertebrobasilar ischemia include: Dizziness, diplopia, dysarthria, dysphagia, ataxia, gait disturbances, numbness, nystagmus
- Classified as asymptomatic, oligosymptomatic (only neurologic symptoms or upper limb ischemia is present), or complete (both symptoms)

PHYSICAL EXAM

- Absent or diminished pulses in ipsilateral arm:
  - Compare carotid, subclavian, brachial, radial, and ulnar pulses.
  - Using a handheld continuous wave Doppler, a monophasic or reduced biphasic pulse may be heard distal to the lesion.
- A brachial systolic pressure difference of >15 mm Hg is >90% specific for subclavian stenosis (only ~50% sensitive).
- Auscultation of carotid and suprascapular bruits
- On physical exam, we can subdivide subclavian stenosis as moderate (difference >15 and <25 mm Hg) or severe (difference >25 mm Hg). This correlates with long-term prognosis (2).
- Compression–decompression test (hyperemia test): Inflate a BP cuff above the systolic BP for 3 minutes. Vertebrobasilar symptoms may be reproduced by rapid decompression.
- Perform Allen's test bilaterally

DIAGNOSTIC TESTS & INTERPRETATION

Lab

- No lab findings are pathognomonic for subclavian steal syndrome.
- Noninvasive measurement of BP in upper extremities
- Pulse volume recording of upper extremities
- If Takayasu arteritis is suspected:
  - ESR (elevated)
  - CBC (thrombocytosis)
  - ECG (ischemic pattern)
  - Chest x-ray (CXR) (widening of thoracic aorta)

Imaging

- Duplex scanning of extracranial vessels
- Magnetic resonance angiography
- Arteriogram of arch vessels with delayed films of vertebral arteries

Diagnostic Procedures/Surgery

- Arteriography
- Doppler ultrasound may be used as screening test.
- According to the hemodynamics, there are 4 subtypes:
  - Vertebrovertebral
  - Carotid–basilar
  - External carotid–vertebral
  - Carotid–subclavian (can only occur on the right side with brachiocephalic occlusion proximal to the origin of the carotid artery)

DIFFERENTIAL DIAGNOSIS

- Vascular: Intracranial vascular disease, carotid artery disease, vertebral artery disease
- Neurogenic: Brain tumor, seizures, subdural hematoma
- Cardiac arrhythmias

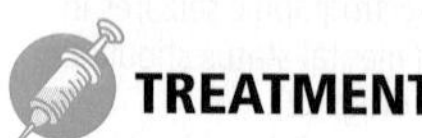

TREATMENT

ADDITIONAL TREATMENT

General Measures

- Antiplatelet therapy with aspirin (or clopidogrel if intolerant of aspirin), especially in patients with concomitant coronary artery disease
- Reduce cholesterol levels, if appropriate, using diet or medication (statin drugs) with a goal low-density lipoprotein (LDL) <100.
- Cessation of smoking.

Issues for Referral

- In symptomatic patients, consider consulting vascular medicine and cardiovascular surgery.
- Potential indications for subclavian artery intervention include:
  - Vertebrobasilar ischemia
  - Disabling upper limb ischemia: rest pain and digital embolization
  - Angina in a patient with a left internal mammary artery (LIMA) graft
  - Leg claudication in patient with axillofemoral graft
  - To increase flow before CABG using the internal mammary artery (IMA) or before creation of dialysis arteriovenous fistula
  - Subclavian artery repair prethoracic endovascular aortic repair (TEVAR). Controversial (3).

SURGERY/OTHER PROCEDURES

Treatment options include:

- Balloon angioplasty: Stent insertion increases long-term patency rates (4)[B]:
  - The 8–10-year primary patency is 83–95% (5):
    - Long-term patency can be aided with antiplatelet agents.
  - Complications occur in up to 10% of the cases and include:
    - Femoral pseudoaneurysm
    - Embolic stroke (0.9–1.4% complication rate)
    - Distal embolism
- Carotid–subclavian bypass
- Carotid–subclavian transposition:
  - To be considered if there is distal embolization from the subclavian artery lesion
  - The reported patency is 100% at 10 years compared with 74% for carotid bypass.
- Axilloaxillary bypass: 12-year graft occlusion of 10% and 0.4% periprocedural mortality
- Carotid endarterectomy
- Subclavian arterectomy

IN-PATIENT CONSIDERATIONS

Aggressive management of cardiovascular risk factors

Initial Stabilization

Outpatient care unless vascular surgery is anticipated

Admission Criteria

Stroke, critical limb ischemia

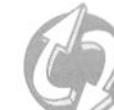

ONGOING CARE

FOLLOW-UP RECOMMENDATIONS

- Poststenting follow-up at 1-, 6-, and 12-month intervals initially, then yearly thereafter
- Frequent neurologic review of systems and subclavian Doppler ultrasound for patients who become symptomatic or have a BP difference of >10 mm Hg between arms.

Patient Monitoring

Annual physical examination including BP reading in both arms in patients with known stenosis

DIET

Low-cholesterol diet, if appropriate

PATIENT EDUCATION

- Prevent injury to arm.
- Reduce exercise of arm.

PROGNOSIS

- The presence of subclavian stenosis recently has been defined as an independent risk factor for cardiovascular death (2).
- After angioplasty of the subclavian artery, younger age and stenting are independent predictors of restenosis-free survival (4).

COMPLICATIONS

Completed stroke

REFERENCES

1. Hwang HY, Kim JH, Lee W, et al. Left subclavian artery stenosis in coronary artery bypass: Prevalence and revascularization strategies. *Ann Thorac Surg*. 2010;89:1146–50.
2. Aboyans V, Criqui MH, McDermott MM, et al. The vital prognosis of subclavian stenosis. *J Am Coll Cardiol*. 2007;49:1540–5.
3. Kotelis D, Geisbüsch P, Hinz U, et al. Short and midterm results after left subclavian artery coverage during endovascular repair of the thoracic aorta. *J Vasc Surg*. 2009;50:1285–92.
4. Sixt S, Rastan A, Schwarzwälder U, et al. Long term outcome after balloon angioplasty and stenting of subclavian artery obstruction: A single centre experience. *Vasa*. 2008;37:174–82.
5. Wang KQ, Wang ZG, Yang BZ, et al. Long-term results of endovascular therapy for proximal subclavian arterial obstructive lesions. *Chin Med J*. 2010;123:45–50.
6. Bicknell CD, Subramanian A, Wolfe JH. Coronary subclavian steal syndrome. *Eur J Vasc Endovasc Surg*. 2004;27:220–1.

ADDITIONAL READING

Brott TG, Halperin JL. 2011 ASA/ACCF/AHA/AANN/AANS/ACR/ASNR/CNS/SAIP/SCAI/SIR/SNIS/SVM/SVS guideline on the management of patients with extracranial carotid and vertebral artery disease: Executive summary. *JACC*. 2011;57(8):1002–44.

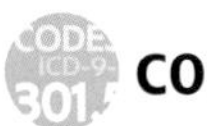

CODES

ICD9

435.2 Subclavian steal syndrome

CLINICAL PEARLS

- Takayasu arteritis/vasculitis is most common in young females. The aorta and its branches are the major vessels affected by inflammation, thrombus formation, and aneurysmal dilatation. Subclavian steal syndrome is thought to be relatively common in this disorder (6).
- The left upper extremity is affected more frequently, perhaps because subclavian steal occurs when the obstruction is proximal to the origin of the vertebral artery, and this distance is shorter on the right than on the left.
- The physical findings associated with subclavian steal syndrome are lower BP, decreased pulse, and bruit (supraclavicular) on the affected side.
- Subclavian artery stenosis should be detected before bypass surgery when a LIMA graft is planned. If present, a stenosis may present later on as coronary–subclavian steal syndrome

S

SUBCONJUNCTIVAL HEMORRHAGE

Jaye Cole, MD
Kelly Bennett, MD

BASICS

DESCRIPTION

- Subconjunctival hemorrhage (SCH) is bleeding from small blood vessels underneath the conjunctiva, the thin clear skin covering the sclera of the eye.
- SCH is diagnosed clinically (1):
  - Demarcated areas of extravasated blood can be seen just under the surface of the conjunctiva of the eye (red patch of blood sign) (1).
- Typically, SCH resolves spontaneously within 1–2 weeks (1).

EPIDEMIOLOGY

- Study of 8,726 encounters in an outpatient eye clinic had a 3% rate of diagnosis of SCH (2).
- Male = Female, no gender predilection found (2)

Incidence

Incidence increases:

- With increasing age (3,4)
- In contact lens wearers (3)
- With systemic diseases such as diabetes, hypertension, and coagulation disorders (3)
- During summer months, possibly due to trauma (2)

RISK FACTORS

- Age
- Contact lens wearer
- Systemic diseases
- Bleeding disorders (3)
- Recent cataract surgery

GENERAL PREVENTION

- Correct cleaning and maintenance of contact lenses
- Protective eyewear in sports and hobbies
- Control of high BP
- Optimizing control of systemic diseases, such as diabetes and atherosclerotic disease
- Control of prothrombin time (PT)/international normalized ratio (INR) in patients on Coumadin therapy (1)

PATHOPHYSIOLOGY

- Direct trauma to the blood vessels of the conjunctiva from blunt or penetrating trauma (5)
- Direct trauma to the conjunctiva from improper contact lens placement or improper cleaning
- Increased BP in the vessels of the conjunctiva from hypertension or from the temporary increase in BP from a Valsalva type maneuver (such as vomiting) (5)
- Damaged vessels from diabetes and atherosclerotic disease (5)
- Increased bleeding tendencies from either thrombocytopenia, elevated PT/elevated INR (5)

ETIOLOGY

- Trauma to the eye
- Valsalva maneuvers such as coughing, vomiting, straining, and pushing of a laboring patient
- Hypertension
- Atherolsclerotic disease and diabetes (5)
- Bleeding factors such as thrombocytopenia, elevated prothrombin time (from either disease or medication side effects)

DIAGNOSIS

HISTORY

- Generally asymptomatic; usually the patient noticed the redness in the mirror or another person mentions it to them
- There should be little to no pain involved (1).
- Obtain history of trauma.
- Obtain history of contact lens usage or cataract surgery (3).
- Comprehensive past medical history to evaluate if at risk for systemic diseases or treatments

PHYSICAL EXAM

- Evaluate BP to assess control (2).
- Measure visual acuity because it should be normal in a simple SCH (1).
- Verify that the pupils are equal and reactive to light and accommodation; this should be normal with an SCH (1).
- There should be no discharge or exudate noted (1).
- Look at sclera for a bright-red demarcated patch:
  - Demarcated area is most often on inferior aspect of eye due to gravity (4).
- If penetrating trauma is a consideration, do a gentle digital assessment of the integrity of the globe (5).

Geriatric Considerations

In older adults, the area of SCH will be more widespread across the sclera (4).

DIAGNOSTIC TESTS & INTERPRETATION

If a foreign body is suspected, perform a fluorescein exam:

- Fluorescein exam of a patient with a SCH should show no uptake of staining (1).

Lab

Typically none, as SCH is a clinical diagnosis.

Follow-Up & Special Considerations

If history and physical exam suspicious for a bleeding etiology (1):

- CBC
- Prothrombin time (PT)/International ratio (INR)

Imaging

If suspect an orbital fracture, may obtain plain facial bone films or CT scan (5)

ALERT

If suspect a penetrating injury, may obtain a CT scan of the orbits but not an MRI (if object may be metal) (5)

DIFFERENTIAL DIAGNOSIS

- Conjunctivitis (viral, bacterial, allergic, chemical)
- Foreign body to conjunctiva
- Penetrating trauma
- Acute angle glaucoma
- Iritis (1)

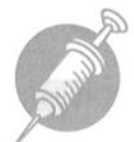

TREATMENT

MEDICATION

No prescription medications are useful in treatment of SCH.

ADDITIONAL TREATMENT

- Warm compresses
- Eye lubricants (1)

General Measures

- Control BP.
- Control blood glucose.
- Control INR (1).
- Protective eyewear

Issues for Referral

- If you suspect a penetrating eye injury, send the patient to the emergency room for emergent ophthalmology consultation (1).
- If the patient complains of any decreased visual acuity or visual disturbances, refer to an ophthalmologist as soon as possible.
- If there is no resolution of SCH within 2 weeks, patient may need referral to an ophthalmologist.

ONGOING CARE

FOLLOW-UP RECOMMENDATIONS

- Follow up only if the area does not resolve within 2 weeks.
- If SCH recurs, then work up patient for systemic sources such as bleeding disorders (1).

PATIENT EDUCATION

- Reassurance of the self-limited nature of the problem and typical time frame for resolution.
- Education to return to clinic if the area does not heal or recurs.
- Correct cleaning and maintenance of contact lenses
- PubMed Health: Subconjunctival hemorrhage at www.ncbi.nlm.nih.gov/pubmedhealth/PMH0002583/
- WebMD: Subconjunctival hemorrhage at www.webmd.com/eye-health/bleeding-in-the-eye

PROGNOSIS

Excellent

COMPLICATIONS

Rare

REFERENCES

1. Cronau H, Kankanala RR, Mauger T, et al. Diagnosis and management of red eye in primary care. *Am Fam Physician*. 2010;81:137–44.
2. Fukuyama J, Hayasaka S, Yamada K, et al. Causes of subconjunctival hemorrhage. *Ophthalmologica*. 1990;200:63–7.
3. Mimura T, Usui T, Yamagami S, et al. Recent causes of subconjunctival hemorrhage. *Ophthalmologica*. 2010;224:133–7.
4. Mimura T, Yamagami S, Usui T, et al. Location and extent of subconjunctival hemorrhage. *Ophthalmologica*. 2010;224:90–5.
5. Wirbelauer C, et al. Management of the red eye for the primary care physician. *Am J Med*. 2006;119: 302–6.

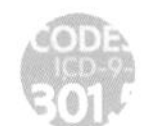

CODES

ICD9

372.72 Conjunctival hemorrhage

CLINICAL PEARLS

- Subconjunctival hemorrhage (SCH) is a clinical diagnosis. The condition is typically asymptomatic and will resolve spontaneously in 1–2 weeks.
- Always check BP in a patient with SCH, as hypertension is a risk factor (2).
- Indications for immediate referral to an ophthalmologist: Eye pain, change in vision, and/or penetrating eye trauma
- Reassurance and comfort measures are key.
- Contact lens wearers should not wear contacts until the SCH resolves completely.

SUBDURAL HEMATOMA

Ryan F. Coughlin, MD
Richard P. Moser, MD, FACS

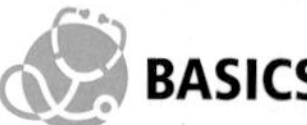

BASICS

DESCRIPTION

- Acceleration-deceleration brain injury leading to tearing of bridging vessels. Blood collects in potential space between dura mater and arachnoid mater.
- Acute: ≤14 days; more severe than chronic; often associated with parenchymal brain injury; diagnosis with CT scan and treated with surgery
- Chronic: >2 weeks; often seemingly trivial injury in older patients, e.g., fall from standing; good prognosis after surgery; recurrence is common.

EPIDEMIOLOGY

Predominant age (1):

- Acute: Predominant age group 30–50 years
- Chronic: Predominant age group >50 years

Incidence

- Acute: 1–2 per 100,000 per year; male > female; acute subdural hematoma is present in 5–22% of episodes of severe head trauma.
- Chronic: 3.4 per 100,000 <65 years; 8–58 per 100,000 ≥65 years (prevalence is increasing with aging population)

Prevalence

As many as 1 in 2,000 patients from general population may have incidental subdural hemorrhage seen on MRI (2).

RISK FACTORS

- Acute: Severe head trauma (e.g., MVAs, falls, child abuse)
- Chronic: Cerebral atrophy, chronic alcoholism, dementia, falls, minor trauma, epilepsy, coagulopathy/anticoagulation therapy, antiplatelet drugs, low ICP, hemodialysis, child abuse (1)

ALERT

Cerebral atrophy due to age or alcoholism predisposes to subdural hematomas. Never forget nonaccidental trauma in children!

GENERAL PREVENTION

- Acute: Seatbelt, bicycle/motorcycle helmet, construction hard hat
- Chronic: Alcoholism treatment, PT, epilepsy treatment, cautious prescription of anticoagulation therapy, shunts in hydrocephalus patients

PATHOPHYSIOLOGY

- Acute:
  - Bleed (e.g., from tearing of bridging veins; most common cause), injury to small cortical arteries (rare), low CSF pressure causing reduced brain buoyancy
  - Fibroblasts proliferate, wall off hematoma, and migrate into hematoma.
  - Bleeding usually is tamponaded by compression due to increasing ICP or direct compression by the clot itself
  - Phagocytes cause liquefaction of the hematoma, which eventually resolves if the bleed is slow enough. If unable to reabsorb, it becomes chronic.
- Chronic:
  - Hematoma not entirely reabsorbed; alternatively, recurrent bleeding at least as fast as body's resorption rate. The membrane encapsulating the clot may calcify over time (1).

ETIOLOGY

- Acute:
  - Young adult: 56% MVAs; 12% falls
  - Elderly: 22% MVAs; 56% falls
  - Trauma from high-velocity acceleration-deceleration brain injury
  - Blunt trauma often leads to subdural bleeds on coup side of brain as opposed to epidural bleeds, which tend to occur on contre-coup side.
- Chronic:
  - Geriatric patients: Trivial head injury (e.g., fall from standing)
  - Children: May be caused by nonaccidental head trauma, unrecognized/unreported trauma, or, rarely, birth trauma

ALERT

Both acute and chronic subdural bleeds can occur without physical impact!

COMMONLY ASSOCIATED CONDITIONS

- Acute: Brain contusion or subarachnoid hemorrhage (most common); epidural hematoma, diffuse axonal injury, facial fractures; cervical spine injury (1)
- Chronic: Subdural hygroma (extracranial collection of CSF), seizure disorder, coagulopathy, CSF shunt, birth trauma, child abuse, metastatic carcinoma (rare)

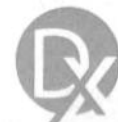

DIAGNOSIS

HISTORY

- Acute:
  - Assess for risk factors: head trauma, anticoagulation medications, falls
  - Loss of consciousness; lucid interval 12–38%
  - Headache, nausea, vomiting, nuchal rigidity, ataxia
  - 85% of children with subdural hematoma from nonaccidental head trauma will have other signs of abuse (e.g., bruises or fractures) (3).
- Chronic: 30–50% have no history of trauma. Symptoms include progressive headache, confusion, lightheadedness, personality changes. Alcoholics frequently present with acute on chronic SDHs owing to frequent trauma and coagulopathies associated with chronic alcohol abuse.

PHYSICAL EXAM

- Acute:
  - GCS <8 (comatose): 37–80%; altered level of consciousness: 99%
  - Pupillary irregularity (usually ipsilateral to hematoma): 47–53%; hemiparesis (usually contralateral to hematoma): 34–47%
  - Decerebrate posturing or flaccid motor exam: 47%; papilledema: 16%; cranial nerve VI palsy: 5%
- Chronic:
  - Altered mental status: 50–70% in elderly; confusion, delirium, psychiatric manifestations, coma
  - Hemiparesis: 45–58%; onset often is insidious and gradually progressive; most commonly contralateral
  - Headache: Less common among the elderly
  - Falls may be a presenting symptom
  - Papilledema: 24%; cranial nerve III abnormality: 11%; hemianopsia: 7%
  - Seizure: Most commonly in patients with large hematomas and focal neurological deficits
  - Atypical presentations: Parkinsonism, vertigo, nystagmus, Gerstmann syndrome
  - Infants: Accelerated increase in head size, irritability, poor feeding, occasional vomiting, tension of anterior fontanelle, seizures

DIAGNOSTIC TESTS & INTERPRETATION

Consider EEG for seizures (patients may have nonconvulsive seizures).

Lab

Initial lab tests

PT, INR, type and screen, CBC, chem-7, glucose, blood alcohol level, urine toxicology screen, anticonvulsant levels in epileptics

ALERT

Make sure to type and cross patients receiving anticoagulation therapy in case there is need for emergent reversal of coagulopathy (e.g., fresh frozen plasma for supratherapeutic INR).

Imaging

- CT scan (without contrast) is test of choice because of shorter exam time. Acute subdural hematoma: Hyperdense, extra-axial, crescent-shaped collection. Subacute: Isodense lesion (difficult to identify and may require MRI for elucidation). Chronic: Hypodense lesion (usually takes 3 weeks to evolve). Bilateral chronic SDH: Medial compression of ventricles, narrow slit-like ventricle termed *squeezed ventricle*
- MRI more sensitive than CT head scan; aids in diagnosis of hematomas isodense with brain due to mixture of chronic hematoma with recurrent hemorrhage. Helpful in diagnosing lesions located in base of skull, posterior fossa, and vertex because CT scan emits large shadow effect

Pathological Findings

- Acute: Fresh hemorrhage
- Chronic: Liquefied hematoma; outer membrane beneath dura after 1 week; inner membrane between hematoma and arachnoid after 3 weeks. On rare occasions, cytology examination may reveal association between metastatic carcinoma cells and hemorrhage.

DIFFERENTIAL DIAGNOSIS

Epidural hematoma, cerebral contusion, dementia, depression, stroke/TIA, subdural empyema, meningitis, concussion, hypoxia, intoxication/withdrawal, shock, seizure, hypoglycemia, hypertensive crisis, myxedema coma, neoplasm/metastasis, subdural hygroma

TREATMENT

MEDICATION

First Line

- Acute (note that emergent surgical craniotomy is often the treatment of choice):
  - Phenytoin (Dilantin) 1,000 mg load (50 mg/min IV) with ECG monitoring, followed by 100 mg IV q8h or as needed to maintain therapeutic blood levels (10–20 μg/mL [40–79 μmol/L]). Convert from IV to PO ASAP to avoid cardiovascular complications of IV phenytoin (hypotension, bradycardia, arrhythmia).

- Logic: Start antiseizure prophylaxis with phenytoin ASAP in adults following severe traumatic brain injury (i.e., prolonged loss of consciousness or amnesia, intracranial hematoma or brain contusion on CT scan, and/or a depressed skull fracture) to decrease the risk of posttraumatic seizures occurring within first 7 days (4). Convulsions may exacerbate systemic injuries, and status epilepticus has high fatality in this population. Prophylaxis does not prevent future development of epilepsy.
  - Mannitol 20% solution 0.5–1 g/kg, followed by 0.25–0.75 g/kg q4–6h:
    - Logic: Management of cerebral edema and elevated ICP
- Chronic:
  - Small hematomas that are asymptomatic or mildly symptomatic (e.g., headache) may be appropriately treated conservatively with observation because some chronic SDHs have been known to resolve spontaneously:
    - Steroids (e.g. prednisone) may be helpful for symptomatic treatment in these patients if not otherwise contraindicated.

Second Line

- Acute:
  - Loop diuretic can be used to augment Mannitol's effect. Administer furosemide (Lasix) 0.5 mg/kg IV.
  - Hypertensive saline: 7.2% NaCl/HES 200/0.5 solution at 1.4 ml/kg. May be more effective than mannitol at reducing ICP and improving cerebral blood flow. If risk of central pontine hyalinosis, exclude hyponatremia prior to administration
  - Check serum osmolality every 8 hours and serum electrolytes at least daily.
- Chronic:
  - Medical management alone for large SDHs or in patients with significant neurologic signs is frequently unsuccessful and entails risks of neurologic deterioration. Seizure prophylaxis currently not recommended for chronic SDH because conclusive evidence lacking.

ADDITIONAL TREATMENT

General Measures

- Acute (medical management):
  - Maintenance of adequate airway and ventilation and support of cardiovascular system to promote normal cerebral perfusion. Goals: PaO_2 >60 mm Hg (5) and SBP >90 mm Hg (5)
  - ICP management:
    - Monitor ICP in all patients with GCS <8 (5)[B]; target: ICP <20 mm Hg (5)[B]
    - Ventriculostomy with external gauge transducer is most accurate and cost-effective method of monitoring ICP.
    - Elevate head of bed to reduce ICP and promote venous outflow from head.
    - Cerebral perfusion pressure (CPP): CPP = mean arterial pressure – ICP. Target CPP = 60 mm Hg (5)[B]. Avoid CPP >70 mm Hg due to risk of adult respiratory distress syndrome, and avoid CPP <50 mm Hg because of risk of cerebral ischemia
  - Treat multisystem injuries. Spine precautions: As appropriate to injury until spine injury ruled out

ALERT

Avoid hyperventilation in first 24 hours after injury. This may reduce ICP but can also induce secondary cerebral ischemia (5).

SURGERY/OTHER PROCEDURES

- Acute: Emergent craniotomy is often treatment of choice. Other surgeries: Burr hole trephination, decompressive craniectomy, large decompressive hemicraniectomy. Choice of surgery mostly dependent on neurosurgeon's preference (1)
- Indications for surgery:
  - Hematoma thickness >10 mm or midline shift >5 mm by CT (1)[C]
  - Coma patient (GCS score <9), even if thickness <10 mm or shift <5 mm, if: Decrease in GCS score >2 points since admission, asymmetric pupils or fixed and dilated pupils, ICP >20 mm Hg
  - Timing of intervention: Surgery should be performed within 2–4 hours after clinical deterioration (1).
  - Other factors influencing decision to perform surgery: History (age, comorbidities, neurological deterioration), physical exam, GCS score, ICP
- Subacute:
  - If patient is neurologically stable, surgery may be delayed until hematoma matures and becomes chronic, at which time burr-hole drainage can be performed.
  - In a setting of mass effect, neurologic deficit, and solid (nonliquefied) clot, SDH may require craniotomy for complete evacuation.
- Chronic (6):
  - Patients with small SDHs may not require surgery.
  - Several techniques available: Burr-hole drainage (2 approaches) with bedside twist drill vs. operation with burr holes and irrigation; both have been shown effective in prospective, randomized trial and prospective, nonrandomized series (6)[C]

IN-PATIENT CONSIDERATIONS

IV Fluids

Normal saline with 20 mEq/L KCl as needed

ALERT

Refrain from using hypotonic fluids or fluids with glucose because they may cause increased ICP.

ONGOING CARE

FOLLOW-UP RECOMMENDATIONS

Patient Monitoring

- Patients with chronic subdural hematomas should have a follow-up CT scan 1–2 months after surgery to confirm interval improvement.
- Patients requiring anticoagulation should resume this medical treatment when risk of hemorrhage is low; this decision is made on individualized patient basis.

DIET

- Acute: Most patients require enteral or total parenteral nutrition initially if decreased mental status. Patients should be fed to full caloric replacement by day 7 after injury (5)[C].
- Chronic: Depending on the level of consciousness, patients usually can have diet advanced to regular food as tolerated. Consider swallow evaluation in patients with neurologic change.

PROGNOSIS

Outcome is highly dependent on neurologic status before surgery:

- Acute: Mortality: 40–60% requiring surgery; 57–68% comatose at presentation (1)
- Chronic: Mortality: 15.6%; postsurgical intervention, mortality 6.5%. Most predictive prognostic indicator: Neurological status on admission

COMPLICATIONS

- Postoperative complications: New or recurrent hematoma; elevated ICP and cerebral edema; cortical injury secondary to drill procedures; infection (subdural empyema, meningitis); tension pneumocephalus (air trapped in cranial cavity causing midline shift); seizures (in 11–33% of patients); there is benefit of seizure prophylaxis in period immediately after acute head trauma (7 days); no proven benefit for long-term seizure prophylaxis
- Chronic: Recurrent SDH in up to 50% of patients (reduced with use of drainage catheter) s/p burr hole: 9.2–26.5%. Delirium, intracranial hemorrhage (rare), subdural hygroma, seizures in up to 10% of patients (1)

REFERENCES

1. Bullock MR, Chesnut R, Ghajar J, et al. Surgical management of acute subdural hematomas. *Neurosurgery*. 2006;58:S16–24; discussion Si–iv.
2. Vernooij MW. Incidental findings on brain MRI in the general population. *NEJM*. 2007;357: 1821–28.
3. Hobbs C. Subdural hematoma and effusion in infancy. *Arch Dis Child*. 2005;90:952–55.
4. Chang BS, Lowenstein DH. Practice parameter: Antiepileptic drug prophylaxis in severe traumatic brain injury. Report of the Quality Standards Subcommittee of the American Academy of Neurology. *Neurology*. 2003;60:10–6.
5. Brain Trauma Foundation, American Association of Neurological Surgeons, Congress of Neurological Surgeons, et al. Guidelines for the management of severe traumatic brain injury. *J Neurotrauma*. 2007;24(Suppl 1):S1–106.
6. Muzii VF, Bistazzoni S, Zalaffi A, et al. Chronic subdural hematoma: Comparison of two surgical techniques. Preliminary results of a prospective randomized study. *J Neurosurg Sci*. 2005;49:41–6; discussion 46–7.

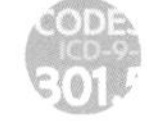

CODES

ICD9

- 432.1 Subdural hemorrhage
- 852.25 Subdural hemorrhage following injury without mention of open intracranial wound, with prolonged [more than 24 hours] loss of consciousness without return to pre-existing conscious level

CLINICAL PEARLS

- Elderly patients, alcoholics, or infants <2 years old are most susceptible to acute SDH.
- Consider chronic SDH in elderly patient with progressive symptoms of headache, personality changes, and/or functional decline.
- SDH can occur without physical impact to head.
- Non–contrast-enhanced CT scan is test of choice for acute SDH demonstrating a hyperdense, crescent-shaped, extra-axial lesion.
- Recurrence is a common complication in chronic SDHs.

SUBSTANCE USE DISORDERS

S. Lindsey Clarke, MD, FAAFP

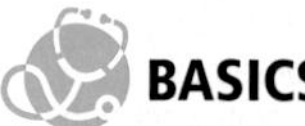

BASICS

DESCRIPTION

A substance use disorder manifests as any pattern of substance use causing significant physical, mental, or social dysfunction:

- Substances of abuse include:
  - Alcohol
  - Amphetamines
  - Anabolic steroids
  - Barbiturates
  - Benzodiazepines
  - Cannabinoids (hashish, marijuana)
  - Club and designer drugs (mostly methamphetamine derivatives)
  - Cocaine
  - Flunitrazepam
  - Gamma-hydroxybutyrate
  - Heroin (diacetylmorphine)
  - Inhalants (gasoline, glue, paint thinners, nitrous oxide)
  - Ketamine
  - Lysergic acid diethylamide (LSD)
  - Mescaline, psilocybin (mushrooms, peyote)
  - Methadone
  - Methamphetamines
  - Methaqualone
  - Methylphenidate
  - Nicotine
  - Opium
  - Opioids (codeine, fentanyl, hydrocodone, hydromorphone, meperidine, morphine, oxycodone, propoxyphene, others)
  - Phencyclidine
- For current listing of street terms, see drug charts at www.nida.nih.gov/drugpages/.
- System(s) affected: Cardiovascular; Endocrine/Metabolic; CNS
- Synonym(s): Drug abuse; Drug dependence; Substance abuse

Geriatric Considerations

- Alcohol is the most commonly abused substance, and abuse often goes unrecognized.
- Higher potential for drug interactions

Pregnancy Considerations

Substance abuse may cause fetal abnormalities, morbidity, and fetal or maternal death.

EPIDEMIOLOGY

Incidence

- Predominant age: 16–25 years
- Predominant sex: Male > Female

Prevalence

- 21.8 million, or 8.7%, of Americans reported use of illicit substance in last month in 2009.
- Rates: 10% for ages 12–17 years; 21.2% for ages 18–25 years
- 1 in 6 males aged 18–25 years uses marijuana.

RISK FACTORS

- Male gender, young adult
- Depression, anxiety
- Other substance use disorders
- Family history
- Peer or family use or approval
- Low socioeconomic status
- Unemployment
- Accessibility of substances of abuse
- Family dysfunction or trauma
- Antisocial personality disorder
- Academic problems, school dropout
- Criminal involvement

Genetics

Substances of abuse affect dopamine, acetylcholine, gamma-aminobutyric acid, norepinephrine, opioid, and serotonin receptors. Variant alleles may account for susceptibility to disorders.

GENERAL PREVENTION

Early identification and aggressive early intervention improve outcomes.

ALERT

Screening: A single question: "How many times in the past year have you used an illegal drug or used a prescription medication for nonmedical reasons?": In primary care setting, resulted in sensitivity of 100% and specificity of ~75% (1)[B].

ETIOLOGY

Multifactorial, including genetic, environmental

ALERT

Prescription narcotic overdose is the leading cause of accidental death between the ages of 35 and 55 in the US; this correlates with the increase in prescription of long-acting oxycodone (www.cdc.gov/injury/wisqars/pdf/Unintentional_2007_BW-a.pdf).

COMMONLY ASSOCIATED CONDITIONS

- Depression
- Personality disorders
- Bipolar affective disorder

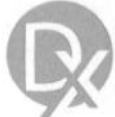

DIAGNOSIS

- Substance abuse: A maladaptive pattern of substance use manifested by 1 or more of the following:
  - Failure to fulfill major obligations at work, school, or home
  - Recurrent use in hazardous situations
  - Recurrent substance-related legal problems
  - Continued substance use despite substance-related social or interpersonal problems
- Substance dependence: A maladaptive pattern of substance use manifested by 3 or more of the following:
  - Tolerance (decreased response to effects of drug due to constant exposure)
  - Withdrawal (physical or psychological response following the abrupt drug discontinuation)
  - Using the substance more than intended
  - Persistent desire or attempts to cut down or stop
  - Much time spent obtaining, using, or recovering from the substance
  - Social, occupational, or recreational activities sacrificed for substance use
  - Continued use despite substance-related physical or psychological problems

HISTORY

- History of infections (e.g., endocarditis, hepatitis B or C, TB, STI, or recurrent pneumonia)
- Social or behavioral problems, including chaotic relationships and/or employment
- Frequent visits to emergency department
- Criminal incarceration
- History of blackouts, insomnia, mood swings, chronic pain, repetitive trauma
- Anxiety, fatigue, depression, psychosis
- Sexual assault related to use of GBH or Rohypnol

PHYSICAL EXAM

- Abnormally dilated or constricted pupils
- Needle marks on skin
- Nasal septum perforation (with cocaine use)
- Cardiac dysrhythmias, pathologic murmurs
- Malnutrition with severe dependence

DIAGNOSTIC TESTS & INTERPRETATION

- CRAFFT questionnaire is superior to CAGE for identifying alcohol use disorders in adolescents and young adults; sensitivity is 94% with 2 or more "yes" answers:
  - C—Have you ever ridden in a *c*ar driven by someone (including yourself) who was "high" or who had been using alcohol or drugs?
  - R—Do you ever use alcohol or drugs to *r*elax, feel better about yourself, or fit in?
  - A—Do you ever use alcohol or drugs while you are *a*lone?
  - F—Do you ever *f*orget things you did while using alcohol or drugs?
  - F—Do your family or *f*riends ever tell you that you should cut down on your drinking or drug use?
  - T—Have you gotten into *t*rouble while you were using alcohol or drugs?
- TICS (2-item conjoint screen): ≥1 positive response is 79% sensitive, 78% specific for current substance use disorder:
  - In the past year, have you ever drunk or used drugs more than you meant to?
  - Have you felt you wanted to cut down on your drinking or drug use in the past year?

Lab

- Blood alcohol concentration
- Urine drug screen (Order qualitative UDS and, if specific drug is in question, a quantitative analysis for specific drug; confirmatory serum tests if you suspect false positive.)
- Approximate detection limits:
  - Alcohol: 6–10 hours
  - Amphetamines and variants: 2–3 days
  - Barbiturates: 2–10 days
  - Benzodiazepines: 1–6 weeks
  - Cocaine: 2–3 days
  - Heroin: 1–1.5 days
  - LSD, psilocybin: 8 hours
  - Marijuana: 1 day–4 weeks
  - Methadone: 1 day–1 week
  - Opioids: 1–3 days
  - PCP: 7–14 days
  - Anabolic steroids: Oral, 3 weeks; injectable, 3 months; nandrolone, 9 months
- Liver transaminases
- HIV, hepatitis B and C screens

Imaging

- Echocardiogram for endocarditis
- Head CT scan for seizure, delirium, trauma

DIFFERENTIAL DIAGNOSIS

- Depression, anxiety, or other mental states
- Metabolic delirium (hypoxia, hypoglycemia, infection, thiamine deficiency, hypothyroidism, thyrotoxicosis)
- ADHD
- Medication toxicity

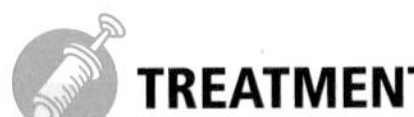

TREATMENT

Determine substances abused early (may influence disposition).

MEDICATION

- Alcohol withdrawal: See "Alcohol Abuse and Dependence" and "Alcohol Withdrawal."
- Benzodiazepine or barbiturate withdrawal:
  - Gradual taper preferable to abrupt discontinuation
  - Substitution of longer-acting benzodiazepine or phenobarbital
- Nicotine withdrawal: See "Tobacco Use and Smoking Cessation."
- Opioid withdrawal:
  - Buprenorphine: 2–16 mg/d sublingually; use restricted to licensed clinics and certified physicians (2)[A]
  - Methadone: 20–35 mg/d PO; use restricted to inpatient settings and specially licensed clinics (3)[A]
  - Clonidine: 0.1–0.2 mg PO t.i.d. for autonomic hyperactivity (4)[A]
- Stimulant withdrawal:
  - No agent with clear benefit for cocaine
  - Naltrexone: 50 mg PO twice weekly reduces amphetamine use in dependent patients (5)[B].
  - Methylphenidate ER: 54 mg/d PO might enhance abstinence in amphetamine-dependent patients.
- Adjuncts to therapy:
  - Use all medications in conjunction with psychosocial behavioral interventions.
  - Antiemetics, nonaddictive analgesics for opioid withdrawal
  - Nonhabituating antidepressants, mood stabilizers, anxiolytics, and hypnotics for comorbid mood and anxiety disorders and insomnia that persist after detoxification
- Contraindications:
  - Buprenorphine in lactation
  - Naltrexone in pregnancy, liver disease
- Precautions: Clonidine can cause hypotension.
- Significant possible interactions:
  - Buprenorphine and ketoconazole, erythromycin, or HIV protease inhibitors
  - Naltrexone and opioid medications (may precipitate or exacerbate withdrawal)

ADDITIONAL TREATMENT

General Measures

- Nonjudgmental, medically oriented attitude
- Motivational interviewing and brief interventions can overcome denial and promote change.
- Behavioral and cognitive therapy
- Community reinforcement
- Interventional counseling
- Self-help groups to aid recovery (Alcoholics Anonymous, other 12-step programs)
- Support groups for family (Al-Anon and Alateen)

Issues for Referral

- Consider addiction specialist, especially for opioid and polysubstance abuse.
- Maintenance therapy for opioid dependence (e.g., methadone) only in licensed clinics
- Psychiatry for comorbid psychiatric disorders
- Social services

IN-PATIENT CONSIDERATIONS

Initial Stabilization

Look for signs of severe infection (e.g., bacterial endocarditis).

Admission Criteria

- Indications for inpatient detoxification:
  - History of withdrawal symptoms (e.g., seizures)
  - Disorientation
  - Threat of harm to self or others
  - Obstacles to close monitoring (follow-up)
  - Comorbid medical illness
  - Pregnancy
- For narcotic addiction and withdrawal

IV Fluids

Maintenance until patient is taking fluids well by mouth

Nursing

- Take frequent vital signs during withdrawal.
- Monitor for signs of drug use in the hospital.

Discharge Criteria

Detoxification complete

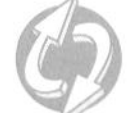

ONGOING CARE

FOLLOW-UP RECOMMENDATIONS

Restricted if dangerous, psychotic, or disoriented

Patient Monitoring

Verify patient's compliance with the substance abuse treatment program.

DIET

Patients often are malnourished.

PATIENT EDUCATION

- Center for Substance Abuse Treatment: (800) 662-HELP or http://findtreatment.samhsa.gov (facility locator)
- Substance Abuse and Mental Health Services Administration: http://ncadi.samhsa.gov
- Alcoholics Anonymous: Contact local chapter or www.aa.org
- Narcotics Anonymous: www.na.org

PROGNOSIS

- Patients in treatment for longer periods of time (≥1 year) have higher success rates.
- Behavioral therapy and pharmacotherapy are most successful when used in combination.

COMPLICATIONS

- Hepatitis, HIV, tuberculosis, syphilis
- Subacute bacterial endocarditis
- Malnutrition
- Social problems, including arrest
- Poor marital adjustment and violence
- Depression, schizophrenia
- Serious harm to self and others: Accidents, violence
- Sexual assault related to use of GHB, Rohypnol
- Overdoses resulting in seizures, arrhythmias, cardiac and respiratory arrest, coma, death

REFERENCES

1. Smith PC, Schmidt SM, Allensworth-Davies D, et al. A single-question screening test for drug use in primary care. *Arch Intern Med*. 2010;170:1155–60.
2. Gowing L, Ali R, White JM, et al. Buprenorphine for the management of opioid withdrawal. *Cochrane Database Syst Rev*. 2009;CD002025.
3. Mattick RP, Breen C, Kimber J, et al. Methadone maintenance therapy versus no opioid replacement therapy for opioid dependence. *Cochrane Database Syst Rev*. 2009;CD002209.
4. Gowing L, Farrell M, Ali R, et al. Alpha2-adrenergic agonists for the management of opioid withdrawal. *Cochrane Database Syst Rev*. 2009;CD002024.
5. Jayaram-Lindström N, Hammarberg A, Beck O, et al. Naltrexone for the treatment of amphetamine dependence: A randomized, placebo-controlled trial. *Am J Psychiatry*. 2008;165(11):1442–8.

ADDITIONAL READING

- Department of Health and Human Services, Substance Abuse and Mental Health Services Administration, Office of Applied Studies. Results from the 2009 national survey on drug use and health. Accessed July 4, 2011, at http://oas.samhsa.gov.
- Griswold KS, Aronoff H, Kernan JB, et al. Adolescent substance use and abuse: Recognition and management. *Am Fam Physician*. 2008;77:331–6.

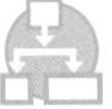

See Also (Topic, Algorithm, Electronic Media Element)

Alcohol Abuse and Dependence; Alcohol Withdrawal; Tobacco Use and Smoking Cessation

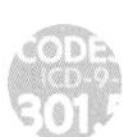

CODES

ICD9

- 305.1 Tobacco use disorder
- 305.20 Nondependent cannabis abuse, unspecified use
- 305.90 Other, mixed, or unspecified drug abuse, unspecified

CLINICAL PEARLS

- Substance use disorders are prevalent, serious, and often unrecognized in clinical practice. Comorbid psychiatric disorders are common.
- Substance abuse is distinguished by family, social, occupational, legal, or physical dysfunction that is caused by persistent use of the substance. Dependence is characterized by tolerance, withdrawal, compulsive use, and repeated overindulgence.
- The CRAFFT questionnaire is preferred for identifying alcohol and substance use disorders in adolescents and young adults.
- Motivational interviewing, brief interventions, and a nonjudgmental attitude can help to promote a willingness to change behavior.

SUDDEN INFANT DEATH SYNDROME (SIDS)

Fern R. Hauck, MD, MS

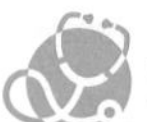

BASICS

- Leading cause of death in infants 1–12 months of age
- Third leading cause of infant mortality overall
- There has been a reduction of SIDS deaths by over 50% in the US and other countries that have introduced risk-reduction campaigns, heavily focused on back sleeping for infants (1).
- The condition still remains mysterious, and the exact cause is unknown.

DESCRIPTION

- The sudden death of an infant <1 year of age that remains unexplained after a thorough case investigation, including performance of a complete autopsy, examination of the death scene, and review of the clinical history
- Sudden infant death syndrome (SIDS) was first formally defined in 1969. The definition was revised in 1989.
- System(s) affected: Cardiovascular; Endocrine/Metabolic; Nervous; Pulmonary
- Synonym(s): Crib death; Cot death

EPIDEMIOLOGY

- SIDS can affect any infant, but some infants are at higher risk than others, including African Americans and American Indians/Native Americans, males, infants whose mothers smoked or used illegal drugs during pregnancy, and several others described below.
- There is a characteristic age pattern, with deaths peaking at 2–4 months, and more deaths occurring during the colder seasons.

Incidence

- For 2007: All races: 0.57/1,000 live births (2,461 cases/yr):
  - White non-Hispanic: 0.58/1,000 live births (1,341 cases/yr)
  - Black non-Hispanic: 1.08/1,000 live births (677 cases/yr)
  - Hispanic: 0.29/1,000 live births (310 cases/yr)
  - Native American: 1.42/1,000 live births (70 cases/yr)
- Predominant age: Uncommon in first month of life; peak occurs between 2 and 4 months of age; 90% of deaths occur by 6 months of age.
- Predominant sex: Male > Female (52–60% male)

Pediatric Considerations

Occurs only in infants

RISK FACTORS

- While some infants may die from SIDS who have no apparent risk factors, most have 1 or more of the following risk factors associated with SIDS:
  - Race: African Americans and Native Americans have highest incidence.
  - Season: Late fall and winter months
  - Time of day: Between midnight and 6 a.m.
  - Activity: During sleep
  - Low birth weight; intrauterine growth retardation (IUGR)
  - Poverty
- Maternal factors:
  - Younger age
  - Decreased education
  - Maternal use of cigarettes or drugs (e.g., cocaine, opiates) during pregnancy
  - Higher parity
  - Inadequate prenatal care
- Respiratory or GI infection in recent past
- Sleep practices:
  - Prone and side sleep positions
  - Overheating from heavy clothing and bedding and/or elevated room temperature
  - Soft bedding
  - Bed sharing
  - No room sharing
- Passive cigarette smoke exposure after birth
- No pacifier use
- No breast-feeding

Genetics

Emerging evidence for genetic risk factors, especially related to impaired brain-stem regulation of breathing or other autonomic control, impaired immune responses, and cardiac ion channelopathies associated with long QT syndrome and fatal arrhythmia

GENERAL PREVENTION

Because a SIDS death is sudden and the cause is unknown, SIDS cannot be "treated." However, there are some measures that may be effective in reducing the risk of SIDS (2)[B]:

- Maternal avoidance of cigarette smoking and illicit drug use during pregnancy
- Avoidance of passive cigarette smoke exposure
- Avoidance of the prone (face-down) and side sleep positions, excessive bed clothing, and soft bedding such as pillows and comforters or a soft mattress
- Avoidance of overheating
- A crib, bassinet, or cradle conforming to federal safety standards is the recommended sleeping location.
- Avoidance of bed sharing with the infant, particularly by adults other than the parent(s) or by other children. Bed sharing should be avoided if the mother or father has used cigarettes, drugs, or alcohol. Bed sharing on couches is very dangerous and should never be done.
- Infants who sleep in the same room as their parents (without bed sharing) have a lower risk of SIDS. It is recommended that infants sleep in a crib or bassinet in their parents' bedroom, which when placed close to their bed will allow for more convenient breast-feeding and contact.
- Breast-feeding is associated with a decreased risk of SIDS and is recommended for all infants (3)[B].
- Pacifier use is associated with a reduced risk of SIDS:
  - Consider offering a pacifier at bedtime and nap time.
  - Delay the introduction of the pacifier among breast-fed infants until 1 month of age (4)[B].
  - Pacifier use has not been found to be detrimental to breast-feeding if it is introduced after the baby is 1 month of age, when breast-feeding is well established (5)[A].
- Avoidance of commercial devices marketed to reduce the risk of SIDS
- It is critical that all people caring for infants, including daycare providers, be instructed in these risk-reduction measures.
- Newborn nurseries should implement these recommendations well before discharge so parents see appropriate practices modeled.

PATHOPHYSIOLOGY

Strong evidence for a respiratory pathway that includes the following stages:

- A life-threatening event causes severe asphyxia and/or brain hypoperfusion. This can include rebreathing exhaled carbon dioxide in a face-down position.
- The vulnerable infant doesn't wake up or turn his head in response to asphyxia, resulting in further rebreathing and inability to recover from apnea.
- Progressive apnea leads to hypoxic coma.
- Bradycardia and hypoxic apnea occur.
- Autoresuscitation fails, resulting in prolonged apnea and death (6).

ETIOLOGY

- There are many theories. There may be subtle developmental abnormalities resulting from pre- and/or perinatal brain injury, which make the infant vulnerable to SIDS.
- Possible causes:
  - Abnormalities in respiratory control and arousal responsiveness
  - Central and peripheral nervous system abnormalities
  - Cardiac arrhythmias
  - Rebreathing in face-down position on soft surface, leading to hypoxia and hypercarbia
  - SIDS may occur when 1 or more environmental risk factors interact with 1 or more genetic risk factors.

COMMONLY ASSOCIATED CONDITIONS

Infants are generally well, or may have had a mild febrile illness (i.e., gastroenteritis or an upper respiratory infection) prior to death.

DIAGNOSIS

The diagnosis of SIDS is made by trained medical examiners or coroners when the death is believed to be from natural causes and after thorough reviews of the medical history, death scene investigation, and postmortem examination do not produce an explanation of the death.

HISTORY

Infant usually found unresponsive by parent or other caregiver without any warning

PHYSICAL EXAM

- These babies generally appear healthy or may have had a minor upper respiratory or GI infection in the last 2 weeks before death.
- Complete postmortem exam to look for signs of possible trauma/child abuse or other cause of death

DIAGNOSTIC TESTS & INTERPRETATION

Standardized postmortem protocols have been proposed. While testing varies across sites, common diagnostic tests include electrolytes, toxicology, and microbiology.

Lab

- Pneumocardiograms have been abandoned in the workup.
- Postmortem laboratory tests are performed to rule out other causes of death (e.g., electrolytes to rule out dehydration and electrolyte imbalance). No consistently abnormal laboratory tests are found.

Imaging

X-rays to rule out possible child abuse

Diagnostic Procedures/Surgery

Because the diagnosis of SIDS is often one of "exclusion," it is crucial to do a thorough death scene investigation and case review in addition to the autopsy and laboratory tests.

Pathological Findings

Characteristic findings on postmortem examination:

- Frothy discharge, sometimes blood tinged, from nostrils and mouth
- Petechiae on surface of lungs, heart, and thymus gland in 50–85% (but not unique to SIDS)
- Pulmonary congestion and edema often present
- Morphologic markers of hypoxia: Increased gliosis in brain stem, retention of periadrenal brown fat, and hematopoiesis in the liver:
  - Present to varying degrees; not confirmed by all studies

DIFFERENTIAL DIAGNOSIS

- Suffocation/accidental asphyxia
- Abnormalities of fatty acid metabolism (e.g., deficiency of medium-chain acyl-coenzyme A dehydrogenase or of carnitine)
- Dehydration/electrolyte disturbance
- Homicide

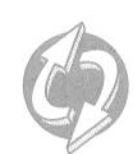

ONGOING CARE

General recommendations for positioning infants:

- Infants frequently should be placed on their bellies when awake and observed by responsible adults to prevent head flattening (plagiocephaly) that can result from infants sleeping supine.
- Avoid placing infants for extended periods in car seat carriers or "bouncers."
- Upright "cuddle time" should be encouraged.
- Alter the side to which the infant places his or her head during sleep.
- Swaddling infants may aid in sleeping more comfortably in the supine position. Infants should never be swaddled if sleeping in the prone position.

FOLLOW-UP RECOMMENDATIONS

- Safe sleep and SIDS risk-reduction messages should be delivered at all well-child checks and by all health professionals in a consistent manner.
- Parents often change from the recommended practices as the baby gets older, often during the peak SIDS incidence period. Thus, it is important to ask about infant care practices at each well-child check.

Patient Monitoring

Although some authorities recommend cardiopulmonary monitoring in siblings of prior SIDS victims, there is no evidence that the use of monitors prevents SIDS, and they should not be prescribed for that purpose (7)[B].

PATIENT EDUCATION

- Family counseling (see "Prognosis")
- Back to Sleep Information Line, (800) 505-CRIB (2742) (sponsored by the Eunice Kennedy Shriver National Institute of Child Health and Human Development, the Maternal and Child Health Bureau, and other organizations to provide information to parents and health providers about their recommendation to place infants on their backs, and general information about SIDS)
- National SIDS/Infant Death Resource Center, McLean, VA; (866) 866-SIDS (7437)
- Association of SIDS and Infant Mortality Programs, Lansing, MI; (800) 930-SIDS (7437)
- First Candle/SIDS Alliance, Baltimore, MD; (800) 221-SIDS (7437)
- CJ Foundation for SIDS, Hackensack, NJ; 8CJ-SIDS (7437)
- SIDS Network, Ledyard, CT; (800) 560-1454
- Cribs for Kids, Pittsburgh, PA; (888) 721-CRIB (2742)

PROGNOSIS

- SIDS deaths have a powerful impact on families and their functioning. Physicians play an important role in providing immediate information about SIDS and sensitive counseling to limit parents' misinformation and feelings of guilt.
- Counseling needs of families vary from the short term to long term:
  - Support groups are helpful to many couples.
  - Physicians need to be familiar with resources available in their communities to help families mourning a SIDS death.
- Follow-up counseling, including review of the autopsy report with the family after some time has passed, is important to help with understanding this condition and to alleviate the tremendous guilt these families experience.
- Parents need to be counseled about subsequent pregnancies:
  - Genetic testing and counseling may be indicated to rule out a metabolic or other genetically acquired disorder.
  - Parents need to be advised of the most current recommendations regarding sleep position and other infant care practices during subsequent pregnancies.

S

REFERENCES

1. Mitchell EA. SIDS: Past, present and future. *Acta Paediatr*. 2009;98:1712–9.
2. Task Force on Sudden Infant Death Syndrome. American Academy of Pediatrics. SIDS and other sleep-related infant deaths: Expansion of recommendations for a safe infant sleeping environment. *Pediatrics*. 2011 (in press).
3. Hauck FR, Thompson JMD, Tanabe KO, et al. Breastfeeding and reduced risk of sudden infant death syndrome: A meta-analysis. *Pediatrics* 2011;128:103–10.
4. Hauck FR, Omojokun OO, Siadaty MS. Do pacifiers reduce the risk of sudden infant death syndrome? A meta-analysis. *Pediatrics*. 2005;116. Available at: www.pediatrics.org/cgi/content/full/116/5/e716.
5. O'Connor NR, Tanabe KO, Siadaty MS. Pacifiers and breastfeeding: A systematic review. *Arch Pediatr Adolesc Med*. 2009;163:378–82.
6. Kinney HC, Thach BT. The sudden infant death syndrome. *N Engl J Med*. 2009;361:795–805.
7. Committee on Fetus and Newborn. American Academy of Pediatrics. Apnea, sudden infant death syndrome, and home monitoring. *Pediatrics*. 2003;111:914–7.

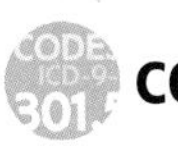

CODES

ICD9

798.0 Sudden infant death syndrome

CLINICAL PEARLS

- Although the exact cause of SIDS is unknown, there are several risk-reduction measures that will significantly reduce an infant's chance of dying from SIDS.
- SIDS incidence has decreased by more than 50% just by placing infants in a supine position to sleep.
- Breast-feeding is recommended for all infants.
- Safe sleeping arrangements and pacifier use after the age of 1 month are other ways to reduce the risk of SIDS.

SUICIDE

Irene C. Coletsos, MD
Harold J. Bursztajn, MD

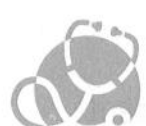

BASICS

DESCRIPTION

Suicide and attempted suicide are significant causes of morbidity and mortality.

EPIDEMIOLOGY

- Predominant sex:
  - Women *attempt* suicide 1.5× more often than men. Men *complete* suicide 4× more often than women. Men are more likely to choose a means with high lethality.
- Predominant age: Adolescent and geriatric population
- Predominant race: 84% of people who complete suicides are White, non-Hispanic. Native Americans have the next highest rate in the US. Whites have twice the risk of suicide compared to African Americans.
- Marital status: Single > Divorced; widowed > married
- Worldwide, in 1/3 of all countries, youths (ages 10–24) are the highest risk group.

Incidence

- In 2009, 11th leading cause of death in adults in the US. There are an estimated 480 attempted suicides every day. Military service is associated with increased risk: In 2008, there were 20.2 suicides/100,000 active-duty personnel (with a higher rate of 24/100,000 among Marines) versus 19.5/100,000 in a similar demographic (CDC data). In 2009 and 2010, more soldiers died of suicide than in active duty in those years, according to a congressional study.
- Worldwide, suicide is the third leading cause of death.

RISK FACTORS

- "Human understanding is the most effective weapon against suicide. The greatest need is to deepen the awareness and sensitivity of people to their fellow man." –Edwin Schneidman, PhD, American Association of Suicidology
- Overall, Schneidman says that health providers should be alert to a combination of "perturbation" (increased emotional disturbance) and "lethality" (having the potential tools to cause death) (see "Treatment").
- Most people (80%) who complete suicides had a previous attempt.
- 1 study shows that 90% who complete suicide meet *Diagnostic and Statistical Manual* criteria for Axis I or II disorders:
  - Substance use (especially alcohol): Schizophrenia; borderline and antisocial personality disorders; anorexia nervosa; panic disorder
  - Family history of suicide
  - Physical illness
  - Despair: The patient feels unendurable emotional pain *and* has "given up" on himself or herself, feels without hope and, consciously or unconsciously, unworthy of help.
- Psychological:
  - Recent loss: What may seem to be a small loss (to a medical provider) may be a devastating loss to the patient. *Patient-specific* factors need to be taken into account; social isolation; anniversaries and holidays. Patients who attempt suicide also seem to have impaired decision-making skills and risk awareness, and increased impulsivity, compared to patients who have never made such an attempt, according to 2 studies on adults and elders (1,2).
- If a patient is incompetent (e.g., too delusional) to inform providers about the potential for suicide, that puts the patient at increased risk, and the treating clinician should consider hospitalizing the patient.
- Access to lethal means: Firearms, poisons (including prescription and nonprescription drugs)

GENERAL PREVENTION

- Know how to access resources 24/7 within and outside of the health care institution.
- Suicide is a rare event, and there is no definitive method of predicting who will attempt suicide. However, it can be foreseeable and, one hopes, preventable. Screen for risk factors, and consider the overall clinical picture.
- Screen all patients for suicide risk. Potential screening instruments include the Patient Health Questionnaire-2, the modified PHQ-2 (see "Diagnosis" section), the PHQ-9, Beck's Scale for Suicidal Ideation, Linehan's Reasons for Living Inventory, and Risk Estimator for Suicide. Treat underlying mental illness and substance abuse. Screen for possession of means of harm, including prescription and nonprescription drugs and firearms (encourage these patients to remove guns from their homes and to relinquish gun licenses).
- Create a safety plan for patients at risk for suicide and their families, including education about how to access emergency care 24 hours a day.
- Promote public education about how to help others access emergency psychiatric care. Sometimes suicidal people will first confide in those they trust outside health care (e.g., family members, religious leaders, community elders, "unofficial" community leaders such as "healers," hairdressers, and bartenders).
- In developing world countries, pesticide ingestion is a common method of suicide. Strategies that limit free access to this chemical have led to reductions in the suicide rates, according to the World Health Organization (WHO).

DIAGNOSIS

HISTORY

- Depressed patients should be asked about ideation and about a plan:
  - "Have you ever felt that life isn't worth living? Do you ever wish you could go to sleep and not wake up? Are you having thoughts about killing yourself?"
- In a mental health setting, use psychodynamic formulation, which combines mental-state exam (i.e., behavior, mood, mental content, judgment); past history (i.e., what resources has the patient used in the past for support, and are they currently available?); and history of current illness. If the patient is experiencing a loss, is under stress, and does not have access to a previously sustaining resource (e.g., a significant other, a pet, sports ability, a job), that patient is under increased risk for suicide.
- Prior attempts: What precipitated the event, lethality, intent to die, precautions taken to avoid being rescued, reaction to survival (a patient who is upset that the suicide was not completed is at increased risk)
- Detailed history of psychiatric symptoms, substance abuse. Also note strengths, such as a patient's reasons to live, hopes for future, social supports. A patient without these is at increased risk.
- Collateral history is important (from friends, family, physicians). It may be appropriate to break confidentiality if patient is at imminent risk of suicide.

PHYSICAL EXAM

- Medical conditions: Delirium, intoxication, withdrawal, medication side effects (which can be risk factors)
- Psychosis: Observe for signs of/ask about command auditory hallucinations to kill oneself, delusional guilt, and persecutory delusions.
- Observe for signs of hopelessness/despair (see "Risk Factors").

DIFFERENTIAL DIAGNOSIS

Differentiate between patients and pseudopatients (i.e., those who are using suicide threats and gestures to manipulate others). Consider a psychiatric consult. All decisions regarding treatment must be carefully documented and communicated to all involved health care providers.

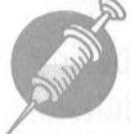

TREATMENT

MEDICATION

- Patients are at increased risk of suicide at the outset of antidepressant treatment and if/when medications are discontinued. Consider tapering/switching medical therapies rather than sudden discontinuation if at all possible. Careful monitoring is needed at these times.
- Anxiety, agitation, and delusions crescendoing in intensity are risk factors for suicide and should be treated aggressively.
- In patients with mood disorders, a meta-analysis of randomized, controlled trials found that lithium reduced the risk of death by suicide by 60% (3)[A]. Long-term treatment for psychosis with clozapine shows some benefit for reducing rate of suicide (4)[A]. Agitated or combative patients may require sedation with IV or IM benzodiazepines and/or antipsychotics. Clinical response is typically seen within 20–30 minutes if given IM/IV.

Pediatric Considerations

The FDA has issued a black box warning for antidepressants in the pediatric population after increased suicidality was noted. If risk of untreated depression is sufficient to warrant treatment with antidepressants, children must be monitored very closely for suicidality.

First Line

Obtain baseline ECGs before prescribing or continuing antidepressants or antipsychotics. Certain drugs are associated with QT prolongation and sudden cardiac death.

ADDITIONAL TREATMENT

General Measures

- Patients expressing active suicidal thoughts or who made an attempt require an examination for suicide risk factors, mental status examination, and competency (to determine if they are able or willing to inform treatment team about ongoing/changing suicidal intentions), as well as a formal psychiatric consultation.
- Cognitive therapy decreased reattempt rate in prior suicide attempters by half (5)[B].
- Psychotherapy with suicidal patients is a challenge even for the most experienced clinicians. The countertransference, a clinician's feelings toward a patient, can evolve into wanting to be rid of the patient. If the patient detects this, the risk of suicide is seriously heightened. The clinician can avoid this by recognizing his or her countertransference and bearing it within so well that the patient remains unaware of it (6).

IN-PATIENT CONSIDERATIONS

Initial Stabilization

- Determine appropriate level of care: Inpatient hospitalization if patient is suicidal with a plan to act or is otherwise at high risk; if immediate risk for self-harm, may be hospitalized involuntarily
- Immediately after a suicide attempt, treat the medical problems resulting from the self-harm before attempting to initiate psychiatric care.
- Order lab work (e.g., solvent screen, blood and urine toxicology screen, aspirin and acetaminophen levels). Patients may not disclose ingestions if they wish to succeed in their attempt or if they are undergoing mental status changes.
- Risk for self-harm continues even in hospital setting. Ensure patient safety by least restrictive method (i.e., remove potentially dangerous objects, provide 1-to-1 constant observation, medication). Use mechanical restraints if deemed necessary for patient safety. Trained staff should search patient for dangerous objects as soon as the patient enters the hospital.
- The period after transfer from involuntary to voluntary hospitalization is also a time of high risk.

Discharge Criteria

- No longer considered a danger to self/others
- Clinicians should be aware that a patient may *claim* that he or she is no longer suicidal in order to facilitate discharge—and complete the act. Look for clinical and behavioral signs that the patient truly is no longer in despair and is hopeful, such as improved appetite, sleep, engagement with staff, and group therapy. Clinicians should check with family and ancillary staff to assess patients' conditions because they may share more information with those contacts than with doctors (7).
- Provide information about resources that are available in a crisis. Patients and those in their support system must be aware of, and willing to, access services 24/7 to enhance patient safety.

ONGOING CARE

FOLLOW-UP RECOMMENDATIONS

Patient Monitoring

- Increase monitoring at the beginning of treatment, when changing medication regimens, and on discharge. These are times of increased risk.
- Educate family members and other close contacts/confidants to the warning signs of suicidality. For adults: Despair/hopelessness, isolation, discussing suicide, stating that the world would be a "better place" without them, losses in areas key to the patient's self-worth. For youths: May exhibit the same signs and symptoms, but one should be aware of these additional risks: History of abuse (e.g., sexual, physical), bullying in person or via electronic media (such as text messages or social Web sites), family stress, changes in eating and sleeping patterns, suicidality of friends, and giving away treasured items.
- Make sure that the patient is willing to accept the type of follow-up offered. Do not assume that just setting it up is protection enough.
- Curtail access to firearms.
- Limiting the number of pills may also be appropriate for an impulsive patient. However, clinicians may believe that by simply limiting the number of pills they prescribe, they are preventing further suicide attempts, an example of "magical thinking." Clinicians who find themselves thinking this way, can take it as a warning sign that their patients may actually be at increased risk of suicide.

PATIENT EDUCATION

Patients who feel they are in danger of hurting themselves should consider one or several of these options:

- Call 911.
- Go directly to an emergency room.
- If already in counseling, contact that therapist immediately.
- Call the National Suicide Prevention Hotline at 1-800-273-TALK (8255).
- Servicemen and servicewomen and their families can call 1-800-796-9699; if there is no immediate answer, call 1-800-273-8255.

PROGNOSIS

The key to a favorable course and prognosis is early recognition of risk factors, early diagnosis and treatment of a psychiatric disorder, and appropriate intervention and follow-up.

COMPLICATIONS

- The sequelae of attempted and completed suicides can be lifelong for family members and close friends.
- According to the American Association of Suicidality (AAS), the grief process for significant others of suicide victims can be lifelong and can be expressed in emotions ranging from anger to despair. Survivors often attempt to shoulder the burden on their own because of the added guilt and shame of the nature of the attempted death or death.
- The AAS recommends:
  - Counseling: Could include short-term behavioral therapy as well as psychotherapy; some therapy should focus on the survivors' relationships to their current and future significant others. An expert on the lives of adult children of parents/close family members who completed suicides reports that these survivors often seek out life partners as "replacements" for those they lost. This may prevent the survivor from completing his or her mourning (8).
  - Sympathetic listening by friends of the survivors
  - Special support at holiday times, when the loneliness intensifies
  - A Web site with links to resources and self-help strategies is www.survivorsofsuicide.com.

S

REFERENCES

1. Clark L, Dombrovski AY, Siegle GJ, et al. Impairment in risk-sensitive decision-making in older suicide attempters with depression. *Psychol Aging*. 2011;26:321–30.
2. Jollant F, Bellivier F, Leboyer M, et al. Impaired decision making in suicide attempters. *Am J Psychiatry*. 2005;162:304–10.
3. Cipriani A, Pretty H, Hawton K, et al. Lithium in the prevention of suicidal behavior and all-cause mortality in patients with mood disorders: A systematic review of randomized trials. *Am J Psychiatry*. 2005;162:1805–19.
4. Hennen J, Baldessarinin RJ. Suicide risk during treatment with clozapine: A meta-analysis. *Schizophr Res*. 2004;73:139–45.
5. Brown GK, et al. Cognitive therapy for the prevention of suicide attempts: A randomized controlled trial. *JAMA*. 2005;295:563–70.
6. Maltsberger JT, Buie DH. Countertransference hate in the treatment of suicidal patients. *Arch Gen Psychiatry*. 1974;30:625–33.
7. Simon S, Gutheil TG. Sudden improvement among high-risk suicidal patients: Should it be trusted? *Psychiatric Services*. 2009;60:387–9.
8. William J. Massicotte Faculty, Canadian Institute of Psychoanalysis Chair, National Scientific Program Committee, Canadian Psychoanalytic Society. *Personal correspondance*, April 24, 2009.

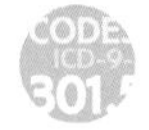

CODES

ICD9

V62.84 Suicidal ideation

CLINICAL PEARLS

- The most important preventative measure is to listen to a patient and take steps to keep him or her safe. This could include immediate hospitalization. The most important questions to explore not only include, "Are you thinking of killing yourself?" but also, "Who do you have to live for?" and "What has to change, or what needs to change, for you to live with your suffering?"
- Clozapine, lithium and cognitive-behavioral therapy are proven to reduce the risk of suicide.
- Resources for clinicians: www.suicidology.com; www.suicideassessment.com
- Family members and contacts of people who have attempted or committed suicide suffer from reactions ranging from rage to despair. Their grief is often longer lasting and less well treated because of the shame and guilt associated with the act. Encourage them to discuss this and consider counseling.

SUPERFICIAL THROMBOPHLEBITIS

Kelly J. Alberda, MD

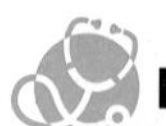

BASICS

DESCRIPTION

- Superficial thrombophlebitis is an inflammatory condition of the veins with secondary thrombosis.
- Traumatic thrombophlebitis types:
  - Injury
  - IV catheter related
  - Intentional (i.e., sclerotherapy)
- Septic (suppurative) thrombophlebitis types:
  - Iatrogenic, long-term IV catheter use
  - Infectious, mainly syphilis and psittacosis
- Aseptic thrombophlebitis types:
  - Primary hypercoagulable states: Disorders with measurable defects in the proteins of the coagulation and/or fibrinolytic systems
  - Secondary hypercoagulable states: Clinical conditions with a risk of thrombosis
- Mondor disease:
  - Rare presentation of anterior chest/breast veins of women
- System(s) affected: Cardiovascular
- Synonym(s): Phlebitis; Phlebothrombosis

Geriatric Considerations

Septic thrombophlebitis is more common; prognosis is poorer.

Pediatric Considerations

Subperiosteal abscesses of adjacent long bone may complicate the disorder.

Pregnancy Considerations

- Associated with increased risk of aseptic superficial thrombophlebitis
- NSAIDs are contraindicated.

EPIDEMIOLOGY

- Predominant age:
  - Traumatic/IV related has no predominate age/sex
  - Aseptic primary hypercoagulable state:
    - Childhood to young adult
  - Aseptic secondary hypercoagulable state:
    - Mondor disease: Women, ages 21–55 years
    - Thromboangiitis obliterans onset: Ages 20–50 years
- Predominant sex:
  - Suppurative: Male = Female
  - Aseptic:
    - Mondor: Female > Male (2:1)
    - Thromboangiitis obliterans: Female > Male (1–19% of clinical cases)

Incidence

- Septic:
  - Incidence of catheter-related thrombophlebitis is 88/100,000 persons.
  - Develops in 4–8% if cutdown is performed
- Aseptic primary hypercoagulable state: Antithrombin III and heparin cofactor II deficiency incidence is 50/100,000 persons.
- Aseptic secondary hypercoagulable state:
  - In pregnancy, 49-fold increased incidence of phlebitis
  - Superficial migratory thrombophlebitis in 27% of patients with thromboangiitis obliterans

Prevalence

- Superficial thrombophlebitis is common.
- 1/3 of patients in a medical ICU develop thrombophlebitis that eventually progresses to the deep veins.

RISK FACTORS

- Nonspecific:
  - Immobilization
  - Obesity
  - Advanced age
  - Postoperative states
- Traumatic/septic:
  - IV catheter (plastic > coated)
  - Lower extremity IV catheter
  - Cutdowns
  - Cancer, debilitating diseases
  - Burn patients
  - AIDS
  - Varicose veins
- Aseptic:
  - Pregnancy
  - Oral contraceptives
  - Surgery, trauma, infection
  - Hypercoagulable state, i.e., factor V, protein C or S deficiency, others
- Thromboangiitis obliterans: Persistent smoking
- Mondor disease:
  - Breast cancer or breast surgery

Genetics

Not applicable other than hypercoagulable states

GENERAL PREVENTION

- Avoidance of lower extremity cannulations/IV
- Insertion under aseptic conditions, securing cannulas, and replacing q72h
- Avoiding stasis or using usual DVT prophylaxis in high-risk patients (i.e., ICU, immobilized)

PATHOPHYSIOLOGY

- Similar to DVT and Virchow triad. A combination of vessel trauma, stasis, and hypercoagulability whether it is genetic, iatrogenic, or idiopathic.
- Mondor disease pathophysilogy not completely understood

ETIOLOGY

- Septic:
  - *Staphylococcus aureus, Pseudomonas, Klebsiella, Peptostreptococcus* sp.
  - *Candida* sp.
- Aseptic primary hypercoagulable state:
  - Due to inherited disorders of hypercoagulability
- Aseptic secondary hypercoagulable states:
  - Malignancy (Trousseau syndrome: Recurrent migratory thrombophlebitis): Most commonly seen in metastatic mucin or adenocarcinomas of the GI tract (pancreas, stomach, colon, and gallbladder), lung, prostate, and ovary
  - Pregnancy
  - Oral contraceptives
  - Behçet, Buerger, or Mondor disease

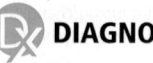

DIAGNOSIS

HISTORY

Pain along the course of a vein

PHYSICAL EXAM

- Swelling, tenderness, redness along the course of a vein or veins
- May look like localized cellulitis or erythema nodosa
- Fever in 70% of patients in septic phlebitis
- Sign of systemic sepsis in 84% of suppurative cases

DIAGNOSTIC TESTS & INTERPRETATION

Lab

Initial lab tests

Often none necessary if afebrile, otherwise healthy

Follow-Up & Special Considerations

- If suspicious for sepsis:
  - Blood cultures (bacteremia in 80–90%)
  - Consider culture of the IV fluids being infused.
  - CBC demonstrates leukocytosis.
- Aseptic: Evaluation for coagulopathy if recurrent or without another identifiable cause. (e.g., protein C and S, lupus anticoagulant, anticardiolipin antibody, factor V and VIII, homocysteine)
- In migratory thrombophlebitis, have a high index of suspicion for malignancy.

Imaging

- Small or distal veins (i.e., forearms or below the knee): No recommended imaging
- Venous Doppler ultrasound to assess extent of thrombosis and rule out DVT

Follow-Up & Special Considerations

Repeat venous ultrasound to assess effectiveness of therapy:

- If thrombosis is extending, more aggressive therapy required

Pathological Findings

The affected vein is enlarged, tortuous, and thickened with endothelial damage and necrosis.

DIFFERENTIAL DIAGNOSIS

- Cellulitis
- DVT
- Erythema nodosa
- Cutaneous polyarteritis nodosa

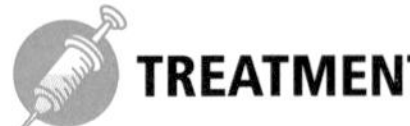

TREATMENT

MEDICATION

First Line

Localized, mild (usually self-limited):

- NSAIDs, ASA for inflammation/pain

Second Line

- Septic/suppurative:
  - May present or be complicated by sepsis
  - Requires IV antibiotics (broad spectrum initially) and anticoagulation
- Large or involving long saphenous vein are at risk for progression into DVT; consider pharmacologic preventive therapies:
  - To prevent venous thromboembolism (VTE), 4 weeks of LMWH; such as enoxaparin (1)[A]
  - 45 days of fondaparinux was found to reduce DVT and VTE by 85% (relative risk reduction) in one study (2)[B].
- Superficial thrombophlebitis related to inherited or acquired hypercoagulable states will need to be prevented by treating the related disease.

ADDITIONAL TREATMENT

General Measures

- Suppurative: Consultation/evaluation for urgent surgical venous excision
- Local, mild:
  - Nonmedication management crucial, antibiotics not useful:
    - For varicosities:
      - Compression stockings, maintain activities
    - Catheter/trauma associated:
      - Immediately remove IV and culture tip,
      - Elevate with application of warm compresses.
      - If slow to resolve, consider antimicrobials or LMWH.
- Large, severe, or septic thrombophlebitis:
  - Inpatient care or bedrest with elevation and local warm compress
  - When the patient is ambulating, then start compression stockings or Ace bandages.

Issues for Referral

Varicosities, severely inflamed, or very large phlebitis should be evaluated for excision.

SURGERY/OTHER PROCEDURES

- Septic:
  - Consult/evaluate for excision of the involved vein segment and all involved tributaries.
  - Drainage of contiguous abscesses
  - Remove all associated cannula and culture tips.
- Aseptic: Management of underlying conditions:
  - Evaluation for saphenous vein ligation to prevent deep vein extension
  - Consider referral for varicosity excision.

IN-PATIENT CONSIDERATIONS

Initial Stabilization

- Septic: Inpatient
- Aseptic: Outpatient

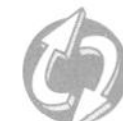

ONGOING CARE

FOLLOW-UP RECOMMENDATIONS

Patient Monitoring

- Septic:
  - Routine WBC count and differential and culture-based treatment
- Severe aseptic:
  - Repeat venous Doppler ultrasound in 1–2 weeks to ensure no DVT and assess treatment effectiveness:
    - Don't expect resolution, just nonprogression.
  - Repeat of blood studies for fibrinolytic system, platelets, and factors
- Local, mild: Per clinician judgement, usually PRN if not resolving

DIET

No restrictions

PATIENT EDUCATION

Importance of local care, elevation, and use of compression hose for acute treatment and prevention of recurrence

PROGNOSIS

- Septic/suppurative:
  - High mortality (50%) if untreated
  - Depends on treatment delay or need for surgery
- Aseptic:
  - Usually benign course; recovery in 2–3 weeks
  - Depends on development of DVT and early detection of complications
  - Aseptic thrombophlebitis can be isolated, recurrent, or migratory.
  - Recurrence likely if related to varicosity or if severely affected vein not removed

COMPLICATIONS

- Septic: Systemic sepsis, bacteremia (84%), septic pulmonary emboli (44%), metastatic abscess formation, pneumonia (44%), subperiosteal abscess of adjacent long bones in children
- Aseptic: DVT, VTE, thromboembolic phenomena

REFERENCES

1. Wichers IM, Di Nisio M, Büller HR, et al. Treatment of superficial vein thrombosis to prevent deep vein thrombosis and pulmonary embolism: A systematic review. *Haematologica*. 2005;90:672–7.
2. Decousus H, Prandoni P, Mismetti P, et al. Fondaparinux for the treatment of superficial-vein thrombosis in the legs. *N Engl J Med*. 2010; 363:1222–32.

ADDITIONAL READING

- Di Nisio M, Wichers IM, Middeldorp S. Treatment for superficial thrombophlebitis of the leg. *Cochrane Database Syst Rev*. 2007;CD004982.
- Gillet JL, French P, Hanss M, et al. [Predictive value of D-dimer assay in superficial thrombophlebitis of the lower limbs.] *J Mal Vasc*. 2007;32(2):90–5.
- Samlaska CP, James WD. Superficial thrombophlebitis. II. Secondary hypercoagulable states. *J Am Acad Dermatol*. 1990;23:1–18.
- Samlaska CP, James WD. Superficial thrombophlebitis. I. Primary hypercoagulable states. *J Am Acad Dermatol*. 1990;22:975–89.

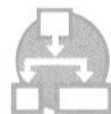

See Also (Topic, Algorithm, Electronic Media Element)

Deep Vein Thrombosis (DVT)

CODES

ICD9

- 451.0 Phlebitis and thrombophlebitis of superficial vessels of lower extremities
- 451.9 Phlebitis and thrombophlebitis of unspecified site
- 451.82 Phlebitis and thrombophlebitis of superficial veins of upper extremities

CLINICAL PEARLS

- Mild disease is self-limiting.
- Severe or saphenous disease may need anticoagulation to prevent DVT.

S

SUPERIOR VENA CAVA SYNDROME

Sandra Cuellar, PharmD, BCOP
Kelly Valla, PharmD
Amber Seba, MD

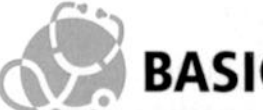

BASICS

DESCRIPTION
- Partial or complete obstruction of the superior vena cava (SVC):
  - 90% from neoplasm (most frequently lung cancer)
  - 20–40% from placement of intravascular devices and thrombosis
- Usual course: Acute; usually 2 weeks from onset of symptoms to diagnosis
- Synonym(s): Superior mediastinal syndrome; Superior vena cava obstruction

EPIDEMIOLOGY
- Predominant age: All ages, less commonly children and young adults (16–30 years old)
- Predominant sex: Male > Female

Incidence
15,000 new cases/yr in the US

RISK FACTORS
- Uncontrolled primary cancer
- History of mediastinal tumor
- Previous invasive procedures

GENERAL PREVENTION
No preventive measures known

PATHOPHYSIOLOGY
Increased pressure in the venous system draining into the superior vena cava. This obstruction of the venous drainage system of the upper chest and neck may result in the rapid development of cerebral edema, intracranial thrombosis, and death.

ETIOLOGY
- Malignancy:
  - In adults, obstruction may be related to primary tumor or lymph node metastasis:
    - Most common primary tumor is lung cancer.
    - Second most common primary malignancy is lymphoma.
    - Lymph node metastases are most commonly from breast and testicular cancers.
  - In children, most common after cardiac surgical procedures
- Fungal infections
- Iatrogenic (intravascular devices)
- Thyroid goiter
- Thrombosis of SVC
- Pericardial constriction
- Idiopathic sclerosing mediastinitis

COMMONLY ASSOCIATED CONDITIONS
- Malignancy:
  - Common: Lung, lymphoma, and metastatic breast
  - Less common: Germ-cell tumors
- Hyperthyroidism
- Infections: Tuberculosis, histoplasmosis, syphilis
- Recent cardiac procedure

DIAGNOSIS

Superior vena cava (SVC) syndrome is a constellation of symptoms caused by the impairment of blood flow through the SVC to the right atrium. In the absence of tracheal obstruction, treatment of SVC syndrome can be delayed until histologic diagnosis has been determined. Following investigations are useful in establishing the diagnosis:
- Radiologic studies, like chest x-ray and CT scan of thorax, to look for mediastinal masses and associated pleural effusion, lobar collapse, or cardiomegaly
- Venography, MRI, and ultrasound to assess the site and nature of the obstruction
- Biopsy of the tumor

HISTORY
- Dyspnea
- Facial swelling and head fullness
- Cough
- Arm swelling
- Chest pain
- Dysphagia
- Headaches
- Visual symptoms
- *Of note: Symptoms may be exacerbated by lying down or bending forward.*

PHYSICAL EXAM
- Accessory venous drainage: Venous distention of neck and chest wall
- Facial edema
- Plethora of face (excess RBCs)
- Cyanosis
- Horner syndrome
- Swelling of arms
- Confusion

DIAGNOSTIC TESTS & INTERPRETATION

Lab

Initial lab tests
- Made on clinical grounds in nearly all cases
- Diagnostic testing should be done prior to treatment, assuming patient is stable.
- If done, increased central venous pressure; usually 20–40 mm Hg
- Sputum cytology can provide diagnosis with malignant cells.

Imaging

Initial approach
- Confirmed by imaging, usually CT scan
- Abnormal chest x-ray
- Contrast-enhanced CT or MRI usually adequate to establish diagnosis
- Venography (if stent or surgery planned)

Follow-Up & Special Considerations
Severity of symptoms is important in determining urgency of intervention. The following grading system has been proposed; see algorithm for management (1):
- Grade 0: Asymptomatic: Radiographic superior vena cava obstruction in the absence of symptoms
- Grade 1: Mild: Edema in head or neck (vascular distention), cyanosis
- Grade 2: Moderate: Edema in head or neck with functional impairment (dysphagia, cough, impairment of head movements, visual disturbances)
- Grade 3: Severe: Mild or moderate cerebral edema (headache, dizziness) or laryngeal edema or diminished cardiac reserve
- Grade 4: Life-threatening: Significant cerebral edema (confusion, obtundation) or severe laryngeal edema or significant hemodynamic compromise
- Grade 5: Fatal: Death

Diagnostic Procedures/Surgery

- Percutaneous stenting:
  - For immediate relief, if needed
- Percutaneous needle biopsy used to establish histologic diagnosis; should be prior to initiation of therapy
- Open biopsy may be necessary; however, these patients are at increased risk for cardiorespiratory compromise under general anesthesia.
- Bronchoscopy, thoracentesis, thoracotomy, lymph node biopsy as indicated

Pathological Findings

Sputum cytology, occasionally thoracentesis, bone marrow, lymph node biopsy, bronchoscopy, or thoracotomy confirms malignant cells.

DIFFERENTIAL DIAGNOSIS

- SVC blood clot
- Syphilitic aneurysm
- Tuberculosis mediastinitis
- Fungal infections

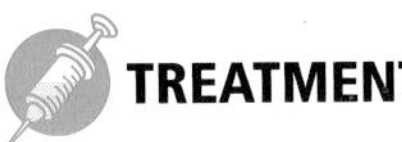

TREATMENT

MEDICATION

- Supportive therapy:
  - Corticosteroids:
    - Often debated and no clear evidence of benefit, but may provide symptomatic relief
    - May interfere with diagnosis of suspected lymphoma if administered prior to diagnostic procedures
    - Most commonly referenced steroid is dexamethasone
  - Diuretics:
    - Loop diuretics also have no clear evidence of benefit, but may provide symptomatic relief.
- Anticoagulation:
  - Not routinely recommended, especially as initial therapy
  - Use of thrombolytics may be useful in cases of superior vena cava thrombosis.
  - Use of aspirin postpercutaneous stent placement may also be considered to prevent thrombosis of stent.
- Chemotherapy:
  - Dependent on etiology/diagnosis

ADDITIONAL TREATMENT

General Measures

- Depends on etiology and etiology's sensitivity to treatment (2)[B]
- Percutaneous stenting (for immediate relief) (3)
- Chemotherapy (treatment of choice for small-cell lung cancer and germ-cell tumors)
- Radiotherapy (once the treatment of choice; now used for radio-sensitive tumors)
- Neoadjuvant chemoradiotherapy and then resection (Pancoast tumors)
- Anticoagulation or fibrinolytic therapy
- Benign causes usually respond to medical therapy, including diuretics, upright positioning, and fluid restriction, until adequate collateral circulation is established and clinical regression is noted.

SURGERY/OTHER PROCEDURES

- Radiotherapy mainly in non–small-cell lung cancer and non-Hodgkin lymphoma
- Tissue confirmation, especially for lymphomas that require tumor architecture
- Superior vena cava reconstruction for benign processes may be considered, but is rarely done.

IN-PATIENT CONSIDERATIONS

Initial Stabilization

- Inpatient, intensive care as clinically indicated
- Institute supportive therapy:
  - Bed rest
  - Elevate head
  - Oxygen
- Steroids (see "Medication" section)
- Diuretics (see "Medication" section)

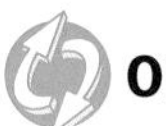

ONGOING CARE

FOLLOW-UP RECOMMENDATIONS

- Bed rest, and elevate patient's head to decrease the hydrostatic pressure.
- SVC syndrome is often associated with terminal illness; discuss advance directives: www.caringinfo.org/i4a/pages/index.cfm?pageid=3289

Patient Monitoring

- Severity of clinical symptoms
- If malignant, monitor response to radiotherapy or chemotherapy.
- If infectious, monitor for evaluation of antimicrobial treatment.

DIET

As tolerated; possibly salt restriction

PROGNOSIS

- High probability of initial response
- Linked to cause:
  - Lung cancer: 1-year survival 20%
  - Lymphoma: 2-year survival 50%
- Neoplastic cases: 85% better in 3 weeks with radiation therapy, but symptoms usually recur

COMPLICATIONS

Complications of underlying disease

REFERENCES

1. Yu JB, Wilson LD, Detterbeck FC. Superior vena cava syndrome–a proposed classification system and algorithm for management. *J Thorac Oncol*. 2008;3:811–4.
2. Rowell NP, et al. Steroids, radiotherapy, chemotherapy and stents for superior vena caval obstruction in carcinoma of the bronchus: A systematic review. *Clin Oncol*. 2002;14:338–51.
3. Hochrein J, Bashore TM, O'Laughlin MP, et al. Percutaneous stenting of superior vena cava syndrome: A case report and review of the literature. *Am J Med*. 1998;104:78–84.
4. Thirlwell C, Brock CS. Emergencies in oncology. *Clin Med*. 2003;3:306–10.

ADDITIONAL READING

- Wan JF, Bezjak A, et al. Superior vena cava syndrome. *Hematol Oncol Clin North Am*. 2010;24:501–13.
- Wilson LD, Detterbeck FC, Yahalom J. Clinical practice. Superior vena cava syndrome with malignant causes. *N Engl J Med*. 2007;356:1862–9.

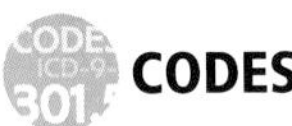

CODES

ICD9

459.2 Compression of vein

CLINICAL PEARLS

- Lung cancer is the leading cause of SVC syndrome; other leading malignant causes include lymphoma and metastatic breast cancer (4).
- Percutaneous stenting can provide immediate relief.
- Current treatment is disease-specific, so pathologic confirmation is vital (see treatment algorithm for management).
- Radiotherapy mainly useful in non–small-cell lung cancer and non-Hodgkin lymphoma
- Chemotherapy for small-cell lung cancer and germ-cell tumors

SURGICAL COMPLICATIONS

Anne Granfield, MD
Mitchell A. Cahan, MD

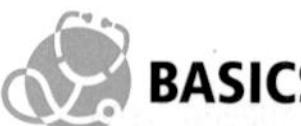

BASICS

DESCRIPTION

- Broadly defined: Any negative outcome perceived either by surgeon or patient
- A lack of consensus exists about how to define complications.
- Multiple classification systems exist based on severity.

EPIDEMIOLOGY

Incidence

Incidence of complications can vary with type of operation, operative time, hospital, surgeon, and patient characteristics, amongst other factors:

- Mortality rate in general and among vascular surgery patients is 3.5–6.9% (1).
- Overall complication rate in general and among vascular surgery patients is 24.6–26.9% (1).
- Postoperative fever is very common. Incidence ranges widely (14–91%) depending on definition and patient population (2).
- In 2000: ~8.96 postoperative pulmonary emboluses per 1,000 surgical discharges in the US (3)
- In 2000: ~2.057 postoperative abdominal wound dehiscences per 1,000 abdominopelvic surgeries in the US (3)
- Emergent cases are associated with more post op complications versus nonemergent cases (22.8% vs. 14.2%) and have a higher mortality rate (6.5% vs. 1.4%) (4)
- Surgical infection incidence varies with type of operation:
  - 1–2% clean operative site (e.g., hernia repair)
  - 5–15% clean contaminated (e.g., cholecystectomy)
  - 10–20% contaminated (e.g., colectomy)
  - 50% dirty operative site

RISK FACTORS

- People at increased operative risk include those with:
  - Poorly controlled diabetes
  - Heart disease (especially MI and heart failure)
  - Bleeding disorders
  - Malnutrition
  - Renal failure
  - Liver disease
  - Pulmonary disease
  - Obesity
  - Smoking history
  - Immunosuppression
  - Malignancy
- Other risk factors:
  - Prolonged surgery
  - Immobility following surgery
  - Emergency surgery

Genetics

- Malignant hyperthermia:
  - Incidence: 1 in 50–100,000; treated with dantrolene
- Bleeding disorders, including hemophilia

GENERAL PREVENTION

Preventive measures span entire perioperative period:

- Imaging to delineate anatomy and recognize aberrancy
- Appropriate fluid/blood resuscitation
- Assessment of underlying risk factors
- Preoperative antibiotics when appropriate
- Sterile technique
- Warming during surgery
- Clip hair instead of shaving preoperatively (5)[B]

PATHOPHYSIOLOGY

- Fever caused by pyrogens (mediated by interleukin-1): Bacteria, viruses, antigen-antibody complexes
- Wound dehiscence: Poor wound healing (malnutrition) or increased abdominal pressure
- Deep vein thrombosis: blood clot formation in deep vein attributed to 1 of 3 factors described in Virchow triad:
  - Hypercoagulability
  - Hemodynamic changes (stasis, turbulence)
  - Endothelial injury/dysfunction
- Renal failure:
  - Drug toxicity (commonly antibiotics)
  - Inadequate resuscitation leading to poor perfusion (catecholamine release during surgery and activation of renin-angiotensin-aldosterone system) results in ATN.
- Respiratory:
  - Decreased vital capacity leads to atelectasis, pneumonitis, and ARDS.
  - Aspiration can occur at any time. Stomach acid/particulate matter cause an inflammatory reaction, leading to cyanosis or death.
  - Pulmonary edema due to fluid transudation to alveolus from fluid overload or heart failure
  - Pulmonary mechanics are compromised postoperatively. Precipitating factors include pain and altered mental status.
- Cardiac:
  - Postoperative MI generally occurs within 3 days of surgery and is caused by anesthetics and blood loss (loss of as little as 500 cc can cause shock).
  - Arrhythmia is due to destabilization of cardiac membranes or prolongation of conduction.
- Small bowel obstruction: Intra-abdominal adhesive bands (scar tissue) can form and constrict the bowel, even decades after surgery.
- Urinary retention: Men affected more frequently than women, impaired coordination between α-receptors in the bladder neck and parasympathetic stimulation to the bladder

ETIOLOGY

- Fever in the first 24 hours is usually due to atelectasis. Consider the 5 Ws:
  - Wind—atelectasis, PNA, aspiration
  - Water—UTI
  - Walking—DVT
  - Wound—surgical site infection; *C. perfringens* or Group A *Streptococcus*
  - Wonder drugs—drug fever
- *Staphylococcus aureus* is the most common cause of wound infection. Others include *Pseudomonas*, *Proteus*, and *Klebsiella*.
- Hematoma: Inadequate hemostasis/bleeding
- Seroma: Disruption of lymphatics
- UTI: Related to indwelling catheter
- Dehiscence: Increased abdominal pressure, inadequate fascial closure, malnutrition, contamination, and chemotherapy are contributory.
- Renal failure: Hypovolemia, drug toxicity (commonly due to antibiotics or IV contrast).
- Respiratory: Volume overload, aspiration, and decreased vital capacity lead to decreased diffusion capacity. Pulmonary embolism formation is another possible postoperative etiology.
- Pulmonary embolism: Generally due to thromboembolism from the deep veins of the legs; more rarely from air, fat, or amniotic fluid.
- Cardiac: Arrhythmia occurs due to electrolyte abnormalities, catecholamine release (from pain), hypercapnia, and digitalis.
- Small bowel obstruction: Adhesive bands (scar tissue) form intra-abdominally and can constrict the bowel; occurs remotely after abdominal surgery.
- Fistula/intestinal leak: Generally occurs at the site of bowel anastomosis due to suture line breakdown
- Stomal complications:
  - More common in obese patients
  - Include fibrosis of bowel at stoma, necrosis, retraction, skin breakdown, and stomal stricture
  - Most complications are due to technical errors at the time of operation.
- Urinary retention: Due to anesthetics

COMMONLY ASSOCIATED CONDITIONS

- Adrenal insufficiency when on chronic steroids preoperatively
- Liver failure in patients with pre-existing disease
- Delirium tremens in alcoholics
- Thyroid storm in patients with undiagnosed hyperthyroidism
- Parotitis in the elderly
- Depression

Pediatric Considerations

Operative procedures can lead to severe anxiety in children, with lasting emotional disturbance in 20%, and is most pronounced in patients 1–2 years old.

Geriatric Considerations

90% of patients >65 years experience depression after surgery, with activities of daily living impaired in 50%. Increase human contact to prevent withdrawal and reduce symptoms.

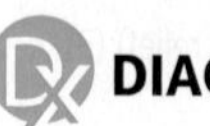

DIAGNOSIS

HISTORY

- Wound infection: History of surgery several days prior to presentation with pain, warmth, redness, or drainage at site of incision
- Expanding mass is consistent with seroma or hematoma. Hematoma more likely if surgery within 2–3 days; seroma more likely if interval is longer.
- Dehiscence/hernia: Some patients feel sutures "pop." They may complain of a palpable bulge. Attributed to increased abdominal pressure (e.g., coughing, Valsalva maneuver)
- DVT: Pain, swelling, and redness of leg in immobilized patient or with hypercoagulability
- Renal failure: Oliguria or anuria, fatigue

- Pulmonary: Lack of incentive spirometry, narcotics, fluid retention, age >65, shortness of breath, chest pain
- Cardiac: Elderly, cardiac dysfunction; chest pain in 27% of perioperative MI (most are pain-free)
- Ileus or small bowel obstruction: Progressive nausea, bilious vomiting, inability to tolerate PO intake, abdominal pain, cessation of flatus
- Fistula or intestinal leak: Severe abdominal pain (leak), fever, nausea/vomiting
- Stomal complications: Pain at stoma site, change in color of stoma
- Urinary retention: Inability to void, suprapubic pain

PHYSICAL EXAM

- Low fevers are not significant until 48 hours postop. Wound infection is most common cause of fever after 72 hours.
- High fever, mental status changes, hypotension, and rigors are associated with severe wound complications or intestinal leak.
- Dolor, tumor, rubor, and calor may indicate a wound infection, as do pus or foul-smelling discharge. The patient may be febrile.
- Hematoma is an expanding, tender mass. Seroma is a slowly expanding, nontender mass.
- Dehiscence/hernia: Salmon-colored drainage on postop days 4–5, evisceration, or later as ventral hernia; may see open incision or palpable fascial edge, rarely tender
- Renal failure: Persistent oliguria; can have pericardial rub, bleeding/hematoma if uremic
- Pulmonary: Dyspnea, cough, fever, basilar crackles, poor inspiratory effort, egophony, dullness to percussion at bases
- Cardiac: Peripheral edema, irregularly irregular heartbeat
- Ileus/small bowel obstruction: "Tinkling" or absent bowel sounds, tympanitic abdomen, tenderness to palpation, occasionally guarding
- Fistula/intestinal leak: Feces protruding from skin opening, acute or firm abdomen, fever, guarding, peritoneal signs, hypotension
- Stomal complications are evident when the ostomy appliance is removed: Skin irritation, black/discolored intestinal mucosa, retracted ostomy
- Urinary retention: Suprapubic pain, palpable bladder

DIAGNOSTIC TESTS & INTERPRETATION

Lab

Initial lab tests

- CBC with differential, blood culture and sensitivity (C/S), chemistries, BUN/creatinine, UA, urine C/S, ABG, CXR
- Elevated WBC count is seen in wound infections, atelectasis, pneumonia, infected hematoma/seroma, bowel leak, and stomal complications.
- Renal failure: BUN, creatinine, urine chemistries and FE_{NA}
- Pulmonary: Hypoxia, hypercarbia on ABG
- Cardiac: Elevated troponins, creatine kinase (CK), CK-MB
- UTI: UA, urine C/S
- DVT: D-dimer

Imaging

Initial approach

- SC gas can be seen in necrotizing fasciitis on x-ray or CT.
- CT or ultrasound can be used to diagnose hernia or fascial disruption.
- Small bowel obstruction/ileus: Upright abdominal film shows air-fluid levels, dilated small bowel; transition point may be seen on CT.
- Fistula: Fistulogram aids in diagnosis and is critical for treatment planning.
- Intestinal leak: CXR reveals free air under the diaphragm; CT shows fluid collection in abdomen.
- Bladder scan can help diagnose urinary retention if diagnosis in doubt.
- Duplex ultrasound to diagnose DVT.
- Pulmonary: CXR, CT pulmonary angiography more sensitive test for suspected pulmonary embolism.

Diagnostic Procedures/Surgery

- Exploratory laparotomy/laparoscopy if the patient is extremely ill or septic and diagnosis is unknown but abdominal cause is suspected.
- Dehiscence is considered a surgical emergency.
- Intra-abdominal abscesses frequently can be drained percutaneously.
- Cardiac: ECG shows signs of ischemia or dysrhythmia.

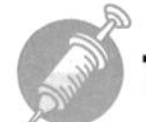

TREATMENT

MEDICATION

- Opiates for pain control.
- Broad-spectrum antibiotics for sepsis or severe infection (piperacillin/tazobactam and vancomycin).
- Simple wound infections and stomal complications: First- or second-generation cephalosporins
- Intestinal leak: Gram-negative and gram-positive coverage (levofloxacin and metronidazole)
- Pneumonia should be treated empirically with antibiotics to cover local flora.
- Cardiac complications can be avoided or treated with β-blockade for rate control.
- Urinary retention: α-blockers (tamsulosin)

ADDITIONAL TREATMENT

General Measures

- Drain pathologic fluid collections.
- Tamponade: Ligate or repair vessel for uncontrolled bleeding.

Issues for Referral

Organ injuries require consultation with their associated specialists (e.g., urology, gynecology), even when repaired by the surgeon at the time of injury.

SURGERY/OTHER PROCEDURES

- Wound infections may need surgical debridement if they are not responsive to antibiotics.
- Hematomas may need re-exploration and hemostasis if they are large and progressing.
- Dehiscence/hernia should be repaired. Evisceration is a surgical emergency.
- Small bowel obstruction that fails to resolve with nasogastric decompression should be explored; adhesions should be lysed.
- Intestinal leak is a surgical emergency for immediate exploration and repair. Fistulas generally need surgical intervention to resolve.
- Some stomal complications (necrosis, retraction) need surgical revision.

IN-PATIENT CONSIDERATIONS

Initial Stabilization

- Fluid resuscitation as needed
- Broad-spectrum antibiotics if the patient is septic
- IV antibiotics for infections

Admission Criteria

- Need for IV fluids/antibiotics
- Need for surgical procedure
- Need for nasogastric decompression

Discharge Criteria

- Infection resolved/responding to antibiotics
- Able to tolerate PO intake
- Patient has bowel function

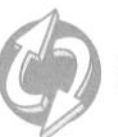

ONGOING CARE

DIET

Nothing by mouth for patients with fistula, intestinal leak, or small bowel obstruction.

PROGNOSIS

With appropriate treatment, most patients with complications return to baseline status.

REFERENCES

1. Ghaferi A, et al. Variation in hospital mortality associated with inpatient surgery. *N Engl J Med*. 2009;361:1368–75.
2. Pile JC, et al. Evaluating postoperative fever: A focused approach. *Cleve Clin J Med*. 2006; 73(Suppl 1):S62–6.
3. US Department of Health and Human Services, Agency for Healthcare Research and Quality. *National Healthcare Quality Report*, 2003. Full Report. Rockville, MD: AHRQ. www.ahrq.gov/qual/nhqr03/fullreport/index.htm.
4. Becher RD, Hoth JJ, Miller PR, et al. A Critical assessment of outcomes in emergency versus nonemergency general surgery using the American College of Surgeons National Surgical Quality Improvement Program Database. *Am Surg*. 2011;77:951–9.
5. Tanner J, et al. Preoperative hair removal to reduce surgical site infection. *Cochrane Database Syst Rev*. 2006;3.

CODES

ICD9

- 998.11 Hemorrhage complicating a procedure
- 998.30 Disruption of wound, unspecified
- 998.59 Other postoperative infection

CLINICAL PEARLS

- Surgical site infections are decreased by clipping to remove hair rather than shaving.
- Appropriate antibacterial preparation should be utilized to decrease bacterial counts.
- Amputation sites heal faster with plaster casting than with gauze. There is no difference in healing rates with foam versus gauze dressings, but patients prefer foam.
- 50% of all wound infections are identified after the patient is discharged.
- Treatment of some complications related to hospitalization will no longer be reimbursed by payers, including wrong-site surgery and central venous catheter infections.

SYNCOPE

Santiago O. Valdes, MD
Ricardo A. Samson, MD

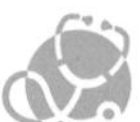

BASICS

DESCRIPTION

- Transient loss of consciousness characterized by unresponsiveness, loss of postural tone, and spontaneous recovery usually caused by cerebral hypoxemia
- System(s) affected: Cardiovascular; Nervous

EPIDEMIOLOGY

Incidence

- Up to 20% of adults will have ≥1 episode by age 75; 15% of children <18 years of age
- Accounts for 1–6% of hospital admissions and ~3% of emergency room visits

Prevalence

In institutionalized elderly (>75 years), 6%

RISK FACTORS

- Heart disease
- Dehydration
- Drugs:
  - Antihypertensives
  - Vasodilators (including calcium channel blockers, ACE inhibitors, and nitrates)
  - Phenothiazines
  - Antidepressants
  - Antiarrhythmics
  - Diuretics

Genetics

Specific cardiomyopathies and arrhythmias may be familial (i.e., long QT syndrome, hypertrophic cardiomyopathy).

GENERAL PREVENTION

See "Risk Factors."

PATHOPHYSIOLOGY

- In some cases, vagal response leads to decreased heart rate.
- Systemic hypotension secondary to decreased cardiac output and/or systemic vasodilation leads to a drop in cerebral perfusion and resulting loss of consciousness.

ETIOLOGY

- Cardiac: Obstruction to outflow:
  - Aortic stenosis
  - Hypertrophic cardiomyopathy
  - Pulmonary embolus
  - Anomalous coronary artery origin resulting in cardiac ischemia
- Cardiac arrhythmias:
  - Sustained ventricular tachycardia (VT)
  - Supraventricular tachycardia (atrial fibrillation, atrial flutter, re-entrant SVT)
  - Second- and third-degree AV block
  - Sick-sinus syndrome
  - Pacing-induced infranodal block
  - H-V interval >100 ms
- Noncardiac:
  - Reflex-mediated vasovagal (neurocardiogenic/neurally mediated), situational (micturition, defecation, cough)
  - Orthostatic hypotension
  - Drug-induced
  - Neurologic: Seizures; transient ischemic attack (can in theory cause syncope, but presentation usually markedly clinically different from pure syncope)
  - Carotid sinus hypersensitivity
  - Psychogenic

COMMONLY ASSOCIATED CONDITIONS

See "Etiology."

DIAGNOSIS

HISTORY

- Careful history, physical exam, and an ECG are more important than other investigations in determining the diagnosis (1)[A]. Syncope associated with physical exertion suggests a potential cardiac etiology.
- Make sure that the patient or witness (if present) is not talking about vertigo (i.e., sense of rotary motion, spinning, and whirling), seizure, or causes of fall without loss of consciousness.
- Even after careful evaluation, including diagnostic procedures and special tests, the cause will be found in only 50–60% of the patients.
- Onset of syncope is usually rapid, and recovery is spontaneous, rapid, and complete. Duration of episodes are typically brief (<60 seconds). The presence of underlying cardiac or neurologic conditions provides the key to diagnosis.

PHYSICAL EXAM

- BP and pulse, both lying and standing
- Check for cardiac murmur or focal neurologic abnormality.

DIAGNOSTIC TESTS & INTERPRETATION

History and physical examination should guide laboratory testing.

Lab

Initial lab tests

Consider (not all indicated in all individuals):

- CBC
- Electrolytes, BUN, creatinine, glucose (rarely helpful: <2% have hyponatremia, hypocalcemia, hypoglycemia, or renal failure causing seizures).
- Cardiac enzymes
- D-dimer (for pulmonary embolism workup)
- HCG

Follow-Up & Special Considerations

- If history and physical suggest ischemic, valvular, or congenital heart disease:
  - ECG
  - Exercise stress test (if syncope with exertion)
  - Echocardiogram
  - Cardiac catheterization
- If CNS disease suspected:
  - EEG
  - Head CT scan
  - Head MRI/MRA when vascular cause is suspected
  - Do not order these tests unless there are hints of CNS disease on history or physical exam.
- ECG monitoring, either in hospital or ambulatory (Holter):
  - Useful in 4–15% of patients
  - Should be done in patients with heart disease or recurrent syncope
  - Arrhythmias frequently documented, but not always associated with syncope
- Electrophysiologic studies:
  - Have been positive in 18–75% of patients
  - Induction of VT and dysfunction of His-Purkinje system are the 2 most common abnormalities.
  - Should be done in patients with heart disease or recurrent syncope, although they may not show whether arrhythmia noted or induced during study is cause of syncope
- Carotid hypersensitivity evaluation:
  - Carotid hypersensitivity should be considered in patients with syncope during head turning, especially while wearing tight collars, and with neck tumors and neck scars.
  - The technique is not standardized; 1 side at a time is compressed gently at a time for 20 seconds with constant monitoring of pulse and BP/ECG.
  - Atropine should be readily available.
- Tilt-table testing ± isoproterenol infusion:
  - Provocative test for vasovagal syncope
  - Perform if cardiac causes have been excluded; role in workup of patients with syncope of unknown origin
  - Not standardized but has been reported positive (symptomatic hypotension and bradycardia) in 26–87% of patients; also positive in up to 45% of control subjects
- Psychiatric evaluation: Anxiety, depression, and alcohol and drug abuse can be associated with syncope.

Imaging

- ECG
- Echocardiogram if clinically indicated

Initial approach

Lung scan or helical CT scan of thorax if history and physical exam suggest pulmonary embolism (PE)

Diagnostic Procedures/Surgery

Patient-activated implantable loop recorders can record 4–5 minutes of retrograde ECG rhythm. Helpful in recurrent syncope, with yield of 24–47%.

Pathological Findings

Depends on etiology and presence of underlying cardiac or neurologic conditions

DIFFERENTIAL DIAGNOSIS

- Drop attacks
- Coma
- Vertigo
- Seizure disorder

TREATMENT

Maintaining good hydration status and normal salt intake are initial therapy. Educate patients of the premonitory signs of syncope.

MEDICATION

First Line

- Geared toward specific underlying cardiac or neurologic abnormalities
- In cases of recurrent vasovagal/neurocardiogenic/neurally mediated syncope:
  - β-Adrenergic blockers
  - Mineralocorticoids (fludrocortisone)
  - α-Adrenergic agonists (midodrine)

Second Line

- SSRIs (paroxetine, sertraline, fluoxetine)
- Vagolytics (disopyramide)

ADDITIONAL TREATMENT

General Measures

- Patients with heart disease should be admitted to the hospital for evaluation.
- Elderly patients without previously recognized heart disease should be admitted if the physician thinks that the cause of syncope is likely cardiac.
- Patients without heart disease, especially young patients (<60 years old), can be worked up safely as outpatients.
- Prescribe antiarrhythmics for documented arrhythmias occurring simultaneously with syncope or symptoms of presyncope. Asymptomatic arrhythmias do not necessarily require treatment.
- The decision to treat patients on basis of arrhythmias or conduction abnormalities provoked or detected during EPS is even more problematic: Does the arrhythmia or conduction abnormality have anything to do with the patient's symptoms?
- Most would treat patients with provoked sustained VT with an antiarrhythmic drug that suppressed arrhythmia during study.
- Rationale for such treatment: Recurrent syncope is less frequent in patients with positive EPS who are treated than it is in those who have negative EPS.

Issues for Referral

When cardiac or neurologic etiologies are suspected, appropriate expert consultation is indicated.

COMPLEMENTARY AND ALTERNATIVE MEDICINE

St. John's wort has been used in cases of recurrent noncardiac syncope.

SURGERY/OTHER PROCEDURES

- ICD placement for patients with cardiac conditions with high risk of sudden death and/or recurrent syncope on medications (i.e., long QT syndrome, hypertrophic cardiomyopathy)
- Many recommend pacemaker implantation in patients with
  - Second- (Mobitz type II) and third-degree heart block
  - H-V intervals >100 ms
  - Pacing-induced infranodal block
  - Sinus node recovery time $\geq$3 seconds

IN-PATIENT CONSIDERATIONS

Initial Stabilization

- Support ABCs.
- Stabilize heart rate and BP, typically with IV fluids.

Admission Criteria

Patients with heart disease should be admitted to the hospital for evaluation.

IV Fluids

Use isotonic crystalloid fluids for fluid resuscitation if needed.

Nursing

Close monitoring of BP, heart rate during initial presentation

Discharge Criteria

- Attainment of hemodynamic stability
- Satisfactory completion of workup for etiology
- Adequate control of specific arrhythmia or seizure, if present

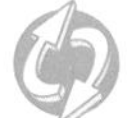

ONGOING CARE

FOLLOW-UP RECOMMENDATIONS

Patient Monitoring

- Frequent follow-up visits for patients with cardiac causes of syncope, especially patients on antiarrhythmics
- Patients with an unknown cause of syncope rarely (5%) are diagnosed during the follow-up.

DIET

- No specific diet unless the patient has heart disease
- Increased fluid and salt intake to maintain intravascular volume in cases of recurrent vasovagal syncope

PATIENT EDUCATION

- Reassure the patient that most cardiac causes of syncope can be treated, and patients with noncardiac causes do well, even if the cause of syncope is never discovered.
- The physician and patient should carefully consider whether the patient should continue to drive while syncope is being evaluated. Physicians should be aware of pertinent laws in their own states.

PROGNOSIS

- Cumulative mortality at 2 years:
  - Low (25%): Young patients (<60 years) with noncardiac or unknown cause of syncope
  - Intermediate (20%): Older patients (>60 years) with noncardiac or unknown cause of syncope
  - High (32–38%): Patients with cardiac cause of syncope
- Independent predictors of poor short-term outcomes:
  - Abnormal ECG
  - Shortness of breath
  - Systolic BP <90 mm Hg
  - Hematocrit <30%
  - Congestive heart failure

COMPLICATIONS

- Trauma from falling
- Death (see "Prognosis")

REFERENCE

1. Kessler C, Tristano JM, De Lorenzo R. The emergency department approach to syncope: Evidence-based guidelines and prediction rules. *Emerg Med Clin North Am*. 2010;28:487–500.

ADDITIONAL READING

- European Heart Rhythm Association (EHRA); Heart Failure Association (HFA) et al. Guidelines for the diagnosis and management of syncope (version 2009): The Task Force for the Diagnosis and Management of Syncope of the European Society of Cardiology (ESC). *Eur Heart J*. 2009;30(21): 2631–71.
- Goble MM, Benitez C, Baumgardner M, et al. ED management of pediatric syncope: Searching for a rationale. *Am J Emerg Med*. 2008;26:66–70.
- Kuriachan V, Sheldon RS, Platonov M. Evidence-based treatment for vasovagal syncope. *Heart Rhythm*. 2008;5:1609–14.
- Parry SW, Tan MP. An approach to the evaluation and management of syncope in adults. *BMJ*. 2010;340:c880.
- Reed MJ, Newby DE, Coull AJ, et al. The ROSE (risk stratification of syncope in the emergency department) study. *J Am Coll Cardiol*. 2010;55: 713–21.
- Romme JJ, Reitsma JB, Go-Schön IK, et al. Prospective evaluation of non-pharmacological treatment in vasovagal syncope. *Europace*. 2010;12:567–73.
- Strickberger SA, Benson DW, Biaggioni I. AHA/ACCF scientific statement on the evaluation of syncope: From the American Heart Association Councils on Clinical Cardiology, Cardiovascular Nursing, Cardiovascular Disease in the Young, and Stroke, and the Quality of Care and Outcomes Research Interdisciplinary Working Group; and the American College of Cardiology Foundation in Collaboration with the Heart Rhythm Society. *J Am Coll Cardiol*. 2006;47:473–84.

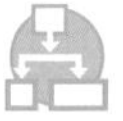

See Also (Topic, Algorithm, Electronic Media Element)

- Aortic Valvular Stenosis; Atrial Septal Defect (ASD); Carotid Sinus Hypersensitivity; Idiopathic Hypertrophic Subaortic Stenosis (IHSS); Patent Ductus Arteriosus; Pulmonary Arterial Hypertension; Pulmonary Embolism; Seizure Disorders; Stokes-Adams Attacks
- Algorithms: Syncope; Transient Ischemic Attack and Transient Neurologic Deficit

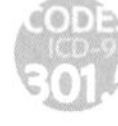

CODES

ICD9

780.2 Syncope and collapse

CLINICAL PEARLS

- A careful history and physical are key to a diagnosis.
- Use the ECG/event-recorder to evaluate for cardiac conditions.
- True neurologic causes of syncope are very rare; cardiac causes by far are more common.
- Fewer than 2% of cases are caused by hyponatremia, hypocalcemia, hypoglycemia, or renal failure causing seizures.

SYNCOPE, NEURALLY MEDIATED

Sana Syed, MD
Martina Vendrame, MD, PhD

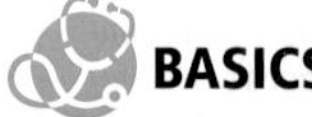

BASICS

Syncope is a reversible loss of consciousness and postural tone secondary to systemic hypotension and cerebral hypoperfusion due to vasodilation and/or bradycardia (rarely tachycardia) with spontaneous recovery and no neurologic sequelae. The term syncope excludes seizures, coma, shock, or other states of altered consciousness.

DESCRIPTION

- Derived from the Greek term "syncopa," meaning "to cut short"
- Sudden, transient loss of consciousness characterized by unresponsiveness, falling, and spontaneous recovery
- Common cause of syncope in all age groups, especially in patients with no evidence of neurologic or cardiac disease
- 4 types: Vasovagal or neurocardiogenic syncope, carotid sinus syncope, situational syncope, and glossopharyngeal/trigeminal neuralgia syncope (uncommon) (1)

EPIDEMIOLOGY

- Mortality: Cardiac-related syncope 20–30% and 5% in idiopathic syncope
- Age: Any age

Incidence

- Ranges from 7.5% in children <18 years of age and 15–18% in adults >70 years of age (1)
- 36–62% of all syncopal episodes

Prevalence

22% in the general population (1)

RISK FACTORS

- Low resting BP
- Age: Older age
- Prolonged supine position with resulting deconditioning of autonomic control

Genetics

- Vasovagal syncope: Strong heritable component to the etiology of over 20% of cases
- Orthostatic hypotension: Gene polymorphisms include:
  - Endothelin-1 gene (insertion variant in the 5′UTR)
  - B1-adrenergic receptor gene (polymorphism beta1Gly49)
  - Human norepinephrine transporter gene (polymorphism Ala457Pro)
  - Gs protein alpha-subunit (polymorphism T131C)
  - G-protein beta 3 subunit (polymorphism C825T)
  - SCNN1G gene encoding the gamma subunit of the amiloride-sensitive epithelial sodium channel
  - Presence of multiple point mutations in the mitochondrial DNA (mtDNA) in 3 families with orthostatic hypotension

GENERAL PREVENTION

Avoidance of precipitating events or situations. Optimization of (DM) control, elastic stockings, adequate hydration. Limited evidence suggests that polydipsia may reduce recurrences.

PATHOPHYSIOLOGY

Cause: An abnormal interaction of the normal mechanisms for maintaining BP and upright posture:

- In normal individuals, upright posture results in venous pooling and transient decrease in BP.
- Neurally induced syncope may result from a cardioinhibitory response, a vasodepressor response, or a combination of the 2.
- Cardioinhibitory response results from increase in parasympathetic tone and may cause bradycardia
- Vasodepressor response results from decrease in sympathetic tone and may cause hypotension (2)

ETIOLOGY

- Vasovagal syncope usually has a precipitating event, often related to fright, pain, panic, or exercise. Also common in pregnancy when changing from supine to lateral decubitus or upright position (2).
- Carotid sinus syncope is precipitated by position change, turning head, or wearing a tight collar. (Possible neck tumors or surgical scarring.)
- Situational syncope is related to micturition, defecation, or coughing.
- Glossopharyngeal syncope is related to throat or facial pain (1).

COMMONLY ASSOCIATED CONDITIONS

- Cardiopulmonary disorders: CHF, MI, arrhythmias, HOCM, HTN, PE
- Neurologic disorders: Autonomic dysfunction, Shy-Drager, PD, MSA, TIA, VBI, PN
- Psychiatric disorders:
  - Generalized anxiety disorder
  - Panic disorder
  - Major depression
  - Alcohol dependence

DIAGNOSIS

History and physical and 12-lead ECG are preliminary tests.

HISTORY

- Evaluation of syncope and presyncope are the same.
- Important first to rule out cardiac syncope
- Neurally mediated syncope is preceded by blurred vision, palpitations, nausea, warmth, diaphoresis, or lightheadedness, or there may be history of nausea, warmth, diaphoresis, or fatigue *after* syncope (3).
- Vasovagal syncope:
  - 3 phases: Prodrome, loss of consciousness, and postsyncope
  - Precipitating event or stimulus is usually identified, such as panic, fright, pain, or exercise.
  - Athletes may have after exertion (diagnosis of exclusion)
  - Position: *Can be preceded by prolonged standing, but can occur from any position; generally resolves when the patient becomes supine:*
    - Preceding events: As discussed above
    - Prodrome: As listed above for neurally mediated syncope
  - Duration: Generally brief (seconds–minutes)
  - Recovery: May be prolonged with persistent nausea, pallor, and diaphoresis but without neurologic change or confusion
- Carotid sinus syncope is precipitated by position change, after turning head, or wearing a tight collar.
- Situational syncope is related to micturition, defecation, or coughing.
- Glossopharyngeal syncope (less common) is related to throat or facial pain (1):
  - Precipitating events or situations may include panic, pain, exercise, micturition, defecation, coughing, or swallowing.

PHYSICAL EXAM

- Vital signs, including orthostatics and bilateral BP
- Cardiac exam: Volume status, murmurs, rhythm, carotid bruits
- Neurologic exam: Signs of focal deficit
- Assess for occult blood loss, including guaiac.
- Dix Hallpike to rule out benign paroxysmal vertigo

DIAGNOSTIC TESTS & INTERPRETATION

As indicated by history and physical

Lab

Includes basic tests to rule out the 3 main reasons for syncope: Hypoglycemia, arrhythmia, and anemia

Initial lab tests

- Blood sugar
- ECG should be ordered for all patients (6). Abnormal ECG findings are common in patients with cardiac syncope.
- CBC to rule out anemia

Follow-Up & Special Considerations

- 24-hours Holter monitoring only in patients with a high probability of cardiac cause of syncope and/or abnormal ECG findings
- A low hemoglobin without obvious cause of bleed would warrant a guaiac, CT abdomen, CT head to rule out retroperitoneal bleed, SAH.

Imaging

Head CT, MRI/MRA, carotid ultrasound only in patients whose history or physical exam suggests a neurologic cause of syncope

Initial approach

- The 2007 ACEP Guidelines for diagnostic testing for syncope are as follows:
- *Level A recommendations:* Standard 12-lead ECG
- *Level B recommendations:* None specified
- *Level C recommendations:* Laboratory testing and investigations, including echocardiography or head CT, to be performed only if indicated by specific findings in the history or physical examination

Follow-Up & Special Considerations

- Negative imaging will prompt workup for alternative causes.
- Stroke, bleed, or carotid stenosis will require appropriate disease-oriented management.
- EEG only when history or physical exam is very suggestive of seizure activity

Diagnostic Procedures/Surgery

- Head-up tilt-table testing:
  - Contraindicated in patients with known cardiac or neurovascular disease or in pregnancy
  - Indicated for recurrent syncope or single episode accompanied by injury or risk to others (e.g., pilots, surgeons, etc.)
  - Uses positional changes to reproduce symptoms
  - Positive tests are diagnostic for vasovagal syncope.
- Carotid sinus massage, only in a monitored setting (i.e., BP and HR monitoring, IV access):
  - Contraindicated in patients with carotid disease (careful auscultation prior to massage is essential)
  - Pressure at the angle of the jaw for 5 seconds with simultaneous ECG monitoring
  - Positive tests (causing syncope or cardiac pause >3 seconds) are diagnostic of carotid sinus syncope.
- Psychiatric evaluation: To rule out anxiety, depression, and alcohol abuse

DIFFERENTIAL DIAGNOSIS
- Seizure
- Hypoglycemia
- Cardiac syncope
- Cerebrovascular syncope
- Orthostatic hypotension
- Drop attacks
- Psychiatric illness

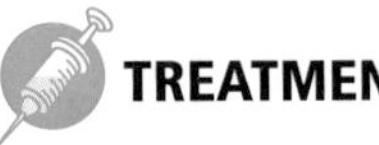

TREATMENT

Therapy is primarily for recurrent syncope. Situational syncope will not warrant any treatment.

MEDICATION
Medical management is based on small nonrandomized clinical trials.

First Line
- Nonpharmacologic treatment:
  - Includes patient counseling:
    - Development of coping skills
    - Increased salt and fluid intake
  - Moderate exercise training
  - Tilt-table training
- Pharmacologic treatment: β-blockers: Metoprolol, atenolol, or pindolol (if bradycardia develops) are used:
  - Block peripheral vasodilators and ventricular mechanoreceptor stimulation
  - Stabilization of HR and BP
  - Side effects: Hypotension and bradycardia (with worsening of syncope), fatigue, depression, and sexual dysfunction
  - Contraindicated in asthma

Second Line
- α-agonists: Midodrine is commonly used. It increases peripheral vascular resistance and venous return. Side effects include hypertension, paresthesia, urinary retention, "goose bumps," hyperactivity, dizziness, tremor, and nervousness.
- SSRIs: Paroxetine, fluoxetine, and sertraline are SSRIs useful in treating neurally mediated syncope (NMS):
  - Serotonin induces vagally mediated bradycardia and hypotension.
  - Side effects include weight gain, nausea, anxiety, sexual dysfunction, and insomnia.
- Mineralocorticoids: Fludrocortisone has been found helpful mainly in pediatric groups:
  - Helpful in renal sodium absorption and increasing the vasoconstrictive peripheral vascular response.
  - Adverse reactions include fluid retention, HTN, CHF, peripheral edema, and hypokalemia.
- Anticholinergics: These include disopyramide, scopolamine, and propantheline:
  - Decreases vagal tone
  - Side effects include dry mouth, constipation, urinary retention, confusion, and blurred vision (2).

ADDITIONAL TREATMENT

General Measures
Recognition and avoidance of precipitating events or situations

Issues for Referral
Neurology or cardiology as needed

Additional Therapies
- Increased salt and fluid intake: May include salt tablets or electrolyte/sports drinks
- Moderate exercise training
- Tilt-table training: Involves periods of prolonged, forced upright posture
- Use of support/pressure stockings
- Leg crossing, hand grip, or arm tensing
- Clonazepam may be effective in refractory neurally mediated syncope (4).

COMPLEMENTARY AND ALTERNATIVE MEDICINE
These include treatments for underlying heart disease or precipitating factors like anxiety:
- Nutrition and supplements: Omega-3 fatty acids, multivitamin, CoQ10, acetyl-L-carnitine, alpha-lipoic acid, and L-arginine
- Herbs: Green tea (*Camellia sinensis*), bilberry (*Vaccinium myrtillus*), ginkgo (*Ginkgo biloba*)
- Homeopathy: Carbo vegetabilis, opium, sepia
- Acupuncture: An analysis of 102 serious cases showed improvement in majority cases. It may precipitate fainting.

SURGERY/OTHER PROCEDURES
Pacemaker placement may be of use in patients with frequent cardioinhibitory syncope or mixed carotid sinus syncope (class I–II, level B) (2):
- Prevents prolonged bradycardia
- Long-term effect
- Invasive placement procedure (2)

IN-PATIENT CONSIDERATIONS

Initial Stabilization
IV fluids to stabilize HR and BP

Admission Criteria
2007 ACEP Guidelines mandate that the patient be admitted if:
- *Level B recommendations:*
  - Admit patients with syncope and evidence of heart failure or structural heart disease.
  - Admit patients with syncope and high-risk factors.
- High-risk stratification is based on following factors:
  - Older age and associated comorbidities
  - Abnormal ECG, hematocrit (Hct) 30 (if obtained)
  - History or presence of heart failure, coronary artery disease, or structural heart disease
- Additional causes to admit:
  - Syncope occurring during exercise
  - Syncope causing severe injury
  - Family history of sudden death

IV Fluids
Isotonic crystalloids as needed

Nursing
Vital sign monitoring

Discharge Criteria
Hemodynamically stable and workup satisfactory

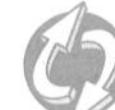

ONGOING CARE

DIET
- Increased salt intake may be helpful if not contraindicated (2).
- Maintain fluid intake.

PATIENT EDUCATION
- To identify and avoid precipitating events or situations
- Avoid dehydration, alcohol consumption, warm environments, tight clothing, and long periods of standing motionless.
- Recognize presyncopal symptoms.
- Use behaviors, such as lying down, to avoid syncope.

PROGNOSIS
May be recurrent but not life-threatening

COMPLICATIONS
May result in injury from fall

REFERENCES

1. Chen-Scarabelli C, et al. Neurocardiogenic syncope. *Br Med J*. 2004;329:336.
2. Nair N, et al. Pathophysiology and management of neurocardiogenic syncope. *Am J Managed Care*. 2003;9:327–34.
3. Chen LY, Benditt DG, Shen WK. Management of syncope in adults: An update. *Mayo Clin Proc*. 2008;83:1280–93.
4. Márquez MF, Urias-Medina K, Gómez-Flores J, et al. [Comparison of metoprolol vs clonazepam as a first treatment choice among patients with neurocardiogenic syncope]. *Gac Med Mex*. 2008; 144:503–7.

ADDITIONAL READING

- Huff S, Decker W. Clinical policy: Critical issues in the evaluation and management of adult patients presenting to the emergency department with syncope. *Ann Emerg Med*. 2007;49:431–44.
- Lelonek M, et al. [Genetics in neurocardiogenic syncope] *Prz Lek*. 2006;63:1310–2.
- Syncope. www.umm.edu/altmed/articles/syncope-000059.htm.

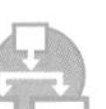

See Also (Topic, Algorithm, Electronic Media Element)

Algorithms: Syncope; Transient Ischemic Attack and Transient Neurologic Deficit

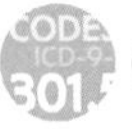

CODES

ICD9
- 337.01 Carotid sinus syndrome
- 780.2 Syncope and collapse

CLINICAL PEARLS

- History should include a careful analysis of the events preceding the attack.
- It is important to rule out cardiologic or neurologic pathology.
- Prodrome is often present.
- Recovery may be prolonged, with persistent symptoms but no neurologic deficit or confusion.
- Patient counseling to avoid precipitating situations or events is first-line treatment.

SYPHILIS

Melissa Badowski, PharmD, BCPS, AAHIVE
Mahesh Patel, MD

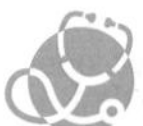

BASICS

DESCRIPTION

- A chronic, systemic infectious disease caused by *Treponema pallidum*
- Transmitted sexually, maternal–fetal, contact with an active lesion, and via blood transfusions
- Untreated disease progresses through a series of 4 overlapping stages:
  - Primary: Usually single painless chancre at point of entry; appears in 10–90 days; chancre heals without treatment in 3–6 weeks
  - Secondary: Appears 2–8 weeks after primary chancre. Nonpruritic rash on palms or soles of feet, mucous membrane lesions, headache, fever, lymphadenopathy
  - Latent: Seroreactive without evidence of disease:
    - Early latent: Acquired within the last year
    - Late latent: Exposure >12 months prior to diagnosis
  - Tertiary (late): Serology may be negative (though FTA-ABS is positive almost 100%):
    - Refers to gumma and cardiovascular and late neurosyphilis; may be lethal
  - Neurosyphilis: represents *any* type of CNS involvement with syphilis and can occur at *any* stage:
    - Psychosis, delirium, dementia
- Ability to affect nearly every organ/tissue in the body has led to it being called "the great imitator."

Pediatric Considerations

In noncongenital cases, consider child abuse

Pregnancy Considerations

- All pregnant patients should have VDRL or RPR test at first prenatal visit (1). If high exposure risk, repeat the tests at 28 weeks and at delivery.
- The same nontreponemal test for initial diagnosis also should be used for follow-up tests.

EPIDEMIOLOGY

Incidence

- Syphilis rate decreased until 2000, increasing primarily in men since then (2).
- In 2009: 4.6/100,000 population (an increase of 5% from 2008) (3):
  - Highest in both men and women aged 20–24 years
    - Men: 7.8/100,000
    - Women: 1.4/100,000
  - Congenital: 10 cases/100,000 live births
- Race/Ethnicity (2):
  - White, non-Hispanic: 2/100,000
  - African American: 14/100,000
  - Hispanic: 4.3/100,000
  - Asian/Pacific Islander: 1.2/100,000
  - Native American/Alaska native: 4.3/100,000

Prevalence

- Predominant sex: Male > Female (6:1)
- Increasing male:female ratio (was 1.2:1 in 1996) suggests greatest syphilis increase in men having sex with men (MSM).

RISK FACTORS

MSM, multiple sexual partners, exposure to infected body fluids, IV drug use, transplacental transmission, adult inmates, high-risk sexual behavior, HIV positive

GENERAL PREVENTION

Education; condoms reduce but do not eliminate transmission (4)[A].

ETIOLOGY

Treponema pallidum subspecies *pallidum*, spirochete

COMMONLY ASSOCIATED CONDITIONS

HIV infection, hepatitis B, other STDs

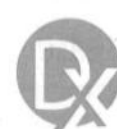

DIAGNOSIS

HISTORY

Previous sexual contact with partner with known infection or partner with high-risk sexual behavior

PHYSICAL EXAM

Signs/symptoms depend on stage:

- Primary: Single (occasionally multiple), usually painless ulcer (chancre) in groin or at other point of entry
- Secondary:
  - Rash: Skin or mucous membranes
    - Rough, red–brown macules, usually on palms and soles
    - May appear with chancre or after it has healed
  - Nonspecific symptoms: Fever, adenopathy, malaise, headache

DIAGNOSTIC TESTS & INTERPRETATION

Lab

Initial lab tests

- Dark-field microscopy demonstrating *T. pallidum* spirochetes in lesion exudate or tissue biopsy: Gold standard, but difficult and not very sensitive
- Nontreponemal tests (VDRL or RPR):
  - Primary screening test: Positive within 7 days of exposure
  - Nonspecific, false-positive results common; must confirm diagnosis with treponemal tests.
  - Positive test should be quantified and titers followed at regular intervals after treatment (5).
    - Titers usually correlate with disease activity. 4-fold change demonstrates clinical significant difference (5).
    - Titer decreases with time or treatment; following adequate treatment for primary or secondary, a 4-fold decline should be noted after 6 months.
    - Absence of 4-fold decline indicates failure of treatment.
    - Titers eventually should be negative (see "serofast reaction" below).
    - Titers of patients treated in latent stages decline gradually.
  - Prozone phenomenon: Negative results from high titers of antibody; test diluted serum
  - Serofast reaction: Persistently positive results years after successful treatment; new infection diagnosed by 4-fold rise in titer.
  - Disorders that may alter lab results (noting that all stages of syphilis can have a false-negative RPR, especially in primary syphilis):
    - Pregnancy, autoimmune disease, mononucleosis, malaria, leprosy, viral pneumonia, presence of cardiolipin antigens, injection drug use, acute febrile illness, HIV infection, elderly can have false-positive results
- Treponemal tests (*confirmatory test after positive nontreponemal screening test*): FTA-ABS, TP-PA:
  - FTA-ABS (fluorescent treponemal antibody absorbed), TP-PA (*T. pallidum* particle agglutination)
  - Confirmatory test; not used for screening
  - Usually positive for life after treatment
  - Titers of no benefit
  - 15–25% of patients treated during the primary stage revert to being serologically nonreactive after 2–3 years
- Lumbar puncture:
  - Indicated if clinical evidence of neurologic involvement or has syphilitic ocular or auditory manifestations
  - Some experts advise in all secondary and early latent cases without neurologic symptoms
  - In some HIV-positive patients with late latent or latent of unknown duration
  - In select patients with late latent or latent of unknown duration or when nonpenicillin therapy is planned
  - In treatment failures
  - If other evidence of active tertiary syphilis is present (e.g., aortitis, gumma, iritis)
  - In children with syphilis, after the newborn period, and to rule out neurosyphilis
  - VDRL, not RPR, used on CSF; may be negative in neurosyphilis; highly specific but insensitive
  - Send fluid for protein, glucose, and cell count
  - Monitor resolution by cell count at 6 months along with serologies as recommended (see "Patient Monitoring")
  - Negative FTA-ABS or MHA-TP on CSF excludes neurosyphilis (highly sensitive)
  - Positive FTA-ABS or MHA-TP on CSF not diagnostic because of high false-positive rate
  - Bloody tap, tuberculosis (TB), pyogenic or aseptic meningitis can result in false-positive VDRL

DIFFERENTIAL DIAGNOSIS

- Primary:
  - Chancroid, lymphogranuloma venereum, granuloma inguinale, condyloma acuminata, herpes simplex, Behçet syndrome, trauma, carcinoma, mycotic infection, lichen planus, psoriasis, fungal infection
- Secondary:
  - Pityriasis rosea, drug eruption, psoriasis, lichen planus, viral exanthema, Stevens-Johnson syndrome
- Positive serology, asymptomatic:
  - Previously treated syphilis
  - Other spirochetal disease (yaws, pinta)

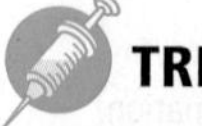

TREATMENT

MEDICATION

Parenteral penicillin G is drug of choice for all stages (5)[A]. Choice of formulation is determined by the disease stage and clinical manifestations.

ALERT

- Bicillin L-A should be used and *not* Bicillin C-R (combination benzathine–procaine penicillin) when penicillin G benzathine is indicated (5)[A].
- Primary, secondary, and early latent <1 year:
  - Benzathine penicillin G, 2.4 million units IM for 1 dose (5)[A]

- Penicillin-allergic patients: Doxycycline, 100 mg PO b.i.d. × 2 weeks, or tetracycline, 500 mg PO q.i.d. × 2 weeks, or ceftriaxone, 1 g IM or IV daily × 10–14 days:
  - Azithromycin, 2 g PO × 1 dose (early syphilis only; should not be used in MSM or pregnancy):
    - Resistance and treatment failures have been noted in several geographical locations in the US.
- Late latent or latent of unknown duration and tertiary without evidence of neurosyphilis:
  - Benzathine penicillin G, 2.4 million units IM weekly × 3 doses (5)[A]
  - Penicillin-allergic patients: Attempt desensitization and treatment with penicillin, or doxycycline, 100 mg PO 2 b.i.d. × 28 days, or tetracycline, 500 mg PO q.i.d.× 28 days; compliance may be an issue
- Neurosyphilis:
  - Aqueous crystalline penicillin G, 3–4 million units IV q4h or continuous infusion × 10–14 days
  - Procaine penicillin G, 2.4 million units IM daily in conjunction with probenecid, 500 mg PO q.i.d. × 10–14 days (if compliance can be ensured) (5)[A]
  - Penicillin-allergic patients: Attempt desensitization (ONLY if patient does NOT have a history of type I IgE-mediated hypersensitivity to penicillin) and treat with penicillin; ceftriaxone, 2 g/d IM or IV × 10–14 days
  - If late latent, latent of unknown duration, or tertiary in addition to neurosyphilis, consider also treating as recommended for late latent after completion of neurosyphilis treatment.
- Congenital:
  - Aqueous crystalline penicillin G, 50,000 units/kg/dose IV q12h × first 7 days of life and q8h thereafter for a total of 10 days, or procaine penicillin G, 50,000 units/kg/dose IM daily × 10 days (5)[A]
  - If negative CSF serologies, normal physical exam, and titer: Maternal titer, then 50,000 units/kg benzathine penicillin G IM in single dose is also alternative (5)[A]
  - If >1 day of drug is missed, restart course.
  - Children (after newborn period): Aqueous crystalline penicillin G, 50,000 units/kg/dose IV q4–6h × 10 days; late latent, [MJB2] 50,000 units/kg IM as 3 doses at 1-week intervals (5)[A]
  - Epidemiologic treatment for contacts without symptoms: Treat as primary after serologies.
  - HIV-infected and pregnant patients may show poor response to recommended IM doses. Use IV therapy for all treatment failures in these patients.
  - Do not give benzathine or procaine penicillins IV.
- Children (after newborn period): Aqueous crystalline penicillin G, 50,000 units/kg/dose IV q4–6h × 10 days; late latent, [MJB2] 50,000 units/kg IM as 3 doses at 1-week intervals (5)[A]
- Pregnancy:
  - Treatment same as for nonpregnant patients
  - Some specialists recommend second dose of 2.4 million units benzathine penicillin G 1 week after initial dose in third trimester or with primary, secondary, or early latent syphilis
  - Penicillin sensitivity: No proven alternatives to penicillin exist for treatment during pregnancy; consider desensitization and treatment with penicillin (5)[A]
  - Epidemiologic treatment for contacts without symptoms: Treat as primary after serologies.
  - HIV-infected and pregnant patients may show poor response to recommended IM doses. Use IV therapy for all treatment failures in these patients.
  - Do not give benzathine or procaine penicillins IV.
- Epidemiologic treatment for contacts without symptoms: Treat as primary after serologies.
- Precautions:
  - HIV-infected and pregnant patients may show poor response to recommended IM doses. Use IV therapy for all treatment failures in these patients.
  - Do not give benzathine or procaine penicillins IV.

ADDITIONAL TREATMENT

General Measures

- Advise patients to avoid intercourse until treatment is complete and keep track of partners.
- All persons who have syphilis should be tested for HIV.
- Management of sexual contacts:
  - Those exposed within 90 days of diagnosis, treat presumptively
  - Those exposed more than 90 days before diagnosis should be treated presumptively if serologic test results are not available immediately and follow-up is uncertain.
  - Those exposed to a patient diagnosed with syphilis of unknown duration and who have high treponemal titers (>1:32) should be treated presumptively.
  - Long-term sex partners of patients with latent infection should be evaluated clinically and serologically and treated on the basis of findings.

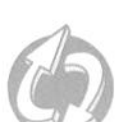

ONGOING CARE

FOLLOW-UP RECOMMENDATIONS

- Clinical and serologic evaluation at 6 and 12 months after treatment; if >1 year's duration, check at 24 months also.
- In HIV-infected persons, clinical and serologic evaluation at 3, 6, 9, 12, and 24 months after therapy

Patient Monitoring

- Use VDRL or RPR test to monitor therapy: 4-fold rise in titer indicates new infection, whereas failure to decrease 4-fold in 6 months is considered treatment failure (although definitive criteria for cure not established); titers not consistent between tests; always use same test, preferably same lab, as initially performed.
- Retreat for persistent clinical signs or recurrence, 4-fold rise in titers, or failure of initially high titer to decrease 4-fold by 6 months.
- Labs titer tests to final endpoint (e.g., not report as ">1:512") to make best use of results in monitoring therapy response
- Neurosyphilis: Repeat lumbar puncture every 6 months to check for normalization of CSF cell count (± CSF-VDRL and protein evaluation).

PATIENT EDUCATION

No sexual contacts until 4-fold titer drop

PROGNOSIS

- Excellent in all cases except patients with late-syphilis complications and with HIV infection
- Syphilis in HIV-infected patient:
  - Treatment same as for HIV-negative patients
  - More often false-negative treponemal and nontreponemal tests or unusually high titers
  - Response to therapy less predictable
  - Early syphilis: Increased risk of neurosyphilis and higher rates of treatment failure
  - Late neurosyphilis: Harder to treat; can occur up to 20 years after infection

COMPLICATIONS

- Cardiovascular
- Membranous glomerulonephritis
- Paroxysmal cold hemoglobinemia
- Meningitis and tabes dorsalis
- Irreversible organ damage
- Jarisch-Herxheimer reaction:
  - Fever, chills, headache, myalgias, new rash
  - Common when starting treatment (of primary or secondary disease; less common with tertiary) owing to lysis of treponemes
  - Should not be confused with drug reaction
  - Managed with analgesics and antipyretics

REFERENCES

1. U.S. Preventive Services Task Force. Screening for syphilis infection in pregnancy: U.S. Preventive Services Task Force reaffirmation recommendation statement. *Ann Intern Med*. 2009;150:705–9.
2. Centers for Disease Control and Prevention. *Sexually Transmitted Disease Surveillance 2007 Supplement, Syphilis Surveillance Report*. Atlanta, GA: U.S. Department of Health and Human Services, Centers for Disease Control and Prevention, March 2009.
3. Centers for Disease Control and Prevention. *2009 Sexually Transmitted Diseases Surveillance*. Atlanta, GA, November 2010.
4. Koss CA, Dunne EF, Warner L, et al. A systematic review of epidemiologic studies assessing condom use and risk of syphilis. *Sex Transm Dis*. 2009;36: 401–5.
5. CDC Sexually Transmitted Diseases Treatment Guidelines, 2010. *MMWR Weekly*. 2010; 59(RR-12):26–36.

ADDITIONAL READING

- Blank LJ, Rompalo AM, Erbelding EJ, et al. Treatment of syphilis in HIV-infected subjects: A systematic review of the literature. *Sex Transm linfect*. 2011;87(1):9–16.
- Farhi D, Dupin N, et al. Management of syphilis in the HIV-infected patient: Facts and controversies. *Clin Dermatol*. 2010;28:539–45.

See Also (Topic, Algorithm, Electronic Media Element)

Chlamydial Sexually Transmitted Diseases; Gonococcal Infections

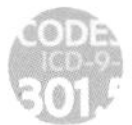

CODES

ICD9

- 091.2 Other primary syphilis
- 091.9 Unspecified secondary syphilis
- 097.9 Syphilis, unspecified

CLINICAL PEARLS

All patients with high-risk activity or HIV-positive status should be screened for syphilis.

SYSTEMIC LUPUS ERYTHEMATOSUS (SLE)

Katherine Tromp, PharmD
Jill A. Grimes, MD

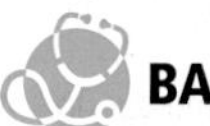

BASICS

DESCRIPTION

- Multisystem autoimmune inflammatory disease characterized by a chronic relapsing/remitting course; can be mild to severe and may be life-threatening (CNS and renal forms)
- System(s) affected: Mucocutaneous; Musculoskeletal; Renal; Nervous; Pulmonary; Cardiac; Hematologic; Vascular; Gastrointestinal
- Synonym(s): SLE; Lupus

ALERT

Women with SLE have a 7–50-fold increased risk of coronary heart disease and may present with atypical or nonspecific symptoms.

EPIDEMIOLOGY

Predominant age: 15–45 years

Incidence

- Per year, 1.6–7.6/100,000
- Most common: African American women (8.1–11.4/100,000 per year)
- Least common: Caucasian men (0.3–0.9/100,000 per year)

Prevalence

Occurs in 30–50/100,000

RISK FACTORS

- Race: African Americans, Hispanics, Asians, and Native Americans
- Females > Males (8:1)
- Environmental factors may include UV light, infectious agents, stress, diet, drugs, hormones, and cigarette smoke.

Genetics

- Identical twins: 24–58% concordance
- Fraternal twins and siblings: 2–5% concordance
- 8-fold risk if first-degree relative with SLE
- Major histocompatability complex associations: HLA-DR2, HLA-DR3
- Deficiency of early complement components, especially C1q, C2, and C4
- Immunoglobulin receptor polymorphisms: FCγR2A and FCγR3A
- Polymorphism in genes associated with regulation of programmed cell death, protein tyrosine kinases, and interferon production

PATHOPHYSIOLOGY

- Skin: Photosensitivity; scaly erythematous, plaques with follicular plugging, dermal atrophy, and scarring; nonscarring erythematous psoriasiform or annular rash; alopecia; mucosal ulcers
- Musculoskeletal: Nonerosive arthritis; ligament and tendon laxity, ulnar deviation, and swan neck deformities; avascular necrosis
- Renal: Glomerulonephritis
- Pulmonary: Pleuritis, pleural effusion, alveolar hemorrhage, pneumonitis, interstitial fibrosis, shrinking lung, pulmonary hypertension, PE
- Cardiac: Nonbacterial verrucous endocarditis, pericarditis, myocarditis, atherosclerosis
- CNS: Thrombosis of small intracranial vessels ± perivascular inflammation resulting in micro/macroinfarcts ± hemorrhage
- PNS: Mononeuritis multiplex, peripheral neuropathy
- GI: Pancreatitis, peritonitis, colitis
- Hematologic: Hemolytic anemia, thrombocytopenia, leukopenia, lymphopenia
- Vascular: Vasculitis, thromboembolism

ETIOLOGY

- Most cases are idiopathic.
- Genetic and environmental factors
- Drug-induced lupus: Hydralazine, quinidine, procainamide, minocycline, isoniazid, TNF-alpha inhibitors, etc.

COMMONLY ASSOCIATED CONDITIONS

- Overlap syndromes: Rheumatoid arthritis (RA), Sjögren syndrome, scleroderma
- Antiphospholipid syndrome
- Coronary heart disease
- Nephritis
- Depression

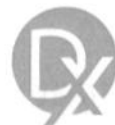

DIAGNOSIS

Consider SLE in multisystem disease including fever, fatigue, and signs of inflammation.

HISTORY

- Fever, fatigue, malaise, weight loss, headache
- Rash (butterfly rash), photosensitivity, alopecia
- Oral or nasal ulcers (usually painless)
- Arthritis, arthralgia, myalgia, weakness
- Pleuritic chest pain, cough, dyspnea, hemoptysis
- Stroke, seizure, psychosis, cognitive deficits
- Proteinuria, cellular casts
- Hemolytic anemia, leukopenia, lymphopenia, thrombocytopenia
- Abdominal pain, anorexia, nausea, vomiting
- Raynaud phenomenon

PHYSICAL EXAM

- Vital signs: Fever, hypertension
- Malar, discoid, psoriasiform, or annular rash, alopecia
- Oral or nasal ulcers
- Lymphadenopathy, splenomegaly
- Acrocyanosis
- Inflammatory arthritis, tenosynovitis
- Pleural or pericardial rub, heart murmur
- Bibasilar rales
- Cranial or peripheral neuropathies

DIAGNOSTIC TESTS & INTERPRETATION

Lab

Initial lab tests

- Antinuclear antibody (ANA):
  - High sensitivity (98%), low specificity
  - False-positive rate of 5–30%: Elderly, autoimmune thyroid/liver disease, chronic infection, etc.
  - Low titers <1:160 of limited clinical utility
- Anti–double-stranded DNA (dsDNA) and anti-Smith antibodies: High specificity for SLE:
  - Correlates with disease activity
- RNA protein antibodies (anti-RNP, anti-Ro, anti-La): Less specific for SLE
- False-positive VDRL: High sensitivity, low specificity. Surrogate marker of cardiolipin antibody presence.
- Low serum complement levels: C3, C4, Ch50
- ESR: Nonspecific, often high in active disease
- CBC: Hemolytic anemia, thrombocytopenia, leukopenia, or lymphopenia
- Serum creatinine: Elevated in lupus nephritis
- Urinalysis: Proteinuria, hematuria, cellular cast
- Phospholipid antibodies: Cardiolipin IgG/IgM, lupus anticoagulant, beta 2 glycoprotein IgG/IgM
- Anti-P (ribosomal autoantibodies) are associated with SLE arthritis and disease activity

Follow-Up & Special Considerations

- Hemolytic anemia: Elevated reticulocyte count and indirect bilirubin, low haptoglobin, positive direct Coombs test
- Confirm positive phospholipid antibodies results in 12 weeks
- 24-hour urine collection or spot protein/creatinine to quantify proteinuria
- Histone antibodies present in >95% of drug-induced lupus (vs. 80% of idiopathic SLE)
- Fasting lipid panel and glucose
- Follow vitamin D25OH levels and replenish as needed

Imaging

Initial approach

- Initial imaging is highly dependent on presenting symptoms
- Radiograph of involved joints
- Chest x-ray: Infiltrates, pleural effusion, low lung volumes
- Chest CT scan, V-Q scan, duplex ultrasound (US) for PE or deep vein thrombosis
- Head CT scan: Ischemia, infarct; hemorrhage
- Brain MRI: Focal areas of increased signal intensity
- Echocardiogram: Pericardial effusion, valvular vegetations, pulmonary hypertension
- Contrast angiography for medium-size artery vasculitis: Mesenteric or limb ischemia, CNS symptom

Diagnostic Procedures/Surgery

- Renal biopsy to diagnose lupus nephritis
- Skin biopsy with immunofluorescence on involved and uninvolved non–sun-exposed skin (*lupus band test*) may help differentiate SLE rash from others
- Lumbar puncture in patients with fever and CNS or meningeal symptoms
- EEG for seizures or global CNS dysfunction
- Neuropsychiatric testing for cognitive impairment
- EMG/NCS for peripheral neuropathy and myositis
- Nerve and/or muscle biopsy
- ECG, cardiac enzymes, stress tests
- American College of Rheumatology classification (not diagnostic) criteria: Any 4 of the 11 listed (95% specificity and 85% sensitivity):
  - Malar (butterfly) rash
  - Discoid rash
  - Photosensitivity: By patient history or physician observation
  - Oral/nasopharyngeal ulcers
  - Nonerosive arthritis: Involving 2 or more peripheral joints
  - Pleuritis OR pericarditis
  - Renal disorder: Proteinuria (>0.5 g/d or >3+) or cellular casts (red cell, hemoglobin, granular, tubular, or mixed)
  - Neurologic disorder: Psychosis or seizures
  - Hematologic disorder: Hemolytic anemia, leukopenia (<4,000/mm^3 on ≥2 tests),

lymphopenia (<1,500/mm^3 on ≥2 tests), thrombocytopenia (<100,000/mm^3)
  - Immunologic disorder: Anti-DNA, anti-Sm, anticardiolipin IgG/IgM, lupus anticoagulant, or false-positive VDRL
  - Positive ANA in absence of drugs known to cause positive ANA

Pathological Findings

- Skin: Vascular/perivascular inflammation, immune-complex deposition at dermal–epidermal junction, mucinosis, basal layer vacuolar changes:
  - Similar findings seen in other connective tissue disorders such as dermatomyositis
- Renal: Mesangial hypercellularity or matrix expansion, subendothelial/subepithelial immune deposits, glomerular sclerosis, fibrous crescents
  - Vary depending on degree of involvement
- Vascular: Immune-complex deposition in vessel walls with fibrinoid necrosis and perivascular mononuclear cell infiltrates, intraluminal fibrin thrombi

DIFFERENTIAL DIAGNOSIS

Undifferentiated connective tissue disease, Sjögren syndrome, fibromyalgia, RA, vasculitis, idiopathic thrombocytopenia purpura, antiphospholipid antibody syndrome, drug-induced lupus, and so on

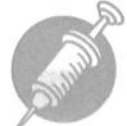

TREATMENT

MEDICATION

First Line

- *Antimalarial agents and NSAIDs are first-line therapy for patients with mild SLE* (1)[A]:
  - Hydroxychloroquine for constitutional and musculoskeletal symptoms, rash, mild serositis; may reduce flares and increase long-term survival (2,3)[A]. Chloroquine also is effective; however, it is associated with more side effects (3)[A].
  - NSAIDs for musculoskeletal manifestations, mild serositis, headache, and fever (2,4)[C]
- Systemic glucocorticoids (prednisone or equivalent):
  - Low dose (<0.5 mg/kg) for minor disease activity not responsive to NSAIDs or when NSAIDs are contraindicated (2)[A]
  - High dose (1–2 mg/kg/d) (2)[A] or IV pulse methylprednisolone (4)[C] for organ-threatening disease, particularly CNS and renal; often combined with immunosuppressive agent (2)[A]
- Topical or intralesional glucocorticosteroids for skin manifestations

Second Line

- Methotrexate (2)[A], azathioprine (2)[B] mycophenolate mofetil (2)[C], or leflunomide as steroid-sparing agent for persistent active disease or to maintain remission:
  - Require periodic laboratory monitoring for toxicity
- Belimumab as adjunct for preventing flares (5)[A]
- Biologic treatments under investigation: Rituximab, epratuzumab, abatacept, interferon-α inhibitors, abetimus sodium (LJP 394), prasterone (4)
- Immunosuppressive agents for severe disease:
  - Cyclophosphamide (2)[A]: Ensure adequate hydration to reduce risk of hemorrhagic cystitis
  - Mycophenolate mofetil (2)[A]: More efficacious for lupus nephritis (1)[A]

ADDITIONAL TREATMENT

General Measures

- Education, counseling, and support
- Influenza/pneumococcus vaccines are safe; avoid live vaccines in immunocompromised patients.
- Low-estrogen oral contraceptives safe in mild SLE (2)[A]

COMPLEMENTARY AND ALTERNATIVE MEDICINE

Biofeedback, visual imagery, cognitive therapy

SURGERY/OTHER PROCEDURES

Renal transplant for end-stage renal disease (2)[B]

IN-PATIENT CONSIDERATIONS

Initial Stabilization

- Difficult to differentiate SLE flare from infection; may need to treat both pending full evaluation
- IV pulse Solu-Medrol 1 g/d × 3–5 days for life- or organ-threatening disease (2)[A]

Admission Criteria

- Severe acute or rapidly progressive disease involving any organ system
- Fever, sepsis; acute coronary syndrome

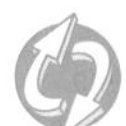

ONGOING CARE

FOLLOW-UP RECOMMENDATIONS

Patient Monitoring

- Clinical evaluation for signs and symptoms:
  - Weekly to monthly for active disease
  - Every 3–6 months for mild or inactive disease
- Measures of disease activity and damage: Systemic Lupus Erythematosus Disease Activity Index, British Isles Lupus Assessment Group Index, European Consensus Lupus Activity Measure
- Laboratory studies:
  - CBC with differential
  - Serum creatinine, urinalysis
  - Declining C3 or C4 and rising DS-DNA and ESR may correlate with disease activity (2)[B].
- Monitor for adverse effects of treatment:
  - NSAIDs: GI bleeding and/or ulceration
  - Glucocorticoids: Glucose, lipids, bone density
  - Hydroxychloroquine: Ophthalmologic exam every 6–12 months
  - Methotrexate: CBC, creatinine, albumin, AST, ALT every 2 months
  - Azathioprine and mycophenolate mofetil: CBC every 1–3 months
  - Cyclophosphamide:
    - CBC, creatinine, urinalysis every 2 weeks and liver function tests monthly during treatment
    - Urinalysis every 6–12 months for life

DIET

- No special diet unless for complications, such as renal failure, diabetes, hyperlipidemia (2)[C]
- Adequate calcium/vitamin D intake in patients on corticosteroids (2)[A]

PATIENT EDUCATION

- Avoid UV light exposure: Sunscreens (SPF ≥30), protective clothing (2)[B]
- Weight control, smoking cessation, exercise (2)[C]
- Stress avoidance/management

PROGNOSIS

- Permanent treatment-free remission is uncommon.
- 5-year survival after diagnosis is 95%.
- Poor prognostic factor: Major organ involvement
- Drug-induced lupus resolves within weeks to months after discontinuation of the offending drug.

COMPLICATIONS

Infections, neoplasms, cardiac disease, nephritis, neuropsychiatric lupus

Pregnancy Considerations

- Exacerbations during pregnancy are less common when in remission for 6 months prior to conception.
- Fetal loss is increased, especially in those with active lupus or antiphospholipid antibodies.
- There is a 2% risk of congenital heart block if anti-SS-A (Ro) or anti-SS-B (La) antibodies are present.
- See "Antiphospholipid Antibody Syndrome" for recommendations regarding use of aspirin and heparin to prevent pregnancy complications.

REFERENCES

1. Yildirim-Toruner C, Diamond B, et al. Current and novel therapeutics in the treatment of systemic lupus erythematosus. *J Allergy Clin Immunol*. 2011;127.
2. Bertsias G, Ioannidis JP, Boletis J. EULAR recommendations for the management of systemic lupus erythematosus. Report of a Task Force of the EULAR Standing Committee for International Clinical Studies Including Therapeutics. *Ann Rheum Dis*. 2008;67:195–205.
3. Ruiz-Irastorza G, Ramos-Casals M, Brito-Zeron P. Clinical efficacy and side effects of antimalarials in systemic lupus erythematosus: A systematic review. *Ann Rheum Dis*. 2010;69(1):20–8.
4. Kalunian K, Joan TM. New directions in the treatment of systemic lupus erythematosus. *Curr Med Res Opin*. 2009;25:1501–14.
5. Sandra V , Navarra SV, Guzman RM, et al. Efficacy and safety of belimumab in patients with active systemic lupus erythematosus: A randomised, placebo-controlled, phase 3 trial. *Lancet*. 2011;377:721–31.

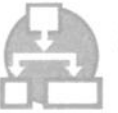

See Also (Topic, Algorithm, Electronic Media Element)

Antiphospholipid Antibody Syndrome

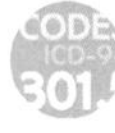

CODES

ICD9

- 710.0 Systemic lupus erythematosus
- E947.9 Unspecified drug or medicinal substance causing adverse effects in therapeutic use

CLINICAL PEARLS

- SLE is a multisystem inflammatory autoimmune disease that preferentially affects women during the child-bearing years.
- Atherosclerotic and atheroembolic complications are the major cause of death, so identify and treat risk factors.
- ANA has 5–30% false positives; low titers <1:160 of limited clinical utility

TARDIVE DYSKINESIA

Lawrence E. Udom, MD, MPH

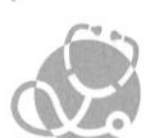

BASICS

DESCRIPTION

- A neurologic syndrome with the essential features of abnormal, involuntary movements of the tongue, lips, face, trunk, and extremities
- Most commonly associated with long-term treatment with dopamine receptor antagonists, (e.g., neuroleptic medications and metoclopramide.)
- Movements can include grimacing, sticking out the tongue, and smacking and sucking the lips. Within a given patient, movements have choreiform characteristics (i.e., rapid, jerky, or nonrepetitive), athetoid characteristics (i.e., slow, sinuous, continual), or rhythmic characteristics.
- Tardive dyskinesia (TD) symptoms can begin during treatment with neuroleptics or within 4 weeks of discontinuing neuroleptics. TD can be mild, moderate, or severe.
- System(s) affected: Nervous; musculoskeletal
- Synonym(s): Orofacial dyskinesia

EPIDEMIOLOGY

TD rates for patients beginning treatment with conventional antipsychotics in their fifth decade or later are 3–5 times those found for younger patients, despite treatment with lower doses.

Incidence

- Predominant age: Occurs in all ages; however, advanced age is a major risk factor for TD.
- Predominant sex: Male = Female, until advanced years, when female > male
- In studies that used haloperidol as predominant classical antipsychotic:
  - Younger patients (<55 years) taking classic antipsychotics have a 5% incidence of developing TD per year of use, with a 50–60% incidence of development over their lifetime.
  - Older patients (>60 years) have a ~20% incidence rate after 1 year of exposure, moving to 30% and nearly 50% at 2- and 3-year exposures, respectively.
  - Annualized incidence of TD was 3.9% for those taking second-generation antipsychotics and 5.5% for those taking first-generation antipsychotics.

Prevalence

Overall estimated prevalence of 15–25% of TD within 5 years of continuous classic antipsychotic use

RISK FACTORS

- Use of classic antipsychotics:
  - Haloperidol (Haldol)
  - Chlorpromazine (Thorazine)
  - Fluphenazine (Permitil, Prolixin)
  - Thioridazine (Mellaril)
  - Perphenazine (Trilafon)
  - Trifluoperazine (Stelazine)
  - Pimozide (Orap)
  - Thiothixene (Navane)
  - Molindone (Moban)
  - A few of the new class of atypical antipsychotics have been linked to TD, although in lower incidences than noted with the older medications:
    - Quetiapine (Seroquel)
    - Olanzapine (Zyprexa)
    - Risperidone (Risperdal)
- Length of neuroleptic use
- Older age: The most significant risk factor
- Postmenopausal women
- Mental retardation
- Alcoholism and substance abuse
- Extrapyramidal symptoms early in the course of neuroleptic treatment
- Presence of other movement disorders
- Diabetes mellitus
- Mood disorders (particularly major depressive disorder)

Geriatric Considerations

Occurs in all ages; however, advancing age is a major risk factor for TD.

Genetics

- No definitive data indicate a genetic basis for TD; however, recent research suggests a possible association with a polymorphic variant of the Ser9Gly *DRD3* gene and severe TD.
- Also, the absence of a glutathione *S*-transferase gene was associated with TD, particularly among white women (1).
- There have been associations with the polymorphism of the *dopamine receptor* D_2 gene, *TaqI A* and *TaqI B,* and associated haplotypes that may contribute to the development of TD (2).

GENERAL PREVENTION

- Choosing an atypical neuroleptic as first-line therapy statistically reduces the risk of developing TD (3)[A].
- If traditional neuroleptics must be used, limit long-term use and use the lowest effective doses with frequent patient assessments.

PATHOPHYSIOLOGY

- The mechanism by which TD occurs is still under debate. Antipsychotics (both traditional and atypical) have a high affinity for the D_2 receptors. It is postulated that the long-term blockade of these receptors leads to an upregulation in the number and sensitivity of D_2 receptors in the striated region of the brain (which controls muscle coordination). This upregulation is associated with involuntary movements and hence TD.
- It also has been postulated that the depletion of gamma-aminobutyric acid (GABA) in the substantia nigra may lead to orofacial dyskinesia, as may excess free radicals.

ETIOLOGY

Prolonged use of dopamine antagonist drugs:

- Traditional antipsychotics
- Atypical antipsychotics
- Metoclopramide (Reglan), prochlorperazine (Compazine), antiemetics with potent D_2 antagonism
- Antimalarials (Chloroquine)
- Antiparkinson agents (bromocriptine, levodopa, and combined levodopa and carbidopa [Sinemet])
- Lithium
- Stimulants (amphetamine, methylphenidate, caffeine)

COMMONLY ASSOCIATED CONDITIONS

- Presence of movement disorder
- Psychiatric disorders commonly treated with neuroleptics

DIAGNOSIS

HISTORY

- Diagnosis of TD is clinical, upon exclusion of other etiologies; there must be a history of dopaminergic blockade (most commonly antipsychotics), use for at least 3 months (or 1 month if individual's age ≥60 years), and the presence of dyskinetic or dystonic involuntary movements.
- TD must be distinguished from other movement disorders.
- Abnormal movements must not be due to a neurologic condition or other general medical conditions (e.g., Huntington disease, Sydenham chorea, spontaneous dyskinesia, hyperthyroidism, heavy-metal poisoning, Wilson disease), ill-fitting dentures, or exposure to other medications that can cause acute reversible dyskinesia (e.g., L-dopa, bromocriptine, amantadine, Sinemet, Adderall, Ritalin, and Compazine).
- Other neuroleptic-induced movement disorders must be ruled out (e.g., tardive tourettism, blepharospasm, tardive akathisia, tardive myoclonus, tardive tremor, and tardive dystonia), as well as spontaneous dyskinesias and mental disorders.
- Question patient about a history of neurologic disorders that may involve the basal ganglia (e.g., cerebrovascular accident, encephalitis, head trauma, neoplasms).
- Attempt to elicit a family history for hereditary dyskinesias (e.g., Huntington disease).
- Ask about medication usage, particularly aforementioned medications. *Note:* Neuroleptics can mask TD, thus explaining onset after discontinuation of medication.

PHYSICAL EXAM

- Abnormal, involuntary movements of the tongue, lips, and extremities; facial grimacing; and swaying movements of the trunk or hips
- In 1 major report:
  - 75% of individuals with TD had orofacial dyskinesia.
  - 50% had limb dyskinesia.
  - 25% had axial dyskinesia.
  - 10% had total-body involvement.
- Orofacial dyskinesia is common in the ≥60 population.
- Limb + axial dyskinesia is more common in the younger population (1,3).
- These signs and symptoms must occur while taking neuroleptics or within 4 or 8 weeks of withdrawal from an oral or depot neuroleptic medication, respectively.
- The signs typically are minimal to mild in nature and progress in severity with prolonged use.

DIAGNOSTIC TESTS & INTERPRETATION

Lab

Only used to rule out other causes

Initial lab tests

- Rule out Wilson disease: Low serum ceruloplasmin due to an abnormal copper transporter gene and elevated 24-hour urine copper collection; in addition, liver function tests and liver transaminases may be abnormal, along with elevated hepatic copper levels. Also, check the copper transporter gene in patients in whom Wilson disease is suspected.
- Thyroid-stimulating hormone, calcium, syphilis serology
- Connective-tissue disease screening tests (CBC, ESR, urinalysis, chemistry panel, rheumatoid factor, antinuclear antibodies) are useful to exclude systemic lupus erythematosus and other vasculitides.
- Obtain RBC counts to exclude polycythemia rubra vera.

Imaging

May be done to rule out other causes

Diagnostic Procedures/Surgery

Screen for dyskinetic movements before initiating antipsychotics, at regular scheduled intervals (e.g., every 6 months). Several questionnaires elicit this information and rate TD on a severity scale; the most commonly used is the Abnormal Involuntary Movement Scale.

DIFFERENTIAL DIAGNOSIS

- Huntington disease
- Sydenham chorea
- Spontaneous dyskinesia
- Wilson disease
- Thyrotoxicosis
- Blepharospasm
- Tardive akathisia
- Tardive dystonia
- Physical signs may point the way to another diagnosis:
  - Tachycardia, sweating, and a goiter suggest thyrotoxicosis.
  - Jaundice, hepatomegaly, or Kayser-Fleischer rings suggest a workup for Wilson disease.
- Dementia in addition to the movement disorder (chorea) and postural instability requires a workup for Huntington disease.

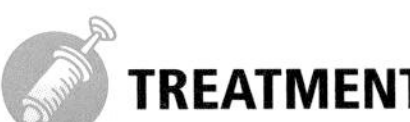

TREATMENT

MEDICATION

First Line

Cessation of neuroleptic or metoclopramide use upon identifying TD. Therapies have produced no more than a modest improvement in TD symptoms, so prevention and early detection are the best treatment options.

Second Line

- No definitive treatment for TD
- Replace any traditional antipsychotic with an atypical (Risperdal, olanzapine, quetiapine, ziprasidone, and clozapine) (4).
- Some evidence suggests that the use of clozapine has been effective in diminishing involuntary movements in patients with TD:
  - Some studies have shown remission of TD in up to 34% of patients after treatment with clozapine for 6–12 months (5)[A]. This improvement in symptoms possibly is secondary to the downregulation of sensitized D_2 receptors.
  - However, the side effect of clozapine (i.e., agranulocytosis) prevents it from being a first-line medication.
- As a last resort, the clinician may resume the antipsychotic agent in an attempt to suppress TD; this usually is done in those patients with life-threatening or permanent TD that has been shown to be treatment resistant.

ADDITIONAL TREATMENT

Use of Zofran (Ondansetron), a selective 5-hydroxytryptamine-3 antagonist, has been shown to help some individuals with TD (6)[B].

COMPLEMENTARY AND ALTERNATIVE MEDICINE

- Vitamin E, a free-radical scavenger, has been found in a number of studies to reduce the severity of TD, though more recent studies suggest it is indicated primarily for newly diagnosed TD (7)[A].
- Benzodiazepines provide GABA agonistic effects. This helps in some patients with TD; however, it can be sedating and has abuse potential.
- Branched-chain amino acids mix (Tarvil) was shown in 1 study to be superior to placebo in treating TD at a dosage of 222 mg/kg t.i.d.
- Botulinum toxin has been recommended for localized forms of TD such as cervical dystonia, blepharospasm, or retrocollis. This is not without its own adverse effects (e.g., excessive muscle weakness) and should avoided in patients with neuromuscular conditions.

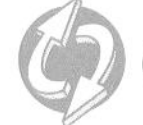

ONGOING CARE

FOLLOW-UP RECOMMENDATIONS

Patient Monitoring

- Instruct patients and family members to watch for the subtle early signs.
- Warn that TD may be exacerbated by stimulant use (Ritalin, Adderall), neuroleptic withdrawal, and anticholinergics.
- Symptoms are affected by emotional states and stress.

PROGNOSIS

TD can be mild to moderate, with resolution of symptoms after a period of discontinuation from the offending drug. In rare incidences, TD may be severe and irreversible.

REFERENCES

1. de Leon J, Susce MT, Pan RM, et al. Polymorphic variations in GSTM1, GSTT1, PgP, CYP2D6, CYP3A5, and dopamine D2 and D3 receptors and their association with tardive dyskinesia in severe mental illness. *J Clin Psychopharmacol*. 2005;25: 448–56.
2. Liou YJ, Lai IC, Liao DL, et al. The human dopamine receptor D2 (DRD2) gene is associated with tardive dyskinesia in patients with schizophrenia. *Schizophr Res*. 2006;86:323–5.
3. American Psychiatric Association. *DSM-IV-TR 2000: Diagnostic & Statistical Manual of Mental Disorders*, 4th ed. Washington DC: American Psychiatric Publishing; 2000.
4. Caroff SN, Mann SC, Campbell EC, et al. Movement disorders associated with atypical antipsychotic drugs. *J Clin Psychiatry*. 2002;63(Suppl 4):12–9.
5. Lieberman JA, Saltz BL, Johns CA, et al. The effects of clozapine on tardive dyskinesia. *Br J Psychiatry*. 1991;158:503–10.
6. Zullino DF, Eap CB, Voirol P. Ondansetron for tardive dyskinesia. *Am J Psychiatry*. 2001;158: 657–8.
7. Pham DQ, Plakogiannis R, et al. Vitamin E supplementation in Alzheimer's disease, Parkinson's disease, tardive dyskinesia, and cataract: Part 2. *Ann Pharmacother*. 2005;39: 2065–72.
8. Correll CU, Schenk EM. Tardive dyskinesia and new antipsychotics. *Curr Opin Psychiatry*. 2008;21: 151–6.

ADDITIONAL READING

- Ormerod S, McDowell SE, Coleman JJ, et al. Ethnic differences in the risks of adverse reactions to drugs used in the treatment of psychoses and depression: A systematic review and meta-analysis. *Drug Saf*. 2008;31:597–607.
- Woerner MG, Alvir JM, Saltz BL, et al. Prospective study of tardive dyskinesia in the elderly: Rates and risk factors. *Am J Psychiatry*. 1998;155:1521–8.

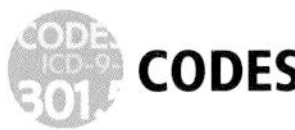

CODES

ICD9

- 333.82 Orofacial dyskinesia
- 333.85 Subacute dyskinesia due to drugs

CLINICAL PEARLS

- Second-generation antipsychotics have a lower incidence of TD than first-generation medications (8)[A].
- Ensure that oral dyskinesias are not triggered by ill-fitting dentures.
- The older the patient, the higher the risk for TD from antipsychotics.
- Remember that TD can begin after the discontinuation of antipsychotics (up to 4 weeks).
- Use the minimum effective dosage and duration.

TARSAL TUNNEL SYNDROME

Chris Graves, MD
Douglas A. Pepple, MD

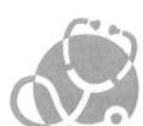

BASICS

DESCRIPTION

Tarsal tunnel syndrome is a compression neuropathy of the posterior tibial nerve as it passes under the flexor retinaculum in the medial ankle; a region commonly known as "the tarsal tunnel."

Pregnancy Considerations

- Tarsal tunnel syndrome can occur during pregnancy, typically secondary to local compression caused by fluid retention and volume changes.
- Care usually is supportive until after delivery because many cases resolve after pregnancy.

EPIDEMIOLOGY

Women are slightly more affected than men (56%). Individuals in all postpubescent ages can be affected.

RISK FACTORS

Several authors have associated tarsal tunnel syndrome with certain occupations and activities, especially those that involve repetitive weight bearing on the foot and ankle, like jogging (1) or dancing (2).

PATHOPHYSIOLOGY

- Tarsal tunnel syndrome is caused by compression of the tibial nerve, resulting in decreased blood flow and ischemic damage.
- Increased pressure in the confined space of the tarsal tunnel is caused by a variety of mechanisms, both mechanical and biochemical, all of which result in increased pressure on the posterior tibial nerve.
- Chronic compression can destroy endoneurial microvasculature, leading to edema and eventually fibrosis and demyelination (3).

ETIOLOGY

- The specific cause is identifiable in only 60–80% of patients (4); causes can be grouped into 3 categories: Trauma, space-occupying lesion, and deformity.
- Most common causes include (4):
  - Trauma
  - Varicosities
  - Hindfoot varus or valgus
  - Fibrosis of the perineurium
- Other causes of compression include ganglia, lipoma, neurilemmoma, inflammatory synovitis, pigmented villonodular synovitis, tarsal coalition, and accessory musculature.

DIAGNOSIS

Frequently misdiagnosed because of poorly localized and variable symptoms

HISTORY

- Often have history of trauma to foot, including trivial trauma that precipitated pain
- Classically, pain and paresthesia on plantar aspect of foot
- Pain usually worsens during standing or activity
- Pain can radiate proximally up medial leg (Valleix phenomenon) in 33% of patients with severe compression or distally along the path of involved nerves (4).
- Some patients have substantial night pain, which may be related to venostasis.
- Symptoms improve with rest, wearing loose footwear, and elevation.

ALERT

Other neuropathies due to systemic causes such as diabetes, alcoholism, HIV, or drug reactions can present with similar symptoms.

PHYSICAL EXAM

- Perform a complete foot and ankle examination.
- Foot alignment:
  - Examine for hindfoot varus or valgus abnormalities.
  - Exaggerating heel dorsiflexion, inversion, or eversion may reproduce symptoms by stretching or compressing the nerve.
- Palpate the tarsal tunnel and the course of the tibial nerve for:
  - Tenderness
  - Swelling consistent with a space-occupying lesion
- Tinel sign: Percussion over the course of the tibial nerve may produce paresthesias and distal symptoms.
- Cuff test: Using a pneumatic cuff to create a venous tourniquet may cause engorgement of varicosities and reproduce symptoms.
- Compression test: Applying pressure to the tarsal tunnel for 60 seconds may reproduce symptoms.
- Sensory examination:
  - The medial calcaneal nerve usually is spared, but numbness and altered sensation may be present in the distribution of the medial plantar nerve or lateral plantar nerve).
  - 2-point discrimination is decreased early in the disease process.
- Motor examination:
  - Intrinsic weakness is difficult to assess.
  - Rarely, weakness of toe plantarflexion may be present.
  - Atrophy of the abductor hallucis or abductor digiti minimi may be seen late in the disease process.

DIAGNOSTIC TESTS & INTERPRETATION

Lab

Routine laboratory tests can be used to rule out other conditions that may mimic tarsal tunnel syndrome, including diabetic neuropathy, thyroid dysfunction, or other systemic illnesses (5).

Imaging

- Routine weight-bearing radiographs, followed by CT if necessary to assess for fracture or structural abnormality
- Consider evaluation of lumbar spine x-ray if "double-crush" (injury to lumbar nerve results in compensatory injury to posterior tibial nerve) is suspected (5).
- MRI: Can be helpful in assessing the tarsal tunnel for masses or other sources of nerve compression before surgery (4)
- Ultrasound: Alternatively, ultrasound can be used to check for synovitis or ganglia (5).

Pediatric Considerations

MRI is recommended for evaluating pediatric tarsal tunnel syndrome because compression by a neoplastic mass is not uncommon.

Follow-Up & Special Considerations

Postoperative management includes:

- Non–weight-bearing splint until incision heals (2–3 weeks), followed by progressively increased weight-bearing and range of motion exercises
- RICE protocol (rest, ice, compression, elevation) to limit swelling

Diagnostic Procedures/Surgery

Electrodiagnostic studies (4):

- According to a systematic review in 2005, electromyography (EMG) can be used only to confirm the diagnosis of tarsal tunnel syndrome because there is a large percentage of asymptomatic people with abnormal results.
- It is important to evaluate for proximal nerve compression, including a lumbar radiculopathy or a double-crush phenomenon.

Pathological Findings

At the time of surgical exploration, the following may be found:

- Focal swelling, scarring, or nerve abnormalities
- A pathologic source of compression

DIFFERENTIAL DIAGNOSIS

- Peripheral neuropathies (diabetes, alcoholism, HIV, or drug related)
- Inflammatory arthritis (rheumatoid arthritis) (6)
- Morton neuroma
- Metatarsalgia
- Subtalar joint arthritis
- Tibialis posterior tendinitis/dysfunction
- Plantar fasciitis
- Plantar callosities
- Peripheral vascular disease
- Lumbar radiculopathy
- Proximal injury or compression of the tibial branch of the sciatic nerve

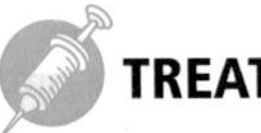

TREATMENT

Conservative management is recommended, except for tarsal tunnel syndrome of acute onset or in the setting of a known space-occupying lesion:

- Rest/immobilization
- Taping and bracing
- Orthotics or shoe modification
- Anti-inflammatories (steroid injections vs. NSAIDs)
- Medications to alter neurogenic pain (antidepressants, antiepileptic drugs, nerve blocks)
- Physical therapy for desensitization (stretching, ultrasound, massage, icing)
- Physical therapy to strengthen the intrinsic and extrinsic muscles of the foot and to restore the medial longitudinal arch
- Compression stockings to decrease swelling
- Weight loss in obese patients

MEDICATION

Initially, nonoperative management is recommended, except for acute tarsal tunnel syndrome or in the setting of a known space-occupying lesion (excluding synovitis):

- Rest/immobilization
- Orthotics
- Anti-inflammatories, including steroid injections and nonsteroidal drugs
- Medications that alter neurogenic pain (tricyclic antidepressants, antiepileptic drugs, nerve blockers)
- Physical therapy (desensitization)
- Compression stockings
- Weight loss

SURGERY/OTHER PROCEDURES

- Surgery is indicated (3,4,7):
  - If nonoperative measures fail following a 3–6-month trial
  - In the setting of acute tarsal tunnel syndrome
  - If a space-occupying lesion is identified
- The surgical outcome is dependent on technique and postoperative management. The ability to achieve a good to excellent outcome ranges from 50–95%.

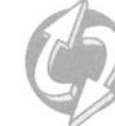

ONGOING CARE

PATIENT EDUCATION

An outline of the conservative care modalities available should be presented. Use of each of these therapies will depend on patient circumstance. A decision about surgical intervention should be made with a clear understanding of limitations of this treatment and the potential adverse outcomes.

PROGNOSIS

The most symptomatic improvement with surgery is expected for (4):

- Young patients
- Short duration of symptoms
- Localized space-occupying lesion identified (7)
- No motor neuron involvement
- Surgical outcomes are dependent on technique and postoperative management.

COMPLICATIONS

- The main adverse outcome is unsuccessful surgical intervention: No improvement, partial/incomplete improvement, or temporary improvement with recurrence of symptoms (4)
- Causes for a failed tarsal tunnel release:
  - Incorrect diagnosis
  - Incomplete release
  - Adhesive neuritis (external scar formation)
  - Intraneural damage (systemic disease, direct nerve injury)
  - Failure to treat all sources of nerve compression in a double-crush phenomenon
- Electrodiagnostic studies are rarely helpful in determining the cause of a failed tarsal tunnel release.
- Revision surgery results are poorer than for the primary surgical release.

REFERENCES

1. Shapiro BE, Preston DC. Entrapment and compressive neuropathies. *Med Clin North Am*. 2009;93:285–315, vii.
2. Kennedy JG, Baxter DE. Nerve disorders in dancers. *Clin Sports Med*. 2008;27:329–34.
3. Dellon AL. The four medial ankle tunnels: A critical review of perceptions of tarsal tunnel syndrome and neuropathy. *Neurosurg Clin N Am*. 2008;19: 629–48.
4. Lau JT, Daniels TR. Tarsal tunnel syndrome: A review of the literature. *Foot Ankle Int*. 1999;20: 201–9.
5. Franson J, Baravarian B. Tarsal tunnel syndrome: A compression neuropathy involving four distinct tunnels. *Clin Podiatr Med Surg*. 2006;23:597–609.
6. Campbell WW, Landau ME. Controversial entrapment neuropathies. *Neurosurg Clin N Am*. 2008;19:597–608.
7. Sung KS, Park SJ, et al. Short-term operative outcome of tarsal tunnel syndrome due to benign space-occupying lesions. *Foot Ankle Int*. 2009;30: 741–5.

ADDITIONAL READING

- Allen JM, Greer BJ, Sorge DG, et al. MR imaging of neuropathies of the leg, ankle, and foot. *Magn Reson Imaging Clin N Am*. 2008;16:117–31.
- Patel AT, Gaines K, Malamut R, et al. Usefulness of electrodiagnostic techniques in the evaluation of suspected tarsal tunnel syndrome: An evidencebased review. *Muscle Nerve*. 2005;32:236–40.

T

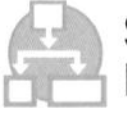

See Also (Topic, Algorithm, Electronic Media Element)

Algorithm: Foot Pain

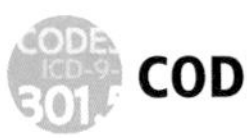

CODES

ICD9

355.5 Tarsal tunnel syndrome

CLINICAL PEARLS

- Tinel sign: Percussion over the course of the tibial nerve produces paresthesias and distal symptoms over the plantar aspect of the foot (most sensitive and specific test) (3).
- Conservative management is recommended, except for tarsal tunnel syndrome of acute onset or in the setting of a known space-occupying lesion.
- EMG abnormality alone cannot be used to diagnose tarsal tunnel syndrome; it may only be used to confirm clinical diagnosis.

TEETHING

Jennifer E. Frank, MD

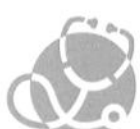

BASICS

DESCRIPTION

- Teething is the eruption of the primary or deciduous teeth, which most children experience without difficulty. It is a natural, gradual, and predictable process, with normal variation among infants.
- Primary (deciduous) teeth:
  - Primary tooth eruption usually begins at 5–7 months of age.
  - The order of primary tooth eruption and average age is:
    - Central mandibular incisors (5–7 months)
    - Central maxillary incisors (6–8 months)
    - Lateral mandibular incisors (7–10 months)
    - Lateral maxillary incisors (8–11 months)
    - Cuspids (16–20 months)
    - First molars (10–16 months)
    - Second molars (20–30 months)
  - Delayed eruption may be familial or due to systemic syndromes or nutritional deficiencies. Delayed eruption may also be seen with cleft palate (1) and lower birth weight (2,3).
  - Tooth eruption in premature infants occurs according to postconceptual age rather than age since birth (chronological age).
  - Natal/neonatal teeth:
    - Natal teeth (present at birth) occur in 1/2,000 neonates.
    - Neonatal teeth erupt in the first month of life.
    - Natal/neonatal teeth are most often prematurely erupted primary (deciduous) teeth, but may be supernumerary.
    - 15–20% of cases are familial; also may be secondary to a syndrome or congenital anomalies of the head and neck.
    - Natal/neonatal teeth may be loose, but most are the normal deciduous lower central incisors and can persist.
    - Natal/neonatal teeth may be removed if there is an aspiration risk or if they cause trauma to the infant or to the mother (breast-feeding).
- System(s) affected: Gastrointestinal

EPIDEMIOLOGY

Incidence

Predominant age: Birth–3 years of age

RISK FACTORS

Genetics

Both premature and delayed tooth eruption may be familial. Primary failure of eruption has been linked to mutations of the PTHR1 gene (4).

COMMONLY ASSOCIATED CONDITIONS

Teething may be coincident with other conditions, such as common childhood illnesses (e.g., roseola, viral gastroenteritis, upper respiratory infection) and serious bacterial infections, causing local or systemic signs and symptoms (e.g., fever, GI disturbance, fussiness, drooling, rash, and sleep disturbance).

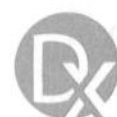

DIAGNOSIS

HISTORY

- Biting
- Drooling
- Rubbing of gingivae
- Sucking
- Irritability
- Wakefulness
- Ear rubbing
- Facial rash
- Decreased appetite for solid foods

PHYSICAL EXAM

- Infants may have no signs or symptoms of teething, although symptoms are present in a majority of children (5).
- Excessive drooling and chewing on fingers begins at 3–4 months of age. This is also the time that normal hand–mouth stimulation increases salivation.
- Discomfort may be observed more commonly with the eruption of the first tooth, the molars, and/or with the simultaneous eruption of multiple teeth.
- Minor signs and symptoms of biting or chewing, drooling, irritability, facial rash, and low-grade fever (<38.9°C) have been reported in association with teething, although no evidence identifies specific signs/symptoms caused by teething (6)[B].
- Serious signs and symptoms (e.g., fever >38.9°C, dehydration) are not caused by teething and warrant evaluation for organic disease (6,7,8,9)[B].
- A small red or white spot may appear over the swollen gingivae just prior to tooth eruption.
- Local inflammation, swelling, or hematoma (bluish swelling) can be found on the involved gingivae overlying the erupting tooth.

DIAGNOSTIC TESTS & INTERPRETATION

Imaging

Radiographs can distinguish prematurely erupted primary teeth from supernumerary teeth.

DIFFERENTIAL DIAGNOSIS

Herpetic gingivostomatitis: Infants with fever, irritability, sleeplessness, and difficulty feeding may have underlying infection caused by herpes simplex virus. Some infants with positive culture may not have evidence of inflammation or ulceration expected in gingivostomatitis.

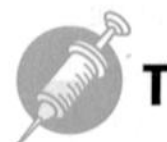

TREATMENT

MEDICATION

First Line

For an infant with low-grade fever, irritability, and/or inflamed gingivae (where other comforting measures have not been of help), acetaminophen in proper doses (15 mg/kg/dose q4–6h PRN) can be used.

Second Line

- Topical analgesics are commonly used by parents (5).
- Over-the-counter preparations for teething, such as lidocaine (Xylocaine 2%, Baby Ora-Gel, Num-zit Gel, Num-zit Liquid, Baby Anbesol), should be used with caution. Misuse, overuse, toxicity, and sensitivity have been reported (10):
  - These are of questionable benefit because they are washed off quickly by saliva, and the benefit may be due in part to the pressure placed on the gingivae when applied (11).
  - If used, care should be taken to select the infant formulation, because some products also come in adult strength.

Pediatric Considerations

Recently, the FDA issued a warning about a possible effect of benzocaine, found in over-the-counter teething gels, causing methemoglobinemia (12).

ADDITIONAL TREATMENT

Infants can be taught not to bite or chew while breast-feeding.

General Measures

- Education of mothers regarding common symptoms of teething and management options resulted in decreased use of pharmacologic treatment and increased use of other methods such as rubbing the gums (13).
- Treatment includes reassurance and symptomatic treatment.
- Provide the infant with a safe, 1-piece teething ring, clean cloth, or pacifier for gumming.
- Apply pressure over involved swollen gingivae with a clean finger or piece of wet gauze.
- May use cool (but not frozen) fluids, cold teething rings, or cold vegetables such as a peeled cucumber
- Avoid the use of alcohol (historically rubbed on gingivae for an analgesic effect).
- Gingival hematomas that erupt appear as blue cysts. Most do not require medical intervention. Be sure there are no other signs of a bleeding disorder.
- Avoid:
  - Dipping a pacifier or teething ring in sugar or honey
  - Giving an infant a bottle in bed
  - Using fluid-filled teething rings (contents may leak)
  - Using frozen foods or teething rings (these could cause thermal damage to the tissues)
  - Tying a teething ring around infant's neck

Issues for Referral

If tooth eruption is significantly delayed, consider referral to pediatric dentist.

COMPLEMENTARY AND ALTERNATIVE MEDICINE

Homeopathy is used to treat teething. Calcarea carbonica (i.e., calcium carbonate) is one recommended treatment (14).

IN-PATIENT CONSIDERATIONS

Initial Stabilization

Outpatient

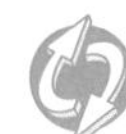

ONGOING CARE

FOLLOW-UP RECOMMENDATIONS

No restrictions

DIET

Breast-feeding can continue during and after teething. Otherwise, no special diet.

PATIENT EDUCATION

- Parents should be cautioned not to misinterpret teething as the cause of any systemic manifestation. The health provider should be consulted for any systemic complaints.
- American Dental Association, *For the Dental Patient: Tooth Eruption, the Primary Teeth,* 2005; www.ada.org
- Teething Tots: http://kidshealth.org/parent/pregnancy_newborn/common/teething.html

PROGNOSIS

Normal progression through the teething process without illness

REFERENCES

1. Kobayashi TY, Gomide MR, Carrara CF. Timing and sequence of primary tooth eruption in children with cleft lip and palate. *J Appl Oral Sci*. 2010;18:220–4.
2. Aktoren O, Tuna EB, Guven Y, et al. A study on neonatal factors and eruption time of primary teeth. *Community Dent Health*. 2010;27:52–6.
3. Sajjadian N, Shajari H, Jahadi R, et al. Relationship between birth weight and time of first deciduous tooth eruption in 143 consecutively born infants. *Pediatr Neonatol*. 2010;51:235–7.
4. Stellzig-Eisenhauer A, Decker E, Meyer-Marcotty P, et al. Primary failure of eruption (PFE)–clinical and molecular genetics analysis. *J Orofac Orthop*. 2010;71:6–16.
5. Feldens CA, Faraco Jr. IM, Ottoni AB, et al. Teething symptoms in the first year of life and associated factors: A cohort study. *The J Clin Pediatr Dent*. 2010;34:201–6.
6. Tighe M, Roe MF. Does a teething child need serious illness excluding? *Arch Dis Child*. 2007;92:266–8.
7. Macknin ML, Piedmonte M, Jacobs J, et al. Symptoms associated with infant teething: A prospective study. *Pediatrics*. 2000;105:747–52.
8. Ashley MP. It's only teething. . . A report on the myths and modern approaches to teething. *Br Dental J*. 2001;191:4–8.
9. Frank J, Drezner J. Is teething in infants associated with fever or other symptoms? *J Fam Pract*. 2001;50:257.
10. Williams GD, Kirk EP, Wilson CJ, et al. Salicylate intoxication from teething gel in infancy. *Med J Austr*. 2011;194:146–8.
11. McIntyre GT, McIntyre GM. Teething troubles? *Br Dental J*. 2002;192:251–5.
12. FDA Drug Safety Communication: Reports of a rare, but serious and potentially fatal adverse effect with the use of over-the-counter (OTC) benzocaine gels and liquids applied to the gums or mouth. Available at: www.fda.gov/Drugs/DrugSafety/ucm250024.htm.
13. Plutzer K, Spencer AJ, Keirse MJ. How first-time mothers perceive and deal with teething symptoms: A randomised controlled trial. *Child Care Health Dev*. 2011 Mar 6 (Epub).
14. Bergguist P. Therapeutic Homeopathy. In: *Integrative Medicine*, 2nd ed. Philadelphia: Saunders; 2007:1181.

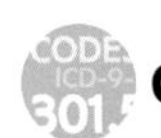

CODES

ICD9

520.7 Teething syndrome

CLINICAL PEARLS

- Teething is the natural, gradual, and predictable process of eruption of the primary or deciduous teeth, which most children experience without difficulty.
- Teething may cause discomfort, but does not cause significant fevers.
- Teething babies can still breast-feed. Babies can be taught not to bite, and breast-feeding may continue past 12 months of age without difficulty.

T

TEMPOROMANDIBULAR JOINT (TMJ) SYNDROME

Scott A. Fields, MD

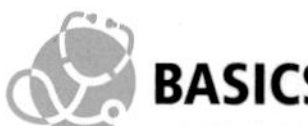

BASICS

DESCRIPTION

- Syndrome characterized by the following:
  - Pain and tenderness in jaw muscles
  - Sound and/or pain over temporomandibular joint (TMJ) with movement
  - Limitation of mandibular movement
- System(s) affected: Musculoskeletal
- Synonym(s): Myofascial pain–dysfunction syndrome; Bruxism

EPIDEMIOLOGY

Incidence

- Predominant age: Symptoms more common in ages 30–50 years
- Predominant sex: Female > Male (3:1)

Prevalence

Symptoms of TMJ dysfunction are present in up to half the population, but only 5–25% seek treatment.

RISK FACTORS

- Chronic oral habit, such as clenching or grinding of the teeth
- Osteoarthritis, rheumatoid arthritis
- Dental malocclusion
- Fibrositis
- Psychosocial stress

GENERAL PREVENTION

- Elimination of tension-relieving oral habits
- Reduction in overall muscle tension

ETIOLOGY

May be categorized according to origin of pain:

- Articulatory disorders primarily involving the joint:
  - TMJ synovitis
  - TMJ disk derangement
  - Hyper- or hypomobile TMJ
  - TMJ trauma
  - Condylar fractures
  - Osteoarthritis of the TMJ
- Muscle disorders involving the muscles of mastication:
  - Occlusomuscular dysfunction (bruxism)
  - Masticatory muscle spasm
  - Poorly fitting dentures

COMMONLY ASSOCIATED CONDITIONS

Craniomandibular disorders

DIAGNOSIS

Several research classification systems exist. Most share several of the below history and physical findings.

HISTORY

Facial and/or TMJ pain; locking or catching of jaw; TMJ noises: clicking, grinding, popping; headache; earache; neck pain

PHYSICAL EXAM

- Test jaw range of motion (opening, closing, lateral, protrusive) and masticatory muscle strength. Maximal (pain-free) jaw opening with interincisal distance <40 mm is suggestive if accompanied by other signs and symptoms.
- There may be tenderness over the TMJ.
- Palpation of muscles of mastication may produce tenderness
- Clicking of jaw with opening

DIAGNOSTIC TESTS & INTERPRETATION

Imaging

This is a clinical diagnosis based primarily on history and physical examination. Consider the following:

- Single-contrast video arthrography: Demonstrates joint dynamics and disk movement
- Panoramic dental radiographs
- MRI: Noninvasive study for disk position; information gained helps in deciding conservative vs. surgical management.

Pathological Findings

- Condylar head displacement
- Anterior disk displacement
- Posterior capsulitis
- Loosening of disk and capsular attachments
- Chondroid metaplasia of disk leading to disk perforation and degeneration

DIFFERENTIAL DIAGNOSIS

- Condylar fracture/dislocation
- Trigeminal neuralgia
- Dental or periodontal conditions
- TMJ neoplasm

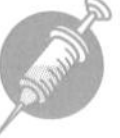

TREATMENT

- Jaw rest
- Local heat therapy
- Anti-inflammatory medications
- Muscle relaxants
- Analgesics
- Correction of malocclusion with orthodontic appliance (3)[A]
- Stress reduction
- Behavior modification to eliminate tension-relieving oral habits
- Buccal separator orthodontic appliance
- Linearly polarized, near-infrared irradiation

MEDICATION

First Line

- NSAIDs: No drug more efficacious than another (1)[C]
- Botulinum toxin (2)[C]

Second Line

- Analgesic agents (1)[C]
- Muscle relaxants (1)[C]

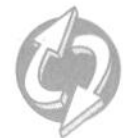

ONGOING CARE

FOLLOW-UP RECOMMENDATIONS

- Be aware of any teeth-clenching or grinding habits.
- Relax jaw by disengaging teeth.
- Avoid wide, uncontrolled opening, such as yawning.
- Stress management and behavior-modification counseling may be helpful.

Patient Monitoring

- Ongoing assessment of clinical response to conservative therapies (NSAIDs, behavior modification, occlusal splints) is necessary.
- Surgical procedure to correct disk displacement or replace a damaged disk may be indicated only if the patient has not responded to conservative treatment.

DIET

Soft diet to reduce chewing

PROGNOSIS

- With conservative therapy, symptoms resolve in 75% of cases within 3 months.
- Patients benefit most from a comprehensive treatment approach, including the following:
  - Correction of occlusal discrepancies
  - Restoration of normal muscle function
  - Pain control
  - Stress management
  - Behavior modification

COMPLICATIONS

- Secondary degenerative joint disease
- Chronic TMJ dislocation
- Loss of joint range of motion
- Depression and chronic pain syndromes

REFERENCES

1. Cooper BC, Kleinberg I. Establishment of a temporomandibular physiological state with neuromuscular orthosis treatment affects reduction of TMD symptoms in 313 patients. *Cranio*. 2008; 26(2):104–17.
2. Gonzalez YM, Greene CS, Mohl ND. Technological devices in the diagnosis of temporomandibular disorders. *Oral Maxillofac Surg Clin North Am*. 2008;20(2):211–20, vi.
3. Koh H, Robinson P. Occlusal adjustment for treating and preventing temporomandibular joint disorders. *Cochrane Database Sys Rev*. 2003;1:CD003812.

ADDITIONAL READING

- Al-Ani MZ, Davies SJ, Gray RJM, et al. Stabilisation splint therapy for temporomandibular pain dysfunction syndrome. *Cochrane Database Sys Rev*. 2004;1:CD002778.
- Scrivani SJ, Keith DA, Kaban LB. Temporomandibular disorders. *N Engl J Med*. 2008;359:2693–705.

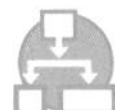

See Also (Topic, Algorithm, Electronic Media Element)

Headache, Tension

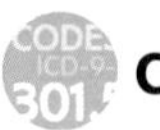

CODES

ICD9

524.60 Temporomandibular joint disorders, unspecified

CLINICAL PEARLS

- The condition called TMJ syndrome actually designates a number of potential underlying joint and muscle conditions involving the jaw.
- Characteristic of all are pain and functional limitation.
- Cognitive-behavioral therapy reduces pain, depression, and limitation of function.
- Other treatments such as splinting, NSAIDs, acupuncture, and botulinum toxin injection have some evidence of efficacy.

TENDINOPATHY

Mathew J. Devine, DO
Mark H. Mirabelli, MD

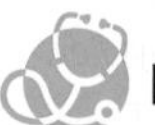

BASICS

DESCRIPTION

- Inflammation or tissue degeneration of a tendon and/or tendon sheath
- System(s) affected: Musculoskeletal

ALERT

- The term *tendinopathy* has replaced the term *tendinitis* as a generic descriptor of clinical conditions associated with pain, swelling, and impaired performance in and around tendons, arising from overuse. The labels *tendinitis* and *tendinosis* are reserved for the condition after histologic exam is performed (1).
- Tendinopathies can be pathologically classified as:
  - Tendinitis: Acute inflammation of the tendon
  - Tendinosis: Chronic degeneration of the tendon; also can be related to partial tendon rupture
  - Tenosynovitis: Inflammation of the tendon sheath
- Common sites of overuse tendon injuries:
  - Knee: Patella or jumper's knee, medial plica, and pes anserine
  - Shoulder: Rotator cuff muscles
  - Ankle: Achilles and posterior tibialis
  - Hip: Hamstring muscles and iliotibial tract
  - Elbow: Lateral epicondylitis or tennis elbow, medial epicondylitis or golfer's or thrower's elbow, and triceps (2)

EPIDEMIOLOGY

Incidence

- Predominant age: Adolescent and middle-aged groups; common in rotator cuff, Achilles tendon, and patellar injuries
- Predominant sex: Male = Female
- Overuse injuries are more common among high-risk populations (e.g., athletes and geriatric populations).
- Blood type O is related to chronic tendon problems.

Pediatric Considerations

Tendons in children tend to be more stable than the epiphyseal plate. Therefore, consider growth plate avulsion fractures versus overuse apophysitis following trauma in children (2). Tendinopathy is uncommon in children with open growth plates.

Prevalence

Tendinopathy/tendinitis is common.

RISK FACTORS

- Extrinsic factors:
  - Training errors (most common)
  - Footwear and equipment (second most common)
  - Training surfaces
  - Environmental conditions
- Intrinsic factors:
  - Malalignment
  - Limb length discrepancy
  - Muscular imbalance
  - Muscular insufficiency

GENERAL PREVENTION

Preparticipation screening, warm-up sessions, core and supporting muscle strengthening, safe environment, protective equipment using braces or taping, and health education have been shown to be useful for prevention of future injuries.

PATHOPHYSIOLOGY

- Overuse injuries involve incomplete and disorganized repair mechanisms. These result in a defective repaired tendon that lacks extracellular tissue organization and has decreased strength, making the tendon more susceptible to further injury (1). This tendon disorganization is the basis for chronic tendinopathy.
- Healing response of an acute tendon injury has a triphasic response of inflammation, proliferation, and maturation.

ETIOLOGY

- Increased repetitive stress and force on the tendon cause an increased risk of injury. Over time, with intrinsic and extrinsic factors, the above-listed tendinopathies can develop.
- Causes are still unknown and only have been theorized (3).

COMMONLY ASSOCIATED CONDITIONS

- Bursitis (common)
- Arthritis
- Apophysitis

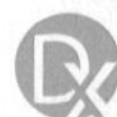

DIAGNOSIS

HISTORY

- Among the general population, history of repetitive use with onset of pain in area of muscle origin or insertions
- History of overuse or overtraining in the case of an athlete
- Pain at the specific point of the affected tendon is the most common symptom.
- Reproducible pain on muscle group activity
- Thickening of tendon(s) involved
- Decreased active range of motion (ROM) of the muscle group involved

ALERT

- With excessive posttraumatic tension or pain in a lower extremity, must consider urgent care for acute compartment syndrome
- With excessive swelling in traumatic injury, also must consider muscular tendon rupture

PHYSICAL EXAM

- Precise physical exam is key to the diagnosis
- Palpable pain over muscle tendon unit
- Warmth and redness in acute tendinopathies
- Note asymmetry and tendon thickness in chronic tendinopathies.
- Pain may limit ROM.
- Full musculoskeletal exam
- Neurologic exam as needed
- Snowball or creaky crepitus

DIAGNOSTIC TESTS & INTERPRETATION

Lab

If inflammatory arthritis suspected: ESR (or C-reactive protein; both are *not* necessary); if elevated, check antinuclear antibodies, rheumatoid factor

Imaging

Initial approach

- Imaging only to be used as adjunct as needed
- Ultrasound:
  - Can measure tendon width, water content within the tendon and peritendon, and collagen integrity
  - Abnormal tendons on ultrasound have the following findings: Increased tendon diameter, focal hypoechoic intratendinous areas, localized tendon swelling and thickening, collagen discontinuity, and tendon sheath swelling of calcifications (4).

Follow-Up & Special Considerations

MRI:

- Indicated only in specific causes
- Reveals tendon thickening and increased signal of tendons
- Areas of mucoid degeneration seen as high intensity on T1- and T2-weighted images

ALERT

- Areas of increased signal on MRI must be correlated with clinical pathology because these could represent asymptomatic areas of degeneration.
- MRI is unreliable in changes of paratendinitis.

Pathological Findings

Refer to tendinopathy pathology classification.

DIFFERENTIAL DIAGNOSIS

- Knee:
  - Patellofemoral pain syndrome: Lateral tracking of patella, causing irritation and abrasion of the cartilage of the patella and resulting in pain
  - Exertional compartment syndrome: A reversible ischemia secondary to a noncompliant osseofascial compartment that is unresponsive to the expansion of muscle volume that occurs with exercise (1); most common in the anterior compartment of lower extremities
  - Stress fractures: Partial or complete bone fracture from repeated force less than the force required to fracture the bone in a single loading; most common areas are the tibia, metatarsals, and fibula (1)[A]
- Shoulder:
  - Bursitis: Often is present with a tendinopathy
  - Adhesive capsulitis
  - Arthritis: An inflammation within a specific joint of the body; should be differentiated from tendinopathy, which is isolated to the muscle insertion site and not within the joint spaces (5)
  - Cervical radiculopathy
- Ankle:
  - Rupture: Achilles rupture is uncommon and is not a cause of tendinitis.
  - Sprains: In acute sprains, tendinitis can develop if too much stress is placed on noninjured musculature.

- Hip: Stress fracture: With excessive pain during internal rotation of hip, place the patient on crutches until femoral fracture is ruled out.

ALERT

There are many tendons in the body; the most common were selected in the "Differential Diagnosis" section.

Pediatric Considerations

- Osgood-Schlatter tibial apophysitis (common)
- Sever disease: Calcaneal apophysitis
- Pelvic apophysitis
- Little League elbow/Little League shoulder

TREATMENT

MEDICATION

First Line

NSAIDs provide good analgesic effects:

- Naprosyn: Over the counter (OTC), 500 mg b.i.d. with food
- Ibuprofen: OTC, up to 800 mg t.i.d. with food (adjust NSAIDs by weight for pediatric patients) (6)[B]
- Meloxicam: 7.5–15 mg/d
- Piroxicam (Feldene): 10–20 mg/d

Second Line

- Corticosteroids (4)[C]:
  - Oral corticosteroids (prednisone, others); PO
  - Injectable:
    - Methylprednisolone (Depo-Medrol): 40 mg used with 1% or 2% lidocaine (Xylocaine) 4–6 mL
    - Contraindication: Tendons never should be injected with local anesthetic and/or cortisone to allow participation in an athletic event. This can lead to complete rupture of the tendon.
- Topical: Research in progress

ALERT

- Some of the COX-2 inhibitors have been removed from the market. Current literature supports the use of celecoxib for tendinopathy in individuals a low cardiovascular risk.
- Contraindication: Do not use NSAIDs in patients with recent history of GI bleed or ulcer.
- Precautions: Compare medications for any drug interactions. See the manufacturer's profile of each drug.
- Use caution with renal disease.
- A rare side effect of fluoroquinolones has been tendon rupture and tendinopathy (7)[C].

ADDITIONAL TREATMENT

General Measures

- Avoid extrinsic factors.
- During acute phase: Rest of tendon involved
- Treat as outpatient.

Issues for Referral

Orthopedics/sports medicine referral in cases of highly competitive athletes, continued pain >4 weeks, radiologic finding of avulsion/stress fractures, or uncertainty of diagnosis

Additional Therapies

- Icing very beneficial in treatment (1)[C]
- Physical therapy

ALERT

- Muscle strengthening and intrinsic factor recognition are critical to continue the healing process.
- Using eccentric exercises aimed at structurally improving the musculotendinatous unit to protect it from increased stresses and therefore try and prevent injury (8)[C].
- Patient progress should be monitored with pain threshold. If pain continues, then the activity needs to be decreased (1)[C].

COMPLEMENTARY AND ALTERNATIVE MEDICINE

- Orthotics: OTC or prescription as needed
- Current research shows no benefit to using laser therapy or other radiotherapies (3)[C].

SURGERY/OTHER PROCEDURES

- For chronic tendinopathy, surgical treatment is an option if conservative treatment fails after 4–6 months. Patellar tendinitis is operated on most commonly (3)[C].
- Long-standing tendinopathies are associated with poorer surgical outcomes.

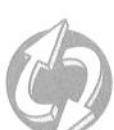

ONGOING CARE

FOLLOW-UP RECOMMENDATIONS

- Advise patient of susceptibility of exacerbation of injury up to 3 weeks after resolution of symptoms with increased activity.
- Treatment plans vary based on site of injury.
- Most plans include rest, medications, cryotherapy, and physical therapy.
- Follow-up at the discretion of the provider and patient.

Patient Monitoring

Follow-up at the discretion of the provider and patient.

PATIENT EDUCATION

- Increase activity in stepwise fashion as long as the patient remains pain free.
- Scales such as the Victorian Institute of Sports Assessment for patellar and Achilles tendons may provide some quantification of progress (5).
- Strengthening and stretching of muscle groups are involved.

PROGNOSIS

Symptoms usually subside with rest and proper therapy. Most tendinopathies improve without any major complications.

COMPLICATIONS

Exacerbation of pain in affected area

REFERENCES

1. Wilder RP, Sethi S. Overuse injuries: Tendinopathies, stress fractures, compartment syndrome, and shin splints. *Clin Sports Med*. 2004;23:55–81.
2. Maffulli N, Wong J, Almekinders LC. Types and epidemiology of tendinopathy. *Clin Sports Med*. 2003;22:675–92.
3. Sharma P, Maffulli N. Tendon injury and tendinopathy: Healing and repair. *J Bone Joint Surg Am*. 2005;87:187–202.
4. Warden SJ, Brukner P. Patellar tendinopathy. *Clin Sports Med*. 2003;22:743–59.
5. New Zealand Guidelines Group. *Diagnosis and Management of Soft Tissue Shoulder Injuries and Related Disorders*. New Zealand Guidelines Group, 2004.
6. Cook JL, Purdam CR. Rehabilitation of lower limb tendinopathies. *Clin Sports Med*. 2003;22:777–89.
7. Pantalone A, Abate M, D'Ovidio C, et al. Diagnostic failure of ciprofloxacin-induced spontaneous bilateral Achilles tendon rupture: Case-report and medical-legal considerations. *Int J Immunopathol Pharmacol*. 2011;24:519–22.
8. Maffulli N, Longo UG, Denaro V, et al. Novel approaches for the management of tendinopathy. *J Bone Joint Surg Am*. 2010;92:2604–13.

ADDITIONAL READING

Crowson CS, Rahman MU, Matteson EL, et al. Which measure of inflammation to use? A comparison of erythrocyte sedimentation rate and C-reactive protein measurements from randomized clinical trials of golimumab in rheumatoid arthritis. *J Rheumatol*. 2009;36:1606–10.

CODES

ICD9

727.00 Synovitis and tenosynovitis, unspecified

CLINICAL PEARLS

- Consider tendinopathy in cases of muscle or joint pain associated with overuse activity.
- Signs and symptoms include swelling, tenderness at site, and possibly erythema.
- Recommend rest of affected muscle–tendon unit and liberal use of ice and NSAIDs for acute tendonitis.
- Recommend ice, stretching, and eccentric exercises for treatment of more chronic tendinopathies.
- Muscle strengthening and intrinsic factor recognition are critical to continue the healing process.

TESTICULAR MALIGNANCIES

Satya B. Allaparthi, MRCS, MD

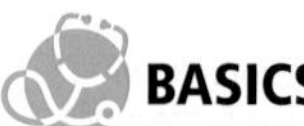

BASICS

DESCRIPTION

- Testicular cancer accounts for 1% of all cancers in men and is the most common solid malignancy in men aged 15–35 years; ~8,480 new cases will be diagnosed in the US in 2010
- Is one of the most curable solid-organ cancers (95.9%, 5-year survival)
- Arise from any testicular or adnexal cell; divided into germinal cell (GC) (~95%) and nongerminal tumors (~5%). GC divided into seminomatous and nonseminomatous types.

Pediatric Considerations

- 1–2% of all solid tumors in childhood; incidence of 0·5–2 per 100,000; 74% of primary testis tumors in prepubertal children were benign.
- Bimodal distribution, peak in young adults and smaller peak in the first 3 years of life
- The peak age at presentation: 2 years, 60% of tumors present earlier; median age for presentation of yolk-sac tumors is 16 months; and for teratomas, 13 months
- Cryptorchidism is risk factor for testicular cancer; ~10% occurs in this setting. Correct by 9–15 months with orchiopexy; this does *not* completely eliminate the risk of cancer.

RISK FACTORS

- Cryptorchidism: The only proven risk factor, with 4- to 10-fold increased risk
- Intratubular germ cell neoplasia: Left untreated, the risk of progression to invasive malignancy is ~50% in 5 years.
- Caucasian race, especially Scandinavian and Swiss
- Family history (1–3% with affected first-degree relative)
- Increased maternal estrogen, infertility, preterm birth, atrophy, trauma, other: (i.e., Klinefelter syndrome, XY dysgenesis, Down syndrome)

Genetics

- Nearly all cases of germ cell tumors (GCTs) show chromosome 12p abnormalities; exact genes involved are not yet defined; however, familial clustering observed.
- Increased expression of p53 protein is found in many GCTs; mutations in *TP53* gene not demonstrable.
- Role of telomerase activity: Highest levels of expression are seen in embryonal carcinomas. Telomerase is absent in mature teratomas, and contributes to their limited proliferative capacity.

PATHOPHYSIOLOGY

- Testicular cancer can arise from testicular GCTs or from sex chord stromal cells (Sertoli or Leydig cells).
- GCTs are pure seminomas, nonseminomas, or a mix of the 2. Nonseminoma is the more clinically aggressive tumor. Nonseminomas can be yolk-sac tumors, choriocarcinomas, embryonal tumors, teratomas, or a mixture of these. Teratomas are considered to be either mature or immature, and immature depending on if adult-type differential cell types or partial somatic differentiation, similar to that present in the fetus.
- Adults: 95% are GCTs; children, 65% GCTs. 60% of GCTs are seminomatous; 40% nonseminomatous. Seminomas rare before 10 and after 60, but are most common histologic type overall.

COMMONLY ASSOCIATED CONDITIONS

Cryptorchidism, testicular atrophy, Klinefelter syndrome, Down syndrome

DIAGNOSIS

HISTORY

- In adults:
  - Testicular nodule/painless swelling/enlarged testicle (most common presentation)
  - Dull ache/heavy sensation (30–40%), hydrocele (10–20%)
  - Acute pain (10%) related to hemorrhage/infarction; often mistaken for epididymitis
  - Gynecomastia (5%) systemic endocrine manifestation of testicular neoplasm
- In children: Painless testicular mass is the most common.

PHYSICAL EXAM

- Testicular exam: For size, consistency, and nodules; masses do not transilluminate.
- Supraclavicular nodes, inguinal nodes, abdominal masses, and gynecomastia

DIAGNOSTIC TESTS & INTERPRETATION

Lab

Initial lab tests

- CBC, BUN, electrolytes, liver function tests
- Tumor markers: α-fetoprotein (AFP), β-human chorionic gonadotropin (β-hCG), lactate dehydrogenase (LDH):
  - Markers used to stage disease, monitor response, prognosis, and detect recurrence
  - Levels should be drawn preoperatively and postoperatively.
  - AFP:
    - Increased in yolk-sac tumors, teratomas, embryonal carcinomas (or combination)
    - If >10,000 ng/mL, almost exclusively in patients with nonseminoma GCTs and hepatocellular carcinoma
    - Not increased in pure choriocarcinoma or pure seminoma
  - β-hCG: Increased in pure choriocarcinoma and 5–10% of pure seminomas
  - LDH: Reflects "tumor burden"; not specific, but a proven prognostic factor
  - Drugs that may alter lab results:
    - AFP elevated with chemotherapy, anesthetics, antiepileptics, and alcohol abuse
    - β-hCG may be elevated by marijuana use.
  - Disorders that may alter lab results:
    - AFP altered by liver damage: Drugs, viral hepatitis, alcohol abuse, liver conditions
    - β-hCG altered by hypogonadism and malignancies of pancreas, stomach, kidney, breast, or bladder

Imaging

Initial approach

- Scrotal ultrasound is gold standard; any hypoechoic area within tunica albuginea is suspicious. Biopsy if a hypoechoic mass or macrocalcification is identified. If only microcalcifications, testicular biopsy is not necessary (1).
- If an intratesticular mass is identified, measure serum AFP, LDH, hCG, and CXR.
- For staging:
  - CT scan of the abdomen and pelvis. If + abdominal CT or abnormal chest x-ray (2)[B].
  - MRI of brain if β-hCG >10,000 or >10 metastases in lungs
  - Bone scan for patients with metastasis or elevated alkaline phosphatase

Diagnostic Procedures/Surgery

- Radical inguinal orchiectomy: Definitive procedure for pathologic diagnosis
- Transscrotal biopsy/orchiectomy: Contraindicated, as lymphatic drainage is violated and leaves inguinal portion of spermatic cord
- If testicular atrophy, consider contralateral testicle biopsy if patient is >30 years or testicle is <12 mL in volume

Pathological Findings

Clinical staging (based on 1997 AJCC TNMS):

- Stage 0: Carcinoma in situ
- Stage Ia: Tumor limited to testis and epididymis without vascular/lymphatic invasion; normal serum tumor markers
- Stage Ib: Tumor limited to testis and epididymis, vascular/lymphatic invasion or tumor extending through tunica albuginea and involvement of tunica vaginalis; normal tumor markers
- Stage Is: Any tumor with elevated markers but no nodal involvement or metastasis
- Stage IIa: Any tumor with lymph node mass/masses <2 cm
- Stage IIb: Any tumor with lymph node mass/masses 2–5 cm
- Stage IIc: Any tumor with lymph node mass >5 cm
- Stage IIIa: Any tumor/lymph node presence with nonregional nodal or pulmonary metastases
- Stage IIIb: Any tumor/lymph node presence with moderately elevated serum tumor markers
- Stage IIIc: Any tumor/lymph node presence with greatly elevated serum tumor markers
- Risk stratification of metastatic GCT:
  - Based on International Germ Cell Cancer Collaborative Group, divided into good-, intermediate-, and poor-risk groups based on primary site of the GCT, metastatic sites of involvement, and levels of serum tumor markers
  - Seminoma: Good vs. intermediate risk based on whether extrapulmonary metastases. Serum β-hCG and LDH not used in assigning risk status
  - Good risk: Any primary site; no nonpulmonary visceral metastases; normal serum AFP (any elevation of AFP is inconsistent with the diagnosis of seminoma, patient should receive therapy for nonseminomatous GCT, even if pathology fails to identify these elements)
  - Intermediate risk: Any primary site; nonpulmonary metastases present; normal serum AFP
  - Nonseminomatous GCT: Good risk: Testicular or retroperitoneal primary tumor; no nonpulmonary visceral metastases; serum AFP <1,000 ng/mL, β-hCG <5,000 million IU/mL; LDH <1.5× upper limit of normal
  - Intermediate risk: Testicular or retroperitoneal primary tumor; no nonpulmonary visceral metastases; intermediate level of any of following: Serum AFP 1,000–10,000 ng/mL; β-hCG 5,000–50,000 million IU/mL; LDH 1.5–10× upper limit of normal

- Poor risk: Mediastinal primary site ± metastases; nonpulmonary visceral metastases (e.g., with liver or brain metastases); marked elevation in: Serum AFP >10,000 ng/mL; serum β-hCG >50,000 million IU/mL; LDH >10× upper limit of normal

DIFFERENTIAL DIAGNOSIS

- Epididymitis, hernia, hydrocele, hematoma, spermatocele, syphilitic gumma, varicocele
- Children: Epidermoid/dermoid cyst, paratesticular rhabdomyosarcoma, macroorchidism, torsion

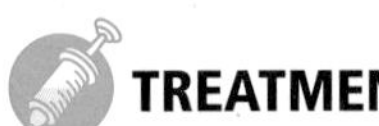

TREATMENT

MEDICATION

First Line

- Primary chemotherapy regimens:
- EP : Etoposide 100 mg/m^2 IV on days 1–5, cisplatin 20 mg/m^2 IV on days 1–5; repeat every 21 days (2)[A]
- BEP: Etoposide 100 mg/m^2 IV on days 1–5, cisplatin 20 mg/m^2 IV on days 1–5; bleomycin 30 units IV weekly on days 1, 8, and 15 repeat every 21 days (2)[A]
- VIP: Etoposide 75 mg/m^2 IV on days 1–5, ifosfamide 1,200 mg/m^2 on days 1–5, cisplatin 20 mg/m^2 IV on days 1–5, repeat every 21 days (2)[A]
- Patients who cannot tolerate BEP (low pulmonary reserve) should receive 4 courses of EP (etoposide, cisplatin) or VIP (vincristine or etoposide, ifosfamide, cisplatin).

Second Line

- Carboplatin, etoposide, paclitaxel, ifosfamide are used in various combinations as second-line conventional chemotherapy (2)[A].
- Gemcitabine, oxaliplatin are used in palliative chemotherapy regimens (2).

ADDITIONAL TREATMENT

General Measures

- Tumors with both seminomatous and nonseminomatous components managed as nonseminoma
- Surgery:
  - Radical inguinal orchiectomy for all patients; prosthesis can be inserted at this time.
- Seminoma:
  - Classified based on risk
  - Low risk: Tumor <4 cm and absence of rete testis invasion: Low relapse risk of 12%
  - High risk: Tumor >4 cm and presence of rete testis invasion: 32% risk of relapse
  - Carcinoma in situ: Surveillance versus radiotherapy depends on patient's preference
  - Low-risk stage I: 5-year surveillance with regular abdominal imaging vs. treatment as for high-risk stage I
  - High-risk stage I: Carboplatin × 1 cycle vs. radiotherapy; have similar relapse risk and long-term survival. Radiotherapy carries long-term risk of second malignancy.
  - Stage IIA–B: Radiotherapy, optional chemotherapy as per stage IIC
  - Stage IIC–III: BEP chemotherapy × 3–4 cycles; need for bleomycin must be addressed in patients >40 years of age with poor lung volumes due to risk of pneumonitis
  - Relapse after radiotherapy: Chemotherapy × 4 cycles of BEP lower dose of etoposide:
    - Stage II–III: CXR and CT 1 month after chemotherapy to evaluate response
    - Follow-up of metastatic disease: Normal posttreatment scan: Follow up as for stage I; abnormal: Repeat CT scan every 6 months until stabilized; PET scan may be considered for residual active cancer
    - Biopsy or resection for large residual or growing masses
- Nonseminoma:
  - Stage I:
    - Low risk (no vascular invasion): 20% relapse rate; surveillance protocol
    - High risk (vascular invasion present): 40–50% relapse rate; BEP ×2 cycles
  - Stage II–IV:
    - Good prognosis: BEP × 3 cycles
    - Poor prognosis: BEP × 4 cycles vs. VIP × 4 cycles

Additional Therapies

- Retroperitoneal lymph node dissection (RPLND) in patients with residual disease within 4 weeks of CT scan and 7–10 days of markers (2)[B]
- Sperm cryopreservation considered for patients intended for chemo/radiotherapy

SURGERY/OTHER PROCEDURES

- RPLND is the standard approach to the surgical management of NSGCT in both primary and postchemotherapy setting.
- A template dissection or a nerve-sparing approach should be considered to minimize the risk of ejaculatory disorders.

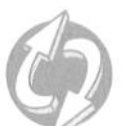

ONGOING CARE

FOLLOW-UP RECOMMENDATIONS

- A 10-fold decrease in or normalization of the serum β-hCG concentration (half-life 18–36 hours) over 2 weeks or serum AFP (half-life, 5–7 days) over 25–30 days is indicative of an appropriate decline, whether following surgery or chemotherapy.
- Postoperative tumor markers drawn only in nonseminomatous cases:
  - Seminoma:
    - No tumor markers reliably serve as indicators of disease recurrence in seminomas, so tumor markers are checked every 6 months, a less frequent schedule than for nonseminomatous GCT.
    - Surveillance: Every 4 months for first 3–4 years; 6 months for 4–7 years; 12 months for 8–10 years
  - Nonseminoma:
    - Surveillance/no adjuvant chemotherapy: Tumor markers monthly for first year, and then every 2 months for second year, every 4 months for third year, and then every 6 months until fifth year; CT scan of abdomen at 3 and 12 months
    - After chemotherapy: Tumor markers every 2 months for first year, then every 3 months for second year, then every 6 months until fifth year, then annually; CT scan as clinically indicated
- Follow-up imaging based on histology of tumor and cancer staging:
  - Seminoma:
    - Stage IA, IB: H&P, AFP, LDH, HCG, CXR, exam every 3–4 months for years 1–3, then every 6 months for years 4–7, then annually (2)[B]
    - Stage IIA, IIB: H&P, AFP, LDH, HCG, CXR exam every 3–4 months for years 1–3, then every 6 months for year 4, then annually
    - Stage IIC, III: H&P, AFP, LDH, HCG, CXR exam every 2 months for year 1, every 3 months for year 2, every 4 months for year 3, every 6 months for year 4, then annually
    - Metastatic: If posttreatment CT scan is normal, follow-up as for stage 1; if abnormal posttreatment CT scan, repeat CT scan every 6 months until stable
    - PET scan helps to identify patients who have residual active cancer.
    - Nonseminoma:
      - Stage IA, IB surveillance: CXR, clinical exam done at same time that serum tumor markers are drawn every month during first year, and then every 2 months during second year. See lab follow-up above; CT scan at 3, 6, 9, 12, and 24 months.

PROGNOSIS

- 5-year survival rate >96% for all stages and >70% for men with distant metastases
- Low-, intermediate-, and poor-risk disease 5-year survival rates: 91%, 79%, and 48%, respectively

COMPLICATIONS

- Orchiectomy: Intrascrotal hematoma, retroperitoneal hematoma
- RPLND: Intraoperative hemorrhage, lymphocele, loss of seminal emission/infertility
- Radiation: Radiation enteritis, nephritis

REFERENCES

1. Motzer RJ, Agarwal N, Beard C, et al. NCCN clinical practice guidelines in oncology: Testicular cancer. *J Natl Compr Canc Netw*. 2009;7:672–93.
2. National Comprehensive Cancer Network guidelines for testicular cancer 2011. http://www.nccn.org/professionals/physician_gls/f_guidelines.asp#site

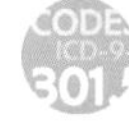

CODES

ICD9

- 186.0 Malignant neoplasm of undescended testis
- 186.9 Malignant neoplasm of other and unspecified testis

CLINICAL PEARLS

- Testicular cancer is the most common solid-organ tumor in males aged 20–34 years.
- Ultrasound is initial imaging of choice for testicular pathology.
- Radical orchiectomy is used for both diagnosis and treatment.
- >95% overall survival

TESTICULAR TORSION

Timothy L. Black, MD

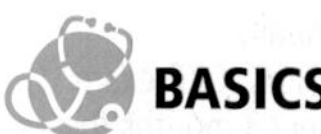

BASICS

DESCRIPTION

- Twisting of testis and spermatic cord, resulting in acute ischemia:
  - Intravaginal torsion: Occurs within tunica vaginalis
  - Extravaginal torsion: Involves twisting of testis, cord, and processus vaginalis (especially in newborns) and in undescended testes
- System(s) affected: Reproductive

Geriatric Considerations

Rare in this age group

Pediatric Considerations

Peak incidence at age 14 years

EPIDEMIOLOGY

Incidence

- ~1/4,000 males before age 25 years (1)
- Predominant age:
  - Occurs from newborn period to seventh decade
  - 2/3 of cases occur in second decade, with peak at age 14 years (2)[C].
  - Second peak in neonates (in utero torsion usually occurs around week 32 of gestation)

RISK FACTORS

- May be more common in winter
- Paraplegia
- Previous contralateral testicular torsion

Genetics

- Unknown
- Familial testicular torsion, although previously rarely reported, may involve as many as 10% of patients (3)[C]

PATHOPHYSIOLOGY

- The most common anatomic anomaly is a high insertion of the tunica vaginalis on the spermatic cord, resulting in increased testicular mobility:
  - This anomaly is bilateral in nearly 80% of patients.
- There is no clear anatomic defect associated with extravaginal testicular torsion.

ETIOLOGY

- Torsion is usually spontaneous and idiopathic.
- History of trauma in 20% of patients
- 1/3 have had prior episodic testicular pain.
- Contraction of cremasteric muscle or dartos may play a role and is stimulated by trauma, exercise, cold, and sexual stimulation.
- Possible alterations in testosterone levels during nocturnal sex response cycle; possible elevated testosterone levels in neonates
- Testis must have inadequate, incomplete, or absent fixation within scrotum.
- Torsion may occur in either clockwise or counterclockwise direction (1)[C].

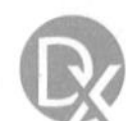

DIAGNOSIS

HISTORY

- Acute onset of pain, often during period of inactivity
- Prior history of multiple episodes of testicular pain with spontaneous resolution may indicate intermittent testicular torsion (2).

PHYSICAL EXAM

- Scrotum is enlarged, red, edematous, and painful.
- The first symptom is pain (usually sudden but may have a gradual onset with subsequent increase in severity).
- Nausea and vomiting are common.
- Fever may occur but is not typical.
- Testicle is exquisitely tender.
- Testis may be high in scrotum with a transverse lie.
- Absence of cremasteric reflex
- Tender, swollen, erythematous testicle

DIAGNOSTIC TESTS & INTERPRETATION

Lab

Urinalysis usually not helpful

Imaging

Doppler ultrasound may confirm testicular swelling but is diagnostic by demonstrating lack of blood flow to the testicle.

Diagnostic Procedures/Surgery

- Doppler US flow detection demonstrates absent or reduced blood flow with torsion and increased flow with inflammatory process (reliable only in first 12 hours) (1)[C].
- Radionuclide testicular scintigraphy with technetium-99m pertechnetate demonstrates absent/decreased vascularity in torsion and increased vascularity with inflammatory processes (including torsion of appendix testes).
- In boys with intermittent, recurrent testicular torsion, both Doppler ultrasound and radionuclide scintigraphy will be normal (4)[C].

Pathological Findings

- Venous thrombosis
- Tissue edema and necrosis
- Arterial thrombosis

DIFFERENTIAL DIAGNOSIS

- Epididymo-orchitis
- Incarcerated/strangulated inguinal hernia
- Acute hydrocele
- Traumatic hematoma
- Idiopathic scrotal edema
- Torsion appendix testis (this may account for 35–67% of all cases of acute scrotal pain in children) (5)[B]
- Acute varicocele
- Epididymal hypertension (venous congestion of testicle or prostate due to sexual arousal that does not end in orgasm)
- Testicular tumor
- Henoch-Schönlein purpura
- Scrotal abscess
- Leukemic infiltrate

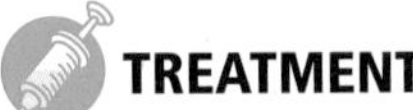

TREATMENT

- Manual reduction: Best performed by experienced physician; may be successful, facilitated by lidocaine 1% (plain) injection at level of external ring; always must be followed by orchidopexy
- Surgical exploration via scrotal approach with detorsion, evaluation of testicular viability, orchidopexy of viable testicle, orchiectomy of nonviable testicle
- In boys with a history of intermittent episodes of testicular pain, scrotal exploration is warranted with testicular fixation if abnormal testicular attachments are confirmed (4)[C].

ADDITIONAL TREATMENT

General Measures

Early exam is crucial because necrosis of the testicle usually occurs after 6–8 hours.

SURGERY/OTHER PROCEDURES

Operative testicular fixation of the torsed testicle after detorsion and confirmation of viability:

- At least 3–4-point fixation with nonabsorbable sutures between the tunica albuginea and the tunica vaginalis
- Excision of window of tunica albuginea with suture to dartos fascia
- Any testis that is not clearly viable (and obvious) should be removed.
- Testes of questionable viability that are preserved and pexed invariably atrophy.
- Requires general anesthesia
- Usually can be done on outpatient basis
- Bilateral testicular fixation is recommended by many surgeons.
- Contralateral testicle frequently has similar abnormal fixation.

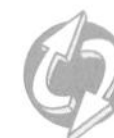

ONGOING CARE

FOLLOW-UP RECOMMENDATIONS

Patient Monitoring

- Postoperative visit at 1–2 weeks
- Yearly visits until puberty may be needed to evaluate for atrophy.

DIET

Regular

PATIENT EDUCATION

Possibility of testicular atrophy in salvaged testis with depressed sperm counts

PROGNOSIS

- Testicular salvage:
  - Salvage is related directly to duration of torsion (85–97% if <6 hours, <10% if >24 hours)
  - The degree of torsion is related to testicular salvage (5)[B]:
    - The median degree of torsion is <360 in patients who are explored and orchidopexy performed.
    - The median degree of torsion is 540 in patients who undergo exploration and require orchiectomy.
- 80–94% may have depressed spermatogenesis related to duration of ischemic injury (possibly related to autoimmune-mediated injury).
- As many as 2/3 of salvaged testicles may atrophy in first 2–3 years after torsion.

COMPLICATIONS

- Possible testicular atrophy
- Abnormal spermatogenesis
- Infertility (5)[B]:
  - Nearly 36% of patients who experience torsion have sperm counts <20 million/mL.
  - Antisperm antibodies and inhibin B may be useful following testicular function.

REFERENCES

1. Sessions AE, Rabinowitz R, Hulbert WC, et al. Testicular torsion: Direction, degree, duration and disinformation. *J Urol*. 2003;169:663–5.
2. Van Glabeke E, Khairouni A, Larroquet M, et al. Acute scrotal pain in children: Results of 543 surgical explorations. *Pediatr Surg Int*. 1999;15: 353–7.
3. Cubillos J, Palmer JS, Friedman SC, et al. Familial testicular torsion. *J Urol*. 2011;185:2469–72.
4. Eaton SH, Cendron MA, Estrada CR, et al. Intermittent testicular torsion: Diagnostic features and management outcomes. *J Urol*. 2005;174: 1532–5; discussion 1535.
5. Kapoor S. Testicular torsion: A race against time. *Int J Clin Pract*. 2008;62:821–7.

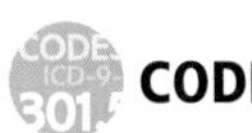

CODES

ICD9

608.20 Torsion of testis, unspecified

CLINICAL PEARLS

- The diagnosis of testicular torsion is usually made by physical exam. Patients with suspected torsion should be taken to the operating room without delay. If diagnosis is in question, a testicular Doppler ultrasound may be done to evaluate blood flow.
- Testicular necrosis present within 6–8 hours of symptom onset
- Infertility can be a problem even if the testicle is viable. Autoimmune antibodies may be produced, and they may affect subsequent fertility.

TESTOSTERONE DEFICIENCY

Janice E. Daugherty, MD, FAAFP, ABIHM

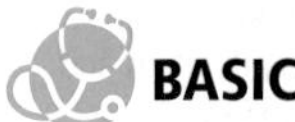

BASICS

DESCRIPTION

- FDA definition: Testosterone <300 ng/dL
- Testosterone is essential for normal sexual development and function.
- Testosterone levels may decline with aging and certain disease states.
- Low androgen levels increase the risk of low-trauma fractures and are associated with a decline in sexual function, sense of well-being, muscle mass, and strength.
- System(s) affected: Body Composition and Strength; Bone; Cardiovascular; Reproductive; Mood; Central Nervous System; Hematologic
- Synonym(s): Hypogonadism; Hypoandrogenism; androgen deficiency in the aging male syndrome

EPIDEMIOLOGY

Incidence

- 12.3 per 1,000 person-years in the US
- Late-onset hypogonadism: 481,000 new cases in US men 40–69 years old

Prevalence

- 2–4 million men in US; because of problems of definition, the prevalence in women is undetermined.
- 12% of men in their 50s; 28% between 70 and 79 years of age; 49% in men ≥80 years of age

RISK FACTORS

- Obesity, type 2 diabetes, chronic obstructive pulmonary disorder
- Medications that affect testosterone production or metabolism
- Stress
- Undescended testicles
- Trauma; infection; radiation or tumors of testis, pituitary, hypothalamus; chemotherapy
- Exposure to environmental endocrine modulators
- Chronic infections or inflammatory disease

Genetics

Some chromosomal disorders are inherited:

- Klinefelter: XXY karyotype (small testis, eunuchoid body habitus, gynecomastia)
- Kallmann: Abnormal gonadotropin-releasing hormone (GnRH) secretion due to abnormal hypothalamus development (micropenis, anosmia)

GENERAL PREVENTION

General health maintenance, such as prevention and treatment of obesity

PATHOPHYSIOLOGY

- Normal hypothalamic–pituitary–testis axis:
  - Hypothalamus produces GnRH, which stimulates pituitary to produce follicle-stimulating hormone (FSH) and luteinizing hormone (LH).
  - LH stimulates the testis to produce testosterone.
  - Testosterone inhibits production of LH through negative feedback.
- Primary testosterone deficiency: Testes produces insufficient amount of testosterone; FSH/LH levels are elevated.
- Secondary testosterone deficiency (also known as *hypogonadotropic hypogonadism*): Low testosterone from inadequate production of LH

ETIOLOGY

- Congenital syndromes: Undescended testicles
- Orchiectomy; testicular trauma
- Infectious: Mumps orchitis, HIV/AIDS, tuberculosis
- Systemic:
  - Cushing syndrome
  - Hemochromatosis
  - Autoimmune
  - Granulomatous
  - Severe illness (e.g., renal disease, cirrhosis)
  - Sickle-cell disease
- Obesity; obstructive sleep apnea
- Drugs that decrease production: Corticosteroids, ethanol, ketoconazole, spironolactone, marijuana, opioids, cimetidine
- Elevated prolactin:
  - Prolactinoma
  - Dopamine antagonists block inhibitory dopamine effects on prolactin secretion: Neuroleptics, metoclopramide, etc.
- Idiopathic hypogonadotropic hypogonadism
- Chemotherapy
- Radiation to the testis

COMMONLY ASSOCIATED CONDITIONS

- Infertility, low sperm count, erectile dysfunction
- Osteopenia/osteoporosis
- Diabetes, dyslipidemia, depression: Increased incidence and shorter time to diagnosis (1)
- Increased ratio of fat to lean body mass
- Free testosterone levels are lower in those with Alzheimer disease (2).

DIAGNOSIS

Test populations who may be at increased risk of testosterone deficiency due to congenital conditions or environmental exposures; broad-based population screening for testosterone deficiency is not recommended

HISTORY

- Congenital and developmental abnormalities
- Infertility
- Sexual function issues, including decreased libido, erectile dysfunction
- Depression, fatigue, difficulty with concentration/attention
- Decreased beard growth (increased interval between shaving), decreased muscle strength, energy level
- Increase in body fat, development of diabetes
- Bone fractures from relatively minor trauma
- Testicular trauma, infection, radio- or chemotherapy
- Decrease in testicle size or consistency
- Headaches or vision changes suggesting pituitary dysfunction
- Use of medications for associated conditions increases risk of low testosterone

PHYSICAL EXAM

- Infancy: Ambiguous genitalia
- Puberty:
  - Impaired growth of penis, testicles
  - Lack of secondary male characteristics
  - Gynecomastia, eunuchoid habitus
- Adulthood:
  - Note whether muscular development, hair patterns on face and body, and fat distribution are consistent with age.
  - Presence of gynecomastia
  - Dermatologic changes to suggest hemochromatosis, corticosteroid excess
  - Eunuchoid habitus: Lower body >2 cm longer than upper, arm span >2 cm longer than height
  - Kyphosis, loss of height, especially more than expected for age
- Testicular exam on Prader orchidometer:
  - Normal testis: 20–30 cc
  - Normal volume but soft and atrophic suggests postpubertal hypogonadism
  - Volume <5 cc suggests prepubertal causes.
  - Small and firm testis suggests Klinefelter.

DIAGNOSTIC TESTS & INTERPRETATION

Lab

An accurate diagnosis is based on the level of *bioavailable* testosterone; with aging, illness, or certain other exposures (e.g., tobacco smoke) levels of sex hormone-binding globulin may increase and total testosterone level may not reflect hormone that is actually available to the tissues.

Initial lab tests

- In symptomatic individuals, morning total testosterone level as initial test (3)[B]
- Opinions differ regarding utility and whether to measure or calculate free testosterone value:
  - Total testosterone reference range: 300–1,200 ng/dL (350 in younger men); free: 9–30 ng/dL; bioavailable testosterone at least 70 ng/dL.
  - Repeat the test in the morning if screening results are low (3)[B].
  - Diagnosis should not be made during an acute or subacute illness (3)[B].

Follow-Up & Special Considerations

- If testosterone is low or low-normal, check LH:
  - High LH level: Primary hypogonadism
  - Low or normal LH: Secondary hypogonadism:
    - Check prolactin: High level inhibits GnRH.
    - Check TSH: Hypothyroidism
    - Transferrin saturation: Hemochromatosis
    - Dexamethasone suppression test (Cushing)
- Karyotype if Klinefelter suspected

Imaging

Imaging is not helpful in the initial diagnosis of testosterone deficiency.

Follow-Up & Special Considerations

If pituitary causes are suspected, CT or MRI may be used to evaluate structural lesions.

Diagnostic Procedures/Surgery

Dual-emission x-ray absorptiometry bone scan to evaluate bone density

DIFFERENTIAL DIAGNOSIS

- Ambiguous genitalia; micropenis
- Cryptorchidism
- Delayed puberty
- Obesity (lower total testosterone; assess bioavailable testosterone to confirm)
- Normal aging

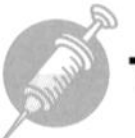

TREATMENT

Testosterone replacement is recommended for symptomatic men with low testosterone levels.

MEDICATION

First Line

Testosterone gel (AndroGel, Testim):
- 5–10 g containing 50–100 mg of testosterone applied daily

ALERT

- Must avoid transfer of testosterone gel to female partner or children
- Improvements in sexual function, mood, lean body mass, bone density have been reported (4)[C].
- Oral therapy is not recommended:
  - May cause liver toxicity
  - Physiologic levels are difficult to maintain.
  - Not beneficial in older men

Second Line

- Delatestryl (testosterone enanthate) or Depo-Testosterone (testosterone cypionate) injection:
  - 100 mg/wk or 200 mg every 2 weeks
  - Inexpensive
  - Levels high immediately after injection, fall to very low before next injection is due; may cause mood swings
- Transdermal patch (Androderm, Testoderm):
  - More expensive
  - May cause skin irritation
  - Scrotal patch:
    - Applied daily; delivers 6 mg
    - Need to shave scrotum
    - Dihydrotestosterone levels are higher than normal.
  - Nonscrotal patch: 1–2 patches daily
  - Rotate sites to avoid irritation.
- Transbuccal bioadhesive tablets (Striant):
  - 30 mg b.i.d.
  - Gum-related events in 16% of men
- SC pellets (Testopel) or compounded:
  - Last 3–6 months
  - May be difficult to adjust dose; easier to customize with compounded formulation.
  - Requires surgical insertion, which can be done in the office with local anesthesia.

ADDITIONAL TREATMENT

General Measures

- Pretreatment labs: CBC, lipid profile, liver function tests, and prostate-specific antigen (PSA).
- Baseline physical exam (including digital rectal exam and prostate exam)
- For secondary testosterone deficiency, correction of underlying cause may be necessary.
- If fertility is not an issue, testosterone replacement therapy is recommended in symptomatic men with androgen deficiency who have low testosterone levels to induce and maintain secondary sex characteristics and to improve their sexual function, sense of well-being, muscle mass and strength, and bone mineral density (3)[B].
- Testosterone therapy is contraindicated in patients with breast or prostate cancer, palpable prostate nodule or induration, PSA >3 ng/mL without further urologic evaluation, hematocrit >50, hyperviscosity, untreated obstructive sleep apnea, severe lower urinary tract symptoms with an International Prostate Symptom Score >19, or class III or IV heart failure (3)[B].
- Testosterone therapy is not recommended for:
  - Mood or strength improvement in otherwise healthy older men (5)[C]
  - Asymptomatic men with low testosterone measurements (3)[B]
- Testosterone-deficient men with HIV infection or receiving high doses of glucocorticoid treatment may benefit from short-term testosterone therapy to promote preservation of lean body mass and bone density (3)[B].

Issues for Referral

- In prepubertal patients, starting hormonal therapy at the appropriate age is of paramount importance:
  - In hypogonadotropic hypogonadism, testosterone therapy does not confer fertility or stimulate testicular growth.
  - Pulsatile LH–releasing hormone or human chorionic gonadotropin therapy is an option.
- Elevated PSA; abnormal prostate exam

COMPLEMENTARY AND ALTERNATIVE MEDICINE

Dehydroepiandrostenedione supplementation has not been studied adequately in humans to define potential risks vs. benefits (6).

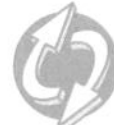

ONGOING CARE

Monitoring the effectiveness of therapy as well as surveillance for adverse effects of replacement is necessary every 6–12 months.

FOLLOW-UP RECOMMENDATIONS

Patient Monitoring

Monitor replacement therapy for 2–4 months initially and then 6–12 months thereafter:
- Digital prostate exam, PSA, lipid profile, CBC, serum glutamic pyruvic transaminase before initiating therapy and at least annually thereafter
- Testosterone levels until stabilized

DIET

- Calcium 1,200 mg daily, vitamin D 800 IU daily
- Hypocaloric diet to reduce weight if obese

PATIENT EDUCATION

- Testosterone deficiency is a chronic condition that is likely to need lifelong replacement therapy.
- Women and children must not be allowed to come in contact with testosterone replacement products.

PROGNOSIS

- Sustained reversal of symptoms is the goal of therapy when adequate serum levels of testosterone are achieved.
- Hypogonadotropic hypogonadism may be reversed successfully in 10% of patients (7).
- Androgen supplementation does not seem to improve any aspects of age-related frailty (6).

COMPLICATIONS

- Decreased sexual desire, muscle mass, bone density, loss of secondary sexual characteristics
- Complications of testosterone replacement:
  - Benign prostate hyperplasia exacerbation
  - Gynecomastia
  - Acne
  - Aggressive behavior
  - Polycythemia
  - Exacerbation of sleep apnea
  - Possible increased risk for cardiovascular events (8)
  - Hepatotoxicity with prolonged use
  - Exacerbation of metastatic prostate cancer

T

REFERENCES

1. Shores MM, Sloan KL, Matsumoto AM, et al. Increased incidence of diagnosed depressive illness in hypogonadal older men. *Arch Gen Psychiatry*. 2004;61(2):162–7.
2. Moffat SD, Zonderman AB, Metter EJ, et al. Free testosterone and risk for Alzheimer disease in older men. *Neurology*. 2004;62(2):170–1.
3. Bhasin S, Cunningham GR, Hayes FJ, et al. Testosterone therapy in adult men with androgen deficiency syndromes: An Endocrine Society clinical practice guideline. *J Clin Endocrinol Metab*. 2006;91(6):1995.
4. Wang C, Cunningham G, Dobs A, et al. Long-term testosterone gel (AndroGel) treatment maintains beneficial effects on sexual function and mood, lean and fat mass, and bone mineral density in hypogonadal men. *J Clin Endocrinol Metab*. 2004;89(5):2085–98.
5. Lawrence D. US panel urges caution on testosterone therapy. Large-scale trials of efficacy and safety are needed before widespread use can be recommended. *Lancet*. 2003;362(9397):1725.
6. Muller M, van den Beld AW, van der Schouw YT, et al. Effects of dehydroepiandrosterone and atamestane supplementation on frailty in elderly men. *J Clin Endocrinol Metab*. 2006;91:3988–91.
7. Raivio T, Falardeau J, Dwyer A, et al. Reversal of idiopathic hypogonadotropic hypogonadism. *N Engl J Med*. 2007;357:863–73.
8. Haddad RM, Kennedy CC, Caples SM, et al. Testosterone and cardiovascular risk in men: A systematic review and meta-analysis of randomized placebo-controlled trials. *Mayo Clin Proc*. 2007;82:29–39.

CODES

ICD9

- 257.2 Other testicular hypofunction
- 758.7 Klinefelter's syndrome

CLINICAL PEARLS

- Every man presenting with a complaint of erectile dysfunction or with a low-trauma fracture should be assessed for the presence of hypogonadism.
- Initial test of choice is a morning total testosterone; if low, repeat morning total testosterone.

TETANUS

Zerlina Wong, MD
Thomas Germano, MD

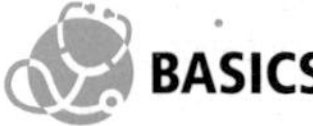

BASICS

Tetanus, or "lockjaw," was first described by Hippocrates nearly 30 centuries ago. Its etiology was discovered in 1884 by Carle and Rattone. Nocard developed passive immunization in 1897, which was used during World War I. Tetanus toxoid was developed by Descombe in 1924 and has been used for vaccination since.

DESCRIPTION

- Severe toxic bacterial infection by *Clostridium tetani* characterized by acute onset of hypertonia and intermittent tonic spasms of voluntary muscles—usually of the jaw and neck
- 4 types:
  - Generalized (most common, most severe)
  - Localized (generally mild)
  - Cephalic (affects cranial nerves)
  - Neonatal (very high mortality, rare in the US)
- Usual course is acute, 3–6 weeks duration; may be fatal
- Severity determined by frequency of spasms, presence of opisthotonus, and autonomic dysfunction (1)
- System(s) affected: Nervous

Pediatric Considerations

- Mortality high in young
- Majority present at 6–8 days
- Infection most commonly enters through umbilical cord

Pregnancy Considerations

- Must treat vigorously despite pregnancy
- Infection may enter uterus postpartum.
- Tetanus toxoid in second and third trimesters of pregnancy if indicated/higher risk will reduce neonatal tetanus deaths (2)[A]

EPIDEMIOLOGY

Incidence

- Rare in the US due to vaccination:
  - 0.10 per 1 million annually in the US
  - Near elimination of neonatal tetanus attributable to childhood vaccination and improved childbirth practices (3)
- 700,000–1,000,000 cases annually worldwide

Prevalence

- Age (median 49 years):
  - Persons >65 years of age are less likely to have had a vaccine booster (3).
- Gender: Male > Female
- Predominantly affects low- and medium-income countries of Asia and sub-Saharan Africa:
  - Neonates are the most vulnerable group.

RISK FACTORS

- Lack of vaccination or up-to-date booster:
  - Unknown vaccination history (i.e., immigrants, elderly)
- Age >65 years
- IV drug use
- Recent acute wound:
  - Puncture wounds
  - Crush injuries
  - Surgical wounds
- Diabetes (skin ulcers)
- Chronic wounds/wounds predisposed to anaerobic conditions
- Exposure of open wounds to soil/animal feces
- Newborn (umbilical entry, circumcision)
- Early postpartum with an infected uterus
- Burns
- Tattooing/multiple piercings

GENERAL PREVENTION

- Active immunization with tetanus toxoid:
  - DTaP (diphtheria, tetanus toxoid, and acellular pertussis): For children 6 weeks to 7 years of age:
    - Primary series of 4 doses at 2, 4, 6, and 15–18 months. Follow with booster at 4–6 years.
  - Tdap (tetanus, diphtheria, acellular pertussis): Give 1 dose at 11–12 years if completed the recommended childhood DTP/DTaP series:
    - Important for health care workers and people in contact with infants <12 months
    - Recent recommendations encourage Tdap administration if necessary, regardless of interval since last tetanus- or diphtheria-toxoid containing vaccine (4)
  - Td (tetanus and diphtheria toxoid) boosters every 10 years for general health maintenance (2)
  - Toxoid immunization given to pregnant women at least 4 weeks apart reduces neonatal tetanus by 94% (5).
- Wound debridement/decontamination
- Benzathine penicillin/penicillin G/erythromycin

ALERT

Postexposure prophylaxis (6):

- Passive immunization with tetanus immunoglobulin (TIG): 250 units IM
- Active immunization with tetanus toxoid
- If both TIG and tetanus toxoid are indicated, use separate syringes and separate injection sites.
- In setting of unknown vaccination history, consider patient unvaccinated: Administer Tdap (or Td if ≥65 years)

PATHOPHYSIOLOGY

- *C. tetani* is a gram-positive obligate anaerobic rod. The organism is sensitive to heat and oxygen, but its spores are heat-resistant and may survive contact with most antiseptics.
- Tetanus is transmitted by tetanus spores, which enter the body through a contaminated wound.
- Following inoculation, spores germinate under anaerobic conditions to produce the toxins tetanospasmin and tetanolysin, which disseminate through blood and lymphatics:
  - Tetanospasmin causes the symptoms of tetanus.
  - Tetanolysin causes hemolysis, but plays no major role otherwise.
- Incubation period generally 4–14 days after injury.
- Tetanospasmin enters the CNS peripherally, travels centrally to the brain and sympathetic nervous system, and acts at motor neuron end-plates to alter neurotransmitter release.
- Tetanospasmin blocks inhibitory neurons and results in unopposed muscle contraction/spasm/seizure.
- Affects newborns born to mothers who were not properly vaccinated. Transplacental transfer of antitoxin generally protective for first 1–2 months of life (5).

COMMONLY ASSOCIATED CONDITIONS

See "Risk Factors."

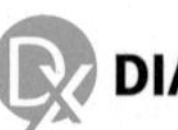

DIAGNOSIS

HISTORY

- Penetrating injury
- IV drug use
- History of contamination, especially soil/manure
- In neonates:
  - Poor umbilical hygiene
  - Lack of maternal immunization

PHYSICAL EXAM

- Painful tonic convulsions
- Autonomic instability
- Opisthotonos
- *Risus sardonicus* (fixed smile)
- Stiffness of the jaw (lockjaw, trismus)
- Dysphagia/drooling
- Hyperreflexia
- May also see:
  - Asphyxia
  - Convulsions
  - Glottal/laryngeal spasms
  - Hydrophobia
  - Hyperhidrosis
  - Hyperpyrexia
  - Irritability
  - Muscular rigidity/nuchal rigidity/spasticity
  - Pain at wound site

DIAGNOSTIC TESTS & INTERPRETATION

Diagnosis is based on clinical features. Laboratory tests may be performed to rule out other conditions that may mimic or complicate tetanus.

Lab

Initial lab tests

- CBC: Polymorphonuclear (PMN) leukocytosis
- *C. tetani* not generally visible on Gram stain/wound culture:
  - Culture positive in ~30%
  - Umbilical stump cultures usually negative
- CSF generally normal (no findings)

Diagnostic Procedures/Surgery

- ECG: Tachy- or bradyarrhythmia
- Antitoxin assay (not readily available) levels >0.01–0.015 IU/mL are protective—tetanus less likely (5)[B]
- Spatula test:
  - Touch oropharynx with tongue blade.
  - Test negative if gag reflex elicited as patient tries to expel blade
  - Test positive if patient bites down on blade due to masseter reflex spasm
  - 94% sensitive; 100% specific

DIFFERENTIAL DIAGNOSIS

- Acute dystonic reaction:
  - Phenothiazines
  - Metoclopramide
- Neuroleptic malignant syndrome (NMS)
- Rabies
- Meningoencephalitis

- Seizure disorder
- Hypocalcemic tetany
- Strychnine poisoning
- Alcohol withdrawal
- Amyotrophic lateral sclerosis

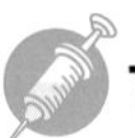

TREATMENT

MEDICATION

First Line

- Diazepam to treat muscle rigidity; combined anticonvulsant and muscle relaxation action, sedative, and anxiolytic effect (1)[A]:
  - 5–10 mg PO q4–6h PRN for mild spasms, IV for moderate spasms
  - Mix 50–100 mg in 500 mL D5W and infuse at 40 mg/hr for severe spasms.
- Tetanus toxoid in a previously immunized patient
- TIG confers passive immunity: 3,000–6,000 units IM
- Intrathecal immunoglobulin (1,000 U lyophilized human immunoglobulin) reduces spasms, hospital stay, and respiratory assistance (number needed to treat [NNT] 4.2) (7)[A].
- Metronidazole may decrease mortality; some reviews consider it drug of choice:
  - 500 mg PO q6h OR
  - 1 g IV q12h not to exceed 4 g/d
- Penicillin G: 2 million U IV q6h; traditionally considered drug of choice
- If penicillin-allergic:
  - Doxycycline 100 mg q12h OR clindamycin 150–300 mg IV q6h

ALERT

- Benzodiazepines (BZD) are the mainstay of treatment.
- Giving diazepam alone or supplementing with conventional anticonvulsants found to shorten hospitalization and produce milder clinical course (1)[A]
- Caution with high doses of BZDs; may cause respiratory depression
- Do not use TIG IV. Administer IM in different location than toxoid to avoid reaction.
- Antibiotic course should be given for 7–10 days.

Second Line

- Equine tetanus antitoxin: 500–1,000 IU/kg given IM/IV, but only if TIG (human) is not available
- Chlorpromazine/phenobarbitone for muscle rigidity:
  - Higher mortality and longer, more severe clinical course than diazepam (1)[A]

ADDITIONAL TREATMENT

General Measures

- Rest and observation
- Adequate caloric supply
- Deep vein thrombosis and ulcer prophylaxis

Issues for Referral

- Supportive care and airway considerations require ICU care
- Consult pulmonologist if severe respiratory symptoms
- Consult anesthesia if considering intrathecal therapy/airway control

Additional Therapies

Physical therapy once spasms resolve

SURGERY/OTHER PROCEDURES

- Wound debridement
- Tracheostomy if needed

IN-PATIENT CONSIDERATIONS

Initial Stabilization

- Intubation: Consider prophylactic intubation for moderate/severe symptoms:
  - Prepare for emergency surgical airway due to reflex laryngospasm.
  - Caution if using succinylcholine; risk of hyperkalemia later in course of disease
- Anticonvulsants for muscle spasms and/or rigidity

Admission Criteria

Diagnosis of tetanus

Nursing

Maintain quiet, dark environment and minimize manipulation/procedures to avoid triggering spasm

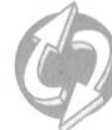

ONGOING CARE

FOLLOW-UP RECOMMENDATIONS

- Tetanus immunization series is necessary:
  - Infection does NOT confer immunity.
- Sequelae after infection are rare.

Patient Monitoring

Admit to ICU due to possible cardiac arrhythmias, autonomic dysfunction, and respiratory failure

DIET

NPO until well, feed by nasogastric (NG)/ percutaneous endoscopic gastrostomy (PEG) tube

PATIENT EDUCATION

Importance of tetanus immunization

PROGNOSIS

- 25–50% mortality
- Poor prognostic factors:
  - Autonomic system involvement
  - Form of tetanus:
    - Neonatal > Generalized > Cephalic > Localized
  - Rapid onset of symptoms
  - Extremes of age
  - Severity of symptoms
- Recovery is complete if patient survives.

COMPLICATIONS

- Respiratory arrest/airway obstruction
- Cardiac failure
- Pulmonary emboli
- Bacterial infection
- Dehydration
- Vertebral fractures
- Urinary retention
- Constipation
- Aspiration pneumonia
- Rhabdomyolysis/acute renal failure
- Complications of vaccination: Local adverse reaction (erythema/edema), local lymphadenopathy, hives, anaphylaxis, Guillain-Barré syndrome, peripheral neuropathy

REFERENCES

1. Okoromah CN, Lesi FE. Diazepam for treating tetanus. *Cochrane Database Syst Rev*. 2004; CD003954.
2. Demicheli V, Barale A, Rivetti A. Vaccines for women to prevent neonatal tetanus. *Cochrane Database Syst Rev*. 2008;1:CD002959.
3. Centers for Disease Control and Prevention (CDC), et al. Tetanus surveillance—United States, 2001–2008. *Morb Mortal Wkly Rep*. 2011;60: 365–9.
4. Centers for Disease Control and Prevention (CDC), et al. Updated recommendations for use of tetanus toxoid, reduced diphtheria toxoid and acellular pertussis (Tdap) vaccine from the Advisory Committee on Immunization Practices, 2010. *Morb Mortal Wkly Rep*. 2011;60:13–5.
5. Blencowe H, Lawn J, Vandelaer J, et al. Tetanus toxoid immunization to reduce mortality from neonatal tetanus. *Int J Epidemiol*. 2010; 39(Suppl 1):i102–9.
6. Chapman LE, Sullivent EE, Grohskopf LA, et al. Postexposure interventions to prevent infection with HBV, HCV, or HIV, and tetanus in people wounded during bombings and other mass casualty events—United States, 2008: Recommendations of the Centers for Disease Control and Prevention and Disaster Medicine and Public Health Preparedness. *Disaster Med Public Health Prep*. 2008;2:150–65.
7. Miranda-Filho Dde B, Ximenes RA, Barone AA, et al. Randomised controlled trial of tetanus treatment with antitetanus immunoglobulin by the intrathecal or intramuscular route. *BMJ*. 2004;328: 615.

ADDITIONAL READING

- Poudel P, Budhathoki S, Manandhar S, et al. Tetanus. *Kathmandu Univ Med J (KUMJ)*. 2009;7: 315–22.
- Tetanus. Epidemiology and Prevention of Vaccine-Preventable Diseases. *CDC Web site*. 2008.

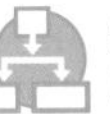

See Also (Topic, Algorithm, Electronic Media Element)

Lockjaw, Tetanus Neonatorum, Anaerobic and Necrotizing Infections; Immunizations; Meningitis, Bacterial

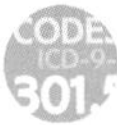

CODES

ICD9

037 Tetanus

CLINICAL PEARLS

- Tetanus is caused by *C. tetani*; can be severe and life-threatening.
- Infection is associated with contaminated wounds and unclear vaccination history.
- Immunization is essential to prevention. Inadequate vaccination and wound prophylaxis continue to be the most important risk factors associated with tetanus.
- Diagnosis is clinical and must be considered in patients with muscle spasms despite often negative lab results.
- Age >65 greatly increases the risk for a fatal disease course.
- Treatment involves neutralizing toxin, vaccinating, and providing antibiotics; however, supportive care is the mainstay of therapy to prevent complications.

THALASSEMIA

Herbert L. Muncie, Jr., MD

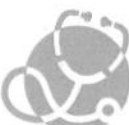

BASICS

DESCRIPTION

- A group of inherited hematologic disorders that affect the synthesis of adult hemoglobin tetramer (HbA) (1)
- β-thalassemia is due to a deficient synthesis of β-globin chain, whereas α-thalassemia is due to a deficient synthesis of α-globin chain:
  - The synthesis of the unaffected globin chain proceeds normally.
  - This leads to inadequate hemoglobin production and unbalanced accumulation of globin chains, which then results in hypochromic, microcytic RBCs and hemolytic anemia.
- Thalassemia is prevalent in the Mediterranean region, the Middle East, Southeast Asia, and among ethnic groups originating from these areas.
- β-thalassemia is increased in patients of African and Southeast Asian descent, whereas α-thalassemia is more common in persons of Mediterranean, African, and Southeast Asian descent.
- Types:
  - Thalassemia (minor) trait (α or β): Absent or mild anemia with microcytosis and hypochromia. No transfusion therapy is needed.
  - α-thalassemia major with hemoglobin Barts usually results in fatal hydrops fetalis.
  - α-thalassemia intermedia with hemoglobin H (hemoglobin H disease): Hemolytic anemia and splenomegaly
  - β-thalassemia major: Severe anemia, growth retardation, hepatosplenomegaly, bone marrow expansion, and bone deformities. Transfusion therapy is necessary to sustain life.
  - β-thalassemia intermedia: Milder form. Transfusion therapy may not be needed or may be needed later in life.
- Varieties common in Southeast Asians include hemoglobin H disease (a more severe form of α-thalassemia) and hemoglobin E/β-thalassemia, which often mimics α-thalassemia major in its severity.
- System(s) affected: Hematologic/Lymphatic/Immunologic; Cardiac; Hepatic
- Synonym(s): Mediterranean anemia; Hereditary leptocytosis; Thalassemia major and minor; Cooley anemia

Pediatric Considerations

- β-thalassemia major causes symptoms during early childhood, usually starting at 6 months of age, and requires periodic transfusions to sustain life.
- Newborn's cord blood or heel stick should be screened for hemoglobinopathies with hemoglobin electrophoresis or comparably accurate test, although this primarily detects sickle cell disease.

Pregnancy Considerations

- Genetic counseling is advised for couples at risk for having a child with thalassemia and for parents or other relatives of a child with thalassemia (2,3)[A].
- During the first trimester, a chorionic villus sample at 10–11 weeks' gestation or an amniocentesis at 15 weeks' gestation to detect point mutations or deletions with polymerase chain reaction (PCR) technology

EPIDEMIOLOGY

Incidence

- Occurs in ~4.4/10,000 live births
- Predominant age: Symptoms start to appear 6 months after birth with β-thalassemia major.
- Predominant sex: Male = Female

Prevalence

- Worldwide ~200,000 people are alive with β-thalassemia major and <1,000 patients are affected in the US.
- The prevalence of thalassemia trait within the involved ethnic groups ranges from 5–30%.

RISK FACTORS

Family history

Genetics

- Inherited in an autosomal recessive pattern
- α-thalassemia results from the deletion of $\geq$1 of the 4 genes, 2 on each chromosome 16, responsible for α-globin synthesis. Nondeletional forms do occur rarely. 4-gene deletion results in hemoglobin Barts causing fatal hydrops fetalis. 3-gene deletion results in hemoglobin H, 2-gene deletion is the trait, and 1-gene deletion is a silent carrier state.
- β-thalassemia is caused by any of >200 point mutations and, very rarely, deletions on chromosome 11, although probably 20 alleles account for >80% of the mutations.
- Significantly disparate phenotype with the same genotype occurs because β-globin chain production can range from near normal to absent.

GENERAL PREVENTION

- Prenatal information: Genetic counseling regarding partner selection and information on the availability of diagnostic tests in the event of pregnancy
- Complication prevention:
  - For offspring of adult thalassemia patients, an evaluation for thalassemia by 1 year of age
  - Severe forms:
    - Avoid exposure to sick contacts.
    - Keep immunizations up to date, including pneumococcal vaccine and annual influenza vaccine.
  - Promptly treat bacterial infections (after splenectomy, patients should maintain a supply of an appropriate antibiotic to take at the onset of symptoms of a bacterial infection).
  - Dental checkups every 6 months
  - Avoid activities that could increase the risk of bone fractures.
- Genetic counseling

ETIOLOGY

Genetic

COMMONLY ASSOCIATED CONDITIONS

See "Complications."

DIAGNOSIS

Thalassemia trait has no signs or symptoms.

HISTORY

- Poor growth
- Excessive fatigue
- Cholelithiasis
- Pathologic fractures
- Shortness of breath

PHYSICAL EXAM

- Pallor
- Splenomegaly
- Jaundice
- Maxillary hyperplasia
- Dental malocclusion

DIAGNOSTIC TESTS & INTERPRETATION

Special tests:

- Bone marrow aspiration to evaluate for other causes of microcytic anemia is rarely needed
- Multiple indices have been evaluated to discriminate β-thalassemia trait from iron deficiency anemia, yet none is sensitive enough to exclude β-thalassemia trait (4).

Pediatric Considerations

For children, calculate Mentzer index (mean corpuscular volume/RBC count):

- <13: Thalassemia more likely
- >13: Iron deficiency more likely

Lab

- Hemoglobin: Usual range 10–12 g/dL with thalassemia trait and 3–8 g/dL with β-thalassemia major before transfusions
- Hematocrit:
  - 28–40% in thalassemia trait
  - May fall to <10% in β-thalassemia major
- Peripheral blood:
  - Microcytosis
  - Hypochromia
  - High percentage of target cells
  - Reticulocyte count elevated
- Red cell distribution width (RDW):
  - A normal RDW with a microcytic hypochromic anemia is almost always thalassemia trait.
  - While the RDW will almost always be elevated in iron-deficiency anemia, it can be elevated in ~50% of thalassemia trait patients.
- Hemoglobin electrophoresis:
  - In β-thalassemia trait, elevated HbA_2 levels (>4%) may be present but are usually normal (5).
  - In β-thalassemia major or intermedia, elevated HbA_2, elevated HbF, reduced or absent HbA
  - In α-thalassemia trait, no recognizable electrophoretic pattern occurs in adults.
  - The presence of hemoglobin H or hemoglobin Barts at birth confirms α-thalassemia.
  - If HbA_2 is below normal (<2.5%) and a normal HbF level, the diagnosis is α-thalassemia intermedia (HbH disease)
- DNA analysis:
  - DNA analysis with PCR can definitely diagnosis α-thalassemia, but is not routinely done due to the high cost.

Pathological Findings
- Bone marrow erythroid hyperplasia
- Iron deposits in heart muscle
- Hepatic siderosis

DIFFERENTIAL DIAGNOSIS
- Iron deficiency
- Other hemolytic anemias
- Hemoglobinopathies

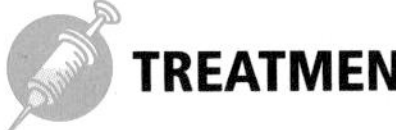

TREATMENT
- Outpatient for mild cases
- Inpatient for transfusion therapy

MEDICATION
- Antibiotics for bacterial infections
- Thalassemia intermedia and major: Folic acid supplements (1 mg daily)

First Line
β-thalassemia major:
- Iron chelation with deferoxamine (Desferal):
  - SC or continuous IV infusion, 20–40 mg/kg over 8–12 hours daily
  - Usually started before 5–8 years of age
  - Treatment lasts 3–5 years to reach serum ferritin <1,000 ng/mL.
- Deferasirox (Exjade) 20–30 mg/kg/d PO acceptable alternative; approved in the US (6)

Second Line
Deferiprone 75–100 mg/kg/d PO acceptable alternative for patients unable to receive deferoxamine; not approved in the US

ADDITIONAL TREATMENT
β-thalassemia intermedia:
- Hydroxyurea may improve hemoglobin 1–2 g/dL (7).

General Measures
- Mild cases require no therapy.
- Thalassemia intermedia: Normally, no therapy is necessary unless hemoglobin falls to a level that causes symptoms; then transfusion therapy may be needed. Decision is based primarily on patient's quality of life.
- Thalassemia major:
  - Maintain a mean hemoglobin level of at least 9.3 g/dL (1.4 mmol/L) with a regular transfusion schedule.
  - Folate supplementation daily (1 mg)
  - Treat bacterial infections promptly.
- Iron overload:
  - Patients receiving transfusion therapy increase total-body iron 4× over the normal amount.
  - Therapy is iron chelation.

Issues for Referral
Thalassemia major usually requires hematology consult.

Additional Therapies
Psychological support seems appropriate for this chronic disease. However, no conclusions can be made regarding specific psychological therapies.

SURGERY/OTHER PROCEDURES
- Splenectomy:
  - May be needed if hypersplenism causes a marked increase in the transfusion requirements (>180–200 mg/kg/yr) (8)
  - Defer surgery until patient is at least 4 years of age (due to increased infection risk).
  - Administer pneumococcal polyvalent-23 vaccine 1 month before splenectomy. Children should complete their pneumococcal conjugate vaccine series.
  - Daily penicillin prophylaxis, 250 mg b.i.d., after splenectomy for 2 years for all patients and for children until age 16.
- Bone marrow transplantation in childhood: Only curative therapy for β-thalassemia major, and generally excellent outcome for low-risk patients

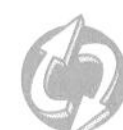

ONGOING CARE

FOLLOW-UP RECOMMENDATIONS
- Thalassemia trait requires no restrictions.
- β-thalassemia major:
  - Avoid strenuous activities (e.g., football, soccer).
  - Acceptable activity levels will be determined on an individual basis depending on the severity of the disorder.

Patient Monitoring
- Thalassemia-trait patients require no special follow-up.
- For β-thalassemia major, lifelong monitoring is necessary because the therapy and disease progression have numerous potential complications.

DIET
- Thalassemia trait requires no restrictions.
- β-thalassemia major:
  - Limit intake of iron-rich foods (e.g., red meats such as liver and some cereals).

PATIENT EDUCATION
Printed patient information available from Cooley Anemia Foundation, 330 7th Ave. Suite 900, New York, NY 10001; www.thalassemia.org or www.cooleysanemia.org

PROGNOSIS
- Outlook varies depending on type.
- Thalassemia-trait patients live a normal life span.
- β-thalassemia major patients live an average of 17 years and usually die by age 30.
- Iron overload causes most of the morbidity and mortality:
  - Cardiac events are the primary cause of death.
  - Effective iron chelation is improving longevity.

COMPLICATIONS
- Chronic hemolysis
- Susceptibility to infections after splenectomy
- Infections from blood transfusion
- Jaundice
- Leg ulcers
- Cholelithiasis
- Osteoporosis and low-trauma fractures
- Impaired growth rate
- Delayed or absent puberty
- Hypogonadism
- Hepatic siderosis
- Splenomegaly
- Cardiac disease from iron overload
- Thromboembolic phenomenon
- Aplastic and megaloblastic crises

REFERENCES

1. Muncie HL, Campbell J. Alpha and beta thalassemia. *Am Fam Physician*. 2009;80:339–44.
2. ACOG Committee on Obstetrics. ACOG Practice Bulletin No. 78: Hemoglobinopathies in pregnancy. *Obstet Gynecol*. 2007;109:229–37.
3. Tamhankar PM, Agarwal S, Arya V, et al. Prevention of homozygous beta thalassemia by premarital screening and prenatal diagnosis in India. *Prenat Diagn*. 2009;29:83–8.
4. Ehsani MA, Shahgholi E, Rahiminejad MS, et al. A new index for discrimination between iron deficiency anemia and beta-thalassemia minor: Results in 284 patients. *Pak J Biol Sci*. 2009;12:473–5.
5. Mosca A, Paleari R, Ivaldi G, et al. The role of haemoglobin A(2) testing in the diagnosis of thalassaemias and related haemoglobinopathies. *J Clin Pathol*. 2009;62:13–7.
6. Taher A, El-Beshlawy A, Elalfy MS, et al. Efficacy and safety of deferasirox, an oral iron chelator, in heavily iron-overloaded patients with beta-thalassemia: The ESCALATOR study. *Eur J Haematol*. 2009;82:458–65.
7. Dixit A, Chatterjee TC, Mishra P, et al. Hydroxyurea in thalassemia intermedia–a promising therapy. *Ann Hematol*. 2005;84:441–6.
8. Galanello R, Origa R. Beta-thalassemia. *Orphanet J Rare Dis*. 2010;5:11.

ADDITIONAL READING

Disler PB, Lynch SR, Charlton RW, et al. The effect of tea on iron absorption. *Gut*. 1975;16:193–200.

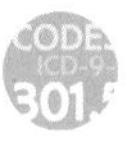

CODES

ICD9
- 282.49 Other thalassemia
- 282.5 Sickle-cell trait
- 282.60 Sickle-cell disease, unspecified

CLINICAL PEARLS
- A hemoglobin electrophoresis is not required to make the diagnosis of thalassemia minor when evaluating a patient with mild hypochromic, microcytic anemia, and normal serum ferritin. Unless there is a need for genetic counseling, a hemoglobin electrophoresis is not required.
- Thalassemia is a genetic condition; hemoglobin will not improve over time.
- The anemia from thalassemia minor is not due to inadequate iron availability or iron storage. Therefore, giving iron supplements will not improve the anemia, and could be potentially harmful due to GI distress and iron overload. If coexisting iron deficiency is proven, then iron therapy would be appropriate.

THORACIC OUTLET SYNDROME

William A. Tosches, MD
Daniel Mandell, MD

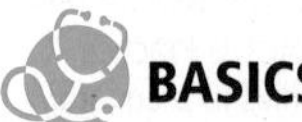

BASICS

DESCRIPTION

- A constellation of symptoms that affect the head, neck, shoulders, and upper extremities caused by compression of the neurovascular structures (i.e., brachial plexus and subclavian vessels) at the thoracic outlet, specifically in the area superior to the first rib and posterior to the clavicle
- 3 forms of thoracic outlet syndrome (TOS) have been described: Neurogenic, vascular (containing venous and arterial symptoms), and nonspecific (includes traumatic and secondary to certain provocative movements).
- Synonym(s): Scalenus anticus syndrome; Cervical rib syndrome; Costoclavicular syndrome

Pregnancy Considerations

Generalized tissue fluid accumulations and postural changes may aggravate symptoms.

EPIDEMIOLOGY

Incidence

- Predominant age:
  - Neurogenic type (95%): 20–60 years
  - Venous type (4%): 20–35 years
  - Arterial type (1%; atherosclerosis): Young adult or >50 years
- Predominant sex:
  - Neurogenic type: Female > Male (3.5:1)
  - Venous type: Male > Female
  - Arterial type: Male = Female
- No objective confirmatory tests available to measure true incidence
- Estimated 3–8/1,000 cases for neurogenic type
- Incidence of other TOS types is unclear.

RISK FACTORS

- Trauma especially to the shoulder girdle
- Presence of a cervical rib
- Posttraumatic, exostosis of clavicle or first rib, postural abnormalities (e.g., drooping of shoulders, scoliosis), body building with increased muscular bulk in thoracic outlet area, rapid weight loss with vigorous physical exertion and/or exercise, pendulous breasts
- Occupational exposure: Computer users; musicians; repetitive work involving shoulders, arms, hands
- Young, thin females with long necks and drooping shoulders

GENERAL PREVENTION

Consider observation or further evaluation in patients with cervical ribs.

PATHOPHYSIOLOGY

The interscalene triangle area is reduced in TOS and may become smaller during certain shoulder and arm movements. Fibrotic bands, cervical ribs, and muscle variations may further narrow the triangle. Trauma or provocative movements affecting the lower brachial plexus have strong implications in TOS pathogenesis.

ETIOLOGY

- 3 known causes of TOS: Anatomic, traumatic/repetitive-movement activities, and neurovascular entrapment
- Anatomic: Variations in the anatomy of the neck scalene muscles may be responsible for presentations of the neurologic type of TOS, and may involve the superior border of the first rib. Cervical ribs also have been implicated as a cause of neurologic TOS, with subsequent neuronal fibrosing and degeneration associated with arterial hyalinization in the lower trunk of the brachial plexus. Fibrous bands to cervical ribs are often congenital.
- Trauma or repetitive-movement activities: Motor vehicle accidents with hyperextension injury and resulting fibrosis, including fibrous bands to the clavicle; musicians who maintain prolonged positions of shoulder abduction or extension may be at increased risk.
- Neurovascular entrapment: Occurring in the costoclavicular space between the first rib and the head of the clavicle

COMMONLY ASSOCIATED CONDITIONS

- Paget–von Schrötter syndrome: Thrombosis of subclavian vein
- Gilliatt-Sumner hand: Neurogenic atrophy of abductor pollicis brevis

DIAGNOSIS

HISTORY

- Neurologic type, upper plexus (C4–C7):
  - Pain and paresthesias in head, neck, mandible, face, temporal area, upper back/chest, outer arm, and hand in a radial nerve distribution
  - Occipital and orbital headache
- Neurologic type, lower plexus (C8–T1):
  - Pain and paresthesias in axilla, inner arm, and hand in an ulnar nerve distribution, often nocturnal
  - Hypothenar and interosseous muscle atrophy
- Venous type: Arm claudication, cyanosis, swelling, distended arm veins
- Arterial type: Digital vasospasm, thrombosis/embolism, aneurysm, gangrene

PHYSICAL EXAM

- Positive Adson maneuver (head rotation to the affected side with cervical extension and then deep inhalation); test is positive if paresthesias occur or if radial pulse is not palpable during maneuver.
- Tenderness to percussion or palpation of supraclavicular area
- Worsening of symptoms with elevation of arm, overhead extension of arms, or with arms extended forward (e.g., driving a car, typing, carrying objects); prompt disappearance of symptoms with arm returning to neutral position
- Morley test:
  - Brachial plexus compression test in the supraclavicular area from the scalene triangle
  - Positive with reproduction of an aching sensation and typical localized paresthesia
- Hyperabduction test: Diminishment of radial pulse with elevation of arm above the head
- Military maneuver (i.e., costoclavicular bracing): When patient elevates chin and pushes shoulders posteriorly in an extreme "at-attention" position, symptoms are provoked.
- 1-minute Roos test:
  - A thoracic outlet shoulder girdle stress test
  - Shoulders and arms are braced in a 90° abducted and externally rotated position; patient is required to clench and relax fists repetitively for 1 minute.
  - A positive test reproduces the symptom.

DIAGNOSTIC TESTS & INTERPRETATION

Lab

Initial lab tests

CBC, ESR, and C-reactive protein (CRP) determination may rule out underlying inflammatory conditions.

Imaging

Initial approach

- Radiograph (chest, C-spine, shoulders) (1) may reveal elongated C7 transverse process or a cervical rib, Pancoast tumor, or healed clavicle fracture.
- Nerve conduction studies and electromyography (EMG)
- CT scan or MRI, although MRI is the method of choice when searching for nerve compression
- Evidence is insufficient to use MR angiography (2).
- Doppler and duplex ultrasound if vascular obstruction is suspected.
- Arteriogram and venogram have limited roles; useful when symptoms suggestive of arterial insufficiency or ischemia, or in planning surgical intervention (3)

Diagnostic Procedures/Surgery

No indicated procedures; anesthetic anterior scalene block may relieve pressure by scalene muscles on the brachial plexus, making this type of block diagnostic and potentially therapeutic, but it poses the risk of procedural damage to the brachial plexus.

Pathological Findings

Systematic results of biopsy have not been reported. There is no indication for biopsy unless to investigate another underlying condition.

DIFFERENTIAL DIAGNOSIS

Cervical disk syndrome, carpal tunnel syndrome, orthopedic shoulder problems (shoulder strain, rotator cuff injury, tendonitis), cervical spondylitis, ulnar nerve compression at elbow and hand, multiple sclerosis, spinal cord tumor/disease, angina pectoris, migraine, complex regional pain syndromes, C3–C5 and C8 radiculopathies

TREATMENT

MEDICATION

- No firm evidence exists for any approach to the 4 types of TOS.
- Physical therapy is first-line treatment (4)[B].
- Anti-inflammatory (ibuprofen):
  - Adult dose: 400–800 mg PO q8h; not to exceed 3,200 mg/d
  - Pediatric dose:
    - <12 years: Not recommended
    - >12 years: As in adults
  - Contraindications: Documented hypersensitivity; active PUD; renal or hepatic impairment; recent use of anticoagulants; hemorrhagic conditions
- Neuropathic pain: Carbamazepine, gabapentin, phenytoin, pregabalin; muscle relaxants such as baclofen, methocarbamol or tizanidine may be helpful
- Severe pain: Consider opiates for brachial plexus nerve block, steroid injections

ADDITIONAL TREATMENT

General Measures

- Conservative management usually involves approaches to reduce and redistribute pressure and traction through the use of physiotherapy or prosthesis.
- Interscalene injections of botulinum toxin have been shown to decrease symptoms of suspected neurogenic TOS.
- Physical therapy will develop strength in pectoral girdle muscles and achieve normal posture (1)[C].
- Severe cases may use taping, adhesive elastic bandages, moist heat, TENS, or ultrasound but should not substitute active exercise and correction of posture and muscle imbalance (4)[B].

Issues for Referral

- Neurologic, anesthesiologic, orthopedic, vascular surgery referral(s) may be indicated depending on the type of pathologic condition.
- Physical and rehabilitation physicians

SURGERY/OTHER PROCEDURES

- Operative if vascular involvement is present and/or loss of function or lifestyle occurs secondary to severity of symptoms and if conservative therapy fails after 2–3 months (1)[C]
- Transaxillary first rib resection (TFRR) may provide better pain relief than supraclavicular neuroplasty of the brachial plexus (SNBP), while overall both treatment options have generally positive outcomes (5)[B].
- Resection of first rib or cervical ribs via transaxillary (preferred with good to excellent outcome 80% of patients), supraclavicular (good to excellent outcome 80% of patients), posterior approaches (reserved for complicated TOS due to necessity of large muscle incision)
- Excision of adhesive bands, anterior scalenectomy (6)[B]

IN-PATIENT CONSIDERATIONS

Initial Stabilization

Conservative, outpatient, nonpharmacologic treatment is reasonable first-line therapy except in cases of thromboembolic phenomena and acute ischemia, symptoms of chronic vascular occlusion, stenosis, arterial dilatation, or progressive neurologic deficit (4)[A].

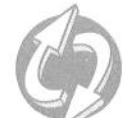

ONGOING CARE

FOLLOW-UP RECOMMENDATIONS

Correct improper posture, practice proper posture, exercises to strengthen shoulder elevator and neck extensor muscles, stretching exercises for scalene muscles, support bra for women with pendulous breasts, breast reduction surgery in selected cases; sleep with arms below chest level, avoid/reduce prolonged hyperabduction.

Patient Monitoring

Office follow-up visits every 3–4 weeks

PATIENT EDUCATION

Physical therapy, postural exercises, ergonomic workstation

PROGNOSIS

Follow-up from surgery at mean of 7.5 years showed that functional results were excellent, good, fair, and poor in 87 (49.4%), 61 (34.6%), 14 (8%), and 14 (8%) procedures, respectively (7)[C].

COMPLICATIONS

- Postoperative shoulder, arm, hand pain, and paresthesias in 10%
- Patients who will have symptomatic recurrences at 1 month to 7 years postoperatively (usually within 3 months): 1.5–2%
- Patients who will have brachial plexus injury, probably due to intraoperative traction: 0.5–1%
- Reoperation is indicated for symptomatic recurrence with long posterior remnant of first rib (posterior approach) or with disrupted fibrous adhesions (transaxillary approach).
- Venous obstruction or arterial emboli; usually responds to thrombolytics

REFERENCES

1. Huang JH, Zager EL. Thoracic outlet syndrome. *Neurosurgery*. 2004;55:897–902; discussion 902–3.
2. Estilaei SK, Byl NN. An evidence-based review of magnetic resonance angiography for diagnosing arterial thoracic outlet syndrome. *J Hand Ther*. 2006;19:410–20.
3. Sanders RJ, Hammond SL, Rao NM. Diagnosis of thoracic outlet syndrome. *J Vasc Surg*. 2007;46:601–4.
4. Vanti C, Natalini L, Romeo A. Conservative treatment of thoracic outlet syndrome. A review of the literature. *Eura Medicophys*. 2007;43:55–70.
5. Sheth RN, Campbell JN. Surgical treatment of thoracic outlet syndrome: A randomized trial comparing two operations. *J Neurosurg Spine*. 2005;3:355–63.
6. Urschel HC, Kourlis H. Thoracic outlet syndrome: A 50-year experience at Baylor University Medical Center. *Proc (Bayl Univ Med Cent)*. 2007;20:125–35.
7. Degeorges R. Thoracic outlet syndrome surgery: Long-term functional results. *Ann Vas Surg*. 2004;18(5):558–65.

ADDITIONAL READING

- Demondion X, Herbinet P, Van Sint Jan S. Imaging assessment of thoracic outlet syndrome. *Radiographics*. 2006;26:1735–50.
- Jordan SE, Ahn SS, Freischlag JA. Selective botulinum chemodenervation of the scalene muscles for treatment of neurogenic thoracic outlet syndrome. *Ann Vasc Surg*. 2000;14:365–9.
- Jordan SE, Machleder HI. Diagnosis of thoracic outlet syndrome using electrophysiologically guided anterior scalene blocks. *Ann Vasc Surg*. 1998;12:260–4.
- Nakatsuchi Y. Conservative treatment of thoracic outlet syndrome using an orthosis. *J Hand Surg*. 1995;20(1):34–9.
- National Institute of Neurological Disorders and Stroke (NINDS). Information page on TOS.
- Novak CB, Collins ED, Mackinnon SE. Outcome following conservative management of thoracic outlet syndrome. *J Hand Surg [Am]*. 1995;20:542–8.
- Povelson B, Belzberg A, Hansson T, et al. Treatment for thoracic outlet syndrome. *Cochrane Database Sys Rev*. 2010;1.

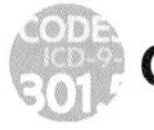

CODES

ICD9

353.0 Brachial plexus lesions

CLINICAL PEARLS

- Consider breast reduction for patients with pendulous breasts.
- Avoid opiate dependence.
- Consider pain clinic referral if there are nonsurgical causes.

THROMBOANGIITIS OBLITERANS (BUERGER DISEASE)

Alfonso J. Tafur, MD, RPVI
Felix B. Chang, MD

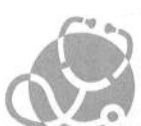

BASICS

DESCRIPTION

- Nonatherosclerotic vasculitis of small and medium-sized arteries and veins resulting in segmental occlusion
- Characterized clinically by an inflammatory and vaso-occlusive phenomenon, rest pain, unremitting ischemic ulcerations, and gangrene of the digits of hands and feet
- Occurs primarily in men who smoke
- System(s) affected: Cardiovascular
- Synonym(s): Buerger disease

EPIDEMIOLOGY

- The prevalence has decreased in North America over the last 30 years.
- Worldwide, but most prevalent in Eastern Europe, Mediterranean, and Asian countries

Incidence

- 11–30/100,000 persons/yr
- Predominant age: 20–40 years
- Predominant sex: Male > Female; increasing numbers of women are being diagnosed, possibly due to increased smoking (1)

Prevalence

- Estimates range from as low as 0.5–5.5% in Western Europe, to 45–63% in India, to 80% in Israel among Jews of Ashkenazi ancestry.
- Accounts for 5% and 16% of patients hospitalized for arterial occlusive disease in Europe and Japan, respectively
- 13/100,000 US population
- The overall occurrence is decreasing worldwide (2).

Geriatric Considerations

Not common in this age group

Pediatric Considerations

It should be considered in the differential diagnosis of the young patient with claudication.

RISK FACTORS

- Smoking tobacco. The degree of dependence is similar to that in subjects with coronary artery disease. Occasional cases in users of smokeless tobacco and snuff.
- *C. sativa* and *C. indica* have been considered as risk factors.
- Chronic anaerobic periodontal infection also may play a role in the development of Buerger disease.

Genetics

- Greater prevalence of HLA-A54, HLA-A9, and HLA-B5
- HLA-B12 antigen may be associated with disease resistance.
- Familial cases reported rarely

GENERAL PREVENTION

Never smoke. Tobacco and smoking cessation is the only way to prevent recurrence of disease.

PATHOPHYSIOLOGY

- Impaired endothelium-dependent vasorelaxation and decreased peripheral sympathetic outflow
- Segmental infiltration of inflammatory cells in vessel wall leads to thrombotic occlusion of vessel.
- Highly cellular and inflammatory thrombus with relative sparing of the blood vessel wall

ETIOLOGY

- Idiopathic
- Smoking
- Genetic factors
- Autoimmune disorder with cell-mediated sensitivity to types I and III human collagens (both are normal constituents of blood vessels)
- Impaired peripheral endothelium-dependent vasodilation. Nonendothelial mechanisms of vasodilation are intact.
- Arsenic content of tobacco
- Chronic anaerobic periodontal infection

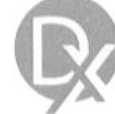

DIAGNOSIS

- Point scoring systems may help to clarify clinical diagnosis. Many diagnostic tools are available.
- The criteria proposed by Olin is one of the most widely accepted:
  - Smoking history
  - Onset before the age of 50 years
  - Infrapopliteal arterial occlusions
  - Either upper limb involvement or phlebitis migrans
  - Absence of atherosclerotic risk factors other than smoking
  - Disease diagnosis may be made only when all 5 requirements have been fulfilled.
- Symptoms tend to wax and wane in early disease and often are asymmetric. Symptoms may be gradual or have a sudden onset related to impaired vasculature. Usually more than 1 limb is involved.

HISTORY

- Foot or arch claudication may be the presenting manifestation (rarely hand, forearm) and is often mistaken for an orthopedic problem.
- Cold sensitivity
- Paresthesias (e.g., numbness, tingling, burning, hypoesthesia) of feet and/or fingers
- Persistent extremity pain (may be worse at rest); pain may be disabling
- Paroxysmal "electric shock" pain of ischemic neuropathy
- Migratory superficial phlebitis

PHYSICAL EXAM

- 76% of patients had ischemic ulcerations at the time of presentation.
- Allen test should be performed.
- Ulceration of digits
- Raynaud phenomenon (~20% of patients)
- Postural color changes: Pallor on elevation; rubor on dependency
- "Buerger color": Cyanosis of hands and feet
- Tender skin nodules on extremities
- Impaired distal pulses
- Proximal pulses normal; Allen test may be abnormal.
- Foot edema
- Gangrene

DIAGNOSTIC TESTS & INTERPRETATION

Lab

- There is no specific lab finding relevant for thromboangiitis obliterans (TAO).
- Noninvasive vascular studies, including TCPO2, ankle brachial index, and simultaneous brachial pressures
- In order to rule out diseases in the differential diagnosis, consider CBC, liver function tests, creatinine, fasting glucose, ESR, antinuclear antibodies (ANA), rheumatoid factor (RF), anticentromere antibody, and SCL70, as well as a hypercoagulability screen.
- Autoantibodies to collagen and circulating immune complexes may be present, but the significance is still to be determined.
- Increased levels of antiendothelial cell antibodies are seen in patients with active disease.
- Anticardiolipin antibodies may be associated with TAO and may worsen the thrombotic event (3)[A].
- Homocysteine may be elevated but lacks specificity.
- Toxin screen when appropriate: Cocaine, amphetamines, and cannabis ingestion can mimic TAO.

Follow-Up & Special Considerations

- The Westergren sedimentation rate and serum C-reactive protein are usually normal.
- Commonly measured autoantibodies (e.g., ANA and RF) are normal or negative.
- Circulating immune complexes, complement levels, and cryoglobulins are normal despite an immune reaction in the arterial intima.

Imaging

- Doppler ultrasound (not specific)
- Arteriogram or digital-subtraction angiography:
  - Multiple areas of segmental occlusion of small to medium-sized arteries of arms and legs
  - The disease is confined most often to the distal circulation and is almost always infrapopliteal in the lower extremities and distal to the brachial artery in the upper extremities.
  - "Skip" areas may be demonstrated.
  - Numerous collateral vessels around occluded segments may give a characteristic corkscrew appearance (Martorell sign):
    - Classification by size and pattern has been proposed:
      - Type I, artery diameter >2 mm, large helical sign
      - Type II, diameter >1.5 mm and ≤2 mm, medium helical sign
      - Type III, diameter ≥1 mm and ≤1.5 mm, small helical sign
      - Type IV, diameter <1 mm, tiny helical sign (4)
  - Larger arteries are spared. More serious disease occurs distally.
  - No apparent source of emboli

Follow-Up & Special Considerations

The prevalence of ischemic ulcers is significantly higher in patients who have small corkscrew patterns (type III and IV) in distal segments of limb collaterals than in patients who have large corkscrew collaterals (4).

Diagnostic Procedures/Surgery
- History and physical examination
- Echocardiography (to exclude emboli)
- Biopsy only indicated if there are unusual features:
  - Age >45 years at onset
  - Disease in unusual location
  - Proximal disease
  - CNS disease
  - Tobacco history is not consistent with diagnosis.

Pathological Findings
- Segmental inflammatory thrombosis of both arteries and veins
- Histologic findings may vary between acute, intermediate, and chronic stages of the disease.
- Histologic sine qua non: Granulomas with collections of neutrophils in the organizing thrombus:
  - The vessel wall is relatively spared.
  - Wall sparing distinguishes TAO from arteriosclerosis and other systemic vasculitides, which show striking wall disruption.
- Acute lesions show occlusive, highly cellular, inflammatory thrombi with less inflammation in vessel wall. Polymorphonuclear neutrophils, microabscesses, and multinucleated giant cells may be present.
- Intermediate lesions show organizing thrombus.
- Chronic lesions show recanalized thrombus and perivascular fibrosis.

DIFFERENTIAL DIAGNOSIS
- Peripheral neuropathy, peripheral atherosclerotic disease, arterial embolus and thrombosis, idiopathic peripheral thrombosis
- Takayasu arteritis; CREST syndrome (calcinosis, Raynaud phenomenon, esophageal dysfunction, sclerodactyly, telangiectasia)
- Hypercoagulable states; systemic lupus erythematosus; scleroderma
- Occupational trauma; acrocyanosis; frostbite; neurotrophic ulcers
- Reflex sympathetic dystrophy; metatarsalgia; gout

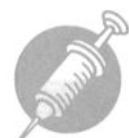

TREATMENT

MEDICATION

First Line
- Discontinue smoking or tobacco use in any form.
- Antibiotics for infected digital ulcers and osteomyelitis
- Urokinase or streptokinase selectively infused into occluded artery
- IM endothelial growth factor gene therapy

Second Line
- If vasospasm is present, trial of dihydropyridine calcium channel blocker such as amlodipine or nifedipine
- Iloprost, a prostacyclin analogue, promotes ulcer healing and decreases analgesic requirement.
- IM gene transfer of vascular growth factors

ADDITIONAL TREATMENT
Initiate a walking program.

General Measures
- Stop smoking (mandatory).
- Protect against trauma (poorly fitting shoes) and infections.
- Protect against vasoconstriction from cold or drugs.
- Eliminate exposure to thermal and chemical damage (e.g., iodine, carbolic acid, salicylic acid).
- Thrombolytic therapy of occlusive thrombus and angioplasty are experimental.

Issues for Referral
Consider referral to nicotine-addiction clinics.

Additional Therapies
- Intermittent pneumatic compression has been shown to enhance calf and may serve as adjunctive therapy in patients who are not candidates for revascularization.
- Foot care
- Lubricate skin with moisturizer.
- Lamb's wool between toes
- Avoid trauma (e.g., heel protectors, orthotics for shoes, vascular boots).

COMPLEMENTARY AND ALTERNATIVE MEDICINE
Hyperbaric oxygen therapy and autologous bone marrow transplant of mononuclear cells are alternative therapy modalities, with very small studies suggesting potential utility.

SURGERY/OTHER PROCEDURES
- Amputation:
  - For nonhealing ulcers, gangrene, or intractable pain
  - Should preserve as much limb as possible
- Omental autotransplantation has been successful in treating ulcers.
- Infrainguinal bypass
- In severe disease, a lumbar sympathectomy to increase blood supply to the skin (5)[A]
- Surgical revascularization is not usually a viable alternative due to the diffuse segmental involvement and extreme distal nature of the disease.

IN-PATIENT CONSIDERATIONS
Inpatient nicotine-dependence treatment is an alternative for recidivist smokers.

Initial Stabilization
- Inpatient if surgery needed for gangrene
- Inpatient for dorsal or lumbar sympathectomy if indicated

Admission Criteria
Critical limb ischemia

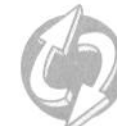

ONGOING CARE

FOLLOW-UP RECOMMENDATIONS
- Restricted by symptoms
- Use a bed cradle (nonheated) to prevent pressure from bed linens.

Patient Monitoring
Frequent history and physical examinations

PATIENT EDUCATION
- Remove possibilities of exposure to others in the environment who smoke.
- Nicotine replacement may keep the disease active.
- Use heel pads or foam rubber boots.

PROGNOSIS
- Average death age 52 ± 8.9 years; significantly lower than matched US population (6)
- In the Cleveland Clinic series, 94% of patients who quit smoking remained free of amputation, whereas 43% of patients who continued smoking required at least 1 amputation (1).
- Data from Mayo Clinic showed an amputation rate of 25% at 5 years and 38% at 10 years of follow-up (6).
- The risk of amputation is eliminated after 8 years of smoking cessation.

COMPLICATIONS
- Ulcerations, gangrene, need for amputation
- Rare occlusion of cerebral, coronary, renal, splenic, mesenteric, pulmonary, iliac arteries, and aorta

REFERENCES

1. Olin JW, Shih A. Thromboangiitis obliterans (Buerger's disease). *Curr Opin Rheumatol*. 2006; 18:18–24.
2. Maecki R, Zdrojowy K, Adamiec R, et al. Thromboangiitis obliterans in the 21st century–a new face of disease. *Atherosclerosis*. 2009;206: 328–34.
3. Pereira de Godoy JM, Braile DM. Buerger's disease and anticardiolipin antibodies. *J Cardiovasc Med (Hagerstown)*. 2009;10(10):792–4.
4. Fujii Y, Soga J, Nakamura S, et al. Classification of corkscrew collaterals in thromboangiitis obliterans (Buerger's disease). *Circ J*. 2010;74(8):1684–8.
5. Bozkurt AK, Köksal C, Demirbas MY, et al. A randomized trial of intravenous versus lumbar sympathectomy in the management of Buerger's disease. *Int Angiol*. 2006;25(2):162–8.
6. Cooper LT, Tse TS, Mikhail MA, et al. Long-term survival and amputation risk in thromboangiitis obliterans (Buerger's disease). *J Am Coll Cardiol*. 2004;44:2410–1.

ADDITIONAL READING

Grotenhermen F, et al. Cannabis-associated arteritis. *VASA*. 2010;39:43–53.

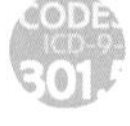

CODES

ICD9
443.1 Thromboangiitis obliterans (Buerger's disease)

CLINICAL PEARLS
- No form of medical treatment has been proven effective for the treatment of TOA. Medications are not a substitute for discontinuing smoking.
- Measurement of urinary nicotine and cotinine should be performed if the disease is still active despite patient's claims of tobacco cessation.
- A vascular biopsy is usually not necessary unless patients present with unusual characteristics such as large-artery involvement or age >45 years.
- ~94% of patients who quit smoking avoid amputation compared with 43% who continue smoking.

THROMBOPHILIA AND HYPERCOAGULABLE STATES

Priscilla Merriam, MD
Nancy J. Freeman, MD

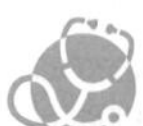

BASICS

DESCRIPTION

- A heritable or acquired disorder of the coagulation system predisposing an individual to thromboembolism (the formation of a venous or less commonly arterial clot) (1)
- Venous thrombosis typically manifests as deep venous thrombosis (DVT) of the lower extremity and pulmonary embolism (PE) (1).
- System(s) affected: Cardiovascular; Nervous; Pulmonary; Reproductive; Hematologic
- Synonym(s): Hypercoagulation syndrome

EPIDEMIOLOGY

- An inherited thrombophilic defect or risk can be detected in some 50% of patients with venous thromboembolism (VTE).
- Factor V Leiden is the most common inherited thrombophilia (half of all currently characterizable inherited thrombophilia cases involve the factor V Leiden mutation), and it is present in its heterozygous form in up to ~20% of patients with a first VTE.
- Heterozygous prothrombin G20210A mutation, the second most common inherited thrombophilia, is present in up to ~8% of patients with VTE.

Incidence

First-time thromboembolism:

- ~100 per 100,000 per year among the general population
- <1 per 100,000 per year in those <15 years old
- ~1,000 per 100,000 per year in those ≥85 years old

Prevalence

- 40–80% of lower extremity orthopedic procedures are complicated by VTE (calf or proximal) unless prophylaxis is used.
- VTE accounts for ~1.2–4.7 deaths per 100,000 pregnancies.

RISK FACTORS

- Acquired risk factors:
  - Immobilization
  - Trauma
  - Surgery, especially orthopedic
  - Malignancies (especially pancreatic, ovarian, brain, and lymphoma)
  - Pregnancy
  - Exogenous female hormones/oral contraceptives
  - Obesity
  - Nephrotic syndrome
  - Antiphospholipid syndrome (APS) and lupus anticoagulant
  - Myeloproliferative disorders (polycythemia vera, essential thrombocythemia)
  - Hyperviscosity syndromes (sickle cell, paraproteinemias)
  - Hyperhomocysteinemia secondary to vitamin deficiencies (B_6, B_{12}, folic acid)
  - Tamoxifen, thalidomide, lenalidomide, bevacizumab, L-asparaginase, erythropoietic stimulating agents
  - Previous thromboembolism
- Established genetic factors:
  - Factor V Leiden
  - Prothrombin G20210A mutation
  - Protein C deficiency
  - Protein S deficiency
  - Antithrombin III deficiency
- Rare genetic factors:
  - Dysfibrinogenemia
  - Hyperhomocysteinemia (methylene tetrahydrofolate reductase mutation)
- Indeterminate factors:
  - Elevated factor VIII
- Age
- Gender: Men
- Race: Incidence is higher among African Americans.

Genetics

- The most common genetic thrombophilias (factor V Leiden, prothrombin G20210A, proteins C and S, and antithrombin III deficiency) are inherited in an autosomal-dominant pattern.
- Homozygous mutations generally have a higher risk of VTE.
- Factor V Leiden/activated protein C (aPC) resistance is the most common inherited thrombophilia:
  - 2–5% prevalence among whites; rare in African Americans, Asians
  - aPC does not cleave factor Va, and thrombin formation continues.
  - Other acquired risks are synergistic (2).
- Prothrombin gene mutation G20210A: Prevalence 6% among whites. Heterozygous carriers have increased risk of thrombosis.
- Hyperhomocysteinemia: 5–6% among the general population. Increases risk of coronary artery disease/myocardial infarction, cerebrovascular accident, DVT/PE. Acquired in those with folate, vitamin B_{12}, and vitamin B_6 deficiencies.
- Antithrombin deficiency: <0.2% incidence among the general population; produced in the liver; acquired deficiency in disseminated intravascular coagulation (DIC), sepsis, liver disease, nephrotic syndrome.
- Protein C and S deficiencies: 0.5% and 1% incidences, respectively, among the general population. Homozygotes and heterozygotes are hypercoagulable. Vitamin K-dependent, produced in the liver. Protein C inactivates Va and VIIIa. Protein C may become an acquired deficiency in liver disease, sepsis, DIC, acute respiratory distress syndrome, and after surgery. Protein S is a cofactor for protein C, and it may become an acquired deficiency with oral contraceptive pill (OCP) use, pregnancy, liver disease, sepsis, DIC, HIV, and nephrosis.

GENERAL PREVENTION

- Prophylaxis with medications should be considered in any hospitalized patient with VTE risk factors, and hospitalized patients should be encouraged to become mobile as soon as possible (3)[A].
- Mechanical prophylaxis may be considered in patients at low risk for VTE or those in whom anticoagulation may be contraindicated.
- Consider prophylaxis with low-molecular-weight heparin (LMWH) + aspirin in pregnant patients with APS or other thrombophilia.
- Prophylaxis with unfractionated heparin or LMWH should be considered in patients with genetic or acquired risks of thrombosis and an anticipated additional risk, such as the immobilization associated with surgery.
- Use caution with procoagulant medicines (e.g., OCPs) in asymptomatic individuals who have a known hereditary predisposition.

PATHOPHYSIOLOGY

- Virchow hypothesis to explain the cause of VTE evolved to include the triad of blood stasis, vascular endothelial injury, and abnormalities in circulating blood constituents (i.e., hypercoagulability)
- An imbalance between the hemostatic and fibrinolytic pathways leads to thrombus formation; this may be too much of a prothrombotic protein or too little of an antithrombotic protein.
- VTE is considered to be the result of genetic tendencies (measurable or not) with other acquired risks.
- Upper extremity DVT: >60% are associated with venous catheters. Malignancy is an additional significant risk (4).

COMMONLY ASSOCIATED CONDITIONS

Advanced age, cancer, pregnancy, obesity, prior history of thrombosis, surgery, immobilization

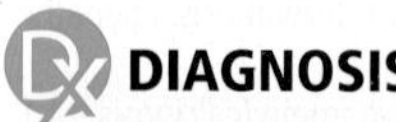

DIAGNOSIS

HISTORY

Consider prothrombotic assessment for:

- Unprovoked thrombosis at age <45–50 years
- Thrombosis at an unusual anatomic site or recurrent thromboses
- Family history suggesting multiple individuals affected with VTE
- Thrombosis with recent immobilization, travel, hospitalization, surgery
- Recurrent pregnancy loss or thrombosis with OCP use

PHYSICAL EXAM

- Physical findings may be unreliable for DVT.
- Swelling, pain, warmth, and redness, usually of one extremity
- Dyspnea, pleurisy, hemoptysis, hypoxia in PE
- Superficial phlebitis: Red, painful cord palpable along the path of thrombosed vein
- Postthrombotic syndrome: Pain, swelling, pigmentation, and/or ulceration

DIAGNOSTIC TESTS & INTERPRETATION

Lab

Testing for heritable thrombophilia in all patients presenting with a first episode of VTE is not indicated (4)[B].

Initial lab tests

- CBC
- aPC resistance: 95–100% are factor V Leiden positive; false-positive in pregnancy or with use of OCPs) → can confirm with factor V Leiden mutation testing or can consider factor V Leiden mutation testing upfront:
  - aPC resistance may be unreliable while taking LMWH or unfractionated heparin (UFH)

- Prothrombin G20210A genetic assay
- ATIII functional assay:
  - Will be low with acute thrombosis and on heparin therapy
- Protein C functional assay:
  - May be low with acute thrombosis; will be lower on warfarin
- Protein S antigen and functional assay and free S:
  - May be low with acute thrombosis; will be lower on warfarin
- Antiphospholipid antibodies → phospholipid-dependent tests and anticardiolipin antibodies, lupus anticoagulant:
  - May be unreliable on heparin
- Consider homocysteine level → although treatment of hyperhomocysteinemia (vitamins B_{12} and B_6, folate) does not alter the thrombophilic risk

Follow-Up & Special Considerations

Dysfibrinogenemia and plasminogen deficiency are very rare causes of thrombophilia.

DIFFERENTIAL DIAGNOSIS

Lower extremity VTE:

- Edema from other causes (congestive heart failure, medicines)
- Baker cyst
- Cellulitis
- Lymphedema
- Chronic venous insufficiency

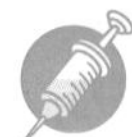

TREATMENT

MEDICATION

First Line

- LMWH has largely replaced UFH as first-line therapy for VTE:
  - Enoxaparin (Lovenox) 1 mg/kg SC b.i.d. for at least 5 days (with concomitant warfarin orally), until international normalized ratio (INR) has reached 2 for at least 24 hours
  - Enoxaparin is preferred in patients with active cancer for a minimum of 3 months (and can be at 1.5 mg/kg SC daily), after which time the patient can be re-evaluated to continue enoxaparin or transition to warfarin.
  - Adverse reactions: Bleeding, heparin-induced thrombocytopenia (HIT) <0.5% incidence, bone loss (uncommon)
  - Reversal: Stop LMWH
  - UFH: Dose, 80 U/kg or 5,000-unit IV bolus, then 18 U/kg/hr or 1,300 U/hr to target the activated partial thromboplastin time (aPTT) to a corresponding anti-Xa level of 0.3–0.7 U/mL. The first aPTT should be checked 6 hours after initial therapy and adjusted per standard heparin nomograms, aiming for an adequate level within 24 hours. Transition to warfarin is similar to the recommendations for enoxaparin.
  - Adverse reactions: Bleeding, HIT 3% incidence, bone loss (long-term use)
  - Reversal: Stop heparin, protamine
- Oral anticoagulation:
  - Warfarin (Coumadin) 5 mg/d initially and adjusted to INR 2–3 for at least 3 months, potentially indefinitely for patients with high risk of recurrence, or recurrent, or unprovoked VTE.
  - Warfarin requires careful and frequent monitoring because there are many drug–drug and drug–diet (e.g., vitamin K) interactions.
  - Adverse reactions: Bleeding, skin necrosis (rare and early in course); cannot be used in pregnancy
  - Reversal: Fresh frozen plasma and/or vitamin K
- Pregnancy (controversial): Low-dose aspirin and/or LMWH or UFH; warfarin is contraindicated

Second Line

Usually indicated when contraindication to heparin or LMWH, such as heparin-associated thrombosis and thrombocytopenia, if there is an inability to use IV drugs, or renal failure:

- SC UFH is another alternative and can be given as 5000 units IV (once) followed by 250 U/kg SC b.i.d., or 250 U/kg bolus followed by 250 U/kg b.i.d. (monitored as for IV UFH), or 333 U/kg once followed by 250 U/kg SC b.i.d. (unmonitored).
- Indirect factor Xa inhibitor (ATIII inhibitor):
  - Representative drug: Fondaparinux: Efficacious for prevention and treatment of acute VTE, postoperative prophylaxis, PE (FDA-approved indications).
    - Dose: Acute VTE/PE. Weight <50 kg: 5 mg/d SC; weight 50–100 kg: 7.5 mg/d SC; weight >100 kg: 10 mg/d SC; use for 5–9 days until oral anticoagulation is therapeutic
    - Prophylaxis: 2.5 mg/d SC
    - Dose adjustments: Needed for renal insufficiency; if creatinine clearance is <30 mL/min, use is contraindicated
- Direct thrombin inhibitors: Most commonly used for anticoagulation in HIT. Representative drugs include:
  - Lepirudin: Excreted by kidneys, crosses the placenta; dosing based on creatinine clearance; therapeutic dose based on aPTT.
  - Argatroban: Liver metabolized; may be dose adjusted in liver dysfunction; therapeutic dose based on aPTT.
  - Dabigatran is an oral direct thrombin inhibitor, the only current FDA indication for which is for thromboembolic prophylaxis in patients with nonvalvular atrial fibrillation (not inferior to warfarin).

SURGERY/OTHER PROCEDURES

- Catheter extraction/thrombectomy for extreme emergencies (e.g., massive PE where thrombolysis not feasible)
- Inferior vena cava filter:
  - Reduces short-term risk of PE (e.g., GI bleeding and inability to anticoagulate)
  - May increase long-term risk of recurrent DVT
  - Use for patients with multiple episodes of recurrent thromboembolism despite therapeutic anticoagulation.

ONGOING CARE

FOLLOW-UP RECOMMENDATIONS

Avoid significant risk for trauma (e.g., contact sports, climbing a ladder).

Patient Monitoring

Monitor warfarin as frequently as needed to maintain an INR goal of 2–3 (through an anticoagulation clinic).

DIET

Vitamin K-stable diet if patient is taking warfarin

PATIENT EDUCATION

- Assume that any drug may enhance or attenuate the warfarin effect.
- Increase the frequency of monitoring following any medication change to ensure therapeutic anticoagulation and to avoid overanticoagulation.
- Many drugs may modulate warfarin effect: Alcohol, antibiotics, aspirin, NSAIDs, acetaminophen

PROGNOSIS

- Patients with a provoked VTE (i.e., surgery, hospitalization) not receiving chronic anticoagulation have a risks of recurrence of 7% (year 1), 16% (year 5), and 23% (year 10).
- Patients with an unprovoked VTE not receiving chronic anticoagulation have risks of recurrence of 15% (year 1), 41% (year 5), and 53% (year 10).
- Currently there is no data from randomized controlled trials or controlled clinical trials about the benefits of thrombophilia testing to decrease the risk of recurrent VTE (1).

COMPLICATIONS

Venous or arterial thrombosis; bleeding in anticoagulated patients

REFERENCES

1. Cohn D, Vansenne F, de Borgie C, et al. Thrombophilia testing for prevention of recurrent venous thromboembolism. *Cochrane Database Syst Rev*. 2009;CD007069.
2. Anderson JA, Weitz JI. Hypercoagulable states. *Clin Chest Med*. 2010;31:659–73.
3. Hill J, Treasure T, National Clinical Guideline Centre for Acute and Chronic Conditions, et al. Reducing the risk of venous thromboembolism in patients admitted to hospital: Summary of NICE guidance. *BMJ*. 2010;340:c95.
4. Baglin T, Gray E, Greaves M, et al. Clinical guidelines for testing for heritable thrombophilia. *Br J Haematol*. 2010;149:209–20.

ADDITIONAL READING

Hirsh J, Bauer KA, Donati MB, et al. Parenteral anticoagulants: American College of Chest Physicians Evidence-Based Clinical Practice Guidelines (8th Edition). *Chest*. 2008;133:141S–59S.

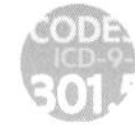

CODES

ICD9

- 281.4 Protein-deficiency anemia
- 286.9 Other and unspecified coagulation defects
- 289.81 Primary hypercoagulable state

CLINICAL PEARLS

- Factor V Leiden (resistance to aPC) is the most common inherited thrombophilia, with a prevalence of 2–7% in the white US population.
- Test patients <50 years of age with a history of venous thrombosis, and consider testing first-degree relatives.
- Rule out malignancy, especially in those older than age 50.

THROMBOTIC THROMBOCYTOPENIC PURPURA

Kellie A. Sprague, MD
Carol Curtin, MSW, LICSW

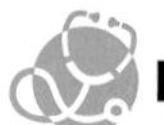

BASICS

DESCRIPTION

- An acute syndrome hallmarked by microangiopathic hemolytic anemia (MAHA) and consumptive thrombocytopenia with deposition of hyaline thrombi in terminal arterioles and capillaries leading to ischemic multiorgan damage
- Thrombotic thrombocytopenic purpura (TTP) is characterized by MAHA and thrombocytopenia, with or without the following signs and symptoms (1):
  - Neurologic symptoms
  - Renal dysfunction
  - Fever
  - Most patients do not show the historic pentad of MAHA, thrombocytopenia, renal dysfunction, neurologic abnormalities, and fever, because treatment is initiated before the pentad can develop.

EPIDEMIOLOGY

Incidence

- Predominant age: 30–60 years. Rare under age 20.
- Predominant sex: Female > Male (2:1)
- Incidence ratio in blacks to nonblacks is 3:1
- The age–sex–race standardized incidence of clinically suspected TTP/hemolytic-uremic syndrome (HUS) is 11/million/yr in the US.

RISK FACTORS

- Pregnancy and oral contraceptives
- AIDS and early symptomatic HIV infection
- Autoimmune disease:
  - Antiphospholipid antibody syndrome
  - Systemic lupus erythematosus
  - Scleroderma
- Cancer
- Hematopoietic stem cell transplantation
- Drug toxicity:
  - Cancer chemotherapy:
    - Mitomycin C and gemcitabine
    - Bleomycin and cisplatin
  - Calcineurin inhibitors:
    - Tacrolimus and cyclosporine
  - Immune-mediated:
    - Quinine and quinidine
    - Ticlopidine and clopidogrel

Genetics

TTP is most often an acquired disorder. A congenital form of inherited TTP (Schulman-Upshaw syndrome) is due to a mutation at the ADAMTS13 metalloproteinase gene locus on chromosome 9q34. This rare form of TTP has an autosomal recessive pattern of inheritance (3).

PATHOPHYSIOLOGY

- In TTP, the aggregating agent responsible for platelet thrombi is unusually large von Willebrand factor (UL vWF) multimers, which are far larger than those found in normal plasma.
- A metalloproteinase, ADAMTS13, which normally enzymatically cleaves UL vWF multimers to prevent clumping within vessels, is deficient, defective, or absent, allowing UL vWF to react with platelets. This leads to the endothelial cell damage and disseminated thrombi characteristic of TTP.
- Arterioles most often affected are in the brain, kidney, pancreas, heart, and adrenal glands. Lungs and liver are relatively spared.

ETIOLOGY

- In familial TTP, patients have low or absent levels of ADAMTS13.
- In acquired idiopathic TTP, some studies have demonstrated IgG autoantibodies made to the metalloproteinase ADAMTS13 to receptors on the surfaces of platelets or to the surface of the endothelial cell. The trigger is unknown (4)[A].
- Endothelial injury, either directly from a drug/toxin or indirectly via platelet/neutrophil activation, has been proposed as a cause of secondary TTP, especially in those without ADAMTS13 deficiency:
  - Drug-induced (see "Risk Factors")
  - Hematopoietic cell transplantation

COMMONLY ASSOCIATED CONDITIONS

- TTP and HUS have similar presentations with MAHA and thrombocytopenia and multiorgan involvement.
- TTP generally presents with minimal renal involvement and may have neurologic abnormalities, whereas the opposite tends to be more characteristic of HUS.
- However, patients with HUS and TTP may have both prominent renal and neurologic manifestations, often making the distinction unclear, leading to the hybrid name "TTP-HUS."
- ADAMTS13 levels are diminished in adults with familial or acquired idiopathic TTP but are normal in children diagnosed with HUS following infection with *E. coli* (particularly type O157:H7) so-called "typical HUS."

DIAGNOSIS

- Most common symptoms are nonspecific: Nausea, vomiting, weakness, abdominal pain, fatigue, fever
- Related to thrombocytopenia:
  - Easy bruising, purpura, or petechiae
  - Epistaxis, menorrhagia, bleeding gums
  - GI bleeding
  - Intracranial hemorrhage
  - Visual symptoms due to retinal hemorrhage
- Related to hemolytic anemia (MAHA): Jaundice, fatigue
- Related to end-organ ischemia:
  - Neurologic: CNS symptoms occur in 50%:
    - Often fluctuating symptoms
    - Headache
    - Altered mental status: Spectrum runs from behavioral/personality changes to obtundation/stupor or coma.
    - Seizures
    - Stroke
  - Renal: Hematuria, oliguria, or anuria
  - Cardiac: Arrhythmia, myocardial infarction, heart failure

HISTORY

- Generally acute onset of symptoms but subacute in about 1/4 of patients
- It is important to assess for potential underlying causes or risk factors (see above).

PHYSICAL EXAM

- Fever
- Mental status/neurologic: Confusion, coma, stupor, weakness
- HEENT: Retinal hemorrhage, scleral icterus, epistaxis
- Abdomen/GI: Nonspecific tenderness
- Skin: Jaundice, petechiae, purpura, ecchymoses

DIAGNOSTIC TESTS & INTERPRETATION

Lab

Initial lab tests

- CBC:
  - Hemoglobin (decreased):
    - Average is 8–9 g/dL; <6 g/dL in 40%
  - Platelets decreased
- Reticulocyte count (increased)
- Peripheral smear:
  - Schistocytes (prominent)
  - Helmet cells, RBC fragments
  - Nucleated RBCs
  - Polychromasia (reticulocytosis)
- Coagulation studies:
  - Normal in most; mild elevation in 15%
  - Fibrinogen normal
- Coombs test: Negative direct Coombs test
- Electrolytes, BUN/creatinine: Mild elevation of BUN and creatinine (creatinine <3 mg/dL)
- Liver function studies: Increased indirect bilirubin (hemolysis)
- Lactate dehydrogenase (LDH): 5–10 × normal
- Haptoglobin decreased (hemolysis)
- Urinalysis:
  - Proteinuria, microscopic hematuria
  - Positive dipstick for large blood, but minimal RBCs on microscopic exam
- ECG: Sinus tachycardia, heart block
- No utility of ADAMTS13 assay in diagnosis and decision to initiate therapy at presentation, but assay is helpful for confirmation of idiopathic or familial TTP.

Imaging

Head CT scan: Performed if mental status changes are present to rule out possible intracranial hemorrhage or ischemic changes

Pathological Findings

Biopsy of affected organs shows platelet thrombi within or beneath damaged endothelium. However, biopsy is rarely obtained because the diagnosis is made on clinical grounds and laboratory findings.

DIFFERENTIAL DIAGNOSIS

- HUS (see "Associated Conditions")
- Antiphospholipid antibody syndrome: Prolonged partial thromboplastin time (PTT) and presence of lupus anticoagulant
- Systemic lupus erythematous
- Malignant hypertension (HTN): Diastolic >130 mm Hg, papilledema, retinal hemorrhages
- Pregnancy-associated preeclampsia/eclampsia or HELLP: Low ATIII levels
- Disseminated intravascular coagulation:
  - Prolonged prothrombin time (PT)/PTT, low fibrinogen
  - Low factors V and VIII
  - Secondary to sepsis/shock or widely disseminated malignancy

- Idiopathic thrombocytopenic purpura:
  - No hemolysis, normal LDH and bilirubin
  - Presence of antiplatelet antibodies
- Malignancy-associated microangiopathy
- Evan syndrome (autoimmune hemolytic anemia and thrombocytopenia): Positive direct Coombs test
- Sclerodermal kidney
- 90% mortality without treatment

TREATMENT

- Prompt treatment is necessary due to the high mortality (90%).
- In the absence of another apparent cause, the dyad of MAHA and thrombocytopenia is sufficient to begin treatment for TTP while the workup proceeds (4)[B]:
  - Plasma exchange transfusion (PEX) is the cornerstone of treatment of classic TTP (4)[A].
  - PEX is thought to replace a deficient or defective metalloproteinase (ADAMTS13) and remove UL vWF and antimetalloproteinase antibodies.
  - 1–1.5 plasma volumes/day should be begun immediately and continued daily.
  - Continue daily until LDH, platelets, neurologic symptoms, and renal function normalize (4)[A].
  - Fresh frozen plasma (4)[A]: Temporary measure until PEX can be initiated.

MEDICATION

First Line

Glucocorticoids may be of benefit in some patients. British guidelines recommend its use for all patients (4)[C]:

- Steroids may work by suppressing the autoantibodies inhibiting ADAMTS13 activity.
- Utility may be in patients with severe ADAMTS13 deficiency, in the setting of exacerbation when PEX is stopped or in relapse after remission.
- There is little benefit of steroids when used as monotherapy.
- Doses: Prednisone 1 mg/kg/d and taper once in remission (4,5)[C] or methylprednisolone 1 g/d IV × 3 days (4)[C]

Second Line

The following medications are used in refractory cases:

- Rituximab (6)[C]
- Vincristine, cyclophosphamide, cyclosporin
- IVIG

ADDITIONAL TREATMENT

Issues for Referral

- Hematology or blood bank for plasma exchange transfusion
- Nephrology for dialysis
- Cardiology for presence of significant heart block
- Neurosurgery for intracranial hemorrhage

SURGERY/OTHER PROCEDURES

Splenectomy is reserved for severe, refractory cases with ambiguous results.

IN-PATIENT CONSIDERATIONS

Initial Stabilization

- ABCs, oxygen, IV access, telemetry
- Volume resuscitation if hypotensive/actively bleeding
- Packed RBCs can be transfused safely
- Platelet transfusion may be used for the prevention and treatment of hemorrhage (7)[B].

Discharge Criteria

On normalization and stabilization of neurologic symptoms, LDH, platelets, and renal function

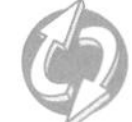

ONGOING CARE

FOLLOW-UP RECOMMENDATIONS

- No maintenance therapy is required. After PEX is discontinued, blood counts should be monitored over a few months. If testing remains normal, testing interval can be lengthened (8)[C].
- Promptly evaluate any symptoms of relapse.

PATIENT EDUCATION

- On discharge, advise patients to self-monitor for signs of relapse (e.g., fever, headache, bruising).
- Patients should be advised about prolonged periods of fatigue following the acute phase.
- www.nhlbi.nih.gov/health/dci/Diseases/ttp/TTP'WhatIs.html

PROGNOSIS

- Most patients recover fully from idiopathic TTP when treated promptly:
  - 30-day mortality is 10% in those who receive PEX.
  - 70% respond within 14 days; 90% respond within 28 days.
  - 80% survival in patients with idiopathic TTP treated with PEX (9)
- Initial LDH and platelet counts are not predictive of the patient's response to treatment.
- Final platelet count and LDH or the length or intensity of treatment does not predict relapse.
- Low levels of ADAMTS13 activity during remission are associated with higher risk of relapse (10,11).
- In patients with severe ADAMTS13 deficiency, the risk of relapse is estimated to be 41% at 7.5 years, with the greatest risk being in the first year (9).

COMPLICATIONS

- Patients may experience mild cognitive impairments in attention, concentration, and memory following 1 or more episodes of TTP (12).
- Complications of PEX include:
  - Central line infections and hemorrhage
  - Citrate toxicity
  - Hypersensitivity reactions to frequent plasma

REFERENCES

1. Sadler JE. Von Willebrand factor, ADAMTS13, and thrombotic thrombocytopenic purpura. *Blood*. 2008;112:11–8.
2. Terrell DR, Williams LA, Vesley SK, et al. The incidence for thrombotic thrombocytopenic purpura-hemolytic uremic syndrome: All patients, idiopathic patients, and patients with severe ADAMTS13 deficiency. *J Thromb Heamost*. 2005;3(7):1432–6.
3. Levy GG, Nicholas WC, Lian EC, et al. Mutations in a member of the ADMATS gene family cause thrombotic thrombocytopenic purpura. *Nature*. 2001;413(6855):488–94.
4. George JN. Clinical practice. Thrombotic thrombocytopenic purpura. *N Engl J Med*. 2006;354:1927–35.
5. Allford SL, Hunt BJ, Rose P, et al. Guidelines on the diagnosis and management of the thrombotic microangiopathic haemolytic anaemias. *Br J Haematol*. 2003;120:556–73.
6. Ling HT, Field JJ, Blinder MA. Sustained response with rituximab in patients with thrombotic thrombocytopenic purpura: A report of 13 cases and review of the literature. *Ann J Hematol*. 2009;84(7):418–21.
7. Swisher KK, Terrell DR, Vesely SK, et al. Clinical outcomes after platelet transfusion in patients with thrombotic thrombocytopenia purpura. *Transfusion*. 2009;49(5):873–87.
8. George JN. How I treat patients with thrombiv thrombocytopenic purpura: 2010. *Blood*. 2010;116(20):4060–69.
9. Kremer Hovigna JA, Vesley SK, et al. Survival and relapse in patients with thrombotic thrombocytopenic purpura. *Blood*. 2010;115(8):1500–11.
10. Jin M, Casper C, Cataland SR, et al. Relationship between ADAMTS13 activity in clinical remission and the risk of TTP relapse. *Br J Haematol*. 2008;141(5):651–58.
11. Peyvandi F, Lavoretano S, Palla R, et al. ADAMTS13 and anti-ADAMTS13 antibodies are markers for recurrence or acquired thrombotic thrombocytopenia purpura during remission. *Haematologica*. 2008;93:69–76.
12. Kennedy AS, Lewis QF, Scott JG, et al. Cognitive deficits after recovery from thrombotic thrombocytopenic purpura. *Transfusion*. 2009;49:1092–101.

ADDITIONAL READING

Sadler JE, Moake JL, Miyata T, et al. Recent advances in thrombotic thrombocytopenic purpura. *Hematol Am Soc Hematol Educ Program*. 2004;407–23.

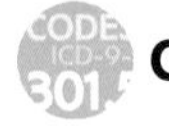

CODES

ICD9

446.6 Thrombotic microangiopathy

CLINICAL PEARLS

- The diagnosis of TTP is made clinically; common symptoms are nonspecific: Nausea, vomiting, weakness, abdominal pain, fatigue, fever and easy bruising, purpura, or petechiae
- The historical pentad of fever, neurologic symptoms, renal dysfunction, MAHA, and thrombocytopenia is not present in most patients.
- The dyad of MAHA and thrombocytopenia is sufficient to initiate treatment with PEX.
- Do not wait for results of ADAMTS13 determination to initiate therapy.

T

THYROGLOSSAL DUCT CYST

Felix B. Chang, MD

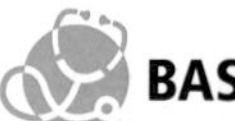

BASICS

Cyst composed of epithelial remnants of the thyroglossal tract

DESCRIPTION

- Usually midline neck mass at the level of the thyrohyoid membrane, closely associated with the hyoid bone
- Within 2 cm of the midline
- Single, smooth, nontender, and mobile
- 65% infrahyoid type
- 20% suprahyoid
- 15% juxtahyoid
- 10% suprasternal
- Intralaryngeal very rare: Suprasternal notch, superior mediastinum
- Endolaryngeal cyst (ectopic location): Extremely rare
- System(s) affected: Endocrine/Metabolic; Skin/Exocrine

EPIDEMIOLOGY

- The most common form of congenital cyst in the neck
- Accounts for 2–4% of all neck masses

Incidence

- Most patients are children or adolescents.
- Up to 1/3 are aged 20 years or older.
- Predominant age: 50% <10 years, 65% <20 years
- Predominant sex: Male = Female
- White race

Prevalence

- Thyroglossal duct cysts were found in 7% of adults in 1 autopsy study.
- Thyroglossal duct anomalies are the second most common pediatric neck mass, behind adenopathy in frequency.

RISK FACTORS

Genetics

- Usually sporadic; if familial, autosomal dominant is most common mode of inheritance (1).
- Familial occurrence is extremely rare (2).

PATHOPHYSIOLOGY

- Cystic expansion of a remnant of the thyroglossal duct tract
- Persistence of the epithelial tract, the thyroglossal duct, during the descent of the thyroid from the foramen cecum to its final position in the anterior neck
- The thyroglossal duct tract usually atrophies and disappears by the 8th to 10th week of gestation.
- Portions of the tract and remnants of thyroid tissue associated with it may persist at any point between the tongue and the thyroid.
- The wall of a thyroglossal duct is the second most common site for ectopic thyroid tissue.

ETIOLOGY

- Failure of the thyroglossal duct to atrophy and involute after descent of the thyroid in the fourth to seventh week of gestation
- Hypothesis: Lymphoid tissue associated with the tract hypertrophies at the time of a regional infection, thereby occluding the tract with resulting cyst formation.

COMMONLY ASSOCIATED CONDITIONS

- Often the patient has a history of a recent upper respiratory tract infection.
- Ectopic thyroid tissue is found in 50% of patients.
- If thyroid gland fails to descend to orthotopic site, an ectopic thyroid gland results. Most ectopic thyroid glands are lingual. Many patients with ectopic thyroid gland are hypothyroid.

DIAGNOSIS

May be located and can track anywhere from the thyroid cartilage up the base of the tongue

HISTORY

- Most often asymptomatic, midline upper neck mass that is cystic
- Swelling
- Painful or only slightly tender
- Redness
- Neck mass
- 1/4 of patients present with a draining sinus.
- Foul taste in the mouth if the spontaneous drainage occurred by way of the foramen cecum
- Rare presentations: Severe respiratory distress or sudden infant death syndrome from lesions at the base of the tongue, a lateral cystic neck mass, an anterior tongue fistula, or coexistence with branchial anomalies

PHYSICAL EXAM

- Midline neck mass, usually within 2 cm of the midline
- Nontender or slightly tender, unless infected
- Rises in the neck with tongue protrusion and swallowing
- 80% adjacent to the hyoid bone
- Infected thyroglossal duct cyst may manifest as tender mass with associated dysphagia, dysphonia, draining sinus, fever, or increasing neck mass.
- Airway obstruction is possible, especially with intralingual cysts.
- ~1/3 present with a concurrent or prior upper respiratory tract infection.
- Cyst below the thyrohyoid membrane is rare

DIAGNOSTIC TESTS & INTERPRETATION

The preoperative evaluation for a patient who has a suspected thyroglossal duct cyst includes a complete history and physical examination, preoperative ultrasound, and a screening thyroid-stimulating hormone (TSH) determination.

Lab

Initial lab tests

Assess thyroid function.

Imaging

- Ultrasound or CT scan to confirm diagnosis, identify thyroid, and demonstrate relationship to hyoid bone
- Patients with elevated TSH levels suggesting hypothyroidism or a solid mass should undergo scintiscanning to rule out a median ectopic thyroid.
- Thyroid scan if midline ectopic thyroid or thyroid nodule is suspected
- Small roll under shoulders allows exposure of neck in infants.
- Occasionally, if the cyst is infected, hemorrhagic, or has a high protein content, it may appear as hyperdense on CT scan, as an area of high signal intensity on T1- and T2-weighted MRI, and have an internal echo on ultrasound.
- Malignancy may be suspected if a soft tissue component exists within or around the cyst.

Follow-Up & Special Considerations

- If a solid mass is encountered during excision of a suspected thyroglossal duct cyst, it should be sent for frozen section to rule out a median ectopic thyroid.
- Fine-needle aspiration (FNA) biopsy is the most reliable method for preoperative diagnosis of thyroid carcinoma, especially if done with ultrasound guidance.
- FNA can be helpful to decrease cyst size, and in some cases may lead to identification of thyroglossal duct cyst carcinoma if solid elements of the lesion can be sampled.

Diagnostic Procedures/Surgery

- FNA for preoperative evaluation of thyroglossal duct cysts may reveal colloid, neutrophils, macrophages, lymphocytes, and ciliated columnar cells. It is often used to exclude other diagnoses.
- If cyst is infected, antibiotic treatment may be required prior to definitive resection.
- Incision and drainage with resulting scarring may complicate resection.

Pathological Findings

- Cyst lined with stratified squamous or pseudostratified ciliated columnar epithelium
- Thyroid tissue is seen in 10–45% of cysts.
- Reports show traces of the thyroglossal duct located near the hyoid bone, superior to the thyroid isthmus, or lingually.
- Fewer than 1% of thyroglossal duct cysts have malignant tissue, usually well-differentiated thyroid carcinoma.

DIFFERENTIAL DIAGNOSIS

- Ectopic midline thyroid
- Dermoid cyst
- Thyroid adenoma of isthmus or pyramidal lobe
- Lymphadenitis
- Cervical thymic cyst
- Sebaceous (epidermal) cysts
- Medial branchial cleft cyst
- Salivary gland tumor
- Lymphatic malformations
- Lipoma
- Hypertrophic pyramidal lobes of the thyroid

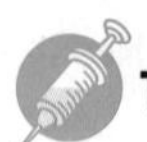

TREATMENT

Elective surgical excision is the treatment of choice for uncomplicated thyroglossal duct cysts to prevent infection of the cyst.

MEDICATION

- All thyroglossal duct cysts should be surgically removed.
- Infected cysts or sinuses are first managed by treating the infection.

- The most common organisms are *Haemophilus influenzae, Staphylococcus aureus,* and *S. epidermidis.*
- Antibiotics directed toward these organisms should be started. Successful treatment requires broad-spectrum antibiotics.

First Line

For infected cyst: Cephalexin 500 mg PO q6h, amoxicillin-clavulanate 500 mg/125 mg PO q8h, or clindamycin 600 mg PO q8h.

Second Line

- Coverage against methicillin-resistant *Staphylococcus aureus* is not recommended, unless identified by culture.
- For severe infections: Cefazolin 1–1.5 g IV q8h in combination with clindamycin (600–900 mg IV) q8h

ADDITIONAL TREATMENT

General Measures

IV antibiotics for severe infections

Additional Therapies

Sclerotherapy: Percutaneous ethanol injection is an alternative approach in patients who are not surgical candidates if the presence of malignancy can be excluded. It is effective in 1/3 of patients.

SURGERY/OTHER PROCEDURES

- Sistrunk procedure: Removal of the center portion of the contiguous hyoid bone and resection of a core of tissue from the hyoid upwards toward the foramen cecum
- Recurrence is rare after the Sistrunk procedure and is treated with excision of a core of tissue from the hyoid to the foramen cecum to remove any superior tract arborization (3).
- Suture-guided transhyoid pharyngotomy modification of the Sistrunk operation has also been proposed, but is not recommended at this time.
- If the cyst is infected, infection should be treated with antibiotics and local heat and/or drainage prior to surgery. After resolution of the inflammation, excision should be performed (1,4)[C].

IN-PATIENT CONSIDERATIONS

Admission Criteria

- If incision and drainage are necessary, the incision should be placed so that it can be excised completely with an ellipse at the time of definitive resection.
- Formal incision and drainage should be avoided.

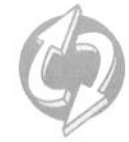

ONGOING CARE

If a thyroglossal duct is not removed, as many as half become infected.

FOLLOW-UP RECOMMENDATIONS

- Unrestricted
- Infection before surgery is a well-described cause of recurrence.

Patient Monitoring

1–2 weeks after resection

DIET

Unrestricted

PATIENT EDUCATION

Reassure family about absence of malignancy (if appropriate).

PROGNOSIS

- Recurrence after complete excision using Sistrunk procedure is reported to be 2.6–5% (5).
- Increased risk of recurrence:
  - Failure to completely excise the cyst
  - In children <2 years of age, intraoperative cyst rupture and presence of a cutaneous component
  - Preoperative or concurrent infection of the cyst at the time of the surgery
- After excision, thyroglossal cyst has a high risk for recurrence (20–35%) and requires a wider en bloc resection.
- Most cases of thyroglossal duct cyst carcinoma are treated adequately by Sistrunk procedure, with a reported cure rate of 95%.

COMPLICATIONS

- Infection occurs in up to half of cysts if not excised.
- Malignant degeneration may occur (1–2%) if cyst is not excised.
- Most common tumor type is papillary carcinoma (6)
- Malignancy is not usually suspected prior to discovery on histologic examination.
- FNA is most reliable for preoperative diagnosis of malignancy, but yield is low due to low incidence of malignancy.
- Unless tumor is invasive (which is rare), Sistrunk procedure is usually curative.
- Must rule out primary thyroid carcinoma if thyroglossal duct cyst carcinoma is found
- Reports demonstrate that lingual location of thyroglossal duct cysts can cause not only various respiratory problems but also infant death.
- Wide local excision is a valuable extension of the Sistrunk operation for the management of recurrent disease (3)[C].
- Patient may require thyroid medication for life if ectopic midline thyroid is mistakenly removed.
- If the cyst ruptures, it may go on to form a thyroglossal duct sinus or a thyroglossal duct fistula that exits through the overlying skin.

REFERENCES

1. Kaselas Ch, Tsikopoulos G, Chortis Ch, et al. Thyroglossal duct cyst's inflammation. When do we operate? *Pediatr Surg Int.* 2005;21:991–3.
2. Schader I, Robertson S, Maoate K, et al. Hereditary duct cyst. *Pediatric Surg Int.* 2005;21(7):593–4.
3. Patel NN, Hartley BE, Howard DJ. Management of thyroglossal tract disease after failed Sistrunk's procedure. *J Laryngol Otol.* 2003;117:710–2.
4. Ostlie DJ, Burjonrappa SC, Snyder CL, et al. Thyroglossal duct infections and surgical outcomes. *J Pediatr Surg.* 2004;39:396–9; discussion 396–9.
5. Sistrunk WE. The surgical treatment of cysts of the thyroglossal tract. *Ann Surg.* 1920;71:121–2.
6. Heshmati HM, Fatourechi V, van Heerden JA, et al. Thyroglossal duct carcinoma: Report of 12 cases. *Mayo Clin Proc.* 1997;72:315–9.

ADDITIONAL READING

- Albayrak Y. A case of papillary carcinoma in a thyroglossal cyst without a carcinoma in the thyroid gland. *Diagn Cytopathol.* 2011;39(1):38–41.
- Min-Ho P, Jun-Ha Y. Papillary thyroglossal duct cyst carcinoma with synchronous occult papillary thyroid microcarcinoma. *Yonsei Med.* 2010;J51(4): 609–11.
- Rosenberg TL. Evaluating the adult patient with a neck mass. *Med Clin North Am.* 2010;94(5): 1017–29.
- Sistrunk's operation for the treatment of thyroglossal cyst. *Mymensingh Med J.* 2010;19(4):565–8.

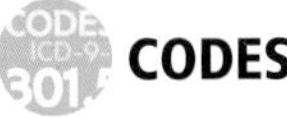

CODES

ICD9

759.2 Anomalies of other endocrine glands, congenital

CLINICAL PEARLS

- Malignancy may be suspected if a soft tissue component exists within or around the cyst or in those cases with clinical changes.
- Thyroglossal duct cysts should be removed surgically, but surgery is usually elective unless the cyst is obstructing the airway.
- Sistrunk procedure is performed once all inflammation has resolved.
- FNA biopsy is the most reliable method for preoperative diagnosis of thyroid cancer, especially if done with ultrasound guidance.
- If the cyst is found to contain thyroid carcinoma, the surgeon must be sure that the carcinoma arose from within the cyst and is not a cystic metastasis to a midline lymph node from a primary thyroid carcinoma.
- When possible, cultures should be obtained with a fine-needle aspirate for Gram stain, aerobic and anaerobic culture, fungal stain and culture, acid-fast stain, and mycobacterial culture.
- The carcinoma is considered to have originated in the thyroglossal duct cyst if there is histologic evidence of columnar or squamous epithelial lining in the cyst, normal thyroid follicles in the cyst wall, and complete absence of lymph node tissue, and there is ultrasonographic evidence of a normal thyroid gland.

THYROID MALIGNANT NEOPLASIA

James P. Miller, MD
Timothy L. Black, MD

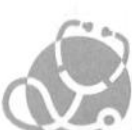

BASICS

DESCRIPTION

Thyroid malignant neoplasia is an autologous growth of thyroid nodules with potential for metastases.

- Papillary carcinoma:
  - Most common variety, 60–70% of thyroid tumors
  - Peak incidence in the third and fourth decades
  - 3× more common in women
  - May be associated with radiation exposure
  - Tumor contains psammoma bodies.
  - Metastasizes by lymphatic route (30% at time of diagnosis)
  - Multicentric in 20% or more, especially in children
- Follicular carcinoma:
  - 10–20% of thyroid tumors
  - Peak incidence in fifth decade of life
  - Incidence has been decreasing since the addition of dietary iodine.
  - Metastasizes by the hematogenous route
- Hürthle cell carcinoma:
  - Usually in patients >60 years of age
  - Radioresistant
  - Composed of distinct large eosinophilic cells with abundant cytoplasmic mitochondria
  - Variant of follicular carcinoma with worse prognosis
- Medullary thyroid carcinoma (MCT):
  - Arises from parafollicular cells, C cells
  - Multiple endocrine neoplasia (MEN) syndromes 2A & 2B occur within the first 2 decades of life.
  - 3–4% of all thyroid tumors
  - 25–35% are associated with MEN syndromes (2A more common than 2B), which can be familial or sporadic.
  - Calcitonin is a chemical marker.
  - RET proto-oncogene mutation is screen.
- Anaplastic carcinoma:
  - 3% of thyroid tumors
  - Usually in patients >60 years of age
- Other: Lymphoma, sarcoma, or metastatic (renal, breast, or lung)
- System(s) affected: Endocrine/Metabolic
- Synonym(s): Follicular carcinoma of the thyroid; Papillary carcinoma of the thyroid; Hürthle cell carcinoma of the thyroid; Anaplastic cell carcinoma of the thyroid

Geriatric Considerations

Risk of malignancy increases at >60 years of age.

Pediatric Considerations

>60% of thyroid nodules are malignant.

EPIDEMIOLOGY

Incidence

- 10/100,000 per year in the US
- Deaths: 6/1 million/yr in the US
- In 2011, estimated 48,020 new cases and 1,740 deaths from thyroid cancer in the US
- Predominant age: Usually >40 years
- Predominant sex: Female > Male (2.6:1).

RISK FACTORS

- Family history
- Neck irradiation (6–2,000 rads): Papillary carcinoma
- Iodine deficiency: Follicular carcinoma
- Multiple endocrine neoplasia syndrome: Medullary carcinoma
- Previous history of subtotal thyroidectomy for malignancy: Anaplastic carcinoma
- Asian race

Genetics

- Familial polyposis of the colon, Turcot syndrome, and Gardner syndrome with the *APC* gene, 5q21
- Medullary: Autosomal dominant with MEN syndrome
- *BRAF* mutation
- *RET* oncogene

GENERAL PREVENTION

- Physical exam in high-risk group
- Calcium infusion or pentagastrin stimulation test screening in high-risk MEN patients
- Screen for RET proto-oncogene in groups at risk for MCT.

ETIOLOGY

Unknown

COMMONLY ASSOCIATED CONDITIONS

Medullary carcinoma: Pheochromocytoma, hyperparathyroidism, ganglioneuroma of the GI tract, neuromata of mucosal membranes

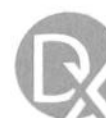

DIAGNOSIS

HISTORY

- Change in voice (hoarseness)
- Positive family history
- Neck mass
- Dysphagia
- Dyspnea
- Cough

PHYSICAL EXAM

- Neck mass: If fixed to surrounding tissue, this finding suggests advanced disease.
- Cervical adenopathy

DIAGNOSTIC TESTS & INTERPRETATION

- Medullary carcinoma: Calcitonin level (normal <30 pg/mL [300 ng/L]), pentagastrin stimulation test and RET proto-oncogene
- Thyroglobulin (TG) level: Postoperative tumor marker
- DNA content of tumors from biopsy specimen: Diploid content has a better prognosis.

Lab

Thyroid function tests usually normal

Imaging

- Thyroid scan: Cold nodules are more suspicious of malignancy.
- Ultrasound: Solid mass and microcalcifications are more suspicious of malignancy.
- CT scan and MRI can be useful to evaluate large substernal masses and recurrent soft tissue masses.
- ^{18}F-FDG positron-emission tomographic scan can help if the cytology is inconclusive; helpful with recurrent disease when patient has a negative ^{131}I scan and an elevated TG level (1)[C].

Diagnostic Procedures/Surgery

- Fine-needle aspiration (FNA)
- Surgical biopsy/excision
- Laryngoscopy if vocal cord paralysis is suspected

Pathological Findings

- Papillary: Psammoma bodies, anaplastic epithelial papillae
- Follicular: Anaplastic epithelial cords with follicles
- Hürthle cell: Large eosinophilic cells with granular cytoplasm
- Medullary: Large amounts of amyloid stroma
- Anaplastic: Small-cell and giant-cell undifferentiated tumors

DIFFERENTIAL DIAGNOSIS

- Multinodular goiter
- Thyroid adenoma
- Thyroglossal duct cyst
- Thyroiditis
- Thyroid cyst
- Ectopic thyroid
- Dermoid cyst

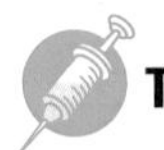

TREATMENT

MEDICATION

Postoperatively, will require thyroid hormone replacement. Goal is to keep TSH <0.1 mU/L:

- Levothyroxine (T_4, Synthroid) 100–200 μg/d, *or*
- Liothyronine (T_3, Cytomel) 50–100 μg/d

ADDITIONAL TREATMENT

Additional Therapies

- ^{131}I thyroid remnant ablation
- External-beam radiation for advanced disease

SURGERY/OTHER PROCEDURES

- Papillary carcinoma: Lobectomy with isthmectomy (if lesion <1.5 cm) or total thyroidectomy and removal of suspicious lymph nodes
- Follicular carcinoma and Hürthle cell: Total thyroidectomy and removal of suspicious lymph nodes
- Medullary carcinoma: Total thyroidectomy with central node dissection; unilateral or bilateral modified radical neck dissection if lateral nodes are histologically positive
- Anaplastic carcinoma: Aggressive en bloc thyroidectomy; tracheostomy often required. Not responsive to ^{131}I.

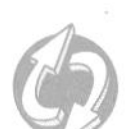

ONGOING CARE

FOLLOW-UP RECOMMENDATIONS

Patient Monitoring

- Thyroid scan at 6 weeks and administration of ^{131}I for any visible uptake; any evidence of residual thyroid tissue (after total thyroidectomy) or lymph node disease noted on scan is treated with radioactive iodine.
- At 6 months and then yearly, the patient should have a thyroid scan and chest x-ray.
- Papillary and follicular: A thyroglobulin (TG) level should be done yearly. Recombinant human thyroid-stimulating hormone (rhTSH)–stimulated TG level may be more sensitive (2,3)[B].
- Medullary: Calcitonin level should be done yearly with pentagastrin stimulation.
- The thyroid scan and TG level should be done with the patient in the hypothyroid state induced by 6-week withdrawal of levothyroxine or 2–3-week withdrawal of liothyronine.

DIET

Avoid iodine deficiency.

PATIENT EDUCATION

National Cancer Institute, Building 31, Room 101-18, 9000 Rockville Pike, Bethesda, MD 20892; (301) 496-5583; www.cancer.gov

PROGNOSIS

- Papillary carcinoma: Overall mortality 3–8%
- Follicular carcinoma: Overall 80% 5-year survival rate, 77% 10-year survival rate; histologically, microinvasive tumors parallel papillary tumor results, whereas grossly invasive tumors do far worse.
- Hürthle cell carcinoma: 93% 5-year survival rate and 83% survival rate overall; grossly invasive tumor survival <25%.
- Medullary carcinoma: Negative nodes, 90% 5-year survival rate and 85% 10-year survival rate; with positive nodes, 65% 5-year survival rate and 40% 10-year survival rate. Prognosis worse for MEN 2B compared to MEN 2A.
- Anaplastic carcinoma: Survival unexpected

COMPLICATIONS

- Recurrence of tumor
- Hoarseness from tumor invasion or operative injury to recurrent laryngeal nerve
- Hypoparathyroidism from operative injury to parathyroid glands

REFERENCES

1. Wang W, Larson SM, Fazzari M, et al. Prognostic value of [18F]fluorodeoxyglucose positron emission tomographic scanning in patients with thyroid cancer. *J Clin Endocrinol Metab*. 2000;85: 1107–13.
2. Blamey S, Barraclough B, Delbridge L, et al. Using recombinant human TSH for the diagnosis of recurrent thyroid cancer. *ANZ J Surg*. 2005;75: 10–20.
3. Haugen BR, Pacini F, Reiners C, et al. A comparison of recombinant human thyrotropin and thyroid hormone withdrawal for the detection of thyroid remnant or cancer. *J Clin Endocrinol Metab*. 1999;84:3877–85.

ADDITIONAL READING

- Burns WR, Zeiger MA. Differentiated thyroid cancer. *Semin Oncol*. 2010;37:557–66.
- Cox AE, LeBeau SO. Diagnosis and treatment of differentiated thyroid carcinoma. *Radiol Clin North Am*. 2011;49:453–62, vi.
- Marsh DJ, Gimm O. Multiple endocrine neoplasia: Types 1 and 2. *Adv Otorhinolaryngol*. 2011;70: 84–90.
- Pitt SC, Moley JF. Medullary, anaplastic, and metastatic cancers of the thyroid. *Semin Oncol*. 2010;37:567–79.

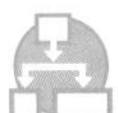

See Also (Topic, Algorithm, Electronic Media Element)

Multiple Endocrine Neoplasia (MEN)

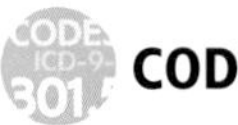

CODES

ICD9

193 Malignant neoplasm of thyroid gland

CLINICAL PEARLS

- Standard workup for a patient suspected of having a thyroid cancer is a physical exam, TSH level, neck US, and FNA.
- Thyroglobulin levels can be elevated in several thyroid disorders. Its usefulness comes once the diagnosis of cancer has been made. It serves as a better marker for recurrent disease.
- ~2% of the normal population will have a positive ^{18}F-FDG positron-emission tomographic scan, so it is more useful for postresection follow-up.

T

THYROIDITIS

Michelle A. Tinitigan, MD

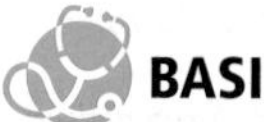

BASICS

DESCRIPTION

Inflammation of the thyroid gland that may be painful or painless:

- Thyroiditis with thyroid pain:
  - Subacute granulomatous thyroiditis (nonsuppurative thyroiditis, de Quervain thyroiditis, or giant cell thyroiditis): Self-limited; caused by a viral or postviral inflammatory process
  - Infectious/suppurative thyroiditis:
    - Bacterial, fungal, mycobacterial, or parasitic infection of the thyroid
    - Most commonly associated with *Streptococcus pyogenes*, *Staphylococcus aureus*, and *Streptococcus pneumoniae*.
  - Radiation-induced thyroiditis: From radioactive iodine therapy (1%) or external irradiation for lymphoma and head or neck cancers
- Thyroiditis with no thyroid pain:
  - Hashimoto (autoimmune) thyroiditis (chronic lymphocytic thyroiditis): Most common etiology of chronic hypothyroidism; autoimmune disease; 90% of patients with high-serum antithyroid peroxidase (TPO) antibodies
  - Postpartum thyroiditis: Occurs within 1 year postpartum (or after spontaneous/induced abortion)
  - Painless (silent) thyroiditis (subacute lymphocytic thyroiditis): Mild hyperthyroidism, little or no thyroid enlargement, and no Graves ophthalmopathy or pretibial myxedema
  - Riedel (fibrous) thyroiditis: Rare, extensive fibrosis of the thyroid gland and adjacent tissue; presents as a firm mass in the thyroid commonly associated with compressive symptoms. The presence of dyspnea, dysphagia, hoarseness, and aphonia, caused by local pressure or in- filtration of the advancing fibrotic process, is classically described (1).
  - Drug-induced thyroiditis: Interferon-alfa, interleukin-2, amiodarone, or lithium

EPIDEMIOLOGY

- Subacute granulomatous thyroiditis: Most common cause of thyroid pain; peaks during summer; affects women more than men; common among those 40–50 years of age
- Suppurative thyroiditis: Commonly seen with pre-existing thyroid disease or immunocompromise
- Hashimoto thyroiditis: Peak age of onset, 30–50 years; increases with age; can occur in children; primarily a disease of women (sex ratio 7:1)
- Postpartum thyroiditis: 5–7% of postpartum women; occurs in 25% with type 1 diabetes mellitus
- Painless (silent) thyroiditis: Women affected 4 times more than men
- Reidel thyroiditis: Women are 4 times more affected than men; highest prevalence among those age 30–60 years

RISK FACTORS

- Hashimoto disease: Family history of thyroid or autoimmune disease, personal history of autoimmune disease (type 1 diabetes, celiac disease), high iodine intake, cigarette smoking, selenium deficiency
- Subacute granulomatous thyroiditis: Recent viral respiratory infection
- Suppurative thyroiditis: Congenital abnormalities (persistent thyroglossal duct or piriform sinus fistula), greater age, immunosuppression
- Radiation-induced thyroiditis: High-dose irradiation, younger age, female sex, pre-existing hypothyroidism
- Postpartum thyroiditis: Smoking, history of spontaneous or induced abortion
- Painless (silent) thyroiditis: Iodine-deficient areas

Genetics

Autoimmune thyroiditis is associated with the CT60 polymorphism of cytotoxic T-cell lymphocyte–associated antigen 4. Also associated with human leukocyte antigen (HLA)-DR4, -DR5, and -DR6 in whites.

GENERAL PREVENTION

Selenium may decrease inflammatory activity in pregnant women with autoimmune hypothyroidism and may reduce postpartum thyroiditis risk in those positive for TPO antibodies (2).

ETIOLOGY

Hashimoto disease: Antithyroid antibodies may be produced in response to an environmental antigen and cross-react with thyroid proteins (molecular mimicry). Precipitating factors include infection, stress, sex steroids, pregnancy, iodine intake, radiation exposure.

COMMONLY ASSOCIATED CONDITIONS

Postpartum thyroiditis: Family history of autoimmune thyroid disease; HLA-DRB, -DR4, and -DR5.

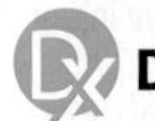

DIAGNOSIS

HISTORY

- Hypothyroid symptoms (e.g., constipation, heavy menstrual bleeding, dry skin, hair loss)
- Hyperthyroid symptoms (e.g., weakness, fatigue, irritability, heat/cold intolerance, increased sweating, palpitations, disturbed sleep, stare, and lid retraction)
- Subacute granulomatous thyroiditis: Sudden or gradual onset with preceding upper respiratory infection/viral illness (fever, fatigue, malaise, anorexia, and myalgia are common); pain may be limited to thyroid region or radiate to upper neck, jaw, throat, or ears

PHYSICAL EXAM

- Examine thyroid for size, symmetry, and palpable nodules:
  - Hashimoto disease: 90% have a symmetrical, diffusely enlarged, painless gland with a firm, pebbly texture; 10% have thyroid atrophy.
  - Postpartum thyroiditis: Painless, small, nontender, firm goiter (2–6 months after delivery)
  - Reidel thyroiditis: Rock-hard, woodlike, fixed, painless goiter, often accompanied by symptoms of esophageal or tracheal compression (stridor, dyspnea, a suffocating feeling, dysphagia, and hoarseness)
- Signs of hypothyroid: Delayed relaxation phase of deep tendon reflexes, nonpitting edema, dry skin, alopecia, bradycardia
- Signs of hyperthyroid: Moist palms, hyperreflexia, tachycardia/atrial fibrillation

DIAGNOSTIC TESTS & INTERPRETATION

Lab

- Thyroid-stimulating hormone (TSH), anti-TPO antibodies
- Hashimoto disease:
  - High titers of anti-TPO antibodies
- Subacute granulomatous thyroiditis:
  - High T_4, T_3; low TSH during early stages and elevated later
  - High thyroglobulin; normal levels of anti-TPO and antithyroglobulin antibodies
  - Elevated ESR (usually >50 mm/hr) and C-reactive protein; mild anemia and slight leukocytosis; liver function tests frequently abnormal during initial hyperthyroid phase and resolve over 1–2 months
- Suppurative thyroiditis:
  - In the absence of pre-existing thyroid disease, thyroid function normal but hyperthyroidism or hypothyroidism may occur
  - ESR is elevated, and WBCs generally show a marked increase with a left shift.
  - Fine-needle aspiration (FNA) of the lesion with Gram stain and culture is the most useful diagnostic test.
- Postpartum thyroiditis:
  - High or high-normal T_4 and T_3, low TSH 2–10 months after delivery with recovery over the next 2–3 months. Hypothyroidism occurs between 2 and 12 months after delivery, most commonly at 6 months (3).
  - Most patients (80%) have normal thyroid function at 1 year; 30–50% of patients develop permanent hypothyroidism within 9 years (3).
  - High anti-TPO antibodies and thyroglobulin; normal ESR
- Painless (silent) thyroiditis:
  - Hyperthyroid state in 5–20%: Averages 3–4 months, and total duration of illness is <1 year, followed by hypothyroidism and then a return to normal state; some have primary or subclinical hypothyroidism.
  - Half of patients have anti-TPO antibodies
- Reidel thyroiditis:
  - Hypothyroidism because of extensive replacement of the gland by scar tissue. Anti-TPO antibodies are present in 2/3 of patients and low radioactive iodine uptake (RAIU).
- Drug-induced thyroiditis:
  - Hyperthyroidism or hypothyroidism, low RAIU, and variable presence of anti-TPO antibodies
- Drugs that may alter lab results: Thyroid hormones, corticosteroids, iodine-containing drugs and contrast media, lithium, amiodarone
- Disorders that may alter lab results: Iodine deficiency, nonthyroidal illness

Imaging

- Ultrasonography
- Thyroid RAIU scan: Decreased in all forms of thyroiditis, but usually is not helpful in establishing diagnosis of Hashimoto disease. High RAIU in hashitoxicosis, Graves disease.

- Random urine iodine measurement may be helpful to distinguish this disease from other causes of low RAIU:
  - Urine iodine <500 μg/L (subacute granulomatous thyroiditis)
  - Urine iodine >1,000 μg/L (in patients with exposure to excess exogenous iodine/radiocontrast material)

Diagnostic Procedures/Surgery

- Hashimoto with a dominant nodule should undergo FNA to rule out thyroid carcinoma.
- Open biopsy is necessary for a definitive diagnosis of Reidel thyroiditis.

Pathological Findings

- Hashimoto disease: Lymphocytic infiltration with formation of Askanazy (Hürthle) cells, oxyphilic changes in follicular cells, fibrosis, thyroid atrophy
- Subacute granulomatous thyroiditis: Giant cells, mononuclear cell infiltrate
- Postpartum thyroiditis: Lymphocytic infiltration, occasional germinal centers, disruption and collapse of thyroid follicles
- Painless thyroiditis: Lymphocytic infiltration but without fibrosis, Askanazy cells, and extensive lymphoid follicle formation (3)

DIFFERENTIAL DIAGNOSIS

Simple goiter; iodine-deficient or lithium-induced goiter; Graves disease; lymphoma; acute infectious thyroiditis; hemorrhage into a thyroid nodule/cyst; infections of oropharynx and trachea; subacute systemic illness; subacute granulomatous thyroiditis; thyroid cancer

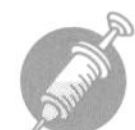

TREATMENT

MEDICATION

- Hashimoto disease:
  - If hypothyroid or goitrous: Levothyroxine (1.7 μg/kg/d for adults <50 years). If no cardiac complications and no adrenal insufficiency, halve replacement dose and increase to full replacement in 10 days:
    - If >50 years of age or heart disease and/or adrenal insufficiency, begin with 25 μg/d and titrate to TSH of lower limit normal range.
  - If thyrotoxic and symptomatic: Propylthiouracil and propranolol
  - An elevated TSH level in a woman who is pregnant or attempting to become pregnant is an indication for thyroid replacement (4).
- Subacute granulomatous thyroiditis:
  - Pain: Analgesics for 2–8 weeks (NSAIDs or aspirin).
  - Symptomatic hyperthyroidism: β-Blockers while thyrotoxic (propranolol 40–120 mg/d, propranolol LA 80 mg/d, or atenolol 25–50 mg/d)
  - Symptomatic hypothyroid phase: Levothyroxine as above, target TSH in the normal range
  - Pain with no improvement in 2–3 days after NSAID use: Prednisone 40 mg/d; should result in pain relief in 1–2 days; if not, question diagnosis
  - Severe pain: Prednisone 40–60 mg/d gradually discontinued over 4–6 weeks. If pain recurs, increase dose for several weeks and then taper.
- Suppurative thyroiditis:
  - Parenteral empiric, broad-spectrum antibiotics and surgical drainage
- Painless thyroiditis:
  - No treatment because thyroid dysfunction usually is mild, transient
  - If symptomatic during hyperthyroid state, treat with β-blocker, as above
  - Prednisone shortens the period of hyperthyroidism. TSH should be monitored every 4–8 weeks to confirm resolution.
  - Treat hypothyroid symptoms and asymptomatic patients with TSH >10 mU/L with levothyroxine (50–100 μg/d), to be discontinued after 3–6 months.
  - Up to 20% will develop permanent hypothyroidism.
- Postpartum thyroiditis:
  - Treat symptomatic hyperthyroid/hypothyroid state. The majority do not need treatment.
  - Caution in breast-feeding mothers because β-blockers are secreted into breast milk.
  - For symptomatic hypothyroidism, treat with levothyroxine. Otherwise, remonitor in 4–8 weeks. Taper replacement hormone after 6 months to determine if thyroid function has normalized.
- Reidel thyroiditis:
  - Corticosteroids in early stages, but controversial thereafter. Prednisone 10–20 mg/d for 4–6 months is recommended, possibly continued thereafter if effective (1).
  - Tamoxifen 10–20 mg monotherapy or in conjunction with prednisone can significantly reduce mass size and clinical symptoms.
  - Methotrexate has been used, with some success.
  - Reduction of goiter seen with a combination of mycophenolate mofetil (1 g b.i.d.) and 100 mg prednisone daily.
  - Debulking surgery is limited to isthmusectomy to relieve constrictive pressure when total thyroidectomy is not possible (1).
- Drug-induced thyroiditis:
  - Discontinue offending drug
- Contraindications: Propylthiouracil: Allergy or hypersensitivity to analgesics/narcotics; propranolol: Insulin therapy, asthma; prednisone: Adverse reactions; levothyroxine: None.
- Significant possible interactions: Sucralfate (Carafate) and iron preparations may decrease levothyroxine availability.

ADDITIONAL TREATMENT

General Measures

Analgesics for pain; corticosteroids for severe granulomatous thyroiditis

SURGERY/OTHER PROCEDURES

Enlarged thyroid with pain or tracheal/esophageal compression

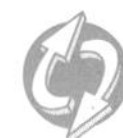

ONGOING CARE

FOLLOW-UP RECOMMENDATIONS

Patient Monitoring

- Hashimoto disease: Repeat thyroid function tests every 3–12 months.
- Subacute granulomatous thyroiditis: Repeat thyroid function tests every 3–6 weeks until euthyroid; check every 6–12 months.
- Postpartum thyroiditis: Patients who have antithyroid peroxidase antibodies have a 70% risk of recurrence following a subsequent pregnancy. Measure TSH annually, particularly within 5–10 years of initial diagnosis.
- Reidel thyroiditis: CT of cervical mediastinal region is recommended.
- Drug-induced thyroiditis: Monitor TSH every 6 months in patients taking amiodarone.

Pregnancy Considerations

- Avoid radioisotope scanning if possible.
- Keep TSH maximally suppressed.
- If using RAIU scan, discard breast milk for 2 days because RAI is secreted in breast milk.

PROGNOSIS

- Hashimoto disease: Persistent goiter; eventual thyroid failure
- Granulomatous thyroiditis: Eventual return to normal over; remission may be slower in the elderly
- Postpartum thyroiditis: Women may be euthyroid or continue to be hypothyroid at the end of first postpartum year (5). Recurrence is likely after future pregnancies; there is substantial risk for later development of hypothyroidism or goiter.

REFERENCES

1. Hennessey JV. Clinical review: Riedel's thyroiditis: A clinical review. *J Clin Endocrinol Metab*. 2011;96:3031–41.
2. Duntas LH. Selenium and the thyroid: A close-knit connection. *J Clin Endocrinol Metab*. 2010;95:5180–8.
3. Bindra A, Braunstein GD. Thyroiditis. *Am Fam Physician*. 2006;73:1769–76.
4. Reid SM, Middleton P, Cossich MC, et al. Interventions for clinical and subclinical hypothyroidism in pregnancy. *Cochrane Database Syst Rev*. 2010;7:CD007752.
5. Stagnaro-Green A, Schwartz A, Gismondi R, et al. High rate of persistent hypothyroidism in a large-scale prospective study of postpartum thyroiditis in southern Italy. *J Clin Endocrinol Metab*. 2011;96:652–7.

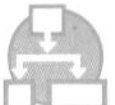

See Also (Topic, Algorithm, Electronic Media Element)

Hyperthyroidism; Hypothyroidism, Adult

CODES

ICD9

- 245.0 Acute thyroiditis
- 245.8 Other and unspecified chronic thyroiditis
- 245.9 Thyroiditis, unspecified

CLINICAL PEARLS

- TSH elevation above the normal range indicates a hypothyroid state; suppressed TSH indicates hyperthyroid state. Follow up with free T_3/T_4 determination.
- Follow patients on thyroid replacement with periodic TSH levels.

TINEA (CAPITIS, CORPORIS, CRURIS)

Elisabeth L. Backer, MD

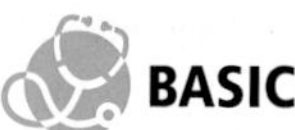

BASICS

DESCRIPTION

- Superficial fungal infections of the skin or scalp; the names relate to the particular area affected:
  - Tinea cruris: Infection of crural fold and gluteal cleft
  - Tinea corporis: Infection involving the face, trunk, and/or extremities:
    - Often presents with ring-shaped lesions, hence the misnomer *ringworm*
  - Tinea capitis: Infection of the scalp and hair:
    - Affected areas of the scalp can show characteristic black dots resulting from broken hairs.
- Infections result from contact with infected persons or animals:
  - Zoophilic infections are acquired from animals.
  - Anthropophilic infections are acquired from personal contact (e.g., wrestling) or fomites.
  - Geophile infections are acquired from the soil.
- System(s) affected: Skin/Exocrine
- Synonym(s): Jock itch; Ringworm

EPIDEMIOLOGY

Incidence

- Tinea cruris:
  - Predominant age: Any age; rare in children
  - Predominant sex: Male > Female
- Tinea corporis:
  - Predominant age: All ages
  - Predominant sex: Male = Female
- Tinea capitis:
  - Predominant age: 3–9 years; almost always occurs in young children
  - Predominant sex: Male = Female

Prevalence

Common

Pediatric Considerations

- Tinea cruris is rare prior to puberty.
- Tinea capitis is common in young children.

Geriatric Considerations

Tinea cruris more common in the geriatric population due to an increase in risk factors.

Pregnancy Considerations

Tinea cruris and capitis are rare in pregnancy.

RISK FACTORS

- Warm climates; summer months and/or copious sweating; wearing wet clothing or multiple layers (tinea cruris)
- Daycare centers/schools/confined quarters (tinea corporis and capitis)
- Depression of cell-mediated immune response (e.g., individuals with atopy or AIDS)
- Obesity (tinea cruris and corporis)
- Direct contact with an active lesion on a human, an animal, or rarely, from soil; working with animals (tinea corporis)

Genetics

Evidence suggests a genetic susceptibility in certain individuals.

GENERAL PREVENTION

- Avoidance of risk factors, such as contact with suspicious lesions
- Fluconazole or itraconazole may be useful in wrestlers to prevent outbreaks during competitive season (1)[A].

PATHOPHYSIOLOGY

Superficial fungal infection of skin/scalp

ETIOLOGY

- Tinea cruris: Source of infection is usually the patient's own tinea pedis, with agent being transferred from the foot to the groin via the underwear when dressing; most common causative dermatophyte is *Trichophyton rubrum*; rare cases caused by *Epidermophyton floccosum* and *T. mentagrophytes*.
- Tinea corporis: Most commonly caused by *T. rubrum*; *Microsporum canis* can cause multiple lesions
- Tinea capitis: *T. tonsurans* found in 90% and *Microsporum* sp. in 10% of patients

COMMONLY ASSOCIATED CONDITIONS

Tinea pedis, tinea barbae, tinea manus

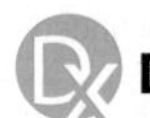

DIAGNOSIS

HISTORY

- Lesions range from asymptomatic to pruritic.
- In tinea cruris, acute inflammation may result from wearing occlusive clothing; chronic scratching may result in an eczematous appearance.
- Previous application of topical steroids, especially in tinea cruris and corporis, may alter the overall appearance, causing a more extensive eruption with irregular borders and erythematous papules. This modified form is called *tinea incognito*.

PHYSICAL EXAM

- Tinea cruris: Well-marginated, erythematous, half-moon–shaped plaques in crural folds that spread to upper thighs; advancing border is well defined, often with fine scaling and sometimes vesicular eruptions. Lesions are usually bilateral and do not include scrotum or penis (unlike with *Candida* infections) but may migrate to perineum, perianal area, and gluteal cleft and onto the buttocks in chronic/progressive cases. The area may be hyperpigmented on resolution.
- Tinea corporis: Scaling, pruritic plaques characterized by a sharply defined annular pattern with peripheral activity and central clearing (ring-shaped lesions); papules and occasionally pustules/vesicles present at border and less commonly in center
- Tinea capitis: Commonly begins with round patches of scale (alopecia less common). In its later stages, the infection frequently takes on patterns of chronic scaling with either little or marked inflammation and alopecia. Less often, patients will present with multiple patches of alopecia and the characteristic black-dot appearance of broken hairs. Extreme inflammation results in kerion formation (exudative, pustular nodulation).

DIAGNOSTIC TESTS & INTERPRETATION

Wood lamp exam reveals no fluorescence in most cases (*Trichophyton* sp.); 10% of infections, those caused by *M. rubrum*, will fluoresce with a green light.

Lab

Initial lab tests

- Potassium hydroxide (KOH) preparation of skin scrapings from dermatophyte leading border shows characteristic translucent, branching, rod-shaped hyphae
- Arthrospores can be visualized within hair shafts.

Follow-Up & Special Considerations

- Re-evaluate to assess response, especially in resistant or extensive cases.
- Fungal culture using Sabouraud dextrose agar or dermatophyte test medium

Pathological Findings

- Skin scrapings show fungal hyphae in epidermis.
- Arthrospores found in hair shafts

DIFFERENTIAL DIAGNOSIS

- Tinea cruris:
  - Intertrigo: Inflammatory process of moist opposed skin folds, often including infection with bacteria, yeast, and fungi; painful longitudinal fissures may occur in skin folds.
  - Erythrasma: Diffuse brown, scaly, noninflammatory plaque with irregular borders, often involving groin; caused by bacterial infection with *Corynebacterium minutissimum;* fluoresces coral red with Wood lamp
  - Seborrheic dermatitis of groin
  - Psoriasis of groin ("inverse psoriasis")
  - Candidiasis of groin (typically involves the scrotum)
  - Acanthosis nigricans
- Tinea capitis:
  - Psoriasis
  - Seborrheic dermatitis
  - Pyoderma
  - Alopecia areata and trichotillomania
  - Aphasia cutis congenital
- Tinea corporis:
  - Pityriasis rosea
  - Eczema (nummular)
  - Contact dermatitis
  - Syphilis
  - Psoriasis
  - Seborrheic dermatitis
  - Subacute lupus erythematosus (SLE)
  - Erythema annulare centrifugum
  - Erythema multiforme; erythema migrans
  - Impetigo circinatum
  - Granuloma annulare

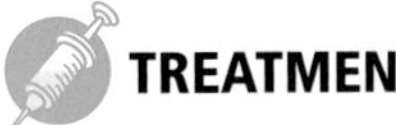

TREATMENT

MEDICATION

First Line

- Tinea cruris/corporis:
  - Topical azole antifungal compounds (2)[C]:
    - Econazole (Spectazole), ketoconazole (Nizoral): Usually applied b.i.d. × 2–3 weeks
    - Terbinafine (Lamisil): Over-the-counter (OTC) compound; can be applied once or b.i.d. × 1–2 weeks
    - Butenafine (Mentax): Applied once daily × 2 weeks; also very effective
    - Mycostatin (Nystatin): Not effective for tinea cruris or corporis
  - To prevent relapse, use for 1 week after resolution (3)[C].
- Tinea capitis:
  - Oral griseofulvin (4,5)[A] for *Trichophyton* and *Microsporum* sp.; microsized preparation available; dosage 125 mg/d in patients weighing 10–20 kg; 250 mg/d if weight is 20–40 kg; 500 mg/d if weight is >40 kg; taken b.i.d. or as a single dose daily × 6–12 weeks
  - Oral terbinafine (4,5)[A] can be used for *Trichophyton* sp. at 62.5 mg/d in patients weighing 10–20 kg; 125 mg/d if weight 20–40 kg; 250 mg/d if weight >40 kg; use for 4–6 weeks
  - Oral itraconazole (5)[A] can be used for *Microsporum* sp. and matches griseofulvin's efficacy while being better tolerated. Dosage of 3–5 mg/kg/d, but most studies have used 100 mg/d × 6 weeks in children >2 years of age.

Second Line

Tinea cruris/corporis:

- Oral antifungal agents are effective but not indicated in uncomplicated tinea cruris or corporis cases. They can be used for resistant and extensive infections or if the patient is immunocompromised. If topical therapy fails, one may consult a dermatologist for possible oral therapy. Griseofulvin can be given 500 mg/d for 1–2 weeks.
- The following oral regimens have been reported in medical literature as being effective but currently are not specifically approved by the FDA for tinea cruris:
  - Oral terbinafine (Lamisil): 250 mg/d × 1 week
  - Oral itraconazole (Sporanox): 100 mg b.i.d. once and repeated 1 week later (6)
  - Oral fluconazole (Diflucan): 150 mg once per week × 4 weeks
- Topical terbinafine 1% solution has been studied recently and appears effective as a once-daily application for 1 week.
- Contraindications:
  - Oral itraconazole (Sporanox): Contraindicated with astemizole (Hismanal), triazolam (Halcion), lovastatin (Mevacor), simvastatin (Zocor). Pravastatin (Pravachol) can be given with itraconazole.
- Oral antifungals can interact with warfarin, BCPs, alcohol; contraindicated in pregnancy. Monitor for liver toxicity when using oral antifungals.

ADDITIONAL TREATMENT

General Measures

- Careful hand washing and personal hygiene; laundering of towels/clothing of affected individual; no sharing of towels/clothes/headgear
- Evaluate other family members, close contacts, or household pets.
- Avoid predisposing conditions such as hot baths and tight-fitting clothing (boxer shorts are better than briefs) (5)[C].
- Keep area as dry as possible (talcum/powders may be beneficial) (5)[C].
- Itching can be alleviated by OTC preparations such as Sarna or Prax.
- Topical steroid preparations should not be used (see "Tinea Incognito") (2)[C].
- Avoid contact sports (e.g., wrestling) temporarily while starting treatment.

Issues for Referral

Refer if disease is nonresponsive or resistant, especially in immunocompromised host.

Additional Therapies

Treatment of secondary bacterial infections

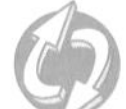

ONGOING CARE

FOLLOW-UP RECOMMENDATIONS

Re-evaluate response to treatment.

Patient Monitoring

Liver function testing prior to therapy and at regular intervals during course of therapy for patients requiring oral terbinafine, fluconazole, itraconazole, and griseofulvin

PATIENT EDUCATION

Explanation of the causative agents, predisposing factors, and prevention measures

PROGNOSIS

- Excellent prognosis for cure with therapy in tinea cruris and corporis
- In tinea capitis, lesions will heal spontaneously in 6 months without treatment, but scarring is more likely.

COMPLICATIONS

- Secondary bacterial infection
- Generalized, invasive dermatophyte infection

REFERENCES

1. Kohl TD, Martin DC, Berger MS. Comparison of topical and oral treatments for tinea gladiatorum. *Clin J Sport Med*. 1999;9:161–6.
2. Bonifaz A. Comparative study between terbinafine 1% emulsion-gel versus ketoconazole 2% cream in tinea cruris and corporis. *Eur J Derm*. 2000;10:107.
3. Lesher JL. Butenafine 1% cream in the treatment of tinea cruris: A multicenter, vehicle-controlled, double-blind trial. *J Am Acad Dermatol*. 1997; 36(2 pt 1):S20–4.
4. Elewski BE, Cáceres HW, DeLeon L. Terbinafine hydrochloride oral granules versus oral griseofulvin suspension in children with tinea capitis: Results of two randomized, investigator-blinded, multicenter, international, controlled trials. *J Am Acad Dermatol*. 2008;59:41–54.
5. Gonzalez U, Seaton T, Bergus G, et al. Systemic antifungal therapy for tinea capitis in children. *Cochrane Database Sys Rev*. 2007:CD004685.
6. Sanmano B, Hiruma M, Mizoguchi M. Abbreviated oral itraconazole therapy for tinea corporis and tinea cruris. *Mycoses*. 2003;46:316–21.

ADDITIONAL READING

- Akinwale SO. Personal hygiene as an alternative to griseofulvin in the treatment of tinea cruris. *Afr J Med Sci*. 2000;29:41.
- Fuller LC, Smith CH, Cerio R. A randomized comparison of 4 weeks of terbinafine vs. 8 weeks of griseofulvin for the treatment of tinea capitis. *Br J Dermatol*. 2001;144:321–7.
- Gupta AK, Cooper EA. Update in antifungal therapy of dermatophytosis. *Mycopathologia*. 2008;166: 353.
- Nozickova M, Koudelkova V, Kulikova Z. A comparison of the efficacy of oral fluconazole, 150 mg/week versus 50 mg/day, in the treatment of tinea corporis, tinea cruris, tinea pedis, and cutaneous candidosis. *Int J Dermatol*. 1998;37:703–5.

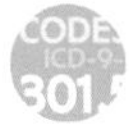

CODES

ICD9

- 110.0 Dermatophytosis of scalp and beard
- 110.2 Dermatophytosis of hand
- 110.3 Dermatophytosis of groin and perianal area

CLINICAL PEARLS

- Tinea corporis is characterized by scaly plaque, with peripheral activity and central clearing.
- Tinea cruris is characterized by erythematous plaque in crural folds, usually sparing the scrotum.
- Tinea capitis is a fungal infection of the scalp, affecting hair growth.

TINEA PEDIS

Elisabeth L. Backer, MD

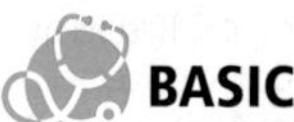

BASICS

DESCRIPTION
- Superficial infection of the feet caused by dermatophytes
- Most common dermatophyte infection encountered in clinical practice
- Often accompanied by tinea manuum, tinea unguium, and tinea cruris
- 2 clinical forms: Acute and chronic
- System(s) affected: Skin/Exocrine
- Synonym(s): Athlete's foot

EPIDEMIOLOGY
- Predominant age: 20–50 years, although can occur at any age
- Predominant gender: Male > Female

Prevalence
4% of population

Pediatric Considerations
Rare in younger children; common in teens

Geriatric Considerations
Elderly are more susceptible to outbreaks because of immunocompromise and impaired perfusion of distal extremities.

RISK FACTORS
- Hot, humid weather
- Occlusive/tight-fitting footwear
- Immunosuppression
- Prolonged application of topical steroids

Genetics
No known genetic pattern

GENERAL PREVENTION
- Good personal hygiene
- Wearing rubber or wooden sandals in community showers, bathing places, locker rooms
- Careful drying between toes after showering or bathing; blow-drying feet with hair dryer may be more effective than drying with towel
- Changing socks and shoes frequently
- Applying drying or dusting powder
- Applying topical antiperspirants
- Putting on socks before underwear to prevent infection from spreading to groin

PATHOPHYSIOLOGY
Superficial infection caused by dermatophytes that thrive only in nonviable keratinized tissue

ETIOLOGY
- *Trichophyton mentagrophytes* (acute)
- *Trichophyton rubrum* (chronic)
- *Trichophyton tonsurans*
- *Epidermophyton floccosum*

COMMONLY ASSOCIATED CONDITIONS
- Hyperhidrosis
- Onychomycosis
- Tinea manuum/unguium/cruris/corporis

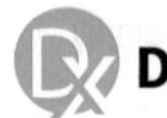

DIAGNOSIS

HISTORY
- Itchy, scaly rash on foot, usually between toes; may progress to fissuring/maceration in toe web spaces
- May be associated with onychomycosis and other tinea infections

PHYSICAL EXAM
- Acute form: Self-limited, intermittent, recurrent; scaling, thickening, and fissuring of sole and heel; scaling or fissuring of toe webs; or pruritic vesicular/bullous lesions between toes or on soles
- Chronic form: Most common; slowly progressive, pruritic erythematous erosion/scales between toes, in digital interspaces; extension onto soles, sides/dorsum of feet (moccasin distribution). If untreated, may persist indefinitely.
- Other features: Strong odor, hyperkeratosis, maceration, ulceration

DIAGNOSTIC TESTS & INTERPRETATION
Wood lamp exam will not fluoresce unless complicated by another fungus, which is uncommon; *M. furfur* (yellow to white), *Corynebacterium* (red), or *Microsporum* (blue–green).

Lab
Initial lab tests
- Direct microscopic examination (potassium hydroxide)
- Culture (Sabouraud medium)

Pathological Findings
- Potassium hydroxide preparation: Septate and branched mycelia
- Culture: Dermatophyte

DIFFERENTIAL DIAGNOSIS
- Interdigital type: Erythrasma, impetigo, pitted keratolysis, candida intertrigo
- Moccasin type: Psoriasis vulgaris, eczematous dermatitis, pitted keratolysis
- Inflammatory/bullous type: Impetigo, allergic contact dermatitis, dyshidrotic eczema, bullous disease

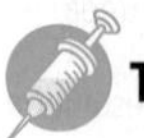

TREATMENT

Treatment is generally with topical antifungal medications for up to 4 weeks (1)[A]:
- Acute treatment:
  - Aluminum acetate soak (Burow solution; Domeboro, 1 pack to 1 quart warm water)
  - Antifungal cream of choice b.i.d. after soaks
- Chronic treatment:
  - Antifungal creams twice daily, continuing for 3 days after the rash is resolved: Clotrimazole 1%, econazole 1%, ketoconazole 2%, tolnaftate 1%, etc. (1)[A].
  - May try systemic antifungal therapy; see below (consider if concomitant onychomycosis or after failed topical treatment)

MEDICATION
First Line
- Systemic antifungals (2)[A]:
  - Itraconazole (Sporanox) 200 mg PO b.i.d. for 14 days (cure rate >90%)
  - Terbinafine (Lamisil) 250 mg PO daily for 14 days
- If concomitant onychomycosis:
  - Itraconazole 200 mg PO b.i.d. for first week of month for 3 months. Monitoring liver function testing is recommended.
  - Terbinafine 250 mg PO daily for 12 weeks, or pulse dosing: 500 mg PO daily for first week of month for 3 months. Not recommended if creatinine clearance <50 mL/min.

- Pediatric dosing options:
  - Griseofulvin 10–15 mg/kg/d or divided
  - Terbinafine 10–20 kg: 62.5 mg/d:
    - 20–40 kg: 125 mg/d
    - >40 kg: 250 mg/d
  - Itraconazole 5 mg/kg/d
  - Fluconazole 6 mg/kg/d
- Contraindications: Itraconazole, pregnancy Category C
- Precautions: All systemic antifungal drugs may have potential hepatotoxicity.
- Significant possible interactions: Itraconazole requires gastric acid for absorption; effectiveness is reduced with antacids, H_2 blockers, proton pump inhibitors, etc. Take with acidic beverage such as soda if on antacids.

Second Line

- Systemic antifungals:
  - Fluconazole 150 mg, 1 tablet every week for 1–4 weeks. (Noted in 1997 Sanford Guide: 70% cure; however, not an FDA-approved indication.)
  - Griseofulvin 250–500 mg of microsize b.i.d. daily for 21 days
- Contraindications: Griseofulvin:
  - Patients with porphyria, hepatocellular failure
  - Patients with history of hypersensitivity to griseofulvin
- Precautions: Griseofulvin:
  - Should be used only in severe cases
  - Periodic monitoring of organ-system functioning, including renal, hepatic, and hematopoietic
  - Possible photosensitivity reactions
  - Lupus erythematosus, lupuslike syndromes, or exacerbation of existing lupus erythematosus has been reported.
- Significant possible interactions: Griseofulvin:
  - Decreases activity of warfarin-type anticoagulants
  - Barbiturates usually depress griseofulvin activity.
  - May potentiate effect of alcohol, producing such effects as tachycardia and flush

ADDITIONAL TREATMENT

General Measures

- Soak with aluminum chloride 30% or aluminum subacetate for 20 minutes b.i.d.
- Careful removal of dead/thickened skin after soaking or bathing
- Chronic or extensive disease or nail involvement requires oral antifungal medication and systemic therapy.

Issues for Referral

If extensive or resistant disease, especially in immunocompromised host

Additional Therapies

- Treatment of secondary bacterial infections
- Treatment of eczematoid changes

ONGOING CARE

FOLLOW-UP RECOMMENDATIONS

Avoid sweating feet.

Patient Monitoring

Evaluate for response, recognizing that infections may be chronic/recurrent.

DIET

No restrictions

PATIENT EDUCATION

See "General Prevention."

PROGNOSIS

- Control, but not complete cure
- Infections tend to be chronic with exacerbations (e.g., in hot weather).
- Personal hygiene and preventive measures such as open-toed sandals, careful drying, and frequent sock changes are essential.

COMPLICATIONS

- Secondary bacterial infections (portal of entry for streptococcal infections, producing lymphangitis/cellulitis)
- Eczematoid changes

REFERENCES

1. Crawford F. Athlete's foot and fungally infected toe nails. *Clin Evid*. 2002;(7):1458–66.
2. Bell-Syer SE, Hart R, Crawford F, et al. Oral treatments for fungal infections of the skin of the foot. *Cochrane Database Syst Rev*. 2002: CD003584.

ADDITIONAL READING

Gupta AK, Nolting S, de Prost Y, et al. The use of itraconazole to treat cutaneous fungal infections in children. *Dermatology*. 1999;199:248–52.

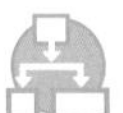

See Also (Topic, Algorithm, Electronic Media Element)

Dermatitis, Contact; Dyshidrosis

CODES

ICD9

110.4 Dermatophytosis of foot

CLINICAL PEARLS

- Treatment is generally with topical antifungal medications for up to 4 weeks (1)[A].
- Often is recurrent/chronic in nature
- Careful drying between toes after showering or bathing helps prevent recurrences. (Blow drying feet with hair dryer may be more effective than drying with towel.)
- Socks should be changed frequently. Put on socks before underwear to prevent infection from spreading to groin (tinea cruris).
- Dusting and drying powders (containing antifungal agents) may prevent recurrences.

T

TINEA VERSICOLOR

Elisabeth L. Backer, MD

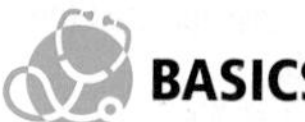

BASICS

DESCRIPTION
- Rash due to a common superficial mycosis with a variety of colors and changing shades of color, predominantly present on trunk and proximal upper extremities; macules usually hypopigmented, light brown, or salmon-colored; fine scale often apparent.
- System(s) affected: Skin/Exocrine
- Synonym(s): Pityriasis versicolor

EPIDEMIOLOGY
Incidence
- Common, especially in tropical climates
- Predominant age: Teenagers and young adults
- Predominant sex: Male = Female

Pediatric Considerations
Usually occurs after puberty (except in tropical areas); facial lesions are more common in children.

Geriatric Considerations
Not common in the geriatric population

RISK FACTORS
- Hot, humid weather
- Use of topical skin oils
- Hyperhydrosis
- HIV infection/immunosuppression (1)[C]
- High cortisol levels (Cushing, prolonged steroid administration)
- Pregnancy
- Malnutrition
- Oral contraceptives

Genetics
No known genetic pattern

GENERAL PREVENTION
- Recheck and treat again each spring prior to tanning season.
- Avoid skin oils.

PATHOPHYSIOLOGY
Inhibition of pigment synthesis in epidermal melanocytes, leading to hypomelanosis; in the hyperpigmented type, the melanosomes are large and heavily melanized.

ETIOLOGY
- Saprophytic yeast: *Pityrosporum orbiculare* (also known as *P. ovale, Malassezia furfur,* or *M. ovalis*), which is a known colonizer of all humans
- Variations in skin lipid formation

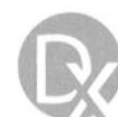

DIAGNOSIS

HISTORY
- Asymptomatic scaling macules on trunk
- Possible mild pruritus
- More prominent in summer
- Sun tanning accentuates lesions because infected areas do not tan.
- Periodic recurrences common

PHYSICAL EXAM
- *Versicolor* refers to the variety and changing shades of colors.
- Sun-exposed areas: Lesions usually white/hypopigmented
- Covered areas: Lesions often brown or salmon-colored
- Distribution (sebum-rich areas): Chest, shoulders, back (also face and intertriginous areas)
- Appearance: Small individual macules that frequently coalesce
- Scale: Fine, more visible with scraping

DIAGNOSTIC TESTS & INTERPRETATION
Wood lamp: Yellow to yellow–green fluorescence or pigment changes

Lab
Initial lab tests
- Direct microscopy of scales with 10% potassium hydroxide (KOH) preparation to visualize hyphae and spores ("spaghetti and meatballs" pattern)
- Routine lab tests usually not necessary
- Fungal culture not useful

Pathological Findings
- Short, stubby, or Y-shaped hyphae
- Small, round spores in clusters on hyphae

DIFFERENTIAL DIAGNOSIS
Other skin diseases with discolored macules and plaques, including:
- Pityriasis alba/rosea
- Vitiligo (presents without scaling)
- Seborrheic dermatitis (more erythematous; thicker scale)
- Nummular eczema
- Secondary syphilis

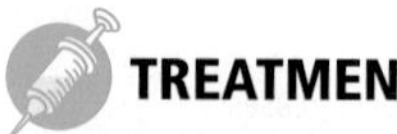

TREATMENT

MEDICATION
Topical antifungal therapy is the treatment of choice in limited disease.

First Line
- Ketoconazole 2% shampoo applied to damp skin and left on for 5 minutes × 1–3 days *OR*
- Selenium sulfide shampoo 2.5% (Selsun):
  - Allowed to dry for 10 minutes prior to showering: Daily × 1 week *OR*
  - Allowed to remain on body for 12–24 hours prior to showering: Once a week × 4 weeks *OR*

- Clotrimazole topical (Lotrimin) b.i.d. × 2–4 weeks *OR*
- Miconazole (Micatin, Monistat) b.i.d. × 2–4 weeks *OR*
- Ketoconazole 2% (Nizoral) cream b.i.d. × 2–4 weeks *OR*
- Terbinafine (Lamisil) 1% solution b.i.d. × 1 week *OR*
- Terbinafine (Lamisil Derm Gel) once daily × 1 week
- Cure rates of topical antiyeast preparations typically 70–80%; healing continues after active treatment. Resumption of even pigmentation may take months.
- Contraindications: Ketoconazole is contraindicated in pregnancy.
- Newer preparations: 2.25% Selenium sulfide foam; ketoconazole gel

Second Line
- Use for extensive disease or nonresponders
- Oral ketoconazole (rarely needed and has significant adverse reactions) 400 mg in single dose or 200 mg/d for 1 week; cure rate >90%
- Itraconazole 200 mg/d PO × 1 week; cure rate >90% (2)[C]

ADDITIONAL TREATMENT
General Measures
- Apply prescribed topical medications to affected skin with cotton balls.
- Pigmentation may take months to fade or fill in.
- Repeat treatment each spring prior to sun exposure.

Issues for Referral
- If resistant to treatment
- If extensive disease occurs in immunocompromised host

ONGOING CARE

- Ketoconazole 2% or selenium sulfide 2.5% shampoo can be used weekly for maintenance or monthly for prophylaxis.
- Itraconazole 400 mg once monthly during the warmer months of the year can also reduce recurrences.

FOLLOW-UP RECOMMENDATIONS
Warn patients that whiteness will remain for several months after treatment.

Patient Monitoring
- Recheck and treat again each spring prior to tanning season.
- Failure to respond should prompt reassessment or dermatology referral.
- Resistance to treatment, frequent recurrences, or widespread disease may point to immunodeficiency.

PATIENT EDUCATION
For patient education materials favorably reviewed on this topic, contact American Academy of Dermatology, 930 N. Meacham Road., P.O. Box 4014, Schaumberg, IL 60168-4014; (708) 330-0230.

PROGNOSIS
- Duration of lesions months/years
- Recurs almost routinely, since this yeast is a known human colonizer

REFERENCES

1. Güleç AT, Demirbilek M, Seçkin D, et al. Superficial fungal infections in 102 renal transplant recipients: A case-control study. *J Am Acad Dermatol*. 2003; 49:187–92.
2. Köse O, Bülent Taştan H, Riza Gür A, et al. Comparison of single 400 mg dose versus a 7 day 200 mg daily dose of itraconazole in the treatment of tinea versicolor. *J Dermatolog Treat*. 2002; 13(2):77–9.

ADDITIONAL READING

- Bhogal CS, Singal A, Baruah MC. Comparative efficacy of ketoconazole and fluconazole in the treatment of pityriasis versicolor: A one year follow-up study. *J Dermatol*. 2001;28:535–9.
- Faergemann J, Gupta AK, Al Mofadi A, et al. Efficacy of itraconazole in the prophylactic treatment of pityriasis (tinea) versicolor. *Arch Dermatol*. 2002; 138:69–73.
- Hu SW, Bigby M. Pityriasis versicolor: A systematic review of interventions. *Arch Dermatol*. 2010;146: 1132.
- Morishita N, Sei Y. Microreview of Pityriasis versicolor and Malassezia species. *Mycopathologia*. 2006;162:373–6.

CODES

ICD9
111.0 Pityriasis versicolor

CLINICAL PEARLS

- Noncontagious macules of varying colors, with fine scale
- Recurrence in summer months
- More apparent after tanning. Skin areas with fungal infection do not tan; thus, hypopigmented areas become more visible.
- Warn patients that whiteness will remain for several months after treatment.

TINNITUS

David M. Holmes, MD

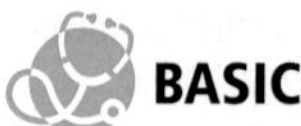

BASICS

DESCRIPTION

- Tinnitus is the perception of sound in the absence of an acoustic stimulus; may be a buzz, ring, roar, chirp, whistle, or hiss. Tinnitus is derived from the Latin word *tinnire* meaning "to ring."
- Subjective tinnitus: Heard only by the patient
- Objective tinnitus: Heard through a stethoscope placed near the patient's ear
- Tinnitus for >6 months is considered chronic.

EPIDEMIOLOGY

Prevalence

- Predominant age: 40–70 years (prevalence increases with age)
- Predominant sex: Males > Females; men traditionally have greater noise exposure in military, occupational, and recreational activities.
- ~16% of the US population, or ~50 million people in the US; 25–30% of US population >65 years of age have chronic tinnitus
- Interferes with daily activities in 12 million people (~4%) in the US, and 25% of those with tinnitus consider it to be a significant problem.
- Rare in children with normal hearing; occurs in 33–64% of children who have severe hearing loss

RISK FACTORS

- Advanced age
- Pregnancy
- Excessive noise exposure
- Hearing loss
- Use of ototoxic medications
- Renal or hepatic impairment
- White
- Male sex

Genetics

There is a possible genetic predisposition, but a tinnitus gene has not yet been discovered. Genes have been identified for temporomandibular joint (TMJ) dysfunction, Ménière disease, and acoustic neuroma.

GENERAL PREVENTION

Avoid prolonged exposure to loud noises, wear hearing protection when loud noises cannot be avoided (e.g., lawn mower, power tools), and avoid overuse of ototoxic medications.

PATHOPHYSIOLOGY

- Moderate sounds cause tiny movements of the stereocilia, which are attached to hair cells in the cochlea. This triggers neuronal transmission in CN VIII. Loud sounds (≥85 dB) cause the stereocilia to bend more than they should. Hair cells that respond to higher-frequency sounds are located at the base of the cochlea and are the first to be damaged. This causes high-pitched ringing. If loud noise exposure is excessive, then stereocilia cannot recover and permanent damage occurs. This results in hearing loss and possibly tinnitus.
- Other causes of hearing loss or damage to the auditory system also can cause tinnitus.
- Tinnitus has many similarities with the symptoms of central neuropathic pain and paresthesias, and it may be related to these neurological disorders (1).

ETIOLOGY

- Subjective tinnitus (My AAA NOISE PAIN):
  - *M*edications and heavy metals that cause or exacerbate tinnitus: Aspirin, aminoglycosides, benzodiazepines, calcium channel blockers, chloroquine, cisplatin, erythromycin, fluoroquinolones, lead, lidocaine, loop diuretics, mercury, methotrexate, NSAIDs, proton pump inhibitors, quinine, sertraline, tetracycline, tricyclic antidepressants, valproate, vancomycin
  - *M*énière disease (estimated 1% prevalence in the US) or other forms of endolymphatic hydrops (abnormally high inner ear pressure)
  - *A*ging-related hearing loss (presbycusis)
  - *A*nemia
  - *A*rterial problems (hypertension, arteriosclerosis, cerebral aneurysm, cerebrovascular accident)
  - *N*oise (chronic exposure to loud noise or acoustic trauma due to acute exposure to very loud noise)
  - *O*tosclerosis and osteogenesis imperfecta
  - *I*nfections (otitis, meningitis, Lyme disease, neurosyphillis, rubella) or impaction (cerumen)
  - *S*clerosis (multiple sclerosis)
  - *E*ndocrine (diabetes mellitus, thyroid)
  - *P*sychogenic (depression, anxiety, psychosis)
  - *A*utoimmune disease of inner ear
  - *I*njury (head and neck) and idiopathic
  - *N*eoplasms (acoustic neuroma or cholesteatoma)
- Objective tinnitus (<1% of all cases of tinnitus; CAGED PETS):
  - Vascular abnormalities:
    - *C*arotid stenosis/CAD
    - *A*rteriovenous shunt/fistula
    - *G*lomus jugulare
    - *E*xisting stapedial artery
    - *D*ehiscent jugular bulb or a vascular loop
  - Mechanical abnormalities:
    - *P*alatal myoclonus
    - *E*ustachian tube abnormally patent
    - *T*MJ disorder
    - *S*tapedial muscle spasticity

COMMONLY ASSOCIATED CONDITIONS

- Hearing loss (~90% of chronic tinnitus is associated with sensorineural hearing loss):
  - Causes of sensorineural hearing loss: Loud noise, presbycusis, ototoxic medications, Ménière disease, acoustic neuroma
  - Causes of conductive hearing loss: Cerumen, ear infection/effusion, trauma, tumor
- TMJ dysfunction
- Depression, anxiety, insomnia, fibromyalgia (40–60% of patients with tinnitus also have major depressive disorder)
- Psychological disorders can contribute to the distress of tinnitus. Some patients with severe tinnitus contemplate suicide.

DIAGNOSIS

HISTORY

- Onset and duration: Gradual (presbycusis), sudden (recent loud noise exposure)
- Location: Unilateral (cerumen impaction, otitis media), unilateral plus hearing loss (acoustic neuroma, CVA)
- Pattern: Continuous (hearing loss), episodic (Ménière disease), pulsatile (vascular)
- Pitch: Low-pitch, rumbling (Ménière disease), high-pitched (sensorineural hearing loss)
- Severity: Use 1–10 scale (10 = most severe), Visual Analog Scale, Tinnitus Severity Index, or Tinnitus Handicap Inventory.
- Exacerbated by: Fatigue, stress, noise exposure, medications
- Alleviated by: Lying down with head in dependent position, medications, masking sounds
- Sudden hearing loss in 1 ear that progresses to the other ear (autoimmune)
- Hearing loss (type: congenital, sensorineural, conductive, or mixed)
- Vertigo (Ménière disease)
- Facial muscle paralysis (cholesteatoma)
- Vertigo (Ménière disease)
- Vestibular disturbances
- Symptoms of depression or anxiety; suicidal thoughts
- Insomnia, difficulty concentrating
- Noise exposure >85 dB (traffic = 85 dB)
- Upper respiratory infection, sinusitis, ear infection, allergic rhinitis
- Otalgia
- Otorrhea
- Head trauma
- Surgery
- Family history of hearing loss or tinnitus
- Medical history or symptoms of: Hypo- or hyperthyroidism, HTN, DM, arteriosclerosis, autoimmune disorders
- Medications (prescription and OTC)
- Exposure to heavy metals (lead or mercury)
- Psychosocial history: Employment, recreational activities, insomnia, anxiety, depression, obsessive–compulsive disorder, psychosis, fibromyalgia

PHYSICAL EXAM

- Otoscopy: Otitis externa/media, cerumen
- Auscultation close to ear for objective tinnitus
- Auscultation of neck (bruits, venous hum)
- Tinnitus of venous origin is suppressed by compression of ipsilateral jugular vein
- Examine TMJ
- Air and bone conduction testing with 512- or 1,024-Hz tuning fork (Weber and Rinne tests)
- Neurologic exam: Romberg test, Dix-Hallpike maneuver (if patient has vertigo), gait testing, cranial nerves
- Test hearing (audiology)

DIAGNOSTIC TESTS & INTERPRETATION

- **Audiometry**
- Tympanometry
- Auditory brain stem response (retrocochlear pathology such as acoustic neuroma)
- Electrocochleography (endolymphic hydrops)
- Electronystagmography (vestibular disorders)

Lab

- Lab investigation is not indicated in all patients; use clinical judgment.

Initial lab tests
Consider:
- CBC
- BUN/creatinine
- Fasting glucose
- Fasting lipid profile
- Thyroid-stimulating hormone

Follow-Up & Special Considerations
Consider HIV, rapid plasma reagin, autoimmune panel

Imaging
- A full clinical evaluation should precede radiologic studies.
- Gadolinium-enhanced MRI (if tinnitus is continuous)
- Contrast-enhanced CT scan or MRI (if tinnitus is pulsatile)
- Sonography, angiography, or MRA (to asses vascular abnormalities in the neck)
- SPECT may be more sensitive than CT scan, MRI, or MRA, and it identifies dynamic changes within the brain at the neurotransmitter level.
- PET scan: Increased activity in the auditory cortex suggests that transcranial magnetic stimulation may effectively treat the tinnitus.

DIFFERENTIAL DIAGNOSIS
Auditory hallucinations

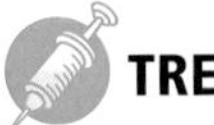

TREATMENT

MEDICATION
New-onset tinnitus often is associated with hearing loss; steroid pulse or standard-dose therapy is indicated with idiopathic sudden sensorineural hearing loss (ISSHL)

First Line
Antidepressants (SSRIs or TCAs such as amitriptyline): If patients are depressed/anxious or have severe tinnitus; no evidence that one antidepressant works best. Caution: Tinnitus can be a side effect of antidepressant medications.

Second Line
- Antihistamines
- Baclofen
- Benzodiazepines
- Hyperbaric oxygen may help to improve hearing of those with early presentation of ISSHL.
- Anticonvulsants, such as gabapentin, are used occasionally, but research has shown that they do not significantly reduce tinnitus (2).

ADDITIONAL TREATMENT

General Measures
- Management depends on the severity of tinnitus and may require multiple treatment strategies.
- Treat the underlying cause.
- Discontinue ototoxic medications.
- Anxiety, insomnia, and depression may exacerbate tinnitus, which, in turn, may exacerbate the anxiety, insomnia, and/or depression. Treat to stop this vicious cycle.
- Hearing aids/cochlear implants
- Hearing protection during noise exposure
- Compression of myofascial trigger points (3)[B]

Issues for Referral
- Refer patients to a comprehensive tinnitus management program (audiologist).
- Otolaryngologist, neurologist, and/or neurosurgeon, depending on etiology

Additional Therapies
- Cognitive-behavioral therapy: There is no evidence that it decreases loudness of tinnitus, but it does improve depression and quality of life (4)[A].
- Transcranial magnetic stimulation (TMS) and repetitive TMS: A noninvasive method to stimulate neurons in the brain by rapidly changing magnetic fields. This is a new and effective technique to reduce tinnitus, and is effective even with patients who have long-term symptoms that are resistant to medications. It also may help treat migraine headaches, strokes, Parkinson disease, dystonia, major depression, and auditory hallucinations (5)[B].
- Acoustic therapy: Listening to relaxing sounds through headphones when the environment is too quiet.
- Biofeedback and stress reduction: Relaxation techniques may help to reduce the severity of the tinnitus.
- Neurofeedback: Many patients with tinnitus have abnormal oscillatory brain activity. Neurofeedback helps to normalize this and treat tinnitus.
- Tinnitus retraining therapy: Uses counseling and sound enrichment to help patients stop their negative reaction to tinnitus and then reduce and eventually end their perception of it (6)[B].
- Sound therapy (masking): Patients wear low-level noise generators to mask the tinnitus noise; commonly used but effectiveness is unknown; may require 1–2 years of therapy

COMPLEMENTARY AND ALTERNATIVE MEDICINE
- Zinc: In 1 small study zinc 50 mg daily for 2 months decreased severity of subjective tinnitus
- Botulinum toxin
- Acamprosate (a medication used to treat alcohol dependence)
- Hypnosis (7)[B]
- Acupuncture (unknown effectiveness)
- Low-power laser to mastoid bone (unknown effectiveness)
- Gingko biloba, melatonin, lecithin (all are ineffective)

SURGERY/OTHER PROCEDURES
- Otosclerosis: Stapedectomy surgery with implantation of ossicular prosthesis
- Severe Ménière disease or other forms of endolymphatic hydrops that are not alleviated by medications: Installation of endolymphatic shunt, labyrinthectomy, or vestibular neurectomy
- Auditory neoplasms: Surgical resection or radiation
- Vascular pulsatile tinnitus due to atherosclerotic carotid artery disease: Carotid endarterectomy

IN-PATIENT CONSIDERATIONS

Admission Criteria
Hospitalization is rarely indicated.

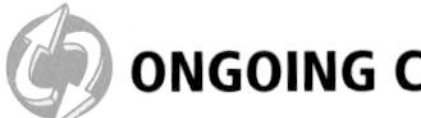

ONGOING CARE

FOLLOW-UP RECOMMENDATIONS
- Audiologist: For complete evaluation and therapy; specialists as indicated
- Family physician: 1–2 months after therapy initiated and periodically thereafter

PATIENT EDUCATION
- Help patients to understand that tinnitus is a perception of sound and is not a threat to their physical health.
- Sources of information for patients:
  - American Tinnitus Association: (800) 634-8978; www.ata.org
  - National Institute on Deafness and Other Communication Disorders: (800) 241-1044; www.nidcd.nih.gov
  - American Academy of Otolaryngology: (703) 836-4444; www.entnet.org

PROGNOSIS
Most cases of chronic tinnitus cannot be cured because of association with irreversible sensorineural hearing loss. Therefore, focus is on managing the tinnitus and reducing its severity, not curing it.

REFERENCES

1. Møller AR. Tinnitus and pain. *Prog Brain Res*. 2007;166:47–53.
2. Hoekstra CE, Rynja SP, van Zanten GA, et al. Anticonvulsants for tinnitus. *Cochrane Database Syst Rev*. 2011:CD007960.
3. Rocha CA, Sanchez TG. Myofascial trigger points: Another way of modulating tinnitus. *Prog Brain Res*. 2007;166:209–14.
4. Martinez Devesa P, Waddell A, Perera R et al. Cognitive behavioural therapy for tinnitus. *Cochrane Database Syst Rev*. 2007: CD005233.
5. Anders M, Dvorakova J, Rathova L et al. Efficacy of repetitive transcranial magnetic stimulation for the treatment of refractory chronic tinnitus: A randomized, placebo controlled study. *Neuroendocrine Letters*. 2010;31(2):238–49.
6. Phillips JS, McFerran D. Tinnitus Retraining Therapy (TRT) for tinnitus. *Cochrane Database Syst Rev*. 2010:CD007330.
7. Cope TE. Clinical hypnosis for the alleviation of tinnitus. *Int Tinnitus J*. 2008;14:135–8.

ADDITIONAL READING

- Hoare DJ, Kowalkowski VL, Kang S, et al. Systematic review and meta-analyses of randomized controlled trials examining tinnitus management. *Laryngoscope*. 2011;121:1555–64.
- Savage J, Cook S, Waddell A, et al. Tinnitus. *Clin Evid (Online)*. 2009;2009.

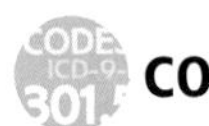

CODES

ICD9
- 388.30 Tinnitus, unspecified
- 388.31 Subjective tinnitus
- 388.32 Objective tinnitus

CLINICAL PEARLS
- Tinnitus is rare in children with normal hearing but common in children with severe hearing loss.
- To keep tinnitus from getting worse, avoid loud noises, reduce stress, control BP, get enough sleep, decrease alcohol and caffeine, and do not smoke.
- People have different levels of tolerance to tinnitus. It may affect sleep, concentration, and emotional state. ~50% of patients with chronic tinnitus also have major depressive disorder.

TOBACCO USE AND SMOKING CESSATION

S. Lindsey Clarke, MD, FAAFP

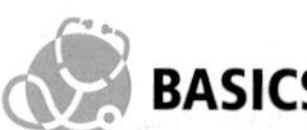

BASICS

DESCRIPTION

- Tobacco use is the leading cause of preventable morbidity and mortality worldwide:
  - 443,000 deaths annually in the US
  - 4.2 million premature deaths/yr worldwide
  - Major risk factor for:
    - Atherosclerotic cardiovascular disease
    - Lung cancer
    - Chronic obstructive pulmonary disease (COPD)
- Nicotine is highly addictive.
- Smoking damages nearly every organ in the human body.
- Second-hand exposure to cigarette smoke is associated with a 20% greater risk of lung cancer and coronary heart disease.
- Quitting smoking has both immediate and long-term health benefits.

EPIDEMIOLOGY

Incidence

- 2.5 million new smokers annually in the US (initiation rate = 2.8%) (2009 data)
- 59% of new smokers are <18 years of age (6% initiation rate for teens).

Prevalence

- 70 million Americans (27.7%) currently use tobacco (2009 data).
- Highest among those aged 18–25 years (41.6%); peak age of tobacco use is 22 years
- Predominant race: Prevalence highest among American Indians/Alaskan Natives (41.8%) and lowest among Hispanics (23.2%) and Asians (11.9%)
- Predominant sex: Male (33.5%) > Female (22.2%)
- Inversely proportional to education level

RISK FACTORS

- Presence of a smoker in the household
- Easy access to cigarettes
- Perceived parental approval of smoking
- Comorbid stress and psychiatric disorders
- Low self-esteem and self-worth
- Poor academic performance
- Boys: High levels of aggression and rebelliousness
- Girls: Preoccupation with weight and body image

GENERAL PREVENTION

- Most first-time tobacco use occurs before high school graduation, so educational interventions should target students in grade school and middle school, and must address both the health consequences and the psychosocial aspects of smoking.
- The American Academy of Family Physicians' Tar Wars program has targeted fourth and fifth graders successfully.
- Other helpful measures include:
  - Smoking bans in public areas and workplaces
  - Restriction of minors' access to tobacco
  - Restrictions on tobacco advertisements
  - Raising prices through taxation
  - Media literacy education
  - Tobacco-free sports initiatives

PATHOPHYSIOLOGY

- Addiction due to nicotine's rapid stimulation of the brain's dopamine system (teenage brain especially susceptible)
- Atherosclerotic risk due to adrenergic stimulation, endothelial damage, carbon monoxide, and adverse effects on lipids
- Direct airway damage from cigarette tar
- Carcinogens in all tobacco products

COMMONLY ASSOCIATED CONDITIONS

- Coronary artery disease
- Cerebrovascular disease
- Peripheral vascular disease
- Abdominal aortic aneurysm
- COPD
- Cancer of the lip, oral cavity, pharynx, larynx, lung, esophagus, stomach, pancreas, kidney, bladder, cervix, and blood
- Pneumonia
- Osteoporosis
- Periodontitis
- Alcohol use
- Depression and anxiety
- Reduced fertility

Pregnancy Considerations

- 15.3% of pregnant women smoke.
- Women who smoke or who are exposed to 2nd-hand smoke during pregnancy have increased risks of miscarriage, placenta previa, placental abruption, premature rupture of membranes, preterm delivery, low-birth-weight infants, and stillbirth.

Pediatric Considerations

- Second-hand smoke increases the risk of the following in infants and children:
  - Sudden infant death syndrome
  - Acute upper and lower respiratory tract infections (1)[A]
  - More frequent and more severe exacerbations of asthma
  - Otitis media and need for tympanostomies
- Nicotine passes through breast milk, and its effects on the growth and development of nursing infants are unknown.

DIAGNOSIS

HISTORY

- Screen for tobacco use and second-hand smoke exposure at every physician encounter.
- Type and quantity of tobacco used
- Pack years = packs/day × years
- Awareness of health risks
- Assess interest in quitting
- Identify triggers for smoking
- Prior attempts to quit: Method, duration of success, reason for relapse

PHYSICAL EXAM

- General: Tobacco smoke odor
- Skin: Premature wrinkling of the face
- Mouth: Nicotine-stained teeth; inspect for suspicious mucosal lesions
- Lungs: Crackles, wheezing, increased or decreased volume
- Vessels: Carotid or abdominal bruits, abdominal aortic enlargement, peripheral pulses, stigmata of peripheral vascular disease

DIAGNOSTIC TESTS & INTERPRETATION

Imaging

- Chest x-ray for patients with pulmonary symptoms or signs of cancer but not for screening
- US Preventative Services Task Force recommends 1-time screening ultrasound for abdominal aortic aneurysm in men ≥65 years who ever have smoked (number needed to screen to prevent 1 AAA = 500)

Diagnostic Procedures/Surgery

Pulmonary function testing for smokers with chronic pulmonary symptoms such as wheezing and dyspnea

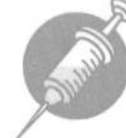

TREATMENT

Identify and address triggers by recommending alternative agents (e.g., gum, hard candy, cough lozenges, etc.).

MEDICATION

First Line

- Varenicline (Chantix): 0.5 mg/d PO × 3 days, then 0.5 mg b.i.d. × 4 days, then 1 mg b.i.d. (2,3)[A]:
  - Start 1 week prior to smoking cessation, and continue for 12–24 weeks.
  - Superior to placebo and to bupropion; number needed to treat = 7
  - Side effects: Nausea, insomnia, headache, depression, suicidal ideation; safety not established in patients with psychiatric illness; not well studied in adolescents; pregnancy Category C

Second Line

- Bupropion (Zyban): 150 mg PO × 3 days, then 150 mg b.i.d. (4)[A]:
  - Start 1 week prior to smoking cessation, and continue for 7–12 weeks.
  - Twice as effective as placebo
  - Side effects: Tachycardia, headache, nausea, insomnia, dry mouth; drug of choice for depressed patients; contraindicated in patients who have seizure disorders or bipolar affective disorder; pregnancy Category C
- Nortriptyline: 25–75 mg/d PO or in divided doses (4)[A]:
  - Start 10–14 days prior to smoking cessation, and continue for at least 12 weeks.
  - Efficacy similar to bupropion, but side effects more common; pregnancy Category D

- Nicotine replacement therapy (e.g., patch, gum, lozenge, inhaler, nasal spray) (5,6)[A]:
  - Improves quit rates by 50–70% compared with placebo
  - Various forms have equivalent efficacy.
  - Over the counter (OTC)
  - Patch (NicoDerm CQ, others): 21, 14, and 7 mg:
    - 1 patch q24h
    - Start with 21 mg if smoking ≥10 cigarettes/d; otherwise, start with 14 mg.
    - 6 weeks on initial dose, then taper
    - 2 weeks each on subsequent doses
    - No proven benefit beyond 8 weeks
  - Gum (Nicorette): 2 and 4 mg:
    - Use 4 mg if smoking ≥25 cigarettes/d.
    - Chew 1 piece q1–2h × 6 weeks, then 1 q2–4h × 3 weeks, then 1 q4–8h × 3 weeks.
  - May use in combination with bupropion, but monitor for hypertension
  - Side effects: Headache, pharyngitis, cough, rhinitis, dyspepsia; all mainly with inhaler and spray forms
  - Pregnancy Category D, but probably safer than continued smoking during pregnancy

ADDITIONAL TREATMENT

General Measures

- The 5 As of smoking cessation:
  - Ask about tobacco use at every office visit.
  - Advise all smokers to quit.
  - Assess the patient's willingness to quit.
  - Assist the patient in his or her attempt to quit.
  - Arrange follow-up.
- It might help for patients to have a quitting partner, such as a spouse, friend, or coworker, to provide mutual encouragement.
- Patients desiring to quit should dispose of all smoking paraphernalia (such as lighters) on their quit dates to make relapse more difficult.
- Patients should try to anticipate situations that they associate with smoking and should have a plan for dealing with their urge to smoke.

Additional Therapies

The following interventions have been shown to be effective in helping patients quit smoking:

- Brief physician advice at every visit:
  - "The best thing you can do for your health right now is to stop smoking."
- Advice from nurses, especially in hospital
- Individual counseling and group therapy
- Telephone counseling (see "Patient Education")
- Web-based cessation programs
- Exercise (limited data)
- "Electronic cigarettes" are type of nicotine delivery system; controversial; FDA has decided to regulate them as tobacco products.

COMPLEMENTARY AND ALTERNATIVE MEDICINE

Acupuncture and hypnosis have not been proven to enhance long-term smoking cessation.

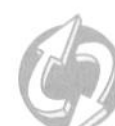

ONGOING CARE

FOLLOW-UP RECOMMENDATIONS

- Follow up soon after scheduled quit date and regularly thereafter.
- Refraining from tobacco products for the first 2 weeks is critical to long-term abstinence.

Patient Monitoring

- Short-term withdrawal symptoms include irritability, anxiety, insomnia, and poor concentration.
- Longer-term risks of smoking cessation include weight gain (4–5 kg on average) and depression.
- Quitting also is associated with exacerbations of ulcerative colitis and worsening of cognitive function in patients with schizophrenia.

DIET

Healthy eating is important for limiting weight gain following smoking cessation.

PATIENT EDUCATION

- 1-800-QUIT-NOW: Free counseling, resources, and support for quitting
- www.smokefree.gov

PROGNOSIS

- Smoking cessation by age 40 is associated with significant preservation of life expectancy.
- Measurable cardiovascular benefits of smoking cessation begin as early as 24 hours after quitting and continue to mount until the risk is reduced to that of nonsmokers by 5–15 years.
- People who quit smoking after a heart attack or cardiac surgery reduce their risk of death by at least 1/3.
- Relapse rates initially >60% but decrease to 2–4% per year after completing 2 years of abstinence.

COMPLICATIONS

- Disability and premature death due to heart attack, stroke, cancer, COPD
- Smoking more than doubles the risk of coronary artery disease and almost doubles the risk of stroke.
- Smokers are 12–22× more likely than nonsmokers to die from lung cancer.
- Smokers die an average of 14 years earlier than nonsmokers.

REFERENCES

1. Jones LL, Hashim A, McKeever T, et al. Parental and household smoking and the increased risk of bronchitis, bronchiolitis and other lower respiratory infections in infancy: Systematic review and meta-analysis. *Respir Res*. 2011;12:5.
2. Cahill K, Stead LF, Lancaster T. Nicotine receptor partial agonists for smoking cessation. *Cochrane Database Syst Rev*. 2011;(2):CD006103.
3. Hays JT, Ebbert JO. Varenicline for tobacco dependence. *N Engl J Med*. 2008;359:2018–24.
4. Hughes JR, Stead LF, Lancaster T, et al. Antidepressants for smoking cessation. *Cochrane Database Syst Rev*. 2007;CD000031.
5. Moore D, Aveyard P, Connock M, et al. Effectiveness and safety of nicotine replacement therapy assisted reduction to stop smoking: Systematic review and meta-analysis. *BMJ*. 2009;338:b1024.
6. Stead LF, Perera R, Bullen C, et al. Nicotine replacement therapy for smoking cessation. *Cochrane Database Syst Rev*. 2008;CD000146.

T

ADDITIONAL READING

- Clinical Practice Guideline Treating Tobacco Use and Dependence 2008 Update Panel, Liaisons, and Staff. A clinical practice guideline for treating tobacco use and dependence: 2008 update. A U.S. Public Health Service report. *Am J Prev Med*. 2008;35(2):158–76.
- Department of Health and Human Services, Substance Abuse and Mental Health Services Administration, Office of Applied Studies. Results from the 2009 national survey on drug use and health. Accessed July 4, 2011, at http://oas.samhsa.gov.
- Rosen IM, Maurer DM. Reducing tobacco use in adolescents. *Am Fam Physician*. 2008;77:483–90.

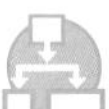

See Also (Topic, Algorithm, Electronic Media Element)

Nicotine Addiction; Substance Use Disorders

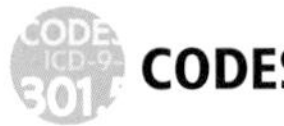

CODES

ICD9

- V15.82 Personal history of tobacco use
- 305.1 Nondependent tobacco use disorder

CLINICAL PEARLS

- Tobacco use is a major cause of mortality and morbidity due to atherosclerotic cardiovascular disease, lung cancer, COPD, and other health problems.
- Varenicline (Chantix) is the single most effective prescription aid to smoking cessation. Other proven therapies include bupropion, nortriptyline, and OTC nicotine replacement systems.
- Smokers die an average of 14 years earlier than nonsmokers
- Brief physician advice and telephone counseling have been shown to be effective in helping patients to quit smoking. 1-800-QUIT-NOW is a free patient resource for counseling and support for quitting smoking.

TORCH INFECTIONS

Kendall Johnson, MD
Timothy Gibson, MD

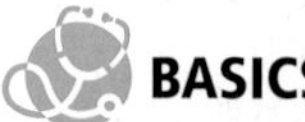

BASICS

DESCRIPTION

- An acronym describing a group of infections that are acquired prenatally or during the birth process and have similar physical findings, including skin and ocular manifestations:
  - *T*oxoplasmosis: Protozoan parasite, *Toxoplasma gondii* (1,2)
  - *O*ther (syphilis): Spirochete, *Treponema pallidum* (3)
  - *R*ubella: Virus (4,5)
  - *C*MV: Cytomegalovirus (6)
  - *H*erpes: Herpes simplex virus (HSV) (7,8)
- System(s) affected: Skin/Exocrine; HEENT; Nervous; Gastrointestinal; Lymphatic/Heme; Renal; Cardiac; Pulmonary
- Synonym(s): CMV infection also known as cytomegalic inclusion disease (CID) or cytoplasmic inclusion body disease

EPIDEMIOLOGY

- Predominant age: Prenatal to infants
- Predominant sex: Male = Female

Incidence

- Toxoplasmosis: 1.1 per 1,000 live births
- Syphilis: 10.1 per 100,000 live births
- Rubella: No longer endemic in the US; rare cases seen with emigrating mothers
- CMV: 1 per 100 live births; defects present in 10% of infected infants
- Herpes: 1 per 5,000 live births

RISK FACTORS

- General: Inadequate prenatal care
- Toxoplasmosis: Effects more severe with first- or second-trimester infection; increased risk with maternal history as southeast Asian refugee; exposure to raw meat or cat feces
- Rubella: Inadequate maternal vaccination
- CMV: Care for preschool-aged children during pregnancy; initial sexual activity <2 years prior to pregnancy; STD during pregnancy; maternal age <25 years
- Herpes: Positive HSV serology at delivery *and* vaginal delivery; invasive monitoring; initial episode of HSV; premature labor; maternal age <21 years

GENERAL PREVENTION

- Toxoplasmosis: Avoid handling of cat litter; keep cats indoors and fed canned foods; wear rubber gloves for meat preparation and gardening
- Syphilis: Screen with VDRL or RPR test at first prenatal visit, confirm with FTA-ABS:
  - Give previously untreated pregnant women penicillin G IM, dose 2.4 million units once for primary, secondary, or early latent; 2.4 million units weekly every 3 weeks for late latent (9)
- Rubella: Test IgG titers to determine immunity at initial prenatal visit
- CMV: Prenatal antibody titers to determine serologic status; avoid prolonged exposure to young children during pregnancy
- Herpes: Insufficient evidence for antiviral prophylaxis decreasing neonatal herpes incidence, although it does decrease viral shedding, clinical lesions, and number of cesarean sections.
  - Prophylactic treatment with acyclovir 200 mg q.i.d. or 300 mg t.i.d. starting at 36 weeks' gestation.

PATHOPHYSIOLOGY

- All infections transmitted vertically, either transplacentally or through maternal genital tract
- Toxoplasmosis: *T. gondii* protozoan results in cyst dissemination throughout tissues and host cell death
- Syphilis: Spirochetes cause inflammatory damage to most organ systems
- Rubella: Mechanism of damage unclear, possibly secondary to vasculitis
- CMV: Immunosuppressive virus replicates in leukocytes, secretory glands, and kidneys.
- Herpes: Virus replicates in sensory ganglion; inability to control replication results in disseminated infection

ETIOLOGY

Acquired vertically due to maternal infection during pregnancy

COMMONLY ASSOCIATED CONDITIONS

Of newborns with CMV, 17–41% also have chorioretinitis.

DIAGNOSIS

HISTORY

- Toxoplasmosis: No maternal symptoms or history of flulike syndrome
- Syphilis, rubella, and CMV: Maternal history of fever and rash
- Herpes: Infant may present with fever, change in mental status, or seizures

PHYSICAL EXAM

- Toxoplasmosis: Growth retardation, jaundice, maculopapular rash, microcephaly, chorioretinitis, ascitis, hepatosplenomegaly
- Syphilis: Most infants asymptomatic; early signs are snuffles (rhinitis), poor feeding and hepatosplenomegaly; rash varies from red macular to bullous; chronic infection may present with neurosyphilis (tabes dorsalis, deafness), Hutchinson incisors, mulberry molars, saddle nose deformity, or uveitis
- Rubella: Classic triad involves sensorineural hearing loss, ocular abnormalities (cataracts, glaucoma, retinopathy) and congenital heart disease (PDA); also see intrauterine growth restriction and jaundice
- CMV: Most infected infants are asymptomatic; 10% with symptoms including IUGR, hepatosplenomegaly, petechiae and purpura (blueberry muffin rash), microcephaly, deafness, chorioretinitis
- Herpes: Clustered vesicular lesions (50%), fever, irritability, gingivitis, nuchal rigidity, focal neurologic symptoms

DIAGNOSTIC TESTS & INTERPRETATION

Lab

Initial lab tests

- Toxoplasmosis: Newborn serum testing of IgM and IgA antibodies; may also test maternal blood prenatally
- Syphilis: Newborn screen with VDRL or RPR test, confirm with FTA-ABS; CBC with differential and liver function tests
- Rubella: Viral isolation by PCR preferred over serologic testing
- CMV: Viral culture from bodily fluid
- Herpes: Viral isolation; tissue culture or CSF

Imaging

Initial approach

- Toxoplasmosis: Ultrasound at 20–24 weeks' gestation to evaluate for hydrocephalus
- Syphilis: Chest x-ray (CXR) (pneumonia alba); long-bone x-ray (onion-skinning, rat bite tibia)
- Rubella: CXR if respiratory symptoms present
- CMV: Head CT (periventricular calcifications)
- Herpes: Head CT or MRI if concern for encephalitis (temporal lobe abnormalities)

Follow-Up & Special Considerations

- Toxoplasmosis: Head CT (ring-enhancing lesions)
- Rubella: ECHO to diagnose heart defects; head CT may show intracranial calcifications

Diagnostic Procedures/Surgery

Syphilis: Obtain CSF in all infected infants >1 month to evaluate for neurosyphilis

Pathological Findings

- Toxoplasmosis: Tissue with tachyzoites definitive for active infection
- CMV: Presence of inclusion giant cells
- Herpes: Multinucleate giant cells

DIFFERENTIAL DIAGNOSIS

- Congenital lymphocytic choriomeningitis virus
- Encephalopathies
- Meningitis
- Parvovirus B19
- Bacterial sepsis
- HIV
- Varicella
- Epstein-Barr virus

TREATMENT

MEDICATION

First Line

- Toxoplasmosis: Pyrimethamine (1 mg/kg/d PO daily for 6 months, then MWF for 6 months; max 25 mg/d) and sulfadiazine (100 mg/kg/d PO q12h) for 12 months in both symptomatic and asymptomatic infants. Folinic acid (5–10 mg 3 times a week) to reduce hematologic toxicity.
- Syphilis: Aqueous crystalline penicillin G 50,000 units/kg IV q12h for 7 days, then q8h for total treatment of 10 days. Desensitize patient if penicillin allergic.
- Rubella: No specific antiviral agent indicated
- CMV: Ganciclovir may be useful for acutely ill infants.
- Herpes: Insufficient evidence to evaluate antiviral use in neonates; recommended treatment is acyclovir 10–20 mg/kg IV q8h for 14–21 days

Second Line

- Toxoplasmosis: Clindamycin if sulfadiazine is not tolerated; corticosteroids for ocular and CNS complications
- Syphilis: Procaine penicillin G 50,000 units/kg IM daily for 10 days

ADDITIONAL TREATMENT

General Measures

- Nutritional and respiratory support
- Rubella: Vision and hearing screening in asymptomatic infants; phototherapy for hyperbilirubinemia.

Issues for Referral

Consider consultation based on organ systems involved (ophthalmology, cardiology, neurology, orthopedics)

SURGERY/OTHER PROCEDURES

- Possibility of gastrostomy placement based on nutritional needs
- Rubella: Repair of congenital heart defects

IN-PATIENT CONSIDERATIONS

Initial Stabilization

Respiratory support

Admission Criteria

Infected neonates to remain inpatient from birth

IV Fluids

Indicated if oral feeding is inadequate; determined by weight-based calculations

Discharge Criteria

Once stable and treatment is completed or arranged on outpatient basis; infants infected with rubella must remain hospitalized in isolation until 2 cultures taken 1 month apart are negative

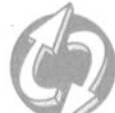

ONGOING CARE

FOLLOW-UP RECOMMENDATIONS

Patient Monitoring

- Continue to follow neurologic and developmental status.
- Toxoplasmosis: Follow up every 2 weeks until stable, then monthly while being treated; CBC every week for 1 month, then every 2 weeks
- Syphilis: Serologic testing every 2–3 months until nonreactive for 4-fold decrease. If CSF is abnormal, repeat LP every 6 months until normal.
- Rubella: Vision and hearing screens

DIET

Normal diet as tolerated

PATIENT EDUCATION

- An infected mother should be informed of potential harm to the fetus.
- Pregnant women should avoid contact with those infected with rubella.

PROGNOSIS

- Toxoplasmosis: Development and behavior normal with adequate treatment; chorioretinitis in 26% of treated infants (2)
- Syphilis: 6.4% mortality rate
- Rubella: Poor outcome with significant organ damage
- CMV: Normal development if 12-month exam within normal limits; chorioretinitis untreatable
- Herpes: 50% mortality, mostly disseminated disease; good outcome with treated mucocutaneous infections

COMPLICATIONS

- Toxoplasmosis: Meningoencephalitis with hydrocephalus, seizure disorder, vision impairment, deafness, mental retardation
- Syphilis: Pneumonia alba, stillbirth, multiple-organ damage
- Rubella: Deafness, vision impairment, skeletal defects, congenital heart defects
- CMV: Hearing loss, chorioretinitis, thrombocytopenia
- Herpes: Seizures, pneumonia, adrenal involvement, respiratory distress, liver dysfunction, eczema herpeticum

REFERENCES

1. Jones J, Lopez A, Wilson M, et al. Congenital toxoplasmosis. *Am Fam Physician*. 2003;67: 2131–8.
2. McLeod R, Boyer K, Karrison T, et al. Outcome of treatment for congenital toxoplasmosis, 1981–2004: The National Collaborative Chicago-Based, Congenital Toxoplasmosis Study. *Clin Infect Dis*. 2006;42:1383–94.
3. French P. Syphilis. *BMJ*. 2007;334:143–7.
4. Banatvala JE, Brown DW. Rubella. *Lancet*. 2004;363:1127–37.
5. Control and prevention of rubella: Evaluation and management of suspected outbreaks, rubella in pregnant women, and surveillance for congenital rubella syndrome. *MMWR Recomm Rep*. 2001;50: 1–23.
6. American College of Obstetrics and Gynecologists. ACOG practice bulletin. Perinatal viral and parasitic infections. Number 20, September 2000. (Replaces educational bulletin number 177, February 1993). *Int J Gynaecol Obstet*. 2002;76:95–107.
7. Anzivino E, Fioriti D, Mischitelli M, et al. Herpes simplex virus infection in pregnancy and in neonate: Status of art of epidemiology, diagnosis, therapy and prevention. *Virol J*. 2009;6:40.
8. Corey L, Wald A. Maternal and neonatal herpes simplex virus infections. *N Engl J Med*. 2009;361: 1376–85.
9. Workowski KA, Berman S, Centers for Disease Control and Prevention (CDC), et al. Sexually transmitted diseases treatment guidelines, 2010. *MMWR Recomm Rep*. 2010;59:1–110.

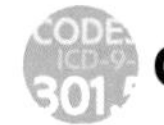

CODES

ICD9

771.89 Other infections specific to the perinatal period

CLINICAL PEARLS

- Adequate prenatal care is paramount for prevention of TORCH infections.
- Initial workup includes thorough maternal history and indicated lab tests (CBC, antibodies, viral culture).
- Infants with altered mental status need brain imaging to evaluate for intracranial lesions, hydrocephalus, or other abnormalities.
- After treatment, infants should be regularly monitored for potential sequelae.

TORSION, OVARIAN

Ruth Levesque, MD
Dawn S. Tasillo, MD

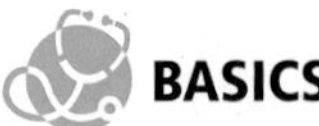

BASICS

DESCRIPTION

- Twisting of adnexal components by at least one complete turn
- Most commonly, it is the ovary and fallopian tube rotating together around the broad ligament, but it can also be twisting of the ovary or the fallopian tube individually around either the mesovarium or mesosalpinx, respectively.
- Torsion can lead to impedance of blood flow to and from the ovary, potentially evolving into necrosis of the ovary.
- Torsion of a normal ovary can occur. However, upwards of 94% of cases of ovarian torsion involve a mass in the ovary such as a cyst or neoplasm.

EPIDEMIOLOGY

Prevalence

Fifth most common gynecological emergency (2.7%), accounts for 15% of all surgically treated adnexal masses (1)

RISK FACTORS

- At least 60% of all torsions occur on the right side, likely because the right utero-ovarian ligament is longer than the left and the sigmoid colon on the left side decreases the space for movement and torsion of the left ovary (1,2).
- Benign masses are more common than ovarian cancers because malignant tumors often invade nearby tissues and/or cause adhesions, therefore decreasing the rate of torsion. Enlarged ovaries like polycystic ovaries or those with benign cystic teratomas are more vulnerable to torsion (2).
- The rate of malignancy seen with ovarian torsion is between 2% and 15% (2).
- Torsed ovaries were 5 cm or greater in 89% of cases (3). Ovaries >~6 cm typically rise out of the true pelvis due to their size and, therefore, have an increased rate of torsion because the bony constraints of the pelvis are no longer preventing them from moving freely (4).
- Patients with ligated uterine tubes have increased risk of ovarian torsion possibly due to electrocoagulation damage to the tube, which increases laxity and/or hydrosalpinx due to the tube no longer being able to drain secretions effectively.
- Ovarian stimulation (as with fertility treatments) causes an increased risk of torsion due to the increased volume and weight of the ovary.

Genetics

Congenitally long ovarian ligaments increase mobility of ovaries and fallopian tubes leading to increased risk of torsion, even in a normal ovary.

GENERAL PREVENTION

- Diagnosis and treatment of ovarian masses can decrease the rate of torsion. Awareness of the risk of torsion is important for patients undergoing ovarian stimulation for IVF treatments and for patients with known ovarian masses.
- Patients with known masses are often cautioned to avoid vigorous activity (running, intercourse) until the mass has resolved.

PATHOPHYSIOLOGY

- Adnexal blood supply comes from both the uterine and ovarian vessels.
- Torsion commonly cuts off blood supply from one source. However, the ovary often continues to be perfused by the other source.
- While the venous drainage from the ovaries is a very low-pressure system, the arterial supply to ovaries is a high pressure system.
- Therefore, torsion can cause venous drainage to stop while arterial supply into the ovary remains unchanged. This causes congestion and swelling of the ovary but prevents immediate infarction.

Pregnancy Considerations

- Signs and symptoms of ovarian torsion in the pregnant patient are similar to those seen in a nonpregnant patient.
- Rates of torsion have been cited at between 0.6% and 6% in pregnancies obtained by ovarian stimulation, and the rate of torsion increases to between 7.5% and 16% in patients presenting with ovarian hyperstimulation syndrome (1,5).
- ~82% of cases of ovarian torsion in pregnancy occur in the first trimester.
- Of pregnant women with a diagnosed ovarian torsion, 19.5% have a future reoccurrence (5).
- Of all torsions, 8–25% of cases occur in pregnant patients (2,4).
- Most commonly, the corpus luteum cyst is the causative etiology of the torsion.
- Management of ovarian torsion in the pregnant woman is similar to that of the nonpregnant patient.
- Laparoscopic treatment of the torsion is considered safe in pregnancy with studies reporting between 2% and 5% risk of loss of the pregnancy following surgery, and an 8% rate of preterm labor (5).
- If the corpus luteum is removed prior to 10 weeks' gestation, progesterone replacement is recommended in order to maintain the pregnancy; this will need to be initiated soon after surgery. Several dosing regimens are available. Consultation with an obstetrics provider prior to surgery (or immediately after) is recommended.

Pediatric Considerations

- Adnexal torsion most commonly presents in perimenarchal and early teenage years (6).
- The most common symptoms of ovarian torsion in the pediatric population are pain, nausea, and vomiting.
- ~15% of cases of ovarian torsion occur during infancy and childhood (6).
- Ovarian torsion may be present within an incarcerated inguinal hernia; 27% of girls with an incarcerated hernia had ovarian torsion and infarction of their ovaries (6).
- Children with torsion and no underlying ovarian pathology had an 11.4% risk of asynchronous torsion of the other ovary (6).
- Incidence of underlying ovarian pathology in children with torsion ranges from 64–82% with the most common pathological findings being benign cystic teratomas or hemorrhagic or follicular cysts (6).
- In a recent review, only 2 cases of ovarian torsion with associated ovarian malignancy were reported in the pediatric population (6).
- The role of oophoropexy in the treatment of children with ovarian torsion is unclear at this time.

ETIOLOGY

- Increased mass and size of ovary causing increased risk of torsion because the ovary is able to swing on its vascular pedicle more readily.
- Predominant sex: Female only

COMMONLY ASSOCIATED CONDITIONS

Pregnancy and ovarian stimulation

DIAGNOSIS

HISTORY

- The most common symptom is pelvic pain (96%) (2). Women commonly complain of sharp lower abdominal pain, usually sudden in onset, worsening over several hours to days, and often radiating to the flank and thighs.
- Pain is localized to the involved side but may radiate across the lower pelvis.
- Associated nausea and vomiting for 42–70% of patients
- Fever is not a common symptom of ovarian torsion (8%). However, it can be seen in advanced cases when necrosis has started.
- Pain may subside or resolve in an unresolved torsion, due to necrosis of pain fibers.

PHYSICAL EXAM

- Adnexal mass is found in 41–98% of cases (1,2,7)
- Bilateral adnexal pain during pelvic exam found in 26% of cases (1)

DIAGNOSTIC TESTS & INTERPRETATION

Lab

Initial lab tests

- No lab work required for diagnosis
- CBC: Elevated WBC count seen in 20% of cases (7)

Imaging

Initial approach

- Torsion remains a clinical diagnosis.
- Ultrasound is the most useful for evaluation of possible torsion with a positive predictive value of 87.5% and specificity of 93.3% (8).
- Torsion can also mimic ectopic pregnancy, tubo-ovarian abscess, hemorrhagic ovarian cyst, or endometrioma (8)
- Specific ultrasound findings associated with ovarian torsion include multiple follicles rimming an enlarged ovary, which reflects ovarian congestion and edema; a bull's-eye target shape, whirlpool, or snail shell appearance, all of which are suggestive of a twisted pedicle (8).
- Between 9% and 26% of cases of torsion occur on normal adnexa and show no signs of abnormality on sonography (1).

- Doppler imaging potentially adds information about the presence or lack of arterial and venous blood flow to and from the ovary. However, there is disagreement as to the usefulness of Doppler imaging and it does not provide a definitive diagnosis. Studies have reported 60% of cases of torsion were missed by Doppler imaging while noting a positive predictive value of 100% (7,8).
- Another study reports loss of venous blood flow was noted in 81.3% of patients with confirmed torsion (2).
- MRIs and CTs are not routinely used and carry an increased cost compared to ultrasound or clinical diagnosis.

Follow-Up & Special Considerations

Definitive diagnosis of adnexal torsion is by direct visualization with surgery—either with a laparotomy or laparoscopy.

Diagnostic Procedures/Surgery

- Both a laparotomy and laparoscopy are diagnostic and therapeutic.
- A laparoscopy is preferred due to shorter recovery time and complication rates.

DIFFERENTIAL DIAGNOSIS

- Ectopic pregnancy
- Appendicitis
- Endometriosis
- Mittelschmerz
- UTI
- Pelvic inflammatory disease
- Diverticulitis
- Ovarian cyst
- Ruptured ovarian cyst

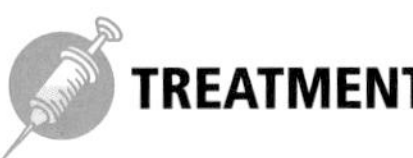

TREATMENT

MEDICATION

- Medication is not a first- or second-line treatment for ovarian torsion.
- Pain relief can be obtained with medication; however, surgical detorsion is the only definitive treatment.

ADDITIONAL TREATMENT

General Measures

Surgery is the definitive treatment of choice.

SURGERY/OTHER PROCEDURES

- Torsion must be evaluated by either a laparoscopy or laparotomy.
- Conservative treatment involves untwisting the adnexa, and it is now the accepted treatment of choice for children and women of reproductive age (1,3,9). Blue–black appearance of the ovary is common, yet 91–93% will recover follicular function after detorsion (9). Removal of the affected adnexa is recommended if the patient is postmenopausal, or if the ovary is completely replaced by pathologic lesion.
- Previously, the affected ovary was always removed for fear that detorsing the ovary could cause a thromboembolic event secondary to release of a thrombus from the adnexal veins. However, recent studies have shown the rate of thromboembolic event to be 0.2% and not increased after untwisting of the adnexa (1,3,7,9).
- The lesion that causes torsion is commonly a functional cyst (3). Concerning ovarian lesions should be excised; however, some studies recommend delaying cystectomy for 6–8 weeks after the primary intervention to reduce risk of injury to the ovary. If during the initial procedure, ovarian cancer is suspected, frozen sections should be obtained to allow confirmation of malignancy (1). If left in situ, decompressing any remaining cysts may decrease risk of recurrent torsion (9).
- Average ovarian mass size for torsion treated with laparotomy (9.9 cm) was greater than average mass size of torsion treated with laparoscopy (8 cm) (7). The choice of procedure type depends on the surgical judgment of the operator.
- There is an increased rate of laparotomy in pregnant patients (12%) vs. nonpregnant patients (4%) due to advanced gestational age or large sized cystic ovary (5).
- Ovariopexy or plication of the utero-ovarian ligament has been proposed by some authors and has indications including malformation or excessive length of the utero-ovarian ligament, torsion of a solitary adnexa, torsion of a normal ovary in childhood, or contralateral pexy after torsion leading to adnexectomy of the other ovary (1).

IN-PATIENT CONSIDERATIONS

Initial Stabilization

A patient should remain in the hospital until torsion has been resolved, pain has been controlled, patient is ambulating on her own, and she is able to maintain a regular diet.

IV Fluids

IV fluid repletion is often necessary as patients in pain have inadequate oral intake. IVF hydration should be maintained in preparation for surgical exploration and treatment.

Discharge Criteria

- Previously, patients had an average hospital stay of 7.4 days after treatment of torsion by laparotomy. (1)
- Laparoscopy treatment of ovarian torsion is more commonly done today, and no difference was found in rate of complications; however, patients who underwent laparoscopy had much shorter hospital stays (1).

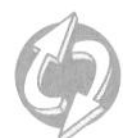

ONGOING CARE

FOLLOW-UP RECOMMENDATIONS

Patient Monitoring

- Because of more conservative treatments, the rate of repeat torsions is likely to increase.
- Patients with cystic lesions managed conservatively at the time of torsion diagnosis may require additional surgical intervention if those lesions do not resolve.
- Ovariopexy is a follow-up option for patients with a single ovary, patients with repeat torsion, or patients with adnexectomy of the contralateral ovary (1).
- Routine laboratory testing or imaging to confirm return of ovarian function is usually unnecessary.

PROGNOSIS

- Ovarian function is likely to recover after detorsion (3).
- Recurrent torsion of the treated or opposite ovary is possible.

COMPLICATIONS

- Surgical complications, including infection or hemorrhage
- Repeat torsion if conservative treatment performed
- Infertility (due to adhesions or removal of ovarian tissue)
- Peritonitis and systemic infection if ovary becomes necrotic and is not removed

REFERENCES

1. Huchon C, Fauconnier A. Adnexal torsion: A literature review. *Eur J Obstet Gynecol Reprod Biol*. 2010;150:8–12.
2. Balci O, Icen MS, Mahmoud AS, et al. Management and outcomes of adnexal torsion: A 5-year experience. *Arch Gynecol Obstet*. 2011;284(3): 643–6.
3. Oelsner G, Cohen SB, Soriano D, et al. Minimal surgery for the twisted ischaemic adnexa can preserve ovarian function. *Hum Reprod*. 2003; 18(12):2599–602.
4. Houry D, Abbott JT. Ovarian torsion: A fifteen-year review. *Ann Emerg Med*. 2001;38:156–9.
5. Hasson J, Tsafrir Z, Azem F, et al. Comparison of adnexal torsion between pregnant and nonpregnant women. *Am J Obstet Gynecol*. 2010;202(6):536.e1–6.
6. Cass DL. Ovarian torsion. *Semin Pediatr Surg*. 2005;14(2):86–92.
7. Lo LM, Chang SD, Horng SG, et al. Laparoscopy versus laparotomy for surgical intervention of ovarian torsion. *J Obstet Gynaecol Res*. 2008; 24(6):1020–5.
8. Chang HC, Bhatt S, Dogra VS, et al. Pearls and pitfalls in diagnosis of ovarian torsion. *RadioGraphics*. 2008;28:1355–68.
9. Oelsner G, Shashar D. Adnexal torsion. *Clin Obstet Gynecol*. 2006;49(3):459–63.

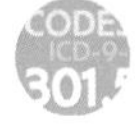

CODES

ICD9

620.5 Torsion of ovary, ovarian pedicle, or fallopian tube

CLINICAL PEARLS

- Ovarian torsion is the rotation of the ovary, fallopian tube, or both, leading to pain and increased risk of necrosis of these organs.
- Torsion of a normal ovary can occur. However, upwards of 94% of cases of ovarian torsion involve a mass in the ovary such as a cyst or neoplasm.
- Risk of torsion is increased during pregnancy, especially with ovarian stimulation.
- Surgery is both diagnostic and definitive; treatment can be accomplished by either a laparoscopic or open approach.
- Conservative treatment with detorsion and ovarian preservation is preferred in premenarchal girls and women of reproductive age.

TORTICOLLIS

Bryan C. Bordeaux, DO, MPH

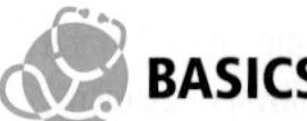

BASICS

DESCRIPTION

- Torticollis is a spectrum of disorders characterized by head tilt with rotation or involuntary movement.
- Pediatric disorders include:
  - Congenital muscular torticollis (CMT): 80% of all infants presenting with torticollis are found to have CMT. CMT is seen at birth or early infancy and results from unilateral fibrosis and shortening of the sternocleidomastoid (SCM) muscle.
  - Acquired torticollis
- Adult disorders include:
  - Acquired torticollis (also known as wryneck), which is usually self-limited
  - Spasmodic torticollis, also known as cervical dystonia, is caused by recurrent involuntary muscular contractions.
- Other forms (oculogyric, gastroesophageal reflux, arthritis-related, scoliosis-related, and hysterical torticollis) are not discussed.
- System(s) affected: Musculoskeletal; Nervous
- Synonym(s): Acute wryneck; Idiopathic generalized torticollis; SCM torticollis; Neonatal torticollis; Idiopathic cervical dystonia; Focal dystonia; Nuchal dystonia

EPIDEMIOLOGY

- ~90% of cases occur in individuals ages 31–60 years.
- Predominant age: CMT: Newborn and infants; pediatric acquired torticollis: <10 years; adult acquired torticollis: 30–60 years; spasmodic torticollis: 30–50 years (mean age of 40–43 years) (1).
- Predominant sex: Spasmodic torticollis: Female > Male (1.6:1); Congenital muscular: Male > Female (3:2) (2).

Incidence

Congenital: Up to 1/250 births (2); spasmodic: estimated at 1/100,000; overall incidence for torticollis is 24/1 million persons.

Prevalence

All focal dystonias combined: 295/1 million persons; no reliable data for pediatric and adult acquired torticollis

RISK FACTORS

- CMT: Intrauterine crowding, breech position, ischemia, birth injury
- Pediatric acquired torticollis: Soft tissue inflammation or infection, neurologic conditions, visual disturbances, trauma
- Adult acquired torticollis: Stress, unusual positioning (particularly when sleeping), exposure to cold drafts of air, medications, trauma, infection
- Spasmodic: Family history of dystonia, soft tissue inflammation or infection, neurologic conditions, visual disturbances, trauma

Genetics

Some forms may have genetic basis, such as spasmodic torticollis (1).

ETIOLOGY

- CMT:
  - Intrauterine malpositioning may lead to trauma of the SCM and fibrosis.
  - Birth trauma such as a clavicular fracture
- Pediatric acquired torticollis: Pain, spasm, decreased range of motion without trauma
- Adult acquired torticollis:
  - Emotional stress, postural factors (e.g., work, sleep, lying while reading or watching TV, prolonged unusual positioning of neck), or exposure to cold. Many cases are idiopathic.
  - Medication reactions (e.g., amphetamines, haloperidol, chlorpromazine, ketamine)
- Spasmodic torticollis:
  - Muscular damage from inflammatory or infectious diseases
  - Cervical spine injuries and spondylosis
  - Ocular disorders
  - Organic CNS disorders
  - Psychogenic
  - Tumors
  - Vestibular dysfunction

Pediatric Considerations

Congenital: Associated with birth injury that, without treatment, becomes a fibrous cord and may be associated with persistent craniofacial deformities

COMMONLY ASSOCIATED CONDITIONS

- Over 80% of infants with CMT also present with craniofacial asymmetry, deformational plagiocephaly of varying degrees, and developmental hip dysplasia.
- Congenital and pediatric acquired torticollis: Consider Klippel-Feil syndrome (congenital fusion of cervical vertebrae).
- Pediatric and adult acquired torticollis: Spinal abnormalities
- Spasmodic torticollis: Treatment of psychiatric disorders

DIAGNOSIS

HISTORY

- Abnormal head posture, neck pain, headache, neck muscle stiffness, restricted neck range of motion (ROM), neck mass or swelling
- Birth history in children
- Family history focusing on dystonias
- Medication history
- Recent cervical spine trauma

PHYSICAL EXAM

- Normal ROM: Flexion 60°; extension 75°; rotation 90°; sidebending 45°.
- It can present in rotational (twisting), anterocollis (flexion), laterocollis (side bending), and retrocollis (extension) positions with the head tilting to the affected side (80%, to right side) and the chin rotating to the opposite side.
- Intermittent painful spasms of trapezius, SCM, and other neck muscles
- There may be tenderness over affected SCM
- Neck mass, lymphadenopathy in some cases
- Craniofacial asymmetry (plagiocephaly) indicates congenital or chronic torticollis.
- Phasic jerking or tremor of antagonist muscles
- Sensory tricks (*geste antagoniste*) such as touching face reduce severity in most patients (pathognomonic for spasmodic torticollis) (1,3).
- Ocular irregularities such as diplopia
- Spinal abnormality: Short neck with low posterior hairline may indicate occipitocervical synostosis.
- Structural abnormalities of the hips or feet
- Common presentations:
  - CMT: At birth there may be firm, nontender, palpable enlargement of the SCM (2). However, the SCM may appear normal at birth with swelling and tightness developing weeks later.
  - Pediatric and adult acquired torticollis: Unilateral neck stiffness, pain, or decreased ROM
  - Spasmodic torticollis may initially present with neck stiffness progressing to pain, head jerking, and neck spasms (1).

DIAGNOSTIC TESTS & INTERPRETATION

Lab

Lab studies are generally not helpful and are only needed to evaluate an underlying primary cause.

Follow-Up & Special Considerations

All pediatric patients should have a complete eye exam.

Imaging

Initial approach

- Radiographs should be taken to rule out spinal pathology in traumatic and congenital cases.
- Consider MRI or CT scan of cervical spine for patients with neurologic deficits.
- CMT can be confirmed with ultrasonography of the involved SCM muscle.

Diagnostic Procedures/Surgery

For pediatric-acquired torticollis, response to low-dose levodopa (100–300 mg) with carbidopa suggests that torticollis is secondary to a dopa-responsive dystonia.

DIFFERENTIAL DIAGNOSIS

- Osseous:
  - Atlantoaxial rotatory subluxation
  - Atlanto-occipital subluxation
  - Posttraumatic fracture or dislocation
  - Cervical disc disease
  - Congenital scoliosis
  - Klippel-Feil syndrome
  - Occipitocervical synostosis
  - Grisel syndrome (subluxation of C1 on C2, associated with head or neck infection)
  - Syringomyelia
  - Arnold-Chiari malformation
- Nonosseous:
  - Myositis involving cervical muscles
  - Soft-tissue trauma
  - Neoplastic: Spinal cord tumor, acoustic neuroma, osteoblastoma, orbital tumor, fibromatosis, metastasis
  - Infection: Upper respiratory infection, cervical lymph node abscess, epidural abscess, retropharyngeal abscess, vertebral osteomyelitis
  - Vestibular disorders
  - Essential head tremor
  - Basal ganglion diseases
  - Cranial nerve palsy
  - Psychiatric disorders
  - Drugs or toxins
  - Down syndrome
  - Sandifer syndrome (association of gastroesophageal disease with spastic torticollis and dystonic body movements)
  - Myasthenia gravis

TREATMENT

MEDICATION

Treatment for spasms:

- Botulinum toxin: Type A and B injections may be more effective than anticholinergic drugs for cervical dystonia (1)[B]. EMG may be useful in guiding the injection site:
  - Congenital muscular: Botulinum toxin type A was found effective in a case series (2),(4)[C].
  - Cervical dystonia: Botulinum toxin type A was found effective and safe for treating adults (≥16 years of age) with cervical dystonia (1)[B].
    - Botox: Botulinum toxin type A:
      - Adult: Initial 1.25–2.5 units (0.05–0.1 mL) IM into most active neck muscles; repeat every 3–4 months; not to exceed 200 units cumulative dose in 1-month period.
      - Pediatric (<12 years of age): Not established; >12 years: administer as for adults.
    - Myobloc: Botulinum toxin type B:
      - Adult: 2,500–5,000 units IM divided among affected muscles in patients treated previously with any type of botulinum toxin; use lower dose in untreated patients.
      - Pediatric: Not established
- Diazepam:
  - Adult: 2–10 mg PO b.i.d./q.i.d.
  - Pediatric: 1–2.5 mg PO t.i.d./q.i.d.; increase gradually as needed or tolerated.
- Diphendydramine or diazepam can be used for torticollis caused by medications (1)[C].
  - Diphendydramine:
    - Adult: 25–50 mg PO q6–8h PRN, not to exceed 400 mg/d; 10–50 mg IV/IM q6–8h PRN, not to exceed 400 mg/d
    - Pediatric: 12.5–25 mg PO t.i.d./q.i.d. *or* 5 mg/kg/d *or* 150 mg/m^2/d divided t.i.d./q.i.d. PRN, not to exceed 300 mg/d; 5 mg/kg/d IV/IM *or* 150 mg/m^2/d, divided q.i.d. PRN, not to exceed 300 mg/d
- Anticholinergics may relieve acute muscle spasms (1)[C]. High doses are usually necessary, and benefit is often delayed by several weeks.
- Carbidopa-levodopa (1)[C] for focal dystonia of unknown cause: Trial might be warranted although some non–dopa-responsive-dystonias improve and equal numbers have symptoms worsen.

Treatment for pain:

- Analgesics are useful for acquired torticollis and may be helpful in other cases. Consider NSAIDs and acetaminophen for most cases and opiates for only the most severe pain.

ADDITIONAL TREATMENT

General Measures

- CMT:
  - >90% of children achieve good outcome with conservative treatment when therapy is initiated in first 12 months of life.
  - Conservative treatment for CMT includes positioning, environmental adaptations, passive and active stretching of the tight SCM muscle, strengthening of weak neck and trunk muscles, and movement therapy.
  - Physical therapy and aggressive stretching should be started before ages 3–6 months (2)[B].
  - Place television/toys on opposite side of bed from rotational deformity to encourage use of affected muscles.
  - Surgery is occasionally indicated for refractory cases.
- Pediatric acquired torticollis:
  - Place a television on opposite side of bed from rotational deformity.
- Adult and pediatric acquired torticollis:
  - Conservative management includes soft cervical collar, intermittent heat or ice, and bed rest.
  - Analgesics are helpful for pain relief.
- Spasmodic:
  - Conservative: Soft cervical collar, intermittent heat or ice, and bed rest.
  - Selective peripheral nerve denervation is a safe procedure with infrequent and minimal side effects that is indicated exclusively for cervical dystonia.
  - Pallidal deep brain stimulation is a good alternative for cervical dystonia after medication or botulinum toxin has failed to provide adequate improvement.

Issues for Referral

- Emergently refer potentially life-threatening conditions including retropharyngeal abscesses, epiglottitis, spinal epidural abscesses, and cervical spine fractures or dislocations.
- Refer prolonged symptoms of idiopathic spasmodic torticollis to a neurologist.
- Fixed deformities in children may require surgical referral.
- CMT: Referrals if: Visual dysfunction (ophthalmology), failed hip screen (orthopedics), abnormal neurologic exam (neurology), patient has plagiocephaly (plastic surgery), patient presents with bony end feel (orthopedics) (5,6).

Additional Therapies

- Osteopathic manipulation may be useful including the following techniques:
  - Direct myofascial stretching of cervical region with attention to the SCM
  - Occipital-atlantal release
  - V-spread of the occipitomastoid suture on the side of restriction
  - Muscle energy and/or functional positional release at the cervical region
- Physical therapy may be beneficial for acquired childhood and adult torticollis
- If detected early, 90% of CMT responds to stretching exercises.

COMPLEMENTARY AND ALTERNATIVE MEDICINE

Acupuncture may also provide benefit.

SURGERY/OTHER PROCEDURES

CMT: Surgical release if physical therapy is unsuccessful by 1 year of age

ONGOING CARE

FOLLOW-UP RECOMMENDATIONS

- Infants with CMT should be monitored at 2–4-week intervals.
- Screen for depression, since this is a common complication in protracted cases.

PROGNOSIS

- CMT: Good for correctable pathologies:
  - 50–70% resolve spontaneously by first year.
  - Over 90% of children achieve good to excellent outcome with conservative treatment when therapy is instituted during the first 12 months of life.
- Pediatric acquired torticollis: Good when the underlying pathology is discovered
- Adult acquired torticollis: Excellent and generally resolves in a few days to weeks
- Spasmodic: May wax and wane for years, even with treatment

COMPLICATIONS

- Facial asymmetry in congenital cases
- Dental malocclusion
- Degenerative osteoarthritis of the cervical spine, hypertrophy of the SCM muscle, and paresthesia due to compressed nerve roots
- Depression

REFERENCES

1. Tarsy D, Simon DK. Dystonia. *N Engl J Med*. 2006;355:818–29.
2. Do TT. Congenital muscular torticollis: Current concepts and review of treatment. *Curr Opin Pediatr*. 2006;18:26–9.
3. Consky EA, et al. Clinical assessments of patients with cervical dystonia. In: Jancovic J, et al., eds. *Therapy with Botulinum Toxin*. New York: Marcel Dekker; 1994:211–37.
4. Benecke R, Dressler D. Botulinum toxin treatment of axial and cervical dystonia. *Disabil Rehabil*. 2007;29:1769–77.
5. Lee IJ, Lim SY, Song HS, et al. Complete tight fibrous band release and resection in congenital muscular torticollis. *J Plast Reconstr Aesthet Surg*. 2010;63:947–53.
6. van Vlimmeren LA, Helders PJ, van Adrichem LN, et al. Torticollis and plagiocephaly in infancy: Therapeutic strategies. *Pediatr Rehabil*. 2006; 9:40–6.

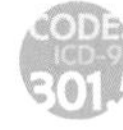

CODES

ICD9

- 723.5 Torticollis not otherwise specified
- 754.1 Congenital musculoskeletal deformities of sternocleidomastoid muscle
- 847.0 Sprain of neck

CLINICAL PEARLS

- Suspect torticollis in patients with head tilt, chin lift, and restricted movement of the neck.
- Be vigilant for secondary causes in both children and adults.
- Most adult cases of torticollis are self-limiting and resolve within days to weeks.
- Physical therapy, manual treatment, and acupuncture may be helpful adjuncts.
- In congenital and acquired pediatric cases, rearranging the child's environment by placing items of interest (e.g., TV, toys) on the opposite side of the bed is often beneficial.

TOURETTE SYNDROME

Evan R. Horton, PharmD
Kimberly A. Pesaturo, PharmD
Jill A. Grimes, MD

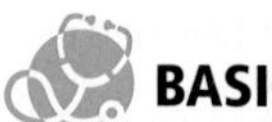

BASICS

DESCRIPTION

- A childhood-onset neurobehavioral disorder characterized by the presence of multiple motor and at least 1 phonic tic (see "Physical Exam" section):
  - Tics are sudden, brief, repetitive, stereotyped motor movements (motor tics) or sounds (phonic tics) produced by moving air through the nose, mouth, or throat.
  - Tics tend to occur in bouts.
  - Tics can be simple or complex; motor tics precede vocal tics, and simple tics precede complex tics.
  - Tics often are preceded by sensory symptoms, especially a compulsion to move; patients are able to suppress their tics, but voluntary suppression is associated with an inner tension that results in more forceful tics when suppression ceases.
- System(s) affected: Nervous

EPIDEMIOLOGY

Incidence

- Predominant age:
  - Average age of onset: 7 years (3–8 years)
  - Tic severity is greatest at ages 7–12 years, with 96% presenting by age 11.
  - 50% of children with Tourette syndrome (TS) will experience complete resolution of symptoms by age 18 (based on self-reporting).
- Predominant sex: Male > Female (3:1)
- Predominant race/ethnicity: Clinically heterogeneous disorder, but non-Hispanic whites 2:1 compared with Hispanics and/or blacks

Prevalence

Estimated at 3:1,000 in children ages 6–17 years

RISK FACTORS

- Risk of TS among relatives ranges between 9.8% and 15%.
- First-degree relatives of individuals with TS have a 10–100-fold increased risk of developing TS compared with the general population.

Genetics

- Predisposition, frequent familial history of tic disorders and obsessive–compulsive disorder (OCD)
- Precise pattern of transmission and genetic origin are unknown. Recent studies suggest polygenic inheritance with evidence for a locus on chromosome 17q; sequence variants in *SLITRK1* gene on chromosome 13q also are associated with TS.
- Higher concordance in monozygotic compared with dizygotic twins; wide range of phenotypes

PATHOPHYSIOLOGY

Research suggests that abnormalities of dopamine neurotransmission and receptor hypersensitivity, most likely in the ventral striatum, play a primary role in the pathophysiology.

ETIOLOGY

- Abnormality of basal ganglia development
- Mechanism uncertain; may involve dysfunction of basal ganglia–thalamocortical circuits, likely involving decreased inhibitory output from the basal ganglia, which results in an imbalance of inhibition and excitation in the motor cortex
- Controversial pediatric autoimmune neuropsychiatric disorder association with *Streptococcus* (PANDAS) (1):
  - TS/OCD cases linked to immunologic response to previous group A β-hemolytic streptococcal infection (GABHS)
  - Thought to be linked to 10% of all TS cases
  - 5 criteria:
    - Presence of tic disorder and/or OCD
    - Prepubertal onset of neuropsychosis
    - History of sudden onset of symptoms and/or episodic course, with abrupt symptom exacerbation, interspersed with periods of partial or complete remission
    - Evidence of a temporal association between onset or exacerbation of symptoms and a prior streptococcal infection
    - Adventitious movements during symptom exacerbation (e.g., motor hyperactivity)

COMMONLY ASSOCIATED CONDITIONS

- ADHD and OCD are most common.
- Depression and anxiety are also concerns due to disruptive behavior problems that can lead to social difficulties and learning disorders.
- Impairments of visual perception, sleep disorders, restless leg syndrome, and migraine headaches are higher than in the general population.

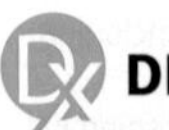

DIAGNOSIS

HISTORY

Diagnosis of TS is based on history and clinical presentation (i.e., observation of tics with or without presence of coexisting disorders).

PHYSICAL EXAM

- Typically, the physical exam is normal.
- Motor and vocal tics are the clinical hallmarks.
- Tics fluctuate in type, frequency, and anatomic distribution over time.
- Multiple motor tics include facial grimacing, blinking, head or neck jerking, tongue protruding, sniffing, and touching.
- Vocal tics include grunts, snorts, throat clearing, barking, yelling, and hiccupping.
- Tics are exacerbated by anticipation, emotional upset, anxiety, or fatigue.
- Tics subside when patient is concentrating or absorbed in activities.
- Motor and vocal tics may persist during all stages of sleep, especially light sleep.
- Blink-reflex abnormalities may be observed.
- No clinical measures are known to reliably predict children who will continue to express tics in adulthood; severity of tics in late childhood is associated with future tic severity.
- *Diagnostic and Statistical Manual* (DSM) criteria:
  - Both multiple motor and $\geq$1 vocal tics have been present at some time during the illness, although not necessarily concurrently.
  - Tics occur many times a day (usually in bouts) nearly every day or intermittently throughout a period of >1 year, with no tic-free period of >3 consecutive months.
  - Onset occurs before age 18 years.
  - Tics are not due to the direct physiologic effects of a substance (e.g., stimulants) or a general medical condition (e.g., Huntington disease or postviral encephalitis).
- The World Health Organization and Tourette Syndrome Classification Group also have classification systems.

DIAGNOSTIC TESTS & INTERPRETATION

Lab

Initial lab tests

- No definitive lab tests diagnose TS.
- Thyroid-stimulating hormone (TSH) should be measured because of association of tics with hyperthyroidism.

Imaging

Initial approach

- No imaging studies diagnose TS.
- EEG shows nonspecific abnormalities; useful only to differentiate tics from epilepsy.

Pathological Findings

- Smaller caudate volumes in TS patients
- Striatal dopaminergic terminals are increased, as is striatal dopamine transporter (DAT) density.

DIFFERENTIAL DIAGNOSIS

- Chronic motor or vocal tic disorder
- Transient tic disorder
- Tic disorder not otherwise specified
- Huntington disease
- Stroke
- Lesch-Nyhan syndrome
- Wilson disease
- Sydenham chorea
- Multiple sclerosis
- Postviral encephalitis
- Head injury
- Dystonia
- Myoclonus
- Drug effects (e.g., dopamine agonists)

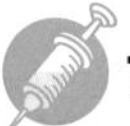

TREATMENT

MEDICATION

First Line

α_2-adrenergic receptor agonists:
- *First-line agents because they have no long-term serious side effects, but suboptimal efficacy*
- Clonidine 0.1–0.3 mg/d given b.i.d. or t.i.d. (2)[A]:
  - Side effects: Sedation and hypotension frequently an issue; need to initiate therapy gradually and taper when discontinuing to avoid cardiac adverse events:
    - 50–75% of subjects report little or no improvement in tics.
- Guanfacine 1–3 mg/d given daily or b.i.d.:
  - Less sedating and has a longer duration of action than clonidine
  - Need to initiate therapy gradually and taper when discontinuing to avoid cardiac adverse events
  - Shown to improve motor or vocal tics by 30% in some studies, no better than placebo in others (2)[A]

Second Line

- Neuroleptics:
  - Dopamine receptor antagonists:
    - Typical antipsychotics (3)[A]:
      - Haloperidol: 0.5–5 mg at bedtime; side effects, including extrapyramidal symptoms (EPS), may limit use
      - Pimozide: Initiate 0.5 mg/d and titrate 0.5 mg/week up to 1–8 mg at bedtime; prolonged QT interval limits use; must be given under ECG monitoring; long-term use may induce sedation, weight gain, depression, pseudoparkinsonism, and akathisia; found to work better in long-term control of tics versus acute exacerbations
    - Atypical antipsychotics (4)[A]:
      - Risperidone: 1–2 mg b.i.d.; side effects include weight gain, sedation, and to a lesser extent, EPS
    - Anticonvulsants (5)[B]:
      - Topiramate: 100 mg/d
- Benzodiazepines:
  - Clonazepam: 0.5–1 mg t.i.d.: Side effects include sedation, weight gain, irritability, oppositional behavior, mood changes, and cognitive impairment. May induce Tourette-like disorder in exceptional cases.
- Treatment of ADHD in patients with tics (6)[A]:
  - Stimulants:
    - Methylphenidate: 2.5–30 mg/d
    - Dextroamphetamine: 5–30 mg/d; comorbid tic disorder is not a serious contraindication, as previously held; exacerbation of tics is neither clinically significant nor common
  - α_2-adrenergic agonists:
    - Guanfacine
    - Clonidine: The combination of methylphenidate and clonidine has shown efficacy in treating both ADHD and tic symptoms in 1 trial.
  - Other medications:
    - Atomoxetine
    - Desipramine
- Treatment of OCD in patients with tics (1)[B]:
  - SSRIs:
    - Fluoxetine: 10–80 mg/d
    - Fluvoxamine: 50–300 mg/d
    - Sertraline: 50–200 mg/d
    - Side effects include nausea, insomnia, sexual dysfunction, headache, and agitation .
    - First-line treatment of OCD
    - Comorbid tic disorder not a contraindication; exacerbation of tics neither clinically significant nor common
    - Some risk of suicidality noted with SSRIs and other antidepressants
  - Tricyclic antidepressants:
    - Clomipramine: 25–200 mg/d; can be used in refractory SSRI patients or to augment SSRIs in partial responders; side effects: Weight gain, dry mouth, lowered seizure threshold, and constipation; ECG changes, including QTc interval prolongation and tachycardia

ADDITIONAL TREATMENT

General Measures

- Educate that tics are neither voluntary nor psychiatric.
- Many patients require no treatment; patient should play active role in treatment decisions.
- Educate patient, family, teachers, and friends to identify and address psychosocial stressors and environmental triggers.
- No cure for tics: Treatment is purely symptomatic, and multimodal treatment usually is indicated.
- Neurologic and psychiatric evaluation may be useful for other primary disorders and comorbidities (especially ADHD, OCD, and depression).
- TS clusters with several comorbidities; each disorder must be evaluated for associated functional impairment because patients often are more disabled by their psychiatric conditions than by the tics; choice of initial treatment depends largely on worst symptoms (tics, obsessions, or impulsivity).
- Monotherapy is preferred to polytherapy.

COMPLEMENTARY AND ALTERNATIVE MEDICINE

Nonpharmacologic therapy:
- Reassurance and environmental modification
- Identification and treatment of triggers
- Behavioral therapy: Awareness or assertiveness training, relaxation therapy, habit-reversal therapy, and self-monitoring
- Hypnotherapy
- Biofeedback
- Acupuncture

SURGERY/OTHER PROCEDURES

Thalamic ablation and deep brain stimulation have been used experimentally.

IN-PATIENT CONSIDERATIONS

Nursing

Habit-reversal training provides a viable tic suppression treatment: Works equally for motor and vocal tics

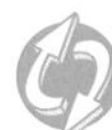

ONGOING CARE

FOLLOW-UP RECOMMENDATIONS

Patient Monitoring

Observe for associated psychiatric disorders.

PROGNOSIS

Based on self-reporting, in 1/2–2/3 of children with TS, severity of tics attenuates during adolescence, often remitting completely by early adulthood. However, OCD symptoms tend to increase.

REFERENCES

1. Lombroso PJ, Scahill L. Tourette syndrome and obsessive-compulsive disorder. *Brain Dev*. 2008;30:231–7.
2. Eddy CM, Rickards HE, Cavanna AE, et al. Treatment strategies for tics in Tourette syndrome. *Ther Adv Neurol Disord*. 2011;4:25–45.
3. Pringsheim T, Marras C. Pimozide for tics in Tourette's syndrome. *Cochrane Database Syst Rev*. 2009;(2):CD006996.
4. Shekelle P, Maglione M, Bagley S. *Comparative effectiveness of off-label use of atypical antipsychotics*. Comparative effectiveness review No. 6. (Prepared by the Southern California/RAND Evidence-based Practice Center under contract No. 290-02-0003.) Rockville, MD: Agency for Healthcare Research and Quality. January 2007. Available at: www.effectivehealthcare.ahrq.gov/reports/final.cfm.
5. Jankovic J, Jimenez-Shahed J, Brown LW, et al. A randomised, double-blind, placebo-controlled study of topiramate in the treatment of Tourette syndrome. *J Neurol Neurosurg Psychiatr*. 2010;81:70–3.
6. Pringsheim T, Steeves T. Pharmacological treatment for attention deficit hyperactivity disorder (ADHD) in children with co-morbid tic disorders. *Cochrane Database Syst Rev*. 2011;(4):CD007990.

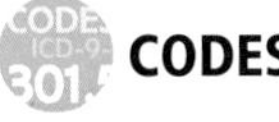

CODES

ICD9

307.23 Tourette's disorder

CLINICAL PEARLS

- TS is diagnosed by history and witnessing tics; have parent video patient's tics if not present on exam in your office.
- 50% of children with TS will have resolution of their symptoms by age 18.
- Nearly 50% of children with tics also have ADHD. Stimulants may be used as first-line treatment for ADHD (tics are not a contraindication, as previously believed).

TOXOPLASMOSIS

Jonathan MacClements, MD

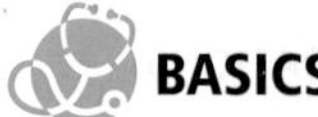

BASICS

- Obligate intracellular protozoan parasite *Toxoplasma gondii*
- Most common latent protozoan infection
- Usually dangerous only in pregnancy or in an immunocompromised patient

DESCRIPTION
- Acute self-limited infection if immunocompetent
- Acute symptomatic or reactivated latent infection in immunocompromised persons
- Congenital toxoplasmosis (acute primary infection during pregnancy)
- Ocular toxoplasmosis

Pediatric Considerations
- The earlier fetal infection occurs, the more severe the disease.
- Risk of perinatal death is 5% if infected first trimester

Pregnancy Considerations
- Immunocompromised and HIV-infected women should undergo serologic testing in pregnancy (1)[C].
- Seronegative pregnant women should emphasize prevention.
- Serologic testing during pregnancy is controversial.

EPIDEMIOLOGY
Incidence
- Birth prevalence of congenital toxoplasmosis in the US: 10–100/100,000 live births
- Predominant age: All ages
- Predominant sex: Male > Female

Prevalence
- In the US, 11% aged 6–49 years are seropositive.
- Age-adjusted prevalence in the US is 22.5%.
- Seroprevalence among women in the US is 15%.

RISK FACTORS
- Immunocompromised states, including HIV infection with CD4 cell count $<100/\mu L$
- Primary infection during pregnancy; risk of transmitting infection to the fetus increases with gestational age at seroconversion, although transmission in the first trimester is associated with more severe consequences.
- Chronically infected pregnant women who are immunocompromised have an increased risk of congenital toxoplasmosis.

Genetics
Human leukocyte antigen (HLA) DQ3 is a genetic marker of susceptibility in AIDS.

GENERAL PREVENTION
Prevention is important in seronegative pregnant women and immunodeficient patients:
- Avoid eating undercooked meat. Meat should be cooked to 152°F (66°C) or frozen for 24 hours at –12°C or lower.
- Avoid drinking unfiltered water. Wash fruits and vegetables.
- Strict hand hygiene after touching soil.
- Wear gloves while handling and wash hands after handling raw meat or cat litter.
- Avoid eating shellfish; it can be infected with *Toxoplasma* cysts.

PATHOPHYSIOLOGY
Transmission to humans:
- Ingestion of raw or undercooked meat, food, or water containing tissue cysts or oocytes; usually from soil contaminated with feline feces
- Transplacental to fetus from infected mother; risk of transmission is 30% on average
- Blood product transfusion and solid-organ transplantation

ETIOLOGY
T. gondii, an obligate intracellular sporozoan

COMMONLY ASSOCIATED CONDITIONS
Chorioretinitis; self-limiting, febrile lymphadenopathy; mononucleosislike illness

DIAGNOSIS

HISTORY
- Congenital toxoplasmosis:
  - Clinical presentation varies widely; 80% of patients are asymptomatic at birth.
  - Classic triad *uncommon:* Chorioretinitis, hydrocephalus, cerebral calcifications
  - Manifestations may include prematurity, intrauterine growth retardation (IUGR)
  - Anemia, thrombocytopenia, jaundice, rash
  - Mental retardation, seizures, visual defects, spasticity, sensorineural hearing loss
- Ocular toxoplasmosis:
  - Chorioretinitis: Focal necrotizing retinitis
  - Yellowish white elevated cotton patch
  - Congenital disease usually bilateral; acquired, unilateral
  - Symptoms include blurred vision, scotoma, pain, and photophobia.
- Acute toxoplasmosis (immunocompetent host):
  - ~90% of patients are asymptomatic.
  - Most common manifestation is bilateral, symmetric, nontender cervical lymphadenopathy.
  - Constitutional symptoms such as fever, chills, and sweats are usually mild.
  - Headaches, myalgias, pharyngitis, hepatosplenomegaly, and diffuse nonpruritic maculopapular rash may occur.
  - Atypical lymphocytosis
  - Pregnant women are often asymptomatic. If symptomatic: Monolike illness with lymphadenopathy.
- Acute or reactivation in immunocompromised host:
  - Most common site is CNS with toxoplasmic encephalitis.
  - Headache; focal neurologic deficits and seizures
  - Fever usually present
  - Extracerebral toxoplasmosis: Pneumonitis, chorioretinitis, and rarely: GI system, liver, musculoskeletal system, heart, bone marrow, bladder, and orchitis

PHYSICAL EXAM
- In adults: Fever, lymphadenopathy, nonpruritic rash
- In newborns: Hydrocephalus, neurologic abnormalities, hepatosplenomegaly, chorioretinitis, microcephaly, anemia, thrombocytopenia, mental retardation

DIAGNOSTIC TESTS & INTERPRETATION
Lab
- Serology interpretation:
  - In acute infection, IgM antibodies appear within the first week.
  - Diagnosis can be made if initial test demonstrates positive IgM and negative IgG, with both tests becoming positive 2 weeks later.
  - If follow-up IgG remains negative 2–4 weeks later but IgM is still positive, it is likely a false-positive result.
  - Negative IgG rules out prior infection because it remains detectable for life.
- Types of serologic tests:
  - ELISA: Standard test used by most labs
  - Sabin-Feldman dye test: Gold standard against which all other serologic assays are compared
  - IFA test: More readily available in commercial labs
  - ISAGA: Widely available commercially; more sensitive and specific than IFA for detecting IgM antibodies
  - Avidity testing: Confirmatory test to establish whether positive IgM/IgG reflects recent or chronic infection
- PCR: *T. gondii* DNA amplification in blood or amniotic fluid; used for diagnosis of fetal infection
- Culture: Organism can be isolated either by cell culture or by mouse inoculation; rarely performed but may be considered in neonates

Initial lab tests
- Diagnosis of primary infection is usually serologic.
- *Toxoplasma*-specific IgG and IgM are first determined from 1 serum sample.
- According to the result of IgM test, the avidity of IgG may be determined.
- Diagnosis of maternal infection and congenital toxoplasmosis:
  - Pregnant women who have mononucleosislike illness but negative heterophile test should be tested for toxoplasmosis.
  - Maternal infection accurately diagnosed when based on 2 blood samples at least 2 weeks apart showing seroconversion
  - High avidity of IgG during first trimester is a strong indicator against maternal primary infection.
  - Real-time PCR analysis for *T. gondii* on amniotic fluid provides an accurate tool to predict fetal infection and to decide on appropriate treatment and surveillance (2).
  - Fetal ultrasound for prognostic information
  - Routine screening is not recommended.
- Diagnosis of congenital toxoplasmosis after birth:
  - May require several serum samples for IgM and IgA antibodies for serologic diagnosis
  - Sampling of the cord or peripheral blood should be done within the first 2 weeks because sensitivity declines thereafter.
  - Ophthalmologic, auditory, and neurologic examinations, as well as lumbar puncture and CT scan of the head, should be performed.
- Diagnosis of toxoplasmic encephalitis:
  - Serology for IgG
  - Imaging: MRI more sensitive than CT scan for identification of multiple ring-enhancing brain lesions

Imaging
- MRI: For identifying multiple ring-enhancing brain lesion in AIDS patients with cerebral toxoplasmosis
- SPECT and PET scans: Can be useful in distinguishing toxoplasmosis from CNS lymphoma

Diagnostic Procedures/Surgery
- Lymph node biopsy showing characteristic pathologic triad
- Brain biopsy in CNS disease
- Amniocentesis with PCR (risk of false negatives and false positives)
- Isolation of *Toxoplasma* from placenta is diagnostic.

Pathological Findings
- Confirmatory, meningocerebritis ± abscesses with necrosis, Giemsa
- Lymph node histology shows triad of:
  - Reactive follicular hyperplasia
  - Irregular clusters of epithelioid histiocytes on and blurring margins of germinal centers
  - Distension of sinuses with monocytoid cells
- Sensitivity of triad 62.5%, specificity 91.3%

DIFFERENTIAL DIAGNOSIS
Syphilis, lymphoma, progressive multifocal leukoencephalopathy, cryptococcal meningitis, congenital TORCH infections, *Listeria* infection, tuberculosis (TB), erythroblastosis fetalis

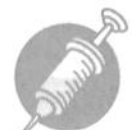

TREATMENT

MEDICATION
First Line

ALERT

Important to note: All pyrimethamine-containing regimens should include leucovorin (folinic acid 10–25 mg/d PO) to prevent drug-induced hematologic toxicity. Treatment in immunocompromised hosts:

- Initial drug regimen of choice is pyrimethamine 200-mg loading dose PO, followed by 75 mg/d plus sulfadiazine 6–8 g/d PO in 4 divided doses; for those intolerant or allergic to sulfadiazine, clindamycin 600–1,200 mg IV or 450 mg PO q.i.d. can be used instead.
- Alternative regimens for patients intolerant to sulfadiazine and clindamycin include:
  - Pyrimethamine 200-mg loading dose PO, followed by 75 mg/d plus azithromycin 1,200–1,500 mg PO once daily
  - Pyrimethamine 200-mg loading dose PO, followed by 75 mg/d plus atovaquone 750 mg PO q.i.d.
  - Sulfadiazine 1,500 mg q.i.d. plus atovaquone 1,500 mg b.i.d.
  - Trimethoprim-sulfamethoxazole 10/50 mg/kg/d PO or IV divided b.i.d. (for 30 days) may be an effective alternative in resource-poor settings.
- Duration of therapy: Typically 6 weeks, following which decrease to lower doses for secondary prophylaxis
- Adjunctive steroids should be used in patients with signs of increased intracranial pressure.
- Anticonvulsants if there is a history of seizures
- Prophylaxis in immunocompromised patients:
  - Primary prophylaxis: Indicated for patients with HIV infection and CD4 count <100 cells/μL who are *T. gondii* IgG–positive. Trimethoprim-sulfamethoxazole-DS 1 tablet PO daily. Alternative for sulfa allergy is dapsone 50 mg PO daily plus pyrimethamine 50 mg PO weekly plus leucovorin 25 mg PO weekly or atovaquone 1,500 mg PO daily.
  - Secondary prophylaxis: Following 6 weeks of therapy, administer lower doses of drugs.
- Sulfadiazine 2–4 g/d in 2–4 divided doses plus pyrimethamine 25–50 mg/d is the first choice.
- Alternative regimens include clindamycin 600 mg PO q8h plus pyrimethamine 25–50 mg/d PO or atovaquone 750 mg PO b.i.d.–q.i.d. ± pyrimethamine 25 mg PO daily.
- Prenatal treatment in pregnant women diagnosed with toxoplasmosis: Lack of evidence on whether antenatal treatment reduces congenital transmission; however, prenatal treatment is usually offered.
- Pregnant women who become infected: Treat immediately with spiramycin 1 g PO q8h without food.
- Pyrimethamine and sulfadiazine should be considered only if fetal infection is documented.
- Different dosing regimens:
  - 3-week course of pyrimethamine 50 mg once per day PO or 25 mg b.i.d. plus sulfadiazine 3 g/d PO divided into 2–3 doses, alternating with 3-week course of spiramycin 1 g PO t.i.d. until delivery
  - Pyrimethamine 25 mg once PO and sulfadiazine 4 g/d divided into 2–4 doses continuously until term
- Treatment of infected newborns: Treat irrespective of the presence or absence of clinical manifestations:
  - Pyrimethamine (2 mg/kg/d × 2 days, then 1 mg/kg/d × 2–6 months, then 1 mg/kg on Monday, Wednesday, and Friday), sulfadiazine <100 mg/kg/d divided b.i.d.), and leucovorin (5–10 mg on Monday, Wednesday, and Friday)
- Treatment in immunocompetent nonpregnant patients: Generally do not require treatment unless symptoms are severe or prolonged; 1 of the following 2 regimens can be used:
  - Pyrimethamine 100-mg loading dose PO, followed by 25–50 mg/d plus sulfadiazine 2–4 g/d in 4 divided doses
  - Pyrimethamine 100-mg loading dose PO, followed by 25–50 mg/d plus clindamycin 300 mg PO q.i.d.

Second Line
- Clindamycin: 900–1,200 mg t.i.d. IV used for ocular and CNS toxoplasmosis alone and in combination with pyrimethamine; as effective as the sulfadiazine-pyrimethamine but fewer adverse effects (3)[C]
- Corticosteroids (prednisone 1–2 mg/kg/d) are added for macular chorioretinitis or CNS infection.
- Alternatives: Atovaquone (Mepron), azithromycin (Zithromax), clarithromycin (Biaxin), or dapsone plus pyrimethamine and leucovorin
- Trimethoprim-sulfamethoxazole appears to be equivalent to pyrimethamine-sulfadiazine in AIDS patients with CNS disease (4)[C].

ADDITIONAL TREATMENT
General Measures
Immunocompetent patients with *Toxoplasma* lymphadenopathy usually require no treatment.

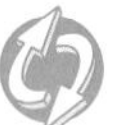

ONGOING CARE

FOLLOW-UP RECOMMENDATIONS
Patient Monitoring
- Precautions:
  - Monitor for bone marrow, renal, or liver toxicity. Test citation.
  - Good hydration: Sulfadiazine is poorly soluble and may crystallize in the urine.
  - Watch for diarrhea on clindamycin.
- Sulfonamides may increase phenytoin, warfarin, or oral hypoglycemic agents.

T

PATIENT EDUCATION
- See "Prevention."
- www.aafp.org/afp/20030515/2145ph.html
- http://familydoctor.org/online/famdocen/home/women/pregnancy/illness/180.html

PROGNOSIS
- Immunodeficient patients often relapse if treatment/suppression therapy is stopped.
- Treatment may prevent the development of untoward sequelae in all infants with congenital toxoplasmosis.

REFERENCES

1. Montoya JG, Liesenfeld O. Toxoplasmosis. *Lancet*. 2004;363:1965–76.
2. Wallon M, Franck J, Thulliez P, et al. Accuracy of real-time polymerase chain reaction for *Toxoplasma gondii* in amniotic fluid. *Obstet Gynecol*. 2010;115:727–33.
3. *Toxoplasmosis gondii*. In: Drugs for Parasitic Infections. *Treat Guidel Med Lett*. 2010; 8(Suppl):57.
4. Guidelines for prevention and treatment of opportunistic infections in HIV-infected adults and adolescents. *MMWR*. 2009;58(RR-4):1.

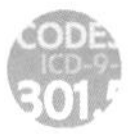

CODES

ICD9
- 130.7 Toxoplasmosis of other specified sites
- 130.9 Toxoplasmosis, unspecified
- 771.2 Other congenital infections specific to the perinatal period

CLINICAL PEARLS

- Newborn screening for congenital toxoplasmosis is feasible, but studies do not indicate clear benefits in children.
- Prevention is important, especially for seronegative pregnant women and immunodeficient patients.
- Immunologically normal patients may not need treatment.

TRACHEITIS, BACTERIAL

Mary Cataletto, MD

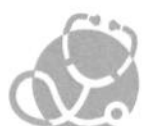

BASICS

DESCRIPTION

- Acute, potentially life-threatening infraglottic bacterial infection following a primary viral infection, usually parainfluenzae or influenza viruses:
  - Direct laryngoscopy reveals marked subglottic edema and thick mucopurulent secretions, sometimes causing pseudomembranes.
- System(s) affected: Pulmonary
- Synonym(s): Laryngotracheobronchitis; Pseudomembranous croup; Bacterial croup

EPIDEMIOLOGY

Incidence

- Estimated incidence: 0.1/100,000
- First cases described prior to 1950; resurgence of cases has been noted since 1979
- Peak incidence in children: Fall and winter
- Predominant age: 6 months to 8 years; mean age 4 years (similar to croup)
- Infections in adolescents and adults have been reported.
- Predominant sex: Male > Female (2:1)
- Accounts for 5–14% of upper-airway obstruction in children requiring critical-care services

Prevalence

- Rare illness
- Most common potentially life-threatening upper-airway infection in children
- Methicillin-resistant *S. aureus* (MSRA) may contribute to changing epidemiology and virulence.

RISK FACTORS

- Periods of increased seasonal activity of respiratory viruses
- Reports following adenoidectomy, with chronic tracheal aspiration, with evidence of other concurrent infections, including sinusitis, otitis, pneumonia, or pharyngitis

Genetics

No known genetic predisposition

GENERAL PREVENTION

- Standard precautions with scrupulous attention to hand washing, especially when caring for tracheostomy patients
- Vaccination against viruses that may predispose to bacterial tracheitis

ETIOLOGY

- *Staphylococcus aureus* (most common pediatric cause): Consider MRSA
- *Haemophilus influenzae* type b
- *Streptococcus pyogenes* group A
- *Streptococcus pneumoniae*
- *Moraxella catarrhalis* (associated with higher intubation rate; more frequent in younger children)
- Often polymicrobial

COMMONLY ASSOCIATED CONDITIONS

- Consider anatomic abnormalities or foreign body as well as recent pharyngeal or laryngeal surgery.
- Predisposing: Down syndrome, immunodeficiency, subglottic hemangioma, tracheoesophageal fistula repair, tracheobronchomalacia
- Viral coinfection may occur

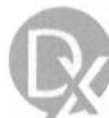

DIAGNOSIS

- May present with fever and systemic toxicity or as more localized disease
- Careful history and physical examination are the best method to distinguish bacterial tracheitis from croup and other rare causes of upper-airway obstruction (1).

HISTORY

- Prodromal upper respiratory tract symptoms
- Gradual progression of mild upper airway symptoms over 1 hour to 6 days to acute, febrile phase of rapid respiratory decompensation
- No drooling
- No response to aerosolized epinephrine

PHYSICAL EXAM

- Fever >38°C
- Child usually lying flat
- May be toxic looking
- Variable degree of respiratory distress:
  - Tachypnea
  - Inspiratory stridor
- Voice and cry usually normal
- Barking "brassy" cough
- Drooling uncommon

DIAGNOSTIC TESTS & INTERPRETATION

- Routine laboratory studies are not required to make the diagnosis.
- Radiographs are neither definitive nor diagnostic.
- Endoscopy provides a definitive diagnosis.

Lab

Initial lab tests

- Bacterial cultures of tracheal secretions are required for culture isolates and sensitivities.
- Routine laboratory studies may not be helpful.
- CBC results may vary:
  - WBC count may show marked leukocytosis or may be normal.
  - Increased band cell counts
- Blood cultures rarely positive
- Rapid antigen testing

Imaging

- Radiographs may be normal, but exudates may mimic the findings in foreign-body aspiration.
- Pneumonic infiltrates are common.
- Anteroposterior (AP) and lateral neck x-rays show subglottic and tracheal narrowing (i.e., steeple sign on AP film) with haziness and radiopaque linear or particulate densities (crusts).
- In patients with risk of acute respiratory obstruction, either do not obtain x-rays or monitor carefully.

Follow-Up & Special Considerations

Follow chest film if suspect pneumonia.

Diagnostic Procedures/Surgery

- Direct laryngoscopy and tracheoscopy is diagnostic and demonstrates:
  - Normal supraglottic structures
  - Marked subglottic erythema and edema
  - Ulcerations
  - Epithelial sloughing
  - Copious mucopurulent secretions ± plaques or pseudomembranes
- Obtain Gram stain and aerobic, anaerobic, and viral cultures of tracheal secretions during the procedure.

Pathological Findings

- Tracheal biopsy is rarely indicated, but may be considered in immunodeficient child or child with ulcerative colitis.
- Diffuse inflammation of larynx, trachea, and bronchi
- Mucopurulent exudate
- Semiadherent membranes (containing numerous neutrophils and cellular debris) may be identified within the trachea.

DIFFERENTIAL DIAGNOSIS

- Severe croup (viral)
- Spasmodic croup
- Diphtheria
- Retropharyngeal abscess
- Epiglottitis
- Pneumonia
- Asthma
- Foreign-body aspiration

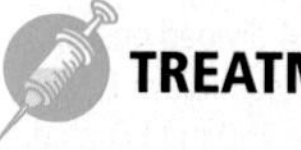

TREATMENT

- Treat as potentially life-threatening airway emergency.
- Children with suspected or actual bacterial tracheitis should be cared for in a pediatric ICU.
- Assess and monitor respiratory status
- Airway protection and support as necessary (at least 50% require intubation; some studies report up to 100%)
- Intermittent positive-pressure breathing (IPPB) may be required.
- Suctioning
- Different clinical course in previously healthy children compared with those with artificial airway

MEDICATION

- Empiric therapy should cover the most common pathogens until sensitivities are available: Antistaphylococcal agent (Vancomycin or Clindamycin) and a third-generation cephalosporin (e.g., Ceftriaxone or Cefotaxime)
- In the case of technology-dependent children with tracheostomy, make initial antibiotic choices based on previous tracheal culture.
- Narrow regimen when pathogens and sensitivities available
- Contraindications: Refer to the manufacturer's literature for each drug.
- Precautions: Refer to the manufacturer's literature for each drug. Avoid aminoglycosides in patients with previous hearing loss.
- Significant possible interactions: Refer to the manufacturer's literature for each drug.
- Airway obstruction is not relieved by nebulized epinephrine or corticosteroids.

ADDITIONAL TREATMENT

Issues for Referral

All children with suspect or actual bacterial tracheitis should be cared for in a pediatric ICU by a pediatric critical-care team that may include the following subspecialists: Pediatric intensivist, infectious-disease specialist, pulmonologist, and/or otolaryngologist.

Additional Therapies

- At present there is a lack of evidence to establish the effect of heliox inhalation in the treatment of group in children (2).
- For technology-dependent children with artificial airway:
  - Initial antibiotic choices should cover most recent tracheal aspirate isolates and then be refined according to culture and sensitivity results.
  - Adjunctive aerosol therapy may be helpful, particularly when multidrug-resistant organisms are present.

SURGERY/OTHER PROCEDURES

- Tracheostomy may be necessary.
- Therapeutic bronchoscopy may be necessary to facilitate removal of inspissated secretions.
- Tracheal membranes may require removal.

IN-PATIENT CONSIDERATIONS

- Aggressive supportive care and airway protection are paramount.
- Initial treatment of choice for bacterial tracheitis is broad-spectrum antibiotic coverage.
- Children with tracheitis and artificial airways present unique challenges: Tracheoscopy is important in establishing diagnosis in this population.
- Be vigilant for possible MRSA.

Initial Stabilization

Pediatric Considerations

- True pediatric emergency
- Admission to ICU
- Maintain airway: Often difficult due to copious secretions:
  - Endotracheal or nasotracheal intubation usually needed, especially in infants and children <4 years of age
  - Much less likely to need intubation if child >8 years of age
  - Advantage of intubation is ability to clear trachea and bronchi of secretions and pseudomembranes.
- Vigorous pulmonary toilet to clear airway of secretions
- Hydration, humidification, antibiotics

Admission Criteria

- Suspected or confirmed diagnosis of tracheitis
- Respiratory distress
- Artificial airway

Nursing

- Provide calm, quiet environment for child once endoscopy and cultures are done.
- Airway monitoring
- Frequent suctioning
- Monitor fluid balance
- Establish and maintain open lines of communication with child and parents.

Discharge Criteria

No longer in need of acute care

ONGOING CARE

FOLLOW-UP RECOMMENDATIONS

Patient Monitoring

Children with artificial airways will require ongoing follow-up.

DIET

Varies with clinical situation

PATIENT EDUCATION

Keep immunizations up to date.

PROGNOSIS

- Intubation generally 3–11 days
- Usually requires 3–7 days of hospitalization
- With effective early recognition and management, complete recovery can be expected.
- Cardiopulmonary arrest and death have occurred.

COMPLICATIONS

- Cardiopulmonary arrest
- Hypotension
- Acute respiratory distress syndrome (ARDS)
- Pneumonia
- Formation of pseudomembranes

REFERENCES

1. Bjornson CL, Johnson DW. Croup. *Lancet*. 2008; 371:329–39.
2. Vorwerk C, Coats T. Heliox for croup in children. *Cochrane Database Syst Rev*. 2010;2: CD006822.

ADDITIONAL READING

- Graf J, Stein F. Tracheitis in pediatric patients. *Semin Pediatr Infect Dis*. 2006;17:11–13.
- Hopkins A, Lahiri T, Salerno R, et al. Changing epidemiology of life threatening upper airway infections: The reemergence of bacterial tracheitis. *Pediators*. 2006;118:1418–21.
- Huang YL, Peng CC, Chiu NC, et al. Bacterial tracheitis in Pediatrics: 12 year experience at a medical ceter in taiwan, *Pediatr Int*. 2009;51:110.
- Loftis L. Acute infectious upper airway obstructions in children. *Semin Pediatr Infect Dis*. 2006;17:5–10.
- Rotta AT, Wiryawan B. Respiratory emergencies in children. *Respir Care*. 2003;48:248–58; discussion 258–60.
- Salamone FN, Bobbitt DB, Myer CM, et al. Bacterial tracheitis reexamined: Is there a less severe manifestation? *Otolaryngol Head Neck Surg*. 2004; 131:871–6.
- Shah S, Pediatric respiratory infections. *Emerg Med Clin N Am*. 2007;25:961–79.
- Taussig LM, Landau LI, et al (ed). Bacterial Tracheitis. In: *Pediatric Respiratory Medicine*. Philadelphia: Mosby Elsevier: 2008:477–8.
- Tebruegge M, Pantazidou A, Thorburn K, et al. Bacterial tracheitis: A multicentre perspective. *ScandJ Infect Dis*. 2009;41(8):548–57.

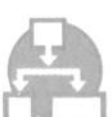

See Also (Topic, Algorithm, Electronic Media Element)

Croup (Laryngotracheobronchitis); Epiglottitis

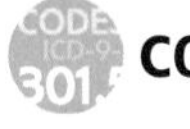

CODES

ICD9

- 464.10 Acute tracheitis without mention of obstruction
- 464.11 Acute tracheitis with obstruction

CLINICAL PEARLS

- Bacterial tracheitis is an acute, potentially life-threatening, infraglottic bacterial infection following a primary viral infection that accounts for 5–14% of upper-airway obstructions in children requiring critical-care services.
- Children with suspected or actual bacterial tracheitis should be cared for in a pediatric ICU.
- Endoscopy provides a definitive diagnosis.
- Initial treatment of choice for bacterial tracheitis is broad-spectrum antibiotic coverage, aggressive airway protection, and supportive care.

TRANSIENT ISCHEMIC ATTACK (TIA)

Abir O. Kanaan, PharmD, RPh
Kristin A. Tuiskula, PharmD, RPh
George Abraham, MD, MPH, FACP

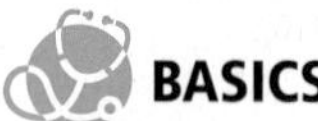

BASICS

DESCRIPTION
- A transient episode of neurological dysfunction due to focal brain, retinal, or spinal cord ischemia without acute infarction
- Most important predictor of stroke
- System(s) affected: Nervous
- Synonym(s): Ministroke

EPIDEMIOLOGY
Currently, there are 6.5 million stroke survivors in the US, and 700,000 new cases per year.

Incidence
- The incidence is underestimated as some patients do not report symptoms.
  - About 68.2/100,000/yr
  - First ever TIA incidence is 44.1/100,000/yr
- Predominant age: Risk increases >55 years of age; highest in seventh and eighth decades
- Predominant sex: Male > Female (3:1)
- Predominant race/ethnicity: African Americans > Hispanics > Caucasians

RISK FACTORS
- Hypertension (HTN)
- Atrial fibrillation
- Cardiac disease
- Cigarette smoking
- Diabetes
- Antiphospholipid antibodies
- Hypercholesterolemia

Genetics
Inheritance is polygenic, with tendency to clustering of risk factors within families

GENERAL PREVENTION
- Lifestyle changes, including smoking cessation, diet modification, and increasing physical activity
- Strict control of medical risk factors (e.g., diabetes, HTN, hyperlipidemia, cardiac disease)
- Antiplatelet therapy
- ACE inhibitors
- HMG-CoA reductase inhibitors (known as statins)
- Anticoagulation when high risk of cardioembolism (e.g., atrial fibrillation, mechanical valves)

PATHOPHYSIOLOGY
Temporary reduction or cessation of cerebral blood flow adversely affecting neuronal function

ETIOLOGY
- Carotid or vertebral atherosclerotic disease:
  - Artery-to-artery thromboembolism
  - Low-flow ischemia
- Small, deep vessel disease associated with HTN: Lacunar infarcts
- Cardiac disease
- Embolism secondary to:
  - Valvular (mitral valve) pathology
  - Mural hypokinesias or akinesias with thrombosis (acute anterior myocardial infarctions or congestive cardiomyopathies)
  - Cardiac arrhythmia (atrial fibrillation)
- Hypercoagulable states:
  - Antiphospholipid antibodies
  - Deficiency of protein S, protein C
  - Presence of antithrombin III
  - Oral contraceptives
  - Pregnancy and parturition
- Arteritis:
  - Noninfectious necrotizing vasculitis
  - Drugs
  - Irradiation
  - Local trauma
- Sympathomimetic drugs (e.g., cocaine)
- Other causes: Spontaneous and posttraumatic (e.g., chiropractic manipulation) arterial dissection
- Fibromuscular dysplasia

ALERT
There is an ~5–20% risk of stoke within 5 days of first TIA. Close follow-up and secondary prevention are essential.

Geriatric Considerations
- Older patients have a higher mortality rate than younger patients.
- Atrial fibrillation is a frequent cause among the elderly.
- Highest incidence in seventh and eighth decades

Pediatric Considerations
- Congenital heart disease is a common cause among pediatric patients.
- Other causes inlcude:
  - Metabolic: Homocystinuria, Fabry disease
  - Central nervous system (CNS) infection
  - Clotting disorders
  - Marfan syndrome
  - Moyamoya disease

COMMONLY ASSOCIATED CONDITIONS
- Atrial fibrillation
- Uncontrolled HTN
- Carotid stenosis

DIAGNOSIS

HISTORY
- Carotid circulation (hemispheric): Monocular visual loss, hemiplegia, hemianesthesia, neglect, aphasia, visual field defects (amaurosis fugax); less often, headaches, seizures, amnesia, confusion
- Vertebrobasilar (brain stem or cerebellar): Bilateral visual obscuration, diplopia, vertigo, ataxia, facial paresis, Horner syndrome, dysphagia, dysarthria; also headache, nausea, vomiting, and ataxia
- Obtain witness accounts with emphasis on symptom onset, progression, and recovery
- Past medical history, baseline functional status

PHYSICAL EXAM
- BP
- Thorough neurologic and cardiac exams

DIAGNOSTIC TESTS & INTERPRETATION
Lab
Initial lab tests
- In all patients:
  - International normalization ratio (INR) and partial thromboplastin time (PTT)
  - CBC
  - Glucose
  - Electrolytes
  - Cardiac enzymes
  - Oxygen saturation
- Consider toxicology/alcohol screen and pregnancy tests in selected patients

Follow-Up & Special Considerations
- Duplex carotid ultrasonography: Obtain promptly if carotid embolic source possible
- ECG
- Angiography:
  - Cerebral
  - Carotid arterial stenosis
- Transthoracic echocardiography; if normal and cardiac source is suspected, follow with transesophageal ECHO.
- Holter monitoring: If suspected arrhythmia
- MR angiography: Brain and blood vessels
- EEG: If seizure suspected

Imaging
Initial approach
- CT scan of head, noncontrast: Acute phase
- Multimodal CT and MRI may provide additional information to improve diagnosis: MRI with diffusion weighted imaging is the most sensitive and specific imaging modality in the detection of acute ischemia, and therefore, can help exclude mimics or confirm the diagnosis

DIFFERENTIAL DIAGNOSIS
- Migraine (hemiplegic)
- Focal seizure (Todd paralysis)
- Hypoglycemia
- Bell palsy
- Evolving stroke
- Neoplasm of brain
- Subarachnoid hemorrhage
- Intoxication

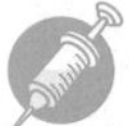

TREATMENT

MEDICATION
Choice of antiplatelet agent should be individualized based upon patient comorbidities, tolerance, preferences, and costs of therapy. It is uncertain whether switching therapy in patients who have additional ischemic attacks while on one therapy is beneficial.

First Line
- Enteric-coated aspirin: 50–325 mg/d PO (1)[A]:
  - Contraindications: Active peptic ulcer disease, hypersensitivity to aspirin or NSAIDs
  - Precautions: May aggravate pre-existing peptic ulcer disease; may worsen symptoms of asthma
  - Significant possible interactions: May potentiate effects of anticoagulants and sulfonylurea analogues
- Clopidogrel (Plavix): 75 mg/d PO (1)[B]:
  - Has fewer side effects than ticlopidine. Likely as effective as aspirin.
  - Can be used in patients who are allergic to aspirin (1)[C]
  - Precautions: TTP can occur and increased risk of bleeding when combined with aspirin

- Dipyridamole–aspirin (Aggrenox): 1 capsule PO b.i.d. (1,2)[B]:
  - Each capsule contains 200 mg of extended-release dipyridamole and 25 mg of immediate-release aspirin
  - May be very slightly more effective than aspirin alone; much more expensive and more side effects than aspirin.
- Warfarin (INR-adjusted dose) (1,3)[A]: For patients with atrial fibrillation and cardioembolic stroke:
  - Contraindications: Intolerance or allergy, active liver disease, active bleeding, pregnancy
  - Significant possible interactions: Antibiotics, antiepileptics, antifungals, and many others
- Heparin: Dose and regimen vary based on goal; may be used primarily as bridge for long-term warfarin anticoagulation (4)[B].

Second Line

- Ticlopidine (Ticlid): 250 mg PO b.i.d. has fallen out of favor due to unfavorable side effect profile. The 2011 AHA/ASA guidelines do not mention ticlopidine:
  - Contraindications: Known hypersensitivity to the drug, presence of hematopoietic or hemostatic disorders, conditions associated with active bleeding, severe liver dysfunction
  - Precautions:
    - 2.4% of patients develop neutropenia (0.8% severe), which is reversible with cessation of the drug. Monitor blood counts every 2 weeks for first 3 months.
    - TTP can occur.
  - Significant possible interactions: Digoxin plasma levels decreased 15%; theophylline half-life increased from 8.6–12.2 hours

ADDITIONAL TREATMENT

- Venous thromboembolism (VTE) prophylaxis may be provided using:
  - Compression devices
  - Unfractionated heparin 5,000 units SC q8h or q12h
  - Enoxaparin: 40 mg SC q24h; dose needs to be adjusted with a CrCl <30 mL/min
- Patients with TIA or ischemic stroke should be started on a statin (1,5)[A]
- BP should be reduced when appropriate. ACEIs have shown to be of benefit (1)[A]
- Dietary modifications should be considered: Salt restriction, diet rich in fruit and vegetables

General Measures

- TIA is a neurologic emergency. Immediate medical attention should be sought within 24–48 hours of symptom onset.
- Current evidence suggests that patients with high-risk TIAs require rapid referral and 24-hour admission.
- Acute phase:
  - Inpatient for surgery and high-risk groups
  - Outpatient investigations may be considered based on patient's stroke risk, arrangement of follow-up, and social circumstances.
- Antithrombotic therapy for VTE prophylaxis
- Treatment or control of underlying associated conditions

Issues for Referral

- Neurology for ongoing workup and treatment
- Cardiology if cardiac cause suspected
- Vascular surgery if carotid endarterectomy appropriate

Additional Therapies

Secondary prevention of TIA should be initiated

SURGERY/OTHER PROCEDURES

Carotid endarterectomy may be considered in patients with high degree of carotid artery stenosis (1)[A]

IN-PATIENT CONSIDERATIONS

Initial Stabilization

Fluid and electrolyte imbalances should be corrected.

Admission Criteria

- Ongoing symptoms
- Uncertain diagnosis

Discharge Criteria

- Consider safety at home if another incident occurs.
- History of TIAs with current appropriate treatment

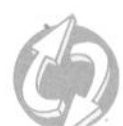

ONGOING CARE

FOLLOW-UP RECOMMENDATIONS

Patient Monitoring

- Follow up every 3 months for first year; then yearly
- ABCD^2 stroke risk score stratifies patients with TIA on 5 criteria (6)[A]:
  - Age ≥60 = 1
  - Systolic BP (SBP) ≥140 mm Hg and/or diastolic BP (DBP) ≥90 mm Hg = 1
  - Clinical: Unilateral weakness = 2 or speech impairment without weakness = 1
  - Duration ≥60 minutes = 2 or 10–59 minutes = 1
  - Diabetes: Present = 1
- Risk score with associated 2-day stroke risk (%):
  - Low risk <4 (1%)
  - Medium risk = 4 or 5 (4.1%)
  - High risk >5 (8.1%)
- Validated stroke risk score protocols may be beneficial in predicting future strokes and choosing the most appropriate follow-up care (6)[A].

DIET

As appropriate for underlying medical problems

PATIENT EDUCATION

Education regarding condition, complications, and drug therapy should be provided.

PROGNOSIS

- The risk of stroke on the ipsilateral side within 90 days and cumulative thereafter is 5–20%.
- Frequency increases with the addition of multiple risk factors and severity of carotid stenosis.
- The major cause of death in the first 5 years is cardiac disease.

COMPLICATIONS

- Stroke
- Functional impairment

REFERENCES

1. Furie KL, Kasner SE, Adams RJ, et al. Guidelines for the prevention of stroke in patients with stroke or transient ischemic attack. A guideline for healthcare professionals from the American Heart Association/American Stroke Association. *Stroke*. 2011;42:227–76.
2. De Schryver EL, Algra A, van Gijn J. Dipyridamole for preventing stroke and other vascular events in patients with vascular disease. *Cochrane Database Syst Rev*. 2007;CD001820.
3. Aguilar MI, Hart R, Pearce LA. Oral anticoagulants versus antiplatelet therapy for preventing stroke in patients with non-valvular atrial fibrillation and no history of stroke or transient ischemic attacks. *Cochrane Database Syst Rev*. 2007;CD006186.
4. Albers GW, Amarenco P, Easton JD, et al. Antithrombotic and thrombolytic therapy for ischemic stroke: American College of Chest Physicians Evidence-Based Clinical Practice Guidelines (8th ed). *Chest*. 2008;133:630S–69S.
5. Manktelow BN, Potter JF. Interventions in the management of serum lipids for preventing stroke recurrence. *Cochrane Database Syst Rev*. 2009;CD002091.
6. Tsivgoulis G, Stamboulis E, Sharma VK. Multicenter external validation of the ABCD2 score in triaging TIA patients. *Neurology*. 2010;74:1351–7.

ADDITIONAL READING

Wallis A, Saunders T. Imaging transient ischaemic attack with diffusion weighted magnetic resonance imaging. *BMJ*. 2010;340:c2215.

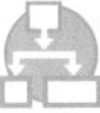

See Also (Topic, Algorithm, Electronic Media Element)

Algorithms: Stroke; Transient Ischemic Attack and Transient Neurologic Deficit

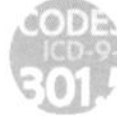

CODES

ICD9

435.9 Unspecified transient cerebral ischemia

CLINICAL PEARLS

- Primary prevention is important, stressing smoking cessation and control of HTN, hyperlipidemia, and diabetes.
- Antiplatelet therapy (e.g., aspirin or clopidogrel or aspirin-dipyridamole) should be initiated.
- Warfarin should be initiated in patients with atrial fibrillation based on risk factors.
- There is a 30% risk of stroke within 5 years of a TIA.

TRANSIENT STRESS CARDIOMYOPATHY

Timothy P. Fitzgibbons, MD
Gerard P. Aurigemma, MD

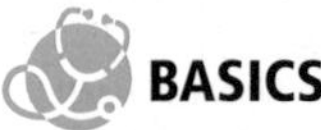

BASICS

DESCRIPTION

- Transient stress cardiomyopathy (TSC) is a unique cause of reversible left ventricle (LV) dysfunction with a clinical presentation indistinguishable from the acute coronary syndromes, particularly ST-segment elevation myocardial infarction (MI).
- Typically, the patient is a postmenopausal woman who presents with acute chest pain or dyspnea after an identifiable "trigger" (i.e., an acute emotional or physiologic stressor).
- First reported by authors from Japan (1,2), TSC was known initially as the *Takotsubo syndrome* because the typical LV morphology (i.e., apical ballooning) resembled that of a Japanese octopus trap, or *takotsubo*.
- Presenting clinical features include:
  - Chest symptoms and/or dyspnea
  - ECG changes, including ST-segment elevations or diffuse T-wave inversions
  - Mild elevation in cardiac biomarkers (creatine kinase [CK], troponin)
  - Transient wall motion abnormalities that may involve the base, midportion, and/or lateral walls of the LV
  - The apex of the right ventricle (RV) may be affected in up to 25% of cases (4).
- Clinical features may vary on a case-by-case basis, and formal diagnostic criteria have not been established.
- Authors from the Mayo Clinic have proposed that 3 of the 4 following criteria establish the diagnosis (5):
  - Transient akinesis or dyskinesis of the LV apical and midventricular segments with regional wall motion abnormalities extending beyond a single epicardial vascular distribution
  - Absence of obstructive coronary artery disease (CAD) or angiographic evidence of acute plaque rupture
  - New ECG abnormalities, either ST-segment elevation or T-wave inversion
  - Absence of:
    - Recent significant head trauma
    - Intracranial bleeding
    - Pheochromocytoma
    - Obstructive epicardial CAD
    - Myocarditis
    - Hypertrophic cardiomyopathy
- Synonym(s) (3): Takotsubo cardiomyopathy; Apical ballooning syndrome; Stress cardiomyopathy; Broken heart syndrome; Ampulla cardiomyopathy

EPIDEMIOLOGY

Incidence

- TSC accounts for a small percentage (1–3%) of acute coronary syndromes (3).
- In a recent prospective evaluation of patients admitted to the intensive care unit, as many as 28% of patients had apical ballooning, often in association with sepsis (3).
- Predominant sex: 82–100% of cases occur in women (5).
- Predominant age: Mean age of patients is 62–75 years.

Prevalence

2.2% of patients presenting to a referral hospital with ST-segment MIs were found to have TSC (5).

RISK FACTORS

- Female sex
- Postmenopausal state
- Emotional stress (i.e., argument, death of family member)
- Physiologic stress (i.e., acute medical illness)

Genetics

No genetic associations have been described to date.

PATHOPHYSIOLOGY

- The exact pathophysiology is not known.
- It has been speculated that overwhelming activation of the sympathetic nervous system incites a cascade of events, including:
  - Catecholamine-induced LV dysfunction: Increased β-receptor density at the cardiac apex may explain apical sympathetic hypersensitivity.
  - Endothelial dysfunction: Prolonged thrombolysis in MI (TIMI) frame counts in all 3 coronary vascular beds have been observed by some authors in the acute phase of this syndrome.
  - Multivessel epicardial spasm:
    - Diffuse multivessel spasm was reported in 15% of cases from Japan.
    - More recent studies have not supported this hypothesis.
  - Cellular metabolic injury:
    - Myocardial norepinephrine release
    - Calcium overload
    - Contraction band necrosis

COMMONLY ASSOCIATED CONDITIONS

Death from TSC is rare, and most cases resolve rapidly, within 2–3 days. Reported complications include:

- Left-sided heart failure
- Pulmonary edema
- Cardiogenic shock and hemodynamic compromise
- Dynamic LV outflow tract gradient complicated by hypotension
- Mitral regurgitation
- Ventricular arrhythmias
- LV thrombus formation
- LV free wall rupture
- Death (rare, 0–8%)

DIAGNOSIS

Because TSC often is indistinguishable from an acute coronary syndrome, it should be treated initially as such:

- Activate emergency medical services or report to emergency department.
- Oxygen, IV access, and ECG monitoring
- Urgent cardiology consultation

HISTORY

- Exposure to a "trigger event":
  - Emotional stress: Argument, death of family member, divorce, public speaking, etc.
  - Physiologic stress: Acute medical condition such as head trauma, asthma attack, seizure, etc.
- Acute onset of dyspnea or chest pain
- Palpitations
- Syncope

PHYSICAL EXAM

Exam may be unremarkable or may include any of the following:

- Tachypnea
- Tachycardia
- Hypotension
- Jugular venous distension
- Bibasilar rales
- S_3 gallop
- Systolic ejection murmur due to dynamic LV outflow tract gradient
- Holosystolic murmur of mitral regurgitation

DIAGNOSTIC TESTS & INTERPRETATION

ECG should be done urgently and may show:

- Diffuse ST-segment elevations
- Diffuse and often dramatic T-wave inversions
- QTc interval prolongation
- Q waves

Lab

Laboratory tests typically reveal a mild elevation in cardiac biomarkers, such as:

- CK (rarely >500 U/mL)
- Troponin I
- B-type natriuretic peptide

Imaging

- Chest radiograph:
  - Cardiomegaly
  - Pulmonary edema
- Echocardiogram:
  - Reduced LV systolic function
  - Abnormal diastolic function, including evidence of increased filling pressures
  - Regional wall motion abnormalities in 1 of the following patterns:
    - Classic or "Takotsubo-type" ballooning of the apex with a hypercontractile base
    - "Reverse Takotsubo": Apical hypercontractility with basal akinesis
    - "Midventricular" akinesis with apical and basal hypercontractility
    - Focal or localized akinesis of an isolated segment
  - Dynamic intracavitary LV gradient
  - Mitral regurgitation
  - Variable involvement of the right ventricle
- Cardiac MRI:
  - Reduced LV function
  - Wall motion abnormalities as described for transthoracic echocardiography
  - Absence of delayed hyperenhancement with gadolinium

Diagnostic Procedures/Surgery

- Because ST-segment elevation MI is the diagnosis of exclusion, patients typically are referred for urgent cardiac catheterization.
- Coronary angiography:
  - Nonocclusive CAD
  - Rarely, epicardial coronary spasm
  - Endothelial dysfunction, as measured by fractional flow reserve or TIMI frame counts
- Left-sided heart catheterization: Increased LV end-diastolic pressure
- Ventriculography: Wall motion abnormalities as described for transthoracic echocardiography
- Right-sided heart catheterization:
  - Increased pulmonary capillary wedge pressure
  - Secondary pulmonary hypertension
  - Increased right ventricular filling pressures
  - Reduced cardiac output or cardiogenic shock (cardiac index <2 and mean arterial pressure [MAP] <60 mm Hg)

Pathological Findings

Characteristic pathologic findings of involved myocardium have not been described.

DIFFERENTIAL DIAGNOSIS

- Acute ST-segment elevation MI
- Pulmonary embolism
- Myopericarditis
- Pheochromocytoma
- Hypertrophic cardiomyopathy
- Subarachnoid hemorrhage or stroke

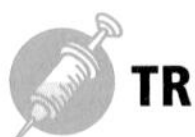

TREATMENT

- Activation of emergency medical services
- Advanced cardiac life support therapies as needed
- Oxygen
- IV access
- ECG monitoring

MEDICATION

After diagnostic cardiac catheterization, empirical treatment goals are:

- Management of hypotension: Differentiation between cardiogenic shock or dynamic LV cavity gradient
- Management of increased filling pressures and congestive states
- Attenuation of sympathetic drive

First Line

- Consideration should be given to β-blockers in all patients (e.g., metoprolol 12.5–75 mg PO b.i.d. or carvedilol 6.25–25 mg PO b.i.d.) if tissue perfusion is adequate.
- If there is evidence of congestive heart failure (CHF) or pulmonary edema, consider:
  - Furosemide 20–40 mg IV b.i.d. as needed to reduce LV filling pressures and dyspnea
  - ACE inhibitors: Lisinopril 10–40 mg/d PO or equivalent

Second Line

Short-term anticoagulation should be considered in patients with severely reduced LV function to prevent LV thrombus formation. Unfractionated heparin 80 U/kg IV bolus followed by 18 U/kg/hr IV or Lovenox 1 mg/kg SC b.i.d.

ADDITIONAL TREATMENT

Issues for Referral

All patients with TSC generally should be comanaged with cardiology while inpatient and referred to cardiology as an outpatient.

Additional Therapies

- Urgent cardiology consultation and consideration of cardiac catheterization
- Hypotension may require:
  - Vasopressors (e.g., dopamine or Levophed) if there is no LV outflow tract gradient
  - Phenylephrine and IV fluids to increase afterload in the presence of an LV outflow tract gradient
  - Cardiogenic shock that is not due to a LV outflow tract gradient may require placement of an intraaortic balloon pump.

IN-PATIENT CONSIDERATIONS

Initial Stabilization

- 12-lead ECG
- Chest radiograph
- Laboratory testing
- Echocardiography

Admission Criteria

Patients with TSC usually are admitted for observation because the differential diagnosis includes ACS.

IV Fluids

Normal saline infusion to support BP, if necessary, and no evidence of heart failure

Discharge Criteria

Generally considered after exclusion of acute coronary syndrome and resolution of:

- Congestive state
- Hypotension
- Profound impairments of systolic function

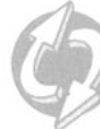

ONGOING CARE

FOLLOW-UP RECOMMENDATIONS

- Impairments in systolic function typically resolve in 2–3 days, but may last as long as 1 month.
- Patients should follow up with cardiology and serial echocardiography to document improved LV function.

PROGNOSIS

- Prognosis is excellent. Inpatient mortality is rare and ranges from 0–8%.
- Recurrence is rare; it also has been reported in 0–8% of patients.

REFERENCES

1. Dote K, Sato H, Tateishi H, et al. [Myocardial stunning due to simultaneous multivessel coronary spasms: A review of 5 cases]. *J Cardiol*. 1991;21:203–14.
2. Tsuchihashi K, Ueshima K, Uchida T, et al. Transient left ventricular apical ballooning without coronary artery stenosis: A novel heart syndrome mimicking acute myocardial infarction. Angina Pectoris-Myocardial Infarction Investigations in Japan. *J Am Coll Cardiol*. 2001;38:11–8.
3. Aurigemma GP. Acute stress cardiomyopathy and reversible left ventricular dysfunction. *Cardiol Rounds*. 2006;10(10).
4. Fitzgibbons TP, Madias C, Seth A, et al. Prevalence and clinical characteristics of right ventricular dysfunction in transient stress cardiomyopathy. *Am J Cardiol*. 2009;104:133–6.
5. Bybee KA, Kara T, Prasad A, et al. Systematic review: Transient left ventricular apical ballooning: A syndrome that mimics ST-segment elevation myocardial infarction. *Ann Intern Med*. 2004;141:858–65.

ADDITIONAL READING

- Bybee KA, Prasad A. Stress-related cardiomyopathy syndromes. *Circulation*. 2008;118:397–409.
- Madias C, Fitzgibbons TP, Alsheikh-Ali AA, et al. Acquired long QT syndrome from stress cardiomyopathy is associated with ventricular arrhythmias and torsades de pointes. *Heart Rhythm*. 2011;8:555–61.
- Wittstein IS, Thiemann DR, Lima JA, et al. Neurohumoral features of myocardial stunning due to sudden emotional stress. *N Engl J Med*. 2005;352:539–48.

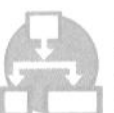

See Also (Topic, Algorithm, Electronic Media Element)

Algorithm: Chest Pain/Acute Coronary Syndrome

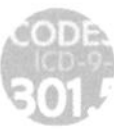

CODES

ICD9

429.83 Takotsubo syndrome

CLINICAL PEARLS

- TSC is a cause of reversible LV dysfunction with a clinical presentation indistinguishable from the acute coronary syndromes, particularly ST-segment elevation MI.
- Echocardiography may strongly suggest the diagnosis.
- Treatment is supportive and should include β-blockers in most patients, and diuretics and ACE inhibitors in patients with CHF.

TRICHOMONIASIS

Teresa M. Robb, MD

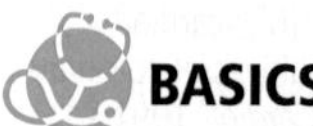

BASICS

DESCRIPTION

- Sexually transmitted urogenital infection caused by a pear-shaped, parasitic protozoan
- A cause of nongonococcal urethritis (NGU) in men
- System(s) affected: Genitourinary
- Synonym(s): Trich; Trichomonal urethritis

EPIDEMIOLOGY

Incidence

- Estimated 7.4 million new cases annually in the US among men and women
- 10–25% of vaginal infections
- 1–17% of cases of NGU; reported prevalence rates among men without urethritis have ranged from 0–8%.
- Predominant age: Young and middle-aged adults:
  - Rare until onset of sexual activity
  - Not uncommon in postmenopausal women; age is not protective, and long-term carriage is possible.
- Predominant sex: Male = Female, but women are more commonly symptomatic.

Pediatric Considerations

Rare in prepubertal children; confirmed diagnosis should raise concern of sexual abuse

Prevalence

- 2.3% of young adults:
  - 2.8% of women
  - 1.7% of men
- 3.1% of all US women
- Racial disparity exists (1):
  - 1.3% of white, non-Hispanic women
  - 1.8% of Mexican American women
  - 13.3% of black, non-Hispanic women

RISK FACTORS

- Multiple sexual partners
- Unprotected intercourse
- Lower socioeconomic status
- Other STIs
- Untreated partner with previous infection

Genetics

No known genetic considerations

GENERAL PREVENTION

- Use of male or female condoms
- Reducing exposure by limiting numbers of partners
- Male circumcision may be protective (2).

ETIOLOGY

- *Trichomonas vaginalis*: A pear-shaped, flagellated, parasitic protozoan
- Grows best at 35–37°C in anaerobic conditions at pH of 5.5–6
- STI
- Transmission via a nonvenereal route is possible because the organism survives for several hours in a moist environment.

COMMONLY ASSOCIATED CONDITIONS

- Other STIs, including HIV
- Bacterial vaginosis

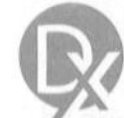

DIAGNOSIS

HISTORY

- Women:
  - Yellow–green, malodorous vaginal discharge
  - Vulvovaginal pruritus
  - Dysuria
  - 50–75% are asymptomatic.
- Men:
  - Dysuria
  - Urethral discharge
  - 80% are asymptomatic.

PHYSICAL EXAM

- Women:
  - Vaginal erythema
  - Yellow–green, frothy, malodorous vaginal discharge
  - Petechiae on cervix (strawberry cervix; seen in ~10% of patients)
- Men: Penile discharge, spontaneous and with expression

DIAGNOSTIC TESTS & INTERPRETATION

Lab

Initial lab tests

- Wet mount of vaginal or urethral discharge (3)[A]: Direct visualization of motile trichomonads:
  - Sensitivity of 60–70%
  - Specificity of 99.8%
- Gram stain
- Culture: Sensitivity >95%; can take 4–7 days:
  - ELISA and direct fluorescent antibody tests: Sensitivity of 80–90%
  - Rapid diagnostic kits using polymerase chain reaction DNA probes: Sensitivity of 97%, specificity of 98%

Follow-Up & Special Considerations

Detection on Papanicolaou smear (3)[A]:

- Sensitivity of 57–98%
- Specificity of 97%

DIFFERENTIAL DIAGNOSIS

- Women (other vaginitides):
  - Bacterial vaginosis
  - Vaginal candidiasis
  - Chlamydial infection
  - Gonorrheal infection
  - Mixed vaginitis
- Men (other urethritides):
  - Chlamydial infection
  - Gonorrheal infection

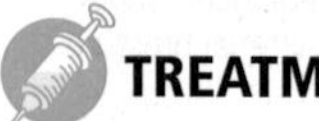

TREATMENT

- Symptomatic individuals require treatment.
- Asymptomatic partners should be treated presumptively.
- Complete screening for other STIs should be considered part of required treatment.

MEDICATION

First Line

- Metronidazole 2 g PO, 1 dose (4)[A]
- Metronidazole 1.5 g PO, 1 dose:
  - FDA pregnancy risk Category B
  - American Association of Pediatrics recommends abstaining from breast-feeding during treatment and for 12–24 hours after last dose, but this is an old recommendation that is not supported by current evidence (5).
- Tinidazole 2 g PO, 1 dose:
  - FDA pregnancy risk Category C
  - Abstain from breast-feeding during treatment and for 3 days after the dose.

Second Line

- Only if still symptomatic after initial treatment
- Metronidazole 500 mg PO b.i.d. for 7 days (4)[A]

Pregnancy Considerations

No evidence supports the use of metronidazole in asymptomatic patients because adverse outcomes are not prevented by treatment (6)[A].

ADDITIONAL TREATMENT

General Measures

If metronidazole resistance is suspected, use tinidazole.

Issues for Referral

- Multidrug-resistant organism
- Patient allergy to metronidazole: Desensitization to metronidazole is possible.

Additional Therapies

- Men:
  - None currently available in the US
- Women (4)[A]:
  - Clotrimazole 100 mg PO b.i.d. for 7 days
  - Sulfanilamide-aminacrine-allantoin vaginal suppositories b.i.d. for 7 days
  - Nonoxynol 9
  - Povidone-iodine douche

COMPLEMENTARY AND ALTERNATIVE MEDICINE

Not enough adequately investigation to be recommended

IN-PATIENT CONSIDERATIONS

Admission Criteria

Admission may be necessary for resistant organisms because IV therapy provides higher tissue concentrations.

Discharge Criteria

Clearance of infection

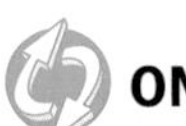

ONGOING CARE

FOLLOW-UP RECOMMENDATIONS

- If symptoms persist after initial treatment, reculture and/or repeat wet mount.
- No need for test of cure in asymptomatic individuals (4)[A]

DIET

Abstain from alcohol while being treated with 5-nitroimidazole derivatives due to disulfiramlike reaction.

PATIENT EDUCATION

Education about the sexually transmitted aspect of the infection:

- Inform partner so that partner can be treated.
- Discuss safe sex during health maintenance visits.
- Abstain from intercourse while undergoing treatment; use condoms if abstention is not feasible/possible.
- Avoid alcohol during treatment with metronidazole or tinidazole.
- Condom use can prevent recurrence.

PROGNOSIS

- Excellent
- Usually treated after 1 course, but increasing number of metronidazole-resistant cases

COMPLICATIONS

Pregnancy Considerations

Linked to low birth weight, preterm/premature rupture of membranes, and preterm birth (6)

REFERENCES

1. Sutton M, Sternberg M, Koumans EH, et al. The prevalence of *Trichomonas vaginalis* infection among reproductive-age women in the United States, 2001–2004. *Clin Infect Dis*. 2007;45: 1319–26.
2. Sobngwi-Tambekou J, Taljaard D, Nieuwoudt M, et al. Male circumcision and *Neisseria gonorrhoeae, Chlamydia trachomatis* and *Trichomonas vaginalis:* Observations after a randomised controlled trial for HIV prevention. *Sex Transm Infect*. 2009;85: 116–20.
3. Wiese W, Patel SR, Patel SC, et al. A meta-analysis of the Papanicolaou smear and wet mount for the diagnosis of vaginal trichomoniasis. *Am J Med*. 2000;108:301–8.
4. Forna F, Gülmezoglu AM. Interventions for treating trichomoniasis in women. *Cochrane Database Syst Rev*. 2003:CD000218.
5. Hale T. Medications and Mothers Milk: A Manual of Lactational Pharmacology (Medications and Mother's Milk), 14th ed. Amarillo, TX: Pharmasoft Medical Pub, 2009.
6. Gülmezoglu AM, Azhar M. Interventions for trichomoniasis in pregnancy. *Cochrane Database Syst Rev*. 2011:CD000220.

ADDITIONAL READING

- Allsworth JE, Ratner JA, Peipert JF, et al. Trichomoniasis and other sexually transmitted infections: Results from the 2001–2004 National Health and Nutrition Examination Surveys. *Sex Transm Dis*. 2009;36:738–44.
- Centers for Disease Control and Prevention, Workowski KA, Berman SM. Sexually transmitted diseases treatment guidelines, 2006. *MMWR Recomm Rep*. 2006;55:1–94.
- Centers for Disease Control and Prevention. Tichomoniasis. Available at: www.cdc.gov/std/trichomonas.
- Helms DJ, Mosure DJ, Secor WE, et al. Management of *Trichomonas vaginalis* in women with suspected metronidazole hypersensitivity. *Am J Obstet Gynecol*. 2008;198:370e1–370e7.
- Klebanoff MA, Carey JC, Hauth JC, et al. Failure of metronidazole to prevent preterm delivery among pregnant women with asymptomatic Trichomonas vaginalis infection. *N Engl J Med*. 2001;345: 487–93.
- McClelland RS, Sangare L, Hassan WM, et al. Infection with *Trichomonas vaginalis* increases the risk of HIV-1 acquisition. *J Infect Dis*. 2007;195: 698–702.
- Miller M, Liao Y, Gomez AM, et al. Factors associated with the prevalence and incidence of *Trichomonas vaginalis* infection among African American women in New York city who use drugs. *J Infect Dis*. 2008;197:503–9.
- Saperstein AK, Firnhaber GC. Clinical inquiries. Should you test or treat partners of patients with gonorrhea, chlamydia, or trichomoniasis? *J Fam Pract*. 2010;59:46–8.
- Wendel KA, Workowski KA. Trichomoniasis: Challenges to appropriate management. *Clin Infect Dis*. 2007;44(Suppl 3):S123–9.

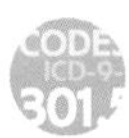

CODES

ICD9

- 131.00 Urogenital trichomoniasis, unspecified
- 131.01 Trichomonal vulvovaginitis
- 131.9 Trichomoniasis, unspecified

CLINICAL PEARLS

- Both partners need to be treated for trichomoniasis.
- Test of cure is unnecessary.
- Avoid alcohol during treatment with standard agents.
- Treatment does not improve risk of adverse pregnancy outcomes.
- Male circumcision may be protective.

T

TRICHOTILLOMANIA

Christine Tam, MD
Frank J. Domino, MD

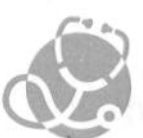

BASICS

- Trichotillomania is an impulse control disorder that involves pulling out an individual's own hair, usually causing variable severity of hair loss.
- Trichotillomania is classified as a type of anxiety disorder. According to DSM IV, trichotillomania is considered an impulse-control disorder. It can also be considered an obsessive–compulsive disorder because many individuals experience a sense of relief once the hair is pulled, resolving their internal tension.

DESCRIPTION

- Trichotillomania usually presents in childhood or early adolescence.
- Symptoms of trichotillomania consist of hair pulling, but denial of hair pulling and associated increased stress/anxiety.
- Trichotillomania causes uncontrollable hair pulling from anywhere on the body, though the scalp is the most common area followed by the eyelashes, eyebrows, pubic/perirectal area, axilla, and face.
- There are multiple subtypes of trichotillomania.
- Trichotillomania usually results in variable degrees of alopecia.
- When trichotillomania is associated with trichophagia, it may also result in GI complaints secondary to bezoars.

EPIDEMIOLOGY

- It is difficult to assess the exact number of individuals affected by trichotillomania due to the social stigma associated with it. Smaller studies have estimated a range of 1–3.5% of adolescents and young adults affected by it.
- It is possible that up to 1 out of 50 individuals are affected by trichotillomania at least once in their lifetime.
- According to DSM IV, the mean age of onset is at 13.
- During childhood, males and females are equally affected by trichotillomania. During adulthood, females are more affected than males.

RISK FACTORS

- Positive family history
- Other psychiatric disorders: Depression, obsessive–compulsive disorder, anxiety, PTSD, eating disorders, nail biting, skin picking

Genetics

There is no concrete evidence that genetics has a strong relationship with trichotillomania; however, it has been seen that individuals with a strong family history are predisposed to trichotillomania.

ETIOLOGY

- Serotonin deficiency
- Lenticular abnormalities
- Tension relief
- Habit

COMMONLY ASSOCIATED CONDITIONS

- Depression
- Anxiety
- Obsessive–compulsive disorder
- Eating disorders
- Posttraumatic stress disorder (PTSD)

DIAGNOSIS

Trichotillomania may be difficult to diagnose because individuals may deny it because of the social stigma and embarrassment (1).

HISTORY

- Trichotillomania most commonly manifests as hair pulling from any part of the body, resulting in alopecia of variable severity.
- The scalp is the most common area from which hair is pulled, but can also involve other parts of the body such as eyebrows and eyelashes.
- Individuals may deny the hair pulling because of embarrassment, making it hard to diagnose because the hair pulling may be done in private and is unwitnessed by others (2).
- Trichotillomania may also cause social isolation because individuals may withdraw from friends and family to engage in hair-pulling behavior.
- If trichotillomania is associated with trichophagia (compulsive eating of hair), it may present with various GI symptoms with variable severity, from acute generalized abdominal pain to a bowel obstruction picture secondary to a trichobezoar.
- Trichotillomania is not always associated with anxiety and stress, but it is commonly precipitated by highly stressful situations. The action of hair pulling may be associated with tension relief.

PHYSICAL EXAM

- The most common manifestation of trichotillomania is alopecia.
- The severity of the alopecia is variable, from isolated areas of hair loss to complete baldness.
- Hair loss can be from any part of the body.
- The Friar Tuck sign may be seen, which consists of hair loss seen in a circular pattern with varying lengths of broken hairs (1).
- There are also a lack of dermatologic abnormalities associated with the hair loss.
- In addition to the hair loss, hair abnormalities consisting of damaged hair follicles, broken hairs of varying lengths.
- When trichotillomania is associated with trichophagia and consequently, trichobezoars, which may cause symptoms of abdominal pain, nausea, vomiting, obstructive jaundice, bowel obstruction symptoms, and anemia (2)

DIAGNOSTIC TESTS & INTERPRETATION

Imaging

Ultrasound or CT scan for trichobezoar detection

Diagnostic Procedures/Surgery

- Trichotillomania Scale for Children
- Trichotillomania Diagnostic Interview
- National Institute of Mental Health Trichotillomania Questionnaire
- Premonitory Urge for Tics Scale (2)

Pathological Findings
- Punch biopsy: High frequency of telogen hairs; deformed, noninflamed catagen hairs; melanin pigment casts
- Trichogram

DIFFERENTIAL DIAGNOSIS
- Alopecia areata
- Tinea capitis
- Traction alopecia
- Loose anagen syndrome
- Obsessive–compulsive disorder
- Schizophrenia or other psychotic disorders
- Stereotypic movement disorders
- Factitious behaviors

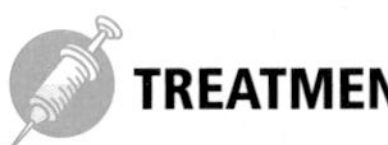

TREATMENT

Treatment of trichotillomania involves both pharmacologic treatment and psychological methods.

MEDICATION
First Line
SSRIs:
- Fluoxetine (Prozac): 20–80 mg/d
- Sertraline (Zoloft): 50–200 mg/d
- Paroxetine (Paxil): 10–50 mg/d
- Citalopram (Celexa): 20–60 mg/d
- Escitalopram (Lexapro): 10–20 mg/d

Second Line
- Tricyclic antidepressants
- Atypical neuroleptics
- Opioid blockers
- Glutamate modulators

ADDITIONAL TREATMENT
Psychological treatment of trichotillomania is needed in addition to pharmacologic treatment.

Additional Therapies
- Habit reversal training
- Competing reaction training
- Relaxation training
- Psychotherapy
- Hypnosis
- Treatment of comorbid psychiatric condition

SURGERY/OTHER PROCEDURES
Surgery is only warranted for removal of trichobezoars.

IN-PATIENT CONSIDERATIONS
Inpatient admission is usually not due to trichotillomania itself, but either treatment of comorbid psychiatric conditions or bowel obstruction picture secondary to trichobezoar.

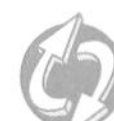

ONGOING CARE

DIET
No special diet required for trichotillomania

PATIENT EDUCATION
- Trichotillomania is a multifactorial condition. Not only do medications aid in the treatment of TTM, but psychological therapies have a benefit as well.
- Online resource: www.trich.org

PROGNOSIS
Trichotillomania tends to be a chronic disorder; however, trichotillomania can be transient in childhood.

COMPLICATIONS
- Trichobezoars
- Alopecia

REFERENCES

1. Springer K , Brown M, Stulberg DL, et al. Common hair loss disorders. *Am Fam Physician*. 2003;68: 93–102.
2. Franklin ME , Zagrabbe K, Benavides KL, et al. Trichotillomania and its treatment: A review and recommendations. *Expert Rev Neurother*. 2011;11: 1165–74.

ADDITIONAL READING

- Duke DC, Keeley ML, Geffken GR, et al. Trichotillomania: A current review. *Clin Psychol Rev*. 2010;30:181–93.
- Trichotillomania Learning Center: www.trich.org.

CODES

ICD9
312.39 Other disorders of impulse control

CLINICAL PEARLS

- Etiology of trichotillomania is multifactorial and differs among individuals. It is important to distinguish between different etiologies.
- Patients benefit from both medications and psychological therapy.
- It is important to realize that TTM is underreported and underdiagnosed because of the social stigma.

TRIGEMINAL NEURALGIA

Noah M. Rosenberg, MD
Stacy E. Potts, MD, MEd

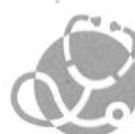

BASICS

DESCRIPTION

- Disorder of the sensory nucleus of the trigeminal nerve (cranial nerve [CN] V) that produces episodic, paroxysmal, severe, lancinating facial pain lasting seconds to minutes in the distribution of ≥1 divisions of the nerve
- Often precipitated by stimulation of well-defined, ipsilateral trigger zones: Usually perioral, perinasal, and occasionally intraoral (e.g., by washing, shaving)
- System(s) affected: Nervous
- Synonym(s): Tic douloureux; Fothergill neuralgia; Trifacial neuralgia; Prosopalgia

EPIDEMIOLOGY

Incidence

- 4.3 per 100,000 per year
- Women: 5.9 per 100,000 per year
- Men: 3.4 per 100,000 per year
- >70 years of age: ~25.6 per 100,000 per year
- Predominant age:
  - >50 years; incidence increases with age
  - Rare <35 years of age (consider another primary disease; see "Etiology").
- Predominant sex: Female > Male (~2:1)

Prevalence

16 per 100,000

Pediatric Considerations

Unusual during childhood

Pregnancy Considerations

Teratogenicity limits medical therapy during the first and second trimesters.

RISK FACTORS

Unknown

PATHOPHYSIOLOGY

- Demyelination around the compression site seems to be the mechanism by which compression of nerves leads to symptoms.
- Demyelinated lesions may set up an ectopic impulse generation causing erratic responses: Hyperexcitability of damaged nerves and transmission of action potentials along adjacent, undamaged, unstimulated sensory fibers.

ETIOLOGY

- Compression of trigeminal nerve by anomalous arteries or veins of posterior fossa, compressing trigeminal root
- Etiologic classification:
  - Idiopathic (classic)
  - Secondary: Cerebellopontine angle tumors (e.g., meningioma); tumors of CN V (e.g., neuroma, vascular malformations), trauma, demyelinating disease (e.g., multiple sclerosis [MS])

COMMONLY ASSOCIATED CONDITIONS

- Sjögren syndrome
- Rheumatoid arthritis
- Chronic meningitis
- Acute polyneuropathy
- MS
- Hemifacial spasm
- Charcot-Marie-Tooth neuropathy
- Glossopharyngeal neuralgia

DIAGNOSIS

HISTORY

Paroxysms of pain in the distribution of the trigeminal nerve

PHYSICAL EXAM

All exam findings typically are negative due to the paroxysmal nature of the disorder.

DIAGNOSTIC TESTS & INTERPRETATION

- The International Headache Society diagnostic criteria for classic trigeminal neuralgia:
  - Paroxysmal attacks of pain lasting from a fraction of 1 second to 2 minutes, affecting 1 or more divisions of the trigeminal nerve
  - Pain has at least an intense, sharp, superficial, or stabbing characteristic or is precipitated from trigger areas or by trigger factors.
  - Attacks are stereotyped in the individual patient.
  - There is no clinically evident neurologic deficit.
  - Not attributed to another disorder
- Secondary trigeminal neuralgia is characterized by pain that is indistinguishable from classic trigeminal neuralgia but is caused by a demonstrable structural lesion other than vascular compression.

Imaging

Indicated in all first-time presenting patients to rule out secondary causes

Initial approach

- MRI vs. CT scan: MRI with and without contrast offers more detailed imaging; preferred if not contraindicated
- Routine head imaging identifies structural causes in up to 15% of patients.
- No positive findings are significantly correlated with diagnosis.

Pathological Findings

- Trigeminal nerve: Inflammatory changes, demyelination, and degenerative changes
- Trigeminal ganglion: Hypermyelination and microneuromata

DIFFERENTIAL DIAGNOSIS

- Other forms of neuralgia usually have sensory loss. Presence of sensory loss nearly excludes the diagnosis of trigeminal neuralgia (if younger patient, frequently MS).
- Neoplasia in cerebellopontine angle
- Vascular malformation of brain stem
- Demyelinating lesion (MS is diagnosed in 2–4% of patients with trigeminal neuralgia)
- Vascular insult
- Migraine, cluster headache
- Giant cell arteritis
- Postherpetic neuralgia
- Chronic meningitis
- Acute polyneuropathy
- Atypical odontalgia
- SUNCT syndrome (short-lasting, unilateral, neuralgiform pain with conjunctival injection)

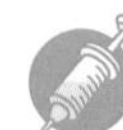

TREATMENT

MEDICATION

Persistent lack of randomized controlled trials regarding treatment of symptomatic trigeminal neuralgia (TN)

First Line

- Carbamazepine (Tegretol) (1)[A]: Start at 100–200 mg b.i.d.; effective dose usually 200 mg q.i.d.; maximum dose 1,200 mg/d:
  - 70–90% of patients respond initially.
  - By 3 years, 30% are no longer helped (number needed to treat [NNT] = 1.8) (1)[A].
  - Most common side effect: Sedation
- Contraindications: Concurrent use of monoamine oxidase inhibitors (MAOIs)
- Precautions: Caution in the presence of liver disease
- Significant possible medication interactions: macrolide antibiotics, oral anticoagulants, anticonvulsants, tricyclics, oral contraceptives, steroids, digitalis, isoniazid, MAOIs, methyprylon, nabilone, nizatidine, other H_2 blockers, phenytoin, propoxyphene, benzodiazepines, and calcium channel blockers
- Oxcarbazepine (Trileptal): Start at 150–300 mg b.i.d.; effective dose usually 375 mg b.i.d.; maximum dose 1,200 mg/d:
  - Efficacy similar to carbamazepine (1)[B],(2)[A]
  - Faster, with less drowsiness and fewer drug interactions than carbamazepine
  - Decreases serum sodium
  - Most common side effect: Sedation

Second Line

- Nonantiepileptics: Insufficient evidence from randomized controlled trials to show significant benefit from nonantiepileptic drugs in trigeminal neuralgia (3)[A]
- Phenytoin (Dilantin) 300–400 mg/d (synergistic with carbamazepine):
  - Potent P450 inducer (enhanced metabolism of many drugs)
  - Various CVS side effects (sedation, ataxia)
- Baclofen (Lioresal) 10–80 mg/d; start at 5–10 mg t.i.d. with food (as an adjunct to phenytoin or carbamazepine); side effects: drowsiness, weakness, nausea, vomiting
- Gabapentin (Neurontin): Start at 100 mg t.i.d. or 300 mg at bedtime; can increase dose up to 300–600 mg t.i.d.–q.i.d. Can be used as monotherapy or in combination with other medications and reduces the cost of illness.
- Lamotrigine: Titrate up to 200 mg b.i.d. over weeks; side effect: 10% experience rash
- Chlorphenesin carbamate (Maolate): 800–2,400 mg/d (as an adjunct to phenytoin and/or carbamazepine); side effect: Drowsiness
- Antidepressants, including amitriptyline, fluoxetine, trazodone:
  - Used especially with anticonvulsants
  - Particularly effective for atypical forms of trigeminal neuralgia

- Clonazepam (Klonopin) frequently causes drowsiness and ataxia.
- Sumatriptan (Imitrex) 3 mg SC reduces acute symptoms and may be helpful after failure of conventional medical therapy.
- Capsaicin cream topically
- Botulinum toxin injection into zygomatic arch
- Valproic acid (Depakene, Depakote)

ADDITIONAL TREATMENT

General Measures

- Outpatient
- Drug treatment is first approach.
- Invasive procedures are reserved for patients who cannot tolerate, fail to respond to, or relapse after chronic drug treatment.
- Avoid stimulation (e.g., air, heat, cold) of trigger zones, including lips, cheeks, and gums.

Issues for Referral

Initial treatment failure or positive findings on imaging studies

Additional Therapies

- Radiotherapy
- Stereotactic radiosurgery such as gamma knife radiosurgery has been shown to be effective after drug failure:
  - Produces lesions with focused gamma knife radiation
  - Therapy aimed at the proximal trigeminal root
  - Minimal clinically effective dose: 70 Gy
  - 75% of patients achieve complete relief within 3 months; by 3 years, 50% maintain complete relief (NNT = 2).
  - Most common side effect: Sensory disturbance (corneal numbness)
  - Viable treatment option for patients who have not had prior invasive procedures because rates of failure are higher in patients with past invasive procedures (4)

COMPLEMENTARY AND ALTERNATIVE MEDICINE

Acupuncture, moxibustion (herb): Poor evidence

SURGERY/OTHER PROCEDURES

- Microvascular decompression of CN V at its entrance to (or exit from) brain stem:
  - 98% of patients achieve initial pain relief; by 33 months, 73% maintain complete relief (NNT = 1.3).
  - Surgical mortality across studies was 0.3–0.4% (5)[B]
  - Most common side effect: Transient facial numbness and diplopia, headache, nausea, vomiting
  - Mean hospital stay was 3.4–4.3 days (5)
  - Pain relief after procedure strongly correlates with the type of TN pain: Type 1 (shocklike pain) results in better outcomes than type 2 (constant pain) (6).
- Peripheral nerve ablation (multiple methods):
  - Higher rates of failure and facial numbness than decompression surgery
  - Radiofrequency thermocoagulation
  - Neurectomy
  - Cryotherapy: High relapse rate
  - Partial sensory rhizotomy
- 4% tetracaine dissolved in 0.5% bupivacaine nerve block (only a few case reports to date; ropivacaine)
- Alcohol block or glycerol injection into trigeminal cistern: Unpredictable side effects (dysesthesia and anesthesia dolorosa); temporary relief
- Peripheral block or section of fifth nerve proximal to Gasserian ganglion
- Balloon compression of Gasserian ganglion
- The evidence supporting destructive procedures for benign pain conditions remains limited (7)[A].

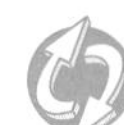

ONGOING CARE

FOLLOW-UP RECOMMENDATIONS

Regular outpatient follow-up to monitor symptoms and therapeutic failure

Patient Monitoring

- Carbamazepine and/or phenytoin serum levels
- If carbamazepine is prescribed: CBC and platelets at baseline, then weekly for a month, then monthly for 4 months, then every 6–12 months if dose is stable (regimens for monitoring vary)
- Reduce drugs after 4–6 weeks to determine whether condition is in remission; resume at previous dose if pain recurs. Withdraw drugs slowly after several months, again to check for remission or if lower dose of drugs can be tolerated.

DIET

No special diet

PATIENT EDUCATION

- Instruct patient regarding medication dosage and side effects, risk–benefit ratios of surgery or radiation therapy.
- After having microvascular decompression surgery, most patients wish they had undergone the procedure sooner (73%; NNT = 1.4) (8)[A].
- Trigeminal Neuralgia Association: www.endthepain.org

PROGNOSIS

- 50–60% eventually fail pharmacologic treatment (1)[B].
- Of those, relapse is seen in ~50% of stereotactic radiosurgeries and ~27% of surgical microvascular decompressions (1)[B].

COMPLICATIONS

- Mental and physical sluggishness; dizziness with carbamazepine (1)
- Paresthesias and corneal reflex loss with stereotactic radiosurgery
- Surgical mortality and morbidity associated with microvascular decompression

REFERENCES

1. Beniczky S, Tajti J, Tímea Varga E, et al. Evidence-based pharmacological treatment of neuropathic pain syndromes. *J Neural Transm*. 2005;112: 735–49.
2. Attal N, Cruccu G, Baron R, et al. EFNS guidelines on the pharmacological treatment of neuropathic pain: 2010 revision. *Eur J Neurol*. 2010;17: 1113–e88.
3. Yang M, Zhou M, He L, et al. Non-antiepileptic drugs for trigeminal neuralgia. *Cochrane Database Syst Rev*. 2011;1:CD004029.
4. Dhople AA, Adams JR, Maggio WW, et al. Long-term outcomes of Gamma Knife radiosurgery for classic trigeminal neuralgia: Implications of treatment and critical review of the literature. Clinical article. *J Neurosurg*. 2009;111:351–8.
5. Sekula RF, Frederickson AM, Jannetta PJ, et al. Microvascular decompression for elderly patients with trigeminal neuralgia: A prospective study and systematic review with meta-analysis. *J Neurosurg*. 2011;114:172–9.
6. Miller JP, Acar F, Burchiel KJ, et al. Classification of trigeminal neuralgia: Clinical, therapeutic, and prognostic implications in a series of 144 patients undergoing microvascular decompression. *J Neurosurg*. 2009;111:1231–4.
7. Zakrzewska JM, Akram H. Neurosurgical interventions for the treatment of classical trigeminal neuralgia. *Cochrane Database Syst Rev*. 2010;8:CD007312.
8. Cetas JS, Saedi T, Burchiel KJ. Destructive procedures for the treatment of nonmalignant pain: A structured literature review. *J Neurosurg*. 2008;109:389–404.

ADDITIONAL READING

- Borges A, Casselman J. Imaging the trigeminal nerve. *Eur J Radiol*. 2010;74:323–40.
- Gronseth G, Cruccu G, Alksne J, et al. Practice parameter: The diagnostic evaluation and treatment of trigeminal neuralgia (an evidence-based review): Report of the Quality Standards Subcommittee of the American Academy of Neurology and the European Federation of Neurological Societies. *Neurology*. 2008;71:1183–90.
- van Kleef M, van Genderen WM, Narouze S, et al. World Institute of Medicine. *Trigeminal Neuralgia Pain Pract*. 2009;9(4):252–9.

CODES

ICD9

350.1 Trigeminal neuralgia

CLINICAL PEARLS

- Patients with TN typically have a normal physical exam.
- The long-term efficacy of pharmacotherapy for TN is 40–50%.
- If pharmacotherapy fails, stereotactic radiosurgery or surgical microvascular decompression often is successful.

TRIGGER FINGER (DIGITAL STENOSING TENOSYNOVITIS)

Alan M. Ehrlich, MD
Robert A. Yood, MD

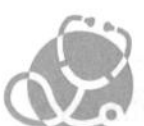

BASICS

DESCRIPTION
Trigger finger manifests in a clicking, snapping, or locking of a finger or thumb after full flexion ± associated pain.

EPIDEMIOLOGY
Incidence
- Adult population: 28/100,000/yr; rare in children
- Diabetics have up to 4 times the risk of the general population (1)[B].
- Predominant age:
  - Childhood form presents typically with thumb involvement in the first decade of life.
  - Adult form typically presents in the fifth and sixth decades of life.
- Predominant sex:
  - Children: Female = Male
  - Adults: Female > Male (6:1)

Prevalence
Lifetime prevalence in the general population is 2.6%.

Pediatric Considerations
- The thumb is more commonly involved in children (2)[C].
- When children have a trigger finger instead of a trigger thumb, surgery is often more complicated. Release of the A1 pulley alone is often insufficient, and other procedures may be necessary at the time of surgery.

RISK FACTORS
- Diabetes mellitus (DM)
- Rheumatoid arthritis (RA)
- Hypothyroidism
- Mucopolysaccharide disorders
- Amyloidosis

GENERAL PREVENTION
Most cases are idiopathic, and no known prevention exists. There is no clear association with repetitive movements.

PATHOPHYSIOLOGY
- Narrowing of the A1 pulley usually is due to either thickening from inflammation or protein deposits or thickening of the tendon per se; with prolonged inflammation, fibrocartilaginous metaplasia of the tendon sheath occurs.
- The flexor tendon may become distorted with nodule formation, which can give rise to the triggering because the nodule has difficulty passing through the area of narrowing. Because flexors are stronger than extensors, the finger can get stuck in the flexed position.

ETIOLOGY
- Most cases are idiopathic, and no known prevention exists.
- No clear association with repetitive movements

COMMONLY ASSOCIATED CONDITIONS
- De Quervain tenosynovitis
- Carpal tunnel syndrome
- Dupuytren contracture (usually occurs in fourth or fifth digit; thickening of palmar connective tissue results in a flexion contraction of the distal digit)
- DM
- RA
- Hypothyroidism
- Amyloidosis

DIAGNOSIS

Diagnosis is based on clinical presentation.

HISTORY
History of clicking, snapping, or locking of a finger or thumb after full flexion ± associated pain

PHYSICAL EXAM
- A palpable nodule may be present.
- Snapping or locking may be present, but neither is necessary for the diagnosis.
- Tenderness to palpation is variable.

DIAGNOSTIC TESTS & INTERPRETATION
Pathological Findings
- Thickening of the A1 pulley with fibrocartilaginous metaplasia
- Thickening or nodule formation of flexor tendon

ONGOING CARE

FOLLOW-UP RECOMMENDATIONS
- Follow-up is needed only if symptoms persist or if complications of surgery develop.
- Splinting of the affected digit to minimize flexion/extension of the MCP joint can lead to resolution of symptoms (1)[B],(3)[C].

PROGNOSIS
Prognosis for resolution of symptoms is excellent with either conservative or surgical intervention. Recurrence following corticosteroid injection is more likely for patients with type 1 DM, younger age, involvement of multiple digits, and history of other upper-extremity tendinopathies (4)[C].

COMPLICATIONS
- Complications from surgery include infection, bleeding, digital nerve injury, and persistent pain and loss of range of motion of the affected finger. The rate of major complications is low (3%) but the rate of minor complications (including loss of range of motion) can be significantly higher (up to 28%) (5).
- Injury to the A2 pulley may result in bowstringing, which is a bulging of the flexor tendon in the palm with flexion. This can be associated with pain.
- Diabetic patients may have significantly increased blood sugar levels for up to 5 days following steroid injection.

TREATMENT

- Splinting the metacarpophalangeal (MCP) joint at 10–15° of flexion for 6 weeks with the distal joints free to move has been reported to be effective. Splinting is more effective for treating fingers than thumbs (70% vs. 50%). This is less effective with severe symptoms, symptoms >6 months, and multiple digits involved (1)[B].
- Long-acting corticosteroids may be injected several times to achieve relief of symptoms, although subsequent injections often are less likely to work than the initial injection.

MEDICATION

First Line

Steroid injection of the tendon sheath or surrounding SC tissue has 57–90% success rate (4)[B],(6)[C]. Injection in surrounding tissues is as efficacious as injecting into the tendon sheath (1,7)[B]. Higher success rates are associated with a shorter duration of symptoms.

Second Line

NSAIDs may reduce pain and discomfort, but they have not been shown to improve the underlying cause. They do not reduce symptoms of snapping or locking.

ADDITIONAL TREATMENT

General Measures

Splinting or steroid injection should be tried before surgery.

Issues for Referral

Refer to a hand surgeon if the patient is not responding to splinting and/or steroid injections.

Additional Therapies

Physiotherapy has been used in the treatment of trigger digits in children.

SURGERY/OTHER PROCEDURES

- Surgical release can be done as an open procedure or percutaneously (8).
- Success rates with either procedure are very high (8).
- Most hand surgeons still prefer the open release because of concern about avoiding nerve injury with the blind procedure.

IN-PATIENT CONSIDERATIONS

Admission Criteria

Day surgery for trigger finger release

Discharge Criteria

Absence of complications

REFERENCES

1. Akhtar S, Bradley MJ, Quinton DN. Management and referral for trigger finger/thumb. *BMJ*. 2005;331:30–3.
2. Cardon LJ, Ezaki M, Carter PR. Trigger finger in children. *J Hand Surg*. 1999;24A:1156–61.
3. Ryzewicz M, Wolf JN. Trigger digits: Principles, management, and complications. *J Hand Surg*. 2006;31A:135–46.
4. Rozental TD, Zurakowski D, Blazar PE. Trigger finger: Prognostic indicators of recurrence following corticosteroid injection. *J Bone Joint Surg Am*. 2008;90:1665–72.
5. Will R, Lubahn J. Complications of open trigger finger release. *J Hand Surg Am*. 2010;35(4):594–6.
6. Fleisch SB, Spindler KP, Lee DH. Corticosteroid injections in the treatment of trigger finger: A level I and II systematic review. *J Am Acad Orthop Surg*. 2007;15:166–71.
7. Kazuki K, Egi T, Okada M. Clinical outcome of extrasynovial steroid injection for trigger finger. *Hand Surg*. 2006;11:1–4.
8. Bamroongshawgasame T. A comparison of open and percutaneous pulley release in trigger digits. *J Med Assoc Thai*. 2010;93:199–204.

ADDITIONAL READING

Moore JS. Flexor tendon entrapment of the digits (trigger finger and trigger thumb). *J Occup Environ Med*. 2000;42:5.

CODES

ICD9

727.03 Trigger finger (acquired)

CLINICAL PEARLS

- This condition is narrowing of the A1 pulley usually due to either thickening from inflammation or protein deposits or thickening of the tendon per se; with prolonged inflammation, fibrocartilaginous metaplasia of the tendon sheath occurs.
- Splinting the MCP joint at 10–15° flexion for 6 weeks with the distal joints free to move has been reported to be effective. Splinting is more effective for treating fingers than thumbs (70% vs. 50%). This is less effective with severe symptoms, symptoms >6 months, and multiple digits involved (1)[B].
- Long-acting corticosteroids may be injected several times to achieve the relief of symptoms, although subsequent injections often are less likely to work than the initial injection.
- Both open and percutaneous surgery have high success rates with a low risk of complications (8).
- Most hand surgeons still prefer the open release because of concern about avoiding nerve injury with the blind procedure.

TROCHANTERIC BURSITIS (GREATER TROCHANTERIC PAIN SYNDROME)

David W. Kruse, MD
Mohammad Shahsahebi, MD

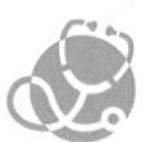

BASICS

The name *trochanteric bursitis* has been used in the historical literature to refer to pain at the lateral hip with tenderness over the greater trochanter. As more continues to be understood about potential sources of pain at the lateral hip and the discovery that many patients lack an inflammatory process, this condition has been referred to as *greater trochanteric pain syndrome* (GTPS) in the more recent literature (1).

DESCRIPTION

- Bursae are fluid-filled sacs that are found at bony protuberances, typically at tendon attachment sites. Multiple bursae are described in the area of the greater trochanter of the femur. These bursae correspond to the tendons of the gluteus muscles, iliotibial band (ITB), and tensor fasciae latae. The subgluteus maximus bursa is implicated most commonly in lateral hip pain (1).
- Other structures that surround the lateral hip include the ITB, tensor fasciae latae, gluteus maximus tendon, gluteus medius tendon, gluteus minimus tendon, quadratus femoris muscle, vastus lateralis tendon, and piriformis tendon.
- *Bursitis* refers to inflammation of the bursa.
- *Tendinopathy* refers to any abnormality of a tendon, inflammatory or degenerative.

EPIDEMIOLOGY

Incidence

- In primary-care setting: 1.8 patients/1,000 persons/yr
- Predominant age: All ages; peak incidence in fourth to sixth decades

Prevalence

- Predominant sex: Female > Male
- Sports:
  - Running
  - Contact sports: Football, rugby, soccer

RISK FACTORS

Multiple factors have been implicated (1,2):

- Female
- Obesity
- Tight hip musculature or ITB
- Direct trauma
- Total hip arthroplasty
- Abnormal biomechanics or gait:
  - Leg-length discrepancy
  - Sacroiliac (SI) joint dysfunction
  - Knee or hip osteoarthritis
  - Abnormal foot mechanics (e.g., pes planus, overpronation)
  - Neuromuscular disorder

Genetics

No known genetic factors

GENERAL PREVENTION

- Maintain ITB, hip, and lower-back flexibility and strength.
- Avoid direct trauma (use of appropriate padding in contact sports).
- Avoid banked running.
- Appropriate shoe wear
- Weight loss, if appropriate

PATHOPHYSIOLOGY

- Acute: Abnormal gait or poor muscle flexibility and strength lead to:
  - Friction on bursa, causing inflammatory response
  - Tendon overuse and inflammation
  - Direct trauma from contact or frequently lying with body weight on hip can cause an inflammatory response.
- Chronic:
  - Fibrosis and thickening of bursal sac due to chronic inflammatory process
  - Tendinopathy due to chronic overuse and degeneration: Gluteus medius and minimus (1)

ETIOLOGY

See "Risk Factors" and "Pathophysiology" sections.

COMMONLY ASSOCIATED CONDITIONS

- Many biomechanical factors can be associated with this condition (1):
  - Tight ITBs
  - Leg-length discrepancy
  - SI joint dysfunction
  - Pes planus
- Other associated pathology (1):
  - Low-back pain
  - Knee and hip osteoarthritis
  - Obesity

DIAGNOSIS

HISTORY

General historical points on presentation (1)[C]:

- Pain localized to the lateral aspect of the hip or buttock
- May radiate to groin or lateral thigh (pseudoradiculopathy)
- Exacerbated by:
  - Prolonged walking or standing
  - Rising after prolonged sitting
  - Sitting with legs crossed
  - Lying on affected side
- Other possible points:
  - Direct trauma to affected hip
  - Chronic low-back pain
  - Chronic leg/knee/ankle/hip pain
  - Recent increase in running distance or intensity
  - Change in running surfaces

PHYSICAL EXAM

- Point tenderness with direct palpation over the lateral hip is the most characteristic sign for GTPS (1)[B].
- Other exam tests have been described but lack sensitivity (1)[B]:
  - May have pain with extremes of passive rotation, abduction, or adduction
  - Pain with resisted hip abduction and external or internal rotation
  - Trendelenburg sign
- Other testing to evaluate for associated conditions:
  - Positive Patrick-FABERE (flexion, abduction, external rotation, extension) testing for SI joint dysfunction
  - Ober test for ITB pathology
  - Flexion and extension of hip for osteoarthritis
  - Leg-length measurement
  - Foot inspection for pes planus or overpronation
  - Lower extremity neurologic assessment for lumbar radiculopathy or neuromuscular disorders

DIAGNOSTIC TESTS & INTERPRETATION

Lab

No routine lab testing is recommended.

Follow-Up & Special Considerations

If there is a concern for a septic bursitis, then aspiration or incision and drainage may be necessary.

Imaging

Diagnosis can be made by history and exam, but radiologic imaging can be helpful to evaluate for other associated conditions.

Initial approach

If imaging is ordered:

- Anteroposterior and frog-leg views of affected hip
- Consider lumbar spine radiographs if back pain is thought to be a contributing factor.
- Musculoskeletal ultrasound also can provide accurate imaging of potential pathology.

Follow-Up & Special Considerations

Advanced imaging rarely necessary; detection of abnormalities on MRI is a poor predictor of GTPS (3)[B].

DIFFERENTIAL DIAGNOSIS

Multiple conditions should be considered (1)[C]:

- ITB syndrome
- Gluteus medius or minimus tendinopathy
- Osteoarthritis or avascular necrosis of the hip
- Lumbosacral osteoarthritis/disc disease causing nerve root compression
- If associated trauma: Fracture or contusion of the hip or pelvis
- Stress reaction/fracture of femoral neck, especially in female runners
- Septic bursitis/arthritis

TREATMENT

- Weight loss (if applicable)
- Minimize aggravating activities such as prolonged walking or standing.
- Avoid lying on affected side.
- Runners:
  - May need to decrease distance and/or intensity of runs
  - May need a period of cessation of running
  - Should avoid banked tracks or roads with excessive tilt

MEDICATION

- NSAIDs (1)[B]:
  - Naprosyn 500 mg PO b.i.d.
  - Ibuprofen 800 mg PO t.i.d.
- Corticosteroid injection is effective for pain relief (4)[C]. In certain cases, injection can be considered first-line therapy:
  - Dexamethasone 4 mg/mL *or*
  - Kenalog 40 mg/mL 1–2 mL
  - Consider adding a local anesthetic (short- and/or long-acting) for more immediate pain relief.
  - Can be repeated for recurrence with similar effect if original treatment showed a strong response

ADDITIONAL TREATMENT

Issues for Referral

- Septic bursitis
- Recalcitrant bursitis

Additional Therapies

- Ice
- Physical therapy to address underlying dysfunction and rebuild atrophic muscle mass
- Focus on achieving flexibility of hip musculature, particularly the ITB.
- Correct pelvic/hip instability.
- Correct lower limb biomechanics.
- Address contributing factors:
  - Low-back flexibility
  - If leg-length discrepancy, may need heel lift
  - If pes planus or overpronation, may need arch supports or custom orthotics

COMPLEMENTARY AND ALTERNATIVE MEDICINE

Other techniques have been described for the treatment of chronic fibrosis and tendinopathy and may play a role in the treatment of GTPS. These include acupuncture, prolotherapy, growth factor injection techniques, and low-energy extracorporeal shock wave therapy.

SURGERY/OTHER PROCEDURES

- Rarely requires surgery
- If surgery is indicated, potential options include:
  - Arthroscopic bursectomy (5,6)[B]
  - Release of the ITB

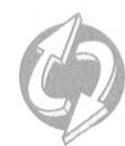

ONGOING CARE

FOLLOW-UP RECOMMENDATIONS

4 weeks posttreatment, sooner if significant worsening

PATIENT EDUCATION

- Avoid lying on affected side.
- Minimize prolonged standing or walking.
- Maintain hip musculature flexibility, including ITB.
- Correct issues that may cause abnormal gait:
  - Low back pain
  - Knee pain
  - Leg-length discrepancy
  - Foot mechanics
- Gradual return to physical activity

PROGNOSIS

Depends on chronicity and recurrence, with more acute cases having an excellent prognosis

COMPLICATIONS

Bursal thickening and fibrosis

REFERENCES

1. Williams BS, Cohen SP. Greater trochanteric pain syndrome: A review of anatomy, diagnosis and treatment. *Anesth Analg*. 2009;108:1662–70.
2. Farmer KW, Jones LC, Brownson KE, et al. Trochanteric bursitis after total hip arthroplasty: Incidence and evaluation of response to treatment. *J Arthroplasty*. 2010;25:208–12.
3. Blankenbaker DG, Ullrick SR, Davis KW, et al. Correlation of MRI findings with clinical findings of trochanteric pain syndrome. *Skeletal Radiol*. 2008;37(10):903–9.
4. Stephens MB, Beutler AI, O'Connor FG. Musculoskeletal injections: A review of the evidence. *Am Fam Physician*. 2008;78:971–6.
5. Baker CL, Massie RV, Hurt WG, et al. Arthroscopic bursectomy for recalcitrant trochanteric bursitis. *Arthroscopy*. 2007;23:827–32.
6. Pretell J, Ortega J, García-Rayo R, et al. Distal fascia lata lengthening: An alternative surgical technique for recalcitrant trochanteric bursitis. *Int Orthop*. 2009;33:1223–7.

CODES

ICD9

726.5 Enthesopathy of hip region

CLINICAL PEARLS

- One of the most common complaints from a patient with GTPS is inability to lie on the affected side.
- Thorough knowledge of associated conditions ensures accurate diagnosis and effective treatment.
- Corticosteroid injection can be considered first-line therapy for some patients.
- Aggressive use of physical therapy in treatment to address underlying dysfunction and rebuild weakened muscle mass

TUBERCULOSIS

Swati B. Avashia, MD

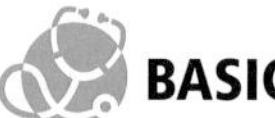

BASICS

DESCRIPTION

- Usually contracted from a person with active TB by inhalation of airborne bacilli. Bacilli multiply in alveoli and are carried by macrophages, lymphatics, and blood to distant sites. 3 possible outcomes:
  - Eradication: Tissue hypersensitivity halts the infection within 10 weeks.
  - Primary infection: Disease from initial infection
  - Latent infection: Asymptomatic with positive PPD, negative chest radiograph, noninfectious
- Active tuberculosis:
  - Develops from primary infection or reactivation of latent infection
  - Occurs in 10% of infected individuals without preventive therapy
  - Risk increases with immunosuppression and is highest the first 2 years after infection
  - Well-described forms: Miliary (disseminated), meningeal, abdominal, and pulmonary:
    - 85% of cases are pulmonary, which are contagious.
    - Abdominal TB more common in the third or fourth decade in women

Pediatric Considerations

- Disseminated TB is more common in infants; treat with 4 drugs.
- Children <4 are at increased risk for disseminated TB (lower-lobe infections more common); also more likely to have immediate clinical or radiographic signs.
- Older children and adolescents develop upper-lobe infiltrations; can have recurrence in adulthood.

EPIDEMIOLOGY

Incidence

TB incidence in 2008: US 4.2/100,000; worldwide 139/100,000 (1,2)

Prevalence

- 1/3 of world's population infected with latent TB
- 2 million people worldwide die each year from TB (1).

RISK FACTORS

- For infection:
  - Homeless, minority, residents and employees in institutionalized settings; close contact with infected individual; persons from areas with a high incidence of active tuberculosis (Asia, Africa, Latin America, former Soviet Union states); health care workers; frequent or prolonged visits to areas with a high prevalence of TB; and populations with locally increased incidence (e.g., medically underserved, low income, substance abusers)
- For development of disease once infected:
  - HIV; lymphoma; silicosis; diabetes mellitus; chronic renal failure; cancer of head, neck, or lung; children <5 years of age; malnutrition; systemic corticosteroids, immunosuppressive drugs; IV drug abuse, alcohol abuse, cigarette smokers; <2 years since infection with *M. tuberculosis*; history of gastrectomy or jejunal bypass; <90% of ideal body weight

GENERAL PREVENTION

- Treat latent TB infection.
- Report to health department for treatment, identification, and testing of all close contacts.
- Bacille Calmette Guérin (BCG) vaccine: Live attenuated *Mycobacterium bovis:*
  - Used more in countries with endemic TB
  - Prevents 50% of pulmonary disease; 80% of meningitis and miliary disease in children
  - In the US, consider BCG for children with negative PPD and HIV tests with unavoidable high risk and for health care workers at high risk for drug-resistant infection.

PATHOPHYSIOLOGY

- Cell-mediated response by the body causes accumulation of activated T lymphocytes and macrophages to form a "granuloma" that limits replication of organism. Destruction of the macrophages produces early "solid necrosis." In 2–3 weeks, "caseous necrosis" develops, establishing latency.
- In people with intact immunity, granuloma undergoes "fibrosis" and calcification; in people with less effective immune systems, primary progressive tuberculosis develops.

ETIOLOGY

Mycobacterium tuberculosis, M. bovis, or *M. africanum*

COMMONLY ASSOCIATED CONDITIONS

HIV infection (emphasize direct observed therapy [DOT]); most recommendations remain the same

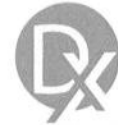

DIAGNOSIS

HISTORY

- Known exposure
- HIV status/risk factors
- Signs and symptoms:
  - General: Fever, night sweats, weight loss, malaise, painless adenopathy
  - Pulmonary TB: Cough, hemoptysis, pleuritic chest pain
  - Abdominal TB: Acute presentation often as surgical emergencies, such as peritonitis or acute abdomen, obstruction, or perforation; chronic presentation may be doughy abdomen, vague abdominal symptoms, abdominal mass
  - Meningitis: See "Tuberculosis, CNS."
  - Miliary: See "Tuberculosis, Miliary."

PHYSICAL EXAM

- Often entirely normal; specific findings vary based on organ involvement and might include adenopathy, rales on lung exam, or hepatosplenomegaly
- Late findings: Renal, bone, or CNS disease

DIAGNOSTIC TESTS & INTERPRETATION

Lab

Initial lab tests

- Persons with TB should be tested for HIV; if positive, get CD4 count at baseline.
- Baseline CBC, creatinine, AST, ALT, bilirubin, alkaline phosphatase, visual acuity, and red–green color discrimination
- If high risk: Test for hepatitis B and C (injection drug users, Africa or Asia born, HIV infected).
- If extrapulmonary suspected: Urine, CSF, bone marrow, and liver biopsy for culture as indicated

Follow-Up & Special Considerations

Nonspecific laboratory findings include:

- Anemia, monocytosis, thrombocytosis, hypergammaglobulinemia, SIADH, sterile pyuria

Imaging

Initial approach

- Chest radiograph:
  - With primary TB: Infiltrate with or without effusion, atelectasis, or adenopathy
  - With recrudescent TB: Cavitary lesions and upper-lobe disease with hilar adenopathy
  - HIV: Atypical findings with primary infection, right upper-lobe atelectasis
- CT chest: Good sensitivity

Diagnostic Procedures/Surgery

- Tuberculin skin test (TST) (e.g., PPD): 5 U (0.1 mL) intermediate-strength intradermal injection into volar forearm. Measure induration at 48–72 hours:
  - PPD positive if induration:
    - >5 mm and HIV infection, immunosuppressed, recent TB contact, evidence of disease on chest film
    - >10 mm and age <4 years or other risk factors
    - >15 mm and age >4 years and no risk factors
    - 2-step test if no recent PPD, age >55, nursing home resident, prison inmate, or health care worker. Place second test 1–3 weeks after initial test; interpret as usual.
  - Treatments that may alter PPD results:
    - False positive: Steroids or BCG (unreliable, should not affect decision to treat)
    - False negative: HIV, gastrectomy, alcoholism, renal failure, sarcoidosis, malnutrition, hematologic or lymphoreticular disorder
- 3 different morning sputum samples for acid-fast bacilli (AFB) stain and culture; use aerosol induction, gastric aspirate (children), or bronchoalveolar lavage if needed:
  - If positive AFB, begin treatment immediately. Culture and sensitivity guide treatment.
- Interferon gamma release assays (IGRAs) measure interferon release after stimulation in vitro by *M. tuberculosis* antigens (3):
  - Lack of cross-reaction with BCG and most nontuberculous mycobacteria:
    - Preferred for testing persons who have had BCG (vaccine or for cancer therapy)
  - Can be used in all settings in which skin testing is recommended with exceptions below:
    - TST is preferred in children <5 years old.

Pathological Findings

- AFB stains: Positive
- Biopsy: Granulomas with central caseating necrosis

DIFFERENTIAL DIAGNOSIS

Other pneumonias, malignancies, fungal infections, other atypical *Mycobacteria* or *Nocardia*

TREATMENT

MEDICATION

- Ideal body weight should be used to dose antitubercular drugs.
- DOT required for children, institutionalized patients, risk for nonadherence, and nondaily regimens. DOT strongly recommended for all regimens.

First Line

- Regimen 1 (preferred) (4):
  - Initial phase:
    - Isoniazid (INH) 5 mg/kg, rifampin (RIF) 10 mg/kg, pyrazinamide (PZA) 15–30 mg/kg, and ethambutol (EMB) 15–20 mg/kg once daily for 8 weeks
    - OR, INH/RIF/PZA/EMB 5 days/wk for 8 weeks
  - Continuation phase:
    - INH/RIF daily for 18 weeks; or, if DOT, INH/RIF 5 days/wk for 18 weeks (recommended for HIV + with CD4 <100 cells/mm^3 due to increased risk of resistance)
    - Or, INH/RIF 2–3 times a week for 18 weeks (not recommended if HIV+ with CD4 <100; may be associated with increased risk of relapse)
    - Or INH/rifapentine once weekly for 18 weeks (acceptable alternative only for HIV– patients without cavitary disease but may have increase risk of relapse) (4)
- Regimen 2:
  - Initial phase:
    - INH/RIF/PZA/EMB daily for 2 weeks then twice weekly for 6 weeks
    - OR INH/RIF/PZA/EMB 5 days/wk for 2 weeks then twice weekly for 6 weeks
  - Continuation phase:
    - INH/RIF 2–3 times a week for 18 weeks (not recommended if HIV+ with CD4 <100; may have increased risk of relapse)
    - Or INH/rifapentine once weekly for 18 weeks (acceptable alternative only for HIV– patients without cavitary disease; may have increase risk of relapse) (4)
    - Treat TB in pregnancy with INH, RIF, and EMB; supplement with pyridoxine 25 mg/d.

Pregnancy Considerations

Streptomycin: Caution—ototoxic and nephrotoxic; do not use in pregnancy. Pyrazinamide is not usually used in pregnant women in the US.

- Congenital infection: May occur with maternal miliary or endometrial TB. If suspected, get PPD, CXR, lumbar puncture, and culture placenta. Start treatment promptly.
- Breast-feeding: OK while taking TB drugs; supplement with pyridoxine 25 mg/d
- Children: Ethambutol is not used:
  - Children on medication may attend school.
  - Maximum drug doses: INH 300 mg daily or 900 mg 2–3 times/wk, RIF 600 mg all regimens, PZA 2,000 mg daily or 4,000 mg 2 times/wk, EMB, 600 mg daily or 4,000 mg 2 times/wk

ALERT

- If patient doesn't receive PZA during entire first 2 months, extend treatment to 9 months.
- *M. bovis* is resistant to PZA, must be treated 9 months
- Continue EMB until determine drug susceptibility to INH+RIF

Second Line

Steroids: Recommended for TB meningitis or pericarditis, use only with concomitant anti-TB therapy (5)[B].

ADDITIONAL TREATMENT

General Measures

- If clinical suspicion, treat immediately
- Prescribing physician responsible for treatment completion
- Ambulatory patients use mask and tissues
- Not infectious if favorable clinical response after 2–3 weeks of therapy and 3 negative AFB smears

Issues for Referral

ALERT

Refer drug-resistant TB and HIV+ patients on antiretroviral therapy.

COMPLEMENTARY AND ALTERNATIVE MEDICINE

Vitamin D deficiency may increase susceptibility to tuberculosis and conversion from latent to active tuberculosis. Supplementation may be beneficial in infected individuals with insufficient levels of vitamin D (6).

SURGERY/OTHER PROCEDURES

For extrapulmonary complications (e.g., spinal cord compression, intestinal obstruction, constrictive pericarditis)

IN-PATIENT CONSIDERATIONS

- Place in an airborne infection isolation.
- Use personal sealed respirators.
- 3 negative sputum AFB smears from different days for release from isolation

Discharge Criteria

Once the diagnosis of TB is ruled out or when the patient is being treated and has met the following:

- The patient is on effective therapy and making clinical improvement.
- An outpatient appointment has been arranged with a provider who will manage TB.
- Case management from the local public health department is involved and agrees with plan.
- The patient is in possession of sufficient anti-TB medication (not just prescriptions) to last until outpatient appointment.

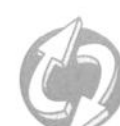

ONGOING CARE

FOLLOW-UP RECOMMENDATIONS

Patient Monitoring

- Assess monthly for treatment adherence and adverse effects.
- HIV+ need labs every 1–3 months: CD4 count, CBC, and liver enzymes
- Liver enzymes monthly if chronic liver disease, alcohol use, pregnant, or postpartum. Temporarily discontinue medications if asymptomatic and enzymes are ≥5 times normal or if symptomatic and enzymes as ≥3 times normal.
- Visual acuity and red–green color discrimination monthly if on ethambutol more than 2 months or doses >20 mg/kg/d
- If culture is positive after 2 months of therapy, reassess drug sensitivity and initiate DOT.
- Chest radiograph at 3 months

PATIENT EDUCATION

- Emphasize importance of adherence to drug therapy.
- Identify patient contacts to notify.
- Let patient know that you are obligated to inform the local health department.
- CDC Questions and Answers about TB, 2009. Available at: www.cdc.gov/tb/publications/faqs/default.htm

PROGNOSIS

Generally few complications and full resolution of infection if drugs taken for full course as prescribed. If untreated, can lead to multiple complications, including death.

COMPLICATIONS

- Cavitary lesions can become secondarily infected.
- Drug resistance declining in the US. At risk for drug resistance if HIV+, or treatment taken improperly, or if from an area with high incidence of resistance.

REFERENCES

1. Global Tuberculosis Control: A short update to the 2009 report. WHO; 2009.
2. Pratt R, Robinson V, Navin T. Trends in tuberculosis 2008. *MMWR*. 2009;58(10):249–53.
3. Mazurek GH, Jereb J, Vernon A, et al. Updated Guidelines for using interferon gama release assays to detect *Mycobacterium tuberculosis* infection–United States. *MMWR Recomm Rep*. 2010;59(RR05):1–25.
4. Hall RG, Leff RD, Gumbo T. Treatment of active pulmonary tuberculosis in adults: Current standrads and recent advances. *Pharmacotherapy*. 2009;29(12):1468–81.
5. Golden MP, Vikram HR. Extrapulmonary tuberculosis: An overview. *Am Fam Physician*. 2005;72:1761–8.
6. Luong KVQ, Nguyen LTH. Impact of vitamin D in the treatment of tuberculosis. *Am J Med Sci*. 2011;341(6):493–8.
7. Jacob JT, Mehta AK, Leonard MK. Acute forms of tuberculosis in adults. *Am J Med*. 2009;122:12–7.

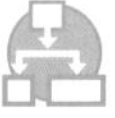

See Also (Topic, Algorithm, Electronic Media Element)

- Tuberculosis, CNS; Tuberculosis, Latent; Tuberculosis, Miliary
- Algorithm: Weight Loss

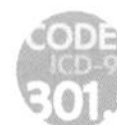

CODES

ICD9

- 011.90 Unspecified pulmonary tuberculosis, confirmation unspecified
- 018.90 Miliary tuberculosis, unspecified, unspecified
- 795.51 Nonspecific reaction to tuberculin skin test without active tuberculosis

CLINICAL PEARLS

- Have high suspicion for TB in patients with chronic cough and 1 additional risk factor
- Patients ≥65 have few classic clinical and laboratory features of TB.
- Consider acute TB in critically ill patients with enigmatic acute respiratory distress syndrome, shock, or disseminated intravascular coagulation (7).

TUBERCULOSIS, CNS

Raul Davaro, MD
Sumanth Gandra, MD, MPH

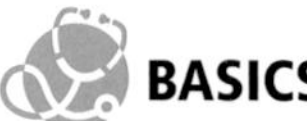

BASICS

DESCRIPTION

- Tuberculosis (TB) of the CNS is a granulomatous infection of the brain, meninges, or spinal cord caused by *Mycobacterium tuberculosis* (1).
- Includes tuberculous meningitis, intracranial or spinal tuberculoma, and spinal tuberculous arachnoiditis

EPIDEMIOLOGY

Incidence

- US: Incidence of TB is 3.6/100,000
- CNS TB accounts for 1% of all TB, but kills and disables more than any other type of TB (1).

Prevalence

Over 9 million cases of active tuberculosis annually worldwide

RISK FACTORS

- Very young or old, HIV-infected, diabetics, treatment with steroids or other immunosuppressive agent
- History of pulmonary TB or exposure
- Malnutrition, recent measles in children, alcoholism, malignancies
- Latent TB infection
- Immigrants from TB-endemic areas

Genetics

TB meningitis development is influenced by host factors: Polymorphisms of toll-like receptors and the *Mycobacterium* tuberculosis genotype.

GENERAL PREVENTION

- Direct observed antitubercular therapy to improve treatment success and minimize drug resistance
- Childhood BCG vaccination in areas with high incidence of tuberculosis disease may protect against tuberculous meningitis (TBM) (2)[B].

PATHOPHYSIOLOGY

Spreads hematogenously to the CNS, generally from a pulmonary focus

ETIOLOGY

M. tuberculosis: History elicited in only 10% of infected adults

COMMONLY ASSOCIATED CONDITIONS

HIV infection

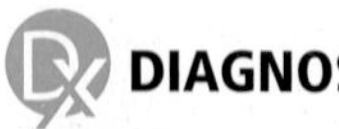

DIAGNOSIS

HISTORY

- Malaise, fever, headache, vomiting
- Confusion, seizures, altered mental status

PHYSICAL EXAM

- Neurologic exam:
  - Meningismus
  - Confusion/lethargy
  - CN palsy
  - Coma
  - Hemiparesis
- Signs of extracranial TB
- Meningitis: 3 phases:
  - Prodrome: 2–3 weeks of malaise, headache, low-grade fever
  - Meningitic: Headache, vomiting, lethargy, CN, and long-tract signs
  - Paralytic: May accelerate rapidly; confusion developing into stupor and coma, seizure, hemiparesis
- Untreated, will result in death in 5–8 weeks of illness onset

DIAGNOSTIC TESTS & INTERPRETATION

Lab

Initial lab tests

- CSF examination
- Purified protein derivative tuberculin skin test may be of limited value in many patients because active TB infection may suppress reactivity (anergy).

Follow-Up & Special Considerations

Drugs that may alter lab results:

- Steroids may alter CSF and give false-negative skin test results.
- Antituberculous therapy

Imaging

Initial approach

- CXR: Active TB is found on 30–50% patients.
- CT scan of head with contrast material:
  - Hydrocephalus
  - Tuberculomas
  - Cerebral edema
  - Basilar meningeal involvement
  - Response to treatment
  - Normal in 30% of stage I meningitis patients, especially the elderly
  - CT evidence of basilar meningeal enhancement and hydrocephalus is strongly suggestive of TBM.
- MRI:
  - In tuberculous meningitis, contrast-enhanced MRI is more sensitive in demonstrating early infarcts or brain stem, midbrain, and basal ganglion lesions than CT scan.
  - Solid tuberculomas are seen as round/lobulated masses with irregular walls, homogeneous/ring-enhancing lesions; typically found in the frontal/parietal lobes, with the magnitude of surrounding edema inversely proportional to the age of the lesion.

Diagnostic Procedures/Surgery

- Lumbar puncture:
  - CSF study in tuberculous meningitis:
    - Moderate elevation in protein (100–500 mg/dL usually, but may increase to 2–6 g/dL)
    - Lymphocytic predominance
    - Low glucose: <45 mg/dL in 80% of patients
    - Cell count 100–500/μL
    - Nucleic acid amplification of CSF has a sensitivity of 56% and a specificity of 98%.
    - Tubercle bacilli found on direct smear in 20% depending on specimen quality and quantity
    - Large volumes of CSF increase the diagnostic yield for smear and nucleic acid amplification.
    - Cultures grow in 4–8 weeks, but DNA probes may provide preliminary identification better than cultures.
  - CSF study in tuberculomas: Isolated from subarachnoid space due to thick capsule, so rarely are CSF changes seen
- Biopsy: CT-guided stereotactic brain biopsy is helpful in differentiating tuberculomas from other space-occupying lesions.

Pathological Findings

- In tuberculous meningitis:
  - Thick tubercular exudates seen in the basal cisterns and sylvian fissures
  - Hydrocephalus common
  - Exudates in basal cisterns compress vessels, with subsequent ischemia
- In tuberculoma:
  - Well-defined avascular lesions composed of a necrotic caseous center surrounded by tuberculous granulation tissue; TB bacilli can be present in this granulation tissue
  - Surrounding brain shows edema.
  - Occurs at any site; may adhere to dura
  - Usually solitary lesions

DIFFERENTIAL DIAGNOSIS

- Tuberculous meningitis:
  - Meningitis (e.g., chronic, viral, fungal, bacterial, carcinomatous)
  - Sarcoidosis, lymphoma, viral encephalitis
- Intracranial tuberculoma:
  - Granulomas (e.g., sarcoid, fungal)
  - Pyogenic abscess, metastasis, glioma
- Spinal tuberculoma:
  - Intramedullary tumors, syringomyelia, spinal abscess, myelitis

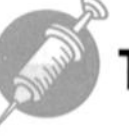

TREATMENT

- An early diagnosis before the onset of coma and neurologic deficits is the greatest contribution in improving the outcome of patients with CNS TB.
- Treatment must be started empirically if clinical suspicion is high.

MEDICATION

First Line

- **Antituberculous medications:**
  - Isoniazid (INH): Adults: 5 mg/kg/d PO or IM (maximum 300 mg/d); children: 10–15 mg/kg/d PO or IM (maximum 300 mg/d)
  - Rifampin (RIF): Adults: 10 mg/kg/d PO or IV (maximum 600 mg/d); children: 10–20 mg/kg/d PO or IV (maximum 600 mg/d)
  - Ethambutol (EMB): Adults: Body weight (BW) 40–55 kg: 800 mg/d PO; BW 56–75 kg: 1,200 mg/d PO; BW 76–90 kg: 1,600 mg/d PO; children: 15–20 mg/kg/d (maximum 1,000 mg/d)

- Pyrazinamide (PZA): Adults: BW 40–55 kg: 1,000 mg/d PO; BW 56–75 kg: 1,500 mg/d PO; BW 76–90 kg: 2,000 mg/d PO; children: 15–30 mg/kg/d (maximum 2,000 mg/d)
- Usual regimen: INH + RIF + EMB + PZA for 2 months, followed by INH + RIF for 7–10 months

- Corticosteroids:
  - Steroids are recommended for patients with meningitis (3)[A] or tuberculoma, or those whose diagnosis is inconclusive.
  - Dexamethasone dosing (IV or PO):
    - Adults and children >25 kg: 12 mg/d
    - Children <25 kg: 8 mg/d
  - Continue full-dose steroids for 3 weeks, followed by taper over 3 more weeks.
- Anticonvulsants:
  - High incidence of seizures in tuberculomas requires the routine use of anticonvulsants.
- Diuretics:
  - Furosemide or acetazolamide used for communicating hydrocephalus (4)[C]
- Contraindications:
  - INH: Acute liver disease, previous INH-associated hepatitis
  - RIF: Concomitant use of some HIV antiretrovirals (may need to change antiretrovirals), hypersensitivity to RIF
  - EMB: Optic neuritis, patients unable to report visual adverse effects (e.g., young children)
  - PZA: Severe hepatic dysfunction
- Side effects:
  - INH: Peripheral neuropathy, rash, abnormal LFTs, psychosis, lupuslike syndrome, hepatitis, seizures, optic neuritis
  - RIF: Hepatotoxicity, red-orange-colored body fluids, GI distress
  - EMB: Optic neuritis (color blindness, decreased visual acuity), rash, dizziness, hyperuricemia
  - PZA: Transient rash, hyperuricemia, hepatotoxicity, arthralgias
- Significant possible interactions:
  - INH inhibits the metabolism of phenytoin, carbamazepine, warfarin, and theophylline, resulting in elevated serum concentrations of these drugs; decreases efficacy of levodopa and itraconazole; monitor closely
  - RIF has numerous significant drug interactions due to its potent hepatic enzyme–inducing effects. Consult prescribing information for details.
  - Antacids decrease the absorption of EMB.

Second Line

- Ethionamide, kanamycin, capreomycin, cycloserine, and fluoroquinolones
- Reserved for patients with resistant TB or intolerance to first-line agents (5)[C]

Pregnancy Considerations

- Streptomycin not recommended
- Breast-feeding is not contraindicated.

ADDITIONAL TREATMENT

Corticosteroids should be routinely used in HIV-negative people with tuberculous meningitis to reduce death and disabling residual neurologic deficit among survivors. However, there is not enough evidence to support or refute a similar conclusion for those who are HIV positive (3).

Issues for Referral

Consult infectious disease specialist.

SURGERY/OTHER PROCEDURES

Reserved for treatment failures or when the diagnosis is in doubt:

- Tuberculous meningitis: Surgical diversion of CSF when tuberculous meningitis associated with symptomatic elevated ICP and noncommunicating hydrocephalus (ventriculoperitoneal shunt or external drainage preferred) (6)[B]
- Tuberculoma:
  - Surgical intervention for decompression or debulking of large, symptomatic tuberculomas is required (7)[C]
  - Surgery is considered for treatment failures or to relieve elevated ICP. Antituberculous therapy is continued to prevent seeding of meninges.
- Tubercular abscess: Puncture, continuous drainage, fractional drainage, repeat aspiration through burr hole, stereotactic aspiration, or total excision of the abscess

IN-PATIENT CONSIDERATIONS

Initial Stabilization

- Appropriate restraint if seizures are present
- Isolation only if pulmonary disease is present or until the patient has 3 negative sputum smears for AFB

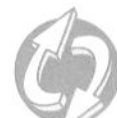

ONGOING CARE

FOLLOW-UP RECOMMENDATIONS

- Look for other foci of infection.
- Institute seizure precautions.
- Neuropsychological surveillance is essential.
- Treat concurrent HIV infection, if present.

Patient Monitoring

- Assessment of peripheral neuropathy, hepatotoxicity
- Monthly visual acuity and red–green color discrimination testing if receiving EMB
- Attention to possible drug–drug interactions
- Contrast-enhanced CT scan in patients with tuberculoma on medical treatment every 3–6 months until complete resolution of symptoms and stabilization of lesions
- Hormonal evaluation (e.g., TSH, cortisol, prolactin) in pituitary TB

DIET

Pyridoxine supplementation (25 mg/d) in patients may prevent neuropathy (poor nutritional status, diabetes, HIV infection, pregnancy, alcohol use), especially if taking isoniazid

PATIENT EDUCATION

Emphasize importance of adherence to drug therapy, adverse effects, and drug interactions.

PROGNOSIS

- Adults:
  - Stage/grade I: Alert and oriented without focal neurologic deficits; mortality rate is 18%
  - Stage/grade II: GCS 14–11 or 15 with focal neurologic deficits; mortality rate is 34%
  - Stage/grade III: GCS 10 or less; mortality rate of 72%
- Children:
  - Stage/grade I: Nonspecific constitutional symptoms (headache, nausea, fussiness, fever; mortality rate is 0%
  - Stage/grade II: CN palsies (especially CN III, VI, VII) and signs of meningeal irritation; mortality rate of 12%
  - Stage/grade III: Altered mental status with signs of increased ICP; mortality rate of 49%

COMPLICATIONS

Visual deterioration, focal deficits, cognitive deterioration, paraplegia, hormonal deficiencies, shunt block or infection, or side effects of therapy

REFERENCES

1. Thwaite G, Schoeman J. update on tuberculosis of the central nervous system: Pathogenesis, diagnosis and treatment. *Clin Chest Med*. 2009;30:745–54.
2. Trunz B, Fine P, Dye C. Effect of BCG vaccination on childhood tuberculous meningitis and miliary tuberculosis worldwide: A meta-analysis and assessment of cost-efectiveness. *Lancet*. 2006;367: 1173–80.
3. Kadhiravan T, Deepanjali S. Role of corticosteroids in the treatment of tuberculosis: An evidence-based update. *Indian J Chest Dis Allied Sci*. 2010;52: 153–8.
4. Donald PR, Schoeman JF. Tuberculous meningitis. *N Engl J Med*. 2004;351:1719–20.
5. Yew W, Leung C. Management of multidrug resistant tuberculosis. *Respirology*. 2008;13:21–46.
6. Thwaites GE, Tran TH. Tuberculous meningitis: Many questions, too few answers. *Lancet Neurol*. 2005;4:160–70.
7. Jain SK, Kwon P, Moss WJ. Management and outcomes of intracranial tuberculomas developing during antituberculous therapy: Case report and review. *Clin Pediatr*. 2005;44:443–50.

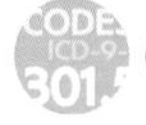

CODES

ICD9

- 013.00 Tuberculous meningitis, unspecified
- 013.20 Tuberculoma of brain, unspecified
- 013.90 Unspecified tuberculosis of central nervous system, unspecified

CLINICAL PEARLS

- Initial treatment should include 4-drug therapy with isoniazid, rifampin, pyrazinamide, and ethambutol for 2 months, followed by isoniazid and rifampin for 7–10 months.
- Adjunctive dexamethasone is recommended for tuberculous meningitis and tuberculoma.

TUBERCULOSIS, LATENT

Kay A. Bauman, MD, MPH

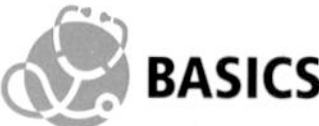

BASICS

DESCRIPTION

- Tuberculosis (TB) is a common infection transmitted by inhaling airborne bacilli from a person with active TB. The bacilli multiply in the alveoli and are carried by macrophages, lymphatics, and blood to distant sites (e.g., lung, pleura, brain, kidney, bone). Tissue hypersensitivity halts infection within 10 weeks.
- Latent TB infection (LTBI) is asymptomatic, noninfectious, and usually detected by a positive skin test (i.e., purified protein derivative [PPD]) or chest x-ray (CXR), which is evidence of prior TB infection; acid-fast bacilli smear and culture are negative, and CXR does not suggest active TB.
- TB: Active disease occurs in 5–10% of infected individuals without preventive therapy. Chance of disease increases with immunosuppression and is highest for all individuals within 2 years of infection; 85% of the cases are pulmonary, which is infectious.
- LTBI treatment is a key component of the TB elimination strategy of the US. For example, an estimated 4,000–11,000 active TB cases were prevented by LTBI treatment in 2002 (1).
- System(s) affected: Asymptomatic

EPIDEMIOLOGY

- High-risk groups include immigrants from Asia, Latin America, Africa, and the Pacific Basin; homeless persons; persons with a history of drug use or history of incarceration; HIV-infected individuals.
- Also at high risk are those newly exposed, including the pediatric population

Prevalence

- In the US, ~4% of the population has latent TB infection.
- Worldwide, it is estimated that 1/3 of the population harbors latent TB.
- Predominant gender: Male > Female

RISK FACTORS

- HIV infection, immunosuppression
- Immigrants (from Asia, Africa, Latin America, Pacific Islands, or area with high rate of TB), including migrant workers
- Close contact with infected individual
- Institutional environment (e.g., prison, nursing home)
- Use of illicit drugs
- Lower socioeconomic status or homeless
- Health care workers
- Chronic disease such as diabetes mellitus (DM), end-stage renal disease, cancer, or silicosis; organ transplant
- Persons with fibrotic changes on CXR consistent with previous TB infection (2)
- Recent TB skin test (TST) converters (2)
- Personnel from mycobacteriology laboratories
- Patients with organ transplants

GENERAL PREVENTION

Treatment of LTBI is preventive: The goal is to decrease the incidence of active TB in the individuals treated and to decrease the risk to close contacts should active TB occur.

ETIOLOGY

Mycobacterium tuberculosis, M. bovis, and *M. africanum*

COMMONLY ASSOCIATED CONDITIONS

- HIV infection (see "Tests")
- Immune suppression

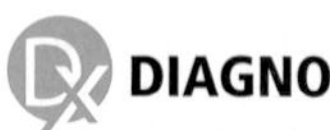

DIAGNOSIS

HISTORY

History of immigration from a high-risk area, history of IV drug use and/or drug treatment, HIV, homelessness, recent incarceration

PHYSICAL EXAM

No signs of infection

DIAGNOSTIC TESTS & INTERPRETATION

Lab

Initial lab tests

- None routinely recommended
- In higher-risk patients: Liver profile, hepatitis C virus (HCV) and hepatitis B virus (HBV) screening
- HIV test recommended to assess risk for active TB in men who have sex with men or persons with a history of IV drug use

Imaging

Initial approach

- CXR required to rule out TB in asymptomatic infected persons
- CT scan of the chest has good sensitivity.

Diagnostic Procedures/Surgery

- PPD: 5 U (0.1 mL) intermediate-strength intradermal volar forearm. Measure induration at 48–72 hours:
  - Positive if induration is:
    - >5 mm and patient has HIV infection (or suspected) (2), is immunosuppressed, had recent close TB contact, or has clinical evidence of active or old disease on CXR.
    - >10 mm and patient <4 years old or has other risk factors noted above
    - >15 mm and patient >4 years old and has no risk factors (2)
  - Negative if induration <5 mm on initial test and, if indicated, on second test
  - Use the 2-step test (administer a second intradermal test 1–3 weeks after initial test; measure and interpret as usual) if patient has had no recent PPD and is >55 years old or is a nursing home resident, prison inmate, or health care worker (3).
- The interferon-γ blood test or QuantiFERON-TB and QuantiFERON-TB GOLD measure the release of interferon-γ by sensitized lymphocytes when exposed to antigens of *M. tuberculosis*. It is unaffected by prior BCG vaccination, requires only 1 patient visit, and has improved sensitivity and specificity, but is costly (1).
- Special considerations:
  - Steroids: False-negative skin test
  - Measles vaccine: May suppress tuberculin activity; simultaneous PPD and measles vaccine recommended; if not simultaneous, defer PPD 4–6 weeks after measles vaccine.
  - The multiple-puncture tine test is not recommended.
  - Do not use BCG vaccination as a reason to ignore a positive PPD in adults and forego recommendation for treatment.
  - Disorders that may alter results and give a false-negative skin test:
    - Recent viral infection
    - New (<10 weeks) infection
    - Severe malnutrition
    - HIV
    - Anergy
    - Age <6 months
    - Overwhelming TB

DIFFERENTIAL DIAGNOSIS

Fungal infections; atypical mycobacteria or *Nocardia*

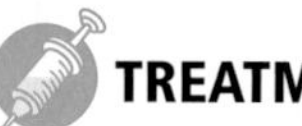

TREATMENT

MEDICATION

First Line

INH scored tablets: 100 mg, 300 mg, or syrup 10 mg/mL:

- Daily: Adult 300 mg; pediatric 10–15 mg/kg (maximum 300 mg) (3,4)
- Twice weekly: Adult 15 mg/kg; pediatric 20–30 mg/kg (maximum 900 mg) (3,4)
- Treatment for 9 months
- Precautions:
  - Follow liver function if the patient has history of alcoholism, HBV, HCV or other liver dysfunction, or new signs of liver injury.
  - INH: Peripheral neuritis and hypersensitivity are possible. Consider pyridoxine (3).
  - INH: An idiosyncratic drug reaction that results in INH-associated severe liver injury has been reported by the CDC in 17 patients in years 2004–2008. These included 15 adults and 2 children. 5 underwent liver transplantation and 5 subsequently died (one of the liver transplant recipients). Thus, monitoring of patients while on treatment is recommended looking for symptoms of liver injury (all were symptomatic!), and not be limited to laboratory monitoring. The rate of this reaction is difficult to calculate, as unknown numbers of patients are treated for LTBI, but 1 estimate is 291,000–433,000 per year in the US (5).

Second Line

- Rifampin alone: Adults 600 mg/d for 4 months; children 10–20 mg/kg/d for 6 months. Less data exists for efficacy of this regimen, but can be considered for contacts of INH-resistant TB or patient with INH contraindications. In 1 study, the 4-month course increased compliance from 52.6% with INH to 71.6% with rifampin (6).

- On the horizon (TB Trials Consortium Study 26): Rifapentine, a rifampinlike drug used to treat active TB, 900 mg weekly and INH, 15–25 mg/kg weekly for 3 months. This new and shorter treatment had increased rates of completion compared to 9 months of INH, more adverse effects, and was more costly (approximately $160 vs. $6 for course of treatment). Contraindications to rifapentine: Alcoholism, renal failure, HIV infection, pregnancy. Can cause hyperuricemia and hematuria (7).

ADDITIONAL TREATMENT

Pediatric Considerations

- Protocol for newborn with mother/household contact with infection or disease
- If mother or household contact has LTBI, skin test all household contacts and treat any with positive PPD.
- If contact has abnormal CXR, separate infant until infectious status known; if not contagious, monitor infant PPD (4).
- If mother has disease and is possibly contagious, evaluate infant for congenital TB and test for HIV; separate newborn until mother is noninfectious (4).
- If congenital TB is suspected, treat.
- If there is no congenital disease, start isoniazid (INH) and repeat PPD after 3–4 months. If positive, reassess infant and finish 9 months of INH. If PPD is negative and source is noninfectious, stop INH and monitor infant (4).

General Measures

- Must exclude active TB
- Treatment for LTBI is crucial to control and eliminate TB disease in the US because it both decreases the risk of active TB in those treated and decreases risks to those potentially infected by those same people (2).
- Treat LTBI at any age if patient has HIV, has had close TB contact, is a recent converter (<2 years), is an IV drug user, has an abnormal CXR, has a high-risk medical condition, or is in another high-risk group:
  - Use INH for 9 months.
  - Preferred: INH 300 mg/d or 900 mg twice weekly × 9 months (2)
  - Acceptable alternative: INH 300 mg/d or 900 mg twice weekly × 6 months (2)
  - Directly observed therapy (DOT) is recommended if patient adherence is not assured.
- Treat LTBI during pregnancy if patient has recent infection or is HIV positive (use INH with pyridoxine and monitor liver enzymes); otherwise, treatment may be postponed until postpartum (2).
- Special considerations for HIV infection and suspected INH resistance (2)
- *Note:* Because of severe liver injury and death associated with rifampin and pyrazinamide, these medications are no longer recommended for LTBI (2).
- Exclusions: Cirrhosis, active hepatitis, history of excessive alcohol consumption (2)

Additional Therapies

BCG vaccine, live-attenuated *M. bovis*: Used more commonly in developing countries in children to prevent complications of TB

IN-PATIENT CONSIDERATIONS

Geriatric Considerations

- Before entering a chronic-care facility, patients should have a PPD using 2-step protocols.
- INH side effects are more pronounced.

Discharge Criteria

- Activity as tolerated
- No isolation required

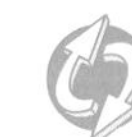

ONGOING CARE

FOLLOW-UP RECOMMENDATIONS

Patient Monitoring

- During preventive therapy for LTBI: Initial monthly visits to assess adherence to regimen and to monitor for hepatitis and neuropathy; if stable, can monitor less frequently.
- If patient remains asymptomatic, repeat CXR is not needed.
- Check liver enzymes if patient is symptomatic, is HIV positive, has chronic liver disease, uses alcohol, or is pregnant or postpartum, and modify drugs if needed.

DIET

Regular; consider pyridoxine supplement, 10–50 mg/d.

PROGNOSIS

- Generally there are few complications and treatment is effective if drugs are taken for full course as prescribed.
- Retreatment is not necessary.

COMPLICATIONS

Recrudescent TB

REFERENCES

1. Campos-Outcalt D. When, and when not, to use the interferon-gamma TB test. *J Fam Pract*. 2005;54: 873–5.
2. Centers for Disease Control and Prevention. Guidelines for preventing the transmission of *Mycobacterium* TB in health-care settings, 2005. *MMWR Recomm Rep*. 2005;54(RR-17):53–5.
3. Blumberg HM, Leonard MK, Jasmer RM. Update on the treatment of tuberculosis and latent tuberculosis infection. *JAMA*. 2005;293:2776–84.
4. American Academy of Pediatrics. *Report of the Committee on Infectious Diseases (Red Book)*. Elk Grove Village, IL: American Academy of Pediatrics; 2003.
5. Centers for Disease Control and Prevention (CDC), et al. Severe isoniazid-associated liver injuries among persons being treated for latent tuberculosis infection—United States, 2004–2008. *Morb Mortal Wkly Rep*. 2010;59:224–9.
6. Page KR, Sifakis F, Montes de Oca R, et al. Improved adherence and less toxicity with rifampin vs isoniazid for treatment of latent tuberculosis: A retrospective study. *Arch Intern Med*. 2006;166: 1863–70.
7. London S. Shorter combo therapy effective for latent TB. *FP News*. 2011;(7).

ADDITIONAL READING

- Centers for Disease Control and Prevention (CDC), American Thoracic Society. Update: Adverse event data and revised American Thoracic Society/CDC recommendations against the use of rifampin and pyrazinamide for treatment of latent tuberculosis infection–United States, 2003. *Morb Mortal Wkly Rep*. 2003;52:735–9.
- Young DB, Gideon HP, Wilkinson RJ. Eliminating latent tuberculosis. *Trends Microbiol*. 2009;17(5): 183–8.

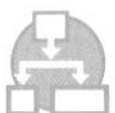

See Also (Topic, Algorithm, Electronic Media Element)

Tuberculosis; Tuberculosis, Miliary

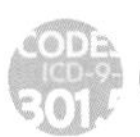

CODES

ICD9

795.51 Nonspecific reaction to tuberculin skin test without active tuberculosis

CLINICAL PEARLS

- Treatment for latent TB is crucial to control and eliminate TB disease in the US, and an estimated 4% of the US population has LTBI.
- Test household contacts of PPD-positive patients.
- History of BCG vaccination, especially >10 years before PPD testing, should not be considered to be the cause of a positive PPD. The interferon-γ blood test is unaffected by prior BCG vaccination.
- Treat all HIV-positive patients with latent TB with a prophylactic regimen.

T

TUBERCULOSIS, MILIARY

Kevin C. Shannon, MD, MPH, FAAFP

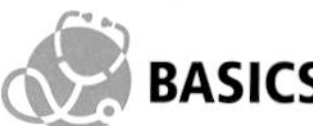

BASICS

DESCRIPTION

- Clinical disease from widespread hematogenous dissemination of *Mycobacterium tuberculosis*. Originally named for "millet seed" appearance of nodules often found in lungs. 3 types:
  - Acute: Usually with primary infection; rapidly progressive; more severe type
  - Late generalized: Occurs after years of latent infection; chronic, more indolent course
  - Anergic: Rare; microabscesses form in place of granulomas; reactivation of old disease; older patients
- Multiorgan failure and acute respiratory distress syndrome (ARDS) are also known to occur.
- System(s) affected: Most commonly Pulmonary; Lymphatic; Central Nervous System (TB meningitis); Hepatic; Splenic; Bone Marrow
- Synonym(s): Disseminated TB

EPIDEMIOLOGY

Incidence

- 1–3% of all TB cases
- Worldwide incidence: 9.4 million new cases of TB in 2009 (137/100,000 population)(WHO), out of which 1–3% may be miliary TB (1)
- In the US in 2009, total new TB cases were estimated at 13,000 (4.1/100,000) (1).
- Predominant sex: Male > Female (as in all types of TB)

Prevalence

Global TB prevalence: 14 million, corresponding to 164/100,000 population (1)

RISK FACTORS

Within TB-infected population, risk factors for miliary disease include HIV/AIDS, young age (especially <1 year) or old age, iatrogenic immunosuppression (i.e., organ transplant patients, chronic corticosteroid use, tumor necrosis factor inhibitors), diabetes mellitus (DM), pregnancy, chronic renal failure, protein malnutrition, alcohol abuse, and immigration from higher-prevalence regions.

GENERAL PREVENTION

- Bacille Calmette-Guérin (BCG) vaccine:
  - 78% effective at preventing severe meningeal and miliary TB in children (2)[B]
  - The effects of BCG do not increase with a second dose (3)[A].
- Treatment of latent TB infection with isoniazid (INH) (see "Tuberculosis, Latent")

PATHOPHYSIOLOGY

- Lymphatic, then hematogenous spread from a local focus, with failure of the body to halt infection by granulomatous encapsulation
- Predilection for more vascular organs (i.e., spleen, liver, brain, bone marrow); in a vast majority of cases, many organs are affected.
- Iatrogenic disease is also reported after solid-organ transplants, urethral catheterization, and cardiac valve transplants.

ETIOLOGY

Mycobacterium infection in the context of impaired cell-mediated immunity:

- Primary infection in immunocompromised host or recrudescent infection in once-healthy host with new health impairment; or immature immune system (majority of cases in children <5 years of age)
- Iatrogenic infection as above

COMMONLY ASSOCIATED CONDITIONS

HIV/AIDS, malignancy, pregnancy, malnutrition

DIAGNOSIS

HISTORY

- Ask about risk factors and exposures. Need high index of suspicion based on these; 1/5 of cases are undiagnosed antemortem even with full testing modalities available.
- Most common symptoms are nonspecific: Night sweats (>90%), fatigue/malaise (>90%), anorexia (>80%), weight loss (>75%)
- Late generalized miliary TB has mean duration of symptoms of 2 months before diagnosis.

PHYSICAL EXAM

Presentation extremely variable, but may include:

- Fever (>90%)
- Tachypnea, tachycardia (>75%)
- Cough, dyspnea (>60%)
- Pulmonary: Rales (>50%)
- Hepatomegaly (>40%)
- Generalized lymphadenopathy (>40%)
- Neurologic/HA/mental status changes (>25%)
- Meningeal signs (meningitis) in 20% (found in 50% miliary TB cases postmortem)
- Single or multiorgan failure
- Severe disease resulting in septic shock and ARDS has been reported.
- Choroidal tubercles on dilated funduscopic exam (found in 50% miliary TB cases postmortem)

DIAGNOSTIC TESTS & INTERPRETATION

Lab

Initial lab tests

- Purified protein derivative (PPD) test positive in <50% of patients
- Sputum for acid-fast bacillus (AFB) smear and culture
- Smears should be sent for acid-fast fluorochrome dye, auramine-O rather than traditional Ziehl-Nielson stain, because the former is more sensitive.
- QuantiFERON-TB gold test (4)[B]: Preferred for patients not likely to return for PPD reading and for those who have had BCG
- Gastric washings (especially in children), blood cultures, or bone and liver biopsy also for smear and culture; liver biopsy most likely to be (+), and CSF least likely (so only get CSF smear if symptoms/signs)
- Test for HIV and hepatitis B and C.
- Baseline liver enzymes, bilirubin, creatinine, CBC
- Nonspecific laboratory findings include: Anemia, monocytosis, pancytopenia (but leukocytosis and thrombocytosis seen too); hypergammaglobulinemia; syndrome of inappropriate antidiuretic hormone (SIADH); sterile pyuria; elevated ESR; elevated transaminases

Follow-Up & Special Considerations

- AFB smears and cultures to monitor response
- False-negative skin test more likely on steroids

Pediatric Considerations

May need to culture samples from infected adult contact because samples can be difficult to obtain in pediatric patients

Imaging

- CXR: Faint reticulonodular infiltrate, uniform distribution; often mediastinal/hilar adenopathy; only in 50%
- Chest CT scan: Numerous 2–3-mm nodules scattered throughout lungs in >85% of patients; chest CT scan, especially high-resolution CT (1-mm cuts), more sensitive than CXR (5)[B].
- Abdominal/pelvic CT scan: If suspicious of other organ involvement
- Brain MRI: Cerebral nodules or tuberculoma; only if neurologic symptoms present

Diagnostic Procedures/Surgery

- See "Tuberculosis."
- Collect samples for AFB/culture. Sampling fluids from multiple sites greatly improves yield for AFB smear and culture:
  - Sputum culture positive in 62% (smear in 33%)
  - Bronchial lavage (BAL) culture positive in 55% (smear in 27%)
  - Gastric aspirate culture positive in nearly 100% (smear in 43%)
  - CSF culture positive in 60% (smear in 8%)
- Biopsy organs based on symptoms.

Pathological Findings

- Caseating granulomas on tissue biopsy (liver most common site)
- Microabscesses with neutrophilic response in acute type
- Can see mycotic aneurysms if disease affects aorta
- TB pericarditis diagnosed by pericardial biopsy

DIFFERENTIAL DIAGNOSIS

- Other pneumonias (and other etiologies of ARDS)
- Lymphoma; lymphangitic spread of cancer
- Metastatic carcinoma
- Sarcoidosis
- Sepsis
- Addison disease
- Ascites (other etiologies)
- Various HIV-related opportunistic infections

TREATMENT

- Diagnosis is often hampered by low clinical suspicion and delay in collecting fluid/tissue samples for AFB smear and culture; empiric therapy is often indicated, as early initiation of therapy improves survival.
- Once patient receives several weeks of effective treatment, feels much better, and sputum smears are negative, it is still not certain that patient is not contagious; tight adherence to regimen is necessary.
- Duration for all forms of TB should be tailored to the patient: Those with miliary TB are likely to be at the extremes of age, have a higher incidence of underlying disease, and a larger burden of organism. Thus, it is often appropriate to extend the duration of therapy beyond the minimum.

MEDICATION

- All drug regimens are the same as those for general TB.
- Adherence extremely important to prevent drug resistance; directly observed therapy (DOT) important for nondaily regimens

First Line

- Regimen 1 (preferred):
  - Initial phase: Isoniazid (INH), rifampin (RIF), pyrazinamide (PZA), and ethambutol (EMB) once daily × 8 weeks
  - Continuation phase: INH/RIF daily × 18 weeks *or* INH/RIF twice weekly × 18 weeks (only use for HIV+ patients if CD4 >100) *or* INH/rifapentine once weekly × 18 weeks (acceptable alternative for HIV–patients only) (6)[A]
- Regimen 2:
  - Initial phase: INH/RIF/PZA/EMB daily × 2 weeks, then twice weekly × 6 weeks
  - Continuation phase: INH/RIF twice weekly × 18 weeks (HIV+ patients only if CD4 >100) *or* INH/rifapentine once weekly × 18 weeks (acceptable alternative for HIV patients only) (6)[A]
- Regimen 3 (acceptable alternative):
  - Initial phase: INH/RIF/PZA/EMB daily × 8 weeks
  - Continuation phase: INH/RIF 3× weekly × 18 weeks (6)[A]
- Regimen 4 (only when unable to give preferred regimen):
  - Initial phase: INH/RIF/EMB daily × 8 weeks
  - Continuation phase: INH/RIF daily or twice weekly × 31 weeks (6)[B]
- No studies proving efficacy of 5× weekly regimen, but clinical evidence suggests it (6)[C].
- DOT required for nondaily regimens (6).
- Dosing (for alternate dosing less frequently than daily, see "Tuberculosis"):
  - INH: Adult 5 mg/kg/d (maximum 300 mg); pediatric 10–15 mg/kg/d (maximum 300 mg)
  - RIF: Daily or twice-weekly dose: Adult and pediatric 10–20 mg/kg (maximum 600 mg)
  - PZA: Adults 40–55 kg: 18–25 mg/kg/d, maximum 1 g; 56–75 kg: 20–27 mg/kg/d, maximum 1.5 g; >75 kg: 22–26 mg/kg/d, maximum 2 g. Pediatric 15–30 mg/kg/d (maximum 2 g).
  - Rifabutin (Mycobutin): Daily or twice weekly: Adult 5 mg/kg, maximum 300 mg
  - Rifapentine (Priftin): For continuation phase only. HIV adults: 600 mg once weekly, given with INH; not effective if HIV+ (6)[A]
  - EMB: Adults 40–55 kg: 15–20 mg/kg/d, maximum 800 mg; 56–75 kg: 16–22 mg/kg/d, maximum 1.2 g; >75 kg: 22–26 mg/kg/d, maximum 2.6 g. Pediatrics: 15–20 mg/kg/d, maximum 1 g.
- Contraindications:
  - RIF: Avoid if patient taking antiretrovirals
  - EMB: May cause optic neuritis; avoid unless patient is old enough to cooperate for visual acuity and color testing
- Precautions:
  - INH, RIF, PZA: May cause hepatitis; caution if liver disease
  - RIF: Colors urine, tears, and secretions orange; can stain contact lenses
  - INH: Peripheral neuritis and hypersensitivity possible; treat with pyridoxine.
  - PZA: May increase uric acid; unclear safety during pregnancy (6)[C]
- Significant possible interactions: Rifamycins alter level of phenytoin, antivirals, and other drugs metabolized by liver and may inactivate birth control pills (recommend a barrier method).

Second Line

- Corticosteroids: Use only with concurrent anti-TB therapy. Recommended for TB meningitis, pericarditis, or severe miliary disease (2)[B]: Reduce fluid reaccumulation in pericarditis, but no proven mortality benefit (6)[B]
- Streptomycin: Caution: Ototoxic and nephrotoxic; do not use in pregnancy.

ADDITIONAL TREATMENT

General Measures

- Respiratory isolation if pulmonary disease; TB mask when out of hospital room or in contact with others at home (if still deemed contagious)
- Nutrition: Attention to good nutrition is important, and many miliary TB patients are debilitated and malnutrition can weaken the immune system.

Issues for Referral

Infectious disease specialist is helpful for patients also on antiretrovirals because doses may need adjusting.

Pregnancy Considerations

Streptomycin cannot be used in pregnancy.

SURGERY/OTHER PROCEDURES

- Location- and patient-specific
- Medical treatment unresponsiveness may rarely require surgical intervention; there is some evidence for the role of surgical therapy in select cases of drug-resistant TB (7).

IN-PATIENT CONSIDERATIONS

Place initially in isolation/negative-pressure room. Miliary TB is usually somewhat less contagious than other TB forms. If patient lives at home with someone at increased risk of acquiring TB (e.g., with HIV infection), then keep hospitalized until several consecutive sputum smears are negative and significant clinical improvement.

ONGOING CARE

FOLLOW-UP RECOMMENDATIONS

- General TB follow-up; most states require department of public health notification.
- Identify and test any close contacts.

Patient Monitoring

See "Tuberculosis."

DIET

Some evidence suggests that high-cholesterol diet accelerates sterilization of sputum in pulmonary TB patients. In all patients, it is important to attend to specific malnutrition correction.

PATIENT EDUCATION

As for general TB

PROGNOSIS

- Mortality: Untreated, approaching 100%; 16–38% on average; with early and appropriate treatment, <10%
- Nutritional deficit (assessed by 4 measures: Very low BMI, low serum albumin and cholesterol, and lymphocytopenia) is an independent risk factor for acute respiratory failure in miliary TB (8).
- Relapse rate: <5% with adequate, directly observed therapy

COMPLICATIONS

- ARDS with refractory hypoxemia can occur.
- Multidrug-resistant TB is rare in the US but increasing elsewhere.

REFERENCES

1. World Health Organization. Global tuberculosis control—epidemiology, strategy, financing WHO Report 2010. Available at: www.who.int/tb/publications/global_report/2010/en/index.html.
2. Colditz GA, Brewer TF, Berkey CS, et al. Efficacy of BCG vaccine in the prevention of tuberculosis. Meta-analysis of the published literature. *JAMA*. 1994;271:698–702.
3. Pereira SM, Dantas OM, Ximenes R, et al. [BCG vaccine against tuberculosis: Its protective effect and vaccination policies]. *Rev Saude Publica*. 2007;41(Suppl 1):59–66.
4. Mazurek GH, Jereb J, Vernon A, et al. Updated guidelines for using interferon gamma release assays to detect *Mycobacterium tuberculosis* interferon—United States, 2010. *MMWR Recomm Rep*. 2010;59(RRO5):1–25.
5. Optican RJ. High-resolution computed tomography in the diagnosis of miliary tuberculosis. *Chest*. 1992;102(3):941–3.
6. Potter B. Management of active TB. *Am Fam Physician*. 2005;72(11).
7. Kang MW, Kim HK, Choi YS, et al. Surgical treatment for multidrug-resistant and extensive drug-resistant tuberculosis. *Ann Thorac Surg*. 2010;89:1597–602.
8. Kim DK, Kim HJ, Kwon SY, et al. Nutritional deficit as a negative prognostic factor in patients with miliary tuberculosis. *Eur Respir J*. 2008;32:1031–36.

ADDITIONAL READING

Trends in tuberculosis—United States 2007. *MMWR*. 2008;57(11):281–85.

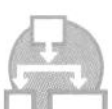

See Also (Topic, Algorithm, Electronic Media Element)

Tuberculosis; Tuberculosis, CNS

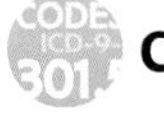

CODES

ICD9

- 018.00 Acute miliary tuberculosis, unspecified
- 018.80 Other specified miliary tuberculosis, unspecified
- 018.90 Unspecified miliary tuberculosis, unspecified examination

CLINICAL PEARLS

- Chest CT scan is more sensitive than CXR for detecting miliary disease in the lung.
- PPD is positive in <50% of patients.
- Empiric therapy usually appropriate: To increase likelihood of survival, when miliary TB is probable, do not withhold treatment pending test results.

TUBEROUS SCLEROSIS COMPLEX

Michele Roberts, MD, PhD

BASICS

DESCRIPTION

- Tuberous sclerosis complex (TSC) is a genetic neurocutaneous syndrome (phakomatosis). Many organ systems are affected, with the formation of multiple hamartomas.
- Manifestations may be subtle but can include lesions of the CNS, skin, retina, heart, lung, viscera, kidney, bone, teeth, liver, and nails.
- System(s) affected: Cardiovascular; Musculoskeletal; Nervous; Pulmonary; Renal/Urologic; Skin/Exocrine
- Synonym(s): Bourneville disease

Pregnancy Considerations

Prenatal diagnosis by mutational analysis is possible when a molecular cause is known.

EPIDEMIOLOGY

Incidence

- 1 per 5,000 to 1 per 10,000 live births
- Predominant age: Clinical expression is variable; usually is diagnosed during the first decade of life.
- Predominant gender: Male = Female, but autism is more common in men.

RISK FACTORS

- Family history.
- Expressivity is variable, even within a family.
- If neither parent meets criteria for TSC, the recurrence risk is 1–2% per child (parental germ-line mosaicism).

Genetics

- Autosomal dominant with complete penetrance and variable expressivity (Online Mendelian Inheritance in Man no. 191100).
- 2/3 of cases result from new mutations. Somatic mosaicism occurs in 2–10% of de novo TSC.
- 2 chromosomal loci have been mapped: *TSC1* (9q34) and *TSC2* (16p13.3).
- Clinical phenotype of *TSC1* mutations generally is milder than that of *TSC2* mutations, but genotype–phenotype correlation is not established.

GENERAL PREVENTION

Genetic counseling

PATHOPHYSIOLOGY

- Mutations in either of 2 genes—*TSC1* and *TSC2*—that code for the tumor growth-suppressor proteins hamartin and tuberin, respectively
- The hamartin–tuberin complex is involved in cell proliferation and differentiation.
- Mutations may result in decreased production of these proteins and excessive cell proliferation, resulting in tuber formation. Loss of gene function is associated with enhanced mammalian target of rapamycin signaling (1).

ETIOLOGY

Some hamartomas in patients with TSC show loss of heterozygosity in the chromosomal region 9q34 or 16p13.3:

- This implies that the patient has inherited a mutation or a deletion in 1 copy of the gene, but the patient develops a lesion only when there is a somatic mutation in the other copy.
- This 2-hit mechanism seems to apply to cardiac rhabdomyomas, renal angiomyolipomas, and subependymal giant cell tumors (SGCTs), but not to cerebral tubers.

COMMONLY ASSOCIATED CONDITIONS

- Mental retardation (60–70%): Usually associated with history of seizures
- Seizures (80%): 25% of patients with infantile spasms have TSC
- Autism (10–20%)
- Cardiac arrhythmias
- Renal insufficiency

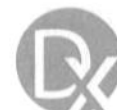

DIAGNOSIS

- Physical examination and imaging are most useful, although molecular diagnostics may be useful when clinical criteria are not met or for family members of affected patients.
- Most common presenting signs include seizures, infantile spasms, cardiac rhabdomyomas, hypopigmented macules; although most patients are diagnosed before age 10, the diagnosis is frequently missed at first presentation (2).
- Diagnostic criteria for TSC (3) (approximate percentage of patients affected):
  - Major criteria:
    - Facial angiofibromas (80%) or forehead plaques
    - Shagreen patch (connective tissue nevus)
    - 3 or more hypomelanotic macules (50%)
    - Nontraumatic ungula or periungual fibromas (20%)
    - Lymphangioleiomyomatosis (<10%; also known as *lymphangiomyomatosis*), predominantly in premenopausal women
    - Renal angiomyolipoma
    - Cardiac rhabdomyoma (50%; mostly in newborns)
    - Multiple retinal nodular hamartomas (50–80%)
    - Cortical tuber
    - Subependymal nodules
    - Subependymal giant cell astrocytoma
  - Minor criteria:
    - Confetti skin lesions (multiple 1–2-mm hypomelanotic macules)
    - Gingival fibromas
    - Multiple randomly distributed pits in dental enamel
    - Hamartomatous rectal polyps
    - Multiple renal cysts (50–80%)
    - Nonrenal hamartomas (liver hamartoma in 10%)
    - Bone cysts
    - Retinal achromic patch
    - Cerebral white matter radial migration lines
- Definite TSC: 2 major *or* 1 major and 2 minor criteria
- Probable TSC: 1 major *and* 1 minor criterion
- Possible TSC: 1 major *or* 2 minor criteria
- 95% of patients with TSC may have a seizure disorder.
- Although epilepsy and mental retardation are more common in patients with TSC, they are not included among diagnostic criteria because they are common among the general population (4).
- Hypomelanotic macules often can be seen in newborns, especially with Wood lamp examination.
- When a new diagnosis is made in a child with no family history of TSC, careful evaluation of the parents should include:
  - A comprehensive dermatologic examination (in room light and with a Wood lamp)
  - Ophthalmologic examination
  - Cranial CT scan or MRI
  - Renal ultrasound

HISTORY

- Family history of TSC stigmata; about 1/3 of patients with TSC have a positive family history.
- Assess for seizures and developmental delay in children.
- Patients with TSC are at increased risk for brain tumors and may present with symptoms of obstructive hydrocephalus, including headaches, vomiting, and neurologic deficits (including loss of vision). Children with obstructive hydrocephalus may present with nonspecific symptoms, including fatigue, decreased appetite, depression, and increased frequency of seizures.

PHYSICAL EXAM

- Dermatologic:
  - 96% of patients with TSC have characteristic skin lesions (5):
    - Hypopigmented macules (ash-leaf spots, usually elliptical); are not usually present before age 5 years
    - Angiofibromas (formerly, and incorrectly, *adenoma sebaceum*); typically involve the malar regions of the face (butterfly distribution); usually appear later than hypopigmented macules.
    - Shagreen patches, most common on the lower trunk
  - A brown, fibrous plaque on the forehead may be the first recognized feature of TSC during physical examination of infants.
  - Periungual and ungual fibromas may appear during adolescence or adulthood.
- Ophthalmologic:
  - Funduscopic evaluation:
    - Retinal hamartomas: Hamartoma may be a flat, translucent lesion (most common) or a multilobular mulberry lesion (with calcification), or it may have features of both.
    - Retinal giant cell astrocytoma, secondary retinal detachment
    - Chorioretinal depigmentation (punched-out appearance)
    - Papilledema or visual loss: Suggestive of brain tumors
    - An abnormal red reflex should not be mistaken for retinoblastoma.
  - Angiofibromas of the eyelids, nonparalytic strabismus, colobomas, and sector iris depigmentation
  - Refractive errors not different from those of the general population
- Dental: Multiple, randomly distributed pits in enamel
- Neurologic: Focal deficits may indicate growth of brain tumors.

DIAGNOSTIC TESTS & INTERPRETATION

Lab

Molecular diagnostics:

- Mutations detected in 75% of patients who meet the diagnostic criteria for TSC.
- Mutations in the *TSC2* gene are about 3 times as common as those of the *TSC1* gene (6).
- Identification of a mutation in *TSC1* or *TSC2* can confirm the diagnosis in a child whose clinical evaluation is suggestive but not diagnostic of TSC.
- A negative result in molecular testing cannot rule out TSC in a patient with a clinical diagnosis of TSC.
- Mutational analysis is useful for prenatal diagnosis and for evaluation of relatives of those with a known mutation.

Imaging

Initial approach

- Cranial MRI before age 2, with gadolinium enhancement
- Fetal cardiac rhabdomyomas may be seen on ultrasound or MRI during late gestation.
- CT scan or ultrasound of kidneys
- Pulmonary CT scan or chest imaging of the lungs, as indicated, in women beginning at age 18; pulmonary pathology is uncommon in men.

Diagnostic Procedures/Surgery

- Ash-leaf spots more readily seen with a Wood lamp
- Biopsy of questionable lesions
- Clinical neuropsychological evaluation may reveal attentional deficits in children and adolescents with TSC, even when they have normal intellectual abilities and no seizures or disruptive behaviors (7)[B].

Pathological Findings

- Lesions may be sparse at birth. Facial angiofibromas, ungual fibromas, and renal angiomyolipomas may develop months or years after birth.
- Brain lesions:
  - Cortical tubers (glioneural hamartomas): Disorganized neuronal and glial elements with astrocytosis (possibly epileptogenic)
  - White matter heterotopia: Dysplastic and dysmyelinated white matter
  - Subependymal nodules: Hamartomas comprising atypical enlarged glial and neuronal cells may transform to giant cell astrocytomas.
  - SGCT of mixed glioneuronal lineage.
  - Calcification of subependymal lesions may not occur until several months after birth.
  - Extensive anatomic abnormalities may be seen in gray and white matter, even in patients with normal intelligence.
- Renal lesions (50–80%): Angiomyolipomas, benign cysts, and lymphangiomas; may adversely affect renal function
- Pulmonary lesions: 1% of patients with TSC may present with pulmonary lymphangioleiomyomatosis, usually women of reproductive age.
- Cardiac rhabdomyoma (50–70% of infants), usually asymptomatic

DIFFERENTIAL DIAGNOSIS

- Non-TSC polycystic kidney disease
- Other causes of seizure disorders, mental retardation, autistic behavior
- Traumatic ungual fibromata
- Other phakomatoses: Neurofibromatosis, Sturge-Weber syndrome, von Hippel-Lindau syndrome

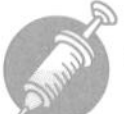

TREATMENT

MEDICATION

- Anticonvulsants for seizure control
- No drugs are used routinely, although the biochemical rationale for the potential use of rapamycin has been described, with clinical trials suggesting that this agent may be useful to treat TSC (8).

ADDITIONAL TREATMENT

Issues for Referral

- Multidisciplinary team evaluation: Genetics, neurology, ophthalmology, nephrology, surgery, dermatology, neurosurgery, radiology, and plastic surgery
- Physical therapy, occupational therapy, and speech therapy; social workers for home care; vocational training support

SURGERY/OTHER PROCEDURES

Surgery may be necessary for hydrocephalus, increased intracranial pressure, rapidly growing SGCT (1), malignant tumors, and seizure control.

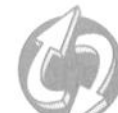

ONGOING CARE

FOLLOW-UP RECOMMENDATIONS

Patient Monitoring

- Pediatric:
  - Annual physical examination, growth assessment, ophthalmologic examination
  - Annual developmental testing and review of school progress, neuropsychologic evaluation, and intelligence quotient testing, if indicated.
  - Echocardiography: Pediatric cardiologist should follow children with cardiac rhabdomyoma. Cardiac rhabdomyomas typically develop in utero, regress spontaneously in early childhood, and involute completely by adulthood.
- EEG: For seizure management
- Renal ultrasound: Every 1–3 years beginning in adolescence; abdominal MRI or CT scan for evaluation of large angioleiomyomas
- Chest CT scan: For pulmonary dysfunction
- Screening MRI without contrast: Every 1–3 years for children and adolescents, less frequently in adults; if SGCT is identified, surgery is performed, if appropriate. Otherwise, repeat cranial MRI every 3–6 months

PATIENT EDUCATION

Tuberous Sclerosis Alliance: info@tsalliance.org; www.tsalliance.org

PROGNOSIS

Variable; shortened longevity in individuals with complications

COMPLICATIONS

- In addition to benign tumors associated with TSC (e.g., angiofibromas, hamartomas, rhabdomyomas, and angiomyolipomas), there is an 18-fold increase in risk of malignancy, especially of the kidney, brain, and soft tissues.
- Rhabdomyosarcoma, although rare, has increased incidence in TSC.
- 1–2% of adults develop renal cell carcinoma 25 years earlier than in general population.
- CNS complications, including epilepsy, cognitive impairment, behavioral problems, hyperactivity, self-injurious behavior, and autism, occur in 85% of children and adolescents with TSC.
- Neuropsychologic attention deficits may be greater than intellectual impairment.
- Causes of death: Neurologic disease is most common (SGCT and status epilepticus), renal disease, pulmonary disease
- SGCTs are benign but may undergo malignant transformation or may grow rapidly or hemorrhage.

T

REFERENCES

1. Moavero R, Pinci M, Bombardieri R, et al. The management of subependymal giant cell tumors in tuberous sclerosis: A clinician's perspective. *Childs Nerv Syst*. 2011;27:1203–10.
2. Staley BA, Vail EA, Thiele EA. Tuberous sclerosis complex: Diagnostic challenges, presenting symptoms, and commonly missed signs. *Pediatrics*. 2011;127:e117–25.
3. Roach ES, Gomez MR, Northrup H. Tuberous sclerosis complex consensus conference: Revised clinical diagnostic criteria. *J Child Neurol*. 1998;13:624–8.
4. Roach ES, Sparagana SP. Diagnosis of tuberous sclerosis complex. *J Child Neurol*. 2004;19:643–9.
5. Webb DW, Clarke A, Fryer A, et al. The cutaneous features of tuberous sclerosis: A population study. *Br J Dermatol*. 1996;135:1–5.
6. Au KS, Williams AT, Roach ES, et al. Genotype/phenotype correlation in 325 individuals referred for a diagnosis of tuberous sclerosis complex in the United States. *Genet Med*. 2007;9:88–100.
7. de Vries PJ, Gardiner J, Bolton PF, et al. Neuropsychological attention deficits in tuberous sclerosis complex (TSC). *Am J Med Genet A*. 2009;149A:387–95.
8. Orlova KA, Crino PB. The tuberous sclerosis complex. *Ann N Y Acad Sci*. 2010;1184:87–105.

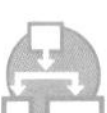

See Also (Topic, Algorithm, Electronic Media Element)

Neurofibromatosis

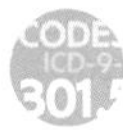

CODES

ICD9

759.5 Tuberous sclerosis

CLINICAL PEARLS

Hypopigmented areas (e.g., ash-leaf spots), mainly on the trunk and extremities, are often the first sign and are present at birth or shortly after (50%). These are best seen with a Wood lamp. Diagnosis of TSC is frequently missed.

TURNER SYNDROME

Michele Roberts, MD, PhD

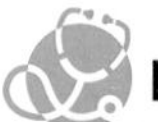

BASICS

DESCRIPTION

- Turner syndrome (TS) is a condition characterized by ovarian dysgenesis and short stature in phenotypic females who have only 1 sex chromosome, an X; although a partial second sex chromosome, X or Y, may be present
- The most common sex chromosome abnormality syndrome in females
- System(s) affected: Cardiovascular; Reproductive; Endocrine/Metabolic; Musculoskeletal; Nervous; Renal/Urologic
- Synonym(s): Ullrich-Turner syndrome; Bonnevie-Ullrich syndrome; Monosomy X; Sexual infantilism; Gonadal dysgenesis

EPIDEMIOLOGY

Incidence

- Occurs in 1/2,500 live female births
- ~1–3% of all conceptuses affected, of whom fewer than 1% will survive to term
- Accounts for 15% of all spontaneously aborted fetuses
- Predominant sex: Female only

Prevalence

Estimated 50,000–75,000 females in the US

RISK FACTORS

Genetics

- 50% of patients have 45,X karyotype (sporadic nondisjunction). Translocations involving the X chromosome may result in TS.
- 80% of girls with 45,X have maternal X, although phenotype is identical if X is paternal.
- TS occurs with a deletion of the *SRY* segment of the Y chromosome in 46,XY karyotype, with resulting female phenotype (5–6%)
- It is important to identify Y chromosomal material because of increased risk of gonadoblastoma (7–10%) if Y material is present. FISH or PCR may be necessary to identify Y material.
- Also may be mosaic for 45,X/46,XY; 45,X/46,XX; or 45,X/47,XXX

PATHOPHYSIOLOGY

Haploinsufficiency of the *SHOX* gene (short stature homeobox-containing gene), located in the pseudoautosomal region of the X chromosome, is thought to be responsible for short stature and skeletal abnormalities in TS.

ETIOLOGY

Monosomy for all or part of the X chromosome can result in features of TS. Genes involved are located mainly in Xp11.2–p22.1.

COMMONLY ASSOCIATED CONDITIONS

- Very frequent (>50%):
  - Gonadal dysgenesis (infertility 98%)
  - Short stature (virtually 100%)
  - Hearing loss (50%), otitis media (70–100%)
- Frequent (>5–10% but <50% of individuals):
  - Cardiovascular abnormalities, including coarctation of the aorta (15–30%), aortic valvular disease (1/3 have bicuspid aortic valve), mitral valve prolapse (25%), aortic root dilatation (8–29%), aortic dissection
  - Renal abnormalities
  - Hypertension (>30%)
  - Glucose intolerance
  - Hyperlipidemia
  - Ocular abnormalities
  - Hypothyroidism, autoimmune thyroiditis
  - GI vascular malformations
  - Glucose intolerance
  - Gonadoblastoma in 8% of individuals with Y chromosomal material
- Occasional:
  - Inflammatory bowel disease, celiac disease
  - Colon cancer
  - Neuroblastoma
  - Juvenile rheumatoid arthritis
  - Liver disease, especially cirrhosis

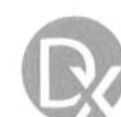

DIAGNOSIS

HISTORY

- Edema of hands and feet and redundant skin of the neck (webbing) are presenting features during infancy.
- 50% of girls are less than fifth percentile in height by 1.5 years; 75% by 3.5 years
- During adolescence, primary amenorrhea, short stature, and infantile secondary sex characteristics are presenting features.
- Diagnosis of TS should be considered in any girl with an unexplained short stature

PHYSICAL EXAM

Frequencies are for classic 45,X and vary with other chromosomal abnormalities associated with TS (1):

- Intelligence is usually normal.
- Very frequent (>50% of individuals):
  - Short stature: Use the Turner growth chart.
  - Lymphedema of hands and feet present at birth, and may recur
  - Deep-set hyperconvex nails
  - Unusual shape and rotation of ears
  - Narrow maxilla and dental crowding
  - Micrognathia
  - Low posterior hairline
  - Broad chest with widely spaced, inverted, or hypoplastic nipples
  - Cubitus valgus
  - Short fourth metacarpals and/or metatarsals
  - Tibial exostosis
  - Tendency to obesity
  - Recurrent otitis media
  - Frequent (<50% of individuals):
    - Pigmented nevi
    - Webbed neck
    - Keloid formation
    - Scoliosis (10–12%), hip dysplasia
  - Occasional (<5% of individuals): Kyphosis, lordosis

DIAGNOSTIC TESTS & INTERPRETATION

Lab

Initial lab tests

- Chromosome analysis: A buccal smear is not adequate to rule out TS. An analysis of at least 20–30 cells is required. Analysis of 2 cell types (e.g., blood and skin) may be necessary.
- Thyroid function tests, celiac screening

Follow-Up & Special Considerations

- At puberty, follicle-stimulating hormone (FSH) and luteinizing hormone levels may approach levels consistent with the absence of ovaries. FSH may be transiently high in infancy.
- The high incidence of thyroid problems should prompt annual evaluation of thyroid function.

Imaging

Initial approach

- Magnetic resonance aortography in addition to echocardiography to evaluate cardiovascular system (2)
- Renal ultrasound to evaluate structural renal abnormalities

Diagnostic Procedures/Surgery

- Upper and lower extremity BP
- ENT/audiology: Hearing test
- Assess for congenital hip dislocation

Pathological Findings

- Ovarian dysgenesis (>90%): Streak gonads, atretic follicles, or no follicles present
- Renal: Horseshoe kidney, double collecting system (60%)
- Cardiac (20–40% of patients): Coarctation of the aorta, bicuspid aortic valve, valvular aortic stenosis (70% of TS patients with heart defects also have coarctation), hypertension
- Bone dysplasia (>50%), osteoporosis
- Gonadoblastomas in patients with X/XY mosaicism
- Ocular abnormalities: Amblyopia, ptosis, strabismus, red/green color blindness
- GI: Increased incidence of celiac disease
- Central nervous system abnormalities: ADHD, decreased visuospatial organization, impaired social cognition (3)

DIFFERENTIAL DIAGNOSIS

- Short stature:
  - Noonan syndrome: A genetic condition that shares some facial and other physical characteristics with TS (but is unrelated to TS); has been described inaccurately as "male TS"
  - Hypothyroidism
  - Familial short stature
  - Dyschondrosteosis (Léri-Weill syndrome)
  - Brachydactyly E
  - Growth hormone deficiency
  - Glucocorticoid excess
  - Klippel-Feil anomaly
  - Short stature due to chronic disease
- Amenorrhea or delayed puberty:
  - Pure gonadal dysgenesis
  - Polycystic ovary syndrome (Stein-Leventhal syndrome)
  - Primary/secondary amenorrhea
- Lymphedema:
  - Hereditary congenital lymphedema
  - Milroy disease
  - Lymphedema with recurrent cholestasis
  - Lymphedema with intestinal lymphangiectasia
- Other:
  - Multiple pterygium syndrome
  - Pseudohypoparathyroid syndrome

TREATMENT

MEDICATION

- Recombinant human growth hormone (rhGH):
- Treat when there is any evidence of growth failure (4)[C]; height falls below the fifth percentile by 18 months of age. Adult height is maximized if growth hormone is initiated at a young age:
  - 0.375–0.400 mg/kg/wk
  - Anabolic steroids in conjunction with GH.
- Estrogen:
  - Due to accelerated follicular atresia, most girls with TS undergo ovarian failure prior to or around the time of puberty. Treat gonadal failure in girls who do not enter puberty spontaneously:
  - Replacement therapy: Starting at age 13–14 years, continuing to age 50. Begin with 1–2 years of low-dose estrogen, followed by larger-dose estrogens cycled with progesterone. Do not delay puberty to promote statural growth (2).
  - Promotes sexual development and bone maturation, optimizes peak bone mass
  - May benefit cognitive development in young girls (3)

ADDITIONAL TREATMENT

Pregnancy Considerations

- Although pregnancy is rare, sexually active girls and women should receive contraception counseling.
- Infertility is the general rule; <2% of pregnancies are achieved without medical assistance:
  - In vitro fertilization and embryo transfer may be options.
  - Successful ovarian transplants have been reported in teenage girls with Turner syndrome.
  - Ovarian hyperstimulation and oocyte cryopreservation to preserve fertility in mosaic Turner.
  - High risk of maternal mortality secondary to cardiac complications, especially aortic dissection during pregnancy. Aortic root dimensions must be monitored throughout pregnancy by echo (5).

Issues for Referral

- Genetics
- Congenital heart disease, bicuspid aortic valve, coarctation of the aorta, aortic dissection (especially with valvular abnormalities or coarctation, or systemic hypertension) (2). Close cardiology follow-up in pregnancy.
- Pediatric endocrinologist for ghGH and estrogen
- Orthodontic evaluation
- Psychiatric/educational: May have problems in nonverbal areas such as evaluating objects in relationship to one another. Evaluate school performance. Patients may be at risk for ADHD or impaired social cognition (3).

SURGERY/OTHER PROCEDURES

- Removal of gonads is recommended in patients with X/XY mosaicism due to risk of gonadoblastoma.
- Angioplasty or surgical correction of coarctation of the aorta
- Physical appearance may be enhanced by reconstructive surgery.

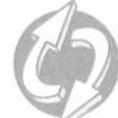

ONGOING CARE

FOLLOW-UP RECOMMENDATIONS

Patient Monitoring

- For complete health supervision guidelines, see Frias et al. (1).
- Regular cardiac exams; ultrasound/MRI at pubertal induction
- Every 4–6 months (6):
  - Height, weight, BP
  - Pubertal staging (after age 10)
- Every 12–18 months:
  - Thyroid function and IGF-1
  - Bone age
  - Hearing and vision assessment
- Every 3–5 years: Dual-energy x-ray absorptiometry scan for bone density
- FSH, liver function tests (LFTs), and pelvic ultrasound prior to pubertal induction
- Regular visits to primary care physicians are recommended. Be aware of the social and emotional problems associated with issues such as short stature and infertility.
- Adults with TS should be monitored for cardiovascular disease, including hypertension and valve disease.
- Cardiac imaging (preferably MRI) every 5–10 years for aortic root dilatation/aortic dissection. Frequent imaging during pregnancy.
- Adults also should be monitored yearly for thyroid disease, liver and kidney abnormalities, diabetes, and dyslipidemia.

PATIENT EDUCATION

- Families and patients need a thorough explanation of the condition and its management, especially about sexual development and growth. Support groups may be helpful.
- Turner Syndrome Society of the United States: (800) 365-9944; www.turnersyndrome.org. "Turner Syndrome: A Guide for Families" (2002) is downloadable from this site.
- Magic Foundation: www.magicfoundation.org
- Human Growth Foundation: www.hgfound.org

PROGNOSIS

- Most girls with TS lead reasonably normal lives with appropriate medical management; however, mortality was found to be 3-fold higher in women with TS than in the general population. Medical follow-up is important in adulthood; some deaths are preventable.
- Infertility: Most women with TS are infertile; however, pregnancy without medical assistance has been documented (but is rare). Successful pregnancy following oocyte donation is well described, although a thorough cardiovascular evaluation should be performed because the risk of aortic dissection is greatly increased during pregnancy.
- The overall risk of cancer is not increased in women with TS; however, in addition to increased risk of gonadoblastoma in individuals with 45,X/46,XY mosaicism, risk may be increased for meningioma, childhood brain tumors, and possibly bladder cancer, melanoma, and uterine cancer in individuals with TS when compared with that of the general population. Women with TS have a decreased risk of breast cancer.

REFERENCES

1. Frías JL, Davenport ML. Committee on Genetics and Section on Endocrinology. Health supervision for children with Turner syndrome. *Pediatrics*. 2003; 111:692–702.
2. Bondy CA, Turner Syndrome Study Group. Care of girls and women with Turner syndrome: A guideline of the Turner Syndrome Study Group. *J Clin Endocrinol Metab*. 2007;92:10–25.
3. Hong DS, Dunkin B, Reiss AL, et al. Psychosocial functioning and social cognitive processing in girls with turner syndrome. *J Dev Behav Pediatr*. 2011; 32:512–20.
4. Davenport ML. Approach to the patient with Turner syndrome. *J Clin Endocrinol Metab*. 2010;95: 1487–95.
5. Boissonnas CC, Davy C, Marszalek A, et al. Cardiovascular findings in women suffering from Turner syndrome requesting oocyte donation. *Hum Reprod*. 2011;26(10):2754–62.
6. Donaldson MDC. Optimising management in Turner syndrome: From infancy to adult transfer. *Arch Dis Child*. 2006;92:513–20.

ADDITIONAL READING

- Collett-Solberg PF. Update in growth hormone therapy of children. *J Clin Endocrinol Metab*. 2011; 96:573–9.
- Grote FK, Oostdijk W, De Muinck Keizer-Schrama SM, et al. The diagnostic work up of growth failure in secondary health care: An evaluation of consensus guidelines. *BMC Pediatr*. 2008;8:21.

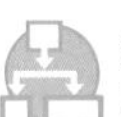

See Also (Topic, Algorithm, Electronic Media Element)

Amenorrhea; Coarctation of the Aorta; Hypothyroidism

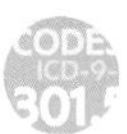

CODES

ICD9

758.6 Gonadal dysgenesis

CLINICAL PEARLS

- TS is the most common sex chromosome abnormality syndrome in females.
- Edema of the hands and feet and redundant skin of the neck (webbing) are presenting features during infancy. In school-aged girls, the triad of short stature, social issues, and frequent ear infections should be investigated. During adolescence, primary amenorrhea, short stature, and infantile secondary sex characteristics are presenting features.
- Much of the treatment provided to individuals with TS is not evidence-based, and consequently, there are many areas of controversy, especially with regard to hormone replacement therapy.

TYPHOID FEVER

Douglas W. MacPherson, MD, MSc(CTM), FRCPC

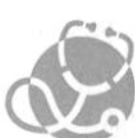

BASICS

- Typhoid fever is a rare enteric infectious syndrome in the US.
- Most cases reported in the US are imported from endemic areas of the world; in particular, South and Southeast Asia.

DESCRIPTION

- Typhoid fever is an acute systemic illness in humans caused by *Salmonella typhi*. It is a classic example of enteric fever caused by the *Salmonella* bacterium.
- Enteric fevers due to *S. paratyphi* can present in a similar manner as classic typhoid fever.
- Typhoid is endemic in some developing nations where sanitation is poor. Most cases in North America and other developed nations are acquired after travel to disease-endemic areas.
- "Visiting family or friends" travelers may be at greater risk of typhoid.
- Mode of transmission is fecal–oral through ingestion of contaminated food (commonly poultry, water, and milk).
- Incubation period varies from 7–21 days.
- System(s) affected: Gastrointestinal; Pulmonary; Skin/Exocrine
- Synonym(s): Typhoid; Typhus abdominalis; Enteric fever

Geriatric Considerations

Disease is more serious in the elderly.

Pediatric Considerations

Disease is more serious in infants, but may be milder in children.

EPIDEMIOLOGY

Although typhoid outbreaks have been described in the US, most cases are reported in international travelers who have been exposed in endemic transmission zones (in particular, South and Southeast Asia, parts of Latin America):

- Predominant age: All ages
- Predominant sex: Male = Female

Incidence

In the US, 300–500 new cases per year

RISK FACTORS

Must be considered in any patient presenting with fever after tropical travel or exposure to a chronic carrier

GENERAL PREVENTION

- Food and water consumption precautions are paramount in the prevention of all enteric infections, including typhoid fever.
- Avoid tap water, salad/raw vegetables, unpeeled fruits, and dairy products in tropical travel.
- Avoid poultry or poultry products left unrefrigerated for prolonged periods.
- For high-risk travel to an endemic area, consider vaccination against typhoid (1)[A]:
  - Parenteral ViCPS or capsular polysaccharide typhoid vaccine (Typhim Vi) *or*
  - Ty21a or live oral typhoid vaccine (Vivotif Berna), particularly if traveler will be at prolonged risk (>4 weeks)
- Consider vaccination for workers exposed to *S. typhi* or those with household or intimate exposure to a carrier of *S. typhi*.
- Occupational health and safety precautions, including screening of domestic and commercial food handlers, may be considered in some situations.

PATHOPHYSIOLOGY

- Acute typhoid and other enteric fevers are seen most commonly in international travelers to endemic *S. typhi* regions of the world.
- The initial infection is transmitted via the fecal–oral route with a GI source of the bacterium resulting in bacteremia and sepsis. Involvement of the bowel wall (Peyer patch) rarely may be associated with bleeding from the bowel or bowel perforation.
- *S. typhi* chronic carrier state may occur with shedding of the bacterium in the stools. Potential for person-to-person transmission may occur. In a chronic carrier state, *S. typhi* appears to locate in the biliary tract and in particular the gallbladder. Chronic suppressive antimicrobials may clear a carrier state. In extreme cases, cholecystectomies have been performed to attempt to clear carriage of *S. typhi*.

ETIOLOGY

Salmonella typhi

DIAGNOSIS

Assessment of the clinical presentation and exposure history, including endemic zone travel and known chronic *S. typhi* carrier exposure

HISTORY

Patient presentation: Fever, headache, constipation with:

- Travel history to an endemic region and exposure to contaminated food or water
- Exposure to a chronic *S. typhi* carrier

PHYSICAL EXAM

- Fever
- Headache
- Malaise
- Abdominal discomfort/bloating/constipation
- Diarrhea (less common)
- Dry cough
- Confusion/lethargy
- Rose spot (transient erythematous maculopapular rash in anterior thorax or upper abdomen)
- Splenomegaly
- Hepatomegaly
- Cervical adenopathy
- Relative bradycardia
- Conjunctivitis
- Constitutionally unwell, fever, relative bradycardia, rose spots, abdominal pain, hepatosplenomegaly

DIAGNOSTIC TESTS & INTERPRETATION

Due to the rarity of enteric fevers/typhoid syndromes in the US, a high level of clinical suspicion must be present. A travel history to a known typhoid endemic zone or exposure to a known chronic carrier of *S. typhi* will contribute to the clinical and laboratory diagnosis of typhoid fever.

Lab

- Definitive diagnosis is by culture of *S. typhi* from blood
- Isolation of *S. typhi* in sputum, urine, or stool is a presumptive diagnosis in typical clinical presentation.
- Serology is nonspecific and usually not useful.
- If there are multiple negative blood cultures, or in patients with prior antibiotic therapy, diagnostic yield is better with bone marrow culture.
- Anemia, leukopenia (neutropenia), thrombocytopenia, or evidence of disseminated intravascular coagulopathy are supportive. Elevated liver enzymes are common.
- Drugs that may alter lab results:
  - Prior antibiotic therapy
  - Vaccination

Imaging

Consider serial plain abdominal films for evidence of intestinal perforation.

Diagnostic Procedures/Surgery

- Bone marrow aspirate for culture of *S. typhi* has been reported to be more sensitive than blood cultures, but is rarely indicated as a primary investigation.
- A bone marrow aspiration may be done for evaluation of a persistent fever in a clinically suspect situation with negative cultures or for investigation of a pyrexia of unknown origin.

Pathological Findings

Classically, mononuclear proliferation involving lymphoid tissue of intestinal tract, especially Peyer patch in terminal ileum

DIFFERENTIAL DIAGNOSIS

- Malaria
- "Enteric feverlike" syndrome caused by *Yersinia enterocolitica*, pseudotuberculosis, and *Campylobacter* spp.
- Enteric fever caused by nontyphoid *Salmonella* spp.
- Infectious hepatitis
- Atypical pneumonia
- Infectious mononucleosis
- Subacute bacterial endocarditis
- Tuberculosis
- Brucellosis
- Q fever
- Toxoplasmosis
- Viral infections: Epstein-Barr virus (EBV), cytomegalovirus (CMV), viral hemorrhagic agents

TREATMENT

Awareness of emerging drug-resistant *S. typhi* strains globally and the epidemiology of the patient's exposure may direct primary therapy. Knowledge of local resistance patterns for presumptive treatment or laboratory sensitivity should guide therapy. Fluoroquinolone-resistant *S. typhi* is becoming common in Asia.

MEDICATION

See below for treatment recommendations for acute typhoid fever and chronic carrier states.

First Line

- Chloramphenicol: Pediatric 50 mg/kg/d PO q.i.d. × 2 weeks; adult dose 50 mg/kg/d divided q6h for 2 weeks *or*
- Ampicillin: Pediatric 100 mg/kg/d q.i.d. PO × 2 weeks; adults 500 mg q6h for 2 weeks *or*
- Ciprofloxacin: 500 mg PO b.i.d. × 2 weeks, indicated in multiple-drug-resistant typhoid (has been used successfully and safely in children) *or*
- Ceftriaxone: 1–2 g IV once daily × 2 weeks *or*
- Furazolidone: 7.5 mg/kg/d PO × 10 days; in uncomplicated multiple-drug-resistant typhoid; safe in children; efficacy >85% cure
- Chronic carrier state:
  - Ampicillin: 4–5 g/d plus probenecid 2 g/d q.i.d. × 6 weeks (for patients with normally functioning gallbladder without evidence of cholelithiasis)
  - Ciprofloxacin: 500 mg PO b.i.d. for 4–6 weeks is also efficacious. Chloramphenicol resistance has been reported in Mexico, South America, Central America, Southeast Asia, India, Pakistan, Middle East, and Africa.
- Contraindications: Refer to manufacturer's profile for each drug.
- Precautions: Rarely, Jarisch-Herxheimer reaction appears after antimicrobial therapy.
- Significant possible interactions: Refer to manufacturer's profile for each drug.

Second Line

Trimethoprim–sulfamethoxazole

Pregnancy Considerations

Ciprofloxacin therapy is relatively contraindicated in pregnant patients.

ADDITIONAL TREATMENT

General Measures

- Fluid and electrolyte support
- Strict isolation of patient's linen, stool, and urine
- Monitor clinically, and consider serial plain abdominal films for evidence of perforation, usually in the third to fourth week of illness.
- Indications and contraindications for specific treatment of typhoid disease and chronic carrier states must be determined on an individual basis. Factors to be considered are age, public health and occupational health risk (e.g., food handler, chronic care facilities, medical personnel), intolerance to antibiotics, and evidence of biliary tract disease.
- For hemorrhage: Blood transfusion and management of shock

Issues for Referral

Complications of sepsis, bowel perforation

SURGERY/OTHER PROCEDURES

- Complications: Bowel perforation
- Cholecystectomy may be warranted in carriers with cholelithiasis, relapse after therapy, or intolerance to antimicrobial therapy.

IN-PATIENT CONSIDERATIONS

Initial Stabilization

- Inpatient if acutely ill
- Outpatient for less ill patient or for carrier

Admission Criteria

Clinical severity

Nursing

Observe enteric precautions.

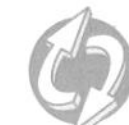

ONGOING CARE

FOLLOW-UP RECOMMENDATIONS

Bed rest initially, then activity as tolerated

Patient Monitoring

See "General Measures."

DIET

If abdominal symptoms are severe, NPO. With improvement, begin normal low-residue diet, possibly high-calorie.

PATIENT EDUCATION

- Discuss chronic carrier state and its complications.
- For family members, travelers, or workers at risk, provide hygiene education and possibly vaccination.

PROGNOSIS

Overall prognosis is good with therapy; <2% mortality rate; 15% relapse rate with some antibiotic treatments; 3% bowel perforation

COMPLICATIONS

- Intestinal hemorrhage and perforation in distal ileum
- Patients may become chronic carriers (up to 3%), defined as persistent stool excretor of *S. typhi* for >1 year.
- Predilection for seeding in the biliary tract exists and may become a focus for relapse of typhoid fever: Most common in females and older patients (>50 years)
- Osteomyelitis is found especially in patients with sickle cell anemia, systemic lupus erythematosus, and hematologic neoplasms, as well as in immunosuppressed hosts.
- Endovascular infection in the elderly and in patients with a history of bypass operation or aneurysm
- Rarely, endocarditis or meningitis

REFERENCES

1. Typhoid Immunization Recommendations of the Advisory Committee on Immunization Practices (ACIP). *MMWR*. 1994;43(RR14):1–7. Available at: www.phppo.cdc.gov/cdcRecommends/showarticle.asp?a_artid=M0035643&TopNum=50&CallPg=AdvCDC.

ADDITIONAL READING

- Basnyat B. Typhoid fever in the United States and antibiotic choice. *JAMA*. 2010;303:34; author reply 34–5.
- Bhutta ZA. Current concepts in the diagnosis and treatment of typhoid fever. *Br Med J*. 2006;333: 78–82.
- Butler T. Treatment of typhoid fever in the 21st century: Promises and shortcomings. *Clin Microbiol Infect*. 2011;17(7):959–63.
- Centers for Disease Control and Prevention. Vaccines and preventable diseases: Typhoid. Available at: www.cdc.gov/vaccines/vpd-vac/typhoid/default.htm.
- Centers for Disease Control and Prevention. *The Pre-travel Consultation. Travel-Related Vaccine Preventable Diseases*. Chapter 2. Typhoid and Paratyphoid Fever. Available at: wwwnc.cdc.gov/travel/yellowbook/2010/chapter-2/typhoid-paratyphoid-fever.htm.
- Centers for Disease Control and Prevention. Typhoid fever. Available at: www.cdc.gov/ncidod/dbmd/diseaseinfo/typhoidfever_g.htm.
- Clark TW, Daneshvar C, Pareek M, et al. Enteric fever in a UK regional infectious diseases unit: A 10 year retrospective review. *J Infect*. 2010;60: 91–8.
- Crump JA, Mintz ED. Global trends in typhoid and paratyphoid fever. *Clin Infect Dis*. 2010;50: 241–6.
- Kroger AT, Atkinson WL, Marcuse EK, et al. General recommendations on immunization. Recommendations of the Advisory Committee on Immunization Practices (ACIP). *MMWR*. 2006; 55(RR15):1–48.
- Lynch MF, Blanton EM, Bulens S, et al. Typhoid fever in the United States, 1999–2006. *JAMA*. 2009; 302:859–65.

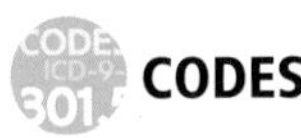

CODES

ICD9

002.0 Typhoid fever

CLINICAL PEARLS

- Along with malaria and other regionally defined exotic infections, including dengue, enteric fevers, and others, typhoid should be considered as a possible diagnosis for any febrile traveler from endemic areas such as Latin America, sub-Saharan Africa, or South Asia.
- Routine blood cultures will detect *S. typhi*, but may be negative if antibiotics have been taken prior to testing.
- A history or documentation of vaccination against *S. typhi* does not exclude the diagnosis of typhoid fever.

TYPHUS FEVERS

Douglas W. MacPherson, MD, MSc(CTM), FRCPC

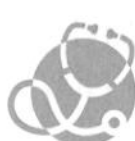

BASICS

Typhus is an infectious disease syndrome caused by several bacterial organisms resulting in acute, chronic, and recrudescing disease.

DESCRIPTION

- Acute infectious diseases caused by 3 species of *Rickettsiae*:
  - Epidemic typhus: Human-to-human transmission by body louse vector. Primarily in circumstances such as refugee camps, war, famine, and disaster. Recrudescent disease, occurring years after initial infection, can be a source of human outbreak. Flying squirrels are also a reservoir.
  - Endemic (murine) typhus: Infection by rodents to humans by rat flea bite
  - Scrub typhus: Infection and infestation of chiggers and of rodents to humans by the chigger; primarily in Asia and Western Pacific areas
- System(s) affected: Endocrine/Metabolic; Hematologic/Lymphatic/Immunologic; Pulmonary; Skin/Exocrine
- Synonym(s): Louse-borne typhus; Brill-Zinsser disease; Murine typhus

EPIDEMIOLOGY

- Epidemic and endemic typhus: Rare in the US (outside of south Texas)
- Scrub typhus: Travelers returning from endemic areas only (rare)

Incidence

Endemic typhus: <100 cases annually, primarily in states around the Gulf of Mexico, especially south Texas; underreporting suspected

RISK FACTORS

Exposure to vectors (e.g., during travel to countries where endemic)

Geriatric Considerations

Elderly may have more severe disease.

GENERAL PREVENTION

Avoid vectors for each disease:

- Scrub typhus: Wear protective clothing and use insect repellents.
- Endemic typhus: Practice ectoparasite and rodent control.
- Epidemic typhus: Delousing and cleaning of clothing; vaccine may be considered for those at high risk of exposure (typhus vaccine production has been discontinued in the US).

ETIOLOGY

- Epidemic typhus by *R. prowazekii*
- Endemic typhus by *R. typhi*
- Scrub typhus by *R. tsutsugamushi*

DIAGNOSIS

Given the rarity of typhus syndromes in the US, a high level of clinical suspicion is necessary to make the diagnosis.

HISTORY

Travel or other risk exposure

PHYSICAL EXAM

- General:
  - Acute onset
  - Fever
  - Chills
  - Headache
  - Myalgia
  - Malaise
  - Diffuse organ involvement (e.g., intestine, liver, heart, kidneys, brain)
- Epidemic typhus:
  - Incubation period ~1 week
  - Macular or maculopapular rash beginning on trunk ~fifth day of illness
  - Nonproductive cough
  - Pulmonary infiltrates
- Endemic typhus:
  - Incubation period 1–2 weeks
  - Macular or maculopapular rash beginning on trunk third to fifth day of illness
- Scrub typhus:
  - Incubation period 1–3 weeks
  - Eschar at bite site
  - Regional lymphadenopathy
  - Generalized lymphadenopathy
  - Splenomegaly
  - Macular or maculopapular rash beginning on trunk approximately fifth day of illness
  - Relative bradycardia early in disease
  - Ocular pain
  - Conjunctival injection

DIAGNOSTIC TESTS & INTERPRETATION

- Specific serologic test showing a rising antibody titer
- Isolation of *Rickettsia* should be undertaken only in special laboratories to minimize the risk of laboratory-acquired infection.

Lab

- Leukocyte findings usually normal
- Abnormalities reflecting the particular organs affected
- Weil-Felix serologic reaction may be positive; test value hampered to midillness or after, and by low sensitivity and nonspecificity; epidemic and endemic typhus, 4-fold titer rise or titer >1/320 to OX-19; scrub typhus, 4-fold rise in titer to OX-K
- Hyponatremia in severe cases
- Hypoalbuminemia in severe cases
- Drugs that may alter lab results: Prior antibiotic use

Pathological Findings

Diffuse vasculitis

DIFFERENTIAL DIAGNOSIS

- Any acute febrile disease
- Rocky Mountain spotted fever
- Meningococcemia
- Bacterial meningitis
- Mediterranean spotted fever (boutonneuse fever) (*R. conorii*)
- Measles
- Rubella
- Toxoplasmosis
- Leptospirosis
- Typhoid fever
- Dengue
- Malaria
- Relapsing fever
- Secondary syphilis
- Viral syndromes: Mononucleosis, acute retroviral syndrome

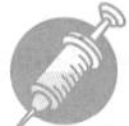

TREATMENT

Treatment should be started based on strong epidemiologic risk assessment and clinical presentation.

MEDICATION

First Line

- Treatment should begin when diagnosis is reasonably likely and continue until the patient's state is improved and the patient is afebrile for a minimum of 48 hours; usual treatment course: 5–7 days.
- Children ≥8 years of age and adults:
  - Tetracycline: 25 mg/kg PO initially, then 25 mg/kg/d in equally divided doses q6h
  - If severely ill, may use doxycycline IV: Adults 100 mg q12h, children ≥8 years of age 5 mg/kg in 24 hours (maximum of 200 mg/24 hours)
- Children ≤8 years of age, pregnant women, or if typhoid fever is possible cause of illness:
  - Chloramphenicol: 50 mg/kg PO initially, then 50 mg/kg/d in equally divided doses q6h
  - If severely ill, chloramphenicol sodium succinate: 20 mg/kg IV initially, infused over 30–45 minute, then 50 mg/kg/d infused in equally divided doses q6h until orally tolerable
- Precautions: Refer to the manufacturer's profile for each drug.
- Significant possible interactions: Refer to the manufacturer's profile for each drug.

Second Line

- Doxycycline: Single oral dose of 100 or 200 mg for those in refugee camps, victims of disasters, or in the presence of limited medical services
- Isolated reports indicate that erythromycin and ciprofloxacin are effective.
- Azithromycin 3-day course is effective for scrub typhus; better tolerated than doxycycline but more expensive (1)[B]
- Rifampin may be effective in areas where scrub typhus responds poorly to standard antirickettsial drugs (2)[A].

ADDITIONAL TREATMENT

General Measures

- Protect agitated patient from injury.
- Skin and mouth care
- Supportive care for the severely ill, directed at complications

Issues for Referral

Due to the rarity of typhus syndromes in the US, a tropical medicine or infectious disease consultation may be required if the diagnosis or management is uncertain.

IN-PATIENT CONSIDERATIONS

Initial Stabilization

Outpatient care unless severely ill

Admission Criteria

Severely ill or constitutionally unstable (e.g., shock)

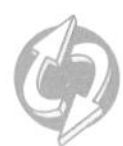

ONGOING CARE

FOLLOW-UP RECOMMENDATIONS

Bed rest during acute stages; otherwise, as tolerated

Patient Monitoring

- Severely ill patients should be admitted and observed regularly in the hospital.
- Outpatients should be checked periodically until clinically improving.

DIET

As tolerated

PATIENT EDUCATION

Provide prevention information to travelers.

PROGNOSIS

- Recovery is expected if treatment is instituted before the onset of complications.
- Relapses may follow treatment, especially if initiated within 48 hours of onset (this is *not* an indication to delay treatment). Relapses are treated the same as primary disease.
- Without treatment, the mortality rate of typhus is 40–60% for epidemic, 1–2% for endemic, and up to 30% for scrub.
- Mortality higher among the elderly

COMPLICATIONS

- Consequences of specific organ-system involvement in the second week (e.g., azotemia, meningoencephalitis, seizures, delirium, coma, myocardial failure, hyponatremia, hypoalbuminemia, hypovolemia, and shock)
- Death

REFERENCES

1. Phimda K, Hoontrakul S, Suttinont C, et al. Doxycycline versus azithromycin for treatment of leptospirosis and scrub typhus. *Antimicrob Agents Chemother*. 2007;51:3259–63.
2. Panpanich R, Garner P. Antibiotics for treating scrub typhus. *Cochrane Database Syst Rev*. 2002; CD002150.

ADDITIONAL READING

- Adjemian J, Eremeeva ME, Dasch, GA. Rickettsial (spotted and typhus fevers) and related infections (anaplasmosis and ehrlchiosis). Chapter 5. Other infectious disease related to travel. Available at: wwwnc.cdc.gov/travel/yellowbook/2010/chapter-5/rickettsial-and-related-infections.htm.
- Botelho-Nevers E, Raoult D. Host, pathogen and treatment-related prognostic factors in rickettsioses. *Eur J Clin Microbiol Infect Dis*. 2011;30:1139–50.
- Graham J, Stockley K, Goldman RD. Tick-borne illnesses: A CME update. *Pediatr Emerg Care*. 2011;27(2):141–7; quiz 148–50.
- Green JS, Singh J, Cheung M, et al. A cluster of pediatric endemic typhus cases in Orange County, California. *Pediatr Infect Dis J*. 2011;30:163–5.
- Hendershot EF, Sexton DJ. Scrub typhus and rickettsial diseases in international travelers: A review. *Curr Infect Dis Rep*. 2009;11:66–72.
- Jensenius M, Fournier PE, Raoult D. Rickettsioses and the international traveler. *Clin Infect Dis*. 2004;39:1493–9.
- Molina N. Borders, laborers, and racialized medicalization Mexican immigration and US public health practices in the 20th century. *Am J Public Health*. 2011;101:1024–31.
- Walker DH, Paddock CD, Dumler JS, et al. Emerging and re-emerging tick-transmitted rickettsial and ehrlichial infections. *Med Clin North Am*. 2008;92: 1345–61, x.

CODES

ICD9

- 080 Louse-borne (epidemic) typhus
- 081.1 Brill's disease
- 081.9 Typhus, unspecified

CLINICAL PEARLS

- Along with malaria or dengue, consider a typhus diagnosis with any febrile traveler from endemic areas, including sub-Saharan Africa and Asia.
- Rickettsial infections typically present within 2–14 days, so febrile illnesses onset >18 days after travel are unlikely to be rickettsial.
- Routine blood cultures will not detect *Rickettsia* bacteria.
- Vaccination against travel diseases does not exclude the diagnosis of typhus.
- Severe headache is often intractable and not eased by the standard drugs.
- Report case to appropriate health department or other agency.

ULCER, APHTHOUS

Cary D. Douglass, MD

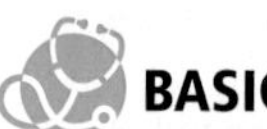

BASICS

DESCRIPTION

Self-limited, painful ulcerations of the oral mucosa that are typically recurrent; they occur on nonkeratinized mucosa inside the mouth: The inner side of the lips and cheeks, the back and floor of the mouth, and under the tongue.

EPIDEMIOLOGY

- The first episode of aphthous stomatitis usually occurs during the first or second decade of life. The incidence then begins to decrease after the third decade. It affects 10–15% of the US population (1).
- Aphthous ulcers may be categorized into 3 types:
  - Minor aphthous ulcers:
    - 70–90% of all aphthae
    - $<$10 mm in diameter
    - Up to 5 appear at a time.
    - Heal in 7–10 days
    - Nonscarring
  - Major aphthous ulcers (also called Sutton disease):
    - 10–15% of all aphthae
    - $>$10 mm in diameter
    - 1–10 ulcers at a time
    - Take weeks to months to heal
    - Scarring may occur.
  - Herpetiform aphthous ulcers:
    - 7–10% of all aphthae
    - Between 1 and 3 mm in diameter
    - Multiple (tens to hundreds) in small clusters
    - Last 7–30 days
    - Scarring may occur.

RISK FACTORS

- Trauma
- Stress
- Vitamin, iron, or folic acid deficiency
- Immunodeficiency
- Smoking
- Toothpastes containing sodium lauryl sulfate
- Celiac disease (2)

Genetics

Possible familial correlation

ETIOLOGY

Unknown etiology; likely multifactorial with some correlation with:

- Immunologic dysfunction
- Activation of cell-mediated immune system:
  - Infection
  - Food hypersensitivities
  - Vitamin deficiency
  - Pregnancy
  - Menstruation
  - Psychological and genetic factors

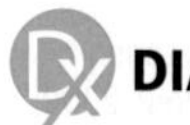

DIAGNOSIS

Diagnosis is made by history and clinical presentation.

HISTORY

- Prodrome of burning or pricking sensation of oral mucosa 1–2 days prior to appearance of ulcers
- Inquire about family history of systemic lupus erythematosus (SLE), inflammatory bowel disease (IBD), or Behçet disease.
- Inquire about patient medical history of SLE, HIV, IBD, Behçet disease, or cancer.

PHYSICAL EXAM

- Round or ovoid ulcerations generally $<$10 mm in size, with inflammatory halo
- Look for signs of dehydration.
- Vital signs should be within normal limits.
- Evaluate for signs of secondary infection.

DIAGNOSTIC TESTS & INTERPRETATION

Lab

Lab workup rarely helpful unless atypical presentation suggests underlying systemic disease such as Behçet or Crohn disease. Consider testing for celiac disease. Other tests if suggested by history and exam:

- CBC
- Rapid plasma reagin test
- Antinuclear antibody (ANA) test
- Tzanck stain (herpesvirus)
- Celiac disease serology IgA-TTG (see "Celiac Disease")
- Vitamins B_6 and B_{12}
- Serum iron and folate
- HIV

Diagnostic Procedures/Surgery

- Biopsy: Multinucleated giant cells (cytomegalovirus)
- Fungal cultures: *Cryptosporidium*

DIFFERENTIAL DIAGNOSIS

- Consider oral manifestation of systemic disease.
- Trauma:
  - Biting
  - Dentures
- Drug exposure:
  - NSAIDs
  - Nicorandil

- Infection:
  - Herpesvirus:
    - Vesicular lesions
    - Ulcers on attached mucosa
  - Cytomegalovirus: Immunocompromised patient
  - Varicella virus: Characteristic skin lesions
  - Coxsackievirus:
    - Ulcers preceded by vesicles
    - Hand, foot, buttock lesions
  - Syphilis: Other skin or genital lesions
  - Erythema multiforme:
    - Lip crusting
    - Lesions on attached and unattached mucosa skin lesions
  - *Cryptosporidium* infection, mucormycosis, histoplasmosis
  - Necrotizing gingivitis
- Underlying disease:
  - Behçet syndrome:
    - Genital ulceration
    - Uveitis
    - Retinitis
  - Reiter syndrome:
    - Uveitis
    - Urethritis
    - HLA-B27–associated arthritis
  - Sweet syndrome:
    - Fever
    - Erythematous skin plaques/nodules
    - In conjunction with malignancy
  - IBD:
    - Bloody or mucous diarrhea
    - GI ulcerations
  - SLE: Malar rash
  - Bullous pemphigoid/pemphigoid vulgaris:
    - Vesiculobullous lesions on attached and unattached mucosa
    - Diffuse skin involvement
  - Cyclic neutropenia: Periodic fever
  - Squamous cell carcinoma:
    - Chronicity
    - Head/neck adenopathy
  - Immunocompromised patient:
    - HIV
    - Agranulocytosis

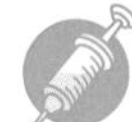

TREATMENT

MEDICATION

- Analgesia:
  - Debacterol (available over the counter [OTC]), a topical treatment, chemically cauterizes the oral lesion, eliminating pain associated with the lesion.
  - 5-aminosalicylic acid 5% cream: 3× daily × 2 weeks
  - Dyclonine HCl 1% solution: 5-mL rinse q.i.d.
  - Magnesium hydroxide/diphenhydramine hydrochloride: 5 mg/5 mL in 1:1 mix; swish and swallow q.i.d.
  - Sucralfate: 10 mL; swish and swallow or swish and spit q.i.d.
  - Viscous lidocaine 2%: Apply to ulcer as needed q.i.d.
  - Topical OTC preparations (e.g., Orabase, Anbesol)
- Promote ulcer healing/prevent recurrence (first-line agents):
  - Triamcinolone 0.1% in Orabase: Apply to ulcer 2–4× daily until healed.
  - Amlexanox 5% paste: 0.5 cm applied to ulcer q.i.d. after meals
  - Clobetasol 0.05%: 0.5 cm applied to ulcer 2× daily
  - Fluocinonide 0.05% gel: 0.5 cm applied to ulcer up to 5× daily
- Second-line agents:
  - Prednisone tablets: 40 mg/d PO × 7 days
  - Thalidomide: 200 mg/d PO × 4 weeks

ADDITIONAL TREATMENT

Issues for Referral

Follow up with otolaryngologist if lesions have not resolved within 2 weeks.

Additional Therapies

Vitamin and iron supplementation

IN-PATIENT CONSIDERATIONS

Admission Criteria

- Unable to eat or drink after appropriate analgesia
- Abnormal vital signs or evidence of dehydration

Discharge Criteria

- Tolerating fluids
- Adequate analgesia
- Normal vital signs

REFERENCES

1. Chattopadhyay A, Shetty KV. Recurrent aphthous stomatitis. *Otolaryngol Clin North Am*. 2011;44:79–88, v.
2. Pastore L, Carroccio A, Compilato D, et al. Oral manifestations of celiac disease. *J Clin Gastroenterol*. 2008;42:224–32.

ADDITIONAL READING

Messadi DV, Younai F. Aphthous ulcers. *Dermatol Ther*. 2010;23:281–90.

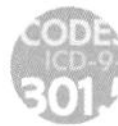

CODES

ICD9

- 528.00 Stomatitis and mucositis, unspecified
- 528.2 Oral aphthae

CLINICAL PEARLS

- Risk of recurrence decreases with quitting smoking.
- Use of toothpastes without the ingredient sodium lauryl sulfate may reduce or even prevent recurrences.
- Avoid oral trauma from aggressive toothbrushing or foods with sharp edges.
- Risk factors include: Trauma; stress; vitamin, iron, or folic acid deficiency; immunodeficiency, smoking; toothpastes containing sodium lauryl sulfate; celiac disease
- Most are self-limiting; treat symptoms with topical agents like: Debacterol, Triamcinolone 0.1% in Orabase, others

ULCER, STASIS

Kelly J. Alberda, MD

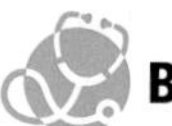

BASICS

DESCRIPTION

Stasis ulcer, or venous ulcer, is an ulceration of the skin of the lower leg or ankle related to disease of insufficiency of the venous system.

EPIDEMIOLOGY

Incidence

Up to 1% of population throughout lifetime

Prevalence

6–7 million people affected at any given time in the US

RISK FACTORS

- Prior leg injury
- Elderly
- Obesity
- Phlebitis or DVT
- Varicosities
- Prolonged sitting or standing

GENERAL PREVENTION

- Avoiding prolonged sitting or standing by taking breaks that include walking to induce the calf-muscle-venous pump.
- Stockings for men and women are available that provide compression, promote venous return, and prevent blood pooling in the lower extremities. The best have a gradient compression that provides increased compression at the foot compared to ankle and calf areas.

PATHOPHYSIOLOGY

Primary mechanisms are unclear. Most sources describe a combination of lower extremity venous incompetence and associated venous stasis and hypertension that leads to capillary dilatation and inflammation. The subsequent intracellular edema leads to skin breakdown and poor wound healing. It is also unclear why some patients have more severe disease or a poor response to treatment.

ETIOLOGY

Must differentiate between venous ulcers, which are largely due to venous disease, and other causes of skin ulceration, namely arterial or ischemic ulcers, neuropathic (diabetic) ulcers, and pressure ulcers.

COMMONLY ASSOCIATED CONDITIONS

- Edema
- Varicosities and telangiectasias
- Venous dermatitis
- Lipodermatosclerosis (hardening of SC adipose tissue)

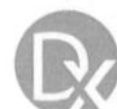

DIAGNOSIS

HISTORY

- Symptoms:
  - Leg pain, aching, or heaviness
  - Skin that is dry, irritated, or eczematous
  - Edema that improves with elevation
- Signs:
  - Ulcers usually over bony prominences (medial malleolus)
  - History of or current varicose veins

PHYSICAL EXAM

Venous stasis ulcers are typically shallow and the skin will generally not be erythematous. Border is flat and irregular. Hyperpigmentation and chronic, changes are common as is granulation tissue.

DIAGNOSTIC TESTS & INTERPRETATION

Venous/stasis ulcers are generally a clinical diagnosis, but additional studies can be helpful if other disease processes are suspected such as cirrhosis, thrombosis, vasculitis, or diabetes.

Lab

CBC, LFTs, and glucose can be considered.

Imaging

- Venous duplex sonography should be done if there is any suspicion of a DVT. It can also clarify the extent of venous incompetency.
- Venography can be considered. Usually done with consultation of vascular specialist

Diagnostic Procedures/Surgery

Ankle-brachial index helpful to rule out arterial disease:

- Classification can be helpful to communicate to specialists the severity of chronic venous disorders based on CEAP score (1).
- C: Clinical classification:
  - 0–6, no visible signs of venous disease to active ulcer
- E: Etiology:
  - Congenital, primary, or secondary (DVT)
- A: Anatomic:
  - Superficial, perforator, or deep veins
- P: Pathophysiologic:
  - Reflux, obstructive, or both

DIFFERENTIAL DIAGNOSIS

- Nonvenous ulcers as listed above
- Skin malignancy
- Vasculitis

TREATMENT

- Conservative: Elevation and compression are considered standard of care.
  - Elevation: Ideally done for 30 minutes 3–4 times per day above heart level
  - Compression therapy: Elastic, multilayer compression appears more effective than nonelastic or single-layer therapy (2). Intermittent pneumatic compression is not recommended:
    - Inelastic: Provides no resting pressure. Most common (Unna boot) contains zinc oxide and hardens after application (2)[A].
    - Elastic: Ace wraps are not recommended; gradient compression stockings (provide higher compression at foot than ankle or calf, [e.g., Jobst]) better than other stockings (nongradient) or bandages.
    - Multilayer elastic (e.g., Profore): May be the most effective compression option, but need skilled application or wound care therapist
  - Dressings: No proven advantage of 1 type over another. Low-cost nonadherent dressings were not inferior to others in meta-analysis (3).
- Example application:
  - First layer: Nonadherent bandage, hydrocolloid (DuoDerm), Vaseline-gauze (Adaptic), or Xeroform
  - Second layer: Foam wrap
  - Third layer: Preferable to use *gradient* compression stocking over elastic bandage or wrap. If using wrap, must also wrap the foot so as not to block venous return.

MEDICATION

Oral medication is usually considered in more severe disease as adjuvant treatment.

First Line

- Pentoxifylline (Trental) inhibits platelet aggregation, 400 mg 3× daily:
  - Effective as adjuvant therapy, but cost-effectiveness not clearly established
- Aspirin 1× daily generally recommended in addition to compression and elevation

ADDITIONAL TREATMENT

Systemic or topical antibiotics and antiseptics are not useful (as these wounds may be colonized), unless treating a cellulitis, per a Cochrane review (4).

Issues for Referral

- Complicating and moderate-to-severe venous insufficiency/varicosities
- Nonhealing or worsening ulcers

Additional Therapies

- Hyperbaric oxygen therapy has limited data in venous ulcers.
- Vacuum-assisted closure generally not used due to lack of good clinical data, cost, and difficulty in application.

COMPLEMENTARY AND ALTERNATIVE MEDICINE

Oral zinc

SURGERY/OTHER PROCEDURES

- Surgical débridement is not commonly needed in venous ulcer disease; more commonly needed in other caused of lower extremity ulcers
- Skin grafting in selected, severe cases
- For patients who have underlying venous insufficiency (i.e., varicose veins), surgical options should be considered.

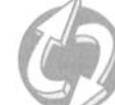

ONGOING CARE

FOLLOW-UP RECOMMENDATIONS

- Frequent follow-up (once or twice weekly) necessary for large lesions until proven to respond to therapy. Consider wound therapist referral, if available, to assist in treating and monitoring.
- Chronic lesions are usually followed less frequently if stable or improving.

PATIENT EDUCATION

Adherence to elevation and application of compression are difficult for most; therefore, the importance of these 2 treatment modalities should be stressed. As with most chronic disease, the medication prescribed may be the least important part of the wound-healing treatment.

PROGNOSIS

- Obviously, prognosis depends on severity, but success rates in compression and elevation studies range from 30 to 60 days in 6 months. Up to one quarter will persist at 1 year.
- Large (>6 cm) and prolonged duration (>3 months) are poor prognostic factors (1).

REFERENCES

1. Eklöf B, Rutherford RB, Bergan JJ, et al. Revision of the CEAP classification for chronic venous disorders: Consensus statement. *J Vasc Surg*. 2004;40:1248–52.
2. O'Meara S, Cullum NA, Nelson EA, et al. Compression for venous leg ulcers. *Cochrane Database Syst Rev*. 2009:CD000265.
3. Palfreyman S, Nelson EA, Michaels JA, et al. Dressings for venous leg ulcers: Systematic review and meta-analysis. *BMJ*. 2007;335:244.
4. O'Meara S, Al-Kurdi D, Ologun Y, et al. Antibiotics and antiseptics for venous leg ulcers. *Cochrane Database Syst Rev*. 2010:CD003557.

ADDITIONAL READING

- Collins L, Seraj S. Diagnosis and treatment of venous ulcers. *Am Fam Physician*. 2010;81:989–96.
- Etufugh CN, Phillips TJ. Venous ulcers. *Clin Dermatol*. 2007;25:121–30.

CODES

ICD9

454.0 Varicose veins of lower extremities with ulcer

CLINICAL PEARLS

- Must differentiate from non-venous ulcers
- Elevation and compression are considered standard of care.
- Topical antibiotics and antiseptics generally not helpful
- Medications (i.e., pentoxifylline and aspirin) considered adjuvant therapy, not as monotherapy

ULCERATIVE COLITIS

Michele L. Matthews, PharmD, CPE, RPh
Craig Lubin, MD

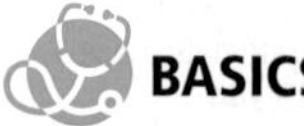

BASICS

DESCRIPTION
- An idiopathic inflammatory disease of the colonic mucosa that can affect any section of the colon from the rectum to the cecum
- >95% of patients have rectal involvement, with 50% of cases limited to rectum and sigmoid.
- 20% have pancolitis.

EPIDEMIOLOGY
Incidence
- US: 9–12 new cases/100,000 persons/yr
- Predominant age: 15–35 years; second and smaller peak in the seventh decade
- Predominant sex: Female > Male (slight)

Prevalence
205–240/100,000 persons

Pediatric Considerations
20% of patients are ≤21 years of age.

Pregnancy Considerations
- Similar to general population; 1 study showed 30% with inactive disease at onset of pregnancy relapsed.
- Treatment with sulfasalazine does not seem to affect outcome of pregnancy.
- Recommend that patients delay pregnancy until time when disease is inactive.

RISK FACTORS
- Better sanitation, artificial work environments (e.g., indoors), and fatty foods increase risk.
- NSAIDs can activate disease.
- Appendectomy is protective against later development of disease.
- Negative association with smoking: Relative risk of smokers is 40% of nonsmokers.

Genetics
- Family history in 5–10% in population surveys and 20–30% in referral-based studies
- More common in the Jewish population

GENERAL PREVENTION
- Patients with long-term disease who do not have colectomy are at increased risk for colon cancer.
- Aspirin (≥300 mg/d), sclerosing cholangitis, and ursodeoxycholic acid (10 mg/kg) have been shown to be preventive.

Pediatric Considerations
Breast-feeding may be protective for pediatric inflammatory bowel disease (IBD).

ETIOLOGY
Unknown; hypotheses include allergy to dietary components and abnormal immune responses to bacterial or "self" antigens; final outcome is mucosal inflammation secondary to immune cell infiltration (1)[B].

COMMONLY ASSOCIATED CONDITIONS
- Extracolonic manifestations in 10–15%
- Arthritic conditions including large joint arthritis, sacroiliitis, and ankylosing spondylitis
- Pyoderma gangrenosum
- Episcleritis and uveitis
- Sclerosing cholangitis
- Asymptomatic fatty liver (common); occasional hepatomegaly
- Primary sclerosing cholangitis: 1–4%
- Cirrhosis of liver: 1–5%
- Bile duct carcinoma
- Thromboembolic disease: 1–6%

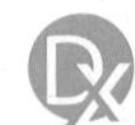

DIAGNOSIS

HISTORY
Bloody diarrhea (watery stool accompanied by blood, pus, and mucus); tenesmus; abdominal pain (tenderness in severe disease); rectal urgency, occasional fecal incontinence; weight loss; arthralgias

PHYSICAL EXAM
- Arthralgias and arthritis: 15–40% (2)[A]
- Spondylitis: 3–6%
- Ocular: 4–10%; include uveitis, cataracts, keratopathy, and central serous retinopathy
- Erythema nodosum
- Pyoderma gangrenosum
- Aphthous ulcers of mouth: 5–10%

DIAGNOSTIC TESTS & INTERPRETATION
Lab
- Anemia (chronic disease ± iron deficiency from blood loss)
- Leukocytosis during exacerbation
- Elevated ESR and CRP
- Electrolyte abnormalities, especially hypokalemia
- Hypoalbuminemia, elevated LFTs
- Perinuclear antineutrophil cytoplasmic antibody (p-ANCA) is elevated in 85% of cases of ulcerative colitis.
- Anti-*Saccharomyces cerevisiae* antibodies (ASCA) or perinuclear antineutrophil cytoplasmic antibodies (pANCA) can diagnose but not rule out inflammatory bowel disease.
- Antiglycan antibody is elevated in 75% of Crohn disease and 5% of ulcerative colitis cases.

Imaging
- Plain abdominal films:
  - Obtain immediately in patients with significant abdominal tenderness, fever, and leukocytosis. Permits the early diagnosis of toxic megacolon and perforation and treatment planning
- Barium enema:
  - Mucosal irregularities, effacement of haustra, pseudopolyposis
  - Upper GI series with small bowel follow-through to rule out Crohn disease
- Ultrasound, MRI, scintigraphy, and CT may have similar accuracy in diagnosis of IBD (3)[A].

Diagnostic Procedures/Surgery
- Sigmoidoscopy (4) (may include biopsy): Should be sufficient to make initial diagnosis
- Colonoscopy (4) (may include biopsy):
  - For evaluation of premalignant features; to differentiate from Crohn disease; to investigate suspected stricture or mass; to define the extent and location of involvement and specific segments
- Full colonoscopy contraindicated in severely active disease or colonic dilatation because of risk of perforation.

Pathological Findings
Inflammation of the colonic mucosa with ulcerations:
- Ulcerations are hyperemic and hemorrhagic.
- Rectum is involved 95% of the time.
- The inflammation can extend proximally in a continuous fashion.
- May affect terminal ileum, so-called backwash ileitis
- Colonic strictures are rare with ulcerative colitis.

DIFFERENTIAL DIAGNOSIS
- Other sources of rectal bleeding: Hemorrhoids, neoplasms, colonic diverticula, arteriovenous malformation, Crohn disease
- Infectious diarrhea, including bacterial (enterotoxigenic *Escherichia coli*), *Clostridium difficile* colitis, and parasitic (*Entamoeba histolytica*)
- Herpes simplex, *Chlamydia trachomatis, Cryptosporidium, Isospora belli*, cytomegalovirus
- Radiation proctitis
- Ischemic colitis

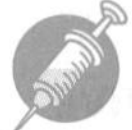

TREATMENT

Management involves acute treatment of inflammatory symptoms, followed by maintenance of remission; therapeutic approach is determined by the symptom severity and the degree of colonic involvement:

- 5-aminosalicylic acid (5-ASA) therapies are effective in inducing remission in mild-to-moderately active disease (NNT = 6) and are very effective at preventing relapse in quiescent disease (NNT = 4) (4)[A]:
  - Topical mesalamine agents are superior to oral aminosalicylates or topical steroids (4)[A].
  - Combination of oral and topical aminosalicylates is more effective than either alone (4)[A].
- Corticosteroid therapies are effective at inducing remission in active disease (NNT = 3) (4)[A].
- Azathioprine or 6-mercaptopurine (6-MP) are not recommended for inducing remission in active disease but are effective at preventing relapse in quiescent disease (4)[C].
- Methotrexate is not recommended for inducing remission in active disease or for preventing relapse in quiescent disease (4)[C]. (MTX is only indicated in Crohn disease.)
- Maintenance of remission in mild-to-moderate distal disease with the use of the following: Mesalamine suppositories for proctitis or enemas for distal colitis, sulfasalazine, balsalazide, or combination oral and topical mesalamine (4)[A]
- Maintenance of remission in mild-to-moderate extensive disease with the use of the following: Sulfasalazine, olsalazine, mesalamine, and balsalazide (4)[A]
- Infliximab is effective at inducing remission in ambulatory patients with moderate-to-severely active disease (4)[A] and for symptomatic improvement of hospitalized patients with severely active disease (4)[C].

MEDICATION

First Line

- Sulfasalazine:
  - Uncoated tablets. Adults: Initial: 1 g PO q6–8h; maintenance: 500 mg PO q6h. Children ≥6 years: Initial: 40–60 mg/kg/d PO in 3–6 divided doses; maintenance: 30 mg/kg/d PO divided q6h (maximum = 2 g/d)
  - Enteric-coated tablets. Adults: Initial: 3–4 g/d PO in divided doses; maintenance: 2 g/d PO in divided doses. Children ≥6 years: Initial: 40–60 mg/kg/d PO in 3–6 divided doses; maintenance: 30 mg/kg/d PO in 4 divided doses (maximum = 2 g/d)
- Mesalamine:
  - Oral delayed-release tablets (Asacol) for induction of remission. Adults: 800 mg PO t.i.d. × 6 weeks
  - Oral controlled-release tablets (Pentasa) for maintenance of remission. Adults: 1 g PO q.i.d.
- 5-ASA (such as mesalamine) enemas and suppositories can be used to treat proctitis or proctosigmoiditis:
  - Suppositories: Adults: 500 mg per rectum b.i.d., retained in the rectum for >1–3 hours (can increase to 3× daily if inadequate response after 2 weeks) *or* 1,000 mg per rectum once daily q.h.s. may be used for 3–6 weeks or until remission
  - Enemas: Adults: 4 g per rectum, retained for 8 hours each night; use for 3–6 weeks or until remission is achieved
- Balsalazide: Adults: 2,250 mg PO t.i.d. for total daily dose of 6.75 g for 8–12 weeks. Children/adolescents: 2,250 mg PO t.i.d. for total daily dose of 6.75 g or 750 mg PO t.i.d. for total daily dose of 2.25 g for 8 weeks
- Olsalazine: Adults: 500 mg PO b.i.d. (up to 3 g/d). Children/adolescents: 30 mg/kg/d in 2 divided doses (up to 2 g/d), primarily used for maintenance

Second Line

- Prednisone for severe exacerbations: Adult dosage: Initial: 40–60 mg/d PO (maximum = 1 mg/kg/d) × 7–10 days; taper over 2–3 months; can be given IV in hospitalized patients
- Infliximab is effective in patients whose disease is refractory to conventional treatment (4,5)[A]:
  - Adult dose: 5 mg/kg IV at weeks 0, 2, and 6 for induction, then maintenance of 5 mg/kg IV is given every 8 weeks

Pediatric Considerations

- Infliximab can increase the risk of cancer in children and adolescents; weigh risks vs. benefits prior to use.
- Immunomodulators can be used in patients unresponsive to steroids and aminosalicylates, or who cannot be weaned from high-dose steroids:
  - Daily plain films of the abdomen are obtained until improvement occurs.
  - If dilatation of colon increases or treatment has failed to attain reversal in 72 hours, emergency colectomy is indicated.

ADDITIONAL TREATMENT

General Measures

Control inflammation, prevent complications, and replace nutritional losses and blood volume.

COMPLEMENTARY AND ALTERNATIVE MEDICINE

Probiotics added to standard therapy may provide modest benefits in patients with mild-to-moderately severe ulcerative colitis (6)[B].

SURGERY/OTHER PROCEDURES

- Emergency surgery for massive hemorrhage, perforation, and toxic dilatation of the colon
- Surgery indicated for cancer, multisite mucosal dysplasia, and patients refractory to all other forms of therapy
- Total colectomy with ileostomy is curative. An alternative is total colectomy with ileoproctostomy.
- Regular proctoscopic surveillance is required if a colonic mucosal cuff is retained, thereby leaving a risk of future cancer development.

IN-PATIENT CONSIDERATIONS

Initial Stabilization

- Obtain imaging studies to assess disease activity.
- Initiate IV corticosteroids.

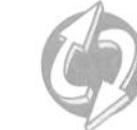

ONGOING CARE

FOLLOW-UP RECOMMENDATIONS

Patient Monitoring

- Colonoscopy for cancer surveillance with biopsy every 1–2 years after the disease has been present for 7–8 years
- Low-grade dysplasia warrants more frequent evaluation (e.g., every 3–6 months), and high-grade dysplasia (or low-grade dysplasia within a mass) warrants consideration of colectomy.
- Magnification chromoendoscopy may detect significantly more intraepithelial neoplasias than conventional colonoscopy.
- Annual liver tests
- Cholangiography for cholestasis

Pediatric Considerations

Cancer surveillance is important because occurrence of cancer relates to the duration and extent of disease, whether frequently symptomatic or not.

DIET

- NPO during acute exacerbations
- Lactose-free diet is often recommended; evidence-based support is lacking without an associated lactase deficiency.
- Omega-3 fatty acids, seal and cod liver oil, dietary lactulose, wheat grass juice, and diets with decreased meat and alcohol have been recommended to reduce relapses and improve systemic symptoms (evidence is conflicting).

PATIENT EDUCATION

- Discuss the importance of adherence to drug therapy to induce and maintain remission.
- Self-help organizations such as Crohn's and Colitis Foundation of America (CCFA): www.ccfa.org

PROGNOSIS

- Variable; mortality for initial attack is ~5%; 75–85% experience relapse; and up to 20% eventually require colectomy.
- Colon cancer risk is the single most important risk factor affecting long-term prognosis.
- Left-sided colitis and ulcerative proctitis have favorable prognoses with probable normal lifespan.

Geriatric Considerations

Increased mortality if first presentation occurs after 60 years of age

COMPLICATIONS

- Perforation
- Toxic megacolon
- Liver disease
- Stricture formation (<Crohn disease)
- Colon cancer

REFERENCES

1. Hanauer SB. Inflammatory bowel disease: Epidemiology, pathogenesis, and therapeutic opportunities. *Inflamm Bowel Dis*. 2006; 12(Suppl 1):S3–9.
2. D'Incà R, Podswiadek M, Ferronato A, et al. Articular manifestations in inflammatory bowel disease patients: A prospective study. *Dig Liver Dis*. 2009.
3. Horsthuis K, Bipat S, Bennink RJ, et al. Inflammatory bowel disease diagnosed with US, MR, scintigraphy, and CT: Meta-analysis of prospective studies. *Radiology*. 2008;247:64–79.
4. Talley NJ, Abreu MT, Achkar JP, et al. An evidence-based systematic review on medical therapies for inflammatory bowel disease. *Am J Gastroenterol*. 2011;106:S2–S2.
5. Lawson MM, Thomas AG, Akobeng AK. Tumour necrosis factor alpha blocking agents for induction of remission in ulcerative colitis. *Cochrane Database Syst Rev*. 2006;3:CD005112.
6. Mallon P, McKay D, Kirk S, et al. Probiotics for induction of remission in ulcerative colitis. *Cochrane Database Syst Rev*. 2007:CD005573.
7. Mack DR, Langton C, Markowitz J, et al. Laboratory values for children with newly diagnosed inflammatory bowel disease. *Pediatrics*. 2007;119: 1113–9.

See Also (Topic, Algorithm, Electronic Media Element)

Algorithm: Hematemesis (Bleeding, Upper GI)

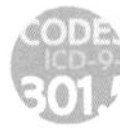

CODES

ICD9

- 556.1 Ulcerative (chronic) ileocolitis
- 556.8 Other ulcerative colitis
- 556.9 Ulcerative colitis, unspecified

CLINICAL PEARLS

- Smokers have 1/2 the risk of nonsmokers for developing ulcerative colitis
- Patients with proctitis should be treated with 5-ASA suppositories instead of oral therapy
- Surgical removal of colon and rectum is curative
- Indications for surgery include intractability, dysplasia, carcinoma, massive bleeding, toxic megacolon
- Normal screening lab tests (ESR, hemoglobin, platelets, and albumin) do NOT rule out inflammatory bowel disease, regardless of disease severity (7)

UPPER RESPIRATORY INFECTION

Lisa M. Schroeder, MD
Puja Sharma, MD

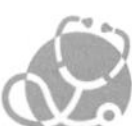

BASICS

Upper respiratory infections (URIs) are the second most common medical diagnosis, contributing to nearly 20 million office visits per year.

DESCRIPTION

- Inflammation of nasal passages resulting from infection with various respiratory viruses
- Most cases are self-treated.
- Usually mild to moderate severity, self-limited
- System(s) affected: ENT; Pulmonary

EPIDEMIOLOGY

- Symptoms usually peak in 1–3 days and stop in 7 days. However, a cough can persist.
- Most infections occur in the winter months.

Incidence

- Predominant age: Children > Adults:
  - Preschool children: 6–10 colds/yr
  - Kindergarten: 12/yr
  - Schoolchildren: 7/yr
  - Adolescents/adults: 2–4/yr
- Predominant sex: Male = Female

RISK FACTORS

- Exposure to infected people
- Touching one's nose or conjunctiva with contaminated fingers
- Allergic disorders
- Smoking
- Immunosuppression

GENERAL PREVENTION

- Frequent hand washing, especially in children (1)[A]
- Limiting exposure to infected persons/children

PATHOPHYSIOLOGY

Rhinoviruses infect the ciliated epithelium lining the nose, resulting in edema and hyperemia of nasal mucous membranes.

ETIOLOGY

- Usually due to 1 of 200 virus strains from 6 virus families; many strains present within the same geographic region or patient family:
  - Rhinovirus, with >200 serotypes
  - Influenzavirus types A, B, C
  - Parainfluenza viruses
  - Respiratory syncytial viruses
  - Coronaviruses
  - Adenoviruses
- *In 40% of cases, no pathogen is identified.*

COMMONLY ASSOCIATED CONDITIONS

- Pharyngitis
- Sinusitis
- Otitis media
- Bronchitis
- Bronchiolitis
- Pneumonia
- Croup
- Asthma

DIAGNOSIS

HISTORY

- Nasal stuffiness and/or obstruction (80–100%)
- Sneezing (50–70%)
- Scratchy throat (50%)
- Cough (40%)
- Hoarseness (30%)
- Malaise (20–25%)
- Headache (25%)
- Fever exceeding 100°F (37.7°C) (0–1%)

PHYSICAL EXAM

- Low-grade temperature or afebrile
- Stable vital signs
- Rhinorrhea (clear, yellow, or green)
- Inflamed mucosa
- Postnasal drainage
- Erythema of the throat
- Dull tympanic membranes

DIAGNOSTIC TESTS & INTERPRETATION

Lab

Initial lab tests

- No routine lab testing is needed.
- For pharyngitis, use a lab test (rapid strep antigen or culture) to rule out group A strep infection.
- Rapid flu test if influenza suspected

Follow-Up & Special Considerations

Patients should contact the primary care physician's office for fever >101°F associated with systemic symptoms, difficulty breathing, or purulent drainage >2 days.

Imaging

Initial approach

Not necessary

Pathological Findings

- Exudation of serous and mucinous fluid containing immunoglobulins
- Histology: Edema of subepithelial connective tissue and a scanty cellular infiltrate containing neutrophils, plasma cells, lymphocytes, and eosinophils
- Rhinovirus causes a "nondestructive" inflammation of the mucous membranes.
- Influenza and parainfluenza denude epithelium to the basement membrane.

DIFFERENTIAL DIAGNOSIS

- Allergic rhinitis
- Acute sinusitis
- Strep pharyngitis
- Infectious mononucleosis
- The "flu" (caused by influenza viruses): Systemic symptoms, including myalgias, malaise, severe headache, and ocular symptoms, overshadow respiratory complaints
- H1N1 influenza
- Pertussis

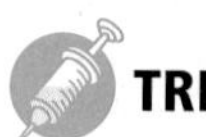

TREATMENT

MEDICATION

- Primarily for supportive therapy
- No cure or practical preventive measures

First Line

- NSAIDs for relieving discomfort or pain caused by the common cold (2)[A]:
  - Naproxen can also be administered to help decrease cough in this setting. American College of Chest Physicians (ACCP Grade A)
- Topical decongestants (sympathomimetics) reduce edema and swelling of the nasal mucosa, promote drainage, and reduce nasal airflow resistance. These are preferred over oral types because of minimal systemic effects. Sprays are preferred over drops in patients >6 years old:
  - Oxymetazoline:
    - Adults and children aged 6–12 years: 0.05% solution, 2–3 sprays in each nostril b.i.d.
    - Children aged 2–6 years: 0.025% solution, 2–3 drops in each nostril b.i.d.
    - Rebound congestion (rhinitis medicamentosa) unlikely if used <5 days
- Inhaled anticholinergics:
  - Ipratropium inhaler: A bronchodilator; recommended by the American College of Chest Physicians for use as a cough suppressant in URIs (ACCP Grade A):
    - Adults and children age >14: 2 sprays (17 mcg/spray) 4 times per day.
- Topical anticholinergics control rhinorrhea but do not relieve nasal congestion or sneezing:
  - Ipratropium: Adults and children >11 years old: 0.06% solution, 2 sprays to each nostril t.i.d. × 4 days
  - The combination of ipratropium and xylometazoline has been shown to provide greater relief from rhinorrhea and congestion when compared with placebo and single-ingredient treatments. Combination treatments are safe. Adverse events are limited to epistaxis, nasal passage irritation, nasal dryness, and mucus tinged with blood (3)[A].
- Oral decongestants (sympathomimetic) advantages over topical decongestants: Longer duration of action, lack of local irritation, and no risk of rebound congestion:
  - Pseudoephedrine: Potential for abuse/misuse for methamphetamine production:
    - Adults: 60 mg q4–6h (120 mg sustained-release q12h) superior to placebo in short-term use (4,5)[A]
    - Children aged 6–12 years: 30 mg q4–6h; 2–5 years: 15 mg q4–6h
  - Acute cough, postnasal drip, and throat clearing associated with the common cold can be treated with a first-generation antihistamine/decongestant preparation (brompheniramine and sustained-release pseudoephedrine). (ACCP Grade A)

- A single oral dose of phenylephrine 10 mg is an effective decongestant in adults with acute nasal congestion associated with the common cold (6)[A].

- Antihistamines: Safe and mildly effective for sneezing and rhinorrhea. Only first-generation (sedating) antihistamines recommended for cough:
  - Chlorpheniramine:
    - Adults: 4 mg q.i.d., 8 mg t.i.d., 12 mg b.i.d.
    - Children age 6–12: 2 mg q4–6h
    - Children age 2–6: 1 mg q4–6h
  - Brompheniramine
- Cough suppressants: Not recommended for use by the American College of Chest Physicians (ACCP Grade D) due to limited efficacy:
  - Codeine: Side effects of sedation and GI upset:
    - Adults: 10–20 mg q4–6h PRN
  - Dextromethorphan:
    - Adults: 10–30 mg q4–6h
    - Children age 6–12: 15 mg q4–6h
    - Children age 2–6: 2.5–7.5 mg q4–6h
- Expectorants:
  - Guaifenesin (no evidence in children, some evidence in adults):
    - Adults: 100–400 mg q4hrs
    - Children age 6–12: 100–200 mg q4hrs
    - Children age 2–6: 50–100 mg q4hrs
- Common combinations: Most cold medicines come in combinations, multiple OTC, and prescription variations: Not recommended for use by ACCP (Grade D):
  - Dextromethorphan/phenylephrine/guaifenesin: 10/5/100 mg, peds: 5/2.5/50
  - Dextromethorphan/guaifenesin: 10/100 mg
  - Acetaminophen/chlorpheniramine/dextromethorphan/phenylephrine: 160/1/5/2.5 mg
  - Chlorpheniramine/dextromethorphan/phenylephrine: 4/15/12.5 mg
  - Chlorpheniramine/dextromethorphan: 1/7.5 mg

Pediatric Considerations

In 2007, the FDA issued a warning on all cough and cold preparations for children 2 and younger due to risk of overdose.

Second Line

- Many mouthwashes, gargles, and lozenges are promoted to relieve the pain of sore throat. The demulcent effects of hard candy, gargling with warm saline, and products with anesthetics (benzocaine or phenol) may provide pain relief.
- Aromatic oils (menthol, camphor, eucalyptus), in topical or lozenge form, produce a sensation of increased airflow in the absence of a significant change in airflow resistance.
- Saline nasal irrigation is safe for adults and children.
- *Antibacterials are of no value.*

ADDITIONAL TREATMENT

General Measures

- Smoking cessation
- Vaporizer/humidifier

COMPLEMENTARY AND ALTERNATIVE MEDICINE

- Zinc prevents viral replication in vitro, but the efficacy of lozenges remains unproved:
  - Avoid intranasal preparations of zinc: Risk of potential permanent loss of smell
- Echinacea has not proven effective for treatment of common cold symptoms (7)[A].
- Probiotics may decrease severity and duration of URIs but not the incidence (8)[A].
- Vitamin C (ascorbic acid):
  - No preventive effects; 23% reduction in severity and duration of symptoms
  - Precipitation of urate, oxalate, or cystine stones has been seen. Urine glucose monitoring may be inaccurate in people taking large doses of vitamin C.
  - High-dose vitamin C prophylaxis has proven beneficial in those exposed to heavy exertion and cold stress.
- Zinc and high-dose vitamin C prophylaxis and treatment should *not* be recommended for the general population (9).

Geriatric Considerations

Cold medications, especially decongestants, commonly produce adverse effects in older people.

Pregnancy Considerations

- Ipratropium is category B.
- Decongestants: No clear association has been determined between use of this drug group and congenital defects.
- Antihistamines: No clear association has been confirmed between use of this drug group and congenital defects.
- Codeine: Indiscriminate use during pregnancy may pose a risk to the fetus.

ONGOING CARE

FOLLOW-UP RECOMMENDATIONS

Contact the primary care physician's office for fever, difficulty breathing, or symptoms persisting beyond expected course.

DIET

Encourage fluids and adequate hydration (10)[C]

PATIENT EDUCATION

- Discuss with patients the difference between viral and bacterial infections; instruct about appropriate and inappropriate antibiotic use.
- Frequent hand washing (1)[A]
- Symptomatic treatment; no cure
- Patient information: www.niaid.nih.gov/factsheets/cold.htm

PROGNOSIS

Excellent; expect full recovery. Usual duration 5–7 days. For smokers, 3–4 additional days.

COMPLICATIONS

Small percentage may develop worsening symptoms leading to otitis media, sinusitis, bronchitis, or pneumonia.

REFERENCES

1. Jefferson T, Del Mar CB, Dooley L, et al. Physical interventions to interrupt or reduce the spread of respiratory viruses. *Cochrane Database Syst Rev.* 2011;CD006207.
2. Kim SY, Chang YJ, Cho HM. Non-steroidal anti-inflammatory drugs for the common cold. *Cochrane Database Syst Rev.* 2009;CD006362.
3. Eccles R, Pedersen A, Regberg D, et al. Efficacy and safety of topical combinations of ipratropium and xylometazoline for the treatment of symptoms of runny nose and nasal congestion associated with acute upper respiratory tract infection. *Am J Rhinol.* 2007;21:40–5.
4. Eccles R, Jawad MS, Jawad SS. Efficacy and safety of single and multiple doses of pseudoephedrine in the treatment of nasal congestion associated with common cold. *Am J Rhinol.* 2005;19:25–31.
5. Taverner D, Latte J, Draper M. Nasal decongestants for the common cold. *Cochrane Database Syst Rev.* 2004; Issue 3. Art No CD001953.
6. Kollar C, Schneider H, Waksman J. Meta-analysis of the efficacy of a single dose of phenylephrine 10 mg compared with placebo in adults with acute nasal congestion due to the common cold. *Cl Therapeutics.* 2007;29(6):1057–70.
7. Linde K, Barrett B, Wolkart K, et al. Echinacea for preventing and treating the common cold. Cochrane Acute Respiratory Infections Group. *Cochrane Database Syst Rev.* 2006; 4.
8. Vouloumanou EK, Makris GC, Karageorgopoulos DE. Probiotics for the prevention of respiratory tract infections: A systematic review. *Int J Antimicrob Agents.* 2009;34(3):197.e1–10.
9. Douglas RM, Hemila H, Chalker E, et al. Vitamin C for preventing and treating the common cold. Cochrane Acute Respiratory Infections Group. *Cochrane Database Syst Rev.* 2006; 4.
10. Guppy MPB, Mickan SM, Del Mar CB, et al. Advising patients to increase fluid intake for treating acute respiratory infections. *Cochrane Database Syst Rev.* 2011;2.

ADDITIONAL READING

- FDA advisory on decongestants. *Morb Mortal Wkly Rep.* 2007;56(1):1–4.
- National Guideline Clearinghouse. 2008 diagnosis and treatment of respiratory illness in children and adults. Available at: www.guideline.gov.
- National Guideline Clearinghouse. Cough suppressant and pharmacologic protussive therapy: ACCP evidence-based clinical practice guidelines and cough and the common cold. Available at: www.guideline.gov.

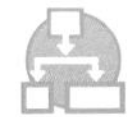

See Also (Topic, Algorithm, Electronic Media Element)

Bronchitis, Acute; Pharyngitis; Rhinitis, Allergic

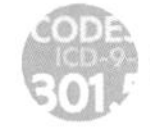

CODES

ICD9

465.9 Acute upper respiratory infections of unspecified site

CLINICAL PEARLS

- Supportive therapy is mainstay.
- If pharyngitis is the primary complaint, diagnose group A strep with lab testing.
- Limit unnecessary use of antibiotics.
- Patient education is key.

URETHRITIS

Janelle M. Evans, MD

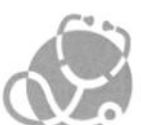

BASICS

DESCRIPTION

- Urethral inflammation marked by painful urination, pruritus, hematuria, and/or discharge
- Usually a result of an STI or, less commonly, autoimmune disorders (Reiter syndrome), trauma, or chemical irritation
- Complications such as urethral stricture in men or pelvic inflammatory disease (PID) in women may occur if untreated.
- System(s) affected: Renal/urologic

EPIDEMIOLOGY

Incidence

- In 2007, 1.1 million new cases of chlamydia and 355,000 new cases of gonorrhea were reported by the CDC. Prevalence varies by region, with 5 times more cases of chlamydia and gonorrhea in the southern US. Racial discrepancies include an 8 times higher rate for African Americans and a 2.9 times higher rate for Hispanic patients compared with whites.
- Predominant age: 15–24 years, sexually active, following trends for STI
- Predominant sex: Men report symptoms more frequently, but similar incidence is likely.

RISK FACTORS

- Multiple sexual partners and unprotected intercourse
- African American, Native American, or Hispanic ethnicity
- History of STIs, bacterial vaginosis, recurrent candidiasis
- Excessive use of chemical lubricants or powders

GENERAL PREVENTION

- Safer sex techniques and treatment of all partners
- Abstinence
- Avoidance of excessive lubricants, powders, or chemical irritants

ETIOLOGY

- Predominantly *Neisseria gonorrhoeae* and *Chlamydia trachomatis* infection, increased transmission among HIV-positive persons
- Less common infectious agents, including:
  - *Ureaplasma urealyticum*
  - *Trichomonas vaginalis*
  - Herpesvirus
  - *Mycoplasma genitalium*
- Noninfectious causes (generally rare): Foreign bodies, soaps, shampoos, douches, spermicides, urethral instrumentation

COMMONLY ASSOCIATED CONDITIONS

Other STIs: Patients should be urged strongly to undergo testing for syphilis, hepatitis B and C, *Trichomonas,* and HIV.

DIAGNOSIS

- Important to take detailed sexual and travel history; increased incidence seen with travel to some regions
- In men:
  - Abrupt onset of dysuria symptoms 3–14 days after exposure to an infected sexual partner
  - Urethral discharge: May be profuse and purulent in acute gonorrhea
  - Urethral itching or tenderness
  - Proctitis, pharyngitis, and conjunctivitis also may be present (sexual history is important).
- In women: Classic urethral syndrome often is not present:
  - Tenderness, edema, and inflammation of the urethral meatus, especially in women
  - Dyspareunia
  - Vaginitis, cystitis, cervicitis
- Fever is not part of the syndrome and suggests another diagnosis.
- Bloody discharge: Rarely seen and suggests another diagnosis
- Suprapubic or abdominal pain suggests another diagnosis or presence of complications (e.g., PID, prostatitis, or cystitis).

Pediatric Considerations

In pediatric patients, proven cases of gonorrhea, chlamydia, and trichomoniasis require evaluation for sexual abuse.

DIAGNOSTIC TESTS & INTERPRETATION

- For patients who present without symptoms and state that a sexual partner was treated for this problem, obtain specimens for lab tests, but immediate treatment is recommended.
- Evidence is insufficient to recommend for or against screening in asymptomatic men at increased risk.

ALERT

The US Preventative Services Task Force recommends screening all sexually active women until age 25 years and all women at increased risk of infection

Lab

- Gram stain of discharge: ≥5 WBCs per high-power field (HPF) indicates urethritis. Intracellular gram-negative diplococci strongly indicate gonorrhea.
- Cultures of the intraurethral/endocervical swabs:
  - Gonorrhea and chlamydia cultures should be obtained in all symptomatic patients.
  - Culture may be performed on urethral exudates if they are present.
- Nucleic acid amplification test (NAAT) using polymerase chain reaction assay on urine is very sensitive and specific but costly. Be sure to test for other, less common pathogens if negative.
- Urinalysis:
  - Usually normal in cases of simple urethritis
  - First-void urine often is positive for leukocyte esterase and should have ≥10 WBCs per HPF in urethritis.
  - Men should not have urinated for at least 4 hours prior.
- Urine culture: Performed only if gram stain of discharge is unremarkable or unobtainable
- Wet prep: May reveal *Trichomonas;* trichomoniasis, bacterial vaginosis, and *Candida* infection; need to be evaluated for persistent symptoms after antibiotic course
- Syphilis, HIV, and hepatitis B serology as indicated to rule out concomitant STIs

Initial lab tests

ALERT

When an STI is suspected, provide informed consent and recommend HIV testing at initial presentation.

Follow-Up & Special Considerations

Test of cure for chlamydia and gonorrhea recommended in pregnant women or when treatment noncompliance is suspected.

Diagnostic Procedures/Surgery

Urethrocystoscopy for cases with suspected foreign body, intraurethral warts, urethral stricture

Pathological Findings

Urethral strictures (untreated gonorrhea), intraurethral lesions (venereal warts, congenital anomalies), PID, or tubo-ovarian abscesses possible

DIFFERENTIAL DIAGNOSIS

- Other genitourinary tract diseases:
  - Cystitis/urinary tract infection
  - Painful bladder syndromes
  - Epididymitis
  - Prostatitis
  - PID
  - Pyelonephritis
- Vaginal atrophy, especially in postmenopausal women
- Stevens-Johnson syndrome
- Reiter syndrome: Arthritis, uveitis, and urethritis (can't see, can't pee, can't climb a tree)
- Wegener granulomatosis

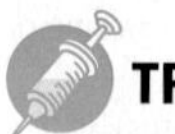

TREATMENT

MEDICATION

First Line

- Gonorrhea (1,2)[C]:
  - Ceftriaxone: 250 mg IM single dose
  - Cefixime: 400 mg PO single dose (higher resistance rates vs. Ceftriaxone)
  - If patient cannot tolerate cephalosporin, consider Azithromycin 2 g PO single dose (high rate of GI side effects)

- Chlamydia:
  - Azithromycin: 1 g PO single dose
  - Doxycycline: 100 mg PO b.i.d. for 7 days
- Trichomoniasis: Metronidazole 2 g PO single dose or 250 mg t.i.d. for 7 days
- Recurrent and resistant urethritis: Metronidazole 2 mg PO single dose *plus*:
  - Erythromycin 500 mg PO q.i.d. for 7 days and valacyclovir 400 mg PO t.i.d. for 5 days if herpes simplex virus (HSV) suspicious
- Contraindications: Sensitivity to any of the indicated medications
- Precautions: Patients taking tetracyclines may have increased photosensitivity.
- Significant possible interactions:
  - Tetracyclines should not be taken with milk products or antacids.
  - Oral contraceptives may be rendered less effective by oral antibiotics. Patients and partners should use a backup method of birth control for the remainder of the cycle.

Pregnancy Considerations

- Tetracyclines and quinolones are contraindicated.
- Avoid erythromycin estolate because of an increased risk of cholestatic jaundice; otherwise, use the standard treatment recommendations.
- Single-dose therapy is recommended.

Second Line

- Gonorrhea:
  - Because of the spread of quinolone-resistant *N. gonorrhoeae* from the Pacific, Hawaii, California, and Asia, quinolones no longer are recommended treatments for individuals who have acquired gonorrhea from that area (3)[C].
  - Resistance to penicillin and tetracycline has been reported in up to 1/3 of isolates of *N. gonorrhoeae*.
  - Ciprofloxacin: 500 mg PO single dose (3)[C]
  - Ofloxacin: 400 mg PO single dose (1)[C]
  - Levofloxacin: 250 mg PO single dose (1)[C]
  - Other drugs are available but offer no particular advantage over the drugs of choice.
- Chlamydia:
  - Erythromycin base: 500 mg PO q.i.d. for 7 days
  - Erythromycin ethylsuccinate: 800 mg PO q.i.d. for 7 days; if intolerant of high-dose erythromycin: Erythromycin base 250 mg PO q.i.d. for 14 days or erythromycin ethylsuccinate 400 mg PO q.i.d. for 14 days
  - Ofloxacin: 300 mg PO b.i.d. for 7 days
  - Levofloxacin: 500 mg PO daily for 7 days

ADDITIONAL TREATMENT

General Measures

All sexual partners who came in contact with the patient within 60 days should be evaluated, tested, and treated for both gonorrhea and chlamydia.

IN-PATIENT CONSIDERATIONS

Initial Stabilization

- Most cases can be treated in the outpatient setting.
- Single-dose regimens, directly observed in office for noncompliant or high-risk patients
- Antibiotics should not be withheld from symptomatic patients until culture results are known if there is a convincing clinical presentation.
- Treatment should cover both gonorrhea and chlamydia and any other suspected pathogens.
- Patients with persistent symptoms and signs after adequate treatment should be:
  - Evaluated and/or treated for trichomoniasis
  - Retreated with the original regimen if not compliant or re-exposed
  - Retreated with an alternative regimen for 14 days if *Ureaplasma urealyticum* is suspected (tetracycline resistance in <10% of isolates)
  - Evaluated for HSV

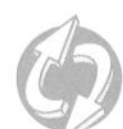

ONGOING CARE

FOLLOW-UP RECOMMENDATIONS

- Full activity
- Sexual activity should be avoided until both partners complete treatment and are symptom-free or 7 days after single-dose therapy.

Patient Monitoring

Instruct patients to return if symptoms persist or recur after completing treatment. Test-of-cure cultures usually are not required unless the patient is pregnant.

DIET

Avoid alcohol when taking metronidazole.

PATIENT EDUCATION

Most important to emphasize the need for compliance with therapy, treatment of sexual partners, and use of safer sex practices; patients should be urged to undergo screening for other STIs.

PROGNOSIS

If the diagnosis is firmly established, appropriate medications are prescribed, and the patient is compliant with treatment, relief of symptoms occurs within days, and the problem will resolve without sequelae.

COMPLICATIONS

- Stricture formation
- Epididymitis
- Prostatitis
- Proctitis
- PID in women
- Disseminated gonococcal infection
- Gonococcal meningitis
- Gonococcal endocarditis
- Perinatal transmission (chlamydial conjunctivitis, chlamydial pneumonia, ophthalmia neonatorum)
- Reiter syndrome

REFERENCES

1. Berg AO. Screening for chlamydia infections: Recommendations and rationale. *Am J Prev Med*. 2001;20:90–4.
2. Centers for Disease Control and Prevention. Sexually transmitted diseases treatment guildeines, 2010. Gonococcal infections. Available at: www.cdc.gov/std/treatment/2010/gonococcalinfections.htm.
3. Centers for Disease Control and Prevention. Sexually transmitted diseases treatment guidelines. *MMWR*. 2006;55(No. RR-11).

ADDITIONAL READING

- Ansart S, Hochedez P, Perez L, et al. Sexually transmitted diseases diagnosed among travelers returning from the tropics. *J Travel Med*. 2009;16: 79–83.
- Centers for Disease Control and Prevention. *Sexually Transmitted Disease Surveillance, 2007*. Atlanta, GA: U.S. Department of Health and Human Services; December 2008.
- Groseclose SL, Brathwaite WS, Hall PA, et al. Summary of notifiable diseases–United States, 2002. *Morb Mortal Wkly Rep*. 2004;51:1–84.
- Wetmore CM, Manhart LE, Lowens MS, et al. *Ureaplasma urealyticum* is associated with nongonococcal urethritis among men with fewer lifetime sexual partners: A case-control study. *J Infect Dis*. 2011;204:1274–82.

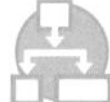

See Also (Topic, Algorithm, Electronic Media Element)

- Chlamydial Sexually Transmitted Diseases; Epididymitis; Gonococcal Infections; Pelvic Inflammatory Disease (PID); Prostatitis; Urinary Tract Infection in Females; Urinary Tract Infection in Males; Vulvovaginitis, Estrogen Deficient; Vulvovaginitis, Prepubescent
- Algorithms: Dysuria; Genital Ulcers; Urethral Discharge

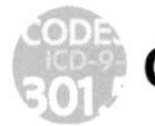

CODES

ICD9

- 098.0 Gonococcal infection (acute) of lower genitourinary tract
- 099.41 Other nongonococcal urethritis, chlamydia trachomatis
- 597.80 Urethritis, unspecified

CLINICAL PEARLS

- Urethral inflammation marked by painful urination, pruritus, hematuria, and/or discharge
- Usually a result of an STI or, less commonly, autoimmune disorders (Reiter syndrome), trauma, or chemical irritation
- Complications such as urethral stricture in men or PID in women may occur if untreated.

URINARY TRACT INFECTION (UTI) IN FEMALES

Akhil Das, MD, FACS
Leonard G. Gomella, MD, FACS

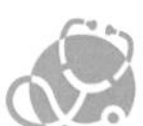

BASICS

DESCRIPTION

- Presence of pathogenic microorganisms within the urinary tract with concomitant symptoms
- This topic refers primarily to infectious cystitis; other urinary tract infections (UTIs), such as pyelonephritis, are discussed elsewhere.
- Uncomplicated UTI: Uncomplicated UTI occurs in patients who have a normal, unobstructed genitourinary tract, who have no history of recent instrumentation, and whose symptoms are confined to the lower urinary tract. Uncomplicated UTIs are most common in young, sexually active women.
- Complicated UTI: Complicated UTI is an infection of the lower or upper urinary tract in the presence of an anatomic abnormality, a functional abnormality, or a urinary catheter.
- Recurrent UTI: Recurrent UTIs are symptomatic UTIs that follow resolution of an earlier episode, usually after appropriate treatment:
  - No single definition of the frequency of recurrent UTI exists, but a pragmatic definition is 3 or more infections per year.
  - Most recurrences are thought to represent reinfection rather than relapse.
  - There is no evidence that recurrent UTIs lead to health problems such as hypertension or renal disease, in the absence of anatomic or functional abnormalities of the urinary tract (1).
- System(s) affected: Renal/Urologic
- Synonym(s): Cystitis; Infectious cystitis

EPIDEMIOLOGY

Incidence

- Accounts for 8 million doctor visits and 1 million emergency room visits, and contributes to >100,000 hospital admissions each year
- 11% of women have UTIs in any given year.
- Predominant age: Young adults and older
- Predominant sex: Female > Male

Prevalence

- >50% of females have at least 1 UTI in their lifetime.
- 1 in 4 women have recurrent UTIs.

RISK FACTORS

- Previous UTI
- Diabetes mellitus (DM)
- Pregnancy
- Sexual activity
- Use of spermicides or diaphragm
- Underlying abnormalities of the urinary tract, such as tumors, calculi, strictures, incomplete bladder emptying, urinary incontinence, neurogenic bladder
- Catheterization
- Recent antibiotic use
- Poor hygiene
- Estrogen deficiency
- Inadequate fluid intake

Genetics

In women with HLA-3 and nonsecretor Lewis antigen, there is an increased bacterial adherence, which may lead to an increased risk in UTI.

GENERAL PREVENTION

- Maintain good hydration.
- Women with frequent or intercourse-related UTI should empty bladder immediately before and following intercourse; consider postcoital antibiotic.
- Avoid feminine hygiene sprays and douches.
- Wipe urethra from front to back.
- Cranberry juice (not cranberry juice cocktail) consumption may prevent recurrent infections.

PATHOPHYSIOLOGY

- Bacteria and subsequent infection in the urinary tract arise chiefly via ascending bacterial movement and propagation.
- Pathogenic organisms (*Escherichia coli*) possess adherence factors and toxins that allow initiation and propagation of genitourinary infections:
  - Type 1 and *P. pili*
  - Lipopolysaccharide

ETIOLOGY

- Most UTIs are caused by bacteria originating from bowel flora:
  - *E. coli* is the causative organism in 80% of cases of uncomplicated cystitis.
  - *Staphylococcus saprophyticus* accounts for 15% of infections.
  - Enterobacteriaceae (i.e., *Klebsiella, Proteus, Enterobacter, Pseudomonas)* also contribute.
- *Candida* is associated with nosocomial UTI.

COMMONLY ASSOCIATED CONDITIONS

See "Risk Factors."

Geriatric Considerations

- Elderly patients are more likely to have underlying urinary tract abnormality.
- Acute UTI may be associated with incontinence or mental status changes in the elderly.

DIAGNOSIS

HISTORY

Note: Any or all may be present:

- Burning during urination
- Pain during urination (dysuria)
- Urgency (sensation of need to urinate often)
- Frequency
- Sensation of incomplete bladder emptying
- Blood in urine
- Lower abdominal pain or cramping
- Offensive odor of urine
- Nocturia
- Sudden onset of urinary incontinence
- Dyspareunia

PHYSICAL EXAM

- Suprapubic tenderness
- Urethral and/or vaginal tenderness
- Fever or costovertebral angle tenderness indicates upper UTI.

DIAGNOSTIC TESTS & INTERPRETATION

Lab

Initial lab tests

- Urinalysis:
  - Pyuria (>10 neutrophils/high-power field [HPF])
  - Bacteriuria (any amount on unspun urine, or 10 bacteria/HPF on centrifuged urine)
  - Hematuria (>5 RBCs/HPF)
- Dipstick urinalysis:
  - Leukocyte esterase (75–96% sensitivity, 94–98% specificity, when >100,000 colony-forming units [cfu])
  - Nitrite tests useful with nitrite-reducing organisms (e.g., Enterococci, *S. saprophyticus, Acinetobacter*)
- Urine culture: *Only* indicated if diagnosis is unclear or patient has recurrent infections and resistance is suspected:
  - Presence of 100,000 cfu/mL of organism indicates infection.
  - Suspect a contaminated specimen when culture shows multiple types of bacteria.

Follow-Up & Special Considerations

- In nonpregnant, premenopausal women with symptoms of UTI, positive urinalysis, and no risks for complicated infection, empirical treatment without obtaining a urine culture may be given.

- Some argue that dipstick urinalysis is unnecessary with characteristic symptoms (i.e., high pretest probability).

Imaging

Initial approach

Imaging studies are often not required in most cases of UTI.

Follow-Up & Special Considerations

- Imaging may be indicated for UTIs in men, infants, immunocompromised patients, febrile infection, signs or symptoms of obstruction, failure to respond to appropriate therapy, and in patients with recurrent infections.
- CT scan and MRI provide the most complete anatomic data in adults.

Pediatric Considerations

For infants and children, obtain ultrasound; if ureteral dilatation is detected, obtain either voiding cystourethrogram or isotope cystogram to evaluate for reflux.

Diagnostic Procedures/Surgery

- Urethral catheterization to obtain urine specimen from children and adults if voided urine is suspected of being contaminated
- Suprapubic bladder aspiration or urethral catheterization to obtain specimen from infants
- Cystourethroscopy may be indicated for patients with recurrent UTIs and previous anti-incontinence surgery or hematuria.

DIFFERENTIAL DIAGNOSIS

- Vaginitis
- Asymptomatic bacteruria
- STDs causing urethritis or pyuria
- Hematuria from causes other than infection (e.g., neoplasia, calculi)
- Interstitial cystitis
- Psychological dysfunction

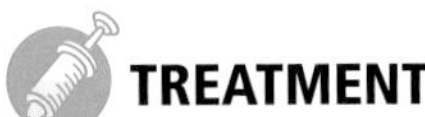

TREATMENT

MEDICATION

First Line

- Uncomplicated UTI (adolescents and adults who are nonpregnant, nondiabetic, afebrile, immunocompetent, and without genitourinary anatomic abnormalities) (2):
  - TMP-SMZ (Bactrim) 160/800 mg PO b.i.d. × 3 days, where resistance of *E. coli* strains <20% (3)[C]
  - 5-day course of nitrofurantoin or 3-day fluoroquinolone course should be used in patients with allergy to TMP-SMZ and in areas where *E. coli* resistance to TMP-SMZ >20% (3)[C].
- UTI in pregnancy:
  - Nitrofurantoin (Macrobid) 100 mg PO b.i.d. × 7 days (4)[C]
  - Cephalexin (Keflex) 500 mg PO b.i.d. × 7 days (4)[C]
- Postcoital UTI: Single-dose TMP-SMX or cephalexin may reduce frequency of UTI in sexually active women.
- Complicated UTI (pregnancy, diabetes, febrile, immunocompromised patient, recurrent UTIs): Extend course to 7–10 days of treatment with antibiotic chosen based on culture results; may begin with fluoroquinolone, TMP-SMX, or cephalosporin while awaiting results:
  - Fluoroquinolones are not safe during pregnancy or for treatment of children.
  - TMP-SMX use in pregnancy is not desirable (especially in third trimester), but is appropriate in some circumstances.

Second Line

- Uncomplicated UTI:
  - Ciprofloxacin 250 mg PO b.i.d. × 3 day; should be reserved for complicated UTIs
  - Fosfomycin (Monurol) 3 g PO single dose
- Chronic UTIs:
  - Women with recurrent symptomatic UTIs can be treated with continuous or postcoital prophylactic antibiotics [A]. Treatment duration guided by the severity of patient symptoms and by physician and patient preference: Consider 6 months of therapy, followed by observation for reinfection after discontinuing prophylaxis (1):
    - Continuous antimicrobial prophylaxis involves daily administration of low-dose TMP-SMX 40/200 mg or nitrofurantoin 50–100 mg, among others (1,5).
  - Another treatment option is self-started antibiotics.

Pediatric Considerations

Long-term antibiotics appear to reduce the risk of recurrent symptomatic UTI in susceptible children, but the benefit is small and must be considered together with the increased risk of microbial resistance (6).

ADDITIONAL TREATMENT

General Measures

- Maintain good hydration.
- Maintain good hygiene.
- 1/4 of women with uncomplicated UTI experience a second UTI within 6 months and 1/2 at some time during their lifetime.
- Avoid sexual intercourse while symptomatic.

Issues for Referral

Men with uncomplicated UTI and most other patients with complicated UTI should be referred to a urologist for evaluation.

Pediatric Considerations

UTI in children, especially <1 year of age, should prompt workup for urinary tract anomalies.

COMPLEMENTARY AND ALTERNATIVE MEDICINE

- Preliminary studies indicate that *Vaccinium macrocarpon* (cranberry) juice may help to prevent and treat UTIs by inhibiting bacterial adherence to the bladder epithelium.
- Cranberry juice may decrease the number of symptomatic UTIs over a 1-year period, particularly for women with recurrent UTIs [A]. The optimum dosage or method of administration (e.g., juice, tablets, or capsules) is still unclear (7).

SURGERY/OTHER PROCEDURES

- Urinary tract obstruction with urosepsis requires drainage of obstructed system.
- Patients with emphysematous pyelonephritis or pyonephrosis may need immediate surgical intervention.

IN-PATIENT CONSIDERATIONS

Outpatient treatment, except for complicated or upper tract infections

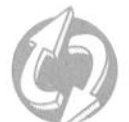

ONGOING CARE

FOLLOW-UP RECOMMENDATIONS

- First or rare UTI: In young or middle-aged, nonpregnant adult females, no follow-up is required if cured after 3-day therapy.
- If persistently symptomatic after 2–3 days of therapy, obtain culture/sensitivity and change antibiotic accordingly.

Pregnancy Considerations

- UTI during pregnancy always requires culture/sensitivity and usually requires a 10–14-day treatment.
- Following the treatment of acute infection, pregnant women warrant surveillance urine cultures every trimester. They may receive prophylactic antibiotics for the remainder of pregnancy for recurrent or upper tract disease.

PATIENT EDUCATION

- Although there are no controlled studies to support this intervention, postcoital voiding is commonly advised.
- FamilyDoctor.org at http://familydoctor.org/online/famdocen/home/women/gen-health/190.html

PROGNOSIS

Symptoms resolve within 2–3 days of antibiotic treatment in almost all patients.

COMPLICATIONS

- Pyelonephritis or sepsis
- Renal abscess
- Acute urinary outlet obstruction

Pregnancy Considerations

Pregnant females, infants, and young children with cystitis are at higher risk of pyelonephritis.

REFERENCES

1. Kodner CM, Thomas Gupton EK, et al. Recurrent urinary tract infections in women: Diagnosis and management. *Am Fam Physician*. 2010;82: 638–43.
2. Litza JA, Brill JR. Urinary tract infections. *Prim Care*. 2010;37:491–507, viii.
3. Warren JW, Abrutyn E, Hebel JR, et al. Guidelines for antimicrobial treatment of uncomplicated acute bacterial cystitis and acute pyelonephritis in women. Infectious Diseases Society of America (IDSA). *Clin Infect Dis*. 1999;29:745–58.
4. Mehnert-Kay SA. Diagnosis and management of uncomplicated urinary tract infections. *Am Fam Physician*. 2005;72:451–6.
5. Stapleton A, Stamm WE. Prevention of urinary tract infection. *Infect Dis Clin N Am*. 1997;11:719–33.
6. Williams G, Craig JC. Long-term antibiotics for preventing recurrent urinary tract infection in children. *Cochrane Database Syst Rev*. 2011: CD001534.
7. Jepson RG, Craig JC. Cranberries for preventing urinary tract infections. *Cochrane Database Syst Rev*. 2008:CD001321.

ADDITIONAL READING

- Car J, Sheikh A. Recurrent urinary tract infection in women. *BMJ*. 2003;327:1204.
- Fihn SD. Acute uncomplicated urinary tract infection in women. *N Engl J Med*. 2003;329(3):259–66.

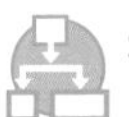

See Also (Topic, Algorithm, Electronic Media Element)

Algorithm: Dysuria

CODES

ICD9

- 595.9 Cystitis, unspecified
- 599.0 Urinary tract infection, site not specified

CLINICAL PEARLS

- Uncomplicated UTIs cause a significant morbidity but generally do not cause renal damage.
- Treatment of uncomplicated UTIs reduces morbidity, but the risk of recurrence stays the same.
- Most UTIs are caused by bacteria originating from bowel flora.
- The combination of bacteriuria and WBCs in the urine gives us a presumptive diagnosis of UTI.
- >100,000 cfu/mL on a urine culture confirms a symptomatic UTI.
- Imaging studies are not required for most women with UTIs.
- Uncomplicated UTIs should be treated for 3 days.
- All pregnant women with bacteriuria should be treated.

U

URINARY TRACT INFECTION (UTI) IN MALES

Scott A. Fields, MD

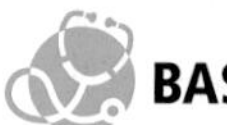

BASICS

DESCRIPTION

- Cystitis is an infection of the lower urinary tract, usually resulting from a single gram-negative enteric bacteria. (See "Prostatitis," "Pyelonephritis," and "Urethritis.")
- System(s) affected: Renal/Urologic
- Synonym(s): Urinary tract infection (UTI); Cystitis

EPIDEMIOLOGY

Incidence

- Predominant age: Increases with age
- Uncommon in men <50 years of age
- 8 infections per 10,000 men aged 21–50 years

Prevalence

Not common

RISK FACTORS

- Benign prostatic hypertrophy (BPH)
- Cognitive impairment
- Fecal incontinence
- Urinary incontinence
- Anal intercourse
- Recent urologic surgery, catheterization
- Infection of the prostate or kidney
- Urinary tract instrumentation
- Immunocompromised host
- Outlet obstruction

GENERAL PREVENTION

- Prompt treatment of predisposing factors
- Use a catheter only when necessary; if needed, use aseptic technique and closed system, and remove as soon as possible.

ETIOLOGY

- *Escherichia coli* (80% of infections)
- *Klebsiella*
- *Enterobacter*
- *Proteus*
- *Pseudomonas*
- *Serratia*
- *Streptococcus faecalis* and *Staphylococcus* sp.

COMMONLY ASSOCIATED CONDITIONS

- Acute bacterial pyelonephritis
- Chronic bacterial pyelonephritis
- Urethritis
- Prostatitis
- Prostatic hypertrophy
- Prostate cancer

Geriatric Considerations

Bacteriuria is common among the elderly, seems to be related to functional status, and usually is transient. If asymptomatic bacteriuria is noted, no treatment is needed.

Pediatric Considerations

Usually associated with obstruction to normal flow of urine, such as vesicoureteral reflux

DIAGNOSIS

Urologic investigations are necessary to rule out other disorders.

HISTORY

- Urinary frequency
- Urinary urgency
- Dysuria
- Hesitancy
- Slow urinary stream
- Dribbling of urine
- Nocturia
- Suprapubic discomfort
- Low back pain
- Hematuria

PHYSICAL EXAM

Systemic symptoms (chills, fever) present with concomitant pyelonephritis or prostatitis.

DIAGNOSTIC TESTS & INTERPRETATION

Lab

- Pyuria
- Bacteriuria
- Urine dipstick leukocyte esterase (75–90% sensitivity, 95% specificity) and nitrate (35–85% sensitivity, 70% specificity)
- Urine culture: 10 high-power colonies of pathogens (or counts >100,000 bacteria/mL of urine) confirm diagnosis (*E. coli, Klebsiella, Pseudomonas,* other agents). Lower counts also may be indicative of infection, especially in the presence of pyuria (1)
- Nucleic acid amplification tests: DNA probes of urine to identify gonococcal and chlamydia infections
- Segmented bacteriologic localization cultures:
  - Variable block (VB) 1: Collect 5–10 mL of urine from patient's initial void.
  - VB2: Then a sample of sterile midstream urine is obtained.
  - Expressed prostatic secretion (EPS): Prostatic massage is performed, and EPS is collected from the meatus.
  - VB3: Patient completes voiding, and fourth sample is collected.
  - Cultures and sensitivity are collected from each specimen.
- Consider differentiating UTI from STD based on history and risk factors, and, if present, test and treat for *Chlamydia* and *Neisseria gonorrhoeae.*
- Drugs that may alter lab results: Antibiotics prior to culture

Imaging

- IV pyelography
- Cystoscopy
- Ultrasound

Pathological Findings

Depends on site of infection

DIFFERENTIAL DIAGNOSIS

- Anatomic or functional pathology
- Urethritis/STIs
- Infections in other sites of the genitourinary tract (e.g., epididymis)

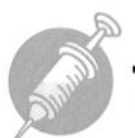

TREATMENT

MEDICATION

First Line

- Acute infection, first infection, no risk factors for treatment: Prescribe 7–10 days of oral antibiotics, either empirically or based on culture and sensitivity results. For empirical therapy, trimethoprim-sulfamethoxazole DS (SMX-TMP, Bactrim DS, Septra DS, others) b.i.d. usually will treat the most likely pathogens (2,3)[C].
- Complicated or recurrent infection: Prescribe 14–21 days of antibiotics based on antimicrobial sensitivities with repeat urine check after the treatment (2,3)[C].

Second Line

According to culture and sensitivity results and patient's history

ADDITIONAL TREATMENT

General Measures

- Hydration; analgesia if required
- Discontinue sexual activity until cured.
- Patient with indwelling catheters:
  - If asymptomatic bacterial colonization, there is no need to treat (sterilization of urine is not possible, and resistant organisms may take up residence).
  - If symptomatic of acute infection, institute treatment.

IN-PATIENT CONSIDERATIONS

Admission Criteria

- Inability to tolerate oral medications
- Acute renal failure
- Suspected sepsis

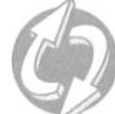

ONGOING CARE

FOLLOW-UP RECOMMENDATIONS

Patient Monitoring

- Close follow-up until clinically well
- Repeat urinalysis after treatment.

DIET

Encourage adequate fluid intake.

PATIENT EDUCATION

- For patient education materials about this topic that have been reviewed favorably, contact the National Kidney Foundation, 30 E. 33rd Street, Suite 1100, New York, NY 10016;(212):889–2210.
- Push fluids, especially those that acidify the urine.

PROGNOSIS

Clearing of infections with appropriate antibiotic treatment

COMPLICATIONS

- Pyelonephritis
- Ascending infection
- Recurrent infection

REFERENCES

1. van Pinxteren B, van Vliet SM, Wiersma TJ, et al. [Summary of the practice guideline 'Urinary-tract infections' (second revision) from the Dutch College of General Practitioners]. *Ned Tijdschr Geneeskd.* 2006;150:718–22.
2. Finn SD. Urinary tract infections—diagnosis and treatment in women and men. *Consultant.* 1992; 10:43–58.
3. Naber KG, Bergman B, Bishop MC, et al. EAU guidelines for the management of urinary and male genital tract infections. Urinary Tract Infection (UTI) Working Group of the Health Care Office (HCO) of the European Association of Urology (EAU). *Eur Urol.* 2001;40:576–88.

ADDITIONAL READING

Lipsky BA. Managing urinary tract infections in men. *Hosp Pract (Off Ed).* 2000;35:53–59, discussion 59–60.

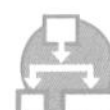

See Also (Topic, Algorithm, Electronic Media Element)

- Prostate Cancer; Prostatic Hyperplasia, Benign (BPH); Prostatitis; Pyelonephritis; Urethritis
- Algorithms: Dysuria; Urethral Discharge

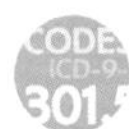

CODES

ICD9

- 595.0 Acute cystitis
- 595.9 Cystitis, unspecified
- 599.0 Urinary tract infection, site not specified

CLINICAL PEARLS

- Cystitis is an infection of the lower urinary tract, usually resulting from a single gram-negative enteric bacteria. (See "Prostatitis," "Pyelonephritis," and "Urethritis.")
- Risk factors/causes: BPH, cognitive impairment, fecal incontinence, urinary incontinence, anal intercourse, recent urologic surgery, catheterization, infection of the prostate or kidney, urinary tract instrumentation, immunocompromised host, outlet obstruction
- Evaluation: Urinalysis, urine culture, STD testing (gonorrhea, chlamydia, etc., by culture or DNA probe)

UROLITHIASIS

Janelle M. Evans, MD

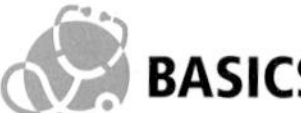

BASICS

DESCRIPTION

- Stone formation within the urinary tract: Urinary crystals bind to form a nidus, which grows to form a calculus (stone).
- Range of symptoms: Asymptomatic to obstructive; febrile morbidity if result of infection

EPIDEMIOLOGY

- The worldwide epidemiology differs according to both geographic area (higher prevalence in hot, arid, or dry climates) and socioeconomic conditions (dietary intake and lifestyle). Radiolucent stones and stones secondary to infection are less influenced by environmental conditions.
- Vesical calculosis (bladder stones) due to malnutrition during early life is frequent in Middle Eastern and Asian countries.
- Incidence in industrialized countries seem to be increasing, probably due to improved diagnostics as well as to increasingly rich diets.
- Increased incidence in patients with surgically induced absorption issues such as Crohn disease and gastric bypass surgery (1)[B]

Incidence

- In industrialized countries: 100–200 per 100,000 per year (2)
- Predominant age: Mean age is 40–60 years.
- Predominant sex: Male > Female (~2:1)

RISK FACTORS

- White > African American in regions with both populations
- Family history
- Pregnancy
- Diet rich in protein, refined carbohydrates, and sodium
- Occupations associated with a sedentary lifestyle or with a hot, dry workplace
- Incidence rates peak during summer secondary to dehydration
- Obesity
- Surgically or medically induced malabsorption (Crohn, gastric bypass, celiac)

Genetics

- Up to 20% of patients have a family history. However, spouses of those who form stones have higher calcium excretion rates than controls, suggesting strong dietary–environmental factors.
- Autosomal dominant: Idiopathic hypercalciuria
- Autosomal recessive:
  - Cystinuria, Lesch-Nyhan syndrome, hyperoxaluria types I and II
  - Ehlers-Danlos syndrome, Marfan syndrome, Wilson disease, familial renal tubular acidosis

GENERAL PREVENTION

- Hydration (3)[A]
- Decrease salt and meat intake.
- Avoid oxalate-rich foods.

Pediatric Considerations

Rare: More common in men; those with low socioeconomic status

Pregnancy Considerations

- Pregnant women have the same incidence of renal colic as do nonpregnant women.
- Majority of symptomatic stones occur during the second and third trimesters, heralded by symptoms of flank pain or hematuria.
- Most common differential diagnosis is physiologic hydronephrosis of pregnancy. Use ultrasound to avoid irradiation. Noncontrast-enhanced CT scan also is diagnostic.
- Treatment goals:
  - Control pain, avoid infection, and preserve renal function until birth or stone passage.
  - 30% require intervention such as stent placement.

PATHOPHYSIOLOGY

- Supersaturation and dehydration lead to high salt content in urine, which congregates.
- Stasis of urine:
  - Renal malformation (e.g., horseshoe kidney, ureteropelvic junction obstruction)
  - Incomplete bladder emptying (e.g., neurogenic bladder, prostate enlargement, multiple sclerosis)
- Crystals may form in pure solutions (homogeneous) or on existing surfaces such as other crystals or cellular debris (heterogeneous).
- Balance of promoters and inhibitors: Organic (Tamm-Horsfall protein, glycosaminoglycan, uropontin, nephrocalcin) and inorganic (citrate, pyrophosphate)

ETIOLOGY

- Calcium oxalate and/or phosphate stones (80%):
  - Hypercalciuria:
    - Absorptive hypercalciuria: Increased jejunal calcium absorption
    - Renal leak: Increased calcium excretion from renal proximal tubule
    - Resorptive hypercalciuria: Mild hyperparathyroidism
  - Hypercalcemia:
    - Hyperparathyroidism
    - Sarcoidosis
    - Malignancy
    - Immobilization
    - Paget disease
- Hyperoxaluria:
  - Enteric hyperoxaluria:
    - Intestinal malabsorptive state associated with irritable bowel disease, celiac sprue, or intestinal resection
    - Bile salt malabsorption leads to formation of calcium soaps.
  - Primary hyperoxaluria: Autosomal recessive, types I and II
  - Dietary hyperoxaluria: Overindulgence in oxalate-rich food
- Hyperuricosuria:
  - Seen in 10% of calcium stone formers
  - Caused by increased dietary purine intake, systemic acidosis, myeloproliferative diseases, gout, chemotherapy, Lesch-Nyhan syndrome
  - Thiazides, probenecid
- Hypocitraturia:
  - Caused by acidosis: Renal tubular acidosis, malabsorption, thiazides, enalapril, excessive dietary protein
- Uric acid stones (10–15%): Hyperuricemia causes as above
- Struvite stones (5–10%): Infected urine with urease-producing organisms (most commonly *Proteus* species)
- Cystine stones (<1%): Autosomal-recessive disorder of renal tubular reabsorption of cystine
- In children: Usually due to malnutrition

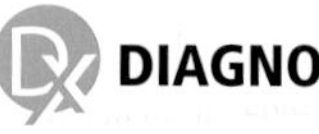

DIAGNOSIS

- Pain:
  - Renal colic: Acute onset of severe groin and/or flank pain
  - Distal stones may present with referred pain in labia, penile meatus, or testis.
- Microscopic or gross hematuria occurs in 95% of patients.
- Nonspecific symptoms of nausea, vomiting, tachycardia, diaphoresis
- Low-grade fever without signs of infection
- Infectious origin: Associated with high-grade fevers
- Frequency and dysuria especially occur with stones at the vesicoureteric junction (VUJ).
- Asymptomatic: Nonobstructing stones within the renal calyces

PHYSICAL EXAM

Tender costovertebral angle with palpation/percussion and/or iliac fossa

DIAGNOSTIC TESTS & INTERPRETATION

Lab

- Urinalysis for RBCs, leukocytes, nitrates, pH (acidic urine <5.5 is associated with uric acid stones; alkaline >7 with struvite stones)
- Midstream urine for microscopy, culture, and sensitivity
- Blood: Urea, creatinine, electrolytes, calcium, and urate; consider CBC.
- Parathyroid hormone only if calcium elevated
- Stone analysis if/when stone passed

Imaging

- Noncontrast-enhanced CT scan of the abdomen and pelvis has replaced IV pyelogram as the investigation of choice (4)[A]:
  - Stone is found most commonly at levels of ureteric luminal narrowing: Pelviureteric junction, pelvic brim, and VUJ
  - Acute obstruction: Proximal ureter and renal pelvis are dilated to the level of obstruction, and perinephric stranding is possible on imaging.
- X-ray of kidneys, ureter, and bladder to determine if stone is radiopaque or lucent:
  - Calcium oxalate/phosphate stones are radiopaque.
  - Uric acid stones are radiolucent.
  - Staghorn calculi (that fill the shape of the renal calyces) are usually struvite and opaque.
  - Cystine stones are faintly opaque (ground-glass appearance).
- US has low sensitivity and specificity but is often the first choice for pregnant women.

DIFFERENTIAL DIAGNOSIS
- Appendicitis
- Ruptured aortic aneurysm
- Musculoskeletal strain
- Pyelonephritis (upper UTI)
- Pyonephrosis (obstructed upper UTI; emergency)
- Perinephric abscess
- Ectopic pregnancy
- Salpingitis

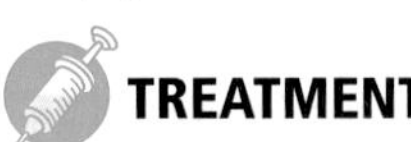

TREATMENT

MEDICATION
- Medical expulsive therapy: α_1-Antagonists (e.g., terazosin) and calcium channel blockers (e.g., nifedipine) improve likelihood of spontaneous stone passage with a number needed to treat (NNT) of ~5.
- Class C in pregnancy

ADDITIONAL TREATMENT
General Measures
- 75% of patients are successfully treated conservatively and pass the stone spontaneously.
- Stones that do not pass usually require surgical intervention.
- 30–50% of patients will have recurrent stones.

Issues for Referral
- Urgent referral of patients with UTI/sepsis or acute renal failure/solitary kidney
- Early referral of pregnant patients, large stones (>8 mm), chronic renal failure, children
- Refer patients if there is no passage at 2–4 weeks or poorly controlled pain.

Additional Therapies
- Uric acid stone dissolution therapy:
  - Alkalinize urine with potassium citrate; keep pH >6.5.
  - Allopurinol 100–300 mg/d PO
- Cystine stone dissolution/prevention:
  - Alkalinize urine with potassium citrate; keep pH >6.5
  - Chelating agents: Captopril, α-mercapto propionylglycine, D-penicillamine
- Consider altering medications that increase risk of stone formation: Probenecid, loop diuretics, salicylic acid, salbutamol, indinavir, triamterene, acetazolamide.
- Treat hypercalciuria with thiazides on an acute basis only.
- Treat hypocitraturia with potassium citrate and high-citrate juices (orange, lemon, etc.).
- Treat enteric hyperoxaluria with oral calcium or magnesium, cholestyramine, and potassium citrate.

SURGERY/OTHER PROCEDURES
- Immediate relief of obstruction is required for patients with the following conditions:
  - Sepsis
  - Renal failure (obstructed solitary kidney, bilateral obstruction)
  - Uncontrolled pain despite adequate analgesia
- Emergency surgery for obstruction:
  - Placement of a retrograde stent (i.e., endoscopic surgery, usually requires an anesthetic)
  - Radiologic placement of a percutaneous nephrostomy tube
- Elective surgery for stone treatment:
  - Extracorporeal shock-wave lithotripsy
  - Ureteroscopy with basket extraction or lithotripsy (laser or pneumatic)
  - Percutaneous nephrolithotomy
- Open surgery is uncommon.

IN-PATIENT CONSIDERATIONS
Initial Stabilization
- Analgesia:
  - Combination of NSAIDs, ketorolac 30–60 mg) and oral opiate
  - Parenteral narcotic if vomiting or if preceding fails to control pain (morphine 5–10 mg IV or IM q4h)
  - Antiemetic if required or prophylactically with parenteral narcotics
- Septic patients with pyonephrosis may require IV fluids and, in severe cases, cardiorespiratory support in intensive care during recovery.

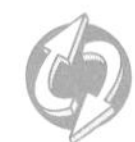

ONGOING CARE

FOLLOW-UP RECOMMENDATIONS
- Patients with ureteric stones who are being treated conservatively should be followed until imaging is clear or stone is visibly passed:
  - Strain urine and send stone for composition.
  - Tamsulosin and nifedipine in selected patients to speed passage
  - Present to the hospital if pain worsens or signs of infection.
  - If pain management is suboptimal or stone does not progress or pass within 2–4 weeks, patient should be referred to a urologist and imaging should be repeated.
- Patients with recurrent formation of stones should have follow-up with a urologist for metabolic workup: 24-hour urine for volume, pH, creatinine, calcium, cystine, phosphate, oxalate, uric acid, magnesium

DIET
- Increased fluid intake for life cannot be overemphasized for decreasing recurrence. Encourage intake of 2–3 L/d; advise patient to have clear urine rather than yellow.
- Patients who form calcium stone should minimize high-oxalate foods such as green leafy vegetables, rhubarb, peanuts, chocolates, and beer.
- Decrease protein and salt intake.
- Lowering calcium intake is inadvisable and even may increase urine calcium excretion.

PROGNOSIS
- Spontaneous stone passage depends on stone location (proximal vs. distal) and stone size (<5 mm, 90% pass; >8 mm, 10% pass).
- Stone recurrence: 50% of patients at 10 years

REFERENCES

1. Matlaga BR, Shore AD, Magnuson T, et al. Effect of gastric bypass surgery on kidney stone disease. *J Urol*. 2009;181:2573–7.
2. Tiselius HG. Epidemiology and medical management of stone disease. *BJU Int*. 2003;91: 758–67.
3. Qiang W, Ke Z. Water for preventing urinary calculi. *Cochrane Database Sys Rev*. 2004;3:CD004292.
4. Worster A, Preyra I, Weaver B, et al. The accuracy of noncontrast helical computed tomography versus intravenous pyelography in the diagnosis of suspected acute urolithiasis: A meta-analysis. *Ann Emerg Med*. 2002;40:280–6.

ADDITIONAL READING

Penniston KL, Jones AN, Nakada SY, et al. Vitamin D repletion does not alter urinary calcium excretion in healthy postmenopausal women. *BJU Int*. 2009;104: 1512–6.

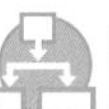

See Also (Topic, Algorithm, Electronic Media Element)

Algorithms: Dysuria; Renal Calculi; Urethral Discharge

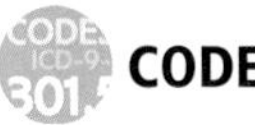

CODES

ICD9

592.9 Urinary calculus, unspecified

CLINICAL PEARLS

- Incidence in industrialized countries seems to be increasing, probably due to improved diagnostics as well as to increasingly rich diets.
- Vesical calculosis (bladder stones) due to malnutrition during early life is frequent in Middle Eastern and Asian countries.
- Medical expulsive therapy: α_1-Antagonists (e.g., terazosin) and calcium channel blockers (e.g., nifedipine) improve likelihood of spontaneous stone passage with NNT of ~5.
- Increased fluid intake for life cannot be overemphasized for decreasing recurrence. Encourage 2–3 L/d intake; advise patient to have clear urine rather than yellow.
- Patients who form calcium stone should minimize high-oxalate foods such as green leafy vegetables, rhubarb, peanuts, chocolates, and beer.
- Decrease protein and salt intake.
- Lowering calcium intake is inadvisable and even may increase urine calcium excretion.

U

URTICARIA

M. Tye Haeberle, MD
William B. Adams, MD

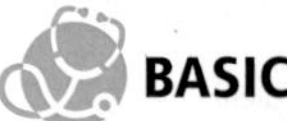

BASICS

DESCRIPTION

- A cutaneous lesion involving transient edema of the epidermis and/or dermis characterized by the acute onset of a polymorphic lesion with central pallor and edema with an erythematous flare ranging in size from millimeters to centimeters
- Pathophysiology is primarily mast cell degranulation and subsequent histamine release
- Lesions subside within 24 hours, whereas angioedema, a dermal lesion of similar pathophysiology, may take up to 72 hours to remit.
- Pruritus and burning are more commonly associated with urticaria; pain more often with angioedema
- Commonly referred to as hives or wheals
- Spontaneous urticaria:
  - Acute: Persists <6 weeks:
    - Specific extrinsic triggers commonly are the cause although there is a vast number of possibilities (e.g., drugs, foods, infections [esp *Streptococci*], envenomation, allergens)
    - Underlying etiology may be difficult to pinpoint
  - Chronic: Persists >6 weeks with >2 episodes/wk off treatment:
    - Unlike acute urticaria, 80% of cases have no obvious external stimulus.
    - If symptoms occur less than twice a week, this is more likely recurrent acute urticaria and should be approached as such.
    - For those with chronic urticaria, 40% have concurrent angioedema.
    - Chronic infection, pseudoallergy, malignancy including mastocytosis, autoimmunity (especially thyroid), and medications may underlie the remaining 20%.
    - Half of those with chronic idiopathic urticaria have sera positive for IgG that releases histamine through binding of IgE or its receptor.
    - The other 50% are truly idiopathic.
  - Physical urticaria: Urticaria due to mechanical stimuli
    - Dermatographism: "Skin writing" or the appearance of linear wheals at the site of friction, scratching, or any type of irritation. This is the most common physical urticaria.
    - Cold urticaria: Wheals occur within minutes of rewarming after cold exposure; 95% idiopathic but can be due to infections (mononucleosis, HIV), neoplasia, or autoimmune diseases
    - Delayed pressure urticaria: Urticaria occurs 0.5–12 hours after pressure to skin (e.g., from elastic or shoes), may be pruritic and/or painful, and may not subside for several days
    - Solar urticaria: From sunlight exposure, usually UV; onset in minutes; subsides within 2 hours
    - Heat urticaria: From direct contact with warm objects or air; rare
    - Vibratory urticaria/angioedema: Very rare; secondary to vibrations (e.g., motorcycle)
  - Special forms of urticaria:
    - Cholinergic urticaria: Due to brief increase of core body temperature from exercise, baths, or due to emotional stress; small pin-sized (5- to 10-mm) wheals surrounded by an erythema, but also can have larger wheals. This is the second most common form.
    - Adrenergic urticaria: Also caused by stress; extremely rare; vasoconstricted, blanched skin around pink wheals as opposed to cholinergic's erythematous surrounding
    - Contact urticaria: Wheals at sites where chemical substances contact the skin, may be either IgE dependent (e.g., latex) or IgE independent (e.g., stinging nettle)
    - Aquagenic and solar urticaria: Small wheals after contact with water of any temperature or UV light, respectively; rare
    - Urticarial vasculitis: Urticaria >24 hours and more painful than pruritic. A leukocytoclastic vasculitis; may be palpable and purpuric; arthralgias

EPIDEMIOLOGY

Incidence

- Equally distributed across all ages: Children more likely to have acute while adults and elderly predisposed to chronic urticaria
- Predominant gender: Female predilection; 2:1 in chronic urticaria
- In 20% of patients, chronic urticaria lasts >10 years.

Prevalence

- Affects anywhere from 5–25% of the population
- Of people with urticaria, 40% have no angioedema, 40% have urticaria and angioedema, and 20% have angioedema with no urticaria (1)
- Up to 3% of the population at some point has chronic idiopathic urticaria
- Chronic urticaria affects only 0.1–3% of children.

RISK FACTORS

- Atopic diseases, asthma, allergic rhinitis, other allergies
- Of patients, >50% possess an atopic disease, >40% with allergic rhinitis, and >15% have atopic dermatitis or allergic asthma in chronic urticaria (1)

Genetics

No consistent pattern known: Chronic urticaria has increased frequency of HLA-DR4 and HLA-D8Q MHC II alleles

GENERAL PREVENTION

Treatment of any underlying atopic or other disease, avoidance of known triggers

PATHOPHYSIOLOGY

- Mast cell degranulation with release of inflammatory reactants, which leads to vascular leakage, inflammatory cell extravasation, and dermal (angioedema) and/or epidermal (wheals/hives) edema
- Histamine, cytokines, leukotrienes, and proteases are main active substances released
- Mast cell degranulation may be caused by allergen cross-linkage of IgE, autoimmune activation of FcϵRI (IgE receptor), substance P, C5a, opiates, or physical stimuli

ETIOLOGY

- Spontaneous acute urticaria:
  - Bacterial infections: Strep throat, sinusitis, otitis, urinary tract
  - Viral infections: Rhinovirus, rotavirus, hepatitis B, mononucleosis, herpes
  - Foods: Peanuts, tree nuts, seafood, milk, soy, fish, wheat, and eggs; tend to be IgE-mediated; pseudoallergenic foods, such as strawberries, tomatoes, preservatives, and coloring agents contain histamine.
  - Drugs: IgE-mediated (e.g., penicillin and other antibiotics), direct mast cell stimulation (e.g., aspirin, NSAIDs, opiates)
  - Inhalant, contact, ingestion, or occupational exposure (e.g., latex, cosmetics)
  - Parasitic infection; insect bite or sting
  - Transfusion reaction
- Spontaneous chronic urticaria:
  - Chronic subclinical allergic rhinitis, eczema, and other atopic disorders
  - Chronic indolent infections: *H. pylori*, fungal, parasitic (*Anisakis simplex*, strongyloidiasis), and chronic viral infections (hepatitis)
  - Collagen-vascular disease (cutaneous vasculitis, serum sickness, lupus)
  - Thyroid autoimmunity, especially Hashimoto's
  - Hormonal: Pregnancy and progesterone
  - Autoimmune antibodies to the IgE receptor α chain on mast cells and to the IgE antibody
  - Chronic medications (e.g., NSAIDs, hormones, ACE inhibitors, etc.)
  - Malignancy
  - Physical stimuli (cold, heat, vibration, pressure) in physical urticaria

COMMONLY ASSOCIATED CONDITIONS

- Angioedema
- Anaphylaxis

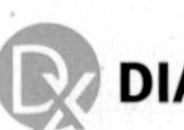

DIAGNOSIS

HISTORY

- Duration, timing (onset/offset) and distribution of lesions; exacerbating and alleviating factors, and history of atopy and/or autoimmune diseases
- Potential trigger exposure
- Concomitance of angioedema: Pruritus in urticarial wheals vs. pain in angioedema
- Urticaria may be an initial symptom of a generalized anaphylactic reaction.
- Fast onset; resolves in <24–48 hours

PHYSICAL EXAM

- Single or multiple raised, polymorphic indurated plaques with central pallor and edema with an erythematous flare
- Variably sized: 1–20 cm or larger
- Evaluation for underlying conditions including thyroid abnormalities (nodules), bacterial, viral, or fungal infection (fever, etc.)
- Often, lesions have cleared and patient's photographs may be useful

DIAGNOSTIC TESTS & INTERPRETATION

Lab

- Acute urticaria: Testing should be directed by clinical suspicion of underlying cause:
  - Full lab workups provide little except in cases of a failed trial of antihistamines, lesions that last >24 hours, lesions that do not blanch on pressure or leave pigmentary changes

- – Allergy skin tests and RAST for inhaled allergens, insects, drugs, or foods
- – Infection: Pharyngeal culture, liver function tests (LFTs), mononucleosis test, urinalysis
- Chronic urticaria:
  - – Often not indicated in mild cases that respond to therapy
  - – CBC with differential, ESR, and/or CRP are recommended by most guidelines
  - – Thyroid function tests, LFTs, and urinalysis are recommended by several guidelines.
  - – Allergy skin tests and RAST for inhaled allergens, insects, drugs, or foods, total IgE level
  - – Autoimmune: ESR, ANA, RF, complement (such as CH50, C3, C4), cryoglobulins in urticarial vasculitis
  - – Tests for *H. pylori* (e.g., antibodies) in dyspeptic patients, stool for ova and parasites
  - – Autologous serum skin testing: Injection of serum under skin to test for presence of IgE receptor-activating antibodies
  - – Measurement of antibodies to FcRI
  - – Malignancy workup, including serum protein electrophoresis and immunofixation

Imaging

Indicated only if clinical suspicion for underlying indolent infections or malignancy

Diagnostic Procedures/Surgery

- Food and drug reactions: Elimination of or challenges with suspected agents
- Physical and special forms of urticaria: Challenge tests:
  - – Dermatographism: Stroke skin lightly with rounded object and observe for surrounding urticaria
  - – Cold urticaria: Ice cube test: Place ice cube on skin for 5 minutes; observe for 10–15 minutes.
  - – Cholinergic: Exercise to the point of sweating or partial immersion in 42°C bath for 10 minutes
  - – Solar: Exposure to different wavelengths of light
  - – Delayed pressure: Apply 5 lb. sandbag to back for 20 minutes, observe 6 hours later.
  - – Aquagenic: Apply water at various temperatures.
  - – Vibratory: Apply vibration 4–5 minutes with a lab mixing device; observe.
- Skin biopsy to rule out urticarial vasculitis in cases of lesions lasting >24 hours

Pathological Findings

- Early lesions: Dermal edema with intravascular margination of neutrophils
- Late lesions: Scant polymorphous perivascular and interstitial infiltrate, with no expansion of cell walls or fibrin deposition

DIFFERENTIAL DIAGNOSIS

- Anaphylaxis (may present with urticaria)
- Morbilliform or fixed drug eruptions
- Erythema multiforme
- SLE, vasculitis, and polyarteritis
- Angioedema without urticaria
- Urticaria pigmentosa/systemic mastocytosis
- Bullous pemphigoid (urticarial stage)
- Arthropod bite
- Atopic or contact dermatitis
- Viral exanthem

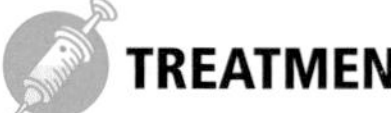

TREATMENT

MEDICATION

First Line

- Second-generation antihistamine (H1) blockers are the first-line treatment of any urticaria in which avoidance of stimulus is impossible or not feasible (2,3,4)[A]:
  - – Fexofenadine (Allegra): 180 mg/d
  - – Loratadine (Claritin): 10 mg/d; only medication studied for safe use in pregnancy
  - – Desloratadine (Clarinex): 5 mg/d
  - – Cetirizine (Zyrtec): 10 mg/d
  - – Levocetirizine (Xyzal): 5 mg/d; requires weight-based dosing in children
  - – Rupatadine: Novel H1 antagonist with antiplatelet activating factor activity
- First-generation antihistamines (H1; for patients with sleep disturbed by itching) (2,3,4)[A]:
  - – Older children and adults: Hydroxyzine or diphenhydramine 25–50 mg q6h
  - – Children <6 years old: Diphenhydramine 12.5 mg q6–8h (5 mg/kg/d) or hydroxyzine (10 mg/5 mL) 2 mg/kg/d divided q6–8h
- H2-specific antihistamines (beneficial as adjuvants) (2,3,4)[C]:
  - – Cimetide, ranitidine, nizatidine, famotidine
- Precautions and notes:
  - – Drowsiness and dry mouth and eyes in first-generation H1 blockers (elderly)
  - – Higher than typical second-generation H1 blocker dosages may obviate the need for first-generation H1 blockers or H2 blockers

Second Line

- Corticosteroids: Prednisolone 2 × 20 mg/d × 4 days; avoid chronic use (3)[C]
- Doxepin: Tricyclic antidepressant with strong H1- and H2-blocking properties; 10–30 mg at bedtime; sedation limits usefulness; useful in treating concomitant depression (2,3)[C].
- Mirtazapine: Tetracyclic antidepressant with H1 antagonist properties; may be helpful in delayed-pressure urticaria (2,3)[C]
- Leukotriene antagonists (montelukast, zileuton, and zafirlukast): Safe and worth trying in chronic, unresponsive cases; useful alone but best used in addition to antihistamines (2,3)[C]
- Nifedipine: Calcium channel blocker potentially useful in patients with hypertension (2,3)[C]
- Cyclosporine: Well-studied, effective (2.5–5 mg/kg/d), may be used in combination with antihistamines; significant renal side effects (2)[C]
- Omalizumab: Anti-IgE; expensive (3)[C]
- UV therapy decreases number of mast cells; has shown promise in the treatment of mastocytosis-induced urticaria (2)[C]
- IVIG, plasmapheresis, sulfasalazine, dapsone, danazol, colchicine, calcium channel blockers, tacrolimus, methotrexate, hydroxychloroquine, warfarin, and mycophenolate mofetil have been reportedly successful, although data remain sparse.

ADDITIONAL TREATMENT

General Measures

- Calamine or 1% topical menthol may be useful.
- Avoid the eliciting stimulus (e.g., diet modification).
- NSAIDs and alcohol may exacerbate symptoms.
- Cold and heat urticaria: Avoid sudden changes in temperature.
- Dermatographic and delayed-pressure urticaria: Avoid pressure applied to the skin.
- Solar urticaria: Avoid the sun; use sunscreen.
- Cholinergic urticaria: Avoid sudden changes in body temperature.

Issues for Referral

Referral to an allergist, immunologist, or dermatologist for recalcitrant cases, complex management, testing for potential triggers, and anaphylaxis

IN-PATIENT CONSIDERATIONS

Admission Criteria

- Educating patient on use of EpiPen as pathophysiology similar
- If the airway is threatened, immediate consult to evaluate for laryngeal edema and need for airway access

ONGOING CARE

FOLLOW-UP RECOMMENDATIONS

Patient Monitoring

A diary of potential triggers (foods, activities, etc.) may help in recalcitrant or persistent cases

PROGNOSIS

- Resolution of acute symptoms: 70% <72 hours.
- Of patients with chronic urticaria, 35% will be symptom-free in a year, while another 30% will see symptom reduction (5).
- Not life threatening but 18% of those with chronic urticaria will have decreased quality of life (1)

REFERENCES

1. Zuberbier T, Balke M, Worm M, et al. Epidemiology of urticaria: A representative cross-sectional survey. *Clin Exp Dermatol*. 2010;35:869–73.
2. Poonawalla T, Kelly B. Urticaria: A review. *Am J Clin Dermatol*. 2009;10(1):9–21.
3. Zuberbier T, Asero R, Bindsley-Jensen C, et al. EAACI/GA²LEN/EDF/WAO guideline: Management of urticaria. *Allergy*. 2009;64:1427–43.
4. Oranje AP. Management of urticaria and angioedema in children: New trends. *G Ital Dermatol Venereol*. 2010;145:771–4.
5. Schaefer P. Urticaria: Evaluation and treatment. *Am Fam Physician*. 2011;83(9):1078–84.

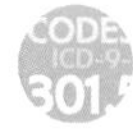

CODES

ICD9

- 708.1 Idiopathic urticaria
- 708.8 Other specified urticaria
- 708.9 Unspecified urticaria

CLINICAL PEARLS

- "Chronic urticaria" with <2 episodes per week should be approached as acute.
- Antihistamines are the best studied and most efficacious therapy.
- Lesions lasting >24 hours should be evaluated for urticarial vasculitis.

UTERINE MYOMAS

Eric L. Jenison, MD
Michael P. Hopkins, MD, MEd
Stephen J. Bacak, DO, MPH

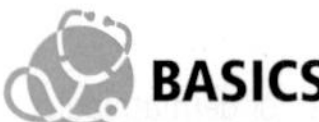

BASICS

DESCRIPTION

- Uterine leiomyomas are well-circumscribed, pseudoencapsulated, benign monoclonal tumors composed mainly of smooth muscle with varying amounts of fibrous connective tissue (1,2,3).
- 3 major subtypes:
  - Subserous: Common; external; may become pedunculated
  - Intramural: Common; within myometrium; may cause marked uterine enlargement
  - Submucous: ~5% of all cases; internal, evoking abnormal uterine bleeding and infection; occasionally protruding from cervix
- Rare locations: Broad, round, and uterosacral ligaments
- System(s) affected: Reproductive
- Synonym(s): Fibroids, myoma, fibromyoma, myofibroma, fibroleiomyoma

EPIDEMIOLOGY

Incidence

- Cumulative incidence is 70% (4)
- Incidence increases with each decade during reproductive years
- Highest incidence in perimenopausal age group
- Not seen in premenarchal females
- Predominant sex: Females only
- 3 times more frequent and occurs earlier in African Americans

Prevalence

- 4–11% of all women
- 20–40% of women in reproductive years (3)

RISK FACTORS

- African American heritage
- Early menarche (<10 years)
- Nulliparous
- Hypertension
- Familial predisposition
- Obesity
- Alcohol

Genetics

- ~50% of leiomyomas have an abnormal karyotype (1).
- Most common cytogenetic abnormalities are deletions on chromosome 7.

PATHOPHYSIOLOGY

Enlargement of benign smooth muscle tumors that may lead to symptoms affecting the reproductive, GI, or genitourinary system

ETIOLOGY

Complex multifactorial process involving transition from normal myocyte to abnormal cells and then to visibly evident tumor (monoclonal expansion):

- Hormones (2): Increases in estrogen and progesterone are correlated with myoma formation (i.e., rarely seen before menarche):
  - Estrogen receptors in myomas bind more estradiol than normal myometrium (3).
- Growth factors (2):
  - Increased smooth muscle proliferation (transforming growth factor β [TGF-β], basic fibroblast growth factor [bFGF])
  - Increase DNA synthesis (epidermal growth factor [EGF], PDGF)
  - Stimulate synthesis of extracellular matrix (TGF-β)
  - Promote mitogenesis (TGF-β, EGF, IGF, prolactin)
  - Promote angiogenesis (bFGF, VEGF)
- Vasoconstrictive hypoxia (2): Proposed, but not confirmed, mechanism of myometrial injury during menstruation

COMMONLY ASSOCIATED CONDITIONS

Endometrial and breast cancer also associated with high unopposed estrogen stimulation.

DIAGNOSIS

HISTORY

- Usually asymptomatic, ~30% present with abnormal symptoms (3)
- Symptoms include:
  - Abnormal uterine bleeding, usually heavy or prolonged menses
  - Pain: Infrequent, usually associated with torsion of pedunculated myoma, degeneration, or cervical dilation by submucous myoma near cervical os
  - Pressure on bladder: Suprapubic discomfort, urinary frequency or obstruction
  - Pressure on rectosigmoid: May cause low back pain, constipation
  - Infertility: Rare, estimated 1–2.5% (3). Usually from submucous myoma distorting the uterine cavity or interference with implantation.

ALERT

Rapid growth, particularly in perimenopausal or postmenopausal patients, may indicate sarcoma. Extremely rare, 0.1–0.3% of cases (3).

PHYSICAL EXAM

- Usually incidental finding on abdominal and pelvic exam
- Firm, smooth nodules or masses arising from uterus
- Masses are mobile without tenderness

DIAGNOSTIC TESTS & INTERPRETATION

Lab

Initial lab tests

- Pregnancy test
- Hemoglobin

Follow-Up & Special Considerations

Consider CA-125: May be slightly elevated in some cases of uterine myoma but generally more useful in differentiating myomas from various gynecologic adenocarcinomas

Imaging

Initial approach

- Pelvic ultrasound: Shows characteristic hypoechoic appearance (5)[B]
- Saline-infusion hysterosonography: Helps to distinguish submucosal myomas (5)[B]
- Hysterosalpingogram: Evaluates the contour of the endometrial cavity (5)[B]
- CT scan or MRI: May help to differentiate complex cases or used when uterine artery embolization is planned (5)[B]

Follow-Up & Special Considerations

- IV pyelogram: If suspect ureteral distortion (5)[B]
- Barium enema

Diagnostic Procedures/Surgery

- Fractional dilation and curettage: Aids in ruling out cervical or uterine carcinomas when clinically suspicious
- Hysteroscopy: Helps to diagnose submucosal or intracavitary myomas
- Laparoscopy: Useful in complex cases and to rule out other pelvic diseases or disorders

Pathological Findings

- Myomas are usually multiple and vary in size and location; have been reported up to 100 lb.
- Gross pathology: Firm tumors with characteristic whorl-like trabeculated appearance; a thin pseudocapsular layer is present
- Microscopic: Bundles of smooth muscle mixed with varying amounts of connective tissue elements running in different directions
- Cellular variant has a preponderance of muscle cells. Mitoses are rare.
- May undergo various types of degeneration:
  - Hyaline degeneration: Very common
  - Calcification: Late result of circulatory impairment to myomas
  - Infection and suppuration: Most common with submucosal myomas
  - Necrosis: Most common with pedunculated myomas secondary to torsion
  - Sarcomatous changes: Incidence 0.1–0.3% of clinically apparent myomas (3)[B]

DIFFERENTIAL DIAGNOSIS

- Intrauterine pregnancy
- Ovarian or uterine cancer
- Leiomyosarcoma/malignancy
- Cecal or sigmoid tumor
- Appendiceal abscess
- Diverticulitis
- Pelvic kidney
- Urachal cyst

TREATMENT

- Treatment must be individualized
- Medical therapy may be of benefit
- Patients with minimal symptoms may be managed with iron preparations and analgesics.
- Conservative management of asymptomatic myomas:
  - Pelvic exams and ultrasounds at 3-month or longer intervals if size remains stable
  - Substantial regression usually occurs after menopause
- Surgical options should be considered if symptomatic or worrisome myomas are unresponsive to conservative or medical management.

MEDICATION

- Progestins may reduce overall uterine size (5)[B]:
  - Norethindrone 10 mg/d
  - Medroxyprogesterone (Depo-Provera) 200 mg IM monthly
  - Levonorgestrel intrauterine device (3)[B]
- Combination oral contraceptives: May help prevent development of new fibroids:
  - Contraindications: History of thromboembolic events: See manufacturer's profile.
  - Adverse reactions and significant interactions: See manufacturer's profile.
- Luteinizing hormone–releasing hormone:
  - Nafarelin (Synarel Nasal Spray), goserelin (Zoladex Depot), and leuprolide (Lupron Depot)
  - Induces abrupt artificial menopause; may reduce myoma symptoms dramatically; induces atrophy of myomas by up to 40% in 2–3 months (5)[B]
  - May be valuable as preoperative adjunct to myomectomy or hysterectomy by allowing recovery of anemia, donation of autologous blood, and possibly converting abdominal to vaginal hysterectomy, thereby decreasing postoperative pain, hospitalization, and morbidity (5)[B]
  - Not recommended for use >6 months because of osteoporosis risk
  - Following discontinuation, myomas return within 60 days to pretherapy size
- Mifepristone:
  - Antiprogesterone
  - Shown to have similar reduction in myoma size as gonadotropin-releasing hormone agonists (6)[B]

ADDITIONAL TREATMENT

General Measures

Patients not desiring pharmacologic therapy or surgery may consider:

- Uterine artery embolization: Averages 50% shrinkage of myomas (5)[A]; painful and may cause ovarian failure (1–2%), amenorrhea, or other complications; shorter hospital stay and quicker recovery but no difference in satisfaction compared with hysterectomy (3,7)[B]
- MRI-guided focused ultrasound: Noninvasive, ultrasound transducer passes through abdominal wall and causes coagulative necrosis of fibroid. Up to 98% reduction in myoma volume and symptoms. Not appropriate for some types of myomas (3)[B]. Efficacy may be comparable with other hysterectomy-sparing procedures (6)[B].

Issues for Referral

- Medical therapy may be initiated by a primary care physician or gynecologist. Adequate pelvic examination must be performed initially.
- Surgical considerations may be pursued with gynecologic consultation.
- Uterine embolization may be discussed with an interventional radiologist.

SURGERY/OTHER PROCEDURES

- Surgical management is indicated in the following situations (5)[B]:
  - Excessive uterine size or excessive rate of growth (except during pregnancy)
  - Submucosal myomas when associated with hypermenorrhea
  - Pedunculated myomas that are painful or undergo torsion, necrosis, and hemorrhage
  - If a myoma causes symptoms from pressure on bladder or rectum
  - If differentiation from ovarian mass is not possible
  - If associated pelvic disease is present (endometriosis, pelvic inflammatory disease)
  - If infertility or habitual abortion is likely due to the anatomic location of the myoma
- Surgical procedures:
  - Preliminary pelvic examination, Pap smear, and endometrial biopsy should be performed to rule out malignant or premalignant conditions.
  - Hysterectomy: May be performed vaginally, laparoscopically, robotically, or by laparotomy:
    - Effective in relieving symptoms and improving quality of life (6)[B]
  - Abdominal, laparoscopic, or robotic myomectomy may be performed in younger women who want to maintain fertility (5)[B].
  - Hysteroscopic or laparoscopic cautery or laser myoma resection can be performed in selected patients.
  - Endometrial ablation: For small submucosal myomas

IN-PATIENT CONSIDERATIONS

Initial Stabilization

- Usually outpatient
- Inpatient for some surgical procedures

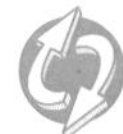

ONGOING CARE

FOLLOW-UP RECOMMENDATIONS

Patient Monitoring

- Pelvic examination and ultrasound: Every 2–3 months for newly diagnosed symptomatic or excessively large myomas
- Hemoglobin and hematocrit: If uterine bleeding is excessive
- Once uterine size and symptoms stable, monitor every 6–12 months

DIET

No restrictions

PATIENT EDUCATION

- Medline Plus: www.nlm.nih.gov/medlineplus/uterinefibroids.html
- JAMA Patient Page on uterine fibroids: http://jama.ama-assn.org/cgi/reprint/301/1/122.pdf
- Society of Interventional Radiology: http://sirweb.org/patients/uterine-fibroids/
- US Department of Health and Human Services: http://womenshealth.gov/faq/uterine-fibroids.cfm
- American Congress of Obstetricians and Gynecologists (ACOG): www.acog.org

PROGNOSIS

- Resection of submucosal fibroids has been associated with increased fertility (6)[B].
- Laparoscopic myomectomy does not have any difference in clinical pregnancy rate and live-birth rate than laparotomy (8)[B].
- At least 10% of myomas recur after myomectomy; however, most women will not require further treatment (6)[B].

COMPLICATIONS

- May mask other gynecologic malignancies (e.g., uterine sarcoma, ovarian cancer)
- Degenerating fibroids may cause pain and bleeding
- May rarely prolapse through the cervix

Pregnancy Considerations

- Rapid growth of fibroids is common.
- Pregnant women may need additional fetal testing if placenta is located over or near fibroid.
- Complications during pregnancy: Abortion, premature labor, second-trimester rapid growth leading to degeneration and pain, and third-trimester fetal malpresentation and dystocia during labor and delivery
- Previous myomectomy patients may develop uterine rupture during labor. Cesarean section is recommended if the endometrial cavity was entered during previous myomectomy.

Geriatric Considerations

In postmenopausal patients with newly diagnosed uterine myoma or enlarging uterine myomas, have a high suspicion of uterine sarcoma or other gynecologic malignancy.

REFERENCES

1. Okolo S. Incidence, aetiology and epidemiology of uterine fibroids. *Best Pract Res Clin Obstet Gynaecol*. 2008;22(4):571–88.
2. Parker WH. Etiology symptomatology, and diagnosis of uterine myomas. *Fertil Steril*. 2007;87:725–36.
3. Duhan N, Sirohiwal D. Uterine myomas revisited. *Eur J Obstet Gynecol Reprod Biol*. 2010;152: 119–25.
4. Laughlin SK, Schroeder JC, Baird DD, et al. New directions in the epidemiology of uterine fibroids. *Semin Reprod Med*. 2010;28:204–17.
5. Wallace EE, Vlahos NF. Uterine myomas: An overview of development, clinical features and management. *Obstetrics Gynecol*. 2004; 104(2):393–406.
6. Parker WH. Uterine myomas: Management. *Fertil Steril*. 2007;88:255–71.
7. Freed MM, Spies JB. Uterine artery embolization for fibroids: A review of current outcomes. *Semin Reprod Med*. 2010;28:235–41.
8. Agdi M, Tulandi T. Minimally invasive approach for myomectomy. *Semin Reprod Med*. 2010;28: 228–34.

ADDITIONAL READING

Istre O. Management of symptomatic fibroids: Conservative surgical treatment modalities other than hysterectomy and abdominal or laparoscopic myomectomy. *Best Pract Res Clin Obstet Gynaecol*. 2008;22(4):571–88.

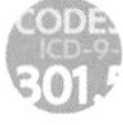

CODES

ICD9

- 218.0 Submucous leiomyoma of uterus
- 218.1 Intramural leiomyoma of uterus
- 218.9 Leiomyoma of uterus, unspecified

CLINICAL PEARLS

- Uterine myomas are benign smooth muscle tumors composed mainly of fibrous connective tissue.
- Usually incidental finding on pelvic exam or ultrasound, but may cause pelvic pain and pressure, abnormal uterine bleeding, and/or infertility
- Management ranges from conservative to medical to surgical.

UTERINE PROLAPSE

Eric L. Jenison, MD
Michael P. Hopkins, MD, MEd
Cameron J. Codd, DO

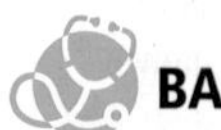

BASICS

DESCRIPTION

- Uterine prolapse occurs when the integrity of pelvic supporting structures is lost. This allows the uterus to descend into the vagina. In advanced cases, complete protrusion with inversion of the vagina occurs, known as procidentia.
- Before menopause, the degree and severity of prolapse are usually related to the number of pregnancies and the difficulty of childbirth. After menopause, atrophy and loss of tissue integrity can lead to further prolapse.
- System(s) affected: Gastrointestinal; Renal/Urologic; Reproductive
- Synonym(s): Uterine prolapse; Genital prolapse; Genital relaxation; Uterine descensus; Total or partial procidentia; Dropped uterus

Geriatric Considerations

This is largely a disease of aging, and incidence will be much higher as the median age of the population increases.

Pediatric Considerations

Prolapse in newborns has been reported, but it is rare and usually associated with congenital disorders and neuropathies.

EPIDEMIOLOGY

Incidence

- Annual incidence ~2%
- Predominant age: Perimenopausal and postmenopausal women
- Predominant sex: Female only

Prevalence

~30–50% of women experience some degree of prolapse.

RISK FACTORS

- Childbirth, particularly multiple parity
- Vaginal delivery, especially operative vaginal delivery
- Advancing age
- Caucasian or Hispanic (4–5-fold increased risk compared to African Americans)
- Tobacco use
- Occupations requiring heavy lifting
- Various connective tissue and neurogenic disorders
- Conditions resulting in increased intra-abdominal pressure (e.g., obesity, abdominal or pelvic tumors, pulmonary disease with chronic coughing, chronic constipation)
- Estrogen-deficient state

Genetics

- More common among Caucasians
- Less common among Asians and African Americans, and particularly uncommon in South African Bantus and West Africans

GENERAL PREVENTION

- Kegel exercises increase the strength of the pelvic diaphragm muscles and may provide some pelvic support.
- Weight loss and proper management of conditions that increase abdominal pressure help to prevent prolapse.
- Tobacco cessation
- Postmenopausal estrogen replacement therapy

ETIOLOGY

- Advancing age and vaginal childbirth are the most important factors.
- Incidence of prolapse increases with frequency and difficulty of vaginal deliveries (e.g., operative vaginal delivery); <2% of prolapse occurs in nulliparous women.
- Although this disorder in large part results from the distension and distortion of supporting tissues with vaginal childbirth, pregnancy, regardless of mode of delivery, may contribute to prolapse.
- Other less common causes of prolapse include connective tissue disorders with lax tissue (e.g., Marfan syndrome), neurogenic disorders (e.g., multiple sclerosis), cloacal agenesis, chronic constipation, pelvic tumors or ascites, and chronic coughing resulting from chronic lung disease.
- Patients who have undergone radical vulvectomy with loss of the external supporting structures have a higher rate of prolapse.

COMMONLY ASSOCIATED CONDITIONS

Cystocele, rectocele, enterocele, and vaginal vault prolapse are often associated with uterine prolapse.

DIAGNOSIS

HISTORY

- Patients are often asymptomatic. They may experience the following:
  - Pelvic pressure and low back pain
  - Bulging sensation in vagina or at introitus
  - Dyspareunia
  - Difficulty with urination or defecation
  - Symptoms often worsen following long periods of standing
  - Vaginal bleeding (mucosal irritation)
- Inquiry should be made as to:
  - The number of pregnancies, mode of deliveries, episiotomies, extent and repair of vaginal/perineal lacerations
  - Previous pelvic surgery
  - Congenital abnormalities
  - Medical conditions that chronically increase intra-abdominal pressure (e.g., chronic obstructive pulmonary disease [COPD])

PHYSICAL EXAM

- Diagnosis is confirmed by a pelvic exam. With coughing and straining, the cervix will prolapse toward introitus or beyond.
- Use only 1 blade of speculum during pelvic examination to better appreciate prolapse.

ALERT

- The patient needs to be examined while standing as well as lying down to confirm diagnosis.
- Severity of symptoms and degree of prolapse are not strongly correlated.
- Can use 1 of many evaluation systems to describe extent of prolapse
- Baden-Walker system (1):
  - Grade 0: Normal position
  - Grade 1: Descent halfway to the hymen
  - Grade 2: Descent to the hymen
  - Grade 3: Descent halfway past the hymen
  - Grade 4: Maximum possible descent
- Pelvic Organ Quantification (POP-Q) system also used, but it is more complex and used primarily in research settings

DIAGNOSTIC TESTS & INTERPRETATION

Lab

- Evaluation of renal function (BUN and creatinine) to rule out ureteral obstruction
- Urinalysis to rule out UTI

Imaging

- IV pyelogram to rule out ureteral obstruction in complete uterine prolapse (optional)
- Pelvic ultrasound or CT scan to rule out other pelvic pathology, if suspected (optional)

Diagnostic Procedures/Surgery

- If surgical correction is planned, urodynamic studies should be performed to evaluate for potential urinary incontinence masked by the prolapse (2)[B].
- If ulceration or bleeding is present, Pap smears and appropriate cervical and endometrial biopsies should be done to rule out concomitant malignancies.

Pathological Findings

Hyperkeratosis of the cervical and vaginal tissues occurs with prolapse beyond the introitus due to chronic irritation and drying. As the irritation becomes more pronounced, bleeding and ulceration occur.

DIFFERENTIAL DIAGNOSIS

- Other pelvic organ prolapse (e.g., cystocele, rectocele, enterocele)
- Pelvic mass, benign or malignant

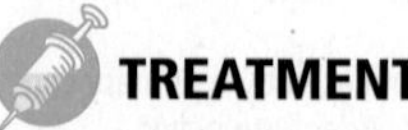

TREATMENT

MEDICATION

- Vaginal estrogen therapy can increase blood supply to the vagina and supporting tissue, which may improve tissue strength; may also be beneficial for mild urinary incontinence.
- This is especially important in postmenopausal women using pessaries or undergoing reconstructive pelvic surgery (2)[B].

- Progestin therapy or monitoring of endometrial status in a woman with an intact uterus is not necessary with vaginal estrogen therapy.
- Estrogen therapy should be used in the lowest possible dose for the shortest time. However, women may need long-term therapy due to the chronic nature of uterine prolapse.
- 3 forms of vaginal estrogen therapy:
  - Vaginal cream (Premarin conjugated equine estrogen or estradiol cream): Insert via applicator each night × 14 days and then 2–3 times/wk.
  - Vaginal estradiol tablet: Insert via preloaded applicator each night × 14 days and then 2–3 times/wk.
  - Estradiol-containing vaginal ring: Insert into vagina and replace every 3 months.
- Contraindications:
  - Breast- or estrogen-dependent carcinoma
  - Undiagnosed vaginal bleeding
  - Thromboembolic disorders
  - Thrombophlebitis
  - Pregnancy
- Precautions: Any abnormal vaginal bleeding must be evaluated.

ADDITIONAL TREATMENT

General Measures

- Treatment depends on multiple variables, including the severity of prolapse, age, sexual activity, associated pelvic pathology, and desire for future fertility.
- Treatment of grade I or II prolapse is expectant unless patient is symptomatic.
- Conservative therapies include vaginal estrogen replacement, pessary use, and physical therapy (3)[C].
- Pessaries are indicated for women who are unfit for, or decline, surgery. Proper fitting and maintenance are required (4)[C].
- Pessaries also may be used in the preoperative evaluation of prolapse (4)[C].
- Surgery is indicated for women who fail conservative therapies and/or desire definitive treatment (2)[B].

Issues for Referral

Urogynecology evaluation for patients who may be surgical candidates

Additional Therapies

Physical therapy, including biofeedback, electrical stimulation, and pelvic muscle training (Kegels), may be an option for women with mild prolapse and/or those wishing conservative therapy (4)[C].

SURGERY/OTHER PROCEDURES

- Surgical candidates without additional pelvic pathology: Vaginal or abdominal hysterectomy ± enterocele, cystocele, rectocele, paravaginal repair, urethral suspension, and culdoplasty depending on coexisting pelvic organ prolapse (2)[B]
- Incontinence procedure often done at same time as prolapse repair although almost 1/3 of women relieved of stress urinary incontinence by prolapse surgery alone (5)[B]
- Vault suspension is typically necessary with hysterectomy:
  - Vaginal procedures include sacrospinous ligament fixation, uterosacral ligament fixation, and endopelvic fascial suspension.
  - Sacral colpopexy can be performed via laparoscopic or open abdominal approach.
  - The abdominal approach (sacral colpopexy) has decreased risk of recurrent apical prolapse and less postoperative dyspareunia and stress incontinence compared with the vaginal approach (sacrospinous ligament fixation). However, the abdominal approach is associated with longer operative time and recovery time (6)[A].
- Uterine suspension is an option for patients who desire to maintain reproductive function (2)[B].
- In elderly women, uterine conservation with sacrospinous fixation is comparable to vaginal hysterectomy but with fewer postoperative complications (7)[B].
- Older women who are not sexually active can be treated with colpocleisis or vaginal obliteration procedure.

IN-PATIENT CONSIDERATIONS

Initial Stabilization

- Outpatient
- Inpatient when surgery is necessary

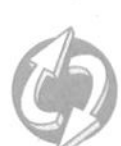

ONGOING CARE

FOLLOW-UP RECOMMENDATIONS

- Heavy lifting, sexual intercourse, and other activities that increase intra-abdominal pressure should be avoided for 6–12 weeks after surgical correction.
- Maintain ideal body weight.

Patient Monitoring

- Expectant management is appropriate, with periodic follow-up exams.
- If a pessary is placed, it should be removed, cleaned, and replaced every 3–6 months (4)[C].

DIET

Avoid constipation by increasing dietary fiber and fluid intake.

PATIENT EDUCATION

- Kegel exercises when applicable
- American College of Obstetricians and Gynecologists (ACOG), 409 12th St., SW, Washington, DC 20024-2188; (800) 762-ACOG; www.acog.org

PROGNOSIS

- It is expected that the incidence and severity of prolapse will increase as patients age.
- Although surgical correction is usually successful initially, reoperation rate is ~29% (2)[B].

COMPLICATIONS

- Ureteral obstruction and renal failure
- Incarceration of bowel herniations
- Pessary use may not always be effective and may cause discomfort, ulcers, and infection.

REFERENCES

1. Baden WF, et al. Fundamentals, symptoms and classification. In Baden WF, et al., eds. *Surgical Repair of Vaginal Defects*. Philadelphia: Lippincott, 1992;14.
2. Thakar R. Regular review: Management of genital prolapse. *Br Med J*. 2002;324:1258–62.
3. Fox WB. Physical therapy for pelvic floor dysfunction. *Med Health R I*. 2009;92:10–1.
4. Trowbridge ER, Fenner DE. Conservative management of pelvic organ prolapse. *Clin Obstet Gynecol*. 2005;48:668–81.
5. Borstad E, Abdelnoor M, Staff AC. Surgical strategies for women with pelvic organ prolapse and urinary stress incontinence. *Int Urogynecol J Pelvic Floor Dysfunct*. 2010;21:179–86.
6. Maher C, Feiner B, Baessler K. Surgical management of pelvic organ prolapse in women. *Cochrane Database Syst Rev*. 2010;4:CD004014.
7. Hefni M, El-Toukhy T. Sacrospinous cervicocolpopexy with uterine conservation for uterovaginal proplapse in elderly women: An evolving concept. *Am J Obstet Gynecol*. 2003; 188:645–50.

ADDITIONAL READING

- Doshani A, Teo RE, Mayne CJ, et al. Uterine prolapse. *BMJ*. 2007;335:819–23.
- Farrell S. The detection and management of vaginal atrophy. *Int J Gynecol Obstet*. 2005;88:222–8.

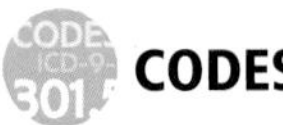

CODES

ICD9

- 618.1 Uterine prolapse without mention of vaginal wall prolapse
- 618.2 Uterovaginal prolapse, incomplete
- 618.3 Uterovaginal prolapse, complete

CLINICAL PEARLS

- Uterine prolapse occurs when the integrity of pelvic supporting structures is lost.
- Advancing age and vaginal childbirth (including the number of pregnancies and the difficulty of childbirth) are the most important factors that contribute to uterine prolapse.
- Conservative therapies include vaginal estrogen replacement, pessary use, and physical therapy.
- Surgery is indicated for women who fail conservative therapies and/or desire definitive treatment.

UTERINE SYNECHIAE

Young-Me Chung, MD
Heidi L. Gaddey, MD

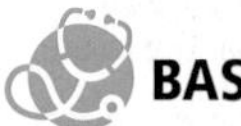

BASICS

DESCRIPTION

- Presence of intrauterine adhesions causing symptoms of secondary amenorrhea, pelvic pain, recurrent miscarriages, and/or infertility in a female of child-bearing age
- Disease ranges from mild to moderate to severe depending on degree of adhesions (e.g., number, density, thickness, quality) .
- 7 different classification systems to categorize disease severity:
  - Each system includes consideration of adhesion characteristics on hysteroscopy (1).
  - Important to classify severity since has prognostic value for fertility (1)[B]; however, currently no single uniform system that can be endorsed
  - Variety of systems also makes comparing different studies difficult (1)[C]
- Synonym(s): Intrauterine adhesions (IUAs); Asherman syndrome (= pain, menstrual disturbance, subfertility in any combination of 3 PLUS presence of IUAs., i.e., "asymptomatic" IUAs technically does NOT equal Asherman syndrome) (1,2)

EPIDEMIOLOGY

Incidence

1.5% of all hysterosalpingographies (4)

Prevalence

- Varies with geography, population profile, availability of diagnostic devices
- Asymptomatic population: 0.3% incidental finding of uterine adhesions
- After postpartum curettage: 22% (2)
- After postabortion curettage: 37% (4)

RISK FACTORS

- Postpartum curettage, especially after initial 48 hours postpartum (2,4)
- 37% of postabortion curettage develop IUA (2,4)
- Postpartum hemorrhage (2,4)
- Recurrent miscarriages (2,4)
- Cesarean section (2,4)
- Pelvic radiation (2,4)
- Trauma to nonpregnant uterus, e.g., polypectomy, IUD insertion, diagnostic curettage, myomectomy (2,4)
- Pelvic infection—controversial (2,4)

Genetics

To date, not significant contributor to pathophysiology

GENERAL PREVENTION

- Expectant or medical management rather than surgical management (curettage) of miscarriages, blighted ovum
- Minimize intrauterine operative interventions while fertile and desiring pregnancy.

PATHOPHYSIOLOGY

- Endometrial injury stimulates fibrosis.
- Stroma and glands are replaced with fibrous tissue with decreased vascularity.
- End effect of atrophic and inert endometrial lining (2)

ETIOLOGY

- Any damage to endometrium: Primarily trauma to pregnant uterus, especially postpartum curettage, e.g., in setting of incomplete abortion (2)
- Infection is a potential culprit, e.g., endometrial tuberculosis or pelvic inflammatory disease, but much rarer than traumatic causes; hence, controversial (2).

COMMONLY ASSOCIATED CONDITIONS

Recurrent miscarriage (2)

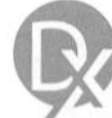

DIAGNOSIS

HISTORY

- Infertility (2)
- Menstrual abnormalities: Amenorrhea/hypomenorrhea (2)
- Hematometra, hematosalpinx (2)
- Recurrent miscarriage (2)
- Cyclical pelvic pain (2)

PHYSICAL EXAM

- Usually no abnormalities (1,2)
- Occasionally cervical obstruction may be present on blind transcervical uterine sounding (1,2).

DIAGNOSTIC TESTS & INTERPRETATION

Lab

Initial lab tests

- Labs do not play key role in diagnosis of uterine synechiae.
- More critical for work-up to evaluate for other causes of infertility, menstrual abnormalities, recurrent miscarriages.
- See particular topics for suggested lab workups of those complaints.

Follow-Up & Special Considerations

Other role for labs is in management of uterine synechiae, which is primarily surgical:

- Routine preoperative labs: CBC, electrolytes, coagulation panel

Imaging

Initial approach

- Hysteroscopy is "criterion standard" for diagnosis, as it allows direct visualization of adhesions for diagnosis, classification, and therapy (1,2) [B].
- If hysteroscopy unavailable, hysterosalpingogram and hysterosonography reasonable alternatives, especially as interim diagnostic sources of information to decide whether to refer if hysteroscopy not readily available locally (1)[B].
- Hysteroscopy compared to other diagnostic sources (1,2):
  - Hysterosalpingography: Sensitivity 75–81%, specificity 80%, PPV 50%, high false-positive rate (up to 38%)
  - Sonohysterography/saline infusion sonography: Sensitivity 75%, specificity 43%
  - Transvaginal ultrasound: Sensitivity 52%, specificity 11%
  - 3D ultrasound: Compared to 3D sonohystography (not to gold-standard hysteroscopy): Sensitivity 87%, specificity 45%
  - MRI: Not recommended since limited by cost, availability, and unknown sensitivity

Follow-Up & Special Considerations

- Assess patient's goals for fertility and/or pelvic pain control to counsel on benefits and risks of pursuing hysteroscopy for definitive diagnosis.
- Once diagnosis made, counsel on benefits and risks of expectant management vs. medical intervention

Diagnostic Procedures/Surgery

Hysteroscopy is the criterion standard for diagnosis:

- Allows direct visualization of adhesions for diagnosis and classification
- Convenient that diagnosis and therapy can be achieved with same procedure (1,2)[B]

Pathological Findings

Diagnosis confirmed by:

- Visualization of intrauterine adhesions
- Volume and quality of adhesions
- Areas of occlusion (e.g., fundus, ostia, portion of uterine cavity)
- Quality of endometrial lining

DIFFERENTIAL DIAGNOSIS

Differential diagnosis for amenorrhea, infertility, recurrent miscarriage, and cyclic pelvic pain all apply.

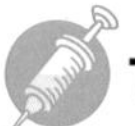

TREATMENT

MEDICATION

First Line

No role for medical treatments in absence of primary surgical intervention (1)

ADDITIONAL TREATMENT

General Measures

Counsel on option of expectant management (observation): Limited data without formal RCTs for expectant vs. hysteroscopic lysis (1)[C]:

- Spontaneous return of menses in 78% within 7 years
- Spontaneous pregnancy in 46%

Issues for Referral

Referral to gynecologist with expertise in hysteroscopy should be offered (1)[C].

SURGERY/OTHER PROCEDURES

Hysteroscopy with adhesiolysis = gold standard (1,2)[B]:

- No RCTs to compare adhesiolytic techniques under hysteroscopy; therefore, cannot recommend any as superior
- Hysteroscopy with myometrial scoring (1)[C]: For severe IUAs where hysteroscopic adhesiolysis cannot be safely performed
- Open laparotomy followed by hysterotomy and subsequent blunt dissection of adhesions with finger or curette (used rarely in severe cases) (1)[C]
- Alternative visualizing methods such as fluoroscopy, transabdominal ultrasound, laparoscopy have been described but with higher rates of uterine perforation and cost
- Postoperative follow-up:
  - Mild-to-moderate disease: Adhesion recurrence rate 1 in 3 women
  - Severe disease: Adhesion recurrence rate 2 of 3
  - Thus, need to reassess with repeat hysteroscopy or hysterosalpingogram, usually 2–3 menstrual cycles after adhesiolytic hysteroscopy (1)[B]
- No randomized control trials (RCTs) of any treatment vs. expectant management or any other treatment (1)
- Ancillary treatments following surgery (1):
  - Estrogen ± progestin (1,2)[C]
  - IUD (Lippes loop—no longer widely commercially available, pediatric Foley catheter, amnion graft, adhesion barrier films with hyaluronic acid) (1)[C]:
    - IUDs such as Mirena or copper IUD are NOT appropriate for posthysteroscopy IUD management. They are proinflammatory and surface area is too small for goal of providing physical barrier between uterine walls.
  - Hyaluronic acid barrier films/gels: Promising but cannot be recommended to use currently outside of research until further studied (1)[C]
  - Nonhormonal medications to increase vascular flow to endometrial flow such as aspirin, nitroglycerin, sildenafil—only use in research with rigorous protocols (1)[C]

IN-PATIENT CONSIDERATIONS

N/A: Typically managed as outpatient same-day surgery in absence of complications

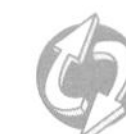

ONGOING CARE

FOLLOW-UP RECOMMENDATIONS

- Routine visits at 2 and 6 weeks after surgery
- Repeat hysteroscopy, or second-line hysterosalpingography, at 2–3 months after surgery to assess for adhesion recurrence

Patient Monitoring

Routine same-day surgery

DIET

- Routine same-day surgery care: Advance diet as tolerated to preoperative baseline.
- No restrictions

PATIENT EDUCATION

Review pathophysiology with patient to counsel on general guidelines for patient decision making on future elective invasive gynecologic procedures (e.g., incomplete abortion/anembryonic ovum—expectant or medical management vs. operative) in context of patient's future pregnancy goals.

PROGNOSIS

1–2 out of 3 women will need multiple hysteroscopic lysis of adhesions because of high recurrence rate.

COMPLICATIONS

For hysteroscopy:

- Uterine perforation
- Recurrence of adhesions
- Visceral organ injury

REFERENCES

1. AAGL practice report: Practice guidelines for management of intrauterine synechiae. *AAGL Advancing Minimally Invasive Gynecology Worldwide*. 2010;17(1):1–7.
2. Deans R, Abbott J. Review of intrauterine adhesions. *J Minim Invasive Gyencol*. 2010; 17(5):555–6.
3. Socolov, R. The endoscopic management of uterine synechiae. A clinical study of 78 cases. *Chirurgia*. 2010;105(4):515–8.
4. Dawood A, Al-Talib A, Tulandi T. Predisposing factors and treatment outcome of different stages of intrauterine adhesions. *J Obstet Gynaecol Can*. 2010;32(80):767–77.

ADDITIONAL READING

Thomson AJ, Abbott JA, Deans R, et al. The management of intrauterine synechiae. *Curr Opin Obstet Gynecol*. 2009;21:335–34.

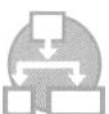

See Also (Topic, Algorithm, Electronic Media Element)

Algorithm: Amenorrhea, Secondary; Infertility; Pelvic Pain

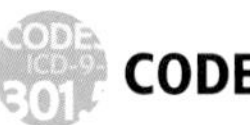

CODES

ICD9

621.5 Intrauterine synechiae

CLINICAL PEARLS

- Severe disease is usually due to curettage in postpartum/postabortion setting.
- Typical presentations: Secondary amenorrhea, infertility, recurrent miscarriages, cyclic pelvic pain
- Hysteroscopy is the standard for both diagnosis (adhesion visualization) and therapy (adhesion lysis).
- Posthysteroscopy oral hormone supplementation, perioperative antibiotics, and/or placement of intrauterine device such as a pediatric Foley catheter are adjuncts to hysteroscopy commonly practiced with goal to decrease risk of recurrence, but no high-quality evidence such as RCTs to recommend such practice (1)[C]

UVEITIS

Shailendra K. Saxena, MD, PhD
Mikayla Spangler, PharmD, BCPS

BASICS

DESCRIPTION

- A nonspecific term used to describe any intraocular inflammatory disorder.
- Symptoms vary, depending on depth of involvement and associated conditions.
- The uvea is the middle layer of the eye between the sclera and retina. The anterior part of the uvea includes the iris and ciliary body. The posterior part of the uvea is the choroid:
  - Anterior uveitis: Refers to ocular inflammation limited to the iris (iritis) alone or iris and ciliary body (iridocyclitis)
  - Intermediate uveitis: Refers to inflammation of the structures just posterior to the lens (pars planitis or peripheral uveitis)
  - Posterior uveitis: Refers to inflammation of the choroid (choroiditis), retina (retinitis), or vitreous near the optic nerve and macula
- System(s) affected: Nervous
- Synonym(s): Iritis; Iridocyclitis; Choroiditis; Retinochoroiditis; Chorioretinitis; Anterior uveitis; Posterior uveitis; Pars planitis; Panuveitis. Synonyms are anatomic descriptions of the focus of the uveal inflammation.

Geriatric Considerations

The inflammatory response to systemic disease may be suppressed.

Pediatric Considerations

- Infection should be the primary consideration.
- Allergies and psychologic factors (depression, stress) may serve as a trigger.
- Trauma is also a common cause in this population.

Pregnancy Considerations

May be of importance in the selection of medications

EPIDEMIOLOGY

- Predominant age: All ages
- Predominant sex: Male = Female, except for HLA-B27 anterior uveitis: Male > Female (2.5:1)

Incidence

Anterior uveitis most common (8.2 cases/100,000 annual incidence)

Prevalence

Iritis is 4 times more prevalent than posterior uveitis.

RISK FACTORS

- No specific risk factors.
- Higher incidence seen with specific associated conditions

Genetics

- No specific pattern for uveitis in general
- Iritis: Of patients, 50–70% are HLA-B27–positive.

ETIOLOGY

- Infectious: May result from viral, bacterial, parasitic, or fungal etiologies
- Suspected immune-mediated: Possible autoimmune or immune-complex–mediated mechanism postulated in association with systemic (especially rheumatologic) disorders
- Isolated eye disease
- Idiopathic (~25%)
- Autoimmune uveitis (AIU) patients should be referred to an ophthalmologist for local treatment.
- Masquerade syndromes: Diseases such as malignancies that may be mistaken for primary inflammation of the eye

COMMONLY ASSOCIATED CONDITIONS

- Viral infections: HIV, herpes simplex, herpes zoster, cytomegalovirus
- Bacterial infections: Tuberculosis (TB), leprosy, propionibacterium infection, syphilis, leptospirosis, brucellosis, Lyme disease, Whipple disease
- Parasitic infections: Toxoplasmosis, acanthamebiasis, toxocariasis, cysticercosis, onchocerciasis
- Fungal infections: Histoplasmosis, coccidioidomycosis, candidiasis, aspergillosis, sporotrichosis, blastomycosis, cryptococcosis
- Suspected immune-mediated: Ankylosing spondylitis, Behçet disease, Crohn disease, drug or hypersensitivity reaction, interstitial nephritis, juvenile rheumatoid arthritis, Kawasaki disease, multiple sclerosis, psoriatic arthritis, Reiter syndrome, relapsing polychondritis, sarcoidosis, Sjögren syndrome, systemic lupus erythematosus, ulcerative colitis, vasculitis, vitiligo, Vogt-Koyanagi (Harada) syndrome
- Isolated eye disease: Acute multifocal placoid pigmentary epitheliopathy, acute retinal necrosis, bird-shot choroidopathy, Fuchs heterochromatic cyclitis, glaucomatocyclitic crisis, lens-induced uveitis, multifocal choroiditis, pars planitis, serpiginous choroiditis, sympathetic ophthalmia, trauma
- Masquerade syndromes: Leukemia, lymphoma, retinitis pigmentosa, retinoblastoma

DIAGNOSIS

HISTORY

- Decreased visual acuity
- Pain, photophobia, blurring of vision:
  - Usually acute
- Anterior uveitis (~80% of patients with uveitis):
  - Generally acute in onset
  - Deep eye pain
  - Photophobia (consensual)
- Intermediate and posterior uveitis:
  - Unresolving floaters
  - Generally insidious in onset
  - More commonly bilateral

PHYSICAL EXAM

Slit-lamp exam and indirect ophthalmoscopy are necessary for precise diagnosis:

- Anterior uveitis (~80% of patients with uveitis):
  - Conjunctival vessel dilation
  - Perilimbal (circumcorneal) dilation of episcleral and scleral vessels (ciliary flush)
  - Small pupillary size of affected eye
  - Hypopyon or hyphema (WBCs or RBCs pooled in the anterior chamber)
  - Frequently unilateral (95% of HLA-B27–associated cases)
  - Bilateral involvement and systemic symptoms (fever, fatigue, abdominal pain) may be associated with interstitial nephritis.
  - Systemic disease is most likely to be associated with anterior uveitis (in 1 study, 53% of patients found to have systemic disease).
- Intermediate and posterior uveitis:
  - More commonly bilateral
  - Posterior inflammation will generally cause minimal pain or redness unless associated with an iritis.

DIAGNOSTIC TESTS & INTERPRETATION

Lab

No specific test for the diagnosis of uveitis. Tests for etiologic factors or associated conditions should be based on history and physical exam.

Initial lab tests

- CBC, BUN, creatinine (interstitial nephritis)
- HLA-B27 typing (ankylosing spondylitis, Reiter syndrome)
- Antinuclear antibody, ESR (systemic lupus erythematosus, Sjögren syndrome)
- Venereal disease research laboratory (VDRL) test, fluorescent titer antibody (syphilis)
- Purified protein derivative (PPD) tuberculin skin test (TB)
- Lyme serology (Lyme disease)
- Disorders that may alter lab results: Immunodeficiency

Imaging

- Chest x-ray (sarcoidosis, histoplasmosis, TB, lymphoma)
- Sacroiliac radiograph (ankylosing spondylitis)

Diagnostic Procedures/Surgery

Slit-lamp exam

Pathological Findings

- Keratic precipitates
- Inflammatory cells in anterior chamber or vitreous
- Synechiae (fibrous tissue scarring between iris and lens)
- Macular edema
- Perivasculitis of retinal vessels

DIFFERENTIAL DIAGNOSIS

- Conjunctivitis
- Episcleritis
- Scleritis
- Keratitis
- Acute angle-closure glaucoma

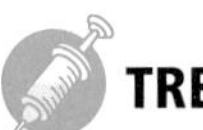

TREATMENT

MEDICATION

First Line

- The treatment depends upon the etiology, location, and severity of the inflammation.
- Homatropine hydrobromide (Isopto) 5% ophthalmic solution: 1–2 drops to the affected eye b.i.d., or as often as q3h if necessary; *plus*
- Prednisolone acetate 1% ophthalmic suspension: 2 drops to the affected eye q1h initially, tapering to once a day with improvement (1,2)[C]:
  - Contraindications:
    - Hypersensitivity to the medication or component of the preparation
    - Cycloplegia is contraindicated in patients known to have, or be predisposed to, glaucoma.
    - Topical corticosteroid therapy is contraindicated in uveitis secondary to infectious etiologies, unless used in conjunction with appropriate anti-infectious agents (3)[C].
  - Precautions:
    - Homatropine hydrobromide may produce adverse systemic antimuscarinic effects. Use extreme caution in infants and young children because of increased susceptibility to systemic effects.
    - Topical corticosteroids may increase intraocular pressure. Prolonged use may cause cataract formation and exacerbate existing herpetic keratitis, which may masquerade as iritis.
  - Significant possible interactions
  - Refer to manufacturer's profile for each drug.

Second Line

- Cycloplegia: Scopolamine hydrobromide 0.25% (IsoptoHyoscine) up to t.i.d. or cyclopentolate hydrochloride 1% (Cyclogyl) or Atropine 1% (2)[C]
- Anti-inflammatory: Prednisolone sodium phosphate 1% (Ocu-Pred Forte), dexamethasone sodium phosphate 0.1% (OU-Dex), dexamethasone suspension, rimexolone 1% (Vexol), and loteprednol etabonate 0.5% (Lotemax) (2)[C]
- Rimexolone 1% (Vexol) may be equally effective as prednisolone acetate 1% for short-term treatment of anterior uveitis (4)[B].
- Loteprednol etabonate (Lotemax) may not be as effective as prednisolone acetate 1%, but may be less likely to increase intraocular pressure in cases of acute anterior uveitis (4)[B].
- Systemic NSAIDs may provide some benefit (2)[C].

ADDITIONAL TREATMENT

General Measures

- Outpatient care with urgent ophthalmologic consultation
- Medical therapy best initiated following full ophthalmologic evaluation
- Treatment of underlying cause, if identified
- Anti-inflammatory therapy

Issues for Referral

Caution should be used when using empiric treatment; referral to an ophthalmologist is recommended in most cases.

ONGOING CARE

FOLLOW-UP RECOMMENDATIONS

Patient Monitoring

- Complete history and physical to evaluate for associated systemic disease
- Ophthalmologic follow-up as recommended by consultant

PATIENT EDUCATION

- Instruct on proper method for instilling eye drops.
- Wear dark glasses if photophobia is a problem.

PROGNOSIS

- Depends on the presence of causal diseases or associated conditions
- Uveitis resulting from infections (systemic or local) tends to resolve with eradication of the underlying infection.
- Uveitis associated with seronegative arthropathies tends to be acute (lasting <3 months) and frequently recurrent.

COMPLICATIONS

- Cycloplegia: Paralysis of the ciliary muscle of the eye, resulting in a loss of accommodation
- Loss of vision as a result of the following:
  - Keratic precipitate deposition on the corneal or lens surfaces
  - Increased intraocular pressure, acute angle-closure glaucoma
  - Formation of synechiae
  - Cataract formation
  - Vasculitis with vascular occlusion, retinal infarction
  - Macular edema
  - Optic nerve damage

REFERENCES

1. Audio PA. A review of evidence guiding the use of corticosteroids in the treatment of intraocular inflammation. *Oculi Immunol Inflame*. 2004;12(3): 169–92.
2. American Optometric Association. Optomeric clinical practice guideline: Care of the patient with anterior uveitis. Available at: http://www.aoa.org/documents/CPG-7.pdf.
3. McCluskey PJ, Towler HM, Lightman S. Management of chronic uveitis. *BMJ*. 2000; 320(7234):555–8.
4. Jabs DA. Treatment of ocular inflammation. *Ocular Immunol Inflame*. 2004;12(3):163–8.

ADDITIONAL READING

- Levy RA, de Andrade FA, Foeldvari I, et al. Cutting-edge issues in autoimmune uveitis. *Clin Rev Allergy Immunol*. 2011;41:214–23.
- Patel H, Goldstein D. Pediatric uveitis. *Pediatr Clin North Am*. 2003;50(1):125–36.
- Schiffman RM, Jacobsen G, Whitcup SM. Visual functioning and general health status in patients with uveitis. *Arch Ophthalmol*. 2001;119(6):841–9.
- Smith JR, Rosenbaum JT. Management of uveitis: A rheumatologic perspective. *Arthritis Rheum*. 2002;46(2):309–18.

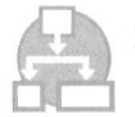

See Also (Topic, Algorithm, Electronic Media Element)

Conjunctivitis, Acute; Glaucoma, Primary Closed-Angle; Scleritis

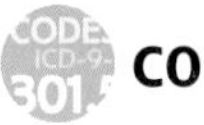

CODES

ICD9

- 363.20 Chorioretinitis, unspecified
- 364.3 Unspecified iridocyclitis

CLINICAL PEARLS

Severe or unresponsive uveitis may require therapy, including periocular injection of corticosteroids, systemic corticosteroids, cytotoxic agents, immunosuppressive agents, immunomodulatory agents, or tumor necrosis factor inhibitors.

VAGINAL ADENOSIS

Michael P. Hopkins, MD, MEd
Jonna M. Quinn, DO

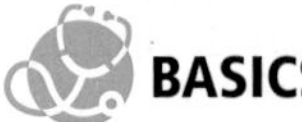

BASICS

DESCRIPTION

- The normal vagina is lined by squamous epithelium. Adenosis is characterized by the presence of columnar epithelium or glandular tissue in the wall of the vagina.
- At about the 15th week of embryologic development, the Müllerian system, which forms the upper 2/3 of the vagina, fuses with the invaginating cloaca or urogenital sinus to form the lower 1/3 of the vagina. Squamous metaplasia from the cloacal region then produces a squamous epithelium through the vagina.
- Adenosis occurs when this squamous epithelium fails to epithelialize the vagina completely.
- 3 main types of adenosis epithelium described:
  - Endocervical
  - Endometrial
  - Tubal
- System(s) affected: Reproductive

Geriatric Considerations

- Adenosis is a disorder of the young female. By menopause, the vagina and cervix should be completely epithelialized.
- The presence of glandular epithelium in the postmenopausal patient is an indication for excision and close evaluation for the possibility of a well-differentiated adenocarcinoma.

Pregnancy Considerations

Pregnancy produces a wide eversion of the transformation zone of the cervix. This occasionally will become so widely everted that it will extend onto the vaginal fornices, leading to the impression of adenosis. This will resolve after the pregnancy is completed.

EPIDEMIOLOGY

Incidence

- While the incidence of vaginal adenosis is unknown, the incidence of cloacal malformations is 1/20,000 to 1/25,000 live births.
- Predominant age:
  - Teenage years: Epithelialization occurs from puberty to ~20 years of age.
  - By age 30 years, it is extremely rare for adenosis to be present.

Prevalence

In the US: Adenosis is relatively common, affecting 10–20% of young females studied. As maturation progresses with puberty, epithelialization occurs (1)[C].

RISK FACTORS

Adenosis of the vagina/cervix in female offsprings is significantly higher in those exposed to diethylstilbestrol (DES) before birth (2).

GENERAL PREVENTION

None: Last DES exposure in the 1970s

PATHOPHYSIOLOGY

- In the vast majority of young females, the etiology is incomplete squamous metaplasia or epithelialization. This occurs as a natural phenomenon and resolves with age.
- Described as congenital or acquired (3):
  - Congenital: Proliferation of the remnant Müllerian epithelium in the vagina due to exposure to DES in utero
  - Acquired: Trauma and inflammation causing spontaneous de novo changes or changes in an acquired lesion in the vaginal epithelium:
    - Trauma: Carbon dioxide laser, 5-fluorouracil, vaginal packs, chronic pessary use
    - Proliferation of the glandular cells in the remnant Müllerian epithelium of the vagina due to sex hormones
    - Idiopathic spontaneous change in epithelium, no cause has been identified

ETIOLOGY

In DES-exposed females, the incidence of adenosis is higher; the etiology presumably is from the effect of the DES on the developing embryologic system.

COMMONLY ASSOCIATED CONDITIONS

DES exposure:

- Adenosis from DES exposure should lead to an evaluation of other DES-related abnormalities.
- Müllerian tract anomalies associated with DES exposure include cervical hood, cervical ridge, shortened cervix, incompetent cervix, and T-shaped uterine cavity.
- Patients with known DES exposure should have the reproductive tract evaluated prior to conception.
- The vast majority of patients with adenosis have not been DES exposed and do not require evaluation of the reproductive system.
- DES was last used to prevent spontaneous abortion in the US in 1971; therefore, it is decreasing in clinical significance.

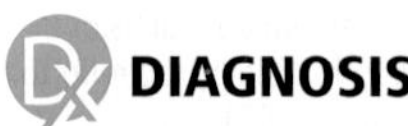

DIAGNOSIS

HISTORY

- Maternal DES exposure
- Complaints of:
  - Profuse mucoid vaginal discharge from the glandular epithelium
  - Pruritus
  - Pain/soreness of the vaginal introitus
  - Postcoital bleeding
  - Dyspareunia

PHYSICAL EXAM

On pelvic exam, adenosis appearance is varied: Patchy or diffuse red stippling, granularity or nodularity, single or multiple cysts, erosions, ulcers, or warty protuberances that may even extend to vulva

DIAGNOSTIC TESTS & INTERPRETATION

Lab

Initial lab tests

4-quadrant Pap smear should be used liberally to isolate quadrants of the vagina that may contain abnormalities.

Follow-Up & Special Considerations

Pap smear can be followed by colposcopy and biopsy.

Imaging

Initial approach

None unless diagnosed with underlying malignancy

Diagnostic Procedures/Surgery

Colposcopy should be used to outline areas of adenosis to ensure that no malignancy is present.

Pathological Findings

- Biopsy will show benign glandular epithelium.
- Biopsies in the areas of ongoing squamous metaplasia will be typical for this process (3)[C].

DIFFERENTIAL DIAGNOSIS

- Erosive lichen planus
- Fixed drug eruption
- Erythema multiforme
- Bullous skin disease
- Adenocarcinoma:
  - A thorough evaluation for adenocarcinoma of the vagina arising in adenosis should be done.
  - A biopsy may be necessary to ensure that the process represents only benign adenosis.

TREATMENT

ADDITIONAL TREATMENT

General Measures

- Unless malignancy is present, conservative treatment is indicated.
- In the vast majority of young females with this condition, it will resolve with expectant management (4)[C].
- Treatment is warranted in women with severe subjective symptoms that impair the quality of life (5).

Issues for Referral

Malignancy found on biopsy warrants referral to gynecologic oncology specialist.

SURGERY/OTHER PROCEDURES

- Aggressive therapy such as laser or surgical excision is necessary if premalignant or malignant changes arise (3)[C].
- Symptomatic treatment with carbon dioxide laser coagulation, unipolar coagulation, or, lastly, vaginal resection (4)

IN-PATIENT CONSIDERATIONS

Admission Criteria

Outpatient management

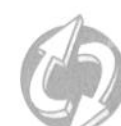

ONGOING CARE

FOLLOW-UP RECOMMENDATIONS

Patient Monitoring

If the initial colposcopy is normal, a yearly 4-quadrant Pap smear of the vagina and Pap smear of the cervix are all that is necessary.

DIET

No special diet

PATIENT EDUCATION

- No limitations
- It is not necessary to avoid intercourse or placing objects in the vagina.
- The patient should be educated to keep annual pelvic and Pap smear appointments. In the vast majority of situations, this is benign, and expectant management is all that is necessary.
- www.acog.org

PROGNOSIS

- It is expected that the vast majority of patients will have squamous metaplasia and epithelialization with complete resolution of the adenosis.
- The rare patient, 1/1,000–1/10,000, may develop adenocarcinoma in the adenosis and will require definitive therapy as for vaginal cancer.

COMPLICATIONS

- Infertility with DES association
- Adverse pregnancy outcome with DES association
- Adenocarcinoma of vagina

REFERENCES

1. Sandberg EC. The incidence and distribution of occult vaginal adenosis. *Am J Obstet Gynecol*. 1968;101:322–34.
2. Bamigboye AA, Morris J. Oestrogen supplementation, mainly diethylstilbestrol, for preventing miscarriages and other adverse pregnancy outcomes. *Cochrane Database Syst Rev*. 2003:CD004271.
3. Chattopadhyay I, Cruickshan DJ, Packer M. Non diethylstilbestrol induced vaginal adenosis–A case series and review of literature. *Eur J Gynaecol Oncol*. 2001;22(4):260–2.
4. Kranl C, Zelger B, Kofler H, et al. Vulvar and vaginal adenosis. *Br J Dermatol*. 1998;139:128–31.
5. Cebesoy FB, Kutlar I, Aydin A. Vaginal adenosis successfully treated with simple unipolar cauterization. *J Natl Med Assoc*. 2007;99(2): 166–7.

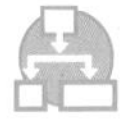

See Also (Topic, Algorithm, Electronic Media Element)

Vaginal Malignancy; DES Exposure

CODES

ICD9

623.8 Other specified noninflammatory disorders of vagina

CLINICAL PEARLS

- Adenosis is characterized by the presence of columnar epithelium or glandular tissue in the wall of the vagina.
- Adenosis is more common among women exposed to DES in utero.
- Adenosis is rarely associated with an underlying vaginal malignancy.

V

VAGINAL BLEEDING DURING PREGNANCY

Virginia VanDuyne, MD
Tracy Kedian, MD

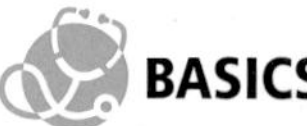

BASICS

DESCRIPTION

- Vaginal bleeding during pregnancy has many causes and ranges in severity from benign with normal pregnancy outcome to life threatening for both infant and mother.
- Bleeding can vary from scant to excessive, from brown to bright red, and can be painless or painful.
- Etiology can be from the vagina, cervix, and uterus; fetus; placenta; or mother. The differential diagnosis is guided by the gestational age of the fetus.

EPIDEMIOLOGY

Prevalence

- In early pregnancy: 7–25% of patients (1)
- In late pregnancy, 0.3–2% of patients (2,3,4)

RISK FACTORS

See specific etiologies below

GENERAL PREVENTION

- Address modifiable risk factors, such as domestic violence and tobacco and drug use.
- If placenta or vasa previa, nothing per vagina

ETIOLOGY

- Many times the cause is unknown.
- Anytime in pregnancy:
  - Cervicitis (infectious or noninfectious)
  - Vaginal or cervical trauma (including postcoital)
  - Cervical lesion or neoplasia
  - Hyperemia of cervix (increased blood flow from pregnancy)
- Early pregnancy:
  - For up to 50% of early pregnancy bleeding, no cause is ever found (5).
  - Ectopic pregnancy: Leading cause of first-trimester maternal death in the US (6). Risk factors: Previous ectopic, trauma to fallopian tubes (tubal surgery, infection, congenital anomaly, tumor), in utero DES exposure, current use of IUD, history of infertility, tobacco use (7).
  - Spontaneous abortion: Risk factors: AMA, alcohol use, tobacco use, anesthetic gas, heavy caffeine use, cocaine use, chronic maternal diseases (poorly controlled DM, celiac disease, autoimmune diseases such as antiphospholipid syndrome), short interconceptional time (3–6 months), IUD in place, maternal infection (e.g., HSV, gonorrhea, chlamydia, toxoplasmosis, listeriosis, HIV, syphilis, malaria), medications (e.g., retinoids, methotrexate, NSAIDs), multiple previous therapeutic abortions, previous spontaneous abortion, toxins (arsenic, lead, polyurethane), uterine abnormalities (congenital, adhesions, fibroids) (8).
  - Implantation bleeding: Benign, about 6 days after fertilization (6)
  - Uterine fibroids
  - Subchorionic bleed: Occurs in late first trimester (6)
  - Low-lying placenta
  - Gestational trophoblastic disease: Hydatidiform mole (most common), choriocarcinoma, or placental-site trophoblastic tumors (6)
- Late pregnancy:
  - Bloody show of labor
  - Placenta previa: Painless bleeding. Occurs in 0.4% deliveries in the US. Risk factors: Previous history of placenta previa, previous uterine surgery (cesarean section, D&C), chronic hypertension, multiparity, multiple gestation, tobacco use, AMA (9).
  - Placental abruption: Painful bleeding. Occurs in 1–2% deliveries in the US. Risk factors: Previous placental abruption, first-trimester bleeding, hypertension, preeclampsia, multiple gestation, tobacco, cocaine or methamphetamine use, unexplained elevated maternal alpha-fetal protein, poly- or oligohydramnios, AMA, trauma to abdomen, sudden uterine decompression, premature rupture of membranes, thrombophilia, short umbilical cord, chorioamnionitis, nutritional deficiency, male fetus (3,9).
  - Vasa previa: Minimal bleeding with fetal distress. Rare (1:2,500 deliveries). Risk factors: In vitro fertilization, multiple gestation, placental abnormalities (low-lying position, bilobate, succenturiate lobe, velamentous insertion of umbilical cord) (5,10).
  - Placenta accreta, increta, percreta: Risk factors: Uterine scar (e.g., from cesarean section, endometrial ablation or D&C), current placenta previa, AMA, tobacco use, multiparity, uterine anomalies, uterine fibroids, hypertension (2).
  - Uterine rupture: Vaginal bleeding, abnormal fetal heart rate, and disordered or hypertonic uterine contractions with or without pain. Risk factors: Previous cesarean section (most common), trauma, use of oxytocin or prostaglandins, multiparity, external cephalic version, placental abruption, shoulder dystocia, placenta percreta, Müllerian duct anomalies, history of pelvic radiation (5,10,11).

DIAGNOSIS

HISTORY

- Anytime in pregnancy: Quality of pregnancy dating, context (e.g., following bowel movement, during voiding, after intercourse, drug use or trauma including domestic violence), amount of bleeding, obstetrical history
- Early pregnancy: Severe nausea/vomiting (can be associated with molar pregnancy), amount of bleeding, pelvic pain or suprapubic cramping (e.g., spontaneous abortion, ectopic), complications in previous pregnancies (e.g., spontaneous abortion, abruption, first-trimester vaginal bleeding)
- Late pregnancy: Contractions (labor), abdominal pain especially between contractions (abruption), presence or absence of fetal movement, rupture of membranes
- See "Etiology" for additional pertinent history.

PHYSICAL EXAM

- Vital signs: Signs of hemodynamic instability are: First, tachycardia and tachypnea, then hypotension and thready pulse (10,11).
- Abdominal exam for uterine tenderness, fundal height
- Speculum exam to visualize cervix, identify source of bleeding.
- Sterile vaginal exam to assess for cervical dilation. Required to assess for labor, but should not perform if vaginal bleeding late pregnancy until placenta is located with ultrasound.
- Fetal heart tones in early pregnancy. If gestational age is >26 weeks, do external fetal monitoring.

DIAGNOSTIC TESTS & INTERPRETATION

Lab

Initial lab tests

- CBC
- Blood type and screen; if significant hemorrhage, type and cross-match
- Quantitative β-human chorionic gonadotropin (β-hCG):
  - Used in early pregnancy when ultrasound is not able to diagnose cause; transvaginal ultrasound should be able to see an intrauterine pregnancy (IUP) when the qualitative β-hCG > 2,000.
  - Prior to 12 weeks, levels can be followed serially every 2 days with following trends:
    - Doubles in 48 hours in normal pregnancy
    - Falls in spontaneous abortion
    - Extremely high in molar pregnancy
    - Rises gradually (<50% in 48 hours) or plateaus in ectopic pregnancy
- Other lab tests based on clinical scenario:
  - Fetal fibronectin, wet mount, gonorrhea/chlamydia, Pap smear
  - Progesterone level: For determination of viability in spontaneous abortion (<5 indicates not viable, >25 indicates viability, 5–25 is equivocal) (8)
  - Bleeding time, fibrinogen, and fibrin split products: If suspect coagulopathy or abruption
  - Kleihauer-Betke: Low sensitivity and specificity for abruption; helpful for dosing RhoGAM (3)
  - Apt test: For vasa previa; alkaline denaturation test on blood sample from vaginal vault to determine presence of fetal blood (9)

Imaging

Initial approach

Ultrasound is the preferred imaging modality:

- Early pregnancy:
  - Gestational sac seen at 5–6 weeks. Fetal heartbeat observed by 8–9 weeks.
  - Diagnostic of ectopic with nearly 100% sensitivity when β-hCG level 1,500–2,000 mIU/mL. If no IUP is present and ultrasound does not confirm ectopic pregnancy, serial quantitative β-hCG values should be followed (12).
- Late pregnancy:
  - Confirm fetal presentation and placental position prior to cervical exam.
  - Proceed to rule out:
    - Placenta previa with ultrasound
    - Labor with serial cervical exams
    - Abruption with external fetal monitoring
  - Ultrasound is *not* used to diagnose or exclude placental abruption.

DIFFERENTIAL DIAGNOSIS

- Hematuria from UTI, kidney stones
- Rectal bleeding

TREATMENT

MEDICATION

First Line

- Treat underlying cause of bleeding, if identified.
- If mother is Rh negative: Give Rho(d) immunoglobulin (RhoGAM) to prevent autoimmunization. In late pregnancy, dose according to the amount of estimated fetomaternal hemorrhage.
- Consider tocolytics in preterm labor (typically contraindicated in placental abruption) (9).
- Consider betamethasone for fetal lung maturity if fewer than 34 completed weeks gestation.

SURGERY/OTHER PROCEDURES

- Cesarean section if indicated for recurrent or uncontrolled bleeding with placenta or vasa previa
- If ectopic is diagnosed, immediate surgical treatment may be needed. Some early ectopic pregnancies can be treated medically if certain criteria are met (7,12).
- Surgical uterine evacuation necessary for molar pregnancy due to malignant potential (6).
- Incomplete or inevitable spontaneous abortion: Management is patient-centered. In the absence of infection, patient may elect expectant, medical or surgical management. If expectant management, typically wait 2 weeks for patient to complete abortion; most complete by 9 days. If at 2 weeks abortion is not completed or medical management has failed, surgical intervention (D&C or aspiration) generally indicated. Send tissue to pathology to confirm (8,13).

IN-PATIENT CONSIDERATIONS

Admission Criteria

- Heavy bleeding with abdominal pain in early pregnancy
- In late pregnancy, if significant bleeding and presence of maternal or fetal compromise
- In late pregnancy with trauma, if more than 2 contractions in 10 minutes

IV Fluids

If heavy bleeding, maintain IV hydration and IV access:

- Give 3mL IV isotonic solution per 1 mL blood lost (10).

Discharge Criteria

- In case of trauma in late pregnancy, may discharge home after normal fetal heart tracing for at least 4 hours with fewer than 2 contractions in 10 minutes (3).
- In late pregnancy, may discharge when bleeding has stopped; labor, previa, and abruption have been ruled out; and fetal heart tracing is normal.

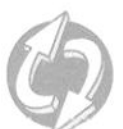

ONGOING CARE

PATIENT EDUCATION

- Patient should be instructed to report any increase in the amount or frequency of bleeding and to seek immediate care if experiencing abdominal pain or sudden increased bleeding. She should save any tissue passed vaginally for examination (6).
- Nothing per vagina
- American Academy of Family Physicians (AAFP): www.familydoctor.org
- American College of Obstetricians & Gynecologists (ACOG): www.acog.org

PROGNOSIS

- Prognosis depends on the etiology of vaginal bleeding, the severity of bleeding, and the rapidity of diagnosis.
- Maternal mortality is 31.9 deaths/100,000 ectopic pregnancies (14).
- Half of patients with early pregnancy bleeding miscarry. If fetal heart tones are present in first-trimester bleed, there is <10% chance of pregnancy loss (1,8).
- Heavy bleeding in early pregnancy, particularly when accompanied by pain, is associated with higher risk of spontaneous abortion. Spotting and light episodes are not, especially if lasting only 1–2 days (1).
- Subchorionic hemorrhage has about 2–3-fold increased risk of spontaneous abortion. Smaller hemorrhage and presence of viable fetal heart rate confer lower risk of loss. Most resolve spontaneously (6).
- Women with early pregnancy bleeding have an increased risk of preterm delivery, premature rupture of membranes, manual removal of placenta, placental abruption, elective cesarean delivery, and term labor induction later in the same pregnancy. Also they have an increased risk of adverse pregnancy outcomes, including hyperbilirubinemia, congenital anomalies, NICU admission, and reduced neonatal birth weight (4,15).
- Women with early pregnancy bleeding also have an increased risk of recurrence of early pregnancy bleeding and other complications in the subsequent pregnancies (16,17).
- Bed rest has not been shown to affect the outcome of bleeding in early pregnancy, but may be indicated in bleeding in late pregnancy with placenta or vasa previa or with maternal hypertension.

COMPLICATIONS

- Anemia
- Infection
- Preterm delivery with associated complications
- Choriocarcinoma or invasive mole in the case of hydatidiform mole
- Coagulopathy: 10% of cases of placental abruption will develop coagulopathy (Mercier).
- Maternal renal failure, shock
- Fetal hypoxia
- Fetal or maternal death

REFERENCES

1. Hasan R, Baird DD, Herring AH, et al. Association between first-trimester vaginal bleeding and miscarriage. *Obstet Gynecol*. 2009;114:860–7.
2. Publications Committee, Society for Maternal-Fetal Medicine, Belfort MA, et al. Placenta accreta. *Am J Obstet Gynecol*. 2010; 203:430–9.
3. Oyelese Y, Ananth CV. Placental abruption. *Obstet Gynecol*. 2006;108:1005–16.
4. Magann EF, Cummings JE, Niederhauser A, et al. Antepartum bleeding of unknown origin in the second half of pregnancy: A review. *Obstet Gynecol Surv*. 2005;60:741–5.
5. Mercier FJ, Van de Velde M. Major obstetric hemorrhage. *Anesthesiol Clin*. 2008;26:53–66, vi.
6. Snell BJ. Assessment and management of bleeding in the first trimester of pregnancy. *J Midwifery Womens Health*. 2009;54:483–91.
7. Mukul LV, Teal SB. Current management of ectopic pregnancy. *Obstet Gynecol Clin North Am*. 2007;34:403–19, x.
8. Griebel CP, Halvorsen J, Golemon TB, et al. Management of spontaneous abortion. *Am Fam Physician*. 2005;72:1243–50.
9. Sakornbut E, Leeman L, Fontaine P. Late pregnancy bleeding. *Am Fam Physician*. 2007;75: 1199–206.
10. Zeltzer JS. Vaginal bleeding in late pregnancy. In: Bope ET, Kellerman RD, eds. *Conn's Current Therapy*. Philadelphia: Elsevier; 2011.
11. Walfish M, Neuman A, Wlody D, et al. Maternal haemorrhage. *Br J Anaesth*. 2009;103(Suppl 1): i47–56.
12. Deutchman M, Tubay AT, Turok D, et al. First trimester bleeding. *Am Fam Physician*. 2009;79: 985–94.
13. Trinder J, Brocklehurst P, Porter R, et al. Management of miscarriage: Expectant, medical, or surgical? Results of randomised controlled trial (miscarriage treatment (MIST) trial). *BMJ*. 2006;332:1235–40.
14. Grimes DA. Estimation of pregnancy-related mortality risk by pregnancy outcome, United States, 1991 to 1999. *Am J Obstet Gynecol*. 2006;194:92–4.
15. Dadkhah F, Kashanian M, Eliasi G. A comparison between the pregnancy outcome in women both with or without threatened abortion. Early Hum. *Dev*. 2010;86:193–6.
16. Lykke JA, Dideriksen KL, Lidegaard O, et al. First-trimester vaginal bleeding and complications later in pregnancy. *Obstet Gynecol*. 2010;115:935–44.
17. Wijesiriwardana A, Bhattacharya S, Shetty A, et al. Obstetric outcome in women with threatened miscarriage in the first trimester. *Obstet Gynecol*. 2006;107:557–62.

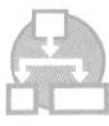

See Also (Topic, Algorithm, Electronic Media Element)

Abnormal Pap and Cervical Dysplasia; Abortion, Spontaneous (Miscarriage); Abruptio Placentae; Cervical Malignancy; Cervical Polyps; Cervicitis, Ectropion, and True Erosion; Chlamydial Sexually Transmitted Diseases; Ectopic Pregnancy; Placenta Previa; Preterm Labor; Trichomoniasis; Vaginal Malignancy

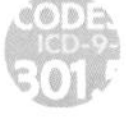

CODES

ICD9

- 640.00 Threatened abortion, unspecified as to episode of care or not applicable
- 640.93 Unspecified hemorrhage in early pregnancy, antepartum
- 641.93 Unspecified antepartum hemorrhage

CLINICAL PEARLS

- Obtain blood type and screen on all women presenting with vaginal bleeding in pregnancy and administer Rho(d) immunoglobulin (RhoGAM) to all Rh-negative patients.
- For up to 50% of early pregnancy bleeding, no cause is ever found.
- Always consider ectopic pregnancy in first-trimester bleeding.
- Do not perform digital exam in late pregnancy bleeding until placenta has been located on ultrasound.

VAGINAL MALIGNANCY

Michael P. Hopkins, MD, MEd
Eric L. Jenison, MD
Michael S. Guy, MD

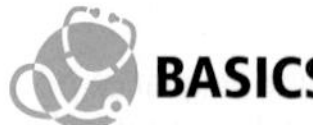

BASICS

DESCRIPTION

- Vaginal cancer is rare and comprises ~2–3% of gynecologic cancers.
- Vaginal intraepithelial neoplasia (carcinoma in situ): A premalignant phase with full-thickness neoplastic changes in the superficial epithelium; however, no invasion occurs through the basement membrane.
- Invasive malignancies: Vaginal malignancies include squamous cell carcinoma (85–90%), adenocarcinoma (5–10%), sarcoma (2–3%), and melanoma (2–3%). Clear cell carcinoma is a subtype of adenocarcinoma.
- To be classified as a vaginal malignancy, only the vagina can be involved. If the cervix or vulva is involved, then the tumor is classified as a primary cancer arising from the cervix or the vulva.
- Most vaginal malignancies are metastatic (e.g., cervix, vulva, endometrium, breast, ovary).
- System(s) affected: Reproductive
- Synonym(s): Bowen disease; Vaginal intraepithelial neoplasia (VAIN)

Geriatric Considerations

Older patients, many with a long history of smoking, are at a higher risk for malignancies requiring surgical treatments.

Pediatric Considerations

Childhood sarcomas can be treated in a conservative fashion with multimodality therapy. This avoids the loss of the young child's bladder and/or rectum.

Pregnancy Considerations

This malignancy is not associated with pregnancy.

EPIDEMIOLOGY

Incidence

- 2,300 new cases in 2010 in the US
- Predominant age:
  - Carcinoma in situ: Mid-40s–60s
  - Invasive squamous cell malignancy: Mid-60s–70s
  - Adenocarcinoma: Any age; 50s is mean age. The most common vaginal malignancy occurs in patients under 20 years of age.
  - Clear cell adenocarcinoma occurs most often in females <30 years old with a history of exposure to diethylstilbestrol (DES) in utero.
  - Mixed Müllerian sarcomas and leiomyosarcomas in the adult population: Mean age 60 years
  - Sarcoma botryoides and embryonal sarcomas are pediatric conditions: Mean age 3 years

Prevalence

In the US, it is one of the rarest of all gynecologic malignancies (2–3%).

RISK FACTORS

- Similar risk factors as cervical cancer
- Age
- African American
- Smoking
- Multiple sex partners, early age of first sexual intercourse
- History of squamous cell cancer of the cervix or vulva
- Human papillomavirus (HPV) infection (70% of invasive vaginal malignancies)
- Vaginal adenosis
- Vaginal irritation
- DES exposure in utero

Genetics

No known genetic pattern

ETIOLOGY

- Women with a history of cervical malignancy have a higher probability of developing squamous cell malignancy in the vagina after hysterectomy.
- HPV has been associated with vulvovaginal, cervical, adenocarcinoma, and squamous cell carcinoma.
- Smokers have a higher incidence.
- Clear cell adenocarcinoma of the vagina in young women has been associated with DES exposure. The incidence, however, is exceedingly rare, estimated at 1/1,000–1/10,000 DES-exposed females.
- Metastatic lesions can involve the vagina from the other gynecologic organs.
- Although rare, renal cell carcinoma, lung adenocarcinoma, GI cancer, pancreatic adenocarcinoma, ovarian germ cell cancer, trophoblastic neoplasm, and breast cancer can all metastasize to the vagina.

COMMONLY ASSOCIATED CONDITIONS

Due to the field effect, patients with vaginal cancer are more likely to develop malignancy in the cervix or vulva and should be followed closely.

DIAGNOSIS

HISTORY

- Abnormal bleeding is the most common symptom.
- Postcoital bleeding can result from direct trauma to the tumor.
- Vaginal discharge
- Dyspareunia
- Urinary symptoms, including hematuria and increased frequency
- Constipation
- Pain along with symptoms and signs of hydroureter are late findings when the tumor has spread into the paravaginal tissues and extends to the pelvic sidewall.

Pediatric Considerations

In children, sarcomas can present either as a mass protruding from the vagina or as abnormal genital bleeding.

PHYSICAL EXAM

Pelvic examination:

- The vagina, uterus, adnexae (fallopian tubes and ovaries), bladder, and rectum should be evaluated for unusual changes.
- Vaginal malignancies are found most commonly on the posterior wall in the upper 1/3 of the vagina.

DIAGNOSTIC TESTS & INTERPRETATION

Lab

Initial lab tests

- PAP smear may incidentally detect asymptomatic lesions.
- Biopsy suspicious lesions.

Imaging

Initial approach

- CXR: To evaluate for metastatic disease
- IV pyelogram (IVP) to evaluate for ureteral obstruction
- CT scan and MRI to evaluate the liver and retroperitoneum, especially the lymph nodes in the pelvic and periaortic area
- Barium enema to rule out rectal invasion
- Positron-emission tomographic (PET) scan detects primary and secondary metastatic lesions more often than CT scan.

ALERT

PET scan correlation with CT scan lesions strongly suggests malignancy.

Follow-Up & Special Considerations

Lymphangiography has been useful for evaluation of the lymph node status (1)[B].

Diagnostic Procedures/Surgery

- Colposcopy with directed biopsies for small lesions
- Wide excision under anesthesia of superficial disease may be necessary to ensure that invasive cancer is not present.
- Cystoscopy to rule out bladder invasion
- Sigmoidoscopy to rule out rectal invasion

Pathological Findings

Tumors are staged clinically:

- Stage 0: Carcinoma in situ/vaginal intraepithelial neoplasia (VAIN)
- Stage I: Infiltrative tumor not involving the paravaginal tissues (26%)
- Stage II: Carcinoma involves the paravaginal tissues but not the pelvic wall (37%)
- Stage III: Carcinoma extended to the sidewall (24%)
- Stage IVA: Tumor involving the bladder or the rectum, or true pelvis (13% stage IVA and IVB)
- Stage IVB: Spread to distant organs

DIFFERENTIAL DIAGNOSIS

- VAIN involves premalignant changes that do not infiltrate beyond the basement membrane.
- Adequate biopsies ensure that invasive lesions are not overlooked. Invasive lesions penetrate the basement membrane and cannot be treated conservatively.
- Other malignancies such as endometrial, cervix, bladder, or colon cancer can invade directly into the vagina or metastasize to the vagina.
- In the child-bearing years, trophoblastic disease should be considered:
  - The vagina is a common site of metastases.
  - Biopsy usually will provide a clue to the primary site.

TREATMENT

MEDICATION

- With 1 exception, there are no chemotherapeutic agents that have shown a survival advantage. The exception is childhood sarcomas, which have been treated with combinations of:
  - Vincristine
  - Dactinomycin (actinomycin-D)
  - Cyclophosphamide (Cytoxan)
  - Cisplatin
  - Etoposide (VP-16)
- Patients with advanced squamous cell carcinoma or adenocarcinoma receive concurrent irradiation and cisplatin-based chemotherapy (2)[B].
- Neoadjuvant chemotherapy followed by radical surgery may benefit select patients (3)[C].
- Intraepithelial neoplasia of the vagina (VAIN) can be treated with topical chemotherapy (5-fluorouracil cream) (4)[C].
- Treating VAIN with imiquimod has led to complete response in certain patients (5)[C].
- Contraindications:
  - The diagnosis must be established with certainty prior to treatment.
  - If there is any doubt that a process beyond in situ disease exists, vaginectomy must be performed. These patients are often elderly, and aggressive therapy is limited by the patient's performance status and ability to tolerate radical surgery, chemotherapy, or radiation.

ADDITIONAL TREATMENT

General Measures

- Outpatient or inpatient care, depending on specific treatments
- Carcinoma in situ can be treated by a variety of methods:
  - Laser vaporization under microscopic guidance
  - Fluorouracil (Efudex) intravaginal cream
  - Partial vaginectomy
- In most tumor types, metastatic disease from the vagina to other sites is only minimally responsive to chemotherapy.

Issues for Referral

Patients should be treated by a gynecologic oncologist and/or a radiation oncologist.

Additional Therapies

- Treatment with radiotherapy depends on the stage of disease. This treatment option should be discussed with physicians experienced with this malignancy (4)[C].
- It is common to use radiotherapy and chemotherapy (chemoradiation) for better cancer control.
- Early-stage primary squamous cell carcinoma treated with radiation alone has shown good results (6)[A].
- Stage III vaginal cancer may benefit from combined radiation and hyperthermia (7)[C].

SURGERY/OTHER PROCEDURES

- Whenever there is a doubt as to the presence or absence of invasive disease, vaginectomy must be performed.
- Invasive lesions usually are treated by radiation therapy, but stage I lesions can be treated with radical hysterectomy or radical vaginectomy with pelvic lymph node dissection (8)[A].
- If the lesion involves the lower vagina, inguinal node dissection also must be done because cancer involving the lower vagina can metastasize to the groin region.
- Premenopausal women who desire to retain ovarian function are better candidates for radical surgery for early-stage disease with vaginal reconstruction possible afterward.
- Patients who have not completed their family occasionally can be treated with limited resection and localized radiation to the area.
- Sarcomas are treated by radiation therapy followed by pelvic exenteration if persistent disease is present.
- Childhood sarcomas:
  - Are treated with chemotherapy followed by local resection
  - Are responsive to multiagent combination chemotherapies

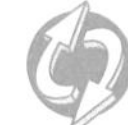

ONGOING CARE

FOLLOW-UP RECOMMENDATIONS

- Patients are usually ambulatory and able to resume full activity by 6 weeks after surgery.
- Most patients are fully active while receiving chemotherapy and radiation therapy.

Patient Monitoring

- Pelvic examination and Pap smear every 3 months for 2 years, then every 6 months for the next 3 years, and then yearly thereafter
- Annual CXR

PATIENT EDUCATION

- Printed patient information available from American College of Obstetricians and Gynecologists, 409 12th St., SW, Washington, DC 20024–2188; (800) 762–ACOG; www.acog.org
- American Cancer Society: www.cancer.org
- Medline Plus: www.nlm.nih.gov/medlineplus/vaginalcancer.html

PROGNOSIS

Stage and 5-year survival:

- I: 77.6%
- II: 52.2%
- III: 42.5%
- IVA: 20.5%
- IVB:12.9%

COMPLICATIONS

- Those typically associated with major abdominal surgery or radiation therapy
- Common complications of treatment include rectovaginal or vesicovaginal fistulas, rectal/vaginal strictures, radiation cystitis, and/or proctitis.

REFERENCES

1. Frumovitz M, Gayed IW, Jhingran A, et al. Lymphatic mapping and sentinel lymph node detection in women with vaginal cancer. *Gynecol Oncol*. 2008;108(3):478–81.
2. Dalrymple JL, Russell AH, Lee SW, et al. Chemoradiation for primary invasive squamous carcinoma of the vagina. *Int J Gynecol Cancer*. 2004;14:110–7.
3. Benedetti Panici P, Bellati F, Plotti F, et al. Neoadjuvant chemotherapy followed by radical surgery in patients affected by vaginal carcinoma. *Gynecol Oncol*. 2008;111:307–11.
4. Creasman WT. Vaginal cancers. *Curr Opin Obstet Gynecol*. 2005;17:71–6.
5. Iavazzo C, Pitsouni E, Athanasiou S, et al. Imiquimod for treatment of vulvar and vaginal intraepithelial neoplasia. *Int J Gynaecol Obstet*. 2008;101:3–10.
6. Tran PT, Su Z, Lee P, et al. Prognostic factors for outcomes and complications for primary squamous cell carcinoma of the vagina treated with radiation. *Gynecol Oncol*. 2007;105:641–9.
7. Franckena M, van der Zee J. Use of combined radiation and hyperthermia for gynecological cancer. *Curr Opin Obstet Gynecol*. 2010;22:9–14.
8. Tjalma WA, Monaghan JM, de Barros Lopes A, et al. The role of surgery in invasive squamous carcinoma of the vagina. *Gynecol Oncol*. 2001;81: 360–5.

ADDITIONAL READING

Gray HJ. Advances in vulvar and vaginal cancer treatment. *Gynecol Oncol*. 2010;118:3–5.

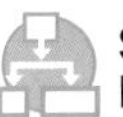

See Also (Topic, Algorithm, Electronic Media Element)

Algorithm: Metrorrhagia (Intermenstrual Bleeding)

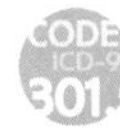

CODES

ICD9

- 184.0 Malignant neoplasm of vagina
- 233.31 Carcinoma in situ, vagina
- 623.0 Dysplasia of vagina

CLINICAL PEARLS

- Vaginal cancer is rare; 85–90% of vaginal cancers are squamous cell.
- Vaginal malignancies are found most commonly on the posterior wall in the upper 1/3 of the vagina.
- Most vaginal malignancies are metastatic (from cervix, vulva, endometrium, breast, or ovary).

VAGINISMUS

Stephanie Yu-hsuan Chen, MD

BASICS

Vaginismus is a clinical syndrome that consists of overlapping elements of hypertonic pelvic floor muscles (recurrent or persistent involuntary contractions), pain, and avoidance of sexual intercourse leading to difficulty in vaginal penetration.

DESCRIPTION

- It is defined as the recurrent or persistent difficulties of a woman to allow vaginal entry of a penis, a finger, and/or an object, despite the woman's expressed wish to do so (1).
- Classified as a sexual pain disorder, along with dyspareunia and noncoital sexual pain disorder:
  - Experience of pain is not required for the diagnosis of vaginismus, though in most women with vaginismus there is anticipation or fear of pain.
- Primary vaginismus is present when a woman has never been able to experience vaginal penetration without difficulty.
- Secondary vaginismus occurs when a woman who has previously been able to achieve penetration develops vaginismus.
- Can be complete (difficulty with attempts to insert anything into vagina) or situational (tampons or pelvic exams permitted)
- Etiology is often multifactorial.
- Women with vaginismus often avoid intercourse and may avoid appropriate health care.
- Treatment is based on the patient's goals and is focused on patient education, therapy, and behavioral exercises.

Pregnancy Considerations

- Pregnancy can occur in patients with vaginismus when ejaculation occurs on the perineum.
- Vaginismus is an independent risk factor for cesarean delivery (2)[C].

EPIDEMIOLOGY

Incidence

- The incidence of vaginismus is thought to be about 1–17% worldwide (3).

Prevalence

- True prevalence is unknown due to limited data/reporting.
- Population-based studies report prevalence rates of 0.5–30% (3).
- Affects women in all age groups

RISK FACTORS

- Though the exact role in the condition is unclear, many women report a history of abuse or sexual trauma (4)[C].
- Often associated with other sexual dysfunctions

ETIOLOGY

- Most often multifactorial in both primary and secondary vaginismus
- Primary:
  - Psychologic and psychosocial issues:
    - Negative messages about sex and sexual relations in upbringing may cause phobic reaction.
    - Poor body image and limited understanding of genital area
    - History of sexual trauma
  - Abnormalities of the hymen
- Secondary:
  - Vaginal infection
  - Inflammatory dermatitis
  - Surgical or postdelivery scarring
  - Endometriosis
  - Inadequate vaginal lubrication
  - Pelvic radiation
  - Estrogen deficiency
  - Conditioned response to pain from physical issues previously listed

COMMONLY ASSOCIATED CONDITIONS

- Marital stress, family dysfunction
- Anxiety
- Dyspareunia
- Vulvodynia/vestibulodynia

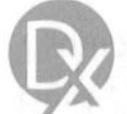

DIAGNOSIS

Vaginismus is a clinical diagnosis.

HISTORY

- Complete medical history
- Full psychosocial and sexual history, including:
  - Relationship difficulty
  - Inability to allow vaginal entry for different purposes:
    - Sexual (penis, digit, object)
    - Hygiene (tampon use)
    - Health care (pelvic examination)
  - Infertility
  - Past traumatic experiences
  - Religious beliefs
  - Views on sexuality

PHYSICAL EXAM

- Pelvic examination is necessary to exclude structural abnormalities or organic pathology.
- Educating the patient about the examination and giving her control over the progression of the examination is essential, as genital/pelvic examination may induce varying degrees of anxiety in patients.
- Referral to a gynecologist or other providers specializing in the treatment of sexual disorders may be appropriate.
- Lamont classification system aids in the assessment of severity:
  - First degree: Perineal and levator spasm relieved with reassurance
  - Second degree: Perineal spasm maintained throughout the pelvic exam
  - Third degree: Levator spasm and elevation of buttocks
  - Fourth degree: Levator and perineal spasm and elevation with adduction and retreat (5)

DIAGNOSTIC TESTS & INTERPRETATION

Lab

No laboratory tests indicated

Imaging

None indicated

Pathological Findings

- Rarely found in primary vaginismus except for hymenal anomalies
- May be varied in secondary vaginismus, such as endometriosis or scarring

DIFFERENTIAL DIAGNOSIS

- Dyspareunia
- Vaginal infection
- Vulvodynia/vestibulodynia
- Vulvovaginal atrophy
- Urogenital structural abnormalities
- Interstitial cystitis

TREATMENT

- Vaginismus may be successfully treated.
- Outpatient care is appropriate.
- Treatment of physical conditions is first-line if present (see "Secondary" under "Etiology").
- Role for pelvic floor physical therapy and myofascial release

- Some evidence suggests that cognitive-behavioral therapy may be effective (6)[C]:
  - Includes desensitization techniques such as gradual exposure, aimed at decreasing avoidance behavior and fear of vaginal penetration
- Evidence suggests that Masters and Johnson sex therapy may be effective (7)[C]:
  - Involves Kegel exercises to increase control over perineal muscles
  - Stepwise vaginal desensitization exercises:
    - With vaginal dilators that the patient inserts and controls
    - With woman's own finger(s) to promote sexual self-awareness
    - Advancement to partner's fingers with patient's control
    - Coitus after achieving largest vaginal dilator or 3 fingers; important to begin with sensate-focused exercises/sensual caressing without necessarily a demand for coitus
    - Female superior at first; passive (nonthrusting); female-directed
    - Later, thrusting may be allowed.
- Topical anesthetic with desensitization exercises may be considered.
- Patient education is an essential component of treatment (see "Patient Education" section).

MEDICATION

Botulinum neurotoxin type A injections may improve vaginismus in patients who do not respond to standard cognitive-behavioral and medical treatment for vaginismus:

- Dosage: 20, 50, and 100–400 units of botulinum toxin type A injected in the levator ani muscle have been shown to improve vaginismus (8)[C].

ADDITIONAL TREATMENT

Issues for Referral

For diagnosis and treatment recommendations, the following resources may be consulted:

- Obstetrics/gynecology
- Pelvic floor physical therapy
- Psychiatry
- Sex therapy
- Hypnotherapy

COMPLEMENTARY AND ALTERNATIVE MEDICINE

- Biofeedback
- Functional electrical stimulation

SURGERY/OTHER PROCEDURES

Contraindicated

ONGOING CARE

FOLLOW-UP RECOMMENDATIONS

Desensitization techniques of gentle, progressive, patient-controlled vaginal dilation

Patient Monitoring

General preventive health care

DIET

No special diet

PATIENT EDUCATION

- Education about pelvic anatomy, nature of vaginal spasms, normal adult sexual function
- Handheld mirror can help the woman to learn visually to tighten and loosen perineal muscles
- Important to teach the partner that spasms are not under conscious control and are not a reflection on the relationship or a woman's feelings about her partner
- Instruction in techniques for vaginal dilation
- Resources:
  - American College of Obstetricians & Gynecologists (ACOG), 409 12th St., SW, Washington, DC 20024-2188; (800) 762-ACOG. www.acog.org
  - Valins L. *When a Woman's Body Says No to Sex: Understanding and Overcoming Vaginismus*. New York: Penguin; 1992.

PROGNOSIS

Favorable with early recognition of the condition and initiation of treatment

REFERENCES

1. Basson R, Wierman ME, van Lankveld J. Summary of the recommendations on sexual dysfunctions in women. *J Sex Med*. 2010;7:314–26.
2. Goldsmith T, Levy A, Sheiner E, et al. Vaginismus as an independent risk factor for cesarean delivery. *J Matern Fetal Neonatal Med*. 2009;22(10):863–6.
3. Wimons JS, Carey MP. Prevalence of sexual dysfunctions: Results form a decade of research. *Arch Sex Behav*. 2001;30:177–217.
4. Reissing E, Binik Y, Khalife S, et al. Etiological correlates of vaginismus: Sexual and physical abuse, sexual knowledge, sexual self-schema, and relationship adjustment. *J Sex Marital Ther*. 2003;29:47–59.
5. Lamont J. Vaginismus. *Am J Obstet Gynecol*. 1978;131:632–6.
6. ter Kuile MM, van Lankveld JJDM, de Groot E, et al. Cognitive behavioral therapy for women with lifelong vaginismus: Process and prognostic factors. *Behav Res Therapy*. 2008;45:359–73.
7. Jeng CJ, Wang LR, Chou CS. Management and outcome of primary vaginismus. *J Sex Marital Ther*. 2006;32:379–87.
8. Bertolasi L, Frasson E, Cappelletti JY. Botulinum neurotoxin type A injections for vaginismus secondary to vulvar vestibulitis syndrome. *Obstet Gynecol*. 2009;114:1008–16.

ADDITIONAL READING

- Crowley T, Goldmeier D, Hiller J. Diagnosing and managing vaginismus. *BMJ*. 2009;338:b2284.
- Lahaie MA, Boyer SC, Amsel R, Khalifé S, et al. Vaginismus: A review of the literature on the classification/diagnosis, etiology and treatment. *Womens Health (Lond Engl)*. 2010;6:705–19.

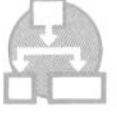

See Also (Topic, Algorithm, Electronic Media Element)

Dyspareunia; Sexual Dysfunction in Women

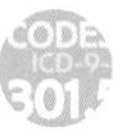

CODES

ICD9

- 306.51 Psychogenic vaginismus
- 625.1 Vaginismus

CLINICAL PEARLS

- In a patient with suspected vaginismus, a complete medical history, including a comprehensive psychosocial and sexual history, and a patient-centric, patient-controlled educational pelvic exam should be conducted.
- Vaginismus can be treated effectively.
- Cognitive-behavioral therapy may be effective for the treatment of vaginismus.
- Botox injection therapy is in the experimental stages but looks promising for the treatment of vaginismus.

V

VAGINITIS AND VAGINOSIS

Marie Ellen Caggiano, MD, MPH

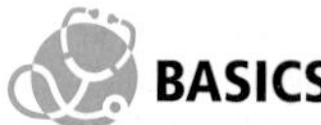

BASICS

DESCRIPTION

- Vulvovaginal candidiasis (VVC): Inflammation of the vagina and vulva caused by infection with *Candida* sp.
- Bacterial vaginosis (BV): A syndrome in which the hydrogen peroxide–producing lactobacilli normally found in the vagina are replaced by other bacteria, usually anaerobes:
  - VVC and BV are not generally considered STIs.
- Other causes of vaginitis include allergic and contact dermatitis from feminine hygiene products (fragrances, creams, douches, lubricants, and their preservatives).
- A number of dermatoses, such as lichen planus, lichen sclerosus, and psoriasis, may mimic vaginitis symptoms.
- System(s) affected: Reproductive; Skin/Exocrine
- Synonym(s): VVC: Monilial vulvovaginitis; Vaginal yeast infection; BV: *Gardnerella* vaginosis; Nonspecific vaginitis; *Haemophilus* vaginitis; *Corynebacterium* vaginitis

EPIDEMIOLOGY

- Both VVC and BV are common among reproductive-age females.
- Most cases of VVC are related to *C. albicans*, but may be caused by other *Candida* sp. (e.g., *C. glabrata*).
- VVC related to *C. glabrata* may be more common among diabetic women.

Prevalence

- VVC: Second most common cause of vaginitis after BV:
  - 75% of women diagnosed at least once with VVC; up to 45% diagnosed more than once
  - <5% of females are diagnosed with recurrent VVC (defined as 4 or more episodes of VVC in 1 year).
  - Studies have shown that up to 72% of females may be colonized with yeast but do not exhibit symptoms of vaginitis.
- BV: Prevalence varies based on age, race/ethnicity, and socioeconomic status:
  - Most common vaginal infection among reproductive-aged women
  - NHANES data reported an overall prevalence of 29%, with the highest rates (50%) among black women.

Pediatric Considerations

VVC and BV are less common before the onset of puberty and after menopause.

RISK FACTORS

- VVC:
  - Diabetes mellitus (DM) with poor glycemic control
  - Antibiotic therapy
  - Immunosuppression (e.g., corticosteroid therapy, HIV infection)
  - High-estrogen states (e.g., pregnancy, oral contraceptive use, hormone-replacement therapy); *C. albicans* accounts for 85–90% of vaginitis cases in pregnancy.
- BV:
  - Black race
  - Lower socioeconomic status
  - Smoking
  - New or multiple sex partner(s)
  - Female sex partners
  - Spermicide use
  - Vaginal douching

GENERAL PREVENTION

- Vulvar hygiene (see "General Measures"); avoid implicated feminine hygiene products.
- Maintenance therapy for recurrent cases
- Treatment of sexual partners generally is not recommended, but may be considered in recurrent cases.

ETIOLOGY

- VVC: Overgrowth of yeast in the vagina
- BV: Shift from a healthy lactobacilli-based endogenous flora to an anaerobically based endogenous flora, including *G. vaginalis*, *Mobiluncus* sp., *Mycoplasma hominis*, *Peptostreptococcus*, *Prevotella*, *Bacteroides*, and *Atopobium vaginae*; the rectum may be a reservoir of organisms leading to autoinfection.
- Aerobic vaginitis has been described in which lactobacilli are decreased in number and aerobic organisms including *E. coli*, group B streptococci, and *S. aureus* predominate (1).

COMMONLY ASSOCIATED CONDITIONS

- STIs
- Balanitis in male partners may occur rarely.
- Research is limited in same-sex partners. Symptomatic partners should be evaluated.

DIAGNOSIS

HISTORY

- VVC:
  - Vaginal and vulvar pruritus
  - Vulvar pain, external dysuria, and dyspareunia
  - Thick, curdlike vaginal discharge
- BV:
  - 50% of women are asymptomatic.
  - Unpleasant musty or fishy vaginal odor, exacerbated by intercourse
  - 10–30% may have vaginal/vulvar irritation.
  - Thin gray–white or frothy vaginal discharge

PHYSICAL EXAM

- VVC:
  - Thick, curdlike vaginal discharge
  - Vulvar erythema and edema
  - Vulvar fissures and excoriations
  - Normal vaginal pH (<4.5)
- BV:
  - 10–30% may have vaginal/vulvar irritation.
  - Thin gray–white vaginal discharge is mildly adherent to vaginal walls.
  - 10% have frothy discharge.
  - pH >4.5

DIAGNOSTIC TESTS & INTERPRETATION

Lab

- Wet mount: Prepare 2 slides, both with fresh vaginal discharge: 1 with NaCl and 1 with 10% KOH:
  - The presence of budding yeasts and hyphae consistent with VVC (may be more easily seen on KOH prep)
  - Clue cells >20% of total epithelial cells considered clinically significant for diagnosis of BV (saline)
  - WBCs are not numerous in BV but may be present in large numbers in candidiasis.
- Amsel criteria for BV (need 3 out of 4): Clue cells, characteristic vaginal discharge, vaginal pH >4.5, and positive "whiff test" (transient but potent amine or fishy odor with the addition of 10% KOH); vaginal pH also may suggest need for testing for *Trichomonas*. In cases of aerobic vaginitis, clue cells may be <20%.
- Consider vaginal culture for VVC when characteristic symptoms are present, vaginal pH is normal, and no yeast are present on wet mount or to identify species if no improvement with treatment or relapse occurs within 2 months.
- Positive culture for *Candida* sp. or other yeast species may only indicate colonization; clinical correlation is required.
- VVC or BV: May be noted on cytology but must be correlated with clinical symptoms; asymptomatic women generally do not need treatment.
- DNA probe–based tests are available (Affirm VP III, Becton Dickinson, Sparks, MD), but it is unclear that identification of the presence of yeast (or low numbers of *G. vaginalis*) indicates that the organism is the cause of symptoms. Use may not be cost-effective.

DIFFERENTIAL DIAGNOSIS

- Physiologic discharge and cervical ectropion
- Trichomoniasis
- Contact dermatitis
- Mechanical/chemical irritation
- Cervicitis (chlamydial or gonococcal)
- UTI
- Atrophic vaginitis
- Dermatoses: Lichen sclerosus, lichen planus, seborrheic dermatitis, psoriasis

TREATMENT

MEDICATION

First Line

- VVC (2):
  - Short-course therapy with topical azoles is effective in 80–90% of patients.
  - Many topical therapies are available over the counter:
    - Butoconazole 2% cream 5 g intravaginally × 3 days
    - Clotrimazole 1% cream 5 g intravaginally × 7–14 days or 2% cream 5 g intravaginally × 3 days
    - Miconazole 2% cream 5 g intravaginally × 7 days or 4% cream 5 g intravaginally × 3 days or 100 mg vaginal suppository, 1 suppository × 7 days or 200 mg vaginal suppository, 1 suppository × 3 days or 1,200 mg vaginal suppository, 1 suppository × 1 day
    - Tioconazole 6.5% ointment 5 g intravaginally in a single application
  - Prescription therapies include:
    - Butoconazole 2% cream (single dose bioadhesive) 5 g intravaginally × single application
    - Nystatin 100,000-unit vaginal tablet, 1 tablet × 14 days
    - Terconazole 0.4% cream 5 g intravaginally × 7 days or 0.8% cream 5 g intravaginally × 3 days or 80 mg vaginal suppository, 1 suppository × 3 days

  - Fluconazole 150 mg PO once; use with caution in patients with liver disease and with coadministration of other drugs.
- BV (2):
  - Metronidazole (Flagyl): 500 mg PO b.i.d. × 7 days *or*
  - Metronidazole vaginal gel: 0.75% 5 g intravaginally daily × 5 days *or*
  - Clindamycin: 2% vaginal cream 5 g intravaginally daily × 7 days
  - 85–90% of women respond to initial treatment; however, recurrence rates may be as high as 80%.
  - Antibiotic resistance against clindamycin and metronidazole has been reported and may be responsible for some cases of recurrent BV (1).

ALERT

Oil-based preparations may weaken latex condoms.

Second Line

- VVC:
  - Recurrent VVC: Obtain cultures. Infections associated with *C. glabrata* (5–15%) are less responsive to first-line therapies (3,4).
  - Consider longer-duration therapy (7–14 days of topical or oral fluconazole every third day for a total of 3 doses).
  - Suppressive maintenance therapy (oral fluconazole weekly × 6 months or topical treatments weekly) (5)
  - Women with recurrent candidiasis may benefit from fluconazole 150 mg/wk plus cetirizine 10 mg/d (6)[B] for allergy or itching.
  - Boric acid: 600-mg gelatin capsule inserted vaginally daily × 2 weeks (indicated for non-*Albicans* disease; 70% clinical and mycologic cure rate) (4)
- BV:
  - Metronidazole: 2 g PO single dose (less effective than alternative regimens)
  - Clindamycin: 300 mg PO daily × 7 days
  - Clindamycin ovules: 100 g intravaginally at bedtime × 3 days
  - Tinidazole: 1 g daily × 5 days or 2 g PO × 1 dose. Vaginal application of tinidazole has also been studied and may be effective.
  - Regimens for treating recurrent BV involve use of metronidazole gel twice weekly. Small studies have shown possible benefit from the addition of probiotics and vaginal boric acid although larger, randomized controlled (7) trials are needed (8).

ALERT

Avoid any alcohol-containing product while taking metronidazole.

Pregnancy Considerations

- VVC: Topical therapy preferred over oral therapy
- BV: Associated with preterm delivery; however, it is unclear whether the treatment of BV prevents preterm delivery. All symptomatic women should be treated, screening reserved for women at high risk for preterm delivery. Avoid creams; metronidazole 500 mg PO b.i.d. × 7 days or clindamycin 300 mg PO b.i.d. × 7 days. Package labeling of metronidazole indicates that it is contraindicated in the first trimester of pregnancy, but this is not supported by recent meta-analyses of available data.

ADDITIONAL TREATMENT

General Measures

- Avoid douching, use of panty liners, pantyhose, occlusive pants, and undergarments.
- Regular use of condoms may help to prevent BV, as exposure to semen may trigger symptoms for some women.

Issues for Referral

Treating male sexual partners does not reduce symptoms or prevent recurrence, but this may be considered in patients who have recurrent infection.

COMPLEMENTARY AND ALTERNATIVE MEDICINE

- A Cochrane analysis reviewed the use of probiotics for BV and found inconclusive evidence to recommend probiotics as primary treatment or as a preventive strategy. Further study was recommended (7).
- Acidification of the vagina has not been proven beneficial.

ONGOING CARE

FOLLOW-UP RECOMMENDATIONS

- Delay sexual relations until symptoms clear/discomfort resolves.
- Use of condoms may reduce recurrence of BV.

Patient Monitoring

- Generally, no specific follow-up needed; if symptoms persist or recur within 2 months, repeat pelvic exam and culture.
- Consider suppressive therapy for women with recurrent infection.

DIET

Reduction of sugar intake has been recommended but is not supported by evidence.

PATIENT EDUCATION

American College of Obstetricians and Gynecologists (ACOG), 409 12th St., SW, Washington, DC 20024-2188; (800) 762-ACOG; www.acog.org

PROGNOSIS

VVC: 80–90% of uncomplicated cases cured with appropriate treatment; 30–50% of recurrent infections return after discontinuation of maintenance therapy; there is a relatively high spontaneous remission rate of untreated symptoms as well.

COMPLICATIONS

- VVC may occur following treatment of BV.
- BV has been associated with an increased risk of acquisition and transmission of STIs, including HIV.
- BV has been associated with increased risk of pregnancy complications, including preterm birth, chorioamnionitis, postpartum and postabortal endometritis, and pelvic inflammatory disease (PID).

REFERENCES

1. Donders G. Diagnosis and management of bacterial vaginosis and other types of abnormal vaginal bacterial flora: a review. *Obstet Gynecol Surv*. 2010;65:462–73.
2. Workowski KA, Berman S, Centers for Disease Control and Prevention (CDC), et al. Sexually transmitted diseases treatment guidelines, 2010. *MMWR Recomm Rep*. 2010;59:1–110.
3. Owen MK, Clenney TL. Management of vaginitis. *Am Fam Physician*. 2004;70:2125–32.
4. Ray D, Goswami R, Banerjee U, et al. Prevalence of *Candida glabrata* and its response to boric acid vaginal suppositories in comparison with oral fluconazole in patients with diabetes and vulvovaginal candidiasis. *Diabetes Care*. 2007;30:312–7.
5. Pappas PG, Kauffman CA, Andes D, et al. Clinical practice guidelines for the management of candidiasis: 2009 update by the Infectious Disease Society of America. *Clin Infect Dis*. 2009;48(5):503–35.
6. Neves NA, Carvalho LP, Lopes AC, et al. Successful treatment of refractory recurrent vaginal candidiasis with cetirizine plus fluconazole. *J Low Genit Tract Dis*. 2005;9:167–70.
7. Senok AC, Verstraelen H, Temmerman M, et al. Probiotics for the treatment of bacterial vaginosis. *Cochrane Database Syst Rev*. 2009;4:CD006289.
8. Reichman O, Akins R, Sobel JD, et al. Boric acid addition to suppressive antimicrobial therapy for recurrent bacterial vaginosis. *Sex Transm Dis*. 2009;36:732–4.

V

ADDITIONAL READING

- Frey Tirri B. Antimicrobial topical agents used in the vagina. *Curr Probl Dermatol*. 2011;40:36–47.
- Quan M. Vaginitis: Diagnosis and management. *Postgrad Med*. 2010;122:117–27.
- Summers PR. Topical therapy for mucosal yeast infections. *Curr Probl Dermatol*. 2011;40:48–57.

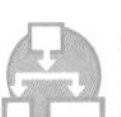

See Also (Topic, Algorithm, Electronic Media Element)

Algorithm: Discharge, Vaginal

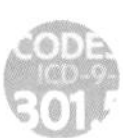

CODES

ICD9

- 041.9 Bacterial infection, unspecified, in conditions classified elsewhere and of unspecified site
- 112.1 Candidiasis of vulva and vagina
- 616.10 Vaginitis and vulvovaginitis, unspecified

CLINICAL PEARLS

- Clinical symptoms, signs, and microscopy have relatively poor performance compared with so-called gold standards such as culture and DNA probe assays, but these more sensitive assays may detect organisms that may not be causing symptoms.
- Most women experience relief of symptoms with therapy chosen without such gold standard tests, and even when the treatment does not correspond with the underlying infection.
- Vaginal pH is underused as a diagnostic tool for evaluation of vaginitis.
- Treatment of sexual partners is not currently the standard of care for either BV or VVC.

VARICOSE VEINS

Joseph A. Florence, MD

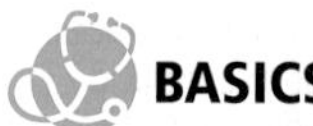

BASICS

DESCRIPTION
- Superficial venous disease causing a permanent dilatation and tortuosity of superficial veins, usually occurring in the legs and feet; caused by systemic weakness in the vein wall, and may result from congenitally incomplete valves or valves that have become incompetent
- Affects legs where reverse flow occurs when dependent
- Truncal varices involve the great and small saphenous veins; branch varicosities involve the saphenous vein tributaries.
- Categorized as (1):
  - Uncomplicated (cosmetic)
  - With local symptoms (pain confined to the varices, not diffuse)
  - With local complications (superficial thrombophlebitis, may rupture causing bleeding)
  - Complex varicose disease (diffuse limb pain, swelling, skin changes or ulcer)
- System(s) affected: Cardiovascular; Skin

ALERT
Ulceration of varicose veins has a high rate of infection, which can lead to sepsis.

Geriatric Considerations
- Common; usually valvular degeneration but may be secondary to chronic venous deficiency
- Elastic support hose and frequent rests with legs elevated rather than ligation and stripping

Pregnancy Considerations
- Frequent problem
- Elastic stockings are recommended for those with a history of varicosities or if a great deal of standing is involved.

EPIDEMIOLOGY
Incidence
- Predominant age: Middle age
- Predominant gender: Female > Male (5:1)
- National Women's Health Information Center estimates that 50% of women have varicose veins.

RISK FACTORS
- Increasing age
- Pregnancy, especially multiple pregnancies
- Occupations that require prolonged standing, restrictive clothing (e.g., very tight girdles)
- Obesity
- History of phlebitis
- Family history

Genetics
Familial, dominant, X-linked

PATHOPHYSIOLOGY
- Varicose veins are caused by venous insufficiency from faulty valves in ≥1 perforator veins in the lower leg, causing secondary incompetence at the saphenofemoral junction (valvular reflux).
- Valvular dysfunction causing venous reflux and subsequently venous hypertension (HTN)
- Failed valves allow blood to flow in the reverse direction (away from the heart), from deep to superficial and from proximal to distal veins.
- Deep thrombophlebitis
- Increased venous pressure from any cause
- Congenital valvular incompetence
- Trauma (consider arteriovenous fistula; listen for bruit)
- Presumed to be due to a loss in vein wall elasticity with failure of the valve leaflets

COMMONLY ASSOCIATED CONDITIONS
- Stasis dermatitis
- Large varicose veins may lead to skin changes and eventual stasis ulceration.

DIAGNOSIS

HISTORY
- Symptoms range from minor annoyance or cosmetic problem to a lifestyle-limiting problem.
- Localized symptoms: Pain, burning, itching
- Generalized symptoms:
  - Leg muscular cramp, aching
  - Leg fatigue or swelling
- Pain if varicose ulcer develops
- Symptoms often worse at the end of the day, especially after prolonged standing
- Women are more prone to symptoms due to hormonal influences: Worse during menses
- No direct correlation with the severity of varicose veins and the severity of symptoms

PHYSICAL EXAM
- Inspect lower extremities while the patient is standing. Varicose veins in the proximal femoral ring and distal portion of the legs may not be visible when the patient is supine.
- Varicose veins are:
  - Dilatated, tortuous, superficial veins, chiefly in the lower extremities
  - Dark purple or blue in color, raised above the surface of the skin
  - Often twisted, bulging, and can look like cords
  - Most commonly found on the posterior or medial lower extremity
- Edema of the affected limb may be present.
- Skin changes may include:
  - Eczema
  - Hyperpigmentation
  - Lipodermatosclerosis
- Spider veins (idiopathic telangiectases):
  - Fine intracutaneous angiectasis
  - May be extensive/unsightly
- Neurologic sensory and motor exam:
  - Peripheral arterial vasculature; pulses
  - Musculoskeletal exam for associated rheumatologic or orthopedic issues

DIAGNOSTIC TESTS & INTERPRETATION
- Trendelenburg test for varicose veins (2):
  - Patient lies on back and raises leg to empty the veins.
  - Tourniquet is applied just below the saphenous opening, around the upper thigh.
  - Patient stands and the tourniquet is removed in 60 seconds.
  - Normally, the vein should fill from below within 35 seconds with the tourniquet on. Earlier filling indicates incompetence of a communicating vein. If on release the veins fill rapidly from above, there are incompetent saphenofemoral valves.
- Perthes test for assessing the patency of the deep femoral veins (2):
  - With the patient standing and veins filled, a tourniquet is placed around the midthigh, and the patient walks for 5 minutes.
  - If the saphenous veins collapse below the tourniquet, the deep veins are patent, and the communicating veins are competent; if unchanged, both saphenous and communicating veins are incompetent; and if the veins increase in prominence and pain occurs, the deep veins are occluded.

Imaging
Duplex ultrasound: Formal noninvasive imaging of the venous system with duplex ultrasound will confirm the etiology, anatomy, and pathophysiology of segmental venous reflux.

Diagnostic Procedures/Surgery
- Tourniquet tests have been replaced by ultrasound techniques for assessing varicose veins before treatment.
- Duplex scanning, venous Doppler study, photoplethysmography, light-reflection rheography, air plethysmography, and other vascular testing should be reserved for patients who have venous symptoms and/or large (>4 mm in diameter) vessels or large numbers of spider telangiectasia indicating venous HTN.

Pathological Findings
- Medial fibrosis of veins
- Disappearance or atrophy of valves

DIFFERENTIAL DIAGNOSIS
- Nerve root compression
- Arthritis
- Peripheral neuritis
- Telangiectasia: Smaller, visible blood vessels that are permanently dilated
- Deep vein thrombosis
- Inflammatory liposclerosis

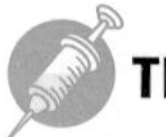

TREATMENT

- Ambulatory, conservative, hemodynamic management of varicose veins is more effective than stripping with clinical marking or stripping with duplex marking to treat varicose veins (3)[B].
- Conservative therapy (e.g., elevation, external compression, weight loss) may be helpful (4)[A].
- Endovenous laser ablation, radiofrequency ablation, foam sclerotherapy, and surgical stripping for great saphenous varicose veins are all efficacious (5)[A].
- Long-term safety and efficacy of surgery for varicose veins is supported by low-quality evidence; short-term studies support the efficacy of less invasive treatments that are associated with less periprocedural disability and pain (6)[A].
- There is insufficient evidence to recommend preferentially sclerotherapy or surgery (7)[A].
- Endovenous ablation has improved the treatment profile: Easily administered, well-tolerated, ambulatory treatment (8)[B]
- Sclerotherapy may be used to improve the symptoms and cosmetic appearance of varicose veins (9)[B], but it is associated with a high recurrence rate.

- Technical failure rate is highest after foam sclerotherapy; both radiofrequency ablation and foam are associated with faster recovery and less postoperative pain than endovenous laser ablation and stripping (5)[A].

MEDICATION

Superficial thrombophlebitis is not an infective condition and does not require antibiotic treatment.

ADDITIONAL TREATMENT

General Measures

Patients with unsightly varicose veins often seek treatment for cosmetic reasons.

Issues for Referral

Referral guidelines from National Institute for Health and Clinical Excellence (10)[A]:

- Emergency: Bleeding from a varicosity that has eroded the skin
- Urgent: Varicosity that has bled and is at risk for bleeding again
- Soon: Ulcer that is progressive or painful despite treatment
- Routine:
  - Active or healed ulcer or progressive skin changes that may benefit from surgery
  - Recurrent superficial thrombophlebitis
  - Troublesome symptoms attributable to varicose veins, or patient and provider feel that the extent, site, and size of the varicosities are having a severe impact on quality of life

Additional Therapies

- Apply elastic stockings before lowering legs from the bed
- Activity:
  - Frequent rest periods with legs elevated
  - If standing is necessary, frequently shift weight from side to side.
  - Appropriate exercise routine as part of conservative treatment
  - Walking regimen after sclerotherapy is important to help promote healing.
  - Never sit with legs hanging down.
- Physical therapy

SURGERY/OTHER PROCEDURES

- Surgery:
  - Challenge to balance a cosmetically acceptable result with a low incidence of recurrence and complications
  - Surgery is indicated if there is pain, recurrent phlebitis, or skin changes/ulceration, or for cosmetic improvement for severe cases.
  - Minimally invasive techniques include:
    - Radiofrequency ablation (RFA)
    - Endovenous laser therapy
    - Transilluminated power phlebectomy
    - Ambulatory phlebectomy has a lower risk of recurrence than sclerotherapy (11)[A].
  - Traditional surgical methods include:
    - Ligation and stripping of the varicose vein
    - Stab avulsion phlebectomy
  - Surgical treatment of clinically symptomatic varicose veins involves treatment of the saphenous vein reflux as well as the varicosities.
- Sclerotherapy:
  - Randomized, controlled trials suggest that the choice of sclerosant, dose, formulation (foam vs. liquid), local pressure dressing, and degree and length of compression has no significant effect on the efficacy of sclerotherapy (12)[A].
  - Sclerosing solution is injected into varicosities, causing vein walls to swell, adhere, and scar; 50–90% improvement can be expected.
  - Ultrasound-guided sclerotherapy combined with saphenofemoral ligations was less expensive, involved a shorter treatment time, and resulted in more rapid recovery than saphenofemoral ligation, saphenous stripping, and phlebectomies (13)[B].
- Radiotherapy:
  - RFA takes longer to perform but has better early outcome than conventional surgery in patients with great saphenous varicose veins (14)[B].
  - Radiofrequency and laser treatments replace "stripping"; however, most varicosities still require phlebectomy or sclerotherapy.

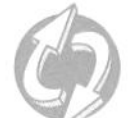

ONGOING CARE

DIET

- No special diet
- Weight-loss diet is recommended if obesity is a problem.

PATIENT EDUCATION

- Avoid long periods of standing and crossing legs when sitting.
- Exercise (walking, running) regularly to improve leg strength and circulation.
- Maintain an appropriate weight.
- Wear elastic support stockings.
- Avoid clothing that constricts legs.
- Surgery or sclerotherapy may not prevent development of varicosities and the procedure may need to be repeated in later years.
- National Heart, Lung and Blood Institute, Communications and Public Information Branch, National Institutes of Health, Building 31, Room 41–21, 9000 Rockville Pike, Bethesda, MD 20892; (301) 496-4236.

PROGNOSIS

- Usual course: Chronic
- Favorable with appropriate treatment
- Quality of surgical treatment is less satisfactory if significant deep venous reflux, history of ulceration, or congenital arteriovenous malformation exists.

COMPLICATIONS

- Petechial hemorrhages
- Chronic edema
- Superimposed infection
- Varicose ulcers
- Pigmentation
- Eczema
- Recurrence after surgical treatment
- Scarring or nerve damage from stripping technique

REFERENCES

1. Raju S, Neglén P. Clinical practice. Chronic venous insufficiency and varicose veins. *N Engl J Med*. 2009;360:2319–27.
2. Kim J, Richards S, Kent PJ. Clinical examination of varicose veins–a validation study. *Ann R Coll Surg Engl*. 2000;82:171–5.
3. Parés JO, Juan J, Tellez R, et al. Varicose vein surgery: Stripping versus the CHIVA method: A randomized controlled trial. *Ann Surg*. 2010;251:624–31.
4. Palfreyman SJ, Michaels JA. A systematic review of compression hosiery for uncomplicated varicose veins. *Phlebology*. 2009;24(Suppl 1):13–33.
5. Rasmussen LH, Lawaetz M, Bjoern L, et al. Randomized clinical trial comparing endovenous laser ablation, radiofrequency ablation, foam sclerotherapy and surgical stripping for great saphenous varicose veins. *Br J Surg*. 2011;98:1079–87.
6. Murad MH, Coto-Yglesias F, Zumaeta-Garcia M, et al. A systematic review and meta-analysis of the treatments of varicose veins. *J Vasc Surg*. 2011;53:49S–65S.
7. Rigby KA, Palfreyman SJ, Beverley C, et al. Surgery versus sclerotherapy for the treatment of varicose veins. *Cochrane Database Syst Rev*. 2004:CD004980.
8. Lane TR, Pandey VA, Davies AH, et al. Superficial venous disease treatment–is there still a role for open surgery in 2011? *Acta Chir Belg*. 2011;111:125–9.
9. Jones RH, Carek PJ. Management of varicose veins. *Am Fam Physician*. 2008;78:1289–94.
10. National Institute for Clinical Excellence. *Referral Advice for Varicose Veins*. London: NICE; 2001.
11. Sadick NS. Advances in the treatment of varicose veins: ambulatory phlebectomy, foam sclerotherapy, endovascular laser, and radiofrequency closure. *Dermatol Clin*. 2005;23:443–55, vi.
12. Tisi PV, Beverley C, Rees A. Injection sclerotherapy for varicose veins. *Cochrane Database Syst Rev*. 2006:CD001732.
13. Bountouroglou DG. Varicose veins and their management. *BMJ*. 2006;533:287–92.
14. Subramonia S, Lees T. Randomized clinical trial of radiofrequency ablation or conventional high ligation and stripping for great saphenous varicose veins. *Br J Surg*. 2010;97:328–36.

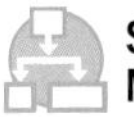

See Also (Topic, Algorithm, Electronic Media Element)

Dermatitis, Stasis; Hemorrhoids

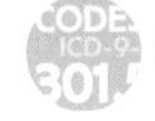

CODES

ICD9

454.9 Asymptomatic varicose veins

CLINICAL PEARLS

- Insufficient evidence exists to prefer sclerotherapy over surgery (7)[A].
- The efficacy of sclerotherapy is not significantly affected by the choice of sclerosant, dose, formulation (foam vs. liquid), local pressure dressing, or degree and length of compression (12)[A].

V

VASCULITIS

Irene J. Tan, MD

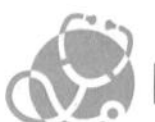

BASICS

DESCRIPTION

Vasculitis is an inflammatory disease of the blood vessels:

- Clinical features result from the destruction of blood vessel walls, with subsequent thrombosis, ischemia, bleeding, and/or aneurysm formation.
- Consists of a large, heterogeneous group of diseases classified by the predominant size, type, and the location of the blood vessels involved:
  - Small-vessel vasculitis:
    - Churg-Strauss syndrome
    - Wegener granulomatosis
    - Microscopic polyangiitis
    - Henoch-Schönlein purpura
    - Essential cryoglobulinemic vasculitis
    - Hypersensitivity vasculitis
    - Viral-/retroviral-associated vasculitis
    - Connective tissue disorder–associated vasculitis
  - Medium-vessel vasculitis:
    - Polyarteritis nodosa
    - Kawasaki disease
    - Isolated CNS vasculitis
  - Large-vessel vasculitis:
    - Takayasu arteritis
    - Giant cell arteritis
- Occurs as primary disorders or secondary to infection, a drug reaction, malignancy, or connective tissue disorder
- Protean features often delay the diagnosis.

EPIDEMIOLOGY

Highly variable, depending on the vasculitic syndrome:

- *Hypersensitivity vasculitis is the most commonly encountered vasculitis in clinical practice.*
- Kawasaki disease, Henoch-Schönlein purpura, dermatomyositis are more common in children.
- Takayasu arteritis is most prevalent in young Asian women.
- Wegener granulomatosis, microscopic polyangiitis, and Churg-Strauss syndrome are more common in middle-aged males.
- Giant cell arteritis occurs exclusively in those >50 years of age and is rare in the black population.

Incidence

The annual incidence in adults unless otherwise specified:

- Hypersensitivity vasculitis: Depends on drug exposure patterns
- Connective tissue disorder–associated vasculitis: Variable
- Henoch-Schönlein purpura: 200–700/1 million in children <17 years of age
- Giant cell arteritis: 170/1 million
- Kawasaki disease: Depends on race/age; ~170/1 million
- Polyarteritis nodosa: 2–33/1 million
- Wegener granulomatosis: 4–15/1 million
- Microscopic polyangiitis: 1–24/1 million
- Churg-Strauss arteritis: 1–3/1 million
- Viral-/retroviral-associated vasculitis: Unknown; >90% of cases of cryoglobulinemic vasculitis are associated with hepatitis C.
- Polyarteritis nodosa: 2–33/1 million
- Takayasu arteritis: 2/1 million

RISK FACTORS

A combination of genetic susceptibility and environmental exposure is presumed to play a role in disease onset.

Genetics

A number of the vasculitic syndromes have been linked to candidate genes. No single gene has been found to be sufficient to cause vasculitis.

GENERAL PREVENTION

None. Early identification is the key to prevent irreversible organ damage in severe forms of systemic vasculitis.

PATHOPHYSIOLOGY

3 major immunopathogenic mechanisms have been proposed:

- Immune-complex formation: Systemic lupus erythematosus (SLE), polyarteritis nodosa, and essential mixed cryoglobulinemia
- Antineutrophil cytoplasmic antibodies (ANCAs): Wegener granulomatosis, microscopic polyangiitis, and Churg-Strauss syndrome
- Pathogenic T-lymphocyte response: Giant cell arteritis and Takayasu arteritis

ETIOLOGY

Not well understood in most forms of vasculitis, except where known drug triggers have been identified (e.g., antibiotics, sulfonamides, and hydralazine)

COMMONLY ASSOCIATED CONDITIONS

Hepatitis C (essential cryoglobulinemic vasculitis), hepatitis B (polyarteritis nodosa [PAN]), SLE, rheumatoid arthritis (RA), Sjögren's, mixed connective tissue disease (MCTD), dermatomyositis, ankylosing spondylitis, Behçet disease, relapsing polychondritis (CTD-associated vasculitis), HIV, cytomegalovirus (CMV), Epstein-Barr virus (EBV), hepatitis B and C (viral-/retroviral-associated vasculitis), respiratory tract methicillin-resistant *Staphylococcus aureus* (MRSA) (Wegener granulomatosis [WG]).

DIAGNOSIS

HISTORY

- Consider patient's age, sex, and ethnicity.
- Note the organs affected and estimate the size of blood vessels involved.
- Use the pattern of demographics, clinical features, and the predominant vessel size/organ involvement to narrow down the specific type of vasculitis.

PHYSICAL EXAM

- Constitutional symptoms: Fever, weight loss, malaise, fatigue, diminished appetite, sweats
- Skin findings: Palpable purpura, livedo reticularis, nodules, ulcers, gangrene, nail bed capillary changes
- CNS findings: Mononeuritis multiplex, polyneuropathy, headaches, visual loss, tinnitus, stroke, seizure, encephalopathy
- Heart/lung findings: Myocardial infarction, cardiomyopathy, pericarditis, arrhythmia, cough, chest pain, hemoptysis, dyspnea
- Renal manifestations: Hypertension, proteinuria, hematuria, renal insufficiency
- GI manifestations: Abdominal pain, hematochezia, perforation
- Musculoskeletal manifestations: Arthralgia, myalgia
- Miscellaneous: Unexplained ischemic or hemorrhagic events, chronic sinusitis, scleritis, episcleritis, and recurrent epistaxis

DIAGNOSTIC TESTS & INTERPRETATION

ALERT

Clinically silent kidney involvement warrants both a routine serum creatinine and urinalysis with microscopy for underlying glomerulonephritis.

Lab

Labs are required to exclude alternate diagnosis, which has major treatment implications:

- Routine tests: CBC, liver enzymes, serum creatinine, urinalysis with microscopy
- Serology: Antinuclear antibodies (ANA), rheumatoid factor (RF), rapid plasma reagin/venereal disease reaction level (RPR/VDRL), Rocky Mountain spotted fever (RMSF titer, Lyme test, complements C3,C4, ANCA titer, hepatitis screen for B and C, antiglomerular basement membrane titer, HIV, serum protein electrophoresis.
- Miscellaneous: Drug screen, ESR, C-reactive protein, creatine kinase (CK), blood culture, ECG

Imaging

Chest x-ray (CXR), CT scan, MRI, and arteriography may be required to delineate extent of organs involved.

Diagnostic Procedures/Surgery

- Electromyography with nerve conduction studies may be useful for documenting neuropathy and to target affected nerve for biopsy.
- Biopsy of the affected tissue/organ is essential to substantiate diagnosis (e.g., temporal artery, sural nerve, renal biopsy, etc).
- If biopsy is not practical, angiography may be diagnostic for large- and medium-vessel vasculitides.
- Bronchoscopy may be required to differentiate pulmonary infection from potentially life-threatening hemorrhagic vasculitis in patients with hemoptysis.

Pathological Findings

Immune cell infiltration into the blood vessel wall layers with varying degrees of necrosis and granuloma formation, depending on the type of vasculitis

DIFFERENTIAL DIAGNOSIS

- Fibromuscular dysplasia
- Embolic disease (atheroma, cholesterol emboli, atrial myxoma, mycotic aneurysm with embolization)
- Vasospasm, drug-induced (cocaine, amphetamines, ergots)
- Thrombotic thrombocytopenic disorders (disseminated intravascular coagulation [DIC], thrombotic thrombocytopenic purpura [TTP], antiphospholipid syndrome, heparin or warfarin-induced thrombosis)
- Systemic infection (infective endocarditis, fungal infections, disseminated gonococcal infection, lyme, syphilis, RMSF, bacteremia)
- Malignancy (lymphomatoid granulomatosis, angioimmunoblastic T-cell lymphoma, intravascular lymphoma)
- Miscellaneous (Goodpasture syndrome, sarcoidosis, amyloidosis, Whipple disease, congenital coarctation of aorta)

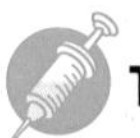

TREATMENT

MEDICATION

First Line

Corticosteroids are the initial systemic anti-inflammatory agent (1)[A],(2)[C] with rapid onset of action.

Second Line

Cytotoxic medications (e.g., cyclophosphamide (3,4,5)[A], methotrexate, azathioprine (4)[A], mycophenolate mofetil, and rituximab) are often required in combination with corticosteroids for rapidly progressive vasculitis with significant organ involvement or inadequate response to corticosteroids.

ADDITIONAL TREATMENT

General Measures

- Discontinue the offending drug for hypersensitivity vasculitis.
- Simple observation for mild cases of Henoch-Schönlein purpura.

Issues for Referral

- Rheumatology referral for complicated cases where newer or more toxic treatments are required.
- Nephrology referral for persistent hematuria or proteinuria, rising creatinine, or a positive ANCA titer
- Pulmonary referral for persistent pulmonary infiltrate unresponsive to antibiotic therapy or gross hemoptysis

Additional Therapies

- IVIG and aspirin for Kawasaki disease, but corticosteroids are contraindicated.
- Plasma exchange appears to improve recovery of patients with severe acute renal failure secondary to vasculitis (5,6)[A] and pulmonary hemorrhage.

SURGERY/OTHER PROCEDURES

Rarely, corrective surgery is required to repair tissue damage as a result of aggressive vasculitis.

IN-PATIENT CONSIDERATIONS

Initial Stabilization

Initial therapy is guided by the organ system involved:

- If pulmonary hemorrhage is present, life-saving measures may include mechanical ventilation, plasmapheresis, and immunosuppression.
- If acute renal failure is present, electrolyte and fluid balance as well as plasma exchange and immunosuppression should be considered.
- If signs of intestinal ischemia, patient should be NPO and be considered for plasmapheresis, immunosuppression, and parenteral nutrition.

Admission Criteria

Hemoptysis, acute renal failure, intestinal ischemia, any organ-threatening symptoms or signs, and/or need for biopsy

Discharge Criteria

Stabilization or resolution of potential life-threatening symptoms

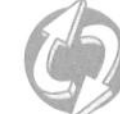

ONGOING CARE

FOLLOW-UP RECOMMENDATIONS

If significant coronary artery disease is involved in Kawasaki disease, there may be benefit from a moderate activity restriction.

Patient Monitoring

Frequent clinical follow-up supported by patient self-monitoring is the key to the timely identification of disease relapse.

DIET

Special diet for patients with renal involvement, or ones with hyperglycemia/dyslipidemia as a result of therapeutic corticosteroids

PROGNOSIS

Prognosis is good, particularly vasculitis with limited organ involvement. Relapsing courses, renal or extensive lung involvement portend the worst prognosis.

COMPLICATIONS

- Varying degrees of persistent organ dysfunction may be the result of the disease, medications, or scarring in the more serious forms of vasculitis.
- Early deaths are due to active vasculitic disease, and late deaths may be from complications of therapy (corticosteroids and cytotoxic medications).

REFERENCES

1. Weiss PF, Feinstein JA, Luan X, et al. Effects of corticosteroid on Henoch-Schönlein purpura: A systematic review. *Pediatrics*. 2007;120:1079–87.
2. Wood L, Tulloh R. Kawasaki disease: Diagnosis, management and cardiac sequelae. *Expert Rev Cardiovasc Ther*. 2007;5:553–61.
3. Bertsias G, Ioannidis JP, Boletis J, et al. EULAR recommendations for the management of systemic lupus erythematosus. Report of a Task Force of the EULAR Standing Committee for International Clinical Studies Including Therapeutics. *Ann Rheum Dis*. 2008;67:195–205.
4. Bosch X, Guilabert A, Espinosa G, et al. Treatment of antineutrophil cytoplasmic antibody associated vasculitis: A systematic review. *JAMA*. 2007;298: 655–69.
5. Walters G, Willis NS, Craig JC. Interventions for renal vasculitis in adults. *Cochrane Database Syst Rev*. 2008:CD003232.
6. Walters GD, Willis NS, Craig JC. Interventions for renal vasculitis in adults. A systematic review. *BMC Nephrol*. 2010;11:12.

ADDITIONAL READING

Appel GB, Contreras G, Dooley MA, et al. Mycophenolate mofetil versus cyclophosphamide for induction treatment of lupus nephritis. *J Am Soc Nephrol*. 2009;20(5):1103–12.

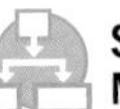

See Also (Topic, Algorithm, Electronic Media Element)

- National Heart Lung and Blood Institute Diseases and Conditions Index: Vasculitis: www.nhlbi.nih.gov/health/dci/Diseases/vas/vas_whatis.html
- The Vasculitis Foundation: www.vasculitisfoundation.org/

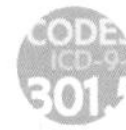

CODES

ICD9

- 446.0 Polyarteritis nodosa
- 446.1 Acute febrile mucocutaneous lymph node syndrome [MCLS]
- 447.6 Arteritis, unspecified

CLINICAL PEARLS

- Suspect a vasculitic process in patients with unexplained ischemia or multiorgan involvement, particularly presence of palpable purpura, glomerulonephritis, pulmonary-renal syndrome, intestinal ischemia, or mononeuritis multiplex.
- Look for clinically silent kidney involvement with serum creatinine and urinalysis with microscopy.
- Vasculitis tends to be "skip" lesions, so a generous specimen may be needed for diagnostic biopsy.
- A pitfall in vasculitis is the failure to exclude a primary process such as infection, thrombosis, or malignancy.

VENOUS INSUFFICIENCY ULCERS

Barbara Provo, MSN, APNP, CWOCN, FNP-BC
Irina Shakhnovich, MD, MS

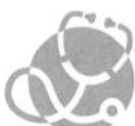

BASICS

- Venous insufficiency disorders include simple spider veins, varicose veins, and leg edema.
- Venous leg ulcers are the most serious consequence of venous insufficiency.
- ~500,000 people in the US have chronic venous ulcers, with an estimated treatment cost exceeding $3 billion per year.

DESCRIPTION

- Full-thickness skin defect with surrounding pigmentation and dermatitis
- Most frequently located in ankle region of lower leg ("gaiter region")
- Present for >30 days and fail to heal spontaneously
- May only have mild pain unless infected
- Other signs of chronic venous insufficiency include edema/brawny edema and chronic skin changes (i.e., hyperpigmentation and/or fibrosis).

EPIDEMIOLOGY

Up to 80% of leg ulcers are caused by venous disease; arterial disease accounts for 10–25%, which may coexist with venous disease.

Incidence

- Overall incidence of venous ulcers is 18 per 100,000 person-years, respectively.
- Women > Men (20.4 vs. 14.6 per 100,000 for venous ulcer); increased with age for both sexes

Prevalence

- Seen in about 1% of adult population
- Prevalence studies only available for Western countries.
- Point prevalence underestimates the extent of the disease because ulcers often recur.
- 70% of ulcers recur within 5 years of closure.

RISK FACTORS

- History of leg injury
- Obesity
- Congestive heart failure (CHF)
- History of deep venous thrombosis (DVT)
- Failure of calf pump (e.g., ankle fusion, inactivity) is a strong independent predictor of poorly healing wounds.
- Previous varicose vein surgery
- Family history

GENERAL PREVENTION

- Primary prevention (1)[A] after symptomatic DVT shown in randomized, controlled trials (RCTs): Prescribe compression hose to be used as soon as feasible for at least 2 years (≥20–30 mm Hg compression).
- Secondary prevention of recurrent ulceration includes compression, correction of the underlying problem, and surveillance. Circumstantial evidence from 2 RCTs showed those who stopped wearing compression were more likely to recur (2)[A].
- Since most ulcers develop following some type of trauma, avoidance of lower leg trauma may help to prevent ulceration.

PATHOPHYSIOLOGY

- In a diseased venous system, venous pressure in the deep system fails to fall with ambulation, causing venous hypertension.
- Venous hypertension comes from:
  - Venous obstruction
  - Incompetent venous valves in the deep or superficial system
  - Inadequate muscle contraction (e.g., arthritis, myopathies, neuropathies) so that the calf pump is ineffective
- Venous pressure transmitted to capillaries leading to venous hypertensive microangiopathy, extravasation of RBCs and proteins (especially fibrinogen)
- Increased RBC aggregation leads to reduced oxygen transport, slowed arteriolar circulation, and ischemia at the skin level, contributing to ulcers.
- Leukocytes aggregate to hypoxic areas and increase local inflammation.
- Factors promoting persistence of venous ulcers:
  - Prolonged chronic inflammation
  - Bacterial infection, critical colonization

COMMONLY ASSOCIATED CONDITIONS

Up to 50% of patients have allergic reactions to topical agents commonly used for treatment:

- Contact sensitivity was more common in patients with stasis dermatitis (62% vs. 38%).
- Avoid neomycin sulfate in particular (including triple antibiotic).

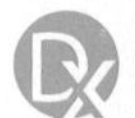

DIAGNOSIS

A diagnosis of venous reflux or obstruction must be established by an objective test beyond the routine clinical examination of the extremity.

HISTORY

- Family history of venous insufficiency and ulcers
- Recent trauma
- Nature of pain: Achy (better with leg elevation)
- Wound drainage
- Duration of wound and treatments already attempted, over the counter (OTC)
- History of DVTs (especially factor V Leiden mutation; strongly associated with ulceration)
- Family history of venous insufficiency and ulceration
- History of leg edema that improves at night. Edema that does not improve at night is more likely lymphedema.

PHYSICAL EXAM

- Look for evidence of venous insufficiency:
  - Pitting edema
  - Hemosiderin staining (red and brown spotty or diffuse pigment changes)
  - Stasis dermatitis
  - White lesions (atrophie blanche)
  - Lipodermatosclerosis ("bottle neck" narrowing in the lower leg from fibrosis and scarring)
- Look for evidence of significant lymphedema (i.e., dorsal foot or toe edema, edema that doesn't resolve overnight or with elevation). This may require referral for special comprehensive lymph therapy.
- Examine for palpable pulses.

ALERT

- Examine wound for:
  - Diameter and depth, to monitor wound healing rate
  - Presence of necrotic tissue
  - Presence of infection: Purulent material in the wound, spreading cellulitis, fever and chills
  - Extent and type of drainage
- Get initial and interim girth measurements (at ankle and midcalf) to monitor edema.
- Important to rule out poor arterial circulation:
  - Compression dressings cannot be used in patients with ankle brachial index (ABI) <0.8.

DIAGNOSTIC TESTS & INTERPRETATION

Lab

- Consider prothrombin time (PT)/international normalization ratio (INR) and partial thromboplastin time (PTT) if patient is anticoagulated.
- Consider biopsy of leg ulcers that fail to heal or have atypical features.
- Consider factor V Leiden mutation; strongly associated with venous ulcers
- Test for diabetes as necessary with fasting glucose

Imaging

Initial approach

Use duplex imaging to diagnose anatomic and hemodynamic abnormalities with venous insufficiency. It also will identify any DVT present.

Diagnostic Procedures/Surgery

- Check ABI for evidence of significant arterial disease.
- An ABI <0.8 is a relative contraindication to compression therapy.
- With concomitant severe arterial insufficiency, refer to a vascular surgeon for revascularization.

Pathological Findings

Strongly consider biopsy on wounds with atypical locations, failure to heal, or any suspicion of malignancy.

DIFFERENTIAL DIAGNOSIS

- Arterial insufficiency ulcer
- Neuropathic ulcer
- Malignancy
- Sickle cell ulcer
- Vasculitic ulcer
- Calciphylaxis
- Cryoglobulinemia
- Pyoderma gangrenosum
- Collagen vascular disease
- Leishmaniasis
- Cutaneous tuberculosis

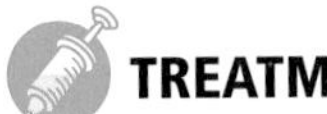

TREATMENT

MEDICATION

- No role for systemic drugs
- Effective compression management is the cornerstone of therapy (2)[A].
- Diuretics may help to reduce edema, but compression is the mainstay.
- Pentoxifylline 400 mg PO t.i.d., in addition to local care and compression, improves cure rates. There is some response even without compression. GI side effects are common (3).

ADDITIONAL TREATMENT

- Edema management: Reduce venous hypertension and improve venous return to reduce inflammation and pain and improve healing:
  - Compression therapy for edema management is the cornerstone of treatment for venous insufficiency ± ulcers (2)[A].
  - Short-stretch multilayer bandages are ideal for acute phase, until edema is stable, and the patient can be fitted for compression hose.
  - Long-term compression hose are helpful (have these fit once edema is reduced). Aim for a minimum pressure 20–30 mm Hg, preferably 30–40 mm Hg.
  - Elevation of legs to heart level for 30 minutes 3–4 times/d.
  - Exercise to strengthen calf muscle pump is also effective.
- Infection control:
  - Debride necrotic tissue.
  - Treat cellulitis (usually gram-positive bacteria) with bactericidal systemic antibiotics. Suspect local infection when there is pain or no improvement in the wound after 2 weeks of compression. Consider quantitative swab or tissue biopsy for culture.
  - Treat critical colonization with topical antimicrobials, especially cadexomer iodine (4)[A]. (Silver dressings are widely used, but definitive data are lacking.)

General Measures

Dressings: All wounds need some kind of a dressing underneath the compression system:

- Wound dressings: No single type of dressing proven superior (5)[B]
- Maintain moist wound environment: Not excessively wet or dry
- Wounds are often exudative until edema is decreased: Use absorptive dressings (calcium alginate or absorptive pads). Both super-absorbent diapers and female protection pads are cost-effective alternatives.
- Consider using barrier ointment/cream to prevent maceration of surrounding skin.
- If wound tends to be dry, use a hydrogel or a hydrocolloid dressing.

Issues for Referral

- With prominent toe or foot edema, consider lymphedema. Refer to certified lymphedema therapist (CLT).
- Refer to a wound clinic for complex or poorly healing ulcers.
- Use home health nurses to help with immobile patients needing frequent wrapping/dressing changes.

Additional Therapies

- For venous ulcers resistant to healing with wound care and compression, consider adding an intermittent compression pump 1–4 hr/d (6)[B].
- Encourage exercise (e.g., activation of calf muscle pump with ankle flexion and extension) with leg compression.
- Vacuum-assisted closure (VAC) dressings may be beneficial, but Cochrane Review indicates no clear benefit over optimal traditional wound care (7)[A].

COMPLEMENTARY AND ALTERNATIVE MEDICINE

- Chestnut seed extract (50 mg b.i.d.) is effective for venous insufficiency but not ulceration.
- Topical medicinal honey used on wounds shows no evidence of improved healing.

SURGERY/OTHER PROCEDURES

- Necrotic tissue impedes healing:
  - Consider sharp débridement.
  - Other methods include enzymatic ointments (collagenase), low-frequency ultrasound, and wet-to-dry dressings.
  - Avoid using collagenase with silver dressings because silver inactivates the enzyme.
- Allografts made of synthetic skin bilayer with living keratinocytes and fibroblasts improves healing at 6 months; but insufficient evidence to support use of autografts

IN-PATIENT CONSIDERATIONS

For those with acute significant cellulitis

Admission Criteria

Infected wounds requiring IV antibiotics, especially in diabetics

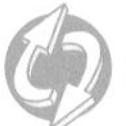

ONGOING CARE

- Venous insufficiency is a lifelong issue.
- After resolution of an ulcer, edema management must be maintained lifelong.

FOLLOW-UP RECOMMENDATIONS

When ulcers are nearly healed and edema is controlled, switch from compression bandages to compression hose:

- Insurance may not reimburse for compression hose unless an ulcer is present.
- Referral for hose fitting must be done while the ulcer is still present.

Patient Monitoring

Monitor the ulcer for healing by measuring its area. Expect at least 10% reduction every 2 weeks.

DIET

- Obese patients may benefit from weight loss.
- Low-salt diets help fluid retention.

PATIENT EDUCATION

- Patient education for understanding of underlying mechanism is important for long-term management:
  - Develop long-term plan for edema management and instruction on compression therapy.
  - Instruct the patient on topical wound therapy.
  - Teach early recognition and treatment of new ulcers or cellulitis.

PROGNOSIS

- Ulcers recur frequently. Early identification and immediate treatment are essential.
- Ongoing diligence, with edema control, avoiding infections, and avoiding trauma, are important.

REFERENCES

1. O'Brien JF, Grace PA, Perry IJ, et al. Randomized clinical trial and economic analysis of four-layer compression bandaging for venous ulcers. *Br J Surg*. 2003;90:794–8.
2. O'Meara S, Cullum NA, Nelson EA. Compression for venous leg ulcers. *Cochrane Database Syst Rev*. 2009:CD000265.
3. Jull A, Arroll B, Parag V, et al. Pentoxifylline for treating venous leg ulcers. *Cochrane Database Syst Rev*. 2007:CD001733.
4. O'Meara S, Al-Kurdi D, Ovington LG. Antibiotics and antiseptics for venous leg ulcers. *Cochrane Database Syst Rev*. 2008:CD003557.
5. Palfreyman SJ, Nelson EA, Lochiel R, et al. Dressings for healing venous leg ulcers. *Cochrane Database Syst Rev*. 2006;3:CD001103.
6. Kearon C, Kahn SR, Agnelli G, et al. Antithrombotic therapy for venous thromboembolic disease: American College of Chest Physicians Evidence-Based Clinical Practice Guidelines (8th Edition). *Chest*. 2008;133:454S–545S.
7. Ubbink DT, Westerbos SJ, Evans D, et al. Topical negative pressure for treating chronic wounds. *Cochrane Database Syst Rev*. 2008;CD001898.

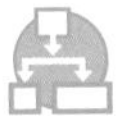

See Also (Topic, Algorithm, Electronic Media Element)

Algorithm: Leg Ulcer

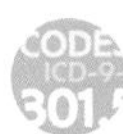

CODES

ICD9

- 459.81 Venous (peripheral) insufficiency, unspecified
- 707.8 Chronic ulcer of other specified sites

CLINICAL PEARLS

- Initial diagnostic workup should include venous duplex scan and arterial evaluation.
- Refer patients with ABI <0.8 to vascular surgery specialist.
- Refer patients with recurrent or poor healing venous ulcers to venous specialist.
- Compression is essential for edema management ± wounds.
- Treat critical colonization with topical antimicrobials (avoid neomycin).
- Make sure that the diagnosis is correct, and biopsy when in doubt.

VENTRICULAR SEPTAL DEFECT

Jessica E. Haley, MD
Brent J. Barber, MD

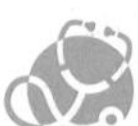

BASICS

DESCRIPTION

- Congenital or acquired defect of the interventricular septum that allows communication of blood between the left and the right ventricles
- Other than bicuspid aortic valve, this is the most common congenital heart malformation reported in infants and children. It also occurs as a complication of acute myocardial infarction (MI).
- Blood flow across the defect typically is left to right and depends on the size of the defect and the pulmonary vascular resistance (PVR).
- Prolonged shunting of blood can lead to pulmonary hypertension (HTN) and eventually reversal of flow across the defect, as well as to cyanosis (Eisenmenger complex).
- System(s) affected: Cardiovascular

Geriatric Considerations

In this population, almost entirely associated with MI

Pediatric Considerations

Congenital

ALERT

- Pregnancy may exacerbate symptoms and signs of a ventricular septal defect (VSD).
- Tolerated during pregnancy if the septal defect is small
- May be associated with an increased risk of preeclampsia in women with an unrepaired VSD (1)

EPIDEMIOLOGY

Incidence

- Predominant sex: No gender predilection
- Males are affected more than females if associated with MI.
- Occurs in ~2 of 1,000 live births (2)

Prevalence

In the US:

- Acute MI: Estimated to complicate 1–3%
- Lowered prevalence in adults due to spontaneous closure of defects

RISK FACTORS

- Congenital:
  - Risk of sibling being affected: 4.2%
  - Risk of offspring being affected: 4%
- Postacute MI:
  - First MI
  - Limited coronary artery disease
  - HTN
  - Most frequent within first week after MI
  - Occurs in 1–3% of MIs, most commonly after anterior MI

Genetics

Multifactorial etiology; autosomal-dominant and -recessive transmissions have been reported.

GENERAL PREVENTION

For adults, avoid risk factors for MI and obtain evaluation before pregnancy.

ETIOLOGY

- Congenital
- In adults, secondary to MI

COMMONLY ASSOCIATED CONDITIONS

- Congenital:
  - Tetralogy of Fallot
  - Aortic valvular deformities, especially aortic insufficiency and bicuspid aortic valve
  - Down syndrome (trisomy 21), endocardial cushion defect
  - Transposition of great arteries
  - Coarctation of aorta
  - Tricuspid atresia
  - Truncus arteriosus
  - Patent ductus arteriosus
  - Atrial septal defect
  - Pulmonic stenosis
  - Subaortic stenosis
- Adult: Coronary artery disease

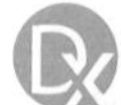

DIAGNOSIS

HISTORY

- Depends on the degree of shunting across the defect; may be completely asymptomatic with small defects
- Respiratory distress, tachypnea, tachycardia
- Diaphoresis with feeds, poor weight gain in infants

PHYSICAL EXAM

- Small defect:
  - Harsh holosystolic murmur loudest at left lower sternal border
  - Detected after pulmonary vascular resistance drops at 4–8 weeks of life
- Moderate defect:
  - Harsh holosystolic murmur at left lower sternal border associated with a thrill
  - Forceful apical impulse with lateral displacement
  - Increased intensity of P_2
  - Diastolic rumble at apex due to increased flow across the mitral valve
- Large defect:
  - Holosystolic murmur heard throughout the precordium with diastolic rumble at apex, although large defects may have little or no murmur initially
  - If congestive heart failure (CHF) exists: Tachycardia, tachypnea, and hepatomegaly
  - If pulmonary HTN exists: Cyanosis with exertion
  - If Eisenmenger complex is present: Cyanosis and clubbing

DIAGNOSTIC TESTS & INTERPRETATION

Lab

Initial lab tests

- A 12-lead ECG may suggest severity of VSD. Initially, left ventricular hypertrophy and left atrial enlargement may be evident. With pulmonary HTN, right ventricular hypertrophy and right atrial enlargement may be seen.
- After surgical repair, right bundle-branch block is common.

Follow-Up & Special Considerations

Weight and hematocrit check

Imaging

Initial approach

- A chest x-ray (CXR) may demonstrate increased pulmonary vascularity and/or cardiomegaly.
- A 2D echocardiogram for visualization of location and size of defect
- Color-flow Doppler for direction and velocity of ventricular septal defect jet; may be used to estimate right ventricular pressure

Follow-Up & Special Considerations

Cardiac catheterization performed occasionally for perioperative planning or assessing need for closure of defect

Diagnostic Procedures/Surgery

- Cardiac catheterization (left and right sides of heart) can confirm the diagnosis, document number of defects, quantify ratio of pulmonary blood flow to systemic blood flow (Qp/Qs), and determine pulmonary vascular resistance.
- Demonstration of an oxygen saturation step-up from the right atrium to the distal pulmonary artery

Pathological Findings

- Congenital VSD (4 major anatomic types):
  - Membranous (70%)
  - Muscular (20%)
  - Atrioventricular canal type (5%)
  - Supracristal (5%; higher in Asians)
- Post-MI VSD predominantly involves muscular septum.

DIFFERENTIAL DIAGNOSIS

- Any defect with left-to-right shunt, such as patent ductus arteriosus, atrial septal defect
- Children: Tetralogy of Fallot
- Adults: Mitral regurgitation

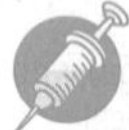

TREATMENT

- Start diuretic therapy if overload signs present.
- Minimize IV fluids.
- Consider ACE inhibitor and/or digoxin.
- Nasogastric feeds
- Correct anemia via iron supplementation or a possible RBC transfusion.

MEDICATION

First Line

- Endocarditis antibiotic prophylaxis is no longer recommended for most VSDs. Antibiotic prophylaxis is recommended for VSDs associated with complex cyanotic heart disease, during the first 6 months after surgical repair, or for residual VSDs located near the patch following surgery (3).
- Pediatric: Medications aim to control pulmonary edema, decrease work of breathing, and allow for growth:
  - Furosemide: 1–2 mg/kg PO/IV once to twice a day (4)[A]
  - Digoxin: Infants <2 years of age: 10 mg/kg/d PO divided b.i.d.; children, 2–10 years of age: 5–10 mg/kg/d PO divided b.i.d.; children >10 years of age: 2–5 mg/kg/d PO divided b.i.d.
  - Spironolactone: 1–2 mg/kg/d divided b.i.d.
  - Captopril: 0.1–0.4 mg/kg PO given q6–24h (maximum 6 mg/kg/24 hr)
- Adults: Digoxin and diuretics may be beneficial in some circumstances.
- Side effects:
  - Drugs that increase systemic vascular resistance may increase left-to-right shunting and cause signs and symptoms of pulmonary overcirculation.
  - Hypotension

Second Line

- Surgical closure is generally indicated if the pulmonic-to-systemic flow is >2:1 or with poorly controlled pulmonary overcirculation despite maximal medical and dietary interventions.
- If an infant with a VSD has persistent pulmonary HTN, surgical repair generally is recommended prior to 6 months of age even if patient is asymptomatic.
- In the post-MI setting, afterload reduction, inotropic support, intra-aortic balloon pump, and left ventricular assist device may be used to stabilize the patient prior to surgery.

ADDITIONAL TREATMENT

General Measures

- Appropriate health care
- Outpatient, until surgical repair is indicated
- Inpatient in setting of acute MI
- Inpatient for treatment of severe CHF

Issues for Referral

Close follow-up of a congenital VSD is necessary until primary intracardiac repair is performed to ensure that significant pulmonary HTN does not develop.

Additional Therapies

- Caloric requirements up to 150 kcal/kg/d for adequate weight gain
- Treatment of iron-deficiency anemia to increase oxygen-carrying capacity

SURGERY/OTHER PROCEDURES

- Surgical correction with either a VSD patch or repair is commonly utilized. Postsurgical outcomes for isolated VSD are excellent. Complications are rare and include reoperation for residual VSD, extended hospital stay, arrhythmias, valve injury, depressed ventricular function, and heart block (5).
- Percutaneous transcatheter device closure of muscular defects is an option (6). The closure of membranous defects with septal occluders is currently under research protocols. Complications include embolization of the device, residual defects, and complete heart block.
- Periventricular device closure of isolated VSDs without cardiopulmonary bypass is feasible and safe under transesophageal echocardiographic (TEE) guidance. However, further evaluation of intermediate and long-term results is necessary.

IN-PATIENT CONSIDERATIONS

Initial Stabilization

- Stabilize airway.
- Reduce temperature stress.

Admission Criteria

- Failure to thrive
- Pulmonary overcirculation/CHF

Nursing

Frequent vital sign monitoring; daily weight and calorie counts

Discharge Criteria

CHF stabilization, weight gain, or successful repair

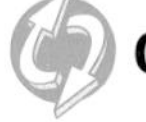

ONGOING CARE

FOLLOW-UP RECOMMENDATIONS

- Small VSDs without evidence of CHF or pulmonary HTN generally can be followed every 1–5 years after the neonatal period.
- Moderate to large VSDs require more frequent follow-up.
- Potential complications of VSDs include right ventricular outflow obstruction and aortic valve prolapse.

Patient Monitoring

- Physical growth and development monitoring
- Influenza vaccine for children >6 months of age
- Palivizumab to children <2 years of age with hemodynamically significant lesions

DIET

- Low-sodium in heart failure
- High-calorie in failure to thrive

PATIENT EDUCATION

- No activity restriction in absence of pulmonary HTN
- Parents need support and instructions for prevention of complications until the child is ready for surgery.

PROGNOSIS

- Congenital:
  - Course is variable depending on the size of the VSD
  - Small VSD: 25–45% will close spontaneously by age 3 years. Muscular defects are more likely to close spontaneously.
  - Large VSD: CHF or failure to thrive in infancy necessitating surgical repair
  - 20-year survival rate for isolated VSD: 98.3% (7)
  - Progressive pulmonary vascular disease and pulmonary HTN are the most feared complications of VSD caused by left-to-right shunting and may eventually lead to reversal of the shunt (Eisenmenger complex). Death usually occurs in the fourth decade of life if untreated.
- Post-MI:
  - With medical management alone, 80–90% mortality in the first 2 weeks
  - Prognosis worse with inferior MI compared with anterior MI

COMPLICATIONS

- CHF
- Aortic insufficiency
- Sudden death
- Hemoptysis
- Cerebral abscess
- Paradoxical emboli
- Cardiogenic shock
- Heart block rarely may accompany surgical closure.
- Pulmonary HTN

REFERENCES

1. Yap S-C, Drenthen W, Pieper P. Pregnancy outcome in women with repaired versus unrepaired isolated ventricular septal defect. *BJOG*. 2010;117:683–9.
2. Mitchell SC, Korones SB, Berendes HW. Congenital heart disease in 56,109 births: Incidence and natural history. *Circulation*. 1971;43:323–32.
3. Wilson W. Prevention of infective endocarditis. Guidelines From the American Heart Association. A guideline From the American Heart Association Rheumatic Fever, Endocarditis, and Kawasaki Disease Committee, Council on Cardiovascular Disease in the Young, and the Council on Clinical Cardiology, Council on Cardiovascular Surgery and Anesthesia, and the Quality of Care and Outcomes Research Interdisciplinary Working Group. *Circulation*. 2007;116(15):1736–54.
4. Faris R, Flather MD, Purcell H. Diuretics for heart failure. *Cochrane Database Sys Rev*. 2006: CD003838.
5. Scully BB, Morales DL, Zafar F, et al. Current expectations for surgical repair of isolated ventricular septal defects. *Ann Thorac Surg*. 2010;89:544.
6. Knauth AL, Lock JE, Perry SB. Transcatheter device closure of congenital and postoperative residual ventricular septal defects. *Circulation*. 2004;110: 501–7.
7. Tennant PW, Pearce MS, Bythell M, et al. 20-year survival of children born with congenital anomalies: A population-based study. *Lancet*. 2010;375:649.

ADDITIONAL READING

- Chang RK, Chen AY, Klitzner TS. Factors associated with age at operation for children with congenital heart disease. *Pediatrics*. 2000;105:1073–81.
- Mehta AV, Chidambaram B. Ventricular septal defect in the first year of life. *Am J Cardiol*. 1992;70:364–6.
- Patanè F, Centofanti P, Zingarelli E. Potential role of the Impella Recover left ventricular assist device in the management of postinfarct ventricular septal defect. *J Thorac Cardiovasc Surg*. 2009;137: 1288–9.
- Quansheng X, Silin P, Zhongyun Z. Minimally invasive perventricular device closure of an isolated perimembranous ventricular septal defect with a newly designed delivery system: Preliminary experience. *J Thorac Cardiovasc Surg*. 2009;137: 556–9.

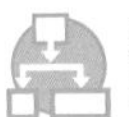

See Also (Topic, Algorithm, Electronic Media Element)

Down Syndrome; Myocardial Infarction, Non–ST-Segment Elevation (NSTEMI); Myocardial Infarction, ST- Segment Elevation (STEMI); Tetralogy of Fallot

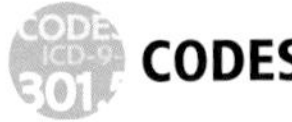

CODES

ICD9

745.4 Ventricular septal defect

CLINICAL PEARLS

- A loud 2–3/6 low-pitched harsh holosystolic murmur at the left lower sternal border is typical.
- A diastolic rumble at the apex indicates moderate-to-large VSD or Qp:Qs > 2:1.
- Disappearance of the murmur could be secondary to spontaneous closure of the defect or the development of pulmonary HTN.
- Development of a new murmur of semilunar valve insufficiency should be further evaluated. Pulmonary regurgitation may occur as PVR increases, and the development of aortic regurgitation usually will require early surgery.

V

VERTIGO

Michele L. Matthews, PharmD, CPE, RPh
Kristy Kedian Brown, DO

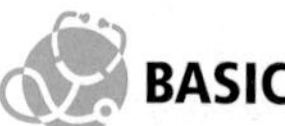

BASICS

DESCRIPTION

- Sensation of movement ("room spinning") when no movement is actually occurring; results from peripheral or central causes, or may be induced by medications or anxiety disorders
- Important to distinguish between vertigo and presyncope (patient feels lightheaded; vision and hearing may become obscured)
- System(s) affected: Nervous
- Synonym(s): Dizziness; Acute vestibular neuronitis; Labyrinthitis; Benign paroxysmal positional vertigo (BPPV)

EPIDEMIOLOGY

Incidence

- Accounts for 54% of cases of dizziness reported in primary care; >90% of these patients are diagnosed with peripheral causes, such as BPPV
- Predominant sex: Female = Male; women are more likely to experience central causes, particularly vertiginous migraine

Geriatric Considerations

Patients who are elderly and have risk factors for cerebrovascular disease (CVD) are more likely to experience central causes.

Prevalence

- Ranges from 5–10% within the general population
- Lifetime prevalence for BPPV is 2.4%

RISK FACTORS

- History of migraines
- History of CVD or risk factors for CVD
- Use of ototoxic medications
- Trauma or barotrauma
- Perilymphatic fistula
- Heavy weight bearing
- Psychosocial stress/depression
- Exposure to toxins

Genetics

Family history of CVD or migraines may indicate higher risk of central causes.

GENERAL PREVENTION

- Precautions to avoid injuries from falls that may occur secondary to imbalance
- If due to motion sickness, consider pretreatment with anticholinergics such as scopolamine

PATHOPHYSIOLOGY

Dysfunction of the rotational velocity sensors of the inner ear results in asymmetric central processing. This is related to the combination of sensory disturbance of motion and malfunction of the central vestibular apparatus.

ETIOLOGY

- Peripheral causes: Acute labyrinthitis, acute vestibular neuronitis, BPPV, herpes-zoster oticus, cholesteatoma, Ménière disease, otosclerosis
- Central causes: Cerebellar tumor, CVD, migraine, multiple sclerosis
- Drug causes: Psychotropic agents (antipsychotics, antidepressants, anxiolytics, anticonvulsants, mood stabilizers), aspirin, aminoglycosides, furosemide, amiodarone
- Other causes: Cervical, psychological

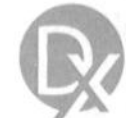

DIAGNOSIS

HISTORY

- Determine whether true vertigo exists vs. other causes of dizziness by asking the patient if he or she feels lightheaded or sees the world spinning around during a dizzy spell (1). Spinning is indicative of true vertigo.
- Ask about the presence of the following symptoms: Dizziness, rotary illusions, nystagmus, nausea and vomiting, hearing loss, diaphoresis, pain, neurologic symptoms (e.g., ataxia)
- Factors that may help to distinguish between peripheral and central causes:
  - Timing and duration:
    - Seconds–minutes: Peripheral
    - Minutes–hours: Peripheral or central
    - Days: Peripheral or central
    - Weeks: Central or psychological
  - Provoking factors:
    - Changes in head position: Peripheral or central
    - Spontaneous episodes: Peripheral or central
    - Recent upper viral respiratory infection: Peripheral
    - Stress: Central or psychological
    - Immunosuppression: Peripheral
    - Changes in ear pressure: Peripheral
  - Associated symptoms:
    - Rotary illusions with nausea and vomiting: Peripheral
    - Horizontal and rotational nystagmus: Peripheral
    - Horizontal, vertical, or rotational nystagmus: Central
    - Hearing loss: Peripheral
    - Neurologic symptoms: Central
- Obtain medical and medication history:
  - Recent use of ototoxic medications (e.g., aminoglycosides)
  - History of alcohol, nicotine, and caffeine use
  - Sexual history
  - History of CVD or risk factors for CVD

PHYSICAL EXAM

- Neurologic (1): Cranial nerves for signs of palsies, nystagmus
- Balance:
  - Peripheral: Mild to moderate, able to walk
  - Central: Severe, unable to walk
- Dix-Hallpike maneuver (PPV 83%, NPV 52%):
  - If induced symptoms subside after repeated maneuvers, consider peripheral causes.
  - If induced symptoms do not subside, consider central causes.
- Head and neck (1): Tympanic membranes:
  - Vesicles: Herpes-zoster oticus
  - Cholesteatoma
- Cardiovascular (1): Orthostatic changes in BP, dehydration or autonomic dysfunction

DIAGNOSTIC TESTS & INTERPRETATION

Lab

Initial lab tests

Consider CBC/chemistry panel in the absence of clinical findings pointing to specific cause. Not routinely necessary.

Imaging

Initial approach

Consider MRI in the presence of other neurologic symptoms, risk factors for CVD, or progressive unilateral hearing loss

Diagnostic Procedures/Surgery

Audiometry if acoustic neuroma or Ménière disease is suspected

DIFFERENTIAL DIAGNOSIS

- Acoustic neuroma
- Anxiety disorder
- BPPV
- Cerebellar degeneration, hemorrhage, or tumor
- Labyrinthitis or labyrinthine concussion
- Ménière disease
- Multiple sclerosis
- Perilymphatic fistula
- Syphilis
- Vascular ischemia
- Vertiginous migraine
- Vestibular neuronitis or ototoxicity

TREATMENT

- Epley maneuver for BPPV (2)[A]
- Modified Epley maneuver for BPPV (3)[B]
- Vestibular exercises for acute vestibular neuronitis (3)[B]
- Low-salt diet and diuretics for Ménière disease (3)[B]
- Migraine prophylaxis, migraine abortive medications, and vestibular exercises for vertiginous migraines (3)[B]
- SSRIs when associated with anxiety disorders (3)[B]
- Vestibular-suppressant medications for symptom relief in acute vestibular neuronitis (3,4)[C]

MEDICATION

Avoid use of medication in mild cases. Use for acute phase only (few days at most) as longer-term use may impair adaptation/compensation by the brain. Medications not recommended for BPPV:

- Meclizine: 12.5–50 mg PO q4–8h (3,4)[C]
- Dimenhydrinate: 25–100 mg PO, IM, or IV q4–8h (3,4)[C]:
  - Precautions: Concomitant use of CNS depressants, prostatic hyperplasia, glaucoma
  - Adverse effects: Sedation, xerostomia
  - Interactions: CNS depressants
  - Prochlorperazine: 5–10 mg PO or IM q6–8h; 25 mg rectally q12h; 5–10 mg by slow IV over 2 minutes (3,4)[C]:
    - Contraindications: Blood dyscrasias, age <2 years, severe hypotension
    - Precautions: Children with acute illness, glaucoma, history of breast cancer, impaired cardiovascular function, pregnancy, prostatic hyperplasia
    - Adverse effects: Sedation, xerostomia, hypotension, extrapyramidal effects
    - Interactions: Phenothiazines, tricyclic antidepressants
  - Metoclopramide: 5–10 mg PO q6h, 5–10 mg slow IV q6h:
    - Contraindications: Concomitant use of drugs with extrapyramidal effects, seizure disorders
    - Precautions: History of depression, Parkinson disease, hypertension
    - Adverse effects: Sedation, fluid retention, constipation
    - Interactions: Linezolid, cyclosporine, digoxin, levodopa
  - Benzodiazepines (3,4)[C]:
    - Diazepam: 2–10 mg PO or IV q4–8h
    - Lorazepam: 0.5–2 mg PO, IM, or IV q4–8h:
      - Contraindications: Acute angle-closure glaucoma, age <6 months
      - Precautions: Concomitant use of CNS depressants, hepatic insufficiency, pregnancy
      - Adverse effects: Sedation, respiratory depression, hypotension
      - Interactions: CNS depressants

Geriatric Considerations

Use vestibular-suppressant medications with caution due to increased risk of falls and urinary retention.

Pregnancy Considerations

Meclizine and dimenhydrinate are pregnancy category B.

ADDITIONAL TREATMENT

General Measures

- Provide an explanation and offer assurance to avoid anxiety that may exacerbate symptoms.
- Treatments depend on cause:
  - BPPV: Epley maneuver or modified Epley maneuver (2)[A]
  - Vestibular neuronitis and labyrinthitis:
    - Vestibular-suppressant medications (3,4)[C]
    - Vestibular rehabilitation exercises (3)[B]
  - Ménière disease (see separate topic):
    - Low-salt diet (<1–2 g/d) (3)[B]
    - Diuretics such as hydrochlorothiazide (3)[B]
  - Vascular ischemia: Prevention of future events through BP reduction, lipid lowering, smoking cessation, antiplatelet therapy, and anticoagulation if necessary
  - Vertiginous migraines: Dietary and lifestyle modifications, vestibular rehabilitation exercises, prophylactic and migraine abortive medications (3)[B]
  - Drug-induced vertigo: Discontinue causative agent
  - Psychological: SSRIs (3)[B]

Issues for Referral

Consider referral to otolaryngologist, ENT specialist, vestibular rehabilitation therapist, or neurologist if patient requires further care.

Additional Therapies

- Epley maneuver or modified Epley maneuver for BPPV to displace calcium deposits in the semicircular canals (2)[A]:
  - Effective for short-term symptomatic improvement and for converting patient from positive to negative Dix-Hallpike maneuver
  - Video demonstrations of technique available at www.youtube.com
  - Contraindications: Carotid stenosis, unstable cardiac disease, severe neck disease
- Vestibular rehabilitation exercises (3)[B]: Ball toss, lying-to-standing, target-change, thumb-tracking, tightrope, walking turns

ONGOING CARE

FOLLOW-UP RECOMMENDATIONS

Balance exercises should be adhered to for symptom improvement and return to normal activities of daily living (ADLs).

Patient Monitoring

After 1–2 weeks, assess for the following:

- Recurrence of symptoms
- New-onset symptoms
- Medication-related adverse effects
- Relief from vestibular rehabilitation exercises

DIET

- Restricted salt intake for Ménière disease
- Dietary modifications for vertiginous migraine

PATIENT EDUCATION

- Reduce sodium intake (Ménière disease).
- Avoid triggers such as caffeine or alcohol (vertiginous migraine).

PROGNOSIS

Dependent upon diagnosis and response to treatment

COMPLICATIONS

- Anxiety
- Depression
- Disability
- Injuries from falls

REFERENCES

1. Labuguen RH. Initial evaluation of vertigo. *Am Fam Physician*. 2006;73:244–51.
2. Hilton M, Pinder D. The Epley (canalith repositioning) maneuver for benign paroxysmal positional vertigo. *Cochrane Database Syst Rev*. 2007;(3):CD003162.
3. Swartz R, Longwell P. Treatment of vertigo. *Am Fam Physician*. 2005;71:1115–22.
4. Hain TC, Uddin M. Pharmacological treatment of vertigo. *CNS Drugs*. 2003;17:85–100.

ADDITIONAL READING

- Bhattacharyya N, Baugh RF, Orvidas L. Clinical practice guideline: Benign paroxysmal positional vertigo. *Otolaryngol Head Neck Surg*. 2008;139: S47–81.
- Fife TD, Iverson DJ, Lempert T. Practice parameter: Therapies for benign paroxysmal positional vertigo (an evidence-based review): Report of the Quality Standards Subcommittee of the American Academy of Neurology. *Neurology*. 2008;70:2067–74.

See Also (Topic, Algorithm, Electronic Media Element)

- Ménière Disease, Motion Sickness
- Algorithm: Vertigo

CODES

ICD9

- 386.2 Vertigo of central origin
- 386.11 Benign paroxysmal positional vertigo
- 386.19 Other peripheral vertigo

CLINICAL PEARLS

- Risk factors that should be assessed in a patient with suspected vertigo include history of migraines, history of CVD or risk factors for CVD, use of ototoxic medications, trauma or barotrauma, perilymphatic fistula, heavy weight bearing, psychosocial stress, and exposure to toxins.
- The Dix-Hallpike maneuver is performed by rapidly moving the patient from a sitting position to the supine position with the head turned 45° to the right. After waiting ~20–30 seconds, observing for nystagmus, the patient is returned to the sitting position. If no nystagmus was observed, the procedure then is repeated on the left side. The presence of nystagmus indicates a positive test, implying that peripheral causes should be investigated.
- The Epley maneuver is recommended for the treatment of BPPV; this maneuver repositions calcium debris within the semicircular canals to provide relief from vertigo; a modified version of the maneuver can be performed at home. Medications are not recommended for BPPV.

VERTIGO, BENIGN PAROXYSMAL POSITIONAL (BPPV)

Janet O. Helminski, PT, PhD
Mark A. Sanders, DO, JD, MPH, LLM, FACOFP
Tinh Le, DO, MBA

BASICS

DESCRIPTION

BPPV is a mechanical disorder of the inner ear characterized by a brief period of vertigo experienced when the position of the patient's head is changed relative to gravity. The brief period of vertigo is caused by abnormal stimulation of one or more of the 3 semicircular canals of the inner ear, with the posterior canal most commonly affected. BPPV is the single most common cause of vertigo (26% of all cases) (1).

EPIDEMIOLOGY

- The lifetime prevalence of BPPV is 2.4% and the 1-year incidence is 0.6% (2). The age of onset is most commonly between the fifth and seventh decades of life, and the incidence of BPPV increases with each decade of life, peaking in the sixth and seventh (2). BPPV affects women more than men (2).
- BPPV affects the quality of life of elderly patients and is associated with reduced activities of daily living scores, falls, and depression (3).

PATHOPHYSIOLOGY

In BPPV, calcite particles (otoconia) that normally weight the sensory membrane of the maculae become dislodged and settle into the canals, changing the dynamics of the canals. Reorientation of the canal relative to gravity causes the otoconia to move to the lowest part of the canal, creating a drag on the endolymph and activating the primary afferent sensory apparatus. This results in the generation of nystagmus and the associated sensation of vertigo.

ETIOLOGY

BPPV may be idiopathic (50%), posttraumatic (17%), and associated with viral neurolabyrinthitis (17%) (4).

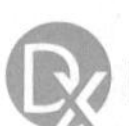

DIAGNOSIS

The diagnosis is established based on history and findings on positional testing (5,6). Positional tests place the plane of the canal being tested into the plane parallel with gravity.

HISTORY

- Brief episodes of vertigo associated with:
  - Rolling over in bed
  - Getting out of bed
  - Looking up (referred to as top shelf syndrome)
  - Bending forward
  - Quick head movements
- Patients may also complain of lightheadedness or feeling "off balance." Frequently patients complain of nausea and, if severe enough, vomiting.

PHYSICAL EXAM

- The Dix-Hallpike Test (DHT) is used to diagnosis BPPV (5,6)[A]. The test provokes the characteristic nystagmus associated with the symptoms of vertigo.
- To perform the DHT, the patient is positioned in long-sitting on the examination table with the knees extended. If testing the right posterior canal, the head is rotated 45° to the right. The patient is then lowered into supine with the head 20° below the horizontal, over the edge of the examination table. The position is maintained for 45 seconds. The patient is then returned to the seated position. The procedure is repeated toward the left.
- For each position, the clinician notes the direction of the fast phase of the nystagmus and the latency and duration of the nystagmus. For posterior canal BPPV, in the head hanging position, the superior pole of the eye beats and rotates toward the lower-most ear, the involved ear. On return to the seated position, the eye reverts and the rotation reverses direction. The latency of onset of nystagmus is 1–45 seconds, and the duration is usually <1 minute. The nystagmus fatigues (reduction in the severity of symptoms) with repeated positioning. For anterior canal BPPV, in the head hanging position, the eye will beat toward and rotate toward the involved ear. For lateral canal BPPV, a directional changing positional nystagmus is observed. The eye will beat horizontally toward the lower-most ear in the head left and right position or will beat away from the floor.
- Alternative positional tests are available if the patient is unable to assume the test positions (side-lying test) or if the lateral canal is involved (supine roll test).
- No further testing is indicated unless the diagnosis is uncertain or there are additional symptoms and signs unrelated to BPPV that warrant testing (5).

DIFFERENTIAL DIAGNOSIS

- Orthostatic hypotension and other disorders that cause low BP. Symptoms usually occur when the patient stands up.
- Damage to the brain stem or cerebellum can cause positional vertigo, but is accompanied by other neurologic signs and usually has a different pattern of nystagmus.
- Low spinal fluid pressure may cause positional symptoms that are worse when lying down.
- Migraine-associated vertigo

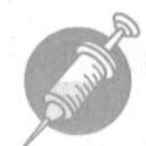

TREATMENT

- The Canalith Repositioning Procedure (CRP) or Epley maneuver is effective in the treatment of posterior canal BPPV (5,6)[A]. A number of illustrative videos are available on www.youtube.com. The clinician moves the patient through a series of positions. With each position, the otoconia settles to the lowest part of the canal. The debris is moved around the arc of the canal into the vestibule. In randomized controlled trials, the average short-term success rate of the CRP following 1 treatment session is 80 ± 9% (6)[A]. Contraindications are carotid stenosis, unstable cardiac disease, and severe neck disease. If the CRP is ineffective, the self-administered CRP is performed at home (5,6)[A]. The patient performs the CRP on the bed over the edge of the pillow. Better outcomes are achieved with a combination of the CRP + the self-administered CPR (6).

- CRP illustrated for right PC-BPPV (see figure on Web site). The clinician moves the patient through a series of 4 provoking positions, starting with the placement of the involved canal in the head-hanging position of the DHT. The head is then rotated 90° toward the uninvolved side. Maintaining 45° of head rotation, the patient is rolled onto the uninvolved side with the head slightly elevated from the supporting surface. The patient then sits up. Each position is maintained for a minimum of 45 seconds. The procedure is repeated 3 times.
- Postmaneuver activity restrictions are often advocated (6). For 1 week following the maneuver, patients should avoid lying on the involved side, use 2 pillows to sleep slightly elevated, and avoid up-and-down movements of the head.
- Vestibular suppressant medications are not recommended for treatment of BPPV, other than for the short-term management of vegetative symptoms (5)[C]. Antiemetics such as ondansetron (Zofran) may be considered for prophylaxis for patients who have had severe nausea or vomiting with the DHT. Vestibular suppressants such as benzodiazepines and antihistamines should be avoided because they may suppress nystagmus during the DHT and treatment and prevent accommodation of the brain.
- Consider a referral to a specialist if BPPV is unresponsive to treatment or if the patient is diagnosed with atypical BPPV involving the anterior or lateral canal. Other maneuvers are available for treatment of typical and atypical BPPV. Consider referring to a physical therapist, ENT specialist, or neurologist.

ADDITIONAL TREATMENT

- Brandt-Daroff exercises are not as effective as the self-administered CRP (6). At 1 week, the average success rate for the Brandt-Daroff exercise is 23–24% compared to 90% for the self-administered CRP (6).
- Surgical intervention is rarely indicated, except for refractory BPPV, and includes posterior canal occlusion and singular neuroectomy.

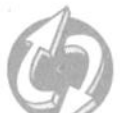

ONGOING CARE

FOLLOW-UP RECOMMENDATIONS

The patient should follow up within a week after treatment to ensure resolution.

PROGNOSIS

- BPPV may effectively be treated with particle repositioning maneuvers (5,6).
- 30% of patients diagnosed with BPPV will spontaneously resolve within 1 week.
- BPPV often recurs. Of patients treated successfully, 25% redevelop BPPV within 1 year and 44% redevelop BPPV within 2 years.

COMPLICATIONS

During the maneuvers, a canal conversion may occur. The debris from the canal being treated may reflux into another canal.

REFERENCES

1. Baloh RW, Sloane PD, Honrubia V. Quantitative vestibular function testing in elderly patients with dizziness. *Ear Nose Throat J*. 1989;68(12): 935–9.
2. von Brevern M, Radtke A, Lezius F, et al. Epidemiology of benign paroxysmal positional vertigo: A population based study. *J Neurol Neurosurg Psychiatry*. 2007;78(7):710–5.
3. Oghalai JS, Manolidis S, Barth JL, et al. Unrecognized benign paroxysmal positional vertigo in elderly patients. *Otolaryngol Head Neck Surg*. 2000;122(5);630–4.
4. Baloh RW, Honrubia V, Jacobson K. Benign positional vertigo: Clinical and oculographic features in 240 cases. *Neurology*. 1987;37(3): 371–8.
5. Bhattacharyya N, Baugh RF, Orvidas L, et al. Clinical practice guideline: Benign paroxysmal positional vertigo. *Otolaryngol Head Neck Surg*. 2008;139(5 Suppl 4):S47–81.
6. Helminski JO, Zee DS, Janssen I, et al. Effectiveness of particle repositioning manuevers in the treatment of benign paroxysmal positional vertigo: A systematic review. *Phys Ther*. 2010;90(5):663–78.

ADDITIONAL READING

- Epley JM. The canalith repositioning procedure: For treatment of benign paroxysmal positional vertigo. *Otolaryngol Head Neck Surg*. 1992;107(3): 399–404.
- Fife TD, Iverson DJ, Lempert T, et al. Practice parameter: Therapies for benign paroxysmal positional vertigo (an evidence-based review): Report of the Quality Standards Subcommittee of the American Academy of Neurology. *Neurology*. 2008;70(22):2067–74.
- Radtke A, von Brevern M, Tiel-Wilck K, et al. Self-treatment of benign paroxysmal positional vertigo: Semont maneuver vs Epley procedure. *Neurology*. 2004;63(1):150–2.

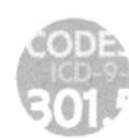

CODES

ICD9

386.11 Benign paroxysmal positional vertigo

CLINICAL PEARLS

- The diagnosis of BPPV is based on history and findings on positional testing (Dix-Hallpike test)
- BPPV may effectively be treated with particle-repositioning maneuvers.
- Vestibular suppressant medications are not recommended for treatment of BPPV, other than for the short-term management of symptoms.

VITAMIN B_{12} DEFICIENCY

Jennifer Gao, MD
Edward Feller, MD

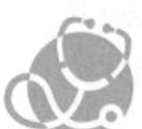

BASICS

Vitamin deficiency related to inadequate intake or inability to absorb cobalamin (vitamin B_{12})

DESCRIPTION

Normal B_{12} absorption:

- B_{12} present in animal-source foods (meat, fish, eggs, milk) and foods fortified with B_{12}
- Dietary vitamin B_{12} (cobalamin) bound to food cleaved by acids in stomach and bound to R-proteins
- Duodenal proteases cleave B_{12} from R-proteins.
- In duodenum, B_{12} binds to intrinsic factor (IF) secreted by gastric parietal cells.
- B_{12}-IF complex absorbed by terminal ileum into portal circulation.
- Body's B_{12} stored in liver = 50%:
  - B_{12} secreted into bile from liver recycled via enterohepatic circulation
  - Delay 5–10 years from onset of B_{12} deficiency to clinical symptoms due to hepatic stores and enterohepatic circulation
- Typical Western diet: 3–30 mcg daily (1):
  - Recommend 2.4 mcg/d for adults and 2.6–2.8 mcg/d during pregnancy.

EPIDEMIOLOGY

Prevalence

- Endemic area: Northern Europe, including Scandinavia
- Prevalence 5–20% in developed countries (1):
  - 12% in elderly living in community
  - 30–40% in elderly in institutions, sick, or malnourished
  - 5% patients in tertiary reference hospitals
- Prevalence by age group (2):
  - 20–39 years old: Prevalence 3%
  - 40–59 years old: Prevalence 4%
  - >70 years old: Prevalence 6%

RISK FACTORS

Genetics

Imerslund-Grasbeck disease (juvenile megaloblastic anemia): Inadequate uptake of B_{12}-IF complex

GENERAL PREVENTION

Recognition of risk factors and adequate supplementation

PATHOPHYSIOLOGY

- Pernicious anemia: Autoimmune attack on gastric IF
- Chronic atrophic gastritis: Autoimmune attack on gastric parietal cells causing decreased IF production
- *H. pylori* infection: Impairs release of B_{12} from bound proteins
- Intestinal disorders: Ileal malabsorption
- PPIs, H_2 antagonists, antacids: B_{12} stays bound to dietary protein with decreased acidity.
- Pancreatic insufficiency: Pancreatic proteases are required to cleave the vitamin B_{12}–R factor bond to allow vitamin B_{12} to bind to intrinsic factor.
- Nutritional deficiency: Strict vegetarians uncommonly develop deficiency because only 1 mg/d is needed with adequate amounts in legumes.
- Hereditary (rare):
  - Imerslund-Grasbeck disease (juvenile megaloblastic anemia)
  - Congenital deficiency of transcobalamin
  - Severe methylene tetrahydrofolate reductase deficiency
  - Abnormalities of methionine synthesis

ETIOLOGY

Causes:

- Food-cobalamin malabsorption syndrome (1):
  - 53% of cases
  - Primary cause in elderly
  - Pathophysiology: Inability to release cobalamin from food or binding protein, especially if in the setting of hypochlorhydria
  - Causes: Atrophic gastritis, long-term ingestion of antacids and biguanides, possible relationship to *H. pylori* infection
- Pernicious anemia (1,3):
  - 33% of cases
  - Second most common cause in elderly after food-cobalamin malabsorption syndrome
  - Autoimmune disease with destruction of gastric fundal mucosa cells via a cell-mediated process
  - Antigastric parietal cell antibodies: Sensitivity >90%, specificity 50%; use for screening test
  - Anti-intrinsic factor antibodies: Sensitivity 50%
  - Associated with other autoimmune diseases
- Insufficient dietary intake (1):
  - 2% of cases
- Intestinal causes (1,3,4):
  - 1% of cases
  - Gastrectomy: Due to decreased production of intrinsic factor
  - Gastric bypass: Appears 1–9 years after surgery, prevalence 12–33%
  - Ileal resection or disease
  - Fish tapeworm
  - Severe pancreatic insufficiency
- Undetermined etiology (1):
  - 11% of cases

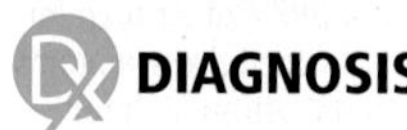

DIAGNOSIS

Symptoms and physical exam findings:

- Asymptomatic patients may be diagnosed by the incidental finding of an elevated mean corpuscular volume (MCV) during routine testing or evaluation of unassociated disorders.
- Hematological (1):
  - Frequent: Macrocytosis, hypersegmentation of neutrophils, spinal cord medullar megaloblastosis (blue spinal cord)
  - Rare: Isolated thrombocytopenia and neutropenia, pancytopenia
  - Very rare: Hemolytic anemia, thrombotic microangiopathy with schistocytes
- Neuropsychiatric (1):
  - Frequent: Sensitive polyneuritis, ataxia, positive Babinski sign, paresthesias, weakness, mild gait unsteadiness
  - Classic: Spinal cord sclerosis
  - Under investigation: Dementia, stroke, atherosclerosis, parkinsonian syndromes, depression, multiple sclerosis
- Digestive (1):
  - Classic: Hunter glossitis, jaundice, and high LDH and bilirubin
  - Possible: Abdominal pain, dyspepsia, nausea, vomiting, diarrhea
  - Rare: Mucocutaneous ulcers

- Other (1):
  - Frequent: Fatigue, anorexia
  - Under investigation: Chronic vaginal and urinary infections, atrophy of vaginal mucosa, hypofertility, venous thromboembolism, angina, miscarriages
  - Commonly insidious and nonspecific; thus, delay in diagnosis is common.

HISTORY

Falls (due to diminished proprioception), loss of sensation in "stocking-glove" distribution, glossitis/loss of sense of taste, other subtle, nonspecific neurologic symptoms

DIAGNOSTIC TESTS & INTERPRETATION

Lab

- Check for folate deficiency and other causes of anemia.
- CBC: Low hemoglobin and hematocrit, mean corpuscular volume (MCV) > 95–100 fL
- MCV may be normal, decreased, or increased if vitamin B_{12} deficiency coexists with other forms of anemia, such as iron deficiency or hemolysis.
- Peripheral blood smear:
  - Macrocytic RBCs
  - Hypersegmented neutrophils
- Serum cobalamin (1):
  - <150 pmol/L and clinical features and/or hematologic anomalies
  - <150 pmol/L on 2 separate occasions
  - <150 pmol/L and total serum homocysteine >130 umol/L or methylmalonic acid >0.4 umol/L (with no concomitant renal failure, folate deficiency, or vitamin B_6 deficiency)
  - Serum holotranscobalamin <35 pmol/L
- Homocysteine and methylmalonic acid (MMA):
  - Elevated in B_{12} deficiency secondary to decreased metabolism
  - If both are normal, B_{12} deficiency is effectively ruled out.
  - If both are increased, B_{12} deficiency is ruled in with a sensitivity and specificity of 94% and 99%, respectively.
  - If MMA is normal and homocysteine is increased, think folate deficiency.
- Pernicious anemia:
  - Check antibody to intrinsic factor → positive test is confirmatory for PA.

ALERT

- Renal insufficiency may cause falsely low percent excretion of radiolabeled B_{12}.
- Macrocytosis may be due to reticulocytosis, medications, bone marrow dysplasia, hypothyroidism, or be masked by concomitant microcytic anemia.

Imaging

Patient may present with encephalopathy or myelopathy. MRI may be required.

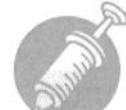

TREATMENT

MEDICATION

- Consider giving folate and vitamin B_{12} repletion together.
- IM cyanocobalamin (1):
  - 1,000 mcg daily for 7 days, then
  - 1,000 mcg weekly for 4 weeks, then
  - 1,000 mcg monthly for life
- Sublingual 2,000 mcg/d for 7–12 days a possible alternative (1)
- Open studies for oral B_{12} repletion underway as an alternative to IM injections

ALERT

Folic acid without vitamin B_{12} in patients with PA is contraindicated; will not correct neurologic abnormalities.

IN-PATIENT CONSIDERATIONS

Initial Stabilization

Consider blood transfusion for severe anemia.

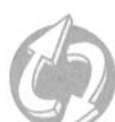

ONGOING CARE

FOLLOW-UP RECOMMENDATIONS

Patient Monitoring

- Hematologic:
  - Reticulocytosis in 3–4 days
  - Rise in hemoglobin beginning at 10 days; usually will return to normal in ~8 weeks
  - Monitor potassium in profoundly anemic patients (hypokalemia due to potassium utilization).
- Neurologic: Symptoms largely irreversible

DIET

Meat, animal protein, and legumes unless contraindicated

REFERENCES

1. Dali-Youcef N, Andres E. An update on cobalamin deficiency in adults. *QJMed*. 2009;102:17–28.
2. Allen L. How common is vitamin B-12 deficiency? *Am J Clin Nutr*. 2009;89(Suppl):693S–6S.
3. Fernandez-Banares F, Monzon H, Forne M. A short review of malabsorption and anemia. *World J Gastroenterology*. 2009;15(37):4644–52.
4. Lahner E, Annibale B. Pernicious anemia: New insights from a gastroenterological point of view. *World J Gastroenterology*. 2009;15(41): 5121–8.

ADDITIONAL READING

Langan RC, Zawistoski KJ. Update on vitamin B_{12} deficiency. *Am Fam Phys*. 2011;83:1425–1430.

CODES

ICD9

- 266.2 Other B-complex deficiencies
- 281.0 Pernicious anemia
- 281.3 Other specified megaloblastic anemias not elsewhere classified

CLINICAL PEARLS

- The Schilling test, the classic procedure to diagnose PA, is no longer available in many parts of the country; in the vast majority of cases, diagnosis can be made by anti-intrinsic factor antibodies, increased serum gastrin, and elevated pepsinogen.
- Consider monitoring B_{12} levels annually if on metformin.
- Vitamin B_{12} deficiency can coexist with other causes of anemia, including iron deficiency or hemolysis; thus, mean corpuscular volume (MCV) can be normal, decreased, or increased.

VITAMIN D DEFICIENCY

Frank J. Domino, MD
Samir Malkani, MD

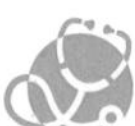

BASICS

This topic covers the commonly acquired vitamin D deficiency and not type II vitamin D–resistant rickets or type I pseudo vitamin D–resistant rickets (both rare autosomal-recessive disorders).

DESCRIPTION

- Vitamin D is both a hormone and a vitamin. Cholecalciferol (D3) is synthesized in the skin by exposure to ultraviolet B (UVB) radiation. Ergocalciferol (D2) and D3 are present in foods.
- D2 and D3 are hydroxylated in the liver to 25 vitamin D (calcidiol), its major circulating form.
- Calcidiol is further hydroxylated in the kidney to the active metabolite 1,25 vitamin D (calcitriol).
- Hypocalcemia stimulates parathyroid hormone (PTH) to be secreted, which prompts the increased conversion of 25 vitamin D to 1,25 vitamin D, which decreases renal calcium and phosphorus excretion, increases intestinal calcium and phosphorus absorption, and increases osteoclast activity. These actions of 1,25 vitamin D serve to increase plasma calcium.

EPIDEMIOLOGY

- Unclear in general population
- In the community, a cohort study of asymptomatic adolescents in Boston found 24.1% were deficient, with 4.6% severely deficient (1).
- A study of hospitalized patients in Massachusetts found 57% vitamin D–deficient (VDD) (2).
- Women with history of osteoporosis or osteoporotic fracture have high prevalence of VDD (3)[A].
- A cross-sectional study of patients with persistent, nonspecific pain in an urban Minneapolis primary care clinic found 93% deficient and 28% severely deficient (4).
- A cohort study in Arizona found over 25% of adults were VDD; highest rates among blacks and Hispanics (5).
- A randomized clinical trial to study VDD and depression in obese adults found treating low serum levels had significant benefit on Beck Depression Inventory at 1 year (6).

Pediatric Considerations

NHANES data found 70% of children did not have sufficient 25 OH vitamin D serum levels (9% deficient and 61% insufficient), which was associated with an increase in BP and decrease in HDL cholesterol (7)[B].

RISK FACTORS

- Inadequate sun exposure
- Female
- Dark skin
- Immigrant populations
- Low socioeconomic status
- Latitudes higher than 38°
- Elderly
- Institutionalized
- Depression
- Medications (phenobarbital, phenytoin)

Genetics

Numerous rare genetic disorders can induce hypoparathyroidism (DiGeorge syndrome).

GENERAL PREVENTION

- Adequate exposure to sunlight and dietary sources of vitamin D (plants, fish); many foods are fortified with D2 and D3.
- Recommended daily allowance from the 2010 Institute of Medicine Report is minimally 600 IU/d for those ≥70 years old and 800 IU/d for those >70 years. Up to 4,000 IU/d is safe in healthy adults without risk of toxicity (8)[C].
- Higher intake of vitamin D recommended for ages >50
- 2005 and 2009: Meta-analysis demonstrated for ages 51–70, minimally recommended supplementation is 800 IU/d to prevent nonvertebral fractures (9,10)[A].

Pediatric Considerations

The American Academy of Pediatrics recommends all breast-fed babies receive 400 IU/d of vitamin D beginning "within the first few days of life."

PATHOPHYSIOLOGY

- Insufficient dietary intake of vitamin D and/or lack of UVB exposure results in low levels of vitamin D. This limits calcium absorption, causing excess PTH to be released.
- PTH stimulates osteoclast activity, which raises calcium and phosphorous but results in osteomalacia.

ETIOLOGY

- Dietary deficiency:
  - Inadequate vitamin D intake
  - Macrobiotic diet
- Inadequate sunlight exposure:
  - Institutionalized patients
  - Hospitalized patients
  - Chronic illness
  - Liver or kidney disease
- Malabsorptive states

COMMONLY ASSOCIATED CONDITIONS

- Osteomalacia, osteoporosis
- Premenstrual syndrome
- Rickets
- Celiac disease
- Gastric bypass
- Chronic renal disease
- Bacterial vaginosis in pregnant women
- Hypertension
- All-cause mortality (11)[B]

DIAGNOSIS

- Nonspecific musculoskeletal complaints
- Weak antigravity muscles
- Fracture with minimal trauma

HISTORY

- Senior citizens at risk of falling
- Renal disease
- GI (malabsorption) disorders
- Liver dysfunction
- Immigration from tropical to colder climates
- Dark-skinned or veiled individuals
- Housebound patients
- Women at perimenopause

PHYSICAL EXAM

- Numerous neurologic signs: Numbness, proximal myopathy, paresthesias, muscle cramps, laryngospasm
- Chvostek sign: Contraction of the muscles of the eye, mouth, or nose by tapping along the facial nerve
- Trousseau phenomenon: Carpal spasms and paraesthesia produced by pressure on nerves and vessels of the upper arm
- Tetany
- Seizures

DIAGNOSTIC TESTS & INTERPRETATION

Lab

- 25 OH vitamin D (most sensitive measure of vitamin D status)
- Vitamin D deficiency:
  - <20 ng/mL
- PTH elevation (normal in early vitamin D deficiency), not routinely obtained unless severe deficiency
- Low-normal or low calcium and phosphorous
- Elevated alkaline phosphatase (in later disease)

Imaging

- Plain radiographs: If atypical fracture, radiographs may show osteomalacia (pseudofractures or Looser zones) in pelvis, femur, and fibula.
- Osteoporosis screen (12)[C]:
  - Women ≥65 years with no risk factors
  - Women ≥60 years at risk: Body weight <70 kg (best predictor)
  - Less evidence: Smoking, low body mass index, family history, decreased activity, alcohol, or caffeine use
  - African American women have higher bone density than Caucasians.

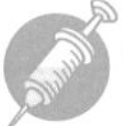

TREATMENT

Treatment goals remain unclear, but current "normal" 25 OH vitamin D levels are based on suppression of PTH.

Geriatric Considerations

In senior citizens, serum 25 OH vitamin D of 50 nmol/L resulted in optimal hip and greater trochanter BMD, and in best physical performance scores (13).

MEDICATION

- Vitamin D sufficiency:
  - Vitamin D 800–4,000 IU/d D2 or D3
  - D3 (animal derived) may be slightly more effective than D2 (plant derived), but clinical significance is uncertain.
  - Calcium supplementation: Unclear benefit and may increase some CHD risk in patients with normal kidneys. No supplementation currently required (see below).
- Vitamin D deficiency:
  - Ergocalciferol 50,000 IU/wk for 8–12 weeks, followed by 2-4,000 IU/d of vitamin D3
- Calcium: Meta-analysis data support:
  - Dietary intake of ~700 mg/d leads to best outcomes; higher doses did NOT decrease risk of osteoporotic fractures (14)[A].
  - Higher doses of daily calcium were associated with an increased risk of myocardial infarction (15)[A].

ADDITIONAL TREATMENT

Issues for Referral

Endocrinology if no response to treatment

Additional Therapies

Aggressive calcium in ICU patients with ionized calcium <3.2 mg/dL or if symptomatic (tetany, seizures, QT prolongation, bradycardia, or hypotension, or ventilated patient with decreased diaphragmatic function)

IN-PATIENT CONSIDERATIONS

Admission Criteria

- Symptoms of severe hypocalcemia *or*
- Malabsorption syndromes

ONGOING CARE

FOLLOW-UP RECOMMENDATIONS

Follow-up of abnormal 25 OH vitamin D not currently required.

DIET

- Cod liver oil is most potent source of vitamin D and has ~1,300 IU vitamin D/Tbs
- Fatty fish (tuna, salmon)
- Fortified milk (100 IU/8 oz), cereal, and foods

PROGNOSIS

- Systematic review of 63 observational studies found adequate 25 vitamin D levels correlated with lower rates of colon, breast, and prostate cancer (16)[A].
- Cohort study found that vitamin D deficiency is correlated with increased risk of all-cause mortality (11)[B].

ALERT

Meta-analysis of 57,000 patients found supplementation of >500 IU/d lowered the risk of all-cause mortality (17)[A].

REFERENCES

1. Gordon CM, DePeter KC, Feldman HA, et al. Prevalence of vitamin D deficiency among healthy adolescents. *Arch Pediatr Adolesc Med*. 2004;158:531–7.
2. Thomas MK, Lloyd-Jones DM, Thadhani RI, et al. Hypovitaminosis D in medical inpatients. *N Engl J Med*. 1998;338:777–83.
3. Gaugris S, Heaney RP, Boonen S, et al. Vitamin D inadequacy among post-menopausal women: A systematic review. *QJM*. 2005;98:667–76.
4. Plotnikoff GA, Quigley JM. Prevalence of severe hypovitaminosis D in patients with persistent, nonspecific musculoskeletal pain. *Mayo Clin Proc*. 2003;78:1463–70.
5. Jacobs ET, Alberts DS, Foote JA, et al. Vitamin D insufficiency in southern Arizona. *Am J Clin Nutr*. 2008;87:608–13.
6. Jorde R, Sneve M, Figenschau Y, et al. Effects of vitamin D supplementation on symptoms of depression in overweight and obese subjects: Randomized double blind trial. *J Intern Med*. 2008;264:599–609.
7. Kumar J, Muntner P, Kaskel FJ, et al. Prevalence and associations of 25-hydroxyvitamin D deficiency in US children: NHANES 2001–2004. *Pediatrics*. 2009;124(3):e362–70.
8. Ross AC, Manson JE, Abrams SA, et al. The 2011 report on dietary reference intakes for calcium and vitamin D from the Institute of Medicine: What clinicians need to know. *J Clin Endocrinol Metab*. 2011;96:53–8.
9. Bischoff-Ferrari HA, Willett WC, Wong JB, et al. Fracture prevention with vitamin D supplementation: A meta-analysis of randomized controlled trials. *JAMA*. 2005;293:2257–64.
10. Bischoff-Ferrari HA, Willett WC, Wong JB, et al. Prevention of nonvertebral fractures with oral vitamin D and dose dependency: A meta-analysis of randomized controlled trials. *Arch Intern Med*. 2009;169:551–61.
11. Melamed ML, Michos ED, Post W, et al. 25-hydroxyvitamin D levels and the risk of mortality in the general population. *Arch Intern Med*. 2008;168:1629–37.
12. Available at: www.ahrq.gov.
13. Kuchuk NO, Pluijm SM, van Schoor NM, et al. Relationships of serum 25-hydroxyvitamin D to bone mineral density and serum parathyroid hormone and markers of bone turnover in older persons. *J Clin Endocrinol Metab*. 2009;94:1244–50.
14. Warensjö E, Byberg L, Melhus H, et al. Dietary calcium intake and risk of fracture and osteoporosis: Prospective longitudinal cohort study. *BMJ*. 2011;342:d1473.
15. Bolland MJ, Avenell A, Baron JA, et al. Effect of calcium supplements on risk of myocardial infarction and cardiovascular events: Meta-analysis. *BMJ*. 2010;341:c3691.
16. Garland CF, Garland FC, Gorham ED, et al. The role of vitamin D in cancer prevention. *Am J Public Health*. 2006;96:252–61.
17. Autier P, Gandini S. Vitamin D supplementation and total mortality: A meta-analysis of randomized controlled trials. *Arch Intern Med*. 2007;167:1730–7.

ADDITIONAL READING

CDC Monograph: www.cdc.gov/breastfeeding/recommendations/vitamin D.htm.

CODES

ICD9

268.9 Unspecified vitamin D deficiency

CLINICAL PEARLS

- Risk factors for VDD: Senior citizen, renal disease, GI (malabsorption) disorders, liver dysfunction, immigration from tropical to colder climates, dark-skinned or veiled individuals, housebound patients, perimenopause
- Diagnosis: 25 OH vitamin D (most sensitive measure of vitamin D status)
- Vitamin D deficiency: <20 ng/mL
- Up to 4,000 IU/d is safe in healthy adults without risk of toxicity.
- Meta-analysis showed supplementing with at least 500 IU/d resulted in lower all-cause mortality.
- 2005 and 2009: Meta-analysis demonstrated for ages 51–70 minimally recommended supplementation is 800 IU/d to prevent nonvertebral fractures (9,10)[A].
- The American Academy of Pediatrics recommends all breast-fed babies receive 400 IU/d of vitamin D beginning within a few days of birth.

VITAMIN DEFICIENCY

Neil A. Gilchrist, PharmD
David B. Gilchrist, MD

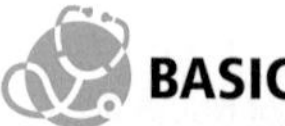

BASICS

DESCRIPTION

- Vitamins are essential micronutrients required for normal metabolism, growth, and development.
- Specific vitamin deficiencies can lead to medical conditions and health complications.
- Deficiencies are rarely diagnosed or documented in the Western world. Regulations mandating vitamin supplementation in food products, adequate food supply, availability of vitamin supplements, and lack of physician awareness all play a role.
- Fat-soluble vitamins (A, D, E, K) and water-soluble vitamins (B)

EPIDEMIOLOGY

Incidence

- Predominant age:
  - Affects mainly geriatric population
  - Occurs in select adult demographics: Pregnant women, chronic disease states (see "Etiology")
- Travelers spending extended time in developing nations
- Very low for isolated vitamin deficiencies in Western world; true incidence unknown
- Vitamin levels are rarely measured (exceptions include vitamin B_{12} [risk increases >50] and folate [risk increases with specific states: Pregnancy, antiepileptic drugs, neoplastic processes, alcoholism])

Prevalence

Varies by age groups, comorbid conditions, geography, and setting (i.e., urban, rural)

RISK FACTORS

Poverty, malnutrition, chronic disease states, advanced age, dietary restrictions, bariatric surgery, and exclusively breast-fed infants

Genetics

- Cystic fibrosis
- Rare genetic predisposition:
  - Autoimmune disease (e.g., pernicious anemia)
  - Congenital enzyme deficiencies (e.g., biotinidase deficiency)
  - Transcobalamin II deficiency
  - Ataxia and vitamin E deficiency (AVED)
- A-β-lipoproteinemia

GENERAL PREVENTION

- No data exist that demonstrate that use of a multivitamin decreases risk of any disease.
- Ingesting large and varied amounts of vitamins increases risk of toxicity and drug–drug interactions.
- Use of antioxidants to prevent cancer has had no beneficial effect on cancer incidence, and in some studies has increased risk of death (1)[A].
- Adequate intake of a balanced diet containing carbohydrates, proteins, and fats
- Avoidance of fad diets
- Vitamin or nutrition supplementation, when appropriate

ALERT

Use of multivitamins has not resulted in decreased risk of cancer, heart disease, stroke, or all-cause mortality (2)[A].

PATHOPHYSIOLOGY

Deficiencies usually related to disease can develop under healthy conditions and generally occur by 1 of 5 mechanisms:

- Reduced intake
- Diminished absorption
- Increased utilization
- Increased demand
- Increased excretion

ETIOLOGY

- Chronic disease states: HIV, malabsorption, chronic liver and kidney disease, alcoholism, pernicious anemia, etc.
- Gastric surgeries: Gastric bypass, gastrectomy, small or large bowel resection, etc.
- Predisposition related to certain medicines: Prednisone, phenytoin, isoniazid, protease inhibitors, proton pump inhibitors, chronic antibiotic use, penicillamine, hydralazine, etc. (3)
- Malnutrition, imbalanced nutrition, eating disorders: Obesity, bulimia/anorexia, fad diets, extreme vegetarianism
- Dialysis
- Parasitic infestation

COMMONLY ASSOCIATED CONDITIONS

Osteoporosis, anemia, neuropathies, Hartnup disease

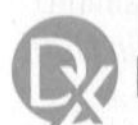

DIAGNOSIS

HISTORY

- Dietary intake
- Night blindness
- Macular degeneration
- Decreased visual acuity
- Poor wound healing
- Hyperkeratosis of skin
- Neuropathy
- Abnormal food cravings (pica)
- Osteomalacia or history of fracture
- Spina bifida
- Previous GI or gastric bypass surgery
- Prior or current medical conditions:
  - Tuberculosis (TB)
  - HIV infection
  - Hepatitis
  - Neoplastic condition
  - Hypermetabolic state:
    - Thyrotoxicosis
    - Second- or third-degree burns
    - Wound healing
    - Any systemic infection
  - Any chronic disease requiring steroids or immunosuppressants
  - Any malabsorption or chronic GI disorder: Celiac disease, sprue, Crohn disease, ulcerative colitis
- Parenteral or enteral nutrition via tube feeding
- Pregnancy
- Medications
- Supplements
- Food allergies or intolerances

PHYSICAL EXAM

- Breakdown of skin integrity
- Coarse or thinning hair
- Reduced visual acuity
- Beefy red tongue
- Angular cheilitis (perlèche)
- Poor dentition and gingivitis
- Cognitive impairment
- Bruising and/or petechiae
- Sensory and motor neuropathies
- Ataxic gait

DIAGNOSTIC TESTS & INTERPRETATION

Lab

Initial lab tests

- None needed unless a specific deficiency is suspected; screening with "routine" labs is not recommended
- CBC
- If clinical characteristics are present, consider:
  - 25 OH vitamin D
  - Prothrombin time (PT)/partial thromboplastin time (PTT)
  - Vitamin B_{12} and folate levels
  - Serum homocysteine and methylmalonic acid levels if high suspicion of vitamin B_{12} deficiency with normal serum B_{12} level
- Ancillary tests include:
  - BUN
  - Albumin
  - Calcium
  - Phosphorous
  - Magnesium
  - Liver function tests (LFTs)

Follow-Up & Special Considerations

Bariatric surgery patients are at risk for select nutritional deficiencies:

- Cyanocobalamin
- Thiamine
- Folic acid
- Calcium
- Vitamin D
- Iron
- Zinc

Imaging

Initial approach

- X-ray of long bones and spine
- Bone densitometry: Indicated in:
  - Women >65 years
  - Men >70 years
  - Patients <65 years with risk factors for osteoporosis, including patients with chronic disease requiring long-standing steroids or immunosuppressants, patients on thyroid medicine and antiepileptic drugs (see topic "Osteoporosis")

Pathological Findings

- Vitamin A (retinol):
  - Decreased visual acuity, Bitot spots
  - Advanced disease: Keratomalacia and blindness
- Vitamin B_1 (thiamine):
  - Wernicke encephalopathy: Memory disturbance, truncal ataxia, nystagmus, ophthalmoplegia
  - Korsakoff syndrome: Anterograde and retrograde amnesia, confabulation
  - Dry beriberi: Symmetric motor and sensory peripheral neuropathy, paresthesias, loss of reflexes
  - Wet beriberi: Cardiovascular symptoms of peripheral vasodilation, high-output failure, dyspnea, and tachycardia

- Vitamin B_2 (riboflavin): Glossitis, stomatitis, cheilitis
- Vitamin B_3 (niacin): Pellagra: Dermatitis, dementia, and diarrhea
- Vitamin B_6 (pyridoxine): Dermatitis, cheilitis, atrophic glossitis, neuropathy
- Vitamin B_{12} (cobalamin): Pernicious anemia, subacute combined degeneration, gait disturbance, cognitive impairment, neuropathy
- Vitamin C (ascorbic acid): Scurvy: Ecchymoses, bleeding gums
- Vitamin D (calciferol): Rickets, osteomalacia, osteopenia/osteoporosis
- Vitamin K: Ecchymosis, mucosal bleeding

DIFFERENTIAL DIAGNOSIS

Many medical conditions may lead to symptoms and signs that mimic vitamin deficiencies, including diabetes mellitus (DM), hyperparathyroidism, thyroid disorders, heart failure, Alzheimer disease, multiple sclerosis, substance abuse, toxic ingestions and overdose, and hematologic disorders/malignancies.

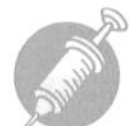

TREATMENT

MEDICATION

- Encourage patients to bring in vitamin and supplement bottles for personal review by a physician or knowledgeable health care practitioner or pharmacist.
- Folic acid and vitamin B_6/B_{12} therapy has been shown to lower homocysteine levels; however, there is no data showing benefit of this therapy re: Cognitive impairment or risk of developing diabetic nephropathy, retinopathy, and CHD/vascular diseases (4).

COMPLEMENTARY AND ALTERNATIVE MEDICINE

- Patients should be asked specifically about herbal and dietary supplements as part of a complete medication history.
- Prescribers should assess for possible adverse drug effects and drug interactions (5).

IN-PATIENT CONSIDERATIONS

Initial Stabilization

- Provide daily B-vitamin complex (folate, B_6, B_{12}), including thiamine supplementation (dose = 100 mg) via oral or parenteral route, to all patients with chronic medical conditions admitted to hospital or in postoperative state at risk for alcohol withdrawal (6)[B].
- If thiamine deficiency suspected, give thiamine replacement prior to IV fluids containing glucose to prevent precipitation of Korsakoff psychosis.
- Consider obtaining dietician/nutrition consult.
- There is currently no consensus practice guideline for recommending supplement dosing regimens after bariatric surgery. Dosing of supplements should be guided by patient symptoms and serum levels when appropriate.

Geriatric Considerations

- Vitamin B_{12} deficiency: 25% of the general population ≥65 years has borderline or low levels of vitamin B_{12} necessitating supplementation. Treatment of symptomatic or severe deficiency should consist of cyanocobalamin 1,000 μg/d IM × 1 week and then weekly × 1 month. Prevention of recurrence or treatment of mild deficiency may include a regimen of oral B_{12} 1,000–2,000 μg/d or IM B_{12} 100–1,000 μg every 3 months.
- A large percentage (>40%) of elderly patients in the community setting in the US are deficient in vitamin D. The percentage is even higher in the hospitalized elderly.

Pediatric Considerations

- Hemorrhagic disease of the newborn:
  - Deficiency of vitamin K may be seen in neonates because they require 1 week of life to establish their intestinal flora (intestinal bacteria manufacture vitamin K) and because breast milk is a poor source of vitamin K.
  - Peaks 2–10 days after birth; presents with bleeding from the umbilical stump and/or circumcision site along with generalized bruising and GI hemorrhage
  - Routine injection of newborns with vitamin K (1 mg) prevents hemorrhagic disease.
- Vitamin D deficiency: Vitamin D supplementation (400 IU/d) is recommended in all exclusively breastfed infants starting in the first few days of life (AAP recommendations) to prevent rickets.
- Many vitamin deficiencies lead to developmental delay in children.
- Supplemental vitamins in otherwise healthy children, although encouraged, are not mandated by medical authorities.

Pregnancy Considerations

Folate and pregnancy: All pregnant women and women of child-bearing age considering pregnancy should be strongly encouraged to take a multivitamin containing 0.4 mg folic acid daily to prevent neural tube defects.

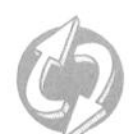

ONGOING CARE

DIET

- Monitor nutrient intake.
- Supplemental enteral nutrition (i.e., Ensure, Boost, Sustacal, etc.) if anorexic or if difficulty eating solids

PATIENT EDUCATION

- One-a-day vitamins are generally safe for all patients but are of no value in the Western world, and caution should be exercised about taking vitamins with some medications to minimize drug–drug interactions.
- Toxicity can occur with many vitamins, most commonly the fat-soluble vitamins (A, D, E, K). Refer to the Recommended Dietary Allowance (RDA) for specific intake guidelines.

PROGNOSIS

- Most vitamin deficiencies are fully reversible if treated without undue delay.
- Vitamin repletion or supplementation may be required short term (<3 months) or long term (>3 months), depending on cause of deficiency.

COMPLICATIONS

- Vitamin toxicities:
  - Liver failure (vitamins A, D, E, K)
  - Desquamation of skin (vitamin A)
  - Neuropathy (vitamin B_6)
  - Kidney stones (vitamin C)
  - Hypercoagulability (vitamin K)
  - Pseudohyperparathyroidism (vitamin D)
  - Masking of pernicious anemia (folic acid)
- Any vitamin can be taken to excess; refer to the Recommended Dietary Allowance (RDA) for specific intake guidelines.

REFERENCES

1. Bjelakovic G, Nikolova D, Gluud LL, et al. Antioxidant supplements for prevention of mortality in healthy participants and patients with various diseases. *Cochrane Database Syst Rev*. 2008:CD007176.
2. Neuhouser ML, Wassertheil-Smoller S, Thomson C, et al. Multivitamin use and risk of cancer and cardiovascular disease in the Women's Health Initiative cohorts. *Arch Intern Med*. 2009;169: 294–304.
3. Felipez L, Sentongo TA. Drug-induced nutrient deficiencies. *Pediatr Clin North Am*. 2009;56: 1211–24.
4. House AA, Eliasziw M, Cattran DC, et al. Effect of B-vitamin therapy on progression of diabetic nephropathy: A randomized controlled trial. *JAMA*. 2010;303:1603–9.
5. Haller CA. Clinical approach to adverse events and interactions related to herbal and dietary supplements. *Clinical Toxicology*. 2006;44:605–10.
6. Thomson AD, Marshall EJ. The treatment of patients at risk of developing Wernicke's encephalopathy in the community. *Alcohol Alcohol*. 2006;41:159–67.

ADDITIONAL READING

- Davies DJ, Baxter JM, Baxter JN. Nutritional deficiencies after bariatric surgery. *Obes Surg*. 2007; 17:1150–8.
- Rosen CJ. Clinical practice. Vitamin D insufficiency. *N Engl J Med*. 2011;364:248–54.

CODES

ICD9

269.2 Unspecified vitamin deficiency

CLINICAL PEARLS

- Take a thorough dietary history to assess for possible vitamin deficiencies, especially if physical exam findings suggest a vitamin deficiency.
- All pregnant women and women of child-bearing age should be counseled to take a multivitamin with 0.4 mg folic acid.
- All exclusively breast-fed infants should be given 400 IU vitamin D supplementation starting in the first few days of life and continued until weaned to formula or, if >12 months, taking 32 oz of fortified cow's milk daily.

VITILIGO

Julia K. Anderson, MD
Diane L. Whitaker-Worth, MD

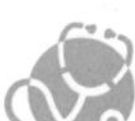

BASICS

DESCRIPTION

An acquired depigmentation of skin, which correlates with a loss of epidermal melanocytes. There are 3 clinical variants, each with subtypes:

- Localized: Often in childhood, rapid onset, then stabilizes. Involvement of hair is common early in the course. Lacks associated autoimmune diseases:
  - Focal: Few lesions, random distribution
  - Segmental: Lesions follow Blaschkoid lines or dermatome (mostly trigeminal).
  - Mucosal: On mucosal surfaces
- Generalized/Nonsegmental (most common variant): Up to 90% of cases, 30% of childhood. Progressive, with flares, commonly associated with autoimmunity. Locations are sites sensitive to pressure/friction (Koebner phenomenon):
  - Vulgaris: Most common subtype. Scattered macules, often symmetric, mostly hands, axillae, and groin
  - Acrofacial: On distal extremities and face
  - Mixed: Coexistence of above
- Universal: Involves >80% of the body surface area (BSA). Most likely to have family history, comorbidities are common, and associated with poorest quality-of-life (QOL) scores.
- Other rare variants:
  - Ponctué: Discrete confettilike macules
  - Trichrome: Tan zone is present between normal and depigmented skin.
  - Quadrichrome: As above but with marginal/perifollicular hyperpigmentation
  - Blue: Dermal melanophages give blue hue.
- System(s) affected: Skin
- Synonym(s): Leukoderma

EPIDEMIOLOGY

- 50% begin before age 20, peak in females: First decade; males: Fifth decade (1). Onset earlier with positive family history. Can appear as early as 6 weeks old (1).
- Predominance: Men = Women; more frequently reported in women.
- No race or socioeconomic predilection

Incidence

Worldwide ~1%. Peak incidence 10–30 years old

Prevalence

~1% in the US and Europe and 0.1–8% in the world; highest in Gujarat, India at 8.8% (1)

RISK FACTORS

- Family history of vitiligo/autoimmune disorders
- Personal history of associated conditions

Genetics

- Most cases are sporadic, but family clustering in polygenic/multifactorial inheritance
- 20% of patients report affected relative, but monozygotic twins have only 23% concordance (1).
- HLA haplotypes, small nucleotide polymorphisms, and specific genes are all possible contributors.

ETIOLOGY

Most likely a spectrum of disorders with a common phenotype, and multiple mechanisms contribute to the pathology (convergence theory).

- Genetic: See above.
- Autoimmune: Humoral autoantibodies and skin-homing T cells
- Neural: Local or systemic dysregulation leading to excess neurotransmitters
- Oxidative stress from elevated H_2O_2 and decreased catalase

COMMONLY ASSOCIATED CONDITIONS

- Most common:
  - Endocrine: Thyroid disease and hypoparathyroidism, Addison disease, insulin-dependent diabetes
  - Dermatologic: Psoriasis, atopic dermatitis, alopecia areata, chronic urticaria, halo nevi, ichthyosis
  - Pernicious anemia, hypoacusis, rheumatoid arthritis
  - Ocular abnormalities in up to 40%
- Less common:
  - Systemic lupus erythematosus
  - Inflammatory bowel disease
  - Melanoma (may be a sign of positive outcome of melanoma) and other skin cancers
  - Syndromes: Alezzandrini, MELAS (mitochondrial encephalomyopathy, lactic acidosis, and stroke-like episodes), Schmidt, and autoimmune polyendocrinopathy-candidiasis-ectodermal dysplasia (APCED)
- Age >50 at onset should prompt investigation for associated conditions.

Pediatric Considerations

Associated with Hashimoto thyroiditis in a significant portion of children. Screening at onset and possibly annually may be beneficial (2).

DIAGNOSIS

HISTORY

- Inquire about recent history of sunburns, pregnancy, skin trauma, or emotional stress.
- Family history of premature graying, vitiligo, and autoimmune disorders (3)
- Review of systems for related associated conditions
- Ascertain psychological impact on QOL, Dermatology Life Quality Index (DLQI).

PHYSICAL EXAM

- Full-body skin exam with Wood's lamp to accentuate lesions and determine depigmentation from hypopigmentation
- Lesions are well demarcated, uniform, white macules, and patches.
- Look for evidence of repigmentation (most commonly at hair follicles).

DIAGNOSTIC TESTS & INTERPRETATION

Lab

Initial lab tests

- TSH,CBC, ANA (1)
- Antithyroid peroxidase and antithyroglobulin antibodies, if family/patient history of autoimmune disease (1)

Follow-Up & Special Considerations

- Monitor for disease progression/flares.
- Monitor for symptoms of related conditions.

Diagnostic Procedures/Surgery

- Skin biopsy rarely needed. Highest yield is with comparison of lesional/perilesional biopsies.
- Consider ophthalmologic and audiologic evaluation.

Pathological Findings

Few/no epidermal melanocytes. At margins, melanocytes may be larger, vacuolated, and dendritic. Early lesions show inflammation, and later, degeneration, including of adnexa and nerves.

DIFFERENTIAL DIAGNOSIS

- Infectious:
  - Tinea versicolor, leprosy, leishmaniasis, onchocerciasis, treponematoses(pinta/syphilis)
- Postinflammatory hypopigmentation:
  - Psoriasis, atopic dermatitis, pityriasis alba, systemic lupus erythematosus
- Inherited hypomelanoses:
  - Piebaldism, tuberous sclerosis, Waardenburg, hypomelanosis of Ito, Vogt-Koyanagi-Harada
- Malformations:
  - Nevus anemicus, nevus depigmentosus
- Paraneoplastic:
  - Mycosis fungoides, melanoma-associated leukoderma
- Occupational and chemical induced:
  - Occupational: Phenolic/catecholic derivatives and arsenic-containing compounds
  - Chemical: Numerous, including cosmetics, cleansers, insecticides, and even medications
- Melasma: Normal skin may be confused as vitiligo in the setting of surrounding hyperpigmentation.
- Halo nevi
- Lichen sclerosis et atrophicus
- Idiopathic guttate hypomelanosis
- Progressive acquired macular hypomelanosis

TREATMENT

- Absence of a standardized scoring system makes comparison of different treatments difficult.
- The variant of vitiligo may affect response.
  - If untreated, progression is the natural course for those with mucosal involvement, family history, koebnerization, and nonsegmental.
  - Lesions that respond best are on the face, of recent onset, in darker skin type, and in younger patients.

MEDICATION

- Individualize therapy depending on age, extent, distribution, and rate of progression.
- Many therapies are not FDA approved for vitiligo, although they are often considered first-line therapy.
- Corticosteroids: Topical corticosteroids (TCS) are the most effective monotherapy. The combination of light therapy and TCS is the most effective treatment overall. Systemic corticosteroids can be helpful but dosage and safety parameters are not fully evaluated (4):
  - High potency has proven more beneficial, such as clobetasol propionate ointment, BID for a max of 50 g/wk for 2 weeks, then break. Do not use on face/axilla/groin; do not occlude except under close monitoring. Pediatric: As above, for children >12 years old. Consider decreased potency.

- Topical calcineurin inhibitors: Slightly inferior to TCS as monotherapy but better side effect profile (4)[A]. Can be used as adjunctive to light therapy. Carries a controversial black box warning for a theoretical risk of lymphoma or skin cancer. Extensive safety profiling has not revealed any evidence for this in children or adults using topical calcineurin inhibitors (4):
  - Tacrolimus 0.03% or 0.1% ointment b.i.d. Pediatric: 0.03% strength b.i.d., in children >2 years old.
  - Pimecrolimus 1% cream b.i.d. Pediatric: As adults, for children >2 years old.
- Vitamin D3 analogs: Less effective than TCS alone but in combination with TCS can shorten time until, and improve stability of, repigmentation (4):
  - Calcipotriene ointment 1–2 times per day. Pediatric: Not defined.
  - Available as a combination formulation, betamethasone dipropionate 0.064%/calcipotriene 0.005% ointment daily, max dose of 100 g/wk for 4 weeks, not for >30% BSA, not for face/axilla/groin. Pediatric: not defined.
- Phototherapy: Narrow band UVB (NBUVB) is superior to UVA. Psoralens and khellin enhance the effect of light. Psoralen plus UVA (PUVA) may increase incidence of skin cancers. L-phenylalanine can be used topically and orally as a photosensitizer for natural or artificial light (4).
- Laser therapy: Excimer laser (308 nm) is superior to other light therapy. Helium neon laser works for segmental vitiligo (4).
- Antioxidants: May have protective role in preventing melanocyte degradation from reactive oxygen species (4)
- Surgical therapy: See below.
- New concepts: Tumor necrosis factor-alpha inhibitors, minocycline, and immunosuppressants are currently being evaluated (4).

First Line

- Recommended: TCS alone (4)[A] or in combination with a topical vitamin D_3 analog (4)[A]
- Alternatively:
  - Topical calcineurin inhibitors (preferred for face, neck, axilla, and groin) (4)[A]
  - Systemic steroids (4)[B]
  - Topical L-phenylalanine (4)[B]
  - Topical antioxidants and mitochondrial stimulating cream (4)[B]
  - Natural sunlight with oral khellin (4)[B]
  - For rapidly progressive vitiligo, consider systemic corticosteroids (4)[B].
  - For treatment-resistant lesions on the extremities, consider topical tacrolimus under occlusion (4).
  - Camouflage and psychotherapy should be offered to all patients at any stage (4).

Second Line

- Recommended: NBUVB with topical calcineurin inhibitors (4)[B] or TCS (4)[B]
- Alternatively:
  - NBUVB with oral antioxidants (4)[B], oral steroids (4)[B], polypodium leucotomos (4)[B]
  - UVA with psoralens (4)[B], oral steroids (4)[B], topical vitamin D_3 analogs (4)[B], oral khellin (4)[B], oral L-phenylalanine (4)[B]

Third Line

- Recommended: 308 nm laser with topical steroids (4)[B]
- Alternatively: 308 nm laser with topical calcineurin inhibitors (4)[A]
- For segmental vitiligo: All of above and consider helium neon laser (4)[B]

Fourth Line

- Blister graft (4)[C]
- Split-thickness skin graft (4)[C]
- Punch graft (4)[C]
- Autologous melanocyte suspension transplant (4)[A]

ADDITIONAL TREATMENT

General Measures

- Sunscreen to decrease sunburn and prevent accentuation of uninvolved skin
- Corrective camouflage as cover-up (Cover FX, Dermablend)

Issues for Referral

- Dermatologist: For facial/widespread vitiligo or when advanced therapy necessary
- Ophthalmologist: For ocular symptoms, or monitoring of TCS near eyes
- Endocrinologist: Evaluation/management of associated conditions
- Psychologist: For severe distress
- Medical geneticist: When associated conditions are present

Additional Therapies

- Dihydroxyacetone (DHA) is the most frequently used self-tanning agent (3)[C].
- Depigmentation therapy with monobenzone, hydroquinone, or Q-switched ruby laser (4)[B]: For extensive vitiligo recalcitrant to therapy
- Cosmetic tattooing for localized stable vitiligo

COMPLEMENTARY AND ALTERNATIVE MEDICINE

Ginkgo biloba 40 mg PO t.i.d. may stop slowly spreading vitiligo (5)[B].

SURGERY/OTHER PROCEDURES

- Goal is to transport melanocytes from other areas of the skin. Methods include punch, blister or split-thickness skin grafting, or transplantation of autologous melanocytes.
- Patients who koebnerize or form keloids may be worse, and permanent scarring is a risk for all patients (4).

ONGOING CARE

FOLLOW-UP RECOMMENDATIONS

Patient Monitoring

- Monitor for symptoms of related conditions.
- With topical steroids, follow at regular intervals to avoid steroid-atrophy, telangiectasia, and striae distensae.

DIET

No restrictions

PATIENT EDUCATION

- Discussion of disease course, progression, and cosmesis
- Education regarding trauma/friction and Koebner phenomenon

PROGNOSIS

- Vitiligo may remain stable, or may slowly or rapidly progress.
- Spontaneous repigmentation is uncommon.
- Generalized vitiligo is often progressive, with flares. Focal vitiligo often has rapid onset, then stabilizes.

COMPLICATIONS

- Adverse effects of each treatment modality
- Psychiatric morbidity: Depression, adjustment disorder, low self-esteem, and embarrassment in relationships:
  - Different cultures may have different perceptions/social stigmas about vitiligo. Some believe it to be contagious or related to infection. Women with vitiligo may have difficulty getting married and have low self-esteem (1).

REFERENCES

1. Alikhan A, Felsten LM, Daly M, et al. Vitiligo: A comprehensive overview Part I. Introduction, epidemiology, quality of life, diagnosis, differential diagnosis, associations, histopathology, etiology, and work-up. *J Am Acad Dermatol*. 2011;65:473–91.
2. Kakourou T, Aghia S. Vitiligo in children. *World J Pediatr*. 2009;5(4):265–8.
3. Taïeb A, Picardo M. Clinical practice. Vitiligo. *N Engl J Med*. 2009;360:160–9.
4. Felsten LM, Alikhan A, Petronic-Rosic V, et al. Vitiligo: A comprehensive overview Part II: Treatment options and approach to treatment. *J Am Acad Dermatol*. 2011;65:493–514.
5. Szczurko O, Boon HS. A systematic review of natural health product treatment for vitiligo. *BMC Dermatol*. 2008;8:2.

ADDITIONAL READING

Whitton ME, Pinart M, Batchelor J, et al. Interventions for vitiligo. *Cochrane Database Syst Rev*. 2010; CD003263.

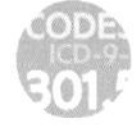

CODES

ICD9

709.01 Vitiligo

CLINICAL PEARLS

- Vitiligo can be a psychologically devastating skin disease.
- Screen for associated diseases, particularly if onset occurs later in life.
- Treatment should be individualized based on BSA, skin type, and patient goals.
- Dermatology consultation when extensive disease, facial involvement, and when advanced treatments are considered

V

VON WILLEBRAND DISEASE

Aaron S. Mansfield, MD

BASICS

DESCRIPTION

- von Willebrand disease (vWD) is a bleeding disorder caused by a defect in or deficiency of a blood-clotting protein called *von Willebrand factor* (vWF).
- vWF is a protein critical to the initial stages of blood clotting.
- vWD primarily manifests as mucocutaneous or perioperative bleeding.
- vWD can be an inherited or acquired condition.

EPIDEMIOLOGY

Prevalence

- The prevalence of the inherited forms of vWD is about 1–2% of the general population.
- The prevalence of the acquired forms of vWD is about 0.1% of the general population.
- Acquired vWD is secondary to some malignancies (lymphoma, leukemia, multiple myeloma), autoimmune disorders (systemic lupus erythematosus [SLE]) and other conditions (hypothyroidism, aortic stenosis, ventricular septal defects [VSDs]), and some medications.
- Up to 21% of individuals with aortic stenosis have acquired vWD.
- 1/3 of patients with polycythemia vera have acquired vWD.

Pediatric Considerations

Many cases of vWD are diagnosed in childhood, including during initial years of menstruation.

Pregnancy Considerations

Although levels of vWF increase during pregnancy, women with vWD are most likely to experience an increased incidence of obstetric complications that manifest with bleeding.

RISK FACTORS

Genetics

- The gene for vWF is located on chromosome 12.
- >250 mutations have been identified.
- Type 1 follows an autosomal-dominant inheritance pattern with variable expressivity.
- Type 2 varies, but primarily follows an autosomal-dominant inheritance pattern.
- Type 3 follows an autosomal-recessive inheritance pattern and is usually due to a frameshift or nonsense mutation in the gene causing lack of expression.

PATHOPHYSIOLOGY

- vWF is a large multimeric protein that is released by endothelial cells and carried within platelets. It mediates platelet plug formation by the attraction and aggregation of platelets at sites of endothelial injury.
- vWF is also a carrier for factor VIII (FVIII) and stabilizes this factor from degradation. A deficiency in vWF results in lower levels of FVIII.
- When vWF is deficient or dysfunctional, primary hemostasis is compromised, resulting in increased mucocutaneous and postprocedural bleeding.
- There are 3 major categories of inherited vWD:
  - Type I is the most common and mildest form, representing 60–80% of cases:
    - Mild-to-moderate quantitative deficiency of vWF and concordant deficiency of FVIII
    - Generally a mild bleeding disorder
  - Type 2 accounts for 10–30% of cases and is divided into multiple subtypes:
    - In type 2, vWF itself has an abnormality.
    - Type 2A is noted for defective platelet-dependent functions and lack of large multimers.
    - Type 2B is noted for increased binding affinity for platelets and is associated with thrombocytopenia, low ristocetin cofactor activity, and few large multimers.
    - Type 2M is noted for defective platelet-dependent functions but not multimer defects.
    - Type 2N demonstrates defective binding to FVIII.
  - Type 3 represents 1–5% of cases:
    - Most severe form
    - Low-to-undetectable levels of vWF and FVIII
- There is also an increasingly recognized acquired form of vWD secondary to multiple conditions such as aortic stenosis, dysproteinemias, lymphoproliferative disorders, myeloproliferative disorders, solid tumors, hypothyroidism, autoimmune disorders, and medication use (e.g., ciprofloxacin, valproic acid, griseofulvin). The pathophysiology of the acquired form is related to the underlying condition:
  - In aortic stenosis, vWF deficiency may result from enhanced A Disintegrinlike and Metalloproteinase with Thrombospondin (ADAMTS)13-mediated proteolysis due to increased shear stress.
  - Adsorption of vWF has been demonstrated by certain tumor cells and by activated platelets in essential thrombocythemia.

ETIOLOGY

- >250 mutations have been identified in the inherited forms.
- Some mechanisms of the acquired forms are described above.

COMMONLY ASSOCIATED CONDITIONS

- Aortic stenosis
- Myeloproliferative disorders
- Lymphoproliferative disorders

DIAGNOSIS

HISTORY

- Most patients with an inherited type have a family history of vWD; however, patients with mild forms of vWD and their families may be unaware of their disease. Those with acquired vWD often have no family history of this disorder.
- The most important component of diagnosis is the hemostatic history (history of bleeding after procedure).
- Common symptoms are those of mucocutaneous (recurrent epistaxis, menorrhagia, ecchymosis) or postprocedural bleeding.
- A history of 3 distinct hemorrhagic symptoms is specific diagnostic criterion for vWD (1)[B].
- Hemarthrosis is rare but does occur with severe types.

PHYSICAL EXAM

- Physical exam may be entirely normal, although there may be some ecchymoses.
- Findings suggestive of other causes of increased bleeding should be sought out (liver disease, skin laxity, or telangiectasia).

DIAGNOSTIC TESTS & INTERPRETATION

More than 1 test may be needed to make the correct diagnosis.

Lab

Initial lab tests

- The most specific tests for vWD include: vWF antigen, ristocetin cofactor activity (if unavailable: collagen-binding activity); these tests should be ordered when suspicion for vWD is high. Other tests include CBC, prothrombin time (PT)/international normalized ratio (INR), partial thromboplastin time (PTT), bleeding time:
  - Platelet count is often normal, except in type 2B or when there is an underlying myeloproliferative disorder.
  - Platelet function assay is usually prolonged but may be normal in mild disease.
  - PT/INR is normal, unless there is concurrent liver disease or Coumadin use.
  - Activated PTT may be prolonged because a decrease in FVIII accompanies vWD.
  - Bleeding time is usually prolonged but may be normal in mild disease. This test has been discontinued at many institutions.
- Specific tests for vWD:
  - vWF antigen testing is done via immunologic methods:
    - vWF antigen testing has a positive predictive value (PPV) of 33% for detecting significant FVIII deficiency and a PPV of 80% for detecting ristocetin cofactor activity abnormalities (2)[C].
    - The levels of antigen may be normal in type 2 vWD.
  - Ristocetin cofactor activity is a functional assessment of vWF. Ristocetin promotes binding of platelets to vWF, and this activity is reduced in most forms of vWD.
  - Collagen-binding activity is another functional assessment of vWF, and is reduced in most forms of vWD.
  - vWF multimer analysis is performed by electrophoresis on agarose gel. This test identifies patients with type 2 vWD who have normal vWF antigen levels and decreased ristocetin cofactor activity.
  - FVIII-vWF binding assay activity is low in patients with type 2N vWD.

Follow-Up & Special Considerations

- Unless patients have severe forms of vWD or are undergoing treatment, follow-up laboratory studies are not usually obtained.
- Patients with blood group O have 20–30% lower levels of vWF antigen and ristocetin cofactor activity.
- vWF is an acute-phase reactant, so elevations may be seen in inflammatory conditions, liver disease, during pregnancy (which may correct mild deficits), or with estrogen use.

DIFFERENTIAL DIAGNOSIS

- Primary hemostatic disorders:
  - Congenital thrombocytopenia
  - Coagulation factor deficiencies
- Secondary hemostatic disorders:
  - Liver disease
  - Uremia
  - Connective tissue disorders
  - Coagulation factor inhibitors

TREATMENT

MEDICATION

First Line

- Desmopressin (DDAVP):
  - Enhances release of vWF from endothelial cells
  - Primarily effective for type 1 vWD
  - Not effective in severe deficiencies, in types of vWD with defective vWF, or for prophylaxis prior to major procedures
  - 0.3 mcg/kg IV/SC or 300 mcg/d intranasally
  - Common side effects: Flushing, tachycardia, water retention
  - Obtain repeat testing of ristocetin cofactor activity and FVIII 1 and 4 hours after infusion to evaluate peak response and clearance of DDAVP (3)[C].
  - Tachyphylaxis may develop with repeat doses.
- Fresh frozen plasma (FFP) and cryoprecipitate:
  - FFP contains the components of the coagulation, fibrinolytic, and complement systems and proteins that maintain oncotic pressure and modulate immunity.
  - Cryoprecipitate contains FVIII, fibrinogen, vWF, factor XIII, and fibronectin.
  - Both contain both vWF and FVIII.
  - Not considered as safe as the virus-inactivated plasma concentrates below
- vWF and FVIII concentrates:
  - Humate-P and Alphanate are commercial concentrates of vWF and FVIII that are given in doses of 25–50 IU/kg/d based on clinical situation:
    - Humate-P is the only treatment for urgent bleeding that has been validated in prospective, open-label studies (4)[B]. Dose may be adjusted for FVIII levels and ristocetin cofactor activity.
    - These concentrates are the mainstay of treatment for patients who do not respond to DDAVP and may be used in acquired forms, but have a shortened half-life.
    - FVIII levels should be monitored when providing these replacements in order to avoid supranormal levels and possible venous thromboembolism (VTE).
    - Contraindicated if patient develops alloantibodies to vWF
- Antifibrinolytics:
  - Useful for mucosal bleeding
  - Contraindicated in patients with hematuria due to risk of retention of large blood clots in the renal collecting system
  - Given as adjunct to desmopressin
  - Aminocaproic acid may be given at 50–60 mg/kg q4–6h IV or PO
  - Tranexamic acid may be given at 50–60 mg/kg q8–12h IV or PO
- Recombinant FVIII:
  - Used for patients who develop alloantibodies to vWF
  - Given as bolus of 90 mcg/kg q2h or 20 mcg/kg every hour until hemostasis is achieved

Second Line

- Platelets may be given as an adjunct to factor concentrates if hemostasis has not been achieved.
- IVIG has been useful in some patients with monoclonal gammopathy of undetermined significance.
- Oral contraceptives may have a role in the treatment of chronic menorrhagia.
- Recombinant FVIIa has been used effectively in patients with type 3 vWD.

ADDITIONAL TREATMENT

General Measures

- Most patients with type 1 vWD do not require activity restrictions.
- Patients with type 3 vWD should avoid contact sports.
- An emergency ID bracelet may be useful.

Issues for Referral

The diagnosis of vWD is not always straightforward. It may be useful to consider consultation with a coagulation laboratory and/or a hematologist for the interpretation of testing results and treatment decision making.

SURGERY/OTHER PROCEDURES

Aortic valve replacement may be curative for acquired vWD in aortic stenosis.

IN-PATIENT CONSIDERATIONS

Initial Stabilization

- For patients with major bleeds or those undergoing major surgical procedures, levels of ristocetin cofactor activity need to be restored and then maintained above 50% for 3–5 days. FVIII levels need to be maintained above 40% for 10–14 days.
- For patients undergoing minor surgical procedures, maintain FVIII levels >30 IU/dL for 5–7 days.
- For patients delivering or in need of epidural anesthesia, obtain FVIII levels >50 IU/dL.

ONGOING CARE

FOLLOW-UP RECOMMENDATIONS

Patients should be seen by a hematologist prior to invasive procedures for determination of perioperative management or advice regarding delivery.

Patient Monitoring

Patients with mild disease do not require monitoring.

DIET

No restrictions are recommended.

PATIENT EDUCATION

National Hemophilia Foundation: www.hemophilia.org/NHFWeb/MainPgs/MainNHF.aspx?menuid=182&contentid=47&rptname=bleeding

PROGNOSIS

Most patients with vWD have a normal life expectancy.

COMPLICATIONS

- Significant perioperative bleeding may occur.
- Patients with type 3 vWD can have bleeding complications similar to patients with hemophilia A, such as hemarthrosis and intracranial hemorrhage.
- Patients with aortic stenosis and acquired vWD are known to have higher rates of GI blood loss.
- Multiple transfusions may result in alloantibodies against vWF.
- VTE may result from supranormal levels of FVIII.

REFERENCES

1. Rodeghiero F, Castaman G, Tosetto A, et al. The discriminant power of bleeding history for the diagnosis of type 1 von Willebrand disease: An international, multicenter study. *J Thromb Haemost*. 2005;3:2619–26.
2. Lippi G, Franchini M, Salvagno GL, et al. Correlation between von Willebrand factor antigen, von Willebrand factor ristocetin cofactor activity and factor VIII activity in plasma. *J Thromb Thrombolysis*. 2008;26:150–3.
3. Hanebutt FL, Rolf N, Loesel A, et al. Evaluation of desmopressin effects on haemostasis in children with congenital bleeding disorders. *Haemophilia*. 2008;14:524–30.
4. Thompson AR, Gill JC, Ewenstein BM, et al. Successful treatment for patients with von Willebrand disease undergoing urgent surgery using factor VIII/VWF concentrate (Humate-P). *Haemophilia*. 2004;10:42–51.

ADDITIONAL READING

- Kessler CM. Diagnosis and treatment of von Willebrand disease: New perspectives and nuances. *Haemophilia*. 2007;13(Suppl 5):3–14.
- Kumar S, Pruthi RK, Nichols WL. Acquired von Willebrand disease. *Mayo Clin Proc*. 2002;77:181–7.
- Mannucci PM. Treatment of von Willebrand's disease. *N Engl J Med*. 2004;351:683–94.
- Robertson J, Lillicrap D, James PD. Von Willebrand disease. *Pediatr Clin North Am*. 2008;55:377–92, viii–ix.
- Rodeghiero F, Castaman G, Tosetto A, et al. How I treat von Willebrand disease. *Blood*. 2009;114:1158–65.
- Sciscione AC, Mucowski SJ. Pregnancy and von Willebrand disease: A review. *Del Med J*. 2007;79:401–5.

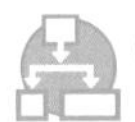

See Also (Topic, Algorithm, Electronic Media Element)

Algorithms: Bleeding Gums; Ecchymosis

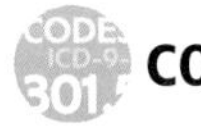

CODES

ICD9

286.4 Von Willebrand's disease

CLINICAL PEARLS

- vWD can vary from a minor to a severe bleeding disorder, and affects 1–2% of the US population.
- It is important to determine the exact type of vWD (1, 2, or 3) a patient has to guide effective treatment.
- There should be suspicion for acquired vWD in patients with acquired bleeding disorders.

VULVAR MALIGNANCY

Michael P. Hopkins, MD, MEd
Eric L. Jenison, MD
Michael S. Guy, MD

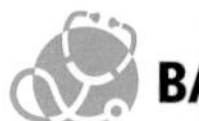

BASICS

DESCRIPTION

- Carcinoma in situ (Bowen disease): Premalignant changes involving the squamous epithelium of the vulva
- Squamous cell carcinoma: Invasive squamous cell carcinoma is the most common malignancy involving the vulva (90% of patients) (1). The malignancy can be well, moderately, or poorly differentiated.
- Other invasive cell types include melanoma, Paget disease, adenocarcinoma, adenoid cystic carcinoma, small cell carcinoma, verrucous carcinoma, and sarcomas. Sarcomas are usually leiomyosarcoma and probably arise at the insertion of the round ligament in the labium major.
- System(s) affected: Reproductive

Geriatric Considerations

- Older patients with associated medical problems are at high risk from radical surgery. The surgery, however, is external, usually well tolerated, and is the treatment of choice. Patients who are not surgical candidates can be treated with primary radiotherapy.
- In the very elderly, palliative vulvectomy provides relief of symptoms for ulcerating symptomatic advanced disease.

EPIDEMIOLOGY

Incidence

- In the US, invasive vulvar malignancy is the fourth most common gynecologic malignancy, accounting for ~3,500 new cases in 2010.
- Predominant age:
  - In situ disease: Mean age 40s
  - Invasive malignancy: Mean age 60s, with a range of 20s–90s

RISK FACTORS

- VIN or CIN
- Smoking
- Lichen sclerosus (vulvar dystrophy)
- HPV infection
- Autoimmune processes

Genetics

No known genetic pattern

GENERAL PREVENTION

- Human papillomavirus (HPV) vaccination has the potential to decrease vulvar cancer by 1/3 (1).
- Abstinence from smoking/smoking cessation counseling

ETIOLOGY

- Patients with cervical cancer are more likely to develop vulvar cancer at a later date. This is due to the so-called "field effect" with a carcinogen involving the lower genital tract.
- HPV has been associated with squamous cell abnormalities of the cervix, vagina, and vulva but has not been proven to be the causative agent. 60% of vulvar cancers are attributable to oncogenic HPV.
- Smoking is associated with squamous cell disease of the vulva, possibly from direct irritation of the vulva by the transfer of tars and nicotine on the patient's hands or from systemic absorption of carcinogen.

COMMONLY ASSOCIATED CONDITIONS

- Patients with invasive vulvar cancer are often elderly and have associated medical conditions.
- High rate of other gynecologic malignancies; patients should be evaluated for these.

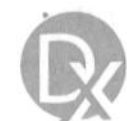

DIAGNOSIS

HISTORY

Complaints of pruritus or raised lesion in the vaginal area

PHYSICAL EXAM

- In situ disease: A small raised area associated with pruritus
- Invasive malignancy: An ulcerated, nonhealing area; as lesions become large, bleeding occurs with associated pain and foul-smelling discharge.
- In far-advanced disease: The patients can develop rectal bleeding or urethral obstruction.
- Large involved inguinal lymph nodes are also associated with advanced disease.

DIAGNOSTIC TESTS & INTERPRETATION

Lab

Initial lab tests

- Hypercalcemia can occur when metastatic disease is present.
- Squamous cell antigen can be elevated with invasive disease.

Follow-Up & Special Considerations

- Any woman complaining of symptoms related to the vulva should have a close examination and biopsies of appropriate areas.
- The vulva can be washed with 3% acetic acid to highlight areas. Areas of white, raised epithelium should be biopsied.
- Patients with new onset of pruritus should be biopsied in the area of pruritus.
- Liberal biopsies must be used to diagnose in situ disease prior to invasion and to diagnose early invasive disease.
- The patient should not be treated for presumed benign conditions of the vulva without full exam and biopsy.
- When symptoms persist, re-examination and rebiopsy should be undertaken.
- The treatment of benign condyloma of the vulva has not been shown to decrease the eventual incidence of in situ or invasive disease of the vulva.

Imaging

Initial approach

- CXR to evaluate for metastatic disease
- CT scan to evaluate pelvic and periaortic lymph node status

Diagnostic Procedures/Surgery

Office vulvar biopsy is done to establish the diagnosis.

Pathological Findings

A surgical staging system is used for vulvar cancer (International Federation of Obstetrics and Gynecology Classification):

- Stage I: Tumor confined to the vulva:
  - Stage IA: Lesions ≤2 cm in size, confined to the vulva or perineum, and with stromal invasion ≤1 mm, no node metastasis
  - Stage IB: Lesions >2 cm in size or with stromal invasion >1 mm, confined to the vulva or perineum, with negative nodes
- Stage II: Tumor of any size with extension to adjacent perineal structures (1/3 lower urethra, 1/3 lower vagina, anus) with negative nodes
- Stage III: Tumor of any size with or without extension to adjacent perineal structures (1/3 lower urethra, 1/3 lower vagina, anus) with positive inguinofemoral lymph nodes:
  - Stage IIIA:
    - With 1 lymph node metastasis (≥5 mm), or
    - 1–2 lymph node metastasis(es) (<5 mm)
  - Stage IIIB:
    - With 2 or more lymph node metastases (≥5 mm), or
    - 3 or more lymph node metastases (<5 mm)
  - Stage IIIC: With positive nodes with extracapsular spread
- Stage IV: Tumor invades other regional (2/3 upper urethra, 2/3 upper vagina) or distant structures
  - Stage IVA: Tumor invades any of the following:
    - Upper urethral and/or vaginal mucosa, bladder mucosa, rectal mucosa, or fixed to pelvic bone or
    - Fixed or ulcerated inguinofemoral lymph nodes
  - Stage IVB: Any distant metastasis, including pelvic lymph nodes

DIFFERENTIAL DIAGNOSIS

- The definitive diagnosis for vulvar lesions is made by biopsy. Infectious processes can present as ulcerative lesions and include syphilis, lymphogranuloma venereum, and granuloma inguinale.
- Crohn disease can present as an ulcerative area on the vulva.
- Rarely, lesions can metastasize to the vulva.

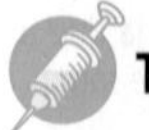

TREATMENT

There are no curative drugs.

MEDICATION

- As an adjuvant therapy, fluorouracil (Efudex) cream for in situ disease can produce occasional results, but is not well tolerated because of irritation of the vulva.
- Chemoradiotherapy with cisplatin and 5-fluorouracil has been successful in advanced or recurrent disease, although local morbidity is increased (2)[B].
- Adjuvant chemotherapy has not proven to be effective in this disease (3)[A].

- Contraindications: Elderly patients: If chemotherapeutic agents are used, pay close attention to the patient's performance status and ability to tolerate aggressive chemotherapy.
- Precautions: The usual precautions for chemotherapy agents. Refer to manufacturer's literature for each drug.

ADDITIONAL TREATMENT

General Measures

- Wide excision can be performed for carcinoma in situ, and any lesion about which there is doubt should be further excised for definitive diagnosis to ensure that invasive disease is not coexistent with the carcinoma in situ.
- Cystoscopy and sigmoidoscopy should be performed if there is a question of invasion into the urethra, bladder, or rectum.

Issues for Referral

Patients may need care from a gynecologic oncologist and/or a radiation oncologist.

Additional Therapies

- Radiation therapy is used as adjuvant therapy for patients with positive inguinal lymph nodes.
- Preoperative radiation/chemotherapy may allow for a less radical surgical procedure in patients with advanced disease (4,5)[B].
- Postoperative radiation as an adjuvant treatment decreases recurrence frequency and may improve survival (4)[B].
- Radiation is contraindicated with verrucous carcinoma because it induces anaplastic transformation and increases metastases.

SURGERY/OTHER PROCEDURES

- In situ disease can be treated with wide excision or laser vaporization of the affected area. Laser vaporization is preferable in the younger patient, whereas wide excision is preferable in the elderly patient, in whom the risk of invasive disease is also higher.
- 0.5 mm of negative margin is adequate for in situ disease (2)[C].
- Stage IA: radical local excision without lymph node dissection because lymph node metastases are <1% (2)[C].
- Stage IB: Radical local excision with lymph node dissection because the risk of metastases increases to 8% (2)[C]
- Stage II: Modified radical vulvectomy and groin node dissection are recommended (2)[C].
- Stage III and IVA: Radical vulvectomy and bilateral inguinal lymph node dissection are recommended (2)[C].
- Bulky advanced-stage lesions are often treated initially with chemoradiation followed by less radical surgery (5)[B].
- Adjuvant radiation therapy is recommended with microscopically positive lymph nodes (2)[C].
- Pelvic exenteration after radiation provides effective therapy for advanced or recurrent malignancies involving the bladder or rectum.
- More limited surgery:
  - Has been undertaken for early invasive lesions, especially in young patients, to preserve the clitoris and sexual function
  - Sentinel lymph node (SLN) biopsy also has been advocated in early invasive lesion; however, data show lower accuracy compared to complete dissection (6)[C].
  - Radical vulvectomy with bilateral groin node dissection through separate incisions provides better cosmetic results than the en bloc technique.
  - Radical hemivulvectomy and unilateral groin node dissection also can be used for smaller unilateral lesions.

IN-PATIENT CONSIDERATIONS

Typically inpatient for treatment

Initial Stabilization

In advanced malignancy involving the urethra and rectum, concomitant cisplatin/5-fluorouracil (5-FU) chemotherapy with radiation produces a significant decrease in size of the primary tumor, usually obviating the need for pelvic exenteration.

ONGOING CARE

FOLLOW-UP RECOMMENDATIONS

Patient Monitoring

- Clinical exam of the groin nodes and vulvar area every 3 months for 2 years; then every 6 months for 3 years
- Annual CXR

DIET

Unrestricted, unless undergoing radiation

PATIENT EDUCATION

- American College of Obstetricians and Gynecologists (ACOG), 409 12th St., SW, Washington, DC 20024-2188; (800) 762-ACOG; www.acog.org
- American Cancer Society: www.cancer.org
- Medline Plus: www.nlm.nih.gov/medlineplus/vulvarcancer.html

PROGNOSIS

The 5-year survival is based on stage:

- Stage I: 78.5%
- Stage II: 58.8%
- Stage III: 43.2%
- Stage IV: 13%

COMPLICATIONS

- The major complications from radical vulvectomy and groin node dissection are:
  - Wound breakdown
  - Lymphocysts
  - Lymphedema
  - Urinary stress incontinence
  - Psychosexual consequences
- 2 common complications with radical vulvectomy and bilateral groin node dissection:
  - In the immediate postoperative period, ~50% of patients experience breakdown of the wound. This requires aggressive wound care by visiting nurses as often as twice a day. The wounds usually granulate and heal over a period of 6–10 weeks.
  - ~15–20% of patients experience some form of mild-to-moderate lymphedema after the groin node dissection. These patients should be instructed in the use of leg elevation and support hose. <1% of patients experience severe, debilitating lymphedema.

REFERENCES

1. Smith JS, Backes DM, Hoots BE, et al. Human papillomavirus type-distribution in vulvar and vaginal cancers and their associated precursors. *Obstet Gynecol*. 2009;113:917–24.
2. de Hullu JA, van der Zee AG. Surgery and radiotherapy in vulvar cancer. *Crit Rev Oncol Hematol*. 2006;60:38–58.
3. Shylasree TS, Bryant A, Howells RE. Chemoradiation for advanced primary vulval cancer. *Cochrane Database Syst Rev*. 2011;(4):CD003752.
4. Montana GS. Carcinoma of the vulva: Combined modality treatment. *Curr Treat Options Oncol*. 2004;5:85–95.
5. de Hullu JA, van der Avoort IA, Oonk MH, et al. Management of vulvar cancers. *Eur J Surg Oncol*. 2006;32(8):825–31.
6. Radziszewski J, Kowalewska M, Jedrzejczak T, et al. The accuracy of the sentinel lymph node concept in early stage squamous cell vulvar carcinoma. *Gynecol Oncol*. 2010;116:473–7.

ADDITIONAL READING

- CDC. Quadrivalent human papillomavirus vaccine: Recommendations of the advisory committee on immunization practices. *MMWR*. 2007; 569(No.RR02).
- Crosbie EJ, Slade RJ, Ahmed AS, et al. The management of vulval cancer. *Cancer Treat Rev*. 2009;35:533–9.

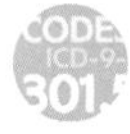

CODES

ICD9

- 184.1 Malignant neoplasm of labia majora
- 184.4 Malignant neoplasm of vulva, unspecified
- 233.39 Carcinoma in situ, other female genital organ

CLINICAL PEARLS

- 60% of vulvar cancers are attributable to oncogenic HPV. Therefore, HPV vaccination has the potential to decrease vulvar cancer by 1/3.
- Biopsy all suspicious or nonhealing vulvar lesions.

VULVODYNIA

Pamela L. Grimaldi, DO
Kathryn Wilson, MD

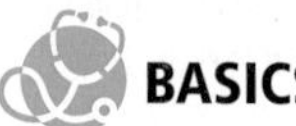

BASICS

DESCRIPTION

- Vulvar discomfort, often described as "burning," for at least 3 months; occurs in the absence of relevant visible findings or a clinically identifiable neurologic disorder
- Classification is based on whether pain is generalized or localized and whether it is provoked, spontaneous, or mixed:
  - Generalized: Involvement of majority of the vulva; persistent pain, often spontaneous but sometimes provoked (by physical contact) or mixed
  - Localized: Severe pain of certain vulvar areas, such as the vestibule (AKA *vestibulodynia*), upon touch or attempted vaginal entry; thought to be the leading cause of painful intercourse among premenopausal women
    - Primary: Introital dyspareunia from first episode of intercourse or first insertion of tampon or vaginal speculum
    - Secondary: Introital dyspareunia developing after a period of painless intercourse, tampon use, or speculum exams

EPIDEMIOLOGY

- Most women diagnosed between the ages of 20 and 50
- More likely to have a history of candidal vulvovaginitis
- Patients are psychologically comparable to asymptomatic controls and have similar marital satisfaction.
- No more likely to have been abused

Incidence

- Recent retrospective study estimates annual rate of new onset vulvodynia to be 1.8% (1).
- Evidence indicates lifetime cumulative incidence approaches 15%, suggesting nearly 14 million US women will experience persistent vulvar discomfort at some point in their lives (2).

Prevalence

- Reports between 3.1% and 15%; nonclinic-based studies approximate a prevalence of 7% with validation by exam.
- Studies show Hispanics more likely to present with vulvar pain compared with whites and African Americans.

RISK FACTORS

- Vulvovaginal infections: Vulvovaginal candidiasis and bacterial vaginosis
- Hyperoxaluria: Increased urinary oxalate excretion suggested as possible vulvar irritant
- Allergy: Vaginal fluid specimens reveal increased IgE levels; mast cells have also been noted in biopsy specimens.
- Hormonal factors: Controversial evidence proposes increased risk with use of OCPs; early age at first use of OCPs and longer duration of use have been associated with increased risk. Strong association between this disorder and the postpartum period also has been identified.
- Pelvic floor dysfunction: Increased instability of pelvic floor muscles may perpetuate vulvar tissue inflammation, leading to vascular changes and histamine release.
- Comorbid interstitial cystitis and painful bladder syndrome; potentially related to common embryological origin of structures.
- Abuse: Increased risk of vulvodynia if childhood physical or sexual abuse by a primary family member; causal relationship remains unclear (2)

Genetics

Proposed genetic deficiency impairing one's ability to stop the inflammatory response triggered by infection or chemicals; homozygosity of the 2 alleles of the IL1 receptor antagonist occurs in 25–50% of vestibulodynia patients, compared to fewer than 10% in controls (3).

GENERAL PREVENTION

- Wear 100% cotton underwear in the daytime and no underwear to sleep.
- Avoid douching and other vulvar irritants such as perfumes, dyes, detergents.
- Clean the vulva with water only and pat area dry after bathing.
- Avoid use of hairdryers in the vulvar area.
- Use adequate lubrication during intercourse.
- Apply cool gel packs to vulvar area.
- Apply preservative-free emollient (petrolatum) topically to trap moisture and improve barrier function.

PATHOPHYSIOLOGY

- Vulvodynia is likely to be neuropathically mediated:
  - Allodynia and hyperalgesia are thought to result from neurogenic inflammation leading to sensitization of primary afferents by inflammatory peptides, prostaglandins, cytokines. Impulses transmitted to CNS, where reinforcing signals sustain pain loop.
  - In recent investigations of vulvar biopsy specimens, increased neuronal proliferation and branching in vulvar tissue are evident when compared with tissue of asymptomatic women (3).
- Pelvic floor pathology also should be considered:
  - In one study, the vulvodynia group showed an increase in pelvic floor hypertonicity at the superficial muscle layer, less vaginal muscle strength with contraction, and decreased relaxation of pelvic floor muscles after contraction (2).

ETIOLOGY

Lack of standard criteria to describe sexual pain syndromes and interchangeable descriptors for vulvar pain make it difficult to characterize causes. However, below is a list of proposed etiologies:

- Recurrent vulvovaginal candidiasis
- Chemical exposure (trichloroacetic acid)
- High level of urinary oxalates
- Reduced estrogen receptor expression/changes in estrogen concentration
- CNS etiology, similar to other regional pain syndromes

COMMONLY ASSOCIATED CONDITIONS

Higher incidence of chronic pain syndromes associated with vulvodynia, including:

- Trigonitis
- Chronic cystitis
- IBS
- Fibromyalgia
- Migraines
- Depression
- Endometriosis
- TMJ syndrome

DIAGNOSIS

- Vulvodynia is a clinical diagnosis and should be suspected in any women with chronic pain at the introitus and vulva (3)[B].
- Pain should be characterized using a standard measure such as the McGill Pain Questionnaire; duration and nature of the pain should be established. Physical exam used to rule out other causes of vulvovaginal pain. Negative fungal culture, along with relevant history and positive cotton swab test (see below), confirm diagnosis.

HISTORY

Adequate sexual, social, and pain history should be taken to assess degree of symptoms. Visual pain scales and pain diaries may be helpful (4)[C]:

- Onset of vulvodynia often sudden and without precedents.
- Pain often described as generalized, unprovoked
- Specific skin complaints may suggest alternate Dx; a history of allergies may suggest vulvar dermatitis.
- Assess for precipitants of vulvar pain: Tight garments, bicycle riding, tampon use, prolonged sitting, perfumed or deodorant soaps, douching
- Assess for complaints of dyspareunia:
  - Presence of vaginismus (involuntary vaginal muscle spasm), adequate lubrication, anorgasmia, partner problems, abuse
  - Psychosexual morbidity significantly higher in patients with vulvodynia; counseling may complement medical interventions.

PHYSICAL EXAM

- Mouth and skin exams to assess for lesions suggestive of lichen planus or lichen sclerosis
- Vaginal exam should be done to exclude other causes of vulvovaginal pain:
  - The vulva may be erythematous, especially at the vestibule. Discomfort with separation of the labia minora is common.
  - Spontaneous or elicited pain at the lower 1/2 of anterior vaginal wall suggests bladder etiology.
- Bulbocavernosus and anal wink reflexes should be checked to assess for peripheral neuropathy.

DIAGNOSTIC TESTS & INTERPRETATION

Cotton swab or Q-tip test:

- Vulva tested for localized areas of pain beginning at thighs and continuing medially toward vestibule. 5 distinct positions (2, 4, 6, 8, and 10 o'clock) surveyed using light palpation. Pain rated on a scale from 0 (none) to 10 (most severe). Posterior introitus and posterior hymenal remnants most common sites of increased sensitivity.
- If pain confirmed, fungal culture obtained. Lack of sensitivity in all of the designated areas unusual among women with vulvodynia.

Lab

Initial lab tests

- Vaginal pH, wet mount, Gram stain, and yeast culture are recommended to rule out vaginitis.
- Gonorrhea and chlamydia testing done at physician's discretion

- HPV screening is unnecessary; no association has been identified between HPV and vulvodynia.

Follow-Up & Special Considerations

Varicella-zoster and herpes simplex virus should be considered if ulcers or vesicular eruptions are present.

Diagnostic Procedures/Surgery

Colposcopy can be helpful if epidermal abnormalities are present. This should be done with caution as acetic acid worsens vulvar pain.

Pathological Findings

- No specific histologic features are associated with vulvodynia, although reactive squamous atypia has been observed. Biopsies are unnecessary for diagnosis.
- Presence of rash/altered mucosa is not consistent with vulvodynia; this requires further evaluation (4)[C].

DIFFERENTIAL DIAGNOSIS

- Infections: Candidiasis, herpes, HPV, bacterial vaginosis, dermatophytes
- Inflammation: Lichen planus, immunobullous disorder, allergic vulvitis, lichen sclerosis
- Neoplasia: Paget disease, vulvar intraepithelial neoplasia, squamous cell carcinoma
- Neurologic/muscular: Herpes neuralgia, spinal nerve compression, vaginismus

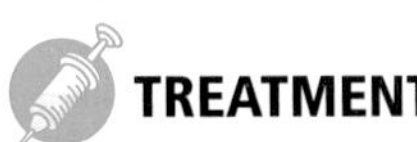

TREATMENT

Tricyclics, venlafaxine, and gabapentin all have been used as off-label interventions for the treatment of vulvodynia.

MEDICATION

- Oral therapies:
  - TCAs: First-line treatment for unprovoked vulvodynia (4)[B]; do not stop use abruptly; contraindicated in patients with cardiac abnormalities and those taking MAOIs; fatigue, constipation, and weight gain are most common side effects:
    - Amitriptyline, Nortriptyline: Most widely studied; start at 10 mg daily; dose should be titrated to pain control. Average effective dose is 60 mg daily. In one study a 47% complete response rate was recorded (5)[B].
  - SSRIs/SNRIs: Not commonly used; however, have been helpful in those who cannot tolerate TCAs:
    - Venlafaxine is currently being prescribed more frequently with good results.
  - Gabapentin: Started at 300 mg daily and increased by 300 mg every 3 days. Maximum recommended dose is 3,600 mg daily. Dosing regimen limits popularity.
  - Narcotics/NSAIDs: Consistently have not been helpful in relieving vulvar pain
- Topical therapies: A trial of local anesthetics may be recommended for all patients who present with vulvodynia symptoms. Use judiciously to avoid increased irritancy; ointments are preferred (4)[C]:
  - Lidocaine gels/ointments: For provoked vestibulodynia; application advised 15–20 minutes prior to intercourse. Penile numbness and possible toxicity with ingestion can occur:
    - In one study, lidocaine 5% ointment was left in vestibule overnight (average of 8 hours) for a period of 6–8 weeks; at follow-up, up to 76% of women reported no discomfort with intercourse (2)[C].
  - Cromolyn cream (4%): Decreases mast cell degranulation in vulvar tissue; recommended application t.i.d. (3)[C]
  - Capsaicin (0.025%): Decreases in discomfort and increases in frequency of intercourse with 20-minute daily application (2)[B]
  - 2% topical amitriptyline combined with 2% baclofen is helpful in patients with comorbid vaginismus.
  - Topical corticosteroids and testosterone creams have not been shown to alleviate symptoms of vulvodynia.
  - Gabapentin ointment 3% or 6%
  - Topical nitroglycerin side effect: Headaches
- Injectable therapies:
  - Triamcinolone acetonide 0.1%: No more than 40 mg should be injected monthly; is best when combined with 0.25–0.5% bupivacaine.
  - Submucosal methylprednisone and lidocaine: Reports of up to 68% response rate with weekly injections (4)[B]
  - Interferon alpha: Useful in treatment of vestibulodynia. Side effects (myalgias, fever, malaise) limit use.
  - Botulinum toxin A injectable

ADDITIONAL TREATMENT

- Biofeedback/physical therapy: Useful with concomitant vaginismus. Treats both generalized and localized vulvar pain; treatment value for unprovoked pain remains unclear. Most studies report an average of 12–16-week treatment time. Decrease in pelvic floor spasms and improved pelvic neuromuscular functioning seen in those with vestibulodynia:
  - Surface electromyography (sEMG): Efficacious for pelvic floor rehabilitation. Patients are more likely to endure pain-free sexual intercourse after sEMG. Significant reductions seen on pain measures at long-term follow-up.
- Cognitive-behavioral therapy (CBT): One randomized trial revealed that CBT is associated with a 30% decrease in vulvar discomfort with sexual intercourse. CBT is the recommended treatment for patients who present with dyspareunia as a main complaint (3)[B].

General Measures

Combining treatments should be encouraged when treating women with vulvodynia (4)[C]:

- Various studies reveal that patients respond better to surgical interventions when combined with psychosexual treatments.
- Various reports looking at use of combination of medical treatments, psychotherapy, and dietary intervention reveal women do significantly better compared with those who receive medication only.

Issues for Referral

A team approach is recommended for most effective management. Triage to psychosexual medicine, psychology, and pain management teams should be strongly considered (4)[B].

COMPLEMENTARY AND ALTERNATIVE MEDICINE

Acupuncture: Small studies of women with unprovoked vulvodynia who did not respond to conventional treatment reported significant decreases in pain severity with acupuncture; treatment value with provoked pain is unknown (4)[C].

SURGERY/OTHER PROCEDURES

- Surgery may be considered for patients who have failed to respond to other measures. Use of surgical treatment is not recommended for generalized vulvodynia (4)[B].
- 60–80% of women who undergo surgery report a significant improvement in pain symptoms; however, when surveyed, patients prefer behavioral therapies to surgical intervention.
- A 3-armed randomized trial in 2001 found that women who underwent surgical intervention were more satisfied than those treated with biofeedback or CBT (3)[B].
- All patients who are considering surgical intervention should be tested for vaginismus. Vestibulectomy is less successful in this subgroup.
- Surgical approaches:
  - Local excision: Precise localization of painful areas; tissue closed in elliptical fashion
  - Total vestibulectomy: Incision os made and tissue is removed from Skene ducts to perineum. The vagina is then brought down to cover defect.
  - Perineoplasty: Vestibulectomy + removal of perineal tissue; incision usually terminated above the anal orifice; reserved for severe cases (3)[B]

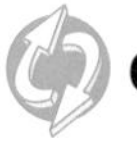

ONGOING CARE

PATIENT EDUCATION

Patients should be reassured that this condition is not infectious, nor does it predispose to cancer (4)[C].

PROGNOSIS

Traditionally viewed as a chronic pain disorder, new evidence of remission has been documented; recent 2-year follow-up study revealed 1 in 10 vulvodynia patients reported remission.

REFERENCES

1. Reed B, Haefner H, Sen A, et al. Vulvodynia incidence and remission rates among adult women: A 2-year follow-up study. *Obstet Gynecol*. 2008;112:231–7.
2. Boardman L, Stockdale C. Sexual pain. *Clin Obstetrics and Gynecology*. 2009;52:682–90.
3. Reed B. Vulvodynia: Diagnosis and management. *Am Fam Physician*. 2006;73:1231–9.
4. Mandal D, Nunns M, Byrne J, et al. Guidelines for the management of vulvodynia. *BJD*. 2010;162:1180–5.
5. Haefner H, Collins M, Davis G, et al. The vulvodynia guideline. *J Low Genit Tract Dis*. 2005;9:40–51.

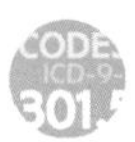

CODES

ICD9

- 625.70 Vulvodynia, unspecified
- 625.71 Vulvar vestibulitis
- 625.79 Other vulvodynia

CLINICAL PEARLS

Vulvodynia is a clinical diagnosis and should be suspected in any woman with chronic pain at the introitus and vulva.

VULVOVAGINITIS, ESTROGEN DEFICIENT

Maria de La Luz Nieto, MD
Danielle Patterson, MD, MSc

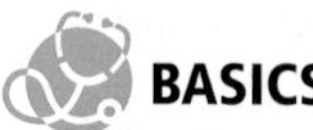

BASICS

DESCRIPTION

- Vaginal atrophy is due to decreased blood flow to vaginal epithelium, resulting in thinning of the female genital tissues.
- Estrogen deficiency affects all tissues in the female body; however, the genital tissues are especially hormone-responsive and are most affected, leading to atrophy.
- Patients with estrogen-deficient vulvovaginitis may present with urinary incontinence, increased urinary frequency, or recurrent UTIs.
- System(s) affected: Reproductive

EPIDEMIOLOGY

Incidence

- Predominant age: Postmenopausal females:
  - The average age of menopause in the US is 51.3 years.
- May affect lactating women.
- Predominant sex: Female only
- May occur in younger women with premature ovarian failure.

Prevalence

- Most postmenopausal women are affected to some degree.
- Up to 40% of postmenopausal women experience symptoms severe enough to seek treatment.

RISK FACTORS

Estrogen-deficient states

Genetics

No known pattern

PATHOPHYSIOLOGY

- Decreased estrogen levels in the vagina and vulva result in decreased blood flow and decreased lubrication of vaginal and vulvar tissue.
- Vaginal and vulvar tissues become thin secondary to decreased vaginal cell maturation.
- Decreased cellular maturation results in decreased glycogen stores, which affects the normal vaginal flora and pH.

ETIOLOGY

Estrogen deficiency due to:

- Menopause (surgical or natural)
- Premature ovarian failure (chemotherapy, irradiation, autoimmune, anorexia, genetic)
- Postpartum, lactation
- Medications that alter hormonal concentration such as gonadotropin-releasing hormone agonists, and antiestrogens such as tamoxifen and danazol
- Elevated prolactin from hypothalamic-pituitary disorders

COMMONLY ASSOCIATED CONDITIONS

- Urge and stress urinary incontinence
- Pelvic organ prolapse
- Frequent UTIs
- Bacterial vaginosis or yeast infections

DIAGNOSIS

HISTORY

- All female patients should be asked about symptoms because many women are embarrassed to discuss these issues with their health care providers:
  - Vaginal dryness
  - Dyspareunia
  - Pruritus
  - Burning
  - Pressure
  - Tenderness
  - Malodorous discharge
  - Urinary symptoms: Dysuria, hematuria, frequency, infections, stress and urge urinary incontinence
- Ask about self-treatment and products used.
- Determine exposure to irritants (e.g., soaps, feminine sprays, lotions, lubricants, constant pad use).

PHYSICAL EXAM

Evidence for the diagnosis includes the following (1)[C]:

- Loss of pubic hair
- Decreased vulvar and vaginal fullness
- Decreased vulvar SC fat and moisture
- Pale-appearing, shiny, smooth vaginal and urethral epithelium
- Vaginal shortening, intolerance to speculum exams
- Loss of vaginal rugation
- Pelvic organ prolapse

DIAGNOSTIC TESTS & INTERPRETATION

Lab

As vulvovaginitis is a clinical diagnosis, labs are not always necessary.

Initial lab tests

However, the following labs may be obtained as corroborative of clinical impression:

- Check follicle-stimulating hormone (FSH) and estrogen levels. FSH rises and estrogen drops with menopause.
- Evaluate for infections via wet preparation and vaginal pH (usually >5).
- Urine dip and urinalysis if suspected concomitant UTI
- Perform cytology for maturation index: Higher proportion of parabasal cells and lower proportion of intermediate and superficial cells indicate decreased maturation index.

Follow-Up & Special Considerations

Drugs that may alter lab results:

- Estrogen therapy will alter the maturation index.
- Digoxin has estrogenlike properties.
- Tamoxifen may produce menopausal-type symptoms, but also may act on genital tissues as a weak estrogen agonist.
- Progestins, danazol, and gonadotropin-releasing hormone agonists may produce a reversible pseudomenopause state.

Pathological Findings

- Thinning of the cornified squamous layer of both the vulva and the vagina
- Increased parabasal cells
- Compact underlying collagenous tissue

DIFFERENTIAL DIAGNOSIS

- Malignancy
- Dermatologic conditions of vulva and vagina:
  - Dermatitis
  - Lichen sclerosis
  - Lichen planus
- Bacterial or yeast vulvovaginitis

TREATMENT

MEDICATION

- Vaginal estrogen can reverse atrophic changes and help to alleviate symptoms (2,3)[A]:
  - Vaginal cream 1 g (conjugated equine estrogens or estradiol cream): Insert via applicator each night × 14 days and then 2–3×/wk.
  - Vaginal estradiol 10 μg tablet: Insert via preloaded applicator each night × 14 days and then 2–3×/wk.
  - Estradiol-containing vaginal ring 2 mg: Insert into vagina, and replace every 3 months.
- Estrogen therapy should be used in the lowest possible dose for the shortest duration of time.
- Long-term therapy may be necessary owing to the chronic nature of estrogen-deficient vulvovaginitis.
- Systemic therapy typically is used as hormonal treatment of vasomotor symptoms and not for the primary treatment of estrogen-deficient vulvovaginitis.
- Contraindications:
  - Breast or estrogen-dependent carcinoma
  - Undiagnosed vaginal bleeding
  - Thromboembolic disorders
  - Thrombophlebitis
  - Pregnancy
- Precautions: Any abnormal vaginal bleeding must be evaluated.

ADDITIONAL TREATMENT

General Measures

- Wear loose-fitting, undyed cotton underwear.
- Avoid prolonged pad use, especially scented pads.
- Avoid feminine deodorant sprays and douching.
- Use over-the-counter water-based lubricants as needed.
- Symptomatic relief if needed (e.g., cool baths or compresses)

Issues for Referral

- Refer to urogynecologist for evaluation if symptomatic due to pelvic organ prolapse and/or stress and urge urinary incontinence.
- Recurrent UTIs should be referred to Urogynecology and/or Urology for evaluation.

IN-PATIENT CONSIDERATIONS

Initial Stabilization

Outpatient treatment

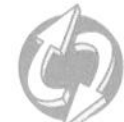

ONGOING CARE

FOLLOW-UP RECOMMENDATIONS

No restrictions

Patient Monitoring

Instruct the patient that symptoms should improve within 30–60 days. If they do not, re-evaluate and re-examine for other causes.

DIET

No special diet

PATIENT EDUCATION

- American College of Obstetricians and Gynecologists (ACOG), 409 12th St., SW, Washington, DC 20024-2188; (800) 762-ACOG; www.acog.org
- Lactating postpartum women with high levels of prolactin are in a hypoestrogenic state. These women should be instructed to use lubrication for symptoms of dyspareunia and reassured that the symptoms will resolve when they are no longer breast-feeding.

PROGNOSIS

The prognosis is excellent. The vast majority of symptoms will be alleviated with vaginal estrogen replacement therapy.

COMPLICATIONS

- Recurrent UTIs may occur in women with vaginal atrophy.
- Vaginal atrophy predisposes patients to vaginal infections.

REFERENCES

1. Johnston SL, Farrell SA, Bouchard C, et al. The detection and management of vaginal atrophy. *J Obstet Gynaecol Can*. 2004;26(5):503–15.
2. Suckling J, Lethaby A, Kennedy R. Local oestrogen for vaginal atrophy in postmenopausal women. *Cochrane Database Sys Rev*. 2006;4:CD001500.
3. Farquhar CM, Marjoribanks J, Lethaby A, et al. Long-term hormone therapy for perimenopausal and postmenopausal women. *Cochrane Database Sys Rev*. 2005;3:CD004143.

ADDITIONAL READING

- Ibe C, Simon JA. Vulvovaginal atrophy: Current and future therapies (CME). *J Sex Med*. 2010;7: 1042–50; quiz 1051.
- Mehta A, Bachmann G. Vulvovaginal complaints. *Clin Obstet Gynecol*. 2008;51:549–55.

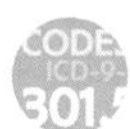

CODES

ICD9

- 616.10 Vaginitis and vulvovaginitis, unspecified
- 627.3 Postmenopausal atrophic vaginitis
- 794.6 Nonspecific abnormal results of other endocrine function study

CLINICAL PEARLS

- Estrogen-deficient vulvovaginitis affects virtually all postmenopausal women to some degree.
- This disorder is often associated with urinary incontinence, increased urinary frequency, and recurrent UTIs.
- Lab tests are generally unnecessary to make the diagnosis.
- Vaginal estrogen preparations, rather than systemic preparations, should be first-line therapy in a woman whose primary complaint is associated with vaginal atrophy.

VULVOVAGINITIS, PREPUBESCENT

Katherine M. Callaghan, MD
Dawn S. Tasillo, MD

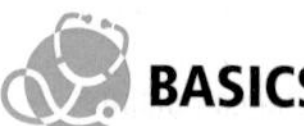

BASICS

DESCRIPTION

- Vulvitis is inflammation of the external genitals.
- Vaginitis, often associated with vaginal discharge, is inflammation involving the vaginal mucosa.
- In premenarchal girls, vulvitis is usually primary with secondary extension into the vagina.
- System(s) affected: Reproductive; Skin/Exocrine
- Synonym(s): Vaginitis; Vulvitis

EPIDEMIOLOGY

Incidence

Unknown

Prevalence

Most common gynecologic problem in prepubertal girls

RISK FACTORS

- Prepubertal girls are particularly susceptible due to behavioral and anatomic reasons:
  - Inadequate hand washing or perineal cleansing after urination and defecation
  - Tight-fitting clothing
  - Proximity of the vagina to the anus, lack of protective hair, and labial fat pads
  - Trauma
- Obese girls are also susceptible to nonspecific vulvovaginitis (1).

Genetics

Understudied

GENERAL PREVENTION

- Good perineal hygiene (including wiping from front to back)
- Urination with legs spread apart and labia separated
- Avoidance of tight-fitting clothing and nonabsorbent underwear
- Avoidance of irritants such as harsh soaps and bubble baths

PATHOPHYSIOLOGY

- In the prepubertal child, the levels of estrogen are low.
- Due to the low levels of estrogen, the vaginal epithelium is thin, immature, and fragile.
- The absence of pubic hair and a well-developed labia as well as close proximity of the anus and vagina make contamination more likely.
- The prepubertal child also has an absence of lactobacilli, creating a neutral-to-alkaline vaginal pH.
- The neutral pH, atrophic mucosa, and moist environment of the vagina increases the risk of infection.

ETIOLOGY

- Most cases of pediatric vulvovaginitis are nonspecific inflammation.
- The specific infections that occur are typically respiratory, enteric, or sexually transmitted.
- Nonspecific vulvovaginitis:
  - Poor perineal hygiene
  - Nonspecific chemical irritants (bubble baths, scented soaps, shampoos)
  - Tight-fitting clothing
- Specific vulvovaginitis:
  - The most common respiratory pathogen is *Streptococcus pyogenes*. Vulvitis may occur in the absence of respiratory symptoms.
  - Shigella vaginitis is associated with mucopurulent bloody discharge and likewise is not always accompanied by a history of diarrhea.

Respiratory	Enteral	Sexually Transmitted
Streptococcus pyogenes	*Shigella*	*Neisseria Gonorrhoeae*
Staphylococcus aureus	*Yersinia enterocolitica*	*Chlamydia trachomatis*
Haemophilus influenzae		*Trichomonas vaginalis*
Moraxella catarrhalis		*Papilloma virus*
Streptococcus pneumoniae		*Herpes virus*
Neisseria meningitidis		

- Enterobius vermicularis (pinworms)
  - Very common in young children and certain populations
  - Should be considered in children with vaginal itching and irritation
  - Most common symptom is nocturnal perineal itching
- Foreign body
  - Presents with foul-smelling, bloody, or brown discharge from the vagina
  - Should be considered with recurrent vulvovaginitis where other causes have been eliminated
- Other
  - With chronic vulvovaginitis, anatomic abnormalities or systemic disease should be considered:
    - Anatomic abnormalities include double vagina with fistula, ectopic ureter, and urethral prolapse.
  - Systemic disease (inflammatory diseases)
  - Other conditions such as lichen sclerosus, vitiligo, psoriasis, and atopic dermatitis should be considered.

ALERT

Cultures of sexually transmitted organisms in prepubertal children warrant investigations of sexual abuse.

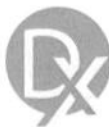

DIAGNOSIS

HISTORY

- Irritation and erythema of vulva
- Itching
- Bleeding
- Vaginal discharge
- Unpleasant odor
- Dysuria
- Soreness

PHYSICAL EXAM

- Look for evidence of chronic illness or dermatologic disease.
- Inspect the genital area in the supine position:
  - Excoriation of the genital area
  - Inflammation (erythema, swelling) of the introitus
  - Inspect the vagina and cervix in the knee–chest position
  - Perform rectal exam if vaginal bleeding or abdominal pain

DIAGNOSTIC TESTS & INTERPRETATION

Lab

Initial lab tests

- Culture for bacteria, fungi (yeast), or viruses (herpes)
- Tape exam for pinworms
- Potassium hydroxide and saline smears of vaginal discharge, if present

Follow-Up & Special Considerations

The exploration of the vagina for a foreign body may be necessary in cases of persistent, recurrent vulvitis.

Imaging

- If an anatomic abnormality is suspected, imaging may be necessary to confirm.
- Consider consultation with a pediatric or adult gynecologist to determine the most appropriate imaging study.

Diagnostic Procedures/Surgery

If blood or foul-smelling discharge is present, visualization is mandatory:

- Place the child in the knee–chest position for best results. Hold the buttocks apart and slightly upward.
- Visualization of the vagina may be necessary by using a nasal speculum or infant laryngoscope.
- If available, consider referral to a provider with specific training/experience in this specialized exam.

DIFFERENTIAL DIAGNOSIS

- Contact dermatitis
- Eczema
- Psoriasis
- Lichen sclerosus

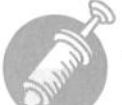

TREATMENT

- The definitive diagnosis of bacterial vulvitis requires a culture of vulva and vaginal secretions.
- The typical colony count and bacterial mix are unknown in prepubescent girls. Antibiotic use should be directed against the species with the highest colony count.
- General hygiene always should be recommended, particularly in cases of a retained foreign body (such as toilet paper).

MEDICATION

First Line

- To break the itching–scratching–infection cycle, use a low-dose topical hydrocortisone cream for a limited time (2).
- Estrogen deficiency with labial adhesion/agglutination: Estrogen cream, 0.625 mg to fused area nightly for 2 weeks (3).
- The use of antibiotics should be restricted to cases of bacterial infection only (2).
- For empirical treatment of suspected bacterial infection, use amoxicillin, 20 mg/kg/d for 7 days (3).
- Specific organisms on culture:
  - Group A *Streptococcus*, *S. pneumoniae*: Penicillin V (Pen Vee K), 250 mg PO b.i.d–t.i.d. for 10 days (4)
  - *H. influenzae*: Amoxicillin, 20–40 mg/kg/d PO for 7 days (4)
  - *S. aureus*: Cephalexin, 25–50 mg/kg/d PO q.i.d. for 7–10 days *or* Dicloxacillin, 25 mg/kg/d for 7–10 days *or*, amoxicillin-clavulanate, 20–40 mg/kg/d for 7–10 days (4)
  - S. pyogens: Amoxicillin, 50 mg/kg/d PO divided into 3 doses per day for 10 days (2)
  - *Candida* sp.: Topical nystatin (Mycostatin), miconazole, clotrimazole, or terconazole
  - *Shigella*: Trimethoprim/sulfamethoxazole or ampicillin for 5 days
  - Pinworms: Mebendazole, 100 mg PO, repeated in 2 weeks
  - Chlamydia trachomatis: ≤45 kg: Erythromycin, 50 mg/kg/d t.i.d. for 14 days; ≥45 kg: Azithromycin, 1 g PO or Doxycycline 100 mg b.i.d. for 7 days (4)
  - Neisseria gonorrhoeae: ≤45 kg: Ceftriaxone, 125 mg IM plus medication for chlamydia if not ruled out (4); >45 kg: Ceftriaxone, 250 mg IM × 1
  - Trichomonas: Metronidazole, 15 mg/kg/d t.i.d. (max 250 mg t.i.d.) for 7 days (4)
- Contraindications: Allergy to proposed treatment
- Precautions: Avoid potential allergens and topical sensitizers if possible.

ADDITIONAL TREATMENT

General Measures

- Appropriate health care: Outpatient (except where systemic illness requires hospital care)
- Soak the vulva/perineum in a small amount of clear, warm water for 15 minutes b.i.d.
- If smegma is present in the labial folds, clean the area gently with a mild soap (1).

Issues for Referral

- Suspected sexual abuse
- Suspected anatomic abnormality (except minor labial agglutination)
- Persistent, severe, or recurrent infections

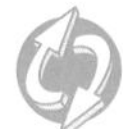

ONGOING CARE

FOLLOW-UP RECOMMENDATIONS

Patient Monitoring

Monitor for fever, pruritus, and vaginal discharge.

DIET

- Healthy balanced diet, high in fiber to prevent constipation
- Adequate fluid intake

PATIENT EDUCATION

Hygiene:

- Wipe front to back after elimination.
- Avoid bubble baths and other irritating products.
- Clean daily with mild soap and water and dry gently with soft towel or cool hair dryer.
- Apply bland ointments for protection of the skin, if necessary.

PROGNOSIS

Excellent

COMPLICATIONS

- If an STI is identified and not treated effectively, the patient is at risk for pelvic inflammatory disease (PID).
- Vaginismus

REFERENCES

1. Van Eyk N, Allen L, Giesbrecht E, et al. Pediatric vulvovaginal disorders: A diagnostic approach and review of the literature. *J Obstet Gynaecol Can.* 2009;31:850–62.
2. Dei M, DiMaggio F, DiPaolo G. Vulvovaginitis in childhood. *Best Pract Res Clin Obstet Gynaecol.* 2010;24:129–37.
3. Sultan C. Pediatric and adolescent gynecology: Evidence-based clinical practice. *Endocr Dev* 2004;7:1–8 [PMID: 15045783].
4. Emans JS. Vulvovaginal problems in the prepubertal child. *Pediatric & Adolescent Gynecology*, 5th ed. Philadelphia: Lippincott Williams & Wilkins; 2005: 83–99.

ADDITIONAL READING

- Jasper JM, Ward MA. Shigella vulvovaginitis in a prepubertal child. *Pediatr Emerg Care.* 2006;22: 585–6.
- Joishy M. Do we need to treat vulvovaginitis in prepubertal girls? *Br Med J.* 2005;22:330(7484): 186–8.
- Kokotos F. Vulvovaginitis. *Pediatr Rev.* 2006;27: 116–7.
- Merkley K. Vulvovaginitis and vaginal discharge in the pediatric patient. *J Emerg Nurs.* 2005;31:400–2.
- Sticker T. Vulvovaginitis. *Ped Child Health.* 2009;20: 143–5.
- Stricker T, Navratil F, Sennhauser FH. Vulvovaginitis in prepubertal girls. *Arch Dis Child.* 2003;88:324–6.

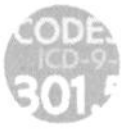

CODES

ICD9

616.10 Vaginitis and vulvovaginitis, unspecified

CLINICAL PEARLS

- Vulvovaginitis is the most common gynecologic problem in prepubescent girls.
- The hypoestrogenic state and prepubescent anatomy may increase susceptibility to vulvar and vaginal infection.
- Treatment is typically supportive (avoid scratching, warm soaks) but may require antibiotics if a bacterial infection is suspected.
- Isolating an infection with known sexual transmission should prompt further investigation.
- Recurrent or persistent vulvitis, especially with foul-smelling discharge, should prompt a skilled exam of the vagina for a retained foreign body.
- Good perineal hygiene will limit this condition.

WARTS

Herbert P. Goodheart, MD

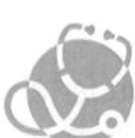

BASICS

- Warts (verrucae) are benign growths that are confined to the epidermis. All warts are caused by the human papillomavirus (HPV). Warts can appear on any area of the skin or mucous membranes. Common warts are predominantly seen in children and young adults.
- Clinically, warts are rather arbitrarily described as:
  - Common warts (verrucae vulgaris)
  - Plantar warts (verrucae plantaris)
  - Flat warts (verrucae plana)
  - Venereal warts (condyloma acuminatum)
  - Epidermodysplasia verruciformis is a rare, lifelong hereditary disorder characterized by chronic infection with HPV.
- System(s) affected: Skin/Exocrine

DESCRIPTION

- Common warts are most often found at sites subject to frequent trauma, such as the hands and feet. Since warts often vary widely in shape, size, and appearance, the various descriptive names for them generally reflect their clinical appearance, location, or both.
- For example, filiform (fingerlike) warts are threadlike, planar warts are flat, and plantar warts are located on the plantar surfaces (soles) of the feet.
- Genital warts, or condyloma acuminata, may be large and cauliflowerlike, or they may consist of small papules.
- Warts on mucous membranes (mucosal papillomas), such as those in the mouth or vagina, tend to be white in color due to moisture retention.

EPIDEMIOLOGY

Incidence

- Predominant age: Young adults and children
- Female = Male

Prevalence

- ~7–10% of the US population
- Common warts appear ~2 times as frequently in whites as in blacks or Asians.

RISK FACTORS

- HIV/AIDS and other immunosuppressive diseases (e.g., lymphomas)
- Immunosuppressive drugs that decrease cell-mediated immunity (e.g., prednisone, cyclosporine, and chemotherapeutic agents)
- Pregnancy
- Handling raw meat, fish, or other types of animal matter in one's occupation (e.g., butchers)
- Previous wart infection

GENERAL PREVENTION

There is no known way to prevent them.

ETIOLOGY

- HPV is a double-stranded, circular, supercoiled DNA virus.
- The virus infects epidermal keratinocytes, which stimulates cell proliferation.
- Various strains of DNA HPV: To date, >150 different subtypes have been identified.
- Common warts: HPV types 2 and 4 (most common), followed by types 1, 3, 27, 29, and 57
- Palmoplantar warts: HPV type 1 (most common), followed by types 2, 3, 4, 27, 29, and 57
- Flat warts: HPV types 3, 10, and 28
- Butcher warts: HPV type 7
- The virus is passed primarily through skin-to-skin contact or from the recently shed virus kept intact in a moist, warm environment.

DIAGNOSIS

- Most often made on clinical appearance
- Skin biopsy, if necessary

PHYSICAL EXAM

- Distribution of warts is generally asymmetric, and lesions are often clustered or may appear in a linear configuration due to scratching (autoinoculation).
- Common wart: Rough-surfaced, hyperkeratotic, papillomatous, raised, skin-colored to tan papules, 5–10 mm in diameter; several may coalesce into a cluster (mosaic wart) 1–3 cm in diameter; most frequently seen on hands, knees, and elbows; usually asymptomatic but may cause cosmetic disfigurement or tenderness
- Filiform warts: These are long, slender, delicate, fingerlike growths, usually seen on the face around the lips, eyelids, or nares.
- Plantar warts often have a rough surface and appear on the plantar surface of the feet in children and young adults:
  - Can be tender and painful, and extensive involvement on the sole of the foot may impair ambulation, particularly when present on a weight-bearing surface.
  - Most often seen on the metatarsal area, heels, and toes in an asymmetric distribution (pressure points)
  - Pathognomonic "black dots" (thrombosed dermal capillaries); punctate bleeding becomes more evident after paring with a no. 15 blade
  - Both common and plantar warts generally demonstrate the following clinical findings:
    - A loss of normal skin markings (dermatoglyphics) such as finger, foot, and hand prints
    - Lesions may be solitary or multiple, or they may appear in clusters (mosaic warts).
- Flat warts: Slightly elevated, flat-topped, skin-colored or tan papules, small (1–3 mm) in diameter:
  - Commonly found on the face, arms, dorsa of hands, shins (women)
  - Sometimes exhibit a linear configuration caused by autoinoculation
  - In men, shaving spreads flat warts.
  - In women, they often occur on the shins, where leg shaving spreads lesions.
- Epidermodysplasia verruciformis (rare): Widespread flat, reddish brown pigmented papules and plaques that present in childhood with lifelong persistence on the trunk, hands, upper and lower extremities, and face are characteristic.

DIAGNOSTIC TESTS & INTERPRETATION

Diagnosis

Lab

- HPV cannot be cultured, and lab testing is rarely necessary.
- Definitive HPV diagnosis can be achieved by:
  - Electron microscopy
  - Viral DNA identification employing Southern blot hybridization used to identify the specific HPV type present in tissue
  - Polymerase chain reaction may be used to amplify viral DNA for testing.

Imaging

Follow-Up & Special Considerations

Skin biopsy if unusual presentation or if diagnosis is unclear

Pathological Findings

- Histopathologic features of common warts include digitated epidermal hyperplasia, acanthosis, papillomatosis, compact orthokeratosis, hypergranulosis, dilated tortuous capillaries within the dermal papillae, and vertical tiers of parakeratotic cells with entrapped red blood cells above the tips of the digitations.
- In the granular layer, HPV-infected cells may have coarse keratohyaline granules and vacuoles surrounding wrinkled-appearing nuclei. These koilocytic (vacuolated) cells are pathognomonic for warts.

DIFFERENTIAL DIAGNOSIS

- Molluscum contagiosum
- Seborrheic keratosis
- Epidermal nevus
- Acrochordon (skin tag)
- Solar keratosis and cutaneous horn
- Acquired digital fibrokeratoma
- Squamous cell carcinoma (SCC)
- Keratoacanthoma
- Subungual SCC can easily be misdiagnosed as a subungual wart or onychomycosis.
- Corns/calluses:
  - Corns (clavi) are sometimes difficult to distinguish from plantar warts. Like calluses, corns are thickened areas of the skin and most commonly develop at sites subjected to repeated friction and pressure, such as the tops and the tips of toes and along the sides of the feet:
    - They are usually hard and circular, with a polished or central translucent core, like the kernel of corn from which they take their name.
    - Corns do not have "black dots," and skin markings are retained except for the area of the central core.

ALERT

- A melanoma on the plantar surface of the foot can mimic a plantar wart.
- Verrucous carcinoma, a slow-growing, locally invasive, well-differentiated SCC, also may be easily mistaken for a common or plantar wart.

TREATMENT

The abundance of therapeutic modalities described below is a reflection of the fact that none of them are uniformly effective. The method of treatment depends on:

- The age of the patient
- Cosmetic and psychological considerations
- Relief of symptoms
- The patient's pain threshold
- The type of wart
- The location of the wart

MEDICATION

First Line

- Self-administered topical therapy: Keratolytic (peeling) agents: The affected area(s) should be hydrated first by soaking in warm water for 5 minutes before application. Most over-the-counter agents contain salicylic acid and/or lactic acid; agents such as Duofilm, Occlusal-HP, Trans-Ver-Sal, and Mediplast (1)[A].
- Office-based:
  - Cantharidin, an extract of the blister beetle that causes epidermal necrosis and blistering
  - Combination cantharidin: 30% salicylic acid, 2% podophyllin, and 19% cantharidin in flexible collodion; applied in a thin coat, occluded 4–6 hours, then washed off

Second Line

- Home-based:
  - Imiquimod (Aldara) 5% cream, a local inducer of interferon, is applied at home by the patient. It is approved for external genital and perianal warts, and is used off-label and may be applied to warts under duct-tape occlusion. It is applied at bedtime and washed off after 6–10 hours. Applied to flat warts without occlusion.
  - Topical retinoids (e.g., tretinoin 0.25%–0.1% cream or gel) for flat warts
- Immunotherapy: Induction of delayed-type hypersensitivity with:
  - Diphenylcyclopropenone (DCP)
  - Dinitrochlorobenzene (DNCP)
  - Squaric acid dibutylester (SADBE): There is possible mutagenicity and side effects with this agent.
- Intralesional injections:
  - Mumps or *Candida* antigen
  - Bleomycin: Intradermal injection is expensive and usually causes severe pain.
  - Interferon-α-2b
- Oral therapy:
  - Oral high-dose cimetidine: Possibly works better in children (2)
  - Acitretin (an oral retinoid)
- Other treatments (all have all been used with varying results):
  - Dichloroacetic acid, trichloroacetic acid, podophyllin, formic acid, aminolevulinic acid in combination with blue light (3), 5-fluorouracil, silver nitrate, formaldehyde, levamisole, topical or IV cidofovir for recalcitrant warts in the setting of HIV, and glutaraldehyde

ADDITIONAL TREATMENT

General Measures

- There is no ideal treatment.
- In children, most warts tend to regress spontaneously.
- In many adults and immunocompromised patients, warts are often difficult to eradicate.
- Painful, aggressive therapy should be avoided unless there is a need to eliminate the wart(s).
- For surgical procedures, especially in anxious children, pretreatment with anesthetic cream such as EMLA (emulsion of lidocaine and prilocaine)

COMPLEMENTARY AND ALTERNATIVE MEDICINE

- Duct tape: Cover wart with waterproof tape (e.g., duct tape). Leave the tape on for 6 days, and then soak, pare with emery board, and leave uncovered overnight; then reapply tape cyclically for 8 cycles; 85% resolved compared with 60% efficacy with cryotherapy (4,5).
- Hyperthermia: Safe and inexpensive approach; immerse affected area into 45°C water bath for 30 minutes 3× per week
- Hypnotherapy (6)
- Raw garlic cloves have demonstrated some antiviral activity.
- Vaccines are currently in development.

Pregnancy Considerations

The use of some topical chemical approaches may be contraindicated during pregnancy or in women who are likely to become pregnant during the treatment period.

SURGERY/OTHER PROCEDURES

- Cryotherapy with liquid nitrogen (LN_2) may be applied with a cotton swab or with a cryotherapy gun (Cryogun) (7):
  - Best for warts on hands; also during pregnancy and breast-feeding
  - Fast; can treat many lesions per visit
  - Painful; not tolerated well by young children
  - Freezing periungual warts may result in nail deformation.
  - In darkly pigmented skin, treatment can result in hypo- or hyperpigmentation.
- Light electrocautery ± curettage:
  - Best for warts on the knees, elbows, and dorsa of hands
  - Also good for filiform warts
  - Tolerable in most adults
  - Requires local anesthesia
  - May cause scarring
- Photodynamic therapy: Topical 5-aminolevulinic acid is applied to warts followed by photoactivation.
- CO_2 or pulse-dye laser ablation: Expensive and requires local anesthesia
- For filiform warts: Dip hemostat into LN_2 for 10 seconds, and then gently grasp the wart for 10 seconds and repeat. Wart sheds in 7–10 days.

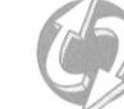

ONGOING CARE

FOLLOW-UP RECOMMENDATIONS

Patient Monitoring

1/3 of the warts of epidermodysplasia may become malignant.

PROGNOSIS

- More often than not (especially in children), warts tend to "cure" themselves over time.
- In many adults and immunocompromised patients, warts often prove difficult to eradicate.
- Rarely, certain types of lesions may transform into carcinomas.

COMPLICATIONS

- Autoinoculation (pseudo-Koebner reaction)
- Scar formation
- Chronic pain after plantar wart removal or scar formation
- Nail deformity after injury to nail matrix

REFERENCES

1. Gibbs S, Harvey I. Topical treatments for cutaneous warts. *Cochrane Database Syst Rev.* 2006;3: CD001781.
2. Rogers CJ, Gibney MD, Siegfried EC, et al. Cimetidine therapy for recalcitrant warts in adults: Is it any better than placebo? *J Am Acad Dermatol.* 1999;41:123–7.
3. Ohtsuki A, Hasegawa T, Hirasawa Y, et al. Photodynamic therapy using light-emitting diodes for the treatment of viral warts. *J Dermatol.* 2009;36:525–8.
4. de Haen M, Spigt MG, van Uden CJ, et al. Efficacy of duct tape vs placebo in the treatment of verruca vulgaris (warts) in primary school children. *Arch Pediatr Adolesc Med.* 2006;160:1121–5.
5. Wenner R, Askari SK, Cham PM, et al. Duct tape for the treatment of common warts in adults: A double-blind randomized controlled trial. *Arch Dermatol.* 2007;143:309–13.
6. Ewin DM. Hypnotherapy for warts (verruca vulgaris): 41 consecutive cases with 33 cures. *Am J Clin Hypn.* 1992;35:1–10.
7. Keogh-Brown MR, Fordham RJ, Thomas KS, et al. To freeze or not to freeze: A cost-effectiveness analysis of wart treatment. *Br J Dermatol.* 2007;156: 687–92.

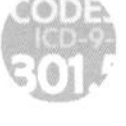

CODES

ICD9

- 078.10 Viral warts, unspecified
- 078.12 Plantar wart
- 078.19 Other specified viral warts

CLINICAL PEARLS

- No single therapy for warts is uniformly effective or superior; thus, treatment involves a certain amount of trial and error.
- Since most warts in children tend to regress spontaneously within 2 years, benign neglect is often a prudent option.
- Conservative, nonscarring, least painful, least expensive treatments are preferred.
- Freezing and other destructive treatment modalities do not kill the virus, but merely destroy the cells that harbor HPV.
- For filiform warts, a small mosquito hemostat dipped into LN_2 for 10 seconds and then used to gently grasp the wart for 10 seconds is a relatively painless treatment option.

W

WARTS, PLANTAR

Kaelen C. Dunican, PharmD
Robert A. Baldor, MD

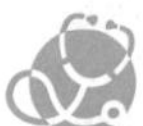

BASICS

DESCRIPTION

- Form of cutaneous wart caused by the human papillomavirus (HPV)
- Appears as discrete or grouped firm keratotic masses on the plantar surface of the foot, usually at pressure points such as the heel, forefoot, or under toes
- System(s) affected: Skin/Exocrine
- Synonym(s): Verruca plantaris

EPIDEMIOLOGY

Incidence

- In the US: Widespread: Estimated 2% of population
- Predominant age: Any age, although more common in children and young adults
- Predominant sex: Female > Male (slightly)

Prevalence

Cutaneous warts are estimated to occur in about 7–10% of the population.

RISK FACTORS

- Immunosuppression, including HIV/AIDS, lymphomas, use of immunosuppressive drugs
- Use of public facilities while barefoot, such as gyms and swimming pools
- Previous wart infection

GENERAL PREVENTION

- Use rubber footwear in communal shower areas.
- Once infected, maintain proper foot hygiene (see "Patient Education").

ETIOLOGY

- Infection with HPV, a double-stranded DNA virus, results in proliferation of epidermal keratinocytes.
- Most common cause is HPV subtypes 1, 2, 4, 27, and 57
- Transmitted by direct person-to-person contact or via fomites
- Minor trauma to the skin and maceration may facilitate transmission of the virus to basal keratinocytes.
- Autoinoculation can occur.

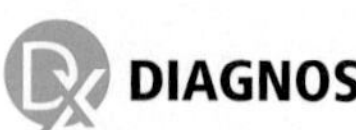

DIAGNOSIS

Most often made on clinical appearance (1)[C]

HISTORY

- Complaints of thickened skin on sole of foot
- May be painless, depending on location
- May cause leg or back pain (distortion of posture)

PHYSICAL EXAM

- Discrete or grouped keratotic lesions on sole of foot with disruption of normal skin markings
- Rough, hyperkeratotic surface with brown–black dots (thrombosed capillaries): May bleed when pared down; helps to distinguish warts from corns or calluses
- Callus formation surrounding wart core
- Warts generally occur at pressure points
- Moderate discomfort to severe pain with deep penetration
- Many warts may coalesce to form "mosaic warts."

DIAGNOSTIC TESTS & INTERPRETATION

Diagnostic Procedures/Surgery

- Inspection usually confirms the diagnosis.
- If you cannot distinguish between callus and wart, examine with a magnifying lens. The wart should demonstrate a highly organized mosaic pattern.
- When pared down, warts have a soft central core and bleeding points (unlike calluses).

Pathological Findings

Acanthotic epidermis with hyperkeratosis, papillomatosis, and parakeratosis

DIFFERENTIAL DIAGNOSIS

- Corns (clavi)
- Calluses
- Black heel (ruptured capillaries)
- Lichen planus
- Epidermal nevus
- Molluscum contagiosum
- Squamous cell carcinoma

TREATMENT

MEDICATION

- No universally effective agent or cure exists.
- Topical salicylic acid therapy has the best evidence available (1,2)[A].
- Cryotherapy with liquid nitrogen is no more effective than salicylic acid with increased adverse effects (3)[B].

First Line

Salicylic acid: Pooled efficacy 73% (1)[A]:

- Available over the counter (OTC) as 17% liquid in a flexible collodion base (Compound W, Occlusal-HP), 15% patch (Trans-Ver-Sal), and 40% salicylic acid plasters/patches (Mediplast, Duofilm)
- Prior to each application, the wart should be soaked in warm water and pared down with an emery board or pumice stone.
- Patches/plasters: Supplied in various sizes of sheets/pads, which are cut to the size of the wart, and the sticky surface is applied to the wart. They are removed every 1–2 days, the white keratin is peeled, and a fresh plaster is applied.
- Liquids: Apply a few drops directly to the wart daily. Applying a ring of petrolatum to the skin around the wart will protect the healthy skin tissue.
- May require weeks to months of treatment
- Side effects: Minor skin irritation, contact dermatitis
- Precautions: Poor circulation, peripheral neuropathy

Second Line

- Cryotherapy and pulse dye laser therapy are appropriate as second line (2,4)[A] (see "Surgery/Other Procedures").
- Intralesional immunotherapy with *Candida* skin test antigen can be used as second-line therapy (2)[B]:
  - Injected every 3 weeks until cleared or a total of 3 treatments
  - Not approved by the FDA for warts.
  - Side effects: Pain and itching at injection site, flulike symptoms
- Third line: Bleomycin (Blenoxane) injected into wart every 3–4 weeks until cleared; inconsistent evidence (2)[B]:
  - Dosing: 0.2 unit injected under the base of the wart, or 0.001 unit multiple punctures with bifurcated needle, or drops applied directly to the wart and then pricked into the wart using a fine needle
  - Not approved by the FDA for warts.
  - Side effects: Injection-site burning and pain (may be severe), erythema, scarring, change in pigmentation
  - Contraindications: Pregnancy, children, immunosuppressed patients, and patients with vascular disease
- Imiquimod (Aldara) 5% cream: Apply daily after soaking. It may be more effective when occluded and when in combination with other treatments such as cryotherapy or keratolytics. (Insufficient evidence to recommend at this time (2)[B]; reserved for recalcitrant warts. Not approved by the FDA for warts.)
- Cimetidine: 20–40 mg/kg PO daily may be effective in children (5)[C]. Not approved by the FDA for warts.

ADDITIONAL TREATMENT

General Measures

- If warts are asymptomatic, no treatment is necessary, and may be an option for patients to consider; however, patient may be at risk for spread of warts.
- Warm soaks followed by patient's paring of the top layer of skin on repeated occasions may speed disappearance.
- Patient may use pumice stone, emery board, or a blade to pare down the wart.
- Use of a heel bar or appropriate padding to relieve pressure points where warts tend to aggregate

Additional Therapies

Hyperthermia: Hot water immersion (113°F) 30–45 minutes 2–3 times/wk × 16 treatments is effective for some patients.

COMPLEMENTARY AND ALTERNATIVE MEDICINE

Duct tape: Cut a piece to the size of the wart and apply continuously for 6 days, remove, pare the wart, and then repeat for up to 2 months (4,6)[C]. Not approved by the FDA for warts.

SURGERY/OTHER PROCEDURES

- Cryotherapy:
  - Liquid nitrogen or dimethyl ether and propane (Wartner OTC)
  - The wart is frozen for 10–30 seconds until a 1–2-mm halo surrounds the wart; repeated every 2–3 weeks.
  - It usually requires at least 4 applications at weekly or biweekly intervals.
  - Aggressive cryotherapy may cause blistering or even scarring; light applications with 2 freeze–thaw cycles and paring are preferred.
  - Side effects: Prolonged pain, scarring, hypo- or hyperpigmentation, tendon or nerve damage (with aggressive therapy)
  - Caution: When treating patients with poor circulation
- Pulse dye laser (vascular lesion laser) therapy:
  - Repeated 2–3 times
  - Side effects: Pain, scarring, discoloration lasting 10–14 days
- Blunt dissection: A simple surgical procedure is effective and usually nonscarring. It requires inserting a blunt dissector between the wart and normal skin and separating the wart using a short, firm stroke.
- Carbon dioxide laser surgery: Used for recalcitrant warts
- Chemotherapy with trichloroacetic acid (not approved by the FDA for warts): Callus is pared, and the surrounding skin is protected by a ring of petrolatum. Each wart is coated with acid, which then is worked into the wart with a sharp toothpick. Procedure should be repeated at weekly intervals.
- Other (not approved by the FDA for warts):
  - Podophyllin: 25% solution; apply to wart 3–5 times/d.
  - 5-fluorouracil (5-FU): 5% topical cream applied b.i.d. with occlusion
  - Formaldehyde soaks
- Combination therapies: Salicylic acid plus imiquimod ± cryotherapy

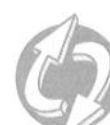

ONGOING CARE

FOLLOW-UP RECOMMENDATIONS

Patient Monitoring

With any treatment modality, follow up weekly until resolution (return of normal dermatoglyphics).

PATIENT EDUCATION

- Review treatment regimen, including proper application and persistence (it may take weeks to months for resolution).
- Prevent spread to others and autoinoculation:
  - Wear footwear or cover securely before walking barefoot.
  - Wash socks and towels that may have come in contact with the wart in hot water.
  - Wash hands before and after treating/touching wart.
- Web sites for patient information:
  - American Podiatric Medical Association: www.apma.org/s_apma/doc.asp?cid=146&did=9430
  - Mayo Clinic: www.mayoclinic.com

PROGNOSIS

The course of plantar warts is like that of other varieties of warts (i.e., highly variable). Most resolve spontaneously in weeks to months.

COMPLICATIONS

- Scarring with overly aggressive treatment
- Leg and back pain
- Warts can cause considerable morbidity at times and significantly affect quality of life.
- A rare type of verrucous carcinoma, epithelioma cuniculatum, is thought to arise from these warts.

REFERENCES

1. Gibbs S, Harvey I. Topical treatments for cutaneous warts. *Cochrane Database Syst Rev*. 2006:3.
2. Bacelieri R, Johnson SM. Cutaneous warts: An evidence-based approach to therapy. *Am Fam Physician*. 2005;72:647–52.
3. Cockayne S, Hewitt C, Hicks K, et al. Cryotherapy versus salicylic acid for the treatment of plantar warts (verrucae): A randomised controlled trial. *BMJ*. 2011;342:d3271.
4. Lipke MM. An armamentarium of wart treatments. *Clin Med Res*. 2006;4:273–93.
5. Paquette D, Rothe MJ. Unapproved dermatologic indications for H2 receptor antagonists, cromolyn sodium, and ketotifen. *Clin Dermatol*. 2000;18: 103–11.
6. Focht DR. The efficacy of duct tape vs. cryotherapy in the treatment of verruca vulgaris. *Arch Pedatr Adolesc Med*. 2002;156:971–4.

ADDITIONAL READING

- Ciconte A, Campbell J, Tabrizi S. Warts are not merely blemished on the skin: A study of the morbidity associated with having viral cutaneous warts. *Aus J Derm*. 2003;44:169–75.
- Keogh-Brown MR, Fordham RJ, Thomas MO. To freeze or not to freeze: A cost-effectiveness analysis of wart treatment. *Br J Dermatol*. 2007;156:687–92.

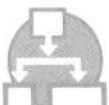

See Also (Topic, Algorithm, Electronic Media Element)

Condyloma Acuminata; Warts

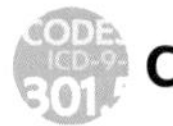

CODES

ICD9

078.12 Plantar wart

CLINICAL PEARLS

- If the wart is painless, therapy is not necessary. Most untreated warts will resolve spontaneously in a few weeks to months, although they can last for years.
- Treating plantar warts requires diligence with proper application and adherence to the treatment regimen.
- Salicylic acid is the least expensive pharmacotherapeutic option and has the best evidence of efficacy.
- To reduce pain, care should be taken to avoid excessive contact with normal skin when using keratolytics or chemotherapy.
- Proper foot hygiene is the key to preventing transmission.

WEGENER GRANULOMATOSIS

Christopher M. Wise, MD

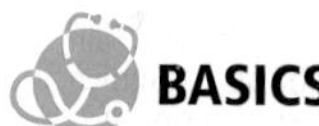

BASICS

DESCRIPTION

- A disease characterized by granulomatous vasculitis involving multiple organs
- The characteristic triad of involvement includes the upper airway (e.g., otitis, sinusitis, nasal mucosa), lungs, and kidneys.
- Other organ systems involved include the skin, joints, and nervous system (peripheral or central).
- As the condition progresses untreated, upper airway erosions, necrotic pulmonary nodules, and renal failure are common.
- Without treatment, mortality rate is high. With treatment, survival rate is ~75% at 5 years (1).
- System(s) affected: Upper Airways (sinusitis, otitis); Cardiovascular; Gastrointestinal; Nervous; Pulmonary; Renal/Urologic; Skin/Exocrine
- Alternative names:
  - ANCA-associated vasculitis (to include patients with Wegener and microscopic polyangiitis)
  - Granulomatosis with polyangiitis

EPIDEMIOLOGY

Incidence

- Estimated at ~0.4–1.0/100,000 persons per year and possibly increasing over the past decade
- Predominant age: Mean age of onset is the mid-40s, but the disease has been described in all age groups.
- Predominant gender: Male > Female (3:2)

Prevalence

3/100,000 persons

RISK FACTORS

Genetics

Increased presence in HLA-B8 and HLA-DR2

ETIOLOGY

- The etiology is unknown.
- Autoimmune phenomena and immune-complex deposition in arterial walls are implicated, and the activation of neutrophils by bacteria or other infectious agents may be important as well:
  - The role of antibodies directed against neutrophils is currently being investigated.
- A specific triggering infectious agent has not been identified.

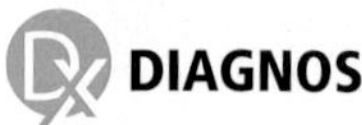

DIAGNOSIS

HISTORY

- Fever: 34% (2)
- Weight loss: 16%
- Cough: 34%
- Arthralgia/arthritis: 44%
- Epistaxis: 11%
- Hemoptysis: 18%
- Rash: 13%
- Chest pain, anorexia, proptosis, dyspnea, oral ulcers, hearing loss, headache: All <10%

PHYSICAL EXAM

- Ocular inflammation: 16%
- Otitis: 25%
- Sinusitis: 67%
- Rhinitis: 22%
- Rash: 13%

DIAGNOSTIC TESTS & INTERPRETATION

Lab

Initial lab tests

- CBC: Anemia, leukocytosis, and thrombocytosis common during active phases of disease
- ESR usually markedly elevated (75%)
- Rheumatoid factor present in low-to-moderate titers in up to 50%
- Hematuria and/or cellular casts with moderate-range proteinuria
- Renal failure (11%): Renal insufficiency, mild to moderate at first; frequently progresses to end-stage renal disease

Follow-Up & Special Considerations

- Antibodies to neutrophilic cytoplasmic antigens with a cytoplasmic pattern of staining (c-ANCAs) are detected in 60–90% of patients. c-ANCAs are highly specific (90%+); immunoblotting techniques or ELISA may detect antibodies to PR3 or MPO (anti-PR3 antibodies are more specific).
- Perinuclear staining (p-ANCAs) is nonspecific and is seen with other vasculitic syndromes or isolated necrotizing glomerulonephritis.

Imaging

Initial approach

- Upper airways: Chronic otitis and sinusitis, often with evidence of erosion into bony structures—seen on plain radiographs
- Pulmonary infiltrates (71%): Lung radiographs show nodular pulmonary densities, often with central necrosis and cavitation. Local infiltrates or more diffuse interstitial involvement is also described, as are radiographic findings of pulmonary hemorrhage.

Follow-Up & Special Considerations

CT scan may show mucosal and bony involvement in sinuses and better define pulmonary lesions.

Diagnostic Procedures/Surgery

- Sinus or upper airway mucosal biopsy is often helpful, although findings are often nonspecific.
- Open lung biopsy is most likely to confirm granulomatous arteritis.
- Renal biopsy may give findings consistent with diagnosis, although it is not always definitive.
- Diagnosis is best made by demonstration of granulomatous arteritis of involved organ, although a compatible renal lesion in the setting of chronic destructive sinusitis and/or pulmonary nodules may make a presumptive diagnosis.
- A positive serologic test for c-ANCAs in the proper clinical setting is often diagnostic.

Pathological Findings

- Upper airways: Granulomatous inflammation is seen frequently, although it is not specific unless showing actual vasculitis.
- Lung: Granulomatous arteritis involving vessels; classically medium-sized arteries
- Kidney: Necrotizing and crescentic glomerulonephritis without immunofluorescent staining (pauci-immune) is common; granulomatous vasculitis is seen rarely.
- Skin: Vasculitic lesions from leukocytoclastic vasculitis of small vessels; granulomatous arteritis is seen occasionally.

DIFFERENTIAL DIAGNOSIS

- Otitis media and sinusitis (bacterial or fungal)
- Midline granuloma or upper airway malignancy
- Relapsing polychondritis
- Fungal or tuberculous pulmonary infections
- Goodpasture syndrome
- Other vasculitic syndromes (including polyarteritis nodosa, microscopic polyangiitis, lymphomatoid granulomatosis, Churg-Strauss vasculitis, and overlap vasculitis syndromes)
- Any disease associated with necrotizing and crescentic glomerulonephritis, sarcoidosis

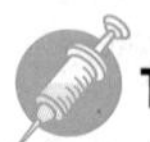

TREATMENT

- Patients with significant renal involvement or serious pulmonary disease require cyclophosphamide for optimal initial control in most cases, but may be converted to methotrexate, azathioprine, mycophenolate, or other agent after several months of inactive disease.
- Rituximab appears to be one of the more promising potential therapies for patients with serious active disease refractory to cyclophosphamide, and may have a role in initial therapy as an alternative to cyclophosphamide.
- An occasional patient without serious renal or pulmonary involvement may respond to methotrexate as initial immunosuppressive therapy without requiring cyclophosphamide therapy.

MEDICATION

First Line

- Prednisone (3)[C],(4)[A]:
  - Given initially in high doses (60–100 mg/d)
  - After the first 2–4 weeks, may be tapered to alternate-day regimen then gradually discontinued over 2–6 months in most patients, depending on clinical course
  - Maintaining chronic low dose (5–10 mg/d) may reduce the risk of relapse
- Cyclophosphamide:
  - In critically ill patient, may be given initially at a dose of 4 mg/kg/d IV × 2–3 days, then at 2 mg/kg/d PO
  - In stable patient, start at 2 mg/kg/d PO
  - Dosage may need to be adjusted based on patient response and toxicity (usually bone marrow suppression).
  - Usually continued for 6–24 months after patient is felt to be in remission; then tapered slowly, with careful monitoring for reactivation of disease
  - Give dose in morning to decrease amount of drug present overnight in bladder
- Methotrexate 15–25 mg/wk PO has been shown in a recent trial to be successful in maintaining remission in patients treated with cyclophosphamide. Methotrexate may be used in place of cyclophosphamide in some patients without pulmonary or renal involvement (3)[B].
- Azathioprine 2 mg/kg/d may be useful in maintaining remission in patients treated with cyclophosphamide, and a recent study showed that it was comparable in efficacy with methotrexate for this purpose (5)[B].
- No absolute contraindications, although diabetes, hypertension, and metabolic bone disease are relative contraindications to prednisone.

- Precautions:
  - Carefully monitor a patient taking corticosteroids.
  - Consider reducing dose of cyclophosphamide with baseline leukopenia or renal insufficiency.
  - Methotrexate contraindicated in patients with renal insufficiency
- Significant possible interactions:
  - Prednisone may interfere with hypoglycemics and antihypertensives.
  - Cyclophosphamide may increase risk of bone marrow toxicity.

Second Line

- Azathioprine or mycophenolate: For patients with history of severe bone marrow toxicity or hemorrhagic cystitis from cyclophosphamide; may be useful in maintaining remission in patients with stable disease after remission is obtained
- Trimethoprim-sulfamethoxazole (TMP-SMX) has been used alone with success in some patients with limited (usually upper airway) disease and has some potential as an adjunctive therapy with prednisone and cyclophosphamide.
- Methotrexate: For some patients without renal involvement; may be useful in maintaining remission in patients with stable disease, as an alternative to chronic cyclophosphamide therapy
- Rituximab has been shown in prospective studies to be useful in patients with relapsing disease, and has potential as a part of the initial treatment regimen (6)[A].
- IVIG has been reported to be useful in case reports of patients with disease relapses.
- Etanercept does not appear to be of benefit, and other TNF antagonists have not been adequately evaluated.

ADDITIONAL TREATMENT

Issues for Referral

Rheumatology, Otolaryngology (ENT), ophthalmology, pulmonology, nephrology, and dermatology consultants are often needed initially to evaluate and/or manage ongoing organ-specific problems.

SURGERY/OTHER PROCEDURES

Surgery is indicated for diagnostic purposes only.

IN-PATIENT CONSIDERATIONS

Initial Stabilization

- Adequate fluid balance and exclusion of alternative pathology for renal disease
- Intensive pulmonary monitoring may be needed for patients with severe pulmonary involvement with hemoptysis and/or pulmonary hemorrhage.

Admission Criteria

- Pulmonary hemorrhage or hemoptysis
- Respiratory failure
- Unstable renal function

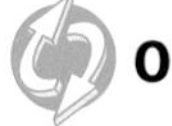

ONGOING CARE

FOLLOW-UP RECOMMENDATIONS

Patient Monitoring

- Early, careful monitoring of upper airway, pulmonary, and renal manifestations
- BP, glucose, and potassium for steroid effects
- CBC with differential every 2–4 weeks to monitor for bone marrow toxicity from cyclophosphamide. Leukopenia is most common. Dose must be reduced if peripheral WBC count $<3{,}000/mm^3$.
- Urinalysis for potential of hemorrhagic cystitis from cyclophosphamide; consider cystoscopy for persistent or recurrent hematuria.
- Acute-phase reactants (erythrocyte sedimentation rate, C-reactive protein) and serum c-ANCA levels may be useful in monitoring disease activity during follow-up.

DIET

- Vigorous nutritional support may be needed early in the illness.
- Calorie and salt reduction in patients on prednisone
- High fluid intake to prevent hemorrhagic cystitis from cyclophosphamide

PATIENT EDUCATION

- Nutritional and drug counseling when patient is able to return home
- Vasculitis Foundation (formerly the Wegener Granulomatosis Association), PO Box 28660, Kansas City, MO 64188, www.vasculitisfoundation.org and www.wegenersgranulomatosis.net

PROGNOSIS

- Without treatment, almost uniformly fatal, with a 10% 2-year survival; mean survival of 5 months
- With aggressive treatment, survival improved to 75–90% at 5–10 years.
- Severe renal and pulmonary disease are the most prominent risk factors for death.
- Survival has improved significantly over the past 30–40 years, and limitation of cyclophosphamide therapy has resulted in decrease in treatment-related morbidity (7)[A].
- Relapses may occur in 40–50% of patients over 2–5 years of follow-up.
- Treatment-related toxicity is significant, especially from long-term cyclophosphamide. After a 6-month to 1-year disease-free interval, cyclophosphamide is usually changed to methotrexate, azathioprine, or mycophenolate, although some patients may demonstrate disease reactivation.

COMPLICATIONS

- Disease-related:
  - Destructive nasal lesions with "saddle nose" deformity
  - Deafness from refractory otitis
  - Necrotic pulmonary nodules with hemoptysis
  - Interstitial lung disease
  - Renal failure
  - Foot drop from peripheral nerve disease
  - Skin ulcers, digital and limb gangrene from peripheral vascular involvement
  - Deep vein thrombosis, pulmonary embolism, and other thromboembolic events are more common in patients with long-standing disease.
- Drug-related:
  - Prednisone: Weight gain, hyperglycemia, hypertension, hypokalemia, skin thinning and bruising, infection, osteoporosis
  - Cyclophosphamide: Bone marrow suppression (especially leukopenia, neutropenia), alopecia, hemorrhagic cystitis, mucosal membrane irritation, sterility and premature gonadal failure, secondary malignancies (especially leukemias) with long-term therapy; risk of bladder cancer is 5% (10 years) and 16% (15 years) after first treatment and is related to previous cystitis.

REFERENCES

1. Phillip R, Luqmani R. Mortality in systemic vasculitis: A systematic review. *Clin Exp Rheumatol*. 2008;26:94–104.
2. Weeda LW, Coffey SA. Wegener's granulomatosis. *Oral Maxillofac Surg Clin North Am*. 2008;20: 643–9.
3. Specks U. Methotrexate for Wegener's granulomatosis: What is the evidence? *Arthritis Rheum*. 2005;52:2237–42.
4. Walsh M, Merkel PA, Mahr A, et al. The effects of duration of glucocorticoid therapy on relapse rate in anti-neutrophil cytoplam antibody associated vascultitis: A meta-analysis. *Arthritis Care Res*. 2010;62:1166–73.
5. Pagnoux C, Mahr A, Hamidou MA, et al. Azathioprine or methotrexate maintenance for ANCA-associated vasculitis. *N Engl J Med*. 2008;359:2790–803.
6. Stone JH, Merkel PA, Spiera R, et al. Rituximab versus cyclophosphamide for ANCA-associated vasculitis. *N Engl J Med*. 2010;363:221–32.
7. Holle JU, Gross WL, Latza U, et al. Improved outcomes in 445 patients with Wegener's granulomatosis in a German vascultis center over four decades. *Arthritis Rheum*. 2011;63:257–66.

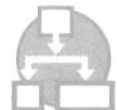

See Also (Topic, Algorithm, Electronic Media Element)

Polyarteritis Nodosa; Microscopic Polyangiitis; ANCA-Associated Vasculitis, Granulomatosis with Polyangiitis

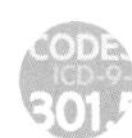

CODES

ICD9

446.4 Wegener's granulomatosis

CLINICAL PEARLS

- Biopsies of mucosal lesions, skin lesions, lung, or kidney typically are needed to confirm a diagnosis of Wegner granulomatosis, but tissue diagnosis is often difficult unless an open lung biopsy is done.
- A positive c-ANCA (or anti-PR3 antibody) test in the setting of a patient with 2 of 3 classic areas of involvement (i.e., nephritis, pulmonary lesions, sinusitis/otitis) may be sufficient for a clinical diagnosis.
- Aggressive therapy with potent immunosuppressive/cytotoxic therapy is needed for most patients with Wegener granulomatosis. Patients with severe renal or pulmonary manifestations usually require cyclophosphamide for initial disease control.
- After initial remission, most patients should be continued on methotrexate, azathioprine, or mycophenolate as maintenance therapy to reduce the risk of later exacerbation.
- Rituximab appears to be useful for patients with relapsing disease and may eventually be an appropriate initial therapy for many patients.
- Mortality rates are falling as a result of more effective intervention but remain elevated substantially in severe disease.

WILMS TUMOR

Timothy L. Black, MD

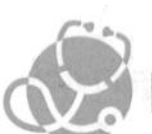

BASICS

DESCRIPTION

- An embryonal renal neoplasm containing blastema, stromal, or epithelial cell types, usually affecting children <5 years of age
- Most common renal tumor in children; fifth most common pediatric malignancy
- Staging: In the US, National Wilms Tumor Study Group (NWTSG) staging is done pretreatment based on radiographic imaging and surgery, whereas in Europe/Asia, Société Internationale d'Oncologie Pédiatrique (SIOP) staging is done *after* neoadjuvant chemotherapy is administered (1):
  - I: Tumor limited to kidney; completely excised
  - II: Tumor extends beyond kidney; completely excised
  - III: Residual nonhematogenous tumor confined to abdomen (lymph nodes positive, spillage of tumor, peritoneal implants, extension beyond resection region)
  - IV: Hematogenous metastases
  - V: Bilateral renal involvement
- System(s) affected: Renal/Urologic
- Synonym(s): Nephroblastoma

Pediatric Considerations

- Occurs only in children
- Most common renal malignancy in childhood

EPIDEMIOLOGY

Incidence

- Frequency rarer in East Asian populations than whites
- Frequency higher in black children than in whites
- Predominant age: Median age of 36.5 months
- Predominant sex: Female > Male (1.1:1)
- Represents 6–7% of all childhood cancers:
  - More than 80% are diagnosed before 5 years of age (median age is 3.5 years at diagnosis).

Prevalence

US: 0.69/100,000; 7.6 cases/1 million children <15 years

RISK FACTORS

- Familial occurrence (1–2%):
  - These patients tend to have earlier age of onset.
  - Familial patients have greater risk of bilateral disease.
- Parental occupation (machinists, welders, motor vehicle mechanics, auto body repairmen)
- Maternal exposure to pesticides prior to child's birth (2)[B]
- High birth weight or preterm birth (2)[B]
- Compared with first born, being a second or later birth may be associated with significantly decreased risk of Wilms tumor (2)[B].

Genetics

- Several congenital anomalies are known to be associated with Wilms tumor. A 2-stage mutational model has been proposed: Occurrence in either hereditary form or sporadic form. Patients with aniridia have a deletion of the short arm of chromosome 11 (11p13).
- Abnormalities of chromosome 11 at the 11p15 locus are associated with Beckwith-Wiedemann syndrome.
- Wilms tumor-suppressor gene (*WT1*) has been identified, as well as additional candidates for another suppressor gene (*WT2*).
- Chromosome band 17q12–21 has been linked to 2 kindreds with Wilms tumor, and other kindreds are associated with a Wilms tumor predisposition gene at 19q13.3–q13.4.
- Loss of heterozygosity at chromosomes 16q and 1p is associated with adverse outcome (1)[C].

GENERAL PREVENTION

Routine surveillance in patients with syndromes associated with Wilms tumor

ETIOLOGY

- Hereditary or sporadic forms of genetic mutation
- Familial form: Autosomal-dominant trait with incomplete penetrance (1%)
- Potential of parental occupational exposure (machinists, welders, motor vehicle mechanics, auto body repairmen)

COMMONLY ASSOCIATED CONDITIONS

- Aniridia (partial or complete absence of iris) 600× >normal risk
- Hemihypertrophy (100× >normal risk)
- Cryptorchidism
- Hypospadias
- Duplicated renal collecting systems
- Wiedemann-Beckwith syndrome
- Denys-Drash syndrome (nephropathy, renal failure, male pseudohermaphroditism, Wilms tumor)
- Klippel-Trénaunay syndrome
- WAGR complex (Wilms tumor, aniridia, genitourinary malformations, and mental retardation)
- Beckwith-Wiedemann syndrome (visceromegaly, macroglossia, omphalocele, hyperinsulinemic hypoglycemia)

DIAGNOSIS

- Symptoms of pain, anorexia, vomiting, malaise in 30% (1)[C]
- Over 90% present with asymptomatic abdominal mass (3)[B].

HISTORY

- History of increasing abdominal size
- Usually asymptomatic

PHYSICAL EXAM

- Palpable upper abdominal mass
- Abdominal pain
- Fever
- Anemia
- Rarely, signs of acute abdomen with free intraperitoneal rupture
- Cardiac murmur
- Hepatosplenomegaly
- Ascites
- Prominent abdominal wall veins
- Varicocele
- Gonadal metastases
- Aniridia (present in 1.1% of Wilms tumor patients)
- Hypertension (20–65%) (1)[C]

DIAGNOSTIC TESTS & INTERPRETATION

Lab

- Urinalysis (occasional hematuria, proteinuria)
- CBC (anemia)
- Lactate dehydrogenase
- Plasma renin (rarely helpful)
- Urine catecholamines
- Serum creatinine and calcium
- Coagulation factors

Imaging

- Chest radiograph
- Kidney, ureter, and bladder (presence of linear calcifications)
- Abdominal ultrasound (with Doppler imaging): Gives best information about tumor extension into inferior vena cava
- CT scan (with IV and oral contrast material) of chest and abdomen (12–15% have lung metastases at diagnosis) (1)
- IV pyelogram rarely helpful

Diagnostic Procedures/Surgery

Occasionally, bone marrow aspiration necessary to distinguish from neuroblastoma

Pathological Findings

- Favorable findings (mortality of 7%):
  - Bulky lesion, well encapsulated
  - Focal areas of hemorrhage and necrosis
  - Absence of anaplasia and sarcomatous cell types
  - Presence of blastema, stomal, and epithelial elements (3)[B]:
    - Predominance of epithelial elements usually are less aggressive when diagnosed early, but tend to be resistant to treatment when diagnosed late.
    - Predominance of blastemal elements indicate more aggressive tumors.
- Unfavorable histology (mortality rate of 57%):
  - Anaplasia: Markedly enlarged and multipolar mitotic figures, 3-fold enlargement of nuclei in comparison with adjacent similar nuclei, hyperchromasia of enlarged nuclei; anaplasia may be diffuse or focal
  - Sarcomatous changes: Now considered to be separate from Wilms, not subtypes (mortality 64%)
  - Rhabdoid tumor of the kidney: Now considered to be separate tumor from Wilms
- Nephroblastomatosis: Considered premalignant
- Nephrogenic rests (3)[B]:
  - These are precursor lesions found in 25–40% of Wilms.
  - Found in 1% of infants at autopsy, but most do not develop into malignancy

DIFFERENTIAL DIAGNOSIS

- Neuroblastoma
- Hepatic tumor
- Sarcoma
- Rhabdoid tumor
- Cystic nephroma
- Renal cell carcinoma (generally occurs in older children)

- Mesoblastic nephroma:
  - Distinguished only by histology
  - Age usually <6 months
  - Essentially benign, although metastases have been reported; tends to be locally invasive
  - Operative spillage may lead to recurrence.
  - No chemotherapy or radiotherapy is needed with complete excision.
- Nephroblastomatosis: Considered premalignant; may present as nodularity of 1 or both kidneys; treated with biopsy and local excision (renal tissue sparing)

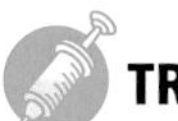

TREATMENT

MEDICATION

First Line

- Dactinomycin (Actinomycin-D)
- Vincristine
- Doxorubicin
- Cyclophosphamide (Cytoxan)
- Iphosphamide
- Etoposide

Second Line

- Doxorubicin (Adriamycin)
- Cyclophosphamide

ADDITIONAL TREATMENT

General Measures

- Appropriate health care: Inpatient workup and treatment until stable postoperative and induction chemotherapy completed
- Chemotherapy; some recommend pretreatment with neoadjuvant chemotherapy (1):
  - May decrease incidence of intraoperative tumor rupture (debatable)
  - May result in inappropriate treatment with chemotherapeutic agents of non-Wilms tumors (5%) or benign lesions (1.6%)
  - Results in the inability to directly compare treatment results worldwide
- Radiation therapy in stage II (unfavorable histology), stage III, and stage IV

SURGERY/OTHER PROCEDURES

- Exam (visual and manual) of contralateral kidney
- Radical nephroureterectomy and biopsies as needed to provide precise staging information
- Sampling of any enlarged lymph nodes (absence of any lymph nodes in the surgical specimen mandates treatment as stage III disease) (3)[B]
- Identification of any retained tumor with titanium clips
- Tumor should be given to pathologist fresh, not in formalin.
- Vertical midline incision if tumor extension to right atrium present (possible use of cardiopulmonary bypass)
- Bilateral Wilms tumors (represent 4–6% of Wilms) (3)[B]:
  - Preoperative chemotherapy with re-evaluation by CT or MRI after 6 weeks (some are biopsied prior to chemotherapy)
  - Renal sparing operation at 6 weeks if good response to chemotherapy:
    - Partial nephrectomy or wedge excision of tumor preferred, but only if it does not compromise tumor resection
    - Kidney with lowest tumor burden is addressed first. If successful resection accomplished, radical nephrectomy can be done on the contralateral kidney. Bilateral partial nephrectomy may be possible in some cases.
- Preoperative treatment also generally is accepted in a solitary kidney, horseshoe kidneys, intravascular extension of tumor above the intrahepatic vena cava, and in the case of respiratory distress from extensive metastatic tumor.

ONGOING CARE

FOLLOW-UP RECOMMENDATIONS

Patient Monitoring

- Multidrug chemotherapy every 3–4 weeks for 16 weeks–15 months depending on stage
- Every 4 months for 1 year, every 6 months for second to third year, yearly after that
- CBC, CT of chest and abdomen with each visit
- Patients at high risk for developing Wilms tumor should be monitored with renal ultrasound every 3–4 months until 5 years of age. Patients with Beckwith-Wiedemann syndrome or Simpson-Golabi-Behmel syndrome should have yearly ultrasound until 7 years of age (4)[C].

PATIENT EDUCATION

- Possibility of second malignancy (up to 12% by age 50)
- Side effects of chemotherapy, radiation therapy

PROGNOSIS

- With favorable histology (1):
  - Children <2 years of age and stage I, favorable histology: 98% survival in NWTSG 1–3 studies
  - Children with stage III, favorable histology tumor: Overall survival of 89% in NWTSG 3–4 studies
- With diffuse anaplasia (1):
  - Children with stage I, diffuse or focal anaplasia: Overall survival 82.6%
  - Stage II tumors with anaplasia: Overall survival 81.5%
  - Stage III tumors with anaplasia: Overall survival 66.7%
  - Stage IV tumors with anaplasia: Overall survival 33.3%
- With bilateral involvement (stage V): 4-year survival 81.7% (1)
- With rhabdoid features: 19% 3-year survival

COMPLICATIONS

- Complication rate of 6–10%
- 1–2% will develop 2nd malignant neoplasms (leukemia, lymphoma, hepatocellular carcinoma, soft tissue sarcoma): 12.2% by 50 years of age
- High risk of delivering low-birth-weight infants, perinatal mortality in offspring of female survivors of Wilms tumor
- Chest is usual site of recurrence.
- Occurrence of second malignant neoplasms in 2% of patients 7–34 years after treatment:
  - Bone and soft tissue sarcomas, breast cancer, hepatocellular carcinoma, lymphoma, gastrointestinal tract tumors, melanoma, leukemias
- Surgical complications (5)[B]:
  - Postoperative small bowel obstruction (5–7%)
  - Tumor rupture with spillage in 15.3% according to NWTSG-5; this may be spontaneous or surgical and results in upstaging the tumor. Only 2.7% of spills are considered avoidable (6)[B]. Incidence of tumor spillage is reported as 2.2% by SIOP following preoperative neoadjuvant chemotherapy (3)[B].
- Local tumor recurrence:
  - Abdominal tumor recurrence after tumor spillage is reduced by radiation therapy (10 or 20 Gy) (7)[B]
- Renal failure
- Cardiomyopathy (usually related to doxorubicin and radiation therapy)
- Impaired pulmonary function (radiation therapy)

REFERENCES

1. Sonn G, Shortliffe LM. Management of Wilms tumor: Current standard of care. *Nat Clin Pract Urol*. 2008;5:551–60.
2. Chu A, Heck JE, Ribeiro KB, et al. Wilms' tumour: A systematic review of risk factors and meta-analysis. *Paediatr Perinat Epidemiol*. 2010;24:449–69.
3. Ko EY, Ritchey ML. Current management of Wilms' tumor in children. *J Pediatr Urol*. 2009;5:56–65.
4. Scott RH, et al. Surveillance for Wilms Tumour in at-risk children: Pragmatic recommendations for best practice. *Arch Dis Child*. 2006;91:995–9.
5. Ritchey ML, Shamberger RC, Haase G, et al. Surgical complications after primary nephrectomy for Wilms tumor: Report from the national Wilms tumor study group. *J Am Coll Surg*. 2001;192:63–8.
6. Ehrlich PF, Ritchey ML, Hamilton TE, et al. Quality assessment for Wilms tumor: A report from the national Wilms study-5. *J Ped Surg*. 2005;40:208–12.
7. Kalapurakal JA, Li SM, et al. Intraoperative spillage of favorable histology Wilms tumor cells: Influence of irradiation and chemotherapy regimens on abdominal recurrence. A report from the National Wilms Tumor study group. *Int J Radiat Oncol Biol Phys*. 2010;76:201–6.

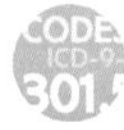

CODES

ICD9

189.0 Malignant neoplasm of kidney, except pelvis

CLINICAL PEARLS

- Wilms is most common renal tumor in children; it is an embryonal renal neoplasm containing blastema, stromal, or epithelial cell types, usually affecting children <5 years of age.
- Risks include parental occupation (machinists, welders, motor vehicle mechanics, auto body repairmen) and maternal exposure to pesticides prior to child's birth.
- Nephrectomy performed as soon as possible after completing radiographic evaluation is the major component in tumor staging.

W

ZINC DEFICIENCY

Adarsh K. Gupta, DO, MS

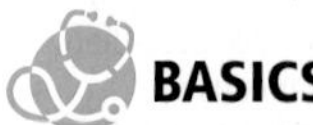

BASICS

DESCRIPTION
- Condition whose manifestations may involve growth retardation; hypogonadism; cell-mediated immune dysfunction; poor wound healing; poor appetite; hair loss; depression; and increased incidence of infection, anorexia, diarrhea, and eye and skin lesions related to decreased zinc levels (1)
- System(s) affected: Endocrine/Metabolic; Nervous; Skin/Exocrine; Hematologic/Oncologic; Gastroenterologic

Geriatric Considerations
- Zinc deficiency may cause poor night vision, leading to falls; poor wound healing or chronic ulcer; or loss of smell and taste, which may cause worsening nutrition.
- Elderly persons living in institutions may have low zinc intake.

Pediatric Considerations
Zinc deficiency may cause failure to thrive and diarrhea, and may impair growth and development of secondary sexual characteristics (2).

Pregnancy Considerations
Requirements increase; deficiency may cause spontaneous abortion, inadequate weight gain

EPIDEMIOLOGY
Prevalence
- In the US: Rare in general population
- High prevalence in developing countries
- Predominate age: All ages
- Predominant sex: Male = Female

RISK FACTORS
- Drugs: Diuretics, penicillamine, sodium valproate, and ethambutol
- Low socioeconomic status
- Malabsorption syndromes
- Living in developing nations
- Hyperalimentation with zinc supplementation
- Thermal burns
- Strict vegetarian diet
- Alcoholism
- Chronic renal failure patients on hemodialysis

Genetics
Usually acquired, but rarely caused by acrodermatitis enteropathica (autosomal recessive) and associated with sickle cell anemia (autosomal recessive)

GENERAL PREVENTION
- Adequate diet
- Supplementation when indicated (see "Medication")

ETIOLOGY
- Increased requirements:
  - Pregnancy
  - Lactation
  - Rapid growth phase in childhood
  - Burns
  - Major trauma
- Increased losses:
  - Diabetes
  - Cirrhosis
  - Renal disease
  - Malabsorption states (e.g., inflammatory bowel diseases)
  - Sickle cell anemia
  - Diuretics: Thiazides, chlorthalidone
- Decreased absorption:
  - Acrodermatitis enteropathica, an autosomal-recessive deficiency in the enzyme required for intestinal absorption
  - Geophagia
  - Chelating agents
  - Parasitism
  - Diet high in phytates (plant fiber)
  - Drugs: Penicillamines, tetracyclines, quinolones, bisphosphonates
- Insufficient dietary intake:
  - Vegetarianism
  - Parenteral hyperalimentation without zinc supplementation
  - Breast-feeding
  - Suboptimal zinc conditions in diet (rare)
  - Alcoholism

COMMONLY ASSOCIATED CONDITIONS
- Sickle cell anemia
- Malabsorption
- Parenteral hyperalimentation
- In the older patient: Those taking diuretics, those with diabetes mellitus, cirrhosis
- In hemodialysis patients, zinc deficiency is associated with depression.

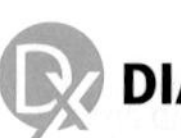

DIAGNOSIS

HISTORY
- Mild deficiency:
  - Hypogeusia (lack of taste)
  - Decreased dark adaptation
  - Decreased lean body mass

- Moderate deficiency:
  - All of the above
  - Diarrhea
  - Growth retardation
  - Hypogonadism (especially male)
  - Mental lethargy
  - Anergy
  - Rough skin
  - Delayed wound healing
  - Glucose intolerance
  - Impaired cell-mediated immunity
- Severe deficiency:
  - All of the above
  - Bullous pustular dermatitis
  - Weight loss
  - Dwarfism
  - Emotional instability
  - Tremors
  - Ataxia
  - Alopecia
  - Death

PHYSICAL EXAM
- Depends on level of deficiency
- Acrodermatitis enterohepatica: Erythema, scales, erosions, and/or vesiculobullous eruptions often quite dramatic in diaper area

DIAGNOSTIC TESTS & INTERPRETATION
Lab
- Plasma zinc levels decreased (in moderate-to-severe zinc deficiency). Levels <60 g/L are strongly suggestive, but correction may be needed for low albumin because most serum zinc is bound to albumin.
- Erythrocyte or leukocyte zinc levels more adequately reflect tissue stores, but are not widely available.
- Hair and fingernail levels are not useful.

DIFFERENTIAL DIAGNOSIS
- Congenital dwarfism
- Failure to thrive in infants
- Multiple micronutrient deficiencies
- Primary hypogonadism
- Mental retardation

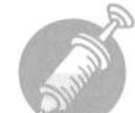

TREATMENT

MEDICATION
- Zinc supplements (take at least 1 hour before or 2 hours after meals high in calcium, fiber, and phytates)
- Oral form: Zinc gluconate (lozenges, tablets), zinc sulfate (capsules, tablets, extended-release tablets)
- Injectable form: Zinc chloride, zinc sulfate
- Use the recommended dietary allowance (RDA) as a guideline for dosing (see "Diet").
- In adult patient, 4–6 mg/d of elemental zinc added to hyperalimentation; may increase to 12 mg q.i.d. if suspect ongoing heavy zinc losses (e.g., burns or major trauma)
- Precautions: Avoid large (>20 mg elemental zinc) parenteral doses.

ONGOING CARE

FOLLOW-UP RECOMMENDATIONS
Full activity

Patient Monitoring
Clinical status such as improved energy, weight gain, resolution of symptoms

DIET
- Balanced omnivorous diet or vegetarian diet with supplementation
- Avoid excessive intake of foods with high phytate content (e.g., raw cereals, but ready-to-eat cereal may be the richest source of zinc from a plant product).
- Lean beef and pork, oysters, poultry, soybeans, pumpkin, sunflower seeds, seafood, milk, eggs, grains, legumes, nuts, and wheat bran are rich in zinc.
- RDA for zinc:
  - Men: 15 mg/d
  - Women: 12 mg/d
  - Pregnant women: 15 mg/d
  - Breast-feeding women: 19 mg/d

PROGNOSIS
Immediate improvement in clinical status with treatment; full resolution in signs and symptoms

REFERENCES

1. http://ods.od.nih.gov/factsheets/zinc.asp#en2.
2. Lukacik M, Thomas RL, Aranda JV. A meta-analysis of the effects of oral zinc in the treatment of acute and persistent diarrhea. *Pediatrics*. 2008;121: 326–36.

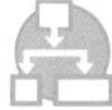

See Also (Topic, Algorithm, Electronic Media Element)

Alcohol Abuse and Dependence; Anemia, Sickle Cell; Failure to Thrive (FTT)

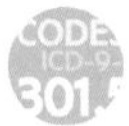

CODES

ICD9
269.3 Mineral deficiency, not elsewhere classified

CLINICAL PEARLS
- Zinc deficiency is uncommon in the US.
- Elderly living in long-term facilities may have diets deficient in zinc.
- Zinc deficiency may cause poor wound healing; consider supplementation when treating chronic skin ulcers.

ZOLLINGER-ELLISON SYNDROME

Douglas S. Parks, MD

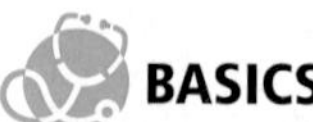

BASICS

DESCRIPTION

- Zollinger-Ellison Syndrome triad:
  - Markedly elevated gastric acid secretion
  - Peptic ulcer disease
  - A gastrinoma or non-β islet cell tumor of the pancreas or duodenal wall that produces gastrin
- Gastrinomas (at the time of diagnosis) may be single or multiple (1/2–2/3), large or small, benign or malignant (2/3), sporadic (70–75%) or associated with MEN1 (*Multiple Endocrine Neoplasia type 1*) (25–30%).
- System(s) affected: Endocrine/Metabolic; Gastrointestinal
- Synonym(s): Z-E syndrome; Pancreatic ulcerogenic tumor syndrome; Multiple endocrine neoplasia, partial; Ulcerogenic islet cell tumor

EPIDEMIOLOGY

Incidence

- 1–3 per million per year
- Predominant age: Middle age (30–65 years)
- Predominant sex: Male > Female (1.3:1)

Pediatric Considerations

Very aggressive cases have been reported in teenagers.

Pregnancy Considerations

Cases reported; influences medication choices and surgical timing

RISK FACTORS

- MEN1
- Family history of ulcer disease

Genetics

~25–30% of cases occur in association with the MEN1 syndrome.

GENERAL PREVENTION

Screen first-degree relatives of patients with MEN1.

ETIOLOGY

- Gastrinoma is equally distributed between the head of the pancreas and the first or second portion of the duodenum; if in the pancreas, the lesion is more likely to metastasize to the liver.
- Also may be found rarely in the mesentery, peritoneum, spleen, skin, or mediastinum (possibly metastasis with primary not identified)

COMMONLY ASSOCIATED CONDITIONS

- MEN1: Hyperparathyroidism, prolactinomas, other pituitary tumors
- Insulinoma
- Carcinoid tumors

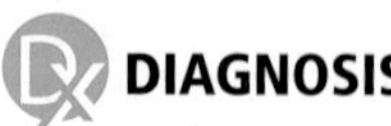

DIAGNOSIS

HISTORY

Average of 5 years of symptoms, including recurrent ulcers before diagnosis is made:

- Abdominal pain (80%)
- Diarrhea, including while fasting (70%)
- Heartburn (60%)
- Nausea (30%)
- Reflux esophagitis
- Vomiting that is unresponsive to standard therapy
- Weight loss
- Steatorrhea

PHYSICAL EXAM

- Peptic ulcer disease
- Hepatomegaly with metastasis
- Endoscopic findings, including esophagitis, duodenal ulceration with multiple ulcers, and prominent gastric and duodenal folds
- Complications of severe peptic ulcer disease, including hemorrhage, perforation, and obstruction
- Signs of MEN1 are hypercalcemia, hyperparathyroidism, and Cushing syndrome.

Geriatric Considerations

- Consider the diagnosis in a patient with persistent or recurring peptic ulcer disease; it is a less aggressive disease if it appears >65 years.

DIAGNOSTIC TESTS & INTERPRETATION

- Preferred test is secretion stimulation test: Gastrin level >100 pg/mL (>100 ng/L) (1)[A],(2)[B]
- Gastric secretory studies: Basal acid output
- Alternative test is calcium infusion test: Gastrin level >400 pg/mL (test is less specific and more dangerous because of IV calcium infusion)

Lab

- Elevated serum gastrin fasting level: >1,000 pg/mL with ulcers diagnostic; >200 pg/mL with ulcers suggestive
- Elevated basal gastric acid output: >15 mEq/hr (>15 mmol/hr)
- Gastric pH <2 with elevated gastrin
- Check serum calcium, phosphorus, cortisol, and prolactin to rule out MEN1.
- Drugs may alter lab results:
  - Histamine (H_2)-blockers and proton-pump inhibitors (PPIs) may increase gastric pH and serum gastrin.
  - Hold PPIs 7 days and H_2-blockers 2 days prior to drawing gastrin level.

Imaging

- Used to localize tumor for possible resection
- Much more likely to find tumors >3 cm (95%) than <1 cm (<15%) (3)[B]
- Abdominal CT scan: Most useful for pancreatic tumors and metastasis >3 cm
- Abdominal ultrasound: Not useful except in large tumors
- Abdominal angiography: Not useful except in large tumors
- Endoscopic ultrasound: Finds 24–38% of primary tumors
- Abdominal magnetic resonance imaging: Not very useful except in large tumors
- Somatostatin receptor scintigraphy (SRS): More sensitive than radiologic studies but still only finds 30% of small tumors
- Portal venous sampling and selective venous sampling for gastrin can localize the area of tumor and metastasis (80–90% sensitivity).
- Sella turcica imaging may help if MEN1 is suspected in order to look for pituitary tumors.
- Because pancreatic tumors are most likely to be large and to metastasize to the liver, which worsens prognosis, it is suggested to get SRS and an abdominal CT scan to look for resectable tumors. Both studies are much more sensitive for pancreatic tumors, and surgical resection may improve prognosis considerably (4)[B].

Diagnostic Procedures/Surgery

Endoscopy may reveal tumors in the duodenal wall; multiple ulcers, including jejunal ulcers; and prominent gastric and duodenal folds.

Pathological Findings

- 90% of gastrinomas are found in the gastric triangle (the borders are the bile duct, the junction of second and third portions of the duodenum, and the junction of the head and body of pancreas).
- Almost 50% of gastrinomas are in the head of the pancreas (more likely >3 cm, metastasis to liver).
- Almost 50% of gastrinomas are in the wall of the first or second portion of duodenum (more likely to be small, solitary).
- 2/3 of gastrinomas are malignant in both sites (defined by tendency for metastasis).
- 50% of gastrinomas stain positive for adrenocorticotropic hormone (ACTH), vasoactive intestinal polypeptide, insulin, or neurotensin (in decreasing order of incidence).
- 1/3 of patients have metastasis on presentation with regional nodes > liver > bone, rarely to peritoneum, spleen, skin, and mediastinum.
- Duodenal, jejunal, and gastric ulcers; often multiple
- Gastric and duodenal mucosal fold thickening
- Hyperplasia of antral gastrin-producing cells
- Histology similar in appearance to carcinoid

DIFFERENTIAL DIAGNOSIS

- Elevated serum gastrin with hypochlorhydria/achlorhydria:
  - Atrophic gastritis
  - Drug-induced (associated with PPIs)
  - Gastric cancer
  - Pernicious anemia
  - Postvagotomy
- Elevated serum gastrin with normal or increased gastric acid:
  - Antral G-cell hyperfunction
  - Chronic renal failure
  - *Helicobacter pylori* infection
  - Gastric outlet obstruction
  - Retained gastric antrum
- Consider gastrinoma in all patients with the following symptoms:
  - Recurrent or refractory ulcer disease
  - Gastric hypertrophy and ulcers
  - Duodenal and jejunal ulcers
  - Ulcers and diarrhea
  - Ulcers and kidney stones
  - Hypercalcemia and ulcers
  - Pituitary disease
  - Family history of ulcer disease or endocrine tumors suggestive of MEN1

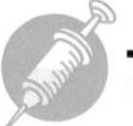

TREATMENT

MEDICATION

- Drugs heal 80–85% of ulcers.
- Although medications heal ulcers, the ulcers nearly always recur. Although doses may be adjusted, the patient should plan on lifelong use of medication.
- Dosages frequently exceed usual doses for treatment of ulcers by 4–8-fold. Start at a lower recommended dose given below, and titrate up to resolution of symptoms or the maximum listed subsequently.
- If hyperparathyroidism is present because of MEN1, hypercalcemia must be corrected.
- PPIs are the first-line treatment; H_2-blockers may need to be added.

First Line

- PPIs:
  - Omeprazole: 60–120 mg/d
  - Lansoprazole: 60–180 mg/d (doses >120 mg need to be divided b.i.d.)
  - Rabeprazole: 60–100 mg/d up to 60 mg b.i.d.
  - Pantoprazole: 40–240 mg/d PO; 80–120 mg q12h IV
- H_2-blockers:
  - Cimetidine: 300 mg q6h up to 1.25–5 g/d
  - Ranitidine: 150 mg q12h up to 6 g/d
  - Famotidine: 20–800 mg at bedtime
- Contraindications:
  - Known hypersensitivity to the drug
  - H_2-blockers: Androgen effects, drug interactions due to cytochrome P450 stimulation
  - PPIs: None
- Precautions:
  - Adjust the doses for renal and geriatric patients depending on the drug.
  - Gynecomastia has been reported with high-dose cimetidine (>2.4 g/d).
  - PPIs may induce a profound and long-lasting effect on gastric acid secretion, thereby affecting the bioavailability of drugs depending on low gastric pH (e.g., ketoconazole, ampicillin, iron).
- Significant possible interactions: Refer to the drug manufacturers' literature.

Second Line

- Octreotide appears helpful in slowing the growth of a liver metastasis, and it may produce regression in some cases. Octreotide LAR can be given every 28 days (3)[B].
- Chemotherapy regimens of streptozocin, 5-fluorouracil, and doxorubicin show only limited response.
- Interferon shows a limited response but may be useful in combination with octreotide.

ADDITIONAL TREATMENT

General Measures

- Advanced imaging initially to assess for possible resection
- Surgical removal when primary tumor can be identified and as an adjunct to symptom control
- Medical treatment for symptom control when primary tumor is not found or metastasis is present on diagnosis

SURGERY/OTHER PROCEDURES

- Laparotomy to search for resectable tumors (especially in the pancreas and duodenal wall), unless patient has liver metastasis on presentation or MEN1; improves outcome (5)[B]
- Definitive therapy: Removal of gastrinomas when found (surgery finds 95% of tumors; 5-year cure is 40% when all can be removed)
- Total gastrectomy was formerly used to stop acid production before pharmacologic therapy became available; now it is seldom done.
- In MEN1, parathyroidectomy, by lowering calcium, may decrease acid production and decrease antisecretory drug use. Gastrinomas are generally small, benign, and multiple and not usually cured by surgery.

IN-PATIENT CONSIDERATIONS

Initial Stabilization

- Advise daily care based on symptoms.
- Appropriate surveillance of basal gastric acid output to monitor antacid secretory therapy
- Appropriate surveillance postoperatively to look for metastasis

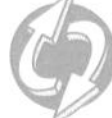

ONGOING CARE

FOLLOW-UP RECOMMENDATIONS

Patient Monitoring

- The patient must be monitored over time for evidence of metastasis.
- Careful dose titration of medical therapy is necessary to control symptoms.
- Gastric acid analysis to maintain basal gastric acid output to <10 mEq/hr (<2 mEq/hr if patient has complications such as perforation or esophagitis)

DIET

Restrict foods that aggravate symptoms.

PATIENT EDUCATION

Inform patients as to the nature of disease and prognosis.

PROGNOSIS

- Overall survival rate: 5–10 years: 69–94%
- The prognosis improves if complete surgical removal of the tumor is possible.
- If liver metastasis is present on initial surgery, 5-year survival is 30–40%; 10-year survival is 25%.
- Mortality directly related to liver metastasis associated with larger tumors and pancreatic tumors (3,4)[B]

COMPLICATIONS

- Complications of peptic ulcer disease (bleeding, perforation, obstruction)
- 2/3 of gastrinomas are malignant with metastasis.
- A tumor may produce other substances, such as ACTH (5–8% of patients), with resulting Cushing syndrome.
- Decrease in vitamin B_{12} levels are possible with long-term PPI use (6)[B].

REFERENCES

1. Berna MJ, Hoffmann KM, Long SH, et al. Serum gastrin in Zollinger-Ellison syndrome: II. Prospective study of gastrin provocative testing in 293 patients from the National Institutes of Health and comparison with 537 cases from the literature. evaluation of diagnostic criteria, proposal of new criteria, and correlations with clinical and tumoral features. *Medicine (Baltimore)*. 2006;85:331–64.
2. Kuiper P, Biemond I, Masclee AA, et al. Diagnostic efficacy of the secretin stimulation test for the Zollinger-Ellison syndrome: An intra-individual comparison using different dosages in patients and controls. *Pancreatology*. 2010;10:14–8.
3. Hoffmann KM, Furukawa M, Jensen RT. Duodenal neuroendocrine tumors: Classification, functional syndromes, diagnosis and medical treatment. *Best Pract Res Clin Gastroenterol*. 2005;19:675–97.
4. Jensen RT. Gastrinomas: Advances in diagnosis and management. *Neuroendocrinology*. 2004; 80(Suppl 1):23–7.
5. Morrow EH, Norton JA. Surgical management of Zollinger-Ellison syndrome; state of the art. *Surg Clin North Am*. 2009;89:1091–103.
6. Hirschowitz BI, Worthington J, Mohnen J, et al. Vitamin B12 deficiency in hypersecretors during long-term acid suppression with proton pump inhibitors. *Aliment Pharmacol Ther*. 2008;27: 1110–21.

ADDITIONAL READING

- Hirschowitz BI, Fineberg N, Wilcox CM, et al. Costs and risks in the management of patients with gastric acid hypersecretion. *J Clin Gastroenterol*. 2010;44: 28–33.
- Mortellaro VE, Hochwald SN, McGuigan JE, et al. Long-term results of a selective surgical approach to management of Zollinger-Ellison syndrome in patients with MEN-1. *Am Surg*. 2009;75:730–3.
- Smallfield GB, Allison J, Wilcox CM, et al. Prospective evaluation of quality of life in patients with Zollinger-Ellison syndrome. *Dig Dis Sci*. 2010; 55:3108–12.

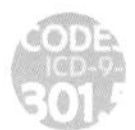

CODES

ICD9

251.5 Abnormality of secretion of gastrin

CLINICAL PEARLS

- ~25–30% of cases of Z-E syndrome occur in association with MEN1.
- Once diagnosed, look for the gastrinoma; gastrinoma location is equally distributed between the head of the pancreas and the first or second portion of the duodenum.
- PPIs heal ulcers, but think of Z-E syndrome if peptic ulcers recur or if high doses are needed to control symptoms/ulcers.

Z

Centers for Disease Control and Prevention

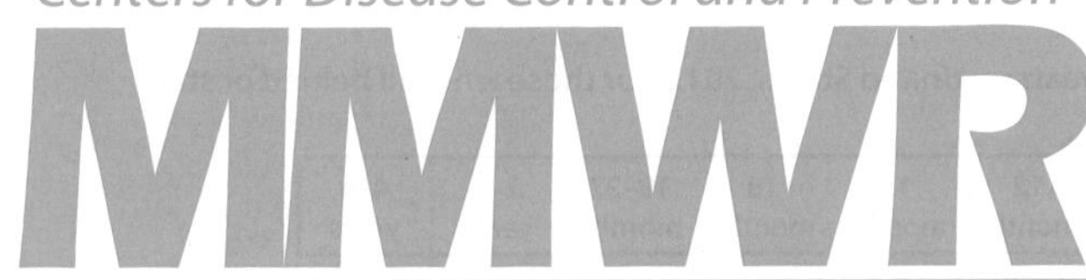

Morbidity and Mortality Weekly Report

QuickGuide / Vol. 61 / No. 5 February 10, 2012

Recommended Immunization Schedules for Persons Aged 0 Through 18 Years — United States, 2012

Each year, the Advisory Committee on Immunization Practices (ACIP) publishes immunization schedules for persons aged 0 through 18 years. These schedules summarize recommendations for currently licensed vaccines for children aged 0 through 6 years and 7 through 18 years and include recommendations in effect as of December 23, 2011.

Vaccination providers are being advised to use all three schedules (Figure 1, Figure 2, and Figure 3) and their respective footnotes together and not separately.

A parent-friendly schedule for children and adolescents is available online at http://www.cdc.gov/vaccines/recs/schedules/child-schedule.htm#printable.

Changes to the previous schedules include the following:

- Updates to Figure 1 ("Recommended immunization schedule for persons aged 0 through 6 years"):
  - — Quadrivalent meningococcal conjugate vaccine (MCV4) purple bar has been extended to reflect licensure of MCV4-D (Menactra) use in children as young as age 9 months.
  - — A wording change has been introduced in the hepatitis A (HepA) vaccine yellow bar; wording now states, "Dose 1." A new yellow and purple bar has been added to reflect HepA vaccine recommendations for children aged 2 years and older.
- Guidance is provided for administration of hepatitis B (HepB) vaccine in infants with birthweights <2,000 grams and ≥2,000 grams. Clarification is provided for doses after administration of the birth dose of HepB vaccine.
- Rotavirus (RV) vaccine footnotes have been condensed.
- *Haemophilus influenzae* type b (Hib) conjugate vaccine footnotes have been condensed, and use of Hiberix for the booster (final) dose has been clarified. Guidance for use of Hib vaccine in persons aged 5 years and older in the catch-up schedule has been updated.
- Pneumococcal vaccine footnotes have been condensed.
- Guidance is provided for use of measles, mumps, and rubella (MMR) vaccine in infants aged 6 through 11 months. Footnotes in the catch-up schedule have been condensed.
- HepA vaccine footnotes have been updated to clarify that the second dose of HepA vaccine should be administered 6–18 months after dose 1.
- MCV4 footnotes have been updated to reflect recent recommendations published in *MMWR.*
- Influenza vaccine footnotes have been updated to provide guidance on live, attenuated influenza vaccine (LAIV) contraindications.
- Influenza vaccine footnotes also have been updated to clarify dosing for children aged 6 months through 8 years for the 2011–12 and 2012–13 seasons.
- Figure 2 ("Recommended immunization schedule for persons aged 7 through 18 years") has been updated to include number of doses for each vaccine. Information regarding the recommended age (16 years) for the booster dose of MCV4 has been added.
- Tdap vaccine recommendations for children aged 7 through 10 years have been updated.
- Human papillomavirus (HPV) vaccine footnotes have been updated to include routine recommendations for vaccination of males.
- Varicella (VAR) vaccine footnotes have been condensed.
- Inactivated poliovirus vaccine (IPV) footnotes have been updated to include upper age limit for routine vaccination. IPV footnotes in the catch-up schedule have been condensed, and relevant wording added to Figure 3 ("Catch-up immunization schedule for persons aged 4 months through 18 years who start late or who are more than 1 month behind").
- In the catch-up immunization schedule, HepA vaccine and HepB vaccine footnotes have been removed. Relevant wording has been added to Figure 3.
- MCV4 vaccine has been added to Figure 3 along with corresponding footnotes.

The recommended immunization schedules for persons aged 0 through 18 years and the catch-up immunization schedule for 2012 are approved by the Advisory Committee on Immunization Practices, the American Academy of Pediatrics, and the American Academy of Family Physicians.

Suggested citation: Centers for Disease Control and Prevention. Recommended immunization schedules for persons aged 0–18 years—United States, 2012. MMWR 2012;61(5).

FIGURE 1. Recommended immunization schedule for persons aged 0 through 6 years — United States, 2012 (for those who fall behind or start late, see the catch-up schedule [Figure 3])

Vaccine ▼ Age ►	Birth	1 month	2 months	4 months	6 months	9 months	12 months	15 months	18 months	19–23 months	2–3 years	4–6 years
Hepatitis B[1]	HepB	HepB					HepB					
Rotavirus[2]			RV	RV	RV[2]							
Diphtheria, tetanus, pertussis[3]			DTaP	DTaP	DTaP		See footnote[3]	DTaP				DTaP
Haemophilus influenzae type b[4]			Hib	Hib	Hib[4]		Hib					
Pneumococcal[5]			PCV	PCV	PCV		PCV				PPSV	
Inactivated poliovirus[6]			IPV	IPV			IPV					IPV
Influenza[7]								Influenza (yearly)				
Measles, mumps, rubella[8]							MMR			See footnote[8]		MMR
Varicella[9]							VAR			See footnote[9]		VAR
Hepatitis A[10]								Dose 1[10]			HepA series	
Meningococcal[11]									MCV4 — See footnote[11]			

Range of recommended ages for all children

Range of recommended ages for certain high-risk groups

Range of recommended ages for all children and certain high-risk groups

This schedule includes recommendations in effect as of December 23, 2011. Any dose not administered at the recommended age should be administered at a subsequent visit, when indicated and feasible. The use of a combination vaccine generally is preferred over separate injections of its equivalent component vaccines. Vaccination providers should consult the relevant Advisory Committee on Immunization Practices (ACIP) statement for detailed recommendations, available online at http://www.cdc.gov/vaccines/pubs/acip-list.htm. Clinically significant adverse events that follow vaccination should be reported to the Vaccine Adverse Event Reporting System (VAERS) online (http://www.vaers.hhs.gov) or by telephone (800-822-7967).

1. **Hepatitis B (HepB) vaccine.** (Minimum age: birth)
   At birth:
   - Administer monovalent HepB vaccine to all newborns before hospital discharge.
   - For infants born to hepatitis B surface antigen (HBsAg)–positive mothers, administer HepB vaccine and 0.5 mL of hepatitis B immune globulin (HBIG) within 12 hours of birth. These infants should be tested for HBsAg and antibody to HBsAg (anti-HBs) 1 to 2 months after receiving the last dose of the series.
   - If mother's HBsAg status is unknown, within 12 hours of birth administer HepB vaccine for infants weighing ≥2,000 grams, and HepB vaccine plus HBIG for infants weighing <2,000 grams. Determine mother's HBsAg status as soon as possible and, if she is HBsAg-positive, administer HBIG for infants weighing ≥2,000 grams (no later than age 1 week).

   Doses after the birth dose:
   - The second dose should be administered at age 1 to 2 months. Monovalent HepB vaccine should be used for doses administered before age 6 weeks.
   - Administration of a total of 4 doses of HepB vaccine is permissible when a combination vaccine containing HepB is administered after the birth dose.
   - Infants who did not receive a birth dose should receive 3 doses of a HepB-containing vaccine starting as soon as feasible (Figure 3).
   - The minimum interval between dose 1 and dose 2 is 4 weeks, and between dose 2 and 3 is 8 weeks. The final (third or fourth) dose in the HepB vaccine series should be administered no earlier than age 24 weeks and at least 16 weeks after the first dose.
2. **Rotavirus (RV) vaccines.** (Minimum age: 6 weeks for both RV-1 [Rotarix] and RV-5 [Rota Teq])
   - The maximum age for the first dose in the series is 14 weeks, 6 days; and 8 months, 0 days for the final dose in the series. Vaccination should not be initiated for infants aged 15 weeks, 0 days or older.
   - If RV-1 (Rotarix) is administered at ages 2 and 4 months, a dose at 6 months is not indicated.
3. **Diphtheria and tetanus toxoids and acellular pertussis (DTaP) vaccine.** (Minimum age: 6 weeks)
   - The fourth dose may be administered as early as age 12 months, provided at least 6 months have elapsed since the third dose.
4. ***Haemophilus influenzae* type b (Hib) conjugate vaccine.** (Minimum age: 6 weeks)
   - If PRP-OMP (PedvaxHIB or Comvax [HepB-Hib]) is administered at ages 2 and 4 months, a dose at age 6 months is not indicated.
   - Hiberix should only be used for the booster (final) dose in children aged 12 months through 4 years.
5. **Pneumococcal vaccines.** (Minimum age: 6 weeks for pneumococcal conjugate vaccine [PCV]; 2 years for pneumococcal polysaccharide vaccine [PPSV])
   - Administer 1 dose of PCV to all healthy children aged 24 through 59 months who are not completely vaccinated for their age.
   - For children who have received an age-appropriate series of 7-valent PCV (PCV7), a single supplemental dose of 13-valent PCV (PCV13) is recommended for:
     — All children aged 14 through 59 months
     — Children aged 60 through 71 months with underlying medical conditions.
   - Administer PPSV at least 8 weeks after last dose of PCV to children aged 2 years or older with certain underlying medical conditions, including a cochlear implant. See *MMWR* 2010:59(No. RR-11), available at http://www.cdc.gov/mmwr/pdf/rr/rr5911.pdf.
6. **Inactivated poliovirus vaccine (IPV).** (Minimum age: 6 weeks)
   - If 4 or more doses are administered before age 4 years, an additional dose should be administered at age 4 through 6 years.
   - The final dose in the series should be administered on or after the fourth birthday and at least 6 months after the previous dose.
7. **Influenza vaccines.** (Minimum age: 6 months for trivalent inactivated influenza vaccine [TIV]; 2 years for live, attenuated influenza vaccine [LAIV])
   - For most healthy children aged 2 years and older, either LAIV or TIV may be used. However, LAIV should not be administered to some children, including 1) children with asthma, 2) children 2 through 4 years who had wheezing in the past 12 months, or 3) children who have any other underlying medical conditions that predispose them to influenza complications. For all other contraindications to use of LAIV, see *MMWR* 2010;59(No. RR-8), available at http://www.cdc.gov/mmwr/pdf/rr/rr5908.pdf.
   - For children aged 6 months through 8 years:
     — For the 2011–12 season, administer 2 doses (separated by at least 4 weeks) to those who did not receive at least 1 dose of the 2010–11 vaccine. Those who received at least 1 dose of the 2010–11 vaccine require 1 dose for the 2011–12 season.
     — For the 2012–13 season, follow dosing guidelines in the 2012 ACIP influenza vaccine recommendations.
8. **Measles, mumps, and rubella (MMR) vaccine.** (Minimum age: 12 months)
   - The second dose may be administered before age 4 years, provided at least 4 weeks have elapsed since the first dose.
   - Administer MMR vaccine to infants aged 6 through 11 months who are traveling internationally. These children should be revaccinated with 2 doses of MMR vaccine, the first at ages 12 through 15 months and at least 4 weeks after the previous dose, and the second at ages 4 through 6 years.
9. **Varicella (VAR) vaccine.** (Minimum age: 12 months)
   - The second dose may be administered before age 4 years, provided at least 3 months have elapsed since the first dose.
   - For children aged 12 months through 12 years, the recommended minimum interval between doses is 3 months. However, if the second dose was administered at least 4 weeks after the first dose, it can be accepted as valid.
10. **Hepatitis A (HepA) vaccine.** (Minimum age: 12 months)
    - Administer the second (final) dose 6 to18 months after the first.
    - Unvaccinated children 24 months and older at high risk should be vaccinated. See *MMWR* 2006;55(No. RR-7), available at http://www.cdc.gov/mmwr/pdf/rr/rr5507.pdf.
    - A 2-dose HepA vaccine series is recommended for anyone aged 24 months and older, previously unvaccinated, for whom immunity against hepatitis A virus infection is desired.
11. **Meningococcal conjugate vaccines, quadrivalent (MCV4).** (Minimum age: 9 months for Menactra [MCV4-D], 2 years for Menveo [MCV4-CRM])
    - For children aged 9 through 23 months 1) with persistent complement component deficiency; 2) who are residents of or travelers to countries with hyperendemic or epidemic disease; or 3) who are present during outbreaks caused by a vaccine serogroup, administer 2 primary doses of MCV4-D, ideally at ages 9 months and 12 months or at least 8 weeks apart.
    - For children aged 24 months and older with 1) persistent complement component deficiency who have not been previously vaccinated; or 2) anatomic/functional asplenia, administer 2 primary doses of either MCV4 at least 8 weeks apart.
    - For children with anatomic/functional asplenia, if MCV4-D (Menactra) is used, administer at a minimum age of 2 years and at least 4 weeks after completion of all PCV doses.
    - See *MMWR* 2011;60:72–6, available at http://www.cdc.gov/mmwr/pdf/wk/mm6003.pdf, and Vaccines for Children Program resolution No. 6/11-1, available at http://www.cdc.gov/vaccines/programs/vfc/downloads/resolutions/06-11mening-mcv.pdf, and *MMWR* 2011;60:1391–2, available at http://www.cdc.gov/mmwr/pdf/wk/mm6040.pdf, for further guidance, including revaccination guidelines.

This schedule is approved by the Advisory Committee on Immunization Practices (http://www.cdc.gov/vaccines/recs/acip), the American Academy of Pediatrics (http://www.aap.org), and the American Academy of Family Physicians (http://www.aafp.org).

FIGURE 2. Recommended immunization schedule for persons aged 7 through 18 years — United States, 2012 (for those who fall behind or start late, see the schedule below and the catch-up schedule [Figure 3])

Vaccine ▼ Age ▶	7–10 years	11–12 years	13–18 years
Tetanus, diphtheria, pertussis[1]	1 dose (if indicated)	1 dose	1 dose (if indicated)
Human papillomavirus[2]	*See footnote*[2]	3 doses	Complete 3-dose series
Meningococcal[3]	See footnote[3]	Dose 1	Booster at age 16 years
Influenza[4]	Influenza (yearly)		
Pneumococcal[5]	See footnote[5]		
Hepatitis A[6]	Complete 2-dose series		
Hepatitis B[7]	Complete 3-dose series		
Inactivated poliovirus[8]	Complete 3-dose series		
Measles, mumps, rubella[9]	Complete 2-dose series		
Varicella[10]	Complete 2-dose series		

Range of recommended ages for all children

Range of recommended ages for catch-up immunization

Range of recommended ages for certain high-risk groups

This schedule includes recommendations in effect as of December 23, 2011. Any dose not administered at the recommended age should be administered at a subsequent visit, when indicated and feasible. The use of a combination vaccine generally is preferred over separate injections of its equivalent component vaccines. Vaccination providers should consult the relevant Advisory Committee on Immunization Practices (ACIP) statement for detailed recommendations, available online at http://www.cdc.gov/vaccines/pubs/acip-list.htm. Clinically significant adverse events that follow vaccination should be reported to the Vaccine Adverse Event Reporting System (VAERS) online (http://www.vaers.hhs.gov) or by telephone (800-822-7967).

1. **Tetanus and diphtheria toxoids and acellular pertussis (Tdap) vaccine.** (Minimum age: 10 years for Boostrix and 11 years for Adacel)
   - Persons aged 11 through 18 years who have not received Tdap vaccine should receive a dose followed by tetanus and diphtheria toxoids (Td) booster doses every 10 years thereafter.
   - Tdap vaccine should be substituted for a single dose of Td in the catch-up series for children aged 7 through 10 years. Refer to the catch-up schedule if additional doses of tetanus and diphtheria toxoid–containing vaccine are needed.
   - Tdap vaccine can be administered regardless of the interval since the last tetanus and diphtheria toxoid–containing vaccine.
2. **Human papillomavirus (HPV) vaccines (HPV4 [Gardasil] and HPV2 [Cervarix]).** (Minimum age: 9 years)
   - Either HPV4 or HPV2 is recommended in a 3-dose series for females aged 11 or 12 years. HPV4 is recommended in a 3-dose series for males aged 11 or 12 years.
   - The vaccine series can be started beginning at age 9 years.
   - Administer the second dose 1 to 2 months after the first dose and the third dose 6 months after the first dose (at least 24 weeks after the first dose).
   - See *MMWR* 2010;59:626–32, available at http://www.cdc.gov/mmwr/pdf/wk/mm5920.pdf.
3. **Meningococcal conjugate vaccines, quadrivalent (MCV4).**
   - Administer MCV4 at age 11 through 12 years with a booster dose at age 16 years.
   - Administer MCV4 at age 13 through 18 years if patient is not previously vaccinated.
   - If the first dose is administered at age 13 through 15 years, a booster dose should be administered at age 16 through 18 years with a minimum interval of at least 8 weeks after the preceding dose.
   - If the first dose is administered at age 16 years or older, a booster dose is not needed.
   - Administer 2 primary doses at least 8 weeks apart to previously unvaccinated persons with persistent complement component deficiency or anatomic/functional asplenia, and 1 dose every 5 years thereafter.
   - Adolescents aged 11 through 18 years with human immunodeficiency virus (HIV) infection should receive a 2-dose primary series of MCV4, at least 8 weeks apart.
   - See *MMWR* 2011;60:72–76, available at http://www.cdc.gov/mmwr/pdf/wk/mm6003.pdf, and Vaccines for Children Program resolution No. 6/11-1, available at http://www.cdc.gov/vaccines/programs/vfc/downloads/resolutions/06-11mening-mcv.pdf, for further guidelines.
4. **Influenza vaccines (trivalent inactivated influenza vaccine [TIV] and live, attenuated influenza vaccine [LAIV]).**
   - For most healthy, nonpregnant persons, either LAIV or TIV may be used, except LAIV should not be used for some persons, including those with asthma or any other underlying medical conditions that predispose them to influenza complications. For all other contraindications to use of LAIV, see *MMWR* 2010;59(No.RR-8), available at http://www.cdc.gov/mmwr/pdf/rr/rr5908.pdf.
   - Administer 1 dose to persons aged 9 years and older.
   - For children aged 6 months through 8 years:
     — For the 2011–12 season, administer 2 doses (separated by at least 4 weeks) to those who did not receive at least 1 dose of the 2010–11 vaccine. Those who received at least 1 dose of the 2010–11 vaccine require 1 dose for the 2011–12 season.
     — For the 2012–13 season, follow dosing guidelines in the 2012 ACIP influenza vaccine recommendations.
5. **Pneumococcal vaccines (pneumococcal conjugate vaccine [PCV] and pneumococcal polysaccharide vaccine [PPSV]).**
   - A single dose of PCV may be administered to children aged 6 through 18 years who have anatomic/functional asplenia, HIV infection or other immunocompromising condition, cochlear implant, or cerebral spinal fluid leak. See *MMWR* 2010:59(No. RR-11), available at http://www.cdc.gov/mmwr/pdf/rr/rr5911.pdf.
   - Administer PPSV at least 8 weeks after the last dose of PCV to children aged 2 years or older with certain underlying medical conditions, including a cochlear implant. A single revaccination should be administered after 5 years to children with anatomic/functional asplenia or an immunocompromising condition.
6. **Hepatitis A (HepA) vaccine.**
   - HepA vaccine is recommended for children older than 23 months who live in areas where vaccination programs target older children, who are at increased risk for infection, or for whom immunity against hepatitis A virus infection is desired. See *MMWR* 2006;55(No. RR-7), available at http://www.cdc.gov/mmwr/pdf/rr/rr5507.pdf.
   - Administer 2 doses at least 6 months apart to unvaccinated persons.
7. **Hepatitis B (HepB) vaccine.**
   - Administer the 3-dose series to those not previously vaccinated.
   - For those with incomplete vaccination, follow the catch-up recommendations (Figure 3).
   - A 2-dose series (doses separated by at least 4 months) of adult formulation Recombivax HB is licensed for use in children aged 11 through 15 years.
8. **Inactivated poliovirus vaccine (IPV).**
   - The final dose in the series should be administered at least 6 months after the previous dose.
   - If both OPV and IPV were administered as part of a series, a total of 4 doses should be administered, regardless of the child's current age.
   - IPV is not routinely recommended for U.S. residents aged18 years or older.
9. **Measles, mumps, and rubella (MMR) vaccine.**
   - The minimum interval between the 2 doses of MMR vaccine is 4 weeks.
10. **Varicella (VAR) vaccine.**
    - For persons without evidence of immunity (see *MMWR* 2007;56[No. RR-4], available at http://www.cdc.gov/mmwr/pdf/rr/rr5604.pdf), administer 2 doses if not previously vaccinated or the second dose if only 1 dose has been administered.
    - For persons aged 7 through 12 years, the recommended minimum interval between doses is 3 months. However, if the second dose was administered at least 4 weeks after the first dose, it can be accepted as valid.
    - For persons aged 13 years and older, the minimum interval between doses is 4 weeks.

This schedule is approved by the Advisory Committee on Immunization Practices (http://www.cdc.gov/vaccines/recs/acip), the American Academy of Pediatrics (http://www.aap.org), and the American Academy of Family Physicians (http://www.aafp.org).

FIGURE 3. Catch-up immunization schedule for persons aged 4 months through 18 years who start late or who are more than 1 month behind — United States, 2012

The figure below provides catch-up schedules and minimum intervals between doses for children whose vaccinations have been delayed. A vaccine series does not need to be restarted, regardless of the time that has elapsed between doses. Use the section appropriate for the child's age. **Always use this table in conjunction with the accompanying childhood and adolescent immunization schedules (Figures 1 and 2) and their respective footnotes.**

Vaccine	Minimum age for dose 1	Minimum interval between doses			
		Dose 1 to dose 2	Dose 2 to dose 3	Dose 3 to dose 4	Dose 4 to dose 5
Persons aged 4 months through 6 years					
Hepatitis B	Birth	4 weeks	8 weeks and at least 16 weeks after first dose; minimum age for the final dose is 24 weeks		
Rotavirus[1]	6 weeks	4 weeks	4 weeks[1]		
Diphtheria, tetanus, pertussis[2]	6 weeks	4 weeks	4 weeks	6 months	6 months[2]
Haemophilus influenzae type b[3]	6 weeks	4 weeks if first dose administered at younger than age 12 months 8 weeks (as final dose) if first dose administered at age 12–14 months No further doses needed if first dose administered at age 15 months or older	4 weeks[3] if current age is younger than 12 months 8 weeks (as final dose)[3] if current age is 12 months or older and first dose administered at younger than age 12 months and second dose administered at younger than 15 months No further doses needed if previous dose administered at age 15 months or older	8 weeks (as final dose) This dose only necessary for children aged 12 months through 59 months who received 3 doses before age 12 months	
Pneumococcal[4]	6 weeks	4 weeks if first dose administered at younger than age 12 months 8 weeks (as final dose for healthy children) if first dose administered at age 12 months or older or current age 24 through 59 months No further doses needed for healthy children if first dose administered at age 24 months or older	4 weeks if current age is younger than 12 months 8 weeks (as final dose for healthy children) if current age is 12 months or older No further doses needed for healthy children if previous dose administered at age 24 months or older	8 weeks (as final dose) This dose only necessary for children aged 12 months through 59 months who received 3 doses before age 12 months or for children at high risk who received 3 doses at any age	
Inactivated poliovirus[5]	6 weeks	4 weeks	4 weeks	6 months[5] minimum age 4 years for final dose	
Meningococcal[6]	9 months	8 weeks[6]			
Measles, mumps, rubella[7]	12 months	4 weeks			
Varicella[8]	12 months	3 months			
Hepatitis A	12 months	6 months			
Persons aged 7 through 18 years					
Tetanus, diphtheria/tetanus, diphtheria, pertussis[9]	7 years[9]	4 weeks	4 weeks if first dose administered at younger than age 12 months 6 months if first dose administered at 12 months or older	6 months if first dose administered at younger than age 12 months	
Human papillomavirus[10]	9 years	Routine dosing intervals are recommended[10]			
Hepatitis A	12 months	6 months			
Hepatitis B	Birth	4 weeks	8 weeks (and at least 16 weeks after first dose)		
Inactivated poliovirus[5]	6 weeks	4 weeks	4 weeks[5]	6 months[5]	
Meningococcal[6]	9 months	8 weeks[6]			
Measles, mumps, rubella[7]	12 months	4 weeks			
Varicella[8]	12 months	3 months if person is younger than age 13 years 4 weeks if person is aged 13 years or older			

1. **Rotavirus (RV) vaccines (RV-1 [Rotarix] and RV-5 [Rota Teq]).**
   - The maximum age for the first dose in the series is 14 weeks, 6 days; and 8 months, 0 days for the final dose in the series. Vaccination should not be initiated for infants aged 15 weeks, 0 days or older.
   - If RV-1 was administered for the first and second doses, a third dose is not indicated.
2. **Diphtheria and tetanus toxoids and acellular pertussis (DTaP) vaccine.**
   - The fifth dose is not necessary if the fourth dose was administered at age 4 years or older.
3. ***Haemophilus influenzae* type b (Hib) conjugate vaccine.**
   - Hib vaccine should be considered for unvaccinated persons aged 5 years or older who have sickle cell disease, leukemia, human immunodeficiency virus (HIV) infection, or anatomic/functional asplenia.
   - If the first 2 doses were PRP-OMP (PedvaxHIB or Comvax) and were administered at age 11 months or younger, the third (and final) dose should be administered at age 12 through 15 months and at least 8 weeks after the second dose.
   - If the first dose was administered at age 7 through 11 months, administer the second dose at least 4 weeks later and a final dose at age 12 through 15 months.
4. **Pneumococcal vaccines.** (Minimum age: 6 weeks for pneumococcal conjugate vaccine [PCV]; 2 years for pneumococcal polysaccharide vaccine [PPSV])
   - For children aged 24 through 71 months with underlying medical conditions, administer 1 dose of PCV if 3 doses of PCV were received previously, or administer 2 doses of PCV at least 8 weeks apart if fewer than 3 doses of PCV were received previously.
   - A single dose of PCV may be administered to certain children aged 6 through 18 years with underlying medical conditions. See age-specific schedules for details.
   - Administer PPSV to children aged 2 years or older with certain underlying medical conditions. See *MMWR* 2010:59(No. RR-11), available at http://www.cdc.gov/mmwr/pdf/rr/rr5911.pdf.
5. **Inactivated poliovirus vaccine (IPV).**
   - A fourth dose is not necessary if the third dose was administered at age 4 years or older and at least 6 months after the previous dose.
   - In the first 6 months of life, minimum age and minimum intervals are only recommended if the person is at risk for imminent exposure to circulating poliovirus (i.e., travel to a polio-endemic region or during an outbreak).
   - IPV is not routinely recommended for U.S. residents aged 18 years or older.
6. **Meningococcal conjugate vaccines, quadrivalent (MCV4).** (Minimum age: 9 months for Menactra [MCV4-D]; 2 years for Menveo [MCV4-CRM])
   - See Figure 1 ("Recommended immunization schedule for persons aged 0 through 6 years") and Figure 2 ("Recommended immunization schedule for persons aged 7 through 18 years") for further guidance.
7. **Measles, mumps, and rubella (MMR) vaccine.**
   - Administer the second dose routinely at age 4 through 6 years.
8. **Varicella (VAR) vaccine.**
   - Administer the second dose routinely at age 4 through 6 years. If the second dose was administered at least 4 weeks after the first dose, it can be accepted as valid.
9. **Tetanus and diphtheria toxoids (Td) and tetanus and diphtheria toxoids and acellular pertussis (Tdap) vaccines.**
   - For children aged 7 through 10 years who are not fully immunized with the childhood DTaP vaccine series, Tdap vaccine should be substituted for a single dose of Td vaccine in the catch-up series; if additional doses are needed, use Td vaccine. For these children, an adolescent Tdap vaccine dose should not be given.
   - An inadvertent dose of DTaP vaccine administered to children aged 7 through 10 years can count as part of the catch-up series. This dose can count as the adolescent Tdap dose, or the child can later receive a Tdap booster dose at age 11–12 years.
10. **Human papillomavirus (HPV) vaccines (HPV4 [Gardasil] and HPV2 [Cervarix]).**
    - Administer the vaccine series to females (either HPV2 or HPV4) and males (HPV4) at age 13 through 18 years if patient is not previously vaccinated.
    - Use recommended routine dosing intervals for vaccine series catch-up; see Figure 2 ("Recommended immunization schedule for persons aged 7 through 18 years").

Clinically significant adverse events that follow vaccination should be reported to the Vaccine Adverse Event Reporting System (VAERS) online (http://www.vaers.hhs.gov) or by telephone (800-822-7967). Suspected cases of vaccine-preventable diseases should be reported to the state or local health department. Additional information, including precautions and contraindications for vaccination, is available from CDC online (http://www.cdc.gov/vaccines) or by telephone (800-CDC-INFO [800-232-4636]).

Centers for Disease Control and Prevention

MMWR

Morbidity and Mortality Weekly Report

QuickGuide / Vol. 61 / No. 4

February 3, 2012

Recommended Adult Immunization Schedule — United States, 2012

Each year, the Advisory Committee on Immunization Practices (ACIP) reviews the recommended adult immunization schedule to ensure that the schedule reflects current recommendations for licensed vaccines. In October 2011, ACIP approved the adult immunization schedule for 2012, which includes several changes from 2011. A footnote directing readers to links for the full ACIP vaccine recommendations and where to find additional information on specific vaccine recommendations for travelers is now included. In addition, a **Table** summarizing precautions and contraindications was added. This table is based on the corresponding table in the 12th edition of Epidemiology and Prevention of Vaccine-Preventable Diseases and is included to provide ready access to key safety information for adult vaccine providers (*1*).

Changes to the footnote for tetanus, diphtheria, and acellular pertussis (Tdap) and tetanus, diphtheria (Td) vaccines were made to update recommendations. Tdap vaccine is recommended specifically for persons who are close contacts of infants younger than 12 months of age (e.g., parents, grandparents, and child-care providers) and who have not received Tdap previously. Before 2011, vaccination postpartum was preferred for women who had not had a previous adult Tdap dose. However, in 2011, ACIP recommended pregnant women preferentially receive Tdap vaccination during later pregnancy (>20 weeks gestation). Other adults who are close contacts of children younger than 12 months of age continue to be recommended to receive a one-time dose of Tdap vaccine.

Updates to the footnotes and figures also were made for human papillomavirus (HPV) and hepatitis B vaccines based on recommendations made at the October 2011 ACIP meeting. The HPV vaccine recommendation has been updated to include routine vaccination of males 11–12 years of age, with catch-up vaccination recommended for males 13–21 years of age. HPV vaccine also is recommended for previously unvaccinated males 22–26 years of age who are immunocompromised, or who test positive for human immunodeficiency virus (HIV) infection, or who have sex with men.

ACIP also voted in October 2011 to recommend hepatitis B vaccine for adults <60 years of age who have diabetes, as soon as possible after diabetes is diagnosed. In addition, hepatitis B vaccination is recommended at the discretion of the treating clinician for adults with diabetes who are 60 years or older based on a patient's likely need for assisted blood glucose monitoring, likelihood of acquiring hepatitis B, and likelihood of immune response to vaccination.

A notation was included for zoster vaccine to acknowledge that the vaccine was recently approved by the Food and Drug Administration (FDA) for administration to persons 50 years of age and older; however, ACIP continues to recommend that vaccination begin at age 60 years. The influenza vaccine footnote was revised to specify age indications for the different licensed formulations of trivalent inactivated influenza vaccine (TIV). The footnote for the measles, mumps, rubella (MMR) vaccine was simplified to focus only on routine use of this vaccine in adults; information on use of the vaccine for outbreak control was removed. Readers are referred to the ACIP MMR recommendations and to the ACIP recommendations for the immunization of health-care personnel regarding the use of MMR vaccine in outbreak settings. Additional information on the use of quadrivalent meningococcal conjugate vaccine (MCV4) and meningococcal polysaccharide vaccine (MPSV4) for specific age and risk groups was added. Minor clarifications also were made to the footnotes for HPV vaccine, varicella vaccine, and pneumococcal polysaccharide vaccine (PPSV).

Additional information is available as follows: 1) immunization schedule (in English and Spanish) at http://www.cdc.gov/vaccines/recs/schedules/adult-schedule.htm; 2) information regarding adult vaccination at http://www.cdc.gov/vaccines/default.htm; 3) ACIP statements for specific vaccines at http://www.cdc.gov/vaccines/pubs/acip-list.htm; and 4) reporting of adverse events at http://www.vaers.hhs.gov or by telephone, 800-822-7967. This schedule also has been presented to the American Academy of Family Physicians, the American College of Physicians, the American College of Obstetricians and Gynecologists and the American College of Nurse-Midwives for approval and publication in their respective journals.

The recommended adult immunization schedule has been approved by the Advisory Committee on Immunization Practices, the American Academy of Family Physicians, the American College of Obstetricians and Gynecologists, the American College of Physicians, and the American College of Nurse-Midwives.

Suggested citation: Centers for Disease Control and Prevention. Recommended adult immunization schedule—United States, 2012. MMWR 2012;61(4).

Footnote changes for 2012

- A new footnote (1), "Additional information," has been added to the beginning of the footnotes. This footnote provides links to the full ACIP vaccine recommendations and information on travel requirements that might have been referred to previously in subsequent footnotes.
- The "Influenza vaccination" footnote (2) was revised to clarify that all persons aged 6 months and older can receive TIV and that health-care personnel (HCP) who care for persons requiring a protected environment should receive TIV. HCP younger than 50 years who do not have a contraindication may receive either the live attenuated influenza vaccine or TIV. In addition, age indications for two recently licensed formulations of TIV were included. The link to additional information regarding influenza vaccination has been removed because a link now is provided in footnote 1.
- The "Human papillomavirus (HPV) vaccination" footnote (5) now clarifies that although HPV vaccination is not specifically recommended for HCP, HCP should receive the HPV vaccine if they are in the recommended age group. This footnote also was changed to reflect the recommendation of the quadrivalent human papillomavirus (HPV4) vaccine for males at age 11 or 12 years and catch-up vaccination for males 13 through 21 years of age. Males 22 through 26 years of age may be vaccinated with HPV4 vaccine.
- The "Zoster vaccination" footnote (6) now indicates that while zoster vaccination is not specifically recommended for HCP, HCP should receive the vaccine if they are in the recommended age group. This footnote also acknowledges that the vaccine is FDA-approved for use in persons 50 years and older; however, ACIP continues to recommend that vaccination begin at age 60 years.
- The link in the "Measles, mumps, rubella (MMR) vaccination" footnote (7) that directs the reader to more information about evidence of immunity has been removed. In addition, the information about the use of MMR vaccine in outbreak settings has been removed. Readers are referred to the ACIP MMR recommendations and to the ACIP recommendations for the immunization of health-care personnel regarding the use of MMR vaccine in outbreak settings.
- The "Pneumococcal polysaccharide (PPSV) vaccination" footnote (8) has been revised to include additional examples of functional and anatomic asplenia. Language is included for persons with asymptomatic or symptomatic HIV infection and persons undergoing cancer chemotherapy or who are on other immunosuppressive therapy.
- The "Revaccination with PPSV" footnote (9) has been revised to clarify guidance for those aged 65 years and older who had been vaccinated with PPSV23 before age 65 and for whom at least 5 years has passed since their previous dose.
- The "Meningococcal vaccination" footnote (10) has been revised to include military recruits in the group recommended to receive a single dose of meningococcal vaccine. The language about college students has been clarified to indicate that first-year college students up through age 21 years who are living in residence halls should be vaccinated if they have not received a dose on or after their 16th birthday. Language regarding travel to sub-Saharan Africa and travel to Mecca has been removed, and readers are referred to the footnote on information about vaccines for travelers (1).
- The "Hepatitis B vaccination" footnote (12) has been revised to include persons with diabetes younger than 60 years old and persons 60 years and older based on need for assisted blood glucose monitoring.
- Finally, all footnotes were changed from paragraph form to a bulleted format to provide for greater ease in use of the recommendations.

Figures

- For Figure 1, the bar for Tdap/Td for persons 65 years and older has been changed to a yellow and purple hashed bar to indicate that persons in this age group should receive 1 dose of Tdap if they are a close contact of an infant younger than 12 months of age. However, other persons 65 and older who are not close contacts of infants may receive either Tdap or Td.
- The 19–26 years age group was divided into 19–21 years and 22–26 years age groups. The HPV vaccine bar was split into separate bars for females and males. The recommendation for all males 19–21 years to receive HPV is indicated with a yellow bar, and a purple bar is used for 22–26 year old males to indicate that the vaccine is only for certain high-risk groups.
- For Figure 2, a new column was added for men who have sex with men (MSM) to note in the figure that MSM is an indication for HPV, hepatitis A, and hepatitis B vaccines.
- In addition, the diabetes indication was moved to the same column as chronic kidney disease to accommodate the new recommendation for hepatitis B vaccination of persons with diabetes.
- Because pregnant women not previously vaccinated with Tdap are now preferentially recommended for vaccination with Tdap during later pregnancy (>20 weeks gestation), the yellow bar has been extended across all risk groups.
- The HPV vaccine bar was separated into a bar for females and one for males. The bar for females is unchanged from the previous year except that the bar was extended to include HCP to clarify that HCP who are in the recommended age group for receipt of HPV vaccine are recommended for vaccination.
- Lastly, the HPV vaccine bar for males was added and indicates that all males through age 26 should be vaccinated if they are immunocompromised, have HIV, or are MSM. However, the age indication is through age 21 for males with or without these risk factors.

Reference

1. CDC. Epidemiology and prevention of vaccine-preventable diseases. Atkinson W, Wolfe S, Hamborsky J, eds. 12th ed. Washington DC: Public Health Foundation; 2011.

FIGURE 1. Recommended adult immunization schedule, by vaccine and age group[1] — United States, 2012

VACCINE ▼ AGE GROUP ►	19–21 years	22–26 years	27–49 years	50–59 years	60–64 years	≥65 years
Influenza[2,*]	1 dose annually					
Tetanus, diphtheria, pertussis (Td/Tdap)[3,*]	Substitute 1-time dose of Tdap for Td booster; then boost with Td every 10 years					Td/Tdap[3]
Varicella[4,*]	2 doses					
Human papillomavirus (HPV)[5,*] Female	3 doses					
Human papillomavirus (HPV)[5,*] Male	3 doses					
Zoster[6]					1 dose	
Measles, mumps, rubella (MMR)[7,*]	1 or 2 doses			1 dose		
Pneumococcal (polysaccharide)[8,9]	1 or 2 doses					1 dose
Meningococcal[10,*]	1 or more doses					
Hepatitis A[11,*]	2 doses					
Hepatitis B[12,*]	3 doses					

* Covered by the Vaccine Injury Compensation Program

For all persons in this category who meet the age requirements and who lack documentation of vaccination or have no evidence of previous infection

Recommended if some other risk factor is present (e.g., on the basis of medical, occupational, lifestyle, or other indications)

Tdap recommended for ≥65 if contact with <12 month old child. Either Td or Tdap can be used if no infant contact

No recommendation

FIGURE 2. Vaccines that might be indicated for adults, based on medical and other indications[1] — United States, 2012

INDICATION ► / VACCINE ▼	Pregnancy	Immunocompromising conditions (excluding human immunodeficiency virus [HIV])[4,6,7,14]	HIV infection[4,7,13,14] CD4+ T lymphocyte count <200 cells/μL	HIV infection[4,7,13,14] CD4+ T lymphocyte count ≥200 cells/μL	Men who have sex with men (MSM)	Heart disease, chronic lung disease, chronic alcoholism	Asplenia[13] (including elective splenectomy and persistent complement component deficiencies)	Chronic liver disease	Diabetes, kidney failure, end-stage renal disease, receipt of hemodialysis	Health-care personnel
Influenza[2,*]	1 dose TIV annually				1 dose TIV or LAIV annually	1 dose TIV annually				1 dose TIV or LAIV annually
Tetanus, diphtheria, pertussis (Td/Tdap)[3,*]		Substitute 1-time dose of Tdap for Td booster; then boost with Td every 10 years								
Varicella[4,*]	Contraindicated			2 doses						
Human papillomavirus (HPV)[5,*] Female		3 doses through age 26 years				3 doses through age 26 years				
Human papillomavirus (HPV)[5,*] Male		3 doses through age 26 years				3 doses through age 21 years				
Zoster[6]	Contraindicated				1 dose					
Measles, mumps, rubella[7,*]	Contraindicated			1 or 2 doses						
Pneumococcal (polysaccharide)[8,9]		1 or 2 doses								
Meningococcal[10,*]	1 or more doses									
Hepatitis A[11,*]	2 doses									
Hepatitis B[12,*]	3 doses									

* Covered by the Vaccine Injury Compensation Program

For all persons in this category who meet the age requirements and who lack documentation of vaccination or have no evidence of previous infection

Recommended if some other risk factor is present (e.g., on the basis of medical, occupational, lifestyle, or other indications)

Contraindicated

No recommendation

NOTE: The above recommendations must be read along with the footnotes on pages 4–5 of this schedule.

1. **Additional information**
   - Advisory Committee on Immunization Practices (ACIP) vaccine recommendations and additional information are available at: http://www.cdc.gov/vaccines/pubs/acip-list.htm.
   - Information on travel vaccine requirements and recommendations (e.g., for hepatitis A and B, meningococcal, and other vaccines) available at http://wwwnc.cdc.gov/travel/page/vaccinations.htm.
2. **Influenza vaccination**
   - Annual vaccination against influenza is recommended for all persons 6 months of age and older.
   - Persons 6 months of age and older, including pregnant women, can receive the trivalent inactivated vaccine (TIV).
   - Healthy, nonpregnant adults younger than age 50 years without high-risk medical conditions can receive either intranasally administered live, attenuated influenza vaccine (LAIV) (FluMist), or TIV. Health-care personnel who care for severely immunocompromised persons (i.e., those who require care in a protected environment) should receive TIV rather than LAIV. Other persons should receive TIV.
   - The intramuscular or intradermal administered TIV are options for adults aged 18–64 years.
   - Adults aged 65 years and older can receive the standard dose TIV or the high-dose TIV (Fluzone High-Dose).
3. **Tetanus, diphtheria, and acellular pertussis (Td/Tdap) vaccination**
   - Administer a one-time dose of Tdap to adults younger than age 65 years who have not received Tdap previously or for whom vaccine status is unknown to replace one of the 10-year Td boosters.
   - Tdap is specifically recommended for the following persons:
     — pregnant women more than 20 weeks' gestation,
     — adults, regardless of age, who are close contacts of infants younger than age 12 months (e.g., parents, grandparents, or child care providers), and
     — health-care personnel.
   - Tdap can be administered regardless of interval since the most recent tetanus or diphtheria-containing vaccine.
   - Pregnant women not vaccinated during pregnancy should receive Tdap immediately postpartum.
   - Adults 65 years and older may receive Tdap.
   - Adults with unknown or incomplete history of completing a 3-dose primary vaccination series with Td-containing vaccines should begin or complete a primary vaccination series. Tdap should be substituted for a single dose of Td in the vaccination series with Tdap preferred as the first dose.
   - For unvaccinated adults, administer the first 2 doses at least 4 weeks apart and the third dose 6–12 months after the second.
   - If incompletely vaccinated (i.e., less than 3 doses), administer remaining doses.

   Refer to the ACIP statement for recommendations for administering Td/Tdap as prophylaxis in wound management (See footnote 1).
4. **Varicella vaccination**
   - All adults without evidence of immunity to varicella (as defined below) should receive 2 doses of single-antigen varicella vaccine or a second dose if they have received only 1 dose.
   - Special consideration for vaccination should be given to those who
     — have close contact with persons at high risk for severe disease (e.g., health-care personnel and family contacts of persons with immunocompromising conditions) or
     — are at high risk for exposure or transmission (e.g., teachers; child care employees; residents and staff members of institutional settings, including correctional institutions; college students; military personnel; adolescents and adults living in households with children; nonpregnant women of childbearing age; and international travelers).
   - Pregnant women should be assessed for evidence of varicella immunity. Women who do not have evidence of immunity should receive the first dose of varicella vaccine upon completion or termination of pregnancy and before discharge from the health-care facility. The second dose should be administered 4–8 weeks after the first dose.
   - Evidence of immunity to varicella in adults includes any of the following:
     — documentation of 2 doses of varicella vaccine at least 4 weeks apart;
     — U.S.-born before 1980 (although for health-care personnel and pregnant women, birth before 1980 should not be considered evidence of immunity);
     — history of varicella based on diagnosis or verification of varicella by a health-care provider (for a patient reporting a history of or having an atypical case, a mild case, or both, health-care providers should seek either an epidemiologic link to a typical varicella case or to a laboratory-confirmed case or evidence of laboratory confirmation, if it was performed at the time of acute disease);
     — history of herpes zoster based on diagnosis or verification of herpes zoster by a health-care provider; or
     — laboratory evidence of immunity or laboratory confirmation of disease.
5. **Human papillomavirus (HPV) vaccination**
   - Two vaccines are licensed for use in females, bivalent HPV vaccine (HPV2) and quadrivalent HPV vaccine (HPV4), and one HPV vaccine for use in males (HPV4).
   - For females, either HPV4 or HPV2 is recommended in a 3-dose series for routine vaccination at 11 or 12 years of age, and for those 13 through 26 years of age, if not previously vaccinated.
   - For males, HPV4 is recommended in a 3-dose series for routine vaccination at 11 or 12 years of age, and for those 13 through 21 years of age, if not previously vaccinated. Males 22 through 26 years of age may be vaccinated.
   - HPV vaccines are not live vaccines and can be administered to persons who are immunocompromised as a result of infection (including HIV infection), disease, or medications. Vaccine is recommended for immunocompromised persons through age 26 years who did not get any or all doses when they were younger. The immune response and vaccine efficacy might be less than that in immunocompetent persons.
   - Men who have sex with men (MSM) might especially benefit from vaccination to prevent condyloma and anal cancer. HPV4 is recommended for MSM through age 26 years who did not get any or all doses when they were younger.
   - Ideally, vaccine should be administered before potential exposure to HPV through sexual activity; however, persons who are sexually active should still be vaccinated consistent with age-based recommendations. HPV vaccine can be administered to persons with a history of genital warts, abnormal Papanicolaou test, or positive HPV DNA test.
   - A complete series for either HPV4 or HPV2 consists of 3 doses. The second dose should be administered 1–2 months after the first dose; the third dose should be administered 6 months after the first dose (at least 24 weeks after the first dose).
   - Although HPV vaccination is not specifically recommended for health-care personnel (HCP) based on their occupation, HCP should receive the HPV vaccine if they are in the recommended age group.
6. **Zoster vaccination**
   - A single dose of zoster vaccine is recommended for adults 60 years of age and older regardless of whether they report a prior episode of herpes zoster. Although the vaccine is licensed by the Food and Drug Administration (FDA) for use among and can be administered to persons 50 years and older, ACIP recommends that vaccination begins at 60 years of age.
   - Persons with chronic medical conditions may be vaccinated unless their condition constitutes a contraindication, such as pregnancy or severe immunodeficiency.
   - Although zoster vaccination is not specifically recommended for health-care personnel (HCP), HCP should receive the vaccine if they are in the recommended age group.
7. **Measles, mumps, rubella (MMR) vaccination**
   - Adults born before 1957 generally are considered immune to measles and mumps. All adults born in 1957 or later should have documentation of 1 or more doses of MMR vaccine unless they have a medical contraindication to the vaccine, laboratory evidence of immunity to each of the three diseases, or documentation of provider-diagnosed measles or mumps disease. For rubella, documentation of provider-diagnosed disease is not considered acceptable evidence of immunity.

   Measles component:
   - A routine second dose of MMR vaccine, administered a minimum of 28 days after the first dose, is recommended for adults who
     — are students in postsecondary educational institutions;
     — work in a health-care facility; or
     — plan to travel internationally.
   - Persons who received inactivated (killed) measles vaccine or measles vaccine of unknown type from 1963 to 1967 should be revaccinated with 2 doses of MMR vaccine.

   Mumps component:
   - A routine second dose of MMR vaccine, administered a minimum of 28 days after the first dose, is recommended for adults who
     — are students in postsecondary educational institutions;
     — work in a health-care facility; or
     — plan to travel internationally.
   - Persons vaccinated before 1979 with either killed mumps vaccine or mumps vaccine of unknown type who are at high risk for mumps infection (e.g., persons who are working in a health-care facility) should be considered for revaccination with 2 doses of MMR vaccine.

   Rubella component:
   - For women of childbearing age, regardless of birth year, rubella immunity should be determined. If there is no evidence of immunity, women who are not pregnant should be vaccinated. Pregnant women who do not have evidence of immunity should receive MMR vaccine upon completion or termination of pregnancy and before discharge from the health-care facility.

   Health-care personnel born before 1957:
   - For unvaccinated health-care personnel born before 1957 who lack laboratory evidence of measles, mumps, and/or rubella immunity or laboratory confirmation of disease, health-care facilities should consider routinely vaccinating personnel with 2 doses of MMR vaccine at the appropriate interval for measles and mumps or 1 dose of MMR vaccine for rubella.
8. **Pneumococcal polysaccharide (PPSV) vaccination**
   - Vaccinate all persons with the following indications:
     — age 65 years and older without a history of PPSV vaccination;
     — adults younger than 65 years with chronic lung disease (including chronic obstructive pulmonary disease, emphysema, and asthma); chronic cardiovascular diseases; diabetes mellitus; chronic liver disease (including cirrhosis); alcoholism; cochlear implants; cerebrospinal fluid leaks; immunocompromising conditions; and functional or anatomic asplenia (e.g., sickle cell disease and other hemoglobinopathies, congenital or acquired asplenia, splenic dysfunction, or splenectomy [if elective splenectomy is planned, vaccinate at least 2 weeks before surgery]);
     — residents of nursing homes or long-term care facilities; and
     — adults who smoke cigarettes.
   - Persons with asymptomatic or symptomatic HIV infection should be vaccinated as soon as possible after their diagnosis.

- When cancer chemotherapy or other immunosuppressive therapy is being considered, the interval between vaccination and initiation of immunosuppressive therapy should be at least 2 weeks. Vaccination during chemotherapy or radiation therapy should be avoided.
- Routine use of PPSV is not recommended for American Indians/Alaska Natives or other persons younger than 65 years of age unless they have underlying medical conditions that are PPSV indications. However, public health authorities may consider recommending PPSV for American Indians/Alaska Natives who are living in areas where the risk for invasive pneumococcal disease is increased.

9. Revaccination with PPSV

- One-time revaccination 5 years after the first dose is recommended for persons 19 through 64 years of age with chronic renal failure or nephrotic syndrome; functional or anatomic asplenia (e.g., sickle cell disease or splenectomy); and for persons with immunocompromising conditions.
- Persons who received PPSV before age 65 years for any indication should receive another dose of the vaccine at age 65 years or later if at least 5 years have passed since their previous dose.
- No further doses are needed for persons vaccinated with PPSV at or after age 65 years.

10. Meningococcal vaccination

- Administer 2 doses of meningococcal conjugate vaccine quadrivalent (MCV4) at least 2 months apart to adults with functional asplenia or persistent complement component deficiencies.
- HIV-infected persons who are vaccinated should also receive 2 doses.
- Administer a single dose of meningococcal vaccine to microbiologists routinely exposed to isolates of *Neisseria meningitidis*, military recruits, and persons who travel to or live in countries in which meningococcal disease is hyperendemic or epidemic.
- First-year college students up through age 21 years who are living in residence halls should be vaccinated if they have not received a dose on or after their 16th birthday.
- MCV4 is preferred for adults with any of the preceding indications who are 55 years old and younger; meningococcal polysaccharide vaccine (MPSV4) is preferred for adults 56 years and older.
- Revaccination with MCV4 every 5 years is recommended for adults previously vaccinated with MCV4 or MPSV4 who remain at increased risk for infection (e.g., adults with anatomic or functional asplenia or persistent complement component deficiencies).

11. Hepatitis A vaccination

- Vaccinate any person seeking protection from hepatitis A virus (HAV) infection and persons with any of the following indications:
  - — men who have sex with men and persons who use injection drugs;
  - — persons working with HAV-infected primates or with HAV in a research laboratory setting;
  - — persons with chronic liver disease and persons who receive clotting factor concentrates;
  - — persons traveling to or working in countries that have high or intermediate endemicity of hepatitis A; and
  - — unvaccinated persons who anticipate close personal contact (e.g., household or regular babysitting) with an international adoptee during the first 60 days after arrival in the United States from a country with high or intermediate endemicity. (See footnote 1 for more information on travel recommendations). The first dose of the 2-dose hepatitis A vaccine series should be administered as soon as adoption is planned, ideally 2 or more weeks before the arrival of the adoptee.
- Single-antigen vaccine formulations should be administered in a 2-dose schedule at either 0 and 6–12 months (Havrix), or 0 and 6–18 months (Vaqta). If the combined hepatitis A and hepatitis B vaccine (Twinrix) is used, administer 3 doses at 0, 1, and 6 months; alternatively, a 4-dose schedule may be used, administered on days 0, 7, and 21–30 followed by a booster dose at month 12.

12. Hepatitis B vaccination

- Vaccinate persons with any of the following indications and any person seeking protection from hepatitis B virus (HBV) infection:
  - — sexually active persons who are not in a long-term, mutually monogamous relationship (e.g., persons with more than one sex partner during the previous 6 months); persons seeking evaluation or treatment for a sexually transmitted disease (STD); current or recent injection-drug users; and men who have sex with men;
  - — health-care personnel and public-safety workers who are exposed to blood or other potentially infectious body fluids;
  - — persons with diabetes younger than 60 years as soon as feasible after diagnosis; persons with diabetes who are 60 years or older at the discretion of the treating clinician based on increased need for assisted blood glucose monitoring in long-term care facilities, likelihood of acquiring hepatitis B infection, its complications or chronic sequelae, and likelihood of immune response to vaccination;
  - — persons with end-stage renal disease, including patients receiving hemodialysis; persons with HIV infection; and persons with chronic liver disease;
  - — household contacts and sex partners of persons with chronic HBV infection; clients and staff members of institutions for persons with developmental disabilities; and international travelers to countries with high or intermediate prevalence of chronic HBV infection; and
  - — all adults in the following settings: STD treatment facilities; HIV testing and treatment facilities; facilities providing drug-abuse treatment and prevention services; health-care settings targeting services to injection-drug users or men who have sex with men; correctional facilities; end-stage renal disease programs and facilities for chronic hemodialysis patients; and institutions and nonresidential daycare facilities for persons with developmental disabilities.
- Administer missing doses to complete a 3-dose series of hepatitis B vaccine to those persons not vaccinated or not completely vaccinated. The second dose should be administered 1 month after the first dose; the third dose should be given at least 2 months after the second dose (and at least 4 months after the first dose). If the combined hepatitis A and hepatitis B vaccine (Twinrix) is used, give 3 doses at 0, 1, and 6 months; alternatively, a 4-dose Twinrix schedule, administered on days 0, 7, and 21–30 followed by a booster dose at month 12 may be used.
- Adult patients receiving hemodialysis or with other immunocompromising conditions should receive 1 dose of 40 μg/mL (Recombivax HB) administered on a 3-dose schedule or 2 doses of 20 μg/mL (Engerix-B) administered simultaneously on a 4-dose schedule at 0, 1, 2, and 6 months.

13. Selected conditions for which *Haemophilus influenzae* type b (Hib) vaccine may be used

- 1 dose of Hib vaccine should be considered for persons who have sickle cell disease, leukemia, or HIV infection, or who have anatomic or functional asplenia if they have not previously received Hib vaccine.

14. Immunocompromising conditions

- Inactivated vaccines generally are acceptable (e.g., pneumococcal, meningococcal, and influenza [inactivated influenza vaccine]), and live vaccines generally are avoided in persons with immune deficiencies or immunocompromising conditions. Information on specific conditions is available at http://www.cdc.gov/vaccines/pubs/acip-list.htm.

These schedules indicate the recommended age groups and medical indications for which administration of currently licensed vaccines is commonly indicated for adults ages 19 years and older, as of January 1, 2012. For all vaccines being recommended on the adult immunization schedule: a vaccine series does not need to be restarted, regardless of the time that has elapsed between doses. Licensed combination vaccines may be used whenever any components of the combination are indicated and when the vaccine's other components are not contraindicated. For detailed recommendations on all vaccines, including those used primarily for travelers or that are issued during the year, consult the manufacturers' package inserts and the complete statements from the Advisory Committee on Immunization Practices (http:// www.cdc.gov/vaccines/pubs/acip-list.htm).

Report all clinically significant postvaccination reactions to the Vaccine Adverse Event Reporting System (VAERS). Reporting forms and instructions on filing a VAERS report are available at http://www.vaers.hhs.gov or by telephone, 800-822-7967.

Information on how to file a Vaccine Injury Compensation Program claim is available at http://www.hrsa.gov/vaccinecompensation or by telephone, 800-338-2382. Information about filing a claim for vaccine injury is available through the U.S. Court of Federal Claims, 717 Madison Place, N.W., Washington, D.C. 20005; telephone, 202-357-6400.

Additional information about the vaccines in this schedule, extent of available data, and contraindications for vaccination also is available at http://www.cdc.gov/vaccines or from the CDC-INFO Contact Center at 800-CDC-INFO (800-232-4636) in English and Spanish, 8:00 a.m. to 8:00 p.m., Monday through Friday, excluding holidays.

Use of trade names and commercial sources is for identification only and does not imply endorsement by the U.S. Department of Health and Human Services.

U.S. Department of Health and Human Services • Centers for Disease Control and Prevention

TABLE. Contraindications and precautions to commonly used vaccines in adults[1*†]

Vaccine	Contraindications	Precautions
Influenza, injectable trivalent (TIV)	Severe allergic reaction (e.g., anaphylaxis) after previous dose of any influenza vaccine or to a vaccine component, including egg protein.	Moderate or severe acute illness with or without fever. History of Guillain-Barré syndrome (GBS) within 6 weeks of previous influenza vaccination.
Influenza, live attenuated (LAIV)[2]	Severe allergic reaction (e.g., anaphylaxis) after previous dose of any influenza vaccine or to a vaccine component, including egg protein. Immune suppression. Certain chronic medical conditions such as asthma, diabetes, heart or kidney disease.[3] Pregnancy.	Moderate or severe acute illness with or without fever. History of GBS within 6 weeks of previous influenza vaccination. Receipt of specific antivirals (i.e., amantadine, rimantadine, zanamivir, or oseltamivir) 48 hours before vaccination. Avoid use of these antiviral drugs for 14 days after vaccination.
Tetanus, diphtheria, pertussis (Tdap); tetanus, diphtheria (Td)	Severe allergic reaction (e.g., anaphylaxis) after a previous dose or to a vaccine component. For Tdap only: Encephalopathy (e.g., coma, decreased level of consciousness, or prolonged seizures) not attributable to another identifiable cause within 7 days of administration of a previous dose of Tdap or diphtheria and tetanus toxoids and pertussis (DTP) or diphtheria and tetanus toxoids and acellular pertussis (DTaP) vaccine.	Moderate or severe acute illness with or without fever. GBS within 6 weeks after a previous dose of tetanus toxoid--containing vaccine. History of arthus-type hypersensitivity reactions after a previous dose of tetanus or diptheria toxoid–containing vaccine; defer vaccination until at least 10 years have elapsed since the last tetanus toxoid–containing vaccine. For Tdap only: Progressive or unstable neurologic disorder, uncontrolled seizures, or progressive encephalopathy until a treatment regimen has been established and the condition has stabilized.
Varicella,[2]	Severe allergic reaction (e.g., anaphylaxis) after a previous dose or to a vaccine component. Known severe immunodeficiency (e.g., from hematologic and solid tumors, receipt of chemotherapy, congenital immunodeficiency, or long-term immunosuppressive therapy[4] or patients with human immunodeficiency virus (HIV) infection who are severely immunocompromised). Pregnancy.	Recent (≤11 months) receipt of antibody-containing blood product (specific interval depends on product).[5] Moderate or severe acute illness with or without fever. Receipt of specific antivirals (i.e., acyclovir, famciclovir, or valacyclovir) 24 hours before vaccination; if possible, delay resumption of these antiviral drugs for 14 days after vaccination.
Human papillomavirus (HPV)	Severe allergic reaction (e.g., anaphylaxis) after a previous dose or to a vaccine component.	Moderate or severe acute illness with or without fever. Pregnancy.
Zoster	Severe allergic reaction (e.g., anaphylaxis) to a vaccine component. Known severe immunodeficiency (e.g., from hematologic and solid tumors, receipt of chemotherapy, or long-term immunosuppressive therapy[4] or patients with HIV infection who are severely immunocompromised). Pregnancy.	Moderate or severe acute illness with or without fever. Receipt of specific antivirals (i.e., acyclovir, famciclovir, or valacyclovir) 24 hours before vaccination; if possible, avoid use of these antiviral drugs for 14 days after vaccination.

See table footnotes on page 7.

TABLE. (Continued) Contraindications and precautions to commonly used vaccines in adults[1*†]

Vaccine	Contraindications	Precautions
Measles, mumps, rubella (MMR)[2]	Severe allergic reaction (e.g., anaphylaxis) after a previous dose or to a vaccine component. Known severe immunodeficiency (e.g., from hematologic and solid tumors, receipt of chemotherapy, congenital immunodeficiency, or long-term immunosuppressive therapy[4] or patients with HIV infection who are severely immunocompromised). Pregnancy.	Moderate or severe acute illness with or without fever. Recent (within 11 months) receipt of antibody-containing blood product (specific interval depends on product).[6] History of thrombocytopenia or thrombocytopenic purpura. Need for tuberculin skin testing.[7]
Pneumococcal polysaccharide (PPSV)	Severe allergic reaction (e.g., anaphylaxis) after a previous dose or to a vaccine component.	Moderate or severe acute illness with or without fever.
Meningococcal, conjugate, (MCV4); meningococcal, polysaccharide (MPSV4)	Severe allergic reaction (e.g., anaphylaxis) after a previous dose or to a vaccine component.	Moderate or severe acute illness with or without fever.
Hepatitis A (HepA)	Severe allergic reaction (e.g., anaphylaxis) after a previous dose or to a vaccine component.	Moderate or severe acute illness with or without fever. Pregnancy.
Hepatitis B (HepB)	Severe allergic reaction (e.g., anaphylaxis) after a previous dose or to a vaccine component.	Moderate or severe acute illness with or without fever.

1. Vaccine package inserts and the full ACIP recommendations for these vaccines should be consulted for additional information on vaccine-related contraindications and precautions and for more information on vaccine excipients. Events or conditions listed as precautions should be reviewed carefully. Benefits of and risks for administering a specific vaccine to a person under these circumstances should be considered. If the risk from the vaccine is believed to outweigh the benefit, the vaccine should not be administered. If the benefit of vaccination is believed to outweigh the risk, the vaccine should be administered.
2. LAIV, MMR, and varicella vaccines can be administered on the same day. If not administered on the same day, these live vaccines should be separated by at least 28 days.
3. See CDC. Prevention and control of influenza with vaccines: recommendations of the Advisory Committee on Immunization Practices (ACIP), 2010. MMWR 2010;59(No. RR-8). Available at http://www.cdc.gov/vaccines/pubs/acip-list.htm.
4. Substantially immunosuppressive steroid dose is considered to be ≥2 weeks of daily receipt of 20 mg or 2 mg/kg body weight of prednisone or equivalent.
5. Vaccine should be deferred for the appropriate interval if replacement immune globulin products are being administered.
6. See CDC. General recommendations on immunization: recommendations of the Advisory Committee on Immunization Practices (ACIP). MMWR 2011;60(No. RR-2). Available at http://www.cdc.gov/vaccines/pubs/acip-list.htm.
7. Measles vaccination might suppress tuberculin reactivity temporarily. Measles-containing vaccine may be administered on the same day as tuberculin skin testing. If testing cannot be performed until after the day of MMR vaccination, the test should be postponed for ≥4 weeks after the vaccination. If an urgent need exists to skin test, do so with the understanding that reactivity might be reduced by the vaccine.

* Adapted from CDC. Table 6. Contraindications and precautions to commonly used vaccines. General recommendations on immunization: recommendations of the Advisory Committee on Immunization Practices. MMWR 2011;60(No. RR-2):40-41 and from Atkinson W, Wolfe S, Hamborsky J, eds. Appendix A. Epidemiology and prevention of vaccine preventable diseases. 12th ed. Washington, DC: Public Health Foundation, 2011. Available at http://www.cdc.gov/vaccines/pubs/pinkbook/default.htm.

† Regarding latex allergy: some types of prefilled syringes contain natural rubber latex or dry natural latex rubber. Consult the package insert for any vaccine administered.

More information on vaccine components, contraindications, and precautions also is available from specific vaccine package inserts and ACIP recommendations for specific vaccines, and is summarized in Atkinson W, Wolfe S, Hamborsky J, eds. Epidemiology and prevention of vaccine preventable diseases. 12th ed. Washington, DC: Public Health Foundation, 2011. Available at http://www.cdc.gov/vaccines/pubs/pinkbook/default.htm.

INDEX

F

O

V

W

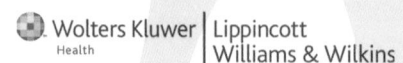

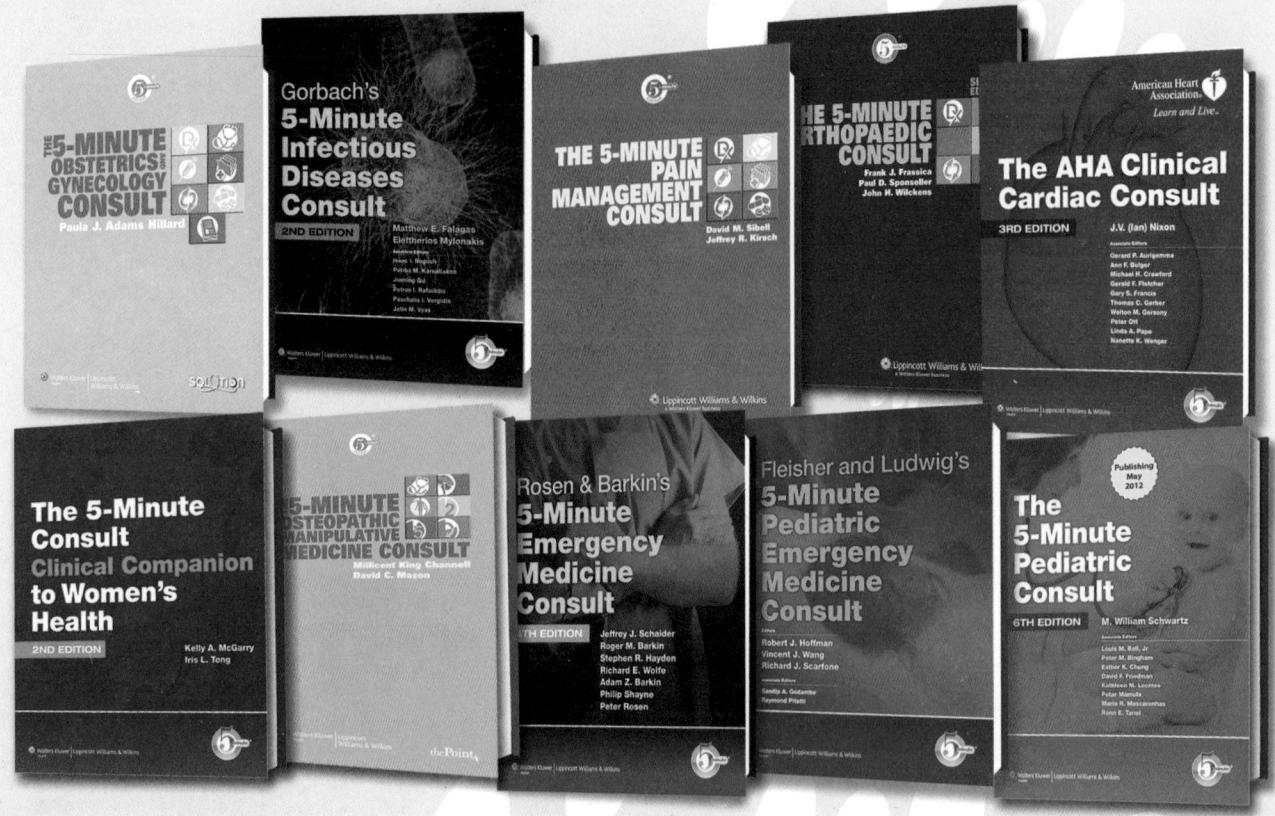